Success in the Classroom, in Clinicals, and on the NCLEX-RN®

Classroom

- Detailed lecture notes organized by learning outcome
- Suggestions for classroom activities
- Guide to relevant additional resources
- Comprehensive PowerPoint™ presentations integrating lecture, images, animations, and videos
- Classroom Response questions
- Image Gallery
- Video and Animation Gallery
- Online course management systems complete with instructor tools and student activities available in a variety of formats

PEARSON mynursinglab

- Saves instructors time by providing quality feedback, ongoing formative assessments and customized remediation for students.
- Provides easy, one-stop access to a wealth of teaching resources, such as test item files, PowerPoint™ slides, and video suggestions.
- A built-in electronic gradebook tracks students' progress on assessment and remediation activities.

Clinical

- Suggestions for Clinical Activities and other clinical resources organized by learning outcome

Real Nursing Simulations Facilitator's Guide: Institutional Edition

- 25 simulation scenarios that span the nursing curriculum
- Consistent format includes learning objectives, case flow, instructions for set up, student debriefing questions and more!
- Companion online course cartridge with student exercises, activities, videos, skill checklists, and reflective questions also available for adoption

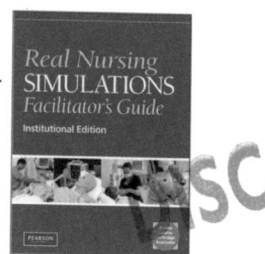

NCLEX-RN®

- Test Item Files with NCLEX®-style questions and complete rationales for correct and incorrect answers mapped to learning outcomes. *available in TestGen, Par Test, and MS Word*

Instructor Resources

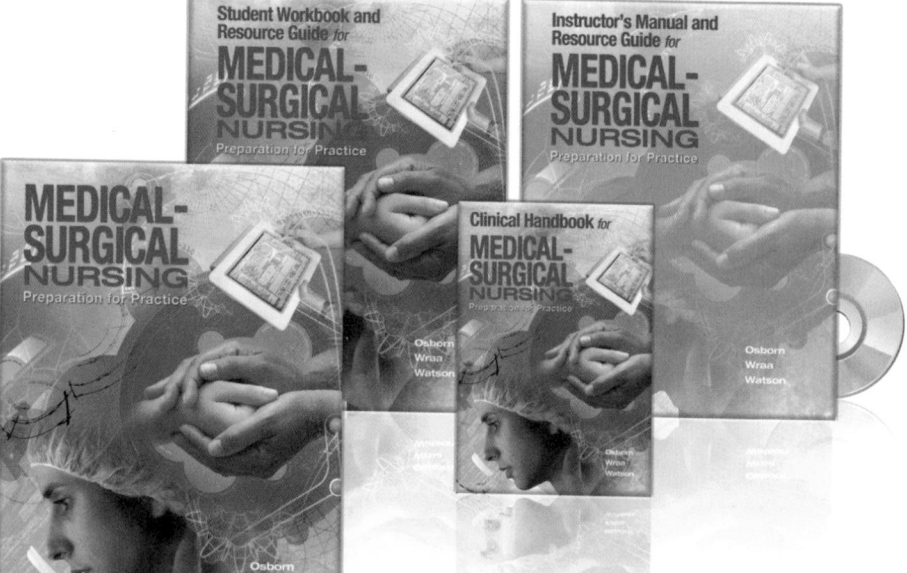

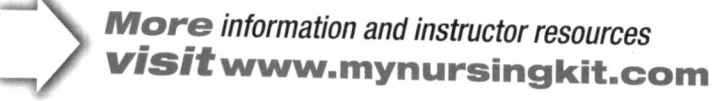

BRIEF CONTENTS

Your steps to success.

 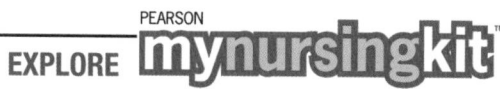
STEP 1: Register

All you need to get started is a valid email address and the access code below. To register, simply:

1. Go to **www.mynursingkit.com**.
2. Select "**Student**".
3. Find and click on the appropriate book cover. Cover must match the textbook edition being used for your class.
4. On the new page click "**I have an access code**".
5. Read the **License Agreement** and **Privacy Policy**. If you accept, click "**I Accept**."
6. Leave "**No**" selected under "Do you have a Pearson account?"
7. Using a coin scratch off the silver coating below to reveal your access code. Do not use a knife or other sharp object, which can damage the code.
8. Enter your access code in lowercase or uppercase.
9. Follow the on-screen instructions to complete registration.

During registration, you will establish a personal login name and password to use for logging into the Website. You will also be sent a registration confirmation email that contains your login name and password. Be sure to save this email. You must respond to the confirmation e-mail to activate the account correctly.

Your Access Code is:

*Note: If there is no silver foil covering the access code, it may already have been redeemed, and therefore may no longer be valid. In that case, you can purchase access online using a major credit card. To do so, go to www.mynursingkit.com. Click "Students" under "First Time Users," find the cover of your textbook, then click "**Buy Access**," and follow the on-screen instructions.*

STEP 2: Log in

1. Go to **www.mynursingkit.com** and click "**Students**".
2. Find and click on the appropriate book cover. Cover must match the textbook edition being used for your class.
3. Enter the login name and password that you created during registration. If unsure of this information, refer to your registration confirmation email.
4. Click "**Login**."

Got technical questions?

Customer Technical Support: To obtain support, please visit us online anytime at http://247pearsoned.custhelp.com where you can search our knowledgebase for common solutions, view product alerts, and review all options for additional assistance.

SYSTEM REQUIREMENTS

For the latest updates on System Requirements, go to www.mynursingkit.com. Click "**Support**" and choose "**System Requirements**". Click on "**Need help**" at bottom of page for site requirements and other frequently asked questions.

Important: Please read the Subscription and End-User License agreement, accessible from the book website's login page, before using the *mynursingkit* website. By using the website, you indicate that you have read, understood, and accepted the terms of this agreement.

0-13-178102-2

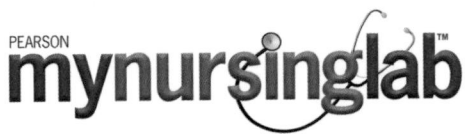
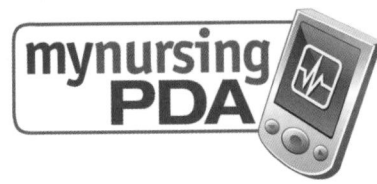

MEDICAL-SURGICAL NURSING
Preparation for Practice

Kathleen S. Osborn, RN, MS, EdD
California State University
Sacramento, California

Cheryl E. Wraa, RN, MSN
University of California, Davis Medical Center
California State University
Sacramento, California

Annita B. Watson, RN, MS, DNSc
California State University
Sacramento, California

DATE DUE

BRODART, CO.   Cat. No. 23-221

Pearson
Boston Columbus Indianapolis New York San Francisco Upper Saddle River
Amsterdam Cape Town Dubai London Madrid Milan Munich Paris Montreal Toronto
Delhi Mexico City Sao Paulo Sydney Hong Kong Seoul Singapore Taipei Tokyo

Library of Congress Cataloging-in-Publication Data

Osborn, Kathleen S.

 Medical-surgical nursing: preparation for practice/Kathleen S. Osborn, Cheryl E. Wraa, Annita B. Watson.
  p. ; cm.
 Includes bibliographical references and index.
 ISBN-13: 978-0-13-178102-3
 ISBN-10: 0-13-178102-2
 1. Nursing. 2. Surgical nursing. I. Wraa, Cheryl E. II. Watson, Annita B., III. Title.
 [DNLM: 1. Perioperative Nursing—methods. 2. Nurse's Role. 3. Nursing Care—methods. WY 161 081m 2010]
 RT41.068 2010
 610.73—dc22

                                                                                       2009002926

Publisher: Julie Levin Alexander
Publisher's Assistant: Regina Bruno
Editor-in-Chief: Maura Connor
Executive Acquisitions Editor: Pamela Fuller
Development Editor: iD8 Publishing Services, Marion Waldman
Editorial Assistant: Jennifer Aranda
Managing Production Editor: Patrick Walsh
Production Liaison: Cathy O'Connell
Production Editor: Emily Bush, S4Carlisle Publishing Services
Manufacturing Manager: Ilene Sanford
Creative Director: John Christiana, Design Development Services
Interior and Cover Design: Mary Siener, Design Development Services
Cover and Interior Illustration: A.k.A., Anthony Robinson
Director of Marketing: Karen Allman
Senior Marketing Manager: Francisco Del Castillo
Marketing Specialist: Michael Sirinides
Marketing Assistant: Crystal Gonzalez
Digital Media Product Manager: Travis Moses-Westphal
Media Project Manager: Deb O'Connell, All Things Media
Media Project Manager: Rachel Collett
Manager, Rights and Permissions: Zina Arabia
Manager, Visual Research: Beth Brenzel
Image Permission Coordinator: Fran Toepfer
Composition: S4Carlisle Publishing Services
Printer/Binder: Courier/Kendallville
Cover Printer: Lehigh-Phoenix Color/Hagerstown
Cover Photos: A.k.A., Anthony Robinson, Shayle Keating

Notice: Care has been taken to confirm the accuracy of information presented in this book. The authors, editors, and the publisher, however, cannot accept any responsibility for errors or omissions or for consequences from application of the information in this book and make no warranty, express or implied, with respect to its contents.

The authors and publisher have exerted every effort to ensure that drug selections and dosages set forth in this text are in accord with current recommendations and practice at time of publication. However, in view of ongoing research, changes in government regulations, and the constant flow of information relating to drug therapy and drug reactions, the reader is urged to check the package inserts of all drugs for any change in indications of dosage and for added warnings and precautions. This is particularly important when the recommended agent is a new and/or infrequently employed drug.

www.pearsonhighered.com

10 9 8 7 6 5 4 3 2 1
ISBN-10:   0-13-178102-2
ISBN-13:   978-0-13-178102-3

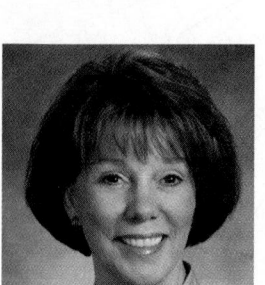

KATHLEEN S. OSBORN

Dr. Kathleen Osborn was first introduced to the profession of nursing at St. Francis School of Nursing in San Francisco, where she received her diploma. She went on to obtain a bachelor's degree in nursing from Sacramento State University, a master of science degree from the University of California, San Francisco, and a doctorate in educational leadership from the University of Southern California. Her clinical practice is in critical care, including cardiac, burn, neurological, and respiratory specialties. She has more than 29 years of experience teaching bachelor and master's degree students, as well as teaching nurses in hospital in-service and continuing education programs. Dr. Osborn's expertise includes program and course development, didactic lecturing, and clinical supervision of undergraduate and graduate students. She also has been actively involved in nursing research and publication throughout her clinical and teaching career. Since 1999, Dr. Osborn has participated as a nurse educator on humanitarian surgical missions to Laos, Africa, Vietnam, Honduras, Bangladesh, and Ecuador. She received the "Heroes in Healthcare" Community Service Award for her humanitarian work from the Coalition for Excellence in Healthcare, a division of the Health Communication Research Institute of Northern California. She also received the Community Service Award from Sacramento State University for her humanitarian work and her service to student development. In 1995, a perpetual faculty award was begun in her honor by the graduating class: The Guiding Light Award for Outstanding Performance by a Nursing Faculty.

This book is dedicated to the important people in my life. I want to thank my husband John for his devotion, patience, and understanding during this project. I also want to thank our children, Christopher and his wife Toni, Patrick, Staci, and Mike for their ongoing understanding of my time away from them. Finally, I want to thank all of the nursing students whom I have had the pleasure of teaching and the patients around the world that I have cared for. You have made my career fulfilling and happy.

—Kathleen Osborn

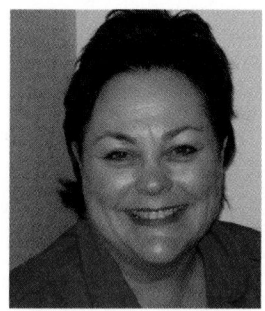

CHERYL E. WRAA

Cheryl Wraa received her nursing diploma from the Kaiser Foundation School of Nursing in Oakland, California. She went on to obtain a bachelor's degree, and master of science degree in nursing from California State University, Sacramento. Her clinical career has focused on critical care nursing, leadership, and education. Ms. Wraa's clinical practice includes the medical intensive care unit, emergency department, and flight nursing. She is currently the trauma program manager at a level 1 trauma center and clinical faculty for advanced medical–surgical nursing students in a baccalaureate program. Ms. Wraa is also an educator for Interplast and has participated on surgical missions to Vietnam, Bangladesh, and Ghana. She has been active in education and publication throughout her career and is currently a senior clinical editor for the *Journal of Emergency Nursing*. She is past president of the Air and Surface Transport Nurses Association, and president-elect of the Trauma Managers Association of California. Ms. Wraa received the Barbara A. Hess Award for her contributions to education in the air medical and ground transport field.

I dedicate this book to my parents for sharing their incredible faith, zest for life, and unconditional love— I miss you. To my mentors for sharing their wisdom— I would not be where I am without you. To my students for keeping the thirst for knowledge alive and, most importantly, to my family and friends for their unending support and love—I would not have survived this without you.

—Cheryl Wraa

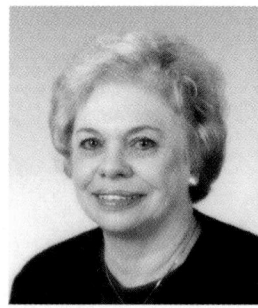

ANNITA B. WATSON

Dr. Annita Watson began her nursing career in Jamestown, New York, at WCA Hospital School of Nursing. She completed her bachelor's degree at Teachers College, Columbia University, and her master's and doctorate in nursing at the University of California, San Francisco. Her graduate focus was medical–surgical nursing and leadership and administration in the service and educational settings. Dr. Watson began her teaching career in 1970 at California State University, Sacramento, where she currently teaches at both the undergraduate and graduate levels. Her areas of practice include medical–surgical nursing, intensive care, long-term care, and community health. Throughout her career, she has served as a national consultant to health care agencies and educational programs on topics related to development of management systems, quality improvement of patient care, curriculum development and evaluation, and implementation of accreditation processes. She has published in like areas, and made numerous professional preparations. Research interests focus on measurement of patient and student outcomes. Currently Dr. Watson assumes a leadership role on several local and regional community boards, focusing on health services for vulnerable populations, for example, children, the elderly, and people who have been abused. Nationally, she serves as an accreditation site evaluator for the Commission on Collegiate Nursing Education. In 2008, she was awarded the Life Time Achievement Award for community service by California State University, Sacramento, recognizing her contributions to the health of the community and her ability to foster community-based learning experiences for students.

To my family, friends, colleagues, and students who supported me in completing this project. Thank you for your existence, endurance, and encouragement. I could not have completed this project without you. Your inspiration and guidance remain in my thoughts and prayers.

—Annita Watson

THANK YOU

We extend a heartfelt thanks to our contributors, who gave their time, effort, and expertise so tirelessly to the development and writing of chapters and resources that helped foster our goal of preparing student nurses for evidence-based practice.

Text Contributors

Jaynce Agruss, PhD, APN/CNP
Coordinator, Family Nurse Practitioner Program
Rush University Medical Center
Chicago, Illinois
Chapter 62

Mary Alexander, MA, RN, CRNI, CAE
Chief Executive Officer
Education Manager
Infusion Nurses Society
Norwood, Massachusetts
Chapter 22

Nancy Ames, RN, MSN, CCRN
Critical Care Clinical Specialist
National Institutes of Health, Clinical Center
Nursing and Patient Care Services
Bethesda, Maryland
Chapter 36

Sue Apple, RN, DNSc
Assistant Professor
School of Nursing and Health Studies
Georgetown University
Washington, D.C.
Chapter 39

Jane Ashley, PhD, RN
Associate Professor
Connell School of Nursing
Boston College
Boston, Massachusetts
Chapters 25 and 27

Laurie Baker, RN, MS, APRN, BC, ANP
Coordinator, Barrow Neurosurgical Spine Assessment Clinic
Barrow Neurosurgical Associates
Phoenix, Arizona
Chapter 34

Patricia Baker, RN
Skills Lab Coordinator
School of Nursing and Health Studies
Georgetown University
Washington, D.C.
Chapters 24 and 32

Doris Ballard-Ferguson, RN, PhD
Professor
School of Nursing
Florida A&M University
Tallahassee, Florida
Chapter 7

Karen Bawel Brinkley, RN, PhD
Associate Professor
Chair, Advanced Medical-Surgical Nursing
School of Nursing
San Jose State University
San Jose, California
Chapter 55

Patricia Benner, RN, PhD, FAAN
Thelma Shobe Endowed Chair in Ethics and Spirituality in Nursing
University of California San Francisco
San Francisco, California
Chapter 2
The Foreword

Deborah Benvenuto, BS, CRNI
Education Manager
Infusion Nurses Society
Norwood, Massachusetts
Chapter 22

Debra Brady, DNP, RN, CNS
Assistant Professor of Nursing
California State University Sacramento
Sacramento, California
Chapters 59 and 60

Krista Margaret Brecht, RN, MSc(A)N
Nurse Specialist
Pain Programs
McGill University Health Centre
Montreal General Hospital
Montreal, QC
Chapter 26

Claudia Campbell, RN, BSN, CCRN
Manager of Pain Services LDS Hospital
Intermountain Healthcare
Salt Lake City, Utah
Chapter 15

Ann Cashion, RN, PhD
Chair and Associate Professor, Acute and Chronic Care Department
Robert Wood Johnson Executive Nurse Fellow
Director, Center for Health Evaluation and Lifestyle Promotion
University of Tennessee Health Science Center
Memphis, Tennessee
Chapter 11

Patricia Caudle, DNSc, CNM, FNP
Faculty
Frontier School of Midwifery and Family Nursing
Heber Springs, Arizona
Chapters 48 and 50

Donna York Clark, RN, MS, CFRN, CMTE
Senior Account Manager
Golden Hour Data Systems
Carmel, Indiana
Chapter 1

Jan Clark, BSN, RN, CWOCN
Wound, Ostomy, Continence Consultant
Wilford Hall Medical Center
Lackland Air Force Base
San Antonio, Texas
Chapter 67

Karen Cooper, RN, MSN, CCRN, CNS, WOCN
Assistant Manager ICU
Kaiser Permanente
Sacramento, California
Chapters 33 and 57

Ellen DeLuca, RN, PhD
Professor of Nursing
Lynchburg College
Lynchburg, Virginia
Chapter 35

Jeromy D. Dyer, PA-C, MPAS
Orthopedic Surgery Specialist
Sutter General Hospital
Sutter Medical Group
Sacramento, California
Chapter 55

Lucie Elfervig, DNS, MSN, BSN, APRN-CS, CRNO, FAAN
Ophthalmic Consultant, Clinician, Researcher, Educator,
and Electrophysiologist
Eye Specialty Group
Memphis, Tennessee
Chapter 71

Peggy Ellis, PhD, RN, ANP, FNP, BC
Associate Professor
Associate Dean, School of Nursing,
Director, DNP Program
Doisy College of Health Sciences
St. Louis University
St. Louis, Missouri
Chapters 20, 65, and 66

Harold Engle, RN, BSN, BS
Program Director
Memorial Hermann Northeast Wound Care Center (R)
Humble, Texas
Chapter 67

Gina Flaharty, RN, BSN, FNP
President & Owner
Passport Health of Northern California
Sacramento, California
Chapter 40

Darlene M. Gilcreast, PhD, RN, MSN, BSN, CLNC
Partner, Diabetes Educator
Gilcreast & Associates, LLC
San Antonio, Texas
Chapter 18

J. Carolyn Graff, PhD, RN, FAAIDD
Associate Professor, College of Nursing
Director, College of Graduate Health Sciences
Chief of Nursing, Boling Center for Developmental Disabilities
University of Tennessee Health Science Center
Memphis, Tennessee
Chapter 11

Michele Grigaitis, MS, FNP-BC, CNRN
Nurse Practitioner, Adult Neurosurgical Services
Barrow Neurological Institute
Phoenix, AZ
Chapter 28

Ginny Wacker Guido, JD, MSN, RN
Associate Dean and Director of Graduate Studies
College of Nursing
University of North Dakota
Grand Forks, North Dakota
Chapter 4

Kori Harder, RN, MS
Clinical Nurse Specialist, Cardiology
Nurse Manager, Cardiovascular
University of California Davis Heart Center
Sacramento, CA
Chapter 40

Ann Harley, EdD, RN
Former Dean/Chair
Nursing Behavioral Health
Carson-Newman College
Jefferson City, Tennessee
Chapter 21

Corinne Harmon, RN, MS, EdD, AOCN
Assistant Professor
Clemson University
Clemson, South Carolina
Chapter 51

Helene Harris, RN, MSN
Instructor
Temple College
Temple, Texas
Chapters 54 and 55

Abby M. Heydman, PhD, RN
Interim President
Samuel Merritt College
Oakland, California
Chapter 52

Reneé Semonin Holleran, RN, PhD, CEN, CCRN, CFRN, CTRN, FAEN
Staff Nurse
Emergency Department
Intermountain Medical Center
Salt Lake City, Utah
Chapters 61 and 73

Rich Keegan, RN, MSN
Lecturer
Division of Nursing
Sacramento State University
Sacramento, California
Chapter 9

Katherine Kelly, RN, MSN, FNP-C, CEN
Lecturer
Sacramento School of Nursing
California State University
Sacramento, California
Chapter 17

Gale Kittle, RN, MPH
Research Nurse Coordinator
Barrow Neurological Institute
Arizona Alzheimer's Center
Phoenix, Arizona
Chapter 30

Dawn Lambie, RN, MSN, CHPN
Clinical Nurse Educator
Clinical Education
Kaiser Permanente
Roseville, California
Chapter 64

Kristine L'ecuyer, MSN, RN
Continuing Nursing Education Director Associate Professor
School of Nursing
Saint Louis University
St. Louis, Missouri
Chapter 37

Joseph Lindsay Jr, MD, FACC
Professor of Medicine
The George Washington University School of Medicine
Director, Emeritus, Division of Cardiology
Washington Hospital Center
Washington, D.C.
Chapter 39

Dawna Martrich, RN, BSN, MSN
Director, Education
MCN Healthcare, Inc.
Denver, Colorado
Chapter 70

Bonnie McCracken, RN, NP
UC Davis Medical Center
Sacramento, CA
Chapter 44

Brenda McCulloch, RN, MSN, CNS
Sutter Heart and Vascular Institute
Sutter Medical Center
Sacramento, California
Chapter 43

Arlene McGory, DNSc, RN
Research Nurse
Massachusetts Eye and Ear Infirmary
Boston, Massachusetts
Chapter 69

Joyce Mikal-Flynn, RN, FNP, EdD
California State University, Sacramento
Sacramento, California
Chapter 7

Barbara Moyer, BSN, MS, EdD
DeSales University
Center Valley, Pennsylvania
Chapter 70

Teri A. Murray, PhD, RN
Doisy College of Health Sciences
St. Louis University
St. Louis, Missouri
Chapters 20, 65, and 66

Krisna Ogerio, RN, BScN, CPN(C)
McGill University Health Centre
Royal Victoria Hospital
Montreal, QC
Chapter 26

John Osborn, MD, FACS
Senior Surgeon, The Plastic Surgery Center
Clinical Professor, Department of Surgery
University of California Davis School of Medicine
Sacramento, California
Chapter 49

M. Miki Patterson, PhD, RN, PNP, ONP-C
Past President-National Association of Orthopedic Nurses
UMass Memorial Orthopedics
North Worcester, Massachusetts
Chapter 56

Laurie Quinn, BSN, MSN, PhD
Clinical Associate Professor
College of Nursing
University of Illinois
Chicago, Illinois
Chapter 53

Kismet Rasmusson, FNP-BC, FAHA
Heart Failure Prevention and Treatment Program, NP-Program Development
Intermountain Healthcare
College of Nursing
University of Utah
Salt Lake City, Utah
Chapter 42

Kathleen Richerson
Chief Nursing Officer
North Bay Healthcare
VacaValley Hospital
Vacaville, California
Chapter 3

Katherine Ricossa, MS, RN
Director of Education
Kaiser Permanente San Jose Medical Center
San Jose, California
Chapter 58

Leslie Rittenmeyer, RN, CNS, PsyD
Associate Professor of Nursing
Purdue University Calumet School of Nursing
Hammond, Indiana
Chapter 13

Carol Robinson, RN, MPA, CNAA, FAAN
Director of Nursing/Chief Patient Care Services Officer
University of California Davis Health System
Sacramento, California
Chapter 5

Denita Ryan, MN, RN, ANP-C, CNRN
Nurse Practitioner, Adult Neurosurgical Service
Barrow Neurological Institute
St. Joseph's Hospital and Medical Center
Phoenix, Arizona
Chapters 29 and 30

Ann Sievers, RN, MA, CORLN
Clinical Nurse Specialist
University California Davis Medical Center
University of California Davis
Sacramento, California
Chapter 34

Karen Silady, RN, MN, CNS, CEN
Staff Nurse
East Jefferson General Hospital
Metairie, Louisiana
Chapter 72

Donna Stanbridge, BScN, MA, CPN(C)
Clinical Nurse Specialist
Minimally Invasive Surgery and Surgical Innovation
McGill University Health Centre
Montreal General Hospital
Montreal, QC
Chapter 26

James Stotts, RN, MS
Director
PCS, Practice and Education
Stanford University Medical Center
Stanford, California
Chapter 40

Douglas Sutton, APRN, EdD
Assistant Professor,
Christine E. Lynn College of Nursing
Florida Atlantic University
Boca Raton, Florida
Chapters 45 and 46

Debera Thomas, DNS, RN, CS, ARNP
Assistant Dean and Associate Professor,
Christine E. Lynn College of Nursing
Florida Atlantic University
Boca Raton, Florida
Chapters 45 and 46

Gail Thurkauf, RN, MS
Director of the Department of Nursing Quality
Georgetown University Hospital
Washington, D.C.
Chapter 19

Eileen Trigoboff, RN, APRN/PMH-BC, DNS, DABFN
Clinical Nurse Specialist
Buffalo Psychiatric Center
Buffalo, New York
Chapter 16

Sheila Tucker, MA, RD
Nutritionist, Dining Services
Part Time Faculty, School of Nursing and Lynch School of Education
Boston College
Boston, Massachusetts
Chapter 14

Danielle Vigeant, MScN, CPN(C)
Nurse Manager
Peri-operative Services
McGill University Health Centre
Royal Victoria Hospital
Montreal, QC
Chapter 26

Laurie Walsh, NP
Kaiser Permanente
Sacramento, CA
Chapter 10

Suzanne Watt, RN, MSc(A), CON(C)
McGill University Health Centre
Royal Victoria Hospital
Montreal, QC
Chapter 26

Kathy Yeates, BSN, RN, CCRN
Mercy General Hospital
Sacramento, California
Chapter 60

Supplement Contributors

Tracy Blanc, RN, BSN
Nursing Instructor
Ivy Tech Community College
Terre Haute, Indiana
Instructor's Resource Manual

Monica G. Cashiotta-Munn, RN, MFT
Instructor
National University
La Jolla, CA
Instructor's Resource Manual

Kim Cooper, RN, MSN
Nursing Department Chair
Ivy Tech Community College
Terre Haute, Indiana
Instructor's Resource Manual
Test Item File

Karlynne Galczyk, RN, MSN, MPH
Lecturer
Widener University School of Nursing
Chester, Pennsylvania
Instructor's Resource Manual
Test Item File

Margaret Gingrich, RN, MSN
Professor
Harrisburg Area Community College
Harrisburg, Pennsylvania
Test Item File

Wanda K. Lawrence, PhD, RNC, MSN
Assistant Professor of Nursing
Winston-Salem State University
Winston-Salem, North Carolina
Instructor's Resource Manual

Andrea R. Mann, MSN, RN
Instructor and Third Level Chair
Frankford Hospital School of Nursing
Philadelphia, Pennsylvania
Test Item File

Dawna Martich, RN, BSN, MSN
Director, Education
MCN Healthcare, Inc.
Denver, Colorado
Test Item File

Joyce Mikal-Flynn
Assistant Professor
Division of Nursing
Sacramento State University
Sacramento, California
Instructor's Resource Manual

Donna Russo, RN, MSN, CCRN, CNE
Nursing Instructor
Frankford Hospital School of Nursing
Philadelphia, Pennsylvania
Test Item File

Barbara Kim Stevens, MSN, RN
Professor of Nursing
University of Rio Grande
Rio Grande, Ohio
Instructor's Resource Manual

Betsy Swinny MSN, RN, CCRN
Critical Care Educator
St. Lukes Baptist Hospital
San Antonio, Texas
Test Item File

REVIEWERS. Our heartfelt thanks go out to our colleagues from schools of nursing across the country who have given their time generously to help create this exciting new medical-surgical nursing textbook. These individuals helped us plan and shape our book and resources by reviewing chapters, art, design, and more. *Medical-Surgical Nursing: Preparation for Practice* has reaped the benefit of your collective knowledge and experience as nurses and teachers, and we have improved the materials due to your efforts, suggestions, objections, endorsements, and inspiration. Among those who gave their time generously to help us are the following:

UNIT REVIEWERS. We are so grateful to our Unit Reviewers, who contributed their valuable time, knowledge, and insight to ensure that the Units are written to the highest standard of accuracy and consistency.

Christi DeLemos, RN, MSN, ACNP-c
UC Davis Medical Center, Department of Neurological Surgery, Sacramento, California
Unit 6

Heidi A. Hotz, RN
Cedars-Sinai Medical Center, Los Angeles, California
Unit 16

Dawn Lambie, RN, MSN, CHPN
Kaiser Permanente, Roseville, California
Immunological, Inflammatory and Hematological Disorders
Units 5, 13, and 14

Mary McDermott, MS, RN
Hospital for Special Surgery, New York, New York
Unit 12

Charlotte Miller, RN
Cool, California
Units 1, 2, and 8

Kim Moody, PhD, RN
University of Southern Maine School of Nursing, Portland, ME
Unit 8

Donna York, RN, MS, CFRN, CMTE
Indiana University School of Nursing, Indianapolis, Indiana
Units 3 and 4

Kelly Karr, BA, MA
Sacramento, California

Academic Reviewers

Faisal H. Aboul-Enein, RN, MSN, MPH, NP, BC
Texas Woman's University College of Nursing, Houston, Texas

Joy Ache-Reed, RN, MSN
Indiana Wesleyan University, Marion, Indiana

Betty N. Adams, PhD
Prairie View A & M University, Houston, Texas

Sheila A. Alexander, RN, PhD
University of Pittsburgh, Pittsburgh, Pennsylvania

Cheryl Alt, RN, MSN
Great Falls College of Technology, Great Falls, Montana

Ella R. Anaya, RN, MSN, CNS
Kent State University, Kent, Ohio

Beverly Anderson, MSN, RN
Salt Lake Community College, Salt Lake City, Utah

Cheryl Anema, RN, MSN
Trinity Christian College, Palos Heights, Illinois

Gail Armstrong, RN, ND
University of Colorado–Denver, Denver, Colorado

Karen Sue Bailey, RN, MSN, APRN-BC-FNP
Marshall University, Huntington, West Virginia

L. Antoinette Bargagliotti, DNSc, RN, ANEF
University of Memphis, Memphis, Tennessee

Shirley Sperinde Baxter, RN, BSN, MSN
University of California Davis Medical Center, Sacramento, California

Randal D. Beaton, PhD, EMT
University of Washington, Seattle, Washington

Julie A. Beck, RN, DEd, CNE
York College of Pennsylvania, York, Pennsylvania

Deborah Becker, PhD, RN, ACNP-BC
University of Pennsylvania, Philadelphia, Pennsylvania

William T. Bester, MSN, RN
The University of Texas at Austin, Austin, Texas

Cynthia Ann Blum, PhD, RN, CNE
Florida Atlantic University, Boca Raton, Florida

Donna W. Bohmfalk, MSN, RN
The University of Texas Medical Branch, Galveston, Texas

Joanne Bonesteel, MS, RN
Excelsior College, Albany, New York

Portia A. Botchway, MSN, RN
Clemson University, Clemson, South Carolina

Sharon McFadden Bradley, MSN, RN, CNL
University of Florida College of Nursing, Gainesville, Florida

Janet Witucki Brown, RN, PhD
University of Tennessee, Knoxville, Knoxville, Tennessee

Cindy L. Brubaker, EdD, RN
Bradley University, Peoria, Illinois

Tammy Bryant, RN, BSN
Southwest Georgia Technical College, Thomasville, Georgia

Kathleen Burke, PhD, RN
Ramapo College, Mahwah, New Jersey

Dorothy Burns, RN, PhD, MS
Hampton University, Hampton, Virginia

Dorothy Stano Carlson, DEd, RN
Edinboro University of Pennsylvania, Edinboro, Pennsylvania

Tracy Carlson, MSN, RN
Kent State University, Kent, Ohio

Monica G. Cashiotta-Munn, RN, MFT, MSN
National University, La Jolla, California

Olivia Catolico, PhD, RN, BC
Dominican University of California, San Rafael, California

Donna York Clark, RN, MS, CFRN, CMTE
Golden Hour Data Systems, San Diego, California

Patricia Clark, RN, PhD
Abraham Baldwin College, Tifton, Georgia

Pamela S. Combs, MSN, RN
University of Louisville, Louisville, Kentucky

Cathy Cormier, PhD, RN
Southeastern Louisiana University, Hammond, Louisiana

Nancy Dentlinger, RN, AS, BS, MS, EdD
Redlands Community College, El Reno, Oklahoma

Susan DeSanto-Madeya, DNSc, RN
University of Massachusetts, Boston, Massachusetts

Patricia Brown Dominguez, RN, MSN
Houston Baptist University, Houston, Texas

Nancy Duffy, RN, CEN, MSN
Medical University of South Carolina, Charleston, North Carolina

Jaibun Earp, FNP, PhD, MA, BSN
Florida Agricultural and Mechanical University, Quincy, Florida

Sandra Eggenberger, PhD
Minnesota State University Mankato, Mankato, Minnesota

Jeanette Embry, RN, MS, PhD
West Texas A&M University, College Station, Texas

Deborah Erickson, PhD, RN
Bradley University, Peoria, Illinois

Geralyn M. Frandsen, EdD, RN
Maryville University, St. Louis, Missouri

Kathy Frum, RN, MSN
West Virginia University at Parkersburg, Parkersburg, West Virginia

Kay E. Gaehle, RN, PhD
Southern Illinois University, Edwardsville, Illinois

Karlynne Galczyk, RN, MSN, MPH
Widener University, Chester, Pennsylvania

Donna Gauthier, PhD, RN, CNE
University of Louisiana, Lafayette, Louisiana

Rebecca Gesler, MSN, RN
Spalding University, Louisville, Kentucky

Margaret M. Gingrich, RN, MSN
Harrisburg Area Community College, Harrisburg, Pennsylvania

Donna Glankler, MSN, RN
College of Mount St. Joseph, Cincinnati, Ohio

Sharron Guillett, PhD, RN
Marymount University, Arlington, Virginia

Susan Sweat Gunby, RN, PhD
Mercer University, Atlanta, Georgia

Polly C. Haigler, PhD, RN
University of South Carolina, Columbia, South Carolina

Lori Rae Hamilton, RN, MSN
Otero Junior College, La Junta, Colorado

Jenny Hamner, DSN
Auburn University, Auburn, Alabama

Chris Hawkins, PhD, RN
Texas Woman's University, Denton, Texas

Connie S. Heflin, MSN, RN, CNE
West Kentucky Community and Technical College, Paducah, Kentucky

Carol Heim, MA, RN
Mount Mercy College, Cedar Rapids, Iowa

Jan Herren, MSN, RNC
Southern Arkansas University, Magnolia, Arkansas

Susan Holmes, RN, MSN, CRNP
Auburn University, Auburn, Alabama

Gail M. Holtzman, MSN, CCRN, CNE
University of Alaska, Anchorage, Alaska

Linda Howe, PhD, CNS, CNE
Clemson University, Clemson, South Carolina

Trinity Ingram, MSN, APRN, CPNP, PCNS
South University and Savannah Technical College, Savannah, Georgia

Pamela B. James, RN, BSN, MSN
Fayetteville Technical Community College, Fayetteville, North Carolina

Cindy K. Jenness, BSN, MAE, MSN
Allen College, Waterloo, Iowa

Michelle Johnson, MSN, RN
Northern Michigan University, Marquette, Michigan

Pam Johnson, MSN, RN, APRN, BC
Viterbo University, LaCrosse, Wisconsin

Karin Jones, RN, PhD
Grambling State University, Grambling, Louisiana

Peggy Kalowes, RN, MSN, CNRN, CNS
California State University, Los Angeles, California

Tamara Kear, MSN, RN, CNN
Gwynedd-Mercy College, Gwynedd Valley, Pennsylvania

Frances Keen, DNSc, RN
Villanova University, Villanova, Pennsylvania

Deborah Kern, MSN, RNCS, FNP
Montana State University, Bozeman, Montana

Joan E. King, PhD, ACNP-BC, ANP-BC
Vanderbilt University, Nashville, Tennessee

Kenn M. Kirksey, RN, PhD, APRN, BC
California State University, Fresno, California

Ina Koerner, RN, MS, PhD
University of Louisiana, Lafayette, Louisiana

Cheryl Lacasse, PhDc, RN, OCN
University of Arizona, Tucson, Arizona

Dawn Lambie, RN, MSN, CHPN
Kaiser Permanente, Roseville, California

R. Shelly Lancaster, MSN, RN
University of Wisconsin, Oshkosh, Wisconsin

Karen M. Lavallee, RNC, CS, ARNP
New Hampshire Technical Institute, Concord, New Hampshire

Wanda K. Lawrence, PhD, RN, MSN
Winston-Salem State University, Winston-Salem, North Carolina

Theresa Gunter Lawson, MS, APRN, FNP-BC
Lander University, Greenwood, South Carolina

Patricia Price Lea, PhD, RNC, MSN, MSEd, BSN
North Carolina Agricultural & Technical State University, Greensboro, North Carolina

Barbara Lee, MSN, RN, BC, MEd, CWOCN
Bellarmine University, Louisville, Kentucky

Elizabeth Lee, MSN, APRN, BC
Harding University, Searcy, Arkansas
Manon Lemonde, RN, PhD, BScN, MScN
University of Ontario Institute of Technology, Ontario, Canada
Linda Lichty, RN
Cosumnes Community Fire Service District, Elks Grove, California
Cynthia A. Logan, PhD, RN
Southeastern Louisiana University, Hammond, Louisiana
Gayla Love, RN, MS, BSN, CCM
Griffin Technical College, Griffin, Georgia
Naomi Lungstrom, MN, FNP
Washington State University, Pullman, Washington
Susan Luparell, PhD, CNS-BC, CNE
Montana State University, Bozeman, Montana
Amy Ma, DNP, APRN, FNP-BC
Long Island University, Brooklyn, New York
Bernadette Madara, BC, EdD, APRN
Southern Connecticut State University, New Haven, Connecticut
Cecilia Jane Maier, MS, RN
Mount Carmel College of Nursing, Columbus, Ohio
Andrea R. Mann, MSN, RN
Frankford Hospital School of Nursing, Philadelphia, Pennsylvania
Bradley J. Manuel, RN, MSN, CNOR(E)
Texas Woman's University, Houston, Texas
Karen S. March, PhD, RN, CCRN, ACNS-BC
York College of Pennsylvania, York, Pennsylvania
Suzanne Marnocha, RN, MSN, PhD, CCRN
University of Wisconsin, Oshkosh, Wisconsin
Janet G. Marshall, PhD, RN
Florida A&M University School of Nursing, Tallahassee, Florida
Brenda Mason, MSN, BSN, RN-FNP
Alderson-Broaddus College, Philippi, West Virginia
Dotti Mathers, MSN, RN
Pennsylvania College of Technology, Williamsport, Pennsylvania
Amy McClune, PhD, RN, BC
Edinboro University of Pennsylvania, Edinboro, Pennsylvania
Emily McClung, RN, MSN
Kent State University College of Nursing, Kent, Ohio
Barbara McGraw, MSN, RN, CNE
Central Community College, Grand Island, Nebraska
Phyllis McKiernan, MSN, APN-C, RN
Hackensack University Medical Center, Hackensack, New Jersey
Melody McKinney, DNS, RN
Indiana State University, Terre Haute, Indiana
Tara McMillan-Queen, RN, MN, APRN, BC
Mercy School of Nursing, Charlotte, North Carolina
Debbie Metzler, MSN, APNP, GNP-BC
Bellin College of Nursing, Green Bay, Wisconsin
Rita Miller, MSN, RN
Idaho State University–Pocatello, Boise, Idaho
Connie Miller, MSN, FNP-C
University of Northern Colorado, Greeley, Colorado
Donna Molyneaux, PhD
Gwynedd-Mercy College, Gwynedd Valley, Pennsylvania
Kimberly Moody, PhD, RN-CS, ANP
University of Southern Maine, Portland, Maine
Judy K. Moren, BM, RN
California State University, Sacramento, California
Martha C. Morris, PhD, RN
The University of Southern Mississippi, Hattiesburg, Mississippi
Deborah R. Murphy, RN, MSN
West Virginia University at Parkersburg, Parkersburg, West Virginia
Janice A. Neil, RN, PhD
East Carolina University, Greenville, North Carolina
Nancy Noble, RN, MSN, ACNS-BC
Marian University, Fond du Lac, Wisconsin
Catherine M. Nosek, RN, PhD
Winona State University, Winona, Minnesota
Elizabeth Palmer, PhD, RN, CNE
Indiana University of Pennsylvania, Indiana, Pennsylvania
Laurie J. Palmer, RN, MS, AOCN
Monroe Community College, Rochester, New York

Denise Panosky, MSN, RN, CCHP
University of Connecticut, Storrs, Connecticut
Barbara Patterson, RN, PhD
Widener University, Chester, Pennsylvania
Jo Ann Pelaez-Fisher, MSHA, BSN, RN
The College of Southern Nevada, Las Vegas, Nevada
Linda Honan Pellico, MSN, PhD, RN
Yale University, New Haven, Connecticut
Sheila Perrault, MSN
Salem State College, Salem, Massachusetts
Kathleen Perrin, PhD, RN, CCRN
Saint Anselm College, Manchester, New Hampshire
Rebecca Phillip, PhD, RN
The University of Oklahoma Health Sciences Center, Oklahoma City, Oklahoma
Jennifer Ponto, RN, BSN
South Plains College, Levelland, Texas
Christopher B. Powe, PhD(c), ACNP
University of Mississippi Medical Center, Jackson, Mississippi
Rorey D. Pritchard, RN, MSN, CNOR
Chippewa Valley Technical College, Eau Claire, Wisconsin
Anne Purvis, RN, MSN
Gordon College, Barnesville, Georgia
Colleen M. Quinn, RN, MSN
Broward College, Pembroke Pines, Florida
Valeria Ramdin, MS, APRN-BC
Northeastern University, Boston, Massachusetts
Carol Delia Ratta, RN, MS, CCRN
Stony Brook University, Stony Brook, New York
Kathleen M. Rayman, PhD, RN
East Tennessee State University, Johnson City, Tennessee
Anita K. Reed, MSN, RN
Saint Joseph's College, Lafayette, Indiana
Joy Reed, MS, BSS, ADN
Indiana Wesleyan University, Marion, Indiana
Mattie L. Rhodes, RN, PhD, CNS
State University of New York at Buffalo, Buffalo, New York
Gwendolyn E. Richardson, APRN, MN
Midlands Technical College, Columbia, South Carolina
Margaret Richbourg, MSN, BSN, ASN, AA
Florida State University, Tallahassee, Florida
Michelle Robnett, BA, BSN, MA, MBA, PhD
University of Iowa, Iowa City, Iowa
Cheryl Ross, MS, RN
Oklahoma City University, Oklahoma City, Oklahoma
Donna Russo, RN, MSN, CCRN, CNE
Frankford Hospital School of Nursing, Philadelphia, Pennsylvania
Arlene Saliba, MS, RNCS
Andrews University, Berrien Springs, Michigan
Buckie Sasser, RN, MSN
South Georgia College, Douglas, Georgia
Jacalyn M. Schaefer, MSN, RN, CNOR
The Ohio State University, Columbus, Ohio
Gisela Schmidt, RN, MA, MS
Andrews University, Berrien Springs, Michigan
Nancy Schoofs, RN, PhD
Grand Valley State University, Grand Rapids, Michigan
Connie J. Schroeder, MS, RN
Danville Area Community College, Danville, Virginia
Jenny Schuessler, RN, DSN
Auburn University School of Nursing, Auburn, Alabama
Lisa A. Seldomridge, PhD, RN
Salisbury University, Salisbury, Maryland
Joanne Farley Serembus, EdD, RN, CCRN, CNE
Drexel University, Philadelphia, Pennsylvania
Laurie J. Singel, MSN, RN, BC
The University of Texas Health Science Center at San Antonio
San Antonio, Texas
Patricia Slesinski, BS, MS
State University of New York, Middletown, New York
Rose Marie Smith, MSN, RN
Platt College North, Oklahoma City, Oklahoma
Soledad M. Smith, RN, PhD
The University of Louisiana at Lafayette, Lafayette, Louisiana

Marilyn Smith-Stoner, RN, PhD, CHPN
California State University, San Bernardino, California
Cheryl Bruick Sorge, RN, MA
Indiana University, Fort Wayne, Indiana
Sharon Souter, RN, PhD, CNE
University of Mary Hardin-Baylor, Belton, Texas
Martha Spies, PhD
Chamberlain College of Nursing, St. Louis, Missouri
Russlyn A. St. John, RN, MSN
St. Charles Community College, Cottleville, Missouri
Annette Smith Stacy, MSN, RN, AOCN
Arkansas State University, Jonesboro, Arkansas
Barbara Kim Stevens, MSN, RN
University of Rio Grande, Rio Grande, Ohio
James Stotts, RN, MS, CNS
Stanford Hospital and Clinics, Stanford, California
Kathleen Stroh, MA, MSN, RN
Edinboro University of Pennsylvania, Edinboro, Pennsylvania
Ardith L. Sudduth, PhD, GNP, FNP-BC
University of Louisiana at Lafayette, Lafayette, Louisiana
Katherine Elizabeth Sullivan, BSN, MA
Rockland Community College, Suffern, New York
Sheila Cox Sullivan, PhD, RN, CNE
Central Arkansas Veterans Healthcare System, Little Rock, Arkansas
Beth Swart, RN, MES
Ryerson University, Toronto, Canada
Marianne F. Swihart, RN, BSN, MEd, MSN, CRNI, CWON, PCCN
Pasco Hernando Community College–West Campus, New Port Richey, Florida
Judith Tanner, RN, MSN
Sacramento City College, Sacramento, California
Marilyn M. Teeter, RN, MSN
Harrisburg Area Community College, Gettysburg, Pennsylvania
Kathleen Thiede, MA, RN
The College of St. Scholastica, Duluth, Minnesota
Scott Thigpen, RN, BSN, MSN, CCRN, CEN
South Georgia College, Douglas, Georgia
Cindy Thomas, PhD, RN
Mesa State College, Grand Junction, Colorado
Loris A.Thomas, PhD, ARNP, ACNP-BC/ANP-BC
University of Florida College of Nursing, Gainesville, Florida
Shirley Thompson, MSN, CNS, RN
Bethune-Cookman College, Daytona Beach, Florida
Janet P. Tracy, RN, PhD
William Paterson University, Wayne, New Jersey
Lise Turner, RNC, MSN
Mercy School of Nursing, Charlotte, North Carolina
Karla Uhde, RN, MSN, CNE
Ivy Tech Community College of Indiana-Southwest, Evansville, Indiana
Carolyn VanCouwenberghe, RN, PhD
California State University, Sacramento, California
Shellye A. Vardaman, RN, BC, MSN
Troy University, Troy, Alabama
Delayne Vogel, MSN, RN
Viterbo University School of Nursing, La Crosse, Wisconsin
Gerry Walker, MSN, RN
Park University, Parkville, Missouri
Susan Walker, PhD, RN, FNP
University of Texas at Arlington, Arlington, Texas
Patricia Walters, RN, ACNP, CCRN, ACLS, BCLS
Hackensack University Medical Center, Hackensack, New Jersey
Carol L. Warner, MSN, RN, CPN, FNP-BC
St. Luke's School of Nursing, Bethlehem, Pennsylvania
Diane Graham Webb, MSN, RN, CNE
Northwestern State University of Louisiana, Natchitoches, Louisiana
Bonnie K. Webster, MSN, RN, BC
University of Texas Medical Branch, Galveston, Texas
Linda B. Wheeler, RN, MSN
University of North Carolina at Greensboro, Greensboro, North Carolina
Ann White, RN, PhD, MBA, CNA, BC
University of Southern Indiana, Evansville, Indiana
Loretta White, DNS
Indiana State University, Terre Haute, Indiana

Barbara Wilder, DSN, CRNP
Auburn University, Auburn, Alabama
Anna Wilson, RN, BS
California State University, San Bernardino, California
Marion E. Winfrey, EdD, RN
University of Massachusetts, Boston, Massachusetts
Karen M. Wood, RN, DNSc, CCRN, CNL
Saint Xavier University, Chicago, Illinois
Lisa Woodley, MSN, RN
University of North Carolina, Chapel Hill, North Carolina
Kathy Woodruff, MSN, CRNP
University of Maryland, Baltimore, Maryland
Wendy Woodward, PhD, RN
Humboldt State University, Arcata, California
Linda Wray, RN, PhD
Eastern Kentucky University, Richmond, Kentucky
Malou Blanco Yarosh, MSN, RN, CNS
University of California, Los Angeles, California

Clinical Reviewers

Carmalita F. Andrus, CNRN, MN, FNP-C
Lafayette General Medical Center, Lafayette, Louisiana
Susan D. Anthony, MN, RN, APRN
South Plains Health Provider Organization, Plainview, Texas
Elizabeth Archer-Nanda, MSN, ARNP, CNS
Louisville Oncology, Louisville, Kentucky
Traci Ashcraft, BSN, RNBC
West Virginia University School of Nursing, West Milford, West Virginia
Kathleen J. Bailey, BSN, MA, MS, RN, CNM
US Army Landstuhl Regional Medical Center, Landstuhl, Germany
Dian Baker, RN, MA, MSN, CPNP
California State University Hospital, Sacramento, California
Brenda J. Baranowski, RN, CMSRN, CHPN
Froedtert Hospital, Milwaukee, Wisconsin
Shirley Sperinde Baxter, RN, BSN, MSN
University of California, Davis Medical Center, Sacramento, California
Megan Brunson, BSN, RN
St. Joseph's Hospital of Atlanta, Atlanta, Georgia
Christine Greiser Chadwell, MSN, APRN, BC, NP-C
Albright Health Center, Highland Heights, Kentucky
Karen Cheng, RN
Stanford University Medical Center, Stanford, California
Patricia G. Christy, MSN, APRN, BC, CFNP
Darian Lake Medical Clinic, Lake Charles, Louisiana
Regina Ciambrone, RN, BSN
Overlook Hospital, Summit, New Jersey
Donna York Clark, RN, MS, CFRN, CMTE
Golden Hour Data Systems, San Diego, California
John A. Collins, RN, CCRN
Lehigh Valley Hospital, Allentown, Pennsylvania
Damon Cottrell, MS, RN, CCNS, CCRN, APRN-BC, CEN
Providence St. Vincent Medical Center, Portland, Oregon
Janice Ann Cousino, RN, MSN, CNS
Hartford Hospital, Hartford, Connecticut
Diane K. Daddario, MSNc, RN, BC, CMSRN
Pennsylvania College of Technology, Williamsport, Pennsylvania
Yvonne D'Arcy, MS, CRNP, CNS
Suburban Hospital, Bethesda, Maryland
Sherri Davidson, RN, MSN, CS, ACNP
Central Texas Neurological Association, Waco, Texas
Christi DeLemos, RN, MSN, ACNP-c
UC Davis Medical Center, Department of Neurological Surgery, Sacramento, California
Lisa Duquette, BSN, CCRN, CEN, CFRN, EMT-P
Hartford Hospital, Hartford, Connecticut
Tracey C. Gaslin, RN, MSN, CRNI, CPNP
University of Louisville, Louisville, Kentucky
Barbara Gercke, MSN, FNP
San Diego State Student Health Services, San Diego, California
Denice E. Gibson, MSN
Banner Good Samaritan Medical Center, Phoenix, Arizona
Jean G. Gisler, RN, MSN, FNP-c, CDE
University of Texas Health Science Center at San Antonio, San Antonio, Texas

Theresa M. Glessner, RN, MSN, NP, BC, CCRN
Rochester General Hospital, Rochester, New York
Karen Diane Groller, MSN, RN, BC, CMSRN
Lehigh Valley Hospital, Allentown, Pennsylvania
Melody H. Hale, MSN, APRN-BC
New River Family Health, Scarbro, West Virginia
Lori Harris, RN, BSN, CNOR, CLNC
Mercy Health Center, Oklahoma City, Oklahoma
Amy Herrington, RN, MSN, CEN, NR-EMT-B
Bluegrass Community and Technical College, Lexington, Kentucky
Ellen S. Kane, MSN, RN, CDE
Banner Good Samaritan Medical Center, Phoenix, Arizona
Mary Knudtson, DNSc, NP
University of California Irvine, Irvine, California
Dawn Lambie, RN, MSN, CHPN
Kaiser Permanente, Roseville, California
Marilyn Leshko, RN
Lehigh Valley Hospital, Allentown, Pennsylvania
Patricia Lewis, MSN, FNP, CVN
Bassett Healthcare, Cooperstown, New York
Lori Kennedy Madden, MS, RN, ACNP, CCRN, CNRN
University of California, Davis, Sacramento, California
Kathleen-McCaffrey, RN, MSN
New York University Medical Center, New York, New York
Mary McDermott, MS, RN, NE-BC, APRN
Hospital for Special Surgery, New York, New York
Phyllis McKiernan, MSN, APN-C, RN
Hackensack University Medical Center, Hackensack, New Jersey
Ann McSwain, RN, MSN, CCRN, APRN, BC
St. Mary's Health Center, Jefferson City, Missouri
Peggy Tidikis Menck, PhD, RN
Independent Consultant
Barry M. Mitchneck, RN, MSN, CEN
Lehigh Valley Hospital, Allentown, Pennsylvania

Judy K. Moren, BM, RN
Nursing Education and Collections Training Manager, BloodSource, Sacramento, California
Maxine L. Morris, BSN
New York Medical Center, New York, New York
Agnes Oblas, ANP-C
Ray Road Medical Center, Phoenix, Arizona
Jaime L. Peters, ADN
Lehigh Valley Hospital, Bethlehem, Pennsylvania
Sherri Reese, RN, BSN, CIC
University of California Davis Medical Center, Sacramento, California
Lory Anne F. Robles, BSN, MSN, RN
Stanford University Hospital, Palo Alto, California
Bonnie Smith Rosario, RN
Assumption Rural Health Clinic, Napoleonville, Louisiana
Sande Rowlee, MS, RN, CNS, ACNP-BC
Sacramento Bariatric Medical Associates, Carmichael, California
Jeremy Sabatino, BSN
Trinitas Hospital, Elizabeth, New Jersey
Debby Skroch, BSN, RN
John C. Lincoln North Mountain Hospital, Phoenix, Arizona
Leonard Sterling, RN, BSN
University of California Davis Medical Center, Sacramento, California
Ann D. Stoltz, PhD, RN
California State University, Sacramento, California
Belinda J. Swearingen, RN, MSN, FNP-C
Corrigan Medical Center, Corrigan, Texas
William E. Trumbore, III, RN, CEN, PHRN, AAS, BSPA
Lehigh Valley Hospital, Allentown, Pennsylvania
Deborah Tuggle, RN, MN, CCNS
Jewish Hospital-St. Mary's Healthcare, Louisville, Kentucky
Patricia Walters, RN, ACNP, CCRN, ACLS, BCLS
Hackensack University Medical Center, Hackensack, New Jersey

Authors Kathleen Osborn, Cheryl Wraa, and Annita Watson and their contributors have written an integrative and comprehensive textbook for preparing basic nursing students for evidence-based practice in medical–surgical nursing. This text places caring practices as conceptualized by the nurse theorist Sr. Simone Roach (1984) at the center of excellent nursing practice. Caring includes six essential components: compassion, competence, confidence, conscience, commitment, and comportment. The authors also place clinical judgment and critical thinking within the context of best evidence-based practice, recognizing that nursing and medicine are subject to ever-changing modes of scientific discovery and validation and that a particular patient may not easily fit into statistical norms. Therefore, the nurse must exercise good clinical reasoning, evaluation of evidence, and critical thinking.

This text invites the student to begin a lifelong journey of learning and clinical knowledge development while providing a clear road map beginning with the general and moving to more complex medical–surgical nursing care. The ability to recognize the nature of an ambiguous, under-determined clinical situation is at the heart of good clinical reasoning and care. The Critical Alert boxes throughout the text help the student focus on essential nursing interventions for attending to a particular patient with specific clinical conditions. Mastering this text will facilitate students' learning so they begin to think like a nurse in a broad range of clinical situations.

The authors are to be commended for fostering a comprehensive and holistic view of nursing practice, as caregiver, patient advocate, educator, researcher, and leader. Clinical vignettes and nurse interviews are included so that the student can develop a clinical imagination for the care of patients with specific clinical conditions and sociocultural characteristics. I highly recommend this book for all nursing students! Studying this text is a great way to gain visions and examples of excellent nursing practice, research, patient advocacy, leadership, and education.

PATRICIA BENNER, RN, PhD, FAAN
Thelma Shobe Endowed Chair in Ethics and Spirituality
University of California, San Francisco,
Department of Social and Behavioral Sciences

As the 21st century evolves, nursing and its place in health care are also evolving. This era is characterized by rapid change, including a growing multicultural population, longer life spans, arrival of new illnesses, and poor health conditions. Explosive advances in technology, ever-changing work settings, and a complex health care environment that is costly and competitive contribute to nursing's evolving environment. The burgeoning level of information affects decision making, and newer, faster modes of communication add to the environment's complexity. The definitions of roles and responsibilities for health care providers are changing; new boundaries are defined in which accountabilities are different, quality indicators are vital, and evidence-based practice is the standard. Ethical considerations must be balanced as nurses are called on to think quickly in establishing short- and long-term goals with the patient and family, in collaboration with the health care team and the community.

Never before in the history of nursing has the profession faced greater challenges to produce enough qualified nurses to practice in such a rapidly changing environment. And at a time when the need for professional nurses is overwhelming, we face a deficit in qualified nurses. Thus, it is time for professional scrutiny, self-determination, and innovation; nursing education is challenged to be innovative in preparing nurses for practice now and in the future. The challenge is to prepare nurses who can provide cognitively skilled care, in a caring manner, with a diverse patient population, and in innovative health care settings.

The authors' vision for this textbook is to meet that challenge. This textbook prepares the learner to be a knowledgeable, caring health care professional. It is a foundation on which to build the nursing practice of today and tomorrow, incorporating the cognitive, affective, and psychomotor skills necessary to practice. This book is not a destination to be achieved, but the beginning of lifelong learning.

Goals

The goal of this book is to expose the learner to concepts basic to the practice of professional nursing, including caring, critical thinking, research, nursing process, and health promotion. Caring is the foundation of nursing practice because of its impact on patients and their families. The authors have adopted Roach's (1984) theory of caring, which includes six components: compassion, competence, confidence, conscience, commitment, and comportment. Within the chapter features the authors have applied these six components when describing the nursing care needed for each of the physical disorders. This helps learners develop their understanding of how to be a caring nurse and makes them aware of these qualities in fellow health care professionals' practice and when advocating for the patient.

The nursing process is used to develop critical thinking and clinical reasoning skills, providing the framework for applying evidenced-based practice. Research is discussed throughout the text, providing opportunities for the reader to examine current research topics and their application to nursing practice.

Health promotion, one of the primary roles of the nurse, is woven throughout the book, so learners will understand the importance of educating the patient/family about healthy habits and lifestyles that prevent illnesses and injuries.

Readers will become active participants in learning about nursing as they progress through the book contents. Learners should be able to demonstrate understanding of the concepts of medical–surgical nursing in a variety of settings by collaborating with the authors in defining requisite content for patient care, arriving at patient diagnoses, and developing plans of care.

The concepts of experiential learning shape the book contents. The intention is that learners will engage in reflective thought and analysis of their practice as they apply the principles and concepts incorporated in the book to clinical practice, using the book as a resource for validating perceptions, expanding their knowledge base, and evaluating their approaches to patient care. The book is organized to introduce learners to the basic concepts of health care in general, and to nursing specifically, before moving on to the concepts underlying health promotion and disease management and the common physiological disorders that are encountered in medical–surgical nursing practice.

The units and chapters are grouped to lead the learner from general concepts to the more complex concepts and challenges of disease management. The information is sequenced to enhance critical thinking skills, thereby promoting the development of clinical judgment.

Knowledge acquisition is enhanced by application, analysis, and evaluation. Thus, this text provides numerous opportunities for learners to participate in activities designed to develop critical thinking and problem-solving skills in collaboration with the nursing experts who have contributed to the book. These learning activities include preparing clinical preparation plans, establishing priorities for care, developing patient care plans, and evaluating knowledge in the affective, cognitive, and psychomotor domains of practice. As learners complete these experiential and interactive activities, they will achieve a holistic, scientific, and caring approach to professional nursing practice for now and the future.

Organization

The book consists of 16 units sequenced from simple, basic concepts to complex, medical–surgical disorders. Units 1 and 2 introduce the reader to general concepts related to health care delivery, followed by basic concepts related to nursing practice. The next two units cover physiological concepts and the theoretical basis of skills that are germane to all areas of nursing practice. Units 5 through 16 focus on physiological disorders common to medical–surgical nursing. Each disorder unit opens with an assessment chapter that provides a template to assess the presenting patient within the specific body system.

THE TEXT FEATURES were designed to highlight the concepts that form the framework for this textbook and that are basic to professional nursing: **caring, research, critical thinking, the nursing process,** and **health promotion.** The capstone feature in each disorders chapter, **Clinical Preparation,** offers learners the opportunity to bring all of the concepts into one summary exercise and thus prepares learners for safe and knowledgeable clinical practice in their future work as professional nurses.

Profiles in Nursing

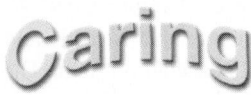
Caring

Profiles in Nursing. Each unit opens with a portrait of a nurse who describes "a day in the life" of working in a given specialty area. This profile includes a snapshot of a typical day and highlights the nurse's application of the six components of caring into his or her specialty. The information helps nursing students learn about the possibilities open to them when they are deciding where to spend concentrated clinical rotations or contemplating a job change.

Heart Failure

Clinical Problem

Heart failure (HF) remains the most common discharge diagnosis in elderly patients, accounting for almost a quarter of all cardiovascular hospitalizations (Stewart et al., 2002). Heart failure patients commonly experience readmissions due to noncompliance, lack of understanding of self-management principles, inadequate treatment, and/or progressive disease. Although a number of pharmacologic treatments have been shown to improve outcomes in patients with HF (Jessup & Brozena, 2003), the prognosis of these patients remains poor (MacIntyre et al., 2000), resulting in frequent readmission to the hospital. Thus, there is a need for other approaches to management.

Research Findings

McAlister, Stewart, Ferrua, & McMurray (2004) conducted a study to determine whether multidisciplinary strategies improve outcomes for HF patients. The researchers searched electronic databases, bibliographies, and contacted experts to find multidisciplinary management programs in HF. Twenty-nine trials (5,039 patients) were identified. The researchers independently reviewed the results of the search strategy and selected all studies reporting the impact of outpatient-based multidisciplinary management strategies on mortality or hospitalization rates in patients with HF. Each type of intervention was then independently assigned to one of four groups: (1) multidisciplinary HF clinic; (2) multidisciplinary team providing specialized follow-up but not in a hospital or practice-based clinic; (3) telephone follow-up or telemonitoring and enhanced communication with primary care physician (including advice to deteriorating patients to see their regular physician); or (4) educational programs designed to enhance patient self-care activities.

The study results reveal that these programs are associated with a 27% reduction in HF hospitalization rates and a 43% reduction in total number of HF hospitalizations. Those strategies that incorporate specialized follow-up by a multidisciplinary team or in a multidisciplinary HF clinic also reduce all-cause mortality by approximately one-quarter and all-cause hospitalizations by one-fifth.

Implications for Nursing Practice

In order to assist the patient in getting ready for discharge from the hospital, it is essential that the nurse have an understanding of the symptoms, diagnosis, and management (medical, device, and self-management). The nurse must stress the importance of compliance with every aspect of care. If the patient has been cared for using a multidisciplinary approach, the nurse typically coordinates each member of the team. The nurse must reinforce teaching and

determine the patient/family's understanding of the disease and its management.

When doing discharge planning, the nurse must ask the patient about her resources and support system. A plan needs to be developed that is realistic and manageable for the patient and family. Assistance for patients who may have difficulties taking or obtaining their medications must be provided. Ensure patients have access to urgent care, outside emergency department settings. It could be beneficial if a system for postdischarge telephone follow-up were instituted for these patients.

Critical Thinking Questions

1. Your patient was discharged from the hospital 3 days ago after a heart failure hospitalization. You are the nurse calling him to see how he is feeling since discharge. He states that his daughter was supposed to pick up his medications, but had a family emergency and forgot. He still does not have his medications, and he was discharged 5 days ago. What do you do?

2. You are the nurse in a clinic, and a patient with heart failure says she is taking her medications appropriately and following a low-salt, fluid-restricted diet. Your patient's weight continues to rise, and symptoms are worsening. What do you do to help this patient?

3. Your patient is readmitted for heart failure 2 weeks after his last heart failure hospitalization. What can you do to understand what went wrong at home, and how you can prevent a third admission?

References

Jessup, M., & Brozena, S. (2003). Medical progress heart failure. *The New England Journal of Medicine, 348,* 2007–2018.

MacIntyre, K., Capewell, S., Stewart, S., et al. (2000). Evidence of improving prognosis in heart failure trends in case fatality in 66,547 patients hospitalized between 1986 and 1995. *Circulation, 102,* 1126–1131.

McAlister, F. A., Stewart, S., Ferrua, S., & McMurray, J. J. (2004). Multidisciplinary strategies for the management of heart failure patients at high risk for admission: A systematic review of randomized trials. *Journal of the American College of Cardiology, 44*(4), 810–819.

Stewart, S., Jenkins, A., Buchan, S., McGuire, A., Capewell, S., & McMurray, J. J. V. (2002). The current cost of heart failure to the National Health Service in the UK. *European Journal of Heart Failure, 4,* 361–371.

EVIDENCE-BASED PRACTICE

Evidence-Based Practice. This feature presents examples of evidence and how the studies impact nursing interventions, patient teaching, skills, and professional guidelines. Learners have an opportunity to test their understanding by responding to the critical thinking questions provided for each Evidence-Based Practice feature.

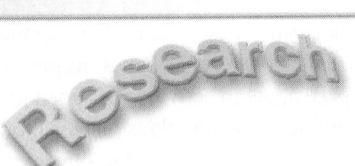
Research

RESEARCH OPPORTUNITIES AND CLINICAL IMPACT RELATED TO CORONARY ARTERY DISEASE	
Research Area	**Clinical Impact**
Stem cell injection after acute myocardial infarction.	Stimulate new growth of myocardial cells and increase myocardial viability.
Gene therapy for chronic CAD patients who have no other alternatives.	Stimulate angiogenesis, thereby decreasing symptoms and increasing quality of life.
Facilitated percutaneous intervention for acute myocardial infarction.	Conjoined mechanical and pharmacologic interventions for AMI will decrease mortality and increase myocardial salvage.
Establish heart-healthy food supplements.	Decrease hyperlipidemia, thereby providing risk factor modification for some predisposed risk factors.
Identify predictors of vulnerable plaque and their impact.	Provide ability to manage plaque and prevent plaque rupture, thus future coronary events.
Establish standard of providing fibrinolytic therapy in the field.	Increase survival for acute myocardial infarction patient.
Effect of community awareness programs on patients with ACS emphasizing early symptom recognition and treatment.	Decrease adverse cardiovascular events and increase survival from out-of-hospital events.
Effect of immediately triaging women with ACS-like symptoms to chest pain unit.	Increase survival in the female population and bring awareness because their symptoms are often missed.
Behavior modification techniques and their effect on CAD and its events.	Lower all modifiable risk factors, thereby decreasing cardiovascular events in a high-risk population.
Effect on established grammar and high school education program teaching about CAD; i.e., signs and symptoms, treatments, outcomes.	Establish an aware and healthier population early on, thereby decreasing total cardiovascular events.

Research Opportunities and Clinical Impact. Current research topics and their clinical impact introduces the learner to prospective research needs that are designed to potentially improve patient care. The purpose is to help the learner focus on future research needs and potential projects to improve patient care.

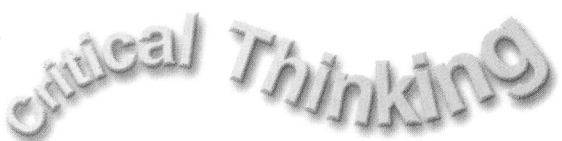
Critical Thinking

ETHICAL ISSUES for Pain Management at End of Life

Management of pain at the end of life is the right of the patient and the duty of the caregiver. Many families state that their loved ones suffered from untreated pain at the end of their life (Jackson & Abrahm, 2005). Failure to treat the pain adequately can arise from the caregiver's fear of violating ethical and moral tenets in the administration of pain medication to the dying patient.

At the end of life, the use of opioids, benzodiazepines, and other medications in doses high enough to control the patient's symptoms may unintentionally hasten death. This is referred to as double effect, where an action may have two possible effects, one good and one bad. The action is not considered immoral if it is undertaken with the intention of achieving the good effect without intending the bad effect, even though it may be foreseen. At the end of life not administering a drug to relieve symptoms because it may hasten death would be viewed as causing the patient harm and increased suffering.

Ethical Issues. This feature highlights the diverse ethical dilemmas that nurses face in clinical practice daily.

GERONTOLOGICAL CONSIDERATIONS Weight Management

Adults over age 65 years can benefit from weight management with improved day-to-day functioning and reduced cardiovascular risk. Before weight loss is recommended or attempted, however, a thorough nutrition assessment should be considered because of the high prevalence of malnutrition among older adults. Improper dieting attempts could unwittingly contribute to increased risk of malnutrition. Patients should be evaluated for their individual risks and benefits associated with potential weight loss. Specific attention should be given to preservation of muscle mass with physical activity. Appropriate referrals should be made for monitoring nutrition and exercise in the elderly.

Gerontological Considerations. The special needs of the fastest growing population are considered in order to help prevent complications and improve the prognoses for elderly patients.

CULTURAL CONSIDERATIONS for Therapeutic Communications

Munoz and Luckmann (2005) provide a rationale for the growing need for transcultural communication. They cite the increasing ethnic, racial, and cultural diversity of the United States; the increase in the number of patients who represent different culturally influenced patterns of health behavior; the different cultural meanings of health care; the different ways in which patients and families respond to health care; the multicultural nature of health care settings; and the nursing profession's commitment to culturally competent humanistic care. They further contend that talking to strangers about deeply personal issues is often difficult and may be particularly so for patients who are from different cultural backgrounds. They identify several behaviors on the part of nurses that are necessary to encourage patients to talk about themselves. Nurses must convey empathy, show respect, build trust, establish rapport, listen actively, provide appropriate feedback, and demonstrate genuine interest (p. 148). They also identify barriers to effective transcultural communication as follows: nurses' lack of knowledge, bias, ethnocentrism, prejudice, and stereotyping. Further, language differences, differences in the understanding of terminology, and differences in perceptions and expectations also create barriers (p. 162).

Cultural Considerations. These topics teach the learner to be sensitive to the needs of patients with different ethnic/cultural backgrounds, religious practices, and beliefs about health care and end of life, thereby enabling the learner to develop a multicultural approach to care.

GENETIC CONSIDERATIONS Implications for Weight Management

Speculation about the genetic implications in weight management has existed for some time. The specific roles of genetics as related to risk of obesity and eating disorders are being investigated. Risk factors for the development of eating disorders have been linked to genetic phenotypes for other disorders, such as the traits for obsessive-compulsive disorder and disturbances of dopamine systems (Kaye et al., 2004; Shinohara et al., 2004).

The role of genetics and the possibility of genetic manipulation have been heavily researched in the hope of identifying obesity risk factors and treatment options. Substances involved in appetite regulation, such as neuropeptide Y and ghrelin, proteins involved in thermogenesis, and leptin, and their relation to obesity are among the areas of research (Campion, Milagro, & Martinez, 2004; Marti, Moreno-Aliaga, Hebebrand, & Martinez, 2004). Although the topic of genetic influence on the development of both eating disorders and obesity is intriguing, it is difficult to draw firm conclusions without further research into these areas (Bulik, Sullivan, Wade, & Kendler, 2000; Kaye et al., 2004).

Genetic Considerations. This box contributes vital information about risk factors, therapies, research, legal implications, and counseling/ screening, as appropriate.

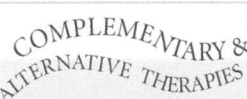
COMPLEMENTARY & ALTERNATIVE THERAPIES   Music Therapy

BEHAVIORAL MEDICINE, psychologists, and nurses have focused on prevention and psychosocial influences of cardiovascular diseases for the past 30 years. Music therapy is a viable collaborative, complementary method in the psychosocial arena for alleviating risks and motivating rehabilitation from cardiac events. For the most part, music is listened to via headphones during hospitalization. Cardiac units should stock headphones, CD or other varieties of players, and a wide selection of musical CDs, ranging from country-western to rock and roll to classical scores. Patients can be encouraged to use their music of choice on an outpatient basis prior to discharge.

Research Support:
Research supports the use of music to modulate heart health measurements such as heart rate and blood pressure, to enhance exercise programs, and to relieve stress symptoms. One study (Metzger, 2004) involved administering a music therapy survey to determine current use and preference for music in a cardiac rehabilitation program. Patients attending sessions in a large city hospital completed a survey on which they rated their level of use of music for exercise, relaxation, and enjoyment. Information was also gathered about musical preferences, musical experiences, and pertinent demographics. Patients, mostly white males over the age of 60, showed positive responses to the aesthetically pleasurable aspects of music. The results suggest that education about and development of music therapy in a cardiac rehabilitation program are warranted.

A German study with coronary patients (Vollert et al., 2003) concluded that music is able to lower stress and fear, contributing to relaxation in spite of physical exercise. Fifteen patients in a coronary sports unit listened to relaxation music while doing their heart-frequency-adapted exercises. Before the exercises and after listening to music, blood pressures were measured and blood was collected for determination of beta-endorphin. Simultaneous to blood collection, the participants had to perform two psychometric tests: the Perceived Stress Questionnaire (PSQ) of Levenstein, to measure the graduation of subjective perceived stress, and the State-Trait Anxiety

Inquiry (STAI) of Spielberger, as an indicator of coping. The whole protocol was performed one week prior to the mean trial, but without listening to music and without blood collections and blood pressure measurements. In the test trial without music, there were no significant changes in PSQ data. In the mean trial, under the influence of music, values in the section "worries" decreased as a sign of lower worries. STAI values were significantly lower as a sign of reduced fear after listening to music. Beta-endorphin concentration and systolic blood pressure decreased significantly after listening to music. These researchers conclude that in worries and fear, patients benefit by the intervention of music (Vollert et al., 2003).

The use of music therapy has been shown to reduce pain, anxiety, and physiological parameters in patients having surgical procedures. One study (Sendelbach et al., 2006) used an experimental design to compare the effects of music therapy versus a quiet, uninterrupted rest period on pain intensity, anxiety, physiological parameters, and opioid consumption after cardiac surgery. A sample of 86 patients was randomized to 1 of 2 groups receiving either 20 minutes of music (intervention) or 20 minutes of rest in bed (control). A significant reduction in anxiety and pain was demonstrated in the group that received music compared with the control group, but no difference was observed in systolic blood pressure, diastolic blood pressure, or heart rate. No reduction in opioid usage occurred in the 2 groups.

References
Metzger, L. K. (2004). Assessment of use of music by patients participating in cardiac rehabilitation. *Journal of Music Therapy, 41*(1), 55–69.
Sendelbach, S. E., Halm, M. A., Doran, K. A., Miller, E. H., & Gaillard, P. (2006). Effects of music therapy on physiological and psychological outcomes for patients undergoing cardiac surgery. *Journal of Cardiovascular Nursing, 21*(3), 194–200.
Vollert, J. O., Stork, T., Rose, M., & Mockel, M. (2003). Music as adjuvant therapy for coronary heart disease. Therapeutic music lowers anxiety, stress and beta-endorphin concentrations in patients from a coronary sport group. *Dtsch Med Wochenschr, 128*(51–52), 2712–2716.

Complementary and Alternative Therapies. The content of this feature introduces the learner to a variety of therapies used by patients that augment mainstream medicine. An understanding of the interactions of these therapies with more traditional therapies is essential for patient safety.

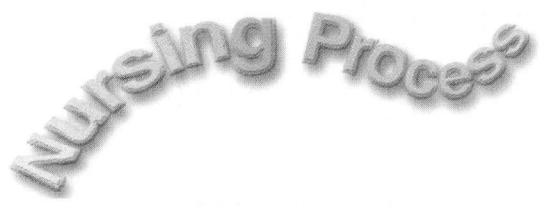

Nursing Process

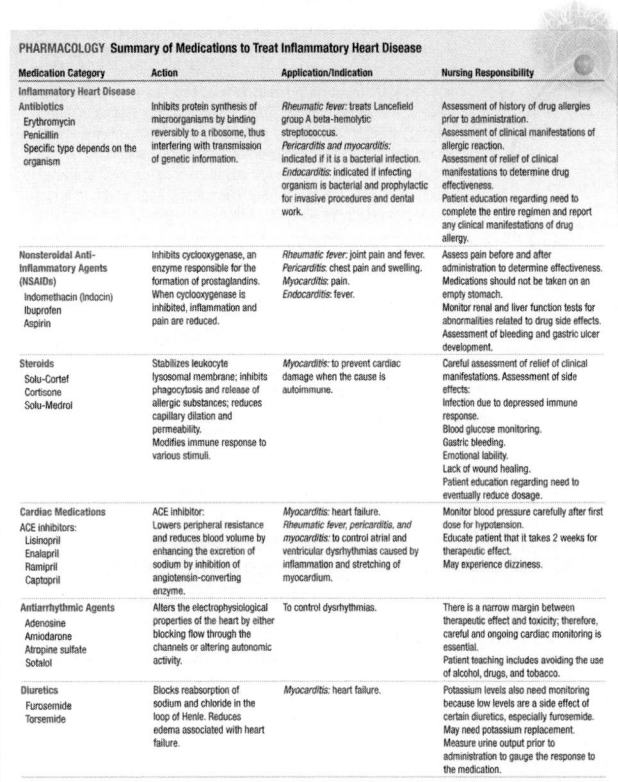

CRITICAL ALERT	
	When teaching patients about dietary control of cholesterol and lipids, it is important for the nurse to inquire about food preferences and cultural factors. The teaching needs to be tailored to include these preferences and cultural considerations in order to increase compliance with the restrictions.

Critical Alerts. This feature alerts the learner to the immediate need for a nursing intervention that will prevent complications and promote learning. The learner will differentiate the critical nature of various clinical situations and determine the need to prioritize interventions.

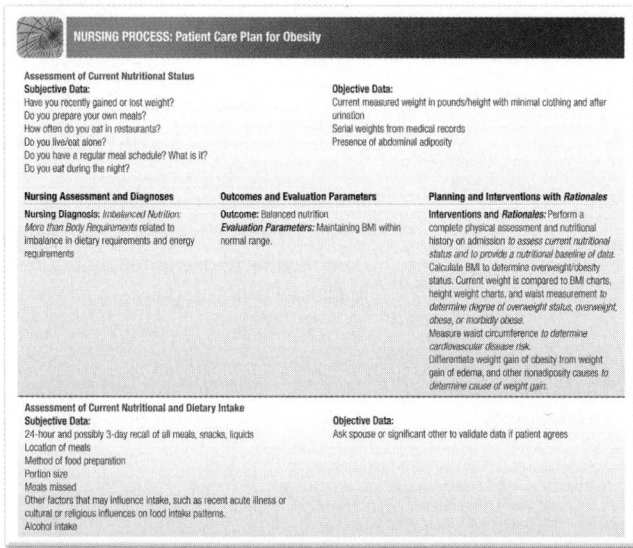

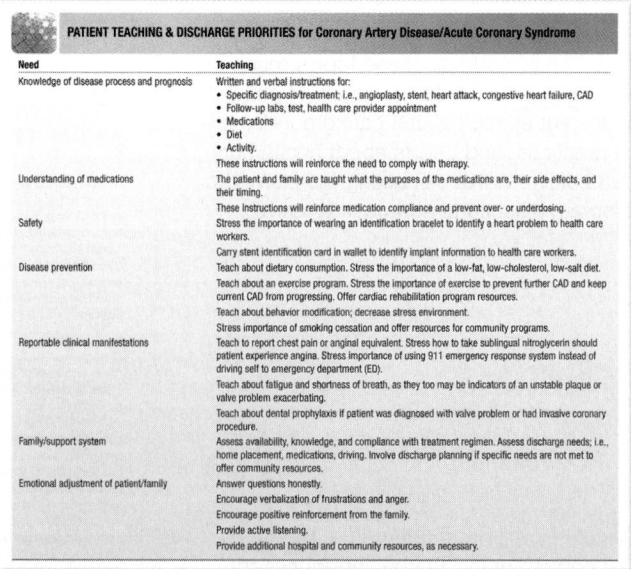

PHARMACOLOGY Summary of Medications to Treat Inflammatory Heart Disease

Medication Category	Action	Application/Indication	Nursing Responsibility
Inflammatory Heart Disease			
Antibiotics Erythromycin Penicillin Specific type depends on the organism	Inhibits protein synthesis of microorganisms by binding reversibly to a ribosome, thus interfering with transmission of genetic information.	*Rheumatic fever:* treats Lancefield group A beta-hemolytic streptococcus. *Pericarditis and myocarditis:* indicated if it is a bacterial infection. *Endocarditis:* indicated if infecting organism is bacterial and prophylactic for invasive procedures and dental work.	Assessment of history of drug allergies prior to administration. Assessment of clinical manifestations of allergic reaction. Assessment of relief of clinical manifestations to determine drug effectiveness. Patient education regarding need to complete the entire regimen and report any clinical manifestations of drug allergy.
Nonsteroidal Anti-Inflammatory Agents (NSAIDs) Indomethacin (Indocin) Ibuprofen Aspirin	Inhibits cyclooxygenase, an enzyme responsible for the formation of prostaglandins. When cyclooxygenase is inhibited, inflammation and pain are reduced.	*Rheumatic fever:* joint pain and fever. *Pericarditis:* chest pain and swelling. *Myocarditis:* pain. *Endocarditis:* fever.	Assess pain before and after administration to determine effectiveness. Medications should not be taken on an empty stomach. Monitor renal and liver function tests for abnormalities related to drug side effects. Assessment of bleeding and gastric ulcer development.
Steroids Solu-Cortef Cortisone Solu-Medrol	Stabilizes leukocyte lysosomal membrane; inhibits phagocytosis and release of allergic substances; reduces capillary dilation and permeability. Modifies immune response to various stimuli.	*Myocarditis:* to prevent cardiac damage when the cause is autoimmune.	Careful assessment of relief of clinical manifestations. Assessment of side effects: Infection due to depressed immune response. Blood glucose monitoring. Gastric bleeding. Emotional lability. Lack of wound healing. Patient education regarding need to eventually reduce dosage.
Cardiac Medications ACE inhibitors: Lisinopril Enalapril Ramipril Captopril	ACE inhibitor: Lowers peripheral resistance and reduces blood volume by enhancing the excretion of sodium by inhibition of angiotensin-converting enzyme.	*Myocarditis:* heart failure. *Rheumatic fever, pericarditis, and myocarditis:* to control atrial and ventricular dysrhythmias caused by inflammation and stretching of myocardium.	Monitor blood pressure carefully after first dose for hypotension. Educate patient that it takes 2 weeks for therapeutic effect. May experience dizziness.
Antiarrhythmic Agents Adenosine Amiodarone Atropine sulfate Sotalol	Alters the electrophysiological properties of the heart by either blocking flow through the channels or altering autonomic activity.	To control dysrhythmias.	There is a narrow margin between therapeutic effect and toxicity; therefore, careful and ongoing cardiac monitoring is essential. Patient teaching includes avoiding the use of alcohol, drugs, and tobacco.
Diuretics Furosemide Torsemide	Blocks reabsorption of sodium and chloride in the loop of Henle. Reduces edema associated with heart failure.	*Myocarditis:* heart failure.	Potassium levels also need monitoring because low levels are a side effect of certain diuretics, especially furosemide. May need potassium replacement. Measure urine output prior to administration to gauge the response to the medication.

Pharmacology Summary Tables. These four-column tables offer a comprehensive overview of the pharmacology for the chapter disorders, organized by drug categories, and include medications, actions, applications and indications, and the nursing responsibilities.

NURSING PROCESS: Patient Care Plan for Obesity

Assessment of Current Nutritional Status

Subjective Data:	Objective Data:
Have you recently gained or lost weight? Do you prepare your own meals? How often do you eat in restaurants? Do you live/eat alone? Do you have a regular meal schedule? What is it? Do you eat during the night?	Current measured weight in pounds/height with minimal clothing and after urination Serial weights from medical records Presence of abdominal adiposity

Nursing Assessment and Diagnoses	Outcomes and Evaluation Parameters	Planning and Interventions with *Rationales*
Nursing Diagnosis: *Imbalanced Nutrition: More than Body Requirements* related to imbalance in dietary requirements and energy requirements	**Outcome:** Balanced nutrition ***Evaluation Parameters:*** Maintaining BMI within normal range.	**Interventions and *Rationales:*** Perform a complete physical assessment and nutritional history on admission *to assess current nutritional status and to provide a nutritional baseline of data.* Calculate BMI to determine overweight/obesity status. Current weight is compared to BMI charts, height weight charts, and waist measurement *to determine degree of overweight status, overweight, obese, or morbidly obese.* Measure waist circumference *to determine cardiovascular disease risk.* Differentiate weight gain of obesity from weight gain of edema, and other nonadiposity causes *to determine cause of weight gain.*

Assessment of Current Nutritional and Dietary Intake

Subjective Data:	Objective Data:
24-hour and possibly 3-day recall of all meals, snacks, liquids Location of meals Method of food preparation Portion size Meals missed Other factors that may influence intake, such as recent acute illness or cultural or religious influences on food intake patterns. Alcohol intake	Ask spouse or significant other to validate data if patient agrees

Nursing Process: Patient Care Plan. The nursing process care plan provides the learner with an easy-to-follow, easy-to-apply, succinct way of organizing nursing care, guided by nursing diagnosis, assessment, intervention, and outcome evaluation. It is designed to assist the learner in developing a plan of care specific to the patient with desired patient outcomes and specific nursing interventions for a given diagnosis.

DIAGNOSTIC TESTS for Cardiac Valve Disease

Test and *Normal Values*	Expected Abnormality	Rationale for Abnormality
Echocardiogram and transesophageal echocardiography (TEE) Echocardiogram (ultrasound): *Normal chamber size and normal cardiac structures*	Abnormal structure and function of heart valves, able to identify thickened valve leaflets, vegetative growths, myocardial function, and chamber size. TEE is particularly useful not only for diagnosing but also for tracking the progression of the disease.	Vegetative growths and infection cause a thinning of valve leaflets leading to abnormal function.
Chest x-ray: *Clear lungs and normal heart size*	Pulmonary congestion, cardiac hypertrophy, chamber and great vessel enlargement, and calcification of the valves.	Abnormal valve function causes a change in blood flow leading to changes in chamber size and valve structure.
Cardiac catheterization: *Normal coronary artery blood flow, chamber size, and valve function*	The size of the valve opening and pressure gradients across valve surfaces is abnormal. Pressure in the heart chambers and pulmonary system is increased. Cardiac output typically is decreased.	Abnormal valve structure causes changes in openings leading to increased pressures in the cardiac chambers and decreased cardiac output.
Electrocardiogram (ECG): *Normal conduction time intervals*	Conduction delays, atrial and ventricular dysrhythmias, and the presence of cardiac ischemia. Is useful in detecting increased ischemia and the presence of life-threatening dysrhythmias.	Changes occur due to diminished blood flow to the myocardium due to decreased cardiac output caused by abnormal valvular function.
Cardiac MRI (CMR): *Normal heart valve function*	Valve size and competence.	Abnormal valve structure causes changes in openings, leading to increased pressures in the cardiac chambers and decreased cardiac output.

Diagnostic Tests. These tables inform the learner about the relevant diagnostic tests for the disorder under discussion. Normal result ranges are included, as well as expected abnormalities with rationales.

PATIENT TEACHING & DISCHARGE PRIORITIES for Coronary Artery Disease/Acute Coronary Syndrome

Need	Teaching
Knowledge of disease process and prognosis	Written and verbal instructions for: • Specific diagnosis/treatment; i.e., angioplasty, stent, heart attack, congestive heart failure, CAD • Follow-up labs, test, health care provider appointment • Medications • Diet • Activity. These instructions will reinforce the need to comply with therapy.
Understanding of medications	The patient and family are taught what the purposes of the medications are, their side effects, and their timing. These instructions will reinforce medication compliance and prevent over- or underdosing.
Safety	Stress the importance of wearing an identification bracelet to identify a heart problem to health care workers. Carry stent identification card in wallet to identify implant information to health care workers.
Disease prevention	Teach about dietary consumption. Stress the importance of a low-fat, low-cholesterol, low-salt diet. Teach about an exercise program. Stress the importance of exercise to prevent further CAD and keep current CAD from progressing. Offer cardiac rehabilitation program resources. Teach about behavior modification; decrease stress environment. Stress importance of smoking cessation and offer resources for community programs.
Reportable clinical manifestations	Teach to report chest pain or anginal equivalent. Stress how to take sublingual nitroglycerin should patient experience angina. Stress importance of using 911 emergency response system instead of driving self to emergency department (ED). Teach about fatigue and shortness of breath, as they too may be indicators of an unstable plaque or valve problem exacerbating. Teach about dental prophylaxis if patient was diagnosed with valve problem or had invasive coronary procedure.
Family/support system	Assess availability, knowledge, and compliance with treatment regimen. Assess discharge needs; i.e., home placement, medications, driving. Involve discharge planning if specific needs are not met to offer community resources.
Emotional adjustment of patient/family	Answer questions honestly. Encourage verbalization of frustrations and anger. Encourage positive reinforcement from the family. Provide active listening. Provide additional hospital and community resources, as necessary.

Patient Teaching & Discharge Priorities. This table helps identify priorities for discharge planning while integrating patient teaching with home and community care.

Health Promotion

Risk Factors. These boxes highlight particular items in the patient history and interview that should alert the nurse to possible problems.

Health Promotion. Found as appropriate in many chapters, Health Promotion sections call the learner's attention to one of the primary roles of the nurse, that of educating the patient and family about healthy habits and lifestyles, thereby preventing or ameliorating unhealthy conditions.

RISK FACTORS for Stress

Younger adults	Stress may go unnoticed in the very young and old.
Women in general	Women may be at higher risk than men for stress-related chest pain, but men's hearts may be more vulnerable to adverse effects from long-term stress.
Working mothers	Working mothers face higher stress levels and possibly adverse health effects, most likely because they bear a greater and more diffuse workload than men or other women.
Caregivers of family members	Caregivers of family members with physical or mental disabilities are at risk for chronic stress. They are particularly vulnerable to stress-related health threats such as influenza, depression, and heart disease.
Less educated individuals	Less educated individuals may be at higher risk because they may not be able to differentiate the causes of stress.
Divorced or widowed individuals	Unmarried people generally do not live as long as their married contemporaries.
The unemployed	Being unemployed is an environmental stressor that threatens security.
Isolated individuals	Such individuals usually lack support systems.
People who are targets of racial or sexual discrimination	Discrimination is an environmental stressor that is beyond individual control.
Those without health insurance	This is a threat to one's health that can lead to stress.
People who live in cities	City dwellers may be more stressed as a result of external stressors beyond their control.

NATIONAL GUIDELINES American Society of PeriAnesthesia Nurses Pain and Comfort Clinical Guidelines

Preoperative Phase

Assessment

1. Vital signs including pain and comfort goals (e.g., 0 to 10 scale).
2. Medical history (e.g., neurological status, cardiac and respiratory, instability, allergy to medication, food and objects, use of herbs, motion sickness, sickle cell, fibromyalgia, use of caffeine/substance abuse, fear, and anxiety).
3. Pain history (e.g., preexisting pain, acute, chronic, pain level, pattern, quality, type of source, intensity, location, duration/time, course, pain effect, and effects on personal life).
4. Pain behaviors/expressions or history (e.g., grimacing, frowning, crying, restlessness, tension, and discomfort behaviors, such as shivering, nausea, and vomiting. Note that physical appearance may not necessarily indicate pain/discomfort or its absence.)
5. Analgesic history: type (i.e., opioid, nonopioid, and adjuvant analgesics), dose, frequency, effectiveness, adverse effects, other medications that may influence choice of analgesics (e.g., anticoagulant, antihypertensive, muscle relaxants).
6. Patient's preferences (e.g., for pain relief/comfort measures, expectations, concerns, aggravating and alleviating factors, and clarification of misconceptions).
7. Pain/comfort acceptable levels (e.g., patient and family, as indicated, agree to plan of treatment/interventions postoperatively).
8. Comfort history (i.e., physiological, sociocultural, psychospiritual, and environment, such as spiritual beliefs/symbols, warming measures, music, comfort objects, privacy, positioning, factors related to nausea/vomiting).
9. Educational needs (i.e., consider age or level of education, cognitive and language appropriateness, and barriers to learning).
10. Cultural language preference, identification of personal beliefs, and resulting restrictions.
11. Pertinent laboratory results (e.g., prolonged prothrombin time, partial thromboplastin time, and abnormal international normalized ratio and platelet count to determine risk for epidural hematoma in patients with epidural catheter).

Interventions

1. Identify patient, validate physician's order and procedure (i.e., correct name of drug, dose, amount, route, and time), and validate type of surgery and correct surgical site as applicable.
2. Discuss pain and comfort assessment (i.e., presence, location, quality, intensity, age, language, condition, and cognitively appropriate pain rating scale [e.g., a 0 to 10 numerical scale or FACES scale] and comfort scale). Assessment method must be the same for consistency.
3. Discuss with patient and family, as indicated, information about reporting pain intensity using a numerical or FACES rating scales and available pain relief and comfort measures. Include discussion of patient's preference for pain and comfort measures; implement comfort measures (i.e., physiological, sociocultural, spiritual, environmental support as indicated by patient).
4. Discuss and dispel misconceptions about pain and pain management.
5. Encourage patient to take a preventive approach to pain and discomfort by asking for relief measures before pain and discomfort are severe or out of control.
6. Educate purpose of intravenous or epidural patient-controlled analgesia (PCA) as indicated; educate about use of nonpharmacologic methods (e.g., cold therapy, relaxation breathing, music).
7. Discuss potential outcomes of pain and discomfort treatment approaches.
8. Establish pain relief/comfort goals with the patient (e.g., a pain rating of less than 4 on a scale of 0 to 10 to make it easy to cough, deep breathe, and turn). Premedicate patients for sedation, pain relief, and comfort (e.g., nonopioid, opioid, antiemetics as ordered; consider needs of chronic pain patients).
9. Arrange interpreter throughout the continuum of care as indicated.
10. Utilize interventions for patients with sensory impairments (e.g., device to amplify sound, sign language, and interpreters).
11. Report abnormal findings including laboratory values (prolonged PT/PTT and abnormal INR and platelet count among epidural patients).
12. Arrange for parents to be present for children.

Expected Outcomes

1. Patient states understanding of care plan and priority of individualized needs.
2. Patient states understanding of pain intensity scale, comfort scale, and pain relief/comfort goals.
3. Patient establishes realistic and achievable pain relief/comfort goals (e.g., a pain rating of less than 4 on a scale of 0 to 10 to make it easier to cough, deep breathe, and turn upon discharge).
4. Patient states understanding or demonstrates correct use of PCA equipment as indicated.
5. Patient verbalizes understanding of importance of using other nonpharmacologic methods of alleviating pain and discomfort (e.g., cold therapy, relaxation breathing, music).

Source: American Society of PeriAnesthesia Nurses. (2003). ASPAN pain and comfort guideline. *Journal of PeriAnesthesia Nursing, 18*(4), 232–236.

National Guidelines. These guidelines are integrated throughout the chapters where appropriate to provide pertinent, specific objectives to increase the awareness of the learner of the need for uniformity of care on national and international levels (i.e., *Healthy People 2010,* HIPAA, and AHA).

Preparation for Practice

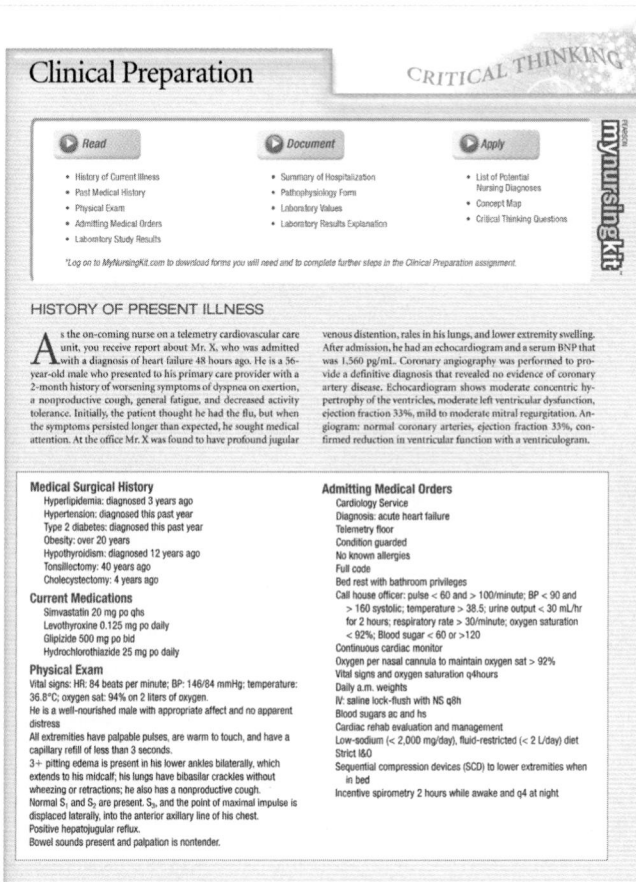

Clinical Preparation

CRITICAL THINKING

Read

- History of Current Illness
- Past Medical History
- Physical Exam
- Admitting Medical Orders
- Laboratory Study Results

Document

- Summary of Hospitalization
- Pathophysiology Form
- Laboratory Values
- Laboratory Results Explanation

Apply

- List of Potential Nursing Diagnoses
- Concept Map
- Critical Thinking Questions

**Log on to MyNursingKit.com to download forms you will need and to complete further steps in the Clinical Preparation assignment.*

HISTORY OF PRESENT ILLNESS

As the on-coming nurse on a telemetry cardiovascular care unit, you receive report about Mr. X, who was admitted with a diagnosis of heart failure 48 hours ago. He is a 56-year-old male who presented to his primary care provider with a 2-month history of worsening symptoms of dyspnea on exertion, a nonproductive cough, general fatigue, and decreased activity tolerance. Initially, the patient thought he had the flu, but when the symptoms persisted longer than expected, he sought medical attention. At the office Mr. X was found to have profound jugular venous distention, rales in his lungs, and lower extremity swelling. After admission, he had an echocardiogram and a serum BNP that was 1,560 pg/mL. Coronary angiography was performed to provide a definitive diagnosis that revealed no evidence of coronary artery disease. Echocardiogram shows moderate concentric hypertrophy of the ventricles, moderate left ventricular dysfunction, ejection fraction 33%, mild to moderate mitral regurgitation. Angiogram: normal coronary arteries, ejection fraction 33%, confirmed reduction in ventricular function with a ventriculogram.

Medical Surgical History

Hyperlipidemia: diagnosed 3 years ago
Hypertension: diagnosed this past year
Type 2 diabetes: diagnosed this past year
Obesity: over 20 years
Hypothyroidism: diagnosed 12 years ago
Tonsillectomy: 40 years ago
Cholecystectomy: 4 years ago

Current Medications

Simvastatin 20 mg po qhs
Levothyroxine 0.125 mg po daily
Glipizide 500 mg po bid
Hydrochlorothiazide 25 mg po daily

Physical Exam

Vital signs: HR: 84 beats per minute; BP: 146/84 mmHg; temperature: 36.8°C; oxygen sat: 94% on 2 liters of oxygen.
He is a well-nourished male with appropriate affect and no apparent distress
All extremities have palpable pulses, are warm to touch, and have a capillary refill of less than 3 seconds.
3+ pitting edema is present in his lower ankles bilaterally, which extends to his midcalf; his lungs have bibasilar crackles without wheezing or retractions; he also has a nonproductive cough.
Normal S_1 and S_2 are present. S_3, and the point of maximal impulse is displaced laterally, into the anterior axillary line of his chest.
Positive hepatojugular reflux.
Bowel sounds present and palpation is nontender.

Admitting Medical Orders

Cardiology Service
Diagnosis: acute heart failure
Telemetry floor
Condition guarded
No known allergies
Full code
Bed rest with bathroom privileges
Call house officer: pulse < 60 and > 100/minute; BP < 90 and > 160 systolic; temperature > 38.5; urine output < 30 mL/hr for 2 hours; respiratory rate > 30/minute; oxygen saturation < 92%; Blood sugar < 60 or >120
Continuous cardiac monitor
Oxygen per nasal cannula to maintain oxygen sat > 92%
Vital signs and oxygen saturation q4hours
Daily a.m. weights
IV: saline lock-flush with NS q8h
Blood sugars ac and hs
Cardiac rehab evaluation and management
Low-sodium (< 2,000 mg/day), fluid-restricted (< 2 L/day) diet
Strict I&O
Sequential compression devices (SCD) to lower extremities when in bed
Incentive spirometry 2 hours while awake and q4 at night

Clinical Preparation. This exercise is presented at the end of each disorder chapter to present the learner with a reality-oriented approach to patient assessment and diagnosis. The learner will complete the assignment on the Web in MyNursingKit.

CRITICAL THINKING QUESTIONS

1. When reviewing Mr. X's orders when coming on shift, list them in order of priority.
2. Why would the patient receive daily a.m. weights?
3. Which laboratory values may require notification to the ordering provider?
4. What should you monitor for after giving lisinopril 2.5 mg PO daily?
5. Why is a beta-adrenergic blocker not listed on the ordered medications?

Clinical Preparation Assignments. The assignment helps the learner develop a problem-solving approach to nursing care. By completing the assignments presented at the end of the chapters, the learner will gain experience in critical thinking skills and develop a systematic method for determining a patient's health problem, devising a plan of care, developing evaluation criteria, and determining expected outcomes. The Clinical Preparation assignments also help the learner articulate the patient's needs and learn how to write effective evaluation statements. This, in turn, significantly improves documentation skills and the ability to communicate with other health care team members to provide the safest, most effective, and holistic care for the patient.

ACKNOWLEDGMENTS

In addition to the individuals mentioned in our dedications, we would also like to thank people who were instrumental in the development of the book. The following people assisted us in bringing this project to fruition:

- Marion Waldman, the development editor, for being the glue that kept the project moving in a positive direction. For listening and being patient with our never ending list of questions. We could not have done it without her.
- Kelly Karr for her editing expertise and for the long hours she dedicated to making sure each chapter was error free.
- Susan Poirier for her exacting work in developing, formatting, and editing the pharmacology tables.
- Charlotte Miller for precise review of units to ensure consistency of content, developing the Kardex format, and placing URLs in the chapters.
- Linda Cooke for developing the clinical preparation framework, hand printing the Kardexs, and patiently guiding the authors to ensure consistency.
- Judy Tanner for her endless support, diligence, and patience in the detailed editing of chapters in the first page proofs.
- Mary Ann Shahdi, Jennifer FitzGerald, Andrea Perry, Sonia Garcia, Kathleen Budesa, and Jolie Tietz, nursing students, who generously shared their thoughts and feelings about caring behavior observed in nurses, presented in Chapter 1.
- Mike Osborn, Maddison Thivierge, and Adam Jonathan Davis for very short notice assistance with finalizing content for the book; it was greatly appreciated.

CONTENTS

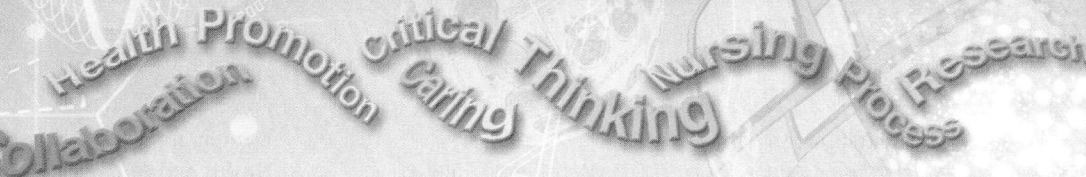

UNIT 5

Nursing Management of the Surgical Patient 584

UNIT 6

Nursing Management of Patients with Neurological Disorders 692

UNIT 9

**Nursing Management of Patients
with Gastrointestinal, Renal,
and Urinary Disorders**   1364

UNIT 10

Nursing Management of Patients with Reproductive Disorders   1502

UNIT 11

Nursing Management of Patients with Endocrine Disorders   1594

UNIT 12

**Nursing Management of Patients
with Musculoskeletal Disorders**   1708

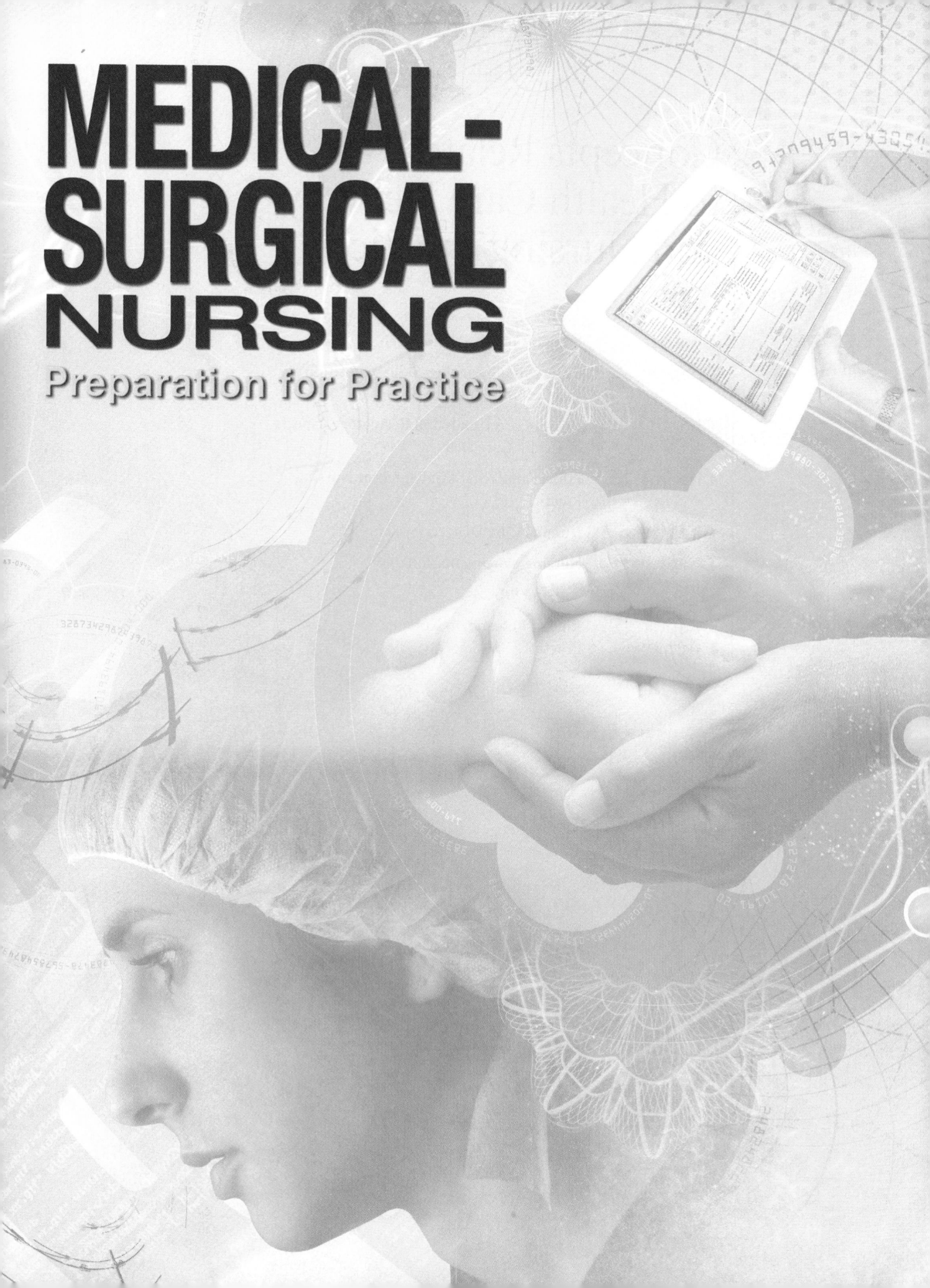

MEDICAL-SURGICAL NURSING

NURSING

Preparation for Practice

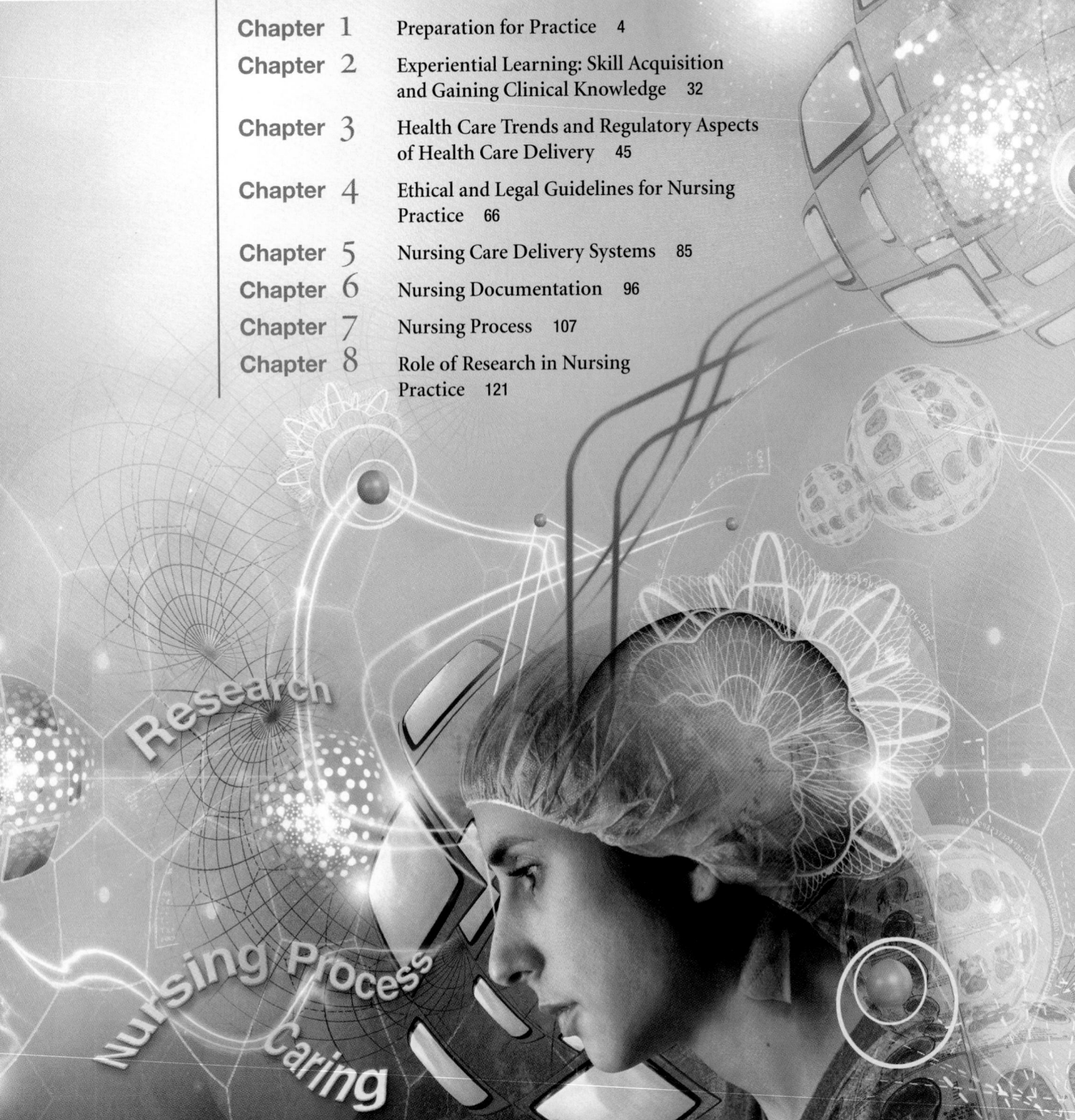

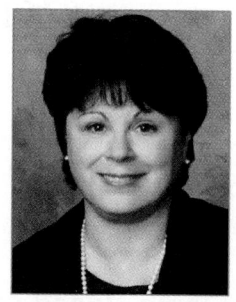

KATHY My name is Kathy and my nursing role is that of senior management leader for nursing services with the title of Vice President, Chief Nursing Officer, for two nonprofit, independent community acute care hospitals that offer a full range of services. I oversee all inpatient nursing units, including emergency/trauma, perioperative, women's/children's, cardiopulmonary, medical–surgical units, and physician hospitalist programs. Specifically I am responsible for staffing/scheduling functions, strategic direction, environment of practice, quality/patient safety, standards of care, and collaborative relationships with other disciplines providing care to patients. I also oversee the financial planning for operating and capital budgets that support the provision of care and the resources needed to meet the demands of our services. This role allows me to interface at many levels including governing board meetings, unit-based staff meetings, medical staff committees, and various state and community forums. One of my essential responsibilities is to ensure high-quality, safe patient care while balancing the financial needs of the organization.

I begin my day catching up on e-mail and voice mail communications because I know it is important for people to get timely responses. I keep my door open when I am in my office for "drop-in" conversations and "face time" with my team. Visibility is a key component of my job because staff, physicians, and the nursing management team need to know that I am listening to their concerns. A technique I use to increase my visibility is that when I need information I go to the person or department to communicate with them directly. This way I can check in with people as I travel the hallways and I can observe the environment. My **commitment** to being available to staff and my leadership team is important to ensure I understand their needs in order to represent them well.

The majority of my work is done in groups and team meetings to discuss, debate, and make decisions on policy and direction for the hospitals. My **comportment** is important in order to adequately represent nurses as credible leaders. I must be knowledgeable about issues such as quality and patient safety standards so I can contribute to discussions for improvement. My individual meetings are with the people who report directly so I can guide and mentor them in their roles.

The hardest part of my day is adjusting to changing priorities and schedules. At any moment a disaster can occur. For example, one day a pipe burst, causing water to be shut down in the main part of the hospital, which caused the closure of the surgery unit and required emergency plans to make sure the needs of staff, patients, and visitors were met. You must be very calm and considerate at these times as people deal with no running water, electricity, or functioning toilets. The **competence** to remain calm and direct the activities of a hospital during crises like this only comes from years of experience. Every situation gives me new insight into how things work and different solutions for unexpected events.

Another aspect of my job is dealing with complaints, which can be related to the quality of care and/or its aftermath, when patients receive their bills. It is very important to show **compassion** and to let the patients or their families know that I value their opinion and am committed to working with them to solve the problem. While care may have been delivered appropriately, if the caregiver failed to have the right attitude it will impact the recipients of that care. One vivid incident I remember was a woman whose husband had died. He had a terminal diagnosis, but they thought they had months to deal with his eventual death. Instead he became septic and died quickly. During the hospitalization she kept trying to get people to understand that she was confused and scared, yet everyone was so busy taking care of him, no one was listening to her. She was devastated by the experience and fearful that her husband's last moments were painful and chaotic. Incidents like these weigh heavy on my **conscience** and I work hard to help the staff know that their behavior and attitude can greatly affect the people they serve.

Working on committees with physicians and other allied health providers has helped me to understand the political dynamics of the hospital and how those dynamics interface with the community. I have to understand the internal workings of these committees, their level of authority to make decisions that affect patient care and nursing practice, and how the members perceive their responsibilities. This is very complex and requires study and preparation to be able to help the process along. First I must be sure that my **clinical reasoning** is sound so that I can debate on an appropriate level. My **critical thinking skills** are used to prepare appropriate responses and to offer solutions.

Although my days are busy, I enjoy the challenges of my job. Working in the global realm of the hospital allows me to use all of the components of the nursing process.

"Every situation gives me new insight into how things work and different solutions for unexpected events."

Preparation for Practice

Kathleen Osborn, Cheryl Wraa, Annita Watson

With contributions by:
Donna York-Clark (Roles of the Nurse)

Outcome-Based Learning Objectives

After studying this chapter, the learner will be able to:

1. Distinguish the characteristics of nursing as defined in the roles of caregiver, advocate, educator, researcher, and leader.
2. Apply the six components of caring as defined by Roach to nursing practice.
3. Describe the roles of the professional nurse within the health care delivery system.
4. Compare and contrast the nursing role in the care delivery models for nursing practice.
5. Explain the importance of cultural competence as defined by Campinha-Bacote.

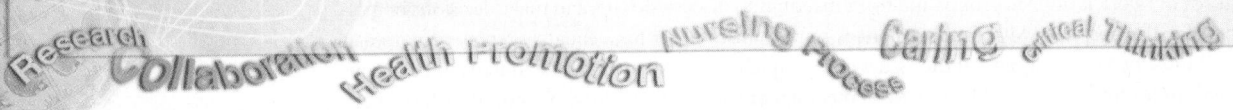

Research · Collaboration · Health Promotion · Nursing Process · Caring · Critical Thinking

THE UNIQUENESS of nursing as a professional career lies in its diversity of practice and the opportunity for lifelong learning. The relatively fluid nature of the profession allows nurses to move from one setting to the next, thereby expanding knowledge, skills, and interest in their profession. The goal of nursing is to mobilize human and environmental resources to support healing, maintain well-being, prevent illness, and promote health. In every setting or specialty, the core of practice is the nursing process: assessment, diagnosis, planning, implementation, and rationales, and evaluation (Carpenito-Moyet, 2007). The American Nurses Association (ANA) states that "the essence of nursing is that nurses combine the art of caring with the science of health care. Nursing places its focus not only on a particular health problem, but on the whole patient and his or her response to treatment. Care of the patient and a firm base of scientific knowledge are indispensable elements" (ANA, 2008, p. 1).

There are approximately 2.8 million licensed nurses in the United States who deliver patient care in all locations where care is provided, including hospitals, ambulatory care centers, nursing homes, private homes, schools, and employee workplaces (Institute of Medicine [IOM], 2004). Patients within the health care system often turn to nurses for assistance, because nurses are the

health care providers the patients are most likely to encounter and the ones with whom the patients spend the greatest amount of time. As America moves forward to improve the health care delivery system, nurses will contribute in many ways. The ANA publication **Nursing's Agenda for the Future** (2002) states:

> Nursing is the pivotal health care profession, highly valued for its specialized knowledge, skill and caring in improving the health status of the public and ensuring safe, effective, quality care.
>
> The profession mirrors the diverse population it serves and provides leadership to create positive changes in health policy and delivery systems.

As health care in America changes, nurses must have a strong voice in cultivating a stable workforce and be key participants in developing a viable health care system.

◼ Medical–Surgical Nursing

The Academy of Medical–Surgical Nurses (AMSN) is a professional organization committed to promoting nursing practice in the areas of health promotion and prevention of illness in adults. Within its position statement, *Identification of the Registered Nurse in the Workplace* (AMSN, 2004), the organization offers a description of medical–surgical nursing:

> The nurse provides leadership for the provision of [medical surgical] care based on current research, nursing judgment, and careful analysis of each individual patient's unique situation. The nursing process is the decision-producing model for the selection of nursing interventions. The nurse as a direct or indirect practitioner selects, executes, performs, delegates, directs and supervises, and evaluates nursing actions. It is in the performance of these activities that the nurse is distinguished from other health care professionals.

Nurses play a pivotal role in health care, and research is beginning to document that how well patients are cared for by nurses affects their health (IOM, 2004). Advances in health care and technology have allowed more patients to receive care in venues other than the hospital. However, the acuity of patients within the hospital setting has risen. Patients who would have been cared for in an intensive care unit a few years ago are now being cared for on medical–surgical floors or in the home (American Association of Critical Care Nurses [AACN], 2004).

Nurses develop a partnership with the patient and assist patients in learning how to cope with circumstances in order to develop an environment that promotes health, prevents illness, and facilitates recovery (Figure 1–1 ■). One of the stated goals of the ANA (2004a) is to "implement new ways in which nursing services can be delivered to respond to current and future demands for cost-effective, quality health care."

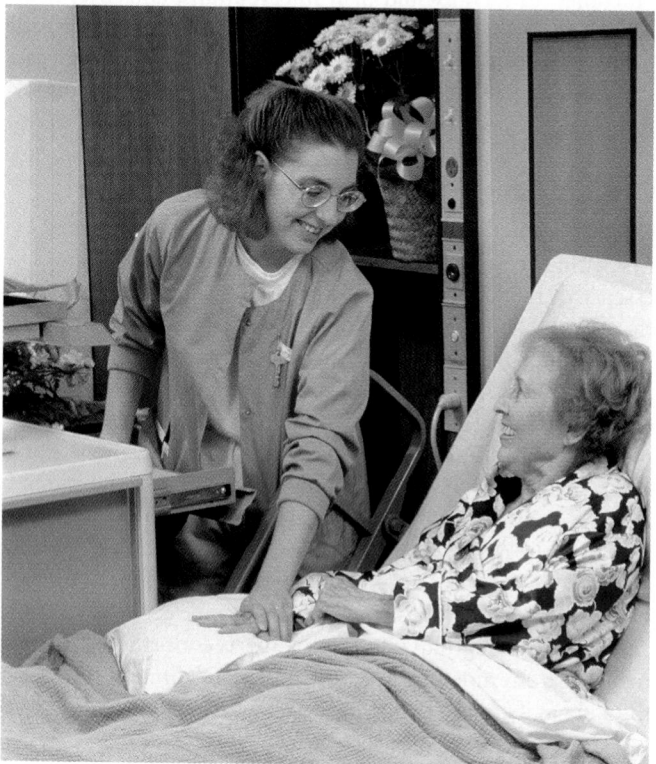

FIGURE 1–1 ■ The nurse–patient partnership is critical to help the patient cope with illness.
Source: Chip Henderson/Photolibrary.com

Components of the Nursing Role

Certain commonalities are a part of every nursing role. The commonalities included in the nursing role are as follows: caregiver, advocate, educator, researcher, and leader. Each of these components is discussed next.

Caregiver

The nurse provides care based on current research, nursing judgment, and careful analysis of each individual patient's unique situation. The nursing process is the decision-producing model for the selection of nursing interventions (AMSN, 2004). Caring is the most central and unifying concept in nursing. In 1988, Jean Watson identified human care as an intersubjective human process and a moral ideal for nursing. She stated that the necessary conditions for caring to occur are knowledge and awareness about the need for care, an intention to act, action's based on knowledge, and a positive change that results from caring (Watson, 1988).

Advocate

As patients enter the health care system, they are often overwhelmed and unprepared to make informed decisions regarding their care. Also, patients may be so ill that they are unable to communicate their wishes. Part of the nurse–patient relationship is the nurse's assessment of the patient's and family's understanding regarding the diagnosis and plan of care, identification of educational needs, and communicating with other members of the health care team to advocate for the patient's rights to autonomy, free choice, and the ability to make informed decisions.

Nurses play a key role by serving as change agents within the health care system. Advocacy is more than just understanding an issue; it requires involvement and collaboration to provide a strong unified voice for nursing through legislative and regulatory representation. The American Nurses Association has federal and state advocacy web pages that track the status of current issues that are affecting health care. The ANA has also developed the Nurses Strategic Action Team (N-STAT). N-STAT is a grassroots network for nurses that alerts members to the progress of key bills as they move through Congress and who to contact regarding support or opposition (ANA, 2007a). The nurse as advocate supports excellence of care through patient, family, and community education, communication with other health care team members, and participation in health policy formulation.

Educator

The nurse not only provides education for patients and families, but also participates in the education of the community. Health education determines how well patients, families, and communities are able to develop behaviors that are beneficial to optimal self-care. The ANA's *Standards of Clinical Nursing Practice* (1998) and all state nurse practice acts include teaching as a function of nursing practice.

The emphasis in nursing education is on health promotion and maintenance. Nurses promote health by teaching, by modeling lifestyles that promote wellness, and by providing information regarding the characteristics and consequences of diseases, including risk factors and ways to decrease health risks. The U.S. Department of Health and Human Services (DHHS) has published national health objectives for the year 2010 (DHHS,

2000). The focus areas represent an opportunity for healthy lifestyle choices and encourage clinicians to incorporate prevention into their practice. An overview of the focus areas of *Healthy People 2010* occurs later in this chapter.

Researcher

The American Nurses Association (1997) believes that nurses from all levels of educational preparation are capable of participating in research activities, from the design of the study to interpretation of results. Nurses not only investigate issues of relevance to the practice of nursing, but also participate in interdisciplinary collaborations to research common health care issues. Collaborative and interdisciplinary research fosters communication and mutual respect and enhances collaborative practice. The National Institute of Nursing Research (NINR, 2001) believes that with more interdisciplinary collaborations, nursing can provide a more comprehensive approach to research in health promotion, illness, and disabling conditions. Chapter 8 explores the role of research in nursing practice.

Leader

There are many definitions of the word *leadership*. One example states that leadership refers to the use of personal traits and personal power to constructively and ethically influence patients, families, and others toward an end point vision or goal (Yoder-Wise, 2008). All nurses are leaders as they model time management, priority setting, patient and family teaching, evaluation of the quality of care, precepting of students, mentoring of colleagues, and development of community outreach programs. A leader has the ability to tie together the support, collaboration, and enthusiasm of people to meet specific goals and objectives, whether it is a patient and his family or an entire organization.

Throughout this book, the learner is presented with a body of knowledge and skills that, with experience, will assist the nurse to create relationships and environments that are healing, humane, and caring. Professional nurses practice with compassion and respect for the inherent dignity, worth, and uniqueness of every individual, despite social or economic status, personal attributes, or the nature of health problems.

■ Framework for Nursing Practice

The framework for nursing practice is that it is an evidence-based profession that is guided by the ANA Code of Ethics for nurses (ANA, 2001a). The practice of nursing requires knowledge, critical thinking skills, and clinical judgment, and uses the nursing process to apply these concepts to patient care situations. All aspects of nursing practice are shaped and guided by a caring approach to patient care. Additionally, nurses have a responsibility to promote health and wellness for individuals and communities. Nursing as a profession was one of the first to understand the need for primary health care and prevention. As gaps in health care have occurred over the years, nurses have been able to fill them and provide high-quality service. This is true in all areas of nursing: acute care, specialty nursing, advanced practice, community nursing, and education. The nursing profession also has actively cared for disadvantaged socioeconomic groups. Because the breadth of nursing practice is so great, the profession is in a good position to impact health care policy and decisions. In this time of tremendous health care transition, nurses must rise to the challenge of providing accessibility to quality patient care. The tenets of the framework for nursing practice are discussed next.

Nursing Process

The **nursing process** is a thinking and doing approach to patient care that provides the nurse with a systematic means of identifying, preventing, and treating actual and potential health problems (Carpenito-Moyet, 2007). According to the American Nurses Association (2007b), the nursing process is defined as a variation of scientific reasoning and is used to diagnose and to treat human responses to potential and actual health problems. The nursing process provides a patient-centered approach to care that is an essential part of the patient care plan. It is the framework that provides nurses with a concise method of organizing patient care. The nursing process promotes communication and collaboration with the health care team because it is an established approach that is understood and used by nurses to identify and treat patients' problems.

The nursing process includes the following steps: assessment, diagnosis, outcome identification, planning, implementation, and evaluation. These steps are ordered to facilitate the process of identifying patient problems and desired outcomes in an efficient, consistent manner. Each step depends on the activity of the previous step. In practice, the steps of the nursing process overlap with each other. For example, while performing interventions, the nurse continues to assess the patient. The new data that result from the assessment are used to determine desired outcomes, to identify and plan interventions, and to evaluate them. The evaluation phase overlaps all phases of the nursing process because the nurse is constantly evaluating nursing care (Wilkinson, 2009). Chapter 7 contains an in-depth discussion of the nursing process.

Critical Thinking

Nursing is a highly complex and challenging profession that exists within a rapidly changing health care environment. The essence of nursing lies not in the special environments or amid the special equipment, but in the nurse's decision-making process and willingness to act on these decisions. In other words, the nurse must have the ability to think critically, possess sound clinical judgment, and effectively apply these concepts in multiple health care arenas and complex patient care situations. Critical thinking is not a separate body of knowledge to be learned, but, like reading and writing, critical thinking is a process that occurs in all areas of life and learning. Critical thinking is typically described as a purposeful, two-dimensional, goal-directed, self-regulatory process that is context bound (Lipe & Beasley, 2006). An international group of nursing experts consisting of 72 participants from nine countries developed a definition of critical thinking as it applies to nursing:

Critical thinking in nursing is an essential component of professional accountability and quality nursing care. Critical thinkers in nursing exhibit these habits of the mind: confidence, contextual perspective, creativity, flexibility, inquisitiveness, intellectual integrity, intuition, open-mindedness, perseverance, and reflection. Critical thinkers in nursing practice the cognitive skills of analyzing, applying standards, discriminating, information seeking, logical reasoning, predicting and transforming knowledge. (Gendrop & Eisenhauer, 1996)

Two dimensions are necessary for the development of critical thinking: the cognitive, which entails reflective, reasoned thinking, and the affective, which consists of being open-minded to divergent perspectives and having an inquisitive spirit (Lipe & Beasley, 2006). In addition to the cognitive and affective abilities, effective critical thinking skills evolve with time, knowledge, professional practice, and structured feedback (Benner, Tanner, & Chesla, 1996). Critical thinking skills develop in tandem with intellectual and ethical development (L'Eplattenier, 2001). Chart 1–1 identifies key critical thinking skills.

Critical thinking is necessary to begin the problem solving necessary for complex patient care situations. Critical thinking, however, is not *just* problem solving; it is also an application of logic that evolves from an understanding of the need to question conventions and habits and to base decisions on sound reasoning (D'Amico & Barbarito, 2007; Lipe & Beasley, 2006). Critical thinking is cultivated by questioning the norms and avoiding an acceptance of the biases. According to D'Amico and Barbarito, five essential elements are involved in the critical thinking process:

- Collection of information
- Analysis of the situation
- Generation of alternatives
- Selection of alternatives
- Evaluation.

Critical thinking skills are needed in order to observe, gather, organize, and analyze data accurately because interpretation of patient's symptoms can be complex and diverse. When applied to patient care situations critical thinking promotes health and assists the patient to achieve the desired outcomes of care (Fesler-Birch, 2005).

The process of developing critical thinking skills begins during the nurse's education process. The American Association of Colleges of Nursing (2007) requires that critical thinking be reflected within academic nursing programs as a core competency for pro-

---

| CHART 1–1 | **Critical Thinking Skills** |

- Be inquisitive by asking pertinent questions.
- Assess what information is necessary to determine a solution to the problem.
- Gather the facts and validate the information.
- Consider available options.
- Be flexible and open-minded about all options.
- Draw on past experiences and knowledge.
- Formulate creative decisions and test their effectiveness.
- Be open-minded to dissonance and ambiguity.

---

gram accreditation. However, the evolution and refinement of critical thinking continue as the nurse gains experience through practice (Brunt, 2005). To think critically, the nurse needs to apply experience and knowledge to patient care situations. Benner (2001) asserts that as nurses gain experience and knowledge in practice they progress through five distinct stages of skill acquisition, from novice to expert nurse. A complete description of these stages is discussed as outlined in Chapter 2 ☁.

The goal of nursing education is to holistically prepare the learner for the profession by not only providing the necessary critical thinking skills, but also by providing socialization to the role of nursing. Central to role socialization is the development of **clinical judgment**, which is defined as a complex skill involving several cognitive phases and integrative processes. Critical thinking skills overlap with the conceptual boundaries of clinical judgment (Fesler-Birch, 2005).

Christine Tanner (1983), an identified expert in the study of clinical judgment, defines clinical judgment skills as follows:

- Making decisions regarding what to observe in the patient situation
- Making inferential decisions by deriving meaning from data observed
- Making decisions regarding actions to be taken that will be of optimal benefit to the patient.

After reviewing more than 200 studies on clinical judgment, Tanner (2006) identified five conclusions about a nurse's ability to develop and refine clinical judgment skills:

- Clinical judgment is more influenced by what nurses bring to the situation than the objective data about the situation at hand.
- Sound clinical judgment rests to some degree on knowing the patient's typical pattern of responses, as well as an engagement with the patient and her concerns.
- Clinical judgments are influenced by the context in which the situation occurs and the culture of the nursing care unit.
- Nurses use a variety of reasoning patterns alone or in combination.
- Reflection on practice is often triggered by a breakdown in clinical judgment, and therefore is critical in the development of clinical knowledge and improvement in clinical reasoning skills.

Tanner (2006) states that nurses' backgrounds, the context of situations, and nurses' relationships with their patients are central to what nurses notice and how they interpret findings, respond to those findings, and reflect on their responses. Assumptions basic to an integrated critical thinking model for clinical judgment development are that it is a multidimensional concept and that every act of clinical judgment in nursing has diagnostic, therapeutic, and ethical dimensions. Therefore, sound clinical judgment, which is a requirement for expertise in nursing, is derived from an ability to think critically.

Development of Critical Thinking Skills

As stated earlier, the acquisition of both critical thinking and subsequent clinical judgment skills begins with the education process. During all phases of nursing education, learners are initially taught theory in the classroom followed by psychomotor skill demonstrations, which are practiced in simulated situations. To further refine decision-making and problem-solving skills, the student must then transfer and apply the theoretical knowledge to the clinical setting in a variety of patient care situations (Walsh & Seldomridge, 2006). It is imperative for the nurse to reflect on attitudes such as curiosity, fair-mindedness, humility, courage, and perseverance, which facilitate critical thinking in each patient care situation. Additionally, it is beneficial to reflect on previous patient care situations in which decisions were made and then assess the outcome of those decisions. This reflective thinking process identifies areas of strengths and weaknesses in a given situation, and gives direction to the nurse for future development and refinement of critical thinking and clinical judgment skills. Being open-minded to dissonance and ambiguity is essential if the nurse is going to expand critical thinking skills. If possible, any final decision should be suspended until all sides of an issue have been evaluated; note, however, that emergency situations do not allow for delay. This is why experienced nurses typically function more effectively in emergent situations—they have the thinking and judgment skills to effectively function with minimal delay.

Creating an environment where critical thinking is encouraged and nurtured is the responsibility of the nursing leadership. Differences in opinions and examination of various solutions must be tolerated and encouraged. Independent, individual, and divergent thinking skills are necessary to avoid "group thinking" and the pressure to defer to group decisions. If nurses are aware of their critical thinking skills, while they are doing the *thinking*, they can detect errors in judgment. Experiencing both negative and positive outcomes promotes the development of these skills. One example of clinical setting analysis occurs in some trauma centers where emergency resuscitation situations are videotaped and subsequently analyzed by the staff to determine the effectiveness of the resuscitation efforts. This is an excellent way of reflecting on the thinking and decision making that was done in a high-stress, complex patient care situation. The purpose of this reflective effort is to promote more effective patient care outcomes. But, it also presents an opportunity to enhance and refine high-level critical thinking and clinical judgment skills through experience.

Six Components of Caring

When a family member is being treated, families often do not remember the medications and the machines as much as they remember the caring spirit of the nurses. Nursing is a caring discipline with a foundation of nursing science guided by the application of moral and ethical principles of care and responsibility. **Caring**, which is directly derived from the ethical principle of beneficence, is the core of nursing and constitutes the essence of nursing regardless of the level at which nursing is practiced and conceptualized. Caring represents the unique aspect of nursing and is reflected in conscience, confidence, compassion, commitment, competence, and comportment (Roach, 1984). Without these components, nursing is a scientific and technical skill-based body of knowledge. Adding the components of caring to this body of knowledge enables nursing to be identified as a holistic profession. Without caring the nurse will not see the psychological and spiritual sufferings of the patient (DeWolf-Bosek & Savage, 2007). The definition of each component of caring is outlined here:

- *Conscience* is possessing a moral sense of what is right and wrong. The nurse's conscience guides the nurse's practice and serves as a strong deterrent to providing minimal or inappropriate care. Conscience is not easily displayed, but every action is led by the conscience. The conscience helps nurses decide right from wrong and guides the *care* nurses give to patients.
- *Confidence* is defined as having a full belief in the trustworthiness or reliability of a person. Confidence in oneself is the belief in your own knowledge and skills and the ability to use them when necessary. Confidence in a fellow nurse means that you are totally secure in the accuracy and efficiency of your colleague. Being confident in both yourself and your colleagues minimizes conflict and provides an optimal working environment that ultimately benefits the patient.
- *Compassion* is having a sympathetic feeling for another with an aspiration to help that individual. This is not just a feeling one possesses; it is accompanied by an action to do good. Effective holistic nursing requires a feeling of compassion for people who are sick and injured.
- *Commitment* means being obligated to see something through to completion. Nurses must value their profession and be committed to delivering the highest level of nursing care. Professional commitment is manifested in different ways. To achieve positive outcomes, nurses must be committed to their patients as well as their institution. The institution also has a duty to be supportive of its nurses, to assist them in increasing their knowledge and skills, and to provide current monitoring equipment that promotes a safe patient care environment.
- *Competence* refers to being capable and qualified to perform a job. Caring as it relates to nursing is not simply a matter of good intentions or warm regard; there also must be a foundation of knowledge. The nurse has a responsibility to the patient to be knowledgeable about the disease process and about the skills necessary to ensure safe patient care.
- *Comportment* means that one is aware of one's conduct and behavior around others. Professional comportment is an essential aspect of nursing because it is representative of the level of professionalism being exhibited. Additionally, it instills confidence in the patient and provides an atmosphere that alleviates anxiety. Nurses must conduct themselves professionally with their patients as well as their fellow health care workers. Being respectful of each other is germane to creating a positive work environment that promotes team building (Roach, 1984).

The nurse manifests caring as she assists health care consumers in preventing or adapting to actual and potential health problems. Without caring, nursing becomes mechanical and lacking in warmth. It takes much skill and devotion on the nurse's part to ensure that every patient is afforded the components just listed to make certain that patient care is as nurturing and positive as possible. The manner in which nurses choose to implement the six components of caring in clinical practice greatly influences how well the patient is able to adapt to the environment. Caring "sets up the conditions of trust that enables the [patient] to accept the help offered and to *feel* cared for" (Benner & Wrubel, 1989, p. 4).

Development of Caring Skills

During the educational process it is essential that learners perceive caring as critical to their socialization to the professional nursing field. Therefore, it is incumbent on educators to incorporate the concept of caring with its component parts in all aspects of the curriculum. It is not enough to incorporate the content of caring into didactic materials; the concept also must be communicated as a guide for practice and modeled by the faculty. Caring must become a measurable outcome of learner performance comparable to the measurement of scientific knowledge and psychomotor skills. To illustrate this point, excerpts from learners' clinical assignments in which they were asked to observe an example of nurses demonstrating caring behaviors are listed here:

- **Conscience**

  An example of staff working by their conscience during my shift was when a young patient came in and we had to treat him. He was brought in after driving drunk, hitting a car, and fleeing the scene. After hitting the first car, he hit a second car and attempted to flee that scene as well and was finally caught. We knew the damage he had done and we knew that when he was released, he was being released to the police and placed under arrest. However, this did not stop us from providing him with the best treatment we could. We did a full assessment, cleaned him up and controlled his pain just as we did with all of the other patients that we cared for.

  Source: Courtesy of Jennifer Fitzgerald, Sacramento, CA

- **Confidence**

  In the emergency department all of the nurses displayed confidence in their skills and procedures. The nurse established a level of trust right from the beginning. A patient displayed confidence in the nurse when he asked for something and the nurse answered that she could not do that. The patient was not happy with the answer but he had confidence in the nurse to know that she knew what needed to be done for his treatment, and he accepted the answer without question.

  Source: Courtesy of Sonia Garcia

- **Compassion**

  Possibly one of the most important components of caring is compassion. As a medical professional it may become easy to simply detach oneself from the plight of patients in pain or in need; however remaining compassionate is crucial to good patient care. It is the best way to build trust with your patient and to facilitate a caring environment, which is especially important in the emergency department where patients are often afraid and in severe pain. I saw many people exhibit compassion throughout the shift; for example, when a patient complained of severe leg pain that did not respond to the two doses of morphine his nurse had already given him, the RN went to the physician and requested a stronger pain medicine which finally put the patient at ease.

  Source: Courtesy of Maryam Shahdi, Sacramento, CA

- **Commitment**

  The nurse that I worked with in the Post Anesthesia Care Unit (PACU) had actually been called in that day after another nurse had called in sick. I guess he had been called in because nobody from the night shift wanted to stay and they were anticipating a very busy day in surgery. Since the level of acuity is so high in the PACU, it is necessary to have plenty of nurses on every shift. He told me he did not mind coming in on his day off though, because he really enjoyed his job and liked to come to work. One could say with absolutely no hesitation that this employee was very committed to his job and to his patients.

  Source: Courtesy of Jolie Tietz, Sacramento, CA

- **Competence**

  The nurse I was assigned to in the emergency department had four patients within a half hour that needed IVs placed. In previous experiences, I have seen nurses try three or four times, wiggling the needle around in the poor patient's arm before finding a vein. However, this nurse efficiently and almost painlessly started the IVs one after the other. I know the patients appreciated her accuracy, and she probably did not even think about how simply she had started the things.

  Source: Courtesy of Andrea Perry

- **Comportment**

  The Post Anesthesia Care Unit (PACU) nurse I worked with showed comportment to our patients, especially when they were first waking up. When the patient with a nasopharyngeal tube became more awake, he began to move and flail his arms around. He then began to try to take out the nasopharyngeal tube. The nurse and I carefully took his arms and held them so he would not pull out any lines or hurt himself. My nurse very calmly explained to the patient that the surgery was over, that it went well, and that he was in the PACU. He also explained who we were, what time it was, and why there was a tube in his nose. The nurse's demeanor helped the patient to calm down. The nurse also explained to the patient that the "spacey feeling" he was having was due to the anesthesia because of the fact that our bodies are not used to it. He reassured the patient that the feeling would soon wear off. My nurse handled the situation beautifully, and his caring behavior positively impacted the patient.

  Source: Courtesy of Kathleen Budesa, Sacramento, CA

Health and Wellness Promotion

In the last two decades, the concept of health and wellness promotion has come to the forefront of health care issues. The focus has shifted from disease treatment to a holistic approach of disease prevention and promotion of wellness. People are more aware than ever before how the relationship between healthy lifestyles and habits impacts disease prevention. For example, most individuals regularly monitor their cholesterol and triglycerides and understand that lifestyle changes are necessary when the levels become elevated. Regular exercise programs and a well-balanced healthy diet have become a way of life for many individuals.

In 1979 the surgeon general's office published its first health promotion and disease guidelines in *Healthy People*. This first report was followed in 1990 by a second edition, titled *Healthy People 2000,* which emphasized health promotion, health protection, and preventive service strategies (DHHS, 1991). The report was once again updated in the year 2000. This current report, *Healthy People 2010,* outlines a 10-year strategy for promoting health, preventing illness, disability, and premature death

(DHHS, 2000). The report also identified two major goals that are reflective of the changing demographics in the United States:

- Increase quality and years of healthy life.
- Eliminate health disparities.

Healthy People 2010 outlines 27 focus areas for improving health and meeting these two major objectives (Chart 1–2).

Healthy People 2010 also outlined the leading health concerns for the beginning of the 21st century, as listed in Chart 1–3. These indicators illuminate individual behaviors, physical and social environmental factors, and important health system issues that greatly affect the health of individuals and communities. Indicators are identified to help in the development of action plans for dealing with each indicator (DHHS, 2000, p. 24). For each leading health indicator, specific objectives have been identified that can be used to track progress and provide a snapshot of the health of the nation. The goal is to improve the health of both the individual and the community.

CHART 1–2 *Healthy People 2010:* Focus Areas for Improving Health

- Access to quality health care services
- Arthritis, osteoporosis, and chronic back conditions
- Cancer
- Chronic kidney disease
- Diabetes
- Disability and secondary conditions
- Educational and community-based programs
- Environmental health
- Family planning
- Food safety
- Health communication
- Heart disease and stroke
- HIV
- Immunization and infectious diseases
- Injury and violence prevention
- Maternal, infant, and child health
- Medical product safety
- Mental health and mental disorders
- Nutrition and overweight
- Occupational safety and health
- Oral health
- Physical activity and fitness
- Public health infrastructure
- Respiratory diseases
- Sexually transmitted infections
- Tobacco use
- Vision and screening

Source: U.S. Department of Health and Human Services. (1991). *Healthy people 2000: National health promotion and disease prevention objectives* (DHHS Publication No. 91-5021). Washington, DC: U.S. Government Printing Office; U.S. Department of Health and Human Services. (2000). *Healthy people 2010.* Retrieved May 1, 2004, from http://www.health.gov/healthpeople.

A vital part of the nurse's role today is to promote health and wellness through teaching and modeling of healthy behaviors based on the health indicators. For consistency and comprehensiveness, it is helpful to develop a template for health education. The components of this template include an understandable description of the cause of the disease or disorder, what habits will slow or stop progression, medication actions, side effects, and prognosis. As part of the plan, the nurse should provide written material and other resources such as websites and support organizations. It is important to provide the patient and family with an opportunity to ask questions and air feelings about the diagnosis. The nurse also needs to tailor the education to be culturally sensitive. This is especially true when it comes to dietary teaching, because food selection is heavily dependent on cultural customs. In summary, teaching as a function of the nursing role is included in the ANA's *Standards of Clinical Nursing Practice* (1998) and in all state nurse practice acts (ANA, 2004b).

Standards of Nursing Practice

Nurses are accountable to the public for their practice. Therefore, the ANA has developed standards for nursing practice and articulated the scope of practice (DeWolf-Bosek & Savage, 2007). **Standards of nursing practice** are authoritative statements by which the nursing profession describes the common level of performance or care by which the quality of practice can be determined, and responsibilities for which its practitioners are accountable (ANA, 2004b, p. 1). There are two parts to the standards of practice: standards of care and standards of professional performance. Charts 1–4 (p. 12) and 1–5 (p. 13), respectively, outline the ANA standards of care and standards of professional performance. In addition to the general standards the ANA also publishes standards for many specialty areas. The **standards of care** are guidelines for nursing practice and are general to any setting or specialty, and follow the nursing process with the broad categories of assessment, diagnosis, outcomes identification, planning, implementation, and evaluation (ANA, 2004b). **Standards of professional performance** address the professional nursing role with regard to education, ethics, research, collegiality, and resource utilization (ANA, 2004b). Standards of practice and performance focus on the nurse as the provider of patient care. They are process oriented and relate to what is expected of the provider. Each state has its own nurse practice act that defines the scope of nursing practice in that state. They have evolved as criteria against which care is measured for quality purposes.

It is essential that institutions where nurses practice provide an environment that is conducive to safe nursing practice and facilitates nurses' abilities to adhere to the standards of practice. Nurses are required to maintain currency in the knowledge and skills needed to practice in a given setting. This is accomplished in part by reading current professional journals, attending education classes related to their area of practice, and collaborating with fellow colleagues to share knowledge. Many states mandate continuing education classes in order to retain licensure. Professional organizations offer programs and conferences that nurses can attend to maintain currency.

CHART 1–3	*Healthy People 2010* Leading Health Indicators

Leading Health Indicator	Rationale
Physical activity	Regular physical activity throughout life is important for maintaining a healthy body, enhancing psychological well-being, and preventing premature death.
Overweight and obesity	Overweight and obesity are major contributors to many preventable causes of death. On average, higher body weights are associated with higher death rates. The number of overweight children, adolescents, and adults has risen over the past four decades.
Tobacco use	Cigarette smoking is the single most preventable cause of disease and death in the United States. Smoking results in more deaths each year in the United States than AIDS, alcohol, cocaine, heroin, homicide, suicide, motor vehicle crashes, and fires—combined.
Substance abuse	Alcohol and illicit drug use are associated with many of this country's most serious problems, including violence, injury, and HIV infection. The annual economic costs to the United States from alcohol abuse were estimated to be $167 billion in 1995, and the costs from drug abuse were estimated to be $110 billion.
Responsible sexual behavior	Unintended pregnancies and sexually transmitted infections (STIs), including infection with the human immunodeficiency virus that causes AIDS, can result from unprotected sexual behaviors. Abstinence is the only method of complete protection. Condoms, if used correctly and consistently, can help prevent both unintended pregnancy and STIs.
Mental health	Approximately 20 percent of the U.S. population is affected by mental illness during a given year; no one is immune. Of all mental illnesses, depression is the most common disorder. More than 19 million adults in the United States suffer from depression. Major depression is the leading cause of disability and is the cause of more than two-thirds of suicides each year.
Injury and violence	More than 400 Americans die each day from injuries due primarily to motor vehicle crashes, firearms, poisonings, suffocation, falls, fires, and drowning.
Environmental quality	An estimated 25 percent of preventable illnesses worldwide can be attributed to poor environmental quality. In the United States, air pollution alone is estimated to be associated with 50,000 premature deaths and an estimated $40 billion to $50 billion in health-related costs annually. Two indicators of air quality are ozone (outdoor) and environmental tobacco smoke (indoor).
Immunization	Vaccines are among the greatest public health achievements of the 20th century. Immunizations can prevent disability and death from infectious diseases for individuals and can help control the spread of infections within communities.
Access to health care	Strong predictors of access to quality health care include having health insurance, a higher income level, and a regular primary care provider or other source of ongoing health care. Use of clinical preventive services, such as early prenatal care, can serve as indicators of access to quality health care services.

Source: U.S. Department of Health and Human Services. (2000). *Healthy people 2010.* Retrieved May 1, 2004, from http://www.health.gov/healthpeople.

Code of Ethics for Nurses

A **code of ethics** is a formal statement by a group that expresses the group's ideals and values. A code of ethics for an organization is a set of ethical principles that have been agreed on by the organization's members that reflect their moral judgments, define expectations, and serve as a standard for their professional actions (DeWolf-Bosek & Savage, 2007). Codes of ethics, although not legally enforceable, typically have more stringent requirements than legal standards. Codes of ethics must not be stagnant; they must be revised as a given profession changes and evolves.

The purposes of nursing's code of ethics include the following:

- Inform the public about the minimum standards of the profession and help them understand professional nursing conduct.
- Provide a sign of the profession's commitment to public service.
- Outline the major ethical considerations of the profession.
- Provide ethical standards for professional behavior.
- Guide the profession in self-regulation.

- Remind nurses about the special responsibility they assume when caring for the sick.

Fundamental to the practice of nursing is a respect for human dignity and the uniqueness of each patient, without regard for social and economic status, the cause of the illness, or personal attributes. Therefore, it is the responsibility of every educator to ensure that an integral part of socializing the learner to the profession of nursing is to incorporate the code of ethics into the learner's value set (DeWolf-Bosek & Savage, 2007). The principles contained within the code serve to guide the learner in formulating the ethical values necessary for practicing nursing.

Values are freely chosen beliefs or attitudes about the worth of an individual or object. Values influence decisions and actions including ethical decision making. A value set is an internal group of beliefs that have been formulated and prioritized based on past experiences, education, and influences from others. This system of values gives direction to life and determines behavior, especially when decisions and choices are required. When learners enter a professional nursing program they do so with an

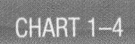 **American Nurses Association Standards of Care**

STANDARD I. ASSESSMENT

The Nurse Collects Patient Health Data

Measurement Criteria

1. Data collection involves the patient, family, and other health care providers as appropriate.
2. The priority of data collection is determined by the patient's immediate condition or needs.
3. Pertinent data are collected using appropriate assessment techniques and instruments.
4. Relevant data are documented in a retrievable form.
5. The data collection process is systematic and ongoing.

STANDARD II. DIAGNOSIS

The Nurse Analyzes the Assessment Data in Determining Diagnoses

Measurement Criteria

1. Diagnoses are derived from the assessment data.
2. Diagnoses are validated with the patient, family, and other health care providers, when possible and appropriate.
3. Diagnoses are documented in a manner that facilitates the determination of expected outcomes and plan of care.

STANDARD III. OUTCOME IDENTIFICATION

The Nurse Identifies Expected Outcomes Individualized to the Patient

Measurement Criteria

1. Outcomes are derived from the diagnoses.
2. Outcomes are mutually formulated with the patient, family, and other health care providers, when possible and appropriate.
3. Outcomes are culturally appropriate and realistic in relation to the patient's present and potential capabilities.
4. Outcomes are attainable in relation to resources available to the patient.
5. Outcomes include a time estimate for attainment.
6. Outcomes provide direction for continuity of care.
7. Outcomes are documented as measurable goals.

STANDARD IV. PLANNING

The Nurse Develops a Plan of Care that Prescribes Interventions to Attain Expected Outcomes

Measurement Criteria

1. The plan is individualized to the patient (e.g., age appropriate, culturally sensitive) and the patient's condition or needs.
2. The plan is developed with the patient, family, and other health care providers, as appropriate.
3. The plan reflects current nursing practice.
4. The plan provides for continuity of care.
5. Priorities for care are established.
6. The plan is documented.

STANDARD V. IMPLEMENTATION

The Nurse Implements the Interventions Identified in the Plan of Care

Measurement Criteria

1. Interventions are consistent with the established plan of care.
2. Interventions are implemented in a safe, timely, and appropriate manner.
3. Interventions are documented.

STANDARD VI. EVALUATION

The Nurse Evaluates the Patient's Progress toward Attainment of Outcomes

Measurement Criteria

1. Evaluation is systematic, ongoing, and criterion based.
2. The patient, family, and other health care providers are involved in the evaluation process, as appropriate.
3. Ongoing assessment data are used to revise diagnoses, outcomes, and the plan of care, as needed.
4. Revisions in diagnoses, outcomes, and the plan of care are documented.
5. The effectiveness of interventions is evaluated in relation to outcomes.
6. The patient's responses to intervention are documented.

Source: American Nurses Association. (2004b). *Nursing: Scope & Standards of Practice.* Silver Spring, MD: Nursebooks pp. 21–31. Reprinted with permission from American Nurses Association, Nursing: Scope and Standards of Practice, © 2004 nursesbooks.org, Silver Spring, MD.

inherent set of values. It is the responsibility of the education system to assist learners in socializing to the nursing profession and adopting its code of ethics and values. This also is true of the nurse practicing in a health care organization where comparable values are essential. The organization has its own set of values, as does the nurse, and those values must be compatible in order for the nurse to provide appropriate and comprehensive patient care.

Codes of ethics have been established by international, national, and state nursing associations. Nursing's first code of ethics is believed to be the Florence Nightingale pledge that was written by Lystra Gretter in 1893 (Chart 1–6, p. 14). It is apparent even in that early code that nurses understood the impor-

tance of patient privacy that is still stressed today in health care, although it is also apparent in that first code that there was a dependence on physicians. Today, nursing has become more autonomous, which is why codes of ethics are revised to keep pace with current practice. It is essential that codes of ethics be updated as situations change with time (Tschudin, 2006). An updated code of ethics was not adopted until 1950 (DeWolf-Bosek & Savage, 2007). The code of ethics was again revised in 1956, 1960, 1968, 1976, and 2001.

The ANA represents the interests of the nation's registered nurses through its 54 constituent state and territorial associations. The ANA advances the nursing profession by fostering high standards of nursing practice, promoting the economic

CHART 1–5	American Nurses Association Standards of Professional Performance

STANDARD I. QUALITY OF CARE

The Nurse Systematically Evaluates the Quality and Effectiveness of Nursing Practice

Measurement Criteria

1. The nurse participates in quality of care activities as appropriate to the nurse's education and position. Such activities may include:
   - Identification of aspects of care important for quality monitoring.
   - Analysis of quality data to identify opportunities for improving care.
   - Development of policies, procedures, and proactive guidelines to improve quality of care.
   - Identification of indicators used to monitor quality and effectiveness of nursing care.
   - Collection of data to monitor quality and effectiveness of nursing care.
   - Formulation of recommendations to improve nursing practice or patient outcomes.
   - Implementation of activities to enhance the quality of nursing practice.
   - Participation on interdisciplinary teams that evaluate clinical practice or health services.

2. The nurse uses the results of quality of care activities to initiate changes in nursing practice.

3. The nurse uses the results of quality of care activities to initiate changes throughout the health care delivery system, as appropriate.

STANDARD II. PERFORMANCE APPRAISAL

The Nurse Evaluates One's Own Nursing Practice in Relation to Professional Practice Standards and Relevant Statutes and Regulation

Measurement Criteria

1. The nurse engages in performance appraisal on a regular basis, identifying areas of strength as well as areas for professional development.

2. The nurse seeks constructive feedback regarding one's own practice.

3. The nurse takes action to achieve goals identified during performance appraisal.

4. The nurse participates in peer review as appropriate.

5. The nurse's practice reflects knowledge of current professional practice standards, laws, regulations.

STANDARD III. EDUCATION

The Nurse Acquires and Maintains Current Knowledge and Competency in Nursing Practice

Measurement Criteria

1. The nurse participates in ongoing educational activities related to clinical knowledge and professional issues.

2. The nurse seeks experience to maintain current clinical skills and competence.

3. The nurse acquires knowledge and skills appropriate to the specialty area and practice setting.

STANDARD IV. COLLEGIALITY

The Nurse Interacts with, and Contributes to, the Professional Development of Peers and Other Health Care Providers as Colleagues

Measurement Criteria

1. The nurse shares knowledge and skills with colleagues.

2. The nurse provides peers with constructive feedback regarding their practice.

3. The nurse acquires knowledge and skills appropriate to the security area and practice setting.

4. The nurse contributes to an environment that is conductive to clinical education of nursing learners, other health care learners, and other employees, as appropriate.

5. The nurse contributes to a supportive and healthy work environment.

STANDARD V. ETHICS

The Nurse's Decisions and Actions on Behalf of Patients Are Determined in an Ethical Manner

Measurement Criteria

1. The nurse's practice is guided by the *Code for Nurses.*

2. The nurse maintains patient confidentiality within legal and regulatory parameters.

3. The nurse acts as a patient advocate and assists patients in developing skills to advocate for themselves.

4. The nurse delivers care in a nonjudgmental and nondiscriminatory manner that is sensitive to patient diversity.

5. The nurse delivers care in a manner that preserves patient autonomy, dignity, and rights.

6. The nurse seeks available resources to formulate ethical decisions.

STANDARD VI. COLLABORATION

The Nurse Collaborates with the Patient, Family, and Other Health Care Providers in Providing Patient Care

Measurement Criteria

1. The nurse communicates with the patient, family, and other health care providers regarding patient care and nursing's role in the provision of care.

2. The nurse collaborates with the patient, family, and other health care providers in the formulation of overall goals, the plan of care, and decisions related to care and the delivery of services.

3. The nurse consults with other health care providers for patient care, as needed.

4. The nurse makes referrals, including provisions for continuity of care, as needed.

(continued)

| CHART 1–5 | **American Nurses Association Standards of Professional Performance—*Continued*** |

STANDARD VII. RESEARCH

The Nurse Uses Research Findings in Practice

Measurement Criteria

1. The nurse utilizes available research to develop the plan of care and interventions.

2. The nurse participates in research activities as appropriate to the nurse's education and position. Such activities may include:
   - Identifying clinical problems suitable for nursing research.
   - Participating in data collection.
   - Participating in a unit, organization, or community research committee or program.
   - Sharing of research activities with others.
   - Conducting research.
   - Critiquing research for application to practice.
   - Using research findings in the development of policies, procedures, and practice guidelines for patient care.

STANDARD VIII. RESOURCE UTILIZATION

The Nurse Considers Factors Related to Safety, Effectiveness, and Cost in Planning and Delivering Patient Care

Measurement Criteria

1. The nurse evaluates factors related to safety, effectiveness, availability, and cost when choosing between two or more practice options that would result in the same expected patient outcome.

2. The nurse assists the patient and family in identifying and securing appropriate and available services to address health-related needs.

3. The nurse assigns or delegates tasks as defined by the state nurse practice act and according to the knowledge and skills of the designated caregiver.

4. If the nurse assigns or delegates tasks, the delegation is based on the needs and conditions of the patient, the potential for harm, the stability of the patient's condition, the complexity of the task, and the predictability of the outcome.

5. The nurse assists the patient and family in becoming informed consumers about the cost, risks, and benefits of treatment and care.

Source: American Nurses Association. (2004b). *Nursing: Scope & Standards of Practice.* Silver Spring, MD: Nursebooks pp. 33–44. Reprinted with permission from American Nurses Association, Nursing: Scope and Standards of Practice, © 2004 nursesbooks.org, Silver Spring, MD.

| CHART 1–6 | **Florence Nightingale Pledge** |

I solemnly pledge myself before God and in the presence of this assembly, to pass my life in purity and to practice my profession faithfully. I will abstain from whatever is deleterious and mischievous, and will not take or knowingly administer any harmful drug. I will do all in my power to maintain and elevate the standard of my profession, and will hold in confidence all personal matters committed to my keeping and all family affairs coming to my knowledge in the practice of my calling. With loyalty will I endeavor to aid the physician, in his work, and devote myself to the welfare of those committed to my care.

Source: Retrieved October 29, 2007, from http://www.countryjoe.com/nightingale/pledge.htm.

and general welfare of nurses in the workplace, projecting a positive and realistic view of nursing, and by lobbying the Congress and regulatory agencies on health care issues affecting nurses and the general public. The most recent revision of the ANA code of ethics was adopted in July 2001 and is shown in Chart 1–7.

Guiding Ethical Principles

Ethical principles guide nurses in making determinations about what is and is not ethical in nursing and medicine (DeWolf-Bosek & Savage, 2007; Guido, 2006; Mathes, 2005a). There are four cornerstone principles of bioethics from which many other ethical principles can be derived. These principles do not always exist in harmony and there is not a generally accepted ranking system (DeWolf-Bosek & Savage, 2007). These principles are used by nurses as tools for moral reflection and to aid them in decision making when controversy exists. The four cornerstone principles are (1) nonmaleficence, (2) beneficence, (3) autonomy, and (4) justice. These and other ethical principles are discussed in detail in Chapter 4.

■ Roles of the Nurse

As stated, the professional nurse embodies many roles. Throughout history, nursing has continuously adapted to the ever-changing needs of patients and the health care delivery system. There are roles that interface with patients throughout the entire health care continuum and these roles continue to grow. The spectrum of nursing roles includes practice in acute and nonacute care, advanced practice, and practice in a number of new and evolving arenas. All nursing practice roles rely on the nursing process as a framework for patient care delivery.

Acute Care Nurses

Acute care nurses practice in the hospital setting. These nurses care for patients with actual and potential health problems related to any body system and any age group. The types of patients an acute care nurse works with will vary depending on the individual hospital's mission, goals, and specialty areas provided.

Staff Nurse

The staff nurse has the primary responsibility to care for a specific patient or group of patients for an assigned period of time. Patient care assignments vary among organizations depending on the nursing care delivery model being used. The nursing care delivery models are discussed in Chapter 5. These models define the workload distribution and job description for each member of the nursing health care team. Organization and coordination are inherent in the role of the nurse regardless of the type of patient care delivery model due to the variety of diagnoses and complexity of patient care. Therefore, the staff nurse uses critical nursing judgments in determining patient interventions according to assigned responsibilities. Regardless of which care delivery model is used, certain components are common to all of them, including nursing management and administration, which are described next.

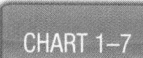

American Nurses Association Code of Ethics for Nurses

CHART 1–7

1. The nurse in all professional relationships practices with compassion and respect for the inherent dignity, worth, and uniqueness of every individual, unrestricted by considerations of social or economic status, personal attributes, or the nature of health problems, and restoration of health; the prevention of illness; and the alleviation of suffering in the care of clients.

2. The nurse's primary commitment is to the patient, whether an individual, family, group, or community.

3. The nurse promotes, advocates for, and strives to protect the health, safety, and rights of the patient.

4. The nurse is responsible and accountable for individual nursing practice and determines the appropriate delegation of tasks consistent with the nurse's obligation to provide optimum patient care.

5. The nurse owes the same duties to self as to others, including the responsibly to preserve integrity and safety, to maintain competence, and to continue personal and professional growth.

6. The nurse participates in establishing, maintaining, and improving health care environments and conditions of employment conducive to the provision of quality health care and consistent with the values of the profession through individual and collective action.

7. The nurse participates in the advancement of the profession through contributions to practice, education, administration, and knowledge development.

8. The nurse collaborates with other health professionals and the public in promoting community, national, and international efforts to meet health needs.

9. The profession of nursing, as represented by associations and their members, is responsible for articulating nursing values, for maintaining the integrity of the profession and its practice, and for shaping social policy.

Source: Reprinted with permission from American Nurses Association, Code of Ethics for Nurses with Interpretive Statements, © 2001 nursesbooks.org, Silver Spring, MD.

Nurse Manager

The role of nurse managers is to coordinate and ensure the delivery of quality nursing care in their area of responsibility. Their role encompasses personnel management, staff development, and ensuring the availability of supplies, other resources, and processes that allow the nurses they manage to provide care. In most settings a nurse manager has 24-hour accountability for a specific patient care arena.

Nurse Administrator

Nurse administrators have a greater scope of responsibility than nurse managers. The ultimate role of a nurse administrator is to support the achievement of the standards that the organization has set for nursing practice and the guidelines of care that outline how care is to be delivered in a setting.

Nurse Researcher

Research is the never-ending quest for information and validation that lead to evidenced-based nursing practice. Nurse researcher

roles are multifaceted and involve many aspects of pharmaceutical, medical, and nursing research. Nurses serve as investigators, monitors, auditors, data managers, clinical coordinators, or research professionals. Research nurses monitor patient responses and other critical parameters.

Factors to consider as a research nurse are regulatory developments and trends, clinical research management, protocol design and implementation, and ethical issues in human research. Educational preparation varies depending on the role and setting in which one practices. Some nurses involved in research may be educationally prepared as ADN, diploma, or BSN nurses. Some nurses accomplish PhD preparation and serve as primary scientific investigators. Chapter 8 ⊛ provides a complete description of the role of nurses in research.

Nurse Educator

Nurse educators are a critical component to the success of nurses and their patients. The role of educator varies from organization to organization and department to department. Many in-hospital educator roles include responsibilities such as teaching of patients and staff, research, and direct patient care. Core competencies for the role of educator are strong clinical skills and effective teaching skills.

The nurse educator may be responsible for developing educational content for presentation, written delivery, or multimedia applications. Nurse educators also participate in the evaluation of learners (staff or patients) and serve as consultants to staff and patients. The ultimate goal of a nurse educator is to ensure quality patient care by providing education to patients and nurses and assessing the competency of those who practice.

Nonacute Care Nursing

Nonacute nurses practice outside of a hospital setting. For example, nurses perform a variety of roles in the community setting. Each role requires special training and expertise, which can be acquired through formal education and on-the-job training. With the goal of providing nursing care and preventive health care, nurses in these settings have to be flexible and creative when providing their nursing care. Examples of common nonacute nursing roles are discussed in the following subsections.

Community-Based Home Health Nurse

Community-based home health nurses are employed by government agencies, private enterprises, hospitals, and a myriad of other clinics or health care–focused organizations. These nurses provide care to patients in the community by making home visits to patients, operating mobile clinics, and staffing various types of health screening events. Home health nurses concentrate on providing care and educating patients and their significant others regarding health care issues.

These nurses may be specialists who focus on specific populations or generalists who work with families to improve the overall health of communities. Each agency operates with the concepts of disease prevention, nutrition, and child care and elder care as constructs on which to build healthy communities. Home health nurses integrate into the community and work in concert with community leaders, teachers, parents, and physicians to promote community health education.

Parish Nurse

Parish nursing is a form of community nursing that concentrates on the population of a church and the members of the congregation. The health care provided by a parish nurse is very similar to that provided by a home health/community health nurse. The parish nurse serves as a consultant and facilitator for the health care needs of the parish's congregation. Many parish nurse programs provide preventive health screening such as blood pressure and cholesterol clinics.

Long-Term Care Nurse

Long-term care is not a subset of acute care; it is a distinct entity with special needs, functions, and care providers. A variety of medical and social services are provided to help people who have disabilities or chronic care needs. Services may be short or long term and may be provided in a person's home, in the community, or in residential facilities (e.g., nursing homes or assisted living facilities). Care is provided in the form of medical and support services to persons who have lost some or all of the capacity to function due to an illness or disability. Most long-term care clients are older and require care due to diagnoses such as stroke or Alzheimer's disease. However, long-term care is not limited to those who are elderly. Younger patients may require long-term care for a chronic disease such as multiple sclerosis or conditions resulting from trauma such as spinal cord injury or traumatic brain injury. A source for more information on long-term care is the American Society for Long-Term Care Nurses.

Assisted Living Nurse

Assisted living is defined as a setting in which patients are provided long-term assisted care in a residential setting. Assisted living settings provide care to patients who have needs that are beyond the scope of home care, but do not require the level of services provided in nursing homes. Assisted living programs take on many forms; however, the most encompassing description is any group residential program not licensed as a nursing home that provides care to residents through trained staff available to respond to unscheduled calls for assistance.

Assisted living services support the resident in all activities of daily living (ADLs). Examples of activities where staff assist residents include bathing, grooming, taking medications, transferring assistance, and toileting. The assisted living setting provides a "homey" environment for people requiring or potentially requiring assistance with ADLs, but for which 24-hour nursing care is not a necessity.

Nurses' roles in assisted living facilities are multifaceted. Nurses provide direct care in some, oversee medication administration, and participate with the staff in evaluating and planning to meet the needs of residents. Unlike their acute care counterparts, nurses who care for residents in assisted living facilities are often called on to participate in decisions that impact the quality of care and quality of life of the resident (Day, 2005).

Occupational Health and Industrial Nurse

Occupational health and *industrial nursing* are terms that have been used interchangeably. This practice integrates concepts of public health nursing theory, holistic evaluation, primary prevention, surveillance, and compliance. The American Association of Occupational Health Nurses describes occupational nursing as a practice that focuses on promotion and restoration of health, prevention of illness and injury, and protection from work-related and environmental hazards.

The occupational health nurse has two primary objectives: (1) participating in the management of workers' health to mitigate health issues that may adversely affect work productivity and (2) ensuring that the employer's practices are compliant with the requirements of the Occupational Safety and Health Act.

The occupational health nurse practices in many settings, including factories, corporations, or hospitals. This type of nurse may provide direct nursing care to employees, manage workers' compensation records, conduct environmental surveillance for health hazards, and provide health education or counsel employees.

School Nurse

School nursing practice strives to advance the well-being, academic performance, and lifelong achievement of students. School nurses interact with students to foster positive responses to normal growth and development and promote health and safety practices. School nurses get involved with actual and potential health problems. In some situations a school nurse may be called on to provide case management services. These nurses actively collaborate with the student, administration, teachers, parents, and legal entities to build student and family capacity for adaptation to health care needs and self-management of issues, to promote self advocacy, and to foster learning of health-related concepts. A source of information regarding school nursing is the National Association of School Nurses.

Clinic Nurse

Clinic nurses provide patient care and support within the setting of an office building, a clinic, or a surgery center. They are routinely responsible for preparing patients for examination, administering injections, and performing clerical duties. Clinic nurses are the physician's most important professional adjunct. In this role, nurses facilitate the delivery of care to patients and manage the daily operation of the office. A source of information regarding clinic nursing is the American Association of Office Nurses.

Hospice Nurse

Hospice nurses provide care for the physical and emotional needs of dying patients and their significant others. Interventions may include pain management, palliative care, symptom management, and emotional support. A source of information regarding hospice nursing is the Hospice and Palliative Nurses Association. Chapter 17 ☻ provides a detailed description of the role of hospice nurses.

Gerontologic Nurse

Gerontologic nurses provide for the physical and psychosocial needs of older adults both in the acute care and community setting. These specialized nurses work with their patient's insurance carrier, such as health maintenance organizations, to maximize functional ability while working with the patient to maintain and restore the patient's physical and mental health. The arena of gerontologic nursing is growing because older adults have begun to represent an increasingly greater component of the population.

Age-related health issues and typically a limited ability to navigate the health care system could result in inadequate health maintenance, especially for the frail elderly. Gerontologic nurses are specially trained to deal with the special needs of this population. This training can be either in the form of an advanced degree or on-the-job training. Care specific to the elder patient is discussed in Chapter 10 ⊙ . One source of information regarding gerontologic nursing is the National Gerontological Nurses Association.

Advanced Practice Nursing Roles

Advanced practice nursing roles have grown in response to a societal need to improve the distribution of health care services and to decrease the costs of health care. The development of advanced practice roles such as nurse practitioners, clinical nurse specialists, certified nurse midwives, certified registered nurse anesthetists, and academic nurse educators occurred as a direct response to patient needs, specifically the need for access and cost-effective care.

Research has demonstrated that the use of advanced practice nurses has improved patient outcomes and reduced health care costs. Key factors that led to this success were the interpersonal skills of the nurse, knowledge and expertise in the area of practice, and a level of trust when working with physicians, nursing staff, vendors, pharmacists, insurance companies, and other health care providers. Successful enactment of the role required being a facilitator for patients and families with the health care team (Canam, 2005; MacDonald, Herbert, & Thilbeault, 2006).

These nurses provide direct care to patients through independent practice, practice within a health care agency, or in collaboration with a health care provider. As in all professions, advancements in technology and the incredible access to information have resulted in the various advanced practice roles becoming more and more specific. The most rapidly growing sectors of advanced practice nursing are the roles of nurse practitioner and clinical nurse specialist.

Nurse Practitioner

Nurse practitioners (NP) focus on individualized care. Nurse practitioners interact with patients of all ages as they examine the impact of illness on the lives of patients and their support networks. NPs practice in both acute and nonacute care settings, are eligible for Medicare reimbursement, and, in some states, have prescriptive authority.

NPs formulate their actions and interventions with a focus on prevention, wellness, and patient education. The impact of these priorities often results in fewer prescriptions and potentially less expensive medical care. NPs collaborate with their patients by fostering the acquisition of knowledge and encouraging participation in decision making related to their health care needs. The role of the NP is not limited to the delivery of health care; many are active participants in research, whereas others are active in patient advocacy work, such as development of support groups for a specific diagnosis.

Nurse practitioner programs classically specialize in an area such as family practice, internal medicine, or women's health. The advanced practice degree can be granted by a number of academic institutions. The variety of educational paths for NPs is a result of the historical development of the role. In 1965, the profession of nurse practitioner was introduced with a requirement of a master's degree. After successful completion of the education program, the NP candidates must achieve licensure in the state in which they plan to practice. The state boards of nursing regulate nurse practitioners, and each state has its own licensing and certification criteria. In general, the criteria include completion of an accredited advanced practice program and clinical experience. Depending on the requirements of the various state boards, nurse practitioners may have to fulfill additional requirements such as certification by the American Nurses Credentialing Center (ANCC) or a specialty nursing organization. Terms of licensure also vary from state to state.

Clinical Nurse Specialist

The National Association of Clinical Nurse Specialists (NACNS) defines a clinical nurse specialist (CNS) as a licensed registered nurse who has graduate preparation (master's degree or doctorate) in nursing as a CNS. CNS practice usually takes place in a hospital setting and involves interactions with patients all across the health care continuum. CNSs practice within a prescribed area of care, and define their role as having five components: clinical practice, education, management, consultation, and research. These advanced practice nurses deliver direct patient care, educate staff and patients, consult with other health care professionals, do research, and provide leadership and supervision in the workplace. Depending on the state in which they practice, the institutional policies, and the clinical specialty they choose, clinical nurse specialists may have extended scope of practice authority.

CNSs are expert nurses in a specialized area of clinical practice. According to the NACNS, the specialty may be identified in different ways. The CNS practice may be focused on a specific type of problem (e.g., pain, wounds, and stress), a defined patient population (e.g., pediatrics, geriatrics, women's health), or a setting (e.g., critical care, emergency department). Other practice focuses include medical subspecialty (e.g., diabetes, oncology) and types of care (e.g., psychiatric, rehabilitation). Although most CNSs do practice in the hospital setting, some practice in other health care settings.

In addition to providing direct patient care, the CNS influences care outcomes by providing expert consultation for nursing staff and by implementing improvements in health care delivery systems. The practice of a CNS integrates expert nursing practice, which focuses on assisting patients in the prevention or resolution of illness, with a medical diagnosis and treatment of disease, injury, and disability. It is believed that CNSs improve outcomes such as better pain management, reduced medical complications in hospitalized patients, and reduced frequency of emergency visits.

As advanced practice roles continue to grow, more need for clarification of roles and responsibilities has been required. Many states have amended their nurse practice acts to authorize nurses to perform functions that were previously restricted to the practice of physicians. Examples of these expanded functions include diagnosis, treatment, performance of selected invasive procedures, and prescription of medications and treatments. Each state regulates practices differently. In all states, the board of nursing controls these functions.

The differences in the role of nurse practitioner and clinical nurse specialist are often unclear, especially in hospital settings. This lack of distinction is very confusing to the health care consumer, other health care providers, and nurses. There is a need for clear universal definitions of the roles and responsibilities of advanced practice nurses. Nurses who pursue these roles often discuss the benefits in terms of interdependent function with other health care professionals and the establishment of peer relationships with physicians. As health care systems continue to develop, the roles of these advanced practice nurses will continue to adapt and change.

Nurse-Midwife

A nurse-midwife is defined as a nurse who has undergone special training and has received certification on child birthing (labor and delivery). Nurse-midwives can perform most of the same tasks as physicians, although they typically have emergency physician backup when they deliver a baby.

Nurse-midwives have been contributing to the birth process of millions of women and families during the past 300 years. The American College of Nurse-Midwives (ACNM) reported in 2005 that there were 6,200 nurse-midwives in clinical practice and 43 accredited ACNM nurse-midwifery programs in the United States. Of these programs, 4 are postbaccalaureate certificate programs and 39 are graduate degree programs. This advanced practice role is lawful in all 50 states and in the District of Columbia. According to an ACNM fact sheet (2005) more than 50% of certified nurse-midwives list physician practices or hospitals as their principal employer.

Certified Registered Nurse Anesthetist

The American Association of Nurse Anesthetists (2007) states "Nurse anesthesia is an advanced clinical nursing specialty. As anesthesia specialists, certified registered nurse anesthetists (CRNA) administer approximately 65% of the 26 million anesthetics given to patients in the United States each year." CRNAs provide care to patients in collaboration with other health care professionals including anesthesiologists, surgeons, and dentists.

The consistent functions of a CRNA include providing care of a patient's anesthesia needs before, during, and after surgery or the delivery of a baby. The CRNA's responsibilities are to assess, participate in operative teaching, prepare the operative area for anesthetic management, administer anesthesia, and maintain anesthesia during the operative procedure.

A CRNA is a registered nurse who is prepared through a formal nurse anesthesia didactic and clinical program. This education process prepares the CRNA candidate to sit for a national certification examination. This exam is administered by the Council on Certification of Nurse Anesthetists (CCNA). The mission of CCNA is to protect the public by ensuring that individuals who are credentialed have met predetermined qualifications or standards for providing nurse anesthesia services. All nurse anesthesia programs are graduate or postgraduate degree programs.

It is clear that initial care, ambulatory health care, and anticipatory guidance are all becoming increasingly important in nursing practice. Advanced practice roles enable nurses to function interdependently with other health care professionals and to establish a more collegial relationship with physicians. As changes in health care delivery continue, the role of advanced practice nurses, especially in primary care settings, is expected to increase in terms of scope, responsibility, and recognition.

Academic Nurse Educator

College and continuing education nursing instruction must be provided by nurses prepared at the master's or doctoral level. All **academic nurse educators** practice as faculty in colleges, universities, hospital-based schools of nursing or technical schools, or as staff development educators in health care facilities. The continuum of students these educators instruct ranges from entry into nursing practice, professional nurses in pursuit of advanced degrees, and practicing nurses interested in expanding their knowledge and skills related to care of individuals, families, and communities (*Nurses for a Healthier Tomorrow*, 2007).

Nursing Care Delivery Models

The assignment of nursing care staff to patients is a basic activity of health care systems. **Assignment** is defined as the transfer of a task and the accountability for the outcome (Huber, 2006). Assignments are the method by which the division of labor is accomplished within the structure of a health care system. A determination of the parts of an assignment that will be transferred from an RN to an assistant is *delegation*. Organizations use the concept of delegation in nursing when determining the nursing care model, or system of nursing care delivery, that will be established for the work unit.

Nurses deliver and coordinate patient care within the framework of the organizational structure and model of the nursing care delivery system. The model of care selected has a direct correlation to the allocation of control over decisions about patient care. This, in turn, has implications for job satisfaction, the character of professional practice, and the amount of authority that is actually transferred to the staff (Huber, 2006).

A nursing care model is the method of organizing and delivering nursing care to meet patients' needs. The basic elements of nursing care delivery models are work allocation, clinical decision making, communication, and management. These are fully described in Chapter 5 😊 for the four traditional models of nursing care delivery: case method, functional nursing, team nursing, and primary nursing. The practice model also may be thought of as a link between the problems presented by the patient population, the purposes of professional occupations, and the purposes of health care organizations.

For any practice model, there needs to be consistency between the degree of integration of the nursing care given to a patient, the degree of continuity in assignment of care to a patient, and the type of coordination used to plan or organize the patient's care based on general patient characteristics, available nursing resources, and the organizational support available to nursing (Huber, 2006). There is no one correct way of structuring patient care delivery. All models have advantages and disadvantages. Any specific model may be better suited to one set of environmental circumstances than another. It is, therefore, important to have an understanding of the models of patient care delivery.

Models of Organizing Patient Care

The four primary means of organizing nursing care for patient care delivery are (1) case method, (2) functional nursing, (3) team and modular nursing, and (4) primary nursing. (Marquis & Huston, 2007). Each of these basic types has undergone many modifications, often resulting in new terminology. For example, *primary nursing* now is frequently referred to as a *professional practice model*, and *team nursing* often is termed *partners in care* or *patient service partners* or other similar names.

When closely examined many of the newer models of patient care delivery systems are recycled, modified, or retitled versions of older models. In fact, it is difficult to find a "pure" delivery model; the models have become blended with most having parts of others in their design. Choosing the most appropriate organizational mode to deliver patient care for each unit or organization depends on the skill and expertise of the staff, the availability of RNs, the economic resources of the organization, the acuity of the patients, and the complexity of the tasks to be completed. These factors may change over time within an organization contingent on external environmental factors (e.g., the nursing shortage, technological advances, population factors), in which case, the nursing care delivery model also may change.

We discuss the four primary means of organizing patient care mentioned above, along with some other methods and new methods, in the following subsections.

Case Method

Case method is the oldest model of organizing care. In this method nurses assume total responsibility for meeting all of the needs of assigned patients during their time on duty. Initially, case method, sometimes referred to as case management, was provided in the patient's home, and the nurse was responsible for cooking, house cleaning, and other activities specific to the patient and family, in addition to traditional nursing care (Nelson, 2000). This type of care also was called *private duty nursing*. When people could no longer afford home care, during the depression of the 1930s, they began using hospitals for care that had been performed by private duty nurses in the home. As hospitals grew during the 1930s and 1940s, case method continued as the primary means of organizing patient care.

As mentioned above, case method nursing is sometimes referred to as a total patient care assignment because patients were assigned as cases—much like contemporary private duty nursing is carried out. Nurses are responsible for the care of a patient but only for the hours in which that specific nurse is present. The distinguishing feature of case method is the shift-only accountability for care. The term has come to mean the assignment of each patient to a nurse who plans and delivers care during a typical 8- to 12-hour per shift workweek. Within this context case method has been termed a "form of primary nursing" (Marquis & Huston, 2007). This method of assignment still is widely used in hospitals and home health agencies. Its uses and advantages and disadvantages are discussed in Chapter 5 .

Functional Nursing

Functional nursing has been defined as work assignment by functions or tasks, such as passing medications, doing dressing changes, giving baths, or doing vital signs. Philosophically, functional nursing is not oriented to individualized and holistic patient care, but is more oriented to task accomplishment, as patterned after the industrial concepts of scientific management. Under functional nursing the nurse identifies the tasks to be done for a shift. The work is divided up and assigned to personnel who focus on completing the assigned tasks. Functional nursing has the advantage of being efficient for taking care of the tasks related to handling a large number of patients. It is also

considered to be an economical means of providing care with efficiency (Marquis & Huston, 2007). The historical development of functional nursing and the advantages and disadvantages of this care delivery model are discussed in Chapter 5 .

Team Nursing/Modular Nursing

Team nursing is a care model that involves a group of people led by a knowledgeable nurse. It was developed in the 1950s in an effort to decrease the problems associated with the functional organization of patient care, the intent being to reduce the fragmentation that accompanied functional nursing. In team nursing, ancillary personnel collaborate in providing care to a group of patients under the direction of a professional nurse. As the team leader, the nurse is responsible for knowing the conditions and needs of all patients assigned to the team and for planning individual care.

This care delivery model usually is associated with democratic leadership, and allows team members to contribute their own special expertise. Group members are given as much autonomy as possible when performing assigned tasks, although the team shares responsibility and accountability collectively. Team leaders should use their knowledge about each member's abilities when making patient assignments. Recognizing each member's worth and giving team members autonomy results in high job satisfaction. The advantages and disadvantages of team nursing are discussed in Chapter 5 . Recent attempts to refine and improve team nursing have resulted in the concept of "modular" nursing, as discussed next (Marquis & Huston, 2007).

Modular Nursing

Modular nursing is a type of team nursing that involves a small team of two to three persons. It is predicated by a facility's layout and actual structural and spatial changes that enable nurses to stay near the bedside. Nurses are stationed near their patients, and a wider range of responsibility is delegated to them. The open designs and convenient access architectures of modular nursing provide for geographic decentralization of care delivery and enhanced communication (Huber, 2006).

Primary Nursing

Primary nursing was developed in the early 1970s to overcome the discontent associated with the emphasis of the functional and team nursing methods on tasks and discrete functions. Primary nursing uses some of the concepts of case method to bring the registered nurse back to the bedside to provide clinical care (Marquis & Huston, 2007). This goes along with a societal trend toward accountability and nursing's rising level of professionalism. As originally designed, primary nursing requires a nursing staff comprised totally of RNs. The RN primary nurse assumes 24-hour responsibility for planning the care of one or more patients from admission or the start of treatment to discharge or the treatment's end.

Although designed for use in hospitals, the structure lends itself well to home health nursing, hospice nursing, and other health care delivery systems. An integral responsibility of the primary nurse is to establish clear communication among the patient and family, the physician, associate nurses, and other team members. Although the primary nurse establishes the plan of care, input is sought from others in coordinating the patient's care. Clear and consistent communication among the group and consistent, direct patient care by relatively few nursing staff allows for holistic, high-quality patient care. The primary nursing care delivery model is discussed in Chapter 5 ⊘, including its advantages and disadvantages.

New Types of Care Delivery Models

Evolving or new types of nursing care delivery models can be found in the literature. In general, these new types are mixed models, revisited primary care, or professional practice models that emphasize outcomes management, collaboration, use of a variety of caregivers with variable competencies and preparation, and integrated practice. "The terms *case management* and *managed care* are joined with concepts of accountability, cost containment, effectiveness, seamless continuum of care, integration, multidisciplinary collaboration, new roles, alteration in skill mix, and new assignment systems" (Huber, 2003, p. 525). All seek to reconfigure nursing's work within resource constraints, care needs, and current ideas about professional nursing practice.

Among the new types of models are partnership models such as interdisciplinary teams and patient-focused care. These models are designed to meet the needs of organizations that are reengineered to be more cost effective and competitive. Due to the nature of complex knowledge, work models are needed that enhance the professional practice of all disciplines, clarify accountability for outcomes, and focus decision making at the point of service. As organizations integrate, partnership concepts become important as a way to create relationships and horizontal links that will make the system effective. Teams are no longer a mechanism for assigning work. Nor are they even composed of just nursing personnel. Rather, they form the core strategy for managing interdependency to address the complexity of health care service delivery.

Patient-Centered Care

The **patient-centered care** model, also referred to as *patient-focused care*, is part of a redesign effort to realign the structure and processes involved in delivering care to center around the patient to improve efficiency and resource use. This approach adopts the perspective of the person receiving care and strives to establish mutual goals to meet unique needs. The advantage of patient-centered care redesigns is that they center systems and services closer to the patient. This strong customer focus tends to increase patient satisfaction, which can conserve resources (Marquis & Huston, 2007).

Case Management

Case management is the latest work design proposed to meet patient needs. It is a collaborative process that assesses, plans, implements, coordinates, monitors, and evaluates options and services to meet an individual's health needs through communication and available resources to promote quality, cost-effective outcomes (Cesta & Tahan, 2003; Huber, 2006; Marquis & Huston, 2007). The focus in case management is on individual patients, not populations of patients. Case managers handle each case individually, identifying the most cost-effective providers, treatments, and care settings for insured individuals (Finkelman, 2001).

Some health care organizations use the term *case management* to define a patient-centered model of care. The American Nurses Association first defined nursing case management as a system of health assessment, planning, service procurement, service delivery, service coordination, and monitoring through which the multiple service needs of clients are met (ANA, 1988). Case management within the hospital setting is seen as a way to incorporate the strengths of earlier care models yet provide a professional practice model. Case management in acute care hospital nursing has been defined as a system of patient care delivery that focuses on the achievement of patient outcomes within effective and appropriate time frames and resources (Marquis & Huston, 2007). It focuses on an entire episode of illness, crossing all sections in which the patient receives care. A case manager directs care; however, the case manager may or may not be a nurse.

Community-Based Care

A community is a "locally-based entity composed of formal organizations reflecting societal institutions, informal groups, and aggregates. These components are interdependent, and function to meet a wide variety of collective needs" (Schuster & Goeppinger, 1996, p. 290). The community is considered to be the client when the nursing focus is on the collective or common good rather than the health of an individual. Thus, **community-based care**, also called *community-based nursing practice*, is directed toward health changes for the whole community's benefit. The unit of service may be individuals, families, groups, aggregates, institutions, or communities, but the purpose is to affect the entire community. The term *community* denotes a local entity, whereas the term *population* refers to an aggregate with any common characteristic, not necessarily tied to a place.

Within this context community-based nursing describes a setting for practice and a philosophy of care applicable to all nurses in all settings. It reflects how nursing care is provided, is typically not confined to one practice setting, is directed toward individuals and families within any community setting, and is designed to assist patients as they move among health care settings. Community-based nursing occurs in places where people spend their time, for example, in the home, in shelters, in long-term care residences, at work, in senior citizen centers, in ambulatory settings, and in hospitals (Berman, Snyder, Kozier, & Erb, 2008).

Legislative, regulatory, and social changes in the health care system as a result of health care reform initiatives of the 1990s have increased the need to move services out of the hospital and into community-based alternative health care settings. The numbers and kinds of agencies that provide care in the home and community have expanded because of the increasing needs of patients. As more health care delivery shifts into the community, more nurses are working in public health and community-based settings.

Community-based nurses are challenged as patients with complex nursing care needs are discharged from acute care settings early in the recovery process. Such patients include those who are elderly and have multiple-system problems. Medical technologies that were once thought to be useful in the hospital setting only have been adapted to the home and community settings. As a result, the community-based care setting is becoming one of the largest practice areas for nursing.

Within these settings nurses often deliver care without direct supervision or the support of other health care personnel. They must be self-directed, flexible, adaptable, and tolerant of various lifestyles and living conditions. Expertise in independent decision making, critical thinking, assessment, health education, and competence in basic nursing care are essential to function effectively in community-based settings.

Community Health Nursing

The phrase *community-based nursing* often is interchanged with *community health nursing*, but a distinction should be made. The phrase **community health nursing** has generally been equated with *public health nursing,* a specialty focused on special populations although care may be given to individuals. The term *community health* means meeting the collective needs of a group by identifying problems and managing interactions both within the community and among communities that make up the larger society. Community-based nursing is broader and may incorporate community health/public health nursing.

Population-Based Care

Population-based care is focused on aggregates and communities. Williams (1996) defined a population as "a collection of individuals who have in common one or more personal or environmental characteristics" (p. 25). Also called an aggregate, the members of a community are defined in terms of geography, special interest, disease state, or other common characteristics. The research-related term is target population. In community health, population-focused practice is directed toward care for defined populations or subpopulations as opposed to care for individual patients. Population-based case management is defined as the integration and coordination of health services for a specified population. This concept is implemented by providing a continuum of care from many health care organizations, and it is sometimes referred to as disease management.

Disease Management

More typically, the term *disease management* refers to a comprehensive, integrated approach to care and reimbursement based on a disease's natural course. The goal is to address the disease condition with maximum effectiveness and efficiency. Huber (2006) describes this as addressing a high-cost, chronic illness or condition, such as diabetes, with maximum efficiency across treatment settings regardless of typical reimbursement patterns. Thus, a continuum of chronic illness care is established that includes early detection and early intervention. This prevents or reduces exacerbation of the disease, acute episodes, and the use of expensive resources such as hospital inpatient care. Prevention and proactive case management are two major aspects of disease management programs. Additionally, disease management programs include comprehensive tracking of patient outcomes. Thus, the goals for disease management are focused on integrating components and improving long-term outcomes (Marquis & Huston, 2007).

Community-Based Care Versus Acute Care

Although there are noted differences between community-based care and acute care, there also are similarities. Practice in the acute care setting, where the patient is defined by disease or condition, typically takes place in specialized units where family access and patient autonomy are regulated by agency policies. Health is viewed as the opposite of illness, and the focus of care

is to eliminate illness. Nursing activities are geared toward short-term interventions. In the community setting, the patient is seen within the context of family and social network, and is treated in one's own environment, typically where the patient is more at ease. Illness is seen as a part of life, and the purpose of care is to limit patient disability and to improve functional capacity and quality of life. Nursing practice in the community has greater autonomy with therapeutic interventions, usually defined by clinician and patient who hold the patient's values central to the care performed.

Although traditional values and ways in which we think about each area of practice differ, nursing does not require widely different skills and knowledge. In both settings, nurses apply principles of interpersonal communication and caring skills to the patient, family, and other caregivers. Similarly, in each setting, nurses use leadership skills to plan, organize, coordinate, delegate, and evaluate care of patients. In both, nurses provide effective physical care. General principles of community-based care include advocating self-care; focusing on prevention; family, culture, and community; and continuity of care. Within the framework of these principles, when patient self-care, prevention, collaboration, continuity, and care within the context of family, culture, and community are emphasized, the nurse is participating in community-based nursing. It truly becomes a philosophy of care about *how* nurses practice—not *where* they work—and it can be incorporated into any type of work setting.

The Future and Workplace Design

The preceding discussion allows one to conclude that there is no one single way to organize patient care delivery systems. The method of workplace design depends on the internal and external environmental factors currently in play. They are not static, but in a constant state of flux.

It is well known that forces and pressures outside of nursing influence nursing care delivery models; however, it is not known which form is the best care model for each setting (Marquis & Huston, 2007). Although we have knowledge about the advantages of different model types, there is a lack of research evidence about which setting is most appropriate for which care model, where each is most cost effective, or which one is going to produce a higher quality of care delivery. Restructuring today means looking at new care models as they relate to a cost–quality balance. In the restructuring process, the desired outcomes are that patient care be delivered more efficiently, people be more satisfied, and costs be minimized. What is clear is that with all models, nurses must collaborate with each other and other members of the health care team in order to provide health care to the current and future generations.

Collaborative Care

Collaboration among health care professionals becomes increasingly important as the roles and boundaries change and merge. Some practitioners have begun to specialize in progressively more narrow areas of expertise, whereas others have taken on the role of generalist. Over time the legal scope of practice of each health care profession may change. To deliver optimum comprehensive care to the patient, nurses must work as a member of a team, collaborating in a collegial manner with other health care providers. This requires discussing patients' diagnoses and cooperating in the management and delivery of care (ANA, 1992).

Nurses as collaborators in patient care delivery also may be involved in determining and resolving bioethical issues, speaking out on legislation, participating in health-related research, and working with professional organizations. In fulfilling a collaborative role, nurses need to assume accountability and increased authority in practice areas. Key elements necessary for collaboration include effective communication skills, mutual respect, trust, and a decision-making process.

Some institutions use the collaborative practice model. Nurses, physicians, and ancillary health personnel function within a decentralized organizational structure and collaborate when making clinical decisions. A joint practice committee, with representation from all care providers, may function at the unit level to monitor, support, and foster collaboration (Berman et al., 2008; Marquis & Huston, 2007). The collaborative model of care, or some variation of it, should be a primary goal for nursing. This model promotes shared participation, responsibility, and accountability in a health care environment that is striving to meet the complex health care needs of the public with an increasing array of health care workers.

Influences in Health Care Delivery

The health care delivery system of the 21st century is undergoing a major transformation. A new system is emerging in response to the social, economic, technological, scientific, and political forces challenging the century. Among the most significant of these changes are the changing population demographics, changes in health care needs, and changing expectations of the consumers of health care.

The characteristics of the 21st-century health care system include short-term stays, fast patient turnover, advanced technology, flexibility, early engagement, mobility, and the involvement of family members as primary caregivers. These changes along with the environmental changes previously discussed will influence how nursing care is delivered, as well as who will deliver the care and when this will occur (Huber, 2006; Sullivan & Decker, 2005; Yoder-Wise, 2008).

Population Demographics

Population changes in general are having a direct impact on health care delivery. The 2000 U.S. census data indicated that the United States population is 281.4 million people. This figure indicates that people are living longer, possibly due to improved health services and improved nutrition. In 2004, the U.S. Census Bureau completed an estimate of general demographic characteristics. At that time the total U.S. population was estimated to be 299,398,484, with a small majority being female.

Most sources agree that not only is the population increasing and living longer, but it is also changing in composition. The decline in birth rate and the increase in life span attributed to improved health care have resulted in fewer school-age children and more senior citizens, most of whom are women. People re-

side in areas dictated by age and ethnicity. Much of the population resides in highly congested urban areas, with a steady migration of minority groups to the inner cities and migration of middle-class people to suburban areas. The culturally diverse population is growing, as is the homeless population.

These population shifts, joined by major concerns about emerging infectious diseases, trauma, and bioterrorism, are changing the focus of health care and, therefore, the roles of health care providers. The focus is shifting more to prevention, health promotion, and management of chronic conditions than in the prior century. This shift in focus coincides with a nationwide emphasis on cost control and resource management directed toward providing cost-effective and efficient health services for all (Dower, 2002).

Aging Population

Advances in technology, discoveries of cures for diseases, new treatment modalities, and the push for wellness have all had an impact on life span, significantly increasing the proportion of the population who grow to old age. According to some projections, by the year 2010, the baby boomers will turn 65 plus. In the next decade the proportion of society over 65 years of age will nearly double, and the health of older Americans will become a critical health care issue during this century (Administration on Aging [AoA], 2004). However, as the population of older adults dramatically increases, a few signs indicate that adequate resources will not be available to meet the challenge of providing health care and good quality of life for these older adults and their families. The aging population currently accounts for 12.4% of the entire U.S. population. The projection by the year 2030 is that the older U.S. population will double to about 71 million and account for 20% of the population (AoA, 2004). The "oldest-old" Americans, those 85 years and older, are the fastest growing group in the United States. This population is projected to increase from 4.6 million in 2002 to 9.6 million in 2030 (National Center for Health Statistics, 2007).

Although demographic projections for the coming decades include growth in the population of older adults, particularly those over age 85, a decrease in younger age groups is projected, a reflection of lower fertility rates and delayed childbearing among baby boomers. The dependency ratio often is cited as a determining factor in care for older adults, and is projected to reach unprecedented heights, having grown from 9.1 older adults per 100 workers in 1930 to 35.7 in 2030 (Centers for Disease Control and Prevention [CDC], 2004; U.S. Census Bureau, 2000). The concern is that this will create a functional scarcity among younger generations, with higher demand on fewer people for informal caregiving and proportionately lower contributions to Social Security benefits (AoA, 2004).

Other trends may also influence the availability of family caregivers. For example, fewer women are at home to provide care because of the growing number of female heads of households and two-income families. In the future there will be more childless elders, based on a higher percentage of currently childless women in the 40- to 45-year-old age group. It is important to consider that the oldest-old individuals are most likely to have disabilities, use multiple medications, or need consistent caregiving. Also important to note is that many older adults will be from ethnically diverse cultures. Hispanic elders, now 5.6% of the elderly population, will increase to 16.4% of the elderly population in the next 50 years (CDC, 2004). These trends are important to those planning health care services for the future because they suggest an increasing demand on formal services, a pattern already in evidence during the past decade. The health care needs of the aging, availability of health care resources, and the nurse's role in caring for the aging are discussed in detail in Chapter 10 ⊕.

Informed Consumers

In addition to age, other demographic factors are developing that will affect health care in the 21st century. The majority of the consumers of health care will be well educated and, hence, better able to obtain and use the information needed for maintaining health (Baker, Wagner, Singer, & Bundorf, 2003). They will be able to use the Internet to assist them in learning about their illness or health issues, and they will be better able to make informed decisions regarding their health care. Consumers also will be more diverse, requiring a multicultural sensitivity.

The roles of women and the family will change. There will be an increase in single-parent families and an increase in multiple-family combinations. Parents will be older with fewer children. More women will work outside the home and choose to remain in the workplace after having children. Society will place a higher value on children. Such demographic variables have a significant impact on health care, economics, public policy, and quality of life, including the delivery of health care (Dower, 2002; Getzen, 2006; Mechanic, Rogut, & Colby, 2005; Shortell & Kaluzny, 2005).

Cultural Diversity

Diversity is a word that means something different to each and every person. **Cultural diversity** refers to the variations among groups of people with respect to the habits, values, preferences, beliefs, taboos, and rules determined to be appropriate for individuals and social interaction (Huber, 2006). It represents the variety and differences in the customs and practices of defined social groups. The changing demographics and economics of our growing multicultural world and the long-standing disparities in the health status of people from culturally diverse backgrounds have challenged health care providers and organizations to consider cultural diversity as a priority.

As with aging, cultural diversity is increasing at a rapid speed (U.S. Census Bureau, 2002). Some projections indicate that by 2030 racial and ethnic minority groups will comprise 40% of the U.S. population. With increased immigration, this figure could rise to 50% by the year 2030. As the cultural composition of the population changes, it becomes increasingly important to address cultural considerations in the delivery of health care. Patients from diverse sociocultural groups bring different health care beliefs, values, and practices to the health care setting, as well as different risk factors for some disease conditions. They also respond to treatment uniquely. These factors significantly affect the way one responds to health care problems or illness, to those who provide the care, and to the care itself. It is understood that an appreciation of the diverse characteristics and needs of individuals from varied ethnic and cultural backgrounds is important in health care and nursing. Unless these

factors are understood and respected by health care providers, the care delivered may be ineffective and health care outcomes may be negatively affected.

In addressing cultural diversity, health care providers must realize that it goes beyond knowing the values, beliefs, customs, and practices of racial groups, such as African Americans, Asians, Hispanics/Latinos, Native Americans, and Pacific Islanders. Religious affiliation, language, physical size, gender, sexual orientation, age, disability, political orientation, socioeconomic status, occupational status, and geographic location also represent a few of the faces of diversity (Campinha-Bacote, 2003).

To understand cultural diversity, it is necessary to understand **culture**. Culture refers to a complex of learned patterns of behavior, beliefs, and values that can be attributed to a particular group of people. These learned behaviors, beliefs, and values guide thinking, decisions, and actions. Included among the many characteristics that distinguish cultural groups are the manner of dress, language spoken, values, rules or norms of behavior, gender-specific practices, economics, politics, laws and social control, artifact, technology, dietary practices, and health beliefs and practices. Health promotion, illness prevention, causes of sickness, treatment, coping, caring, dying, and death are all a part of the health-related component of every culture. Individuals have a unique belief and value system, which has, in part, been shaped by their cultural environment. This value system influences and guides the individual's response to illness and to health care. It is incumbent on the health care delivery system to consider these individual needs by providing practitioners who are culturally competent and providing organizational structures that are sensitive to cultural diversity.

Cultural Competence

Health care service policies, protocols, and regulations call for **cultural competence**, which is the act of providing care effectively to persons from a multiplicity of cultures. Cultural competence is an ongoing evolution of knowing, respecting, and incorporating the values of others. It means being open to the cultural beliefs and behaviors of others. It is a crucial link to practicing empathy, understanding, communicating, valuing, and caring in health care.

To achieve cultural competence one must possess a set of congruent behaviors, attitudes, and policies that come together in a system, agency, or among professionals and enables that system, agency, or those professionals to work effectively in cross-cultural situations. The word *competence* implies having the capacity to function effectively (Campinha-Bacote, 2003). Because cultural differences are learned, cultural sensitivity and competence also can be learned. The four identified components needed to become more culturally competent are cultural awareness, cultural knowledge, cultural skill, and cultural encounters.

Campinha-Bacote (2003) believes that all people belong to the same human race, with all of the same basic needs. However, she stresses that it is important to remember that these needs may be expressed differently, and that quality health care services may mean something different to each person. It is critically important for the health care delivery system to recognize the increasing diversity of those who seek care and make provisions for those who practice in the system to become culturally competent. It is equally important for health care professionals to apply the concepts of cultural competence to the patients they care for. Because every person comes from a unique and different background, the individual needs and values must be taken into account to make hospital stays as comfortable as possible. For example, the nurse should consider which room numbers mean bad luck to Asian Americans, what foods are comfort foods to Hispanics, or how to bring comfort and caring to a Muslim individual. Cultural competence will enable the health care system to improve the quality of care as measured by patient outcomes and to meet state and national licensure and accreditation standards.

Changing Disease Patterns

The health problems of Americans have changed significantly during the past 50 years. Many infectious diseases have been controlled or eradicated; others, such as tuberculosis, acquired immunodeficiency syndrome (AIDS), and sexually transmitted infections are on the rise. An increasing number of infection agents are becoming resistant to antibiotics. Conditions that once were treated easily have become complex and difficult to treat—some have even become life threatening.

The increasing life span of the general population is contributing significantly to the increase in chronic disease and disability (CDC, 2004). Also, the successful treatment options for conditions such as cancer and human immunodeficiency virus (HIV) allow people with these conditions to live decades longer than in earlier years. People with chronic illnesses are the largest group of health care consumers in the United States (CDC, 2004). Due to the heavy incidence of chronic conditions, many people are learning how to protect and maximize their health within the constraints of chronic illness and disability. As chronic conditions increase, health care broadens from a focus on cure and eradication of disease to include the prevention or rapid treatment of exacerbations of chronic conditions. The shifting changes in disease patterns support the need for increased emphasis on community-based care, rather than acute care.

In discussing changing disease patterns, it is necessary also to address globalization and health for all. Those entering the United States through travel and immigration are bringing many new diseases with them. Current society exists in a world where global infectious disease cannot be controlled by border patrols. One of the new diseases, West Nile virus, was first detected in the United States in 1999. By 2002, West Nile virus had spread to most of the continental United States. The first human case of this virus was reported in early July 2003, with three deaths due to the virus reported by August. In 2005 alone, there were 3,000 human cases and 119 deaths linked to infection, up from 2,539 cases and 100 deaths in 2004 (Medline Plus, 2006). Severe acute respiratory syndrome (SARS) is another example of a new viral disease that was first identified in China, Hong Kong, and Vietnam in 2003. This disease has spread to the United States, and at the time of this writing, there were more than 200 suspected cases in the United States (National Institute of Allergy and Infectious Diseases, 2005). According to the World Health Organization, 8,098 people worldwide became

sick with SARS during the 2003 outbreak. Of these, 774 died. In the United States only 8 people had laboratory evidence of SARS-CoV infection; no deaths were reported (CDC, 2006).

Now, society is faced with the avian flu and methicillin-resistant *Staphylococcus aureus* (MRSA). Avian influenza virus refers to influenza A viruses found chiefly in birds, but infections with these viruses can occur in humans. Although the risk for human infection is low, confirmed cases of human infection from several subtypes of avian influenza infection have been reported since 1997. Most cases of avian influenza infection in humans have resulted from contact with infected poultry (e.g., domesticated chicken, ducks, and turkeys) or surfaces contaminated with secretion/excretions from infected birds.

Of the few avian influenza viruses that have crossed the species barrier to infect humans, H5N1 has caused the largest number of detected cases of severe disease and death in humans. However, it is possible that those cases in the most severely ill people are more likely to be diagnosed and reported, while milder cases go unreported (CDC, 2007). Of the human cases associated with the ongoing H5N1 outbreaks in poultry and wild birds in Asia and parts of Europe, the Near East, and Africa, more than half of those people reported infected with the virus have died. Most cases have occurred in previously healthy children and young adults and have resulted from direct or close contact with H5N1-infected poultry or H5N1-contaminated surfaces.

Although there has been some human-to-human spread of H5N1, it has been limited, inefficient, and unsustained. Nonetheless, because all influenza viruses have the ability to change, scientists are concerned that one day the H5N1 virus could be able to infect humans and spread easily from one person to another. Because these viruses do not commonly infect humans, there is little or no immune protection against them in the human population. If the H5N1 virus were to gain the capacity to spread easily from person to person, an influenza pandemic (worldwide outbreak of disease) could begin. No one can predict when a pandemic might occur. However, experts from around the world are watching the H5N1 situation in Asia and Europe very closely and are preparing for the possibility that the virus may begin to spread more easily and widely from person to person.

MRSA joins avian flu, West Nile virus, SARS, and HIV as a potentially deadly infectious disease that seems to be becoming more prevalent (Mayo Clinic, 2007). Worldwide, an estimated 2 billion people carry some form of *S. aureus*; of these, up to 53 million (2.7% of carriers) are thought to carry MRSA. In the United States, 95 million carry *S. aureus* in their noses; of these, 2.5 million (2.6% of carriers) carry MRSA.

Increasing numbers of outbreaks of community-acquired MRSA colonization and infection through skin contact in locker rooms and gymnasiums, even among healthy populations, have been reported. MRSA causes as many as 20% of *S. aureus* infections in populations that use intravenous drugs. These out-of-hospital strains, or community-acquired (CA)-MRSA, are more easily treated, even though they are more virulent, than hospital-aquired (HA)-MRSA. CA-MRSA apparently did not evolve *de novo* in the community but represents a hybrid between MRSA that spread from the hospital environment and strains that were once easily treatable in the community. Most of the hybrid strains also acquired a factor that increases their virulence, resulting in the development of deep tissue infections from minor scrapes and cuts, as well as many cases of fatal pneumonia.

The spread of HIV/AIDS and other catastrophic illnesses threatens both personal and political viability. Lack of access to safe reproductive health puts hundreds of millions of people at risk and also contributes to the burgeoning global population growth and migration. Poor child health and nutrition rob future generations of human potential and years of life. Health for all continues to be a call for equity and social justice, a global issue that must be dealt with at the local level in communities around the world.

Complementary and Alternative Therapy

Health care in the 21st century requires that nurses not only care for the critically ill, elderly, and infirm, but also that they recognize and incorporate new and evolving methods to enhance the health of those who choose alternative or complementary therapies. This evidence-based, integrative style of care originates from holistic nursing, a precursor and philosophical framework for many of the now popular alternative and complementary therapies. Holistic nursing is simply defined as caring for the whole person—body, mind, and spirit—in an ever-changing environment.

Complementary or Alternative: What Is the Difference?

The words *complementary* and *alternative* are sometimes used interchangeably, but they are not the same. **Complementary therapy** refers to a therapy used in addition to a conventional therapy. For example, a nurse might use touch therapies, music, or guided imagery for pain control in addition to the prescribed drug therapy.

Alternative therapy, sometimes called *unconventional therapy*, refers to a therapy used instead of conventional or mainstream therapy. An example is the use of acupuncture instead of analgesics.

Integration of Complementary and Alternative Systems into Traditional American Health Care

Until recently, in North America, the primary system of medicine was simply called *medicine*, although some refer to it as **allopathic medicine**. In the past two decades a number of schools of thought and philosophies have become intertwined with traditional medicine. The most frequently seen new systems include Ayurvedic, Chinese, chiropractic, naturopathic, Native American, and osteopathic medicine. Each of these systems can stand alone, or be used in combination with other systems (Chart 1–8, p. 26).

Safety and Effectiveness of Alternative Therapies

Safety generally is interpreted to mean "freedom from danger" in which the benefits of alternative therapy outweigh the risks. If the patient is interested in using an alternative or complementary therapy, the nurse should first counsel the person about the benefits and risks and advise her to ask the practitioner of the therapy about the safety and effectiveness of the treatment.

Complementary and alternative medicine (CAM) therapies can be dangerous if used improperly. As for any medical endeavor, practitioners must be trained and, with some therapies, licensed or certified. The most prevalent deficit of CAM therapies is seen when patients use them instead of conventional therapy and do not seek traditional diagnosis and treatment. People who choose CAM therapies first and continue to use them for symptom treatment may delay diagnosis of treatable cancers as well as a huge array of curable conditions. Thus, most CAM therapies are best used alongside conventional medicine. The positive effects of these therapies used to augment allopathic medicine are presented in the Complementary and Alternative Therapies feature boxes that appear in most of the forthcoming disorder chapters in this text.

When assessing patients the nurse should ask if they use any nontraditional therapies and, if so, what their response is to them. The nurse should try to eliminate any preconceived notions she may have about a certain therapy. Patients typically will feel more comfortable discussing nontraditional therapies if they feel the nurse understands the treatment and why they have decided to use it. If patients are unfamiliar with alternative or complementary therapies (Chart 1–9, p. 27), they may ask the nurse questions about specific treatments or therapies. Following are some sample questions that patients may ask:

- What will this therapy do for me?
- What are the advantages of this therapy?
- What are the disadvantages?
- Are there side effects?
- What risks are associated with this therapy?
- How much will it cost?
- How long will it take? How many treatments will be necessary?
- How will it interact with my other therapies?

The use of alternative and complementary therapies is proliferating. Nurses who have additional training in specific CAM therapies can use many of them to provide better care for patients. When patients use complementary therapies, nurses should consider the usage an attempt to increase potential health benefits and not as signs of distress or dissatisfaction with their current care. Throughout this text in the chapters that cover disorders, Complementary and Alternative Therapies features highlight single or occasionally multiple therapies that will work with one of the conditions referred to in the chapter. These boxed features may be used as an example of how nurses can incorporate CAM into their care.

Advances in Technology and Genetics

Advances in technology and genetics have occurred with greater frequency in the last several decades than ever before. They are causing changes in all health care settings and in the roles and responsibilities of all health care providers.

Technological Changes

Biomedical technology, information technology, telecommunications, and the Internet have changed the delivery of health care into a national and even international system. The previous state of the art is being replaced by new high-tech developments at an ever-increasing rate. The advances have enabled practitioners to make faster diagnoses, treat illnesses more quickly,

CHART 1–8	Systems of Health Care Services

System	Description
Allopathic/Western medicine	The most common name for allopathic medicine is *Western medicine*. Other terms for Western medicine are *conventional medicine* and *mainstream medicine*. Many people have not heard the term *allopathic* because most health care professionals do not refer to themselves or their practice with this name. Practitioners of other systems of medicine more often use the term when referring to what can be called Western medicine or mainstream medicine. Allopathy is a method of treating disease with remedies that produce effects different from those caused by the disease itself. This system of medicine uses scientific data to determine the validity of a diagnosis and the effectiveness of treatment. It is evidence-based medicine. Practitioners use a variety of therapies including drugs, surgery, and radiation therapy. Western medicine practitioners have made most of the significant advances and developments in modern medicine.
Ayurvedic medicine	Ayurveda is the ancient Hindu system of medicine from India. Its main goals are to maintain the health of healthy people and cure the illnesses of sick people. Ayurveda maintains that illness is the result of falling out of balance with nature. Diagnosis is based on three metabolic body types call *doshas*. The Ayurvedic doctor determines the doshas type as vata, pitta, and kapha. Treatment usually involves prescribing a diet, herbal remedies, breathwork, physical exercise, yoga, meditation, massage, and a rejuvenation or detoxification program.
Traditional Chinese medicine	Traditional Chinese medicine is thousands of years old and involves such techniques and practices as acupuncture, acupressure, herbs, massage, and qi gong. The diagnosis and treatment of disturbances of qi (pronounced "chee")—or vital energy—are distinctive characteristics of Chinese medicine. Acupuncturists, one type of traditional Chinese medicine practitioner, access patients' health by checking pulses, looking at the color of the tongue, checking facial color, assessing voice and smell, and asking a variety of questions. To treat patients, acupuncturists insert a needle(s) along the meridians (pathways) where qi flows. Many acupuncturists also prescribe herbs.
Chiropractic	The main treatment modality of chiropractors is manual adjustment and manipulation of the vertebral column and the extremities. They use direct hand contact and mechanical and electrical treatment methods in the course of treatment. Chiropractors primarily treat back pain, neck pain, and headaches. They do not perform surgery, nor do they prescribe drugs.
Homeopathic medicine	Homeopathy is based on the principle that "like cures like," in which tiny doses of a substance that create the symptoms of disease in a healthy person will relieve those symptoms in a sick person.
Naturopathic medicine	Naturopathy primarily uses natural therapies such as nutrition, botanical medicine, hydrotherapy, counseling, physical medicine, and homeopathy to treat disease, promote healing, and prevent illness. Naturopathic physicians have a doctor of naturopathy (ND) degree and must be licensed.
Native American healing	Native American medicine practices vary from tribe to tribe. In general, Native American medicine is a community-based system with rituals and practices: the sweat lodge, use of herbal remedies, the medicine wheel, sacred hoop, the "sing," and shamanistic healing. For example, an ill person may be placed in a small, enclosed sweat lodge. While singing or chanting is done outside the lodge, it is believed that toxic substances will come out in the sweat of the person inside the lodge. After the ceremony, the ill person may be placed on a cot outside and be prayed over.
Osteopathic medicine	This practice of medicine emphasizes the interrelationship of the body's nerves, muscles, bones, and organs. The osteopathic philosophy involves treating the whole person, recognizes the body's ability to heal itself, and stresses the importance of diet, exercise, and fitness with a focus on prevention.

make decisions faster, and communicate more quickly and effectively with all members of the health care team.

Biomedical Technology

Biomedical technology is used for physiological monitoring, diagnostic testing, drug administration, and therapeutic treatments. Developments in biomedical technology include the use of implantable devices such as automated defibrillators, artificial organ transplants, gene therapy, and the use of robotics for people who have disabilities. Biomedical technologies also have revolutionized surgery, making it convenient and cost effective for many surgical procedures to be performed on an outpatient basis. Robotic inventions have invaded health care settings. They currently are being used in surgery, and in some institutions they provide patient care.

The health care industry also has benefited from the advanced technologies developed for space travel. These technologies have been adapted to produce health care aids such as Viewstar (an aid for people with visual impairments), the insulin infusion pump, the voice-controlled wheelchair, magnetic resonance imaging, laser surgery, filtering devices for intravenous fluid control devices, and monitoring systems for intensive care.

Information Technology

Information technology refers to those systems used to manage and process information. This involves the computer, other equipment, and processes used to store, organize, retrieve, and communicate data with accuracy and speed. Most health care delivery systems use computers and computer programs to pro-

CHART 1–9 Categories and Types of Alternative and Complementary Therapies

Category of Therapy	Types of Individual Therapies
Herbal medicine and nutritional supplements	Herbal medicine Nutrition and special diet therapies Nutritional supplements
Mind–body therapies	Psychology Art therapy Music/sound therapies Guided imagery Hypnosis and hypnotherapy Meditation and relaxation
Posture and mobility	Movement therapies T'ai chi and qi gong Yoga
Touch therapies and body work	Massage and related massage therapies Acupressure
Energetic therapies	Biofeedback Healing touch Magnet therapy Polarity therapy Reiki Spiritual healing Therapeutic touch
Miscellaneous therapies	Aquatherapy/hydrotherapy Aromatherapy Chanting Chelation therapy Colon therapy Kinesiology Light therapy Pet therapy

vide accounting, clinical, and administrative functions. Clinical nursing information systems and medical information systems manage clinical information required for the practice of nursing and medicine, respectively.

The use of information technology is growing at an exponential rate, in part because the federal government and third-party payers are supporting new technologies to reduce costs. Much of the growth in information technology has been spearheaded by an executive order that created the Office of the National Coordinator for Health Information Technology (DHHS, 2004). A 10-year plan was developed to transform the delivery of health care by building a new health information infrastructure, including electronic health records and a new network to link health records nationwide. Health information technology is believed to improve quality of care and reduce medical errors, even as it lowers administrative costs (DHHS, 2004).

The use of health information technology is really just getting started, with much growth anticipated in the next 10 years, resulting in many changes in the way health care is implemented, documented, and monitored. However, the phenomenon of information overload also can develop. According to some the adoption of information technology (IT) has been slow and the results have been mixed. If not implemented correctly, IT systems without well-conceived process improvements can hinder the efficiency, accuracy, and effectiveness of the health care system, leading to critical delays or mistakes (Klein, 2006). Another potential problem to be considered is "information overload." It is possible to move from a century in which there was a deficit of patient information to a century in which there is a surplus of patient information. The question is raised, "Can health care workers assimilate the volume of information becoming available to them?"

Longitudinal computerized patient records, telecommunications, and devices that store health history data are technologies that will grow in the future. Computerized charting and scheduling of procedures already are the norm. Hospital reimbursement systems have resulted in the redesign of patient care plans to clinical pathways that detail the interventions needed day by day to achieve the outcomes of discharge by the final approved day. Data from the clinical pathway form the basis of the episode of care in the computerized patient record. The federal government has mandated use of a computerized patient record. Credit card–like devices called smart cards store a limited number of pages of data on a computer chip. The implementation of computer-based health information systems will lead to computer networks that will store health records across local, state, national, and international boundaries. The smart card serves as a bridge between the clinician terminal and the central repository, making patient information available to the caregiver quickly and cheaply at the point of service because the patients bring it with them. This will help coordinate care, improve quality of care decisions, and reduce risk, waste, and duplication of effort (Sullivan & Decker, 2005). The challenge for nurses is to use data to create information and then change information into knowledge, which will improve the health outlook for all. This emerging body of knowledge is known as informatics.

Informatics Informatics is a combination of computer science, information science, and health care science that is designed to assist in the management and delivery of health care. Nursing informatics facilitates the integration of data, information, and knowledge and is used to assist the nurse in decision making in all roles and settings. This support is accomplished through the use of information structures, information processes, and information technology (ANA, 2001b). According to the ANA, the beginning nurse "is expected to have fundamental information management and computer literacy skills" (p. 25). Nurses must be proficient in the use of computer hardware and software. They may participate in computer utilization at varying levels of competency, although it is recognized that the level of skill needed may vary among nurses.

In many health care settings nurses will be expected to use integrated delivery systems as facilities become paperless (Huber, 2006; Marquis & Huston, 2007). The move toward increased use of information technology systems is supported strongly by The Joint Commission.

Telecommunications

Telecommunications and systems technology facilitate clinical oversight of health care via telephone or cable lines, remote monitoring, information links, and the Internet. Telehealth is the use of modern telecommunications and information technologies for the provision of health care to individuals at a distance and the transmission of information to provide that care.

This is accomplished through the use of two-way interactive videoconferencing and high-speed telephone lines, fiber-optic cable, and satellite transmissions. Patients sitting in front of the teleconference camera can be diagnosed, treated, monitored, and educated by nurses and physicians. Electrocardiograms and x-ray films can be viewed and transmitted. Sophisticated electronic stethoscopes and dermascopes allow nurses and physicians to hear heart, lung, and bowel sounds and to look closely at wounds, eyes, ears, and skin. Ready access to expert advice and patient information is available no matter where the patient or information is located, which is of particular benefit to patients in rural areas and prisons.

Advances in telemedicine already can be evidenced by home monitoring systems, where the sound of a patient's heart or a patient's blood pressure readings are transmitted over telephone lines to off-site physicians; by transmission of x-ray images over a modem to specialized physicians in other states; and by videoconferencing in which physicians consult with patients or other physicians. Telecommunications also are being used to teach physicians and nurses how to treat patients and how to provide patient care.

Internet

Another vehicle for health information is the Internet. The Internet can provide health education and health information. Health care providers and patients alike can use it to retrieve and share information. The Internet also provides a system of communication between health care provider and patients and can be a very effective means of delivering health services to people (Baker et al., 2003).

Future Projections

Technological advances in the future health care environment will stress wellness, health promotion, illness management, and the linking of local and global communities. Care in this era will focus on empowering patients and their families through information and education. Clinicians will move beyond the traditional walls of health care facilities to become skilled with wellness maintenance activities and prevention methods as well as direct care delivery. Technology will become the bond that links people and information. Nurses need to prepare for this future in which developments and refinements such as portable computers, handheld terminals, voice input, videodisc technology, expert systems, artificial intelligence, and more advanced decision support and modeling systems will continue to augment their practice. There will be greater connectedness and outreach linkages. Matching payment strategies with the technology evolution will continue to challenge the heath care system.

Nurses will be using information technology for effective outcome measurement and for capturing information at the point of care that is then distributed instantly to other users. Systems can then be mined in real time for data on quality and cost targets. Point-of-care technology can transform nurses' work processes. For example, wireless or radio frequency technology, tablet personal computers, locking/docking stations, and barcode readers constitute technological advances for nursing (Huber, 2006; Marquis & Huston, 2007).

Not only do nurses need to know how to use this technology and to access data in order to do their jobs, they need to function as information brokers and advocates for patients. As more people use the computer and the Internet to access health-related information, it becomes incumbent on the nurse to assist them in sorting out relevant, valid, and reliable information. This becomes a part of the nurse educator role. The nurse also must assume the ethical responsibility of safeguarding the integrity and confidentiality of patient information, which is now mandated by the 1996 Health Insurance Portability and Accountability Act (HIPAA) (Sullivan & Decker, 2005). HIPAA is discussed in Chapters 3, 4, & 6 😊 as it relates to the specific content area.

Genetics

Within the last decade the body of knowledge called genetics has exploded, largely due to the result of identifying the human genome through the Human Genome Project (HGP). The HGP was funded by Congress in 1988, and is the result of a collaborative, coordinated research effort in human genetics planned by the Department of Energy and the National Institutes of Health (Drell & Adamson, 2003). The HGP has been instrumental in fostering a multidisciplinary approach to research with an expectation of openness and sharing of discoveries via information technology. The achievement of uncovering the full genome sequence is regarded as a historic scientific event. The HGP has provided knowledge and insights into many diseases and development of improved methods for diagnosis and prevention.

As the pace of genetic knowledge continues to progress at a rapid rate, the private and public sectors have become increasingly interested. The private sector is interested in building markets on the information available from the HGP and offering commercialization of genetic diagnostics and services. Molecular medicine and information-based targeted health care are attracting entrepreneurial companies to consider the role of proactive prediction and prevention of disease risk based on an individuated genetic profile. Optimum goals of the HGP for the 2009 and beyond include a catalog of variations in the human DNA sequence, faster/cheaper technology, a focus on gene function, and continued attention to the implications of such knowledge for society.

The new discoveries in genetics are being publicized in all forms of mass media. Health care consumers are becoming more aware of gene-based tests and therapies and the technologies that make them possible. As genetic-based testing becomes more commonplace, individuals and their families will approach health care providers with questions about testing, resources for having testing done, interpretation of results, and requests for specialized services in genetic centers. Because nurses are widely accessible to the public, they are regarded as a group of health care providers who can begin to provide basic information and referrals for appropriate assistance. The ANA (1999) has adopted the position that the nurse, as "a provider in all health settings must have a strong knowledge base in genetics to be able to accurately assess, provide information, and make referrals for patients and families with genetic concerns" (p. 1). Chapter 11 😊 contains a complete discussion of genetics.

Economics

During the past 20 years, health care costs in the United States have skyrocketed and are expected to continue to rise. It is projected that by 2010 they will consume 13% of the gross domestic product, the highest percentage among the five other industrialized nations (Congressional Budget Office, 2003). Health care spending continues to outstrip inflation and be a source of concern for insured and uninsured alike. New medical technology, expanding insurance coverage, increased spending for prescription drugs, and the aging of the population account for the greatest increases in spending in recent years. As overall health care costs have spiraled upward, so have employers' health care costs, thereby causing many employers to decrease the coverage provided for employees or increase the amount that employees must contribute toward their health care.

With rising costs and an unstable economy, the number of uninsured Americans continues to grow (Dower, 2002; Sullivan & Decker, 2005). Studies have shown that those who are uninsured often go without necessary medical care and are more likely to be sicker and in an emergency room when they do seek care. Hospitals must cope with higher indigent medical care expenses, additional regulatory fees, and escalating equipment and supply costs. These factors have led to higher patient care charges, which means higher costs for third-party payers. This, in turn, means higher health care insurance premiums, which then leads to a greater number of uninsured.

Demand for health services has expanded along with medical costs (U.S. Census Bureau, 2002). This is occurring at a time when there is a shortage of many health care personnel to provide needed services, and when patient expectations of medical care also are at higher levels. Patients want access to the latest and greatest technology, the most modern prescription drugs available, and all forms of alternative medicine. They expect services to be provided in a timely manner. If a health care facility cannot offer such services, patients may choose to go elsewhere. It has been found that health care corporations that achieve positive patient satisfaction results do so because they have created a customer service culture and infrastructure that enables them to respond to the ever-changing demands of customers (Marquis & Huston, 2007). Patient satisfaction is significant because health care organizations are operating in an extremely competitive environment, and patient satisfaction has become key to gaining and maintaining market share. Though employers, legislators, insurers, and health care providers continue to collaborate in efforts to resolve the issues affecting the costs of health care, a solution has not yet been found. A comprehensive discussion of health care economics is found in Chapter 3 ☞.

Demand for Quality Care

With rising health care costs, consumers and third-party payers alike are questioning the quality of service provided by health care providers and organizations. The general public has become increasingly aware of health care options and health promotion. An increased knowledge base has been generated by television, magazines, periodicals, newspapers and other communications media, and by political debate. Consumers have become more active in pursuing health care in an organization that measures and reports quality of care behaviors and outcomes. Regulatory agencies and third-party payers also are basing approval and acceptance behaviors on the ability of health care organizations to produce quality of care indicators and outcomes. The demand for quality from a consumer and regulatory perspective is fully discussed in Chapter 3 ☞.

■ Summary

Nursing offers a career path in which opportunity abounds for all interested. As the population ages and the need for nurses continues to sky rocket, the practice of nursing will grow and evolve. The work of nurses will continue to change. Many hypothesize that nurses will become much more active in the fields of prevention and health screening as they reach further out into the fabric of the community in which patients live. Others suggest that nursing will continue to grow in the technology of interventional patient care, translating the high-tech information and educating those involved to care for those who have received these interventions in the home environment.

This also is a time of incredible tension as the need for change in the U.S. health care delivery system continues to expand. What will nursing be in 10 years? Advancements in the science of clinical practice, including imaging, pharmaceutical agents, and technology, keep adding to the demands of nursing. These advancements also result in changes in patients' expectations and knowledge. Nurses continue to serve the role of integrator of patients into health care systems. Their practice will be based on scientific and caring concepts, and they will develop from novice to expert through experiential learning as discussed in Chapter 2 ☞.

The future is unclear, but the diversity and adaptability of nursing is a constant. There is one certainty: Nurses will continue to be a critical component of health care delivery and the opportunities are limitless for those who join the ranks of the nursing profession.

REVIEW QUESTIONS

1. One of the characteristics of nursing is defined in the role of nursing education. In providing information regarding the characteristics and consequences of disease, promoting and modeling healthy lifestyle, the professional nurse is emphasizing which of the following?

   1. Health promotion and maintenance
   2. Advocacy
   3. Complementary therapies
   4. Physiological adaptation

2. Roach identified six components of caring that are reflected in conscience, confidence, commitment, competence, and comportment. Without caring, the nurse will not see what type needs of the client?

   1. Physical and comfort
   2. Psychological and spiritual
   3. Physiological
   4. Ethics and moral

3. When deciding on a delivery model for nursing practice, nursing administration determined that a method of assignment with nurses having accountability for a specific 'case load' of patients for a defined shift was appropriate for the department.

   This describes which delivery model?

   1. Functional nursing
   2. Modular nursing
   3. Primary care nursing
   4. Total patient care nursing

4. The staff nurse has the primary responsibility to care for a specific patient or group of patients for an assigned period. Organization and coordination are inherent in the role due to which of the following?

   1. The need to support the achievement of practice standards
   2. Patient advocacy
   3. Variety of client diagnoses and complexities of patient care
   4. The requirement for 24-hour accountability

5. Cultural competence will enable the health care system to improve the quality of care as measured in patient outcomes. Campinha-Bacote defines four components of this model. They are cultural awareness, cultural knowledge, cultural skills, and

   1. Cultural encounters
   2. Cultural studies
   3. Cultural diversity
   4. Culture

Answers for review questions appear in Appendix D

KEY TERMS

academic nurse educator *p.18*
acute care nurse *p.14*
advanced practice nursing *p.17*
allopathic medicine *p.25*
alternative therapy *p.25*
assignment *p.18*
assisted living *p.16*
caring *p.8*
clinical judgment *p.7*

code of ethics *p.11*
community-based care *p.20*
community health nursing *p.21*
complementary therapy *p.25*
cultural competence *p.23*
cultural diversity *p.23*
culture *p.23*
information technology *p.26*

nursing process *p.6*
Nursing's Agenda for the Future p.4
patient-centered care *p.20*
population-based care *p.21*
standards of care *p.10*
standards of nursing practice *p.10*
standards of professional performance *p.10*
values *p.11*

PEARSON
EXPLORE **mynursingkit**™

MyNursingKit is your one stop for online chapter review materials and resources. Prepare for success with additional NCLEX®-style practice questions, interactive assignments and activities, web links, animations and videos, and more!

Register your access code from the front of your book at
www.mynursingkit.com

REFERENCES

Academy of Medical–Surgical Nurses. (2004). *Identification of the registered nurse in the workplace*. Retrieved May 23, 2004, from http://www.medsurgnurse.org/position/workprnt.htm

Administration on Aging. (2004). *Statistics: Aging into the 21st century*. Retrieved October 10, 2007, from http://www.aoa.gov/prof/Statistics/future_growth/aging21/summary.asp

American Association of Colleges of Nursing. (2007). *The essentials of baccalaureate education for professional nursing practice (draft)*. Retrieved October 9, 2007, from http://www.aacn.nche.edu/Education/pdf/BEdraft8-1-07.pdf

American Association of Critical Care Nurses. (2004). *About critical care nursing*. Retrieved May 31, 2004, from http://www.aacn.org

American Association of Nurse Anesthetists. (2007). *About AANA*. Retrieved April 8, 2008, from http://www.aana.com

American College of Nurse-Midwives. (2005). *About ACNM*. Retrieved from http://www.midwife.org/about.cfm

American Nurses Association. (1988). *Nursing case management* (Publication No. NS-32). Kansas City, MO: Author.

American Nurses Association. (1992). *House of delegates report: 1992 convention, Las Vegas, Nevada* (pp. 104–120). Kansas City, MO: Author.

American Nurses Association. (1997). *Education for participation in nursing research*. Retrieved May 31, 2003, from http://www.ana.org

American Nurses Association. (1998). *Standards of clinical nursing practice* (2nd ed.). Silver Spring, MD: Author.

American Nurses Association. (1999). *House of delegates action report: Nursing and genetics*. Retrieved April 22, 2004, from http://www.ana.org

American Nurses Association. (2001a). *Code of ethics for nurses with interpretive statements*. Washington, DC: American Nurses Publishing.

American Nurses Association. (2001b). *Scope and standards of nursing informatics practice*. Washington, DC: American Nurses Publishing.

American Nurses Association. (2002). *Nursing's agenda for the future*. Retrieved May 23, 2004, from http://www.ana.org

American Nurses Association. (2003). *Nursing's social policy statement 2003*. Washington, DC: American Nurses Publishing.

American Nurses Association. (2004a). American nurses association (ANA) & you: Nursing on the move. In *ANA Stakeholders Report*. Silver Spring, MD: Author.

American Nurses Association. (2004b). *Nursing scope & standards of practice*. Silver Spring, MD: Author.

American Nurses Association. (2007a). *Let's make nurses' voice heard! Sign up for N-STAT today*. Retrieved April 8, 2008, from http://rnaction.org/politicalpower/join.html

American Nurses Association. (2007b). *The nursing process: A common thread amongst all nurses*. Retrieved September 16, 2007, from http://nursingworld.org/EspeciallyForYou/StudentNurses/Thenursingprocess.aspx

American Nurses Association. (2008). *What is nursing*. Retrieved April 18, 2008 from http://nursingworld.org/EspeciallyForYou/StudentNurses/WhatisNursing.aspx

Baker, L., Wagner, T. H., Singer, S., & Bundorf, K. (2003). Use of the Internet and e-mail for health care information. *Journal of the American Medical Association, 289*(19), 2400–2406.

Benner, P. (2001). *From novice to expert: Excellence and power in clinical nursing practice. A commemorative edition.* Upper Saddle River, NJ: Pearson Prentice Hall.

Benner, P., Tanner, C., & Chesla, C. (1996). *Expertise in nursing practice; Caring, clinical judgment, and ethics.* New York: Springer.

Benner, P., & Wrubel, J. (1989). *The primacy of caring: Stress and coping in health and illness.* Menlo Park, CA: Addison-Wesley.

Berman, A., Snyder, S. J., Kozier, B., & Erb, G. (2008). *Kozier & Erb's fundamentals of nursing: Concepts, process, and practice* (8th ed.). Upper Saddle River, NJ: Pearson Prentice Hall.

Brunt, B. A. (2005). Models, measurement, and strategies in developing critical-thinking skills. *Journal of Continuing Education in Nursing, 36*(6), 255–262, 283–284.

Campinha-Bacote, J. (2003). Many faces: Addressing diversity in health care. *Online Journal of Issues in Nursing, 8*(1). Retrieved April 8, 2008, from http://nursingworld.org/MainMenuCategories/ANAMarketplace/ANAPeriodicals/OJIN/TableofContents/Volume82003/Num1Jan31_2003/AddressingDiversityinHealthCare.aspx

Canam, C. (2005). Illuminating the clinical nurse specialist role of advanced practice nursing: A qualitative study. *Canadian Journal of Nursing Leadership, 18*(4), 70–89.

Carpenito-Moyet, L. J. (2007). *Nursing diagnosis: Application to clinical practice* (12th ed.). Philadelphia: Lippincott Williams & Wilkins.

Centers for Disease Control and Prevention. (2004). *Health care in America: Trends in utilization* (DHHS Publication No. 2004-1031). Washington, DC: U.S. Government Printing Office.

Centers for Disease Control and Prevention. (2006). *Severe acute respiratory syndrome* (SARS). Retrieved July 28, 2006, from http://www.cdc.gov/NCIDOD/SARS/factsheet.htm

Centers for Disease Control and Prevention. (2007). *Key facts about avian influenza (bird flu) and avian influenza A (HRN1).* Retrieved October 24, 2007, from http://www.cec.gov/flu/avian/gen-info/facts.htm

Cesta, T. G., & Tahan, H. A. (2003). *The case manager's survival guide: Winning strategies for clinical practice* (2nd ed.). St. Louis: Mosby.

Congressional Budget Office. (2003, March 20). Testimony to the Senate Special Committee on Aging.

D'Amico, D., & Barbarito C. (2007). *Health and physical assessment in nursing.* Upper Saddle River, NJ: Pearson Prentice Hall.

DeWolf-Bosek, M. S., & Savage, T. A. (2007). *The ethical component of nursing education.* Philadelphia: Lippincott Williams & Wilkins.

Dower, C. (2002). *Status of changes in patient care delivery: How can we meet demand for health care workers?* San Francisco: Center for the Health Professions, University of California, San Francisco.

Drell, D., & Adamson, A. (2003). *Fast forward to 2020: What to expect in molecular medicine.* Retrieved January 20, 2008, from http://www.ornl.gov/sci/ techsourcexews/Human+Genome/ medicine/tnty.shtml

Fesler-Birch, D. M. (2005). Critical thinking and patient outcomes: A review. *Nursing Outlook, 53,* 59–65.

Finkelman, A. W. (2001). *Managed care: A nursing perspective.* Upper Saddle River, NJ: Pearson Prentice Hall.

Gendrop, S., & Eisenhauer, L. (1996). A transactional perspective on critical thinking. *Scholarly Inquiry into Nursing Practice: International Journal, 10,* 329–342.

Getzen, T. E. (2006). *Health economics and financing* (3rd ed.). Indianapolis: John Wiley & Sons.

Guido, G. W. (2006). *Legal and ethical issues in nursing* (4th ed.). Upper Saddle River, NJ: Pearson Prentice Hall.

Huber, D. (2003). *Leadership and nursing care management* (2nd ed.). Philadelphia: W. B. Saunders.

Huber, D. (2006). *Leadership and nursing care management* (3rd ed.). Philadelphia: W. B. Saunders.

Institute of Medicine. (2004). *Keeping patients safe: Transforming the work environment of nurses.* Washington, DC: National Academies Press.

Klein, M. (2006, May 15). Will technology improve healthcare delivery? *Wisconsin Technology Network.* Retrieved July 23, 2006, from http://wistechnololgy.com/printarticle.php?id+2961

L'Eplattenier, N. (2001). Tracing the development of critical thinking in baccalaureate nursing learners. *Journal of the New York Nurses Association, 32*(2), 27–32.

Lipe, S., & Beasley, S. (2006) *Critical thinking in nursing: A cognitive skills workbook.* Philadelphia: Lippincott Williams & Wilkins.

MacDonald, J. A., Herbert, R., & Thilbeault, C. (2006). Advanced practice nursing: Unification through a common identity. *Journal of Professional Nursing, 22*(3), 172–179.

Marquis, B. L., & Huston, C. J. (2007). *Leadership roles and management functions in nursing theory & application* (5th ed.). Philadelphia: Lippincott Williams & Wilkins.

Mathes, M. (2005a). Ethical decision making and nursing. *Dermatology Nursing, 17*(6), 444–458.

Mayo Clinic Staff. (2007). *MRSA infection.* Retrieved January 20, 2008, from http://www.mayoclinic.com/health/mrsa/DS00735

Mechanic, H., Rogut, L., & Colby, D. C. (2005). *Policy challenges in modern health care.* Piscataway, NJ: Rutgers University Press.

Medline Plus. (2006). West Nile laying low, so far. *Scout News.* Retrieved July 28, 2006, from http://www.nlkn.nih.gov/medlineplus/news/fullstory_36096.html

National Center for Health Statistics. (2007). *Professional vital statistics for April 2007 Released.* Retrieved January 20, 2008, from http://www.ced.gov/nchs

National Institute of Allergy and Infectious Diseases. (2005). *NIAID research on severe acute respiratory syndrome (SARS).* Retrieved January 20, 2008, from http://www.niaid.nih.gov/factsheets/sars.htm

National Institute of Nursing Research. (2001). *Mission statement.* Retrieved May 31, 2004, from http:// www.nih.gov/ninr/research/diversity/mission.html

Nelson, J. W. (2000). Models of nursing care: A century of vacillation. *Journal of Nursing Administration, 30*(4), 156, 184.

Nurses for a Healthier Tomorrow. (2007) Retrieved June 29, 2007, from http://www.nursesource.org/nurse-educator.html

Roach, M. (1984). *Caring the human mode of being: Implications for nursing.* Toronto, Canada: University of Toronto Press.

Shortell, S., & Kaluzny, A. D. (2005). *Health care management: Organization design and behavior* (5th ed.). Clifton Park, NY: Delmar Cengage Learning.

Sullivan, E. J., & Decker, P. J. (2005). *Effective leadership & management in nursing* (6th ed.). Upper Saddle River, NJ: Pearson Prentice Hall.

Tanner, C. (1983). Research on clinical judgment. In W. Holzemer (Ed.), *Review of research in nursing education.* Thorofare, NJ: Charles B. Slack.

Tanner, C. (2006). *Thinking like a nurse: A research-based model of clinical judgment in nursing. Journal of Nursing Education, 45*(6).

Tschudin, V. (2006). How nursing ethics as a subject changes: An analysis of the first 11 years of publications of the journal of nursing ethics. *Nursing Ethics, 13*(1), 65–75.

U.S. Census Bureau. (2000). *Profile of older Americans: 2000. Population projections of the United States by age, sex, race, and Hispanic origin 1995–2050* (Current Population Reports, P25-1130). Washington, DC: Author.

U.S. Census Bureau. (2002). *National population projections summary tables.* Retrieved May 19, 2004, from: http://www.census.gov/population/www/projections/natproj.html

U.S. Department of Health and Human Services. (1991). *Healthy people 2000: National health promotion and disease prevention objectives* (DHHS Publication No. 91-5021). Washington, DC: U.S. Government Printing Office.

U.S. Department of Health and Human Services. (2000). *Healthy people 2010.* Retrieved May 1, 2004, from http://www.health.gov/healthpeople

U.S. Department of Health and Human Services. (2004, July 21). *Thompson launches decade of health information technology.* Press release retrieved July 28, 2006, from http://www.hhs.gov/news/press//2004pres/20049721a.html

Walsh, C. M., & Seldomridge, L. A. (2006). Critical thinking: Back to square two. *Journal of Nursing Education, 45*(6), 212–219.

Watson, J. (1988). *Nursing: Human science and human care. A theory of nursing.* New York: National League for Nursing.

Wilkinson, J. (2009). *Nursing process and critical thinking* (3rd ed.) Upper Saddle River NJ: Pearson Prentice Hall.

Williams, C. A. (1996). Community-based population-focused practice: The foundation of specialization in public health nursing. In M. Stanhope & J. Lancaster (Eds.), *Community health nursing: Promoting health of aggregates, families, and individuals* (4th ed., pp. 21–33). St. Louis: Mosby.

Yoder-Wise, P. S. (2008). *Leading and managing in nursing* (4th ed.). St. Louis: Mosby.

Experiential Learning: Skill Acquisition and Gaining Clinical Knowledge

Patricia Benner

Outcome-Based Learning Objectives

After studying this chapter, the learner will be able to:

1. Recognize and describe their own clinical learning in the form of an experience-near first person narrative account.
2. Give at least three examples of practical and theoretical knowledge related to adult medical-surgical nursing.
3. Give two examples of clinical interventions that can be standardized and two examples of clinical interventions that cannot be standardized.
4. Give an example of phronesis or clinical judgment that illustrates adjusting to transitions in the patient's clinical condition, or the clinician's understanding of the patient's clinical condition.
5. Give two clinical examples of how the nurse's relationship with the patient may alter the nurse's clinical judgment.
6. Explain how and why the nurse's moral agency might change with experience, according to the Dreyfus Model of Skill Acquisition.
7. Characterize three distinct differences between competent and expert clinical nursing practice.

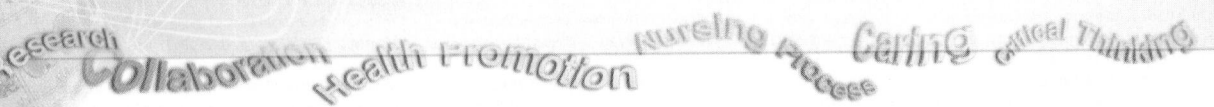

Nursing like medicine, involves a rich, socially embedded clinical know-how that encompasses perceptual skills, transitional understandings across time, and understanding of the particular in relation to the general. Clinical knowledge is a form of engaged reasoning that follows modus operandi thinking, in relation to patients' and clinical populations' particular manifestations of disease, dysfunction, response to treatment and recovery trajectories. Clinical knowledge is necessarily configurational, historical (by historical, I mean the immediate and long-term histories of particular patients and clinical populations), contextual, perceptual, and based upon knowledge gained in transitions. . . . [Through articulation], clinical understanding becomes increasingly articulate and translatable at least by clinical examples, narratives and puzzles encountered in practice. (Benner, 1994, p. 139)

BECOMING A NURSE requires more than mastery of technical and scientific knowledge. It also requires ongoing experiential learning, reflection on practice, and continuous improvement in practice as science and technology and experiential knowledge change. A metaphor of "mastery" is somewhat misleading in any professional endeavor because it projects the imagined possibility that the field is stable and can be completely "mastered" or learned at any one point in time. Fields like nursing and medicine, however, are constantly changing, self-correcting, and the study of these fields never completely covers what actually might be encountered in clinical practice. Another way of saying this is that clinical practice is open ended and un-

derdetermined. Underdetermined here, means that more than one thing may be going on, and more than one or two outcomes may occur, and that the situation is practical and necessarily ambiguous and historical. For example, the nurse's action may well alter the course and outcome of the situation in ways that are not necessarily predetermined, or uninfluenced by the patient's response, and the timing of the intervention. Clinical practice knowledge includes learning experientially and directly by engaging in practice situations. Relational knowledge (skills of engaging with patients and patient situations), skilled know-how in actual practice situations, and patient interventions based on patients' responses to their illnesses and therapies are all examples of experiential clinical learning.

Types of Knowledge and Learning Experiences

Clinical knowledge (a type of phronesis), which includes recognizing signs and symptoms of physiological and emotional distress and changes in a patient's vital signs and knowing how to titrate an intravenous (IV) rate, **clinical judgment**, and many more aspects of engaging in nursing are all forms of **practical knowledge**. For example, having a sense of **salience**, that is, having some things stand out as more or less important in a practical situation, is a form of practical knowledge that is learned after having many concrete clinical experiences in which a range of relevant clinical issues stand out as high priority, such as reestablishing IV access in a critically ill patient whose IV has become occluded or attending to opening an airway and providing respiration for a patient who is not breathing. The preceding two examples work well because they are obvious, but with experience other clinical aspects will stand out as salient—not just as one more fact among many equally relevant facts. With time, any highly salient clinical demands begins to seem obvious to the expert clinician.

Skills of engagement with both patients and their families and with clinical problems are learned experientially and are also forms of practical knowledge. For example, learning how to be attuned to a patient's emotional responses and concerns and knowing when and how to communicate about concerns and feelings associated with illness and recovery require experiential learning of **skills of involvement**. The skill of perceiving, that is, noticing relevant changes or nuances in clinical situations, also is experientially learned and forms part of a nurse's practical clinical knowledge.

Practical knowledge is shaped by a nurse's knowledge of the discipline and practice, the science and technology relevant to the situation at hand. But scientific, formal knowledge is not sufficient for good clinical practice, whether the discipline is law, medicine, nursing, teaching, or social work. Practitioners still have to learn when and how to use scientific knowledge in practical situations.

Clinical reasoning, a form of practical knowledge, also is distinct from scientific reasoning even though it draws on science. Clinical judgment requires clinical reasoning across time about a particular patient. Clinical judgment is very different from the scientific reasoning used in doing clinical or bench research. Scientific experiments use formal criteria to develop "yes" and "no" judgments under controlled circumstances at specific points in time. Scientific reasoning is closer to static snapshot reasoning than clinical reasoning, which is reasoning across time about the particular situation through changes in the clinician's understanding or changes in the patient's condition (Taylor, 1993). Practical knowledge may be compared to, though not completely separated from, theoretical knowledge. For example, knowledge of growth and development are essential to developing practical knowledge about working with young children, just as normal physiology and pathophysiology are essential for understanding clinical signs and symptoms. Discovery and experiential learning favor the prepared knowledgeable practitioner who is engaged in learning both practical and theoretical knowledge.

Because nurses are involved in assisting patients and families as they cope with the demands of an illness in the context of their social world (lifeworld), nurses need to learn much practical knowledge about human concerns and functioning in diverse social worlds. Learning how patients and families cope and how to assist them with specific transitions in recovery and rehabilitation or even as they face death requires both practical and theoretical learning in nursing. The nurse can learn much from each patient's concerns and strategies in dealing with an illness and recovery, as well as what illness and recovery trajectories look like in different patients. This kind of experiential learning of nurses in caring for many patients needs to be captured and made accessible for reflection and study. The practice of nursing gives many unique windows on a large range of human experience that remain sources of experiential learning to the curious and reflective nurse.

Given the range of practical knowledge and experiential learning required in nursing, one begin's to understand why reducing rationality to the kind offered by scientific experiments is too narrow. **Rationality** includes reasoning across time with changes in the patient's condition and concerns. Practical rationality, as illustrated in clinical judgment, includes noticing subtle changes and informed emotional responses, such as those that happen when a patient's condition changes, but the changes are not limited to explicit vital signs and may not show up immediately in the vital sign trends. For example, in early impending shock due to blood loss, the patient usually compensates at first, so the actual changes in vital signs are delayed and are best detected by assessing the patient's distress and following vital sign trends, rather than an isolated finding.

A contrast also can be made between what can be standardized and replicated, described by the early Greeks as **techne** (the know-how and skill of producing things), and what requires productive thinking, adjustment, and judgment in particular cases. Aristotle called the latter *practice* or *praxis* that requires *phronesis,* something qualitatively distinct from techne. Clinical judgment is a prime example of phronesis. This distinction is similar to the distinction between scientific and clinical reasoning. Scientific experiments must be capable of replication under precise conditions, whereas clinical reasoning is applied to a practice that occurs in real time, is uncontrolled, often about a single case, and is almost always underdetermined. The professions of nursing, medicine, and law all require a socially embedded form of knowledge that has notions of the good internal to the practice. For example, holding the patient's best interests and choices as central to clinical decisions is internal to the practice of nursing and medicine. Aristotle's example of the use of phronesis was that of a statesman who had to develop character, skilled know-how, practical reasoning, and comportment, all of which include appropriate emotional responses and relationships.

This contrast form of rationality and skill-based character, called **phronesis**, is a good example of clinical judgment and stands in contrast to rational-technical thinking. A rational-technical mode (techne), sometimes called rational technicality, separates means and ends and focuses on achieving prespecified outcomes. Rational-technical thought is a powerful strategy for those areas of science and technology that can be standardized and routinized. Nursing and medicine use techne, such as blood pressure measurements and dosage ranges for medication, but when clinical judgment, relationship, perception (or noticing), timing, and skilled know-how are involved, then more than techne or rational calculation is required. Guignon (1983) points out that separating means and outcomes often devalues or does violence to the means, especially where means and ends are closely interwoven. For example, it is not sensible to separate means and ends in human situations such as birth, comfort, health promotion, or end-of-life care. In each of these caring practices, means and ends are not separable. The picture is further complicated by the fact that most often there are multiple means and ends at stake in any clinical encounter.

As an example, consider caregiving relationships. Such relationships may open up possibilities or close them down. But even with the best intentions and comportment, the person cared for may not be able to respond to care. "Outcomes" in caregiving relationships are necessarily interdependent and mutual. Some types of influence are morally unacceptable. Manipulation, coercion, or misuse of professional influence in persuading a patient to accept a treatment is unethical. When things go well and the patient or family is able to respond to caring practices, the practitioner cannot attribute the good outcome solely to the efficacy of some technique she may have used. The focus on "prespecified outcomes" and identifying and evaluating nursing outcomes in case management are based on the premise that only technique is involved in health care, that one knows the outcomes to expect, and that all things can be "fixed." The problem is further complicated by institutional constraints to good caregiving. Meeting and responding to the patient or family may clash with the bureaucratic goals of care for the many in the most cost-efficient manner. For all of these reasons, developing moral agency and the skills of involvement that are required for the development and use of good clinical judgment present ongoing demands for experiential learning and character development in nursing. Viewing nursing as a basic human encounter and as a practice that requires phronesis has major implications for nursing education and the moral development of practitioners.

Technical care and restorative care are not mutually exclusive for the nurse or physician. One way to create more equal partners between technical medicine and human lifeworlds is to understand medicine, nursing, and other health care practices as *practices* that encompass more than the science and technologies that they use to effect cures.

The Nature of Practice: A Socially Embedded Form of Knowledge

As noted earlier, a socially organized practice such as nursing has notions of *good* internal to the practice (Dreyfus, 1992). For example, attentiveness, not neglect, and recognition practices, not depersonalization, are notions of good internal to the practice of nursing. A nurse educated to be an excellent nurse can recognize, in most instances, good and poor nursing care, even though it would be impossible to formally list all of the precise behaviors and comportments of excellent nursing care.

In philosophy, the inability to make explicit or formal all elements of a social practice is called the **limits of formalization** (Dreyfus, 1992). Likewise, the practical knowledge embedded in the traditions of science cannot be made completely formal and explicit (Benner, Tanner, & Chesla, 1996; Lave & Wenger, 1991). Every complex social practice has a foreground of focused attention and a background of comportment, practical skills, and understanding of the social practice. Science and technology have

extensive traditions of formalizing the reasoning and knowledge associated with scientific experiments. Consequently, it can appear to the naïve scientific practitioner that thinking within a particular scientific discipline is restricted to what can be formalized. However, as Thomas Kuhn (1970) demonstrated through historical examples, every science has nonrational (not *irrational*) aspects of thinking such as the use of metaphors, understandings about what constitutes an interesting scientific problem, and skillful know-how in conducting experiments. The practice of a particular discipline such as nursing or a science such as crystal growing or genomics contains the **ethos** or notions of what counts as good nursing or good scientific practice. In practice disciplines such as nursing and medicine, the ethos of the practice shapes and is shaped by relevant science. Knowledge development occurs in science and in experiential learning directly from practice. Practice is a way of knowing in its own right, in this nontechnological understanding of what constitutes a practice (Benner & Wrubel, 1982; Dunne, 1997).

To make good clinical judgments, the nurse must be skillful in moral and clinical perception (Benner & Wrubel, 1982; Dunne, 1997; Vetleson, 1994). Although conceptual knowledge is essential, it is not sufficient to ensure that the nurse will form relationships with patients that lead to salient disclosures, or that the nurse will notice and correctly identify an instance of pulmonary edema, despair, or pain when the nurse sees it, even though the nurse may know conceptually what the formal characteristics of these patient conditions are in principle. Perceptual recognition skills, skills of involvement, and moral agency are required for good clinical judgment and acting on behalf of the patient based on one's judgment.

In the practice of medicine and nursing, science and technology are used to increase certainty about the measurement of signs and symptoms. The practice of objective measurement of signs and symptoms reduces errors and improves clinical judgment. No one would recommend going back to guessing body temperatures by palpation alone. However, even the most formal measurements cannot replace the perceptual skill of the clinician in recognizing when a measurement is relevant or the meaning of a particular measurement. Also, following the course of a patient's development of signs and symptoms (the trajectory or evolution of signs and symptoms) improves the clinician's understanding of the meaning of the signs and symptoms. This may seem patently obvious to any practicing clinician, yet current strategies for applying algorithms or making particular clinical judgments based on aggregate outcomes data alone ignore the clinical know-how, relational skills, and need for clinical judgment as reasoning across time (Halpern, 2001).

Good nursing practice requires ongoing development of clinical knowledge through experiential learning. Experiential learning is not automatic. It requires openness, attentiveness, reflection on practice, and active engaged learning on the part of the practitioner. Here a distinction is being made between detached, disengaged reflection and engaged thinking-in-action (Guignon, 1983). Standing outside of a situation and reflecting back on it is a powerful critical-thinking strategy for improving practice, especially in situations of breakdown and error (Schon, 1987). However, being emotionally attuned to the patient and family and the demands of the situation in the immediate moment is also required for well-timed expert performance (Figure 2–1 ■).

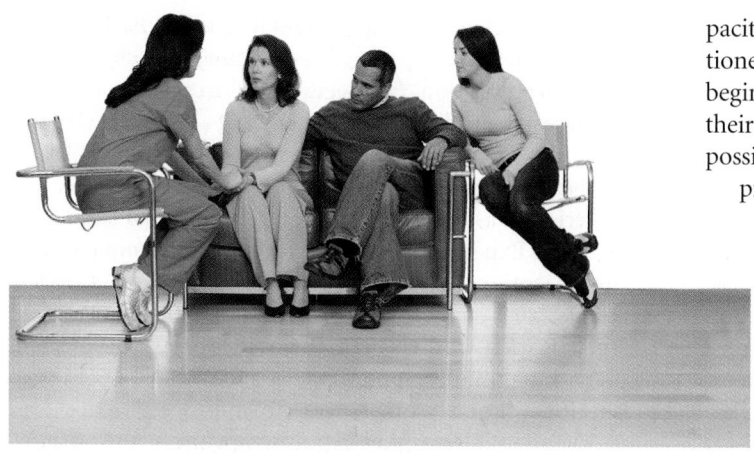

FIGURE 2–1 ■ A nurse must always be emotionally attuned to the demands of a specific situation.
Source: © Timothy Tadder/CORBIS All Rights Reserved

Doctoring and nursing particular patients require relational and communication skills and art. The relationship between the patient and nurse, for example, determines what will be disclosed by the patient, what can be thought about and talked about together, and what level of acceptance and endorsement of the therapies will be acceptable to patients and clinicians alike. Patients often rehearse their most fearful concerns with nurses who they expect to be more approachable than a physician and also effective in helping them communicate with physicians. Technique alone cannot address the interpersonal and relational responsibilities, discernment, and situated possibilities required when caring for persons made vulnerable by illness and injury. Phronesis (clinical judgment and the ability to act on good clinical judgment) is required. Means and ends are inextricably related when caring for people who are ill. Clinician and patient bend and respond to the other so that new horizons appear or are reconstituted, leading to the emergence of new possibilities. On the patient's side, healing and recovery of one's embodied relationship with the world is lived rather than mastered and requires relationship, openness, and trust.

The clinician must always intelligently appraise the relevance of the best evidence for a particular patient in addition to critically evaluating the "best evidence" itself. Qualitative distinctions must be made about the patient's concerns, actual responses to therapies, and the disease or injury processes. Clinical judgment, when not requiring instantaneous action (e.g., titrating a vasopressor IV medication to keep the patient's blood pressure within safe parameters), must be communicated and adjudicated by other clinicians. If a nurse recognizes early signs of deterioration in a patient's clinical condition, she must be able to document and communicate the evidence for the changes. This requires social skills and experiential wisdom in communicating with other clinicians so that the evidence can be verified.

Dreyfus Model of Skill Acquisition

The **Dreyfus model of skill acquisition** is based on determining the level of practice evident in particular situations (Benner, 1984, 2001; Dreyfus, 1979; Dreyfus & Dreyfus, with Athanasiou, 1986). It elucidates strengths as well as problems. Situated practice ca-

pacities are described rather than traits or talents of the practitioners. At each stage of experiential learning (novice, advanced beginner, competent, proficient, expert), clinicians can perform at their best. For example, one can be the best advanced beginner possible, typically during the first year of practice. However, no practitioner can be beyond experience regardless of the level of skill acquisition in most clinical situations and despite the necessary attempts to make practice as clear and explicit as possible. If the nurse has never encountered a particular clinical situation, experiential learning is required. For example, referring to critical pathways is not the same as recognizing when and how these pathways are relevant or must be adapted to particular patients. Experiential learning that leads to individualization and clinical discernment is required to render the use of critical pathways sensible and safe. Such individualization requires clinical discernment based on experience with past whole concrete clinical situations. This ability to make clinical comparisons between whole concrete clinical cases without decomposing the whole situation into its analytical components is a hallmark of expert clinical nursing practice (Benner & Wrubel, 1982; Ruddick, 1989).

A renewing, coherent, recognizable identity requires that practitioners develop notions of good that are constantly being worked out and extended through experiential learning in local and larger practice communities. Practice is a way of knowing, as well as a way of being in the world (Dunne, 1997; Ruddick, 1989; Taylor, 1993, 1994). A self-renewing practice directs the development, implementation, and evaluation of science and technology. Clinical judgment requires **moral agency** (defined as the ability to effect and influence situations), relationship, perceptual acuity, skilled know-how, and narrative reasoning across time about particular patient transitions (Benner & Wrubel, 1982; Guignon, 1983). As Joseph Dunne notes:

> A practice is not just a surface on which one can display instant virtuosity. It grounds one in a tradition that has been formed through an elaborate development and that exists at any juncture only in the dispositions (slowly and perhaps painfully acquired) of its recognized practitioners. (Dunne, 1997, p. 378)

The Dreyfus model of skill acquisition has illuminated ongoing research on skill acquisition and articulation of knowledge embedded in expert practice in nursing (Dreyfus, 1982; Dreyfus & Dreyfus, 1977, 1979, 1980). The Dreyfus model is developmental, based on situated performance and experiential learning. Three studies of skill acquisition in nursing that were guided by the Dreyfus model of skill acquisition have been conducted. Hubert and Stuart Dreyfus served as consultants in each of these three studies (Benner, 1982, 1984; Benner, Hooper-Kyriakidis, & Stannard, 1999; Benner, Tanner, & Chesla, 1992).

The first study, conducted from 1978 to 1981 (Benner, 1982, 1984), was based on 21 paired interviews with newly graduated nurses and their preceptors. In addition, interviews or participant observations were conducted with 51 additional experienced nurse clinicians, 11 newly graduated nurses, and 5 senior nursing students to further delineate and describe characteristics of nurse performance at different levels of education and experience. The small-group and individual interviews were conducted in six hospitals: two private community hospitals, two community teaching hospitals, one university medical center, and one inner-city general hospital.

A second study of skill acquisition and clinical knowledge of critical care nurses was conducted between 1988 and 1994 (Benner et al., 1992; Benner, Tanner, Chesla with Dreyfus and Dreyfus and Rubin 1996). The study population was made up of 130 nurses practicing in intensive care units and general floor units from eight hospitals, seven of which are located in two far Western and one in the Eastern region of the country. Small-group narrative interviews, individual interviews, and participant observation were used as data collection strategies. The two aims of the study relevant to this discussion were to (1) describe the nature of skill acquisition in critical care nursing practice and (2) delineate the practical knowledge embedded in expert practice.

The third study was an extension of this study, conducted from 1996 to 1997 to include other critical care areas (including emergency departments, flight nursing, home health, the operating room, and postanesthesia care units; $N = 75$ nurses) and enlarge the sample of advanced practice nurses.[1] This chapter synthesizes the findings of these three studies using data from each of the studies.

Nursing, like other practice disciplines, is not merely an "applied" field in the sense that the practice is complex, varied, and underdetermined. Good practice requires that the nurse develop skillful ethical comportment as a practitioner and that the nurse use good clinical judgment informed by scientific evidence and technological development. The sciences of medicine and nursing are broad and multidisciplinary and require translation into the particular practice situation. Basic sciences such as biochemical; physical, biological, and physiological processes; research and development of specific therapies and technologies; and finally clinical trials and more make up a broad range of relevant science used in the practice of medicine and nursing.

Monitoring the quality of care and preventing imminent breakdown in practice quality require social communication skills and effective moral agency, both of which are the patient's frontline defense against errors and the hazards of hospitalization. For example, in the operating room (OR), it is the requirement of anyone in the OR to immediately and verbally identify a break in sterile technique, just as it is the nurse's job to provide early warnings of changes in a patient's clinical condition. Moral agency requires more than the intent to do good or to *be* a good practitioner; it requires the experiential skill to recognize when an ethical breach in practice has occurred and the social and communication skills to effectively intervene on behalf of the patient.

Skill Acquisition and Experiential Learning

The clinician's capacity for moral agency literally changes with the growth of clinical judgment, perceptiveness, communication skills, and skillful comportment. The skill of involvement

both with the patient and engagement with the clinical situation are also learned developmentally over time and change with level of skill acquisition. The stages of skill acquisition as uncovered in research on clinical nursing practice are described in this chapter with a focus on the development of the relational skills of involvement and the skills of moral agency in the clinician.

Experience, as defined here, is an active process (Gadamer, 1960/1975). **Experiential learning** requires a turning around of preconceptions, or an adding of nuances to one's understanding. Experiential learning also requires the stance of an engaged learner, rather than the stance of one expert in techne who skillfully applies well-established knowledge in prespecified clear circumstances. To improve practice over time, experiential learning requires openness and responsiveness by the learner. The learner who develops an attuned, response-based practice learns to recognize whole situations in terms of past concrete experiences as pointed out by the Dreyfus model.

The researchers found that recognizing the situation as an "instance of particular concerns" is central to the logic of excellent practice. For example, consider a situation of heart "pump" failure or fluid depletion (Benner, 2001; Benner, Hooper-Kyriakidis & Stannard, 1999). Deciding which intervention to implement depends on clarifying and confirming the nature of the clinical situation at hand. The skillful practitioner learns to keep background understandings fluid or semipermeable so that he can recognize when these tacit expectations are not met. For example, a nurse with expertise in detecting heart arrhythmias on a unit where all patients' cardiac functioning is monitored will only notice aberrations in sound patterns, rather than attending to the familiar sounds in the foreground of attention. Recognizing the unexpected, that is, recognizing when tacit global expectations of patients' recovery are not met, is a hallmark of expert practice.

Major Shifts in the Style of Practice with the Development of Expertise

As noted earlier, the nurse's capacity for effective moral agency changes with developing practice skills and insights from experience. Also the skills of problem and person engagement grow more attuned. The development of moral agency and skills of involvement should be considered at each stage of skill acquisition, from novice to expert. The nurse increasingly is able to recognize when she does not have a good grasp of the clinical situation, and this lack of a sense of understanding guides the nurse's questioning and problem solving. Over time, an increased grasp of the nature of particular clinical situations, including opportunities and constraints, guides the nurse's actions and interactions. Consequently, responses to patients become more contextualized and attuned.

Recognition of clinical situations moves from abstract textbook accounts of general features to comparisons with past whole concrete cases. These real comparisons can include qualitative distinctions and more subtle variations. Having a grasp of the situation, with all of its various possibilities and constraints, enables the nurse to move from rule-governed thinking to an intuitive grasp of the situation (Dreyfus & Dreyfus with Athanasiou, 1986). This intuitive grasp is experienced based and not based on "extrasensory" powers or wild hunches. It is situated in

[1]The first study was sponsored by a grant from the U.S. Department of Health and Human Services, Public Health Service, Division of Nursing, Bureau of Health Professions (Grant No. 7 D10 NU 29104-03). The second and third studies were funded by the Helene Fuld Health Trust.

the clinician's grasp of the situation based upon experience with prior similar situations. Improved skills of involvement create disclosive spaces where all patients and families express their concerns, and allow the nurse to notice and respond to the most plausible actions to be discovered and taken in particular situations. Relational skills are schooled by learning to be "at home" in a highly differentiated clinical world where some actions are plausible and effective, and others are experienced as "ill timed" or implausible. A sense of salience develops over time so that some things stand out as more plausible and appropriate than others.

The practitioner develops a richer sense of the possibilities of practice based on shared notions of good practice within the profession (Rubin, 1996). Because the Dreyfus model of skill acquisition is a situated and descriptive phenomenological account of the development of skill over time, it does not point to isolated competencies nor enabling traits or talent. Consequently, a practitioner may be at different levels of skill in different areas of practice based on the particular practitioner's background experience and knowledge. For example, a practitioner skilled in caring for adults at an expert level will not be at that level of skill when caring for young children or premature infants. The patient populations that nurses care for determine the nurses' opportunities for experiential learning. Chart 2–1

lists the stages of skill acquisition in the Dreyfus model. The stages are also discussed in the following subsections.

Novice: First Year of Education

The novice stage of skill acquisition occurs in areas where the student has no experiential background on which to base an understanding of clinical situations. For example, the art and skill required for a range of medical and nursing interventions on particular patients will be new. The educator must offer good descriptions of features and attributes of the situation that the novice can recognize. For example, to determine fluid balance students are given clear parameters and guidelines:

> To determine fluid balance, check the patient's morning weights and daily intake and output for the past three days. Weight gain and an intake that is consistently greater than 500 mls could indicate water retention, in which case fluid restriction should be started until the cause of the imbalance can be found. (Benner, 1984, p. 21)

An experienced clinician can immediately think of the many situations where this evaluation would be inappropriate or too stringent. But the novice is given clear directions about safe ways to proceed until the significance of fluid balance for different clinical conditions can be learned.

CHART 2–1   **Major Characteristics of Dreyfus Model of Skill Acquisition Found in Nursing**

NOVICE: BEGINNING NURSING STUDENT

- Little or no experiential background understanding
- Recognizes attributes and features
- Requires rules and broad guidelines to organize task world
- Matches actual cases with textbook descriptions

ADVANCED BEGINNER, NEWLY GRADUATED NURSE

- Developing a perspective on clinical patient situations
- Legitimizing and evaluating the discomfort of patients
- Establishing boundaries of the role and expectations of the nurse
- Finding credible sources of information and teaching

COMPETENT STAGE—ONE TO TWO YEARS OF PRACTICE

- A time of planning and analysis
- Limit the unexpected through planning and prediction
- Anxious times now more tailored to situation
- Clinical forethought and clinical grasp developing
- Cushion of inexperience, cannot know what you don't know
- Work world can seem like a bunch of Multiple and competing tasks
- Matching examples with textbook accounts with new kinds of patients
- Limits of formal knowledge; Now knows that not everything is in procedure book or text books
- Choosing a perspective for clinical work is now required for organization
- Pattern recognition based upon experience developing
- Encountering the patient anew; now recognizes patient's plight and suffering anew

PROFICIENCY: A TRANSITION TO EXPERTISE

- A QUALITATIVE LEAP in way work is organized
- Sees the "big" picture of the patient's world and clinical situation
- Takes situated action, as orderly as the situation requires
- Gains a differentiated world of practice
- Recognizes changing relevance where changes in treatment goals or patient's clinical condition changes the meanings and interpretation of signs and symptoms
- Situation speaks to practitioner. Practice is becoming more situated, patient-response based
- Gains differentiated skill of involvement based on differing concerns and needs of patient

EXPERTISE...PRACTICE NOW EXCELLENT

- Uses both techne and phronesis appropriately
- Practice takes up theories and ends of practice in multiple ways that fit the situation
- Attunement; Skilled know-how is related to particular patients
- Skill of involvement varied and suited to individual patients need
- The particularities of clinical situations now more discernible
- New clinical knowledge is developed from practice
- Makes qualitative distinctions about patients' conditions, signs, and symptoms
- Moral dilemmas are articulated and made more visible to the work group

Source: Adapted from Benner, P., Tanner, C. A., Chesla, C. A. *Expertise in nursing practice: Caring, clinical judgment, and ethics.* New York: Springer Publishers. 1996.

Note that the rules and guidelines must not require prior experience for their recognition. They must provide a safe beginning point for specific, situated learning in a clinical situation. Fluid balance is salient, but what must be learned is the particular salience for particular patients. The rule-governed behavior of the novice is extremely limited and inflexible. The student is coached in comparing and matching textbook examples with actual clinical cases. Skills that are performed easily on a mannequin in a skills lab require adaptation along with communication and reassurance skills when performed on patients whose attitudes range from calm to highly anxious. Students have a limited ability to forecast immediate futures because they have not yet lived through many of them; usually they must instead rely on textbook forecasts.

The best clinical educators are good ethnographers who can give students access to the culture and expectations of the clinical units where they are gaining clinical experience. Clinical educators should offer broad guidelines and timelines to guide their students' understanding of the task world and the expectations of a particular unit (Figure 2–2 ■). Good informants are identified as resources for the new students on the unit. In addition, the clinical supervisor is "on call" to deal with questions or emergencies encountered by the student.

Advanced Beginner: New Graduate

The newly graduated nurse has usually functioned very close to the level of a beginning staff nurse in his final year of nursing education. Typically, newly graduated nurses will not have functioned in any administrative or managerial functions, though they will have studied principles and practices related to these roles. The striking change for the newly graduated nurse is that she now has full legal and professional responsibility for patients. This new level of responsibility and entitlement brings with it changes in the way nurses experience themselves and the practice environment. They no longer feel that they can always look to other nurses to tell them what to do or to bear their responsibility. This level of individual and team professional responsibility heightens new nurses' sense of engagement with patients and their clinical problems. Nurses look to patients and family members to fill in expectations of them in their newly forming role. This heightened and qualitatively different kind of engagement encourages experiential learning and spurs the development of a sense of moral agency in the professional role (Benner et al., 1996, p. 93).

The quality of learning is quite different for new as opposed to more experienced nurses. Beginners have a level of trust in the environment and in the legitimacy of coworkers' knowledge, which allows them to absorb information as fact. This trust sets up qualities of freedom and exhilaration in learning that are probably only available to those who do not yet comprehend the contingent nature of both the situation and what is known about it. This freedom in learning is furthered because advanced beginners do not yet feel responsible for managing clinical situations with which they are unfamiliar.

In what follows, an advanced beginner evidences this "lightness of being" about learning as he describes a postoperative patient who had undergone complex gastrointestinal (GI) surgery. His entire statement was delivered in an excited, enthusiastic tone:

> I had learned so much. There are two clinical nurse specialists involved right now. There are people on the unit who are CNII's and CNIII's who are just really knowledgeable on major GI surgery on infants. I talked to all these people and pediatric surgery were really helpful, and our attendings and fellows were . . . I mean, I just learned so much in the last three days, I couldn't even tell you. (Benner et al., 1996, p. 52)

Advanced beginners have a heightened awareness of any feedback on performance and pay close attention to the practice of colleagues. They actively search for credible sources of good and useful information. In the preceding situation, clinical nurse specialists assisted with the care of the infant but also engaged in intensive teaching of the new nurse.

The advanced beginner can experience each situation as a myriad of competing tasks, all of which may feel of equal priority to the new nurse. Anxiety and excessive fatigue are frequently experienced by new nurses. Worry and anxiety tend to be more global because the advanced beginner does not yet have a sense of salience in a range of situations, and the anxiety of learning to perform new tasks is ever present:

> And I just talked to myself and I had a great night because this was the first time I did it. . . . I was (saying to myself) "Okay. Just take it one step at a time. You're only human, do one thing then go onto the next thing. It will all get done, it will get done easier if you're calm and because you think better that way." . . . And the shift went great. (Benner et al., 1996, p. 50).

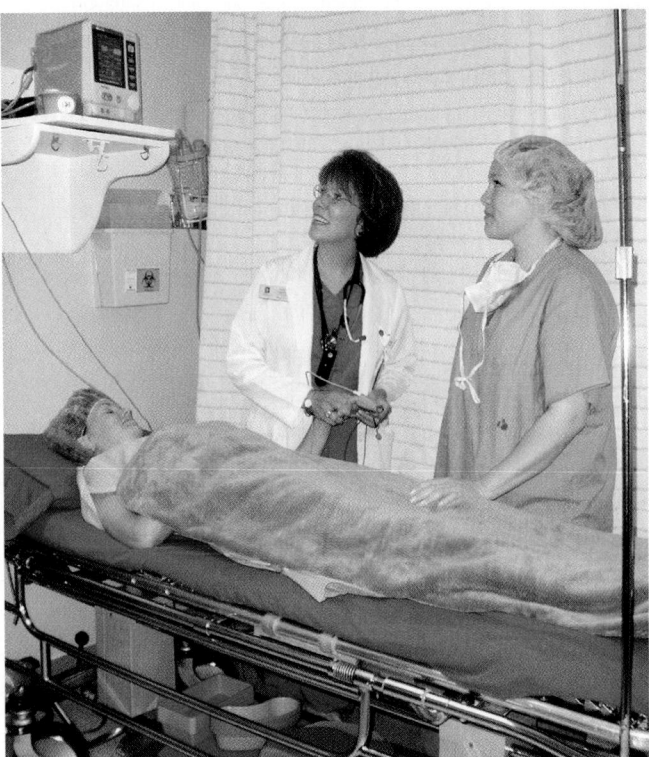

FIGURE 2–2 ■ A clinical educator presents a broad overview of the experiences students can expect in a particular unit.
Source: John M. Osborn, M.D, FACS

Much of the experiential learning required of an advanced beginner has to do with developing a perspective on particular situations and developing a sense of salience in particular clinical assignments and situations. In coaching an advanced beginner, strategies for keeping anxiety at bay and staying calm enhance performance capacity because the anxiety is so general. The sense of foreboding and anxiousness over particular clinical situations is not yet very attuned to the demands, possibilities, and constraints of the situation simply due to a lack of experience.

Anxiety is also ameliorated by this very lack of attunement and sense of salience. Advanced beginners have a secondary ignorance, or "cushion of inexperience," in that they have few past high-warning situations. Consequently, the advanced beginner in a new clinical setting may feel less concerned over lack of knowledge of specific clinical situations than an expert nurse transferring to a novel practice setting where the expert nurse is keenly aware of missing practice knowledge and lack of knowledge of resources.

Advanced beginners rely on textbook accounts of patient signs and symptoms related to diseases, injuries, and therapies, but they may have difficulty recognizing subtle variations. In addition, they cannot gauge the level of severity based on past experiences simply because they have not had enough experiences. For example, advanced beginners collect their assessment data carefully and then consult about the meanings of the numbers and signs and symptoms in a particular case. They will need to ask "Is this the usual amount of bleeding or is this a frank hemorrhage in a postoperative or obstetrical patient? Drainage from wounds and tubes must be evaluated in relation to the "usual" quantities and qualities. But the "usual" quantities may vary with specific procedures, patient conditions, and characteristics. The range and variations cannot be captured fully in textbooks. (Remember the discussion earlier in this chapter of the "limits of formalism.")

The perceptual skills associated with recognizing fuzzy or "family resemblances," qualitative distinctions, and real-life presentations complete with their range of manifestations cannot be captured in textbooks or single case presentations. The difficulty in recognizing fuzzy resemblances and the need for situated coaching from clinical mentors is vividly illustrated in the following nursing student's account of a clinical emergency:

> This man is a very pleasant fellow, very bright, very alert and awake, and was unfortunately requiring tracheal suctioning approximately every hour to two hours for moderate amounts of tracheal secretions which were relatively tenacious in character, relatively white tannish in color. He unfortunately did not tolerate the suctioning extremely well. It was relatively uncomfortable for him, caused a moderate amount of cough and gag reflex, which in turn caused a transient increase in blood pressure. Following suctioning on one occasion, as I was replacing his tracheal mist mask, he began coughing up very copious amounts of bright red blood per mouth. I mildly panicked, called for help from the nurse next door, placed him in a moderate Trendelenburg position, opened his I.V. to a rapid rate, and continued to experience mild panic. Perhaps more like moderate panic. (Benner, 1984, p. 19)

This advanced beginner nurse performed well considering the enormity of the situation. The student wonders tacitly whether his suctioning technique was too traumatic and, therefore, caused the bleeding. But notice that the advanced beginner cannot know this because he has had little experience with patients with similar compromised situations and with the skill of suctioning itself. The story is told with extraneous details, and the language is couched in textbook terms. The student's account responds to the immediate situation with little or no forecasting of the future. He gives a full account of his own anxiety in the situation that results in part from his lack of experiential knowledge about what can be done in the situation. Like the novice, the advanced beginner is dependent on others to provide them with experience-based comparisons, interpretations, and qualitative distinctions. In a later section, this episode is contrasted with the account from the expert's perspective.

Competent Stage: 1 to 2 Years of Practice

Developing skill and clinical judgment in particular cases is dependent on experiential learning. Consequently, how fast someone can gain competence depends on how varied and complex his patient population is. Obviously, nurses working in a high-volume heart surgery center where the patient population is the same will gain more experience sooner about typical patterns in a specific patient population than a nurse working on a general medical–surgical floor. But even in the high-volume center, it is usually some time before the newer nurse is assigned complete responsibility for complicated postoperative patients.

Competence with particular patient populations will develop unevenly depending on experience with that population and with the quality of clinical teaching available in the institution. The competent stage of skill acquisition is typically a time of heightened planning for what are now more predictable immediate futures. The competent nurse tries to limit the unexpected through planning and analysis and by forecasting the needs and contingencies of the immediate future. Anxiety is no longer just general anxiety; it is now more attuned to the particular situation as illustrated in the following example in which a nurse describes her discovery (experiential learning) that a post–heart transplant surgery patient could not maintain good oxygenation when placed on the nonoperative side, a physiological principle that the new graduate would probably recognize in a formal, written test, but which is more ambiguous to her in the actual situation:

> I was being a good nurse and turning him every two hours and he had really bad breath sounds on his left side. So I gave him P.T., elevated his left side so he could drain, had him cough. But it took me a couple of times to realize that when I turned him on his left side, with his bad lung down and his good lung up, his oxygen saturations showed great readings and his heart rate was wonderful, and then I would turn him on his back, or turn him up on his right side and within a few minutes, he would go into bursts of SVT [*supraventricular tachycardia*] and his [*oxygen*] saturations would drop. I had called the doctors and they didn't seem too concerned about it. They said: "Relax, he has a healthy heart." I said, if he has a healthy heart, why is he doing this? It spontaneously resolved after I turned him off his side. And I said okay, now I know what's going on. I'll keep him off that side. It was just a hypoxic reaction because he wasn't oxygenating well enough with his bad lung... It could be a bad situation if we left this so now we

know that we just have to work on that lung and get it back aerating again, and he did fine. He's out walking around. (Benner et al., 1996, p. 155)

In reflecting on the above experiential learning, the competent level nurse comments:

Nurse: It kind of humbles you. At one point, I'm feeling like I have things straight now, and I can handle the situations, and when something like this happens, I think, well, I still have a lot of learning to do. I can handle the situations that are status quo; it's the unexpected that I have to learn to deal with now. But then I think back to situations when I was brand new. Things that are status quo now weren't back then. Things I can troubleshoot and solve now were much different back then. I usually needed help. (Benner et al., 1996, p. 172)

This nurse's anxiety is now more tailored to the particular situation. Coaching at this point should encourage a competent-level nurse to follow through on her sense that things seem out of the ordinary or even her vague feelings of foreboding or anxiety. The nurse now has an experiential base from which these emotional responses serve to activate a "fuzzy" recognition of similar or dissimilar past clinical situations.

Nurses at this stage feel exhilarated when they perform well, and remorse when they recognize that their performance could have been more effective or more prescient. These emotional responses are the formative stages of aesthetic appreciation of good practice. Feelings of satisfaction and uneasiness with performance act as a moral compass that guides experiential ethical and clinical learning. There is a built-in tension between the strategies of organizing, planning, and prediction and the development of a more response-based practice as pointed out in our study of critical care nurses:

Not needing help, ordering the task world, and planning based on goals and predictions structure what the nurse notices, and what are considered issues. It is not accidental that this vision of performance and agency is institutionally rewarded and encouraged as "standard."

Structuring the day by goals and plans, however, interferes with perceiving the demands of the situation and with timing interventions in response to the patient's responses and readiness. The competent nurse seldom sees changing relevance in a clinical situation. Their skill of seeing is hampered by the need to organize data collection and to achieve goals. Inevitably the clinical situation intrudes by not matching the goals and plans and the nurse must adapt. Conceptual descriptions do not automatically lead to recognition of actual signs, and varied responses require time to assimilate and interpret. Slavishly following one's plans and holding on to preset expectations can limit perceptual grasp of when the situation has changed significantly. This was illustrated in the nurse's discovery of the cause of the heart transplant patient's supraventricular tachycardia.

The nurse's lack of prior experience with this particular situation calls for new experiential learning in order for her to realize that turning the patient so that his good or less compromised lung was compressed from lying on his right side, and his left lung (compromised lung) when placed up, was not able to com-pensate for the loss of aeration from the right long (Benner et al., 1996, pp. 155–172). In the future, no doubt, this common problem with post operative heart patients will be more recognizable to this nurse.

Experiential learning based on past patient care enables the nurse to develop a greater sense of salience. As illustrated in the preceding nurse's statement, there is an increasing sense of when the nurse has or does not have a good clinical grasp of the situation. Nurses can use their sense of confusion or questioning to propel their understanding of the clinical situation. Because they have now lived through more clinical futures, they can now better predict immediate likely events and the resulting patient needs and better plan for them.

Toward the upper limits of competent performance, nurses may begin to apprehend the limits of formal and practical knowledge. Nurses can now recognize that not everyone is a proficient or expert clinician, just at the point that they realize that they must develop a perspective on the situation in order to perform well in the situation. They typically buy more comprehensive reference works and medical and nursing textbooks at this point because loss of confidence in the advice of specific others may be overgeneralized and, consequently, the nurse may feel hyper-responsible. This inability to trust colleagues can be aggravated if incompetence, accompanied by a lack of social integration and informal coaching, is encountered on a particular clinical unit.

Proficiency: The Transition to Expertise

It is the felt crisis in the limits of formalism, the limits of planning and prediction, and an enhanced ability to read a situation that may propel the nurse into the proficient stage of performance. Whereas skill development up until this point has been incremental, now, in order to progress, learners must make a qualitative leap in the way they engage and perform in any given situation. They must literally learn to situate themselves differently in relation to their work. At this stage, experience-near first-person narratives (Geertz, 1987) often take the form of describing changes in their perspectives on a situation. The narrative structure is often something like "I went into the situation thinking that I knew what was going on or that this particular thing was going on," only to have it disconfirmed by the patient's responses to their assessment. This is evidence for developing the ability to let reading the situation guide their patient assessment:

Nurse: You're with the patient, you take care of them and you see them hour to hour exactly. [The physicians] don't see every little drop in the blood pressure or every little change in the rhythm. They just kind of get an overview, [whereas] you are in there constantly.... They [The physicians] can go read the chart; you're in there. You're turning this patient, you're doing this, and you're seeing every little aspect.

This excerpt illustrates a new level of skill of seeing and interpreting patient responses. The interviewer asks the nurse quoted above:

Interviewer: Can you give a specific example of when you saw something very differently?

Nurse: [The physicians] come in and look at the flow sheet and we don't, you can't write every, every change you know.

Everyone always says, you may take hourly signs that you put on the chart, but if we had a little computer in our head that really wrote down every little blood pressure or heart rate we looked at for the day, it might be just fine. So they might come in and say, "He looks stable, why don't we take him off the dopamine." And we say, well, wait a minute, I didn't write everything down. I turned him and his blood pressure dropped.

You don't know that. "Let's give him some Lasix." "No, he's not ready for that." . . . I notice that [the physicians are] good about talking to you before making decisions.

The nurse is now synthesizing the meaning of the patient's responses through time. She imagines that a computer could capture all of her readings, but she fails to recognize that her understanding of the patient is now situated and based on a practical understanding of the patient's responses and qualitative changes made over time rather than a collection of data points. The clinician struggles with articulating this practical grasp:

Nurse: I had drawn a [blood] gas on a person and the gas was pretty poor and I took another gas to the house officer and he looked at it and said: "I don't believe this gas, the patient hasn't changed. And at that point—it takes a while to get to this point, but I felt comfortable in saying to him: "What do you mean, this patient hasn't changed?" This patient's blood pressure has gone up to 200, and I presented him with a picture of this patient that he had obviously overlooked. It takes a while to get to the point where you can feel comfortable saying this to the doctor and feeling comfortable, feeling that you can go with your instincts.

Interviewer: What happened in that situation?

Nurse: I was right. . . .

Interviewer: How did you learn that the objective signs that you were seeing were correlated with blood gas?

Nurse: Just experience and seeing different patients and different breathing patterns and knowing by looking at the patient that this breathing pattern is effective and this one isn't, knowing whether there is air exchange there or not. These breaths aren't effective and he's wearing himself out and that could be the cause of his deterioration in his gas, and just experience and seeing different cases and how people adjust to physical things that are going on.

Though difficult to articulate, this practical grasp is not mystical. It reflects the skill of seeing the practical manifestations of changed physiological states and patient responses and engaging in practical reasoning about these changes. The nurse actively interprets the direction of the change and keeps track of what can be ruled in or ruled out. Practical grasp is perceptually grounded and response based and requires being open to correction and to having one's thinking disconfirmed as the situation unfolds. The clinician is always in the situation with some practical understanding, and it is that practical understanding that is revised or confirmed.

In situations where patterns and trends are clear and have definitive interventions associated with the clinical trend, the practitioner can make quick decisive responses. When the practitioner's grasp of the patient's clinical situation is jarred by changes or un-

expected patient responses, the practitioner searches for a new grasp and, if all goes well, experiential clinical learning occurs. Engaged reasoning through transitions requires being open to correction and disconfirmation. The ethos of openness, rather than prediction and control, and fidelity to what one sees and hears, rather than excessive suggestibility and confusion, are embodied and linked to emotional responses to the situation. Thus, one's skilled emotional responsiveness guides perceptual acuity *and* responsiveness to changes in the situation (Benner et al., 1996, pp. 116–117).

The nurse operates in a much more differentiated world of practice at the proficient level. The nurse feels increasingly at home in the situation and can now recognize changing relevance. The following excerpt demonstrates this new comfort level by describing open heart surgery patients' trajectories:

Nurse: I feel pretty comfortable, and you learn when they're warming to start giving the volume and when to stop because now maybe they need a little bit of Levophed to keep their blood pressure up, when to shut off the Levophed because they're waking up and you know their catecholamines have kicked in and that kind of thing. It's almost routine, whereas before it took a lot of trial and asking questions.

This change is based on procedural knowledge and protocols, but the transition being described is the flexible recognition of patient changes in particular situations. These decisions cannot be based on quantitative physiological measures alone, but must be based on understanding the relationship between the numbers and the way the patient looks and responds. This form of response-based action is crucial for performing well in a rapidly changing emergency (Benner et al., 1996, p. 232).

Because the proficient-level nurse is learning to adjust her responses to the situation more, the skill of both problem and person engagement becomes more differentiated and attuned. Observing nurses across situations reveals that they vary their relationships with patients and families based on their understanding of what the situation requires. Timing becomes much more refined, and recognizing opportunities in the situation for patient learning or for supporting a patient is now more attuned to the needs and concerns of the patient.

Nurse: Transplant patients become so dependent on you for everything—Can I brush my teeth now? Do you think I should do this? And you have to really encourage them to take control back. It's a hard concept for a lot of them because they need to be dependent—because it's safe for them to be dependent. . . . I've learned how to give them control back slowly and how to encourage them to take that control back over their own [lives].

Qualitative distinctions are laden with tone, emotional and attitudinal qualities as well as action and contextual qualities. In the context of extreme fatigue or the beginning of rejection or infection, the transplant patient may have to relinquish most independence, but with astute coaching the patient can often retain control over information and participation in decision making may be retained even in extreme periods of dependency (Benner et al., 1996, pp. 125–126). Once begun, the proficient nurse usually continues to refine his reading of particular situations.

Expertise: Phronesis

Once a nurse has progressed to proficiency, the style of being a more situated, response-based performer propels experiential learning and the ability to switch from taking for granted tacit expectations to focusing on aspects of the situation that are changing and creating an altered sense of the situation. The expert nurse is response based in using techne and phronesis. The expert is able to take up theories and ends or goals and notions of *good* in the practice in multiple ways, often creating new possibilities (Taylor, 1991). These situated practical innovations seem intuitively obvious to the practitioner and might not be captured easily in a narrative description of the situation. This is why observation and informal interviewing in actual situations are required to discover and describe all levels of practice, but particularly proficient and expert levels of practice. As noted in our research, ways of seeing the situation increasingly just call for appropriate actions.

Intuitive links develop between seeing and responding to the most relevant issues. This is revealed by observing the nurse in the situation, and is partially captured in the following account of an emergency situation in which a patient who was hemorrhaging stopped breathing. The links between the patient's condition and action are sufficiently strong that the nurse attends primarily to actions rather than assessment of signs and symptoms. This is reasonable since, in extreme circumstances, the possible responses are fewer, but experience is required to make this shift in performance:

> *Nurse:* So we didn't even call the code. We just called the doc[tor] stat [emergency] and got him up there. [They had sufficient people available to resuscitate the patient, so no formal page for additional help was needed.] I looked at his heart rate and I said: "O.K. he is bradying down. Someone want to give me some atropine?" I just started calling out the drugs that I needed to get for this guy, so we started to push these drugs in. In the meantime, I said, "Can we have some more blood?" I was just barking out this stuff [the things that were needed and had to be done]. I can't even tell you the sequence. I was saying, "We need this." I needed to anticipate what was going to happen and I could do this because I had been through this a week before with this guy and knew what we had done [and what had worked]. The anesthesiologist came in and did a good intubation. He asks: "What kind of [IV] lines do we have?" I said, we have a triple lumen and we have blood. All [IV] ports are taken. We need another kind of line. He's got no veins left." He goes, "O.K., fine, give me a cut-down tray. . . .

The recognition and assessment language are minimal, in part, because the number of actions per problem are limited, but also because recognition and assessment language become so linked with actions and outcomes that they become self-evident or "obvious" for the expert practitioner. In this situation, the response was fluid and knowing because this nurse had taken care of this patient during a previous successful resuscitation where she had learned, firsthand, what worked and what did not. This is not just a rote repetition of the previous resuscitation; rather her responses are based on the understanding gained in the previous situation (Benner et al., 1996, pp. 142–143).

Based on enriched experiential learning spawned by an increasing ability to read the current situation in terms of past whole concrete cases, nurses develop a sense of whether or not they have a good (better or poorer) grasp of the situation. They describe the frustrating situation of "chasing a problem" and never being quite "in synch" with the situation when they do not have a good perceptual grasp of the situation at hand (Benner et al., 1996, pp. 146–147; 1999, pp. 23–87). Skilled "know-how" now allows for more fluid and rapid performance of procedures. Narratives often focus on new clinical learning or troubling moral dilemmas or conflicts in the situation. Qualitative distinctions associated with nuanced responses allow nurses to know and do more than they can tell or think to describe (Polanyi, 1958/1962).

Attunement allows for flexible fusion of thought, feeling, and action. Seeing the unexpected based on having a rich set of expectations as well as a rich sense of the particular situation requires engagement with the patient, openness to noticing when things do not go as implicitly expected, and evidence that disconfirms one's assumptions (Benner et al., 1999, pp. 85–86). Exhibiting the relational skill of attunement to the patient's concerns and clinical situation creates the possibility that patients and family members will disclose or reveal their concerns and fears to the nurse and allows for the nurse to notice changes in the patient/family across time (transitions). The qualities of attentiveness and relationship literally create different disclosive spaces and moods for the patient and family so that different clinical issues are noticed based on qualitatively different disclosive possibilities.

Now, let's return to the example in the advanced beginner discussion in which a patient developed a carotid hemorrhage. Now compare the expert's narrative of the event with the advanced beginner's version:

> I had worked late and was just about ready to go home, when a nurse preceptor said to me, "Jolene, come here." Her voice had urgency in it, but not Code Blue. I walked in and I looked at the patient and his heart rate was about 120, and he was on the respirator and breathing. And I asked her: "What's wrong?" There was a new graduate taking care of him. And he just pointed down to the patient who was lying in a pool of blood. There was a big stream of blood drooling out of his mouth. This man's diagnosis was mandibular cancer, which had been resected, and about a week previous to that he had had a carotid bleed from external carotid, which had been ligated secondary to radiation erosion. That wound had become septic and he had developed respiratory failure and he was in the ICU for that. So I looked at the dressing and it was dry, the blood was coming out of his mouth. The man had a tracheostomy because of the type of surgery that had been done. He also had an NG tube in for feedings, and I got to thinking that it might be the innominate or the carotid artery that had eroded. So we took him off the ventilator to see if anything was going to pump out of his trach. There was a little blood, but it looked mostly like it had come down from the pharynx into the lungs. So we began ventilating him, trying to figure what was inside his mouth that was pumping out this tremendous amount of blood. . . . (Benner, 1984, p. 17).

This nurse went on to describe her quick actions to draw blood for a cross-match and typing and preparing the man for an immediate transfer to the OR after marshalling all of the resources for the surgical team. She gives us an immediate, direct grasp of the nature of the situation. Action, thought, and feeling are fused. She evaluates the resistance in the lungs by hand ventilating the patient. Fortunately, because of her rapid responses, the patient survived the hemorrhage.

Expert practice by its very nature is comprised of local specific knowledge, know-how, and technical and scientific knowledge, which are transferable to other practice contexts. Because practice is a way of knowing through experiential learning and embodied know-how, it is highly valuable to study and articulate the knowledge embedded in complex practices such as nursing and medicine. Articulation of the knowledge embedded in proficient and expert practice, plus articulation of the range of practical knowledge learned by beginning practitioners in local settings creates the possibility of self-improving practice based on making experiential learning public and, therefore, open to development so that experiential learning and practical wisdom become cumulative and shared.

Summary

Nursing is a practice discipline that is comprised of both practical and theoretical knowledge. Nursing, like medicine, is an underdetermined complex practice that requires clinical judgment and discernment in particular situations. Clinical reasoning calls for reasoning across time about changes in the patient and changes in the clinician's understanding of the situation. Nursing and medicine cannot be reduced to techne (or technique), but must include phronesis, wise skillful judgment, and practice by excellent practitioners.

Every professional nurse is engaged in ongoing experiential learning, clinical inquiry, and clinical knowledge development. Clinicians need to keep track of their experiential learning over time, reflect on it, and make it public and accessible for examination and further studies. Clinical practice is a way of knowing in its own right, but this experiential clinical knowledge development needs to be made accessible to others, and extended by further studies and confirmation in diverse clinical situations.

Each of the studies on skill acquisition conducted by Benner and colleagues was based on extensive experience-near first-person narrative accounts of clinical situations that stood out in the participants' minds. In addition a subsample of participants was observed and informally interviewed in their practice. The nurse researchers deliberately sampled nurses with a range of experience and reported skillfulness, and interviewed nurses with like backgrounds in small-group narrative interviews. They created an open dialogue with the tenets of the Dreyfus model of skill acquisition and the philosophical basis for this model. The researchers found that the model was predictive and descriptive of distinct stages of skill acquisition in nursing practice, and added nuances to the model in terms of the development of moral agency and the influence of emotional engagement with the person and the problem, as well as emotional climate on skill acquisition. They found that nurses who had some difficulty with understanding the ends of practice, and difficulty with their skills of interpersonal and problem engagement did not go on to become expert nurses.

The model was also useful in helping articulate knowledge and skill embedded in the practice of nursing. The rational-technical vision of performance is that of a practitioner or technical expert developing mastery of a body of knowledge and applying that knowledge in prespecified ways to arrive at prespecified outcomes. The rational-technical model does not account for development of relational, perceptual, or skillful comportment over time. It also does not account for the role of experiential learning in learning to practice in a dynamic, underdetermined, and complex practice such as nursing and medicine. A strict technical application of knowledge does not take into account the skills required for discerning the nature of the situation and its possibilities and constraints. Even the expert in the Dreyfus model of skill acquisition must stay attuned to the situation and remain open to the unexpected. Practitioners must remain open to experiential learning and reading changes in transitions in fast-paced, open-ended environments. In the Dreyfus model, the practitioner is assumed to dwell with increasing skill and finesse in a meaningful, intelligible but changing world.

REVIEW QUESTIONS

1. After assisting with care for a patient with a sudden gastrointestinal bleed, the nurse states "I learned so much from watching all of the other nurses and doctors help this patient." Which of the following levels of experience is this nurse most likely to be?
    1. Novice
    2. Advanced Beginner
    3. Competent
    4. Proficient

2. The nurse provides oxygen at 2 liters via nasal cannula to a patient whose pulse oximetry measurement is 95% on room air. One reason for this administration of oxygen would be:
    1. The patient requested oxygen.
    2. The patient expressed anger for being admitted to the hospital.
    3. The patient's glucose level is elevated.
    4. The patient's hemoglobin and hematocrit levels are low.

3. While being transferred from the bed to a chair, a patient who is day 2 total knee replacement experiences a gush of bright red blood from the incision site. The nurse, following the care map for a total knee replacement, should:
    1. Place the patient in the chair.
    2. Return the patient to the bed.
    3. Measure the patient's blood pressure once situated in the chair.
    4. Reinforce the dressing once the patient is situated in the chair.

4. A newly admitted patient repeatedly responds inappropriately to health related questions. Which of the following should the nurse do first to assist this patient?
    1. Contact the physician and suggest a neurological evaluation for a stroke.
    2. Repeat the questions to evaluate the patient's hearing.
    3. Determine if the patient is becoming combative and apply wrist restraints per organizational policy.
    4. Measure the patient's blood pressure and heart rate.

5. A patient, admitted with a sudden onset of lower extremity edema and multiple spontaneous leg wounds, demonstrated breathlessness when asking for the bedpan. Which of the following should the nurse do first?

1. Culture the leg wound exudate.

2. Elevate the patient's legs.

3. Further explore the patient's breathlessness.

4. Ambulate the patient to the bathroom.

Answers to review questions appear in Appendix D

KEY TERMS

clinical judgment *p.32*
clinical knowledge *p.32*
Dreyfus model of skill acquisition *p.35*
ethos *p.34*
experience *p.36*

experiential learning *p.36*
limits of formalization *p.34*
moral agency *p.35*
phronesis *p.33*
practical knowledge *p.32*

rationality *p.33*
salience *p.32*
skills of involvement *p.33*
techne *p.33*

PEARSON
EXPLORE **mynursingkit**™

MyNursingKit is your one stop for online chapter review materials and resources. Prepare for success with additional NCLEX®-style practice questions, interactive assignments and activities, web links, animations and videos, and more!

Register your access code from the front of your book at
www.mynursingkit.com

REFERENCES

Benner, P. (1982). From novice to expert. *American Journal of Nursing, 82*, 402–407.

Benner, P. (1984). *From novice to expert: Excellence and power in clinical nursing practice.* (Commemorative ed.) Menlo Park, CA: Addison-Wesley.

Benner, P. (1994). The role of articulation in understanding practice and experience as sources of knowledge in clinical nursing. In J. Tully (Ed.), *Philosophy in an age of pluralism: The philosophy of Charles Taylor in question* (pp. 136–155). New York: Cambridge University.

Benner, P. (2001). *From novice to expert: Excellence and power in clinical nursing practice.* (Commemorative ed.) Menlo Park, CA: Addison-Wesley.

Benner, P., Chelsa, C., Dreyfus, H. L., Dreyfus, S. E., and Rubin, J. (1996). *Expertise in Nursing Practice: Caring, Clinical Judgment & Ethics.* New York, NY: Springer Publishing Company.

Benner, P., Hooper-Kyriakidis, P., & Stannard, D. (1999). *Clinical wisdom and interventions in critical care: A thinking-in-action approach.* Philadelphia: W. B. Saunders.

Benner, P., Tanner, C., & Chesla, C. (1992). From beginner to expert: Gaining a differentiated clinical world in critical care nursing. *Advances in Nursing Science, 14*(3), 13–28.

Benner, P., Tanner, C. A., & Chesla, C. A. (1996). *Expertise in nursing practice: Caring, clinical judgment, and ethics.* New York: Springer.

Benner, P., & Wrubel, J. (1982). Clinical knowledge development: The value of perceptual awareness. *Nurse Educator, 7*, 11–17.

Dreyfus, H. L. (1979). *What computers can't do: The limits of artificial intelligence.* (Rev. ed.) New York: Harper & Row.

Dreyfus, H. L. (1992). *What computers still can't do: A critique of artificial reason.* Cambridge, MA: The MIT Press.

Dreyfus, H. L., & Dreyfus, S. E. (1977, March). *Uses and abuses of multi-attribute and multi-aspect model of decision making.* Unpublished manuscript, Department of Industrial Engineering and Operations Research, University of California at Berkeley.

Dreyfus, H. L., & Dreyfus, S. E., with Athanasiou, T. (1986). *Mind over machine, the power of human intuition and expertise in the era of the computer.* New York: The Free Press.

Dreyfus, S. E. (1982). Formal models vs. human situational understanding: Inherent limitations on the modeling of business expertise. *Office: Technology and People, 1*, 1133–1155.

Dreyfus, S. E., & Dreyfus, H. L. (1979, February). *The scope, limits, and training implications of three models of aircraft pilot emergency response behavior.* Unpublished report supported by the Air Force Office of Scientific Research, USAF (Grant AFOSR-78-3594), University of California at Berkeley.

Dreyfus, S. E., & Dreyfus, H. L. (1980, February). *A five-stage model of the mental activities involved in directed skill acquisition.* Unpublished report supported by the Air Force Office of Scientific Research, USAF (Contract F49620-79-C-0063), University of California at Berkeley.

Dunne, J. (1997). *Back to the rough ground, practical judgment and the lure of technique.* Notre Dame, IN: University of Notre Dame Press.

Gadamer, H. (1960/1975). *Truth and method* (G. Barden & J. Cumming, Trans.). New York: Seabury.

Geertz, C. (1987). Deep play: Notes on the Balinese cockfight. In P. Rabinow & W. Sullivan (Eds.), *Interpretive social science: A second look.* Berkeley, CA: University of California.

Guignon, C. B. (1983). *Heidegger and the problem of knowledge.* Indianapolis, IN: Hackett.

Halpern, J. (2001). *From detached concern to empathy. Humanizing medical care.* Oxford: Oxford University Press.

Kuhn, T. S. (1970). *The structure of scientific revolutions* (2nd ed.). Chicago: University of Chicago Press.

Lave, J., & Wenger, E. (1991). *Situated learning: Legitimate peripheral perspectives (Learning in doing: Social, cognitive and computational perspectives.)* Cambridge, UK: Cambridge University Press.

Polanyi, M. (1958/1962). *Personal knowledge: Towards a post-critical philosophy.* Chicago: University of Chicago Press.

Rubin, J. (1996). Impediments to the development of clinical knowledge and ethical judgment in critical care nursing. In P. Benner, C. Tanner, & C. Chesla (Eds.), *Expertise in nursing practice, caring, clinical judgment and ethics* (pp. 170–192). New York: Springer.

Ruddick, S. (1989). *Maternal thinking: Toward a politics of peace.* New York: Ballantine.

Schon, D. (1987). *The reflective practitioner: How professionals think in action.* New York: Basic Books.

Taylor, C., (1991). *Ethnics of authenticity.* Cambridge, MA: Harvard University Press.

Taylor, C. (1993). Explanation and practical reason. In M. Nussbaum & A. Sen (Eds.), *The quality of life.* Oxford: Clarendon Press.

Taylor, C. (1994). Philosophical reflections on caring practices. In S. S. Phillips & P. Benner (Eds.), *The crisis of care: Affirming and restoring caring practices in the helping professions* (pp. 174–187). Washington, DC: Georgetown University Press.

Vetleson, A. J. (1994). *Perception, empathy, and judgment: An inquiry into the preconditions of moral performance.* University Park, PA: Pennsylvania State University Press.

Health Care Trends and Regulatory Aspects of Health Care Delivery

Kathleen Richerson
With contributions by: Annita Watson

Outcome-Based Learning Objectives

After studying this chapter, the learner will be able to:

1. Discuss how major trends in health care quality and patient safety are related to nursing practice.
2. Compare the differences between the types of managed care plans: health maintenance organizations, preferred provider organizations, Medicare, and Medicaid.
3. Describe the key components of the budget process for hospitals and health care systems.
4. Explain the nurse's role in assisting patients with insurance and financial issues.
5. Differentiate between the three types of standards used to measure quality in health care settings.
6. Compare and contrast the impact of licensure, regulation, and accreditation on health care delivery systems.
7. Differentiate between the types of advance directives for health care and describe the nurse's responsibility in advocating and documenting the patient's wishes related to an advance directive.
8. Explain the patient's rights with regard to his or her medical record according to the legal principles of documentation in the patient's medical record.
9. Identify the three main components of the Health Insurance Portability and Accountability Act.
10. Identify the components of case management in the hospital and the associated acute care nursing responsibilities.

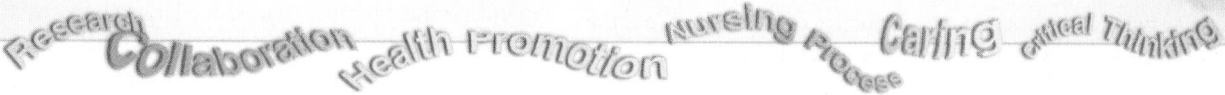

HEALTH CARE at the federal and state level is highly regulated to ensure that care is delivered safely, access to care is available, and patient rights are secure. Consumer demand for assurances about the quality of the care they receive and the right to choose their care providers has greatly influenced legislation regarding health care funding and programs. It is important for nurses to understand from a global perspective the forces at work in the health care environment that affect nursing practice, patient care, delivery of service, and advancements in science and technology. As discussed in Chapter 5 ☺ nurses play a vital role in managing these challenges by providing leadership in the management of patient care and design of patient care delivery models.

This chapter provides an overview of legal, financial, and social forces that influence the way health care is provided in organizations and how it is delivered to patients. The issues discussed directly and indirectly affect the practice of nursing, the way in which nurses contribute to the health of patients, the organizations for which they work, and the communities in which they live.

■ Health Care Delivery Systems

A **health care delivery system** is a set of services designed to deliver professional health care and to promote health and wellness to constituents in a given society (Barber et al., (1998). Basically, it is all the activities of a society that are designed to protect or restore health, whether directed at the individual, society, or the environment. These activities include services from personnel engaged in medical occupations, physical plants, capital, and other goods and services.

Health care delivery systems in the United States have evolved significantly during the past two decades. Historically, people in the United States received health care through personal physicians and locally owned and operated community hospitals. However, highly competitive, expanding health care delivery systems are replacing that model. This transformation of the health care industry is being molded by increasing delivery costs, changing reimbursement requirements, standardization of diagnoses and treatment methods, contracted care, rising liability issues, and emerging technologies. Other influencing factors include increased severity of illness in inpatient facilities, major cost reductions and restructuring, emerging new illnesses, changing population demographics, and an exploding global community.

Within the context of these changes, delivery systems have moved from a horizontal organizational model to a vertically integrated model and more recently are evolving into a model of virtual networks. In **horizontal organizational models**, hospitals were aligned to form multiple-hospital systems, with a focus on traditional acute care services. With the transition to **vertically integrated models**, services have been aligned to provide a continuum of care. This model includes the integration of physician, hospital, and ancillary services. Integrated systems can offer a broad range of services pre- and post-hospitalization from primary care to long-term care (Wolper, 2004).

Health care delivery models have most recently evolved into networks of integrated systems and services that are virtually connected by relationships through contracts rather than ownership. Within the virtually integrated model, technology plays a critical part in linking the network. The concept of e-health, which provides a computer-based framework for communication and a central repository for data and information, has been introduced. This central framework allows virtual patient access. For instance, patient-specific health information is available at any time to providers within the network and to the patients themselves (Harris et al., 2003). As this model develops, patients and their families will begin to rely on nurses to assist them with accessing care within these complex systems. Linking to resources such as financial counseling, social services, and case management may be required to provide specific support for patients. Such links are especially important when preparing the patient for discharge and transition to other care and services outside the hospital.

Future Delivery Implications

High consumer demand and increasing health care costs are dominant forces influencing the future structure of health care delivery. Joining these prevailing forces is a heightened scrutiny around the quality and safety of care delivered to patients as well as how patients access that care. Evidence of this influence is the growth of agencies that provide ratings and benchmarking for health care systems locally, regionally, and nationally, most of which are publicly available and Internet-based for easy access. Consumers can use ratings information to evaluate the services and quality outcomes of organizations before making choices about health plans or providers. This major trend is driving health care organizations to shift to consumer-directed service cultures (Scalise, 2005).

In the future, health care providers will be challenged to incorporate new advances in technology and treatment. This challenge will come primarily from consumers and payers seeking new services and cost-effective care. Traditional inpatient hospital services are evolving into more sophisticated outpatient-focused services that will allow more consumer control in terms of the selection of treatments and services (Abramson & Tyler, 2006). One such example of the transition from inpatient to outpatient is general surgery laparoscopic procedures.

Hospital Organizations

Currently, according to the American Hospital Association (2006) there are four categories of hospital organizations: general acute care, specialty, rehabilitative, and psychiatric. General acute care hospitals provide diagnostic and therapeutic services for a range of health conditions. General acute care hospitals range from small rural facilities to large multicampus academic medical centers. The types of services vary depending on community needs, competition with other organizations in the immediate market area, and the specific mission of the organization.

Specialty organizations focus on specific medical conditions or procedures. Some specialty organizations provide outpatient services only or short-stay 24-hour service. Some examples of organizations in this category are cardiovascular, orthopedic, plastic/cosmetic surgery, and women's services (McKinley, 2005). Rehabilitative and chronic disease facilities provide care for people who have disabilities. Their patients receive restorative or adjustive care on either a short-term or long-term basis. Examples of these types of agencies include Alzheimer and memory loss care centers and skilled nursing or long-term care centers. Finally, psychiatric care facilities provide inpatient and outpatient care for psychiatric-related illnesses (American Hospital Association [AHA], 2007). These are freestanding facilities that may or may not be associated with an acute care facility. Chart 3–1 outlines the various types of hospital organizations. Each type of health care organization is subject to increasing health care costs and survival as a health care delivery system.

■ Health Care Costs

Health care costs have steadily increased during the past two decades, spiraling to a higher figure than that spent on national defense (California HealthCare Foundation, 2004). Costs are expected to continue their unparalleled growth in the future. As a result of these increasing costs, many employers have decreased the coverage provided to employees or increased the amount that employees contribute toward their health care costs, thereby contributing to the numbers of uninsured Americans. On the other hand, even as health care costs have escalated, so have patients' demands for health care services, due largely in part to the growing numbers of elderly and the request for the latest technological and pharmaceutical advances in medical care (U.S. Census Bureau, 2002). Health care organizations are striving to meet patients' expectations in order to survive in a very competitive marketplace.

Historical Development of Health Care Economics

The current economics of health care have developed as a result of the historical impact of social, cultural, political, and economic issues in the United States. Prior to the 1940s, the U.S. government's role in health care delivery was limited to the local level. Almshouses and poorhouses were built for those with insurance, people who had chronic disabilities, and people who were mentally ill. Other individuals requiring health care paid their local doctor out of pocket and they usually were cared for in their homes. Private-duty nurses often were hired to provide nursing care at home because there was little insurance to pay for hospital care. Care was provided under a fee-for-service arrangement; the patient or the insurer paid for the type and amount of care provided based on a cost reimbursement system.

Since the 1940s, several major legislative acts have led to an increased role for the federal government. Market forces also have helped to replace fee-for-service plans with prospective contracted insurance plans, referred to as managed care, for most working Americans. Enacted in 1946, post–World War II,

| CHART 3-1 | **Hospital Organizations** |

Type of Hospital Organization	Description
General acute care	Functions to provide patient care, diagnostic and therapeutic services for a variety of medical conditions. Includes • Diagnostic imaging • Clinical laboratory • Operating rooms.
Specialty	Functions to provide diagnostic and treatment services for specified medical conditions. Includes • Appropriate diagnostic and treatment services for the specialty • Clinical laboratory capable of providing tissue diagnosis when offering pregnancy termination services.
Rehabilitative	Functions to provide diagnostic and treatment services to individuals with handicaps or disabilities who require restorative and adjustive care. Includes • Arrangements for diagnostic imaging services • Arrangements for clinical laboratory services • Arrangements for operating room services if required • Physical therapy service • Occupational therapy service • Psychological and social work services on a regular basis • Arrangements for educational and vocational services on a regular basis • Transfer agreements with a general acute care hospital for transfer of patients requiring a higher level of care.
Psychiatric	Functions to provide diagnostic and treatment services for patients who have psychiatric-related illnesses. Includes • Arrangements for clinical laboratory services • Arrangements for diagnostic imaging services • Psychiatric, psychological, and social services • Arrangements for electroencephalograph services on a regular basis • Transfer agreements with a general acute care hospital for transfer of patients requiring a higher level of care.

Source: American Hospital Association. (2007). Guide to the health care field—2007 edition.

the Hill-Burton program was established to fund the construction of hospitals. The program required facilities that were receiving federal funds to make their services available to all persons residing in the facility's service area without discrimination. Although the program meant that health care services would be available to all who lived in that community, it did not dictate how hospitals would charge for their services or how people would pay for them (Grohar-Murray & DiCroce, 2003).

In the 1960s Medicare and Medicaid legislation was passed as an amendment to the Social Security Act. The **Medicare** portion of the act provides insurance for people over age 65 and payment for their hospitalization, physicians' fees, and diagnostic tests. Medicare also provides coverage for persons with disabilities and those with permanent kidney failure. As an entitlement for older adults, Medicare essentially provides universal coverage for hospitalization and outpatient care. Together these services account for more than half of all Medicare expenditures (Centers for Medicare & Medicaid Services [CMS], 2007). The other portion, **Medicaid**, funds health care to the dependent population and is administered by each state. The state determines eligibility and level of coverage, establishes the rate of payment for services, and retains the right and power to determine the type, amount, duration, and scope of services.

The role of insurance companies as third-party payers evolved as a part of these new reimbursement procedures. Employers began providing health care benefits to workers as part of a total employment package, and organized labor aggressively negotiated for better packages. The relationship between hospitals, physicians, and patients changed, as everyone became aware that the insurance companies, rather than the patients, were paying most health care bills.

Because the medical world was aware that the insurance companies and government would pay for all reasonable costs of health care, expenses skyrocketed in the early 1980s. Abuses and fraud have been widely publicized, especially those involving Medicare and Medicaid. Also, rapid technological advances contributed to the increased cost of care, as more knowledgeable patients came to expect the latest and best of diagnostic and interventional care. Malpractice fears also influenced the diagnostic test-ordering practices of primary care providers and the cost of health care. Although the overall quality of life of the elderly population has improved, the goal of providing cost-effective health care through these programs has not been achieved.

In the 1980s public attention became focused on the spiraling costs of health care. The philosophy that all citizens had the right to comprehensive quality health care prompted governmental concerns about the spiraling costs and the wide variation in charges among providers. The government was no longer able to pay for care that was delivered without defined limits or costs (Sullivan & Decker, 2005). In the face of huge budget deficits, the federal government moved to gain control of spiraling Medicare costs by enacting legislation to change Medicare payments from retrospective fee-for-service schedules to prospective fee schedules based on diagnostic categories. A payment system was adopted, based on diagnostic-related groups, that organizes diagnoses- and procedure-related conditions into categories or groups. Payment is based on national averages for cost and length of stay for these groups. *Length of stay* refers to the number of days a patient is hospitalized.

Managed Care and the Current Status of Reimbursement Practices

Within the complex American health care system, changes in reimbursement practices have led to changes in the way health care is delivered or "managed." *Managed care* is a generic term for a system that attempts to control and influence the way health care is financed and delivered. Managed care has affected the health care industry significantly since the early 1980s by changing the standards, the cost structure of medical care, and many aspects of access to care. The development of managed care has been aimed at balancing the three elements of access, cost, and quality. Under the fee-for-service system, health care costs increased dramatically due to high utilization of services. Other factors that have continued to contribute to high costs include new technology, cost shifting, the aging population, legal pressures, and administrative costs (Wolper, 2004).

Discussions and debate over time have tried to determine the effect of managed care plans on the quality of health care in light of managed care's cost-cutting strategies and tight controls on utilization of services. The National Committee for Quality Assurance (NCQA) found that plans do vary in their approach to prevention and treatment, but that performance of the plans in contrast to fee-for-service plans was equivalent or better under managed care. In addition, patients may be more likely to comply with the health risk screenings and preventive treatments that are the focus of managed care. They also reported that patients are satisfied with the actual care, but complain about the administrative services (NCQA, 2006). The managed care system and health plans will continue to evolve along with the dynamics of social and environmental change. Consumers are demanding more choice in selection of health care providers and seem to be willing to pay higher premiums for this flexibility.

It is important to understand the basic plan designs that provide coverage for health care within the United States. Plans differ in the aspects of care that are covered and funding for that care. Chart 3–2 defines the types of insurance plans that are common throughout the country.

Forms of Managed Care

A number of abbreviations are used to describe the various types of managed care. These include HMO, IPA, PPO, and EPO. An HMO refers to a health maintenance organization, IPA refers to an independent/individual practice association, PPO refers to a preferred provider organization, and EPO refers to an exclusive provider organization. An EPO has a contract with a single entity or group of physicians rather than a network of independent providers as seen in a PPO. Chart 3–3 outlines the most common forms of managed care.

The HMOs and PPOs pay a fixed rate per day per patient for providing care, regardless of equipment, supplies, or number of procedures or services required. Per case or per stay reimburses providers a fixed sum regardless of the length of stay. Capitation arrangements pay the hospital a fixed amount each month per member enrolled.

Many managed care organizations, regardless of whether the member uses the hospital, physician, or other services, have in-

CHART 3–2 Definitions of Health Insurance Plans

Type of Health Plan	Definition
Traditional insurance	*Indemnity:* The insured individual is indemnified against financial losses for health care costs. The insured is not restricted in terms of which providers they can access and they are reimbursed directly for any costs. *Service plans:* The plan contracts with providers to accept payment based on a fee schedule. The insured may have some restrictions on providers, and the provider is paid directly by the plan.
Government programs	*Medicare:* National health insurance program for individuals age 65 or older, under age 65 with disabilities, and those with end-stage renal disease. *Medicaid:* Medical assistance for individuals and families with low incomes. Each state will set regulations about eligibility and services. Military, civil service, federal employees, and veterans programs also fall under this category.
Self-funded plans	Under the Employee Retirement Income Security Act companies can cover their employees for medical costs instead of providing commercial insurance plans.
Health maintenance organization (HMO)	The organization provides comprehensive health care to individuals who prepay through premiums for the coverage. A primary care physician generally directs care within a network of providers.
Preferred provider organization (PPO)	The organization has a network of providers under contract. The insured can use the network providers or—for a higher deductible—access providers outside the network.

Sources: Data from HCAB, 2003; Grohar-Murray, M. E., & DiCroce, H. R. (2003). *Leadership and management in nursing.* Upper Saddle River, NJ: Pearson Prentice Hall; Wolper, L. F. (2004). *Health care administration: Planning, implementing, and managing organized delivery systems* (4th ed.). Sudbury, MA: Jones and Bartlett.

CHART 3–3	Common Forms of Managed Care
Health maintenance organization (HMO)	A group health care agency that provides basic and supplemental health maintenance and treatment services to voluntary enrollees. A fee is set without regard to the amount or kind of service provided.
Independent practice association (IPA)	A group of physicians who are in practice for themselves join together to form an associate offering a full spectrum of services to managed care organizations. IPAs will take capitated payment from HMOs and distribute a fee-for-service arrangement within the association. IPAs provide an opportunity for physicians who want to remain in individual practices to form an association that can interact and negotiate with HMOs.
Preferred provider organization (PPO)	Consists of a group of physicians, and perhaps a health care agency, that provide an insurance company or an employer with health services at a discounted rate. Employers and insurance companies set up standards and criteria for practices. When joining the organization the physician agrees to abide by those standards and abide by the reimbursement structure. An advantage of a PPO is that it provides the patient with a choice of health care providers and services.
Exclusive provider organization (EPO)	The physician organization becomes the exclusive provider of care. Participants are not allowed to receive coverage from any other providers. By developing an exclusive provider situation, an exclusive employer provider can negotiate better rates because the system can guarantee a certain volume of business.

ducements for maintaining wellness through health screenings and patient education. This emphasis is believed to decrease the number of inpatient hospital days per admission and can have a positive effect on a hospital margin.

Another way in which managed care plans control costs is to require prior approval for many types of care. Referrals by an individual's primary care provider also are often required. Although "true emergencies" are covered, many visits to the emergency department fall into nonemergent categories and coverage for these visits can be denied. The issue of prior approval also can arise before a patient can receive prescription drug benefits for certain drugs. Formularies of lists of drugs that are covered actually help to decrease skyrocketing drug costs by providing therapeutic, cost-effective choices for the practitioner. However, these limits also may delay care in an attempt to get approval for non-formulary drugs and patients may be required to pay any costs not covered by the insurance plan. These additional costs are based on the contract prices and selections health care providers have negotiated with the pharmaceutical distributors. Additionally, practitioners in groups often are given financial incentives for keeping their members healthy and out of the hospital.

Managed care today is in the mode of creating a delivery system that manages both costs and care along with methods of documenting cost-effective care. As such, quality improvement activities are now mandated, and health care organizations must meet the standards of the NCQA with the Health Plan Employer Data and Information Set.

Health Maintenance Organization

Health maintenance organizations (HMOs) were the earliest form of managed care, and are now the most common. HMOs deliver comprehensive health services for fixed, prepaid fees or capitation. Comprehensive health care usually includes procedures that focus on preventive care and early detection, such as annual physicals, mammography, proctoscopy, immunizations, and well-baby visits. HMOs manage services and costs through utilization review/management, restriction of access to a specific network of providers, and incentives for physicians.

Various HMO models and structures are available based on the relationship of the HMO and the providers. A group model

is one in which a medical group or organization contracts to provide care exclusively to the HMO's members. In return, the HMO pays the medical group on a capitated basis, which is a set amount per member per month. An example of this model is Kaiser Permanente. In a network model, the HMO has a nonexclusive contract with two or more physician groups and allows the physicians to treat HMO as well as non-HMO patients (HCAB, 2003b).

Independent Practice Association

An **independent practice association (IPA)** contracts on the behalf of individual physicians or groups of physicians to provide health care to the members of an HMO. In this model the physicians remain independent contractors with separate practices. Another model is a staff model in which the HMO employs physicians to provide care to its members (HCAB, 2003b).

Preferred Provider Organization

A **preferred provider organization (PPO)** differs from an HMO in several ways. PPOs provide a coordinated care plan that provides medical care by contracting with a network of providers. These providers agree to accept a set reimbursement rate for care covered by the plan. PPOs also provide reimbursement for covered care to noncontracted providers, but the level of reimbursement may differ from their contracted providers, and the member may have to pay a higher deductible.

PPOs also differ from HMOs in that they do not rely on strict utilization management and other controls common with HMOs (Grohar-Murray & DiCroce, 2003). Instead, they usually attempt to contain costs by negotiating with individual providers and health care organizations to provide certain kinds of health care at an agreed-on price. This price is usually lower than the price that a patient would pay for the same medical services outside of the PPO.

Government Programs

The Medicare and Medicaid programs were established by the Social Security Act in 1965. Medicare is the national health insurance program that covers people 65 years or older, some people under 65 years with disabilities, and people with end-stage renal disease. In the mid-1980s Congress adopted a prospective payment system based on the use of diagnosis-related groups

(DRGs) as a reimbursement method for hospitalized Medicare patients. A DRG refers to a like classification of diagnoses. The hospital is paid a certain capped amount per DRG category. A fixed payment has been predetermined for more than 470 possible diagnostic categories, covering the majority of medical diagnoses of all patients admitted to the hospital.

The switch to the DRG payment schedule effectively predetermined the amount that a hospital is reimbursed for the treatment of a Medicare patient diagnosed with a particular condition. DRGs shifted the payment unit from total charges or "days in the hospital" to the patient's diagnosis. The purpose of the DRG was, and still is, to ease the burden of Medicare financing and to control delivery of care. The advent of DRGs has served as an incentive for hospitals to place greater emphasis on reducing costs, utilization of services, and length of patient stay.

Under the DRG prospective payment system, hospitals and extended care facilities have had to develop length-of-stay (LOS) estimates for a variety of diagnoses. These estimates help determine, on average, the LOS beyond which the facility will not be reimbursed for the patient's care. A subspecialty of nursing, called *discharge planners,* has evolved to help plan patient discharges in a timely manner. Discharge planning nurses also help provide some assurance that the patient's needs will be met after discharge. At discharge, arrangements are made for family teaching, home care, or extended care.

With an emphasis on patient days, discharge planners have focused on care management and clinical pathways. Consequently, patient acuity levels in hospitals are now higher, and those discharged are sicker than ever before (Dower, 2002; Shortell & Kaluzny, 2005). Patients are sometimes discharged to their homes before it is appropriate, and equipment and services are not always adequate to meet all of their needs. This situation has led to the emergence of subacute, transitional rehabilitation units in long-term care facilities. These facilities have had to train their staff to care for much sicker patients than they usually care for, patients who often require intravenous therapy and complex nursing interventions previously provided only in the acute care setting. Also, it is not unusual for those patients who have returned home to be treated with intravenous therapy, respiratory care, wound care, and various rehabilitation therapies. Much of the home care is dependent on the availability of family members, who may have to take unpaid time from work to care for their loved ones. The care that family and friends provide is not without cost, even though it is not reimbursed. Critics of the DRG system believe that while prospective payment may ease the burden of Medicare financing, it does not necessarily reduce the overall cost of health care, especially when these costs are calculated from the point of view of society as a whole. It is worth noting that high hospital readmission rates are seen in cases of patients sent home too early or those sent home without appropriate care and support. To guarantee Medicare reimbursement for the readmission, these patients are sometimes readmitted with a different diagnosis than the initial admission (Dower, 2002).

Medicaid is a state-administered program that provides medical assistance for certain individuals and families (dependents) with low incomes and resources. The federal agency that is responsible for oversight of the programs is the Centers for Medicare and Medicaid Services. CMS also establishes guidelines for state Medicaid programs; however, program requirements are set by the individual state and administration of the state program may differ by county. These coverage plans may be administered by a managed care contract through an HMO or PPO to provide care for patients (CMS, 2006).

Future Economic Projections

Managed care as a model for health care delivery is not going to go away (Marquis & Huston, 2007; Rosenbaum, 1998). It permeates the current health care delivery system and is likely to grow in magnitude regarding the number of subscribers to its plans as well as its impact on the entire health care system. Although managed care continues to dominate markets, it is evolving in ways that have diminished its potential to control costs and promote quality. As health care premiums continue to rise and labor markets slacken, consumers are likely to face growing financial burden for the cost of care. These developments could have the positive effect of making consumers more cost conscious in their use of health care services. Conversely, they may result in increased disparities in the health system, with further stratification based on the ability to pay and greater burden on those who have chronic illnesses for the cost of their care (Dower, 2002; Marquis & Huston, 2007; Shortell & Kaluzny, 2005).

Currently, Americans spend more on their health care than any other Western industrialized nation. The United States is the only one of this group of nations that does not offer basic benefits globally to all citizens (Woolf, Johnson, & Geiger, 2006). The many barriers created by the current health care system affect access to care for individuals and specific population groups such as the elderly and rural residents. According to the American Hospital Association, consumers worry about insurance cost increases, that their income will not keep pace with these rising costs, and that insurance plans may decrease health care quality and access to cut their operating expenses. There is further concern that as these issues go unchecked, consumers may be influenced to go without insurance or the care they need. Inappropriate use of hospital emergency departments and the inability of patients to pay increased costs for health care is forcing hospitals to offset these losses by raising prices for services, drugs, and supplies. The consequences of these trends may include higher rates of chronic illnesses, more frequent and severe disease complications, and overall adverse effects on access to health care for children (Woolf et al., 2006).

It is expected that out-of-pocket costs, or those expenses not covered by health plans, will grow rapidly for consumers. This is primarily due to higher premiums for health plan coverage, which are based on higher medical care costs. These higher premiums have forced employers to share the added burden with their employees. To combat these competing cost structures, which seem to be increasing without end, reform initiatives are being proposed on many fronts. Certainly the government is looking at reducing expenses within the Medicare and Medicaid programs. Additionally, coverage programs are being developed to give consumers more choice about what their health plan will include and to align incentives among all parties to focus on access, appropriate care, and reduced costs (Samuel, Raleigh, Hower, & Schwartz, 2003).

Nurses should assess their patient's health care coverage or insurance plan for potential referrals for financial assistance or counseling. Patients may be concerned about their current coverage or may lack coverage altogether. This concern can cause significant stress that may affect the patient's ability to rest and recover. Referrals may be made to the hospital's financial department or social services to assist in resolving any payment or coverage issues.

The cost and financing of health care will continue to drive the development of health care delivery models based on the premise that more should be provided for less. This focus will influence how health care professionals, including nurses, are used in the future. This pressure will continue until the consumers (individual, employer, and insurance provider) are comfortable that the health care product (service) they are receiving is balanced by its availability and cost. Along with changes in health care finances and managed care, other important trends are affecting the future of health care delivery systems and the financial configuration of health care organizations.

Financial Aspects of Health Care Organizations

Health care organizations, especially hospitals, are structured financially in one of two ways. **For-profit or proprietary organizations** focus their mission and structure on earning a profit from their operations. The profits are then distributed to the owners of the organization or the investors who have purchased shares of the organization (Finkler & Kovner, 2000). The excess earnings of a **not-for-profit organization** must be used for public rather than private gain. The mission of the not-for-profit organization is to earn a profit, but those profits are generally used to improve the physical facility and services offered by the agency (Wolper, 2004).

Regardless of whether a hospital uses a for-profit or not-for-profit structure, it cannot turn patients away who require emergency care services and it cannot refuse to care for patients. The **Emergency Medical Treatment and Labor Act (EMTALA)** was enacted in 1986 to ensure public access to emergency services regardless of patients' ability to pay. When patients are not able to pay for care, they fall under the hospital's charity care policy. Charity care is accounted for in annual budgets based on the organization's history and the demographic projections for the population they serve. Charity care is considered a loss from the organization's operations. Programs are available to assist hospitals that are adversely affected by their patient population's inability to pay; however, this assistance does not cover all costs incurred by the organization. Charity care can contribute to higher costs for insured or self-pay patients if the hospital has to structure its financial plan to make up for large losses. Chapter 73 ⊕ includes an in-depth discussion of emergency department regulations.

Budgeting Process for Health Care Institutions

Budgets have three main components:

• Revenue is the money an organization receives or is entitled to receive to cover the costs of providing services or goods.

• Expenses are costs of operating the organization and include salaries, benefits, supplies, utilities, purchased services, and administrative costs.

• Capital refers to equipment purchased by the organization or construction projects.

Chart 3–4 (p. 52) outlines the basic structure of a hospital-based budget.

A budget is basically a plan for a future period that is defined in measurable terms and expected outcomes. The process begins with the forecasting of revenue and expense projections for the next budget period. This period is referred to as a fiscal year and is generally a calendar year, but may begin at any time during the year, and lasts for 12 consecutive months. For instance, some organizations budget January through December, whereas others may define their fiscal year as July through June.

Forecasting involves a review of the organization's assets, which includes their property, equipment cash on hand, and the amount of money calculated as outstanding from billing. Organizations will next look at the trends in reimbursement for services and population demographics for growth or change. Reimbursement is the payment received for health or medical care from a health plan (insurance) or payer source. The amount of payment is often discounted from the actual charges for the service. Historical data also are reviewed for volume trends and patterns of service that may be seasonal in nature such as higher patient admissions during winter months.

All of this information is calculated to provide a projection for potential revenue, which must be compared to the estimated expenses. The comparison takes into account the bottom line or the outcome of revenue divided by expense. Usually this is a positive outcome, but at times organizations will project a loss or a break-even scenario based on their analysis of all of these factors. The administration and the governing body of the organization generally approve budgets before they are implemented. The budget is monitored continuously throughout the year and appropriate adjustments are made as necessary.

Capital budgets determine the organization's ability to purchase equipment and to upgrade or expand facilities. The capital budget is based on a calculation from the operating budget, or an estimate of what the organization can afford. Projections range from the next fiscal year to multiple years out into the future. Capital equipment needs generally fall into the categories of needing replacement, upgrading of existing equipment or systems, or purchasing of a new business or service opportunity. Facility needs usually are based on the age of the building, technology, and expansion for population growth or new services (Wolper, 2004).

Funding for the capital budget comes from the estimated revenue from operations or a percentage of expected income or loans. Some capital equipment can be leased to avoid an outright purchase if purchasing funds are not available. Some leases allow the organization to rent equipment with an option to buy at the end of a set period for a discounted price or to allow payments for large pieces of equipment to be billed over several years.

Nursing professionals play an important part in the budget process through their observations of the environment, equipment, and changing needs of patients. Their input to the management structure provides important information for making

CHART 3–4	**Hospital Budget Components**	
Major Category	**Component**	**Definition**
Revenue	Volume	Volume for hospitals overall is based on units of service. The overall hospital generally looks at patient days, and departments look at relative statistics for the type of work they do. *Examples:* Inpatient unit = patient days Surgery = surgery minutes Respiratory therapy = procedures or treatments Laboratory = tests or procedures Emergency department = patient visits
	Charges	Charges are based on the cost of supplies or services. They take into consideration the price paid to the vendor and a markup for processing, staff time, and organizational overhead.
	Deductions from revenue	These deductions are any decrease in revenue from charity care or payer contracts.
	Nonoperating revenue	Includes adjustments that may come from investment income or legal actions in favor of the organization.
Operating expenses (controllable expenses)	Salaries/wages	These expenses include regular salaries for staff, premium pay such as overtime, benefits, and temporary labor. Benefits can include medical care coverage, vacation/sick time, training/orientation, and travel reimbursement.
	Supplies	Examples include disposable and reusable supplies, minor medical equipment, and office supplies.
	Purchased services	Examples include maintenance agreements for large equipment, equipment rentals, repair costs, and vendor contracts for services.
Non-Discretionary expenses	Overhead	This category covers system costs for depreciation of the buildings and equipment, administrative positions and expenses, and interest on loans. Administrative costs are for nonrevenue-generating departments such as finance, human resources, and housekeeping.

Sources: Data from Finkler, S. A., & Kovner, C. T. (2000). *Financial management for nurse managers and executives.* Philadelphia: W. B. Saunders; Wolper, L. F. (2004). *Health care administration: Planning, implementing, and managing organized delivery systems* (4th ed.). Sudbury, MA: Jones and Bartlett.

decisions about the allocation of resources, the control of expenses, and planning for future growth. It is also important for nurses to take an active role in containing costs through judicial use of supplies, awareness of equipment safety and maintenance, and appropriate adjustments to staffing and workload.

Health Care Trends

Several major trends are affecting and changing health care in the United States:

- Evidence-based practice guidelines and research are creating a shift in approach to care that is more systematic and clear.
- Quality and patient safety standards have been a main focus of consumer watchdog groups and regulatory bodies and are influencing the purchase of health care insurance and the selection of medical care providers.
- Threats of potential major events such as bioterrorism attacks or widespread epidemics are requiring health care organizations to set priorities and plan their responses.
- Advancements in technology and science are enhancing medical care now and in the future.

These and other trends are discussed in the following subsections.

Evidence-Based Practice

Evidence-based practice can be described broadly as an approach that integrates current research evidence with clinical expertise and patients' needs. Evidence-based practice has come about as a response to the demand for grounded clinical decision making that critically examines the benefits and costs of treatments and interventions.

Factors that form a framework for decision making with this approach include understanding patients' needs, their concerns, and their values, building on the clinical expertise or experience of the professional nurse, and seeking relevant clinical data and best practices (Malloch & Porter-O'Grady, 2006). Best practices are defined as proven processes that produce consistent, high-quality results. In nursing there are many sources of knowledge that guide critical thinking about care, including the applicability of nursing interventions and intuition about approaches and interactions with patients. Data and research are also becoming more available through the use of Internet resources in the practice arena. Internet resources provide instant access for caregivers. Information systems used in health care organizations often provide immediate access to concise resources and guidelines for practice. It is important for nurses to keep current with relevant literature in their area of practice and be competent in accessing available resources.

Hospital Report Cards

Consumer-oriented hospital report cards are available to the public through periodicals and on the Internet. They provide a wealth of information on quality outcome measurements and the experience of organizations in providing care (Richard, Rawal, & Martin, 2005). The development of these tools was intended to help improve the quality of care by providing feedback and benchmarking practice standards. Benchmarking offers qualitative or quantitative measurement of specific data related to reported outcome information. Benchmark information often is displayed as a range and includes the best practice reported by participants. This can be of interest to patients or patient groups with specific health problems or chronic diseases who are making a selection of physicians or health care institutions (Werner & Asch, 2005).

Patient Safety Standards

There is heightened awareness in the United States regarding the safety of patients in the health care environment. Major efforts are under way to focus on measuring, reporting, and improving patient safety. Organizations conducting such research include the Institute of Medicine, the Leapfrog Group, and the Joint Commission.

The **Institute of Medicine (IOM)** provides science-based advice on medicine and health in an effort to improve health. It provides unbiased, evidence-based, and authoritative information to policy makers, professionals, and the public at large (IOM, 1999). In 1999 IOM produced the study, *To Err Is Human: Building a Safer Health System*, which indicated that preventable errors in hospitals are the eighth leading cause of death in the United States. Following the recommendations of the IOM report, hospitals were required to assess their practices and institute changes to ensure the reduction of preventable errors. Reports from the investigation of medical errors found that errors were not necessarily the result of carelessness, but were instead the result of systems and processes that did not provide the appropriate checks to prevent the errors (Leapfrog Group, 2006).

The **Leapfrog Group** was established by a coalition of public and private organizations that provide health care benefits. The group focuses on collecting data about medical errors and setting standards that will reduce errors. In addition, information is provided to consumers that assist them in making more informed choices about hospitals and health care systems. The Leapfrog Group has developed platforms for improving patient safety including (1) computer physician order entry (CPOE), (2) evidence-based hospital referral, (3) intensive care unit (ICU) physician staffing or the use of intensivists, and (4) National Quality Forum–endorsed safe practices.

CPOE is aimed at eliminating errors from the process of transcribing physician orders that are handwritten or given verbally. CPOE requires that the prescribing physician or allied health care provider personally enter orders into the computer system. It is well known that illegible handwriting has been one of the root causes of medication and therapy error. According to the Leapfrog Group, if this practice were implemented in all urban hospitals in the United States as many as 907,600 serious medication errors could be prevented each year. In addition, CPOE has been shown to reduce patient length of stay and du-

plicate orders for procedures and tests (Leapfrog Group, 2006). Computer system software programs are also available that help to prevent prescribing errors by providing alerts to incompatibilities with medications.

Evidence-based hospital referral is aimed at guiding patients to hospitals and clinical teams that are more likely to produce better outcomes for specific treatments and procedures. Information provided on Leapfrog Group web pages offers data on hospital volume, geographic specifics, risk-adjusted outcomes, and benchmarking among providers. Currently the Leapfrog Group collects data on eight high-risk conditions or procedures and three maternal high-risk delivery outcomes.

The group also advocates for dedicated physician staffing in ICUs. This type of program provides physicians who specialize in critical care and managing complex patients. Studies have shown that when this system is in place there is a 30% reduction in overall hospital mortality and a 40% reduction in mortality in the intensive care environment (Leapfrog Group, 2006). These intensivist programs in the ICU can also be used to provide remote monitoring of acutely ill patients (Nathans et al., 2006). Remote coverage is provided via computer monitoring of clinical data from specific diagnostic equipment and the ongoing review of test results and recorded documentation. Some systems provide video surveillance of the patient from the bedside linked to intensivists at a central location. Benefits of using an intensivist model include reduced mortality rates, reduced inappropriate admissions, shorter ICU stays, faster weaning from mechanical ventilators, early detection of hemodynamic complications, fewer consultations with other specialists, and an overall reduction in hospital costs (Fuchs, Berenholtz, & Dorman, 2005).

The National Quality Forum is a public–private partnership created to develop and implement a national strategy for health care quality measurement and reporting. The organization has established an agenda to implement proven patient safety practices (National Quality Forum, 2006). National patient safety goals and practices have been endorsed by other organizations such as the Joint Commission and the Leapfrog Group who have formed a partnership to collaborate on patient-safety standards. In addition, the CMS (2006) is also joining with the Leapfrog Group to provide information for their consumers about the initiatives and hospital-specific ratings that are now available.

The Joint Commission (**Joint Commission**), the accrediting body for hospitals and health care organizations, is an independent, private, not-for-profit organization. The Joint Commission focuses on setting standards for patient care and safety, competency of staff, and responsibilities of the administration and governing board. It evaluates and certifies or accredits health care organizations and programs in the United States. The Joint Commission's patient safety standards took effect in July 2001 and are generally updated or expanded on an annual basis. Hospitals must take all of these standards and initiatives into consideration as they plan quality activities and develop policies and procedures (Joint Commission, 2006).

Emergency Preparedness

Hospitals must develop disaster or emergency preparedness plans to ensure that the organization can respond rapidly and function under extreme conditions. These plans are required by licensing and accreditation agencies. Accreditation agencies evaluate and certify organizations on specific standards or regulations. The plans must address fire, utility failures, terrorism, and natural disasters. A committee generally oversees the development and periodic revision of the plan, as well as the conduction of drills to test the training and readiness of the staff to respond (Wolper, 2004).

Nurses have a vital role in the response to these emergency situations. Patients in the hospital may need to be evacuated to a safe area or triaged based on their current status. Triage involves skilled evaluation of the patient's condition, stability, and ongoing need for treatment. In a community-wide disaster, beds in the acute care hospital will need to be made available for patients with immediate life-threatening needs. To ensure maximum bed capacity, patients may be discharged to lower levels of care or be sent home to recover. Assessment of the patient's home environment and evaluation of the competency of surrogate caregivers are essential functions of the nurse in these instances.

With the advent of the September 11, 2001, terrorist attacks in New York City and Washington, D.C., and the events surrounding the mailing of anthrax to citizens, the standards for hospital emergency planning changed dramatically:

- Hospitals have been engaged in training and readiness planning for all types of bioterrorism, which include threats of biological, chemical, or radiological exposures (Zinkovich, Malvey, Hamby, & Fottler, 2005).

- Community-wide and institutional drills are required to test and train staff members on the current plans to ensure readiness on an ongoing basis.

- Hospitals must be able to identify infections such as anthrax, smallpox, plague, and other communicable diseases as part of heightened surveillance.

- Hospitals must be aware of the worldwide concern for potential pandemics from diseases such as influenza and avian flu.

- Natural disasters, such as floods, earthquakes, fires, and storms, will trigger similar responses.

Procedures have also been put in place to handle mass casualties and to lock down facilities to prevent contamination from the environment should a chemical or radiological event occur. In the future hospitals will be required to have advanced systems and processes in place to provide for staff, patient, and community safety (Hsu et al., 2006). Disasters and bioterrorism are discussed in detail in Chapter 72 .

Scientific and Technical Advancements
Telemedicine
Telemedicine refers to systems or programs that use video or computer-based equipment to link providers or to monitor patients electronically. Telemedicine was actually first given a trial in the 1930s when television technology began. Now it is used throughout the world to provide videoconferencing in a variety of health care settings. This technology is used to improve access to higher levels of care for advice and direction, especially in rural areas, prison health care, psychiatry, and home health.

Telecommunication capabilities for diagnostic imaging examinations, such as digital x-rays and computerized tomogra-phy (CAT) scans, are common in institutions. These capabilities are particularly useful for emergency departments to link physicians remotely to diagnose patient conditions or obtain specialty consultations (Heinzelmann, Lugn, & Kvedar, 2005).

Other applications for telemedicine include its use in accessing consultations in distant clinic settings, which saves the patient time and expense for travel to specialists. Through videoconferencing, physicians and technicians can engage in assessment, view procedures, and review data concurrently while communicating directly with the patient. The use of telecommunications is discussed at length in Chapter 1 .

Minimally Invasive Surgery
Minimally invasive surgery depicts a surgical technique that uses laparoscopic or video equipment to perform procedures without directly opening the body's cavities. Small incisions are made to introduce probes, video devices, and instruments. The technique has been described as telemanipulation, because the surgeon is physically separated from the surgical site and operates equipment using tactile cues and intuitive dexterity (Darzi & Mackay, 2002). It has been estimated that in the near future 70% of all surgical procedures will involve minimally invasive techniques. Surgeries now being performed in this manner include removal of esophageal tumors, treatment of morbid obesity, excision of malignant liver tumors, removal of gallbladders and colon tumors, and a variety of gynecologic procedures (Fuchs, 2002). Benefits of minimally invasive surgery include reduced pain, quicker return to oral intake, and less scarring. This results in shorter hospitalizations and an increased use of outpatient centers for these procedures (Robinson & Stiegmann, 2004).

Robotics
Robotics used in surgery is described as computer-controlled manipulators that have artificial sensory abilities. These manipulators can be programmed to perform surgical tasks using tools or instruments (Satava, 2004). Surgical robots are used passively to consistently hold a position or to actively move instruments in the surgical area. Benefits of the use of robotics include minimized surgical trauma, improved precision, decreased invasiveness, and fewer complications. It is also estimated that patients recover faster following the use of robotics techniques than other traditional or open procedures. Surgical procedures can be performed long distance, and the same type of robotics have been used to perform nonsurgical procedures in space (Chandra & Frank, 2003).

Robotics also is being used to perform internal examinations through the use of pills or capsules that contain video cameras and light sources. One such device, a video pill, can perform endoscopic examinations for the small and large bowel (Baines, 2003). Lastly, according to Marketing Health Services (2003), a robot has been developed to assist with some aspects of patient care. The robot can provide mobile communication and videoconferencing and will be able to transport patients and eventually to take temperatures and draw blood.

Gene Therapy
Genes are located in the nuclei of all cells and control hereditary traits and cell functions. Genes are attached end to end in long, double-stranded helical molecules of DNA. The study of genes

has been aimed at identifying them individually, their functions, how they work, and what happens when they do not work. Scientists have been able to identify the human genetic code and the sequencing of 100% of the human genome (Human Genome Project, 2008). This research is helping to determine gene function and even how to stop a gene from functioning if it produces disease or adverse conditions. Ongoing studies are focused on understanding the other elements of the biological processes of genes (Medem Medical Library, 2006).

Ethical and legal issues surround the field of gene therapy and the ongoing research in this area. Patients undergoing gene research face social dilemmas, especially if there is the potential to predict a debilitating disease. Personal conflicts may arise when disease is detected, but not yet manifested. Although gene therapy will continue to be a major part of future health research, it is extremely expensive and thus questions arise about access to therapy and payment for associated services. See Chapter 11 💿 for a complete discussion on genetics.

Inpatient to Outpatient Shift

As mentioned earlier, one overall trend in health care service is a shift from inpatient care to outpatient care settings for many procedures and treatment modalities. Even though the predicted growth of inpatient bed needs is 10% to 15% during the next decade (HCAB, 2003c) the need for more outpatient beds is even more crucial. Factors affecting this growth include population growth, aging of the population, new technologies to manage chronic diseases, and less invasive procedures, which will reduce length of stay. Specialty centers are becoming more prevalent and are offering alternatives to the acute care hospital. Outpatient settings have advantages over the hospital in that they provide increased efficiency and reduced costs per procedure. Outpatient specialty centers have been developed for spine surgery, incontinence treatment, diagnostic testing, endoscopic procedures, surgical specialties like orthopedics, and cardiac services (HCAB, 2003c).

Health Care Worker Shortages

Shortages of physicians, nurses, and other health care–related specialists are affecting the delivery of care and services in the United States and elsewhere in the world. In hospitals shortages of nurses, radiology technicians, pharmacists, medical record personnel, housekeepers, and food service personnel are becoming severe. A report released by the American Hospital Association (2006) indicated that the many open nursing positions in hospitals in the United States equate to an 8.5% vacancy rate. Nursing education programs turned away 147,000 qualified applicants in 2005 due to shortages of faculty (American Association of Colleges of Nursing [AACN], 2006).

Factors affecting the recruitment and retention of health care workers include aging of the workforce, workload concerns, pay and benefits, and the work environment (Buerhaus et al., 2005). In 2006 *Nursing Management* magazine's Aging Workforce Survey indicated that 55% of the respondents were planning on retiring before 2020. The Health Resources and Services Administration (HRSA) further indicated in an April 2006 survey it conducted that the shortfall of registered nurses will be 17% in 2010 and will grow to 36% in 2020. Hospitals are implementing strategies to retain and recruit health care staff; however, the benefits and overall effect of these strategies will not be felt for years. In addition, nursing education programs and health care service organizations are collaborating on new models for boosting the enrollment in and graduation from nursing schools (AACN, 2006; HRSA, 2006).

Hospitalist Programs

Inpatient hospital care has become a specialty for physicians, called **hospitalists**, who concentrate their practice in the acute care environment. The use of hospitalists is designed to provide 24-hour coverage for patients. Hospitalists may be contracted to provide care to inpatients by primary care physicians who do not provide inpatient care or by patients who do not have a physician at the time of hospitalization. Internists and family practice physicians are turning the care of their patients who need hospitalization over to these specialists (Freed, 2004).

The benefits of using a hospitalist program include decreases in length of stay, improved outcomes, and enhanced efficiency (Cowan et al., 2006). Continuity of care is improved, and there is increased development and adherence to clinical pathways and guidelines because the hospitalist is readily available to assess the patient's progress and make adjustments to the medical plan of care. These benefits also help to reduce inpatient costs and provide a higher level of inpatient care. Hospitalists become assimilated as part of the hospital staff, working well with the nursing staff and other providers to develop relationships and trust (Amin & Owen, 2006).

Information Technology

The growth of information management technology in health care has been an ongoing trend. New systems span the continuum of care and provide resources that are immediately available to practitioners and patients. Electronic medical records and clinical information systems that integrate departmental functions and facilitate reporting and tracking of data and observations are being increasingly used. Clinical information systems also link providers to individual patient data and appropriate clinical reference material (Harrison & Palacio, 2006). Some of these systems allow patients to schedule appointments for therapy and follow-up and also communicate with health care professionals regarding their questions or concerns.

Connections through the Internet or a telephone also are used to monitor and interact with patients who have chronic disease disorders such as heart failure and diabetes. Disease management programs are successful in reducing emergency department visits and acute admissions to the hospital. In the future most data collection and documentation will be electronic and integrated for use in caring for patients. Integrated electronic documentation is expected to improve quality, reduce costs, and enhance work flow. It also creates better clinical collaboration and fosters evidence-based decision making and the use of best practices (Halamka, 2006). Chapter 6 💿 discusses the use of electronic medical records and documentation in detail.

Demand for Quality Care

Four driving forces underlie health care system policies and decisions: cost, equity, access, and quality. Thus, quality is an important factor in public policy regarding health care delivery. Quality, the definition and interpretation of such, has become critically important as the general public has become increasingly aware of health care options and as health care moves forward in the 21st century (Marquis & Huston, 2007).

Quality Defined

Quality refers to the characteristics of and the pursuit of excellence. Excellence may be established by determining whether the outcomes compare favorably to the standards that were set. **Quality of care** is the degree to which health services for individuals and populations increase the likelihood of desired health outcomes and are consistent with current professional knowledge. Donabedian (1980) has defined health care–related quality as the balance of health benefits and harms to a patient. Quality also may be defined in terms of effectiveness and efficiency, benefits and harm, or appropriateness of care, as is the case in a service setting. It has been described as consisting of two interdependent parts: quality in fact and quality in perception. **Quality in fact** is defined as conforming to standards and meeting one's own expectations. **Quality in perception** is meeting the customer's expectations. Within the framework of continuous quality improvement, quality is defined as meeting or exceeding customer requirements. The Joint Commission has considered quality to increase the probability of desired outcomes and reduce the probability of undesired outcomes (Huber, 2006; Joint Commission, 2007).

Quality processes in which health care delivery systems engage have been categorized as quality assurance programs, quality improvement programs, total quality management, and continuous quality improvement. Each of these terms and the current state of utilization are described next in order to understand the impact of quality demands on health care delivery systems:

- Quality assurance generally refers to an organization's effort or ability to provide services according to accepted professional standards and in a manner acceptable to the patient. Quality assurance builds on quality assessment, the measurement of quality, taking evaluative action to ensure a designated level of quality (Huber, 2006). Thus, quality assurance activities are intended to guarantee or ensure quality of care. Most health care organizations do not use this interpretation of quality anymore because they do not endorse the concept that quality can be assured. The term *quality assurance* has been replaced with *quality assessment, improvement,* or *management.*

- Quality improvement programs function as organizational umbrellas that extend into many areas for the purpose of accountability to the consumer and payer. The program is a continuous, ongoing measurement and evaluation process that includes structure, process, and outcomes. The quality improvement process uses preestablished criteria and standards and then follows the evaluation of care with an appropriate change for the purpose of improvement. Thus, quality improvement is a process of attaining a new level of performance that is superior to the previous level (Marquis & Huston, 2007). Many health care organizations have endorsed the concept of quality improvement and have adopted standards of care designed to improve quality of care.

- Total quality management (TQM), sometimes called the total quality process, is a way to ensure customer satisfaction by involving all employees in the improvement of the quality of every product or service. All systems and processes are evaluated and improved. The goal of TQM is to reduce the waste and cost of poor quality. TQM has been defined as a structured system for involving an entire organization in a continuous quality improvement process targeted to meet and exceed customer expectations (Marquis & Huston, 2007; Sullivan & Decker, 2005). Many health care systems subscribe to this process of defining and measuring quality.

- Continuous quality improvement (CQI) is a process of continuously improving a system by gathering data on performance and using multidisciplinary teams to analyze the system, collect measurements, and propose changes. The four main principles are (1) a customer focus, (2) the identification of key processes to improve quality, (3) the use of quality tools and statistics, and (4) the involvement of all people and departments in problem solving (Huber, 2006; Sullivan & Decker, 2005). CQI is endorsed by many health care agencies.

With the paradigm shift from the assurance of quality to quality assessment, there has been a value shift from a focus on the provider's values to a focus on the customer's (patient's) values. At the level of the individual nurse and patient, the quality improvement process is an appraisal of how the nurse is performing in taking care of patients. At the unit level, concurrent and retrospective audits, clinical pathway variances, and other data analyses may be used to examine the process and outcomes of care (Huber, 2006).

Regulatory Agency Impact

Standard setting occurs outside the professional arena in three areas: (1) federal and state government regulation (via Medicare and Medicaid reimbursement regulations), (2) state licensure, and (3) private accreditation. All are concerned with quality, usually at a minimum level. Federal reimbursement regulations for Medicare are administered through the Centers for Medicare and Medicaid Services. Individual states promulgate Medicaid rules and regulations. They also regulate segments of the health care system, such as skilled nursing facilities or capital expenditures. Since the Joint Commission's founding in 1951, it has become the principal, but not exclusive, standard setter for health care facilities (Joint Commission, 2007).

Other major accreditation initiatives are those of the National Committee for Quality Assurance. The NCQA is the not-for-profit accrediting body for managed care organizations. The NCQA has developed a core set of 60 health plan performance measures. These measures that cover the areas of quality access, patient satisfaction, membership, utilization, and finance, as found in the 1993 version of the Health Plan Employer Data and Information Set (HEDIS). HEDIS represents a major effort to standardize and systematize the quality measurement process, thereby allowing for national comparison of performance and benchmarking. Technical quality of care, access to services, and enrollee satisfaction are measured. HEDIS measures are evaluated every 3 years, and new standards are added as appropriate. NCQA has a national database for comparison and benchmarking, referred to as the Quality Compass (NCQA, 2006).

The CMS has mandated the use of the standardized Outcome and Assessment Information Set (OASIS) for home health care for both Medicare and non-Medicare patients. OASIS is a series of questions for collecting data on the quality of home care. Clinical, financial, and administrative data are included. For all of the accreditation and regulation systems, the goals are to improve the quality of care and collect data for comparisons.

Quality Measurement

The measurement of quality is founded on several principles: Quality can be measured; quality measures results against a standard or some degree of excellence; and excellence is determined either by validating standards of care or by measuring professional actions in caring for patients. Standards essentially define quality, against which outcomes and performance are measured. Because standards establish the baseline against which an evaluation is conducted, they need to be reliable and valid. Standards take three different approaches or forms: structure, process, and outcomes (Huber, 2006):

- **Structure standards**, or measures, focus on the internal characteristics of the organization and its personnel. They answer the questions "Is a structure in place that will allow quality to exist?" and "Is the structure of the organization set up to allow quality of care?"

- **Process standards** focus on whether the activities within an organization are being conducted appropriately. Process measures focus on the behaviors of the provider of care. Process standards look at activities, interventions, and the sequence of caregiving events.

- **Outcome standards** refer to whether the services provided by the organization make any difference. They answer questions about the services that nurses provide and whether they make a difference to the patients or to the health status of the population. Outcome standards address physical health status, mental health status, social and physical functioning, health attitudes/knowledge/ behavior, utilization of services, and the patient's perception of quality care. Outcome refers to a change in the current or future health status attributed to antecedent health care and patient attributes of health care. Outcomes present the possibility of measuring the effectiveness, quality, and time allocated for care.

In measuring quality, both structure and process parameters are important, but they are not sufficient in determining whether the care made a difference or whether the patient learned, recovered, or improved his health status. It is important for the care to make a difference and that the care is not above a certain cost. In addition, measuring nursing care outcomes as related to cost would assist in establishing the value of nursing care. Chart 3–5 provides a definition of the three types of standards and examples corresponding to each.

Quality Improvement and Research Studies

Research and quality assessment/management both rely on evaluation and are applications of the problem-solving process. However, they are distinct and separate processes. Highly controlled experimental research is on one end of the spectrum, and day-to-day quality assessment evaluation is on the other. Research studies manipulate variables, may introduce new nursing

CHART 3–5	Quality Standards and Measurement Examples
Type of Standard	**Measurement Example**
Structure standards focus on the internal characteristics of the organization and its personnel. These standards regulate the environment to ensure quality and answer the question "Is a structure in place that will allow quality to exist?"	Nursing department provides in-service opportunities for staff development. Agency will staff at least one RN for every six patient visits.
Process standards focus on whether the activities within an organization are being appropriately conducted. These standards target behaviors, activities, interventions, and the sequence of caregiving events.	A nursing assessment will be completed on each patient within 2 hours of admission. Vital signs will be taken every hour.
Outcome standards refer to whether the services provided make any difference. These standards address physical health status, mental health status, social and physical function, health attitudes/knowledge/behavior, utilization of services, and the patient's perception of care.	Ambulates without assistance. Breath sounds are clear, free of rales and rhonchi.

procedures, and may not have an immediate application to practice. In contrast, quality improvement studies do not withhold an intervention to see if it made a difference. In a quality improvement study an intervention that is not commonly accepted would not be introduced.

Quality improvement studies are necessary for the institution's patient care management. They are not designed to manipulate variables, withhold interventions, or introduce new techniques. They are designed for measuring what exists with the idea of determining how it measures against standards, so that patient care can be managed and improved. The purpose of nursing research is generalizable knowledge; the purpose of quality improvement is determining effectiveness, efficiency, and appropriateness of care. Research utilization and other research activities can contribute to quality improvement, whereas the contribution of quality assessment to the research process is through problem identification. A key challenge for the future is to integrate research, clinical practice, and evaluation methods. Chapter 8 ☞ includes a complete description of research and quality assessment.

▮ Licensure, Regulations, and Accreditation of Health Care Organizations

Licensure refers to the process for approving a health care organization to provide medical care and services. Licensing is generally accomplished at the state level through a department of health services. The purpose of the licensure process is generally to ensure access to care and the quality of the care provided. Regulations on licensure differ from state to state as does the process for credentialing an organization. Requirements generally cover business practices, building codes, facility maintenance, aspects of safety, evaluation and planning activities, and delivery of care including the credentials and competency of employees. States also determine licensure for professionals and describe the scope of practice for various levels of caregivers.

The state agency responsible for licensing will survey the organization periodically for compliance with regulations. Regulations are rules or laws that govern delivery of care or maintenance of the facility or work environment. A compliance survey focuses on all aspects of the facility's operations in addition to the quality improvement program. State agencies are enforcement bodies that can levy fines and other restrictions on health care organizations that do not meet the intent of the regulations or show a history of deficiencies or noncompliance with requirements or the organization's own policies.

Federal and state governmental agencies regulate the delivery of health care in specific areas such as safety, facility structural requirements, and disease prevention and control. These agencies have some jurisdiction over hospitals and other health care delivery organizations to ensure compliance with standards and to assist with problems that may occur in those environments.

Occupational Safety and Health Administration

The **Occupational Safety and Health Administration (OSHA)** is an agency that oversees environmental safety. It was established under the U.S. Department of Labor by the Occupational Safety and Health Act of 1970. This agency works through federal and state partnerships to inspect and enforce safety standards in the workplace. OSHA oversees numerous health and safety requirements within health care facilities. Examples of this oversight include bloodborne pathogen control programs, control of biological hazards, ergonomic health/safety issues, and chemical and radiological safety. It also is concerned with medical equipment, mechanical maintenance, food and laundry services, and housekeeping standards.

OSHA produces guidelines and reports that help hospitals and other care facilities meet state and national regulatory standards. OSHA personnel provide consultation services on health and safety issues, and they survey or inspect facilities if complaints are received regarding regulations under their jurisdiction. If facilities do not meet OSHA regulations, the organization can be fined or have its licensure affected (OSHA, 2006).

Fire and Life Safety Standards

Health care facilities must also meet fire and life safety standards and regulations. These regulations vary by state and community. Inspections are generally made on a routine basis by the fire marshal, or other appropriate officials, to check for building code compliance and the training of staff to respond to emergency situations. Inspections also occur whenever new regulations or standards are enacted, during construction and remodeling, or after any significant structural damage. Facilities must maintain compliance with regulations or be subject to evacuation of employees and patients and possibly closure of affected areas.

Infection and Disease Control

The **Centers for Disease Control and Prevention (CDC)** is an agency under the U.S. Department of Health and Human Services. This agency focuses on protecting the health and safety of people within and outside of health care environments. The CDC accomplishes this charge through the development and application of disease prevention and control, promotion of environmental health, and education. The CDC provides guidelines and alerts, which are communicated to health care organizations usually through the infection control department of a health agency. These communications are aimed at assisting organizations with policy development, screening of patients, and reporting requirements if specific diseases are detected. The CDC responds to significant outbreaks and threats to assist health care organizations in taking appropriate actions (CDC, 2006). Chapter 20 ⚭ provides a full discussion of infection control policies and procedures.

Professional Practice Oversight

Certain agencies oversee the practice of professionally licensed care providers. For example, there are professional licensing boards for physicians, nurses, pharmacists, and radiology and laboratory technicians. These boards will set the specific requirements for initial licensure, ongoing or continuing education hours and courses, the scope of practice for the particular discipline, and the disciplinary action processes should a professional act outside of the scope of practice or behavioral requirements.

The requirements may differ from state to state as to the curriculum and number of clinical hours required from educational programs and the acceptable scores for passing licensing examinations. Compliance with licensing standards is reviewed with the professional's periodic recertification or renewal of license and during surveys of the organization by regulatory and accreditation agencies. Professional practice oversight is discussed in more detail in Chapter 4 ⚭.

Accreditation

Accreditation is the process of evaluating actual care delivered to patients, performance of the hospital as an organization, and the outcomes of treatment for patients. The leading accreditation body for health care providers in the United States is the Joint Commission. The Joint Commission accredits about 80% of the nation's health care organizations, which includes hospitals, home health agencies, health care networks, ambulatory care facilities, long-term care facilities, behavioral health agencies, and clinical laboratories (Joint Commission, 2006).

The concept of accreditation for health care agencies dates back to 1910 when Ernest Codman, MD, proposed a process to evaluate the outcomes of ineffective treatments. He called this concept the "end result system of hospital standardization." Several years later the American College of Surgeons (ACS) adopted this methodology to develop minimum standards for hospitals, which included on-site surveys. In 1952 the ACS forwarded this responsibility to a new organization called the Joint Commission on Accreditation of Hospitals. This organization evolved during the next 30 years and transitioned to the current expanded form of the Joint Commission (Joint Commission, 2006).

An approved accrediting body must certify hospitals and other health care organizations that want to participate in the federal Medicare and state Medicaid programs. This requirement from the CMS is termed *conditions of participation.* Through the accreditation process, organizations must develop and maintain a quality assessment and performance improvement program. Organizations also must provide ongoing monitoring of key clinical indicators and be able to demonstrate assessment of the data and appropriate actions taken to improve results (*Federal Register*, 2003).

The Joint Commission generally conducts accreditation surveys every 3 years. Prior to 2004 these surveys were prescheduled and consisted of reviewing written material provided by the health care organization on policies, procedures, and data regarding compliance with standards, and a site inspection of the organization to look at current practice and retrospectively review past practice. Beginning in 2004 a new process was implemented using a "tracer" methodology, which is designed to monitor a specific patient through his or her hospitalization and evaluate policies along with the patient's interactions and experience with all services. In 2005 the survey process initiated unannounced survey visits (Joint Commission, 2006). Standards are organized into functions of the organization, which delineate specific criteria that must be met. Chart 3–6 outlines the functional areas for which the Joint Commission has developed standards.

Hospitals also are held to the Joint Commission patient safety standards and national indicators called *core measures.* Hospital-specific data regarding compliance with these criteria are incorporated into the survey process. Hospitals are required to collect data and report performance outcomes from sets of identified core measures. Examples of current core measures categories set by the Joint Commission include acute myocardial infarction, heart failure, community-acquired pneumonia, and pregnancy and related conditions. These core measures are part of the Joint Commission's initiative focusing on the integration of outcomes and performance measurement into the accreditation process (Joint Commission, 2006).

The Joint Commission also publishes sentinel event alerts that advise hospitals of process or system failures that have resulted in significant errors. **Sentinel events** are unexpected occurrences that have the potential to cause, or actually result in, death or serious physical or psychological injury. Serious injury specifically includes loss of limb or function. The hospital must review the sentinel event alerts, then address their own policies and procedures to be sure they have measures in place to reduce risk. Examples of recent alerts from the Joint Commission include prevention of fires in surgical areas, misadministration of concentrated potassium chloride, and prevention of ventilator-related infections and deaths. The alerts contain a root-cause analysis that defines actual causes of errors or events that threaten patient and staff safety. Risk reduction strategies are provided to assist hospitals with policy and procedure development to prevent error (Joint Commission, 2006).

Legal Aspects of Health Care

Having an understanding of the legal aspects of health care is important for the staff nurse's role of advocacy for patients and their families. Laws and regulations that guide practice and guard the rights of patients can be complex and change frequently. Nurse practice acts that define the scope of nursing responsibility and expectations for the delivery of care support the nurse's role in meeting legal requirements for communication with patients/families, reporting and recording of observations related to patients' conditions and their safety, and the limitations of practice for each discipline caring for the patient.

Nurses are held accountable for their performance within the scope of their practice. It is imperative that nurses be familiar with the policies and procedures of their organization and maintain competency as defined by those standards. Should a nurse fail to perform appropriately, the nurse could be held subject to malpractice or negligence claims. Health care organizations provide malpractice insurance to cover staff performing under the professional standards of those of the organization. It is generally recommended that professionals also carry personal malpractice insurance to cover any risks outside of their employment area. Chapter 4 ⬡ includes a discussion of the legal principles that guide nursing practice.

Nurses also have a role in the management of problems or risk in the health care environment. **Risk management** encompasses the identification of real or potential risks to employees, patients, and the public. Real or potential risks usually are formally identified through the use of incident or unusual occurrence reports. These reports are submitted by any individual who identifies a problem or risk. The forms used assist with gathering important data about the issue and help with follow-up investigation and resolution of the issue. Hospitals have formalized risk management programs that create comprehensive

CHART 3–6	**The Joint Commission's Hospital Standards**
Section	**Standards**
1. Patient-focused functions	• Ethics, rights, and responsibilities
	• Provision of care, treatment, and services
	• Medication management
	• Surveillance, prevention, and control of infection
2. Organization functions	• Improving organization performance
	• Leadership
	• Management of the environment of care
	• Management of human resources
	• Management of information
3. Structures with functions	• Medical staff
	• Nursing

Source: © Joint Commission Resources (2006). Hospital Accreditation Standards. Oakbrook Terrace, IL: Joint Commission on Accreditation of Healthcare Organizations. Available at http://www.jointcommission. Accessed October 21, 2006. Reprinted with permission.

plans for preventing risk and taking appropriate actions when adverse events take place. Risks to an organization can also be financial in nature related to business failures, property damage, and the resulting liability for negative patient outcomes (Grohar-Murray & DiCroce, 2003).

Advance Directives

Advance directives are instructions individuals can give, in advance of a health problem, to guide caregivers in the event the individuals are no longer able to speak for themselves. Advance directives were enhanced with the federal Patient Self-Determination Act of 1989, which was implemented in December 1991. This act requires that individuals under Medicare and Medicaid be provided with information about their rights to determine health care decisions. It was the intention of this legislation to increase the use of advance directives, thus improving appropriateness of care and ensuring the patient's right to make decisions (American Medical Association, 2006; Salmond & David, 2005).

With advancements in medical knowledge and technology, end-of-life decisions have become more and more complex. For patients who are considering making decisions regarding medical care, there are three possible goals: cure, stabilization of functioning, and preparing for a comfortable and dignified death. These goals may change over a person's lifetime depending on the status of the individual's health and age. Advance directives can be used at any time to establish a plan to meet goals regarding medical care. For example a young, healthy person may establish an advance directive to guide decisions should she suffer an irreversible condition following a catastrophic event. Another person who has been diagnosed with a potentially terminal disease may document choices about pain management, terminal care, or life-sustaining measures. Advance directives can be changed as the individuals needs and goals change. Chart 3–7 discusses the differences between the various types of advance directives.

Patient and Caregiver Issues and Concerns

The nurse should be aware of certain issues and concerns for patients establishing advance directives and the ability to have them carried out. First, not all health care professionals are comfortable or knowledgeable about advance directives and sometimes fail to discuss this aspect of care with the patient. The nurse should query patients regarding any discussions or decisions they may have made. If a patient has not dealt with this issue, it should be brought to the attention of the attending health care professionals. A lack of formal education, barriers to communication, or personal opinions may also interfere with the process. Not all patients wish to be fully informed about their diagnosis or condition. It may be helpful to determine the patient's preferences for receiving information (Keating, Nayeem, Gilmartin, & O'Keeffe, 2005). The patient or family can be given a referral to appropriate resources such as social services to aid them in understanding these issues.

Second, cultural or situational factors may influence an individual's decision about executing an advance directive. This seems to be more prevalent in the younger, healthy population than in the elderly or those dealing with disabilities or chronic illness (Rosnick & Reynolds, 2003). Although considerable information has been presented to the public about advance directives, a significant number of individuals have not followed

CHART 3–7	Types of Health Care Advance Directives
Type of Directive	**Key Points**
Health care advance directive	Documented instructions about your health care if you cannot speak for yourself. *Written:* Witnessed document, which requires the individual's signature and those of the witnesses. *Oral:* Instructions given to the individual's physician during the course of treatment, illness, or stay in a hospital. This directive is documented in the patient's medical record.
Living will	Formal written documents that communicate the wishes of the individual about life-sustaining medical treatments should she become terminally ill. They are dependent on the caregiver's willingness to follow the wishes stated and they may have no legal effect.
Health care power of attorney, durable health care power of attorney	Legal document that establishes a surrogate decision maker to make medical treatment decisions for the individual should he become incapacitated.
Do-not-resuscitate order	Organizations will usually have policies that describe resuscitation orders and options. These can be implemented by the patient surrogate or family telling the physician, by an advance directive, or by a durable power of attorney for health care.

Sources: Data from American Association of Colleges of Nursing. (2006). *Nursing shortage resource.* Retrieved December 15, 2006, from http://www.aacn.nche.edu; Healthguide. (2006). *Advance directives.* Retrieved October 21, 2006, from http://www.healthguide.org; Stein, J. (2003). The ethics of advance directives: A rehabilitation perspective. *American Journal of Physical Medicine and Rehabilitation, 82*(2), 152–157.

through to complete the process. For those dealing with disabilities or chronic illness, knowledge about treatments and alternatives is necessary before the individual can articulate appropriate choices, including the desire to have an advance directive. For example, an individual may need to choose among palliative care, aggressive chemotherapy, or refusing treatment altogether. In the latter case, an advance directive should be executed.

Third, the advance directive may not be present at the time it is needed due to an emergency situation, or the patient may not have given a copy of it to the health care provider. Patients should be encouraged to have documents readily available in their home to guide prehospital caregivers, such as emergency medical technicians (EMTs), should they respond to an emergency situation for the patient. The documentation contained within the patient's medical record and the placement of the advance directive in the record affect the ability of the physician and other caregivers to use the information at critical times (Williams & Haywood, 2003).

In some situations family members may disagree with the treatment plan and the patient's stated wishes. This can present an ethical dilemma for the nurse in advocating for the patient and assisting the family through appropriate decision making. At this point the nurse should seek consultation with the health care provider and an administrative representative of the organization regarding a plan of action.

If the patient is not able to advocate for himself, the case may need to be referred to social services or the appropriate committee within the organization for discussion and counsel. Bioethics or biomedical ethics involves obtaining relevant factual information, assessing its reliability, identifying moral problems, and recommending alternative solutions to problems that have been identified. In medicine this specifically relates to problems identified with making decisions about a patient's care and treatment. The bioethics process in most hospital organizations includes a committee or an ad hoc group that can quickly assemble to review a case and provide advice and counsel on a course of action. A case conference with the caregivers, family, and patient, if appropriate, can be called to discuss openly all of the facts. Nurses can be integral to this process because they may have firsthand knowledge of the patient's wishes or can offer information regarding the patient's present condition. Health care providers are obligated to follow an advance directive or the patient's wishes regarding care and treatment. If there is any doubt or conflict it should be referred to the appropriate authority for resolution (Williams & Haywood, 2003).

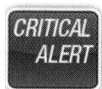

- *It is the nurse's responsibility to know the policies and procedures for identifying and referring a bioethical issue.*
- *The nurse must manage disputes regarding the patient's care and treatment plan and assist to diffuse situations that may be detrimental to the patient's immediate environment.*
- *The nurse should notify the health care provider and the organizational leadership when disputes arise.*
- *The nurse must be prepared to participate in conferences to discuss a case and advocate for the patient per her assessment and knowledge of the patient's wishes.*

Documentation and Legal Requirements

Health care directives are legal in all states, but the requirements for their content and authorization may differ. An advance directive has two parts: appointment of an agent or surrogate decision maker and specific instructions about care and treatment preferences. The patient has the option to complete either or both parts. Most states have legal forms and witnessing requirements. An advance directive can be canceled or changed at any time. If an advance directive is changed, all copies of the previous directive should be destroyed and replaced with the new ones to avoid confusion. In the acute care setting, the nurse has a key role in ensuring that documentation has been done regarding the presence of a directive, actions taken if no directive is available, and any ongoing issues regarding the status of the patient's wishes.

Nursing responsibilities include:

- *Query the patient regarding the existence of an advance directive.*
- *Document the existence in the medical record:*
  a. *If there is a prestanding directive from a previous admission, the nurse should query the patient regarding any changes and confirm the date of the directive.*
  b. *If the patient is submitting the document to a health care provider for the first time, it should be placed in the medical record per policy.*
  c. *If the patient has a directive, but did not bring it with him, it should be documented as such and efforts should be made to have the document brought in as soon as possible.*
- *If the patient wishes to make an oral directive, the health care provider should be notified.*
- *After discussion with the patient, the health care provider must document in the medical record the results of the discussion with the patient.*
- *If the patient does not have a directive, information should be given to the patient and, if appropriate, a referral made to a resource such as social services. The actions taken should be clearly documented in the medical record.*

Legal Aspects of Documentation

Documentation of patient care and interactions is important for many aspects of health care. For example, it provides a vehicle for communication between health care providers, promotes continuity of care, meets insurance requirements, ensures compliance with regulations, and helps create a health history for the patient. Clear documentation also assists with accurate coding of the patient's care and treatment process for appropriate billing and maximum reimbursement for the organization. Chapter 6 🔗 provides detailed information on nursing documentation.

Nursing documentation is critical from a legal perspective to describe the care the patient received and the actions taken by the caregivers. It is estimated that nurses spend 13% to 28% of their time on documentation (Clancy, Delany, Morrison, & Gunn, 2006). Studies have shown, however, that nursing documentation sometimes fails to provide a clear record due to the following reasons:

- Lack of understanding of the importance of documentation for medical and legal reasons
- Time constraints on care delivery and the time needed for documentation
- Discrepancies between observations and their interpretation from the patient's, nurse's, or other caregiver's perspectives.

Other documentation issues include the redundancy of information on multiple forms and the location of records in multiple places, inconsistent and irregular systems, and a lack of standardization in how information is written (Taylor, 2003).

Trends in Documentation

To address concerns with documentation, several initiatives have been advanced over time, including charting by exception, interdisciplinary assessment forms, and computerized documentation systems. These models or systems are aimed at saving nursing time and reducing redundancy in the patient's medical record.

One major trend in health care documentation is the implementation of clinical information systems. These systems allow documentation by multiple providers to be retrieved from a central database or repository. Information is consistent and readily available 24 hours a day, 7 days per week. Systems can also allow care to be summarized and trends in data to be detected over time. An additional benefit is the ability to conduct quality and outcome studies concurrently and retrospectively directly from the data repository (Doyle, 2006).

The Medical Record

The patient's medical record is a legal document that is the property of the institution providing care and services to the patient. Patients do, however, have a right to view and copy their records and enter their own information into them as they see fit. Care providers are legally required to compile and maintain an accurate record of a patient's care and treatment. This is important to guide ongoing care needs and to support decisions and actions taken should litigation occur.

Health care licensing agencies and accreditation bodies have established standards and requirements for adequacy and completeness of records as well as where they are stored and how long they must be kept. During health care organizational surveys to evaluate performance, the legibility, currency, and completeness of medical records are scrutinized (Wolper, 2004). The content and sequencing, or order, of medical records fall under general guidelines that are organization specific. Documentation or entries in the medical record should accurately reflect the care provided and any events that occur during the course of hospitalization or treatment.

- *The patient should be clearly identified on each record form or upon accessing the record electronically. This will prevent errors in charting that could lead to care decisions that may harm the patient.*
- *Observations should be objective and factual. Opinions regarding care or decisions are not appropriate for the legal record.*
- *Entries should be accurate and legible using only approved terms and abbreviations. It is essential that other caregivers be able to translate the information and for the caregiver to be able to accurately recall the information he has entered.*
- *Observations should be entered as close to the time they occurred as possible. This prevents loss of information and makes critical information available to others who may assume care of the patient.*
- *All entries should be authenticated with the name and title of the caregiver.*

Health Insurance Portability and Accountability Act

The **Health Insurance Portability and Accountability Act (HIPAA)** became law in 1996. The intent of this act was to improve health insurance portability and continuity of coverage for individuals. The three central goals of this law are (1) to create standards and a framework for health information, (2) to prevent inappropriate access to health information, and (3) to give patients control over their health information and how it is used.

In December 2001 the Administrative Simplification Compliance Act became law. Its goal is to add administrative efficiencies into the transmission of health information by standardizing electronic transactions. These laws affect almost every aspect of health care and have required organizations to make significant changes in the way they conduct business and provide patient care (Banks, 2006; Department of Health and Human Services [DHHS], 2006).

Impact of HIPAA Standards

Organizations must take the implementation of and compliance with HIPAA standards seriously. Penalties for noncompliance—whether intentional or unintentional—are assessed. Unintentional violations may result in fines of up to $25,000 for each incident. Intentional violations can result in imprisonment of up to 10 years and fines of $250,000 (HIPAAcomply, 2007).

The implementation of HIPAA impacts the delivery of nursing care in many ways. Nurses must be educated regarding the details of the regulations and the policies governing their specific health care organization. All health care providers are held individually responsible for preventing indiscriminate or unauthorized review or disclosure of personal information, medical or otherwise, from any source the patient has expressly prohibited. The guiding principle for caregivers is the "minimum necessary" rule, which means that the information disclosed will be only that which is minimally required for the specified purpose. Patients will be asked to make known their preferences about disclosure at the time of admission or when beginning a relationship with a health care provider (DHHS, 2006).

Case Management

Case management is an approach to coordinating care for patients in the hospital or in an outpatient setting. The Case Management Society of America (CMSA) defines case management as a collaborative process that assesses, plans, implements, coordinates, monitors, and evaluates the options and services required to meet an individual's health needs, using communication and available resources to promote quality, cost-effective outcomes. This occurs across a continuum of care and addresses ongoing individual needs (CMSA, 2006). Acute care hospitals generally have case management services that provide oversight and management of discharge planning, social services, and utilization review. Chart 3–8 provides an overview of key functions of the components of hospital-based case management.

CHART 3–8	**Components of Hospital-Based Case Management**
Component	**Key Functions**
Discharge planning	• Assess discharge needs.
	• Coordinate referrals.
	• Assign expected length of stay.
	• Evaluate progress toward discharge.
	• Provide consultation to the patient and family on placement alternatives if appropriate.
	• Arrange for health assistance or durable medical equipment and supplies as necessary.
Social services	• Assess referral needs.
	• Assist with application for aid if needed.
	• Provide links to financial counseling/consultation.
	• Evaluate discharge environment and caregiver support.
Utilization review	• Track length-of-stay data.
	• Review resources and services used.
	• Evaluate appropriate placement and level of care.

Sources: Centers for Medicare and Medicaid Services. (2006). *Programs, guidelines and regulations.* Retrieved December 15, 2006, from http://www.cms.gov; Cohen, E. L., & Cresta, T. (2004). *Nursing case management: From essentials to advanced practice applications* (4th ed.). St. Louis: Mosby; HCAB (2003b) *HMOs' impact on health care quality.*

Focus of Case Management in the Hospital

Hospital case managers focus on potential admissions for their appropriateness in the acute care setting and on length of stay (LOS). LOS is an important measure because it is an indicator of quality and risk, and many payers limit reimbursement by benchmarked standards for hospital stays. Many institutions have implemented case management in the emergency department to assist with determining appropriate placement of patients either to admit them to the hospital or transfer them to other hospitals or levels of care. A benefit of this approach is that potentially high-risk patients can be identified early and tracked for utilization of services and special referral needs (Bristow & Herrick, 2002). Case managers also work closely with physicians and other care providers to determine ongoing needs for the patient and potential modifications to their lifestyle and home environment after discharge. This includes identifying the need for caregivers to assist the patient at home and the ability of the patient's support system to provide needed care.

Staff Nurse Case Management Responsibilities

Case managers interface with the nursing staff to help assess discharge needs and to establish a plan for discharge. Discharge planning begins when the patient is admitted and continues to be evaluated throughout the patient's stay. The interface between the staff nurse providing direct care and the case manager is crucial in assessing the need for referral to specialty services and in determining financial concerns for ongoing care and progress toward the discharge goals.

Another form of case management is performed by or on the part of the payer source for patients' medical care. It is focused on continuity of care and **repatriation**, or the return of patients to appropriate levels of care or contracted institutions. Patients with long-term needs for care such as mental health services, chronic disease management, or rehabilitation are also assigned case managers who are agents of the payer source or a contracted service for the payer (Cohen & Cresta, 2004).

Case Management by Health Plans

Case review from these nonhospital-based managers may be accomplished by telephone from a central office or by on-site reviewers. The reviewers ensure that the patient's case is progressing as expected. If the patient is not progressing, the manager may authorize continued or additional care. If the reviewer determines that the patient no longer needs hospitalization at a specific level of care, he will issue a denial of payment for services (Wolper, 2004). The institution and the payer will work through these issues via a process of case review and appeals to determine a financial outcome.

Summary

It is evident from both historical and current perspectives that social and economic forces influence the types and availability of health care delivery systems. Consumers are not only vulnerable to these influences, but also are in a position to dictate and determine how the future of health care should be delivered. The new consumer-driven health care model that is emerging focuses on the quality of services as well as their costs. In developing new models of health care delivery, nurses will play a key role in determining how the future evolution of health care will meet the needs of a changing society.

REVIEW QUESTIONS

1. A nurse is planning the care for a patient using the best practice approach. Which of the following best describes this approach?
   1. It integrates current research evidence with clinical expertise and patient's needs.
   2. It is a proven process that produces consistent high quality results.
   3. It offers qualitative or quantitative measurement of specific data related to reported outcome information.
   4. It focuses on collecting data about medical errors and setting standards that will reduce errors.

2. A nurse is analyzing the revenue category of the annual budget. Which of the following is a component of this category?
   1. Salaries/wages
   2. Supplies
   3. Overhead
   4. Volume

3. When preparing to change a patient's dressing, the nurse has several choices for supplies. Which of the following would be the most cost effective choice for the nurse to make?
   1. Use some supplies that have already been charged to another patient.
   2. Select supplies that can be used over a period of time for less cost.
   3. Select the supplies the patient needs making sure there are supplies left over for the next dressing change.
   4. Create a dressing changing area within the patient's room that is fully stocked with multiple supply items so everyone can use the supplies at any time.

4. Individuals from an accrediting body arrive at a health care organization, requesting to conduct a "tracer" visit. The accrediting body is most likely:
   1. OSHA.
   2. The Joint Commission.
   3. The CDC.
   4. The state board of nursing.

5. A patient tells the nurse that he has a paper that says that his wife is supposed to make decisions about his health care if he becomes unable to do so himself. This patient is describing:
   1. Living will.
   2. Oral advance directive.
   3. Health care power of attorney.
   4. Written advance directive.

Answers for review questions appear in Appendix D

KEY TERMS

accreditation *p.58*
case management *p.62*
Centers for Disease Control and Prevention (CDC) *p.58*
Emergency Medical Treatment and Labor Act (EMTALA) *p.51*
evidence-based practice *p.52*
for-profit (proprietary) organization *p.51*
health care delivery system *p.45*
Health Insurance Portability and Accountability Act (HIPAA) *p.62*
health maintenance organization (HMO) *p.49*

horizontal organizational model *p.46*
hospitalist *p.55*
independent practice association (IPA) *p.49*
Institute of Medicine (IOM) *p.53*
Joint Commission *p.53*
Leapfrog Group *p.53*
licensure *p.57*
Medicaid *p.47*
Medicare *p.47*
not-for-profit organization *p.51*
Occupational Safety and Health Administration (OSHA) *p.58*
outcome standards *p.57*

preferred provider organization (PPO) *p.49*
process standards *p.57*
quality *p.56*
quality in fact *p.56*
quality in perception *p.56*
quality of care *p.56*
repatriation *p.63*
risk management *p.59*
robotics *p.54*
sentinel event *p.59*
structure standards *p.57*
telemedicine *p.54*
vertically integrated models *p.46*

PEARSON

EXPLORE **mynursingkit**™

MyNursingKit is your one stop for online chapter review materials and resources. Prepare for success with additional NCLEX®-style practice questions, interactive assignments and activities, web links, animations and videos, and more!

Register your access code from the front of your book at
www.mynursingkit.com

REFERENCES

Abramson, S. M., & Tyler, D. (2006). Margin alert: Time to revisit your outpatient strategy. *Healthcare Financial Management, 60*(4), 106–108, 110, 112–113.

American Association of Colleges of Nursing. (2006). *Nursing shortage resource.* Retrieved December 15, 2006, from http://www.aacn.nche.edu

American Hospital Association. (2006). *Healthcare consumer research.* Retrieved December 10, 2006, from http://www.aha.org

American Hospital Association. (2007). *Guide to the health care field—2007 edition* (page A3). Chicago: Author.

American Medical Association. (2006). *Resources/standards, policy statement on provision of life-sustaining medical treatment.* Retrieved December 15, 2006, from http://www.ama-assn.org

Amin, A. N., & Owen, M. M. (2006). Productive interdisciplinary team relationships: The hospitalist and the case manager. *Lippincott's Case Management, 11*(3), 160–164.

Baines, E. (2003, April 14). Pill-sized robot is reinventing endoscopy. *General Practitioner.*

Banks, D. L. (2006). The Health Insurance Portability and Accountability Act: Does it live up to the promise? *Journal of Medical Systems, 30*(1), 45–50.

Barber, J., Koch, K. E., Parente, K., Mark, J., Davis K. M. (1998). Evolution of an Integrated Health System: A Life Cycle Framework. *Journal of Healthcare Management, 43*(4), 361–375.

Bristow, D. P., & Herrick, C. A. (2002). Emergency department case management: The dyad team of nurse case manager and social worker improve discharge planning and patient and staff satisfaction while decreasing inappropriate admissions and costs: A literature review. *Lippincott's Case Management, 7*(6), 243–251.

Buerhaus, P. I., Donelan, K., Ulrich, B. T., Norman, L., Williams, M., & Dittus, R. (2005). Hospital RNs' and CNOs' perceptions of the impact of the nursing shortage on the quality of care. *Nursing Economics, 23*(5), 214–221.

California HealthCare Foundation. (2004). *Preventing unnecessary hospitalizations in Medi-Cal: Comparing fee-for-service with managed care.* Retrieved February 13, 2007 from University of California San Francisco's Primary Care Research website: http://www.chef.org/topics/medi-cal

Case Management Society of America. (2006). *What is case management?* Retrieved February 13, 2007, from http://www.cmsa.org

Centers for Disease Control and Prevention. (2006). *Guidelines and alerts.* Retrieved December 15, 2006, from http://www.cdc.gov

Centers for Medicare and Medicaid Services. (2006). *Programs, guidelines and regulations.* Retrieved December 15, 2006, from http://www.cms.gov

Centers for Medicare and Medicaid Services. (2007). *Brief summaries of Medicare*Medicaid, Title XVIII and Title XIX of the Social Security Act as of November 1, 2007.* Retrieved January 23, 2008, from http://search.cms.hhs.gov/search?q=Expenditures+2002+reference&site=cms_collection&…

Chandra, A., & Frank, Z. D. (2003). Use of robotics in health procedures—Are we ready for it? *Hospital Topics, 81*(1).

Clancy, T. R., Delany, C. W., Morrison, B., & Gunn, J. K. (2006). The benefits of standardized nursing languages in complex adaptive systems such as hospitals. *Journal of Nursing Administration, 36*(9), 426–434.

Cohen, E. L., & Cresta, T. (2004). *Nursing case management: From essentials to advanced practice applications* (4th ed.). St. Louis: Mosby.

Cowan, M. J., Shapiro, M., Hays, R. D., Afifi, A., Vazirani, S., Ward, C. R., et al. (2006). The effect of a multidisciplinary hospitalist/physician and advance practice nurse collaboration on hospital costs. *Journal of Nursing Administration, 36*(2), 79–85.

Darzi, A., & Mackay, S. (2002). Recent advances in minimal access surgery. *British Medical Journal, 324*(7328).

Donabedian, A. (1980). *Explanations in quality assessment and monitoring: The definition of quality and approaches to its assessment* (Vol. 1). Ann Arbor, MI: Health Administration Press.

Dower, C. (2002). *Status of changes in patient care delivery: How can we meet demand for health care workers?* San Francisco: The Center for the Health Professions, University of California, San Francisco.

Doyle, M. (2006). Promoting standardized nursing language using an electronic medical record system. *AORN Journal, 83*(6), 1336–1342.

Federal Register. (2003). Medicare and Medicaid programs; hospital conditions of participation: Quality assessment and performance improvement final rule. *68*(16), 3435–3455.

Finkler, S. A., & Kovner, C. T. (2000). *Financial management for nurse managers and executives.* Philadelphia: W. B. Saunders.

Freed, D. H. (2004). Hospitalists: Evolution, evidence, and eventualities. *Health Care Management, 23*(3), 238–256.

Fuchs, K. H. (2002). Minimally invasive surgery. *Endoscopy, 3*(42), 154–159.

Fuchs, R. J., Berenholtz, S. M., & Dorman, T. (2005). Do intensivists in ICU improve outcomes? *Best Practice and Research. Clinical Anaesthesiology, 19*(1), 125–135.

Grohar-Murray, M. E., & DiCroce, H. R. (2003). *Leadership and management in nursing.* Upper Saddle River, NJ: Pearson Prentice Hall.

Halamka, J. (2006). The perfect storm for electronic health records. *Journal of Healthcare Information Management, 20*(3), 25–27.

Harris, C. M., Burns, J., Gregorich, T., Kall, G., Piar, P. M., Miller, H. D., et al. (2003). Managing technology in a complex healthcare delivery system. *Journal of Healthcare Information Management, 17*(2), 37–41.

Harrison, J. P., & Palacio, C. (2006). The role of clinical information systems in health care quality improvement. *Health Care Management, 25*(3), 206–212.

Health Care Advisory Board. (2003b, March 25). *HMOs' impact on health care quality* (pp. 1–4).

Health Care Advisory Board. (2003c, July 9). *Rising costs place financial burden on patients and employers.*

Health Resources and Services Administration. (2006). *What is behind HRSA's projected supply, demand, and shortage of registered nurses?* Retrieved December 15, 2006, from http://hrsa.gov

Heinzelmann, P. J., Lugn, N. E., & Kvedar, J. C. (2005). Telemedicine in the future. *Journal of Telemedicine and Telecare, 11*(8), 384–390.

HIPAAcomply. (2007). *HIPAA FAQs.* Retrieved February 13, 2007, from http://www.hipaacomply.com

Hsu, E. B., Thomas, T. L., Bass, E. B., Whyne, D., Kelen, G. D., & Green, G. B. (2006, March 20). Healthcare worker competencies for disaster training. *Biomedical Central Medical Education,* pp. 6–19.

Huber, D. (2006). *Leadership and nursing care management* (3rd ed.). Philadelphia: W. B. Saunders.

Human Genome Project. (2008). Frequently Asked Questions. Retrieved April 26, 2008, from http://www.ornl.gov

Institute of Medicine. (1999). *To err is human: Building a safer health system.* Retrieved October 21, 2006, from http://www.iom.edu

Joint Commission on Accreditation of Healthcare Organizations. (2006). *Hospital accreditation standards.* Retrieved October 21, 2006, from http://www.jointcommission

Joint Commission on Accreditation of Healthcare Organizations. (2007). *Setting the standard.* Oakbrook Terrace, IL: Author.

Keating, D. T., Nayeem, K., Gilmartin, J. J., & O'Keeffe, S. T. (2005). Advance directives for truth disclosure. *Chest, 128*(2), 1037–1039.

Leapfrog Group. (2006). *Patient safety initiatives.* Retrieved October 21, 2006, from http://www.leapfroggroup.org

Malloch, K., & Porter-O'Grady, T. (2006). *Introduction to evidence-based practice in nursing and healthcare.* Sudbury, MA: Jones and Bartlett.

Marketing Health Services. (2003). *Robots to the Rescue,* Summer 2003: 23(2).

Marquis, B. L., & Huston, C. J. (2007). *Leadership roles and management functions in nursing theory & application* (5th ed.). Philadelphia: Lippincott Williams & Wilkins.

Medem Medical Library. (2006). *Gene therapy.* Retrieved December 15, 2006, from http://medem.com

McKinley, A. (2005, December 31). Health care providers and facilities: Health facilities—2005 (End of year issue brief). *Issue Brief Health Policy Tracking Service,* pp. 1–10.

Nathans, A. B., Rivara, F. P., Mackenzie, E. J., Maier, R. V., Wang, J., Egleston, B., et al. (2006). The impact of an intensivist-model ICU on trauma-related mortality. *Annals of Surgery, 244*(4), 545–554.

National Committee for Quality Assurance. (2006). *Measurement improves healthcare quality for 70 million American's, but gaps remain.* Retrieved November 2, 2006, from http://ncqa.org

National Quality Forum. (2006). *Health care quality measurement and reporting.* Retrieved October 21, 2006, from http://www.qualityforum.org

Occupational Safety and Health Administration. (2006). *Safety and health regulations and guidelines.* Retrieved December 15, 2006, from http://www.osha.gov

Richard, S. A., Rawal, S., & Martin, D. K. (2005). An ethical framework for cardiac report cards: A qualitative study. *BioMedical Central Medical Ethics, 28*(6), E3.

Robinson, T. N., & Stiegmann, G. V. (2004). Minimally invasive surgery. *Endoscopy, 36*(1), 48–50.

Rosenbaum, S. (1998). Negotiating the new health system: Purchasing publicly accountable managed care. *American Journal of Preventive Medicine, 14*(3S), 67–71.

Rosnick, C. B., & Reynolds, S. L. (2003). Thinking ahead: Factors associated with executing advance directives. *Journal of Aging and Health, 15*(2), 409–429.

Salmond, S. W., & David, E. (2005). Attitudes toward advance directives and advance directives completion rates. *Orthopaedic Nursing, 24*(2), 117–127.

Samuel, T. W., Raleigh, S. G., Hower, J. M., & Schwartz, R. W. (2003). The next stage in the health care economy: Aligning the interests of patients, providers, and third-party payers through consumer driven health care plans. *American Journal of Surgery, 186*(2),117–124.

Satava, R. M. (2004). Future trends in the design and application of surgical robots. *Seminars in Laparoscopic Surgery, 11*(2),129–135.

Scalise, D. (2005). Building a consumer-directed service culture. *Hospitals and Health Networks, 79*(12), 53–59.

Shortell, S., & Kaluzny, A. D. (2005). *Health care management: Organization design and behavior* (5th ed.). Clifton Park, NY: Delmar Cengage Learning.

Sullivan, E. J., & Decker, P. J. (2005). *Effective leadership & management in nursing* (6th ed.). Upper Saddle River, NJ: Pearson Prentice Hall.

Taylor, H. (2003). An exploration of the factors that affect nurses' record keeping. *British Journal of Nursing, 12*(12), 751–754, 756–758.

U.S. Census Bureau. (2002). *National population projections summary tables.* Retrieved May 19, 2004, from http://www.census.gov/population/www/projections/natproj.html

U.S. Department of Health and Human Services. (2006). *Medical privacy—National standards to protect the privacy of personal health information.* Retrieved December 15, 2006, from http://www.hhs.gov

Werner, R. M., & Asch, D. A. (2005). The unintended consequences of publicly reporting quality information. *Journal of the American Medical Association, 293*(10), 1239–1244.

Williams, M. A., & Haywood, C., Jr. (2003). Critical care research on patients with advance directives or do-not-resuscitate status: Ethical challenges of clinician-investigators. *Critical Care Medicine, 31*(3), 167–171.

Wolper, L. F. (2004). *Health care administration: Planning, implementing, and managing organized delivery systems* (4th ed.). Sudbury, MA: Jones and Bartlett.

Woolf, S. H., Johnson, R. E., & Geiger, H. J. (2006, October 31). The rising prevalence of severe poverty in America, a growing threat to public health. *American Journal of Preventive Medicine,* No. 4, pp. 332–341.

Zinkovich, L., Malvey, D., Hamby, E., & Fottler, M. (2005). Bioterror events: Preemptive strategies for healthcare executives. *Hospital Topics, 83*(3), 9–15.

Ethical and Legal Guidelines for Nursing Practice

Ginny Wacker Guido and Annita Watson

Outcome-Based Learning Objectives

After studying this chapter, the learner will be able to:

1. Explain how ethical theories and principles influence nursing practice in a clinical setting.
2. Identify and apply the steps of the MORAL model in ethical decision making.
3. Compare and contrast the three distinct structures that ethics committees demonstrate in health care institutions.
4. Explain how the state nurse practice act governs and guides nursing practice.
5. Distinguish among the types of laws that typically affect nursing practice: common, civil, tort, contract, and criminal.
6. Identify the six elements of malpractice law as described in the chapter.
7. Discuss the importance of standards of care and how they are differentiated between internal and external standards.
8. Distinguish between regional and national norms.
9. Identify the three most common intentional torts and three most common quasi-intentional torts seen in health care settings and explain the defenses against them.
10. Explain the doctrine of informed consent as it relates to the use of implied consent in nursing settings.
11. Explain actions that the nurse may take to avoid or prevent possible liabilities.

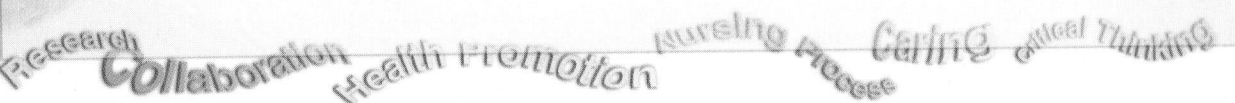

Research   Collaboration   Health Promotion   Nursing Process   Caring   Critical Thinking

---

THIS CHAPTER highlights the continuing influence that ethical and legal concepts have on the professional practice of nursing. Professional accountability and responsibility continue to gather additional prominence, especially as nurses become more autonomous and practice settings expand from acute care facilities to community, ambulatory, and long-term settings and as consumers of health care become more knowledgeable about their rights and options for care.

It is not sufficient, though, to know and understand ethical and legal concepts. Nurses must blend these important aspects with competent, skilled nursing diagnoses and interventions. To perform this high-quality nursing care, nurses must also understand the concepts of critical thinking and clinical judgment, for without these latter concepts one is not able to fully appreciate the application of legal and ethical concepts in professional practice settings. Thus, this chapter first explores ethics and legal concepts and issues that impact professional nursing practice and concludes with a section on critical thinking and clinical judgment. Knowing about and using these concepts and issues moves nursing from merely a "hands-on" skills performance role to that of a truly professional practice.

Ethics and Nursing

Ethics is the science relating to moral actions and individual value systems. It is the systematic study of what a person's conduct and actions ought to be with regard to self, other human beings, and the environment. Many nurses envision ethics as dealing with principles of morality and what is right or wrong (Yoder-Wise, 2007). Applied ethics requires application of normative ethical theory to everyday problems. Normative ethical theory for each profession provides the foundation and filter from which ethical decisions are made (Marquis & Huston, 2006). Thus, from a nursing perspective, a broader conceptual definition of ethics is that ethics is concerned with motives and attitudes and the relationship of these attitudes to the overall care of the individual. It is the justification of what is right or wrong, and the study of what one's life and relationships ought to be, not what they are (Marquis & Huston, 2006).

Morality concerns the social nature of the community, codes of behavior, and community expectations (Hall, 2000; Perle, 2004). Morality provides the means for ascertaining if certain actions are right or wrong and whether the consequences of actions are good or bad. Thus, morals are ways of behaving to accomplish ethical practices. Ethics is the broader, more reflective endeavor and begins when a person goes beyond the acceptance and internalization of traditional rules, or normative behaviors, of the social group. The ultimate goal of ethics is to provide a reasoned and best solution to situations that arise in everyday clinical practice.

As a beginning step in the application of ethics to everyday clinical practice, nurses should first determine the essential or underlying issue. Does the issue concern a situation that the patient or the patient's family views as wrong, such as the discontinuance of nonextraordinary life-support measures? For many, the removal of a feeding tube that is delivering to the patient essential fluids and nutritional support would be considered a violation of a moral duty. Or does the issue involve a treatment or therapy that could or could not be instituted, such as whether to initiate full life-support measures in a geriatric patient who is terminally ill?

The implementation of ethics is internal to one's self, looks to the good of an individual rather than society as a whole, and concerns the "why" of one's actions. Ethics asks questions about motives and actions. Why did the person act as she did and what was the final outcome of acting as she did? Was the outcome satisfactory to the individual?

Ethical Theories

Many different ethical theories have evolved to justify existing moral principles. These theories are considered normative because they describe the norms or standards of behavior and value that are ultimately applied to daily life. Normative ethics concerns human actions and the outcomes of those actions. Most normative approaches to ethics fall under the three broad theoretical categories discussed next.

Deontological Theories

Deontological (from the Greek *deon*, or "duty") **theories** derive norms and rules from the duties human beings owe to one another by virtue of commitments made and roles assumed. Generally, deontologists hold that a sense of duty consists of rational respect for the fulfilling of one's obligations to other human beings, rather than looking at the rewards of one's actions. The greatest strength of this theory is its emphasis on the dignity of human beings. Deontological theory looks not to the end or consequences of an action, but to the intention of the action. It is one's good intentions, the intentions to do a moral duty that ultimately determine the praiseworthiness of the action.

Duty-based, rights-based, and intuitionist ethical reasoning derive their framework from deontological theory. Deontological ethics have sometimes been subdivided into situation or "love" ethics, wherein the decision making takes into account the unique characteristics of each individual, the caring relationship between the person and the caregiver, and the most humanistic course of action given the circumstances (Butts & Rich, 2005). Examples of this theory in action in the health care setting abound when making these types of decisions:

- Decisions about forgoing life-sustaining treatment that may conflict with religious beliefs

- Decisions not to pursue aggressive treatment while waiting to see what outcome God wants or trusting that conservative treatment will work if God so intends

- Decisions to bow to a higher order, given by divine command, such as in the case of Jehovah's Witnesses, who do not ingest blood and, therefore, refuse blood transfusions even if they will lose their lives or the lives of their children (DeWolf-Bosek & Savage, 2007).

Teleological Theories

Teleological (from the Greek *telos*, for "end") **theories** derive norms or rules for conduct from the consequences of actions. Right consists of actions that have good consequences, and wrong consists of actions that have bad consequences. Teleologists disagree, though, about how to determine the goodness or badness of the consequences of actions. Teleological theories support decisions that favor the common good. An alternate way of viewing this theory is that the usefulness of an action is determined by the amount of happiness it brings. An example of a decision using this approach is that of allowing individual family members to make the difficult choices for their loved ones rather than mandating that all patients in persistent vegetative states must be given parenteral nutrition.

This theory frequently is referred to as utilitarianism; what makes an action right or wrong is its utility, and useful actions bring the greatest amount of happiness and satisfaction into existence (Butts & Rich, 2005). Teleological theories are used to support utilitarianism. Utilitarian ethics can be subdivided into rule and act utilitarianism. Rule utilitarianism seeks the greatest happiness for all; it appeals to public agreement as a basis for objective judgment about the nature of happiness. Act utilitarianism tries to determine in a particular situation which course of action will bring about the greatest happiness, or the least harm and suffering, to a single person. As such, act utilitarianism makes happiness subjective, basing decisions on what is the best for the greatest number of people (Guido, 2006; Marquis & Huston, 2006).

Principlism

A third ethical theory has slowly been evolving over the past 25 years and, although not yet given the full status of a theory, it does assist nurses and health care providers who are struggling with difficult ethical issues. Called **principlism**, this emerging theory incorporates existing ethical principles and attempts to resolve conflicts by applying one or more of those ethical principles (Beauchamp & Childress, 2001). Ethical principles actually control ethical decision making much more than do ethical theories, since principles encompass the basic premises from which rules are developed. Principles are moral norms that nurses demand and strive to implement daily in clinical settings. In the case of principlism, four principles form the basis for decision making: respect for autonomy, nonmaleficence, beneficence, and justice. Each of the principles can be used individually, although it is much more common to encounter two or more ethical principles used in concert or to see two or more principles coming into conflict in a specific patient situation.

Ethical theories are important because they form the essential base of knowledge from which to proceed. Without ethical theories, decisions revolve around personal emotions. Because most health care providers do not ascribe to either deontology or teleology exclusively, principlism is growing in popularity among health care professionals in today's society.

Ethical Principles

There are eight ethical principles that nurses encounter when making decisions in clinical settings. Chart 4–1 outlines these principles and gives a short definition for each principle.

Autonomy

The principle of **autonomy** addresses personal freedom and the right to choose what will happen to one's own person. The legal doctrine of informed consent is a direct reflection of this principle. Autonomy involves health care deliverers' respect for patients' rights even if the health care deliverer does not agree with the decisions made. For example, autonomy issues often arise when parents of young children refuse immunizations. Most health care deliverers would advocate for their need in preventing possible complications should the child later be exposed to what could have been a preventable disease.

Beneficence

The principle of **beneficence** states that the actions a person takes should promote good. In caring for patients, good can be defined in many ways, including allowing a person to die without advanced life support and in the company of loved ones. Good may prompt the nurse to encourage the patient to undergo extensive, painful treatment procedures especially if these procedures will increase both the quality and quantity of life. Good also may extend to the patient's family by prompting family members to leave a patient's bedside so that they can get some needed rest.

Nonmaleficence

The corollary of beneficence, the principle of **nonmaleficence**, states that a person should do no harm. Many nurses find it difficult to follow this principle when performing treatments and procedures that bring discomfort and pain to patients. Health care providers often use the concept of a detrimental-benefit analysis when the issue of nonmaleficence is raised. Using this analysis, the focus of the projected treatment or procedure is on the consequences of the benefits to the patient and not on the harm that occurs at the time of the intervention. For example, the nurse may use this analysis when medicating a postoperative patient. Even though the injection causes some level of discomfort and suffering, the overall benefit is less postoperative pain. A second example is the need to change and reapply dressings for patients who have sustained severe burns. Though extremely painful, not performing this needed intervention would cause more serious complications for the patient. Thus, the principle of nonmaleficence may be chosen because even pain and suffering can bring about a desirable outcome for the patient.

Veracity

Veracity concerns truth telling and incorporates the concept that individuals should always tell the truth. This principle also compels that the truth be told completely. Nurses and other health care providers exemplify this principle when they give all of the facts of a situation truthfully and then assist patients and their loved ones to make appropriate decisions. For example, patients must be told of all options in terms that they can understand and then be allowed to make their own decisions.

The principle of veracity compels health care members to fully inform patients about all aspects of care, both the desirable effects as well as the more negative effects. Without the entire truth, patients cannot make informed choices. This also is true of nursing management. For instance, a manager who believes deception is morally acceptable if it is done with the objective of beneficence may tell all rejected job applicants that they were highly considered, whether they had been or not. Another management example is that of the nurse manager who, in the event of a low patient census (i.e., a slow period on a unit), relays all of the options to staff and lets them make their own decisions about floating to other units, taking vacation time, or taking a day without pay, contingent on agency policy.

Justice

Justice concerns the issue that persons should be treated equally and fairly. This principle usually arises in times of short supplies or when there is competition for resources or benefits. This principle most often is considered when patient census is high and two patients are equally qualified to be cared for in a specific unit, such as an intensive care or cardiac care unit, or when there is an organ available for transplantation and two patients are equally appropriate candidates for the organ transplant.

Justice also demands that the same quality of care be given to all patients, regardless of their ethnicity, socio-economic status, or lifestyle. Thus, the health care team must be vigilant concerning decisions that are made about why one candidate would be the more appropriate recipient of an available transplant organ and how the care of the second potential recipient will be delivered. Acceptable reasons for selecting one candidate over a second potential recipient could be compliance with recommended therapies and the supportive role of family members.

Paternalism

The principle of **paternalism** sometimes referred to as parentialism, allows one to make decisions for another and often has been viewed as a negative or undesirable principle. Used appropriately, however, paternalism assists persons to make decisions when they do not have sufficient data or expertise to make a decision. Staff members frequently use some degree of paternalism when they assist patients and their family members to decide if surgical procedures should be undertaken or if medical management is a better option. Paternalism becomes undesirable when the entire decision is taken from the patient or family member.

CHART 4–1	**Ethical Principles**

Principle	Definition
Autonomy	Personal freedom, right of self-determination
Beneficence	Duty to perform good actions
Nonmaleficence	Duty to prevent harm from occurring
Veracity	Truth-telling
Justice	Fairness, treating all equally
Paternalism	Allows another to make decisions for individual patients
Fidelity	Duty to keep one's promises and commitments
Respect for others	Duty to treat all respectfully and without prejudice

Fidelity

Fidelity means keeping one's promises or commitments. Staff members know not to make promises to patients that they may not be able to keep, such as assuring the patient that no code will be performed before consulting with the patient's physician for such an order or that the patient will be able to return home at a specific time frame. Fidelity also prevents health care deliverers from promising that the patient will be given sufficient pain medication after a surgical procedure so that the patient is totally pain free. Rather, nurses reinforce that such freedom from pain is a goal that the health care team will work to achieve.

Hamric (2002) suggests that it is helpful to view the "nurse in the middle" phenomenon from a fidelity perspective. Although nurses have multiple fidelity duties to the patient, physician organization, profession, and self that at times may conflict with one another, the American Nurses Association (ANA) Code of Ethics is clear than one duty "dominates" over all others, namely, the nurse's commitment to the patient.

Respect for Others

Many think the principle of **respect for others** is the highest principle and incorporates all other principles. Respect for others acknowledges the right of individuals to make decisions and to live by these decisions. Respect for others also transcends cultural differences, gender issues, and racial concerns. Nurses positively reinforce this principle daily when giving competent nursing care to all patients for whom they care. Nurses also reinforce these principles when they incorporate Watson's (2003) theory of caring into their interactions with patients and peers. For example, caring for a very demanding, verbally abusive patient is difficult, and nurses might elect not to be as attentive to her needs as a patient who is pleasant and cooperative. The principle of respect for others, however, demands that appropriate and competent care be given to both patients.

Ethical Decision Making

In clinical practice, ethical principles differ among the individuals involved in patient care settings. Frequently, the ethical principles and values of family members differ from patients' values or from health care providers' values. For example, an elderly, but independent patient may value his independence and ability to remain in an independent living situation (autonomy), whereas his fam-

ily and the staff caring for him may feel that he needs closer supervision and desire that the patient be relocated to an assisted living center (beneficence). Resolving such issues is the goal of understanding ethical dilemmas and ethical decision making.

Ethical Dilemma

When such disagreements occur, an ethical dilemma emerges. **Ethical dilemmas** by definition involve two or more unfavorable alternatives to a given situation. For example, in the preceding scenario, the elderly gentleman may be at risk for injury when living by himself at his home, but his ability to be independent will be hampered by living at an assisted living center. One means of addressing such situations is to use ethical decision-making models. **Ethical decision making** involves asking the following questions:

1. Who should make the choices?
2. What are the possible options or courses of action?
3. What are the available and reasonable alternatives?
4. What are the consequences, both positive and negative, of all possible options?
5. Which rules, obligations, and values should direct the choices?
6. What are the desired goals and outcomes in the given situation?

When making decisions, health care providers must use an orderly, systematic, and objective method to find the best solution. Various ethical decision-making models are available to assist with ethical decision making. These models are based on a process of steps and vary from 5 to 20 steps, depending on the specific model. The decision maker moves from step to step in an attempt to decide the best course of action given the specifics of the situation. Perhaps one of the easiest ethical decision-making models to use in clinical settings is the **MORAL model** (Thiroux, 1977). The MORAL model was developed by Thiroux (1977) and then subsequently, applied to nursing situations. Since that time, the MORAL model has been further refined and utilized by Crisham (1990). The MORAL model of decision making is shown in Chart 4–2.

Ethical decision making is always a process and the steps of the process remain fluid and flexible. As health care providers

CHART 4–2	**MORAL Model of Ethical Decision Making**	

The letters of the acronym remind users of the steps of the model

Acronym Request	Example	
M	Massage the dilemma.	Issues are identified and defined, taking into consideration the value systems and principles of all major players in the dilemma.
O	Outline the options.	Options are fully examined, including those that are less realistic.
R	Resolve the dilemma.	Issues and options are reviewed and basic ethical principles are applied to each of the identified options. A decision is made concerning the plan of action that will be taken.
A	Act by applying the chosen option.	Requires implementation by all members of the health care team and family members.
L	Look back and evaluate.	Process of reviewing and reexamining whether desired outcomes were attained and whether new options need to be implemented.

move through any model's various steps, they may find that they need to return to a previous step and redefine the issue or that a major player's values were not taken into consideration when making the final decision. Sufficient time must be allowed for making decisions so that all players in the dilemma reach a conclusion that they can support.

Accountability and responsibility for making ethical decisions varies depending on the dilemma encountered. For the ethical decisions that must be addressed on a daily basis, such as helping family members understand the full extent of their loved one's prognosis or assisting a patient with understanding why a nurse cannot give more pain medication when the patient continues to have pain, the nurses working directly with the patients are generally responsible for these ethical dilemmas. For issues that involve the entire health care team, such as assisting family members to determine if a feeding tube should be placed for nutritional support in an elderly patient who is terminal, the hospital ethics committee is generally responsible for making such decisions.

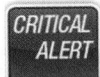 *It is not uncommon in the practice of nursing to encounter situations in which a patient and family members must make decisions about lifesaving measures: Should they or should they not be used? The resulting conflict may compromise how nurses choose to provide care to the patient/family and how that care is rendered, keeping in mind that the nurse has an ethical duty to provide the minimum standard of care. It is essential that nurses know what resources are available to them in the agency where they work to help them solve this dilemma and meet the normal standard of care for the given situation.*

Ethics Committees

With the increasing complexity of ethical issues in health care, ethics committees have been created to assist in making ethical decisions in clinical settings. Ethical committees can:

1. Provide structure and guidelines for potential problems.
2. Serve as an open forum for discussion and debate.
3. Function as a patient advocate by placing the patient at the core of the committee's deliberations.

Committee Structures

Ethics committees generally follow one of three distinct structures, though in some institutions these structures are blended. The autonomy model facilitates decision making for the competent patient. The patient benefit model uses **substituted judgment** (what the person would have done if she were capable of making a decision) and facilitates decision making for the incompetent patient. The social justice model considers broad social issues that may arise within the institution; in this model, many ethics committees hold ethical grand rounds.

Ethical grand rounds usually are conducted on a monthly basis and allow staff members to begin to be more involved in ethical decision making by presenting cases that involve a variety of ethical issues. The purpose of ethical grand rounds is to assist health care providers with future ethical decision making by making them more knowledgeable about ethical principles and the MORAL model. For example, presenting the case of the elderly gentleman who desires to remain in his own home rather than move to an assisted living center helps nurses to fully ex-

amine both sides of the issue. The nurses are then able to more quickly and competently address this same type of issue in the future. Such case presentations also allow nurses to become more fully versed on both sides of controversies and better understand their own ethical values and principles.

■ Legal Concepts in Nursing

Legal concepts are equally important as ethics concepts in forming a framework for practice in health care settings. A general definition of **law** is that it concerns rules and regulations by which a society is governed. These rules and regulations are made by individuals and are capable of being changed or modified. Legal issues differ from ethical issues in that laws are external to the individual because they entail the rules and regulations of society as a whole, and laws are concerned with one's conduct and actions as opposed to the motives and values of the individual. The question asked is "What did the person do or fail to do?" rather than "Why did the person act as he did?" Finally, the enforcement of laws is much stronger that enforcement of ethics; laws are enforced through courts of law, statutes, and state boards of nursing.

Sources of Law

The most basic source of law is constitutional law, which is a system of fundamental laws or principles for the governance of a nation, society, or other aggregate of individuals. Statutory laws are those rules and regulations enacted by the legislative branch of the government. Nurses are usually familiar with this source of law because the nurse practice act is an example of statutory law. Administrative laws are enacted through the decisions and rules of administrative agencies, which are specific governing bodies charged with implementing selected legislation. When statutory laws are enacted, administrative agencies are given the authority to implement the specific intentions of the statutes, creating rules and regulations that enforce the statutory law. Boards of nursing are examples of administrative law agencies. Finally, judicial laws are created by courts of law, interpreting legal issues that are in dispute.

All laws, regardless of origin, are subject to change. Constitutional laws may be amended; statutory laws may be amended, repealed, or expanded; administrative agencies may be dissolved, expanded, or redefined; and judicial laws may be modified or completely altered by subsequent court decisions.

Nurse Practice Acts

An example of statutory and administrative law is the state nurse practice act. The state **nurse practice act** is the single most important piece of legislation for nursing because the practice act affects all aspects of nursing practice. The act defines nurses' **scope of practice**, those actions and duties that are allowable by a profession, and establishes standards for nurses in a given state or territory. Requirements for licensure and entry into practice, empowerment of a board of nursing to oversee practice, and means for disciplinary action are part of the nurse practice act. The act is the law within the state or territory, and state boards of nursing cannot grant exceptions, waive the act's provisions, or expand practice outside the act's specific provisions.

Nurse practice acts typically define three categories of nurses: licensed practical or vocational nurses, licensed registered nurses, and advanced practice nurses. The nurse practice act, in concert with common law, sets educational and examination requirements, provides for licensing by individuals who have met these requirements, defines the functions of each category of nurse, and may include a section on mandatory continuing education hours for renewal of licenses. Additionally, nurse practice acts state any exceptions that may occur, such as that nursing students may function in clinical settings as an exception to required licensure. The state nurse practice act also may include help for those affected by addiction, for example, diversion programs for registered nurses with drug and alcohol and mental illness problems. Many acts also provide assistance for nurses undergoing rehabilitation for a chemical dependency.

Individual differences in nurse practice acts among states are seen. For instance, some states have separate acts for licensed practical or vocational nurses and some states do not define advanced practice roles. Five states have separate boards for the licensing of practical or vocational nurses and registered nurses: California, Georgia, Louisiana, Texas, and West Virginia.

Each state practice act establishes a board of nursing. This board ensures enforcement of the act, regulation of those who come under its provisions and prevention of those not addressed by the act from practicing nursing, and protection of the public. Qualifications for board members, terms of office, and specific duties of board members are defined in the state practice act.

Although the nurse practice act is a statutory law, judicial law may become involved in its application. The application of judicial law actually helps define the meaning of the act for practicing nurses. In selected court decisions, the interpretation of the nurse practice act has assisted nurses in understanding the full application of the law. For example, landmark court cases in 1983 upheld the right of nurses to practice as advanced nurse practitioners (*Sermchief v. Gonzales*) and in 1985 allowed a board of nursing to set educational standards for advanced nurse practitioners (*Bellegie v. Board of Nurse Examiners*).

Nurses should be aware that when courts or legislatures expand the nurse's role, the legal accountability of nurses also increases. Thus, nurses have an obligation to continually remain current on issues that affect their practice. Means of remaining current include reading professional nursing journals, accessing the state board of nursing website for changes in the state nurse practice act, and being active in professional nursing organizations. Many states require mandatory continuing education in order to renew the registered nurse license.

Divisions or Types of Law

There are different types or divisions of law that affect nursing practice. Each type or division of law uses different processes to determine guilt or innocence.

Common and Civil Law

Common law, which initiated in England, is a system of law that is derived from judges' decisions (which arise from the judicial branch of the government), rather than statutes or constitutions (which are derived from the legislative branch of government) (Garner, 2004). Common law is derived from principles rather than rules and regulations. Common law is based on justice, reason, and common sense. It represents law made by judges through decisions in specific cases. These case-by-case decisions are used again and again in similar cases, thereby becoming customary or "common" to all people living under the authority of the court of law. Common law in modern America continues to be the product of generations of judicial decisions. Principles that govern the use of human subjects in research and the composition and function of an institutional review board are examples of common law (DeWolf-Bosek & Savage, 2007).

Civil law, or continental law, is the predominant system of law in the world. In contrast to common law, civil law was promulgated after the French Revolution in France and is based on rules and regulations that became normative principles. These normative principles are codified in codes and statutes. In countries with civil law, legislation is seen as the primary source of law. By default, courts thus base their judgments on the provision of codes and statutes from which solutions in particular cases are to be derived. The terms *common law* and *civil law* often are used interchangeably to describe law that affects individuals rather than state entities. However, the main difference is that common law draws abstract rules from specific cases, whereas civil law starts with abstract rules, which judges must then apply to the various cases before them (Guido, 2006). Common and civil law are divided into a variety of legal specializations, including tort law and contract law (Guido, 2006).

Tort Law

Nurses are more likely to become involved in civil litigation rather than criminal litigation. Such litigation usually comes under the category of tort law. A tort is a wrongful act committed against another person or the person's property. These wrongful acts result in an injury or harm, thereby, constituting the basis for a claim by the injured party. Although some torts are crimes punishable by imprisonment, the primary aim of **tort law** is to provide relief for the damages incurred and to deter others from committing the same harms. The injured person may sue for an injunction to prevent the continuation of the tortuous conduct or for monetary damages (Stanford Encyclopedia of Philosophy, 2003). Examples of such tort actions include negligence, malpractice, assault and battery, false imprisonment, defamation, invasion of privacy, and breach of confidentiality. Each of these types of actions is covered in subsequent sections.

Lawsuits involving tort law usually are broken down into intentional, nonintentional, or quasi-intentional wrongs. **Intentional torts** are those that occur when the person acting knew or should have known a wrong would result from his conduct. A **nonintentional tort** is a wrong that would result from a person's negligent conduct. A tort becomes **quasi-intentional** when intent is lacking, but there is a volitional or willful action and direct causation.

Contract Law

Contracts are promises that the law will enforce. Contract law is that which governs the formation of these promises or agreements between two or more parties, in relation to a particular subject. Contracts can cover a broad range of matters, including the sale of goods or real property, the terms of employment or of an independent contractor relationship, the settlement of a dispute, and ownership of intellectual property developed as part of a work for hire (Larson, 2003). The law provides remedies if a promise is breached or recognizes the performance of a promise as a duty. Contracts arise when a duty does or may come into existence because of a promise made by one of the parties. To be legally binding as a contract, a promise must be exchanged for adequate consideration. Adequate consideration is a benefit or determinant that a party receives which reasonably and fairly induces them to make the promise (i.e., contract).

Contracts are mainly governed by state statutory and common (judge-made) law and private law. Private law principally includes the terms of the agreement between the parties who are exchanging promises. This private law may override many of the rules otherwise established by state law. Statutory law may require some contracts to be put in writing and executed with particular formality. In certain situations, the parties may enter into a binding agreement without signing a formal written document. Typically, in order to be enforceable, a contract must involve the following elements: mutual consent, offer and acceptance, mutual consideration, performance or delivery, good faith, and no violation of public policy. Given these stipulations it is important to remember that an agreement, or contract, between parties can be a verbal agreement. This is referred to as an oral contract.

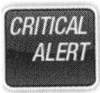 *Though an oral contract is legal, it can be very difficult to prove that an oral contract exists. Absent proof of the terms of the contract, a party may be unable to enforce the contract or may be forced to settle for less than the original bargain.*
Thus, even when there is no opportunity to draft a formal contract, it is always good practice to put something in writing, signed by both parties, to capture the key terms of an agreement.

 Because contracts are promises that the law will enforce, the law provides remedies if a promise is breached or the court recognizes the performance of a promise as a duty. Consider these very good reasons to avoid breaching a contract:

- *Your business or professional reputation could be damaged.*
- *You could sever your business or professional relationship with the other party.*
- *You could be sued. If sued, you could be forced to spend valuable time away from your business or practice in order to respond to factors of litigation: discovery requests, depositions, court appearances.*
- *You could incur legal fees.*
- *You could be ordered by the court to perform your obligations under the contract. If you do not obey the court's order, you could be held in contempt of court, fined, and/or imprisoned.*
- *You could be forced to pay money damages to the nonbreaching party, in an amount that puts that party in as good a position as it would have been in were it not for the breach.*
- *You could be forced to pay punitive damages, which are not limited by the amount of the other party's losses and can be very significant.*
- *You could end up spending much more time, money, and mental and physical energy resolving the breach than you would have spent performing your obligations under the contract.*

Criminal Law

Criminal law, sometimes called public law, refers to laws that affect the state in its political capacity and that affect society as a whole. Criminal law involves prosecution by the government of a person for an act that has been classified as a crime. This is in contrast to a civil case, which involves individuals and organizations seeking to resolve legal disputes. In a criminal case, the state, through a prosecutor, initiates the suit; whereas in a civil case, the victim brings the suit. A crime is any act or omission to act that violates public law either in forbidding or commanding it. Most crimes are established by local, state, and federal governments; thus, criminal laws vary from state to state. Criminal law may be divided into misdemeanors, or lesser crimes, and felonies, or more serious crimes that involve fines of more than $1,000 and are punishable by prison terms of greater than 1 year or death.

Sources of Civil and Criminal Litigation for Nurses

Nurses and other health care professionals may become involved with either the civil or criminal justice systems. The most frequent means by which a nurse incurs criminal action is by failure to renew one's nursing license in a timely manner. Once a nursing license has expired, the nurse is then practicing nursing without a license, which is a direct violation of state nurse practice acts. Other actions against nurses that are examples of criminal law frequently involve substance abuse, particularly if the nurse is illegally acquiring medications from clinical settings (e.g., when patients' prescribed narcotics are diverted to support a nurse's substance abuse and the patients are given placebos instead). Less frequently, nurses have been charged with either intentionally or unintentionally causing the death of a patient.

Negligence and Malpractice

Negligence and malpractice are the common terms for nonintentional torts. **Negligence** is the commission of an act that a reasonable and prudent person would not perform or the omission of something that a reasonable and prudent person would do in a given situation. In these situations reasonableness is described as acceptable and according to common sense or normal practice. It connotes sensibility and rational thought. Negligence thus denotes conduct that is lacking in care and is usually seen as carelessness on the part of the care provider.

Malpractice, sometimes referred to as professional negligence, evolves from negligence law and the premise that all individuals are responsible for the consequences of their actions or inactions (Negligence, 2007). It refers to any misconduct or lack of skill in carrying out professional responsibilities in a reasonable and prudent manner. Issues of malpractice have become increasingly important to the nurse as the authority, accountability, and autonomy of nurses have increased. As roles have expanded, nurses have begun performing duties traditionally reserved for medical practice. As a result of an increased scope of practice, many nurses now carry individual malpractice insurance, which is considered by some to be a double-edged sword. Nurses need malpractice insurance because of their expanded role, but they also incur a greater likelihood of being sued if they have malpractice insurance, because insured parties tend to seek damages from as many individuals with financial resources as possible (Marquis & Huston, 2006). The National Practitioner Data Bank reveals that the number of malpractice payments made by nurses has increased during the past several years and the trend shows no sign of stopping (Croke, 2003).

In all liability suits, there is a plaintiff and a defendant. In malpractice cases, the plaintiff is the injured party and the defendant is the professional who is alleged to have caused the injury. Essentially, six elements must be presented in a successful malpractice suit; all of these factors must be proven before the court will find liability against the nurse and/or institution (Guido, 2006). These six elements are duty owed the patient, breach of the duty owed the patient, foreseeability of harm, causation, injury, and damages. Chart 4–3 outlines these elements in greater detail and each of these elements is further expanded in the subsections that follow.

Elements of Malpractice

To understand how the law applies each element of malpractice to specific court cases, we use the following scenario: A nurse employed by a state medical center has been assigned to care for Mr. Gee, a patient admitted for a right hip replacement. Mr. Gee is 89 years old, weighs 255 pounds, is in relatively good health, and is competent mentally. He is to have surgery tomorrow and requires assistance in ambulating to and from the bathroom. While caring for Mr. Gee, the nurse fails to obtain the assistance of a second person when walking Mr. Gee to the bathroom, and he falls. Mr. Gee sustains a broken left hip and a mild concussion. He will be hospitalized for several additional days because he must now undergo bilateral hip replacement and physical therapy. Additionally, he will spend 2 days in the neurological step-down unit because of the concussion.

Duty Owed the Patient

The first element of malpractice is duty owed the patient and involves both the existence of the duty and the nature of the duty. That a nurse owes a duty of care to a patient is usually not hard to establish. Often this is established merely by showing the valid employment of the nurse within the institution. The more difficult part is the nature of the duty, which involves standards of care that represent the minimum requirements that define acceptable practice (internal standards). In the preceding scenario,

the applicable standard of care is taken from the institution's policy and procedure manual and concerns the standard of care owed the elderly patient regarding safety issues. In this instance, the specific standard of care relates to the need for two attendants to safely assist Mr. Gee to the bathroom. Standards of care are established by reviewing the institution's policy and procedure manual, the individual's job description, and the practitioner's education and skills, as well as the pertinent standards as established by professional organizations, journal articles, standing orders and protocols, and national and community expectations (or standards) for this type of care.

Several sources can be used to determine the applicable standard of care. The American Nurses Association, as well as a cadre of specialty organizations, publishes standards for nursing practice. The overall framework of these external standards is the nursing process. In 1988, the ANA first published its standards for nurse administrators, a series of nine standards incorporating the responsibilities of nurse administrators across all practice settings. Since that time, additional standards have been published that describe nursing care for a variety of patient populations and in selected nursing settings (ANA, 2001). A list of current ANA nursing practice standards is shown in Chart 4–4 (p. 74). Accreditation standards, especially those published yearly by the Joint Commission (2007), also assist in establishing the acceptable standards of care for health care facilities.

Breach of the Duty Owed the Patient

The second element of malpractice is breach of the duty of care owed the patient, or failure to meet the standard of care. Once the standard of care has been established, the breach of or failure to provide the standard of care is often easy to show. But establishing the standard of care may be difficult because the various parties to the suit may not be able to agree on the applicable standard of care, depending on whether the injured party or the hospital's attorney is trying to establish the standard of care for the given circumstances. The injured party will attempt to show that the acceptable standard of care is a higher standard

CHART 4–3 **Elements of Malpractice and Examples of Nursing Actions That May Result in Malpractice**

Element	Explanation	Examples of Nursing Actions
Duty owed the person	Care should be given under the circumstances (what the prudent nurse would have done).	Failing to monitor a patient for postoperative bleeding
Breach of duty owed the patient	Not giving the care that should be given under the circumstances.	Failing to observe and report changes in a patient's condition
Foreseeability of harm	The nurse must have reasonable access to information about whether the possibility of harm exists.	Failing to act as a patient advocate, for example, the drug handbook specifies that the wrong route of dosage may cause injury. The nurse acts on behalf of the patient to clarify the correct route of administration.
Causation (a direct relationship exists between failure to meet the standard of care and injury and can be proven)	Patient is harmed because proper care is not given.	Failing to question an inappropriate order
Injury	Actual harm results to patient.	Failing to provide patient education and discharge planning
Damages	Based on pain and suffering, expenses, emotional damages, or malicious damages.	Giving the patient incorrect medications

| CHART 4–4 | **ANA Nursing Standards** |

- Corrections Nursing: Scope and Standards of Practice
- Faith Community Nursing: Scope and Standards of Practice
- Genetics/Genomics Nursing: Scope and Standards of Practice
- HIV/AIDS Nursing: Scope and Standards of Practice
- Holistic Nursing: Scope and Standards of Practice
- Home Health Nursing: Scope and Standards of Practice
- Hospice and Palliative Nursing: Scope and Standards of Practice
- Intellectual and Developmental Disabilities Nursing: Scope and Standards of Practice
- Legal Nurse Consulting: Scope and Standards of Practice
- Neonatal Nursing: Scope and Standards of Practice
- Nursing Informatics: Scope and Standards of Practice
- Nursing: Scope and Standards of Practice
- Pain Management Nursing: Scope and Standards of Practice
- Plastic Surgery Nursing: Scope and Standards of Practice
- Psychiatric–Mental Health: Scope and Standards of Practice
- Public Health Nursing: Scope and Standards of Practice
- Radiology Nursing: Scope and Standards of Practice
- School Nursing: Scope and Standards of Practice
- Scope and Standards for Nurse Administrators, Second Edition
- Scope and Standards of Addictions Nursing Practice
- Scope and Standards of Diabetes Nursing Practice (2nd Edition)
- Scope and Standards of Gerontological Nursing Practice, 2nd Edition
- Scope and Standards of Neuroscience Nursing Practice
- Scope and Standards of Practice for Nursing Professional Development
- Scope and Standards of Vascular Nursing Practice

Source: Nursing World/Nurses online Bookstore: ANA Nursing Standards. Retrieved May 18, 2007 from http://nursingworld.org/books/pdescr.cfm?cnum=15. American Nurses Association. ANA Nursing standards, April 14, 2008 from www.nursingworld.org

of care than that shown by the defendant hospital and staff. Each of these two sides to the dispute help determine the standard of care through the testimony of expert witnesses. Expert witnesses give testimony in court to determine the applicable and acceptable standard of care on a case-by-case basis and to assist the judge and jury in understanding nursing standards of care. In the scenario involving Mr. Gee, the injured party's expert witness would quote the institution's policy manual, and the nurse's expert witness would note any viable exceptions to the stated policy.

An example case that remains the standard for the distinction in standards of care is *Sabol v. Richmond Heights General Hospital* (1996). In *Sabol*, a patient was admitted to a general acute care hospital for treatment after attempting suicide by drug overdose. While in the acute care facility, the patient became increasingly paranoid and delusional. A nurse sat with the patient and tried to calm him. Restraints were not applied because the staff feared this would compound the situation by raising his level of paranoia and agitation. The patient got out of bed, knocked down the nurse who was in his room, fought his way past two nurses in the hallway, ran off the unit, and jumped from a third-story window, fracturing his arm and sustaining other relatively minor injuries.

Expert witnesses for the patient introduced standards of care pertinent to psychiatric patients, specifically those patients hospitalized in psychiatric facilities or in acute care hospitals with separate psychiatric units. The court ruled that the nurses in this general acute care situation were not negligent in this patient's care. The court stated that the nurses' actions were consistent with basic professional standards of practice for medical–surgical nurses in an acute care hospital. They did not have, nor were they expected to have, specialized psychiatric nursing training and would not be judged as if they did.

Foreseeability of Harm

The third element of malpractice, **foreseeability of harm**, involves the concept that certain events may reasonably be expected to cause specific results. The nurse must have prior knowledge or information that failure to meet a standard of care may result in harm. The challenge is to show what was foreseeable given the facts of the case at the time of the occurrence, not when the case finally comes to court. In the given scenario, it was foreseeable that the patient could fall and harm himself if fewer than two people attempted to assist with ambulation.

Causation

The fourth element of malpractice is causation, which means that the nurse's action or lack of action directly caused the patient's harm and not merely that the patient had some type of harm. There must be a direct relationship between the failure to meet the standard of care and the patient's injury. Stated differently, causation means that it is not sufficient that a patient was harmed (Guido, 2006; Nursing malpractice, 2003)—the patient must be able to show that the nurse's action or lack of action was the direct reason for the injury that resulted. In the given scenario, Mr. Gee suffered a broken hip and a concussion as a result of his fall.

Injury

The resultant injury, the fifth element of malpractice, must be physical, not merely psychological or transient. In other words, the patient must incur some physical harm before malpractice will be found against the health care provider. In the given scenario, Mr. Gee came to harm as a direct result of ambulating to the bathroom, and he incurred the physical injuries of both a broken hip and a concussion.

Damages

Finally, the injured party must be able to prove damages, the sixth element of malpractice. The term *damages* refers to financial harm incurred by the injured party. The ability to prove damages is vital in a malpractice suit because malpractice is nonintentional and unintended. Thus, the patient must show financial harm before the courts will allow a finding of liability against the defendant nurse and/or hospital. Mr. Gee, in the given scenario, would be able to show damages that include additional hospital costs related to the second hip replacement surgery, physical therapy needs, and admission to the step-down unit. Further medical needs may arise based on these injuries, such as a need for long-term physical therapy and temporary admission to a skilled nursing facility.

Liability for Negligence by Students

Nursing students have the ultimate responsibility for their own actions and may be liable for their own negligence. Student liability holds true even if the student is not an adult under state law. The often used adage that a student practices under the instructor's license is not a true or valid statement because only the individual awarded the license practices on the license. The individual student always retains accountability, and nurse practice acts allow students to perform professional actions without being awarded a license to practice nursing, thus according them the opportunity to learn how to practice nursing.

The standard of care to which the nursing student is held is the same as that for the reasonably prudent practicing professional nurse. As such, the student and the instructor must know hospital policies and procedures and remain current in medical and nursing knowledge. The licensure exception further requires that unprepared nursing students or those who need additional supervision inform the faculty instructor of their special needs or lack of preparedness for clinical practice. Thus, nursing students remain accountable for their knowledge and skills, and faculty or staff may become accountable for individual student incompetence or lack of preparedness (Guido, 2006).

Regional and National Norms for Standards of Care

Sometimes the issue of whether standards of care follow a **regional (locality) rule** or national norm becomes an issue in courts of law. **National standards of care** are based on reasonableness and are the average degree of skill, care, and diligence exercised by members of the same profession. Such national standards mean that nurses in all settings, urban and rural, must meet the same standards when caring for patients in clinical settings.

National standards of care have slowly replaced the previously used regional or locality standard of care, which allowed the standard of care to be viewed from the perspective of care within a given geographical area or "similar community." There are two important reasons for national standards of care. With the advent of educational programs and videos, a better ability to transport individuals to national conferences or to consult in small, more rural areas, and the use of telemedicine and virtual diagnostics, all areas with health care delivery systems have access to the same information and educational opportunities. A second reason is that all patients have the right to quality health care, whether hospitalized in a small community setting or in a major medical center.

Intentional Torts

Nurses also may be found liable for intentional torts, which are generally defined as actions that violate another person's rights. In such actions, the nurse's actions must intend to interfere with the patient or property, the nurse must intend to bring about the consequences of the act, and the act must be a substantial factor in bringing about the consequences or outcomes. Note that, unlike negligence and malpractice, no actual harm is necessary for this tort; it is the violation of another person's rights that creates the cause of action. The more commonly seen intentional torts in

health care settings are assault, battery, and false imprisonment (Guido, 2006; Nursing malpractice, 2003), as discussed next.

Assault, Battery, and False Imprisonment

Assault places the patient in apprehension of being touched in an offensive, insulting, or physically injurious manner, such as when one threatens the patient with an injection or the placement of a nasogastric tube. **Battery** is the actual contact with another person or the person's property. Examples of batteries include forcing patients to ambulate against their wishes and restraining a patient so that a procedure can be implemented. For assault or battery to occur, there must be an absence of legal consent on the part of the patient.

 With assault, no actual touching of the person is required; it is the fear or apprehension of being touched that constitutes the intentional tort. Thus, a nurse cannot assault a sleeping or unconscious patient, because no matter how angry or violent the nurse might be or how irrational the nurse's actions might be, the patient has no knowledge of the potential contact and is, therefore, not apprehensive of the potential contact.

With battery, however, a single touch, regardless of how fleeting or faint, is sufficient for a tort to have occurred. The patient does not need to experience any harm, injury, or pain in order for battery to occur. Also, in contrast to assault, the patient need not be aware of the battery for tort to have occurred. Taking the pulse of a sleeping person could be considered battery. The nurse also may commit battery by the unwarranted touching of the patient's clothes or an article held by the patient, such as a purse or suitcase. For purposes of battery, anything that is connected with the patient's person is viewed as part of the person.

False imprisonment is the unjustified detention of a person without the legal right to confine the person, such as when one prevents a patient from leaving against medical advice or when nurses restrain a person in a confined space. Use of medications that alter a patient's ability to leave the health care setting can also create this tort. As with assault and battery, consent is a vital element in this tort; patients who are compromised mentally and are restrained to prevent their harm are not falsely imprisoned because consent is implied (Guido, 2006).

 The patient must be aware of the detention or restraint (the act) for a successful false imprisonment lawsuit. False imprisonment also may occur if the act is directed at the patient's family or possessions, such as keys, clothing, or a purse. Sedated patients who are incapable of realizing their confinement do not have a suit for false imprisonment. Likewise, future threats are not enough to sustain the tort of false imprisonment. It is, however, prudent to realize that state law must be followed to the letter when a person's liberty is at stake; if it is not the citizen can sue for false imprisonment.

Quasi-Intentional Torts

Tort law also recognizes quasi-intentional torts. The difference between quasi-intentional and intentional torts is that there is no intent to injure or cause distress to another person; there is, however, an intentional (volitional) action that causes injury or distress. Two quasi-intentional torts are recognized in health care settings: defamation of character and invasion of privacy, which includes the subset of breach of confidentiality.

Defamation of Character

Defamation of character, also known as libel and slander, is harming another's reputation by diminishing the esteem, respect, goodwill, or level of confidence that others have for that person. Individuals have the right to their good name. Defamation often occurs in medical record documentation, and nurses are cautioned about what and how to record patient data and descriptions in the medical record. For example, charting that a patient is a prostitute or acts "crazy" may raise potential liability issues for the nurse and agency. If there is no reason to include a statement, such as the comment about a person's lifestyle or occupation, then it should not be included in the official record. If, however, a record is needed to validate a patient's mental state or actions, the nurse should chart actual patient behaviors or statements rather than making a subjective appraisal of the patient. The nurse should state exactly what the patient said and not the nurse's interpretation of the statement. A rule that assists nurses in this area is to write in the medical record as though the patient and her family will be reading the record. The documentation should always be truthful (Nursing malpractice, 2003).

Invasion of Privacy

Invasion of privacy is a violation of a person's right to protection against unreasonable and unwarranted interference with his personal life. To show that invasion of privacy has occurred, the person must show that the nurse intruded on the patient's privacy, the intrusion would be objectionable to a prudent and reasonable person, the intrusion concerns private or unpublished facts or pictures of a private nature, and that public disclosure of private facts was made. Examples of invasion of privacy include the taking of photographs without the patient's permission, disclosure of medical facts to persons not entitled to those facts, and publishing information that misrepresents the patient's condition.

Breach of Confidentiality

Breach of confidentiality, a part of invasion of privacy, concerns facts that are presented in the medical record. The majority of the cases concerning breach of confidentiality concern privileged conversations that are included in the patient's medical record and the faxing or electronic conveyance of medical records. Health care professionals are cautioned to have procedures in place that allow for the disclosure of confidential data; the patient's written authorization to reveal selected information prevents a cause of action concerning invasion of privacy and breach of confidentiality.

Health Insurance Portability and Accountability Act (HIPAA)

A newer application of invasion of privacy is the recently enacted Health Insurance Portability and Accountability Act of 1996 (HIPAA; Public Law 104-191), which is further elaborated on in Chapters 3, 6, and 8 💿 . The HIPAA regulations greatly expand the patient's right to confidentiality in all health care settings. Prior to the enforcement of this act, federal law did not protect patient confidentiality in the medical record and individual states offered only limited protection of these records.

The HIPAA legislation includes comprehensive standards regarding the transmission of medical data, administrative records, and financial records. Significant fines and penalties are included to enable enforcement of the act against those who violate its provisions, so organizations must take the implementa-

tion of and compliance with HIPAA standards seriously. Unintentional violations may result in fines of up to $25,000 for each incident. Intentional violations can result in imprisonment of up to 10 years and fines of $250,000 (HIPAAdvisory, 2006). Only "covered entities" come under the HIPAA regulations and such covered entities include health care plans that employ greater than 50 participants and who transmit health care information in an electronic format (45 *Code of Federal Regulations*, Sections 160.102 and 160.103, 1996).

One of the most important reasons for this act was the concept that patients retained a right to their medical information. Before HIPAA was enacted, information could be shared with other entities; now, patients have the right to either allow the disclosure or deny the disclosure. To ensure that medical information is protected, the act defines protected health information (PHI), which includes 18 possible identifiers that relate to the past, present, or future physical or mental health of the person. PHI includes the following: names of the individual or initials; addresses, including street, e-mail, and Internet addresses; dates, including birth dates and dates of services received; telephone and fax numbers; Social Security or other personal identification numbers; medical record numbers; health plan identification numbers; license or certificate numbers; medical device identifiers; biometric identifiers such as fingerprints or photographic images; or any other unique identifying characteristic or code (45 *Code of Federal Regulations*, Section 160.103, 1996).

The HIPAA standards limit how information will be used or shared, mandate safeguards for the protection of health information, and shift control of health information from providers to the patient. Covered health care facilities must provide patients with a document entitled Notice of Privacy Practices, which explains how the PHI will be used or shared with other entities. The document also alerts patients to the process for complaints if they determine that their information rights were violated. Chart 4–5 provides a concise overview of the components of the HIPAA.

Consent

Generally, the health care provider's right to treat a patient, barring true emergency conditions or unanticipated occurrences, is based on a contractual relationship that arises through the mutual consent of parties to the relationship. This relationship is formed when the health care provider performing the therapy or treatment provides the patient with needed information and the patient voluntarily consents to the therapy or treatment. This fulfills the provisions of contracts: (1) agreements made between two or more persons or entities for the performance of an action; (2) mutual understanding of the terms and meanings of the contract; (3) compensation in the terms of something of value; and (4) fulfillment of a lawful purpose (Guido, 2006). This concept is discussed under the previous section on contract law and in Chapter 6 💿 .

Consent is the voluntary authorization by a patient or the patient's legal representative to do something to the patient. It is based on the mutual consent of all parties involved, and the key to true and valid consent is patient comprehension. Consent may be given orally or in writing. Unless state law mandates written consent, the law views oral and written consent as

| CHART 4–5 | Overview of HIPAA |

Provision	Requirements
Electronic data interchange	• Implement standardized transactions, which includes forms and content. • Implement use of standard code sets for documenting care, drugs, and services. • Implement use of individual and unique identifiers for the patient, the provider, and the insurance plan.
Security	• Develop administrative policies and procedures. • Provide physical safeguards for health information. • Provide technical security and mechanisms for health information.
Privacy	• Limit disclosure of information to appropriate sources. • Define information use and authorization for access to health information. • Establish business associate agreements.

Sources: HIPAA privacy rule and public health. Guidance from CDC and the U.S. Department of Health and Human Services. (2003). *Morbidity and Mortality Weekly Report, 5*(2; Suppl), 1–17; Indian Health Service. (2008). HIPAA. Retrieved April 18, 2008, from http://www.ihs.gov/Adminmngrresources/HIPAA/index.cfm.

| CHART 4–6 | Information Necessary for Informed Consent |

1. A brief, but complete explanation of the treatment or procedure to be performed.
2. The name and qualifications of the person who will perform the procedure and, if others will assist, the names and qualifications of those assistants.
3. An explanation of any serious harm that may occur during the procedure, including death if that is a realistic outcome. Pain and discomforting side effects both during the procedure and following the procedure also should be discussed.
4. An explanation of alternative therapies to the procedure or treatment, including the risk of doing nothing at all.
5. An explanation that the patient can refuse the therapy or procedure without having alternative care or support discontinued.
6. The fact that the patient can still refuse, even after the procedure or therapy has begun. For example, all of the suggested radiation treatments need not be completed.

Informed Consent

Consent, technically, is an easy yes or no: "Yes, I will allow the surgery" or "No, I want to try medications first, then maybe I will allow the surgery." The law concerning consent in health care situations is based on informed consent. The doctrine of **informed consent** has developed from negligence law as the courts began to realize that although consent may have been given, not enough information was imparted to form the foundation of an informed decision. Informed consent mandates to the physician or independent health care provider the separate legal duty to disclose needed material facts in terms that the patient can reasonably understand so that the patient can make an informed choice. There should also be a description of the available alternatives to the proposed treatment and the risks and dangers involved in each alternative. Failure to disclose the needed facts in understandable terms does not negate the consent, but it does place potential liability on the practitioner for malpractice. To be informed, the patient must receive, in terms he can understand and comprehend, specific information (American Medical Association, 2007), as shown in Chart 4–6.

Nurses may become involved in the process of obtaining informed consent in one of several ways. When one realizes that consent must be obtained for all procedures and treatments, not just medical procedures, one realizes the vast impact of this doctrine. This does not mean that nurses have to obtain written consent each time they give an injection or turn a patient. Most nursing interventions rely on oral expressed consent or implied consent that may be readily inferred through the patient's actions.

What the doctrine of informed consent means is that nurses must continually communicate with patients. What it also means is that the patient's refusal to allow a certain procedure must be respected. If the patient is unable to communicate, permission may be derived from the patient's admission to the hospital or obtained from the patient's legal representative.

A second way to enhance understanding is to allow time between the actual giving of information and when the patient

equally valid. As a precaution, health care providers should recognize that oral consent is much more difficult to prove should consent or lack of consent become a legal issue. As a convenience and to prevent such court issues, most health care institutions require written consent, primarily for invasive procedures, surgical interventions, and selected medication regimes.

Consent becomes an important issue from a legal perspective in that the patient may sue for a battery (unconsented touching) if she does not consent to the procedure or treatment and the health care provider goes ahead with the procedure or treatment. This means that the patient may bring a lawsuit and be awarded damages even if the patient was helped by the procedure or treatment. The more current trend, though, is to argue consent under a negligence or malpractice cause of action because generally the patient has given consent for the procedure, an adverse outcome has occurred, and the issue of consent is argued secondary to the adverse outcome (harm) that occurred.

The right to consent and the right to refuse consent are based on a long-recognized, common law right of persons to be free from harmful or offensive touching of their bodies. Consent is not contingent on a request for information or clarification by the patient, but must be actively given by health care providers.

Consent may be obtained in a variety of ways. Perhaps the easiest means of obtaining informed consent is when the consent is expressed. Expressed consent is consent given by direct words, either written or oral. For example, after the nurse informs the patient that she is going to start an intravenous infusion, the patient says, "Okay, but could you put the needle in my left hand, as I am right-handed?" As a rule, expressed consent is the type most often sought and received by health care providers, particularly nurses.

must make a decision. Such time intervals allow patients to consider what has been suggested, to put into words their questions and concerns, and then make the final decision and sign the informed consent forms.

Implied Consent

Implied consent is consent that may be inferred by the patient's conduct or that may legally be presumed in emergency situations. Many patients hold out their arm and roll up their sleeve when the nurse approaches with a stethoscope and blood pressure cuff. This is an example of implied consent because a reasonable person would infer by the patient's action that she is consenting to the procedure. Or the patient extends his left shoulder for an injection after the nurse explains why the medication is being given. Nurses most often obtain implied consent for minor procedures and routine care.

Implied consent may be presumed to exist in true emergency situations and is known as the **emergency doctrine**. For such consent, the patient must not be able to make his wishes known, and a delay in providing care would result in the loss of life or limb. An important element in allowing emergency consent is that the health care provider must not have any reason to know or believe that consent would *not* be given were the patient able to deny consent. For example, a health care provider cannot wait until a patient loses consciousness to order treatment that the patient had previously refused, such as a blood transfusion for a patient who is known to be a Jehovah's Witness. Implied consent is frequently relied on during surgery or in critical care units when an untoward event occurs and an immediate decision must be made to prevent further injury to the patient.

Revocation of Consent

The nurse also has an important role if the patient subsequently wishes to revoke his or her prior consent or if it becomes obvious that the patient's already signed, informed consent form does not meet the institution's standards for informed consent. Most nurses have been faced with the problem of what to do when it becomes all too clear that the patient does not understand the procedure to be performed or believes that there are no major risks or adverse consequences inherent to the procedure. It is important to remember that the nurse and the hospital may incur liability if there is reason to know that the standards of informed consent have not been met. In such a case, it is the nurse's responsibility to contact his immediate supervisor and the responsible physician. Both entities need to be informed of the patient's change of mind or lack of comprehension.

Signing of a Consent Form

Equally as important as the patient being given all material facts needed on which to base an informed choice is that the correct person(s) consent to the procedure or therapy. Informed consent becomes a moot point if the wrong signature is obtained. The basic rule is that if the patient is a competent adult according to state law, only that adult can give or refuse consent. Most states recognize 18 as the age at which one becomes an adult, although some actions might serve to classify the person as an adult prior to the legal age, for example, marriage or termination of parental rights. The adult giving or refusing consent must be competent to either sign or refuse to sign the necessary

consent forms. Competency at law means that (1) the court has not declared the person to be incompetent and (2) the person is generally able to understand the consequences of her actions. There is a strong legal presumption of continuing competency.

Some persons are never adjudicated or judged to be incompetent by a court of law, but they become incompetent to give informed consent based on their current medical condition. Many states allow the patient's family members to make decisions for the incompetent patient. For example, an automobile accident may render the patient incapable of making decisions and giving consent, and the physician will frequently ask the family about medical matters for the unconscious patient. The order of selection for most states usually is (1) spouse, (2) adult children or grandchildren, (3) parents, (4) grandparents, (5) adult brothers and sisters, and (6) adult nieces and nephews.

Most states recognize the child under 18 as a minor. Parental or guardian consent is necessary for medical therapies unless (1) the emergency doctrine applies, (2) the individual is an emancipated (liberated) minor or mature minor, (3) there is a court order to proceed with the therapy, or (4) the law recognizes the minor as having the ability to consent to the therapy. Some states also follow the *in loco parentis* doctrine, which refers to the ability of a person or the state to stand in the place of the parents. Look to the individual state statutory laws to see who may consent in the absence of a parent and what constitutes emancipated status because there is no general consensus on these issues. Such laws can be accessed through the individual state governmental website. If there is a family consent doctrine, it will generally be a grandparent, adult brother or sister, or adult aunt or uncle.

Emancipated minors are persons under the legal age of an adult who are no longer under their parent's control and regulation and who are managing their own financial affairs. Some states require the parent to completely surrender the right of care and custody of the child to prevent runaways from coming under this classification. Such emancipated minors may validly consent for their own medical therapies. Examples of emancipated minors are married persons, underage parents, or those in the armed service of their country. In some states pregnant adolescents are considered emancipated for the purposes of giving or refusing medical treatment for themselves and their fetuses. However, after the infant is born, the adolescent mother may only make decisions for the infant or for herself unless she is married. Some states allow college students living away from their parents to fall in the category of emancipated minor. Individual nurses should consult agency policies and state regulations for information regarding emancipated minors.

Mature minors also may consent to some medical care. The concept of a mature minor is a relatively new one that is gaining legal recognition (DeWolf-Bosek & Savage, 2007; Driggs, 2002; Guido, 2006). The mature minor is a minor between the ages of 14 and 17 who is able to understand the nature and consequences of the proposed therapy, is making his own decisions on a daily basis, and is independent. The health care provider is encouraged to seek parental consent along with the consent of the mature minor in most circumstances. Such a practice aids in limiting potential liability and encourages family involvement. It is necessary to consult agency policy for further information regarding this concept and the state statutes that govern the interpretation of mature minors.

The law also recognizes the right of the minor to consent to some selected therapies without informing parents of the treatment. The reason for these exceptions is to encourage the minor to seek needed treatment. Informing the parents of the treatment might prevent the minor from receiving the necessary therapy. Instances for which the minor may give valid consent include (1) diagnosis and treatment of infectious, contagious, or communicable diseases; (2) diagnosis and treatment of drug dependency, drug addiction, or any condition directly related to drug usage; (3) obtaining birth control devices; and (4) treatment during a pregnancy as long as the care concerns the pregnancy.

 There is no foolproof method for determining maturity among minors. It is a subjective and arbitrary process depending to a great degree on the perceptions of the evaluator. Also, state courts are inconsistent in the use of a standard of proof that is required for application of the mature minor doctrine.

Preventing Possible Liability

Nurses and other health care providers often ask what they can do to prevent potential lawsuits. Understanding and applying the legal concepts involved are two means of preventing possible liability. For example, ensuring that standards of care are fully implemented each time a nurse administers nursing care will help prevent potential lawsuits. Two other areas where nurses can have the most impact in reducing their potential legal liability involve the nurse–patient relationship and patient rights.

Nurse–Patient Relationship

One of the most fundamental aspects of malpractice law involves relationships. For a duty to be owed the patient, one must first establish that a nurse–patient relationship exists. This may be accomplished by showing that a reliance relationship exists: One person (the patient) is depending on another person (the nurse) for competent, quality nursing care.

The core of any reliance relationship is trust and communication. Establishing rapport with a patient, informing patients honestly and openly of all aspects of their care, and allowing patients to make decisions for themselves have always been credited to nurses as one means of preventing potential liability. Nursing is a caring profession; part of caring is maintaining communications and ensuring that trust is established and continues throughout the interactions between the nurse and the patient.

Patient Rights

Health care providers are becoming increasingly more aware and respective of patient rights. In 1959, the National League for Nursing wrote one of the earliest statements regarding patients' rights (National League for Nursing, 1959). In the early 1970s, the American Hospital Association (AHA) published *A Patient's Bill of Rights*, enumerating 12 rights that were to be afforded all hospitalized patients. These rights primarily concerned the patient's right to considerate and respectful care; informed consent concepts, including making treatment decisions based on informed choice; considerations of privacy; the right to know who will provide care; and the right to information about advance directives. The docu-

ment was revised in 1992, and more recently in 2003, and now presents patients' rights, expectations, and responsibilities. The latest document (2003) emphasizes a collaborative approach to patient care in which the patients' responsibilities are explicit. In return, patients may expect a certain level of care delivery. This statement is entitled The Patient Care Partnership: Understanding Expectations, Rights, and Responsibilities, and an abridged version is shown in Chart 4–7 (p. 80). The full text may be obtained from the American Hospital Association. See Chart 4–7 (p. 80) for the current provisions of *A Patient's Bill of Rights* (AHA, 2003).

Today, nurses are much more cognizant of the rights of patients, including those not enumerated on the various published documents. For example, the patient has the right to be cared for in a facility that ensures the safety rights of the patients. Observing and enforcing these patient rights prevents possible lawsuits. In this regard, nurses serve as patients' advocates by defending their legal and ethical rights.

Nursing has identified three models of advocacy that are employed in clinical practice settings. The rights protection model is perhaps the best known model of advocacy. Nurses assist patients in asserting their autonomy rights; for example, a nurse might help an individual patient successfully convince health care providers that he does not desire surgical intervention for coronary artery disease, but will comply with medical management. The third principle in the ANA's Code of Ethics (2001) reinforces this mandate: "The nurse promotes, advocates for, and strives to protect the health, safety, and rights of the patient."

A second approach to advocacy is the values-based decision model. Using this approach, the nurse assists the patient by discussing her needs and desires and helps the patient make choices that are most consistent with the patient's values, lifestyle, and desires. This model is predicated on sharing information and assisting the individual to become empowered to speak on her own behalf. Using this approach, the patient is assisted to exert her right to autonomy and self-determination.

The third model is the respect for persons model, which is sometimes known as the patient-advocate model. This approach centers on the inherent human dignity that is deserving of respect. In this model, the nurse acts to protect the rights, dignity, and choices of the patient. If the patient cannot assist in making decisions about his care and treatments, the nurse advocates for the best interests of the patient. The ultimate goal of this model is to promote the autonomy and individual uniqueness of the patient.

Defenses Against Torts

In the event that a legal claim or lawsuit is filed, nurses and other health care providers can use certain legal defenses to negate liability. Defenses are arguments in support of or arguments used for justification. Defenses may be based on statutory law, common law, or the doctrine of precedent, in which decisions are left to stand based on prior decisions made by a court (Guido, 2006). Defenses also can be classified by the type of cause of action, or tort, filed against the health care personnel: intentional, quasi-intentional, or nonintentional.

Defenses Against Intentional Torts

Defenses against intentional torts are most commonly consent, self-defense, defense of others, and necessity. Consent, as

---

CHART 4–7　**The Patient Care Partnership: Understanding Expectations, Rights and Responsibilities**

Our goal is for you and your family to have the same care and attention we would want for our families and ourselves. The sections explain some of the basics about how you can expect to be treated during your hospital stay. They also cover what we will need from you to care for you better. If you have questions at any time, please ask them. Unasked or unanswered questions can add to the stress of being in the hospital.

WHAT TO EXPECT DURING YOUR HOSPITAL STAY

- **High quality hospital care.** Our first priority is to provide you the care you need, when you need it, with skill, compassion, and respect. Tell your caregivers if you have concerns about your care or if you have pain. You have the right to know the identity of doctors, nurses and others involved in your care.

- **A clean and safe environment.** We use special policies and procedures to avoid mistakes in your care and keep you free from abuse or neglect. If anything unexpected and significant happens during your hospital stay, you will be told what happened, and any resulting changes in your care will be discussed with you.

- **Involvement in your care.** Please tell your caregivers if you need more information about treatment choices. When decision-making takes place, it should include:
  - *Discussing your medical condition and information about medically appropriate treatment choices.* To make informed decisions with your doctor, you need to understand:
    - The benefits and risks of each treatment, and whether the treatment is experimental or part of a research study.
    - What you can reasonably expect from your treatment and any long-term effects it might have on your quality of life.
    - What you and your family will need to do after you leave the hospital.
    - The financial consequences of using uncovered services or out-of-network providers.
  - *Discussing your treatment plan.* When you enter the hospital, you sign a general consent to treatment. In some cases, such as surgery or experimental treatment, you may be asked to confirm in writing that you understand what is planned and agree to it.

- *Getting information from you.* Your caregivers need complete and correct information about your health and coverage so that they can make good decisions about your care. That includes:
  - Past illnesses, surgeries or hospital stays; past allergic reactions; any medicines or dietary supplements (such as vitamins and herbs) that you are taking; and any network or admission requirements under your health plan.

- *Understanding your health care goals and values.* Make sure your doctor, your family and your care team know your wishes.

- *Understanding who should make decisions when you cannot.* If you have signed a health care power of attorney stating who should speak for you if you become unable to make health care decisions for yourself, or a "living will" or "advance directive" that states your wishes about end-of-life care; give copies to your doctor, your family and your care team.

- **Protection of your privacy.** State and federal laws and hospital operating policies protect the privacy of your medical information. You will receive a Notice of Privacy Practices that describes the ways that we use, disclose and safeguard patient information and that explains how you can obtain a copy of information from our records about your care.

- **Preparing you and your family for when you leave the hospital.** The success of your treatment often depends on your efforts to follow medication, diet and therapy plans. You can expect us to help you identify sources of follow-up care and to let you know if our hospital has a financial interest in any referrals. You can also expect to receive information and, where possible, training about the self-care you will need when you go home.

- **Help with your bill and filing insurance claims.** Our staff will file claims for you with health care insurers or other programs, such as Medicare and Medicaid. If you have questions about your bill, contact our business office. If you need help understanding your insurance coverage or health plan, start with your insurance company or health benefits manager. If you do not have health coverage, we will try to help you and your family find financial help or make other arrangements.

---

previously discussed, may be oral, implied by law, or expressed. Self-defense and defense of others may be justifiable to protect oneself and others from harm, for example, in the case of a combative patient. Defense of others can be extended to include the patient as well. The overriding caveat is that one can only use reasonable force—that which is necessary to defend oneself or others from injury. Necessity allows the nurse to interfere with the patient's property rights to avoid threatened injury, for example, an attack with a knife. The two overriding caveats in this situation are that a defense of necessity (1) does not allow the nurse the right to search the patient's property and (2) stipulates that the patient's property must be the threatening factor.

Defenses Against Quasi-Intentional Torts

The primary defenses against quasi-intentional torts are consent, truth, privilege, qualified privilege, and disclosure statutes. Consent

may be a defense against the quasi-intentional torts of defamation and invasion of privacy as well as to the intentional torts. Truth is a valid defense against defamatory statements; however, nurses should be aware that in using this defense the entire statement must be true, not merely parts of the statement (Guido, 2006).

Privilege is a disclosure that might otherwise be considered defamatory under different circumstances, however, such disclosure may be allowable to protect or further private or public interests recognized by law. An example of such would be the legal mandate to report persons with certain diagnoses or diseases or those suspected of abusing others. Qualified privilege prevails when the person making the allegedly defamatory statements has a legal duty to do so, as in the case of a manager reporting the professional performance of an employee. Qualified privilege legally negates any inference of malice because of the overriding public policy interest. When the quality of medical care is at issue, the reputation rights of health care professionals may concede to the greater social need. Liability will not be imposed, even if the communications are false, as long as there is no malice and the communications are made in good faith to those persons who need to know such facts. Three caveats of qualified privilege need to be observed: The communication must be made through appropriate channels to persons needing the information, liability may be granted for untruthful communications released with malice, and the communications should be worded in objective and observable behavioral terms rather than judgmental descriptions.

Both federal and state laws require the reporting of certain types of health-related information to protect the public at large. These laws are referred to as disclosure statutes. These statutes require that health care providers submit certain information to the proper agency. The most common example of reporting statutes is vital statistics. All states require births and deaths to be reported, and a majority of states require an accounting of neonatal deaths and abortions. Public health agencies may require a variety of disease states to be reported, for example, communicable and venereal disease must be reported to protect the public. In addition, some states require that patients suffering any type of seizure disorder be reported to the state driver's licensing agency. Also, cancer and other related diseases are to be reported in some states. If providers disclose only the limited information they are required to disclose by law, there is no liability for the disclosure under either a defamation or invasion of privacy lawsuit. Thus, the statutes serve as a defense against both defamation and invasion of privacy (Guido, 2006).

Defenses Against Nonintentional Torts

Defenses against nonintentional torts or negligent actions include release, contributory or comparative negligence, assumption of the risk, unavoidable accident, defense of the fact, and immunity statutes. A release may be signed during the process of settling a claim to prevent any and all future claims arising from the same incident. Once signed, the release bars future suits. In medical malpractice claims, a release is frequently a part of the "out-of-court" settlement. Effectively, the plaintiff states that the agreed-on settlement is the only compensation for the negligent action. Contributory and comparative negligence serve as defenses and in essence hold injured parties accountable for their part in the injury. Such fault by the plaintiff may occur for failure to follow prescribed treatments or if incorrect treatment is given based on the patient's false information to the physician. Similarly, the assumption of risk defense states that plaintiffs are partially responsible for consequences if they understood the risk involved when they proceeded with the action (Guido, 2006).

The defense of unavoidable accident comes into play when nothing other than an accident could have caused the person's injury. An unavoidable accident is an inevitable occurrence that cannot be foreseen or prevented by vigilance, care, and attention and not occasioned by or contributed to in any manner by an act or omission of the party claiming the accident was unavoidable (Dawson, 2007; Guido, 2006). The defense of the fact is used when there is no indication, direct or otherwise, that the health care provider's actions were the cause of the patient's injury or untoward outcome (e.g., the patient who receives an injection in his right arm and then begins to experience numbness and tingling in his left leg). There is no connection between the two events; thus, the defense is defense of fact.

Immunity

Immunity statutes have been enacted in some states that serve to dismiss certain causes of action. A good example of a state immunity statute is the Good Samaritan statute. Because of these laws, negligent actions against health care providers at scenes of accidents are rare. Good Samaritan laws are enacted to allow health care personnel and citizens who are trained in first aid to deliver needed medical care in an emergency without unnecessary fear of incurring criminal and civil liability (Garner, 2004). Most states require that the care be given in good faith and that it be gratuitous. Guidelines that govern the interpretation of Good Samaritan laws are shown in Chart 4–8 (p. 82).

Critical Thinking, Decision Making, and Clinical Judgment

Nurses in today's professional world must do more than merely understand legal and ethical concepts. Nurses must blend these important aspects with competent, skilled nursing diagnoses and interventions. To perform such high-quality nursing care, nurses must understand the concepts of critical thinking and clinical judgment, for without these latter concepts one is not able to fully appreciate the application of legal and ethical concepts in professional practice settings. For this reason, the concepts of critical thinking, decision making, and clinical judgment are discussed in depth in Chapters 1, 2, and 7 ⊘. National guidelines that may be used in assisting nurses with making legal and ethical decisions are shown in the National Guidelines box. Research possibilities for ethics and legal concepts are suggested in the Research Opportunities and Clinical Impact box (p. 82).

CHART 4–8 **Good Samaritan Laws**

1. Make your decision quickly as to whether you will stay and help. There is no common law duty to stop and render aid; however, once you begin to provide care, you incur the legal duty to maintain a standard of reasonable emergency care.

2. Ask the injured person or family members for permission to help. Do not force your services once refused.

3. Care for the injured party where you can do so safely, in the vehicle or at the exact site where the victim is found. Only move the injured party if you must do so without causing further harm and as needed to prevent further harm.

4. Apply the rules of first aid. Assess for and prevent major bleeding, assess for the need to initiate cardiopulmonary resuscitation, cover the injured party with a blanket or coat, and so forth.

5. Assess and reassess the person continuously for additional injuries, and communicate findings of your assessment to the injured person and family.

6. Have someone call or go for additional help while you stay with the injured person.

7. Stay with the injured person until equally or more qualified help arrives. Prevent unskilled persons from treating or moving the injured party.

8. Provide the police or emergency medical personnel with as complete a description as possible of the care that you have rendered so that continuity of care exists. Give family members or police any personal items such as dentures, eyeglasses, and the like.

9. Do not accept any compensation of any kind offered by the injured party or family members as this may change your status into a fee-for-service situation and cause you to lose your Good Samaritan protection.

10. Should you choose not to stop and render aid, stop at the nearest phone and report the accident to proper authorities so that the injured party may be aided.

Source: Guido, G. W. *Legal and ethical issues in nursing* (4th ed.) © 2006. Electronically reproduced by permission of Pearson Education Inc., Upper Saddle River, New Jersey.

NATIONAL GUIDELINES for Interpretation of Ethical and Legal Issues

- American Hospital Association *A Patient's Bill of Rights* (1992)
- American Medical Association statement of informed consent (2007)
- American Nurses Association Code of Ethics (2001)
- American Nurses Association Nursing Practice Standards (1998)
- Health Insurance Portability and Accountability Act (HIPAA) (1996)
- Joint Commission *Accreditation Manual for Hospitals* (2007)

RESEARCH OPPORTUNITIES AND CLINICAL IMPACT RELATED TO PROFESSIONAL CONCEPTS

Research Opportunity	Clinical Impact
Ethical Concepts	
Means by which nurses make ethical decisions	Improve the knowledge base of nurses concerning ethical principles so that they can make more effective ethical decisions in clinical practice settings.
Identification of ethical dilemmas by nurses in clinical practice settings	
Knowledge base of nurses regarding ethical principles	Explore why nurses are not on ethics committees and the vital need to include nurses in this aspect of patient care.
Involvement of nurses in institutional ethics committees	
Legal Concepts	
Knowledge base of practicing nurses regarding legal issues	Understand the extent of lawsuits filed against nurses, the causes of actions in the filed lawsuits, and the legal knowledge of practicing and student nurses to hopefully prevent further lawsuits.
Numbers of malpractice lawsuits in which nurses are named as defendants	
Numbers of legal courses in schools of nursing	
Critical Thinking, Decision Making, and Clinical Judgment	
Descriptive and qualitative studies on how nurses make decisions and their critical thinking abilities	Improve nurses' decision-making and critical thinking skills with the goal of improving patient outcomes.
Use of clinical pathways and clinical judgment in multiple clinical practice settings	Determine the effectiveness of critical pathways currently being used and the need for modifications, as applicable.
Patient outcomes studies to determine the effectiveness of clinical pathways	

REVIEW QUESTIONS

1. During the course of one day, a nurse will support one patient's decision to not receive a particular medication, suggest family members of another patient go home to get rest, promise one patient that the injection will only pinch for a second, and will spend equal amounts of time with each patient on her assignment. Which ethical theory is this nurse demonstrating?

   1. Deontology
   2. Principlism
   3. Rule utilitarianism
   4. Act utilitarianism

2. The hospital ethics committee is currently studying all of the options available to them to address an ethical dilemma. In which step of the MORAL model is this committee functioning?

   1. Identify issues
   2. Resolve
   3. Options
   4. Evaluate

3. The Ethics Committee schedules Ethics Grand Rounds to be held the Friday of every month. This committee is demonstrating which type of ethics committee structure?

   1. Autonomy model
   2. Social justice model
   3. Fidelity model
   4. Patient benefit model

4. A nurse that just recently passed the state board examination has questions about what she can and cannot do regarding patient care. This nurse should:

   1. Read the state nurse practice act.
   2. Study the organization's standards of patient care.
   3. Contact the school in which she earned her nursing education.
   4. Assume she can provide all aspects of care since she did pass the state board examination.

5. A patient cannot find his dentures and claims the nurse threw them away when they were left on a meal tray. In which of the following types of laws would this situation be addressed?

   1. Common
   2. Civil
   3. Contract
   4. Tort

Answers for review questions appear in Appendix D

KEY TERMS

assault *p.75*
autonomy *p.68*
battery *p.75*
beneficence *p.68*
breach of confidentiality *p.76*
civil law *p.71*
common law *p.71*
criminal law *p.72*
defamation of character *p.75*
deontological theories *p.67*
emancipated minors *p.78*
emergency doctrine *p.78*
ethical decision making *p.69*
ethical dilemma *p.69*
ethics *p.66*

false imprisonment *p.75*
fidelity *p.69*
foreseeability of harm *p.74*
implied consent *p.78*
informed consent *p.77*
intentional torts *p.71*
invasion of privacy *p.76*
justice *p.68*
law *p.70*
malpractice *p.72*
mature minors *p.78*
MORAL model *p.69*
morality *p.66*
national standards of care *p.75*

negligence *p.72*
nonintentional torts *p.71*
nonmaleficence *p.68*
nurse practice acts *p.70*
paternalism *p.68*
principlism *p.67*
quasi-intentional torts *p.71*
regional (locality) rule *p.75*
respect for others *p.69*
scope of practice *p.70*
substituted judgment *p.70*
teleological theories *p.67*
tort law *p.71*
veracity *p.68*

EXPLORE PEARSON mynursingkit™

MyNursingKit is your one stop for online chapter review materials and resources. Prepare for success with additional NCLEX®-style practice questions, interactive assignments and activities, web links, animations and videos, and more!

Register your access code from the front of your book at
www.mynursingkit.com

REFERENCES

American Hospital Association. (1992). *A patient's bill of rights.* Chicago, IL: Author.

American Medical Association. (2007). Informed consent. *AMA Legal Issues.* Retrieved June 3, 2007, from http://www.ama-assn.org/ama/pub/category/print/4608.html

American Nurses Association. (2001). *Code of ethics with interpretive statements.* Silver Spring, MD: Author.

Beauchamp, T. L., & Childress, J. G. (2001). *Principles of biomedical ethics* (5th ed.). New York: Oxford University Press.

Butts, J. B., & Rich, K. L. (2005). *Nursing ethics across the curriculum and into practice.* Sudbury, MA: Jones and Bartlett.

Crisham, N. (1990). Living wills: Controversy and certainty. *Journal of Professional Nursing, 6*(6), 321.

Croke, F. M. (2003). Nurses, negligence, and malpractice. *American Journal of Nursing, 103*(9), 54–64.

Dawson, J. (2007). *Negligence oversimplified.* Retrieved June 3, 2007, from University of Vermont website: http://asci.uvm.edu/equine/law/articles/neg12.htm

DeWolf-Bosek, M. S., & Savage, T. A. (2007). *The ethical component of nursing education.* Philadelphia: Lippincott Williams & Wilkins.

Driggs, A. E. (2002). *The mature minor doctrine: Do adolescents have the right to die?* Columbus, OH: Case Western Reserve University School of Law.

Garner, B. A. (2004). *Black's law dictionary* (8th ed.). Berkeley, CA: West Group Publishing.

Guido, G. W. (2006). *Legal and ethical issues in nursing* (4th ed.). Upper Saddle River, NJ: Pearson Prentice Hall.

Hall, R. T. (2000). *An introduction to health care organizational ethics.* New York: Oxford University Press.

Hamric, A. B. (2002). Bridging the gap between ethics and clinical practice. *Nursing Outlook, 50*(5), 176–178.

HIPAAdvisory. (2006). *Status of HIPAA regulations compliance calendar.* Retrieved November 8, 2007, from http://www.hipaadvisory.com/Regs/com;loiancecal.htm

Joint Commission. (2007). *Accreditation manual for hospitals.* Oak Terrace, IL: Author.

Larson, A. (2003). *Contract law—An introduction, expert law.* Retrieved May 9, 2007, from http://www.expertlaw.com/library/business/contract_law.html

Marquis, B. L., & Huston, C. J. (2006). *Leadership roles an management functions in nursing* (5th ed.). Philadelphia: Lippincott Raven Publishers.

National League for Nursing. (1959). *Patients' rights.* New York: Author.

Negligence. (2007). *The Columbia Electronic Encyclopedia* (6th ed.). New York: Columbia University Press.

Nursing malpractice: Understanding the risks [Special issue]. (2003, June). *Travel Nursing 2003,* pp. 7–12.

Perle, S. (2004). Morality and ethics: An introduction.11(4). Retrieved April 29, 2008 from The American Academy of Anti-Aging Medicine, In. website: http://www.chiroweb.com/archives/22/06/16.html

Sabol v. Richmond Heights General Hospital, 676 N.E.2nd 958 (Ohio App. 1996).

Stanford Encyclopedia of Philosophy (2003). Theories of Tort Law. Retrieved August 14, 2008 from http://plato.stanford-edu/entries/tort-theories/

Thiroux, J. (1977). *Ethics: Theory and practice.* Philadelphia: Macmillan.

Watson, J. (2003, July–September). Love and caring: Ethics face and hand—An invitation to return to the heart and soul of nursing and our deep humanity. *Nursing Administration Quarterly, 27*(3), 197–202.

Yoder-Wise, P. S. (2007). *Leading and managing in nursing* (4th ed.). St. Louis: Mosby.

45 Code of Federal Regulations, Sections 160.102 and 160.103. (1996). General Adminstrative Requirements. Retrieved August 14, 2008 from http://www. hhs.gov/OCR/regtext.html.

Nursing Care Delivery Systems

Carol Robinson

Outcome-Based Learning Objectives

After studying this chapter, the learner will be able to:

1. Identify the four types of nursing care delivery systems most commonly used in health care settings.
2. Analyze the influences of each nursing care delivery system on professional nurse satisfaction, patient satisfaction, and quality of care delivered.
3. Explain the delegation responsibilities of the registered nurse for each nursing care delivery system.
4. Distinguish among the economic variables influencing the selection of a nursing care delivery system.
5. Differentiate the roles of advanced practice nurses and case managers within the context of the four nursing care delivery systems identified in this chapter.

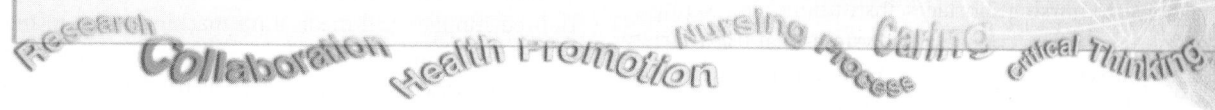

Research · Collaboration · Health Promotion · Nursing Process · Caring · Critical Thinking

NURSING AND hospital administrators have struggled for more than 100 years with the question of how to deliver appropriate nursing care to patients in an efficient and effective manner. **Nursing care delivery systems** were developed to describe a structure for the organization of nursing work, to identify the types of health care workers providing the nursing care, and to define the boundaries for the delegation of authority.

Nursing Care Delivery Systems: Past to Present

Registered nurses work in several different settings and have many different job titles, responsibilities, and credentials. (As new roles for nurses develop in the health care setting, many nursing professionals describe these innovations in care modalities as nursing care delivery systems.) This chapter will discuss the innovations and advancements in health care delivery as evolutionary adaptations of the four basic nursing delivery systems using Marie Manthey's (1990) definition of a nursing care delivery system. Manthey describes nursing care delivery systems as ". . . a set of concepts defining four basic organizational elements. The definitions of these elements are based on principles that are in turn based on fundamental values. These fundamental values will ultimately determine the quality of the product. These four fundamental values or elements are clinical decision making, work allocation, communication, and management" (Manthey, 1990, p. 203). Marie Manthey's definitions of nursing care delivery systems published in 1990 are still widely accepted (Tiedeman & Lookinland, 2004).

Historical Influence

Nursing care delivery systems are complex and subject to the economic, social, political, and technological influences of the time period. World wars, the Industrial Revolution, the Great Depression, the development of diagnosis-related groups (DRGs), and managed care have sparked changes in health care delivery and challenged the way the profession of nursing is practiced (Marquis & Huston, 2006). (See Chapter 1.)

The pressure to reduce unnecessary costs resulted in the development of several different types of managed care organizations such as the health maintenance organization (HMO). Managed care is a form of health care delivery that uses financial incentives to direct patients to the most cost-effective and efficient treatment center. HMOs focus resources on prevention of illness and the avoidance of the use of costly hospital resources. Managed care has resulted in shorter lengths of stay for hospitalized patients. Conversely, it has caused more patients to require home health services and utilize outpatient clinics, and it has created a dire need for the coordination of care (Roussel, 2006). The complexity of how health care is financed has a great impact on who delivers the care and how the care delivery is organized (Finkler & Kovner, 2000). Chapter 3 ⊚ discussed health care finance issues.

Current Influence

The nursing shortage has historically influenced the types of nursing care delivery systems used in many health care settings, and the shortage continues to drive the search for the ideal nursing care delivery system. It is predicted that there may be a shortage of as many as 800,000 nurses by the year 2020, and an unprecedented shortage of registered nurses by 2030 if dramatic interventions are not taken (Buerhaus, Donelan, Ulrich, Norman, & Dittus, 2006). The decision to implement a particular nursing care delivery system will increasingly depend on the complexity and variability within the health care setting. The availability of the labor pool, the acuity of patients, and the financial health of the institution are important variables to consider when selecting a nursing care delivery system. The term **acuity** refers to the measurement of patient severity of illness and the amount of nursing care required by the patient (Finkler & Kovner, 2000). It is an important variable that must be considered when determining the skill level needed to provide appropriate care, and it takes into account patients' needs, technology required to care for patients, and the amount of interdisciplinary support needed by the nurse (Hinshaw & McClure, 2002; Ritter-Teitel, 2004).

In response to nursing shortages, institutions tend to implement or modify nursing care delivery systems that use a variety of licensed nurses and unlicensed assistive personnel (UAP) (Formella & Rovin, 2004). Because RN salaries have increased due to the decreased supply of nurses and the increased demand for nurses, many health care institutions have changed the skill mix by hiring UAP in an effort to reduce labor costs. Organized labor unions have responded to managements' cost savings efforts by introducing legislation in several states to enact mandatory staffing ratios as a patient safety initiative and to force hospitals to increase the number of licensed nurses. In January 2004 California was the first state to mandate licensed nurse staffing ratios (Clarke & Aiken, 2003; Haugh, 2005). A literature review in 2004 of more that 490 articles and a detailed analysis of 43 articles revealed that there is "... no support for specific, minimum nurse–patient ratios for acute care hospitals, especially in the absence of adjustments for skill and patient mix. ..." This study found probable relationships between richer RN staffing and nurse satisfaction, lower failure to rescue rates, lower inpatient mortality, and shorter lengths of stay" (Lang, Hodge, Olson, Romano, & Kravitz, 2004, p. 326). The legislation by the state of California has opened debate and fueled a call for more research to clearly identify the relationship of quality patient outcomes to skill mix. In the meantime, many states have legislation pending in an attempt to attract and retain RNs in the face of increasing acuity and the nursing shortage. The Joint Commission on Accreditation of Healthcare Organizations, the national accrediting body for hospitals and health systems, has set standards for nurse staffing and assignment of patient care. These must be adhered to in order to maintain accreditation

> **NATIONAL GUIDELINES for The Joint Commission**
>
> The Joint Commission is an accrediting body for hospitals and health systems. Information on staffing requirements can be found in the September 2006 document titled *Comprehensive Accreditation Manual for Hospitals, The Official Handbook, Update 2,* but can only be accessed through an organization that has purchased the reference. Limited free information can be found on the Joint Commission's official website: http://www.jointcommission.org.

and to meet quality of care standards. These guidelines are described in the National Guidelines box.

The physical design of the patient care areas and the experience and competency of the personnel might also influence the choice or modification of a nursing care delivery system (Daditch, 2003). Nursing units designed in circles, squares, or rectangles with central or decentralized medication and supply services may require different configurations of staff to safely provide observation and care. The creation of smaller sections where patient care is delivered may increase the ability of staff to obtain assistance when needed (Kalisch & Begeny, 2005). The American Institute of Architects (AIA) published design standards in 2006 that emphasize safety for patients and staff. These guidelines recommend a unit layout that can reduce the time nurses spend walking and thereby reduce the fatigue factor that leads to errors (AIA, 2006). The National Guidelines box provides more information about the AIA guidelines. Units designed to have decentralized supplies and medication machines close to the patient care activities are referred to as modular units (Ulrich & Quan, 2004). Increased support from ancillary departments is critical for modular units to succeed. "The intent behind any nursing unit design must be to reduce time spent performing non-nursing tasks" (Institute of Medicine [IOM], 2004, p. 101).

Evidenced-Based Management Practices

Traditional delivery systems form a framework that can be modified to meet the uniqueness of the particular agency setting; however, measuring the effectiveness of such a system is complex and difficult. The efficiency and effectiveness of any system usually is evaluated by measuring four factors: quality patient care, patient satisfaction, nursing job satisfaction, and cost effectiveness for the health care organization. The Joint Commission (2006) has adopted a standard definition of quality patient care as "the degree to which health services for individuals and populations increase the likelihood of desired health outcomes and

> **NATIONAL GUIDELINES for the American Institute of Architects**
>
> *Guidelines for Design and Construction of Health Care Facilities* is a publication of the American Institute of Architects. The guidelines were developed in 2006 with the assistance of the U.S. Department of Health and Human Services. Federal agencies, the Joint Commission, and 42 states use this information to plan and guide new construction or remodels of patient care areas.

are consistent with current professional knowledge" (p. GL-20). Desired outcomes that might be measured include fewer medication errors and fewer pressure ulcers. Undesired outcomes might be the failure of the RN to rescue the patient before the patient's condition causes irreparable harm or death (Huber, 2006; IOM, 2004).

The California Nursing Outcomes Coalition is a self-funded organization that was created by the Association of California Nurse Leaders and the American Nurses Association. The purpose of this organization is to develop a database of patient outcomes and hospital statistics. Data on nurse staffing, patient days, patient falls, pressure ulcer prevalence, and patient satisfaction scores are captured, and the data are used to provide evidence for practice changes (Brown, 2002). There is potential for future research as more hospitals elect to contribute to this database.

The outcome variable of patient satisfaction measures the degree of coordination of care, the degree to which emotional and spiritual needs are met, and the degree of safety in the care provided. The outcome variable of nurse job satisfaction measures the degree to which nursing care delivery systems acknowledge, nurture, and protect the practice of the professional nurse. Common indicators of nurse job satisfaction are the degree of job autonomy, the accountability of the professional nurse, and the presence of meaningful work (Aiken, Clarke, Sloane, Sochalski, & Silber, 2002; Deutschendorf, 2003; Kramer & Schmalenberg, 2002).

The cost-effective measurement of nursing care delivery systems is difficult to achieve. Identifying the best care for the lowest cost may be deemed a cost-effective choice (Finkler & Kovner, 2000). Deutschendorf (2003) studied care delivery, but concluded that all models need to be uniquely developed while balancing fiscal responsibility. A review of the research in the Institute of Medicine's 2004 report *Keeping Patients Safe* did not identify a particular nursing care delivery system that stood out from all others. The complexity of the nursing work environment today involves leadership resources, availability of technology, culture, and measures of workload. Nursing researchers are still testing nursing care delivery systems, but have not achieved success in identifying specific cost-effective systems.

Houser (2003) tested a model of demands on nursing in an attempt to measure the multivariate nature of the nursing work environment. This research was a first step toward evaluating the complex issues of maintaining a competent, satisfied workforce and providing acceptable patient care at a reasonable cost. Further evidence relating nursing workload to patient outcomes is needed to make the management decisions necessary to achieve the desired results. Nursing researchers such as Aiken, Buerhaus, Kramer, and Needleman have contributed to a body of knowledge about work hours, work environment, satisfaction, patient outcomes, and educational preparation that begins to answer some of management's questions about professional practice, but falls short of identifying effective delivery systems. Citing the lack of evidence to support a specific delivery system, the IOM and others support the selection of care delivery system models that can be tailored to the unit's unique design, availability of resources, and quality of professional staff (Deutschendorf, 2003; Formella & Rovin, 2004; IOM, 2004). Subsequent to the IOM report, Needleman and Buerhaus (2006) found that increases in the proportion of nurses while keeping the number of hours of care the same can reduce unnecessary deaths and shorten lengths of stay.

Integration of RN Roles in Care Delivery Systems

There are four well-defined and widely used traditional nursing care delivery systems encountered in acute, outpatient, and long-term health care settings. Each of these systems—the case method, functional nursing, team nursing, and primary nursing—takes advantage of a variety of caregivers with licenses or certifications and different education levels. Different roles for **registered nurses (RNs)** have been developed over the years to complement and support nurses and physicians delivering care at the bedside (Bryant-Lukosius, DiCenso, Browne, & Pinelli, 2004). These roles include the advanced practice nurse, certified registered nurse anesthetist, clinical nurse specialist, certified nurse midwife, nurse practitioner, and the new role of clinical nurse leader. These roles are discussed within the context of each of the delivery systems.

An **advanced practice nurse (APRN)** is a registered nurse with advanced education, knowledge, and skills. APRNs might also have additional certifications, and their practice can vary depending on the scope of practice defined by the state board of registered nursing in which they work. APRNs are increasingly being used in the clinical setting and may be used in all nursing care delivery systems without changing the basic structure or philosophy of the delivery system. Advanced practice nurses include nurses with the titles **certified registered nurse anesthetist (CRNA), clinical nurse specialist (CNS), certified nurse midwife (CNM),** and **nurse practitioner (NP).** Economic, social, political, and technologic factors influence the acceptability and demand for these roles in much the same way as nursing care delivery models are influenced (Bryant-Lukosius et al., 2004). Chapter 1 ⊙ includes an in-depth discussion of advanced practice roles.

A new role for an RN at the bedside is currently being evaluated. The role of **clinical nurse leader (CNL)** is intended to manage patient services across multidisciplinary boundaries at the bedside and to be a resource to the bedside nurse. The American Association of Colleges of Nursing (AACN) determined that a new role was needed to differentiate the education of nurses and entry levels into nursing without differentiating existing practice levels. CNLs are envisioned as coordinators of care and leaders with the authority to function as part of the clinical health care team. CNLs, by virtue of their advanced education and ability to manage complex systems of care, would be responsible for evaluating outcomes and leading change at the point of care (AACN, 2005; Drenkard & Cohen, 2004). Several institutions are piloting this role; however, research is not complete as to the effectiveness of such a role (Begun, Hamilton, Tornabeni, & White, 2006). Another, more widely accepted approach to coordinating and managing complex systems has been the delegation of these responsibilities to administrative nurses without direct clinical care duties.

The introduction of managed care in the early 1990s resulted in a new position being created within the health care setting titled **case manager.** Managed care requires close coordination of care across all health care settings and therefore affects the role of the RN in the delivery of care. Some institutions, however, do not always use RNs (Huber, 2006). The chief function of the case manager is to collaboratively plan, coordinate, and evaluate services in a cost-effective manner. Nurse case managers interact with health care team members to reduce fragmentation and improve outcomes. In many settings, case managers do not provide direct patient care (American Nurses Credentialing Center, 2006; White & Hall, 2006). In others, case management is considered to be a care delivery model.

Care Delivery Models

The delivery of health care to the patient is a multidisciplinary process that must take into account the availability of resources, the educational preparation of the nurse, the competencies of staff, the needs of the patient, and the cost implications for the institution or health system (McCauley & Irwin, 2006). Models of care delivery are continually being modified to adjust for the many variables in the health care setting. The traditional models are presented next to provide a baseline understanding of the structured work of nursing in a health care setting.

Case Method

The **case method** of delivering nursing care is simply defined, and sometimes referred to as **total patient care.** The RN is responsible for the patient and has total care responsibility for the patient during the shift worked.

Work Allocation

All patients have an RN assigned to them, and this type of delivery system requires exclusive use of an all RN staff (Figure 5–1 ■). There is no assignment requirement that the RN have the same patient day after day nor is there a consistent coordinator to ensure continuity of care during the course of the hospitalization (Tomey, 2004). The case method is frequently practiced in the intensive care setting or in the home health setting (Huber, 2006).

Clinical Decision Making

The RN assumes responsibility for the total care of the patient and may have several assigned patients. In addition to being responsible for the nursing process, the RN is responsible for all indirect and direct patient care functions. Care planning and goal setting occur between family, patient, and nurse during the specific shift. The charge nurse may have a patient load or may assist where needed. The role of the charge nurse is to manage the shift activities, provide consultation to staff, and make patient assignments according to the resources available.

Communication

The RN communicates changes, needs, and requests for assistance to the charge nurse. The RN is generally expected to communicate with physicians and other disciplines regarding patient care needs. Communication and coordination of care between shifts is dependent on the efforts of the individual shift nurse.

Management

The advantages of the case method are considered to be holistic and comprehensive care delivered by a registered nurse. The cost of RNs, the lack of continuity between shifts, and the dependence on an adequate supply of nurses are considered to be disadvantages of this system (Daditch, 2003).

The disadvantages to the case method of nursing care delivery can be mitigated through the use of advanced practice nurses and case managers. Advanced practice nurses typically work side by side in settings where the case method is implemented. The clinical nurse leader would serve to coordinate care between the other disciplines in this delivery care system. The use of the CNS or NP in the intensive care unit may provide specialty expertise and education for the nursing staff or extend the physician's capabilities and provide additional consultative support for the bedside nurse (Whitcomb et al., 2002). The use of advance practice nurses as part of the health care team provides continuity of care and can reduce the length of stay and mortality rate (Cowan et al., 2006). Case managers may place patients with a specific diagnosis on a clinical pathway. In situations where case managers are used, the planning, coordinating, and evaluating of the care responsibilities of the bedside nurse are assumed by the case manager. The bedside nurse then is responsible for the assessment and intervention components of patient care (Marquis & Huston, 2006). A collaborative effort between the bedside nurse, the case manager, and the physician ensures continuity of care for the patient as the patient progresses to different levels of care. This collaborative partnership is outcome

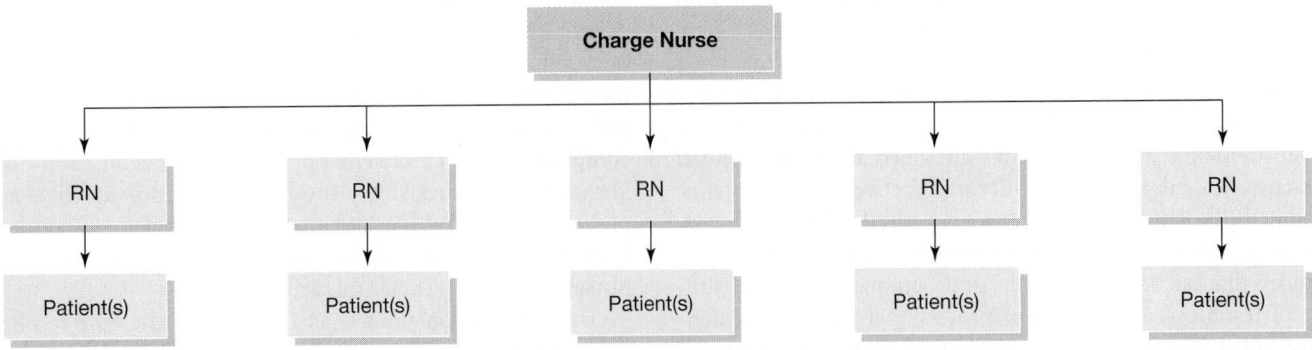

INTENSIVE CARE SETTING

FIGURE 5–1 ■ Sample staffing assignments for the case method of nursing care delivery.

driven and offers the added benefit of providing care to a defined group of patients with limited resources (Cortes, Noyes, & Brennan, 2000). (Case management is discussed in more detail in Chapter 3 .)

Functional Nursing

The functional nursing care delivery system was first developed in response to the increasing demand for hospital nursing in the late 1800s and it resurfaced due to the sporadic nursing shortages resulting from World War II (Daditch, 2003). A **functional nursing** care delivery system is defined as a task-oriented system in which individual caregivers are not given patient assignments, but are expected to perform specific assigned tasks within their capability for all patients in a given area. This method of providing care to the patient involves both licensed nursing staff and unlicensed assistive personnel. "**Unlicensed assistive personnel** are health care personnel who are not licensed and may be technicians or certified nurses' aides or nursing assistants" (Daditch, 2003 p. 255). Several variations may be used in health care settings today, but all functional models depend on a hierarchical structure that requires strict definition of roles and responsibilities and control of tasks (Tomey, 2004).

Work Allocation

Figure 5–2 ■ shows a standard flowchart for the functional nursing care delivery system. The charge nurse may be responsible for both administrative and clinical functions such as taking orders, contacting physicians for patient needs, assisting personnel with difficult or emergent patient care needs, adjusting staffing schedules, and evaluating or orienting staff. The task of medication administration is usually assigned to an RN in the role of **medication nurse.** The use of a medication nurse is not a common practice in acute care facilities today, but it is a useful function in long-term care facilities. This role may be assigned in

acute care settings, however, during disasters or other emergent situations when the patient-to-staff ratio is higher than usual.

In situations where there is a shortage of RNs, a **licensed vocational/practical nurse (LVN/LPN)** may be assigned to administer oral and parenteral medications while the charge RN administers the IV medications (Daditch, 2003). LVN/LPNs receive 1 to 2 years of practical training to deliver basic nursing care and are licensed according to state practice acts.

A treatment nurse is assigned the responsibility of providing treatments. This nurse is frequently an LVN/LPN and the assignment of tasks is dependent on the scope of practice of the LVN/LPN and the complexity of patients' needs. The scope of practice may change according to state law and regulations. It also is dependent on agency policy, wherein the agency may be more restrictive than the law allows.

UAP are assigned to take vital signs, assist the patients with basic hygiene tasks, and provide comfort measures. This variation in the functional delivery system may work well in skilled nursing facilities or facilities with lower acuity patients (Tomey, 2004).

Clinical Decision Making

In a typical functional model, an RN is assigned to be in charge and coordinate the care of all patients. The clinical decision making for all patients rests with the charge nurse since that individual is responsible for collecting all pertinent information about the patients. The RN is responsible for delegating tasks to personnel consistent with the applicable state nurse practice act. **Delegation** is defined as being accountable for outcomes of work that is shared with others (Daditch, 2003). "To delegate is to transfer authority to a competent individual for completing selected nursing tasks/activities/functions" (National Council of State Boards of Nursing [NCSBN], 2005).

CRITICAL ALERT | *Delegation by an RN requires clinical judgment and knowledge of the applicable state's nurse practice act, which authorizes the scope of responsibility and grants the authority to delegate. All RNs must know how to prioritize patients' needs and assign tasks based on the competency of the personnel, but they also must know how to supervise the personnel and intervene when necessary.*

The RN must consider qualifications, job descriptions, and competency when delegating tasks to various caregivers. Qualifications are generally determined by state licensure or certification, and the RN may reference hospital policies and procedures, job descriptions, published state practice acts, or unit guidelines if unfamiliar with specific qualifications (Koloroutis, 2004). For instance, an LVN/LPN may be permitted by license to draw blood in some states. In other states the LVN/LPN must have an additional certification to draw blood.

State practice acts address these qualifications in published regulations, and hospital job descriptions delineate the roles and responsibilities of individuals within a specific agency. Many workers may be unlicensed and have only basic training in health care. The nurse needs to be familiar with each job description and confident about the competency of the worker before assigning tasks. The authority and accountability for the outcome of the worker's performance still rests with the RN (Potter & Grant, 2004). (The functions of state nursing practice acts are discussed in more detail in Chapter 4 .)

MEDICAL OR SURGICAL 30 BED UNIT

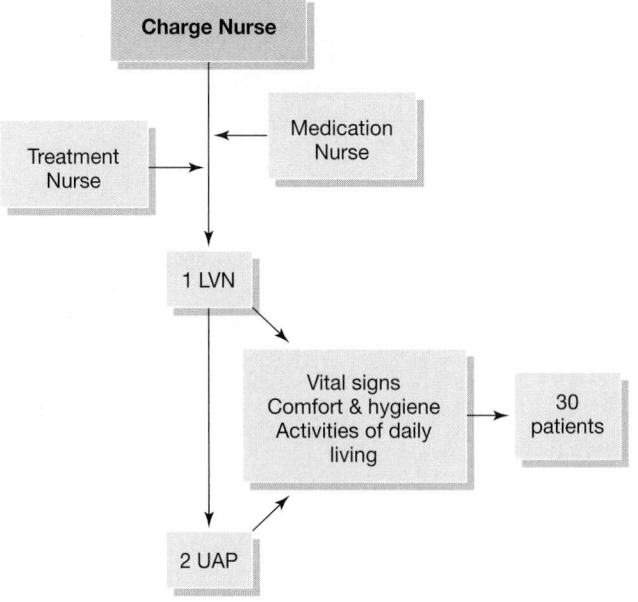

FIGURE 5–2 ■ Sample staffing assignments for the functional method of nursing care delivery.

Competency to perform a task or procedure may be measured by tests, clinical observation, or certification by a training facility. Nursing assistants may be certified by the state or may have a certificate from a training facility. Certifications specifically identify the types of procedures or tasks that the individual has been trained to perform. RNs and LVN/LPNs also may be certified to perform specific procedures. The RN must be knowledgeable about the competence of the individual before delegating tasks, and the hospital must keep records documenting the competence of the individuals performing those tasks.

Delegating a task to an individual who is not competent has serious implications for the RN, the RN's license, and the institution should the patient suffer an adverse outcome. The RN should assess the patients' needs and consider situations where the outcome is uncertain or the potential for harm is high. Tasks should not be delegated under those circumstances. Nursing assessment and judgment may not be delegated. In addition to considering qualifications, job descriptions, competence, and patient needs, the RN must evaluate the effectiveness of the delegation and whether the desired outcome was achieved (Corbo, 2006; NCSBN, 2005).

Communication

The members of the staff are responsible for communicating changes to the charge nurse. It is the charge nurse's ultimate responsibility to communicate patient needs and coordinate the care with other disciplines. On busy or large patient care units, there is a possibility that patient needs will be overlooked (Huber, 2006). The increased number of personnel performing specific tasks for the individual patient intentionally fragments care. The functional nursing model is an industrial efficiency model that demands a high level of coordination and communication. The overall assessment of the patient from beginning to end may be incomplete and cause critical changes to go unnoticed (Daditch, 2003).

Management

Functional care delivery systems are implemented by management when the desired outcomes for nursing are efficiency in completing a large number of tasks. The ability to train unskilled personnel to complete limited specific tasks and to avoid high labor costs by using lower paid workers are incentives for health care facilities interested in the industrial model of efficiency (Huber, 2006). Institutions that embrace the industrial model of efficiency do not tend to modify the nursing care delivery system to provide better coordinated care by using advanced practice nurses or case managers. Nurse practitioners or nurse midwives might be used as physician extenders in these facilities.

The disadvantages of functional nursing are fragmented patient care, low job satisfaction, and low patient satisfaction. Nurses report a lack of satisfaction with their work because tasks are boring or because there is difficulty identifying the effect of their work on their patients. Functional nursing resembles assembly-line tasking and the fragmentation of tasks results in a perceived lack of accountability and increased frustration (Tiedeman & Lookinland, 2004; Tomey, 2004). Reduced patient satisfaction is linked to fragmented care and the resultant lack of confidence in the caregivers (Huber, 2006).

Charge nurses working with a functional nursing care delivery system must be knowledgeable about the RN and LVN/LPN practice laws in the state in which they are practicing. The delegation of tasks must be consistent with the state training and licensure or certification regulations. The UAP performing patient care tasks may face misdemeanor charges or penalties for practicing nursing without a license in states where mandatory licensure protects the title of registered nurse and the actions are protected by the state nursing practice act (Guido, 2006; NCSBN, 2005). The nursing practice act and its functions as related to regulations are discussed at length in Chapter 4 ☺.

Team Nursing

Team nursing was developed in the early 1950s in response to complaints that functional nursing created a fragmented care delivery system and resulted in nursing and patient dissatisfaction with care (Marquis & Huston, 2006). In the team nursing care delivery system, patients are assigned to a nursing team, which usually is led by an RN. The team may include RNs, LVN/LPNs, respiratory therapists, dieticians, and UAP. Small teams may be assigned to care for patients. These teams include an LVN/LPN and UAP. These types of teams may be called care partners, modular teams, patient-focused teams, or any name that incorporates the concept of a work redesign with the skill mix intended to be used.

Work Allocation

A typical unit with 30 patients may have a charge nurse, two team leaders, and usually two to four team members per team (Figure 5–3 ■), but no more than five members per team (Marquis & Huston, 2006). Assignments are based on the acuity of the patients and the skill level and experience of the caregivers (Huber, 2006). The team leader assigns all patients to team members and may delegate additional tasks according to the team members' competence (Daditch, 2003). The team assign-

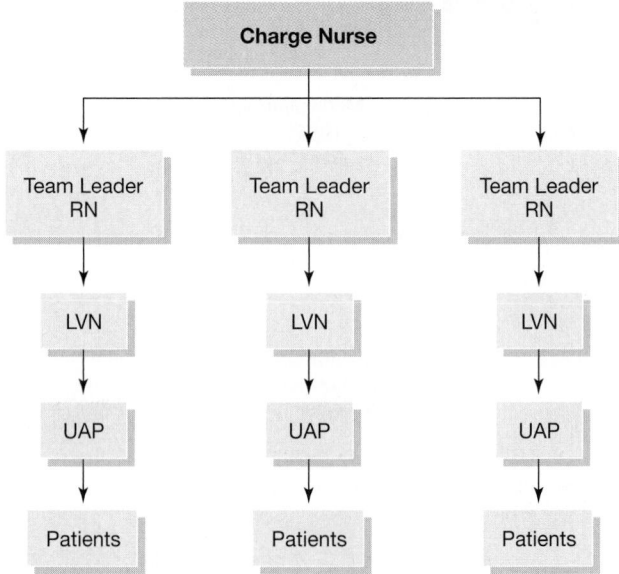

MEDICAL OR SURGICAL UNIT

FIGURE 5–3 ■ Sample staffing assignments for the team method of nursing care delivery.

ments may sometimes mirror a functional approach to care when the team leader is the only RN or licensed person on the team (Marquis & Huston, 2006). The team leader would assume responsibility for administering all medications and IV solutions to patients on the team and delegate remaining responsibilities to the team members.

Clinical Decision Making

The charge nurse is responsible for assigning groups of patients and caregivers to the team leaders and for facilitating communications between multidisciplinary caregivers. Decision making is delegated to several team leaders versus a single charge nurse, and team members work collaboratively toward common goals. Team leaders are responsible for making the individual patient assignments to their team members. Team leaders plan the care, delegate tasks, and monitor the work of the team to ensure quality. As time permits, the team leader may coordinate care conferences for patients with complex health care needs. Daily conferences are the ideal, but frequently time constraints prevent completion of conferences.

Communication

Team nursing is difficult to implement without extensive team communication (Daditch, 2003). Nursing shortages and high turnover among unlicensed assistive personnel can make communication between ever-changing team members a challenge. Research has documented RN dissatisfaction with communication and teamwork when UAP are used. Research also suggests that how personnel are assigned may mitigate these concerns (Potter & Grant, 2004). Experienced RNs with good communication, organization, and leadership skills are necessary (Marquis & Huston, 2006). Numerous formal and informal structures for communication among team members are available. Written care plans, written assignment responsibilities, and team conferences encourage coordinated care (Yoder-Wise, 2007).

Management

Team nursing has advantages because it uses individual team members' strengths to the greatest advantage for a large number of patients (Huber, 2006). Responsibility for the delegation of tasks remains the same as in the functional nursing care delivery system. Unlicensed assistive personnel may not practice nursing without a license, and nursing responsibilities are delineated in the state nursing practice act. All team members need specific role definition and communication skills to ensure that care is not fragmented, because fragmentation of care may decrease job satisfaction and contribute to decreased quality of care. It also has been reported that high-level teams working toward common goals and focused missions can experience increased job satisfaction (Kalisch & Begeny, 2005).

Complex, time-intensive training is essential to ensure that team members can function within a team structure and effectively communicate. Clinical nurse specialists and nurse practitioners can provide consultative support in a team nursing care delivery system. The clinical nurse leader role could be useful in this type of delivery system because the CNL would provide coordination within multidisciplinary teams and provide consistent information to the patient as well as the team. The use of APRNs can complement nursing care of patients with complex

needs and provide advanced educational support (Deutschendorf, 2003).

Primary Nursing

Primary nursing was developed as a nursing care delivery system in the late 1960s or early 1970s in response to the unhappiness of the professional nurse with the lack of autonomy and the declining quality of patient care (Daditch, 2003). **Primary nursing** is defined as a system in which each patient is assigned to a nurse who has 24-hour responsibility for the nursing care delivered to the patient (Tomey, 2004).

Work Allocation

Figure 5–4 ■ (p. 92) shows a typical flowchart for the primary nursing care method. The primary nurse is responsible for planning for the patient's care and delegating the care during the hours that the nurse is not present and also is accountable for the coordination and continuity of care from admission to discharge. The nurse who assists the primary nurse during off-duty hours is called an **associate nurse** or **associate caregiver.** The associate nurse follows the plan of care, communicates pertinent information or changes in the patient status to the primary nurse, and provides direct patient care when the primary nurse is not present. An associate caregiver may be an LVN/LPN or UAP (Manthey, 2002). A nurse may be a primary nurse for a small caseload of patients and also may be an associate nurse for other patients.

Clinical Decision Making

The three major responsibilities of the primary nurse can be simplified into (1) clear communication among all care disciplines, (2) development of a plan of care using the nursing process, and (3) discharge planning from the time of admission to discharge (Marquis & Huston, 2006). The primary nurse is held accountable for collecting and communicating important patient information during the patient's hospitalization. The primary nurse provides direct patient care because this nurse is in the best position to plan the care (Manthey, 2002; Roussel, 2006). Involving the patient in the collection of information, eliciting patient expectations for the outcomes of care, and encouraging participation in the development of goals is a significant part of the process (Daditch, 2003).

The nurse develops the plan of care using whatever documentation method the health care facility may have developed to direct all care providers. Instruments such as Kardex care plans, care pathways, care maps, nursing admission forms, guidelines, and multidisciplinary education forms can be used. Planning for the discharge of the patient is facilitated by the process of fulfilling the first two responsibilities: identifying the expected outcomes on admission and keeping the health care team on target with the plan of care (Manthey, 2002; Roussel, 2006). The primary nurse may use institutional resources such as discharge planning nurses, case managers, or social services to assist the patient in discharge from the health care facility.

Communication

Consistent and accurate communication of information between shifts and appropriate delegation of care planning activities between associate nurses and primary nurses eliminate the charge nurse from the communication chain between physician

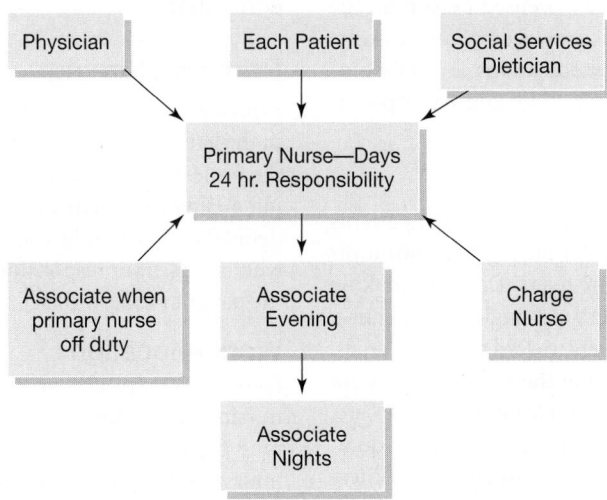

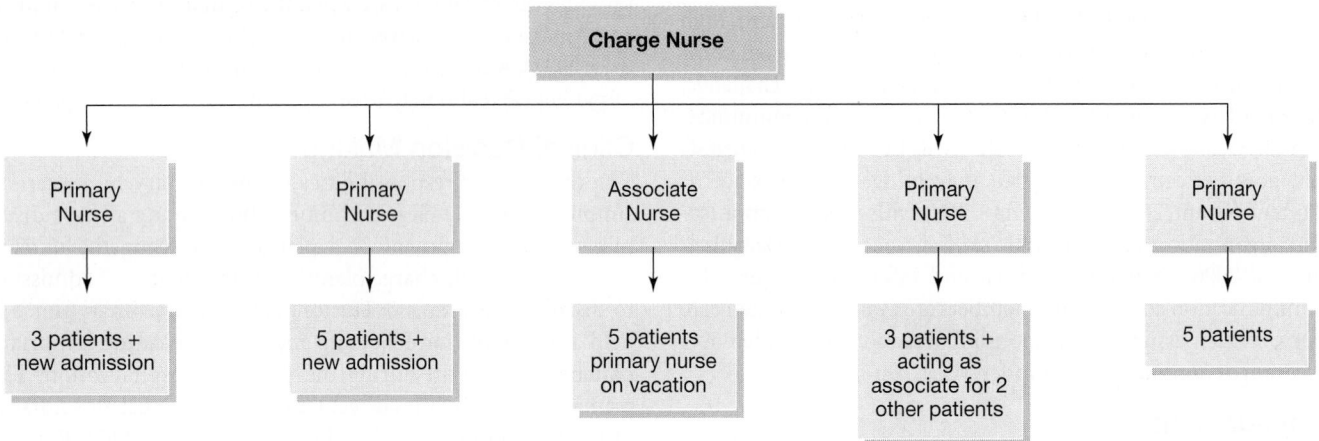

FIGURE 5–4 ■ Sample staffing assignments for the primary nursing method of nursing care delivery.

and caregiver (Roussel, 2006; Swansburg & Swansburg, 2002). Direct communication improves the rapport and trust between the primary nurse, the patient, and the physician, creating a therapeutic relationship. The charge nurse is then able to support the activities of the unit and provide consultation for the primary nurse.

Management

The use of an associate caregiver is not inconsistent with the intent of the primary nursing care delivery system, which is to provide patient-focused care in an environment where the professional nurse is held accountable for practice. The associate caregiver may be task focused, but the care continues to be coordinated and monitored on a 24-hour basis by the primary nurse.

The advantages of the primary nursing care delivery system are the increased nurse perception of autonomy, the continuity of care, and the patient focus. Research also suggests that the outcomes of care are better and nurse satisfaction is higher (Tomey, 2004). Although the research does not support a spe-

cific patient care delivery model, many studies suggest that richer RN staffing levels result in lower lengths of stay, fewer patient deaths, and lower failure-to-rescue rates (Aiken, Clarke, & Sloane, 2000; Needleman et al., 2002; Sovie et al., 2000). Patient satisfaction has been correlated with nurse satisfaction and quality of care in several basic studies (Hegyvary & Haussman, 1976; Weisman & Nathanson, 1985). Recent studies suggest a link between nurse burnout and decreased patient satisfaction (Vahey, Aiken, Sloane, Clarke, & Vargas, 2004). Other research suggests that there are higher levels of nurse satisfaction, greater continuity of care, positive patient outcomes, and improved nurse retention with the use of primary nursing care delivery systems (Huber, 2006; Kramer & Schmalenberg, 2002).

The primary nursing care delivery system uses many hospital resources, but places the control and authorization of such resources in the hands of the primary nurse. The primary nurse is responsible for developing the plan of care and prioritizing the daily activities to achieve the mutually agreed-on goals in the plan. For instance, because the primary nurse understands the sleeping and eating preferences of a particular patient who has cancer, routines and treatments can be adjusted to meet the patient's basic needs. If the patient and family need complex information from the physicians or other members of the health care team about the prognosis and treatment options of chemotherapy and radiation, the primary nurse may coordinate a care conference and identify the desired outcomes to realize a productive meeting. The primary nurse may advocate for scheduling placement of central lines for chemotherapy with patient and family schedules. Chemotherapy treatments may be managed to coincide with family support. All of these activities are the responsibility of the primary nurse providing care at the bedside.

Nurse practitioners can function within this system as physician extenders and consultants to the primary nurse. Clinical nurse specialists are valuable in providing clinical expertise and education to the primary nurse. The use of case managers may be redundant because of the primary nurse's accountability for the entire patient experience. This also may be true of the clinical nurse leader role, depending on the interpretation of primary nursing used, since the primary nurse is responsible for all of the functions that a clinical nurse leader normally would assume in one of the other types of nursing care delivery models. This may not be true in all agencies, depending again on the interpretation and usage of primary nursing.

A primary nursing care delivery system may not be the preferred system during downturns in the economy and cyclical nursing shortages. There is a perception that labor costs are high because primary nursing requires a large number of RNs, although cost studies have disputed this perception (Daditch, 2003). Additional research is needed to determine whether a primary nursing care delivery system shields an institution from the impact of a nursing shortage by attracting and retaining nurses and improving patient outcomes.

Relationship-Based Care

Primary care is enjoying renewed popularity as a nursing care delivery system because of an evolution described as *relationship-based care*. Relationship-based care incorporates the structure of primary nursing with the principles and values of a professional nursing practice environment. "The purpose of relationship-based care is to establish a therapeutic relationship between nurses, patients, and their families during their episode of care, to accomplish essential nursing interventions, and to maximize collaborative interdisciplinary practice" (Person, 2004, p. 159).

The professional nursing practice environment is best defined by research conducted in the early 1990s by Linda Aiken, Margaret McClure, Margaret Sovie, Marlene Kramer, Donna Havens, Heather Laschinger, and others. A professional nursing practice environment facilitates professional autonomy and control over individual practice, while encouraging collaborative relationships. These researchers and many others identified specific professional nursing practice attributes in hospitals that were successful in retaining and attracting nurses. These hospitals were labeled **magnet hospitals.** Research on magnet hospitals indicates that there is improved quality of care, improved patient satisfaction, and improved nursing satisfaction within hospitals meeting the magnet standards (Aiken, 2002; Kramer & Schmalenberg, 2004). The national standards for magnet hospitals are shown in the National Guidelines box.

The primary nursing care delivery system that has evolved using the principles of relationship-based care reinforces the professional practice environment. This system builds on healing relationships that can be tailored to individual units with varying staffing patterns or standardized health care settings to meet the unique needs of patients and families. This structure may be attractive to health care settings trying to attract and retain nurses while improving the quality of care, improving patient satisfaction, and improving patient safety. There is increasing pressure from third-party payers to reduce medical errors, hospital-acquired infections, patient falls, and pressure ulcers, and the search has begun to discover the links between the environment and the safe delivery of health care.

■ Providing Safe Patient Care

The IOM published its report *Keeping Patients Safe: Transforming the Work Environment of Nurses* in 2004. It speaks to the importance of providing safe patient care in a complex health system. Safe patient care depends on evidence-based nursing

---

NATIONAL GUIDELINES for Magnet Hospitals

Hospitals are recognized and formally designated by the American Nurses Credentialing Center as magnet hospitals when they have demonstrated, to the satisfaction of specially trained external appraisers, that the 14 forces of magnetism or standards are evident throughout the facility. Designation is valid for 4 years and hospitals must provide annual documentation of continued compliance with the forces.

The 14 forces of magnetism are listed below:

1. Quality of nursing leadership
2. Organizational structure
3. Management style
4. Personnel policies and programs
5. Professional models of care

6. Quality of care
7. Quality improvement
8. Consultation and resources
9. Autonomy
10. Community and the hospital
11. Nurses as teachers
12. Image of nursing
13. Interdisciplinary relationships
14. Professional development

Detailed information on the magnet recognition program can be found at the following website: http://www.nursecredentialing.org/magnet/forces.html.

care delivery systems. Nurses are critical elements of the overall health system and how care is organized, how work is designed, how much staffing is allocated, and how the multidisciplinary teams work together will determine whether quality care can be delivered with minimal errors to the patient (IOM, 2004).

Four nursing care delivery systems have historically provided a basic structure for organizing and delivering nursing care, but the research appears to support a model that uses a richer mix of RNs. The primary nursing model discussed in this chapter uses a richer mix of RNs, with its emphasis on relationship-based care, and creates new possibilities for collaborative success. Leaders in health care are searching for the components and processes to make patient care safe, and the ability of the RN to coordinate, communicate, and manage the multidisciplinary team of health care workers will be very important.

REVIEW QUESTIONS

1. A nurse is responsible for providing total care to a patient during the entire scheduled shift. The nurse is functioning within which of the following care delivery systems?
   1. Case method
   2. Functional
   3. Team
   4. Primary

2. Which of the following statements best describes the quality of care patients receive on a unit that utilizes functional nursing?
   1. Holistic and comprehensive
   2. Maximum use of individual caregivers' strengths for a large number of patients
   3. Better care outcomes and greater nurse satisfaction
   4. Intentional fragmentation of care

3. In a functional nursing care delivery system, a registered nurse is in charge and is responsible for delegating activities and tasks to unlicensed assistive personnel. This same approach to delegating tasks to unlicensed assistive personnel is seen in which of the following care delivery systems?
   1. Case Method
   2. Team
   3. Primary
   4. Primary Care

4. An organizational committee is considering changing the current care delivery system to one that is more cost-effective. Which of the following characteristics should be considered when selecting a cost-effective method to provide patient care?
   1. Highest quality for the lowest cost
   2. Amount of job autonomy
   3. Nurse accountability
   4. Patient acuity

5. Which of the following care areas would be the least likely to utilize advance practice nurses or case managers to assist with patient care needs?
   1. Case method
   2. Functional
   3. Team
   4. Primary

Answers for review questions appear in Appendix D

KEY TERMS

acuity *p.86*
advanced practice nurse (APRN) *p.87*
associate caregiver *p.91*
associate nurse *p.91*
case manager *p.87*
case method *p.88*
certified nurse midwife (CNM) *p.87*
certified registered nurse anesthetist (CRNA) *p.87*

clinical nurse leader (CNL) *p.87*
clinical nurse specialist (CNS) *p.87*
delegation *p.89*
functional nursing *p.89*
licensed vocational/practical nurse (LVN/LPN) *p.89*
magnet hospital *p.93*
medication nurse *p.89*

nurse practitioner (NP) *p.87*
nursing care delivery systems *p.85*
primary nursing *p.91*
registered nurse (RN) *p.87*
team nursing *p.90*
total patient care *p.88*
unlicensed assistive personnel *p.89*

EXPLORE PEARSON mynursingkit™

MyNursingKit is your one stop for online chapter review materials and resources. Prepare for success with additional NCLEX®-style practice questions, interactive assignments and activities, web links, animations and videos, and more!

Register your access code from the front of your book at
www.mynursingkit.com

REFERENCES

Aiken, L. H. (2002). Superior outcomes for magnet hospitals: The evidence base. In M. McClure & A. S. Hinshaw (Eds.), *Magnet hospitals revisited* (pp. 61–81). Washington, DC: American Nurses Association.

Aiken, L. H., Clarke, S. P., & Sloane, D. M. (2000). Hospital restructuring: Does it adversely affect care and outcomes? *Journal of Nursing Administration, 30,* 457–465.

Aiken, L. H., Clarke, S. P., Sloane, D. M., Sochalski, J., & Silber, J. H. (2002). Hospital nurse staffing and patient mortality, nurse burnout, and job dissatisfaction. *Journal of the American Medical Association, 288*(16), 1987–1993.

American Association of Colleges of Nursing. (2005). *Fact sheet: The clinical nurse leader.* Retrieved January 15, 2007, from http://www.aacn.nche.edu/Media/FactSheets/CNLFactSheet

American Institute of Architects. (2006). *Private rooms are new standard in guidelines for design and construction of health care facilities.* Retrieved January 15, 2007, from http://www.aia.org/release_071906_healthcare

American Nurses Credentialing Center. (2006). Retrieved January 15, 2007, from http://www.nursingworld.org/ancc/cert/eligibility/CaseMgmt

Begun, J. W., Hamilton, J. A., Tornabeni, J., & White, K. R. (2006). Opportunities for improving patient care through lateral integration: The clinical nurse leader. *Journal of Healthcare Management, 51*(1) 19–25.

Brown, D. (2002). *Linking quality measurement and evidence-based practice research for hospitals and long-term care.* CalNOC Director's Report. Retrieved February 28, 2007, from http://nurseweb.ucsf.edu/conf/cripc/calnocDirRep.html

Bryant-Lukosius, D., DiCenso, A., Browne, G., & Pinelli, J. (2004) Advanced practice nursing roles: Development, implementation and evaluation. *Journal of Advanced Nursing, 48*(5), 519–529.

Buerhaus, P. I., Donelan, K., Ulrich, B. T., Norman, L., & Dittus, R. (2006). State of the register nurse workforce in the United States. *Nursing Economics, 24*(1), 6–12.

Clarke, S. P., & Aiken, L. H. (2003). Failure to rescue: Needless deaths are prime examples of the need for more nurses at the bedside. *American Journal of Nursing, 103*(1), 42–47.

Corbo, S. A. (2006). Delegation defined: Examining the principles of this tool as both an art and a science. *Advance for Nurses, 8*(16), 21.

Cortes, T., Noyes, B., & Brennan, E. (2000). Is now the time to design new care delivery models? *Journal of Nursing Administration, 30*(9), 403–404.

Cowan, M. J., Shapiro, M., Hays, R. D., Afifi, A., Vasirani, S., Ward, C. R., et al. (2006). The effect of a multidisciplinary hospitalist/physician and advanced practice nurse collaboration on hospital costs. *Journal of Nursing Administration, 36*(2), 79–85.

Daditch, K. (2003). Care delivery strategies. In P. S. Yoder-Wise (Ed.), *Leading and managing in nursing* (3rd ed.). St. Louis: Mosby.

Deutschendorf, A. L. (2003). From past paradigms to future frontiers: Unique care delivery models to facilitate nursing work and quality outcomes. *Journal of Nursing Administration, 33*(1), 52–59.

Drenkard, K., & Cohen, E. (2004). Clinical nurse leader: Moving toward the future. *Journal of Nursing Administration, 34*(6) 257–269.

Finkler, S. A., & Kovner, C. T. (2000). *Financial management for nurse managers and executives* (2nd ed.). Philadelphia: W. B. Saunders.

Formella, N., & Rovin, S. (2004). Creating a desirable future for nursing, part 2: The issues. *Journal of Nursing Administration, 34*(6), 264–267.

Guido, G. W. (2006). *Legal and ethical issues in nursing* (4th ed.). Upper Saddle River, NJ: Pearson Prentice Hall.

Haugh, R. (2005 , February). California: Can this sinking ship be saved? *Hospitals and Health Networks,* pp. 54–60.

Hegyvary, S. T., & Haussman, R. K. (1976). Correlates of the quality of nursing care. *Journal of Nursing Administration, 6*(9), 22–27.

Hinshaw, A. S. (2002). Building magnetism into organizations. In M. McClure & A. S. Hinshaw (Eds.), *Magnet hospitals revisited* (pp. 83–102). Washington, DC: American Nurses Association.

Houser, J. (2003). A model for evaluating the context of nursing care delivery. *Journal of Nursing Administration, 33*(1), 39–47.

Huber, D. (2006). *Leadership and nursing care management* (3rd ed.). Philadelphia: W. B. Saunders.

Institute of Medicine. (2004). *Keeping patients safe: Transforming the work environment of nurses.* Washington, DC: National Academies Press.

Joint Commission. (2006, September). *Comprehensive accreditation manual for hospitals: The official handbook. Update 2.* Retrieved on February 27, 2007, from http://www.Jointcommission.org

Kalisch, B. J., & Begeny, S. M. (2005). Improving nursing unit teamwork. *Journal of Nursing Administration, 35*(12), 550–556.

Koloroutis, M. (2004). Professional nursing practice. In M. Koloroutis (Ed.), *Relationship-based care* (pp. 117–158). Minneapolis, MN: Creative Health Care Management.

Kramer, M., & Schmalenberg, C. (2002). Staff nurses identify essentials of magnetism. In M. McClure & A. S. Hinshaw (Eds.), *Magnet hospitals revisited* (pp. 25–55). Washington, DC: American Nurses Association.

Kramer, M., & Schmalenberg, C. (2004). Development and evaluation of essentials of magnetism tool. *Journal of Nursing Administration, 34*(7/8), 365–378.

Lang, T. A., Hodge, M., Olson, V., Romano, P. S., & Kravitz, R. L. (2004). Nurse–patient ratios: A systematic review on the effects of nurse staffing on patient, nurse employee, and hospital outcomes. *Journal of Nursing Administration, 34*(7/8), 326–337.

Manthey, M. (1990). Definitions and basic elements of a patient care delivery system with an emphasis on primary nursing. In G. G. Mayer, M. J. Madden, & E. Lawrenz (Eds.), *Patient care delivery models* (pp. 201–211). Rockville, MD: Aspen Publishers.

Manthey, M. (2002). *The practice of primary nursing* (2nd ed.). Boston: Blackwell Scientific Publications.

Marquis. B. L., & Huston, C. J. (2006). *Leadership roles and management functions in nursing* (5th ed.). Philadelphia: Lippincott Williams & Wilkins.

McCauley, K., & Irwin, R. S. (2006). Changing the work environment in ICUs to achieve patient-focused care. *Chest, 130*(5), 1571–1578.

National Council of State Boards of Nursing. (2005). *Working with others: A position paper.* Retrieved January 15, 2007, from http://www.NCSBN.org/pdfs/workingwithothers.pdf

Needleman, J., & Buerhaus, P. (2006). Nurse staffing in hospitals: Is there a business case for quality? *Health Affairs, 25*(1), 204–211.

Needleman, J., Buerhaus, P. I., Mattke, S., Stewart, M., Zelevinsky, K. (2002). Nurse staffing levels and the quality of care in hospitals. *New England Journal of Medicine, 346,* 1715–2722.

Person, C. (2004). Patient care delivery. In M. Koloroutis (Ed.), *Relationship-based care* (pp. 159–182). Minneapolis, MN: Creative Health Care Management.

Potter, P., & Grant, E. (2004). Understanding RN and unlicensed assistive personnel working relationships in designing care delivery strategies. *Journal of Nursing Administration, 34*(1), 19–25.

Ritter-Teitel, L. (2004). Registered nurse hours worked per patient day. The key to assessing staffing effectiveness and ensuring patient safety. *Journal of Nursing Administration, 34*(4), 167–169.

Roussel, L. (2006). Conceptualization of nursing administration: Theory and concepts. In L. Roussel (Ed.) with R. C. Swansburg & R. J. Swansburg, *Management and leadership for nurse administrators.* Sudbury, MA: Jones and Bartlett.

Sovie, M. D., Gift, A., Jawad, A. F., Stratton, L., Wallace, PL., Aiken, L. (2000). *Hospital restructuring's impact on outcomes. Final report* (NIH Grant 5 R01 NR04285-03). Bethesda, MD: National Institute of Nursing Research.

Swansburg, R. C., & Swansburg R. J. (2002). *Introduction to management and leadership for nurse managers* (3rd ed.). Sudbury, MA: Jones and Bartlett.

Tiedeman, M. E., & Lookinland, S. (2004). Traditional models of care delivery. What have we learned? *Journal of Nursing Administration, 34*(6), 291–297.

Tomey, A. M. (2004). *Guide to nursing management and leadership* (6th ed.). St. Louis: Mosby.

Ulrich, R., & Quan, X. (2004). *The role of the physical environment in the hospital of the 21st century: A once-in-a-lifetime opportunity. The Center for Health Design for Designing the 21st Century Hospital Project.* Princeton, NJ: Robert Wood Johnson Foundation.

Vahey, D. C., Aiken, L. H., Sloane, D. M., Clark S. P., & Vargas, D. (2004). Nurse burnout and patient satisfaction. *Medical Care, 42*(2), 11-57–11-66.

Weisman, C. S., & Nathanson, C. A. (1985). Professional satisfaction and client outcomes. *Medical Care, 23*(10) 1179–1192.

Whitcomb, R., Wilson, S., Chang-Dawkins, S., Durand, J., Pitcher, D., Lauzon, C., et al. (2002). Advanced practice nursing: Acute care model in progress. *Journal of Nursing Administration, 32*(3), 123–125.

White, P., & Hall, M. E. (2006). Mapping the literature of case management of nursing. *Journal of the Medical Library Association, 94,* E99–E106.

Yoder-Wise, P. S. (2007). Delegation: An art of professional practice. In P. S. Yoder-Wise (Ed.), *Leading and managing in nursing* (4th ed.). St. Louis: Mosby.

Nursing Documentation

Cheryl Wraa

Outcome-Based Learning Objectives

After studying this chapter, the learner will be able to:

1. Explain regulatory and professional standards for patient care documentation.
2. List general principles that guide documentation.
3. Differentiate advantages and disadvantages of different documentation systems.
4. Apply the nursings process to the Preparation for Practice exercises.

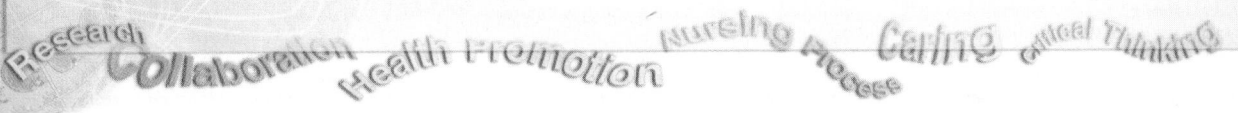

NURSES COLLECT data from multiple sources that they analyze and integrate to formulate nursing care plans, implement care decisions, evaluate patient response, and communicate the information to other members of the health care team. The most familiar way in which the information is conveyed is through the patient's **medical record,** which is the legal document for all information regarding a patient's hospital course and evidence for the extent of care provided and the outcome of that care. The medical record also describes anticipated treatment and educational needs (Austin, 2006; Lee, 2005). The patient's medical record is not only used to verify the care given, but to convey the quality of care, ensure continuity of care, assist with reimbursement, demonstrate compliance with regulations and policies, provide evidence in a court of law, and provide data for research and education (Austin, 2006; Childers, 2005).

Documentation Standards

Accrediting organizations, federal and state agencies, and professional organizations and institutions all set standards that guide nursing documentation in the particular places in which nurses practice.

Accreditation Standards

Nursing documentation must comply with the standards established through accrediting and licensing organizations, such as the Joint Commission, formerly known as the Joint Commission on Accreditation of Healthcare Organizations or JCAHO. The commission surveys facilities to measure compliance with its standards for safe health care. This accreditation could be jeopardized by inadequate or poor documentation. Loss of accreditation can affect reimbursement eligibility for Medicare, Medicaid, and managed care plans. The Joint Commission's standards do not require traditional nursing care plans, but do require documentation of an individualized plan of care for each patient. Here are some selected standards that should be reflected within the nursing documentation:

- Staff members integrate the information from various assessments of the patient to identify and assign priorities to their care needs.
- A registered nurse assesses the patient's need for nursing care in all settings where nursing care is provided.
- The assessment process for an infant, a child, or an adolescent patient is individualized.
- The assessment process addresses the special needs of patients who are receiving treatment for alcoholism or other drug dependencies.
- The assessment process addresses the special needs of patients who are receiving treatment for emotional or behavioral disorders.

- The assessment process addresses the special needs of patients who are possible victims of abuse.
- Each patient is reassessed at points designated in hospital policy.
- Care is planned and provided in an interdisciplinary, collaborative manner by qualified individuals.
- Care, treatment, and rehabilitation are planned to ensure that they are appropriate to the patient's needs and severity of disease, condition, impairment, or disability.
- The patient's progress is periodically evaluated against care goals and the plan of care and, when indicated, the plan or goals are revised.
- Continuing care at the time of discharge is based on the patient's assessed needs.
- Functional rehabilitation status is assessed to determine the current level of functioning, self-care, self-responsibility, independence, and quality of life.
- Restraint or seclusion use is limited to situations with adequate, appropriate, clinical justification.
- Patients are educated about pain and pain management.

Accrediting organizations will periodically review medical records to ensure that the standard of care is consistent throughout. The Joint Commission currently uses a *tracer methodology* during accreditation visits. The site surveyor will choose a patient who is currently hospitalized and use the patient's clinical record as a "road map." The surveyor reviews the care documented to determine if the organization has complied with standards and systems for providing care. The Joint Commission also requires that health care facilities regularly monitor, evaluate, and explore ways to improve the quality of care given to patients.

Each year the Joint Commission publishes patient safety goals that need to be addressed by health care facilities to improve patient care (Joint Commission, 2008). They are listed on the Joint Commission website for the current year. One example of a patient safety goal is the 2008 goal to "improve the effectiveness of communications among caregivers," which includes a standardized list of abbreviations, acronyms, symbols, and dose designations that are *not* to be used throughout the organization. The Joint Commission (2008) has stated that the following abbreviations are banned from use:

Abbreviation	Alternative
• U	unit(s)
• IU	international unit(s)
• QD	daily
• QOD	every other day
• Always use leading zero	Use 0.X mg (example: 0.5 mg)
• Never use a trailing zero	Use X mg (example: 5 mg)
• MS	Morphine sulfate or morphine
• MSO$_4$	Morphine sulfate or morphine
• MgSO$_4$	Magnesium sulfate

State, Federal, and Professional Standards

Documentation must also follow guidelines set by state and federal agencies such as the Health Care Financing Administration (HCFA), insurance companies, professional organizations such as the American Nurses Association, and the policies of the institution where the nurse is employed. In general, they require documentation to include initial and ongoing assessments, any change in the patient's condition, therapies given and the patient's response, patient teaching, and relevant statements made by the patient (Duclos-Miller, 2004).

State boards of nursing control the practice of nursing by development of state **nurse practice acts** that establish guidelines to ensure safe practice. The standards set by the practice acts are based on the nursing process, which is a systematic method of planning and providing care to the patient, and requires compliance as evidenced in documentation. State nurse practice acts are revised frequently and, as such, documentation requirements may also change. What the nurse documents in the medical record shows compliance with the standards set by the health care facility, state law, and professional organizations (Austin, 2006).

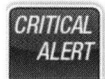 *It is important to be familiar with the nurse practice act of the state in which you work. Most state boards of nursing have a website for reference.*

Health Insurance Portability and Accountability Act

The Health Insurance Portability and Accountability Act (HIPAA) of 1996 requires the Department of Health and Human Services (DHHS) to adopt standards for electronic health care transactions. DHHS published a Privacy Rule in December 2000 that became effective on April 14, 2001. The Privacy Rule set national standards for the protection of health information. It was modified in March 2002 and again in August 2002. Further information is found in Chapter 3 ⊘.

The rule affects documentation in that only the patient or those health care team members involved with the patient's care have a legal right to review the medical record. Release of patient information without the consent of the patient is a violation of the patient's privacy and a violation of HIPAA. If a health care facility is found to be in violation of HIPAA, the facility must pay a fine and is in jeopardy of losing Medicare and Medicaid funding. The person responsible for the violation may face immediate dismissal.

▮ Documentation Principles

To be effective, documentation needs to be systematic, timely, and accurate and give a clear account of the nursing care that was provided. The standards and guidelines for documentation differ among health care facilities and specific patient populations, but certain fundamental principles guide all forms of documentation:

- Write legibly.
- Date and time each entry.
- Use only approved abbreviations.

- Document in chronological order.
- Document information promptly.
- Document all observations objectively.
- Use institutional policy to correct written errors.
- Ensure that documentation is complete, concise, and accurate.
- Sign all documents per your institutional policy and include your professional credentials.

Complete, Concise, and Accurate

It is important to document your observations as clearly as possible. Document only facts: what you see, hear, and do. Describe what you see and do not be vague. For example, "Drainage from the surgical wound soaked three 4×4s in 10 minutes. Surgeon notified" is more accurate than "Drainage from surgical wound increased."

Chart relevant information that relates to the patient's care and the nursing process. The documentation should clearly differentiate the nurse's actions from those of the other health care team members. It should reflect nursing actions and the patient outcomes indicating the progress of the patient. Incomplete documentation negates the purpose of documentation. If incomplete, the document cannot stand as sound evidence in a court of law, quality of care cannot be evaluated, continuity of care may be broken, coordination of care may be compromised, and reimbursements may be rejected. The patient record is a legal document, so the nurse should never:

- Document procedures or medication administration in advance.
- Chart for another person without signing his name.
- Add information at a later date unless the nurse indicates that he did so.
- Add inaccurate information.
- Refer to staff conflicts or staffing problems.
- Document that you filed an "incident report."
- Destroy records.

 **CRITICAL ALERT** *In a court of law, the general rule is if it was not documented, it was not done.*

Objectivity

Document accurately what happened and your findings. Describe the factual occurrences that you can see, hear, smell, or touch. Be objective and avoid vague statements that are subjective. Instead of documenting that a patient "appears short of breath" or "breathing appears labored," document statements such as these:

- Patient is complaining of shortness of breath.
- Patient is able to speak only in 1- or 2-word sentences.
- Inspiratory and expiratory wheezes heard.

The example "patient appears short of breath" is subjective and could be manipulated later should your treatment or judgment be challenged. Instead of using the word "appears" as a shortcut, fac-

tually describe what you see that makes you come to the conclusion that the patient "appears" short of breath. For example, "Patient noted to have increased respiratory rate with use of accessory muscles and nasal flaring."

Any information you obtain from the patient or family should be documented in that context to preserve your credibility. For example, if the nurse writes "Patient fell from standing position," but did not observe this actually happening, it is not accurate. It should be documented as follows "Per patient (or witness), patient walking on uneven surface, fell from standing position." Complete, factual, accurate documentation is difficult to misinterpret and will give a clear account of the patient's care.

Timeliness

Documentation should flow so that the person reading it can picture exactly what is occurring. Timeliness includes these aspects: (1) Document as soon as possible after an observation is made or care is provided. Documentation that is done concurrently with the care provided is more likely to be accurate and complete. (2) Document date and time of each entry. Documenting the sequence of events and changes in patient condition is essential. Timed occurrences followed by nursing actions and patient response can help prevent misinterpretation. Failure to act or improper action can lead to a malpractice suit. The expectation is that you practice at the same level as any other competent registered nurse in the same situation. Deviation from the standard of care or poor documentation of care can lead to allegations of negligence. Frequent, accurate updates verify the nursing care that was given. If you have forgotten to document something, or need to add important information, add the entry on the first available line and record the current date and time, label it *late entry,* and record the date and time when the entry should have been made.

Military time is used by many facilities to alleviate confusion over a.m. and p.m. entries. Military time is expressed in 24 one-hour-long periods per day, rather than two sets of 12 one-hour periods. Chart 6–1 compares military time to regular time.

CHART 6–1	**Military Time**		
Military Time	**a.m.**	**Military Time**	**p.m.**
0100 hours	1 a.m.	1300 hours	1 p.m.
0200 hours	2 a.m.	1400 hours	2 p.m.
0300 hours	3 a.m.	1500 hours	3 p.m.
0400 hours	4 a.m.	1600 hours	4 p.m.
0500 hours	5 a.m.	1700 hours	5 p.m.
0600 hours	6 a.m.	1800 hours	6 p.m.
0700 hours	7 a.m.	1900 hours	7 p.m.
0800 hours	8 a.m.	2000 hours	8 p.m.
0900 hours	9 a.m.	2100 hours	9 p.m.
1000 hours	10 a.m.	2200 hours	10 p.m.
1100 hours	11 a.m.	2300 hours	11 p.m.
1200 hours	12 noon	2400 hours	12 midnight

Legibility

One of the main purposes of the patient medical record is to communicate with other members of the health care team. Documentation that is sloppy or difficult to read wastes time and puts the patient in jeopardy because critical information may be missing or misinterpreted. Incorrect grammar and misspelled words can create the same negative impression as sloppy handwriting. Even if you gave excellent care to the patient, the attorney or jury in a court of law may interpret it as below the acceptable standard of care if the documentation is sloppy or incomplete (Austin, 2006; Childers, 2005).

The medical record is a legal, permanent document and should be completed in colored ink that is easily photocopied. If a nurse's cursive writing is difficult to read, then the nurse should print instead.

Abbreviations

Accrediting bodies and state regulation stipulate that health care facilities must develop an approved list of abbreviations to be used for documentation. Use of unapproved abbreviations can lead to serious errors. For instance, what does the abbreviation "BS" mean? Are you documenting information regarding the patient's breath sounds or their bowel sounds? Does "pt" stand for patient, physical therapy, or prothrombin time?

 *Be sure that you know and use your institution's approved abbreviations. If you are not sure the abbreviation is correct, spell the word out.*

Corrections

Documentation errors may occur. When a nurse has made a documentation error, she should correct it immediately by drawing a single line through the entry, identifying it as an error, and adding the date, time, and her signature. The nurse should never try to obliterate the error with ink or correction fluid because this appears as if she is trying to hide something.

If you are documenting on a computerized record, follow the protocol developed by your facility for correction of entries. As with handwritten entries, once notes are entered into the computerized record, they become a part of that permanent record and should not be deleted or changed without explanation, date, time, and signature. If using an electronic medical record, the date, time, and signature will be placed automatically.

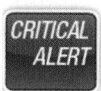 *Changing a patient care record in any way is illegal and constitutes tampering.*

Effective documentation is clear, concise, objective recording of the care given, including any significant events, presented in a legible, organized manner that is representative of the nursing process.

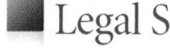 Legal Situations

Certain procedures or legal situations in which the nurse is involved require special documentation. You should be aware of these and know how to document them.

Consent Forms

Prior to most procedures or treatments, the procedure must be explained to the patient and the patient must agree to have the procedure or treatment. Included in this explanation are the risks and benefits. Most facilities have a standard form that is used to obtain consent. The legal responsibility for obtaining informed consent is with the physician, but the nurse may be asked to witness the consent. The requirement for obtaining informed consent can be waived in two situations: (1) if the patient who is mentally competent states that he does not want to hear the details of the treatment or procedure (2) if the patient is in extremis and an immediate medical or surgical treatment is needed to save her life.

If the patient asks questions after the physician has explained the procedure, answer only those questions that fall within your scope of practice. Document the information that you gave the patient. When you witness a consent, it is important to evaluate the patient to make sure the person is competent, awake, alert, and aware of what he is being told.

 *Patients who have received sedation or pain medication should never be allowed to sign an informed consent. The patient may not be able to understand the risks and benefits associated with the procedure, and the consent will be invalid, putting the institution and the nurse at legal risk.*

Advance Directives

The Patient Self-Determination Act requires that health care facilities provide information about the patient's right to refuse treatment. It is the nurse's responsibility to document that the patient received the information. The facility is also required to ask if the patient has advance directives, which are legal documents that state the patient's wishes regarding life-sustaining medical care. If the patient has advance directives, the nurse should ascertain if the patient brought them to the hospital. Whenever a patient has an advance directive, a copy should be placed in the patient's medical record. Common types of advance directives include durable powers of attorney for health care, living wills, and do-not-resuscitate orders.

Using Restraints

Most facilities have special forms for physical restraint orders. Such orders must contain the date and time of the order, reason for restraint use, duration of restraint use, type of restraint, and the physician's signature. The order must be reviewed and renewed every 24 hours. It is the nurse's responsibility to observe the patient frequently for any problem that might be related to the restraint, such as skin breakdown or decreased distal circulation. Additionally, the nurse should perform range-of-motion exercises on all extremities, and document observations and care.

Leaving Against Medical Advice

A patient who is mentally competent has the right to refuse treatment and leave the hospital at any time. If a patient chooses to leave, it should be clearly documented that the patient has been advised that she is leaving against medical advice (AMA), understands the risks of leaving, and understands that she can come back.

An AMA form should be signed by the patient and includes this information:

- Names of those notified of the patient's decision
- The risks of leaving as told to the patient
- Name of person accompanying the patient and any discharge instructions given
- The patient's destination, if known.

This protects the facility, physician, and nurse if problems arise after the patient leaves. If the patient refuses to sign or leaves without telling anyone, an incident report should be completed.

Incident Reports

Whenever an adverse event occurs, an incident report should be completed. An incident report is not part of the patient's medical record; it is a mechanism for informing administration about an incident. The incident report can alert the administration to a potential claim and, therefore, the need to gather more detail. It also assists the administration in identifying possible areas for performance improvement. Only those who witnessed the incident should complete and sign the form, and each witness should file a separate form. When completing the form, include, in quotes, any statements made by the patient or family members regarding the incident.

Documentation of the incident in the patient's medical record should be factual and include follow-up treatment and the patient's response. Do not document in the patient record that an incident report was completed, because this negates the confidential nature of the report. Most facilities have specific forms for legal situations. If you are not familiar with the form, be sure to ask for assistance in order to protect yourself and the facility.

Nursing Process

The nursing process is a systematic method of planning and providing care to patients and is the foundation for nursing documentation. It is also the basic organizing system for the National Council Licensure Examination for registered nurses (NCLEX-RN®). The nursing process contains six phases or steps: assessment; nursing diagnosis, which describes an actual or potential health problem that a nurse can legally manage; outcome identification; planning; implementation; and evaluation (Hendler, Kovach, & Sciarra, 2005; White, 2003). (Note that one of the steps discussed here, outcome identification, is often considered part of the diagnosis phase; see further discussion in Chapter 7 .)The steps build on each other, but are not linear. Steps overlap and the process changes as new information is gathered and the patient's responses are evaluated. The nursing process requires critical thinking skills to evaluate findings, identify assumptions, examine alternatives, and understand various points of view. Critical thinking is an integral part of each step of the nursing process.

The steps in the nursing process are briefly discussed next. Chapter 7 covers the nursing process in more detail.

Assessment

Assessment initiates the nursing process. It begins when the patient arrives at the facility and continues throughout the hospi-

talization. During the assessment, important information is collected from various sources to assist the nurse in formulating nursing diagnoses.

Documentation of assessment findings is very important because it serves as a communication tool for the other health care team members.

Nursing Diagnosis

A nursing diagnosis differs from a medical diagnosis in that doctors are licensed to diagnose and treat illnesses, and nurses are licensed to diagnose and treat the patient's response to illness and need for education. Nursing diagnosis should be documented in order of priority with the highest priorities being those related to immediate physical care needs.

Outcome Identification

The goal is to assist the patient to reach the highest functional level possible. Expected outcomes should be realistic, measurable, and documented with target dates. When documenting outcome statements, the following should be included:

- The desired behavior that is to be observed
- Criteria for measuring the behavior
- The conditions under which the behavior should occur
- When the behavior should occur.

Planning

The plan of action or nursing care plan is developed to help deliver quality patient care. The plan includes nursing diagnoses, expected outcomes, and nursing interventions. The documented plan of care becomes a permanent part of the medical record, and often guides daily documentation of the patient's progress.

> **CRITICAL ALERT** *Patients' problems can change during their hospitalization. Review the plan of care often and make changes as needed.*

In some specialized areas, such as intensive care units, the nursing care plan has been replaced by plans that are developed by multidisciplinary teams. These plans, called **critical pathways,** are comprehensive plans of care for specific patient situations or disease processes. Critical pathways include nursing interventions, medical interventions, and expected timelines for patient outcomes. The critical pathway is placed on a flow sheet for documentation purposes. A sample critical pathway is provided on the accompanying Student CD-ROM.

Implementation

Implementation refers to the actual nursing interventions delivered. The interventions must be directed toward the "related to" clause of the identified nursing diagnoses. To write interventions clearly, state when and how the intervention is to be performed. Be sure the intervention fits the patient's age, condition, developmental level, and values. Also, keep the patient's safety in mind, consider other health care activities, and use available resources. Documentation should be outcome oriented, so it is important to document when an intervention has been performed and the patient's response.

Evaluation

Documentation standards include an evaluation of the patient's progress toward the expected outcomes within the plan of care. An evaluation statement is one that includes the details of the care provided, with objective evidence of the patient's response. The evaluation should indicate whether the expected outcome criterion from the plan of care was achieved.

The nursing process allows for an organized method of planning and delivering nursing care. Using the nursing process for the basis of your documentation demonstrates that the standard of care has been met.

◼ Documentation Systems

Health care facilities select documentation systems to meet the needs of their specific patient care areas and to comply with legal and regulatory requirements. An acute care facility may have multiple systems in different areas of the hospital. Chart 6–2 provides brief comparisons of the different documentation systems.

Narrative System

Narrative documentation is used across most health care settings. It consists of narrative progress notes that describe a chronologi-
cal account of the patient's status, interventions performed, and response to interventions. Advantages to narrative documentation are that it is flexible, descriptive and gives the reader a picture of what has occurred over an extended period of time. Key elements of this system are knowing when to document, what to document, and how to organize the data. A disadvantage to narrative documentation is the tendency to chart everything that happens. This can make the documentation long and repetitive.

Flow sheets are often used in conjunction with narrative documentation. They are used to document routine observations such as assessments. This allows the reader to observe significant changes or trends. Samples that you can use to practice your documentation skills are located in the Student CD-ROM Toolbox. Please go to the accompanying CD-ROM to access this useful information.

Problem-Oriented Medical Record

The problem-oriented medical record (POMR) is most effective in acute and long-term settings. This system consists of five components that are discussed further: baseline data, a problem list, a plan of care for each problem, multidisciplinary progress notes, and a discharge summary. This system was developed by physicians and later adapted by nurses.

CHART 6–2 Documentation Systems Comparison

System	Parts of Record	Description	Nurse's Notes Format
Narrative	Nurse's notes Flow sheets to supplement care plan	Each discipline writes narrative progress notes in segregated areas of the medical record.	Narration with time of entry
Problem-oriented medical record (POMR)	Nurse's notes Database Nursing care plan Problem list Discharge summary	Consists of gathering baseline data and creating a problem list and plan of care for each identified problem.	SOAP, SOAPIE, or SOAPIER
Problem, intervention, evaluation (PIE)	Nurse's notes Assessment flow sheets Problem list	Uses a problem, intervention, evaluation format to describe patient problems, intervention, and evaluation of responses to interventions.	Problem Intervention Evaluation
Focus	Nurse's notes Flow sheets Checklists	Uses a data–action–response format to identify focus areas of concern, plan care, and evaluate response to care.	Data Action Response
Charting by exception (CBE)	Nurse's notes Flow sheets with patient teaching records and discharge notes Care plan Graphic record	Only requires documentation of abnormal or significant findings and events.	SOAPIE or SOAPIER
Flow sheet, assessment, concise, timely (FACT)	Nurse's notes Flow sheets Assessment sheet	Uses a baseline assessment and data, action, response format to evaluate problems identified in the nursing diagnosis care plan.	Data Action Response
Electronic medical record (EMR)	Nurse's notes Flow sheets Nursing care plan Database Teaching plan	Uses a database, outcome-based plan of care.	Evaluative statements Expected outcomes Learning outcomes

Source: From Duclos-Miller, P. A. (2004). Managing documentation risk: A guide for nurse managers. Marblehead, MA: HCPro, Inc.

Database

Nurses most commonly complete the database or admission assessment. This initial assessment is very important, because it is the basis for the patient's plan of care. The database includes the reason for hospitalization, past medical history, allergies, current medications, physical assessment, psychosocial findings, self-care abilities, educational needs, and discharge planning needs. From this information, the problem list is formed.

Problem List

The problem list contains the patient's current medical problems in chronological order of when each was identified, not in order of acuteness or priority. The list provides the nurse with an overview of the patient's health status. Each problem is then given a number. Documentation on the initial plan, progress notes, and discharge summary will correspond to these numbers. When a problem has been resolved, the problem remains on the list, but is then highlighted to show that it has been resolved.

Initial Plan

From the problem list, an initial plan is developed that includes expected outcomes, plans for further data collection, patient care, and teaching plans. The nurse should include the patient in goal setting as the plan is developed.

Progress Notes

Progress notes are written using the SOAP, SOAPIE, or SOAPIER format. This format documents the following information for each problem:

- **S–subjective data:** Information that the patient or significant others tell the nurse. It can be stated as a complaint or an impression if not from the patient.
- **O–objective data:** Measurable information the nurse gathers during the assessment, such as vital signs, laboratory test results, and signs and symptoms noted.
- **A–assessment data:** This is stated as the patient problem or nursing diagnosis that the nurse derived from the subjective and objective data that was gathered. This is a dynamic process and will change as more information is gathered.
- **P–plan:** The plan describes the interventions planned to resolve each problem. The plan should include short-term and long-term goals.
- **I–interventions:** This documents the measures that are taken to achieve an expected outcome. Teaching and documentation of the patient's understanding of the plan would be placed here.
- **E–evaluation:** Evaluation of the patient's response to the interventions.
- **R–revision:** Documentation of any change of plan for a particular problem.

Discharge Summary

The discharge summary notes whether each problem on the list is resolved. This is the place in the SOAPIE note for the nurse to discuss unresolved problems and document the plan for addressing the problem after discharge. It is also the place to note any communication with an outside facility, agency, or the patient's family.

CHART 6–3	Sample of SOAPIE Documentation

1/12/09 0800

S: The patient states "I am having chest pain."

O: Patient in telemetry bed, skin pale and moist, monitor shows sinus rhythm with elevated T waves and occasional unifocal PVCs. Blood pressure 170/98, heart rate 66, respiratory rate 24, patient rates pain at a 6.

A: Patient appears in moderate distress

P: Follow physician orders for chest pain, page primary physician.

1/12/09 0810

I: Placed patient on oxygen at 2L per nasal cannula, 4 mg of morphine given IV, 12-lead ECG completed, Dr. Johnson at bedside.

E: Patient states pain has decreased to a 3. Skin now dry with good color. Monitor shows sinus rhythm without ectopy, T waves remain elevated.

A sample of documentation using the SOAPIE method is shown in Chart 6–3.

One disadvantage of the problem-oriented system is that it lists the problems in chronological order, rather than by priority.

Problem, Intervention, Evaluation System

The problem, intervention, evaluation (PIE) system works well in areas where the patient's condition can change rapidly. This system lists the patient's problem first, followed by the interventions taken to alleviate the problem, and last, the evaluation of the patient's response to the intervention. This system organizes the information according to the patient's problems and integrates the plan of care into the progress notes. A daily assessment flow sheet is used to document routine care and monitoring measures, with detailed information documented in the progress note. Chart 6–4 shows an example of PIE documentation.

Problem

After an initial assessment is done, nursing diagnoses are identified and form the "problem" piece of the documentation system. Most facilities will develop a list of accepted nursing diagnoses that usually correspond to those approved by the North American Nursing Diagnosis Association (NANDA). Each problem is then numbered for future reference.

CHART 6–4	Sample of PIE Nursing Progress Notes

1/12/09 2200

P#1: Pain related to fractured femur

IP#1: Pain identified as 8 out of 10. Pain medication given per physician orders. Reassess pain level at 2230. Continue to assess pain every 4 hours using pain scale.

1/12/09 2230

EP#1: Pain identified as 4 out of 10.

Intervention

Nursing actions that are taken to alleviate a problem are documented for each nursing diagnosis. Each "I" should be labeled with the corresponding problem number.

Evaluation

Following the interventions, the patient's responses should be documented. As with the interventions, the "E" should be labeled with the corresponding problem number.

One disadvantage of the PIE system is that each problem needs to be evaluated once each shift. The PIE system also does not document the planning step in the nursing process, which addresses expected outcomes.

Focus System

The Focus system includes a detailed patient assessment leading to the development of patient-centered problems or foci of concern. Each problem is written as a nursing diagnosis or may refer directly to a specific sign or symptom, patient behavior, or significant event such as an invasive procedure. The Focus system is flexible, centers on the nursing process, and allows the reader to easily locate information about a specific problem. A daily assessment flow sheet is used to document routine care and monitoring measures.

The Focus documentation is completed in the progress notes in a data–action–response format, as shown in Chart 6–5. The problem focus is identified and then followed by:

- **D–data:** The data include both subjective and objective information regarding the problem.
- **A–action:** The action includes current and future nursing actions based on the assessment of the patient.
- **R–response:** The response describes the patient's response to the action.

Charting by Exception System

Charting by exception (CBE) is used to eliminate lengthy or repetitive documentation. It departs from traditional types of systems by documenting only significant or abnormal findings. To use the CBE system, the nurse must be using critical pathway or interdisciplinary plans of care that address every possible patient problem. The format contains baseline data and a problem-oriented plan of care. Preprinted guidelines are prepared for each body system and the initial and ongoing assessments are documented only as exceptions to these guidelines. Flow sheets provide a normal assessment to chart against. For each body system the nurse would document within normal limits or document what is not normal. The different types of flow sheets needed for the CBE system are:

- Physician's order flow sheet
- Nursing order flow sheet
- Graphic form
- Patient teaching record
- Patient discharge note
- Supplemental nurse's progress notes.

The CBE system saves time and decreases the amount of documentation needed. The flow sheets are nursing focused and improve documentation because the format highlights care interventions and requires a documented evaluation of the patient's response. A disadvantage of the CBE system is the time it takes to develop the guidelines and standards of care. These must be in place and taught to all nursing staff for this system to be effective.

FACT System

The FACT system uses assessment and action flow sheets with nursing progress notes. The flow sheets may be patient specific or follow the CBE format of normal assessment parameters for each body system. The nursing progress notes use the data–action–response format discussed earlier. The FACT acronym stands for the four key elements of the system:

- **F**–Flow sheets that are individualized to specific services
- **A**–Assessment features that are standardized with baseline parameters
- **C**–Concise, integrated nursing progress notes and flow sheets that document the patient's condition and response to treatments
- **T**–Timely entries that can be documented when care is given.

As with CBE, the FACT system eliminates repetition and promotes consistent language. It encourages immediate recording of data because the system is readily accessible. Disadvantages include the time commitment needed to develop the standards and the training needed to implement the system.

Electronic Medical Record

One of the most significant recent changes in documentation has been the introduction of computerized charting systems. The ability to have universal access to patient records is necessary to the delivery of safe and effective health care. For example, a patient's medication history is readily accessible throughout the health care system and each change can be updated whether the change is made by telephone or via an office visit. The electronic medical record (EMR) is legible, decreases recording time and costs, decreases errors, improves communication between health care providers, and provides better access to medical data for patient care, education, performance improvement activities, and

| CHART 6–5 | Sample of Focus Charting |

Date	Time	Focus	Nursing Progress Notes
1/12/09	1000	Pain	D: Patient complains of pain to abd. incision. Rates pain as 6 out of 10. Abdominal incision clean dry and intact. No redness or drainage noted. Abdomen soft with moderate tenderness near the incision. A: Patient given pain medication per physician order.
1/12/09	1030		R: Patient states pain is now 3 out of 10.

research (Duclos-Miller, 2004). Another advantage to the EMR is the use of standard terminology, which promotes better communication among providers.

As just stated, the EMR allows a patient's medication history to be accessible throughout the health care system. Complications from drug reactions account for approximately 4.7% of admissions to hospitals in the United States with the estimated associated costs being $3.8 million per hospital per year (Varkey et al., 2007). Because of these adverse reactions, the Institute for Healthcare Improvement's 100,000 Lives Campaign and the Joint Commission identified the prevention of adverse drug reactions as a priority for national action and have required institutions to perform **medication reconciliation,** which is the process of identifying an accurate list of all medications the patient is taking and using this list to provide correct medications for the patient anywhere in the health care system. The initial list is developed by either the primary care provider or on admission to the hospital. When a patient is admitted to the hospital, any new medication prescribed is added to the EMR or any medication stopped during the hospitalization is marked as deleted. The EMR medication list is then reconciled by the health care team daily. It is of great importance to reconcile the medication list prior to the patient's discharge. The nurse will review and be sure that the patient understands all changes.

Depending on the type of computer and software that is used by a facility, patient information may be accessed by voice recognition, a keyboard, light pen, touch screen, or mouse. Most facilities place computers or terminals at workstations or patient bedsides to allow quick access by the health care team to patient information.

Privacy rights and confidentiality need to be addressed through institutional policies specific to the EMR. Security can be monitored by assigning electronic log-in names to each user and creating audit trails.

Nursing Care Documentation

Most EMRs provide a menu of words and phrases from which to choose to document in a standard format. You can further elaborate on a problem or clarify flow sheet documentation in the comment section of the form.

Nursing information systems (NIS) software programs have been developed that allow you to select and record nursing actions in the EMR. These systems contain most of the components of the nursing process and therefore adhere to the Joint Commission standards for documentation. Most NIS have features that allow customization of forms to allow specific institutional requirements. Some newer systems are interactive and, as data are entered, will prompt you with questions and suggestions regarding your data. These systems will also suggest nursing diagnoses for the care plan based on the assessment data that were entered.

The advantages of an EMR are the ability to retrieve information quickly and easily. It helps to link different sources of patient information such as clinic notes, laboratory results, consults, and diagnostic results. The EMR uses standard terminology and the documentation is legible, which improves communication among health care providers. Disadvantages are that not all health care providers are comfortable with computer

technology and extensive training may be necessary; lack of security measures can threaten patient confidentiality; if the system is "down," then information is unavailable unless hard copies are used and readily accessible; and initial implementation of the system is expensive.

Regardless of the system that is used where you practice, knowing the components of that system and understanding the basic principles of documentation are essential. The patient's medical record demonstrates that the care given was based on accepted professional and regulatory standards. When you complete your documentation, ask yourself the following questions:

- Is it factual?
- Does it document all the care given?
- If it is read 2 years from now, will it demonstrate that the care given met the standard of care?
- Does it show the sequence of events accurately, including the patient's response to treatment?
- Does it contain subjective statements or personal opinions?
- Does it clearly identify when information was obtained from the patient, family, or other caregivers?
- Is it legible?
- Are errors corrected in the approved manner?

Your documentation will show the quality of the care given, the outcome of that care, and collaboration among the members of the health care team and also describe future interventions and education needed. Documentation that is accurate and complete protects both the patient and the caregiver.

Preparation for Practice

As stated earlier, the development of a nursing plan of care using the nursing process requires critical thinking skills to evaluate findings, identify assumptions, examine alternatives, and understand various points of view. Critical thinking is an integral part of each step of the nursing process. To assist you in the development of your critical thinking skills, each chapter that covers a disorder has a real-life vignette at the end, followed by several questions to stimulate critical thinking. Using the same vignette, you will proceed to the accompanying MyNursingkit to view:

1. **The patient care Kardex.** The Kardex contains information regarding the patient's name, age, religion, medical diagnoses, past medical history, surgeries and major procedures since admission, current medications, treatments, diet, intravenous therapy, diagnostic tests, and procedures. The Kardex will also include the permitted level of activity, functional limitations, and assistance that may be needed.

2. **Three days of laboratory results.** This will allow you to look for abnormal values and trends.

From this information you will be asked to complete several forms that would assist you in preparing to care for the patient:

- **Summary of hospitalization.** This includes pertinent information regarding the patient such as age, admitting diagnosis, past medical history, surgeries or major procedures since admission, history of current illness or injury, vital signs and physical findings from the previous 24 hours, and the basic nursing care needed for the patient.

- **Pathophysiology.** This includes detailed pathophysiology for the current illness. Included are common signs and symptoms, and possible complications. This will help you to anticipate the patient's needs, possible complications, and knowledge deficits.

- **Laboratory results explanations.** All abnormal lab values or significant trends should be listed. Next to the result you will write a brief explanation of what the cause of the abnormality might be for this patient and the significance of the finding. This will help you to become familiar with trends for specific disease processes and hone your interpretive skills.

- **Medication administration record.** This form includes the usual dose, route, frequency, class, and action of the drug, the rationale for administration, side effects with nursing implications, and assessment data that indicate effectiveness. This will help you to become familiar with different classes of drugs, the nursing interventions and assessments necessary for safe administration, and the evaluations necessary to determine effectiveness.

- **Concept map.** The concept map assists the learner in the development of the nursing plan of care using the nursing process. The primary and secondary diagnoses are listed. For the primary diagnosis, list the critical assessments that are a priority for the patient. Follow the primary and secondary nursing diagnoses with high-risk potential problems. For each nursing diagnosis, list all assessment findings that sup-

port the diagnosis such as vital signs, lab results, and physical assessment findings. Then list medical and nursing interventions aimed at improving the problem. Following the nursing process, list the knowledge deficits and educational needs for the patient and family. In the last section, describe what the patient must be able to do before discharge or transfer, including appropriate community referrals.

The assignment assists the learner in the development of a problem-solving approach to nursing care. By doing this, the learner will gain experience in critical thinking skills and develop a systematic method for determining a patient's health problem, devising a plan of care, developing evaluation criteria, and knowing expected outcomes. The Preparation for Practice assignments will also help the learner to articulate the patient's needs and learn how to write effective evaluation statements. This, in turn, will significantly improve documentation skills and the ability to communicate with other health care team members to provide the safest most effective and holistic care for the patient.

Summary

Accurate, concise documentation takes practice. Remember, the patient's medical record is not only used to verify the care given, but to convey the quality of care. The record ensures continuity of care, assists with reimbursement, demonstrates compliance with regulations and policies, provides evidence in a court of law, and provides data for research and education. The patient's medical record is a powerful communication tool. Developing the ability to articulate the patient's condition and potential problems assists in creating a collaborative plan of care.

REVIEW QUESTIONS

1. The nurse is reviewing the latest National Patient Safety Goals. The regulatory body that publishes these goals is:
   1. Medicare.
   2. Medicaid.
   3. The Joint Commission.
   4. The State Board of Nursing.

2. The nurse makes a mistake while documenting in a patient's medical record. What should this nurse do?
   1. Rip out the page in the record and start over.
   2. Draw a single line through the entry, write the word error, date, time, and sign the entry.
   3. Use liquid paper to white out the entry.
   4. Use heavy black ink to darken the entry.

3. The nurse is documenting, using the narrative method. One disadvantage of using this method is:
   1. The time needed to develop standards.
   2. Problems are listed in chronological order.
   3. Problems need to be evaluated once per shift.
   4. There is a tendency to document everything.

4. Which of the following tools helps the nurse prepare a plan of care using the nursing process?
   1. Kardex
   2. Concept Map
   3. Medication Administration Record
   4. Past Medical History

Answers for review questions appear in Appendix D

KEY TERMS

critical pathways *p.100*
medical record *p.96*

medication reconciliation *p.104*
nurse practice act *p.91*

EXPLORE PEARSON **mynursingkit**

MyNursingKit is your one stop for online chapter review materials and resources. Prepare for success with additional NCLEX®-style practice questions, interactive assignments and activities, web links, animations and videos, and more!

Register your access code from the front of your book at
www.mynursingkit.com

REFERENCES

Austin, S. (2006). Ladies and gentlemen of the jury, I present the nursing documentation. *Nursing 2006, 36*(1), 56–62.

Childers, K. P. (2005). Paying a price for poor documentation. *Nursing 2005, 35*(11).

Duclos-Miller, P. A. (2004). *Managing documentation risk: A guide for nurse managers*. Marblehead, MA: HCPro, Inc.

Hendler, C., Kovach, P., & Sciarra, J. (Eds.). (2005). *Charting made incredibly easy* (3rd ed.). Philadelphia: Springhouse.

Joint Commission. (2008). *Facts about the 2008 national patient safety goals*. Retrieved April 22, 2008, from http://www.jointcommission.org/PatientSafety/NationalPatientSafetyGoals/08_npsg_facts.htm

Lee, T. (2005). Nursing diagnoses: Factors affecting their use in charting standardized care plans. *Journal of Clinical Nursing, 14,* 640–647.

Varkey, P., Cunningham, J., O'Meara, J., Bonacci, R., Desai, N., & Sheeler, R. (2007). Multidisciplinary approach to inpatient medication reconciliation in an academic setting. *American Journal of Health-System Pharmacists, 64*(8), 850–854.

White, L. (2003). *Documentation & the nursing process*. New York: Thomson.

Nursing Process

Doris Ballard Ferguson, Annita Watson
With contributions by: Joyce Mikal-Flynn

Outcome-Based Learning Objectives

After studying this chapter, the learner will be able to:

1. Differentiate between the roles in nursing as specified by the American Nurses Association.
2. Explain the five steps of the nursing process and their relationship to each other.
3. Describe the cognitive, affective, and psychomotor skills necessary to conduct a comprehensive nursing assessment.
4. Differentiate between nursing diagnoses and collaborative problems.
5. Explain the relationship between critical thinking and the nursing process.

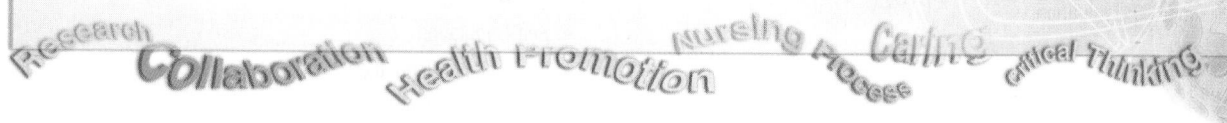

Research Collaboration Health Promotion Nursing Process Caring Critical Thinking

FOR THE PAST 30 YEARS, the American Nurses Association (ANA) has published many standards of nursing practice. These standards and the social policy statement adopted by the ANA (2003) serve as national guidelines for nursing practice. A topical overview of both is shown in Chart 7–1 (p. 108).

In nursing practice, nurses' roles are defined as *independent, interdependent, and dependent* (ANA, 2004). **Independent activities** are those that nurses perform, prescribe, and or delegate based on their education and skills. Examples of independent activities are assessing, analyzing and diagnosing, planning, implementing, and evaluating. **Interdependent activities** are those activities that overlap with the activities of other health team members, physicians, social workers, pharmacists, nutritionists, and therapists (physical, speech, occupational) and require coordination and planning with these various health team members. **Dependent activities** are those prescribed by the physician and carried out by the nurse. They include implementing the physician's orders to administer medications or treatments. The nursing process, a concept coined in 1967 by Yura and Walsh (1988) and subsequently adopted by the ANA (2004), enhances each of the three roles for the patient's benefit and is the means for nurses to demonstrate accountability and responsibility to patients.

Nursing Process

The **nursing process** is defined as a variation of scientific reasoning and is used to diagnose and to treat human responses to potential and actual health problems (ANA, 2007). As the operational framework for nursing practice, the nursing process is the vehicle through which the nurse applies knowledge and skills in a systematic, goal-directed fashion to achieve the outcomes desired for the patient (ANA, 2007; King, 1971). By using the nursing process, the nurse approaches and responds to clinical situations consciously and deliberately. Such an approach avoids nursing care based on imitation ("That's how the others do it"), intuition ("This seems like a good way to do it"), or tradition ("We've always done it that way").

Nurse–Patient Relationship

The **nurse–patient relationship** is the means for applying the nursing process. This relationship is the mechanism by which the nurse works with the patient (Carpenito-Moyet, 2007; Orlando, 1961; Peplau, 1952; Rogers, 1970; Wilkinson, 2006). Three attributes are necessary to a successful nurse–patient relationship: (1) genuineness, the ability to be aware of one's own feeling, or being real; (2) respect for and acceptance of the other unconditionally;

CHART 7–1 **National Guidelines for Nursing Practice**

NURSING SCOPE AND STANDARDS OF PRACTICE

Scope of Nursing Practice

- Definition of Nursing
- Evolution of Nursing Practice
- Integrating the Science and Art of Nursing
- The Professional Registered Nurse
- Advanced Practice Registered Nursing
- Registered Nurses in Role Specialties
- Settings for Nursing Practice
- Continued Commitment to the Profession
- Professional Trends and Issues

Standards of Practice

- Standard 1. Assessment
- Standard 2. Diagnosis
- Standard 3. Outcomes Identification
- Standard 4. Planning
- Standard 5. Implementation
  Standard 5a. Coordination of Care
  Standard 5b. Health Teaching and Health Promotion
  Standard 5c. Consultation
  Standard 5d. Prescriptive Authority and Treatment
- Standard 6. Evaluation

Standards of Professional Performance

- Standard 7. Quality of Practice
- Standard 8. Practice Evaluation
- Standard 9. Education
- Standard 10. Collegiality
- Standard 11. Collaboration
- Standard 12. Ethics
- Standard 13. Research
- Standard 14. Resource Utilization
- Standard 15. Leadership

NURSING'S SOCIAL POLICY STATEMENT

Introduction

- The Social Context of Nursing
- Values and Assumptions of Nursing's Social Contract

Definition of Nursing

Knowledge Base for Nursing Practice

- Scope of Nursing Practice
- Specialization in Nursing
- Advanced Practice Registered Nurses
- Additional Advanced Roles

The Regulation of Nursing Practice

- Self-Regulation
- Professional Regulation
- Legal Regulation

Sources: American Nurses Association. (2004). *Standards of clinical nursing practice.* Washington, DC: Nursebooks.org; American Nurses Association. (2003). *Nursing's social policy statement* (2nd ed.). Washington, DC: Nursebooks.org.

---

and (3) a continuing desire to understand and empathize with the other. Effective nurse–patient relationships can be obtained when nurses are willing to look at their own values, prejudices, strengths, and limitations. Nurses must be open to the discovery of their own motivation and feelings through experience and relationships with others (Peplau, 1952; Rogers, 1970; Wilkinson, 2006).

Steps of the Nursing Process

The steps of the nursing process are progressive and successive— each step builds on previous steps and influences subsequent steps. For example, the nurse cannot develop a plan of care and se- lect nursing interventions from that plan until valid nursing diag- noses have been formulated from an adequate database, which includes the patient's perspective and input (Carpenito-Moyet, 2007; Johnson, 1980; Orem, 1971). The nurse cannot evaluate outcomes of care unless the desired outcomes have been specified as patient goals or objectives in the care plan.

The nursing process generally consists of five successive and interrelated steps: (1) assessment, (2) diagnosis, (3) planning, (4) implementation, and (5) evaluation (Carpenito-Moyet, 2005). In 1999, however, the ANA added "outcome identification" as a discrete step of the process, although this component of the

process often is incorporated into the diagnosis phase and is pre- sented as such in this chapter. The components of the five steps in the nursing process follow:

1. Assessment
   - Data collection
   - Analysis/synthesis of data
   - Nursing diagnosis
2. Nursing diagnosis and outcome identification
3. Planning of goals and objectives
   - Plans
   - Priorities
   - Scientific rationale
4. Implementation
5. Evaluation

These five steps and their components are depicted in more de- tail in Figure 7–1 ■, which illustrates the dynamic, cyclical, inter- dependent, and often overlapping nature of the steps of the nursing process. For example, while the nurse implements a planned intervention, such as pain relief measures, additional data may be collected that further validate and support the nurs-

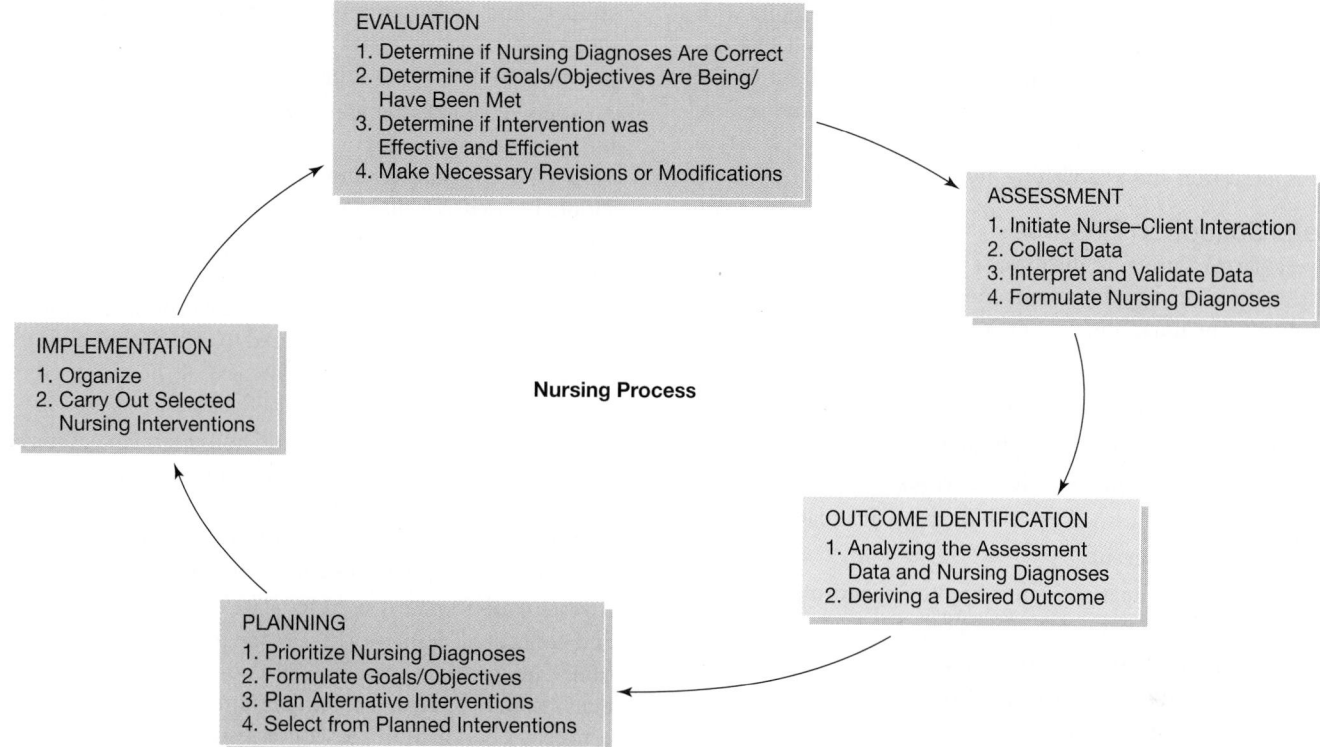

Nursing Process

EVALUATION
1. Determine if Nursing Diagnoses Are Correct
2. Determine if Goals/Objectives Are Being/
   Have Been Met
3. Determine if Intervention was
   Effective and Efficient
4. Make Necessary Revisions or Modifications

ASSESSMENT
1. Initiate Nurse–Client Interaction
2. Collect Data
3. Interpret and Validate Data
4. Formulate Nursing Diagnoses

IMPLEMENTATION
1. Organize
2. Carry Out Selected
   Nursing Interventions

OUTCOME IDENTIFICATION
1. Analyzing the Assessment
   Data and Nursing Diagnoses
2. Deriving a Desired Outcome

PLANNING
1. Prioritize Nursing Diagnoses
2. Formulate Goals/Objectives
3. Plan Alternative Interventions
4. Select from Planned Interventions

FIGURE 7–1 ■ The nursing process.

ing diagnosis of pain, while also leading to the development of additional nursing diagnoses, such as a disturbance in the patient's usual sleeping patterns. Thus, during any nurse–patient interaction, the nurse is continuously collecting data that may then be helpful in planning, implementing, evaluating, or revising nursing care.

The nursing process is flexible and is, therefore, capable of being adapted to a variety of situations (Levine, 1973). It may be used in any type of clinical setting and with patients of varying ages, health status, and cultural backgrounds (Carpenito-Moyet, 2007; Leininger, 1991; Spector, 2004; Stanton, Paul, & Reeves, 1980; Wilkinson, 2006). The nursing process also can be used with families and communities as well as with individual patients. Each phase (step) of the nursing process is discussed next.

Assessment

In general terms, **assessment** is defined as the act of evaluating or appraising. Yura and Walsh (1988) provide a clear, concise, and useful definition of assessment as it relates to nursing: "The act of reviewing a situation for the purpose of diagnosing the patient's problems" (p. 110). Assessment actions include "examining the patient and identifying cues, collecting and analyzing the data, and reaching conclusions" (p. 110).

The nursing assessment begins the moment the nurse establishes initial contact with a patient. Data are collected through formal and informal interviews and a variety of other methods including observation, inspection, palpation, percussion, auscultation, and consultation with the patient and other health care providers. Data collection is a foundation of the nursing process; therefore, the nurse must strive for accuracy, completeness, and objectivity. An accurate assessment leads to identification of the patient's health status, concerns, and nursing diagnoses.

The purpose of data collection is to identify and obtain pertinent data about the patient. Nurses should consider patients in a multidimensional way; that is, the biophysical, psychological, spiritual, and sociocultural elements of the patient must be considered to ensure a comprehensive and accurate assessment (Henderson, 1966; Johnson, 1980; Watson, 1988, 2003).

Data Sources

The nurse uses two kinds of data sources: primary and secondary. The primary source of data is the patient. Secondary data sources include family, friends, other health care professionals, the patient's current health care record, and the nurse's own knowledge base. These secondary data sources should be viewed as a supplement to the data supplied by the primary source, the patient. The usefulness of information obtained from secondary sources is in clarifying, amplifying, or substantiating the data the nurse obtains from the patient.

Data Types

The nurse gathers two types of data: subjective data and objective data (Carpenito-Moyet, 2007; Wilkinson, 2006). **Subjective data** is the information that can be perceived only by the patient and not by the observer. One of the primary sources of subjective data is the nursing or health history. Because the patient is the informant, the information collected while taking a health history is subjective. **Objective data** consist of behaviors, activities, and events that can be observed or measured by another person using the five senses. Objective data are factual; they can be seen, heard, touched, smelled, or tasted. Vital signs, laboratory reports, rashes, and body posture are some examples of objective data.

Objective and subjective data are equally important in a comprehensive nursing assessment. When assessing a patient, the nurse should try to elicit objective data that correspond with the subjective data, and subjective data that correspond with objective data. By categorizing data as subjective and objective, the nurse is better able to validate data and to identify and resolve discrepancies and accurately report information to assist in communication and establishing nursing diagnoses.

Data Collection Process

Several factors influence the process of data collection: how the data are presented by the patient and how they are perceived by the nurse. The nurse and patient are influenced by their respective:

- Physical, mental, and emotional states and needs
- Cultural, social, and philosophical backgrounds
- Number and functional ability of senses
- Past experiences associated with the present situation
- Meaning of the event
- Interest, preoccupations, preconceptions, and motivational levels
- Knowledge or familiarity with the situation
- Environmental conditions and distractions
- Presence, attitudes, and reactions of others.

These factors create a situation in which both patient and nurse automatically assign personal meaning or interpretations to situations. Problems arise when the nurse's perception or interpretation is used as fact. The nursing diagnosis is the end product of the nursing assessment. The nurse analyzes the data gathered and reaches a conclusion about the health status. A patient may have one or more nursing diagnoses. Once the diagnoses have been formulated, the nurse is ready to develop a plan of care. Therefore, skill is needed in differentiating actual data from personal interpretation. The nurse's interpretation must be validated with the patient. Chart 7–2 provides examples of objective data versus personal interpretation of them.

CRITICAL ALERT *The nurse's interpretation of the patient's problem (diagnosis) always must be validated with the patient.*

Guidelines for Data Collection

The ANA *Standards of Clinical Nursing Practice* (2004) are the guidelines for data collection. The recommended guidelines are as follows:

- Data that are collected are comprehensive and multifocal. The data need to reflect the life experiences of the patient and should consider biophysical, psychological, spiritual, socio-cultural, and socioeconomic influences. The nurse must use judgment in focusing data collection on areas that are most pertinent to the patient situation.
- A variety of sources are used for data collection. The patient is the primary source for data collection, but because perceptions of events and circumstances can vary, other sources should be used as well. Some general examples of sources are family, significant others, health care personnel, and written records.
- Appropriate tools are used for data collection. At least two data collection tools should be used to ensure the validity of the data obtained. The appropriateness of the tool used depends on the patient's age and health status.
- The data collected are objective and nonjudgmental. Data are collected through the use of observation, measurement, and interaction with the patient. Personal interpretations or perceptions of a situation may lead to further data collection, but must never be stated as data themselves.
- A systematic format is used for data collection. Theoretical and conceptual frameworks provide guides for data collection. The nurse begins data collection by assessing the patient's major concern, including multifocal influences on the concern. Then a more general assessment of the patient's health status is included as appropriate.
- The data collected reflect updating of information. Data collection is continuous in nature. The data should reflect appropriate updating of information obtained from a variety of data sources. As new data are obtained any changes in the health concerns or status of the patient must be noted.
- The data collected are recorded and communicated appropriately. Data collection is useless unless it is communicated appropriately in the patient's record. Therefore, information must be kept in a retrievable record-keeping system.

Data Collection and the Patient's Health Record

The patient's health record is a document containing (1) the medical history; (2) the findings from the physical examination; (3) the reports of laboratory tests; (4) the findings and conclusions from special examinations; (5) the findings and diagnoses of consultants; (6) the diagnoses of the responsible physician; (7) notes on treatment, including medication, surgical operations, radiation, and physical therapy; and (8) progress notes by physicians, nurses, and others. The purpose of the patient's medical record is to assist all health care providers (nurses, physicians, and others) with accurate communication and information, thus, improving the care and treatment of the patient (White, 2003). The health record also is discussed in Chapter 6 .

Sequence of Components in the Health Record

The parts of the health history follow a standardized sequence, differing only in small details from one institution to another. The sequence shown in Chart 7–3 is an example used for adult patients. A different order is usually preferred by pediatricians, who set the birth history and the past history ahead of the present illness. Health history guidelines also are shown in Chapter 9 .

CHART 7–2	Objective Data Versus Personal Interpretation	
Objective Data		**Personal Interpretation**
"I'd rather be left alone."		Patient is angry
Shoulder-length dark brown hair		Long, dirty brown hair
Blood pressure: 130/76		Normal blood pressure
Smiles frequently		Appears to be happy

<table>
<tr><td>

CHART 7–3   **Sequence for Taking a Health History**

</td></tr>
</table>

I.   Identification and vital statistics

II. Informant, relation to the patient

III. Chief complaints (CC)

IV. Present illness (PI)

V.   Medications and allergies

VI. Past history (PH)
   A. General health
   B. Infectious diseases
   C. Operations and injuries
   D. Previous hospitalizations
   E. Review of systems (ROS)
      1. Integument
      2. Lymph nodes
      3. Bones, joints, and muscles
      4. Hematopoietic system
      5. Endocrine system
      6. Allergic and immunologic history
      7. Head
      8. Eyes
      9. Ears
      10. Nose
      11. Mouth
      12. Throat
      13. Neck
      14. Breasts
      15. Respiratory system
      16. Cardiovascular system
      17. Gastrointestinal system
      18. Genitourinary system
      19. Nervous system
      20. Psychiatric history

VII. Social history (SH)

VIII. Family history (FH)

IX.   Physical examination

X.   Laboratory

XI.   Summary

Frameworks for Data Collection

Frameworks for data collection include a health history, a physical format and functional instrument such as a growth and development chart for pediatric patients, activities of daily living (ADLs), and instrumental ADLs for older adults. Some examples of data collection tools for ADLs are provided in Charts 7–4 and 7–5 (p. 112).

Nursing Diagnosis and Outcome Identification

The assessment process is applicable to all groups of patients: individuals, families, and communities. After all data have been collected, they are sorted, organized, interpreted, and validated, and conclusions are then drawn about the patient's health status. These conclusions are called **nursing diagnoses.** Nursing diagnoses are clinical judgments about an individual, family, or community response to actual or potential health problems and life processes (North American Nursing Diagnosis Association [NANDA], 2007).

Nursing diagnoses are different from **collaborative problem**s such as medical diagnoses (diabetes, hypertension, coronary artery disease) because nurses' accountability differs for nursing diagnoses and collaborative problems. Nurses ultimately are accountable for formulating nursing diagnoses and intervening appropriately. With regard to a collaborative problem, the nurse is accountable for monitoring changes in the status of the problem and initiating the appropriate interventions, either nurse prescribed or physician prescribed. Nursing diagnoses and collaborative problems are equally important and are determined by the severity of the patient's illness at a particular point in time (Carpenito-Moyet, 2007). According to Carpenito-Moyet, there are four types of nursing diagnoses: actual, high risk, wellness, and syndrome. Each type has a specific purpose and unique components as shown in Chart 7–6 (p. 113).

Outcome Identification

Outcome identification is accomplished by analyzing the assessment data and the nursing diagnosis and deriving a desired outcome for a given problem. The **outcome** is a statement of how the patient's status will change once interventions have been successfully instituted. It is an individual measurable patient objective, or measurable criterion, that specifically indicates that the patient care objective has been met.

Planning

Once nursing diagnoses are formulated, the **planning** phase begins. The nurse is seldom able to resolve all of the patient's nursing diagnoses simultaneously; therefore, these diagnoses must be prioritized. Several factors must be considered when establishing the priority of the patient's nursing diagnoses. These include the patient's needs for biological survival and functioning, the urgency of the need, the patient's perceptions and values, and the nature of the nurse–patient relationship (Carpenito-Moyet, 2007; Wilkinson, 2006).

Certain basic human needs, such as oxygenation, fluid and electrolyte balance, temperature regulation, pain avoidance, nutrition, elimination, and protection from injury take precedence over needs such as activity, sexual needs, emotional security, attachment, and self-esteem. Basic survival needs are based on Maslow's hierarchy of needs (Maslow, 1954). For example, the needs of a patient with burn injuries for a patent airway, prevention of hypovolemic shock, and pain control must be attended to immediately. Concerns about the patient's alteration in body image and possible interferences with sexuality and self-esteem are dealt with when the patient's physiological functioning has been stabilized.

The urgency of the nursing diagnosis also must be considered. The potential threat to safety of an infant whose crib rail has been left down or to an elderly disoriented patient who tries to leave a nursing home unattended takes precedence (at least temporarily) over the infant's nutritional needs or the elderly patient's nursing diagnosis of pain resulting from arthritis.

The patient's perceptions and values are important determinants in setting priorities for nursing care—when the patient's

CHART 7–4 **Activities of Daily Living**

TOILETING

_____ Cares for self at toilet completely; no incontinence (lack of bladder/bowel control).

_____ Needs to be reminded or needs help in cleaning self, or has rare (weekly at most) accidents.

_____ Soiling or wetting while asleep more than once a week.

_____ Soiling or wetting while awake more than once a week.

_____ No control of bowel or bladder.

FEEDING

_____ Eats without assistance.

_____ Eats with minor assistance at mealtimes and/or with special preparation of food; helps cleaning up after meals.

_____ Feeds self with moderate assistance for all meals.

_____ Requires extensive assistance for all meals.

_____ Does not feed self at all and resists efforts of others to feed him/her.

DRESSING

_____ Dresses, undresses, and selects clothes from own wardrobe.

_____ Dresses and undresses self with minor assistance.

_____ Needs moderate assistance in dressing or selection of clothes.

_____ Needs major assistance in dressing, but cooperates with efforts of others to help.

_____ Needs total grooming care, but can remain well groomed after help from others.

PHYSICAL WALKING

_____ Goes about grounds or city.

_____ Walks with assistance of (check one—none may apply):

_____Another person _____Railing _____Cane _____Walker

_____ Uses a wheelchair (gets in and out without help).

_____ Uses a wheelchair (needs help getting in, out).

_____ Sits unsupported in chair or wheelchair, but cannot propel self without help.

_____ Bedridden more than half the time.

BATHING

_____ Bathes self (tub, shower, sponge bath) without help.

_____ Bathes self with help getting in and out of tub.

_____ Washes face and hands only, but cannot bathe rest of body.

_____ Does not wash self, but is cooperative with those who bathe him/her.

_____ Does not try to wash self, and resists efforts to keep himself/herself clean.

CHART 7–5 **Instrumental Activities of Daily Living**

ABILITY TO TELEPHONE

_____ Operates telephone on own initiative (looks up and dials numbers, etc.).

_____ Dials a few well-known numbers.

_____ Answers telephone, but does not dial.

_____ Does not use telephone at all.

SHOPPING

_____ Takes care of all shopping needs independently.

_____ Shops independently for small purchases.

_____ Needs to be accompanied on any shopping trip.

_____ Completely unable to shop.

FOOD PREPARATION

_____ Plans, prepares, and serves adequate meals independently.

_____ Prepares adequate meals if supplied with ingredients.

_____ Heats and serves prepared meals, or prepares meals but does not maintain adequate diet.

_____ Needs to have meals prepared and served.

HOUSEKEEPING

_____ Maintains house alone or with occasional assistance (i.e., heavy work done by others).

_____ Performs light daily tasks such as dish washing and bed-making.

_____ Performs light daily tasks, but cannot maintain acceptable level of cleanliness.

_____ Needs help with all home maintenance tasks.

_____ Does not participate in any housekeeping tasks.

LAUNDRY

_____ Does personal laundry completely.

_____ Launders small items: rinses socks, stockings, etc.

_____ All laundry must be done by others.

MODE OF TRANSPORTATION

_____ Travels independently on public transportation or drives own car.

_____ Arranges own travel via taxi, but does not otherwise use public transportation.

_____ Travels on public transportation when assisted or accompanied by another.

_____ Travels limited to taxi or automobile, with assistance of another.

_____ Does not travel at all.

RESPONSIBILITY FOR OWN MEDICATION

_____ Is responsible for taking medication in correct dosages at correct time.

_____ Takes responsibility if medication is prepared in advance in separate dosages.

_____ Is not capable of dispensing own medication.

ABILITY TO HANDLE FINANCES

_____ Manages financial matters independently (budgets, writes checks, pays rent and bills, goes to bank).

_____ Manages day-to-day purchases but needs help with banking, major purchases, etc.

_____ Incapable of handling money.

CHART 7–6	Types of Nursing Diagnoses		
Actual	**High Risk**	**Wellness**	**Syndrome**
A state that has been clinically validated by identifiable major defining characteristics having four components: label, definition, defining characteristics, and related factors.	A clinical judgment that a patient is more vulnerable to develop the problem than are others in the same or similar situation having four components: label, definition, risk factors, and related factors.	A patient's clinically validated desire to move from a specific level of wellness to a higher level of wellness having only one component: the label.	A cluster of actual or high-risk nursing diagnoses that are predicted to be present because of a single event or situation having one component: the label which contains the etiology or contributing factors to the diagnosis.

perceptions of priority are ignored, the desired outcomes of care are not likely to be achieved. For example, a mother brings her toddler child in for a health checkup. The nurse observes the child drinking cola from a baby bottle and validates with the mother that the toddler consumes about three 8-ounce bottles a day. Although this is a pressing nutritional concern, the mother's chief concern is not being able to control the child's aggressive behavior. Unless the nurse focuses first on the mother's perceived priority need, success in changing the child's nutritional habits will be thwarted.

The nature of the nurse–patient relationship also will determine the order in which the nurse attempts to deal with the patient's diagnoses (Fawcett, 2005; Peplau, 1952). For example, suppose the patient's problem is interpersonal or sexual. Effective intervention will depend on a close and trusting relationship between the nurse and the patient. Such relationships take time to develop. Consequently, the nurse may assign these nursing diagnoses a lower priority until mutual rapport, trust, and respect have developed.

After nursing diagnoses have been assigned priorities, patient goals and objectives are established to clearly outline expected outcomes of care. A **goal** is a broad statement of purpose that describes the aim of nursing care; for example, "To alleviate pain and promote comfort" or "To facilitate adequate oxygenation" or "To promote acceptance of altered body image." Objectives for the individual patient should then be formulated for each goal, in terms of changes in patient behaviors that should result from nursing interventions. Objectives should include measurable criteria that provide parameters for determining whether objectives have been achieved. For example, if a hospitalized patient's nursing diagnosis is "Sleep disturbance related to environmental noise and interruptions for nursing care," the goal may be "To promote adequate rest and sleep." The objective (or outcome), then, may state, "The patient will sleep for at least two uninterrupted periods of 3 hours each during the night." It is important to formulate patient objectives that are both measurable and realistic. An objective that specifies a hospitalized patient will sleep for an 8-hour uninterrupted period is probably quite unrealistic. A realistic objective must take into account the patient's usual pattern and motivation; the health care setting; resources available to the patient and nurse; and the patient's age, cultural background, and health status. Goals and objectives that are inconsistent with the patient's cultural practices, for example, will probably not be achieved (Spector, 2004).

 CRITICAL ALERT *Goals for patient care are set based on the nurse's perspective and are differentiated from measurable objectives or outcomes, which are the patient's response to care. To assess the patient's response to care or the outcome, evaluation parameters must be identified that can be observed and measured.*

Objectives may be short term or long term. Short-term objectives can facilitate ongoing evaluation of the patient's progress toward long-term objectives. For example, a long-term objective for an obese woman might be "Patient will lose 50 pounds in 1 year." A short-term statement might be "Patient will lose approximately 1 pound per week."

Objectives are useful and effective when they are:

- Mutually acceptable to nurse, patient, and family
- Appropriate in terms of nursing and medical diagnoses and therapy
- Realistic in terms of patient's capabilities, time, energy, and resources
- Specific enough to be understood clearly by the patient and other nurses
- Measurable enough to facilitate evaluation.

Once goals and objectives have been identified, the next step is to formulate interventions for achieving the stated goals and objectives. Interventions are planned nursing actions that are likely to facilitate desired outcomes. For example, alternatives for a postoperative patient experiencing pain may include distraction and relaxation techniques, positioning for comfort, or administration of a prescribed analgesic.

After identifying nursing actions (interventions), the nurse then selects from the alternatives. In a sense, selection of nursing actions parallels the process of prioritizing the nursing diagnoses. The actions the nurse selects, and the order in which they are implemented, depend on the following factors:

- Patient preferences
- Known effectiveness of the action (based on prior knowledge, experience, and evidence)
- Time and resources available
- Possible side effects of treatments or medications.

In the case of pain relief, for example, the nurse might decide to help the patient learn conscious relaxation techniques. This action requires time, however, and if the patient is having acute, intense pain and is requesting "a pain medication" the nurse probably will choose to administer the prescribed analgesic first and then teach the patient relaxation techniques once pain relief has been achieved. This will help the patient cope with recurrence of the pain; for instance, if the pain recurs, the nurse may select distraction as the first alternative nursing action.

Implementation

Implementation is the "doing" or intervening phase of the nursing process. It involves organization and actual delivery of nursing care, which leads to achievement of stated goals and objectives. Nursing **interventions** are actions designed to facilitate achievement of positive patient outcomes. They must be purposeful and must be supported by a rationale. A sound rationale is derived from the nurse's knowledge base, prior experience, and the individualized assessment of the patient. Safe and effective nursing interventions are based on a through assessment and individualized care plan (Abdellah, Beland, Martin, & Matheney, 1960; ANA, 2007). NANDA has developed standardized nursing interventions, referred to as the Nursing Intervention Classification (NIC), that correspond with the NANDA nursing diagnoses (Ackley & Ladwig, 2007; Johnson et al., 2006; Lunney, 2001; NANDA, 2007).

Standards of care are based on research and provide an efficient method for identifying predicted problems that occur in a particular situation. Critical pathways are examples of implementation tools that anticipate and describe (in advance) the care of patients within a specified timeline (Carpenito-Moyet, 2007). The critical pathway is based on research and consists of evidence-based or benchmark practices. These practices provide rationales for care and serve to assist nurses in providing answers to the patients' questions as to why proposed interventions are the best approach to their health care. Critical pathways are discussed in Chapter 6 🔗 .

Evidence-Based Practice

Evidence-based practice (EBP) is the recommended standard in health care used by nurses (DiCenso, Guyatt, & Ciliska, 2005; Malloch & Porter-O'Grady, 2006; Melnyk & Fineout-Overholt, 2004). Omery and Williams (1999) have defined EBP as "the careful and practical use of current best evidence to guide health-care decisions" (p. 51). With this definition "current best evidence" includes clinical practice guidelines developed nationally by expert researchers, clinicians, and theorists in their areas of excellence. EBP involves the interpretation and implementation of these clinical guidelines by health care providers based on their clinical expertise, the needs and views of the patient and family, and the resources of the health care system. Thus, EBP is essential in establishing nursing interventions as part of the nursing process. As a problem-solving approach to clinical decision making, it is inherent in the nursing process and incorporates a search for the best and latest evidence, clinical expertise and assessment, and a patient's preferences and values within a context of caring (Benner & Leonard, 2005). Chapter 8 🔗 includes further discussion about EBP.

Evaluation

Evaluation focuses on a patient's behavioral changes and compares them with the criteria stated in the objectives. It consists of both the patient's status and the effectiveness of the nursing care. Both must be evaluated continuously, with the care plan modified as needed (ANA, 2007). Thus, evaluation is ongoing through all phases of the nursing process. As the nurse works with a patient, the patient's responses to the nursing interventions are appraised to determine if the desired outcomes (objectives) have been achieved. For example, if the example states that the patient "will ambulate with assistance for 15 minutes four times a day," this intervention can easily be evaluated by confirming it with the patient and reviewing the nurses' notes. However if the objectives are not achieved, the nurse must determine:

- If the nursing diagnosis was correct
- If the goals and objectives were realistic and reasonable
- If nursing interventions were appropriate
- If any revisions and modifications in the plan are indicated.

It may be that a faulty nursing diagnosis was made from incomplete or inaccurate data or that the goals and objectives were unacceptable to the patient (unreasonable) or unrealistic in terms of the patient's usual patterns and lifestyles, and available resources (Johnson et al., 2006). Nursing interventions must be evaluated in terms of their effectiveness. If the selected intervention did not achieve the intended outcome, another should be attempted.

Patient Care Plan

The **patient care plan** is a documented record of the nursing process. Nursing diagnoses, outcomes with evaluation parameters, and interventions with supporting rationales are recorded on the care plan to communicate with the health care team and to guide patient care. The care plan also should be evaluated on the basis of information obtained from the patient evaluation. Evaluation of the patient care plan is necessary to follow a patient's increased or decreased ability to provide self-care, thus allowing for appropriate modifications. An example of how the nursing process is used with a patient care plan is shown in the Nursing Process box (p. 116). The steps of the nursing process are summarized in Chart 7–7.

◼ Critical Thinking and the Nursing Process

Critical thinking and the nursing process are interrelated aspects of judgment and clinical reasoning. These processes influence and empower the nurse to demonstrate accountability to the patient through the independent, interdependent, and dependent roles inherent in nursing practice.

Critical Thinking

Critical thinking has become a popular phrase in nursing circles during the past decade. Essentially, **critical thinking** is a different way of viewing the information that one knows or learns. Critical thinking demands that one examine information in a variety of ways, exploring means of considering what is important and why some information is more important than other aspects of

- **Assessment** is the collection of both objective and subjective data about the patient. The nurse collects physical evidence, for example, lung sounds, blood pressure, and presence or absence of peripheral pulses. The subjective data are derived from talking with the patient and family about the clinical manifestations that necessitated the need for health care. These data also include the medical history, allergies, and significant previous medical or surgical interventions. Both the subjective and objective data are then organized and documented on the patient's medical record and the patient care plan.

- **Nursing diagnoses** are derived from an analysis of the data collected during the assessment of the patient. Diagnoses include both actual and potential health problems. These diagnoses are then prioritized and categorized into those that can be managed independently by nursing and those that require a collaborative approach to management. Nurses are pivotal in coordinating the other health care professionals who contribute to positive patient outcomes.

- **Outcome identification**, often considered a part of the diagnosis step, consists of analyzing the assessment data and nursing diagnoses and deriving a desired outcome for a given problem. The outcome is a statement of how the patient's status will change once the interventions have been successfully instituted. A group of nurses from Iowa published a standardized vocabulary and classifications of nursing outcomes as they relate specifically to nursing interventions—the Nursing Outcomes Classification (NOC) (Johnson, Maas, & Moorhead, 2000).

- **Planning** is the phase of the nursing process in which interventions are planned that will achieve the identified outcomes associated with each nursing diagnosis. The interventions need to be prioritized to ensure patient safety. The planning phase may or may not be documented in the patient record. Often it is a mental process of choosing the appropriate interventions.

- **Implementation** is the carrying out of the plan identified in the previous step of the nursing process. Communication is a critical piece of the implementation process. This phase requires that the nurse identify which interventions can be accomplished independently and which require collaboration with other members of the health care team. The nurse needs to ensure that all members have received clear communication about the patient's needs. There also is a standardized classification of nursing interventions referred to as the Nursing Interventions Classifications (NIC) (Wilkinson, 2006). These standards provide a list of interventions associated with each nursing diagnosis. The final step of the implementation phase is recording the interventions on the patient record.

- **Evaluation** requires that the nurse compare the patient status to the desired outcomes. If the outcome is unmet, the care plan is revised and the process begins again until positive outcomes are achieved if at all possible.

information, and then taking what is most important and using that information to make decisions and solve problems.

Critical thinking is organized, purposeful, and disciplined. It entails the examination of elements of thought implicit in all reasoning: purpose, problem or question at issue, assumptions, concepts, reasoning leading to conclusions, implications, and consequences (Paul, 2004). Using critical thinking, the individ-

ual systematically and habitually imposes criteria and intellectual standards on the thinking process. During this process, the individual is aware of and takes charge of the thinking process, guiding his thinking to arrive at new and innovative conclusions (Paul, 2004). Critical in this respect does not mean that one is eager to find fault, but rather that one is judging carefully and competently. "Critical thinking in nursing entails purposeful, goal-directed thinking; aims to make judgments based on fact rather than guesswork; is based on principles of science and scientific method; and requires strategies that maximize human potential and compensate for problems caused by human nature" (Alfaro-LeFevre, 1995, p. 9).

At the center of critical thinking is one's ability to look at information in different ways, to question the information and assimilate it in new ways. With critical thinking comes the ability to apply new knowledge, often taken from fields outside nursing, create new options and means of implementing appropriate nursing care, and question why certain interventions give better patient outcomes. Some of the aspects of being a critical thinker are that one continually seeks new knowledge, remains open minded and receptive to new possibilities rather than merely accepting or rejecting ideas without examination, and strives to develop more innovative and effective ways to improve her decision-making capabilities. Characteristics of a critical thinker are that the individual is reflective, uses healthy, constructive skepticism, is autonomous in that he is not easily manipulated but thinks independently, is fair in his assessments, and focuses on what to do or believe.

Critical thinkers use a variety of cognitive skills in their thought processes. They are able to differentiate fact from opinion, evaluating within themselves the credibility of information sources and seeking additional sources to better evaluate the information that has been gathered. They clarify concepts, question assumptions, and ensure that the assumptions on which they base decisions and actions are accurate.

Critical thinking is essential to competent, skillful nursing care. When caring for patients, especially in stressful situations, critical thinking enables nurses to recognize important cues, respond quickly, and adapt interventions as needed. Nurses accomplish this outcome by (1) analyzing the situation to discover what issues are involved and what actions are appropriate, (2) applying standards according to established personal and professional rules, (3) discriminating by recognizing the similarities and differences among patients and diagnoses, (4) seeking additional information by searching for knowledge and gathering relevant data about the patient and her condition or diagnosis, (5) drawing conclusions that are supported by the data, (6) creating a plan of action, and (7) transforming knowledge into action. It is essential when analyzing each situation that nurses consider the ethical and legal principles involved.

Decision Making

The application of critical thinking is for decision making and effective clinical judgment. A subset of problem solving, decision making is the art of determining the best course of action to take in a given situation. In decision making, the individual selects a course of action from among two or more choices, using a variety of strategies to determine the best course of action.

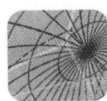

NURSING PROCESS: Patient Care Plan Example

Nursing Assessment of Pain

Subjective Data:

What is your pain level at, using the 1–10 scale? A 1 is very little pain and a 10 is the worst imaginable pain.

What is your experience with pain?

Do you routinely take pain medications at home; if so, what for and what kind?

Are you allergic to any pain medication?

Do you have any cultural or religious beliefs that impact your pain control?

Objective Data:

Grimacing upon movement

Restlessness and irritability

Taut facial expression

Nursing Assessment and Diagnosis	**Outcomes and Evaluation Parameters**	**Planning and Interventions with Rationales**
Nursing Diagnosis: Acute pain related *to bilateral knee replacement therapy, physical therapy, and movement*	**Outcome:** Comfort level maintained. **Evaluation Parameters:** Able to communicate pain level and therapies that help alleviate it. On a scale of 10, reported pain will remain at 3 or less throughout hospitalization. Absence of pain behaviors such as grimacing. Nonpharmacological method of control is effective as evidenced by patient report and no pain behaviors. Reports satisfaction with pain management program.	**Interventions and *Rationales:*** Use pain scale (0–10) to quantify pain level. *Quantifying pain increases consistency.* Instruct patient to inform nurse if pain is not relieved. *Indicates need to change pain management plan.* Assess cultural and religious impact on patient's responses. *Different cultures and religions respond differently to pain.* Correct misconceptions about risk of addiction and overdose. *Decreases anxiety related to medication addiction.* Explain, prepare, and medicate patient for painful procedures (dressing change, ambulation, physical therapy) and anticipated discomforts. *Controls increased pain level related to procedure.* Provide a supportive environment in which patient is able to express pain level. *Opens communication and facilitates pain management.* Use pain control measures before it becomes severe. *Increases comfort and decreases need for medication.* Teach nonpharmacologic method of control (i.e., guided imagery, massage, and breathing exercises). *Augments pain relief.* Maintain proper positioning of affected leg. *Proper positioning reduces pain and enhances pain relief.* Provide rest periods between procedures to assist with coping with ongoing pain. *Decreases the fatigue related to long-term pain.* Revise pain management plan as wounds heal and pain decreases. *To prevent overmedication.* Plan diversional activities: relaxation, alternative sensory stimulation such as music, massage, heat/cold, movies, TV, reading, and breathing techniques. *Augments pain relief measures.*

As such, decision making is synonymous with the act of choosing, of converting information into action.

Decision making may or may not be the result of an immediate problem, but is initiated as part of an immediate problem. Elements in decision making include (1) identification of a problem, (2) establishment of criteria to evaluate potential solutions, (3) a search for alternative solutions or actions, (4) evaluation of alternative choices, and (5) selection of a course of action. The four phases of decision making are deliberation, judgment, choice, and evaluation of the effectiveness of the outcomes. Perhaps the most time-consuming phase is the deliberation phase when one determines that there is a decision to be made, begins to establish criteria for evaluating the effectiveness of potential solutions, and searches for possible solutions. The judgment phase involves a thorough understanding of the possible choices at hand and evaluation of these choices. Once these two phases have been explored, the third phase involves the selection and implementation of what has been determined to be one's best choice of action. Finally, evaluation of the effectiveness of the outcomes occurs, which may begin the process anew if desired outcomes are not attained.

A nurse can employ any of several strategies when deciding the best course of action to take. These strategies include trial-and-error methods, pilot projects, brainstorming, group input, cost–benefit analyses, cause and effect, worst-case scenarios, and the more recently endorsed EBP model (see earlier discussion). Depending on the immediacy of a needed solution and the seriousness of outcomes if an alternate course of action is taken, some of these listed strategies may not be the most appropriate strategies for decision making in different instances.

Critical Pathways

Newer forms of decision making in clinical areas include the development of critical pathways. Critical pathways identify key events of patient care and expected time frames. Their advantages include improved patient outcomes, streamlined charting, facilitation of quality assessment, improved patient education, and enhanced communication among health care providers. Again, many critical or clinical pathways are developed as a result of research and identified as one source for evidence-based practice (see Chapters 6 and 8 ☺).

National Standards and Guidelines

National standards and guidelines also assist with decision making in clinical areas and reducing variance in professional practice patterns. National standards and guidelines have been promulgated by regulatory agencies and professional organizations. The Joint Commission promotes the use of appropriate, measurable clinical indicators in clinical settings. These measures promote quantitative measures to monitor and evaluate the quality of care. Professional organizations such as the American Association of Critical Care Nurses or the Emergency Nurses Association promote standards of care for patients served in various types of practice settings. Other standards promote care for a specialization, such as the ANA's standards of care for hospice nursing or its standards of care for ambulatory nursing care (ANA, 2004).

Clinical Judgment

Clinical judgment, sometimes referred to as reflective thinking or clinical reasoning, is the process of drawing conclusions based on a comparison of the patient's current data with specific outcome data and giving meaning to data based on that comparison. For example, clinical judgment is involved when a nurse notes that the patient's potassium level is 6.8 compared to a "normal" potassium level of 3.6 to 5.0. Thus, clinical judgment involves comparing the patient's current health status to the expected or desired status and deciding which measures are the most appropriate given that comparison. If the comparison is essentially the same, the nurse can conclude that current interventions are successful. If the comparison varies, the nurse can conclude that further interventions are required. The nurse would then use critical thinking and decision making to determine the next course of action.

Using Critical Thinking with the Nursing Process

The use of critical thinking with the nursing process enhances the validity, reliability, and effectiveness of outcomes to patients. Critical thinking is essential in nursing when the nurse is assessing, diagnosing, implementing, and evaluating the patient and developing the care plan (Wilkinson, 2006). Chart 7–8 depicts the relationship between critical thinking and the nursing process.

Critical thinking requires developing characteristics of critical thinkers as shown in Figures 7–2 ■ and 7–3 ■ (p. 118). Because critical thinking is contextual, it changes depending on circumstances. However, because the decisions nurses make affect people's lives, their judgment must be sound, precise, and disciplined. Critical thinking promotes accuracy and depth of data collection and seeks to identify the needs of the patient. This controlled thinking is essential to help people avoid illness and its complications and to help people gain optimal independence, a sense of well-being, and/or a peaceful death as appropriate.

Twelve aspects of critical thinking were initially identified by Ennis in 1962, reaffirmed in 1996, and reiterated in recent publications (Ennis, 2003, 2004). These aspects of critical thinking are shown in Chart 7–9 (p. 118) and are consistent with the definition and explanation of critical thinking as presented in Chapter 1 ☺ of this text. In essence, critical thinking focuses on deciding what to believe or do. It is relevant not only to the formation and checking of beliefs, but also to deciding on and evaluating actions. It involves creative activities such as formulating hypotheses and plans. Critical thinking is reflective and reasonable (Ennis, 1996). As such it is a critical element in using the nursing process.

CHART 7–8 **Critical Thinking, Nursing Process Actions, and Nursing Process Phases (Steps)**

Critical Thinking	Nursing Process Action	Nursing Process Phase
Get a better understanding of something or someone else.	Initiate nurse–patient interaction. Collect data. Interpret and validate data.	Assessment
Identify actual and potential problems.	Formulate nursing diagnosis. Derive a desired outcome.	Nursing diagnosis and outcome identification
Make decisions about an action.	Prioritize nursing diagnosis. Formulate goals/objectives. Select planned interventions.	Planning
Reduce risk of getting undesirable results.	Organize interventions. Carry out selected nursing interventions.	Implementation
Increase likelihood of achieving beneficial results.	Determine if nursing diagnosis is correct. Determine if goals/objectives are/have been met. Make necessary revisions and modifications.	Evaluation
Find ways to improve (even when no problem exists).	Repeat the process to gain optimal independence, sense of well-being, or peaceful death.	Nursing process continues

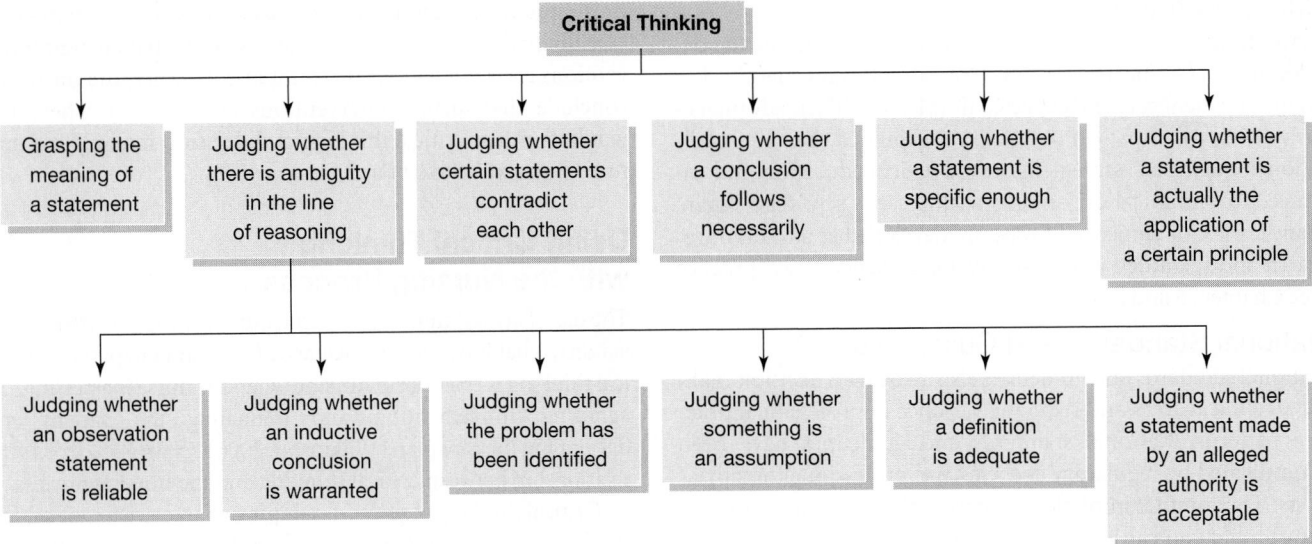

FIGURE 7–2 ■ Critical thinking.

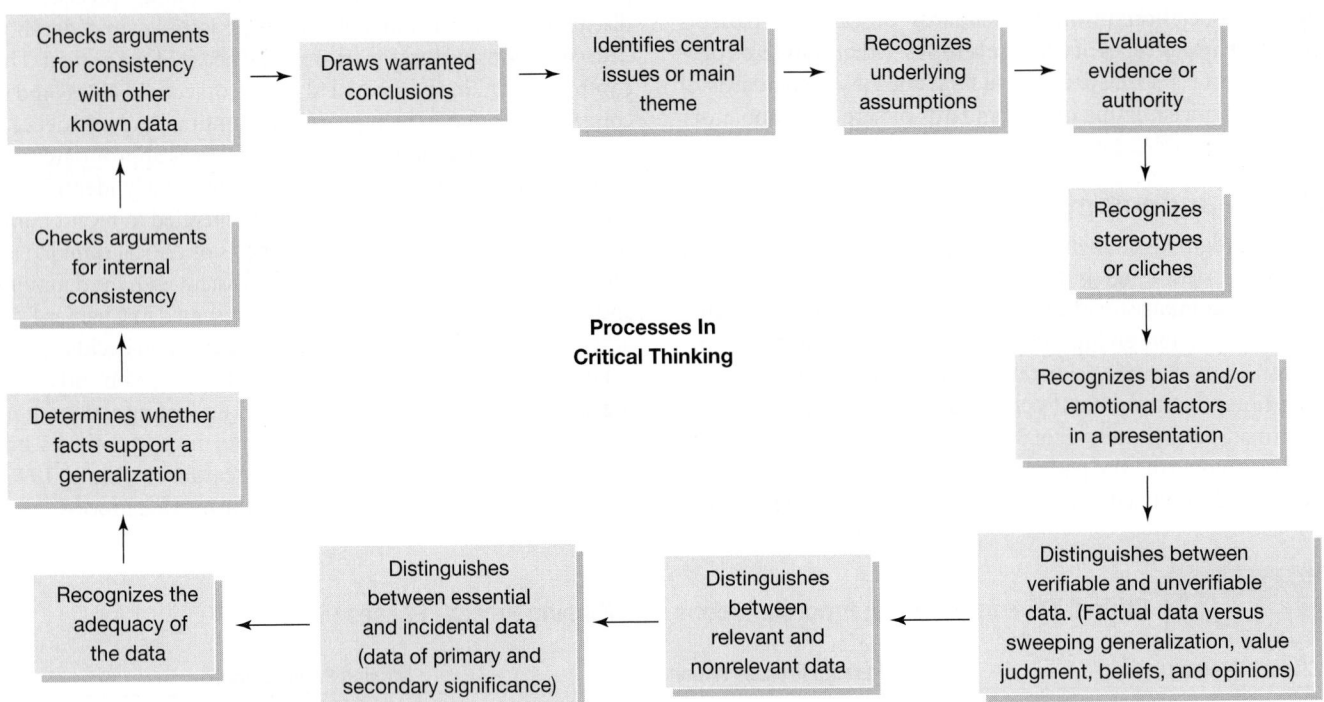

FIGURE 7–3 ■ Processes in critical thinking.

CHART 7–9 **Twelve Aspects of Critical Thinking**

1. Grasping the meaning of a statement

2. Judging whether there is ambiguity in the line of reasoning

3. Judging whether certain statements contradict each other

4. Judging whether a conclusion follows necessarily

5. Judging whether a statement is specific enough

6. Judging whether a statement is actually the application of a certain principle

7. Judging whether an observation statement is reliable

8. Judging whether an inductive conclusion is warranted

9. Judging whether the problem has been identified

10. Judging whether something is an assumption

11. Judging whether a definition is adequate

12. Judging whether a statement made by an alleged authority is acceptable

Sources: From Robert H. Ennis, "A Concept of Critical Thinking," *Harvard Educational Review,* 32:1 (Winter 1962), pp. 84. Copyright © by the President and Fellows of Harvard College. All rights reserved. For more information, please visit www.harvardeducationalreview.org; Ennis, R. H. (1996). *Critical thinking.* Upper Saddle River, NJ: Pearson Prentice Hall.

Summary

The nursing process is a patient-centered method for structuring the delivery of nursing care. As such, it is the common thread that unites different types of nurses who work in varied areas; it serves as the essential core of practice for the registered nurse (ANA, 2007). The nursing process is the vehicle through which the nurse applies intuitive and scientific knowledge, critical thinking, and nursing skills in a systematic, goal-directed fashion to achieve the outcomes desired for the patient. The nursing process entails gathering and analyzing data in order to identify patient strengths, potential or actual problems, and goals, and developing and evaluating a plan of nursing interventions to achieve mutually agreed-on outcomes. At every stage of the five-step process, the nurse works closely with the patient to individualize care and build a relationship of mutual respect.

REVIEW QUESTIONS

1. The nurse is conducting an independent nursing activity with a patient. Which of the following would this nurse be doing?
   1. Assessing a wound
   2. Documenting intake on a calorie count form
   3. Assisting the patient to use a walker
   4. Administering medication

2. The nurse is reviewing a patient's situation in order to diagnose the patient's problems. This nurse is conducting which phase of the nursing process?
   1. Assessment
   2. Planning
   3. Implementation
   4. Evaluation

3. The nurse does a finger stick to check a patient's current blood glucose level. The nurse is utilizing which skill for conducting this assessment?
   1. Cognitive
   2. Affective
   3. Psychomotor
   4. Psychosocial

4. At the completion of a patient's assessment, the nurse creates a clinical judgment about a potential health problem. This clinical judgment is considered:
   1. Goal setting.
   2. Planning interventions.
   3. Determining collaborative problems.
   4. Determining a nursing diagnosis.

5. The nurse is making a decision about a future action with patient care. This critical thinking activity is equated with which of the following steps of the nursing process?
   1. Assessment
   2. Planning
   3. Implementation
   4. Evaluation

Answers for review questions appear in Appendix D

KEY TERMS

assessment *p.109*
collaborative problems *p.111*
critical thinking *p.114*
dependent activities *p.107*
evaluation *p.114*
goal *p.113*

implementation *p.114*
independent activities *p.107*
interdependent activities *p.107*
intervention *p.114*
nurse–patient relationship *p.107*
nursing diagnosis *p.111*

nursing process *p.107*
objective data *p.109*
outcome *p.111*
patient care plan *p.114*
planning *p.111*
subjective data *p.109*

REFERENCES

Abdellah, F. G., Beland, K. K., Martin, A., & Matheney, R. J. (1960). *Patient centered approaches to nursing.* New York: Macmillan.

Ackley, B. J., & Ladwig, G. B. (2007). *Nursing diagnosis handbook: an evidence-based guide to planning care* (8th ed.). St Louis: Mosby.

Alfaro-LeFevre, R. (1995). *Critical thinking in nursing: A practical approach.* Philadelphia: W. B. Saunders.

American Nurses Association. (2003). *Nursing's social policy statement* (2nd ed.). Washington, DC: Author.

American Nurses Association. (2004). *Standards of clinical nursing practice.* Washington, DC: Author.

American Nurses Association. (2007). *The nursing process: A common thread amongst all nurses.* Retrieved September 16, 2007, from http://nursingworld.org/ExpeciallyForYou/StudentNurses/Thenursingprocess.aspx

Benner, P., & Leonard, V. W. (2005). Patient concerns and choices and clinical judgment in EBP. In B. Melnyk & E. Fineout-Overholt (Eds.), *Evidence-based practice in nursing and healthcare: A guide to best practices.* Philadelphia: Lippincott.

Carpenito-Moyet, L. J. (2005). *Understanding the nursing process: Concept mapping and care planning for students.* Philadelphia: Lippincott Williams & Wilkins.

Carpenito-Moyet, L. J. (2007). *Nursing diagnosis: Application to clinical practice* (12th ed.). Philadelphia: Lippincott Williams & Wilkins.

DiCenso, A., Guyatt, G., & Ciliska, D. (2005). *Evidence-based nursing: A guide to clinical practice.* Philadelphia: Elsevier.

Ennis, R. H. (1962). A concept of critical thinking. *Harvard Educational Review, 32,* 81–111.

Ennis, R. H. (2003). Critical thinking assessment. In C. Fasko (Ed.), *Critical thinking and reasoning: Current theories, research, and practice.* Cresskill, NJ: Hampton.

Ennis, R. H. (2004). Applying soundness standards to qualified reasoning. *Informal Logic, 24*(1), 23–39.

Fawcett, J. (2005). *Contemporary nursing knowledge: Analysis and evaluation of nursing models and theories* (2nd ed.). Philadelphia: F. A. Davis.

Henderson, V. (1966). *The nature of nursing.* New York: Macmillan.

Johnson, D. E. (1980). The behavioral system model for nursing. In J. P. Riehl & C. Roy (Eds.), *Conceptual models for nursing practice* (2nd ed.). New York: Appleton-Century-Crofts.

Johnson, M., Bulechek, G. M., Butcher, H., Dochterman, J. M., Maas, M., Moorhead, S., et al. (2006). *NANDA, NOC and NIC linkages: Nursing diagnoses, outcomes and interventions* (2nd ed.). Philadelphia: Elsevier.

Johnson, M., Maas, M., & Moorhead, S. (2000). *Nursing outcomes classification* (NOC) (2nd ed.). St. Louis: Mosby.

King, I. M. (1971). *Toward a theory of nursing; General concepts of human behavior.* New York: John Wiley & Sons.

Leininger, M. M. (1991). *Culture care diversity and universality: A theory of nursing.* New York: National League of Nursing Press.

Levine, M. (1973). *Introduction to clinical nursing* (2nd ed.). Philadelphia: F. A. Davis.

Lunney, M. (Ed.). (2001). *Critical thinking and nursing diagnosis: Case studies and analysis.* Philadelphia: North American Nursing Diagnosis Association.

Malloch, K., & Porter-O'Grady, T. (2006). *Introduction to evidence-based practice in nursing and health care.* Sudbury, MA: Jones and Bartlett.

Maslow, A. H. (1954). *Motivation and personality.* New York: Harper and Row Publishers.

Melnyk, B. M., & Fineout-Overholt, E. (Eds.). (2004). *Evidence-based practice nursing and healthcare: A guide to best pratice.* Philadelphia: Lippincott Williams & Wilkins.

North American Nursing Diagnosis Association. (2007). *Nursing diagnoses: Definitions & classification 2007–2008.* Philadelphia: Author.

Omery, A., & Williams, R. P. (1999). An appraisal of research utilization across the United States. *Journal of Nursing Administration, 29,* 50–56.

Orem, D. (1971). *Nursing concepts of practice.* New York: McGraw-Hill.

Orlando, I. J. (1961). *The dynamic nurse–patient relationship: Function, process, and principles.* New York: G. P. Putnam's Sons.

Paul, R. (2004). *Defining critical thinking.* Retrieved October 22, 2006, from http://www.criticalthinking.org/aboutCT/definingCT.shtml

Peplau, H. E. (1952). *Interpersonal relations in nursing.* New York: G. P. Putnam's Sons.

Rogers, M. E. (1970). *The theoretical basis of nursing.* Philadelphia: F. A. Davis.

Spector, R. E. (2004). *Cultural diversity in health & illness.* Upper Saddle River, NJ: Pearson Prentice Hall.

Stanton, J., Paul, C., & Reeves, J. S. (1980). An overview of the nursing process. In *Nursing theories: The base for professional nursing practice.* Englewood Cliffs, NJ: Prentice Hall.

Watson, J. (1988). New dimensions of human caring theory. *Nursing Science Quarterly, 1*(4), 175–181.

Watson, J. (2003). *Jean Watson and the theory of human caring.* Retrieved on February 14, 2003, from http://ww2.uchsc.edu/son/caring/content/sct.asp

White, L. (2003). *Documentation and the nursing process: A review.* Clifton Park, NY: Delmar.

Wilkinson, Judith M. (2006). *Nursing process & critical thinking* (4th ed.). Upper Saddle River, NJ: Pearson Prentice Hall.

Yura, H., & Walsh, M. B. (1988). *The nursing process* (5th ed.). New York: Appleton-Century-Crofts.

Role of Research in Nursing Practice

Annita Watson

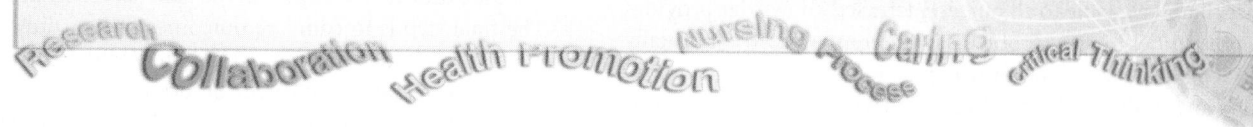

Outcome-Based Learning Objectives

After studying this chapter, the learner will be able to:

1. Differentiate between basic and applied research.
2. Differentiate between quantitative and qualitative research.
3. Identify three types of quantitative and three types of qualitative research.
4. Describe the first step of the research process.
5. Determine how a research design is selected.
6. Differentiate between research utilization and evidence-based practice.
7. Describe the three ethical principles that guide research studies.
8. Describe the impact of HIPAA on nursing research studies.
9. Explain the four stages of completing a quantitative research critique.

Research is a formal, systematic, and organized method used to answer a question or solve a problem. It is defined as a "diligent, systemic inquiry or study that validates and redefines existing knowledge and develops new knowledge" (Burns & Grove, 2003, p. 3). Though researchers frequently attach different meanings to the term *research,* there is consensus that the term implies a formal, rigorous, and precise process intended to discover new knowledge and relationships and find solutions to problems or questions. This type of scientific inquiry provides a forum to facilitate the ongoing process of questioning and evaluating practice, informs practice based on available data, and guides new practices through research and experimental learning. As such, research is essential for defining the nursing profession, providing a mechanism for ascertaining best practices, and advancing the science of nursing practice. This chapter focuses on the process and outcomes of research and the manner in which it is used by nurses to promote clinical practice. Specific examples of research intended to change and improve medical–surgical nursing practice are discussed in the specific disorder chapters within the text.

Nursing Research

Nursing research is similar to research conducted by other professional groups or disciplines in that the same rigorous steps must be followed, and the research design and method of investigation must be appropriate to the problem or question being studied. Gillis and Jackson (2002) suggest, however, that nursing research is distinguished by the diversity of the human experience. When compared to other fields, nursing practice requires greater flexibility in the definition and interpretation of research, thereby providing for the variations that occur across professional practice settings. This has become particularly evident as globalization of the world community has highlighted the differences in nursing practice and contexts across countries.

Defining nursing research requires determining the relevant knowledge for nursing. Since Florence Nightingale's era, nurses have been expanding their professional practice foundation through research efforts designed to develop and test knowledge. In 1976, the American Nurses Association (ANA) adopted the following definition, which remains broad enough today to encompass globalization of the world community:

> Nursing research is investigation into the area of knowledge in which the physical and behavioral sciences meet and influence one another in an effort to study how health problems relate to human behavior and how behavior relates to health and illness. It addresses the human and behavioral questions that arise in the treatment of disease, in the prevention of illness, and in the promotion and maintenance of health. (ANA, 1976, p. 1)

Nursing research also may be viewed as research into phenomena that are predominantly and appropriately the responsibility of nurses in their professional practice (Gillis & Jackson, 2002). Nurses are responsible for provision of patient care, administration of nursing and health care services, and education of practitioners. Therefore, research in nursing encompasses systematic inquiry into each of these areas. With this interpretation nursing research not only adds to the knowledge base of nursing, but also influences changes for patients, their futures, and their environments. It also impacts the health care delivery system and related costs of health care.

The world is constantly changing. Much of nursing knowledge is not generated through research. Nurses typically draw on knowledge from a variety of sources, each offering something unique to holistic nursing practice. These include tradition, authority, trial and error, personal experience, intuition, and logical reasoning. However, nurses can no longer rely on the assumptions that come only from experience and trial and error. Information that is supported by data is critical to improving the clinical care provided to patients. The difficulty with non–research-based knowledge is that it has limited scientific predictability and cannot be used to justify nursing actions or provide new scientific information to direct practice.

Evidence from research must be applied to nurses' practices to assure patients that they have the best knowledge available for safe and compassionate care. In addition, research findings must be shared with others in order to broaden the current knowledge base that is available to all nurses. Increased knowledge provides opportunities to solve problems in different ways, to continually challenge the status quo of why practice is performed in a certain way, and to understand phenomena that occur in the professional sphere. In this era of rapid change it is critical for research to be used as a tool to provide caring, compassionate, and scientific care.

Basic and Applied Research

The general purpose of nursing research is to answer questions or solve problems relevant to the nursing profession. In terms of the intent of the research, a distinction can be made between basic and applied research. **Basic research,** as traditionally defined, is undertaken to extend the knowledge base in a discipline or to formulate or refine a theory. **Applied research** focuses on finding solutions to existing problems. For example, a study to determine the effectiveness of a nursing intervention to ease pain would be applied research. The specific purposes of nursing research include identification, description, exploration, explanation, prediction, and control (Polit & Beck, 2008). Practicing nurses are most apt to be involved in applied research. This, then, becomes the focus of this chapter.

Although this chapter highlights the current status of research in nursing, particularly as it relates to the development of evidence-based practice, it is necessary to understand the research process before one can participate in it. A description of the research process, the conditions under which research is undertaken, and the types of research typically used by nurses and other health care professionals provides the groundwork for the discussion of research utilization and evidence-based practice.

◼ The Research Process

The **research process** is very similar to the nursing process in that it proceeds through discrete steps in order to answer a question. Thus, the steps of the research process should not be totally new to the learner because nurses perform similar activities every day when they engage in critical thinking, reflect on their practice, and apply the nursing process. For example, nurses engage in data collection about patients when they read the patient's chart; receive reports; and engage in dialogue with colleagues, the patient, and the family. Based on this information and observations, the nurse formulates a diagnosis of the patient's health needs. This stage is similar to naming, classifying, or identifying problems. Next, the nurse develops a plan of care specific to the patient's identified needs. This step is similar to the methodology plan that the researcher develops after the problem statement is clearly defined. The plan is based on an expectation that certain interventions produce intended outcomes for the patient. This is similar to prediction in the quantitative research process.

The nurse then evaluates the effect of the interventions on the patient's outcomes and recommends modifications to the plan as new evidence becomes available. This is similar to interpretation of findings and the recommendation stage of the research process (Gillis & Jackson, 2002). For example, a problem/question is identified, a literature search is conducted, a method or research design is selected to answer the question, data are collected and analyzed about the responses to the problem/question, and conclusions are drawn based on what the data demonstrate.

The final step is to compare outcomes of the study. The researcher asks "Do the outcomes of the study reflect current practice, is more research indicated, or does practice need to be changed from the evidence of the study?" A caution is that practices should not be changed only on the basis of one study. A research study should be replicated (repeated) in different settings, with different patients, to be sure the results are similar and that they can be generalized to other populations and settings.

A relationship between problem solving and research also can be drawn, because problem solving is the basis of the nursing process. For some, the assimilation of the research process is easier when presented in the context of problem solving and the nursing process. Chart 8–1 shows the similarities and differ-

CHART 8-1	Problem Solving and Research: Similarities and Differences
SIMILARITIES	**DIFFERENCES**
Critical thinking	Unique language
Complex reasoning	Rigorous application of research methods
Information is gathered	Broader focus: groups versus individuals
Observations are made	Stronger theoretical base
Problems are identified	Greater precision, rigor, and control
Plans are developed	Outcomes shared with a larger audience
Actions are taken	Research process is more complex
Effectiveness and efficiency are evaluated	
Outcomes are determined	

ences between problem solving versus research. Chart 8–2 shows a comparison of the nursing process to the problem-solving process and the research process.

Conducting Research

Discrete steps must be taken in order to conduct research. The order and progression of these steps vary depending on whether one is conducting quantitative or qualitative research. However, some of the basic elements of the process apply to both types of research approaches, including identifying the problem and purpose, conducting a literature review, collecting and analyzing data, and drawing conclusions. These steps may or may not progress in a linear way depending on the type of research being conducted, quantitative or qualitative, and are discussed under the respective topics of quantitative and qualitative research; commonalities, however, are presented next.

Research Problem and Purpose

The first step in any research process is to identify a researchable problem. A researchable problem is a situation in need of a solution, alteration, or improvement. It is an area of concern for a particular population that requires investigation and it is derived from a topical area. Not all problems are researchable. For instance, problems or questions of a moral or ethical nature are incapable of being researched because there is no right or wrong answer, only points of view that reflect one's values.

The problem concept or topical area of concern typically is very broad and generally contains numerous potential research problems. The actual research problem is a very small piece of the entire topical area. This may be thought of as a very small piece of a large puzzle or a very small slice of a very large pie. For example, pain is a general research topic/concept, and one researchable question (problem) related to pain is "Does fatigue exacerbate pain in cancer patients?" Figure 8–1 ■ (p. 124) reflects

---

CHART 8–2	Comparison of Steps of the Nursing Process, the Problem-Solving Process, and Stages of Nursing Research	

Nursing Process	Problem-Solving Process	Stages of Nursing Research
1. Assess to determine the degree of discrepancy between what is and what should be in relation to the optimum health of an individual patient.	1. Identify a particular problem or condition of the patient or family or a problem in the setting that requires change.	1. Identify a research problem, from clinical observations or from the literature and current theoretical thought, or from a combination of the two. Delineate the problem clearly and delimit the problem to a manageable research question or hypothesis.
2. Intervene by refining the nursing diagnoses to behavioral goals in collaboration with the patient, formulating the desired outcomes for problem resolution in the form of behavioral objectives, generating and selecting an alternate course of actions, and implementing the action alternatives.	2. Analyze the various aspects of the problem (e.g., the need for immediate or long-term change), the type of approach that is needed, the need to involve other people in the problem-solving process, and the resources that are available.	2. Collect essential facts pertaining to the problem. Review the literature, validate the significance of the problem selected, or develop the theoretical or conceptual underpinnings for the problem to explain it and its possible solution(s).
3. Evaluate to appraise the degree to which the actual outcomes match the desired outcomes (the behavioral objectives).	3. Collect data about the patient or family, the setting, related facets of the problem, and possible solutions to the problem through the use of observations, interviews, discussion with experts, and a review of the literature.	3. Create a theoretical or conceptual framework and operationalize the concepts under consideration. Develop tentative solutions to be tested in the form of hypotheses or develop the general approach that will provide the desired information in the form of research question(s).
4. Revise the plan by redesigning the behavioral objectives that have not been attained; by selecting and implementing other action alternatives; and by collecting and analyzing more data to evolve new nursing diagnoses, new behavioral objectives, and other action alternatives, all in collaboration with the patient.	4. Analyze the information collected using the analysis as a guide for appropriate actions. Establish a plan for change and a means for evaluating the success of the change.	4. Develop an appropriate design to answer the question(s) or test the hypotheses, which includes measuring instruments, setting, sample, protocol, methodology, and statistical analysis design and the rationale for each.
	5. Implement the plan of change.	5. Collect the essential data.
	6. Evaluate the effects of the change as determined by the evaluation plan developed. If the actions fail to solve the problem, begin again, looking for alternative solutions to the problem.	6. Analyze the data, interpret the findings, and generalize the results in terms of the framework, the theoretical perspective, and the sampling rationale.
		7. Disseminate the research findings.

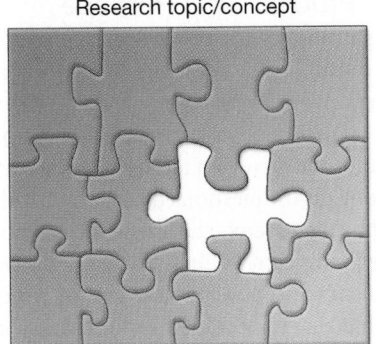
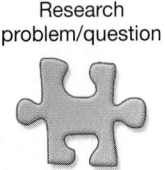
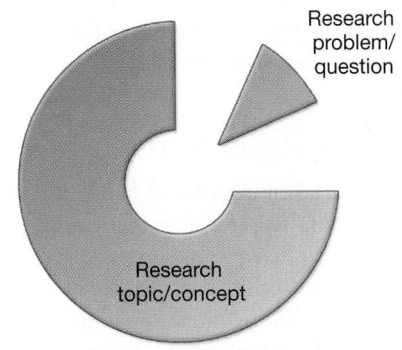

Research topic/concept

Research problem/question

Research problem/question

Research topic/concept

FIGURE 8–1 ■ The problem concept or topical area of concern typically is very broad, whereas the actual research problem is a very small piece of the entire topical area. This may be thought of as a very small piece of a large puzzle or a very small slice of a very large pie.

the minuteness of the research problem in relation to the problem topic. The study or **research problem** is a very specific and precise statement of the phenomenon to be studied. The study problem also may be phrased as a **research question**. Examples of research topics/concepts with related research problems are shown in Chart 8–3.

Research problems may be developed from a variety of sources, such as nursing practice, researcher and peer interactions, literature review, theory, and research priorities identified by funding agencies and specialty groups. The researcher should keep in mind that the problem selected must meet four criteria. The problems must be:

- Significant to nursing (someone must benefit from the evidence that is produced)
- Researchable (amenable to scientific inquiry)
- Feasible to address (time to complete, available study participants, cooperation of others, faculties and equipment, money, experience of the researcher, and ethically sound)
- Of interest to the researcher (genuine interest in and curiosity about the problem).

CRITICAL ALERT

Select a research problem that:

1. *Is researchable.*
2. *Has significance to nursing practice.*
3. *Is feasible to address.*
4. *Is of genuine interest to the researcher.*

Research Purpose

The **research purpose** is generated from the problem. It identifies the goal or goals of the study and directs the development of the study. In the research process, the purpose usually is stated after the problem has been determined, because the problem identifies the gap in knowledge in a selected area and the purpose clarifies the knowledge to be generated by a study. The purpose clearly identifies the goals of the study. In quantitative research, the problem identifies an area of concern and the purpose reflects the type of study to be conducted: descriptive, correlational, quasi-experimental, or experimental. Problems formulated for qualitative studies also identify an area of concern, and the purpose indicates the focus of the investigation: a subjective concept, an event, a phenomenon, or a fact of a culture or society (Polit & Beck, 2008).

CHART 8–3 **Research Topics/Concepts and Related Research Problems/Questions**

Research Topic/Concept	Research Problem/Question
Pregnancy in teenage girls	Adaptation to pregnancy in teenage girls varies according to ethnic culture.
Quality of life among Alzheimer patients' caregivers.	Quality of life among Alzheimer patients varies according to the amount of social support received.
Testicular cancer	Instruction on testicular self-exam in adolescents is predictive of performing self-exams as an adult.
Informatics	Educational level of the registered nurse influences the use of computers in the clinical setting.
Discharge planning in acute care settings	What is the role of the staff nurse in discharge planning?
Falls in acute care setting	Fall prevention programs affect the number of falls in acute care settings.
Competence in elders	Level of competence in those over age 85 determines the ability to live independently by self.
Evidence-based practice	The use of evidence-based practice is influenced by level of education of the registered nurse.
Staffing in acute care settings	Staffing in acute care settings affects patient outcomes.
Breast cancer screening	Living in rural areas versus the city influences frequency of mammograms and other breast cancer screening mechanisms.

Literature Review

After a researchable problem has been identified and stated or posed as a research question, a **literature review** is completed. This is a critical step, and one that can be quite time consuming. It is, however, essential, and serves several purposes, one of the primary functions being to further clarify the problem identified for study. The review also helps to specify the study problem and set limits for the target population. Another function of the literature review is to verify that this is an important clinical problem, which needs answering in order to improve patient care. Thus, the literature review should be used to determine (1) if other studies similar to the one to be conducted have been done previously, (2) if prior findings would be helpful in defining the proposed study, and (3) if it would be possible to replicate a prior study. Other purposes of the literature review include finding gaps in existing knowledge that can help fill out the current study design, selecting a research design and identifying instruments to measure the central aspects of the design, and helping the researcher interpret the findings from the study.

Literature searches may be conducted by reviewing references in a library, and by conducting computer searches, which is the most common method today. Computer searches may unveil vast amounts of data, so it will be necessary to limit the search to a reasonable time period. The search also may be limited by using primary sources as the major literature source. Primary resources are those written by investigators who conducted the studies. Secondary sources are those in which a writer describes or summarizes studies done by others. Review articles are an example of secondary literature sources. They can be valuable in guiding one to primary literature. They also may be helpful in reviewing theoretical or conceptual material that assists the researcher in establishing a design and methodology.

Research Design

The third major step in the research process is selecting the type of research that will answer the question and the concomitant **research design**. The design is the overall plan or blueprint for the study and should be described in detail, including the methods used for data collection and analysis. There are a number of research design strategies that may be employed to answer the research question that has been posed. The one that will help maximize the possibilities of achieving accurate information in the results should be used. The design for the study is dictated by the research problem/question, also known as a **hypothesis,** and assumptions of the theoretical framework.

It is helpful to begin the design section by writing an overview in which the theoretical or conceptual framework is stated if one is used. The overview is an extension of the research problem. It states how and where the study will be conducted and who is going to be studied and also how the study question(s) will be evaluated (measured). Different designs would be used for describing phenomena, exploring relationships, or searching for effects of **variables**. The study design may represent qualitative or quantitative research.

Types of Research Design: Quantitative and Qualitative

There are various types of nursing research, but the most common types are quantitative and qualitative. The following descriptions provide broad distinctions between these two main types of research.

Quantitative Research   **Quantitative research** is characterized by the collection of numerical values, under a controlled situation, that yield data, which can be generalized. Quantitative designs typically are descriptive, correlational, quasi-experimental, and experimental. **Descriptive research designs** often search for associations among certain variables. A **correlational research design** is aimed at examining linear relationships between two or more variables. The term **quasi-experimental** indicates a research design with an intervention, but one in which it is difficult to manipulate or control the setting, subjects, or variables as needed for a true experimental study. An **experimental research design** is used to determine the effects of an intervention, and it is highly controlled. Experimental research most often occurs in a laboratory setting, and is used to determine the effects of an intervention or of the manipulation of an independent variable. In contrast, a **nonexperimental research design,** which is not a specific type of design, consists of studies in which the researcher collects data without introducing an intervention. Quantitative research uses subjects that represent certain groups.

Research is not value free; that is, the background and biases of the researcher have an influence on study outcomes. In quantitative studies, the researcher strives to control as much bias as possible through design decisions. Understanding what biases can influence certain design decisions can be useful in the data analysis phase of the study.

In a quantitative study, the researcher moves from the beginning point of a study (posing a research question) to the end point (finding an answer). The researcher passes through five phases from the beginning to the end of the study: the conceptual phase, the design and planning phase, the empirical phase, the analytic phase, and the dissemination phase (Polit & Beck, 2008). The conceptual phase consists of thinking about the study and discussing the possibility of the study with colleagues. During this phase, the researcher calls on creativity and deductive reasoning to arrive at a researchable problem. During the second phase, the design and planning phase, the researcher develops methods to be used in conducting the study and to gather data. The third phase, the empirical phase, involves the collection of research data and the preparation of those data for analysis. During the fourth phase, the analytic phase, the data are analyzed and interpreted. Questions posed in the first phase of the study are answered. The fifth and final stage of the process is the dissemination phase. The results of the study are disseminated. This phase should include recommendations regarding how the results of the study could be incorporated into the practice of nursing. The sequential steps that occur during each phase of the research process are shown in Chart 8–4 (p. 126).

Qualitative Research   **Qualitative research** describes events as they occur naturally. Qualitative research involves the use of a systematic, subjective approach to describe life experiences and give them meaning (Burns & Grove, 2005). Thus, compared to quantitative research, qualitative research uses methods that are more subjective, a smaller sample size, and fewer research controls. Qualitative research studies generally use phenomenology,

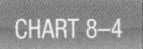

Steps in the Quantitative Research Process

CHART 8–4

PHASE 1: THE CONCEPTUAL PHASE

1. Identify a researchable problem.
2. Establish a purpose for the study.
3. Conduct a literature review.
4. Develop a theoretical/conceptual framework.
5. Formulate research objectives, questions, and hypotheses.

PHASE 2: THE DESIGN AND PLANNING PHASE

6. Select a research design.
7. Identify population to be studied.
8. Design the sampling plan.
9. Specify methods to measure the research variables.
10. Finalize and review the research plan.
11. Conduct a pilot study (if possible) and make revisions.

PHASE 3: THE EMPIRICAL PHASE

12. Collect the data.
13. Prepare the data for analysis.

PHASE 4: THE ANALYTIC PHASE

14. Analyze the data.
15. Interpret the results.

PHASE 5: THE DISSEMINATION PHASE

16. Communicate the findings.
17. Use the findings.

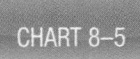

Activities Inherent in Qualitative Research

CHART 8–5

PHASE 1: CONCEPTUALIZING AND PLANNING THE STUDY

1. Clarify the topic area.
2. Proceed with a broad research question that may be delineated after the study is under way.
3. Conduct a literature review.
4. Identify a study site.

PHASE 2: CONDUCTING THE STUDY

5. Develop a sampling plan.[a]
6. Collect data.[a]
7. Analyze and interpret the data.[a]
8. Identify themes and categories.
9. Confirm that findings accurately reflect the feelings and experiences of participants.

PHASE 3: DISSEMINATING THE FINDINGS

10. Share findings with other nurses and health care specialists.

[a]These activites are cyclical and may be revised as the study progresses. Analysis and interpretation are ongoing and concurrent activites, used to guide the people to sample next and the questions or observations to make. Sampling also is guided by the data.

grounded theory, or ethnography to explore personal meaning within a given context.

Phenomenology describes the meaning of a lived experience through the perspective of the participant. **Grounded theory** refers to the idea that conclusion of a qualitative study should be grounded in the data, that is, based on direct and careful observations of everyday life within the group. **Ethnography** focuses on the culture of a group of people, with an effort to understand the world view of those under study.

This type of research is important when little is known about a topic because it can identify factors of influence. Often the discoveries of qualitative research generate hypotheses to be used in quantitative research. Many times a combination of the two methods yields a better understanding of human phenomena as seen every day in nursing. The design of the qualitative study is not specified in advance as it is in quantitative research; instead the design tends to evolve over time during the study. Decisions about the best ways to gather data, how to schedule and record data, how many subjects will be used in the study, and so on, are all decisions made during the study. This has been called an emergent design—one that becomes clear during the study as the researcher makes decisions about what she has learned (Colling, 2003). Because qualitative studies involve researchers directly and personally, and because the design emerges during the study, the biases of the researcher must be carefully examined before the study begins.

Qualitative studies do not follow the same linear progression of quantitative studies. The process tends to resemble a circle more than a line. The researcher is continually examining and interpreting data and making decisions about how to proceed based on what has already been discovered. There are, however, some major activities in which the researcher engages, and these too occur in phases similar to those described for quantitative research: phase 1, conceptualizing and planning the study; phase 2, conducting the study; and phase 3, disseminating the findings. These activities are discussed further in Chart 8–5.

Research Setting

The **setting** in which the study is conducted also will influence the type of research design selected. This is an important consideration when planning a study, because the setting and the dynamics within the setting can greatly influence the outcomes. Settings can be natural, in which no attempt is made to control elements of the setting; partially controlled, meaning that the setting has been modified in some way to strengthen the research design; or highly controlled, in which case a laboratory setting is usually used, such as when animal research is conducted. Many research studies use quasi-natural settings such as hospitals, clinics, or other care facilities.

Sample Selection Studies rarely gather information from an entire **population** of interest. A population is the entire aggregation of cases in which a researcher is interested, for example, all registered nurses with a master's degree in nursing who are currently practicing nursing in northern California. Instead, a sample is selected. **Sampling** is the process of selecting a portion of the population to represent the entire population. A **sample,** then, is a subset of the population.

A major concern when selecting a sample is how representative the sample is of the population; that is, how closely the sample mirrors the characteristics of the entire population of interest. A representative sample is one whose key characteristics closely approximate those of the population. Sampling strategies are classified as either probability sampling or nonprobability sampling (Polit & Beck, 2008). **Probability sampling** involves random selection when choosing the elements. **Nonprobability sampling** means that the elements are selected by nonrandom methods. Six common sampling strategies are explained in this chapter and are shown in Chart 8–6.

Convenience Sampling   With **convenience sampling,** the most available persons or units are selected for inclusion in the study. This also is referred to as accidental sampling (Polit & Beck, 2008). This type of sampling is easy and usually inexpensive. However, it is a weak strategy to use unless no other alternatives are possible or one is doing a **pilot study** (a small preliminary study prior to conducting a larger study). The researcher has no control over the characteristics of this sample, which may mean that the sample may be quite different from the population to which the study results are expected to be relevant. Thus, if this sampling strategy is used, it is wise to build in some limiting characteristics that the sample population must possess. Consider factors that might influence the outcome of the study, for example, socioeconomic status, gender, age, and cultural differences, and decide whether these should be included or excluded.

Quota Sampling   **Quota sampling** involves nonrandom selection of the participants in which the researcher prespecifies characteristics of the sample to increase its representation. Dividing a convenience sample into two subgroups in order to increase the potential for the sample to be representative of the total population may achieve this.

Purposive Sampling   **Purposive sampling** implies that certain people or elements are deliberately selected for the study. This type of sampling is used particularly in qualitative studies. Subjects, also called participants or informants in qualitative studies, are purposively selected for qualitative studies. They are individuals experiencing a common problem or sharing a common circumstance. Usually very few participants are needed since data collection is done through extensive interviews and observations.

Network Sampling   In **network sampling** participants refer other participants to the study. Polit and Beck (2008) also refers to network sampling as snowball sampling. This type of sampling works well for hard-to-find participant groups.

Simple Random Sampling   The **simple random sampling** strategy gives each person in a population an equal chance of being selected for the study. For example, if one were going to study a set of characteristics of breast cancer patients seen in a clinic during the past 2 years, the entire population who meet the study criteria would be listed. A sample from this population would then be randomly selected.

Random samples may be selected in a number of ways. One way is to put names or patient record numbers in a container and draw the names or numbers randomly. Another way is to flip a coin. If the toss is heads, the person is selected; if it is tails, the person is not selected. A more sophisticated method is to use a table of random numbers. Random number tables may be found in most research books. Random sampling greatly strengthens the design of the study by reducing potential selection biases.

There is a difference between random sample and random assignment that should be noted. As has been explained, a random sample means that every person within the category has an equal chance of being in the study. A **random assignment,** however, means that subjects are randomly assigned to treatment versus control groups. For example, if the category was "all cancer patients in California" and every patient in California had an equal chance of being in the study, it would be constitutive random sampling. However, in this example as in many cases this would be a too costly and time-consuming way in which to establish a random sample. Therefore, a random assignment of subjects may be done. For example, every other woman diagnosed with breast cancer in the clinic could be assigned to the treatment group for an educational intervention and every other woman assigned to the control group. Of course, random assignment would not be possible in some cases, for example, if the control group was in another location, or if ethical issues were involved.

Stratified Random Sampling   **Stratified random sampling** means that the population is first divided into two or more

| CHART 8–6 | **Examples of Sampling Strategies** |

Type of Sampling Strategy	Explanation
Convenience sampling	The researcher uses the most conveniently available people as study participants; participants are selected because they are in the right place at the right time.
Quota sampling	The researcher identifies population strata and determines how many participants are needed from each stratum; inclusion of participants is based on predetermined characteristics; a type of convenience sampling.
Purposive sampling	Based on the belief that researchers' knowledge about the population can be used to handpick sample members; also referred to as judgmental sampling.
Network sampling	Participants are referred by other participants; also called snowball sampling.
Simple random sampling	All members of a population are enumerated and then the sample is selected from the sampling frame using random procedures; the most basic type of probability sampling design.
Stratified random sampling	The population is first divided into two or more strata, and then the sample is randomly selected from the homogeneous subsets of the sample.

strata or subpopulations, for example, participants younger than 30 years of age, those between 30 and 45, and those 46 years or older. As with quota sampling the aim is to enhance representation. Polit and Beck (2008) note that stratified sampling designs subdivide the population into homogeneous subsets from which an appropriate number of elements are selected at random. Stratification often is based on such demographic attributes as age, gender, and income level.

Regardless of the sampling strategy used, it is essential to keep a careful record of the sampling decisions and identify how many people began the study, how many completed the study, and why subjects left the study before completing it. It also is important to keep a record of those who refused to participate in the study. These records are very helpful in identifying potential biases in the study results and a clear narrative of the sampling strategy, as well as to interpret the study findings more precisely.

Sample Size Determining sample size is a major consideration in developing a research study. If subjects are hard to get or expensive to enroll in the study, it is prudent to use as few as possible to still have a credible study. However, too few subjects could result in sampling error. Studies with too few subjects to reliably "determine" an effect have low "power," meaning that tests of **statistical significance** are less likely to indicate significance even if the study has a real effect. This is particularly true if the effect is small relative to the variability of the sample. For instance, suppose that the researcher is planning a chart review study to determine if men who had prostate surgery under the age of 65 had as much postsurgery incontinence as those who were over 65. Twenty charts of those under age 65 and 20 of those over 65 are selected. From the literature review, it is expected that the incidence in older men, those over 65, will be much higher than in the younger, under age 65 men. When a test for the significance is applied, the statistic is not significant. Thus, even though there was an effect, the number of subjects was too low to be statistically significant. It is likely that with so few subjects, the variability was too homogeneous and may not have reflected the true rate of incontinence in the entire population. However, the findings from this study could lead to an examination of other factors as to why the incidence of incontinence among these men is lower than what the literature would lead one to expect.

Computing a power analysis is the gold standard in determining sample size. A **power analysis** builds on the concept of an effect size, which expresses the strength of the relationships among research variables. It increases the probability that the results are true results. Conducting a power analysis requires some knowledge of statistics, and the learner is referred to a research or statistical text for further information on power analyses.

There are no simple formulas that can advise how large a sample is needed in a given quantitative study; however, Polit and Beck (2008) suggest using the largest sample possible. The larger the sample, the more representative of the population it is likely to be. Because practical constraints such as time, subject availability, and resources often limit sample size, many nursing studies are based on relatively small samples. In many cases a small sample can lead to misleading or inconclusive results. Thus, the learner is cautioned to consider the generalizablity of

the findings based on the sample size. If there is reason to believe that the population is relatively homogeneous, a small sample may be adequate. For clinical studies that deal with biophysiological processes in which variation is limited, a small sample may adequately represent the population. However, for most nursing studies it is safer to assume a fair degree of heterogeneity, unless there is evidence from prior research to the contrary. The process of drawing a sample may vary according to the type of research design employed. Polit and Beck (2008) have, however, developed a general outline of procedures that may be employed: (1) identify the population, (2) specify the eligibility criteria, (3) specify the sample plan, and (4) recruit the sample. These steps with limited explanation are shown in Chart 8–7.

Qualitative studies almost always use small, nonrandom samples. Whereas quantitative research is concerned with measuring attributes and therefore a representative sample is needed to ensure that the measurements accurately reflect and can be generalized to the population, the aim of qualitative studies is to discover meaning and to uncover multiple realities. Thus, generalizability is not a guideline. A critical first step in qualitative sampling is selecting settings with high potential for information richness. The qualitative researcher may begin with the following types of sampling questions in mind: Who would be an information-rich data source for my study? Who should I talk to or what should I observe first, so as to maximize my understanding of the phenomenon? There are no criteria or rules for sample size in qualitative research. Sample size is largely a function of the purpose of the inquiry, the quality of the informants, and the type of sampling strategy used. Samples are usually small, probability sampling is almost never used, and final sampling decisions usually take place in the field during data collection (Polit & Beck, 2008). The main consideration for sample size is

CHART 8–7	Sampling Steps for Quantitative Studies
Identify the population.	Identify an accessible population, and then decide how best to define the target population.
Specify the eligibility criteria.	The criteria should be as specific as possible with respect to characteristics that might exclude potential subjects (e.g., inability to read Spanish).
Specify the sampling plan.	Once the accessible population has been identified, decide the method for drawing the sample and how large it will be. If possible, perform a power analysis to determine the desired number of subjects. If probability sampling is an option for selecting a sample, it should be exercised.
Recruit the sample.	Recruit prospective study participants according to the plan and after needed institutional permissions have been obtained.

Source: Polit, D.G. & Beck, C.T. (2008) *Nursing research: generating and assessing evidence for nursing practice* (8th ed.). Philadelphia: Wolters Kluwer/Lippincott Williams & Wilkins. Pages 351 and 352. http://lww.com

data saturation, which refers to sampling to the point at which no new information is obtained and redundancy is achieved (Polit & Beck, 2008). Saturation depends on a number of factors. For example, the broader the scope of the research question, the more participants will likely be needed. Data quality also affects sample size. If participants are able to reflect on their experiences and communicate effectively, saturation can be achieved with a relatively small sample. If longitudinal data are collected, few participants may be needed, because each provides a greater amount of information.

In qualitative studies, the sampling plan is evaluated in terms of adequacy and appropriateness. Adequacy refers to the sufficiency and quality of data retrieved. An appropriate sample is one in which the participants can best supply the information according to the conceptual requirements of the study. There are similarities and differences among the various qualitative approaches with regard to sampling. The similarities include the following: Sample size is generally small, probability sampling is almost never used, and final sampling decisions usually take place in the field during data collection. The differences in sampling related to qualitative approaches and tradition are shown in Chart 8–8.

◼ Research Utilization and Evidence-Based Practice

Florence Nightingale probably was the first nursing researcher because she wrote down her observations of nursing care during the formative years of the nursing profession. In her writings, she documented her research approach. She observed what was going on, developed hypotheses, collected and analyzed the data, and then reached conclusions (Burns & Grove, 2003). Essentially, she used the research process to decrease the loss of lives from disease. Based on her skillful analyses of the factors affecting soldier mortality and morbidity during the Crimean War, she was successful in effecting some changes in nursing care and, more generally, in public health. Her landmark publication, *Notes on Nursing* (1859) described her early research interest in environmental factors that promote physical and emotional well-being, an interest of nurses that continues today, nearly 150 years later. For many years after Nightingale's work, there was little reference to research in the nursing literature. It was not until the early 1900s that nursing research began to emerge with a focus primarily on nursing education: characteristics of nurses, the supply and demand of nurses, and the amount of time required in performing certain nursing activities. A shift in focus emerged in the 1950s, accelerating the development of nursing research in the direction of clinical nursing problems. In the 1960s practice-oriented research emerged in the literature.

The advance of nursing research has continued through the last several decades, highlighted by several publications including *Advances in Nursing Science, Research in Nursing & Health, Nursing Research,* the *Western Journal of Nursing Research,* and the *Journal of Advanced Nursing.* These journals contribute to the dissemination and use of nursing research and the increased emphasis on improvement of patient care through research.

Research Utilization

The need for a systematic approach for using research to change practice was recognized in the early 1970s, leading to publication of the first model for research utilization by Stetler and Marram (Stetler, 1994). Subsequently, through the next several decades, much of the progress in using research in practice was based on that model and on work completed by the Western Interstate Commission for Higher Education's Regional Program for Nursing Research Development and the Conduct and Utilization of Research in Nursing (CURN) Project (Burns & Grove, 2005; Polit & Beck, 2008). The major emphasis of the CURN project was to increase the use of research results by direct-care nurses through facilitating organizational change. Since

MyNursingKit | National Institute of Nursing Research

CHART 8–8	**Sampling Differences Related to Qualitative Approaches and Tradition**
Qualitative Research Approach	**Sampling Guidelines**
Ethnography (focuses on the culture of a group of people, with an effort to understand the worldview of those under study)	Initially, researchers may contact as many members of the culture under study as possible, yet researchers rely heavily on a smaller number of key informants. Key informants are chosen purposively, as guided by the theoretical underpinnings of the study. Researchers (ethnographers) must decide on not only who to sample, but what to sample as well: observation of activities and events, examining records and artifacts, and exploring places.
Phenomenology (focuses on the lived experiences of humans)	Researchers tend to rely on a very small sample size, typically 10 or fewer. All participants must have experienced the phenomenon under study and must be able to articulate what it is like to have lived that experience. This is an example of criterion-referenced sampling.
Grounded theory (designed to develop theories and theoretical propositions grounded in real-world observations)	Theoretical sampling is done to create a sample size of 20 to 30 people. The goal is to select people who can best contribute to the evolving theory; thus, the first cases solicited may be purposive, convenient, or gained through networking. Sampling, data collection, data analysis, and theory construction occur simultaneously, so study participants are selected serially and contingently until saturation is reached (Polit & Beck, 2008).

that time there has been a growing emphasis on using research findings to improve nursing practice. This emphasis has grown in importance with the push in the United States to achieve cost-effective, high-quality patient care based on sound scientific evidence coupled with the global emphasis on quality. Though nursing has a long history of using research to make practice decisions, this process has not been well used, nor has it been well documented or labeled evidence-based practice.

The formation and adoption of the position of the National Institute of Nursing Research (NINR) in 1993 solidified the recognition of nursing research as a major component of nursing practice and moved nursing into the mainstream research path enjoyed by other health disciplines (Polit & Beck, 2008). At present, **research utilization** (RU) is perceived as the purposeful application of research findings to the clinical setting to improve patient care by using the findings from a disciplined study or set of studies in a practical, or real-world, application. Research utilization is important for the bedside nurse whose patients may benefit from implementation of research findings. Nurses in direct patient care also are the best resource for determining if a change of practice will be successful on their respective nursing unit and benefit the patients they serve. Because they are the individuals taking care of patients, nurses must use the newest research findings to keep their practice current, as well as to provide the highest standard of care to patients. Thus, research utilization is one method or source for achieving evidence-based practice.

Evidence-Based Practice

In some settings evidence-based practice and research utilization are used interchangeably; however, there are some distinct differences (Polit & Beck, 2008). **Evidence-based practice (EBP),** in contrast to research utilization, is a broader concept and relies on more than research to support and improve practice. It extends beyond research utilization and involves making clinical decisions on the basis of the best possible evidence. Though the best evidence usually comes from rigorous research, EBP also uses other sources of credible information. Some experts have differentiated between RU and EBP by explaining that RU is part of EBP and is a prescribed task of summarizing and using research findings to address a particular practice problem. In contrast, EBP is "the careful and practical use of current best evidence to guide health care decisions" (Omery & Williams, 1999, p. 51). As seen in both examples of differentiation cited earlier, EBP is broader than RU and is the interpretation chosen by most agencies adopting EBP as a practice model.

The definition of EBP posed by Omery and Williams (1999) asserts that current best evidence includes clinical practice guidelines that usually are developed nationally by expert researchers, clinicians, and theorists in their areas of excellence. EBP involves the interpretation and implementation of these clinical guidelines by health care providers based on their clinical expertise, the needs and views of the patient and family, and the resources of the health care system.

Although evidence-based practice has been emphasized in medicine for years, and expert researchers, clinicians, and theorists have developed numerous evidence-based guidelines for the prevention of illness and diagnosis and management of chronic and acute illnesses (Burns & Grove, 2005), it is in its initial stages of development in the nursing field. As the new recommended standard in health care and nursing, it is important to understand EBP and how it is used to de-emphasize ritual, isolated clinical experiences, ungrounded opinions, and tradition as a basis for nursing practice. Not only does it stress the use of research findings, it also stresses, as appropriate, the use of quality improvement data, other operational and evaluation data, the consensus of recognized experts, and affirmed experience to substantiate practice (Stetler, 1994). EBP calls for nurses to question their practice, looking to reliable evidence to improve and evaluate specific outcomes, rather than simply doing things as they have always done.

EBP is, in effect, a problem-solving approach to clinical decision making that incorporates a search for the best and latest evidence, clinical expertise and assessment, and a patient's preferences and values within a context of caring. This decision-making approach integrates clinical expertise with the best available evidence from systematic research in contrast to opinion-based health care decision making that is based primarily on values and resources. Factors that form a framework for decision making with this approach include understanding the patient's needs, concerns, and values; building on the clinical expertise or experience of the professional nurse; and seeking relevant clinical data and best practices (Malloch & Porter-O'Grady, 2006). Best practices are those proven processes that produce consistent, high-quality results.

Development of Evidence-Based Practice

Five steps are involved in developing evidence-based nursing practice: (1) defining the question, (2) collecting evidence, (3) making a critical appraisal, (4) integrating the evidence and patient factors to make and carry out the decision, and (5) evaluating the whole process (McKibbon, Eady, & Marks, 1999; Stuart, 2001). Also, five levels of evidence used in practice have been identified (Stuart, 2001). The lowest and least powerful evidence is provided by opinions of reviewers that are based on their experience and knowledge and constitute clinical practice guidelines. Somewhat stronger evidence is derived from opinions that come from well-known experts and respected authorities. Even more compelling evidence comes from the results of research studies. Three levels of evidence are derived from research. These are listed in order of increasing strength: nonrandomized controlled studies or cohort studies, small randomized controlled trials, and large randomized controlled trials. Large randomized controlled trials and meta-analyses of studies providing evidence in a specific area are considered the "gold standards" as they furnish the strongest and most powerful evidence for clinical practice.

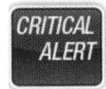

1. *Define the question.*
2. *Collect evidence.*
3. *Make a critical appraisal.*
4. *Carry out the decision by integrating evidence and patient factors.*
5. *Evaluate the whole process.*

As a problem-solving approach to clinical decision making, EBP incorporates a search for the best and latest evidence, clinical expertise and assessment, and patient preferences and values within a context of caring. The search for evidence in an attempt to answer a burning clinical question related to the effectiveness of a clinical intervention or treatment should begin with databases that contain systematic reviews of randomized controlled trials. Critical appraisal of these reviews for validity, strength of the findings, and applicability is a necessary step in evidence-based decision making and quality patient care.

Implementation of Evidence-Based Practice

Government mandates, consumer demands for accountability, professional efforts to improve quality, and organization requirements for fiscally responsible patient care have all helped develop EBP. Alarming reports of medical errors and the consequences of poor safety practices have inspired a social and professional mandate to improve care quality. In response, a number of health care institutions are seeking to implement evidence-based nursing practice, often including it in strategic plans—with many linking it to the national accrediting body, the Joint Commission. However, two questions remain: Are health care agencies ready to provide the resources that enable nurses to participate in this promising, best-practices model, and are nurses ready to meet the challenge?

Barriers to Evidence-Based Practice

Although a laudable and critical goal, EBP within the health care setting is not easily accomplished due to human and organizational barriers. Nurses often act on experiential knowledge, rather than research evidence, in their day-to-day clinical decision making. They tend to rely most frequently on information learned about the patient, personal experience, manuals, information learned in nursing school, fellow nurses, and nonresearch nursing journals and texts. Nurses' reluctance to use research is compounded by lack of time, access, and skills (Ciliska, Pinelli, DeCenso, & Cullum, 2001; Malloch & Porter-O'Grady, 2006). Although many agencies have incorporated computer usage into the normal work environment, many nurses still have difficulty using computers to conduct database searches. The principal obstacles to nurses' progress in using computers to assist them in retrieving research data are a hectic work environment and lack of time to practice database searching. Nurses' primary responsibility rightfully remains patient care, so taking time away from the bedside to perform literature searches or participate in research projects is not only challenging, but also may be discouraged by peers and managers—especially in a time of staffing shortage.

Other types of barriers to implementing EBP may be categorized as human and institutional barriers. Nurses are attached to historical practice, for example, waking patients during the night to weigh them on standing scales versus using the hospital's newly acquired bed scales because the nurses judge them to be inaccurate. Absence of other clinicians' buy-in constitutes a barrier as does lack of manager/director support. Lack of manager support may result in the unit manager going to the hospital education session to foster staff nurses' interest in research and keeping the staff on the unit. Institutional structure and processes (i.e., red tape) are also a big obstacle. For example, a staff nurse pursuing new, evidence-based protocol on the time of an antibiotic administration must first gain approval from numerous agency committees and administrative personnel. Lack of funding for research projects constitutes another barrier in many agencies, particularly in light of attempts to reduce health care costs.

Also to be considered is the role and support of the nurse researcher, if there is one, present in the agency. The nurse researcher position often becomes one of isolation in which the researcher lacks peer and mentor support. This isolation coupled with weak, or lack of, leadership support prohibits effective use of the nurse researcher and often leads to the nurse researcher leaving the agency; thereby, absenting a role model and coordinator for nursing research. Finally, the nurse's skills, or lack thereof, may lead to the collection of unreliable data. For instance, if the unit is participating in a study on skin integrity using the Braden scale, nurses collecting the data must know how to code pressure ulcers correctly using the scale. If they do not the data are compromised.

From the barriers identified, it is obvious that research-based practice initiatives need dedicated expertise, leadership support, and grassroots enthusiasm to thrive. In many situations this means changing an organization's culture of practice.

Strategies to Promote Evidence-Based Practice

Numerous strategies to overcome the barriers of using research and clinical evidence in practice are noted in the literature. Establishing a research committee is one suggestion. A research committee could explore and adopt a research critique tool and discuss issues of concern. Another approach is to survey nurses to determine their interest in research activities. After areas of interest are established, collaborative research groups can identify research topics for investigation. A group also could be formed to look at inconsistencies in practice and varied patient outcomes, to improve patient care, and to increase the research base of practice by defining a standard protocol. Information gained from such a group could be used to develop assessments and protocols.

Other mechanisms for increasing staff participation in EBP are by forming research clubs where research studies are reviewed systematically, much like a book club. Continuing education and in-service programs also are good ways to teach nurses about research utilization. Nursing forums that focus on the research process or on research results can give nurses an increased understanding of the research utilization process. Other methods that might be useful include independent self-study packets, a newsletter, a journal club, community research groups, informal research promotion, and, of course, changes in nursing education. The main key is to stimulate interest and enthusiasm in nurses so they will want to understand and use research. It is necessary to captivate their interest and engage them in seeing the excitement of changing practice through research.

In the future, EBP should increase. Many nursing students are being taught to use research findings as a basis for interventions. Thus, the emphasis is no longer limited to research conduction. It is well known that perceptions of priority and attitudes about research influence the use of research in practice.

MyNursingKit | Evidence-Based Practice Centers

If the nurse does not perceive research findings to be important or relevant to his particular work setting, he will not be as likely to read research or seek out research-related outcomes to improve practice. It is absolutely necessary that nurses know that the nursing administration and the health care organization endorse the concept of EBP. Only then is it probable that the perceptions of priority will change for the nurse.

Lack of access to information is perhaps the most difficult barrier to overcome. Internet access and current literature databases must be available. Personal digital assistants can provide quick reference, but are not yet practical for most nurses, although they are becoming more useful. An on-site library is helpful, but it is not the entire solution. Information must be available and easy to access at the point of care. This will only become available when nurses start to demand it and incorporate it into their practice. Research has shown that using best practices is cost effective and reduces both complications and lengths of stay. When nurses demand tools that support their own best practice, the tools will be provided.

Practicing nurses must strive to base their practices on research in order to improve patient outcomes. Nursing manuals, policies, procedures, and protocols should reflect current research-based knowledge. It is probable that, in the future, accrediting agencies will require that nursing care interventions be research based. It follows that research utilization should be actively promoted in all health care agencies. Examples of ways in which research and clinical evidence have been used to change practice are shown in Chart 8–9.

As of December 2007, there were 15 evidence-based practice centers (EPCs) across the United States and in Canada funded by the Evidence-based Practice Program of the Agency for Healthcare Research and Quality (AHRQ). These agencies are funded to review all relevant scientific literature on clinical, behavioral, organizational, and financing topics to produce evidence reports and technology assessments. The EPCs also conduct research on methodologies to determine the effectiveness of their implementation, to provide technical assistance in translating the reports and assessments into quality improvement tools, and to help inform coverage policies.

The 15 centers as of December 2007 are listed here:

- Blue Cross and Blue Shield Association, Technology Evaluation Center (TEC), Chicago, Illinois
- Duke University, Durham, North Carolina
- ECRI Institute, Plymouth Meeting, Pennsylvania
- Johns Hopkins University, Baltimore, Maryland
- McMaster University, Hamilton, Ontario, Canada
- Minnesota Evidence-based Practice Center, Minneapolis
- Oregon Health & Science University, Portland
- RTI International University of North Carolina at Chapel Hill
- Southern California Evidence-based Practice Center–RAND, Santa Monica
- Stanford University, Stanford, and University of California, San Francisco
- Tufts-New England Medical Center, Boston, Massachusetts
- University of Alberta
- University of Connecticut, Farmington, CT
- University of Ottawa
- Vanderbilt University, Nashville, Tennessee

Evidence-based report topics and disease category listings may be obtained via the Internet by going to www.ahrq.gov/clinic/epcindex.htm. To date, more than 80 reports have been released (AHRQ, 2007).

■ Research and Ethics in Health Care

The practice of ethics guides health care professionals when they are making decisions concerning life and death situations. The term *ethics* refers to the goodness and badness of human actions or to principles of what is right and wrong in conduct. The intent of ethics is to develop methods for clarifying confusing questions even if final solutions remain elusive. Ethics deals with concerns for good behavior among people and struggles to resolve ethical differences among members of society. The ethical codes and oaths of professionals do not always help, because personal feelings are often involved in each situation. Nurses and physicians often are put in a situation of conflict. Such a position may occur when participating in nursing research. A full discussion of ethical principles that guide nursing practice is given in Chapter 4 .

At every stage of the research process, there are ethical considerations for nurse researchers to consider. This consideration may start with the selection of a research problem; from an ethical viewpoint, should the problem be studied or not? For example, should subjects with mental impairments who may not be able to give informed and voluntary consent be studied? As more and more nurses participate in research activities, it is imperative for the profession to operate from a sound ethical knowledge base. Because research is central to the evolution of nursing care, the avoidance of conducting nursing research might be considered unethical. Similarly, the failure to engage in

---

CHART 8–9	**Examples of Ways in Which Research and Clinical Evidence Have Changed Practice**

- Development of a heart failure center (Crowther, 2003)
- Use of saline versus heparin to maintain patency of peripheral intravenous access (DeBourgh, 2001)
- Use of Trendelenburg position for hypotension in emergencies. (DeBourgh, 2001)
- Frequency of ventilator circuit tubing change (DeBourgh, 2001)
- Use of normal saline when suctioning endotracheal tubes (DeBourgh, 2001)
- Music as an intervention in hospitals (2001)
- Maintaining oral hygiene in older people (2001)
- Assessing and managing pain in older adults (Ardery, Herr, Titler, Sorofman, & Schmittet, 2003)
- Fall risk assessment, prevention, and management (Poe, Cvach, Gartrell, Radzik, & Joy, 2005)

evidence-based practice—in other words, to base practice decisions solely on tradition or intuition rather than on empirical finding—denies patients access to the best available care and, thus, also might be considered unethical.

Nurses are involved in a variety of research efforts, including research specific to nursing, multidisciplinary research, and research of other disciplines on patients receiving nursing care. In all of these situations, nurses are expected to engage in ethical research behavior. With this expectation arises the question of how nurse researchers can make ethical decisions. What are the characteristics of ethical research? What are the rights of those participating in the study, and how does the nurse researcher guard those rights? An exploration of ethical decision making addresses these questions.

Ethical Frameworks

Two ethical frameworks have been proposed in Western society to assess the ethical acceptability of a research project. These are the utilitarian and the deontological perspectives (Gillis & Jackson, 2002). Each of these perspectives articulates ethical norms that transcend disciplinary boundaries.

Utilitarian Perspective

The utilitarian perspective suggests that ethical judgments about a research project should be made by evaluating its consequences for the participants, for society, and for the academic discipline. This view entails the belief that the good of a research project is defined by the consequences of the results. The well-known philosopher John Stewart Mill proposed that actions should be taken to promote the greatest good for the greatest number. The utilitarian perspective considers that the end justifies the means. Based on this perspective, a research project is judged ethical if it produces the greatest good for the greatest number; the problem is in determining what is good. Small-scale studies with little ability for generalization of findings to the larger society may be judged to be unethical from a utilitarian perspective. For example, research into liver transplantation that has the potential to influence quality of life for a small number of participants who receive this costly medical intervention may not be considered ethical unless it can be shown that the results will benefit a large number of people in the future. In contrast, research into the prevention of liver disease through lifestyle change is justifiable from a utilitarian perspective because lifestyle change is more likely to benefit many more people than will costly surgical procedures available to only a few. When discussing the utilitarian perspective, it is necessary to recognize that each researcher may have a different definition of what is good for the majority.

Deontological Perspective

The deontological approach to research ethics proposes absolute moral imperatives that must never be violated. In taking the deontological view, one might propose absolutes such as never using deception, never making participants' identity known, and never putting any pressure on respondents to participate in a study. Rather than assessing the consequences of a given research procedure, the deontological approach may propose, in its most extreme form, that deception in experiments is never justified, regardless of what the positive contributions to one's knowledge might be. Immanuel Kant, a well-known deontologist, supported the categorical imperative; that is, basic laws apply without exception. For example, telling an untruth is always wrong, regardless of the consequences, or the welfare of the patient must always be placed above the integrity of the research if a conflict exists. Some deontologists take a more flexible approach, accepting more than one basic law and considering context and circumstances in determining priority. Some argue that types of harm can be distinguished: harm to a participant's interest, wrongdoing, and a moral harm. Still others argue that although harms can be compensated for, wrongs cannot be, the argument being that if doing a wrong is essential to conducting a research project, then the project should be banned (Holden, 1979).

Codes and Guidelines for Ethical Decision Making

Throughout its history, the field of nursing has been sensitive to the ethical dimension of doing nursing research. Thus, many professional organizations have developed codes of ethics to guide nurses in their research endeavors. These codes articulate the level of ethical behavior expected of nurse researchers and provide a standard for nurses working through ethical conflicts that may arise in research. They also provide guidance on ethical decision making in clinical practice, education, and administration.

During the past four decades, largely in response to human rights violations, various codes of ethics have been developed. One of the first internationally recognized efforts to establish ethical standards is referred to as the Nuremberg code, which was developed after the Nazi atrocities of World War II were made public in the Nuremberg trials. Several other international codes of ethics have been developed since then, the most notable being the Declaration of Helsinki. This declaration was adopted in 1964 by the World Medical Association and was most recently revised in 2000. Most disciplines have established their own code of ethics, as has nursing.

The American Nurses Association's Code of Ethics was adopted in 1985, and is shown in Chapter 1 ⬡. The ANA also put forth a document in 1995 entitled *Ethical Guidelines in the Conduct, Dissemination, and Implementation of Nursing Research.* This document presents nine ethical principles used to guide nursing research. These nine principles are shown in Chart 8–10 (p. 134).

In 1978, an important code of ethics was adopted in the United States that was created by the National Commission for the Protection of Human Subjects of Biomedical and Behavioral Research (1978). The commission issued a report that served as the basis for regulations affecting research sponsored by the federal government. The report, sometimes referred to as the Belmont report, also served as a model for many of the guidelines adopted by specific disciplines. The Belmont report articulated three primary ethical principles on which standards of ethical conduct in research are based: respect for persons, beneficence, and justice. Information about various codes of ethics and ethical requirements for government-sponsored research can be found in the Web links for this chapter on MyNursingkit.

CHART 8–10   Ethical Principles in Nursing Research

The Investigator . . .

1. Respects autonomous research participants' capacity to consent to participate in research and to determine the degree and duration of that participation without negative consequences.

2. Prevents harm, minimizes harm, and/or promotes good to all research participants, including vulnerable groups and others affected by the research.

3. Respects the personhood of research participants, their families, and significant others, valuing their diversity.

4. Ensures that the benefits and burdens of research are equitably distributed in the selection of research participants.

5. Protects the privacy of research participants to the maximum degree possible.

6. Ensures the ethical integrity of the research process by use of appropriate checks and balances throughout the conduct, dissemination, and implementation of the research.

7. Reports suspected, alleged, or known incidents of scientific misconduct in research to appropriate institutional officials for investigation.

8. Maintains competency in the subject matter and methodologies of his or her research, as well as in other professional and societal issues that affect nursing research and the public good.

9. Involved in animal research maximizes the benefits of the research with the least possible harm or suffering to the animals.

Source: From Silva, M.C. (1995). *Ethical guidelines in the conduct, dissemination, and implementation of nursing research (pp. v-vi.)* Washington, DC. American Nurses' Association. Printed in Polit & Beck, (2004). *Nursing research: Principles and methods (7th ed.).* Philadelphia: Lippincott Williams & Wilkins. http://lww.com

Principles of Ethical Research

At times ethical theories such as deontology or utilitarianism may not be adequate to guide nurses in ethical decision making. In these situations, ethical principles rather than theories may prove more helpful. The three principles from the Belmont report just discussed and elaborated on next are useful for ethical decision making.

Respect for Persons

Inherent in the principle of respect for persons are the concepts of autonomy, dignity, uniqueness, freedom, and choice. This principle forms the foundation of the participants' rights to informed consent, privacy, and confidentiality, and involves respecting people's autonomy or right to choose freely for themselves. Participants have choices based on their own values and beliefs and to be free from undue pressure or coercion by others. They must be made fully aware of any risks and benefits of the study. This principle requires that the participants' confidentiality and anonymity be safeguarded.

Beneficence

Two concepts are inherent in the principle of beneficence: nonmalfeasance, or the ability to not inflict physical or emotional harm, and beneficence, or the duty to promote or do good. To apply the concepts of beneficence, researchers must provide a standard of care. Standards of care usually are established by society and by professional role expectations. Nurses' duties to act as patient advocates require that nurses intervene if a research intervention produces more harm than benefit to a patient.

It is the researcher's responsibility to minimize risks and maximize benefits to participants; not doing so would contravene the ethical principle of beneficence. When a nurse researcher is a care provider, the potential for conflict between the duty to care and the duty to advance knowledge may be imminent. Some refer to this as the research imperative, advancement of knowledge versus the duty to care (Gillis & Jackson, 2002). Sometimes it is difficult to determine at what point the therapeutic imperative is being compromised by the research imperative. When doubt is evident, the therapeutic imperative must take precedence over the research imperative for the nurse as caregiver. This is due to the fact that the nurse must always act as the patient's advocate.

Justice

The principle of justice requires that people be treated fairly. The protection of participants from incompetence and the right to receive research treatments are expectations of the justice principle. Justice is an important principle to follow in the selection of subjects for research studies. The risks and benefits of a study should be fairly distributed among participants based on the subjects' efforts, needs, and rights. If possible, random selection of participants avoids potential sources of bias and unfairness in sample selection.

Nurses involved in any aspect of the process have a responsibility to see that research complies with the principles of respect for persons, beneficence, and justice. This is true for nurses' own research as well as for research conducted by others that affects their patients.

Methods of Protecting Human Subjects

Two methods of protecting human subjects have been developed during the past three decades. These include obtaining informed consent and the review of research proposals by an ethics committee or an institutional review board.

Informed Consent

Informed consent is based on the principle of respect for persons and incorporates the ethical concept of autonomy or the client's right to self-determination. The key elements of informed consent include disclosure of sufficient and appropriate information, understanding of information, and voluntary participation. Comprehension of information is essential to informed consent. The researcher must determine that the participants understand the information provided to them. It is incumbent on the researcher to make sure that the participants understand the risks involved as well as the benefits. They also must be fully informed about the research protocol so that they can make informed choices. Voluntary participation implies that participants agree to be part of a study of their own free will without coercion of any kind.

In obtaining informed consent, always:

- *Provide participants adequate information about the research.*
- *Make sure participants are capable of comprehending information.*
- *Make sure participants have the power of free choice.*
- *Document the informed consent.*

In qualitative investigations, the idea of process consent is suggested rather than a traditional consent. In process consent, the researcher renegotiates the consent with participants as unforeseen circumstances arise. This allows the participants to be part of the decision making as the study unfolds, and is in contrast to traditional consent, which is signed at the beginning of a study and not reconsidered.

Institutional Review Boards

Research involving humans should be submitted for approval to an ethics committee, commonly referred to as an institutional review board (IRB) or an ethics review committee. The purpose of the review is to ensure that ethical principles are appropriately applied to research involving human subjects. Most institutions, hospitals, governmental agencies, and universities in which research involving human subjects is carried out require specific information to make informed and responsible decisions regarding the ethical acceptability of a proposal. Chart 8–11 describes the type of information that should be included in a submission to an IRB (Gillis & Jackson, 2002). Additional information on IRBs is included in agency policy and also may be found in research texts.

Rules for Conducting Ethical Research

There are ethical rules that serve as guidelines for conducting research. They are organized around two themes: (1) nurse researchers' ethical responsibility to participants and (2) nurse researchers' responsibility to the discipline of nursing and society (Gillis & Jackson, 2002). These rules include the following, and are summarized in Chart 8–12 (p. 136):

1. Protect the confidentiality of participants.
2. Do not place pressure on participants.
3. Make the subjects' participation painless and free from discomfort and harm.

4. Identify sponsors.
5. Disclose the basis on which participants have been selected.
6. Place no hidden identification codes on questionnaires.
7. Honor promises to provide participants with research reports.
8. Informed consent is a key concern.
9. Debrief subjects.

Rules for Socially Responsible Nursing Research

Not only do nurses have ethical responsibilities to the participants but also to society at large and the nursing discipline in particular. Research-minded practitioners, educators, administrators, nursing students, and other health care professionals expect nurse researchers to do ethical research. The end result of nursing studies is to shape nurses' practice and promote excellence in nursing care. To this end, researchers should conduct unbiased studies and report results in trustworthy manners; seven rules guide this process. Researchers should:

1. Distinguish between science and advocacy.
2. Not hunt through data looking for pleasing findings.
3. Be aware of potential sources of bias.
4. Represent research literature fairly.
5. Do the best research possible.
6. Acknowledge all sources.
7. Seek advice on ethical issues.

These rules are shown and explained in Chart 8–13 (p. 136).

Privacy and the Health Insurance Portability and Accountability Act

One of the rules of conducting ethical research is that of maintaining the privacy and confidentiality of participants. Privacy is the right an individual has to determine the time, extent, and general circumstances under which personal information will be shared with or withheld from others (Burns & Grove, 2005). Such information consists of one's attitudes, beliefs, behaviors, opinions, and records. The research subject's privacy is protected if the subject is informed and consents to participate in a study and voluntarily shares private information with the researcher. An invasion of privacy occurs when private information is shared without an individual's knowledge or against her will. An invasion of privacy occurs most frequently during the data collection phase of the research process. This may occur when invasive questions are asked during an interview, an interview is taped without the subject's consent, or hidden cameras or mirrors are used to observe the subjects.

The Privacy Act of 1974 was enacted to safeguard subjects' privacy rights, and has led to scrutiny of data collection methods by an IRB or committee formed to review all research proposals. Improvements in technology also were a precipitating factor for the Privacy Act as it became so easy to collect and transmit data without the knowledge or control of the subject. With the advent of the Internet and increased access to information on individuals, including health information, the federal

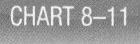

CHART 8–11 **Information to Be Included in Submission to an IRB**

- The purpose of the study and its significance to health research
- The study design and methodology
- Potential research participants and a description of the selection process
- Risk and benefits to the participants
- Steps to ensure participant choice, confidentiality, and anonymity protection
- Areas of potential conflict of interest

Source: From Gillis, A., & Jackson, W. (2002). *Research for nurses: Methods and interpretation.* Philadelphia: F. A. Davis, page 336.

CHART 8-12	**Rules for Conducting Ethical Research**

Rule	Interpretation
Protect the confidentiality of participants.	Confidentiality is to be treated as a sacred trust, based on the ethical principle of respect for persons. If researchers need to identify individuals' names with particular questionnaires, then number codes, rather than names, should be used. If data are released to other researchers, steps should be taken to mask the individual identities of participants.
Do not put pressure on participants.	No pressure should be put on participants to cooperate in the study. Respondents must feel free to refuse participation, to withdraw at any time, or to refuse to answer any particular question. This rule is based on the principle of respect for persons.
Make the subjects' participation painless and free from discomfort.	Researchers must not expose participants to needlessly long experimental trials or questionnaires or ask questions that pry unnecessarily into personal matters; only relevant information should be collected. Maintaining the comfort, and safety, and self-esteem of the participants should be a central concern of researchers. This is based on the principle of beneficence, which requires that one should do good and, above all, do no harm.
Identify sponsors.	Participants must be informed about who is doing the study.
Disclose the basis on which participants have been selected.	Participants have the right to know how they were selected for participation in a study. Respondents need to know if the selection was made by means of a probability sampling procedure or if it was based on special characteristics related to the research problem or phenomenon under investigation (e.g., age, health status, medical diagnosis). Selection of participants is based on the ethical principle of justice.
Place no hidden identification codes on questionnaires.	Do not place hidden identification codes on questionnaires to aid in the identification of those who have or have not returned questionnaires. If individuals are to be identified, this information should be placed directly on the questionnaire and discussed in a cover letter. The identification corresponding to participant names should be kept in a secure area to protect the identity of participants. Only the researcher should have access to this information.
Honor promises to provide participants with research reports.	When a promise to provide participants a copy of the research report is made, this promise should be fulfilled. This reinforces the idea of a reciprocal contract between the researcher and the participant.
Informed consent is a key concern.	In dealing with competent adults, participation should be based on informed consent; potential participants must be informed about the nature of the study, what kinds of issues will be explored, how participants were selected, what the risk and benefits to the participants are, and who is sponsoring the research. Prospective participants also should be informed about confidentiality and anonymity, and they should feel free to withdraw from the study at any time without prejudice if they wish to do so. Any time selective nondisclosure of information or deception is used in a research study, the researcher must question how acceptable it is to do so. With deception, the risks to the participants should be minimal and outweighed by the benefits.
Debrief subjects.	When experiments or field studies involve deception, subjects should have the study explained to them after the session. They should be told what deception was used and why it was necessary.

CHART 8-13	**Rules for Socially Responsible Nursing Research**

Rules	Interpretation
Researchers should distinguish between science and advocacy.	Nurses should distinguish between citizen-advocate roles and researcher roles. As a citizen-advocate, it is legitimate to comment on the evidence of others and to produce evidence that is appropriate to the issue under dispute. However, that information is being presented from the perspective of a citizen-advocate, not from that of an expert nurse scientist (Gillis & Jackson, 2002).
Do not hunt through data looking for pleasing findings.	The surest way to be guilty of misrepresentation is to search for support of one's views. To do so would be both bad science and unethical behavior.
Be aware of potential sources of bias.	Researchers have an ethical responsibility to avoid bias as much as possible.
Represent research literature fairly.	Portray the body of literature accurately. Reporting findings selectively is not acceptable.
Do the best research possible.	Always seek to do the best research possible; do research with care; strive to be competent and impartial, and report results objectively.
Acknowledge all sources.	Acknowledge people who have played a role in the research and acknowledge all literature sources that have directly influenced the study; site each literature source used.
Seek advice on ethical issues.	If ethical issues arise, seek the advice of appropriate professional bodies or institutions involved in the project.

government enacted the Health Insurance Portability and Accountability Act (HIPAA) of 1996 (Olsen, 2003). Under federal law, HIPAA's privacy requirements are intended to guarantee individuals new rights and protections against the misuse or unauthorized disclosure of their health records. Though the law does not target research, it does affect the manner in which research is conducted.

The HIPAA privacy regulations constitute an extensive reform of the way health care information is handled. Disclosures of health information for research are allowed but regulated beyond the common-rule regulations currently monitored by IRBs. HIPAA is a concern for anyone conducting or reviewing nursing research. There are three points at which the HIPAA privacy regulations will impact nursing research: (1) assessing data from a covered entity (e.g., reviewing medical records of subjects), (2) creating data (e.g., an intervention study), and (3) disclosing data (e.g., with a colleague from another institution).

- *Accessing data:* It is the covered organization's obligation not to disclose information improperly when a researcher seeks data that includes private health information. A covered organization is one that "transmits information in an electronic form, and includes health plans, health care clearing houses, and health care agencies. All covered entities are required to comply with the Privacy Rule (Connor, Smaldone, Bratts, & Stone, 2003). Researchers will be expected to work closely with clinical agencies used as research sites to ensure that both sides meet HIPAA obligations. Individually identifiable health information (IIHI) data may be accessed for research under specific conditions; the pertinent access terms and explanations for IIHI are presented in Chart 8–14.

- *Creating data:* Researchers also may be creating IIHI data. If the researcher is part of a covered entity, any protected health information obtained by any means is covered by HIPAA, and the researcher and his or her institution are bound by HIPAA regulations. When obtaining IIHI directly from the subject, the subject must authorize the use of the information. Essential elements of disclosure must be included in the authorization: who will be receiving the information, what further disclosures the researcher anticipates, and what information will be disclosed to the researcher.

- *Disclosing data:* Nurse researchers should be aware that sharing data with colleagues and students might constitute disclosures of IIHI, according to HIPAA regulations. The researcher is the holder of the IIHI and can disclose it only under appropriate conditions. When the researcher creates and holds IIHI, he must track any further disclosures made through waiver of authorization or in a review preparatory for research for 6 years and be prepared to report these to the former patient (Olsen, 2003).

 *HIPAA governs privacy in accessing data, creating data, and disclosing data.*

One may conclude that privacy of health information is widely accepted as an essential element of the researcher's obligation to respect the autonomy of subjects. To do this effectively, the nurse must understand HIPAA and its privacy provisions. They are of critical importance for current investigations as well as future research endeavors. The primary focus of HIPAA modifications in research protocols is in the areas of

---

CHART 8–14 **Disclosure Rules for Individually Identifiable Health Information for Research Purposes**

Condition of Information Disclosure	Explanation
Information pertains only to deceased persons	Information gathered about living persons from the records of the deceased, e.g., relatives, must be obtained in accordance with HIPAA.
Review preparatory to research	Allows researchers to assess the feasibility of projects by examining the information recorded in patients' records or the interventions currently in place without authorization from the potential subject or the permission of an IRB or privacy board. However, the information cannot be removed from the covered entity. The holder of the IIHI must determine how to monitor researchers' activity in this area.
Deidentification	All information that acts as an identifier as defined in the HIPAA regulations has been removed. Such information can be shared freely because it is no longer IIHI. This would include identifiers such as name, address, and date of birth. HIPAA regulations also state that IIHI can be deidentified if a person with appropriate credentials in statistics determines that the risk is very small that the information could be used to identify an individual.
Authorization	An organization, or covered agency, may disclose IIHI if the researcher presents an authorization signed by the patient. The authorization may be signed as part of the informed consent or as a separate document. Researchers also may be granted access to IIHI if an IRB or privacy board has waived the need for authorization. There are special conditions under which this waiver may be granted, and the IRB or privacy board should be contacted for this information.
Recruitment	Researchers also need to access data from the organization, or covered entity for recruitment. Under the HIPAA regulations it is inappropriate for a covered entity to disclose potential subjects for a researcher to contact. There are two alternatives. Personnel at the covered entity can make potential subjects aware of the protocol and then obtain an authorization to disclose the potential subject to the researcher, or the researcher can obtain a partial waiver of authorization from the IRB.

Source: U.S. Department of Health and Human Services, Office for Civil Rights. (2003). Standards for privacy of individually identifiable health information. *Code of Federal Regulations,* Title 45, Parts 160 & 164. Retrieved June 13, 2007 from http://www.hhs.gov/ocr/hipaa/privruletxt.txt

informed consent. Additional information on HIPAA can be obtained from the HIPAA website. HIPAA also is discussed at length in Chapter 4 ⊕.

Informatics

As has been noted, evidence-based practice is characterized by using the best available information when making clinical decisions, in lieu of intuition and unmethodical clinical experience. It is the new recommended standard in health care. Many agree that EBP has the potential to improve patient care and outcomes, yet, in order to be effective, information must be available and accessible, and practitioners must be skilled at using resources such as computers. Government mandates, consumer demands for accountability, professional efforts to improve quality, and organizational requirements for fiscally responsible patient care have all helped develop evidence-based practice. However, the questions, as previously posed, remain: "Are health care facilities ready to provide the resources that will enable nurses to participate in this promising, best-practices model? And, if so, are nurses ready to meet the challenge?" This is best answered by the acknowledgment that both health care facilities and health care providers must become skilled in informatics in order to effectively participate in evidence-based practice.

Informatics can be interpreted as a combination of computer science, information science, and health care science designed to assist in the management and delivery of health care. It is the knowledge necessary to use the computer and programs effectively to retrieve, input, and use knowledge to assist in decision making. In the case of nursing research, informatics is used to retrieve information to support an identified problem, conduct a literature review, input data for analysis, complete statistical analyses, and share findings with colleagues. The computer and specific research-oriented programs may be used to analyze both quantitative and qualitative data. Research texts typically identify computer programs that may be used for data analysis

(Burns & Grove, 2005; Gillis & Jackson, 2002; Polit & Beck, 2008). Every nurse is expected to have fundamental information management and computer literacy skills, although it is recognized that the level of skill needed may vary among nurse researchers. These levels have been defined by Staggers, Gassert, and Curran (2002) and are shown in Chart 8–15.

1. *All nurses are expected to have fundamental information management and computer literacy skills.*
2. *All nurses must know how to use the computer to retrieve data, input data, and use knowledge for decision making.*

The Research Critique

Applying research findings to practice is now recognized as essential to developing scientifically based nursing practice. A key step in this process is the ability of nurses to read nursing research studies and determine the usefulness of their findings for practice. To determine if the research is useful and applicable, the nurse must evaluate the completed research, identifying areas of adequacy and inadequacy, virtues as well as faults. This **research critique** is an intellectual process of a careful, complete examination of a study to judge its strengths, weakness, logical links, meaning, and significance. The critique involves a high level of critical thinking and analysis of each component of the study. A quality study focuses on a significant problem, demonstrates sound methodology, produces credible findings, and is easily replicated by other researchers. A critique appraisal involves judging whether or not a research study meets these quality standards and is described clearly and comprehensively enough to decide if the findings and implications are logical and believable and should be considered seriously in practice.

Generally research is critiqued to broaden understanding, summarize knowledge for use in practice, and provide a base for the conduct of a study (Polit & Beck, 2008). Research critiques are performed by nursing students, nursing instructors, practicing nurses, and nurse researchers. Each may have a different in-

CHART 8–15	Definitions for Levels of Nurses' Computer Competency Skills

Level	Competency
Level 1: Beginning nurses	Have fundamental information management and computer technology skills and use existing information systems and available information to manage their practice.
Level 2: Experienced nurses	Have proficiency in their domain of interest (e.g., public health, acute care, education, administration). These nurses are highly skilled in using information management and computer technology skills to support their major area of practice. Experienced nurses use current information systems, but collaborate with information specialists to suggest system improvements.
Level 3: Informatics specialists	Informatics specialists usually are registered nurses prepared at least at the baccalaureate level who possess additional knowledge and skills specific to information management and computer technology. They focus on information needs for the practice of nursing, which includes education, administration, research, and clinical practice. Informatics specialists' practices are built on the integration and application of information science, computer science, and nursing science. In their practice, informatics specialists use the tools of critical thinking, data management skills, and computer skills.
Level 4: Informatics innovators	Informatics innovators are educationally prepared to conduct informatics research and to generate informatics theory. These nurses lead the advancement of informatics practice and research.

Source: From Staggers, N., Gassert, C. A., & Curran, C. (2002). A delphi study to determine informatics competencies for nurse levels of practice. *Nursing Research, 51*(6), 383–390. http://lww.com

tent and focus; however, they all basically follow a similar process. For example, in nursing education, a critique often is seen as the first step in learning the research process. By conducting research critiques, students develop critical thinking skills, strengthen their knowledge base, and increase their use of research findings in practice. Critiques of studies by practicing nurses are essential for the implementation of evidence-based practice. These critiques tend to focus on the scientific merit of the study and on its implications for nursing practice. Educators conduct research critiques to expand their knowledge base and improve the educational process, and researchers conduct critiques to plan and implement a study. This section focuses on the general guidelines that can be used by any group to conduct a research critique.

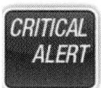 • *Applying research findings to practice is essential.*
• *Nurses must know how to read research studies and determine the usefulness of findings for practice.*

Elements of a Research Critique

Specific elements must be considered when critiquing a research study. The results of both quantitative and qualitative studies are used to improve nursing practice, so critique methods for both are discussed.

Quantitative Research Critique

Gillis and Jackson (2002) suggest the following criteria for evaluating quantitative research studies:

1. Relevant and clearly articulated statement of purpose
2. Consistency between explicitly stated purpose and problem statement or question or hypothesis
3. Comprehensive literature review identifies gaps in the research area and logically leads to the research questions under study
4. Theoretical framework provides a rationale for the study
5. Congruent match between the purpose, design, and method
6. Appropriate sample and sample selection procedures
7. Statistical procedures appropriate to the type of data collected and research questions posed
8. Adequate reliability and validity to accept findings and generalize to appropriate populations
9. Significance of study for nursing is apparent. (p. 614)

The actual review of a quantitative study uses the criteria just set forth and divides the critique into four stages of review (Gillis & Jackson, 2002; Polit & Beck, 2008):

• Stage 1 refers to a review of the purpose, problem statement, and congruency with design and methodology. The reviewer must gain a clear understanding of the meaning of the purpose and problem statement of a study, and determine if the research design and methodology are consistent with the study purpose.

• Stage 2 focuses on the conduct of the research. This refers to studying the manner in which the research was conducted

and includes determining if the methodology was applied correctly.

• Stage 3 refers to studying the findings of the research and assessing if the outcomes and conclusions are believable and supported by the findings. The focus is on the outcomes of the study.

• Stage 4 summarizes the overall quality of the study, identifying the strengths and limitations of the study, and evaluating the contributions of the study to nursing. At this point the reviewer also looks for suggestions for improving the work of the researcher.

Chart 8–16 summarizes the criteria used in each of the stages of appraising quantitative research reports. Chart 8–17 (p. 140) shows key questions that can be asked by the reviewer when critiquing quantitative designs.

Qualitative Research Critique

Critical evaluation of qualitative studies uses different standards than those of quantitative due to the nature of the study. Qualitative studies emerge from the naturalistic-inductive paradigm and as such are based on a different set of assumptions and a different worldview, and have a different purpose than quantitative studies. Qualitative research hopes to promote understanding of phenomena. A scholarly critique of qualitative studies includes a balanced evaluation of a study's strengths and weaknesses. Five

CHART 8–16	**Stages of the Critiquing Process and Components of a Quantitative Research Project**
Stage of Critique Process	**Review Components**
Stage 1: Purpose, problem statement, and congruency with design and methodology	• Study purpose • Problem statement • Theoretical framework • Literature review • Hypothesis or research question • Research design • Sampling procedures • Data collection procedures • Instruments • Data analysis
Stage 2: Conduct of the research	• Protection of participants' rights • Ethics of research • Consistency and integrity of procedures
Stage 3: Outcomes of the research process	• Statistical significance of results • Clinical significance of results • Discussion of findings • Implications for practice, education, and research
Stage 4: Overall quality of study	• Conclusions

Source: From Gillis, A., & Jackson, W. (2002). *Research for nurses: Methods and interpretation.* Philadelphia: F. A. Davis Co.

| CHART 8–17 | **Key Questions for Critiquing Quantitative Designs** |

STAGE 1 QUESTIONS: CRITICAL APPRAISAL OF PURPOSE, PROBLEM STATEMENT, AND CONGRUENCE WITH DESIGN AND METHODOLOGY

Purpose or Problem Statement

- Is the study problem and purpose statement clearly articulated?
- Are the reasons for conducting the study stated?
- Is the study's potential contribution to nursing knowledge stated?
- Are the research objectives or research questions or hypotheses stated clearly and researchable (answerable through the collection of empirical data)?
- Are terms defined conceptually and operationally?

Literature Review

- Does the literature review or theoretical framework provide evidence that the researcher has synthesized the classic and current literature and placed the research question in the proper context?
- Does the literature review identify gaps in knowledge, suggest how the current study extends the knowledge base in this area, and point out contradictions in the current knowledge base?
- Does the researcher summarize the literature review, provide a rationale for the current study, and show how this study will extend previous research?

Design

- Is the study design specified, including its advantages and limitations for the research problem?
- Is there evidence that a pilot study had been conducted and the findings were used to enhance the design?
- Is the design (overall plan of research) appropriate to the research purpose and capable of answering the research question?
- How does the design control for extraneous variables?

Sample

- Was probability or nonprobability sampling used and the reason for the choice specified?
- Is the population to whom results will be generalized described?
- Are precautions taken to avoid collecting a biased sample (see Chapter 9) that would limit generalizability of the findings?
- Are the demographic characteristics of the sample described?
- Is the sample representative of the population?
- Are inclusion and exclusion criteria identified?
- Is the sample size appropriate to meet assumptions of statistical tests?

Data Collection

- Are data collection methods appropriate to meet the study purpose and answer the questions or hypotheses?
- What evidence is provided that data collection procedures are valid and reliable?
- Are adaptations to data collection tools described?
- Are data collection instruments described in sufficient detail to enable readers to ascertain method of scoring and range of values and what a particular score means?

Data Analysis

- Are data analysis procedures described?
- Are the statistical techniques appropriate for the study methodology (i.e., the type of data collected and analysis)?

- Do the statistical tests answer the research questions and specify the level of significance?
- If results are nonsignificant, is a power analysis conducted to explore nonsignificant findings?

STAGE 2 QUESTIONS: CRITICAL APPRAISAL OF THE CONDUCT OF RESEARCH

Human Rights

- How are rights of research participants protected?
- Are ethical issues anticipated and handled appropriately?

Procedures

- Are techniques used to ensure that there is consistency in the data collection process?
- What procedures were used to keep research conditions the same for all participants?
- Are there strategies to limit errors in data collection, recording, and analysis?
- Did any unplanned circumstances influence the results?
- In experimental designs, is there evidence of manipulation of independent variables, randomization in selection of sample and assignment to experimental and control groups, and control of extraneous variables?

STAGE 3 QUESTIONS: CRITICAL APPRAISAL OF RESEARCH OUTCOMES

Findings

- Are the findings presented clearly and correctly and are they related to the theoretical framework?
- Is there a clear statement of whether or not the data support the hypotheses or answer each research question?
- Are tables and graphs clearly labeled, easy to comprehend, and congruent with results presented in text form?
- Are findings presented in an unbiased manner?

Discussion

- Are alternative approaches offered for the findings?
- Does the researcher discuss both clinical and statistical significance of findings?
- Does the researcher overgeneralize the findings beyond the appropriate population?
- Are limitations of the study such as sample size, inadequate instruments, sources of bias, and so on identified and their implications discussed?

Implications and Conclusions

- Does the researcher identify important implications of the study for practice, education, or research (if appropriate)?
- How do the findings of the study advance nursing knowledge?
- Do new research questions emerge from the study?

STAGE 4 QUESTIONS: CRITICAL APPRAISAL OF THE OVERALL STUDY

Overall Quality

- What are the major strengths of the study?
- What are the major limitations of the study?
- Was the study described in sufficient detail to facilitate a replication study?
- What are the major contributions of this study to knowledge development in nursing?
- What suggestions might enhance the study and correct the limitations?

Source: From Gillis, A., & Jackson, W. (2002). *Research for nurses: Methods and interpretation.* Philadelphia: F. A. Davis Co.

standards have been proposed to evaluate qualitative studies (Burns & Grove, 2005):

- **Standard 1: descriptive vividness**—With **descriptive vividness,** the site, participants, experience of collecting data, and the thinking of the researcher are described so clearly that the reader has the sense of personally experiencing the event.

- **Standard 2: methodological congruence**—**Methodological congruence** has four dimensions: documentation rigor, procedural rigor, ethical rigor, and auditability (Burns & Grove, 2005). All elements of the study must be clearly documented, for example, the study subject, significance, purpose, research questions, assumptions, ethical implications, sampling methods, data gathering and analysis strategies, theoretical development, conclusions, and implications for practice. Documentation regarding these study elements must be clear and complete. Procedural rigor should be evident in that the researcher should clearly state the steps taken to ensure that data were accurately recorded and that the data obtained were representative of the data as a whole. Ethical rigor is reflected in the discussion by the researcher of the ethical implications related to the study, informed consent, and protection of participants' rights. Auditability refers to a decision trail. The research report should be sufficiently detailed to allow a second reader, using the original data and the decision trail, to arrive at conclusions similar to those of the original researcher.

- **Standard 3: analytical preciseness**—**Analytical preciseness** requires the researcher to make the effort needed to identify and record the decision-making processes through which concrete data are transformed into a theory or explanation of the phenomenon being studied.

- **Standard 4: theoretical connectedness**—**Theoretical connectedness** requires that the theoretical schema developed from the study be clearly expressed, logically consistent, reflective of the data, and compatible with the practice of nursing.

- **Standard 5: heuristic relevance**—The results of the study should have **heuristic relevance** for the reader. "This value is reflected in the reader's ability to recognize the phenomenon described in the study, its theoretical significance, its applicability to nursing practice, and its influence on future research" (Burns & Grove, 2003, p. 432). Dimensions of relevance include intuitive recognition, relationship to the existing body of knowledge, and applicability.

Key questions, developed by Burns and Grove (2005), can be used to critique a qualitative research report. They are grouped in four stages consistent with a review of quantitative research and are shown in Chart 8–18 (p. 142).

■ Future of Perspectives of Nursing Research

Research is critical to the practice of nursing, now and in the future. It is of vital importance to nursing in developing and acquiring new knowledge. This knowledge is changing practice, education, and health policy, and will continue to do so. Application of research findings to practice helps ensure the highest possible quality care that can be delivered in a cost-effective manner. This is critical to the future of nursing and health care.

Because knowledge is the foundation of professional practice, all nurses can and should develop and apply research skills in practice. As a professional nurse, the level of educational preparation will influence the role one plays in research. Though the trend is toward an expanded researcher role with advanced education, nurses at all levels of roles and responsibilities assume a role when it comes to nursing research. The ANA (1994) has defined these roles, which serve as national guidelines for education preparation, as follows:

1. **Associate degree in nursing.** Graduates of associate degree programs have several important roles to play in research. They need to develop an appreciation for research and can:
   - Help to identify clinical problems in nursing practice.
   - Assist in the collection of data within a structured format.
   - In conjunction with nurses holding more advanced credentials, appropriately use research findings in clinical practice.

2. **Baccalaureate degree in nursing.** Graduates of baccalaureate programs have an important role to play as consumers of research. This assumes that they have an intimate understanding of the research process; an ability to critically read, analyze, and critique research studies; and the judgment to interpret and evaluate research findings for application to practice. They participate in research by:
   - Identifying clinical problems
   - Assisting experienced investigators gain access to clinical sites
   - Influencing the selection of appropriate methods of data collection
   - Collecting and implementing nursing research findings.

   Baccalaureate-level nurses are prepared to understand the research protocols of other disciplines and to participate in data collection or other aspects of research.

3. **Master's degree in nursing.** Graduates of master's programs also play important roles in nursing research. They have a rich understanding of clinical practice and usually an in-depth perspective on nursing problems specific to various practice settings. This enables the researcher to identify clinically relevant problems and provide expert clinical advice on ways that services should be delivered and projects conducted. They are skilled in assisting others to use research findings appropriately. They help to create a climate in the practice setting that supports scholarly inquiry, and collaborate with others in proposal development, data collection, and data analysis and interpretation.

4. **Doctoral education.** Doctorally prepared nurses contribute to nursing knowledge through the conduct of research aimed at theory generation or theory testing. Graduates of doctoral programs are best prepared to appraise, design, and conduct research. According to the

CHART 8–18	**Key Questions for Critiquing Qualitative Designs**

STAGE 1 QUESTIONS: CRITICAL APPRAISAL OF PURPOSE, STATEMENT OF RESEARCH PHENOMENON, AND CONGRUENCE WITH DESIGN AND METHODOLOGY

Purpose or Statement of the Phenomenon of Interest

- Is the research phenomenon of interest clearly stated?
- Is rationale provided for approaching the study in an inductive, qualitative manner?
- Is the philosophy of the research tradition described?
- Is a statement of self-understanding included?
- Is there a single broad research question? Are their subquestions?
- Does the initial question become more focused as data are collected and analyzed?
- Is the study purpose clearly stated (e.g., discovery, description, theory building, and so on)?

Literature Review

- Does the qualitative method used call for a literature review before data collection?
- Does the review indicate that the researcher has expertise in the chosen area, know where gaps exist, and show how this study will eliminate such gaps?
- If a review is appropriate only after data collection, is there evidence that this is done?
- Is a framework appropriate? If so, is it presented clearly?

Design

- Is the design (i.e., overall plan for the research) appropriate to the research purpose?
- Is there congruency between the methodology and the research question?
- Is the context for the study adequately described?
- Is the researcher–participant relationship understood?

Sample

- Is purposive sampling used?
- Are informants capable of informing the study?
- Is the selection of participants appropriate to allow for saturation of data?

Data Collection

- Is data collection congruent with the study purpose, research question, and qualitative tradition selected?
- Are prolonged engagement and persistent observation in the field used to build trust with participants and ensure validity of data collection?
- Are data collection strategies and procedures described in sufficient detail?

Data Analysis

- Are data analysis procedures clearly described and appropriate to the research tradition?
- What evidence is provided that data collection and analysis are concurrent and ongoing?
- Is there evidence of decision rules for analyzing data, and does the researcher remain true to the rules?

- What evidence is there of narrowing the coding as categories are systematically discarded when they are unsupported by the data and the researcher becomes more focused on data collection and analysis?
- Is there evidence of "theoretical saturation?"

STAGE 2 QUESTIONS: CRITICAL APPRAISAL OF THE CONDUCT OF THE RESEARCH

Human Rights

- How are the rights of research participants protected?
- Are ethical issues anticipated and handled appropriately?

Procedures

- What evidence is provided that research meets the criteria of rigor (credibility: findings must be understood and viewed as credible by the informants; trustworthiness: one can believe the findings are true; and usefulness: findings shed light on an important phenomenon)?
- Creswell (1998) identifies eight procedures for testing the truth value (appropriate representation of multiple realities) and notes that researchers should use at least two of these in any given study. The critic should ask which of these the researcher uses.

  1. Prolonged engagement and persistent observation in the field to build trust with participants, learn about the culture and context, and correct distortions introduced by the researcher's presence

  2. Triangulation for purpose of corroborating evidence from different sources to shed light on a theme or perspective

  3. Peer review as an external check of the research process; this person asks hard questions about the method, meanings, and interpretations and keeps the researcher honest

  4. Negative case analysis, in which the researcher reworks the hypothesis until all cases fit it

  5. The researcher articulates researcher bias so that the reader knows what prejudices, biases, or past experiences have shaped the researcher's approach to the study

  6. Member checks to solicit informants' opinions of the accuracy and credibility of the findings and conclusions. Some methods, however, such as hermeneutic analysis, do not always conduct member checks because their emphasis is on the interpretation of meaning by the research team of the experience of the participants in the research project

  7. External audits in which a consultant examines both the process and product of the qualitative study to assess accuracy and determine if the findings, interpretations, and conclusions are supported by the data

  8. Rich, in-depth descriptions of participants and setting are provided so that the reader can make decisions regarding transferability of findings to other settings

STAGE 3 QUESTIONS: CRITICAL APPRAISAL OF THE RESEARCH OUTCOMES

Findings

- Are the findings contextualized (i.e., presented within the context of the circumstances that influence their interpretation)?
- Do readers of the report recognize the phenomenon or vicariously experience it?

> **CHART 8–18**   **Key Questions for Critiquing Qualitative Designs—*Continued***
>
> - Are the findings true to the data?
> - Do the themes, categories, or theoretical statements present a comprehensive, plausible, and meaningful picture of the phenomenon?
> - If models, diagrams, or figures are used, are they effective?
> - Are the findings compatible with the field of nursing's knowledge base?
> - Are reasons for incompatible findings explored by the researcher?
>
> **Discussion, Implications, and Conclusions**
>
> - Does the researcher identify implications of the study for nursing (i.e., in practice, theory building, instrument development, education, and research)?
>
> - Is a context provided in which to use the findings?
> - Do the implications and conclusions follow logically from the findings?
> - Do new research questions emerge from the findings?
>
> **STAGE 4 QUESTIONS: CRITICAL APPRAISAL OF THE OVERALL QUALITY OF THE STUDY**
>
> - What are the major strengths of the study?
> - What are the major limitations of the study?
> - What are the major contributions of this study to knowledge development in the field of nursing?
> - What suggestions might enhance the study and correct the limitations?

Source: Gillis, A., & Jackson, W. (2002). *Research for nurses: Methods and interpretation.* Philadelphia: F. A. Davis Co.

> **CHART 8–19**   **Research Themes for the Future**
>
> 1. Changing lifestyle behaviors for better health
> 2. Managing the effects of chronic illness to improve health and quality of life:
>   - Health care practice
>   - Self-management of chronic illness symptoms and treatment
>   - Informal (family) caregiving.
> 3. Identifying effective strategies to reduce health disparities
> 4. Harnessing advanced technologies to serve human needs
> 5. Enhancing the end-of-life experience for patients and their families

Source: National Institute of Nursing Research. (2003). *Research themes for the future.* Bethesda, MD: National Institutes of Health.

ANA (1994), they develop nursing knowledge through original research and theory development. They also conduct funded independent research projects.

The vision for nursing in the 21st century is to narrow the gap between research and practice by helping nurses base their decisions and practice strategies on the best available evidence, thereby improving nursing care and patient outcomes. As the levels of sophistication and complexity in nursing increase, use of the scientific process to improve patient care and outcomes becomes more crucial, as does the educational preparation for engaging in research activities. Thus, research utilization, the process of transforming knowledge obtained from research into clinical practice, is a critical step in improving nursing care and ultimately patients' outcomes. It is, therefore, incumbent on all nurses to understand and use the research process, and to participate in the critical process of research review and utilization. This chapter has presented the basic guidelines for assisting learners to garner that knowledge, and has provided a background for interpreting research findings and future research goals presented throughout the book.

Future Research Goals

The research themes for the future as determined by the NINR are shown in Chart 8–19. Each of the five themes includes specific research goals. The themes and goals in their entirety may be found on the NINR website.

REVIEW QUESTIONS

1. The nurse is planning a study using basic research. This nurse is most likely going to be studying:
   1. The effectiveness of a type of wound dressing.
   2. The frequency of side effects from one particular medication.
   3. How Orem's theory can be applied to the nursing process.
   4. The effectiveness of teaching self-insulin administration to a patient diagnosed with diabetes mellitus.

2. The nurse researcher is conducting a quantitative research study. Which of the following will most likely be done during this study?
   1. Change the study as information is collected.
   2. Approach the process in a circular method rather than a straight line.
   3. Collect numerical values within a controlled situation.
   4. Use a small sample size.

3. The nurse researcher is planning an experimental quantitative research project. This project will most likely be conducted:

   1. On a general medical–surgical unit.

   2. In the emergency room.

   3. In the intensive care unit.

   4. In a laboratory.

4. The Quality Improvement Committee is planning to conduct a research study. Which of the following should this committee do first?

   1. Determine the patients who will participate in the study.

   2. Identify the problem to be studied.

   3. Assign data collection roles to specific committee members.

   4. Figure out how long the study will take to complete.

5. A nurse researcher is determining the best design to use for a research project. Which of the following can be used as a guide for this design?

   1. Methods used to collect data

   2. Approaches used to analyze the data

   3. Determine if the study is a quantitative or qualitative research.

   4. Write out the research problem or question.

Answers for review questions appear in Appendix D

KEY TERMS

analytical preciseness *p.141*
applied research *p.122*
basic research *p.122*
convenience sampling *p.127*
correlational research design *p.125*
data saturation *p.129*
descriptive research design *p.125*
descriptive vividness *p.141*
ethnography *p.126*
evidence-based practice (EBP) *p.130*
experimental research design *p.125*
grounded theory *p.126*
heuristic relevance *p.141*
hypothesis *p.125*
informatics *p.138*
literature review *p.125*

methodological congruence *p.141*
network sampling *p.127*
nonexperimental research design *p.125*
nonprobability sampling *p.127*
phenomenology *p.126*
pilot study *p.127*
population *p.126*
power analysis *p.128*
probability sampling *p.127*
purposive sampling *p.127*
qualitative research *p.125*
quantitative research *p.125*
quasi-experimental research design *p.125*
quota sampling *p.127*
random assignment *p.127*
research *p.121*

research critique *p.138*
research design *p.125*
research problem *p.124*
research process *p.122*
research purpose *p.124*
research question *p.124*
research utilization (RU) *p.130*
sample *p.126*
sampling *p.126*
setting *p.126*
simple random sampling *p.127*
statistical significance *p.128*
stratified random sampling *p.127*
theoretical connectedness *p.141*
variables *p.125*

REFERENCES

Agency for Healthcare Research and Quality. (2007). *Evidence-based practice centers.* Retrieved December 14, 2007, from http://www.ahrq.gov/clinic/epc

American Nurses Association. (1976). *Preparation for nurses for participation research.* Kansas City, MO: Author.

American Nurses Association. (1994). *Education for participation in nursing research.* Retrieved June 10, 2007 from http://www.AmericanNursesAssociaton.org

Ardery, G., Herr, K. A., Titler, M. G., Sorofman, B. A., & Schmitt, M. G. (2003). Assessing and managing acute pain in older adults: a research base to guide practice. *MedSurg Nursing, 12*(il), 7, 13.

Burns, N., & Grove, S. K. (2003). *Understanding nursing research* (3rd ed.). Philadelphia: W. B. Saunders.

Burns, N., & Grove, S. K. (2005). *Understanding nursing research* (5th. ed.). Philadelphia: W. B. Saunders.

Ciliska, D., Pinelli, J., DeCenso, A., & Cullum, N. (2001). Resources to enhance evidence-based nursing practice. *AACN Clinial Issues, 12*(4), 520–528.

Colling, J. (2003). Desiging clinical research studies: (Demystifying clinical research studies: sample size. *Urologic Nursing, 23*(8), This article was published prior to Part 1, and was not labeled as such.

Connor, J. A., Smaldone, A. M., Bratts, T., & Stone, P. W. (2003). Ask an expert: HIPAA in 2003 and its meaning for nurse researchers. *Applied Nursing Research, 16,* 291–293.

Creswell, J. (1998). *Qualitative inquiry and research design: Choosing among five tradtions.* London: Thousand Oaks, Sage Publications.

Crowther, M. (2003). Evidence-based development of a hospital based heart failure centre. *Evidence-Based Nursing, 6,* 4–6.

DeBourgh, G. A. (2001). Champions for evidence-based practice: A critical role for advanced practice nurses. *AACN Clinical Issues, 12*(4), 491–508.

Gillis, A., & Jackson, W. (2002). *Research for nurses: Methods and interpretation.* Philadelphia: F. A. Davis.

Holden, C. (1979). Ethics in social science research. *Science, 206,* 537–540.

Malloch, K., & Porter-O'Grady, T. (2006). *Introduction to evidence-based practice in nursing and health care.* Sudbury, MA: Jones and Bartlett.

McKibbon, A., Eady, A., & Marks, S. (1999). *PDQ: Evidence-based principles and practice.* (PDQ series) Hamilton, Ont.; London: B.C. Decker.

National Commission for the Protection of Human Subjects of Biomedical and Behavioral Research (1978). *Belmont report: Ethical principles and guidelines for research involving human subjects.* Washington, DC: U.S. Government Printing Office.

Nightingale, F. (1859). *Notes on nursing: What it is and what it is not.* Philadelphia: J. B. Lippincott.

Olsen, D. P. (2003). HIPAA privacy regulations and nursing research. *Nursing Research, 52,* 344–348.

Omery, A., & Williams, R. P. (1999). An appraisal of research utilization across the United States. *Journal of Nursing Administration, 29,* 50–56.

Poe, S. S. Cvach, M. M., Gartrell, D. G., Radzik, B. R., & Joy, T. L. (2005). *Journal of Nursing Care Quality, 20*(2), 107–116.

Polit, D. F., & Beck, C. T. (2008). *Nursing research: Principles and methods* (8th ed.). Philadelphia: Lippincott Williams & Wilkins.

Staggers, N., Gassert, C. A., & Curran, C. (2002). A delphi study to determine informatics competencies for nurse levels of practice. *Nursing Research, 51*(6), 383–390.

Stetler, C. B. (1994). Refinement of the Stetler/Maram model for application of research findings into practice. *Nursing Outlook, 42,* 15–35.

Stuart, J. (2001). Evidence-based psychiatric nursing practice: Rhetoric or reality, *Journal of American Psychiatric Nurses* Association, *7,* 103–114.

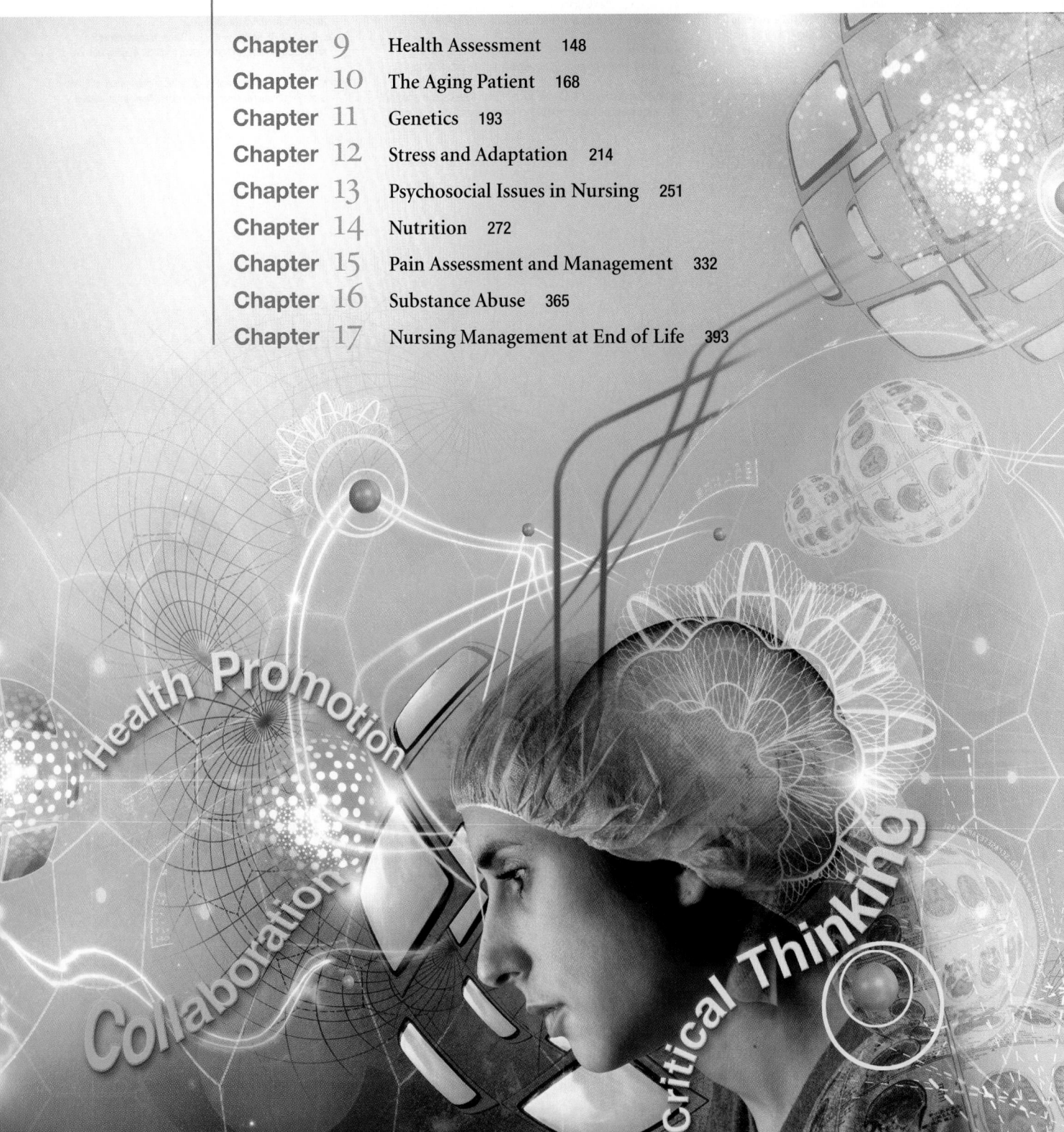

Health Promotion

Collaboration

Critical Thinking

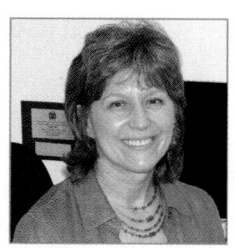

TERI Throughout my baccalaureate nursing program at California State University, Sacramento, I knew I wanted to work with the older population. I am sure this desire was fueled by the close relationship I had with my grandparents and the social interactions with many of their older friends as I grew up. While attending nursing school, I decided the skilled nursing facility (SNF) setting might be a good fit for me. Contrary to many negative perceptions of geriatric nursing, I saw it as a growing and challenging field. I could be at the forefront of exciting changes as the complexity and diversity of the aging population increased. I was driven by the sense that I could learn from my patients' life experiences and possibly make a difference in this last stage of their lives.

After graduation, I became a charge nurse on a 40-bed skilled nursing unit. I was responsible for the total care of 20 elderly residents, most of whom had been admitted for a short stay of 2 weeks or less for rehabilitation and others who presented with multiple diagnoses affecting their quality of life. I was responsible for administering medications, completing treatments, and documenting the patient's care regimen. I worked with the unit manager to keep the residents, their families, and the physicians apprised of all changes and to continually update the plan of care. My days were challenging, demanding, satisfying, and never boring!

After a short period of time, I was promoted to unit manager. It was in this position that my passion for geriatric nursing grew. I supervised licensed nurses and certified nursing assistants on all shifts and worked closely with the interdisciplinary team, physicians, and families to ensure that quality care was provided at all times. A sense of ownership and accomplishment was felt by all staff on the unit when our quality measures compared well to state and national averages. But more importantly, there was a sense of *family* between staff, residents, and their family members. It was easy to become emotionally attached to residents as we cared for them daily over the years, advocating for them as they negotiated the health care system. It was this **commitment** to residents, staff, and families and a hope for innovative health care for seniors that kept me excited about going to work each day.

Attending physicians in SNFs are required to see their patients within 72 hours of admission and then monthly thereafter. This lack of constant physical presence by physicians provides the SNF nurse with a great measure of autonomy in his or her practice combined with the awesome responsibility of accurate clinical assessments. The SNF nurse must be **confident** in his or her assessment and be able to demonstrate **competence** in geriatric physiology and overall assessment of the older patient in order to work with the physician in prescribing medications and treatments. I remember admitting an elderly woman, Mrs. G, following surgery for a fractured hip. Because her recovery was not as quick and complete as she had hoped, neither her interdisciplinary health team nor I could in good **conscience** recommend discharge to her home without additional help. A meeting was scheduled with the team, Mr. and Mrs. G, and the physician to discuss in an open and honest manner the team's reservations regarding a safe discharge and the resident's right and desire to go home without assistance. By demonstrating our respect for the resident's wishes and presenting a forum for open communication, Mrs. G's husband was able to express some of his own anxiety over the pending discharge. Ultimately, Mrs. G made the decision to allow home health to send a RN to her home for follow-up after discharge. Through a collaborative process and the team's professional **comportment** and **compassion**, an atmosphere of trust was built in which the resident's wishes were respected and the team was able to demonstrate their caring for the resident's continued well-being.

My experiences in skilled nursing motivated me to pursue advanced education at the master's and doctoral level in geriatrics, gerontology, and health administration. Being a geriatric nurse allows me to use a wide range of my nursing skills from medical–surgical to community health. It has led me to my current position as Director of Quality and Compliance for a large multiservice agency based in Northern California. As director, I am able to continue working with the elderly across a wide continuum of care from independent living to skilled nursing care and to become involved in making policy decisions in our community as well as statewide. I am able to influence the direction of geriatric care by precepting new nurses and gerontology students, by participating in community and government projects, and by providing input into policy development designed to improve the quality of life for this population. It is this search for the best senior care that keeps me motivated to learn more about aging and excited about my role in caring for this growing population.

"It was this **commitment** to residents, staff, and families and a hope for innovative health care for seniors that kept me excited about going to work each day."

Health Assessment

Rich Keegan, Cheryl Wraa, Kathleen Osborn
With contributions by: Annita Watson

Outcome-Based Learning Objectives

After studying this chapter, the learner will be able to:

1. Describe the components of the health assessment.
2. Explain the steps of the patient interview for the health history.
3. Compare and contrast verbal and nonverbal responses that enhance the collection of information.
4. Explain how the techniques of inspection, palpation, percussion, and auscultation can be applied to the physical assessment of the major body systems.
5. Differentiate between the steps of the critical thinking component as it relates to health assessment.

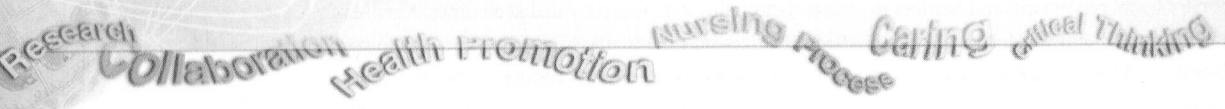

Research   Collaboration   Health Promotion   Nursing Process   Caring   Critical Thinking

THE FOCUS of health care in the United States is evolving beyond treatment of illness and injury to also include prevention and promotion of wellness. This newer model requires the development of a comprehensive plan of care that will guide the patient and family toward a healthy lifestyle and away from risk factors that can increase illness and injury. The nurse takes an active role in care plan development and execution. The nursing process guides the nurse when gathering and analyzing information. It is an effective method of problem solving and provides a framework on which to make informed decisions regarding the patient's plan of care.

Assessment, the first step of the nursing process, is when the nurse gathers initial data. It is a systematic process that assists the nurse in identifying current health status, actual and potential problems, and areas that need health promotion. It also provides a baseline on which future comparisons can be made. The assessment includes data about the physical, emotional, mental, spiritual, and cultural factors that impact health. It consists of both **objective data** (collected by using the senses: observation, palpation, auscultation, percussion, and smell) and **subjective data** (information the patient or caretaker tells the nurse). Both types of data are used to formulate a nursing diagnosis. The nursing diagnosis, which evolves from the assessment data, describes conditions treated by nurses (North American Nursing Diagnosis Association, 2007). Ultimately, a thorough health assessment al-

lows the nurse to collaborate with the health care team in developing a plan that integrates personal health care with prevention efforts to reach the national goal to increase quality and years of healthy life.

As a member of the health care team, nurses must adhere to the current legislation that is in place to protect the confidentiality of the individual patient. As a nurse, it is unethical and against federal and state statutes to disclose a patient's medical information without the patient's express consent. Note, however, that in the course of providing care to a patient, health care professionals can share information in order to formulate a plan of care to meet the patient's needs. Regulatory issues are covered in detail in Chapter 3 ☉.

■ National Guidelines: *Healthy People 2010*

Healthy People 2010: Understanding and Improving Health (U.S. Department of Health and Human Services [DHHS], 2000) is a 10-year strategy developed by the DHHS to recognize preventable threats to health and to identify and establish national goals to reduce these threats. *Healthy People 2010* has two distinct goals:

Goal 1: Increase quality and years of healthy life.

Goal 2: Eliminate health disparities.

The *Healthy People 2010* Leading Health Indicators

In addition to the two goals, 10 **leading health indicators** have been identified that reflect the major public health concerns of the 21st century for Americans: (1) physical activity, (2) overweight and obesity, (3) tobacco use, (4) substance abuse, (5) responsible sexual behaviors, (6) mental health, (7) injury and violence, (8) environmental quality, (9) immunization, and (10) access to health care. To achieve the goals and address the leading health indicators, *Healthy People 2010* is supported by specific objectives in 28 focus areas, as shown in the National Guidelines box. The nurse's role in assisting patients to achieve these goals requires an in-depth understanding of the patient's current health status. This understanding begins with a thorough health assessment.

Physical Activity

Regular physical activity helps maintain physical and psychological well-being. It also plays a significant role in reducing the incidence of many diseases including cardiovascular disease, diabetes mellitus, hypertension, colon cancer, depression, and anxiety. Physical activity is important at all ages to maintain muscle strength and decrease body fat, and it is an important component of weight control.

Physical activity is any bodily movement produced by skeletal muscles that results in an expenditure of energy. Physical fitness is defined as a set of attributes a person has with regard to a person's ability to perform physical activities that require aerobic fitness, endurance, strength, or flexibility and is determined by a combination of regular activity and genetically inherited ability. A pattern of physical activity is regular activities that are performed:

- Most days of the week, preferably daily;
- Five or more days of the week if moderate-intensity activities (in bouts of at least 10 minutes for a total of at least 30 minutes per day); or
- Three or more days of the week of vigorous-intensity activities (for at least 20 to 60 minutes per session) (Centers for Disease Control and Prevention [CDC], 2008).

One measurement of the level of exercise intensity is the **metabolic equivalent level (MET)**. The MET establishes the amount of oxygen used for physical activity, and it increases as physical activity increases. A second method of determining physical activity intensity is the Borg Rating of Perceived Exertion (RPE). Perceived exertion is how hard an individual feels like his or her body is working. It is based on the physical sensations a person experiences during physical activity, including increased heart rate, increased respiration or breathing rate, increased sweating, and muscle fatigue. Although this is a subjective measure, a person's exertion rating may provide a fairly good estimate of the actual heart rate during physical activity. The third method for measuring physical activity intensity is by determining the number of calories burned.

According to the CDC (2008), adults should strive to meet either moderate-intensity physical activity or vigorous-intensity physical activity. Moderate-intensity physical activity refers to a level of effort in which a person should experience one or more of the following:

- Some increase in breathing or heart rate
- A "perceived exertion" of 11 to 14 on the Borg RPE scale (e.g., the effort a healthy individual might expend while walking briskly, mowing the lawn, dancing, swimming, or bicycling on level terrain)
- Three to 6 METs
- Any activity that burns 3.5 to 7 Calories per minute (kcal/min).

Vigorous-intensity physical activity may be intense enough to represent a substantial challenge to an individual and refers to a level of effort in which a person should experience one or more of the following:

- A large increase in breathing or heart rate (conversation is difficult or "broken")
- A "perceived exertion" of 15 or greater on the Borg RPE scale (e.g., the effort a healthy individual might expend while jogging, mowing the lawn with a nonmotorized pushmower, participating in high-impact aerobic dancing, swimming

NATIONAL GUIDELINES for *Healthy People 2010* Focus Areas

Access to Quality Health Services	Injury and Violence Prevention
Arthritis, Osteoporosis, and Chronic Back Conditions	Maternal, Infant, and Child Health
Cancer	Medical Product Safety
Chronic Kidney Diseases	Mental Health and Mental Disorders
Diabetes	Nutrition and Overweight
Disability and Secondary Conditions	Occupational Safety and Health
Educational and Community-Based Programs	Oral Health
Environmental Health	Physical Activity and Fitness
Family Planning	Public Health Infrastructure
Food Safety	Respiratory Diseases
Health Communication	Sexually Transmitted Diseases
Heart Disease and Stroke	Substance Abuse
HIV	Tobacco Use
Immunization and Infectious Diseases	Vision and Hearing

continuous laps, bicycling uphill, carrying more than 25 lbs up a flight of stairs, standing or walking with more than 50 lbs)
- Greater than 6 METs
- Any activity that burns more than 7 kcal/ min (CDC, 2008).

Overweight and Obesity

Overweight and obese persons have a significant increased risk for heart disease, diabetes mellitus, stroke, arthritis, and serious sleep disorders. The number of obese persons has risen dramatically since the 1980s and has become a leading health problem in the United States. Obesity is more prevalent among women and proportionately higher in African American and Mexican women (D'Amico & Barbarito, 2007). Nutrition and exercise training are important factors in preventing weight gain and maintaining a healthy weight. Nutrition related to weight maintenance is discussed in detail in Chapter 14 ⊙.

Tobacco Use

Cigarette smoking is responsible for more deaths in the United States than are HIV/AIDS, drug abuse, homicide, suicide, automobile crashes, and fire combined. In addition, smoking is a risk factor associated with a number of prevalent diseases such as cardiovascular, respiratory, and cancer. Secondary smoke accounts for an increased incidence of asthma and bronchitis in children and heart and lung disease in adults (D'Amico & Barbarito, 2007). Staying away from people while they are smoking and making a choice to not smoke are two effective ways of not exacerbating these diseases.

Guidelines have been developed for professionals who are working with patients who smoke, but want to stop. For smokers who have expressed a desire to stop smoking, the guidelines include the five "A's":

- **A**sk about smoking at every visit.
- **A**dvise (that is, urge) all smokers to stop.
- **A**ssess the client's willingness to stop.
- **A**ssist or aid the patient in quitting. Work with the patient to develop a plan while providing counseling, recommending pharmacotherapy, and providing resource materials.
- **A**rrange for follow-up to determine progress or need for further assistance.

Substance Abuse

Substance abuse of alcohol and illicit drugs has been linked to many health problems, including injuries from accidents, sexually transmitted infections, cardiac and liver disease, violence, and a disruption of families. Abuse also is occurring with prescription drugs such as pain relievers, sedatives, tranquilizers, and stimulants.

Identification and diagnosis of drug abuse begins with a screening assessment. A questionnaire developed by Ewing (1984) uses the mnemonic CAGE to help professionals remember these four screening questions:

- Have you ever wanted to **C**ut down on alcohol/prescription drug use?
- Have you ever felt **A**nnoyed when remarks are made about alcohol/prescription drug use?
- Have you ever felt **G**uilty about alcohol/prescription drug use?

- Have you **E**ver used alcohol/prescription drugs as a way to change your mood or feeling of energy?

Questions about the amount and type of alcohol/prescription drug used are included in the social history section of a health assessment (Figure 9–1 ■).

Responsible Sexual Behaviors

Unprotected sexual activity increases the risk for sexually transmitted infections (STIs) and pregnancy. According to *Healthly People 2010*, individuals must understand how STIs are transmitted in order to increase the probability that this awareness will change risky behaviors. Chapters 49 and 50 ⊙ discuss the transmission of the various STIs.

Health care providers have a pivotal role in assessing behaviors and educating individuals about prevention. Effective questions for a health assessment include the following:

- Are you sexually active?
- When was the last time you had sexual activity (oral, vaginal, anal)?
- When you had sexual activity was a condom used?
- Do you now have or have you ever had more than one sexual partner?
- Have you ever been treated for STIs?
- Have you ever had sexual activity with a partner who used intravenous drugs?

Mental Health

Mental illness affects not only individuals, but families, and even communities. According to *Healthy People 2010*, one-fifth of the people in the United States are affected by mental illness each year (D'Amico & Barbarito, 2007). Mental disorders include depression, schizophrenia, bipolar disorder, obsessive compulsive disorder, and panic disorder. Depression accounts for the majority of these cases and significantly contributes to disability and suicide. Screening for depression may be difficult because the common symptoms such as fatigue, sleep disorders, and pain are vague and can be related to many conditions. Screening for depression is accomplished through patient interviews and the use of screening questions such as these:

- Have you felt down, depressed, or hopeless in the last two weeks?
- Have you had little interest or pleasure in doing things?

When a patient answers yes to one or both of these questions, to confirm the diagnosis of depression, the nurse needs to inquire about the presence of the symptoms outlined here:

- Significant weight loss or gain
- Disturbed sleep patterns
- Agitation or slowness
- Fatigue
- Feelings of guilt or worthlessness
- Inability to concentrate or make decisions
- Thoughts of death or suicide.

If the patient answers yes to the presence of four or more of these symptoms, a diagnosis of depression is confirmed. The nurse should then assess for a family history of depression or

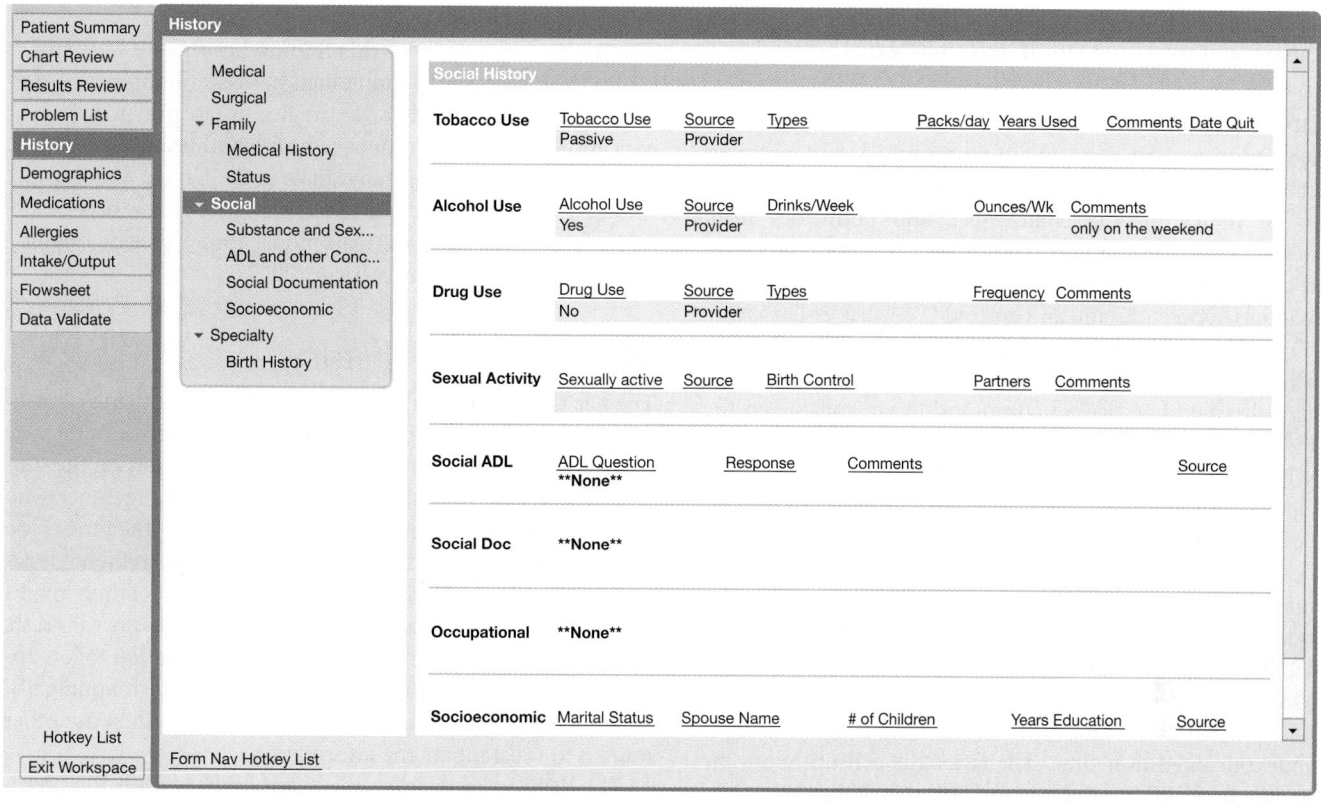

FIGURE 9–1 ■ Social history section of a health assessment.

other mental disorders, two or more chronic illnesses, stress in the home or at work, and loss of interest in sexual activity.

Injury and Violence

Serious injuries occur as a result of motor vehicle and motorcycle crashes, falls, drowning, fires, poison, guns, and knives. Other types of injury include child abuse and homicides from firearms. The greatest number of injuries occurs from motor vehicle crashes, with the greatest number of deaths occurring in individuals between 17 and 24 years old (D'Amico & Barbarito, 2007). Alcohol has been associated with almost half of all motor vehicle fatalities. Increased use of safety equipment and decreased driving after alcohol consumption are considered the best ways to decrease fatalities.

When assessing the patient who admits to drinking after driving it is important to stress how much alcohol can be consumed and still be able to drive. The amount of alcohol in the bloodstream is referred to as blood alcohol level (BAL). The BAL is recorded in milligrams of alcohol per 100 milliliters of blood, or milligrams percent. For example, a BAL of 0.10 means that 1/10 of 1 percent (or 1/1,000) of the total blood content is alcohol. BAL depends on (1) the amount of blood in the individual (which will increase with weight) and (2) the amount of alcohol consumed over time. The faster the consumption, the higher the BAL, because the liver can only metabolize about one drink per hour—the rest builds up in the bloodstream. If a person has a BAL of greater than 0.08%, most states' laws consider that person to be drunk. Disposable breathalyzers may be helpful in monitoring BAL before driving. Encourage individuals to never drive after drinking alcohol. Ask them to consider alternatives such as a taxicab or some form of public transportation.

Environmental Quality

The environment includes the physical air, water, and soil. The social environment includes housing, transportation, land use, development, and agriculture. Health risks related to the physical environment include exposure to chemical, biological, and physical agents that lead to respiratory and cardiovascular diseases and cancer. Health risks associated with the social environment include the ones in the physical environment as well as stress, injury, and violence.

Government programs and laws have been enacted that dictate standards for water treatment, food safety, and waste management. Policies vary and are more stringent in some areas such as urban settings as apposed to rural areas. When assessing patients, it is important to determine risks they may face based on their physical and social environments. *Healthy People 2010* provides information about environmental issues.

Immunization

When immunizations are consistently given to a population, they can prevent diseases, disabilities, and the spread of infection. Recommendations for childhood immunizations have been developed and when followed will reduce the incidence of many childhood illnesses. Immunizations such as pneumonia and influenza are considered an effective way to decrease death or complications from infectious diseases in older adults. Chapter 20 🔗 includes an in-depth discussion of immunizations.

Access to Health Care

The major component of this leading health care indicator is health insurance. When individuals have health insurance, they tend toward regular and preventive health care practices. Higher education and income influence health and health promotion. A significant number of individuals in the United States under the age of 65 are without health insurance, and those between 18 and 24 years old are most commonly found to lack ongoing health care (D'Amico & Barbarito, 2007).

■ The Health History

The health history is a detailed account of the patient's perception of his current and past health in his own words. In the case of a young child or infant, the nurse will have to rely on the subjective perceptions of the patient's adult family member who cares for the child. In the case of an adult who at the time is too ill to give an accurate account of her health history, then it is acceptable to rely on the subjective perceptions of a family member or close friend. In some instances, such as a severe car crash, total strangers may be the only source of information for an unconscious patient. To ensure the accuracy of information gathered under these circumstances, the nurse must then use other sources to substantiate the information.

The detailed nursing health history differs from the physician's medical history in that nurses are focusing on what effect the patient's current health status will have on being able to function independently in providing for activities of daily living (ADLs). For example, if an elderly patient were to be admitted for a hip fracture, the physician would be concerned with the surgical intervention needed to repair the fracture. The nurse would be focused on what the patient would need to be able to perform his ADLs while in the hospital and once cleared for discharge. The nurse would ascertain what the patient's level of functioning was before the event and apply the new limitations into a plan of care for this patient. Issues such as whether the patient requires assistive devices and whether the patient has family members or friends who are able to provide assistance once the patient goes home would all need to be assessed. The nurse must teach the caretakers all aspects of care as well as when it is appropriate to seek medical attention.

Conducting the Health Interview

When beginning the interview, nurses should address patients using their surnames and then introduce themselves and their role in the agency. They should state if they are a student. Finally, nurses should tell patients the purpose for the interview.

During the data collection phase of the interview, the nurse uses two types of questions: open ended and direct or closed. **Open-ended questions** ask for narrative information by stating the topic in general terms. This type of question is useful for introducing a subject such as "What brought you to the hospital?" A **direct question** is used to elicit specific information. Direct questions can be used to clarify specific details. For instance, if the patient stated that she is experiencing abdominal pain, a direct question would be "Is the pain sharp or dull?"

To encourage free expression, it is important for the nurse to listen carefully, not cut the patient off, and respond in a way that encourages the patient to provide more information. Responses that are helpful include the following:

- *Silence:* This allows the patient time to think and allows the nurse to observe for nonverbal cues.
- *Facilitation:* Comments such as "please continue" or nodding one's head encourages the patient to tell the nurse more.
- *Explanation:* Using factual information to explain an issue helps to clarify it for the patient. For example, telling the patient how a specific procedure is performed may decrease the patient's anxiety regarding the test.
- *Interpretation:* Interpretive responses link events or imply cause. "From what you have told me, it appears that whenever you have a meal high in fat you begin to have abdominal pain."
- *Clarification:* If patients describe an issue using ambiguous language, the nurse should ask them to clarify, such as "Please describe for me what 'feeling weird' means."
- *Empathy:* Acknowledging patients' feelings with a statement of understanding helps patients to feel accepted and more comfortable discussing the issue. An example of an empathetic response is "Not being able to do your normal activities must be frustrating for you."
- *Summary:* At the end of the interview, the nurse summarizes his perceptions of the patient's health problem from what he has learned during the interview. This acknowledges agreement between the nurse and the patient regarding the patient's health status.

Responses that are nonproductive and should be avoided by the nurse include providing false reassurance, using authoritarian language, giving unwanted advice and not allowing the patient to make decisions regarding their own solution, talking too much, using professional jargon that the patient will not understand, and using avoidance language or euphemisms to avoid reality.

An awareness of body language is an important factor during the interview. Positive nonverbal messages enhance the relationship with the patient and show attentiveness and acceptance. Examples of positive nonverbal messages are a professional appearance, a relaxed open posture, appropriate eye contact, equal-status seating, a moderate tone of voice and rate of speech, and appropriate touch. Examples of negative nonverbal messages are a tense posture, critical gestures such as pointing or finger-tapping, yawning, speaking too quickly, avoiding eye contact by focusing on notes, and inappropriate touch. Note, that it is important for the nurse to understand the different cultural norms regarding appropriate eye contact and appropriate touch as well as other related issues. Various communication norms for different cultures are discussed in the Cultural Considerations box (p. 154).

The components of the health history are consistent from one health care agency to another. The six main components of the health history include (1) biographical data; (2) present health/illness, including health patterns and beliefs; (3) past medical history, including a medication history; (4) family history; (5) psychosocial history; and (6) a review of body systems (i.e., physical assessment) (Rhodes, 2006).

Biographical Data

Biographical data, which provides baseline information about the patient, contains the following elements:

- *Name and address:* This is usually the first biographical data to be obtained. By having the patient state her name, the professional nurse is able to hear the patient speak. This assessment of whether the patient can hear and then respond appropriately helps to determine her level of consciousness.
- *Age and date of birth:* By establishing the chronological age of the patient, the nurse is then able to assess certain characteristics that occur over the age continuum. A 20-year-old male will exhibit a developed musculature and his skin will be smooth and without wrinkles, whereas a 70-year-old male will exhibit aging skin with wrinkling and will have muscle wasting secondary to inactivity.
- *Gender:* The gender of the patient in association with his or her age gives the nurse clues as to physical development and the presence of secondary sex characteristics. Adult males will typically have greater muscle mass and possess facial hair, whereas a female of the same age will not have these characteristics.
- *Birthplace:* A patient's birthplace can provide the nurse with evidence of environmental or cultural factors that may have contributed to the patient's current state of health. For example, a patient born and raised in the Central Valley of California may have signs and symptoms of reactive airway disease as a result of exposure to pesticides and dust in the region.
- *Geography:* A patient's geography refers to the country, region, section, community, or neighborhood in which he was born and raised or currently resides. Where someone was raised affects family life and general customs practiced by the individual. The availability of community resources including schools, churches, health care facilities, social systems, transportation, and support services differs depending on the region. Urban areas typically offer more services than rural areas.
- *Marital status:* By determining if the patient is single, married, widowed, or divorced, the nurse can establish whether or not there is a significant person involved in this patient's life. It is also important to ask the patient if she has ever been in a committed relationship; this encourages a response for same-gender relationships.
- *Race:* By determining the patient's race, the nurse can assess for certain characteristics that are known about certain races in the United States. Caucasians have less melanin than Hispanics or African Americans and are, therefore, more prone to skin cancers. There are also certain health-related characteristics associated with race. For example, Mexican Americans have a higher rate of adult-onset diabetes than other races (Kaushik et al., 2007).
- *Religion:* Determining the religious affiliation to which the patient ascribes is an important part of an assessment. Belonging to a religious faith can dictate whether a patient will accept the medical/nursing interventions offered. For example, a devout Jehovah's Witness will not permit blood transfusions. Persons belonging to the Jewish or Muslim faiths may not eat pork. Patients who are Roman Catholic may not eat meat on Fridays during the period of Lent.
- *Occupation:* By determining the patient's occupation, the nurse can determine if there are health-related conditions

CULTURAL CONSIDERATIONS for Communication Customs

Native American	Family may request spiritual healers. Loud voice may be associated with aggression. Avoiding eye contact is respectful.
Cambodian	It is inappropriate to touch the head without permission. Consider it impolite to disagree so may say "yes" but not mean it. Very important to speak softly and be polite.
Chinese	Eye contact with authority figures avoided as sign of respect. Chinese language is expressive and loud. Need to assess understanding of conversations because the patient or family may not ask questions as a sign of respect. Privacy very important.
Gypsies	Important to establish trust. Very respectful of elder authority, therefore will have greater respect for older health care providers and dismiss younger team members. Tone of voice is commonly loud and argumentative. Very modest; never ask personal questions in mixed company.
Hmong	Very polite and aware of disrespectful and prejudicial behavior. Prolonged eye contact considered disrespectful. Communication may be indirect; will not say "no" but may say "I will think about it." Interpreters employed by the hospital are considered to be loyal to the institution and therefore not trusted. The family may request a bilingual family member be present during discussions. Language structure is different; make sure the interpreter understands the intent of the discussion. The Hmong language has almost no medical terms. Have great respect for authority. Elders of the family will meet to make decisions regarding the patient's care. Immediate family members and female relatives may not have exclusive decision-making power.
Japanese	May not ask questions; defer to health care team to provide care. Illness not discussed outside of family. Soft voice considered polite with direct conflict avoided. Facial expressions are controlled and prolonged direct eye contact is considered disrespectful. Promptness very important. Cleanliness of body is important, as is modesty and preservation of dignity.
Mexican	Direct eye contact with authority figures is avoided. Silence may show lack of agreement with the plan of care. Touching by a stranger is considered disrespectful, although therapeutic touch is an integral part of traditional healing.
Russians	Direct eye contact is used. Respectful of elders. Tone of voice may be loud.
South Asians (India, Pakistan, Bangladesh, Sri Lanka, Nepal, Fiji, East Africa)	Touching not common; caring expressed through eyes. Prolonged direct eye contact considered rude. Modesty, humility, tolerance, and silence emphasized. Tone of voice should be soft. Loudness is considered disrespectful.
Vietnamese	Head may be considered sacred and feet profane; do not touch the feet and then the head. Avoiding eye contact is a sign of respect. Using both hands when giving a person something shows respect. Tone of voice should be soft. A loud voice or pointing of the finger is a sign of disrespect.

inherent in the type of work the patient performs. If a patient works in a factory around loud machines, there may be resultant hearing loss from repeated exposure to noise. Occupation can also be a socioeconomic indicator of the patient. Some jobs for unskilled workers often do not pay enough for the patient to have adequate housing, insurance for health care, and adequate nutrition.

• *Health insurance:* Although information about health insurance is often obtained by the registration staff, it is an important assessment of the nurse. The type of health insurance the patient has can often be a predictor of the type of health-seeking behaviors the patient may or may not have. Patients who are enrolled in a health maintenance organization (HMO) are usually aware of the preventive aspect of the insurance and the focus on healthy lifestyle and the emphasis on regular health screenings along the age continuum.

- *Source of information:* As part of the data collection process, the person providing the information must be identified. If it is the patient who is providing the health information, then this is considered the primary source. A person other than the patient who provides health information about the patient is considered a secondary source. If an interpreter is used in obtaining the health history, then that should be noted on the questionnaire. In either case, it is the responsibility of the nurse to determine the reliability of the person giving the information.

Present Health/Illness

The history of the present illness includes information about what brought the patient to the health care provider. By using open-ended questioning, the nurse can obtain the reason why the patient is seeking care. The reason is usually written verbatim in the health record and often becomes the **chief complaint**. A leading question is "Why did you come in today?" The nurse then writes down the specific responses from the patient, such as "I have lost fifteen pounds in the last two weeks." The nurse can then ask further questions to gather more subjective data from the patient, such as "How has your appetite been?"

Health Patterns

It is important for the nurse to assess the health patterns of the patient because this can be a determinant of his or her current state of health. Health patterns such as sleep can determine whether or not the patient is achieving the norm for his demographic. Open-ended questions can be used to gather this information: "How much sleep do you normally get each night?" "Is your sleep interrupted during the night?" "How many times do you have to get up to go to the bathroom during the night?" The responses that the patient provides will be a good predictor of whether or not he is getting the required 8 to 10 hours of sleep each night. Sleep patterns will usually be addressed in the neurological portion of the body system review.

Other health patterns to assess are the patient's access to preventive health maintenance. Questions such as "When was the last time you had an eye examination?" "How often do you see a dentist?" "When was your last physical exam?" "How often do you exercise?" will assist the nurse in determining the normal routine or preventive measures of the patient.

Health Beliefs and Practices

An individual's belief about health is based on knowledge, heritage, and experiences. Culture also influences these beliefs. Today with information so readily available in the mass media and on the Internet, people tend to be better informed about health issues. An increase in information about preventive medicine has made people better informed about lifestyles and habits that promote health.

The following questions and statements will assist the nurse in learning more about the patient's health care beliefs:

- What do you think it means to be healthy?
- Tell me about your own health.
- Do members of your family have the same beliefs about health as you do?

- What do you do to remain healthy?
- Do you have any behaviors that you believe are unhealthy?
- Where do you get your health information?
- Do you have a regular health care provider?
- How often do you have a complete physical examination?
- Do you have any home remedies that you use regularly?

Past Medical History

The past medical history is a timeline of the patient's health that includes childhood illnesses, immunizations, allergies, surgeries, hospitalizations, labor and deliveries, injuries, major illnesses, and any mental, emotional, or psychiatric illnesses. It is important with a chronic illness to establish when it first occurred, what has been the progression of the illness to this point, and whether there are any **sequelae** (residual problems as a result of the illness) (Zator-Estes, 2006). By determining this, the nurse can establish what effect the chronic illness has had on the patient's ability to live a "normal" life. Repeated hospitalizations, numerous doctor visits requiring invasive tests, and multiple medications can affect the patient's perception of her quality of life when living with a chronic illness such as diabetes. The past medical history is also the place to discuss whether the patient uses tobacco, alcohol, or drugs. Typical questions include these:

- Are you currently under the supervision of a health care provider for a medical condition?
- What diseases have you experienced, beginning with childhood?
- Have you ever been hospitalized? If so, tell me why, when, for how long?
- Have you been told you have any diseases that are not curable?
- Have you experienced any complications (sequelae) from diseases or injuries?
- Do you have any disabilities or special needs? If so, please describe.
- Have you ever been involved in an accident in which you were injured? If so, please describe.
- Have you ever had a blood transfusion? If so, when and where?
- Has any disease or injury affected your ability to lead a normal life?
- Have you ever suffered from any mental illnesses, such as depression?

Medications

It is necessary to obtain a complete medication history for every patient. The medication history must include both prescription and nonprescription, or over-the-counter (OTC), medications that the patient may be taking. It is important to get the name, dose, and dosage times for each medication and why the patient is taking that particular medication.

While obtaining the medication history from the patient, the nurse can determine from the responses of the patient how much he knows about the medication regime. The more complete and precise the obtained answers, the greater the indication that the patient has a comprehensive understanding of his medications. It also is important during this time to determine if the patient is taking any home remedies, vitamins, or herbs. Because many medications have the potential for reacting adversely when taken simultaneously, it is important to have a complete and accurate medication history from the patient. General questions about the safe handling of medications also are important to ascertain. Consider these sample questions:

- How long do you save unused drugs and are you aware of discard dates?
- How do you dispose of unused, outdated drugs?
- Where do you keep or store your medications?
- Do you check to see if the medication needs refrigeration?
- Do you take the entire prescription of antibiotics when prescribed?
- Do you share medications or needles with anyone?

Family History

Obtaining a detailed family history from the patient is important because this history can serve as a predictor of potential health problems that the patient may encounter later in life. If, for example, the family history reveals that the parents and all of the siblings have diabetes, the nurse could then question the patient about potential signs and symptoms of diabetes; weight loss, hunger, frequent urination.

Because many conditions occur more frequently in specific ethnic backgrounds, the family history must also include information about the ethnic background. Examples include thalassemia in Southeast Asian's and Tay-Sachs in Ashkenazi Jewish populations (Gene Clinics, 2008). Some familial illnesses do not occur in every generation; therefore, it is important to ask the patient about relatives in other generations. Typical questions that will illicit the needed information include the following:

- Please tell me about your family members and their health, including your spouse, children, siblings, parents, aunts, uncles, and grandparents.
- Do any of these individuals have medical illnesses or diseases? If so, what are they?
- Have there been any deaths in the immediate family? If so, what was the cause?
- How old were your relatives when they died and what was the cause?

Psychosocial History

Assessing behaviors of the patient during the health assessment will give the nurse *cues* to the patient's sense of self-esteem. Assessing the patient's dress, body language, and tone of voice during the interview can aid the nurse in determining the patient's emotional state at that particular time. Note, however, that the nurse must be careful not to formulate a conclusion based solely on one factor such as how the patient dressed for the interview; instead any conclusions should be based on a variety of factors. The nurse will assess for presence of eye contact during the interview and posture while seated: Was it relaxed or did the patient appear tense? Did the patient show signs of anxiety about answering the health assessment questions?

The psychosocial history includes information about the patient's occupational history, level of education, financial history, familial roles, relationships and interdependent relationships, cultural identity, and self-concept. The information gathered regarding a patient's occupational history, level of education, and financial history will alert the nurse to possible health risks both present and future. For example, a patient who is of low socioeconomic status may work in jobs that have actual or potential health hazards associated with them such as a farmworker who has worked in the fields and has been exposed to prolonged ultraviolet radiation from the sun and pesticides used on the crops.

By obtaining information regarding the patient's level of education, the nurse will gain insight into whether the patient can read and understand prescriptions or instructions given to her by a health care provider. Questions regarding the patient's financial background will give the nurse opportunities to determine the patient's health-seeking behaviors. For example, a patient who is financially secure often will have an established health care provider who is seen on a regular basis versus a patient who may be working two or more low-paying jobs and is without basic health coverage and who only seeks health care when ill.

In determining the patient's perception of role and family identity, the nurse might ask, "Is there someone significant in your life?" This "support" person may be a spouse, significant other, or a trusted friend. At this time, the nurse then can ask about siblings and other family members that the patient may be close to. Depending on the patient's chronological age, the list of significant family members may be lengthy or very short if the person is in the later stages of life. The nurse needs to inquire about the presence of family and the patient's level of participation in family life.

A patient's self-concept can be elicited by such open-ended questions as "How are you feeling about yourself?" or "Where do you see yourself in the next five years?" By gathering subjective and objective data to either support or refute a patient's perception of his self-concept, the nurse can determine if the patient has a good or a distorted view. An example would be a patient who states verbally that he has a good self-concept, yet his appearance is unkempt, he is poorly dressed, he does not maintain eye contact with the nurse, and he is slouched down in the chair during the screening interview. All of these observable signs will point toward a person who has a low self-concept. When patients have a positive self-concept, they often will have coping mechanisms in place to deal with stressors in their lives. A leading question by the nurse can be "How do you handle stress?"

Sexuality also is another component of a person's self-concept. Patients who are in a committed relationship and have a strong self-concept usually will report that their sexuality is complete or strong. The issue of sexuality is a delicate topic that patients may be reluctant to talk about, so it is important for the nurse to establish a very trusting and supportive rapport with the patient before attempting to discuss issues pertaining to sexuality. Once a level of trust and rapport has been established between the nurse and patient, such open-ended questions as "Are you dating?" or "Are you and your spouse engaging in sexual intimacy on a regular basis?" can be asked of the patient.

One final question that the nurse is required to ask of patients is whether or not they have been at risk for abuse. This may be difficult for a patient to answer if a family member or spouse is in the exam room with the patient. For this question, the nurse may need to ask the question while performing the physical exam or while alone with the patient and the patient is able to be more forthright when answering.

Stress and Coping

Stress is a physical or psychological stressor and coping is the individual's physical and emotional response to the stressor. Stress is not the event itself, but the meaning of the event to the individual. What may be a stressor for one person is not for another. The immediate physical response to acute stress is the fight-or-flight response, which is due to catecholamine release. This produces a variety of manifestations such as sweaty palms and a pounding heart. The manifestations of long-term stress are different, including habitually cold hands and suppressed immune function. Emotional reactions may include difficulty sleeping, inability to concentrate, and anxiety.

The nurse should assess the patient for the physical signs of stress including:

- Increased and pounding heart rate
- Decreased blood clotting time
- Increased rate and depth of respirations
- Dilated pupils
- Elevated glucose levels
- Dilated skeletal blood vessels
- Elevated blood pressure.

Stress in and of itself is not always bad and in fact can be a motivator to enhance performance. It is the coping skills or strategies that an individual uses that determine the impact and long-term effect. Coping is a learned behavior that develops over a person's lifetime. Chapter 12 💿 provides a complete discussion of stress and adaptation.

Cultural Beliefs and Practices

When inquiring about the patient's cultural identity, the nurse can open with a leading question such as "What culture do you identify with most?" Cultural identity can determine how patients view themselves and how they seek health services. Patients who identify themselves as Hispanic may have a strong sense of family and will be guided by familial desires when making health care decisions. Hispanics may also have a strong sense of spirituality and will resort to prayer for their concerns. Patients' ethnic identities might also influence their dietary habits. For example, many Asian cultures will have rice as a component with each meal.

Most Americans, when ill, seek out a health care practitioner and then comply with the traditional "Western medicine" approach to treatment. As the influx of emigrants from countries where the traditional Western model of medicine is foreign increases, it is important for the nurse to assess what health-seeking beliefs and behaviors the patient may favor. For example, when a Southeast Asian patient is ill, it is a common practice for the family to perform a "coining" ritual by rubbing a coin forcefully over the person's body in order to rid them of the spirit causing the ailment. Chinese emigrants may use herbalists to treat many ailments. Those of the Hispanic cultures may use a *curandera* (folk healer) to cast the evil from the body of the ill person.

Some leading questions that the nurse can use to determine if a patient uses alternative forms of medicine to treat illnesses are:

- Do you use any cultural or religious practices to treat illnesses?
- Do you use any home remedies to treat illnesses?
- Do you use any holistic remedies, such as meditation, yoga, or herbs, to treat illnesses?

It is then necessary to document any alternative practices that the patient may use on the health assessment (Spector, 2004).

National standards for culturally and linguistically appropriate services (CLAS) have been issued by the DHHS's Office of Minority Health. These standards are aimed at helping individuals who enter the health care system receive equitable and effective treatment in a culturally and linguistically appropriate manner.

Spiritual Beliefs

As nurses continually strive to assist patients and families with their health needs, they must also attend to their spiritual needs, because one cannot truly assess a patient/family without assessing its spirituality (Tanyi, 2006). The purpose of obtaining information about spiritual beliefs is to better understand the patient and the impact, if any, that these beliefs have on their health. As the interview is being conducted, the nurse should be alert for spiritual clues. For example, if the patient says she is a vegetarian (Hindu) or her hair has never been cut (women: Orthodox Jews), it is a good time to inquire about the basis for these practices.

While obtaining the spiritual history, the nurse should also inquire about an advance directive (living will or durable medical power of attorney). The patient's answer may involve spiritual beliefs. An example would be a patient who believes that it is up to God to decide when he dies, not anyone else.

Components of the Physical Assessment

Prior to conducting the physical assessment, the nurse should make sure that the examination area allows for privacy and the physical environment is comfortable and conducive to developing a rapport with the patient. For example, the temperature in the area should be at a comfortable level; lighting should be sufficient to see, but not glaring; distracting objects should be removed; the noise level should not be loud or distracting; and the room should be large enough to allow for 4 or 5 feet of space between the nurse and the patient.

In reviewing the body systems, a head-to-toe approach is one method used for obtaining data about each body system. Usually this is done by asking the patient a series of questions from a preprinted questionnaire regarding each body system. The assessment questionnaire will include a review of biophysical systems such as integument, head and neck, respiratory, cardiovascular, musculoskeletal, neurological, genitourinary (female/male), and reproductive (female/male).

Finally, it is important for the nurse to consider the age of the patient when performing a physical assessment. For example, aging patients' body weight will decrease during their 70s and 80s, and the distribution of fat changes with the subcutaneous fat being lost in the face and forearms and additional fat deposited in the abdomen.

Functional Assessment

The functional assessment uses observation to gather data while the patient is performing common or routine activities (D'Amico & Barbarito, 2007). As a part of the general survey, the nurse will observe such things as how patients enter the exam room; their dress, how they seat themselves and their arm movements when straightening their clothing once seated; their hand gestures while talking; and facial expressions and facial symmetry. All of the above will be interpreted by the nurse as she begins to formulate assessment data on this patient.

Physical Assessment

In conducting the physical assessment, the nurse starts with a general survey that begins at the time he first encounters the patient and then moves on to a specific examination of the body systems. The general survey is one in which the nurse observes the patient while performing the interview (described earlier) during the health assessment (Rhodes, 2006). As the nurse is asking questions, he is observing the patient and formulating a mental picture of the patient. The nurse can observe any distinguishing features such as presence or absence of facial hair in an adult male (secondary sex characteristics). During this time, the nurse will observe all that can be seen, heard, or smelled while conducting the interview. This will then set the course for the nurse when performing the physical examination. The major components of the survey are physical appearance, nutritional status, mental status, mobility, and behavior of the patient.

Physical Appearance

By looking at the patient, the nurse can formulate various facts related to the patient. If the patient looks older than her stated age, this is an important observation. The patient who appears emaciated suggests intentional or unintentional weight loss, which could be related to an underlying pathology. By looking at the patient, body symmetry can be ascertained. Does the patient's upper and lower torso have the same distance from head to pelvis as pelvis to feet? Does the patient's head appear to be in proportion to the rest of her body? By observing body shape and size, the nurse can determine whether there could be any potential disorders such as overeating or anorexia.

Nutritional Assessment

A component of the health assessment is a nutrition assessment. Such leading questions as "How many meals do you normally eat each day?" "What time do you eat your last meal of the day?" and "Do you have any dietary restrictions?" will give the nurse some insight into the patient's dietary habits. A more reliable nutrition assessment is obtained, however, by having the patient fill out a journal of the eating times and amount and type of food eaten for a 3-day period. This requires that the patient be able to write and makes the assumption that he will be honest in keeping and recording the food diary. This technique requires a subsequent visit by the patient so the diary can be added to his health assessment. Nutrition is discussed in detail in Chapter 14 ⊕.

Mental Status

The nurse can assess the patient's mental status while the patient is responding to the various questions during the health history.

While asking the health questions, the nurse will be noting the patient's affect, mood, and demeanor. At this time the nurse will be able to determine if the patient is oriented to person, place, and time by virtue of how the patient responds to the questions. If the patient appears confused, the nurse can further determine the patient's mental status by asking such questions as "Do you know what day it is today?" or "What time is it?" If the patient has difficulty answering these questions, then the nurse will need to conduct a more detailed work-up.

Mobility

The nurse can observe how the patient moves when the patient enters the office area: Are the patient's movements fluid and purposeful? Is her posture erect and is she moving with a steady stride? The nurse can observe for deviations in movement and assess whether or not the patient has full range of motion in her extremities. An elderly female with advanced osteoporosis may walk with a "stooped over" posture and it may appear that the patient is having pain or is laboring to perform movements. Relative to mobility, the nurse also observes whether the patient is using any ambulatory aids such as a walker, cane, wheelchair, leg braces, or special orthotic shoes.

Behavior

The nurse can observe the patient's affect and response to questions. Is it an appropriate response, or does the patient under- or overreact to the situation. For example, if the patient is telling the nurse about the death of someone close, is there an emotional response? Lack of an appropriate response referred to as "flat affect" and should be documented in the medical record. At the other end of the spectrum, is the patient overreacting or visibly uncomfortable with unemotional queries.

Measuring Height and Weight

Height and weight are measured by the nurse as a means of obtaining baseline data about the patient. In obtaining the actual height and weight, the nurse can account for any differences in what the patient may have subjectively told the nurse during the health questioning.

The most common method of obtaining an adult patient's height and weight is with the platform scale. Once the weight is obtained, the patient turns with his back to the scale. The nurse then slides a height bar up above his head, folds out the right-angled arm and lowers it until it barely touches the patient's head, and takes the height measurement.

Many standard height and weight charts for both men and women have been developed by insurance companies and the DHHS. The nurse should make sure to use the chart that is approved by her health system. A common measure of weight to height is the body mass index (BMI). BMI is a person's weight in kilograms divided by the square of his height in meters giving a measure of kg/m^2. The BMI ranges are as follows:

- Normal range: <18.5– 24.9
- Overweight: 25.0–29.9
- Obese: >30.

Weight as it is related to cardiac risk factors is discussed in Chapter 40 ⊕.

Measuring Vital Signs

Temperature, pulse, respirations, blood pressure, and pain level are the **vital signs** that the nurse will measure during the health assessment. Temperature is often obtained with an electronic thermometer and recorded in either degrees Fahrenheit or Celsius. The most common route for obtaining a temperature is via the oral cavity. Other routes are rectal, axillary (under the arm), and tympanic (ear).

Obtaining the pulse of the adult patient is most commonly done by palpating the radial artery and counting the pulse for 15 seconds and then multiplying by 4 to arrive at a 60-second pulse rate. During the assessment the apical, bilateral radial, and bilateral pedal pulses are evaluated (Figure 9–2 ■). At the same time that the nurse is recording the pulse rate, he will also be assessing the character of the patient's pulses for such descriptors as

weak, thready, bounding, regular, or irregular. If there are irregularities in the pulse rate, then the nurse should check the pulse rate for a full 60 seconds to get an accurate pulse rate. Abnormalities related to the pulse are discussed in Chapter 37 ⊘.

The respiratory rate is usually obtained while obtaining the pulse rate. Once the nurse has obtained the pulse rate, she will observe the patient's chest movement and count the number of times the patient inhales in a 15-second interval and again multiply this by 4 to achieve a 1-minute respiratory rate. The nurse should also be observing the character and movement of the patient's chest while obtaining the respiratory rate. She will be observing for a rhythmic inhalation and exhalation and for nasal flaring or use of accessory muscles in taking a breath. A more detailed examination of the patient's breathing will occur when auscultating the lungs with a stethoscope. The detailed respiratory examination is further explained in Chapter 33 ⊘.

The blood pressure is obtained by using a cuff, sphygmomanometer, and a stethoscope. The patient is placed in a sitting position. It is important for the nurse to select a cuff that is the appropriate size for the circumference of the patient's upper arm. The width of the cuff should equal 40% of the circumference of the extremity used, and the length of the cuff should equal 80% of the circumference. Using a cuff that is too narrow will give a falsely high blood pressure. The nurse must also palpate the brachial artery (Figure 9–2 ■) and align the arrows of the cuff so that they are over the artery.

Once the cuff is secure on the patient, the nurse places the bell of the stethoscope over the area where he palpated the brachial pulse. Slowly the nurse begins to inflate the cuff by squeezing the bulb and listening for the brachial pulse to be obliterated. A standard is to pump the cuff to 30 mm over the number where the pulse was first lost. The nurse then slowly releases the pressure and observes the needle of the manometer, which should be decreasing at a rate of about 2 to 3 mmHg per second. The nurse notes the manometer readings while listening. The first sound and corresponding number on the manometer will be the systolic measurement, and the last sound and corresponding number will be the diastolic measurement. Once the diastolic reading has been obtained, the nurse releases the pressure from the cuff, removes the cuff from the patient's arm, and records the findings. Abnormalities related to blood pressure are discussed in Chapters 21, 40, and 61 ⊘.

Pain

The assessment of pain, often referred to as the fifth vital sign, is essential for the nurse to obtain with each assessment of the patient (D'Amico & Barbarito, 2007). The presence of pain—whether acute or chronic, severe or mild—is a subjective experience solely unique to that individual. A pain history includes the following data:

- *Location:* The nurse asks the patient to point to the location of the pain source. Often the nurse will also use a body diagram and ask the patient to use the diagram to locate the pain. The nurse then identifies the locus of the pain using the nearest anatomic landmarks (e.g., sharp pain in right patellar region posterior and medial).

- *Intensity:* The nurse asks the patient to rate the level of pain that she is experiencing using a pain scale. For most adults, a

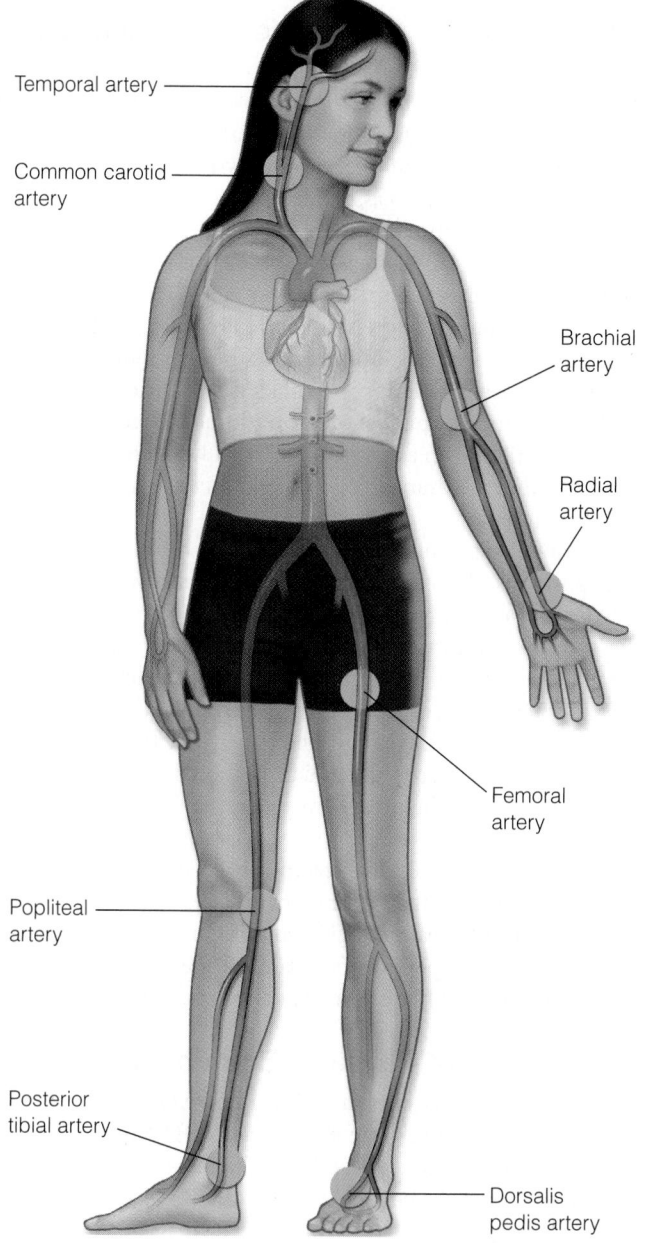

Temporal artery

Common carotid artery

Brachial artery

Radial artery

Femoral artery

Popliteal artery

Posterior tibial artery

Dorsalis pedis artery

FIGURE 9–2 ■ Apical, bilateral radial, and bilateral pedal pulse locations.
Source: From D'Amico, Barbarito, Health and Physical Assessment in Nursing (2007). Pearson Education. pp. 115 Figure 7.10

numerical pain scale of 0 to 10 can be used where 0 is no pain and 10 is the highest level of pain.

- *Quality:* Asking the patient to describe the pain as either dull, throbbing, sharp, piercing, aching, etc., gives the nurse a sense of the quality of the pain that the patient is experiencing. When using the patient's exact words to describe the quality of the pain, the nurse puts the patient's words in quotation marks.

- *Pattern:* The onset and duration of pain is noted as the pattern. The nurse assesses whether the pain is constant or intermittent. If the pain is intermittent, the nurse also asks about duration, that is, when the pain subsides and returns. Again, the nurse records the patient's response in the narrative.

- *Precipitating factors:* The nurse attempts to learn from the patient what brings on the pain. A precipitating factor could be, for example, ascending three flights of stairs (after which the patient experiences substernal chest pain).

- *Relief methods:* Along with assessing for the presence of pain, the nurse also asks the patient what she has done to attempt to relieve the pain. Here the nurse lists all prescription treatments and OTC remedies that the patient may have utilized, as well as any alternative health providers such as an herbalist, massage therapist, chiropractor, or acupuncturist. The nurse also notes which of these methods has helped in relieving the pain and for how long (duration).

- *Impact on ADLs:* By assessing how the pain is impacting the patient's ability to perform her ADLs, the nurse can obtain a clearer picture of how the pain may be affecting this particular patient and ultimately the quality of her life.

- *Coping strategies:* Coping strategies include yoga, meditation, relaxation exercises, prayer, support groups, or withdrawal. Each of these strategies is unique to the individual patient and will also be a reflection of the patient's age, culture, and belief system.

Refer to Chapter 15 for a thorough discussion of pain.

Documentation of the Health History

In the acute care setting, specific forms or page screens on an electronic medical record (EMR) help guide the nurse in documentation of the health history. Figure 9–3 ■ shows examples of EMR screens for documentation of a health history in the acute care setting. Of note is the importance of documenting *who* is answering the questions. Detailed information on documentation is discussed in Chapter 6 .

■ Physical Examination

There are two types of physical exams. The **comprehensive exam** (head-to-toe exam) is usually performed on new patients who will be seen on a routine basis by various clinicians. A **focused exam** is performed in emergent or urgent situations and is focused on a specific problem (Rhodes, 2006). Regardless of the type of exam to be done, an organized and systematic examination is necessary to obtain pertinent data in the shortest amount of time. An organized approach creates trust and encourages the cooperation of the patient. The information that was gathered during the health history will help to guide aspects of the physical examination. At all times during the exam, the patient's physical

and psychological comfort is taken into consideration. It is important to explain all aspects of the examination to the patient; this will enhance the patient's experience and decrease his anxiety during the examination.

Incorporating the head-to-toe examination into a nurse's routine takes practice and repeated examinations in order for the process to flow in a natural manner that is comfortable to both the nurse and the patient (Rhodes, 2006). It is important for the nurse to develop a routine that will become comfortable and will not omit any pertinent data during the examination. Expertise comes with practice, and the ability to interpret findings develops with experience. There is no one correct way to perform the head-to-toe examination. The main goal is to have a sequence that flows smoothly and allows for patient comfort and privacy. The examination of specific systems is discussed in detail throughout the book in each unit's assessment chapter.

Preparation for the Physical Examination

The environment where the physical examination is to take place must be private, quiet, and a comfortable temperature. The room needs to have adequate lighting. The nurse needs to use standard precautions throughout the entire physical examination. The equipment should all be assembled in the room prior to the beginning of the examination. It is helpful to assemble the equipment in order of use. Figure 9–4 ■ (p. 162) shows the instruments used for a physical examination.

The patient must be prepared both physically and psychologically for the physical examination. Before beginning, ask the patient if she needs to empty her bladder. If a urine specimen is needed, instruct the patient on the technique for collection. Provide the patient with a gown and instruct her to remove all necessary clothing. A drape is left in the room to be used during the examination.

During the examination the patient will have to assume various positions to facilitate the assessment and will need to be draped properly with each position change (Figure 9–5 ■, p. 163). Be sure to consider any limitations the patient may have that would prevent the usual positioning. These include arthritis, weakness, fractures, or joint deformities.

To psychologically prepare the patient for the examination, the nurse should assume a calm, professional demeanor and explain each step of the process in general understandable terms. Be sensitive to any discomfort created by exposing various parts of the body. Be culturally sensitive when dealing with people from cultures other than your own. In some cultures women are restricted from revealing their bodies to males other than their husbands. When a person of the same gender is requested for an examination, if at all possible, that request should be honored.

Techniques of Physical Examination

During the physical examination the nurse will utilize each of his senses while examining the patient. Such techniques as inspection, palpation, percussion, and auscultation are implemented to objectively assess the patient (Rhodes, 2006).

Inspection

Inspection is the deliberate, systematic examination of the patient using both sight and smell. It begins with the first encounter and continues the entire time the nurse is with the

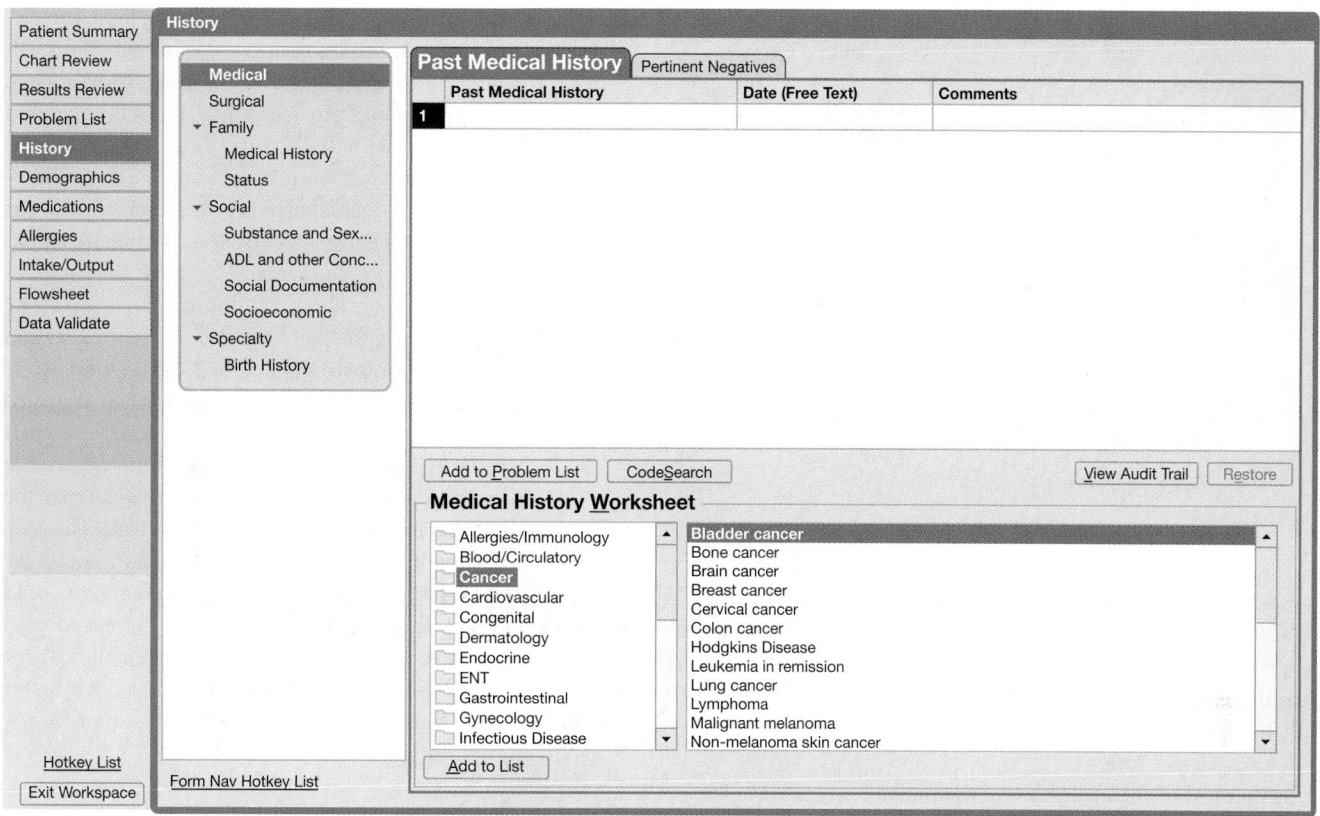

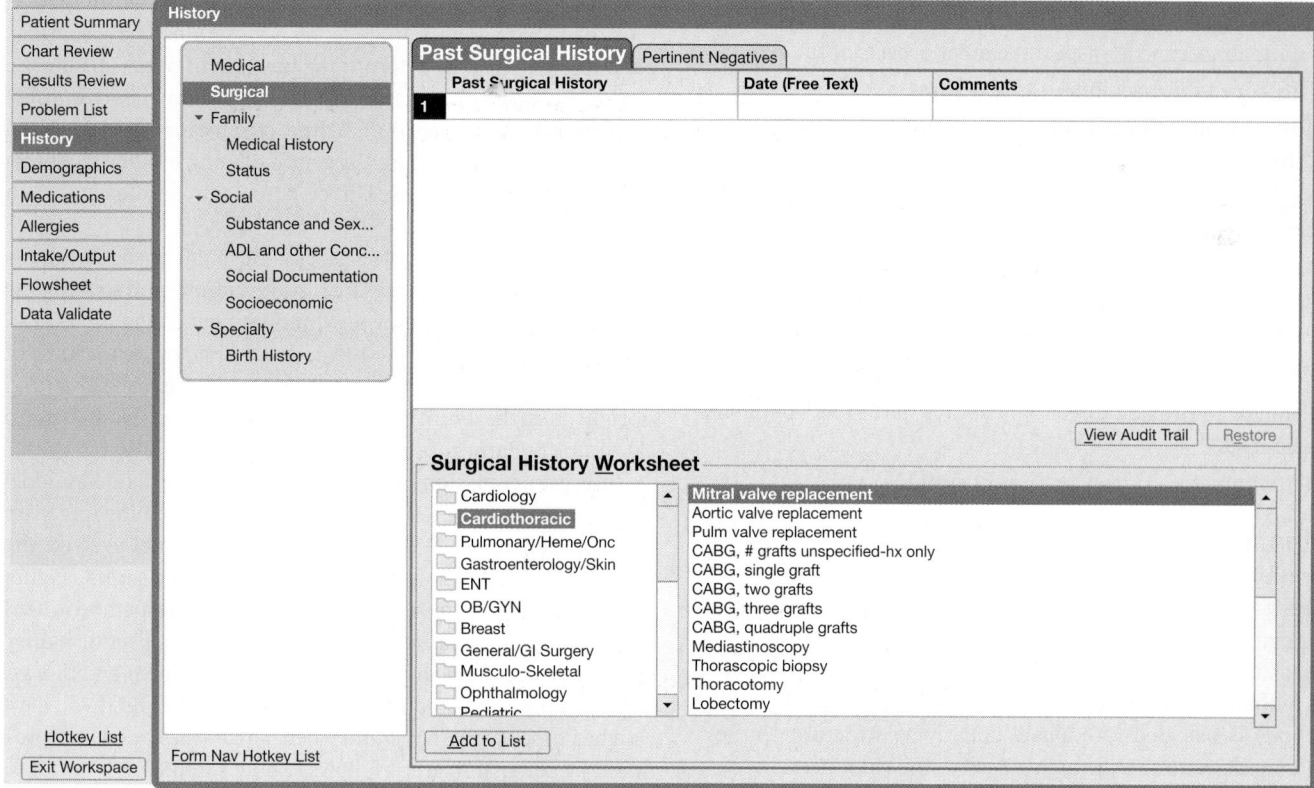

FIGURE 9–3 ■ Past medical history.

patient. The nurse observes gait, mannerisms, stature, and other physical attributes. The inspection begins by assessing the patient's appearance and comparing the right and left side of the body for symmetry. Inspection of each region of the body includes observing color, warmth, size, symmetry, contour, move-

ment, or drainage (D'Amico & Barbarito, 2007). For example, the color of the nail beds and the temperature of the fingers are assessed on each side and then a comparison of the right versus left is done. Under normal conditions the finger temperature and nail bed color are the same in both hands. A cold dusky blue

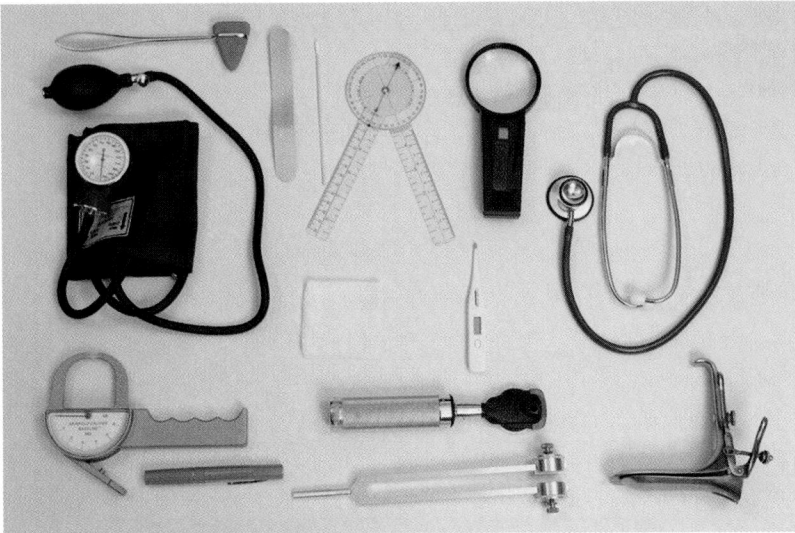

FIGURE 9–4 ■ Equipment used for physical assessment.
Source: From D'Amico, Barbarito, Health and Physical Assessment in Nursing (2007). Pearson Education. pp. 101 Table 6.1

appearance of only one hand indicates a problem with the blood supply to that area. The nurse also should note any unusual odor and determine its cause.

During most of the inspection of the patient, no instruments are needed, but some parts of the assessment require special tools that will assist the nurse. The instruments include the following:

- Ophthalmoscope to inspect the inner aspects of the eye
- Otoscope to inspect inner ear structures
- Tongue blade to inspect the inside of the mouth, tongue, and throat
- Vaginal speculum to dilate the vaginal canal and inspect the cervix
- Vision chart to test near- and farsightedness
- Stethoscope to listen to lungs, bowel sounds, and blood pressure
- Blood pressure cuff
- Penlight to provide direct light source and to test pupillary responses
- Thermometer to check body temperature

Palpation

Palpation uses touch in order to collect data to determine specific characteristics of the body (Rhodes, 2006). Such characteristics as temperature, texture, moisture, tenderness, pain, vibrations, and edema are assessed using palpation. Additionally, the size, shape, and mobility of a body part can be palpated. Each specific area of the body is palpated to evaluate underlying structures, pulses, lymph nodes, and specific organs such as the kidney and liver.

In palpating, the nurse will use the fingertips, finger pads, base of the fingers, palmar surface of the fingers, and the dorsal and ulnar surfaces of the hands (D'Amico & Barbarito, 2007) (Figure 9–6 ■, p. 164). The nurse's hand is moved slowly and intentionally and discomfort can be minimized by warming the hands, having nails cut short, and not wearing any jewelry. Gloves may be worn when there are open or exposed areas. When using latex gloves it is necessary to ask patients if they have any allergies to latex.

Palpation is characterized as being light, moderate, or deep. The nurse always begins with light palpation and culminates with deep palpation to evaluate such organ structures as the kidney and liver. The use of light palpation first will aid the nurse in assessing the texture, temperature, and any painful or reddened area on the surface of the patient's skin (Figure 9–7 ■, p. 164). Moderate palpation is used to assess major areas of the patient's anatomy especially the abdominal organs. The nurse will use the palmar aspect of the fingers and gently press down about 1 to 2 centimeters while rotating the fingers in a circular motion (D'Amico & Barbarito, 2007) (Figure 9–8 ■, p. 164). Deep palpation is used by the nurse to assess an organ that lies deep within the abdominal cavity, such as the liver and or kidneys (Figure 9–9 ■, p. 164). The level of palpation is usually 2 to 4 cm. The nurse must explain the procedure to the patient because deep palpation could cause some discomfort if the patient already experienced pain upon light to moderate palpation. It is important for the patient to be relaxed during palpation of the soft tissue areas. It is better to use the dominant hand when possible because it is more sensitive than the nondominant one.

Percussion

Percussion is the creation of sound vibrations by pushing, tapping, or using a device to generate a vibration. The vibrations produced will help in determining position of organ structures. The three types of percussion are direct, blunt, and indirect (D'Amico & Barbarito, 2007). **Direct percussion**, used to examine such areas as the sinuses, is gentle tapping to illicit the presence or absence of fluid. Direct percussion results in a dull sound (Figure 9–10 ■, p. 164).

Blunt percussion involves placing the palm of the nondominant hand over a body area (such as the kidney) and striking the palm with the closed fist of the dominant hand (Figure 9–11 ■, p. 165). This method is used to assess for pain or tenderness of the liver, gallbladder, or kidneys. The patient is usually sitting upright and the blunt percussion is performed from behind (D'Amico & Barbarito, 2007).

Indirect percussion involves using the hyperextended middle finger of the nondominant hand (pleximeter) and the finger tip of the middle finger of the dominant hand (plexor) to strike the pleximeter by using a wrist action that will elicit a sound (Figure 9–12 ■, p. 165) (D'Amico & Barbarito, 2007). This method is used to determine the location of an organ such as the liver or kidney and also to determine fluid air levels in the abdomen and thorax. Organs will produce a dull sound, whereas air and fluid will have a higher, more tympanic sound when percussed. The sounds produced by percussion are as follows (Rhodes, 2006):

- **Tympany** is a high-pitched, drum-like tone of medium duration. It is commonly heard over the air-filled intestines.
- **Resonance** is a loud hollow tone of long duration. It is commonly heard over the lungs.
- **Hyperresonance** is a loud low tone with a longer duration than resonance. It is heard when air is trapped in a space such as the lungs.

POSITION	AREAS EXAMINED	RATIONALE	CONTRAINDICATIONS
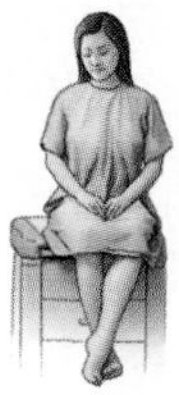 Sitting	Vital signs, head and neck, back, posterior and anterior thorax and lungs, breasts, axillae, heart, upper and lower extremities, reflexes	Sitting upright allows for full lung expansion and better visualization of upper body symmetry.	Older and weak clients may be unable to sit without support. An alternate position is supine with the head of the bed elevated.
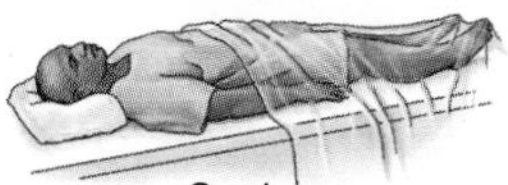 Supine	Vital signs, head and neck, anterior thorax and lungs, breasts, axillae, heart, abdomen, extremities, peripheral pulses	This is a relaxed position for most clients. It provides access to pulse sites and prevents contracture of abdominal muscles, especially if a small pillow is placed under the knees.	Clients with cardiovascular and respiratory problems may be unable to lie flat without becoming short of breath. An alternate position is to raise the head of the bed. Clients with lower back pain may be unable to lie flat without flexing the knees.
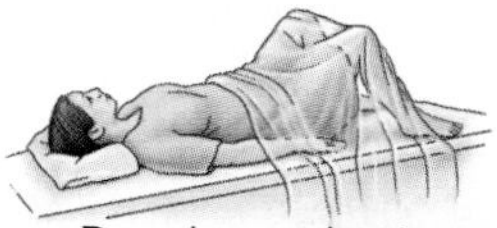 Dorsal recumbent	Abdomen and external genitalia	Flexed knees reduce tension on lower back and abdominal muscles and increase client comfort.	Same as for supine. The client should not raise the arms over the head or clasp the hands behind the head because this increases contraction of the abdominal muscles.
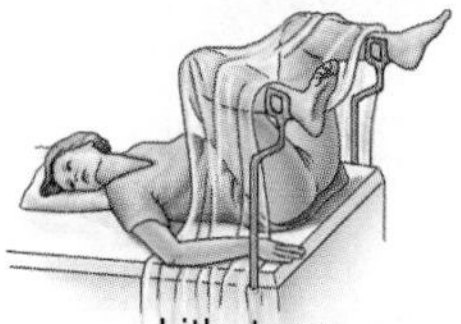 Lithotomy	Female genitalia, reproductive tract, and rectum	This position maximally exposes the genitalia and facilitates the insertion of a vaginal speculum.	This position is assumed immediately before it is needed because it is embarrassing and uncomfortable. The client is kept draped. Clients with arthritis or joint deformity may be unable to assume this position. Alternate positions are dorsal recumbent and Sims'.
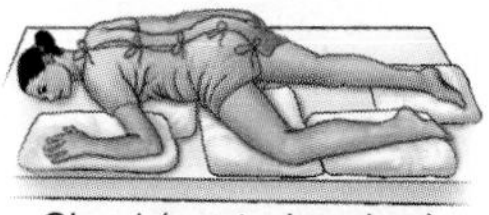 Sims' (posterior view)	Rectum, vagina	Flexion of the upper hip and knee improves exposure of the rectal area.	Clients with deformities of the hip or knee may be unable to assume this position. Older and obese clients may be uncomfortable.
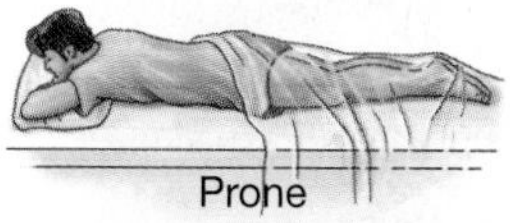 Prone	Posterior thorax, hip movement, popliteal pulses	This position is used to assess hip extension. Sometimes popliteal pulse palpation is facilitated in this position.	This position is not well tolerated by older clients or clients with cardiovascular or respiratory problems.
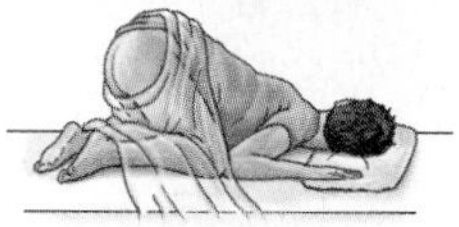 Knee-chest	Rectum, prostate	This position provides maximal exposure of the anal and rectal areas and facilitates insertion of instruments into the rectum.	Poorly tolerated by clients with cardiovascular or respiratory problems. Clients with difficulty flexing hips or knees may be unable to assume this position.
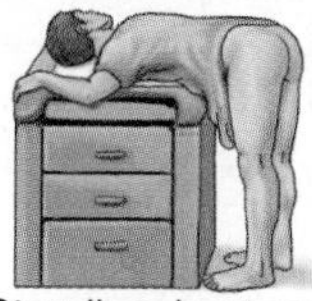 Standing, bent over examining table	Rectum, prostate	This is a more comfortable position than knee-chest and allows for palpation of the prostate gland.	This position is assumed immediately before it is needed because it is embarrassing. Clients with back problems may need assistance.

FIGURE 9–5 ■ Patient positioning during physical examination.

- **Dullness** is a high-pitched tone of short duration and is soft in quality. It is heard over the large organs such as the liver and kidney.
- **Flatness** is a soft, high-pitched tone with a short duration. It is heard over muscle and bone.

Percussion sounds have characteristic features that the nurse must become familiar with through experience and practice. These features include intensity, pitch, duration, and quality. *Intensity* is the amplitude or the loudness and softness of the sound. The intensity is influenced by the amount of air and the ability of the structure to vibrate. *Pitch* refers to the frequency of vibrations of sound per second. Slow vibrations produce a low-pitched sound, whereas fast vibrations produced a high-pitched sound. The length of time that the sound can be heard is referred to as *duration*, and it can be very short to very long. *Quality* refers to the type of sound and is described as clear, hollow, muffled, or dull (D'Amico & Barbarito, 2007).

Auscultation

Auscultation is the technique of listening to body sounds (Rhodes, 2006). The nurse must use both the unassisted sense of hearing and, where needed, a stethoscope. Body sounds that can be heard unassisted include speech, coughing, respirations, and the percussion tones just described. The stethoscope (Figure 9–4 ■) is used to assess the lungs, heart, and abdomen. The stethoscope

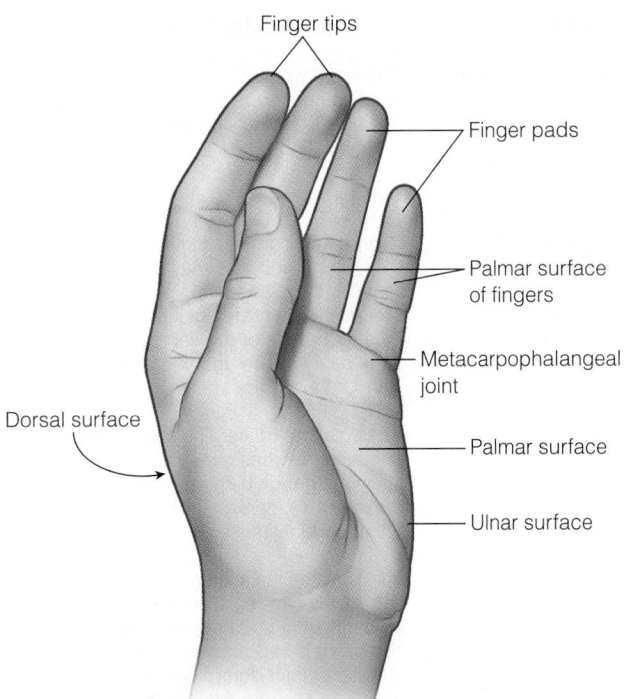

FIGURE 9–6 ■ Palpation.
Source: From D'Amico, Barbarito, Health and Physical Assessment in Nursing (2007). Pearson Education. pp. 97 Figure 6.2

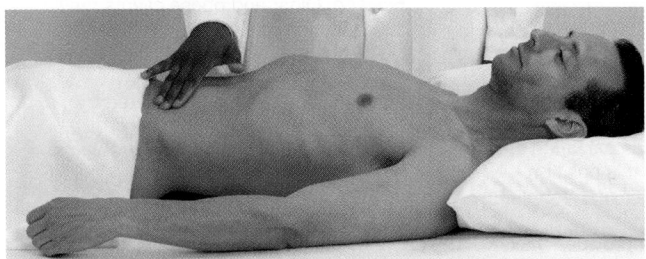

FIGURE 9–7 ■ Light palpation.
Source: From D'Amico, Barbarito, Health and Physical Assessment in Nursing (2007). Pearson Education. pp. 97 Figure 6.3

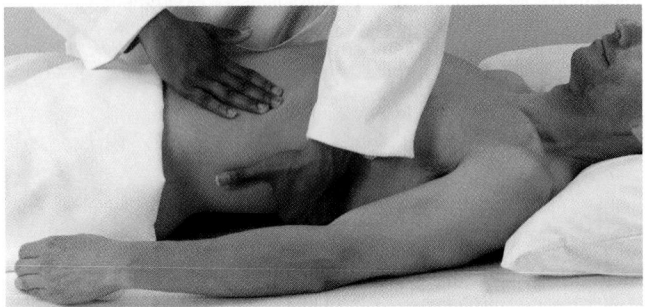

FIGURE 9–8 ■ Moderate palpation.
Source: From D'Amico, Barbarito, Health and Physical Assessment in Nursing (2007). Pearson Education. pp. 98 Figure 6.4

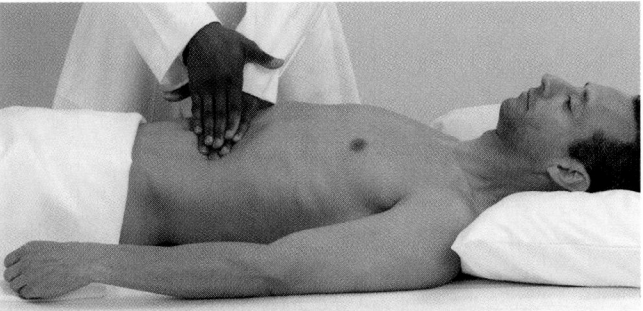

FIGURE 9–9 ■ Deep palpation.
Source: From D'Amico, Barbarito, Health and Physical Assessment in Nursing (2007). Pearson Education. pp. 98 Figure 6.5

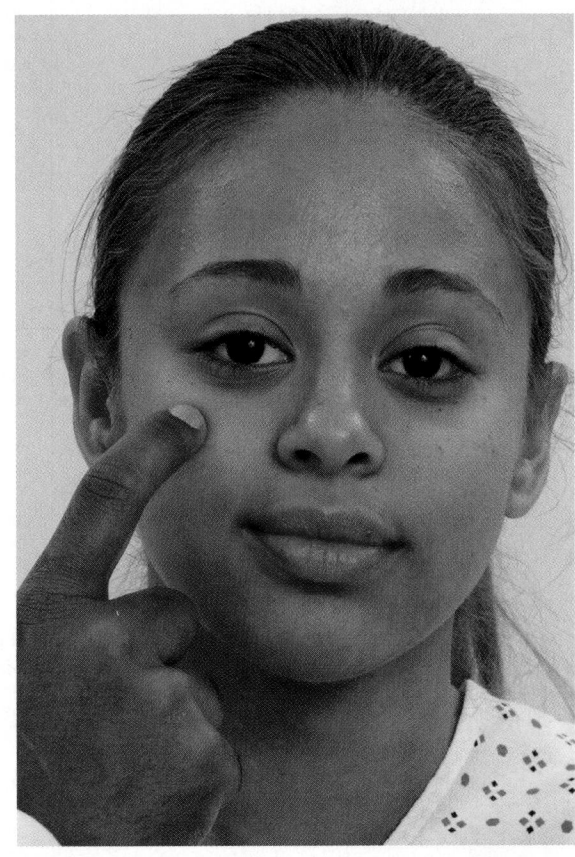

FIGURE 9–10 ■ Direct percussion.
Source: From D'Amico, Barbarito, Health and Physical Assessment in Nursing (2007). Pearson Education. pp. 99 Figure 6.6

ultrasound waves to detect sounds such as fetal heart tones and peripheral pulses. Interference with the Doppler can be eliminated by applying gel to the skin.

 CRITICAL ALERT *Do not press the bell end piece of the stethoscope into the skin. This causes the skin to act as a diaphragm and will reduce audible vibratory sensations.*

When listening with the stethoscope, the environment should be as quiet as possible. Rubbing against the patient's clothing or the bed sheets or touching the stethoscope tubing will produce sounds that will interfere with body sounds. While listening, it is important to focus on only one sound at a time. Closing the eyes often assists the nurse to focus. Sounds are described in the same terms as the percussion sounds described earlier: intensity, pitch, duration, and quality.

has two end pieces, a bell, and a diaphragm. The bell has a cuplike shape and is best for hearing low-pitched sounds, such as heart murmurs. The diaphragm or flat end piece is best for high-pitched sounds such as bowel, lung, and normal heart sounds. The diaphragm should be held firmly against the patient's skin. When sounds are very soft and difficult to hear with a normal stethoscope, a Doppler ultrasound stethoscope is useful. It uses

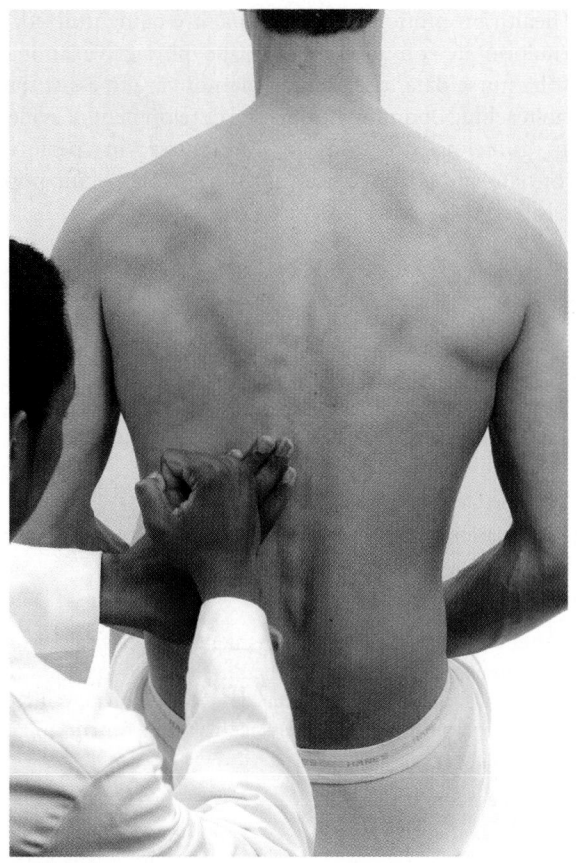

FIGURE 9–11 ■ Blunt percussion.
Source: From D'Amico, Barbarito, Health and Physical Assessment in Nursing (2007). Pearson Education. pp. 99 Figure 6.7

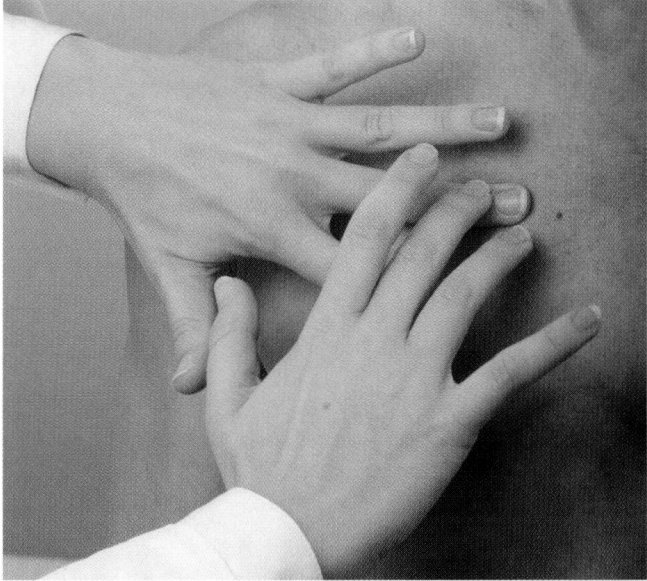

FIGURE 9–12 ■ Indirect percussion.
Source: From D'Amico, Barbarito, Health and Physical Assessment in Nursing (2007). Pearson Education. pp. 99 Figure 6.8

■ Critical Thinking

Critical thinking is a cognitive skill that is needed for every aspect of a health assessment. The nursing process provides an effective framework for applying critical thinking to patient care situations. Critical thinking helps the nurse resolve problems and develop ways to manage situations. Critical thinking requires that the nurse apply logic, question the norm, and problem solve in patient care situations. The nurse must learn to recognize the relative significance of the visual, auditory, or palpable *cues* that occur during the assessment. Cues are bits of information that may hint at the possibility of a health problem. Taking advantage of the information offered by these cues necessitates the development of critical thinking skills.

The five components of critical thinking related to health assessment include collection of information, analysis of the situation, generation of alternatives, selection of alternatives, and evaluation. *Collection of information* begins with the interview and continues throughout the entire health assessment. The collection of subjective and objective data must be done in an organized manner. As the nurse is refining assessment skills, it is helpful to develop a consistent manner in which every health assessment is conducted. For example, the nurse might always use a head-to-toe approach. This helps in both the organization of data and ensures that no piece of the assessment is missed. If the patient is in acute distress, critical thinking skills will assist the nurse to alter the assessment as appropriate to maintain patient safety. For example, if the patient is in respiratory distress, it is imperative that airway management and oxygenation be assessed first.

As the nurse is collecting data, she must verify the reliability of the information. This is done by determining the ability of the patient to be a reliable historian. The nurse should look for inconsistencies and inappropriate information. This is the component where the nurse applies logic and critically assesses information. If concerned, it is sometimes helpful to ask the same question twice during the interview, and if possible check with family members for verification (D'Amico & Barbarito, 2007).

The second skill is *analysis of the situation*. During this phase the nurse must distinguish normal from abnormal. The patient's age, gender, genetic background, and culture affect the analysis. The nurse must utilize laboratory findings, diagnostic tests, charts, and measures related to development and aging. For example, some findings may be normal for an 80-year-old male but not for a 30-year-old female. When using critical thinking skills, the nurse clusters related information to assist in identifying patterns in the information. It is at this point that the nurse identifies missing information and retrieves it (D'Amico & Barbarito, 2007).

Generation of alternatives includes identifying options and establishing priorities. It begins with identification of options and then the nurse and patient work together to establish the priorities. The nurse needs to assess the patient's understanding of the situation and provide more information about the advantages and disadvantages of each option so the patient can make an informed decision.

Once informed about options, the next step is the *selection of alternatives*. The critical thinking skills needed for this step are the ability to develop outcomes and plans. The outcome is the final result of what the patient will attain, and the plan is the activities that will lead to that outcome. Some components of the plan are developed in conjunction with the health care team, whereas others are done by the patient independently.

The last step in critical thinking is *evaluation*. Evaluation requires the nurse to determine if the expected outcomes have been achieved. Each step of critical thinking is used here to determine if any omissions or misinterpretations occurred. It is essential to ensure that decisions were based on all of the facts and that reliable recourses were used (D'Amico & Barbarito, 2007).

■ Summary

Health assessments allow the nurse to gather information regarding the patient's past and current state of health, along with health promotion behaviors that are being utilized. This information in conjunction with the physical examination gives the nurse data to develop a plan of care to assist the patient in reaching optimum health. The development of evidence-based guidelines that assist the nurse in performing appropriate and effective health histories for specific populations is key.

NCLEX® REVIEW

1. The nurse is conducting a health assessment with a newly admitted patient. Which of the following should be included in this assessment?
   1. Subjective data only
   2. Data about the patient's physical, social, cultural, environmental, and emotional statuses
   3. Objective data only
   4. The patient's adherence to *Healthy People 2010* initiatives

2. The nurse is preparing to conduct a patient interview. Which of the following should the nurse do first?
   1. Introduce him/herself.
   2. Measure the patient's vital signs.
   3. Assist the patient into a hospital gown.
   4. Address the patient including the surname.

3. During an interview, the patient asks the nurse if she thinks he has cancer. Which of the following should the nurse make in response?
   1. Probably because your hemoglobin is low and you are exsanguinating from your rectal orifice.
   2. What makes you think that you have cancer?
   3. I'm not the doctor but I will tell you this, it's a good thing you came into the hospital while you still could because you never know what they are going to find with all of their tests and procedures.
   4. What a silly thing to say! You know, if you believe you have cancer you probably do!

4. A patient walks with two canes but is stable when ambulating and changing clothes. Which of the following assessment techniques was used to collect this data?
   1. Auscultation
   2. Palpation
   3. Inspection
   4. Percussion

5. After completing a health assessment and physical examination with a patient, the nurse begins to review the information and group similar data into clusters. Which step of the critical thinking process is this nurse functioning?
   1. Analysis of the situation
   2. Generation of alternatives
   3. Selection of alternatives
   4. Evaluation

Answers for review questions appear in Appendix D

KEY TERMS

auscultation *p.163*
blunt percussion *p.162*
chief complaint *p.155*
comprehensive exam *p.160*
direct percussion *p.162*
direct question *p.152*
dullness *p.163*
flatness *p.163*

focused exam *p.160*
hyperresonance *p.162*
indirect percussion *p.162*
inspection *p.160*
leading health indicators *p.149*
metabolic equivalent level (MET) *p.149*
objective data *p.148*

open-ended questions *p.152*
palpation *p.162*
percussion *p.162*
resonance *p.162*
sequelae *p.155*
subjective data *p.148*
tympany *p.162*
vital signs *p.159*

REFERENCES

Centers for Disease Control and Prevention. (2008). *Physical activity for everyone.* Retrieved May 6, 2008 from http://www.cdc.gov/nccdphp/dnpa/physical/everyone/recommendations/index.htm

D'Amico, D., & Barbarito C. (2007). *Health and physical assessment in nursing.* Upper Saddle River, NJ: Pearson Prentice Hall.

Ewing, J. A. (1984). Detecting alcoholism: The CAGE questionnaire. *Journal of the American Medical Association, 252,* 1905–1907.

Gene Clinics. (2008). *Gene tests.* Retrieved February 3, 2008, from http://www.geneclinics.org

Kaushik, V. P., Snih, S. A., Ray, L. A., Raji, M. A., Markides, K. S., & Goodwin, J. S. (2007). Factors associated with seven-year incidence of diabetes complications among older Mexican Americans. *International Journal of Experimental, Clinical, and Behavioral Gerontology, 53*(4).

North American Nursing Diagnosis Association. (2007). *Nursing diagnoses: Definitions and classifications 2007–2008.* Philadelphia: Author.

Rhodes, J. (2006). *Advanced health assessment and diagnostic reasoning.* New York: Lippincott Williams & Wilkins.

Spector, R. E. (2004). *Cultural diversity in health and illness.* Upper Saddle River, NJ: Pearson Prentice Hall.

Tanyi, R. A. (2006). Spirituality and family nursing: Spiritual assessment and interventions for families. *Journal of Advanced Nursing, 53*(3), 287–294.

U.S. Department of Health and Human Services http://www.cdc.gov/nccdphp/dnpa/physical/everyone/recommendations/index.htm. (2000). *Healthy people 2010: Understanding and improving health.* Retrieved February 5, 2008, from http://www.healthypeople.gov

Zator-Estes, M. (2006). *Health assessment and physical examination* (3rd ed.). Clifton Park, NY: Thompson Delmar Learning.

The Aging Patient

Laurie Walsh and Annita Watson

Outcome-Based Learning Objectives

After studying this chapter, the learner will be able to:

1. Identify normal age related changes of the head, neck, respiratory, cardiovascular, gastrointestinal, genitourinary, musculoskeletal, integumentary, and neurological systems when completing a nursing assessment.

2. Explain the rationale for recommended immunizations and screening exams as proposed by the U.S. Preventive Services Task Force and as stated in the chapter for the patient over 65 years of age.

3. Discuss medications contraindicated in the aging patient as identified by the Beers criteria.

4. Recognize signs and symptoms of elder mistreatment to determine appropriate referrals.

5. Differentiate between residential, assisted living, and skilled nursing care in accordance with the type of patient care services provided.

6. Provide direction and advice to the elderly by describing available innovative housing options.

7. Explain the implications of technological advancements in providing care to the elderly.

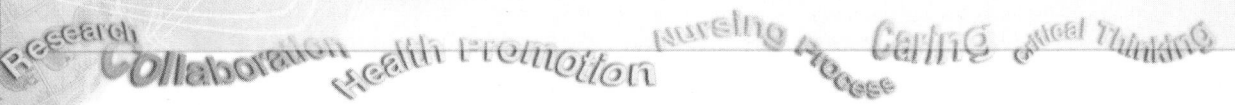

THIS CHAPTER focuses on nursing care of the aging patient, a cohort of individuals projected to represent 20% of the total population by 2030 (Experience CORPS, 2007). As this population grows it is incumbent on nursing and society as a whole to recognize this group's unique needs and provide special consideration to the care of these individuals. It is the intent of this chapter to present the distinctive characteristics of the aging population and to provide goals for care of the older adult. The chapter discusses the physiological and behavioral changes that occur with aging, methods of assessing for these changes, and available health care options including future innovations in caring for the elderly.

   Aging is defined as the process of growing old or maturing. An individual is a composite of his chronological, physiological, and functional age. Chronological age is the number of years lived. Physiological age is the determination of age by body function, and functional age is the ability to contribute to society and to benefit self and others. An elder in some cultures is an individual who has gathered wisdom over a lifetime; an individual to be respected. The legal definition of an elder is any individual 65 years of age and older. However, many people would define an older person as "twenty years older than what I am." In other words, just because an individual has advanced in chronological age does not mean that mentally they have aged.

■ Theories of Aging

How a person ages largely remains a mystery in spite of frequent television infomercials offering the next new "secret" to living to a healthy old age. Factors often considered include what the person eats, where she lives, her chosen occupation, and how much she exercises. Sometimes aging is attributed to what a person inherits at birth. Although no single theory can answer all of the questions, two aging theories—biological and psychosocial—attempt to explain the physical and emotional changes that take place as an individual progresses through life.

Biological Aging Theories

Biological aging theories fall into two groups: programmed theories and error theories. The **programmed theory of aging** proposes that aging follows a biological timetable. It supports the notion that every organism is programmed to live for a certain number of years. An example of a programmed theory is the **immunologic theory of aging.** This theory asserts that the aging body is less able to distinguish its own cells from foreign cells. Alterations in B and T cells result in attacks on and eventually destruction of one's own body cells. The aging patient can boost immune function through a healthy diet and lifestyle, along with preventive health measures such as a yearly flu vaccination.

The **cross-linking theory of aging** is based on the finding that as one ages, proteins, DNA, and other molecules of the body develop inappropriate attachments to one another. These attachments cause decreased elasticity of proteins and other molecules, and prevent enzymes from breaking down proteins. As a result, damaged and unnecessary proteins are left in the system, causing problems. For example, cross-linking of collagen in the skin has been shown to be partially responsible for wrinkling. Another theory, the **rate of living theory of aging,** is based on the premise that humans possess a finite amount of a "vital substance," and when that substance is exhausted, the person dies. In other words, a human is predisposed to take only a certain number of breaths, and a human's heart is programmed to beat only a set number of times. However, this theory does not explain why some individuals live to the age of 100 and beyond (Gavrilov & Gavrilov, 2002).

Error theories of aging propose that environmental factors negatively impact the human body, causing destruction and damage. Two examples of error theories are the **free radical theory of aging** and the **wear-and-tear theory of aging.** The free radical aging theory, also called the *autoimmunity aging theory,* is based on the idea that certain chemical compounds in the body do damage that accumulates to produce aging; for example, unstable free oxygen radicals cause chromosomal changes, pigment accumulation, and collagen alteration. Cells, and eventually organs, lose function and reserve. The use of antioxidants and vitamins is thought to help slow this process. This theory, also sometimes referred to as the homeostatic theory of aging, relates to the age-related accumulation of damage produced by oxidative stress, which reduces the *homeostatic capacity of the organism* (Novoseltsev, Novoseltseva, & Yashin, 2001). The wear-and-tear aging theory compares the human body to a machine that simply wears out as a result of constant use; exposure to internal and external stressors results in the death of cells. Cellular function slows as an individual ages and becomes less efficient in responding to environmental assaults to the body (Tabloski, 2006).

Within the realm of biological theories is the genetic theory of aging, which proposes that lifespan is largely determined by the genes that one inherits. According to this theory, one's potential age is primarily determined at the moment of conception. According to Stibich (2007a), genes can explain a maximum of 35% of lifespan. The other determinants are one's behaviors, exposures, and just plain luck. Another biological theory of aging is the somatic mutation theory. The somatic mutation theory of aging purports that an important part of aging is determined by what happens to genes after they are inherited Stibich (2007b). Each time a cell divides, there is a chance that some of the genes will be copied incorrectly and result in a mutation. Additionally, exposures to toxins, radiation, or ultraviolet light can cause mutations in genes. Eventually the mutated cells accumulate, copy themselves, and cause problems in the body's functioning related to aging. The somatic mutation theory of aging is different from the genetic theory in that the genetic theory is only concerned with the genes in sperm and egg cells, whereas somatic mutations are changes in the genes that occur after they have been inherited, but they cannot be passed down to children, as can the genes in sperm and egg cells.

Psychosocial Theories of Aging

Psychosocial theories of aging describe the changes that take place emotionally and socially as one enters the later years of life. These changes tend to involve roles and social relationships. Three examples of psychosocial theories are activity theory, disengagement theory, and continuity theory. The **activity theory of aging** proposes that the more active elderly persons are, the greater their satisfaction with life; decreased activity leads to meaninglessness and life dissatisfaction. To maintain a positive sense of self, elderly persons must substitute new roles for those lost in old age, thus successful aging is achieved by staying active and extending activities enjoyed in middle age. Life care communities and senior retirement communities are designed to promote the activity theory. Such amenities as golf courses, swimming pools, and clubhouses that provide activity groups not only help support healthy aging, but also help bring individuals together to develop new relationships and interests.

The **disengagement theory of aging,** introduced in 1961, contradicts the activity theory (Tabloski, 2006). It asserts that later in life, age-related changes bring about a mutual and reciprocal withdrawal of the individual and society. In the past, mandatory retirement at age 65 with full Social Security retirement benefits may have promoted such withdrawal. With the movement toward later and more flexible retirement dates, this theory may no longer be as valid. For example, an individual born in 1937 or earlier could retire at age 65 with full benefits, whereas an individual born in 1960 or later will not be able to collect full benefits until age 67 (U.S. Social Security Administration, Office of Policy, 2007).

The **continuity theory of aging** asserts that in order to age successfully, one should substitute new roles for lost ones, and continue to maintain typical ways of adapting to the environment. One should maintain values, habits, and behaviors from his or her adult life. Older age should not be a time for major life changes, but instead one should maintain the usual activities, but at a slower pace as needed. Some older individuals would never consider a life care community or senior community because of the major changes of such a move. These adults choose to live in their established homes, along with the diversity of a neighborhood that houses both younger and older individuals, rather than living in an "all over age 65" environment (Lundell & Morris, 2004; Tabloski, 2006).

Other social theories related to aging include role theory, which maintains that role loss accompanies the aging process and could be associated with the loss of identity and esteem. Also of note are the age stratification theory, modernization theory, and the exchange theory of aging (Darkwa, 2007). Age stratification examines the movement of successive birth cohorts across time, known as *cohort flow.* Each cohort is unique in that it has its own characteristics (e.g., size, gender, and social class distribution). Each cohort experiences particular historical events that affect its members' attitudes and behaviors (Schaffer, 2006). Modernization theory argues that the role and status of the aged are inversely related to the level of societal industrialization. This tends to have a distinctly negative impact on the status of the elderly. This theory supports the premise that the more industrialized the society, the less support is given to the elderly; material family support tends to diminish (Aboderin, 2004).

Lastly, exchange theory indicates that elderly people have less power in relation to younger people because they possess fewer resources, and continued interaction with the younger population becomes more costly. Social interaction between the old and the young tends to decrease because older people have fewer resources to bring to the exchange—lower income, poorer health, and less education. Declining resources strain their possibilities for continued interaction with others (Roy & Russell, 2005).

Demographics of the Aging Population

In 2005, 15% of adults in the United States were over the age of 65. Elders were fairly evenly distributed throughout the United States. In Alaska, 6.5% of the population was comprised of adults age 65 and older. This was the smallest percentage for any state. Florida had the largest percentage of seniors age 65 and older, with 16.6% of the population falling into this age group. This large percentage is attributed to the many seniors who move there for the sunshine and mild climate. The percentage of adults age 65 and older fell somewhere between these two ranges for all of the other states (U.S. Census Bureau, 2005).

Women have always outlived men in the past, and the trend continues among all age groups age 65 and older. For those ages 65 to 74, there are 83 men per 100 women. For those ages 75 to 84, there are 67 men per 100 women. In the age 85 and over age group, there are 46 men per 100 women. These numbers correlate with percentages of women who are widowed. Forty one percent of women ages 65 to 84 are widowed; 79% of women age 85 and older are widowed. In the 2005 Census Bureau survey, 80% of adults ages 65 to 74 identified themselves as white; 86% of those ages 75 to 84 considered themselves white, and 87% of those ages 85 and older answered that they were white (U.S. Census Bureau, 2005).

Older Americans have attained higher levels of education than the generation before them, and this trend continues. In 1950, 17% of older adults had a high school education; only 3% had at least a bachelor's degree. By 2003, 72% were high school graduates, and at least 17% had a bachelor's degree (Administration on Aging [AOA], n.d.). Trending data indicate that advances in medicine will provide an opportunity for individuals to live a longer chronological life, however, it remains unknown as to whether a longer life will be free of disease and disability. Taking advantage of medical advances also will be influenced by educational background and finances, both of which limit one's ability to freely seek health care when it is needed. It is certain that nurses today will have a firsthand opportunity to observe how changes in medical technology affect the graying of America (Strunk, Ginsburg, & Banker, 2006).

Health Assessment of the Aging Patient

The nurse should view the health assessment of the aging patient as not just an opportunity to gather needed medical information, but as an opportunity to become acquainted with an individual who possesses a lifetime of experience. The health assessment includes both the health history and physical examination.

Interviewing the Older Patient to Obtain a Health History

Interviewing an older patient to collect patient health data is identified by the American Nurses Association (ANA) as a standard for clinical gerontological nursing care. See Chart 10–1 for an interpretation of the standards. The interview, as part of a comprehensive health assessment, is essential to developing a comprehensive plan of care for the aging adult (Congdon et al., 2001).

Interviewing and obtaining a health history from the aging patient can be both a challenging and rewarding experience. The experience can be challenging for a number of reasons related to complexity of the health history, as well as the impact of normal changes of aging, such as hearing and visual deficits. Eliciting a health history from an individual with memory deficits presents special challenges. The *National Health Interview Study 1989–91* revealed that 72% of the population over age 65 rated themselves in excellent or good health, yet 10% rated their health as poor (AOA, n.d.). Obtaining information from this group, who are more likely to be encountered during hospitalization, can be time consuming, yet it is essential to providing quality nursing care.

Cultural Considerations

Cultural considerations must also be taken into account when interviewing and obtaining a health history from the aging patient. Many times the nurse will become involved in the hospital setting with patients and families whose cultures are different and whose traditions seem strange and foreign. It is important for the nurse to be sensitive to the needs and customs of the patients in any health care setting. Cultural variances that nurses who work with aging patients should be aware of are discussed in the following subsections and the Cultural Considerations box.

African Americans

The family is very important in African American history and values related to the family are rooted in African traditions (Willis, 1998). The elderly are highly valued in African American families.

Asian

In Asian families family authority and structure are defined by family position, which is defined by age and gender. Older family members have higher status than younger ones, and males

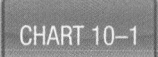 **CHART 10–1** **Scope and Standards of Gerontological Nursing Practice**

One of the responsibilities of the American Nurses Association (ANA) is to define the scope and standards of nursing practice. The *Standards of Clinical Nursing Practice* published in 1998 apply to all professional nurses. The *Scope and Standards of Gerontological Nursing Practice* contain criteria for expectations and competent care associated with the basic and advanced clinical practice of gerontological nursing. This includes nursing care demonstrated through assessment, diagnosis, outcome identification, planning, implementation, and evaluation. These processes form the foundation of clinical decision making that applies to all gerontological nurses.

Source: American Nurses Association. (2004). *Scope and standards of gerontologic nursing practice* (2nd ed.). Washington, DC: Author.

CULTURAL CONSIDERATIONS for Aging Patients

Culturally competent health care systems are those that provide culturally and linguistically appropriate services. An inability to communicate with a patient or insensitivity to cultural differences can result in a compromise in the quality of health care (Anderson, Scrimshaw, Fullilove, Fielding, & Normand, 2003). It is extremely important for the nurse to be cognizant of the cultural values of the patient and family related to aging. It is crucial that, as health care professionals, nurses understand that cultural values often are the driving forces guiding daily behavior. Cultural norms of family life and the role of elderly family members will have an impact on how the elderly are treated within society and the family. Cultural competence demands that nurses look at patients through both their own eyes and the eyes of patients and family members.

hold higher positions than females. Mutual support, cooperation, and interdependence also characterize the family, which is patriarchal in nature. Problems generally are solved within the family, and a sense of family honor and pride limits the amount and type of information to be shared with counselors or other professionals. Elders are venerated in Asia, assuming a place of great respect. As Asian immigrants grow older in the United States, they are exposed to a health care system that is very different from how they were socialized. It is a more demanding task to age in a society where their contributions are devalued, compared to a society where elders are treated with deference (Kao & Lam, 1995).

Hispanic/Latino

The Hispanic/Latino population also is a very diverse ethnic group. The family is of paramount value, which is influenced by both the Spaniards' Catholic religion as well as the values stemming from the indigenous people of the Americas. The family is an extended system that includes more than just blood relations and those related by marriage; it also includes fictive kin adopted through relationships. It is not uncommon to transfer children from one family to another during times of hardship and crises, and mutual help, protection, and caregiving are provided. In the Hispanic/Latino culture, self-sufficiency is not expected for the elderly. Children are obligated to provide care and to respect their elderly parents (Falicov, 1998).

Native American

Native Americans encompass people with many different languages, religions, organizations, and relationships with the U.S. government. The family is regarded as the cornerstone for emotional, social, and economic well-being for individuals (Red Horse, 1981). Extended family members assume very different roles. The primary relationship is not necessarily with the parents, but instead with the grandparents who assume the caregiver and disciplinarian role. Elderly family members are highly regarded. The aged are believed to be the repository of wisdom, and their role is to teach the young the traditions, customs, legends, and myths of the tribe. Consequently, in their old age they are taken care of by the tribe. Consensus often is the goal, and in decision-making processes, individuals often spend a lot of time trying to achieve consensus and harmony.

One can conclude from the brief discussion of four different cultures and the role of society in each one of them that their re-

sponse to aging and health care may be quite different. The role of the family, the environment, and manner of caring for patients vary (Mazanec & Tyler, 2003). A full discussion of cultural competence and the role of the health care provider is discussed in Chapter 1.

People over the age of 65 in the United States account for more than one-third of all hospital stays. Most nurses will care for an aging patient on a typical medical–surgical nursing unit, necessitating the need for obtaining a health history in the hospital environment. It is useful to initially inquire about the individual's present health problem, which usually is the reason the individual has been hospitalized. It is important to determine the patient's perceptions of his health status and then obtain corroborating information from the medical record. It is important to find out how the hospitalization and illness have affected the aging patient's life, as well as the lives of family members.

Past Medical History

The next step is to interview the individual to obtain the past medical history. Collecting patient health data is essential to developing a comprehensive plan of care as identified by the ANA scope and standards of gerontological nursing care, which were shown earlier in Chart 10–1 (Congdon et al., 2001). If the patient is unable to give her medical history, the information from the medical record may be referenced and family members interviewed to fill in the "information gaps." In addition to recording medical diagnoses, obtaining information as to the length of time an individual has had a medical condition is useful. For example, the nursing management and teaching of a patient who is newly diagnosed with diabetes and has been prescribed oral medications are quite different than the management and teaching of an individual who is hospitalized with diabetic complications and has been on insulin for more than 20 years. When obtaining the past medical history, the following questions are useful to ask:

- What medical problems do you have?
- How long have you had these problems?
- What treatment have you sought in the past?
- Have you had any past surgeries? If so, when (the date), and were they successful?
- What medications are you taking?
- Do you have any history of communicable diseases such as TB, hepatitis, HIV?

Psychosocial History

Because psychosocial issues impact one's health status, a psychosocial history is an essential component of the health history. The nurse should keep in mind that education and socioeconomic status may play a role in a patient's vocabulary, self-expression, ability to comprehend, and ability to learn (Lesser, Hughes, Jemelka, & Kumar, 2005). Some questions a nurse might ask when obtaining the psychosocial history include the following:

- Where do you live? Do you live alone? Are you married?
- Do you have any history of accidents or falls?
- If you require assistance with your grooming, hygiene, or other activities of daily living (ADLs), who is available to help you?

- If you had an emergency such as falling or feeling ill, who would you contact?
- What did you do for employment when you were younger?
- Do you have children? Where do they live? Are they involved in your life/care?

Health habits must be explored as well. Questions to ask may include the following:

- Do you currently smoke tobacco? How many packs per day for how many years?
- If you have quit smoking, what was the date you quit? Have you ever had any abnormal chest x-rays?
- Do you drink alcohol? If so, how much and how often?
- Do you exercise? If so, how much and how often?
- Do you have any problems sleeping at night?
- Do you have any problems with your bowels or urinary incontinence?

Physical Assessment of the Older Patient

Nursing assessments in the elderly, as with all adults, are best carried out using a systematic approach to the physical examination. This may be done using the head-to-toe approach or by body systems. Whatever approach is chosen, it is best to stay with the same method during every assessment, so that critical elements are not overlooked and in order to identify trends in changes more clearly.

General Impression

When assessing the elderly patient, it is important to get an overall picture of the individual by looking at his general appearance:

- Is the individual clean; thin or obese?
- Is his behavior and affect appropriate?
- Does the individual seem easily angered, restless, or agitated?
- Do the facial expressions match his speech? It is known that many illnesses may affect one's facial expressions so it is important to identify a correlation, or lack thereof, of expression with speech. For example, people with Parkinson's disease often display a "masked facies," which means that their expression looks as if they are wearing a mask. People who have a long history of use of neuroleptic drugs may exhibit lip smacking, tongue thrusting, and other facial dystonias. These are irreversible side effects attributed to a history of prolonged use of this class of medications. When the medications are discontinued, these movements often remain. Such abnormal facial muscle movements also are seen in individuals with a wide variety of neurological conditions, such as Huntington's disease, Wilson's disease, head injury, and tumors (Tovey, 2007).

Assessment of the Head and Neck

When assessing the head and neck, typical changes may be found with the aging adult. Hair becomes thinner and finer with age, but the size and shape of the skull do not change. The eyes undergo many changes as the body ages. The eyelids relax, often giving the eyes a droopy appearance. When assessing the pupils for light reflex response, one may note a thin grayish-white ring at the margins of the cornea. This normal finding is called arcus senilis. The lens become less transparent and the eyelids may appear dry due to decreased lacrimal duct production. The cornea clouds with aging, and individuals lose peripheral vision. Chapter 71 ⊘ describes eye disorders in detail.

Changes in the ears are related to normal age-related hearing losses. The auricle of the ear becomes less elastic; the lobes elongate and often develop linear wrinkles. Increased hair growth is seen in the auditory canals of males. The tympanic membrane may appear dull, and atrophy of the membrane itself may make the landmarks more prominent appearing. Cerumen may be harder and drier, occluding the auditory canal. A decreased sense of smell is commonly seen, along with reduced taste sensation, in advanced old age due to atrophy of papillae on the outer edges of the tongue.

Age-Related Disorders of the Head, Neck, and Mouth

Common eyelid problems seen in the elderly include ptosis, where the eyelids partially or completely cover the pupil. The lower eyelid can turn inward, called an entropion, or may turn extremely outward, called an ectropion, exposing the tissue of the conjunctiva. Because this pinkish red tissue is normally not visible, when an ectropion develops it is often misinterpreted as an eye infection. If the lower eyelid becomes excessively dry, irritated, or infected, the ectropion can be surgically repaired. Decreased tear production may cause dry eyes, which are easily treated with artificial eyedrops or lubricants. Cataracts also are common and are caused by clouding of the crystalline lens, and can be surgically repaired if they impair vision. Vision problems, even with glasses or contact lenses, affect nearly 20% of the older population (AOA, n.d.). See Chapter 71 ⊘ for more information on disorders of the eye.

Relative to the ears, cerumen impaction can become a chronic problem in the aging patient if not addressed on a routine basis. Impacted cerumen can cause hearing loss as well as vertigo. Therefore, removal should be facilitated using a softening agent, such as Debrox or regular mineral oil, and irrigation by medical personnel if wax cannot be removed during showering with warm water. Accurate hearing tests cannot be conducted unless canals are free of cerumen and the tympanic membrane is readily visualized using an otoscope. Scarring and chronic perforation of the tympanic membrane resulting from years of occupational exposure to loud sounds and ear infections contribute to hearing loss as well. In 2002, almost one-half of all older men and one-third of older women reported trouble hearing without a hearing aid (AOA, n.d.). With the increase in use of personal music players with ear buds inserted into ear canals, the need for hearing aids in the next generation is expected to increase.

Dry oral mucosa along with cheilosis (dry scaling) of the mouth can be indicative of dehydration, vitamin deficiencies, poorly fitting dentures, or the result of medication side effects. Oral assessments should always include removal of dentures, because this is an area where cancerous lesions can appear.

Respiratory Assessment

Structural changes of the thoracic cavity are often seen with aging and can affect respiratory function. **Kyphosis,** which gives the patient a "stooped over" appearance, is caused by osteoporosis and collapse of vertebrae. The chest wall becomes less compliant, and changes in the breathing pattern are seen. Inspiration tends to be shallower, and expiration requires the use of accessory muscles. As a result, the measured vital capacity is decreased, and increased residual capacity will be seen if pulmonary function tests are conducted. The ciliary function of the lungs is reduced, producing a decreased cough reflex.

Age-Related Disorders of the Respiratory System

Some common disorders of the respiratory system seen in the elderly include chronic obstructive pulmonary disease (COPD), pulmonary edema due to congestive heart failure, and pulmonary emboli. Due to physiological changes, the normal PaO_2 should be corrected for age using the formula $109 - 0.43 \times$ patient's age. The PaO_2 and pH may be outside the normal range, but the response to such change is blunted. See Chapter 36 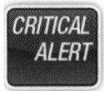 for information on complex respiratory disorders.

An increase in **sleep apnea** and sleep disorders is common. Although older adults need as much sleep as younger people, the sleep they get occurs during the lighter stages of sleep. This sleep is not as restorative as sleep that occurs during the deeper stages of sleep (Gehrman, Diana, & Impastato, 2006). The most common sleep disorder in the older adult is **insomnia**, defined as difficulty falling asleep or staying asleep with a negative impact on daytime alertness. Sleep apnea is a sleep disorder with partial or complete obstruction of airflow. The patient must awaken to resume breathing. Diagnosis is usually made after an overnight sleep study. Treatment involves wearing a nasal positive airway pressure mask at night to keep airways open and facilitate unobstructed airflow while sleeping. Sleep apnea is discussed at length in Chapter 34 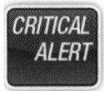.

Cardiovascular Assessment

The heart of the aging patient undergoes normal, age-related changes. A slower heart rate often is seen due to a decrease in the normal number of pacemaker cells, and may be asymptomatic. The heart valves become thicker and more rigid, along with decreased elasticity and increased rigidity of the heart muscle itself. The point of maximal impulse (PMI) may be displaced and palpated at the fifth or sixth left intercostal space at the midclavicular line. Murmurs in the older patient do not necessarily produce symptoms, and are caused by heart valves that become stiff from fibrosis and calcification. These murmurs are best heard at the base of the heart or the aortic area. The arterial walls are more irregular in size and shape, with an increase in calcium and collagen deposits. The walls themselves are thicker, less distensible, and less pliable.

Age-Related Disorders of the Cardiovascular System

Cardiovascular disorders are not specific to the elderly; however, heart disease is the number one cause of death in older people (Tabloski, 2006). Disorders commonly seen may include systolic hypertension, valvular disease (most commonly aortic stenosis), coronary artery disease with acute myocardial infarction (MI), congestive heart failure, arrhythmias, and stroke. These specific disorders are discussed at length in Unit 8 of this text.

CRITICAL ALERT *Atrial fibrillation is the most common sustained arrhythmia seen in the older patient. New-onset atrial fibrillation can be caused by other illnesses such as hyperthyroidism, electrolyte disturbances, or a myocardial infarction. Any patient reporting "palpitations" or "skipped beats" while hospitalized should be reported to the health care provider for further evaluation.*

Gastrointestinal Assessment

Some of the normal age-related changes in the gastrointestinal system contribute to the perception that the elderly are fixated on their bowels. For example, the abdominal muscles of the aging patient weaken and peristalsis decreases. The liver itself becomes smaller in size and storage capacity is reduced. Alterations in insulin release often are seen as well.

Age-Related Disorders of the Gastrointestinal System

Some of the age-related disorders in digestion are caused by *dysphagia,* difficulty swallowing. Dysphagia may be caused by poorly fitted or absent dentures. Even tooth decay can cause difficulty swallowing, resulting in decreased oral intake, weight loss, and undernutrition. Dyspepsia, gastroesophageal reflux disease (GERD), and upper gastrointestinal malignancies occur more often after age 55, and affect about one in four elderly patients (Talley, 2005). GERD is caused by the backflow of gastric or duodenal contents or both into the esophagus and past the lower esophageal sphincter. The reflux causes acute epigastric pain that can radiate to the chest or arm. Pain usually occurs after meals or when the patient lies down—the increased abdominal pressure causes reflux (Moreau, 2006). Upper endoscopy is recommended for elderly patients with symptoms that trigger an alarm, new-onset GERD, or long-standing disease. Elderly patients are at risk for more severe complications from GERD. Based on safety profiles and success in general, proton pump inhibitors (PPIs) are considered to be the first-line medication treatment for GERD in the elderly (Bacak, Patel, Tweed, & Danis, 2006).

Constipation is partially caused by the decreased peristalsis mentioned earlier, but it is also caused by many other contributing factors. A decreased thirst sensation leads to decreased fluid intake, and the use of narcotics for chronic pain management leads to slowed peristalsis, all of which results in constipation. Prolonged constipation can lead to intestinal obstruction, a medical emergency due to the potential for bowel perforation. Constipation also may be caused by a tumor. The incidence of colon cancer affects men and women equally, most commonly between the ages of 60 and 80 years (Tovey, 2007).

Genitourinary Assessment

Unlike the portrayals often seen on television, not all individuals over the age of 65 are incontinent, requiring bladder pads and incontinent briefs. The incontinence product market, however, is estimated to be a billion dollar industry, some of which can be attributed to a few of the disorders seen in the aging genitourinary system. As one ages, the pubic hair thins and grays, and the bladder capacity decreases. In females, vaginal mucosa atrophies from a decrease in estrogen, which also results in a decrease in size and elasticity of the vagina and a decrease in vaginal secretions. In males, slight testicular atrophy is seen, while the prostate gland enlarges. The scrotal sac elongates as well.

Age-Related Disorders of the Genitourinary System

Common disorders of the genitourinary system seen in the aging patient include urinary tract infections (UTIs) and urinary incontinence. More frequent UTIs are thought to be caused by changes in the urinary tract. Urinary incontinence can be caused by stress incontinence, urge incontinence, overflow incontinence, or any

Management of Bowel Routines

Clinical Problem

Management of bowel routines in the acute care setting often is inadequate. Establishing bowel routines also may be complicated if the patient has dementia. Nurses need to determine that if the patient with dementia is agitated, could the agitation be related to constipation?

Research Findings

Leonard and colleagues (2006) examined the records of more than 100,000 nursing home residents living in five states in 2002. All participants were over 60 years old and diagnosed with dementia. It was found that nearly 7% of the residents had been physically aggressive in the week before the assessment, and 10.5% had been verbally aggressive in the week before assessment. It was found that physical and verbally aggressive behavior was associated with depression, delusions, and hallucinations. Physical aggression, including hitting, shoving, scratching, or engaging in sexual abuse was also associated with constipation. The study did not find significant associations with factors such as respiratory tract infections, urinary tract infections, fever, or reported pain.

Implications for Nursing Practice

Although this study took place in nursing homes, constipation is a problem often overlooked in the acute care setting as well. The nurse can play a role in intervention through advocating for preprinted bowel care orders, as well as thorough documentation and tracking of bowel movements during hospitalization. Such simple interventions may reduce the incidence of physical aggression in elderly patients with dementia.

Critical Thinking Questions

1. If a nonverbal patient with dementia who is unable to verbalize symptoms has not had a bowel movement in 3 days even with routine bowel care, what is the best way to assess for constipation?

2. What adjustments to the bowel care regimen should be considered when a nurse receives a new order to give the patient a narcotic for pain relief?

3. If a patient is having frequent small smears of liquid stool, could the patient still be constipated?

Answers to Critical Thinking Questions appear in Appendix D.

Reference

Leonard, R., Tinetti, M. E., Allore, H. G., & Drickamer, M. A. (2006). Potentially modifiable resident characteristics that are associated with physical or verbal aggression among nursing home residents with dementia. *Archives Internal Medicine, 166,* 1295–1300.

combination of the three. Stress incontinence, the result of weakened bladder muscles, is most commonly seen. Urge incontinence, the second most common cause, is the result of bladder spasms, a syndrome often referred to as *overactive bladder,* which can be treated with medication. Overflow incontinence is the result of a bladder that is no longer able to contract efficiently to release urine. Incontinence occurs when urine exceeds the bladder capacity. Atrophic vaginitis, the result of decreased estrogen in the vaginal tissues, can be treated with hormone replacement, although controversial. Application of estrogen vaginal cream to the labia also is sometimes helpful.

The prostate enlarges as a normal part of aging due to a decrease of androgen and increase of estrogen, resulting in an imbalance. The increased estrogen receptors trigger the androgen receptors in the prostate gland to increase. An overgrowth of normal cells begins around the urethra and can cause partial bladder neck obstruction (Moreau, 2006). The result is urinary frequency and retention. Medications in the alpha$_1$ blocker drug class work by relaxing smooth muscle in the bladder neck and prostate. The result is an improvement in urine flow. If the prostate becomes too enlarged, surgical intervention using a transurethral approach may be indicated.

Musculoskeletal Assessment

In the aging patient, one will see normal age-related changes of the musculoskeletal system. A slower reaction time, along with poorer coordination and decreased muscle strength, can all contribute to difficulties with gait. A loss of bone beginning during the fourth decade of life can affect posture and place an individual at risk for developing osteoporosis.

Age-Related Disorders of the Musculoskeletal System

Age-related disorders of the musculoskeletal system include disabilities caused by osteoarthritis, rheumatoid arthritis, gout, osteoporosis, bunions, and hammertoes. Osteoarthritis is the most common type of arthritis, affecting women more than men, with joints of the hand being the most common site affected (Figure 10–1 ■). Hip joints and knee joints also can be affected. Rheumatoid arthritis affects women and men over the age of 65 equally,

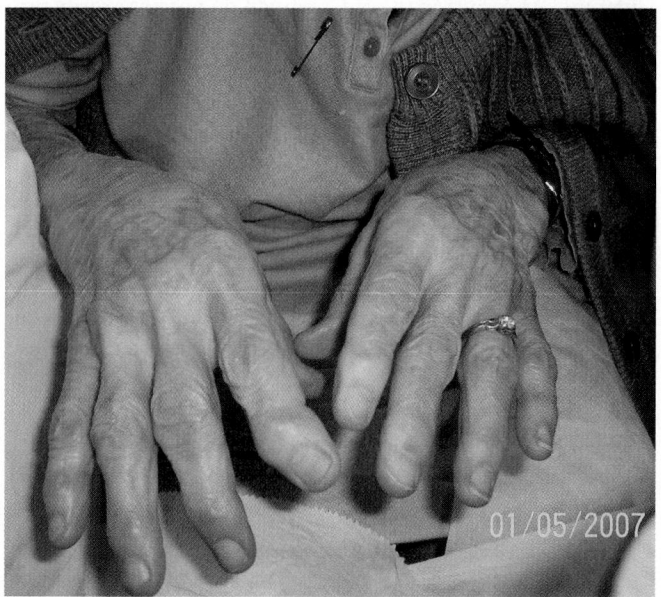

01/05/2007

FIGURE 10–1 ■ Osteoarthritic hands.

and complications can affect mobility and one's ability to carry out ADLs, such as feeding.

Gout is a syndrome caused by deposition of urate crystals in joints and the skin. It causes acute monoarthritis and crystal deposits, called tophi, in the skin. It is more common in older people, and more common in men. Other risk factors include nonwhite ethnicity; obesity; consumption of alcohol, meat, and fish; and use of diuretics. The Mayo Clinic reported that among black men, the annual incidence of gout was 3.1/1,000 versus 1.8/1,000 in white men. Colchicine has been used for many years to treat acute gout, yet it is unknown whether this treatment is effective. The effectiveness of allopurinol in reducing the risk of recurrent attacks compared to placebo or other treatments is unknown as well (Mayo Clinic, 2007a, 2007b; Tovey, 2007).

Osteoporosis is a skeletal disorder characterized by compromised bone strength that places an individual at increased risk for fracture (National Institutes of Health Consensus Development Panel, 2001). Fractures due to osteoporosis can permanently affect function and quality of life. With the advent of bone mineral density (BMD) screening studies, health care providers are able to diagnose osteoporosis before a fracture occurs. The **U.S. Preventive Services Task Force (USPSTF),** sponsored by the Agency for Healthcare Research and Quality (AHRQ), is an independent panel of private sector experts in prevention and primary care. This panel develops recommendations about which preventive services should be incorporated routinely into primary medical care and for which populations. These are considered to be the "gold standards" for clinical preventive services based on documented evidence regarding effectiveness and outcomes of screening, counseling, and preventive medications. The USPSTF recommends bone mineral density screening at least once at age 65, with no recommendations as to how often the test should be repeated (National Guideline Clearing House, 2007). The universal recommendations for management of osteoporosis include oral calcium 1,200 mg/day, oral vitamin D 800 international units/day, fall prevention, tobacco avoidance, weight-bearing exercise, and no more than moderate alcohol consumption. Pharmacologic management should be considered based on risk factors for osteoporosis and BMD screening results. Bisphosphonates also have been shown to increase bone mineral density in the spine and hip (Reuben et al., 2007).

Bony deformities of the feet often are seen as a result of years of poorly fitting footwear and in women, years of wearing tight-fitting, high-heeled shoes. It has been said that "feet only get uglier with age." Bunions are seen in the aging patient from years of the bones in the toes being pushed to fit into tight shoes (Figure 10–2 ■). The bones of the toes take on an angled appearance, and in severe cases, the first toe of the foot will be permanently pushed over the second and third toe. These deformities can only be corrected surgically, where the bones of the feet are essentially "broken" and recast and reset into their proper alignment.

Skin Assessment

Assessment of the skin in the aging patient requires the same techniques one would use in assessing any patient, including in-

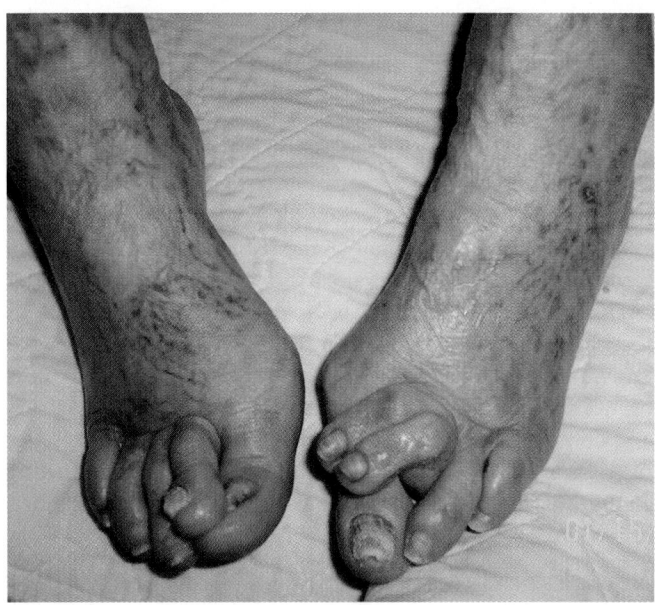

FIGURE 10–2   ■   Bunion feet.

spection of the scalp, head, neck, trunk, and limbs. The skin should be palpated to determine temperature, moisture, thickness, texture, and turgor. The amount of subcutaneous tissue present below the surface of the skin in the aging patient is decreased; thus, skin turgor may not be a reliable indicator for hydration status. Common skin changes in the aging patient include the presence of seborrheic or senile keratoses (Figure 10–3 ■), senile lentigines also known as "liver spots," cherry angiomas, and development of skin tags. Assessment of the skin is discussed more in Chapter 65 ⊘.

Age-Related Disorders of the Integumentary System

The most common skin disorders in the elderly are skin cancers, which are the result of many years of unprotected skin exposure to the sun. Many older individuals grew up on farms or worked

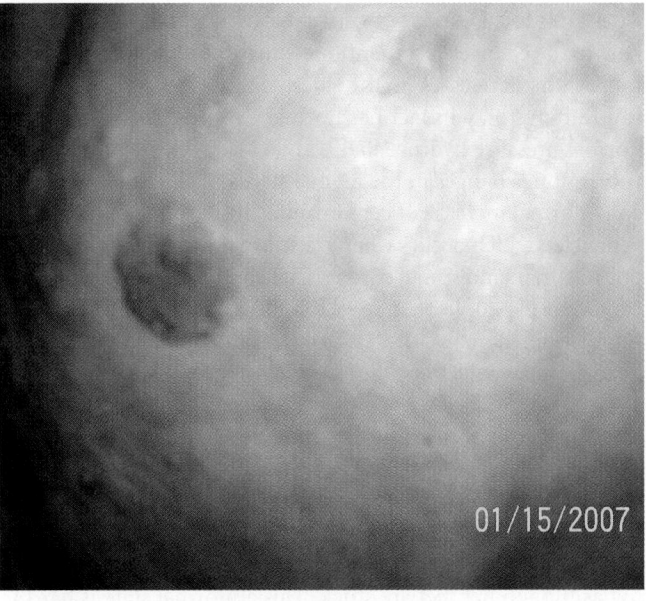

FIGURE 10–3   ■   Seborrheic keratoses.

many years doing physical labor under direct exposure to the sun's rays, without the benefit of topically applied sunscreen. Thus, in their older years, many aging patients present with skin cancers, such as basal cell cancers, or precancerous lesions, such as actinic keratoses. Treatment includes surgical excision, or removal via desiccation for precancerous lesions. Herpes zoster, which produces blistering lesions along a specific dermatome, also is more commonly found in the aging patient. The USPSTF recommends a yearly skin exam in individuals aged 65 and older (AHRQ, 2007).

Dry skin is estimated to be present in approximately 75% of individuals 75 years and older (Mac-Mary, Sainthillier & Humbert, 2004). It is worse during the winter when the air is drier, and develops when the skin loses water to the air. Keratosis and pruritus are chronic problems for many aging patients, fueling an industry that sells lotions, creams, and ointments to treat dry, itchy skin.

Neurological Assessment

Contrary to common myths regarding aging, it is not routine for older people to become senile or demented. However, by age 85, the risk of developing Alzheimer's disease, a type of dementia, is nearly 50% (Alzheimer's Association, 2006). Neurological assessment is covered in detail in Chapter 28 ⬡. However, there are normal changes seen in the aging patient that must be taken into consideration. The brain atrophies with age, but there are no relationships between shrinkage and change in cognition. The sense of taste and smell decrease in the aging patient. Sometimes there is a lack of awareness about food that has spoiled. This predisposes individuals to nutritional problems. Changes in reflexes include decreased deep tendon reflexes in the legs and increased reflexes in the arms, with decreased vibratory sense. There is some decrease in position sense as well. There are many medical conditions associated with pain in the older adult, but certain types of pain may be less severe than others. This may explain why a younger adult experiencing a myocardial infarction will report crushing chest pain, and the aging patient may report vague symptoms of discomfort, such as heartburn (Tabloski, 2006).

Age-Related Disorders of the Neurological System

Due to the changes just mentioned, neurological disease may be more difficult to assess in the elderly. Some abnormal neurological findings may in fact be "normal." Some disorders, such as normal pressure hydrocephalus (NPH) and dementia, may involve subtle changes in the mental status of the patient. NPH is an abnormal increase of cerebrospinal fluid (CSF) in the brain's ventricles, which occurs when the normal flow of CSF throughout the brain and spinal cord is blocked in some way. While this can occur in people of any age, it is most common in the elderly population. It may result from a subarachnoid hemorrhage, head trauma, infection, tumor, or complications of surgery. It also may occur when none of these factors is present; in these cases the cause of the disorder is unknown. Symptoms of NPH include progressive mental impairment and dementia, problems with walking, and impaired bladder control, leading to urinary frequency and/or incontinence. The person also may have a general slowing of movements, with some complaining of feeling as though her feet are stuck. This abnormal state is hard to diagnose because the symptoms often resemble other neurolog-

ical disorders, such as Alzheimer's disease, Parkinson's disease, and Creutzfeldt-Jakob disease (National Institute of Neurological Disorders and Stroke, 2007). Treatment for NPH involves surgical placement of a shunt in the brain to drain excess CSF into the abdomen where it can be absorbed. If not treated, the symptoms of NPH usually get worse over time. The success of treatment with shunts varies, but is generally favorable. Early diagnosis and treatment improves the chance of a good recovery.

The term **dementia** describes a group of symptoms that are caused by changes in brain function (destruction of brain cells) that seriously affect a person's ability to carry out daily activities (National Institute on Aging, 2006). It becomes hard for a person to remember, learn, and communicate, and the condition progresses to the point where it is hard for the person to take care of himself. Presenting symptoms include:

- Asking the same questions repeatedly
- Becoming lost in familiar places
- Being unable to follow directions
- Getting disoriented about time, people, and places
- Neglecting personal safety, hygiene, and nutrition.

Dementia also may change a person's mood and personality. At first, memory loss and trouble thinking clearly may bother the person who has dementia. Later, disruptive behavior and other problems may start, but the person who has dementia may not be aware of these problems.

People with dementia lose their abilities at different rates. It is caused by many conditions some of which are reversible and some are not. Reversible conditions can be caused by a high fever, dehydration, vitamin deficiency and poor nutrition, medication reactions, thyroid problems, or a minor head injury. Sometimes older people have emotional problems that can be mistaken for dementia. Feeling sad, lonely, worried, or bored may be more common for older people facing retirement or coping with the death of a spouse. Emotional problems and the medical problems previously noted should be professionally addressed. Family support also is critical to the care of people with dementia.

The two most common forms of dementia in older people are Alzheimer's disease (AD) and multiple-infarct dementia, sometimes referred to as vascular dementia. These types of dementia are irreversible. Alzheimer's disease is discussed in detail in Chapter 31 ⬡ as a chronic neurological disease.

With multiple-infarct dementia, a series of strokes or changes in the brain's blood supply may result in the death of brain tissue. The location in the brain where the strokes occur and the severity of the strokes determine the seriousness of the problem and the symptoms that arise. Symptoms usually begin abruptly and progress in a stepwise fashion with repeated strokes. Strokes are fully discussed in Chapter 30 ⬡.

Delirium is a sudden, fluctuating, and usually reversible cognitive disorder characterized by a disturbance in consciousness with decreased attention and a change in cognition or development of a perceptual disturbance that develops over a short period of time and tends to fluctuate throughout the day (American Psychiatric Association, 1994; Reuben et al., 2007). This change in cognition often manifests itself in disruptive behaviors in the hospital setting, such as disrobing, pulling out IV lines, striking out at caregivers, and resisting nursing care. Its incidence in the hospital setting is about 20%, with postoperative incidence up to 72%. It is an abnormal mental state, not a disease, and usually a sign of a newly developed disorder, which affects about one-third of hospitalized people age 70 or older.

Detection of delirium is difficult but identification is critical. The Confusion Assessment Method (CAM) is a standardized tool any clinician can use to identify delirium quickly and accurately (Inouye et al., 1990). The short version consists of four features found to have the greatest ability to distinguish delirium from other types of cognitive impairment. It identifies the presence or absence of delirium but does not assess the severity. The first two features that must be present for delirium to be diagnosed are evidence of an acute change in mental status from the patient's baseline or a fluctuation in behavior throughout the day and difficulty focusing attention. The presence of these features and either evidence of disorganized thinking, such as rambling or illogical conversation or an altered level of consciousness, must be present for diagnosis (Waszynski, 2007).

Once delirium is diagnosed, causative factors such as infection or metabolic derangement must be identified and treated. Urinary tract infections in the elderly are the most common cause of delirium, and polypharmacy is the second most common cause (Voyer, Cole, McCusker, & Belzile, 2006). Metabolic disorders such as hypo- or hypernatremia must be corrected as well. Delirium is self-limiting once the underlying problem has been corrected, and usually resolves after 5 days. In extreme cases symptoms can last 3 to 6 months (Mezey, Fulmer, Abraham, & Zwicker, 2003). If confusion and disorientation persist, other neurological disorders such as dementia must be considered. Dementia is diagnosed within 3 years in 60% of hospitalized patients with delirium (Voyer et al., 2006).

The USPSTF recommends cognitive impairment screening annually for the individual age 65 and older (AHRQ, 2007). The **Folstein Mini-Mental State Exam** is one common screening tool used by clinicians in evaluating dementia. It is easily administered after some training. The scoring ranges from 0 to 30 points, with 0 to 10 points typically scored for an individual with advanced dementia, 10 to 20 for moderate dementia, 21 to 26 points seen in mild dementia, and 27 to 30 considered normal, with adjustments made for levels of education (Folstein, Folstein, & McHugh, 1975).

Within the last 10 years, there has been increasing recognition of the elderly experiencing late-onset schizophrenia and bipolar disorders (Howard et al., 2000; Jeste, Paulsen, & Harris, 2000; Wetherell & Jeste, 2004). Late-onset schizophrenia is being diagnosed more frequently in old age and represents a sizable minority of patients diagnosed with schizophrenia (Wetherell & Jeste, 2004). This tends to be attributed to organic factors. Late-onset schizophrenia often is characterized by bizarre delusion and auditory hallucinations. Systematized delusions of physical or mental influence are seen in many of the patients, with grandiose, erotic, or somatic delusions occurring in some cases. Depressive symptoms also may be present. Persons with late-onset schizophrenia tend to have a family history of schizophrenia and have often been considered by others to be eccentric, reserved, and suspicious (Jeste et al., 2000).

Bipolor disorders in the elderly are clinically heterogeneous and present with various courses, switching from recurrent depression to mania, early onset or late bipolar disorders (Aziz, Lorberg, & Tampi, 2006). They can take on uncommon symptoms such as depressive or mixed behaviors, psychosis, mental confusion, or dementia. The prognosis of bipolar disorders in the elderly is poor due to the high prevalence of recurrences, associated somatic disorders, reduced survival, and severe handicap. As with late-onset schizophrenia, there is an immediate need for collaboration between patients, families, and clinicians to provide health care services for this population.

Parkinson's disease is a neurodegenerative disorder associated with asymmetrical bradykinesia, hypokinesia, and rigidity. More information on this disorder is presented in Chapter 31 🔗. It occurs equally in both sexes, and has a mean age onset of 65 years, with the greatest prevalence at 3.5% in the 85- to 89-year-old age group. It currently is incurable; however, dopamine agonists are used to reduce dyskinesias and motor fluctuation, and levodopa is being used to improve motor function. In patients with later onset Parkinson's disease, pallidal surgery has been associated with a high incidence of adverse effects (Tovey, 2007).

Stroke, also discussed under multiple-infarct dementia, is one of the neurological disorders affecting the elderly that can result in the greatest degree of disability. It is defined as loss of cerebral function lasting more than 24 hours or leading to death, with no apparent cause other than that of vascular origin. Ischemic stroke is caused by vascular insufficiency, often from a thromboembolism; hemorrhagic stroke is caused by a hemorrhage of a vessel. Strokes and the ramifications for nursing care are discussed in Chapter 30 🔗.

▪ Health Care Promotion and Preventive Care

The USPSTF is one of several groups that make recommendations for appropriate preventive services and screening exams in adults age 65 and older. As mentioned earlier, the USPSTF is comprised of an independent panel of experts in primary care and preventive care that systematically reviews the evidence and effectiveness of clinical preventive services and develops recommendations (AHRQ, 2007). However, such recommendations do not specifically address the appropriateness of such testing in the frail aging patient with multiple medical problems, functional decline, and a limited life expectancy. When interpreting the guidelines, it is the responsibility of the aging patient and her health care provider to discuss which recommendations are appropriate, taking all of the above factors and the individual's personal wishes into consideration.

Immunizations

Immunizations are one way the aging adult can proactively prevent potential debilitating illnesses. Hospitalization provides an opportunity for patients to update their immunizations. Many hospitals have preprinted order sheets to increase the incidence of immunization in the elderly population. Vaccines in the aging adult are about 50% to 60% effective in preventing hospitalizations from pneumonia and 80% effective in preventing death (Kaldy, 2006). Pneumococcal infections cause an estimated

MyNursingKit | Medicare

MyNursingKit | Healthy People 2010 Number 14 Objective 29

40,000 deaths each year in the United States, causing more deaths than any other vaccine-preventable bacterial disease (Vlassova & Jackson, 2005). Influenza, which typically affects individuals during the winter months, has been associated with approximately 36,000 deaths per year in the United States during the time period from 1990 to 1999 (Smith et al., 2006).

Pneumococcal Vaccine

Streptococcus pneumonia is the organism responsible for pneumococcal pneumonia. All adults over 65 years old are candidates for initial vaccination, with a recommendation for revaccination for adults at age 65 who may have received the vaccination at an earlier age due to chronic health conditions. The USPSTF recommends a pneumonia vaccination once at age 65, and suggests people in that age group consider repeating the vaccine every 6 to 7 years (AHRQ, 2007). The vaccine is administered intramuscularly in the deltoid muscle or subcutaneously. It can be given with the influenza vaccine via a separate injection in the other arm without an increase in the severity of reactions or by affecting antibody response.

Influenza Vaccine

Influenza vaccines contain three virus strains: two type A and one type B. During the influenza season, selected federal "sentinel reporters" who are health care providers submit nasal swabs of individuals who present to health care institutions with influenza-type symptoms. These data are used to develop the influenza vaccine for the upcoming year. In this way, the vaccine should represent the most common viruses to which individuals will likely be exposed in the upcoming influenza season. The influenza vaccine will not always prevent the aging patient from contracting the flu; studies have shown the vaccine prevents severe illness, complications such as the development of pneumonia, and death (Kaldy, 2006). The USPSTF recommends annual influenza immunization in all individuals age 65 and older (AHRQ, 2007). The *Healthy People 2010* strategy for adult immunizations is outlined in the National Guidelines box.

The influenza vaccine is made from egg-grown viruses that are not infectious. Patients cannot get the flu from the vaccination; however, it is absolutely contraindicated in those who have a hypersensitivity to egg protein. The live attenuated influenza nasal vaccine should not be administered to seniors.

Tetanus Vaccine

Many older adults are not aware that they need a tetanus immunization, and others have poor recollection of their immunization history (Fernandes, Flynn, & Masaki, 2003). Immunization against tetanus is recommended every 10 years in adults over 65 years of age (AHRQ, 2007). The vaccine is usually available in multiple-dose vials as tetanus-diphtheria toxoid (Td). The dosage for adults is 0.5 mL administered intramuscularly. The vaccine must be kept in the refrigerator to maintain potency of the vaccine.

Herpes Zoster Vaccine

Herpes zoster virus vaccine is used to prevent herpes zoster virus, also known as shingles, in people over age 60. It contains live, attenuated varicella-zoster virus in a dose 14 times greater than the varicella (chickenpox) vaccine. This larger dose is needed to boost immunity against shingles in older persons. Herpes zoster virus vaccine decreases the occurrence of herpes zoster by about half, and for those who do get herpes zoster, it reduces the severity and risk of developing postherpetic neuralgia. This is important because the pain that is associated with postherpetic neuralgia can be debilitating and persist long after the zoster rash has resolved.

About 50 million people are candidates to receive this vaccine. The cost of the vaccine is approximately $186 per dose, and is reimbursable under Medicare Part D. A single dose of zoster vaccine is recommended for adults age 60 or older whether or not they report a prior episode of herpes zoster. The Advisory Committee on Immunization Practices voted to recommend use of the vaccine for the prevention of postherpetic neuralgia in this same age group (DeYoung & Baty, 2007).

Screening Exams

Addressing screening exams in the aging patient can be a challenge for several reasons. First, unlike children who require certain exams and immunizations both to ensure normal growth and development as well as to enter school, there are no such requirements for seniors. Screening recommendations for seniors are not mandated, and must take into account the comorbidities and functional status of the individual. Second, when considering screening exams, the health care provider needs to know what will be done with the information obtained from the exam. If a patient indicates that he would not pursue treatment if cancer were found as a result of a screening test, ordering the test is most likely unnecessary. Finally, a factor that must be considered is whether the benefit of the test outweighs the burden of administering the test itself. All of these decisions require the health care provider to fully discuss the screening exam with the patient in order to make informed decisions while taking the individual's wishes into account.

Vision

The USPSTF recommends visual screening and full eye exam on an annual basis for all individuals age 65 and older (AHRQ, 2007).

NATIONAL GUIDELINES *Healthy People 2010*

Healthy People 2010 has identified an increase in adults vaccinated as one of its goals. In 1998, 64% of community-dwelling adults ages 65 and older had received the influenza vaccine, and 46% had received the pneumococcal vaccine. The 2010 targets for vaccination are as follows: 90% target for both the influenza and pneumococcal vaccine.

In the institutionalized adult (i.e., a person living in a nursing home), 59% received the influenza vaccine in 1997, and only 25% had received the pneumococcal vaccine. *Healthy People 2010's* targets for vaccination are 90% for both vaccines—the same target as for community-dwelling adults ages 65 and older.

Source: U.S. Department of Health and Human Services. (2000). Increase in adults vaccinated (Objectives 14-29a–f). In *Healthy People 2010: Understanding and improving health.* Retrieved February 11, 2007, from http://www.healthypeople.gov/document/html/objectives/14-29.htm

Visual impairment is defined as visual acuity 20/40 or worse. Legal blindness is defined as 20/200 or worse. Such screening is important because some visual changes occur slowly over many years. The aging patient may not be aware that visual acuity has declined. Acuity testing and tonometry can identify refractive problems, cataracts, age-related macular degeneration, diabetic retinopathy, and glaucoma (Reuben et al., 2007). Mobile optometrists are available in some communities to travel to private homes, senior communities, and long-term care settings to evaluate individuals who are unable to travel to a traditional medical office. This is especially useful for evaluating individuals with dementia who may need eyeglasses but become agitated when moved from their familiar environment.

Hearing

Hearing loss is the most common sensory impairment in the older adult. The USPSTF recommends hearing impairment screening on a yearly basis for all individuals age 65 and older (AHRQ, 2007). The canals must be free of cerumen for reliable testing. Evaluation consists of screening for hearing problems (medical history, questionnaire) and audiometry, which documents the decibel loss across frequencies along with the pattern of loss. Based on the findings, augmentation with hearing aids may be considered (Reuben et al., 2007). Hearing aids can cost up to $5,000 per pair. On admission, history relating to hearing should be collected as part of the initial assessment. As the nurse develops a plan of care relating to the patient's hearing deficits, directions for the management of the patient's hearing aids must be relayed to all care providers. Developing a plan of care is one of the components of the ANA standards of clinical gerontological nursing care (Congdon et al., 2001). The ANA standards are shown earlier in the chapter in Chart 10–1 (p. 170).

Breast Exams/Breast Cancer Screening

The USPSTF recommends monthly breast self-exams and mammograms every 1 to 2 years up to the age of 70. For those over the age of 70, mammography should be continued for those who have a "reasonable life expectancy" (AHRQ, 2007). However, the term *reasonable life expectancy* has not been defined, and it is not clear as to who determines whether an individual has a reasonable life expectancy.

Pap Smears

The USPSTF recommends a Pap smear at least every 3 years in women age 65 and older. However, Pap smears may be stopped after age 65 if there is one negative Pap smear at age 65 and the woman is low risk (USPSTF, n.d.). A woman at low risk is one with an established sexual partner, history of consistent prior screening, and no history of abnormal Pap smears. Women without a cervix should not have Pap smears (Reuben et al., 2007; USPSTF, n.d.).

Prostate Exam/Prostate Cancer Screening

Prostate cancer is the most common cancer other than skin cancers that affects men. About 1 in 6 men will be diagnosed with prostate cancer during their lifetime, but only 1 in 34 will die from it (American Cancer Society, n.d.). The USPSTF recommends a yearly prostate surface antigen (PSA) test and a digital rectal exam (DRE) in males age 65 and older. However, it has been noted that men over the age of 75 with a negative DRE rarely die from prostate cancer, fueling the debate as to who should be screened in this population (Tabloski, 2006).

Prostate cancers tend to be slow growing in older patients, and for those with multiple comorbidities there is a greater chance death will occur from a disease process other than

---

Mammogram Screenings in Elderly Patients

Clinical Problem

When considering health promotion and disease prevention, it is debatable as to who over the age of 70 should receive screening mammograms. The recommendation for those over 70 is to only screen those with a "reasonable life expectancy," yet there is no definition of what "reasonable life expectancy" means. What criteria should be used when referring for a mammogram?

Research Findings

Schonberg and colleagues (2004) surveyed 882 women ages 80 and over to examine the relationship between health status and screening mammograms in the previous 2 years. They found that more than half of the women over age 80 in the United States receive screening mammograms. Of women likely to have life expectancies of less than 5 years due to poor health, nearly 40% received screening mammography.

Implications for Nursing Practice

When addressing the need for a mammogram, the nurse must not just consider the exam itself, but consider the aging patient's overall condition. If the patient is bedbound or unable to participate due to inability to remain still or follow instructions, a mammogram may not be appropriate. For patients with cognitive disorders or chronic

illnesses, the nurse needs to ask this question: "If an abnormality were found, would the patient seek treatment?"

Critical Thinking Questions

1. A patient refused mammograms when she was mentally alert and now has advanced dementia. Her daughter requests you schedule her for a mammogram. What should you do?

2. You are performing your usual nursing admission assessment on a medical–surgical floor on an elderly female with advanced dementia. You note a palpable golf ball–sized mass on the right breast. The patient's daughter is out in the waiting room. What should you do?

3. Your patient is only able to stand for short periods of time, but otherwise requires a wheelchair. Is she able to obtain a mammogram?

Answers to Critical Thinking Questions appear in Appendix D.

Reference

Schonberg, M. A., McCarthy, E. P., Davis, R. B., Phillips, R. S., & Hamel, M. B. (2004). Breast cancer screening in women aged 80 and older: Results from a national survey. *Journal of the American Geriatrics Society, 52,* 1688–1695.

EVIDENCE-BASED PRACTICE

prostate cancer. Older men should discuss this subject with their primary care provider. PSA levels can be falsely elevated when obtained during hospitalization due to catheterization and infection, thus they should not routinely be obtained during hospitalization.

Colon Cancer Screening

Colorectal cancer is the fourth most common cancer in the United States and the second leading cause of death from cancer (AHRQ, 2007). The USPSTF recommends colon cancer screening consisting of fecal occult blood testing (FOBT), sigmoidoscopy, and colonoscopy starting at age 50 for those at average risk for colorectal cancer. Those at high risk, for example, an individual with a first-degree relative diagnosed with colon cancer before age 60, may consider screening at an earlier age. For those age 65 and older, FOBT is recommended yearly, sigmoidoscopy every 5 years, and colonoscopy every 10 years. The appropriate age to discontinue colorectal cancer screening is not known. Most screening studies have restricted enrollees to those less than 80 years of age. The burden of screening may outweigh potential benefits in patients with advanced age and comorbid conditions that limit life expectancy. Thus, the aging patient needs to discuss benefits and potential harms associated with each screening test with a health care provider before deciding on a screening strategy (AHRQ, 2007).

■ Pharmacology and the Aging Patient

There has been a major emphasis in the health care community on appropriate medications for the aging patient with a focus on prevention of complications from medications inappropriately prescribed (Beers, 1997; Bonk, Krown, Matuszewski, & Oinonen, 2006; Fick et al., 2003; Maio et al., 2006). This focus evolved from publication in 1991 of criteria identifying inappropriate medication use in the nursing home population. These criteria were initially developed to aid researchers in evaluating the quality of prescribing, drug utilization systems, and educational efforts in the nursing home setting. Further updates have identified medications or medication classes that should generally be avoided in persons 65 or older for two reasons. First, there are medications that are either ineffective or pose unnecessarily high risk for older persons and a safer alternative is available. Second, there are medications that should not be used in older persons known to have specific medical conditions (Fick et al., 2003). These criteria, now known as the *Beers criteria,* have been expanded to apply to older individuals living in the community, because inappropriate prescribing by health care providers has been shown to occur in both inpatient and outpatient settings (Beers, 1997; Maio et al., 2006). An adult over the age of 65 takes an average of 5.7 medications each day (American Society of Health-System Pharmacists, 2006). Often these medications may be unnecessary or inappropriately prescribed. Five percent to 15% of hospital admissions in elderly patients may be linked to drug-related problems or toxic drug effects (Mezey et al., 2003). In one study, a greater number of medications taken were associated with weight loss and impaired balance in elderly patients, after adjustment for chronic illness (Agostini, Han, & Tinetti, 2004).

Adverse drug reactions (ADRs) or **adverse drug events (ADEs)** can occur when a patient takes a medication that has been appropriately or inappropriately prescribed. An ADE is defined as "noxious and unintended patient events, such as symptoms, signs, and laboratory abnormalities caused by a drug" (Roehl, Talati, & Parks, 2006). Studies have shown that at least one inappropriate medication had been prescribed for 40% of nursing home residents and 21% of elderly living in the community (Bonk et al., 2006; Liu & Christensen, 2002; Maio et al., 2006).

Ethnic background also may place an individual at risk for ADEs. One meta-analysis of studies found this to be the case for cardiovascular medications in various ethnic groups. For example, black patients taking angiotensin converting enzyme (ACE) inhibitors are three times more likely to experience angioedema compared with nonblack patients. East Asian patients are more likely to experience cough due to ACE inhibitors compared to white patients. Black patients have a higher risk of moderate or severe bleeding following thrombolytic therapy compared to nonblack patients. Thus, ethnic background must be considered in individuals experiencing ADEs (McDowell, Coleman, & Ferner, 2006).

 One method to ensure that patients are not re-prescribed medications that previously caused an adverse reaction is to enter those medications in the allergy section of the patient's chart or electronic medical record, along with the reactions the patient experienced. Although not a true drug allergy, listing drug intolerances along with their adverse reaction as part of the medical record will direct providers to choose another medication for a particular condition when prescribing.

Polypharmacy

Polypharmacy is one of the major medication issues affecting the aging patient. **Polypharmacy** is defined as the administration of many drugs together, and the administration of excessive medications (*Polypharmacy,* 2007). However, the definition itself is controversial and varies from study to study, making application of research results in the clinical setting challenging. In the clinical setting, polypharmacy occurs when an individual is using more medications than is clinically indicated. This includes prescription medications, over-the-counter (OTC) medications, and nontraditional medications. This phenomenon called polypharmacy can occur in the acute care setting, in a structured care setting such as an assisted living facility, or at home.

A thorough nursing assessment on admission to the hospital provides an opportunity to identify and eliminate polypharmacy. The following information should be collected:

- Medical diagnoses and self-diagnosed health problems
- Known drug allergies
- History of previous adverse drug reactions
- All prescribed medications taken
- All OTC medications taken
- All nontraditional medications taken
- Length of time each medication has been taken
- Actual amounts of each medication taken and how often
- Reason for taking each medication, any adverse effects
- Any problems with taking the medication in its prescribed form (*Medication Assessment,* 2005).

Medication Administration Principles for the Aging Patient

Medication administration principles for the aging patient go beyond practicing the "five rights" of medication administration. With regard to dosing, the adage to "start low, and go slow" should be followed. Often a nurse is given a choice of a range of doses for an as-needed medication. In the aging patient, the nurse should start with a lower dose than might be typically administered to a younger patient. The aging patient takes longer to metabolize and excrete medications due to decreased renal and hepatic function. Some medication reference guides list geriatric doses, which is helpful. For medications excreted renally, the nurse can calculate the estimated creatinine clearance. Serum creatinine does not accurately reflect renal function in the aging patient due to decreased lean body mass. The Cockcroft-Gault formula is used to estimate creatinine clearance (CrCl):

$$Creatinine\ clearance = \frac{(140 - age) \times weight\ (kg)}{Plasma\ creatinine\ (mg/dl) \times 2.72} (\times\ 0.85\ for\ women)$$

For drugs excreted via the kidneys, dosage adjustments may be necessary if CrCl < 60 (Roehl et al., 2006).

Many hospitalized patients have impaired swallowing or are unable to swallow medications in the traditional pill form due to altered cognition with agitation. These patients present a challenge for the nurse who must be knowledgeable about other possible methods for medication administration. For example, a patient requiring long-term pain management who is unable to swallow or take pain medications on a consistent basis may be appropriate for medication delivery via a transdermal patch (Figure 10–4 ■, p. 182). A transdermal patch delivers a continuous amount of pain medication and only requires changing every 72 hours. This method of medication delivery also may reduce caregiver burden. Chart 10-2 (p. 183) lists some of the medications with potential adverse outcomes for the aging patient.

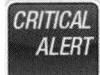 **CRITICAL ALERT** *Medications with an enteric coating as well as sustained-release medications cannot be crushed. If the patient requires her medications to be crushed or administered via nasogastric or gastrostomy tube, notify the physician or health care professional so that the equivalent short-acting medication may be ordered and crushed. Remember, if the medication is difficult to crush, there is a reason why!*

Medication Administration for Aging Patients

Clinical Problem

With all of the various mechanisms in which medications are metabolized in the elderly, how is a nurse to know which ones are not appropriate in this population? Specifically, which medications should nurses tell their aging patients to avoid?

Research Findings

The number of controlled studies on medication use in the aging patient is limited, yet the toxic effects of medications in this population can have profound consequences. The use of consensus criteria is one way to develop reliable and explicit criteria for safe medication use when precise clinical information is lacking (Fick et al., 2003). In 1991, the first research was published identifying inappropriate medication use in nursing home patients. From this original research, the Beers report update in 1997 became the accepted criteria for evaluating appropriate medication use in frail nursing home patients (Beers, 1997). By 1999, the criteria had been adopted by the Centers for Medicare & Medicaid Services for nursing home regulation. In 2003, the criteria were updated to generalize the criteria to older patients regardless of their residence. The Beers criteria identify medication or medication classes that should generally be avoided in persons 65 or older because they are ineffective or pose unnecessarily high risk for this group and safer alternatives exist.

Implications for Nursing Practice

Any nurse caring for elderly patients needs to become familiar with the Beers criteria. In addition, most medication programs that can be installed on a personal digital assistant include a section on special considerations for the elderly. In addition, any hospitalized aging patients who are exhibiting signs of delirium should have their medications reviewed to determine if adverse side effects of the medications are contributing to the delirium.

Critical Thinking Questions

1. Your 95-year-old patient had hip surgery 3 days ago and has now been admitted to your skilled nursing facility for rehabilitation. The patient is reporting aching hip pain. The x-rays are negative for any changes in the alignment of the hip. You call the on-call physician for pain medication orders and are told to give the patient "One Darvocet every four hours for moderate pain, and two Darvocet every four hours for severe pain." How would you respond to the physician?

2. An 85-year-old male on your medical floor has been receiving diphenhydramine nightly to help him sleep as was prescribed by his physician. After 3 days on your floor, he reports he is having difficulty urinating, even though he has made multiple trips to the bathroom. What do you think might be causing his problems with urination?

3. On admission to your unit, you review the admitting medication orders with your alert 90-year-old female patient. She confides in you that she has been taking diazepam 5 mg three times a day for several years that was prescribed by another physician in the community for her "nerves." Her primary care physician is not aware of her diazepam use, but she wants her medication. What should the nurse do?

Answers to Critical Thinking Questions appear in Appendix D.

References

Beers, M. H. (1997). Explicit criteria for determining potentially inappropriate medication use by the elderly. *Archives of Internal Medicine, 157,* 1531–1536.

Fick, D. M., Cooper, J. W., Wade, W. E., Waller, J. L., Maclean, J. R., & Beers, M. H. (2003). Updating the Beers criteria for potentially inappropriate medication use in older adults. *Archives of Internal Medicine, 163,* 2716–2724.

EVIDENCE-BASED PRACTICE

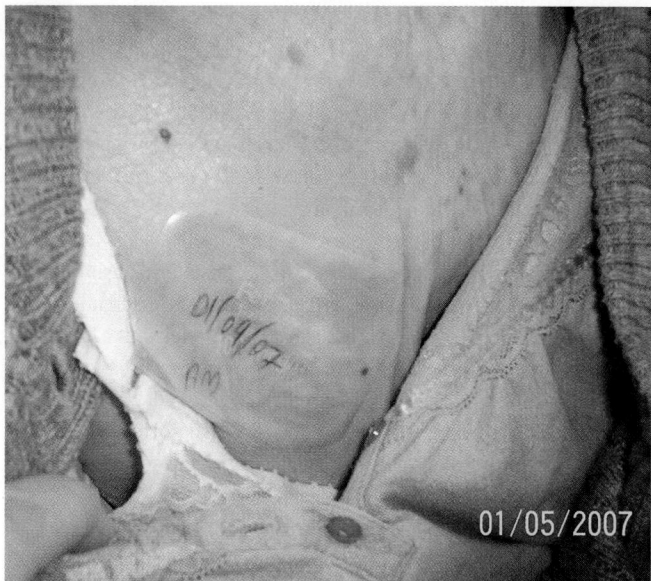

01/05/2007

FIGURE 10–4 ■ Fentanyl patch.

Resources for Caring for an Aging Population

When the aging patient can no longer live alone independently, all viable alternative resources should be explored. Twenty-four-hour-a-day care may be needed in a board and care facility, an assisted living facility, or a nursing home. Contrary to popular belief, Medicare does not cover private home care, board and care, assisted living, or custodial nursing home care. Custodial care residents typically live in a nursing home for an extended period of time due to their need for 24-hour-a-day supervision, nursing care, and assistance with activities of daily living. ADLs include bathing, toileting, eating, and dressing. Generally, Medicare covers skilled nursing care when an individual has been hospitalized and requires a high level of nursing care or therapy at least daily. Examples of skilled nursing care include intravenous (IV) therapy, complicated wound care, and nutrition administered via a feeding tube. Examples of therapy include daily physical, occupational, or speech therapy.

Board and care, assisted living, and many nursing homes cost between $4,000 and $7,000 per month depending on location and amenities offered. Individuals often exhaust their personal life savings paying for such care, and then rely on Medicaid to pay for their care for the remainder of their life. Some nursing homes will not accept Medicaid patients due to concerns that financial reimbursements for these patients have not kept pace with the cost of the care delivered. In fact, in many facilities, private-pay patients pay twice the amount per day that the state reimburses for Medicaid patients.

Medicare and Medicaid

A person's financial means directly affects a patient's ability to pay for housing, food, and medical care. Medical care is of special interest as funding mechanisms have changed drastically in the past 50 years. Prior to the advent of Medicare, health care was primarily a fee-for-service industry. When an individual interacted with the health care system, the provider of care was paid directly for services provided. Medicare, a federally funded health care program for individuals over the age of 65, those under the age of 65 who are disabled, and those with end-stage renal disease, was signed into law in 1965 by President Johnson. Currently Medicare pays for 54% of overall health care costs for its enrollees age 65 and over. Medicare Part A covers hospital stays, pints of blood for transfusions, home health services, hospice care, and some skilled nursing care (after a qualifying hospital stay). Most people or their spouses paid Medicare taxes while working, and will automatically receive Medicare Part A coverage without having to pay a monthly premium. Medicare Part B covers medical services such as medical care by a doctor, nurse practitioner, or physician's assistant; outpatient care; and other medical services not covered by Part A. Enrollment in Part B is optional and there is a monthly premium to pay. Part B deductible must be paid each year before Medicare begins to pay a share of Part B expenses. Some examples of services that fall under Medicare Part B are ambulance services, cardiovascular screenings, bone density measurements, mammogram screenings, and clinical laboratory services.

Individuals enrolled in Medicare can add drug coverage if they join a Medicare prescription drug plan. These plans are offered by private companies that work with Medicare to provide medication coverage. Premiums, copays, and yearly deductibles vary by plans. Each Medicare drug plan has a formulary. A formulary is a list of covered drugs. The list must include at least two drugs in all classes of drugs commonly prescribed to individuals age 65 and older. For more details review Chapter 3 of this text.

Some individuals choose to purchase a supplemental insurance policy to cover extra health care costs not covered by Medicare. This insurance, called a "Medigap" policy, is sold by private insurance companies to fill in the gaps in Medicare coverage. Typically Medigap policies help pay a share of coinsurance, copayments, or deductibles of the costs of Medicare-covered services. Usually when one buys Medigap insurance, both Part A and Part B are covered.

For those who are low income, Medicaid provides financial coverage for health care expenses. Medicaid is a federal program enacted in 1965 at the same time President Johnson enacted Medicare. It is administered individually by each state. Eligibility is based on income and assets. Medicaid covers 10% of overall health care costs for those age 65 and over. In 2006, new rules came into effect requiring Americans to show proof of citizenship or risk losing their Medicaid benefits. This can be challenging for elderly people who lack family support systems and suffer from dementia or mental illness (Centers for Medicare & Medicaid Services [CMS], n.d.). The nurse can assist patients by identifying resources within the hospital setting that can help elderly patients submit the necessary paperwork.

Some individuals enroll in Medicare advantage plans. With these plans, their Medicare is assigned to a preferred provider organization (PPO) or health maintenance organization (HMO), which is responsible for overseeing and coordinating care. Chapter 3 discusses these types of health plans in detail.

CHART 10–2	**Selected Medications with Potential Adverse Outcomes for the Aging Patient**	

Medication Class	Medication	Rationale for Avoiding Medication in the Aging Patient
Muscle relaxants, anticholinergics, and antihistamines	Methocarbamol Carisoprodol Cyclobenzaprine Oxybutynin Chlorpheniramine Hydroxyzine Promethazine Diphenhydramine	Are very anticholinergic and produce toxic effects in the elderly such as cardiac arrhythmias, dry mouth and eyes, and urinary retention. Should be avoided in the elderly, or limited to use for 7 days or less. Diphenhydramine may cause confusion and sedation; should not be used as a sleeping agent; use smallest dose possible if needed to treat an allergic reaction.
Psychotropics and antidepressants	Amitriptyline	Has strong anticholinergic and sedating properties; better antidepressants are available such as selective serotonin reuptake inhibitors (SSRIs) other than fluoxetine.
	Fluoxetine	Has a long half-life and risk of producing excessive central nervous system (CNS) stimulation, with sleep disturbances and agitation. Other antidepressants are available for the elderly that have fewer side effects, such as other SSRIs, atypicals, or bicyclic antidepressants.
	Diazepam, flurazepam	Have a long half-life in the elderly—medications sometimes do not clear system for several days. Produce prolonged sedation, increased risk of falls and fractures. Short- and intermediate-acting benzodiazepines are preferred if needed such as low-dose lorazepam.
	Short-acting benzodiazepines at doses greater than: lorazepam, 3 mg; oxazepam, 60 mg; alprazolam, 2 mg; temazepam, 15 mg; and triazolam, 0.25 mg	Smaller doses in the elderly are effective and safer due to patients' increased sensitivity to these drugs.
Analgesics	Indomethacin	Produces the most CNS side effects of all nonsteroidal anti-inflammatory medications (NSAIDS).
	Ketorolac	Should be avoided because many elderly people have asymptomatic pathologic GI conditions.
	Long-term use of full dosage, longer half-life, non-co-oxygenase (COX) selective NSAIDS such as naproxen and piroxicam	Potential to induce GI bleeding, renal failure, high blood pressure, and heart failure.
	Meperidine	CNS effects; breakdown product can cause convulsions. Safer alternatives exist, such as acetaminophen and a short-acting opiate if necessary.
	Propoxyphene	Limited analgesic advantage over acetaminophen, but has the adverse effects of other narcotic drugs.
Cardiac medications	Digoxin > 0.125 mg/day	Doses greater than 0.125 mg should be avoided because decreased renal clearance leads to increased risk of toxic effects. Doses greater than 0.125 mg, however, can be used to treat atrial arrhythmias.
	Clonidine	Potential for hypotension and CNS effects.
	Amiodarone	Not effective in older adults; risk of torsades de pointes and QT interval problems.
	Disopyramide	Highly anticholinergic; may induce heart failure.
	Doxazosin	Can cause hypotension, dry mouth, and urinary problems.
	Methyldopa	Can cause bradycardia and exacerbate depression; alternative antihypertensives should be considered.
Miscellaneous medications	Ticlopidine	Aspirin is better in preventing clotting than ticlopidine and less toxic.
	Trimethobenzamide	Is one of the least effective antiemetic drugs; can cause extrapyramidal side effects.

Sources: Adapted from Bonk, M. E., Krown, H., Matuszewski, K., & Oinonen, M. (2006). Potentially inappropriate medications in hospitalized senior patients. *American Journal of Health System Pharmacists, 63,* 1161–1165; Beers, M. H. (1997). Explicit criteria for determining potentially inappropriate medication use by the elderly. *Archives of Internal Medicine, 157,* 1531–1536.

Medicare advantage plans provide all of the coverage of Part A and Part B and must cover medically necessary services. Medicare pays an amount every month to these private health plans, whether or not services were used in that particular month. These organizations offer benefits greater than what Medicare alone covers, thus their popularity in certain parts of the United States, such as California.

Long-Term Care Insurance

Long-term care insurance has evolved as one mechanism to ensure that individuals needing long-term care, particularly in a nursing home, will not become financially bankrupt when their time of need for care arises. Nursing home costs vary somewhat throughout the United States. The 2005 average daily rate for a private room in a nursing home was $203, and it cost an average $176 per day for a semiprivate room. Thus, the cost of living in a nursing home for a year would range from $64,240 to $74,095 (MetLife, 2005).

The aging patient has a 50% chance of spending some time in a nursing home. With more than 100 insurance companies offering long-term care insurance policies, one might think that protecting oneself from spending a lifetime of assets on nursing home care is the prudent thing to do. However, only 5% of those over 65 years of age have purchased long-term care insurance. Policies vary widely, many with restrictions, loopholes, and premiums that become unaffordable to maintain. Premiums can range from $2,000 to $10,000 per year, with annual increases. For this reason, only 5 people out of 100 who are 60 years of age or older who take out long-term care insurance policies still have the policy at age 80, when they are most likely to need it (Alexander, 2006). It is recommended that any individual considering long-term care insurance have an attorney review the policy to determine if it will indeed be useful if the time arises when care is needed.

Legal and Ethical Issues of Aging

It is often difficult and challenging for the nurse to discuss legal and ethical concerns with a patient or family member. Many nurses have little experience in this area, and bringing up issues such as elder abuse or advance directives can feel awkward and unsettling. However, such difficult conversations become easier as a nurse gains experience and becomes knowledgeable about legal and ethical issues.

Elder Mistreatment (Abuse)

Elder mistreatment or *abuse* is a broad term that describes the outcome of abuse, neglect, exploitation, or abandonment of older adults. There are three categories of elder mistreatment: domestic, institutional, and self-neglect. Domestic mistreatment occurs in the aging patient's home and involves significant others such as a child, spouse, or relatives. Institutional mistreatment occurs when an individual has a contractual agreement with a care facility such as a nursing home and is abused. Self-neglect occurs when an individual who is capable of making decisions and understanding consequences engages in behavior that threatens his or her safety or well-being (Tabloski, 2006). The seven major types of elder abuse are as follows:

- *Physical abuse* is the use of physical force that may result in injury, pain, or impairment. Some examples of physical abuse are acts of violence such as striking, slapping, kicking, or pinching. Other nonviolent examples include misuse of drugs, force feeding, or use of restraints.
- *Sexual abuse* is nonconsensual sexual contact of any kind with an elderly person. If a person is incapable of giving consent due to cognitive impairment such as dementia, sexual contact also is considered sexual abuse. Some examples include unwanted touching and all forms of sexual assault and battery, such as rape and sodomy.
- *Emotional* or *psychological abuse* involves inflicting pain or distress through verbal or nonverbal means. Insults, threats, and forced social isolation would be considered emotional/psychological abuse.
- *Neglect* is the refusal or failure to fulfill duties to an elder. Examples of neglect include failing to provide necessary personal care for a dependent adult, or failing to hire someone to provide the needed care.
- *Abandonment* is defined as desertion of an elderly person by an individual deemed responsible for the elder's care. An example is a caregiver leaving a dependent elderly person alone for a week while the caregiver takes a vacation out of town.
- *Financial* or *material exploitation* is defined as misuse of an elder's money, property, or assets. Examples of financial exploitation include tricking a dependent elder into signing checks for a caregiver's personal use and stealing money or possessions.
- *Self-neglect* is the refusal or failure of an elderly person to provide himself with adequate food, water, shelter, and health care to the point that personal health or safety is threatened. An example of self-neglect is when an individual with a cognitive impairment uses all of his money to buy cat food for 50 cats and fails to buy food for himself and becomes undernourished as a result (National Center on Elder Abuse [NCEA], 2007c).

It is important for nurses to become knowledgeable regarding elder abuse reporting laws as well as an awareness of possible signs and symptoms of elder mistreatment. Forty-four states and the District of Columbia have laws providing that individuals who care for the elderly are considered mandatory reporters and must report suspected elder abuse or mistreatment. A **mandatory reporter** is a person required by law to report allegations and/or suspicions of abuse. A nurse is a mandatory reporter. Thirty-eight state statutes specify a penalty for mandatory reporters who fail to report when they should (Daly, Jogerst, Brinig, & Dawson, 2004).

In most states, Adult Protective Services (APS) caseworkers are the first responders to reports of abuse, exploitation, and neglect. Their role for the elderly is to ensure the safety and well-being of those who are unable to take care of themselves and have no one to assist them. These caseworkers receive reports of elderly abuse, exploitation, or neglect; investigate the report; and provide case planning including emergency shelter, medical care, legal assistance, and supportive services if indicated, and monitoring and evaluation (NCEA, 2007b). On a national level, the NCEA, directed by the U.S. Administration on Aging, serves as a resource for policy makers, health care professionals, families, and others interested in ensuring that older Americans live free of abuse, neglect, and exploitation (NCEA, 2007a). Chart 10–3 lists possible signs and symptoms of elder mistreatment.

CHART 10–3	Possible Signs and Symptoms of Elder Mistreatment

Type of Mistreatment	Possible Signs and Symptoms
Physical/sexual abuse	• Multiple trips to the emergency room • A patient's report of being hit, slapped, or mistreated • Unexplained fractures or bruises in various stages of healing • Trauma or bleeding in the genital area • Unexplained veneral disease
Emotional/ psychological abuse	• Withdrawn or non-communicative patient, reluctant to answer questions with family member present • A patient who is emotionally upset or agitated • Family members who are or act irritable or refuse to allow patient to answer questions
Neglect/ abandonment	• Unexplained skin rashes, irritation, or ulcers • Family exhibits poor follow-through in obtaining needed medications and medical care for family member • Patient reports being left in unsafe situation for periods of time
Self-neglect	• Poor hygiene in an elder that impacts the individual's health • Dehydration; malnutrition; unexplained weight loss
Financial exploitation	• Discovery that patient's signature was forged • Sudden changes in a patient's financial condition • Unexplained loss of Social Security or pension checks • Visiting family members, especially previously uninvolved ones, are asking someone incapable of making decisions to sign checks or other documents, or financial activity the patient couldn't have done • Unusual interest on the part of caregivers in the patient's assets

Source: Adapted from AGS Foundation for Health in Aging. (2002). *Elder mistreatment.* Retrieved January 25, 2007, from http://www.healthinaging.org; Jaffe-Gill, E., de Benedictis, T., and Segal, J. (2008). *Elder Abuse: Types, Signs, Symptoms, Risk Factors and Prevention.* Retrieved February 8, 2009, from http://www.helpguide.org/mental/elder_abuse_physical_emotional_sexual_neglect.htm; National Center on Elder Abuse (2007). *Major Types of Elder Abuse.* Retrieved February 6, 2009, from http://www.ncea.aoa.gov/ncearoot/Main_Site/FAQ/Basics/Types_Of_Abuse.aspx.

Advance Directives

Advance directives provide a mechanism for individuals to place into writing their wishes regarding treatment should they become ill. Individuals typically execute such a document when they are well and able to think through the various scenarios they might experience as they age. Chapter 17 describes in detail the two forms of advance directives: living wills and durable powers of attorney for health care (DPAHC). Aging patients are encouraged to draft both a living will and a DPAHC while they are healthy and able to discuss wishes re-

garding care and treatments. Once an individual is cognitively impaired and no longer has the capacity to make informed decisions, that person is not legally able to execute a living will or DPAHC. A court-appointed conservator should be pursued to allow a legally designated individual to make decisions on behalf of the patient with a cognitive impairment.

In the nursing home setting, a preferred intensity of care (PIC) or preferred intensity of treatment (PIT) form is used as an additional tool to enable patients or their designated representative to clarify treatment wishes (Figure 10–5 ■, p. 186). Depending on the facility, such forms include yes/no boxes to check to address a number of medical interventions available in the nursing home, such as CPR, nasogastric or artificial feeding methods, IV antibiotics, and transfers to the hospital.

Care Options for the Aging Patient

For many aging patients, hospitalization represents a sentinel event, triggering a downward spiral of health and function (Mezey et al., 2003). Social issues as well as medical issues are brought to light when a frail patient is hospitalized. However, once the crisis of hospitalization has arrived, the nurse needs to look ahead toward discharge planning. Some discussion of post-hospitalization plans should even take place at the time of admission. When the subject of post-hospitalization discharge planning is broached, many older patients oppose returning to anywhere but home. Many envision nursing homes, which in the past were referred to as "rest homes" or "convalescent homes," as dingy, dark places where people go to die. Children and family members make promises that they may not be willing or able to keep, such as "Mom will never go to a nursing home." Fortunately, a variety of housing and care options exist for the aging patient as outlined in the following subsections.

Independent Living

The aging patient has many options for independent living that go beyond remaining in one's home. Life care communities or continuing care retirement centers offer an independent living option, with an opportunity to "age in place" if the individual requires more care as time progresses. Often the independent living area offers apartment or town home living, with or without meals. Support such as housekeeping and activities are available. Such facilities also offer assisted living and skilled nursing care, usually in separate buildings, that the person can take advantage of when it is finally needed. Health plans and Medicare do not cover the expense of life care communities, unless the individual resides in the skilled nursing facility and is receiving rehabilitative services. Such facilities often require a *buy-in,* which can range from thousands to hundreds of thousands of dollars and is in addition to the monthly living expenses. The benefits of such communities are many. Most importantly, residents may move back and forth between levels of care as their health needs dictate, and couples with differing levels of health needs can be accommodated within one building.

Senior supported housing can vary from low-income apartment complexes for seniors subsidized by the government to privately paid apartments that provide some or all meals, housekeeping, and laundry services, along with social activities

---

ACKNOWLEDGMENT OF RECEIPT
ADVANCE DIRECTIVES/MEDICAL TREATMENT DECISIONS

This is to acknowledge that I have been informed in writing in a language that I understand of my rights and all rules and regulations to make decisions concerning medical care, including the right to accept or refuse medical or surgical treatment and the right to formulate and to issue Advance Directives to be followed should I become incapacitated.

☐ I have chosen to formulate and issue the following Advance Directives.

Initial Choices	Yes	No		Yes	No
Resuscitate	___	___	Other _____	___	___
Feeding tube(s) (N/G, G-tube)	___	___	_____	___	___
Antibiotic Therapy	___	___	_____	___	___
Intravenous Therapy	___	___			
Transfer to acute hospital	___	___	_____	___	___
If no, state exceptions _____					

☐ I do not choose to formulate or issue any Advance Directives at this time.
  I want efforts made to prolong my life and I want life-sustaining treatment to be provided.

Resident/Client _____ Date _____

Surrogate Decision Maker _____ Date _____

If Surrogate Decision Maker Signed, Complete the Following:

_____   _____
Print Name   Relationship to Resident

Witness _____ Date _____

— —

If Resident Unable to Sign Name, State Medical Reason:

_____

I have discussed the pertinent diagnosis (ses) and prognosis of the resident and the consequences of withdrawing or withholding life-sustaining services and other health care decisions made with: _____

FIGURE 10–5 ■ Preferred intensity of care form.

and transportation. Health plans and Medicare do not cover the expense of senior supported housing.

Adult Day Health Care and Adult Day Care

Adult day health care offers a program of health services such as nursing care and therapy, meals, social and recreational activities, and social work services in a structured daytime program. Individuals who require health services, social interaction, or supervision during the day can attend while continuing to live at home or in another care setting. Some programs offer transportation; Medicaid may pay for this program.

Adult day care, based on a social model, offers few or no health services. The emphasis of the social day care program is fostering socialization among older adults. These programs aim to keep seniors as active and healthy as possible. These programs offer respite for families and caregivers who need some time away from the caregiver role. Often these programs receive a financial subsidy and charge a daily fee. Private health plans and Medicare do not cover this program.

Residential Care Facilities

A residential care facility is the formal name for the type of facility commonly referred to as "board and care" living. Their licensing oversight varies by state, falling under the department of health. These facilities provide on-site unlicensed caregivers 24 hours a day and assistance with ADLs such as bathing, dressing, and feeding. They provide three meals a day, social activities, housekeeping, laundry services, and limited transportation. Some facilities provide medication supervision by unlicensed personnel and are not medically focused. Many are operated by individual families. Some board and care facilities are six-bed private homes; others may be larger homes designed for such clients with both private and semiprivate rooms (Kaiser Permanente, 2005).

Assisted Living Facilities

Assisted living facilities also are licensed as residential care facilities, but tend to be larger in size, often with 50 to 200 residents, and many are part of a corporation that operates assisted living facilities throughout the country. Most require individuals to be ambulatory, use a walker, or be able to propel their wheelchairs to a common dining area. Rarely are they able to accommodate special diets requiring modified food textures or special liquid consistencies. For example, rarely will an assisted living facility provide a puree diet with honey-thick liquid drinks. Some facilities will only accept an incontinent resident if that individual is able to manage their incontinence products independently.

These facilities cannot accommodate individuals who are bedbound. If an individual requires daily nursing care for problems such as pressure ulcers or an indwelling urinary catheter, the facility must apply for a special waiver to allow the person to remain in the facility. With such large variances in amenities, family members are encouraged to thoroughly examine what the assisted living facility will provide or allow in the way of services before placing a deposit. All types of residential care facilities are licensed by the department of health in the state where they are located.

Intermediate/Skilled Nursing Care

There are times when a frail aging patient has health needs that are beyond what can be provided in a home, board and care, or assisted living facility. Long-term care in an intermediate care or skilled nursing facility might be the best and, in some cases, the only option. A skilled nursing facility may also be called a nursing facility, a nursing home, a convalescent home or hospital, or occasionally a rest home.

Intermediate care facilities (ICFs) and skilled nursing facilities (SNFs) are licensed by the department of health in the state where they are located. They may also be certified to receive payment from Medicare and Medicaid. Approximately 1.6 million people live in the more than 16,000 nursing homes in the United States (Hamilton, 2005). ICFs care for people who are moderately independent but require 24-hour-a-day supervision and assistance, along with intermittent licensed nursing care. ICFs can provide special diets and moderate help with ADLs such as bathing and dressing. They cannot accept individuals who are nonambulatory, incontinent, or require skilled nursing care. ICFs tend to cost less than SNF care, reflecting a lower level of staffing and personal assistance.

Skilled nursing care is usually needed for a short period of time to recover from an acute illness or injury, often following hospitalization. Skilled nursing care is care that must be delivered by a licensed nurse, such as IV therapy, complicated wound care, or nasogastric or gastrostomy tube feedings. Individuals requiring daily physical, occupational, or speech therapy also would qualify for skilled therapy services. Health plans and Medicare cover skilled services and pay for nursing home days that meet established criteria.

Most residents in nursing homes receive custodial care. Custodial care residents live in a nursing home for an extended period of time, sometimes for the remainder of their lives. Some individuals recover enough to move to a less intensive level of care. For those who do not, custodial care provides a higher level of 24-hour-a-day supervision and assistance with ADLs. Licensed nursing staff are on site 24 hours a day to administer medications and deliver other nursing care. Residents who require walkers or wheelchairs for mobility and those who are bedbound or incontinent can be cared for in this setting. Some nursing homes are secured with perimeter fencing and a locked entrance/exit gate to enable those individuals with dementia who are prone to wandering to ambulate freely without becoming injured.

Medical management in the nursing home is handled on site by a physician and often a nurse practitioner who see residents at the facility. This nurse practitioner may be a **gerontological nurse practitioner (GNP),** a registered nurse with a master's degree from a nurse practitioner program specializing in the care of older adults. GNPs are educated to diagnose and manage acute and chronic diseases, using a holistic approach to address the medical, psychosocial, and functional needs of older adults. Any patient discharged from an acute care hospital to a nursing home requires the following forms: history and physical, discharge summary, and nursing home physician orders with indications or diagnoses for all medications ordered. Without these documents, the nursing home cannot admit the patient.

Home Care

Older adults who choose to live independently in their homes for as long as possible can turn to supportive services, such as home care, to provide the needed assistance. Two types of home care are available: home health care and private duty care. The main difference between the two is who pays for the service.

Traditional hospital care involving IV therapy, tube feedings, some forms of dialysis, wound vacuums for pressure ulcer management, and oxygen therapy are now administered in the home. This is partially in response to individuals' preference for care in the home and, in some cases, in response to hospitals' efforts to reign in costs (Matthews, 2006).

ETHICAL ISSUES Regarding Care of MS Patients with Urinary Retention Issues

Many patients with multiple sclerosis (MS) who are ambulatory and able to independently carry out most of their ADLs develop some degree of urinary retention due to their MS. Often, these individuals live in an assisted living settings to maximize their independence. Most assisted living facilities will not accept residents with indwelling catheters. What should the nurse do when the individual develops moderate to significant urinary retention resulting in multiple urinary tract infections and hospitalization for urosepsis?

Some options include:

- Discuss with the resident the risk/benefit of long-term catheter use; insist the resident consent to an indwelling catheter and move to a nursing home.

- Act as a patient advocate and discuss with the assisted living facility the possibility of obtaining a waiver to allow the individual with an indwelling catheter to remain living there.

- Discuss the risk/benefits of long-term urinary retention such as further damage to the bladder, antibiotic-resistant urinary tract infections, and the potential for urosepsis.

- Discuss treating the complications of urinary retention such as urinary tract infections when they occur.

- Discuss the goals of care with the patient given the progressive nature of the multiple sclerosis diagnosis, and whether the benefits of living in assisted living rather than a nursing home outweigh the risks of urinary retention and probable recurrent sepsis with hospitalization and death.

Home health may be covered by an individual's health plan, Medicare, or Medicaid if a physician determines the individual needs intermittent care by at least one professional, such as a registered nurse, physical therapist, occupational therapist, speech therapist, or social worker. A home health aide may be used if requested by the nurse or therapist coordinating the care.

The nurse's role as part of discharge planning during the patient's hospitalization is to determine if the patient or a willing and able caregiver is capable of administering such care in the home environment with support from the home health nurse. The ANA scope and standards of gerontological nursing practice, shown earlier in Chart 10–1 (p. 170), identify the nurse as the professional whose role it is to develop the discharge plan (Congdon et al., 2001). The nurse should begin the teaching process before the individual leaves the hospital, with home health nurses providing specialized care and reinforcement of teaching. Home health nurses typically deliver intermittent care; they may visit daily, several times a week, or weekly, depending on the individual's needs. If an individual's care needs exceed what the family can provide or a home health nurse can accomplish in a home visit, the individual may need care in a skilled nursing facility setting.

Private duty or continuous care is rendered in the home by registered nurses or nursing assistants, homemakers, or companions with the goal to provide personal care and companionship. Caregivers are hired and paid privately by the individual receiving care or through an agency. Some long-term care insurance policies cover in-home private duty care.

Hospice

Hospice services have been available in the home setting for a number of years. Hospice services have been available in nursing homes for nearly 10 years and are requested by patients and family members seeking hospice personnel's expertise in end-of-life care. Once a patient is determined to be appropriate for hospice services in a nursing home, the expectations change from cure to acceptance that a decline is inevitable and the goals change to that of promoting comfort and quality for the remainder of the patient's life. The hospice team can provide support to the family through involvement of social workers, chaplains, and a hospice nurse. Such support is above and beyond what would usually be available in a nursing home (Sattinger, 2006). See Chapter 17 🌐 for more information on hospice and end-of-life issues.

Palliative Care

There is no national consensus on the definition of palliative care. The definition proposed by the Center to Advance Palliative Care (2001) states that "Palliative care aims to relieve suffering and improve the quality of living and dying. It aims to address physical, psychological, social, spiritual and practical expectations and needs of an individual with an acute or chronic life-threatening illness." Jewish Home and Hospital Lifecare System goes on to say that "Care is a comprehensive approach to helping patients manage serious illnesses. Its main focus is to provide patients relief from pain and other distressing symptoms, along with minimizing suffering."

Palliative care programs continue to grow in the hospital setting, with 1,240 hospitals providing programs in 2005, compared to 632 programs in 2000 (*Hospitals Continue to Implement*, 2006). Palliative care programs in the nursing home are rare, possibly due to the newness of the concept and the large amount of resources necessary to implement a program (Tuch Parrish, and Romer, 2002).

◼ Innovations in Caring for the Aging Patient

Innovations in caring for the aging patient have been slow to evolve, primarily due to lack of funding and lack of mechanisms for reimbursement under traditional Medicare and Medicaid models. Innovations currently under way include primary care in the home, the Program for All-inclusive Care of the Elderly, the Green House Project, and elder cohousing communities.

Team-Based Primary Care in the Home

The idea of health care professionals caring for an individual in the home is not new. Years ago, doctors made house calls to patients' homes. As communities grew, medical clinics emerged, and mechanisms for funding health care changed with the advent of Medicare and Medicaid, the days of house calls by a physician came to an end. The U.S. Department of Veterans Affairs (VA) has supported a program with home visits by a physician, a nurse practitioner, and an interdisciplinary team since its inception in 1972. The VA Home-Based Primary Care (HBPC) program provides comprehensive primary care in the homes of veterans with complex chronic disabling disease. Unlike home care that is focused on episodic, time-limited, and focused skilled care, HBPC provides comprehensive longitudinal care. However, this team-based care is only available for those with veterans benefits (Department of Veterans Affairs, 2007).

The concept of team-based primary care in the home is now moving to the traditional Medicare fee-for-service population through demonstration grants. A 3-year pilot project that was scheduled to end in 2008 is testing the effects of increased access and quality of care to elderly people who are chronically ill through the use of house calls by physicians. Care Level Management, the company conducting the project, utilizes a personal physician house call system of care that provides patients with direct, 24-hour access to a physician who is available to provide in-home care anytime, day or night, as needed. This level of care is designed to improve the quality of care for the most chronically ill, frail patients who represent approximately 2% of Medicare beneficiaries. Selection for the pilot project is by invitation; selection criteria include patients with two chronic illnesses and a history of at least two hospitalizations within the past 12 months. The goal is to reduce unnecessary hospitalizations and emergency department visits, thus reducing costs to the patient and the health care system (*Medicare Adds*, 2006).

Program of All-Inclusive Care for the Elderly

The Program of All-Inclusive Care for the Elderly (PACE) is based on the British day hospital model of care. PACE programs provide preventive, primary, acute, and long-term services for their enrolled members all under one roof. With a nursing focus, PACE programs are responsible for managing the health, mental, and psychosocial needs of each participant. PACE programs include the medical component of care, working from a clinic that is open 5 or 6 days a week where participants receive care from a clinic provider, either a physician or a nurse practitioner, along with specialist services such as audiology, dentistry, optometry, speech, and podiatry. These services are offered along with an adult day care program, where participants gather for socialization, recreation, and nursing care. Transportation is provided, and some PACE programs include a housing component for their participants. In their own homes, PACE participants can receive personal, home health, and respite care. If needed, PACE programs cover hospital and nursing home care (Bonifazi, 2004).

Green House Project

The Green House Project in Tupelo, Mississippi, is comprised of 10 suburban homes that have become an experiment in reinventing the nursing home. They are part of a movement to humanize the care for the aging patient with smaller, more "home-like" settings and a closer sense of community among residents and staff. The Green House model was conceptualized by Eden Alternative pioneer Bill Thomas, MD. The model was developed to address the aging patient's fears of being institutionalized, including anxieties about loss of independence and fears of abuse. In a Green House, meals are served at a communal dining table rather than on trays in a dining hall. Staff members who care for residents answer beepers to minimize the sounds of the never-ending call bells often heard in traditional nursing homes. The advantages of deinstitutionalized models are many, but potentially higher costs of operation have kept them from being widely available (Hamilton, 2005).

Elder Cohousing

Another new and innovative housing option is elder cohousing. The concept is built on a Denmark-inspired, 30-year-old community planning model typically developed for intergenerational populations. In the past few years, it has become a focus for individuals over age 55. Cohousing communities exist in California, Virginia, and Colorado and they exhibit similarities to a townhouse or condominium development run by a homeowners' association. The difference is that the residents are individuals who like living and doing things together. One community has 11 households, and all are represented on the board of directors. Members range in age from 55 to 75, with many professionals; some are retired, others are still working. Such communities are designed with the goal of encouraging aging in place through the use of universal design elements and an emphasis on home care.

As such communities develop, new questions arise. How does the community address members with dementias? How does the community address those who require around-the-clock nursing care? Only the future will tell if cohousing will take off as an option for today's aging baby boomers (*Cohousing*, 2006).

Innovations in Technology for the Aging Patient

Rapid advances in technology are beginning to have an impact on care of the aging patient in both traditional and nontraditional settings. With appropriate applications of technology, seniors who choose to remain at home during their aging years will be able to do so successfully. New technology is making it possible for those who choose to live in board and care and assisted living to remain in those types of less restrictive environments compared to the traditional nursing home. Challenges involving telephone communication, medication administration, and overall patient monitoring can be addressed using new technology.

Telephone Communication

The challenges for the aging patient in using the telephone are numerous, due to hearing and vision difficulties. Traditional methods to address such problems include phones with higher volume and use of a text telephone (TTY) for those whose hearing renders them incapable of hearing speech over the phone. The device allows an individual to type into a TTY keyboard, which generates tones that are converted into letters by another TTY device. Newer "smart" phones provide additional options for the aging patient to communicate. For example, many individuals are moving to the Voice over Internet Protocol, which involves using the Internet rather than traditional phone lines to carry voices. The advantage is that one can communicate in several formats such as voice and text or through streaming video with multiple people at the same time (Vanderheiden, 2006).

Medication Administration Technology

Medication administration has advanced beyond the traditional pill reminder, divided up for time of day and days of the week in the home setting. Traditional methods such as pill reminders or alarm clocks that ring when a medication is due do not ensure the aging patient is taking medications when living at home. For those individuals, greater support is needed in medication administration. Newer technologies offer devices that are the size of a small TV and like an "ATM for patient medications." Such devices are wirelessly connected to software that contains an individual's medication administration record, and can be remotely adjusted by a pharmacist or health care provider. The device reminds patients when to take medications, selects the correct dose, and delivers it from the machine. Medications are loaded via blister packs. Such technology is beneficial for the home-dwelling forgetful patient, for someone with a complex drug regimen, and for someone who has difficulty understanding written directions (INRange Systems, 2006). New "closed door" pharmacies have evolved to serve this population. They deliver blister pack medications for each patient on a monthly basis.

Computer Technology

Computers continue to offer an opportunity for seniors to apply technology in their lives to simplify record keeping, even when they are no longer able to live at home. Many seniors keep track of their medical care and health history using notebooks, filing systems or, in some cases, no particular system. An innovative project at Eskaton Village Carmichael, a continuing care retirement community in Northern California, provides seniors a means to keep track of their health information via computer. The partnership between Intel Corporation and Eskaton Village in this endeavor, called the Internet Health File project, allows residents to enter health information into a secure Internet site so that it is organized and available at all times. If residents choose, they may also allow adult children and community staff members access to their Internet health records (*Intel and Eskaton Team Up*, 2006).

Continuous Body Monitoring Technology

Aging patients who live at home alone may benefit from the use of technology involving continuous body monitoring. One device available is an armband, similar to a wristwatch in size, that is applied and collects continuous data on calories burned, duration and level of physical activity, and sleep–wake cycles. Using wireless transmission and software analysis, family members not living with the aging patient could be notified if, for example, the individual did not get out of bed or fell. Those who might benefit most from such technology are individuals who live alone or have an inability to call for help. Such technology might be useful in collecting accurate data for those with chronic conditions to monitor overall health and physical status over time (Matthews, 2006).

High-technology innovations such as continuous body monitoring may not be the only way to integrate technology into the aging patient's life. Simpler systems may solve the same problems at a much more reasonable cost. Miami University's Scripps Gerontology Center in Oxford, Ohio, conducted a pilot study to evaluate how electronic monitoring could alleviate caregivers' burdens of constantly keeping track of their impaired relatives. Nineteen families caring for older relatives with moderate to severe dementia were enrolled. Each home was outfitted with two video cameras with a controller, one off-the-shelf sensor for each door, a cell phone with text messaging features, and monthly broadband Internet service. The equipment cost $300 and Internet service added $50 to $60 per month. Families reported benefits of such a system, even after various system "glitches" were resolved (Piturro, 2004).

■ Summary

It is often a challenge to motivate new graduate nurses to pursue a nursing specialty in caring for the aged. Geriatrics as a field tends not to hold the same level of excitement as working in an emergency department or an intensive care unit. Helping aging patients with ADLs may not, on the surface, have the same appeal as helping deliver babies in the labor and delivery suite or taking care of children on a pediatric floor. Those nurses who grew up around an older relative or had interactions with a senior prior to becoming a nurse, however, know of the rewards of helping a group of individuals who have lived through world wars and the Depression and have gained a lifetime of wisdom. Hopefully, with some new knowledge about the aging patient, there will be renewed interest in caring for this rapidly growing population group.

NCLEX® REVIEW

1. The nurse understands that which of the following age-related changes noted during a patient's physical assessment may be expected within the elderly population:
   1. Shallow inspirations with accessory muscle use and a decreased residual capacity.
   2. Decreased taste sensation often results from hypertrophy to the tongue's papillae.
   3. Point of maximal impulse may be at the sixth left intercostal space, midclavicular line.
   4. Hyperactive bowel sounds secondary to increased peristalsis and fluid intake.

2. As it relates to recommended immunizations and screening exams by the United States Preventative Services Task Force (USPSTF) for patients over 65 years of age, the nurse understands:
   1. These guidelines strictly outline the healthcare provider recommendations for immunizations and screenings for frail elderly patients and those with functional decline.
   2. Elderly patients who are hospitalized may be immunized according to the recommendations, as this can decrease both pneumonia and its resultant death rates.
   3. The pneumococcal and influenza vaccines should be administered at different times since there is decreased antibody response and increased reaction severity when given together.
   4. Doses of the varicella virus vaccine should be 14 times greater than the vaccine for the varicella-zoster virus in order to boost immunity against shingles and its sequelae.

3. The Beers criteria were established:
   1. Because up to 25% of hospital admissions in elderly patients can be linked to adverse drug reactions or toxic effects.
   2. To provide criteria by which health care providers can assess risk for and decrease the occurrence of polypharmacy.
   3. By a panel of experts to make recommendations about preventative services to be included in primary care.
   4. As an adjunct for researchers to evaluate the quality of drug prescribing, utilization, and education in the nursing home.

4. An elderly patient presents from a nursing home, weeping and complaining of nausea. When placing the blood pressure cuff on the client's arm, the nurse notices a large hand-shaped contusion on the bicep. The nurse should:
   1. Confront the patient about what he or she did to deserve the injury.
   2. Ensure confidentiality and inquire directly about the contusion.
   3. Ignore the contusion because the patient is complaining of nausea.
   4. Call the local news to report the injury and implicate the family.

5. A patient is being discharged from the hospital after recovering from a transient ischemic attack. The patient has no residual paralysis or parasthesias and is ambulatory with a cane. They are continent, able to communicate and maintain some of their own ADLs, but do require assistance with medications. The patient and family want to consider a housing option that will meet the patient's needs and be covered by insurance. Which of the following care options is most appropriate for this patient?

1. Skilled nursing care.
2. Adult day care.
3. Residential care facility.
4. Senior supported housing.

Answers for review questions appear in Appendix D

KEY TERMS

activity theory of aging *p.169*
adverse drug event (ADE) *p.180*
adverse drug reaction (ADR) *p.180*
aging *p.168*
biological aging theory *p.168*
continuity theory of aging *p.169*
cross-linking theory of aging *p.169*
delirium *p.176*
dementia *p.176*
disengagement theory of aging *p.169*

error theories of aging *p.169*
Folstein Mini-Mental State Exam *p.171*
free radical theory of aging *p.169*
gerontological nurse practitioner (GNP) *p.187*
immunologic theory of aging *p.168*
insomnia *p.173*
kyphosis *p.172*
long-term care insurance *p.184*

mandatory reporter *p.184*
polypharmacy *p.180*
programmed theory of aging *p.168*
psychosocial theories of aging *p.169*
rate of living theory of aging *p.169*
sleep apnea *p.173*
U.S. Preventive Services Task Force (USPSTF) *p.175*
wear-and-tear theory of aging *p.169*

PEARSON
EXPLORE mynursingkit™

MyNursingKit is your one stop for online chapter review materials and resources. Prepare for success with additional NCLEX®-style practice questions, interactive assignments and activities, web links, animations and videos, and more!

Register your access code from the front of your book at
www.mynursingkit.com

REFERENCES

Aboderin, I. (2004). Modernisation and ageing theory revisited: Current explanations of recent developing world and historical western shifts in material family support for older people. *Ageing and Society, 24:* 29–50.

Administration on Aging. AOA. (n.d.). *A Profile of Older Americans: 2007.* Retrieved May 19, 2008, from http://www.aoa.gov/PROF/Statistics/profile/2004/profiles2004.asp

Agency for Healthcare Research and Quality, (AHRQ). (2007). *2007 National Healthcare Quality & Disparities Reports.* Retrieved May 19, 2008 from http://www.ahrq.gov/qual/grdr07.htm

Agostini, J. V., Han, L., & Tinetti, M. E. (2004). The relationship between number of medications and weight loss or impaired balance in older adults. *Journal of the American Geriatrics Society, 52,* 1719–1723.

Alexander, R. (Ed.). (2006). *Avoiding fraud when buying long-term care insurance.* Retrieved November 2, 2006, from http://www.consumerlawpage.com

Alzheimer's Association. (2006). *Fact sheet: Alzheimer's disease.* Retrieved January 2, 2007, from http://www.alz.org/Resources/FactSheets/FSADFacts.pdf

American Cancer Society. (n.d.). *What are the key statistics about prostate cancer?* Retrieved January 2, 2007, from http://www.cancer.org

American Psychiatric Association. (1994). *Diagnostic and statistical manual of mental disorders* (4th ed., pp. 123–133). Washington, DC: Author.

American Society of Health-System Pharmacists. (2006). Information retrieved November 1, 2006, from http://www.safemedication.com

Anderson, L. M., Scrimshaw, S. C., Fullilove, M. T., Fielding, J. E., & Normand, J. (2003). Culturally competent healthcare systems. *American Journal of Preventive Medicine, 24,* 68–79.

Aziz, R., Lorberg, B., & Tampi, R.R., (2006). Treatments for late-life bipolar disorder. *American Journal of Geriatric Pharmacotherapy,* 4(4), 347–364.

Bacak, B. S., Patel, M., Tweed, E., & Danis, P. (2006). What is the best way to manage GERD symptoms in the elderly? *Journal of Family Practice, 55,* 251–258.

Beers, M. H. (1997). Explicit criteria for determining potentially inappropriate medication use by the elderly. *Archives of Internal Medicine, 157,* 1531–1536.

Bonifazi, W. L. (2004, November 29). *Set the PACE.* Retrieved January 2, 2007, from http://www.Nursesweek.com/news/featuresNurseweek

Bonk, M. E., Krown, H., Matuszewski, K., & Oinonen, M. (2006). Potentially inappropriate medications in hospitalized senior patients. *American Journal of Health System Pharmacists, 63,* 1161–1165.

Center to Advance Palliative Care. (2001). *CAPC manual: Proposed definition of palliative care.* Retrieved May 3, 2008, from http://64.85.16.230/educate/content/elements/palliativecaredefinition.html

Centers for Medicare & Medicaid Services. (n.d.). *Proof of citizenship.* Retrieved December 30, 2006, from http://www.cms.hhs.gov/MedicaidEligibility/05_ProofofCitizenship.asp

Cohousing: The next senior housing option. Interview with Zev Paiss, Elder Cohousing network. (2006). *Nursing Homes, 55*(3), 30.

Congdon, J. G., DeCamp, J., Fletcher, K., Henningson, B., Kaplan, K., & Resnick, B. (2001). *Scope and standards of gerontological nursing practice* (2nd ed.). Silver Spring, MD: American Nurses Association.

Daly, J. M., Jogerst, G. J., Brinig, M. F., & Dawson, J. D. (2004). Mandatory reporting relationships of APS statute language on state reported elder abuse. *Journal of Elder Abuse and Neglect,15*(2), 1–21.

Darkwa, O. (2007). *Social welfare services for the aged.* Retrieved March 16, 2008, from http://www.uic.edu/classes/socw/socw550/AGIMG/tsld001.htm

Department of Veterans Affairs. (2007). *Home-Based Primary Care Program: VHA handbook 11404.01.* Washington D.C.: Veterans Health Administration.

DeYoung, G. R., & Baty, P. J. (2007). Herpes zoster virus vaccine (Zostavax) for the prevention of shingles. *American Family Physician, 76,* 1843–1846.

Experience CORPS. (2007). *Fact Sheet on Aging in America.* Washington. DC. Experience CORPS.

Falicov, C. J. (1998). *Latino families in therapy: A guide to multicultural practice.* New York: The Guilford Press.

Fernandes, R., Flynn, B., & Masaki, K. (2003). Tetanus immunity in the elderly. *Annals of Long-Term Care, 11*(1), 21–24.

Fick, D. M., Cooper, J. W., Wade, W. E., Waller, J. L., Maclean, J. R., & Beers, M. H. (2003). Updating the Beers criteria for potentially inappropriate medication use in older adults. *Archives of Internal Medicine, 163,* 2716–2724.

Folstein, M. F., Folstein, S. E., & McHugh, P. R. (1975). Mini-Mental State: A practical method for grading the cognitive state of patients for the clinician. *Journal of Psychiatric Research, 12*(3), 189–198.

Gavrilov, L. A., & Gavrilov, N. S. (2002). Evolutionary theories of aging and longevity. *The Scientific World Journal, 2,* 339–356.

Gehrman, P., Diana, G., & Impastato, A. (2006). Wide awake in assisted living. *Assisted Living Consult, 2*(2), 26–29.

Hamilton, W. L. (2005, April 23). The new nursing home, emphasis on home. *The New York Times.* Retrieved April 24, 2005, from http://www.nytimes.com

Hospitals continue to implement palliative care programs. (2006). Retrieved January 21, 2007, from http://www.healthday.com

Howard, R., Rabins, P. V., Seeman, M. V., Jeste, D. V., & and International-Onset, Schizophrenia Group. (2000). Late-onset schizophrenia and very-late-onset schizophrenia-like psychosis: An international consensus. *American Journal of Psychiatry, 157,* 172–178.

Inouye, S., van Dyck, C., Alessi, C., Galkin, S., Siegal, A., & Horwitz, R. (1990). Clarifying confusion: the confusion assessment method. *Annals of Internal Medicine, 113*(12), 941–948.

INRange Systems. (2006). *Remote medication management systems.* Retrieved October 30, 2006, from http://www.inrangesystem.com

Intel and Eskaton team up for health. (2006). *Eskaton Connections, 8*(4), 1.

Jeste, K. V., Paulsen, J. S., & Harris, M. J. (2000). *Late-onset schizophrenia and other related psychoses.* Retrieved January 3, 2008, from http://www.acnp.org/g4GN401000138/CH135.html

Kaiser Permanente. (2005, September). *Kaiser Permanente guide to nursing facilities for members* (pp. 11–13).

Kaldy, J. (2006). Managing influenza in the assisted living facility. *Assisted Living Consult, 2*(2), 14–16.

Kao, R. S., & Lam, M. L. (1995). Asian American elderly. In E. Lee (Ed.), *Working with Asian Americans: A guide for clinicians* (pp. 208–223). New York: The Guilford Press.

Lesser, J. M., Hughes, S. V., Jemelka, J. R., & Kumar, S. (2005). Challenges and strategies for taking a comprehensive history in the elderly. *Geriatrics, 60*(11), 22–31.

Liu, G. G., & Christensen, D. B. (2002). The continuing challenge of inappropriate prescribing in the elderly: An update of the evidence. *Journal of the American Pharmaceutical Association, 42*, 847–857.

Lundell, J., & Morris, M. (2004). Tales, tours, tools, and troupes: A tiered research method to inform ubiquitous designs for the elderly. *British Computer Society Human-Computer Interaction Group, 21*, 165–178.

Mac-Mary, S., Sainthillier, J. M., & Humbert, P. (2004). Dry skin and the environment. *Exogenous Dermatology, 3*, 72–80.

Maio, V., Hartmann, C. W., Poston, S., Liu-Chen, X., Diamond, J., & Arenson, C. (2006). Potentially inappropriate prescribing for elderly patients in 2 outpatient settings. *American Journal of Medical Quality, 31*(3), 162–168.

Matthews, J. T. (2006). Existing and emerging healthcare devices for elders to use at home. *Generations, 30*(2), 13–19.

Mayo Clinic. (2007a). *Colchicine (Systemic).* Retrieved August 17, 2007, from http://222.mayoclnica.cm/health/drug-information/DR202160

Mayo Clinic. (2007b). *Probenecid and colchicine (oral route).* Retrieved August 17, 2007, from http://www.mayoclici.com/health/drug-information/DR600297

Mazanec, P. I., & Tyler, M. K. (2003). Cultural considerations in end-of-life care. *American Journal of Nursing, 103*(3), 50–58.

McDowell, S. E., Coleman, J. J., & Ferner, R. E. (2006). Systematic review and meta-analysis of ethnic differences in risks of adverse reactions to drugs used in cardiovascular medicine. *BMJ, 332* 1177–1181.

Medicare adds nearly 14,000 beneficiaries to doctor house call project with care level management. (2006, August 24). Retrieved January 27, 2007, from http://www.carelevel.com

Medication assessment. (2005, February). Retrieved June 20, 2007 from http://www.geronurseonline.org

MetLife. (2005). *Executive summary: MetLife mature market institute market survey.* (2006). Retrieved January 2, 2007, from http://www.metlife.com

Mezey, M. D., Fulmer, T., Abraham, I., & Zwicker, D. (Eds.). (2003). *Geriatric nursing protocols for best practice* (2nd ed.). New York: Springer.

Moreau, D. (Ed.). (2006). *Pathophysiology made incredibly easy* (3rd ed.). Philadelphia: Lippincott Williams and Wilkins.

National Center on Elder Abuse. (2007a). *About NCEA.* Retrieved October 1, 2007, from http://www.ncea.aoa.gov/ncearott/Main_Site/index.aspx.

National Center on Elder Abuse. (2007b). *Adult protective services.* Retrieved October 1, 2007, from http://www.ncea.aoa.gov/ncearoot/main_site/find_help/APS/About_APS.aspx

National Center on Elder Abuse. (2007c). *Major types of elder abuse.* Retrieved October 1, 2007, from http://www.ncea.aoa.gov/ncearoot/Main_Site/FAQ/Basics/Types_of_abuse.aspx

National Guideline Clearing House. (2007). *Preventive services for adults.* Retrieved May 19, 2008 from http://www.guideline.gov/summry/summary.aspx?doc_id=11699&nbr+0060046&string=P...

National Institute of Neurological Disorders and Stroke. (2007). Normal pressure hydrocephalus information page. Retrieved January 3, 2008 from http://www.ninds.nih.gov/disorders/normal_pressure_hydrocephalus

National Institute on Aging. (2006). *Forgetfulness: It's not always what you think.* U.S. National Institutes of Health. Retrieved December 29, 2007, from http://www.niapublications.org/agepages/forgetfulness.asp

National Institutes of Health Consensus Development Panel. (2001). Osteoporosis prevention, diagnosis, and therapy. *Journal of the American Medical Association, 285*, 785–795.

Novoseltsev, V. N., Novoseltseva, J., & Yashin, A. I. (2001). A homeostatic model of oxidative damage explains paradoxes observed in earlier aging experiments: a fusion and extension of older theories of aging. *Biogerontology, 2*(2), 127–138.

Piturro, M. (2004). Assistive technology in ITC. *Caring for the Ages, 5*(12), 32–34.

Polypharmacy. (2007). Retrieved February 14, 2007, from http://www.Mercksource.com/pp/us/cns_search results.jsp

Red Horse, J. (1981). *American Indian families.* Paper presented at the Conference on American Indian Family Strengths and Stress. Elmsford, NY: Pergamon Press.

Reuben, D. B., Herr, K. A., Pacala, J. T., Pollock, B. G., Potter, J. F., & Semala, T. P. (2007). *Geriatrics at your fingertips: 2007–2008* (9th ed.). New York: American Geriatrics Society.

Roehl, B., Talati, A., & Parks, S. (2006). Medication prescribing for older adults. *Annals of Long-Term Care, 14*(6), 33–39.

Roy, H., & Russell, C. (2005). The *encyclopedia of aging & the elderly.* Iowa City, Iowa: MedRounds Publications.

Sattinger, A. M. (2006). Collaboration helps hospice work in ITC. *Caring for the Ages, 7*(3), 17–18.

Schaffer, S. (2006). "Theory and Theorizing Across Borders: Global Social Thought and Geographic Organic Intellectualism" Paper presented at the annual meeting of the American Sociological Association, Montreal Convention Center, Montreal, Quebec, Canada Online. Retrieved June 27, 2008 from http://www.allacademic.com/meta/p104982_index.html

Smith, N. M., Breese, J. S., Shay, D. K., Uyeki, T. M., Cox, N. J., & Strikas, R. A. (2006, June 28). Prevention and control of influenza. *Morbidity and Mortality Weekly Report*, pp. 1–54.

Stibich, M. (2007a). *The genetic theory of aging.* Retrieved May 15, 2008 from htt://longevity.about.com/od/reserachand medicine//p/age_genetics.htm

Stibich, M. (2007b). *Why we age–theories and effects of aging.* Retrieved May 15, 2008 from http://longevity.about.coj/od/longevity101/a/why_we_age.htm

Strunk, B. C., Ginsburg, P. B., & Banker, M. I. (2006). The effect of population aging on future hospital demand. *Health Affairs, 25*(3), 141–149.

Tabloski, P. A. (2006). *Gerontological nursing.* Upper Saddle River, NJ: Pearson Prentice Hall.

Talley, N. J. (2005). American Gastroenterological Association medical position statement: Evaluation of dyspepsia. *Gastroenterology, 129*, 1753–1780.

Tovey, D. (Ed.). (2007). *Clinical evidence handbook.* London: BMJ Publishing Group.

Tuch, H., Parrish, P., & Romer, A. L. (2002). *Integrating palliative care into nursing homes: An interview with Howard Tuch and Pam Parrish* (Vol. 4). Retrieved January 21, 2007, from http://www.edc.org/lastacts

U.S. Census Bureau. (2005). *2005 Community survey.* Retrieved February 10, 2007, from http://factfinder.census.gov

U.S. Department of Veterans Affairs. (n.d.). *What is home based primary care?* Retrieved January 21, 2007, from http://www1.va.gov/HCBC

U.S. Preventive Services Task Force. (n.d.). *Screening for colorectal cancer.* Retrieved January 1, 2007, from http://www.ahrq.gov/clinic

U.S. Social Security Administration, Office of Policy. (2007). *Fast facts & figures about social security.* Retrieved May 15, 2008 from http:www.socialsecurity.gov/p9olicy/docs/cghartbooks/fast_facts/2007/indes.html

Vanderheiden, G. (2006). Potential impact of new technologies on telecommunication for elders. *Generations, 30*(2), 9–12.

Vlassova, O., & Jackson, A. J. (2005). *December 2002 Kaiser Permanente Colorado Region adult pneumococcal vaccine recommendations.* Retrieved July 29, 2006, from http://cl.kp.org/pkc/co/cpg/cpg/immunization_toolkit/pneumovax_flyer.htm

Voyer, P., Cole, J. G., Mc Cusker, J., & Belzile, E. (2006). Prevalence and symptoms of delirium superimposed on dementia. *Clincal Nursing Research, 15*, 46–66.

Waszynski, C. M. (2007). The confusion assessment method (CAM). *Try This: Best Practices in Nursing Care to Older Adults, 13*, New York University College of Nursing: The Hartford Institute for Geriatric Nursing.

Wetherell, J. L., & Jeste, D. V. (2004). Older adults with schizophrenia. *ElderCare, 3*(2), 8–11.

Willis, W. (1998). Families with African American roots. In E. W. Lynch & M. J. Hanson (Eds.), *Developing cross-cultural competence* (pp. 165–202). Baltimore, MD: Paul H. Brookes Publishing.

Genetics

Carolyn Graff,
Ann Cashion

Outcome-Based Learning Objectives

After studying this chapter, the learner will be able to:

1. Describe the role of genetics in health care and nursing.
2. Discuss events of cell division that result in chromosomal abnormalities.
3. Describe the organization of the human genome and the DNA sequence.
4. Describe the influence of the genome on differences among patients.
5. Identify patterns of inheritance and variables influencing interpretation of inheritance patterns.
6. Discuss the role of nurses in detection, management, and care of patients with genetic disorders.
7. Describe emerging genetic technologies and therapies.

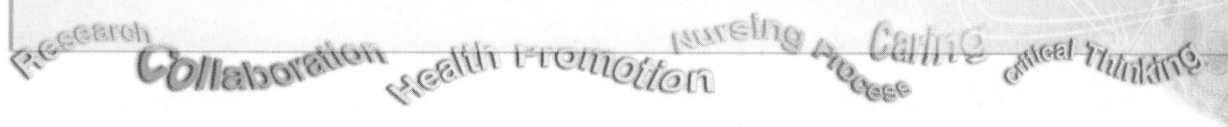

GENETICS FOCUSES on variation and heredity in all living beings. A great deal of genetics information derives from the work of many researchers, including Gregor Mendel, who is attributed with discovering the laws of genetics in 1865, and James Watson and Francis Crick, who described the double-helix structure of DNA (Watson & Crick, 1953). Fifty years after the structure of DNA was described, researchers mapped each human gene and completely sequenced the human **genome,** that is, all of the DNA in human cells. This was accomplished through an international research effort known as the **Human Genome Project (HGP).** The HGP has provided information about and insights into many diseases and development of improved methods for diagnosis and prevention.

The completion of the HGP has been described as the beginning of the genomic era (Collins, Green, Guttmacher, & Guyer, 2003). Integrating genomics into health care is critical because the use of genetic information may improve the health of individuals. **Genomics** is the field of genetics that focuses on translating the knowledge of the human genome into health benefits, including the molecular analysis of the human genome in health and illness. In addition to educating nurses and health professionals about genetic and environmental factors affecting health, findings from genetic research can be used by patients and family members to improve their own health and prevent

illness. Both nurses and patients must be knowledgeable and informed so they can communicate effectively with each other and engage in discussion about the implications of genomics for health.

Foundations for Genetics

An introduction to genetics requires a foundational understanding of cells, chromosomes, and the human genome. More extensive, in-depth information can be found in genetic textbooks, such as those by Klug, Cummings, and Spencer (2005) and Lewin (2000), and appropriate websites.

Cells and Chromosomes

A typical cell has two major parts, the nucleus and the cytoplasm. The nucleus is separated from the cytoplasm by a nuclear membrane and the cytoplasm is separated from the surrounding fluids by a cellular membrane. The nucleus is the primary control center for the cell. It is within the nucleus that **chromosomes,** which house most **deoxyribonucleic acid (DNA),** are located (Figure 11–1 ■, p. 194). Each species can be characterized by its chromosome number and morphology. For example, humans have 23 pairs of chromosomes, whereas dogs have 39 pairs and tomatoes have only 12 pairs. The number of chromosomes is not associated

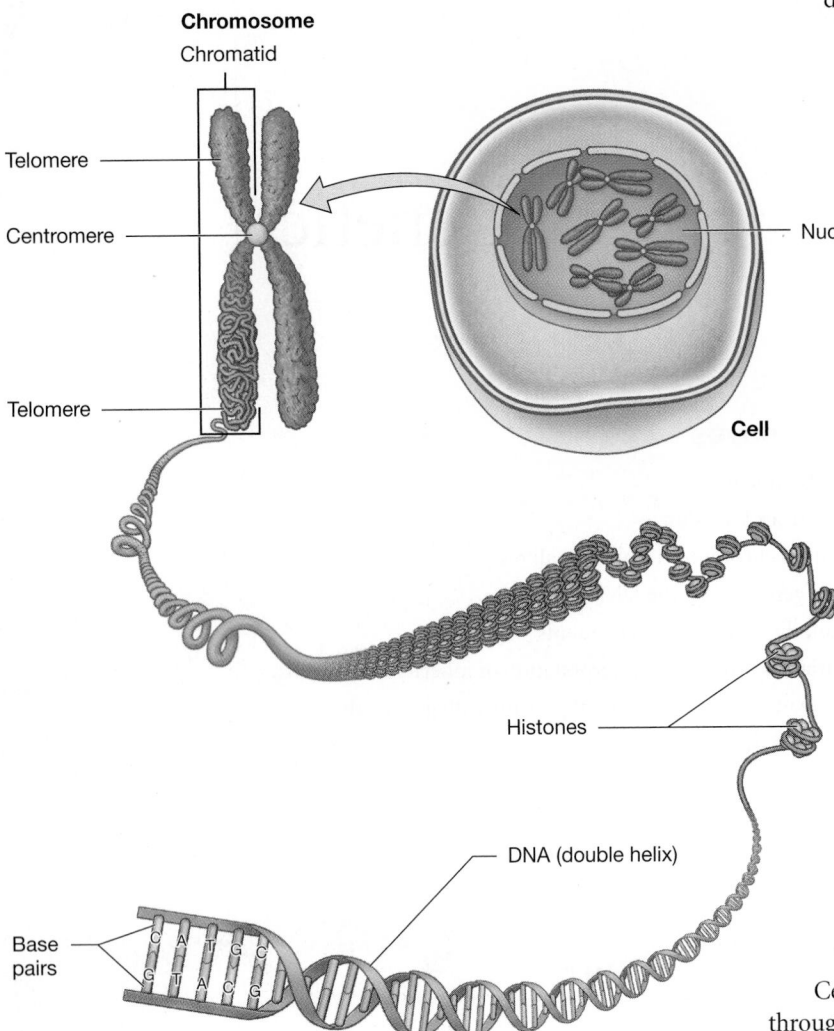

Chromosome

Chromatid

Telomere

Centromere

Telomere

Cell

Nucleus

Histones

DNA (double helix)

Base pairs

C A T G C
G T A C G

FIGURE 11–1 ■ The chromosome.
Source: Courtesy of Darryl Leja, National Human Genome Research Institute, National Institutes of Health, Bethesda, MD.

with intelligence level. The entire chromosome complement within a cell is known as the **karyotype** and is visible microscopically when cells are dividing (Figure 11–2 ■). **Cytogenetics** is the study of chromosomes, their structure, and inheritance.

Chromosomes contain genes organized into linear structural units. **Genes** are the fundamental unit of heredity that carries traits from one generation to the next. Each gene has a specific location, or locus, on the chromosome (Figure 11–3 ■). Each chromosome carries a different subset of genes; however, pairs of chromosomes carry matching genetic information in the same sequence. Because one chromosome of each pair is inherited from each parent, individuals have alternative copies of each gene, called **alleles,** one on each chromosome. For example, if an individual has type AB blood they have an A allele from one parent and a B allele from the other. Alleles are considered **homozygous** when they are the identical (i.e., type AA blood) and **heterozygous** when different (i.e., type AB blood).

Genes are found in the nucleus of almost all human cells, with a notable exception being red blood cells, which have no nucleus. Small subsets of genes are also found in the mitochon-

dria located outside the nucleus in the cytoplasm. Mitochondrial genes exclusively exhibit maternal inheritance, which means an individual can only inherit these genes from his mother.

Chromosomes are divided into two arms by the **centromere,** a constriction in the chromosome (see Figure 11–3 ■). The short or petite arm is designated p and the long arm is designated q. To identify the locus on a chromosome, both the number of the chromosome and the arm are identified. For example, the gene associated with cystic fibrosis is known as the cystic fibrosis transmembrane conductance regulator (*CFTR*) gene and is located at 7q31.2. This means that the gene is located on the long arm (q) of chromosome 7 at locus 31.2. The end of the chromosome is called the **telomere** and is thought to ensure the integrity of the chromosomes during cell division in addition to being associated with the aging process.

Of the 23 pairs of human chromosomes, 22 are classified as **autosomes** and are alike in both males and females. Only one pair is designated as the **sex chromosomes** and these differ by gender: Females have two X chromosomes (XX) and males have an X and a Y chromosome (XY).

Cell Division

Cell reproduction is controlled by DNA and occurs through one of two processes; mitosis or meiosis. Mitosis is the normal replication process used by somatic cells, which are basically all cells in the body excluding **germ line cells** (cells that give rise to egg and sperm reproductive cells). Mitosis begins in the nucleus with the duplication of all DNA in the chromosomes and ends with the formation of two new daughter cells. The daughter cells are exact copies of the parent cell.

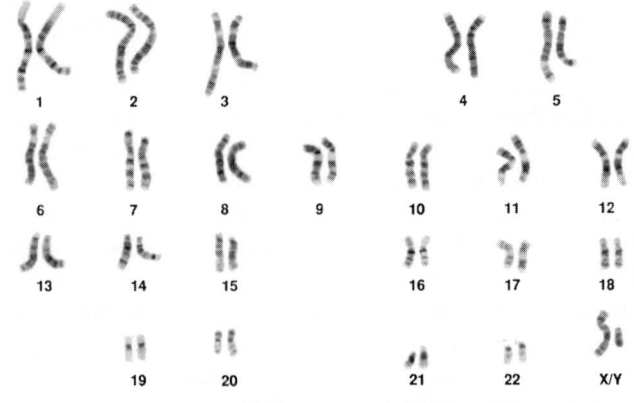

1 2 3 4 5

6 7 8 9 10 11 12

13 14 15 16 17 18

19 20 21 22 X/Y

Normal Karyotype

FIGURE 11–2 ■ Male karyotype, 46xy.
Source: © Mediscan/CORBIS All Rights Reserved

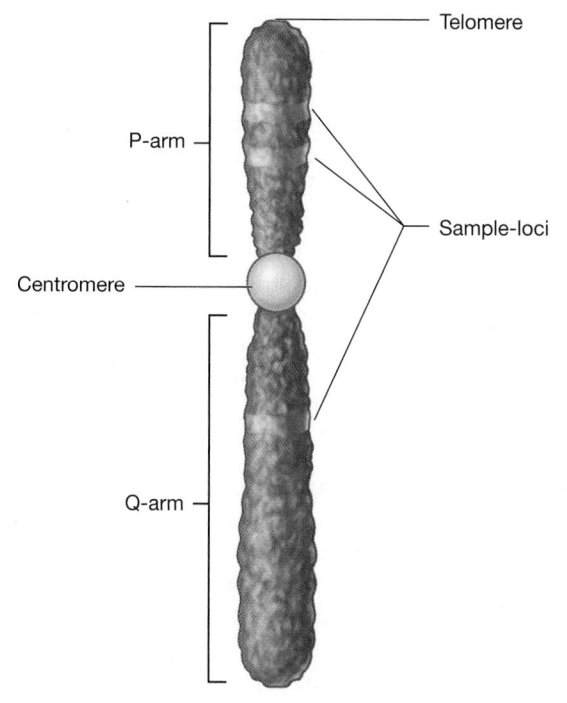

FIGURE 11–3 ■ Structure of a chromosome.

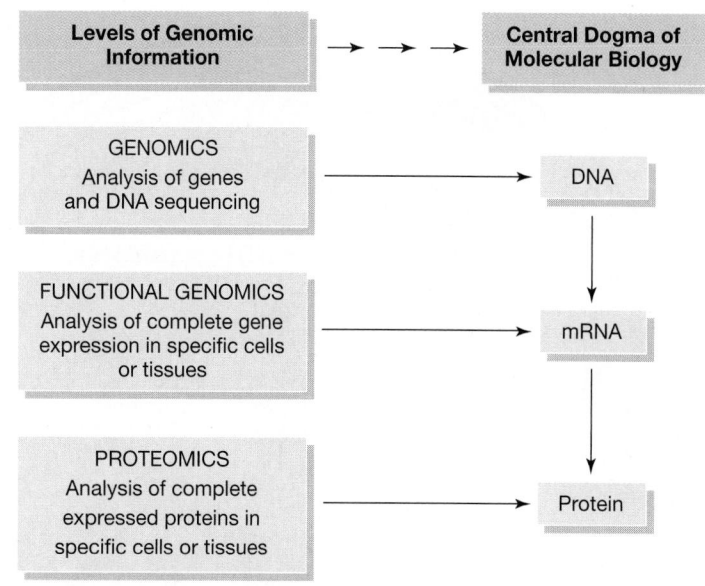

FIGURE 11–4 ■ Framework for genetic technologies.
Source: Loescher, L. J., & Merkle, C. J. (2005). The interface of genomic technologies and nursing. *Journal of Nursing Scholarship, 37*(2), 111–119.

Meiosis is the replication process that occurs in germ line cells. The product of meiosis differs from that of mitosis in that it results in the production of reproductive cells (**gametes**), which have only half the chromosomes of a somatic cell. Gametes have only one of each pair of the 23 chromosomes and are **haploid** (single chromosomes), whereas somatic cells have 46 chromosomes and are considered **diploid** (pairs of chromosomes).

The Human Genome

The **human genome** is the total set of genes carried by an individual. Genes are made of DNA.

DNA and RNA Structure

DNA is composed of four nucleotide bases, adenine (A), cytosine (C), guanine (G), and thymine (T), with the addition of sugar (deoxyribose) and phosphate (refer back to Figure 11–1 ■). The four bases, known as the building blocks of DNA, are of two types: purines and pyrimidines. The purine bases are A and G, and the pyrimidine bases are C and T. In DNA, purines and pyrimidines always pair in a complementary nature so that A always binds to T and C always binds to G. The bases align into two polynucleotide chains to create a double-helix form. Because of the complementary nature of DNA's purines and pyrimidines, the base sequence of each single strand can be deduced from that of its partner. The nature of DNA was originally identified by James Watson and Francis Crick in 1953. Together the DNA macromolecules compose the approximately 20,000 to 25,000 genes in the human genome (International Human Genome Sequencing Consortium, 2004).

The "central dogma" of molecular biology is contained in the flow of genetic information from DNA to RNA to protein (Figure 11–4 ■). More specifically, this means that DNA in the nucleus encodes ribonucleic acid (RNA), which then crosses the nuclear membrane into the cytoplasm where it attaches to ribosomes.

Once attached to ribosomes, proteins are formed using the pattern originally established by DNA. The chemical structure of RNA is similar to that of DNA, except that each nucleotide in RNA has a ribose sugar component instead of the deoxyribose sugar. In addition, uracil (U) replaces thymine as one of the pyrimidine bases.

Gene Expression

Each gene has coding regions known as **exons** and noncoding regions known as **introns.** The coding regions make up less than 10% of the human genome. A primary function of exons is to code for about 60,000 to 80,000 proteins. This is accomplished by two processes known as **transcription** and **translation** (Figure 11–5 ■, p. 196). Transcription occurs when **messenger ribonucleic acid (mRNA)** is formed using DNA as a template. In DNA, each successive section of three nucleotide base pairs forms a **codon.** The codon codes for a single amino acid. The mRNA uses DNA as a template to transfer the genetic information from the DNA to the protein-forming apparatus in the cytoplasm. Once in the cytoplasm, mRNA is decoded, or translated, to produce the protein that has been designated by the gene. Physiologically, when genes increase transcription of mRNA (sometimes known as upregulation), their expression or activity increases, resulting in the production of more proteins.

Clinical and research endeavors are targeted toward quantifying gene activity and subsequent protein formation. Although each cell contains an individual's entire genome, each gene of the genome is not actively expressed by each cell. In fact, most cells only express about 30% of the genes in the genome (Nussbaum, McInnes, & Willard, 2004). For example, neural cells only express the genes needed for normal neural function and kidney cells express genes related to renal function. To determine expression levels of a gene, the mRNA produced by the gene is measured using emerging genetic technologies such as polymerase chain reaction (PCR), real-time PCR, and microarray analysis. These genetic technologies are discussed further in a later section.

MyNursingKit | The Human Genome Project

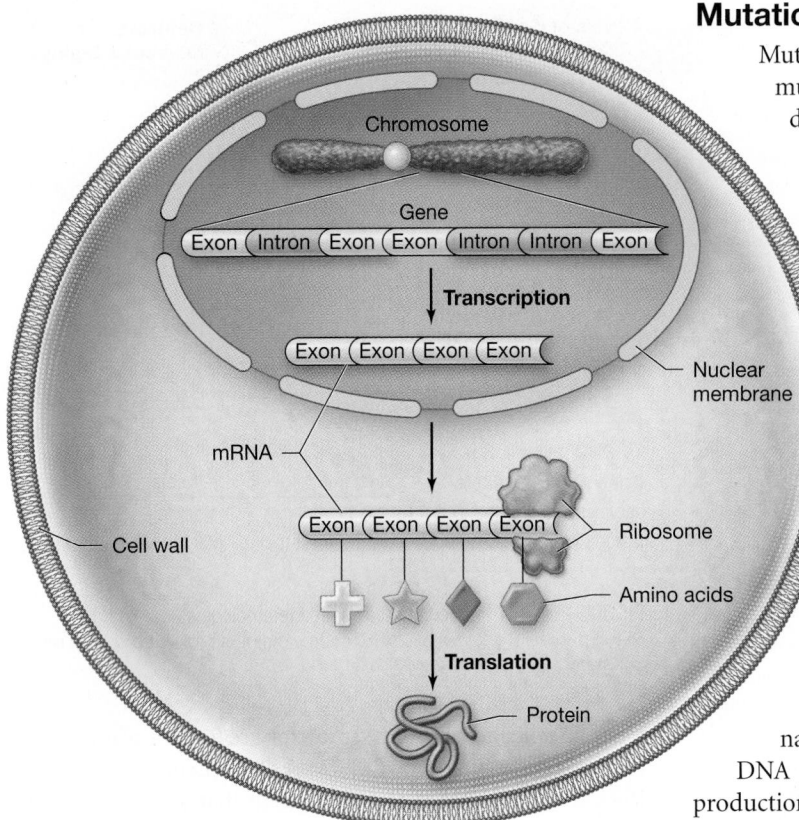

FIGURE 11–5 ■ Transcription and translation.

Polymorphisms and Mutations

During the process of conception, individuals obtain one chromosome from each parent, resulting in cells having matched pairs of chromosomes. Although pairs of chromosomes carry corresponding genetic information in similar sequences, the genetic sequence for each pair of genes may not be identical. Alternative copies of each gene are known as alleles. Each individual will have two alleles (one maternal, one paternal); one on each chromosome. The most common version of an allele is considered "normal" and is called the **wild type.** Alleles that differ from the wild type are known as polymorphisms or mutations. Because molecular genetic technologies are improving, more and more specific alleles are being identified. The genetic makeup of an individual, most specifically the allelic makeup, is that individual's **genotype.**

Polymorphisms

Polymorphisms differ from mutations in that they are observed more frequently in the general population than mutations. Polymorphisms and mutations are key determinants of an individual's observable traits, or **phenotype,** and clinical status. Whether the gene variation is identified as a mutation or polymorphism has more to do with how often the allele is observed instead of whether the allele is harmful or beneficial. A **mutation** is a change in DNA sequence that has been identified in less than 1% of the population. A **polymorphism** is a change in DNA sequence that has been identified in more than 1% of the population and is, thus, more commonly observed than a mutation.

Mutations

Mutations can either be inherited or acquired. Hereditary mutations are germ line mutations that are passed down through families. Examples of diseases caused by hereditary mutations are cystic fibrosis and hemophilia A. Acquired or somatic cell mutations are changes in DNA that develop throughout the life span during normal cell mitosis or through environmental stresses such as radiation. Acquired mutations cannot be inherited, for example, in many instances of cancer. Determining genetic patterns of inheritance can assist in differentiating between somatic and inherited mutations.

Types of Mutations

Mutations can be categorized into several types including missense, nonsense, and frameshift. A **missense mutation** is the most common gene mutation. It occurs when one DNA nucleotide base is substituted for another. This changes the triplet nucleotide coding section (codon) and results in the production of an alternate amino acid. **Nonsense mutations** occur when one DNA nucleotide base is inserted for another and protein production is stopped. Both missense and nonsense mutations are also known as **point mutations** (Figure 11–6 ■). Frameshift mutations are categorized as insertion or deletion mutations. They occur when one or a sequence of nucleotide bases is either deleted or inserted into the gene. As with point mutations, frameshift mutations can alter the nucleotide bases in the coding section and thereby produce a different protein.

Disease-Causing Mutations

In general, disease-causing mutations can be categorized into four groups based on the protein outcome. They result in either (1) loss of protein function, (2) gain of protein function, (3) a new protein function, or (4) expression of the protein at the wrong time or place (Nussbaum et al., 2004). The effect of the mutation on an individual depends on what biochemical role the protein performs in the normal biology of the human body. For example, a mutation in the *HBB* gene causes sickle cell anemia, an autosomal recessive inherited blood disorder characterized by chronic anemia and periodic pain. The gene mutation produces an altered protein, resulting in changes in the structure of the hemoglobin molecule. The hemoglobin molecule functions normally except in conditions of low oxygen tension (i.e., stressful situations), at which time the hemoglobin molecule forms a sickle shape, which can produce a medical emergency.

Individual	DNA sequence	Product	
Person 1	GT**T**ACC ↑		Normal protein
Person 2	GT**A**ACC ↑		Low or nonfunctioning protein

FIGURE 11–6 ■ Point mutations.

Genetic Variance and Phenotype

The associations between **genetic variance** (variations in genotypes) and phenotype are important. Knowledge of which mutation the patient has (genotype) and how that influences the clinical presentation (phenotype) affects nursing management of the patient. When considering genetic variation and its association with disease, a note of caution is required. It is important to differentiate between a gene and a mutation of a gene. It is commonly thought that if a person has the gene associated with a disease, then they are predisposed to the disease. This is not the case. All humans have essentially the same 20,000 to 25,000 genes. Therefore, it is the mutation or polymorphism in the gene, not the gene itself, which predisposes some individuals for disease. For example, each individual has a gene named the cystic fibrosis transference regulator (*CTFR*) gene. Only those who develop cystic fibrosis disease have a mutation in that gene.

 CRITICAL ALERT *Knowledge of which mutation the patient has (genotype) and how that influences the clinical presentation (phenotype) is essential for effective nursing management of the patient.*

Types of Genetic Disorders

Just about any illness is the result of some combination of genetic and environmental activity, but the role of genetics varies from small to large. The disorders caused to some extent by genetic factors are placed into three major categories: single-gene, chromosomal, and complex or multifactorial disorders.

Single-Gene Inheritance Patterns

Single-gene disorders are caused by a mutation in a single gene that may be on one or both chromosomes of a pair. A mutation is a permanent structural change in DNA. Single-gene disorders occur with a frequency of 3.6 per 1,000 by age 25 years; 16.4 per 1,000 after 25 years of age; and 20 per 1,000 over a person's lifetime (Rimoin, Connor, Pyeritz, & Korf, 2002). Commonly identified examples of single-gene disorders include cystic fibrosis, Huntington disease, and Duchenne muscular dystrophy.

Mendelian Inheritance

Single-gene characteristics are called Mendelian in recognition of Gregor Mendel's work. Mendel, an Austrian monk, is attributed with founding the principles of heredity, or Mendel's laws of inheritance. He studied the traits of garden peas and their offspring and conceived the idea of heredity units or "factors" (later called genes) in which one is recessive and the other dominant. He asserted that each individual has two factors for a trait; one factor from each parent. If two factors have identical information, the individual is called homozygous for the trait. If the two factors have different information, the individual is heterozygous.

Mendel believed that a single gene was responsible for one single trait. Today, it is known that individuals inherit genes from their parents and many genes have control over the production of traits. Genes behave as separate units and traits are the product of complex gene–gene and gene–environment interactions.

Online Mendelian Inheritance in Man (OMIM™) is an online version of Victor McKusick's (1998) listing of single-gene phenotypes. OMIM is a continuously updated catalog of human genes that includes primarily inherited genetic disorders and is considered the phenotypic companion to the Human Genome Project. It is an excellent resource for clinicians and researchers.

The patterns of single-gene disorders depend on the chromosomal location of the gene and whether the phenotype is dominant or recessive. The gene may be located on an autosome (autosomal) or the X chromosome (X-linked). The patterns of inheritance for single-gene disorders are autosomal recessive, autosomal dominant, X-linked recessive, and X-linked dominant. (Depictions of the patterns of inheritance for single-gene disorders are presented later in this chapter in Figures 11–8 ■ through 11–11 ■, p. 204.)

Autosomal Recessive Inheritance

With **autosomal recessive inheritance,** the mutant gene is located on an autosome rather than the X chromosome. The most common mechanism for transmitting a single-gene disorder with an autosomal recessive pattern of inheritance is when both parents are heterozygotes or carriers. Each heterozygous parent has one copy of the mutant gene and one copy of the wild-type or normal gene. Parents who are carriers of the mutant gene are usually asymptomatic and have no increased risk for other health problems. When each heterozygous parent gives one copy of the mutant gene to the child, however, the child is affected with a genetic disorder. Risks for the children of heterozygous carriers include the following: (1) They may be affected with the disorder, (2) they can be carriers like their parents, or (3) they can be normal without inheriting the mutant gene. The risk that a child will be affected with the autosomal recessive disorder is 1 out of 4. The risk that phenotypically normal children will be carriers is 2 out of 3. This is true for each pregnancy. Examples of autosomal recessive disorders include cystic fibrosis (CF), phenylketonuria (PKU), and Friedreich ataxia.

Autosomal Dominant Inheritance

With **autosomal dominant inheritance,** the mutant gene is on an autosome and only one copy of the dominant gene is necessary for the effects to be seen. The affected individual is heterozygous and no offspring are carriers. Homozygous individuals, or individuals who have inherited two genes for the disorder, are thought to be so severely affected that they die *in utero* or infancy. The presence of an autosomal dominant disorder in a child may indicate that one parent has the disorder also although this is not always the case. Exceptions to this may include the following: (1) The gene can be present but nonpenetrant, (2) the gene expression may be minimal and go undetected due to variable expression, (3) the disorder can be caused by a new mutation, or (4) the child is not the biological offspring of the parents. A gene is nonpenetrant when an individual carries the mutant gene but does not manifest the disorder caused by the gene.

When a child has one normal parent and one parent with the disorder, the risk for the child to inherit the gene is 50%, regardless of the child's gender. The chance of having a normal child is also 50%. This is true with each pregnancy produced by these parents. Children who are unaffected or normal have no greater risk of having an affected child than the general population, unless nonpenetrance has occurred in the child. If two individuals with the same autosomal dominant disorder have children, the risk is 25% for having a child who is an affected homozygote, 50% for having a child who is an affected heterozygote like the parents, and 25% for having a normal child without the mutant gene. These risks hold true for each pregnancy. The homozygote is usually severely affected and dies *in utero* or infancy. Examples of autosomal dominant disorders are Huntington disease and neurofibromatosis.

X-Linked Inheritance

In X-linked inheritance, the mutant gene is located on the X chromosome. Males have only one X chromosome with no counterpart for its genes. The gene is expressed when it is present in males regardless of whether it is dominant or recessive in the individual's mother. A female receives one X chromosome from each parent for a pair of sex chromosomes, XX. A male receives the X chromosome from his mother and the Y chromosome from his father for a pair of sex chromosomes, XY. Males cannot be carriers of an X-linked disorder.

In **X-linked recessive** disorders, the most common pattern of transmission is when the mother is a heterozygous carrier for the mutant gene. If the father is normal, then the parents have a 25% chance, with each pregnancy, for their child to be either (1) a female carrier like the mother, (2) a normal female without the mutant gene, (3) a normal male without the mutant gene, or (4) a male who is affected with the disorder. A mother who is a carrier usually has no obvious clinical manifestations of the mutant gene, unless X inactivation (inactivation of genes on one X chromosome in somatic cells of females, early in embryonic life) is skewed. In skewed X inactivation, the mutant allele is located on the active X and the normal allele is located on the inactive X. Variation in expression of X-linked disorders is seen commonly in heterozygotes and can range from normal to complete expression. X-linked disorders that are manifesting heterozygotes include color blindness, hemophilia A, hemophilia B, and Duchenne muscular dystrophy.

X-linked dominant disorders are seen less than the other patterns of single-gene inheritance. The mutant gene is dominant, so only one is necessary for the phenotype to manifest. Both males and females can be affected and transmit the gene. Compared to autosomal dominant disorders, in X-linked dominant disorders, an affected male usually has an affected mother because males inherit their X chromosome from their mother; some affected females may be less severely affected than males because of X inactivation; there may be an excess of female offspring in the family because some X-linked dominant genes are lethal in males; and male-to-male transmission is not seen because males transmit their X chromosome only to their daughters, not their sons.

When a female with an X-linked dominant disorder and an unaffected male have offspring, there is a 25% chance for each pregnancy to have either an affected female, an affected male, a normal female, or a normal male. There is a 50% chance that the offspring of each pregnancy will be affected regardless of the child's sex. When a male with an X-linked dominant disorder and normal female have offspring, there is a 50% chance for having an affected female and a 50% chance for having a normal male. If both the male and female had an X-linked dominant disorder, there would be a 25% chance for an affected homozygous female (probably resulting in miscarriage), a 25% chance for an affected heterozygous female, a 25% chance for an af-

fected male, and a 25% chance for a normal male. An example of an X-linked dominant disorder is hypophosphatemic rickets or vitamin D–resistant rickets.

Atypical Patterns of Inheritance

Most patterns of inheritance follow Mendel's laws of inheritance; however, exceptions do occur. Genomic imprinting and mitochondrial mutation inheritance are examples. Originally the sex of the parent was thought to have little effect on the expression of the genes each parent transmits. For some genetic disorders, the expression of the phenotype depends on whether the mutant allele has been inherited from the father or from the mother. Differences in gene expression between the allele inherited from the mother and the allele inherited from the father result from **genomic imprinting.**

Imprinting is caused by an alteration in chromatin that affects the expression of a gene but not its DNA sequence. Examples of genomic imprinting are Prader-Willi syndrome (PWS) and Angelman syndrome. Approximately 70% of individuals with PWS have a deletion of the proximal long arm of chromosome 15 that is inherited from the individual's father only (Prader-Willi Syndrome Association, 2008). Characteristics of PWS include obesity, excessive and indiscriminant eating, small hands and feet, short stature, hypogonadism, and mental retardation. In Angelman syndrome, there is a deletion of approximately the same region on chromosome 15 inherited from the individual's mother. Angelman syndrome is characterized by unusual facial appearance, short stature, severe mental retardation, spasticity, and seizures.

The mitochondrial chromosome (mtDNA) is located in the mitochondrial organelle, not inside the nucleus. The mother's ovum or egg supplies the **zygote,** or fertilized ovum, with its mitochondria. A mother having a mutation in mtDNA passes the mutation to all of her children, and the father carrying the same mutation passes it on to none of his children. Therefore, defects in mtDNA are inherited maternally. With cell division, mtDNA replicates and sorts randomly among newly synthesized mitochondria, which are distributed randomly between the daughter cells. Each daughter cell receives different proportions of mitochondria that carry normal and mutant mtDNA. Mitochondrial function is essential to nearly all cells. The phenotypic expression of a mutation in mtDNA depends on the proportions of normal and mutant mtDNA in the cells of different tissues. Reduced penetrance, variable expression, and multiple phenotypic effects of a single gene or gene pair are typical in mitochondrial disorders. Examples of genetic disorders caused by mtDNA are Leber's hereditary optic neuropathy, Leigh disease, and progressive sensorineural deafness.

Chromosomal Genetic Disorders

Chromosomal disorders are caused by an excess or deficiency of genes contained in whole chromosomes or segments of chromosomes. There is no abnormal individual gene on the chromosome. Chromosome disorders make up a major category of genetic disorders, affect about 7 of 1,000 live-born infants, and account for almost half of all spontaneous first-trimester abortions. The frequency of chromosome disorders is 1.8 per 1,000 before age 25 years; 2 per 1,000 after age 25 years; and 3.8 per 1,000 over a lifetime (Rimoin et al., 2002).

Chromosome abnormalities are related to an abnormal chromosome number or structural rearrangements. They may involve one or more autosomes, sex chromosomes, or both. The most common and clinically significant type is aneuploidy, which occurs in 3% to 4% of all clinically recognized pregnancies. **Aneuploidy** is an abnormal chromosome number due to an extra or missing chromosome. It is usually due to an error during meiosis in which cell division results in a sperm or egg with too many or too few chromosomes.

Most individuals with aneuploidy have trisomy or monosomy, which can be associated with mental or physical developmental problems or both. **Trisomy** refers to the presence of a third or extra chromosome instead of the normal pair of a particular chromosome. **Monosomy** refers to the presence of only one chromosome instead of the normal pair of chromosomes. The most common type of trisomy in infants is trisomy 21 or Down syndrome. The chromosome number and structure seen in 95% of individuals with Down syndrome is 47, XX or 47, XY. Monosomy for an entire chromosome usually results in death, except for Turner syndrome or the monosomy for the X chromosome (45, X).

Nondisjunction

Nondisjunction, or the failure of a pair of chromosomes to separate properly during meiosis, is the most common chromosomal mechanism leading to aneuploidy. Nondisjunction can also occur in a mitotic division after formation of the zygote. A zygote with an additional chromosome 21 might lose the extra chromosome in a mitotic division, resulting in **mosaicism.** Mosaicism occurs when an individual has at least two cell lines that are different in karyotype or genotype. Mosaicism is difficult to study because an individual's karyotype is rarely done without some clinical indication to do so. Because phenotypic effects of mosaicism may not be present, clinically normal mosaic persons are seldom identified. Individuals who are mosaic for Down syndrome or Turner syndrome are usually thought to be less affected than individuals who are nonmosaic.

Deletions

Structural rearrangements of chromosomes may result from **deletions** or loss of a chromosome segment or piece. The loss of a chromosome tip is the most common deletion in humans. Occurring less commonly are two breaks in one chromosome, with rejoining of the two ends and resulting loss of the piece between the two breaks (Nussbaum et al., 2004). If the deletions occur at both ends of the chromosome, the end pieces are lost and the two broken ends unite, forming a ring chromosome. Most deletions are new or individuals with normal chromosomes have a child with a deletion. The chance that these parents will have another child who is affected similarly is probably less than 0.5%. Deletions can be large and detectable by cytogenic methods. Smaller deletions, called microdeletions, are detectable by high-resolution banding methods. Very tiny deletions are detectable only by fluorescence *in situ* hybridization (FISH) or other molecular methods, and submicroscopic ones involving the loss of a single locus are detectable only by molecular methods.

Loss of the short arm of chromosome 5 or 5p– (read "5 p minus") is a cytogenetically visible deletion. It is known as *cri du chat* syndrome or the "cat-cry syndrome" because newborns usually have a high-pitched cry like that of a kitten. Most individuals with 5p– live beyond childhood and have moderate to severe mental retardation. Other syndromes resulting from deletions include Williams syndrome (deletions in 7q) and Prader-Willi syndrome (deletions in 15q).

Translocations

Translocations occur when there are breaks in two or more chromosomes, with reattachments in new combinations. Reciprocal or balanced translocations occur when two chromosomes exchange segments and no chromosomal material is lost. Reciprocal translocations are found in approximately 1 in 600 newborns. They are generally harmless even though these translocations are more common among individuals with intellectual disabilities. Although translocations may not affect an individual's health, carriers of translocations may produce children with an unbalanced amount of chromosome material. These children are at increased risk for mental and physical disabilities, and there is increased risk of spontaneous abortions.

Robertsonian translocations involve the loss of the short arm of chromosomes 13, 14, 15, 21, or 22. Since the short arm (p) is very short on these chromosomes, this loss seems to have little or no effect. Robertsonian translocations are fairly common, occurring in 1 of 900 newborns. Robertsonian translocations between chromosomes 13 and 14 result in trisomy 13 or Patau syndrome, which is characterized by abnormalities of the brain structure and abnormalities in most of the major organ systems (Alvarez, 2006). Translocations between chromosome 14 and 21 can result in trisomy 21 or Down syndrome.

Complex or Multifactorial Disorders

Complex disorders are caused by a combination of small variations in genes that together, with environmental factors, result in or increase the susceptibility to a disorder or illness. These illnesses may be caused by single-gene mutations, yet they are not single-gene disorders. They result from complex interactions between predisposing factors to include the genotype at one or more loci and varied environmental exposures that trigger, increase, or worsen a disease process. The pattern of inheritance of the disorder or illness is not Mendelian, but follows a complex or multifactorial pattern (Nussbaum et al., 2004).

Complex disorders are considered to be disorders of adulthood. The frequency of complex disorders by age 25 years is 46.4 per 1,000; after 25 years is 600 per 1,000; and over an individual's lifetime is 646.4 per 1,000 (Rimoin et al., 2002).

A complex pattern of inheritance is the basis for conditions such as Alzheimer, cancer, cardiovascular disease, diabetes mellitus, and obesity. Although these conditions often occur in more than one member of a family, they do not follow clear Mendelian patterns of inheritance.

Alzheimer Disease

Alzheimer disease (AD) is a neurodegenerative disease characterized by chronic, progressive loss of memory and other intellectual functions. Other traits of AD include personality changes, death of neurons, development of amyloid neuritic plaques, and formation of neurofibrillary tangles within affected neurons. AD is the most common form of dementia in late life, with about 25% of AD being familial. Less than 2% of these families have early-onset familial AD (EOFAD) in which symptoms occur before age 65. Three genes have been identified as a cause of EOFAD:

1. *PSEN1,* located on chromosome 14 (a precursor for presenilin 1)
2. *AD1,* located on chromosome 21 (a precursor for amyloid beta A4 protein)
3. *AD4,* located on chromosome 1 (a precursor for presenilin-2).

EOFAD appears to follow an autosomal dominant transmission.

The majority of familial AD (FAD) occurs after age 65 or is considered to be late-onset FAD. This complex disorder is thought to involve several susceptibility genes. One of these susceptibility genes is the *APOE e4* gene on chromosome 19. Other genes located on chromosomes 2, 9, 10, 12, and 15 are being investigated for contributing to late-onset FAD. Trisomy 21 or Down syndrome appears to be related to AD because essentially all individuals with trisomy 21 will develop signs of AD after age 40. The reason for this is thought to be the lifelong overexpression of the *APP* gene on chromosome 21 (Bird, 1998).

The majority of AD (approximately 75%) is due to unknown causes. This nonfamilial or sporadic AD is thought to be multifactorial and resulting from the combination of aging, genetic predisposition, and exposure to one or more environmental influences. Factors such as head trauma, viruses, and/or toxins have been investigated for their influence on AD but have not been proven to be contributors (Cummings, Vinters, Cole, & Khachaturian, 1998).

Cancer

Cancer, a group of diseases that share common characteristics, is a disease of somatic cells. Specifically, cells experience uncontrolled growth as a result of mutations that affect a limited number of genes. Cancer cells have two characteristics that are not found in normal cells. In normal cells, cell-to-cell contact inhibits further growth and division, a process called contact inhibition. Cancer cells do not have contact inhibition; instead, they continue to grow and divide and may even pile on top of each other. If normal cells are badly damaged or starved for nutrients, they undergo apoptosis, or programmed cell death, and self-destruct. Cancer cells do not undergo apoptosis. Normal cells experience cell senescence or stop dividing in culture after about 50 divisions. Cancer cells in culture divide indefinitely. Additional information about the molecular basis of cancer and conversion of normal somatic cells to cancer cells can be found in Nussbaum et al. (2004) and Hartl and Jones (2004).

About one-third of the 565,650 cancer deaths expected to occur in the United States in 2008 will be related to nutrition, physical inactivity, and obesity or overweight. More than 170,000 cancer deaths are expected to be caused by tobacco use. Although anyone can develop cancer, risks increase as individual's age. About 77% of all cancers are diagnosed in individuals 55 years and older. Cancer researchers refer to the lifetime risk of developing cancer as the probability that an individual will, over the course of his or her lifetime, develop cancer or die from it. Relative risk is a measure of the strength of the relationship between risk factors and a particular cancer. Relative risk compares the risk of developing cancer in individuals with a certain exposure or trait to the risk in persons who do not have this exposure or trait. Male smokers are about 23 times more likely to develop lung cancer than nonsmokers, so their relative risk is 23 (American Cancer Society [ACS], 2008).

About 5% of individuals with cancer have familial cancer or cancer in which there is clear evidence that an inherited gene predisposes the individual to very high risk for a particular cancer (ACS, 2008). The remaining 95% are sporadic or cancers that occur as a result of genetic changes in somatic cells. These changes occur over the lifetime and are due to internal factors such as hormones or digestion of nutrients in cells. They may also be caused by external factors, such as tobacco, chemicals, and sunlight. Inheriting a cancer-causing gene usually does not indicate a 100% chance that cancer will develop, but it may indicate a significant risk that an individual will develop cancer at some point over his or her lifetime. Knowing this, a careful surveillance program can be instituted that will identify cancer early and decrease morbidity and mortality.

Nurses should carefully examine the family history and pedigree for clues associated with an inherited susceptibility to cancer (Chart 11–1). Cancers with a familial basis often occur at a younger age than sporadic cancers; they are usually bilateral in paired organs (e.g., breasts and kidneys), and multifocal, or occur in multiple sites in a single organ. Following analysis of the family history and pedigree, nurses should look for the presence of these clues. If a hereditary syndrome is suspected and if any of the clues are present, the patient and family should be referred to a nurse, physician, or genetic counselor with advanced professional training in cancer genetics (National Cancer Institute, 2004).

Coronary Artery Disease

Coronary artery disease (CAD) is caused by atherosclerosis or thickening and hardening of the inside walls of arteries. Some hardening of the arteries occurs normally as individuals grow older. In atherosclerosis, plaque deposits build up in the arteries. Plaque is made of fat, cholesterol, calcium, and other substances found in the blood. This buildup of plaque can narrow the arteries, resulting in less blood flowing to the heart muscle. This blockage can eventually completely block the arteries and flow of blood. Blood clots may also form and block the arteries. Risk

---

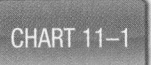 **CHART 11–1** **Clues Suggesting an Inherited Cancer Susceptibility Syndrome**

- Multiple cancers in close relatives
- Early age of onset; younger than 40 to 50 years for adult-onset cancers
- Multiple cancers in a single individual
- Bilateral cancer in paired organs (e.g., breast, kidney)
- Recognition of the known association between etiologically related cancers in the family
- Presence of congenital anomalies or precursor lesions that are known to be associated with increased cancer risk (e.g., presence of atypical nevi and risk of malignant melanoma)
- Recognizable Mendelian inheritance pattern

Source: National Cancer Institute. (2004, September 16). *Elements of cancer genetics risk assessment and counseling.* Last updated October 3, 2006. Retrieved November 12, 2006, from http://www.nci.nih.gov/cancertopics/pdq/genetics/risk-assessment-and-counseling.

factors for CAD include the following: age, family history of early heart disease, high blood cholesterol, high blood pressure, cigarette smoking, diabetes, obesity, and lack of physical activity. All factors except age and family history can be altered by an individual to prevent or delay onset of CAD. Individuals with a family history of early heart disease include those individuals with heart disease diagnosed before age 55 in a father or brother, and before age 65 in a mother or sister.

Single-gene disorders that cause CAD include defects in the apolipoproteins; receptor defects, such as LDL receptor disorder leading to familial hypercholesterolemia; enzyme defects, such as lipoprotein lipase deficiency; and defects in transfer proteins, such as cholesteryl ester transfer protein deficiency. Treatment with appropriate medications and lifestyle changes can reduce cholesterol levels in heterozygous individuals but may not help individuals who are homozygous for the gene contributing to CAD.

Diabetes Mellitus

The two major types of diabetes mellitus are type 1 (insulin-dependent diabetes) and type 2 (non–insulin-dependent diabetes). Of the 20.8 million individuals in the United States who have diabetes mellitus, 5% to 10% have type 1 and approximately 88% have type 2 (American Diabetes Association [ADA], 2008). Both types are complex disorders because both genetic and environmental factors are necessary for their expression.

Type 1 is an autoimmune disorder that is attributed to both an inherited risk and external triggers or factors including viruses, nutrition, and toxins. About 18 regions in the human genome are linked to influencing type 1 diabetes risk. These regions, labeled IDDM1 to IDDM18, each may contain several genes that contribute to risk. The most studied is IDDM1, which contains HLA genes, located on chromosome 6. Inheriting certain alleles of the HLA genes increases the likelihood that immune cells will attack the body's healthy cells. One of the non-HLA genes, *IDDM2,* is the insulin gene, located on chromosome 11. Inheritance of the *IDDM1* HLA genes can account for a greater than 50% genetic risk, and inheritance of the *IDDM2* gene can contribute another 10% genetic risk (Dean & McEntyre, 2004).

Type 2 diabetes has a stronger genetic basis than type 1 and is also affected by environmental factors. Risk factors include obesity and a positive family history of diabetes. Although many genes appear to be involved in the occurrence of type 2 diabetes, they have not been well defined. A rare form of diabetes called maturity-onset diabetes in the young (MODY), whose phenotype is similar to type 2 diabetes, is a single-gene disorder with autosomal dominant inheritance (ADA, 2008).

Obesity

Currently, more than 65% of U.S. adults are overweight or obese, which increases their risk for other chronic diseases such as heart disease and diabetes. In a few rare cases, gene mutations have been found to cause morbid obesity regardless of the environment. However, common forms of obesity are due to susceptibility genes acting within a receptive environment to create an obesity phenotype (Cummings & Schwartz, 2003). According to the "thrifty gene" hypothesis, evolution has favored genes that promote weight gain to protect humans against an environment that was unreliable in providing food. Unfortunately, our thrifty

genes are maladaptive in today's environment of excess foods and diminished physical activity (Hill & Peters, 1998).

Studies of monozygotic and dizygotic twins have shown that estimated inheritability for obesity is 50% to 90% (Froguel & Boutin, 2001). Currently, more than 300 genes and chromosomal regions have been associated with obesity phenotypes. Genes of particular interest include leptin, leptin receptor, melanocortin 4 receptor, and single-minded 1 homologue.

Clinical studies are exploring the genetic determinants of obesity and identifying critical biologic pathways involved in maintaining energy balance. These studies could point the way toward therapeutic interventions and identify those at risk or responsive to environmental modulations.

Hemoglobinopathies

Two hemoglobinopathies, sickle cell disease and thalassemias, are good examples of disorders of hemoglobin. Both are molecular diseases in which the primary disease-causing event is an inherited or acquired mutation. A genetic disease occurs when there is an alteration in the DNA of an essential gene that changes the amount or function or both of the messenger RNA (mRNA) and protein. Single-gene disorders almost always result from mutations that change protein function.

Sickle Cell Disease

Sickle cell disease is an example of a change in the amino acid sequence that causes pathology. This is accomplished by the protein developing a new characteristic, without changing the protein's normal function. It was identified by Linus Pauling and was the first molecular disease to be recognized. The amino acid substitution in sickle cell disease changes the shape of hemoglobin from a round to a distorted sickle shape. The sickled cells' shortened life span (a few weeks compared to four months) results in anemia. Sickle cells become trapped in small blood vessels and cause tissue damage, infections, and periodic episodes of intense pain.

Sickle cell disease is an autosomal recessive disorder occurring most frequently in equatorial Africa and less commonly in the Mediterranean area and India and in countries to which people from these regions have migrated. The sickle cell gene has been described as protecting individuals against malaria, which accounts for its high frequency in areas of the world where malaria occurs. About 1 in 600 African Americans is born with sickle cell disease. Although many individuals die in early childhood, the life span of individuals with sickle cell disease is increasing (National Institutes of Health, 2006).

Thalassemias

Mutations also cause loss of protein function, the most common consequence of mutation. Although the mutations are in the same gene as the mutation that causes sickle cell disease, the red blood cells do not sickle in thalassemia. The severity of the thalassemia that results from loss-of-function mutations is generally related to the amount of function lost. When the thalassemias are grouped together, they are the most common single-gene disorder.

Thalassemia was first discovered in persons of Mediterranean origin. Both alpha- and beta-thalassemia have a high frequency in many populations, although alpha-thalassemia is more prevalent and widely distributed. Thalassemia offers protection against malaria to individuals who are carriers and is found in countries in the Mediterranean, the Middle East, and parts of Africa, India, and Asia.

Nursing Role in Detection, Management, and Care of Individuals with Genetic Disorders

The field of genetics influences all aspects of nursing, from the application of genetic principles in patient care to employing cutting-edge genetic methodologies in research protocols. As may be expected, the specific role played by the nurse depends on several factors, including the patient's needs and the nurse's expertise and knowledge of genetics. Currently, a nationwide effort is underway to increase the genetic content in all health care curricula (e.g., nursing, medicine, and pharmacy). Nurses are on the front line of patient care where the timely integration of genetic knowledge, skills, and attitudes into routine patient care is warranted to provide effective care to individuals and their families. Several organizations, including the International Society of Nurses in Genetics (2007), the National Coalition for Health Professional Education in Genetics (NCHPEG) (2000), and the Consensus Panel on Genetic/Genomic Nursing Competencies (2006), have recommended genetic core competencies and standards for nurses and other health care professionals (Chart 11–2). Principal among these are the abilities to identify who may benefit from genetic services and to make appropriate genetic referrals. As genetic content increases in nursing curricula and as more is learned about genomic determinants of common diseases, nurses will be increasingly involved in the management, interpretation, and decision making related to genetic information and services. In addition, nurses must also consider the ethical, legal, and social issues related to privacy and discrimination of genetic information. These will be discussed in a later section.

Pedigrees

Recognizing patterns of inheritance and clustering of diseases within families is a key skill needed to determine genetic risk assessment. These can be determined based on a thorough family history that is organized into a family tree, called a **pedigree.** Pedigrees enable the health care provider to visualize how diseases and characteristics are clustered within a family and through generations.

Three generational pedigrees are used by geneticists, advanced practice genetic nurses, and genetic counselors, among others, to identify disease risk and to develop a personalized prevention program for chronic conditions as well as single-gene disorders (Consensus Panel on Genetic/Genomic Nursing Competencies, 2006). Once an accurate family history has been established and genetic disorders or health care risks identified, it may be appropriate to refer the client to a geneticist or genetic counselor for follow-up.

Tools have been developed to assist health care providers in conducting a thorough family history and to draw a pedigree

(American Medical Association, 2006; Bennett et al., 1995). For each family member, the most important information to record is the current age (or age at death), ethnicity, and relevant medical conditions with onset or duration. Commonly used pedigree symbols are listed in Figure 11–7 ■ (p. 204) and used in Figures 11–8 through 11–11 ■ (p. 204) as examples of the types of inheritance patterns for single-gene disorders.

Recently, to encourage all Americans to learn more about their family health history, the U.S. Surgeon General in cooperation with other agencies, has launched a national public health campaign called the U.S. Surgeon General's Family History Initiative, My Family Health Portrait. This is a patient-friendly website designed for the general public to create a personalized family health history report from any computer with an Internet connection and an up-to-date web browser. Using the website software, the patient can create a three-generation pedigree that can be printed and shared with health care professionals.

For some disorders, cluster patterns in a pedigree do not appear to follow an autosomal dominant, recessive, or X-linked pattern of inheritance. Occasionally this is due to either incomplete penetrance or varied expressivity. These features are most commonly seen in autosomal dominant conditions. **Penetrance** is the proportion of individuals who have the genotype and actually manifest the disease or trait. It is considered an all-or-none concept. This is because an individual with a specific genotype either will, or will not, be affected with the disorder regardless of environmental or other genetic influences. Some disorders such as myotonic dystrophy, a form of muscular dystrophy characterized by generalized weakness and muscle wasting, have incomplete or reduced penetrance, meaning that some individuals with the genotype are affected and some are not.

Expressivity is the degree to which a person with a specific genotype is affected. For example, two individuals may have the same genotype, but one may have all of the symptoms of the disorder, while the second one has relatively few symptoms. This is known as variable expressivity. Marfan syndrome, an autosomal dominant disorder caused by a mutation in collagen formation, is an example of variable expressivity. Skeletal, optical, and cardiovascular abnormalities range in severity among individuals with Marfan syndrome.

Genetic Testing

The explosion in genetic knowledge and molecular technologies has led to a heightened public awareness of the genetic components of disease. Because of public access to cutting-edge research, patients are approaching their primary health care provider with requests for genetic testing for conditions ranging from rare genetic disorders to colon cancer. In the past, genetic counselors have provided guidance and counseling for genetic testing; however, there are not enough genetic counselors to meet the needs of patients referred for genetic testing. Therefore, it has become the nurses' responsibility to become knowledgeable about genetic testing and the ethical, legal, and social issues pertaining to them.

An accurate family history is a powerful initial method for determining genetic risk and this can be followed up with appropriate laboratory genetic testing. Currently, more than 1,500 diseases can be tested for using genetic tests. Genetic tests include prenatal testing, newborn screening, and carrier, diagnostic, and

CHART 11–2 **Essential Nursing Competencies for Genetics and Genomics**

PROFESSIONAL RESPONSIBILITIES

All registered nurses are expected to engage in professional role activities that are consistent with *Nursing: Scope and Standards of Practice* (American Nurses Association, 2004). In addition, competent nursing practice now requires the incorporation of genetic and genomic knowledge and skills in order to:

- Recognize when one's own attitudes and values related to genetic and genomic science may affect care provided to clients.
- Advocate for client's access to desired genetic/genomic services and/or resources including support groups.
- Examine competency of practice on a regular basis, identifying areas of strength, as well as areas in which professional development related to genetics and genomics would be beneficial.
- Incorporate genetic and genomic technologies and information into registered nurse practice.
- Demonstrate in practice the importance of tailoring genetic and genomic information and services to clients based on their culture, religion, knowledge level, literacy, and preferred language.
- Advocate for the rights of all clients for autonomous, informed genetic- and genomic-related decision making and voluntary action.

PROFESSIONAL PRACTICE DOMAIN

Nursing Assessment: Applying/Integrating Genetic and Genomic Knowledge

The registered nurse:

- Demonstrates an understanding of the relationship of genetics and genomics to health, prevention, screening, diagnostics, prognostics, selection of treatment, and monitoring of treatment effectiveness.
- Demonstrates the ability to elicit a minimum of a three-generation family health history information.
- Constructs a pedigree from collected family history information using standardized symbols and terminology.
- Collects personal, health, and developmental histories that consider genetic, environmental, and genomic influences and risks.
- Conducts comprehensive health and physical assessments which incorporate knowledge about genetic, environmental, and genomic influences and risk factors.
- Critically analyzes the history and physical assessment findings for genetic, environmental, and genomic influences and risk factors.
- Assesses clients' knowledge, perceptions, and responses to genetic and genomic information.
- Develops a plan of care that incorporates genetic and genomic assessment information.

Information

The registered nurse:

- Identifies clients who may benefit from specific genetic and genomic information and/or services based on assessment data.
- Identifies credible, accurate, appropriate, and current genetic and genomic information, resources, services, and/or technologies specific to given clients.
- Identifies ethical, ethnic/ancestral, cultural, religious, legal, fiscal, and societal issues related to genetic and genomic information and technologies.
- Defines issues that undermine the rights of all clients for autonomous, informed genetic- and genomic-related decision making and voluntary action.

Referral Activities

The registered nurse:

- Facilitates referrals for specialized genetic and genomic services for clients as needed.

Provision of Education, Care, and Support

The registered nurse:

- Provides clients with interpretation of selective genetic and genomic information or services.
- Provides clients with credible, accurate, appropriate, and current genetic and genomic information, resources, services, and/or technologies that facilitate decision making.
- Uses health promotion/disease prevention practices that:
  - Consider genetic and genomic influences on personal and environmental risk factors.
  - Incorporate knowledge of genetic and/or genomic risk factors (e.g., a client with a genetic predisposition for high cholesterol who can benefit from a change in lifestyle that will decrease the likelihood that the genetic risk will be expressed).
- Uses genetic- and genomic-based interventions and information to improve clients' outcomes.
- Collaborates with health care providers in providing genetic and genomic health care.
- Collaborates with insurance providers/payers to facilitate reimbursement for genetic and genomic health care services.
- Performs interventions/treatments appropriate to clients' genetic and genomic health care needs.
- Evaluates impact and effectiveness of genetic and genomic technology, information, interventions, and treatments on clients' outcome.

Source: From Consensus Panel on Genetic/Genomic Nursing Competencies. (2006). *Essential nursing competencies and curricula guidelines for genetics and genomics.* Silver Spring, MD: American Nurses Association.

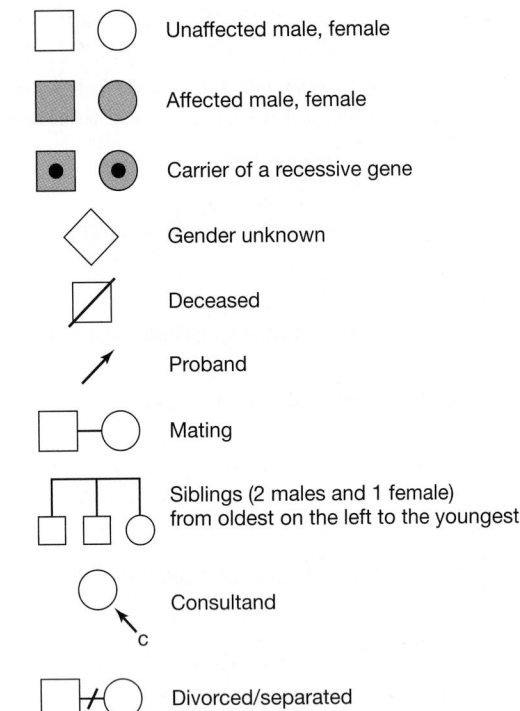

FIGURE 11–7 ■ Pedigree symbols.

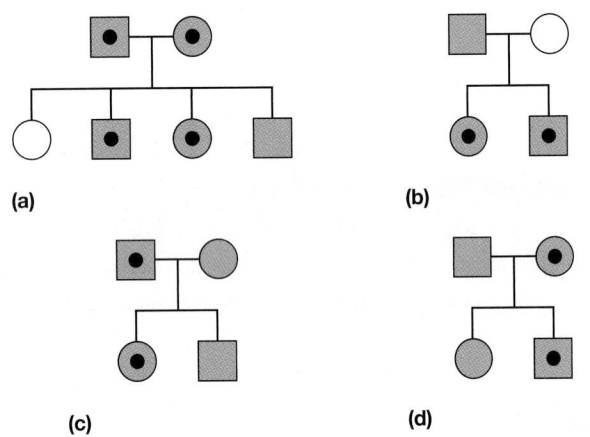

FIGURE 11–8 ■ Autosomal recessive inheritance pedigree.

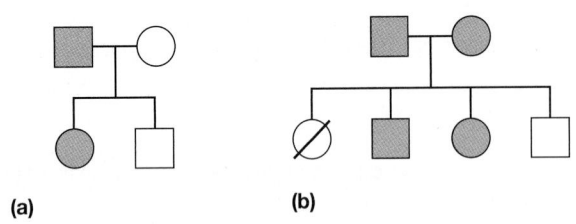

FIGURE 11–9 ■ Autosomal dominant inheritance pedigree.

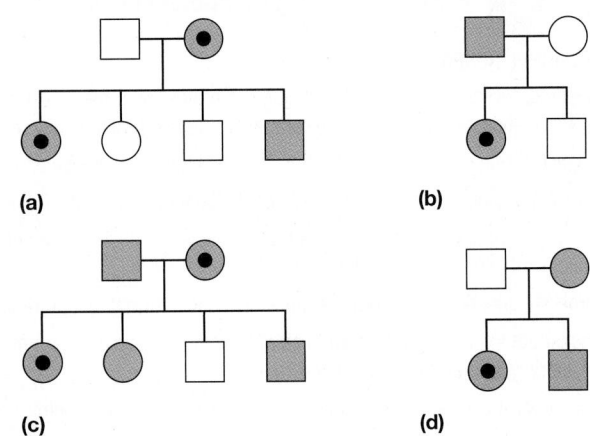

FIGURE 11–10 ■ X-linked recessive inheritance pedigree.

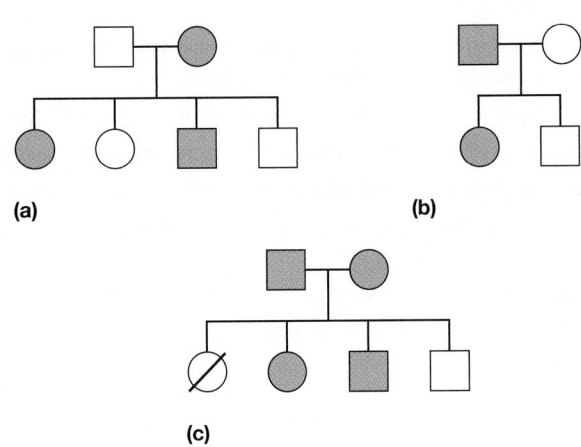

FIGURE 11–11 ■ X-linked dominant inheritance pedigree.

Prenatal Testing and Newborn Screening

Prenatal genetic testing is usually offered when there is increased risk of having a child with a genetic condition. This may be due to maternal age, family history, ethnicity, multiple marker screen, or fetal ultrasound. Biochemical, chromosomal, or molecular-based approaches are used to identify individuals with genetic disorders such as Down syndrome. Because of risks to the fetus and the mother, informed consent is required prior to conducting prenatal testing.

Each year newborns in the United States are screened using heelstick blood spots to detect genetic disorders that can be treated if found early. With the increase in new technologies such as tandem mass spectrometry, many states have expanded their newborn screening programs. The American Academy of Pediatrics Committee on Genetics (Kaye, 2006) describes the status of newborn screening for core conditions including congenital hypothyroidism, congenital adrenal hyperplasia, sickle cell disease, thalassemia, biotinidase, galactosemia, and cystic fibrosis.

Up-to-date information on what tests are required in each state can be located at the National Newborn Screening and Genetic Resource Center website.

Carrier Genetic Tests

Carrier genetic tests are conducted to determine if an unaffected, relatively healthy individual is carrying a disease-causing

predictive testing. Specimens for genetic tests include blood, urine, saliva, stool, body tissues, bone, or hair. Genetic tests include molecular analysis of DNA and RNA, linkage analysis, biochemical testing of certain proteins, and cytogenetic testing on chromosomes (University of Washington, 2006).

gene that could potentially be transmitted to offspring. This can be valuable information in common recessive disorders such as cystic fibrosis and sickle cell disease, or X-linked disorders such as hemophilia A. Knowledge of carrier status in autosomal recessive disorders is important information to use in family planning. If both parents are carriers of a recessive gene, then there is a 25% risk that each child will have the disease and a 50% chance that the child will be a carrier.

Diagnostic Genetic Tests

Diagnostic genetic tests are conducted on symptomatic individuals to identify the genetic disorder and assist with specific treatment and prognosis. For example, if a mother reports to her pediatrician that her 3-year-old son is becoming progressively weak, a DNA test can be conducted to confirm the suspected diagnosis of Duchenne muscular dystrophy. To assist with treatment or prognosis in hereditary cancers, the clinician can test for a mutation in the P53 tumor-suppressor gene. Based on the findings, a decision can be made to treat the cancer more assertively because it is more likely to grow aggressively.

As the clinical validity and utility of genetic testing is demonstrated, increasing numbers of prognostic indicators will be more closely associated with the specific mutation (i.e., BRCA1) instead of the disorder (i.e., breast cancer). Molecular approaches have largely replaced biochemical methodologies for genetic testing. In general, age is not a factor when determining whether or not to conduct a diagnostic genetic test.

Predictive Genetic Tests

Predictive genetic tests are offered to asymptomatic individuals who are at risk for a genetic disorder. The availability of predictive tests is increasing dramatically in association with the explosion in genetic technologies. Predictive tests are categorized into two groups: presymptomatic and susceptibility. Presymptomatic testing is conducted on individuals who will eventually develop the symptoms when the gene mutation is present. An example of this is an individual who has the mutation for Huntington disease, a fatal genetic disorder.

Susceptibility testing is conducted to identify individuals who are predisposed or at risk for developing the genetic disorder, but it is not certain they will develop the disorder even when the mutation is present. An example of this is hereditary nonpolyposis colorectal cancer (HNPCC), which has been associated with mutations in five genes responsible for repairing DNA. Individuals with these mutations have an 80% lifetime risk of developing colorectal cancer. Because of the ethical and psychological issues involved, many genetic laboratories conducting predictive genetic testing require documentation of patient informed consent and counseling.

An inherited gene mutation will be in the DNA of any cells in the body. Therefore, there are many sources from which to obtain samples appropriate for predictive genetic testing of an inherited disorder. DNA analysis is usually conducted using blood specimens, buccal cells (cheek cells), or skin cells because these specimens are relatively easy to obtain via noninvasive means.

Benefits and Limitations of Genetic Testing

Genetic tests differ from other medical tests because they provide genetic information about the health of individuals *and their families* and also identify asymptomatic individuals who are at risk. Benefits can include medical management that is more appropriate for the particular diagnosis and opportunities for counseling and health promotion. Activities to reduce disease risk, increase longevity, and improve quality of life may also be prescribed. Genetic testing results can be useful when making future decisions regarding children, financial planning, career choices, and lifestyle. In addition, for some individuals, knowing the test results may decrease stress and anxiety by eliminating uncertainty—even if the test is positive.

Limitations of genetic testing depend on the type of genetic test conducted. For example, a limitation of predictive testing is that it does not provide a diagnosis; instead, it identifies if the patient is "at risk." Just as a positive result does not always mean that the patient will develop a disease, a negative result does not mean the patient will not develop the disease or disorder. Diagnostic tests may provide a diagnosis, yet there may or may not be a therapeutic intervention for the genetic disorder.

Another significant limitation is that current molecular genetic tests examine for a mutation at a specific locus and do not identify mutations in other areas of the gene or the genome. For example, cystic fibrosis can be diagnosed by a mutation in the cystic fibrosis gene. However, more than 900 different mutations have been identified in that one gene. Additionally, the assay panels commonly test for only 25 of the most frequently identified mutations. Therefore, individuals with one of the other 875 mutations would not be identified and the disorder would go undiagnosed.

Concerns about the effects of information from genetic testing on the patient and family members and implications for the future should be considered. Although universal guidelines have not been developed for genetic testing, all nurses should handle information obtained from genetic testing carefully. Attention should be given to privacy, informed consent, and confidentiality. Patients have the right to privacy regarding test results to avoid future discrimination or questions about employability or insurability. Patients and health care providers should have adequate knowledge of the risks, benefits, and alternatives to genetic testing so that they understand the implications.

Ethical, Legal, and Social Issues of Genetic Information

The Ethical, Legal and Social Implications (ELSI) research program began in 1990 as an essential component of the Human Genome Project. The purpose of the program was to address the implications of the mapping and sequencing of the human genome with regard to the ethical, legal, and social consequences of the mapping and sequencing of the human genome. The intent was to stimulate discussion on these issues and develop policy options that would ensure that the information gained was used to benefit individuals and society. Funds from the National Human Genome Research Institute (NHGRI) are designated to fund ELSI research (NHGRI, 2006). There is a particular emphasis on genetic issues related to discrimination, privacy, psychological impact and stigmatization, and uncertainties associated with interpretation of predictive genetic tests. In addition, issues surrounding the availability and access to testing and treatment and their cost are being addressed.

Genetic discrimination is the concern that genetic information may be used by employers against employees, or to screen potential employees; and by insurance companies to deny or limit insurance. In May of 2008, the Genetic Information Nondiscrimination Act (GINA) was signed into law. The landmark legislation provides protection against discrimination based on an individual's genetic information in health insurance coverage and employment setting and should allow fuller use of genetic testing. In addition, the Health Information Portability and Accountability Act (HIPAA), discussed in Chapter 3 ⊛, addresses privacy issues by affording genetic information increased confidentiality.

Of primary concern is the psychological impact and emotional response of the individual and family to test results. It is important to recognize that an individual's cultural background influences how she will interpret genetic information, make decisions, and adapt to genetic conditions (Greb, 1998). This cultural and ethical context should be considered when preparing the individual and family to receive genetic results. The Cultural Considerations box provides examples of this.

Careful patient assessment, counseling, and follow-up are integral to the nurse's role in the genetic testing process. Genetic information can influence future reproductive decisions and medical treatment. The results may have significant psychological ramifications. For example, it is possible for test results to inadvertently uncover a paternity or adoption issue.

Increasingly, predictive genetic testing for conditions ranging from breast cancer to cardiovascular disease is marketed directly to consumers and is available over the Internet. Because of the complexity of the interpretation of genetic tests, particularly for multifactorial diseases and predictive genetic tests, and the potential lack of counseling and follow-up, there are emerging concerns about these marketing techniques.

■ Emerging Genetic Technologies and Therapies

Emerging genetic technological and methodological advances are based on gene expression (the activity of the gene as measured by the amount of mRNA produced) and the complementary binding nature (A binds to T and C binds to G) of DNA bases. Loescher and Merkle (2005) have described a framework for understanding genomic technologies. Most genetic variation occurs in only 0.1% of the human genome and it is there that researchers test for an association between genetic variation (gene sequence) and disease susceptibility. These technologies allow professionals to identify disease susceptibility genes and monitor gene activity, thus bringing applied genetics to the clinical practitioner (Cashion, Driscoll, & Sabek, 2004). Chart 11–3 (p. 209) gives examples of common genetic technologies and examples of their use.

PCR and Microarrays

Although PCR has been successfully employed since 1983 to replicate, or amplify, as few as one copy of a gene into billions of copies of that gene, real-time PCR and microarrays are emerging technologies. The many exact copies of a gene made by PCR enable researchers and clinicians to identify and study that gene. Real-time PCR allows for the detection and quantification of a small fragment of replicating DNA during the amplification

process. It is an improvement over PCR because it offers more rapid and sensitive quantification of the gene of interest. Clinically, real-time PCR is used to obtain viral load levels of many different viruses including cytomegalovirus and hepatitis C.

Microarray analysis is one of the emerging genetic technologies. Although primarily used in the research setting, it is transitioning into clinical practice, specifically in the area of cancer prognosis and treatment stratification. When conducting a microarray analysis, specialized equipment that uses sophisticated computer programs simultaneously evaluates up to 33,000 genes that have been placed on a small 2.5-cm (1-in.) solid support (usually glass) chip. An application of this would be to identify a genetic pattern that demonstrates which genes are most active in disease states such as leukemia. In addition, clinicians and researchers may use gene expression patterns that emerge to obtain a more specific diagnosis and to better manage patient care (Cashion & Driscoll, 2004).

Gene Therapy and Stem Cell Therapy

Since the 2001 publication of the sequencing of the human genome (Venter et al., 2001), focus has shifted from sequencing the genome to applying this knowledge to treat diseases. **Gene therapy** and stem cell therapies are two applications that are currently in clinical development. Gene therapy is the correction of a genetic mutation by the introduction of DNA into a cell as a treatment modality to improve the patient's health. Gene therapy has been used in clinical research trials to treat X-linked severe combined immune deficiency, a life-threatening disorder of the immune system. However, complications such as the short-lived nature of the treatment and significant adverse effects related to a heightened immune response have arisen in these trials. As a result of the additional research required, no human gene therapy products have been approved for commercial use. Ethical considerations such as those related to general availability of gene therapy due to excessive costs are also issues. For further information on gene therapy, refer to the Human Genome Project Information, Ethical, Legal, and Social Implications website.

In general, stem cells are unspecialized cells that have the potential to divide without limit and to develop into specialized cells. Examples of the specialized cells are nerve, muscle cells, or insulin-producing cells of the pancreas. Research is conducted on embryonic stem cells and adult stem cells. Embryonic stem cells can become all cell types of the body, whereas adult stem cells typically specialize into the cell types based on the tissue in which they originated.

Studies using human embryonic stem cells may provide information about complex aspects of human development including birth abnormalities and diseases such as cancer and Parkinson's. The focus of stem cell research is learning how undifferentiated cells become differentiated. Learning more about this process can lead to an understanding about how these conditions and diseases occur and strategies for treatment. For additional information, visit the Stem Cell Information website, an official National Institutes of Health (NIH) resource for stem cell research. Although there is hope for the treatment potential of stem cell therapies, many ethical and political issues remain to be addressed. The NIH Research Ethics and Stem Cells

CULTURAL CONSIDERATIONS for Genetics

African American	• Greeting and addressing patients should be formal, without using first names unless requested to do so by the patient or family. • Avoid imitating jargon because this may be viewed as ridicule. • Fear of admitting carrier status with sickle cell disease may be a holdover from negative experiences with mass screening in the 1970s when carriers were denied health and life insurance. • Stressing the positive, such as protection against malaria, is important when providing information about sickle cell trait. • Support systems provided by the family may be more important than support systems outside the family. • During the first counseling session, explain the session, follow up, and give suggestions related to the present. Address the future at a later time. (Telfair & Nash, 1996)
Amish	• Introductions of providers should be informal, such as "Dr. Barbara" or "Nurse David." • Decisions are made equally by husband and wife, so provide information directly to both parents. • Because of a strong belief in God, the topics of birth control, DNA storage, abortion, and artificial insemination by a donor are irrelevant. • Carrier screening may be unacceptable. Communities are aware of problems related to consanguinity and may look outside their community for a marriage partner. • Taking photographs of a patient is usually unacceptable, but may be allowed if the patient and family understand its importance in establishing a diagnosis. • Consent for autopsy is usually refused. • A lack of health insurance, which may be common in the community, can result in deciding not to proceed with extensive diagnostic testing. • Written consent may not be well understood because giving one's word is accepted in the community. • Printed visual aids may be helpful in counseling sessions. (Francomano, 1996)
Traditional Asian Indian	• Explain the importance of an in-depth family history. • Explain diagnostic tests thoroughly. Carrier testing can result in discrimination and problems if marriages are arranged. • Because decision making may be done by all family members, schedule two clinic visits so tests can be done at the second visit after family members have made a decision about the suggested tests. • Adoption is well accepted. • Autopsies may be declined by Sikhs and Hindus, whereas Muslims may consent if necessary legally. • Explain informed consent. • Visual aids may be helpful. • Surgical procedures are not readily accepted so detailed information should be given. • Results of tests that Westerners consider bad news may not be as stressful if fatalism is a strong belief. (Patil & Fisher, 1996)
Traditional Chinese	• Family members make decisions in a group and consult other family members if necessary. The oldest male has the most authority in traditional families. • Adoptions are rare. • Autopsies are viewed as irrelevant and expensive. • Carrier testing and use of other technologies may create the potential for blame, especially toward the mother. Stress the importance of "no fault." • The use of visual aids may be appropriate and helpful. • Family histories may be incomplete and mental illness may not be acknowledged or well recognized. (Jung, 1996)
Deaf	• Avoid referring to deafness as a disability because some patients do not consider it to be disabling. When this is the case, giving birth to a child who is deaf will likely not be considered a problem. • Determine how the patient prefers to be referred to (as being deaf, hard of hearing, or hearing impaired) and refer to the patient in that way. • Avoid using terms such as *abnormal* or *affected* when referring to patients who are deaf. Describe genes as altered. • Visual aids can be very helpful. Avoid communicating while the patient is looking at the pictures. • A family history form may need to be sent before clinic visits. The family history may need to be obtained through medical records or hearing family members. (Israel, Cunningham, Thumann, & Arnos, 1996)
Traditional Japanese	• Introductions should include titles with greeting of the patient and family members as Mr. or Mrs. • Adoptions, autopsies, and organ transplants are rare. • Assure the family of confidentiality and privacy. • Explain the need for consent forms. • With carrier testing and other testing, explain the importance of "no fault." • The family needs take precedence over the individual's needs. • The family members may make major decisions so allow time for the family to consult family elders if necessary. • Photographs may be refused, especially if a child has a visible disability. The disability may be viewed as shameful. (Strazaar & Fisher, 1996)

(continued)

Source: Fisher, Nancy L., M.D., M.P.H., ed. Cultural and Ethnic Diversity: A Guide for Genetics Professionals. Pages 32–33, 55, 82–83, 96–97, 111, 127, 153–154, 193–194, 217–218, 235. © 1996 The Johns Hopkins University Press. Reprinted with permission of The Johns Hopkins University Press.

CULTURAL CONSIDERATIONS for Genetics—*Continued*

North American Jewish
- Use of prenatal diagnosis varies widely, depending on the religious orientation.
- In Orthodox families, the male is often the decision maker, but will need to consult with a rabbi. Schedule prenatal testing early enough in the pregnancy to allow for this consultation to occur.
- Orthodox families may have their own internal support groups, whereas less observant Jews may use support groups outside their immediate community.
- Autopsy is usually discouraged unless it is strongly recommended. Discussion with and advice from a rabbi may be necessary. (Greenstein & Bernstein, 1996)

Latino
- The eldest male is greeted first. Shake hands and ask about family to establish rapport.
- Prenatal testing should be offered even though many Latinos are Catholic.
- Disclosure of carrier status or a child's disability to other family members may be viewed as a loss of dignity.
- Couples and patients need time to consult with other family members because family members participate in all decisions.
- Loss of pregnancy is viewed as loss of a child.
- Folk healers and Western physicians may be used by families and couples, so asking what other treatments are being used is important.
- Visual aids may help in explaining genetic concepts.
- If the patient needs to see a counselor more than once, schedule the patient with the same counselor. (Lopez-Rangel, 1996)

Native Americans of the Southwest
- Amniocentesis may be acceptable but because prenatal care may begin later in pregnancy, it is not an option.
- Prenatal procedures may be more acceptable if the health provider's hands are blessed by a native healer before the procedure.
- Adoption for infertile couples occurs along matrilineal lines; the couple adopts a sister's or cousin's child.
- Diagnostic tests such as venipuncture, skin biopsies, and specimen samples usually present no problems.
- Family planning is considered an individual's choice and may be used infrequently.
- Acceptance of carrier testing is not known.
- When greeting the entire family, address the maternal grandmother first.
- The amount of eye contact that is comfortable for a patient may vary, so adjust accordingly.
- Patients may not answer questions immediately, so allow for silence and do not consider it inattentiveness. (Hauck & Knoki-Wilson, 1996)

Countries of Southeast Asia
- If blood tests are done, avoid drawing extra blood. Use microtubes if possible.
- Respect the patient's right to refuse procedures by not assuming that refusal indicates a lack of understanding.
- Ask the patient or family for permission to use visual aids. (Fisher & Lew, 1996)

website provides links and information to explore the issues surrounding the differing views on stem cell research.

As genomic health care expands into the clinical setting, nurses will be required to understand the concepts, principles, and ethical issues underpinning emerging genetic technologies and therapies. Having a basic understanding of these concepts allows the nurse to recognize the benefits, limitations, and applications of each therapy. More importantly, the nurse can translate this knowledge for the patient, thereby improving patient care (Cashion et al., 2004).

Pharmacogenomics

Pharmacogenomics refers to the application of genomic information and methods to pharmacogenetic problems. **Pharmacogenetics** refers to the area of genetics that focuses on the variability of responses to medications due to genetic variation. These genetic variations can alter the ability of the body to absorb, transport, metabolize, or excrete medications or their metabolites. Pharmacogenetics may include any genetically determined variation in response to drugs. It is thought that many of the adverse drug reactions and some fatal adverse reactions may be "largely, if not entirely, genetically determined" (Nussbaum et al., 2004, p. 249).

The origin of polymorphisms for drug response and the mechanisms that maintain them are a challenging problem. The response to medications requires specific biochemical reactions, and the enzymes involved may participate in the metabolism of ordinary food substances. That polymorphisms for drug response may have resulted from the different diets in different populations is supported by the geographical distribution of many of these alleles. Recognizing this normal variation in response to drugs, the "potency" of a drug is defined by the dose that produces a given effect in 50% of the population. This variation is thought to be best explained by a combination of genetic and environmental factors or multifactorial inheritance.

Cytochrome P450 (CYP) enzymes are a family of liver enzymes that help break down more than 30 classes of medications. CYP polymorphisms or DNA variations in genes that code for these liver enzymes affect their ability to metabolize certain medications. When CYP enzymes are less active or inactive in terms of breaking down or eliminating medications from the patient's body, overdose can occur (Human Genome Program, 2006). CYP polymorphisms affect patients' responses to medications that are used to treat depression, psychosis, cancer, cardiovascular disorders, ulcers and gastrointestinal disorders, pain, and seizure disorders (Ingelman-Sundberg, 2004). The research findings that show strong evidence that CYP polymorphisms in genes affect the enzyme CYP2C9 and patient responsiveness to Coumadin may lead to future genotyping for P450 in patients

CHART 11–3	Commonly Used Genetic Methods	
Genetic Method	**Definition**	**Examples of Use**
Fluorescence *in situ* hybridization (FISH)	A physical mapping approach that uses a fluorescent dye to identify variations from normal in metaphase chromosomes	This technique is widely used in cytogenetics to identify deleted or transposed sections of chromosomes.
Genotype	An individual's genetic sequence at a particular locus	To diagnose genetic disease, identify paternity, and in forensic medicine.
Karyotype	A picture of the entire chromosome complement of a cell	To identify individuals with chromosomal disorders such as Down syndrome.
Microarray	Evaluates thousands of genes or gene expression levels simultaneously.	To identify subgroups of cancer to stratify for treatment therapies.
Northern blot	A technique for identifying if a gene is transcribed using electrophoresis, gels, and absorbent sheets	To examine major variations in RNA expression levels in genetic diseases such as hemoglobinopathies.
Polymerase chain reaction (PCR)	Amplifies one copy of a DNA or RNA into billions of copies	PCR has become the standard method for nucleic acid analysis.
Real-time PCR	Allows measurement of replicating DNA or RNA as the amplification process occurs	To determine viral load levels.
Southern blot	A technique for identifying if a gene is present using electrophoresis, gels, and absorbent sheets.	To diagnose genetic diseases such as cystic fibrosis.
Western blot	A technique for identifying protein using electrophoresis, gels, and absorbent sheets.	To determine if dystrophin is present in suspected cases of muscular dystrophy.

receiving Coumadin (Rettie & Tai, 2006). Clinical trials are being conducted by researchers who test for variations in CYP genes to screen and monitor patients. Pharmaceutical companies are screening the chemical compounds in medications to determine how well they are broken down by the various CYP enzymes (Hodgson & Marshall, 1998).

Malignant hyperthermia and serum cholinesterase and succinylcholine sensitivity are two genetics-related concerns that can occur during anesthesia. Malignant hyperthermia is an autosomal dominant condition that occurs in 1 out of 12,000 children and 1 out of 100,000 adults. The ratio of malignant hyperthermia in males to females is 2.5 to 1. The condition results in a dramatic adverse response to inhalational anesthetics such as halothane and muscle relaxants such as succinylcholine chloride, which can lead to death. Individuals can experience a very high temperature, sustained muscle contraction, and accompanying increased catabolism. Most cases of malignant hyperthermia are associated with mutations in a gene called *RYR1*, which maps to chromosome 19. Special precautions must be taken when individuals at risk need anesthesia. Dantrolene sodium prevents or reduces the severity of the response if an unsuspected attack occurs, and alternative anesthetics can be given to patients at risk.

The HGP has led to the understanding that genomic information can be applied successfully to pharmacogenetic problems. Two facets of pharmacogenomics include (1) the likelihood that the design of new drugs will be influenced by knowledge of all genes, and (2) that a pharmacogenetic profile of each individual who is a candidate to receive a medication can be developed, with two possible benefits. The first benefit is that it should be possible to predict those individuals who are likely to have an adverse response to a medication. This may be accomplished even without knowledge of the metabolism of the drug or of the specific alleles that modulate responses to it. A second benefit may come from the development of abbreviated pharmacogenetic profiles such that it should be possible to predict the efficacy of the medication in an individual before the drug is administered.

Overall, the role of drug metabolism in many pathophysiological processes is important. The management of patients with toxic reactions to drugs should include evaluation of the pharmacogenetic status of both the patient and members of the family, and appropriate genetic counseling about potential risks of certain drugs. The application of knowledge from the HGP to pharmacogenetics should usher in an era of "individualized medicine" in which appropriate medications and therapies consider not only the presentation and course of the disease, but also the individual's specific genetic makeup.

Health Promotion

Determining genetic patterns of inheritance can be a powerful way to establish genetic risk and to initiate health promotion activities designed to prevent the onset or lessen the severity of disease. As previously discussed, many diseases of adulthood, such as diabetes and obesity, are a result of gene–gene and gene–environment interactions. Knowing that an individual is susceptible to disease potentially provides motivation for lifestyle changes. In addition, genetic testing provides an opportunity for counseling and health promotion activities that reduce at-risk behaviors. However, for these things to occur, nurses and patients must be knowledgeable and informed so that they communicate effectively with each other and engage in discussion about the identification, monitoring, and treatment of disease using emerging genetic techniques. Refer to the Research Opportunities and Clinical Impact box (p. 210) for research ideas in the area of genetics.

RESEARCH OPPORTUNITIES AND CLINICAL IMPACT RELATED TO GENETICS

Physiological Research

- Translational research to integrate basic science and clinical research
- Pharmacogenomic research to investigate biologic pathways influencing drug metabolism
- Quantifying gene activity and subsequent protein formation in genetic disorders
- Developing animal models to investigate the interaction of genetic and environmental factors on complex disorders

Clinical Impact

- Emerging technologies and treatments would be incorporated into clinical care more rapidly.
- Medications would be individualized based on genotype, and dosage calculated based on genotypic response rather than weight and height.
- Innovative assessment and monitoring methods and treatment therapies would emerge.
- Hypotheses related to biologic pathways in complex disorders would be tested in the animal models and moved more rapidly into human testing.

Psychosocial, Ethical, and Legal Research

- Access and barriers to genetic services
- The public and policy makers use information about a genetic disorder or predisposition to a genetic disorder
- Perceptions of genetics, genetic testing, and the use of genomics by individuals and groups from varied cultural and religious backgrounds
- Strategies for providing information about the risk for complex disorders
- Patient, family, and professional communication about a genetic disorder or predisposition for a genetic disorder

Clinical Impact

- New challenges may be addressing factors such as education, economics, health care resources, values, and beliefs that facilitate or impede access to genetic services.
- Ensure policies are developed and followed that protect patients from stigmatization and discrimination.
- Awareness of the patient perceptions is essential for planning and developing appropriate nursing care with patients and their families.
- Patients should be educated about the risk for complex disorders and recommended behavior or lifestyle changes.
- Patients and their family members should be provided with up-to-date information by appropriately trained professionals to facilitate patient and family communication with themselves and others.

Nursing Management

The nursing management tips in this section were derived from the *Genetics/Genomics Nursing: Scope and Standards of Practice* (International Society of Nurses in Genetics, 2007) and the *Essential Nursing Competencies and Curricula Guidelines for Genetics and Genomics* (Consensus Panel on Genetic/Genomic Nursing Competencies, 2006). The nurse assesses the patient at risk for a genetic disorder and uses assessment data to identify diagnoses and expected outcomes. The nurse then develops interventions to achieve expected outcomes, implements interventions, and evaluates the progress made toward those outcomes. Collaboration among the nurse, patient, family, and health care providers is critical during all phases of the nursing process.

Assessment

The nurse assesses the patient and family at risk for or affected by a genetic disorder to identify risk factors and determine the patient's and family's needs for information, referral, and genetics-related services and interventions. In addition to the routine physical examination and laboratory testing, a physical examination for dysmorphology and genetic laboratory testing may be indicated. The expectations of the patient and family must be taken into consideration. These may include their cultural views, values, and beliefs; environmental risk factors; and the patient's health history. The family history is a critical element in the assessment, which can be organized in a pedigree format that includes at least three generations.

Nursing Diagnosis

The nurse analyzes data collected to identify the nursing diagnoses related to the actual or potential genetic disorder and the patient's and family's responses. Careful attention is given to the patient's knowledge of the risks for and associated with a genetic disorder; the ethical, legal, and social implications of the disorder; and the patient's decisions about managing the genetic disorder. Asking patients to communicate back to the nurse their understanding of a genetic disorder and its implications for the patient and family members can reveal gaps in knowledge, fear of the disorder, and misconceptions about the disorder.

Planning

The nurse and patient work together to develop a plan of care that may include family members, genetic nurses, genetic counselors, geneticists, other specialists, and special laboratories. Clarifying the patient's understanding of the genetic disorder can help ensure that decisions being made for treatment are made with a full understanding of the treatment and related consequences. For example, when genetic testing is pursued, results of the tests can have implications not only for the patient but also for family members.

Interventions

Implementation of interventions may include identifying those persons who have or are at risk for inheriting or transmitting genetic disorders; promoting healthy lifestyles through health teaching; coordinating services to ensure continuity of health care; promoting and maintaining the patient's health; using counseling interventions to assist patients and their family members in adjusting to and using genetic information; and using knowledge of genetic therapeutics to improve the patient's health or prevent health problems and disability.

The ability to effectively carry out interventions is directly related to a nurse's genetic and genomic knowledge. Therefore, the nurse must have current and accurate information and knowledge of resources, services, technologies, and therapeutic interventions for broad and specific genetic disorders.

The nurse considers ethical, legal, cultural, religious, and societal issues surrounding genetic and genomic information and technologies and works to define the issues that undermine the rights of each patient to make an informed decision and voluntarily take action based on that decision. The nurse refers patients as needed for routine and specialized services.

Discussion of the pedigree can lead to mutual identification of the patient's educational needs and opportunities for the nurse to share information about factors that place the patient at increased risk for genetic disorders and risk factors that are associated with the genetic disorder. The nurse considers personal and environmental risk factors, interprets information, and identifies services that are available to each patient. Genetic and genomic risk factors are incorporated into the patient's plan of care and interventions are developed with each patient to improve the patient's outcomes. The plan of care may require collaboration with other health care providers and collaboration with insurance providers/payers to facilitate reimbursement for genetic and genomic health care services.

Advanced practice nurses (APNs) use counseling interventions to promote patients' and families' understandings of the genetic disorder and promote their adjustment to the disorder. APNs who provide genetic counseling services discuss the risk for a genetic disorder, results of genetic testing, and options for genetic therapy when this is feasible. The APN may be the case manager for the patient and provide consultations to the patient and family, other nurses, and other health care providers to ensure that proper care is provided to patients and their families.

Evaluation

The nurse carefully evaluates the impact and effectiveness of genetic and genomic technology, information, interventions, and treatments on the patient's outcomes and reassesses and revises the plan of care as changes occur.

The nurse uses current genetic and genomic information to promote the patient's health, educate the patient and family, prevent illness and injury, and promote informed decision making. The patient and family who understand a genetic disorder can make better use of genetic technology and services and more actively participate in maintaining and promoting their own health. Nurses should continue to increase their knowledge and integrate research findings into practice to assure the patient and family will benefit from advances in genetics and genomics. The nurse should develop a caring relationship with the patient and family that will take into account ethical, legal, and social issues associated with the genetic disorder (International Society of Nurses in Genetics, 2007).

NCLEX® REVIEW

1. Which information best demonstrates a benefit of genetics in health care and nursing?
    1. The information gained through genetic testing can often help individuals diagnosed with the sickle cell trait to find health insurance more easily.
    2. The nurse will be able to counsel parents who are each carriers of phenylketonuria that their children have a 50% chance of being affected.
    3. After a patient has a confirmed diagnosis of Turner syndrome the nurse would be able to explain to the parents about the trisomy cause.
    4. Patients who know they are heterozygous for coronary artery disease can initiate medications and lifestyle changes to help lower cholesterol.

2. A patient asks how chromosomal abnormalities occur. The most appropriate response by the nurse would be:
    1. "With approximately 25,000 genes per chromosome things statistically go wrong."
    2. "There is always either an abundance or deficiency of genes within the chromosome."
    3. "The combination of variation in genes and environmental factors leads to changes."
    4. "There is a hereditary alteration within the DNA sequence of an individual gene."

3. Which of the following statements by the student nurse would indicate the need for further instruction regarding the human genome?
    1. "The primary function of introns is to code for proteins using transcription and translation."
    2. "When genes upregulate the mRNA, their expression also increases and forms more proteins."
    3. "A codon specifies for a single amino acid that will eventually aid in production of protein."
    4. "The alignment of purines and pyrimidines forms polynucleotide chains that form a double helix."

4. Mutations and polymorphisms within the human genome can result in a multitude of disorders. The nurse understands that an example of a condition resultant from a mutant gene located on an autosome, received from parents heterozygous for the mutation and where two mutant copies are required for expression is:
   1. Marfan syndrome.
   2. Cystic fibrosis.
   3. Colorblindness.
   4. Leigh disease.

5. When planning the care of a patient, the nurse understands the importance of obtaining the information contained in a pedigree. Which of the following statements best describes the rationale for utilizing this tool during the planning phase?
   1. To help determine if unaffected or healthy individuals are carriers of disease-causing genes
   2. To locate the genotypic differences among maternal and paternal alleles caused by imprinting
   3. To assist in identifying disease risk and developing a customized prevention program for some conditions
   4. To recognize core genetic disorders that can be treated if found early in patients with increased risk

Answers for review questions appear in Appendix D

KEY TERMS

allele *p.194*
aneuploidy *p.199*
autosomal dominant inheritance *p.197*
autosomal recessive inheritance *p.197*
autosome *p.194*
centromere *p.194*
chromosomal disorder *p.198*
chromosome *p.193*
codon *p.195*
cytogenetics *p.194*
deletions *p.199*
deoxyribonucleic acid (DNA) *p.193*
diploid *p.195*
exon *p.195*
expressivity *p.202*
gamete *p.195*
gene *p.194*
gene therapy *p.206*
genetic variance *p.197*

genome *p.193*
genomic imprinting *p.198*
genomics *p.193*
genotype *p.196*
germ line cells *p.194*
haploid *p.195*
heterozygous *p.194*
homozygous *p.194*
human genome *p.195*
Human Genome Project (HGP) *p.193*
intron *p.195*
karyotype *p.194*
missense mutation *p.196*
monosomy *p.199*
mosaicism *p.199*
messenger ribonucleic acid (mRNA) *p.195*
mutation *p.196*
nondisjunction *p.199*
nonsense mutation *p.196*

pedigree *p.202*
penetrance *p.202*
pharmacogenetics *p.208*
pharmacogenomics *p.208*
phenotype *p.196*
point mutation *p.196*
polymorphism *p.196*
sex chromosome *p.194*
single-gene disorder *p.197*
telomere *p.194*
transcription *p.195*
translation *p.195*
translocation *p.199*
trisomy *p.199*
X-linked dominant *p.198*
X-linked recessive *p.198*
wild type *p.196*
zygote *p.198*

PEARSON
EXPLORE **mynursingkit**™

MyNursingKit is your one stop for online chapter review materials and resources. Prepare for success with additional NCLEX®-style practice questions, interactive assignments and activities, web links, animations and videos, and more!

Register your access code from the front of your book at
www.mynursingkit.com

REFERENCES

Alvarez, N. (2006). Neurology. In I. L. Rubin & A. C. Crocker (Eds.), *Medical care for children and adults with developmental disabilities* (2nd ed., pp. 249–255). Baltimore, MD: Paul H. Brookes.

American Cancer Society. (2008). *Cancer facts & figures 2008.* Atlanta, GA: Author.

American Diabetes Association. (2008). *All about diabetes.* Retrieved May 17, 2008, from http://www.diabetes.org/about-diabetes.jsp

American Medical Association. (2006, June 20). *Family history.* Retrieved November 2, 2006, from http://www.ama-assn.org/ama/pub/category/2380.html

American Nurses Association (2004). *Nursing: Scope and standards of practice.* Washington, DC: Author.

Bennett, R. L. Steinhaus, K. A. Uhrich, S. B., O'Sullivan, C. K., Resta, R. G., Lochner-Doyle, D., et at. (1995). Recommendations for standardized human pedigree nomenclature. Pedigree Standardization Task Force of the National Society of Genetic Counselors. *American Journal of Human Genetics, 56*(3), 745–752.

Bird, T. (1998, October 23). *Alzheimer disease overview.* Last updated February 2, 2005. Retrieved November 12, 2006, from http://www.geneclinics.org

Cashion, A. K., & Driscoll, C. J. (2004). Genetics and kidney dysfunction. *Nephrology Nursing Journal: Journal of the American Nephrology Nurses' Association, 31*(1), 14–18, 29.

Cashion, A. K., Driscoll, C. J., & Sabek, O. (2004). Emerging genetic technologies in clinical and research settings. *Biological Research for Nursing, 5*(3), 159–167.

Collins, F. S., Green, E. D., Guttmacher, A. E., & Guyer, M. S. (2003). A vision for the future of genomics research. *Nature, 422*(6934), 835–847.

Consensus Panel on Genetic/Genomic Nursing Competencies. (2006). *Essential nursing competencies and curricula guidelines for* genetics and genomics. Silver Spring, MD: American Nurses Association.

Cummings, D. E., & Schwartz, M. W. (2003). Genetics and pathophysiology of human obesity. *Annual Review of Medicine, 54,* 453–471.

Cummings, J. L., Vinters, H. V., Cole, G. M., & Khachaturian, Z. S. (1998). Alzheimer's disease: Etiologies, pathophysiology, cognitive reserve, and treatment opportunities. *Neurology, 51*(1, Suppl. 1), S2–S17; discussion, S65–S17.

Dean, L., & McEntyre, J. (2004). *The genetic landscape of diabetes.* Retrieved May 22, 2008, from http://www.ncbi.nlm.nih.gov/books/bv.fcgi?rid=diabetes

Fisher, N. L., & Lew, L. (1996). Culture of the countries of Southeast Asia. In N. L. Fisher (Ed.), *Cultural and ethnic diversity: A guide for genetics professionals* (pp. 113–128). Baltimore, MD: The Johns Hopkins Unviersity Press.

Francomano, C. A. (1996). Amish culture. In N. L. Fisher (Ed.), *Cultural and ethnic diversity: A guide for genetics professionals* (pp. 176–197). Baltimore, MD: The Johns Hopkins University Press.

Froguel, P., & Boutin, P. (2001). Genetics of pathways regulating body weight in the development of obesity in humans. *Experimental Biology and Medicine, 226*(11), 991–996.

Greb, A. (1998). Multiculturalism and the practice of genetic counseling. In D. L. Baker, J. L. Schuette, & W. R. Uhlmann (Eds.), *A guide to genetic counseling* (pp. 171–198). New York: Wiley-Liss.

Greenstein, M. A., & Bernstein, B. A. (1996). Jewish culture in North America. In N. L. Fisher (Ed.), *Cultural and ethnic diversity: A guide for genetics professionals* (pp. 198–219). Baltimore, MD: The Johns Hopkins University Press.

Hartl, D. L., & Jones, E. W. (2004). *Genetics: Analysis of genes and genomes* (6th ed.). Sudbury, MA: Jones and Bartlett.

Hauck, L., & Knoki-Wilson, U. M. (1996). Culture of Native Americans of the Southwest. In N. L. Fisher (Ed.), *Cultural and ethnic diversity: A guide for genetics professionals* (pp. 60–87). Baltimore, MD: The Johns Hopkins University Press.

Hill, J. O., & Peters, J. C. (1998). Environmental contributions to the obesity epidemic. *Science, 280*(5368), 1371–1374.

Hodgson, J., & Marshall, A. (1998). Pharmacogenomics: Will the regulators approve? *Nature Biotechnology, 16,* 243–246.

Human Genome Program. (2006). *Human Genome Project information: Pharmacogenomics.* Retrieved November 12, 2006, from http:// www.ornl.gov/sci/techresources/Human_Genome/medicine/ pharma.shtml

Ingelman-Sundberg, M. (2004). Pharmacogenetics of cytochrome P450 and its applications in drug therapy: The past, present and future. *TRENDS in Pharmacological Sciences, 25,* 193–200.

International Human Genome Sequencing Consortium. (2004). Finishing the euchromatic sequence of the human genome. *Nature, 431,* 931–945.

International Society of Nurses in Genetics and the American Nurses Association. (2007). *Genetics/genomics nursing: Scope and standards of practice.* Silver Spring, MD: American Nurses Association.

Israel, J., Cunningham, M., Thumann, H., & Arnos, K. S. (1996). Deaf culture. In N. L. Fisher (Ed.), *Cultural and ethnic diversity: A guide for genetics professionals* (pp. 220–239). Baltimore, MD: The Johns Hopkins University Press.

Jung, J. H. (1996). Traditional Chinese culture. In N. L. Fisher (Ed.), *Cultural and ethnic diversity: A guide for genetics professionals* (pp. 86–97). Baltimore, MD: The Johns Hopkins University Press.

Kaye, C. I., & Committee on Genetics. (2006). Introduction to newborn screening fact sheets. *Pediatrics, 118,* 1304–1312.

Klug, W. S., Cummings, M. R., & Spencer, C. (2005). *Concepts of genetics and student companion website access card package* (8th ed.). Upper Saddle River, NJ: Pearson Prentice-Hall.

Lewin, B. (2000). *Genes VII.* New York: Oxford University Press.

Loescher, L. J., & Merkle, C. J. (2005). The interface of genomic technologies and nursing. *Journal of Nursing Scholarship, 37,* 111–119.

Lopez-Rangel, E. (1996). Latino culture. In N. L. Fisher (Ed.), *Cultural and ethnic diversity: A guide for genetics professionals* (pp. 19–35). Baltimore, MD: The Johns Hopkins Unversity Press.

McKusick, V. A. (1998). *Mendelian inheritance in man.* Baltimore, MD: The Johns Hopkins University Press.

National Cancer Institute. (2004, September 16). *Elements of cancer genetics risk assessment and counseling.* Last updated October 3, 2006. Retrieved November 12, 2006, from http://www.nci.nih.gov/ cancertopics/pdq/genetics/risk-assessment-and-counseling

National Coalition for Health Professional Education in Genetics. (2000). *Core competencies in genetics essential for all health care professionals,* Retrieved November 12, 2006, from http://www. nchpeg.org

National Human Genome Research Institute. (2006). *ELSI planning and evaluation history.* Retrieved November 2, 2006, from http://www. genome.gov/10001754

National Institutes of Health. (2006). *Sickle cell anemia.* Retrieved February 12, 2006, from http://www.nhlbi.nih.gov/health/dci/ Diseases/Sca/SCA_WhoIsAtRisk.html

Nussbaum, R. L., McInnes, R. R., & Willard, H. F. (2004). *Thompson & Thompson genetics in medicine* (6th ed.). Philadelphia: W. B. Saunders.

Patil, S. R., & Fisher, N. L. (1996). Traditional Asian Indian culture. In N. L. Fisher (Ed.), *Cultural and ethnic diversity: A guide for genetics professionals* (pp. 142–155). Baltimore, MD: The Johns Hopkins University Press.

Prader-Willi Syndrome Association. (2008). *Research on Prader-Willi syndrome.* Retrieved March 26, 2008, from http://www.pwsausa. org/research/index.htm

Rettie, A. E., & Tai, G. (2006). The pharmacogenomics of warfarin. *Molecular Interventions, 6,* 223–227.

Rimoin, D. L., Connor, J. M., Pyeritz, R. E., & Korf, B. R. (2002). Nature and frequency of genetic disease. In D. L. Rimoin, J. M. Connor, R. E. Pyeritz, & B. R. Korf (Eds.), *Emery and Rimoin's principles and practice of medical genetics* (4th ed., pp. 55–59). Edinburgh: Churchill Livingstone.

Strazar, M. D., & Fisher, N. L. (1996). Traditional Japanese culture. In N. L. Fisher (Ed.), *Cultural and ethnic diversity: A guide for genetics professionals* (pp. 98–112). Baltimore, MD: The Johns Hopkins University Press.

Telfair, J., & Nash, K. B. (1996). African American culture. In N. L. Fisher (Ed.), *Cultural and ethnic diversity: A guide for genetics professionals* (pp. 36–59). Baltimore, MD: The Johns Hopkins University Press.

University of Washington. (2006, November 2). *Gene tests.* Retrieved November 2, 2006, from http://www.genetests.org

Venter, J. C., Adams, M. D., Myers, E. W., Li, P. W., Mural, R. J., Sutton, G. G., et al. (2001). The sequence of the human genome. *Science, 291*(5507), 1304–1351.

Watson, J. D., & Crick, F. H. (1953). Molecular structure of nucleic acids; a structure for deoxyribose nucleic acid. *Nature, 171*(4356), 737–738.

Stress and Adaptation

Annita Watson

Outcome-Based Learning Objectives

After studying this chapter, the learner will be able to:

1. Differentiate between internal and external stressors, and provide examples of each.
2. Differentiate between theories of stress as a response, a stimulus, and a transaction.
3. Explain the physiological components of the general adaptation syndrome (GAS).
4. Explain the relationship of oxidative stress to the disease process.
5. Explain ways in which a maladaptive response to stress can increase the risk of illness and cause disease.
6. Describe nursing assessment criteria for patients experiencing stress.
7. Explain the nursing management of patients with physiological stress.

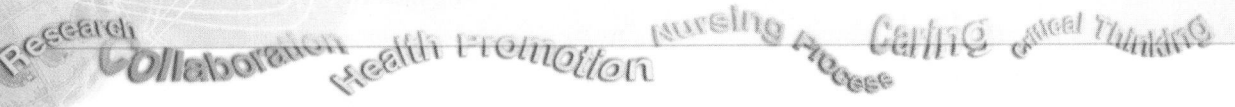

Stress, a universal phenomenon, is considered to be a condition in which people respond physiologically, psychologically, and socially to life changes. These changes may be thought of as a family of related experiences, pathways, responses, and outcomes caused by a range of different events or circumstances, with different people experiencing different aspects and identifying with different definitions of stress (Manktelow, 2003). Keeping in mind that not all stress reactions are negative, the term *stress* also is used to describe a variety of feelings and reactions that accompany actual and perceived threatening or challenging situations. A certain amount of stress is actually necessary for survival. Given the various interpretations of stress, Manktelow concluded that the most commonly accepted definition of stress is that it is a condition or feeling experienced when a person perceives that demands exceed the personal and social resources the individual is able to mobilize, while recognizing that there is an intertwined instinctive stress response to unexpected events. The internal stress response is based, therefore, partly on instinct and partly on the way one thinks.

When an individual experiences an actual or perceived threat or challenge, a physiological stress response occurs. These responses are triggered when the ordinary capacity to adapt to life's demands is strained or taxed. This stress reaction maximizes the expenditure of energy, which helps prepare the body to meet the threatening or challenging situation. The individual tends to mobilize a great deal of effort in order to deal with the event, thereby engaging both the sympathetic/adrenal and pituitary/adrenal systems to aid with the response (Bernard & Krupat, 1994). Within that context stress is viewed as a subset of the concept of adaptation, or the processes of maintaining psychobiological equilibrium during interaction with the environment.

Although a certain amount of stress is necessary for survival, prolonged stress can affect health adversely. Because stress and adaptation are interactive processes by which people respond to daily stimuli, it is important for nurses to understand the concept of stress, its effects on the total person, and how individuals respond to these phenomena.

Stress, Adaptation, and Coping

The human stress response can be viewed from several levels: the sociocultural level, the individual's psychological response (which affects the way the person presents to a health care provider), the biochemical response of the brain and central nervous system, the resulting endochronological response, and the response at the level of the human immune system and, perhaps, concomitantly at the tissue level (Haddy & Clover, 2001). Stress also can be viewed as a sequence of events that begins with a stimulus (**stressor**), which is recognized by the brain (**stress perception**), and that results in the activation of physiological fight/flight/fright systems within the body (**stress response**).

The desired outcome of stress is adaptation. **Adaptation** refers to the reaction to stress that signifies that the person is able to cope with the stressor or change. **Coping** is a compensatory process with physiological and psychological components that allows the individual to adapt to the stressor. From a functional standpoint, stressful conditions are factors that disrupt behavioral organization; distressing feelings are signals that disruption has occurred; and coping responses are efforts to restore behavioral organization and coherence (Van Egeren, 2000).

Coping is adaptive when it involves a realistic evaluation of the situation and determination of what can be done to minimize the impact of the stressor. To be adaptive, one also must deal with the emotional aspects of the situation, and develop emotional tolerance for negative life events, maintaining self-esteem, and keeping emotions in balance. Adaptive coping seeks to preserve important relationships during stressful situations. **Maladaptive coping mechanisms** are those responses to stress that are not effective. These responses generally are chronic, recurrent responses or patterns of response over time that do not promote the goals of adaptation.

The goals of adaptation are somatic or physical health; psychological health, or having a sense of well-being; and enhanced social functioning, which includes work, social life, and positive family relationships. Maladaptive coping responses frequently are cited as precursors to disease. This chapter explores the concepts of stress, adaptation, and coping as they impact the health and well-being of individuals.

Classifications of Stressors

Stress can be caused by internal or external sources (stressors) and can produce adaptive (positive) responses or maladaptive (negative) responses. The defense mechanisms of the body determine the degree to which the responses are healthy and positive or disease provoking and maladaptive. Stress also can be classified as acute or chronic, the variable being the length of time that the individual experiences stress and responds to the stressor. The third mode of classifying stress is according to the type of human response stimulated by the stressor: physical, physiological, and psychosocial. Within this mode stressors are precipitated according to developmental stages and are considered situational.

Internal and External Stressors

Internal stressors originate within a person. They include lifestyle choices, such as the use of caffeine; an overloaded schedule; negative self-talk, such as self-criticism and overanalyzing; mind traps, for example, unrealistic expectations, taking things personally, all-or-nothing thinking, exaggerating, and rigid thinking; and stressful personality traits, for example, being a perfectionist, workaholic, or pleaser. Internal stressors are precipitated by physiological or psychological stimuli, for example, cancer, stroke, depression, and anxiety, occurring within the individual.

External stressors originate outside the body and are precipitated by changes in the external environment. They can be triggered by the actual physical environment, for example, by noise, bright lights, heat, or confined spaces; the social environment, for example, by rudeness, bossiness, or aggressiveness on the part of someone else; the organizational environment, for ex-

ample, rules, regulations, deadlines, and red tape; major life events, such as the birth of a baby or the sudden death of a parent; and by trauma, such as that experienced with severe burns, a motor vehicle crash, or other catastrophic events such as hurricanes, floods, and fires. Daily hassles, such as commuting long distances, misplacing keys, and experiencing mechanical breakdowns, also act as external stressors.

Acute Versus Chronic Stressors

Acute stressors are brief and involve a tangible threat that is readily identified as a stress, whereas chronic stressors have a longer duration and are not readily identified as stressors because they are often ambiguous and intangible. Chronic stressors have become such a part of modern life that they may be taken for granted and can, therefore, pose a serious health risk if they are not recognized and properly managed. Dienstbier (1989) described this phenomenon as physiological toughening. He focused on the concept that stressors vary in their duration and are intermittent in nature, alternating between periods of stress and calm. If an intermittent stressor is viewed as a challenge, it may improve one's physiological resistance to stress by causing repeated, periodic increases in sympathetic arousal, which conditions the body to better withstand subsequent stressors. Emergencies are, therefore, transformed into routine situations, decreasing the intensity of the stressful situation (Mandler, 1982).

Human Response Stressors: Developmental and Situational

Sometimes stressors are classified according to the type of human response they generate: physical, physiological, or behavioral. More often they are considered within the domains of developmental and situational, with stress developing within certain time frames of one's life and according to situations occurring in one's life.

Developmental stressors predictably occur at various points of development throughout the life span. Chart 12–1 (p. 216) depicts stressors associated with developmental stages. **Situational stressors** are precipitated by various situations; examples include illness, a new job, or the death of a child. They are unpredictable, may occur at any time during life, and, again, they may be positive or negative. The effects of the situational stressor may depend on the developmental stage of the individual experiencing the stress.

Coping

Despite the different modes by which sources of stress (stressors) are defined and classified, it is clear that stress provokes a change in the person's homeostatic or balanced state of being. Adaptive mechanisms promote adjustment to these changes, in the form of coping, in order to return the individual to a steady, or balanced, state so that the individual has the energy and resources to meet new demands.

As mentioned earlier, coping is a compensatory process with both physiological and psychological components. It has been defined by Lazarus and Folkman (1984) as constant cognitive and behavioral efforts to manage specific internal and external demands that are appraised as taxing or exceeding the resources of the person. The interpretation and treatment of stress-related

CHART 12–1	Selected Stressors Associated with Developmental Stages
Developmental Stage	**Stressors**
Child	Beginning school
	Establishing peer relationships
	Coping with peer competition
Adolescent	Accepting changing physique
	Developing relationships involving sexual attraction
	Achieving independence
	Choosing a career
Young adult	Getting married
	Leaving home
	Managing a home
	Getting started in an occupation
	Continuing one's education
	Rearing children
Middle adult	Accepting the physical changes of aging
	Maintaining social status and standard of living
	Helping teenage children to become independent
	Adjusting to aging parents
Older adult	Accepting decreasing physical abilities and health
	Accepting changes in residence
	Adjusting to retirement and reduced income
	Adjusting to death of spouse and friends

situations, both adaptive and maladaptive, are contingent on proposed stress theories. Stress theory and the concepts of stress, adaptation, and coping are explored further in this chapter as they relate to an individual's health status and to nurses' management of patients' stress in health promotion, disease prevention, and treatment via the nursing process.

Historical Development of Stress Theories

Stress theory emerged in 1865 when the French physiologist Claude Bernard developed the concept of "constancy in the internal milieu." He defined the internal milieu as the fluid that bathed the cells, and constancy was the balanced internal state maintained by physiological and biochemical processes. Bernard's principle implied a static or fixed process.

Bernard's concept was expanded on by Walter Cannon (1932) when he developed the concept of *homestasy*, physiological equilibrium or homeostasis. Cannon established the existence of the well-known "fight-or-flight" response. He also is credited with determining that the stability of the body's internal environment is coordinated by compensatory processes that respond to changes in the internal environment, thereby causing a compensatory response to minimize the change. These compensatory responses are biologic and seek physiological and chemical balance within the internal milieu. They include blood

oxygen and carbon dioxide levels, blood pressure, body temperature, blood glucose, and fluid and electrolyte balance.

Homeostasis as defined by Cannon (1932) is one of the most typical properties of highly complex open systems, such as the human body or a cell or a large organization. The structure and functions of open systems are maintained by a multiplicity of dynamic equilibriums controlled by interdependent regulation mechanisms. Open systems react to every change in the environment, or to every random disturbance, through a series of modifications of equal size and opposite direction to those that created the disturbance. The goal of these modifications is to maintain the internal balances, or to maintain homeostasis.

Dr. Hans Selye (1936), known as the father of stress theory (Gabriel, 1997), took a different approach from Cannon. Starting with the observation that many different diseases and injuries to the body seemed to cause the same symptoms in patients, he identified a general response with which the body reacts to a major stimulus, the general adaptation syndrome (GAS). While the fight-or-flight response, as identified by Cannon, works in the very short term, the GAS operates in response to longer term exposure to causes of stress.

Selye also recognized the paradox that the physiological systems activated by stress not only can protect and restore, but can damage the body. He applied his theory of stress to the "everyday stress of life" and defined a "code of behavior" to help avoid negative stress and keep an acceptable and necessary level of positive stress. Although Cannon had earlier introduced the term *stress* to medicine, it was Selye who popularized it.

In 1965, Rene Dubos provided further insight into the dynamic nature of the body's internal environment with his theory that two complementary concepts, homeostasis and adaptation, were necessary for homeostatic balance. Dubos noted that homeostatic processes occurred quickly in response to stress, making the necessary adjustments rapidly in order to maintain the internal environment. Dubos, consistent with the concepts set forth by Selye, concluded that acceptable ranges of response to stimuli existed, and these levels of acceptability varied from individual to individual. He concluded that homeostasis and adaptation are both necessary for survival in a changing world.

Contemporary Interpretations of Stress

Current theories typically portray stress in one of three ways: (1) as a stimulus, (2) as a response, and (3) as a transaction or process. As a stimulus, stress typically is generated from three sources: catastrophic events, major life events, and chronic circumstances. As a response, stress refers to how somebody responds to a particular stressor, of which there are two components, physiological and psychological. As a transaction or process, stress is an outcome of a series of interactions and adjustments between the person and the environment. Within the transaction, the person suffering stress is viewed as an active agent who can influence the impact of a stressor through behavioral, cognitive, and emotional strategies.

These three views of stress are complementary in nature and provide the framework in which stress is studied, diagnosed, and, when appropriate, treated. Nurses use these theories to identify the stressor in a particular situation and to predict the individual's responses. They can then use this knowledge to assist patients in strengthening health and coping responses and in adjusting unhealthy, unproductive responses.

Stress as a Response: The General Adaptation Syndrome

As noted earlier, stress as a response was introduced by Selye (1936) in the early 1900s. He is credited with developing the physiologically based theory of stress and adaptation. Selye's theory predicts that stressors from different sources produce a similar physical response pattern. He called these physical responses to stress the **general adaptation syndrome (GAS).** The GAS is composed of three stages: alarm, resistance, and exhaustion. Stressors also are likely to result in a local response called the **local adaptation syndrome (LAS),** which proceeds through the same three stages as the GAS.

Because stress is a state of the body, it can only be observed by noting the changes it produces in the body. This response of the body, the GAS, occurs with the release of certain adaptive hormones and subsequent changes in the structure and chemical composition of the body. Once the stressor or stimulus is integrated into the central nervous system (CNS), multiple responses occur because of activation of the hypothalamic–pituitary–adrenal axis and the autonomic nervous systems. It is necessary to understand these responses in the nervous, endocrine, and immune systems in order to understand the physiological and behavioral changes that occur in an individual experiencing stress.

Body organs affected by stress are the gastrointestinal tract, the adrenal glands, and the lymphatic structures. With prolonged stress, the adrenal glands enlarge considerably; the lymphatic structures, such as the thymus, spleen, and lymph nodes, atrophy; and deep rugae appear in the lining of the stomach. Also, as mentioned, the body can react locally, that is, one organ or part of the body reacts alone. An example of the LAS is inflammation. Figure 12–1 ■ depicts these three stages of adaptation to stress.

Selye also addressed the importance of conditioning factors that may affect the stress response. He coined the term **eustress** to refer to stress associated with positive events such as winning a race or a tennis match. The health consequences of eustress were never fully explained, but the concept is similar to that discussed under the "uplifts" concept proposed by Lazarus when he described stress as a stimulus (see the Hassles and Uplifts section later in this chapter).

Alarm Stage

The first stage of the stress response is the alarm reaction of the GAS, in which the individual experiences a stressor physically or mentally, and the fight-or-flight response is initiated. When the stressor is of sufficient intensity to threaten the steady state of the individual, a reallocation of energy is required so that adaptation can occur. This temporarily decreases an individual's resistance and may even result in disease or death if the stress is

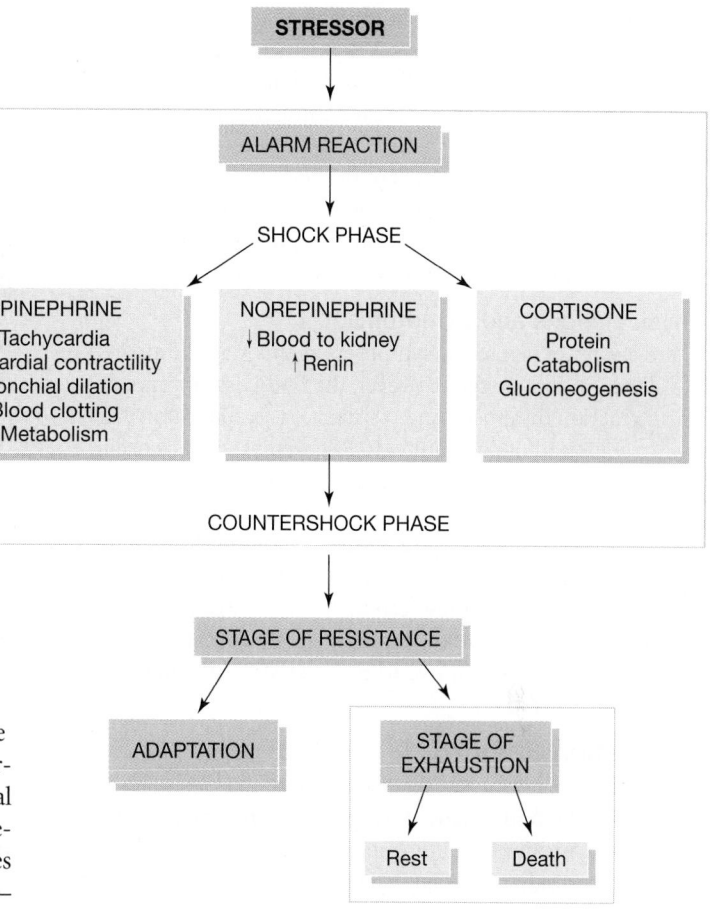

FIGURE 12–1 ■ The three stages of Selye's adaptation to stress model.

prolonged and severe (as in the case of burns or extreme temperature changes). The body has a limited amount of energy available for adapting to a stressor in this acute stage.

The alarm stage can be divided into two parts: the shock phase and the countershock phase (see Figure 12–1 ■) (Selye, 1976). During the shock phase, the stressor may or may not be perceived by the person. The autonomic nervous system reacts, and large amounts of epinephrine (adrenaline) and cortisone are released into the body, accounting for the fight-or-flight syndrome. This primary response is short lived, lasting from 1 minute to 24 hours. During the countershock phase, the changes produced in the body during the shock phase are reversed. Thus, a person is best prepared to react during the shock phase of the alarm reaction.

Physical Signs and Symptoms

Physical signs and symptoms of the alarm reaction generally are those of the sympathetic nervous system stimulation. They include increased blood pressure, increased heart and respiratory rate, decreased gastrointestinal motility, pupil dilation, and increased perspiration. The patient also may complain of such symptoms as increased anxiety, nausea, fatigue, anorexia, and weight loss.

Resistance Stage

The resistance stage reflects the individual's adaptation to the stressor. Ideally the individual moves from the alarm stage to the resistance stage quickly so that physiological forces are used to increase the resistance to stress. At this time, adaptation may occur, involving mediation of the external and internal environments. Resistance is high at this time compared with the normal state. The body attempts to cope with the stressor and to limit the stressor to the smallest area of the body that can deal with it. The amount of resistance varies among individuals, depending on the level of physical functioning, coping abilities, and total number and intensity of stressors experienced.

Physical Signs and Symptoms

There are fewer signs and symptoms at this stage compared to the alarm or acute stage; however, the bodily symptoms of the alarm reaction disappear, and resistance rises above normal. For example, instead of continuing to lose weight, such as occurred in the alarm stage, the person returns to a "normal" weight. Throughout the resistance stage, the person is expanding energy in an attempt to adapt. This adaptive response is limited by the resources of the individual. When resources are adequate, the individual may successfully recover from a stressor such as surgery and return to a normal coping state. If adaptation does not occur, the person may move to the next stage of the GAS, the stage of exhaustion.

Exhaustion Stage

The stage of exhaustion is the final stage of the GAS. The adaptation that the body made during the second stage cannot be maintained, meaning that the means used to cope with the stressor have been exhausted. This stage occurs only if the stress becomes overwhelming or is not removed, or if the individual is ineffective in dealing with it. If adaptation has not overcome the stressor, the stress effects may either rest and return to normal, or death may be the ultimate consequence.

Physical Signs and Symptoms

Physical symptoms of the alarm reaction may reappear briefly as the body makes a final attempt to survive. This is exemplified by a terminally ill person whose vital signs become stronger just before death. The individual in the stage of exhaustion usually becomes ill and may die if assistance from outside sources is not available. Often this stage can be reversed by external sources of adaptive energy such as medication, blood transfusion, and/or psychotherapy. The end of this stage largely depends on the adaptive energy resources of the individual, the severity of the stressor, and the external adaptive resources that are provided.

Interruption Theory as a Response Theory

Mandler (1982) defined stress as an emergency that signals interruption, the basic premise being that autonomic activity results when some organized action or thought process is interrupted. The term *interruption* is used in the sense that any event, whether external or internal to the individual, prevents completion of some action, thought sequence, or plan, and is considered to be interrupted. Interruption can occur in the perceptual, cognitive, behavioral, or problem-solving domains. The consequences of the interruption will always be autonomic activity and will be interpreted emotionally in any number of ways, ranging from the most joyful to the most noxious.

Stress as a Stimulus

According to the stimulus-based theory of stress, stress is defined as a stimulus, a life event, or a set of circumstances that arouses physiological and/or psychological reactions that result in a disrupted response that may increase the individual's vulnerability to illness. Historically, this theory evolved from attempts to develop questionnaires to measure stress in terms of life changes or life events (Holmes & Masuda, 1966; Holmes & Rahe, 1967; Horowitz, Schaefer, Hiroto, Wilner, & Levin, 1977). Two such scales have been developed and are used as the classic foundation for development of this theory: the Social Readjustment Rating Scale (SRRS) and the Schedule of Recent Experiences (SRE). These scales were developed in an attempt to numerically weigh the impact (stress) of various life changes, for example, death of a spouse, divorce, trouble with the boss. In their classic work, *The Social Readjustment Rating Scale*, Holmes and Rahe, with reliability reestablished in 1977 by Horowitz and colleagues, assigned a numerical value to 43 life changes or events. The SRRS is used to document a person's relatively recent experiences. In this view, both positive and negative events are considered stressful.

The Holms and Rahe scale was assigned numerical values by volunteers according to the amount of adjustment required by each event. The highest rated event on the scale was the death of a spouse. Other events were marriage, loss of a job, starting school, bankruptcy, and many others. These researchers placed the items in a questionnaire and scored each according to the rating they got from the first set of volunteers. They gave the questionnaire to people in an emergency room, both to the patients who were sick and to the people who accompanied them; then they compared the scores. The result astounded the world of psychology and medicine: sick people had experienced far more of these life events in the year prior to their illness than the healthy people who brought them to the hospital emergency room. The 43 items included in the Holmes and Rahe Social Readjustment Rating Scale, with assigned numerical values, is shown in Chart 12–2.

It was originally theorized that the greater the number of stressful life events occurring throughout a specific period of time, the greater the vulnerability to illness. Research has demonstrated a significant relationship between number and intensity of life events and the resulting probability of physical and emotional illness following the events (Holmes & Masuda, 1966). However, the relationships often are weak, and findings contrary to these studies also have been reported. Thus, methodological issues regarding additional factors (age, perception, health, previous experiences) must be taken into account when considering life events.

Note also that other factors influence an individual's response to life events. These include cultural influences, personality, clustering of events, biologic variables, socioeconomic status, timing, and interpersonal support systems. Outcomes are another important factor to consider. Disease outcomes often are confused with illness outcomes (total effect of the disease on an individual), leading to inconclusive results. These factors highlight the need to use a holistic approach when assessing the patient.

CHART 12–2 Holmes and Rahe Social Readjustment Rating Scale

LIFE EVENTS SCORE

1. Death of spouse 100
2. Divorce 73
3. Marital separation from mate 65
4. Detention in jail, other institution 63
5. Death of a close family member 63
6. Major personal injury or illness 53
7. Marriage 50
8. Fired from work 47
9. Marital reconciliation 45
10. Retirement 45
11. Major change in the health or behavior of a family member 44
12. Pregnancy 40
13. Sexual difficulties 39
14. Gaining a new family member (e.g., through birth, adoption, oldster moving, etc.) 39
15. Major business readjustment (e.g., merger, reorganization, bankruptcy) 39
16. Major change in financial status 38
17. Death of close friend 37
18. Change to different line of work 36
19. Major change in the number of arguments with spouse 35
20. Taking out a mortgage or loan for a major purchase 31
21. Foreclosure on a mortgage or loan 30
22. Major change in responsibilities at work 29
23. Son or daughter leaving home (e.g., marriage, attending college) 29
24. Trouble with in-laws 29
25. Outstanding personal achievement 28
26. Spouse beginning or ceasing to work outside the home 26
27. Beginning or ceasing formal schooling 26
28. Major change in living conditions 25
29. Revision of personal habits (dress, manners, associations, etc.) 24
30. Trouble with boss 23
31. Major change in working hours or conditions 20
32. Change in residence 20
33. Change to a new school 20
34. Major change in usual type and/or amount of recreation 19
35. Major change in church activities (a lot more or less than usual) 19
36. Major change in social activities (clubs, dancing, movies, visiting) 18
37. Taking out a mortgage or loan for a lesser purchase (e.g., for a car, TV, freezer) 17
38. Major change in sleeping habits 16
39. Major change in the number of family get-togethers 15
40. Major change in eating habits 15
41. Vacation 13
42. Christmas season 12
43. Minor violations of the law (e.g., traffic tickets) 11

SCORING

Less than 150 life change units = 30% chance of developing a stress-related illness

150–299 life change units = 50% chance of illness

More than 300 life change units = 80% chance of illness

Source: Reprinted from the *Journal of Psychomatic Research.* Holmes, T.H. and Rahe, R.H.: The social readjustment rating scale, 11:213–218, Copyright 1967, with permission from Elsevier.

Hardiness and Sense of Coherence

Research has demonstrated that some individuals who experience high scores in terms of changing life events do not experience illness. A mediating factor in this process, that may act as a predictor of illness is the condition termed **hardiness** (Kobasa, Maddi, & Zoda, 1983). The hardy person has (1) a clear sense of personal values and goals, (2) a strong tendency toward interaction with the environment, (3) a sense of meaningfulness, and (4) an internal rather than an external locus of control.

Sense of coherence (SOC) is a closely related concept to hardiness and has been defined and developed by Antonovsky (1987). SOC refers to how an individual sees the world and one's life in it. It is a personality characteristic or coping style rather than a response to a specific situation. The three components of SOC are comprehensibility, manageability, and meaningfulness. Comprehensibility means that stimuli derived from one's internal and external environments are structured, predictable, and explicable. Manageability implies that resources are available to meet the demands posed by these stimuli. Meaningfulness suggests that the demands are challenges worthy of investment and engagement. An individual with a strong SOC has an enduring tendency to see one's life as ordered, predictable, and manageable.

Stress as a Transaction

Transactional theories of stress are based on the work of Lazarus (1966). Lazarus purports that the stimulus and response theories do not consider individual differences. He asserts that neither theoretical approach explains which factors lead some people and not others to respond effectively, nor interprets why some people are able to adapt for longer periods of time than are others. Consequently, Lazarus focused on the person–environment transaction and the cognitive appraisals of demands and coping options (Lazarus & Folkman, 1984). In other words, the way in which a person appraises or interprets (cognition) his relationship with the environment (objects, persons, and situations in the surroundings) determines whether or not the individual perceives the situation as stressful (Lazarus & Folkman, 1984).

According to Lazarus (1966), psychological stress consists of the demands that tax or exceed available resources (internal and external) as perceived by the individual involved. Whether positive or negative (an opportunity for growth or gain versus a damaging or injurious situation), psychological stress does not reside exclusively in either the environment or the person. Instead, stress is generated from the transaction, the mutual influence that occurs between the person and the environment one interacts with during the course of an encounter. Thus, the emphasis is on the process, or dynamics, of what is happening in any given stressful event and how changes are occurring during the event. The transaction is not a static process, but a dynamic one.

Although Lazarus recognized that certain environmental demands and pressures produce stress in substantial numbers of people, he emphasized that people and groups differ in their sensitivity and vulnerability to certain types of events, as well as in their interpretations and reactions. Thus, the Lazarus model takes into account cognitive processes that intervene between the encounter and the reaction and the factors that affect the nature of this process. In contrast to Selye, who focused on physiological responses, Lazarus includes mental and psychological components or responses as part of the concept of stress. His theory encompasses a set of cognitive, affective, and adaptive (coping) responses that arise out of person–environment transactions.

Lazarus proposed that multitudes of internal and external data are received at the neurocognitive level, and that these data are interpreted during the process of cognitive appraisal. Appraisal is a judgment process that includes recognizing the degree of demands, or stressors, placed on the individual. This process also involves the recognition of available resources or options that help when dealing with potential or actual demands. The two major forms of cognitive appraisal are primary and secondary appraisals.

Primary Appraisal

Primary appraisal is the process of evaluating the significance of the transaction as it relates to a person's well-being. During the initial appraisal, a person seeks answers as to the meaning of the situation with regard to his well-being. One of three types of appraisals could be made: (1) It is irrelevant; (2) it is good, or benign-positive; or (3) it is stressful. If demands are appraised as stressful, they can be classified as representing harm or loss, threat, or challenge. Harm or loss demands involve actual damage, and threat demands involve anticipated harm or loss. Challenge demands differ from threat and harm or loss demands because they are viewed as a potential for personal gain or growth. The stress transaction also can be vivacious, such as empathizing with others who are in stress. Therefore, stress is a situation in which demands exceed the individual's adaptive resources. If an adaptive response to those demands does not occur, negative consequences will result (Lazarus & Launier, 1976).

Secondary Appraisal

Secondary appraisal is the process of evaluating the significance of the transaction between the person and her environment as it relates to available coping resources and options. Primary and secondary appraisals often occur simultaneously

and interact with each other in determining stress. They are equally important in the person's cognitive assessment of an event. Figure 12–2 ■ shows a diagram of stress as a transaction. A secondary appraisal can actually cause a primary appraisal. Secondary appraisals include feelings of not being able to deal with the problem.

Cognitive Reappraisal

In addition to primary and secondary appraisal, the act of reappraisal also occurs. **Cognitive reappraisal** develops from the feedback of changes in the person–environment relationship and from reflection about the coping process. Reappraisal allows for changes in the person's evaluation of the event, or a relabeling of the cognitive appraisal. Certain factors influence the labeling of appraisals. Situational factors include the intensity of the external demands, the immediacy of the expected impact, and ambiguity. Person-related factors include motivational characteristics, belief systems, and intellectual resources and skills.

The event may be reappraised and evaluated as nonstressful due to changes in the relationship between the person and the environment. For example, a hospitalization initially may be deemed stressful by the individual, based on primary and secondary appraisal. The event may be reappraised and evaluated as nonstressful, however, because of changes in the relationship between the person and the environment, such as a positive outcome of improved health from the hospitalization.

Hassles and Uplifts

Daily hassle scores have been found to be an important supplement to the life-events approach in predicting health and illness outcomes related to the impact of a stressor. Daily **hassles** are experiences and conditions of daily living that have been appraised as relevant and harmful or threatening to an individual's well-being (Lazarus & Folkman, 1984). The frequency and intensity of daily hassles have a stronger relationship with somatic

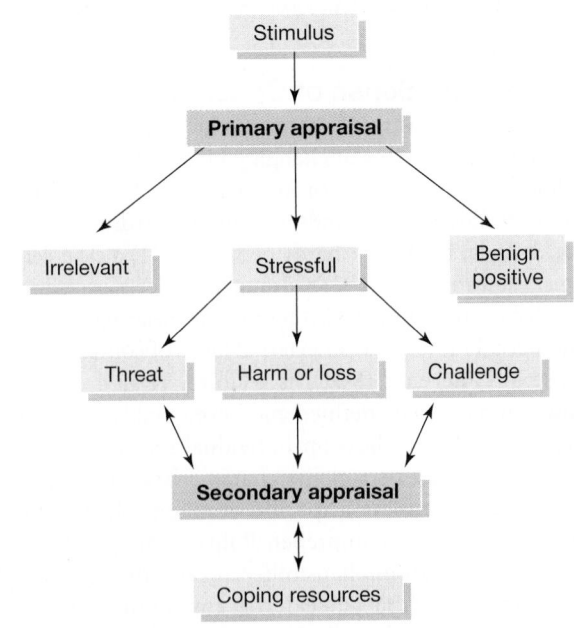

FIGURE 12–2 ■ Stress as a transaction.

illness than with the life-events scale (Lazarus & Folkman, 1984). Items shown on the daily hassles scale reflect work, family, social activities, environment, practical considerations, finances, and health (Lazarus & Folkman, 1984). Examples of daily hassles are shown in Chart 12–3.

Uplifts, the counterpart to hassles, are defined as positive experiences that are likely to occur in everyday life (Lazarus & Folkman, 1984). This concept seems comparable to the eustress described earlier by Selye. Little evaluation has been completed to determine the effects of positive experiences on health outcomes.

Factors That Lead to Stressful Appraisals

Personal factors that lead to stressful appraisals include intellectual, motivational, and personality characteristics. People who have high self-esteem are likely to believe that they have the resources to meet demands. Stressful events are seen as challenging rather than as threatening (Lazarus and Cohen, 1977). In regard to motivation, the more important the threatened goal is, the more stress the person is likely to perceive. Events that involve very strong demands and are imminent tend to be seen as stressful. Life transitions also can be stressful: starting school, moving a household, reaching puberty, starting or changing a career, becoming a parent, losing a spouse, and retiring.

Ambiguity, such as role and harm ambiguity, also can cause stress. Role ambiguity can occur in the workplace, for instance, when people are working without clear guidelines, no standards for performance, and no clear consequences. This is stressful because people are uncertain about what actions and decisions to make. Harm ambiguity occurs when people are not sure what to do to avoid harm. Stress depends on the person's personality, beliefs, and general experience (Lazarus & Folkman, 1984). A person who is seriously ill and does not have clear information might draw hope from this ambiguity, believing that he will get well. Another person in the same situation may believe that people are deliberately giving ambiguous information because the prognosis is poor.

The desirability and controllability of the situation also are important factors. Many of life's events, whether desirable or undesirable, can produce stress. Generally, undesirable events are more likely to be appraised as stressful. People also tend to appraise uncontrollable events as being more stressful than controllable events (Litt, 1988). There are two types of control: behavioral and cognitive. Behavioral control means performing some action, for example, taking a pain control tablet for a headache to make experiencing a headache less stressful. In the case of cognitive control, one can affect the impact of events by using some mental strategy, such as distraction, or by developing a plan to overcome the problem.

Cognition, Emotions, and Stress

A high level of stress impairs people's memory and attention during cognitive activities such as when taking examinations. Disturbing or worrying thoughts can perpetuate stress and make it chronic. Cognitive appraisal processes can influence both the stress and the emotional experience. For example, something that frightens one person, such as running into a black bear on a hike, may make another person feel excited. Fear is a common emotional reaction that can be classified into two categories: phobias and anxiety.

Phobias are intense and irrational fears that are associated with specific events and situations. An example of this would be claustrophobia, a fear of being enclosed in small rooms or crowded conditions. Anxiety is a vague feeling of uneasiness or apprehension. This may be typified by anticipation of impending doom caused by a relatively uncertain or unspecified threat. People may not be aware of situations that seem to arouse anxiety or to know how the "doom" will be manifested. Anxiety also may result from appraisals of low self-worth and the anticipation of a loss of self-esteem.

Another emotional reaction to stress is anger. This often occurs when the person perceives the situation as harmful or frustrating. When stress is accompanied by anger, negative social behaviors tend to increase. Stress-produced anger increases aggressive behavior, and these negative effects tend to continue after the stressful event is over (Helfer & Kempe, 1976). As an example, child abuse often is related to parental stress. Stress may also affect helping behavior. Those experiencing a high level of stress tend not to help others who are experiencing some stressful incident, whereas those experiencing a less stressful event may do so.

Theoretic Summary

Perception is the key to understanding and differentiating between the three major types of stress theories presented. In stress response theory, all demands are stressors with the capacity to elicit a physiological response. Individuals' conditioning factors influence the stress response. In the life-change theory, the perceived stressfulness of the event is not a consideration because all individuals receive the same score on the event scale for a certain stressor. In the transaction theory, the cognitive appraisal process determines whether the demands will be assessed as stressful. Through cognitive appraisal, individuals experience different outcomes in dealing with demands, not only because of conditioning factors, but also as a result of how the demand is perceived and labeled during the person–environment interaction. An event that is stressful to one individual is not necessarily stressful to another individual.

Despite the differentiation made in the types of stress theory, nurses should recognize that stress is ever present, is inevitable,

---

CHART 12–3	**Examples of Daily Hassles**

Concerns about job security

Problems with coworkers

Chronic pain

Difficulties with friends

Marital problems

Inadequate financial resources

Traffic to and from work

Caring for parents

Deadlines

Misplacing or losing things

House repairs

and is a familiar aspect of life as are the stressors that precipitate the stress response. The stressors may, however, originate from different sources, and for some may precipitate stress as a stimulant, whereas for others it becomes a burden. Thus, it is recognized that an integrated stress response consists of the fight-or-flight response, the general adaptation syndrome, and one's mental response to stress as separate mechanisms that fit together in one response.

Stress Research

Traditionally, stress research has been oriented toward studies involving the body's reaction to stressors (biophysiological perspective) and the cognitive processes and transactional processes that appraise the event or interaction/situation as a stressor. However, current social perspectives of the stress response have noted that different people experiencing similar life conditions are not necessarily affected in the same manner. There continues to be a growing interest in the epidemiology of disease thought to result from stress. It has been noted that the incidence of hypertension, cardiovascular ailments, and depression varies with such factors as race, sex, marital status, and income. This kind of socioeconomic variation for disease indicates that the stressors that presumably dispose people toward these illnesses are somehow linked to the conditions that people confront as they occupy their various positions and status in society.

The concept of stress, as recently defined, views the human in an interactive relationship with the environment, with an increasing awareness and emphasis on the social and cultural contexts involved in stress and coping. The biopsychosocial model of stress incorporates a variety of social factors that influence stress reaction and perception. Culture and society may shape what events are perceived as stressful and what coping strategies are acceptable to use in a particular society. As research progresses on a sociocultural perspective of stress, stress may be redefined to reflect both social and cultural differences. The definition of stress may then evolve to be that stress is a set of neurological and physiological reactions that serve an adaptive function in the environmental, social, and cultural values and structures upon which the individual acts. This concept also is used to form the basis for nursing theories that guide nursing practice.

Nursing Theories Based on Systems and Adaptation

Several nursing theories are based on the concepts of stress and adaptation, and are derived from systems theory. Notable among them are those theories credited to Florence Nightingale, Imogene King, Martha Rogers, Betty Neuman, and Sister Callista Roy:

- Florence Nightingale sought to improve nursing by improving the environment. Her *Notes on Nursing* emphasized that a clean environment, warmth, ventilation, and a quiet environment led to good health (Lobo, 2002; Nightingale, 1957).
- Imogene King developed a conceptual model for nursing in the mid-1960s with the idea that human beings are open systems interacting with their environment (Fawcett, 2005;

King, 1971). She based her framework on the premise that there are three interacting systems, with each system having its own distinct group of concepts and characteristics. These systems include personal, interpersonal, and social systems.

- In the 1970s Martha Rogers advanced the theory of the "science of unitary human beings," also known as Rogerian (Fawcett, 2005; Marriner-Tomey & Alligood, 2006; Rogers, 1970). Rogers' model identifies the individual as a unified whole in constant interaction with the environment. Rogers and her colleagues saw human beings as the central phenomenon of interest to nursing, and her model is designed to explain the nature of human beings (Malinski, 2006). In so doing Rogers drew on a vast array of subjects that formed the theoretical underpinning of her framework, including anthropology, astronomy, and mathematics. She focused on treating the whole patient—not just the illness—with the assumption that individuals achieve maximum well-being within their potential.
- Betty Neuman's health care systems model (2002) focuses on the person as a complete system, the subparts being interrelated physiological, psychological, sociocultural, spiritual, and developmental factors (Fawcett, 2005; Polit & Beck, 2008). She defines health as "expanding consciousness," or increasing complexity. The nurse's role is to recognize the person's unique pattern of life and to work within that pattern with the person to achieve the person's goals (George, 2002; Tomey & Alligood, 2005).
- In Sister Callista Roy's adaptation model, humans are purported to be adaptive systems that cope with change through adaptation. Nursing helps to promote client adaptation during health and illness (Fawcett, 2005; Roy, 1990). Both Selye and Lazarus influenced Roy's development of this model. Although the original model was developed in the early 1960s and 1970s, Roy redefined adaptation for the 21st century in 1990. In the latest version of her model, Roy included expanding the adaptive model to include relational persons as well as the individual person, and describing adaptation on three levels of integrated life processes, compensatory processes, and compromised processes (Fawcett, 2005; Roy & Andrews, 2005; Marrner-Tomey & Alligood, 2006).

Nursing theories, such as those just discussed, often form the framework for implementing the nursing process in service settings. Both Neuman and Roy have been used extensively in nursing practice and nursing education as a framework for defining nursing and implementing the nursing process (Parker, 2006).

Physiological Responses to Stress

Physiological responses to stress should be considered within the context of the body as an open living system with an internal and external environment, with information and matter being exchanged continuously between these two environments. Within the internal environment each organ, tissue, and cell is a system unto itself and a subsystem of the whole, with each system exchanging information and matter. Each subsystem also exchanges information and matter in an attempt to maintain a dynamic balance, or a **steady state**, even in the presence of change, so as to maintain harmony with each other; in other words, homeostasis.

When stress occurs that causes a body function to deviate from its stable range, processes are initiated to restore and maintain the dynamic balance. When these compensatory processes are not adequate, the steady state is threatened, function becomes disordered, and pathophysiological mechanisms occur. The pathophysiological mechanisms can lead to disease, thus, becoming a threat to the steady state. Disease is an abnormal variation in the structure or function of any part of the body that occurs within a living system when the sum of stressors acting on that living system exceeds the system's ability to adapt. It disrupts function and therefore limits the person's freedom of action. Because disease may be localized or generalized, it can affect part of the living system or the entire living system (Wilkin, 2005).

The physiological components involved in the stress response include the CNS, the hypothalamus, the sympathetic nervous system, the anterior and posterior pituitary glands, the adrenal medulla, and the adrenal cortex. The physiological components and their secretions (hormones and catecholamines) are responsible for the neuroendocrine response to stressors. The neuroendocrine response involves the nervous system, the endocrine system, and the immune system. Because these three systems are interrelated, the ultimate responses of the person to stress reflect the integration of the three systems. Figure 12–3 ■ depicts the physiological responses to stress.

Nervous System

The body responds physiologically to both actual and symbolic stressors. The hypothalamus participates in both the emotional and physical response to stressors. In addition to the hypothalamus, other parts of the CNS, including the cerebral cortex, limbic system, and reticular formation, are involved in the neural control of emotions and the physiological responses to stress. The functions of these structures are interrelated.

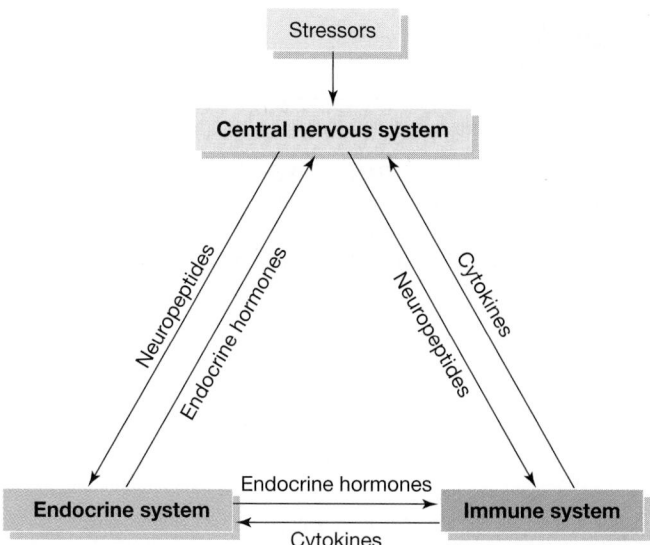

FIGURE 12–3 ■ Neurochemical links among the nervous, endocrine, and immune systems. The communication is bidirectional among the three systems.

Cerebral Cortex

Following an external event, afferent input is sent to the cerebral cortex via sensory impulses from the peripheral nervous system including the eyes and ears. Afferent impulses that travel to the cortex from the periphery via the spinal cord (spinothalamic pathways) also activate the reticular formation in the area of the brainstem. The reticular formation relays input to the thalamus and from the thalamus to the cerebral cortex. This network of neurons, which is involved with arousal and consciousness, is called the **reticular activating system (RAS)**. The RAS functions to maintain wakefulness and alertness.

The somatic, auditory, and visual associative areas of the cerebral cortex receive input from the peripheral sensory fibers, and then interpret them. The prefrontal area serves to reduce the speed of the associative functions so that the person has time to evaluate the information in light of past experiences and future consequences (primary and secondary appraisal) and to plan a course of action. All of these functions are involved in the perception of a stressor. The temporal lobes of the cerebral cortex contain the auditory association areas, which when stimulated produce the sensation of fear. Stimulation of the temporal lobes can result in sounds that seem louder or softer, visual displays that seem nearer or further, and experiences that seem familiar or strange. These effects modify the perception of stress.

Limbic System

The limbic system, lying in the inner midportion of the brain near the base, includes the septum, cingulated gyrus, amygdala hippocampus, and anterior nuclei of the thalamus. It is thought to be primarily responsible for emotions and behaviors. When stimulated, emotions, feelings, and behaviors can occur that ensure survival and self-preservation, such as feeding, sociality, and sexuality. Endorphins are found in structures of the limbic system and are known to reduce the perception of painful stimuli.

Reticular Formation

The reticular formation is located between the lower end of the brainstem and the thalamus. It contains the RAS, which sends impulses contributing to alertness to the limbic system and to the cerebral cortex and thalamus. The RAS also receives impulses from the hypothalamus. When stimulated the RAS increases its output of impulses, leading to wakefulness. Both physiological and perceived stress usually increase the degree of wakefulness.

Hypothalamus

The hypothalamus, which lies just above the pituitary gland, integrates autonomic nervous system mechanisms that maintain the chemical constancy of the internal environment of the body. Together with the limbic system, it regulates emotions and many visceral behaviors necessary for survival, such as eating, drinking, temperature control, reproduction, defense, and aggression. The hypothalamus receives information regarding traumatic stimuli via the spinothalamic pathway, pressure-sensitive input from the baroreceptors via the brainstem, and emotional stimuli via the limbic system.

Because the hypothalamus secretes peptide hormones and factors that regulate the release of hormones by the anterior pituitary, it is central to the connection between the nervous and endocrine systems in responding to stress. Additionally, the hypothalamus regulates the function of both the sympathetic and parasympathetic branches of the autonomic nervous system. Thus, when an individual perceives the presence of a stressor, the hypothalamus mediates both the neural and endocrine responses. It does this by activating the sympathetic nervous system and by releasing corticotropin-releasing hormone (CRH), which stimulates the pituitary to release adrenocorticotropic hormone (ACTH). In response to certain stress conditions, the parasympathetic nervous system is stimulated. This may be manifested as increased gastrointestinal motility, flushing, or bronchial constriction.

Sympathetic Nervous System Response

The sympathetic nervous system response is rapid and short lived, a response to acute stress. Norepinephrine is released at nerve endings that are in direct contact with the respective end organs to cause an increase in function of the vital organs and a state of general body arousal. Heart rate is increased and peripheral vasoconstriction occurs, raising the blood pressure. Blood also is shunted away from abdominal organs in order to provide better blood supply to the vital organs, brain, heart, and skeletal muscles. Blood glucose is increased, supplying a more readily available energy. Pupils are dilated, mental activity is increased, and a greater sense of awareness exists.

Constriction of the blood vessels of the skin limits bleeding in the event of trauma. The person is likely to experience cold feet, clammy skin and hands, chills, palpitations, and a knot in the stomach. Typically, the person appears tense, with the muscles of the neck, upper back, and shoulders tightened, and respirations may be rapid and shallow, with a tense diaphragm. Figure 12–4 ■ depicts the increased sympathetic activity present in a stress response.

Endocrine System

Once the hypothalamus is activated in response to stress, the endocrine system becomes involved. The sympathetic nervous system also stimulates the medulla of the adrenal gland to release the hormones epinephrine and norepinephrine (catecholamines) into the bloodstream. The effect of catecholamines and the sympathetic nervous system, including the adrenal medulla, is referred to as the sympathoadrenal response. These hormones prepare the body for the fight-or-flight response, which is depicted in Figure 12–4 ■. This response is activated by physical stressors such as hypovolemia and hypoxia and emotional states such as anger, excitement, and fear. Catecholamines can be measured in the blood and urine.

The Hypothalamic–Pituitary–Adrenal Response

The hypothalamus releases CHF, which stimulates the anterior pituitary to produce ACTH. ACTH, in turn, stimulates the adrenal cortex to produce glucocorticoids, primarily cortisol. Glucocorticoids, particularly cortisol, are essential for the stress response. Cortisol stimulates protein catabolism, releasing amino acids; stimulates liver uptake of amino acids and their conversion to glucose; and inhibits glucose uptake (antiinsulin action) by many body cells, but not those of the brain or heart. Cortisol also potentiates the action of catecholamines on blood vessels and inhibits the inflammatory response. These cortisol-induced metabolic effects provide the body with a ready source of energy during a stressful situation. These effects are important to consider in relation to people experiencing stress. Any patient who is under stress (perhaps caused by surgery, illness, trauma, or prolonged psychological stress) catabolizes body protein and needs supplements.

In addition to the catecholamines, epinephrine and norepinephrine, and cortisol, other hormones also are released. These are the antidiuretic hormone (ADH) from the posterior pituitary and aldosterone from the adrenal cortex. ADH promotes water reabsorption by the distal and collecting tubules of the kidneys, and aldosterone acts to increase sodium reabsorption in the kidney tubules. As a result, both ADH and aldosterone in-

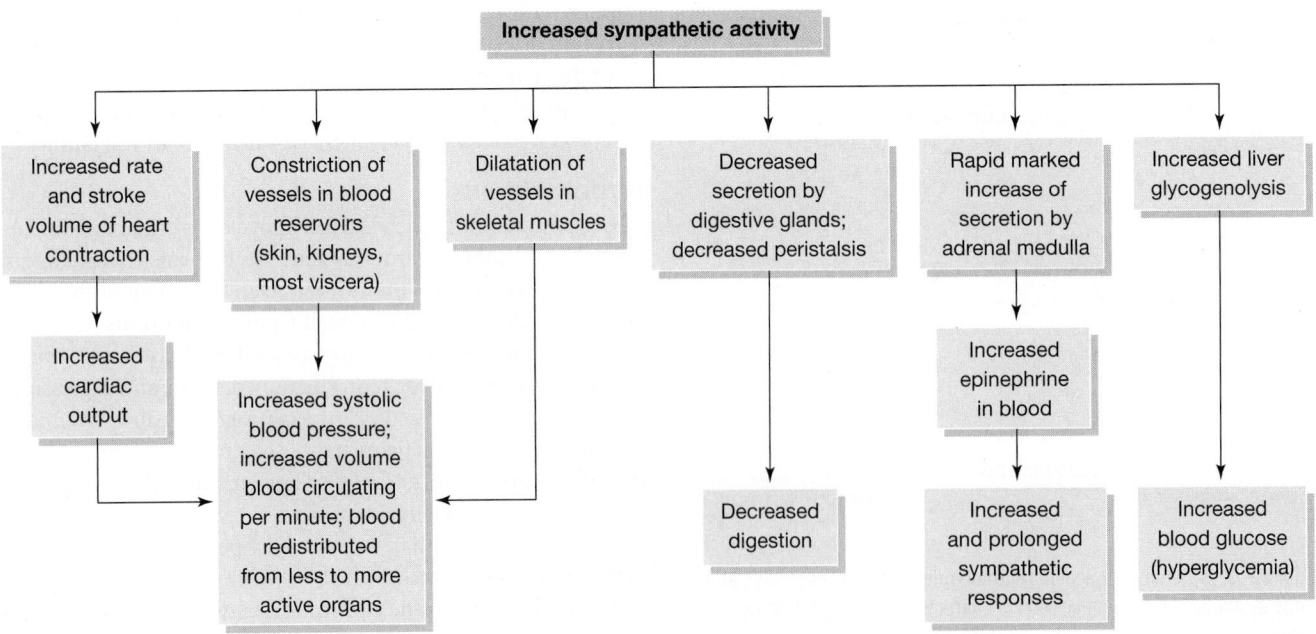

FIGURE 12–4 ■ Alarm reactions resulting from increased sympathetic activity. These responses commonly are referred to as the "fight-or-flight" reaction.

crease extracellular fluid (ECF) by promoting water and sodium retention. This is an adaptive mechanism in the event of hemorrhage or loss of fluids through excessive perspiration.

Stimulation of both the adrenal medulla and cortex results in an increased blood glucose level. This elevation provides the additional fuel for the increased metabolism needed for fighting or fleeing. The increased cardiac output (resulting from the increased heart rate and increased ECF), increased blood glucose levels, and increased metabolic rate make the physical responses possible. Also, the dilation of skeletal muscle blood vessels and resulting increased blood supply to the large muscles and the brain provide for quick movement and increased alertness. The increased blood volume (from ECF and the shunting of blood from the GI system) and increased clotting time function to help maintain adequate circulation to vital organs in case of traumatic blood loss. These responses to stress illustrate the complexity and interrelated nature of the processes involved.

Immune System

The immune system is the body's surveillance system. It detects and battles foreign invaders, such as bacteria, viruses, and tumor cells. The immune system comprises several organs, including bone marrow, spleen, thymus, and the lymph nodes. The most important elements of the immune system are lymphocytes, which are specialized white blood cells that fight bacteria, viruses, and other foreign invaders. Lymphocytes are originally manufactured in the bone marrow and then migrate to the other immune system organs, where they develop and are stored until needed.

Research has demonstrated the connection of the immune system to the neuroendocrine and autonomic systems. Negative stressors lead to alterations in immune function in humans through processes involving the hypothalamic–pituitary–adrenal (HPA) axis and the autonomic nervous system that affect immune function. In return, the immune system also affects endocrine and CNS responses. Both corticosteroids and catecholamines are known to suppress immune function. Figure 12–5 ■ demonstrates the physiological response to stress stimuli originating in the cerebral cortex and ending with the inhibition of the immune system.

Physiological Responses of Acute Versus Chronic Stress

With **acute stress**, as defined under the description of the HPA system or axis, catecholamines suppress activity in areas at the front of the brain concerned with short-term memory, concentration inhibition, and rational thought. This sequence of mental events allows a person to react quickly to the stressful event, to either fight or flee. It also hinders the ability of the person to handle the complex social or intellectual tasks and behaviors associated with the event.

The body actually responds to the stressful event by demonstrated changes in the heart rate, breathing, and blood pressure; the immune system; the skin; and metabolism.

- Breathing becomes rapid and the lungs take in more oxygen. Blood flow increases, sometimes up to 300% to 400%, priming the muscles, lungs, and the brain for added demands, and the spleen discharges red and white blood cells, allowing the blood to transport more oxygen.

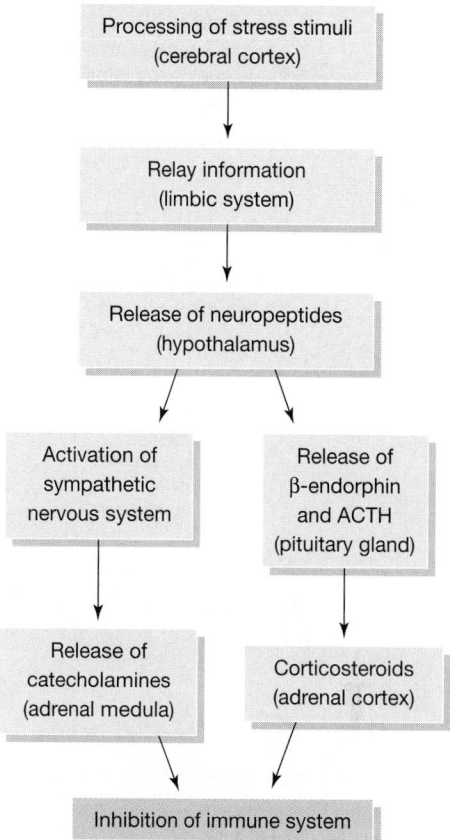

FIGURE 12–5 ■ System progression of the stress response.

- The immune system responds by marshalling a defense to the stress invaders. The steroid hormones diminish parts of the immune system so that infection or other immune molecules can be redistributed. These immune-boosting cells are sent to the injured or infected part of the body (e.g., the skin, the bone marrow, and the lymph nodes).

- The stress effect diverts blood flow away from the skin to support the heart and muscle tissues. The physical effect is cool, clammy, sweaty skin. The scalp also tightens so that the hair seems to stand up.

- Stress shuts down digestive activity, which is considered a nonessential body function during short-term periods of physical exertion or crisis.

Once the threat has passed and the effect has not been harmful, the stress hormones return to normal. This phenomenon is known as the relaxation response.

In contrast, and as previously defined, **chronic stress** is that which occurs on a daily basis and is a result of an ongoing situation. With chronic stress the urge to act (fight or flee) must be suppressed. Chronic stressors include ongoing highly pressured work situations, long-term relationship problems, loneliness, and persistent financial worries. The entire concept of the body's physiological response to stress is shown in Figure 12–6 ■ (p. 226).

Stress at the Cellular Level

Stress also affects the internal milieu of the body at the cellular level, with alterations in cellular structure and function contributing to changes in the steady state. Thus, the processes of

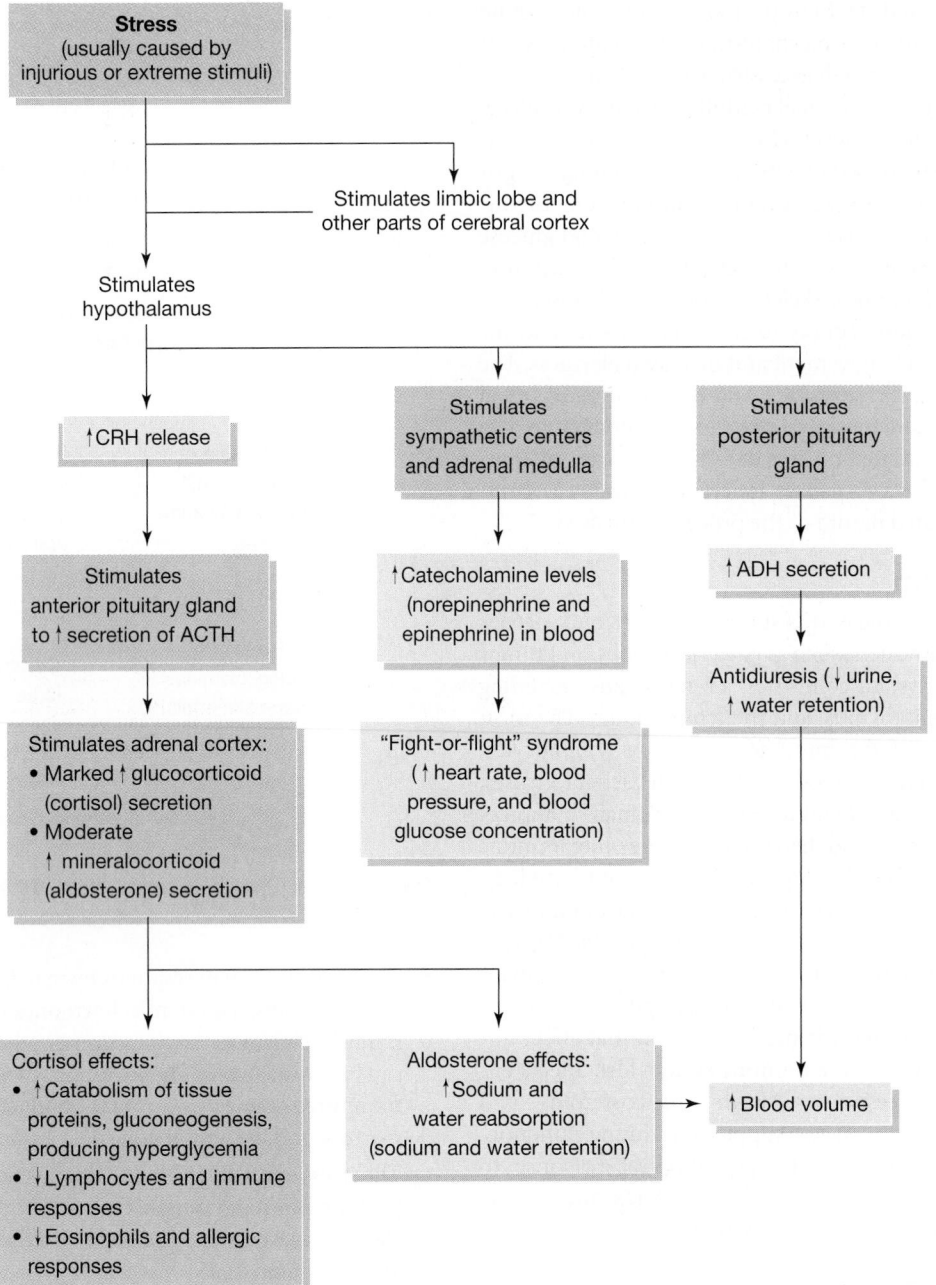

FIGURE 12–6 ■ Current concepts regarding the body's response to stress syndrome. *ACTH,* Adrenocorticotropic hormone; *ADH,* antidiuretic hormone; *CRH,* corticotrophin-releasing hormone.

health and disease or adaptation and maladaptation all can occur at the cellular level.

Cells are complex units that dynamically respond to the changing demands and stresses of daily life. They exist on a continuum of structure and function, ranging from the normal cell, to the adapted cell, to the injured or diseased cell, to the dead cell. Changes from one state to another can occur rapidly and may not be easily discernible.

Cells possess a maintenance function and a specialized function; Goodyear-Bruch & Pierce, 2002; Porth, 2007). The maintenance function refers to activities that the cell must perform with respect to itself; specialized functions are those that the cell performs in relation to the tissues and organs of which it is a part. Individual cells may cease to function without negatively

affecting the organism; however, if the specialized functions of the tissue are altered, the individual's health is threatened.

Cells adapt to environmental stress through structural and functional changes. Some of these adaptations are hypertrophy, atrophy, hyperplasia, dysplasia, and metaplasia:

- **Hypertrophy** and atrophy lead to changes in the size of cells and hence the size of the organs they form. Compensatory hypertrophy is the result of an enlarged muscle mass and commonly occurs in skeletal and cardiac muscles that experience a prolonged, increased workload.

- **Atrophy**, a reduction in size of the cell, can be the consequence of a disease or of decreased use, decreased blood supply, loss of nerve supply, or inadequate nutrition. Disuse of a body part often is associated with aging. Structures primarily affected by the decrease in cell and organ size are the skeletal muscles, the secondary sex organs, the heart, and the brain.

- **Hyperplasia** is the increase in the number of new cells in an organ or tissue. Hyperplasia results when cells multiply and are subjected to increased stimulation; the tissue mass enlarges. This represents a mitotic response to change, but is reversible when the stimulus is withdrawn, thereby distinguishing it from a malignant growth, which continues after the stimulus is removed.

- **Dysplasia** is the change in the appearance of cells after they have been subjected to chronic irritation. Dysplastic cells have a tendency to become malignant. They commonly are seen in epithelial cells in the bronchi of smokers.

- **Metaplasia** is a cell transformation in which a highly specialized cell changes to a less specialized cell. This serves as a protective mechanism because the less specialized cell is more resistant to the stress that stimulated the change.

Examples of these cellular changes are shown in Chart 12–4. These adaptations allow the survival of the organism, and they reflect the changes of the cell in response to stress. If the stress is unremitting, the function of the adapted cell may succumb, and cell injury will occur.

Cellular Injury

Any stressor that alters the ability of the cell or system to maintain optimal balance of its adjustment processes will lead to injury. Structural and functional damage then occurs. This may be reversible, permitting recovery, or irreversible, leading to disability or death. With adaptive changes, compensation occurs and a steady state is achieved, although it may be at new levels. With injury, steady-state regulation is lost, and changes in functioning follow.

Causes of changes in the system (cell, tissue, organ, body) may arise from the internal/external environment and include hypoxia, nutritional imbalance, physical agents, chemical agents, infectious agents, immune mechanisms, genetic defects, and psychogenic factors. The most common are infectious agents, hypoxia, and chemical agents. The presence of one injury

may precipitate another, and it may become a ripple effect. For example, the inadequate oxygenation and nutritional deficiencies make the system vulnerable to infection. These agents act at the cellular level by damaging or destroying the integrity of the cell membrane necessary for ionic balance and the ability of the cell to transform energy, synthesize enzymes and other necessary proteins, and to grow and reproduce.

Hypoxia

Inadequate cellular oxygenation interferes with the cell's ability to transform energy. Hypoxia may be caused by several factors including a decrease in blood supply, decreased hemoglobin, a ventilation/perfusion or respiratory problem, and a problem in the cell's enzyme system that makes it unable to use the oxygen delivered to it. Ischemia is the usual cause. This commonly is seen in myocardial cell injury in which arterial blood flow is decreased because of atherosclerotic narrowing of blood vessels. Ischemia also results from intravascular thrombi or emboli that may form and interfere with blood supply. These commonly result in cerebrovascular accidents (strokes). The amount of time tissues can survive without oxygen varies; however, if the hypoxia is slow and progressive, collateral circulation may develop, whereby blood is supplied to the tissues by other blood vessels. This does not guarantee resolution of the problem. See Chapter 29 🔗 for more information on strokes.

Nutritional Imbalance

Nutritional imbalance refers to a deficiency or excess of one or more essential nutrients. This imbalance results from inadequate nutrition (calories) or too much nutrition (calories). Caloric excess leads to obesity and overloads the cells in the body with lipids. Obesity places a strain on the body because it requires more energy to maintain the extra tissue, and obesity has been associated with the development of disease, especially cardiovascular and pulmonary disease.

Specific diseases can result when an essential nutrient is absent or when there is an imbalance of nutrients. For example, an energy deficit leading to cell injury can occur if there is insufficient glucose or insufficient oxygen to transform the glucose

CHART 12–4	Cellular Adaptation to Stressors	
Stressor	**Adaptation**	**Example**
Increased use (workload)	Hypertrophy—increase in size of cells leading to increase in organ size	Leg muscles of runner Arm muscles in tennis player Cardiac muscle in person with hypertension
Decreased use resulting in decreased blood supply, nutrition, and innervation	Atrophy—reduction in size of cell leading to decreased organ size	Extremity immobilized in cast Secondary sex organ in older adult
Hormonal change	Hyperplasia—increase in number of new cells	Breast changes of a girl in puberty or of a pregnant woman Regeneration of liver cells New red blood cells in blood loss
Reproduction of cells with alteration of size and shape	Dysplasia—change in the appearance of cells subject to chronic irritation	Alterations in epithelial cells of the skin or the cervix could be precursors of a malignancy
Stress applied to highly specialized cells	Reversible transformation of one adult cell type to another	Changes in epithelial cells lining bronchi in response to tobacco irritation (cells become less specialized)

Source: Matthews, B. D., Overby, D. R., Mannix, R., & Ingber, D. E. (2006). Cellular adaptation in mechanical stress: Role of integrins, Rho, cytoskeletal tension and mechanosensitive ion channels. *Journal of Cell Science, 119,* 509–518.

into energy. Conversely, a lack of insulin, or the inability to use insulin, also may prevent insulin from entering the cell from the blood. This occurs in diabetes mellitus. See Chapters 14 and 53 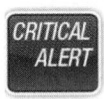, respectively, for more information on nutrition and diabetes.

Physical Agents

Physical agents that can cause injury to the cells include temperature extremes, radiation and electrical shock, and mechanical trauma. Extremely high temperatures precipitate hypermetabolism as manifested by an increase in respiratory rate, heart rate, and basal metabolic rate. With fever induced by infections, the hypothalamic thermostat may be reset at a higher temperature, then returns to normal when the fever goes down. Body temperatures greater than 41°C (106°F) suggest hyperthermia; the physiological function of the thermoregulatory center breaks down and the temperature soars. Eventually, the cell proteins coagulate and the cells die. The local response to thermal or burn injury is similar. There is an increase in metabolic activity and as heat increases, protein coagulates, enzyme systems are destroyed, and, in the extreme, charring or carbonization occurs. See Chapter 68 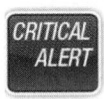 for information on burn injuries.

Low temperature extremes, or cold, cause vasoconstriction. Blood flow becomes sluggish and clots form, leading to ischemic damage in the involved tissues. With still lower temperatures, ice crystals may form and the cells may rupture.

> **CRITICAL ALERT**
> *Extremely high temperatures of 41°C (106°F) cause hyperthermia, which results in cell protein coagulation and cell death. Extremely low temperatures cause vasoconstriction leading to ischemia in involved tissues.*

Radiation and electrical shock, though used for diagnosis and disease treatment, also may cause injury by their destructive action. Radiation decreases the protective inflammatory response of the cell, creating a favorable environment for opportunistic infections. Electrical shock produces burns as a result of the heat generated when electrical current travels through the body. It also may stimulate nerves abnormally, as in cardiac fibrillation.

Mechanical trauma can result in wounds that disturb the cells and tissues. The outcome of mechanical trauma is dependent on the severity of the wound, the amount of blood lost, and the extent of nerve damage.

Chemical Agents

Chemical injuries are caused by poisons that have a corrosive action on epithelial tissues, such as lye, or by heavy metals, such as mercury, arsenic, and lead. Many other chemicals are toxic in specific amounts, in certain people, and in certain tissues. An example of such is excessive amounts of hydrochloric acid, which can damage the stomach lining. Large amounts of glucose can cause osmotic shifts, which affect the fluid and electrolyte balance, and too much insulin can cause subnormal levels of blood glucose and lead to coma.

Drugs also can cause chemical poisoning as can alcohol. The individual's drug tolerance must be carefully assessed when prescribing medications to prevent toxic reactions to the usual or customary dosages. Aging tends to decrease tolerance to medications. Polypharmacy also frequently occurs in the aging pop-

ulation and is a problem due to the unpredictability of medication interactions. Alcohol is a chemical irritant. Alcohol breaks down into acetaldehyde in the body, which has a direct toxic effect on liver cells that leads to a variety of liver abnormalities, including cirrhosis in susceptible individuals. Disordered liver cell function leads to complications in other body organs.

> **CRITICAL ALERT**
>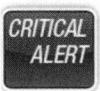
> *The elderly are susceptible to polypharmacy. This potentially is harmful because drug interactions are common with polypharmacy.*

Infectious Agents

Infectious agents known to cause disease in humans are viruses, bacteria, rickettsiae, mycoplasmas, fungi, protozoa, and nematodes. The severity of the infectious disease depends on the number of microorganisms entering the body, their virulence, and the host's defenses (e.g., health, age, immune defenses). Typically, an inflammatory response and immune reaction are the physiological responses of the body to the presence of infection. These processes are discussed at length in Chapters 59, 60, and 61 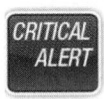.

Cellular Response to Injury

Cells may be injured or killed from the many agents just discussed. When this happens an inflammatory response naturally occurs in the tissues surrounding the injury. **Inflammation** is a defensive mechanism intended to neutralize, control, or eliminate the offending agent to prepare the site for repair. It is a nonspecific response that is meant to serve a protective function. Thus, the mechanism of inflammation basically is the same regardless of the injuring agent. The intensity of the response depends on the extent and severity of injury and on the reactive capacity of the injured person.

Contrary to a popular misconception, inflammation is not the same as infection. Inflammation always is present with infection, but infection is not always present with inflammation. An infection involves invasion of tissues or cells by microorganisms such as bacteria, fungi, and viruses. In contrast, inflammation also can be caused by nonliving agents such as heat, radiation trauma, and allergens. If infection is present, it is from a superimposed invasion of microorganisms. An infectious agent is only one of several agents that may trigger an inflammatory response. An infection exists when the infectious agent is living, growing, and multiplying in the tissues and is able to overcome the body's normal defenses.

> **CRITICAL ALERT**
>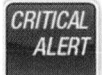
> *Inflammation and infection are not the same thing. Whereas inflammation is always present with infection, infection is not always present with inflammation. Infection is caused by invasion of cells and tissues by an organism (bacteria, fungi, virus). Inflammation also can be caused by heat, radiation, trauma, and allergens. An infection exists when the invading agent is living, growing, and multiplying in the tissues, thereby overcoming the body's defense system.*

The mechanism of inflammation basically is the same regardless of the injuring agent. The intensity of the response depends on the extent and severity of injury and on the reactive capacity of the injured person. The inflammatory response involves changes in the microcirculation, including vasodilation, increased vascular permeability, and leukocytic cellular infiltration. As these changes take place, five cardinal signs of inflammation are produced: redness, heat, swelling, pain, and loss of function. Initially transient vasodilation results in hyperemia, which raises filtration pressure. Vasodilation and chemical mediators cause endothelial cell retraction, which increases capillary permeability. The pain produced is attributed to the pressure of fluids or swelling on nerve endings and to the irritation of nerve endings by chemical mediators released at the site. Bradykinin is one of the chemical mediators suspected of causing pain. Loss of function is most likely related to the pain and swelling; however, the exact mechanism is not known.

Five cardinal signs of inflammation are:

- *Redness*
- *Heat*
- *Swelling*
- *Pain*
- *Loss of function.*

As blood flow increases and fluid leaks into the surrounding tissues, the formed elements (red blood cells, white blood cells, and platelets) remain in the blood, causing it to become more viscous. Leukocytes (white blood cells) collect in the vessels, exit, and migrate to the site of injury to engulf offending organisms and to remove cellular debris in a process called phagocytosis. Fibrinogen in the leaked plasma fluid coagulates, forming fibrin for clot formation, which serves to wall off the injured area and prevent the spread of infection.

Injury initiates the inflammatory response, but chemical substances released at the site induce the vascular changes. Histamine and kinins are foremost among these chemicals. Histamine is responsible for the early stages of vasodilation and vascular permeability. Kinins increase vasodilation and vascular permeability. They also attract neutrophils to the area. Prostaglandins, another group of chemical substances, also are suspected of causing increased permeability.

The inflammatory response often is confined to the site, causing only local signs and symptoms. However, systemic responses also can occur. Fever is the most common sign of a systemic response to injury, and it is most likely caused by endogenous pyrogens released from neutrophils and macrophages. The systemic inflammatory response is discussed fully in Chapter 61 🌐.

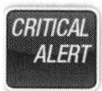

Fever should not be ignored, because it signifies a systemic response to an infectious agent.

Cellular Healing

The reparative process of cellular injury begins at approximately the same time as the injury and is linked with inflammation. Healing progresses after the inflammatory debris has been removed. Healing may occur by regeneration or by replacement. In regeneration, gradual repairs of the defect occur by proliferation of cells of the same type as those destroyed. During replacement, cells of another type, usually connective tissue, fill in the tissue defect and result in scar formation.

The ability of cells to regenerate depends on whether they are labile, permanent, or stable. Labile cells multiply constantly to replace cells worn out by physiological processes, such as the epithelial cells of the skins. Permanent cells include neurons, the nerve cell bodies, not their axons. If normal activity is to return, tissue regeneration must occur in a functional pattern, especially in the growth of several axons. Stable cells have a latent ability to regenerate. If they are damaged or destroyed, they are able to regenerate. These include cells of the kidney, liver, and pancreas.

Healing by replacement may occur through primary intention and/or secondary intention. In primary intention healing, the wound is clean and dry and the edges are approximated, as in a surgical wound. There is little scar formation. In secondary intention, the wound or defect is larger and gaping, and has necrotic or dead material. The wound fills from the bottom upward with granulation tissue. This repair process takes longer and results in more scar formation, with loss of specialized function. For information on wound healing, see Chapter 67 🌐. This is seen in the case of myocardial infarction and is detected on electrocardiographic (ECG) tracings because the electrical signal cannot be conducted through the connective tissue that has replaced the infarcted area. For information on ECGs, see Chapter 38 🌐.

The condition of the host, the environment, and the nature and severity of the injury affect the processes of inflammation and cell repair. Any of the injuries previously discussed can lead to death of the cell. The cell membrane becomes impaired, resulting in a nonrestricted flow of ions. Sodium and calcium enter the cell, followed by water, which leads to edema, and energy transformation ceases. Nerve impulses no longer are transmitted; muscles no longer contract. The cells rupture, lysosomal enzymes that destroy tissues escape, and cell death and necrosis occur. See Chapter 18 🌐 for information on fluid and electrolytes.

Oxidative Stress (OS)

Oxidative stress is rapidly becoming the nutritional and medical buzzword for the 21st century. It is receiving much attention as a way of interpreting the body's physiological response to stress, and it is implicated in a growing list of diseases, from cataracts to cancer. Health conscious people, taking heed of the news about oxygen free radicals, also are taking steps to protect themselves from these active "criminals" that are sabotaging health.

Oxidative stress (OS) is a physiological response to both internal and external stressors. Though in and of itself, it is not a disease, it is a condition that can lead to or accelerate disease development. OS occurs when the available supply of the body's antioxidants is insufficient to handle and neutralize free radicals of different types. The result is massive cell damage, which can result in cellular mutations, tissue breakdown, and immune compromise. The increasing focus on OS makes it increasingly important that nurses understand and appreciate the concept of oxidative stress, both from a treatment perspective and a preventive/educational perspective. The process that allows oxidative stress to occur is discussed next and is related to the physiological development of oxygen-derived free radicals.

Oxygen is necessary for the metabolic production of energy. Mitochondria, through the electron transport chain, use oxygen to oxidize other molecules and generate energy in the form of adenosine triphosphate. During this process oxygen is reduced to water, producing several intermediary **reactive oxygen species (ROS)**. These species are a major contributing factor in diseases in patients who are critically ill. ROSs are controlled by a defense system that depends on the activity of enzymes and other nonenzyme substances. The imbalance between ROSs and the body's defense system is called oxidative stress.

Formation of ROS

During chemical processes, molecules can be reduced or oxidized. A molecule with an unpaired electron can combine with a molecule capable of donating an electron. The donation of an electron is called *oxidation*. The gain of an electron is called *reduction*. During these reactions, the molecule that donates the electron is oxidized and the molecule that accepts the electron is reduced. Reduction and oxidation can leave the reduced molecule unstable and free to react with other molecules to cause damage to cell membranes, proteins, and DNA. These reduced substances are called *free radicals* (Pugliese, 1995).

In homeostasis, the rates of reduction and oxidation are equal. The reduction–oxidation (redox) balance is maintained by physiological defenses such as specialized enzymes and antioxidants. These antioxidants and enzymes remove or inactivate the free radicals. The enzymes and antioxidants can become overwhelmed by an increase in reduced molecules or by a decrease in the defense system, allowing the accumulation of free radicals (Espat & Helton, 2000).

Free radicals are involved in many cellular functions and are a normal part of living. For example, mitochondria within a cell burn glucose for fuel. This process oxidizes the glucose and in so doing generates free radicals. White blood cells also use free radicals to attach and destroy bacteria, viruses, and virus-infected cells. The detoxifying actions of the liver also require free radicals. Although free radicals have useful functions in the body under controlled conditions, they are extremely unstable molecules that can damage cells if left uncontrolled.

Normally, oxygen free radicals are neutralized by antioxidants such as vitamin E or enzymes such as superoxide dismutase. However, in some patients, oxygen free radicals become a problem when either a decrease in the removal of or an overproduction of the radicals occurs. When the body is overwhelmed by increased production of oxidative agents and defense against these agents is decreased, the ensuing damage contributes to cellular derangements, cell injury, and death. The free radicals tend to accelerate aging and contribute to the development of many diseases, such as cancer, ischemia-reperfusion injury, and systemic inflammatory response (Byrnes, 2003).

Evidence-based research confirms the link between oxidative stress and pathophysiological syndromes and diseases, including those mentioned earlier as well as cardiogenic shock, sepsis, acute respiratory distress syndrome (ARDS), diaphragm fatigue, and burns (Goodyear-Bruch & Pierce, 2002). A relationship also has been determined between oxidative stress and septic shock, disseminated intravascular coagulation, multiple organ dysfunction, cardiovascular disease, diabetes mellitus, and trauma, as well as nonhereditary degenerative diseases such as Parkinson's and Alzheimer's (Byrnes, 2003; Emory University Health Sciences Center, 2006).

Poor nutrition in general also contributes to OS. When the body is fed poorly, it slowly starves and all of its systems suffer.

Weak organ systems are prime targets for free radical attack. Even psychological and emotional stress can contribute to OS. When the body is under stress, it produces certain hormones that generate free radicals. Moreover, the liver must eventually detoxify them in a process that also generates free radicals.

Everyone is exposed to free radicals from a variety of sources. Because oxidative stress is associated with a variety and severity of illnesses, the care of patients depends on preventing and controlling production of ROS. Within this realm, collaborative care, which includes nutritional counseling, is an essential component of the patient's care and is focused on removing as many related stressors as possible.

■ Negative (Maladaptive) Effects of Stress

In prehistoric times, the physical changes in response to stress were an essential adaptation for meeting natural threats. Even now in the modern world the stress response can be an asset for raising levels of performance during critical events such as sports activities, an important meeting, or in situations of actual danger or crisis. However, if stress becomes persistent and low level, all parts of the body's stress apparatus (the brain, heart, lungs, vessels, and muscles) become chronically over- or underactivated. This may produce psychological or physical damage over time. Acute stress also can be harmful in certain situations.

Stress-related conditions that are most likely to produce negative physical effects include:

- An accumulation of persistent stressful situations, particularly those that a person cannot easily control (e.g., high-pressure work plus an unhappy relationship)
- Persistent stress following a severe acute response to a traumatic event, such as an automobile crash
- An inefficient or insufficient relaxation response
- Acute stress in people with serious illness, such as heart disease or cancer.

Psychological Effects of Stress

Studies suggest that the inability to adapt to stress is associated with the onset of depression or anxiety (Manktelow, 2003). Some evidence suggests that repeated release of stress hormones produces hyperactivity in the HPA axis and disrupts normal levels of serotonin, the nerve chemical that is critical for feelings of well-being. On a more obvious level, stress diminishes the quality of life by reducing feelings of pleasure and accomplishment, and relationships often are threatened.

Stress and Illness

Stress may increase vulnerability to almost any illness. It has long been suspected to play a role in the etiology of many diseases. (Refer back to the discussion on oxidative stress.) How a stress-provoking event is perceived and how one reacts to it determines its impact on health. When something happens to an individual, she automatically evaluates the situation mentally and decides if it is threatening. She then decides how to deal with the situation and what skills she can use. If she decides that the demands of the situation outweigh the skills she has, the situation is labeled "stressful" and the classic stress response begins. If the individual decides that her coping skills outweigh the demands of the situation, then it is not viewed as stressful.

A threat to one's life or safety is considered stressful and triggers a primal physical response by the body. From deep within the brain, a chemical signal speeds stress hormones through the bloodstream, priming the body to be alert and ready to escape danger. Concentration becomes more focused, reaction time faster, and strength and agility increase. When the stressful situation ends, hormonal signals switch off the stress response and the body returns to normal. But in modern society, fraught with stressful daily events, hassles, and relationships, and also contingent on the individual's hormonal response, stress does not always let up. The stress hormones continue to wash through the system at high levels, never leaving the blood and tissues. Research now shows that long-term activation of the stress system can have a hazardous, even lethal effect on the body, increasing the risk of obesity, heart disease, depression, and a variety of other illnesses. Dr. Gabor Maté (2003) theorized in his treatise *When the Body Says No: Understanding the Stress–Disease Connection* that repressed stressful emotions can interfere with the psychoneuroimmune axis and predispose a person to a variety of diseases—from rheumatoid arthritis to cancer. Manktelow (2003) also has commented on the relationship of stress to disease.

Stress Circuit

The stress response results from the complex interplay between the nervous system and stress hormones, or the hormonal systems known as the **hypothalamic–pituitary–adrenal (HPA) axis** (Figure 12–7 ■). As described earlier, the HPA axis is a feedback loop by which signals from the brain trigger the release of hormones needed to respond to stress. Because of its function the HPA axis also is referred to as the *stress circuit*.

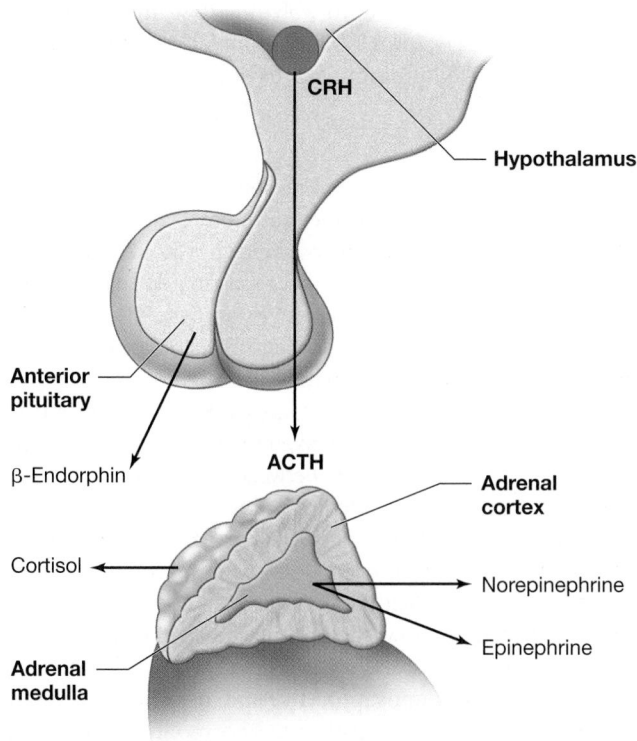

FIGURE 12–7 ■ The hypothalmic–pituitary–adrenal axis (HPA). *ACTH,* Adrenocorticotropic hormone; *CRH,* corticotrophin-releasing hormone.

The stress circuit, or HPA axis, affects systems throughout the body, the autonomic nervous system, regions of the brain, and glandular systems. Short-term response to the stress may be helpful, allowing biochemical resources to be diverted to deal with the threat. Long-term response can result in exacerbations of chronic conditions or major disorders.

The HPA axis also can alter its functioning in response to environmental influences. It may be permanently altered in response to extreme stress during the life cycle—adulthood, adolescence, early childhood, or even in the womb. If a person experiences major stresses in early childhood, the HPA feedback loop becomes stronger and stronger with each new stressful period. This usually results in an adult individual who overreacts hormonally to comparatively minor situations. Thus, from a physiological perspective, it is understandable that chronic and acute events are linked closely to stress. Certain chronic conditions, many of them difficult to treat, have a particularly close link to stress. These include pain and fatigue, mood and anxiety, and addiction and substance abuse. Research also has shown that stress plays an integral part in many disease processes that affect specific organs, body systems, and or behavioral phenomena. Some of these are discussed in the following subsections (Wein, 2000). Figure 12–8 ■ (p. 232) illustrates some disorders that may be caused or aggravated by stress.

Cardiovascular System

An impaired ability to adapt to physiological and psychological stress may contribute to the pathogenesis of cardiovascular disease (Pickering, 2001), because the cardiovascular system is particularly vulnerable to stress (Manktelow, 2003; Schwaertz et al., 2003; Wan, Camandolal, & Mattson, 2003). Excessive exposure to uncontrollable stressors and/or the inability to adapt to stress are implicated in the pathogenesis of several different disorders including hypertension and atherosclerotic vascular disease. Moreover, acute stressors can trigger myocardial infarctions and strokes (Kop, 1999; Manktelow, 2003). Stress is a major trigger for angina as physical stress. Incidents of acute stress have been associated with a higher risk for serious cardiac events, such as heart dysrhythmias and heart attacks, and even death from such events in people with heart disease.

The sympathetic nervous system regulates a broad range of visceral functions and, during extreme emotional or physical states, activates both the cardiovascular and adrenal catecholamine systems for homeostatic adjustments. The CNS neurons responsible for coactivation of these autonomic changes are thought to be governed by a common set of central command neurons that provides dual projections to the sympathetic outflow systems that control the heart and adrenal gland. Stress activates the sympathetic nervous system (the autonomic part of the nervous system that affects many organs, including the heart). The heart may be negatively affected in several ways:

- Sudden stress increases the pumping action and rate of the heart and causes the arteries to constrict, thereby posing a risk for blocking blood flow to the heart.

- The emotional effects of stress alter the heart rhythms and pose a risk for serious arrhythmias in people with existing heart rhythm disturbances.

- Stress causes blood to become stickier (possibly in preparation for potential injury), increasing the likelihood of an artery-clogging blood clot.

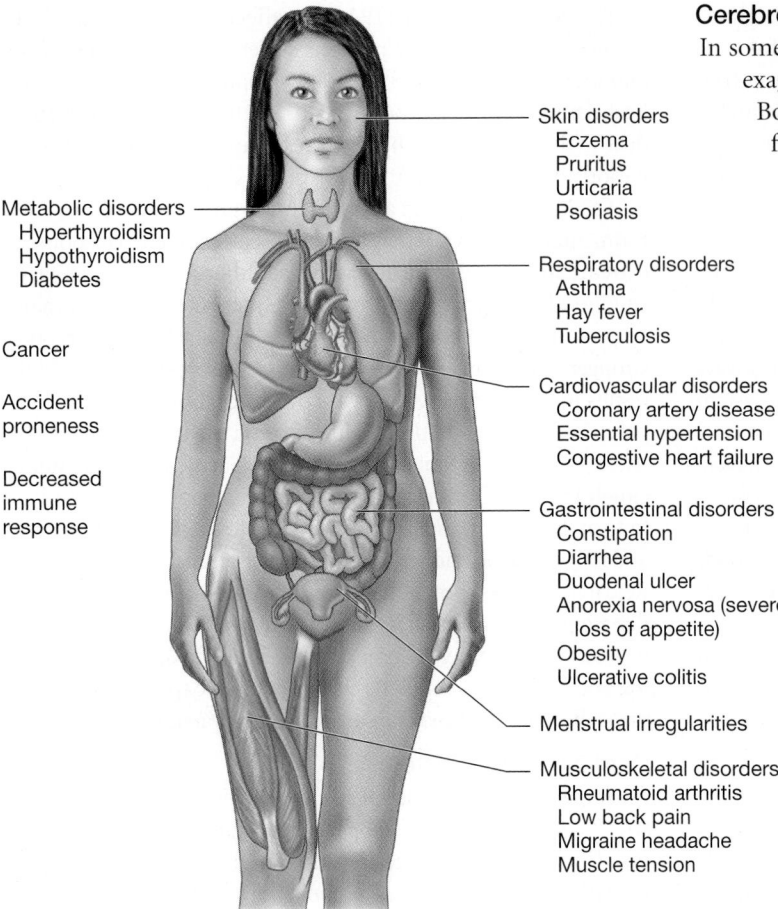

Metabolic disorders
Hyperthyroidism
Hypothyroidism
Diabetes

Cancer

Accident
proneness

Decreased
immune
response

Skin disorders
Eczema
Pruritus
Urticaria
Psoriasis

Respiratory disorders
Asthma
Hay fever
Tuberculosis

Cardiovascular disorders
Coronary artery disease
Essential hypertension
Congestive heart failure

Gastrointestinal disorders
Constipation
Diarrhea
Duodenal ulcer
Anorexia nervosa (severe
loss of appetite)
Obesity
Ulcerative colitis

Menstrual irregularities

Musculoskeletal disorders
Rheumatoid arthritis
Low back pain
Migraine headache
Muscle tension

FIGURE 12–8 ■ Disorders caused or aggravated by stress.

- Stress may signal the body to release fat into the bloodstream, raising blood cholesterol levels, at least temporarily.
- In women, chronic stress may reduce estrogen levels, which are important for cardiac health.
- Stressful events may cause men and women who have relatively low levels of the neurotransmitter serotonin (and, therefore, a higher risk for depression or anger) to produce more of certain immune system proteins, called cytokines, which in high amounts cause inflammation and damage to cells, including possibly heart cells.
- Recent evidence confirms the association between stress and hypertension. People who regularly experience sudden increases in blood pressure caused by mental stress may, over time, develop injuries in the inner lining of their blood vessels.

More research is needed to confirm the actual harm of stress on the heart, although it has been scientifically demonstrated that mentally stressful tasks in patients with coronary artery disease (CAD) can produce acute cardiac effects that are consistent with ischemia, including reductions in left ventricular function, and relative myocardial perfusion (Arrighi et al., 2000). It also is possible that people who work under high-stress conditions try to cope with the situation by resorting to unhealthy habits including high-fat and high-salt diets, tobacco use, alcohol abuse, and a sedentary lifestyle, thereby, contributing to cardiovascular disorders.

Cerebrovascular System

In some people prolonged or frequent mental stress causes an exaggerated increase in blood pressure (Truelsen, Nielsen, Boysen, & Gronbaeck, 2003). A 2001 study linked for the first time a higher risk for stroke in adult Caucasian men and elevated blood pressure during times of stress (Everson et al., 2001).

Gastrointestinal System

Many of the same hormones stimulate the brain and the intestine. Although stress does not cause gastrointestinal problems directly, it can be a trigger (Grumman, 1998; Mayer, Naliboff, & Craig, 2006). The stress circuit influences the stomach and intestines in several ways. The CRH directly hinders the release of stomach acid and emptying of the stomach. The CRH also directly stimulates the colon, speeding up the emptying of its contents. In addition to the direct effects on the stomach, the entire HPA axis, through the autonomic nervous system, also hinders stomach acid secretion and emptying and increases the movement of the colon. Thus, prolonged stress can disrupt the digestive system, irritating the large intestine and causing diarrhea, constipation, cramping, and bloating. Excessive production of digestive acids in the stomach may cause a painful burning. Conditions of the digestive systems strongly related to stress are irritable bowel syndrome, peptic ulcers, and inflammatory bowel disease. According to Levenstein (1998), there is solid evidence that psychological stress triggers many ulcers and impairs responses to treatment. Levenstein (2003) also draws a relationship between stress and ulcerative colitis. Psychological stress probably functions most often as a cofactor with *H. pylori*. It may act by stimulating the production of gastric acid or by promoting behavior that causes a risk to health.

Immune System

As has been noted, physiological responses to stress involve the pituitary–adrenal axis and the autonomic nervous system through the release of corticosteroid hormones and catecholamines, respectively. It has been postulated that the relationship between the immune system and the CNS provides confirmation that the autonomic and physiological pathways through which stress passes can modulate an immune response. According to Glaser and Kiecolt-Glaser (1994) and Segerstrom and Miller (2004), the field of psychoneuroimmunology proposes that a relationship exists between stress, immunological impairment, and health outcomes. The ramifications of this finding are that intense stressors, such as death of a loved one, divorce, and commonplace stressors such as school exams and job stress, adversely affect the immune system. Stress can cause wounds to heal more slowly and people to become more susceptible to infection, colds, and other illness.

Stress can be immunosuppressive and, hence, may be detrimental to health. Glucocorticoid stress hormones are widely regarded as being immunosuppressive and are used clinically as anti-inflammatory agents. The HPA axis interacts with the immune system, increasing vulnerability to colds, flu, fatigue, and infections. In response to an infection or an inflammatory disorder such as arthritis, cells of the immune system produce three substances that cause inflammation: interleukin 1 (IL-1), interleukin 6 (IL-6), and tumor necrosis factor (TNF), working either singularly or in combination to cause the release of CRH. IL-6 also promotes the release of ACTH and cortisol. Cortisol and other compounds then suppress the release of IL-1, IL-6, and TNF, thereby switching off the inflammatory response. Ideally, stress hormones switch off, or dampen, the immune response when it has run its course. However, if the HPA axis is continually running at a high level, the damping down can have a down side, leading to decreased ability to release the interleukins and fight infection.

In some cases, stress can have the opposite effect, making the immune system overreactive. The result is an increased risk of autoimmune diseases, in which the immune system attacks the body's own cells. Stress also can worsen the symptoms of autoimmune disease. For example, stress is one of the triggers for the sporadic flare-ups of symptoms in lupus.

Additionally, the high cortisol levels resulting from prolonged stress could serve to make the body more susceptible to disease by switching off disease-fighting white blood cells. It also has been hypothesized that this same deactivation of white blood cells also might increase the risk for certain types of cancer (National Institutes of Health [NIH], 2004). Conversely, there is evidence to suggest that a depressed HPA axis can result in too little corticosteroid, leading to a hyperactive immune system and increased risk of developing autoimmune diseases (diseases in which the immune system attacks the body's own cells).

The phenomenon of stress has been shown to adversely affect a variety of natural-resistance responses and specific immunological modifications in both animals and men. Although consensus has not been reached on the effects of stress on the immune system, some responses have been validated (Norman, 2003). Stress can have mixed effects on autoimmune diseases (those which are caused by inflammation and damage from immune attacks on the body). It has been shown, for example, that eczema, lupus, and rheumatoid arthritis may demonstrate changes ranging from improvement to deterioration in response to stress. It also has been shown that short-term stress appears to have no negative effect on multiple sclerosis, but chronic stress is a major risk factor for flare-ups.

Susceptibility to Infection   Stress also has been found to impair the immune system. Chronic stress appears to blunt the immune response and increase the risk for infections and may even impair a person's response to immunizations. Studies have shown that subjects experiencing chronic stress have low white blood cell counts and are vulnerable to colds. People who harbor herpes or HIV viruses may be more susceptible to viral activation following exposure to stress. Some research has found that HIV-infected men with high stress levels progress more rapidly to AIDS when compared to those with lower stress levels (Green & Smith, 2004). Stressful events most linked with a higher incidence of infections seem to be interpersonal conflicts, such as those at work or in a relationship (Thomas, Nelesen, Ziegler, Bardwell, & Dimsdale, 2004).

Endocrine System

The endocrine system also has been found to be affected by stress. Chronic stress has been associated with the development of insulin resistance, a condition in which the body is unable to use insulin effectively to regulate glucose (blood sugar). Insulin resistance is a primary factor in diabetes. Stress also can exacerbate existing diabetes by impairing the patient's ability to manage the disease effectively.

Stress and Growth   The hormones of the HPA axis also influence hormones needed for growth. Prolonged HPA activation hinders the release of growth hormone and insulin-like growth factor 1, (IGF-1), both of which are essential for normal growth. According to the NIH (2004), old research also has shown that the stress from emotional deprivation or psychological harassment may result in the short stature and delayed physical maturity of the condition known as psychological short stature (PSS).

Reproductive System

Stress suppresses the reproductive system at various levels. CRH prevents the release of gonadotropin releasing hormone (GnRH), the master hormone that signals a cascade of hormones that direct reproduction and sexual behavior. Similarly, cortisol and related glucocorticoid hormones not only inhibit the release of GnRH, but also inhibit the release of luteinizing hormone, which prompts ovulation and sperm release.

Glucocorticoids also inhibit the testes and ovaries directly, hindering production of the male and female sex hormones testosterone, estrogen, and progesterone. Thus, it has been shown that stress can lead to diminished sexual desire and an inability to achieve orgasm in women. Stress response also can cause temporary impotence in men. Part of the stress response involves the release of brain chemicals that constrict the smooth muscles of the penis and its arteries. This constriction reduces the blood flow into and increases the blood flow out of the penis, which can prevent erection.

Other reactions to stress may manifest as decreased fertility and a higher risk for miscarriage in pregnant women. Stress also has been associated with lower birth weights and an increased incidence of premature births, both of which are risk factors for infant mortality. Stress may cause physiological alterations, such as increased adrenal hormone levels or resistance in the arteries that may interfere with normal blood flow to the placenta.

Conversely, the interaction between the HPA axis and the reproductive system is a two-way reciprocal process. The female hormone estrogen exerts partial control of the gene that stimulates CRH production. This may explain why women, on average, have slightly elevated cortisol levels. In turn, higher cortisol levels, in combination with other, as yet unknown, factors, may be the reason why women are more vulnerable than men to depression, anorexia nervosa, panic disorder, obsessive compulsive disorder, and autoimmune diseases such as lupus and rheumatoid arthritis (Kalantaridou, Makrigiannakis, Zoumakis, & Chrousos, 2004).

It also has been scientifically demonstrated that females under "attack" are less likely to fight or flee and are more apt to attempt to protect their children and seek help from others, particularly other females (Taylor & Klein, et. al, 2000). Taylor and Klein call this pattern of behavior the "tend-and-befriend" response. They suggested an evolutionary explanation for the difference. In many situations it could be disastrous for a woman who is pregnant, nursing, or caring for young children to fight or flee. Befriending, on the other hand, establishes a support system for the mother and child and also helps to defend women against male violence. Taylor and Klein believed that hormones, especially sex hormones and the pituitary hormone oxytocin, are one reason for the difference in response to stress between men and women. Oxytocin, which induces relaxation and lowers anxiety, is released in response to stress by both males and females, but its effects are enhanced by female hormones and reduced by male hormones. In contrast, the fight-or-flight response activates the nervous system and causes the secretion of the stress hormones adrenaline and cortisol. Both sexes release these hormones under stress, but men also release testosterone, which tends to increase hostility and aggression. Because female aggression is less closely linked to nervous system arousal, it has been suggested that their stress is more easily moderated by learning and culture, whereas men tend to do this less easily. Studies on the relationship between oxytocin and stress have concentrated on men, and more research needs to be conducted that also focuses on women.

Cancer

To date, there is no current evidence to support the idea that stress causes cancer. However, Dr. David Spiegel of Stanford University purports that the link between postdiagnosis stress and cancer survival is gaining momentum (Senior, 2001). He has reported that four recent studies have indicated that higher levels of stress hormones lead to more rapid cancer progress. Cortisol concentrations have been found to be a reliable indicator of chronic and severe stress. In one of Dr. Spiegel's most recent studies, he found that patients with abnormally flat cortisol measurements had significantly lower numbers of natural killer cells, which suggests a link between the immune system, stress, and the body's ability to fight breast cancer.

It also has been demonstrated that lack of control over stress (not simply stress itself) has had negative effects on immune function and has contributed to tumor growth in animals. Two small studies on melanoma and breast cancer patients reported improved survival with therapies that offered emotional support (Reuters Health, 2004). More information on cancer can be found in Chapter 64 ⊕.

Pain

Pain and agitation are common in patients who are critically ill. The stress response causes tremendous neurohumoral elevations of plasma catecholamine, cortisol, glucose, ADH, and acute-stage protein levels. These elevations can result in tachycardia, hypertension, vasoconstriction, increased oxygen consumption, salt and water retention, and blunting of the immune response.

The primary goals of sedation and analgesia are to relieve pain and anxiety, attenuate the stress response, and improve compliance with care. In certain situations neuromuscular blocking agents are necessary. Appropriate use of these medications requires a thorough understanding of drug indications, metabolism, side effects, and monitoring techniques. Sedation needs may vary over the course of a patient's stay. In the acute phase, a profound stress response may require deeper sedation and higher doses of analgesics. When a plateau is reached, sedative and analgesic requirements may decrease, but delirium may

emerge. In the recovery phase, sedation and analgesics are tapered and discontinued. Use of agents needs to be tailored to the needs of individual patients; indications, anticipated length of need, and underlying organ system derangements are important considerations (Blanchard, 2002).

Chronic pain caused by arthritis and other conditions may be intensified by stress. Psychological distress also plays a significant role in the severity of back pain. Tension-type headaches are highly associated with stress and stressful events. Some research suggests that tension-type headache sufferers may actually have some biological predisposition for translating stress into muscle contraction. Emotional stress is among the wide range of possible migraine triggers.

Eating Problems

Stress can have varying effects on eating problems and weight. Stress often is related to weight gain and obesity. Many people develop cravings for salt, fat, and sugar to counteract tension and, thus, gain weight. Scientists at the University of California found that comfort foods such as chocolate cake and ice cream literally blunt the body's response to chronic stress (Manisses Communications Group, 2003; SixWise.com, 2006). Eating calorie-rich food seems to calm the nerves, but eating too much can lead to obesity, depression, and more stress.

 *Comfort foods, those rich in calories (e.g., chocolate cake and ice cream), may act as a stress blocker. Too much comfort food, however, leads to obesity, depression, and more stress. Obesity may be a predictor of diabetes and heart problems.*

The weight gained is often abdominal fat, a predictor of diabetes and heart problems. The release of cortisol, a major stress hormone, appears to promote abdominal fat and may be the primary connection between stress and weight gain in people. Rivas (2003) has demonstrated that a hormonal cascade causes hunger. When a stress response is activated, the brain releases CRH, which suppresses the appetite. The adrenal glands then secrete their powerful fight-or-flight stress hormones, adrenaline, and cortisol, which propel sugar into the bloodstream for a short-term energy rush. After that rush, cortisol sparks ravenous hunger for carbohydrates and fat.

If under continuous stress, the result is prolonged, thus elevating cortisol levels that spur the release of insulin, the hormone directs the body to hang on to the fat it has and store more. If one has many stressors, one has many periods of rebound insulin secretion. The cumulative effect is a push toward obesity. Also noted is the fact that the brain's complex appetitive and satiety control system can go haywire under stress. Rivas (2003) contends that most people who overeat when stressed are genetically prone to an imbalance among at least three of the brain's neurotransmitters (serotonins, dopamine, and norepinephrine), which help the body regulate both appetite and mood. When an already short supply of serotonin dwindles further under stress, overeaters launch into desperate forays for sweets because carbohydrates raise serotonin levels (SixWise.com, 2006).

Conversely, some people experiencing stress suffer a loss of appetite and lose weight. In rare cases, stress may trigger hyperactivity of the thyroid gland, stimulating appetite but causing the body to burn up calories at a faster than normal rate. Several eating disorders, such as anorexia nervosa and bulimia, are highly associated with adjustment problems in response to stress and emotional issues.

Sleep Disturbances

The tensions of unresolved stress frequently cause insomnia, generally keeping the stressed person awake or causing awakening in the middle of the night or early morning. Researchers also have theorized that persistent insomnia may result from a disorder of the stress system (NIH, 2004). They found that, when compared to a group of people who did not have difficulty falling asleep, the insomniacs had higher ACTH and cortisol levels, both in the evening and in the first half of the night. The insomniacs with the highest cortisol levels tended to have the greatest difficulty falling asleep. Their ACTH and cortisol levels indicated that the insomniacs had nervous systems that were on overdrive, alert, and ready to deal with a threat, when they should otherwise be quieting down. Thus, the researchers suggested that, rather than prescribing hypnotics to regulate sleep system, the physicians might have more success in prescribing antidepressants to help calm an overactive stress system. Behavior therapy also was recommended.

Memory, Concentration, and Learning

Cognitive changes occur in response to acute, uncontrollable stress. One can become distracted and disorganized, and the working memory abilities worsen, leaving habitual response to control behavior. Neurological research now can begin to explain many of these cognitive changes in response to stress. The neuromodulators called catecholamines (dopamine, norepinephrine, and epinephrine) are released through the peripheral and central nervous systems during stress. Just as catecholamines "turn on" the heart and muscles and "turn off" the stomach to prepare for fight-or-flight responses during stress, similar opposing actions in the brain may turn on a structure called the amygdala and turn off the prefrontal cortex (a higher cognitive center), allowing posterior cortical and subcortical structures to control behavior (Arnsten, 1998). The amygdala is a phylogenetically older structure in the medial temporal lobe, long known to be essential for the expression of emotion and the formation of associations between stimuli and emotions (Aggleton, 1992). In contrast, the prefrontal cortex expands greatly and permits working memory to guide behavior, inhibiting inappropriate responses or distractions and allowing one to plan and organize effectively. High levels of catecholamines exert opposite actions on these brain regions (Arnsten, 1998).

Thus, it can be concluded that stress has substantial effects on the brain, particularly on memory. Typically, one who is experiencing severe stress suffers loss of concentration and may become inefficient at work and home and accident prone. It also has been shown that the immediate effect of acute stress impairs short-term memory, particularly verbal memory. Prolonged exposure to cortisol, the major stress hormone, causes shrinkage in the hippocampus, the center of memory.

Other Disorders

Other disorders precipitated by stress include allergies, skin disorders, hair loss, and periodontal disease, along with depression. Research suggests that stress may actually be a cause of the so-called "sick-building syndrome," which produces allergy-like symptoms, such as eczema, headaches, asthma, and sinus problems (NIH, 2004). Stress also plays a role in exacerbating some skin conditions including hives, psoriasis, acne, rosacea, and eczema. Unexplained itching also may be caused by stress as can unexplained hair loss (alopecia areata). This is hair loss that occurs in localized patches. The exact cause is unknown, but stress is suspected as a player in this condition, for it has been noted that hair loss often occurs during periods of intense stress, such as mourning. Stress also has been implicated in increasing the risk for periodontal disease.

Depression

Evidence suggests that early adverse experiences play a preeminent role in development of mood and anxiety disorders and that a corticotropin-releasing factor (CRF) systems may mediate this association (Heim et al., 2000; Mayer, Naliboff, & Craig, 2006). Melancholic depression has been found to be a major disorder characteristic of an overactive HPA axis. Research has shown that people with depression have a blunted ability to "counterregulate," or adapt, to the negative feedback of increases in cortisol. The body turns on the fight-or-flight response, but cannot turn it off again, thereby, producing anxiety and overreaction to stimulation. This is followed by the paradoxical response called "learned helplessness," in which victims apparently lose all motivation. This form of depression manifests itself as anxiety, loss of appetite, loss of sex drive, rapid heart beat, high blood pressure, and high cholesterol and triglyceride levels. Individuals with this condition tend to produce higher-than-normal levels of CRH, which is probably due to a combination of environmental and hereditary causes, depending on the person affected. However, rather than producing higher amounts of ACTH in response to CRH, depressed people produce smaller amounts of this substance, presumably because their hippocampi have become less sensitive to the higher amounts of CRH.

In an apparent attempt to switch off excess CRH production, the systems of people with melancholic depression also produce high levels of cortisol, the by-products of which are produced in response to high levels of the substance. Thus, these by-products of the cortisol serve as sedatives and perhaps contribute to the overall feeling of depression.

Other conditions also are associated with high levels of CRH and cortisol. These include anorexia nervosa, malnutrition, obsessive-compulsive disorder, anxiety disorder, alcoholism, alcohol and narcotic withdrawal, poorly controlled diabetes, childhood sexual abuse, and hyperthyroidism (NIH, 2004). The excessive amount of the stress hormone cortisol produced in patients with any of these conditions is responsible for many of the observed symptoms. Most of these patients share psychological symptoms including sleep disturbances, loss of libido, and loss of appetite as well as physical problems such as an increased risk for accumulating abdominal fat and hardening of the arteries and other forms of cardiovascular disease. They also may experience suppression of thyroid hormones and of the immune system. Such patients are likely to have their life spans shortened by 15 to 20 years if they remain untreated due to their risk for health problems.

Self-Medication with Unhealthy Lifestyles

People under chronic stress often seek unhealthy means to relieve the stress: drug or alcohol abuse, tobacco use, abnormal eating patterns, or passive activities, such as watching television. The damage caused by these self-destructive habits under ordinary circumstances is exacerbated by the physiological effects of stress itself. The cycle becomes self-perpetuating. A sedentary routine, an unhealthy diet, alcohol abuse, and smoking promote heart disease, interfere with sleep patterns, and lead to increased rather than reduced tension levels.

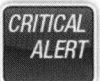

CRITICAL ALERT *Unhealthy lifestyle practices used to reduce stress include alcohol use, tobacco use, abnormal eating patterns, and passive activities.*

Although many disorders result from an overactive stress system, some result from an underactive stress system. This occurs in the case of Addison's disease due to the lack of cortisol. Lack of the hormone CRH also results in the feelings of extreme tiredness common to people suffering from chronic fatigue syndrome. CRH also is central to seasonal affective disorder (SAD), the feelings of fatigue and depression that plague some patients during winter months.

Risk Factors for Stress

At some point in everyone's life, stressful events or conditions develop that overwhelm natural coping mechanisms. Many factors influence susceptibility to stress. People respond differently depending on different factors. These factors have been mentioned before and include early nurturing, personality traits, genetic factors, immune-regulated diseases, and the length and quality of the stressors. Some people are more vulnerable than others to the effects of stress. People who are less emotionally stable or have high anxiety levels tend to experience specific events as more stressful than others. It also has been demonstrated that the lack of an established network of family and friends predisposes one to stress disorders and stress-related health problems, including heart disease and infections (Mayo Clinic, 2006).

CRITICAL ALERT *Stress responses may be influenced by early nurturing or lack thereof, personality traits, genetic factors, immune-related diseases, and length and quality of stressors.*

Work risk factors also must be considered when discussing stress. Job-related stress is particularly likely to become chronic because it is such a large part of daily life (MacDonald, Karasek Punnett, & Scharf, 2001; Parikh, 2004). Stress, in turn, reduces a worker's effectiveness by impairing concentration, causing sleeplessness, and increasing the risk for illness, back problems, accidents, and lost time. Extreme stress, such as harassment or violence on the job, places a burden on the heart and the cardiovascular system.

From a biological perspective, some people exhibit an absent or inadequate relaxation response to stress. Stress hormones remain elevated instead of returning to normal levels. This may occur in highly competitive athletes or people with a history of depression. Scientists also have reported the discovery of a small protein in the brain (orphaninFQ/nocicptin) that plays an important role in the stress response. Animals with a genetic deficiency in this protein are unable to manage stress response and exhibit overanxious behavior in response to new situations. Future research may reveal similar findings in humans (Reuters

Health, 2004). The types of individuals at higher risk for stress are listed in the Risk Factors box.

Coping Strategies for Stress

It has long been understood that how a person adjusts to life stresses is a major component of his ability to lead a fulfilling life. Yet, it was not until the 1980s that coping became a discrete topic of psychological inquiry. Since then, coping has risen to a position of prominence in the modern psychological discourse, especially within the personality, cognitive, and behavioral spheres. As previously discussed the concept of coping has been defined as a compensatory mechanism wherein cognitive and behavioral efforts change constantly to manage specific external or internal demands that are appraised as taxing or exceeding the resources of the person (Lazarus & Folkman, 1984).

RISK FACTORS for Stress

Younger adults	Stress may go unnoticed in the very young and old.
Women in general	Women may be at higher risk than men for stress-related chest pain, but men's hearts may be more vulnerable to adverse effects from long-term stress.
Working mothers	Working mothers face higher stress levels and possibly adverse health effects, most likely because they bear a greater and more diffuse workload than men or other women.
Caregivers of family members	Caregivers of family members with physical or mental disabilities are at risk for chronic stress. They are particularly vulnerable to stress-related health threats such as influenza, depression, and heart disease.
Less educated individuals	Less educated individuals may be at higher risk because they may not be able to differentiate the causes of stress.
Divorced or widowed individuals	Unmarried people generally do not live as long as their married contemporaries.
The unemployed	Being unemployed is an environmental stressor that threatens security.
Isolated individuals	Such individuals usually lack support systems.
People who are targets of racial or sexual discrimination	Discrimination is an environmental stressor that is beyond individual control.
Those without health insurance	This is a threat to one's health that can lead to stress.
People who live in cities	City dwellers may be more stressed as a result of external stressors beyond their control.

Stress and Premature Aging

Clinical Problem

It is well known that stress has a physiological impact on the body and may advance disease and the aging process. Although there has been a deeply held belief that stress leads to premature aging, there has been no hard evidence as to how this might happen until recently. It has now been scientifically demonstrated that prolonged psychological stress affects molecules believed to play a key role in biological aging and, possibly, disease development (Epel et al., 2004; Sapolsky, 2004).

A recent study conducted by Epel and her colleagues (2004) concluded that psychological stress appears to cause cellular damage and premature aging, thereby explaining why intense, long-term emotional strain can make people get sick and grow old before their time. Perceived long-term stress negatively impacts cellular molecules, resulting in increased oxidative stress, lower telomerase activity, and shorter telomere length, all of which are related to cell longevity and disease.

Telomeres are the protective structures (caps) at the end of chromosomes that prevent the DNA strands from unraveling. They also promote genetic stability. Each time a cell divides, the telomeres shorten so that daughter cells have slightly shorter telomeres than their parents and a portion of telomeric DNA dwindles away by a few base parts. After many rounds of cell division, so much DNA has diminished that the aged cell stops dividing. At this point, when the cell stops dividing, it no longer performs its vital functions, and is close to dying. Thus, telomeres play a critical role in determining the health and life span of cells, as well as whatever tissues those particular cells may form.

In effect, chronic stress appears to hasten the shriveling of the tips of the bundles of genes inside cells (the DNA), which threatens their life span and the body's deterioration. The cellular enzyme telomerase acts to replenish a portion of telomeres with each round of cell division, thus protecting these structures. In young people the telomerase is effective in protecting and correcting the cell division process by regenerating the ends. However, as people age, the telomeres shorten significantly and eventually their replication stops all together. Oxidative stress is related to an overabundance of free radical toxins in the body. Free radicals damage lipids, proteins, and DNA, including the DNA of telomeres. Nurses need to understand this degenerative physiological process because it is directly correlated to the perception of high psychological stress. Through assessment and intervention, nurses may be able to help patients cope with stress and mitigate the maladaptive physiological response to stressors, thus, reducing the aging and disease processes.

Research Findings

In 2004 Epel and colleagues at the University of California, San Francisco, conducted a landmark research study in which they found evidence to support the long-suspected association between stress and cellular aging. In a comparison correlational study, they investigated the hypothesis that stress impacts health by modulating the rate of cellular aging through an increase in oxidative stress, lower telomerase activity, and shorter telomere length. They studied both objective (event- or environment-based phenomenon) and subjective (perception-based) stress in 58 healthy premenopausal women who were biological mothers of either a healthy child ($n = 19$, control mothers), or mothers of a child with a chronic illness ($n = 39$, women called caregivers). The latter were predicted to have, on average, environmental exposure to stress. Women in both groups completed a standardized 10-item questionnaire assessing their levels of perceived stress during the past month. This design allowed the researchers to examine the importance of perceived stress and measures of objective stress (caregiving status and chronicity of caregiving stress based on the number of years since a child's diagnosis). They also looked at the chromosomes in the white blood cells of the study participants. Mean telomere length and telomerase activity were measured quantitatively as was oxidative stress.

The research findings did substantiate the proposed hypothesis of the study. As expected, the average perceived stress level was significantly higher in caregivers than in the control group. As a group, caregivers did not differ from controls in telomere length, telomerase activity, or oxidative stress index, but the duration of their chronic stress (number of years spent as a caregiver) varied greatly, from 1 to 12 years. The more years of caregiving, the shorter the length of the telomeres, the lower the telomerase activity, and the greater the oxidative stress level.

The researchers also found significant correlations between perceived stress and all three markers of cellular aging across the entire sample of caregivers and noncaregivers. Notably, telomere length was related to perceived stress in both the control group and the caregiving group. Hence, the relationship between perceived stress and shorter telomeres is not simply because of the severe stress experience by many of the caregivers or because of some biological vulnerability that predisposed their child to have a chronic condition, but rather existed across the continuum of normative stress levels. Although being a caregiver per se was not related to telomere length, the chronicity of caregiving stress was related to telomere length. This finding supported the premise that the perception of being stressed correlated in both the care and control groups with the biological markers.

This correlation held true for oxidative stress as well: The worse the perceived psychological stress, the greater the oxidative stress. In fact, in the most stunning result, the telomeres of women with the highest perceived psychological stress—across both groups—had undergone the equivalent of approximately 10 years of additional aging compared with women across both groups who had lower perceptions of being stressed. The highest stress group also had significantly decreased telomerase activity and higher oxidative stress that the lowest stress group. This was the fist evidence that psychological stress, and how a person perceives stress, may modulate the rate of cellular aging. Further research will explore the relationship of how elevated levels of stress affect the telomeres and telomerase levels by asking the question "Do the chronically elevated levels of stress hormones such as cortisol damage the telomeres and other genes in the body and lower telomerase levels, inhibiting the cells' ability to respond?"

In summary, the study provided evidence that psychological stress, both perceived and chronic, significantly affects cellular integrity and longevity. These findings have implications for understanding how, at the cellular level, stress may promote earlier onset of age-related diseases. This work quantifies a physiological price to feeing highly stressed, drawing on the relationship of mind and body interaction. The researchers concluded that stress is a risk factor—rather than a direct marker—of cell aging. Cell aging, in turn, is a risk factor for later disease. The study also suggests that health care professionals can use these cell markers as a way to monitor health, with very low telomerase or very short telomeres serving as a red flag and indicating the need for professional intervention. Thus,

EVIDENCE-BASED PRACTICE

(continued)

EVIDENCE-BASED PRACTICE

Stress and Premature Aging—*Continued*

the study emphasizes the importance of managing feelings of stress as much as possible in order to give the body a break from the degenerative process. This often means that one has to make life changes that promote a greater sense of well-being.

Implications for Nursing Practice

This study clearly indicates a need for nurses to be aware of the physiological response to chronic stress at the cellular level, which can precipitate or augment disease and aging, particularly in women. Implications for nursing practice begin with the nursing assessment. It is important to specifically question the individual's history and duration of chronic stress. The study emphasizes the importance of having some respite from perceived long-term chronic stress.

It is an inherent responsibility of nurses to determine if the patient perceives chronic stress, to what it is attributable, and how long the perception of high stress has lasted. Following assessment and diagnosis of such, the nurse must be prepared to intervene by providing resources and education to the patient on ways of coping or managing the situation in order to reduce the stress. Most probably this will involve collaborative efforts with the entire health team.

Critical Thinking Questions

1. Explain the relationship of chronic stress to the aging process.

2. Differentiate between the response of young adults and older adults to psychological stress from a physiological and cellular perspective, and explain the relevance of this information to nursing.

3. Classify stress reduction measures that nurses may advise individuals to use when experiencing high psychological stress.

Answers to Critical Thinking Questions appear in Appendix D.

References

Epel, E., & Blackburn, E. H., Lin, J., Dhabhar, F. S., Adler, N. E., Morrow, J. D., et al. (2004). Accelerated telomere shortening in response to life stress. *Proceedings of the National Academy of Sciences of the United States of America,101*(49), 17312–17315.

Sapolsky, R. M. (2004). Organismal stress and telomeric aging: An unexpected connection. *Proceedings of the National Academy of Sciences of the United States of America, 101*(50), 17323–17324.

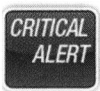 **CRITICAL ALERT** *Coping is influenced by control over the situation. The more control a person has over a situation, the better the person copes. Control is perceived when the stress is internal, transient, and specific. Lack of control stems from stressors that are external, stable, and global.*

Cognitive appraisal and coping are affected by internal characteristics such as health, energy, personal belief systems, commitments or life goals, self-esteem, control, mastery, knowledge, problem-solving skills, and social skills. To date, nursing research has focused on health promotion and hardiness. In many circumstances, it has been found to be more feasible to promote a healthy lifestyle than to alter the stressors. The research often is guided by the transactional model of stress and coping as developed by Glanz, Rimer, & Lewis, 2002. This model provides a framework for evaluating the processes of coping with stressful events. Within this framework stressful experiences are construed as person-environment transactions; these transactions depend on the impact of the external stressor. The impact is mediated by the person's appraisal or perception of the stressor and the individual's availability of social and cultural resources with which to deal with the stressor. Chart 12–5 depicts the key concepts of the Transaction Model of Stress and Coping (Glanz, Rimer, & Lewis, 2002).

Coping strategies, also referred to as stress management, refer to the specific efforts, both behavioral and psychological, that people employ to master, tolerate, reduce, or minimize stressful events (Edelman & Rémond, 2004; MacArthur & MacArthur, 1998; Manktelow, 2003). A distinction that often is made in the coping literature is between active and avoidant coping strategies. Active coping strategies are either behavioral or psychological responses designed to change the nature of the stressor itself or how one

CHART 12–5	**Key Constructs of the Transaction Model of Stress and Coping**

Concept	Definition
Primary appraisal	Evaluation of the significance of a stressful event
Secondary appraisal	Evaluation of the controllability of the stress; a person's coping resources
Coping efforts	Actual strategies used to mediate primary appraisals Strategies directed at changing a stressor.
Problem management, emotional regulation	Strategies aimed at changing the way one feels about a stressful situation
Outcomes of coping	Emotional well-being; functional status

thinks about it, whereas avoidant coping strategies lead people into activities that are considered nonhealthy, for example, alcohol abuse. Generally speaking, active coping strategies, whether behavioral or emotional, are thought to be better ways to deal with stressful events. Avoidant coping strategies appear to a psychological risk factor or marker for adverse responses to stressful life stimuli (Holahan & Moos, 1987) and may become maladaptive. Defense processes, such as denial, also may be included as coping processes, because both defensive and coping processes intertwine and are intrinsic to the psychological integrity of the individual.

Coping resources are defined as characteristics or actions drawn on to manage stress. They include factors in the person or environment that encompass categories such as (1) health, energy, and morale; (2) positive beliefs; (3) problem-solving skills; (4) social skills; (5) social networks; and (6) material networks. According to Lazarus and Folkman (1984), coping mechanisms function in two ways, as problem solving and emotion regulating, being problem focused and emotionally focused. As an individual attempts to deal with demands, internal or environmental, or confront obstacles that create the demands, the person is using the problem-solving method. If, however, the person is concentrating on methods of regulating the emotional response to the problem, the person is using the emotion-focused response to the problem. Coping that is emotion focused seeks to make the person feel better by reducing the emotional distress felt, whereas problem-focused coping aims to make direct changes in the environment so that the situation can be managed more effectively. Oftentimes a combination of problem-focused and emotional-focused coping is used (MacArthur & MacArthur, 1998).

Manktelow's interpretation of stress management is similar to that posed by Lazarus and Folkman, and also can be used as a framework for developing coping strategies. According to Manktelow (2003), three major approaches can be used to manage stress:

- *Action oriented:* in which one seeks to confront the problem causing the stress, often changing the environment or the situation
- *Emotionally oriented:* in which one does not have the power to change the situation, but can manage stress by changing the interpretation of the situation and the way one feels about it
- *Acceptance oriented:* in which something has happened over which one has no power and no emotional control, and where the focus is on surviving the stress.

To be able to take an action-oriented approach, the person must have some power in the situation. If a person does not have the power to change a situation, the situation can be changed by the way the person views it and feels about it. These three approaches to stress management help people to manage the demands placed on them, help people to adjust to perceptions of the situation, and help people survive the situations that they genuinely cannot change.

As a person begins to deal with a stressor, modes of coping may include the following:

- Information seeking (gathering data about the problem and possible solutions to the problem)
- Direct actions (performing concrete acts to alter self or environment)
- Inhibition of action (refraining from an action)
- Intrapsychic processes (reappraising the situation; initiating cognitive activity aimed at improving feelings)
- Obtaining emotional support by turning to others
- Escaping or avoiding.

The choice of coping strategies depends on various factors, such as degrees of uncertainty, threat, or helplessness, and the presence of conflict (Seaward, 2006). If the person is experiencing high uncertainty, direct action is less likely to be selected as a coping strategy. If the degree of threat is severe, more primitive coping modes such as panic are more likely to

occur. In the presence of conflict, an individual may not be able to take direct actions. Helplessness promotes immobilization. The strategy chosen also may be influenced by the outcome of the cognitive appraisal that categorizes the stressor as harm or loss, threat, or challenge. Examples of stress demands and the coping mechanisms people use to handle the stress are shown in Chart 12–6, along with indications of which examples are problem-solving strategies and which are emotion-regulating efforts.

Cultural Considerations

Culture plays a very important role in the choice of a person's coping strategies. Cultures and societies have their own set of rules about what they perceive to be stressful or not. For example, educational systems vary from culture to culture, with some cultures placing greater emphasis on how students do in schools. Access to higher education—and ultimately the better jobs—is determined solely through academic performance. Thus, the stress that the students experience due to this cultural expectation is very high.

People in a monogamous culture will have different responses than those from a polygamous culture. Stressful life events, as described by Holmes and Rahe (1967), will vary among cultures due to different norms and values. Cultural and societal norms must be considered when assisting those from different cultures to identify stressors, stressor resources, and strategies to reduce the stress (Noh & Kaspar, 2003; Wong & Wong, 2006). The Cultural Considerations box (p. 240) discusses two types of cultures, individualist and collectivist, and how they respond to stress.

 *Cultural assessment is instrumental in identifying stressors, stress resources, and coping strategies. Perceptions of stressful life events vary among cultures and are dependent on different norms and values. Nursing interventions must consider cultural norms in order to meet desired outcomes.*

Workplace Culture

Cultural influence also is applicable when discussing work-related stress. Culture has been described as a "defining force" in understanding work habits (Frey-Ridgway, 1997; Parikh, 2004).

CHART 12–6 Examples of Demands and Coping

Demands	Coping
Failing an examination, such as the state board test for nursing	Taking a review course (PS) Studying with friends (PS)
Giving an oral presentation in class for the first time	Practicing in front of a mirror (PS) Taking a walk before class (ER)
Being diagnosed with cancer	Seeking information from a resource library (PS) Discussing with family and friends (ER)
Finding self with insufficient funds to pay monthly bills	Seeking the advice of a financial planner (PS) Exercising daily at the gym (ER)

PS = problem-solving strategy, ER = emotion-regulating strategy.

CULTURAL CONSIDERATIONS Responses by Individualist and Collectivist Cultures to Stress

Individualist cultures (most Western cultures) tend to emphasize personal autonomy and personal responsibility when dealing with problems. They tend to emphasize the importance and value of exerting control over stressful situations. Therefore, members of this type of culture are less likely to seek social support in stressful situations than are people from collectivist cultures (generally Asian and other Eastern countries). Collectivist cultures tend to be more oriented toward their social group, family, or community and toward seeking help with their problems. However, in collectivist cultures, a greater emphasis is placed on controlling one's personal reactions to a stressful situation rather than trying to control the situation itself. It stands to reason then that the learned component of coping, which is arrived at through experiential and reinforcement situations, may stem from cultural and societal values and beliefs.

Each organization or work setting has a unique culture. When there is discord in the work setting or when a person's values and beliefs are at odds with the culture of the setting, stress develops. In fact, work stressors can be identified in almost all aspects of a person's job. Chart 12–7 describes categories and specific components of work-related stressors. The feelings or stressors identified in this chart also can be used as a guided inventory to identify one's own work-related stressors. Difficult interpersonal relationships, discourse with management, and untoward incidents also must be considered as attempts are made to reduce work-related stress.

In most work situations, stress responses cause performance to suffer. As workers become uncomfortably stressed, distractions, difficulties, anxieties, and negative thinking begin to crowd their minds. These thoughts tend to compete with performance of the task for attentional capacity. Concentration suffers, and focus narrows as the brain becomes overloaded. The more overloaded the brain becomes, the more performance can suffer. The more performance suffers, the more new distractions, difficulties, anxieties, and negative thoughts develop.

Research also has shown that stress reduces people's ability to deal with large amounts of information. Both decision making and creativity are impaired because people are unable to take account of all of the information available. This inability accounts for the frequent observation that highly stressed people will persist in a course of action even when better alternatives are available. It also explains why anxious people perform best when they are not put under a lot of additional stress, whereas calm people may need additional pressure to produce a good performance. People perform at their best when they are normally able to concentrate, and focus all of their attention on the important task at hand. It is then that people are sufficiently motivated to resist competing temptations, and anxieties and distractions do not interfere with clear thought (Manktelow, 2003).

Acculturative Stress

In the fast-paced world of today, job-related stress is becoming increasingly recognized as a nontrivial malady that impacts the well-being of both the employees and the organization. Globalization, an irreversible trend of the 21st century, has been widely

acknowledged as having a stress-producing impact on the work setting. The increasing permeability of international borders, cross-border transfers of people and technology, and international mergers and partnerships that fuel globalization are influencing the culture of work settings.

When diverse cultures come together for collective effort in an organization, culture shock could be experienced. This also is known as **acculturative stress**, which can be defined as job-related stress that is exacerbated by cultural differences such as diverse assumptions, values, and beliefs among the participants (Sohmen, 2005). Acculturative stress as a distinct subset of general job-related stress is suggested as a key impediment to personal satisfaction, team morale, and organizational success. Thus, acculturative stress involves multicultural players with more complex, culture-based causes, but with similar symptoms as in job-related stress such as depression, absenteeism, psychosomatic illnesses, low morale, and high turnover (Friedman, Tidd, Currall, & Tsai, 2000).

Gerontological Considerations

It has been found that the ability to achieve a relaxation response after a stressful event becomes more difficult as people age. Elderly people appear to have an impaired resiliency of the HPA axis response to the acute effects of stress (Spencer & Hutchinson, 1999). Conversely, chronic stress may accelerate the aging process by causing overactivity of the HPA axis. Aging may simply wear out the systems in the brain that respond to stress, so that they become inefficient.

Other physiological responses also vary as one ages. It has been scientifically demonstrated that the cardiovascular response to stress is increased in the elderly including such factors as the heart rate, systolic and mean arterial pressure, peripheral resistance and rate pressure product, and lower cardiac output and stroke volumes (Boutcher & Stocker, 1996). In assessing stress among the elderly, the nurse must consider that the elderly very often are exposed to major stressors such as medical problems, the loss of a spouse and friends, a change in a living situation, and financial worries.

 The elderly are affected uniquely by stress. Cardiovascular responses to stress are reflected in changes in:

- *Heart rate*
- *Systolic and mean arterial pressures*
- *Peripheral resistance*
- *Rate pressure product*
- *Lower cardiac output and stroke volume.*

Stress responses also are influenced by lack of coping resources:

- *Social support*
- *Problem-solving skills*
- *Material resources*
- *Medical problems.*

The proposed physiological changes that appear in the elderly also impact their coping responses to stress. Situations perceived as potentially menacing vary throughout life, and consequently, coping styles change. It has been found that coping styles probably vary with age, and that when people age they

CHART 12–7   **Work-Related Stressor Categories and Their Specific Components**

Stressor Category	Specific Components of Category
Disagreement and indecision	Unsure of coworkers' expectations. Unfriendly attitude in coworkers. Job responsibilities go against your better judgment. Cannot satisfy conflicting demands from superiors. Trouble refusing overtime.
Pressure on the job	Overloaded at work, unable to complete tasks during an average day. Too much supervision. Job requirements are taking their toll on your private life. Rushed to complete work or short on time. Too much red tape.
Job description conflict	Uncertainty about your exact job responsibilities. Too much teamwork. Poor flow of information, which makes it difficult to carry out the job. Not enough authority for you to properly do the job. Discomfort in handling unethical assignments.
Communications and comfort with supervisor	Ideas differ from those of the supervisor. Trouble talking to boss. Unable to predict supervisor's reactions. Boss gives little feedback about the work done. Boss is overly critical of the work.
Job-related health concerns	Work conditions are unhealthy. Physical danger exists at workplace. Heavy physical tasks to complete. Hostile threats from coworkers. Sick days are discouraged.
Work overload stress	Cannot consult with others on projects. Coworkers are inefficient. Often take work home to complete. Responsible for too many people/projects. Shortage of help at work.
Work underload stress	Too little responsibility at work. Overqualified for the job. Little chance for growth exists. Trying to "look" busy on job. Feeling unstimulated.
Boredom-induced stress	Performing a repetitive, highly specialized routine. Not learning anything new. Cannot see final outcome of your efforts. Job is too easy. Frequent daydreaming.
Problem of job security	Fear of being laid off or fired. Worry about poor pension. Concern about low wages. Need "pull" to get ahead. Could be fired without cause.
Time pressure	Constant reminders that "time is money." Starting and ending times are rigid. Monotonous pace of work. Not enough break or mealtime. Work pace is too fast.
Job barrier stress	Hope for advancement or raise is limited. Sex/age discrimination exists at job. Not suited to job. Work has no personal meaning. Work goes unrecognized.

Source: American Institute for Preventive Medicine. (2005) Systematic Stress Management Program. www.HealthyLife.com

shift from an active coping style to a more passive one. In addition to the physiological responses to stressors that change, so do some of the cognitive and behavioral responses. Many elderly live alone and many do not have a social support system in place to help them cope. Cognitive problem-solving skills also may be diminished.

Ongoing research in gerontology seeks to examine those situations that elderly adults perceive as potentially menacing, the physical psychosocial implications, and what material resources they have available to face daily demands and establish coping strategies used to diminish the perceived menace. It is critically important for nurses to take these factors into account when assessing the elderly patient and to assist them to evaluate their coping resources and options and to develop effective coping strategies.

Nursing Management

Knowledge of stress, adaptation, and coping theories provides a framework for practice that is applicable to every stage of the nursing process. In caring for patients, the nurse needs to be aware of situations that are likely to be stressful and also to assess and determine the patient's appraisal of the situation and response to the stressor. The nurse also needs to determine the patient's coping resources and strategies as these too impact the patient's physiological and psychosocial response to stressors.

Assessment

Three major areas, previously discussed, serve as a useful guide in the assessment process. These are demands (stressors), the human response to stress, and coping. Although the manifestations of stress vary among individuals, the nurse should assess the patient for the signs and symptoms of the stress that occur as a result of changes in the nervous, endocrine, and immune systems. Also the age of the patient should be considered because many developmental stressors occur at predictable times throughout an individual's life.

Stressors on the patient may include major life changes, events, or situations such as changes in family constellations or daily hassles that the patient is experiencing. The stressors also may be classified as internal and external. Internal demands, aside from perceived tasks and goals, may include physical demands resulting from disease or injury. Additionally, the number of simultaneous demands, the duration of those demands, and previous experience with similar demands should be assessed. It is essential to determine the patient's primary appraisal or perception of the demands to determine if they represent harm or loss, threat, or challenge. Family responses to the patent's demands also should be assessed.

The physiological effects of demands (stressors) that are appraised as stressful are mediated primarily by the sympathetic nervous system and the HPA system. This results in responses such as an increased heart rate, increased blood pressure, loss of appetite, sweating, and dilated pupils. Additionally, the patient may exhibit signs and symptoms related to maladaptation of the immune system or other disorders. Chart 12–8 lists some physiological indicators of stress.

CHART 12–8 Physiological Indicators of Stress

- Pupils dilate to increase visual perception when serious threats to the body arise.
- Diaphoresis increases to control elevated body heat due to increased metabolism.
- Heart rate and cardiac output increase to transport nutrients and by-products of metabolism.
- Skin pales due to constriction of peripheral blood vessels, an effect of norepinephrine.
- Sodium and water retention increase due to release of mineralocorticoids, resulting in increased blood volume.
- Rate and depth of respirations increase because of dilated bronchioles, promotion of hyperventilation.
- Urinary output decreases.
- Mouth may be dry.
- Peristalsis of intestines decreases, resulting in possible constipation and flatus.
- Muscle tension increases in preparation for the fight-or-flight response.
- Blood sugar increases due to the release of glucocorticoids and gluconeogenesis.
- Mental alertness improves with serious threats.

Source: From Kozier, Barbara J.; Erb, Glenora; Berman, Audrey J.; & Snyder, Shirlee J. Fundamentals of Nursing: Concepts, Procedures, & Practices, 7th, © 2004. Electronically reproduced by permission of Pearson Education, Inc., Upper Saddle River, New Jersey.

Behavioral responses include observable actions and cognition of the patient. These may include such behaviors as accident proneness, impaired speech, and anxiety, crying, and shouting. Work-related demands may be manifested in responses such as absenteeism, tardiness, reduced productivity, and job dissatisfaction. Observable cognitive responses include self-reports of excessive demands, inability to make decisions, and forgetfulness. Signs and symptoms of stress are shown in Chart 12–9.

Evaluation of the adequacy and effectiveness of a patient's coping strategies and resources should be assessed. It also is necessary to assess whether or not a certain coping strategy will bring about the desired result. Positive resources might include supportive family members, adequate finances, and the ability to solve problems.

In assessing the individual who seeks health care, it is critical to remember that objective signs and subjective symptoms are the primary indicators of the physiological processes that are occurring. Further signs of change are indicated in diagnostic studies such as computed tomography (CT) and magnetic resonance imaging (MRI). Objective data also may be obtained from laboratory data (e.g., blood glucose, electrolytes, and urinalysis). In making a diagnosis the nurse must relate the symptoms or complaints expressed by the patient to the physical and behavioral signs that are present.

Nursing Diagnoses

Many nursing diagnoses are possible for patients suffering from stress. Anxiety, frustration, anger, and feelings of inadequacy, helplessness, or powerlessness often are emotions associated

CHART 12–9	**Signs and Symptoms of Stress**

General irritability, hyperexcitation, or depression

Dryness of throat and mouth

Urge to cry, scream, or run and hide

Easily fatigued, constantly tired

Floating anxiety

Easily startled

Stuttering

Pacing, moving about, cannot sit still

Gastrointestinal signs and symptoms: "butterflies" in the stomach, diarrhea, vomiting

Changes in menstrual cycle

Loss of or excessive appetite

Increased use of legally prescribed drugs

Injury prone

Disturbed behavior

Pounding of the heart

Emotional instability, impulsive behavior

Inability to concentrate

Feelings of unreality, weakness, or dizziness

Tension

Trembling, nervous tics

Nervous laughter

Grinding of teeth

Insomnia, nightmares, or other sleep difficulties

Excessive perspiration

Frequent urination

Muscle tension and headaches

Pain in the neck or lower back

Increased smoking

Alcohol and drug addiction

Source: This article was published in Stress in health and disease. Selye, H. (1976). Stoneham, MA: Butterworth-Heinemann. Copyright Elsevier, 1976.

CHART 12–10	**Nursing Diagnoses in Coping–Stress–Tolerance Pattern**

Risk Prone Health Behavior

Caregiver Role Strain

Ineffective individual coping:
   Defensive Coping
   Ineffective Denial

Ineffective family coping:
   Coping: Family, Compromised
   Coping: Family, Disabled

Risk for Self-Mutilation

Risk for Other-Directed Violence

Post-Trauma Syndrome

Relocation Stress Syndrome

Coping: Compromised refers to the usually supportive primary person (family member or friend) providing insufficient, ineffective, or compromised support, comfort, assistance, or encouragement that may be needed by the patient to manage the adaptive strategies related to the health challenge (Carpenito, 2007). Specific nursing diagnoses that are derived from the coping–stress–tolerance pattern are shown in Chart 12–10.

NANDA International (formerly the North American Nursing Diagnosis Association) has identified nursing diagnoses related to stress, adaptation, and coping (NANDA, 2007). These are listed below in alphabetical order:

- *Anxiety*: A vague, uneasy feeling of discomfort or dread, the source of which may not be known. It is an alerting signal that warns of impending danger and enables the individual to take measures to deal with a threat.
- *Caregiver Role Strain*: Difficulty in performing the role of caregiver.
- *Compromised Family Coping*: Primary supportive person provides insufficient, ineffective, or compromised support, comfort, or assistance that may be needed by the patient to manage adaptive tasks.
- *Decisional Conflict (Specify)*: Uncertainty about course of action to take when the choice involves risk, loss, or challenge to personal life values.
- *Defensive Coping*: Repeated projection of falsely positive self-evaluation based on a self-protective pattern that defends against underlying perceived threats to positive self-regard.
- *Disabled Family Coping*: Behavior of significant person that disables his or her capacities and the patient's capacities to effectively address tasks essential to adaptation to the health challenge.
- *Fear*: Response to perceived threat that is consciously recognized as a danger.
- *Risk Prone Health Behavior*: Inability to modify lifestyle/behavior in a manner consistent with a change in health behavior.
- *Ineffective Coping*: Inability to form a valid appraisal of the stressors, inadequate choices of practiced responses, and/or inability to use available resources.

with stress. In the presence of these emotions, the customary activities of daily living may be disrupted. For example, a sleep disturbance may be present, activity and eating patterns may be altered, and family processes and roles may be changed.

According to Carpenito (2007), a coping–stress–tolerance pattern has been identified as 1 of 11 functional health patterns. Assessment of the health pattern elicits a description of the coping–stress–tolerance level of a patient, and enables the nurse to identify stressors at the individual or family level. Two overriding diagnoses related to stress have been identified: *Ineffective Coping* and *Compromised, Family Coping*. **Ineffective Coping** is defined as an inability to manage internal or environmental stressors appropriately as a result of inadequate resources (physical, psychological, behavioral, or cognitive). Potential etiologies include disruption of emotional bonds, unsatisfactory support system, sensory overload, and inadequate psychological and physical resources (Carpenito, 2007). **Compromised Family**

- *Ineffective Denial:* Conscious or unconscious attempt to disavow the knowledge or meaning of an event to reduce anxiety/fear, but leading to the detriment of health.
- *Post-Trauma Syndrome:* Sustained maladaptive responses to a traumatic, overwhelming event.
- *Relocation Stress Syndrome:* Physiological and/or psychosocial disturbance following transfer from one environment to another.

Other Nursing Diagnoses
In addition to the examples of nursing diagnoses provided in the preceding section, other applicable diagnoses dealing with stress also include *Social Isolation, Risk for Impaired Parenting, Spiritual Distress, Readiness for Enhanced Family Coping, Situational Low Self-Esteem,* and *Powerlessness.* Because human responses to stress are so varied, as are the sources of stress, arriving at an accurate diagnosis allows interventions and goals to be more specific and leads to improved outcomes.

Outcomes and Evaluation Parameters
Stress management is directed toward reducing and controlling stress and improving coping. The desired patient outcomes of nursing interventions are: illness prevention, improved quality of life as defined by patient, and fewer maladaptive responses to stress. Specific parameters of success in meeting these goals include identification of stressors, identification of stress resources, and use of coping strategies. These serve as measurable parameters on which to evaluate the patient's responses to nursing interventions.

Interventions
Interventions are based on the plans developed in collaboration with the patient, significant support people if possible, and other members of the health care team. They are dependent on the patient's state of health, level of anxiety, support resources, coping mechanisms, and sociocultural and religious affiliation. The nurse and patient need to set goals to change the existing responses to the stressor or stressors.

Although stress is commonplace and occurs daily in one form or another, it also is highly individual. It is, therefore, important to tailor the stress reduction approaches to the individual patient. Interventions that seem to be universal in reducing stress include adequate rest and sleep, time management, optimal nutrition, and physical exercise.

Specific nursing interventions that assist in meeting the goals of stress reduction include the following: promoting a healthy lifestyle, providing stress management education, and recommending support and therapy groups, all of which are discussed next.

Health Promotion
Health and energy aid individuals with their coping strategies; thus, a health-promoting lifestyle provides resources and buffers the impact of stressors. A health risk appraisal may identify lifestyles or habits that place the patient at risk for illness. A health risk appraisal is an assessment method that is designed to promote health by examining an individual's personal habits and recommending changes when a health risk is evident.

Health risk questionnaires estimate the likelihood that a person with a given set of characteristics will become ill. Hopefully, if provided this information, individuals will alter their activities to improve their health. However, research so far has not demonstrated that providing people with such information motivates them to change their behavior. It has been found that the single most important factor for determining health status is social class, and within social class the major factor influencing health is education (Mickler, 1997).

Factors that have been found to be successful in reducing stress include exercise, nutrition, rest and sleep, and time management. Regular exercise promotes both physical and emotional health. Physiological benefits include improved muscle tone, improved cardiopulmonary function, and weight control. Psychological benefits include relief of tension, a feeling of well-being, and relaxation. Good nutrition is essential in increasing the body's resistance to stress. Reducing caffeine, salt, sugar, and fat intake and increasing vitamin and mineral intake will minimize the negative effects of stress, irritability, hyperactivity, and anxiety. Rest and sleep restore the body's energy levels and are an essential element of stress management. Patients may need help in achieving this goal if in pain and they also may need to learn relaxation techniques. People who manage their time effectively usually experience less stress because they feel more in control of their situation. Thus, the nurse may need to help patients prioritize tasks and to consider whether modifications can be made to decrease role demands. This is an important consideration in both inpatient and outpatient settings, particularly as nurses help patients prepare for discharge from acute care to a home environment.

Minimizing anxiety and mediating anger are helpful and appropriate nursing interventions. Nurses carry out measures to reduce patients' anxiety on a daily basis and these activities should be reinforced. These include such measures as explaining procedures before they are performed, administering a massage to help the patient relax, controlling the environment to make it less stressful, providing emotional support to the patient and family, providing an atmosphere of caring and trust, and listening to and validating the patient's perceptions of what is happening and how she is feeling. Mediating anger also is important. Many nurses become upset with the angry patient, who seems irrational, refuses treatment, or becomes verbally abusive. Nurses tend to respond in ways that reduce their own stress, not that of the patient. Fontaine and Fletcher (2003) recommend the following strategies for dealing with patients' anger:

- Know and understand your own response to the feelings and expressions of anger.
- Accept the patient's right to be angry; feelings are real and cannot be discounted or ignored.
- Try to understand the meaning of the patient's anger.
- Ask the patient what contributed to the anger.
- Help the patient "own" the anger; do not assume responsibility for his feelings.
- Let the patient talk about his anger.
- Listen to the patient, and act as calmly as possible.
- After the interaction is completed, take time to process your feelings and your responses to the client with your colleagues.

Always ensure the safety of the patient and others. Do not hesitate to seek help if needed from other staff or security personnel.

 CRITICAL ALERT *Patients may react to stress through anger. The nurse should respond to the angry patient in a constructive manner, not through anger. Always seek help to manage the angry patient when appropriate.*

Using and teaching relaxation techniques are useful mechanisms for stress reduction. Commonly used relaxation techniques include progressive muscle relaxation, meditation, and guided imagery. Specific relaxation techniques that a nurse can teach a patient to help quiet the mind include breathing exercises, massage, biofeedback, yoga, therapeutic touch, music therapy, and humor and laughter. Many agencies have relaxation tapes available for patient use.

Crisis intervention is a short-term helping process of assisting patients to (1) work through a crisis to its resolution, and (2) to restore their precrisis level of functioning. Those in crisis are experiencing an acute, time-limited state of disequilibrium resulting from situational, developmental, or societal sources of stress. They are incapable of coping with or adapting to the stressor by using previous methods of problem solving. They generally have a distorted perception of the event and do not have adequate situational support of coping mechanisms. This is a temporary situation requiring intervention from a professional individual, such as a nurse, physician, psychologist, clergy, or social worker.

The traditional steps of the nursing process closely correspond to the steps of crisis intervention. In the assessment phase, the nurse must focus on the person and the problem, collecting data about the patient, the patient's coping style, the precipitating event, the situational supports, the client's perception of the crisis, and the person's ability to handle the problem. This information provides a basis for future decisions about how and when to intervene and whom to call. An individual's perception of the event and personal response will determine the nursing diagnoses. Diagnoses previously described also are common for people in crisis. Additionally, diagnoses such as *Risk for Self-Directed Violence, Risk for Other-Directed Violence, Rape-Trauma Syndrome,* and *Hopelessness* may be appropriate. Effective planning for crisis intervention must be based on careful assessment and developed in active collaboration with the person in crisis and the significant people in that person's life. Implementation involves crisis counseling and crisis home visits. Crisis counseling focuses on solving immediate problems and it involves individuals, groups, or families. Crisis home visits may be made when telephone counseling does not suffice or when the crisis workers need to obtain additional information by direct observation or to reach a patient who is unobtainable by telephone.

Educating About Stress Management
The goals of nursing educational interventions are to reduce stress and improve the patient's coping ability. These generally are met by providing sensory information and providing procedural information (e.g., preoperative teaching). Teaching structure content, such as a review of cardiovascular anatomy for the cardiac patient or a description of sensations the patient will experience during cardiac catheterization, is one type of preparatory education. This type of education may alter the person–environment relationship such that something that might have been viewed as threatening becomes perceived more positively. Providing patients with information also tends to reduce the emotional response so patients can concentrate and problem solve more effectively.

Enhancing Social Support
As noted, social support has been demonstrated to be effective in mediating life stress. Typically, social support tends to make people feel loved, appreciated, esteemed, and valued. In turn, this tends to elevate the person's sense of self-worth. Those who belong to a social support network share information and make goods and services available to the members on demand. The critical qualities within a social network are the exchange of intimate communications and the presence of solidarity and trust. These social support qualities facilitate an individual's coping behaviors, and create a sense of sharing the stress burden with the individual. The emotions that accompany stress are unpleasant and often increase in a spiraling fashion if relief is not provided. Being able to talk with someone and express feelings openly may help the person gain control of the situation. Nurses can provide this support; however, it is important to identify the person's social support system and encourage its use. Persons who are loners, who are isolated, or who withdraw in times of stress have a high risk of coping failure.

Anxiety also can alter a person's ability to process information, thus, it helps to seek information and advice from others who can assist with analyzing the threat and developing a strategy to manage it. This assists the person in maintaining control and retaining self-esteem. Social networks assist with management of stress by providing the individual with:

- A positive social identity
- Emotional support
- Material aid and tangible services
- Access to information
- Access to new social contacts and new social roles.

Support and Therapy Groups
Support groups are formed for people in similar stressful situations: cancer survivors, people with ostomies, mastectomy patients, parents of autistic children, and those with chronic illnesses and disabilities. There also are groups for drug abusers and alcoholics. Being a member of a group with similar problems or goals generates a releasing effect on a person that promotes freedom of expression and an exchange of ideas. Although not all individuals benefit from membership in such groups, many do. It is the nurse's responsibility, when assessing an individual's stressors and coping resources and strategies, to determine if such an intervention might be helpful to the individual.

Intervention Summary
As noted, a person's psychological and biologic health, internal and external sources of stress management, and relationships with the environment are predictors of health outcomes. These factors are related directly to the individual's health patterns. The nurse plays a significant role in identifying the health patterns of the individual receiving care. If the patient's health patterns are not achieving physiological, psychological, and social

balance, the nurse is obligated, with the consent and assistance of the patient, to seek ways to promote balance through nursing interventions. Many examples of stress reduction techniques, are shown in Chart 12–11. Interventions designed to mediate physiological stress and its effect on the body systems are addressed in greater depth in other chapters of this book.

Evaluation

Desired outcomes provide a guide for evaluating the patient's response to nursing interventions. They serve as indicators of accomplishment or lack of accomplishment in helping the patient reduce the stressors or manage the stressful situation. If outcomes are not achieved, the nurse, patient, support resources, and the health care team need to explore the reasons and revise the interventions as appropriate. Questions such as the following need to be considered:

- How does the patient perceive the problem?
- Is there an underlying problem that has not been identified?
- Were existing coping strategies sufficient to meet intended outcomes?
- How does the patient perceive the effectiveness of new coping strategies?
- Did the patient implement new coping strategies properly?
- Did the patient access and use available resources?
- Have the family and significant others provided effective support?

Additionally, the health care provider should assess physiological values that are indicators of stress. These include vital signs, heart rate, blood pressure, and respiratory rate measurements; level of pain; sleep and rest patterns; and dietary habits.

Collaborative Management

Humans experience stress as an intrinsic part of life and in conjunction with many standard diagnostic, clinical, and experimental manipulations. Unintended stressors, as well as those intended, may significantly affect diagnostic and clinical measures and overall health outcomes. Thus, when conducting clinical, diagnostic, or experimental manipulations, it may be prudent to account for the effects of stress on the specific physiological parameter or health outcome being measured.

Responding to stress signs and symptoms and creating a plan of care require collaboration with all members of the health care team. Depending on the signs and symptoms, the nurse will work with a physician, dietician, physical therapist, respiratory therapist, social worker, and/or home care coordinator. Acute physiological responses to stress in which the patient is experiencing signs and symptoms of critical illness will require close collaboration with the physician in planning, treating, and monitoring care. Other members of the health care team will play an active part in treating respiratory problems, cardiovascular problems, pain, and nutritional imbalances. If stress manifestations are psychological and/or behavioral, it would be prudent for the nurse to collaborate with a psychologist or social worker. The same would hold true for a patient with a nutritional imbalance, or eating habit problems, where the nutritionist or dietician would become a key player.

CHART 12–11 Stress Reduction Techniques	
Maintain a healthy lifestyle by looking after your body.	Maintain regular exercise and a healthy diet rich in a variety of whole grains, vegetables, and fruits, and avoid excessive alcohol, caffeine, and tobacco. Exercise helps by creating a distraction from stressful events and releasing nervous energy.
Discover how to relax.	Relaxation is the polar opposite of the stress response. Deep-breathing exercises may help. If persistently unable to relax, try yoga or t'ai chi. Therapeutic massage also may loosen taut muscles and calm frazzled nerves.
Reduce stress through cognitive-behavioral methods.	Identify sources of stress and question those sources. Whose goals do the stressful activities meet? Can the assumed tasks be reasonably accomplished?
Restructure priorities; add stress-reducing activities.	Shift the balance from stress-producing to stress-reducing activities. Consider as many relief options as possible (e.g., walks, recreation).
Discuss feelings.	Explain your feelings and needs to a trusted individual, in a positive way, or use a journal or letter to express feelings. In return, listen to others.
Keep perspective and look for the positive; shift your outlook.	Focus on positive outcomes; this helps reduce tension and achieve goals. Choose to look at a situation in a more positive way. Step back from the conflict or worry that has put you in knots and ask what part of it is troubling you most. Are you afraid of losing face, or are you so angry that you are in danger of losing self-control. Is your reaction out of proportion? Take a break, talk to someone close and get a different perspective on your troubles.
Use humor.	Use humor and laughter to release pent-up feelings and keep perspective. Laughter also appears to have physical effects that reduce stress hormone levels.
Get help.	Seek professional help from psychiatrists, psychologists, or licensed clinical social workers if unable to change your habitual patterns of thought and behavior that trigger your stress response. Professionals are trained to help you break free of these patterns.

In preparing a patient for discharge from an acute care hospital, the nurse would need to coordinate with, and rely on, the expertise of many other members of the health care team in order to provide a comfortable transition from acute care to the home or extended care environment. And, perhaps most important of all, is the need for the nurse to coordinate with the patient and the patient's family or significant others. As noted throughout the chapter, these people play a key role in providing coping resources and in developing coping strategies. The nurse uses these resources as key elements in implementing the nursing process and developing the plan of care for patients.

Health Promotion

Stress can be a factor in a variety of physical and emotional illnesses, which should be professionally treated. However, many stress symptoms can be managed with over-the-counter medications, for example, aspirin, acetaminophen, or ibuprofen for tension headache, and antacids and antidiarrhea medications for mild stomach distress. However, a physician should be consulted for physical symptoms that are out of the ordinary, particularly those which progress in severity or awaken the patient at night. A mental health professional should be consulted for unmanageable acute stress or for severe anxiety or depression.

In choosing specific strategies for treating stress, several factors should be considered:

- No single method is uniformly successful.
- What works for one person does not necessarily work for someone else.
- Stress can be positive as well as negative. Appropriate and controllable stress can enhance an individual's interest and excitement and motivate the individual to greater achievement. A lack of stress may lead to boredom and depression.
- Stress may play a part in making people vulnerable to illness. A physician or psychologist should be consulted if there are any indications for accompanying medical or psychological conditions, such as cardiac symptoms, significant pain, anxiety, or depression.

Stress Reduction and Impact on Health

An individual's reaction to a specific stressor is different from anyone else's. Some people are naturally laid-back about almost everything, whereas others react strongly at the slightest hint of stress, and most fall somewhere between those extremes. Genetic variations may partly explain the differences. The genes that control the stress response keep most people on a fairly even keel, only occasionally priming the body for fighting or fleeing. Overactive or underactive stress responses may stem from slight differences in these genes. The availability of genetic information and technology enables health care providers to perform screening, testing, and counseling for patients with genetic concerns. Knowledge obtained from the Human Genome Project also has created opportunities for assessing a person's genetic profile and preventing or treating disease.

Life experiences may increase the individual's sensitivity to stress as well. Strong stress reactions sometimes can be traced to early environmental factors. People who were exposed to extreme stress as children tend to be particularly vulnerable to stress as adults.

As explained, stressors develop when the demands of life exceed the ability to cope with them. It follows, then, that stress can be managed by:

- Changing one's environment so that the demands are not so high
- Learning how to better cope with the demands in the environment
- Doing both.

Helpful techniques to accomplish these goals were shown earlier in Chart 12–11.

It is emphasized that treating stress cannot cure medical problems. Stress management is not, therefore, a substitute for standard medical treatments, but it can be an important component in a medical regimen. It has been reported that treatments that reduce psychological distress after a heart attack appear to improve patients' long-term outlooks. It also has been reported that stress management programs may reduce the risk of heart events. Stress management has been found to be effective in coping with anger associated with lowering blood pressure. It also has been found to be effective when used with medications, such as tricyclics, in reducing headaches.

Stress management requires continuous practice as one goes through life and deals with change, often unexpected change. Even if frustrations are taken in stride, the stress response can surge up when dealing with something big, such as illness, job loss, or bereavement. The body's fight-or-flight reaction has strong biological roots. It is there for self-preservation, even if not much help in a demanding job or a difficult relationship. If stress becomes difficult and is potentially causing long-term effects, it is necessary to take action by learning how to recognize the symptoms and by seeking help to mediate the effects of the stress.

▌ Summary

Just as stress is universal, it is a constant factor in caring for patients. The nurse must be able to recognize and treat the physical, psychological, and social manifestations of stress. It is important that nurses recognize the signs and symptoms of stress, both within patients and within themselves, and promote positive adaptive outcomes. To do so, nurses must become familiar with stress theories, understand the physiological, behavioral, and psychosocial responses to stress, and engage in evidence-based practice. Collaborative health care practices are integral to achieving these outcomes and to applying research findings to practices designed to foster improved patient outcomes. Future research opportunities and their impact on clinical practice are shown in the Research Opportunities and Clinical Impact box (p. 248).

RESEARCH OPPORTUNITIES AND CLINICAL IMPACT RELATED TO STRESS

Research	Clinical Impact
Physiological	
Determine types of sedation and analgesics that can best alleviate the stress response and attenuate pain and anxiety.	Provide for appropriate use of sedation and analgesic to improve compliance with care.
Identify the effect of repressed stressful emotions on the psychoneuroimmune axis and the predisposition to illnesses.	Develop treatments specific to the stress-related illnesses. Educate patients about themselves and the body's response to stress.
Determine the effect of stress on wound healing.	Develop wound-healing protocols.
Distinguish between the effects of physical and psychosocial workplace stressors on the etiology of work-related musculoskeletal disorders.	Develop insight into the nature of risk for work-related musculoskeletal disorders.
Identify the possible potentiation of oxidative stress by nursing care activities.	Develop guidelines for care of patients who are critically ill that minimize oxidative stress.
Determine the relationship, if any, between an impaired HPA and axis resiliency during aging.	Realize the affect of stress on aging, and whether or not the HPA axis returns to basal levels after acute stress or to habituate after repeated stress in the elderly.
Explore relationship between postdiagnostic stress and cancer survival.	Provide psychological intervention during the treatment of breast cancer to promote and foster survival.
Explore the relationship between different kinds of abuse at different development stages and potential reversibility of the biological stress vulnerability after psychotherapeutic and psychopharmacological interventions.	Identify implications for the prevention and treatment of mood and anxiety disorders in survivors of early trauma.
Determine if there is a relationship between the clustering of stress indicators and *H. pylori* in the general population.	Treat stress effects on the gastrointestinal system more effectively.
Psychosocial	
Examine social support and its relationship to personality, health, and adjustment	Evaluate the role of social support as a coping resource.
Explore the role that psychosocial factors play in the development of peptic ulcers.	Develop a new paradigm for applying the integrated psychosocial model to medical disorders.
Develop coping measurements.	Expand availability of measurement tools to assess coping.

NCLEX® REVIEW

1. During a focused health interview, a patient identifies a number of external stressors. Which of the following would be considered an external source of stress?
   1. Smoking
   2. Negative self-image
   3. Long commute to work each day
   4. Personal need to work 16 hours each day

2. During a routine health assessment, a patient reports a recent loss of job and divorce however has no health issues to report or discuss. The nurse attributes this patient's ability to handle stress as being:
   1. Disrupted.
   2. Attributed to hardiness.
   3. Able to handle daily hassles.
   4. Situational uplifts.

3. During an assessment, the patient demonstrates physical signs of the alarm phase within the General Adaptation Syndrome. Which of the following is a sign of this phase?
   1. Elevated blood pressure
   2. Normal heart rate
   3. Maintenance of normal weight
   4. Constricted pupils

4. A patient tells the nurse that she needs to be discharged from the hospital soon because she has a job to go to and a family who needs her. The nurse realizes this patient is at risk for additional illnesses because:
   1. She hasn't fully recovered from her current hospitalization.
   2. She shouldn't return to work yet.
   3. The additional stresses of daily life add more stress hormones to the body which can lead to disease.
   4. She isn't focused on her own health.

5. Which of the following would be beneficial to instruct a patient demonstrating signs of oxidative stress?

1. Strive to remove all free radicals from the body.

2. Limit the ingestion of water-based foods.

3. Ingest high doses of vitamin C.

4. Improve nutritional intake including foods containing vitamin E.

6. A patient is demonstrating signs of increasing stress. Which of the following would the nurse assess in this patient?

1. Increased heart rate and blood pressure

2. Cool skin

3. Respiration rate of 12 per minute and regular

4. Bowel sounds present in all quadrants

Answers for review questions appear in Appendix D

KEY TERMS

acculturative stress *p.240*
acute stress *p.225*
acute stressor *p.215*
adaptation *p.215*
atrophy *p.226*
chronic stress *p.225*
cognitive reappraisal *p.220*
Compromised Family Coping p.243
coping *p.215*
developmental stressor *p.215*
dysplasia *p.227*
eustress *p.217*
external stressor *p.215*
general adaptation syndrome (GAS) *p.217*

hardiness *p.219*
hassles *p.220*
homeostasis *p.216*
hyperplasia *p.227*
hypertrophy *p.226*
hypothalamic–pituitary–adrenal (HPA) axis *p.231*
Ineffective Coping p.243
inflammation *p.228*
internal stressor *p.215*
local adaptation syndrome (LAS) *p.217*
maladaptive coping mechanisms *p.215*
metaplasia *p.227*
nutritional imbalance *p.227*

oxidative stress *p.229*
primary appraisal *p.220*
reactive oxygen species (ROS) *p.230*
reticular activating system (RAS) *p.223*
secondary appraisal *p.220*
sense of coherence (SOC) *p.219*
situational stressor *p.215*
steady state *p.222*
stress *p.214*
stress perception *p.214*
stress response *p.214*
stressor *p.214*
uplifts *p.221*

EXPLORE PEARSON mynursingkit™

MyNursingKit is your one stop for online chapter review materials and resources. Prepare for success with additional NCLEX®-style practice questions, interactive assignments and activities, web links, animations and videos, and more!

Register your access code from the front of your book at
www.mynursingkit.com

REFERENCES

Aggleton, J. P. (1992). *The amygdalate.* New York: Wiley-Liss.

Antonovsky, A. (1987). *Unravelling the mystery of health: How people manage stress and stay well.* San Francisco: Jossey-Bass.

Arnsten, A. F. T. (1998). The biology of being frazzled. *Science, 280*(5370), 1711–1712.

Arrighi, J. A., Burg, M., Cohen, I. S., Kao, A. H., Pfau, S., Caulin-Glaser, T., et al. (2000). Myocardial blood-flow response during mental stress in patients with coronary artery disease. *Lancet, 356*(9226), 310–311.

Bernard, L. C., & Krupat, E. (1994). *Health psychology: Biopsychosocial factors in health and illness.* New York: Harcourt Brace.

Blanchard, A. R. (2002). Sedation and analgesia in intensive care: Medications attenuate stress response in critical illness. *Postgraduate Medicine, 3*(2), 59.

Boutcher, S. H., & Stocker, D. (1996). Cardiovascular response of young and older males to mental challenge. *Journals of Gerontology Series B: Psychological Sciences and Social Sciences, 51*(5), P261-P267.

Byrnes, S. (2003). Staying on top of oxidative stress. *The Weston A. Price Foundation modern diseases.* Retrieved January 4, 2007, from http://www.westonaprice.org/moderndiseases/oxidativesterss.html

Cannon, W. B. (1932). *The wisdom of the body.* New York: Norton.

Carpenito, L. J. (2007). *Nursing care plans and documentation: Nursing diagnosis and collaborative problems* (4th ed.). Philadelphia: Lippincott Williams & Wilkins.

Dienstbier, R. A. (1989). Arousal and physiological toughness: Implications for mental and physical health. *Psychological Review, 96*, 84–100.

Edelman, S., Rémond, L. (2004). *Taking charge: A guide for teenagers.* St. Leonards: Foundation for Life Sciences.

Emory University Health Sciences Center. (2006). *Scientists discover possible link between oxidative stress and non-hereditary degenerative disease.* Retrieved January 4, 2007, from http://eurekalert.org/pub_releases/2006-04/euhs-sdp0427-6.php

Espat, N. J., & Helton, W. S. (2000). Oxygen free radicals, oxidative stress, and antioxidants in critical illness. *Support Line, 22*, 11–20.

Everson, S. A., Lynch, J. W., Kaplan, G. A., Lakka, T., Sivenius, J., & Salonen, J. T. (2001). Stress-induced blood pressure reactivity and incident stroke in middle-aged men. *Stroke, 32*, 1263–1270.

Fawcett, J. (2005). *Contemporary nursing knowledge: Analysis and evaluation of nursing models and theories* (2nd ed.). Philadelphia: F. A. Davis.

Fontaine, K. L., & Fletcher, J. S. (2003). *Mental health nursing* (5th ed.). Upper Saddle River, NJ: Pearson Prentice Hall.

Frey-Ridgway, S. (1997). The cultural dimensions of international business. *Collection Building, 16*(1), 12–23.

Friedman, R. A., Tidd, S. T., Currall, S. C., & Tsai, J. C. (2000). What goes around comes around: The impact of personal conflict style on work conflict and stress. *International Journal of Conflict Management, 11*(1), 32–55.

Gabriel, G. (1997). Hans Selye: The discovery of stress. In *Brain Connection.* Oakland, CA: Scientific Learning Corporation. Retrieved December 9, 2006, from http://www.brainconnection.com/topics/printindex.php3?main=fa/Selye

George, J. (Ed.). (2002). *Nursing theories: The base for professional nursing practice.* (5th ed.). Norwalk, CT: Appleton and Lange.

Glanz, K., Rimer, B. K., & Lewis, F. M. (2002). *Health behavior and health education: Theory, research and practice.* San Francisco: Wiley & Sons.

Glaser, G., & Kiecolt-Glaser, J. K. (1994). *Handbook of human stress and immunity.* San Diego: Academic Press.

Goodyear-Bruch, C. & Pierce, J. D. (2002). Oxidative stress in critically ill patients. *American Journal of Critical Care, 11*(6), 543–653.

Green, G., & Smith, R. (2004). The psychosocial and health care needs of HIV-positive people in the United Kingdom: A review. *HIV Medicine, 5*(1), 4.

Grumman, R. (1998). Stomach, digestive system, ulcers, stress. *New Woman, 28*(12), 46–47.

Haddy, R. I., & Clover, R. D. (2001). The biological processes in psychological stress. *Families, System, & Health, 19*(3), 291–302.

Heim, C., Newport, D. J., Heit, S., Graham, V. P., Wilcox, M., Bonsall, R., et al. (2000). Pituitary-adrenal and autonomic responses to stress in women after sexual and physical abuse in childhood. *Journal of American Medical Association, 284*(5), 592–597.

Helfer, R. E., & Kempe, C. H. (1976). *The Abused Child.* Cambridge, MA: Ballinger Publishing Company.

Holahan, C. J., & Moos, R. H. (1987). Risk, resistance, and psychological distress: A longitudinal analysis with adults and children. *Journal of Abnormal Psychology, 96*, 3–13.

Holmes, T. A., Masuda, M. (1966). Magnitude estimations of social readjustments. *Journal of Psychosomatic Research, 11*, 219–225.

Holmes, D., & Rahe, R. (1967). The social readjustment rating scale. *Journal of Psychosomatic Research, 11*, 213–218.

Horowitz, M., Schaefer, C., Hiroto, D., Wilner, N., & Levin, B. (1977). Life event questionnaires for measuring presumptive stress. *Psychosomatic Medicine, 39*(6), 413–431.

Kalantaridou, S. N., Makrigiannakis, A., Zoumakis, E., & Chrousos, G. P. (2004). Stress and the female reproductive system. *Journal of Reproductive Immunology, 62*(1), 61–68.

King, I. (1971). *Toward a theory of nursing: General concepts of human behavior.* New York: John Wiley & Sons, Inc.

Kobasa, S. C., Maddi, S. R., & Zoda, M. A. (1983). Type A and hardiness. *Journal of Behavioral Medicine, 6*(1), 41–51.

Kop, J. J. (1999). Chronic and acute psychological risk factors for clinical manifestations of coronary artery disease. *Psychosomatic Medicine, 61*, 476–487.

Lazarus, R. S. (1966). *Psychological stress and the coping process.* New York: McGraw-Hill.

Lazarus, R. S., & Cohen K. B. (1977). Environmental stress. In I. Altman & J. F. Wohlwill (Eds.), *Human behavior and environment* (Vol. 2). New York: Plenum Press.

Lazarus, R. S., & Folkman, S. (1984). *Stress, appraisal, and coping.* New York: Springer Publishing.

Lazarus, R. S., & Launier, R. (1976). Stress related transactions between person and environment. In L. A. Pervin & M. Lewis (Eds.), *Perspectives in international psychology* (pp. 87–327). New York: Plenum Press.

Levenstein, S. (1998). Stress and peptic ulcer: Life beyond *Helicobacter. British Medical Journal, 316*, 538–541.

Levenstein, S. (2003). Stress and ulcerative colitis: Convincing the doubting Thomases. *American Journal of Gastroenterology, 98*(10), 2203–2208.

Litt, M. D. (1988). Cognitive mediators of stressful experience: self-efficacy and perceived control. *Cognitive Therapy and Research, 12*(3), 241–260.

Lobo, M. L. (2002). Environmental model: Florence Nightingale. In J. B. George (Ed.), *Nursing theories: The base for professional nursing practice* (5th ed., pp. 43–60). Upper Saddle River, NJ: Pearson Prentice Hall.

MacArthur, J. D., & MacArthur, C. T. (1998). *Coping strategies.* Research Network on Socioeconomic Status and Health. Retrieved March 2, 2005, from http://www.maces.ucsf.edu/Reserach/Psychosocial/notebook/coping.html

MacDonald, L. A., Karasek, R. A., Punnett, L., & Scharf, T. (2001). Covariation between workplace physical and psychosocial stressors: Evidence and implications for occupational health research and prevention. *Economics, 44*(7), 696–718.

Malinski, V. M. (2006). Rogerian science-based nursing theories. *Nursing Science Quarterly, 19*, 7–12.

Mandler, G. (1982). Stress and thought processes. In L. Goldgerger and S. Breznitz (Eds.), *Handbook of stress: Theoretical and clinical aspects.* New York: The Free Press.

Manisses Communications Group. (2003). In case you haven't heard. *Mental Health Weekly, 13*(36), 8.

Manktelow, J. (2003). *Stress management techniques from mind tools: Introduction to stress management.* Retrieved December 14, 2006, from http://www.mindtools.com/stress/UnderstandStress/StressIntro.htm

Marriner-Tomey, A., & Alligood, M. R. (2006). *Nursing theorists and their work,* (6th ed.). St. Louis: Mosby.

Maté, G. (2003). *When the body says no: Understanding the stress–disease connection.* Hoboken, New Jersey: Wiley & Sons.

Mayer E. A., Naliboff, B. D., Craig, A. D. (2006). Neuroimaging of the brain-gut axis: from basic understanding to treatment of functional GI disorders. *Gastroenterology, 131*, 1925–42.

Mayo Clinic. (2006). *Reduce stress with a strong social support network.* Retrieved January 5, 2007, from http://www.mayoclinic.com/health/social-support/SR00033

Mickler, M. (1997). *Community organizing and community building for health.* New Brunswick, NJ: Rutgers University Press.

NANDA International. (2007). *NANDA nursing diagnoses: Definitions and classification 2007–2008.* Philadelphia: Author.

National Institutes of Health. (2004). *Stress system malfunction could lead to serious, life threatening disease.* Retrieved November 12, 2004, from http://www.mayoclinic.com/findinformation/conditotncenters/subcenters/cfm

Neuman, B., & Fawcett, J. (2002). *The Neuman systems model* (4th ed.). Upper Saddle River, NJ: Pearson Prentice Hall.

Nightingale, F. (1957). *Notes on nursing.* Philadelphia: J. B. Lippincott. (Original publication in 1859).

Noh, S., & Kaspar, V. (2003). Perceived discrimination and depression: Moderating effects of coping, acculturation, and ethnic support. *American Journal of Public Health, 93*(2), 232–238.

Norman, D. (2003). The effects of stress on wound healing and leg ulceration. *British Journal of Nursing, 12*(21), 1256–1263.

Parikh, P. (2004). Occupational stress and coping in nurses. *Journal of Health Management, 6*(2), 115–127.

Parker, M. E. (2006). *Nursing theories and practice.* Sudbury, MA: Jones and Bartlett.

Pickering, T. G. (2001). Mental stress as a causal factor in the development of hypertension and cardiovascular disease. *Current Hypertension, 3*, 249–254.

Polit, D., & Beck, C.T. (2008). *Nursing research: Generating and assessing evidence for nursing practice* (8th ed.). Philadelphia: Lippincott Williams & Wilkins.

Porth, C. M. (2007). *Essentials of pathophysiology: Concepts of altered health states.* Philadelphia: Lippincott Williams & Wilkins.

Pugliese, P. (1995). The skin, free radicals, and oxidative stress. *Dermatology Nursing, 7*, 316–369.

Reuters Health. (2004). Retrieved January 20, 2004, from http://www.reutershealth.com/wellconnected/doc31.html

Rivas, P. (2003). *Turn off the hunger switch naturally.* Ferndale, WA: Appleton Publishing.

Rogers, M. (1970). *The theoretical basis of nursing.* Philadelphia: F. A. Davis Co.

Roy, C. (1990). Response: conceptual clarification. *Nursing Science Quarterly, 3*, 64–66.

Roy, C., & Andrews, H. A. (2005). *The Roy adaptation model* (3rd ed.). Upper Saddle River, NJ: Pearson Prentice Hall.

Schwaertz, A. R., Gerin, W., Davidson, K. W., Pickering, T. G., Brosschot, J. F., Thayer, J. F., et al. (2003). Toward a causal model of cardiovascular responses to stress and the development of cardiovascular disease. *Psychosomatic Medicine, 65* (1), 22–35.

Seaward, B. L. (2006). *Managing stress: Principles and strategies for health and well-being* (4th ed.). Sudbury, MA: Jones and Bartlett.

Segerstrom, S. C., & Miller, G. E. (2004). Psychological stress and the human immune system: A meta-analytic study of 30 years of inquiry. *Psychological Bulletin, 104*, 601–630.

Selye, H. A. (1936). Syndrome produced by diverse nocuous agents. *Nature, 138*, 32.

Selye, H. (1976). *The stress of life* (rev. ed.). New York: McGraw-Hill.

Senior, K. (2001). Should stress carry a health warning? *Lancet, 357*(9250), 126.

SixWise.com. (2006). *Stress now proven to cause weight gain in women: Five key stress-reduction tips.* Retrieved January 4, 2007, from http://www.sixwise.com/newsletters/05/03/15/stress_now_proven_to_cause_weight_gain_i...

Sohmen, V. (2005). *Acculturative project stress.* Umed School of Business & Economics, Umed University, Sweden. Retrieved December 28, 2006, from http://www.fek.umu.se/~VS

Spencer, R. L., & Hutchinson, K. E. (1999). Alcohol, aging, and the stress response. *Alcohol Research & Health, 23*(4), 272–283.

Taylor, S. E., Klein, L. C., Lewis, B. P., Gruenewald, T. L., Gurung, R. A. R., & Updegraff, J. A. (2000). Biobehavioral responses to stress in females: Tend-and-befriend, not fight-or-flight. *Psychological Review, 107*, 411–429.

Thomas, K. S., Nelesen, R. A., Ziegler, M. G., Bardwell, W. A., & Dimsdale, J. E. (2004). Job strain, ethnicity, and sympathetic nervous system activity. *Hypertension, 44*(6), 891–896.

Tomey, A. M., & Alligoud, M. R. (2005). *Nurse theorists and their work* (6th ed.). Philadelphia: Mosby.

Truelsen, T., Nielsen, N., Boysen, G., & Gronbaeck, M. (2003). Self-reported stress and risk of stroke. *Stroke, 34*, 856–866.

Van Egeren, L. V. (2000). Stress and coping and behavioral organization. *Psychosomatic Medicine, 62*, 451–460.

Wan, R., Camandolal, S., & Mattson, M. P. (2003). Intermittent food deprivation improves cardiovascular and neuroendocrine responses to stress in rats. *The Journal of Nutrition, 133*, 1921–1930.

Wein, H. (2000). *Stress and disease: New perspectives. The NIH Word on Health.* Retrieved March 9, 2006, from http://www.nih.gov/news/WordonHealth/soryol.htm

Wilkin, T. (2005). A definition of disease. *Future Positive.* Retrieved January 4, 2007, from http://futurepositive.synearth.net/eoo5/12/05?print-friendly=true

Wong, P. T. P. , & Wong, L. C. J. (Eds.). (2006). *Cross cultural psychology.* New York: Springer Publishing.

Psychosocial Issues in Nursing

Leslie Rittenmeyer

Outcome-Based Learning Objectives

After studying this chapter, the learner will be able to:

1. Discuss conceptual foundations that inform psychosocial nursing.
2. Define the characteristics of a therapeutic nurse–patient relationship.
3. Utilize culturally competent principles of therapeutic communication for the care of patients and significant others.
4. Apply the principles of teaching and learning to the care of patients and significant others.
5. Identify the dimensions of crisis and the nursing actions that promote adaptive coping.
6. Discuss the impact of illness and hospitalization on patients and significant others.
7. Compare and contrast the psychodynamics of anxiety, frustration, anger, depression, and loss and grief.
8. Utilize the nursing process for patients experiencing loss and grief, anxiety, depression, and anger.

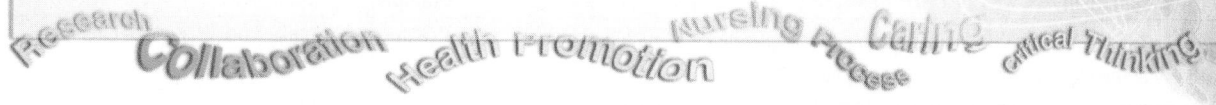

NURSING IS about caring for persons throughout their life span. Nurses are privileged to share some of the most intimate moments in people's lives. They are present for joyful events, like the birth of a child or the successful outcome of a health care crisis, and heartrending events, like the death of a loved one or being presented with a grave prognosis. When nurses care for the whole person, they learn about the rich fabric of their patient's life.

During a person's life span, experiencing periods of both health and illness is inevitable. These experiences influence how people perceive themselves in relation to their own health belief model as well as the health care delivery system. Nurses play a pivotal role in shaping these experiences, and it is often through their influence that patients are able to give meaning to their experiences. In the process patients are empowered to assume more autonomy for their health care decisions. To achieve a positive health care outcome, nurses need to monitor and respond to the holistic needs of patients and their families. This means acknowledging patients as biopsychosocial spiritual beings who are more than the sum of their parts. Developing a knowledge base in the principles of psychosocial nursing helps the nurse apply the nursing process to psychosocial concerns in a holistic way.

Theoretical Foundations

An array of theoretical perspectives informs the practice of psychosocial nursing. Theories provide a scientific basis for practice and further aid in conceptualizing practice situations. Theories also offer a road map for predicting what may happen in a particular practice situation and often provide guidance about what has been effective in the past. A wide variety of theories are applicable to psychosocial nursing. Some of these theories have been borrowed from other disciplines; others are shared theories and have been modified for nursing practice; and yet others are theories specific to the discipline of nursing. This chapter introduces the reader to some of the theories that are most relevant to the practice of psychosocial nursing.

Psychoanalytical Perspective

The psychoanalytical perspective is attributed to the work of Sigmund Freud (1935). The work of Freud was revolutionary for the time, and he was one of the first scientists to suggest a mind–body interaction. He was also one of the first to suggest the importance of the unconscious in mental functioning. He divided aspects of the conscious into three categories. The first category he called the **conscious**, which includes all things that are easily remembered, such as one's mother's name, one's address, or one's favorite food. The second category was termed the **subconscious** and includes those things that have been forgotten but can easily be brought to consciousness, such as an old address, the feelings a man had on his wedding day, or the feeling of wonder at the birth of a first child. The third category was termed **unconscious** and encompasses all of those things that cannot be remembered or brought to conscious thought.

Freud also conceptualized three components of personality. He called these the id, ego, and superego. The **id** represents all of a person's biological and psychological drives. Drives are inborn psychological tensions that call for mental action in order to obtain instant gratification of needs. The id is primitive and instinctual and is often associated with sexual and aggressive impulses. The id does not consider reality or morality as it attempts to reduce psychic tension. The principle of tension reduction is called the **pleasure principle.**

The purpose of the **ego** is to mediate the urges of the id with a dose of reality. It helps individuals make a connection between the realities of the real world and the demands of the id in a way that promotes well-being and survival. An additional function of the ego is to protect the mind against conflict-laden impulses coming from the id. The ego obeys a reality principle.

The ego does not concern itself with morality or social norms. This role is reserved for the **superego.** The superego is really an extension of the ego and represents individuals' early moral training and ideal values imparted by societal norms. The emphasis of superego functioning is not reality but the ideal. To put it simply, the superego tells a person what is right and what is wrong and acts as a control system to help the ego assist the id in choosing objects of gratification that are not immoral.

The concept of anxiety is a thread that runs through the psychoanalytical perspective. Anxiety is conceptualized by Freud as a feeling of discomfort and tension that alerts the ego to a perceived threat or loss of inner control. Once warned, the ego can then undertake a wide variety of rationale defenses to decrease the feelings of discomfort and tension. If, however, the anxiety is overwhelming and the ego is unable to cope, the ego resorts to less rationale coping mechanisms. These processes are called the **ego defense mechanism** and are utilized to alleviate anxiety by denying, distorting, and misinterpreting reality. Although the ego defense mechanisms are helpful for a time, their overuse does not constitute healthy coping. For the most part the ego defense mechanisms operate at an unconscious level. Chart 13–1 provides an explanation of the ego defense mechanisms.

Developmental Perspective

Erik Erikson (1963) is best known for his theory on how humans develop across the life span. He embraced some of Freud's conceptualizations but expanded them to include the influence of culture and society on human development. He felt that the determinants of personality development were not

---

CHART 13–1	**Ego Defense Mechanisms**

Defense Mechanism	Example
Identification: Helps people avoid feeling devalued by adopting the characteristics or behavior of someone who is either feared or respected.	A young girl identifies with her teacher whom she admires.
Introjection: Helps people gain social acceptance by accepting the norms and values of others even if contrary to own beliefs.	A teen who uses drugs tells her brother that it is wrong to use drugs.
Projection: Allows people to avoid acknowledging their own shortcomings by blaming others or the environment for their own unacceptable motives.	A employee who does not do his job blames the incompetence of his boss.
Displacement: Allows people to discharge their emotions on a safer object or person by substituting a less threatening target or person for the recipient of their emotions.	A teenager has a very bad day at school and comes home and fights with her sister.
Rationalization: Allows people to cope with their inability to meet certain goals or standards by justifying behavior that is unacceptable as a socially acceptable rationale.	A man who verbally abuses his wife says "At least I don't hit her."
Denial: Allows people to avoid the full impact of a threatening situation by ignoring or screening the realities of the situation.	A patient who has been told she has a terminal illness is heard making plans for an extended trip abroad.
Repression: Helps people avoid trauma until they have the resources to do so by keeping a threatening thought out of awareness. The repressed material is denied entry into consciousness.	A person who was present at a terrorist attack cannot remember any of the details.
Regression: Helps people to return to a more comfortable time by allowing them to return to a level of functioning that is less demanding.	A very ill patient allows his nurse to nurture and care for him.
Reaction formation: A mechanism that allows people to act the opposite to the way they really feel.	A person who privately likes pornography becomes an advocate of censorship.
Intellectualization: Allows people to protect themselves from hurt by using a rational explanation to remove the personal significance of an incident.	A man's ill father dies and the son says "He wouldn't have wanted to live like that."
Undoing: Allows people to relieve guilty feelings or make amends by acting to annul some act or thought.	A teacher who makes a test too hard curves it so almost everyone passes.
Compensation: Allows people to overcome deficits by emphasizing a more desirable trait or by overachieving in a more comfortable area.	A nonathletic person becomes a sports announcer.
Sublimation: Allows people to avoid acting in socially unacceptable ways by substituting acceptable behavior.	A person with uninhibited sexual drives becomes morally religious.
Substitution: Allows people to keep frustrations to a minimum by replacing a highly valued or nonattainable object with an acceptable or attainable object.	A person wants to write for the *New York Times* but settles for working for her hometown newspaper.

just instinctual and biological as Freud theorized, but social and cultural as well.

Erikson conceptualized eight developmental stages, starting at birth and ending at death. Each of these stages is characterized by a developmental task that must be achieved in order for the person to develop in a healthy manner. Erikson did believe that if a task was not met at an earlier developmental stage, a person could later go backwards and meet the task of that stage successfully. Chart 13–2 provides an explanation of Erikson's developmental stages and tasks and their defining characteristics.

Another developmental theorist who has gained attention is Urie Bronfenbrenner (1979). In his work Bronfenbrenner emphasizes the social contexts in which children develop. A major thesis of his work is that "human abilities and their realization depend in significant degree on the larger social and institutional context of individual activity" (p. 23). His theory of ecological development calls attention to the importance of considering the influences of multiple settings on development. Chart 13–3 (p. 254) provides a summary of Bronfenbrenner's ecological theory.

CHART 13–2	Erikson's Stages of Growth and Development	
Stage	**Developmental Period**	**Explanation**
Trust vs. mistrust	Infancy (first year)	Occurs in the first year of life. The development of trust requires consistent, nurturant caregiving. A positive outcome is the development of feelings of comfort and security attained from having needs met. A sense of mistrust develops when a child is treated negatively and/or is neglected and cannot consistently get her needs met.
Autonomy vs. shame and doubt	Infancy (second year)	Occurs in late infancy and early toddler years. After gaining trust in their caregivers, infants begin to realize that their behavior is their own. It is natural for them to assert their independence and realize that they have a mind of their own. This is how they gain a sense of their own autonomy. If infants are restrained too much (overprotected) or punished too harshly, a sense of shame and doubt occurs.
Initiative vs. guilt	Early childhood (preschool years, ages 3–5)	As young children experience a widening social circle, they are challenged more than they were as infants. To cope with these changes, they need to engage in active, purposeful behavior. In this stage adults expect children to become more responsible and require them to assume more responsibility for taking care of their bodies and belongings. Developing a sense of responsibility increases the child's sense of initiative. Children develop an uncomfortable guilt feeling if they are irresponsible or made to feel too anxious.
Industry vs. inferiority	Middle and late childhood (elementary school years, age 6 to puberty)	The development of initiative in the previous stage brings children into contact with a wealth of new experiences. As they move into the elementary school years, they direct their energy toward mastering knowledge and intellectual skills. At no time are children more enthusiastic about learning than at the end of their childhood, when this imagination is expansive. The danger of this developmental stage is developing a sense of inferiority, unproductiveness, and incompetence.
Identity vs. identity confusion	Adolescence (ages 10–20)	Adolescents try to figure out who they are, what they are about, and where they are going in life. They are confronted with many new roles, some of them adult roles (such as vocational and romantic). Adolescents need to be allowed to explore different paths to attain a healthy identity. It is a time for them to practice the skills they need to become adults. If adolescents do not adequately explore different roles and are not allowed to practice for their adult roles, they develop confusion about their own independence and identity.
Intimacy vs. isolation	Early adulthood (20s and 30s)	The developmental task is to form positive close relationships with others. Erikson describes intimacy as finding one's self but losing one's self in another person. The hazard of this stage is that one will fail to form an intimate relationship with either a romantic partner or through friendship and thus become socially isolated. For such individuals loneliness becomes a looming problem.
Generativity vs. stagnation	Middle adulthood (40s and 50s; later for some)	Generativity means transmitting something positive to the next generation. This can be done through roles of parenting, teaching, or through social activism. Generativity is about leaving a legacy to the next generation. Stagnation is the feeling of having done nothing to help the next generation or failure to leave a legacy.
Integrity vs. despair	Late adulthood	Older adults review their lives, reflecting on what they have done and accomplished. If the retrospective evaluations are positive, a sense of integrity is felt. That is, they can say to themselves "My life was worth living." In contrast, older adults become despairing if, when they look backward, their evaluations are predominantly negative.

Source: Ball, J. W., & Bindler, R. C. (2006) *Child health nursing: Partnering with children & families.* Upper Saddle River, NJ: Pearson Prentice Hall.

CHART 13–3	Bronfenbrenner's Ecological Theory

System	Description
Microsystem	A setting in which the individual spends a lot of time. Most immediate influence on the person. Focus is on face-to-face interactions. Developmental influences include family, peers, school and neighborhood, and religious institutions. Within these microsystems the individual has interaction with parents, teachers, peers, and others. The individual is not a passive recipient of experiences in these settings, but someone who reciprocally interacts with others and helps to construct the setting.
Mesosystem	Links microsystems together. Examples are the connections between family experiences and school experiences, for example, parent–teacher conferences. Experience in one microsystem can affect experiences in another microsystem. For example, an abused child may have difficulty being successful in school.
Exosystem	Setting in which a person does not actually participate but nonetheless exerts an influence. For example, a major layoff by a city's largest employer can affect families. The raising of property taxes by a city council can affects city schools, which in turn affects the individual.
Macrosystem	International and global influences, including the attitudes and ideologies of the culture. Involves the broader culture in which the individual lives, including the society's values and customs. Culture is a broad concept and affects the development of individuals in different ways. For instance, gender roles in one culture are transmitted differently in another culture. Culture includes the roles of ethnicity and socioeconomic factors in development.
Chronosystem	The sociohistorical conditions of an individual's development. For example, children today are living a childhood of firsts: the first day care generation, the first technological generation, the first post–sexual revolution generation. All of these sociohistorical contexts affect the development of individuals.

Source: Paquette, D., & Ryan, J. (2008). Brofenbrenner's ecological theory. National-Louis University. Accessed 5/24/2008 at http://pt3.no.edu/paquetteryanwebquest.pdf

Humanistic Perspective

The work of Abraham Maslow represents what is known as the "third force" in the field of psychology. He wished to provide an alternative to the somewhat mechanistic view of the psychoanalytical and behaviorist perspectives. The humanistic perspective believes that behavior is shaped by people's own perceptions of themselves, their subjective views of the world, and the need of all human beings to experience growth.

Maslow theorized a hierarchy of human needs in which some needs are perceived as more prevailing than other needs. The physiologic needs, such as air, water, and food, are placed on the bottom rung of the hierarchy. The next rung is the need of individuals to feel safe and secure, followed by the need for love and belonging. Further toward the top of the hierarchy is the need for self-esteem. Needs on the first four rungs of the hierarchy are labeled **basic human needs**. Maslow labeled these lower rung needs as *deficit needs*. The next group on the hierarchy is the group of **growth needs**. Maslow identified these as the need to know and understand, aesthetic needs, and self-actualization and transcendence needs. He believed that the higher needs are met only after the lower needs have been satisfied. For example, if a person is without food, it is unlikely that the person will be concerned about her aesthetic needs. Figure 13–1 ■ illustrates Maslow's hierarchy of basic human needs.

Cognitive Development

Jean Piaget (1969) was interested in the cognitive development of children. He theorized that children develop cognitively through their exposure to the world around them. The basic mental structure of Piaget's theory is called a **schema**. Schemas are coordinated patterns of recurring action and are created for the purpose of organizing and interpreting information. As such, children's ability to think matures through two processes, assimilation and accommodation. **Assimilation** occurs when a child incorporates new knowledge into an already existing schema. **Accommodation** occurs when a child must modify an existing schema because the incorporation of new knowledge does not fit into his existing schema (Ball & Bindler, 2006). For example, a child is given a broom to sweep the floor. He has never really swept a floor before, but has watched his father do it and knows that to sweep one has to move the broom back and forth over the floor. He assimilates his behavior into what schemas he already has. But the broom is too big for him and he is holding it up close to the top, so he adjusts his hands lower on the broom handle in order to get a better sweeping action, therefore accommodating adjustments to his existing schema.

Piaget further theorized that children move through stages of cognitive development. The speed at which a child develops cognitively is variable and often depends on a multitude of factors such as genetics and the environment. This information is important to the nurse when considering developmentally appropriate teaching–learning strategies. Chart 13–4 summarizes Piaget's stages of cognitive development.

Cognitive Theory

Cognitive theory has impacted the treatment of a broad range of emotional and mental health disorders. It is based on the premise that mental health symptoms are related to how individuals view themselves and the world around them. Cognitive theory posits that individuals develop a set of core beliefs as a result of interacting with the environment. These beliefs or schemas can be positive or negative. A positive example could be the belief that women are strong and powerful. A negative belief could be the belief that women are weak and helpless. Schemas influence how individuals interpret and evaluate experiences, and behaviors are often the result of these interpretations.

Another construct in cognitive theory is that of the cognitive triad. The cognitive triad is influenced by negative schemas that influence people to (1) see themselves as inadequate, (2) negatively misinterpret an experience, and (3) view the future in a

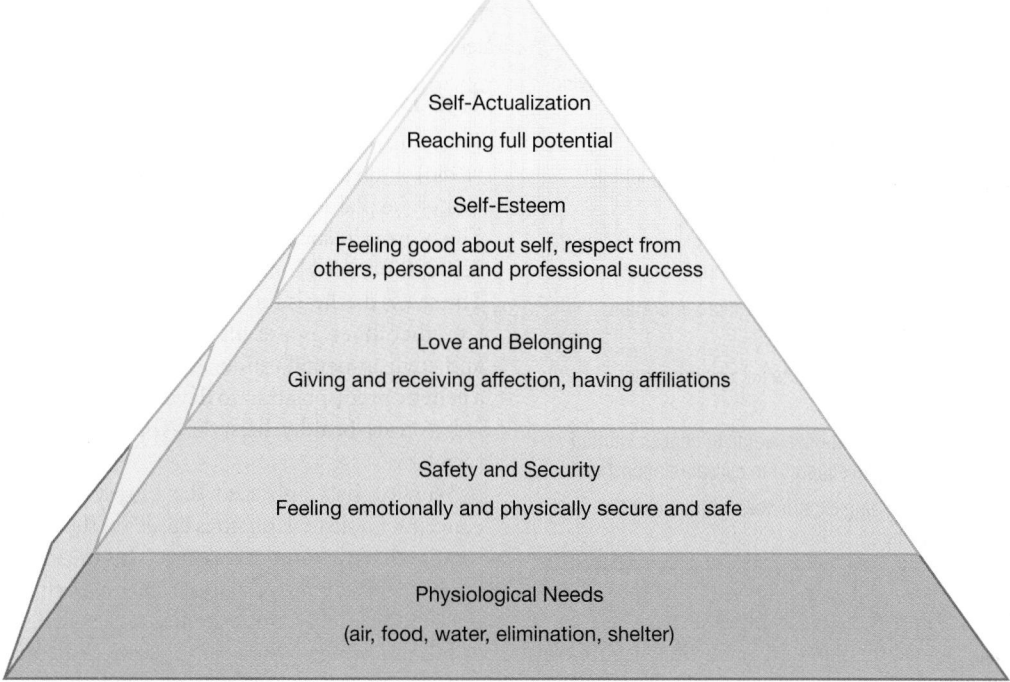

FIGURE 13–1 ■ Maslow's hierarchy of needs.

| CHART 13–4 | Piaget's Stages of Cognitive Development |

Stage	Typical Achievements and Behaviors
Sensorimotor (birth–1½ or 2 years)	Thought is based on action. Infants suck, grasp, look, reach. A child learns about objects through sensory input. These responses become organized into complex activities such as eye–hand coordination and are applied to the environment to solve problems such as reaching for and manipulating objects.
Preoperational (1½–7 years)	Children begin to acquire language and mental imagery. They learn to do symbolic play. They may have difficulty understanding that another person sees, feels, or thinks differently from themselves (egocentrism). Thinking is unidimensionally focused on a single concept. They exhibit precausal (transductive) reasoning, having an incomplete understanding of cause and effect. One manifestation of precausal reasoning is magical thinking, that is, thinking that they can make things happen. Another manifestation is animism, the tendency to attribute human characteristics to inanimate objects. Ability to reason is inconsistent.
Concrete operational (7–11 years)	Children in this stage are capable of mental operations, which follow logical rules for transforming and manipulating information. They develop the ability to classify things. They are no longer fooled by appearances. They can reason effectively about classes of objects and their relationships.
Formal operational (11 years and older)	Adolescents are able not only to imagine but to reason about hypothetical situations. Abstract issues (for example, religion, morality, alternative life styles) can be considered and systematically evaluated. Adolescents are able to think about their own thinking (metacognition). There is a renewed egocentrism, a belief that one is unique and the center of others' attention.

Source: Ball, J. W., & Bindler, R. C. (2006) *Child health nursing: partnering with children & families.* Upper Saddle River, NJ: Pearson Prentice Hall.

negative way. Beck and Freeman (1990) suggest that being stuck in the cognitive triad leads to the development of cognitive distortions, which in return may result in the development of mental health symptoms. See Chart 13–5 (p. 256) for examples of cognitive distortions.

Assessing the cognitive distortions of patients and identifying how their cognitive triads influence the ways in which they are evaluating their health care situation can help the nurse design more effective interventions. One way to challenge cognitive distortions is to provide education that assists patients and

families in examining all available evidence about a situation so that they are informed about options and alternatives. This helps them develop problem-solving strategies that focus away from the most negative extremes of the situation.

Family Systems

In the practice of nursing, it is inevitable that the care of patients will call for inclusion of the family. In today's culture, "family" includes all of those significant others in a person's life such as life partners, friends, or roommates. The family is the mediator

CHART 13–5	**Cognitive Distortions**
Arbitrary inference	Coming to a specific conclusion without having any supporting evidence or in the face of contradictory evidence.
Selective abstraction	Conceptualizing a situation while ignoring contradictory information.
Overgeneralization	Taking specific information and generalizing it broadly to unrelated situations.
Magnification	Seeing something as far more important than it is.
Minimization	Seeing something as far less important than it is.
Personalization	Attributing external events to oneself without evidence to support the causal relationship.
Dichotomous thinking	Categorizing experiences with all-or-none reasoning.

between the individual and society. Family assumes the role of helping its members meet their needs, including health care needs. The family often wishes to be involved in all aspects of health care delivery to its individual members. It is important that nurses acknowledge the importance of patients' families in achieving desirable health care outcomes.

Hospital policies often apply traditional definitions of family to include only those individuals who are related by marriage, blood, or adoption. Although this definition applies to many families, it also serves to exclude those families that have chosen variant family forms. Friedman (1998) provided a broader definition of family that is more inclusive. She defined family as "two or more persons who are joined together by bonds of sharing and emotional closeness and who identify themselves as being part of the family" (p. 9). A more contemporary belief is that family is anyone who the patient says is a family member.

One theoretical approach that has influenced how to look at families is systems theory. Systems theory examines a unit and describes its relationship to a greater whole. Systems theory is concerned with how things interrelate and it creates an umbrella under which other theories may be applied. The major assumption of systems theory is that all matter forms a system that is capable of being studied. Families are considered to be open social systems because they interact with the environment around them. Families also have discrete boundaries that separate them from the environment. These boundaries are porous and serve to allow the family to control how much input the family receives from the environment. For example, if a family member has a major illness, the family may curtail some of its activities in order to better deal with the health care crisis. Families must continually adapt in order to maintain equilibrium. When families are faced with stress, they must mobilize their adaptive resources in order to maintain a steady state. Stress places more strain on the family unit and creates a situation in which they may need help from outside resources in order to maintain equilibrium. Health care problems are stressful for families and the nurse is in a particularly good position in which to offer assistance to encourage healthy adaptations. Systems theory helps

nurses realize that patients and their families are connected to the outside world and what happens to one member has an effect on the whole.

The Biopsychosocial Model

The biopsychosocial model was formalized by George Engel (1980). Engel believed that mental disorders could not be adequately explained by reducing them to biological causations. The biopsychosocial model offered an alternative to the mechanistic, biomedical model and provided a holistic perspective. The stress diathesis model takes this concept further and postulates that illness is a result of both genetic and biological factors and environmental influences. For example, a person may have a genetic predisposition to develop heart disease, but by embracing a heart-healthy lifestyle avoids the development of heart problems.

Nursing has embraced the biopsychosocial model and the concept of holism. **Holism** is based on the premise that the whole is more than the sum of its parts. This means that patients are acknowledged as biopsychosocial spiritual beings that cannot be reduced to a variety of subsystems. It is a belief in the unitary nature of human beings. When nurses care for people holistically, they consider all aspects of their care. The biopsychosocial model and holism are compatible with systems theory. Individuals as open systems are in constant interaction with their environment; therefore, change in one area of their life affects the total system. There is recognition of health as more than the absence of disease and in providing care, nurses should consider not only the individual, but family and social support systems as well. All of this serves to promote the provision of patient-centered care.

The theories just discussed provide a framework within which psychosocial nursing care can be conceptualized. They provide a rationale for the way to frame nursing problems and apply the nursing process for effective patient-centered care. All nursing care takes place in the context of interpersonal relationships and effective communication. It is through the nurse–patient relationship, therapeutic communication, and patient education that persons are empowered to take an active role in their own health care decisions. The following sections provide an overview of the therapeutic nurse–patient relationship, therapeutic communication, and principles of patient education.

◼ The Therapeutic Nurse–Patient Relationship

The word *relationship* suggests human interaction in which the persons involved affect each other in some way. There are differences between social relationships and professional relationships. Professional relationships are meant to be therapeutic. To enter into a professional relationship, specific skills and knowledge are required. The professional or therapeutic nurse–patient relationship sets the stage for application of the nursing process in which assessment, diagnosis, planning, goal setting, intervention, and evaluation are carried out. There is also an emphasis on problem solving and a mandatory duty to accountability, responsibility, and confidentiality. Integral to the nurse–patient relationship is the concept of empowerment. When people are empowered, they are more able to develop the resources needed to make informed decisions about their health care based on their own priorities.

Certain actions foster the nurse–patient relationship. Conveying respect for a person's uniqueness, being nonjudgmental, showing attentiveness, and being empathetic all create the building blocks of a therapeutic nurse–patient relationship. Patients need to feel safe, secure, and understood. Also pivotal is that the nurse is perceived as knowledgeable, trustworthy, sensitive, and unambiguous.

Hildegard Peplau (1952), a nurse theorist, conceptualized the nurse–patient relationship as moving through three phases: introductory (orientation), working, and termination. During each of the phases, particular goals are achieved and particular events take place. The phases, which are often overlapping, are discussed next.

Introductory (Orientation) Phase

The introductory phase begins when the therapeutic relationship is initiated. Introductions take place and the patient is given initial information pertinent to her circumstances. The nurse starts to develop a trusting relationship. It is during this phase that the nurse and the patient establish an agreement—and in some cases a contract—about the purposes and direction of the relationship. This agreement or contract is usually verbal in nature, and in some settings it will be informal and in others more formalized. It is also during this phase that mutual goal setting is initiated. It is important for the goals of the nurse and the goals of the patient to be in alignment.

Another important activity that takes place during this phase is initial assessment. Although assessment takes place throughout the therapeutic relationship, it is essential during the introductory phase because it leads to the initial identification of nursing diagnoses and leads to mutual goal setting. The activities of this stage are built on a foundation of beginning trust and rapport.

Working Phase

The second phase is called the working phase. It is during this phase that a **therapeutic alliance** is established. A therapeutic alliance is one in which the nurse and the patient consciously work together to reach mutually agreed-on goals. Application of the nursing process is continuous during this stage and it is sometimes necessary to seek additional assessment data, realign goals, try new interventions, and reevaluate outcomes. Because new information and unanticipated events sometimes occur, problem solving is also continuous during this phase. Most patient education takes place during the working phase. Trust and rapport continue to grow during this stage. Patients begin to reach clarity and learn to exploit all of the resources that are available to them. Some refer to this as the exploitation phase.

Termination

The third phase of the therapeutic nurse–patient relationship is termination. Depending on the nature, length, and intensity of the therapeutic relationship, the termination phase can be difficult for patients. For this reason termination is introduced during the initial phase and often discussed during the working phase. During this phase the nurse and patient review what occurred during the working phase and what goals have been met

and what progress was made. It is important for the nurse to understand that patients often feel a sense of loss and insecurity during this phase. These feelings on the part of the patient might cause them to present some self-protective behaviors such as displays of hostility or regressing backward in their treatment. This is considered normal during this stage and needs to be worked through. Termination should begin during the introductory phase.

Self-Awareness in the Nurse–Patient Relationship

Hildegard Peplau expressed the importance of each nurse taking on the responsibility of expanding his or her own insight. She believed that the nurse's personality was an important factor in the development of an interpersonal relationship. According to Peplau, a basic task of nursing education should be the development of each nurse as a person who wants to nurse patients in a helpful way with the direction of this development being maturity (Vandemark, 2006).

Caring

The nurse–patient relationship also takes place in a context of caring. Watson (1985) feels that caring is one of the most fundamental attributes in nursing. She believes in general that caring serves to advance health in individual and families and allows for the development of human potential and health autonomy. She has identified 10 carative factors, as listed in Chart 13–6.

Interpersonal relationships between patients and nurses are strengthened when patients perceive the nurse as interpersonally competent. Foshbinder (1994), in a study that analyzed patient perceptions of nursing care, identified four themes that strengthened the perception on the part of patients that the nurse was interpersonally competent. The themes were identified as translating, getting to know you, establishing trust, and going the extra mile. The nursing behaviors that illuminated these themes were when nurses were forthcoming, gave needed information, provided patient teaching, were friendly and interested, took

---

CHART 13–6 Watson's Carative Factors

1. Forming a humanistic-altruistic value system
2. Instilling faith and hope
3. Cultivating sensitivity to oneself and to others
4. Developing a helping, trusting relationship
5. Promoting expression of positive and negative feelings
6. Systematically using the scientific problem-solving method for decision making
7. Promoting interpersonal teaching–learning
8. Providing support of a protective or corrective mental, physical, sociocultural, and spiritual environment
9. Assisting with gratification of human needs
10. Allowing for existential phenomenological forces

Source: Watson, J. (1999). *Nursing: Human science and human care.* Boston: Jones and Bartlett.

charge, appeared to enjoy their work, and provided care beyond expectations. In a study focusing on emotional support provided by nurses to patients with breast cancer, Paisson and Norberg (1995) found that supportive emotional support improved the women's sense of control and, therefore, their sense of well-being.

As nurses enter into therapeutic relationships, they do so with persons of diverse beliefs and values. These beliefs and values are born from cultural and subcultural socialization. Paying attention to cultural influences that may affect the nurse–patient relationship is very important. Providing culturally sensitive care requires a responsible relationship between health care providers and patients, their families, and communities that is based on trust and respect. Nurses are expected to be culturally sensitive and competent. Cultural competence is defined by Camphina-Bacote (1999) as the continual striving by the nurse to provide culturally appropriate care to patients and families. Camphina-Bacote and Munoz (2001) identify five components in their cultural competence model: (1) cultural awareness, (2) adequate cultural knowledge, (3) skill to carry out a cultural assessment, (4) experience with cultural encounters, and (5) the desire to be culturally competent. In a study that looked at culturally diverse nurse–patient interactions, Cioffi (2006) found that relationships between nurses and culturally diverse patients are often tense.

Recommendations from the study suggested better education of nurses and more research in order to develop better models of culturally diverse interaction.

The Office of Minority Health (2001) has developed the *National Standards on Culturally and Linguistically Appropriate Services in Health Care*. These are referred to as the CLAS standards and they are listed in the National Guidelines box. These standards have been cross-referenced to the Joint Commission standards for accreditation of hospitals.

◼ Therapeutic Communication

Having the ability to communicate skillfully is essential to good nursing care. Communication involves both a sender and receiver. It entails a two-way interaction in which a message is sent by the sender, heard and interpreted by the receiver, and a response given. Effective communication calls for active listening skills and allows for feedback and clarification.

Communication also involves nonverbal messages. Nonverbal messages can be delivered through voice tone, rate and volume of speech, the use of silence, the use of touch, and body language. For instance, patients may verbally relate that they feel fine, but they may appear to be very sad. If a verbal and the non-

---

NATIONAL GUIDELINES The CLAS Standards

Standard 1: Health care organizations should ensure that patients/consumers receive from all staff members effective, understandable, and respectful care that is provided in a manner compatible with their cultural health beliefs and practices and preferred language.

Standard 2: Health care organizations should implement strategies to recruit, retain, and promote at all levels of the organization a diverse staff and leadership that are representative of the demographic characteristics of the service area.

Standard 3: Health care organizations should ensure that staff at all levels and across all disciplines receive ongoing education and training in culturally and linguistically appropriate service delivery.

Standard 4: Health care organizations must offer and provide language assistance services, including bilingual staff and interpreter services, at no cost to each patient/consumer with limited English proficiency at all points of contact, in a timely manner during all hours of operation.

Standard 5: Health care organizations must provide to patients/consumers in their preferred language both verbal offers and written notices informing them of their right to receive language assistance services.

Standard 6: Health care organizations must assure the competence of language assistance provided to limited English proficient patients/consumers by interpreters and bilingual staff. Family and friends should not be used to provide interpretation services (except on request by the patient/consumer).

Standard 7: Health care organizations must make available easily understood patient-related materials and post signage in the languages of the commonly encountered groups represented in the service area.

Standard 8: Health care organizations should develop, implement, and promote a written strategic plan that outlines clear goals, policies,

operational plans, and management accountability/oversight mechanisms to provide culturally and linguistically appropriate services.

Standard 9: Health care organizations should conduct initial and ongoing organizational self-assessments of CLAS-related activities and are encouraged to integrate cultural and linguistic competence-related measures into their internal audits, performance improvement programs, patient satisfaction assessments, and outcomes-based evaluations.

Standard 10: Health care organizations should ensure that data on the individual patient's/consumer's race, ethnicity, and spoken and written language are collected in health records, integrated into the organization's management information systems, and periodically updated.

Standard 11: Health care organizations should maintain a current demographic, cultural, and epidemiological profile of the community as well as a needs assessment to accurately plan for and implement services that respond to the cultural and linguistic characteristics of the service area.

Standard 12: Health care organizations should develop participatory, collaborative partnerships with communities and utilize a variety of formal and informal mechanisms to facilitate community and patient/consumer involvement in designing and implementing CLAS-related activities.

Standard 13: Health care organizations should ensure that conflict and grievance resolution processes are culturally and linguistically sensitive and capable of identifying, preventing, and resolving cross-cultural conflicts or complaints by patients/consumers.

Standard 14: Health care organizations are encouraged to regularly make available to the public information about their progress and successful innovations in implementing the CLAS standards and to provide public notice in their communities about the availability of this information.

Source: Office of Minority Health. (2001). *National standards for culturally and linguistically appropriate services in health care. Final report.* Rockville, MD: Author.

verbal message do not match in emotional tone, then the message is said to be incongruent. Incongruent messages are confusing for the receiver and leave interpretation to the imagination.

Therapeutic communication is purposeful communication and is designed to convey openness and caring. Skillful use of therapeutic communication requires the nurse to have an awareness of the feeling environment of the patient. It consists of those words and actions that enhance the nurse–patient relationship and empower patients to make informed choices about their health care. At times, without realizing it, nurses communicate in such ways that create barriers to effective communication. Developing an understanding of therapeutic and nontherapeutic communication techniques helps the nurse avoid communication pitfalls. Chart 13–7 (p. 260) provides a summary of therapeutic and nontherapeutic communication techniques.

Culture also plays a role in therapeutic communication, as discussed in the Cultural Considerations box.

 ## The Teaching–Learning Process

Nurses fulfill many roles as members of the health care delivery team. The nurse as teacher or patient educator is one of those roles. It is often nurses who assume the primary responsibility for patient education. The reality of shorter hospital stays and the fact that many medical problems are treated in outpatient settings create circumstances in which it is essential that patients and families be provided with the necessary patient education. In a meta-analysis study that sampled 116 intervention studies that measured the effects of psychoeducational care provided to adults with cancer, Devine and Westlake (1995) found that psychoeducational care benefited adults with cancer with regard to reducing anxiety, depression, nausea, vomiting, pain, and perceived knowledge.

CULTURAL CONSIDERATIONS for Therapeutic Communications

Munoz and Luckmann (2005) provide a rationale for the growing need for transcultural communication. They cite the increasing ethnic, racial, and cultural diversity of the United States; the increase in the number of patients who represent different culturally influenced patterns of health behavior; the different cultural meanings of health care; the different ways in which patients and families respond to health care; the multicultural nature of health care settings; and the nursing profession's commitment to culturally competent humanistic care. They further contend that talking to strangers about deeply personal issues is often difficult and may be particularly so for patients who are from different cultural backgrounds. They identify several behaviors on the part of nurses that are necessary to encourage patents to talk about themselves. Nurses must convey empathy, show respect, build trust, establish rapport, listen actively, provide appropriate feedback, and demonstrate genuine interest (p. 148). They also identify barriers to effective transcultural communication as follows: nurses' lack of knowledge, bias, ethnocentrism, prejudice, and stereotyping. Further, language differences, differences in the understanding of terminology, and differences in perceptions and expectations also create barriers (p. 162).

Teaching is defined as any deliberate act that involves the planning, implementation, and evaluation of instructional strategies that meet expected learner outcomes. It is a planned method or series of methods used to help someone learn. Learning has occurred when there is a change in behavior (cognitive, affective, or psychomotor) as a result of being exposed to environmental stimuli. It is an internal experience that represents an integration of thoughts, ideas, theory, and experience. Learning is divided into three domains; cognitive, affective, and psychomotor. Cognitive learning involves the storing and recalling of new knowledge and information in the brain. **Affective learning** involves changes in attitudes, values, and feelings. **Psychomotor learning** involves learning that occurs when a physical skill has been acquired.

The teaching–learning process is facilitated by the existence of a therapeutic nurse–patient relationship. The nurse as teacher needs to be able to communicate effectively with individuals, families, and groups. The teaching–learning process can be conceptualized into four steps: assessment of learning needs, developing a teaching plan, implementation of a teaching plan, and evaluation of the teaching plan.

Assessment of Learning Needs

When nurses assess the learning needs of an individual, group, or family, they should use all appropriate information available to them. Patients and families can provide the most accurate information. Unfortunately, there are times when for one reason or another a patient or family member is not a good historian. In such cases, it is necessary to get information from additional sources such as other family members or old medical records. During the assessment process, it is important for the nurse to identify the particular knowledge, skills, and attitudes that are needed by the patient or family. Once this is accomplished the nurse must then assess the emotional and experiential readiness of the patient or family to learn. The following factors should be considered when assessing emotional and experiential readiness to learn:

- The level of emotional health
- Motivation to learn
- Self-concept and body image
- Social and economic stability
- Past experiences with learning
- Attitude toward learning.

Assessing the patient's ability to learn is necessary so an appropriate teaching plan can be designed. The following factors need to be considered:

- Physical condition of the patient and acuity of the illness
- Acuity of the patient's senses
- Developmental considerations
- Level of education
- Literacy
- Communication skills
- Primary language
- Pain level
- Prognosis.

CHART 13–7	**Therapeutic and Nontherapeutic Communication Techniques**

Techniques	Rationale	Examples
Therapeutic Techniques		
Using silence	Gives the patient the opportunity to collect and organize thoughts, to think through a point, or to consider introducing a topic of greater concern than the one being discussed.	When discussing difficult subjects, such as sexual history, or possible abusive situations.
Accepting	Conveys an attitude of reception and regard.	"Yes, I understand what you said." Eye contact, nodding.
Giving recognition	Acknowledging; indicating awareness. Better than complimenting, which reflects the nurse's judgment.	"I see you attended therapy today" or "I see you made your bed."
Offering self	Making oneself available on an unconditional basis increases patient feelings of worth.	"I'll stay with you for awhile," "Let me sit with you awhile," or "I'll be here with you."
Giving a broad opening	Allows the patient to take the initiative in introducing the topic. Emphasizes the importance of the patient's role in the interaction.	"What would you like to talk about today?" or "Tell me what you are thinking."
Offering general leads	Offers the patient encouragement to continue.	"Go on," "Yes, I see," or "And after that?"
Placing the event in time or sequence	Clarifies the relationship of events in time so that the nurse and patient can view them in perspective.	"What seemed to lead up to this," "Was that before or after?" or "When did that happen?"
Making observations	Verbalizing what is observed or perceived. This encourages the patient to recognize specific behaviors and compare perceptions with the nurse.	"You seem tense," "I notice you are pacing a lot," or "You seem uncomfortable."
Encouraging description of perceptions	Asking the patient to verbalize what is being perceived. Often used when a patient is experiencing hallucinations.	"Tell me what is happening now," "Are you hearing the voices now?" or "What do the voices seem to be saying?"
Encouraging comparison	Asking the patient to compare similarities and differences in ideas, experiences, or interpersonal relationships. Helps the patient recognize life experiences that tend to recur as well as aspects of life that are changeable.	"Was this something like. . . ," "How does this compare to the time when. . . ," or "What was your response the last time this situation occurred?"
Restating	The main idea of what the patient has said is repeated. Lets the patient know whether or not an expressed statement has been understood and gives him or her the chance to continue or clarify.	*Pt:* "I can't study. My mind seems to wander." *Nurse:* "You have difficulty concentrating." *Pt:* "I can't take a new job. What if I fail?" *Nurse:* "You are afraid you will fail in this new position?"
Reflecting	Questions and feelings are referred back to the patient so they may be recognized and accepted, and so the patient may recognize that his or her point of view has value. A good technique to use when a patient asks the nurse for advice.	*Pt:* "What do you think I should do about. . . ?" *Nurse:* "It sounds as if you are having difficulty deciding what to do." *Pt:* "My sister won't help a bit towards my mother's care. I have to do it all." *Nurse:* "You feel angry when she doesn't help."
Focusing	Taking notice of a single idea or even a single word. Works well with a patient who is moving rapidly from one thought to another. This technique is not therapeutic for someone who is very anxious. Focusing should not be pursued until the anxiety abates.	"This point seems worth looking at more closely. Perhaps you and I can discuss it together."
Exploring	Delving further into a subject, idea, experience, or relationship. Especially helpful with patients who tend to remain on a superficial level. However, if the patient chooses not to disclose further information, the nurse should refrain from pushing or probing in an area that obviously creates discomfort.	"Please help me understand that situation in more detail" or "Tell me more about that."
Seeking clarification and validation	Striving to explain that which is vague or incomprehensible and searching for mutual understanding. Clarifying the meaning of what has been said facilitates and increases understanding.	"Tell me if my understanding agrees with yours" or "Do I understand correctly that you said. . . ?"

(continued)

CHART 13–7 Therapeutic and Nontherapeutic Communication Techniques—*Continued*

Techniques	Rationale	Examples
Presenting reality	When a patient has a misperception of the environment, the nurse defines reality or indicates his or her perception of the situation for the patient.	"I understand that the voices seem real to you, but I do not hear any voices," or "I can only see you and me in the room right now."
Voicing doubt	Expressing uncertainty as to the reality of the patient's perceptions. Often used with patient's who are experiencing delusional thinking.	"I find that unusual" or "That seems rather doubtful to me."
Verbalizing the implied	Putting into words what the patient has only implied or said indirectly. Can also be used with the patient who is mute or is otherwise experiencing impaired verbal communication. Clarifies what is implicit rather than what is explicit.	*Pt:* "It's a waste of time to be here, I can't talk to you anymore." *Nurse:* "Are you feeling that no one understands?" *Pt:* (Refuses to speak.) *Nurse:* "I'm wondering if you are feeling angry right now."
Attempting to translate words into feelings	When feelings are expressed only indirectly, the nurse tries to "desymbolize" what has been said and find clues to the underlying meaning.	*Pt:* "I feel like I'm adrift in the ocean." *Nurse:* "You must be feeling lonely right now."
Formulating a plan of action	Helping the patient design a plan to deal with an uncomfortable stressful situation using effective coping strategies.	"What could you do to express your anger harmlessly?" or "Next time this comes up what might you do to handle it differently?"

Nontherapeutic Techniques

Techniques	Rationale	Examples
Giving reassurance	Indicates to the patient that there is no cause for anxiety, thereby devaluing the patient's feelings. May discourage the patient from further expressions of feelings if he or she believes that they will only be downplayed.	"I wouldn't worry about that" or "Everything will be all right." Better to say: "We will work on that together."
Rejecting	Refusing to consider or showing contempt for the patient's ideas or behavior. This may cause the patient to discontinue interaction with the nurse for fear of further rejection.	"Let's not discuss. . ." or "Let's not talk about that now." Better to say: "Let's look at that a little closer."
Giving approval or disapproval	Sanctioning or denouncing the patient's ideas or behavior. Implies that the nurse has the right to pass judgment on whether the ideas or behaviors are good or bad, and the patient is expected to please the nurse. The nurse's acceptance of the patient is then seen as conditional depending on the patient's behavior.	"That's good, I'm glad that you. . ." or "That's bad. I'd rather you wouldn't." Better to say: "Let's talk about how your behavior at dinner invoked anger in the other patients."
Agreeing or disagreeing	Indicating accord with or opposition to the patient's ideas or opinions. Implies that the nurse has the right to pass judgment on whether the patient's ideas or opinions are "right" or "wrong." Agreement prevents the patient from later modifying his or her point of view without admitting error. Disagreement implies inaccuracy, provoking the need for defensiveness on the part of the patient.	"That's right, I agree," "I don't believe that," or "I wouldn't do it like that." Better to say: "Let's discuss what you feel is unfair about the new rules."
Giving advice	Telling the patient what to do and how to behave implies that the nurse knows what is best and the patient is incapable of self-direction. Nurtures the patient in the dependent role and discourages independent thinking.	"I think you should" or "I wouldn't do it like that." Better to say: "What do you think you should do."
Probing	Persistent questioning of the patient. Pushing for answers to issues the patient does not wish to discuss. Causes the patient to feel used and valued for only what he or she shares. Causes patient to feel defensive.	"Tell me about your abuse" or "How come you were drinking and driving?"
Defending	Attempting to protect someone or something from verbal attack. To defend what the patient has criticized is to imply that she or he has no right to express ideas, opinions, or feelings. Defending does not change the patient's feelings and may cause the patient to think the nurse is taking sides with those being criticized.	"No one here would lie to you" or "You have a very capable doctor, I'm sure he has your best interest at heart." Better to say: "I will try to answer your questions and clarify some issues regarding your treatment."

(continued)

CHART 13–7	Therapeutic and Nontherapeutic Communication Techniques—*Continued*	
Techniques	**Rationale**	**Examples**
Requesting an explanation	Asking the patient to provide explanations for thoughts, feelings, behavior, and events. Asking "why" a patient did something or feels a certain way can be very intimidating and implies that the patient must defend his or her behavior or feelings.	"Why do you think that?" "Why do you feel that way?" or "Why did you do that?" Better to say: "Describe what you were feeling just prior to this occurrence."
Belittling feelings	When the nurse misjudges the degree of the patient's discomfort, a lack of empathy and understanding may be conveyed. This causes the patient to feel insignificant or foolish. It is no relief to a patient to hear that others are or have been in similar situations.	*Pt:* "I'm so down today." *Nurse:* "Cheer up." *Pt:* "I'm always unhappy." *Nurse:* "Most people are unhappy sometimes." Better to say: "You sound upset. Tell me what you are feeling right now."
Making stereotyped comments	Clichés and trite expressions are meaningless in the nurse–patient relationship. For the nurse to make empty conversation is to encourage a like response from the patient.	"Hang in there," "Keep your chin up," or "It's good for you." Better to say: "Let's talk about your feelings."
Using denial	When the nurse is uncomfortable with a patient's problem and blocks discussion with the patient and avoids helping the patient identify and explore areas of difficulty.	*Pt:* "I've amounted to nothing in my life." *Nurse:* "Everyone has some accomplishments." Better to say: "Let's talk about how you have come to that conclusion."
Interpreting	The nurse attempts to tell the patient the meaning of her or his experience.	"What you really mean is. . ." or "Unconsciously you feel. . . ."
Changing the subject	Changing the subject causes the nurse to take over the discussion. The nurse may do this in order to meet his own agenda or to avoid talking about something he wishes to avoid.	*Pt:* "I think I'm going to die." *Nurse:* "Did you have visitors this weekend?"

Developing a Teaching Plan

The teaching–learning process is more effective when mutual goal setting takes place. Unless the patient values the learning objectives, it is unlikely that much learning will occur. It is also important for all learning goals to be realistic and appropriate for the patient and situation. The following are important steps when designing a teaching plan:

- Identify short- and long-term goals.
- Prioritize the goals.
- Determine who should be included in the teaching.
- Match content with appropriate teaching strategies and learner activities.
- Relate teaching content to the patient's interests, resources, and patterns of everyday living.
- Decide on group versus individual teaching and formal versus informal teaching.
- Design a plan that is realistic for time constraints.

Implementing a Teaching Plan

The implementation of the teaching plan should include varied teaching strategies delivered in an organized manner. The strategies should be appropriate for the type of learning that is desired. Chart 13–8 lists some teaching strategies that might be considered.

CHART 13–8	Suggested Teaching Strategies	
Cognitive Learning	**Affective Learning**	**Psychomotor Learning**
Lecture	Role modeling	Demonstration
Panel discussion	Panel discussion	Self-discovery
Printed materials	Printed materials	Printed materials
AV materials	AV materials	AV materials
Program instruction	Role playing	Practice
Computer instruction	Peer counseling	

Evaluating a Teaching Plan

The mutually set learning goals provide the basis for evaluating whether learning has occurred. This can be accomplished by:

- Direct questioning of the patient
- Observation of behavior
- Return demonstrations
- Paper-and-pencil tests
- Pretests and post-tests
- Patient questionnaires
- Self-evaluation
- Postdischarge follow-up

If the learning objectives have not been met, the learning content and teaching strategies may need to be altered. Further assessment may be needed, new goals agreed on, and the teaching repeated.

■ Psychodynamics of Illness and Hospitalization

Many complex factors can influence a patient's perception of a serious illness or hospitalization. Understanding these different factors and providing appropriate nursing care will improve a patient and family's outlook on health and illness and possibly improve patient outcomes.

Crisis

For many people a serious illness and hospitalization constitute a crisis. A **crisis** can develop when an event or series of events occurs that creates a situation that is perceived as threatening. These events can be personal such as illness or death of a loved one, or more global such as experiencing a terrorist attack. A crisis is said to be maturational when the stressors are related to developmental events. An example of this would be an adolescent who develops an identity crisis. A situational crisis occurs when the stress stems from an unexpected event, such as the development of an acute illness. An adventitious crisis is one that is the result of unexpected natural disasters such as tornadoes or plane crashes.

A crisis develops in response to a series of events. It is not the situation itself that leads to the development of a crisis state, but rather the individual's perception and response to the event. The development stages of a crisis are as follows:

- The individual or family is in a state of homeostasis.
- A stressful event or events occur.
- The event is perceived as a threat.
- Well-known coping skills are applied but fail to reduce the threat.
- A period of disequilibrium occurs with a decrease in problem-solving ability and an increase in feelings of anxiety and depression.
- The problem is either resolved or personal disintegration occurs.

A crisis is also self-limiting. Caplan (1964) found that in a typical crisis state, equilibrium is restored in approximately 4 to 6 weeks. Because of the extreme feelings of disorganization during an active crisis, individuals often need to turn to outside resources in order to return to a state of equilibrium. Nurses are often in contact with individuals and families when they are vulnerable to crisis or already in crisis and therefore become a valuable resource. Early intervention is essential to reduce the effects of the crisis. Providing information and resources sometimes serves to prevent a full-blown crisis from occurring. Intervention should meet the level of disorganization that is felt and should be done as quickly as possible.

Rapport needs to be established quickly. Initially, an assessment should be done to define the problem. Because crisis is about perception of the problem, it is essential that information be described from the patient's perspective. It is important to understand the meaning the event has for the patient. Further, allowing for free expression of feelings can be cathartic in itself. Once these things are accomplished, the nurse can then help the patient clarify the series of events that led to the crisis.

Once the problems have been defined, the nurse and the patient develop an initial plan of action. If the patient is very disoriented, the nurse may need to take a directive role while still allowing for as much input as possible. During this time the nurse can provide practical, concrete help to the patient. The nurse may have to do some things for the patient that under different circumstances the patient would do for himself. It is sometimes helpful to have the patient make a list of his needs and concerns from most important to least important. This can help the nurse plan interventions that will decrease the sense of disequilibrium, reduce feelings of anxiety and depression, and mobilize supportive resources. If there is a concern about self-harm, the patient should be protected and an immediate referral made.

Once the crisis has been stabilized, the nurse can help the patient problem solve and explore alternatives. It is here that new coping skills can be taught. Teaching new coping skills empowers patients to better handle future crisis events. It is for this reason that a crisis is often seen as an opportunity for growth. The nurse provides continual emotional support through this process because the change can be very anxiety producing.

Sick Role Behavior

Illness and hospitalization are often perceived as stressful and make patients more vulnerable to experiencing a crisis. When individuals become ill and must be hospitalized, they are expected to behave in certain ways and assume a sick role. A **sick role** is a set of expectations that people who are ill must meet and which society including caregivers expects of them. When a person enters the hospital, that person is immediately oriented to hospital rules, regulations, policies, and procedures. It is expected that patients and their families will adhere to these rules. The patient is expected to be cooperative, dependent, and nondemanding. Wilson (1963) explains this well:

> The patient comes unbidden to a large organization which awes and irritates him, even as it also nurtures and cares. As he strips off his clothing so he strips off, too, his favored costume of social roles, his favorite style, and his customary identity in the world. He becomes subject to a time schedule and a pattern of activity not of his own making. (p. 70)

Hospitals are bureaucratic entities and services are often fragmented. The hospital is frequently organized for the convenience of the staff and not the patient. Patients are repeatedly the victims of this fragmentation and frequently perceive that they are losing control. This feeling of losing one's autonomy is more disturbing to some patients than to others. The term **locus of control** refers to the perception people have about how much control they exert over the events that happen in their lives. People with an **internal locus of control** orientation believe that events in their lives are controlled by their own actions and decisions. People with an **external locus of control** orientation believe that events in their lives are controlled more by fate, luck, and external circumstances.

Even though health professionals are literally strangers, health care professionals continually ask patients to entrust themselves to their care. Nurses may ask patents to trust their competence, motives, and decision making. Because of a strong need to control their own autonomy, patients with an internal locus of control orientation will find this paternalism in health care bureaucracies frustrating. Patients with an external locus of control orientation will most likely not feel as uncomfortable and actually might need assistance in being more involved in their own health care decision making. Shattel (2004) found that issues such as power, social and cultural contexts, and interpersonal competence influence the nurse–patient relationship. Russell, Daly, Hughes, and op't Hoog (2003) concluded that to provide patient-centered care, power and authority need to be transferred away from health care professionals and to patients. The following are ways in which nurses can demonstrate interpersonal competence and therefore empower patients to be more involved in their health care decisions:

- Answer questions honestly and knowledgeably.
- Do mutual goal setting.
- Inform patients in advance of procedures.
- Prepare the patient for procedures.
- Let patients know what to expect.
- Listen patiently to expressions of concern.
- Do not treat patients as children.

It is important to encourage patients to share their experiences and perceptions with the nurse. Venke, Torjuul, Ross, and Kihigren (2006), in a study that attempted to illuminate the experience of being a "patient," found that patients, even when generally satisfied with their care, made compromises about the things they found as less than optimal. The patients considered this as a necessary part of their experience and did not share their perceptions, therefore making them more vulnerable. Clinical recommendations from the study suggested that nurses need to be aware of the content of their patient's vulnerabilities and act as patient advocates.

Loss and Grief

When patients and significant others are confronted with a serious illness, they often experience feelings of loss and grief. The amount of loss that is perceived by the patient and significant others is individual and should be assessed accordingly. The grieving process can be initiated by any loss. Although impending death represents a major loss, other types of losses can be extremely significant for patients and their significant others and therefore trigger the grieving process. Illness can cause loss of physiological functioning, loss of familiar roles, loss of relationships, loss of financial security, loss of self-esteem, loss of autonomy, and many more losses individual to each situation. How each patient and significant other adapts to their losses depends on their perception of the significance of the loss, their coping skills, their support systems, and the replaceability of the loss. Although each patient and significant others will cope with their losses in an individualized way, each will also go through a grief response process. Chart 13–9 presents the stages of grief response as identified by Kübler-Ross & Kessler (2005).

CHART 13–9	**Kübler-Ross's Stages of Grief and Mourning**
Denial	Individuals react with a shocked "No, not me." This is healthy and allows individuals and significant others time to gather coping resources.
Anger	Individuals say "Why me?" or "Why us?" During this stage people sometimes blame others, including God.
Bargaining	Individuals say "Yes me, but. . . ." or "If you just give me enough time to see my daughter married, I'll be ready."
Depression	Individuals say "Yes me." With this acknowledgment of the reality of the situation comes feelings of depression.
Acceptance	Facing the loss or death peacefully. In the case of death, individuals tend to withdraw into themselves.

Source: Kübler-Ross, E., & Kessler, D. (2005). *On grief and grieving: Finding the meaning of grief through the five stage of loss.* New York: Scribner.

Nursing Management

Nurses are often in the best position to offer support to patients and significant others as they move through the grieving process. It is most important to provide a safe environment for grieving to be expressed. Nurses need to be sensitive to individual differences in expressing grief. Some differences in grieving rituals are culturally influenced. Some people grieve quietly, some loudly, some verbalize a great deal, some not at all, and some are very stoic. Others are very emotional. Nurses provide a quiet acceptance of all grieving practices.

In a systematic review of the effectiveness of palliative care teams in improving the health outcomes of cancer patients, Hearn and Higginson (1998) found that when compared to conventional care, palliative care teams were better able to meet the needs of cancer patients and their families, possibly reducing the overall cost of care.

Assessment

The nurse should answer the following questions when assessing a patient experiencing grief and loss:

- What is the perceived or observable loss as experienced by the individual and/or significant others?
- How does the individual and/or significant others explain or describe the loss?
- Is the individual or significant others able to identify their own feelings about the loss?
- Is the individual or significant others in denial about the loss?
- Is the individual or significant others expressing feelings of helplessness or hopelessness?
- Are there outward expressions of grief such as crying?
- Are there observable symptoms of depression?
- In what stage of the grieving process is the individual or significant others?

Nursing Diagnosis

Possible nursing diagnosis for patients experiencing grief and loss include:

- *Grieving*
- *Coping Ineffective*
- *Spiritual Distress*
- *Knowledge Deficit* related to feelings of loss and grief
- *Hopelessness.*

Planning

The plan of care should facilitate a healthy grieving process.

Outcomes and Evaluation Parameters

An outcome for the grieving patient is the ability to work through the grieving process. This is evaluated by the patient's ability to:

- Verbalize an awareness of the loss.
- Verbalize the significance of the loss.
- Verbalize an awareness of the grieving process.
- Accept support while moving through the grieving process.
- Move toward acceptance of the loss.

Interventions and Rationales

The following interventions and rationales would be appropriate for the patient experiencing loss and grief:

- Assess the individual's and/or significant others' stage in the grief and loss process. *Identifying any issues that may be unresolved facilitates the grieving process. The patient and family members are frequently at different phases of grieving and should be treated appropriately.*
- Provide nonjudgmental support. *Allowing patients to express feelings openly may allow them to move through the phases of grieving more easily. Nonjudgmental listening allows patients to express their feelings without the fear of rejection.*
- Provide a safe environment in which the individual and/or significant others can express all feelings. *When the nurse spends time with the patient and family it may assist with the necessary review and processing of the loss. Being with the patient can decrease feelings of loneliness and reassure them that caregivers perceive the loss as significant.*
- Educate the individual and/or significant others about the grieving process. *Understanding of the grief process allows the patient and significant others to move through the process more easily.*
- Help individuals and/or significant others to identify and reach out to additional support systems. *Assist the patient to identify resources. Referrals to appropriate support groups will help to meet emotional needs.*
- Help individuals and/or significant others problem solve. *Providing the patient and significant others with accurate information prevents misconceptions and may decrease their fears. Allowing patients to make decisions whenever possible enables them to maintain control.*

Evaluation

The patient will be able to move through the grief process in a healthy manner and exhibit effective coping mechanisms.

Depression

Experiencing feelings of depression is a predictable response to illness and hospitalization and often accompanies loss and grief. The DSM-IV-TR (American Psychiatric Association [APA], 2000) provides diagnostic criteria for all of the affective disorders, for example, Major Depressive Disorder, Bipolar Disorder, and Dysthymic Disorder. Specific exploration of these disorders is beyond the scope of this chapter. The focus for this discussion is on depression as a psychological response to the losses associated with illness and hospitalization.

Patients are more vulnerable to developing depressive symptoms when they are experiencing severe, prolonged stress or crisis. The depression can act as a protective mechanism when people exhaust their coping abilities. The ability to adapt to stressors is dependent on the effectiveness of the individuals' coping mechanisms and the amount of perceived stress. Even individuals with excellent coping skills can become overwhelmed when the amount of stressors transcends their ability to cope with them.

Depression is also prevalent with certain diseases. Hackett, Yapa, Parag and Anderson (2005) did a systematic review of the frequency of depression after stroke. Their conclusions were that depression is common among stroke patients and that this needs to be addressed in clinical practice. A study on depression and anxiety as predictors of health outcomes after myocardial infarction found that patients who are worried and unhappy in the hospital are at higher risk for negative psychological and quality-of-life outcomes (Mayou, Gill, and Thompson, 2000). In their conclusions they argue for in-hospital identification and treatment of depression and anxiety.

Sherbourne and colleagues (2000) studied the impact of psychiatric conditions on health-related quality-of-life issues in persons with HIV infection. The results of this study found that comorbid psychiatric conditions predispose patients to impaired functioning and loss of a sense of well-being. Barsevick, Dudley, and Beck (2006) researched cancer-related fatigue, depressive symptoms, and functional status. They found that when fatigue caused patients to have difficulty carrying out routine activities they tended to experience more depressive symptoms. They suggest that interventions should be aimed at reducing the likelihood of impaired functioning that could result in increased depressive symptoms.

◼ Nursing Management

It is often nurses who provide the frontline care for individuals who are experiencing feelings of depression. Intervening with patients who are depressed can sometimes be difficult because dealing with others' pain can be depressing in itself. Because of this, at times there is the tendency to want to avoid depressed patients. It can be hard to find the time to properly intervene, and the fast pace of the hospital environment is counterproductive to the slowed pace of the depressed patient. Sometimes other people view depressed individuals as not doing enough to help themselves. They feel that if depressed people would just try harder, they could pull themselves out of their depressed mood. It is important to understand that depression is a clinical diagnosis and needs to be assessed and treated just like any other disease.

Assessment

Depression is an uncomfortable psychological and physical experience of sadness. To a degree ranging from mild to severe, individuals experience behavioral, physical, affective, and cognitive changes as follows:

Behavioral Changes

- Loss of interest in usually enjoyed activities
- Body posture slumped, dejected looking
- Difficulty making eye contact
- Difficulty carrying out activities of daily living
- Crying.

Physical Changes

- Weight loss or weight gain
- Appetite changes
- Loss of sexual desire
- Somatic symptoms
- Sleep disturbances
- Fatigue
- Lack of energy
- Change in bowel habits.

Affective Changes

- Feelings of emotional sadness
- Low self-esteem
- Labile mood
- Feelings of helplessness or hopelessness
- Pessimistic outlook
- Ambivalence.

Cognitive Changes

- Cognitive distortions
- Slowing of thought processes
- Inability to concentrate
- Indecisiveness
- Loss of memory
- Difficulty problem solving
- Feelings of guilt
- Possible suicidal ideation
- Difficulty looking into the future.

Nursing Diagnosis

Possible nursing diagnoses for a person with depression include:

- *Coping, Ineffective*
- *Impaired Verbal Communication*
- *Social Isolation*
- *Ineffective Health Maintenance*
- *Self-Care Deficits*
- *Sleep Deprivation*
- *Self-Esteem Disturbance*
- *Ineffective Role Performance*
- *Knowledge Deficit*
- *Spiritual Distress*
- *Risk for Self-Directed Violence.*

Planning

Nursing priorities for the patient with depression include establishing rapport and trust, indentifying threat and coping resources, providing interventions to optimize coping skills, and evaluating the effectiveness of interventions.

Outcomes and Evaluation Parameters

Outcomes for the patient with depression include identification of ineffective coping and the ability to participate in developing a plan of care. This will be exhibited by the patient's ability to:

- Identify significant losses.
- Verbalize the significance of losses.
- Verbalize factors that he or she can control.
- Participate in own health care decision making.
- Exhibit reduced symptoms of depression.
- Remain free from self-harm.

Interventions and Rationales

The following interventions and rationales would be appropriate for the patient experiencing depression:

- Validate the presence of the depression. *Acceptance by the nurse allows the patient to feel positive about the therapeutic relationship. This helps with healing, decreases isolation, and increases coping ability.*
- Provide emotional support through empathetic listening. *Empathetic listening helps to build trust and strengthens the therapeutic relationship.*
- Encourage the expression of feelings both positive and negative. *Patients may not fully understand what is happening to them. If they can express feelings freely, the nurse can plan specific actions to assist the patient to see the situation clearly.*
- Avoid excessive cheerfulness and false reassurance. *This will not help patients to work through their problems.*
- Encourage patient to be involved in his or her care. *The ability to control aspects of one's life helps to allay feelings of helplessness.*
- Assist the patient in goal setting and problem solving. *Patients may be overwhelmed by their situation. Assisting them to view the problem in its component parts will reduce anxiety and assist with effective coping behaviors.*
- Assess for suicidal ideation and if present ensure safety and make a referral. *Involve the healthcare team if you suspect that the patient is suicidal.*

- If necessary, refer for psychotherapy and pharmacological intervention. *It is important to ensure safety and prevent patients from harming themselves.*

Evaluation

The nurse should frequently reevaluate the patient's coping mechanism. The patient should be able to describe his or her emotional state, participate in developing a plan of care, and use support offered by caregivers.

Anxiety

Anxiety is a universal psychological response. Without some amount of anxiety, individuals would not be able to accomplish their goals or meet their challenges. When faced with illness and possible hospitalization, most people will experience increased feelings of anxiety. They often become worried about their diagnosis, prognosis, and ability to cope with their illness. Anxiety is a primary emotion from which other emotions such as anger stem. As with depression the DSM-IV-TR (APA, 2000) provides diagnostic criteria for an array of anxiety disorders, for example, Panic Disorder, Generalized Anxiety Disorder, and Posttraumatic Stress Disorder. An explanation of these specific anxiety disorders is beyond the scope of this chapter. The focus for this discussion is on anxiety as a predictable psychological response to the stress of illness and hospitalization.

Anxiety is an uncomfortable feeling of discomfort, dread, apprehension, and unease, the cause of which can be specific or nonspecific. Oftentimes individuals are unable to identify what is making them feel anxious. The symptoms of anxiety are physiological, psychological, and behavioral. Several factors affect the severity of the anxiety: the strength and intensity of the stressors, the duration of the stressors, the individual's coping abilities, and the individual's perceived sense of helplessness. Variables such as culture, religion, education, and past experiences can also influence how well individuals cope with a particular situation. Many variables affect the development of anxiety, including perceived threats to biological integrity, perceived threats to self-esteem, frustration of needs or motives, the inability to control or influence meaningful events, or mental association with previously anxiety-producing events. When patients are exposed to the health care system, events such as hospitalization, waiting for test results, waiting for a diagnosis, needing surgery, and losing time from work, anticipating the outcome of treatment, and experiencing lifestyle changes can all lead to increased anxiety.

Anxiety is both physiological and psychological. This is a very important fact because the mind will perceive a stressor as a threat, but it is the physiological response that causes the feelings of tension and discomfort. This is because the anxiety response is a sympathetic nervous system response, causing symptoms such as increased heart rate, increased respirations, increased blood pressure, and increased glucose. When this occurs individuals want to feel relief from the uncomfortable feelings that the anxiety produces, and if they are unable to apply anxiety-reducing interventions that decrease the physiological arousal the anxiety tends to increase in severity. In the case of chronic anxiety, the increased arousal of the sympathetic nervous system causes dangerous wear and tear on the body. This is why early assessment and intervention to decrease the anxious symptoms is vital.

Anxiety can be conceptualized on a continuum moving from mild to moderate to severe to panic. The higher the level of anxiety the more uncomfortable the symptoms will feel. Immediate interventions that are designed to decrease the physiologic arousal are of utmost importance. The longer the symptoms go unchecked the more anxious the person will feel.

▇ Nursing Management

Nursing interventions to reduce anxiety are variable. Jung-Soon and Kyung-Sook (2001) studied the effects of handholding on anxiety in cataract surgery patients under local anesthesia and found that this cheap noninvasive intervention had potential for reducing anxiety in this group of patients. Vingerhoets (1998) found that patients who go into open heart surgery with high levels of anxiety tend to remain highly anxious after their open heart surgery. In a 1997 study that looked at the effects of relaxation exercises on anxiety and other symptoms of chemotherapy, Arakawa found that patients who received the intervention of relaxation reported less subjective feelings of anxiety. In a systematic review of implementing music in hospitals, Evans (2001) found that the evidence suggests the use of music can reduce anxiety in hospitalized patients. Badger, Segrin, Dorros, Meek, and Lopez (2007) found that phone-delivered psychosocial interventions decreased anxiety and depression in women with breast cancer and their partners.

Assessment

The nurse should assess for the following types of anxiety:

Mild Anxiety

- Alert, attentive, confident
- Open to new experiences
- Good problem-solving abilities
- Perceptual fields open, can deal with more than one thing at a time
- Can apply coping mechanisms.

Moderate Anxiety

- Signs and symptoms are beginning to become noticeable
- Ability to pay attention is narrowed
- Perceptual fields begin to narrow
- Verbalization is increasing
- Problem solving is more rigid
- Increased respiratory rate, heart rate, and muscle tension
- Dry mouth, clammy palms, and sometime palpitations
- General feeling of restlessness.

Severe Anxiety

- Anxiety is obvious
- Cognitive functioning is impaired
- Perceptual fields extremely narrowed
- Can only focus on one detail at a time
- Ability to concentrate decreased significantly

- Learning cannot occur
- Pacing, need for motor activity
- Sweating
- Hyperventilation, tachycardia
- Tremors, numbness, tingling
- Nausea, headache, dizziness.

Panic

- Chest pain, breathlessness, tachycardia
- Feelings of impending death
- Extreme discomfort
- Perceptual fields closed
- Unrealistic distorted perceptions
- Inability to communicate clearly
- Must be resolved quickly.

Planning

Priorities for nursing management for the patient with anxiety should include providing appropriate health information, assisting the patient with applying the information to his or her current health situation, and promoting identification of methods to cope with anxiety. The plan should also identify ways to minimize or prevent the escalation of the patient's anxiety and promote the overall well-being of the patient.

Nursing Diagnosis

Possible nursing diagnoses for the patient experiencing anxiety include:

- *Anxiety*
- *Coping Ineffective*
- *Social Isolation*
- *Sleep Deprivation*
- *Hopelessness*
- *Powerlessness*
- *Knowledge Deficit.*

Outcomes and Evaluation Parameters

The patient will be able to recognize the symptoms of anxiety resulting from identified fears by:

- Acknowledging to the nurse the presence of the anxiety.
- Demonstrating the appropriate use of coping mechanisms.
- Demonstrating increased problem solving.
- Verbalizing feeling less anxious.
- Exhibiting a decrease in the symptoms of anxiety.

Interventions and Rationales

The following interventions and rationales would be appropriate for the patient experiencing anxiety:

- Acknowledge the presence of the anxiety. *Recognition of the anxiety helps the patient to feel accepted and strengthens the therapeutic relationship.*
- Ask the patient to perform deep-breathing exercises. *Deep breathing assists the body to relax and the mind to be focused.*

Learning new techniques allows the patient to participate in promoting personal well-being.

- Offer music. *Music can distract the patient and help to focus his or her thoughts.*
- If possible, identify the stimulus for the anxiety. *Identifying the stimulus helps the patient to clarify realistic and unrealistic perceptions and develop appropriate ways of handling the distress.*
- Provide the patient with needed information. *Written materials give the patient information for discussion with the health care team and significant others. The materials can also be used as a reference when questions arise.*
- Remove anxiety-producing environmental stimuli. *When anxious, the patient may have increased sensitivity to environmental stimuli.*
- Stay with the patient and provide support. *Acceptance by the nurse allows the patient to feel positive about the therapeutic relationship. This helps with healing, decreases isolation, and increases coping ability.*
- Encourage the expression of feelings. *Patients may not fully understand what is happening to them. If they can express feelings freely, the nurse can plan specific actions to assist the patient to see the situation clearly.*
- Explore with the patient usual coping mechanisms. *Understanding the patient's baseline ability starts interventions from the place where the patient is comfortable. It also identifies unhealthy coping skills that need to be changed.*
- Acknowledge to the patient the effective use of coping mechanisms. *Positive reinforcement.*
- Assist the patient in problem solving. *The patient may be overwhelmed by his or her situation. Assisting the patient to view the problem in its component parts will reduce anxiety and assist with effective coping behaviors.*
- Provide opportunities to give the patient more control. *The ability to control aspects of one's life helps to allay feelings of helplessness.*
- Teach the patient relaxation techniques. *Helps the patient to focus.*
- In panic levels of anxiety:
  - Do not leave the patient.
  - Do not ask the patient for explanations.
  - Assure patient you will stay with him or her.
  - Allow patient to rest after attack is over.
  - Refer patient for further evaluation.

Evaluation

It is important for the nurse to assess the effectiveness of the patient's coping strategies. As the patient improves he or she will be able to identify effects of increasing anxiety, understand the sources of his or her anxiety, learn useful coping skills, and differentiate between healthy and unhealthy coping strategies.

Anger

Anger and anxiety are two emotions that are often related. When individuals feel anxious, they also experience accompanying feelings of frustration and helplessness. These feelings can in turn cause individuals to feel powerless to control their own autonomy. Anger develops to a greater or lesser degree as a response to the feelings of powerlessness and helplessness. At least temporarily, anger is a powerful feeling that helps individuals feel more in control. For some people the intolerable feeling of anxiety is replaced with the more powerful feeling of anger. This is effective as a temporary coping mechanism, but not meant to be the only coping strategy. Long-standing anger feelings do not promote health. In fact, Matthews, Gump, Harris, Haney, and Barefoot, (2004) found that long-standing hostility may place people at higher risk for cardiovascular mortality.

In society the open expression of anger is sometimes discouraged and causes others to feel uncomfortable. It is important to recognize that anger is a natural emotion and that the rational expression of angry feelings can be appropriate for some situations. For example, a patient whose diagnostic test results are lost and has to repeat the test would be justified in feeling angry.

Nurses are often the recipients of angry feelings and it is sometimes difficult for them not to personalize their response to these expressions of anger. When patients are angry, nurses can experience feelings of powerlessness and anxiety and respond to the patients' anger with anger of their own. This, of course, only serves to escalate the angry feelings. When anger is conceptualized as anxiety, nurses feel more in control and are able to intervene professionally and rationally.

◼ Nursing Management

The expression of anger can be blatant, for example, when someone yells or throws something, or subtle, such as when someone is a little sarcastic or refuses to speak much. It is important to pick up the early signs of anger because angry feelings tend to increase if the cause for the anger is not dealt with. The earlier the nurse intervenes to reduce the anger and accompanying anxiety, the better the chance for a positive outcome. If a patient's expression of anger is not rationale, the nurse will need to set clear limits. Sometimes patients need to be informed about the types of behaviors that are acceptable and those that are not.

Assessment

Anger can be conceptualized on a continuum ranging from mild, to moderate, to severe, to rage.

Mild Anger

- Feeling tense
- Feeling irritable
- Argumentative
- Difficult to please
- Scowling facial expression
- Sarcasm.

Moderate Anger

- Increasing rumination
- Angry behavior more obvious
- Motor agitation
- Voice pitch increases
- Potential for acting out behavior.

Severe Anger

- Signs of acting-out behavior
- Cursing
- Distinct danger of becoming out of control.

Rage Anger

- Rage is an out-of-control situation and appropriate interventions to protect the safety of the patient and staff must be implemented immediately.

Nursing Diagnosis

Possible nursing diagnoses for an angry person include:

- *Coping Ineffective*
- *Noncompliance* with treatment
- *Social Isolation*
- *Powerlessness*
- *Risk for Other-Directed Violence.*

Planning

Nursing planning begins with establishing rapport and trust with the patient. Following is the identification of the cause of the anger, intervene and identify coping strategies, and evaluate the effectiveness of the interventions.

Outcomes and Evaluation Parameters

The patient will be able to recognize the cause of the anger and use effective coping strategies as evidenced by the ability to:

- Verbalize the presence of anger.
- Demonstrate decreased symptoms of anger.
- Demonstrate decreased symptoms of anxiety.
- Verbalize that he or she feels less angry.

Interventions and Rationales

- Prevention and anger reduction techniques, as listed next, can be useful. *Acceptance by the nurse allows the patient to feel positive about the therapeutic relationship. This helps with healing, decreases isolation, and increases coping ability.*

Prevention

- Listen when patients talk to you.
- Do not dismiss people's concerns.
- Treat each patient as an individual.
- Talk to patients not at them.
- Respect patients' privacy.
- Do not make rules that treat adults as children.
- Recognize when patients are feeling anxious and intervene to reduce the anxiety.

Anger Reduction

- Help patient verbalize angry feelings.
- Validate the patient's anger.
- Avoid defensive responses.
- Use therapeutic communication skills.
- Assist patient to identify the source of anger.

- Allow patient an outlet for angry feelings.
- Do mutual problem solving.
- Allow patient more control over health care decisions.
- Teach patient techniques such as deep breathing and relaxation.

Evaluation

As the patient develops healthy coping strategies he or she should exhibit the ability to describe his or her emotional state to the nurse, articulate an accurate understanding of the current situation, and accept support offered by caregivers.

Summary

This chapter discussed the basic principles and concepts of psychosocial nursing care. They are the concepts that nurses often forget when the pressures exerted by the health care delivery system take precedence. They are also the aspects of nursing care that make nursing a patient-centered and holistic profession.

Several topics for future research are listed in the Research Opportunities and Clinical Impact box.

RESEARCH OPPORTUNITIES AND CLINICAL IMPACT RELATED TO PSYCHOSOCIAL NURSING

Research	Clinical Impact
What interventions will help to relieve the "compassion fatigue" described by nurses?	Developing interventions to relieve the discomfort surrounding care of patients and families will improve the care given to the patients.
What is the best teaching methodology for therapeutic communication?	Best teaching practices would enhance relationship-based care.
What interventions can be done to support culturally appropriate care?	The promotion of cultural customs and rituals surrounding illness can enhance patient care.

NCLEX® REVIEW

1. A patient tells the nurse "I don't have diabetes; just a touch of sugar." The nurse realizes this patient is demonstrating a concept from which of the following theories?
   1. Erikson
   2. Freud
   3. Maslow
   4. Piaget

2. A patient is ambivalent about the types of treatment available for a disease process. Which of the following actions would support a therapeutic nurse–patient relationship?
   1. Encouraging the patient to follow the doctor's orders, without question
   2. Instructing the patient to figure it out and then let the nurse know the decision
   3. Asking the patient if more information is needed to help in the decision-making process
   4. Telling the patient that he has more information about the disease than the nurse

3. A foreign-born patient is trying to explain his current health status. Which of the following would demonstrate culturally sensitive therapeutic communication by the nurse?
   1. Leave the patient alone until he's ready to explain his current health issue.
   2. Sit with the patient and encourage him to explain to the best of his ability.
   3. Stand at the bedside and write down whatever the patient says being careful to avoid eye contact.
   4. Tell the patient he can explain his health problem to the doctor.

4. The nurse is planning to instruct a patient newly diagnosed with diabetes mellitus how to self-inject insulin. Which of the following responses indicates the patient is ready to learn the information?
   1. I will do my best to learn how to do this. I have to.
   2. I don't know why you are doing this. I don't have diabetes.
   3. Wait until my wife comes in. She's the one who will do it.
   4. Can't you do this for me? I don't want to worry about this every day.

5. A patient just learns he has prostate cancer. Which of the following should the nurse do to assist this patient?
   1. Sit with the patient and be prepared to answer any questions.
   2. Leave the patient alone to handle his emotions privately.
   3. Ask the physician to sit with the patient.
   4. Call a social worker to help the patient understand the implications of the diagnosis.

Answers for review questions appear in Appendix D

KEY TERMS

accommodation *p.254*
affective learning *p.259*
assimilation *p.254*
basic human needs *p.254*
conscious *p.251*
crisis *p.263*
ego *p.252*
ego defense mechanisms *p.252*

external locus of control *p.263*
growth needs *p.254*
holism *p.256*
id *p.252*
internal locus of control *p.263*
locus of control *p.263*
pleasure principle *p.252*
psychomotor learning *p.259*

schema *p.254*
sick role *p.263*
subconscious *p.251*
superego *p.252*
teaching *p.259*
therapeutic alliance *p.257*
therapeutic communication *p.259*
unconscious *p.252*

PEARSON
EXPLORE **mynursingkit**™

MyNursingKit is your one stop for online chapter review materials and resources. Prepare for success with additional NCLEX®-style practice questions, interactive assignments and activities, web links, animations and videos, and more!

Register your access code from the front of your book at
www.mynursingkit.com

REFERENCES

American Psychiatric Association. (2000). *Diagnostic and statistical manual of mental disorders, text revision* (4th ed.). Washington, DC: Author.

Badger, T., Segrin, C., Dorros, S. M., Meek, P., & Lopez, A. M. (2007). Depression and anxiety in women with breast cancer and their partners. *Nursing Research, 56*(1), 44–53.

Ball, J. W., & Bindler, R. C. (2006). *Child health nursing: Partnering with children & families.* Upper Saddle River: Pearson Prentice Hall.

Barsevick, A. M., Dudley, W. N., & Beck, S. L. (2006). Cancer-related fatigue, depressive symptoms, and functional status. *Nursing Research, 55*(5), 366–372.

Beck, A. T., & Freeman, A. (1990). *Cognitive theory of personality disorders.* New York: Guilford Press.

Bronfenbrenner, U. (1979). *The ecology of human development: Experiments by nature and design.* Cambridge, MA: Harvard University Press.

Camphina-Bacote, J. (1999). A model and instrument for addressing cultural competence in health care. *Journal of Nursing Education, 38*(5), 203–207.

Camphina-Bacote, J., & Munoz, C. (2001). A guiding framework for delivering culturally competent services in case management. *The Case Manager, 12,* 48–52.

Caplan, G. (Ed.). (1964). *Principles of Preventive Psychiatry.* New York: Basic Books.

Cioffi, J. (2006). Culturally diverse patient–nurse interactions on acute care wards. *International Journal of Nursing Practice, 12,* 319–325.

Devine, E. C., & Westlake, S. K. (1995).The effects of psychoeducational care provided to adults with cancer: Meta-analysis of 116 studies. *Oncology Nursing Forum 22*(9), 1369–1381.

Engel, G. L. (1980). The clinical application of the biopsychosocial model. *American Journal of Psychiatry, 137,* 535–544.

Erikson, E. (1963). *Childhood and society* (2nd ed.). New York: Norton.

Evans, D. (2001). *Music as an intervention for hospital patients: A systematic review.* Adelaide, Australia: Joanna Briggs Institute for Evidence Based Nursing and Midwifery.

Foshbinder, D. (1994). Patient perceptions of nursing care: An emerging theory of interpersonal competence. *Journal of Advance Nursing, 20*(6), 1085–1093.

Freud, S. (1935). *A general introduction to psychoanalysis.* New York: Simon and Schuster.

Friedman, M. (1998). *Family nursing: Research, theory and practice* (4th ed.). Stamford, CT: Appleton and Lange.

Hackett, M. L., Yapa, C., Parag, V., Anderson, C. S. (2005). Frequency of depression after stroke: A systematic review of observational studies. *Stroke, 36*(6):1330–40.

Hearn, J., & Higginson, I. (1998). Do specialist palliative care teams improve outcomes for cancer patients?: A systematic review. *Palliative Medicine, 12*(5), 317–332.

Jung-Soon, M., & Kyung-Sook, C. (2001). The effects of handholding on anxiety in cataract patients under local anesthesia. *Journal of Advanced Nursing, 353*(3), 407–415.

Kübler-Ross, E., & Kessler, D. (2005). *On grief and grieving: Finding the meaning of grief through the five stages of loss.* New York: Scribner.

Mayou, R., Gill, D., & Thompson, D. R. (2000). Depression and anxiety as predictors of outcome after myocardial infarction. *Psychosomatic Medicine, 62,* 212–219.

Matthews, K. A., Gump, B. B., Harris, K. F., Haney, T. L., & Barefoot, J. C. (2004). Hostile behaviors predict cardiovascular mortality among men enrolled in the multiple risk factor intervention trial. *Circulation, 109,* 66–70.

Munoz, C., & Luckmann, J. (2005). *Transcultural communication in nursing.* Clifton Park, NY: Thomson/Delmar Learning.

Office of Minority Health. (2001). *National standards for culturally and linguistically appropriate services in health care. Final report.* Rockville, MD: Author.

Paisson, M. B., & Norberg, A. (1995). Breast cancer patients' experiences of nursing care with the focus on emotional support: The implementation of a nursing intervention. *Journal of Advanced Nursing, 21*(2), 277–285.

Peplau, H. E. (1952). *Interpersonal relations in nursing.* New York: Putnam.

Piaget, J., & Inhelder, B. (1969). *Psychology of the child.* New York: Basic Books.

Russell, S., Daly, J., Hughes, E., & op't Hoog, C. (2003). Nurses and "difficult" patients: Negotiating non-compliance. *Journal of Advanced Nursing, 43*(3), 281–287.

Shatell, M. (2004). Nurse–patient interaction: A review of the literature. *Journal of Clinical Nursing, 13*(6), 714–722.

Sherbourne, C., Hays, R. D., Fleishman, J. A., Benedetto, V., Magruder, K. M., Bing, E. G., et al. (2000). Impact of psychiatric conditions on health related quality of life in persons with HIV infection. *American Journal of Psychiatry, 157,* 248–254.

Vandemark, L. M. (2006). Awareness of self and expanding consciousness: Using nursing theories to prepare nurse-therapists. *Issues in Mental Health Nursing, 27,* 605–615.

Venke, S., Torjuul, K., Ross, A., & Kihigren, M. (2006). Satisfied patients are also vulnerable patients—Narrative from a acute care ward. *Journal of Clinical Nursing, 15*(10), 1240–1244.

Vingerhoets, G. (1998). Perioperative anxiety and depression on open heart surgery. *Psychosomatics, 39,* 30–37.

Watson, J. (1985). *Nursing: Human science and human care.* Norwalk, CT: Appleton-Century-Crofts.

Watson, J. (2004). *Caring science as sacred science.* Philadelphia: F. A. Davis Company.

Wilson, R. (1963). The social structure of a general hospital. *Annals of the American Academy of Political and Social Sciences, 346,* 67–76.

CHAPTER 14

Nutrition

Sheila Tucker

Outcome-Based Learning Objectives

After studying this chapter, the learner will be able to:

1. Explain components of a comprehensive nutrition assessment as part of the nursing care process.
2. Apply the nutritional component of national standards for disease prevention and treatment.
3. Discuss the metabolic effects of physiological stress and the potential impact on nutrition status.
4. Outline the nutrition therapy guidelines for patients with physiological stress, such as postoperative wound healing and burn injury.
5. Differentiate among the principles of medical nutrition therapy in treating general medical conditions.
6. Explain the indications and nursing interventions associated with enteral and parenteral nutrition support.
7. Defend the important role of nursing care in successful medical nutrition therapy.

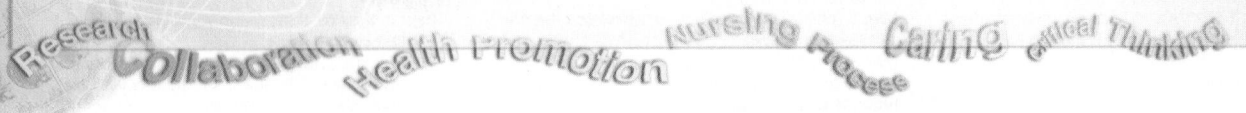

Research   Collaboration   Health Promotion   Nursing Process   Caring   Critical Thinking

NUTRITION PLAYS a crucial role in both the prevention and treatment of disease. Both overnutrition and undernutrition can lead to negative health outcomes. For example, **overnutrition** from excess intake of calories and fat can result in weight gain, elevated blood lipids, and risk of hypertension, diabetes, and some cancers. **Undernutrition,** in which dietary intake is less than the body's requirement, can result in impaired wound healing, poor response to medical treatment, and loss of functional capacity.

Medical nutrition therapy is an integral part of the health care process. Proper nutrition, whether accomplished through a therapeutic diet, nutrition support, or general healthy eating, is associated with positive outcomes. The nurse is uniquely positioned to take an active role in the nutrition care process of medical and surgical patients. The nutrition care process involves assessment, evaluation, and setting of patient goals and objectives in a fashion that can be easily dovetailed into the nursing care process. The registered dietitian is the health care professional with the primary responsibility for overseeing medical nutrition therapy in most settings. However, the nurse's active position on the front line of patient care presents an important opportunity for improving nutritional care with efficient screening and assessment of nutrition status, appropriate and timely referrals, reinforcement of patient education, and close monitoring of nutrition intervention.

■ Nutrition Assessment

The cornerstone of all nutritional care is based on the foundation of a well-done nutrition assessment. Objective and subjective data gathered as part of the nursing assessment can be evaluated to determine a patient's existing or potential risk for undernutrition or overnutrition. Appropriate nursing diagnoses and interventions can then be developed based on findings from the nutrition assessment.

Nutrition Assessment Parameters

No one parameter or single piece of data should be used as an indicator of nutrition status. Data gathered during the physical exam and laboratory assays together with subjective data from the focused interview provide a comprehensive set of information on which to base a nutritional assessment. A nutrition assessment based on limited data has limited clinical value since many parameters used in a nutrition assessment can be influenced by nonnutritional factors. When compiling a nutrition assessment, the nurse should use as many sources of data as are available along with sharp clinical judgment.

Physical Assessment

The physical assessment portion of a nutrition assessment includes the clinical exam along with anthropometric measurements. Pertinent data from the medical history and treatment plan should be considered for any influence on nutrition status because of alterations in physical health. The presence of pain, gastrointestinal symptoms, medication side effects, and impaired cognition or mobility are examples of physical factors that can have negative effects on nutrition status. The Risk Factors chart outlines the potential influences of physical symptoms and health on nutrition status.

Observations from the clinical examination can be incorporated into the nutrition assessment. Nutritional deficiencies can have few, if any, clinical symptoms until nutrient status is compromised for a length of time. The nurse should not dismiss suspicion of poor nutrition health simply because no physical findings are apparent. Physical changes associated with altered nutrition status can also occur for medical or environmental reasons and so deserve further investigation when discovered. Chart 14–1 (p. 274) outlines physical findings that can be indicative of altered nutrition health.

Anthropometric measurements are an important component of the assessment and include any scientific measurement of the body. Measured current weight and height should be obtained during an initial assessment. Weight should be measured at regular intervals thereafter. Self-reported height and weight are not considered accurate and are subject to overreporting and underreporting bias by adults of all ages (Brown, Feng, & Knapp, 2002; Kuczmarski, Kuczmarski, & Najjar, 2001). Use of self-reported weight in a patient with undetected weight loss

will result in an unaddressed clinical change and subsequent delayed intervention. A patient should be weighed with a minimal of clothing and after voiding. Presence of edema or ascites and any unremoved casts or appliances should be noted. Additionally, adjustments in weight should be made for missing limbs following established guidelines (Osterkamp, 1995).

A weight history should also be obtained and confirmed by checking medical records. An unplanned weight loss of >5% in 1 month or >10% in 6 months is clinically significant and warrants attention. Patients who cannot stand to be measured or weighed can be measured using alternative methods. Chair and bed scales can be used to obtain current weight while arm span, knee height, or recumbent measures will provide estimates of height. Recumbent height will yield an overestimation of height by approximately 4 cm (1.5 in.) from changes in spinal compression when standing (American Medical Directors Association, 2001).

Body mass index (BMI) is used to calculate appropriate weight for height using the formula weight (kg)/height^2 (m). Morbidity and mortality statistics have been employed to determine cutoff points to define overweight, obesity, underweight, and healthy weight. Figure 14–1 ■ (p. 275) depicts a table from the National Institute of Health (NIH) that can be used as a tool to determine BMI. Because BMI calculations use simple height and weight measurements, its use does not take into account body composition. Individuals with large bone structure or ample muscle mass can be categorized erroneously as overweight using this single assessment tool. The nurse should discover this discrepancy when conducting a physical exam.

Waist circumference can be used in a nutrition assessment, especially when cardiovascular disease risk is suspected or known. Deposition of excess abdominal fat is considered to be an independent risk factor for heart disease in adults (National Heart Lung, and Blood Institute [NHLBI], 2002). A waist circumference of >102 cm (40 in.) in men or >88 cm (35 in.) in women is associated with risk. Measurement should be made following proper technique with use of bony landmarks. Simply measuring waist circumference just below the umbilicus is not accurate in the obese patient in whom the position of the umbilicus has changed with weight gain (Lean & Han, 2002). Waist circumference measurements are not of nutritional value in patients who are pregnant or have ascites or other fat-free mass increases in abdominal girth because of disease.

Body composition can be tested using a variety of techniques. Skinfold measurements, bioelectrical impedance analysis, near-infrared, and dual x-ray absorptiometry (DEXA) are utilized in different clinical settings to estimate body fat and muscle mass. Bone mineral content and fluid composition can be estimated with more sophisticated technology. Care must be taken to ensure that the most accurate measurements are performed, realizing even then that most methods have a margin of error associated with them. Skinfold measurements are best performed by a practiced clinician, because repeated accurate measurement is difficult. The presence of edema at the measurement site invalidates the findings. Bioelectrical impedance is subject to error caused by changes in hydration. Near-infrared measurements have an increased margin of error when performed on obese subjects (Wagner & Heyward, 1999).

RISK FACTORS for Poor Nutrition Health

Condition	Contributing Symptoms
Chronic disease, acute illness, injury	Disease symptoms (including pain) or treatment can ↓ appetite, ↓ intake, cause malabsorption, or change nutritional requirements
Multiple medications	Gastrointestinal side effects, altered taste, decreased saliva, nutrient interactions
Restrictive eating	Chronic dieting, disordered eating, food beliefs, or faddism can lead to poor intake
Poor oral health	Loose, missing teeth, ill-fitting dentures, gum disease, and mouth sores can ↓ intake
Alcohol abuse	Poor dietary intake and nutrient absorption
Psychosocial issues	Depression, bereavement, social isolation can lead to ↓ intake. Lack of finances or access to adequate food impairs intake. Lack of nutrition knowledge or food preparation skills can yield poor-quality intake
Altered functional status	Immobility, altered cognition can ↓ intake
Sensory changes	Vision, hearing, taste alterations alter ability to prepare or enjoy food or dining

CHART 14–1 **Physical Findings Associated with Altered Nutrition**

	Finding	Potential Altered Nutrient
Hair	Dull, sparse, brittle, dyspigmented	Protein, zinc, biotin
Face	Puffy/moon face, temporal wasting	Protein
	Pallor	Iron
Eyes	Sunken	Water
	Dry mucosa, night blindness	Vitamin A
	Pale conjunctiva	Iron
	Fatty deposits around lids	Elevated serum cholesterol
Mouth	Long tongue furrows	Water
	Cracked corners, lips, magenta tongue	Niacin, vitamin B_6, riboflavin
	Atrophic papillae	Iron
	Spongy, bleeding gums	Vitamin C
	Lack of taste (hypogeusia)	Zinc
Glands	Enlarged thyroid (goiter)	Iodine
Skin	Poor wound healing	Protein, zinc, vitamin C
	Dry, scaly	Vitamin A, zinc, fat
	Bruising	Vitamins C and K
	Pinpoint hemorrhages (petechiae)	Vitamin C
	Photosensitive symmetric rash	Niacin
	Tenting, dry mucous membranes or axillae	Water
Skeleton/trunk	Ascites	Protein
	Beading on ribs, bowed legs	Vitamin D
	Loss of fat, muscle wasting	Protein and calories
Limbs	Edema, loss of muscle, fat	Protein and calories
Nails	Spoon shaped, ridges	Iron
Central nervous system	Confusion, headache, lethargy	Water
	Confabulation, hyporeflexia	Thiamine
	Dementia, ataxia, neuropathy	Vitamin B_{12}
Cardiac	Arrhythmias	Magnesium, potassium

Reference values for all body composition measurements should be current and age and gender specific. The best use of composition measurements is in the serial monitoring of a patient, with the patient's own baseline measures serving as the initial point of reference.

Laboratory Measurements

Laboratory values can be a useful adjunct to other parameters used in a nutritional assessment. No single laboratory value is uniquely indicative of current nutritional status because confounding variables exist for each. Disease, infection, and the inflammatory process can alter laboratory values used in an assessment. Varying half-lives and the body's pool size of plasma proteins will yield differences in the snapshot of nutrition status reflected by their values. Albumin, with its long half-life, provides an older picture of nutrition status than prealbumin with its shorter half-life. Chart 14–2 outlines laboratory testing used in a nutrition assessment.

Nutrition History

A nutrition history can conveniently be incorporated into the focused interview done during a nursing assessment. The nutrition history can include a 24-hour diet recall and a food frequency questionnaire. In the clinical setting where patients receive subsequent monitoring, a food record or diary can be a useful adjunctive tool to evaluate nutrition intervention.

A 24-hour diet recall provides a 1-day snapshot of the patient's intake on which to base an assessment. All meals, snacks, liquids, and nutrition supplements should be recorded with estimates of preparation method and portion size. Because no single day usually illustrates all dietary habits, it is best to ask the patient about other general nutrition habits. A second recall can be performed to improve the type of data, for example, the nurse could query the patient about intake on a workday and a nonworkday. Chart 14–3 (p. 276) outlines data to be considered when conducting a nutrition history.

A food frequency questionnaire can be used to supplement the limited data of a 24-hour recall. The patient can provide information on the frequency of consumption of different food groups by filling out a questionnaire or answering questions during the nutrition history. For example, a nurse may find no fruit intake on the limited recall, but a food frequency questionnaire might reveal that 10 pieces of fruit are eaten a week.

During the nutrition history, the nurse should ask open-ended questions and make no assumptions about types and patterns of intake. Asking a question such as "What did you have for breakfast?" assumes the patient had breakfast or appears to

Body Mass Index Table

	Normal						Overweight					Obese										Extreme Obesity														
BMI	19	20	21	22	23	24	25	26	27	28	29	30	31	32	33	34	35	36	37	38	39	40	41	42	43	44	45	46	47	48	49	50	51	52	53	54
Height (inches)												Body Weight (pounds)																								
58	91	96	100	105	110	115	119	124	129	134	138	143	148	153	158	162	167	172	177	181	186	191	196	201	205	210	215	220	224	229	234	239	244	248	253	258
59	94	99	104	109	114	119	124	128	133	138	143	148	153	158	163	168	173	178	183	188	193	198	203	208	212	217	222	227	232	237	242	247	252	257	262	267
60	97	102	107	112	118	123	128	133	138	143	148	153	158	163	168	174	179	184	189	194	199	204	209	215	220	225	230	235	240	245	250	255	261	266	277	276
61	100	106	111	116	122	127	132	137	143	148	153	158	164	169	174	180	185	190	195	201	206	211	217	222	227	232	238	243	248	254	259	264	269	275	280	285
62	104	109	115	120	126	131	136	142	147	153	158	164	169	175	180	186	191	196	202	207	213	218	224	229	235	240	246	251	256	262	267	273	278	284	289	295
63	107	113	118	124	130	135	141	146	152	158	163	169	175	180	186	191	197	203	208	214	220	225	231	237	242	248	254	259	265	270	278	282	287	293	299	304
64	110	116	122	128	134	140	145	151	157	163	169	174	180	186	192	197	204	209	215	221	227	232	238	244	250	256	262	267	273	279	285	291	296	302	308	314
65	114	120	126	132	138	144	150	156	162	168	174	180	186	192	198	204	210	216	222	228	234	240	246	252	258	264	270	276	282	288	294	300	306	312	318	324
66	118	124	130	136	142	148	155	161	167	173	179	186	192	198	204	210	216	223	229	235	241	247	253	260	266	272	278	284	291	297	303	309	315	322	328	334
67	121	127	134	140	146	153	159	166	172	178	185	191	198	204	211	217	223	230	236	242	249	255	261	268	274	280	287	293	299	306	312	319	325	331	338	344
68	125	131	138	144	151	158	164	171	177	184	190	197	203	210	216	223	230	236	243	249	256	262	269	276	282	289	295	302	308	315	322	328	335	341	348	354
69	128	135	142	149	155	162	169	176	182	189	196	203	209	216	223	230	236	243	250	257	263	270	277	284	291	297	304	311	318	324	331	338	344	351	358	365
70	132	139	146	153	160	167	174	181	188	195	202	209	216	222	229	236	243	250	257	264	271	278	285	292	299	306	313	320	327	334	341	348	355	362	369	376
71	136	143	150	157	165	172	179	186	193	200	208	215	222	229	236	243	250	257	265	272	279	286	293	301	308	315	322	329	338	343	351	358	365	372	379	386
72	140	147	154	162	169	177	184	191	199	206	213	221	228	235	242	250	258	265	272	279	287	294	302	309	316	324	331	338	346	353	361	368	375	383	390	397
73	144	151	159	166	174	182	189	197	204	212	219	227	235	242	250	257	265	272	280	288	295	302	310	318	325	333	340	348	355	363	371	378	386	393	401	408
74	148	155	163	171	179	186	194	202	210	218	225	233	241	249	256	264	272	280	287	295	303	311	319	326	334	342	350	358	365	373	381	389	396	404	412	420
75	152	160	168	176	184	192	200	208	216	224	232	240	248	256	264	272	279	287	295	303	311	319	327	335	343	351	359	367	375	383	391	399	407	415	423	431
76	156	164	172	180	189	197	205	213	221	230	238	246	254	263	271	279	287	295	304	312	320	328	336	344	353	361	369	377	385	394	402	410	418	426	435	443

FIGURE 14–1 ■ BMI table.

Source: From National Institutes of Health website: http://www.nhlbi.nih.gov/guidelines/obesity/bmi_tbl.htm

CHART 14–2 Laboratory Tests Used in Nutrition Assessment

Laboratory Test Normal Finding	Half-life (days)	Expected Abnormality with Mild Malnutrition	Expected Abnormality with Moderate Malnutrition	Expected Abnormality with Severe Malnutrition	Rationale
Albumin 3.5–5 g/L	14–20	2.8–3.4 g/L	2.1–2.7 g/L	<2.1 g/L	↓ w/liver disease, inflammation, infection, renal losses
Transferrin >200 mg/L	8–10	180–200 mg/L	160–180 mg/L	<160 mg/L	↓ w/renal losses, liver disease; ↑ w/infection, inflammation, iron deficiency
Prealbumin 150–350 mg/L	2–3	110–150 mg/L	50–109 mg/L	<50 mg/L	↓ w/liver disease, inflammation, infection, renal losses
Total lymphocytes 2,000–3,500 cells/m^3	NA	1,200–1,500 cells/m^3	800–1,200 cells/m^3	<800 cells/m^3	↓ w/steroid, immunosuppression, cancer treatment

Sources: Beck, F. K., & Rosenthal, T. C. (2002). Prealbumin: A marker for nutritional evaluation. *American Family Physician, 65,* 1575–1578; Omran, M. L., & Morley, J. E. (2000). Assessment of protein-energy malnutrition in older persons, part II: Laboratory evaluation. *Nutrition, 16,* 131–140; Shenkin, A., Cederblad, G., Elia, M., & Isaksson, B. (1996). Laboratory assessment of protein energy status. *Clin Chim Acta, 253,* S5–S59.

CHART 14–3 Nutrition History Data

DIET RECALL AND FOOD FREQUENCY
- All meals and snacks
- All liquids, including alcohol, water, and caffeinated beverages
- Location of meals (home, school, restaurant, car, work, etc.)
- Preparation methods (convenience food, added fat, salt, etc.)
- Portion size
- Meal patterns: number of meals, missed meals

SUPPLEMENT AND MEDICATION USE
- Vitamin and mineral use; include dose, frequency, and ingredients
- Herbal supplement use; include dose, frequency, and ingredients
- Weight loss and sports supplements; include dose, frequency, and ingredients
- Assess over-the-counter and prescription medications for drug–nutrient interactions

FOOD BELIEFS AND PRACTICES
- Use of therapeutic diet for allergy, food intolerance, or medical nutrition therapy
- Lifestyle nutrition choices and food faddism; avoidance of certain foods or food groups, trendy nutrition practices, vegetarianism or vegan diet
- Cultural or religious dietary influences
- Pica: consumption of nonfood items or unusual intake of single foods

OTHER INFLUENCES ON NUTRITION
- Education and literacy as it relates to nutrition knowledge and cooking skills
- Social environment: isolation, food security, access to cooking facilities and refrigeration, presence of substance abuse
- Economics: adequate funds for food
- Functional capacity related to ADLs and I-ADLs: cooking, shopping, self-feeding, meal preparation, general activity level

CULTURAL CONSIDERATIONS in Nutrition Assessment

- Cultural and religious beliefs and traditions can affect dietary habits and practices in many ways. Preparation methods, food choices, and patterns of intake can be based on beliefs of a group or individual interpretation.
- Explore the influence of cultural interpretations and religious beliefs on individual nutrition habits and beliefs. Diversity exists within groups and it is best to discuss an individual's personal practices rather than make assumptions based on generalities.
- Ask about religious dietary laws, food preparation methods, food practices for special occasions (including whether fasting is practiced), and beliefs related to food and health. Medicinal herb use varies among cultures and can play an important role.

the gold standard for evaluating nutrition status in adults. Thus, many tools exist and will continue to be developed. When choosing a tool, it must be validated for use in the intended population. Most assessment tools have cutoff points as part of a scoring system. Because poor nutrition health occurs along a continuum, sharp clinical judgment is a needed accessory to any nutrition assessment tool in order to avoid missed opportunities for intervention and improved outcome.

REAP and WAVE

The Rapid Eating and Activity of Patients (REAP) and Weight, Activity, Variety and Excess (WAVE) validated tools were developed for use by health care providers to improve nutrition assessment and education during clinical encounters (Gans et al., 2003). The tools can be used alone or together to provide assessment and education in less than 9 minutes. The WAVE tool uses the Food Guide Pyramid as a foundation to evaluate a diet recall and the BMI to assess weight and also includes an assessment for risks of overnutrition. The REAP questionnaire can be completed by the patient before the assessment and is meant to supplement the overall assessment. Chart 14–4 (p. 278) depicts the REAP and WAVE tools.

Mini Nutrition Assessment and Subjective Global Assessment

The Mini Nutrition Assessment (MNA) and Subjective Global Assessment (SGA) have both been validated as nutrition assessment tools (Persson, Brismar, Katzarski, Nordenstrom, & Cederholm, 2002). The SGA was developed more than 20 years ago and had been validated in several adult populations since then. The MNA is a newer tool and is specific to older adults (Vellas et al., 1999). The MNA can be incorporated into the nursing assessment or used alone.

Special Considerations Affecting Nutrition Care

Both malnutrition and physiological stress place additional nutritional requirements on the medical–surgical patient. Existing malnutrition can compromise medical treatment and contribute to adverse medical and surgical outcomes. The presence of physiological stress increases nutritional requirements in the patient who may already be at nutritional risk because of a medical condition or disease.

judge that breakfast consumption is expected. This type of questioning can lead the patient to craft an answer to meet the perceived expectations of the nurse rather than answer factually. A better choice to begin the recall would be "What was the first thing you had to drink or eat yesterday? When/what was that?" followed by "When was the next time that you had something?"

Underreporting bias exists in giving a nutrition history. Patients who are seeking the social approval of the interviewer or want to avoid disapproval tend to underreport intake (Novotny et al., 2003). Patients who smoke, are obese, or are of lower socioeconomic or educational level underreport intake more than others. In addition, alcohol intake can be underreported. Cultural influences on the nutrition assessment are outlined in the Cultural Considerations box, and gerontological influences are outlined in the Gerontological Considerations box.

Nutrition Assessment Tools

Data from a nutrition assessment can be gathered following a protocol, the nursing care process, or by using a validated tool. No one screening or assessment tool is universally accepted as

GERONTOLOGICAL CONSIDERATIONS for Nutrition Assessment

Nutrition assessment of the older adult should utilize the same parameters outlined for the general population. However, because of the prevalence of malnutrition in the elderly, specific attention should be paid to assessment of contributing factors to unintentional weight loss and malnutrition.

Physical Exam and Focused Interview
Assess:

- Signs of malnutrition during clinical exam as outlined in Chart 14–1 (p. 274)
- Signs of dysphagia or chewing difficulties; note pocketed food, drooling, mouth sores, dental health, fit of dentures, xerostomia (lack of saliva)
- Cognitive impairment or dependency on others for feeding or meal preparation
- Altered functional status: immobility, loss of strength, fatigue
- Gastrointestinal, appetite, or oral complaints from disease or medication side effects
- Pain
- Psychosocial health: depression, bereavement, isolation, dependency, food security
- Sensory losses and neurological symptoms: vision, hearing, taste, neuropathy, tremors
- Medical conditions or treatment that alter intake, absorption, or nutritional requirements

- Hypermetabolic conditions: fever, infection, sepsis, fracture, wounds, cachexia, burns.

Anthropometric Measurements
Assess:

- Measured height and weight
- Serial weights; check medical record for weight history to confirm
- Body composition measurements must use age and gender-specific references because alterations in skin elasticity, muscle mass, fat distribution, bone density and water content can change with age.

Nutrition History
Assess:

- Nutrition data as outlined in Chart 14–3
- Whether use of therapeutic diet is appropriate
- Use of alcohol
- Access to personal, cultural, or religious food preferences (especially hospitalized or dependent elderly)
- Iatrogenic malnutrition risk: assess days NPO, on clear liquid, or other insufficient diet; inadequate delivery of supplements or tube feedings; overuse of restricted diet resulting in poor intake; insufficient feeding assistance; missed meals for testing.

Malnutrition

Malnutrition can be defined as a deficiency of one or more nutrients. The terms *undernutrition* and *malnutrition* are used interchangeably. A deficiency of macronutrients (carbohydrate, protein, and fat) can result in weight loss from insufficient energy and muscle wasting. Often the general term *malnutrition* is synonymous with the specific term **protein-calorie malnutrition.** Deficiency of any micronutrient may initially be less physically evident than with macronutrient deficiency because a lack of vitamins and minerals can take many weeks or months to manifest clinical symptoms.

Malnutrition occurs because of decreased intake, increased losses, or unmet increased needs for energy or any nutrient. Patients have decreased intake for a number of medical and psychosocial reasons. Nutrient losses can occur from malabsorptive disease or drug interactions. Hypermetabolism during physiological stress, or increased energy needs because of growth, development, and physical activity can cause increased nutritional needs that must be met or malnutrition will develop. The accompanying Risk Factors box (p. 278) outlines the many contributing risk factors to malnutrition.

Malnutrition has adverse consequences such as poor wound healing, risk of decubitus ulcer development, loss of muscle mass (including respiratory and heart) with subsequent loss of strength and functional decline, diminished immunocompetence, and altered pharmacokinetics (Covinsky, 2002; Hoffer, 2001; Holmes, 2003; Sullivan, Bopp, & Roberson, 2002). Weight loss exceeding 40% of body weight is associated with mortality (Hoffer, 2001). Successful treatment of malnutrition is contingent on discovery of the underlying etiology. Provision of adequate nutrition in a well-tolerated form is best based on the recommendations of a registered dietitian who is trained to assess the impact of physiological stress, disease, and alterations in metabolism on baseline nutritional requirements across the life span. Specific nutrition interventions are presented in later discussions in this chapter of medical nutrition therapy.

Physiological Stress

A hypermetabolic response to injury or disease can have significant nutritional ramifications. Major surgery, thermal injury, sepsis, and trauma are examples of **physiological stress**. Unlike periods of inadequate energy intake that result in weight loss and some muscle wasting, a hypermetabolic response because of physiological stress can lead to rapid protein catabolism even when it seems energy and protein intake are sufficient (Hoffer, 2001). The body's response to this metabolic stress leads to a cascade that includes release of catecholamines and cortisol, and a systemic inflammatory response (Hoffer, 2001; Holmes, 2003; Kotler, 2000). Systemic inflammatory response is described in detail in Chapter 61 ☞. The result can be catabolization of skeletal muscle to provide substrate for gluconeogenesis and a degradation of plasma proteins, such as albumin, that are considered acute-phase reactant proteins. Resting energy needs are elevated, which is referred to as **hypermetabolism**. Thus, physiological stress results in hypermetabolism and hypercatabolism. **Hypercatabolism** occurs when catabolism exceeds normal physiological rates. Each of these represents a nutritional challenge that is compounded when present together. The patient who is already malnourished before surgery, injury, or disease will have less available body stores to draw on during a metabolically challenging circumstance. In severe circumstances the rate

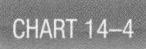

CHART 14–4 REAP and WAVE Tools

WEIGHT

Assess patient's Body Mass Index.*
Patient is overweight if BMI>25.

Height	Body Weight lbs	Height	Body Weight lbs
4'10"	>119	5'8"	>161
4'11"	>124	5'9"	>169
5'0"	>128	5'10"	>174
5'1"	>132	5'11"	>179
5'2"	>136	6'0"	>184
5'3"	>141	6'1"	>189
5'4"	>145	6'2"	>194
5'5"	>150	6'3"	>200
5'6"	>155	6'4"	>305
5'7"	>159		

*Certain pts may require assessment for underweight and/or unintentional weight loss

VARIETY

Is patient eating a variety of foods from important sections of the food pyramid?

Grains (6–11 servings)

Fruits (2–4 servings)

Vegetables (3–5 servings)

Protein (2–3 servings)

Dairy (2–3 servings)

Determine Variety and Excess using one of the following methods:

- Do a quick one-day recall.
- Ask patient to complete a self-administered eating pattern questionnaire.

ACTIVITY

Ask patient about any physical activity in the past week: walking briskly, jogging, gardening, swimming, biking, dancing, golf, etc.

1. Does patient do 30 minutes of moderate activity on most days/wk?
2. Does pt do "lifestyle" activity like taking the stairs instead of elevators, etc.?
3. Does patient usually watch less than 2 hours of TV or videos/day?

If patient answers NO to above questions, assess whether patient is willing to increase physical activity.

EXCESS

Is patient eating too much:

Fat? Saturated fat?

Calories?

Salt?

Sugar?

Alcohol?

- Ask about serving/portion sizes, preparation methods and added fats like butter, mayonnaise, sour cream, salad dressing, etc.
- Does patient eat 4 or more meals from sit-down or take-out restaurants per week?
- Does patient indulge on the weekends?
- *What does patient think are pros/cons of his/her eating pattern?*
- *If patient needs to improve eating habits, assess willingness to make changes.*

Source: Gans, K. M., Ross, E., Barner, C. W., Wylie-Rosett, J., McMurray, J., & Eaton, C. (2003). REAP and WAVE: New tools to rapidly assess/discuss nutrition with patients. *Journal of Nutrition, 133,* 556S–562S.

RISK FACTORS for Malnutrition

Decreased Intake

- Anorexia
- Gastrointestinal symptoms: nausea, vomiting, diarrhea
- Medication side effects
- Pain
- Dysphagia
- Poor dental health or chewing difficulties
- Sensory changes: loss of vision, taste, neuropathy
- Depression, anxiety, cognitive impairment, or other neuropsychological symptoms
- Socioeconomic issues: lack of finances, food insecurity, social isolation, bereavement, dependency on others for food or feeding
- Alcoholism.

Increased Nutrient Losses

- Malabsorptive disease
- Short bowel syndrome
- Alcoholism
- Drug–nutrient interactions.

Increased Nutrient Requirements

- Fever
- Infection or sepsis
- Wounds
- Fracture
- Hypermetabolic disease
- Increased energy expenditure from increased physical activity.

of protein degradation exceeds the body's ability to replenish muscle and plasma stores and, thus, physical and biochemical evidence of malnutrition ensues.

The severe muscle wasting seen with physiological stress is referred to as **cachexia** (Kotler, 2000). When cachexia becomes evident, nutritional repletion is difficult because of the confounding chronic systemic inflammatory response. High energy and protein intake alone often does not overcome the effects. Considerable research has focused on supplementation with so-called "conditionally essential" amino acids, such as glutamine and arginine. Researchers believe that these nonessential amino acids become essential during extreme metabolic stress, such as with trauma or burns (Wilmore, 2001). Amino acid–enhanced nutritional products are available (and prescribed), but their use remains controversial (Buchman, 2001). More recently, resistance training, pharmacological intervention with anabolic agents, cytokine inhibitors, and other metabolic regulators have all been under investigation for a potential role in cachexia treatment (Kotler, 2000; Nerad et al., 2003). Further discussion of the nutritional effects of physiological stress under specific circumstances is provided later in this chapter. The effects of malnutrition on the elderly is presented in the Gerontological Considerations box.

Health Promotion

Health promotion includes nutrition education on both preservation of wellness and disease prevention through diet. The nurse can assist the patient in the development of strategies for lifestyle modifications aimed at improving nutrition health. Several national standards exist with supporting educational tools to guide the nurse in nutrition health promotion.

The *Dietary Guidelines for Americans, 2005 Edition* (U.S. Department of Health and Human Services [DHHS], 2005) are national standards that can be used when advising patients about health maintenance and disease prevention. These science-based general recommendations are targeted to the general population age 2 years and older and serve as the foundation for other federal nutrition guidelines and information, such as the development of the *Healthy People* objectives for the nation (DHHS, 2000). These guidelines are translated for the public into key messages providing diet and physical activity guidance. These messages can become a template for general nutrition education as well as more specific advice about disease prevention. The National Guidelines box outlines the

GERONTOLOGICAL CONSIDERATIONS
Malnutrition

The prevalence of malnutrition among older adults is disproportionately high compared to younger adults. Up to 60% of hospitalized elderly or those under dependent care are malnourished (Singh, Watt, Veitch, Cantor, & Duerksen, 2006; Sullivan, Sun, & Walls, 1999; Thomas et al., 2002). Hospitalized malnourished older adults have twice the 1-year mortality rate after discharge compared to well-nourished older adults (Persson et al., 2002).

Alterations in pharmacokinetics from malnutrition are especially pertinent in the elderly because of the probability of polypharmacy. Low plasma protein levels affect drug binding for certain classes of medications, leaving an increased circulating free fraction of those drugs. Polypharmacy further complicates this when multiple drugs compete for diminished protein binding sites, increasing the likelihood of an adverse drug reaction. Enzymes required for drug metabolism can be affected by inadequate protein and micronutrient status (Holmes, 2003). Malnutrition can affect pharmacokinetics at both the absorptive and cell level for drug and herb metabolism. Unintentional weight loss and signs of malnutrition among the elderly should not be considered a normal part of the aging process and always deserve full consideration and attention to determine the etiology and provide appropriate intervention.

nine major messages of the *Dietary Guidelines for Americans, 2005 Edition.*

Nutrition health promotion also includes the elimination of health disparities that affect nutrition status. The DHHS along with the U.S. Department of Agriculture developed the *Healthy People 2010* document to establish goals and objectives for the nation aimed at improving quality and years of life as well as reducing health disparities (DHHS, 2000). The *Healthy People 2010* objectives can help the nurse to target appropriate interventions for specific population groups. Another National Guidelines box (p. 280) outlines the objectives from *Healthy People 2010* that relate to nutrition health.

Medical Nutrition Therapy for Medical–Surgical Patients

Medical nutrition therapy (MNT) plays a central role in the care of the medical or surgical patient. MNT includes the use of specific nutrition guidelines, nutrients, or therapeutic diets to treat an illness or medical condition. Therapeutic diets are used in the

---

NATIONAL GUIDELINES *Dietary Guidelines for Americans, 2005 Edition*

- Consume a variety of foods within and among the basic food groups while staying within energy needs.
- Control calorie intake to manage body weight.
- Be physically active every day.
- Increase daily intake of fruits and vegetables, whole grains, and nonfat or low-fat milk and milk products.

- Choose fats wisely for good health.
- Choose carbohydrates wisely for good health.
- Choose and prepare foods with little salt.
- If you drink alcoholic beverages, do so in moderation.
- Keep food safe to eat.

Source: U.S. Department of Health and Human Services. (2005). *Dietary guidelines for Americans, 2005 edition.* Retrieved May 17, 2008, from http://www.health.gov/DietaryGuidelines/dga2005/document.

NATIONAL GUIDELINES *Healthy People 2010* Nutrition Objectives

- Increase the proportion of adults who are at a healthy weight.
- Reduce the proportion of adults who are obese.
- Reduce the proportion of children and adolescents who are overweight or obese.
- Reduce growth retardation among low-income children under age 5 years.
- Increase the proportion of persons age 2 years and older who consume at least:
  - Two daily servings of fruit
  - Three daily servings of vegetables, with at least one green or dark orange
  - Six daily servings of grain products, with at least three whole-grain choices
  - And who meet the dietary recommendations for calcium.

- Increase the proportion of people age 2 years and older who consume less than:
  - 10% of calories from saturated fat
  - 30% of calories from total fat
  - 2,400 mg of sodium.
- Reduce iron deficiency anemia among young children and females of childbearing age.
- Reduce low birth weight and very low birth weight.
- Increase the proportion of pregnancies begun with optimum folic acid level.

Source: U.S. Department of Health and Human Services. (2000). *Healthy people 2010: Understanding and improving health.* Retrieved February 5, 2008, from http://www.healthypeople.gov

treatment of many diseases and conditions. Descriptions of specific diets are contained within the discussion of each disease state outlined in this chapter. Nutrition support in the form of tube feedings or intravenous nutrition is a type of MNT and is also discussed. Both hospitals and long-term care institutions are required by accrediting agencies to have a diet manual specific to their organization available in each medical unit. Diet manuals describe the specifics of all therapeutic diets and texture-modified diets offered at the institution. The nurse should refer to this manual to become familiar with the modified diets available for patients.

Many patients may not require a therapeutic diet while hospitalized. A house or regular diet is ordered for such patients. Some patients have a temporary or permanent need for a texture-modified or liquid diet while hospitalized. Clear liquid diets can be used postoperatively or as part of preparation for diagnostic testing. A clear liquid diet contains little in the way of adequate nutrition for the patient and should not be used for more than a day or two without consideration given to additional nutrition intervention. Many institutions require daily renewable prescriptions for a clear liquid diet in the hope it fosters regular reevaluation of the need for the diet. A registered dietitian should be consulted when patients remain on a clear liquid diet as the sole form of nutrition for more than a few days. Difficulties with either chewing or swallowing warrant a nutrition evaluation for the appropriateness of a texture-modified diet. Chart 14–5 outlines various hospital diets prescribed for transitional and texture-modified diets.

Weight Management

Care of the patient who is either overweight or underweight requires a central nutrition component. The approach to medical nutrition therapy in the area of weight management is constantly evolving and requires the need to keep a current knowledge base. Both overweight and underweight states can lead to additional health risks in the medical–surgical patient.

Overweight and Obesity

Overweight and obesity are linked with a multitude of comorbidities, including cardiovascular disease, hypertension, type 2 diabetes, degenerative joint disease, some pulmonary disease, and cancers (NHLBI, 1998). Obesity has been reported to lessen life expectancy, especially in younger adults (Fontaine, Redden, Wang, Westfall, & Allison, 2003). The prevalence of overweight and obesity is increasing among all population groups in the United States, where 63% of all men and 55% of women 20 to 74 years of age are considered overweight or obese (Hedley et al., 2004). Further parental obesity has been reported to more than double the risk of adult obesity among children less than 10 years of age (Whitaker, Wright, Pepe, Seidel, & Dietz, 1997). This worrisome association could lead to future increases in obesity prevalence.

Many factors are postulated as contributing to the prevalence of overweight and obesity. Genetic, metabolic, psychological, and environmental causes have been cited (American Dietetic Association, 2002b; NHLBI, 1998). Hormones, such as leptin, have been hypothesized to have a potential role in the metabolic link to obesity (American Dietetic Association, 2002b). Certain medications, such as psychotropics, can foster weight gain. Medications that block receptors for histamine, serotonin 5-5HT, and dopamine are examples in this category (Devlin, Yanovski, & Wilson, 2000). Although genetic and metabolic contributors to obesity are important, most researchers agree that energy imbalance is a more significant contributor (American Dietetic Association, 2002b). Increased dietary intake, decreased physical activity, or a combination of both can lead to an imbalance in which energy expenditure is less than energy consumption and weight gain follows.

Increased energy consumption occurs for many reasons. One reason is that Americans consume more food outside the home than in the past. Foods prepared outside the home are calorically dense and come in larger portions than in previous years (Harnack & French, 2003; Young & Nestle, 2003). Larger portions are often marketed as a value to the cost-conscious consumer. The consumer may have lost sight of standard food portions with the expansion of market portions between two- and eightfold in the past decades (Young & Nestle, 2003). A sedentary lifestyle can further tip the energy balance equation and contribute to weight gain. More than 25% of U.S. adults are considered sedentary

CHART 14–5	**Transitional and Texture-Modified Diets**			
Diet	**Definition**	**Sample Contents**	**Indications**	**Special Concerns**
Clear liquids	Liquid at room or body temperature and able to be seen through clearly	Clear juices like apple and cranberry, popsicles, gelatin, clear broth, tea	Preparation for diagnostic testing, transition from NPO to reintroduction of oral intake such as after an acute gastrointestinal (GI) event or postoperatively	Provides hydration and some electrolytes and carbohydrate, but nutritionally inadequate. Limit duration of use.
Full liquids	Pourable consistency at room or body temperature	All liquids, including milk and nutrition supplement drinks, ice cream, cooked cereal	Fractured mandible, difficulty chewing or swallowing other consistencies	Ensure safety of this consistency in patients at risk for aspiration, avoid overmodifying texture unnecessarily. Can be modified to exclude lactose-containing foods.
Mechanical soft	Soft or chopped foods without connective tissue, casings, tough skins	Full range of soft foods; can be chopped or mashed	Chewing or swallowing difficulties	Vary texture to patient tolerance. Avoid overly chopped or mashed consistency when not necessary.
Puree	Mechanically blenderized foods to spoon-thick consistency	Mashed potato, pureed hamburger, pureed peas, pudding	Chewing or swallowing difficulties	Avoid more texture modification than is needed. Ensure attractive eating environment to improve visual appeal of diet.
House or regular	All foods	Full choice of available menu items in all food groups	No condition requiring diet modification	Provides complete nutrition. Monitor tolerance and intake.

(Centers for Disease Control and Prevention [CDC], 2001). Reliance on technology, the automobile, and energy-saving devices has made it easier to expend less energy to do work and leisure activities (Nestle & Jacobson, 2000). "Screen time" watching television, videos, or computer games has been linked to obesity in adults and children (Hu et al., 2001; Hu, Li, Colditz, Willett, & Manson, 2003; Shields, 2006).

A nutrition assessment focusing on parameters to measure weight status is an intuitive step before determining treatment interventions for the overweight patient. Overweight is defined as a BMI of 25 to 29.9. Obesity is defined as a BMI greater than 30. Additional stratification exists to denote different classes of obesity. Chart 14–6 lists BMI classifications. Figure 14–1 ■ (p. 275) illustrates BMI calculations and classifications. In the

past, height–weight tables were used to determine appropriate weight and to diagnose overweight. These tables have been replaced by the BMI table in the clinical setting.

Other considerations to include in the assessment process are the presence of obesity risk factors, weight and dieting history (including failures and successes), and patient readiness to attempt weight loss. The nurse needs to assess the patient's readiness for weight loss based on the Stages of Change model. This model can be used to assess readiness for any behavior change and categorizes individuals according to where they are on a spectrum of thinking or action about new behavior using the terms precontemplation, contemplation, action, and maintenance (Kushner, 2003). Patients not ready or unwilling to attempt weight loss should be encouraged to prevent further weight gain (NHLBI, 1998; Serdula, Kettel Khan, & Dietz, 2003). Figure 14–2 ■ (p. 283) shows an algorithm developed by the NIH for weight loss treatment. Chart 14–7 (p. 282) outlines important factors to consider when assessing a patient before weight loss intervention.

The nurse can guide the patient in establishing a reasonable weight loss goal. Generally a goal of 5% to 10% loss of weight is recommended over a 6-month period and is associated with a reduction in health risks associated with obesity (NHLBI, 1998). Many patients wish to attempt a larger weight loss, but this should be discouraged because weight loss maintenance of larger losses can prove frustrating and difficult and lead to weight regain (American Dietetic Association, 2002b; Serdula et al., 2003). The nurse should encourage the patient to attempt weight loss by stressing the associated health benefits with even

CHART 14–6	**BMI Classifications**
BMI	**Classification**
18.5–24.9	Normal
25–29.9	Overweight
30–34.9	Obese class 1
35–39.9	Obese class 2
≥40	Obese class 3

Source: National Heart, Lung, and Blood Institute. (1998). *Clinical guidelines on the identification, evaluation, and treatment of overweight and obesity in adults—the evidence report.* Retrieved February 5, 2004, from www.nhlbi.nih.gov/guidelines/obesity/ob_gdlns.pdf

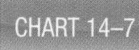

CHART 14–7 — Assessment of Patients Who Are Overweight or Obese for Weight Loss Intervention

Assess for obesity comorbidities.

Assess anthropometrics:
- Weight, weight history, maximum and minimum adult weights
- BMI and waist circumference.

Assess dieting history:
- Amount, frequency, duration, and types of diets
- Use of supplements, devices, or medications for weight loss
- Contributors to weight gain or regain
- Barriers to weight loss or maintenance in past and currently
- Source of information on dieting and nutrition.

Assess current eating according to Chart 14–3.

Assess for symptoms of disordered eating or binge eating.

Assess psychosocial influences:
- Social support
- Financial implications of weight loss treatment
- Readiness, motivation to change.

Assess physical activity frequency, intensity, and duration.

Sources: Kushner, R. F. (2003). *Roadmaps for clinical practice—Case studies in disease prevention and health promotion: Assessment and management of adult obesity—A primer for physicians.* Chicago, IL: American Medical Association. Retrieved December 18, 2003, from http://www.ama-assn.org/ama/pub/category/10931.html; American Dietetic Association 2002; National Institute of Health, National Heart, Lung, and Blood Institute. (NHLBI). (1998). *Clinical guidelines on the identification, evaluation, and treatment of overweight and obesity in adults—The evidence report.* Retrieved February 5, 2004, from http://www.nhlbi.nih.gov/guidelines/obesity/ob_gdlns.pdf; Serdula, M. K., Kettel Khan, L., & Dietz, W. H. (2003). Weight loss counseling revisited. *Journal of the American Medical Association, 289,* 1747–1750.

modest loss. Less than half of obese patients surveyed reported being advised by a health care provider to lose weight (Jackson, Doescher, Saver, & Hart, 2005).

An energy deficit of 500 to 1,000 kilocalories per day can result in weight loss of between 1 to 2 pounds per week. This deficit is best accomplished with a combination of decreased intake and increased energy expenditure (NHLBI, 1998). Any diet with a lower calorie intake than at baseline will produce weight loss. Most current research supports the idea than macronutrient composition (amount of carbohydrate, protein, or fat) does not play a major role, but rather overall calorie deficit does (Freedman, King, & Kennedy, 2001). In published reports of popular low-carbohydrate diets, subjects indeed lost weight but this was reportedly because of an overall reduction in calorie intake and not the carbohydrate content alone (Bravata et al., 2003; Foster et al., 2003; Samaha et al., 2003). Fad and fringe diets may target macronutrient composition or the "magical" combining powers of foods. Those that lead to successful weight loss do so because of calorie reduction and the self-limiting nature of their diet restrictions.

Low-calorie diets occur along a continuum from starvation or fasting to the recommended modest calorie reduction of 500 to 1,000 kilocalories per day. Extreme calorie reduction can lead to unhealthy loss of muscle mass, minerals, electrolytes, and water. In select obese patients, extremely low calorie diets (those with <1,000 kilocalories per day) are used, but with close medical supervision to monitor fluid and electrolyte status as well as general health. Such diets are not recommended for long-term

success (American Dietetic Association, 2002b). Targeting high-fat foods and empty calorie foods with little nutritional content can accomplish a 500- to 1,000-kilocalorie daily reduction in intake. Foods can be replaced with lower calorie foods or omitted. The choices should be realistic and sensible and not contribute to an overall sense of deprivation. Chart 14–8 (p. 284) outlines some examples of lower calorie food swaps.

Some patients want or need the structure of a more formal diet when attempting weight loss. The nurse can educate patients about the components of a healthy diet and guide them in an evaluation of any popular diet they are considering. Chart 14–9 (p. 284) outlines the components of a healthy weight loss diet. Patients who need extensive nutrition guidance and education should be referred to a registered dietitian. Commercial programs are also available for the patient who may benefit from the weekly social support. The nurse can guide the patient to an appropriate individual treatment choice.

Physical activity and a reduction in sedentary activity should be encouraged. Adults with long-term success at weigh loss report ongoing physical activity as a major contributing factor (McInnis, Franklin, & Rippe, 2003). Physical activity has a positive effect on energy balance and can improve body composition and cardiovascular fitness. Weight loss without a physical activity component can lead to loss of lean body mass and a reduced metabolic rate; in contrast, including exercise helps to preserve lean mass (McInnis et al., 2003). The nurse should emphasize the importance of physical activity in preventing weight regain. Exercise can be initiated slowly to eventually accumulate at least 30 minutes of moderate intensity exercise on most days (NHLBI, 1998). Even activities such as walking can replace sedentary activities such as riding an elevator or driving. The nurse can explore any barriers to increasing activity with the patient and offer suggestions tailored to the patient.

Behavior modification is essential for long-term weight loss maintenance and relapse prevention. Weight loss maintenance is a bigger challenge than the initial weight loss for many patients. A lifestyle approach to weight maintenance and healthy social support and coping mechanisms are important. Chart 14–10 (p. 284) outlines behavior modification use in weight loss.

Approved pharmacological treatment for obesity is reserved for patients with a BMI ≥ 30 with no obesity comorbidities or a BMI ≥ 27 if comorbidities exist. Lifestyle diet and exercise modifications should first be attempted for at least 6 months before considering adjunctive medication (NHLBI, 1998; Yanovski & Yanovski, 2002). Pharmacological treatment is not appropriate for cosmetic weight loss attempts.

Bariatric surgery is a treatment option for select clinically severe obese patients (BMI ≥ 40 or >35 with comorbidities). Gastric reduction surgery, including vertical banded gastroplasty, and gastric bypass surgery, such as the Roux-en-Y procedure, are types of bariatric surgery. Weight loss occurs over many months postoperatively. Bypass procedures produce greater weight loss than simpler gastric reduction surgery (American Society for Metabolic and Bariatric Surgery, 2005). Patients undergoing bariatric surgery require intensive presurgical screening and lifelong medical monitoring because of possible short- and long-term health complications (Garza, 2003). Nutrition guidelines following bariatric surgery are discussed later in this chapter.

Treatment Algorithm*

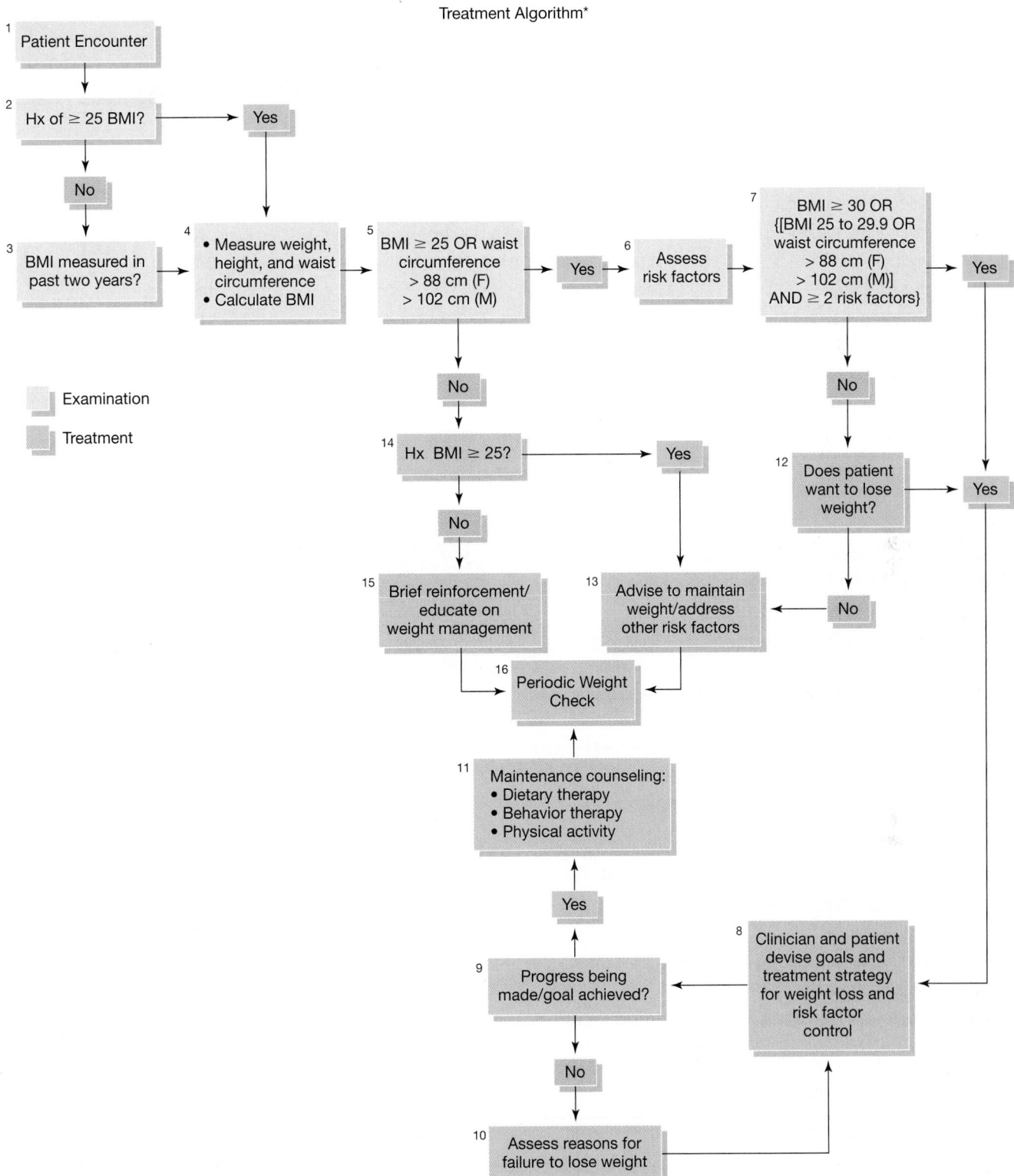

*This algorithm applies only to the assessment for overweight and obesity and subsequent decisions based on that assessment. It does not include any initial overall assessment for cardiovascular risk factors or diseases that are indicated.

FIGURE 14–2 ■ Obesity treatment algorithm.

Source: From National Institutes of Health website: http://www.nhlbi.nih.gov/guidelines/obesity/ob_gdlns.pdf

The nurse should be aware of the many alternative approaches to weight loss that a patient may pursue. Nutrition and herbal supplements, fad diets, and various devices are marketed to the patient as alternative and often "no effort" methods to lose weight. Federal regulation of supplements is minimal because these products are regulated as food and not medicine by the Food and Drug Administration (FDA). The Federal Trade Commission regulates the advertising of such products, however, and

CHART 14–8	Calorie-Saving Examples for Weight Loss Intervention	

Original Food	Alternative Food Suggestion	Approximate Calories Saved
1 C whole milk	1 C skim milk	65
1 C premium ice cream, vanilla	1 C low-fat soft-serve frozen yogurt, vanilla	300
2 TBSP cream cheese	2 TBSP fat-free cream cheese	70
2 TBSP half-and-half coffee creamer	2 TBSP fat-free half-and-half creamer	30
3 oz chicken thigh w/skin, roasted	3 oz chicken breast, skinless, roasted	90
4 oz pork sparerib, braised	4 oz pork tenderloin, trimmed, braised	233
Bagel, 4-1/2-in. diameter	2 English muffin halves	100
Yellow cake, no frosting, 1/12 of 8-in. cake	Angelfood cake, no frosting, 1/12 of 10-in. cake	115
Vanilla crème cookie, 1-3/4 in.	Vanilla wafers, 1 medium	30
1 TBSP oil for sautéing	Cooking spray for sautéing	100
2 TBSP mayonnaise	2 TBSP reduced-calorie mayonnaise	100
2 TBSP Ranch salad dressing	2 TBSP fat-free Ranch salad dressing	100

Note: Not all fat-free or reduced fat foods are lower in calories than the original version. The nurse should instruct patients to compare labels.

Source: USDA Nutrient Data Laboratory http://www.nal.usda.gov/fnic/foodcomp/search

CHART 14–9	Components of a Healthy Weight Loss Diet

- Contains foods from all the major food groups.
- Diet is practical and realistic; can be adhered to without social interruption.
- Fosters no more than a 2 lb per week weight loss on average; higher losses can yield loss of muscle, fluid and electrolytes.
- Emphasis on lean sources of protein: skinless poultry, fish, lean meats, legumes.
- Fruits, vegetables, and whole grains emphasized.
- Intake of 20 to 35 g fiber daily encouraged.
- Adequate low-fat sources of calcium included: nonfat or low-fat milk, yogurt, cheese, or dairy alternatives such as fortified soy milk.
- Adequate water intake of at least 64 oz daily.
- Limited alcohol, if any.
- Minimizes intake of saturated fat, total fat, cholesterol, and sodium.
- Place emphasis on portion sizes.
- No skipped meals; avoids becoming overhungry and overeating as result. Some protein with each meal may satiate longer than an all-carbohydrate meal.
- Physical activity is encouraged.

Sources: Kushner, R. F. (2003). *Roadmaps for clinical practice—Case studies in disease prevention and health promotion: Assessment and management of adult obesity—A primer for physicians.* Chicago, IL: American Medical Association. Retrieved December 18, 2003, from http://www.ama-assn.org/ama/pub/category/10931.html; Jackic, J. M., Clark, K., Coleman, E., et al. (2001). American College of Sports Medicine position stand on the appropriate intervention strategies for weight loss and prevention of weight regain in adults. *Medicine, Science, Sports and Exercise, 33,* 2145–2156; National Institute of Health, National Heart, Lung, and Blood Institute. (2000). *The practical guide: Identification, evaluation and treatment of overweight and obesity in adults.* Retrieved February 5, 2004, from http://www.nhlbi.nih.gov/guidelines/obesity/practgde.htm

CHART 14–10	Behavior Modification in Weight Management

- Allow patient to set goals.
- Encourage self-monitoring of goals; e.g., food diaries and activity logs.
- Identify small steps to take toward daily lifestyle changes.
- Identify environmental cues and contributors to old eating habits. Develop ideas for new cues for exercise and eating habits.
- Discuss and brainstorm coping strategies for relapse prevention: stress management, social support, dealing with boredom or emotions.
- Cognitive restructuring; change self-talk that undermines weight loss or exercise.
- Encourage self-reinforcement; give nonfood rewards when milestones are reached.

Sources: Poston, W. S. C., & Foreyt, J. P. (2000). Successful management of the obese patient. *American Family Physician, 61,* 3615–3622; McInnis, K. J., Franklin, B. A., & Rippe, J. M. (2003). Counseling for physical activity in overweight and obese patients. *American Family Physician, 67,* 1266–1268; National Heart, Lung, and Blood Institute. (1998). *Clinical guidelines on the identification, evaluation, and treatment of overweight and obesity in adults—The evidence report.* Retrieved February 5, 2004, from http://www.nhlbi.nih.gov/guidelines/obesity/ob_gdlns.pdf; National Heart, Lung, and Blood Institute. (2000). *The practical guide: Identification, evaluation and treatment of overweight and obesity in adults.* Retrieved February 5, 2004, from http://www.nhlbi.nih.gov/guidelines/obesity/practgde.htm

Weight management for elderly adults is presented in the Gerontological Considerations box and a patient care plan for obesity is presented in the Nursing Process feature (p. 286).

Disordered Eating

Disordered eating consists of behavioral, psychological, and physical symptoms that surround abnormal perceptions regarding food and body weight. Disordered eating patterns occur along a continuum from minor alterations in food-related behaviors to a clinical eating disorder that meets all established diagnostic criteria. Clinical eating disorders include anorexia nervosa, bulimia nervosa, and eating-disorders-not-otherwise-specified (ED-NOS), which includes binge-eating disorder and disordered eat-

can pursue a manufacturer for flagrantly misleading advertising. Patients need to be educated to view such products with a critical eye. Chart 14–11 outlines examples of alternative products marketed for weight loss, and Chart 14–12 provides educational pointers for evaluating alternative products.

CHART 14–11 Sample Alternative Diet Products (Found Alone or in Combination Products)

Product	Purported Action	Clinical Evidence or Alert
Chitosan	Weight loss from fat "trapping"	Lack of sufficient research. Caution if shellfish allergy. Can alter medication absorption.
Chromium	Lose fat and gain muscle	Deficiency of mineral uncommon. Little evidence products available alter body composition.
Ephedra	Weight loss stimulant	FDA banned the sale of ephedra because of risk of morbidity and mortality from vascular events.
Ginseng	Energy booster	Limited research, little evidence it ↑ energy. Can interact with medication, coagulation.
Hydroxycitric acid or garcinia	Inhibits enzymes of fat metabolism	Controlled trials do not support benefit.
Vanadium	Increase muscle	Limited research showing little to no effect on muscle. Can interact with coagulation.
Mate, guarana, kola nut, green tea	Caffeine-like stimulants of metabolism	Exert caffeine-like effect on central nervous system. Can potentiate other stimulant ingredients. Side effects on blood pressure (BP) and heart rate mimic those of excess caffeine. Labels do not list cumulative "caffeine" equivalent.

Sources: Food and Drug Administration. (2004). *FDA issues regulation prohibiting sale of dietary supplements containing ephedrine alkaloids and reiterates its advice that consumers stop using these products.* News release, retrieved February 6, 2004, from http://www.cfsan.fda.gov/~lrd/fpephed6.html; Morelli, V., & Zoorob, R. J. (2000). Alternative therapies: Part 1. Depression, diabetes, obesity. *American Family Physician, 62,* 1051–1060; Roerig, J. L., Mitchell, J. E., deZwaan, M., Wonderlich, S. A., et al. (2003). The eating disorders medicine cabinet revisited: A clinician's guide to appetite suppressants and diuretics. *International Journal of Eating Disorders, 33,* 443–457; Sarubin Fragakis, A. (2003). *The Health Professional's Guide to Popular Dietary Supplements* (2nd ed.). Chicago, IL: American Dietetic Association.

CHART 14–12 Spotting Quackery in Weight Loss Products

- Weight loss claim is "too good to be true."
- Quick dramatic results are promised with little or no effort.
- Miracle blocking or trapping of fat or carbohydrates is claimed.
- Weight loss occurs while you can eat all you want.
- The product is worn or rubbed on skin and causes weight loss without diet or exercise.
- Pseudomedical jargon is used to infer scientific expertise.
- Anecdotes and testimonials are touted instead of peer-reviewed controlled studies.
- Advertising is condescending to established medical treatment. Claims of hidden medical secret are made.
- Food or groups of foods are labeled as toxic or "poisonous to the system."
- Special powers or attributes are assigned to certain foods (e.g., grapefruit burns fat).

Federal Trade Commission (2003). *Red flag bogus weight loss claims.* Retrieved May 30, 2008 from http://www.ftc.gov/bcp/conline/pubs/buspubs/redflag.pdf

GERONTOLOGICAL CONSIDERATIONS
Weight Management

Adults over age 65 years can benefit from weight management with improved day-to-day functioning and reduced cardiovascular risk. Before weight loss is recommended or attempted, however, a thorough nutrition assessment should be considered because of the high prevalence of malnutrition among older adults. Improper dieting attempts could unwittingly contribute to increased risk of malnutrition. Patients should be evaluated for their individual risks and benefits associated with potential weight loss. Specific attention should be given to preservation of muscle mass with physical activity. Appropriate referrals should be made for monitoring nutrition and exercise in the elderly.

ing not meeting the strict criteria for anorexia or bulimia. Criteria for clinical diagnoses are outlined in the *Diagnostic and Statistical Manual of Mental Disorders, Fourth Edition, Text Revision* (DSM-IV) (American Psychiatric Association [APA], 2000a).

Eating disorders are prevalent in up to 5% of the U.S. population (American Dietetic Association, 2001). Much debate surrounds the etiology of these complex disorders. Biology (including genetics), psychology, and sociocultural influences have all received attention as contributors (Fairburn & Harrison, 2003). More than half of patients with bulimia and almost half of patients with binge-eating disorder have substance abuse disorder. Obsessive-compulsive disorder, anxiety, depression, and other mood disorders are prevalent in all forms of eating disorders (APA, 2000b; American Dietetic Association, 2001; Pritts & Susman, 2003). Chart 14–13 (p. 286) lists population groups felt to be at higher risk for an eating disorder. When conducting a nursing assessment, these groups should be screened for eating disorder signs and symptoms.

Although eating disorders are considered a psychiatric diagnosis, medical and nutritional complications often place the patient in the medical care setting. It is important for the nurse to recognize the physical symptoms when assessing patients and to be involved in the medical and nutritional interventions of any treatment.

Anorexia Nervosa

Patients with anorexia nervosa are at 85% or less of expected body weight yet have an intense fear of gaining weight and a disturbed

CHART 14–13 Populations at Risk for Eating Disorders

Athletes in sports with
- Subjective scoring (e.g., figure skating, gymnastics)
- Performance thinness philosophy (e.g., dance, distance running)
- Contour-revealing clothing (e.g., cheer leading, swim, dance)
- Emphasis on prepubescent body (e.g., gymnastics, figure skating)
- Weight categories (e.g., rowing, wrestling).

Fashion models

People who are obese

Young people with limited diets because of disease (e.g., diabetes)

Family history of mood, anxiety disorder, substance abuse

Family environment of adverse, critical, controlling, or distance parenting; family dieting; comments on physical appearance

Sources: American Dietetic Association. (2001). Position of the American Dietetic Association: Nutrition intervention in the treatment of anorexia nervosa, bulimia nervosa, and eating disorders not otherwise specified (EDNOS). *Journal of the American Dietetic Association, 101,* 810–819; Fairburn, C. G., & Harrison, P. J. (2003). Eating disorders. *Lancet, 361,* 407–416; McNulty, K. Y., Adams, C. H., Anderson, J. M., & Affenito, S. G. (2001). Development and validation of a screening tool to identify eating disorders in female athletes. *Journal of the American Dietetic Association, 101,* 886–892; Rubenstein, S., & Caballero, B. (2000). Is Miss America an undernourished role model? *Journal of the American Medical Association, 283,* 1569.

body image. Weight loss can have occurred as a result of restrictive dieting, excessive exercise, or a combination of both. A BMI ≤17.5 is considered indicative of anorexia (American Dietetic Association, 2001; Becker, Grinspoon, Kilbanski, & Herzog, 1999). Other physical symptoms that may be present on a physical exam are listed in Chart 14–14 (p. 289). During the focused interview, the nurse can use established screening tools to assess for disordered eating or simply rely on informal questions on eating and exercise patterns, dieting behaviors, perception of body weight, and proper nutrition. A vegetarian diet is used by some as a method of masking restrictive eating (Klopp, Heiss, & Smith, 2003). Suspicion of disordered eating accompanied by a new vegetarian lifestyle should be investigated further.

Comprehensive evaluation tools exist but are cumbersome in the primary care setting and best intended for use by mental health professionals (Pritts & Susman, 2003). A quick screening tool appropriate in the medical setting is the SCOFF screening instrument outlined in Chart 14–15 (p. 289) (Morgan, Reid, & Lacy, 1999; Perry et al., 2002). Some patients do not present with symptoms that meet the strict DSM-IV criteria but have abnormal eating or exercise patterns and a significant weight loss history. The nurse should use sound judgment in determining

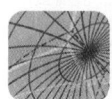

NURSING PROCESS: Patient Care Plan for Obesity

Assessment of Current Nutritional Status

Subjective Data:
Have you recently gained or lost weight?
Do you prepare your own meals?
How often do you eat in restaurants?
Do you live/eat alone?
Do you have a regular meal schedule? What is it?
Do you eat during the night?

Objective Data:
Current measured weight in pounds/height with minimal clothing and after urination
Serial weights from medical records
Presence of abdominal adiposity

Nursing Assessment and Diagnoses	Outcomes and Evaluation Parameters	Planning and Interventions with *Rationales*
Nursing Diagnosis: *Imbalanced Nutrition: More than Body Requirements* related to imbalance in dietary requirements and energy requirements	**Outcome:** Balanced nutrition ***Evaluation Parameters:*** Maintaining BMI within normal range.	**Interventions and *Rationales:*** Perform a complete physical assessment and nutritional history on admission *to assess current nutritional status and to provide a nutritional baseline of data.* Calculate BMI to determine overweight/obesity status. Current weight is compared to BMI charts, height weight charts, and waist measurement *to determine degree of overweight status, overweight, obese, or morbidly obese.* Measure waist circumference *to determine cardiovascular disease risk.* Differentiate weight gain of obesity from weight gain of edema, and other nonadiposity causes *to determine cause of weight gain.*

Assessment of Current Nutritional and Dietary Intake

Subjective Data:
24-hour and possibly 3-day recall of all meals, snacks, liquids
Location of meals
Method of food preparation
Portion size
Meals missed
Other factors that may influence intake, such as recent acute illness or cultural or religious influences on food intake patterns.
Alcohol intake

Objective Data:
Ask spouse or significant other to validate data if patient agrees

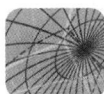

NURSING PROCESS: Patient Care Plan for Obesity—*Continued*

Nursing Assessment and Diagnoses	Outcomes and Evaluation Parameters	Planning and Interventions with *Rationales*
Nursing Diagnosis: *Imbalanced Nutrition: More Than Body Requirements* related to individual factors and patterns in food preparation and eating styles	**Outcome:** Patient lists all foods honestly so that a true intake record is gathered. ***Evaluation Parameters:*** Patient aware of sources of intake and eating habits. Patient states motivation to change unhealthy habits.	**Interventions and *Rationales:*** List food intake for the past 24 hours and the past 3 days *to determine patterns, frequency of certain foods, location of meals, and intake patterns that place patient at high risk for increased nutritional intake.* Observe and identify possible patterns of food intake such as nighttime eating, eating while driving, eating while watching television *to determine total calorie intake and patient's awareness, or lack there of, about the amount of intake.* Keeps a food diary of frequency of intake of high-calorie items *to determine calorie intake.*

Assessment of Disease Risk Factors Influenced by Overweight Status

Subjective Data:

Do you have diabetes?

Is there a history of diabetes in your family?

When was the last time you had your blood sugar tested and what were the results?

Do you have high blood pressure?

When was the last time you had your blood pressure checked and what was the reading?

Do you have any problems with your heart?

When was your last physical examination?

What medications do you take?

Objective Data:

Cholesterol level

Triglyceride level

Blood glucose level

Blood pressure

Medication evaluation

Nursing Assessment and Diagnoses	Outcomes and Evaluation Parameters	Planning and Interventions with *Rationales*
Nursing Diagnosis: Health Maintenance Ineffective risk related to known risk factors for chronic diseases based on overweight status	**Outcomes:** Patient is able to verbalize risk for cardiac disease. Patient establishes a short-term and a long-term weight loss goal that is realistic. ***Evaluation Parameters:*** Verbalization allows the patient to admit that weight is problematic in terms of health status. Verbalizes understanding of impact of excess weight on health status.	**Interventions and *Rationales:*** Ask patient what disease risk factors are related to overweight status. *This question elicits the patient's understanding of how overweight status may affect health status.* Establish a weight goal that is reasonable and achievable *to reduce disease risks.*

Assessment of Changes That Can Be Made in Food Intake to Lower Caloric Intake, Including Patient Readiness to Change Food Intake

Subjective Data:

List the foods you typically eat daily.

Is there a particular food that you eat in excess when you are stressed, sick, or disturbed about something?

What activities do you do when you are stressed?

Do you increase your food intake when stressed?

Do you feel a need to change your dietary habits?

Are you motivated to learn new habits and try instituting them?

Do you have an exercise program?

Are you interested in starting an exercise program?

Objective Data:

Caloric intake per 24 hours based on above food diary

Cholesterol and fat grams in food

Carbohydrate counting

BMI

Daily, weekly, and/or monthly weigh-ins

(continued)

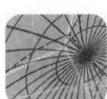 **NURSING PROCESS: Patient Care Plan for Obesity—*Continued***

Nursing Assessment and Diagnoses	Outcomes and Evaluation Parameters	Planning and Interventions with *Rationales*
Nursing Diagnosis: *Impaired Home Maintenance* related to changes in eating patterns that may affect lifestyle, planning, and financial matters	**Outcomes:** Begins and maintains a change in eating habits. Develops healthy choices to deal with stress. **Evaluation Parameters:** Patient can write down changes in food intake that he/she is willing to do in order to lose weight. Keeps weight loss records, measure body circumference area, for progress toward goal. Writes daily weight in a weight loss calendar/diary. Loses 1–2 lb of weight per week.	**Interventions and *Rationales:*** Determine caloric intake for 24-hour period based on patient's size and weight goals. *Weight loss of 7%–10% has been recommended to be a manageable level to achieve and maintain and will also provide a benefit in glucose levels for those who have prediabetes or overt diabetes.* Provide some simple ways to lower caloric counts (e.g., removing skin from chicken, avoiding fried foods, avoiding extra fat and caloric intake such as butter and jelly). *Most nutritious foods can be reduced in terms of calories by the method of preparation and the patient will not feel deprived.* Recommend using a support group *to provide emotional support while losing weight.* Teach patient to eat nutritious foods when hungry at regular times. *This strategy will help patient avoid food items with high caloric value and little to no nutritional value (e.g., cake, donuts, chips, etc.).* Teach the patient who wants a structured diet to count calories, carbohydrates, and/or fat grams in food. *Some patients benefit more from a structured weight loss plan, whereas others prefer less structure.* Teach patient recommendations regarding cholesterol and saturated fat intake. Discuss an exercise program and set realistic goals *to increase calorie burning and promote a healthy lifestyle.* Encourage cues to weight loss action, such as keeping a food diary and putting reminders on the refrigerator regarding physical activity. *Cues to action serve as reminders for health promotion behaviors.* Teach patient to avoid triggers to overeating *to prevent weight gain.* Increase activities that are enjoyable other than eating *to minimize food intake.*

Assessment of Activity Level

Subjective Data:
Do you exercise; if so, what type?
How many times per week do you exercise?
Do you take your pulse during and after exercise?

Objective Data:
Pedometer readings
Documented visits to personal health trainer

Nursing Assessment and Diagnoses	Outcomes and Evaluation Parameters	Planning and Interventions with *Rationales*
Nursing Diagnosis: *Activity intolerance* related to lack of motivation and current health status	**Outcome:** Patient walks at least 30 minutes per day at least four times per week. **Evaluation Parameters:** Activity log shows daily entries of time engaged in activity. Activity levels show a steady increase in time and distance achieved.	**Interventions and *Rationales:*** Encourage 30 minutes of physical activity most days of the week, *which will tone the body and assist in weight loss.* If patient has been physically inactive previously, activity levels should gradually increase *to prevent activity intolerance and cardiac stress.*

Assessment of Knowledge Regarding Surgical Methods of Weight Loss

Subjective Data:
What are your thoughts on surgical intervention for weight loss?
Do you have questions about the various procedures?

Objective Data:
Patient inquires of health provider about suitability of these methods for himself.
Patient attends a surgical information session.

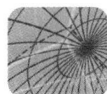

NURSING PROCESS: Patient Care Plan for Obesity—*Continued*

Nursing Assessment and Diagnoses	Outcomes and Evaluation Parameters	Planning and Interventions with *Rationales*
Nursing Diagnosis: *Deficient Knowledge* regarding surgical weight loss methods	**Outcome:** Patient verbalizes knowledge regarding various surgical techniques. ***Evaluation Parameters:*** Patient states will continue to consider surgical means if weight loss is unsuccessful.	**Interventions and *Rationales:*** Discuss the surgical means of weight loss, including lap band surgery and intestinal bypass *to help patient understand the new concepts of surgical intervention.* Discuss the pros and cons of weight loss surgery *to assist the patient in being well informed.* Emphasize the importance of using medical means of weight loss until a decision is reached about the appropriateness of surgery for the patient. *The patient needs to understand that surgical interventions take time to consider and that surgery is more successful with fewer complications if about 10% of body weight has been lost prior to surgery by conventional means.*

CHART 14–14   Symptoms of Eating Disorders

Disorder	Potential Physical Findings
Anorexia/restrictive eating	Alopecia Lanugo (soft light hair growth on body) Dry skin Cold intolerance, loss of subcutaneous fat Hypotension Bradycardia Amenorrhea in nonpregnant women Muscle mass and strength loss Fatigue Pedal edema GI complaints: bloating, constipation
Bulimia/binge–purge behavior	Swollen parotid glands Dental enamel erosion Poor or absent gag reflex Bloodshot eyes, broken blood vessels on face Hoarse voice Scarred knuckle calluses on dorsal surface of hand Weight fluctuations GI complaints: reflux, bloating, constipation

---

CHART 14–15   SCOFF Tool for Screening for Eating Disorders

Do you make yourself **S**ick (induce vomiting) because you feel uncomfortably full?

Do you worry you have lost **C**ontrol over how much you eat?

Have you recently lost more than **O**ne stone (14 lb) in a 3-month period?

Do you feel yourself to be **F**at when others say you are too thin?

Would you say that **F**ood dominates your life?

Scoring: One point for every yes. A score $\geq$ 2 indicates a likely case of anorexia or bulimia.

British Medical Journal, 1999, 319:1467–1468. Morgan J. F. Reid F, Lacey J. H. (1999) The SCOFF questionnaire: Assessment of a new screening tool for eating disorders. Reproduced with permission from the BMJ Publishing Group.

---

whether the patient is at risk for an eating disorder or in need of further evaluation for psychiatric, medical, or nutritional issues.

Anorexia nervosa is treated either in the inpatient or outpatient setting depending on the severity of symptoms. Outpatient care is preferred unless the patient is refractory to treatment with a weight of less than 75% expected or has an emergent mental health event or severe cardiovascular risk, such as bradycardia (<40 beats/min), hypotension (<60 systolic) or hypokalemia (<3 mg/dL). Hypothermia (36°C [<97°F]) is also indicative of need for inpatient treatment (APA, 2000b). A team approach to treatment is recommended because of the complex medical, psychiatric, and nutritional issues; no one clinician or profession is solely able to provide the scope of care required. Goals for treatment include cessation of weight reduction and weight reduction behaviors, weight restoration, improved behaviors related to food and eating, and improvement of any medical or psychiatric conditions (American Dietetic Association, 2001; APA, 2000b).

Nutrition intervention in anorexia initially focuses on cessation of weight loss and then restoration of body weight. Outpatient weight restoration is recommended at 1 to 2 pounds per week; inpatient restoration of 2 to 3 pounds per week can be safely monitored (American Dietetic Association, 2001). Determination of the appropriate meal plan and its progression is the responsibility of the dietitian (American Dietetic Association, 2001; APA, 2000b). The nurse plays an important role in educating the patient on the physiological symptoms and consequences of starvation, reinforcing and monitoring the nutrition plan (including assessing for excessive exercise or squirreling away of uneaten food in the inpatient setting), monitoring for changes in vital signs and body weight, and assessing for symptoms of refeeding syndrome. **Refeeding syndrome** can occur following starvation and reintroduction of fuel in any medical or surgical situation, including eating disorders. As fuel substrate is reintroduced to the body and metabolism increases, fluid and electrolyte shifts can occur. Serum phosphorous levels can become dangerously low as new ATP is generated. The Critical Alert outlines essential assessment data when refeeding begins. The Nursing Process Patient Care Plan (p. 291) outlines nursing management of the weight loss patient.

CRITICAL ALERT *Patients with refeeding syndrome are at risk for cardiac dysrhythmia and sudden death. The nurse needs to assess the patient for the following symptoms (American Dietetic Association, 2001; APA, 2000b; Crook et al., 2001; Ornstein et al., 2003):*

- *Hypophosphatemia*
- *Hypokalemia*
- *Hypomagnesemia*
- *Cardiac dysrhythmia, specifically prolonged QT interval*
- *Edema (can be normal part of refeeding; monitor for presence with other symptoms)*
- *Heart failure.*

Food intake is increased gradually in both the inpatient and outpatient setting to avoid refeeding syndrome and to allow the patient to become comfortable physically and emotionally with increased intake. Use of food, and not tube feedings or parenteral nutrition, is the recommended route for nutrition intervention unless the patient is acutely refusing food (APA, 2000b). This allows for addressing food phobias and assists with eating behavior change. Prescriptive limits or avoidance of exercise is included in the treatment of those patients who exercise excessively. As the patient's condition improves, exercise limitations can slowly be lifted.

The treatment team determines which clinician is most appropriate for monitoring ongoing weight and whether the patient will learn weight measurements or be "blinded" (weighed while standing backwards on the scale). These determinations are made individually. When weighing patients, the nurse should ensure that weights are done in a private setting and not in a common area. The patient should wear minimal clothing and void before the weight measure. Some patients will drink excessive amounts of liquids before being weighed. The voided urine can be assessed for specific gravity to determine if this is happening. An assessment should be done for any hidden weights in or under clothing or undergarments. Weight alone should not be the sole parameter used to determine recovery.

Bulimia Nervosa

Bulimia nervosa is prevalent in 5% of the U.S. population and is characterized by chaotic eating patterns such as binge eating and compensatory purging, and is accompanied by a sense of loss of control as a result (American Dietetic Association, 2001). Patients with bulimia often have a personal set of "rules" governing "good" and "bad" foods and amounts of food. It is not uncommon for patients with bulimia to be restrictive eaters when not bingeing. Binges can be triggered by a perception of breaking such a "rule," hunger from restrictive eating, perceived fullness, or an emotional cause. Compensatory action can be purging with self-induced vomiting, laxative use, diuretic use, or excessive exercise. At-risk

patients should be assessed for use of over-the-counter, prescription, and alternative medicine versions of laxatives and diuretics. Assessment should also include whether syrup of ipecac is used because it has negative cardiovascular effects such as cardiomyopathy (Mehler, 2003). Type, duration, and frequency of exercise should be ascertained as well.

DSM-IV criteria call for binge–purge behavior at least twice a week for 6 months. The nurse may find on assessment that patients engage in this behavior more frequently but not for 6 months duration. Some patients purge up to 10 times in a day (Mehler, 2003). Any binge–purge behavior is deserving of further evaluation. Symptoms of bulimia are subtler than with anorexia. Patients with bulimia are often of normal weight or slightly overweight, making assessment more difficult. Symptomology depends on mode and duration of compensatory purging (Mehler, 2003). Signs and symptoms of bulimia nervosa are listed in Chart 14–14 (p. 289).

Nutrition intervention for bulimia centers on normalizing eating patterns to interrupt the binge–purge cycle. This includes avoidance of hunger and chaotic eating patterns and slow reintroduction of forbidden foods. Generally a more structured eating pattern is prescribed by the dietitian to meet this goal. Finger foods are avoided because portion control is difficult. When excessive exercise is used as a compensatory purging method, prescriptive limits are generally placed on activity. The nurse can be instrumental in reinforcing the meal pattern to encourage avoidance of long time spans between eating. A food record can be helpful to assess this.

Corrections of misconceptions about weight and nutrition are also important. The nurse can educate the patient about normal transient symptoms to expect with the normalization of eating patterns. These include water retention (which will worsen if fluid is restricted or diuretics or laxatives abused) and bloating from delayed gastric emptying or from constipation with laxative reliance. Additionally, the nurse can be effective in counseling the patient who abuses laxatives or diuretics as to the ineffectiveness of those treatments in eliminating calories or fat from the body, in addition to their medical dangers. A high-fiber and high-fluid diet should be encouraged for the patient who is weaning from laxative abuse.

Binge-Eating Disorder

Binge-eating disorder (BED) is prevalent in up to 2% of the U.S. population (American Dietetic Association, 2001). BED is characterized by the same type of binge eating as bulimia nervosa but without the compensatory purging. Most patients with binge-eating disorder are overweight (American Dietetic Association, 2001). Increased focus is pointing to the effects of chronic restrained eating, increased prevalence in some families, and depression and other psychiatric diagnoses as contributing to binge eating (Hudson et al., 2006; Meno, Hannum, Espelage, & Douglas Low, 2008). The nurse should screen obese patients who may be at risk for binge-eating disorder (Striegel-Moore et al., 2003).

Treatment of binge-eating disorder involves medical treatment of any complications of obesity, psychological treatment of any underlying mental health issues, and nutrition treatment to normalize eating patterns. It is under debate whether any attempt at weight loss should occur during binge-eating treatment or be delayed until behaviors are stabilized (American

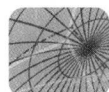

NURSING PROCESS: Patient Care Plan for Malnutrition (Undernutrition)

Assessment of Current Nutritional Status

Subjective Data:

Have you lost weight in the last 3 months, if so how much?

Have you changed your eating habits in the last 3 months?

Do you have any discomfort such as pain or bloating after you eat? Does it occur with any particular type of food?

Ask patient or family how long nutritional intake has been reduced to help determine severity of malnutrition.

Objective Data:

Patient has experienced an unintentional weight loss of >5% or more in 1 month or >10% in 3 months

Current measured weight and height compared to standardized tables of measurement

BMI < 18.5 kg/m²

Gastrointestinal symptoms including constipation, diarrhea, pain or cramping

List of current medications that can cause nutritional side effects (diarrhea, loss of appetite, etc.)

Nursing Assessment and Diagnoses	Outcomes and Evaluation Parameters	Planning and Interventions with *Rationales*
Nursing Diagnosis: *Imbalanced Nutrition: Less Than Body Requirements* related to inability to eat adequate amounts of food to maintain weight	**Outcome:** Normal intake of a balanced diet without side effects. *Evaluation Parameters:* Weight is at recommended level for the height and musculature for the patient. Treatment of gastrointestinal clinical manifestations is effective.	**Interventions and *Rationales:*** Perform a complete physical assessment and nutritional history on admission *to assess current nutritional status and to provide a nutritional baseline of data for plan development.* Instruct patient to weigh daily before breakfast, after urination, using the same scale *to monitor weight gain.* Consult registered dietician *for detailed nutritional analysis and specialized planning.*

Assessment of Current Nutritional and Dietary Intake

Subjective Data:

What is your normal daily dietary intake?

How much alcohol do you drink weekly?

What types of food do you use for snacks?

How many meals a day do you eat and at what time?

Do you use vitamin, herbal, and over the counter (OTC) medications?

Have you taken any weight loss medications or used laxatives for weight loss?

Do you have any difficulty with swallowing or chewing?

Objective Data:

Serial weights from medical records.

Assess muscle wasting.

Assess for acute and/or chronic disease states, e.g., kidney, liver, diabetes, anorexia, cancer.

Test serum albumin level, serum prealbumin level, serum creatinine level, total lymphocyte count, and transferrin level.

Nursing Assessment and Diagnoses	Outcomes and Evaluation Parameters	Planning and Interventions with *Rationales*
Nursing Diagnosis: *Imbalanced Nutrition: Less Than Body Requirements* related to factors inhibiting successful eating patterns to maintain weight	**Outcomes:** Maintain normal nutrition. BMI within normal limits *Evaluation Parameters:* Current weight is compared to BMI charts and height–weight charts to determine level of malnutrition (mild, moderate, or severe). The nurse must use the evaluation parameters that correlate with the etiology of the nutritional deficit. See charts in this chapter for specific deficits in specific disease processes. Food intake is less than energy expenditure.	**Interventions and *Rationales:*** Ask patient/family to list the foods and portion sizes consumed for the last 24 hours and the past 3 days *to assess adequacy of calorie intake.* Explore nutritional beliefs, cultural and religious attitudes toward food, food taboos, use of alcohol, medication and OTC use, and problems with dentition or self-feeding difficulties *to determine factors that impact food intake.* List the calorie count for each food consumed *to determine adequacy of calorie intake.* Measure triceps skinfold, midarm muscle circumference in the younger but not the older patient *to determine baseline for muscle wasting.*

Assessment of Disease Risk Factors That Are Influenced by Underweight Status

Subjective Data:

Do you have any acute or chronic diseases?

When was the last time you had a complete physical examination?

Objective Data:

Assess for cachexia, renal dysfunction, fever, infection, wounds, diabetes mellitus, gastrointestinal pain, and bloating.

(continued)

NURSING PROCESS: Patient Care Plan for Malnutrition (Undernutrition)—*Continued*

Nursing Assessment and Diagnoses	Outcomes and Evaluation Parameters	Planning and Interventions with *Rationales*
Nursing Diagnosis: *Ineffective Health Maintenance* related to disease factors that can result in loss of weight	**Outcome:** Identification and management of disease/s that caused weight loss. ***Evaluation Parameters:*** Prealbumin levels within normal limits. BMI within normal limits.	**Interventions and *Rationales:*** Assess patient for risk factors for malnutrition *to determine problem priority.* Risk factors include acute and chronic illness, depression in the elderly, functional status, polypharmacy, and frailty. Assess patient for signs of impaired wound healing (e.g., pressure ulcers, fistulas), burns, muscle wasting, muscle weakness, loss of calcium, increased risk for falls leading to increased risk for fractures. *These factors indicate patient has high risk for malnutrition.* In oncology patients, assess for weight loss >5%, *which can result in increased mortality, poor response to chemotherapy, and treatment complications.*

Assessment of Changes That Can Be Made in Food Intake to Increase Caloric Intake, Including Readiness to Change Food Intake

Subjective Data:
List the foods you enjoy eating and eat frequently.

Objective Data:
Caloric intake per 24 hr based on above food diary.
Write down each food consumed along with portion size for calculation of food intake by dietician.

Nursing Assessment and Diagnoses	Outcomes and Evaluation Parameters	Planning and Interventions with *Rationales*
Nursing Diagnosis: *Imbalanced Nutrition: Less Than Body Requirements* related to need to increase caloric intake	**Outcomes:** Patient verbalizes changes to increase food intake. ***Evaluation Parameters:*** Weight gain of 1–2 lb per month for 6 months.	**Interventions and *Rationales:*** Reassess hospitalized patients weekly for nutritional status. Encourage balanced nutrition. *To assess progress toward normal BMI.* Measure upper arm and thigh monthly *to assess growth in muscle mass.* Encourage small, frequent meals of foods that patient enjoys. *Potentially increases calorie intake.* *For hospitalized patients:* Monitor tolerance for prescribed tube feedings, total parenteral nutrition (TPN), and other nutritional support as needed including electrolytes and vitamins *to prevent malnutrition.* Provide feeding assistance if needed; if assistance is provided, do not hurry the patient and sit down while feeding *so patient doesn't feel rushed to eat.* Place patient in an upright position while eating and for 30 minutes afterward *to prevent regurgitation.* Provide a pleasant environment for mealtime *to encourage the appetite.* Encourage communal environment for mealtime *to encourage social milieu and appetite.* Avoid prolonged NPO status while inpatient *because this contributes to further loss of intake.*

Dietetic Association, 2001; Goldfein, Devlin, & Spitzer, 2000). The Genetic Considerations box discusses speculation about the roles genetics may play in weight management.

Nutrition and Cardiovascular Disease

Nutrition intervention can have a significant impact on risk reduction with cardiovascular disease. Following lifestyle modifica-

tions, including nutrition recommendations, can help prevent or manage hypertension and coronary artery disease. Medical nutrition therapy is also indicated in the treatment of heart failure.

Hypertension

Lifestyle modifications, including diet, have been shown to have both clinical and public health significance in reduction of blood

GENETIC CONSIDERATIONS Implications for Weight Management

Speculation about the genetic implications in weight management has existed for some time. The specific roles of genetics as related to risk of obesity and eating disorders are being investigated. Risk factors for the development of eating disorders have been linked to genetic phenotypes for other disorders, such as the traits for obsessive-compulsive disorder and disturbances of dopamine systems (Kaye et al., 2004; Shinohara et al., 2004).

The role of genetics and the possibility of genetic manipulation have been heavily researched in the hope of identifying obesity risk factors and treatment options. Substances involved in appetite regulation, such as neuropeptide Y and ghrelin, proteins involved in thermogenesis, and leptin, and their relation to obesity are among the areas of research (Campion, Milagro, & Martinez, 2004; Marti, Moreno-Aliaga, Hebebrand, & Martinez, 2004). Although the topic of genetic influence on the development of both eating disorders and obesity is intriguing, it is difficult to draw firm conclusions without further research into these areas (Bulik, Sullivan, Wade, & Kendler, 2000; Kaye et al., 2004).

CHART 14–16 Lifestyle Modifications for Hypertension

Lifestyle Component	Recommendation
Weight management	Practice weight reduction or management of normal weight.
Diet	Eat a diet rich in fruits, vegetables, and low-fat dairy foods and low in saturated and total fat.
	Reduce sodium intake to not more than 2,400 mg or 6 g NaCl daily.
	Limit alcohol to not more than 2 drinks a day for men and not more than 1 drink a day for women and small men. One drink is 12 oz beer, 5 oz wine, or 1-1/2 oz 80-proof spirits.
Physical activity	Engage in physical activity at least 30 minutes most days.

Sources: Chobanian, A. V., Bakris, G. L., Black, H. R., Cushman, W. C., et al. (2003). The seventh report of the Joint National Committee on Prevention, Detection, Evaluation and Treatment of High Blood Pressure. *Journal of the American Medical Association, 289,* 2560–2572; National Heart, Lung, and Blood Institute. (2004). *The seventh report of the Joint National Committee on Prevention, Detection, Evaluation and Treatment of High Blood Pressure (JNC7).* Retrieved February 5, 2004, from http://www.nhlbi.nih.gov/guidelines/hypertension/express.pdf; Whelton, P. K., He, J., Appel, L. J., Cutler, J. A., Havas, S., Kotchen, T. A., et al. (2002). Primary prevention of hypertension: Clinical and public health advisory from the National High Blood Pressure Education Program. *Journal of the American Medical Association, 288,* 1882–1888.

---

pressure in people with hypertension and those with high normal blood pressure, or prehypertension (Chobanian et al., 2003; Khan et al., 2006; Writing Group of the PREMIER Collaborative Research Group, 2003). The prevalence of hypertension in America is increasing, with almost 29% of all adults exhibiting elevated blood pressure. Of those diagnosed with hypertension and on antihypertensive medication, only 53% had measured blood pressure within the recommended target (Hijjar & Kotchen, 2003). Clearly, improved primary prevention and treatment of hypertension are needed to avoid the negative effects of elevated blood pressure on cardiovascular risk across the life span.

Lifestyle modifications recommended for prevention and management of high blood pressure include several nutrition-centered modifications as well as engaging in regular physical activity. Decades of research have shown the individual and additive effects on blood pressure reduction with weight reduction in overweight people, limiting sodium, alcohol, and total and saturated fat while consuming a diet rich in fruits, vegetables, and low-fat dairy products (Chobanian et al., 2003; Whelton et al., 2002; Writing Group of the PREMIER Collaborative Research Group, 2003). Current national guidelines recommend lifestyle modifications for all people for the primary prevention and management of high blood pressure (Chobanian et al., 2003; NHLBI, 2004; Whelton et al., 2002). Specific guidelines are outlined in Chart 14–16.

The nurse is uniquely positioned to be instrumental in detecting elevated blood pressure and educating patients on prevention and management of hypertension. In addition to weight management methods discussed in this chapter, the nurse can be involved in patient education and monitoring of other nutrition-related lifestyle modifications.

Reduction of dietary sodium intake has been reported to lower systolic blood pressure as a single intervention or in conjunction with other lifestyle modifications or pharmacology (Chobanian et al., 2003; Khan et al., 2006). Further, a low sodium intake compared with usual sodium intake has been reported to reduce the amount of antihypertensive medication needed in

some patients (Mulrow, 2001). The primary source of sodium in the American diet is from packaged, processed, and ready-to-eat food prepared outside the home. Discretionary added sodium in the form of table salt used in the home only accounts for 20% to 30% of sodium consumption (Mulrow, 2001). The nurse should question the patient about eating patterns and preparation methods during the nutrition portion of a nursing assessment. Specifically asking about frequency of restaurant meals and use of convenience products is important to estimate sodium intake. Chart 14–17 lists sources of high-sodium foods.

The NIH's Dietary Approaches to Stopping Hypertension (DASH) diet has taken nutrition intervention for high blood

---

CHART 14–17 Dietary Sources of High Sodium

- In general, processed, preserved, and convenience foods are high in sodium. Terms such as *pickled, cured, dehydrated, smoked, seasoned, ready-to-eat,* and *added sauce* hint at a high sodium content.

- Plain forms of most food have low or moderate sodium content. Fresh fruit, juice, fresh or plain frozen vegetables, plain grains and breads, milk, plain meat, poultry, fish, and dried beans, peas, and lentils are not naturally high in sodium.

- Canned vegetables, frozen vegetables with sauce, canned tomato products, grain mixes, cured or luncheon meats, cheeses, canned meat, fish, beans and poultry, and boxed or frozen meals are higher in sodium than their fresh or plain counterparts.

- Foods labeled "reduced sodium" have 25% less sodium than the original, but may not be low in sodium. Foods labeled "low sodium" have 140 mg sodium or less per serving.

pressure beyond the single low-sodium diet approach. The DASH diet emphasizes fruits, vegetables, nuts, and low-fat dairy while also containing reduced fat and saturated fat levels. The diet is rich in potassium, which has been associated with independent reductions in blood pressure and risk of stroke (Khan et al., 2006). Magnesium and calcium sources are also plentiful in the DASH diet, but results from research on their effects independently or in supplemental form are unclear. Supplemental calcium in amounts of 1,000 to 1,500 mg has had small, inconsistent effects on blood pressure reduction in hypertensive individuals, but this amount is already within recommended levels for intake in the general population (Whelton et al., 2002). The DASH diet recommends the use of foods to attain its goals and remains silent on the use of supplements. Chart 14–18 outlines the DASH diet. The nurse should note that the DASH diet contains various calorie levels that can be used or modified as a weight reduction plan for the overweight patient (NHLBI, 2004).

Alcohol intake above one drink a day for women and lighter weight men or two drinks a day for men has been shown to have a direct negative effect on blood pressure (Chobanian et al., 2003; Khan et al., 2006; Whelton et al., 2002). Although some patients tout the reputed cardioprotective effects of alcohol consumption, intake beyond the recommended limit is not conferring additional benefit. Overweight or obese patients trying to lose weight should be made aware of the significant calorie content that alcoholic beverages can contribute to the diet.

Chapter 21 ✆ includes a complete description of hypertension.

Coronary Heart Disease

Aggressive management of serum lipids is recommended as a primary strategy in the prevention and treatment of cardiovascular disease. Management of elevated serum low-density lipoprotein (LDL) cholesterol should receive priority attention because of its established association with increased risk of coronary heart disease (NHLBI, 2002). Total cholesterol and high-density lipoprotein (HDL) cholesterol levels are also important predictors of cardiac risk. Target values for serum lipid

levels based on the NHLBI's National Cholesterol Education Program (NCEP) are discussed in Chapter 37 ✆.

The general population as well as those patients with established coronary heart disease can benefit from dietary approaches aimed at reducing serum lipids, controlling blood pressure, and managing body weight in an effort to reduce cardiac risk (Lichtenstein et al., 2006). Diet modifications, called **therapeutic lifestyle changes (TLC)**, are recommended as an initial strategy for treating elevated LDL cholesterol or in conjunction with pharmacologic intervention when indicated. Medical nutrition therapy for hyperlipidemia and coronary heart disease targets reduction of both lipid and nonlipid cardiac risk factors. A fat-controlled diet coupled with weight management and increased physical activity comprises the foundation of the therapeutic lifestyle changes. Therapeutic lifestyle changes are outlined in Chart 14–19.

Saturated Fats and Cholesterol

The NCEP guidelines focus on reducing dietary saturated fat and cholesterol. A dose response exists between saturated fat intake and serum LDL cholesterol (NHLBI, 2002). Saturated fats exist primarily in fats from animal-based foods such as fatty meats or whole-milk dairy products. Tropical fats are also saturated fats and include palm oil, coconut oil, and cocoa butter. Hydrogenated and *trans* fats are included in the recommendation to reduce saturated fat intake. These fats originate as *un*saturated oils, but become saturated during food processing when the manufacturer removes hydrogen molecules to make a fat that is more solid at room temperature. Examples include fats used in shortening, stick margarine, and many baked goods and snacks. High intake of dietary cholesterol is associated with increased LDL cholesterol. Dietary cholesterol is present only in foods of animal origin. Fatty and organ meats, egg yolks, and shellfish are among the higher sources of dietary cholesterol.

Unsaturated Fats

Unsaturated fats, which are liquid at room temperature, are not associated with elevated LDL cholesterol. The monounsaturated fats present in olive, peanut, and canola oils and most nuts and

---

CHART 14–18 **DASH Eating Plan: Number of Daily Servings for Other Calorie Levels**

Food Groups	Servings/Day		
	1,600 Calories/Day	2,600 Calories/Day	3,100 Calories/Day
Grains*	6	10–11	12–13
Vegetables	3–4	5–6	6
Fruits	4	5–6	6
Fat-free or low-fat milk and milk products	2–3	3	3–4
Lean meats, poultry, and fish	3–6	6	6–9
Nuts, seeds, and legumes	3/week	1	1
Fats and oils	2	3	4
Sweets and added sugars	0	≤2	≤2

*Whole grains are recommended for most grain servings as a good source of fiber and nutrients.

Source: National Heart, Lung, and Blood Insitute. (2006). *Your guide to lowering your blood pressure with DASH.* Retrieved May 30, 2008 from http://www.nhlbi.nih.gov/health/public/heart/hbp/dash/new_dash.pdf

CHART 14–19 ## Therapeutic Lifestyle Changes for Cardiovascular Disease

Lifestyle Component	Recommendation
Diet	Saturated fat: <7% total daily calorie intake. *Trans* fatty acids should also be limited.
	Monounsaturated fat: up to 20% total daily calorie intake.
	Polyunsaturated fat: up to 10% total daily calorie intake.
	Total fat: 25%–35% total daily calorie intake.
	Cholesterol: <200 mg/day.
	Fiber: 20–30 g/day with consideration given to include 10–25 g soluble fiber daily.
	Carbohydrate: 50%–60% of total daily calorie intake. Emphasize whole grains, fruits, and vegetable sources.
	Protein: approximately 15% of total daily calorie intake.
	Energy intake to maintain desirable weight and prevent weight gain.
Weight management	Maintain desirable weight, avoid weight gain, lose weight if indicated.
Physical activity	Increase physical activity. Energy balance to include at least 200 calories of energy expenditure from moderately intense activity most days.

Source: National Heart Lung and Blood Institute. (2002). *Third report of the National Cholesterol Education Program expert panel on detection, evaluation, and treatment of high blood cholesterol in adults (Adult treatment panel III).* Retrieved February 5, 2004, from http://www.nhlbi.nih.gov/guidelines/cholesterol/atp3full.pdf

avocado have been shown to lower LDL cholesterol when substituted for saturated fats in the diet (NHLBI, 2002). Polyunsaturated fats also can foster a decrease in saturated fats when substituted for saturated fats but can adversely contribute to a small decrease in beneficial HDL cholesterol as well (NHLBI, 2002). Sources of polyunsaturated fats include corn, safflower, sunflower, and soybean oils and are included on Chart 14–20 (p. 296), which lists practical interventions that can be used to make therapeutic lifestyle changes.

Carbohydrate and Fiber

Carbohydrate can be substituted for saturated fat as a strategy for decreasing LDL cholesterol (NHLBI, 2002). However, high carbohydrate intake exceeding 60% of the diet's energy value has been associated with a decrease in HDL cholesterol and an increase in serum triglycerides, neither of which is beneficial to cardiac risk (NHLBI, 2002). Carbohydrate-containing plant foods that contain fiber, specifically soluble fiber, are recommended for their cholesterol-lowering capabilities (Shamliyan, Jacobs, Raatz, Nordstrom, & Keenan, 2006). Soluble fiber is associated with a 3% to 5% reduction of LDL cholesterol when 5 to 10 grams are consumed daily (NHLBI, 2002). Soluble fiber is present in several plant foods such as oats, oat bran,

legumes, and barley. Chart 14–20 (p. 296) lists additional sources of soluble fiber.

Plant Sterol and Stanol Esters

Plant sterol and stanol esters are poorly absorbed derivatives of soybean and wood oils that have been reported to lower total and LDL cholesterol up to 20% with maximum effective intake of 2 g/daily (Lichtenstein et al., 2006). Several brands of margarine and salad dressings exist that have sterol or stanol esters listed as ingredients on the label.

Soy Protein

Soy protein in the diet has been reported to lower plasma LDL cholesterol, especially when consumed with soluble fibers and used to replace animal proteins (Jenkins et al., 2006; Lichtenstein et al., 2006). The mechanism by which soy affects cholesterol and cardiac risk is complex and not fully understood. It may involve both lipid-lowering effects and changes in platelet aggregation and vascular inflammation (Anderson, 2003; Morelli & Zoorob, 2000). Soy protein can be found in soybeans, tofu, soy milk, and many soy "meat" alternatives.

Omega-3 Fatty Acids

Omega-3 fats are associated with decreased risk of cardiac events, specifically cardiac death in people with established coronary heart disease (Gebauer, Psota, Harris, & Kris-Etherton, 2006). Reduction of plasma triglycerides, decreased platelet aggregability, reduction in cardiac dysrhythmias, and improvement in endothelial dysfunction all play a role in the mechanism (Gebauer et al., 2006). The American Heart Association recommends intake of oily fish twice a week for the general adult population and 1 g/day of omega-3 fats from fish or a fish supplement in those with existing atherosclerosis (Lichtenstein et al., 2006). One serving of a fatty fish such as salmon or bluefish has 900 mg of omega-3 fat. Plant sources of omega-3 fats contain smaller amounts of these fats in a serving and include flaxseed and canola oil. The nurse should caution patients who choose to take supplemental forms of omega-3 fats about negative side effects as outlined in the Critical Alert.

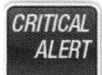 *Omega-3 supplements decrease platelet aggregability. Take care to assess patients for any interaction with medications such as Coumadin or aspirin therapy that potentiate this effect. Additionally, assess for other dietary supplements and herbs with antiplatelet action, such as garlic, feverfew, ginkgo biloba, and vitamin E. Make sure the patient respects proper dosage recommendations of any omega-3 fat supplements.*

Alcohol

A moderate intake of alcohol can reduce the risk of coronary heart disease in adults (Lichtenstein et al., 2006). Moderation is described as no more than one drink per day for a woman and two per day for a man. Wine, specifically red wine, has received great focus when researching the potential cardioprotective effects of alcohol, yet most studies do not support reduced cardiac risk with a specific type of alcohol (Lichtenstein et al., 2006). Red wine is singled out by some because of its antithrombolytic action and antioxidant content perhaps contributing additional benefits over other types of alcohol. Higher intake of alcohol does not confer additional cardioprotection, can be the source of

CHART 14–20	Practical Interventions to Achieve Therapeutic Lifestyle Changes (TLC)

Choose	Limit
Monounsaturated and polyunsaturated fats, oils, and margarines to replace saturated fat ingredients:	Saturated fat and cholesterol sources. Fats that are hard at room temperature tend to be saturated fats:
• Olive oil, canola oil, peanut oil = mono	• Fatty meats, luncheon meats, organ meats
• Sunflower, soybean, safflower, corn, sesame = poly.	• Poultry w/skin
Lower fat and saturated fat protein foods:	• Whole-fat dairy products
• Dried beans, peas, lentils, soy (these also contain soluble fiber)	• Commercial baked goods made with *trans* and hydrogenated fats or lard
• Skinless poultry	• Tropical oils found in processed foods: palm oil, cocoa butter, coconut oil
• Fish	• Stick margarine, shortening, lard.
• Lean, trimmed cuts of meat (round/loin)	High-fat food preparation methods:
• Fat-free and low-fat dairy foods.	• Deep-fat or pan frying
Omega-3 polyunsaturated fat sources:	• Adding sauces, gravies, creams, creamy dressings, or mayonnaise to foods
• Fish: deep, cold-water fish such as salmon, tuna, bluefish, mackerel	• Leaving on poultry skin or visible meat fat on during cooking
• Flaxseed	• Recipes with high oil, butter, margarine, lard, cream, or full-fat cheese content.
• Canola oil	
• Nuts	
• Soy.	
Low-fat food preparation methods:	
• Bake, grill, sauté w/ broth or cooking spray	
• Remove fat/skin from proteins before cooking	
• Use low-fat marinades	
• Substitute low fat ingredients in recipes for high fat version.	
Five or more fruits and vegetables daily. Soluble fiber sources include fruit and vegetables w/edible skins.	
Whole grains, including soluble fiber sources such as oats, oat bran, barley.	

Source: Adapted from National Heart Lung and Blood Institute. (2002). *Third report of the National Cholesterol Education Program expert panel on detection, evaluation, and treatment of high blood cholesterol in adults (Adult treatment panel III).* Retrieved February 5, 2004, from http://www.nhlbi.nih.gov/guidelines/cholesterol/atp3full.pdf

excess calorie intake, and can contribute to an elevated triglyceride level in addition to other medical risks (Lichtenstein et al., 2006). There is little justification to recommend drinking alcohol to patients who do not already do so.

Homocysteine and B-Vitamins

Elevated plasma homocysteine has emerged as a risk factor of cardiovascular disease. It is unclear whether homocysteine is simply a marker of disease or causative in nature (Hackam & Anand, 2003). Homocysteine is an amino acid that is metabolized in the body with the help of folic acid, pyridoxine (vitamin B_6), and vitamin B_{12}. Diets high in folic acid or all three vitamins have been reported to lower plasma homocysteine levels. Whether a reduction of homocysteine levels will lead to a reduction in coronary heart disease remains a matter of debate (Lichtenstein et al., 2006).

Other Supplements and Botanicals

Antioxidant vitamins such as vitamins E and C have been investigated for a possible role in reducing coronary heart disease. To date, observations made in epidemiologic studies regarding these antioxidants have not illustrated a reduction in cardiac risk when investigated in controlled clinical trials (Morris &

Carson, 2003). In several studies of patients with existing cardiovascular disease, antioxidant therapy failed to decrease the risk of future cardiac events or disease. Additionally, antioxidant therapy lessened the interventional effects of a HMG CoA reductase inhibitor (a cholesterol-lowering drug) and nicotinic acid regimen (niacin) (Brown et al., 2001; Waters et al., 2002). The American Heart Association stresses that studies have pointed to the health benefits of diets rich in fruits and vegetables, food sources of antioxidants, but therapeutic use of antioxidant supplements is not recommended because of negative outcomes in research trials (Lichtenstein et al., 2006).

Many other dietary supplements, including herbs, have received attention for possible roles in the reduction of cholesterol or other cardiac risk factors. To date, none has withstood the test of a long-term clinical trial to prove a benefit. Supplemental garlic has been investigated for a mild cholesterol-lowering effect compared to placebo in some trials, but not others (Morelli & Zoorob, 2000; Rahman, 2001; Stevinson, Pittler, & Ernst, 2000). Gugulipid, or guggul gum, has received attention for reported cholesterol-lowering power in clinical trials in India but more recent reports find little effect (Morelli & Zoorob, 2000). Both of these examples serve as a reminder of the uncertainty of using dietary supplements without clinical evidence of efficacy. Controlled research on such supplements is limited, making it difficult to make a good clinical recommendation when queried by patients seeking to avoid or augment the use of pharmacologic therapies. Current lack of research and limited knowledge regarding safety does not support the use of these products in treating coronary heart disease. Additionally, standardization of supplement dosing and ingredients is lacking in the United States, making it a game of roulette when choosing underresearched products. Despite the lack of standardization and research, many consumers are willing to try these supplements and may not volunteer this information to their health care providers. The nurse should assess patients for use of supplements and discuss the lack of clinical studies, any safety concerns, and the potential for drug–supplement interactions.

Weight Management

Overweight and obesity are associated with an increased risk of coronary heart disease, among other comorbid conditions (NHLBI, 2002). Weight management is included in the TLC recommendations for targeting LDL cholesterol reduction. Weight loss of even a few pounds has been reported to reduce LDL cholesterol (NHLBI, 2002). The NCEP and the American Heart Association encourage weight loss through decreased energy intake and increased physical activity. Prevention of weight gain is emphasized (Lichtenstein et al., 2006; NHLBI, 2002). A balanced low-fat diet containing all food groups is stressed for long-term benefit and overall health. A reduction in sedentary time and the addition of moderate physical activity on most days is also encouraged (Lichtenstein et al., 2006). Weight reduction was discussed earlier in the chapter.

Metabolic Syndrome

Recently a cluster of cardiovascular risk factors, referred to as *metabolic syndrome*, has been defined as having three out of the five following conditions: (1) abdominal obesity, (2) high triglycerides, (3) low HDL-C, (4) high blood pressure, and (5) fasting glucose ($\geq$110 mg/dL). The presence of metabolic syndrome can place the overweight patient at additional cardiac risk. Overweight patients with abdominal obesity (apple shape), elevated triglycerides, low HDL cholesterol levels, high blood pressure, or elevated fasting glucose should be assessed for the metabolic syndrome as discussed in Chapters 37 and 40 ⊙. Treatment recommendations begin with a 3-month trial of standard TLCs (see Chart 14–19, p. 295) emphasizing LDL cholesterol reduction and weight loss. If parameters of metabolic syndrome are still present after 3 months, intensified weight loss efforts are indicated. Elevated triglycerides of $\geq$500 mg/dL should be attended to urgently because of an associated risk of pancreatitis (NHLBI, 2002). A very low fat diet ($\leq$15% of daily calorie needs from fat), weight loss, physical activity, and possible pharmacologic intervention are indicated with this level of hypertriglyceridemia (NHLBI, 2002).

Much attention has been given to the concept of carbohydrate-containing foods and elevated postprandial plasma glucose levels, especially in individuals with insulin resistance at risk for metabolic syndrome. Diets that are high in carbohydrate (>60%) are associated with elevated triglyc-

erides and lowered HDL cholesterol. Individuals with metabolic syndrome or insulin resistance can benefit from replacement of dietary saturated fat with unsaturated fats, specifically monounsaturates, as an alternative to adding carbohydrate food sources to replace needed calories (Lichtenstein et al., 2006).

Additionally, the nurse should encourage high-fiber fruits, vegetables, and whole grains as choices for needed carbohydrate sources, nutrient composition, and to promote satiety. Fiber intake has been shown to have benefit in postprandial glycemic control and improvement of blood lipid levels in diabetic patients (American Diabetes Association [ADA], 2003a; Lichtenstein et al., 2006). Some refer to a tool called the glycemic index (GI) that predicts postprandial glucose response to varying foods. The content of individual food constituents such as fiber and fat and the preparation method affect the glycemic response (ADA, 2003a). The GI may prove useful in the future for providing advice to patients with metabolic syndrome and diabetes mellitus. Currently, the tool considers only the glycemic effect of the food when eaten singly and not its consumption in a mixed meal, as would be the usual pattern, making it too cumbersome for practical clinical use (Franz, 2003). The patient who inquires about use of the GI should be encouraged to consume carbohydrates that are unprocessed and retain their original fiber content such as fruits, vegetables, and whole grains. Fruits and vegetables with edible skin or seeds, whole-grain cereals and breads, brown rice, barley, and dried beans are examples.

Heart Failure

A low-sodium diet is prescribed as medical nutrition therapy for cardiac failure. Reduction of dietary sodium along with pharmacologic intervention can help reduce extracellular fluid burden and reduce cardiac workload. Commonly, a 2-g sodium restriction is recommended (see Chart 14–17 (p. 293) for a list of high-sodium foods). A 2-g sodium restriction requires the elimination of table salt use and replacement of high-sodium processed foods with unprocessed versions. The use of low-sodium specialty foods is not necessary to comply with the diet unless the patient's situation requires ongoing use of processed foods.

Advanced cardiac failure can place increased metabolic needs on the patient when lung function becomes compromised and respiration is altered. Increased respiratory rate and use of auxiliary muscles for labored breathing can increase the body's caloric requirement. Fatigue, early satiety, restrictive diet, and medication side effects can hamper appetite and put the patient at further risk for malnutrition. The term *cardiac cachexia* describes the consequences and physical symptoms seen in advanced cardiac failure when nutritional needs go unmet and muscle and fat wasting ensue.

The nurse should monitor patients for signs of weight loss that can be masked by edema. Temporal wasting, loss of adipose muscle, and lack of strength can be indicative of malnutrition. The patient should be encouraged to consume small, frequent meals to minimize early satiety and difficulty with breathing. Nutrient-dense foods high in protein and calories should be encouraged to maximize intake and "make every bite count." In patients consuming insufficient calories, it is prudent to evaluate intake of sodium. Sodium intake may be extremely low because of lack of general intake. Appropriate consideration can be given to allowing intake of some higher sodium foods to promote intake while remaining within the parameters of an overall sodium-restricted diet. Chart 14–21 lists food suggestions for improving intake in patients at risk for cardiac cachexia.

Diabetes Mellitus

Medical nutrition therapy is an essential lifestyle component in the management of diabetes. Nutrition choices and habits following recommended guidelines can improve glycemic control and reduce the risk of diabetic complications such as macrovascular disease in patients with existing disease (Franz et al., 2002). Additionally, lifestyle modifications, including diet, have a positive effect on disease reduction in those with impaired glucose tolerance and at risk for type II diabetes (Diabetes Prevention Program Research Group, 2002). Goals of medical nutrition therapy for diabetes are outlined in Chart 14–22.

The nutrition recommendations for diabetic patients has evolved beyond the old-school "ADA" diet (named for the American Diabetes Association), in which a specific calorie level was prescribed by the health care provider based on an exchange list of foods according to carbohydrate, protein, and fat content. The ADA (2003b) no longer recommends any single type of meal plan for all type I or type II diabetic individuals and urges that this terminology no longer be used.

Current recommendations call for attention to a healthy diet that is mindful of carbohydrate content, matching food choices and consistency of intake to individual needs. The overall diet also should incorporate TLCs known to reduce risk of coronary heart disease through the prevention of dyslipidemia, overweight, and high blood pressure. Rather than provide a blanket recommendation of a specific diet, the focus is now on individual management decisions. The patient is to be included in decision making along with the treatment team. The ADA (2003a)

CHART 14–21	**Suggested Nutrition Interventions for Cardiac Cachexia**
Add "more calories per bite"	Add calorie sources to existing foods: • Butter, gravy,* sauces,* dressings* • Grated cheese* • Powdered milk mixed into regular milk • "Double milk" in baking recipes, desserts, soups,* milkshakes.
Increase intake of nutrient-dense foods	• Encourage more intake at the start of the day or start of the meal when intake is best • Limit mealtime liquids to avoid fullness • High-protein desserts made w/egg or milk such as pudding, custard, ice cream • Frequent snacks of high energy, protein foods like yogurt, peanut butter on crackers,* cheese* • Cream soup* vs. clear soup, juice vs. water.

Monitor overall sodium intake and urge lower sodium versions if intake is high.

CHART 14–22	**Medical Nutrition Therapy Goals for Diabetes**

Attain and maintain optimal metabolic outcomes including:
• Blood glucose levels in the normal range or close to normal to prevent or reduce risk of complications of diabetes.
• A lipid profile that reduces risk of macrovascular disease.
• Blood pressure levels that reduce the risk of vascular disease.
• Prevent and treat chronic complications of diabetes. Modify nutritional intake and lifestyle as appropriate for prevention and treatment of obesity, dyslipidemia, cardiovascular disease, hypertension, and nephropathy.
• Improve health through healthy food choices and physical activity.
• Address individual nutritional needs taking into consideration personal and cultural preferences and lifestyle.

Franz, M. J., Bantle, J. P., Beebe, C. A., Brunzelli, J. D., Chiasson, J., Garg., et al. (2002). Technical review: Evidence-based nutrition principles and recommendations for the treatment and prevention of diabetes and related complications. *Diabetes Care 25,* 148–198. Copyright © 2002 American Diabetes Association From Diabetes Care, Vol. 25, 2002; 148–198. Reprinted with permission from *The American Diabetes Association.*

recommends that the registered dietitian be the treatment team member who provides the medical nutrition therapy, but that all team members are knowledgable about its parameters.

Carbohydrate Recommendations

Carbohydrates are an essential component of a healthy diet. Diabetic patients are urged to include carbohydrates in the form of whole grains, fruits, vegetables, and low-fat milk products. Together with monounsaturated fats, combined intake of carbohydrate and monounsaturated fats should be 60% to 70% of total energy intake (ADA, 2003a). No individual recommendation is given for just carbohydrate intake. The carbohydrate content of the diet and any given meal is determined individually. Some patients with type I diabetes adjust premeal insulin based on the meal's carbohydrate content, whereas others who are on a fixed dose of insulin keep a consistent pattern of day-to-day carbohydrate intake (ADA, 2003a; Franz et al., 2002). Additionally, physical activity can require an adjustment of insulin or carbohydrate intake by some individuals because of increased uptake of plasma glucose by exercising muscle (Franz et al., 2002). The treatment team and patient determine initial parameters for carbohydrate intake based on the registered dietitian's assessment of nutritional needs. Adjustments are made over time to further individualize intake. Patients are educated to read carbohydrate content on food labels and to use a basic system of carbohydrate counting based on a food exchange system. Chart 14–23 provides an example of this system.

It is recommended that patients be educated to recognize their individual glycemic responses to varying foods, levels of activity, and any hypoglycemic agents and to incorporate this into the advice given by the treatment team. The nurse is instrumental is this educational effort.

The ADA (2003a) does not currently support the use of the glycemic index (discussed earlier in this chapter in the Metabolic Syndrome section) in the management of diabetes, citing lack of overall definitive conclusions among limited clinical trials as well as study design criticisms. Much debate has surrounded this topic and varying clinical trials support all sides of the discussion (Brand-Miller, Hayne, Petocz, & Colagiuri, 2003). Glycemic index use is supported by national recommendations in other

CHART 14–23	Sample Carbohydrate Counting for Diabetes Management

Food Group	Serving Size Examples	Grams of Carbohydrate
Starches (grains, breads, cereals, legumes, starchy vegetables)	1/2 cup cooked grain,1-oz slice equivalent (bread, rolls, and buns), 3/4 cup cold cereal	15
Fruit	1 medium peach, 1/2 cup apple juice, 1/2 cup melon	15
Vegetables	1 cup raw or 1/2 cup cooked greens	5
Dairy	1 cup milk or yogurt	12
Miscellaneous foods w/carbohydrate (snack foods, desserts, etc.)	Read label for portion	15

Note: An RD would help determine an individual carbohydrate recommendation for a patient. Patients monitor grams of carbohydrate in their diet or use a system of "carbohydrate choices." One carbohydrate choice is the serving of a food with ≅15 g of carbohydrate. Portions are important to accurately judge intake. Patients learn to manage the diet by reading labels and utilizing the generic exchange system in this chart for carbohydrate-containing foods. Foods not containing carbohydrate (meats, fish, poultry, cheese, fats) must be monitored to avoid cardiovascular risk, but are not part of the carbohydrate-counting system.

Sources: American Diabetes Association & American Dietetic Association. (1995a). *Carbohydrate counting: getting started.* Alexandria, VA, and Chicago, IL: Authors; American Diabetes Association & American Dietetic Association. (1995b). *Exchange lists for meal planning.* Alexandria, VA, and Chicago, IL: Authors; Wheeler, M. L. (2003). Nutrient database for the 2003 exchange lists for meal planning. *Journal of the American Dietetic Association, 103,* 894–920.

countries (Ludwig, 2002). The ADA (2003a) does acknowledge that foods have individual effects on glycemic response, but, given *equal* amounts of carbohydrate, *total amount* of carbohydrate at meals and snacks is more important than *source or type* when considering glycemic response (Franz et al., 2002). Consistent with this message, no type of carbohydrate is prohibited from the diet. Sucrose (table sugar) and other traditionally taboo, empty-calorie "sweets" sources of carbohydrate are allowed, but within the context of an overall healthy diet. The carbohydrate content of these foods should be calculated and considered as is done with all other carbohydrates in the diet. When asked for glycemic index advice by patients, the nurse can encourage intake of recommended plant sources of carbohydrate such as high-fiber fruits, vegetables, and whole grains. High-fiber carbohydrates, especially soluble fiber sources, have been shown to benefit glycemia and a high-fiber diet may be a de facto form of a low-glycemic index diet (Brand-Miller et al., 2003).

Fat Recommendations

Aggressive lipid management and prevention of coronary heart disease are important goals for diabetics (ADA, 2004). Saturated fat and cholesterol intake should be limited to assist with management of LDL cholesterol levels. Guidelines outlined under medical nutrition therapy for coronary heart disease in this chapter should be followed for the patient with diabetes as well. Monounsaturated fats or carbohydrates should be encouraged as calorie replacements for displaced saturated fat in patients seeking to maintain energy balance and body weight. Patients attempting weight loss doubly benefit from reduced saturated fat intake by not replacing saturated fat with equivocal calorie sources and therefore foster a deficit of energy intake. Substitution of monounsaturated fats over carbohydrates is preferred for individuals with elevated triglycerides, elevated postprandial glucose, or low HDL cholesterol. However, this recommendation should be assessed on an individual basis because excess calorie intake from fats and weight gain can ensue if fat is taken *ad libitum* (ADA, 2003a; Franz et al., 2002). Consumption of fatty fish is encouraged for the cardiovascular disease benefits associated with omega-3 fats as discussed earlier.

Vitamin and Mineral Recommendations

The position of the ADA is that no clear evidence exists to support any different advice on vitamin and mineral intake specific to people with diabetes than already exists for the general population. Antioxidants have been researched for their potential effects on clinical outcome with no conclusion specific to people with diabetes. Minerals such as chromium have also been investigated for a role in blood glucose control, but results are limited and seem to apply only to those who have a chromium deficiency, which is uncommon. Thiamine, pyridoxine (B_6), and vitamin B_{12} are used by some to treat diabetic neuropathy, but the efficacy of this is not clear and the ADA does not support this practice (ADA, 2003a; Franz et al., 2002).

Alcohol Recommendations

Like much of the nutritional advice for people with diabetes, alcohol recommendations coincide closely with those for the general adult population. People with diabetes must be aware of the potential hypoglycemic and hyperglycemic effects of alcohol and consume any intake along with food (Franz et al., 2002). Moderate intake is stressed in those who do choose to consume alcohol.

Special Considerations

Additional dietary considerations need to be made for the patient with diabetes who is acutely ill or experiencing other specific circumstances. Changes in diet and insulin needs occur under special circumstances. It is imperative for the nurse to teach the patient and family how to adjust insulin dosages depending on the given circumstance. The most common special considerations are discussed next.

Overweight and Obesity

Patients with diabetes who are also overweight or obese can benefit from weight management. Weight loss specifically in people with type II diabetes can lessen insulin resistance and decrease the risk of coronary heart disease (NHLBI, 2002). The nurse can encourage and support even small amounts of weight loss in these patients. Lifestyle changes for weight reduction outlined earlier in the chapter coincide with recommendations for the patient with diabetes (ADA, 2003a). The use of high-protein, low-carbohydrate diets for weight loss in patients with diabetes is not supported. Long-term effects of high levels of protein intake on the risk of nephropathy development deserve further study. Concern also exists regarding long-term effects of these diets on LDL cholesterol.

Exercise and Type I Diabetes

Glucose uptake is increased by exercising muscle. After consultation with the treatment team, a patient can compensate for this effect by reducing insulin before planned exercise or with consumption of carbohydrate. A registered dietitian could advise the patient on suitable food or beverage choices to fit the intensity, type, and duration of exercise given these parameters for glucose uptake.

Hypoglycemia

Blood glucose levels of ≤50 mg/dL require immediate treatment, whereas those in the range of 60 to 80 mg/dL can follow a decision-making process determined by the health care team (ADA, 2003a). Glucose is the preferred form of carbohydrate replacement to treat hypoglycemia because of its quicker glycemic response compared with other sources, but any carbohydrate source can be used (Franz et al., 2002). Guidelines call for an initial 15- to 20-g ingestion of carbohydrate followed by a reevaluation of blood glucose approximately 60 minutes later (ADA, 2003a). The nurse can guide the patient in pinpointing potential contributors to low blood sugar and suggest interventions to avoid future episodes.

Acute Illness

Symptoms from some acute illnesses can cause eating and diet tolerance to be jeopardized. The need for insulin can persist or be increased despite reduced intake because of the effects of illness on hormone secretion (Franz et al., 2002). Patients with type I diabetes in whom intake is compromised should be encouraged to maintain a carbohydrate intake of 150 to 200 g divided over the day (Franz et al., 2002). Easy-to-tolerate and liquid carbohydrates should be stressed for improved intake and hydration. Clear liquid and full liquid diets should *not* be sugar free (ADA, 2002b). Chart 14–24 outlines examples of appropriate carbohydrate sources to offer a person with diabetes who is ill.

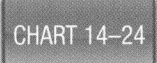 **CHART 14–24** **Sick Day Nutrition Suggestions for Diabetes**

The following foods are approximately 15 g of carbohydrate each or one "carbohydrate choice." Patients should try to approximate normal amount of carbohydrate intake.

Ginger ale, 5 oz	Apple juice, 1/2 cup
Cranberry juice cocktail, 1/3 cup	Fruit juice, frozen bar, 3oz
Sports drink, 1 cup (check labels)	Chicken noodle soup, 1 cup
Gelatin, 1/2 cup	Pudding, 1/4 cup
Sherbert, 1/4 cup	Breakfast bar, 1/2 of a 1-oz bar (check labels)
Canned fruit cocktail in juice, 1/2 cup	Jam, jelly, 1 TBSP
Toast, plain, 1 slice	Rice, plain, 1/3 cup
Noodles, plain, 1/3 cup	

Source: USDA Nutrient Data Laboratory http://www.nal.usda.gov/fnic/foodcomp/search

---

Hospitalized patients with diabetes who require enteral tube feedings or parenteral nutrition support can receive a standard or slightly lower carbohydrate feeding (40% of energy) with close attention paid to glycemic control and hydration. Care must be taken to avoid overfeeding because glycemic control will be adversely affected (Franz et al., 2002). Other parameters used in providing nutrition support also apply to the patient with diabetes.

Special considerations for elderly patients with diabetes are discussed in the Gerontological Considerations box.

Disorders of the Gastrointestinal Tract

Disorders of the gastrointestinal (GI) tract can affect overall health by altering digestion or absorption of food and nutrients. Minor GI complaints are commonplace and may have little impact on nutrition health if short term. Chronic GI conditions or disease can lead to altered intake of food or compromised absorption. Medical nutrition therapy plays a central role in the treatment of most GI diseases.

Swallowing Dysfunction

Dysphagia, or difficulty swallowing, can occur for a number of reasons. Dysphagia is associated with head and neck trauma or disease, neuromuscular disease, stroke, and dementia. Sedation and other medication side effects can impact swallowing directly or indirectly because of diminished saliva production. The patient who experiences dysphagia is at risk for "starvation, dehydration and aspiration" (Palmer, Drennan, & Baba, 2000). Difficulty swallowing can lead to inability to handle oral liquid boluses. Aspiration or loss of fluid volume from drooling or spitting liquids can also lead to dehydration because of diminished intake. Patients can become fearful of drinking liquids and voluntarily self-restrict fluid. Similarly, chewing and swallowing more solid foods can be risky or difficult, so patients may be unable to safely consume adequate nutrition orally.

The nurse should conduct a bedside evaluation to screen for dysphagia. The presence or absence of a gag reflex is not considered an accurate assessment tool (Palmer et al., 2000; Perry, 2001). Screening tools exist that have been validated for use by nurses (Perry, 2001). Warning signs of dysphagia during feeding include drooling or food spilling from the mouth; pocketing of food in the cheek, under the tongue or palate; repeated attempts to swallow a single food bolus; complaint of food sticking or heartburn while eating; frequent throat clearing or coughing while eating (Finestone & Greene-Finestone, 2003; Palmer et al., 2000).

 GERONTOLOGICAL CONSIDERATIONS
Nutrition for Elderly Patients with Diabetes

There is no evidence to support the use of any dietary restrictions in elderly patients with diabetes who reside in long-term care (ADA, 2003b). Long-term care elderly should receive a standard diet individualized to promote adequate intake and prevention of undernutrition, a common risk in older adults (American Dietetic Association, 2002a). In institutionalized elderly, a restricted diet does not provide superior blood glucose control and can lead to diminished intake. The use of "no concentrated sweets" or "no added sugar" diets is generally contraindicated in this population.

Patients with symptoms of dysphagia should be referred to the interdisciplinary team for a thorough evaluation. Speech/language pathologists (SLPs) and advanced practice nurses are the experts in management of swallowing problems and would guide the team in treatment. A dietitian works closely with the team to accommodate appropriate texture modifications to the diet to ensure safe swallowing and provision of adequate fluid and nutrition. The goals of medical nutrition therapy are to reduce choking risk, facilitate independent eating, and enhance enjoyment of eating (Dorner, 2002).

Often, texture modification to the diet can be presented in an unattractive fashion if attention is not given to preparation. Pureed or chopped meals can be made more attractive with sauces, gravies, colorful garnishes, and casseroles rather than being served in lumpy mounds with an ice cream scoop. The nurse should help the patient to have meals in as attractive a surrounding as possible to improve the eating environment. To improve nutrition, whenever possible, the patient should not be interrupted during mealtime for tests or procedures.

When patients with dysphagia are evaluated and transition through various diet modifications, the nurse should monitor the patient for tolerance to texture changes. Foods that form a cohesive bolus are most easily handled and are often attempted first; thin liquids are generally most easily aspirated (Dorner, 2002). The nurse should become familiar with hospital protocol for the dysphagia diet, and learn which foods are permitted with each transitional stage. *Pureed, mechanically altered,* or *mechanical soft* are common terms for food consistency. *Spoon-thick, honey-like, nectar-like,* and *thin* are liquid diet prescriptions (McCallum, 2003). Each patient should have an individualized prescription based on the hospital's dysphagia protocol. An inadvertent mistake in meal delivery could lead to aspiration. The patient should be watched closely for signs of aspiration, food pocketing, or other dysphagia symptoms. Fluid status should be monitored to ensure adequate intake. Commercial products are available to thicken liquids or foods as appropriate. The nurse can also assist the patient with compensatory swallowing techniques or exercises prescribed by the SLP.

Some patients are not able to safely consume adequate food or fluid. Enteral nutrition support with a feeding tube is then indicated. It is important to note that risk of aspiration still exists as do the possibility of gastroesophageal reflux. Nursing interventions to minimize aspiration risk are outlined later in this chapter in the discussion on enteral nutrition support.

Gastroesophageal Reflux Disease, Hiatal Hernia, Esophagitis, and Ulcer Disease

Lifestyle modifications, including dietary manipulation, are used as an adjunct to other treatment throughout the course of therapy for disorders of the upper GI tract. Nutrition therapy is targeted at relief of symptoms from gastroesophageal reflux and mucosal irritation by gastric acid. Additionally, certain foods can precipitate reflux from specific effects on reducing lower esophageal sphincter (LES) pressure in some patients (DeVault, Castell, & Practice Parameters Committee, 1999; Katz, 2003). The nurse should assess the patient for intake of foods or habits that affect LES pressure or intra-abdominal pressure. Chart 14–25

CHART 14–25 Nutrition Therapy for GERD

Limit foods that predispose to ↓ lower esophageal sphincter pressure:
- Fat
- Alcohol
- Coffee, tea, cola
- Chocolate
- Carminatives (mint).

Limit foods that irritate esophagus:
- Citrus
- Tomato
- Spicy.

Limit gastric pressure:
- Avoid tight clothing, belts.
- Avoid large meals and excessive carbonated drinks.
- Avoid recumbency after meals.
- Lose weight if indicated.

Sources: DeVault, K. R., Castell, D. O., & Practice Parameters Committee. (1999). Practice guidelines: Updated guidelines for the diagnosis and treatment of gastroesophageal reflux disease. *The American Journal of Gastroenterology, 94,* 1434–1442; Katz, P. O. (2003). Optimizing medical therapy for gastroesophageal reflux disease: State of the art. *Reviews in Gastroenterological Disorders, 3,* 59–69; National Institute of Diabetes and Digestive and Kidney Diseases. (2003a). *Gastroesophageal reflux.* Retrieved January 13, 2004, from http://digestive.niddk.nih.gov/ddiseases/pubs/gerd/index.htm#4

---

provides general guidelines for adjunctive dietary treatment for gastro-esophageal reflux disease (GERD). Individual patient food intolerances should be added to these guidelines. The nurse should assess the nutritional adequacy of the diet of patients who seem intolerant to many foods or those who have broadly eliminated any major food group assuming intolerance to all of its constituents. An example of this would be the patient who consumes no fruits after poor tolerance of a citrus juice. Such patients need encouragement to try other foods within the food group to ensure adequate intake.

Dumping Syndrome

Dumping syndrome is a condition often resulting from full or partial gastric resection or the removal of the pyloric sphincter. Symptoms include abdominal cramping, diarrhea, sweating, and shakiness following a meal because of rapid emptying of gastric contents into the small intestine. Dumping syndrome can also result following bariatric surgery for morbid obesity. Postoperative nutrition guidelines for bariatric surgical patients are discussed later in this chapter.

The goals of nutrition treatment of dumping syndrome include the prevention of rapid gastric emptying and the reduction of hyperosmolar intestinal contents. Foods high in simple sugars have a concentrated, or hyperosmolar, content that will draw fluid into the gut because of a concentration gradient between plasma and the intestine. This rapid entry of fluid into the gut can contribute to the symptoms of dumping syndrome (NIDDK, 2003). Large meals, fluids with meals, and extreme food temperatures (very hot or very cold) can promote more rapid gastric emptying than usual. Eating smaller meals, avoiding liquids at mealtime, and lying down following a meal can be helpful. Chart 14–26 (p. 302) outlines the guidelines for treatment of dumping syndrome.

| CHART 14–26 | **Nutrition Guidelines for Dumping Syndrome** |

- Limit consumption of simple sugars and carbonated drinks.
- Avoid extremes of hot or cold foods.
- Eat small meals.
- Save liquid for between meals.
- Lie down if needed after eating.

Source: National Heart Lung and Blood Institute. (2002). *Third report of the National Cholesterol Education Program expert panel on detection, evaluation, and treatment of high blood cholesterol in adults (Adult treatment panel III).* Retrieved February 5, 2004, from http://www.nhlbi.nih.gov/guidelines/cholesterol/atp3full.pdf

Lactose Intolerance

Lactose is the principal disaccharide present in milk products that requires the small intestine enzyme lactase for digestion. Insufficient production of lactase can foster maldigestion of lactose-containing foods with resultant intestinal complaints, which can include bloating, cramping, and diarrhea. The nurse should help educate the patient that a lactose intolerance is not an allergy to milk. Lactose maldigestion or intolerance is a common complaint among people with gastrointestinal symptoms. The prevalence of lactose-intolerance symptoms is high among many ethnic groups with the exception of those of Northern European descent (Swagerty, Walling, & Klein, 2002). Several researchers have found that people mistakenly claim they have lactose intolerance when in fact breath hydrogen tests show normal findings, leading some to conclude that the prevalence statistics are overstated (Saltzman et al., 1999). Insufficient lactase production can occur from birth, which is uncommon, or later in life. Secondary lactose intolerance can occur from damage to the small intestine mucosa, such as with infection, small bowel disease, chemotherapy, or intestinal radiation, and may be temporary (Montalto et al., 2006). The degree of lactose intolerance varies among individuals and can be dose dependent (Montalto et al., 2006). Nutrition treatment of lactose intolerance is largely not dependent on the etiology of the intolerance.

A general consensus exists that most people who complain of lactose intolerance are capable of tolerating some lactose in their diets. Additionally, it is believed that tolerance to lactose can be improved with the continual consumption of some lactose-containing foods. Some milk-based foods, such as aged cheeses, naturally contain less lactose than others do. Many yogurts and other fermented dairy products have reduced lactose content and advantageous probiotic bacteria that have a lactase-producing ability that benefits digestion of lactose content (Kopp-Hoolihan, 2001; Montalto et al., 2006; Swagerty et al., 2002).

Because each patient with lactose intolerance has a different ability to produce lactose, medical nutrition therapy occurs along a continuum. The nurse should assess the patient for lactose tolerance among different milk-based foods and under different patterns of consumption. Lactose-containing foods tend to be better tolerated with a meal than when consumed alone (Montalto et al., 2006). The patient's diet should be assessed for adequate calcium and vitamin D sources, especially for those who have broadly eliminated dairy foods from their diets. Chart 14–27 lists suggestions for improving tolerance to lactose and adequate intake of calcium and vitamin D.

| CHART 14–27 | **Nutrition Guidelines for Lactose Intolerance** |

- Try 1/2 to 1 cup milk with meals.
- Gradually increase milk intake in small increments.
- Try cultured and fermented dairy products: yogurt with active cultures, buttermilk, aged cheese.
- Use digestive aides as needed: oral lactase enzyme products or enzyme-incubated milk.
- Monitor diet for adequate calcium and vitamin D intake.
- Be mindful of hidden lactose in baking mixes, processed foods, instant soups, mashed potato mix, cold cuts, commercial sauces, and medicines.
- Read labels for "nonfat milk solids" or "milk by-products" because lactose may be present.

Sources: Montalto, M., Curigliano, C., Santoro, L., Vastola, M., Cammarota, G., & Manna, R. (2006). Management and treatment of lactose malabsorption. *World Journal of Gastroenterology, 12,* 187–191; National Institute of Diabetes, and Digestive Disorders and Kidney Diseases. (2003b). *Lactose intolerance.* Retrieved January 13, 2004, from http://digestive.niddk.nih.gov/ddiseases/pubs/lactoseintolerance; Swagerty, D. L., Walling, A. D., & Klein, R. M. (2002). Lactose intolerance. *American Family Physician, 65,* 1845–1850.

Inflammatory Bowel Disease

A diagnosis of either Crohn's disease or ulcerative colitis can place a patient at risk for malnutrition. Chapter 45 provides a complete description of Crohn's disease. Crohn's patients generally tend to have more extensive nutritional risk factors than do patients with ulcerative colitis because of potential small bowel disease location, severity of symptoms, and fistula formation (Goh & O'Morain, 2003; Jeejeebhoy, 2002a). Active inflammatory bowel disease can cause diminished nutrient intake, increased gut nutritional losses and additional metabolic requirements (Goh & O'Morain, 2003; Jeejeebhoy, 2002a). Together, or singly, these disease consequences present nutritional challenges to the patient and the clinician. Pain, anorexia, fever, and medication side effects can lead to poor intake in the face of the increased metabolic needs required for tissue healing and to compensate for malabsorptive losses. Patients with inflammatory bowel disease require a comprehensive nutrition assessment on which to base the foundation of nutrition therapy. The Risk Factors box lists common nutrition problems association with Crohn's disease.

RISK FACTORS for Malnutrition in Inflammatory Bowel Disease

Risk Factor	Etiology of Malnutrition Risk
Decreased intake	• Nausea, vomiting, diarrhea • Pain or fear of pain • Discomfort associated w/certain foods • Anorexia
Increased nutrient losses	• Malabsorption; depends on disease site • Drug–nutrient interactions (sulfasalazine and folic acid, steroids and calcium, vitamin D) • Iron losses w/bleeding
Increased nutrient needs	• Hypermetabolism from inflammation • Fistula healing requirements

Physical symptoms and disease severity will dictate the nutrition care plan. Small bowel disease in Crohn's can lead to malabsorption of multiple nutrients, depending on the specific location of the disease. Calcium, magnesium, iron, and other minerals are generally absorbed in the proximal small intestine, whereas vitamin B_{12}, fat, and fat-soluble vitamin absorption occur in the ileum. Fat malabsorption can lead to a cascade of other nutritional problems such as vitamin A, D, E, and K and calcium malabsorption, increased absorption of oxalates (with subsequent increased risk of oxalate kidney stones), and loss of the valuable energy derived from fat. Fluid and electrolyte status can also become compromised because of losses from diarrhea. Inadequate absorption of calcium and vitamin D can lead to bone disease and further complicate the nutritional consequences of the steroid therapy often used in these patients (Jeejeebhoy, 2002a).

Anemia from blood losses and poor iron, folate, and vitamin B_{12} absorption can contribute further to the fatigue experienced from inadequate intake and the disease process. Enteric fistula formation can cause intestinal losses of crucial nutrients, as well as fluid and electrolytes. Surgical resection of diseased intestine can result in the loss of crucial absorptive surface and further place the patient at nutritional risk. Short bowel syndrome can be the result and is discussed in a later section. Knowledge of the extent and location of disease, along with a complete nutrition history, is essential to identify nutrition risk and goals.

Nutrition treatment of inflammatory bowel disease focuses on correction of malnutrition and provision of adequate nutrients and energy to promote disease remission. Nutrition plays a central role in disease management and remission but is not the primary treatment (American Gastroenterological Association [AGA] 2001a; Ireton-Jones, 2000; Jeejeebhoy, 2002a). Patients with severe fulminant disease can require nutrition support in the form of a low-fat elemental or polymeric enteral nutrition formula, which is discussed later. These formulas can be taken orally or delivered via a feeding tube. Such formulas require minimal digestion for absorption and can be a better tolerated mode of providing nutrition than a usual diet, though palatability of some formulas is low. A registered dietitian would determine the appropriate type and amount of enteral nutrition support and make a recommendation for treatment.

The nurse should monitor intake and tolerance as described in Chart 14–28 (p. 304). Unless a patient has developed a bowel obstruction, perforation, or severe short bowel syndrome, there is no specific need for parenteral nutrition in disease treatment as compared with enteral support. Achievement of disease remission does not require bowel rest (AGA, 2001a). It is postulated that use of the gut with enteral nutrition provides an additional beneficial effect toward recovery, besides just nutrient content, by preventing intestinal bacterial translocation that can occur when the gut is not used (Goh & O'Morain, 2003; Jeejeebhoy, 2002a).

A low-residue diet with adequate energy and protein is indicated as patients are recovering from a disease flare and transitioning a return to their usual diet (George, Day, & Zeiter, 2000; Ireton-Jones, 2000). Fibrous fruits and vegetables, whole grains, seeds, and nuts are avoided to decrease fecal residue and stool frequency. Patients with stricture should avoid a high-fiber diet to decrease the risk of intestinal obstruction (Jeejeebhoy, 2002a).

Lactose-containing foods may need to be limited in patients for whom secondary lactose intolerance has developed. Due to lack of small bowel involvement, patients with ulcerative colitis are not likely to benefit from altering lactose intake. As the patient improves, the diet can be liberalized as tolerated.

Nutrient supplementation is often indicated for patients unable to tolerate adequate variety in the diet or with active disease. Anemia should be treated with the appropriate dose of iron, folic acid, or vitamin B_{12} depending on anemia type. (Anemia is discussed later in this chapter.) Calcium supplementation to meet the federal Recommended Dietary Allowance (RDA) of 1,000 to 1,200 mg are indicated for patients with a limited diet, steroid therapy, or malabsorption. Adequate vitamin D is needed as well. Zinc is lost when there is high-volume intestinal output as with diarrhea or an enteric fistula. Wound healing, including fistula repair, requires zinc. Zinc replacement of 12 to 15 mg/day per liter of stool output or 20 to 40 mg/day zinc gluconate is recommended (Ireton-Jones, 2000; Jeejeebhoy, 2002b). Magnesium replacement therapy may also be necessary, but care must be used to avoid magnesium salts known to precipitate diarrhea (Jeejeebhoy, 2002b). The nurse should routinely assess patients with inflammatory bowel disease for inadequate or overly restrictive intake and refer appropriate patients for nutritional counseling.

Celiac Sprue

Celiac sprue, or gluten-sensitive enteropathy, is a lifelong condition affecting the small intestine in which the villi morphology is damaged from the presence of gluten in the diet. Gluten is a protein found in grain products, specifically wheat, rye, and barley. The presence of gluten in the intestine leads to villi atrophy and loss of absorptive surface. Diarrhea with malabsorption of most nutrients can follow with risk of weight loss and malnutrition. Individuals vary in their degree of presenting malabsorptive symptoms (AGA, 2001b).

Medical nutrition therapy is essential for resolution of symptoms and return of normal villi morphology (AGA, 2001b). Gluten-containing foods must be avoided to eliminate disease symptoms (NIDDK, 2005a). There is agreement that foods made from wheat, rye, and barley should be eliminated, but considerable debate exists about several other grains. Oats have traditionally been excluded in the diet as well, but more recently evidence exists that oats do not exhibit toxicity and can be well tolerated (NIDDK, 2005a). The AGA permits oat products as part of a gluten-free diet, but warns of the possibility of wheat contamination of oat flour (AGA, 2001b). The chance of wheat contamination has led some to recommend avoidance of oats until disease remission and then only consumption of oat products from a trustworthy source (Farrell & Kelly, 2002). Buckwheat, quinoa, and amaranth are grains recommended by some clinicians and celiac sprue organizations citing different plant taxonomy than offending grains, but they are banned by others because of insufficient information on toxicity (Thompson, 2000b, 2001a). No consensus exists on advice to give patients regarding these three grains. The recommendation regarding wheat-starch faces a similar dilemma in that some recognize it as gluten free, whereas others contend it still has offending protein components (Thompson, 2001b). Distilled vinegar, millet, and wild rice are also debated. Chart 14–29 (p. 305) outlines common dietary sources of gluten.

| CHART 14–28 | **Nursing Interventions in Enteral Nutrition Support** |

Problem	Intervention
Potential for foodborne illness	• Wash hands before handling formula and equipment.
	• Wipe off top of formula container before opening.
	• Label, cover, and store open formula in refrigerator for not >24 hours.
	• Limit "hang time" to 4 hours if water or other additions made to formula. Otherwise 8- to 12-hour hang time allowed if canned formula w/no additives is being used.
Aspiration	• Check gastric residuals. Hold feeding for large volume (>150 mL but treat individually and according to physician's order).
	• Elevate head of bed to at least a 30-degree angle.
	• Avoid bolus feedings.
	• Consider smaller bore or longer tube if nasally intubated. Routinely confirm tube placement.
	• Consider G-tube or J-tube if long-term feeding is required.
Clogged tube	• Administer feeding with pump vs. gravity drip.
	• Administer room temperature feeding. High-temperature storage or heating of formula will cause protein content to coagulate.
	• Follow guidelines for medication administration: 1. Flush tube with 20 to 30 mL water before, between, and after each single medication. 2. Consult pharmacist regarding suitability of crushing medication with a small amount of water and availability of medication elixirs. *Note: If using longer feeding tubes, ensure medication absorption site is not bypassed by tube.*
Diarrhea	• Administer feeding at room temperature. Cold feeding increases gut peristalsis.
	• Consider lactose-free formula.
	• Consider formula with fiber.
	• Consider medications w/cathartic effect: antibiotics, magnesium, potassium, digoxin, theophylline, acetaminophen elixir, and others.
	• Administer continuous drip vs. bolus.
	• Consult registered dietitian regarding temporarily altering formula concentration or rate of delivery.
	• Rule out infection, *Clostridium difficile,* medical etiology.
Constipation	• Consider formula with added fiber.
	• Monitor hydration; ensure adequate intake.
	• Encourage ambulation as indicated.
	• Assess for contributing medications (e.g., narcotics, some antacids).
	• Consider obstruction or medical causes.
Dehydration	• Monitor hydration: weight, intake & output, physical signs.
	• Ensure adequate free water intake. Need 1 mL water per 1 kcal of intake. Most formulas are 50%–75% free water (formula with >1 kcal/mL or high protein content have less free water).

Sources: Rees Parrish, C., & Falls McCray, S. (2003). Nutrition support for the mechanically ventilated patient. *Critical Care Nurse, 23,* 77–80.; Dobson, K., & Scott, A. (2007). Review of ICU nutrition support practices: Implementing the nurse-led enteral feeding algorithm. *Nursing in Critical Care, 12,* 114–123; Swanson, R. W., & Winkelman, C. (2002). Exploring the benefits and myths of enteral feeding in the critically ill. *Critical Care Nursing Quarterly, 24,* 67–75.

The patient with celiac sprue has to be dedicated to label reading and attentive to the diet at all times. Wheat, rye, and barley are present in both obvious and hidden sources in the diet. Some patients with celiac sprue also have secondary lactose intolerance and must adhere to guidelines for that treatment as well. Product reformulation can lead to changes that add or delete ingredients so continued label reading is essential. The nurse should warn patients to be suspect of labels touting "new and improved" versions because ingredients could be altered. The nurse can be empathetic about the need for restrictions and stress the role of diet in avoiding ill health and correcting existing deficiencies.

Gluten-free versions of grain foods can replace the displaced wheat, rye, and barley products. Corn, potato, rice, and soy flours can be used to make alternative breads, pasta, and baked goods. Many stores and online sources sell these products. A local or online celiac sprue support group and a knowledgeable dietitian can provide patients with lists of available products. Wheat flour products are commonly fortified with iron, folic acid, and other B-complex vitamins. Alternative gluten-free products often are not routinely fortified with these nutrients. Alternative sources of iron and B-complex vitamins should be encouraged. The limited diet warrants a recommendation of a gluten-free multivitamin supplement (Thompson, 1999, 2000a).

| CHART 14–29 | **Dietary Sources of Gluten** |

Label reading is essential. In addition to more obvious sources of barley, rye, and wheat, fillers and additives contain hidden sources of gluten that can be discovered by reading ingredient panels. Dietary sources of gluten include:

- Barley including beer, malt beverages, and cereal
- Rye
- Wheat including all wheat flour products (pastas, cereals, baked goods, pizza crust, etc.), wheat or food starch, couscous, spelt, triticale, semolina, distilled vinegar, soy sauce, caramel coloring. Wheat or food starch can be a filler in many products, including instant mixes, sauces, condiments, hot dogs, sausage.

It is under debate whether or not the following grains should be restricted. Patients should be assessed individually and given personal advice:

- Oats
- Buckwheat
- Amaranth
- Quinoa
- Millet
- Sorghum.

Sources: American Gastroenterological Association (AGA). (2001a). Medical position statement: Celiac sprue. *Gastroenterology, 120,* 1761–1778; Farrell, R. J., & Kelly, C. (2002). Celiac sprue. *New England Journal of Medicine, 346,* 180–188; National Institute of Diabetes and Digestive and Kidney Diseases. (2005a). *Celiac disease.* Retrieved November 13, 2006, from http://www.digestive.niddk.nih.gov/ddiseases/pubs/celiac/index.htm; Thompson, T. (2001a). Case problem: Questions regarding the acceptability of buckwheat, amaranth, quinoa, and oats from a patient with celiac disease. *Journal of the American Dietetic Association, 101,* 586–587; Thompson, T. (2001b). Wheat starch, gliadin, and the gluten-free diet. *Journal of the American Dietetic Association, 101,* 1456–1459.

Short Bowel Syndrome

Short bowel syndrome (SBS) describes a set of symptoms that can result from a large surgical resection of any combination of small intestine and colon. Most commonly, the resection is a result of a single or several surgical interventions for inflammatory bowel disease. Bowel infarct, gastric bypass surgery, neoplastic disease treatment, and congenital abnormalities are among other etiology of SBS. In some forms of gastric bypass surgery for morbid obesity, the loss of small intestine absorptive surface is a deliberate attempt to have malabsorption contribute to weight loss efforts. Such surgery and its nutrition intervention are discussed later in the surgical nutrition section of this chapter. Symptoms of SBS can include rapid gut transit time, diarrhea, altered fluid and electrolyte status, malabsorption, and subsequent weight loss and malnutrition (AGA, 2003; Atalay et al., 2003; Jeejeebhoy, 2002b). Loss of absorptive surface and the presence of unabsorbed substrate in the colon are responsible for the symptoms.

A patient with <200 cm (6.5 ft) of small intestine is at risk for short bowel syndrome. Patients with <100 cm (3.3 ft) of remaining small intestine most likely will have some symptoms of this syndrome, especially if losses include the terminal ileum or remaining bowel has disease (AGA, 2003). The terminal ileum is the site of reabsorption of bile salts that are responsible for fat and fat-soluble vitamin absorption. Additionally, vitamin B_{12} and some water and electrolyte absorption occur here. When all of these substances remain unabsorbed and pass into the colon,

their hyperosmolar content draws fluid from the plasma that leads to diarrhea, malabsorption, and altered hydration. If both ileum and colon have been resected, an end jejunostomy is the result and has compromised absorptive ability (AGA, 2003; Jeejeebhoy, 2002b). Postsurgical intestinal adaptation can occur over the course of 1 to 2 years and improve absorptive capability. The ileum can adapt to compensate for the absorptive needs previously met by a resected jejunum, but conversely, the jejunum is less able to compensate for a resected ileum (Jeejeebhoy, 2002b).

Medical nutrition therapy for SBS is essential. Patients must receive adequate nutrition to promote wound healing and prevent malnutrition in the postoperative period. Initially, patients will require at least a 7- to 10-day course of parenteral nutrition to meet fluid, electrolyte, and nutritional demands while potential bowel function begins to return (AGA, 2003). Gradual conversion to enteral nutrition occurs according to patient tolerance. Those patients with more than 100 cm (3.3 ft) of remaining small intestine, especially those with an intact ileum and colon, typically are able to progress to a standard diet, often with few restrictions (Atalay et al., 2003). In contrast, patients with 35 to 100 cm (about 1 to 3.3 ft) of intestinal remnant may progress more slowly from parenteral nutrition to an enteral formula and then to trials of a modified diet over the course of several months to years (AGA, 2003; Atalay et al., 2003). Intestinal absorptive adaptation takes time and requires enteral nutrition in order to occur. Patients with <50 cm (1.6 ft) of remaining intestine present a unique medical challenge because of severely altered absorption and the potential for ongoing disturbances in hydration and electrolyte status and acid–base balance (AGA, 2003; Atalay et al., 2003; Jeejeebhoy, 2002b). Most often these patients require permanent parenteral nutrition to meet their nutritional and fluid and electrolyte requirements, because adaptation is less likely to occur than in cases with larger bowel remnants.

When the patient is hemodynamically stable and bowel sounds return, sips of isotonic liquids can be attempted. Isotonic enteral formula and rehydration solutions are recommended (AGA, 2003). Hypertonic liquids, such as elemental nutrition formula and sugary drinks, or hypotonic liquids (water or overly diluted drinks) are not recommended initially because of potential intestinal fluid and electrolyte shifts compensating for a concentration gradient (AGA, 2003). Sorbitol should be avoided in sugar-free beverages because of its laxative effect. The nurse should monitor fluid intake and tolerance with a careful comparison to measured fluid output. Laboratory values should also be monitored for assessing hydration and electrolyte status, that is, sodium, chloride, potassium, hemoglobin, and hematocrit. Sodium, potassium, magnesium, and zinc losses can be substantial and require replacement (Jeejeebhoy, 2002b). Patients will vary in their ability to successfully attempt this stage of diet transition. Some may require months of parenteral support first.

After several months of tolerance to enteral formula, the patient with SBS can begin the challenging process of further intestinal adaptation with a more solid diet. Patients with <100 cm (3.3 ft) of bowel remnant can require intake of twice their estimated nutrition needs in order to absorb adequate macro- and micronutrients. Protein absorption occurs in the duodenum and generally is not compromised as severely as other nutrients

(Jeejeebhoy, 2002b). A modified diet is encouraged as tolerated following the parameters outlined in Chart 14–30. The diet may be modified to include less lactose and low oxalate content, but not low fat. Altering fat has little effect on symptoms and deprives the patient of needed calories. A lactose-modified diet is recommended only if lactose maldigestion in known. Patients with SBS and an existing colon are at risk for increased absorption of oxalate (AGA, 2003). Oxalate is a substance found in foods such as spinach, chocolate, tea, and rhubarb and normally is bound with calcium and poorly absorbed. However, during fat malabsorption, calcium binds with free fats, leaving oxalates unbound and more apt to be absorbed by the intestine. Eventually such elevated oxalate absorption can lead to calcium oxalate kidney stones (Morton, Iliescu, & Wilson, 2002).

Nutrient supplementation is often necessary if the ileum has been resected. Fat-soluble vitamins A, D, E, and K are needed in a liquid form if **steatorrhea,** or diarrhea from fat malabsorption, is present. This can be confirmed with a Sudan stain of a stool sample. Zinc replacement should correspond with intestinal output. Calcium supplements are needed if a lactose modification is needed or fat malabsorption is present. Calcium supplements can advantageously assist with lessening oxalate absorption. The need for magnesium replacement should also be assessed. Vitamin B_{12} injections are needed in patients without an ileum (AGA, 2003; Jeejeebhoy, 2002b). Patients who experience SBS require long-term monitoring by an experienced health care team to prevent malnutrition, dehydration, and altered electrolyte status.

Constipation

A high-fiber diet is recommended for the treatment of most types of constipation (AGA, 2000). A low-fiber diet and sedentary lifestyle contribute to the occurrence of constipation in adults (Arce, Ermocilla, & Costa, 2002). Fiber is present only in plant foods and can be removed during processing. Adequate fiber intake benefits intestinal motility by contributing to stool bulk and shortening intestinal transit time. The National Academy of Science has set the daily recommendation for fiber at 38 g for men and 25 g for women up to age 50 years. After age 50, the recommendation drops to 30 g and 21 g, respectively (Institute of Medicine [IOM], 2002). The nurse should advise the patient to gradually add fiber to the diet in order to minimize intestinal bloating. Adequate fluid intake is also recommended to both prevent and treat constipation. The established daily adequate intake (AI) of water for men and women is 3.7 and 2.7 liters, respectively (IOM, 2004). Chart 14–31 outlines sources of fiber to recommend.

Diverticular Disease

Patients with uncomplicated diverticulosis should be encouraged to consume adequate fiber to lessen potential symptoms and potentially avoid diverticulitis. Although there is no evidence that a high-fiber diet will decrease intraluminal pressure and subsequent development of diverticula, the recommendation to consume sufficient fiber is felt to be a reasonable approach to amelioration of symptoms of this condition (NIDDK, 2005b; Stollman, Raskin, & Practice Parameters Committee, 1999). Traditionally most fiber sources have been recommended with the exception of seeds and nuts feared to foster diverticulitis when trapped in diverticulum. The AGA does not find sub-

---

CHART 14–30	**Nutrition Therapy for Short Bowel Syndrome**
Early diet	• Use isotonic feedings to minimize diarrhea. • Replace fluid and electrolyte losses. • Determine nutrients at risk for malabsorption based on resection site.
Adaptation	• Maximize intake of energy (including fat) and protein, adjust to tolerance. • Give frequent meals w/liquids separately. • Dilute sugary drinks.
General recommendations	• Limit caffeine, oxalates, lactose, sugar alcohols (such as sorbitol, mannitol). • Monitor and replace electrolytes/minerals, including zinc, potassium, and magnesium. • Replace fat-soluble vitamins and B_{12} if ileum resected/fat malabsorbing.

Sources: Atalay, F., Ozcay, N., Gundogdu, H., Orug, T., et al. (2003). Evaluation of the outcomes of short bowel syndrome and indications for intestinal transplantation. *Transplant Proceedings, 35,* 3054–3056; Jeejeebhoy, K. N. (2002b). Short bowel syndrome. *Canadian Medical Association Journal, 166,* 1297–1302; Stahl, P. (2000). Nutrition protocols for small-bowel transplant patients. *Journal of the American Dietetic Association, 100,* 689.

CHART 14–31	**Fiber Content of Selected Foods***

≤1 g Fiber	2 g Fiber	3 g Fiber	4 g Fiber	≥5 g Fiber
1-oz white bread	1-oz whole-wheat bread	1 med banana	1 C brown rice	1 C bran flake cereal
1 dinner roll, average	2 C popcorn	1 C corn	1/2 C cooked barley	1/2 C dried fruit
1 boiled potato without skin	1 C couscous	1/2 C winter squash	1 C cooked oatmeal	1/2 C cooked beans, peas, or
1 C iceberg lettuce	1 medium peach	1/4 cup soy nuts	1 med apple or pear with skin	lentils
1 C mushrooms	1/2 cup cooked carrots		1 med baked potato with skin	1 C cooked collards
			1 C cooked spinach	1 kiwi
			2 TBSP almonds	

*The nurse should advise the patient that fiber content is listed on "Nutrition Facts" food labels.

Source: USDA Nutrient Data Laboratory http://www.nal.usda.gov/fnic/foodcomp/search

stantial clinical evidence to support this seed and nut restriction (Stollman et al., 1999). The NIH and others still advise against consumption of nuts, popcorn hulls, and seeds (Cunningham & Marcason, 2002; NIDDK, 2005b).

Nutritional management of an episode of diverticulitis requires a short course of a clear liquid diet while medical treatment is given and symptoms abate within a few days (Stollman et al., 1999). Patients who require surgical intervention, an extended course of nil per os (NPO), or more prolonged intake of clear liquids need close nutritional assessment and monitoring with appropriate referral to the registered dietitian as needed. Once diverticulitis is resolved and the patient is free of symptoms, the high-fiber diet should be resumed.

Chronic Diarrhea

Chronic diarrhea can occur for many reasons. Appropriate nutrition intervention is determined by the etiology of the diarrhea, if known. Patients in whom pancreatic exocrine function is compromised may require a low-fat diet as outlined in the nutrition treatment of pancreatic disease. Small bowel disease and lactose intolerance can also result in chronic diarrhea if not adequately treated. (Nutrition therapy for each of these causes was discussed in an earlier section.) The nurse can assess the patient for excessive intake of sugar alcohols, such as sorbitol, which can contribute to diarrhea. The presence of eating disorder symptoms can also be cause to suspect laxative abuse, which can lead to chronic diarrhea. Patients with chronic diarrhea should be routinely assessed for fluid, electrolyte, weight loss, and nutrition depletion. Parenteral nutrition may be required in cases where intestinal losses from the condition exceed enteral ability to compensate and maintain adequate nutrition or fluid balance (AGA, 1999).

Irritable Bowel Syndrome

Irritable bowel syndrome (IBS) is characterized by abdominal pain, constipation, or diarrhea that has no known coexisting organic cause. Nutrition treatment is largely trial and error according to the individual patient's situation. Often a symptom diary is helpful to guide the patient in finding any lifestyle factors, including offending foods, that trigger symptoms (AGA, 2002a). No single food or food group has proven to universally contribute to symptoms though a significant placebo effect was noticed in many research trials. Caffeine, alcohol, fat, and sorbitol are the most commonly mentioned trigger foods. Sorbitol is a sugar alcohol present in dietetic candies and foods that has a laxative effect (Burden, 2001; Viera, Hoag, & Shaughnessy, 2002).

Many patients with IBS can benefit from a psychosocial assessment and appropriate intervention because coexisting stress, coping difficulties, depression, and anxiety occur in these patients (Viera et al., 2002). The nurse can guide the patient in recognizing any individual foods that trigger symptoms and suggest experimenting with limiting caffeine, alcohol, sorbitol, and fat in the diet. Lactose intolerance is often a complaint because of similar symptoms, but can be unfounded. Lactose should be managed only in patients known to have lactase deficiency (Viera et al., 2002).

Liver Disease

The liver performs various functions related to the storage, metabolism, or excretion of most nutrients. Liver disease impacts nutrition status by decreasing nutrient storage and interfering with efficient metabolism. The body's ability to maintain nutritional health is altered when any aspect of nutrient metabolism is compromised by liver disease.

Fatty Liver

Deposition of fatty deposits in the liver can occur from excessive alcohol intake but can also be associated with nonalcoholic etiology. Many cases of fatty liver, or steatosis, are associated with nutritional contributors. Daily intake of more than 20 to 30 g of alcohol, obesity, severe weight loss (as in starvation or following gastric bypass surgery for obesity), total parenteral nutrition, elevated blood triglyceride levels found in type 2 diabetes, and metabolic syndrome are associated with steatosis (AGA, 2002b). Nutrition therapy for fatty liver requires knowledge of the pathogenesis of the condition. Abstinence from alcohol, weight loss if overweight, and control of plasma glucose and lipids are the primary therapies for uncomplicated fatty liver.

Alcohol and Nutrition Status

Malnutrition can be a complication of excessive alcohol intake and is associated with a more dismal prognosis than observed in better nourished people with alcoholic liver disease (Stickel et al., 2003). It is important for the nurse to understand the overall potential impact of alcohol on nutrition status when assessing patients with any type of alcoholic liver disease. Both primary and secondary malnutrition can occur from excessive alcohol intake. Poor-quality food, infrequent food intake, and anorexia are examples of risk factors for primary malnutrition. Secondary malnutrition can occur because of indirect effects such as nutrient malabsorption and altered metabolism. Alcohol contains significant calories (7.1 per gram), which can be a concern in the casual drinker trying to maintain or lose weight. However, when intake of alcohol is excessive, altered and inefficient metabolism of alcohol occurs, resulting in weight loss when significant food calories are replaced by alcohol calories (Santolaria et al., 2000; Stickel et al., 2003). Chart 14–32 (p. 308) lists the contributing causes of both primary and secondary malnutrition with excessive alcohol intake.

A careful assessment of nutrition status should be done when excessive alcohol intake is suspected. Unfortunately, an accurate diet history is difficult to obtain if the patient has suffered periods of altered consciousness. Irregular feeding habits and transient diet quality further make generalizations from a diet recall difficult (Santolaria et al., 2000).

Patients in whom alcohol comprises more than 30% of total calorie intake have been shown to have decreased intake of protein, fat, vitamins A and C, thiamin, calcium, and iron (Lieber, 2000). The altered absorption and metabolism of those nutrients from alcohol can further worsen nutrition health. Physical assessment of the patient should focus on skin integrity, presence of muscle or fat wasting, and edema or ascites. Chapter 46 ⊙ has a complete description of ascites due to liver disease. Altered fluid status can mask changes in body weight, making weight or BMI unreliable assessment tools for nutrition status. If liver disease is present, plasma protein production can be diminished unrelated to nutrition. Malnutrition can also lower serum albumin, prealbumin, or transferrin levels, but it is impossible to differentiate the major cause with the compounded effects of liver disease and poor nutrition status.

CHART 14–32	Effect of Alcohol on Nutrition Status
Primary malnutrition	Replaces nutrient and food intake with alcohol. Appetite can be suppressed.
Secondary malnutrition	Decreased nutrient absorption: • Thiamine • Folate • Vitamin B_{12} • Protein. Increased urinary losses of nutrients: • Folate • Magnesium • Zinc • Nitrogen. Decreased nutrient storage: • Folate • Riboflavin • Vitamin B_6.

Sources: Lieber, C. S. (2000). Alcohol: Its metabolism and interaction with nutrients. *Annual Review Nutrition, 20,* 395–430; Stickel, F., Hoehn, B., & Seitz, H. K. (2003). Nutrition therapy in alcoholic liver disease. *Alimentary Pharmacology Therapy, 18,* 357–373.

Nutrition supplementation is recommended for several nutrients when excessive alcohol intake is suspected or known and nutrition intake is poor. A multivitamin supplement with ample water-soluble vitamins is reasonable, with special attention given to thiamine and folic acid (Stickel et al., 2003). Both nutrients are poorly absorbed in the presence of alcohol. Thiamine supplementation in the alcoholic patient is crucial in order to avoid development of Wernicke-Korsakoff syndrome (Thiamine, 2003). Thiamine is routinely administered on admission to patients suspected or known to abuse alcohol. Trace mineral status should be assessed and deficiencies replaced accordingly. Zinc levels are often diminished from low intake and increased urinary zinc excretion in people with alcoholic liver disease (Lieber, 2000). Abstinence from alcohol is the primary goal.

Hepatitis

Anorexia, fatigue, and gastrointestinal complaints are common symptoms with hepatitis that can place a patient at increased risk for malnutrition. Fever and hypermetabolism require closer than usual attention to energy intake and hydration. Nutrition care of a patient with hepatitis should stress the need for calories and protein to enhance hepatocyte regeneration and prevent weight loss. Patients can require an additional 10% to 40% more calories above normal and up to 1.5 g of protein per kilogram ideal weight (Dietitians of Canada, 2003). Lack of appetite and nausea make meal consumption difficult. Small, more frequent nutrient-dense meals can promote overall increased intake and help with nausea, which is often worsened by an empty stomach. A multivitamin supplement should be considered in patients with poor intake. Importantly, high doses of some vitamins, such as vitamin A and niacin, are hepatotoxic and should be avoided (Riley & Bhatti, 2001).

The nurse should assess the patient for self-prescribed use of supplements and provide education about consuming excesses. Additionally, the patient should be assessed for use of alternative medicine supplements. Many herbal supplements are hepatotoxic. Chaparral, comfrey, and mistletoe are examples of hepatotoxic herbs. Others, like milk thistle, are touted by some for their ability to improve liver function (Riley & Bhatti, 2001). The nurse should consult with a pharmacist knowledgeable about herb safety and review the latest medical research when questions arise. Few recommendations exist on herbal remedies for liver disease and this should not be misinterpreted to mean untested herbs are efficacious or safe.

Cirrhosis

Malnutrition can be a common complication in patients with cirrhosis. Poor nutrition is more likely to occur in cirrhosis from alcoholic liver disease than nonalcoholic liver disease. Nutrition status is related to the etiology of the liver disease as well as its severity. An accurate nutrition assessment is often complicated by the presence of edema and ascites, as well as decreased production of plasma proteins—all secondary to liver disease. Digestion, absorption, metabolism, and storage of nutrients are all negatively affected by cirrhosis. Poor glycogen storage with enhanced breakdown of fat and protein occurs and resembles metabolic alterations seen in short-term starvation. Decreased production of bile salts by the liver can cause energy loss from fat because of steatorrhea. Pancreatic exocrine insufficiency is found in alcoholic liver disease and can impact fat absorption as well (Stickel et al., 2003). Ascites can cause the sensation of early satiety because of abdominal pressure and lead to diminished intake at meals.

Nutrition therapy in cirrhosis should include adequate protein to foster potential hepatic regeneration (Blei, Cordoba, & Practice Parameters Committee, 2001). Frequent meals and snacks should be offered to compensate for hypermetabolism and poor glycogen storage. Hypermetabolism has been reported in some, but not all, patients with cirrhosis. The reason for this increase is not fully understood but can contribute to malnutrition if energy needs go unmet. Energy needs vary individually and are estimated to be between 35 and 40 calories per kilogram dry weight (Kondrup, 2006). Smaller, more frequent meals help if early satiety is an issue. A low-sodium diet (2 g) is indicated in decompensated cirrhosis when ascites or edema is present (Riley & Bhatti, 2001). The nurse should monitor and encourage intake, stressing the importance of the dietary intake to avoid further nutrition risk and compromised health. Malnutrition has been shown to be an independent predictor of survival in patients with cirrhosis (Alberino et al., 2001). Patients with cirrhosis and malnutrition who require liver transplantation or other surgery are considered to be a higher surgical risk than those who are better nourished (Kondrup, 2006).

Hepatic Encephalopathy

Many theories exist as to the pathogenesis of hepatic encephalopathy, but it is agreed that unmetabolized ammonia in the intestinal tract is the major precipitating factor (Blei et al., 2001). Ammonia is normally metabolized by the liver and skeletal muscle, but this can be compromised with liver damage. Elevated ammonia blood levels then lead to sequelae that include altered neurotransmission and encephalopathy. Medical nutrition therapy targeting a reduction in blood ammonia plays a central role in treatment. Ammonia is produced in response to excessive protein from the diet and from metabolism of protein compounds found in the intestine. Intestinal bacteria contribute to this metabolic effect. Constipation, gastrointestinal bleeding, and infection can also increase ammonia production by providing a favorable environment or substrate for intestinal bacteria to produce ammonia. Traditionally, a low-protein diet has been used to treat hepatic encephalopathy, but this approach is now considered to contribute to encephalopathic symptoms when maintained over time (Blei et al., 2001). Protracted restriction of protein can lead to skeletal muscle catabolism and availability of substrate for ammonia production. Additionally, ammonia is normally taken up by skeletal muscle. Catabolism of skeletal muscle can diminish the amount of ammonia that can be taken up by muscle.

Current recommendations for medical nutrition therapy of hepatic encephalopathy call for an initial, short-term protein restriction of 0.5 g/kg ideal weight per day (Blei et al., 2001). This restriction should be prescribed for 1 to 2 days while monitoring the patient for signs of improvement. Depending on the patient's level of consciousness, nutrition can be administered as an oral diet or tube feeding. Enteral feeding is contraindicated in patients with active gastrointestinal bleeding. The diet should then be advanced in small increments to include increasing amounts of protein while monitoring patient tolerance. Ultimate protein intake should reach 1.0 to 1.5 g/kg ideal weight per day (Blei et al., 2001). A 70-kg (about 150-lb) ideal weight patient would need 70 to 105 g of protein. Examples of foods containing protein to meet incremental protein increases are listed in Chart 14–33. Some patients have improved protein tolerance when a portion of their intake is derived from plant protein sources. From 30 to 40 g of plant protein is tolerated without the intestinal side effect of bloating. It is believed that the fiber content of these foods quickens gut transit time and alters the intestinal pH environment by providing substrate for beneficial bacteria action (Blei et al., 2001).

As a last resort in the patient who seems chronically intolerant of protein, enteral formula with enhanced branch chain amino acid (BCAA) content may be tried. BCAA may be better tolerated than other protein sources in some patients. These formulas are expensive and do not contain complete nutrition, but

may be of some benefit in this limited population (Blei et al., 2001). These nutrition-based treatments are used to augment pharmacologic management aimed at lowering ammonia production in the lower GI tract, such as with lactulose or neomycin.

Adequate calorie intake is an essential component of the diet to ensure that energy needs are met. Inadequate energy intake can lead to catabolism of skeletal tissue to provide protein substrate for gluconeogenesis. Altered metabolism of glucose and lipids or overall hypermetabolism compound the difficulty of providing adequate nutrition. Ensuring the delivery of proper nutrition to patients with hepatic encephalopathy can be a challenge for the nurse. Patients have varying levels of somnolence, restlessness, disorientation, agitation, and tremor that can affect their ability to take an oral diet safely. Aggressive or inappropriate behavior in advanced stages of encephalopathy can lead to removal of any feeding tube in place. Family and other visitors who bring gifts of food need to be educated about the incremental protein prescription in order to avoid inadvertent dietary noncompliance that can affect the assessment of protein tolerance. Chapter 46 provides a complete description of hepatic encephalopathy.

Pancreatitis

Most patients who present with acute pancreatitis experience resolution of their symptoms within 5 to 7 days, and do not require aggressive nutritional intervention. However, 20% to 30% of patients exhibit severe disease (≥3 Ranson criteria as described in Chapter 46) and will need multidisciplinary intervention, including nutritional support (Abou-Assi & O'Keefe, 2002). Symptoms of acute pancreatitis such as pain, nausea, and vomiting can preclude oral intake by patients before they seek medical attention. Hypermetabolism and an 80% increase in catabolic rate occur with severe disease because of the local and systemic inflammatory responses by the body (Abou-Assi & O'Keefe, 2002; Alsolaiman, Green, & Barkin, 2003). The combination of inability to consume adequate oral nutrition in the face of a hypermetabolic and hypercatabolic state places these patients at high risk for malnutrition and related complications. The patient who goes on to develop further infection, sepsis, abscess, or pancreatic fistula—all complications of acute pancreatitis—will be at even greater risk.

Medical nutrition therapy for acute pancreatitis centers on the widely held belief that stimulation of the exocrine pancreas needs to be avoided in order to minimize pain and enzyme secretion. Pancreatic rest through bowel rest and provision of nutrition via the parenteral route were treatments of choice for decades. More recently, debate has arisen about the use of enteral versus parenteral nutrition in achieving pancreatic rest, and providing adequate nutrition while minimizing complications. This debate holds only for patients with a functioning gut and not for those in whom an ileus precludes enteral support. It has been demonstrated that most patients with acute pancreatitis tolerate an enteral nutrition formula infused into the jejunum distal to the ligament of Treitz (Abou-Assi & O'Keefe, 2002; McClave, 2004; Olah et al., 2002). Elemental or semielemental small peptide formulas are used that have negligible fat and free amino acids or di- and tripeptides versus intact whole proteins. Such formulas require no pancreatic enzyme secretion for absorption

---

CHART 14–33	**Incremental Protein in Treatment of Hepatic Encephalopathy**

The following foods contain approximately 7 to 10 g of protein per serving listed:

1 egg, whole

1 oz meat, fish, poultry, cheese

1 cup milk or yogurt

1 oz firm tofu

1/2 cup cooked beans, peas, lentils

2 TBSP peanut butter

2 oz nuts, average.

Source: USDA Nutrient Data Laboratory http://www.nal.usda.gov/fnic/foodcomp/search

and do little to stimulate the exocrine pancreas (Abou-Assi & O'Keefe, 2002; Alsolaiman et al., 2003; McClave, 2004; Olah et al., 2002).

Parenteral nutrition also is effective in achieving nutrition goals and pancreatic rest, but it has coincidental risks not associated with enteral nutrition. Studies comparing distal jejunal feeding with parenteral nutrition have illustrated equivocal provision of nutrition, achievement of pancreatic rest, and overall mortality. However, in some studies, but not all, parenteral nutrition was associated with more frequent hyperglycemia, a longer hospital stay, and infection (Abou-Assi, Craig, & O'Keefe, 2002; Jeejeebhoy, 2001). Acute pancreatitis can already cause glucose intolerance because of endocrine pancreas involvement. High glucose parenteral formula can cause greater blood glucose elevations. Catheter-related problems include both local and systemic infections. Those ascribing to the preferential use of the gut for feeding believe that prevention of gut atrophy, maintenance of beneficial gut microflora, and prevention of bacterial translocation are crucial. The theory exists that all of these factors play an important part in preventing changes in gut permeability associated with more advanced complications of pancreatitis (Abou-Assi & O'Keefe, 2002; Olah et al., 2002). Other researchers report that there are insufficient clinical trials supporting either route of nutrition as being superior or preferable, but they are in agreement that nutrition support is a cornerstone of treatment (Jeejeebhoy, 2001).

A reasonable approach to providing nutrition care to the patient with acute pancreatitis is to begin with a jejunal feeding early in the course of severe disease. Patients with evidence of severe disease are most likely to require nutrition support. A small-bore jejunal tube should be placed distal to the ligament of Trietz. After confirmation of tube placement, an elemental or small peptide enteral formula can begin. A registered dietitian should be consulted to recommend the needed volume of feeding and a protocol for advancing the rate and concentration of the formula. Such formulas are hyperosmolar and should not be started at a full-strength concentration or full volume. The nurse should monitor the patient closely for tolerance to the formula and rate changes. An increase in pain, nausea, vomiting, or diarrhea can indicate intolerance and deserves evaluation. Further elevation of the serum pancreatic enzymes, amylase or lipase, indicates intolerance to enteral nutrition. The patient should also be monitored at the bedside with a stethoscope for signs of tube migration. Movement of the tube into the proximal jejunum or duodenum may precipitate pancreatic stimulation and feeding intolerance. A pharmacist should be consulted relative to the administration of medications via a jejunal tube because the site may bypass the point of absorption of many drugs. Additionally, small-bore tubes are prone to clogging and a precipitate from medications could form. Therefore, when administering medication the nurse needs to ensure adequate flushing of the system to maintain patency.

Parenteral nutrition support is indicated when the patient is unable to tolerate enteral support or has an ileus. The nutrition support team will recommend an appropriate parenteral formula to meet the patient's nutritional and fluid and electrolyte needs. The patient should be monitored for hyperglycemia and hypertriglyceridemia because both can occur with pancreatitis and be exacerbated by total parenteral nutrition.

Patients with mild pancreatitis may only require a short period of time NPO and no aggressive nutritional support before resumption of a low-fat oral diet. Fat is minimized to reduce stimulation of the pancreas. Patients transitioning from nutrition support should also receive a low-fat diet.

Chronic pancreatitis can lead to longer term weight loss and malabsorption when the disease affects the majority of the pancreas. Permanent glucose intolerance can also occur. In addition to oral enzyme replacement therapy, many patients will require a modified fat diet and supplementation with a water-miscible, fat-soluble vitamin. Bone disease and clotting abnormalities have been noted from malabsorption of fat-soluble vitamins D and K, respectively. Vitamin B_{12} may also need to be supplemented if insufficient protease production prohibits the cleaving of vitamin B_{12} from its protein. Medium-chain triglycerides do not require pancreatic lipase for absorption and can be prescribed to provide needed calories for patients who have poor intake. Patients with endocrine pancreas dysfunction will also require modification of the carbohydrate content as outlined in the medical nutrition therapy of diabetes. Chapter 45 provides a complete description of pancreatitis.

Renal Disease

The kidney plays an important role in maintaining homeostasis in the body. Regulating nutrition processes and excreting nutrient by-products of metabolism, such as nitrogen, are among the crucial functions performed by the kidney. Kidneys also regulate fluid and electrolyte balance. Additionally, the kidneys are responsible for orchestrating the delicate balance between calcium, phosphorus, and vitamin D in the body. Vitamin D reaches its metabolically active form after being hydroxylated in the kidney.

A complete description of renal disease is provided in Chapter 47 .

Nephrotic Syndrome

Damage to the capillary walls of the glomeruli can cause significant losses of protein in the urine. Following significant proteinuria, decreases in plasma albumin can result with subsequent edema formation. Medical nutrition therapy for nephrotic syndrome focuses on replacement of protein losses to prevent malnutrition, slow the disease progression, and minimize edema. Dietary sodium is limited to control edema (Appel, 2006).

The nurse can educate the patient and reinforce the importance of a low-sodium diet in reducing edema. (A list of high-sodium foods can be found in Chart 14–17 (p. 293) earlier in this chapter). Adequate, but not high, protein is recommended to provide needed protein without contributing to disease progression. A patient should have a 24-hour urine protein assessment to determine the amount of protein replacement needed in addition to the RDA for protein baseline requirement. A registered dietitian would calculate this recommendation for the patient and outline suitable food choices. Adequate nonprotein sources of calories are needed to provide energy and prevent malnutrition because of catabolism of skeletal muscle for gluconeogenesis. If inadequate energy intake occurs, the protein intake will be sacrificed by the body for use as energy instead of as a substrate for anabolic functions.

Renal Failure

Medical nutrition therapy for both acute and chronic renal failure is determined by whether or not dialysis is part of the treatment strategy for the patient. Additionally, current laboratory values, amount of urine production, and any underlying disease will dictate an individualized diet prescription. Uremia results from the buildup of metabolic by-products in the body that is normally excreted via the kidneys. Nitrogenous waste products and inorganic ions are responsible for the clinical manifestations of uremia (National Kidney Foundation [NKF], 2000).Uremia can predispose the patient with renal failure to malnutrition. Anorexia, nausea, and altered taste perception can lead to decreased intake. Medication side effects and a restricted diet can further the potential for nutrition risk.

The short-term goals of medical nutrition therapy are to minimize uremia, manage fluid status, and provide adequate nutrition. Long-term nutrition care is focused on prevention of disease progression and malnutrition. Patients who also have comorbid conditions, such as diabetes or hypertension, must also receive appropriate nutrition intervention for those diseases. Overall, the resultant diet prescription can be quite stringent and patients require close monitoring. The National Kidney Foundation (2000) recommends reassessment and updating of the patient's care plan every 3 to 4 months.

Nutrition assessment is essential before an individualized diet prescription can be tailored to fit established guidelines. Parameters normally used to assess nutrition status can require adjustment in this population. Fluid shifts and resultant weight gain call for use of either a calculated ideal weight or postdialysis edema free body weight in calculating nutritional needs (Wells, 2003).The dietitian will rely on nursing expertise to make a determination of dry weight. Blood pressure monitoring, heart rate, postdialysis symptoms, presence of any hemoconcentration, edema, or increased gastrointestinal losses will all factor into dry weight estimations (Reams & Elder, 2003). Plasma samples obtained to assess albumin or other proteins should be taken before dialysis to avoid the effect of interdialytic protein losses (NKF, 2000). Creatinine index and serum creatinine can be employed to assess for loss of muscle mass or poor protein intake (NKF, 2000; Wells, 2003).

Dietary protein is responsible for the development of nitrogenous by-products during metabolism that contribute to uremia.

Thus, a controlled protein diet is recommended to control uremia. The contribution of a high-protein diet to renal disease progression or, conversely, whether a low-protein diet slows progression is the subject of debate. Following a protein-modified diet is associated with a decreased risk of death associated with renal disease in patients with existing kidney failure (Foque, Laville, & Boissel, 2006). Patients *not* receiving dialysis treatment and with a GFR of <25 mL/min are advised to follow a daily protein restriction of 0.6 g/kg ideal weight (Beto & Bansal, 2004). Some patients are unable to consume this low level of protein without becoming at risk for malnutrition. In such patients, the diet may be liberalized to 0.75 g protein/kg ideal weight (NKF, 2000). Because of protein losses during dialysis, patients receiving hemodialysis or peritoneal dialysis as part of treatment can consume more protein than those not dialyzed. Chart 14–34 outlines recommended protein levels for renal failure.

To achieve the most efficient metabolism, the majority of protein consumed should be of high biological value, having all essential amino acids, such as animal proteins (meats, poultry, fish, dairy) and soy. Use of high biological value proteins is most important for patients consuming low amounts of protein (Beto & Bansal, 2004). Adequate nonprotein calorie intake is essential to support energy needs and not have protein wasted as an energy source. The majority of patients will require 35 calories/kg per day (Beto & Bansal, 2004). The dietitian can recommend appropriate individual adjustments to this recommendation for patients who are sedentary, obese, or hypermetabolic. Additionally, patients receiving peritoneal dialysis can require modification of calorie intake because of the dextrose calories absorbed from the dialysate (Beto & Bansal, 2004).

Nutrition management of altered fluid status and plasma electrolyte and mineral abnormalities also is recommended with renal failure. General guidelines are presented in Chart 14–34, but it should be understood that each patient should have a customized diet prescription that fits his or her individual needs and laboratory parameters (NKF, 2000). A registered dietitian provides this individualized assessment and diet recommendation. Potassium restrictions vary according to treatment mode and laboratory values. Intake of minerals should be matched with excretion (Wells, 2003). The nurse can be instrumental in reinforcing the immediate importance of low-potassium food choices in this

---

CHART 14–34 Medical Nutrition Therapy for Chronic Renal Disease

	Hemodialysis	Peritoneal Dialysis	No Dialysis	Nephrotic Syndrome
Protein (g/kg dry weight)	1.2 g	1.2–1.3 g	0.6–0.75	0.8
Sodium (g)	2–4*	2–4*	2–4*	2–3*
Potassium (g)	2–3*	3–4*	2*	No restriction
Fluid (mL)	500–1,000 + UOP volume	Assess individually	500–1,000 + UOP volume	No restriction
Calories* (kcal/kg)	35 in those < age 65 30–35 in those > age 65	35 in those < age 65 30–35 in those > age 65	35 in those < age 65 30–35 in those > age 65	Assess individually

Note: Emphasis should be placed on individual diet recommendations based on overall renal function, nutrition status, and general health. All parameters outlined in this chart are general and should be adapted to meet patient requirements.

Sources: Beto, J. A., & Bansal, V. K. (2004). Medical nutrition therapy in chronic kidney failure: Integrating clinical practice guidelines. *Journal of the American Dietetic Association, 104*, 404–409; National Kidney Foundation. (2000). *Kidney disease outcomes quality initiative (K/DOQI). Clinical practice guidelines for nutrition in chronic kidney disease.* Retrieved November 16, 2006, from http://www.kidney.org/professionals.doqi/index/cfm; Wells, C. (2003). Optimizing nutrition in patients with chronic kidney disease. *Nephrology Nursing Journal, 30*, 637–646.

population. Noncompliance with a potassium restriction can result in quick deleterious consequences with elevated blood potassium leading to lethal cardiac dysrhythmias and cardiac arrest. Chart 14–35 outlines high potassium foods. Sodium and fluid restrictions correspond to amount of urine production and accumulation of fluid between dialysis treatments. Generally, fluid intake is 500 to 1,000 mL plus volume of 24-hour urine output (Wells, 2003). Patients with acute renal failure who are in the diuretic phase need to have fluid intake reevaluated to match changes in output (see Chapter 47 ⊚). For patients receiving dialysis, large interdialytic fluid gains present medical risk and dialysis difficulties and should be avoided. Interdialytic weight gain should be limited to 2% to 5% of dry weight (Wells, 2003). Compliance with the fluid restriction can be difficult for many patients. The nurse can offer suggestions for helping with thirst, such as mouth care or rinses and sucking on hard candy, and suggest low-potassium fluid choices within restriction parameters.

Chronic renal failure and ongoing dialysis treatment can result in additional nutritional concerns. Water-soluble vitamins are lost in the dialysate and require replacement. Dietary restrictions and poor intake also contribute to poor vitamin status. Formulations are available specifically for renal failure use. Kidney endocrine function becomes compromised and final synthesis of active vitamin D is diminished. Calcitriol, an oral supplement of active vitamin D, is given. Without adequate vitamin D, calcium absorption is lowered, predisposing the patient to bone disease. Plasma phosphorous levels are often elevated and complicate the intricate feedback mechanisms among vitamin D, calcium, and parathyroid hormone. Dietary restriction of phosphorus is indicated but only to the level achieved by the simultaneous protein restriction. Phosphorus is found primarily in milk products, nuts, and legumes. Overreliance on dietary restriction of phosphorus could result in insufficient intake of high-quality protein. Further reduction in plasma phosphorus is achieved with binding medications such as calcium carbonate. These are consumed along with a meal. Erythropoietin production is diminished with resultant anemia because of lowered red blood cell production by the bone marrow (see Chapter 47 ⊚). An erythropoiesis-stimulating agent is given. Additional contributors to anemia should be investigated. Transferrin saturation and ferritin are assessed to determine appropriate intervention for iron deficiency. Intravenous iron replacement is the preferred route of administration in this anemic population (NKF, 2006).

The patient with end-stage renal disease has unique dietary restrictions that make consumption of adequate nutrition a challenge. Patients on low-protein diets without dialysis treatment are at higher risk of malnutrition than those who receive dialysis because of the nature of the diet and disease symptoms (Beto & Bansal, 2004). Restrictions accompanying comorbid conditions such as diabetes present additional considerations. The nurse can provide much needed reinforcement of the importance of dietary compliance in both short-term well-being and long-term disease management.

Renal Stones

Supersaturation of urine favors nucleation and growth of crystals that can cause nephrolithiasis (Bushinski, 2002). Medical nutrition therapy of kidney stones focuses first on adequate fluid intake to promote ample urine volume and flow. Consumption of enough fluid to produce between 2 and 3 L of urine daily is recommended (Morton et al., 2002). Tailoring intake is required with changes in climate when insensible fluid losses increase and urine output is lessened if fluid intake is not adjusted.

Calcium oxalate stones are the predominant type of kidney stone, comprising up to 70% of all stones (Bushinski, 2002; Morton et al., 2002). In the past, a low-calcium diet was recommended in an attempt to decrease hypercalciuria and the likelihood of stone precipitation. However, although this advice resulted in decreased urinary excretion of calcium, it also fostered increased absorption of oxalate from the intestine and increased oxalate in urine. The result was no improvement in relative risk of stone formation and an increased risk of bone disease with insufficient calcium intake (Bushinski, 2002). Current recommendations advise adequate calcium intake, avoidance of excess oxalate intake (spinach, rhubarb, nuts, beets, chocolate, tea, and wheat bran are significant absorbable sources) (Morton et al., 2002). Additionally, excess intake of nondairy animal proteins and sodium has been shown to contribute to stone formation. Excessive animal protein promotes an acid environment in the body to which the body responds by buffering with calcium release from bone. Sodium excretion is associated with calcium excretion in the urine and thus is a target for control of calciuria. A long-term trial of a normal calcium diet that avoided excess sodium and animal protein resulted in a decreased relative risk of stone recurrence when compared with the old calcium-restricted approach (Borghi et al., 2002). Patients at risk for calcium stones should be educated to avoid excess vitamin D and C supplements. Vitamin D causes calcium absorption. Vitamin C promotes increased oxalate, an end product of the metabolism of ascorbate (Massey, Liebman, & Kynast-Gales, 2005; Morton et al., 2002).

Less common uric acid, cystine, and struvite kidney stones require medical management and ample fluid intake to avoid urine supersaturation. Additional dietary manipulations are not common modes of treatment in the prevention of these stones. Purines in meats and organ meats contribute to uric acid formation if consumed in significant quantities on a regular basis. However, management generally involves manipulation of urine pH rather than changes in diet for uric acid nephrolithiasis (Morton et al., 2002).

CHART 14–35 **High Potassium Food Sources**

- Banana
- Dried fruit: apricots, raisins, prunes, dates, figs
- Green leafy vegetables: Swiss chard, spinach, mustard greens
- Legumes: dried beans, peas, lentils
- Melon: cantaloupe, honeydew
- Oranges, orange juice
- Potato
- Tomato
- Whole grains, bran.

Note: Check labels on salt substitutes. Many contain potassium.

Patients at risk for kidney stones should have a nutrition history done to assess for fluid intake and urine output, use of vitamin supplements (vitamins C and D, calcium), and excessive intake of protein and sodium. The nurse should educate the patient to consume adequate fluid to produce between 2 and 3 L of urine daily. Patients who exercise or live in climates where insensible losses are increased should be educated to tailor fluid intake accordingly. Nonnutritional risk factors for kidney stone formation are discussed in Chapter 47 .

Anemias

Nutrition therapy for anemia first requires an established etiology for the hematologic changes. Indiscriminate treatment with vitamin or mineral supplements can mask underlying causes and result in additional negative consequences. This is especially illustrated with macrocytic anemia treatment using folic acid alone, without screening for potential vitamin B_{12} deficiency (Little, 1999). Folic acid therapy can result in improved hematologic indices while masking neurological damage from ongoing deficiency of vitamin B_{12}. Full discussion of anemia testing and treatment is presented in Chapter 63 .

Iron Deficiency

Iron deficiency anemia is the most common nutritional anemia worldwide (CDC, 2002). In addition to the medical etiology of iron deficiency, inadequate diet or poor iron absorption can contribute to the prevalence of this condition. Correction of iron deficiency anemia requires use of iron salt supplementation, but improved iron intake and absorption can facilitate repletion and prevent recurrence once the etiology has been treated. Repletion can take 4 to 6 months unless the patient is experiencing continued abnormal blood loss (Little, 1999).

The nurse can assess the patient for adequacy of iron intake and presence of inhibitors of absorption to facilitate improved iron repletion. Iron is present in animal protein foods such as meats and poultry as well as plant sources. Iron obtained from a "blood source" of iron is called heme iron, and is better absorbed than nonheme sources. Nonheme iron is present in plant sources of iron such as legumes (beans, soy), dried fruit, and iron-fortified products (cereals and pasta, for example). Absorption of iron, especially nonheme iron, can be affected by other dietary substances. Vitamin C sources with a meal enhance iron absorption, whereas consumption of tea, coffee, and calcium during a meal inhibit absorption (Nelson & Poulter, 2004). In patients at risk for iron deficiency, it is recommended that tea consumption in particular be limited to 1 hour outside the mealtime because tea can decrease iron absorption by up to 85%, depending on meal content (Nelson & Poulter, 2004). Chart 14–36 outlines iron content of foods and potential inhibitors and enhancers of iron absorption.

Vitamin B_{12} Deficiency

Adequate stores of vitamin B_{12} can meet nutritional requirements for up to 5 years. Thus, a deficiency of vitamin B_{12} generally occurs following prolonged inadequate intake or absorption (Oh & Brown, 2003). Vitamin B_{12} is present in only foods of animal origin. Any patient following a vegan diet (which contains no animal products) who does not take synthetic vitamin B_{12} to supplement his diet is at risk for deficiency. Plant-based supple-

---

CHART 14–36 **Iron Sources and Absorption**

FOOD SOURCES OF IRON

- Meat, shellfish, dark poultry, dried beans, peas, and lentils
- Green leafy vegetables
- Dried fruit
- Whole grains, fortified cereals, and grain products.

IRON ABSORPTION ENHANCERS

- Vitamin C
- Meat, seafood, poultry.

IRON ABSORPTION INHIBITORS

- Tea
- Coffee
- Binders: oxalates and phytates (e.g., in green leafy vegetables)
- Calcium
- Antacids and other acid reduction medications.

Sources: Hallberg L. & Hulthen, L., (2000). Prediction of dietary iron absorption: An algorithm for calculating absorption and bioavailability of dietary iron. *American Journal of Clinical Nutrition, 71,* 1147–1160.; Little, D. R. (1999). Ambulatory management of common forms of anemia. *American Family Physician, 59,* 1598–1604; Nelson, M., & Poulter, J. (2004). Impact of tea drinking on iron status in the UK: A review. *Journal Human Nutrition Dietetics, 17,* 43–54.

---

ments available on the market are not bioavailable and therefore not recommended (American Dietetic Association & Dietitians of Canada, 2004). Alcoholics or elderly also are at potential risk because of poor intake (Oh & Brown, 2003).

Decreased absorption of vitamin B_{12} can occur for two main reasons. First, an acid environment is required in the stomach to cleave vitamin B_{12} from its protein. Patients with gastric resection, long-term acid suppression treatment, or achlorhydria are at risk of vitamin B_{12} malabsorption because of diminished acid production (Oh & Brown, 2003). Second, intrinsic factor (IF) is required to bind with B_{12} and then be absorbed in the terminal ileum. Lack of IF production by parietal cells, poor binding of IF in the duodenum, and ileal disease or resection all place the patient at risk for malabsorption (Oh & Brown, 2003). Traditionally, an oral supplement of vitamin B_{12} was given to patients with poor acid environment while vitamin B_{12} injections were administered for IF and small bowel related problems (Oh & Brown, 2003). Now, a second passive route of absorption has been recognized and high-dose oral supplementation can be used for many patients to good effect (Nyholm et al., 2003). The nurse can assess patients for risk of vitamin B_{12} deficiency through a diet history and screening for potential factors associated with poor absorption. Patients consuming inadequate vitamin B_{12} need to be advised of important nutritional sources. Animal products, vitamin B_{12}–fortified cereals or milk alternatives, and synthetic supplements are emphasized. Deficiency should resolve within 3 to 4 weeks of treatment unless neurological manifestations have occurred; 6 months or more can pass before any possible neurological improvement is evident (Little, 1999). The risk of vitamin B_{12} deficiency faced by the elderly is discussed in the Gerontological Considerations box (p. 314).

GERONTOLOGICAL CONSIDERATIONS
Associated with Vitamin B$_{12}$ Deficiency

The elderly are at particular risk of vitamin B$_{12}$ deficiency because of age-related atrophic changes in the stomach with resultant achlorhydria. Production of intrinsic factor can also be affected. This alteration in gastric pH and diminished IF production result in decreased absorption of vitamin B$_{12}$. Consideration of routine vitamin B$_{12}$ supplementation is uniquely recommended for adults older than 70 years of age for this reason (IOM, 1998; Russell, Rasmussen, & Lichtenstein, 1999). Adults older than 65 years of age already at risk for poor vitamin absorption who are receiving prolonged acid suppression medication should be assessed for vitamin B$_{12}$ deficiency (Oh & Brown, 2003).

Folate Deficiency

Folate deficiency can occur from decreased intake or absorption, unmet increased needs, or a combination. People with alcoholic liver disease and others with poor-quality diets are at risk for poor folate status. Several medications are folate antagonists or alter absorption; examples include methotrexate, triamterene, phenytoin, sulfasalazine, and corticosteroids (Little, 1999; White & Ashworth, 2000). Folate, which is the name of this B vitamin when found in foods, is present in orange juice, green leafy vegetables, and legumes. It is also present in white flour products as a result of government-mandated folic acid fortification begun in 1996 in the United States. Folic acid is the name used by some to denote supplemental forms of the vitamin.

Generally, a 1-mg dose per day of folic acid is prescribed for deficiency. This is the tolerable upper limit of the vitamin (IOM, 1998). Careful screening to rule out deficiency of vitamin B$_{12}$ is first essential because this level of folic acid repletion can mask a vitamin B$_{12}$ deficiency. Many recommend that unopposed folic acid supplementation at or near the 1-mg dose not be given, but rather complementary vitamin B$_{12}$ also be administered (Fletcher & Fairfield, 2002). The nurse can screen patients for folate intake and the presence of any inhibitory medications. Consumption of good sources of folate should be encouraged. Women of childbearing age should be especially encouraged to consume adequate folate or take a multivitamin supplement with the RDA of 400 mcg folic acid. Adequate maternal folate status is associated with decreased risk of development of neural tube defects in a developing fetus (IOM, 1998).

Acquired Immunodeficiency Syndrome (AIDS)

Nutritional problems, from malnutrition to dyslipidemia, can occur in human immunodeficiency virus (HIV) infection. Malnutrition can occur for a variety of reasons such as opportunistic infection. For example, oral candidiasis can lead to inadequate intake because of pain and dysphagia accompanying inflammation. Other infections can lead to anorexia, fatigue, malabsorption, hypermetabolism from fever and inflammation, nausea and vomiting, or altered cognition and functional status (Nerad et al., 2003).

Pharmacologic treatment of infection can cause gastrointestinal side effects and food and drug interactions. Often, complicated medication schedules and food interactions can make adequate intake a challenge (Nerad et al., 2003). Chemical dependency and socioeconomic issues present additional challenges to nutrition status. These factors in combination or alone can predispose patients with HIV infection to malnutrition. Development of malnutrition can diminish immunocompetence and leave the patient at further risk of opportunistic infection (American Dietetic Association & Dietitians of Canada, 2004). The effectiveness of pharmacologic interventions can be reduced with malnutrition because many medications require critical levels of protein stores or body cell mass for metabolism (American Dietetic Association & Dietitians of Canada, 2004). Many medications require specific food recommendations without which serum drug levels are affected (Gagnon & Therrien, 2006; Nerad et al., 2003). Some patients are unable to tolerate adequate intake, resulting in impaired drug treatment along with poor nutrition status. Thus, a vicious cycle of malnutrition and infection can follow. Weight loss, loss of muscle, adipose, and nutrient deficiencies lead to further negative consequences. Malnutrition in HIV infection is associated with adverse outcomes, such as disease progression and mortality (Grinspoon & Mulligan, 2003; Knox et al., 2003).

Some wasting occurs despite a clear single etiology. In addition to suspected contributors to malnutrition such as inadequate intake and malabsorption, wasting occurs because of changes in metabolism, hypogonadism, and excessive cytokine production associated with HIV (Grinspoon & Mulligan, 2003). No matter what the etiology, the health impact resulting from loss of lean muscle and total body weight is significant.

Current medical treatment of patients with HIV infection using highly active antiretroviral treatment (HAART) has presented clinicians with additional sequelae of potential nutritional problems. Hyperlipidemia, insulin resistance, and body fat redistribution have been associated with the use of protease inhibitors (Dube et al., 2003; Graber, 2001; Nerad et al., 2003). Additionally, length of HIV infection, age, and gender may play a role (Chen, Misra, & Carg, 2002). Limited literature is available to assess the influence of diet on this complication. Patients may present with elevated plasma cholesterol, triglyceride, glucose intolerance, and unique **lipodystrophy**. Lipodystrophy is characterized by adipose loss in the face and extremities and excess fat deposition in the abdomen and over the dorsocervical spine (Chen et al., 2002; Graber, 2001). Such alterations in morphology may lead some patients to alter their diet or medication strategies in an attempt to deal with body image conflicts. This, in turn, may place these patients at risk for poor nutrition or ineffective medication concentration (Nerad et al., 2003). Some patients may experiment with alternative medicine in place of, or in addition to, HAART to counteract the metabolic effects. Not all nutritional and herbal supplements can be safely used by patients with HIV infection and some may compromise effective treatment.

Medical nutrition therapy for HIV infection is based on an up-to-date comprehensive nutrition assessment. It is recommended that a thorough assessment be completed at the time of diagnosis to establish a baseline for later comparison *and* that reevaluation take place up to twice a year in the asymptomatic patient and up to six times a year in patients experiencing HIV-related symptoms (Knox et al., 2003). No nutritional evaluation tool has been validated for exclusive use in assessment of patients with HIV infection. Standard nutrition assessment parameters should all be used, but tailored for specificity with this population. Anthropometric measurements are important to obtain at baseline for potential future estimations of any lipodystrophy. Serial weights should be monitored. Skinfold measurements and waist and hip circumferences are recommended to assess for changes in adipose deposition (Gerrior, Kantaros, Coakley, Labrecht, & Wanke, 2001; Knox et al., 2003).

Weight alone will not suffice for such comparisons because muscle loss and fat gains can mask weight change. Weight alone may also underestimate the presence of malnutrition (Mangili, Murman, Zampini, & Wanke, 2006). Laboratory parameters such as plasma proteins may be reflective of nutrition status or infection-related inflammation and cannot be solely relied on to assess nutrition (American Dietetic Association & Dietitians of Canada, 2004). Serum vitamin B_{12} and zinc levels, among other micronutrients, are often diminished and this has been associated with increased risk of disease progression (American Dietetic Association & Dietitians of Canada, 2004; Baum, Campa, Lai, Lai, & Page, 2003; Fawzi, 2003; Woods et al., 2003).

During the focused interview and the physical examination, the nurse should closely assess the patient for presence of any factor known to influence nutrition health. Knowledge regarding HIV-related nutrition risk factors is important for nurses because the nurse is often first in line to assess a patient. Existing opportunistic infections, oral and digestive symptoms, medication, use of alternative medicines and supplements, and functional status are among the many parameters that are essential to the assessment. Chart 14–37 outlines essential components of the nutritional assessment of patients with HIV infection.

The findings from the nutritional assessment will determine the extent of needed nutrition intervention. Nutrition care and education are central to management of HIV infection. Asymptomatic patients may benefit from general nutrition education about a healthy diet to maintain important muscle mass and body weight. It is important for the nurse to discuss the use of herbal and nutritional supplements that may impact medical management. For example, it has been shown that St. John's wort may decrease crucial therapeutic plasma levels of protease inhibitors (American Dietetic Association & Dietitians of Canada, 2004). Education about the importance of food and water safety is also important to prevent or lessen the risk of foodborne illness. Improperly handled foods and water from unsafe sources each pose a risk to patients who are immunocompromised. Many pathogens identified in patients with opportunistic infection are recognizable as having potentially originated in a food or water source. Salmonella, listeria, cryptosporidia, and *Vibrio vulnificus* are examples (Hayes, Elliot, Krales, & Downer, 2003). Chart 14–38 (p. 316) outlines important aspects of food and water sanitation.

Patients with malnutrition or at risk for malnutrition require quick intervention to prevent further deterioration of nutrition health. Underlying factors responsible for malnutrition must be identified and treated or controlled. Nutrition intervention should be tailored to maximize nutrient repletion while minimizing side effects and symptoms. Chart 14–39 (p. 316) outlines

---

CHART 14–37   **Nutrition Assessment in HIV Infection**

Physical exam/interview	Assess weight, serial weights. Assess baseline body composition and waist-to-hip ratio and monitor serially for muscle wasting or fat redistribution. Assess for risk of ↓ intake: • Oral pain, dysphagia, thrush, oral health • Nausea, vomiting, diarrhea • Food intolerances • Altered cognition • Medication side effects • Complicated food/medicine schedule • Depression, anxiety • Fatigue, shortness of breath • Chemical dependency • Lack of economic resources • Impaired functional status. Assess for risk of ↑ nutrient losses: • Malabsorption because of infection • Enteropathy • Medication interactions. Assess for risk of ↑ nutrient needs: • Active infection/viral load • Fever • Wounds • Other disease.
Laboratory tests	Plasma proteins Lipids Vitamin B_{12} Zinc
Nutrition history	Assess nutrition history data in Chart 14–3 (p. 276). Note use of alternative nutrition therapy, vitamins/minerals, and herbal or other supplements. Assess food and water safety practices.

Sources: American Dietetic Association & Dietitians of Canada. (2004). Position of the American Dietetic Association and Dietitians of Canada: Nutrition intervention in the care of persons with human immunodeficiency virus. *Journal of the American Dietetic Association, 104,* 1425–1441; Knox, T. A., Zafonte-Sanders, M., Fields-Gardner, C., Moen, K., Johansen, D., & Paton, N. (2003). Assessment of nutritional status, body composition, and human immunodeficiency virus-associated morphologic changes. *Clinical Infectious Diseases, 36,* S63–S68; Nerad, J., Romeyn, M., Silverman, E., Allen-Reid, J., Dietrich, D., Merchant, J., et al. (2003). General nutrition management in patients infected with HIV. *Clinical Infectious Diseases, 36,* S52–S62.

---

common causes of malnutrition in HIV infection and sample nutrition strategies the nurse can suggest.

Patients in whom lipodystrophy is evident may require nutrition intervention for any glucose intolerance or hyperlipidemia. Current recommendations advise the prescription of the same diet treatment as for any patient with hyperlipidemia or hyperglycemia (Dube et al., 2003). This area requires more research to determine the efficacy of nutrition therapy in treating these metabolic changes when they occur in this population. Current

CHART 14–38	**Guidelines for Safe Food and Water Handling**

Prepare foods safely:

- Clean surfaces and utensils.
- Wash hands before preparing food and after handling raw meats, poultry, or fish.
- Wash surfaces and utensils after preparing raw meat, poultry, and fish. Use separate cutting board if possible for raw products.
- Cook foods until done and proper temperature; meats, poultry > 165°F internally; fish should be opaque and flaky. Reheat leftovers to 165°F. Bring leftover soup, gravy, or sauce to a boil. Only keep leftovers for 3 to 4 days in refrigerator.

Do not consume raw or undercooked eggs, meat, fish, or poultry:

- Avoid sushi or raw bars, real eggnog, dressings made with raw egg, runny eggs.
- Do not taste test marinades used for tenderizing proteins.

Consume pasteurized juices, milk, and dairy foods.

Wash and peel fruits and vegetables.

Do not drink water from streams, lakes, springs, rivers.

Boil tap water if advised by local health department.

Store foods safely:

- Place raw meat, poultry, and fish in lower shelf of refrigerator to avoid drips onto other food.
- Separate raw products in grocery cart and when bagged in store.
- Keep stored perishable foods out of the 40°–140°F danger zone. Cool hot foods quickly in shallow dish. Keep foods properly refrigerated or frozen.

Sources: Centers for Disease Control. (2007). *Safe food and water.* Retrieved May 30, 2008 from http://www.cdc.gov/hiv/resources/brochures/food.htm; Food and Drug Administration. (2001). *Food safety for you!* Retrieved January 27, 2004, from http://www.cfsan.fda.gov/~dms/fttclean.html; Hayes, C., Elliot, E., Krales, E., & Downer, G. (2003). Food and water safety for persons infected with HIV. *Clinical Infectious Diseases, 36,* S106–S109.

nutrition recommendations are made largely in the absence of data on their use in patients with HIV. Nutrition intervention to alter the effects of fat redistribution or to specifically increase muscle mass in wasting has little reported effect. Strength training and use of pharmacologic interventions are current strategies being suggested (Grinspoon & Mulligan, 2003). A complete description of HIV/AIDS is in Chapter 60 ⬙.

Cancer

Patients diagnosed with cancer are at risk for poor nutrition status because of the effects of the disease as well as the treatment. Anorexia, nausea, and vomiting, changes in taste perception, dysphagia, mucositis, diarrhea, and fatigue can predispose a patient to malnutrition whether the symptoms are caused by tumor effects, radiation, or chemotherapy. Malnutrition that may begin from disease alone may be worsened with treatment side effects. A baseline nutrition assessment at diagnosis followed by reassessment periodically through treatment will allow for early intervention when nutrition risk is evident. The nurse who is part of the treatment team during chemotherapy, radiation, or surgery can be instrumental in identifying symptom changes that prevent adequate intake and planning appropriate intervention. Chart 14–40 lists nutrition interventions that the nurse can recommend to patients and caregivers.

CHART 14–39	**Nutrition Strategies for Common Problems with HIV Infection**

Problem	Nutrition Intervention
Anorexia	Eat small, frequent meals. Choose nutrient dense foods: peanut butter, cheese, meal replacement or breakfast-type drinks, smoothies. See Chart 14–21 (p. 298) for "more calories per bite" food recommendations.
Nausea and vomiting	Nibble on dry carbohydrates: toast, crackers, dry cereal. Eat small meals to avoid empty stomach or feeling too full. Avoid greasy foods, strong odors. Sip flat ginger ale, weak ginger, or mint tea.
Diarrhea	Limit fat, caffeine, and fiber. Assess for lactose intolerance. Replace fluids.
Oral pain or dysphagia	Eat smooth, cool foods: pudding, ice cream, cooled soup, liquid supplement drinks. Avoid citrus, tomato, and hot foods. Use a straw to bypass mouth.
Fatigue	Keep ready-to-eat and convenience foods in stock: microwave or toaster oven items, single-serve pudding, yogurt, hearty soups. Eat nutrient-dense foods early in day and meal when energy level is best.

Patients undergoing treatment with a hematopoietic stem cell transplant require highly specialized nutrition care. Parenteral nutrition is required post-transplant because of treatment-induced mucositis. Nutrition risk is heightened by multiple medications, side effects, and potential graft-versus-host disease (GVHD). GVHD may lead to malabsorptive and liver problems, which in turn alter nutrition requirements and medical nutrition therapy. Treatment of GVHD requires use of medications, such as glucocorticoids, that present additional challenges to maintenance of nutrition health (Roberts & Thompson, 2005). A multidisciplinary care team closely manages medical and nutrition treatment in this population. A complete description of hematopoietic stem cell transplant is included in Chapter 63 ⬙. A description of GVHD is presented in Chapter 59 ⬙.

The nurse should be knowledgeable of current recommendations regarding use of nutritional supplements during active treatment with chemotherapy or radiation. Limited research to date has provided little on which to build the foundation of evidence-based clinical advice. Few studies have investigated the variability in response to conventional treatment when accompanied by use of supplements (Bruemmer, Patterson, Cheney, Aker, & Witherspoon, 2003). A theoretical concern exists that the use of antioxidants during radiation or with certain types of chemotherapy may interfere with the intended cytotoxic effects of those therapies (Norman et al., 2003; Weiger et al., 2002). Antioxidants have been investigated for their potential in minimizing oxidative damage to cells and therefore preventing or slowing cancer. Examples of antioxidant nutrients include beta-carotene (vitamin A precursor), vitamins C and E, and selenium. Patients may take these supplements hoping to minimize disease and spare healthy cells the effects

CHART 14–40	Suggested Nutrition Interventions in Cancer Care

Symptom	Nutrition Intervention
Anorexia or early satiety	Eat small, frequent meals. Eat nutrient-dense foods first. See Chart 14–21 (p. 298) for "more calories per bite" food recommendations.
Nausea	Nibble on dry carbohydrates: toast, crackers, dry cereal. Eat small meals to avoid empty stomach or feeling too full. Avoid greasy foods, strong odors. Sip flat ginger ale. Minimize physical movement before mealtime.
Altered taste	Eat tart candy, juice, or seasonings. Practice good oral care. Eat room temperature or cool foods, especially proteins.
Painful mouth or swallowing	Eat smooth, cool foods: pudding, ice cream, cooled soup, liquid supplement drinks. Avoid citrus, tomato, and hot foods. Use a straw to bypass mouth.
Xerostomia (lack of saliva)	Eat moist foods. Add sauces, gravies, butter, and liquids to foods. Avoid hot foods, alcohol, and dry foods.
Food aversions	To minimize "learned" food aversions from association, avoid favorite foods following treatment when side effects are more likely.

of treatment. The controversy arises in that antioxidants may also theoretically spare diseased tissue from the cytotoxic effects of treatment, thereby diminishing treatment efficacy. Current recommendations are to take only moderate doses of antioxidants, such as in a multivitamin, during treatment until more definitive evidence is available (Norman et al., 2003; Weiger et al., 2002).

Soy supplements are also popular choices of adjuvant therapy in patients who have heard about their natural phytoestrogen content. Phytoestrogens are weak plant estrogens that may possibly have some effect on reproductive cancer risk (Weiger et al., 2002). Until more definitive evidence is available, it is recommended that patients with breast cancer or receiving tamoxifen avoid phytoestrogen supplements (Weiger et al., 2002). Soy isoflavonoids and red clover are examples of phytoestrogens. Essiac tea is often used by patients seeking alternative therapies and can contain red clover (Weiger et al., 2002). Research on soy-based supplementation in prostate cancer is ongoing. The current recommendation is to accept the use of soy supplements by patients with prostate cancer who have chosen to use them (Weiger et al., 2002).

Patients may also choose to use herbal remedies for treatment side effects such as ginger for nausea. The nurse should query the patient for use of all supplements and educate the patient about any known interactions with treatment or medications, possible anticoagulant effects, or other contraindications to use. The safety and efficacy of nutrition and herbal supplement use before, during, and after cancer treatment are areas deserving future research.

Chronic Obstructive Pulmonary Disease and Mechanical Ventilation

Chronic obstructive pulmonary disease (COPD) symptoms such as dyspnea and fatigue can predispose patients to malnutrition by altering diet consumption. Patients may experience shortness of breath that precludes sufficient intake if chewing and swallowing alter breathing patterns and potentially affect arterial oxygen saturation. Early satiety can occur if gastric filling affects perceived or real breathing capacity. **Aerophagia**, or swallowing of air, may occur while eating and lead to bloating and early satiety as well. Fatigue can impair adequate intake when meal preparation and even simple tasks like cutting meats or opening lids prove too exhausting. Medications such as glucocorticoids may cause appetite stimulation but also gastrointestinal upset and altered intake.

COPD may also lead to an increase in energy expenditure due in part to inefficient respiratory mechanics and the increased work of the respiratory muscles. This effect is noted at rest and increases further during activity or exacerbation of respiratory symptoms (Gronberg, Slinde, Engstrom, Hulthen, & Larsson, 2005). Acute treatment with beta-2 agonists and theophylline may elevate energy expenditure (Mallampali, 2004). If the increased need for calories goes unmet, weight loss will occur. Weight loss may occur slowly or be exacerbated during acute disease or infection when nutritional needs are further increased.

Patients with elevated resting energy needs have also been reported to have increased protein turnover in the body, resulting in disproportionate loss of muscle mass or "wasting." Loss of muscle does not spare respiratory muscle; diaphragmatic and auxiliary respiratory muscle can be lost. In some patients this loss of muscle occurs even with maintenance of body weight. The muscle wasting seen in this subpopulation is referred to as pulmonary cachexia (Schols, 2002). Patients with pulmonary cachexia may suffer from loss of respiratory strength and endurance as well as functional capacity. A vicious downward spiral can occur when this in turn leads to further decreased intake and malnutrition. Malnutrition can alter immunocompetence, leaving the patient more susceptible to infection (Cai et al., 2003). A reduced BMI in COPD is associated with reduced survival (Mallampali, 2004).

The goal of medical nutrition therapy for COPD is to prevent malnutrition and weight loss that may occur with advanced disease. In patients who have hypercapnia, nutrition therapy should also focus on minimizing CO_2 production from nutrient metabolism. Each macronutrient produces a given amount of CO_2 for each molecule of O_2 consumed. This is called its **respiratory quotient (RQ)**. Carbohydrates have a higher RQ than do protein and fat and thus have the potential to produce more CO_2 at a given intake. Overfeeding a patient in total calories will also produce more CO_2 than feeding adequate calories (Cai et al., 2003). Providing excess calories or a high carbohydrate load is not recommended for patients with hypercapnia (Cai et al., 2003; Mallampali, 2004).

Nutrition intervention should focus on providing optimal nutrition in a well-tolerated form. For patients with dyspnea, nutrient-dense foods with "more calorie per bite" should be encouraged. When fatigue is a problem, the nurse can encourage intake of higher calorie sources first in the meal (and also earlier in the day) to optimize intake before the patient becomes too tired to eat. The patient should be offered assistance with opening cartons or other tasks when in hospital to conserve energy for eating. Patients experiencing early satiety can be advised to consume many small meals and to minimize filling up on empty-calorie liquids. Supplementation with an oral liquid nutrition supplement may be helpful between meals, but has been found to just replace intake in many studies, resulting in no nutritional improvements (Mallampali, 2004). Chart 14–41 outlines nutrition interventions for the patient with COPD. The patient should be monitored for overall intake and routinely screened for weight loss and muscle wasting. When risk factors exist for malnutrition, the nurse can make suggestions as outlined in Chart 14–41.

Any patient requiring mechanical ventilation and with a functioning gut will require enteral nutrition support. Parenteral nutrition is indicated for patients in whom gut function contraindicates enteral support. Nutrition support of patients on mechanical ventilation should focus on preservation of body weight and muscle, including crucial respiratory muscles essential for weaning from the ventilator. A registered dietitian should assess the patient and determine required nutrition needs and appropriate formula. Generally, standard enteral or parenteral nutrition formulas are used with a focus on not contributing to excess CO_2 production. Overfeeding ventilator patients or prescribing excess carbohydrates is not recommended (Parrish & McCray, 2003). Enteral formulas exist that are higher in fat than standard versions and are marketed for pulmonary use. Current clinical trials do not find that these formulas possess any advantage in duration on ventilation or weaning over standard formulas when overfeeding is avoided (Cook et al., 2001; Parrish & McCray, 2003).

Nutrition and Wound Healing

The presence of a cutaneous wound places metabolic demands on the body that must be met in order for healing to progress. Each stage of wound healing requires adequate nutritional substrate and is contingent on successful outcome of the prior healing phase. Healing phases are described in Chapter 67 ⊕. As a result, delayed wound healing may occur in patients with malnutrition (Casey, 2003). Poor baseline nutrition status prior to wound development or subsequent inadequate intake may predispose a patient to weight loss and poor vitamin, mineral, and protein status that can impact healing and increase the risk for

---

CHART 14–41	**Suggested Nutrition Interventions for COPD**

Dyspnea, early satiety, bloating, and fatigue all contribute to poor intake. Suggested interventions include the following:

- Consume higher calorie, higher protein foods first.
- Get more "calories per bite," especially by adding fat to foods with butter, margarine, mayonnaise, sauces, cream, dressings, and gravy.
- Consume frequent small meals.
- Save liquids for between meals.
- Limit intake of carbonated beverages.
- Keep convenient and ready-to-eat nutrient dense foods available for when fatigued.

---

infection. Inadequate fluid intake offset further by wound exudative fluid losses, fever, diarrhea, or excessive insensible losses can lead to dehydration. Decreased blood volume will not only impair needed oxygen delivery to the wound but also essential nutrients required for tissue repair (Leninger, 2002).

Knowledge of the role of nutrition in wound healing is beneficial to the nurse when completing an assessment of patients with existing wounds or those at risk of pressure ulcers. The early stages of wound healing require adequate protein stores to provide substrate for the inflammatory process. Diminished plasma protein levels before injury may worsen during this acute reaction (Leninger, 2002). Edema can result with decreased plasma proteins and this can impact healing. Collagen synthesis and tissue repair require adequate protein, vitamins C and A, and zinc, among other nutrients (Casey, 2003; Leninger, 2002). Protein is also essential for maintenance of immune function and avoidance of infection risk. Sufficient calorie intake is needed to prevent the use of crucial protein as energy instead of as a building block for tissue repair. Inadequate calorie intake can delay healing and also lead to skeletal muscle catabolism. The dietitian should be consulted to assess calorie, protein, and general nutrition needs. The size of the wound, amount of exudate (which can contribute to protein losses), presence of fever, coexisting injuries or disease, and the patient's baseline nutrition status will all affect nutritional recommendations.

The nurse should assess the patient for baseline nutrition status, paying close attention to protein status, physical signs of malnutrition including overall skin integrity, and diet history. The patient should be monitored for adequate intake of calories, protein, and fluid. The routine use of vitamin supplementation in wound healing is a common practice, yet benefits to this practice have only been reported for those patients who have existing nutritional deficiencies (Casey, 2003; Leninger, 2002). Vitamin C is necessary for collagen formation and is found in many fruits and vegetables, especially citrus or tropical fruit and green leafy vegetables. Zinc supplements are also commonly prescribed based on research that patients who are deficient have delayed reepithelialization of the wound and decreased wound strength (Casey, 2003). Long-term or excessive zinc supplementation can precipitate an imbalance in copper status and gastrointestinal upset (IOM, 2001). Zinc is found in most foods that contain protein, such as meats, poultry, legumes, and nuts. Fluid status should be monitored to provide at least the recommended AI of 2.7 or 3.7 liters of water daily for women and men, respectively (IOM, 2004). Adjustments should be made for excessive fluid losses from the gastrointestinal tract or the wound. Patients managed with an air-fluidized bed should receive an extra 10 to 15mL/kg fluid because of the associated increased insensible fluid losses (Leninger, 2002).

Pressure Ulcers

Malnutrition is among the many potential risk factors for development of a pressure ulcer (Langemo et al., 2006). As with the presence of any wound, adequate nutrition can benefit the healing process by providing necessary nutrients for each phase of tissue repair. Elderly and malnourished patients with a decubitus ulcer require close monitoring to ensure that nutritional needs are met. Individual consideration should be given to the liberalization of any dietary restrictions in these populations to encourage intake. Supplementation with oral nutrition formula may be beneficial if it does not replace normal intake. Multi-vitamin use is reasonable with consideration given to extra vitamin C and zinc in those found to be deficient (Langemo et al., 2006). Pressure ulcers are discussed in detail in Chapter 67 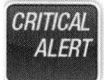.

Burns

Medical nutrition therapy for the patient with a thermal injury focuses on two important management aspects. Both the metabolic response to a burn as well as the healing process require special attention with aggressive nutrition support. Severe burns cause a catabolic response by the body whereby hormonal and inflammatory responses to the injury precipitate tissue losses that compound the burn itself (Andel, Kamolz, Horauf, & Zimpfer, 2003). Patients are also in a hypermetabolic state because of the injury (Demling, DeSanti, & Orgill, 2004). The nutritional requirements for tissue repair must be met in addition to those that result from catabolism and hypermetabolism. With a severe burn, the result is a daily requirement for high levels of calorie and protein intake.

Early enteral feeding is most often recommended for the burn patient (Andel et al., 2003; Demling et al., 2004). Oral nutrition, continuous tube feedings, or supplemental nocturnal tube feedings can be utilized to deliver adequate nutrition in the patient who has a functioning gastrointestinal tract. Patients with gastric stasis may tolerate postpyloric enteral feeding in the duodenum or jejunum rather than via a basic nasogastric tube, because the latter could result in high residual gastric feeding volumes and increase aspiration risk (Andel et al., 2003; Sefton, Boulton-Jones, Anderton, Teahon, & Knights, 2002). Parenteral nutrition may be necessary in patients with ileus or intolerance to sufficient volume of enteral nutrition support. The large dextrose content of parenteral nutrition can supply fodder for bacterial growth; thus, strict aseptic technique is required for the parenteral nutrition intravenous site in order to avoid a disastrous infection.

Nutritional recommendations focus on modulating tissue catabolism and providing sufficient nutrition for tissue repair. Many different equations exist to estimate calorie and protein needs in a burn patient. None is universally accepted due to differences such as technique for factoring the effects of varying degree and percentage of body surface area burned. Typically 35 to 40 calories/kg per day are required for adults; this can be adjusted if **indirect calorimetry** technology is available to estimate energy needs based on oxygen consumption and carbon dioxide production. Up to 2 g protein/kg per day is suggested (Demling et al., 2004). Adjustments can be made based on wound healing progress. Supplemental amino acids in the form of glutamine and arginine may play a role in mediating catabolism post-burn. There have been hopeful research reports resulting in their use by some, but the supplements remain controversial as a standard of care in thermal injury (Andel et al., 2003; Buchman, 2001; Demling et al., 2004; Wilmore, 2001). Supplemental vitamins and minerals are prescribed to support tissue synthesis and the needs of a hypermetabolic state.

The nurse should monitor the patient's tolerance to enteral or parenteral nutrition. Close attention should be given to the amount and type of intake and fluid balance. Serial weights should be monitored to assess for weight loss. Loss of >10% body weight will impair healing. Larger losses of lean muscle mass are associated with increased mortality (Andel et al., 2003). Some patients

are able to tolerate adequate oral intake, whereas others require nocturnal supplementation with a tube feeding. The nurse can help optimize intake by facilitating a comfortable eating environment. Dressing and wound care, venipuncture, and any major repositioning are best avoided near mealtime to minimize discomfort. Optimal pain management during meals is also helpful. Depression, pain, and medication side effects, including sedation, can lead to diminished intake. The patient with a thermal injury requires close monitoring and reevaluation of nutrition status throughout the course of injury and recovery. Chapter 68 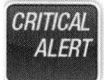 describes the complete care of the burn patient.

Nutrition and the Surgical Patient

Malnutrition is associated with poor surgical outcome and increased postoperative mortality (Howard & Ashley 2003). Impaired wound healing, infection, and reduced strength for postoperative rehabilitation can result because of poor baseline nutrition status. Every effort should be made to ensure that a patient is in good nutritional health preoperatively. Lengthy hospitalization with multiple diagnostic tests requiring withheld or clear liquid feeding can contribute to iatrogenic deterioration of nutrition status. Trauma as a precursor to surgery leads to preoperative metabolic stress with characteristic hypercatabolism and hypermetabolism compromising nutrition status (McKibbin, Cresci, & Hawkins, 2003). Chronic disease existing before surgery, such as organ failure requiring transplantation, can place a patient at risk for malnutrition because of the need for a restrictive diet, medication side effects, and depression and anxiety, as well as a host of other medical symptoms. A nutrition assessment should be routinely included in the preoperative work-up of any patient when possible. Patients found to be at risk for poor nutrition status should receive appropriate referral for further evaluation and intervention. Although it seems intuitive that preoperative improvement in nutrition status will benefit the malnourished patient, it is controversial whether a short course of nutrition support prior to surgery improves operative outcome in this population (Howard & Ashley, 2003).

An assessment of preoperative nutrition and medication use is essential. The nurse should inquire about use of nutrition and herbal supplements during the preoperative nutrition assessment. In one study, up to 34% of patients surveyed reporting using a nutrition or herbal supplement that could interfere with anesthesia or inhibit coagulation (Norred, 2002). Women, people with higher education, and people practicing preventive health measures such as regular exercise, a low-fat diet, and not smoking are more likely to use herbal or nutrition supplements (Gunther, Patterson, Kristal, Stratton, & White, 2004). The Critical Alert outlines herbal and nutritional supplements that should be noted during preoperative screening.

CRITICAL ALERT   *The following supplements can alter coagulopathy or sedation (Fugh-Berman, 2000; Hodges & Kam, 2002; Norred, 2002):*

Borage	Bromelain	Danshen
Devils claw	Dong quai	Evening primrose
Feverfew	Fish oil	Garlic
Ginger	Ginkgo	Ginseng
Kava kava	Papaya	Red clover
St. John's wort	Vitamin E	

Adequate nutrition in the postoperative period is essential to contend with the increased metabolic demands caused by the physiological stress of the surgery. Additionally, wound healing, preservation of nutritional stores, and immunocompetence require sufficient energy, protein, and micronutrient intake. Patients should be transitioned to diet or enteral feeding as quickly as possible. Parenteral nutrition support may be indicated following some surgeries. Prolonged NPO status, reliance on only peripheral dextrose intravenous fluid, or extended use of a clear liquid diet postoperatively will not provide sufficient energy to meet even baseline needs and nutrition health can become compromised beginning with weight loss. The nurse should know that 2 L of a 5% dextrose solution provides only 340 calories! Nurses are uniquely positioned to closely monitor patients for lack of intake or poor intake and to ensure communication of prolonged NPO, clear liquid, and other forms of inadequate intake to the health care provider and nutrition staff. It is not uncommon for hospitalized patients to have periods of continuous or significantly cumulative NPO or poor quality intake to slip by without intervention when good communication patterns have not taken place. Such iatrogenic contribution to malnutrition was reported in one study where hospitalized elderly patients with already poor intake were ordered NPO for 38% of their meals (Sullivan et al., 1999). The reason for the NPO order was not clinically apparent 17% of the time and related to unnecessary delay in returning to a normal diet 20% of the time.

Some specific surgeries require additional postoperative nutrition intervention. Generally a registered dietitian with specialized training in the care of these patients is an active member of the treatment care team. It is important for the nurse to understand the nutrition protocol prescribed and participate in the team effort to ensure adequate nutrition contributes to good surgical outcome.

Bariatric Surgery for Morbid Obesity

Gastroplasty or gastric bypass surgery is indicated for weight loss treatment in some patients with morbid obesity. Gastroplasty is called a gastric restrictive procedure because the goal is to simply reduce gastric volume and therefore limit the amount (and energy content) of intake without causing malabsorption. In contrast, gastric bypass surgery involves reduction of the gastric volume but also causes deliberate malabsorption by bypassing absorptive surface in the small intestine. A Roux-en-Y procedure is the most commonly used bypass configuration; it bypasses the gastric fundus, duodenum, and proximal jejunum (Figure 14–3 ■) (Elliott, 2003). Postoperative care of patients who have undergone bariatric surgery follows careful steps in reintroduction of nutrition. Patients must learn to accommodate the reduction in gastric volume without precipitating nausea, vomiting, or dumping syndrome. Diets are advanced slowly over weeks and months from just liquids to texture modified foods until tolerance improves.

Patients with malabsorptive procedures or protracted vomiting must be closely monitored for nutrition risk. Commonly, supplemental vitamin B_{12}, folic acid, and calcium are prescribed (Elliott, 2003). Individual assessment of iron status may dictate an iron supplement as well since iron may be malabsorbed because of diminished acid production (Elliott, 2003). A chewable multivitamin is often generically recommended (Cunningham & Mar-

Vertical banded gastroplasty

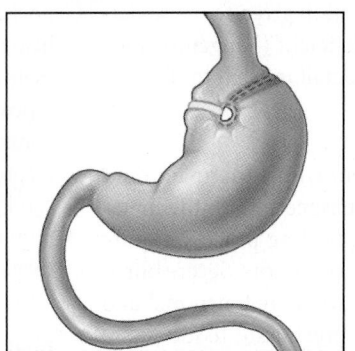

Roux-en-Y gastric bypass

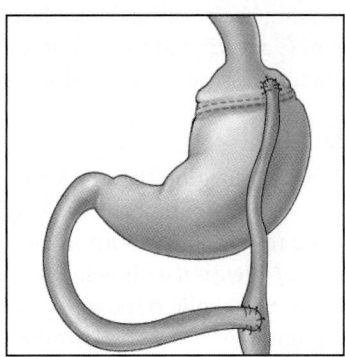

FIGURE 14–3 ■ Gastric bypass line drawing.
Source: National Institutes of Health. (2000). *The Practical Guide: Identification, Evaluation, and Treatment of Overweight and Obesity in Adults.* Retrieved December 10, 2008, from, http://www.nhlbi.nih.gov/guidelines/obesity/prctgd_c.pdf

cason, 2000). Chart 14–42 provides a sample diet recommendation and discharge instructions following bariatric surgery.

Transplant Surgery

Patients presenting for organ, intestinal, or bone marrow transplant are often already nutritionally at risk because of preexisting disease (Weimann et al., 2006). Most will have been closely monitored and have received appropriate nutrition intervention despite the presence of malnutrition. Postoperative recovery requires adequate nutrition for wound healing, repletion of nutrition stores, and support for the hypermetabolic demands of surgery. Patients undergoing renal or hepatic transplantation may have been on a restrictive diet that potentially may be liberalized following surgery when organ function improves. These recommendations are made on an individualized basis according to metabolic changes following surgery (Anbar, Lipa, Zinger, & Mor, 2003). Therapeutic use of immunosuppressive medications requires careful attention to risk factors for infection, including foodborne illness. The patient and family should be instructed about safe food handling (see Chart 14–38, p. 316).

 **CRITICAL ALERT** *Educate patients about the deleterious effects of combining some nutritional and herbal supplements with medications. St. John's wort has been reported to decrease crucial plasma levels of cyclosporine therapy, leading to graft rejection (Henderson et al., 2002).*

Patients undergoing intestinal transplant most commonly have been on some parenteral nutrition support preoperatively because of short bowel syndrome. The postoperative goal is to support the patient with enteral nutrition (Silver & Castellanos, 2000). Patients are closely monitored for return of intestinal motility and function. Enteral nutrition progresses according to patient tolerance and may consist of an oral diet, enteral formula, or a combination of both.

Following allogenic bone marrow transplant, patients routinely receive parenteral nutrition because of treatment-induced mucositis. The ability to take adequate enteral nutrition may not occur for several weeks and requires close monitoring by the team. Better nourished patients have been reported to have a shortened time to engraftment than malnourished patients (Muscaritoli, Grieco, Capria, Iori, & Fanelli, 2002). GVHD can place these patients at higher nutrition risk if malabsorption occurs. Parenteral or enteral supplementation with the amino acid

CHART 14–42 Diet Progression and Discharge Planning Following Bariatric Surgery for Weight Loss

DIETARY CHANGES

Liquids for 1–2 weeks postoperatively:
- Begin with clear liquids and add full liquids as tolerated.
- Avoid sugary beverages.
- Avoid carbonation.
- Slowly work toward intake of 64 oz daily.

Progress to pureed and soft foods 1 month postoperatively:
- Start with 2 TBSP and increase as tolerated per meal.
- Consume many small meals.
- Eat slowly. Eating too much or too fast will cause nausea and vomiting.

Follow guidelines for dumping syndrome if present. Dumping syndrome refers to abdominal pain, nausea, and bloating that occur after eating foods high in sugar, such as ice cream and milkshakes, following a bariatric procedure. Diarrhea, sweating, and fainting can also occur. Avoid foods that could cause this.

Eat slowly and chew well.

Save liquids for between meals.

Drink liquids in smaller amounts than prior to surgery. Continue to drink liquids to prevent dehydration. Signs of dehydration include dry mouth and dark urine.

Use a chewable or liquid multivitamin. Bypass patients require Vitamin B_{12}, iron, folic acid, and fluid and electrolyte monitoring.

ACTIVITY

Keep in mind that recovery takes several weeks.

It is normal to feel tired. Rest as needed.

Walk as often as able. Increase activity slowly.

Do not lift anything heavier than 10 pounds.

Avoid strenuous chores, such as vacuuming or lifting full bags of garbage, until the surgeon says it is safe to do so.

Climb stairs slowly and pause after every few steps.

Start an exercise program 1 week after discharge. You can benefit from simple activities such as walking or gardening. Ask your surgeon how to get started.

Ask your surgeon when you can expect to return to work.

HOME CARE

Continue the coughing and deep-breathing exercises you learned in the hospital.

Shower as needed. But avoid baths, swimming pools, and hot tubs for 2 weeks after going home. This helps prevent infection of the incision site.

Keep the incision clean and dry. Wash the incision gently with mild soap and warm water. Then gently pat the incision dry with a towel.

Follow your surgeon's instructions about caring for the dressing covering your incisions.

If Steri-Strips (small white adhesive strips) were used to close the incision, do not remove them. Let the strips fall off on their own. If they do not come off within 2 weeks after you were sent home, call your surgeon.

Take medications in crushed or liquid form for 3 weeks after surgery and as instructed.

Keep in mind that medications and dosages may need to be adjusted with weight loss.

Do not drive for 2 weeks after surgery.

WHEN TO CALL THE SURGEON

Call the surgeon if these following are present:
- Cloudy or smelly drainage from the incision site
- Fever of 100.4°F or higher, or shaking chills
- Fast pulse
- Night sweats
- Persistent pain, nausea, or vomiting after eating
- Diarrhea beyond the first week after discharge
- Pain in your upper back, chest, or left shoulder
- Persistent hiccups
- Confusion, depression, or unusual fatigue
- Signs of bladder infection (urinating more often than usual; burning, pain, bleeding, or hesitancy when urinating).

Sources: American Society for Metabolic and Bariatric Surgery. (ASBS). (2005). *Rationale for the surgical treatment of morbid obesity.* Retrieved November 21, 2006, from http://www.asbs.org/html/patients/rationale; Cunningham, E., & Marcason, W. (2000). Surgical treatment for obesity. *Journal of the American Dietetic Association, 100,* 1056; University of California, Davis Medical Center. (2007). Discharge instructions for bariatric (obesity) surgery. Davis, CA: Author.

glutamine has been reported to have beneficial effects on mitigating treatment toxicity effects on the GI tract because it is a primary fuel for the enterocyte. This area is deserving of further research (Muscaritoli et al., 2002; Weimann et al., 2006).

Trauma

Patients who sustain major trauma are at nutritional risk because of the hypermetabolic and hypercatabolic metabolic response that follows injury. Blunt or penetrating trauma and head injuries are examples of trauma associated with high nutritional risk. Early and aggressive nutrition support is indicated once the patient is generally hemodynamically stable (McKibbin et al., 2003). Enteral nutrition support is the preferred route unless bowel obstruction or other contraindication exists. The preservation of gut function and potential reduction of bacterial translocation and septic complications are cited as benefits of enteral over parenteral nutrition support in trauma patients (Swanson & Winkelman, 2002). Longer length feeding tubes, such as those used with a jejunostomy, may be required to deliver nutrition in the distal intestine following abdominal surgery or because of altered gastric emptying associated with stress.

Nutrition Support

Nutrition support with enteral or parenteral feeding is indicated when a patient cannot or will not take adequate nutrition to meet their individual needs. Enteral nutrition utilizes the intestinal tract for feeding. Parenteral nutrition is delivered intravenously and is generally reserved for situations where intestinal function is grossly compromised (Weimann et al., 2006).

Enteral Nutrition

Enteral nutrition is the preferred route of delivery for nutrition support. Much has been written on the beneficial effects of maintaining gut integrity and function by continued use of the gastrointestinal tract, even when only small amounts of enteral feeding supplement parenteral nutrition. Increased intestinal permeability and atrophy of intestinal villi occur when the gut is not used (Sun, Spencer, Yang, Haxhija, & Teitelbaum, 2006). Risk of bacterial translocation and sepsis may be reduced when patients receive enteral nutrition support compared to parenteral support or no nutrition support (Olah et al., 2002). Enteral nutrition support is also less costly than parenteral support. Although in the past, many clinicians were quick to institute parenteral nutrition for many gastrointestinal or abdominal conditions, it is now realized that enteral nutrition may be tolerated and beneficial to these patients. Acute pancreatitis, postoperative bowel surgery, and active inflammatory bowel disease are examples of situations where enteral nutrition may be used effectively in most patients, replacing the older practice of using parenteral nutrition. Other indications for enteral nutrition include situations where a patient cannot or will not take an adequate oral diet, but has a functioning GI tract. Anorexia, dysphagia, head and neck surgery or tumor, and mechanical ventilation are examples of conditions that may prevent adequate oral intake. Chapter 45 ⊙ describes GI disorders.

Types of Enteral Formulas

A wide variety of enteral nutrition formulas exist. Most fall into the category of a complete formula, which is one that contains all essential nutrients. Modular feedings are also available that can be used to supplement a complete formula with a single nutrient (for example, fat or protein) or to build a customized formula comprised of all modular components. The latter use is less common.

Complete formulas are further categorized by nutrient composition, density, and form. Some are marketed specifically for a certain disease state, but whether they are superior to generic formulas of similar composition is unknown. Standard complete formulas contain intact nutrients and require full digestive and absorptive ability by the patient. For example, protein is present in its intact form as found in foods, such as soy protein or casein from milk. Some standard formulas contain lactose or added fiber. Fiber in enteral feedings may be beneficial for normal bowel function, especially in patients on long-term feeding. Elemental formulas contain nutrients in a hydrolyzed form such that the patient does not need full digestive or absorptive ability to benefit from the feeding. Instead of whole proteins, an elemental formula may have protein already broken down to amino acids or di- and tripeptides. Generally these formulas have a minimal fat content as well. An elemental formula may be used with a patient with malabsorptive disease, bowel resection, or impaired pancreatic enzyme function. Both standard and elemental formulas contain between 1 and 2 kilocalories/mL. Many are also available in a high-protein version. Higher and lower calorie and protein contents allow for patients with increased or decreased fluid and/or nutritional needs.

When the composition of a 1 kilocalorie/mL formula is made of intact nutrients, the formula is usually isotonic in concentration. An **isotonic formula** has a concentration similar to that of the plasma and therefore should not contribute to an osmotic

draw of fluid into the gut. When fluid is drawn into the gut to dilute a concentrated solution, cramping, bloating, and diarrhea can occur. Other types of formula can be **hypertonic** because they have a higher concentration of electronically active particles, as in the case of elemental formulas that have many small amino acids instead of large protein molecules. Higher calorie or higher protein formulas are also hypertonic because of their increased concentration. Hypertonic formulas may cause an osmotic draw of fluid into the gut in some patients and are often begun at a diluted strength to avoid this consequence initially. The choice of appropriate formula will be driven by whether the patient has full or compromised digestive and absorptive ability and their overall nutrition and fluid requirements.

Routes of Delivery

Enteral nutrition formula may be taken orally or delivered via a small-bore feeding tube of varying lengths. The oral route is used when the patient is able to tolerate liquid intake safely and requires a supplement to the diet, a liquid diet, or an elemental diet. For example, patients with short bowel syndrome may take minimal food and instead consume an elemental formula because of altered absorption. When a tube feeding is indicated, nasogastric, nasoduodenal, or nasojejunal tubes are available. The longer length tubes are used when the upper GI tract is dysfunctional or to reduce risk of aspiration compared with a nasogastric tube. Longer tubes do not remove risk of aspiration, but may lessen risk. The Evidence-Based Practice guidelines discuss the reduction of aspiration risk during tube feeding administration.

Surgical placement of a gastrostomy or jejunostomy feeding tube is used when long-term enteral support is anticipated. Permanent tubes have the advantage of avoiding the irritation and discomfort of a nasal tube. Permanent tubes do not hold open the lower esophageal sphincter or pylorus, which potentially lessens the risk of aspiration. When a feeding tube is placed in the jejunum, an elemental formula must be used because the site of the tube has bypassed the natural sites for digestion of intact nutrients and enzyme secretion. Figure 14–4 ■ demonstrates the various placements and lengths of feeding tubes.

Administration of Feedings

Enteral feedings may be administered in a variety of ways. Bolus feedings can be given several times during the day, mimicking normal food or fluid intake, when the patient is alert and not at risk of aspiration. This would not be unlike a patient consuming an oral diet who consumes a 240-mL cup of a beverage at one sitting. An example of this is a patient with a G-tube secondary to a resected head and neck tumor who is otherwise well and now receiving long-term enteral feedings.

Patients with longer feeding tubes reaching the small bowel will not tolerate bolus feedings because of the osmotic load of the formula. Intermittent or continuous feedings are more common in the acute care setting. Intermittent feedings are delivered at a set rate for intermittent periods of time (for example, all night), whereas continuous feedings are delivered around the clock. Intermittent feedings may be the sole nutrition provided or they may be used to augment oral intake or parenteral nutrition. For example, a patient recovering from burns or a head injury may take an oral diet during the day with no tube feedings to impede appetite, and then receive intermittent feeding during the night in order to meet her high nutritional needs. Slower de-

Reducing Aspiration Risk During Tube Feeding Administration

Clinical Problem

Tube feedings are often stopped or held in patients at high risk of aspiration if gastric residuals are elevated. As a result, the patient does not receive the goal volume of feeding needed to obtain nutritional requirements.

Research Findings

Tube feedings are stopped or held for gastric residual volumes of 150 mL or more out of fear of aspiration. McClave and Snider (2002) report that a cutoff volume for holding feedings can be closer to 400 mL without negative effect on aspiration risk in low-risk patients, or 250 mL in patients at higher risk of aspiration. Saliva and gastric secretions alone amount to almost 190 mL/hr, a factor that deserves consideration when evaluating gastric emptying (McClave & Snider, 2002). An evidence-based review of gastric residual volume urges acceptance of an isolated residual of 250 mL followed by clinical evaluation when two or more consecutive volumes exceed 250 mL (Kattlemann et al., 2006). They report that when single residuals of 250 mL are accepted, greater formula delivery results without altered aspiration risk.

Postpyloric placement of the feeding tube tip has been shown in multiple studies to decrease gastric residual volume and gastric reflux of formula, both risk factors for aspiration (Kattelmann et al., 2006). In turn, patients with postpyloric feeding tube placement are reported to receive formula volume that more closely approximates estimated goals than individuals with gastric placement (Morgan, Dickerson, Alexander, Brown, & Minard, 2004).

Aspiration risk is diminished with proper patient positioning. When possible, elevating the head of the bed to a 45-degree angle during feedings will lessen the risk of reflux of gastric contents (Kattlemann et al., 2006). Positioning patients in this fashion is reported to decrease risk of aspiration pneumonia compared with patients in the supine position during feedings (Collard, Saint, & Mathay, 2003).

Nursing Implications

Critically ill patients are often at high risk of malnutrition. Promoting improved tube feeding tolerance and reduction in risk of aspiration pneumonia through patient positioning and feeding tube placement may offer an additional benefit of increased delivery of crucial nutrition.

Critical Thinking Questions

1. A patient who is sedated and in the supine position has not received any nutrition support because of aspiration risk. What suggestions can the nurse make regarding delivery of nutrition?

2. Sedatives can slow gastric emptying. What parameters should be used for holding any enteral feeding?

Answers to Critical Thinking Questions appear in Appendix D.

References

Collard, H. R., Saint, S., & Mathay, M. A. (2003). Prevention of ventilator-associated pneumonia: An evidence-based systematic review. *Annals of Internal Medicine, 138*, 494–501.

Kattlemann, K. K., Hise, M., Russell, M., Charney, P., Stokes, M., & Compher, C. (2006). Preliminary evidence for a medical nutrition therapy protocol: Enteral feedings for critically ill patients. *Journal of the American Dietetic Association, 106,* 1226–1241.

McClave, S. A., & Snider, H. L. (2002). Clinical use of gastric residual volumes as a monitor for patients on enteral tube feedings. *Journal of Parenteral and Enteral Nutrition, 26*, S43–S48.

Morgan, L. M., Dickerson, R. N., Alexander, K. H., Brown, R. O., & Minard, G. (2004). Factors causing interrupted delivery of enteral nutrition in trauma intensive care unit patients. *Nutrition in Clinical Practice, 19,* 511–517.

EVIDENCE-BASED PRACTICE

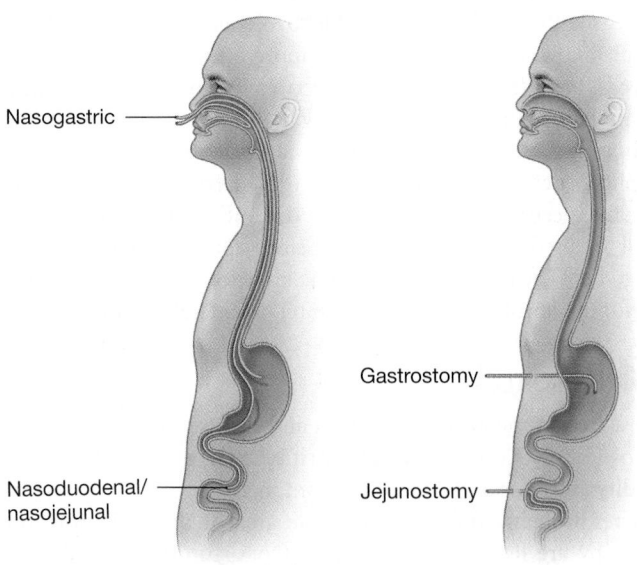

Nasogastric

Nasoduodenal/ nasojejunal

Gastrostomy

Jejunostomy

FIGURE 14–4 ■ Feeding tube placement.

livery of the formula results in avoidance of large gastric or intestinal volumes, minimizing the effect on aspiration risk and intolerance to hypertonic concentration. Feedings may be administered via gravity drip or with a feeding pump. Gravity drip delivery runs the risk of an accidental bolus occurring and should be avoided in patients at risk of aspiration.

The registered dietitian generally will recommend the appropriate formula and volume to meet the patient's needs. Depending on the formula content, the location of the feeding tube, and the patient's medical condition, feedings may be initiated at a diluted concentration or full strength. Isotonic feedings may be initiated at full-strength concentration is some patients, but hypertonic formula routinely are initiated at one-quarter to one-half strength. The concentration is gradually increased to full strength over one or more days depending on patient tolerance. The rate of formula delivery begins at about 50 mL/hr and is also increased as tolerated until recommended volume is achieved. Individual rate and concentration recommendations should be made for each patient.

Nutrition support requires close monitoring by the nurse. Tolerance to formula, amount delivered, and the fluid balance are crucial factors in determining effectiveness of treatment. Starting and stopping feedings for various interventions and repositioning can result in inadequate delivery of feeding and should be monitored for cumulative effect. The nurse must monitor the patient for symptoms such as high gastric residuals of formula, diarrhea, nausea, or vomiting. Severe vomiting or coughing can cause nasal tube displacement and warrants reassessment of placement. Diarrhea is commonly blamed on enteral formula even when other factors contribute more significantly (Parrish & McCray, 2003). Medications including antibiotics, infection, or bowel edema from hypoalbuminemia may be to blame and deserve investigation. Loose stools are to be expected with tube feeding and can be erroneously diagnosed as diarrhea. Formulas with added fiber are helpful in normalizing bowel function in appropriate patients (Swanson & Winkelman, 2002). To minimize risk of aspiration, patients should be fed with the head of the bed up at a 45-degree angle (Kattlemann et al., 2006).

Some medications can be administered through the feeding tube, but not all. Longer tubes may bypass drug absorption sites. Liquid suspension of some medications is not available and crushing medication can alter its action. A pharmacist should be consulted to determine compatibility of medication with tube feeding delivery. Tubes should be flushed before, between, and after medication delivery to avoid formation of precipitates that will clog the tube. A clogged tube or the need to replace a tube will inconvenience both the nurse and the patient. Taking the time to ensure that medication delivery does not lead to tube obstruction is time well spent. Handling of the equipment and formula requires fastidious sanitation to avoid the risk of feeding contamination. Chart 14–28 (p. 304) earlier in the chapter outlines nursing interventions for common problems related to tube feedings.

Parenteral Nutrition

Parenteral nutrition support is indicated in the patient who is unable to tolerate adequate enteral nutrition for more than 1 week (AGA, 2001a). Bowel obstruction, severe intolerance to enteral feeding (such as can occur with short bowel syndrome), and with bone marrow transplant are situations where parenteral nutrition is used. Parenteral formula delivered via a central line is referred to as **total parenteral nutrition (TPN)**. This is indicated in patients requiring support for at least 10 days. Formula delivered via a peripheral vein is called **peripheral parenteral nutrition (PPN)** and must be isotonic. PPN is used as short-term nutrition intervention to offset nutritional requirements until transition to alternative enteral nutrition is initiated. TPN is able to meet most patients' complete nutritional requirements. PPN is limited by the volume of fluid that can be tolerated peripherally and the lower concentration of nutrients that is required to maintain an isotonic concentration. Thus, it may not provide complete nutrition for some patients and is only a short-term solution.

Formula Composition

Parenteral formulas consist of a mix of carbohydrate, protein, fat, micronutrients, and electrolytes in amounts that are individually determined for each patient. Carbohydrate is in the form of dextrose and can be a 5% to 70% solution. Solutions that are more than 10% dextrose are hypertonic and cannot be delivered peripherally. Protein is in the form of amino acids and

begins at concentrations of 5%. A 5% amino acid solution, but not greater, can be tolerated peripherally. Fat can be administered centrally or peripherally and is an important calorie-dense component, a useful benefit when fluid volume is an issue. Both 10% and 20% solutions are available. Vitamins, minerals, and electrolytes are also administered with the formula admixture and can be customized to meet patient needs.

The nutrition support team makes recommendations on formula choice after a thorough assessment of the patient's nutritional, metabolic, and medical needs. Parenteral support is initiated at a low rate (about 50 mL/hr) and increased gradually to reach recommended volume. Maximum rates and volumes for both dextrose and fat administration are individually adjusted to avoid hyperglycemia, poor lipid clearance, and fatty liver. Blood glucose and triglyceride levels are monitored to assess tolerance to formula composition of dextrose and lipid loads, respectively.

The nurse is involved in the close monitoring of parenteral nutrition whether as a member of the nutrition support team or as a staff nurse. Most hospitals or institutions have clinical pathways or protocols that dictate frequency and type of nursing interventions in the care of patients on parenteral support. The nurse should become familiar with the specific protocol. Meticulous care of the access site for parenteral nutrition is imperative to avoid local or systemic infection risk because the high dextrose load of the feeding is fuel for bacteria. Accurate fluid balance calculations along with daily weights are essential. A short-term weight gain of >1 kg is more likely associated with fluid gain than accumulation of lean or adipose tissue. Clinical protocols will also outline metabolic monitoring for hyperglycemia and frequency of required laboratory assays. Close attention is paid to overall fluid and electrolyte status and formula adjustments can be made accordingly.

Patients continuing parenteral nutrition to the home care setting will require regular nursing care and monitoring following modifications of the in-hospital monitoring parameters. Before parenteral nutrition is discontinued, it should be documented consistently that the patient is able to tolerate a diet or enteral formula and consume two-thirds or more of estimated nutritional needs. Parenteral nutrition may be weaned to allow for appetite stimulation. Institutional policy will also outline guidelines for stopping parenteral support. Some advocate substitution of a peripheral dextrose solution to avoid hypoglycemia once a high-dextrose central solution has been discontinued, whereas others call for a reduced rate of delivery before stopping the solution altogether. The nurse should become knowledgeable about the institutional protocol for discontinuing parenteral nutrition.

Research

Research in the area of nutrition and disease can facilitate improved provision of medical nutrition therapy as well as morbidity and mortality outcomes from medical conditions. Topics currently being investigated in the area of medical nutrition therapy are listed in the Research Opportunities and Clinical Impact box. Results of this research can be monitored by reviewing the medical literature referenced through the National Library of Medicine.

RESEARCH OPPORTUNITIES AND CLINICAL IMPACT RELATED TO MEDICAL NUTRITION THERAPY

Research Area	Clinical Impact
Weight Management and Nutrition	
• Specific alterations in dietary carbohydrate, protein, and fat and weight loss efficacy	Improved advice on most effective diet for healthy weight loss
• Effects of significant restricted eating on short- and long-term alterations in brain chemistry and ability of diet to normalize changes.	Better understanding of treatment outcomes in disordered eating management
Coronary Artery Disease and Nutrition	
• Effect of lowering plasma homocysteine levels with diet on disease risk reduction	Potential reduction of disease risk factors
• Effect of antioxidants on disease risk	
• Effect of herbal dietary supplements on disease risk.	
Diabetes Mellitus and Nutrition	
• Use of the glycemic index to improve blood sugar control.	Improved short- and long-term glycemic control
Nutrition and Physiological Stress	
• Use of amino acid supplements, such as glutamine or arginine, in lessening catabolism in burns, trauma, bone marrow transplant, and other conditions	Lessened catabolic response to certain conditions and illnesses
• Use of early enteral nutrition support to prevent bacterial translocation.	
HIV and Nutrition	
• Effect of diet on occurrence and treatment of wasting and lipodystrophy.	Improved maintenance of nutrition status or nutrition repletion in acute care
Nutrition and Cancer	
• Effect of antioxidants on cancer prevention	Decreased incidence and improved treatment of alterations in body composition in HIV patients
• Effect of antioxidants on cancer treatment, including negative effects of antioxidants on chemotherapy or radiation efficacy.	Decreased disease risk
Nutrition and Renal Disease	
• Effect of limiting dietary protein on disease progression in renal failure	Improved treatment response to chemotherapy and radiation
• Effect of high-protein intake on risk of renal disease.	Limited disease progression
	Avoidance of disease risk from excess

Clinical Preparation

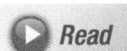

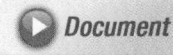 Read

- History of Current Illness
- Past Medical History
- Physical Exam
- Admitting Medical Orders
- Laboratory Study Results

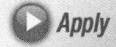 Document

- Summary of Hospitalization
- Pathophysiology Form
- Laboratory Values
- Laboratory Results Explanation

Apply

- List of Potential Nursing Diagnoses
- Concept Map
- Critical Thinking Questions

Log on to MyNursingKit.com to download forms you will need and to complete further steps in the Clinical Preparation assignment.

HISTORY OF PRESENT ILLNESS

A 57-year-old unmarried female office worker was admitted to the telemetry unit through the emergency department (ED) after presenting in the early hours of the morning with a complaint of several hours of severe chest pain. On interview, the patient, Ms. Nance, reports that she was experiencing intermittent, nonradiating chest pain during the late evening after returning home from an elaborate dinner party. She relates that she has had this type of pain in the evening multiple times before during the last year and it eventually goes away on its own; for this reason she tolerated this episode of pain for several hours and it eventually became constant in nature. She then waited several more hours before calling a friend who urged her to seek medical help and drove her to the hospital.

On admission to the ED, she was found to be in sinus tachycardia with no ST segment changes. Initial serial cardiac enzymes were within normal limits (WNL). Nonfasting laboratory values were WNL with the exception of serum cholesterol of 215 mg/dL and blood glucose of 162 mg/dL. Ms. Nance's blood pressure was found to be elevated at 175/110 mmHg and she was begun on antihypertensive medication. The admitting health care provider assessed that her chest pain might be related to gastroesophageal reflux and treated her with a proton pump inhibitor. She was admitted for overnight observation with a diagnosis of acute coronary syndrome due to continued, though milder, chest pain with midepigastric tenderness.

Medical–Surgical History

Her medical history is unavailable because Ms. Nance has not had a physical examination or other health care intervention in more than 20 years. Ms. Nance reports no prior physical complaints. She reports NKA, no prescribed or OTC medications, and no surgical history. Both of her parents died in their mid-70s of CAD.

Physical Exam

On physical examination, significant findings include a blood pressure of 170/105 mmHg and a complaint of moderate midepigastric tenderness. Ms. Nance is 5'5" in height and weighs 198 pounds. Fasting laboratory values reveal serum cholesterol of 209 mg/dL with LDL cholesterol of 151 mg/dL and HDL cholesterol of 35 mg/dL. Her fasting blood glucose is 130 mg/dL. Cardiac enzymes remain normal. You find the following after eliciting her history:

- Ms. Nance is unable to give a good weight history because she does not own a scale, but you discover that her dress

size has climbed by one or two sizes a year for the last 5 years.
- Ms. Nance attempted to lose weight 1 year ago before a nephew's wedding by following a high-protein, very-low-carbohydrate diet. She was able to fit into a dress two sizes smaller after dieting for 6 weeks, but also reported that her chest pain symptoms began while on the diet, leading her to stop adhering to it.
- Her nutrition history reveals that she eats two meals per day, lunch and dinner plus frequent snacks. She has her first meal at work at noon, but does drink several cups of coffee with cream in the morning. She has four or five cups of coffee a day. She buys her lunch at the office, choosing a meat with gravy or other sauce or a stir-fried dish and a potato or fried rice. She does not eat vegetables because she does not like how they are prepared by the office restaurant. Ms. Nance eats dinner out in a restaurant about four times a week with a preference for steak house establishments. Again, she tends to order red meat or chicken and a potato, plus dessert. When home for dinner, she heats a ready-made meal in her microwave or has instant soup. She always has at least one glass of wine with dinner, two if she is at a restaurant. Her snacks consist of chips or pretzels and crackers and cheese. A food frequency assessment reveals that her only fruit intake is orange juice on occasion when she feels she is getting a cold. Her only dairy intake is cream in her coffee. She takes no dietary supplements of any sort.
- Ms. Nance walks to and from her car in the office parking lot five days a week. This is her only exercise and takes approximately 5 minutes each way. On weekends, she remains indoors doing sedentary activities around her apartment and dining out in the evening with friends.

Allergies:	NKA
Medications:	none
Illness:	none reported
Surgeries:	none

Social History

Both parents died in their 70s of CAD. No siblings. Single, never married, lives alone, sedentary office worker. Active social life revolving around dining out with friends.

Physical Exam

Oxygen saturation 94% on RA
BP: 170/105 HR: 90 RR: 20 Temp: 37.1°C (98.9°F)
HEENT: nearsighted, glasses
Skin color: ruddy
Mucous membranes: pink
Sclera: white, no masses
Teeth: partial bridge, no obvious decay
Heart: regular rhythm, with no murmurs/rub, tachycardia
Lungs: clear, reports mild DOE
Abdomen: obese, soft, +BS, mild midepigastric tenderness
Pulses: −1 + radial and pedal
Extremities: no edema, warm and dry, no clubbing of fingers
Neuro exam 1: alert and oriented ×4; speech clear and coherent
Skin: good skin turgor, no rashes, no bruising
ECG: NSR, mild tachycardia, no elevated ST segments

Admitting Medical Orders

Admit to cardiology service
Type of floor: telemetry
Condition: good
Admitting diagnosis: acute coronary syndrome, GERD
Final diagnosis: GERD, HTN, obesity, hypercholesterolemia
No known allergies
Vital signs and oxygen saturation q2h
Activity bed rest, with bathroom privileges
Diet: low fat, saturated fat and cholesterol, 2 g sodium, no caffeine; nutrition consult
Call house officer: Pulse < 60 & > 130/minute; BP < 90 & > 160 systolic; temperature > 38.5°C (101.3°F); urine output < 30 mL/hr for 2 hours; respiratory rate > 30/minute; oxygen saturation < 92%
IV: saline lock; flush with NS q8h
Strict in/out
Sequential compression devices (SCD) to lower extremities
Oxygen 2 L nasal cannula
ECG continuous monitoring
12-lead ECG daily
Daily weight

Scheduled Medications

Omeprazole 20 mg po daily
Vasotec 10 mg po daily

PRN Medications

Phenergan 25 mg IV q6h prn nausea
Triazolam 0.125–0.25 mg q noc, prn sleep
Ativan 0.5–2 mg IV q6–8h prn anxiety (not to exceed 10 mg/24 hours)
Tylenol 650 mg po/pr q4h for pain

Ordered Laboratory Studies

Troponin I q3h × 3
CPK–MB q8h × 3
Chemistry 20 and PO_4 on admission and chemistry 7 q12h for first 2 days, then daily
CBC q a.m.
Mg^{2+} q a.m.
UA

Ordered Diagnostic Studies

Chest x-ray on admission and with adverse changes in O_2 saturation, increased shortness of breath, and/or increasing rales
GI consult for endoscopy

LABORATORY STUDY RESULTS

Test	Day 1	Day 2	Day 3
Sodium	142 mEq/L	137 mEq/L	140 mEq/L
Potassium	4.0 mEq/L	3.5 mEq/L	3.4 mEq/L
Chloride	106 mEq/L	100 mEq/L	102 mEq/L
Calcium	9.5 mg/dL		
Venous carbon dioxide	24 mEq/L	29 mEq/L	29 mEq/L
Blood urea nitrogen (BUN)	15 mg/dL	10 mg/dL	12 mg/dL
Creatinine	1.1 mg/dL	0.6 mg/dL	0.8 mg/dL
Blood glucose	162 mg/dL	130 mg/dL	129 mg/dL
Total proteins	5.2 g/dL		
Magnesium	2.1 mEq/L	2.0 mEq/L	2.1 mEq/L
Phosphorus	3.2 mg/dL		
Troponin I	0.26/0.23/ 0.28 ng/mL		
Myoglobin	0.5 µg/L		
Albumin	4.5 g/dL		
GOT	15 units/L	20 units/L	19 units/L
T. bilirubin	0.5 mg/dL		
CPK total	10 units/L	15 units/L	7 units/L
CPK MB	1.8%		
LDH	80 units/L	90 units/L	87 units/L
WBC	6,000/mm³	5,200/mm³	5,400/mm³
Hemoglobin	16 g/dL	12 g/dL	14 g/dL
Hematocrit	45%	38%	40%
RBC	5/mm³		
Platelets	395/mm³	325/mm³	250/mm³
ABGs			
PO_2	80 mmHg	90 mmHg	91 mmHg
O_2 saturation	94%	97%	97%
pH	7.32	7.40	7.39
PCO_2	35 mmHg	40 mmHg	41 mmHg
HCO_3	22 mEq/L	26 mEq/L	24 mEq/L

CRITICAL THINKING QUESTIONS

1. What are this patient's risk factors for hypertension? Coronary artery disease?

2. What nutrition advice would you give to improve her blood pressure control and decrease her risk of coronary artery disease?

3. What components of the patient's diet may contribute to her symptoms of gastroesophageal reflux?

4. What nutrition advice for cardiac risk reduction should also help with management of reflux symptoms?

Answers to Critical Thinking Questions appear in Appendix D.

NCLEX® REVIEW

1. The nurse should plan to include the following anthropometric measurements when assessing a patient's nutritional status.

   1. Body Mass Index (BMI), weight and waist circumference
   2. Body Mass Index (BMI), blood pressure and pulse
   3. A weight diary and food frequency diary
   4. A twenty-four-hour food recall and blood pressure

2. The nurse should include which nursing intervention when caring for a patient with bulimia?

   1. Offer the patient frequent small servings of finger foods.
   2. Instruct patient to avoid eating unless hungry.
   3. Encourage frequent periods of vigorous exercise.
   4. Explain importance of adhering to scheduled mealtimes.

3. A patient with type I diabetes calls the clinic and reports having nausea and diarrhea secondary to the flu. Which instruction should the nurse provide?

   1. Restrict your intake of proteins and carbohydrates.
   2. Try to eat a lot of sugar-free jello and pudding.
   3. Maintain your carbohydrate intake by eating noodles, toast, and sports drinks.
   4. Do not take your insulin injection until you can eat solid foods.

4. A patient with a large abdominal wound has low albumin levels. The nurse identifies the following condition in the patient will contribute to further protein losses.

   1. The patient is receiving two different antibiotics.
   2. The wound drains large amounts of exudates.
   3. The patient eats a lot of dairy products.
   4. The wound needs surgical debridement.

5. The nurse recognizes the need for intermittent enteral tube feedings may be indicated in the patient recovering from which condition?

   1. Burn injuries
   2. Cholecystitis
   3. Renal transplant
   4. Bulimia

Answers for review questions appear in Appendix D

KEY TERMS

aerophagia *p.317*
anthropometric measurements *p.273*
binge-eating disorder (BED) *p.290*
cachexia *p.279*
celiac sprue *p.303*
dysphagia *p.300*
enteral nutrition *p.322*
hypercatabolism *p.277*
hypermetabolism *p.277*

hypertonic formula *p.322*
indirect calorimetry *p.319*
isotonic formula *p.322*
lipodystrophy *p.314*
malnutrition *p.277*
overnutrition *p.272*
parenteral nutrition *p.324*
peripheral parenteral nutrition (PPN) *p.324*

physiological stress *p.277*
protein-calorie malnutrition *p.277*
refeeding syndrome *p.289*
respiratory quotient (RQ) *p.317*
steatorrhea *p.306*
therapeutic lifestyle changes (TLC) *p.294*
total parenteral nutrition (TPN) *p.324*
undernutrition *p.272*

PEARSON
EXPLORE **mynursingkit**™

MyNursingKit is your one stop for online chapter review materials and resources. Prepare for success with additional NCLEX®-style practice questions, interactive assignments and activities, web links, animations and videos, and more!

Register your access code from the front of your book at
www.mynursingkit.com

REFERENCES

Abou-Assi, S., & O'Keefe, S. J. D. (2002). Nutrition support during acute pancreatitis. *Nutrition, 18,* 938–943.

Abou-Assi, S., Craig, K., & O'Keefe, S. J. D. (2002). Hypocaloric jejunal feeding is better than total parenteral nutrition in acute pancreatitis: results of a randomized, comparative study. *American Journal of Gastroenterology, 97,* 2255–2262.

Alberino, F., Gatta, A., Amodio, P., Merkel, C., et al. (2001). Nutrition and survival in patients with liver cirrhosis. *Nutrition, 17,* 445–450.

Alsolaiman, M. M., Green, J. A., & Barkin, J. S. (2003). Should enteral feeding be the standard of care for acute pancreatitis? *American Journal of Gastroenterology, 98,* 2565–2567.

American Diabetes Association. (2003a). Evidence-based nutrition principles and recommendations for the treatment and prevention of diabetes and related complications. *Diabetes Care, 26,* S51–S61.

American Diabetes Association. (2003b). Translation of the diabetes nutrition recommendations for healthcare institutions. *Diabetes Care, 26,* S70–S72.

American Diabetes Association. (2004). Dyslipidemia management in adults with diabetes. *Diabetes Care, 27,* S68–S70.

American Dietetic Association. (2001). Position of the American Dietetic Association: Nutrition intervention in the treatment of anorexia nervosa, bulimia nervosa, and eating disorders not otherwise specified (EDNOS). *Journal of the American Dietetic Association, 101*, 810–819.

American Dietetic Association. (2002a). Position of the American Dietetic Association: Liberalized diets for older adults in long-term care. *Journal of theA merican Dietetic Association, 98*, 201–204.

American Dietetic Association. (2002b). Position of the American Dietetic Association: Weight management. *Journal of the American Dietetic Association, 102*, 1145–1155.

American Dietetic Association & Dietitians of Canada. (2004). Position of the American Dietetic Association and Dietitians of Canada: Nutrition intervention in the care of persons with human immunodeficiency virus. *Journal of the American Dietetic Association, 104*, 1425–1441.

American Gastroenterological Association (AGA). (1999). Medical position statement: Guidelines for the evaluation and management of chronic diarrhea. *Gastroenterology, 116*, 1461–1463.

American Gastroenterological Association (AGA). (2000). Medical position statement: Guidelines on constipation. *Gastroenterology, 119*, 1522–1525.

American Gastroenterological Association (AGA). (2001a). Medical position statement: Celiac sprue. *Gastroenterology, 120*, 1761–1778.

American Gastroenterological Association (AGA). (2001b). Medical position statement: Parenteral nutrition. *Gastroenterology, 121*, 966–969.

American Gastroenterological Association (AGA). (2002a). Medical position statement: Irritable bowel syndrome. *Gastroenterology, 123*, 2105–2107.

American Gastroenterological Association (AGA). (2002b). Medical position statement: Nonalcoholic fatty liver disease. *Gastroenterology, 123*, 1702–1704.

American Gastroenterological Association (AGA). (2003). Medical position statement: Short bowel syndrome and intestinal transplantation. *Gastroenterology, 124*, 1105–1110.

American Medical Directors Association (AMDA). (2001). *Altered nutritional status: Clinical practice guideline*. Columbia, MD: Author.

American Psychiatric Association (APA). (2000a). *Diagnostic and Statistical Manual of Mental Disorders* (4th ed., text revision). Washington, DC: Author.

American Psychiatric Association (APA). (2000b). Practice guidelines for the treatment of patients with eating disorders. *American Journal of Psychiatry, 157*(s), 1–39.

American Society for Metabolic and Bariatric Surgery. (2005). *Rationale for the surgical treatment of morbid obesity*. Retrieved November 21, 2006, from http://www.asbs.org/html/patients/rationale

Anbar, R., Lipa, R., Zinger, P., & Mor, E. (2003). The role of nutrition support in transplant recipients: Two case reports. *Transplant Proceedings, 35*, 614–616.

Andel, H., Kamolz, L., Horauf, K., & Zimpfer, M. (2003). Nutrition and anabolic agents in burned patients. *Burns, 29*, 592–595.

Anderson, J. W. (2003). Diet first, then medication for hypercholesterolemia. *Journal of the American Medical Association, 290*, 531–533.

Appel, G. B. (2006). Improved outcomes in nephrotic syndrome. *Cleveland Clinic Journal of Medicine, 73*, 161–167.

Arce, D. A., Ermocilla, C. A., & Costa, H. (2002). Evaluation of constipation. *American Family Physician, 65*, 2283–2290.

Atalay, F., Ozcay, N., Gundogdu, H., Orug, T., et al. (2003). Evaluation of the outcomes of short bowel syndrome and indications for intestinal transplantation. *Transplant Proceedings, 35*, 3054–3056.

Baum, M. K., Campa, A., Lai, S., Lai, H., & Page, J. B. (2003). Zinc status in HIV type1 infection and illicit drug use. *Clinical Infectious Diseases, 37*, S117–S123.

Becker, A. E., Grinspoon, S. K., Kilbanski, A., & Herzog, D. B. (1999). Eating disorders. *New England Journal of Medicine, 340*, 1092–1098.

Beto, J. A., & Bansal, V. K. (2004). Medical nutrition therapy in chronic kidney failure: Integrating clinical practice guidelines. *Journal of the American Dietetic Association, 104*, 404–409.

Blei, A. T., Cordoba, J., & Practice Parameters Committee. (2001). Practice guidelines: Hepatic encephalopathy. *The American Journal of Gastroenterology, 96*, 1968–1976.

Borghi, L., Schianchi, T., Meschi, T., Guerra, A., et al. (2002). Comparison of two diets for the prevention of recurrent stones in idiopathic hypercalciuria. *New England Journal of Medicine, 346*, 77–84.

Brand-Miller, J., Hayne, S., Petocz, P., & Colagiuri, S. (2003). Low-glycemic index diets in the management of diabetes. *Diabetes Care, 26*, 2261–2267.

Bravata, D. M., Sanders, L., Huang, J., Krumholz, H. M., Olkin, I., et al. (2003). Efficacy and safety of low-carbohydrate diets: A systemic review. *Journal of the American Medical Association, 289*, 1837–1850.

Brown, J. K., Feng, J., & Knapp, T. R. (2002). Is self-reported height or arm span a more accurate alternative measure of height? *Clinical Nursing Research, 11*, 417–432.

Brown, B. G., Zhao, X., Chait, A., Fisher, L. D., et al. (2001). Simvastatin and niacin, antioxidant vitamins, or the combination for the prevention of coronary disease. *New England Journal of Medicine, 345*, 1583–1592.

Bruemmer, B., Patterson, R. E., Cheney, C., Aker, S., & Witherspoon, R. P. (2003). The association between vitamin C and vitamin E supplement use before hematopoietic stem cell transplant and outcome to two years. *Journal of the American Dietetic Association, 103*, 982–990.

Buchman, A. L. (2001). Glutamine: Commercially essential or conditionally essential? A critical appraisal of the human data. *American Journal of Clinical Nutrition, 74*, 25–32.

Bulik, C. M., Sullivan, P. F., Wade, T. D., & Kendler, K. S. (2000). Twin studies of eating disorders: A review. *International Journal of Eating Disorders, 27*, 1–20.

Burden, S. (2001). Dietary treatment of irritable bowel syndrome: Current evidence and guidelines for future practice. *Journal Human Nutrition Dietetics, 14*, 231–241.

Bushinski, D. A. (2002). Recurrent hypercalciuric nephrolithiasis—Does diet help? *New England Journal of Medicine, 346*, 124–125.

Cai, B., Zhu, Y., Ma, Y., Xu, Z., et al. (2003). Effect of supplementing a high-fat, low-carbohydrate enteral formula in COPD patients. *Nutrition, 19*, 229–232.

Campion, J., Milagro, F. I., & Martinez, A. (2004). Genetic manipulation in nutrition, metabolism and obesity. *Nutrition Reviews, 62*, 321–330.

Casey, G. (2003). Nutrition support in wound healing. *Nursing Standard, 17*, 55–58.

Centers for Disease Control (CDC). (2001). Physical activity trends in the US 1990–1998. *Morbidity and Mortality Weekly Review, 50*, 166–169.

Centers for Disease Control (CDC). (2002). Iron deficiency—United States, 1999–2000. *Morbidity and Mortality Weekly Report, 51*, 897–899.

Chen, D., Misra, A., & Carg, A. (2002). Lipodystrophy in HIV-infected patients. *Journal Clinical Endocrinology Metabolism, 87*, 4845–4856.

Chobanian, A. V., Bakris, G. L., Black, H. R., Cushman, W. C., et al. (2003). The seventh report of the Joint National Committee on Prevention, Detection, Evaluation and Treatment of High Blood Pressure. *Journal of the American Medical Association, 289*, 2560–2572.

Cook, D., Meade, M., Guyatt, G., Butler, R., Aldawood, A., & Epstein, S. (2001). Trials of miscellaneous interventions to wean from mechanical ventilation. *Chest, 120*, 438S–444S.

Covinsky, K. E. (2002). Malnutrition and bad outcomes. *Journal of General Internal Medicine, 17*, 956–957.

Crook, M. A., Hally, V., & Panteli, J. V. (2001). The importance of the refeeding syndrome. *Nutrition, 17*, 632–637.

Cunningham, E., & Marcason, W. (2000). Surgical treatment for obesity. *Journal of the American Dietetic Association, 100*, 1056.

Cunningham, E., & Marcason, W. (2002). What role does fiber play in diverticular disease? *Journal of the American Dietetic Association, 102*, 225.

Demling, R. H., DeSanti, L., & Orgill, D. R. (2004). *Metabolism & nutrition*. Retrieved November 30, 2004, from http://www.burnsurgery.org/index_4x.htm

DeVault, K. R., Castell, D. O., & Practice Parameters Committee. (1999). Practice guidelines: Updated guidelines for the diagnosis and treatment of gastroesophageal reflux disease. *The American Journal of Gastroenterology, 94*, 1434–1442.

Devlin, M. J., Yanovski, S. Z., & Wilson, G. T. (2000). Obesity: What mental health professionals need to know. *American Journal of Psychiatry, 157*, 854–866.

Diabetes Prevention Program Research Group. (2002). Reduction in the incidence of type 2 diabetes with lifestyle intervention or metformin. *New England Journal of Medicine, 346*, 393–403.

Dietitians of Canada. (2003). *Hepatitis C: Nutrition care—Canadian guidelines for healthcare providers*. Retrieved December 18, 2003, from http://www.dietitians.ca/resources/HepatitisC_Guidelines.htm

Dorner, B. (2002). Tough to swallow. *Today's Dietitian*, August, 28–31.

Dube, M. P., Stein, J. H., Aberg, J. A., Fichtenbaum, C. J., Gerber, J. G., Tashima, K. T., et al. (2003). Guidelines for the evaluation and management of dyslipidemia in HIV-infected adults receiving antiretroviral therapy: Recommendations of the HIV Medicine Association and the Infectious Disease Society of America and the Adult AIDS Clinical Trials Group. *Clinical Infectious Diseases, 37*, 613–627.

Elliot, K. (2003). Nutritional considerations after bariatric surgery. *Critical Care Nursing Quarterly, 26*, 135–138.

Fairburn, C. G., & Harrison, P. J. (2003). Eating disorders. *Lancet, 361*, 407–416.

Farrell, R. J., & Kelly, C. (2002). Celiac sprue. *New England Journal of Medicine, 346*, 180–188.

Fawzi, W. (2003). Micronutrients and HIV type 1 disease progression among adults and children. *Clinical Infectious Diseases, 37*, S112–S116.

Finestone, H., & Greene-Finestone, L. S. (2003). Rehabilitation medicine: 2. Diagnosis of dysphagia and its nutritional management for stroke patients. *Canadian Medical Association Journal, 169*, 1041–1044.

Fletcher, R. H., & Fairfield, K. M. (2002). Vitamins for chronic disease prevention in adults: Clinical applications. *Journal of the American Medical Association, 287*, 3127–3129.

Fontaine, K. R., Redden, D. T., Wang, C., Westfall, A. O., & Allison, D. B. (2003). Years of life lost due to obesity. *Journal of the American Medical Association, 289*, 187–193.

Foque, D., Laville, M., & Boissel, J. P. (2006). Low protein diets for chronic kidney disease in nondiabetic adults. *Cochrane Database Review, 19*, CD 001892.

Foster, G. D., Wyatt, H. R., Hill, J. O., McGuckin, B. G., Brill, C., Mohammed, B. S., et al. (2003). A randomized trial of a low-carbohydrate diet for obesity. *New England Journal of Medicine, 348*, 2082–2090.

Franz, M. J., Bantle, J. P., Beebe, C. A., Brunzelli, J. D., Chiasson, J., Garg., et al. (2002). Technical review: Evidence-based nutrition principles and recommendations for the treatment and prevention of diabetes and related complications. *Diabetes Care 25*, 148–198.

Franz, M. J. (2003). The glycemic index: Not the most effective nutrition therapy intervention. *Diabetes Care, 26*, 2466–2468.

Freedman, M. R., King, J., & Kennedy, E. (2001). Popular diets: A scientific review. *Obesity Research 9*, 1S–40S.

Fugh-Berman, A. (2000). Herb-drug interactions. *Lancet, 355*, 134–138.

Gagnon, A. J., & Therrien, R. (Eds.). (2006). *HIV Medication Guide V2.05*. Retrieved January 15, 2004, from http://www.hivmedicationguide.com

Gans, K. M., Ross, E., Barner, C. W., Wylie-Rosett, J., McMurray, J., & Eaton, C. (2003). REAP and WAVE: New tools to rapidly assess/discuss nutrition with patients. *Journal of Nutrition, 133*, 556S–562S.

Garza, S. F. (2003). Bariatric weight loss surgery: Patient education, preparation and follow-up. *Critical Care Nursing Quarterly, 26*, 101–104.

Gebauer, S. K., Psota, T. L., Harris, W. S., & Kris-Etherton, P. M. (2006). N-3 fatty acid dietary recommendations and food sources to achieve essentiality and cardiovascular benefits. *American Journal of Clinical Nutrition, 83*, 1526S–1535S.

George, M. B., Day, L., & Zeiter, T. (2000). Case problem: Medical nutrition therapy for a patient with Crohn's disease. *Journal of the American Dietetic Association, 100*, 474–475.

Gerrior, J., Kantaros, J., Coakley, E., Labrecht, M., & Wanke, C. (2001). The fat redistribution syndrome in patients infected with HIV: Measurements of body shape abnormalities. *Journal of the American Dietetic Association, 101*, 1175–1180.

Goh, J., & O'Morain, C. A. (2003). Nutrition and adult inflammatory bowel disease. *Alimentary Pharmacology Therapy, 17*, 307–320.

Goldfein, J. A., Devlin, J. H., & Spitzer, R. L. (2000). Cognitive behavior therapy for the treatment of binge eating disorder: What constitutes success? *American Journal of Psychiatry, 157*, 1051–1056.

Graber, A. L. (2001). Syndrome of lipodystrophy, hyperlipidemia, insulin resistance and diabetes in treated patients with HIV infection. *Endocrine Practice 7*, 430–437.

Grinspoon, S., & Mulligan, K. (2003). Weight loss and wasting in patients infected with HIV. *Clinical Infectious Diseases, 36*, S69–S78.

Gronberg, A. M., Slinde, F., Engstrom, C. P., Hulthen, L., & Larsson, S. (2005). Dietary problems in patients with severe chronic obstructive pulmonary disease. *Journal of Human Nutrition & Dietetics, 18*, 445–452.

Gunther, S., Patterson, R. E., Kristal, A. R., Stratton, K. L., & White, E. (2004). Demographic and health-related correlates of herbal and specialty supplement use. *Journal of the American Dietetic Association, 104*, 27–34.

Hackam, D. G., & Anand, S. S. (2003). Emerging risk factors for atherosclerotic disease: A critical review of the evidence. *Journal of the American Medical Association, 290*, 932–940.

Harnack, L., & French, S. (2003). Fattening up on fast food. *Journal of the American Dietetic Association, 103*, 1296–1297.

Hayes, C., Elliot, E., Krales, E., & Downer, G. (2003). Food and water safety for persons infected with HIV. *Clinical Infectious Diseases, 36*, S106–S109.

Hedley, A. A., Ogden, C. L., Johnson, C. L., Carroll, M. D., Curtin, L. R., & Flegal, K. M. (2004). Prevalence of overweight and obesity among US children, adolescents and adults. *Journal of the American Medical Association, 291*, 2847–2850.

Henderson, L., Yue, Q. Y., Gerden, B., & Arlet, P. (2002). St. John's wort: Drug interactions and clinical outcomes. *Journal Clinical Pharmacology, 54*, 349–356.

Hijjar, I., & Kotchen, T. A. (2003). Trends in prevalence, awareness, treatment, and control of hypertension in the United States, 1988–2000. *Journal of the American Medical Association, 290*, 199–206.

Hodges, P. J., & Kam, P. C. A. (2002). The perioperative implications of herbal medicines. *Anaesthesia, 57*, 889–899.

Hoffer, L. J. (2001). Clinical nutrition: 1. Protein-energy malnutrition in the inpatient. *Canadian Medical Association Journal, 165,* 1345–1349.

Holmes, S. (2003). Undernutrition in hospital patients. *Nursing Standard, 17,* 45–52.

Howard, C., & Ashley, C. (2003). Nutrition in the perioperative patient. *Annual Review of Nutrition, 23,* 63–82.

Hu, F. B., Leitzmann, M. F., Stampfer, M. J., Colditz, G. A., Willett, W. C., & Rimm, E. B. (2001). Physical activity and television watching in relation to risk for type 2 diabetes mellitus in men. *Archives of Internal Medicine, 161,* 1542–1548.

Hu, F. B., Li, T. Y., Colditz, G. A., Willett, W. C., & Manson, J. E. (2003). Television watching and other sedentary behaviors in relation to risk of obesity and type 2 diabetes mellitus in women. *Journal of the American Medical Association, 289,* 1785–1791.

Hudson, J. I., Lalonde, J. K., Berry, J. M., Pindyck, J. L., Bulik, C. C., Crow, S. J., et al. (2006). Binge-eating disorder as a distinct familial phenotype in obese individuals. *Archives of General Psychiatry, 63,* 313–319.

Institute of Medicine. (1998). *Dietary reference intakes for thiamine, riboflavin, niacin, vitamin B-6, folate, vitamin B-12, pantothenic acid, biotin and choline.* Washington, DC: National Academy Press.

Institute of Medicine. (2001). *Dietary reference intakes for vitamin A, vitamin K, arsenic, boron, chromium, copper, iodine, iron, manganese, molybdenum, nickel, silicon, vanadium and zinc.* Washington, DC: National Academy Press.

Institute of Medicine. (2002). *Dietary reference intakes for energy, carbohydrate, fiber, fatty acids, cholesterol, protein and amino acids.* Washington, DC: National Academy Press.

Institute of Medicine. (2004). *Dietary reference intakes for water, potassium, sodium, chloride and sulfate.* Washington, DC: National Academy Press.

Ireton-Jones, C. (2000). Case problem: Medical nutrition therapy for a patient with Crohn's disease. *Journal of the American Dietetic Association, 100,* 472–474.

Jackson, J. E., Doescher, M. P., Saver, B. G., & Hart, L. G. (2005). Trends in professional advice to lose weight among obese individuals, 1994–2000. *Journal of General Internal Medicine, 20,* 814–818.

Jeejeebhoy, K. N. (2001). Total parenteral nutrition: Potion or poison? *American Journal of Clinical Nutrition, 74,* 160–163.

Jeejeebhoy, K. N. (2002a). Clinical nutrition: 6. Management of nutritional problems of patients with Crohn's disease. *Canadian Medical Association Journal, 166,* 913–918.

Jeejeebhoy, K. N. (2002b). Short bowel syndrome. *Canadian Medical Association Journal, 166,* 1297–1302.

Jenkins, D. J., Kendall, C. W., Faulkner, D. A., Nyguyen, T., Kemp, T., Marchie, A., et al. (2006). Assessment of the longer term effects of a dietary portfolio of cholesterol-lowering foods in hypercholesterolemia. *American Journal of Clinical Nutrition, 83,* 582–591.

Kattlemann, K. K., Hise, M., Russell, M., Charney, P., Stokes, M., & Compher, C. (2006). Preliminary evidence for a medical nutrition therapy protocol: Enteral feedings for critically ill patients. *Journal of the American Dietetic Association, 106,* 1226–1241.

Katz, P. O. (2003). Optimizing medical therapy for gastroesophageal reflux disease: State of the art. *Reviews in Gastroenterological Disorders, 3,* 59–69.

Kaye, W. H., Devlin, B., Barabarich, N., Bulik, C. M., Thornton, L., Bacarus, S., et al. (2004). Genetic analysis of bulimia nervosa. *International Journal of Eating Disorders, 35,* 556–570.

Khan, N. A., McAlister, F. A., Rabkin, S. W., Padwal, R., Feldman, R. D., Campbell, N. R., et al. (2006). The 2006 Canadian Hypertension Education Program recommendations for the management of hypertension: Part II—Therapy. *Canadian Journal of Cardiology, 22,* 583–593.

Klopp, S. A., Heiss, C. J., & Smith, H. S. (2003). Self-reported vegetarianism may be a marker for college women at risk for disordered eating. *Journal of the American Dietetic Association, 103,* 745–747.

Knox, T. A., Zafonte-Sanders, M., Fields-Gardner, C., Moen, K., Johansen, D., & Paton, N. (2003). Assessment of nutritional status, body composition, and human immunodeficiency virus-associated morphologic changes. *Clinical Infectious Diseases, 36,* S63–S68.

Kondrup, J. (2006). Nutrition in end stage liver disease. *Best Practice and Research: Clinical Gastroenterology, 20,* 547–560.

Kopp-Hoolihan, L. (2001). Prophylactic and therapeutic uses of probiotics: A review. *Journal of the American Dietetic Association, 101,* 229–238

Kotler, D. P. (2000). Cachexia. *Annals of Internal Medicine, 133,* 622–634.

Kuczmarski, M. F., Kuczmarski, R. J., & Najjar, M. (2001). Effects of age on validity of self-reported height, weight, and body mass index: Findings from the third National Health and Nutrition Examination Survey 1988–1994. *Journal of the American Dietetic Association, 101,* 28–34.

Kushner, R. F. (2003). *Roadmaps for clinical practice—Case studies in disease prevention and health promotion: Assessment and management of adult obesity—A primer for physicians.* Chicago, IL: American Medical Association. Retrieved December 18, 2003, from http://www.ama-assn.org/ama/pub/category/10931.html

Langemo, D., Anderson, J., Hanson, D., Hunter, S., Thompson, P., & Posthauer, M. E. (2006). Nutritional considerations in wound care. *Advances in Skin and Wound Care, 19,* 297–298, 300, 303.

Lean, M. J., & Han, T. S. (2002). Waist worries. *American Journal of Clinical Nutrition, 76,* 699–700.

Leninger, S. M. (2002). The role of nutrition in wound healing. *Critical Care Nursing Quarterly, 25,* 13–21.

Lichtenstein, A. H., Appel, L. J., Brands, M., Carnethon, M., Daniels, S., Franch, H. A., et al. (2006). Diet and lifestyle recommendations revision 2006: A scientific statement from the American Heart Association. *Circulation, 114,* 82–96.

Lieber, C. S. (2000). Alcohol: Its metabolism and interaction with nutrients. *Annual Review Nutrition, 20,* 395–430.

Little, D. R. (1999). Ambulatory management of common forms of anemia. *American Family Physician, 59,* 1598–1604.

Ludwig, D. S. (2002). The glycemic index: Physiological mechanisms relating to obesity, diabetes and cardiovascular disease. *Journal of the American Medical Association, 287,* 2414–2423.

Mallampali, A. (2004). Nutritional management of the patient with chronic obstructive pulmonary disease. *Nutrition in Clinical Practice, 19,* 550–556.

Mangili, A., Murman, D. H., Zampini, A. M., & Wanke, C. A. (2006). Nutrition and HIV: Review of weight loss and wasting in the era of highly active antiretroviral therapy from the Nutrition for Healthy Living cohort. *Clinical Infectious Diseases, 42,* 836–842.

Marti, A., Moreno-Aliaga, M. J., Hebebrand, J., & Martinez, J. A. (2004). Genetics, lifestyles and obesity. *International Journal of Obesity and Related Metabolic Disorders, 3,* 529–536.

Massey, L. K., Liebman, L. M., & Kynast-Gales, S. A. (2005). Ascorbate increases human oxaluria and kidney stone risk. *Journal of Nutrition, 135,* 1673.

McCallum, S. L. (2003). The national dysphagia diet: Implementation at a regional rehabilitation center and hospital system. *Journal of the American Dietetic Association, 103,* 381–384.

McClave, S. A. (2004). Defining the new gold standard for nutrition support in acute pancreatitis. *Nutrition in Clinical Practice, 19,* 1–4.

McInnis, K. J., Franklin, B. A., & Rippe, J. M. (2003). Counseling for physical activity in overweight and obese patients. *American Family Physician, 67,* 1266–1268.

McKibbin, B., Cresci, G., & Hawkins, M. (2003). Nutrition support for the patient with an open abdomen after major abdominal trauma. *Nutrition, 19,* 563–566.

Mehler, P. S. (2003). Bulimia nervosa. *New England Journal of Medicine, 349,* 875–881.

Meno, C. A., Hannum, J. W., Espelage, D. E., & Douglas Low, K. S. (2008). Familial and individual variables as predictors of dieting concerns and binge eating in college females. *Eating Beahviors, 9,* 91–101.

Montalto, M., Curigliano, C., Santoro, L., Vastola, M., Cammarota, G., & Manna, R. (2006). Management and treatment of lactose malabsorption. *World Journal of Gastroenterology, 12,* 187–191.

Morelli, V., & Zoorob, R. J. (2000). Alternative therapies: Part 1. Depression, diabetes, obesity. *American Family Physician, 62,* 1051–1060.

Morgan, J. F., Reid, F., & Lacey, J. H. (1999). The SCOFF questionnaire: Assessment of a new screening tool for eating disorders. *British Medical Journal, 319,* 1467–1468.

Morgan, L. M., Dickerson, R. N., Alexander, K. H., Brown, R. O., & Minard, G. (2004). Factors causing interrupted delivery of enteral nutrition in trauma intensive care unit patients. *Nutrition in Clinical Practice, 19,* 511–517.

Morris, C. D., & Carson, S. (2003). Routine vitamin supplementation to prevent cardiovascular disease: A summary of the evidence for the US Preventative Services Task Force. *Annals of Internal Medicine, 139,* 56–70.

Morton, A. R., Iliescu, E. A., & Wilson, J. W. L. (2002). Nephrology: 1. Investigation and treatment of recurrent kidney stones. *Canadian Medical Association Journal, 166,* 213–218.

Mulrow, C. (2001). Sound clinical advice for hypertension patients. *Annals of Internal Medicine, 135,* 1084–1086.

Muscaritoli, M., Grieco, G., Capria, S., Iori, A. P., & Fanelli, F. R. (2002). Nutritional and metabolic support in patients undergoing bone marrow tranplantation. *American Journal of Clinical Nutrition, 75,* 183–190.

National Heart, Lung, and Blood Institute. (1998). *Clinical guidelines on the identification, evaluation, and treatment of overweight and obesity in adults—The evidence report.* Retrieved February 5, 2004, from http://www.nhlbi.nih.gov/guidelines/obesity/ob_gdlns.pdf

National Heart, Lung, and Blood Institute. (2002). *Third report of the National Cholesterol Education Program Expert Panel on Detection, Evaluation, and Treatment of High Blood Cholesterol in Adults [Adult Treatment Panel III (ATPIII)].* Retrieved February 5, 2004, from http://www.nhlbi.nih.gov/guidelines/cholesterol/atp3full.pdf

National Heart, Lung, and Blood Institute. (2004). *The seventh report of the Joint National Committee on Prevention, Detection, Evaluation and Treatment of High Blood Pressure (JNC7).* Retrieved February 5, 2004, from http://www.nhlbi.nih.gov/guidelines/hypertension/express.pdf

National Institute of Diabetes and Digestive and Kidney Diseases (2003). *Gastroesophageal reflux.* Retrieved January 13, 2004, from http://digestive.niddk.nih.gov/ddiseases/pubs/gerd/index.htm#4.

National Institute of Diabetes and Digestive and Kidney Diseases. (2005a). *Celiac disease.* Retrieved November 13, 2006, from http://www.digestive.niddk.nih.gov/ddiseases/pubs/celiac/index.htm

National Institute of Diabetes and Digestive and Kidney Diseases. (2005b). *Diverticulosis and diverticulitis.* Retrieved November 13, 2006, from http://www.digestive.niddk.nih.gov

National Kidney Foundation. (2000). *Kidney disease outcomes quality initiative (K/DOQI). Clinical practice guidelines for nutrition in chronic kidney disease.* Retrieved November 16, 2006, from http://www.kidney.org/professionals.doqi/index/cfm

National Kidney Foundation. (2006). *Kidney disease outcomes quality initiative (K/DOQI). Clinical practice guidelines and clinical practice recommendations for anemia in chronic kidney disease.* Retrieved November 16, 2006, from http://www.kidney.org/professionals/kdoqi/guidelines_anemia/index.htm

Nelson, M., & Poulter, J. (2004). Impact of tea drinking on iron status in the UK: A review. *Journal Human Nutrition Dietetics, 17,* 43–54.

Nerad, J., Romeyn, M., Silverman, E., Allen-Reid, J., Dietrich, D., Merchant, J., et al. (2003). General nutrition management in patients infected with HIV. *Clinical Infectious Diseases, 36,* S52–S62.

Nestle, M., & Jacobson, M. F. (2000). Halting the obesity epidemic: A public health policy approach. *Public Health Reports, 115,* 12–24.

Norman, H. A., Butrum, R. R., Feldman, E., Heber, D., et al. (2003). The role of dietary supplements during cancer therapy. *Journal of Nutrition, 133,* 3794S–3799S.

Norred, C. L. (2002). Complementary and alternative medicine use by surgical patients. *AORN, 76,* 1013–1021.

Novotny, J. A., Rumpler, W. V., Riddick, H., Hebert, H., Rhodes, D., Judd, J. T., et al. (2003). Personality characteristics as predictors of underreporting of energy intake on a 24-hour dietary recall interview. *Journal of the American Dietetic Association, 102,* 1146–1151.

Nyholm, E., Turpin, P., Swain, B., Daly, S., et al. (2003). Oral vitamin B-12 can change our practice. *Postgraduate Medical Journal, 79,* 218–221.

Oh, R. C., & Brown, D. L. (2003). Vitamin B-12 deficiency. *American Family Physician, 67,* 979–986.

Olah, A., Pardavi, G., Belagyi, T., Nagy, A., et al. (2002). Early nasojejunal feeding in acute pancreatitis is associated with a lower complication rate. *Nutrition, 18,* 259–262.

Ornstein, R. M., Golden, N. H., Jacobson, M. S., & Shenker, I. R. (2003). Hypophosphatemia during nutritional rehabilitation in anorexia nervosa: Implications for refeeding and monitoring. *Journal of Adolescent Health, 32,* 83–88.

Osterkamp, L. K. (1995). Current perspective on assessment of human body proportions of relevance to amputees. *Journal of the American Dietetic Association, 95,* 215–218.

Palmer, J. B., Drennan, J. C., & Baba, M. (2000). Evaluation and treatment of swallowing impairments. *American Family Physician, 61,* 2453–2462.

Parrish, C. R., & McCray, S. F. (2003). Nutrition support for the mechanically ventilated patient. *Critical Care Nurse, 23,* 77–80.

Perry, L. (2001). Screening swallowing function of patients with acute stroke. Part 1: Identification, implementation and initial evaluation of a screening tool for use by nurses. *Journal of Clinical Nursing, 10,* 463–473.

Perry, L., Morgan, J., Reid, F., O'Brien, A., Luck, A., & Lacey, H. (2002). Screening for symptoms of eating disorders: Reliability of the SCOFF screening tool with written compared to oral delivery. *International Journal of Eating Disorders, 32,* 466–472.

Persson, M. D., Brismar, K. E., Katzarski, K. S., Nordenstrom, J., & Cederholm, T. E. (2002). Nutritional status using Mini Nutritional Assessment and Subjective Global Assessment predict mortality in geriatric patients. *Journal of the American Geriatric Society, 50,* 1996–2002.

Pritts, S. D., & Susman, J. (2003). Diagnosis of eating disorders in primary care. *American Family Physician, 67,* 297–304.

Rahman, K. (2001). Historical perspective on garlic and cardiovascular disease. *Journal of Nutrition, 131,* 977S–979S.

Reams, A. M., & Elder, V. (2003). Dry weight: To be set or not to be. *Nephrology Nursing Journal, 30,* 236.

Riley, T. R., & Bhatti, A. M. (2001). Preventative strategies in chronic liver disease. Part 1: Alcohol, vaccines, toxic medications and supplements, diet and exercise. *American Family Physician, 64,* 1555–1560.

Roberts, S., & Thompson, J. (2005). Graft-vs.-host disease: Nutrition therapy in a challenging condition. *Nutrition in Clinical Practice, 20,* 440–450.

Russell, R. M., Rasmussen, H., & Lichtenstein, A. H. (1999). Modified food guide pyramid for people over 70 years of age. *Journal of Nutrition, 129,* 751–753.

Saltzman, J. R., Russell, R. M., Golner, B., Barakat, S., et al. (1999). A randomized trial of lactobacillus acidophilus to treat lactose intolerance. *American Journal of Clinical Nutrition, 69,* 140–146.

Samaha, F. F., Iqbal, N., Seshadri, P., Chicano, K. L., Daily, D. A., McGrory, J., et al. (2003). A low-carbohydrate as compared with a low-fat diet in severe obesity. *New England Journal of Medicine, 348,* 2074–2081.

Santolaria, F., Perez-Manzano, J. L., Milena, A., Gonzalez-Reimers, E., et al. (2000). Nutrition assessment in alcoholic patients. *Drug and Alcohol Dependence, 59,* 295–304.

Schols, A. M. W. J. (2002). Pulmonary cachexia. *International Journal of Cardiology, 85,* 101–110.

Sefton, E. J., Boulton-Jones, J. R., Anderton, D., Teahon, K., & Knights, D. T. (2002). Enteral feeding in patients with major burn injury: The use of nasojejunal feeding after the failure of nasogastric feeding. *Burns, 28,* 386–390.

Serdula, M. K., Kettel Khan, L., & Dietz, W. H. (2003). Weight loss counseling revisited. *Journal of the American Medical Association, 289,* 1747–1750.

Shamliyan, T. A., Jacobs, D. R., Raatz, S. K., Nordstrom, D. L., & Keenan, J. M. (2006). Are your patients with risk of CVD getting the viscous soluble fiber they need? *Journal of Family Practice, 55,* 761–769.

Shields, M. (2006). Overweight and obesity among children and youth. *Health Reports, 17,* 27–42.

Shinohara, M., Mizushima, H., Hirano, M., Shioe, K., Nakazawa, M., Hiejma, Y., et al. (2004). Eating disorders with binge eating behaviours are associated with the s allele of the 3'-UTR VNTR polymorphism of the dopamine transported gene. *Journal of Psychiatry Neuroscience, 29,* 134–137.

Silver, H. J., & Castellanos, V. H. (2000). Nutritional complications and management of intestinal transplantation. *Journal of the American Dietetic Association, 100,* 680–684.

Singh, H., Watt, K., Veitch, R., Cantor, M., & Duerksen, D. R. (2006). Malnutrition is prevalent in hospitalized medical patients: Are housestaff identifying the malnourished patient? *Nutrition, 22,* 350–354.

Stevinson, C., Pittler, M. H., & Ernst, E. (2000). Garlic for treating hypercholesterolemia: A meta-analysis of randomised clinical trials. *Annals of Internal Medicine, 135,* 420–429.

Stickel, F., Hoehn, B., & Seitz, H. K. (2003). Nutrition therapy in alcoholic liver disease. *Alimentary Pharmacology Therapy, 18,* 357–373.

Stollman, N. H., Raskin, J. B., & Practice Parameters Committee. (1999). Practice guidelines: Diagnosis and management of diverticular disease of the colon in adults. *The American Journal of Gastroenterology, 94,* 3110.

Striegel-Moore, R. H., Dohm, F. A., Kraemer, H. C., Taylor, C. B., Daniels, S., Crawford, B. P., et al. (2003). Eating disorders in white and black women. *American Journal of Psychiatry, 160,* 1326–1331.

Sullivan, D. H., Bopp, M. M., & Roberson, P. K. (2002). Protein-energy undernutrition and life-threatening complications among the hospitalized elderly. *Journal of General Internal Medicine, 17,* 923–932.

Sullivan, D. H., Sun, S., & Walls, R. C. (1999). Protein-energy undernutrition among elderly hospitalized patients. *Journal of the American Medical Association, 281,* 2013–2019.

Sun, X., Spencer, A. U., Yang, H., Haxhija, E. Q., & Teitelbaum, D. H. (2006). Impact of caloric intake on parenteral nutrition-associated intestinal morphology and mucosal barrier function. *Journal of Parenteral and Enteral Nutrition, 30,* 474–479.

Swagerty, D. L., Walling, A. D., & Klein, R. M. (2002). Lactose intolerance. *American Family Physician, 65,* 1845–1850.

Swanson, R. W., & Winkelman, C. (2002). Exploring the benefits and myths of enteral feeding in the critically ill. *Critical Care Nursing Quarterly, 24,* 67–75.

Thiamine. (2003). *Alternative Medicine Reviews, 8,* 59–62.

Thomas, D. R., Zdrowski, C. D., Wilson, M. M., Conright, K. C., Lewis, C., Tariq, S., et al. (2002). Malnutrition in subacute care. *American Journal of Clinical Nutrition, 75,* 308–313.

Thompson, T. (1999). Thiamin, riboflavin and niacin content of the gluten-free diet: Is there cause for concern? *Journal of the American Dietetic Association, 99,* 858–862.

Thompson, T. (2000a). Folate, iron and dietary fiber contents of the gluten-free diet. *Journal of the American Dietetic Association, 100,* 1389–1393.

Thompson, T. (2000b). Questionable foods and the gluten-free diet: Survey of current recommendations. *Journal of the American Dietetic Association, 100,* 463–465.

Thompson, T. (2001a). Case problem: Questions regarding the acceptability of buckwheat, amaranth, quinoa, and oats from a patient with celiac disease. *Journal of the American Dietetic Association, 101,* 586–587.

Thompson, T. (2001b). Wheat starch, gliadin, and the gluten-free diet. *Journal of the American Dietetic Association, 101,* 1456–1459.

U.S. Department of Health and Human Services. (2000). *Healthy people 2010: Understanding and improving health.* Retrieved February 5, 2008, from http://www.healthypeople.gov

U.S. Department of Health and Human Services. (2005). *Dietary guidelines for Americans, 2005 edition.* Retrieved May 17, 2008, from http://www.health.gov/DietaryGuidelines/dga2005/document

Vellas, B., Guigoz, Y., Garry, P. J., Nourhashemi, F., Bennahum, D., Lauque, S., et al. (1999). The Mini Nutritional Assessment and its use in grading the nutritional state of elderly patients. *Nutrition, 15,* 116–122.

Viera, A. J., Hoag, S., & Shaughnessy, J. (2002). Management of irritable bowel syndrome. *American Family Physician, 66,* 1867–1874.

Wagner, D. R., & Heyward, V. H. (1999). Techniques of body composition assessment: A review of laboratory and field methods. *Research Quarterly for Exercise and Sport, 70,* 1–17.

Waters, D. D., Alderman, E. L., Hsia, J., Howard, B. V., et al. (2002). Effects of hormone replacement therapy and antioxidant vitamin supplements on coronary atherosclerosis in postmenopausal women. *Journal of the American Medical Association, 288,* 2432–2440.

Weiger, W. A., Smith, M., Boon, H., Richardson, M. A., et al. (2002). Advising patients who seek complementary and alternative medical therapies with cancer. *Annals of Internal Medicine, 137,* 889–903.

Weimann, A., Braga, M., Harsanyi, L., Laviano, A., Ljungqvist, O., Soeters, P., et al. (2006). ESPEN guidelines on enteral nutrition: Surgery including organ transplantation. *Clinical Nutrition, 25,* 224–244.

Wells, C. (2003). Optimizing nutrition in patients with chronic kidney disease. *Nephrology Nursing Journal, 30,* 637–646.

Whelton, P. K., He, J., Appel, L. J., Cutler, J. A., Havas, S., Kotchen, T. A., et al. (2002). Primary prevention of hypertension: Clinical and public health advisory from the National High Blood Pressure Education Program. *Journal of the American Medical Association, 288,* 1882–1888.

Whitaker, R. C., Wright, J. A., Pepe, M. S., Seidel, K. D., & Dietz, W. H. (1997). Predicting obesity in young adulthood from childhood and parental obesity. *New England Journal of Medicine, 337,* 869–873.

White, R., & Ashworth, A. (2000). How drug therapy can affect, threaten and compromise nutritional status. *Journal Human Nutrition Dietetics, 13,* 119–129.

Wilmore, D. (2001). The effect of glutamine supplementation in patients following elective surgery and accidental injury. *Journal of Nutrition, 131,* 2543S–2549S.

Woods, M. N., Tang, A. M., Jones, C., Hendricks, K., et al. (2003). Effect of dietary intake and protease inhibitors on serum vitamin B-12 levels in a cohort of HIV-positive patients. *Clinical Infectious Diseases, 37,* S124–S131.

Writing group of the PREMIER Collaborative Research Group. (2003). Effects of comprehensive lifestyle modification on blood pressure control. *Journal of the American Medical Association, 289,* 2083–2093.

Yanovski, S., & Yanovski, J. A. (2002). Drug therapy: Obesity. *New England Journal of Medicine, 346,* 591–602.

Young, L. R., & Nestle, M. (2003). Expanding portions sizes in the US marketplace: Implications for nutrition counseling. *Journal of the American Dietetic Association, 103,* 231–234.

Pain Assessment and Management

Claudia E. Campbell, Kathleen Osborn

Outcome-Based Learning Objectives

After studying this chapter, the learner will be able to:

1. Recognize pain as a distinct and frequently encountered human problem in the health care field.

2. Compare and contrast the ethical and legal issues related to pain and pain management.

3. Distinguish the sensory, cognitive, affective, and behavioral components of pain.

4. Apply common pain assessment tools and strategies to elicit details of the multidimensional pain experience.

5. Differentiate between acute, chronic, and cancer-related pain.

6. Describe and give examples of basic pharmacodynamic and pharmacokinetic properties of commonly used pharmacologic therapies, including the role of balanced analgesia in pain management.

7. Examine the usefulness of nonmedication interventions to alleviate pain in clinical practice.

8. Apply nursing pain management techniques in relation to established theories and current research.

9. Specify the major patient-related barriers to adequate pain management and demonstrate effective collaboration as a nurse-member of a multidisciplinary team in the management of pain.

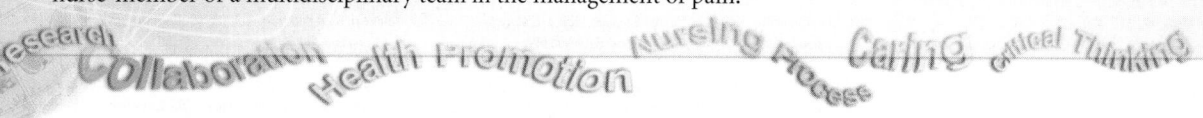

PAIN IS a symptom common to almost every illness, disease, or traumatic injury regardless of a person's age, gender, or socio-economic status. All cultures recognize the experience of pain although it may be expressed and responded to differently. It is pain that alerts an individual to an injury and encourages guarding of the injury to prevent further damage. To most, pain is a transient and unpleasant experience that persists for only moments before becoming an annoyance and then a memory. Pain is a reminder to avoid the activity that caused pain. For most people, the experience of pain leads to a diagnosis of the source of pain, successful treatment, and resolution of pain within a relatively short period of time. For others, pain becomes a complex experience that may not lead to a diagnosis or successful treatment. For some, pain is a disease. These patients are left to live with pain that persists for years and in many cases for the rest of their lives.

Pain is a major health problem of epidemic proportions. Millions of patients are unable to find health care providers who are knowledgeable and willing to treat pain. Pain management specialists are relatively few in number, clinics are generally located only in metropolitan areas, and health care coverage for pain treatment is often limited. Health care professionals, patients, and their family members are oftentimes misinformed so that misconceptions and myths regarding pain and pain treatments abound, creating conflict as patients seek relief from their pain.

In this challenging environment, patients are burdened with navigating an unfriendly health care system at a time when they are in pain, unable to or have a limited ability to self-advocate, and left vulnerable to accepting whatever health care they can easily access. When pain is chronic, patients are likely to experience personal distress from strained relationships, loss of independence, and depression. Patients are often unable to consistently participate in work-related activities, leading to loss of income and financial instability. A survey of chronic pain in America estimated that the annual costs associated with medical care, loss of income, and reduced work productivity are approximately $100 billion (American Pain Society [APS], 2000).

Epidemiology

A national health survey estimates that one-third of the people in the United States experience some type of pain (Lethridge-Cejku & Vickerie, 2005). Although pain management has improved during the past decade, the literature supports the consensus that many patients will experience severe postoperative or post-traumatic pain that is unrelieved (Ferrell et al., 2001). Of those patients experiencing chronic pain, one-half to two-thirds are partially or totally disabled for days, months, years, or even permanently (Bonica & Loeser, 2001). In evaluating the cost of treating pain, both the direct cost (office visits and medications) and the indirect cost (time away from work, reduced productivity, and/or tax revenue) must be considered (Turk, 2006).

Pain is associated with significant personal, economic, and social distress. Research indicates that hospitalized patients suffering unrelieved pain are more likely to experience delayed wound healing, pneumonia, and other postoperative complications (Shea, Brooks, Dayhoff, & Keck, 2002). Pain also is associated with decreased mobility, agitation, sleep deprivation, and postoperative delirium (Pasero & McCaffery, 2001b; Swarm, Karanikolas, & Kalauokalani, 2001). Scientific studies in recent years have just begun to uncover the connection between persistently unrelieved acute pain, subsequent hypersensitivity, and the transition to chronic pain syndromes (APS, 2003; Brookhoff, 2000; Byers & Bonica, 2001). These consequences of unrelieved pain are commonly associated with increased costs of providing health care. They also create financial and personal burdens for patients and underscore the need to make every effort possible to relieve pain in acute stages.

Pain management is associated with legal, ethical, and political concerns. The Joint Commission released pain management standards in 2000 that require accredited health care organizations to educate patients regarding their right to receive appropriate assessment and management of pain (Pasero & McCaffery, 2005). As a result patients are becoming better informed health care consumers who have expectations that their pain will be assessed and managed appropriately. Increased consumer awareness has improved patients' self-advocacy skills so that failure to manage pain is now resulting in increased legal liability for health care institutions, health care providers, and nurses (Pasero & McCaffery, 2001c). More than ever before, nurses must be aware of the importance of statutes and regulations that address the appropriate treatment of pain. Administering excessive amounts of pain medication can lead to sanctions and even criminal penalties for nurses. Now, nurses who do not appropriately treat pain can be investigated and disciplined as well (Frank-Stromborg & Christensen, 2001).

In addition to legal responsibilities, nurses have an ethical obligation to relieve pain. Nurses' ethical responsibilities when caring for patients are outlined in the American Nurses Association (ANA) *Code of Ethics* (ANA, 2001). Additionally, *The ICN Code of Ethics for Nurses* preamble states that nurses have the fundamental responsibility to alleviate suffering (International Council of Nurses [ICN], 2006). The use of placebos in the treatment of pain, treating the patient who has an addiction and pain, and treatment of pain at the end of life are examples of ethical challenges that nurses face in everyday practice. The American Society for Pain Management Nursing (ASPMN) has issued position statements, such as those listed in Chart 15–1, that are useful guides to nurses when they are confronted with difficult ethical situations in the course of managing pain (ASPMN, 2007). The Ethical Issues box discusses additional ethical issues related to pain management.

The science of pain is expanding at an unprecedented pace. The U.S. Congress publicly recognized the need for increased pain research by designating the period beginning January 1, 2001, to December 31, 2010, as the "Decade of Pain Control and Research." With this declaration, Congress recognized that much is still unknown regarding the complexity of pain and that to respond fully to those suffering with unrelenting pain time

---

| CHART 15–1 | **American Society for Pain Management Nursing Position Statements** |

- *Use of Placebos for Pain Management* (Coggins, Arnstein, & Leahy, 2004)
- *Pain Management at the End of Life* (Brown, Phillips, Cusimano, & Osteyee, 2003)
- *Assisted Suicide* (ASPMN, 2007)
- *Pain Management in Patients with Addictive Disease* (Coggins, McCaffery, Pasero, St. Marie, & Nichols, 2002)
- *Authorized and Unauthorized ("PCA by Proxy") Dosing of Analgesic Infusion Pumps* (Wuhrman et al., 2006)
- *The Use of "As-Needed" Range Orders for Opioid Analgesics in the Management of Acute Pain* (Phillips, Gordon, & Frandsen, 2006)
- *Registered Nurse Management and Monitoring of Analgesia by Catheter Techniques* (Primeau, Cowley, Eksterowicz, & Pasero, 2007)

Note: The full position statements are available at www.aspmn.org.

ETHICAL ISSUES in Nonmalignant Pain Management

Chronic nonmalignant pain is not usually proportional to objective disease severity; therefore, confusion about treatment goals and confusion about the reality of pain entangle therapeutic efforts. Doubts about the reality of the pain raise concerns about the issue of medication addiction and often cloud the efforts for relief. The ethical question is not whether chronic nonmalignant pain is real or proportional to objective disease severity, but how it should be managed to optimize the patient's quality of life. Sullivan and Ferrell (2005) proposed patient-centered principles to guide efforts to relieve chronic nonmalignant pain, including these:

- Accept all patient pain reports as valid, but negotiate treatment goals early in care.
- Avoid harming patients.
- Incorporate chronic opioids as one part of the treatment plan if they improve the patient's overall health-related quality of life.

The ban on opioid use in chronic nonmalignant pain is no longer ethically acceptable. Note, however, that ensuring opioids provide overall benefit to patients requires that patients with nonmalignant pain should be assessed and treated for concurrent psychiatric disorders. The presence of a psychiatric diagnosis does not mean that these patients are not entitled to equivalent efforts at pain relief. See the Pharmacology Summary (p. 344) regarding the use of antidepressant medications in the pain management treatment plan.

---

and resources must be dedicated to finding answers. Federal and state legislators are beginning to recognize the importance of pain management in the lives of their constituents. Legislation about issues such as regulatory barriers to appropriate pain management, the use of electronic prescription monitoring programs to monitor for diversion and abuse, establishing intractable pain treatment acts, and mandating pain education for health care professionals is only beginning to address some of the barriers to appropriate pain management (Dahl, 2002). The National Institutes of Health publishes guidelines about pain management, as noted in the National Guidelines box (p. 334).

NATIONAL GUIDELINES for Pain Management

The National Institutes of Health provides a web page with a plan for comprehensive pain management that spans all age groups. Topics covered include:

- Diagnosis/symptoms
- Treatment
- Health check tools
- Alternative therapy
- Coping
- Disease management
- Specific conditions
- Financial issues.

Source: National Institutes of Health. (2008). Retrieved May 28, 2008, from http://medlineplus.nlm.nih.gov/medlineplus/pain.html#fromthenationalinstitutesofhealth

In spite of positive strides, significant barriers prevent the provision of appropriate pain management for many patients. Patients and family members continue to be fearful that the use of opioids to treat pain will, as a singular event, result in addiction. Health care professionals confuse physical dependence and tolerance to opioids as addiction, and consumers are bombarded with inaccurate data and information regarding opioid abuse and diversion. Health care provider, nursing, and pharmacy educational curricula lack evidence-based information regarding pain and pain management, and health care professionals enter their practice without adequate knowledge of pain management principles. Health care institutions and insurance providers continue to provide financial incentives for major procedures or surgeries but fail to provide access to appropriate pain medications, treatments, and health care providers specializing in pain management. See examples of common barriers to appropriate pain management in Chart 15–2.

◼ Definitions of Pain

Discussion of pain is difficult without initially defining the terms commonly used to describe pain. The lack of consistent language is confusing to patients and family members as well as

CHART 15–2 Barriers to Appropriate Pain Management

- Inaccurate consumer education and consumer fears related to addictive disease
- Professional educational curriculums that do not include evidence-based instruction regarding principles of pain management
- Prescribing providers' fears of abuse, diversion, and regulatory scrutiny
- Federal and state laws, policies, and regulations that restrict appropriate access to pain medications and pain management specialists
- Inaccurate media coverage of abuse and diversion of prescription opioids
- Inadequate provider reimbursement for pain management treatments and therapies.

health care providers. Is pain the same as suffering? What is the difference between acute pain and chronic pain? Improved understanding of the principles of pain management begins with learning the terms that are commonly used and then using consistent language in discussions with professional colleagues and when educating patients and families.

Pain is defined as an unpleasant sensory and emotional experience associated with actual or potential tissue damage, or described in terms of such damage (International Association for the Study of Pain [IASP], 1993; Mersky, 1994; Wittbrodt & Tietze, 2004). Pain is always a subjective experience (APS, 2003). It is the subjective nature of pain that creates difficulty for the clinician who feels compelled to prove whether pain is present. Nurses must recognize that the physical assessment is incomplete without assessing patients' understanding of their illness including their pain. In 1968, Margo McCaffery's definition, "Pain is whatever the experiencing person says it is, existing whenever he says it does," described the need to appreciate that behaviors may not be consistent with the experience of pain and the most reliable indicator of the presence of pain is the patient's self-report (McCaffery, 1968; National Institutes of Health [NIH], 1987).

Pain Descriptors

Acute pain is considered to be of relatively short duration and coincides with injury, surgery, or illness. When healing occurs, acute pain decreases and resolves within a relatively predictable period of time (APS, 2003; Pasero, Paice, & McCaffery, 1999). However, it is difficult to classify pain based only on the criterion of duration. Acute pain may persist but still coincide with a high degree of pathology that does not meet the criteria expected for chronic pain. It has been suggested that it may be appropriate to consider pain that is associated with high levels of pathology that can usually be linked to the injury, surgery, or illness as acute regardless of the duration (Turk & Okifuji, 2001).

Acute pain episodes that are relatively short in duration and then completely resolve, leaving the patient pain free for a period of time before pain reoccurs, is defined as **recurrent pain**. This type of pain is usually associated with a chronic disease process that is painless except for episodes of acute pain (e.g., sickle cell disease, pancreatitis, or Crohn's disease). However, recurrent pain also is an appropriate designation when a patient has had multiple surgeries where pain has completely resolved between surgeries that are sequential (Turk & Okifuji, 2001).

When resolution of pain does not occur within the expected time frame, and is persistent beyond 3 to 6 months, it is considered to be **chronic pain**. Chronic pain is sometimes difficult to connect to an injury or illness and may persist for months, years, or even the lifetime of the patient. Chronic pain is associated with low or absent levels of pathology that can be linked to injury, surgery, or illness. The intensity of pain perceived by the patient may appear to be inconsistent with the existing pathology (Sullivan & Ferrell, 2005; Turk & Okifuji, 2001). Common types of chronic pain complaints include headache, low back pain, arthritis pain, or pain resulting from damage to the peripheral nerves or to the central nervous system (CNS) itself. A less common example of chronic pain is when pain is not due to past disease or injury or any visible sign of damage inside or outside the nervous system (psychogenic pain) (National Institute of Neurological Disorders and Stroke [NINDS], 2007a). Untreated chronic pain is currently being recognized as a major health problem in the United States (Sullivan & Ferrell, 2005).

Transient pain is acute pain that is brief and then resolves completely such as the pain associated with a needlestick for phlebotomy or an intramuscular injection. Transient pain is associated with minor tissue damage rather than disease or significant tissue damage.

Breakthrough pain is defined as a "transitory exacerbation of pain that occurs on a background of otherwise stable pain in a patient receiving chronic opioid therapy" (Portenoy & Hagen, 1990). It is referred to as breakthrough pain because the pain "breaks through" the patient's regular pain medication. Breakthrough pain is commonly associated with cancer pain although it can occur with chronic pain as well. Breakthrough pain may be easily confused with the pain caused by a painful procedure (acute pain) or the pain experienced as the effects of analgesic medications decline (end-of-dose failure).

Cancer pain is associated with malignancy and can be acute and chronic in nature. Acute cancer pain is generally caused by disease progression, surgery or procedures, and medications or therapies used in the treatment of cancer. Chronic cancer pain can also occur as a result of nerve injury leading to painful neuropathies (APS, 2005; Turk & Okifuji, 2001). Cancer pain is discussed in detail in Chapter 64 .

Evolution of Pain Theories

Theories on pain have been recorded since ancient times when some believed that pain was punishment as a result of wrongdoing or an expression of mental instability. There are a number of theories to explain the physiological basis of pain (Porth, 2005). The **specificity theory** asserts that pain is directly related to the degree of injury. Once a noxious stimulus has occurred, the message is carried directly to the pain centers in the brain. In 1664, Descartes first described pain as a physical experience using the example of the automatic withdrawal of the injured foot from the fire that burned it (Melzack & Wall, 1983). The **pattern theory** is a group of theories which assert that pain receptors share nerve pathways with other sensory pathways and that the intensity of the stimulus determines the frequency of firing of the receptor (Porth, 2005). Light touch would produce low-frequency firing, whereas intense or painful pressure would produce high-frequency firing of the same receptor, signaling pain. These theories do not account for emotional or learned responses to pain.

The **gate control theory** proposes that the spinal cord has a gating mechanism that either permits or inhibits the transmission of pain information to the brain. The pain is modulated at the substantia gelatinosa in the dorsal horn where there are "gates" that either inhibit or transmit noxious stimuli. Messages are transmitted via either small, nociceptive neurons or by large nonnociceptive neurons. The large neurons transmit nonnoxious stimuli such as massage or electrical stimulation, whereas the small nociceptive neurons transmit painful stimuli. The large nonnociceptive transmissions can inhibit the small transmissions, thereby interrupting the pain transmission. For example, when sudden pain occurs due to a fall, if the area is briskly rubbed the pain diminishes.

The more recent **neuromatrix theory** addresses the brain's role in pain perception as well as other determinants (Melzack, 1999; Porth, 2005). This theory proposes that the brain contains a widely distributed neural network referred to as the *body-self neuromatrix*. This matrix contains somatosensory, limbic, and thalamocortical components whose synaptic architecture is determined by genetics and sensory influences. An individual's matrix integrates multiple sources of input, which results in a multifaceted pain response. This theory is used to explain chronic pain or phantom limb pain where there is no direct relationship. **Phantom limb pain** is felt in the amputated part of the body as a result of the brain misinterpreting the nerve signals as coming from the site of the amputation (Merck, 2007). This theory also helps to explain the highly variable individual perception of painful stimuli (Porth, 2005).

Pain as a Multidimensional Phenomenon

The currently accepted definition of pain and the evolving pain theories of the 20th century all support the rationale that pain is much more than the physical response to tissue damage. Pain is multidimensional and includes the patient's emotions, behaviors, and functionality both physically and mentally in response to the pain. Just as a singular description of pain is not accurate, consideration of all of the dimensions of pain is necessary to fully appreciate the individuality and complexity of the experience of pain. The multiple dimensions of pain discussed in the following subsections are physiological, sensory, affective, cognitive, and behavioral.

Physiological Dimension

Both the peripheral and central nervous systems are involved in processing the perception of pain. The origin of pain can be either nociceptive (tissue) or neuropathic (nerves). Three pathways transmit nociceptive painful stimuli: first-order, second-order, and third-order neurons. First-order neurons, or nociceptors, are nerve endings found in the skin, dental pulp, periosteum, meninges, and some internal organs that exclusively respond to chemical, thermal, and mechanical noxious stimuli. **Nociception**, which means "pain sense," is the process by which **noxious stimuli** (tissue damage) activate sensory neurons to send the message to the CNS, resulting in a **nociceptive pain** response (Porth, 2005).

Nociceptors branch from the skin, sending fibers to local blood vessels, mast cells, hair follicles, and sweat glands. The transmission of pain from these peripheral fibers to the CNS is referred to as **transduction**. Transmission of pain impulses occurs via two types of nerve fibers, fast-conducting A-delta fibers and slower conducting C-fibers. Localized sharp pain is conducted by A-delta fibers, and dull, aching pain is conducted by C-fibers. When noxious stimuli stimulate the nociceptors, histamine is released from the mast cells, causing vasodilation at the injury site. Nociceptors transfer the noxious stimuli into electrical activity, known as action potentials. Once nociception is initiated, the action potentials are transmitted through the peripheral nervous system to the internal organs and the spinal cord (Porth, 2005; Wittbrodt & Tietze, 2004). These action potentials are transmitted via the sensory neurons and converge onto common second-order neurons in the dorsal horn of the spinal cord, where they are processed (Porth, 2005).

The substantia gelatinosa in the dorsal horn is the major site for pain modulation, an individual's perception of the experience.

From the dorsal horn, pain messages are transmitted through the third-order neurons to the thalamus and cerebral cortex where pain is integrated and modulated. The ascending tracts send information about the quality, intensity, and the affective meaning of pain, and will activate the descending pathways. **Endorphins and enkephalins** are endogenous morphine-like substances that reduce or suppress the pain perception in the descending pathways. These descending spinal pathways conduct inhibitory impulses by releasing serotonin, norepinephrine, and endorphins, which reduce nociceptive transmission in the CNS. This process modulates the pain, making it highly personal and individualized (Porth, 2005). Response to pain is dependent on past experience with pain, the concept of the cause of the pain, learned cultural responses, fear, anxiety, age, and individual beliefs.

The second type of pain, neuropathic pain, occurs when there is direct damage to the nerves (Porth, 2005). **Neuropathic pain** is a result of injury or dysfunction in the peripheral nervous system and can progress to the CNS, altering its function and resulting in a chronic painful disease (Backonja, 2001; NINDS, 2007a). Instead of loss of sensation, as would be expected with nerve damage, some injuries are associated with abnormal pain. Normal stimuli such as light pressure may result in significant pain, and normal noxious stimulation such as bumping the affected area produces a supernormal pain response. Traumatic nerve injury, certain diseases (especially shingles and diabetes), and certain toxins (anticancer medications) can cause these painful neuropathies.

The type of injury or disease dictates the origin of the pain. Pain that originates in the skin and subcutaneous tissue is referred to as *superficial*, whereas pain from muscles and bones is *somatic* and pain originating in the organs is *visceral*. Somatic pain is typically described as dull or sharp, and aching, and is most commonly caused by a cut, heat such as a burn injury, ischemia, and bone displacement. Visceral pain typically is described as dull or sharp, aching, and cramping and is caused by distention, ischemia, spasms, and chemical irritants such as medications or spicy food.

Physiological and Pathological Consequences of Unrelieved Pain

Undertreated pain can produce serious adverse physiological, psychological, and immunological effects. Inadequate pain control can stimulate a stress response that involves the cardiovascular, pulmonary, gastrointestinal, metabolic, and neuroendocrine systems (Pasero et al., 1999; Rothley & Therrien, 2002). Pain causes catabolism, which leads to poor wound healing, weakness, and muscle breakdown. Increased heart rate and blood pressure increases the risk of thromboembolic events due to stress hormone effects and decreased mobility. Chapter 12 🔗 describes the relationship of the stress response and pain. Effective respiratory effort is impaired, increasing the risk of infection and hypoxemia. Pain increases salt and water retention, resulting in fluid overload and hypokalemia. Pain also causes decreased gastrointestinal motility and increased blood pressure. Anxiety, depression, and sleep deprivation are commonly associated with pain. Immunologically, pain is associated with reduced natural killer cell counts indicating impaired immune response (APS, 2003; Pasero et al., 1999). Increasing evidence suggests that un-

dertreated acute pain may predispose patients to chronic pain syndromes due to neuronal plasticity (APS, 2003).

Sensory Dimension

The **sensory dimension of pain** includes consideration of the location, intensity, quality, and temporal patterns. An understanding of these factors will influence the diagnosis and ultimately the treatment. Many patients will experience more than one location of pain, and each location may be associated with a different intensity, quality, and pattern. Neuropathic pain, for example, is generally located along the anatomic distribution of the nerve or where the spinal cord is affected. Nociceptive pain may be localized to the injury and the immediate surrounding area. Pain intensity may be described in a variety of ways. Patients can be instructed to use numbers from a scale, select a drawing of a face that best illustrates their pain, or select descriptive words such as *mild* or *severe* (Chart 15–3). If encouraged to describe the quality of their pain, most patients can provide a fairly graphic description using one or two words without coaching. The temporal pattern of pain is generally described in terms of the onset and duration using terms such as *constant* or *steady*, *intermittent*, and *episodic*.

Affective Dimension

The **affective dimension of pain** describes the emotions patients assign to their pain. Patients' emotions can impact the experience of pain both positively and negatively. Postoperative pain for a patient recovering from surgery to remove a mass that was found to be benign would possibly assign different emotions to their pain than another patient would whose tumor was found to be malignant. In addition to the patient's own emotions related to her pain, the emotions and support of friends and family will impact the pain experience. Feeling loved and supported by those who are meaningful in the patient's life can reduce the intensity of pain (Price, Riley, & Wade, 2001). Conversely, patients who do not have a good support system will report greater discomfort. Nurses have long noted that fear, frustration, anger, stress, and anxiety are all associated with increased pain intensity. Descriptive words such as *unbearable*, *punishing*, and *terrifying* convey a different meaning than do *annoying*, *tiring*, and *exhausting*. When negative emotions overwhelm the patient, the term *suffering* is used to describe the unpleasant physical and emotional components of pain. Suffering is hallmarked by feelings of uncontrollability, hopelessness, helplessness, and intolerability that undermine the patient's self-identity and integrity (Turk & Okifuji, 2001).

 *Evaluation of the affective dimension of pain requires the nurse to be attentive to the verbal and nonverbal cues that indicate that the patient's emotions may be negatively impacting his pain.*

Cognitive and Cultural Dimensions

The **cognitive dimension of pain** includes the impact of personal beliefs, attitudes, and meanings attached to pain. Factors such as self-efficacy, self-control, and the locus of control can be beneficial or negative in the experience of pain. Patients who have a history of psychological problems generally report pain

---

CHART 15–3   **Unidimensional Pain Intensity Measurement Tools**

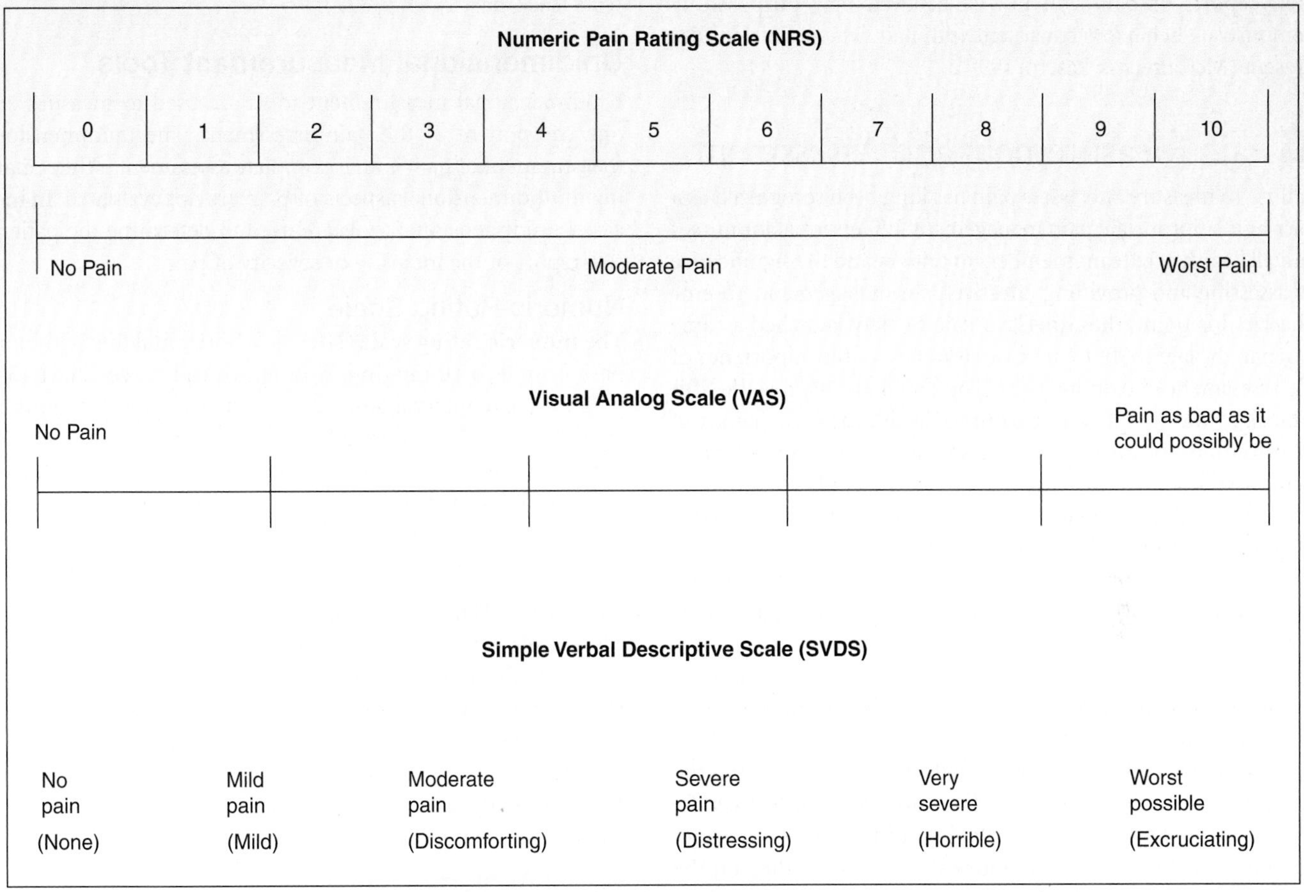

Numeric Pain Rating Scale (NRS)

| 0 | 1 | 2 | 3 | 4 | 5 | 6 | 7 | 8 | 9 | 10 |

No Pain   Moderate Pain   Worst Pain

Visual Analog Scale (VAS)

No Pain   Pain as bad as it
                                                                                could possibly be

Simple Verbal Descriptive Scale (SVDS)

| No pain | Mild pain | Moderate pain | Severe pain | Very severe | Worst possible |
| (None) | (Mild) | (Discomforting) | (Distressing) | (Horrible) | (Excruciating) |

---

that is out of proportion to their physical disability and are prone to a greater degree of disability and depression when pain is chronic (Merck, 2007). Successful treatment of chronic pain often includes assisting the patient to convert unrealistic expectations into willingness to acknowledge and then accept pain as a part of his life. Acceptance enhances the patient's ability to cope and results in improved outcomes and satisfaction with the quality of life (Arnstein, Wells-Federman, & Caudill-Slosberg, 2002). Patients need to be encouraged to develop cognitive control by reducing their focus on pain-related thoughts and shifting to acceptance that meaningful life is possible despite pain. The Cultural Considerations box discusses how spiritual beliefs and culture affect patients' cognitive responses to pain.

Behavioral Dimension

The **behavioral dimension of pain** includes responses to pain that may be situational, developmental, or learned. Behaviors commonly associated with the expression of pain are both verbal and nonverbal. Grimacing or furrowed brow, guarding, agitation, and avoiding required activities are examples of nonverbal expressions of pain. Verbal expressions of pain include crying, moaning, and verbalization. It is appropriate to expect a patient to demonstrate anxiety in situations that are not familiar to him such as treatment in an emergency depart-

CULTURAL CONSIDERATIONS Related to Patient Responses to Pain

Spiritual beliefs, culture, and family affect patients' cognitive responses to pain. A child learns from an early age how to respond to and express pain from observation of her family members. Acceptable responses vary among different cultures. Some cultures believe pain is a punishment for wrongdoing, whereas others feel it is a direct result of a past or future event. Spiritual rituals such as prayer may play an important comforting role in some cultures, whereas other cultures use food rituals to restore balance in the body. Patients may be stoic, remaining silent about their pain, or they may be verbally expressive and prone to pain behaviors such as moaning or crying. In some cultures the patient may remain silent while the head of the family speaks for the patient. Each of these situations and responses plays an important role in the individual's cognitive responses to pain.

ment or hospitalization. Patients who have developmental delays will demonstrate behaviors consistent with the situation and their developmental age. When pain is well controlled, pain behaviors alleviate or resolve and patients appear relaxed, calmer, and are able to participate in daily activities. Participation in required activities of recovery is facilitated.

Failure to respond to a patient's self-report of pain may encourage the development of learned pain behaviors. Patients who come to understand that unless they appear to be uncomfortable their reports of pain will not be believed may purposefully demonstrate behaviors consistent with pain when clinicians are present (McCaffery & Pasero, 1999).

Pain Measurement and Assessment

Failure to measure and assess pain has long been recognized as a barrier to appropriate pain management. It is essential for nurses and all health care team members to understand the significance of assessing and providing effective pain management. To emphasize this point, the American Pain Society launched a campaign in the late 1990s to increase awareness of the importance of the assessment of pain intensity. The statement "Pain is the fifth vital sign" was designed to encourage health care providers and organizations to consider the assessment of pain just as essential as the assessment of the patient's temperature, pulse, blood pressure, and respiratory rate. Pain assessment should be incorporated into routine vital sign assessments (Campbell, 1995).

Not only is it important to regularly assess pain, it is important to assess it correctly and thoroughly to create a pain management plan tailored to meet the individual needs of the patient. Those needs must be based on a unidimensional measurement of pain intensity in addition to the complete assessment of the multidimensional experience of pain.

Assessment and measurement tools have evolved during the past decade such that multiple tools are now available to meet the specific needs of patients with different disease states, ages and developmental stages, and cognitive abilities. Depending on the patient's needs, any one of the tools may be appropriate in a given situation. Regardless of the tool selected, patients should be educated in its use, and the same tool should be used consistently to encourage accurate trending of changes, to facilitate familiarity with the tool, and to ultimately increase the ease of use. Because these tools rely on the patient's ability to understand how to use them properly, patients who speak a language other than that of the health care team should be provided a tool with numbers and descriptors written in their own language to prevent misunderstandings due to language barriers. Whether patients have unique needs or not, assessment tools should always be validated by research and found reliable in the patient population where they will be used. Additionally, tools that are easy for the nurse and the patient to use and document will be more likely to be used routinely.

At times, nurses express frustration over the inability to verify the accuracy of the patient's self-report of pain intensity. Although most patients with pain will not attempt to lie or deceive, some patients will. Regardless, clinicians are required to accept the patient's report of pain (APS, 2003). However, accepting does not require believing. When there is doubt regarding the truthfulness of a patient's response, it is important to recognize that potential of accepting a false report of pain, and responding to that report with an appropriate intervention is justified by the importance of accepting the many reports of pain that are valid and truthful (Pasero & McCaffery, 2001b). Nurses must value the fact that the patient is the only one who

can identify the intensity of pain. Examples of unidimensional tools used to measure pain intensity include the numeric rating scale, the simple verbal descriptive scale, and the visual analog scale (see Chart 15–3, p. 337).

Unidimensional Measurement Tools

Unidimensional measurement tools are used to measure only one component of the pain assessment. The unidimensional measurement of pain is an incomplete assessment if the remaining multidimensional aspects of pain are not evaluated. In most cases, unidimensional tools are used to determine the patient's self-report of the intensity or severity of pain.

Numeric Rating Scale

The **numeric rating scale** (**NRS**) is a horizontal line with numbers from 0 to 10 ranging from left to right (see Chart 15–3, p. 337). Three interval descriptors of pain are located along the scale: "No Pain," "Moderate Pain," and "Worst Pain." Once a patient is instructed on how to use the scale, it is relatively easy to use and assessment can be completed within a few minutes, making it easy for the both the patient and the clinician to use, document, and trend.

Simple Verbal Descriptive Scale

The **simple verbal descriptive scale** (**SVDS**) also uses a horizontal line with numbers from 0 to 10 ranging from left to right. However, interval descriptors of "No Pain," "Mild," "Discomforting," "Distressing," "Horrible," or "Excruciating" pain provide the patient with a few more descriptive options. As with the NRS, this scale is relatively quick and easy for both the patient and the clinician to use.

Visual Analog Scale

The **visual analog scale** (**VAS**) does not have numeric intervals; rather it uses "No Pain" and "Pain as Bad as It Can Possibly Be" as descriptors at either end of a horizontal line measuring 10 centimeters in length. Each centimeter on the scale corresponds to a number from 0 to 10. The patient is instructed to draw a vertical line through the scale to indicate the intensity of their pain. Although this scale is relatively easy for the patient to use, it requires measurement from the start of the scale to the point where the vertical line is drawn to determine the 0 to 10 score. This makes the scale less useful to a busy clinician.

Behavioral Assessment

When patients are unable to provide a self-report of pain intensity, behavioral assessment tools can be used to guide observation for pain-related behaviors. This type of unidimensional tool, often validated for use with preverbal pediatric patients, should be used with caution in adults since pain-related behaviors may be inconsistent (either over- or underemphasized) with actual pain. With the behavioral assessment, the nurse must make an observational judgment that may lead to undermanagement of pain (AHCPR, 1992; APS, 2003).

Patients who are critically ill represent a large population of nonverbal patients. This puts this population at considerable risk for unrelieved pain. One of the primary reasons for inadequate pain relief is the lack of an appropriate pain relief assessment for nonverbal patients (Puntillo, 2007). Nursing researchers are currently studying ways to measure pain in this population (Gelinas, Fortier, Viens, Fillion, & Puntillo, 2004; Puntillo et al., 2004). Pain behaviors in the acutely/critically ill population noted during common painful procedures such as dressing changes included grimacing, rigidity, wincing, shutting of eyes, moaning, verbalization, and clenching of fists.

To date no valid standardized assessment tool exists for use in all populations of critically ill patients. A Critical-Care Pain Observation Tool (CPOT) has been researched and validated in cardiac patients who are critically ill, and it is hoped that this tool and other tools can be further validated in other critically ill populations in the future (Gelinas, Fillion, Puntillo, Viens, & Fortier, 2006). For now, though, nurses need to be aware of the common manifestations of pain in this population in order to assess a patient's specific response. Pasero & McCaffery (2005) recommend the following guidelines for individual nonverbal patient assessment:

- On admission, document reason self-report cannot be used for pain assessment.
- Document underlying conditions, such as chronic pain condition or trauma, as well as any painful activities such as physical therapy and turning.
- Look for individual behaviors that indicate pain.
- Ask caregivers, family, and significant others about behaviors that indicate pain.
- Draw a conclusion about the patient's pain based on the preceding information.
- Devise a pain management plan.
- Initiate an analgesic trial.
- Evaluate response to analgesics.
- Make appropriate adjustments.

Multidimensional Assessment and Measurement Tools

Multidimensional assessment and measurement tools such as the patient interview, the **McGill Pain Questionnaire (MPQ)**, and the **Brief Pain Inventory (BPI)** assess more than one dimension of pain. The MPQ provides 20 sets of words patients can use to describe pain, and scores the responses. Each set of words varies in intensity and measures either the sensory or affective dimension of pain. One set scores the intensity of pain. Patients document the location of pain on a body diagram provided as part of the questionnaire.

The BPI asks multiple questions regarding pain and its impact on patient function and addresses the multidimensionality of the pain experience. Depending on the situation, these tools have advantages and disadvantages that may make them more useful or inappropriate. Most of these tools require the patient to have the cognitive ability to complete the tool, not to mention the time. These two requirements make some of the tools difficult for both the patient and busy nurses to use routinely. However, when pain management is complex, the time spent completing a multidimensional tool can be invaluable.

Patient Interview

The patient interview is the most commonly used multidimensional tool in nursing practice. A unidimensional tool is usually used in addition to the interview questions to determine pain intensity. However, the patient interview can also be combined with any multidimensional tool when appropriate. Prior to conducting an interview, the nurse should review the patient's medical history. Components of the patient's history that are specifically useful in the assessment of pain include:

- Previous experiences with pain including trauma, surgery, or chronic pain
- Medications taken previously or currently to relieve pain
- Significant social history including drug, alcohol, or tobacco abuse
- Comorbid conditions, such as renal insufficiency, pulmonary disease, or hepatic dysfunction, that should be considered when administering analgesics.

During the patient interview, the nurse's demeanor should be supportive and interested. Allow sufficient time for the patient to answer the questions. Patients experiencing moderate to severe pain may have difficulty answering questions. Every effort should be made to make the patient as comfortable as possible before the interview takes place. Interview questions may include the following:

- Where are you having pain?
- Are you having pain anywhere else?
- How intense is the pain?
- What does the pain feel like?
- When did the pain begin?
- How long does the pain last?
- What makes the pain worse?
- Have you had this type of pain before?
- How does your pain affect your daily activities, sleep, mood, and relationships?
- What do you do to reduce the pain?

When asking questions that require the use of an assessment tool, the nurse should first assess the patient's ability to use and understand the tool. Once an appropriate tool has been selected, all members of the health care team should use that same tool consistently to improve the patient's ability to provide self-reports of the details concerning her pain experience.

Location of Pain

Patients may have pain in more than one location due to radiation of the pain, metastases of carcinoma, or multiple injuries, as is often the case with traumatic injuries. Each location of pain may have different characteristics. Unless encouraged to discuss all locations, the patient may not offer this information.

Assist the patient to identify each location of pain. The nurse should then ask all of the interview questions about each location. This will encourage patients to identify sources of pain that may be impacting their level of comfort, but that may be unrelated to the reason they are seeking medical assistance. Locations of pain can be reported verbally or by using a pain assessment tool such as the MPQ as described earlier.

Duration and Pattern of Pain

Pain can be persistent or intermittent. It can occur in a sudden flare of breakthrough pain that resolves quickly, or it may flare and linger, resolving after a period of time, as is the case with recurrent pain. Analgesic medication formulations are becoming more sophisticated and are designed to address the specific durations and patterns of pain. Complementary or alternative treatments may be better suited to relieving pain that is mild in intensity and short in duration. An appropriate treatment plan requires that a thorough assessment of the duration and pattern of the pain be elicited. The nurse can help the patient provide this information by asking the following questions:

- Do you have pain for most of the day and night?
- Does the pain come and go or is it constant?
- Do you have sudden episodes of severe pain that occur without warning or that happen with certain activities?

Pain Intensity

The patient should be instructed in the use of the pain intensity tool. The tool that is used in the assessment should be one that the patient understands and can easily use. The intensity of pain is not generally static regardless of whether the pain is acute or chronic, so a score should be obtained for the least intense pain (usually at rest), the most intense pain (usually with activity), and with sudden flares of breakthrough pain. The nurse can elicit this information with the following questions:

- What is your pain score when you are having the least amount of pain?
- What is your pain score when you are having the most pain?
- Do you have sudden episodes of moderate to severe pain?
- If so, what is your pain score during these episodes?

This level of detail discourages patients from averaging their pain intensity scores to achieve one score that will not provide the information necessary to individualize the treatment plan. More aggressive treatment should be provided during times when pain is the most intense and in anticipation of breakthrough pain episodes. The assessment and reassessment of pain intensity needs to be documented before and after pain interventions to evaluate the effectiveness of pain treatments and to provide trends that will direct adjustments to the pain treatment plan.

Character of Pain

The character of the pain provides clues as to the source of the pain and may indicate which analgesic medication should be used to provide relief. When asked to describe their pain, patients generally use similar terms such as *aching, dull, sharp, stabbing, knife-like, electrical, shooting,* and *burning.* Neuropathic pain is often described as *tingling, shooting, electric,* or *shock-like* and requires different treatments than nociceptive pain, which may be reported as *sharp, stabbing, cutting,* or *throbbing.* As mentioned, the character of the pain may give a clue to its cause. For example, the pain of angina is rarely described as sharp; instead it is described as crushing, pressure, like "an elephant is sitting on my chest." Therefore, if a patient complains of sharp chest pain, the nurse knows to assess for causes other than cardiac ischemia.

Occasionally patients have difficulty describing their pain. They may say "It just hurts." If patients are reluctant to report the characteristic of their pain, the nurse should explain the importance of this information in selecting the medications to be used to treat the pain. For example, incisional pain, cardiac-related chest pain, and neuropathic pain are different in etiology and in treatment. Patients who understand that only *they* can provide this information and that it will be used when determining their treatment are often more willing to try to provide a description of their pain. Provide a few descriptors to give the patient an example of what is needed: Is it sharp, stabbing, burning, sharp-shooting, tight, or pressure pain? Be sure to select a variety of descriptors so that patients can choose one that best represents their pain or can think of one of their own.

Exacerbation of Pain

Assist the patient to identify circumstances when the pain is more intense. Common recovery activities after surgery such as getting in and out of bed, coughing, and walking in the halls may be mentioned. Patients with chronic pain may experience exacerbation of pain with activities of daily living (ADLs). The nurse may help the patient provide information about exacerbation of pain by asking the following questions:

- What do you do that makes your pain more intense?
- What do your doctors and nurses do to you that increases your pain?

When it is known that specific activities or procedures exacerbate pain, the nurse should provide pain treatments prior to the painful event to facilitate the ability to do ADLs, participate in physical therapy, and tolerate medical procedures. If the exacerbation of pain is associated with new pain of a different intensity, location, or character, it may indicate that there is a complication such as infection, that disease is progressing, or that there is a surgical complication. Sudden onset of new pain should be considered an emergency, evaluated, and reported to the health care provider or independent licensed practitioner.

Pain Relief

Encourage the patient to report all nonmedication and medication methods they currently or previously used to relieve the pain. The pain treatment plan should include the patient's preferred methods and medications, whenever it is appropriate. This is especially true when the patient has chronic pain and has a well-established pain management plan that has been effective in relieving their pain. It is important to be specific when questioning the patient to ensure that information about prescription and nonprescription medications is elicited. In addition, the patient should be asked specifically about herbal or dietary supplements so that potential medication interactions can be identified. Sensitive subjects such as abuse of alcohol, prescription medications, or illicit drugs should be approached after developing a rapport with the patient; thus, questions about medications are usually saved until the end of the interview. The nurse should use a nonjudgmental and direct approach and reassure the patient and family that the information they provide will be considered when selecting medications and dosages for the pain treatment plan. The following are examples of questions that can be used to encourage the patient to discuss these sensitive subjects:

- Do you take any pain medications that you can buy without a prescription (e.g., acetaminophen, nonsteroidal anti-inflammatory drugs [NSAIDS])?

- Do you take any pain medications that you buy from the pharmacy with a prescription?

- Do you take any herbal or dietary supplements to relieve your pain?

- Do you drink alcohol daily, weekly, monthly? Do you ever take your pain medications when you are drinking alcohol?

- Have you ever or are you now taking illegal drugs to relieve your pain?

- Have you ever been involved in a drug treatment or methadone program?

- Do you have any concerns regarding addiction?

Impact on Quality of Life and Function

During the interview, observation of the patient and attention to the patient's responses provide information regarding the affective, cognitive, and behavioral dimensions of pain. Observe for expressions of hope or optimism that the pain can be relieved as opposed to hopelessness, helplessness, or even expression of suicidal ideations. Patients may be calm and cooperative or angry, frustrated, anxious, and focused on placing blame. Be watchful for information to be gained from the responses of family members regarding the impact of pain in their personal relationships and the patient's quality of life. Use interviewing techniques such as open-ended questions to encourage the patient and family members to share details about pain and the role it plays in their lives. Patients and family members are observant of the general demeanor of the interviewer and will respond based on the perception that the interviewer is caring and concerned and has time to listen or that time is limited and questions are asked for the purpose of documentation rather than for use in determining a plan for care.

Multidimensional Assessment of At-Risk Patients

Factors such as developmental delays, cognitive impairment, severe emotional disturbance, and critical illness may render patients incapable of providing an accurate report of pain intensity and preclude participation in the patient interview (Puntillo, 2007). Patients who are unable to provide a self-report of pain intensity are at risk for undermanagement of pain (APS, 2003; Herr et al., 2006; Puntillo, 2007). Nurses should take care to avoid erroneously concluding that a patient cannot provide a self-report. Studies have demonstrated that patients with mild to moderate cognitive impairment are able to provide a self-report using unidimensional measurement tools and short versions of some multidimensional assessment tools (Soscia, 2003). Pasero and McCaffery (2000) suggest that five factors be considered to ensure that the patients who are at risk of poor pain management are appropriately managed and plans for pain management care reflect the individual patient's special needs. Chart 15–4 provides steps for assessing patients at risk.

Documentation of Pain Assessment

As the health care team member most likely to spend the greatest amount of time with the patient and family, nurses are pivotal in the appropriate management of pain (McCaffery, Ferrell, & Pasero, 2000). Documentation of assessment findings is a vital part of the patient's medical record. Nurse documentation is

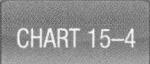

CHART 15–4 **Five Assessment Steps for At-Risk Patients**

1. Be sure that the patient is unable to self-report pain.
2. Consider pathologic conditions and procedures known to be painful.
3. Observe for behaviors consistent with pain.
4. Use a proxy pain rating from close family members or caregivers.
5. Consider physiological measures as a last resort.

Source: Pasero, C., & McCaffery, M. (2000). When patients can't report pain. *American Journal of Nursing, 100,* 22–23.

reviewed by many members of the multidisciplinary team and provides detail that team members may not have had an opportunity to elicit. It is important that details about the pain assessment, treatments, and the patient's response to treatments are accurately and completely documented on the medical record so that decisions regarding the plan of care are made with consideration of the information the nurse has compiled.

Whether recorded on a paper flow sheet, in an electronic medical record (EMR), or written in narrative, the nurse's documentation of pain assessment and measurement creates a baseline by which improvement or negative trends are measured (Campbell, 2006). The Joint Commission standards on pain management require that health care organizations have policies regarding the assessment and management of pain. The nurse must know and understand the contents of policies specific to their workplace, and the nursing documentation should reflect that nursing care was given according to institutional policy.

 Nursing documentation in the legal medical record should reflect topics such as these:

1. *Pain management that was delivered following institutional policy, with consideration of the patient assessment and responses to treatments, and utilizing ordered interventions*

2. *Responses to unrelieved pain, including administration of additional analgesic medications; use of nonmedication treatments; and health care provider or licensed independent practitioner contact and subsequent changes to the patient's pain management plan of care*

3. *The avoidance of labels such as psychotic, whiner, drug seeking, or addict.*

Pain Management

In 1992, the Agency for Health Care Policy and Research (AHCPR) published the first edition of the *Clinical Practice Guideline for Acute Pain Management: Operative or Medical Procedures and Trauma.* A panel of experts completed an exhaustive literature review to establish evidence-based guidelines, and where no evidence was available, best practices were determined (AHCPR, 1992). In 1994, AHCPR published the first edition of the *Clinical Practice Guideline for Management of Cancer Pain* using the same model and goals (Jacox et al., 1994). Nearly a decade later, pain management had not improved significantly. In response, the Joint Commission released new standards on pain management in 1999. These standards are based on the same valid recommendations published in the AHCPR guidelines of 1992 and 1994 and require health care organizations to implement a multidisciplinary team and create an institutional commitment to pain management (Joint Commission, 2002).

Rather than becoming discouraged by the lack of improvement in pain management over the years, nurses are beginning to embrace the potential for improvement by researching the knowledge of student nurses and the relationship between nurses' knowledge and patient outcomes, determining appropriate curriculum components for pain management education in nursing schools, and outlining competency guidelines (Chiu, Trinca, Lim, & Tuazon, 2003; IASP, 1993; Watt-Watson, Stevens, Garfinkel, Streiner, & Gallop, 2001; Wisconsin Cancer Pain Initiative Nursing Education Committee, 1995). However, in spite of these efforts, nursing knowledge and the reported comfort and amount of medication their patients receive continue to be at odds (Watt-Watson et al., 2001). Now is the time for nurses to take the lead professionally by demanding that comprehensive pain management education be provided during professional preparation. Nurses are necessary to the successful implementation of evidence-based pain management practices. In addition, until nurses begin to support improved competency of all health care team members, patients will continue to experience unrelieved pain in spite of the fact that pain can be relieved. Patients with pain must be able to rely on nurses to be knowledgeable regarding pain management principles and practices, professional in the application of pain-relieving treatments, and to advocate on behalf of their patients. No patient should look to the nurse as one of the reasons for his or her unrelieved pain. Management of pain at the end of life is discussed in depth in Chapter 17 🔗.

Acute Pain Management Therapeutic Goals

Acute pain is often the result of surgical procedures, trauma, or burns. Acute pain problems are the most common reason why patients seek medical assistance, and nurses spend a significant portion of their time at the bedside providing pain-relieving treatments and medications (Coda & Bonica, 2001). The plan for pain management provides for organized and rational treatment appropriate to all phases of recovery including the critical or emergent phase, subsequent healing and recovery, and finally rehabilitation.

Management of acute pain is focused on (1) reducing the sympathetic stress response, (2) safely optimizing comfort during treatment and recovery, (3) facilitating participation in recovery and rehabilitation activities, and (4) improving patient outcomes. Nurses educate patients and family members with the goal of improving their understanding of (1) the importance of pain management in the patient's recovery, (2) the role of medications and nonmedication treatment, and (3) the differences between physical dependence, tolerance, and addiction to opioid medications. Establishing comfort and function goals encourages the patient and health care team to work toward meeting a defined pain intensity score and a specific functional goal rather than an elusive or poorly defined therapeutic goal. For example, the patient with acute pain might select a pain intensity score of 3 from the 0–10 NRS and the goal of ambulating three times daily as a postoperative recovery activity.

Chronic Pain Management Therapeutic Goals

The long-term, persistent nature of chronic pain increases the likelihood that psychosocial and environmental factors will contribute to the emotional distress and physical disability that is frequently seen with pain that has limited ongoing pathology. Management of chronic pain is focused on (1) reducing the focus on pain; (2) safely optimizing comfort through appropriate use of analgesic treatments and complementary or alternative strategies; (3) increasing active participation in ADLs, work, and relationships; and (4) restoration of joy and a sense of purpose despite persistent pain (Arnstein, 2003). Nurses educate patients and family members with the goal of improving understanding of (1) the role anxiety, depression, and anger can have in escalation of pain; (2) the role of medications and complementary or alternative treatments in improving function; and (3) the differences between physical dependence, tolerance, and addiction to opioid medications.

When encouraging the patient with chronic pain to establish comfort and function goals, the process is the same as with acute pain, but the scores and functional goals are likely to be very different. Patients who experience moderate to severe pain on a daily basis may consider even a very small reduction in pain intensity as a success. Often functional goals are focused around achieving or maintaining independence in ADLs, work, or relationships and leisure activities. It may be necessary to encourage the patient to identify realistically achievable goals as an intermediate step to his ultimate goals to avoid discouragement.

Cancer Pain Management Therapeutic Goals

The management of cancer pain is a combination of the acute and chronic pain therapeutic goals mentioned previously. Given the dual nature of cancer pain, it is appropriate to have goals that address healing, recovery, and finally rehabilitation for the acute pain associated with surgery and cancer treatments. However, it is also appropriate to consider the role that a potentially lethal diagnosis has on increasing the likelihood of emotional distress and physical disability that is frequently seen with the pain of malignancy. Management of cancer pain is focused on (1) reducing the sympathetic stress response following surgeries or treatments; (2) safely optimizing comfort through appropriate use of analgesic treatments and complementary or alternative strategies; (3) facilitating participation in recovery and rehabilitation activities; (4) increasing active participation in ADLs, work, and relationships; and (5) preservation of a sense of purpose despite a potentially lethal diagnosis.

Nurses educate patients and family members with the goal of improving understanding of (1) the role that anxiety, depression, and anger can have in escalation of pain; (2) the role of medications and complementary or alternative treatments in improving function; and (3) the differences between physical dependence, tolerance, and addiction to opioid medications. When encouraging the patient with cancer pain to establish a comfort and function goal, the process is the same as with acute and chronic pain. Often functional goals are focused around achieving or maintaining independence in daily activities. As with acute and chronic pain, the comfort and function goals should guide the treatment plan. An in-depth discussion of the diagnosis and treatment of cancer is included in Chapter 64 ⊘.

Pharmacologic Strategies

In pain management pharmacology, the multidisciplinary team focus is on establishing a regimen that includes a balance of nonopioid, nonsteroidal anti-inflammatory, adjuvant, and opioid medications whenever possible to optimize the quality of analgesia with minimal medication side effects. This method of managing pain is often referred to as *balanced* or *multimodal analgesia*. The pharmacologic pain management plan is accomplished through the combined efforts of multiple disciplines. The selection of medications requires that the health care provider consider the patient's medical history, including previous and current pain, and the findings of the patient interview and pain assessment as previously discussed. Treatment plans crafted in the absence of this information are often unsuccessful in relieving pain or alternatively more likely to cause adverse effects and potentially patient harm.

Nurses are central to the effectiveness and safety of medication administration with multiple responsibilities at every stage of the prescription process. Prescriptions must be reviewed on the medical record and considered for their appropriateness based on the patient assessment and relevant laboratory studies. If there are questions regarding the prescription, the prescribing health care provider must be contacted for clarification. When it is time to administer the medication, rigorous double checks are completed to ensure the correct prescription is administered to the patient.

Pharmacologic Interventions

When discussing pharmacologic interventions, it is necessary to consider the patient's physiological status in relationship to the pharmacology of each medication that is selected including how it is absorbed, distributed, metabolized or biotransformed, and eventually excreted. In addition, the mechanism of action and therapeutic and adverse effects of each medication should guide the medication selection and monitoring that will be necessary to ensure the patient's safety.

Absorption describes the process by which the medication leaves the site of administration to cross membranes as it journeys to the site of action (Youngkin, Sawin, Kissinger, & Israel, 2005). For example, medications that are administered into the gastrointestinal system absorb from the stomach, small intestine, large intestine, colon, and even the rectum into the systemic circulation for distribution. In contrast, medications that are administered directly into the systemic circulation bypass the absorptive process and are immediately distributed (Youngkin et al., 2005).

Distribution refers to the process of moving the medication into the bloodstream, the extracellular, and the intracellular compartments, as well as in the compartment that is the site of absorption and storage (Youngkin, Sawin, Kissinger, & Israel et al., 2005). Factors that will effect the distribution of a medication are the size of the molecule, the degree to which it binds to protein, and the solubility of the medication. Large molecules and those that bind to protein usually stay in the bloodstream. Hydrophilic drugs, like morphine, are more slowly distributed

in both the bloodstream and the extracellular compartments. Lipid-soluble medications, like fentanyl, are more rapidly absorbed and distributed throughout all three compartments (Miyoshi & Leckband, 2001).

Biotransformation or **metabolism** describes the process of changing a medication's structure in preparation for elimination (Youngkin et al., 2005). Metabolism occurs primarily in the liver, but also the kidneys, and to a very small degree in other organ systems. Once a medication has metabolized, it is no longer the same and effectively discontinues its pharmacologic activity. **Hepatic first-pass metabolism** refers to the reduction of the medication's effect due to partial metabolism in the liver prior to distribution to the ultimate site of action. Medications may produce active metabolites that then exert a pharmacologic action of their own. This is of particular concern when the metabolite has significant adverse effects.

Elimination is the process of excretion from the body and is generally accomplished in the renal system (Youngkin et al., 2005). Elimination can occur after a medication has metabolized or the medication may be eliminated in its primary form. Alterations in the renal system that impair elimination result in prolonging the effects of the primary medication and any metabolites that have been formed, potentially increasing the risks of adverse effects.

Classifying Analgesics

The three-step analgesic ladder designed by the World Health Organization (WHO) outlines recommendations for classes of analgesic medications that would be appropriate for treating mild, moderate, and severe pain (Bajwa, Warfield, & Wootton, 2006; Jacox et al., 1994). Figure 15–1 ■ illustrates the WHO three-step analgesic ladder. This ladder provides a stepped approach based on pain severity. For example, step 1 analgesics include acetaminophen or an NSAID. If the pain persists or worsens despite appropriate dose increases of step 1 drugs, a change to a step 2 or step 3 analgesic is indicated. If the patient presents with moderate to severe pain, step 1 can be skipped (National Cancer Institute, 2007).

It is reasonable to choose the step that most closely describes the patient's pain intensity as a guide in determining a pain

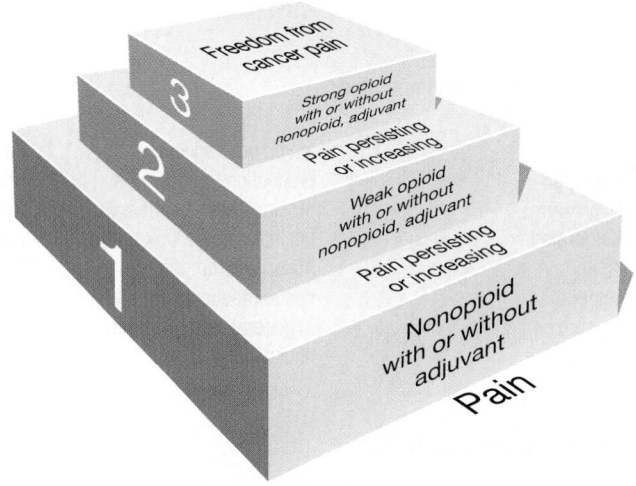

FIGURE 15–1 ■ World Health Organization three-step analgesic ladder.

treatment plan that would provide the best level of analgesia with the fewest potential adverse effects. The steps on the analgesic ladder are additive, meaning as one progresses up the ladder, more medications are added to those already in use to achieve improved analgesia than would be possible with a single medication for a balanced or multimodal approach to pain management. It is important to recognize that when pain is severe, the appropriate step on the analgesic ladder would be at the top and movement through each step to reach the top is not necessary. This method of medication selection has been proven effective in acute, chronic, and cancer pain management. Nurses are vital to the medication administration and monitoring process and so must understand the basic mechanism of action, pharmacology, and adverse effects of each group of medications to function effectively in their role.

Acetaminophen

Acetaminophen is one of the most widely used analgesic medications and is considered a first-line analgesic for treating mild acute and chronic pain (Smith, 2003). It is the first step in the

WHO three-step approach to pain management (APS, 2003; Jacox et al., 1994; Smith, 2003). It is also included as an important medication in steps 2 and 3. The Pharmacology Summary feature includes an in-depth discussion of acetaminophen.

Nonsteroidal Anti-Inflammatory Drugs

NSAIDS effectively reduce inflammation, pain, and fever. More than 20 different NSAIDS are currently available in the United States, and they are one of the most commonly used classes of drugs in the world (Simon, 2003). At equal doses all NSAIDS are equally effective in relieving pain. However, there is an intrapatient variability in response that warrants trying a different NSAID if the desired effect is not achieved on the current NSAID at the maximum recommended dosage (APS, 2003). NSAIDS, along with acetaminophen, are the first step in the WHO analgesic ladder (see Figure 15–1 ■, p. 343) for mild to moderate pain and should be used in conjunction with acetaminophen and opioids on the second and third steps for moderate to severe pain. The Pharmacology Summary includes an in-depth discussion of NSAIDS.

PHARMACOLOGY Summary of Medications Used for Pain Relief

Medication Category	Action	Application/Indication	Nursing Responsibility
Acetaminophen			
First-line analgesic for treating mild acute and chronic pain. Available over the counter in a variety of formulations including liquid, tablets, capsules, caplets, and rectal suppository. Is found in combination with many medications such as the opioids Lortab and Percocet.	Specific action is unclear; thought to be inhibition of the third isoform of the cyclooxygenase (COX-3) pathway only found in the CNS. Absorbed rapidly from the gastrointestinal tract, and its low molecular weight permits easy penetration of the spinal tissues (Smith, 2003).	The first step in the WHO three-step analgesic ladder approach to pain management and included in steps 2 and 3 (see Figure 15–1 ■, p. 343). Used in addition to anti-inflammatory medications, opioids, and adjuvants in the analgesic treatment plan unless contraindicated.	Used with caution in patients who have been fasting for prolonged periods of time or who drink more that three alcoholic beverages per day. The Food and Drug Administration (FDA) now requires acetaminophen to be labeled with warnings for the patient who consumes alcohol on a daily basis and includes cautions for all patients to avoid exceeding eight tablets of 500 mg or a total of 4,000 mg total in 24 hours (Karch & Karch, 2003). Monitor liver function studies. Patients must be educated about potential side effects of overdose to prevent overdose and liver damage.
Nonsteroidal Anti-Inflammatory Drugs (NSAIDS)			
Aspirin Ibuprofen Naproxen Ketoprofen Advil Feldene Celebrex Indocin Motrin Relafen Toradol (only injectable NSAID)	Inhibit prostaglandin production, primarily the prostaglandin E series, via inhibition of the COX enzymes. Absorbed from the gastrointestinal tract and are, in general, highly protein bound.	First step in the WHO three-step analgesic ladder approach to pain (see Figure 15–1). Used alone for mild to moderate pain. Used in conjunction with acetaminophen and opioids on the second and third steps for moderate to severe pain. Aspirin inhibits platelet aggregation for the life of the platelet, therefore, making it useful for preventing thromboembolic events.	Assess character, duration, and intensity of pain prior to administration to determine baseline for effectiveness. Monitor for gastric pain, bleeding, and acute renal failure. Monitor BUN, ALT, AST, creatinine, and hemoglobin before and during continued use. Should be discontinued for several days to 1–2 weeks, if taking aspirin, before surgery or invasive procedures to reduce the risk of bleeding. When using NSAIDS in combination with opioids, frequently the dose of the opioid can be reduced (Bajwa et al., 2006).

PHARMACOLOGY Summary of Medications Used for Pain Relief—*Continued*

Medication Category	Action	Application/Indication	Nursing Responsibility
Opioids			
Codeine Dihydrocodeine Hydrocodone Propoxyphene Oxycodone Morphine Methadone Levorphanol Fentanyl Hydromorphone Meperidine	A natural or synthetic morphine-like substance. Produce their pharmacologic effects and side effects by binding to opioid receptor cells throughout the CNS and peripheral tissues. There are three types of opioid receptors: mu, kappa, and delta. When the mu receptor is stimulated, analgesia, euphoria, reduced gastric motility, sedation, nausea, tolerance, and physical dependence occur.	Third step in the WHO three-step analgesic ladder (see Figure 15–1 ■, p. 343). Symptomatic control of moderate to severe pain and as preanesthetic medication.	Assess character, duration, and intensity of pain prior to administration to determine baseline for effectiveness. Monitor vital signs before and during treatment. Do not administer opioids if the respiratory rate is less than 12 per minute. Monitor level of consciousness and respiratory rate and depth after administration. Obtain allergy history and current and prior drug use. Monitor liver function tests. Document bowel movements. Administer antihistamines (pruritus) and antiemetics (nausea) as ordered. Have a narcotic antagonist (Narcan) readily available if respirations fall below 10 per minute. Monitor urinary output for urinary retention.
Anticonvulsants			
Gabapentin Carbamazepine Phenytoin Diazepam	Limits aberrant nerve firing, leading to neural membrane stabilization.	Neuropathic pain syndrome that is shooting or electrical in nature.	Assess character, duration, and intensity of pain prior to administration to determine baseline for effectiveness. Assess for alteration in vision, concentration, and coordination.
Antidepressants			
Elavil Asendin Tofranil Pamelor Venlafaxine Trazodone Doxepin Amitriptyline Imipramine Venlafaxine	Precise mechanism of analgesic effect unknown. Thought to inhibit the reuptake of serotonin and norepinephrine involved in the descending inhibitory pain pathway. Enhanced endorphin secretion, sodium channel blockade inhibition of substance P, a neuropeptide involved in both pain and depression. Doses for pain relief are lower than doses for depression.	Chronic pain, cancer pain, fibromyalgia, tension migraine headaches, postherpetic neuralgia, diabetic neuropathy, arthritis, low back pain. Most effective in treating burning neuropathic pain.	Assess character, duration, and intensity of pain prior to administration to determine baseline for effectiveness. Monitor for nausea and dry mouth. Gum will help with the dry mouth. Patient education includes time of onset (tricyclics take several weeks to achieve therapeutic effect). Monitor patient for oversedation and insomnia. Educate patient not to discontinue use abruptly. Monitor for orthostatic hypotension. Instruct patient not to rise suddenly from a lying position.
Glucocorticoids			
	Exert anti-inflammatory properties through inhibiting leukotriene and prostaglandin synthesis.	Nerve compression pain, chronic pain.	Assess character, duration, and intensity of pain prior to administration to determine baseline for effectiveness. Due to the impact on certain conditions, prior to therapy the patient needs to be assessed for infection, osteoporosis, diabetes, heart failure, hypertension, and renal disease. Instruct patient to take medication with food and water to prevent gastric irritation. Do not discontinue drug abruptly; therapy needs to be tapered off.

Sources: Adams, M. P., Josephson, D. L., & Holland, L. N. (2005). *Pharmacology for nurses: A pathophysiological approach.* Upper Saddle River, NJ: Pearson Prentice Hall; American Pain Society (APS). (2003). *Principles of analgesic use in the treatment of acute pain and cancer pain* (5th ed.). Glenview, IL: Author; Chandrasekharan, N., Dai, H., Roos, K., Evanson, N., Tomsik, J., Elton, T., et al. (2002). Cox-3, a cyclooxygenase-1 variant inhibited by acetaminophen and other analgesic/antipyretic drugs: Cloning, structure, and expression. *Proceedings of the National Academy of Sciences, 99,* 13926–13931; MacDonald, T., & Wei, L. (2003). Effect of ibuprofen on cardioprotective effect of aspirin. *Lancet, 36,* 542–544; McCaffery, M., & Portenoy, R. K. (1999). Nonopioids. In M. McCaffery & C. Pasero (Eds.), *Pain: Clinical manual* (2nd ed., pp. 129–160). St. Louis, MO: Mosby; Simon, L. S. (2003). Nonsteroidal anti-inflammatory drugs and cyclooxygenase-2 selective inhibitors. In H. S. Smith (Ed.), *Drugs for pain* (pp. 41–54). Philadelphia: Hanley & Belfus; Youngkin, E. Q., Sawin, K. J., Kissinger, J. F., & Israel, D. S. (2005). *Pharmacotherapeutics: A primary care guide* (2nd ed.). Upper Saddle River, NJ: Pearson Prentice Hall.

Opioids

Opioids have long been recognized for their role in relieving pain (Bajwa et al., 2006). The earliest accounts of opioid use date back to the ancient Mesopotamia in Asia Minor in 3500 B.C., where opium was referred to as the *hul gil* or the *joy plant* (Maher & Chaiyakul, 2003). In 1806, Serturner, a German pharmacist, first isolated morphine from the opium extract and named it *morphine* after the god of dreams, Morpheus (Maher & Chaiyakul, 2003). Opioids, morphine-like medications, play a major role in current-day management of moderate to severe pain for acute, cancer, and in certain situations chronic pain. As with all of the analgesic medications, opioids should only be initiated after an assessment of the patient's pain in conjunction with the significant findings of the medical history and physical exam (APS, 2003).

Opioids should be added to nonopioids, NSAIDS, and adjuvants for pain that is not responsive to these analgesics alone (APS, 2003). Unlike acetaminophen and NSAIDS, opioids do not have a ceiling effect and unless combined with acetaminophen or an NSAID (e.g., Lortab, Percocet, Vicoprofen), an opioid dosage can be escalated as needed to relieve pain. The analgesia achieved by opioid administration is dose dependant

and with the appropriate dosing, opioids can usually relieve all intensities of pain (Miyoshi & Leckband, 2001). There is, however, a wide variation in the dosages required by individual patients to achieve pain relief. It is unrealistic to expect the same dose of opioid to be safe and effective for all patients. Opioid dosages should be increased or decreased incrementally to achieve the best level of pain relief with the lowest incidence of opioid-induced side effects.

Major barriers to the effective use of opioid medications are usually centered on misunderstandings regarding tolerance and physical dependence and on unfounded concerns that addiction is inevitable. Opioids require a prescription and are regulated by the Drug Enforcement Administration (DEA) to reduce the risk of abuse and diversion. The challenge of finding a balance between this risk and the need for appropriate management of pain with opioids is an additional barrier. It is of concern that the most significant barriers to effective pain relief using opioid analgesics are not complicated pharmacology or lack of good medications, but bias, regulatory scrutiny, and lack of education (Miyoshi & Leckband, 2001). Discussion of opioid tolerance, physical dependence, addiction, and pseudoaddiction is provided in Chart 15–5.

CHART 15–5   Opioid Tolerance, Dependence, and Addiction

One of the most significant barriers to pain management is the concern that opioid analgesics will cause addiction. *Opiophobia* (Morgan, 1985) is the term that is frequently used to describe the fears that health care providers and patients share: that exposure to opioids will cause addictive disease.

When nurses have insufficient knowledge of the risks and realities of addictive disease, unethical clinical practices such as withholding opioids, administering subtherapeutic dosages when therapeutic dosages are prescribed, administering placebos, and withholding compassionate nursing care may become the hallmark of their professional practice. Nurses play a pivotal role in pain management and are recognized as patient advocates whose professional practice should be based on scientific understanding of addictive disease. They must recognize the important role of opioid therapy in pain management and develop the skills necessary to appropriately provide nursing care and education to patients who have fears regarding opioids, who are recovering from opioid addiction, or who have active addictive disease.

Confusion regarding opioid tolerance, physical dependence, and addiction is common. Defining these conditions and then using these definitions consistently in professional and well as patient interactions is the first step.

- *Tolerance* is "a state of adaptation in which exposure to a drug induces changes that result in a diminution of one or more of the drug's effects over time" (American Academy of Pain Medicine [AAPM], American Pain Society [APS], & American Society of Addiction Medicine [ASAM], (2001).

- *Physical dependence* is "adaptation that is manifested by a drug class specific withdrawal syndrome that can be produced by abrupt cessation, rapid dose reduction, decreasing blood level of the drug, and/or administration of an antagonist" (AAPM/APS/ASAM, 2001).

- *Addiction* is "a primary, chronic, neurobiological disease with genetic, psychosocial, and environmental factors influencing its development and manifestations. It is characterized by behaviors that include one or

more of the following: impaired control over drug use, compulsive use, continued use despite harm and craving" (AAPM/APS/ASAM, 2001).

Tolerance, physical dependence, and addiction are individual conditions, but they are often found in combination. *Pseudoaddiction* is a term used to describe the behaviors that can result from undertreatment of pain such as watching the clock, requesting medications more frequently than allowed or in larger doses (drug seeking), and expressing anger or feelings of being unfairly judged. Pseudoaddiction is commonly mistaken for addiction, but unlike addiction, behaviors will resolve when pain is appropriately relieved (Weissman & Haddox, 1989).

The following are suggestions for the nurse to consider when administering opioids for pain management:

- Assume the patient and family members have concerns regarding the risk of addiction and provide education based on scientific evidence to refute misconceptions.

- Manage pain appropriately and advocate for improvement when pain is unrelieved.

- Recognize that an opioid-tolerant patient will require higher dosages of opioid to achieve pain relief and that this does not equal addiction.

- Respond promptly, with respect and compassion, to requests for pain medications for all patients including those with opioid tolerance, dependence, or addiction.

- Avoid personal biases, labeling of patients, or unethical practices.

Opioids that have modified release formulations to make them long acting are not appropriate for prn dosing (APS, 2003). Controlled-release or sustained-release opioids are designed to provide 12 to 24 hours of analgesia (up to 72 hours of analgesia in the case of transdermal fentanyl patches). Many of these opioids take as long as 4 hours to achieve peak effects and last much longer than short-acting opioids, increasing the risk of oversedation and respiratory depression with prn use.

Sources: Bajwa, Z. H., Warfield, C. A., & Wootton, R. J. (2006). *Overview of treatment for chronic pain*, and Passik, S. D., & Kirsh, K. L. (2003). *Pain management and addiction*. Both retrieved February 25, 2007, from UpToDate website: http://utdol.com/utd/store/index.do.

Opioids are available in two major groups, agonists and agonist-antagonists. **Agonist** opioids are often referred to as morphine-like, or mu, agonists because they bind to the mu, kappa, and delta receptors of the cell, which are located in the CNS, peripheral nervous system, and gastrointestinal tract. Agonist opioids include opioids such as morphine, codeine, meperidine, dihydromorphinone, and methadone. **Agonist-antagonist** opioids are kappa and mu receptor partial agonists and are generally considered to be less efficacious than the pure mu agonists. Of note, a ceiling effect on analgesia has been identified with this group of opioids (Miyoshi & Leckband, 2001). Agonist-antagonist opioids include opioids such as buprenorphine, butorphanol, pentazocine, nalbuphine, and dezocine.

Both agonist and agonist-antagonist effects are reversible with the administration of a pure antagonist such as naloxone. **Antagonists** displace and replace the opioid at the receptor re-versing the opioid's pharmacologic effect and side effects such as respiratory depression. The Pharmacology Summary (p. 344) and Chart 15–6 outline essential information about the mechanism of action and side effects of opioids.

Adjuvant Medications

Medications that are traditionally prescribed and administered for reasons other than pain relief are often used in pharmacologic treatment plans for chronic and cancer pain. Although less commonly used in acute pain, these medications may be of benefit in cases of trauma, burns, and some complex acute pain situations. These medications may enhance the effects of the opioids or NSAIDS, provide analgesia on their own, or reduce the side effects of other analgesic medications (APS, 2003). **Adjuvant medications** by definition are not primarily indicated for treatment of pain (Portenoy & McCaffery, 1999), so the

CHART 15–6	**Side Effects of Opioids**	
Side Effect	**Rationale**	**Nursing Action/Responsibility**
Nausea and vomiting	Very common adverse effect of opioid therapy. Often related to dosages that exceed the patient's individual requirement for pain relief. Physiological explanation for this adverse effect is the stimulation of the chemoreceptor trigger zone in the medulla and vestibular stimulation, which explains the increased nausea associated with the upright position (Miyoshi & Leckband, 2001).	Assess for nausea and vomiting. Reduce the dosage of opioid by 25–50% if patient is comfortable. Consider advocating for an alternative opioid if vomiting persists. Monitor intake and output if vomiting persists. Obtain order for a nonsedating antinausea medication. Use extreme caution when administering a sedating antiemetic such as prochlorperazine. Co-sedation is likely to occur, increasing the risk of respiratory depression. A patient who is compromised by sedation is at risk for aspiration pneumonia, especially after anesthesia. If unable to tolerate food and drink, hold diet and advocate for another route of opioid administration (e.g., IV).
Pruritus	Pruritus, itching without a rash, is most commonly associated with administration of spinal opioids, but may also occur with any route of administration. More likely to occur with dosages that exceed the patient's requirements for pain relief. Usually limited to the face and torso. Increased tolerance to opioids will reduce the incidence of this adverse effect.	Report to health care provider to obtain orders for a nonsedating antipruritic medication. Reduce the dosage of opioid by 25–50% if patient is comfortable. Consider advocating for an alternative opioid if pruritus persists. Antihistamines are used to treat pruritus, however, these medications can be sedating and combined with opioids often lead to significant sedation and respiratory compromise. Assess for skin breakdown. Apply gloves to patient if scratching is causing a loss of skin integrity.
Constipation	Results from the generalized depressant effect of the opioid on the gastrointestinal motility. Slows emptying of gastrointestinal track by reducing peristalsis. This leads to increased absorption of water and drying and compacting of the intestinal contents (Miyoshi & Leckband, 2001). Constipation increases with larger dosages.	Administer a stimulating laxative and stool softener routinely while opioids are administered. Encourage fluid intake. Encourage ambulation if possible. Administer as low a dose of opioid as possible to provide pain relief and ensure patient is receiving acetaminophen and an NSAID if possible to augment pain relief.
Urinary retention	Occurs as a result of increased sphincter tone, making urination difficult or impossible, requiring catheterization of the bladder. This adverse effect decreases as tolerance to opioids develops.	Assess intake and output. Scan bladder to assess retention after urination. Notify health care provider and obtain order for urinary catheter as necessary to prevent retention.

(continued)

CHART 15–6 **Side Effects of Opioids—*Continued***

Side Effect	Rationale	Nursing Action/Responsibility
Sedation	Opioid-induced sedation is more likely to occur when patients are not tolerant to opioids or when opioids are given in doses that exceed the patient's individual requirements. First clinical manifestation is slowed cognition while remaining oriented. May experience drowsiness, drifting into sleep unless stimulated with conversation. Excessive sedation can result in confusion, dizziness, and increased risk for falling. If not treated, may lead to respiratory depression.	Assess for cosedating medications the patient is receiving and eliminate whenever possible. These medications will limit the amount of opioid the patient is able to safely use to relieve pain. Assess level of sedation. Assess breathing and oxygen saturation. If sedation is noted, notify the prescribing health care provider, decrease opioid dosage by 25–50%, and increase the frequency of monitoring until sedation resolves. Provide for patient safety with side rails and close observation. It may be necessary to use an antagonist (naloxone) to reverse significant sedation. Unresponsiveness that is not accompanied by respiratory depression is likely of another etiology and needs to be explored (e.g., cosedating medications, sepsis, and stroke).
Respiratory depression	Opioids reduce the responsiveness of the respiratory center in the pontine and bulbar brainstem to rising carbon dioxide (CO_2) tension, thus depressing the respiratory drive (Maher & Chaiyakul, 2003; Miyoshi & Leckband, 2001). Normally when CO_2 levels increase, the respiratory center responds by stimulating increased respiratory rate to rid the body of the excessive CO_2. Opioids defeat this response and can cause respirations to slow, become irregular, and eventually progress to apnea. Often the cause of undertreatment of pain that could easily be relieved.	Assess rate and depth of respirations and oxygen saturation. Administer oxygen as necessary. Stimulate the patient. Stop opioid administration. Report respiratory depression to the health care provider to obtain further orders. Resume opioid administration at 50% of the previous dosage once sedation and respiratory depression have resolved. Risk of respiratory depression increases when dosages exceed the requirements to achieve adequate pain relief.
Other adverse effects	Opioids impact in the limbic system resulting in euphoria, tranquility, or alternatively dysphoria through mechanisms that are not entirely clear (Miyoshi & Leckband, 2001). Cough suppression may be a desired effect or a potentially harmful adverse effect. Too rapid IV injection can cause chest wall rigidity. Accumulation of opioid and opioid metabolites occurs when renal function is impaired. The development of tolerance to opioids can be considered a benefit or an adverse effect. See discussion of tolerance, physical dependence, and addiction in Chart 15–5 (p. 346). Two very commonly prescribed opioids, meperidine and propoxyphene, both metabolize into active metabolites (normeperidine and norpropoxyphene, respectively) that have long half-lives. Accumulation is a concern with repeated dosing and if excretion is impaired through renal insufficiency (APS, 2003; Maher & Chaiyakul, 2003). As with normeperidine, norpropoxyphene can cause seizures (APS, 2003; Maher & Chaiyakul, 2003). The CNS excitatory effects of normeperidine can cause dysphoria, agitation, and seizures, making meperidine less useful for pain management (APS, 2003; Jacox et al., 1994).	The nurse must consult with the pharmacist as a collaborative resource especially when the patient has multiple disease states, making opioid therapy potentially more likely to result in an adverse effect. Provide patient safety with use of side rails and close observation. Assess oxygen status and lung sounds. Conduct ongoing assessments of renal function studies and report to the health care provider any increase in values. When giving IV, administer slowly and observe for chest rigidity. Assess drug effectiveness and need for increased dosage. Meperidine continues to be useful in small dosages appropriate for treating postanesthetic shivering and rigors. Norpropoxyphene should be limited in its use, especially in the older adult as discussed in this chapter. It is recommended that the use of meperidine be limited to situations where use of an alternative opioid is not possible (e.g., patients who have intolerable side effects with other opioids).

nurse must be aware of the rationale for the specific medication within the context of pain management and be prepared to offer education regarding its use to patients and family members to avoid confusion. Adjuvants may include tricyclic antidepressants, antiepileptic medications, local anesthetics, glucocorticoids, skeletal muscle relaxants, antispasmodic agents, antihistamines, benzodiazepines, caffeine, topical agents, and dextroamphetamine. Bisphosphonates and radionuclides are also useful in the treatment of metastatic bone pain (APS, 2003; Maher & Chaiyakul, 2003).

Routes of Administration

Pain medications are available in a variety of formulations that can be administered via many different routes. This allows the prescribing provider to select a route of medication administration based on the individual needs of the patient given the specific situation. Routes of medication administration provide for a range of absorption times from rapid onset (e.g., transmucosal, intravenous) to delayed onset (e.g., transdermal). Each route of administration has advantages and disadvantages that should be considered. It is appropriate to deliver medications by the least invasive route when possible (APS, 2003).

Oral Route

The oral route of administration is generally preferred because it is the least invasive, most convenient, and often most cost effective. Most analgesic medications come in tablets, capsules, or in a liquid formulation that allow for ease of oral administration. The oral route of administration is preferred in the treatment of chronic and cancer pain because it reduces the need for frequent analgesic administration thus reducing the burden on the patient and caregiver, and it reduces the focus on pain and the "sick role" (APS, 2003). When treating acute pain, the oral route of administration may not be available initially after surgery due to nausea, vomiting, and postoperative ileus. As soon as bowel function is reestablished, transition to the oral route of administration is recommended. The oral route of administration has the disadvantage of slower onset and delayed peak effect. The rate of gastric emptying and intestinal motility can increase or decrease medication absorption (Glen & St. Marie, 2002). Once absorbed, oral analgesics undergo first-pass metabolism in the small intestine and the liver. Gastrectomy and major bowel resection may reduce adequate medication absorption.

Oral Transmucosal Route

The oral cavity provides several locations for medication administration via the vascular mucosal membranes including sublingual, buccal, and gingival. When administering a medication sublingually, the medication is placed under the tongue and held there until it is completely dissolved and absorbed. Buccal administration requires the medication to be placed between the gums of the upper molars and the cheek. Gingival drugs are placed between the gums of the upper incisors and the upper lip (McCaffery & Portenoy, 1999).

Absorption from the oral mucosa is optimal if the medications are lipid soluble and designed specifically for transmucosal delivery. An example is oral transmucosal fentanyl citrate (Actiq). Medications that are less lipid soluble, such as morphine, are not well absorbed by the mucosal membrane. An advantage of transmucosal administration is that the drug is absorbed directly into the venous blood flow going to the superior vena cava with minimal first-pass metabolism by the liver (Glen & St. Marie, 2002).

The nurse should assess the patient's ability to hold the medication under the tongue until completely absorbed. Many patients are unable to either understand or tolerate sublingual administration and instead swallow the medication, resulting in gastric absorption and hepatic metabolism, which reduces the effectiveness of the medication dramatically.

All of the oral transmucosal locations can become irritated with repeated application of a medication. Assessment of the integrity of the mucosa and rotating the site of application from side to side will help reduce this irritation.

Rectal Route

The rectal route of medication administration is generally reserved for use when nausea or vomiting precludes oral administration and in situations where the additional expertise of intravenous administration is not available or desirable. Most medications that can be taken orally may be given rectally with similar dissolution, absorption, and effectiveness. Medications administered into the rectum are absorbed into the superior, middle, and inferior rectal veins through contact with a relatively small area of the rectal wall and without the assistance of digestive enzymes (Glen & St. Marie, 2002; McCaffery & Portenoy, 1999). Relatively rapid systemic absorption and avoidance of hepatic metabolism are possible if the medication is inserted just past the rectal sphincter (Davis, Walsh, LeGrand, & Naughton, 2002). Medications that are formulated or coated so that absorption occurs in the intestine (e.g., enteric coated) are not effective when administered using the rectal route. The pH of the colon is alkaline and enteric-coated medications require the acidic environment of the intestines (McCaffery & Portenoy, 1999). An important disadvantage of the rectal route of administration is the actual placement, which most patients find unpleasant and embarrassing. If medications must be administered frequently, rectal irritation can occur.

Intravenous Route

Intravenous (IV) administration of medications allows for the most rapid onset of effect because medications are delivered directly into the systemic circulation. First-pass hepatic metabolism is avoided. When administering opioids to treat severe pain, IV boluses can be administered by titration (frequent administration of small doses) for rapid control of escalating pain (APS, 2003; McCaffery & Portenoy, 1999; Miyoshi & Leckband, 2001). Because of the rapid onset of effect, the IV route of administration is also associated with the highest level of toxicity. Care must be taken to administer medications slowly or in small doses in order to reduce adverse effects (McCaffery & Portenoy, 1999). Other disadvantages of the IV route of administration include increased risk of infection with vascular access and the expertise required to administer medications aseptically.

The IV route of administration is commonly reserved for acute pain management or in cases of chronic and cancer pain where patients are experiencing severe pain that requires rapid relief or are unable to take oral analgesics due to adverse effects or situations such as disease that impairs gastrointestinal function.

Intramuscular Route

Intramuscular (IM) injection of analgesics should be avoided. The IM route of administration has significant disadvantages. The IM absorption is unreliable with a 30- to 60-minute lag time to peak effect with a rapid falloff of action as compared with oral analgesic administration (APS, 2003; McCaffery & Portenoy, 1999). If the IM route of administration must be used, the deltoid muscles and vastus lateralis muscles have better perfusion, and absorption may be more rapid than with the gluteal muscle (APS, 2003; Glen & St. Marie, 2002). Although hepatic first-pass metabolism is avoided using this route of analgesic administration, the risk of tissue injuries such as sterile abscesses and fibrosis of the muscle and soft tissue as well a nerve injury resulting in persistent neuropathic pain make IM injection a poor choice in pain management situations (APS, 2003; McCaffery & Portenoy, 1999).

Subcutaneous Route

The subcutaneous route of administration is similar to the IM route of administration with the disadvantage of painful injection and variability of absorption based on the location of injection. Hepatic first-pass metabolism is avoided. However, in situations where oral and IV routes of delivery are not available, subcutaneous offers an alternative for administering analgesics. When treating pain in palliative care or end-of-life settings, subcutaneous administration may be an effective option when IV access if difficult. If subcutaneous medications are delivered by continuous infusion, the volume of the medication should be limited to 2 or 3 mL/hour to optimize absorption (APS, 2003; McCaffery & Portenoy, 1999). If higher infusion rates are necessary, the total volume to be infused can be split between two sites to prevent irritation, pain, necrosis, and sloughing at the site (McCaffery & Portenoy, 1999).

Transdermal Route

Transdermal administration of analgesic medications relies on absorption of lipid-soluble medications through the barrier of the intact skin into the local tissues and the systemic circulation. These medications are generally formulated in transdermal patches or topical creams, ointments, or gels. Absorption of the medication can be unintentionally increased with the application of heat or by massaging the skin to increase the blood flow to the area, resulting in rapid absorption and potential overdose (Glen & St. Marie, 2002). Fentanyl, lidocaine, and clonidine are examples of transdermal medications that are commonly used in pain management.

Spinal (Epidural and Intrathecal) Route

Epidural and intrathecal routes of administration are useful for acute pain management for postoperative and trauma pain and also for specific cancer and chronic pain management situations. These routes of medication administration bypass metabolism in the liver and systemic circulation. For this reason, the dosage of medication used to achieve adequate analgesia is very small compared to those administered by other routes.

The epidural space is separated from the spinal cord by the spinal meninges. When opioids, anesthetics, or other medications are administered by the epidural route, they must diffuse across the meninges, into the cerebrospinal fluid (CSF), and subsequently penetrate the spinal cord tissues. Medications injected directly into the intrathecal space have immediate access to the spinal cord tissues without diffusion across the meninges.

Both epidural and intrathecal administration of medications requires access to the spinal tissues through an invasive procedure, either injection through a spinal needle alone or in combination with placement of an indwelling catheter. The epidural or intrathecal catheter is usually temporarily indwelling and can be a potential source of infection. If the intention is to use the epidural or intrathecal route for longer durations, a permanent catheter is tunneled under the subcutaneous tissue to reduce the risk of infection or a fully implanted infusion pump with catheter is placed during a surgical procedure.

Regional Nerve Route

Injection of anesthetic medications into or near a nerve is commonly referred to as regional anesthesia or a nerve block. A variety of regional anesthetic blocks are performed to diagnose nerve pain, as a prognostic prior to a more invasive procedure,

or to relieve chronic and cancer pain. When the anesthetic is injected, it is delivered directly to the nerve tissue. The anesthetic blocks the conduction of both afferent and efferent neural fibers (Buckley, 2001).

Regional anesthetic techniques are often used to diagnose whether pain originates from a peripheral nerve or from the CNS, a technique that is valuable in chronic pain of unknown etiology. Continuous infusion of anesthetics to regional nerves is becoming a very popular option for acute pain management and in situations where it is desirable to reduce the amount of opioid a patient receives throughout the operative and postoperative course (e.g., multiple comorbidities). The nerve block is generally established prior to surgery as a single dose. In some cases a catheter is placed to allow for continuous infusion of anesthetic so that the medication effects continue throughout the operative course and into the postoperative period, improving the quality of pain relief.

Methods of Medication Delivery

Clinical decisions regarding the dosing intervals for the various analgesic medications are based on multiple factors, including the type and intensity of the pain, the pharmacologic attributes of the medication, and the clinical setting. Consideration of the patient's preferences and need for simple dosing schedules is essential. Analgesics may be given as a single dose, multiple intermittent doses, by continuous dosing, or at the patient's request. As with many aspects of pain management, the dosing schedule should be customized to meet the individual needs of the patient to achieve the best results.

Single Dose

Single dosing of analgesic medications is generally a strategy used to treat pain caused by a painful procedure or in some circumstances injury. When premedicating a patient for a painful procedure, the analgesic should be administered so that the peak effects occur just prior to the start of the procedure. For example, a single dose of IV fentanyl administered to the patient just prior to beginning a colonoscopy allows time for the fentanyl to peak and adequately relieve the pain caused by this relatively brief procedure. A single dose of steroid administered into the epidural space may be sufficient to relieve the pain and inflammation associated with an acute low back injury. Single doses of analgesics are sometimes administered as a loading dose in order to rapidly achieve therapeutic blood levels.

Pro re Nata (prn)

Pro re nata (prn), or "as needed," is a common dosing strategy that allows for flexibility in the dosing schedule when pain is intermittent and the analgesic medication is appropriate for intermittent dosing. It is most commonly used for acute pain when pain is not consistent or is expected to decline rapidly as healing occurs. For example, a patient may have a prescription for a short-acting opioid analgesic that can be taken every 4 hours prn, allowing her to take the ordered medication as often as every 4 hours and as infrequently as her pain allows. Disadvantages of the prn dosing schedule are evident when a patient waits too long between doses of medication, allowing the pain to become severe, or when she is experiencing continuous pain that would be best managed with a continuous dosing pattern.

If continuous pain is managed with prn dosing, the patient can be taught to determine the duration of pain relief he experiences with a dose of medication and to then schedule the prn doses at that frequency to be taken routinely. This is an effective strategy for severe acute pain and for chronic or cancer pain. For example, the patient takes the ordered dose of oxycodone and begins to experience the onset of pain after 5 hours of good pain relief. Another dose of medication is taken to avoid the escalation of pain intensity and good pain relief is achieved for another 6 hours. Based on this information, the patient should adjust his prn schedule to a continuous dosing schedule with intervals of every 5 to 6 hours around the clock (ATC).

The use of prn dosing is appropriate when treating breakthrough pain episodes that occur in spite of well-controlled persistent pain. Breakthrough pain is generally unpredictable and severe, requiring the flexibility of a short- or rapid-acting analgesic that can be administered as soon as the breakthrough pain begins. For example, the patient is using a fentanyl transdermal patch once every 72 hours and treats breakthrough pain episodes two to three times daily with oral transmucosal fentanyl citrate (Actiq) units prn.

When the nurse manages prn dosing, the potential for undertreatment of pain becomes a very real concern. Patients often rely on their nurse to know what dosing schedule is best for them, and nurses frequently feel that the patient should ask for medication when they begin to experience the onset of pain. The result is a roller-coaster of severe pain alternating with pain relief. This common scenario is dissatisfying, instills a lack of trust, encourages "clock watching," and increases the risk for undertreatment of pain. Nurses should determine the optimal dosing schedule based on the patient's response to the medication and then offer doses routinely and prior to the onset of severe pain.

At times, the ordered interval for prn dosing is not frequent enough to allow dosing prior to the onset of pain, resulting in undertreated pain if the dosing schedule is followed. The nurse is responsible for conveying this information to the prescribing clinician and advocating for an appropriate dosing interval or an increase in dosage based on assessment findings. Likewise, if the prescribed dosing interval is too frequent to be realistically implemented, it is appropriate for the nurse to contact the prescribing clinician and advocate for an alternative dosing schedule or method. For example, boluses of IV fentanyl every 30 minutes prn for postoperative pain management may be optimally delivered using a continuous infusion or patient-controlled analgesia to avoid missed doses and subsequent undertreatment of pain.

Continuous

When pain is consistently present, analgesic medications should be administered continuously. This dosing strategy is most commonly used for severe pain. The goal of continuous dosing is to maintain a therapeutic level of the medication that provides optimal pain relief without adverse effects. To accomplish continuous dosing, short-acting analgesics may be administered ATC as mentioned or infusion pumps can be used to deliver IV analgesics continuously.

Other analgesic medication formulations have long half-lives or modified delivery to make them long acting and designed specifically for continuous dosing. These medications should be prescribed with a routine dosing interval based on the pharmacology of the medication. For example, controlled-release morphine that is designed so that the medication is released over a period of 24 hours should be prescribed for once-a-day dosing. When the frequency of analgesic dosing is reduced, patients with chronic and cancer pain benefit from the consistent pain relief and a reduced focus on medication administration and the sick role, and they generally experience improved quality of life. Continuous dosing of opioid analgesics should be used with extreme caution when patients are opioid naïve due to increased risk of adverse effects (APS, 2003).

Patient-Controlled Analgesia

Patient-controlled analgesia (PCA) is a dosing strategy that allows patients to request a small dose of analgesic medication when they begin to feel pain. PCA infusion pumps are designed with a patient dose button that the patient can press to activate medication delivery. The prescription includes a dosage and dosing interval that are programmed into the pump so that the patient receives the prescribed dosage no more often than allowed by prescription in spite of the possibility of more frequent button presses to request doses. The PCA can be used successfully to administer analgesic medications by a variety of routes including IV, subcutaneous, epidural, intrathecal, and peripheral nerve. The PCA may be used alone as a prn dose or in combination with a continuous infusion. PCA dosing is generally used in moderate to severe acute pain or in cases of chronic pain where alternate routes of analgesic administration are not available or effective.

The benefits of PCA include increased patient control and participation in pain management. PCA is very effective for acute pain management postoperatively or post-trauma when patients are unable to take oral analgesics and the severity of pain would require an unrealistic frequency of IV medication administration given the nurse's other responsibilities. Reduced time waiting for the nurse to deliver a requested analgesic is another benefit that often makes patients reluctant to relinquish control even when they are able to transition to oral analgesics prn. As mentioned previously, use of continuous dosing of opioids should be used with extreme caution for opioid naïve patients. This is especially true when continuous dosing is combined with PCA dosing.

Complementary and Alternative Therapies

A balanced analgesic medication treatment plan is the foundation of acute and cancer pain management. This is rapidly becoming the case in chronic pain management as well. However, the integration of appropriate complementary therapies is often used to fully treat the multidimensional experience of pain. In spite of the lack of scientific evidence that these therapies are effective in pain relief, the underlying principle of the mind, body, and spirit connection in promoting balance, harmony, and healing is a strong argument for their use (Snyder & Wieland, 2003). Generally, patients use complementary therapies as an additional strategy along with their pharmacologic treatments. However, some patients prefer to use only alternative therapies. Alternative therapies may be attractive to patients who desire to avoid medications and their potential adverse effects or to those who simply have not found medications to be effective in relieving their pain.

The nurse should have a basic understanding of common complementary therapies and include an assessment of the patient's use of complementary therapies in the overall assessment of pain. Patients may be reluctant to discuss their decision to use a complementary or alternative therapy for fear of ridicule or concern that the nurse will attempt to dissuade them from its use (Snyder & Wieland, 2003). The following questions may be used to encourage discussion regarding complementary therapies the patient might be using or desire to learn more about:

- Do you do anything to treat your pain besides taking medications?

- Have you ever used music, massage, or meditation to distract you when you are in pain?

The Complementary and Alternative Therapies feature discusses the use of art in managing pain.

Nursing Management

The nurse's knowledge of the multidimensions of pain management, effective assessment techniques, and common pharmacologic and complementary or alternative strategies is the foundation necessary to provide safe and appropriate nursing care. Consistent with the nursing process, data gathered from the pain assessment is analyzed along with the data gathered from all other aspects of the physical assessment and used in the planning of interventions.

Assessment

The assessment findings related to the physiological dimension should prompt the nurse to recognize the potential harm that unrelieved pain could cause to the patient, especially those who are acutely or critically ill, who are frail or debilitated, or those with multiple disease states that would likely be impacted by a significant stress response.

Specific assessment data includes:

- Type (sharp, dull, burning, pressure)
- Location: including transmission patterns
- Duration
- What brings it on
- What relieves it
- When did it start
- Is it getting worse or better
- Intensity (using a pain scale)

Analysis of the data gathered regarding the sensory dimension of pain provides a baseline that future data may be compared against to determine if the treatment plan is resulting in a positive trend toward adequate pain relief. The quality of the pain will provide some direction in the selection of medications suited to nociceptive or neuropathic pain. The temporal pattern of the pain is important to the selection of formulations and timing of the administration of medications. Sustained-release, modified release, or continuous infusions of analgesics are particularly suited to pain that is constant and persistent and may potentially cause harm when administered for pain that is intermittent or transient. The sudden onset of severe breakthrough pain may require the use of a rapid-acting transmucosal or IV opioid.

COMPLEMENTARY & ALTERNATIVE THERAPIES — Art

Description:

Art therapy is a creative process that uses psychotherapy and visual art to further self-understanding. In the process of art therapy, the patient's created work becomes a reflection of his or her personality, development, abilities, pain, and conflict. This type of therapy includes a range of modalities that include, but are not limited to:

- Painting with oil, acrylic, or water color on canvas or finger painting.
- Basket or loom weaving.
- Sculpturing with wood, metal, marble, or other materials.
- Creating pottery and working with clay.

Research Support:

It is thought that visual creativity consists of not only originality and a special talent, but also sensitivity and even deeper dynamics of the human personality, such as sublimation, reparative-compensating mechanisms, and mental well-being. Art therapy combines all of these capacities and utilizes them in self-healing (Hardi, 2006). Individuals and families use a process of meaning construction to make sense of the world and their experiences. When an individual receives a life-threatening or life-altering illness diagnosis, it often forces the individual to revise his or her "life narrative" and to reconstruct meaning in his or her life. Expressive arts and ritual provide the means by which the individual can create meaning and connection. It is vital for each member of the health care team to help patients and their families express their feelings about their illness and find meaning and purpose at the end of life. Art therapy can allow the relationship among patient, family, and practitioner to be powerfully therapeutic and potentially transformative for all involved (Romanoff & Thompson, 2006).

The goal in art therapy is to facilitate positive change in an individual by engaging with the therapist and the art materials in a safe environment. Art therapy is used with success among all age populations. The therapeutic change occurs during the process of physical involvement with the art materials, such as the process of making of a significant art object, the process of expressing feelings through the created images, and the process of communication with the therapist by means of the art object (Waller, 2006).

Several art therapy programs have been created for use with the elderly population and serve as models for instituting art therapy into nursing practice. For example, The University of Pennsylvania's School of Nursing created a Living Independently for Elderly (LIFE) Program. At a Program of All-Inclusive Care for the Elderly (PACE) site in an urban African American community, art therapy practitioners offer the choice of art media and options for working with elderly clients (Johnson & Sullivan-Marx, 2006).

References

Hardi, I. (2006). Creativity and visual expression. *Psychiatria Hungarica, 21*(4), 268–278.

Johnson, C. M., & Sullivan-Marx, E. M. (2006). Art therapy: Using the creative process for healing and hope among African American older adults. *Geriatric Nursing, 27*(5), 309–316.

Romanoff, B. D., & Thompson, B. E. (2006). Meaning construction in palliative care: The use of narrative, ritual, and the expressive arts. *American Journal of Hospice Palliative Care, 23*(4), 309–316.

Waller, D. (2006). Art therapy for children: How it leads to change. *Clinical Child Psychology and Psychiatry, 11*(2), 271–282.

The affective dimension of pain will yield assessment data that has the potential to undermine even the most carefully planned treatments. The patient's emotions and assignment of meaning to the pain should be considered when prioritizing time spent with the patient. Education and emotional support should be tailored to meet the specific needs of patients who are suffering or have a negative perception of their pain. Involvement of a psychiatric specialist, psychologist, or social worker may be indicated, and based on the analysis of the affective dimension findings, the nurse is in an excellent position to advocate for this on behalf of the patient who may not be able to recognize that this is a concern.

Consideration of assessment findings in the cognitive dimension will assist the nurse in providing for specific religious and cultural needs. In addition, understanding the culturally appropriate response to pain assists the nurse in interpreting pain-related behaviors more accurately. For example, when a patient who is culturally inclined to be quite stoic in the expression of pain becomes more vocal, it should prompt the nurse to consider that pain might be severe in spite of the patient's subdued response. Patients who feel a loss of control might be comforted by having choices in their pain treatment whenever possible. For example, opioids that are ordered to be administered IV prn might be administered using a PCA infusion device, allowing postoperative patients significant control and increasing self-efficacy in their acute pain management.

Assessment of the behavioral dimension of pain is a necessary baseline to determine whether pain-related behaviors are reduced following the implementation of the pain treatment plan for patients who are unable to provide a self-report of pain. The nurse who finds that the patient has developed some unfortunate learned pain behaviors has the opportunity to reduce the use of these behaviors by establishing a trusting relationship, providing pain treatments appropriately as needed rather than waiting until pain behaviors are demonstrated, and reassuring the patient that the health care team is committed to relieving pain and will do everything possible to accomplish that goal. In addition, these findings should prompt the nurse to consider encouraging and assisting patients to develop their skills in using cognitive-behavioral strategies such as meditation, journaling, or redirecting thoughts into a more positive pattern.

Planning

The analysis of assessment findings and planning of interventions should be focused around the therapeutic goals described in this chapter. The baseline assessment of pain intensity and functional ability is matched with the comfort and function goal to establish the means by which progress may be measured. Interventions are defined and initiated using the goals established in the planning phase. Evaluation will determine whether the goals and patient outcomes have been accomplished and redirect the plan if they have not.

Nursing Diagnosis

Nursing diagnoses that may apply to the patient experiencing pain include:

1. Pain, acute
2. Pain, chronic
3. Fatigue
4. Coping ineffective
5. Hopelessness
6. Mobility impaired
7. Powerlessness

Interventions and Rationales

Implementation of interventions, particularly pharmacologic interventions, is multifaceted and focused on patient safety as well as optimizing the potential efficacy of the treatment plan. The nurse uses the knowledge of pharmacologic interventions to review the medications that have been prescribed for the patient. The following questions might be considered:

- Could this medication or dosage cause the patient to experience adverse effects given her physiological status or allergies?
- Is the medication appropriate to treat this patient's source of pain (e.g., neuropathic, nociceptive)?
- Is it likely that this medication and dosage will be able to relieve the intensity of pain this patient is experiencing?
- Is this medication ordered with an appropriate frequency for administration?
- Is the formulation (long-acting, short-acting, etc.) and route of administration appropriate to treat this patient's pattern of pain?
- Does the patient have adequate understanding of how to use the medication to prevent harm through inadvertent misuse?
- Are there other medications that might be appropriate to add to this treatment plan to optimize the effectiveness and safety of pain relief for this patient?

The nurse is the "guardian of patient safety" at the patient's bedside to ensure that when medications are administered they will not cause harm (Campbell, 2006). If there is any concern that the prescribed medication may not be appropriate or ordered in an appropriate dosage or frequency of administration, it is the nurse's responsibility to notify the prescribing clinician and request clarification of the order. The patient's physical condition must be considered when implementing pharmacologic strategies to avoid administration of a medication that has the potential to cause adverse effects or that could result in patient harm and when selecting or implementing complementary or alternative strategies. Because pain medications, particularly opioids, have the potential to cause serious adverse effects, this important nursing role cannot be stressed enough.

Successful implementation of complementary or alternative intervention is based on the selection of a strategy that is embraced by the patient and his family. Some interventions are less demanding of the patient's time and energy (e.g., music, massage), whereas others require the patient to be actively engaged (e.g., meditation, journaling). It is important to consider the selected strategies given the patient's specific needs and to consider alternative strategies if necessary.

Prior to initiating interventions, the patient and family must be educated regarding the goals, rationale, expected outcomes, and potential adverse effects associated with the intervention. Some patients will only be able to understand or desire to learn the most basic concepts regarding their treatments. For these patients, a base of knowledge should be established and then built on with subsequent educational opportunities. Ensure that the patient does not have a cultural barrier to learning such as speaking a language other that of the health care team or having a cognitive impairment (e.g., confusion, sedation). It is important to remember that the presence of severe pain is a barrier to learning and should be relieved as quickly as possible to facilitate the patient's participation in their care. Other patients will want detailed information, and education may have to be provided on multiple occasions to fully answer all of their questions. Educational tools such as diagrams, diaries, audiovisual programs, and demonstrations may provide another avenue of learning for patients who learn more effectively from visual instruction. The education provided must be tailored to meet the specific needs of each patient and their family members.

Equianalgesia

Early studies of the relative potency of various opioids were accomplished by comparing single doses of oral and IV/IM opioids to 10 mg of IV morphine in patients with postoperative and cancer pain (Houde, Wallenstein, & Beaver, 1996). The term *equianalgesia* refers to the ratio derived from these studies that allows selection of a dosage of an opioid that is relatively the same in potency to an opioid that is already in use. For example, a patient receiving IV morphine for postoperative pain can be transitioned to an oral opioid with the goal of providing approximately the same level of pain relief by calculating the equianalgesic dose (Kaplow & Hardin, 2007). An understanding of basic equianalgesia gives the nurse the information necessary to respond appropriately to patients who are rotating to a new opioid and/or new route of administration.

To perform an equianalgesic calculation, the nurse must have access to an equianalgesic chart. Although equianalgesic charts may be published in different formats and with different associated information, the equianalgesic doses are consistent. The nurse should obtain an approved equianalgesic chart from the pharmacy. The opioids listed on the chart will have equianalgesic dosages listed for the IV/IM route of administration and the oral route. A simple calculation allows the nurse to determine the equianalgesic dose:

- First determine the amount of opioid the patient has received in the past 24 hours, being careful to add up all doses given.
- Locate the opioid that has been given in the past 24 hours on the equianalgesic chart and locate the equianalgesic dose under the correct route of administration.
- Divide the 24-hour total dose of opioid by the equianalgesic dose.
- Identify the new opioid's equianalgesic dose on the equianalgesic chart using the new route of administration.
- Multiply the 24-hour total equianalgesic dose by the new opioid equianalgesic dose.
- The answer represents the 24-hour total amount of the new opioid that is relatively equal in potency to the 24-hour total dose of the opioid currently being administered.
- Divide the total 24-hour dose of the new opioid into administration intervals by dividing by the number of doses desired within 24 hours (APS, 2003).

For example, a patient has received IV morphine 1 mg/hr for postoperative pain equaling 24 mg for the past 24 hours. The equianalgesic dose for IV morphine is located on the chart and

is 10. The nurse divides 24 mg by 10 to equal 2.4 equianalgesic dose units. The order for oxycodone (Percocet) has been written and so the nurse locates the equianalgesic dose of 20 for oral oxycodone on the chart. The nurse then multiples the equianalgesic dose units of 2.4 by 20 to equal 48 mg, which is the 24-hour total amount of oxycodone that would be required to provide the same pain relief as 24 mg of IV morphine. As a final step, the nurse then divides 48 mg into 6 equal doses for a q4h administration interval. The 8-mg dose of oxycodone is within the range of the health care provider's order for one to two Percocet (5 mg each tablet) q4h prn. Additionally, the nurse also knows that the patient is likely to need two tablets rather than one tablet given the equialangesic dose.

The nurse should note the following when doing equianalgesic dose calculations:

- If several different opioids or routes of administration are used, the equianalgesic dose units should be determined for each different opioid/route and then added before multiplying by the new opioid equianalgesic dose.
- Patients may have different responses to different opioids and/or routes of administration, so a degree of variability should be expected and monitoring for opioid side effects and pain relief should be increased until the patient is safely transitioned to the new opioid.
- If an order for a new opioid is either too large or too small given the equianalgesic dose calculation, the nurse should request clarification with the prescribing health care provider.
- As a colleague, the pharmacist is generally an excellent resource for assistance with equianalgesic dose calculations.

Management of Unrelieved Pain

As an advocate for change, it falls to the nurse to accurately and concisely communicate the details of the pain assessment, interventions that have been implemented, and the evaluation of the patient's response. Chart 15–7 provides suggestions for using collaborative communication to improve pain management.

Evaluation

Evaluation data is aimed at determining whether pain relief has been achieved. The nurse needs to evaluate each tenant of the plan to determine the most effective interventions. It may not always be realistic to achieve total relief, especially with chronic diseases such as arthritis. The realistic goal may need to be a level of comfort that allows the patient to perform activities of daily living and maintain some quality of life. It is essential that the nurse helps the patient and family identify behaviors that increase the pain and how to avoid these activities.

Reassessment of pain and assessment of the patient's response to interventions is necessary to successfully measure improvement in the quality of pain management as compared to baseline assessments. The reassessment of pain should follow the same pattern used at baseline, including using the same tools to reinforce concepts that were taught during the assessment. Some minor alterations should be made to elicit the details needed to determine if there has been a change after intervention. For example:

- How would you rate your pain intensity on the 0 to 10 scale at rest? With activity? During _____ (the patient's previously identified most painful time)?

CHART 15–7   Collaborative Communication to Improve Pain Management

When collaborating with other members of the health care team to improve pain management, it is vital that the nurse be prepared to concisely, accurately, and knowledgeably convey the details necessary for the health care provider to make a logical and appropriate decision regarding the patient's care. Poorly prepared nurses may actually indirectly cause harm if they communicate inaccurate or incomplete information. Nurses are the eyes, ears, and hands of the other members of the health care team when those members must make decisions away from the patient's bedside (Griffie, 2003). An effective nurse who has the best interests of the patient and the health care team in mind during communications will command a level of trust that encourages support from colleagues and discourages arguments and denial of requests.

Prepare to provide the following:

- Patient name, location, age, and diagnosis or surgery
- Patient's primary health care provider (if speaking with another member of the team)
- Pertinent details of the pain assessment (e.g., pain intensity, location, character)
- Impact of the pain on the patient's function
- Interventions that have been implemented (e.g., medications, therapies)
- The appropriate next step to improve the situation.

The following hypothetical patient scenario provides an example script and rationale for steps that a nurse could follow to improve communication when discussing postoperative pain management with an orthopedic surgeon who is covering for her colleague.

INTRODUCE YOURSELF AND THE PATIENT

"Dr. Smith this is (state your name), I am a nurse here on the medical–surgical unit." Introduce yourself professionally avoiding meaningless chatter. This is an important step that helps the health care provider, in this case, to know whom she is speaking with and their credentials.

"I am caring for Mrs. Jones in Room 246. She is a 78-year-old female who has degenerative arthritis and underwent a total knee arthroplasty yesterday by Dr. Black." This information alerts the health care provider to the fact that this patient is an older adult, recently postanesthetic, and expected to have a significant amount of pain. These are all considerations that will be used in medical decision making. Additionally, this information allows the health care provider time to focus on any information her health care provider colleague may have reported to her and to visualize this patient if she has seen her before.

BRIEFLY REVIEW THE GOALS OF THE PAIN TREATMENT PLAN

"Mrs. Jones' comfort and function goals are a pain score of 4/10 and to be able to participate in her physical therapy two times today." This gives the health care provider a direction and makes the patient's report of pain meaningful in the context of an outcome.

COMMUNICATE THE PERTINENT DETAILS OF THE PAIN ASSESSMENT

"She has reported a pain score of 8/10 for the past 2 hours, and describes the pain as constant, sharp, and throbbing and localized to her left knee.

She has been coping fairly well, but is beginning to express some frustration and anxiety. Her husband is supportive and in the room with her. She grimaces and stiffens up when the continuous passive motion machine reaches its highest and lowest points." This is a concise summary of the sensory assessment (pattern, character, location, and intensity) and the affective and cognitive assessments (emotions and coping), as well as the behavioral assessment (grimacing, stiffening).

DISCUSS THE IMPACT OF THE UNRELIEVED PAIN

"The physical therapist came to take Mrs. Jones to the joint therapy class, but felt she would be unable to participate until her pain was more appropriately relieved." This is strong outcome-based evidence that a change is warranted and validated by two members of the health care team.

REVIEW THE PAIN TREATMENT PLAN AND EVALUATION OF THE PATIENT'S RESPONSE

"Mrs. Jones has IV PCA morphine ordered with settings of zero continuous infusion, 1 mg PCA demand dose, a 15-minute lock-out time, and the hourly limit is set at 4 mg. She has requested an average of three doses to each of the three or four doses she has received since her surgery. She has an ice wrap on her knee. She is alert and oriented. Her respiratory status is stable with good oxygen saturations. She doesn't have any opioid-induced adverse effects." At this point, the health care provider has a very clear direction that is reasonable and based on good physical evidence that a change is not only necessary but will be well tolerated and is prepared to listen to the nurse's request respectfully. In addition, the nurse has established a base of trust through professional communication that will most likely be remembered in future opportunities for collaboration.

MAKE A RECOMMENDATION

"I would like an order to give a bolus of IV morphine 2 mg now and I think it would be helpful to have it available for prn use 10 minutes prior to physical therapy. I think we should decrease the PCA lock-out time to 10 minutes, and increase the hourly limit to 6 mg. As soon as Mrs. Jones is eating, I recommend we start acetaminophen 500 mg PO every 6 hours ATC and celecoxib (Celebrex) 100 mgs PO bid." In approximately 2 to 3 minutes the nurse has conveyed a clear, strong, and appropriate request for a balanced or multimodal approach to acute pain management. The dosages requested reflect an understanding of the patient's potential sensitivity to medication adverse effects due to her age and renal and hepatic function. However, the nurse should be prepared to discuss hepatic and renal function lab results when requesting these medications.

KNOWLEDGEABLY DISCUSS OTHER OPTIONS

"Is there something else you would like for me to try?" Once the nurse's request has been presented, it is important to acknowledge that there may be another equally appropriate change that the health care provider may have in mind or that the health care provider may have information that would make another option more appropriate.

- Is your pain in the same place?
- Do you have any new pain?
- Does your pain feel the same (e.g., aching, burning)?
- Do you feel like the pain treatments are helping to relieve your pain?
- Are you having any nausea, vomiting, itching, or constipation?
- Are you able to urinate? (If opioid analgesics have been administered)
- Do you feel alert and able to keep up with conversations around you when you are not resting?
- Are you able to do _____ (the patient's previously identified goal for function)?

In addition to these assessment questions, the patient's vital signs should be checked with specific attention to respiratory status including depth, quality, and rate of respirations when opioid analgesics have been administered.

If the analgesic treatment plan includes delivery of medications using infusion devices such as a PCA pump, analysis of the data provided by the device becomes an important component of the evaluation process. Review of the pump settings to ensure appropriate programming will prevent errors or encourage rapid identification of an error should one occur. PCA pumps track the number of milligrams, micrograms, or milliliters of medication that is administered to the patient. The PCA pump also tracks the number of times the patient pushes the PCA button to request a dose and the number of times they actually receive a dose. Evaluation of this data can provide important trending information and provide a prompt to initiate a change when necessary.

The frequency of evaluation or reassessment is determined by institutional policies and procedures. However, it is the nurse's obligation to increase the frequency of reassessment if the patient's condition warrants. For example, a patient who is found to be slightly drowsy with a marginal respiratory rate of 10 breaths per minute is scheduled to be reassessed again in 2 hours. Instead, the nurse should identify the potential for significant respiratory depression and reassess the patient more frequently until her respiratory status is stable.

Collaborative Management

A successful pain management plan requires the focused attention of the multidisciplinary team. Nurses are recognized as the team members most likely to spend significant amounts of time with the patient; hence, they play a vital role in the coordination of the care of the multidisciplinary team. It is the nurse's responsibility to assess the ongoing effects and intensity of pain, administer medications and nonmedication treatments, communicate changes in the patient's condition to the other members of the team, and advocate for change. Members of the health care team depend on the knowledge and skill of the nurse to manage the patient's pain adequately facilitating participation in necessary therapies and procedures.

To meet the goals of pain management, the multidisciplinary team draws on the additional support of services such as pain management services, chaplain services, psychologists/psychiatrists, financial assistance, social services, and specific support groups for patients and family members. Pain management services provide expert assistance with complex pain management problems and are skilled in the management of high-technology modalities such as IV PCA, epidural or intrathecal infusion of opioids and anesthetics, and regional anesthetic techniques. Chaplin services, psychologist/psychiatrist, and social services assist with identification and management of concerns in the affective, cognitive, and behavioral dimensions of pain. Financial services assist the patient in meeting immediate needs such as purchasing medications and obtaining specialty pain management care, and providing counseling regarding long-term needs if the patient is unable to return to gainful employment. Finally, specific support groups may be especially beneficial to patients with chronic and cancer pain. Meeting with others who are living with similar challenges allows the patient and family to openly discuss their concerns, exchange ideas, and receive encouragement.

Discharge Planning

Transitioning from one care setting to another can cause a patient and family members to feel anxious, frightened, confused, and even frustrated as they try to understand their pain management plan. Patients and family members should be prepared for discharge throughout the entire course of the admission through the coordinated efforts of all members of the multidisciplinary team. Nurses play a significant role in assessing the needs of the patient and family for discharge.

Initial Discharge Planning

Planning for the pain management regimen should be initiated with consideration of the patent's ability to appropriately use the medications and complementary or alternative strategies. Complex medication plans, although they may provide superior pain relief, may not be appropriate if the patient will not be able to manage the complexity of the plan independently after discharge. Likewise, nonmedication strategies that are difficult to perform without expert skills are less likely to be used after discharge.

Financial considerations such as prescription coverage or ability to pay for prescription medications, if considered during the planning stages, will enhance the patient's willingness and ability to adhere to the medication regimen after discharge. Many patients do not have adequate health care insurance or prescription coverage and the cost of pain medications may be a financial burden. Although it is not always possible, medications should be selected based on the lowest appropriate cost in addition to most appropriately meeting the needs of the patient. However, care must be taken to avoid selecting a less costly medication based on cost alone. A medication that causes side effects that must then be treated with yet another medication will negate any cost savings to the patient.

Some patients have complex pain management needs and the care of a pain management specialist after discharge may be determined to be necessary. In these cases, it is appropriate to begin the process of referral early to facilitate a smooth transition of care after discharge. If a pain management specialist is not available in the patient's community, appropriate follow-up care may be available from a health care provider or licensed independent practitioner in the community. Time will be needed to select a provider and secure an appointment for follow-up care.

Ongoing Discharge Planning

Once a pain management plan is determined, it should be implemented and modified until the best level of pain relief and functionality are achieved with minimal side effects. When pain medications are administered, the patient and family members should be instructed regarding expected onset of relief, side effects that may be experienced, and when additional medication will be provided or should be requested. Treatments of medication side effects should also be reviewed with the patient and family. When assisting a patient with the use of a complementary or alternative strategy, it is imperative to provide adequate opportunity to practice the technique to facilitate the skillful use of the strategy after discharge. Repeated administration of medications and use of nonmedication strategies will allow the patient and family members the opportunity to hear instructions many times before discharge. This approach reduces the stress of having to learn everything on the day of discharge.

Health Promotion

Patient teaching prior to discharge should be a review of the teaching that has been provided during the patient's stay. New information will be very difficult for the patient and family to incorporate this late in their care. Every effort should be made to ensure that the plan for pain management is providing adequate relief of pain and optimal function with minimal side effects so that last minute changes are avoided when possible.

The nurse is the patient's final contact before discharge in most settings. Discharge responsibilities include presenting information in a calm and reassuring manner that will support the patient's need to be confident that he will be able to efficiently continue the plan independent of the support of the health care team.

Determining when to take pain medications can be confusing and requires a thought process that is similar to managing diabetes with insulin injections. Patients must "measure" their pain and its impact on function to determine if additional pain medication is needed and how much. To facilitate optimal understanding, it is important to provide clear and accurate written discharge instructions (AHCPR, 1992; Jacox et al., 1994). Supportive graphics to illustrate the use of each medication may be useful when discussing more complex pain management concepts such as persistent pain and breakthrough pain. Written instructions should include the times that medication was given to the patient while the patient was admitted including when the last dose was taken and when the next dose is due. The nurse should explain how medication administration is recorded to reduce reliance on memory and the chance for errors. Encourage patients to use a similar system to track their own medications after discharge. Patients may find it helpful to use a notebook to document their pain scores, daily function, side effects, and when medications are taken. A written record may provide additional understanding of how much medication they are taking and the impact that pain has on their lives. Patients' and family members' perceptions regarding pain management are occasionally different and a written record may help each to gain an appreciation of the other's perspective.

If the patient participated in a complementary or alternative strategy as part of the pain management plan, written instructions should be provided including when the strategy was used and how it was most effectively executed (e.g., which music was most relaxing). Appropriate referral information should be provided in cases where the strategy requires a specialist (e.g., acupuncture).

The patient and family should be given the opportunity to voice any concerns or questions they may have prior to discharge. In addition, the nurse should review the following concepts:

- Pain management plays an important role in the recovery process.
- Several different pain medications may be prescribed together to relieve pain through different mechanisms.
- When pain is persistent pain medications should be taken routinely.
- Physical dependence and tolerance to opioid pain medications are not addiction.

Many times patients and families are overwhelmed and are not sure what to ask. The nurse should provide the patient and family members with the name of their provider and phone number to contact if they have questions after discharge. Discharge instructions are outlined in the Patient Teaching & Discharge Priorities box (p. 358).

◼ Gerontological Considerations

The older adult patient is at risk for undermanagement of pain due to many barriers unique to the aging population. Myths such as pain is a natural part of aging, older adults are less sensitive to pain, and opioids should be avoided when treating pain are often believed by health care professionals, patients, and their family members. Barriers to appropriate pain management in older adults may include the patient's own reluctance to report pain due to the belief that pain is an expected consequence of aging and disease (Pautex & Gold, 2006). They may have fears about the meaning of pain in terms of disease and the potential impact that it may have on their ability to remain independent. In addition, many patients have fixed incomes and very minimal or no health care benefits. Financial concerns may cause them to delay seeking health care or to choose not to purchase prescribed medications. In addition to these and other age-specific barriers, many patients have multiple medical diagnoses and increased sensitivity to analgesic medications due to altered hepatic and renal function.

Consequences of Unrelieved Pain

The impact of undertreated pain in the older adult is costly on many levels. Older adults with pain may be less active, leading to deconditioning, gait disturbances, and increased risk of falling. Sleep disturbances are common for patients with pain, but have an even greater impact on the older adult, causing decreased energy, depression, and cognitive impairment (Jakcobsson, Klevsgard, Westergren, & Rahm Hallberg, 2003; Pautex & Gold, 2006). As the ability to independently perform daily activities declines, burdens on the health care system, dependence on caregivers, and social isolation increase and exert a negative impact on the quality of life (Weiner & Hanlon, 2001).

Pain Assessment and Measurement

Assessing and measuring the multiple dimensions of pain in the older adult can be accomplished in the same manner as with any adult patient in most cases. The American Geriatrics Society (AGS) has published *The Management of Persistent Pain in Older Persons* as a guide to appropriate pain management (AGS, 2002). It should not be assumed that the older adult would have difficulty with the pain assessment. Instead, the nurse should pay special attention to preparing for the interview so that the best outcomes are possible. The location of the interview should be quiet and free of interruptions. Plan for sufficient time so that the patient is able to take the time needed to answer the questions. Speak clearly while facing the patient and use body language to convey the meaning of the question. Ensure that patients with hearing impairments are wearing their hearing aids if possible. Likewise, ensure that patients are wearing their eyeglasses if vision is impaired. Assessment tools should be enlarged so that the pictures and font of the type are easily visualized.

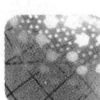

PATIENT TEACHING & DISCHARGE PRIORITIES for Pain Management

Need	Teaching
PRESCRIPTION MANAGEMENT Patient/family	Prescriptions for pain medications should be filled as soon as possible so that the next dosage can be taken on time.
	Secure prescription pain medications to prevent loss or theft.
	Avoid opening medication bottles over the sink or toilet.
	Follow your prescribed pain medication taper plan. • Contact your prescribing health care provider prior to taking extra doses of medication or if dosage needs to be reduced.
	Report unrelieved or new pain to your health care provider.
	If an additional prescription is necessary, notify your prescribing health care provider 2 to 3 days before it is needed.
	Assess pain intensity and ability to perform necessary activities prior to taking pain medications. • Take routine medications on schedule without skipping dosages. • Take "as-needed" medications prior to the onset of severe pain. • Use a notebook or journal to record the pain score, activity at the time of medication, the time and dosage of medication, and notes describing your concerns.
	Assess for pain medication side effects. • Take pain medications with food to prevent nausea. • Take stool softeners and stimulating laxatives routinely if taking opioid pain medications to prevent constipation. • Contact your prescribing health care provider if your opioid pain medication causes excessive sleepiness or heavy snoring.
	Assess knowledge of pain medications and pain management plan.
Family/support system	• Assess knowledge of pain medication side effects and treatments. • Assess knowledge of physical dependence, tolerance, and addiction. • Assess financial needs and resources for prescription coverage. • Provide example of journal or notebook for patient use.
Setting	• Assess discharge referral needs: Pain management specialist/clinic, psychiatrist or psychologist, primary care provider. • Assess need for follow-up appointments.
NONMEDICATION STRATEGY MANAGEMENT Patient/family	Nonmedication strategies that were helpful during admission should continue to be used in addition to pain medications.
	Assess pain intensity and ability to perform necessary activities prior to performing nonmedication strategies. • Record the pain score, activity at the time of the nonmedication strategies, the time, and notes describing your feelings or concerns in the journal or notebook.
Family/support system	Assess knowledge of selected nonmedication strategies role in the pain management plan.
Setting	Assess discharge referral needs: physical therapist, massage therapist, acupuncture practitioner.
	Assess for need for follow-up appointments.
PAINFUL PROCEDURE MANAGEMENT Patient/family Family/support system Setting	Medications that are prescribed for use prior to painful procedures should be taken allowing sufficient time for onset of pain relief prior to beginning procedure.
	Assess pain score prior to, during, and after procedure. • Utilize nonmedication strategies to encourage relaxation or distraction. • Report unrelieved pain during procedures to your prescribing health care provider.
	Assess understanding of the role of premedication in successful procedural pain management.
	Assess knowledge of pain medications and nonmedication strategies to be used prior to and during painful procedures.
	Assess for need for professional home health assistance with procedural pain management.

Many of the common pain intensity measurement tools are valid and acceptable to use when assessing the older adult (AGS, 2002; McDonald, 2006; Pautex & Gold, 2006). It is suggested that the 0–10 numeric rating scale is a good first choice. If the patient has difficulty with the NSR, the nurse should try the simple verbal descriptor scale next, followed by the pain thermometer (a diagram of a thermometer with descriptions that show increasing pain intensity), and then finally the faces pain scale (Herr, 2002). When older adult patients have cognitive impairment (e.g., dementia, Alzheimer's disease, or stroke) assessment of pain can be challenging, as discussed next.

Pain Assessment in Older Adults with Cognitive Impairments

Assessment of pain in an older adult who is cognitively impaired presents a significant nursing challenge. Impairments may range from minor deficits in memory to the advanced stages of Alzheimer's disease. In spite of the difficulty that cognitive impairment presents, studies support the validity of specific pain assessment tools for use in this population and demonstrate that a surprising number of older adults with cognitive impairments are able to use these tools effectively (Soscia, 2003). Just as with cognitively intact patients, the nurse should select a pain assessment tool that specifically meets the needs of the patient. Research findings suggest that the McGill Pain Questionnaire short form is the most reliable and valid for use in the mildly or moderately cognitively impaired older adult patient in the nursing home with only 27% of older cognitively impaired adults being unable to complete the tool (Wynne, Ling, & Remsburg, 2000). Other assessment tools studied were the visual descriptor scale (49% unable to use), the visual analog scale (43% unable to use), and the faces pain scale (39% unable to use) (Wynne et al., 2000). Additional studies suggest that the visual analog scale may be more useful if presented in a vertical form like a thermometer so that patients can relate more intense pain to the rising of the temperature (Herr & Garand, 2001; Herr & Mobily, 1991).

Careful assessment of the behavioral dimension of pain is helpful when the use of most other assessments is not possible. Common pain-related behaviors demonstrated by older adults with cognitive impairment include:

- Aggressiveness
- Restlessness
- Agitation
- Increased or decreased verbalization or vocalization
- Changes in appearance, facial expressions, or body language (AGS, 2002; Parke, 1998).

To fully appreciate the subtle changes that indicate a patient with cognitive impairment is experiencing pain, the nurse must become familiar with the patient's everyday personality, habits, and activities (AGS, 2002; Soscia, 2003). Family members and caregivers can be very helpful in establishing a baseline for the patient's behavior, as well as assisting with identification of changes from baseline (AGS, 2002).

Pain assessment is possible in older adults with cognitive impairments if the nurse recognizes the special assessment needs of this population by selecting the correct assessment tools, utilizing the behavioral assessment, and establishing the patient's normal baseline with the patient's family members or caregiver.

Pharmacologic Considerations

When selecting analgesic medications for the treatment of pain in the older adult, the changes that occur with aging must be considered to reduce the risk of medication side effects. Changes in gastric pH, increased gastric emptying, and decreased intestinal blood flow are common changes that will slow the absorption of medications. When the older adult has decreased lean body mass, increased body fat, decreased body water, and increased plasma protein, the distribution of medications is altered (Smith, 2003; St. Marie & Loeb, 2002). Medications are stored in the tissue longer extending their effects. When hepatic changes such as decreased hepatic mass and blood flow are present, metabolism is impacted, increasing the half-life of medications and reducing clearance or elimination as a result. Older adults also may experience decreased clearance or elimination of medications as a result of decreased glomerular filtration rate, decreased creatinine clearance, and decreased renal blood flow.

The physiological changes that occur with advancing age often result in a more potent effect and longer half-life of medications commonly used to treat pain. Generally those adults who are older than 70, who also have altered absorption, distribution, metabolism, and excretion, should be started on 25% to 50% of the recommended adult starting doses (AHCPR, 1992; APS, 2003). Once the patient's response to the medication is determined, dosages should be slowly increased or decreased as indicated until the desired effects are achieved. Specific medication cautions for the older adult are listed in Chart 15–8.

CHART 15–8	Medication Cautions for the Older Adult
NSAIDS	Highly protein bound NSAIDS, such as aspirin, diflunisal, ibuprofen, naproxen, indomethacin, meclofenamate, and piroxicam are more likely than the younger population to cause toxicities.
Meperidine (Demerol)	The active metabolite normeperidine can cause CNS irritability leading to seizures. Delirium and agitation are more likely when used to treat the postoperative older adult. Metabolite accumulation and toxicity occur when renal function is impaired.
Propoxyphene (Darvon, Darvocet)	The active metabolite norpropoxyphene can make seizures and cardiac arrhythmias more likely to occur. Accumulation and toxicity occur when renal function is impaired.
Pentazocine (Talwin)	More likely to cause seizures, cardiac arrhythmias, and agitation. Analgesia is similar to aspirin.
Tricyclic antidepressants	Anticholinergic effects are often intolerable.
Sedatives, hypnotics, and antiemetics	Long duration of action and sedation side effects make the older adult more prone to delirium, and unstable gait leads to increased risk of falls. Can cause respiratory depression especially when given with opioids.
Antihistamines	Anticholinergic effects are often intolerable. Use should be limited to less than 12 weeks, and in lower dosage ranges.

Sources: American Geriatric Society, Panel on Chronic Pain in Older Persons. (2002). The management of persistent pain in older persons: AGS panel on persistent pain in older persons. *Journal of the American Geriatrics Society, 6*(50), 205–224; St. Marie, B. (2002). Gerontologic pain management. In B. St. Marie (Ed.), *Core curriculum for pain management nursing* (pp. 417–426). Philadelphia: W. B. Saunders; Pasero, C., & McCaffery, M. (2000). When patients can't report pain. *American Journal of Nursing, 100,* 22–23.

RESEARCH OPPORTUNITIES AND CLINICAL IMPACT RELATED TO PAIN MANAGEMENT

Research Area	Clinical Impact
Assessment tools that are culturally sensitive for ethnic minorities who speak English dialects and have low literacy levels	Improved ability to assess pain in this at-risk population of patients
Assessment tools that are disease specific	Improved ability to capture the unique components of pain in diseases such as sickle cell, HIV, or cancer
Outcomes related to high-technology implanted modalities	Improved understanding of when high technology will improve outcomes to facilitate development of clinical guidelines outlining best practices
Neural remodeling as a mechanism of chronic pain	Identification of preventive, management, and restorative treatment possibilities
Use of opioids for the treatment of chronic pain	Improved understanding of the impact of opioids on long-term health to facilitate development of clinical guidelines and consensus on best practice
Gender differences in chronic pain	Improved understanding of sex-related factors and mechanisms that could lead to the development of new medications and management strategies
Clinical trials of complementary and alternative therapies	Establishment of a base of scientific evidence to validate the use of these therapies in specific pain states
Genes that are relevant to pain and inhibitory mechanisms	Development of gene therapy models targeting specific structures within the central nervous system
The role of sleep and circadian variations in perception and modulation of pain	Understand the differences in pain perception and modulation for patients who have unusual sleep/rest/activity needs (e.g., night shift workers, people with insomnia)
Barriers to patient compliance with pain treatment plan	Development of assessments, tools, educational materials, or specific helps that are demonstrated to improve compliance

EVIDENCE-BASED PRACTICE

Pain Management

Clinical Problem

Management of patients' pain is an ongoing nursing challenge. Due to patients' individual perceptions and responses, it can be difficult to quantify the pain. Typically, health care providers order a variety of medications and dosages that can be administered based on the level of pain. Therefore, it is essential that nurses make an accurate assessment of the pain in order to make a decision regarding choice of medication. A number of pain intensity scales, as described earlier in this chapter, have been developed to assist in standardizing pain levels and subsequent management, but the controversy continues about the best method to quantify pain (Pasero & McCaffery, 2005).

Research Findings

McDonald, LaPorta, and Meadows-Olive (2007) conducted a study to determine nurses' responses to patients' reports of pain. The study evaluated three different methods patients used to describe their pain:

Personal description along with a numeric scale

Personal description only

Numeric scale only.

Nurses were randomly assigned to three groups and all were given a vignette about a trauma patient with moderate to severe pain. The vignettes were identical except for the three different methods used by the patients to describe their pain and the patient's age. The results showed that there was no difference in the nurses' responses to the pain management between the three modes. The authors further noted that a relatively small number of pain management strategies were identified by the sample nurses in response to moderately severe pain.

Implications for Nursing Practice

Knowledge of effective pain management is still an evolving area of health care. It is a multifaceted area with issues of effective relief, addiction, and legal ramifications woven into the management decisions. Nurses are in a pivotal position in the pain management arena and therefore must have knowledge of and an appreciation for these issues. Nurses' approach to pain management also requires sensitivity to individual responses to pain. When using the numeric scores it is important to use the appropriate terminology and to further inquire about the reason for the score on the pain scale (Thompson American Health Consultants, 2004). For example, some patients report a pain number and then state they are comfortable with a certain pain level as it relates to their diagnosis and do not require medication, whereas other patients report the same score and are not comfortable and therefore require treatment.

Prior use of both legal and illegal medications also may impact pain scores. Occasionally, patients with illicit drug histories demonstrate "drug-seeking" behaviors such as fabricating pain levels in order to receive medication. Nurses must come to understand individual nuances to effectively manage pain. Use of both personal account and numeric scales provides the nurse with more data when making treatment decisions.

Critical Thinking Questions

1. When a patient reports a pain score what further information is needed to determine the appropriate pain intervention?

2. How would a nurse assess the pain level in a nonverbal patient?

Answers to Critical Thinking Questions appear in Appendix D.

References

Pasero, C., & McCaffery, M. (2005). Pain control: No self-report means no pain-intensity rating: Assessing pain in patients who cannot provide a report. *American Journal of Nursing, 105*(10), 50–53.

Thompson American Health Consultants. (2004). *Managing pain and end of life issues* (Vol. 2). Atlanta: Author.

Research

The science of pain management is expanding with astonishing speed due to the ongoing efforts of scientists, nurses, and other health care providers who have dedicated time and energy to discovery. The "Decade of Pain Research" provides an opportunity to accomplish even more. The Research Opportunities and Clinical Impact feature provides a list of both medical and nursing research topics still under investigation.

Clinical Preparation

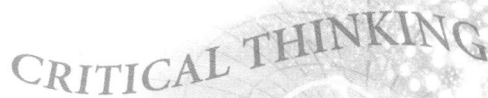

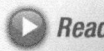 **Read**

- History of Current Illness
- Past Medical History
- Physical Exam
- Admitting Medical Orders
- Laboratory Study Results

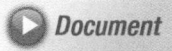 **Document**

- Summary of Hospitalization
- Pathophysiology Form
- Laboratory Values
- Laboratory Results Explanation

 **Apply**

- List of Potential Nursing Diagnoses
- Concept Map
- Critical Thinking Questions

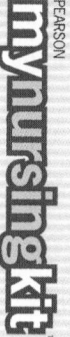

Log on to MyNursingKit.com to download forms you will need and to complete further steps in the Clinical Preparation assignment.

HISTORY OF PRESENT ILLNESS

As the on-coming nurse on the orthopedic nursing unit in a major trauma hospital, you are receiving report about Mr. X, a 27-year-old male who was admitted to the hospital following a motor vehicle collision in which he was the unrestrained driver. Mr. X was ejected from the vehicle, but did not lose consciousness and was able to provide a brief medical history to paramedics at the scene. In the report, the night nurse stated that the patient was now 24 hours post-op following stabilization of an open book pelvic fracture with external fixation. He has multiple lacerations over his arms and legs and a large laceration on his head that the plastic surgeon repaired during surgery.

Medical–Surgical History

His past medical history includes asthma and multiple knee arthroscopies for sports-related injuries.

Social History

Mr. X is married and the father of two children ages 1 and 3. Mr. X's wife and parents are at his bedside. He denies medication allergies, alcohol, smoking, or drug abuse.

Physical Exam

Mr. X is alert, oriented, with no sedation. His respiratory status includes deep, even, respirations at a rate of 14 breaths per minute. He is able to maintain oxygen saturations of 93% to 97% on room air. He has clear breath sounds.

His pulse is regular and strong with an apical heart rate of 68 beats per minute with no extra heart sounds. He has 3+ peripheral pulses with capillary refill < 3 seconds in all extremities. Blood pressure is measured at 132/56.

Bowel sounds are present in all four quadrants of the abdomen and he denies nausea. He has passed flatus and his surgeon has prescribed advancement of diet as tolerated. He has not had a bowel movement since surgery.

A urinary catheter has been placed and is draining approximately 30 mL of dark yellow-brown urine per hour.

Current Pain Assessment

Mr. X reports pain in his lower abdomen bilaterally, right groin, and right shoulder. He rates his pain intensity using the numeric rating scale of 0 to 10 as 7/10 in his abdomen, 9/10 in his right groin, and 5/10 in his right knee. Mr. X describes the pain in his abdomen and right groin as constant, sharp, stabbing with occasional spasms, and the right knee pain as a constant, aching, throbbing pain. He reports his pain is unbearable when he is turned in bed to change the linens.

Mr. X expresses frustration and anger that his pain is unrelieved and that his life is ruined because of the injuries he has sustained. His wife expresses concern that he is not coping as he usually does when faced with difficult circumstances. The hospital chaplain has attempted to visit with Mr. X and his wife on two separate occasions, but each time Mr. X declines the visit stating that he is in too much pain. When Mr. X's wife leaves the room he is calm and watches the sports channel on the TV.

Admitting Medical Orders

Admit to trauma service

Diagnosis: multiple lacerations over arms, legs, and head; rule out internal injuries; open book pelvic fracture

No known allergies

Vital signs every 4 hours

Bed rest

Sequential compression devices (SCD) to lower extremities

Peroxide ½ strength to clean pin sites q12h

Foley catheter

Intake and output

IV: D5½NS plus KCl 20 mEq at 125 hour

NPO

Incentive spirometer q1h while awake and q4h at night

Clean lacerations with ½ strength hydrogen peroxide q8h

Call house officer: Pulse < 60 & > 110/minute; BP < 90 & > 160 systolic; temperature > 38.5; urine output < 30 mL/hr for 2 hours; respiratory rate > 30/minute

Scheduled Medications

IV PCA morphine 1 mg/mL; no continuous infusion, 1 mg PCA demand dose, a 6-minute lockout time, and a 12-mg hourly limit; may bolus with 2 mg every hour prn severe pain

PRN Medications

Phenergan 25 mg IV q6h prn nausea

Ativan 0.5–2 mg IV q6–8h prn anxiety (not to exceed 10 mg/24 hours)

Tylenol 650 mg PR q4h for pain

Benadryl 25–50 mg IV qhs

Ordered Laboratory Studies

CBC q6h times 24 hours, then daily; basic metabolic panel daily, UA ×1 now

Ordered Diagnostic Studies

12-lead ECG

PA and lateral chest x-ray

X-ray of right knee and pelvis post-fixation

LABORATORY STUDY RESULTS

Test	Day 1	Day 2	Day 3
Potassium	4.4 mEq/L	3.8 mEq/L	3.7 mEq/L
Chloride	106 mEq/L	106 mEq/L	111 mEq/L
Sodium	142 mEq/L	141 mEq/L	144 mEq/L
Carbon dioxide (CO_2)	24 mEq/L	24 mEq/L	27 mEq/L
Anion gap	12.4 mEq/L	11.8 mEq/L	7.1 mEq/L
Glucose	97 mg/dL	99 mg/dL	119 mg/dL
Blood urea nitrogen (BUN)	22 mg/dL	22 mg/dL	20 mg/dL
Creatinine	0.8 mg/dL	0.8 mg/dL	1.4 mg/dL
Calcium	8.2 mg/dL	8.2 mg/dL	7.7 mg/dL
Hemoglobin	10/10.2/9.8/10/9.9/10.1 g/dL	10.1 g/dL	10.4 g/dL
Hematocrit	33/33.4/34/32.3/33/34/33/%	33.6 %	34%
Urinalysis			
Appearance and color	Dark amber and clear		
pH	6.2		
Protein	6 mg/dL		
Specific gravity	1.025		
Leukocytes, nitrates, ketones, and bilirubin	All negative		
Urobilinogen	0.02 units/mL		
Crystals and casts	None		
Glucose	None		
WBC and RBC	None		

CRITICAL THINKING QUESTIONS

1. Which dimensions of pain would you consider significant when reviewing your assessment of Mr. X's pain?

2. Which nursing intervention would be appropriate for the change in behavior when Mr. X's wife leaves the room?

3. What additional assessments would be important to consider prior to contacting the prescribing health care provider to advocate for changes to Mr. X's pain medications?

Answers to Critical Thinking Questions appear in Appendix D.

NCLEX® REVIEW

1. After attending a symposium on pain assessment and management, the well-informed nurse understands that pain:

    1. Is a common symptom to most illnesses, disease processes, and traumatic injuries.

    2. Is recognized, expressed, and responded to similarly among all cultures.

    3. Is addressed by a friendly health care system that is willing and able to manage pain.

    4. Is rarely associated with significant personal, social, or economic distress.

2. Confusion about treatment goals and the reality of pain abound, requiring nurses to make many legal and ethical decisions regarding pain and pain management. The nurse implementing a plan of care for the patient with chronic nonmalignant pain should:

    1. Identify that chronic nonmalignant pain is usually directly proportional to objective disease severity.

    2. Exclude the use of chronic opiates when the patient also requires treatment for concurrent psychiatric disorders.

    3. Recognize the fundamental responsibility of all nurses to help alleviate patient suffering and relieve pain.

    4. Acknowledge the patient's own fears of facing criminal penalties for receiving excessive amounts of opiates.

3. The nurse is educating the patient with chronic pain about his condition. The nurse knows the patient has a clear understanding of chronic pain with verbalization of the statement:

    1. "My pain should be brief and then resolve completely."

    2. "The pain I am having coincides with my recent surgery."

    3. "This pain will not last long, but will come back soon."

    4. "My pain may last for months, years, or for my whole life."

4. The nurse recognizes that two of the most accurate multidimensional evaluation methods when assessing a patient's pain would be:

    1. A patient's pain intensity self-report and behavioral assessment.

    2. The McGill Pain Questionnaire and the patient interview.

    3. The numeric rating scale and simple verbal descriptive scale.

    4. A Critical-Care Pain Observation Tool and visual analog scale.

Answers for review questions appear in Appendix D

KEY TERMS

absorption *p.343*
acute pain *p.334*
adjuvant medications *p.347*
affective dimension of pain *p.336*
agonist *p.341*
agonist-antagonist *p.347*
antagonist *p.347*
behavioral dimension of pain *p.337*
biotransformation *p.343*
breakthrough pain *p.335*
Brief Pain Inventory (BPI) *p.339*
cancer pain *p.335*
chronic pain *p.334*

cognitive dimension of pain *p.336*
distribution *p.343*
elimination *p.343*
endorphins *p.336*
enkephalins *p.336*
gate control theory *p.335*
hepatic first-pass metabolism *p.343*
McGill Pain Questionnaire (MPQ) *p.339*
metabolism *p.343*
neuromatrix theory *p.335*
neuropathic pain *p.336*
nociception *p.335*
nociceptive pain *p.335*

noxious stimuli *p.335*
numeric rating scale (NRS) *p.338*
pain *p.334*
pattern theory *p.335*
phantom limb pain *p.335*
recurrent pain *p.334*
sensory dimension of pain *p.336*
simple verbal descriptive scale (SVDS) *p.338*
specificity theory *p.335*
transduction *p.335*
transient pain *p.335*
visual analog scale (VAS) *p.338*

PEARSON

EXPLORE mynursingkit™

MyNursingKit is your one stop for online chapter review materials and resources. Prepare for success with additional NCLEX®-style practice questions, interactive assignments and activities, web links, animations and videos, and more!

Register your access code from the front of your book at
www.mynursingkit.com

REFERENCES

Agency for Health Care Policy and Research, Acute Pain Management Guideline Panel. (1992, February). *Acute pain management: Operative or medical procedures and trauma* (Clinical Practice Guideline, AHCPR Pub. No. 92-0032). Rockville, MD: Author.

American Academy of Pain Medicine, American Pain Society, & American Society of Addiction Medicine. (2001). *Definitions related to the use of opioids for the treatment of pain.* Glenview, IL: American Pain Society.

American Geriatric Society, Panel on Chronic Pain in Older Persons. (2002). The management of persistent pain in older persons: AGS panel on persistent pain in older persons. *Journal of the American Geriatrics Society, 6*(50), 205–224.

American Nurses Association. (2001). *Code for nurses with interpretive statements.* Kansas City, MO: Author.

American Pain Society. (2000). *Principles of analgesic use in the treatment of acute pain and cancer pain* (4th ed.). Glenview, IL: Author.

American Pain Society. (2003). *Principles of analgesic use in the treatment of acute pain and cancer pain* (5th ed.). Glenview, IL: Author.

American Pain Society. (2005). *Guideline for the management of cancer pain in adults and children.* Glenview, IL: Author.

American Society for Pain Management Nursing. (2007). *ASPMN position statement: Assisted suicide.* Retrieved February 12, 2007, from http://www.aspmn.org/pdfs/Assisted%20Suicide.pdf

Arnstein, P. M. (2003). Comprehensive analysis and management of chronic pain. *The Nursing Clinics of North America, 38*(3), 403–417.

Arnstein, P. M., Wells-Federman, C. L., & Caudill-Slosberg, M. A. (2002, August). *Change in self efficacy as a predictor of clinical outcomes and coping skill use at 1 year following participation in a cognitive behavioral pain treatment program.* Paper presented at the 10th World Congress on Pain, San Diego, CA.

Backonja, M. (2001). Painful neuropathies. In J. D. Loeser, S. H. Butler, C. R. Chapman, & D. C. Turk (Eds.), *Bonica's management of pain* (3rd ed., pp. 371–387). Philadelphia: Lippincott Williams & Wilkins.

Bajwa, Z. H., Warfield, C. A., & Wootton, R. J. (2006). *Overview of treatment for chronic pain.* Retrieved February 25, 2007, from UpToDate website: http://utdol.com/utd/store/index.do

Bonica, J. J., & Loeser, J. D. (2001). History of pain concepts and therapies. In J. D. Loeser, S. H. Butler, C. R. Chapman, & D. C. Turk (Eds.), *Bonica's management of pain* (3rd ed., pp. 3–16). Philadelphia: Lippincott Williams & Wilkins.

Brookhoff, D. (2000). Chronic pain: A new disease? *Hospital Practice,* 23–50.

Brown, M., Phillips, P. Cusimano, C., & Osteyee, J. (2003). *ASPMN position statement: Pain management at the end of life.* Retrieved from American Society for Pain Management Nursing website: http://www.aspmn.org

Buckley, P. F. (2001). Regional anesthesia with local anesthetics. In J. D. Loeser, S. H. Butler, C. R. Chapman, & D. C. Turk (Eds.), *Bonica's management of pain* (3rd ed., pp. 1893–1966). Philadelphia: Lippincott Williams & Wilkins.

Byers, M. R., & Bonica, J. J. (2001). Peripheral pain mechanisms and nociceptor plasticity. In J. D. Loeser, S. H. Butler, C. R. Chapman, & D. C. Turk (Eds.), *Bonica's management of pain* (3rd ed., pp. 26–72). Philadelphia: Lippincott Williams & Wilkins.

Campbell, C. E. (2006). The role of nursing in pain management. In M. V. Boswell & B. E. Cole (Eds.), *Weiner's pain management: A practical guide for clinicians* (7th ed., pp. 165–175). Boca Raton, FL: Taylor & Francis Group.

Campbell, J. (1995, November 11). *Pain: The fifth vital sign.* Presidential address presented at the meeting of the American Pain Society, Los Angeles.

Chiu, L. H., Trinca, J., Lim, L. M., & Tuazon, J. A. (2003). A study to evaluate the pain knowledge of two sub-populations of final year nursing students: Australia and Philippines. *Journal of Advanced Nursing, 41,* 99–108.

Coda, B. A., & Bonica, J. J. (2001). General considerations in acute pain. In J. D. Loeser, S. H. Butler, C. R. Chapman, & D. C. Turk (Eds.), *Bonica's management of pain* (3rd ed., pp. 222–254). Philadelphia: Lippincott Williams & Wilkins.

Coggins, C., Arnstein, P., & Leahy, S. (2004). *ASPMN position statement: Use of placebos for pain management.* Retrieved from American Society for Pain Management Nursing website: http://www.aspmn.org

Coggins, C., McCaffery, M., Pasero, C., St. Marie, B., & Nichols, R. (2003). *ASPMN position statement: Pain management in patients with addictive disease.* Retrieved from American Society for Pain Management Nursing website: http://www.aspmn.org

Dahl, J. L. (2002). Working with regulators to improve the standard of care in pain management: The U.S. experience. *Journal of Pain and Symptom Management, 24,* 136–157.

Davis, M. P., Walsh, D., LeGrand, S. B., & Naughton, M. (2002). Symptom control in cancer patients: The clinical pharmacology and therapeutic role of suppositories and rectal suspensions. *Support Care Cancer, 10,* 117–138.

Ferrell, B. R., Novy, D., Sullivan, M. D., Banja, J., Dubois, M. Y., Gitlin, M., et al. (2001). Ethical dilemmas in pain management. *Journal of Pain, 2*(3), 171–180.

Frank-Stromborg, M., & Christensen, A. (2001). A serious look at the undertreatment of pain: Part I. *Clinical Journal of Oncology Nursing, 5*(5), 235–236.

Gelinas, C., Fillion, L., Puntillo, K. A., Viens, C., & Fortier, M. (2006). Validation of the Critical-Care Pain Observation Tool in adult patients. *American Journal of Critical Care, 15*(4), 420–427.

Gelinas, C., Fortier, M., Viens, C., Fillion, L., & Puntillo, K. A. (2004). Pain assessment and management in critically-ill intubated patients: A retrospective study. *American Journal of Critical Care, 13*(2), 126–135.

Glen, V. L., & St. Marie, B. (2002). Overview of pharmacology. In B. St. Marie (Ed.), *Core curriculum for pain management nursing* (pp. 181–202). Philadelphia: W. B. Saunders.

Griffie, J. (2003). Addressing inadequate pain relief. *American Journal of Nursing, 103*(8), 61–63.

Herr, K. (2002). Pain assessment in cognitively impaired older adults. *American Journal of Nursing,102,* 65–67.

Herr, K., Coyne, P. J., Key, T., Manworren, R., McCaffery, M., Merkel, S., et al. (2006). Pain assessment in the nonverbal patient: Position statement with clinical practice recommendations. *Pain Management Nursing, 7*(2), 44–52.

Houde, R., Wallenstein, S., & Beaver, W. (1996). Evaluation of analgesics in patients with cancer pain. In L. Lasagna (Ed.), *International Encyclopedia of Pharmacology and Therapeutics. Section 6, Clinical Pharmacology* (Vol. 1, pp. 59–98). Oxford: Pergamon Press.

International Association for the Study of Pain. (1993). *Outline curriculum on pain for schools of nursing.* Retrieved February 23, 2007, from http://www.iasp-pain.org/nursing_toc.html

International Council of Nurses. (2006). *The ICN code of ethics for nurses.* Geneva, Switzerland: Author.

Jacox, A., Carr, D. B., Payne, R., et al. (1994, March). *Management of cancer pain* (Clinical Practice Guideline No. 9, AHCPR Pub. No. 94-0592). Rockville, MD: Agency for Health Care Policy and Research.

Jakcobsson, U., Klevsgard, R., Westergren, A., & Rahm Hallberg, I. (2003). Old people in pain: A comparative study. *Journal of Pain and Symptom Management, 26,* 625–636.

Joint Commission on Accreditation of Healthcare Organizations. (2002). *Pain assessment and management: An organizational approach.* Retrieved February 26, 2007, from http://www.jointcommission.org

Kaplow, R., & Hardin, S. R. (2007). *Critical care nursing: Synergy for optimal outcomes* (pp. 41–51). Sudbury, MA: Jones and Bartlett.

Karch, A. M, & Karch, F. E. (2003). Acetaminophen's hidden dangers. *American Journal of Nursing, 103,* 101.

Lethridge-Cejku, M., & Vickerie, J. (2005). Summary health for U.S. adults: National health interview survey, 2003. *National Center for Health Statistics, 10,* 225.

Maher, T. J., & Chaiyakul, P. (2003). Opioids (Bench). In H.S. Smith, *Drugs for pain* (pp. 83–96). Philadelphia, PA: Hanley & Belfus, Inc.

McCaffery, M. (1968). *Nursing practice theories related to cognition, bodily pain, and man–environment interactions.* Los Angeles: University of California at Los Angeles Students' Store.

McCaffery, M., & Pasero, C. (1999). Assessment: Underlying complexities, misconceptions, and practical tools. In M. McCaffery & C. Pasero (Eds.), *Pain: Clinical manual* (2nd ed., pp. 35–102). St. Louis, MO: Mosby.

McCaffery, M., & Portenoy, R. K. (1999). Nonopioids. In M. McCaffery & C. Pasero (Eds.), *Pain: Clinical manual* (2nd ed., pp. 129–160). St. Louis, MO: Mosby.

McCaffery, M., Ferrell, B. R., & Pasero, C. (2000). Nurses' personal opinions about patients' pain and their effect on recorded assessments and titration of opioid doses. *Pain Management Nursing, 1*(3), 70–87.

McDonald, D. D. (2006). Postoperative pain management for the aging patient. *Geriatrics Aging, 9*(6), 395–398.

Melzack, R., & Wall, P. D. (1983). *The challenge of pain.* New York: Basic Books.

Melzack, R. (1999). From gate to neuromatrix. *Pain, 6* (Suppl.), S121–S126.

Merck. (2007). Types: Pain. In *The Merck Manual of Medical Information—Home Edition.* Retrieved May 27, 2008, from http://www.merck.com/mmhe/sec06/ch078/ch078b.html?qt=types:%20pain&alt=sh

Mersky, H. (1994). Classification of chronic pain: Descriptions of chronic pain syndromes and definitions of pain terms. *Pain* (Suppl. 3), S215–S221.

Miyoshi, H. R., & Leckband, S. G. (2001). Systemic opioid analgesics. In J. D. Loeser, S. H. Butler, C. R. Chapman, & D. C. Turk (Eds.), *Bonica's management of pain* (3rd ed., pp. 1682–1709). Philadelphia: Lippincott Williams & Wilkins.

Morgan, J. P. (1985). American opiophobia: Customary underutilization of opioid analgesics. *Advances in Alcohol and Substance Abuse, 86*(5), 163–173.

National Cancer Institute. (2007). *Pain PDQ: Pharmacologic management.* Retrieved February 19, 2007, from http://www.cancer.gov/cancertopics/pdq/supportivecare/pain/HealthProfessional/Page3

National Institutes of Health. (1987). The integrated approach to the management of pain. *Journal of Pain and Symptom Management, 2,* 35–44.

National Institute of Neurological Disorders and Stroke. (2007a). *Chronic pain information page.* Retrieved February 19, 2007, from http://www.ninds.nih.gov/disorders/chronic_pain/chronic_pain.htm

National Institute of Neurological Disorders and Stroke. (2007b). *Gene therapy relieves neuropathic pain in rats.* Retrieved February 19, 2007, from http://www.ninds.nih.gov/news_and_events/news_articles/news_article_pain_gene_therapy.htm

Parke, B. (1998). Gerontological nurses' ways of knowing. Realizing the presence of pain in cognitively impaired older adults. *Journal of Gerontological Nursing, 24*(6), 21–28.

Pasero, C., & McCaffery, M. (2000). When patients can't report pain. *American Journal of Nursing, 100,* 22–23.

Pasero, C., & McCaffery, M. (2001b). The patient's report of pain: Believing vs. accepting. There's a big difference. *American Journal of Nursing, 101,* 73–74.

Pasero, C., & McCaffery, M. (2001c). The undertreatment of pain: Are providers accountable for it? *American Journal of Nursing, 101,* 62–65.

Pasero, C., & McCaffery, M. (2005). Pain control: No self-report means no pain-intensity rating: Assessing pain in patients who cannot provide a report. *American Journal of Nursing, 105*(10), 50–53.

Pasero, C., Paice, J. A., & McCaffery, M. (1999). Basic mechanisms underlying the causes and effects of pain. In M. McCaffery & C. Pasero (Eds.), *Pain: Clinical manual* (2nd ed., pp. 15–34). St. Louis, MO: Mosby.

Pautex, S., & Gold, G. (2006) Assessing pain intensity in older adults. *Geriatrics Aging. 9*(6), 399–402.

Phillips, P., Gordon, D., & Frandsen, J. (2006). *ASPMN position statement: The use of "as-needed" range orders for opioid analgesics in the management of acute pain.* Retrieved from American Society for Pain Management Nursing website: http://www.aspmn.org

Portenoy, R. K., & Hagen, N. A. (1990). Breakthrough pain: Definition, prevalence and characteristics. *Pain, 41,* 273–281.

Portenoy, R. K., & McCaffery, M. (1999). Adjuvant Analgesics. In M. McCaffery & C. Pasero (Eds.), *Pain: Clinical manual* (2nd ed., pp. 302). St. Louis, MO: Mosby.

Porth, C. M. (2005). *Pathophysiology: Concepts of altered health states* (7th ed.) Philadelphia: Lippincott Williams & Wilkins.

Price, D. D., Riley, J. L., & Wade, J. B. (2001). Psychological approaches to measurement of the dimensions and stages of pain. In D. C. Turk & R. Melzack (Eds.), *Handbook of pain assessment* (2nd ed., pp. 53–75). New York: Guilford Press.

Primeau, M., Cowley, C., Eksterowicz, N., & Pasero, C. (2007). *ASPMN position statement: Registered nurse management and monitoring of analgesia by catheter techniques.* Retrieved from the American Society for Pain Management Nursing website: http://www.aspmn. org

Puntillo, K. A. (2007). Managing pain, delirium, and sedation. *Critical care nurse* (Suppl.), 8–10.

Puntillo, K. A., Morris, A. B., Thompson, C. L., Stanik-Hutt, J. A., White, L., & Wild, L. J. (2004). Behaviors observed during six common procedures: Results from thunder project II. *Critical Care Medicine, 32*(2), 412–427.

Rothley, B. B., & Therrien, S. R. (2002). Acute pain management. In B. St. Marie (Ed.), *Core curriculum for pain management nursing* (pp. 239–272). Philadelphia: W. B. Saunders.

Shea, R. A., Brooks, J. A., Dayhoff, N. E., & Keck, J. (2002). Pain intensity and postoperative pulmonary complications among the elderly after abdominal surgery. *Heart & Lung, 31,* 440–449.

Simon, L. S. (2003). Nonsteroidal anti-inflammatory drugs and cyclooxygenase-2 selective inhibitors. In H. S. Smith (Ed.), *Drugs for pain* (pp. 41–54). Philadelphia: Hanley & Belfus.

Smith, H. S. (2003). Acetaminophen (bedside). In H. S. Smith (Ed.), *Drugs for pain* (pp. 33–40). Philadelphia: Hanley & Belfus.

Snyder, M., & Wieland, J. (2003). Complimentary and alternative therapies: What is their place in management of chronic pain? *The Nursing Clinics of North America, 38*(3), 495–508.

Soscia, J. (2003). Assessing pain in cognitively impaired older adults with cancer. *Clinical Journal of Oncology Nursing, 7*(2), 174 –177.

St. Marie, B., & Loeb, J. L. (2002). Gerontologic pain management. In B. St. Marie (Ed.), *Core curriculum for pain management nursing* (pp. 417–426). Philadelphia: W. B. Saunders.

Sullivan, M., & Ferrell, B. (2005). *Ethical challenges in the management of chronic nonmalignant pain: Negotiating through the cloud of doubt.* Retrieved February 25, 2007, from American Pain Society, http://www.ampainsoc.org/press/2005_jop/0105.html

Swarm, R. A., Karanikolas, M., & Kalauokalani, D. (2001). Pain treatment in the perioperative period. *Current Problems in Surgery, 38,* 835–920.

Turk, D. C. (2006). Pain hurts—Individuals, significant others, and society. *American Pain Society Bulletin, 16*(1).

Turk, D. C., & Okifuji, A. (2001). Pain terms and taxonomies of pain. In J. D. Loeser, S. H. Butler, C. R. Chapman, & D. C. Turk (Eds.), *Bonica's management of pain* (3rd ed., pp. 17–25). Philadelphia: Lippincott Williams & Wilkins.

Watt-Watson, J., Stevens, B., Garfinkel, P., Streiner, D., & Gallop, R. (2001). Relationship between nurses' pain knowledge and pain management outcomes for their postoperative cardiac patients. *Journal of Advanced Nursing, 36,* 535–545.

Weiner, D. K., & Hanlon, J. T. (2001). Pain in nursing home residents: Management strategies. *Drugs and Aging, 18*(1), 13–19.

Weissman, D. E., & Haddox, J. D. (1989). Opioid pseudoaddiction—An iatrogenic syndrome. *Pain, 36,* 363–366.

Wisconsin Cancer Pain Initiative Nursing Education Committee. (1995). Competency guidelines for cancer pain in nursing education and practice. Retrieved May 27, 2008, from http://www.cityofhope.org/prc/pdf/Competency_Guidelines_ WCPI.pdf

Wittbrodt, E. T., & Tietze, K. J. (2004). *Pain control in the intensive care unit.* Retrieved February 25, 2007, from UpToDate website: http://utdol.com/utd/store/index.do

Wuhrman, E., Cooney, M. F., Dunwoody, C. J., Eksterowicz, N., Merkel, S., & Oakes, L. L. (2006). *ASPMN position statement: Authorized and unauthorized ("PCA by proxy") dosing of analgesic infusion pumps.* Retrieved from American Society for Pain Management Nursing website: http://www.aspmn.org

Wynne, C. F., Ling, S. M., Remsburg, R. (2000). Comparison of pain assessment instruments in cognitively intact and cognitively impaired nursing home residents. *Geriatric Nursing, 21,* 20–23.

Youngkin, E. Q., Sawin, K. J., Kissinger, J. F., & Israel, D. S. (2005). *Pharmacotherapeutics: A primary care guide* (2nd ed.). Upper Saddle River, NJ: Pearson Prentice Hall.

Substance Abuse

Eileen Trigoboff

Outcome-Based Learning Objectives

After studying this chapter, the learner will be able to:

1. Explain the major theories about substance-related disorders.
2. List why some groups are at risk for substance-related disorders.
3. Discuss how the physical, psychological, and withdrawal effects of the major categories of substances manifest themselves.
4. Incorporate nursing assessment components to detect patients who have substance-related disorders.
5. Demonstrate knowledge of a variety of short-term and long-term nursing intervention strategies for clients who have substance-related disorders.
6. Develop outcome criteria for clients who have substance-related disorders.
7. Establish what impact your own feelings and attitudes about clients with substance-related disorders have in your nursing care.

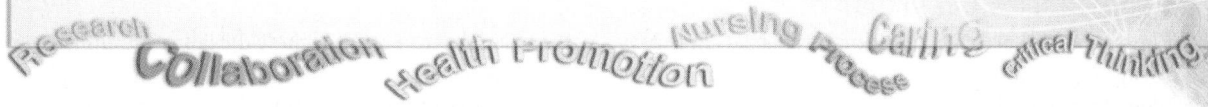

Research Collaboration Health Promotion Nursing Process Caring Critical Thinking

SUBSTANCE ABUSE is the clinical term for people who use or abuse prescription or recreational substances in order to experience one of the following: escape, relief, get a buzz, get away, get in touch, get cushioned, deserve a break, feel high, feel happy, feel numb, feel something, feel normal, feel distant, leave this realm of existence, or any other phrase describing the urge behind the behavior. This behavior is a way for people to cope or escape stress through substance abuse.

Substance abuse affects society as a whole by robbing it of valuable members. It increases the crime rate, automobile crash deaths, number of teenage pregnancies, and the suicide rate, while decreasing the quality of life for individuals and families (National Drug Intelligence Center [NDIC], 2006). There is not a single aspect of a substance abuser's life—social life, family life, community involvement, work productivity, coworker relationships, physical health—that escapes being affected.

The American Nurses Association (ANA) Standards of Addictions Nursing Practice demonstrate how important it is for nurses to understand the implications of addiction. There is an ongoing need for thorough assessment and collaborative treatment with other health care providers. The high incidence of substance abuse in society demands that nurses exhibit competence when treating patients with addictions. See the National Guidelines box for a list of the ANA standards (p. 366).

Definitions and Terminology

Nurses must know the language for this particular area of health care. The terms used to describe substance use and abuse include the names of the various stages of substance use as well as characteristics of behavior within that stage. Accurate nursing assessment is based on a good understanding of these terms.

Substance-Related Disorders

According to the *Diagnostic and Statistical Manual of Mental Disorders*, Fourth Edition, Text Revision (DSM-IV-TR) (American Psychiatric Association [APA], 2000), substance-related disorders are disorders that are (1) a consequence of abusing a drug (such as alcohol), (2) the side effects of a medication (antihistamines, for example), or (3) related to exposure to a toxin (fuel, paint, or other inhalants). Substance-related disorders are divided into two groups:

1. Substance use disorders that include substance dependence and substance abuse
2. Substance-induced disorders (including substance intoxication, substance withdrawal, and substance-induced cognitive disorders and mood disorders).

This chapter focuses on substance abuse. Material in this chapter refers to intoxication and withdrawal issues for some

NATIONAL GUIDELINES ANA Standards of Addictions Nursing Practice

Standard 1: Assessment

The addictions nurse collects patient health data.

Standard 2: Diagnosis

The addictions nurse analyzes the assessment data in determining diagnoses.

Standard 3: Outcome Identification

The addictions nurse identifies expected outcomes individualized to the patient.

Standard 4: Planning

The addictions nurse develops an individualized plan of care that prescribes interventions to attain expected outcomes.

Standard 5: Implementation

The addictions nurse implements the interventions identified in the plan of care.

Standard 5a: Therapeutic Alliance: The addictions nurse uses the "therapeutic self" to establish a therapeutic alliance with the patient and to structure nursing interventions to promote development of insight, coping skills, and motivation for change in behavior that promotes health.

Standard 5b: Health Teaching: The addictions nurse, through health teaching, assists individuals, families, groups, and communities in achieving satisfying, productive, and healthy patterns of living.

Standard 5c: Self-Care and Self-Management: The addictions nurse uses the knowledge and philosophy of self-care and self-management to assist the patient in learning new ways to address stress, maintain self-control, accept personal responsibility, and integrate healthy coping behaviors into lifestyle choices.

Standard 5d: Pharmacological, Biological, and Complementary Therapies: The addictions nurse applies knowledge of pharmacological, biological, and complementary therapies and uses clinical skills to restore the patient's health and prevent consequences from addiction.

Standard 5e: Therapeutic Milieu: The addictions nurse structures, provides, and maintains a therapeutic environment in collaboration with the patient and other health care providers.

Standard 5f: Counseling: The addictions nurse uses counseling interventions to assist patients in promoting healthy coping abilities, preventing addiction, and addressing issues related to patterns of abuse and addiction.

Standard 6: Evaluation

The addictions nurse evaluates the patient's progress toward attainment of expected outcomes.

classes of substances that have traditionally been called psychoactive drugs. Some of the often-abused drugs are listed in the Pharmacology Summary box.

Substance Dependence

Substance dependence is defined as a maladaptive pattern of substance use leading to clinically significant impairment or distress. The hallmarks of this pattern are:

- **Tolerance**, or needing increased amounts of a substance to achieve the desired effect
- **Withdrawal**, or the uncomfortable and maladaptive physiological and cognitive behavioral changes that are associated with lowered blood or tissue concentrations of a substance after an individual has been engaged in heavy use
- Compulsive use
- Needing larger amounts of the substance than intended
- Making unsuccessful efforts to cut down or regulate substance use
- Devoting a great deal of time trying to obtain the substance
- Using the substance or recovering from the effects of the substance
- Continuing to use the substance despite the recognition of associated adverse effects and difficulties (APA, 2000).

This diagnosis can be made for every class of substance except caffeine.

Substance Abuse

Substance abuse is characterized by a pattern of repeated consumption of substances that are used despite harm. Examples of the harm that can result include the failure to fulfill major role obligations (such as parenting), using substances in physically hazardous situations (such as crack houses), and repeated social and relationship problems (domestic violence) (Libby et al., 2006).

Substance Intoxication

Substance intoxication refers to a reversible syndrome of maladaptive physiological and behavioral changes that are due to the effects of a substance on a person's central nervous system (CNS). The syndrome includes disturbances of mood (such as belligerence or mood lability), perception, the sleep–wake cycle, attention, thinking, judgment, and psychomotor as well as interpersonal behavior (Doweiko, 2006).

Substance Withdrawal

Substance withdrawal refers to the development of maladaptive physiological, behavioral, and cognitive changes that are due to reducing or stopping the heavy and regular use of a substance. Some examples include muscle aches, nausea, diarrhea, and increased blood pressure. **Substance withdrawal syndrome** is associated with distress and/or impairment in important areas of social functioning.

Postacute Withdrawal Syndrome

Postacute withdrawal syndrome (PAWS) occurs well after the usual withdrawal symptoms have resolved. It is a physiological state stimulated or stamped on the individual's metabolism and physical responses through drug use. The syndrome is seen as enduring physical remnants of neurotransmitter production and/or receptor site damage. Neurotransmitter production problems, either overproduction or underproduction, affect

PHARMACOLOGY Summary of Medications to Treat Substance-Related Disorders

Medication Category	Action	Application/Indication	Nursing Responsibilities
Replacement Agent/ Anticonvulsant Magnesium sulfate	Anticonvulsant Activities Produced by CNS depression	Magnesium deficiency Seizure treatment and prevention	• Monitor for adverse effects: hypotension, hypothermia, stupor, respiratory depression. • Observe for signs of magnesium toxicity: cathartic effect, profound thirst, sedation, confusion, muscle weakness. Have calcium gluconate available as antidote. • Monitor EKG and vital signs when given IV. • Monitor renal function, magnesium, calcium, and phosphorous levels.
Anxiolytic/Anticonvulsant Diazepam (Valium) Chlordiazepoxide (Librium)	Reduces withdrawal symptoms by action on limbic and subcortical levels of CNS	Symptoms of acute alcohol withdrawal, prophylaxis and treatment of seizures, delirium tremens	• Monitor for adverse effects: drowsiness, fatigue, weakness, ataxia. • Monitor vital signs closely if given parenterally. • Be aware of drug interactions (phenytoin, cimetidine, CNS depressants and others). • Be aware of multiple IV incompatibilities (furosemide, heparin, potassium chloride, and others). • Monitor CBC and liver function if used long term. • Warn patient not to abruptly stop drug.
Antialcohol Agent Disulfiram (Antabuse)	Produces undesirable symptoms as a deterrent to alcohol ingestion by inhibiting acetaldehyde dehydrogenase which normally detoxifies and metabolizes alcohol	Alcohol cessation aid	• Monitor liver function, CBC. • Do not administer unless patient has been alcohol free for a minimum of 12 hours. • Be aware of drug interactions (warfarin, phenytoin, barbiturate, and others). • Warn patient not to consume alcohol in any form including cough and cold preparations, mouthwash, sauces, etc. • Warn patient of potential severe reactions if alcohol ingested while on medication (myocardial infarction, convulsions, respiratory depression, sudden death).
Opiate Antagonist Naltrexone (ReVia)	Reduces euphoria and drug craving by binding with opioid receptors	Adjunct to treatment of narcotic addiction and alcohol dependence	• Give naloxone challenge test before starting naltrexone. • Monitor for adverse effects: nausea, vomiting, abdominal cramps, muscle pain, insomnia, anxiety. • Monitor liver function. • Warn patient to check with physician before using OTC drugs. • Warn patient of risk of overdosing if opiates used.

mood, interpersonal interactions, and cognitive skills. Receptor site damage means that naturally produced neurotransmitters cannot be normally recognized, absorbed, or provide feedback. Therefore, normal functioning is impaired.

Evidence of PAWS is seen as unusual or flattened interpersonal styles, disabilities in functioning within demanding zones such as personal finances and stress, poor occupational/vocational functioning, and difficulties establishing and maintaining relationships. Typical symptoms of PAWS include inability to think clearly, memory problems, emotional overreactions or numbness, sleep disturbances, difficulty with physical coordination, and stress sensitivity. A common reaction from others is to believe that the person who was dependent on a substance and has been abstaining is now using again. This creates social stressors in addition to the physiological and cognitive problems.

Clinicians reporting on their work with alcohol- and substance-dependent individuals anecdotally reported these problems. For a period of time in the 1990s attempts were made to codify these reports in the hope of establishing a verifiable postacute withdrawal syndrome. However, since about 2000 it appears that efforts to accomplish this have been discontinued. It seems likely that the reported aftereffects may be variable enough such that they do not cohere to form a true medical syndrome.

 Etiology

The etiology of substance abuse, or what the causative factor or factors may be, describes how the problem of using substances inappropriately came into being. It is important to determine where and why the problem started in order to develop interventions to address the source.

Biological Theories

The biological explanation of substance abuse has had a great deal of support from recent developments in technology. With the use of magnetic resonance imaging (MRI) and positron emission tomograph (PET) scans, more details about the brain's function can be seen than ever before. Advances in neuroimaging and anatomic discoveries help explain substance abuse in terms of changes in the limbic area of the brain (Heimer & Van Hoesen, 2006). Other studies show biologic explanations of substance abuse and how genes affect the functioning of differential biochemical systems (Serretti et al., 2006), genotypes consistently indicating a relationship with substance abuse problems (Prescott et al., 2006), and the role of family genetics in the development of substance use disorders (Vieten, Seaton, Feiler, & Wilhelmsen, 2004).

Substance abuse prior to conception and pregnancy has such a strong biologic impact that in both males and females it has been validated as damaging to the genetic makeup of the child (Muthen, Asparouhov, & Rebollo, 2006). Research demonstrates that children of people who abuse alcohol have a fourfold risk of becoming alcohol abusers themselves. Even if different families adopt them at birth, identical twins of alcoholic parents have more than a 60% chance of becoming alcoholics; fraternal twins have just under a 30% chance.

Neurobiologic studies clearly support the fact that biologic factors such as genetics shape vulnerability to substance-related disorders and also result from them. Additional biologic foundations can be seen in the treatment of substance abuse. The body's responses to medications with anxiolytic and antidepressant effects used in detoxification and relapse-prevention treatment further support a biologic framework for substance abuse. Genetics may also be involved, as discussed in the Genetic Considerations box.

Psychological Theories

Psychological theories about substance abuse indicate that the psychological underpinnings of experiences and behaviors come together to form the motivations for using substances in a destructive manner. People respond to environmental influences through their underlying neurobiologic system. The remarkable frequency of some disorders—such as bipolar disorder—along with substance abuse further supports how psychological experiences and symptoms affect subsequent maladaptive coping (Albanese, 2005).

Dimensions of a person's personality, up to and including a characterological or personality disorder, can be detected in drug abusers. Routinely identified characteristics include inner dishonesty and self-centeredness, although self-centeredness could be related to the addiction itself. When someone is addicted to a substance, nothing is as important as the drug and the acquiring of it. A number of personality traits, as listed in Chart 16–1, are often associated with disruptive substance abuse.

GENETIC CONSIDERATIONS Related to Substance Abuse

We now have an understanding that a genetic predisposition can provide the base for vulnerabilities to substance abuse, but environment and experiences have an enormous influence on whether those genetics are expressed (Dick & Bierut, 2006). Questions such as whether genes have a substantial influence on adolescent substance abuse are answered considering the variety of contributions to adolescent behavior. Substance use and abuse is not a simple formula with two ingredients but a complex layering and melding of experiences and susceptibilities.

Drug use affects human development on the genetic level because drug use impacts sperm and egg health. Each partner contributes, such as when a male uses a substance and subsequently impregnates a woman, when a woman uses drugs prior to pregnancy, or when a woman uses substances during pregnancy. Birth defects are more commonly linked with paternal DNA damage than with maternal DNA damage (NDIC, 2006). The substance abuse genetics equation is a formula where the preceding circumstances combine to equal a number of physiological consequences for the offspring in addition to an increased risk for the offspring to have substance abuse issues.

Adult alcoholism develops as a result of the considerable role genetics plays when the gene pool has alcohol abusers in it. However, it is acknowledged that family environmental factors do supply a significant platform in terms of how the addiction is allowed to be asserted (Doweiko, 2006). Similarly, adult substance abuse has been examined in those who were adopted and had birth parents who were substance abusers. Again it is supported that having the genes for substance abuse does not, in and of itself, guarantee an addicted adult. The environment must interact with the genetics to create the development of highest risk (Dick & Bierut, 2006).

| CHART 16–1 | **Personality Traits Associated with Substance Abuse** |

It has been hypothesized that people who have substance abuse problems also share certain personality traits. Given that people and adaptive responses, as well as maladaptive responses such as substance abuse, can vary tremendously, this can be a contradictory set of characteristics. Listed below are some personality traits that may be seen in substance abusers:

- Anxiety and tension
- Social conformist
- Impulsive
- Irritable
- More easily fatigued than those without substance abuse
- Less satisfaction with present life situation
- Reports dissatisfaction with childhood experiences
- A tendency to act rashly when distressed
- Extroversion
- A prominence of Cluster B (dramatic, emotional, or erratic) personality patterns
- Choosing a substance when seeking comfort from stress
- Denial of a problem or minimizing the problem
- Projection of feelings onto another person
- Conning, bargaining, feigning
- Rationalization
- A routine of sensation seeking.

Comprehending the psychological infrastructure of substance abuse includes the possible contribution of attachment theory (Shorey & Snyder, 2006). The substance abuser may develop an attachment to the drug much like he would an attachment to another person. The drug becomes the partner in the relationship. The interaction between the person and the drug becomes the primary relationship with experiences and attitudes not unlike any other close bond. This theoretical framework may assist in treatment for this group of patients using support and exploration.

Sociocultural Theories

A sociocultural theoretical framework holds that both the social influences on an individual as well as the culture within that social structure define what has happened to create substance abuse. Poverty and wealth along with youth and age can contribute to the problems that compel some to abuse substances. Some of the sociocultural reasons people may use substances include the following:

- It was learned from the family.
- It was learned from friends.
- It results from a lack of alternative coping skills.
- It helps with anger.
- It helps deal with the side effects of medications.
- It makes them feel better (smarter, interesting, creative, powerful, etc.).

- They think it is normal and usual.
- It helps them cope with the difficulties of life.
- It numbs sexual, physical, emotional trauma.

Neaigus et al. (2006) and Vieten et al. (2004) explored the context of substance abuse and the typical groups at risk for it. After numerous surveys of the population, study summaries maintain that the component parts are the economics of drug use, what place those who are addicted hold in society, how the drug is produced, and what links the sociocultural network together. Learning about the context has been helpful in understanding how epidemics of drug use, such as heroin and methamphetamine, occur.

In a sociocultural framework, the roles different family members play and the importance of family rituals contribute to the problem of substance abuse and its treatment. For example, the family of a person who abuses alcohol may see the annual family reunion as a time when excessive drinking is not only allowed but expected and part of the event's relaxation. Entering a substance abuse treatment program prior to the reunion would be rejected. Similarly, the family of a young man abusing a methamphetamine with cardiac implications may nurse him back to health with each setback. The roles of caretaker may be more important to the family than any other role. Involving the community in substance abuse treatment can take shape in a variety of ways. The National Institute on Alcohol Abuse and Alcoholism has developed several guidelines for effective interventions in dealing with college campus drinking incidents (LaBrie, Pedersen, Lamb, & Bove, 2006). Projects like this target high-risk populations on campus and help students make responsible drinking decisions.

Substance abuse is thought to be created within social and cultural systems, so culture-specific approaches to the treatment of drug addiction would, therefore, be most effective. Treatment approaches that exist vary greatly and exceed the scope of this chapter. However, it is interesting to note that tradition-imbedded practices exist for substance abuse such as the Buddhist temple cure in Thailand, the San Pedro drink therapy (mescaline) for alcoholism in the northern coast of Peru, or the Danshukai groups and the Naikan treatment methods used in Japan.

■ Management of Patients Who Are Substance Abusers

Competent nursing care involves an understanding of the substance of abuse and how to most effectively treat the prioritized problems. This chapter focuses on the main substances of abuse.

Alcohol

Alcohol is a common substance that has just as much destructive power as any other substance of abuse. It is a legal, liquid, recreational drug. Characteristic features seen with abuse of this drug include slurred speech, ataxia, slowed reaction times, disinhibition, and interactions including repetitive argumentativeness or profuse apologizing for drinking. The nurse needs to know how this drug impacts on the patient's physiology. The range of physiological impacts on a patient with blood alcohol levels (BALs) ranging from 0.05 to 0.5 g/dL are presented in Chart 16–2 (p. 370).

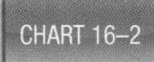

CHART 16–2 Escalating Physiological Impacts of Alcohol

CNS

- Disinhibition (behaviorally and sexually)
- Memory, concentration degradation
- Decrease in reasoning abilities
- Blackouts
- Motor skill degradation
- Labored breathing, severe respiratory depression
- Drowsiness, stupor, unconsciousness, coma, death

MOOD

- Euphoria
- Depression
- Mood lability

BEHAVIOR

- Outbursts
- Ataxia
- Slurred speech
- Incoherent speech
- Vomiting
- Violence

SENSES

- Diplopia

Public figures and famous people are often involved in alcohol-related incidents that the public does not view as being significantly problematic. The same casual attitude seeps into the overall perception of alcoholism in communities; that is, there is a certain level of acceptance about the use of alcohol and alcoholism. Alcohol-related disasters occur in which both the amount of alcohol and the resulting disaster are minimized by those involved: "I only had a couple drinks, of course I could drive." It is not wise to leave the decision to function competently to the person whose judgment is tainted. When those charged with maintaining social order focus on the dangerous combination of alcohol consumption and participation in activities that require judgment and motor skill, the result is a community that is slightly more aware of the problems alcohol consumption creates.

Alcoholism has been, and often still is, viewed as a sign of weakness by those who are unenlightened; note, however, that clinical investigation has redefined alcoholism as a disease. As research about its biochemical aspects has become known, the social stigma attached to alcoholism has decreased and more people have sought help. Professionals, laypeople, students, alcoholics, and nonalcoholics are attending seminars and college courses on alcoholism. Recovery programs are reported widely in the popular media and rehabilitation programs have become common knowledge. Information about alcohol recovery programs is easily accessible on the Internet and in print materials.

It is hard for the person imbibing to see what is happening to her body and quality of life. The devastation is usually seen and felt by others first. Some of the effects of alcoholism include depression; loss of self-respect; alienation from family, friends, and coworkers; malnutrition; decreased competence in self-care; infections; and damaging physiological effects to most body systems. A structured conversation by family and friends with the person who is abusing alcohol may be the first time all of the problems of a person's alcoholism are aired in a matter-of-fact manner.

The patterns of alcohol use vary and include regular daily intake of large amounts of alcohol, regular heavy drinking limited to weekends, or long periods of sobriety interspersed with binges of heavy drinking that last for weeks or months. The pattern does not change the physiological effects or the designation "alcoholic."

The Effects of Alcohol

A sedative anesthetic (CNS depressant), alcohol begins to be absorbed in the mouth, with absorption completed in the stomach and small intestine. Approximately 95% of alcohol is broken down by the liver; the rest is excreted through the lungs, kidneys, and skin. Generally, a person can metabolize 10 mL of alcohol (1 oz of whiskey) every 90 minutes. The rate of absorption varies based on weight, intake of food, liver function, and many other factors. If taken in exceedingly high doses, alcohol can depress respiration and cause death. Intoxication occurs when a person's BAL is 0.10% or more. This blood alcohol level is the legal definition of inebriation in most states, although there is a vigorous trend toward lowering the level to 0.08.

Assessment Aides

Useful, structured assessments around alcohol abuse include the CAGE questionnaire (Chart 16–3). CAGE is an acronym for the main words in the four specific questions about alcohol use. It is quick and direct, and allows professionals in other specialties and nonprofessionals the opportunity to screen for alcohol abuse. Because of its brevity, one of its disadvantages is that it may result in missed opportunities to obtain information. In addition, those particular questions could be offensive and impair communications about substance abuse.

Another quick assessment aid is the World Health Organization's Alcohol Use Disorders Identification Test (AUDIT) test. This is a 10-question assessment developed in 1992 that some consider to be less confrontational than the CAGE. The BEAST acronym (Chart 16–4), described in detail later in this chapter, is used to help addicts avoid taking another drink or drug.

CHART 16–3 CAGE Questions

The CAGE questionnaire is most frequently used for the detection of alcoholism in clinical settings. CAGE is a mnemonic for these four questions:

1. Have you ever felt like you should **C**ut down on your drinking?
2. Have people **A**nnoyed you by criticizing your drinking?
3. Have you ever felt bad or **G**uilty about your drinking?
4. Have you ever had a drink in the morning as an **E**ye-opener to get rid of a hangover?

BEAST Acronym

- **B** is for Boozing Opportunities (weddings, parties, trips, and so on). RR says to be aware of the pitfalls but do not necessarily avoid them. You are not powerless in the face of temptations, and you can choose not to succumb.
- **E** is for Enemy Recognition. Distinguish those thoughts from the Enemy (Beast) that are positive about booze or drugs.
- **A** is for Accuse the Beast of Malice. You can be angry at the Beast for its evil deeds (trying to tempt you), or you can laugh at it. Either way, make clear to the Beast that you have the upper hand and you won't relinquish it.
- **S** is for Self-Control and Self-Worth Reminders. Find ways of showing the Beast you have self-control (like moving your hands in front of your face and holding them there, totally in your control, until the Beast backs down). Find ways of telling yourself that you are a worthwhile person. Choose not to drink for the same reason you drank: to feel good about yourself.
- **T** is for Treasuring Your Sobriety. Focus on the pleasures of life that are attainable only in sobriety (a concept similar to that in AA).

Alcohol Withdrawal Syndrome

Alcohol withdrawal often includes the symptoms described in the following subsections and in Chart 16–5.

Hangover

The term *hangover* is used to describe the unpleasant symptoms of mild alcohol withdrawal occurring approximately 4 to 6 hours after the last alcohol ingestion. These symptoms include:

- Nausea and vomiting
- Gastritis
- Headache
- Fatigue
- Sweating and thirst
- Restlessness
- Irritability
- The "shakes"
- Vasomotor instability.

Chemicals known as congeners are formed during alcohol processing and maturation and increase the likelihood and severity of a hangover. The darker the liquor, the more congeners it contains. The toxins in congeners are distributed throughout the body as the liver breaks down the alcohol. Hangovers change various blood hormone levels that in turn create more symptoms. Alcohol inhibits the antidiuretic hormone, which leads to excessive urination and dehydration. Blood aldosterone and rennin levels increase with a hangover, but how this affects symptoms is unclear. A person is more prone to a hangover if the following circumstances apply:

- Drinks alcohol rapidly
- Mixes different types of alcoholic drinks
- Does not dilute the absorption of liquor with food and non-alcoholic beverages.

Alcohol Withdrawal Symptoms

Symptom	Occurrence Time Frame after Last Drink	Duration Time Frame
Slight at-rest tremors/pronounced and irregular during activities	24 hours	1 week
Diaphoresis	24 hours	3–4 days
Nausea, vomiting, anorexia	24 hours	3–4 days
Increased vital signs	24 hours	3–4 days
Agitation, inner shakiness	24 hours	2 weeks
Insomnia, vivid nightmares	24 hours	At least 2 weeks
Visual hallucinations (usually of disasters during everyday events)	24 hours	3 days
Auditory hallucinations, feeling persecuted, agitation, increased risk for lethality (self and others)	24 hours	3 days to 2 weeks
Delirium tremens (delirium, generalized seizures, disorientation for time and place, visual hallucinations, agitation, panic)	24–48 hours	3–5 days
Rum fits (2–6 generalized seizures)	24–48 hours	3–5 days

The following can help lessen the distressing symptoms of a hangover:

- Sugar and fluids help overcome hypoglycemia and dehydration.
- Anti-inflammatory drugs can reduce headache (aspirin may irritate the stomach; alcohol amplifies the toxic effects of acetaminophen on the liver).

Delirium Tremens

Delirium tremens (DTs), one symptom of withdrawal, is a condition of severe memory disturbance, agitation, anorexia, and hallucinations. Generally, DTs begin a few days after drinking stops and end within 1 to 5 days. They may, however, appear as late as the second week of abstinence from alcohol, especially when there is cross-addiction to other drugs. Additional medical illnesses may be present, such as pneumonia, pancreatitis, and hepatic decompensation.

Medical Detoxification

Medical treatment of alcoholism involves the management of withdrawal symptoms and the use of medication to deter the addicted individual from drinking. Alcohol withdrawal occurs after the individual stops drinking. This syndrome is composed of a constellation of physiological and behavioral symptoms that occur when the alcohol level drops.

Minor Withdrawal

A minor withdrawal from alcohol can occur within 6 to 12 hours after the alcoholic's last drink. Early symptoms include anxiety, agitation, and irritability. As the syndrome progresses other symptoms occur. These include tremor, tachycardia, hypertension, diaphoresis, and hallucinations. Gastrointestinal symptoms of nausea, vomiting, diarrhea, and anorexia may also be present. The appearance of hallucinations (visual, auditory, olfactory, or tactile) and seizures marks the onset of a major withdrawal.

Major Withdrawal

A major withdrawal is the most advanced, potentially life-threatening stage of alcohol withdrawal. Symptoms associated with DTs usually develop 72 hours after the last drink. Physical symptoms of impending DTs include elevated temperature, severe diaphoresis, hypertension, and tachycardia. Behavioral symptoms include confusion and disorientation, agitation, tremors, and alterations in sensory perception (auditory and visual hallucinations). The best treatment for major alcohol withdrawal involves early detection. Medical treatment for withdrawal includes:

1. Monitoring the patient's fluid status. Although some patients are overhydrated, many are dehydrated or have the potential to develop a fluid volume deficit. Fluids should be encouraged, up to 3000 mL/day, if no evidence exists to contraindicate this. Intravenous fluids are indicated if the patient is unable to take fluids by mouth.

2. Many people who abuse alcohol suffer from a magnesium deficiency. Administering magnesium sulfate decreases irritability caused by low magnesium levels and prevents seizures.

3. Administering vitamins, especially thiamine (vitamin B_1), because alcohol interferes with the absorption of B vitamins.

4. Prescribing benzodiazepines, such as diazepam (Valium) or chlordiazepoxide (Librium), to help prevent DTs. Seizures may be treated with IV diazepam, and the patient may be placed on an anticonvulsant.

5. Prescribing disulfiram (Antabuse, an agonist medication). The use of disulfiram may be prescribed in the treatment of patients with alcoholism. Disulfiram inhibits acetaldehyde dehydrogenase, which normally metabolizes acetaldehyde. The mechanism causes acetaldehyde to accumulate if alcohol is consumed. Acetaldehyde is highly toxic, producing nausea and hypotension. Hypotension leads to shock and may be fatal. If the patient uses alcohol, a powerful disulfiram reaction may occur and last for up to 2 weeks. Reaction symptoms include nausea, vomiting, flushing, dizziness, and tachycardia. Because of the potential danger of disulfiram, instruct the patient, orally and in writing, not to use alcohol in any form including alcohol-based cough syrups, cold remedies, or oral hygiene products.

6. Prescribing naltrexone (ReVia, Trexan). Developed in 1984 for treatment of heroin abuse, this drug was approved in January 1994 for blocking the craving for alcohol and the pleasure derived from drinking it. Rather than making the patient sick, it blocks the need to ingest alcohol and the pleasure derived from it, and thus may help prevent relapse when it is combined with long-term support groups and individual counseling. It has had more success as an active treatment mode than the punitive pharmacologic agent disulfiram.

Blackouts

Having **blackouts** is frequently confused with passing out. In fact, passing out refers to unconsciousness, whereas a blackout is anterograde amnesia: loss of short-term memories with retention of remote memories. A person can be fully functional for up to several days—working, talking on the telephone, and driving—yet have absolutely no memory of doing so. To others, the person abusing alcohol may appear normal or "high." Interestingly, alcohol abusers appear unconcerned by the blackouts and eventually learn effective coverups. This appearance of unconcern may be due, in part, to euphoric recall: The alcoholic recalls the feeling that fun or interesting events occurred, but does not recall specific behaviors. Reality is distorted. Some patients find blackouts very disturbing and seek treatment after the first blackout.

Blackouts appearing later in the disease process may indicate physical dependence and are not related to the amount of alcohol consumed. They are unpredictable, and exactly how or why they occur is not clear. One theory holds that blackouts are an acute syndrome caused by dehydration of brain tissue. When assessing a patient who abuses alcohol, determine whether blackouts have occurred.

Fetal Alcohol Syndrome

Fetal alcohol syndrome (FAS) is found in children of women who engage in alcohol consumption during pregnancy. Nurses need to be aware of the harmful effects of alcohol on pregnant women and unborn children. As many as 12,000 infants are born each year in the United States with FAS and three times as many with alcohol-related neurodevelopmental disorder (ARND) and alcohol-related birth defects (ARBD) according to the National Organization on Fetal Alcohol Syndrome. All will suffer varying degrees of effects, ranging from mild learning disabilities to major physical, mental, and intellectual impairment. Physical and mental defects include severe growth deficiency, heart defects, malformed facial features, mental retardation, low birth weight, learning problems, and hyperactivity. If a child has one or two of these characteristics, the condition is called fetal alcohol effects (FAE). Of individuals with FAE between the ages of 12 and 51, many will have mental health problems and disrupted school experiences, as well as trouble with the law and confinement in prison, drug or alcohol treatment centers, or mental institutions. A baby born to an alcoholic mother may need to be withdrawn gradually from alcohol immediately after birth. O'Connor et al. (2006) demonstrated evidence of improvement in the social skills deficits and behavioral problems seen in this population following training involving friendship behavior.

Amphetamines

Amphetamines, also known as "speed," belong to a group of compounds called the sympathomimetics. This group of compounds is comprised of synthetic drugs derived from ephedrine that stimulate the release of adrenaline and do speed up someone's system, thus the common name.

Amphetamines were first synthesized in 1887 and experimental medical use began in the 1920s (McGuinness, 2006). In the 1950s and 1960s, amphetamines were heralded as wonder drugs for depression, management of obesity, and exhaustion. By the 1970s their dangers became known and today they are prescribed less frequently because alternative compounds are available to effectively and safely treat those symptoms. Amphetamines are still used to control appetite and treat depression, narcolepsy, and minimal brain dysfunctions, along with attention deficit hyperactivity disorders in children. Amphetamine abusers are usually teenagers or young adults who are looking for a good time. The uninformed hope for alertness and improved performance through use of these substances, which can lure truck drivers working on long road trips, students during exams, and athletes, among others, into the speed trap.

In small doses, amphetamines cause people to feel energetic, euphoric, and in touch with their surroundings. Users take these CNS stimulants to feel good. A growing number of people who do uppers and downers in a cyclic fashion take amphetamines (the upper) to balance the effects of barbiturates (the downer). Amphetamines are dangerous because they alter judgment and obscure sensations. Taken in high doses or intravenously, amphetamines can have dangerous effects.

Amphetamines act by mimicking two of the brain's most important neurotransmitters, dopamine and norepinephrine. A drug must be able to act on a receptor site or on a number of receptor sites to have an impact. The body may not have a specific amphetamine or cocaine receptor site, so amphetamine and cocaine will take what is called illegal control at the existing receptor sites. Dopamine and dopamine receptor sites are intricately involved in the effects substances of abuse have on the nervous systems of patients. Chronic use of methamphetamines changes the way a person thinks and behaves, because the brain's cortex is no longer activated during decision making. This change in the ability of the brain to transport dopamine to any significant degree creates the clinical characteristics of severe psychiatric symptoms (Kim et al. 2006).

Tolerance develops rapidly, and chronic abusers may suffer a toxic psychosis presenting with the symptoms of paranoid schizophrenia. Argumentativeness, delusions, hallucinations, stereotypic compulsive behavior, increased libido, interpersonal sensitivity, panic, and violence may occur (APA, 2000). Substance abuse with amphetamines means a craving for these drugs and requiring higher and higher dosages. Abusers are rowdy, paranoid, and irritable. A "crash" (depression), often with suicidal symptoms, may last for several weeks. This is so uncomfortable that the user ingests more of the drug in an attempt to feel better and develops a cyclical pattern of abuse and crashing.

Physiologically, the overuse of speed has been tied to stroke and death. Depression, anxiety, and increased stress symptoms are the most common psychological pitfalls in recovering from the use of speed. Changes in neurotransmitter activity increase the patient's sensitivity to stress and may contribute to the spontaneous recurrence of amphetamine and methamphetamine psychosis, called flashbacks. Recurrent flashbacks contribute to recurrent major mood disorders (Barr et al., 2006).

Methamphetamine

The most hypercharged form of speed is methamphetamine (MA). It is less expensive than cocaine and has similar CNS stimulant characteristics. Recently MA has become an enormous public health/substance abuse issue. Recipes to manufacture MA in home drug labs using everyday ingredients (over-the-counter

pseudoephedrine, starter fluids, and drain cleaner) are widely available and have impacted how these products are sold (see the Combat Methamphetamine Epidemic Act of 2005). Lower quality MA is called "speed" or "crank"; higher quality MA is sold in small chunks as "glass" or "ice" because of its crystalline appearance. It is a maximum stimulant with maximum risks.

Exposure to MA is neurotoxic and long-term use leads to extensive neural damage. Physiological changes include cognitive impairments, MA-induced psychosis, inadequate perfusion, and ischemic lesions of the brain. What nurses will see is an inability to competently perform activities of daily living (brush teeth, wash face, etc.), difficulty remembering or problem solving, and delusional accusations or reactions with strong emotional content to something the patient is experiencing (seeing, hearing, feeling). MA morphologically changes the corpus callosum and causes skin lesions, perinatal complications, and hypertension (Arria et al., 2006; Barr et al., 2006; McGuinness, 2006). Each of these impacts has consequences that are far reaching for a person's health and functioning. Before and after photographs of people who use methamphetamine are striking in the differences from weight loss, skin integrity problems, and general poor state of health.

Caffeine

Trimethylxanthine is a drug that keeps one awake and alert with a feeling of goodwill. The drug is caffeine. It is one of the most popular drugs in North America. On average, 90% of adults consume 300 mg of caffeine every day. Chart 16–6 lists the caffeine content of certain beverages and foods.

Caffeine is able to accomplish the physiological effect of stimulation through binding to adenosine receptors; adenosine is a chemical that gives instructions about going to sleep. When adenosine is bound to its receptors, it causes drowsiness by slowing down nerve cell activity in the brain. Caffeine takes illegal control of that receptor so adenosine cannot do its job. When the

CHART 16–6	Caffeine Content of Selected Beverages and Foods
Source	**Approximate Caffeine Content per Average Serving**
Cup of instant coffee	65–100 mg
Mug of drip coffee	115–175 mg
Cup of brewed coffee	80–135 mg
Espresso coffee, 2 oz	100 mg
Decaf coffee, brewed	3–4 mg
Decaf coffee, instant	2–3 mg
Cup of tea	30–60 mg
Green tea	15 mg
Cola drink	Up to 40 mg
Certain carbonated sodas	34–80 mg
Energy drink	Up to 80 mg
Hot cocoa	14 mg
Bar of chocolate	Up to 50 mg

receptors are occupied and controlled by caffeine, the nerve cannot respond to the adenosine. Nerve cell activity speeds up and the patient is not able to relax.

This increased neural firing has an impact on the pituitary gland. Increased neural activity usually accompanies a crisis or stressor and the pituitary gland acts in stressful situations by communicating with the adrenal gland to add adrenaline to the system. This is a survival mechanism to help maintain alertness. Adrenaline causes pupils to dilate, increases the heart rate, and readies skeletal muscles for action. As adrenaline wears off, feelings of fatigue and depression appear. Peak concentrations of caffeine are achieved 30 to 60 minutes after ingestion. The half-life of caffeine is about 6 hours. If a patient drinks caffeine first thing in the morning, another dose would be needed in the afternoon to fight off the fatigue and depression.

Caffeine also increases dopamine levels in the brain. Dopamine is a neurotransmitter that, as discussed later in this chapter, impacts mood and a sense of well-being. The dopamine response is partly responsible for caffeine addiction. Moderate caffeine use is typically defined as up to 300 to 400 milligrams a day; while greater amounts are considered heavy consumption. People who use caffeine use it for its stimulant properties. Typical use is seen upon awakening, during times of low energy or fatigue, and when an external source of comfort is required. Once a pattern of use has been established, individuals continue to use so that they do not suffer withdrawal symptoms (Jones & Lejuez, 2005).

Caffeine is a common substance that is intrinsic to a number of plant products. It is encountered in coffee, tea, chocolate, carbonated beverages, and some pain relievers. The color of a substance is not indicative of its caffeine content—some of the highest caffeine content is found in clear carbonated beverages. Caffeine use—and abuse—has only recently become a health concern. In the United States more than half of the population over the age of 10 drinks coffee. Individuals may have a sensitivity to caffeine that causes physical distress (muscle cramping, cardiac effects, diarrhea). There is evidence that combining alcohol with caffeine, as in popular cocktails, impacts cognition, particularly of those making self-assessments of intoxication (Marczinski & Fillmore, 2006).

The amount of caffeine in tea varies according to the plant variety it is made from and how long it is brewed: The longer it is brewed, the higher the caffeine levels. Coffee also has variable amounts of caffeine depending on its preparation method. For instance, brewed coffee has substantially more caffeine than instant coffee.

If coffee is withdrawn suddenly from people who drink large quantities of brewed coffee (six or more cups a day), they might become irritable and suffer from headaches. Given the stimulant effect of caffeine, it makes sense to advise those who complain of insomnia to switch to decaffeinated coffee or to have their last cup of coffee at least 3 hours before going to bed. Remember, "decaffeinated" does not mean there is no caffeine in the coffee or tea; it means the caffeine content is much reduced but still present. Because tea has much less caffeine per cup than coffee, it does not have as strong a stimulating effect. But if there is a complaint of insomnia, good sleep hygiene demands not drinking large quantities of caffeinated tea just before going to bed in an attempt to minimize stimulation.

A successful strategy for lowering the negative physiological impacts of caffeine is to reduce the harm mode. The individual would decrease overall intake of the substance vehicle (such as coffee or tea), start using decaffeinated mixtures in increasing proportions, then complete the effort with cessation of caffeine ingestion. This process weans the individual from the substance without causing, or at least by minimizing, abrupt and uncomfortable withdrawal symptoms. Health care facilities frequently limit or restrict access to caffeinated beverages so that interference from the stimulating impacts does not complicate health care treatments. Advance planning for alternative behaviors in social and occupational situations is helpful for the patient working on discontinuing this particular form of substance abuse.

Cannabis

Marijuana has been illegal in the United States since 1937, although it has been fairly easy to obtain since the early 1900s. As of this writing, despite a U.S. Supreme Court ruling to the contrary, the federal Drug Enforcement Administration considers it illegal and opposes its use for medical purposes. Legal conflicts remain regarding medical marijuana. A 1996 California law legalized some medical use of it, a federal law prohibits distribution or use of marijuana regardless of state law, and health care providers in seven states are allowed to discuss medical marijuana for pain relief without risking loss of license. But this is a topic, and a treatment, in flux.

Marijuana is the most used illicit drug. It is derived from an Indian hemp plant (*Cannabis sativa*) and contains the psychoactive substance delta 6-3,4-tetrahydrocannabinol (THC). THC is found in the sticky yellow resin secreted by the tops and leaves of the ripe plants.

THC is transformed into metabolites in the body. Unlike alcohol, which is water soluble and leaves the body through urine, breath, and perspiration, THC is stored in the fatty tissues (especially the brain and reproductive system). Consequently, it can be detected in the body for up to 6 weeks. The potency of marijuana has steadily increased over the years. Although marijuana contains more than 400 chemicals, the THC content determines the potency. With an increase in potency comes an increase in health problems. There is compelling evidence that underlying neurochemical mechanisms are at work reinforcing the reward and dependence features of this drug and contributing to addiction (Fride, Perchuk, Hall, Uhl, & Onaivi, 2006).

Researchers have found that marijuana produces a significant analgesic effect and is modestly effective against the nausea and vomiting associated with chemotherapy. Medicinal applications of both THC and cannabidiol for pain have been examined and show significant pain relief (Trossman, 2006). Dronabinol is a synthetic delta-9-tetrahydrocannabinol or delta-9-THC that contains standardized THC content in an FDA-approved pharmaceutical. It is mainly used to treat the weight loss, nausea, and vomiting associated with a number of medical conditions.

Although marijuana does decrease intraocular pressure, it requires high doses and has a short-lived effect, making it inappropriate for the treatment of glaucoma. The cannabinoids of marijuana cross the placental barrier and are distributed to fetal tissues. The risk of fetal death and abnormalities—CNS disturbances, low birth weight, decreased length, and smaller head circumference—increases when the mother uses marijuana. Long-term marijuana smoking is associated with lung damage, increased risk of respiratory cancer, and poorer pregnancy outcomes.

Cocaine

Cocaine is a stimulant extracted from the leaves of the coca plant found in Bolivia and Peru. South Americans chewed coca leaves, enjoying the effects of decreased appetite and increased ability to work at high altitudes, for hundreds of years. Common knowledge held that slaves became more productive when given cocaine. It was an ingredient in the popular soft drink Coca Cola—thus the name—before federal regulations prohibited it in 1903. Today, cocaine is used as a local anesthetic in ear, nose, and throat surgery. When inhaled or injected, cocaine produces alertness and energy and makes users feel sociable and confident. The drug blocks appetite and erases fatigue, which makes it appear to be an ideal performance booster although that is an illusion. Cocaine addicts develop a tolerance to the drug and use amounts that would have been lethal to them earlier.

An estimated 5.7 million Americans chronically use cocaine according to the National Institute on Drug Abuse. Because cocaine abuse has been recognized as a widespread problem, the government invests resources to limit access. Cocaine is purer today than ever before. It is available to all cultural and socioeconomic groups and is used equally by women and men. The cocaine industry is a multibillion dollar illegal drug enterprise that affects every aspect of civilization.

Cocaine's impact is both behavioral and biochemical. It produces a euphoria that diminishes after approximately 5 to 10 minutes. The euphoria, or high, is followed by a terrible letdown called the "postcoke blues" or cocaine abstinence syndrome. Anxiety, depression, and fatigue are part of this syndrome. Cocaine initially increases dopamine (DA) neurotransmission. The cocaine crash, lasting for approximately 30 to 60 minutes, results from depletion of DA, the neurotransmitter responsible for feelings of pleasure and well-being. The development of new dendrites (branches of the nerve cells) to aid in the uptake of the increased amount of DA accounts for the tolerance. Over time, however, cocaine abuse depletes DA in the brain and this depletion may be the basis for the supremely compelling cravings associated with its use (Meyers, Zavala, Speer, & Neisewander, 2006).

Ultimately, cocaine no longer produces pleasure, but not taking it feels even worse. As the DA eventually becomes depleted, the user becomes chronically fatigued, irritable, and anxious. Psychiatric symptoms such as confusion and paranoia emerge. Suicide attempts, accidents, and overdoses are common. The only effect of cocaine that is increased as tolerance develops is its ability to induce a convulsion or seizure. Research with cocaine users indicates that the drug bromocriptine mesylate (Parlodel), a DA receptor agonist, eliminates the craving that users feel after they stop using cocaine.

Although the brain needs to synthesize more DA as a result of the chemical misprogramming from the addiction, it craves more cocaine, which offers immediate relief. The crash intensity appears related to the amount of cocaine used. Addicts often use other drugs, such as alcohol, marijuana, or sleeping pills, during the crash.

When someone is intoxicated with cocaine, the person will be sweating and exhibit dilated pupils, psychomotor agitation, and increased blood pressure and heart rate. Higher doses of cocaine produce high fever, cardiac arrhythmia, seizures, hallucinations, and a paranoid schizophrenic syndrome. Hallucinations typically involve "cocaine bugs," described as feeling like bugs are crawling under the person's skin. The patient may scratch and dig in an attempt to get rid of them. Antipsychotics are used to combat the psychotic symptoms, but the use of those that can further decrease the seizure threshold is avoided.

Detoxification for cocaine abusers depends on the patient's symptoms. Some hospitals use nothing; others administer diazepam (Valium) intravenously 1 to 20 mg at a slow rate (not more than 5 mg/min). Some Valium protocols last approximately 4 days; Valium is decreased from 10 mg q4h PO/IM to 5 mg q8h PO/IM, with additional doses as needed if the patient has withdrawal symptoms. Other hospitals have prn Valium orders only. Another protocol involves the use of phenobarbital in decreasing doses and imipramine hydrochloride (Tofranil).

Because the depression associated with cocaine detoxification is significant, Tofranil or other tricyclic antidepressants may be given for several weeks after the acute detoxification. Tricyclics build up existing levels of neurotransmitters and make them available for transmission.

 **CRITICAL ALERT** *Beta-adrenergic blockers such as propranolol (Inderal) may be used to counteract the tachycardia and hypertension that accompany acute cocaine intoxication. Their use may result in paroxysmal hypertension due to unopposed alpha-adrenergic stimulation. Use cautiously and with constant blood pressure monitoring.*

Synaptic treatment uses tricyclic antidepressants to increase the number of neurotransmitters in the synapse. Postsynaptic treatment for cocaine withdrawal and dependence includes the use of drugs such as bromocriptine (Parlodel) or amantadine (Symmetrel), which increase dopaminergic activity in the synapse and enhance the effects of DA on the postsynaptic receptors. Other medications such as buprenorphine can promote abstinence and there has been success with agonist substitution treatments (Gross, Marsch, Badger, & Bickel, 2006; Lile, 2006). Historically, presynaptic treatment was employed using amino acids such as tryptophan. This was used until 1989, when tryptophan was removed from the market because of several deaths associated with its use. The rationale for instituting presynaptic treatment was based on the body's conversion of amino acids to neurotransmitters. Cocaine abuse depleted neurotransmitters and the tryptophan was thought to replace it to some extent.

Auricular acupuncture for cocaine dependence is widely used (Gates, Smith, & Foxcroft, 2006), but research has not supported its effectiveness. Placing acupuncture needles into specific sites in the ear can promote relaxation and be a stress management technique. This nonpharmacologic intervention requires more robust and reliable research to determine whether it contributes to helping the dependent individual abstain from cocaine use.

Crack

Crack, or "rock" cocaine, recently labeled "the most addictive drug known to man," is a potent form of hydrochloride cocaine

MyNursingKit | National Institute on Drug Abuse

that is mixed with baking soda and water, heated, allowed to harden, and then broken or "cracked" into little pieces and smoked in cigarettes or glass water pipes. Smokable forms of cocaine have effects similar to those of the injectable drug. Crack is more insidious, addictive, and toxic than cocaine. It is not unusual for someone to become addicted after using crack twice.

Crack is cheap and easily acquired. A crack high has a rapid onset and is intensely euphoric, followed by a dramatic crash. Within seconds after the crash, users feel compelled to smoke more crack. Repeatedly smoking cocaine affects the central serotonergic and dopaminergic functions of the brain. The long-lasting and selective disruptions in serotonin pathways following chronic cocaine use may provide a neurochemical basis for the mood changes commonly reported during cocaine withdrawal (Meyers et al., 2006).

Symptoms of crack use include irritability, paranoia, depression, and physical symptoms that go along with the smoking of a toxic chemical, such as wheezing and coughing blood, and black phlegm. Cardiac arrhythmias caused by crack use may lead to death. There is an increase in the number of babies being born to mothers who use crack. These babies are more likely to be premature, have microcephaly, or have low birth weights. They are irritable, and have tremors and muscle rigidity. The children have adjustment problems and are quick to express frustration and have generally disruptive styles of interacting (Dennis, Bendersky, Ramsay, & Lewis, 2006).

Treatment for this addiction is very difficult. Many people seek help only when they can no longer support their habit. That point is much further along than it would be with a more expensive drug, so patients are very debilitated by the time they seek treatment and have usually been coerced by others to do so. It is an extremely problematical drug to stop using. Recidivism is estimated at more than 90%.

Freebase

Freebase is a purified form of cocaine made by applying solvents to ordinary cocaine. Melting the cocaine with a small butane torch helps in the purifying and delivery process. This action alone is dangerous due to the hazard of the solvent exploding. The effects of the freebase are brief but intense, and the short euphoria (3 to 5 minutes) immediately becomes a restless desire for more "base." This sequential abuse of the substance has caused the death of a number of public figures in recent decades.

Hallucinogens

Hallucinogens are synthetic and natural drugs that cause hallucinations and unusual sensory experiences. A variety of plant species have impacts on the CNS that can be exploited as drugs of abuse. Peyote, the active hallucinogen in cactus buttons, is still an integral part of religious rituals of Native Americans in the southwestern United States and Mexico. Psilocybin is the active hallucinogen in certain mushrooms. Recipes using psilocybin mushrooms encompass everyday foods, tea, and honey concoctions. There continues to be controversy around whether psilocybin-containing mushrooms can be smoked to produce a psychoactive effect. People around the world continue to use many species of hallucinogenic plants to achieve distortions in their state of mind (Vaitl et al., 2005). Developed in 1938 for scientific research, LSD (an abbreviation of the German words for

lysergic acid diethylamide) is the drug most commonly identified with the term *hallucinogen* and the most widely used in this class of drugs. It is considered the typical hallucinogen, and characteristics of its action and effects apply to other hallucinogens, including mescaline, psilocybin, and ibogaine.

In the 1960s and 1970s, the U.S. Army experimented with LSD by giving it without informed consent to unsuspecting army employees. One dramatic and much publicized event concerned the army officer who leapt to his death from a window after unknowingly ingesting LSD. At this time the danger of LSD became publicized, as did the unethical research. Physician researchers also were interested in experimenting with the uses of LSD in the treatment of a variety of diseases; however, in 1966 LSD became illegal and could no longer be used in human research.

After a lull in use, LSD ("acid") is again being used because it is cheap ($2 to $5 a "hit") and causes an intense high that lasts 6 to 12 hours. Users today are unacquainted with the horror stories of the 1960s, typically because they are teenagers and young adults. Psychological and physical dependence are unlikely because each experience with a hallucinogen is different. Visual hallucinations, a sense of increased creativity, and revelations regarding the essential meaning of life are the presumed effects of the drugs. If these occur, they are short-lived excursions.

The dangers of hallucinogens include "bad trips" and flashbacks. Users who experience bad trips may appear psychotic and extremely fearful. Reassuring the person and pointing out reality are helpful; occasionally tranquilizers or antipsychotics are given. The symptoms usually disappear within 12 hours but may persist for months.

Flashbacks are a spontaneous reliving of the experiences the person felt while under the influence of the drug, even though the person is currently drug free. The experience may involve perceptual distortions, a variety of physical feelings, and strong emotions such as fear and pleasure. Flashbacks are generally brief, and they occur less frequently over time. Flashbacks may be induced by stress, fatigue, and drug or alcohol ingestion (Vaitl et al., 2005). There exists a clinical concern that hallucinogens pose a particular danger to adolescents in that they may precipitate psychosis. Because teenagers' egos and defenses are weak, they may be especially susceptible to the effects of hallucinogens.

Inhalants

Inhalants are popular among teenagers and school-age children because they are inexpensive, easy to obtain, and are generally typical household items—such as glue, fuels, paints, aerosols, air fresheners, the substance used to resole shoes, and the propellants in canned whipped cream—with the exception of one unusual source: embalming fluid. The abuse of inhalants is increasing at a frightening rate. Their use causes euphoria, light-headedness, and excitement. Children are the most frequent users. Adult users often have a long history of polydrug abuse.

Inhalants are sniffed or inhaled (called "huffing") in a variety of ways. Huffing a rag soaked with the inhalant and placed in a plastic bag or inhaling the gas directly from a tank are the two most common behaviors. Amyl and butyl nitrate (called "poppers") can be easily concealed and passed around a classroom, and paint thinner can be concealed in a soft drink can. Use of these inhalants and solvents can cause ventricular fibrillation, decreased cardiac output, serious brain damage, and sudden death.

Although withdrawal must be managed as with the other substances covered in this chapter, careful assessment, early identification, detoxification, education, and prevention are particularly critical because so many inhalant abusers are children under the age of 12. The appalling consequences of young children's abuse of inhalants cannot be understated (Eaton et al., 2006). Nurses need to be aware of the programs and resources available and should support legislation to make it more difficult for minors to obtain glue and paint products.

Nicotine

Nicotine is the psychoactive stimulating substance found in tobacco. The behavioral and physiological effects of nicotine frequently lead to addiction, and access to this legal drug for adults endangers those under the legal smoking age. Populations with psychiatric conditions and substance abuse problems have higher rates of smoking and show a lack of responsiveness to smoking cessation treatments (Ranney et al., 2006).

Nicotine is a stimulant that acts in the central and peripheral nervous systems on cells that are normally acted on by the neurotransmitter acetylcholine. In the CNS nicotine occupies the receptors for acetylcholine in both dopamine and serotonin neural pathways. This causes the release of both dopamine and norepinephrine. The stimulant nicotine initially increases alertness and cognitive ability, and then has a depressant effect.

Research suggests a role for dopaminergic processes regulating the reinforcing effects of nicotine, making cessation of use more difficult. Dopamine blockers can alter smoking behavior for a limited time, but people compensate for this by then increasing their amount of smoking (Glover, 2006). The usual impact of dopamine being turned over in the system at an increased rate is the reduction of hunger impulses. Once someone tries to quit smoking, hunger impulses return and the person may gain weight.

Smoking rates of the general population have fallen during the past 25 years from 34% in 1980 to close to 22% in 2005 (Hoeppner et al., 2006; Ranney et al., 2006), but are still of concern given the negative physiological impacts of the addiction. Nicotine use is associated with cancer, heart disease, emphysema, hypertension, and death. Smoking cigarettes is an extremely common addiction and is seen routinely despite smoke-free environments and restrictions on cigarette access. Evidence indicates that smoke-free environments protect people from the force of secondhand smoke but do not reduce actual smoking. Instead, smokers will practice anticipatory smoking to ensure their desired level of nicotine is maintained (Doweiko, 2006). There are also socioeconomic differences in smoking rates. The prevalence of smoking in Medicaid recipients is 44% compared to the general population.

Typically, people begin smoking at young ages, during peer pressure contacts, or during times of stress and thereafter find it very difficult to quit successfully. Use of tobacco products can be interrupted briefly during respiratory illnesses, hospitalizations, pregnancy, and following health care provider advice on smoking cessation. Return to tobacco use after a brief time is all too usual. Long-term quit rates range from 10% to 25% including pharmacologic cessation support (nicotine replacement systems, psychopharmacology) (Evans, Blank, Sams, Weaver, & Eissenberg, 2006; Killen et al., 2006).

The most commonly used approach for treating nicotine dependence is nicotine replacement therapy (patch, inhaler, lozenge, gum), which reduces cravings by maintaining the blood level of nicotine. Bupropion (Zyban), an antidepressant, has demonstrated effectiveness in short-term abstinence. Support in a variety of forms is also useful in assisting patients with this difficult addiction. Educational programs targeting the smoking cessation knowledge base of health care providers in prenatal, pediatric, and community health are needed to promote effective treatment of nicotine dependence (Klesges et al., 2006).

Every person trying to make a change in behavior must go through stages before, during, and after the change is made. The transtheoretical model of behavior change (TTM) has been applied successfully to substance abuse as well as co-occurring disorders (Finnell & Osborne, 2006). TTM describes a continuum of five stages of behavior change (see Chart 16–7) and the underpinnings of movement from stage to stage. The beginning of this process is called assessing readiness to change. The entire model describes each of the stages in the process. There is a great deal within the TTM that can be useful to nurses throughout their careers.

CHART 16–7 The Transtheoretical Model of Behavior Change

Any desired change in health care behavior is best understood with a model that explains human behavior. TTM explains the stages of change and the processes of change. Features of change that occur throughout the stages, such as how decisional balance affects the change process, an individual's vision of how effective efforts will be, and how temptation will likely be handled, make this perspective a useful one for promoting change.

Stage	Processes and Principles
Precontemplation	The patient does not intend to change the health behavior in the near future. This stage usually lasts approximately 6 months. What the nurse sees is an avoidance of communications designed to help change occur.
Contemplation	The patient does intend to change the health behavior in the next 6 months. There is awareness of the benefits of change, but the barriers and ambivalence are potent and interfere.
Preparation	The patient intends to make the change within the next month. The patient develops a plan of action with small, important steps taken toward change.
Action	The patient demonstrates modified risky behavior and makes the change. There is significant risk of reverting to previous problematic health behaviors. Healthy action requires considerable time and energy.
Maintenance	Work to prevent relapse occurs in this stage. Temptation gradually diminishes over 6 months to 5 years. This stage is meant to extend through the patient's life.

Source: Reprinted from Addictive Behaviors. Vol 31(8), Hoeppner, B. B., Velicer, W. F., Redding, C. A., Rossi, J. S., Prochaska, J. O., Pallonen, U. E., & Meier, K. S. Psychometric evaluation of the smoking cessation Processes of Change scale in an adolescent sample. Addictive Behaviors, pp. 1363–1372, Copyright 2006, with permission from Elsevier.

Opiates

Opiates as a category of drugs of abuse include heroin and morphine (which are derived from the poppy plant) and synthetic drugs (such as oxycodone, meperidine, codeine, and methadone). Opiates have analgesic qualities and are usually prescribed after a surgical procedure or for chronic pain. They are quite potent and have the ability to decrease awareness of painful stimuli. Depending on the person, the drugs may produce a euphoric high, as it does in drug addicts, but opiates generally cause people to feel drowsy and out of touch with the world (Martin, Loder, Taylor, Almas, & Hilliard, 2005). For information on chronic pain conditions, see Chapter 15 .

Heroin as a drug is not inherently dangerous. Unless there is an accidental overdose, the heroin alone as a substance will not harm the individual. But addiction to heroin exposes the patient to the dangerous and deadly ancillary issues of:

- Diluting agents (which are likely contaminated)
- Needle cleanliness
- Exposure to transmissible diseases such as hepatitis, TB, and HIV
- Overdose
- Malnutrition
- Poisoning by impurities
- Criminal behaviors necessary to support the addiction, which can put the individual at great risk.

These issues and others make the addicted individual of concern to others. The Harrison Narcotics Act of 1914 restricted use of opiates in the United States due to their dangerous impacts. Drugs such as heroin are used for clinical purposes in Europe and the United Kingdom; heroin in particular is used to control pain because it is relatively inexpensive.

Constricted pupils, euphoria, psychomotor retardation, slurred speech, and/or drowsiness indicate opiate intoxication. If a client overdoses, naloxone (Narcan) can be used if it is immediately administered. Abdominal cramps, rhinorrhea, and lacrimation may be treated with belladonna alkaloids or with phenobarbital.

 CRITICAL ALERT *Heroin overdoses, if identified quickly, can be treated with naloxone (Narcan). Naloxone is a fast-acting narcotic antagonist that counteracts respiratory depression. The dose is usually 0.4 to 0.8 mg IV repeated in 5 to 15 minutes.*

Because opiates are physically addictive, withdrawal is a physiological threat. People who use high doses of a drug and who use the drug intravenously are at high risk for severe withdrawal symptoms. Withdrawal symptoms are usually evident within 12 hours after the last dose. The person experiences the most severe withdrawal within 36 to 48 hours with the symptoms decreasing gradually over 2 weeks. Clonidine has been useful in this process. Clonidine blocks the withdrawal symptoms, making the detoxification process less painful. Psychologically, the patient feels less anxious and depressed.

During this stressful withdrawal, the person craves the drug. Babies who are born to addicted mothers must be treated for opiate withdrawal. These babies are irritable, have high-pitched crying, increased respirations, fever, sneezing, yawning, and tremors.

In 1964, methadone was introduced to treat opiate addiction. By the late 1960s and early 1970s, when federal governments allocated money for treatment, methadone maintenance programs mushroomed all over North America. Methadone, a synthetic narcotic, was dispensed daily at clinics to narcotic addicts by prescribers with special licensure to do so. Although addictive, methadone does not produce the ecstatic feeling associated with heroin. Methadone alleviates the addict's craving for narcotics and, therefore, was expected to decrease the illicit drug trafficking, theft, prostitution, and crime necessary to obtain money for the drugs. It was thought that dwindling drug trafficking would allow addicts to lead productive lives. Also, methadone therapy is far less expensive than residential programs or jail. Methadone as a treatment option for these patients has been successful to a certain extent, but has had controversial aspects. The ethics of methadone treatment, as well as the economic aspects of the treatment, are viewed as public health concerns.

Federally controlled substances, including buprenorphine, are alternatives to methadone. Buprenorphine is an opioid mixed agonist and potent analgesic. Buprenorphine, a potential treatment for opiate addiction, is administered under the tongue via a small syringe by specially licensed professionals. Patients do not swallow the medication but allow it to be absorbed through the mucous membranes that line the inside of the mouth (Gross et al., 2006). This medication will not replace methadone therapy that is provided through special methadone treatment facilities, but will provide the office-based prescriber an opportunity to treat patients for addiction to heroin or other opiates, including prescription painkillers. In 1993, LAAM (1-alpha-acetylmethadol) was approved for the management of opiate dependence. Buprenorphine joins methadone, naltrexone, and LAAM as the fourth medication available for treating heroin and other opiate addictions. With most opioid substitution treatment, the patient continues some level of illicit drug use (Carroll, Walsh, Bigelow, Strain, & Preston, 2006).

Phencyclidine

Drugs such as phencyclidine (PCP) and ketamine, which were initially developed as general anesthetics for surgery, distort perceptions of sight and sound and produce feelings of detachment—dissociation—from the environment and self. But these mind-altering effects are not hallucinations. PCP and ketamine are therefore more properly known as "dissociative anesthetics." Dextromethorphan, a widely available cough suppressant, when taken in high doses can produce effects similar to those of PCP and ketamine. The dissociative drugs act by altering distribution of the neurotransmitter glutamate throughout the brain. Glutamate is involved in the perception of pain, responses to the environment, and memory. PCP is considered the typical dissociative drug, and the descriptions of PCP's actions and effects largely apply to ketamine and dextromethorphan as well (Lofwall, Griffiths, & Mintzer, 2006).

PCP was originally used as an anesthetic for humans and as a tranquilizer for animals. Because of its dangerous side effects, it was removed from the market except for veterinary use. However, by the mid-1960s PCP was readily available as a street drug. PCP is inexpensive and easily synthesized by home chemists, making a supply always available.

People who use PCP frequently arrive at the emergency room in a psychotic, violent, and agitated state. The agitation and the sensations experienced by the user generate incredible power and strength. Even a small, slight person can break heavy glass doors or fight several people at once. Some users fluctuate between coma and violence. Hallucinations are common. A differential diagnosis is important but difficult because the symptoms are similar to those of schizophrenia.

A PCP high sets in about 5 minutes after a person takes the drug and lasts 4 to 6 hours. Effects may last up to 48 hours. PCP may be recovered from the blood and urine for 7 to 10 days. While using PCP, a person experiences a wide variety of feelings ranging from euphoria and utter peace to violence, confusion, and disorganization. Distorted sensory perceptions are common. During a "bad trip," anxiety, fear, and paranoia predominate. The dramatic physical and emotional effects of PCP may last for several weeks. Users may suffer from poor impulse control, depression, fatigue, memory loss, and concentration difficulties.

Variable concentrations and questionable purity are vital problems with PCP. Because it is generally manufactured illegally, users never really know what they are buying. Contaminants are often toxic to humans, causing a wide variety of physiological responses including death. PCP is recognized for its potential to cause violence, especially when the drug is taken in high dosages.

Treatment of acute PCP intoxication may include the use of diazepam for muscle spasms, seizures, and agitation. Risperidone or haloperidol may be used for severe psychotic behavior, but phenothiazines should not be used because PCP is anticholinergic. Calcium channel blockers such as verapamil may be given. These drugs are thought to prevent or reverse PCP-induced vasospasms, thereby decreasing the hallucinogenic effects of PCP. This treatment is controversial, however, because some clinicians feel that the use of verapamil may potentiate the effects of PCP. Nursing care during this period should focus on protecting the patient and others from injury and reorienting the person to reality. Providing a quiet, safe environment and addressing the person in a calm, reassuring manner are important.

A substance very similar to PCP is ketamine, a veterinary anesthesia agent also known as Special K, K, Vitamin K, and Cat Valium. It has a much shorter duration of action than PCP and is used recreationally because of its sedative and hallucinogenic properties (Lofwall et al., 2006). It can cause delirium, amnesia, tachycardia, anxiety, and high blood pressure. Ketamine is also used for pediatric conscious sedation.

Sedatives, Hypnotics, and Anxiolytics

Barbiturates are highly addictive sedatives that cause people to feel euphoric, yet relaxed. They are frequently prescribed to reduce anxiety, prevent or relieve pain, and induce sleep but have inherent dangers because of their ability to cause significant CNS depression and lethality if used to overdose. Migraine overuse headache (MOH) can occur when these medications are used too often and requires a withdrawal strategy (Rossi, Di Lorenzo, Faroni, Cesarino, & Nappi, 2006). Overprescribing may be due to health care providers treating the symptoms of anxiety, stress, or insomnia without determining, and then appropriately eradicating, the cause.

Anxiolytic drugs, typically the benzodiazepines (BZDs) and nonbenzodiazepines, began to be widely used because of their ability to reduce anxiety without causing significant CNS depression. These drugs are thought to modify anxiety by altering the balance of neurotransmitters, especially norepinephrine and gamma-aminobutyric acid (GABA) in the brain's limbic system. The limbic system is involved in the regulation of emotion.

BZDs include diazepam (Valium), clorazepate (Tranxene), lorazepam (Ativan), and alprazolam (Xanax). These, and others, are known to produce dependence and withdrawal syndromes. They have a high risk for abuse and physical dependence. When the drug stops working and tolerance builds up, people tend to increase the dosage just "to cope." Even the nonbenzodiazepines such as zolpidem (Ambien) and zaleplon (Sonata) can be used to excess and have dependence issues associated with use.

One type of abuse of these substances involves taking high doses of barbiturates, often in combination with alcohol, to get the "high." The resultant CNS depression makes this practice especially dangerous. "Speed freaks" (amphetamine abusers) use barbiturates to "come down" from a high. Dependence, tolerance, and cross-tolerance to other depressant drugs develop rapidly.

The liver conducts a staged metabolism of barbiturates. Oral ingestion is followed by initial absorption and partial metabolism. The unmetabolized parts of the drug become active metabolites that are stored in the patient's fatty tissues. Taking these drugs over a period of time results in a cumulative effect, unsuspected dependence, and possible overdose. Death from barbiturate overdose commonly occurs when people take alcohol and barbiturates together. While judgment is impaired, they take more pills, thereby unintentionally overdosing. Because alcohol and barbiturates are synergistic, an overdose can occur quickly. Barbiturates are often used in suicide attempts. A deep sleep is followed by decreased respiration, coma, and sometimes death.

Barbiturate withdrawal is unpleasant and life threatening. Babies born to mothers addicted to barbiturates are physically dependent and need to be helped through withdrawal. Withdrawal from BZDs may produce symptoms similar to those of barbiturate withdrawal. The onset of withdrawal symptoms begins within 24 to 72 hours of the last dose, depending on the half-life of the drug used. Symptoms include autonomic hyperactivity (alterations in vital signs and diaphoresis), marked anxiety, agitation, insomnia, depression, and seizures. Medical detoxification can prevent a potentially serious emergency during withdrawal.

Gerontological Considerations

A number of reasons make geriatric substance abuse a major medical concern. People over the age of 65 consume more prescription medications than all other age groups combined. This alone puts this group at risk for deliberate or inadvertent prescription drug abuse. Misunderstandings about what the medication is supposed to accomplish and how exactly it is supposed to be taken combine with poor or slow responses to encourage inaccurate or abusive ingestion. In addition, the medical health of this group is compromised. Overuse or abuse of prescription substances is more dangerous in older people because less-than-optimal liver functioning and other system frailties can potentiate physiological consequences (Oslin, 2005).

The onset of substance abuse late in life may not be the norm for geriatric substance abuse. Lifelong substance abuse that continues into geriatric years occurs frequently and is evident in chronic damage to body systems and concomitant health problems. Typical to substance abuse is the presence of violence that further complicates treatment as support systems are compromised. Addiction to a substance throughout adult milestones has had psychosocial impacts on the patient in profound ways. Wrestling an addiction is not easy at any stage in life; trying to conquer substance abuse after decades is daunting. Specific treatment incorporating gerontology and substance abuse considerations must be put into practice (Mansell, 2005).

Alcohol is the drug of choice in the geriatric patient population. Identifying late-life alcoholism, either sustained from earlier years or as a new addiction, requires a significant knowledge base about alcoholism and aging. Recognizing the effects of alcoholism on the body and developing evidence-based practice and treatments for those effects is vital.

Impaired Health Care Professional

The health care provider with a chemical dependency is not an unusual scenario. Health care workers, in general, work under a great deal of stress, may have physical injuries leading to pain syndromes, and have easy access to drugs. In the midst of daily pain-relieving functions with patients such as administering pain medications, the professional may consider self-medicating. If the professional has a chronic pain condition, it needs to be managed in an effective manner. Performing professional functions is difficult when chronic pain interferes and being able to function and work while being treated for chronic pain (with pain medications) is a proven positive treatment strategy (Turk & McCarberg, 2005). Effective treatment reduces the abusive use of medications in the workplace as a route to pain relief.

Health care providers become substance abusers for the same reasons anyone becomes dependent on or addicted to a substance. And when the substance is abused, the substance becomes more important than anything else in that person's life. Such behavior is dangerous in a health care environment, is a violation of state practice acts and ethical standards of practice, and, depending on the drug and method of obtaining it, may be a criminal offense.

Colleagues of chemically dependent health care workers need to be alert to behavior that suggests a substance abuse problem. They should assess the safety of attempting to talk with the professional who is having difficulty, and if deemed appropriate use the contact to clarify impressions and gather facts. Typical behaviors of impaired health care professionals are listed in Chart 16–8. The nurse's concerns about a colleague should be reported to a supervisor. A coworker relationship, a friendship, family ties, and the nurse's feelings of guilt or fear are not sufficient to neglect protecting patients from exposure to an impaired health care provider.

It is very common to cover up the addicted behavior. Shielding such a health care provider, whatever the professional discipline, puts patients, the health care provider, and the profession at risk and violates professional practice, the code of ethics, and the law in many states. Nurses, however, need to understand that their chemically dependent colleagues have a disease, not a moral problem. This understanding empowers nurses to work together to help each other. Most states have drug treatment or

| CHART 16–8 | **Typical Behaviors Exhibited by Substance-Abusing Health Care Providers** |

- Frequent absenteeism (usually before or after scheduled days off)
- Always working (in order to obtain supply)
- Abrupt mood changes; inappropriate affect
- Sloppy charting and patient care
- On duty when drugs are missing
- Frequent "wasting" of drugs or inaccurate control drug records
- Frequent disappearance from assigned work area
- Offering to give medication to patients not assigned to them
- Patients receiving medications from the health care provider complain of little or no pain relief.

support groups affiliated with the state nurses' association to address the impaired nurse. Disciplinary action, mandated treatment, and determination of suitability to practice all work well in a holistic approach (McKeon, Fogarty, & Hegney, 2006). A humane and rehabilitative approach such as treatment returns competent nursing colleagues to the work force.

Taylor (2004) suggested the following steps to take in supporting a colleague who is in recovery:

- Do not be judgmental or condescending.
- Let your colleague know you will be there for him and be supportive.
- Be available to step in when recovery is in jeopardy.
- Be honest about mentioning troubling behaviors.
- Be ready to intervene if evidence of relapse appears.
- Promote collaborativeness, not an us-against-you attitude.
- Step in and take a stand when others are intolerant.
- If intolerant behavior continues, report it to management.
- Ask questions about recovery, addiction, and relapse.
- Treat the colleague as you would want to be treated.

Remember, a physical injury and a painful rehabilitation can leave any nurse dependent on pain medications and subject to the physical, emotional, and professional problems just discussed (Sinuk & Taylor, 2004).

Nursing Management

Admission to hospitals and clinics for help with intoxication and withdrawal defines the majority of medical–surgical nursing intervention venues for substance abuse. This tends to be a cyclic process; one in which the patient has a negative physiological consequence of the substance abuse, realizes treatment is needed or is forced to participate in treatment, followed by eventual slippage of the drive to abstain and abuse of the substance recurs. Recognizing and accepting that substance abuse problems are chronic, often with remissions and exacerbations, should keep the nurse from succumbing to the frustration felt by many who treat substance abusers who relapse. At stressful times in life, anyone may develop a dependence on drugs or alcohol; however, certain people seem to be predisposed to the illness. The nurse's focus in performing the nursing process with these patients should be on promoting self-awareness, good health, and good interpersonal relationships so that patients can lead healthier, more constructive lives.

Medical–surgical nurses must be prepared to manage patients who have a substance abuse problem in addition to a medical or surgical issue. For example, management of a patient admitted for an extraordinarily painful acute pancreatitis would involve use of the nurse's physical assessment skills, history taking to pinpoint potential contributing factors such as drug abuse, the design and completion of competent pain assessments, provision of pain medications, and incorporation of ongoing assessment of behaviors around pain and its relief.

Assessment

The major approaches to assessing for substance abuse include interviews, questionnaires, and biological measures of biochemical and hematological markers. Nurses must keep up with current trends in drug use to assess and treat competently patients who are substance abusers. This can be accomplished with the knowledge acquired from reading, continuing education programs, and seminars as well as recognition of the realities of drug use in the local community.

The nurse must make an accurate assessment of the substances used and abused to anticipate potential toxic and withdrawal effects. Different substances require different modes of treatment.

Nursing care plans for a patient with chronic alcoholism who is malnourished, exhausted, and depressed include immediate diet regulation, rest, and gradual involvement in a treatment program. The nursing care also involves incorporating the psychosocial and physiological aspects of the disease. The nursing process organizes care from assessment through interventions. The Nursing Process: Patient Care Plan for Chronic Alcoholism box (p. 382) details the assessment of the patient with chronic alcoholism and gives examples of the expected nursing diagnoses. The outcomes of the care as well as the evaluation of the interventions are delineated in addition to the plan for care and the interventions.

People who abuse cocaine or crack are likely to be resistant to treatment and need active staff intervention and a structured program to involve them in treatment. They should not be left alone or purposefully isolated, as might be done with someone who abuses alcohol. The nursing care for a patient with cocaine intoxication focuses on the immediate needs of the patient and the plan for the longer term. As with the chronic alcoholism nursing process care plan, the Nursing Process: Patient Care Plan for Cocaine Intoxication (p. 382) details the assessment of the patient who is intoxicated from cocaine and gives examples of the expected nursing diagnoses, outcomes of the care, and evaluations and rationales. Notice how the focus of one care plan differs from the other.

The nurse should conduct a thorough, nonjudgmental substance use assessment. Some of the interview questions found in Chart 16–9 may be useful. Simply asking "How many drinks do you have at a time?" is insufficient and can minimize the problem if each drink exceeds standard bar amounts of about 2 oz. The CAGE questions discussed earlier in Chart 16–3 (p. 370) are also helpful. Accurate responses to these questions are most

---

> **CHART 16–9** **Substance Abuse Interview Questions**
>
> - How many packs of cigarettes do you smoke daily?
> - Do you take any prescription drugs now?
> - Do you drink alcohol each day? If yes, do you drink a pint or about a quart? (Let the patient correct an overstatement.)
> - Do you drink a pint or quart of alcohol or more on occasion?
> - When was your last drink?
> - Do you have a drug habit?
> - What drugs do you use?
> - What is your daily cost?
> - When did you last drink more than you wanted to?

---

likely when they are part of an interview that includes general lifestyle inquiries about cigarette smoking, coffee consumption, and exercise habits. Experts agree that skillful assessment interviewing of patients and their family members remains the best source of data.

In an emergency situation the patient may be unable to answer key questions such as these:

- What did you take?
- How much did you take?
- When did you take it?
- What have you taken in the last 24 hours? In the last week?

When this happens, the nurse must rely on family or friends as data sources, and then corroborate what is learned with the patient once she is alert.

People who abuse alcohol and other drugs tend to deny they have a problem or minimize the problem by making it appear perfectly normal: "I drink/use every day, but it rarely interferes with my work." Rationalization is common: "I know I shouldn't use, and I'll stop as soon as I get through this problem. It keeps me calm so I can do what I need to do." A detailed assessment generally reveals that the problem is worse than the patient says. Cocaine users tend to project and blame their difficulties on others, often a family member. "I don't need help. My boyfriend's marijuana smoking is the real problem. He can't remember to do anything so I have to stay on the ball to make up for it."

Substance abusers manipulate people and situations to get drugs. The term *drug-seeking behaviors* (DSBs) refers to these manipulations. Examples include feigning illness or an injury to get a drug. It becomes more important to obtain the substance of choice than to function with integrity, honesty, love, or reliability.

An assessment of behavioral changes can cue the nurse to drug use. Less dramatic physical findings that aid in detection may include dry skin, hangnails, malnutrition, ascites, elevated blood pressure, and the smell of alcohol or an inhalant on the patient's breath. As alcoholism progresses, the nurse should be alert to signs and symptoms of liver cirrhosis.

Laboratory Tests

For years, researchers and clinicians have been searching for an objective biologic marker that will reflect problem drinking and make assessment less challenging. Common laboratory tests in

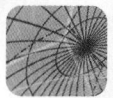

Assessment of Coping Style and Effectiveness

Subjective Data:

What kinds of experiences do you have before you drink alcohol?

What do you consider stressful?

Does stress seem easier to manage when you drink?

How many hours do you sleep at night?

What do you do to promote sleep for yourself?

What do you usually eat throughout the day?

Objective Data:

Inability to manage stress without resorting to substance use

Limited coping skills

Compromised liver function

Insomnia

Poor metabolic health

Malnutrition

Nursing Assessment and Diagnoses	Outcomes and Evaluation Parameters	Planning and Interventions with *Rationales*
Nursing Diagnoses: *Coping, Ineffective* related to alcohol abuse *Sleep Deprivation* related to alcohol abuse *Nutrition, Imbalanced: Less than Body Requirements* related to alcohol abuse	**Outcomes:** Reduction of ineffective and self-destructive coping through alcohol abuse and regular use of more effective coping styles. Sleeping a total of a reasonable number of hours/night indicates successful resolution of sleep deprivation. Patient eats 3 meals every day plus snacks and takes multivitamin as recommended. ***Evaluation Parameters:*** Has begun to substitute effective coping for alcohol use when stressed. Uses sleep-inducing strategies nightly and reports satisfaction with quality of sleep. Reestablishes a consistently healthy sleep routine. Patient identifies and understands relationship between alcoholism and malnutrition. Patient gains weight through a balanced diet.	**Interventions and *Rationales:*** Identify two effective coping mechanisms. *Patients need to have ready choices on how to cope with stress without their addictive substance.* Inventory those situations that challenge patient's abilities to cope. *This prepares the patient for difficulties so rehearsal and skill building can take place.* Rehearse various coping strategies to prepare and select two for regular use. *Rehearsal allows the patient to get familiar with the skill and to learn how to use it.* Teach alternative, healthy coping mechanisms. *Revision of coping styles requires identification of the situations placing the patient at risk, typical problematic responses, and acknowledgment of a need to learn.* Assess for cirrhosis of the liver. *Years of substance abuse may result in cirrhosis.* Assess for depression and feelings of self-reproach and guilt for years of drinking and the effect on others. *Alcohol is a depressant and contributes to deepening existing depressions.* Promote recognition of automatic mechanisms involved in habitually responding to stress with alcohol. *How to cope with stress in adaptive ways will be a new skill.* Consider AA groups, psychiatric treatment, hospitalization, 28-day alcohol treatment programs. *These specialized interventions may be necessary to treat the acute problem.* Evaluate suicide or violence potential. *Alcohol as a depressant certainly raises risk of lethality, plus abstinence may highlight the deep and various life problems the patient has where problem solving sober may seem too big a burden to bear.* Assess for history of insomnia. *Alcohol initially causes somnolence, but chronic use causes insomnia.* Assess current sleep pattern and effective strategies. *Teach and promote healthy sleep hygiene such as warm milk, reading, and other relaxation strategies that counteract ineffective sleep hygiene routines.* Employ effective sleep strategies regularly. *To counteract the alcoholism-disturbed sleep pattern, retraining must take place.* Assess malnourishment from chronic alcoholism. *Vitamins, especially vitamin B, are not metabolized well in an alcoholic's body.* Long-term alcoholism interferes with self-care abilities such as proper nourishment. *Malnutrition from chronic alcoholism can be addressed with a comprehensive nutrition program.* Monitor intake of meals and snacks *to ensure proper intake.* Initiate dietary consult *to explore depth of nutrition problem and educate patient about healthy eating.* Investigate dietary preferences to maximize patient's abilities to expand intake appropriately. *It is easier to reshape a patient's diet when preferences are incorporated.* Educate patient regarding the impact of chronic alcohol ingestion on the digestive tract, metabolism, and overall health. *Alcohol impacts are not commonly known or understood.* Offer frequent food and fluids throughout contacts *to reestablish proper electrolyte, protein, and carbohydrate levels.*

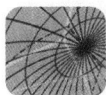

NURSING PROCESS: Patient Care Plan for Cocaine Intoxication

Assessment of Coping Style and Effectiveness

Subjective Data:
What kinds of experiences do you have before you use cocaine?
What do you consider stressful?
Does stress seem easier to manage when you use cocaine?
How are your relationships affected by your cocaine use?

Objective Data:
Inability to manage stress without resorting to substance use
Limited coping skills
Poor social and occupational functioning

Nursing Assessment and Diagnoses	Outcomes and Evaluation Parameters	Planning and Interventions with *Rationales*
Nursing Diagnosis: *Ineffective Coping* related to cocaine abuse	**Outcomes:** Reduction of ineffective and self-destructive coping through cocaine abuse and regular use of more effective coping styles. **Evaluation Parameters:** Has begun to substitute effective coping for cocaine use when stressed. Patient will complete a cocaine detoxification program and will remain free of cocaine. "Clean" urine 72 hours after last use. Replacement of destructive coping with two effective individual coping options.	**Interventions and *Rationales:*** Conduct individual meetings with patient regarding consequences of drug use in work, home, social, and physical arenas. *Defense mechanisms solidly in place throughout the substance abuse period make recognition of self-imposed difficulties difficult.* Discuss prioritization of the work on problem areas. *Immediate medical–surgical concerns take priority over the longer term issues of substance abuse treatment and therapy.* There will be treatment offered for cocaine withdrawal. Arrange access to individual and group therapy. *Team discussions will shape the treatment for the problem in the forefront.* Observe every 1/2 hour. *Withdrawal from cocaine can be a difficult and dangerous time. Lethality risk exists.* Monitor drug-seeking behaviors as an inevitable aspect of this problem. *Long-standing interpersonal styles are not immediately resolved.* When drug-seeking behavior (DSB) commences, interact about patient's feelings and educate about cravings and time frames for resolution. *DSB may be out of patient's awareness and needs to be labeled and addressed.* Help patient recognize the automatic mechanisms involved in turning to cocaine. *Over time the patient sees the connection between stress and demands and the urge to escape through cocaine use.* Identify two effective coping mechanisms. *Patients need to have ready choices on how to cope with stress without their substance.* Help patient rehearse various coping strategies to prepare and select two for regular use. *Revision of coping styles requires learning and practice. Options for coping are more effective and promote resiliency.* Patient begins to substitute effective coping for cocaine use. *Once substitution occurs, there is still the risk of returning to familiar, if maladaptive, responses to stress.* Improve patient's awareness of behaviors, reduce denial, and educate about the addiction. *This intervention serves to supply an educative process that was missing or ineffective before addiction was established.*

which elevated values are associated with excessive alcohol intake are:

- Blood alcohol concentration
- Gamma-glutamyl transferase (GGT)
- Alanine aminotransferase (ALT, formerly SGPT)
- Aspartate aminotransferase (AST, formerly SGOT)
- Lactate dehydrogenase
- Alkaline phosphatase
- Total bilirubin
- Cholesterol
- Triglycerides
- Uric acid
- Mean corpuscular volume (MCV).

These elevated laboratory test values are only one of the alerting factors for problem drinking. (The Diagnostic Tests box provides an overview of the rationale for these tests.) No single test or combination of tests alone to date is appropriate for clinical screening. Confirmation of the excessive use of alcohol in a sensitively conducted assessment interview remains the preferred assessment approach and is considered a prerequisite for successful intervention.

Nursing Diagnosis

Because substance-related disorders are associated with physiological, psychosocial, and spiritual distress, a wide variety of nursing diagnoses are likely to be fundamental to planning comprehensive care. Applicable diagnoses include:

- *Coping, Ineffective*
- *Family Processes, Dysfunctional: Alcoholism*
- *Anxiety*
- *Nutrition Imbalanced: Less than Body Requirements*
- *Decisional Conflict*
- *Pain*
- *Sensory Perception, Disturbed*
- *Social Interaction, Impaired*
- *Thought Processes, Disturbed.*

Outcomes and Evaluation Parameters

When designing care for substance abusers, outcomes must be specifically stated. Although the outcome of total and permanent abstinence may be achievable for some patients with some abuse disorders, for others it may be an unattainable goal. Each situation must be assessed individually. Make sure outcomes can be measured so the treatment team is aware of progress and relapse. Outcome criteria for substance abusers include:

- Coping *as exhibited by goal-directed behavior with resolution of problems.*
- Decision making *as exhibiting patterns of choosing courses of action that meet short- and long-term health-related goals.*
- Impulse control *as exhibited by abstinence.*

See the Patient Teaching & Discharge Priorities box for general guidelines on planning the discharge for these patients.

All of these outcomes impact on sobriety, abstinence from drugs and alcohol, and "getting straight." Further outcomes include risk reduction; improvement of work, family, and social relationships; and lifestyle changes that may include a growing sense of spirituality. No addiction or abuse situation is going to be easy to abandon as a lifestyle. Interventions promote more effectiveness in using new attitudes and behaviors. Although the fear of relapse is always present, over time the craving for chemicals diminishes, and the patient establishes a healthier lifestyle.

Planning and Interventions

Treatment for substance abuse includes promoting adaptive mechanisms and healthy perspectives on self-care and addressing the psychodynamics of drug addiction (Killen et al., 2006; Lile, 2006; Mathias & National Institute on Drug Abuse, 2006). Treatment interventions range from traditional medical interventions and psychiatric care through shamanistic practices. In general, planning care focuses on reducing the harmful use pattern.

Coerced treatment by family, friends, physicians, or the police—a frequent eventuality—inevitably causes the patient to feel anger and resentment. These patients may lash out at people (including the nurse), blame them, and demonstrate resistant or arrogant behavior. In these difficult situations, the nurse must remain detached and nonjudgmental to avoid both power

---

DIAGNOSTIC TESTS for Substance Abuse

Test	Expected Abnormality	Rationale for Abnormality
Liver function profiles	Indications that the liver enzymes are not effective or that the liver would not be able to competently metabolize medications	Alcohol interferes with the liver's abilities to function adequately. Long-standing problems with alcohol cause cirrhosis.
Drug screens (blood and urine)	Evidence of drug in blood or urine	Patient may deny use of substances, but drug screens are able to detect presence.
Breathalyzer	Evidence of alcohol, and the extent of the alcohol, in the expired breath of the patient	Determines the BAL following ingestion of an amount of alcohol.

Sources: Albanese, M. J. (2005). Assessing and treating the bipolar patient with comorbid substance use disorder. *Directions in Psychiatry, 25*(4), 281–290; Kasper, D. L., Braunwald, E., Fauci, A., Hauser, S., Longo, D., & Jameson, J. L. (2007). *Harrison's principles of internal medicine* (16th ed.). New York: McGraw-Hill.

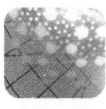

PATIENT TEACHING & DISCHARGE PRIORITIES for Substance Abuse

Need	Teaching
Stabilization of the physiological condition	Patient will be able to demonstrate the need for attention to the physiological demands placed on him as a result of substance abuse.
Involvement in substance abuse treatment	Patient will initiate and continue involvement with substance abuse treatment framework.
Awareness of the substance abuse problem and the necessary treatment	Family members are able to list the signs of substance abuse evident in their relative and the appropriate interventions applicable to the situation.
Contact and linkage with the treatment venue associated with the substance of abuse	The setting of the substance abuse treatment varies depending on the drug of abuse. Alcoholism can be treated via inpatient programs such as a detoxification unit, in a 28-day program, in a halfway house, through self-help such as AA, or as an outpatient.
	Other substances offer a similar array of treatment choices with heroin addiction having an extra component of the methadone clinic as a treatment avenue.

struggles and taking the role of persecutor or rescuer. Interactions are matter of fact: "I know you are [uncomfortable, anxious, afraid, angry] right now. To help you feel better, I need to ask you some questions about your drug use."

General Hospital Care

Substance abusers who are suicidal or acutely ill with DTs, hepatic coma, respiratory depression, or cardiac arrhythmias are often treated in the medical–surgical unit of a general hospital. Life-threatening physiological symptoms are prioritized. When the client is out of danger, the alcoholism or drug addiction issues can be addressed. In this setting, nurses:

- Monitor vital signs and respiratory and cardiovascular support.
- Administer prescribed medications.
- Apply ice packs for fever, such as fever caused by amphetamine intoxication or following cocaine use.
- Decrease stimulation; provide a darkened quiet room.
- Point out reality: "I know you are seeing things, and I know you are frightened. You are in the hospital, and we are caring for you. There are no bugs or monsters here. You are safe and will feel better soon."
- Make sure clients get adequate nutrition and fluids (they are disoriented and generally forget to eat and drink).
- Assess changes in level of consciousness.
- Monitor fluid intake and output.
- Protect skin integrity.
- Offer emotional support and encouragement to the patient and his family.
- Refer patients to community resources for recovery programs.

Other Treatment Settings

Specialized care is given in inpatient hospital units that are geared specifically for the treatment of substance abuse. If the

hospital is equipped with trained personnel and appropriate resources, acutely ill patients, including those who are intoxicated, may be admitted. The physical environment is modified to handle problems with substance abusers. For example, rooms devoid of furniture and potentially harmful materials offer a quiet, unstimulating environment that prevents convulsions and decreases anxiety. A primary nurse may be assigned to decrease confusion and stimulation. Members of the staff are experts in detoxification, education, and treatment. Patients also receive treatment for coexisting medical and psychiatric problems. Staff efforts are geared toward stabilization.

Residential rehabilitation facilities offer inpatients expert care for substance abuse, but in some cases staff members are not skilled in treating medical or psychiatric problems. Extended care facilities provide services for people with physical impairments and a home for recovering alcoholics or drug addicts who have been rejected by their families. Apartments for independent living are useful when available. The nurse working in one of these settings would be aware of each patient's history and propensities around substance use and abuse and be alert to signs and symptoms of relapse to the drug of choice. Impacts on the individual's ability to remain in that health care setting would be a foremost consideration in nursing care.

Outpatient care may consist of daily, weekly, or monthly individual, group, or family therapy in a variety of treatment centers. Daily care is usually given only in intensive programs of limited duration, usually 1 month. Employee assistance programs (EAPs) are now common in many industries and are one example of outpatient care given not in a clinic but in the workplace. Substance abuse outreach counselors work with employees who are chemically dependent.

Self-Help Groups

Self-help groups for addictions have similar goals as other self-help groups: to be a source of mutual aid to individuals who have addictions. Further goals may include serving as a resource to addicts and loved ones as well as increasing awareness of the addiction in the community and its treatment among clinical professionals. Self-help groups may have a specific focus within the support they provide, such as promoting spirituality or helping with a particular addiction. But because longitudinal studies associate self-help group involvement with reduced substance use, improved psychosocial functioning, and lessened health care costs (Guha, 2006), nurses involved in treating addictive processes need to be aware of the benefits of peer groups.

Twelve-Step Programs

In contrast to the previously described treatment programs, Alcoholics Anonymous (AA) and Narcotics Anonymous (NA) are not professionally designed treatment programs. They are spiritual programs based on fellowship among its members. Both are successful self-help groups that meet daily, or more often, in different parts of large cities and weekly in smaller towns in places of worship, schools, town halls, and various mental health treatment facilities. Anyone who has a desire to stop drinking or taking drugs is welcome. This belief pervades both organizations: "Once an alcoholic/addict, always an alcoholic/addict." Members admit they are powerless over chemicals, live "one day at a time," recite the serenity prayer, and believe in "a power greater than man." Members learn to turn their problems over to "the God of my understanding." Their philosophy is revealed in part through their key slogans: "First things first," "Easy does it," and "Let go and let God." Alcoholics learn the "Twelve Steps of AA" (see Chart 16–10).

MyNursingKit | Rational Recovery

CHART 16–10 · Twelve Steps of Alcoholics Anonymous

1. We admitted we were powerless over alcohol—that our lives had become unmanageable.
2. Came to believe that a Power greater than ourselves could restore us to sanity.
3. Made a decision to turn our will and our lives over to the care of God, as we understand Him.
4. Made a searching and fearless moral inventory of ourselves.
5. Admitted to God, to ourselves, and to another human being the exact nature of our wrongs.
6. Were entirely ready to have God remove all these defects of character.
7. Humbly asked Him to remove our shortcomings.
8. Made a list of all people we had harmed, and became willing to make amends to them all.
9. Made direct amends to such people wherever possible, except when to do so would injure them or others.
10. Continued to take personal inventory and when we were wrong, promptly admitted it.
11. Sought through prayer and meditation to improve our conscious contact with God, as we understand Him, praying only for knowledge of His will for us and the power to carry that out.
12. Having had a spiritual awakening as the result of these steps, we tried to carry this message to alcoholics, and to practice these principles in all our affairs.

Source: The Twelve Steps are reprinted with permission of Alcoholics Anonymous World Services, Inc. (AAWS). Permission to reprint the Twelve Steps does not mean that AAWS necessarily agrees with the views expressed herein. AA is a program of recovery from alcoholism only—use of the Twelve Steps in connection with programs and activities, which are patterned after AA but which address other problems, or in any other non-AA context, does not imply otherwise.

Through AA/NA, people learn to change negative attitudes and behaviors into positive ones. A key concept of AA/NA is that total abstinence is essential to recovery. As members become sober or drug free, they begin "sponsoring" (helping) other substance abusers. This offering of support is believed to be vital to recovery, as is regular attendance at AA/NA meetings. Twelve-step recovery programs also emphasize spirituality through meditation and prayer rather than willpower as the means to recovery. Recognizing that AA's 12 steps were written in the 1930s by and for white Christian males may require that the nurse adapt some of the language to a less patriarchal, less religious, and more generally spiritual and culturally relevant usage.

Women for Sobriety

Women for Sobriety (WFS) is another self-help group. Unlike AA/NA, WFS is not based on a spiritual philosophy; instead, the program is based on abstinence. WFS's 13 acceptance statements focus members on new ways of thinking. Women learn to cope and, over time, to change their daily lives. The group recognizes the differences of alcoholism in males and females.

Rational Recovery

Alcoholics and addicts who were not comfortable in AA but were nevertheless determined to become sober have founded Rational Recovery (RR), a self-help approach that rejects the spiritual approach of AA. RR also rejects the notion that alcoholics and addicts are powerless to stop their addictions, suggesting instead that until now they simply have not chosen to do so. Instead of reliance on a higher power (which RR considers another form of dependence), RR members are urged to build on strengths within themselves; the movement inspires independence whenever humanly possible. A constant theme is "Think yourself sober."

In RR, there are no steps, sponsors, moral inventories, making amends to others, or even caring about what others think of you. According to rational emotive therapy, on which RR is based, human beings should love themselves because they are human beings and not because others think well of them. The concept of staying sober one day at a time is rejected in favor of a decision to never drink or use again, period. Sobriety is not supposed to become the cornerstone of one's life. The goal is for members to wean themselves from dependence on alcohol, then from dependence on people, and finally from dependence on the group.

Meetings take place only twice a week, and most people attend for only 1 year, after which they may be pronounced "recovered." They can, however, return to meetings whenever the need arises. Discussions at meetings focus on the here and now rather than past history, and interactive discussion is encouraged.

Whereas AA relies totally on nonprofessionals helping one another, professional coordinators run RR, and each group has volunteer professional advisers available for advice and input. This is necessary because, unlike AA, there are no old-timers around to help newcomers. Advisers attend meetings only occasionally. RR, like AA, offers written materials, the core of which is *Rational Recovery from Alcoholism: The Small Book* (meant to contrast with the Big Book of AA).

RR suggests looking within oneself for strength and direction. Everyone has an inner voice, says RR, that challenges one to go wrong. It is this voice, nicknamed "Beast," that urges one to drink or use drugs, takes over during blackouts, gets one to do terrible things, and speaks louder than one's rational self. It's the voice that tells one things like "You can stop anytime (but not now)" or "You're not really addicted (you just like the taste)" and that tears angrily into those who criticize or try to help. BEAST is an acronym used to help RR members avoid taking another drink or drug. See Chart 16–4 (p. 371) for specifics about the BEAST acronym.

Relapse

Relapse is common among substance abusers, and it seriously complicates treatment. Authorities in the field of alcoholism estimate that 60% to 75% of those who complete treatment programs drink again within the first 90 days. Data suggest that only 10% to 20% of alcoholics remain abstinent for 1 year following treatment, and that only 35% of these are abstinent 5 years later. In fact, recidivism rates are notoriously high across the spectrum of addictive behaviors (Doweiko, 2006; Finnell & Osborne, 2006).

After a successful initial change, the patient experiences perceived control while remaining abstinent. This feeling of perceived control continues until the patient encounters a high-risk situation involving negative emotional states, interpersonal conflict, or social pressure. The patient can avoid relapse by using effective coping responses in the high-risk situation. If, however, the patient cannot cope successfully, an initial "lapse" occurs in which she resorts to the use of a chemical to control stress. The patient then feels less able to exert control and develops a tendency to "give in" to the situation ("It's no use, I can't handle this"). In subsequent high-risk situations, the patient again resorts to the use of chemicals to relieve stress. Repeated lapses set the stage for a return to uncontrolled use (relapse).

Many treatment centers are now incorporating the concept of relapse prevention into their treatment programs. This concept is designed to teach patients how to anticipate relapse. By learning skills to use in high-risk situations, patients gain confidence and the expectation of being able to cope successfully, thus decreasing the probability of relapse.

Research indicates that participation in a 12-step program can help prevent relapse. These programs focus on the patient being "in recovery" and maintaining sobriety, as opposed to having recovered or being cured.

Other Treatment Approaches

Substance abuse is a complex problem, so a single treatment approach is not likely to address the majority of needs. Therefore, a variety of treatments are typically engaged, as discussed in the following subsections.

Complementary and Alternative Therapies

Interest in alternative and complementary treatments has increased and is useful to explore with regard to substance abuse. Treatment for substance abuse is a difficult process prone to failure. The addict must fight the physiological demands of the addiction as well as the psychological repercussions of being in the world without the relief or escape of the drug of choice. Short-lived abstinence can be viewed as a partial success.

Complementary and alternative treatments for substance abuse take on a different form than for other health problems in that an herbal or food supplement substance is not substituted for the pharmaceutical or illicit drug of abuse. As a matter of fact, there are a number of complementary and alternative substances that can be abused for their escapist and stimulating qualities, so suggesting those as a mode of treatment would be counterproductive. Consider the therapeutic impact and the holistic functioning of the person when integrating these aspects of care.

For substance abuse, alternative treatments may include more ethnomedical treatments or those discovered through research on cross-cultural styles rather than substituting a benign botanical for the abused drug. Interventions based on behaviors and beliefs would be alternative to the medical model of drug treatment. Treatments that attend to the cultural aspects of human existence include encouraging traditional values that discourage deviant behaviors such as drug abuse (Gates et al., 2006; Peterson, Mitchell, Hong, Agar, & Latkin, 2006), inducing a relaxation response and thus providing a healthy coping mechanism, or using a nondrug reward for abstinence through the traditional operant behavior analysis style (Turk & McCarberg, 2005).

The use of acupuncture for treating substance abuse is discussed in the Complementary and Alternative Therapies box (p. 388).

Using Confrontation Strategies

Interventions for substance abuse can occur as soon as the problem is identified. Group intervention/confrontation is one strategy that aims to break down the substance abuser's denial. Nurses are often "intervention specialists" and leaders in this process.

Several family members, friends, employers, coworkers, and an alcohol/drug intervention specialist confront the substance abuser in a private meeting. They list the evidence by going around the group, one by one. The family, friends, employer, and so on, following the leader's cues, speak calmly and slowly with minimal emotion. They are presenting the facts, the objective evidence, to the alcoholic/drug abuser. Yelling, blaming, and haranguing are avoided because the alcoholic/drug abuser will inevitably respond by denying the behavior or making excuses. However, confrontation by several people who really care and who persistently present the facts breaks through the denial.

The next step in group intervention/confrontation requires the family, friends, employer, etc., to make clear and direct statements to the alcoholic/drug abuser about the consequences of his behavior:

- "Either you get help now or we will take you off the job."
- "Either you enter a treatment program now or I will move out with the kids."

If the patient agrees to treatment, the caring people agree to remain involved.

Education

Videotapes and talks by recovered substance abusers or experts in the effects of substance abuse are helpful. Education may take place in or out of the hospital, in one comprehensive session or several sessions over time. Nurse-educators should focus on the types of abused substances and their physical, psychological, and social effects. Families are often involved in these sessions because substance abuse is a family problem. The belief underlying such education is that knowledge and awareness may be useful in decreasing self-destructive behavior. But knowledge alone is never enough. Culturally sensitive and relevant educational resources should be used.

Referral and Self-Help Groups

Support and self-help groups are extremely useful in helping patients feel better about themselves and acquire new attitudes and behaviors. Merely being with many people who are suffering in similar ways is beneficial. By observing people who have been sober or drug free for long periods, patients can begin to learn similar behaviors. They can see that there is hope and that recovery is possible. Self-help groups also provide new friends, generally with healthy lifestyles. Patients may choose to attend support groups for the rest of their lives. Some patients who experiment with drugs or alcohol during one period of their lives and who succeed in stopping may attend only during the crisis.

Lifestyle Change

An emphasis on the requirement for a total lifestyle change is necessary. Nurses can help patients discuss ways to alter their destructive habits by suggesting different coping strategies and by encouraging them to discover new interests and capabilities within themselves. Nurses and patients can role-play new responses to old situations. Recognizing that relapse is always a threat, nurses may set up behavioral contracts. For example, there may be an agreement to contact the nurse or an AA/NA sponsor if and when they feel the urge to drink or do drugs. This agreement represents new behaviors that are necessary for a lifestyle change.

Part of a total lifestyle change includes the patients' realization that it is no longer possible to remain abstinent while spending time with friends who are substance abusers or hanging out at places where they used to take drugs or alcohol. The mere sight or smell of paraphernalia or the desired substance is often enough to trigger a relapse. Old ties must be broken; new friends and activities must be pursued. See the Nursing Process: Patient Care Plan (p. 382) earlier in this chapter for specifics on lifestyle changes with cocaine use.

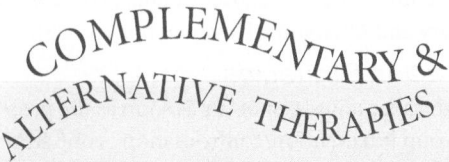

COMPLEMENTARY & ALTERNATIVE THERAPIES — Acupuncture/Acupressure

Description:

Acupuncture is based on the philosophy that Qi (pronounced "chee"), or a person's vital energy, flows through specific energy meridians throughout the body. An acupuncturist inserts very fine needles into the skin to stimulate these energy meridians in order to influence physiological, emotional, and psychological functions of the mind and body. A related CAM therapy, acupressure, uses finger pressure rather than needles along these energy meridians to exert the same influence on the flow of energy. Most acupuncture and acupressure practitioners are health care providers who have chosen to add these therapies to their current practice. These practitioners may choose one or both of the therapies, then pursue certification programs.

Research Support:

A placebo-controlled pilot study was carried out in a community mental health center in a United States–Mexico border city. Most participants were Hispanic males with an average age of 32.8 years. The goal of the study was to examine the effectiveness of acupressure on cravings in drug-addicted individuals. Participants reported an average lifetime use of drug of choice of 14 years. In addition to conventional medical care, participants received specific acupressure treatment once a week for 6 consecutive weeks, and placebo acupressure treatment. Researchers administered the Hopkins Symptom Checklist (SCL-20) Depression Scale to assess changes in emotional distress before and after 6 weeks of treatment. In order to assess changes in craving, researchers used the Brief Substance Craving Scale at baseline and weekly for 6 weeks. The results showed that both specific and placebo acupressure groups experienced a significant reduction in craving at the end of treatment. The specific acupressure group had a greater and more steady reduction in craving. Both specific acupressure and conventional-care-only groups demonstrated a significant reduction in emotional stress (Tian & Krishnan, 2006).

In another study, the effects of acupuncture on 40 HIV-seropositive, cocaine-abusing, methadone-maintained drug users were studied. These participants were randomized to one of two protocols: the standard five-needle National Acupuncture Detoxification Association (NADA) protocol or a reduced, escalating dose (one- to three-needle) protocol. The last 15 of the participants also received a spirituality-focused group therapy intervention in addition to their assigned acupuncture treatments that were offered 5 days per week for 8 weeks. Urine samples from each participant were collected twice weekly and were analyzed for the presence of both cocaine and heroin. Participants' levels of depression and anxiety were assessed both pre- and post-treatment. Results showed that there was no difference in the number of weeks in which urine samples tested negative for heroin and cocaine use between the two acupuncture protocols. However, patients who received the spirituality-focused group therapy in addition to acupuncture treatment showed significantly longer abstinence from heroin and cocaine and greater reductions in depression and anxiety than the patients who did not receive spirituality-focused psychotherapy (Margolin, Avants, & Arnold, 2005).

The goal of another study was to develop an Internet-assisted smoking cessation program accompanied by auricular acupressure. Researchers aimed to compare the abstinence rate and self-efficacy of youth smokers receiving auricular acupressure with and without the Internet-assisted smoking cessation program. Particpants were assigned nonrandomly to two groups. Group 1 received auricular acupressure plus the Internet-assisted smoking cessation program, while group 2 received auricular acupressure only. Researchers collected demographic factors, serum nicotine, quitting rate, nicotine dependence, and self-efficacy data before and after a 4-week intervention. The results showed that after intervention, the abstinence rate was 15.78% in group 1 and 2.56% in group 2. Group 1 showed significantly lower nicotine dependence, nicotine dependence remained unchanged in group 2. Self-efficacy improvement between groups 1 and 2 was significantly different. The combination of auricular acupressure and Internet-assisted smoking cessation program was more effective than auricular acupressure alone in terms of the abstinence rate (Chen, Yeh, & Chao, 2006).

References

Chen, H. H., Yeh, M. L., & Chao, Y. H. (2006). Comparing effects of auricular acupressure with and without an internet-assisted program on smoking cessation and self-efficacy of adolescents. *Journal of Alternative and Complementary Medicine, 12*(2), 147–152.

Margolin, A., Avants, S. K., & Arnold, R. (2005). Acupuncture and spirituality-focused group therapy for the treatment of HIV-positive drug users: A preliminary study. *Journal of Psychoactive Drugs, 37*(4), 385–390.

Tian, X., & Krishnan, S. (2006). Efficacy of auricular acupressure as an adjuvant therapy in substance abuse treatment: A pilot study. *Alternative Therapies in Health and Medicine, 12*(1), 66–69.

Helping the Family

Substance abuse affects the entire family system. Family members often engage in behaviors that enable substance abusers to continue with their substance abuse by protecting them from the consequences of their behavior. Helping family members to be healthier includes clarifying the problem and presenting possible solutions (treatment) and creating a support system for family members. Referring family members to Al-Anon can be a very helpful strategy. Al-Anon is a program for family members and friends whose lives have been affected by a person who abuses alcohol. The program helps them to understand the addiction, the psychological affects of being near someone who abuses alcohol, and to learn coping mechanisms.

In dysfunctional families, the substance abuser often becomes the "identified patient," focusing attention on that individual and away from the other problems in the family. Treatment for the substance abuser may require including some type of family therapy. Family members may need treatment for codependence through group or individual therapy or involvement in a 12-step program such as Al-Anon or Codependents Anonymous (CODA). The Adult Children of Alcoholics (ACOA) support groups could be helpful for those who respond to 12-step self-help groups (Timko, Billow, & DeBenedetti, 2006).

Evaluation

Evaluating nursing interventions for patients who are substance abusers hinges on an evaluation of the patient's abilities to change. Is there evidence of patient honesty, openness, and willingness to take responsibility for his own actions? Regardless of the substance of abuse, once a patient stops blaming others for her use/abuse, treatment has made a positive impact. Another criterion is the amount of substance the patient is placing in his body. Has it decreased? Other indications of positive treatment outcome are increased job stability, improvement in interpersonal relationships with others, and improved problem-solving techniques. Evaluating implementation of the necessary changes in people, places, and things is critical for victory over substance dependence.

Collaborative Management

Treating chronic alcoholism in an effective manner involves nurses, physicians, rehabilitation therapists, and psychotherapists (such as clinical nurse specialists, psychologists, and psychia-

trists), social workers, dieticians, and peer advocacy/support. This disease process is a composite of genetic predisposition, a variety of underlying psychological dynamics, exposure and reactions to stress, and the physiological consequences of the behavior of using alcohol as a coping mechanism.

Each team member will address, in a planned manner, how the patient will move toward recovery from chronic alcoholism. The psychologist can provide psychological testing when there are questions about coexisting psychological problems, and can provide psychotherapy (individual or group) for patients who abuse alcohol whose problems require multifaceted clinical interventions. The dietician will help increase the nutritional status of the patient that has been compromised by malnutrition and the interference of alcohol in metabolizing necessary vitamins and nutrients. The peer support approach of AA has had a significant impact on people addicted to alcohol. The self-help component of this contact is an important factor in the overall success and recovery of an alcoholic. The collaborative team approach offers the best response to the treatment needs of this patient from the day of admission to the ongoing, sustained approach that will help this patient maintain a healthier lifestyle.

Effective treatment of a patient who is intoxicated by cocaine usually involves the same team members used for treating patients with alcoholism. Teams intervene during the intoxication stage and beyond, providing services to enhance the patient's abilities to choose a healthier lifestyle. The rehabilitation counselor provides additional information about the use of cocaine and develops, with the rest of the team, a plan for the patient to maintain cocaine abstinence. As with alcoholism, peer support through Narcotics Anonymous has been proven to be an effective mechanism for recovery. The collaborative team approach offers the best response to the treatment needs of this patient from the day of admission to the ongoing, sustained approach that will help this patient maintain a healthier lifestyle.

Summary

Substance abuse knows no social boundaries. It is important nurses educate themselves and others about the effects of substance abuse. Through the understanding of addiction, the nurse will be able to observe the patient for behaviors or physical symptoms of abuse and report him or her to the health care team. Caring for patients who are substance abusers requires knowledgeable and skilled nursing to develop and implement effective multidisciplinary plans of care.

RESEARCH OPPORTUNITIES AND CLINICAL IMPACT RELATED TO SUBSTANCE ABUSE

Research Area

Standards of Addictions Nursing Practice, Standard XII: Research. This standard states that the nurse contributes to the nursing care of patients with addictions and to the addictions area of practice through innovations in theory and practice and participation in research, and communicates these contributions.

Research demonstrates that children of alcoholics are at higher risk of becoming alcoholics. Even if different families adopt them at birth, identical twins of alcoholic parents have more than a significant chance of becoming alcoholics; fraternal twins have a smaller but still elevated chance (Dick & Bierut, 2006).

Alcoholism clinical investigations have redefined alcoholism as a disease. As research about its biochemical aspects became known, the social stigma attached to alcoholism decreased and more people sought help. Professionals, laypeople, students, alcoholics, and nonalcoholics are attending seminars and college courses on alcoholism. Recovery programs are reported widely in the popular media and rehabilitation programs have become common knowledge. Information about alcohol recovery programs is easily accessible on the Internet and in print materials.

Researchers have found that marijuana produces a significant analgesic effect and is modestly effective against the nausea and vomiting associated with chemotherapy (Trossman, 2006). Dronabinol is a synthetic delta-9-tetrahydrocannabinol or delta-9-THC that contains standardized THC content in an FDA-approved pharmaceutical.

Use of an atypical antipsychotic for the treatment of stimulant abuse and dependence (Stoops et al., 2006) was found to be effective and directs future research for combinations specifically with methamphetamine and cocaine.

Research suggests a role for nicotine replacement in smoking cessation. In time this management option and the only nonnicotine smoking management option approved by the FDA (bupropion SL) may be joined by investigational drugs in the near future (Glover, 2006).

For years, researchers and clinicians have been searching for an objective biologic marker that will reflect problem drinking and make assessment less challenging (Muthen et al., 2006; Prescott et al., 2006; Vieten et al., 2004).

Research indicates that participation in a 12-step program can help prevent relapse. These programs focus on the patient maintaining sobriety, as opposed to having recovered or being cured (Timko et al., 2006).

Clinical Impact

The clinical impact of research in this area of nursing care provides evidence-based practices for addictions and substance abuse treatment providers and deepens one's knowledge base within nursing. When research results are shared throughout the nursing community, patient care is enhanced.

Research into addressing the environments vulnerable children are raised in could ultimately lower the risk factors associated with having genetic predispositions to substance abuse.

Further research into alcoholism would drive the stigma and lack of knowledge into retreat and provide a better venue for the definitions of the illness, effective treatment frameworks, and acceptance of people with alcoholism.

Examination of substances for their beneficial actions contributes to opportunities to capitalize on available treatment and encourage the development of additional compounds to treat clinical problems.

Thorough clinical trials of the biochemistry of substance abuse helps assess the process of abuse, identifies the pathways involved, and can direct clinical interventions more accurately.

Understanding how, when, and why neurochemicals act as they do and how those actions can be translated into human behavior gives treatment providers a scientific basis for care.

Finding an objective biologic marker for alcoholism can be formulated as prevention as well as enhancing treatment.

Clinical research debunked the formerly held view that alcoholics could imbibe moderately as long as they were in control of their consumption. Science showed that the vast majority of alcoholics relapsed quickly with negative consequences if they drank alcohol. Continued research keeps treatment accurately focused.

NCLEX® REVIEW

1. A pregnant patient seen in the clinic informs the nurse she does not consume alcohol or use illicit drugs, but her husband has been abusing cocaine for a few years. When the patient asks, "Will my baby be okay" the nurse explains:

   1. "Since you have abstained from alcohol and drugs, the baby should be fine."
   2. "There is a potential for the baby to have birth defects."
   3. "You should use some form of barrier contraception for the remainder of the pregnancy."
   4. "Sociocultural and environmental factors have a greater influence on substance abuse."

2. The nurse identifies the patient with the following personality traits to be most at risk for disruptive substance abuse:

   1. Outgoing and gregarious
   2. Quiet and studious
   3. Independent and loyal
   4. Impulsive and extroverted

3. The nurse is caring for a patient with a history of alcoholism who has been hospitalized for 48 hours. The nurse suspects the patient is beginning major alcohol withdrawal when the following symptoms are displayed.

   1. Hypothermia
   2. Bradycardia
   3. Diaphoresis
   4. Abdominal pain

4. The nurse caring for a patient in the emergency department who has been sniffing paint solvents places priority on monitoring the patient for:

   1. Cardiac arrhythmias
   2. Suicidal tendencies
   3. Outbursts of rage
   4. Visual hallucinations

5. A patient admitted to the emergency department is displaying symptoms of PCP intoxication. The nurse prepares to administer which drug?

   1. Naloxone, Narcan
   2. Prochloperazine, Phenergan
   3. Diazepam, Valium
   4. Amitriptyline, Elavil

Answers for review questions appear in Appendix D

KEY TERMS

blackouts *p.372*
delirium tremens (DTs) *p.371*
fetal alcohol syndrome (FAS) *p.372*
postacute withdrawal syndrome
   (PAWS) *p.366*

substance abuse *p.366*
substance dependence *p.366*
substance intoxication *p.366*
substance withdrawal *p.366*

substance withdrawal syndrome *p.366*
tolerance *p.366*
withdrawal *p.366*

REFERENCES

Albanese, M. J. (2005). Assessing and treating the bipolar patient with comorbid substance use disorder. *Directions in Psychiatry, 25*(4), 281–290.

American Psychiatric Association. (2000). *Diagnostic and statistical manual of mental disorders* (4th ed., text revision). Washington, DC: Author.

Arria, A. M., Derauf, C., LaGasse, L. L., Grant, P., Shah, R., Smith, L., et al. (2006). Methamphetamine and other substance use during pregnancy: Preliminary estimates from the Infant Development, Environment, and Lifestyle (IDEAL) study. *Maternal and Child Health Journal, 10*(3), 293–302.

Barr, A. M., Panenka, W. J., MacEwan, G. W., Thornton, A. E., Lang, D. J., Honer, W. G., et al. (2006). The need for speed: An update on methamphetamine addiction. *Journal of Psychiatry and Neuroscience, 31*(5), 301–313.

Carroll, C. P., Walsh, S. L., Bigelow, G. E., Strain, E. C., & Preston, K. L. (2006). Assessment of agonist and antagonist effects of tramadol in opioid-dependent humans. *Experimental and Clinical Psychopharmacology, 14*(2), 109–120.

Dennis, T., Bendersky, M., Ramsay, D., & Lewis, M. (2006). Reactivity and regulation in children prenatally exposed to cocaine. *Developmental Psychology, 42*(4), 688–697.

Dick, D. M., & Bierut, L. J. (2006). The genetics of alcohol dependence. *Current Psychiatry Reports, 8*(2) 151–157.

Doweiko, H. F. (2006). *Concepts of Chemical Dependency* (2nd ed.). Washington, DC: American Psychological Association.

Eaton, D. K., Kann, L., Kinchen, S., Ross, J., Hawkins, J., Harris, W. A., et al. (2006). Youth risk behavior surveillance—United States, 2005. *Morbidity and Mortality Weekly Report 9, 55*(Suppl. SS-5), 1–107.

Evans, S. E., Blank, M., Sams, C., Weaver, M. F., & Eissenberg, T. (2006). Transdermal nicotine-induced tobacco abstinence symptom suppression: Nicotine dose and smokers' gender. *Experimental and Clinical Psychopharmacology, 14*(2), 121–135.

Finnell, D. S., & Osborne, F. H. (2006). Stages of change for psychotropic medication adherence and substance cessation. *Archives of Psychiatric Nursing, 20*(4), 166–174.

Fride, E., Perchuk, A., Hall, F. S., Uhl, G. R., & Onaivi, E. S. (2006). Behavioral methods in cannabinoid research. *Methods in Molecular Medicine, 123*, 269–290.

Gates, S., Smith, L. A., & Foxcroft, D. R. (2006). Auricular acupuncture for cocaine dependence. *Cochrane Database of Systematic Reviews*, Issue 1, CD005192. Retrieved from http://www.cinahl.com/cgi-bin/refsvc?jid=s3053&accno=2009359326

Glover, E. D. (2006). Successfully treating nicotine dependence. *American Journal of Health Education, 37*(1), 6–14.

Gross, A., Marsch, L. A., Badger, G. J., & Bickel, W. K. (2006). A comparison between low-magnitude voucher and buprenorphine medication contingencies in promoting abstinence from opioids and cocaine. *Experimental and Clinical Psychopharmacology, 14*(2), 148–156.

Guha, M. (2006). Book reviews (*Review of fleeting pleasures: A history of intoxicants; Cannabis and young people: Reviewing the evidence; Overcoming problem drinking: A self-help guide using cognitive behavioral techniques; Alcohol, gender and drinking problems: Perspectives from low and middle income countries; Substance use among young people in urban environments;* and *Adolescent risk behaviors: Why teens experiment and strategies to keep them safe*). *Journal of Mental Health, 15*(6), 713–716.

Heimer, L., & Van Hoesen, G. W. (2006). The limbic lobe and its output channels: Implications for emotional functions and adaptive behavior. *Neuroscience & Biobehavioral Reviews, 30*(2), 126–147.

Hoeppner, B. B., Velicer, W. F., Redding, C. A., Rossi, J. S., Prochaska, J. O., Pallonen, U. E., et al. (2006). Psychometric evaluation of the smoking cessation Processes of Change scale in an adolescent sample. *Addictive Behaviors, 31*(8), 1363–1372.

Jones, H. A., & Lejuez, C. W. (2005). Personality correlates of caffeine dependence: The role of sensation seeking, impulsivity, and risk taking. *Experimental and Clinical Psychopharmacology, 13*(3), 259–266.

Killen, J. D., Fortmann, S. P., Murphy, G. M., Jr., Hayward, C., Arredondo, C., Cromp, D., et al. (2006). Extended treatment with bupropion SR for cigarette smoking cessation. *Journal of Consulting and Clinical Psychology, 74*(2), 286–294.

Kim, S. J., Lyoo, I. K., Hwang, J., Chung, A., Hoon Sung, Y., Kim, J., et al. (2006). Prefrontal grey matter changes in short-term and long-term abstinent methamphetamine abusers. *International Journal of Neuropsychopharmacology, 9*(2), 221–228.

Klesges, R. C., DeBon, M., Vander Weg, M. W., Haddock, C. K., Lando, H. A., Relyea, G. E., et al. (2006). Efficacy of a tailored tobacco control program on long-term use in a population of U.S. military troops. *Journal of Consulting and Clinical Psychology, 74*(2), 295–306.

LaBrie, J. W., Pedersen, E. R., Lamb, T. F., & Bove, L. (2006). Heads up! A nested intervention with freshmen male college students and the broader campus community to promote responsible drinking. *Journal of American College Health, 54*(5), 301–304.

Libby, A. M., Orton, H. D., Heather, D., Barth, R. P., Webb, M. B., Burns, B. J., et al. (2006). Alcohol, drug, and mental-health specialty treatment services and race/ethnicity: A national study of children and families involved with child welfare. *American Journal of Public Health, 96*(4), 628–631.

Lile, J. A. (2006). Pharmacological determinants of the reinforcing effects of psychostimulants: Relation to agonist substitution treatment. *Experimental and Clinical Psychopharmacology, 14*(1), 20–33.

Lofwall, M. R., Griffiths, R. R., & Mintzer, M. Z. (2006). Cognitive and subjective acute dose effects of intramuscular ketamine in healthy adults. *Experimental and Clinical Psychopharmacology, 14*(4), 439–449.

Mansell, D. (2005). Geriatric substance abuse: An opportunity to improve care. *Substance Abuse, 26*(2), 48.

Marczinski, C. A., & Fillmore, M. T. (2006). Clubgoers and their trendy cocktails: Implications of mixing caffeine into alcohol on information processing and subjective reports of intoxication. *Experimental and Clinical Psychopharmacology, 14*(4), 450–458.

Martin, V. T., Loder, E., Taylor, K., Almas, M., & Hilliard, B. (2005). Eletriptan treatment of migraine in patients switching from barbiturate-containing analgesics: Results from a multiple-attack study. *Cephalalgia, 25*(9), 726–734.

Mathias, M., & National Institute on Drug Abuse. (2006). Alcohol-treatment medication may help reduce cocaine abuse among heroin treatment patients. *NIDA Notes Research Findings, 16*(1), 1–4.

McGuinness, T. M. (2006). Nothing to sniff at: Inhalant abuse & youth. *Journal of Psychosocial Nursing and Mental Health Services 44*(8), 15–18.

McKeon, C. M., Fogarty, G. J., & Hegney, D. G. (2006). Organizational factors: Impact on administration violations in rural nursing. *Journal of Advanced Nursing, 55*(1), 115–123.

Meyers, R. A., Zavala, A. R., Speer, C. M., & Neisewander, J. L. (2006). Dorsal hippocampus inhibition disrupts acquisition and expression, but not consolidation, of cocaine conditioned place preference. *Behavioral Neuroscience, 120*(2), 401–412.

Muthen, B., Asparouhov, T., & Rebollo, I. (2006). Advances in behavioral genetics modeling using Mplus: Applications of factor mixture modeling to twin data. *Twin Research and Human Genetics: The Official Journal of the International Society for Twin Studies, 9*(3), 313–324.

National Drug Intelligence Center. (2006). National drug threat assessment 2006: Product No. 2006-Q0317-001. Johnstown, PA: U.S. Department of Justice. Retrieved from http://www.usdoj.gov/ndic/topics/titles2.htm

Neaigus, A., Gyarmathy, V. A., Miller, M., Frajzyngie, V. M., Friedman, S. R., & Des Jarlais, D. C. (2006). Transitions to injecting drug use among noninjecting heroin users: Social network influence and individual susceptibility. *Journal of Acquired Immune Deficiency Syndromes, 41*(4), 493–503.

O'Connor, M. J., Frankel, F., Paley, B., Schonfeld, A. M., Carpenter, E., Laugeson, E. A., et al. (2006). A controlled social skills training for children with fetal alcohol spectrum disorders. *Journal of Consulting and Clinical Psychology, 74*(4), 639–648.

Oslin, D. W. (2005). Evidence-based treatment of geriatric substance abuse. *Psychiatric Clinics of North America, 28*(4), 897–911.

Peterson, J., Mitchell, S. G., Hong, Y., Agar, M., & Latkin, C. (2006). Getting clean and harm reduction: Adversarial or complementary issues for injection drug users. *Cadernos de Saude Publica, 22*(4), 733–740.

Prescott, C. A., Sullivan, P. F., Kuo, P. H., Webb, B. T., Vittum, J., Patterson, D. G., et al. (2006). Genomewide linkage study in the Irish affected sib pair study of alcohol dependence: Evidence for a susceptibility region for symptoms of alcohol dependence on chromosome 4. *Molecular Psychiatry, 11*(6), 603–611.

Ranney, L., Melvin, C., Lux, L., McClain, E., Morgan, L., & Lohr, K. (2006). *Evidence report on tobacco use: Prevention, cessation, and control* (Evidence Report/Technology Assessment 140, AHRQ Publication 06-E 015). Rockville MD: Agency for Healthcare Research and Quality.

Rossi, P., Di Lorenzo, C., Faroni, J., Cesarino, F., & Nappi, G. (2006). Advice alone vs. structured detoxification programmes for medication overuse headache: A prospective, randomized, open-label trial in transformed migraine patients with low medical needs. *Cephalalgia, 26*(9), 1097–1105.

Serretti, A., Liappas, I., Mandelli, L., Albani, D., Forloni, G., Malitas, P., et al. (2006). Interleukin-1 alpha and beta, TNF-alpha and HTTLPR gene variants study on alcohol toxicity and detoxification outcome. *Neuroscience Letters, 406*(1–2), 107–112.

Shorey, H. S., & Snyder, C. R. (2006). The role of adult attachment styles in psychopathology and psychotherapy outcomes. *Review of General Psychology, 10*(1), 1–20.

Sinuk, P., & Taylor, A. (2004). Nurses' addictions. *American Journal of Nursing, 104*(6), 13.

Stoops, W. W., Lile, J. A. Glaser, P. E. A., & Rush, C. R. (2006). A low dose of aripiprazole attenuates the subject-rated effects of d-amphetamine. *Drug and Alcohol Dependence, 84*(2), 206–209.

Timko, C., Billow, R., & DeBenedetti, A. (2006). Determinants of 12-step group affiliation and moderators of the affiliation-abstinence relationship. *Drug and Alcohol Dependence, 83*(2), 111–121.

Trossman, S. (2006). Issues update. Rx for medical marijuana? Promoting research on and acceptance of this treatment option for patients. *American Journal of Nursing, 106*(4), 77–79.

Turk, D. C., & McCarberg, B. (2005). Non-pharmacological treatments for chronic pain: A disease management context. *Disease Management and Health Outcomes, 13*(1), 19–30.

Vaitl, D., Birbaumer, N., Gruzelier, J., Jamieson, G. A., Kotchoubey, B., Kübler, A., et al. (2005). Psychobiology of altered states of consciousness. *Psychological Bulletin, 131*(1), 98–127.

Vieten, C., Seaton, K. L., Feiler, H. S., & Wilhelmsen, K. C. (2004). The University of California, San Francisco, family alcoholism study. I. Design, methods, and demographics. *Alcoholism: Clinical and Experimental Research, 28*(10), 1509–1516.

Nursing Management at End of Life

Cheryl Wraa, Pamela Coulter, Linda Kelly

Outcome-Based Learning Objectives

After studying this chapter, the learner will be able to:

1. Review ethical theories that influence decisions in end-of-life care.
2. Define advanced directives and their role in end-of-life care.
3. Compare and contrast pharmacological and nonpharmacological therapies used for relief of pain at end of life.
4. Discuss beliefs surrounding death held by various cultures and religions.
5. Identify the need for interdisciplinary collaboration in planning end-of-life care.
6. Identify the role of hospice during end-of-life care.
7. Review the principles of palliative care.

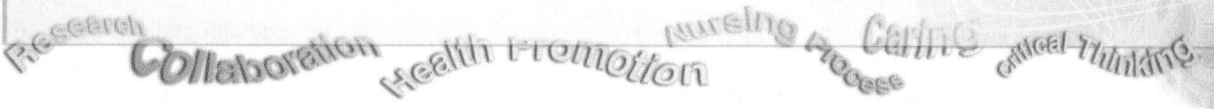

DEALING WITH end-of-life decisions can be an extremely difficult and complex situation for caregivers. This is particularly true in the acute care setting because often the critical nature of the illness or injury is sudden and unexpected. Recent studies report on the dissatisfaction expressed by families with the quality of care their family member received when they died while in the hospital (Heyland et al., 2005; Teno et al., 2004). Family satisfaction depends largely on the information the family receives and the way it is provided.

End of Life in the Acute Care Setting

Palliative care, comprehensive care focused on alleviating suffering and promoting the quality of remaining life of patients living with a chronic, life-threatening, or terminal illness, allows patients and families to guide treatment and set goals for care (National Consensus Project for Quality Palliative Care, 2004). Although palliative care is well defined for patients who are terminally ill, it has not been well defined for patients in the acute care setting who are critically ill.

For health care providers, the transition from providing "curative care" to "comfort care" can be difficult. There are several reasons why making this transition is difficult. First, ethical dilemmas may arise on a daily basis as the choice of extending

life versus postponing death occurs. Second, nurses are influenced by their own values, culture, religion, education, and life experiences. Third, the role of the nurse is to participate as a member of the health care team to assist the patient and families to make fully informed decisions with full knowledge of their options. Finally, it is critical that everyone involved with the patient's care communicate with one another and have consensus prior to discussions with the family. In addition to the normal nursing interventions needed to provide clinical care, there are additional key nursing interventions discussed throughout the chapter that are helpful at end of life. These key nursing interventions include:

- Recognition of autonomy
- Honesty
- Expert communication
- Presence
- Compassion
- Touch
- Assisting in transcendence or developing a sense of meaning and peace with death (Saunders, 2007).

Advances in technology, changes in managed care, and changes in social and family structures have also added to the complexity of end-of-life care (Bednash & Ferrell 2002b). Advances in technology in critical care medicine have added therapeutic options never before available. Today patients who were considered physiologically brittle, including those who are elderly or chronically ill, are receiving operations and complex procedures. Most will survive the operation and recover with few or no complications. Issues arise, however, when complications occur and despite massive resuscitative efforts, the patient continues to deteriorate and further care is deemed futile. The transition from curative to noncurative is particularly difficult for surgeons, due in part to their training (Buchman, Cassell, Ray, & Wax, 2002). An ethnographic study of surgical services completed by C. Bosk at the University of Chicago revealed that one characteristic that sets surgeons apart from their medical colleagues is their sense of accountability for the patient's outcome (Buchman et al., 2002). Surgeons are trained to be heroic, because surgical patients often require immediate decision making and actions. Surgeons' personalities tend to exude confidence and commitment to successful outcomes. This heroic optimism may be a barrier to discussions with families when offering comfort, as opposed to curative care, because the surgeon may view this as a failure on his part. The nurse working in a surgical area may need to assist the family in approaching the surgeon for discussions regarding end-of-life issues.

End of Life in the Intensive Care Unit

Typically, patients who face life-threatening complications are placed in the intensive care unit (ICU) on varying degrees of life support. The ICU is one area where many technological innovations have been developed to prevent death. Therefore, decisions regarding withholding or withdrawing life-sustaining treatment are more consequential than in many other settings. Monitoring in the ICU provides an enormous amount of data regarding the patient's condition—pulse, blood pressure, cardiac output, and oxygen saturation, to name a few. The data may be confusing to the family because one bit of information could bode well at the same time that another bodes poorly. These discordant data make it difficult for a family to comprehend the situation and know how to respond. The Institute of Medicine believes this is especially true because society places a great deal of faith in technology (Buchman et al., 2002). The Institute of Medicine recently asked:

> Are ICU staff, specialty services, and other personnel trained to recognize patients (and families) for whom the goals of curative or life-prolonging care should be reconsidered with particular attention to the goals of physical and emotional comfort and symptom relief? Are procedures in place for arranging appropriate care and consultations? Are the important roles of nurses, social workers, and others recognized and supported? (Buchman et al., 2002, p. 666)

The answer to these questions depends on all members of the health care team being able to acknowledge when rescue attempts are failing.

Nurses spend most of their time at the bedside and are integral to relaying and reinforcing information to patients' families and other members of the health care team. Families in crisis need information repeated or at times explained in a different way. Stud-

ies have demonstrated a significant difference between what clinicians think they said and what patients and families understood (Chaitin & Arnold, 2005). Therefore it is essential that every member of the health care team, especially nurses because of their close and frequent contact with the patient and family, be aware of discussions that are held with the family and the plan of care for the patient. Nurses are instrumental in helping the family not feel abandoned at the end of life. A core nursing function at end of life is to be present and bear witness during the dying process and to help the patient and family find meaning in the experience.

The Study to Understand Prognoses and Preferences for Outcomes and Risks of Treatments (SUPPORT) in 1995 revealed that some physicians have difficulty listening to nurses unless the nurse is responding to a posed question (Buchman et al., 2002). Although physicians in the ICUs believed that their relationships with nurses was collaborative and believed that the information received from nurses was valuable, they tended not to involve them in end-of-life decision-making processes (Buchman et al., 2002). Studies have shown that for families, communication with caregivers is identified as the single most important factor for them during end-of-life care (Chaitin & Arnold, 2005; Heyland et al., 2006). Families, when surveyed, revealed that not just communication but continuity of communication is an essential ingredient (Heyland et al., 2006). As the plan of care shifts from cure to comfort, it is important to repeatedly reassure the family through words and actions that the patient and they will not be ignored or abandoned and that attentive palliative care will be provided. The transition from curative to comfort care is often done gradually and without continuity. For example, at times the patient may be receiving therapies aimed at comfort and others aimed at cure. To bring continuity to the situation, the health care team needs to change to a model focused primarily on symptomatology. In this new model the criteria for an intervention is based on improvement of symptom relief, functional status, or amelioration of emotional, psychological, or spiritual concerns (Chaitin & Arnold, 2005).

Research has shown that nurses in the ICU feel immense frustration about the lack of consensus concerning end-of-life care and that ICUs do not deliver compassionate end-of-life care (Buchman et al., 2002). One way to alleviate this type of frustration is to develop guidelines for end-of-life care in the ICU. Evidenced-based guidelines will assist with health care team continuity and will assist in facilitating discussion regarding a shift from curative to comfort care. Open communication among all members of the health care team will also assist with the psychological and emotional stress incurred by ICU staff when involved in palliating a patient who is dying, as discussed further in the Evidence-Based Practice box.

Oncology nurses who frequently care for patients who are terminally ill are more comfortable with and better understand palliative care (Davidson et al., 2003). Unfortunately, nurses who do not care for patients who are terminally ill on a daily basis usually do not have this knowledge of and familiarity with end-of-life care. A recent exploratory study of the perceptions of palliative care among cardiorespiratory nurses revealed several themes (Davidson et al., 2003). First, nurses felt there was philosophical and cognitive dissonance between acute care and palliative care philosophies. Second, there is a lack of continuity in planning and negotiating with the patient or the family. Often decisions are left

For End-of-Life Care

Clinical Problem

In the hospital setting, conflicts between families and health care providers regarding end-of-life decisions are common. Decisions should be a cooperative effort to achieve treatment goals. When discussions are perceived as conflicts, families often feel misunderstood or isolated, and may doubt the health care providers' commitment to the patient's well-being.

Research Findings

In a study by Breen, Abernethy, Abbott, and Tulsky (2001), health care providers reported that 63% of conflicts with families involved decision making at the end of life. The Center for Gerontology and Health Care Research at Brown Medical School found that many patients and family members of people dying in institutions reported having unmet needs for symptom amelioration, physician communication, emotional support, and being treated with respect (Teno et al., 2004). In Canada, Heyland et al. (2006) conducted a study to describe what seriously ill patients in the hospital and their family members considered to be the key elements of quality end-of-life care. In their results, elements rated as "extremely important" included trust and confidence in their doctors; not to be kept alive when there is little hope for recovery; information regarding their disease being communicated in an honest manner; and preparing for end of life, that is, resolving conflicts, saying good-bye, and life review.

Implications for Nursing Practice

Supportive communication involves active listening and letting the family know that providers are present and are accepting of their strong emotions. For the family, knowing that caregivers listen to and understand what they are going through is therapeutic. The acronym NURSE is a useful tool for how one can be empathetic to families' strong emotions:

Acronym	Request	Example
N	Name *Help the patient or family member understand and give their feelings a name.*	It sounds like you are frustrated.
U	Understanding *Let the family know that you are aware and empathetic of their situation.*	It is hard for me to imagine what it is like to be in this situation.
R	Respect *When a family makes an end-of-life decision, acknowledge how difficult it can be.*	I respect how hard you have tried to follow your loved one's wishes.
S	Support *Let the family know that you are available.*	I am here if you have any questions.
E	Explore *Take time to listen to the family. Help them sort out their feelings.*	Tell me more about what you are thinking.

Critical Thinking Questions

1. After a family meeting with the health care team, you notice that a family member looks confused. How would you approach this person?

2. How will you show support to the patient and family?

Answers to Critical Thinking Questions appear in Appendix D.

References

Breen, C. M., Abernethy, A. P., Abbott, K. H., & Tulsky, J. A. (2001). Conflict associated with decisions to limit life-sustaining treatment in intensive care units. *Journal of General Internal Medicine, 16*, 283.

Heyland, D. K., Dodek, P., Rocker, G., Groll, D., Gafni, A., Pichora, D., et al. (2006). What matters most in end of life care: Perceptions of seriously ill patients and their family members. *Canadian Medical Association Journal, 184*(5), 627–633.

Teno, J. M., Clarridge, B. R., Casey, V., Welch, L. C., Wetle, T., Shield, R., et al. (2004). Family perspectives on end of life care at the last place of care. *Journal of the American Medical Association, 291*(1), 88–103.

EVIDENCE-BASED PRACTICE

to a crisis point and there is poor communication between clinical teams about end-of-life issues. Third, there is discomfort in dealing with death and dying. Fourth, there is a lack of consistency of messages among the health care team. Nurses felt that if the death of the patient had not been managed optimally that it became a critical incident for them. Finally, Davidson and colleagues found that there is a lack of awareness of palliative care philosophies and resources and a need for education on palliative care principles.

Ethical Issues

The transition to end-of-life care in the acute care setting begins with the process of shared decision making to change the focus from care aimed at cure to care aimed at comfort and freedom from pain. When the health care team begins to discuss decisions regarding life-sustaining versus end-of-life interventions, ethical issues and dilemmas are inherent in the discussions. Ethical decision making involves a systematic appraisal of a situation using moral principles and ethical theories to justify the resolution (Gillick, 2004; Jackson & Abrahm, 2005).

Respect for Persons

Fundamental to nursing practice is the respect for the worth, dignity, and rights of every individual. It requires that people be treated as individuals with respect for their human dignity. It is this principle that prevents interference with the plans, privacy, or decisions made by capable adults (Bednash & Ferrell, 2002a).

Privacy

Individuals have a right to privacy and caregivers have a duty to respect the confidentiality of patient information (Saunders, 2007). Any discussion regarding the patient's diagnoses, consultation, examination, and treatment should be conducted discreetly.

Autonomy

Capable adults have the moral and legal right to determine what will be done with their own person. They have the right and ability to determine how they wish to live and to determine what therapies to accept or reject, even if the health care team does not agree. The principle of autonomy is referred to as the right to self-determination (Bednash & Ferrell, 2002a; Gillick, 2004).

 *Caregivers are duty bound to respect patients' choices in all situations unless a choice is overridden by another moral principle of greater weight.*

Veracity

Caregivers have a duty to be truthful. When information is withheld from patients and family or they are not told the truth, they can no longer make informed choices. It is important for the nurse to find out how much and the type of information the patient wants so her goals can be adjusted to fit the time she has left (Bednash & Ferrell, 2002a; Saunders, 2007).

Beneficence

This principle means to do or promote good. It is different from nonmaleficence, or the duty to not inflict harm. It is sometimes difficult when caring for patients to distinguish between preventing harm and providing benefit. When the duty not to inflict harm conflicts with the duty to provide benefit, there is support for the view that the obligation not to injure others is greater than the obligation to benefit them (Bednash & Ferrell, 2002a). Therefore, care given in the acute care setting is focused primarily on the curative model of care. Decisions regarding invasive monitoring, diagnostic tests, or therapeutic interventions are based on whether doing this procedure will contribute to the patient's recovery from the illness. In palliative care, the decision about whether to do an intervention should be based on whether it will improve symptom relief, functional status, or ameliorate emotional, psychological, or spiritual concerns (Peterman & Cella, 2005). Bednash and Ferrell (2002a) state, "Patients at the end of their lives may be particularly vulnerable to harm. They are harmed when they receive unwanted or unnecessary interventions, when they are overtreated with burdensome technological interventions that serve only to prolong dying and when treatments are withdrawn without their consent or agreement. They are most certainly harmed when their pain is not adequately managed due to the nurse's fear that the patient's death might be hastened as a result of pain management with high dose opiates" (p. 4).

The American Nurses Association's Code of Ethics for nurses states "the nurse may provide interventions to relieve symptoms in the dying client even when the interventions entail substantial risks of hastening death" (Bednash & Ferrell, 2002c, p. 75). So at the end of life, not titrating a drug to relieve symptoms because it may hasten death would be viewed as causing the patient harm because it would increase suffering.

Nonmaleficence

Caregivers are required to avoid intentionally causing patients unnecessary harm or pain, both physical and mental (Bednash & Ferrell, 2002a). Health care teams often do procedures that may harm patients in order to benefit them or to prevent a greater harm from occurring. Morally they must decide whether causing the harm is justified.

Justice

This principle is understood as fairness. It involves the determination of what is owed a person or a group. Justice also takes into consideration cultural and religious preferences. Incorporating justice into medical decisions includes the likelihood of medical benefit as well as present and future quality-of-life criteria. Most believe that if a treatment will not benefit a patient, then it is considered futile and, as such, its use is morally and professionally unwarranted. Therefore treatments that are futile should not be suggested or offered to patients or families (Gillick, 2004).

■ Ethical Issues and Dilemmas at End of life

As stated before, the change from "curative care" to "comfort care" can be a difficult transition. Communication among the health care team and family is of great importance during this transition time because a number of ethical issues and dilemmas may arise at the end of life.

Advanced Care Planning

Patients must have the capacity to comprehend information in order to make informed consent. For the patient who is unable to consent for himself, it is important to determine whether he has done any advanced care planning.

Advance Directives

Advance directives lay the groundwork for decision making at the time of acute illness. They are a significant part of the Patient Self-Determination Act and include the living will, the durable power of attorney for health care, and the directive for organ donation (Saunders, 2007). Advance directives give patients peace of mind that their wishes will be followed even if they cannot communicate. The directives give clear directions for significant others and the health care team regarding the patients' wishes. All advance directive statutes contain provisions that grant immunity to health care professionals when they act in good faith and in accordance with state statutes in regard to advance directives.

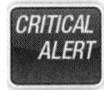 *It is the nurse's responsibility to be aware of a patient's advance directive and to advocate for respecting the patient's wishes.*

Living Wills

Living wills, a form of an advance directive, describe the patient's preferences in case she becomes incapacitated. They usually describe what level of life-prolonging interventions the patient would or would not want and under what circumstances they should be completed, withheld, or withdrawn. Living wills require the signature of two witnesses (Bednash & Ferrell, 2002a; Gillick, 2004).

Durable Power of Attorney

A **durable power of attorney for health care (DPAHC)**, **medical durable power of attorney (MDPA)**, or health care proxy allows the patient to appoint a decision maker in the case of future incapacity. The DPAHC or MDPA specifically states which powers the patient gives to the surrogate. The appointed person responsible for making medical decisions does not need consent from other family members or friends (Bednash & Ferrell, 2002a; Gillick, 2004).

In the ICU setting where initially aggressive lifesaving technology is used, when it is apparent that the patient will not return to his former health, it is often difficult to choose to reject that support. Patients and families may continue to opt for invasive or high-technology therapy out of fear of a painful death or of giving up too soon. When caregivers discuss specific treatments with the patient and family, it is important to explain the potential benefits versus the potential burdens. For the family, it can be emotionally more difficult to withdraw life-sustaining treatments that have been initiated than to withhold them (Gillick, 2004). Health care teams must remember that ethically based medical decisions are a shared process and are based on open communication and a relationship with the patient that respects the patient's privacy and autonomy. Decisions must be made with regard to providing the best recommendation for the patient and not to relieve the stress of any individual in the family or health care team caused by having to make the decision.

Communication During End-of Life Care

Patients and their families have expressed that communication with caregivers is an extremely important factor during end-of-life care (Heyland et al., 2006). Even though health care providers feel overburdened with time constraints, it is important to take the time to sit with the patient and family and communicate with them in an open, genuine manner regarding the patient's illness.

Many critical care clinicians have difficulty initiating a straightforward discussion about death with a patient and/or family because they have been trained to restore health. If the primary goal is to make patients well, then death is often viewed as failure. Adding to the conflict is the question of how certain the health care team is about the patient's prognosis. The team may decide that any further care is futile and suggest withdrawing all life-sustaining treatment and giving comfort care only. On the other hand, it may be decided that there is some chance of survival, but that additional interventions would be burdensome. In this case, conversations would be held regarding continuing the current level of life support, but forgoing additional support in the event of further complications. Another option is a plan that considers each new problem or complication as it arises and weighs the potential burdens and benefits of the treatment that might be administered.

Caring for the acutely ill patient may require that decisions and interventions be made quickly, although the appropriateness of some of these decisions becomes clearer as time passes and as the illness takes its course (Chaitin & Arnold, 2005). If the patient is in a teaching hospital, the family may receive conflicting messages from the multiple teams of physicians caring for the patient. It is better to have a representative from each team present during a family meeting and to ask open-ended questions of the family to ascertain if they clearly understood what was presented. Recom-

mendations are to give information at a ninth-grade level with as little medical jargon as possible. Family members are under stress and their ability to understand large amounts of information is difficult. Experts suggest not giving more than three pieces of information without stopping to check the family members' understanding (Chaitin & Arnold, 2005).

Formal training in end-of-life care skills is not included in most caregivers' education. Most caregivers learn these skills through experience and on-the-job exposure. In Canada, Stevens et al. (2002) completed a study of the perceptions of the limitations of ethics education in end-of-life care for residents. Prior to their ICU rotation, the residents felt that out of 19 determinants considered in the decision for withdrawal of life support, the three factors most important to the decision were patient advance directives, the likelihood of surviving the current illness, and family directives. After completing their ICU rotation, the three most important factors were patient advance directives, the likelihood of surviving the current illness, and the likelihood of long-term survival. Of the 19 determinants, the two that increased the most in importance for the decision to withdraw life support were likelihood of long-term survival and preferences of the attending physicians. From this study, the participating residents recommended more formal and informal education and practical experience in end-of-life issues in the ICU. Specifically they suggested more opportunities to observe senior clinicians during family meetings, discussions on approaches to withdrawal of life support, more patient-centered discussions, and opportunities to lead family meetings to improve their communication skills. The residents felt that formal lectures and grand rounds on the ethical aspects of end-of-life care in the ICU were not of much benefit.

Many clinicians do not feel comfortable with death and are not trained in good communication skills. This combination creates difficult situations for dying patients and their families. The ability to give compassionate, nurturing, end-of-life care is based on the caregiver's ability to be comfortable with death. The structure of tightly organized rounds that occurs in teaching hospitals in the ICU is a wonderful opportunity to include detailed discussion of the goals for care in light of the patient's needs and values. A particular principle that should be taught is that the goals of care should drive the use of technology, not the other way around. These discussions will help caregivers to learn to ask questions such as these: Are the patient's goals and values known? If so, are the treatments the patient is receiving consistent with these goals? If not, why not and what needs to change? Although it is important to be sensitive to the family's wishes, discussions should be guided by respect for what the patient's goals and wishes were.

Additionally, these discussions and having students and nurses accompany the physician team during family meetings give them the opportunity to recognize and deal with the suffering that the family may be experiencing. The ICU also gives caregivers the opportunity to learn the multidisciplinary nature of critical care, collaborative decision making, and effective teamwork.

◼ Ensuring the Patient's Comfort

The transition from curative care to comfort care can be inconsistent with some therapies aimed at comfort and some at cure. In a study done by Heyland et al. (2006), patients and their families identified four issues that were considered extremely important in end-of-life care: (1) trust and confidence in the physicians caring for them, (2) avoiding inappropriate prolongation of death, (3) information about their illness being communicated in an honest manner, and (4) completing things and preparing for life's end.

One suggestion for making the transition from curative to comfort care is to completely rewrite the patient's orders and review the plan of care as if the patient were just now being admitted. Each test or intervention should be reviewed for its need and how it will further the patient's wishes, improve symptom relief, and ameliorate emotional or spiritual concerns. The treatment orders should be organized by symptoms rather than by organ system or disease. The symptom list should be actual and potential and each symptom should be managed separately.

Pain

If the patient is unable to communicate, assessment of pain at the end of life may rely on evaluation of physical signs such as consciousness, breathing pattern, change in blood pressure and heart rate, and facial grimaces.

At the end of life, allowing hypoxia in the face of normocarbia is the fastest path to unconsciousness with the least amount of agitation. Decreased cardiac activity leads to hypoperfusion and decreased cerebral function. Also, lack of oral intake will lead to dehydration, which also decreases cerebral function. This phenomenon has been referred to as *starvation euphoria* and is thought to be related to endogenous opioid production or the analgesic effects of ketosis. So the withdrawal of some treatments may actually assist the patient to be more comfortable.

Environment also plays a factor in the patient's comfort. The hospital is rarely considered a peaceful environment although measures can be taken to enhance the patient's comfort, such as reducing lighting and noise, eliminating unnecessary monitors and machines, removing restraints, and providing room for the patient's significant others. Cultural and spiritual factors such as prayer, ritual, and music can also increase the patient's comfort.

Pharmacologic Therapies

The use of pharmacologic therapies, with attention paid to the pharmacokinetics and pharmacodynamics of the drugs used, can ease many or all of the symptoms the dying patient may experience. The symptoms most often experienced by dying patients are pain, fatigue, dyspnea, excessive respiratory secretions, nausea and vomiting, constipation, and diarrhea (Saunders, 2007). In addition to the specifics discussed in the following subsections, the Pharmacology Summary feature provides more information about the use of medications for a patient who is at the end of life.

Opioids

Opioids are the most common class of drug used for the treatment of pain and suffering in the dying patient. Opioids instill analgesia, sedation, and euphoria by binding to receptor sites in the brain and spinal cord to prevent the release of neurotransmitters involved in pain transmission. The most frequently used opioids are morphine, hydromorphone, and fentanyl. Meperidine is not recommended because its metabolite, normeperidine, produces signs of central nervous system (CNS) excitation such as tremors, and if not excreted, as in the patient with renal insufficiency, is toxic to the CNS and places the patient at risk for seizures (Bednash & Ferrell, 2002c; Jackson & Abrahm, 2005).

Most patients in the acute care setting are already receiving analgesics and may have already developed some tolerance to their effects. For this reason, there is no set dosage for opioids at the end of life. Analgesic drips should be titrated to effect and should not be limited by recommended maximal doses. As stated previously, the increasing of the titration of the opioid is intended to relieve pain and suffering, not to directly cause death (Bednash & Ferrell, 2002c; Jackson & Abrahm, 2005).

 **CRITICAL ALERT** *It is important to document the indication for increasing the dose clearly.*

It is also appropriate to use anticipatory dosing. When withdrawing mechanical ventilation, an increase in dyspnea can be an-

PHARMACOLOGY Summary of Drugs Used in End-of-Life Care

Medication Category	Action	Application/Indication	Nursing Responsibility
Opioid analgesics	Bind with and activate opioid receptors in brain and spinal cord to produce analgesia and euphoria	Treatment of pain and nonpain symptoms associated with dying.	Conduct regular, frequent assessment of pain and nonpain symptoms (e.g., shortness of breath, anxiety). Ensure safe and timely reduction of pain and symptom levels. Address barriers to effective pain management, including inappropriate fears of risk of side effects, addiction, respiratory depressions, or hastening of death.
Benzodiazepines	Produce a calming effect and relax skeletal muscles by increasing the activity of gamma-aminobutyric acid, a major inhibitory neurotransmitter in the brain.	Synergistic sedative effect with opioids. May help prevent development of premorbid seizures.	Same as for opioids.

ticipated. It would not be sufficient to wait for the distress to respond, so adequate medication should be given prior to the withdrawal (Jackson & Abrahm, 2005). Lynn, Lynch Schuster, and Kabcenell (2000) describe a prospective study done by Campbell et al. in 1999 of patient responses during terminal weaning of unconscious patients. The investigators reported that 35% of the patients required no analgesia or sedation at any time during the procedure. Also, there were no significant correlations between the amount of morphine used and the duration of survival after removal from the ventilator. Additionally, when comparing the patients who received morphine and those who did not, there was no difference in length of survival. During this study, the average dose of morphine used was 5.5 mg/hr.

Benzodiazepines

Benzodiazepines have a synergistic sedative effect with opioids, are anticonvulsants, and may help prevent the development of premorbid seizures (Truog et al., 2001). Midazolam, when administered intravenously, changes to a lipophilic (i.e., having an affinity for fat) compound that rapidly penetrates the CNS. The drug is short acting but will have a sustained effect when given by continuous infusion. Starting doses for adult continuous infusion is 1 to 5 mg/hr. Lorazepam is an intermediate-acting benzodiazepine and reaches a peak effect approximately 30 minutes after intravenous infusion. The starting dose for adult continuous infusion is 1 to 8 mg/hr. Further discussion about the use of opioids and benzodiazepines at the end of life is provided in the Ethical Issues box.

Neuroleptics

Neuroleptics, such as haloperidol, may be helpful for patients exhibiting delirium. It is important to try to distinguish between anxiety and delirium, an acute confusional state. The distinction is important because the use of opioids or benzodiazepines can worsen the symptoms of delirium. It has been shown that patients who are given haloperidol for acute delirium require less sedation than with other medications (Truog et al., 2001). Starting doses of haloperidol in adults range from 0.5 to 20 mg. Recommendations are to titrate additional doses at 30-minute intervals until symptoms are controlled. The drug can also be given by continuous infusion ranging from 3 to 25 mg/hr. The use of restraints should be avoided when possible (Truog et al., 2001).

Complementary and Alternative Therapy

Complementary therapies may be helpful to patients who are at the end of life, as discussed in the accompanying Complementary and Alternative Therapies box (p. 400).

Dyspnea

Dyspnea is shortness of breath and can be extremely distressing and frightening. The neuropathways responsible for the sensation are poorly understood (Kuebler, Heidrich, & Esper, 2007). Many patients may be unable to report dyspnea due to their level of consciousness. Physical symptoms that should be considered signs of dyspnea are tachypnea, restlessness, accessory muscle use, grunting at the end of each breath, and nasal flaring. Nonpharmacologic techniques that may lessen the sensation of dyspnea are to elevate the head of the bed to reduce choking sensations and promote expansion of the lungs, and the use of fans that circulate air. Cool air directed gently on the face may reduce the perception of breathlessness (Bednash & Ferrell, 2002c; Truog et al., 2001). The use of oxygen may be effective if the patient is hypoxic, but the use of a face mask may increase the sensation of dyspnea if it makes the patient feel claustrophobic (Truog et al., 2001). Opioids are highly effective in relieving dyspnea by depressing respiratory drive; causing vasodilation, which can reduce pulmonary vascular congestion; and producing sedation and euphoria. The use of opioids for relief of dyspnea in a patient who is near death is considered the standard treatment (Kuebler et al., 2007).

Dyspnea is reported in up to half of dying patients. It is important to educate the family and the patient, if the patient is conscious, regarding the specific symptoms of dyspnea and ways to relieve the sensation and make the patient comfortable (Bednash & Ferrell, 2002c).

Fever

Fevers and infections occur frequently in the acute care setting. For the dying patient, fever can be uncomfortable and antipyretics should be given. Any measure that would cause the patient more discomfort, such as a cooling blanket or alcohol bath, should not be used.

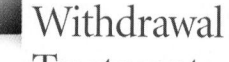

Withdrawal of Life-Sustaining Treatments

The goal of palliative and end-of-life care is to achieve the best quality of life for the patient and her family, consistent with their goals and values, regardless of the location of the patient. Components of palliative care should be offered, discussed, and incorporated into the plan of care at the time of diagnosis of a life-threatening illness. As the disease progresses, the patient or family may decide to forgo or withdraw life-sustaining treatments. When discussing with the family the decision not to initiate cardiopulmonary resuscitation, providing survival statistics to the family can facilitate decision making. Chances of survival to discharge for patients who have suffered an arrest in the hospital range from 6% to 15%, with 30% of survivors suffering a

ETHICAL ISSUES for Pain Management at End of Life

Management of pain at the end of life is the right of the patient and the duty of the caregiver. Many families state that their loved ones suffered from untreated pain at the end of their life (Jackson & Abrahm, 2005). Failure to treat the pain adequately can arise from the caregiver's fear of violating ethical and moral tenets in the administration of pain medication to the dying patient.

At the end of life, the use of opioids, benzodiazepines, and other medications in doses high enough to control the patient's symptoms may unintentionally hasten death. This is referred to as double effect, where an action may have two possible effects, one good and one bad. The action is not considered immoral if it is undertaken with the intention of achieving the good effect without intending the bad effect, even though it may be foreseen. At the end of life not administering a drug to relieve symptoms because it may hasten death would be viewed as causing the patient harm and increased suffering.

significant decrease in quality of life and the ability to be independent (Carney & Meier, 2000).

Discontinuation of mechanical ventilation usually occurs when the burdens of continuing life-prolonging interventions outweigh their benefits. Withdrawal of mechanical ventilation should be planned carefully, ensuring the patient's comfort and allowing the family to be present at the bedside if they wish. Unfortunately, death can be viewed as a failure by the health care team and the antithesis of everything in which they believe. For this reason, the dying patient can become the object of intense effort where death occurs in an arena of machines, tubes, and technicians (Bednash & Ferrell, 2002b). Because the attitudes of both society and members of the health care team can greatly influence the process of dying, it is important to educate all members of the team on the ways in which life-sustaining treatments can be withdrawn (Bednash & Ferrell, 2002a).

Terminal Wean

In 1983 A. Grenvik was the first to describe a systematic approach to ventilator withdrawal by a gradual reduction in the ventilator settings over several hours. The process is a gradual reduction of the fractionated inspired oxygen (FIO_2) and pressure support or control, leading to development of hypoxia and hypercarbia. It is important to remember that in the ICU setting, the sedation and

analgesia adequate for the patient who is currently receiving mechanical ventilation are inadequate to treat his symptoms during terminal weaning. A study done at two San Francisco teaching hospitals by Wilson et al. found that 75% of adult patients from whom life support was withheld or withdrawn received nearly a threefold increase in sedatives, analgesics, or both during the process (Burns et al., 2000). An advantage to terminal weaning is that the patient does not develop any signs of upper airway obstruction and, with the proper administration of sedatives and analgesics, the patient does not develop symptoms of acute air hunger. These advantages promote the comfort of the patient and reduce the anxiety of the family. The disadvantage of terminal weaning is that it may prolong the death by several days and some family members may perceive it as an attempt to have the patient successfully survive separation from the ventilator.

Terminal Extubation

The obvious advantage to terminal extubation is that it does not prolong the dying process and allows the patient to be free from an unnatural tube. It is important to be anticipatory of the distress a patient may experience during terminal extubation. Therefore, the patient should receive anticipatory doses of analgesics and sedatives that are then titrated as necessary to the observed level of the patient's distress.

COMPLEMENTARY & ALTERNATIVE THERAPIES — Journaling

Description:
Many people have found that recording thoughts in a journal helps to relieve pain and emotional suffering. People who are at the end of life, and who create a historical record that lives on after their death often reduce their perception of stress. A diary is the most common form of journaling.

Research Support:
Nursing literature and educational literature frequently discuss journaling as an active technique that can enhance a nurse's reflective practice, which is a means of self-examination. Reflective practice involves looking back over what has happened in practice in an effort to improve, or encourage, professional growth. Some of its benefits include discovering meaning, making connections between clinical experiences and the classroom, instilling values, learning others' perspectives, and developing critical thinking (Blake, 2005). Reflective journaling is also used in the hospice setting, and many hospices now utilize focus groups and reflective journaling with their dying patients (Schaefer & Curley, 2005).

Journaling is reported to have therapeutic benefits by allowing patients a way of making sense of dying in addition to having a strong sense of purpose in sharing their story. This was confirmed when Bingley et al. (2006), a team of English investigators, reviewed samples of narratives written since 1950 by people who were facing death from cancer and other diseases. The investigators' goal was to compare experiences and identify how these experiences relate to broad changes in practice in end-of-life care. The investigators conducted a bibliographic search of libraries, archives, journals, and Internet-based sources. They located English spoken literature, including books, poems, newspapers, journal articles, diaries, and Internet postings of writings by people facing terminal disease. They conducted bibliometric and qualitative content analysis that explored changing authorship, experiences, purpose in writing, and the impact on readers. They applied inclusion/exclusion criteria to the initial search that located a wide range of published and unpublished narratives, which yielded 148 narratives by different authors since 1950. They reviewed a subsample of 63 of these narratives. The investigators found that, over the last 56 years, there have been changes in both the volume of available literature and patterns of writing about the end-of-life experience. The results showed that patients have a clear awareness of social needs when dying. Patients also express issues of communication with medical staff, symptom control, realities of suffering, and spiritual aspects of dying (Bingley et al., 2006).

One component of journaling (or narrative therapy) has been well defined: It allows the patient to externalize problems. One study by Keeling and Bermudez (2006) examined an innovative externalization exercise that combined sculpture and journaling over a period of 4 weeks. Researchers studied the voices and experiences of 17 participants. The principal investigator also engaged in the exercise in an attempt to better understand the participants' experience. The findings were positive: The intervention helped participants express emotions, increase their awareness of personal resources and agency, separate problems from self-decreased symptoms and problem behaviors, and foster a sense of empowerment. This study reveals that physically externalizing problems and interacting with them deliberately over time have potential usefulness as a CAM therapy (Keeling & Bermudez, 2006).

References
Bingley, A. F., McDermott, E., Thomas, C., Payne, S., Seymour, J. E., & Clark, D. (2006). Making sense of dying: A review of narratives written since 1950 by people facing death from cancer and other diseases. *Palliative Medicine, 20*(3), 183–195.

Blake, T.K. (2005). Journaling: An active learning technique. *International Journal of Nursing Education Scholarship, 2,* 7.

Keeling, M. L., & Bermudez, M. (2006). Externalizing problems through art and writing: Experiences of process and helpfulness. *Journal of Marital and Family Therapy, 32*(4), 405–419.

Schaefer, K. M., & Curley, C. (2005). Use of focus groups and reflective journaling in a hospice experience. *Nurse Educator, 30*(3), 93–94.

An issue that may arise during both terminal weaning and terminal extubation is with the patient who is receiving neuromuscular blocking agents. An effort should be made to allow restoration of neuromuscular function before withdrawal of mechanical ventilation. Unfortunately, in some patients with multisystem organ failure, the clearance of the drug may become prolonged and restoration of full neuromuscular function could take days or weeks. Therefore, it may be morally justified to withdraw mechanical ventilation from a patient who is still experiencing the effects of residual blocking agents that were started prior to the decision to forgo life-sustaining measures. This decision must be balanced between the reasons to wait for restoration of neuromuscular function versus the added suffering of continued use of life-sustaining interventions.

Environment

When a patient is dying, it is important to create an environment that facilitates family presence. Discussions with family members regarding end-of-life decisions should not be held in a hallway or in the busy ICU. It is important to schedule a time and find a quiet place where family members can listen and feel comfortable asking questions. Once the decision is made for comfort care only, the patient care area should facilitate comfort for the patient and their family and friends. Rules regarding visiting hours and numbers of persons allowed in the room should be adjusted. Carney and Meier (2000, p. 204) describe a 10-step protocol for patients who are to be withdrawn from the ventilator:

1. Shut off and remove all monitors and alarms from the patient's room.
2. Remove equipment impeding access to hands. Hands are for holding.
3. Remove encumbering, disfiguring devices from the bedside.
4. Invite family to be with patient.
5. Quietly and personally request that vasopressors be turned off and that intravenous lines be set to keep open.
6. Watch for symptoms to develop and treat appropriately.
7. Turn FIO_2 down to 21% and observe patient for respiratory distress.
8. If patient and scene appear comfortable, remove endotracheal tube with clean towel in hand.
9. Educate and debrief house staff and nursing staff about process.
10. Consider contacting family during bereavement period whether by letter or visit.

The goal is to provide a peaceful, pain-free death for the patient and to create a supportive environment for the family.

Cultural Considerations

The manner in which individuals handle death is influenced by their culture, religion, family traditions, and individual preferences (Kuebler et al., 2007). When caring for a patient who is dying, it is important to discuss with the patient and family their cultural beliefs. Cultural practices bring security, integrity, and belonging to the individual. In some cultural groups, the family or a religious representative traditionally prepares the body af-

ter death (Andrews & Boyle, 2003). Most acute care facilities have a standardized procedure for preparation of the body following death. Family members, however, may view this as the facility performing a task that should be done by them. It is important to ask the family about their preferences and to facilitate any ritual that may be important to the patient and to them. Chart 17–1 (p. 402) discusses religious beliefs and traditions relating to end-of-life care.

In addition to religious beliefs, some cultures have specific customs with regard to end-of-life care. Cultural customs may come into play during communication with the patient and their family. Things to be aware of are conversational style and pace, eye contact, personal space, touch, and time orientation (Lipson & Dibble, 2007). The Cultural Considerations box (p. 404) lists known death rituals and communication customs for different cultures.

Grief

At the end of life, loss, grief, and bereavement can affect the family and members of the health care team. Part of the nurse's role at the end of life includes facilitating the grieving process. What is important to understand is that grief is a process an individual must experience to finally accept the reality of the loss (Bednash & Ferrell, 2002a). The grieving process includes a series of stages that the individual must move through to help resolve the grief. The process is not predictable, but fluid and unique to each individual.

There are several theories describing the stages of grief. The stages of grief described by Elizabeth Kubler-Ross are the most well known and are applied to those facing a death as well as those who have experienced a loss. Kubler-Ross identified five stages of grief: denial and isolation, anger, bargaining, depression, and acceptance. The loss of a loved one usually brings with it an intense grief response and may develop into a complicated grief response. Normal grief affects all aspects of a person's being—physical, emotional, cognitive, behavioral, and spiritual.

After a death, the bereaved person is at risk for new illness or worsening of an existing illness during the first year after the loss. Emotional acceptance takes time as the bereaved person feels the pain of the loss. Sadness may lessen at times but returns with reminders of the loved one, such as an anniversary or a photograph. Even if the death was expected at the time, cognitively it will still be a shock. The loss is so intense that the person can hardly believe that the patient is really dead. Behaviorally, the bereaved person gradually returns to daily functioning after the funeral or burial. Maladaptive behaviors may arise such as substance abuse. Spiritual beliefs will affect the way a person grieves. The patient may have held certain religious or cultural beliefs that prescribe certain acts and behaviors after death, but not all significant others may hold those beliefs.

Complicated or abnormal grief response may occur and arises from various internal and external factors. One of these factors is the bereaved person's relationship with the deceased before the death. If the bereaved person still holds unexpressed hostility toward the deceased, then that person is likely to feel anger and guilt, which inhibits the grief process. Chart 17–2 (p. 405) lists characteristics of complicated grief. Nursing care for significant others during end of life includes providing information with sensitivity to what significant others want to know,

CHART 17–1	Religion and End-of-Life Care

Religion	Beliefs	Traditions/Rituals
Christianity • Catholic • Orthodox • Protestant • Amish • Other	Christians believe that Jesus is the messiah.	**Catholic** • Anointing of the sick is done by a priest before the person's death. • Belief in preservation of life but not obligated to take extraordinary means. • Donation of organs is acceptable. • Funerals are generally held 2–3 days after death. **Orthodox** • Last anointing may be conducted before or after death. • Confession and holy communion are important rituals and are conducted by priests. • A memorial service is held on the closest Sunday to the 40th day after death. **Protestant** • There are no last rites. Prayers are given to offer comfort and support. • Some Pentecostal and neocharismatic churches believe in faith healing. **Amish** • Use of narcotic drugs is prohibited. • Prolongation of life and euthanasia are personal matters that may be discussed with the bishop and/or family members. • Autopsy is acceptable in the case of medical necessity or legal requirement. • Prefer to bury the body intact so generally do not donate organs. **Others** • Mormons will administer a sacrament if the patient requests. • Important to Mormons that death be peaceful and dignified. • Jehovah's Witnesses do not believe in sacraments. • Jehovah's Witnesses will be excommunicated if they receive a blood transfusion. • Jehovah's Witnesses do not believe in organ donation. • Christian Scientists rely mostly on spiritual healing. It is unlikely they will seek medical help to prolong life.

Islam	The founder of Islam, Mohammed, received a vision while meditating. This vision later became the Qur'an or Koran. *Allah* is the Arabic word for "God." A follower of Islam is called Moslem or Muslim.	• Second-degree male relatives (cousins or uncles) should be the contact person. They will determine whether the patient and/or family should be told about diagnoses, prognoses, etc.
		• Patients may choose to face Mecca (west or southwest in the United States). The head should be elevated above the body.
		• Discussions about death are not usually welcomed.
		• Stopping medical treatment is viewed as against Allah's will.
		• Grief may be expressed through slapping or hitting the body. Counseling is not well accepted.
		• It is important in Islam to follow prescribed burial procedures:
		  1. Washing of the dead body according to Muslim tradition. Muslim women cleanse a woman's body. Muslim men cleanse a man's body.
		  2. The body is washed three times and then wrapped in three pieces of clean white cloth.
		  3. Special prayers for the dead are required.
		  4. The body should be buried as soon as possible and should be positioned so that the head faces toward Mecca.
		  5. These burial practices are followed for fetuses after a gestational age of 130 days.

CHART 17–1	Religion and End-of-Life Care—*Continued*	

Religion	Beliefs	Traditions/Rituals
Judaism	The Sabbath is celebrated from sunset on Friday to sunset Saturday evening. Sabbath is a day of rest.	• No actions to hasten death are permitted but if a physician states that death is inevitable, no new therapeutic measures that would artificially extend life should be initiated. • A dying person should not be left alone. The exact time of death is noted for the purpose of honoring the deceased the first year after death. • Autopsy and cremation are forbidden. If an autopsy is required, it should be limited to essential organs or systems. All body parts must be returned for burial. • The funeral is usually held the day after death. The body is ritually washed and then clothed in a simple white burial shroud. Embalming and cosmetic treatment of the body are forbidden. • The family mourns for 7 days.
Hinduism	Hindus believe in multiple gods and goddesses, with one great spirit, Brahman. Karma is the working out in this life of events that occurred in a previous life. Reincarnation is a strong belief.	• Life is a perpetual cycle, so death is seen as just one more step toward nirvana. • Rituals include tying a thread around the neck or wrist of the dying person, sprinkling them with water from the Ganges River, or placing a leaf of basil on their tongue. • After death, do not remove sacred threads or wash the body.
Buddhism	The teachings of Buddha included the Four Noble Truths that expound on suffering: the truth of suffering, the truth of the origin of suffering, the truth that suffering can be destroyed, and the way that leads to the cessation of pain. The original teachings also included the Noble Eightfold Way: right views, right intention, right speech, right action, right livelihood, right effort, right mindfulness, and right concentration. Buddhism does not dictate any specific practices so individual differences can be expected and should be respected.	• Buddhist monks should be consulted to offer spiritual support. • A shrine to Buddha may be placed in the patient's room. • "Mindfulness" is an important state of being. Patients may refuse medications because they may alter alertness. • Buddhists generally accept death. • After death, a monk may recite prayers for 1 hour. The prayers need not be said in the presence of the body because it is considered but a shell. • Organ donation is encouraged. • Cremations are common.
Baha'i Faith	Belief is to know and worship God and carry forward an ever-advancing civilization. They believe that all the great religions of the world are divine in origin.	• Baha'is believe that life is unique and precious, so destruction of a human life is not permitted. When natural death has occurred, it is considered in the light of current medical science and legal rulings. • Baha'i law states that the body is not to be embalmed or cremated. • The place of burial must be within 1 hour's travel from the place of death; exceptions are possible.

Sources: Andrews, M., & Boyle, J. (2003). *Transcultural concepts in nursing care* (4th ed.). New York: Lippincott Williams & Wilkins; Bednash, G., & Ferrell, B. (2002a). Ethical and legal issues in end of life care. In *Continuing Education for Nurses* (pp. 21–65). Roseville, CA: CME Resource; Spector, R. (2009). *Cultural diversity in health and illness* (7th ed.). Upper Saddle River, NJ: Pearson Prentice Hall.

providing emotional support, suggesting appropriate referrals to mental health resources, recognizing abnormal grief reactions, and legitimizing the death (Saunders, 2007).

Interventions are designed to help an individual accept the reality of the loss. Interventions may include:

- Presence, active listening, touch
- Providing emotional support
- Encouraging verbalization
- Identifying support systems
- Normalizing the grief process and allowing for individual differences
- Identifying need for additional assistance and making referrals.

To be effective caregivers at end of life, nurses must come to terms with their own views on death and dying. As with patients and their families, nurses' comfort with death is affected by their personality, culture, spiritual belief system, and life experiences. Encouraging nurses to verbalize their feelings and express emotions will help them to process grief and loss and provide quality care at the end of life.

End-of-Life Care for Patients Who Are Terminally Ill

End-of-life care for patients who are terminally ill follows the same principles as those used for patients and families faced

CULTURAL CONSIDERATIONS Communication Customs and Death Rituals

American Indians	• Most embrace the present and avoid contact with the dying. If they feel comfortable being present, they will include immediate and extended family with children. The family will remain positive and even jovial because sadness and mourning are to be done in private. • Family may request spiritual healers. • Loud voice may be associated with aggression. Avoiding eye contact is respectful.
Cambodians	• The family may be quiet and passive. Monks and *aacha* are called to recite prayers, especially on the night of death. • It is inappropriate to touch their heads without permission. • They consider it impolite to disagree so they may say yes but not mean it. • Very important to speak softly and be polite. • After death, the family or monks may wash the body and then shroud it in a white cloth.
Central Americans • Guatemala • Nicaragua • El Salvador	• Spanish language is rich and full of intonations and meanings. It is important to closely observe body language. Loud, boisterous voices are acceptable. • Women are very modest around strangers. • Crosses, rosary beads, or figures of saints may be important. Female children may be protected by wearing red earrings because red is a strong color. Male babies may wear red knitted caps. Both may wear a little red bag (bolsita) of herbs around the neck to protect them from harm. Always check with parents before removing any red item. • If a young person dies it is believed to be a greater loss because of the unfulfilled life. • If the patient can be kept comfortable, they consider prolonged death a relief because it enables more relatives to say their good-byes. • The eldest male in the family should be informed of impending death. • Traditionally family members prepare the body for burial. Nurses should ask if the family wants to prepare the body for the mortuary. • They consider death a spiritual event, so family members need time to say good-bye to the deceased.
Chinese	• Eye contact with authority figures is avoided as a sign of respect. • Chinese language is expressive and loud. • Need to assess understanding of conversations because the patient or family may not ask questions as a sign of respect. • Privacy is very important. • Special amulets and cloths may be placed on the body.
Roma (Gypsies)	• Important to establish trust. • Very respectful of elder authority, therefore will have greater respect for older health care providers and dismiss younger team members. • Tone of voice is commonly loud and argumentative. • Very modest; they never ask personal questions in mixed company. • Moment of death is very significant because the feelings of the dying person at that moment give the family a sense of what will happen in the year after death. The last words of the dying patient are very important and the family will want to hear them.
Hmong	• Very polite and aware of disrespectful and prejudicial behavior. • Prolonged eye contact is considered disrespectful. • Communication may be indirect. Will not say "no" but may say "I will think about it." • Interpreters employed by the hospital are considered to be loyal to the institution and therefore not trusted. The family may request a bilingual family member be present during discussions. • Language structure is different; make sure the interpreter understands the intent of the discussion. The Hmong language has almost no medical terms. • Have great respect for authority. • Elders of the family will meet to make decisions regarding the patient's care. Immediate family members and female relatives may not have exclusive decision-making power. • Traditional beliefs say that at the time of death, the person goes to the next world in the same appearance. It is considered shameful to enter the next world poorly dressed or unclothed. If possible, allow the family to dress the patient in traditional clothing near the time of death. • Do not remove amulets from the dying patient's body.
Japanese	• May not ask questions, deferring to health care team to provide care. • Illness is not discussed outside of the family. • Soft voice is considered polite with direct conflict avoided. • Facial expressions are controlled and prolonged direct eye contact is considered disrespectful. • Promptness is very important. • Family and patient may avoid discussing illness or impending death. The decision not to resuscitate is a difficult one and is decided by the entire family. • Cleanliness of body is important, as is modesty and preservation of dignity.

CULTURAL CONSIDERATIONS Communication Customs and Death Rituals—*Continued*

Mexicans	• Direct eye contact with authority figures is avoided. • Silence may show lack of agreement with the plan of care. • Touching by a stranger is considered disrespectful although therapeutic touch is an integral part of traditional healing. • Family may hang spiritual amulets, religious medallions, or rosary beads near the patient. • After the patient dies, the family will request some time to say good-bye.
Russians	• Direct eye contact is used. • Respectful of elders. • Tone of voice may be loud. • Family members decide whether patients should be told about their condition and prognosis to not burden them. • Tend to use DNR orders for an elderly patient to allow him or her to die comfortably and not on life support. • After death the body is respected and considered sacred.
Asians and Africans • India • Pakistan • Bangladesh • Sri Lanka • Nepal • Fiji • East Africa	• Touching not common; caring is expressed through the eyes. • Prolonged direct eye contact is considered rude. • Modesty, humility, tolerance, and silence are emphasized. • Tone of voice should be soft. Loudness is considered disrespectful. • Family decides whether the patient should be told about his or her condition and prognosis. • Family members will want to be at the bedside at the time of death. Grief will be expressed openly.
Vietnamese	• Head may be considered sacred and feet profane; do not touch the feet and then the head. • Avoiding eye contact is a sign of respect. • Using both hands when giving a person something shows respect. • Tone of voice should be soft. • A loud voice or pointing of the finger is a sign of disrespect. • Family may want to wash the body themselves as the body is highly respected.

Source: Adapted from Lipson, J., & Dibble, S. (Eds.). (2005). *Culture and clinical care.* San Francisco: UCSF Nursing Press.

CHART 17–2 Characteristics of Complicated Grief

Complicated Grief Type	Characteristics
Exaggerated	• Response is out of proportion. • Response is more intense than expected. • The person is disabled with clinical depression or other psychiatric disorders.
Masked	• Feelings are expressed as physical symptoms. • Feelings are expressed as maladaptive behavior. • Feelings are not expressed at all. • The person may not realize that symptoms or behaviors are related to the loss.
Delayed	• Feelings may not arise until another person is lost. • Feelings surrounding the loss are not expressed until the person suffers another loss.
Chronic	• The person never reaches resolution with regard to the loss. • The reaction to the loss is unusually long.

Source: Adapted from Saunders, C. A. (Ed.). (2007). *End of life: A nurse's guide to compassionate care.* Philadelphia: Lippincott Williams & Wilkins, page 235.

with an unexpected death. The main difference is that the patient with a terminal illness has the opportunity to participate in the planning for his death.

Hospice

Hospice is the provision of care at the end of life aimed at comfort instead of cure. It is based on a model that is interdisciplinary and tailored to meet the values and goals of the patient and family. The care is aimed at relieving physical, psychosocial, and spiritual suffering for the patient and to facilitate the grieving and coping strategies of families and caregivers.

Death is an inevitable aspect of the human condition; dying badly is not. (Jennings, Ryndes, D'Onofrio, & Baily, 2003). As the aging of the population continues, more and more individuals will face decisions regarding their end-of-life care. The challenge of end-of-life care will grow during the next three decades because the population of seniors in the United States is projected to more than double during the next 30 years, rising from 34 million in 1997 to more than 69 million by 2030. Despite significant advances in preventive care and treatment modalities that prolong health and life, all but those who die suddenly and unexpectedly will have to make decisions about serious or life-threatening illness.

The History of Hospice

The root word *hospitality* led to the term *hospice*. As far back as medieval times, it originally meant a place for travelers to rest. The first modern hospice established to care for dying patients was founded by Dame Cicely Saunders in 1967 in London. Soon she was lecturing at Yale to medical students and nurses regarding hospice care. This heralded the start of the modern hospice movement.

In 1969, Elizabeth Kubler-Ross published her book *On Death and Dying*, which describes the phases of the dying process and pioneered the concepts of patient choice and self-direction. In 1972 she testified at Senate hearings on aging, which led to an unsuccessful attempt to establish legislation for federal funding of hospice care. In 1979, the Healthcare Financing Administration authorized 26 hospice demonstration projects across America. In 1980, the W. K. Kellogg Foundation awarded a grant to the Joint Commission to develop hospice standards. In 1986 Congress enacted the Medicare Hospice Benefit, which established a reimbursement mechanism for Medicare-eligible beneficiaries. Over the years, Congress has granted several increases and has recommended the incorporation of hospice care into the care of military veterans and Native Americans.

Terminology

Nurses need to have a clear understanding of hospice care, beginning with the customary terminology used. Nurses play a crucial role in assisting patients and families in increasing their knowledge of hospice care and dispelling myths and fears. Hospice care focuses on comfort care versus curative care. An interdisciplinary team of health care providers including physicians, nurses, social workers, spiritual counselors, dieticians, home health aides, and volunteers provides hospice. The care plan encompasses both the patient and family/caregiver as the unit of care, and the care plan is individualized to meet their values and goals. Patients receiving hospice care are generally defined as those patients who have a prognosis of 6 months or less if their terminal disease runs a normal course.

One of the core operating principles of hospice is the ongoing collaboration of the interdisciplinary team to ensure holistic, comprehensive care to meet not only physical needs but psychosocial and spiritual needs. Hospice care is provided to the patient in various settings, although most often this is the patient's home or living facility. According to the National Hospice and Palliative Care Organization (NHPCO, 2006), in 2004, 95.8% of the days of hospice services provided by the nation's hospices were at the home care level. Hospice care is also provided in the inpatient setting. In fact, many hospice programs have dedicated beds or inpatient units to provide hospice care. Inpatient care is generally provided for management of symptoms and periods of caregiver crisis. NHPCO states that, in 2004, 3% of hospice care was provided in an inpatient setting.

Hospices also provide respite care. Respite is care given to a hospice patient by another caregiver so the usual caregiver can rest. Respite care is provided in a hospice facility, hospital, or a skilled nursing facility. Hospices may also provide short-term continuous nursing care in a patient's home to prevent a hospitalization during a period of medical crisis. This allows patients to remain in the comfort of their own home and attain symptom control.

Hospice care also encompasses bereavement services after the death of the patient. These services are available for a minimum of 1 year after the death of the patient and provide support for families and caregivers during the grieving process. Bereavement is provided by telephone and in person, and on an individual or group basis. Most hospice programs also have groups that are available to the community to deal with grief and coping issues.

The term *palliative care* has risen to the forefront in recent years. The World Health Organization's (WHO's) definition of palliative care makes it virtually identical with hospice: "Palliative care is an approach that improves the quality of life of patients and their families facing the problem associated with life-threatening illness, through the prevention and relief of suffering by means of early identification and impeccable assessment and treatment of pain and other problems, physical, psychosocial and spiritual" (2006). From another perspective, however, the two terms are often taken to refer to different caregiving orientations, time frames, and institutional settings. WHO's definition goes on to add "Many aspects of palliative care are also applicable earlier in the course of the illness, in conjunction with anti-cancer treatment." From a medical perspective, then, palliative care may be taken as the broader term, covering all forms of the prevention and treatment of suffering (Jennings et al., 2003).

The concept of comfort care versus curative care is important for nurses who are caring for patients with cancer to fully understand. Comfort care is aimed at improving the quality of life, not necessarily aimed at prolonging the quantity of life. Effective symptom relief may not only improve the quality of life but occasionally will demonstrate some secondary gain in quantity of life. The key to understanding comfort care versus curative care is to ask "What is the primary intent of the treatment intervention?" There are instances where modalities such as chemotherapy and radiation are curative in nature. For example, providing radiotherapy to decrease tumor size may result in less pain. This is different than choosing these therapies in the setting of a more aggressive approach, with the goal being cure.

Most people will progress through the dying process in much the same way that they lived, with a set of values and beliefs that are important to them. The very decision to choose hospice care is rooted in these values and beliefs. For some individuals the concept of hospice means "giving up" and may be in conflict with their core belief system. For those patients who choose hospice, the hospice team individualizes the care plan in collaboration with the patient and family to be sure that the hospice care provided is what they desire. This individualized values-based care allows patients to maintain their independence and have their personal values and preferences respected as they are dying. The majority of Americans have an affinity for as much independence in their lives as possible, even during their final days. Nurses play a pivotal role in providing patients and their families with information about what is happening to them and what options are available to them (Kuebler et al., 2007).

Interdisciplinary care involves interdisciplinary teamwork, which is a hallmark of hospice care. Utilizing the knowledge and expertise of physicians, nurses, social workers, spiritual counselors, dietitians, aides and volunteers, the care is designed to be comprehensive and constantly updated to meet the patient and family needs. Team meetings should be held at regular intervals to discuss all aspects of a patient's care including symptom management, patient and family psychosocial needs, spiritual needs, and the ability to maintain or receive assistance in activities of daily living. All members of the team bring their individual perspectives to the care and have input into care decisions.

Suffering is unrelieved physical, psychological, or spiritual distress. Hospice recognizes the interdependence of all of these factors and relieving these is critical in truly achieving a "good death." An example of *relief of suffering* is resolving psychological or spiritual needs that may be impeding the success of pharmacologic pain control measures. Suffering can also be existential in nature. Existential suffering differs from physical, psychosocial, or spiritual symptoms that may respond to intervention. Existential suffering includes hopelessness, disappointment, remorse, death anxiety, disruption of personal identity, and the meaninglessness of continued life. The goal of hospice is to address all of these needs in an integrated and holistic manner.

Payer Sources

In the United States, hospice care provided at home for patients over the age of 65 or for patients who have been disabled for more than 2 years is covered through Medicare. Most private insurance and health maintenance organizations provide hospice benefits. Hospice care covers physician services, nursing services, social work counseling, dietary instruction, aides and homemakers, volunteers, medical equipment, and drugs prescribed for the terminal illness. Additionally, hospice programs also receive donated funds, most often in memory of one of their patients who has died. These funds may be used to care for patients who do not have medical coverage for hospice care.

Medicare is the largest payer source in America for hospice care. In 1982 the Hospice Benefit was created as part of Medicare. To be eligible for Medicare hospice care, the patient must have Medicare Part A, and the attending physician and the hospice medical director must certify that the patient has a prognosis of 6 months or less if the disease runs its normal course. Patients are reevaluated on an ongoing basis and at intervals defined by Medicare for continued appropriateness for hospice. If the patient's disease does not progress and the patient's condition stabilizes, the patient may be taken off the hospice benefit. Likewise, if a patient changes her mind and wishes to pursue aggressive therapy, the patient may revoke the hospice benefit. However, the patient, in either of these two scenarios, can return to the hospice benefit if disease progression returns and the physician certifies that the patient has a 6-month prognosis. Despite the payer source, most hospice programs model their care under the federal regulations for participation in the Medicare Hospice Program, entitled the Medicare Conditions of Participation.

Access to Hospice Care

NHPCO (2006) estimates that in the year 2004, approximately 3,650 established hospice programs served 1,060,000 patients. Hospice care is provided to patients of all ages; however, the majority of care is provided to those 65 years of age or older.

Hospice care has expanded over the years to include serving patients other than those with cancer diagnoses. Hospices are now caring for patients with other life-threatening, chronic illnesses such as heart disease, respiratory disease, and HIV/AIDS. In 2006, NHPCO reported that in 2004, 46% of hospice patients had a cancer diagnosis. NHPCO reports the top five noncancer causes of death in hospice patients in 2004 as follows: 12.2%, end-stage cardiac disease; 8.9%, dementia; 8.2%, debility; 7.1%, lung disease; and 3.1%, end-stage kidney disease.

Barriers to Hospice Care

With only one in four Americans receiving hospice care at the time of death, it is clear that barriers to hospice care exist. By the year 2030, 20% of Americans will be age 65 or older. One in nine baby boomers is expected to live to age 90, and by 2040, the number of Americans over age 85 will be nearly four times greater than today. The United States already struggles to provide basic primary care to its population; more than 40 million Americans are without consistent, adequate health insurance coverage. Geography plays a significant role in preventing access to services provided by hospice. Patients in inner city, rural, and remote inaccessible areas are likely to be underserved (Jennings et al., 2003).

Physician reluctance to refer to hospice has remained a barrier. Patients depend on their physicians for health care information and guidance; however, many individuals are never introduced to the concept of hospice care by their physicians or health care providers. In a recent study, a significant subgroup of physicians had reservations about the physician being the most appropriate person to introduce the concept of hospice to the patient and was also concerned that discussion of hospice would lead to a sense of hopelessness (Ogle, Mavis, & Wang, 2003).

Information technology has heightened the awareness of patients and their families to promising new treatments and disease-fighting drugs. Consumers are enticed by the media and the Internet to investigate the use of these modalities without much discussion of the associated burden or risk. Patients and families often do not want to hear about hospice, but rather want to avail themselves of every option. Some feel that the regulatory and policy issues represent a barrier to hospice care. As technological options increase for consumers, it is hoped that regulations regarding the requirement that the patient forgo curative treatment will be reevaluated. The ability to expand the types of hospice care provided would benefit patients and families and promote receiving hospice services earlier in their illness.

Nurses will no doubt experience the challenge of end-of-life care more significantly during the next three decades. The lack of available qualified nurses is impacting the ability to provide hospice care in some hospices. The challenge of the shortage will be multiplied by the projected aging of the population.

With the tendency of Americans to deny their mortality, along with physician reluctance and access to increased information regarding new treatments, patients and families are either not referred to or refuse hospice services until very late in their disease course. NHPCO (2006) states the average length of service in 2002 was 51 days, and the median length of stay was 26 days. These short stays do not allow the hospice team to maximize symptom control, to provide psychological and spiritual support, and to begin work on anticipatory grieving. The crucial development of a trusting therapeutic relationship between the patient/family and the hospice team is difficult to achieve in such a limited amount of time.

Diversity

Culture is not the same as race. Culture includes traditions, customs, religious beliefs, and attitudes that occur at a variable pace (Lipson & Dibble, 2007). Language and immigration history also influence cultures. Hospice must work within the culture of each patient and family unit. The hospice team must seek input from the patient and family to develop a plan that is realistic and not in opposition to strongly held cultural beliefs. The Cultural Considerations box (p. 404) discusses details of end-of-life care as it relates to cultural variations.

NHPCO (2006) reports that in 2004, 77.3% of all hospice patients identified themselves as white or Caucasian, 8.1% as black or African American, 6.2% as Hispanic or Latino, 6.4% as multiracial, and 1.7% as Asian or Pacific Islander. The results of a recent study (Colon & Lyke, 2003) indicate that there are significant differences between ethnic groups who use hospice care. Most importantly, the study also determined that African Americans and Latinos are clearly underusing hospice services relevant to their prevalence in the general population.

Identified differences between ethnic groups include age, cultural adaptation, high-risk behaviors, caregivers, and payment method. Hospice programs need to focus on increasing awareness of services within minority communities as well as making the treatment itself more culturally sensitive.

Sexual diversity applies to groups such as lesbians, gays, bisexuals, and transgendered individuals. These groups require special consideration in hospice care due to the fact that, despite advances, social stigmas still exist within certain groups and locales. This may discourage access to hospice care, especially if the terminal illness is associated with lifestyle choices.

The Role of Nursing in Hospice

The professional nurse plays a number of key roles in hospice care. The nurse is critical in not only directing the provision of high-quality, competent care, but also in promoting the hospice concept and advocating for patients and families. Most hospice programs identify the registered nurse as the case manager for a panel of hospice patients. The nurse is accountable for the interdisciplinary collaboration and oversight of the care of the patient and family.

The nurse can play a role in influencing physicians and other health care providers to consider the hospice option for their patients. The nurse can provide knowledge and information, correct myths, and influence the effort for earlier referrals to hospice. The nurse also plays a key role in the education of patients and families about hospice, exploring their concerns and fears, and assisting them in navigating the numerous care options. The nurse is always the patient advocate, ensuring that whatever course is chosen is in alignment with the patient's and family members' values and goals, done with their full knowledge about the options, and the implications of their choices.

Hospice programs have grown tremendously during the past 10 years. NHPCO (2006) reports that in 1992 there were 1,935 hospice programs, growing to 3,650 in 2004. More patients and families are choosing hospice care, up from 246,000 in 1992 to 1,060,000 in 2004. Despite this growth there are challenges. Access issues and barriers to care continue. Hospices are faced with an increasingly diverse population. Physician willingness to refer remains an issue. These challenges exist in a health care system faced with an increasing number of aged Americans, the issues of payer reimbursement, and complex regulations from payers, government agencies, and accrediting organizations. However, there is reason to be optimistic. The hospice movement and the palliative care movements can exist in collaboration to improve

the overall quality of end-of-life care. Structured end-of-life education is being provided to physicians during training and later as continuing education. Education in end-of-life care is being presented to nurses, and increasing numbers of hospice nurses are receiving certification in the specialty of hospice and palliative care. Professional organizations such as NHPCO and state hospice organizations are advocating legislative reforms to increase access to hospice programs, decrease barriers especially with regard to eligibility, and promote increasing the lengths of stay in hospice programs. To provide the impetus for policy and practice changes that will increase access to hospice care, hospice must be re-envisioned as a concept of health care—a new way of thinking about the nature and goals of health care itself, rather than an end-stage form of care (Jennings et al., 2003).

Palliative Care

Palliative care is a relatively new field in nursing. Nurses have traditionally contributed their resources to a health care system that has focused primarily on attempts at curing diseases. Yet, many diseases are incurable including congestive heart failure (CHF), chronic obstructive pulmonary disease (COPD), some cancers, stroke, and dementias, to name a few. Modern medicine continues to overtreat by attempting to cure when cure is no longer possible. Perhaps it is more appropriate to treat death as a natural process rather than an enemy, particularly when the patient's end of life is near.

Palliative care nurses serve patients with incurable illnesses, and their family members, by assisting in the management of their multifaceted symptoms, ultimately enabling them to live within the confines of their illnesses. Traditional disease-centered focus should be aligned with the caring model of nursing, one that focuses on the whole patient, embracing a model that includes the art of caring for ill patients, as well as the science.

Palliative care was recognized as its own field of medicine in 1987, with its roots stemming from hospice, being viewed as active care versus total care (Kuebler et al., 2007). In 1990 the WHO introduced their definition of palliative care as "the active total care of a patient whose disease is manageable but not curable." This includes interventions that:

1. Affirm life and regard dying as a normal process.
2. Neither hasten nor postpone death.
3. Provide relief from pain and other distressing symptoms.
4. Integrate the psychological and spiritual aspects of patient care.
5. Offer a support system to help patients live as actively as possible until death.
6. Offer a support system to help the family cope during the patient's illness and in their own bereavement.

Nurses should be familiar with how palliative care emerged and the types of programs and activities available to patients and their families. It is also important to recognize the barriers those providing palliative care face.

Emergence of Palliative Care

There is a rapidly growing nation movement to improve end-of-life education and the delivery of palliative care. Forces behind the motivation to change have been changes in the delivery of health care in the last century, results of research studies, and the development of programs and projects by renowned organizations.

Changes in the last century in medical science have led to unparalleled progress in the effective treatment of disease, which has, for many, led to prolonged periods of illness, decline, and suffering. Chart 17–3 compares care in the early 20th century to care early in the 21st century, which has been changed tremendously by the advances of modern medicine.

Most people die in the hospital, although surveys indicate that more than 70% of people would prefer to die at home (Solloway, Lafrance, Bakitas, & Gerken, 2005). In a chart review of 782 deaths in hospitals, nursing homes, and hospice/home care in one state, significant differences were found among symptom assessment and provision of emotional and spiritual support for patients and families. Within the hospitals, 56% of deaths were in acute care beds, 30% were in ICUs, and only 4% were in palliative care beds. Nineteen percent of decedents received interventions such as being placed on a ventilator or surgery in the 48 hours preceding death. More than 80% had a do-not-resuscitate (DNR) order, 45% had a DPAHC, and 37% had a living will. Age and setting were significant factors in the presence of advance directives (Solloway et al., 2005). How unfortunate that many Americans die after suffering miserably. Fear of the dying process is a very real emotion for many adults. Many fear the care they will receive during and before end of life, the loss of control they will experience, being attached to machines, dying away from home, and being separated from loved ones.

End-of-life education for health care professionals has been scarce at best. Both medical schools and residency programs devote inadequate efforts to end-of-life care instruction (McPhee, Rabow, Pantilat, Markowitz, & Winker, 2000). Up until recently, nursing textbooks devoted only 2% of the total content to end-of-life care. However, much of the information was found to be inaccurate (Ferrell & Coyle, 2002).

Several organizations are aspiring to better the end-of-life care provided around the country. They are committed to the vision of ensuring a "good death" for patients and their families, where the period prior to death is dignified and comfortable. Included are the Last Acts Campaign of the Robert Wood Johnson (RWJ) Foundation, the Education for Physicians on End of Life Care of the American Medical Association, the Center to Advance Palliative Care, and Americans for Better Care of the Dying. Also, of special mention, are the hospice programs that improve the quality of life for those who are dying and their families (Ditillo, 2002).

The End-of-Life Nursing Education Consortium of the American Association of Colleges of Nursing and the City of Hope National Medical Center is a program funded by the RWJ foundation. It is a 3-day course designed to train nurses who provide continuing education courses and equip them with the resources to integrate end-of-life care into their courses. Renowned researchers, educators, authors, and leaders facilitate the training in the specialty of palliative care. Modules include nursing care at the end of life, pain and other symptom management, cultural issues, ethical/legal considerations, communication, bereavement, and care and preparation for death.

Provision of Palliative Care

As the specialty of palliative care is emerging, so is the evolution of the provision of care. Types of programs are varied, yet many of the activities are common. And, as with all programs, come the inevitable barriers to providing effective care.

Determining the type of palliative care program that would be most effective is very challenging. Many elements need to be considered, and range from selecting the patient population to funding reimbursement. Palliative care units and services can be useful approaches to caring for people who are terminally ill, and include those patients who are chronically ill and may live for years in their disease state.

A palliative care service may include either inpatient and/or outpatient consultations, ranging from comprehensive case management or care coordination to a one-time visit. Types of patients to be seen may include those with chronic illnesses that are incurable and decline over time, such as CHF, COPD, dementia, cancers, and strokes. No single health care provider can successfully meet all of the palliative care needs of patients who have incurable illnesses and the needs of their families. The interdisciplinary team approach is essential because it is comprised of a variety of disciplines that pool their data to reach a consensus about goal setting, and the development of a comprehensive plan of care. Team members may include, but are not limited to, physicians, nurses, social workers, and chaplains. Other ancillary support may be needed depending on the needs of the patient, and include experts in the fields of mental health, physical therapy, nutrition, pharmacy, respiratory therapy, and ethics.

Nurses working in a palliative care program should understand that targeted interventions are common regardless of the program design, and include pain and symptom management, end-of-life care planning, and support that encompasses psychosocial and spiritual needs. The National Guidelines box (p. 410) discusses standards and guidelines for palliative care.

Symptoms will vary according to the disease state and should be monitored and controlled regardless of the proximity to end of life. For patients close to the end of life, symptoms experienced are often distressing and include pain, dyspnea, nausea, constipation, anxiety, restlessness, delirium, fatigue, dehydration, and "death rattles." Palliative care nurses play a pivotal role in accurately assessing, reporting, and ensuring that symptoms are appropriately managed. A patient's quality of life is contingent on an astute, competent nurse who has received thorough education in pain and symptom management and is assertive

CHART 17–3	Effects of Changes in Care: Now and Then	
	1900	**2000**
Average age at death	46 years	78 years
Cause of death	• Infection	• Cancer
	• Accidents	• Heart disease
	• Childbearing	• Stroke
		• Dementias
Location where death occurred	• Home	• Hospital
Prevalence of disability	• Rare	• Average 4 years

NATIONAL GUIDELINES for Quality Palliative Care

In 2002, the Hospice and Palliative Nurses Association and the American Nurses Association developed the *Scope and Standards of Hospice and Palliative Nursing Practice*. Part of the standards follow the nursing process (Saunders, 2007):

Assessment	Collect Patient and Family Data
Diagnosis	Analyze the assessment data and develop diagnoses using an accepted framework that supports hospice and palliative nursing knowledge.
Outcomes	In partnership with a multidisciplinary team, identify expected outcomes relevant to the patient and family.
Planning	In partnership with the patient, family, and multidisciplinary team, develop a plan of care that includes interventions and treatments to attain expected outcomes.
Implementation	Implement the plan of care.
Evaluation	Evaluate the patient's and family's progress in attaining the expected outcomes.

In 2004, the National Consensus Project for Quality Palliative Care, the Center to Advance Palliative Care, and the Last Acts Partnership created the *Clinical Practice Guidelines for Quality Palliative Care* (National Consensus Project for Quality Palliative Care, 2004). More than 100 experts contributed to the evidence-based guidelines. The framework for the clinical practice guidelines include:

- Structure and processes of care
- Physical aspects of care
- Psychological and psychiatric aspects of care
- Social aspects of care
- Spiritual, religious, and existential aspects of care
- Cultural aspects of care
- Care of the imminently dying patient
- Ethical and legal aspects of care.

Source: National Consensus Project for Quality Palliative Care (2004). Clinical practice guidelines for quality palliative care. http://www.nationalconsensusproject.org

enough to advocate for patients in an environment where the proper use of analgesics and adjunct medications may not be understood. Doses often need to be titrated and tailored to a level particular to the individual. Nurses need to recognize that many health care providers lack the expertise to appropriately manage the common and complex symptoms that occur at or near death.

Another key function of the palliative care team is to assist the patient who has an incurable illness to develop a plan of care prior to advancement of his disease process. The plan should be rational and customized to the individualized patient's goals and values. This can be accomplished in an interdisciplinary team setting and should include the patient and key people in his life. A systematic or methodical approach may be very beneficial. It would include a discussion regarding what the patient knows or wants to know about his disease state, and whether or not he is ready to engage in this type of discussion. The provider may then educate the patient regarding the potential trajectory of the illness, and the risk, benefit, and burden measure of each treatment option. Next, the patient would be assisted to set goals of care based on the individual's values.

Remember that any expression of a patient's wishes should be considered valid and binding, whether it is written or oral. Even though it is beneficial for potential agents to witness the patient's statements about what may or may not give meaning and value to one's life, a formal written document signed by the patient helps to avoid ambiguity. The patient should choose a health care agent whom she trusts and is confident would carry out previously discussed wishes, in the event that she cannot speak for herself. The document should be readily available when decisions need to be made. Statute requirements for the state where the patient resides can be determined by contacting the local hospital, state attorney general's office, public health office, local medical society, or state board of nursing.

Paramount to providing good palliative care is the ability of the provider to be absolutely honest with the patient. The concept of truth-telling urges practitioners to overcome the tendency to avoid accurate disclosure when talking to dying patients so they may begin planning for their end-of-life journey (Saunders, 2007). When a curative model of care is offered to a dying patient, it becomes more difficult to allow discussions that are completely truthful in nature. Nurses build relationships with dying patients that allow for discussions centered on shifting the focus of care from curative to more of a palliative model. Staying focused on a curative model fosters false hope and may rob a patient of intimacy and closure at the end of life.

To be effective in providing palliative care for those with terminal illnesses, providers need to be tuned in to the various psychosocial needs of the patient and family. Nurses need to be able to recognize grief and assist with the appropriate interventions to cope, whether that is by nursing actions or consultation with the palliative care team for appropriate referral to psychiatrists, grief counselors, social services, or spiritual counselors. Patients facing incurable and life-threatening illnesses experience losses of function, control, independence, body image, dignity, and of a future.

Spirituality is an inherent and pervasive dimension for persons, particularly those faced with the closure of their lives. Effective palliative care nurses must become comfortable and competent in performing a spiritual assessment. When the nurse queries a patient about spiritual issues, the patient is assisted to reflect on his own humanity. In doing so, the nurse is offering support for patients who naturally grapple with spiritual issues surrounding illness and impending end of life. Last, it is an opportunity for the nurse to be present and witness the sacredness of this life event. Nurses who assist patients may find this involvement in the intimate stories of patients' lives to be an honor, a gift, and a tremendous opportunity for growth as a person.

Barriers to the provision of palliative care are multifaceted. Financial reimbursement to fund palliative care programs is a challenge. Providers have a fear of prescribing controlled substances due to the regulation of narcotics and other medications. There is a general lack of understanding of the services offered by a palliative care team. Providers must overcome the natural tendency to participate in the conspiracy to withhold the facts about prognoses for fear of erasing the patient's hope.

The health care system has the unique opportunity to improve on the services provided to those who are facing chronic, terminal, incurable illnesses. Palliative care programs will no doubt develop and evolve over time, basing changes on the experiences of current-day programs.

Palliative care nurses have been given the honor of assisting patients and their families through a momentous time by alleviating suffering, both physically and emotionally. Caring for those who are preparing the closure of their life provides nurses with a unique challenge—that of being put at a vantage point where one comes face to face with the obviousness of one's own human mortality. In turn, this perspective provides an opportunity to look at the great gift of life, how one might choose to appreciate it and live it well, and how nurses can make an everlasting difference in the death of one and the lives of the remaining.

 # Nursing Management

Variation in the delivery of care to patients is a leading cause of inadequate care. The number of patients who have died in the ICU following a decision to withdraw life support or limit therapy is increasing. Even so, evidence indicates that patients and families are dissatisfied with the care given during end of life (Heyland et al., 2006; Teno et al., 2004). Educating health care professionals in end-of-life care is an important aspect of improving their ability to properly care for dying patients and their families. The goal is to add life to the patient's time, not simply time to the patient's life. A detailed patient care plan for end-of-life care is provided in the Nursing Process box.

 # Collaborative Management

Achievement of a pain-free and meaningful death experience for the patient and family requires a multidisciplinary approach. The nurse is in a pivotal role to bring together the members of

---

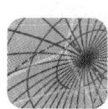

NURSING PROCESS: Patient Care Plan for End-of-Life Care

Assessment of Therapeutic Regimen

Subjective Data:
Are all members of the health care team clear on the plan of care and goals and expected outcomes?
What did the doctor tell you about your family member's prognosis?
Do you know your family member's resuscitation wishes and are you in agreement?
Is there a written advance directive?

Objective Data:
Family and significant others are calm and do not appear surprised by treatment regimen.

Nursing Assessment and Diagnoses	Outcomes and Evaluation Parameters	Planning and Interventions with *Rationales*
Nursing Diagnosis: *Ineffective Therapeutic Regimen Management* related to the acceleration (expected or unexpected) of illness symptoms	**Outcome:** The health care team has a clear understanding of the plan of care. *Evaluation Parameters:* All members of the health care team express understanding regarding: Disease process Rationale for treatment regimen Expectations of regimen Methods to monitor condition Signs or symptoms of complications Honoring the patient's wishes. **Outcome:** The patient and/or family verbalize understanding of the seriousness of the patient's preferences and prognosis. *Evaluation Parameters:* The patient and/or family will verbalize an understanding of the seriousness of the patient's condition. The patient and/or family will be able to verbalize patient's preferences for quality-of-life issues.	**Interventions and *Rationales*:** Request a multidisciplinary meeting with the health care team *to identify concerns and clarify goals and expected outcomes for the patient.* Facilitate multidisciplinary family conference. Be respectful of cultural conversational norms. Listen to identify concerns. Attempt to match expressed needs with services the nurse can provide or facilitate. Demonstrate honesty, consistency, and stability. Maintain preestablished contacts in person or by phone. *To build trust and strength.* Discuss with patient and/or family their understanding of the prognosis; perception of seriousness; perceived level of anxiety; support system; emotional status; and cognitive ability *to identify factors that influence understanding.* Solicit expressions of feelings and questions. Identify if any advance directives were done and/or who will be responsible for care decisions. Encourage patient and family to seek information and make informed decisions. *To promote active participation of the patient and family.*

(continued)

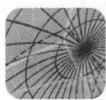

NURSING PROCESS: Patient Care Plan for End-of-Life Care—*Continued*

Assessment of Grieving

Subjective Data:
What is your past experience with loss?
Do you have a support system?
Are there any cultural or religious practices that I can assist you with?

Objective Data:
Observe family interaction with staff and significant others.
Observe the family members' comfort level while in the patient room.
Observe family's ability to cope with the situation.

Nursing Assessment and Diagnoses	Outcomes and Evaluation Parameters	Planning and Interventions with *Rationales*
Nursing Diagnosis: *Grieving*	**Outcome:** Patient/family will demonstrate the ability to make mutual decisions regarding the anticipated death. ***Evaluation Parameters:*** Expresses thoughts, feelings, and spiritual beliefs about the loss. Verbalizes fears/concerns regarding the impending death. Exhibits no somatic distress.	**Interventions and *Rationales:*** When assisting with family discussions, use clear words, such as *death* or *died*, rather than euphemisms. Assist patient/family to verbalize fears/concerns regarding impending loss, including impact on the family unit. *To assist the patient/family to share mutual fears, plans, and concerns with each other.* Teach the patient/family about the normal events of the dying process. Encourage patient/family to implement cultural, religious, and social customs associated with death. Teach the patient/family characteristics of normal and abnormal grieving. *To help the patient and family move through the grieving process.* Arrange equipment and furniture in the patient's room to facilitate family presence and interaction with the patient. Remove as much monitoring equipment and intravenous lines from the patient as possible. Facilitate privacy for the family. Facilitate cultural/religious rituals. *To provide a peaceful, pain-free death for the patient and to create a supportive environment for the family.* Refer to appropriate resources: support groups, legal assistance, financial assistance, social services, and chaplain. *To assist the patient and family with putting the patient's legal affairs in order and to create an environment for emotional closure.*

Assessment of Pain

Subjective Data:
On a scale of 1–10 with one being a little pain and 10 being the worst pain you have ever felt, at what level is your pain?
Do you routinely take pain medication at home? If yes, what is the name of the medication and why do you take it?
Are you allergic to any medications?

Objective Data:
Monitor:
Facial grimacing
Change in breathing pattern
Change in blood pressure and/or pulse rate
Diaphoresis
Agitation

Nursing Assessment and Diagnoses	Outcomes and Evaluation Parameters	Planning and Interventions with *Rationales*
Nursing Diagnosis: *Pain*	**Outcome:** Pain level will be tolerable and the patient will not suffer. ***Evaluation Parameters:*** Patient will not exhibit symptoms of pain or suffering.	**Interventions and *Rationales:*** *Nonpharmacologic:* Reduce lighting and noise, eliminate unnecessary monitors and machines, remove restraints, and provide room for the patient's significant others. Cultural and spiritual factors such as prayer, ritual, and music can also increase the patient's comfort. *Promotes relaxation and comfort.* *Pharmacologic:* Morphine drip: titrate for symptom relief. At end of life, there is no recommended maximal dose. *Titration is intended to relieve pain and suffering.* Benzodiazepines: Midazolam drip: starting dose for adult continuous infusion: 1–5 mg/hr. Titrate for symptom relief. Lorazepam drip: starting dose for adult continuous infusion: 1–8 mg/hr. Titrate for symptom relief. *Benzodiazepines have a synergistic sedative effect with opioids, are anticonvulsants, and may help prevent the development of premorbid seizures.*

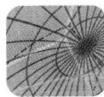

NURSING PROCESS: Patient Care Plan for End-of-Life Care—*Continued*

Assessment of Respiratory Distress

Subjective Data:
If patient is responsive ask if he/she is feeling short of breath.

Objective Data:
Observe nonintubated patient for:
Tachypnea
Restlessness

Accessory muscle use
Grunting at the end of each breath
Nasal flaring

Nursing Assessment and Diagnoses	Outcomes and Evaluation Parameters	Planning and Interventions with *Rationales*
Nursing Diagnosis: *Ineffective Breathing Pattern*	**Outcome:** Breathing pattern will be effective. **Evaluation Parameter:** Patient will not exhibit symptoms of respiratory distress.	**Interventions and *Rationales:*** *Nonpharmacologic:* Elevate the head of the bed. Place a fan in the room that blows gently on the patient's face. *To promote comfort.* *Pharmacologic:* Morphine drip: titrate for symptom relief. At end of life there is no recommended maximal dose. *Titration is intended to relieve pain and suffering.*

Assessment of Body Temperature

Objective Data:
Assess:
Skin temperature
Tachypnea

Tachycardia
Shivering

Nursing Assessment and Diagnoses	Outcomes and Evaluation Parameters	Planning and Interventions with *Rationales*
Nursing Diagnosis: *Imbalanced Body Temperature*	**Outcome:** The patient will not exhibit signs of physical discomfort from a fever. **Evaluation Parameters:** Normal body temperature Free from shivering	**Interventions and *Rationales:*** *Pharmacologic:* Administer an antipyretic *to decrease body temperature. Any measure that would cause the patient more discomfort, such as a cooling blanket, should not be used.*

the team necessary to achieve this objective. It is the nurse's responsibility to ensure that all members of the team are notified regarding the patient and family needs. Additionally, the health care team requires support and assistance to optimally assist the patient and family with this process. Services that may be used include hospital ethics committee, chaplain services, psychologist/psychiatrist, legal services, financial assistance, social services, hospice, and specific support groups for family members.

The ethics committee intervenes when there is conflict among the health care team and/or family regarding the prognosis and continuation of curative care for the patient. Once the decision is made to place the patient on palliative care, the family may need help regarding legal and financial assistance to ensure the patient's affairs are in order. The chaplain, social services, or a psychologist/psychiatrist assists the family to work through the grieving process and bring closure to the situation. If the patient is able to return home to die, hospice services aid the patient and family to facilitate this process in the home setting. Finally, specific support groups will help the family to work through the grieving process both before and after death.

Research Opportunities

There is an abundance of literature and research regarding hospice care for the terminally ill. Unfortunately, little research has been done with regard to end-of-life care when the death is un-

expected. See the Research Opportunities and Clinical Impact box (p. 414) for research topics in this area.

Many hospitals and organizations are working to improve end-of-life care and are committed to ensuring that all patients and families experience a "good death." Unfortunately, though, deciding who is "dying" in the acute care setting can be subjective or more a matter of perspective. Caregivers feel comfortable when pursuing a cure, but once the decision is made that any further care would be futile, caregivers often feel uncomfortable because this is not the "norm." Today's health care system is tailored to handle emergencies and injuries, diagnostic tests, and the most technologically advanced care in the world. It is not designed to accommodate the diverse needs of patients who are dying. Education and care guidelines will help to alleviate the discomfort of caregivers when they end up doing something that is perceived as the opposite of their normal goals.

Summary

As a nurse, one of the most rewarding experiences will be to allow natural death for a patient and to support him or her during this time. Helping the patient and significant others to meet their goals at end of life is challenging and rewarding. We ourselves will come to die and that alone should be reason enough to advocate for a system of care for people at the end of life.

RESEARCH OPPORTUNITIES AND CLINICAL IMPACT RELATED TO END-OF-LIFE CARE

Research Area	Clinical Impact
What interventions will help to relieve the discomfort felt by critical care nurses caring for end-of-life patients?	Developing interventions to relieve the discomfort surrounding end-of-life care will improve the care given to patients at end of life.
Is there a way to measure quality of life as an end point of treatment?	A tool that could accurately measure quality of life would assist in decisions for the end point of treatment.
What interventions can be done to support culturally appropriate end-of-life care?	To promote cultural customs and rituals surrounding end of life.
Compare the efficacy of terminal weaning versus terminal extubation during withdrawal of care.	This research could determine the best approach to withdrawal of ventilatory life support.

NCLEX® REVIEW

1. A family member inquires about the numbers and variety of different health care personnel attending to the patient receiving palliative care. The nurse should inform the patient and family that:
   1. Integrating the goals and expertise of many different disciplines encourages the development of the most comprehensive plan of care.
   2. Increased numbers of health care teams can help to ensure continuity in communication with the patient and family members.
   3. The utilization of an interdisciplinary team decreases the likelihood of civil or criminal liability following new treatment decisions.
   4. A multidisciplinary approach to end-of-life care guarantees that the latest in palliative care technology will guide patient care goals.

2. Which statement made by the student nurse would indicate the need for further instruction regarding end-of-life care?
   1. "The focus of the plan of care should be changed from curative processes to comfort advances."
   2. "The rights of self-determination and confidentiality are essential for all palliative care patients."
   3. "The patient has the right to conclude what treatments or lack of treatments affect his own body."
   4. "The family usually finds it easier to withdraw life-sustaining treatments than to withhold them."

3. The nurse has just completed educating a patient about advanced directives. Which statement made by the patient would indicate the need for further instruction?
   1. "Advance directives will guide the health care team as to my wishes regarding medical treatments should I become incapacitated."
   2. "By signing the advance directive my appointed family member will have the ability to make health care decisions for me if I become ill."
   3. "The advanced directive is supposed to help direct the decision-making process about my intentions for life-sustaining treatments."
   4. "My living will is a type of advanced directive that describes what level of life-prolonging care I desire in the event I become incapacitated."

4. The patient is being admitted for inpatient hospice care. Which instructions should be provided to the patient and his or her family regarding pain control?
   1. "We will continue to increase the pain medication until the symptoms are relieved."
   2. "We are going to limit family visits because the excess stimulation can be detrimental."
   3. "We are planning on reducing the amount of anxiety medication for fear of dependence."
   4. "We feel all the excess lights and noise will help the patient forget all about the pain."

5. A new nurse is being oriented to a hospice position in a culturally diverse area. Which statement made by this new employee would reflect a thorough understanding of cultural diversity as it relates to end-of-life care?
   1. "Many followers of Judaism believe that death is a private matter, and therefore, the dying person should be left alone."
   2. "Some Russians may make their elderly family members a DNR so they will die comfortably and without life-sustaining treatments."
   3. "Believers in the Baha'i faith consider the body as just a shell, so cremations are common and organ donation is encouraged."
   4. "Persons from South Asia may remain positive and upbeat when around the health care team but then mourn in private."

Answers for review questions appear in Appendix D

KEY TERMS

durable power of attorney for health care
   (DPAHC) *p.397*
hospice *p.405*

living wills *p.396*
medical durable power of attorney
   (MDPA) *p.397*

palliative care *p.393*

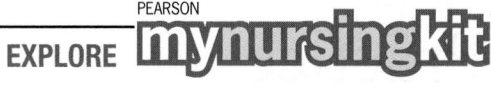

EXPLORE

MyNursingKit is your one stop for online chapter review materials and resources. Prepare for success with additional NCLEX®-style practice questions, interactive assignments and activities, web links, animations and videos, and more!

Register your access code from the front of your book at
www.mynursingkit.com

REFERENCES

Andrews, M., & Boyle, J. (2003). *Transcultural concepts in nursing care* (4th ed.). New York: Lippincott Williams & Wilkins.

Bednash, G., & Ferrell, B. (2002a). Ethical and legal issues in end of life care. In *Continuing Education for Nurses* (pp. 21–65). Roseville, CA: CME Resource.

Bednash, G., & Ferrell, B. (2002b). Nursing care at the end of life. In *Continuing Education for Nurses* (pp. 2–18). Roseville, CA: CME Resource.

Bednash, G., & Ferrell, B. (2002c). Pain and symptom management in end of life care. *Continuing Education for Nurses* (pp. 21–65). Roseville, CA: CME Resource.

Buchman, T., Cassell, J., Ray, S., & Wax, M. (2002). Who should manage the dying patient? Rescue, shame, and the surgical ICU dilemma. *Journal of the American College of Surgeons, 194*(5), 664–673.

Burns, J., Mitchell, C., Outwater, K., Geller, M., Griffith, J., Todres, I., et al. (2000). End of life in the pediatric intensive care unit after the forgoing of life-sustaining treatment. *Critical Care Medicine, 28*(8), 3060–3066.

Carney, M., & Meier, D. (2000). Palliative care and end of life issues. *Anesthesiology Clinics of North America, 18*(1), 183–209.

Chaitin, E., & Arnold, R. (2005). *Communication in the ICU: Holding a family meeting.* Retrieved May 2, 2006, from UpToDate website: http://www.uptodate.com

Colon, M., & Lyke, J. (2003). Comparison of hospice use and demographics among European Americans, African Americans, and Latinos. *American Journal of Hospice and Palliative Care, 20*(3).

Davidson, P., Introna, K., Daly, J., Paull, G., Jarvis, R., Angus, J., et al. (2003). Cardiorespiratory nurses' perceptions of palliative care in nonmalignant disease: Data for the development of clinical practice. *American Journal of Critical Care, 12*(1), 47–53.

Ditillo, B. (2002). The emergence of palliative care: A new specialized field of medicine requiring an interdisciplinary approach. *Critical Care Nursing Clinics of North America, 14*, 127–132.

Ferrell, B. R., & Coyle, N. (2002). An overview of palliative nursing care. *American Journal of Nursing 102*(5), 26–31.

Gillick, M. (2004). *Ethical issues near the end of life.* Retrieved April 24, 2006, from UpToDate website: http://www.uptodate.com

Heyland, D. K., Dodek, P., Rocker, G., Groll, D., Gafni, A., Pichora, D., et al. (2006). What matters most in end of life care: Perceptions of seriously ill patients and their family members. *Canadian Medical Association Journal, 184*(5), 627–633.

Heyland, D. K., Groll, D., Rocker, G., Dodek, P., Gafni, A., Tranmer, J., et al. (2005). End-of-life care in acute care hospitals in Canada: A quality finish? *Journal of Palliative Care, 21*(3), 142–150.

Jackson, V., & Abrahm, J. (2005). *Ethical considerations in effective pain management at the end of life.* Retrieved May 2, 2006, from UpToDate website: http://www.uptodate.com

Jennings, B., Ryndes, T., D'Onofrio, C., & Baily, M. (2003). Access to hospice care: Expanding boundaries, overcoming barriers. *The Hastings Center Report, 33.*

Kuebler, K. K., Heidrich, D. E., & Esper, P. (Eds.). (2007). *Palliative and end of life care.* St. Louis, MO: Saunders.

Lipson, J., & Dibble, S. (Eds.). (2007). *Culture and clinical care.* San Francisco: UCSF Nursing Press.

Lynn, J., Lynch Schuster, J., & Kabcenell, A. (2000). *Improving care for the end of life.* New York: Oxford University Press.

McPhee, S. J., Rabow, M. W., Pantilat, S. Z., Markowitz, A. J., & Winker, M. A. (2000). Finding our way —perspectives on care at the close of life. *JAMA 284*(19), 2502–2507.

National Consensus Project for Quality Palliative Care. (2004). *Clinical practice guidelines for quality palliative care.* Pennsylvania: Author. Retrieved May 31, 2008, from http://www.nationalconsensusproject.org

National Hospice and Palliative Care Organization. (2006). *Facts and figures.* Retrieved August 8, 2006, from http://www.nhpco.org/files/public/Facts_Figures_for2004data.pdf

Ogle, K., Mavis, B., & Wang, T. (2003). Hospice and primary care physicians: Attitudes, knowledge and barriers. *American Journal of Hospice and Palliative Care, 20*(1).

Peterman, A., & Cella, D. (2005). *Evaluation of quality of life.* Retrieved April 24, 2006, from UpToDate website: http://www.uptodate.com

Saunders, C. A. (Ed.). (2007). *End of life: A nurse's guide to compassionate care.* Philadelphia: Lippincott Williams & Wilkins.

Solloway, M., Lafrance, S., Bakitas, M., & Gerken, M. (2005). A chart review of seven hundred eighty-two deaths in hospitals, nursing homes, and hospice/home care. *Journal of Palliative Medicine, 8*(4), 789–796.

Stevens, L., Cook, D., Guyatt, G., Griffith, L., Walter, S., & McMullin, J. (2002). Education, ethics, and end of life decisions in the intensive care unit. *Critical Care Medicine, 30*(2).

Teno, J. M., Clarridge, B. R., Casey, V., Welch, L. C., Wetle, T., Shield, R., et al. (2004). Family perspectives on end of life care at the last place of care. *Journal of the American Medical Association, 291*(1), 88–103.

Truog, R., Cist, A., Brackett, S., Burns, J., Curley, M., Danis, M., et al. (2001). Recommendations for end of life care in the intensive care unit: The Ethics Committee of the Society of Critical Care Medicine. *Critical Care Medicine, 29*(12) 2332–2348.

World Health Organization. (2006). *WHO definition of palliative care.* Retrieved August 8, 2006, from http://www.who.int/cancer/palliative/definition/en

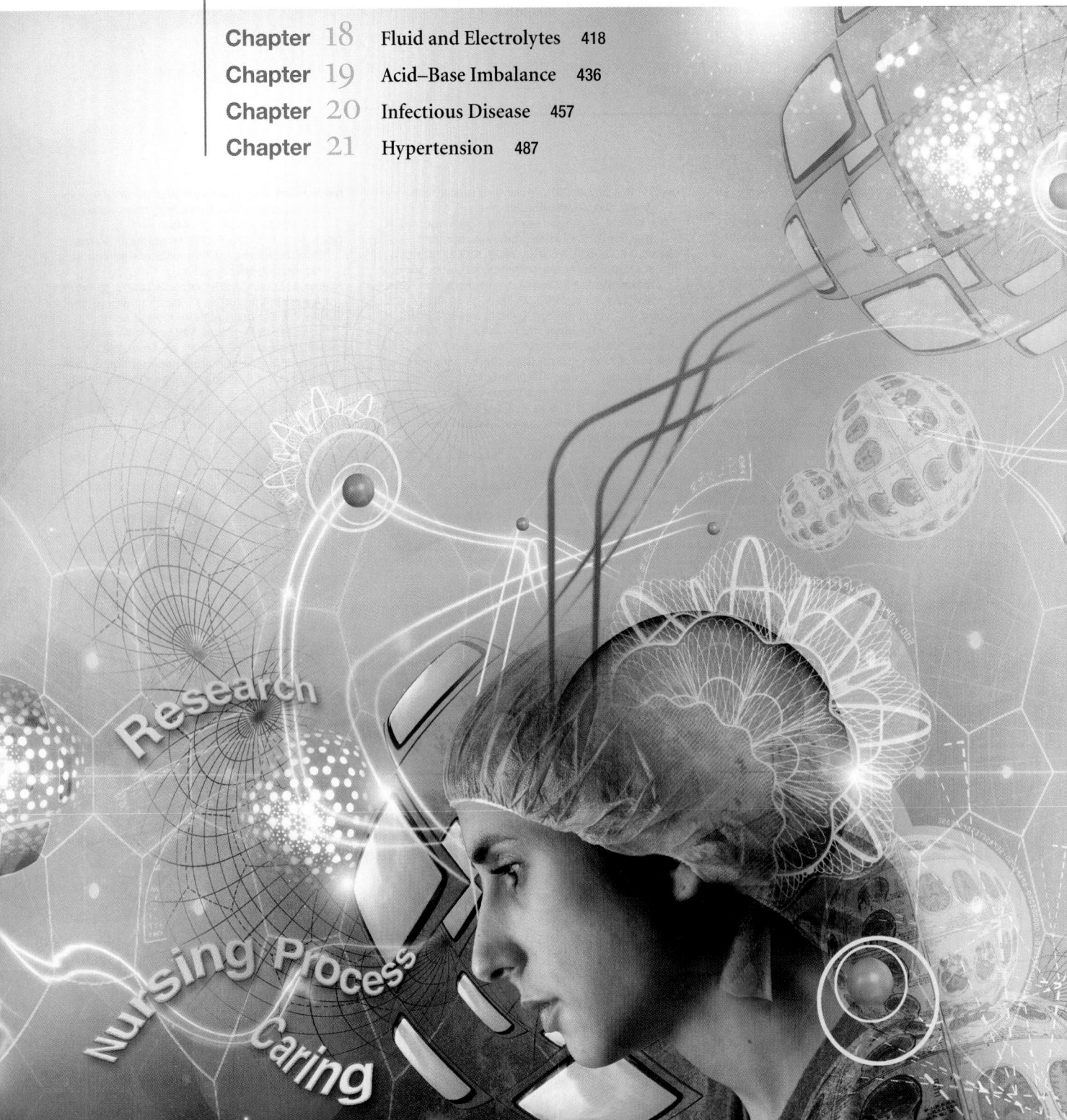

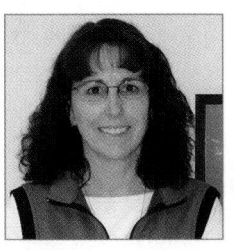

SHERRI My name is Sherri and I am the critical care epidemiologist at a teaching hospital in Northern California. This hospital is a Level 1 trauma center with a Level 3 neonatal intensive care unit (ICU), a burn ICU, and seven other critical care units. I am certified in infection control and my job is to monitor infectious diseases. Much of my time is spent in surveillance for hospital-acquired infections within the critical care units. This surveillance is part of our Infection Control Program and is mandated by the Joint Commission. I perform this surveillance by doing detailed chart reviews monthly. My reports are then sent to the Infection Control Committee and to unit managers as well as unit medical directors. I also make rounds in the ICUs giving the staff an opportunity to ask infection control–related questions. I discuss issues such as patient placement and isolation for those with resistant organisms. At times, I must also interact with the county and state health departments with regard to reporting communicable diseases.

I receive calls from every area of the hospital and clinics requesting information on a variety of subjects related to infection control. I am also called on to collaborate on construction projects that impact critical care especially with regard to dust control and other environmental safety hazards that may pose an infectious disease risk to our patient populations.

In addition, I am involved in studies and interventions designed to reduce or eliminate infections. The most recent initiative is one to eliminate catheter-associated bloodstream infections. The team leading this initiative designed a "Six Step Program to a Cleaner Line" and we have seen the rate of these types of infections decrease dramatically. Daily I review reports showing all microbiology results in order to find potential cases of hospital-acquired infection. I determine which patients have significant culture results and then review the medical record looking for the cause. After reviewing all potential cases, I generate device-related infection rates and present the data at Infection Control Committee meetings to help identify trends and infection control–related problems and to provide evidence of the success or failure of infection control interventions.

Controlling outbreak of infections is another aspect of my position. We monitor microbiology reports for sentinel organisms or for the emergence of the same organism in the cultures of many patients in a single unit. For example, the neonatal ICU had several babies who were positive for *Clostridium difficile* toxin. I worked with the unit manager, the nursing and ancillary staff, physicians, and environmental services to bring the situation to an end. Doing so required isolating and cohorting patients positive for *C. difficile* toxin, repeated cleaning of the environment with a diluted bleach solution, removal of alcohol-based hand rubs from the unit during the outbreak, limiting the movement of patients as much as possible, and touring the unit to look for possible areas of cross contamination. After approximately 15 cases, the outbreak came to an end.

My hospital has participated in the National Nosocomial Infection Surveillance study with the Centers for Disease Control and Prevention, which produced a new data collection system and became the National Health and Safety Network. The system provides specific criteria to help identify hospital-acquired infections.

There are occasions when I am called to help patients and their families in infection control–related situations both via telephone consultation and in person. In one case, a primary care physician called our office and needed help with a patient diagnosed with a pneumonia caused by *Neisseria meningitidis*, the causative organism for meningococcal meningitis. The physician referred him to our department for additional information. In talking with and teaching him about the organism, he was much calmer and felt he could speak intelligently with his close contacts about his situation now that he was armed with information.

Sometimes, the telephone consultation is not enough and intervention in the patient care environment is required. One such case was that of a 2-year-old patient in the pediatric ICU who had trisomy 21 and was currently hospitalized with leukemia. Her microbial flora were changing as she was exposed to antimicrobial therapy, which resulted in the growth of very resistant *Stenotrophomonas maltophilia*. The toddler was appropriately placed in Contact Precautions. I received a call from the unit staff telling me that the patient's family was not complying with the isolation precautions despite multiple reminders. I offered to talk with them in order to take the direct patient caregivers out of the situation so they could concentrate on the care the child required. I approached the family to discuss the resistant organisms and the isolation requirement. They wanted to be able to touch their child without gloves. We discussed options and came to a compromise that worked for everyone. They understood the concepts and I felt sure they would be very careful in their efforts to prevent transmission of the organisms. I gave them my contact numbers and over the subsequent days, I stopped in to chat with the family.

> "Sometimes, the telephone consultation is not enough and intervention in the patient care environment is required."

18

Fluid and Electrolytes

Darlene Gilcreast

Outcome-Based Learning Objectives

After studying this chapter, the learner will be able to:

1. Explain the normal composition of fluids and electrolytes in the body.
2. Describe the normal osmolality of the blood and urine.
3. Define the normal ranges of electrolytes in the body.
4. Discuss various circumstances that place the patient at risk for fluid and electrolyte imbalances.
5. Evaluate fluid status of an adult according to normal fluid and electrolyte values.
6. Identify nursing interventions to restore fluid and electrolyte balance.
7. Explain discharge teaching implications to assist patients to maintain fluid and electrolyte balance.

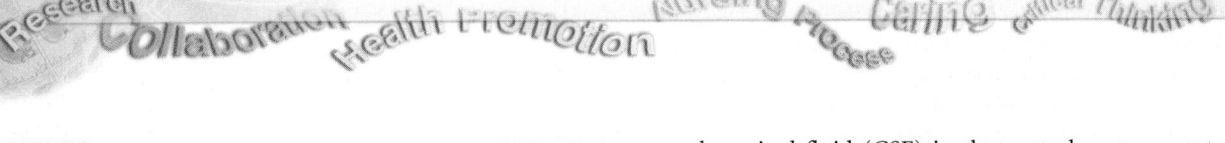

FLUIDS and electrolytes are the basic elements of life. All chemical reactions within the body take place in fluids. The causes of the reactions are electrolytes because they have an electrical charge, negative or positive. The primary fluid of the body is water. Water comprises 70% of living cells, 60% of an average adult's total body weight, and 70% to 80% of body weight in infants (Goyne, 2003). An average healthy person needs about 2 to 2.5 liters of water per day to meet the body's fluid requirements. This is based on the fact that healthy individuals need about 1 to 1.5 ounces of water per kilogram of body weight per day to dissolve and metabolize wastes (Grandjean, Reimers, & Buyck, 2003). Fluids are continually lost through respiration, formation of urine and feces, and perspiration. Most adults produce about 1,500 mL of urine per day (Whitmire, 2003). Additional fluids are lost during illness through **insensible fluid loss**, water that passes through the skin and from the respiratory tract and is lost by evaporation or with fever, wound drainage, vomitus, or diarrhea.

Body Fluid Composition and Function

Basically, there are two body fluid compartments: the **intracellular fluid (ICF)** and the **extracellular fluid (ECF)**. The ICF is all fluids that exist within the cell cytoplasm and nucleus. The ECF is all fluids that exist outside the cell, such as **interstitial fluid** between cells, fluid in the bloodstream (serum), cere-

brospinal fluid (CSF) in the central nervous system, gastrointestinal secretions, sweat, and urine. Two-thirds of the body's water is ICF and one-third is ECF (Felver, 2000). Only 5% of body fluid is normally in the blood (Johnson, 2007; Porth, 2007).

The functions of body fluids are many. Enzymes in saliva and mucus assist the passage of food into the gut and provide mechanisms for hydrolyzing food into elements the body can absorb. ECF in blood and CSF serves as a transport mechanism to deliver electrolytes, oxygen, nutrients, and hormones to tissues. Body fluids also carry immune cells to injury sites for the body's defense. ECF eliminates the body's waste products through the kidneys, bowels, and perspiration. Body functions depend on fluids facilitating the movement of electrolytes from one body compartment to another, often multiple times per minute, to effect an electrochemical action (i.e., the heartbeat, the secretion of a hormone, or a neuromuscular transmission). Another vital function of ECF is the regulation of body temperature through perspiration and capillary dilation to give off excess heat or conserve heat through the skin.

Osmolality

Osmolality is the number of molecules of solute per kilogram of water (Felver, 2000; Hogan, et al., 2006; Mushnick, 2007). The normal osmolality of blood is 275 to 295 milliosmoles per kilogram (mOsm/kg) of body weight. Fluids having osmolalities within this range are known as **isotonic** fluids (Goyne, 2003).

Fluids with osmolalities above 295 mOsm/kg are known as **hypertonic** fluids and fluids with osmolality below 275 mOsm/kg are **hypotonic**.

Electrolytes

Electrolytes are ionized minerals (calcium, chloride, magnesium, phosphorus, potassium, and sodium) that serve as energy transfer mechanisms to cause normal bodily functions by attractions, repulsions, and combinations. Ions either have a positive charge (cations), such as sodium (Na^+), or a negative charge (anions), such as chloride (Cl^-). Electrolytes move from one body compartment to another via the fluids and cause movement of various elements of the body by electrochemical interactions (see Chapter 38 ⊙).

Fluids and electrolytes each have normal ranges in which the body functions well. When elements or fluids are outside normal ranges, dysfunction or decreased performance occurs (Goyne, 2003).

Regulation of Body Fluid

Body fluids are regulated by osmosis, diffusion, and filtration (Goyne, 2003). In **osmosis**, water moves through a semipermeable membrane from an area of lower particle concentration toward one of higher particle concentration. Osmosis is based on the relationship of the molecules of solute (i.e., electrolytes) to water molecules (Goyne, 2003).

Diffusion occurs by movement of molecules from an area of higher concentration to an area of lower concentration. Diffusion depends on the size of the molecules, electrical charges, and pressure gradients. An elevated pressure gradient resists the transfer of elements into the high-pressure area and filters ions from the high-pressure area into a lower pressure area. An example of this process is the filtration done by the kidneys (Goyne, 2003). Pressure gradients are determined by conditions such as blood pressure within arterioles and the surrounding tissues. For example, the kidney juxtaglomerular apparatus exhibits higher pressure in the arterioles than in the renal collecting tubules, thus favoring transfer of fluids and solutes into the renal collecting tubules. Molecules must be small enough to pass through semipermeable membranes. Thus, in the kidney, large protein molecules are not normally filtered. Electrical charges must balance negative and positive ions or move from an area of higher concentration to an area of lower concentration.

Diffusion may be simple or facilitated. An example of simple diffusion is when lipid-soluble molecules pass through the phospholipid bilayers of cellular membranes and through protein channels for lipid-insoluble molecules. Facilitated diffusion requires carrier proteins to carry the substance through the cellular membrane (Porth, 2007). The movement of an ion against an electrochemical gradient is called *active transport* because energy must be used to transfer the molecule (Bond, 2000).

Filtration takes place when molecules from an area of higher concentration move through permeable membranes to an area of lower concentration as a result of hydrostatic pressure (Metheny, 2000). Hydrostatic pressure is the pressure exerted on the surrounding tissues due to the presence of water. Filtration occurs in the body because of hydrostatic pressure generated by the pumping action of the heart. On the arterial side of the capillary, the hydrostatic pressure is 32 millimeters of mercury (mmHg). On the venous side of the capillary, the hydrostatic pressure is about 15 mmHg. This favors movement of fluids from the bloodstream into the tissues on the arterial side of the capillary and back into the bloodstream on the venous side of the capillary after filtering through the tissues and bathing the cells in interstitial fluid (Metheny, 2000).

Filtration is directly opposed by the oncotic pressure of plasma proteins, especially albumin in the bloodstream (Metheny, 2000). **Oncotic pressure** is the influence of plasma proteins on the movement of water into and out of the blood stream based on the fact that plasma proteins maintain a negative ionic charge. Plasma oncotic pressure is about 22 mmHg. In a steady state, the ECF and ICF pressures are equal (Porth, 2007). To maintain homeostasis, fluid loss must equal fluid intake.

Tests for Evaluating Fluid Status

Laboratories routinely test the osmolality of blood. The Diagnostic Tests box (p. 420) lists normal and low and high values for use when evaluating fluid status. The normal range is 275 to 295 mOsm/kg of water (Goyne, 2003). Values above 295 indicate that there are too many molecules of solute per molecule of water, or a water deficit. Values below 275 indicate that there are too few molecules of solute per molecule of water, or a water excess (Goyne, 2003). Both conditions can result in bodily dysfunction. Serum osmolality may be roughly calculated by doubling the serum sodium value (Goyne, 2003; Hogan, et al., 2006).

Another test to evaluate hydration is the serum hematocrit measurement, which is the percentage of blood cells in a given volume of blood. A normal value is ~ 40% to 50%, with males at 42% to 52% and females at 37% to 47%. If the serum is dilute (symbolic of overhydration), the hematocrit will be low with decreased values for sodium, chloride, potassium, and bicarbonate. If the serum is concentrated, the hematocrit, sodium, potassium, chloride, and bicarbonate values will be high. Normal laboratory values for measuring electrolyte and fluid balance are presented in the Diagnostic Tests box (p. 420). Serum concentration can be measured indirectly by measuring the osmolality (**specific gravity** or **SG**) of urine. Normal SG is 1.016 to 1.022. SG will be low when the blood is dilute, and high when the blood is concentrated (Goyne, 2003; Hogan, Gingrich, Ricci, & Overby, 2006) unless other physiological abnormalities are present.

Clinical Manifestations of Overhydration and Dehydration

The body normally does not have excess fluid in the absence of diseases, such as renal failure, congestive heart failure (CHF), or syndrome of inappropriate antidiuretic hormone (Goyne, 2003; Hogan et al., 2006). However, if the blood is dilute, water is redistributed by osmosis from the blood to the ECF and ICF spaces. As a result, cellular edema occurs. Edema between the cells will follow gravity and will be reflected by lower extremity edema in people who are upright and sacral edema in people who are confined to bed. When cells are swollen with water, normal function is slowed or interrupted. Excess fluid volume is common in individuals with reduced renal sodium and water excretion and in patients with liver cirrhosis or CHF (Joy & Hladik, 2007).

DIAGNOSTIC TESTS for Evaluating Fluid Status (Adult Values)

Test and Normal Values	Expected Normal Values	Low (Overhydration)	High (Dehydration)
Urinalysis			
Specific gravity	1.005–1.030	<1.005	>1.030
Urine osmolality	50–1200 mOsm/kg water	>1,200 mOsm/kg	<50 mOsm/kg
Urine electrolytes			
Sodium	40–220 mEq/day	<40 mEq/d	>220 mEq/d
Potassium	25–100 mEq/day	<25 mEq/d	>100 mEq/d
Serum osmolality	285–295 mOsm/kg water	<285 mOsm/kg	>295 mOsm/kg
Hematocrit	Male: 42–52%	Male: <42%	Male: >52%
	Female: 37–47%	Female: <37%	Female: >47%
Serum electrolytes			
Sodium	136–145 mEq/L	<135 mEq/L	>146 mEq/L
Potassium	3.5–5.0 mEq/L	<3.5 mEq/L	>5.0 mEq/L
Chloride	98–106 mEq/L	<98 mEq/L	>106 mEq/L
Bicarbonate	22–26 mEq/L	<22 mEq/L	>26 mEq/L

Sources: Cavanaugh, B. M. (2001). *Nurse's manual of laboratory and diagnostic tests* (3rd ed.). Philadelphia: EA; Davis Company. Ehmann, W.C. (1). ...; Kee, J.L. (2005). *Laboratory and diagnostic tests with nursing implications* (7th ed.). Upper Saddle River, New Jersey: Prentice Hall.

Excess fluid may build up in the lung capillaries and pool in the lung alveoli (air sacs). The fluid can be detected by auscultating the lung bases and hearing "crackles," a sound similar to rubbing the hair between your fingers just in front of your ear. The nurse may also hear an extra heart sound (S_3, just preceding the S_2). This sounds like "pa-lub-dub" instead of the normal "lub-dub" of the heart. Many use the mnemonic "Tennessee" to distinguish this rhythm from the S_4, a "lub-pa-dub" or "Kentucky." The S_3 sound results from the atria of the heart being overly distended by fluid backup in the central venous system and the forcible contraction of the atria (O'Gara & Braunwald, 2001).

The S_3 heart sound is common in children, but not in people over the age of 40 years. The fluid in the alveoli increases the oxygen–carbon dioxide diffusion distance in the pulmonary capillaries and results in less efficient gas exchange. This is exhibited in patients by perceived shortness of breath, reduced blood oxygen levels, higher blood carbon dioxide levels, and a condition known as respiratory acidosis, in which the serum pH is less than 7.35, caused by a buildup of carbonic acid and dissolved carbon dioxide in the blood (O'Gara & Braunwald, 2001). Patients will increase respiratory rates above 24 breaths per minute in an attempt to compensate for reduced gas exchange. Hypervolemia is usually treated with large doses of loop diuretics, such as furosemide, that are efficient in removing free water from the blood via the distal tubules (Joy & Hladik, 2007).

The most common cause of dehydration (pure water deficit) is the excessive loss of free water through urine, such as in people with diabetes insipidus (a condition in which antidiuretic hormone from the pituitary gland is lacking), hyperglycemia (serum glucose above 200 mg/dL and usually above 300 mg/dL) in diabetes mellitus, failure to drink replacement fluids (as may happen in people with altered mental status), or overuse of diuretics (Goyne, 2003; Johnson, 2007). Elderly individuals have decreased perception of thirst due to aging and may not replace fluids appropriately. The elderly are particularly vulnerable to dehydration because many are taking prescription diuretics for high blood pressure. Other causes of fluid deficit may be nausea, vomiting, and diarrhea resulting from gastrointestinal flu, food poisoning, or hyperemesis gravidarum (vomiting related to pregnancy). The elderly are very vulnerable to influenza and contagious diseases because the immune system becomes less effective as the body ages.

Clinical manifestations of dehydration include severe thirst (may be absent in the elderly), dry mouth and tongue, possible cracked and peeling lips, dry skin that "tents" when it is lightly lifted (the skin creates an upward fold that does not return quickly to its original position), and body temperature that may rise one or two degrees (Goyne, 2003; Hogan et al., 2006). Patients will have orthostatic hypotension. Orthostatic hypotension is determined by an increase in pulse of 20 beats/min or blood pressure drop of 20 mmHg or more in the systolic blood pressure or 10 mmHg in the diastolic blood pressure upon changing from the supine to the standing position (Saseen & Carter, 2005). Patients will have tachycardia and weak pulses because of decreased circulating blood volume in dehydration. The extremities may take on a "mottled" (patches of purple and white) appearance due to decreased perfusion (O'Gara & Braunwald, 2001).

■ Nursing Management

Assessing the hydration of patients is part of the initial and ongoing nursing assessments. Assessments, as defined in Chapter 9 🔗, include both the oral history and physical assessments. Many symptoms, such as headache, dizziness, or syncope (faintness), can be reduced with attention to adequate hydration. In the patient with heart failure, overhydration may lead to symptoms of dyspnea, shortness of breath, and intolerance for walking and other activities of daily living (ADLs). Overhydration can lead to orthopnea (difficulty breathing when lying flat), which may necessitate propping up the patient in bed with several pillows or having the patient sit in a recliner chair to sleep (O'Gara & Braunwald, 2001). Sample hydration assessment questions are included in the Nursing Process: Patient Care Plan boxes for dehydration and overhydration (p. 422). The care plans apply the nursing process to relevant nursing diagnoses and provide outcomes and interventions for patients with alterations in hydration.

■ Collaborative Management

To achieve the optimal balance of fluid and electrolytes, patients need a multidisciplinary health care team. The team includes nurses, nursing assistants, physicians, laboratory personnel, dietitians, and dietary assistants. Nurses and physicians assess the patient for alterations in fluids and electrolytes by conducting a thorough history and physical and by maintaining accurate intake and output (I&O) documentation. Nursing assistants often are responsible for maintaining I&O charts, particularly in inpatient settings. However, the nurse, as the supervisor for the nursing assistants, is responsible for the accuracy of the I&O data. Laboratory personnel assist by performing laboratory tests that provide more specific data about the fluid and electrolyte balances of patients. Dietitians and dietary assistants provide appropriate medical nutrition therapy for patients, including appropriate fluids in the right amounts (Goldstein-Fuchs & McQuiston, 2003).

Often, patients need to monitor their fluid status at home. Therefore, a plan for appropriate hydration (avoiding excesses and deficits) may be part of discharge planning. Daily weights may be part of the fluid assessment if patients have a tendency toward overhydration. Daily weights need to be repeated under the same conditions, on the same scale, at the same time of day, dressed in the same clothing (i.e., gown or pajamas), with all drainage tubes empty, for consistency of weighing conditions (Indiana State University, 2007). A weight gain of more than 5 pounds per day indicates that the health care provider should be notified because the retention of 1 pint of fluid results in a gain of 1 pound (Johnson, 2007). Because patients may not prepare their own meals, the person who prepares the meals for the patient must be included in the planning and teaching.

Assessing the frequency and consistency of stools also is a layperson's way of determining the adequacy of hydration. In dehydration, constipation occurs and stools become hard and difficult to pass. When stools are of a normal frequency for the individual, are soft, and easy to pass, it may be assumed that hydration is adequate (Grandjean et al., 2003). Although this may seem a mundane task, monitoring the frequency and quality of patients' bowel movements is important to fluid intake monitoring. If stools become too hard and difficult to pass, patients can induce cardiac dysrhythmias due to excessive internal pressure generated with the Valsalva maneuver, closing the glottis of the throat, and bearing down to pass stools (Ahlquist & Camilleri, 2001). The elderly are more likely to suffer from constipation secondary to decreased physical activity and slowing of bowel activity with aging.

Homeostatic Mechanisms

Serum osmolality is regulated by the osmoreceptors of the hypothalamus. When body water loss is 2% of normal body

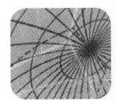

NURSING PROCESS: Patient Care Plan for Dehydration

Assessment of Dehydration

Subjective Data:
Are you feeling thirsty?
Have you had difficulty drinking fluids and keeping them down?
Have you had any nausea, vomiting, diarrhea, or fever lately?
Have you experienced any dizziness on standing?

Objective Data:
Weigh patient and compare weight to usual weight (loss of >2 lb/day indicates dehydration).
Measure temperature (>99°F or 37°C compatible with dehydration), pulse (greater than 100 beats/min), blood pressure (lower than normal, take lying, sitting, standing), and respirations.
Examine mouth for, cracked lips, dried tongue and mucous membranes.
Lift the skin on the back of the hands to assess for "tenting" (skin is slow to return to its normal position).
Obtain urinalysis with specific gravity and serum electrolytes.

Nursing Assessment and Diagnoses	Outcomes and Evaluation Parameters	Planning and Interventions with *Rationales*
Nursing Diagnosis: *Risk for Imbalanced Fluid Volume* related to excessive fluid loss/inability to take fluids as evidenced by low blood pressure, rapid pulse, increased body temperature, and dizziness on standing.	**Outcome:** Adequate fluid balance ***Evaluation Parameters:*** Temperature, pulse, and blood pressures within normal limits. No evidence of dizziness on standing. Able to drink and retain 8 glasses of water per day.	**Interventions and *Rationales:*** Provide a source of fluids that the patient can retain (oral or parenteral). If nausea and vomiting are the source of dehydration, parenteral fluids will be needed. *Inadequate hydration requires restoration of normal circulating volume in order to maintain blood pressure and provide sufficient cardiac output to circulate nutrients to the body. When the fluids cannot be taken and retained orally, a parenteral source of fluids will need to be provided to restore balance.*

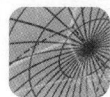

NURSING PROCESS: Patient Care Plan for Overhydration

Assessment of Overhydration

Subjective Data:

Have you had any difficulty urinating lately?

How much fluid have you ingested in the last 24 hours?

Have you eaten a lot of salt or soy sauce?

Have you experienced any shortness of breath with walking or exercise?

Are you able to sleep lying flat? If not, how many pillows do you need for your head?

Do you sleep sitting in a recliner chair?

Objective Data:

Weigh patient and compare weight to usual weight (an increase in weight greater than 2 lb/day indicates fluid retention).

Measure temperature, pulse, blood pressure (higher than normal), and respirations (will be more rapid than normal).

Assess skin on the legs and ankles for dependent edema. If the patient is confined to bed, this will be in the sacral area.

Obtain urinalysis and serum electrolytes.

Nursing Assessment and Diagnoses	Outcomes and Evaluation Parameters	Planning and Interventions with *Rationales*
Nursing Diagnosis: *Risk for Imbalanced Fluid Volume* related to excessive fluid intake/decreased urination as evidenced by high blood pressure, rapid breathing, shortness of breath, and dependent edema.	**Outcome:** Adequate fluid balance ***Evaluation Parameters:*** Temperature, pulse, and blood pressures within normal limits. No evidence of dependent edema. Voiding at least 240 mL/8 hr.	**Interventions and *Rationales:*** Reduce oral fluid and sodium intake as directed by health care provider (about 1 L/day with most taken in the waking hours and <2,000 mg of sodium/day). A fluid-intake schedule is arranged and the patient instructed in fluid restriction. Administer diuretics as prescribed, monitoring serum potassium levels. *Overhydration requires restoration of normal circulating volume to decrease blood pressure and reduce the workload on the heart. When the fluids are excessive, fluids will cross the alveolar capillary barrier and pool fluids in the lungs (pulmonary edema), interfering with oxygen–carbon dioxide diffusion. This reduces blood oxygen levels. When dependent edema is present, it interferes with normal circulation in the tissues resulting in lower tissue oxygen. The patient's cooperation will have to be obtained in order to succeed at fluid restriction. Rapid diuresis will often result in low serum potassium. Serum potassium within the normal range is essential for normal cardiac function.* If the patient is not able to urinate due to renal failure, hemofiltration or dialysis may need to be arranged *to assist in restoration of normal fluid balance.* Additionally, potassium levels will need to be monitored *to ensure the patient is not retaining too much potassium.* Reposition patient every 2 hours *to decrease risk to skin.*

weight, the hypothalamus stimulates the posterior pituitary to secrete **antidiuretic hormone (ADH)**. ADH signals the kidneys to conserve water by reabsorbing water from the distal renal tubules. Additionally, the perception of thirst is stimulated to promote drinking of water to restore normal serum osmolality (Goyne, 2003; Mushnick, 2007).

In the presence of severe dehydration, such as results from vomiting, baroreceptors (pressure-sensitive cells) in the carotid artery sinuses and aorta stimulate the secretion of ADH. Baroreceptors in the afferent glomerular arterioles of the kidneys detect reduced perfusion and secrete renin. Renin causes the conversion of angiotensinogen to angiotensin I, which is converted to angiotensin II in the lungs by angiotensin converting enzyme. Angiotensin II stimulates aldosterone release from the adrenal glands, which promotes retention of sodium (Goldstein-Fuchs & McQuiston, 2003). This mechanism becomes a problem in the elderly. Atherosclerosis narrows the renal arteries in the same fashion as it does the coronary arteries. In response to decreased blood through the kidneys, renin is released stimulating the cascade of sodium and fluid retention. Health care providers address this problem by prescribing angiotensin converting enzyme inhibitors (ACEI) and angiotensin-receptor blocking (ARB) medications (Bomback & Klemmer, 2007).

Electrolyte Balance

Electrolyte balance is the sum of electrolyte intake, absorption, distribution, and electrolyte loss through normal and abnormal routes. Intake is primarily oral, but may include the rectal route if patients use enemas. In the hospital, intravenous fluids are another source of electrolytes for patients (Felver, 2000). Once absorbed, electrolytes are distributed in different ways in the body. For example, the reservoirs for calcium are the teeth and bones, the reservoir for potassium is inside the cells of the body, and sodium and chloride are found primarily in blood. Most electrolytes are lost via the gastrointestinal (GI) tract, urinary tract, and sweat. Other sources of loss may be vomitus, nasogastric suction, wound drainage, or hemorrhage (Felver, 2000).

Electrolyte Imbalances

Because every bodily function is dependent on the electromotive force (the exchange of electrons between molecules), electrolyte imbalances decrease the body's ability to conduct normal activities. These activities include transmission of neural signals, contraction of muscles including the heart, secretion of hormones by secretory glands, and regulation of normal bodily functions, such as oxygenation and metabolization of wastes. The nature of the imbalance is reflected by which electrolyte is out of balance. Often, the complementary electrolyte with which the primary electrolyte combines also is affected. The following sections provide details regarding specific electrolyte imbalances.

Sodium

Sodium is the most numerous cation in the ECF. It maintains ECF volume through osmotic pressure, regulates acid–base balance by combining with chloride or bicarbonate ions, and conducts nerve impulses via the sodium channels of cells. Normal values for sodium are 135 to 145 milliequivalents/liter (mEq/L) (Johnson, 2007). Acid–base balance is discussed thoroughly in Chapter 19 .

Three hormones are responsible for regulating the sodium level in the ECF: (1) **aldosterone**, a hormone secreted by the adrenal cortex; (2) ADH, secreted by the posterior pituitary gland; and (3) **atrial natriuretic peptide (ANP)**, secreted by the atrium of the heart. Aldosterone is secreted in response to low ECF sodium levels, an increase in ICF potassium, low cardiac output, and stress. Aldosterone causes increased retrieval of sodium from the kidney filtrate. Water follows the osmotic attraction of sodium; thus, body ECF is increased. ADH is secreted in response to increased ECF osmolality detected by the osmoreceptors (receptors that detect the osmolality of the serum) in the hypothalamus and causes the reabsorption of water from the kidney distal tubules (Goyne, 2003). When the atria are excessively stretched due to excessive ECF volume in the blood, ANP is secreted as an antagonist to aldosterone to cause increased sodium excretion through the kidneys. As a result, water is also lost into the urine, reducing blood volume and increasing water loss (Porth, 2007).

Hypernatremia (Sodium Excess)

Hypernatremia (sodium above 145 mEq/L) represents a deficit of water in relation to the body's sodium levels. It occurs when there is an excess loss of body fluids that have a lower than normal concentration of sodium so that water is lost in excess of sodium. For example, Cushing's syndrome (aldosterone excess) causes excess sodium retention, or diabetes insipidus causes excessive fluid loss. Initially, fluid moves from the cells into the serum via osmosis to maintain osmolality within the normal parameters (below 295 mOsm/kg) and reduce serum sodium (to 145 mEq/L or below). Thirst is increased due to the increase in serum sodium and osmolality (Johnson, 2003; Porth, 2007).

Clinical symptoms resulting from hypernatremia caused by water loss are largely those of ECG fluid loss and cellular dehydration: thirst, low-grade fever, peripheral and pulmonary edema, and postural hypotension with excess fluid loss (Grogan, 2006; Porth, 2007). A simple test for hypernatremia is whether patients' rings have suddenly become tight on their fingers. This must be closely monitored to make sure that swollen fingers with rings do not threaten the tissue integrity of the fingers. Patients rings should be removed with permission, if they threaten the circulation in the finger. Laboratory values will show increased serum osmolality, elevated serum sodium, and a possible increase in urine specific gravity because of the effect of ADH to conserve water.

Pathophysiologic symptoms of hypernatremia are most likely to occur with sudden onset (Singer & Brenner, 2001). Brain symptoms resulting from hypernatremia are altered mental status, neuromuscular irritability, and occasionally coma or seizures (Singer & Brenner, 2001). One cause of this type of hypernatremia is excess sweating without fluid replacement, such as in heat stroke. Mortality associated with serum sodium levels above 180 mEq/L is very high (Singer & Brenner, 2001).

The brain cells adjust to ECF hypertonicity after 24 hours by moving the excess ions into brain cells. The resulting hyperosmolality inside the cells results in increased hydration inside brain cells to correct cellular dehydration. A potential danger of administering intravenous fluids too aggressively to reduce the osmolality of the blood is that of excess fluids moving into cerebral cells, resulting in cerebral edema (Singer & Brenner, 2001). This can lead to cellular dysfunction in the brain and increased intracranial pressure. Seizures or permanent brain damage could result (Singer & Brenner, 2001). Therefore, the water deficit should be replaced slowly over 48 to 72 hours with oral fluids being the preferred route (Singer & Brenner, 2001).

As mentioned earlier, one possible cause of hypernatremia is Cushing's syndrome. Cushing's syndrome is overactivity of the adrenal glands releasing excess aldosterone, which causes sodium retention. Symptoms of Cushing's syndrome are excess adrenal hormones that include cortisone, aldosterone, and androgens. The person will exhibit truncal obesity (large waist compared to the rest of the body, "apple" figure type) and may have a "buffalo hump" on the nape of the neck, a rounded "moon-shaped" face, fragile skin that bruises easily, muscle wasting of the arms and legs, osteoporosis with possible forward curvature of the spine (kyphosis), mood changes, and increased susceptibility to infections. Females may have excessive facial hair due to excess androgen (male) hormones. Fluid retention secondary to sodium retention results in expanded blood volume with hypertension and subsequent weight gain.

Nursing Management

Treatment requires diagnosis of Cushing's syndrome, possible surgery for tumors of the adrenal or pituitary glands, or drugs to decrease the activity of the adrenal glands (ketoconazole, metyrapone, aminoglutethimide, or mitotane) (Gums & Tovar, 2007). Ketoconazole reduces cortisol in Cushing's syndrome. Ketoconazole, however, can cause gynecomastia and lower testosterone levels. Metyrapone inhibits cortisol synthesis and patients may show an increase in plasma adrenocorticotropic hormone (ACTH). Side effects of metyrapone are nausea, vomiting, vertigo, headache, dizziness, abdominal discomfort, and an allergic rash. Aminoglutethimide inhibits cortisol production and is indicated for short-term use in inoperable Cushing's syndrome with ectopic ACTH production. Mitotane is a cytotoxic drug that reduces the synthesis of cortisol and corticosterone. It selectively inhibits adrenocortical function without causing cellular destruction. Because mitotane can severely inhibit cortisol production, the patient should be hospitalized to initiate therapy (Gums & Tovar, 2007, pp. 1396–1397).

Diabetes insipidus (uncontrolled loss of water in the urine) is due to an absence of ADH related to pituitary damage. This loss of ADH could be due to tumors or possible head injury by accident or as a result of surgery. Because the body lacks ADH, there is decreased water resorption in the distal tubules of the kidneys, resulting in marked increased urinary output with cellular dehydration. Volumes of 5 to 20 L of urine per day are common, with the urine having the appearance of water. The urine specific gravity will be <1.005. The person with diabetes insipidus will have an unquenchable thirst and will drink between 4 and 40 L of fluids per day. The blood osmolality will be high (about 295 mOsm) and serum sodium will be greater than 145 mEq/L because the blood becomes very concentrated due to water deficit (Guin, 2006). Management of diabetes insipidus is the administration of ADH in the form of a drug known as desmopressin acetate, which is administered as a nasal spray (Guin, 2006).

The nursing care of patients with hypernatremia, as outlined in the Nursing Process: Patient Care Plan box, is very important because of the risk for cerebral edema if the serum sodium level is lowered too rapidly. The rate at which sodium is lowered should not exceed 0.5 to 1 mEq/hr (Porth, 2007). To lower it more quickly risks brain dysfunction with neurological problems, such as seizures.

 *Excess sodium is stored in brain cells during hypernatremia to reduce serum sodium. When IV fluids are administered too aggressively, excess fluid may move into cerebral cells, resulting in edema and life-threatening brain dysfunction. Serum sodium should be lowered no faster than 0.5 to 1 mEq/L per hour (Johnson, 2007; Joy & Hladik, 2007).*

Hyponatremia (Low Serum Sodium)

Hyponatremia (serum values below 135 mEq/L) develops with excessive retention of water, inadequate sodium intake, or loss of sodium-rich fluids that are replaced with water. Diuretics, vomiting, diarrhea, GI suctioning, or loss of wound fluids from very large wounds (e.g., burn wounds) may cause sodium deficiency (Johnson, 2007). Excessive use of dextrose 5% intravenous (IV) fluid can result in hyponatremia due to free water being created when glucose is metabolized. In fact, about 2.5% of hospitalized patients experience hyponatremia largely due to IV fluids (Johnson, 2007). Diuretic-induced hyponatremia can result from the administration of thiazide diuretics by the blocking of sodium resorption in the distal tubules. Thus, water is retained in excess of sodium (Joy & Hladik, 2007).

Symptoms of sodium deficit are reduced ability of cells to depolarize and repolarize. Often patients are asymptomatic because both the relative sodium deficit and the rapidity of onset determines symptoms. As sodium levels drop below 120 mEq/L, neurological changes such as lethargy, headache, confusion, personality changes, apprehension, seizures, and even coma could result (Johnson, 2007). Symptoms of hypotension may reduce osmotic pressure in the blood to retain circulating fluid volume. Tissue edema may accompany dilutional hyponatremia caused by inappropriate intravenous fluids. In a syndrome of inappropriate

antidiuretic hormone (SIADH), the urine will be concentrated in spite of hyponatremia due to the lack of ADH. Permanent brain damage, such as central nervous system demyelination, may occur if the serum sodium level drops below 115 mEq/L or is corrected too rapidly (Singer & Brenner, 2001). Symptoms of osmotic demyelination syndrome are flaccid paralysis, dysarthria, and dysphagia. Mortality is high with this syndrome, even in the hospital. People who are most likely to suffer this syndrome are those with chronic hyponatremia (Singer & Brenner, 2001).

SIADH usually occurs as a result of brain trauma that causes increased secretion of ADH despite a normal fluid volume or it may be caused as a side effect of lithium, diuretics, or anticancer drugs (Johnson, 2007). Fluid overload and, hence, delusional hyponatremia are the result. The serum sodium will be less than 135 mEq/L and urine will be concentrated due to fluid retention. Symptoms are bounding pulse, hypertension, pale dry skin, weight gain and edema, renal failure, weakness, confusion, and possible seizures. The cause must be identified and treated to restore fluid and sodium volumes to normal (Johnson, 2007).

■ Nursing Management

The nursing care for a patient with hyponatremia is dependent on the cause. Therapeutic goals are to return serum sodium to near normal (135 mEq/L). Restriction of water intake to 1,000 mL/day is usually implemented to assist sodium increase and to prevent the sodium level from dropping further due to dilution (Johnson, 2007). Foods high in sodium (highly processed foods, such as chips) will be given, unless the patient is NPO (nothing by mouth). Correction of sodium levels may require adjusting other electrolytes to establish balance. Hypertonic saline intravenous fluids are used only in severe cases where seizures have occurred (Johnson, 2007). Overly aggressive correction of chronic hyponatremia could result in permanent brain damage. When hypertonic saline intravenous fluid is given, only sufficient 3% sodium chloride is given to correct symptoms—not to return the sodium to 135 mEq/L (Porth, 2007). See the Nursing Process: Patient Care Plan for hyponatremia (p. 426).

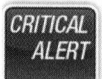 *In hyponatremia, when the sodium level drops to 120 mEq/L, neurological changes occur: lethargy, confusion, personality changes, apprehension, seizures, and coma. Permanent brain damage may occur if the serum sodium level drops below 115 mEq/L or if correction of chronic hyponatremia is overly aggressive due to destruction of myelin (Johnson, 2007; Joy & Hladik, 2007). Hypertonic saline IV fluids are used only in severe cases after seizures have occurred (Johnson, 2007).*

Potassium

Potassium (K+) is an intracellular cation primarily. Ninety-eight percent of potassium is found within cells (Rhyne, 2003b). Small amounts are found in blood (3.5 to 5.0 mEq/L) and bone (Rhyne, 2003b). The function of potassium is to maintain intracellular osmolality and participate in the sodium-potassium exchange that causes cellular depolarization and repolarization. The sodium-potassium-ATPase pump in cellular membranes uses active transport to transport sodium out of the cell and potassium into the cell at a ratio of 3:2 to maintain the appropriate balance (Brophy

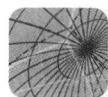

NURSING PROCESS: Patient Care Plan for Hypernatremia (Sodium Excess)

Assessment of Hypernatremia

Subjective Data:

How thirsty have you been lately?

Have you been able to drink water and keep it down?

How much salt or soy sauce have you taken lately?

Objective Data:

Excessive thirst

Low-grade fever (99°F or 38°C)

Peripheral edema

Pulmonary edema (auscultation of S_3 heart sound at left apex and "crackles" in lungs)

Postural hypotension (with large fluid loss)

Cushing's syndrome

Diabetes insipidus

Decreased fluid intake or excessive sodium intake

Laboratory values: increased serum osmolality, sodium, increased urine specific gravity

Nursing Assessment and Diagnoses	Outcomes and Evaluation Parameters	Planning and Interventions with *Rationales*
Nursing Diagnosis: Risk for imbalanced fluid volume with potential for life-threatening cerebral edema related to excess fluid loss or excess sodium retention as evidenced by serum sodium >148 mEq/L	**Outcomes:** Fluid and electrolyte balance Acid–base balance Adequate hydration ***Evaluation Parameters:*** Normal sensorium for patient Serum sodium 135–145 mEq/L Hematocrit: 37–47% for women, 40–50% for men Serum pH 7.35–7.45	**Interventions and *Rationales:*** Monitor fluids and electrolytes, acid–base balance, blood pressure, pulse, temperature *to guide treatment decisions to ensure patient safety.* Administer IV fluids to lower serum sodium slowly at a rate of 0.5–1.0 mEq/L until it reaches 147 mEq/L *to avoid cerebral edema. Chloride follows sodium and chloride is involved in acid–base balance.* Assess level of consciousness every 4 hours. Observe for lethargy, headache, nausea, vomiting, increased blood pressure, or altered sensorium. Notify health care provider of changes. *To recognize the symptoms of cerebral edema early.* Pad bed rails with blankets if seizures are likely *to prevent injury in the event of a grand mal seizure.*

Assessment of Patient's/Family's Knowledge Regarding Cause of Hypernatremia

Subjective Data:

Do you understand how your/the patient's blood levels became out of balance?

What will you be able to do in the future to keep this from happening again?

Do you understand the risks involved with high salt in your blood?

Objective Data:

Patient's/family's answers to above questions and whether they reflect understanding

Rehospitalizations for similar conditions

Nursing Assessment and Diagnoses	Outcomes and Evaluation Parameters	Planning and Interventions with *Rationales*
Nursing Diagnosis: *Deficient Knowledge* on part of patient and family related to cause and treatment of hypernatremia	**Outcomes:** Appropriate knowledge of the definition, causes, and clinical manifestations of hypernatreumia. ***Evaluation Parameters:*** Patient and family member verbalize understanding of causes and treatment of high serum sodium *to reduce likelihood of recurrence* Patient adheres to treatment regimen *to reduce future threats to patient's health and need for hospitalization*	**Interventions and *Rationales:*** Provide discharge instructions to patient and family member on causes and treatment of hypernatremia at an appropriate educational, cultural level *to inform patient/family why hypernatremia occurred, to promote adherence to treatment, and to prevent recurrence.* Provide reminders of adequate fluid intake and treatment adherence for Cushing's syndrome or diabetes insipidus *to prevent future occurrences of hypernatremia.*

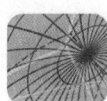

NURSING PROCESS: Patient Care Plan for Hyponatremia (Sodium Deficit)

Assessment of Sodium Deficit

Subjective Data:
How thirsty have you been lately?
Have much water have you been drinking?
How much salt or soy sauce have you taken lately?
Are you having any headaches?
Are you having any difficulty thinking or remembering things?

Objective Data:
Is the patient receiving IV fluids?
Does the patient have psychological problems leading to water intoxication?
Is the patient taking diuretics that may have caused electrolyte imbalance?
Does the patient exhibit neurological changes?
Laboratory values: increased serum osmolality, sodium increased, decreased urine specific gravity

Nursing Assessment and Diagnosis	Outcome and Evaluation Parameters	Planning and Interventions with *Rationales*
Nursing Diagnosis: *Risk for imbalanced body fluids with* potential for life-threatening cerebral edema related to excess fluid retention or sodium deficit as evidenced by serum sodium <135 mEq/L	**Outcomes:** Fluid and electrolyte balance Acid–base balance Adequate hydration ***Evaluation Parameters:*** Patient free from injury with normal sensorium Serum sodium 135–145 mEq/L Hematocrit 38–47% (women), 40–50% (men) Serum pH 7.35–7.45	**Interventions and *Rationales:*** Monitor neurological status (orientation to person, place, time), fluid and electrolytes, and acid–base balance *to determine whether the patient's condition is worsening, improving, or staying constant.* Restrict fluids to <1,000 mL/day *to prevent further dilution of sodium.* Assess blood pressure, dizziness, sensorium *to allow early intervention and maintain normal blood pressure.* Assist patient with ambulation. Maintain bed in lowest position with bed rails up and brakes on *to prevent falls and injury.* Explain to patient and family that disorientation is temporary *to decrease fear.* Use clocks, calendars, and familiar personal items *to reorient the patient and reduce confusion.* Pad the bed rails with blankets if seizures are likely *to prevent injury in the event of a seizure.* If seizures occur, administer hypertonic IV fluids (3% sodium) as ordered *to raise sodium to 135 mEq/L and prevent injury.*

Assessment of Patient's/Family's Knowledge Regarding Cause of Hyponatremia

Subjective Data:
Do you understand how your/the patient's blood levels became out of balance?
What will you do in the future to keep this from happening again?
Do you understand the risks involved with low salt in your blood?

Objective Data:
Patient's/family's answers to above questions reflect whether they understand
Rehospitalizations for similar conditions

Nursing Assessment and Diagnosis	Outcome and Evaluation Parameters	Planning and Interventions with *Rationales*
Nursing Diagnosis: *Deficient Knowledge* on the part of the patient and family related to cause and treatment of hyponatremia	**Outcome:** No future recurrence of low serum sodium ***Evaluation Parameters:*** Patient and family member identify the correct cause of the problem and identify proper treatment *to prevent recurrence*	**Interventions and *Rationales:*** Provide discharge instructions *to identify cause, to teach adherence to treatment, and to prevent future occurrences of hyponatremia.*

& Gehr, 2007). About 70% of intracellular potassium is located in muscle, thus when a person eats meat, potassium is gained. The remaining 30% is in the liver and red blood cells (Brophy & Gehr, 2007). Potassium is essential for cellular integrity, transmission of neuromuscular impulses, acid–base balance, conversion of carbohydrates into energy, and the formation of amino acids into proteins (Rhyne, 2003b). Serum potassium affects the strength and rate of cardiac contraction. Both hypokalemia and hyperkalemia can result in potentially fatal cardiac dysrhythmias because of potassium's essential role in cardiac cell polarization and depolarization (Brophy & Gehr, 2007) (see Chapter 19).

Potassium is gained by eating meat, potatoes, bananas, and other foods (Rhyne, 2003b). (See Chapter 14 for information on nutrition.) Most people consume about 100 mmol/day. Because some potassium is found in most foods, when caloric intake increases, so does the intake of potassium. When the body is in an anabolic state (building new tissue), potassium is stored in the cells. Movement of potassium into the blood occurs (1) with tissue injury or catabolism, when cells are broken down for energy during starvation, or (2) during periods of acidosis, when potassium moves from inside the cell into the blood to allow hydrogen ions to move into the cells to decrease the acidity of the blood (Rhyne, 2003b). Potassium is lost from the body via the kidneys where it is exchanged for sodium and via the GI tract where it is used to buffer hydrochloric acid.

Hyperkalemia

Hyperkalemia (serum potassium greater than 5.0 mEq/L) may occur because of increased potassium intake, decreased urinary excretion, or cellular damage that releases a lot of potassium into the blood (Hogan et al., 2006; Rhyne, 2003b). It may be the result of inappropriate potassium supplementation in IV fluids during hospitalizations or potassium supplementation medication. Decreased potassium excretion, causing hyperkalemia, may be the result of acute or chronic renal failure (urine output less than 30 mL/hr) or potassium-sparing diuretics (amiloride, spironolactone, triamterene) (Brophy & Gehr, 2007). Severe acidosis may greatly increase serum potassium by movement of potassium out of the cells to allow the intracellular storage of hydrogen ion to the buffer blood pH. Cellular release of potassium can occur with surgery, fever, sepsis, or trauma (Rhyne, 2003b). Decreases in the secretion of aldosterone can cause secretion of potassium in exchange for sodium and increase serum potassium levels (Rhyne, 2003b).

Clinical symptoms of hyperkalemia differ based on the degree of potassium elevation. Some common manifestations are muscular weakness and changes in the electrocardiogram (ECG) tracings with progressively widening PR and QRS intervals (Brophy & Gehr, 2007). Because of the increase of potassium inside the cell, potassium cellular repolarization is heightened, resulting in an enlarged or "tented" T wave during repolarization (Brophy & Gehr, 2007). Severe hyperkalemia (>6.0 mEq/L) results in prolonged PR intervals with loss of the P wave at levels above 7.0 mEq/L (complete heart block), wide QRS to a bizarre W configuration, and merging of the QRS and T wave (Brophy & Gehr, 2007) (see Chapter 38). Calcium affects the cellular threshold potential and may compensate for some degrees of hyperkalemia (Brophy & Gehr, 2007; Rhyne, 2003b).

◼ Nursing Management

Nursing management of patients with hyperkalemia includes assessing, planning of interventions, and evaluation.

Assessment

A thorough nursing assessment is essential to identify risks for and symptoms of hyperkalemia. Hyperkalemia is likely in cases of severe cellular injury such as crush injuries or burns, renal disease, insulin deficiency (diabetic ketoacidosis or hyperosmolar hyperglycemic nonketotic syndrome), Addison's disease (hypoaldosteronism), or the use of potassium supplements (Rhyne, 2003b). Symptoms may include irregular pulse, irritability, abdominal distention, cramping, muscle weakness, paresthesia, and diarrhea (Hogan et al., 2006; Rhyne, 2003b). Arterial blood gases (ABGs) may show metabolic acidosis (Brophy & Gehr, 2007).

Outcomes and Evaluation Parameters

Nursing goals are to reduce cardiac risk within 6 hours of admission (Porth, 2007). Positive results are a heart rate within the normal range of 60 to 120 beats/min and an ECG that is reflective of normal rhythm (contains a P wave, QRS is within 0.12 second with normal amplitude, ST segment is no longer depressed, and the T wave is less "tented" in its appearance). See Chapter 38 for more about ECGs.

Planning, Interventions, and Rationales

Treatment for hyperkalemia includes reducing oral or IV intake of potassium while treating the underlying cause of the hyperkalemia by administering potassium reducing agents: Kayexalate enemas (retained for 30 minutes) to exchange potassium for sodium in the gut or oral Kayexalate combined with sorbitol to rapidly remove potassium from the gut via diarrhea (Rhyne, 2003b). Some drugs will temporarily reduce potassium to allow more time for correcting the underlying cause: (1) 1 ampule of 10% calcium gluconate is administered IV, (2) combining administration of IV glucose (dextrose 50%) and IV insulin, (3) beta-adrenergic agonists such as albuterol, or (4) sodium bicarbonate (if the hyperkalemia is due to metabolic acidosis) (Brophy & Gehr, 2007). When these measures are insufficient to reduce the risks associated with hyperkalemia, patients may receive dialysis to remove the potassium (Hogan et al., 2006; Rhyne, 2003b).

When correcting hyperkalemia, the nurse should observe for possible symptoms of hypokalemia due to overcorrection.

 **CRITICAL ALERT** *In hyperkalemia, serum potassium levels greater than 6.0 mEq/L can be life threatening due to decreased ability of the heart to repolarize as evidenced by a "tented" T wave, loss of the P wave, and a wide, bizarre QRS with a depressed ST segment (Brophy & Gehr, 2007; Rhyne, 2003b). Should this occur, stop any potassium supplementation and take measures to reduce serum potassium before life-threatening dysrhythmias occur (Brophy & Gehr, 2007). Measures to reduce serum potassium are Kayexalate enemas, oral Kayexalate given with sorbitol, temporarily moving potassium into cells with the administration of IV glucose and insulin, and beta-adrenergic medications (albuterol). Renal dialysis may be needed (Brophy & Gehr, 2007; Rhyne, 2003b).*

Hypokalemia

Hypokalemia occurs when the serum potassium level is less than 3.5 mEq/L. Average daily losses of potassium are 5 to 10 mEq/L in feces, 0 to 20 mEq/L in sweat, and 40 to 120 mEq/L in urine (Rhyne, 2003b). Lowered serum potassium may or may not be reflective of total body loss of potassium due to the fact that potassium primarily is an intracellular cation. Generally, hypokalemia is not a problem unless people are receiving non–potassium-sparing diuretics, such as furosemide, bumetanide, or ethacrynic acid. Hypomagnesemia also is associated with hypokalemia. In fact, hypomagnesemia should be corrected before potassium is corrected because low magnesium promotes the loss of potassium from the kidneys (Brophy & Gehr, 2007).

Other common causes of low serum potassium are decreased potassium intake, GI and renal disorders, Cushing's disease, potassium-wasting diuretics, and elevated serum insulin (Rhyne, 2003b). Diarrhea may increase excretion of potassium to 200 mEq/day (Rhyne, 2003b). Vomiting or nasogastric suction can increase loss through GI fluids removed. Stress may predispose the body to hypokalemia because of increased aldosterone secretion in response to elevated ADH. This would result in increased sodium retention and increased potassium excretion in the urine. In acidosis serum potassium moves out of the cell to allow hydrogen ions to move intracellular to buffer pH. Hypokalemia can occur when the potassium returns to the ICF and hydrogen ions return to the serum. During the temporary movement of potassium into the ECF to buffer hydrogen ion, potassium may have been lost in the urine, resulting in hypokalemia when the acidosis is corrected (Brophy & Gehr, 2007).

Nursing Management

Nursing management of patients with hypokalemia includes assessing, planning of interventions, and evaluation.

Assessment

Clinical symptoms of hypokalemia are muscle weakness, cramps, nausea, vomiting, decreased bowel sounds with possible ileus (paralysis of the bowels), and paresthesias (Porth, 2007; Rhyne, 2003b). Cardiac manifestations of low serum potassium are a weak, irregular pulse. The ECG shows a flattened T wave followed by a U wave, which is an extra cardiac negative-deflection that is not normally present. Ventricular ectopy may be common due to slow repolarization of the myocardium and could progress to dangerous dysrhythmias, for example, ventricular tachycardia with hemodynamic changes (Rhyne, 2003b).

Planning, Interventions, and Rationales

Nursing interventions are directed at treating the underlying cause and replacing serum potassium as ordered without over-correcting it (Brophy & Gehr, 2007). A diet containing about 50 to 100 mEq of potassium daily should be provided. Vegetables such as spinach, broccoli, carrots, green beans, tomato juice, acorn squash, and potatoes are good sources of potassium (Hogan et al., 2006; Rhyne, 2003b). The usual dosage of intravenous potassium supplementation is 20 to 40 mEq/hr (Rhyne, 2003b). Intravenous potassium is essential if hypokalemia is severe or if the patient is unable to take oral potassium. Potassium is **never** administered IV push! Too rapid administration of potassium can result in hyperkalemia with life-threatening dysrhythmias and death.

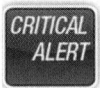 **CRITICAL ALERT**
Potassium is **never** administered IV push! Too rapid administration of potassium can result in life-threatening dysrhythmias. If potassium is replaced too quickly, hyperkalemia may result (Brophy & Gehr, 2007; Rhyne, 2003b).

The IV fluid of choice for replacing potassium is normal saline because dextrose 5% will result in free water once the glucose is utilized. This, in turn, will increase the dilution of potassium in the serum, consequently decreasing the rate of correction (Rhyne, 2003b). IV supplementation usually is reserved for severe cases of hypokalemia (<2.5 mEq/L) and for patients exhibiting cardiac symptoms of hypokalemia via ECG, patients with muscle spasms, or patients unable to take oral therapy (Brophy & Gehr, 2007). "In cases of severe potassium depletion, patients may require as much as 300–400 mEq/day. It is common practice to dilute 40–60 mEq in 1,000 mL of 0.45%

normal saline and infuse at a rate not exceeding 40 mEq/hour" (Brophy & Gehr, 2007, p. 971). It is preferable for this administration to take place under continuous ECG monitoring.

Evaluation

Supplementation of potassium should not be given unless the patient has adequate urinary output (15 to 20 mL/hr). The patient should be monitored for adequate respirations (above 12 per minute) and a peripheral oxygen saturation of >90%. Respirations may be weak due to the weakened muscle contractions present with hypokalemia (Rhyne, 2003b).

Calcium

Calcium (Ca^{2+}) is important for neuromuscular transmission, contraction of muscles, blood clotting, bone and tooth construction, cellular membrane function, and energy conversion (Hogan et al., 2006; Nielson, 2003). Cellular membrane stability relies on calcium. Calcium exerts a sedative effect on nerves (Nielson, 2003). Ninety-eight percent of calcium in the body is found in the bones and teeth. Two percent is in the blood serum (8.5 to 10.5 mg/dL, 50% ionized and 45% bound to albumin) (Nielson, 2003). Ionized calcium, 4.0 to 5.0 mg/dL, is responsible for the physiological actions of calcium, such as blood clotting and muscle contraction. Serum pH greatly affects the level of ionized calcium (Nielson, 2003). Metabolic acidosis decreases calcium binding to albumin, its carrier protein, and causes increased ionized calcium. Metabolic alkalosis has the opposite effect (Joy & Hladik, 2007). Tetany and muscle cramping occur with decreased ionized calcium levels. In the bone, calcium combines with phosphorus to form **hydroxyapatite**, the inorganic hexagonal matrix of bone (Nielson, 2003).

Regulation of calcium serum levels is controlled by vitamin D, calcitonin from the thyroid gland, and parathyroid hormone (PTH) from the parathyroid glands. PTH mobilizes calcium from the bones and causes increased reabsorption of calcium by the kidneys to increase serum calcium levels. Calcitonin inhibits calcium resorption, causes deposition of calcium in the bones and teeth, and increases renal excretion of calcium to lower serum calcium levels (Nielson, 2003). Vitamin D (cholecalciferol), a fat-soluble vitamin, is essential for the absorption of calcium and phosphorus from the gut (Joy & Hladik, 2007). It may be consumed in the diet or manufactured in the skin by ultraviolet light (Nielson, 2003). The kidneys must activate 1,25-dihydroxyvitamin D3 to vitamin D before it is physiologically active (Joy & Hladik, 2007).

Hypercalcemia

Hypercalcemia occurs when serum calcium is greater than 10.5 mg/dL or ionized calcium is greater than 5.5 mg/dL (Nielson, 2003). Symptoms may occur with an increase in total calcium or an increase in ionized calcium because it is the ionized calcium that is active. The latter may occur with acidosis (Nielson, 2003).

Three causes account for 80% of hypercalcemia: primary hyperparathyroidism (dysfunction of the parathyroid gland), bone malignancy, and drug toxicity (from thiazide-related drugs, i.e., thiazide diuretics, lithium carbonate, and vitamins A and D) (Guin, 2006). PTH mobilizes calcium from the bones and causes increased reabsorption of calcium by the kidneys, thus increasing serum calcium levels. Malignancy may involve metastases resulting in bone destruction and the liberation of calcium. Thiazide diuretics can cause renal tubule dysfunction and prevent the excretion of calcium. Vitamins A and D promote the absorption of calcium from the GI tract. Other causes of hypercalcemia are prolonged bed rest causing mobilization of bone calcium, adrenal insufficiency, hyperthyroidism, and rhabdomyolysis (massive muscle destruction resulting in release of myoglobin into the blood with subsequent clogging of the renal glomeruli) (Guin, 2006).

Clinical symptoms of hypercalcemia affect most systems/organs of the body as follows:

1. **Central nervous system**—fatigue, weakness, decreased deep tendon reflexes, headache, impaired concentration, memory defects, personality changes, confusion, lethargy, and depression (Guin, 2006; Joy & Hladik, 2007).

2. **Renal system**—polyuria, kidney stones, acute or chronic renal failure with decreasing urine concentrating ability (Joy & Hladik, 2007).

3. **Gastrointestinal system**—anorexia, nausea, vomiting, pain, constipation; in severe cases, pancreatitis (Joy & Hladik, 2007).

4. **Cardiovascular system**—cardiac dysrhythmias with shortening of the ST segment and QT interval and a prolonged PR interval that can lead to heart block and possible cardiac arrest (Guin, 2006). Hypertension usually is present. "Calcium or calcium-phosphorus complex deposition in blood vessels and multiple organs is a complication of chronic hypercalcemia and/or concomitant hyperphosphatemia and hyperparathyroidism" (Joy & Hladik, 2007, p. 951). These atherosclerotic lesions contribute to heart and vascular disease.

5. **Musculoskeletal system**—muscle weakness, acute arthritis, painful joints, itching, and bony cysts.

6. **Eyes and skin**—conjunctival calcifications leading to conjunctivitis. The severity of the symptoms is proportionate to the level of hypercalcemia. Soft tissue calcifications may occur throughout the body if calcium and phosphorus are elevated simultaneously (Porth, 2007). When excess calcium deposits in the skin, it can cause **calciphylaxis** (Beitz, 2004). Lesions occur primarily in the lower extremities as irregular violet plaques or nodules. They are painful and pruritic and may progress to necrosis and gangrene.

■ Nursing Management

Treatment of hypercalcemia basically is treatment of the underlying cause, that is, partial parathyroidectomy for excess PTH, chemotherapy for malignancy, discontinuation of vitamins A and D and calcium supplementation with a low calcium diet, and discontinuation of thiazide diuretics.

Assessment

As with all electrolyte imbalances, assessment of the patient is critical. Key factors include monitoring the patient's intake and output to prevent fluid overload and ensure adequate kidney function. The patient should be turned carefully to avoid possible pathologic fractures secondary to calcium mobilization from the bones. The nurse also should auscultate breath sounds for "crackles" and rhonchi and heart sounds for the development of an S_3 heart sound with vital signs to detect fluid overload at earliest onset (O'Gara & Braunwald, 2001). In the event that the patient is on digitalis, digitalis toxicity must be considered.

Planning, Interventions, and Rationales

Frequently, normal saline is administered rapidly concurrently with furosemide to dilute the blood and result in increased calcium secretion. Cortisone may be given to compete with vitamin D and decrease calcium absorption (Nielson, 2003). Bisphosphonates can be given to reduce decalcification of the bone in the presence of malignancy. Weight-bearing activity will reduce bone resorption. Calcitonin can be given to promote calcium deposition in the bone and increase calcium excretion. Gallium nitrate may be given to inhibit malignancy-related bone resorption.

 *When treating hypercalcemia, if the patient is also receiving digitalis, monitor for digitalis toxicity (visual green halo around objects, serum level > 2 ng/mL) to avoid the occurrence of lethal dysrhythmias (Joy & Hladik, 2007; Nielson, 2003).*

Hypocalcemia

Hypocalcemia occurs when the serum calcium level is less than 8.5 mg/dL and ionized levels are less than 4.0 mg/dL (Nielson, 2003). Because physiological effects are dependent on ionized calcium, symptoms of hypocalcemia may occur at higher serum levels, especially with a rise in serum pH (Nielson, 2003). Hypocalcemia can occur if the patient receives a large volume of citrated blood because the citrate combines with calcium, thus deactivating it.

Causes of hypocalcemia are reduced calcium intake or absorption (vitamin D deficiency or excessive phosphorous intake), decreased PTH, elevated serum phosphorus, decreased magnesium levels, hypoalbuminemia, and alkalosis. Often, the parathyroid glands are disrupted following thyroid surgery and PTH is reduced. Unless the parathyroid glands were accidentally removed with the thyroid gland, this condition will be temporary (Joy & Hladik, 2007). To monitor this condition, serum calcium concentrations should be checked every 6 hours for 1 to 2 days following thyroid surgery (Joy & Hladik, 2007). On a worldwide basis, vitamin D deficiency is the most common cause of hypocalcemia. Rickets and osteomalacia result (Joy & Hladik, 2007).

Phosphorus and calcium combine in the GI tract under the influence of vitamin D and are exchanged for one another in the kidney. Gastrointestinal surgery, chronic pancreatitis, and small-bowel disease can result in decreased levels of vitamin D and, thus, decrease calcium and phosphorous absorption. Vitamin D supplementation may be needed by an intravenous route (Joy & Hladik, 2007). Renal failure may decrease phosphorous excretion and result in excessive calcium loss. Large calcium losses may occur if the patient is taking loop diuretics (Nielson, 2003). Pancreatitis may cause decreased levels of ionized calcium because of free fatty acids binding calcium (Nielson,

2003). Severe hypomagnesemia also may be associated with severe symptomatic hypocalcemia (Joy & Hladik, 2007).

The faster the drop in serum calcium, the more acute the symptoms become. Symptoms of hypocalcemia are changes in the ECG showing prolonged QT intervals and cardiac contractility that could progress to congestive heart failure (Joy & Hladik, 2007). Dysrhythmias, bradycardia, and hypotension could occur (Joy & Hladik, 2007). Patients with low calcium experience numbness and tingling of the fingers and circumoral area, hyperactive reflexes, muscle cramps, laryngeal spasm, bronchospasm, muscle tetany, confusion, hallucinations, and possible tonic-clonic seizures (Joy & Hladik, 2007; Nielson, 2003). Mental changes can include anxiety, depression, or even psychosis. Pathologic fractures may occur due to calcium-poor bones. Trousseau's sign (carpopedal spasm) or Chvostek's sign may be present. Trousseau's sign is induced by inflating a blood pressure cuff on the upper arm 20 mm above the systolic blood pressure and maintaining the inflation for 3 minutes, resulting in wrist and fingers contracting inward (Nielson, 2003). Chvostek's sign is twitching of the facial muscles obtained by tapping the facial nerve just below the temple on the zygomatic arch. Laryngeal spasm can occur with severe hypocalcemia, resulting in asphyxiation (Nielson, 2003).

◼ Nursing Management

Treatment of hypocalcemia includes oral or IV administration of calcium.

Planning, Interventions, and Rationales

Phosphorous levels should be checked to ensure that hyperphosphatemia is not the cause of the hypocalcemia (Joy & Hladik, 2007). "The elevated levels of calcium and phosphorus product result in precipitation in the arteries, joints, soft tissues and viscera and can result in tissue ischemia termed, calciphylaxis" (Joy & Hladik, 2007, p. 959). For tetany, 10 to 20 mL of 10% calcium gluconate is given IV push at a rate of 0.5 mL/min or by piggyback infusion in 100 mL of 10% calcium gluconate in a 1-L bag of D5W over at least 4 hours (Guin, 2006).

Too rapid administration of calcium can result in cardiac arrest or hypotension. Calcium gluconate is usually preferred over calcium chloride because calcium gluconate is less irritating to veins. "Calcium should not be infused at a rate greater than 60 mg of elemental calcium per minute because severe cardiac dysfunction may result" (Joy & Hladik, 2007, p. 957). Intravenous calcium should be administered with caution in patients taking digitalis glycosides because cardiac dysrhythmias could result. Calcium should not be administered in the same IV line as sodium bicarbonate because a precipitation could result, causing adverse effects (Joy & Hladik, 2007). "The bolus of calcium is usually only effective for one to two hours and should be followed by a continuous infusion of elemental calcium at a rate of 0.5 to 2 mg/kg per hour. Serum calcium concentrations should be monitored every four to six hours during the intravenous infusion" (Joy & Hladik, 2007, p. 958).

Replacement of magnesium should be considered because hypomagnesemia-induced hypocalcemia may recur if calcium is administered alone. Vitamin D should be administered to facili-

tate calcium absorption from the GI tract. Phosphate-binding antacids may be given to reduce phosphorous levels to promote calcium absorption (Nielson, 2003). Oral calcium and vitamin D supplements will be prescribed for patients with chronic hypocalcemia. Discharge instructions include that oral calcium should be taken 30 minutes before meals or at bedtime for maximum absorption. Phosphorous-binding antacids should be taken with meals (Nielson, 2003).

 *With hypocalcemia, sudden drops in blood pressure may occur because of vasodilation and decreased cardiac contractility with rapid administration of IV calcium. Infuse calcium at a rate less than 0.5 to 1 mL/min to avoid hypotension (Joy & Hladik, 2007; Nielson, 2003). Observe closely the type of calcium that is administered because of similarity in packaging. Calcium chloride contains 13.6 mEq of calcium and calcium gluconate contains 4.5 mEq of calcium (both come in 10-mL ampules). To relieve tetany, 10 to 20 mL of 10% calcium gluconate is given IV push or piggyback infusion over at least 4 hours (Joy & Hladik, 2007; Nielson, 2003).*

Magnesium

Magnesium (Mg^{2+}) is an intracellular cation. More than 50% of body magnesium is stored in muscle and bone and only 1% is in the blood (1.4 to 2.1 mg/dL) (Adkins, 2003). Two-thirds of serum magnesium exists in ionized form and one-third is bound to plasma proteins. Forty-five percent of magnesium in the body is intracellular with most of it in the mitochondria where it is a cofactor in enzymatic activities and contributes to neuromuscular interactions, neurotransmission, and cardiac contraction (Adkins, 2003). Magnesium is involved in energy conversion of adenosine triphosphate, carbohydrate metabolism, protein synthesis, and muscular contraction (Adkins, 2003).

Magnesium is absorbed from the diet and excreted by the kidney. The body's requirement for magnesium is 4.5 mg/kg of body weight. In the average diet, 168 to 720 mg of magnesium are consumed each day (Adkins, 2003). The proportion absorbed by the GI tract varies with the amount consumed. Sources of magnesium in the diet are green leafy vegetables, nuts, legumes, seafood, whole grains, bananas, oranges, and chocolate. Magnesium absorption decreases in kidney disease because vitamin D is not activated. Phytates, oxalates, and fat in the diet decrease magnesium absorption. In magnesium-depleted states, absorption of magnesium competes with calcium absorption. When calcium absorption goes up, magnesium absorption goes down (Adkins, 2003). Average daily urinary excretion of magnesium is 100 mg/dL in men and 90 mg/dL in women. The kidney reabsorbs 20% to 30% of filtered magnesium. Excessive magnesium losses occur with diuresis (Adkins, 2003). Alcohol ingestion decreases renal magnesium reabsorption.

Hypermagnesemia

Hypermagnesemia (serum levels greater than 2.1 mg/dL) may occur due to renal failure (Adkins, 2003). It can occur in people with adrenal insufficiency or in obstetrical settings where women receive intravenous magnesium to decrease symptoms of pregnancy-induced hypertension (Adkins, 2003).

Clinical manifestations are related to decreased neuromuscular activity, such as those seen in hyperkalemia. Cardiovascular symptoms are hypotension, bradycardia, flushing and sense of warmth, and possible respiratory or cardiac arrest (Adkins, 2003). Gastrointestinal symptoms are nausea and vomiting; neurological symptoms are mental changes (drowsiness), respiratory depression, and decreased deep tendon reflex (Adkins, 2003). Deep tendon reflexes are usually lost at 8 mg/dL and respiratory failure is likely if the serum level exceeds 10 mg/dL. Coma can occur at a level of 10 mg/dL, and cardiac arrest is possible at levels >15 mg/dL (Porth, 2007).

 ## Nursing Management

Assessment

Nursing assessments should include tendon reflex as well as respiratory status. Both can be compromised with an increased magnesium serum level. The IV site should be monitored closely because extravasated calcium can result in tissue sloughing (Adkins, 2003).

Planning, Interventions, and Rationales

Treatment for serious hypermagnesemia includes immediate cessation of magnesium-containing products, IV push administration of 10 mL of 10% calcium gluconate, or dialysis. If the kidneys are intact, 0.45% normal saline may be given intravenously with diuretics to promote the renal excretion of magnesium (Adkins, 2003).

 CRITICAL ALERT *In hypermagnesemia, the deep tendon reflex is lost at 8 mEq/L and respiratory failure is likely if the serum level exceeds 10 mEq/L (Adkins, 2003; Brophy & Gehr, 2007).*

Complete heart block may occur at levels of more than 15 mEq/L (Adkins, 2003). If this occurs stop magnesium-containing products and provide IV push administration of 10 mL of 10% calcium gluconate or dialysis.

Hypomagnesemia

Hypomagnesemia (serum magnesium of <1.4 mg/dL) occurs because of malnutrition (inadequate intake of magnesium-containing foods) or increased urinary excretion of magnesium due to alcoholism, osmotic diuresis in diabetes, and loop diuretics. It may occur by GI loss with vomiting, diarrhea, or malabsorption syndromes (Adkins, 2003). The most common cause is a combination of factors. Hypomagnesemia, in turn, is a cause of hypertension, cardiac dysrhythmias, and sudden cardiac death (Adkins, 2003; Brophy & Gehr, 2007).

Symptoms of hypomagnesemia are most common when the serum level is ≤1 mg/dL (Adkins, 2003). Severe deficiency may cause confusion, lethargy, seizures, hyperreflexia of deep tendon reflexes, tetany, hallucinations, nausea and vomiting, hypertension, cardiac dysrhythmias, and death (Adkins, 2003). Cardiac symptoms include supraventricular tachycardia, possible coronary artery spasms, and paresthesia (Adkins, 2003). Digitalis toxicity occurs more frequently with low serum magnesium (Adkins, 2003).

 ## Nursing Management

Treatment for hypomagnesemia is parenteral and oral administration of magnesium supplements.

Planning, Interventions, and Rationales

Severe hypomagnesemia is treated with the IV route. IV magnesium must be administered carefully with close observation because of the possibility of developing hypermagnesemia due to overcorrection. Chronic, less severe hypomagnesemia is treated with oral magnesium salts, magnesium-containing antacids, and foods high in magnesium.

 CRITICAL ALERT *When treating hypomagnesemia, IV magnesium must be administered carefully with close observations because of the possibility of developing hypermagnesemia.*

Phosphorus

Eighty-five percent of phosphorus is in a structural matrix with calcium and collagen forming teeth and bones (Rawls & Hogan, 2003). The remainder is found intracellularly and in blood (2.5 to 4.5 mg/dL) (Rawls & Hogan, 2003). **Phosphorus** is essential to carbohydrate, lipid, and protein metabolism and to nerve and muscle function (Rawls & Hogan, 2003). It is part of the basic energy units of the body, adenosine triphosphate (ATP), adenosine diphosphate (ADP), and adenosine monophosphate (AMP). Phosphorus is in phospholipids, which make up the cellular and organelle membranes. It is found in red blood cells in 2,3-diphosphoglycerate, which is a hormone that increases the amount of oxygen carried in red blood cells (Rawls & Hogan, 2003).

About 800 to 1,600 mg of phosphorus is consumed per day and absorbed with the help of vitamin D. Phosphate levels are regulated by calcitonin, parathyroid hormone, and vitamin D in conjunction with calcium regulation (Rawls & Hogan, 2003). PTH blocks the reabsorption of phosphorus. When calcium is reabsorbed from the kidney tubules, phosphate is excreted (Rawls & Hogan, 2003). However, normally 80% to 90% of phosphorus is reabsorbed. Plasma phosphorous levels vary with acid–base balance. The consumption of glucose, insulin, or sugar-containing foods temporarily shifts phosphorus into the cells.

Hyperphosphatemia

Phosphorous balance is regulated primarily by the kidneys (Rawls & Hogan, 2003). Hyperphosphatemia (serum levels greater than 4.5 mg/dL) is due chiefly to renal disease and decreased excretion of phosphorus (Rawls & Hogan, 2003). Other causes may be excessive phosphate replacement or the overuse of phosphate-based enemas (Rawls & Hogan, 2003). Acidosis may cause an extracellular shift of phosphorus because phosphate serves as a buffering anion in acidosis. Cellular destruction, such as with malignancy, chemotherapy, radiation therapy, or rhabdomyolysis, may release large amounts of phosphate because it is mostly an intracellular anion (Rawls & Hogan, 2003). As serum phosphorous levels increase, serum calcium decreases, which may result in hypocalcemia.

The most common complication of hyperphosphatemia is the deposition of calcium phosphate in soft tissues. This occurs when the product of the serum calcium level and serum phosphorous level exceeds 70 mg/dL (Rawls & Hogan, 2003). Deposition of calcium phosphate in the heart muscle could result in cardiac dysrhythmias. Symptoms directly due to hyperphosphatemia are few. Most adverse symptoms relate to the resulting hypocalcemia.

■ Nursing Management

Planning, Interventions, and Rationales

Treatment for hyperphosphatemia is administration of phosphorous-binding antacids, such as calcium carbonate or calcium acetate (Rawls & Hogan, 2003). Phosphorous absorption is reduced and excretion of phosphorus in the feces is increased. Calcium-based antacids are preferred in renal failure because of the potential for hypermagnesemia (Rawls & Hogan, 2003). If hyperphosphatemia is accompanied by hypocalcemia, the correction of the calcium level may reduce the phosphate level (Joy & Hladik, 2007).

 *Deposition of calcium phosphate in soft tissues can occur as a result of hyperphosphatemia when the product of serum calcium and phosphorous levels exceeds 70 mg/dL. In heart muscle, this could result in cardiac dysrhythmias (Joy & Hladik, 2007; Rawls & Hogan, 2003). This phenomenon occurs primarily with renal failure. As serum phosphorus levels increase, there is a simultaneous drop in calcium, resulting in symptoms of hypocalcemia (Joy & Hladik, 2007; Rawls & Hogan, 2003).*

Hypophosphatemia

Hypophosphatemia occurs when the serum phosphate level is less than 2.0 mg/dL (Medline Plus, 2006; Rawls & Hogan, 2003). Common causes are vitamin D deficiency, bowel disorders that lead to malabsorption, excessive use of phosphate-binding antacids (aluminum hydroxide or magnesium hydroxide), alcoholism, or diabetic ketoacidosis. Prolonged respiratory alkalosis can contribute significantly to hypophosphatemia (Joy & Hladik, 2007; Rawls & Hogan, 2003). In acidosis, such as diabetic ketoacidosis, phosphate is consumed as an acid buffer (Rawls & Hogan, 2003). The kidney may fail to reabsorb phosphorus in the presence of elevated PTH. Rhabdomyolysis (breakdown of striated muscle) also may be a source due to heat stroke, viral infections, or catabolic states (Rawls & Hogan, 2003).

Phosphate deficiency commonly impairs neurological function, which may be manifested by confusion, seizures, and coma. Peripheral neuropathy and ascending motor paralysis, similar to Guillain-Barré syndrome, may occur. Extrapontine myelinolysis has been reported (Mailhot, Richard, & Hemphill, 2006).

Hematologic function also may be impaired. The hemolytic anemia associated with severe hypophosphatemia has been attributed to the inability of erythrocytes to maintain integrity of cell membranes in the face of ATP depletion, leading to their destruction in the spleen. Phosphate deficiency also compromises oxygen delivery to the tissues due to decreases in erythrocyte 2,3-DPG and the resulting leftward shift in the oxygen–hemoglobin dissociation curve. Diminished oxygen delivery to the brain may be the cause of some of the neurologic manifestations mentioned earlier (Mailhot et al., 2006).

■ Nursing Management

Assessment

Clinical symptoms of hypophosphatemia are decreased availability of ADP and reduced oxygen-carrying capacity of red blood cells because of 2,3-diphosphoglycerate deficiency with a shift of the oxygen–hemoglobin dissociation curve to the left (greater resistance of oxygen release to the tissues) (Joy & Hladik, 2007; Rawls & Hogan, 2003). Tissue hypoxia can cause dysrhythmias and heart block. If the deficiency is severe, it can result in metabolic encephalopathy syndrome, in which the patient may be irritable, confused and have seizures or chest pain. Respiratory failure is possible due to muscular weakness and diaphragmatic contractile dysfunction (Joy & Hladik, 2007). Thus, phosphate serum monitoring is indicated for patients with respiratory weakness. Neurological symptoms may include apathy, delirium, hallucinations, and paranoia (Joy & Hladik, 2007). Bones may be weakened due to resorption of the bone matrix to salvage phosphate (Rawls & Hogan, 2003). Bone pain and pathologic fractures may occur due to mobilization of phosphate to replace serum losses (Joy & Hladik, 2007).

Planning, Interventions, and Rationales

Treatment of hypophosphatemia is by treating the underlying cause and promoting a high phosphate diet, especially milk, if it is tolerated. Other foods high in phosphate are dried beans and peas, eggs, fish, organ meats (brain, liver, kidney), Brazil nuts and peanuts, poultry, seeds (pumpkin, sesame, sunflower), and whole grains (oats, barley, bran) (Rawls & Hogan, 2003) (see Chapter 14 ✑). Phosphate-binding antacids should be avoided. Mild hypophosphatemia may be corrected by oral supplements, such as Neutra-Phos liquid (sodium and potassium phosphate) or Phospho-Soda (sodium phosphate) (Rawls & Hogan, 2003). Intravenous phosphate salts are not commonly administered to correct hypophosphatemia because of the danger of hyperphosphatemia causing hypocalcemia followed by tetany (Rawls & Hogan, 2003). The IV route is reserved for cases of severe hypophosphatemia or in situations where the bowel is not functioning (Mailhot et al., 2006; Rawls & Hogan, 2003). When intravenous hyperalimentation solutions are administered, 12 to 15 mmol/L of phosphorus should be added (Joy & Hladik, 2007). Acidosis should be corrected, whether metabolic or respiratory.

 *The IV route of phosphate is reserved for cases of severe hypophosphatemia or in situations where the bowel is not functioning because of the danger of hyperphosphatemia (Joy & Hladik, 2007; Rawls & Hogan, 2003). Acidosis should be corrected, whether metabolic or respiratory. Respiratory alkalosis causes serum phosphorus to move into the cells, thereby aggravating hypophosphatemia (Joy & Hladik, 2007; Rawls & Hogan, 2003).*

Chloride

Chloride (Cl$^-$) is the primary anion in the ECF (blood level: 95 to 108 mEq/L) (Covington, 2003). Chloride combines with sodium to create electrical neutrality in the body; therefore, it usually is found in combination with sodium (Covington, 2003). It assists in the reabsorption of sodium in the kidneys (Covington, 2003). Another major function of chloride is to combine with hydrogen ion (H$^+$) to form hydrochloric acid for digestion and hydrolyzing nutrients for absorption in the GI tract. An ample amount of chloride ion is essential for reabsorbing hydrogen ion in the kidneys to buffer alkalosis. Bicarbonate is another major anion in the ECF, and chloride tends to vary inversely with the changes in bicarbonate (Covington, 2003).

When carbon dioxide increases in the blood, chloride moves to the intracellular space to allow bicarbonate into the blood to buffer the carbonic acid. The range of variation of chloride in response to bicarbonate is 10 to 20 mEq/L (Rhyne, 2003a).

Chloride is consumed with sodium in the diet in the form of salt with the recommended daily allowance being 750mg/day. Normal excretion of acid by the kidneys includes the excretion of chloride. Chloride is lost through vomiting, excessive sweating, and in the urine, especially with diuretics (Covington, 2003). Because the serum chloride level usually remains so stable, it is used to calculate the "anion gap" (Rhyne, 2003a). The anion gap is calculated by adding the chloride and bicarbonate levels together and deducting it from the sum of the sodium and potassium levels (Rhyne, 2003a). A normal anion gap is 15 to 30. Anion gaps above 30 indicate excess organic acids, such as lactic acid or ketone acids (Rhyne, 2003a).

Hyperchloremia

Hyperchloremia (serum chloride > 108 mEq/L) may result from metabolic acidosis (arterial pH < 7.35). Common causes are hyperparathyroidism, dehydration, and respiratory alkalosis. Symptoms are increased depth and rate of respiration, lethargy, stupor, disorientation, and coma if the acidosis is not treated (Covington, 2003).

 *Hyperchloremic acidosis occurs when serum Cl^- ion levels are increased, and can develop as the result of abnormal absorption of Cl^- by the kidneys or as a result of treatment with chloride-containing medications (i.e., sodium chloride, amino acid-chloride hyperalimenation solutions, and ammonium chloride). Metabolic acidosis is characterized by a decrease in pH (<7.35) and a decrease in serum HCO_3 levels (<24mEq/L). Though metabolic acidosis seldom is a primary disorder, the nurse should be aware of signs and symptoms of metabolic acidosis that typically begin to appear when plasma HCO_3^- falls to 20mEq/L or less. Acidosis typically produces a compensatory increase in respiratory rate with a decrease in PCO_2. Additional compensatory mechanisms of hyperchloremic acidosis are: hyperkalemia, acid urine, and increased ammonia in urine. Symptomatic manifestations of hyperchloremic acidosis include disorders of the gastrointestinal, nervous, and cardiovascular systems, including anorexia, nausea and vomiting, abdominal pain, weakness, lethargy, confusion, peripheral vasodilation, increased heart rate, and cardiac arrhythmias. The skin also may be warm and flushed (Porth, 2007).*

Hypochloremia

Hypochloremia (95 mEq/L) occurs due to loss of gastric fluids in the form of hydrochloric acid with nasogastric suctioning and severe vomiting (Covington, 2003). Serum chloride will be reduced and bicarbonate significantly elevated (30 to 40 mEq/L). One cause is stomach pyloric obstruction due to duodenal ulcer or prolonged vomiting, possibly due to bowel obstruction (Covington, 2003). Diabetic ketoacidosis may result in chloride loss because of the osmotic diuresis and elevated bicarbonate. A rare condition is Bartter's syndrome, a congenital defect that prevents renal chloride reabsorption (Devarajan, 2006)

Hypochloremia may cause hypochloremic alkalosis with chloride levels < 95 mEq/L and arterial serum pH > 7.45. Bicarbonate will be excessively retained to maintain electrical neutrality and buffer acid–base imbalances (Rhyne, 2003a).

Symptoms of alkalosis are paresthesias of the face and extremities, muscle spasms and tetany, slow and shallow respirations, and dehydration.

 *Hypochloremia results when there is an abnormal depleted level of the chloride into in the blood. It rarely occurs in isolation, but is usually seen in combination with other disorders. Extra renal courses included inadequate sodium chloride intake, loses of certain gastrointestinal fluids (e.g., vomiting and nasogastric suction, or diarrhea as a result of abnormalities in small bowel transport), and loss of fluids through the skin occurring as a result of trauma, e.g., burns. Metabolic alkalosis may result in which case signs of compensation include decreased respirations (rate and depth) with various degrees of hypoxia and respiratory acidosis. Nervous system effects may include: hyperactive reflexes, tetany, confusion, and seizures. Cardiovascular system effects may include hypertension and cardiac arrhythmias (Porth, 2007).*

Collaborative Management

Care of the patient with electrolyte imbalances involves collaboration with a multidisciplinary team. The health care provider directs the patient's care and writes medication, fluid replacement, and laboratory test orders to ascertain the electrolyte status and the outcomes of directed therapies. Pharmacists ensure that the IV fluids and medications administered will bring about the desired change in the patient. Nurses are vigilant at the bedside to notify the health care provider of changes in the patient's clinical condition. Dietitians provide specified diets and nutritional teaching when patients are allowed to eat and are ready for discharge. The team collaboration aspect of care is reflected in the patient care plans included in this chapter.

Research

Opportunities for nursing research related to fluid and electrolyte imbalances are investigations into ways of promoting patient awareness of problems with electrolyte abnormalities and corrective actions to be taken. Because of emphasis on prevention of osteoporosis, nutritional research might address overuse of antacids in combination with high milk ingestion or calcium-supplement therapy. The Research Opportunities and Clinical Impact box (p. 434) outlines research topics on the area of fluid and electrolyte imblances.

Summary

The human body has a complex internal environment that requires cations and anions to balance in the proper fluid volume and space (ICF or ECF). Sodium, potassium, chloride, bicarbonate, calcium, magnesium, and phosphorus have separate roles and precise levels. Cellular life cannot exist outside these boundaries; cellular swelling or shrinkage is fatal. Proper maintenance of electrochemical and neuromuscular activity is dependent on each electrolyte being present in the proper ECF or ICF compartment when it is needed.

When the complexity of the body and human nature is examined, one is amazed by the intricacies of balance that are required to keep bodily systems functioning in normal conditions. Nurses can assist patients by educating them on electrolyte abnormalities that may occur as a result of disease processes and how to avoid health problems.

RESEARCH OPPORTUNITIES AND CLINICAL IMPACT RELATED TO FLUID AND ELECTROLYTE IMBALANCES

Research Area	Clinical Impact
Overuse of antacids in combination with high milk ingestion or calcium-supplement therapy	Prevention of osteoporosis
Low serum magnesium in diabetics due to the diuresis associated with hyperglycemia	Determining what role, if any, this electrolyte abnormality plays in cardiac symptoms in the diabetic population
Assessing the accuracy of bedside monitoring of intake and output reports	Improving the quality of data on patients' intakes and outputs of fluids

NCLEX® REVIEW

1. A patient is experiencing nausea with severe vomiting. The nurse realizes that this patient is at risk for which of the following?
   1. Interstitial fluid volume overload
   2. Intracellular fluid volume deficit
   3. Extracellular fluid volume deficit
   4. Interstitial fluid volume deficit

2. A male patient's hematocrit is 56% with serum sodium of 150 mEq/L and potassium of 5.8 mEq/L. Which of the following would be indicated for this patient?
   1. Prepare to administer a hypertonic intravenous solution.
   2. Prepare to administer a hypotonic intravenous solution.
   3. Prepare to administer an isotonic intravenous solution.
   4. Implement a fluid and sodium restriction for the patient.

3. The nurse is caring for a patient and has just received the laboratory data report. Which of the following results would cause the most concern to the nurse?
   1. Na+: 115 mEq/L
   2. K+: 4.0 mEq/L
   3. Ca+: 9 mg/dL
   4. Mg+: 2.0 mg/dL

4. The nurse is caring for a patient with severe vomiting and diarrhea and a nasogastric tube to low wall suction. The nurse realizes that this patient is at risk for which of the following electrolyte imbalances?
   1. Hypokalemia
   2. Hypercalcemia
   3. Hypermagnesemia
   4. Hypophosphatemia

5. A patient is admitted to the hospital with a fluid volume excess. Which of the following will the nurse most likely assess for this patient?
   1. Dependent edema
   2. Blood pressure: 92/55 mmHg
   3. Respiratory rate 14 breaths/minute and unlabored
   4. Heart rate 86 beats per minute without ectopy

6. The nurse is caring for a patient in renal failure with a serum potassium level of 7.1 mEq/L. Which of the following should the nurse do first to assist this patient?
   1. Assess level of consciousness
   2. Measure urine output hourly
   2. Have arterial blood gases drawn
   4. Obtain an electrocardiogram

7. The nurse is providing discharge instructions to a patient with hypokalemia. Which of the following should the nurse include in these instructions?
   1. Take oral Kaexylate as prescribed.
   2. Limit the intake of spinach and carrots, and green, leafy vegetables.
   3. Eat a balanced diet including tomato juice and potatoes.
   4. Expect muscle cramps and weakness for at least six weeks.

Answers for review questions appear in Appendix D

KEY TERMS

PEARSON
EXPLORE **mynursingkit**™

MyNursingKit is your one stop for online chapter review materials and resources. Prepare for success with additional NCLEX®-style practice questions, interactive assignments and activities, web links, animations and videos, and more!

Register your access code from the front of your book at
www.mynursingkit.com

REFERENCES

Adkins, J. A. (2003). Magnesium balance and imbalances. In M. A. Hogan & D. Wane (Eds.), *Fluids, electrolytes, and acid–base balance: Reviews and rationales* (pp. 113–126). Upper Saddle River, NJ: Pearson Prentice Hall.

Ahlquist, D. A., & Camilleri, M. (2001). Diarrhea and constipation. In E. Braunwald, A. S. Fauci, D. L. Kasper, S. L. Hauser, D. L. Longo, & J. L. Jameson (Eds.), *Harrison's principles of internal medicine* (15th ed., pp. 241–249). New York: McGraw-Hill.

Beitz, J. M. (2004). Wound wise: Calciphylaxis. *American Journal of Nursing, 104*, 36–37.

Bomback, A. S., & Klemmer, P. J. (2007). The incidence and implications of aldosterone breakthrough. *Nature Clinical Practice of Nephrology, 3*(9), 486–492.

Bond, E. F. (2000). Cardiac anatomy and physiology. In S. L. Woods, E. S. Sivarajan Froelicher, & S. A. Underhill Motzer (Eds.), *Cardiac nursing* (4th ed.). Philadelphia: Lippincott Williams & Wilkins.

Brophy, D. F., & Gehr, T. W. B. (2007). Disorders of potassium and magnesium homeostasis. In J. T. DiPiro, R. L. Talbert, G. C. Yee, G. R. Matzke, B. G. Wells, & L. M. Posey (Eds.), *Pharmacotherapy: A pathophysiologic approach* (6th ed., pp. 967–981). New York: McGraw-Hill.

Covington, L. W. (2003). Chloride balance and imbalances. In M. A. Hogan & D. Wane (Eds.), *Fluids, electrolytes, and acid–base balance: Reviews and rationales* (pp. 127–144). Upper Saddle River, NJ: Pearson Prentice Hall.

Devarajan, S. (2006). Bartter Syndrome. *Emedicine*. Retrieved June 14, 2006 from http://www.emedicine.com/PED/topic210.htm

Felver, L. (2000). Fluids and electrolytes balance and imbalance. In S. L. Woods, E. S. Sivarajan Froelicher, & S. A. Underhill Motzer (Eds.), *Cardiac nursing* (4th ed., pp. 132–148). Philadelphia: Lippincott Williams & Wilkins.

Goldstein-Fuchs, D. J., & McQuiston, B. (2003). Renal failure. In L. E. Matarese & M. M. Gottschlich (Eds.), *Contemporary nutrition support practice: A clinical guide* (2nd ed., pp. 460–483). Philadelphia: W. B. Saunders.

Goyne, J. S. (2003). Fluid balances and imbalances. In M. A. Hogan & D. Wane (Eds.), *Fluids, electrolytes, and acid–base balance: Reviews and rationales* (pp. 1–36). Upper Saddle River, NJ: Pearson Prentice Hall.

Grandjean, A. C., Reimers, K. J., & Buyck, M. E. (2003). Hydration: Issues for the 21st century. *Nutrition Reviews, 61*(8), 261–271.

Guin, P. R. (2006). Endocrine disorders. In *Lippincott manual of nursing practice* (8th ed., pp. 873–909). Philadelphia: Lippincott Williams & Wilkins.

Gums, J. G., & Tovar, J. M. (2007). Adrenal gland disorders. In J. T. DiPiro, R. L. Talbert, G. C. Yee, G. R. Matzke, B. G. Wells, & L. M. Posey (Eds.), *Pharmacotherapy: A pathophysiologic approach* (6th ed., pp. 1391–1406). New York: McGraw-Hill.

Hogan, M. A., Gingrich, M. M., Ricci, M. J., & Overby, P. (2006). *Fluids, electrolytes, and acid–base balance* (2nd ed.). Upper Saddle River, NJ: Pearson Prentice Hall.

Indiana State University. (2007). *Nursing management of fluids and electrolytes: Daily weights*. Retrieved November 25, 2007, from http://www.indstate.edu/mary/Fluidlytecf/slide13.htm

Johnson, A. P. (2007). Sodium balance and imbalances. In M. A. Hogan & D. Wane (Eds.), *Fluids, electrolytes, and acid–base balance: Reviews and rationales* (pp. 37–59). Upper Saddle River, NJ: Pearson Prentice Hall.

Joy, M. S., & Hladik, G. A. (2007). Disorders of sodium, water, calcium and phosphorus homeostasis. In J. T. DiPiro, R. L. Talbert, G. C. Yee, G. R. Matzke, B. G. Wells, & L. M. Posey (Eds.), *Pharmacotherapy: A pathophysiologic approach* (6th ed., pp. 937–966). New York: McGraw-Hill.

Mailhot, T., Richard, A. J., & Hemphill, R. R. (2006). *Hypophosphatemia*. Retrieved February 16, 2008, from eMedicine website: http://www.emedicine.com/emerg/topic278.htm

Medline Plus. (2006). *Serum phosphorus*. Retrieved February 16, 2008, from http://www.nlm.nih.gov/medlineplus/ency/article/003478.htm

Metheny, N. M. (2000). *Fluid and electrolyte balance* (4th ed.). Philadelphia: Lippincott Williams & Wilkins.

Mushnick, R. (2007). Osmolality. *Medline Plus*. Retrieved June 14, 2008 from http://www.nim.nih.gov/medlinieplus/ency/article/003463.htm

Nielson, K. A. (2003). Calcium balance and imbalances. In M. A. Hogan & D. Wane (Eds.), *Fluids, electrolytes, and acid–base balance: Reviews and rationales* (pp. 85–112). Upper Saddle River, NJ: Pearson Prentice Hall.

O'Gara, P. T., & Braunwald, E. (2001). Approach to a patient with a heart murmur. In E. Braunwald, A. S. Fauci, D. L. Kasper, S. L. Hauser, D. L. Longo, & J. L. Jameson (Eds.), *Harrison's principles of internal medicine* (15th ed., pp. 207–210). New York: McGraw-Hill.

Porth, C.M. (2007). Essentials *of pathophysiology: Concepts of altered health states*. Philadelphia: Lippincott Williams & Wilkins.

Rawls, M. C., & Hogan, M. A. (2003). Phosphorus balance and imbalances. In M. A. Hogan & D. Wane (Eds.), *Fluids, electrolytes, and acid–base balance: Reviews and rationales* (pp. 145–163). Upper Saddle River, NJ: Pearson Prentice Hall.

Rhyne, L. (2003a). Acid–base balance and imbalances. In M. A. Hogan & D. Wane (Eds.), *Fluids, electrolytes, and acid–base balance: Reviews and rationales* (pp. 165–192). Upper Saddle River, NJ: Pearson Prentice Hall.

Rhyne, L. (2003b). Potassium balance and imbalances. In M. A. Hogan & D. Wane (Eds.), *Fluids, electrolytes, and acid–base balance: Reviews and rationales* (pp. 61–83). Upper Saddle River, NJ: Pearson Prentice Hall.

Saseen, J. J., & Carter, B. L. (2005). Hypertension. In J. T. DiPiro, R. L. Talbert, G. C. Yee, G. R. Matzke, B. G. Wells, & L. M. Posey (Eds.), *Pharmacotherapy: A pathophysiologic approach* (6th ed., pp. 185–218). New York: McGraw-Hill.

Singer, G. G., & Brenner, B. M. (2001). Fluid and electrolyte disturbances. In E. Braunwald, A. S. Fauci, D. L. Kasper, S. L. Hauser, D. L. Longo, & J. L. Jameson (Eds.), *Harrison's principles of internal medicine* (15th ed., pp. 271–282). New York: McGraw-Hill.

Whitmire, S. J. (2003). Fluid, electrolytes, and acid–base balance. In L. E. Matarese & M. M. Gottschlich (Eds.), *Contemporary nutrition support practice: A clinical guide* (2nd ed., pp. 122–144). Philadelphia: W. B. Saunders.

Acid–Base Imbalance

Gail Thurkauf

Outcome-Based Learning Objectives

After studying this chapter, the learner will be able to:

1. Describe the role of hydrogen ions in the determination of plasma pH.
2. Compare and contrast the processes that produce respiratory and metabolic acids in the body and the processes by which they are eliminated.
3. Calculate minute ventilation and explain the effect of minute alveolar ventilation on acid–base balance.
4. Evaluate the process of respiratory compensation for a metabolic abnormality.
5. Discuss the renal handling of hydrogen ion and bicarbonate.
6. Discuss a systematic stepwise process for the interpretation of the arterial blood gas values related to acid–base balance.
7. Relate the major causes, pathophysiology, signs, symptoms, consequences, and medical management for respiratory acidosis and alkalosis and metabolic acidosis and alkalosis.
8. Describe the nursing assessment used in the assessment of acid–base abnormalities.
9. Describe nursing actions to alleviate the symptoms of acid–base abnormalities.

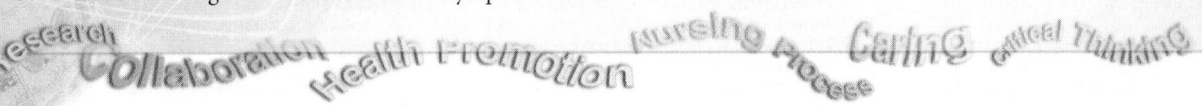

DISORDERS OF THE balance between the acids and the alkali or bases in the body are common clinical problems that result from or accompany a wide variety of pathologic conditions and diseases. A basic understanding of the effect of these imbalances on organ systems is important for nurses when assessing and caring for patients in all clinical settings.

Acid–Base Homeostasis

A **hydrogen ion** is a single charged particle (proton) that is not orbited by any electrons. The hydrogen ion (H⁺) is the smallest ionic particle and it is extremely reactive. Because of this reactivity, the hydrogen ion has a significant effect on physiological functions despite the fact that it is present in very low concentrations. The hydrogen ion combines with alkali/bases or other negatively charged ions at low concentrations. Proteins contain many negatively charged and positively charged groups within their structure. Therefore, even small changes in hydrogen ion concentration can alter protein and enzyme functioning. More extreme changes may totally disrupt the protein's structure, a process referred to as *denaturing* them. Disturbances in hydrogen ion concentration may result in abnormalities of function in many organs such as the pulmonary, renal, or cardiac systems and can also alter such processes as blood clotting and the metabolism of drugs (Schlichtig, 2005).

Plasma **pH** is an indicator of hydrogen ion concentration. It is the negative logarithm of the hydrogen ion concentration measured in nanomoles per liter (nmol/L). A normal pH of 7.40 is equivalent to 40 nmol/L of hydrogen ion. In terms more commonly used, this would be equal to 0.0004 mEq/L. Contrast that with a normal serum potassium level of 4 mEq/L or normal serum sodium of 140 mEq/L. Because it is a *negative* log, as the hydrogen ion concentration increases, the pH decreases. Conversely, as the hydrogen ion concentration goes down, pH goes up. Homeostatic mechanisms work to keep pH within a relatively narrow range of 7.35 to 7.45 for optimal cell functioning. As the pH changes either higher or lower, enzymes may stop functioning, nerve and muscle activity weaken, and, if the change is extreme, all metabolic activity may become deranged. The pH range that is usually considered compatible with life is 6.8 to 7.8.

Acids are compounds that form hydrogen ion in solution. Because of this, they are referred to as proton *donors*. As an example, hydrochloric acid (HCl) gives up H⁺ when added to blood. Strong acids hold their hydrogen ion weakly, so the ion dissociates easily and can then act on other substances. Weak acids hold onto their hydrogen ion more tightly so they do not contribute as much to the free hydrogen ion concentration. Because of this, the solution will have a higher (less acid) pH (Argyle, 2002).

Bases or **alkalis** are compounds that combine with hydrogen ion in solution; they are proton *acceptors*. **Sodium bicarbonate**

(NaHCO$_3^-$) removes hydrogen ion when added to the blood. Acids and bases constantly react with one another to neutralize changes in hydrogen ion concentration.

Carbon dioxide (CO$_2$) can be thought of as a potential acid. When it is dissolved in water, it becomes **carbonic acid**:

$$CO_2 + H_2O \rightarrow H_2CO_3 \text{ (carbonic acid)}$$

Carbonic acid then dissociates into hydrogen ion and bicarbonate:

$$H_2CO_3 \rightarrow H^+ + HCO_3^-$$

In plasma, under normal circumstances, there are 20 parts of bicarbonate to 1 part carbonic acid, a ratio of 20:1. If this 20:1 ratio is altered in either direction, the plasma pH will change (Schlichtig, 2005).

Body metabolism continually produces CO$_2$ (the respiratory acid) and other nonrespiratory acids, called metabolic acids. These acids are released into capillary blood, lowering the pH. Under normal conditions, this pH change is quite small. Blood arrives in the arterioles with a pH of 7.4 (which is equivalent to 40 nmol/L of hydrogen ion) and leaves the venules with a pH of 7.36 (equal to 44 nmol/L of hydrogen ion). Hydrogen ions have been added to the blood from the cell interior, which has a pH of about 7.0, equivalent to 100 nmol/L of hydrogen ion (Grogono, 2006).

The amount of respiratory acid produced is about 288 L/day (Grogono, 2006). This large amount is matched to the lung ventilation, which is its means of excretion. By comparison, very little metabolic acid is produced on a daily basis: about 0.1 mol (100 mEq). The main metabolic acids are lactic acid, pyruvic acid, ketoacids seen in diabetic acidosis, acetoacetic acid, and beta-hydroxybutyric acid. These acids are eliminated by the kidneys or they are metabolized by the liver. The capacity for elimination of these metabolic acids is much less than that of the lungs.

Abnormalities in the balance of acid to base can be grouped into four basic categories:

- **Respiratory acidosis**—excess of carbon dioxide leading to an acid pH
- **Respiratory alkalosis**—lower than normal level of carbon dioxide leading to an alkaline pH
- **Metabolic acidosis**—excess of hydrogen ion or a deficiency in bicarbonate leading to an acid pH
- **Metabolic alkalosis**—excess of bicarbonate leading to an alkaline pH.

Chart 19–1 provides a summary of acid–base terminology. The body's response to changes in acid–base status has three components:

1. **The first defense**—buffering
2. **The second defense**—changing the level of CO$_2$
3. **The third defense**—changing the level of HCO$_3^-$.

Buffer Systems

A **buffer** is a compound that minimizes the change in hydrogen ion concentration and, thus, the change in pH when these ions are added or removed from solution. A buffer acts like a sponge:

CHART 19–1 Acid and Base Terminology

Acidemia/Acidosis	Alkalemia/Alkalosis
Blood pH <7.40	Blood pH > 7.40
Caused by loss of base/alkali; increase of acid	Caused by increase of base/alkali; loss of acid
Lowers the 20:1 bicarbonate-to-carbonic acid ratio	Raises the 20:1 bicarbonate-to-carbonic acid ratio
Less base/more acid	More base/less acid

When there is an excess of hydrogen ion, the sponge soaks up the extra ions. When the level of hydrogen ion is decreased, the sponge can be squeezed out to release hydrogen ions back into the blood. Buffer systems act quickly to prevent excess changes in the pH.

There are buffers within body cells and in the extracellular fluid (ECF). The primary buffers of the extracellular system are carbonic acid and bicarbonate. The concentrations of these two substances are regulated by two independent systems. Carbonic acid is controlled by respiration via the lungs, and bicarbonate is controlled by excretion via the kidneys. Oxidative (aerobic) metabolism of amino acids and the anaerobic metabolism of glucose to lactate and pyruvic acid produce CO$_2$, which, again, can be thought of as a potential acid. Although CO$_2$ does not contain hydrogen ions, it reacts rapidly with water to form carbonic acid, which then dissociates into hydrogen and bicarbonate ions, as noted previously. This reaction can be written:

$$CO_2 + H_2O \rightarrow H_2CO_3^- \leftrightarrow HCO_3^- + H^+$$

This reaction occurs throughout the body and, in certain circumstances such as within red blood cells, can be sped up by the enzyme carbonic anhydrase.

Excess carbon dioxide is exhaled by the lungs as carbon dioxide gas. The concentration of bicarbonate ions is controlled by the kidneys. Under normal circumstances, the kidneys reabsorb and retain all of the bicarbonate presented to them by glomerular filtration. The kidneys also excrete small amounts of acid in the renal tubule. In alkalosis, either respiratory or metabolic, the kidneys retain hydrogen ion and excrete bicarbonate. In contrast, in respiratory acidosis and most cases of metabolic acidosis, the kidneys excrete hydrogen ion and conserve bicarbonate to correct the pH.

The intracellular buffer system is the phosphate buffer system. This system consists of dihydrogen phosphate ion (H$_2$PO$_4$) as the hydrogen ion donor (the acid) and hydrogen phosphate (HPO$_4$) as the hydrogen ion acceptor, the base. These two compounds are in equilibrium with one another inside the cell. When there is excess hydrogen ion in blood plasma, the hydrogen ions cross the cell membrane, enter the intracellular fluid (ICF), and are consumed by reacting with HPO$_4$. If there is extra hydroxide, or base, these compounds enter the intracellular fluid where they react with the H$_2$PO$_4$.

Protein buffers in the blood include plasma proteins and hemoglobin. Hemoglobin (Hgb) is the more important of these because it can bind to both CO$_2$ and H$^+$. Hemoglobin exists in two forms. It leaves the left side of the heart carrying its load of oxygen as oxyhemoglobin. After delivering the oxygen to the cell, the oxygen content is depleted and it has now become de-oxygenated Hgb. Deoxygenated Hgb is a better buffer than oxygenated Hgb because it has a stronger affinity for both the CO_2 and the hydrogen ion. Oxygen unloading at the tissues increases the amount of deoxygenated Hgb, thus producing the superior buffer exactly where it is needed to buffer the additional hydrogen ion being produced by metabolism (Breen, 2001).

At the tissue level, dissolved CO_2 enters the red blood cells (RBCs) where it combines with water to form carbonic acid. Carbonic anhydrase, present in the RBCs, is the enzyme that catalyzes this reaction. The carbonic acid then dissociates into bicarbonate and hydrogen ions. The hydrogen ions then bind to deoxygenated Hgb when they are soaked up by the buffer "sponge." Hemoglobin's buffering capacity is due to a chain within its structure, the imidazole chain. Imidazole can accept an extra proton, the hydrogen ion, or donate it back when the body pH is corrected (Argyle, 2002). The bicarbonate ions formed by the dissociation pass through RBC membranes back into the plasma in exchange for chloride ions (Cl^-). This ensures that there is no gain or loss of negative ions within the RBCs.

When the RBCs reach the lungs, this process is reversed. Hydrogen ions that were bound to the hemoglobin recombine with the bicarbonate to form CO_2, which passes through the RBC membranes into the alveoli so it can be expired. The deoxygenated Hgb combines with oxygen to prepare to return to the tissues. This process is illustrated in Figure 19–1 ■.

In addition to the buffer systems just described, bones also act as a buffer. The carbonate and phosphate salts in bone provide a long-term supply of buffer. They act as a reserve for alkalis. In acute metabolic acidosis, bone can take up hydrogen ion in exchange for calcium (Ca^{2+}), sodium (Na^+), and potassium (K^+). In chronic metabolic acidosis, calcium carbonate is released from bone as bone crystals dissolve. This situation can lead to the osteodystrophy often seen in chronic renal failure, which is a cause of chronic metabolic acidosis (Androgue & Androgue, 2001).

■ The Role of the Lungs

The lungs help to regulate plasma pH on a minute-to-minute basis by regulating the level of carbon dioxide, the respiratory acid. Carbon dioxide is measured as the partial pressure of carbon dioxide in arterial blood, the $PaCO_2$. This level is tightly controlled under normal conditions and kept within a narrow range of 35 to 45 mmHg at sea level. The lungs can either retain or excrete CO_2 by altering the rate and depth of ventilation. The amount of ventilation is generally quantified by how much air the lungs move in 1 minute, referred to as the **minute ventilation**. Minute ventilation is the product of respiratory *rate* and *depth*, referred to as the tidal volume (V_t). Normal resting respiratory rate is about 12 breaths per minute. Normal resting depth tidal volume is about 500 mL. This yields a normal minute ventilation of 6 L/min:

$$12\ breaths/min \times 500\ mL\ V_t = 6{,}000\ mL\ or\ 6\ L$$

The tidal volume refers to the total amount of air inhaled and exhaled with each breath. A portion of that volume, however, is in the large conducting airways such as the trachea and bronchi. That volume, referred to as **anatomic dead space**, does not reach the alveolar airspaces to take part in the exchange of oxygen and carbon dioxide with the blood. The amount of anatomic dead space can be estimated as 1 mL/lb of ideal body weight. Thus, a person with an ideal body weight of 150 pounds has about 150 mL of anatomic dead space.

The remainder of the tidal volume, that portion which *does* reach the alveoli and participates in gas exchange with capillary blood, is termed *alveolar volume*. Minute alveolar ventilation is the volume of alveolar air per minute that takes part in gas exchange, transferring oxygen to the blood and removing carbon dioxide from the blood. It is actually this minute alveolar ventilation that determines the $PaCO_2$. Normal minute alveolar ventilation can be calculated as follows:

$$Tidal\ volume - anatomic\ dead\ space = alveolar\ volume$$

$$500\ mL - 150\ mL = 350\ mL$$

$$Respiratory\ rate \times alveolar\ volume =$$
$$minute\ alveolar\ ventilation$$

$$12\ breaths/min \times 350\ mL = 4{,}200\ mL\ or\ 4.2\ L/min$$

This normal minute alveolar ventilation should yield a normal $PaCO_2$. In clinical practice, the terms *hyperventilation* and *hypoventilation* apply only to alveolar ventilation and its effect on the $PaCO_2$.

Dead space ventilation is that part of the minute ventilation which does not take part in gas exchange; it is actually "wasted ventilation." Dead space ventilation includes the air in the conducting airways, the anatomic dead space as discussed earlier, and the air that *does* reach the alveoli but doesn't take part in gas exchange, typically referred to as **pathologic dead space**. Different disease states such as emphysema can alter this pathologic dead space and affect the ability of the lungs to oxygenate and ventilate.

The respiratory center located in the medulla in the brainstem controls the rate and depth of ventilation in response to the level of arterial CO_2, denoted as $PaCO_2$. Chemoreceptors located on the surface of the medulla are in contact with cerebrospinal fluid (CSF). These receptors are termed "central" because they are located within the central nervous system (CNS). As the level of $PaCO_2$ rises, the arterial $PaCO_2$ reaches equilibrium with the CO_2 in the CSF. That CO_2 in the CSF combines with water to form carbonic acid, as previously described. The carbonic acid dissociates into hydrogen ion and bicarbonate. The CSF hydrogen ion diffuses into the medullary tissue and stimulates the chemorecep-

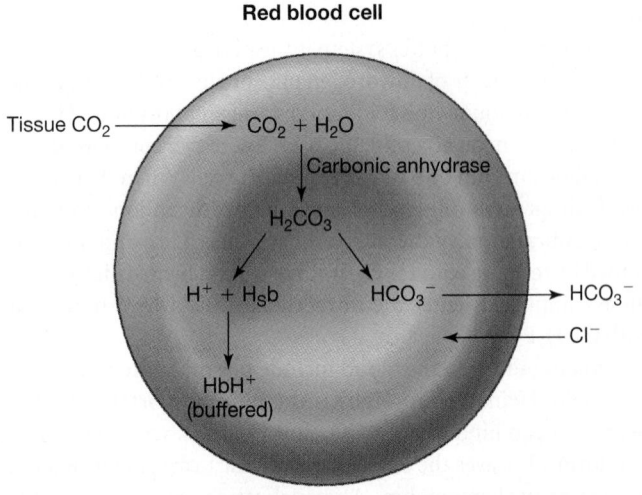

Red blood cell

Tissue CO_2 ⟶ $CO_2 + H_2O$

Carbonic anhydrase

H_2CO_3

$H^+ + Hsb$ HCO_3^- ⟶ HCO_3^-

Cl^-

HbH^+
(buffered)

FIGURE 19–1 ■ Red blood cell.

tors. They, in turn, stimulate the diaphragm and intercostal muscles to increase the rate and depth of ventilation. This increase in minute ventilation will "blow off" excess CO_2, returning it back toward normal, thereby correcting the pH.

The reverse happens when there are abnormally low levels of CO_2. In this state of hyperventilation, the medullary centers slow the rate and depth of ventilation to allow accumulation of CO_2 back toward normal, thereby correcting the pH.

The level of $PaCO_2$, acting on the central chemoreceptors by altering the pH of the CSF, is the most important single determent of ventilation, and is referred to as the **hypercarbic drive**. There are also peripheral chemoreceptors that are responsive to the level of oxygen in the blood and hydrogen ion as well as the $PaCO_2$. These peripheral receptors are located in the carotid arteries at the bifurcation of the common carotid and in the arch of the aorta. The carotid receptors are sensitive to PaO_2, $PaCO_2$, and pH. The aortic receptors are sensitive to PaO_2 and $PaCO_2$ but not pH. Neural impulses from the carotid bodies increase as the PaO_2 falls below about 60 mmHg and stimulate the respiratory centers to increase both rate and depth of ventilation in an attempt to increase the body's oxygen supply. This responsiveness to low oxygen tension, referred to as the **hypoxic drive**, is potentiated by acidosis and hypercapnia.

The hypercarbic drive is a response to *acute* respiratory acidosis. If a person suffers from chronic ventilatory failure, such as a patient with end-stage emphysema that leads to chronically high $PaCO_2$ levels (chronic respiratory acidosis), bicarbonate will cross the blood–brain barrier to buffer the CSF hydrogen ion changes. It takes hours to days for this adaptation to occur. Due to this increased bicarbonate on the brain side of the blood–brain barrier, the central chemoreceptors become less sensitive to changes in the level of CO_2, which results in a decrease in the strength of the ventilatory drive moderated by these central receptors. When this occurs, the only remaining drive to breathe is the stimulation of the peripheral receptors by a low PaO_2, the hypoxic drive.

The terms *hyperventilation* and *hypoventilation* are defined by the $PaCO_2$. Low $PaCO_2$, or hypocapnia, defines the state of **hyperventilation**. A high $PaCO_2$, hypercapnia, defines the state of **hypoventilation**. There is a tendency to describe someone who is breathing rapidly and deeply as "hyperventilating," but this cannot actually be determined without obtaining an arterial blood gas and looking at the $PaCO_2$.

In addition to the level of CO_2, an increase in the arterial hydrogen ion concentration will also stimulate the central chemoreceptors of the respiratory control center, but to a lesser degree because hydrogen ions do not diffuse into the CSF as easily as the lipid-soluble CO_2, so the response is slower. But in a state of metabolic acidosis, such as that which exists during diabetic ketoacidosis, the medullary centers will stimulate the lungs to increase the minute ventilation to blow off CO_2, even if that level is normal. These rapid, deep respirations, referred to as Kussmaul's respirations, are an attempt to correct the arterial pH by decreasing respiratory acid. This process is referred to as **compensation**.

The Role of the Kidneys

The kidneys perform two basic functions to maintain acid–base balance: They secrete hydrogen ions and they restore or reclaim bicarbonate. Bicarbonate ions are freely filtered in the kidneys by glomerular filtration. The level of bicarbonate in the renal tubular fluid is the same as that of plasma. To help make this clear, think of tubular fluid as being outside of the body. During glomerular filtration, plasma, water, and solutes are forced by hydrostatic pressure across the membrane of the glomerular capillaries into the lumen of the tubule. If substances remain in the tubular fluid or other substances are secreted into that fluid, they will eventually leave the body in urine. **Secretion** is the active process of moving substances, such as hydrogen ion, from the blood into the tubular fluid against the concentration gradient. If substances are reabsorbed from the tubular fluid back across the membrane and into the blood, they are being reclaimed back into the body.

The reabsorption of bicarbonate that has been filtered into the tubular fluid occurs primarily in the proximal convoluted tubule of the nephron. Filtered bicarbonate combines with the secreted hydrogen ions to form carbonic acid, which then dissociates into CO_2 and water.

$$HCO_3^- + H^+ \leftrightarrow H_2CO_3 \leftrightarrow CO_2 + H_2O$$

This reaction is catalyzed by carbonic anhydrase, the same enzyme contained in the red blood cells. The CO_2 crosses from the tubular fluid into the cells lining the tubule. Here, the CO_2 recombines with water to again form carbonic acid, which then dissociates to hydrogen ion and bicarbonate. This is the reverse of the preceding equation:

$$CO_2 + H_2O \rightarrow H_2CO_3 \leftrightarrow HCO_3^- + H^+$$

The bicarbonate passes from the cell back across the membrane into the blood while the hydrogen ion passes back into the tubular fluid. This hydrogen ion is exchanged for sodium ion, another positive ion.

In the face of a high load of metabolic acids, the kidneys also increase their production of the urinary buffer, ammonia (NH_4). Under normal circumstances, NH_4 excretion is about 30 mmol/day, or about 0.5 mmol/kg. This excretion can increase to about 280 mmol/day but this response takes several days to be completed (DuBose, 2004).

In the event of respiratory acidosis, where there is an excess of plasma CO_2, and in most cases of metabolic acidosis, the kidneys excrete hydrogen ion and conserve bicarbonate to help restore acid–base balance and return the pH toward normal. In respiratory and metabolic alkalosis, the kidneys retain hydrogen ion and excrete bicarbonate. This metabolic compensation is slow compared to respiratory compensation. It can take hours to days to occur. Note that the average ventilation rate is about 6 L/*minute*, whereas the renal excretion rate is only about 2 L/*day* (Schlichtig, 2005).

▨ Assessment of Acid–Base Balance

Arterial blood gas (ABG) values are most often used to assess acid–base balance, although serum electrolytes will help fine-tune the analysis. The Diagnostic Test box (p. 440) outlines the commonly assessed laboratory values.

Normal ABG values are:

$$pH = 7.40\,(range: 7.35 - 7.45)$$
$$PaCO_2 = 40\,mEq/L\,(range: 35 - 45)$$
$$HCO_3^- = 22 - 28\,mEq/L$$

DIAGNOSTIC TESTS for Acid–Base Imbalances

Test	Expected Abnormality	Rationale for Abnormality
pH	↓'d < 7.35 in uncompensated respiratory or metabolic acidosis ↑'d > 7.45 in uncompensated respiratory or metabolic alkalosis	
$PaCO_2$	>45 mmHg in respiratory acidosis <35 mmHg in respiratory alkalosis	CO_2 is a respiratory acid. An excess will lead to acidosis; a deficiency will lead to alkalosis.
HCO_3^-	<22 mEq/L in metabolic acidosis >28 mEq/L in metabolic alkalosis	HCO_3^- is a base. A deficiency will lead to acidosis; an excess will lead to alkalosis.
Base excess (BE)	> −3 in metabolic acidosis > +3 in metabolic alkalosis	Quantifies the milliequivalents of bicarbonate that are deficient/in excess per liter of ECF.
Serum potassium	↑'d with acidosis	Excess hydrogen ion moves into cells and displaces K^+ out of the cell and into the serum.
Ionized calcium	↓'d in alkalosis	Alkalosis ↑'s the binding of calcium to albumin, resulting in a decrease in free, ionized calcium in the serum.
Anion gap	↑'d above 10–14 in high anion gap acidosis Normal in nonanion gap metabolic acidosis	Indicates an increased anion load (lactic acidosis, ketoacidosis, ingestion of acids, rhabdomyolysis). Loss of bicarbonate (diarrhea, fistula, renal dysfunction) or ingestion of base.

Along with these values, most ABGs also report the **base excess**. This is a calculated value that is based on the bicarbonate level, the $PaCO_2$ and the hematocrit. The base excess refers to the number of milliequivalents of bicarbonate per liter of ECF that one has too much of (base excess) or too little of (base deficit). As an example, a patient has a base excess of +6. This indicates a metabolic alkalosis and quantifies it. Every liter of the patient's ECF has 6 mEq too much bicarbonate or other base. In an opposite example, a patient has a base excess of −10. This indicates a metabolic acidosis and every liter of ECF is deficient in bicarbonate by 10 mEq. This number can help guide clinicians when they are considering how much bicarbonate to administer to a patient with severe metabolic acidosis. (*Note:* Although a positive number indicates a base excess and a negative number indicates a base deficit, in clinical practice, only the term *base excess* is commonly used.) A negative number is referred to as a "base excess of minus *x*." A normal base excess, then, is zero; not too little or too much bicarbonate. The normal range is usually considered to be ±3 mEq. Outlined here is the recommended stepwise approach for the interpretation of ABGs, which is also illustrated in Figure 19–2 ■:

1. **Assess the pH**—is it normal, low, or high? This first step is crucial because it guides the approach to the rest of the values. If the pH is less than 7.35, there is an acidosis. If the pH is greater than 7.45, there is an alkalosis.

2. **Assess the respiratory component**—Is the $PaCO_2$ normal, low, or high? If the cause of an abnormality is a respiratory problem, the $PaCO_2$ and the pH move in opposite direc-

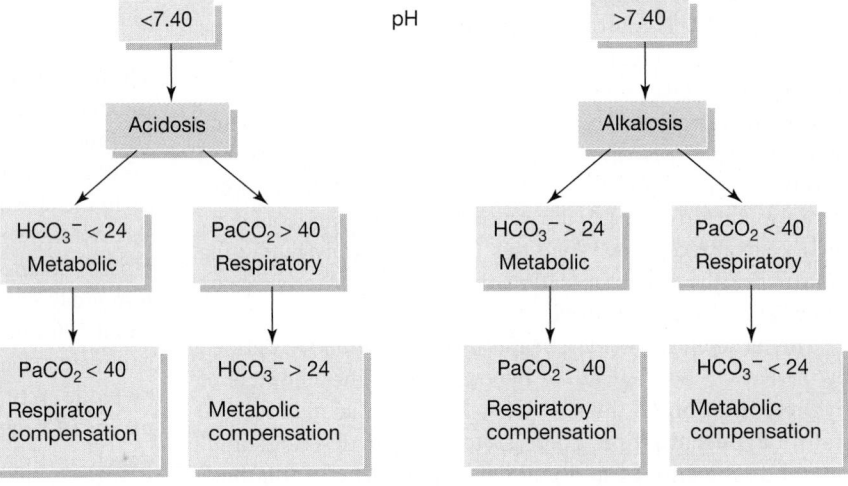

FIGURE 19–2 ■ Stepwise approach to ABG interpretation.

tions. In ventilatory failure, the $PaCO_2$ rises and causes a lowered acid pH. If both the pH and the $PaCO_2$ have moved in the same direction (i.e., both are increased or both are decreased), then the cause of the abnormality is a metabolic one. Refer to the examples in Chart 19–2.

3. **Assess the metabolic component**—Are the bicarbonate and the base excess (BE) normal, low, or high? In a metabolic abnormality, the pH and the bicarbonate move in the same direction. If the bicarbonate is increased, pH will be increased. If the bicarbonate is decreased, the pH will also be lower. Refer to the examples in Chart 19–3.

Steps 2 and 3 will identify the primary problem if there is one. Next, evaluate compensation. Any change in the acid–base equilibrium will cause the system that is *not* the primary cause of the abnormality to respond to attempt to restore the 20:1 ratio of

CHART 19–2 Examples of Abnormalities of the Respiratory Component

Example 1: Mrs. A has a $PaCO_2$ = 56 and a pH = 7.27.
The $PaCO_2$ is increased (16 mmHg above normal). The pH is decreased by 0.13.
In respiratory acidosis, the $PaCO_2$ and the pH move in opposite directions, so:
Mrs. A has a respiratory acidosis.

Example 2: Mr. B has a $PaCO_2$ = 28 and a pH = 7.52.
The $PaCO_2$ is decreased by 12 mmHg. The pH is increased by 0.12.
In respiratory alkalosis, the $PaCO_2$ and the pH move in opposite directions, so:
Mr. B has a respiratory alkalosis.

Example 3: Ms. C has a $PaCO_2$ = 52 and a pH = 7.48.
The $PaCO_2$ is increased. The pH is also increased.
Because both the $PaCO_2$ and the pH are elevated (moving in the same direction), it cannot be a respiratory problem. If it isn't a respiratory problem, then it has to be a *metabolic derangement*. (This is known even though a value for bicarbonate hasn't been given.)

CHART 19–3 Examples of Abnormalities of the Metabolic Component

Example 1: Mr. E has a HCO_3^- of 16 and a pH of 7.24.
Base excess = −6.
The bicarbonate and the pH are both decreased. In a metabolic acidosis, the bicarbonate and the pH move in the same direction.
This is a metabolic acidosis. The base excess of −6 indicates that every liter of Mr. E's extracellular fluid needs 6 mEq of additional bicarbonate to normalize the pH.

Example 2: Mr. F has a HCO_3^- of 34 mEq and a pH of 7.50.
Base excess = +5.
The bicarbonate and the pH are both elevated. In metabolic alkalosis, the bicarbonate and the pH move in the same direction.
This is a metabolic alkalosis. The base excess of +5 indicates that every liter of Mr. F's extracellular fluid has 5 mEq too much bicarbonate or other anion.
(A base excess is not as clinically helpful as a base deficit. A specific number of milliequivalents of bicarbonate cannot be dialyzed or otherwise removed and acids are rarely administered to patients to correct a metabolic alkalosis.)

bicarbonate-to-carbonic acid and bring the pH back toward normal. If the primary problem is a metabolic abnormality, the lungs will increase or decrease total minute ventilation to attempt to bring the pH back toward normal. If the cause of the problem is respiratory, the kidneys will retain or secrete hydrogen ion and/or bicarbonate to restore balance.

Because renal/metabolic compensation is slower, taking hours to days, one can infer whether a respiratory abnormality is an acute problem or a chronic one. If the kidneys have not had enough time to compensate, the problem is acute. If metabolic compensation has taken place, the problem is likely to be a chronic one. Once the primary cause has been identified (CO_2 or HCO_3^-), look at the other value. If that parameter is abnormal, but is moving in a direction that would bring the pH back toward normal, then compensation is occurring. If the pH is in the normal range, then complete compensation has occurred. If the pH is not within the normal range, but moving in the right direction, then partial compensation has occurred. See Chart 19–4 for a summary of the blood gas changes seen in respiratory and metabolic disturbances.

Complex Acid–Base Disorders

Sometimes patients will have combined disorders. For example, a critically ill patient who has recently suffered a cardiac arrest

may have both a respiratory and a metabolic acidosis. It can be helpful, sometimes, to look at the magnitude of the change in the CO_2 or HCO_3^- and compare it to the expected change in the pH. A simple rule of thumb to use is this: For every 10 mmHg change in the $PaCO_2$, there should be a corresponding pH change of 0.08 to 0.1 in the opposite direction. Using the 0.1 is easiest to calculate:

$$Normal\ PaCO_2 = 40;\ normal\ pH = 7.40$$

If the $PaCO_2$ increases to 50 (a change of 10 mmHg from normal), the pH should decrease by 0.10 to 7.30 if there is only a respiratory acidosis. Conversely, if the $PaCO_2$ decreases to 22 (a change of 18 mmHg from normal), the pH should increase to 7.58, a 0.18 increase, if there is only a respiratory alkalosis. However, if the $PaCO_2$ increases to 50 (a change of 10 mmHg), but the pH is 7.15 (a change of 0.25), this change in the pH is much greater than it would be if there was a respiratory acidosis alone. In this case, a concurrent metabolic acidosis must be causing the large drop in pH with a rather moderate increase in the $PaCO_2$.

Acid–Base Imbalances

Imbalances between acids and bases almost always occur as a result of diseases, organ dysfunction, or other pathologic conditions. The following descriptions of the four imbalances

CHART 19–4 Blood Gas Changes in Acid–Base Imbalances

Acid–Base Disorder	pH Normal = 7.35–7.45	$PaCO_2$ Normal = 35–45 mmHg	HCO_3^- Normal = 22–28 mEq/L
Respiratory acidosis	↓	↑	Normal (↑'d if compensating)
Respiratory alkalosis	↑	↓	Normal (↓'d if compensating)
Metabolic acidosis	↓	Normal (↓'d if compensating)	↓
Metabolic alkalosis	↑	Normal (↑'d if compensating)	↑

Note: $PaCO_2$ and pH move in *opposite* directions. HCO_3^- and pH move in the *same* direction.

describe them as distinct abnormalities, but they must be evaluated in the context of the patient's underlying pathology when caring for patients in the clinical setting. Chart 19–5 summarizes the causes of acid–base imbalances.

Respiratory Acidosis

Also referred to as primary hypercapnia, the primary derangement of acid–base balance in this situation is an excess of arterial CO_2 accompanied by a decrease in the pH. The CO_2 is regulated in part by the respiratory rate. When respirations increase, the CO_2 decreases and vice versa with a decreased respiratory rate, thereby increasing the CO_2.

Etiology and Pathophysiology

Whenever excretion of CO_2 via the lungs fails to keep up with the body's CO_2 production, respiratory acidosis will occur. This respiratory system failure may be *acute*, occurring rapidly due to a sudden event. In this situation, the elevation in the $PaCO_2$ results in acidemia and a low pH. Respiratory acidosis may also be *chronic*, where there has been a sustained increase in the $PaCO_2$ that leads to renal compensation and elevated serum bicarbonate. Causes of acute and chronic ventilatory failure are noted in Chart 19–6.

Most of these conditions impair the lung's ability to eliminate CO_2 by impairing ventilation. Conditions that cause alveolar hypoventilation can be categorized as being due to a decreased respiratory drive (patients who "won't breathe") or a decrease in respiratory muscle or chest wall function (patients who "can't breathe"). Normally, an increase in the $PaCO_2$ leads to a marked increase in the ventilatory drive. If there is an abnormality of ventilatory control, there will be an inappropriately low to absent ventilatory drive despite elevations in the $PaCO_2$. This can occur with a neurological event such as cerebral anoxia or from depression of the respiratory centers by drugs such as narcotics.

Another influence on the respiratory drive is the level of CNS arousal. During non–rapid eye movement (NREM) sleep, the ventilatory response to $PaCO_2$ is blunted and the minute ventilation decreases, primarily secondary to a lower tidal volume. The $PaCO_2$ can increase by about 3 to 10 mmHg. This is not clinically a problem unless the person suffers from preexisting hypercapnia, in which case respiratory acidosis may worsen.

Chest wall or respiratory muscle abnormalities can be the result of CNS disorders, neuromuscular disorders, or restrictive lung conditions such as pulmonary fibrosis. These conditions can lead to acute or chronic hypoventilation. A condition worth noting in this category is obesity hypoventilation syndrome. Some people who are morbidly obese, which is defined as having a body mass index (BMI) > 40, have a syndrome that is characterized by chronic hypoventilation and chronic respiratory failure. Chronic respiratory failure develops over a longer period of time, allowing for renal compensation by the retention of bicarbonate. Chapter 36 🔗 discusses the diagnosis and treatment of respiratory failure. These patients have a decreased ventilatory drive and an increased work of breathing. This work of breathing increase is due to a reduction in lung compliance ("stretchiness") and abdominal influences. These persons are prone to the development of obstructive sleep apnea, which causes both hypoventilation and hypoxemia. Chapter 34 🔗 describes obstructive sleep apnea.

| CHART 19–5 | Causes of Acid–Base Disorders |

Acute Respiratory Acidosis	Metabolic Acidosis
CNS Depression	**Excess H+ Production**
Drug overdose	Lactic acidosis due to tissue
Head trauma	hypoxia
Encephalitis	Ketoacidosis: diabetic, alcoholic,
Stroke	starvation
Neuromuscular Disease	**Ingestion of Acids**
Guillain-Barré syndrome	Poisoning with agents such as
Myasthenic crisis	ethylene glycol (antifreeze) or
Spinal cord injury	aspirin
Airway Disease	**Inadequate Acid Excretion**
Status asthmaticus	Renal dysfunction
Upper airway obstruction	Endocrine disturbances (e.g.,
Pleural or Chest Wall Abnormalities	hypoaldosteronism)
	Excessive Loss of Bicarbonate
Pneumothorax	Excessive diarrhea
Large pleural effusion	Acetazolamide

Chronic Respiratory Acidosis

Impaired Central Ventilatory Drive
Central sleep apnea
Obesity hypoventilation

Neuromuscular Disease
Amyotrophic lateral sclerosis
Muscular dystrophy
Poliomyelitis
Multiple sclerosis
Spinal cord injury

Airway and Lung Parenchyma Disease
Emphysema
Chronic bronchitis
Interstitial lung disease

Other:
Kyphoscoliosis
Diaphragmatic paralysis

Respiratory Alkalosis	Metabolic Alkalosis
Central Nervous System	**Excessive Loss of H+**
Pain	Protracted vomiting
Anxiety	Nasogastric suction
Psychosis	**Acid Shifts into Cells**
Fever	Potassium deficiency
Stroke	**Excessive Reabsorption of Bicarbonate**
Meningitis, encephalitis	
Tumor	Hypochloremia
Trauma	Thiazide and loop diuretics
Hypoxemia	
Drugs	
Salicylates, nicotine, progesterone	
Pregnancy	
Sepsis	
Hepatic failure	
Iatrogenic on mechanical ventilation	

CHART 19–6	Causes of Hypercapnic Ventilatory Failure	
Site of Disturbance	**Acute**	**Chronic**
Respiratory center	Drug overdose Trauma Stroke	Tumor
Neuromuscular disease	Guillain-Barré syndrome Myasthenia gravis	Polio Spinal cord injury Amyotrophic lateral sclerosis
Chest wall	Trauma Pleural effusion (large) Pneumothorax	Kyphoscoliosis
Upper airway obstruction	Tumor Laryngeal edema Foreign body	
Peripheral airway obstruction	Asthma (severe)	Emphysema Chronic bronchitis Obesity Hypoventilation

Aside from conditions that cause alveolar hypoventilation, respiratory acidosis can result from an increase in pathologic dead space. The matching of alveolar ventilation to the perfusion of the pulmonary capillaries is most important to the maintenance of normal oxygenation, but it is also important to the maintenance of CO_2 balance. The CO_2 must be delivered from the tissues via the blood to the lungs so it can be excreted. The elimination of CO_2 decreases when perfusion to a segment of the lungs is reduced, such as occurs with a pulmonary embolism or pulmonary vascular disease. This is usually not clinically a problem because the ventilatory centers will increase the rate and depth of ventilation to compensate.

As discussed earlier, anatomic dead space is that portion of the inhaled volume that remains in the large conducting airways and does not take part in the exchange of oxygen and CO_2. The anatomic dead space is a fixed volume, so increase in the tidal volume will increase the alveolar ventilation. Conversely, a decreased tidal volume will result in less air reaching the alveoli and can result in hypercapnia and respiratory acidosis. In acute respiratory failure, patients often resort to a pattern of rapid, shallow breathing that can lead to a higher proportion of dead space to tidal volume. This also is the pattern of breathing seen with neuromuscular disease such as Guillain-Barré syndrome and amyotrophic lateral sclerosis (Priestley & Levine, 2006). Other causes of increased dead space include decreased lung perfusion as noted previously and destruction of pulmonary parenchyma by diseases such as emphysema and pulmonary fibrosis.

In chronic obstructive pulmonary diseases such as emphysema or chronic bronchitis, elevations in the $PaCO_2$ are thought to be a poor prognostic sign. With emphysema, there is decreased surface area for gas exchange that first leads to a decrease in arterial oxygenation, but, in the most severe cases, also leads to chronic hypercapnia. Air trapping in the alveolar airspaces also leads to lung hyperinflation. This hyperinflation flattens out the diaphragm, which, in the relaxed position, is shaped like an upside-down bowl. When the lungs are permanently inflated, this flattened diaphragm impairs the person's ability to generate negative inspiratory pressure, which is needed to pull air into the lungs. This leads to impaired ventilation and greatly contributes to the sensation of breathlessness from which these patients suffer. (Try this yourself: Take a deep breath in and hold it. Now take in more air. Hard, isn't it? And very uncomfortable.)

In some conditions the major problem is increased production of CO_2, rather than impaired elimination. These conditions include exercise, fever, burns, and thyrotoxicosis and catabolic states such as are seen with multiple-organ failure. Using fever as an example, for every degree of temperature elevation, CO_2 production increases by about 13%. Thus, a patient with a fever of 40°C (104°F) must increase alveolar ventilation by about 40% to maintain a normal $PaCO_2$. Increased CO_2 production rarely leads to hypercapnia in otherwise healthy persons because increased production leads to increased ventilation and subsequent CO_2 excretion. Patients with preexisting pulmonary diseases, however, may not be able to increase their ventilation enough to handle the excess CO_2 and their levels will rise.

In acute respiratory acidosis, cellular buffering occurs over minutes to hours. Renal compensation occurs over several days. The kidneys reabsorb bicarbonate and excrete acid. The plasma bicarbonate increases about 3.5 mEq/L for each increase of 10 mmHg in the $PaCO_2$. In acidemia, hydrogen ion moves into cells and displaces K^+ out of the cell into the serum, although respiratory acidosis does not usually cause clinically significant hyperkalemia.

Signs, Symptoms, and Consequences

Acute hypercapnia can be life threatening when it causes severe respiratory acidosis. This usually occurs in conjunction with hypoxemia. Carbon dioxide crosses cell membranes rapidly and leads to a low intracellular pH, which can affect many body systems. CNS symptoms dominate and their severity depends on the magnitude of the increase, the speed with which it occurs, and the accompanying degree of hypoxemia. Carbon dioxide rapidly crosses the blood–brain barrier and lowers CSF pH. The acute effects are cerebral vessel dilation, increased cerebral blood flow, and increased intracranial pressure. Clinical manifestations of these changes include anxiety, irritability, headache, confusion, disorientation, somnolence, and lethargy. Patients may complain of dyspnea. More serious alterations of consciousness such as stupor or coma are rare but are seen when the $PaCO_2$ is markedly elevated, typically more than 70 to 100 mmHg (Priestley & Levine, 2006).

The other major organ system that may be affected in respiratory acidosis is the cardiovascular system. Mild to moderate hypercapnia causes release of the catecholamines epinephrine and norepinephrine and peripheral vasodilation. Catecholamines usually cause peripheral vasoconstriction, but the elevated CO_2 has an inhibitory effect on vascular smooth muscle, which leads to vasodilation. These changes results in an increase in heart rate with normal or elevated blood pressure. Because of the peripheral vasodilation, the patient's skin is often warm, flushed, and diaphoretic.

In chronic hypercapnia, the effects are not as dramatic because organ systems have a chance to adapt and renal compensation has time to occur. The cerebral blood flow returns to normal and the only symptom may be a morning headache, mild irritability, and lethargy. It is important to remember that patients with chronic respiratory failure may develop acute respiratory failure as well. If a patient with a chronically high level of CO_2 presents with an acid pH, he is suffering from acute respiratory failure. See examples in Chart 19–7.

Medical Management

Acid–base disturbances are rarely isolated conditions; they usually accompany other pathophysiologic processes. The main treatment for respiratory acidosis is correction of the underlying disorder that led to its development. This might include a reversal of a drug overdose to counteract respiratory depression, the use of inhaled bronchodilators and steroids to treat the bronchospasm that accompanies acute asthma, or the use of antibiotics to treat pneumonia and improve ventilation, thus correcting the acidosis. Administration of sodium bicarbonate is almost never indicated in the treatment of respiratory acidosis because the bicarbonate will eventually be converted to CO_2. Thus, in the long run, it can actually worsen a respiratory acidosis although, its use may be considered in the situation of cardiac arrest with extremely low pH (<7.0 to 7.1). In this situation, metabolic acidosis is usually combined with respiratory acidosis (Priestley & Levine, 2006). The metabolic acidosis is a lactic acidosis that results from anaerobic metabolism that occurs because of the lack of tissue perfusion during cardiac arrest.

Treatment also is aimed at assisting or increasing ventilation. This can be accomplished invasively through endotracheal intubation and the use of mechanical ventilation or noninvasively through the use of nasal continuous positive airway pressure (CPAP) or nasal bilevel ventilation (BiPAP).

Bilevel Positive Airway Pressure

BiPAP is a noninvasive method of assisting ventilation in children and adults with chronic hypoventilation. The system consists of a blower or compressor attached via tubing to a cushioned nose mask that is held to the face with an elastic headband or a specially designed cap. Patients with sleep-related hypoventilation disorders may only need to use the device at bedtime, whereas others may need the system for longer periods of time. Chapter 36 💬 discusses BiPAP. When positive pressure is applied to the nasopharynx, the soft palate comes in contact with the tongue. These structures are held together and

pushed forward away from the posterior wall of the pharynx, effectively sealing off the oral cavity from the wall of the oropharynx. This prevents air from leaking out through the patient's mouth.

In BiPAP, one level of positive pressure is applied during inspiration and another (lower) level is applied during expiration. In the system, the clinician sets:

- Inspiratory positive airway pressure (IPAP): between 2 and 25 cmH$_2$O
- Expiratory positive airway pressure (EPAP): between 2 and 20 cmH$_2$O
- The frequency of the cycling: usually between 6 and 30 cycle/min
- The percentage of IPAP-to-EPAP: set between 10% and 90%, but is usually around 40%. This means that for 40% of the time of each respiratory cycle, the pressure delivered is the IPAP and 60% of the time it is the EPAP. This percentage of IPAP to EPAP is titrated to achieve the optimum tidal volume with each breath.

The difference between the two pressures is referred to as the *pressure boost* (PB). If the IPAP is 20 cmH$_2$O and the EPAP is 5 cmH$_2$O, then the PB would be 15 cmH$_2$O.

The system does have a backup mode that will kick in if the patient ceases to breathe.

The side effects are few although patients may complain of drying of the nasal mucosa, which can lead to nosebleeds. Pressure through the eustachian tubes can cause "ear popping" discomfort. If the mask is too tight or is not fitted properly, skin breakdown can occur at the bridge of the nose.

Intubation

There are no absolute criteria for deciding when to intubate someone in respiratory distress, but the general rule is that intubation is indicated if the patient has a $PaCO_2$ in the 80- to 90-mmHg range and a pH of less than 7.10 to 7.25. It is often a clinical decision based on the medical team's estimation of whether the patient will be able to keep on or will approach exhaustion. Once the patient is on mechanical ventilation, the patient can be supported while health care clinicians work to correct the underlying pathology. After treating the problem the patient can gradually be weaned off of the ventilatory support.

For patients with chronic hypercarbia, care must be taken when they are placed on mechanical ventilation to correct them slowly. Too efficient ventilation of the patient will correct the $PaCO_2$ too rapidly, and the patient will develop a metabolic alkalosis because of the excess retained bicarbonate. This can alkalinize the CSF and may cause seizures (Priestley & Levine, 2006). Chapter 36 💬 includes a discussion of the various modes of mechanical ventilation.

Supplemental Oxygen

Many patients with hypercapnea are also hypoxemic, so the use of supplemental oxygen may be indicated. It has been shown to decrease mortality and leads to better outcomes. The use of supplemental oxygen in patients with chronic respiratory acidosis, however, must be approached with caution. Because chronic hypercapnea blunts the central hypercarbic drive, these patients'

CHART 19–7	**Acute Ventilatory Failure in the Patient Who Has Chronic Ventilatory Failure**

Example 1: Mr. T has $PaCO_2$ = 60, pH = 7.37, HCO_3^- = 35 mEq/L.
Despite the elevated $PaCO_2$, the pH is normal because the kidneys have retained bicarbonate.
In this patient's case, *Mr. T is at or near his baseline PaCO$_2$.*

Example 2: Ms. Y has $PaCO_2$ = 73, pH = 7.28, HCO_3^- = 35 mEq/L.
The $PaCO_2$ is elevated but the pH is acidic despite the elevated bicarbonate.
This $PaCO_2$ of 73 is higher than the patient's baseline. If it was her baseline, her pH would be at/close to the normal range.
This patient has an *acute respiratory failure superimposed on chronic respiratory failure.*

main stimulus to ventilation is the peripheral hypoxic drive. These patients breathe because their level of PaO_2 goes down. High levels of supplemental oxygen may blunt this hypoxic drive, leading to a further decrease in ventilation and a worsening of hypercapnea. Oxygen should be carefully administered to keep the oxygen saturation level in the low 90% range with a PaO_2 of 60 to 65 mmHg.

 Patients with chronic obstructive pulmonary disease who have chronically elevated levels of $PaCO_2$ may have a blunted hypercarbic drive. Their main stimulus of ventilation is the hypoxic drive. If a person who is a chronic CO_2 retainer receives a high concentration of supplemental oxygen that raises his PaO_2 above the stimulus level, respirations may be depressed. This does not mean that these patients should not receive oxygen if they are hypoxemic. It means clinicians have to be careful and monitor them more closely. (Note: This applies only to persons who are chronic CO_2 retainers. Not all patients who have chronic lung disease retain CO_2.)

Respiratory Alkalosis

This acid–base derangement is characterized by a lower than normal $PaCO_2$ accompanied by an elevated pH. Respiratory rate is a major determinant of the $PaCO_2$ level. Excessively fast or deep ventilation "blows off" the carbon dioxide, decreasing the level and increasing the pH, causing alkalosis.

Etiology and Pathophysiology

Respiratory alkalosis is an acid–base disturbance caused by alveolar overventilation. The overventilation leads to a decreased $PaCO_2$, altering the 20:1 bicarbonate-to-carbonic acid ratio and causing an increased pH. The lungs are removing carbon dioxide faster than the tissues are producing it. This can be an acute or chronic problem. In acute respiratory alkalosis, the pH will be higher than normal. In chronic respiratory alkalosis, the $PaCO_2$ is lower than normal, but the pH is within normal limits because the kidneys have had time to eliminate bicarbonate and normalize the pH. This is renal compensation and it takes about 2 to 4 days to be completed.

Under normal circumstances, a drop in the $PaCO_2$ has an inhibitory effect on the central respiratory centers, but certain disease processes or psychological conditions can stimulate ventilation and lead to hypocapnia. Acute respiratory alkalosis leads to changes in serum electrolytes. Hydrogen ions shift from the intracellular compartment to the plasma. The positively charged hydrogen ions move out of cells in exchange for other positively charged ions, specifically potassium and phosphate, which move into the cells, resulting in hypokalemia and hypophosphatemia. There is also a reduction in free serum calcium because in alkalemia, there is increased binding of Ca^{2+} to serum albumin. Because the only calcium that is physiologically active is the free, nonionized calcium, the patient can develop symptoms of hypocalcemia.

Respiratory alkalosis is often caused by hypoxemia. When the PaO_2 drops, the peripheral chemoreceptors send impulses to the central respiratory control centers. They, in turn, increase ventilation in an attempt to raise the PaO_2. This increased ventilation, however, causes the patient to excrete too much CO_2. This same process occurs in the presence of a metabolic acidosis; the lungs increase ventilation to eliminate CO_2 and normalize the pH.

Neurological conditions such as a stroke, meningitis, encephalitis, head trauma, or tumor can lead to excessive ventilation. Psychological conditions such as anxiety and panic or severe pain can also cause overventilation. During pregnancy, progesterone levels are increased. This situation stimulates the respiratory center and can lead to respiratory alkalosis (Hayes, 2005). It also can be an iatrogenic problem resulting from inappropriate machine settings when the patient is on mechanical ventilation.

Signs, Symptoms, and Consequences

The signs and symptoms of respiratory alkalosis are nonspecific, and often vary according to the underlying illness or cause. Patients may appear anxious; tachycardia and tachypnea are common. CNS effects are due to the cerebral vessel vasoconstriction that occurs with alkalosis. This vasoconstriction causes a significant decrease in cerebral blood flow. Vertigo, anxiety, clumsiness, and forgetfulness are often seen. The cardiovascular effects are nonspecific, but may include tachycardia and atrial and/or ventricular arrhythmias (Hayes, 2005).

Alkalosis of any origin favors the binding of calcium to albumin. When there is increased binding of calcium, there is less free, ionized calcium in the serum. Because only free, ionized calcium is biologically active, any time there is less of it circulating, patients will exhibit signs and symptoms of hypocalcemia. Some of the symptoms seen with respiratory alkalosis symptoms may be the result of hypocalcemia and can include numbness and/or tingling around the mouth or in the hands and fingers. A positive Chvostek's sign or carpopedal (Trousseau's sign) spasm may be seen. Both Chvostek's sign and carpopedal spasm are discussed in Chapter 18 . Muscle cramps also may be experienced.

Medical Management

Treatment is primarily directed at correcting the underlying disorder. This is rarely a life-threatening abnormality and treatment is usually not indicated unless the pH is > 7.50 (DuBose, 2004). If the hypocapnia is secondary to a hypoxemia, supplemental oxygen should be administered. If the patient is on mechanical ventilation, the tidal volume and/or respiratory rate settings should be adjusted to decrease the minute ventilation to the point where the $PaCO_2$ is in the normal range. Chapter 36 includes a discussion of ventilator settings and their impact on the acid–base balance.

Patients with psychological hyperventilation syndromes should benefit from reassurance and methods to decrease stress. During acute episodes, it may be necessary to have them breathe into a paper bag, which causes people to "rebreathe" their CO_2 and minimize loss by ventilation. The nurse plays an important role by maintaining a calm, reassuring demeanor and explaining the reason for the rebreathing. Sedatives should be reserved for patients who do not respond to conservative treatment (Hayes, 2005).

Metabolic Acidosis

This disturbance is characterized by an increase in total body acid, leading to a decreased pH. Any disorder that alters metabolism in the body can contribute to the development of metabolic acidosis.

Etiology and Pathophysiology

Metabolic acidosis is a sign of some underlying disease process. It can be induced in two ways:

- An addition of hydrogen ions or an inability to excrete the H^+ load from dietary metabolism
- A primary decrease in plasma bicarbonate to < 22 mEq/L.

The increased hydrogen ion load can come from numerous sources; lactic acidosis is believed to be the most common cause of metabolic acidosis in the hospitalized patient (Casaletto, 2005). It represents an imbalance between lactate production and utilization. Tissue hypoxia is the most common cause of clinically significant lactic acidosis. The tissue hypoxia is the result of increased oxygen demand or decreased oxygen delivery to body tissues. Without oxygen, tissues resort to anaerobic metabolism. In the face of anaerobic metabolism, body tissues are unable to completely oxidize sugar to CO_2; instead, sugars are partially oxidized to lactic acid. This acid cannot be excreted via the lungs; therefore, it remains in the circulation and causes a metabolic acidosis.

Ketoacidosis from uncontrolled diabetes mellitus, alcoholism, or prolonged starvation can also cause an accumulation of the ketone bodies acetoacetic acid and beta-hydroxybutyric acid. Ingestion of toxins such as a salicylate (aspirin) overdose, methanol, and ethylene glycol (antifreeze) will also cause metabolic acidosis.

A certain amount of acid is produced when dietary proteins are metabolized. These proteins contain sulfate and phosphate groups that, after metabolism, form sulfuric and phosphoric acid. These acids normally amount to about 150 mEq/day and they must be excreted through kidney filtration. If the kidneys fail, acidosis will occur in several days (Casaletto, 2005).

A failure to excrete the hydrogen ion load may be due to renal damage at several sections of the nephron. The term *renal tubular acidosis* refers to a group of renal pathologies that result in diminished hydrogen ion excretion or excess renal loss of bicarbonate. Type 1 renal tubular acidosis (RTA) is referred to as classic RTA or distal RTA because the malfunction is at the level of the distal convoluted tubule. The problem here is an inability to maximally acidify urine. This can be due to an inability of the H^+ pump to work against the osmotic gradient, back-diffusion of the hydrogen ion through leaky tubules, or an insufficient hydrogen ion pumping capacity due to tubular damage. There is low acid secretion and continued excretion of bicarbonate at a time when it should be retained. There is also loss of sodium and potassium in the urine (DuBose, 2004).

Type 2 RTA is also called proximal renal tubular acidosis because the site of damage is the proximal convoluted tubule. The pathology here results in impaired reabsorption of bicarbonate in the proximal tubule. The result is a high urinary bicarbonate loss, a systemic acidosis, and an inappropriately alkaline urine pH. There is accompanying renal loss of potassium that can lead to systemic hypokalemia.

Type 4 RTA is associated with a number of different conditions, but most patients with this pathology have renal failure that results in damage to the renal interstitium and tubules. Here, the defect causes impaired exchange of cations in the distal tubules. This results in reduced secretion of both hydrogen ion and potassium, which may result in hyperkalemia as well as acidosis (DuBose, 2004). (*Note:* There is a Type 3 RTA, but it is a rare variant of Type I RTA seen exclusively in children and not clinically relevant to the discussion here.)

When assessing a patient with metabolic acidosis, it is helpful to calculate the **anion gap**. The anion gap concept is based on the principle of **electroneutrality**. The sum of all of the cationic (positive) charges in the plasma must always be equal to the sum of all of the anionic (negative) charges. However, not all ions are measured and reported by the laboratory. The primary cations that are measured in venous plasma are sodium and potassium; the main anions are chloride and bicarbonate or serum CO_2. Typically, there are more unmeasured anions than cations. This difference is referred to as the anion gap. Several other anions that are not normally measured include phosphates, sulfates, organic ions, and proteins (Bartlett, 2005). Those anions make up the anion gap, which is calculated in one of two ways:

$$(Na^+ + K^+) - (Cl^- + HCO_3^-)$$

or

$$Na^+ - (Cl^- + HCO_3^-)$$

Because the value of potassium is so small, 4 mEq/L, it is sometimes ignored when calculating the anion gap. A normal anion gap is 10 ± 4 when K^+ is not included in the equation, although different sources cite different values for this "normal":

$$(Na^+) - (Cl^- + HCO_3^-)$$
$$140 - (105 + 22) = 13$$

Figure 19–3 ■ graphically depicts the anion gap.

If the anion gap is abnormally large, there are more negative ions than can be explained by the usual unmeasured substances. These extra negative substances are often lactate or the ketone bodies seen with diabetic ketoacidosis: acetoacetic acid and/or

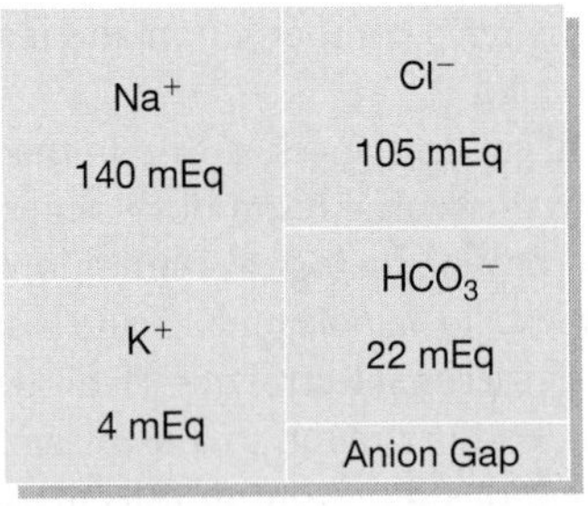

Na$^+$	Cl$^-$
140 mEq	105 mEq
K$^+$	HCO$_3^-$
	22 mEq
4 mEq	Anion Gap

OR

Anions and Cations in Serum

The equivalents of cations in a solution always balances the equivalents of anions

Cations	Anions	
Sodium 140	Chloride 105	
Potassium 4.5	Bicarbonate 24	
Calcium 5	Other = 22	⎤ Anion gap
Magnesium 1.5		⎦
Total = 151	Total = 151	

FIGURE 19–3 ■ Anion gap.

beta-hydroxybutyric acid. In this situation, termed *high anion gap acidosis,* the acid dissociates into hydrogen ion and unmeasured anion. The hydrogen ion is buffered by bicarbonate while the unmeasured ion accumulates in the serum. For example:

$$pH = 7.1 \ Na^+ = 145 \ K^+ = 5 \ Cl^- = 97 \ HCO_3^- = 12$$

$$Gap = 145 - (97 + 12)$$

$$Gap = 36$$

This significant elevation indicates high anion gap acidosis. Sometimes, calculating the anion gap will help identify a metabolic acidosis even when the pH is normal. High anion gap acidosis can also be caused by ingestion of salicylate, methanol, ethylene glycol (antifreeze), or other substances (DuBose, 2004).

If the patient has metabolic acidosis, but the anion gap is within normal limits, the problem is likely to be a loss of bicarbonate rather than an excess of acid. This occurs with gastrointestinal losses of bicarbonate such as that seen with extensive diarrhea or bowel fistulae that cause high output of lower GI fluids. The intestinal fluids beyond the stomach, including pancreatic and biliary secretions, are alkaline and consist of both bicarbonate and other organic anions. When these fluids are absorbed through the intestine, they are converted to bicarbonate in normal metabolism. If these fluids are lost through diarrhea or fistula output, the bicarbonate cannot be reclaimed and pH falls. This scenario also is typically associated with an increase in plasma chloride concentrations. The chloride ions replace plasma bicarbonate. Urinary diversions, such as a ureterosigmoidostomy, can cause hyperchloremic metabolic acidosis in as many as 80% of patients. The colon has an anion exchanger that exchanges HCO_3^- for the high chloride usually found in urine. So, when the urine is diverted to the colon, the urinary chloride is exchanged for bicarbonate, which is then lost in urine. In addition, the colon can directly absorb ammonia (NH_4), which is derived from urine and colonic bacteria. The absorbed NH_4 is converted into NH_3 and hydrogen ion in the liver, leading to hydrogen ion excess (Thomas & Kahled, 2007).

Signs, Symptoms, and Consequences

Patients with metabolic acidosis often complain of dyspnea because of the Kussmaul respirations that occur as the respiratory system tries to compensate. Tachypnea and hyperpnea (deeper than normal respirations) are usually prominent. If the acidosis is severe with a pH < 7.10, patients may develop potentially serious or fatal cardiac dysrhythmias such as ventricular tachycardia. This abnormality may also reduce cardiac contractility and lead to hypotension and heart failure.

Neurological symptoms are nonspecific, but may be manifestations of the underlying cause of the metabolic acidosis, particularly if it is associated with the ingestion of toxic substances such as ethylene glycol or methanol. Patients may complain of headache, visual changes, or mental confusion. Gastrointestinal symptoms include nausea and vomiting, abdominal pain, diarrhea, anorexia, and weight loss (Stavile et al., 2005). Chronic metabolic acidosis such as that associated with uremia or renal tubular acidosis is associated with bone disease due to the buffering of calcium carbonate and increases the risk of fractures in adults.

Laboratory studies used in the evaluation of metabolic acidosis include an ABG, which shows a low pH and low HCO_3^- as well as a base deficit more negative than –3. (Remember that bicarbonate and pH move in the *same* direction.) If the lungs have increased their alveolar ventilation to attempt to compensate for the acidosis, the $PaCO_2$ may also be lower than normal.

A metabolic panel with electrolyte assay is required when assessing patients in metabolic acidosis. The serum sodium, potassium, chloride, and bicarbonate levels are useful when calculating the anion gap. Hyperkalemia often complicates a metabolic acidosis. The excess hydrogen ions cross cell membranes and enter the intracellular space. They, in turn, "bump out" potassium ions, which are in high concentrations inside the cell. Glucose levels will be elevated in the presence of diabetic ketoacidosis; the blood urea nitrogen (BUN) and creatinine will be elevated in uremic acidosis.

Medical Management

The treatment of metabolic acidosis is directed at the correction or treatment of the underlying disorder or cause. The use of alkalinizing therapy is rarely indicated except in the most severe, life-threatening instances. In many cases, the treatment of the underlying cause and the restoration of intravascular volume and arterial oxygenation will be enough to allow for the metabolism of the organic acids (lactate and ketoacids) back to bicarbonate or for the kidney to regenerate new bicarbonate to replace the losses (Black, 2003).

The administration of sodium bicarbonate in acute metabolic acidosis is controversial. Recent studies have shown that giving bicarbonate is ineffective and may actually be detrimental to the patient's welfare (Stavile et al., 2005). The problem is that, when exogenous bicarbonate is administered to a patient who is acidemic, the bicarbonate reacts with hydrogen ions to form carbonic acid. The carbonic acid then dissociates into CO_2 and water, so the $PaCO_2$ rises. When the CO_2 cannot be eliminated, the pH correction will be very slight, or it may become more acidotic.

Metabolic Alkalosis

Metabolic alkalosis is characterized by a primary elevation in the plasma bicarbonate accompanied by an elevated pH. In metabolic imbalances, bicarbonate and pH move in the *same* direction. If bicarbonate is elevated, the pH will be elevated. If bicarbonate is decreased, the pH will decrease. The mortality of severe metabolic alkalosis is quite high, 45% in patients with an arterial pH of 7.55 and 80% when the pH is greater than 7.65 (Yaseen & Thomas, 2006).

Etiology and Pathophysiology

Metabolic alkalosis is caused by pathologic processes that lead to an accumulation of base or a loss of acid in the extracellular fluid. The increase in arterial pH usually causes a depression of the rate and depth of ventilation. This results in an increase in the $PaCO_2$ and a buffering of the alkalemia, which is the respiratory compensation component. Respiratory compensation for metabolic alkalosis is limited, however, because the respiratory center will not depress respiration to the point where oxygenation begins to suffer.

Metabolic alkalosis is a relatively common disorder that is seen with diuretic use or the loss of gastric secretions due to excessive vomiting or nasogastric suction. It also can be caused by alkali administration, loss of hydrogen from extracellular fluid, or depletion of electrolytes such as chloride or potassium, or from intravascular volume depletion.

In addition to the primary pathology, factors must be present that increase the reabsorption of bicarbonate from the kidneys. An excess of bicarbonate or "base loading" is rarely a sole cause of significant persistent metabolic alkalosis because the normal kidney is very efficient at excreting bicarbonate (Yaseen & Thomas, 2006). Transient alkalosis may occur after a patient has received oral or intravenous $NaHCO_3^-$ or a basic/alkaline equivalent such as citrate. Citrate is used as the anticoagulant in transfused blood and fresh frozen plasma. When patients receive multiple blood or plasma transfusions, they receive a significant amount of citrate and this can lead to a metabolic alkalosis. Metabolic alkalosis also may occur temporarily in patients with a chronic respiratory acidosis who have been placed on mechanical ventilation and whose $PaCO_2$ has been corrected too rapidly, before their kidneys have had a chance to excrete the excess bicarbonate.

Loss of hydrogen can occur from the GI tract or in urine. Gastric contents have high concentrations of hydrochloric acid (HCl^-) and a smaller amount of potassium chloride (KCl^-). Gastric hydrogen secretion stimulates, and is matched by, pancreatic bicarbonate secretion. When the acid contents of the stomach pass through the pylorus into the duodenum, they stimulate the pancreas to secrete lytic enzymes and bicarbonate. This bicarbonate neutralizes the acidity of the stomach contents. If the patient suffers excessive vomiting or the gastric secretions are removed by nasogastric suction before they can pass into the duodenum, there is no stimulus to the secretion of bicarbonate and it accumulates.

An excess loss of hydrogen in urine can be caused by a number of pathologic conditions or as a side effect of therapies. An increase in the secretion of the mineralocorticoid aldosterone causes an increased reabsorption of sodium from the kidney tubule back into the kidney interstitium. Under normal conditions, when a person has abnormally low blood pressure, the renin-angiotensin system is stimulated. Angiotensin release stimulates the release of aldosterone, which, in turn, promotes the reabsorption of sodium from kidney tubules. As the sodium is reabsorbed, water follows with it and the intravascular fluid volume increases, thus helping to increase blood pressure. This reabsorption of Na^+, a positive ion, renders the lumen of the tubule more electronegative. Because the lumen is now more negative, hydrogen ion stays in the tubule (again, think of the interior of the kidney tubule as being outside the body). When hydrogen ion reabsorption is inhibited, more of it is lost in the urine. An excess of mineralocorticoids (so named because they affect mineral metabolism) can be seen with primary conditions such as primary aldosteronism or as a secondary problem of many conditions including malignant hypertension or renal cell carcinoma (Black, 2003). Certain classes of diuretics, the loop (so named because they act on the nephron of the kidney at the site of the loop of Henle) or thiazide diuretics, can cause an increased secretion of aldosterone and lead to increased urinary hydrogen secretion as well as decreased intravascular volume.

Chloride helps to maintain the balance of cations to anions in the extracellular fluid to maintain electroneutrality. It does this through its inverse relationship with bicarbonate. If excessive amounts of bicarbonate ions (anions) accumulate, the number of chloride ions (also anions) decreases to maintain the number of negative charges. If sodium ions (cations) increase, the number of chloride ions increases as well, to maintain the balance of positive to negative charges. Chloride and sodium work together; sodium and bicarbonate have an inverse relationship. If serum sodium goes down, chloride also decreases. Chloride losses result in an increase in bicarbonate. Chloride depletion may occur through the loss of gastric secretions, which are rich in chloride ions, or through the kidneys with the loop or thiazide diuretics.

Hypokalemia participates in perpetuating metabolic alkalosis in several ways. When there is a decrease of K^+ in the extracellular fluid, hydrogen ions shift to the intracellular compartment to keep the electrical charge balanced. This makes the inside of the cells acidic. This intracellular acidosis stimulates reabsorption of bicarbonate from the collecting of the kidney. Hypokalemia stimulates an enzyme that promotes potassium ion reabsorption, but the potassium is exchanged for hydrogen ion, the loss of which leads to alkalosis (DuBose, 2004).

When a patient is hypovolemic and has lost relatively large volumes of bicarbonate-free fluid, this can lead to contraction alkalosis. The plasma bicarbonate concentration rises because there is a contraction of the extracellular volume around a relatively constant quantity of bicarbonate. This can occur when a loop diuretic is given to induce rapid fluid removal from a very edematous patient (Rose, 2005). To simplify this, think of a cup of water containing 4 tablespoons of sugar. If one-third cup of the water is poured off, leaving the same 4 tablespoons of sugar, the water will be much sweeter because it has a higher concentration of sugar.

Signs, Symptoms, and Consequences

The symptoms of metabolic alkalosis are difficult to separate from the symptoms of the chloride volume or potassium depletion. The effect on the CNS is the same as with respiratory alkalosis. Cerebral vessels constrict and cerebral blood flow is decreased. This can lead to lethargy, confusion, and/or apathy. If the alkalemia is very severe, coma or seizures may result (Yaseen & Thomas, 2006). The respiratory centers are depressed to attempt compensation, decreasing alveolar ventilation. This decrease in tidal volume can lead to problems with atelectasis and may contribute to the development of pulmonary infection in very ill or immunocompromised patients.

The increased binding of calcium to albumin described in the earlier section about respiratory alkalosis also occurs with metabolic alkalosis. This may lead to neuromuscular irritability resulting in muscle twitching, muscle spasm, and tetany. Positive Chvostek and Trousseau's signs may be present.

Metabolic alkalosis has effects on cardiac function. Myocardial contractility is depressed. Electrocardiogram (ECG) changes include prolongation of the QT interval as well as atrial and ventricular arrhythmias. Hypokalemia and hypomagnesemia often coexist with metabolic alkalosis and these electrolyte imbalances may exacerbate the effect of the alkalosis on cardiac function and rhythm (Yaseen & Thomas, 2006).

The diagnosis of the cause of metabolic alkalosis is usually discerned from the patient's history. A history of vomiting or the use of nasogastric suction or diuretic therapy is easily uncovered during a careful patient history. Sometimes, however, no obvious cause can be found. This may be due to a patient's surreptitious use of diuretics or self-induced vomiting, or to conditions that cause excess mineralocorticoids, usually aldosterone. With vomiting or diuretic use, intravascular volume depletion generally occurs; with hyperaldosteronism, mild volume expansion is usually present.

Medical Management

Once the origin of the metabolic alkalosis is determined, the treatment is quite obvious. Treatment is aimed at correcting the volume depletion, the potassium depletion, or the chloride depletion. In patients with low intravascular volume due to vomiting, gastric suction, or diuretic use, the administration of sodium chloride can correct the dehydration and replete the chloride. Any other electrolyte deficits should be corrected by replacing them. The administration of potassium chloride is important in the correction of metabolic alkalosis. This exogenous (from the outside the body) potassium moves into body cells in exchange for hydrogen ion to maintain electroneutrality. This hydrogen ion buffers excess extracellular bicarbonate in the serum, bringing pH down toward normal. In addition, the correction of intracellular acidosis in renal tubular cells reduces the secretion of hydrogen ion and the reabsorption of bicarbonate (Yaseen & Thomas, 2006).

If the primary cause is an excess of mineralocorticoid, steroids may be used to suppress hormone secretion or the patient may be given the drug spironolactone. Spironolactone is a synthetic steroid with a structure much like that of aldosterone. It acts as a competitive antagonist at the aldosterone receptors in the kidney. This drug is administered until definitive therapy is undertaken to treat the primary disorder (Black, 2003). If the patient is on hemodialysis, the bath solution used for dialysis can be made more acidic. If the patient has posthypercapnic alkalosis, the administration of the drug acetazolamide can speed up the renal elimination of excess bicarbonate.

In very rare cases of severe alkalosis, the administration of intravenous hydrochloric acid may be indicated. This intravenous HCl will buffer excess bicarbonate. This is usually administered over a period of about 24 hours and must be given into a major central vein due to its corrosive nature.

Nursing Management

Disorders of acid–base balance do not exist in a vacuum; instead they are a product of other underlying pathology. The nurse must be aware of patients who are at risk for acid–base disorders. The risk may be from the disorder itself or from a clinical manifestation such as fever, vomiting, diarrhea, age, and sepsis. The risk may be due to a treatment such as diuretics, mechanical ventilation, and total parental nutrition or enteral nutrition that is high in carbohydrates. Finally, the risk could be due to comorbid conditions such as respiratory or cardiac disorders or diabetes. The older adult may have multiple risk factors present from all three categories. The nursing care outlined in Nursing Process: Patient Care Plan for Acid–Base Imbalances (p. 450) must be incorporated into a larger plan of care that addresses the primary pathology or disorder. The Nursing Process: Patient Care Plan box (p. 450) outlines the nursing care required for patients experiencing acid–base disorders. Caring for elderly patients who may have acid–base imbalances is discussed in the Gerontological Considerations box.

GERONTOLOGICAL CONSIDERATIONS: Related to Acid–Base Imbalances in the Elderly

The normal pH range of extra cellular fluid (ECF) is not affected by advanced age. Some changes in respiratory and renal function, however, may affect acid–base balance. These lung and kidney changes are more likely to affect the body's ability to respond to a physiological challenge with compensation may be blunted.

In the lungs, there is uneven ventilation of the alveoli that leads to an altered ventilation/perfusion balance. This causes a drop in arterial oxygen tension, but the $PaCO_2$ remains unchanged. This may be partly due to a drop in the production of CO_2 due to a decrease in the basal metabolic rate that happens during the aging process (Rosenthal & Kavic, 2004). The ability to hyperventilate in response to an acute metabolic acidosis may be blunted and lead to a persistent acidosis.

Renal tubular function is also affected by aging. The ability to conserve sodium and excrete hydrogen ion falls, so the aging kidney may be slower to respond to an acid load (either respiratory or metabolic) and blood pH may take longer to normalize (Marik, 2006). Dehydration is a particular problem because the aging kidney does not respond to fluid and sodium loss by its usual mechanism of increasing sodium retention, thus conserving water (Rosenthal & Kavic, 2004). In addition, many drugs commonly used by elderly people such as salicylates, diuretics, and laxatives may precipitate acid–base disturbances.

Collaborative Care

The care of a patient with a disorder that produces an imbalance of acid–base homeostasis involves nurses and physicians, but may also require respiratory therapy for assistance with bronchodilator therapy or assisted ventilation when treating respiratory causes of imbalance. Other nursing specialists such as dialysis nurses may also be called on for the expertise. Pharmacists may be used as consultants when electrolytes are being administered or when the absorption or action of medications may be altered in the presence of an abnormal pH.

Case managers and discharge planners evaluate placement and discharge needs. They can provide assistance in the arrangement of home nursing and/or respiratory therapy and durable medical equipment such as nebulizers or CPAP or BiPAP machines.

Health Promotion

Many patients with disturbances of acid–base balance suffer from chronic conditions that are the underlying causes of imbalances. Nurses are in a unique position to promote healthy behaviors in the face of chronic illness. These interventions can decrease symptoms and improve quality of life. Several examples are presented here.

Patients with chronic ventilatory failure often experience disabling symptoms such as chronic dyspnea. This can lead to malnutrition because the patient is too short of breath to eat. The nurse can explore the patient's daily routines and make suggestions about switching to five to six small meals per day and limiting mealtime conversation to conserve energy. Dietitians can suggest the best types of foods to conserve energy while supplying adequate nutrition. Subjective feelings of breathlessness can be eased by keeping the environment relatively cool and using fans to create air movement. Positioning for optimal lung expansion may involve the use of a recliner for sleeping and supporting

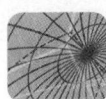

NURSING PROCESS: Patient Care Plan for Acid–Base Imbalances

Assessment of Respiratory Acidosis

Subjective Data:

Do you have a history of shortness of breath or exercise-limiting symptoms?
Do you have a cough? Is it productive? Sputum description?
Any history of sleep-disordered breathing? (Sleeping partner may be aware of excessive snoring.)

Objective Data:

Auscultate breath sounds; be alert for decreases in intensity, diffuse wheezing, stridor
Respiratory rate
Examine fingers for signs of clubbing
Observe for presence of a barrel chest
Laboratory evaluation: ABGs, complete blood count, serum electrolytes, drug screen (if there is suspicion of respiratory depression by drugs)

Nursing Assessment and Diagnoses	Outcomes and Evaluation Parameters	Planning and Interventions with *Rationales*
Nursing Diagnoses: *Impaired Gas Exchange* *Ineffective Airway Clearance*	**Outcomes:** Airway patency will be maintained. Gas exchange will be optimized **Evaluation Parameters:** PaCO$_2$ will return to patient's baseline with a pH in the normal range. Any dyspnea will be relieved as reported by the patient. Patient will return to baseline level of physical activity.	**Interventions and *Rationales*:** Position the patient sitting upright with arms supported on an overbed table. (Positioning in a chair may be preferable to the bed.) *This position helps maximize lung inflation.* Administer any bronchodilators that are ordered. Ensure that the patient is using proper technique if self-administering. *Patients who self-administer metered-dose inhalers (MDI) at home often prefer to continue self-administration while in the hospital as a way to retain control. However, improper technique is a frequent problem in the use of metered-dose inhalers (MDI). Enlist the help of a respiratory therapist.* Encourage the use of an incentive spirometer. Use should be at least every 4 hours while awake. *This is one way to encourage the patient to take deep breaths to help prevent atelectasis.* Encourage early ambulation. Set increasing distance goals with the patient each time. *Helps the patient to avoid complications of immobility.*

Assessment of Respiratory Alkalosis

Subjective Data:

Do you have any shortness of breath, numbness around the mouth, or paresthesias?
Do you have any history of anxiety or acute pain?

Objective Data:

Assess respiratory rate
Laboratory evaluation: ABGs, serum electrolytes, complete blood count

Nursing Assessment and Diagnoses	Outcomes and Evaluation Parameters	Planning and Interventions with *Rationales*
Nursing Diagnosis: *Ineffective Breathing Pattern*	**Outcomes:** Gas exchange will be optimized. Any excess anxiety or pain will be relieved. **Evaluation Parameters:** PaCO$_2$ will return to patient's baseline with a pH in the normal range. Respiratory rate and depth will be within normal parameters.	**Interventions and *Rationales*:** Encourage slow, deep respirations. In the acute stage, this may require the constant presence of the nurse. *A calm, reassuring nurse will help promote relaxation in the patient.* If that is difficult for the patient, the use of a rebreather mask or having the patient breathe into a simple paper bag may be required. *Promotes the rebreathing of exhaled CO$_2$ to help return levels to normal. Explain the reason for the rebreathing to the patient.* Evaluate for the presence of pain using objective criteria such as the visual analog scale. Medicate the patient to a level of pain that is acceptable to the patient. Reassess pain levels 30 minutes after IV medication and 1 hour after oral medication. *Pain can cause an increased respiratory rate. Relief of pain should help return the rate toward normal.* If the cause of the hyperventilation was anxiety or fear, help the patient explore the cause to help identify strategies to avoid future episodes. *Patients may need guidance in stress relief or anticipatory guidance about how to avoid such stress in the future.*

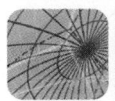

Assessment of Metabolic Acidosis

Subjective Data:

Ask about symptoms that may help determine cause: history of diabetes, renal insufficiency/failure, diarrhea or other loss of intestinal fluids. Ask about dyspnea; count respiratory rate. Observe for Kussmaul respirations.

Objective Data:

Laboratory evaluation:

- ABGs; evaluate pH and HCO_3^-; also examine PaO_2 to evaluate for hypoxemia as a cause of lactic acidosis
- Serum electrolytes; calculate anion gap
- Urine electrolytes, osmolarity
- Blood glucose (to evaluate for uncontrolled diabetes mellitus)
- BUN and creatinine (to evaluate renal function)

Evaluate for physical signs of malnutrition or dehydration

Nursing Assessment and Diagnoses	Outcomes and Evaluation Parameters	Planning and Interventions with *Rationales*
Nursing Diagnoses: *Imbalanced Nutrition: More than body requirements Deficient Fluid Volume*	**Outcomes:** Acid–base balance will be restored. The underlying cause of the acidosis will be identified and treated. Recurrence will be avoided. ***Evaluation Parameters:*** Serum bicarbonate will return to normal levels with a pH within the normal range. Fluid balance will be optimized.	**Interventions and *Rationales:*** *Note:* Much of the nursing care will be directed by the underlying cause of the acidosis. Obtain a baseline weight and weigh the patient frequently during rehydration, if applicable. *An accurate patient weight is a better parameter to measure than is the intake and output measurement. This is particularly true in cases where the cause of any dehydration is excessive diarrhea or fistula output. The patient should be weighed with the same amount of clothing each time.* If the cause of the acidosis is an exacerbation of diabetes or renal failure, it is important to explore the reasons with the patient and family. The problem may be a failure to comply with recommended treatment or may be caused by a concurrent event such as an infection. *An assessment of the patient's knowledge of any underlying disease and its management may help uncover causes of noncompliance or condition exacerbation. Extensive patient and family education or reeducation may be required to help prevent episodes in the future. This may be beyond the scope of the inpatient nurse when hospital stays continue to shorten. Referral to an outpatient facility or consultant such as a diabetes educator may be required.*

Assessment of Metabolic Alkalosis

Subjective Data:

Ask about history that may help identify a cause: vomiting, diarrhea, use of diuretics.
Ask about symptoms of hypokalemia: weakness, muscle aches.
Ask about symptoms of hypocalcemia: tingling around the mouth, muscles cramps.

Objective Data:

Evaluate fluid volume status
Evaluate for signs of hypocalcemia: tetany, Chvostek's sign
Laboratory evaluation:
ABGs; serum electrolytes and calcium, osmolarity; urine electrolytes

Nursing Assessment and Diagnoses	Outcomes and Evaluation Parameters	Planning and Interventions with *Rationales*
Nursing Diagnosis: *Deficient Fluid Volume*	**Outcomes:** Acid–base balance will be restored. The underlying cause of the alkalosis will be identified and treated. Recurrence will be avoided. ***Evaluation Parameters:*** Serum bicarbonate will return to normal levels with a pH within the normal range. Fluid balance will be optimized. Any excess vomiting or gastric suction will be corrected. Any chloride or potassium depletion will be corrected.	**Interventions and *Rationales:*** *Note:* Much of the nursing care will be directed by the underlying cause of the acidosis. Obtain a baseline weight and weigh the patient frequently during rehydration, if applicable. *An accurate patient weight is a better parameter to measure than is the intake and output measurement. This is particularly true in cases where the cause of any dehydration is excessive vomiting. The patient should be weighed with the same amount of clothing each time.* Control any vomiting with antiemetics. If the patient must be on continuous gastric suction, the use of a histamine-2 receptor blocker or a proton pump inhibitor may be indicated. *The goal is to stop the loss of hydrochloric acid from the stomach. The drugs decrease the secretion of acid into the stomach and, hence, stop its loss.* If the alkalemia is severe and the patient's respirations are depressed, encourage frequent deep breathing and the use of an incentive spirometer. *The decrease in tidal volume can lead to atelectasis and may contribute to the development of a pulmonary infection.* If there is no obvious cause for the alkalosis, a sensitive exploration into the possibility of self-induced vomiting or the use of diuretics may be required. *These may be attempts at weight loss or may be symptoms of a disorder such as bulimia.*

the arms on pillows. Patient and family education about the precautions to be taken when oxygen is in use in the home can help to decrease the risk of fire or excess oxygen administration. If the patient uses an oxygen concentrator, a plan about what to do in case of an emergency such as a power outage should be formulated by the patient and the nurse.

Patients with obstructive sleep apnea that leads to respiratory acidosis must be counseled about the dangers of excessive daytime sleepiness. When possible, patients should undergo an outpatient sleep study and evaluation for the use of nasal CPAP to decrease apneic arousal episodes at night and to promote better REM sleep. Patients are often reluctant to use home CPAP machines, and the nurse is in a position to provide encouragement about their use for patient safety. Patients who frequently fall asleep during the day should be counseled about the risks associated with driving because they are prone to accidents.

When patients with diabetes experience an episode of ketoacidosis, the nurse should explore with the patient and family what may have led to the episode. If it is a stressor such as infection, diabetic teaching should be begun or reinforced and the patient counseled to have a "sick day" plan to decrease the chance that blood sugar levels will get out of control. If there is any suspicion that the patient is not following her diabetes management regimen adequately, the nurse will be able to explore the reasons for noncompliance. If the problem is a lack of knowledge, intensive diabetic teaching and reinforcement of previous teaching should be started in the inpatient setting and continued in the outpatient or home care setting.

 ## Research

Current and future research needs to focus on control of symptoms with chronic conditions such as dyspnea and enhancing the quality of life of patients with chronic illnesses. Additionally, improved monitoring systems and treatment measures need to detect and treat symptoms before they progress to cause a debilitating state. The Research Opportunities and Clinical Impact box outlines research topics in the area of acid–base imbalances.

 ## Summary

Acid–base imbalances almost always occur in conjunction with diseases or pathologic conditions that are the primary focus for the nurse caring for the patient. A basic understanding of how these imbalances affect organ systems and blood chemistries will enable nurses to provide focused assessments of the patients in their care and plan nursing interventions accordingly.

RESEARCH OPPORTUNITIES AND CLINICAL IMPACT RELATED TO ACID–BASE IMBALANCES

Research Area	Clinical Impact
Patient Assessment	
• Assessing the severity of dyspnea	Establish a standard measure of dyspnea to measure severity and to gauge the effectiveness of interventions and relief strategies.
• Exploration of ethnic/cultural differences in the description of symptoms such as dyspnea	Enhance cultural sensitivity and ensure that symptoms are recognized and that strategies are undertaken to relieve symptoms.
• Assess accuracy of noninvasive methods of measuring $PaCO_2$	To promote noninvasive methods of assessing the adequacy of ventilation.
• Compare the accuracy of the recording of intake and output vs. accurate patient weight in the assessment of fluid loss/gain	Intake and output recording is time consuming and often inaccurate. Explore more accurate methods of assessment of fluid volume status.
Nursing Intervention Research	
• Effectiveness of interventions to relieve dyspnea	Dyspnea is a strong, subjective experience of physiological distress. Relief of this symptom can enhance quality of life and improve end-of-life care.
• Enhancing quality of life in patients with chronic illness	
• Examine the most effective methods of patient education during short hospital stays	Shorter inpatient hospitalization reduces the time available for patient and family education about disease processes and their management. Evaluation of the most effective methods that can be undertaken in a short time period has a goal of improving comprehension and retention of information.

Clinical Preparation

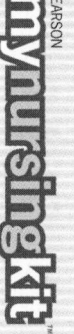

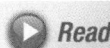 **Read**

- History of Current Illness
- Past Medical History
- Physical Exam
- Admitting Medical Orders
- Laboratory Study Results

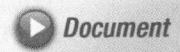 **Document**

- Summary of Hospitalization
- Pathophysiology Form
- Laboratory Values
- Laboratory Results Explanation

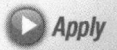 **Apply**

- List of Potential Nursing Diagnoses
- Concept Map
- Critical Thinking Questions

Log on to MyNursingKit.com to download forms you will need and to complete further steps in the Clinical Preparation assignment.

HISTORY OF PRESENT ILLNESS

A.B. is an 82-year-old male who began to feel unwell 2 days prior to presenting to the emergency department (ED). He complained of feeling "achy all over" and developed a cough that was productive of yellowish sputum. He was unable to sleep flat in bed and had begun to try to sleep sitting up in his recliner. The coughing left him short of breath and unable to sleep. He was unable to walk farther than a few steps without becoming increasingly short of breath. Consequently, his wife drove him to the ED. He presented with a complaint of increasing shortness of breath and a productive cough. He had a temperature of 38.2°C and a respiratory rate of 24 breaths/minute with an oxygen saturation of 93% on room air. Chest radiograph showed evidence of pneumonia.

Medical–Surgical History
History of coronary artery disease; two coronary stents placed
  1 year prior to admission
Emphysema
No other significant medical history
Allergies: none known
Drug intolerance: none known

Social History
A.B. lives with his wife independently. He has two sons who live in other states. He depends on friends and neighbors when he needs assistance. He has a 50 pack/year smoking history although the patient stopped smoking 8 years ago after he was told that he had emphysema. Denies use of alcohol.

Physical Exam
The patient appears ill. Vital signs reveal: temperature: 38.2°C; pulse: 112 beats/minute; BP: 156/92; respirations: 24 breaths/minute.

The patient is moderately obese with a barrel chest. On auscultation, coarse rhonchi can be heard throughout. Breath sounds are decreased in the bases and there is a slight expiratory wheeze.

HEENT: PERRLA, ears appear normal; pharynx pink with exudate
Neck: no cervical lymphadenopathy; thyroid nonpalpable
Heart: regular rate and rhythm; no extra heart sounds
Abdomen: bowel sounds present × 4 quadrants; soft and
  nondistended; no tenderness or masses; no hepatomegaly
Pulses: apical, radial, and pedal pulses present and regular
Arterial blood gas: PaO_2: 88 mmHg; $PaCO_2$: 66 mmHg; pH: 7.28;
  HCO_3^-: 34 mEq/L; BE: +5; saturation: 92% on room air

White blood cell count: $14.1 \times 10^3/\mu L$
Chest radiograph revealed a consolidation in the right lower lobe
  but no effusion.
Sputum gram stain showed a few gram-positive cocci in pairs and
  12 to 20 white cells. The culture later grew out *Streptococcus pneumoniae*.

Admitting Medical Orders
Admit to medicine
No known allergies
Diagnosis: exacerbation of COPD and community-acquired
  pneumonia
Vital signs, oxygen saturation every 4 hours
Call house officer: pulse < 60 or > 120/minute; BP < 90 or > 160
  systolic; temperature > 38.5; RR < 10 or > 30; oxygen
  saturation < 92% or patient complaint of increased dyspnea
Activity: bed rest with bathroom privileges tonight. Up ad lib
  tomorrow morning
Diet: AHA (2 g sodium)
Bronchodilator protocol: levalbuterol nebulizer q6h
Oxygen: place patient on least amount of oxygen needed to
  maintain saturation > 92%
Sequential compression devices (SCD) to lower extremities
IV fluids: D5½NS 100 mL/hr
Incentive spirometer q2h while awake
Patient education: obtain spacer; educate patient in use of
  metered-dose inhaler (MDI) and spacer
Case management for discharge planning: possible home oxygen,
  home nebulizer, referral to community pulmonary rehab program

Scheduled Medications

Methylprednisolone sodium succinate (Solu-Medrol) 60 mg IV push q6h

Lasix 40 mg po bid

Ceftazidime 1 g q8h IV

Aspirin 81 mg po/day

Clopidogrel 75 mg po/day

DVT prophylaxis: enoxaparin 30 mg subcutaneously twice a day

PRN Medications

Tylenol 325 mg × 2 po q4h for fever > 38.5°C

Morphine 0.3–5 mg IV q4h prn pain

Temazepam 15-30mg po HS prn insomnia

Droperidol 1.25–2.5mg IV q6h prn nausea

Ordered Laboratory Studies

Chemistry 20 on admission; Chemistry 7 q a.m.

Blood cultures now

CBC w/diff every a.m.

PTT, PT, INR every a.m.

Sputum culture

Ordered Diagnostic Studies

Chest x-ray PA and lateral in a.m.

LABORATORY STUDY RESULTS

TEST	Day 1	Day 2	Day 3
Chemistry			
Sodium	135 mEq/L	137 mEq/L	141 mEq/L
Potassium	4.8 mEq/L	4.0 mEq/L	3.9 mEq/L
Chloride	103 mEq/L	107 mEq/L	105 mEq/L
Carbon dioxide (CO_2)	34 mEq/L	34.5 mEq/L	34.4 mEq/L
Blood urea nitrogen	32 mg/dL	28.8 mg/dL	26 mg/dL
Creatinine	1.7 mg/dL	1.5 mg/dL	1.3 mg/dL
Blood glucose	120 mg/dL	126 mg/dL	118 mg/dL
Calcium	8.8 mg/dL	9.0 mg/dL	9.2 mg/dL
Amylase	110 units/L		
Magnesium	2 mEq/L	2.1 mEq/L	1.8 mEq/L
Phosphorus	3.3 mg/dL		
Alkaline phosphatase	174 units/L		
T. bilirubin	1.0 mg/dL		
CPK total	220 units/L		
LDH	188 units/L		
AST	16 units/L		
ALT	17 units/L		
Hematology			
WBC	14.1/mm³	13.9/mm³	12.8/mm³
Hemoglobin	17.2 g/dL	16.4 g/dL	16.5 g/dL

TEST	Day 1	Day 2	Day 3
Hematocrit	53.5%	50.2%	51.1%
RBC	5.2/mm³	5.0/mm³	5.0/mm³
Platelets	356/mm³		
PTT	29 seconds	31 seconds	28 seconds
PT	11.8 seconds	12.6 econds	14.3 seconds
INR	1.0	1.10	1.14
ABGs			
$\%O_2$	21%	28%	28%
PO_2	88	90	89
O_2 Sat	92%	96%	95%
pH	7.28	7.32	7.33
PCO_2	66	58	56
HCO_3	34	34	31
Miscellaneous			
Digoxin level	Negative		
Toxicology screen	Negative		
Blood alcohol level	Negative		
Sputum culture	*Streptococcus pneumoniae*		
Blood culture	Negative		

CRITICAL THINKING QUESTIONS

1. What does the blood gas indicate in terms of acid–base balance?

2. What were this patient's risk factors for developing pneumonia?

3. What factor(s) contributed to the $PaCO_2$ of 66 mmHg?

4. What nursing measures would help bring the $PaCO_2$ back into normal range?

Answers to Critical Thinking Questions appear in Appendix D.

NCLEX® REVIEW

1. A patient's blood pH is decreasing. The nurse realizes that this patient's hydrogen ion concentration is:
   1. Increasing.
   2. Decreasing.
   3. Being affected by oxygen concentration.
   4. Stabilizing.

2. A patient is admitted with the diagnosis of diabetic ketoacidosis. The nurse realizes that this patient's body will attempt to attain acid–base balance by:
   1. Decreasing the respiratory rate.
   2. Increasing the reabsorption of hydrogen ions.
   3. Increasing the secretion of hydrogen ions.
   4. Decreasing the reabsorption of bicarbonate.

3. A patient has a respiratory rate of 20. The nurse calculates this patient's minute ventilation to be:
   1. 1 L/min.
   2. 2 L/min.
   3. 5 L/min.
   4. 10 L/min.

4. The nurse, admitting a patient with diabetes, believes the patient is attempting to correct an acidotic condition. Which of the following did this nurse most likely observe while assessing this patient?
   1. Slow methodical respirations
   2. Deep rapid respirations
   3. Change in level of consciousness
   4. Intact extraoccular movements

5. The nurse is caring for a patient with metabolic acidosis. The nurse realizes that which of the following laboratory values might be altered for this patient?
   1. Ammonia
   2. Blood-urea-nitrogen
   3. Creatinine
   4. Prothrombin

6. The nurse is reviewing a patient's arterial blood gas results. Which of the following values should the nurse study first?
   1. $PaCO_2$
   2. HCO_3
   3. Compensation
   4. pH

7. The nurse is caring for a patient with pneumonia who has arterial blood gas values of: pH 7.20, $PaCO_2$ 75, HCO_3^- 28, PaO_2 44. Which of the following would be a priority for this patient?
   1. Assist the patient to breathe into a paper bag.
   2. Prepare to administer sodium bicarbonate IV.
   3. Place the patient in high Fowler's position.
   4. Administer the prn sedative available.

8. A patient is admitted in respiratory acidosis secondary to barbiturate overdose. Which of the following will the nurse most likely assess in this patient?
   1. Kussmaul's respirations
   2. Seizures
   3. Slow, shallow respirations
   4. Increased deep tendon reflexes

9. The nurse is providing discharge instructions to a patient with respiratory alkalosis. Which of the following statements indicates the patient understands the instructions?
   1. "I will not take my Lasix without a potassium supplement."
   2. "I will not use Mylanta 5–6 times a day like I used to."
   3. "I will take a stress management class or seek counseling."
   4. "I will call my MD the next time I have diarrhea for a few days."

Answers for review questions appear in Appendix D

KEY TERMS

acids *p.436*
alkalis *p.436*
anatomic dead space *p.438*
anion gap *p.446*
base excess *p.440*
bases *p.436*
buffer *p.437*
carbon dioxide *p.437*

carbonic acid *p.437*
compensation *p.439*
dead space *p.438*
electroneutrality *p.446*
hydrogen ion *p.436*
hypercarbic drive *p.439*
hyperventilation *p.439*

hypoventilation *p.439*
hypoxic drive *p.439*
minute ventilation *p.438*
pathologic dead space *p.438*
pH *p.436*
secretion *p.439*
sodium bicarbonate *p.436*

EXPLORE PEARSON **mynursingkit**™

MyNursingKit is your one stop for online chapter review materials and resources. Prepare for success with additional NCLEX®-style practice questions, interactive assignments and activities, web links, animations and videos, and more!

Register your access code from the front of your book at
www.mynursingkit.com

REFERENCES

Androgue, H. E., & Androgue, H. J. (2001). Acid–base physiology. *Respiratory Care, 46*(4), 328–341.

Argyle, B. (2002). *Blood gas computer program manual.* Retrieved March 10, 2004, from Mad Scientists Software website: http://www. madscientistsoftware.com

Bartlett, D. (2005). Understanding the anion and osmolal gap lab values. *Journal of Emergency Nursing, 31*(1), 109–111.

Black, R. M. (2003). Metabolic acidosis and metabolic alkalosis. In R. Irwin & J. Rippe, *Intensive care medicine* (5th ed., pp. 854–864). Philadelphia: Lippincott Williams & Wilkins.

Breen, P. (2001). ABG and pH analysis. *Anesthesia Clinics of North America, 19*(4), 885–906.

Casaletto, J. (2005). Differential diagnosis of metabolic acidosis. *Emergency Medicine Clinics of North America, 23*(3), 1–12.

DuBose, T. (2004). Acid–base disorders. In B. M. Brenner, *The Kidney* (7th ed.). Philadelphia, Elsevier, Inc.

Grogono, A. (2006). *Acid–base tutorial.* Retrieved April 1, 2007, from http://www.acid-base.com

Hayes, J. A. (2005, June 30). *Respiratory alkalosis.* Retrieved April 6, 2007, from http://www.emedicine.com/topic2009

Marik, P. (2006). Management of the critically ill geriatric patient. *Critical Care Medicine, 34*(9 Suppl.), S176–S182.

Priestley, M., & Levine, G. (2006). *Respiratory acidosis.* Retrieved April 6, 2007, from http://www.emedicine.com/ped/topic16.html

Rose, B. (2005, September 3). *Urine electrolytes in diagnosis of metabolic acidosis.* Retrieved April 1, 2007, from UpToDate website: http://www.utdol.com/application/topic/ topicTest.asp?fil.../18016&type=A&selectedTitle=4~4

Rosenthal, R., & Kavic, S. (2004). Assessment and management of the geriatric patient. *Critical Care Medicine, 32*(4 Suppl.), S92–S105.

Shlichtig, R. (2005). Acid–base balance. In *Textbook of critical care* (5th ed., pp. 829–838). Philadelphia: W. B. Saunders.

Stavile, K. L., et al. (2005). *Metabolic acidosis.* Retrieved April 1, 2007, from http://www.emedicine.com/emerg/topic31.2

Thomas, C., & Khaled, H. (2007, February 1). *Metabolic acidosis.* Retrieved April 6, 2007, from http:///www.emedicine.com/med/ topic1458.htm

Yaseen, S., & Thomas, C. (2006). *Metabolic alkalosis.* Retrieved March 21, 2007, from http://emedicine.com/med/topic1459

Infectious Disease

Teri Murray
Peggy Ellis

Outcome-Based Learning Objectives

After studying this chapter, the learner will be able to:

1. Describe the infectious process and its effects on the body.
2. Identify risk factors for infection.
3. Describe the chain of infection.
4. Describe measures to prevent and control infection.
5. Identify common pathogens causing infection.
6. Differentiate between active and passive immunity.
7. Describe *Healthy People 2010* guidelines for prevention of infection.
8. Identify the assessment and interventions required by a patient with an infection.

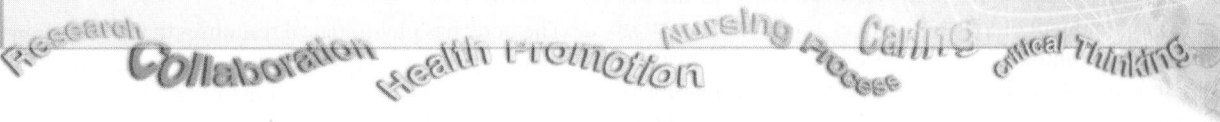

Research   Collaboration   Health Promotion   Nursing Process   Caring   Critical Thinking

INFECTIOUS DISEASE is a major health problem. Infection occurs when a microorganism enters the body and is able to colonize and multiply, leading to an infection and subsequent immune response. A microorganism is a microscopic body such as a bacterium, virus, fungus, or parasite. Some microorganisms live on the human body normally and are beneficial. For example, certain microorganisms live in the intestines and produce enzymes that facilitate digestion. If the immune and inflammatory systems are compromised, as can occur when an individual has a decreased immunity, organisms that usually benefit the body will leave their normal sites and travel to other areas of the body and cause an infection. A microorganism that produces disease is called a pathogen. True pathogens are able to cause disease regardless of the body's normal defenses.

When an infection is acquired outside a health care facility it is considered a **community-acquired infection**. When an infection occurs in a hospitalized patient, it is known as a **nosocomial infection.** Nosocomial infections have been blamed for numerous complications in the hospitalized patient leading to a cost of many lives and billions of health care dollars. Many infections in the hospital are related to the use of invasive devices such as urinary catheters, intravenous catheters, surgical drains, nasogastric tubes, and endotracheal tubes. Because of the increased susceptibility to infection, invasive devices should only be used when necessary for patient care and should be discontinued as quickly as possible. Clean or sterile technique should be used when caring for anyone with invasive devices in order to avoid infection. Patients who develop nosocomial infections are often critically ill with an increased susceptibility to infection.

Nosocomial infections may also occur because the overuse of broad-spectrum antibiotics alters the body's natural defenses and leads to antibiotic resistance in harmful bacteria. Many nosocomial infections are caused by multidrug-resistant organisms (MDROs). The National Nosocomial Infections Surveillance (NNIS) system was formed by the Centers for Disease Control and Prevention (CDC) to create a national database of nosocomial infections. It began in 1970 and is a voluntary, hospital-based reporting system to monitor and accurately describe hospital-acquired infections and provide statistical analysis of those infections. This information aids the infection control practitioner and hospital epidemiologist to develop strategies to reduce nosocomial infection rates. The goals of NNIS are to:

- Collect surveillance data from a sample of acute care hospitals in the United States to permit valid estimation of the magnitude of nosocomial infections (NI) in hospitalized patients.
- Analyze and report NI surveillance data to permit recognition of trends in infection rates, antimicrobial resistance, and nosocomial pathogens.

- Provide hospitals with risk-adjusted NI data that can be used for comparison.
- Assist hospitals in developing surveillance and analysis methods that permit timely recognition of NI problems and prompt intervention with appropriate infection control measures.
- Conduct collaborative research studies with NNIS hospitals (e.g., describe the epidemiology of emerging infections and pathogens, assess the importance of potential risk factors, further characterize nosocomial pathogens and mechanisms of resistance, and evaluate alternative surveillance and prevention strategies).

The NNIS produces a national nosocomial infection database that is used to (1) describe the epidemiology of nosocomial infections, (2) describe antimicrobial resistance trends, and (3) produce NI rates to use for comparison purposes. This information is used to help infection control practitioners and hospital epidemiologists develop guidelines for prevention, timely recognition, and prompt intervention with appropriate infection control measures. The data show that surgical site infections are the leading type of infection in hospitalized patients. The respiratory tract, urinary tract, bloodstream, and surgical wounds are the most common sites and are the most frequently monitored for the occurrence of infection. Although, the rates of infection have decreased during the last 10 years, the prevention of infection in hospitalized patients remains part of the national health objectives for 2010 (U.S. Department of Health and Human Services [DHHS], 2000).

Historically, medicine has made many advances in the prevention and treatment of infection. Potent antibiotics, sanitation programs, and immunizations have been developed to treat and prevent infection. In spite of this, many infectious organisms remain and new varieties and strains are developing. Some of these strains are resistant to antibiotics, making treatment more difficult due to increased susceptibility to infection, which then increases morbidity and mortality and length of hospital stay.

Antimicrobial resistance is becoming an increasingly important problem in health care. It is primarily due to the prolonged or inappropriate use of antibiotics. Bacteria sometimes survive after the use of antibiotics and become able to change their genetic makeup so that the antibiotic is no longer effective. Currently, the most well-known resistant organisms are methicillin-resistant *Staphylococcus aureus* (MRSA), multidrug-resistant tuberculosis (MDR-TB), penicillin-resistant *Streptococcus pneumoniae* (PRSP), vancomycin-resistant enterococci (VRE), vancomycin intermediate-resistant *S. aureus* (VISA), and vancomycin-resistant *S. aureus* (VRSA) (CDC, 2004). Antimicrobial resistance has occurred for a variety of reasons, including but not limited to inappropriate prescribing practices, inconsistent infection control techniques, promotion of antibiotic use by pharmaceutical companies, lack of public knowledge about appropriate antibiotic use, availability of antibiotics without prescription in some parts of the world, and use of antibiotics in agriculture on crops and livestock. Chart 20–1 lists various actions that can be taken to address this problem.

Defense Mechanisms

Most human beings have defenses for prevention of infectious disease including physical, chemical, and immune mechanisms.

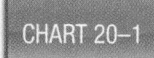

CHART 20–1   Actions to Address Antimicrobial Resistance

- Use antibiotics judiciously. Obtain cultures and do not use antibiotics for prophylactic purposes when the likelihood of infection is low.
- Use the most appropriate narrow-spectrum antibiotic possible. Use a full dose of the antibiotic for the shortest course needed to kill the microorganism.
- Use standard, approved infection control measures. Proper hand hygiene as outlined in Charts 20–3, 20–4, and 20–5 (pp. 462, 463) is essential. Wear gloves when necessary and follow standard precautions for all patients.
- Teach patients the importance of practicing infection control, and when antibiotics are necessary and when they are not.

Whether or not an organism causes disease depends, in part, on the success or failure of these mechanisms. These defense mechanisms include the skin, enzymes that kill microorganisms, structures such as cilia that trap microorganisms and sweep them out of the bronchial tubes, membranes that secrete mucus to prevent the adherence of the organisms, chemical secretions such as hydrochloric acid in the stomach, and the immune system. The immune system produces enzymes, and uses other factors and cells to trap and kill microorganisms. Chart 20–2 depicts human defenses against infection. Chapters 59 and 60 🔗 address immune assessment and immune response.

Inflammation

The body has physiological responses that are designed to eliminate invading organisms and protect against infection. The inflammatory response is a physiological process that attacks, confines, and kills invading organisms. It also allows for tissue repair after damage from an invading organism or from tissue injury and death. The steps in the inflammatory process are di-

CHART 20–2   Defense Mechanisms Against Infection

Mechanism	Purpose
Skin	Offers a protective barrier of five to seven layers with the top layer being shed constantly.
Mucous membranes	Line orifices of body open to the environment, trap microorganisms, contain bacteriostatic agents, secrete IgA, an immunoglobulin that fights infection. Wash out microorganisms and prevent them from adhering to mucosal surfaces.
Respiratory cilia	Trap microorganisms and push them out of the body.
Secretions of oil and moisture from glands	Inhibit penetration of pathogens; inhibit pathogen growth.
Normal flora	Flora that normally exist in the gastrointestinal tract and vagina compete with pathogens for placement.
Chemical secretions	Gastric acid and acidic urine create an atmosphere not conducive to the growth of microorganisms.

agramed in Figure 20–1 ■. The inflammatory process involves a vascular phase and a cellular phase. The vascular phase consists of the following processes, which occur almost simultaneously:

- Temporary vasoconstriction to avoid blood loss after injury
- Vasodilation to increase blood supply to the area, leading to redness and increased warmth of the area
- Increased hydrostatic pressure related to the increase in blood flow
- Increased permeability of blood vessel walls caused by chemical mediators
- Leakage of fluid and cells out of capillaries into interstitial spaces so that toxins are diluted. This leakage of fluid and eventually protein leads to increased osmotic pressure in the interstitial spaces and edema.

The cellular phase involves the response of white blood cells (WBCs) to the cellular injury. It begins as chemotactic substances are released from the tissues by cellular injury and complement is activated. Neutrophils are the first WBCs to arrive at the site and are the main phagocytic cell. The processes involved in the cellular phase are as follows:

- An increased number of WBCs are attracted to the site of injury by chemotactic factors.

- WBCs adhere to the vessel wall during a process called margination.
- WBCs migrate through the vessel wall into the interstitial tissue during a process called diapedesis or emigration.
- WBCs are attracted to the inflamed site by chemotactic factors.
- Neutrophils ingest the bacteria and dead cells through a process of coating microorganisms called opsonization.
- This coating allows the bacteria and dead cells to be easily engulfed and killed by WBCs.
- Neutrophils then die, releasing proteolytic enzymes that liquefy the dead cells and bacteria, resulting in the formation of pus.
- Fibrin is secreted by fibroblasts and serves to wall off the area to prevent the spread of bacteria and lay the groundwork for tissue rebuilding.

The inflammatory phase of wound healing is discussed in Chapter 67 ⬭.

Manifestations of Inflammation

The signs and symptoms related to inflammation can be local and/or systemic depending on the location and severity of the inflammatory response. There are five cardinal local symptoms of inflammation: (1) redness from increased blood flow to the area, (2) heat due to increased blood flow to the area, (3) swelling due

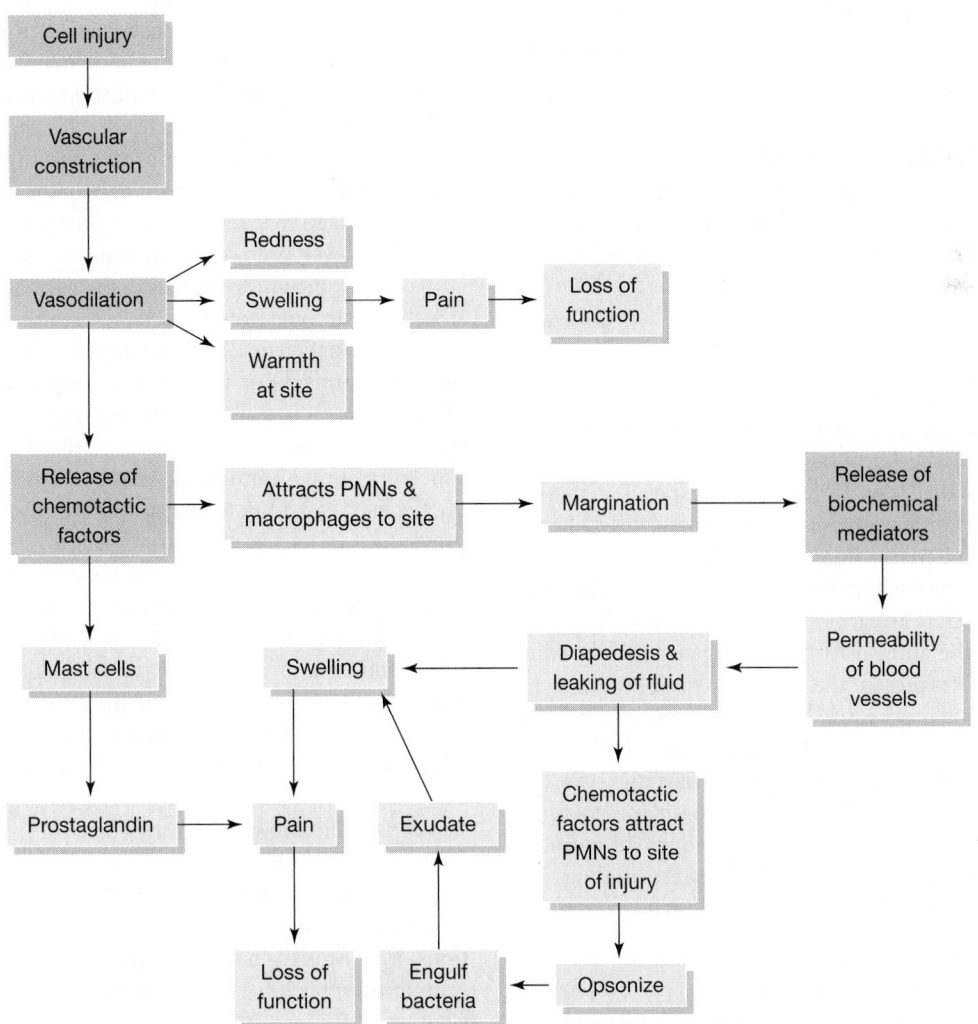

FIGURE 20–1 ■ Steps in the inflammatory process.

to the fluid exudates that form in the interstitial tissue, (4) pain caused by the pressure of the exudates and release of chemicals that irritate nerve endings, and (5) loss of function related to the pain and swelling.

The major systemic symptoms are fever and leukocytosis. Fever occurs because of the release of endogenous pyrogens at the site of inflammation. These endogenous pyrogens consist of substances such as prostaglandins and leukotrienes from injured cells and WBCs that accumulate at the site. These substances are carried to the temperature-regulating center in the hypothalamus where an increased temperature is stimulated. Fever is part of the body's defense mechanism and helps to fight infections.

Leukocytosis is a systemic sign of inflammation that is stimulated by the release of leukopoietins from damaged cells. Leukopoietins stimulate the increased production of WBCs and the release of mature neutrophils by the bone marrow. As inflammation continues the bone marrow releases immature neutrophils known as bands to help meet the body's needs. An increase in the number of bands on a differential WBC count is known as a "shift to the left" and indicates an ongoing acute inflammation. WBC response to infection and inflammation is discussed further in Chapter 61 ⊕.

Immune Responses

The immune responses are specific reactions of the body to invading foreign materials. The body's immune responses are complex and not completely understood. However, it is known that the immune responses work to defend the body against agents that are able to produce infection.

Humoral and Cellular Immunity

The immune responses can be divided into two types: humoral immunity and cellular immunity. The humoral response involves the antigen–antibody reactions, whereas the cellular response involves the reaction of the WBCs. Cellular and humoral defenses against infection also are discussed in Chapter 61 ⊕.

Humoral Immunity

Foreign materials are called antigens and the body responds to antigens by producing antibodies. These antigen–antibody responses are part of the humoral immune response. The humoral response is mediated by activated helper T cells that induce growth and differentiation of B lymphocytes. When B lymphocytes encounter an antigen such as a pathogen, they are stimulated to differentiate into antibody-producing cells called plasma cells that secrete antigen-specific antibodies. These antibodies bind with the antigen-forming antigen–antibody complexes. The antibodies present the antigen to the T lymphocytes for identification and processing. These complexes serve to neutralize the bacterial toxins and viruses, lyse and destroy pathogens, and facilitate phagocytosis. Phagocytic cells can bind, engulf, and digest antigen–antibody complexes more effectively than is possible when the antigen is alone. The antibodies also serve to neutralize a virus by blocking the binding sites on a virus that are used to bind to and infect a cell.

Cellular Immunity

The cellular immune response is a complex process involving an increase in the number of lymphocytes and macrophages in response to the invading organism. T cells mature in the thymus and in the process of growing become able to recognize specific antigens through the growth of antigen-specific receptors. After exposure to the antigens, the production of helper T cells is stimulated. This in turn, increases the production of cytotoxic T cells and natural killer cells that enhance the engulfment and killing of the antigen directly by macrophages.

Increased Susceptibility to Infection

Some known factors make an individual more susceptible to infection. For instance, individuals who are very old or very young have an increased susceptibility to infection. For the very young, the immune system is not fully developed until about the age of 6 months. Susceptibility to childhood infections increases as children are exposed to pathogens at day care facilities and schools. In the elderly, the immune system weakens as a result of decreasing thymus gland function. Changes in lymphocytes may occur as people age, contributing to decreased defenses. It is known that some of the lymphocytes important to immunity become less responsive in the elderly, whereas others function normally.

Defense mechanisms can be improved through lifestyle changes. Good hygiene is important in maintaining strong defense mechanisms. Skin that is unclean serves as a medium for bacterial growth and is more likely to allow invasion of microorganisms. Dust in the environment can serve as a reservoir for pathogens and helps with transportation of pathogens into the body. A balanced diet helps the body maintain an effective immune system by providing the nutrients needed for growth of new, healthy tissue. Protein is needed for the production of antibodies and the functioning of the immune system. Vitamins and minerals are also important to help the body digest and utilize nutrients so that cells can grow and remain strong. Individuals may develop a weakened immune system from chronic stress or chronic illness such as diabetes mellitus or chronic obstructive pulmonary disease.

Immunodeficiencies involve impaired functioning of one or more components of the immune response or inflammatory process. The failure of these defense mechanisms can be caused by a genetic abnormality or by an acquired abnormality such as cancer or human immunodeficiency virus (HIV). An immunodeficiency can lead to abnormal lymphocyte development, prevention of stem cell maturation into T or B cells, or a decrease in the production of a specific class of immunoglobulin. Regardless of the cause, a failure in the immune system will lead to a tendency to develop unusual or recurrent, severe infections. Immunodeficiency should be considered when an individual has frequent severe, documented infections such as otitis media, pneumonia, candidiasis, or meningitis. It should also be suggested when the infections are unusual such as *Pneumocystis carinii*.

People with known immunodeficiencies should be protected from infection. It may be unsafe or even fatal to administer immunizations or perform even simple procedures such as drawing blood. Care should be taken by nurses to avoid transmitting infectious organisms to these individuals. An in-depth discussion of immunosuppression and immunodeficiency is included in Chapter 60 ⊕.

Infectious Process

Infections can range from mild to debilitating or death producing. The severity of the infection depends on the **pathogenicity** or disease-causing potential of the microorganism, the number of invading microorganisms, and the host defenses. The common sequence of events is known as the chain of infection. All links of the chain must be present for infection to occur. The **chain of infection** consists of a causative agent, reservoir, portal of exit, mode of transmission, portal of entry, and a susceptible host (Figure 20–2 ■).

Chain of Infection

A causative agent or microorganism must exist in order for infection to occur. This can be any organism capable of causing disease. This organism must have a **reservoir** or a place where it can survive and may or may not multiply. Humans can serve as reservoirs as can inanimate objects such as soil, water, or equipment. Human reservoirs can be **carriers** or people or animals that do not have symptoms of infection but carry an active pathogenic microorganism. These individuals can be (1) in a period of incubation or before the onset of symptoms, (2) have a subclinical infection, (3) be recovering from an infection, or (4) be chronic carriers of the pathogen.

There must be a **portal of exit** or a path that allows the causative agent to escape from the reservoir. The portal of exit is usually associated with the site where the organism grows. Common human portals of exit include the respiratory system, the gastrointestinal system, the genitourinary (GU) system, and the skin and mucous membranes. Causative agents can be found in blood, sputum, emesis, stool, urine, wound drainage, and genital secretions. The portal of exit will vary depending on the microorganism.

In order for the organism to leave the reservoir, it needs a **mode of transmission,** which is the means by which it travels from the reservoir to a susceptible host. Transmission occurs through one of four modes: *contact, airborne, vehicle,* and *vector-borne.* Contact transmission can occur by direct contact, indirect contact, or droplets. Direct contact occurs when there is actual person-to-person or person-to-source physical contact, such as occurs when a sexually transmitted infection is obtained through sexual activity. Indirect contact involves the susceptible person being exposed to the organism through a contaminated object. An example of indirect contact is exposure to a contaminated dressing or surgical instrument. Droplet transmission occurs when the organism is expelled from its reservoir through the respiratory system in droplets, for instance, when someone sneezes or coughs. These large particles can travel up to 3 feet and can be inhaled by another susceptible person within a 3-foot radius around the person generating the droplets. They set up infection in a new susceptible host by being inhaled.

Airborne transmission occurs when the organism is expelled from the infected person and remains suspended in the air in tiny droplets no larger than 5 microns. These droplets are carried by air currents or on dust and inhaled by the susceptible host. They differ from droplet transmission in that these droplets are small enough to remain suspended in the air for prolonged periods of time. Tuberculosis (TB) is spread by airborne transmission.

Vehicle transmission occurs when the organism's life is maintained on something outside the reservoir until it is passed to the susceptible host. The vehicle is a nonliving object that is not normally harmful but acts as an intermediary for the infectious agent. Pathogenic organisms are contained in contaminated water or food, blood, or other items and transmitted to a susceptible host. This is the method of transmission for hepatitis B, which is transmitted through contaminated blood or blood products or through the salmonella infection.

Vector-borne transmission occurs when a disease-producing organism is carried by a living intermediate host that transfers the organism to a susceptible host. Examples of vectors include mosquitoes that carry West Nile virus and ticks that carry Lyme disease.

A portal of entry is needed to continue the chain of infection. A **portal of entry** is the path by which the infective organism enters the new susceptible host. These sites are usually the same as those for the portal of exit. Once the organism enters a host, the host must be susceptible to infection before an infection will occur. As long as the body's defenses against infection function normally, no infection will occur, but if the body has weakened defenses and is at increased risk, infection can occur.

Stages of the Infectious Process

Once the organism enters the susceptible host, the infectious disease develops in four stages. The first stage is the incubation period. During the incubation period the organism is establishing itself. It is replicating and spreading to other organs or tissues in the body but not yet causing symptoms. This stage can

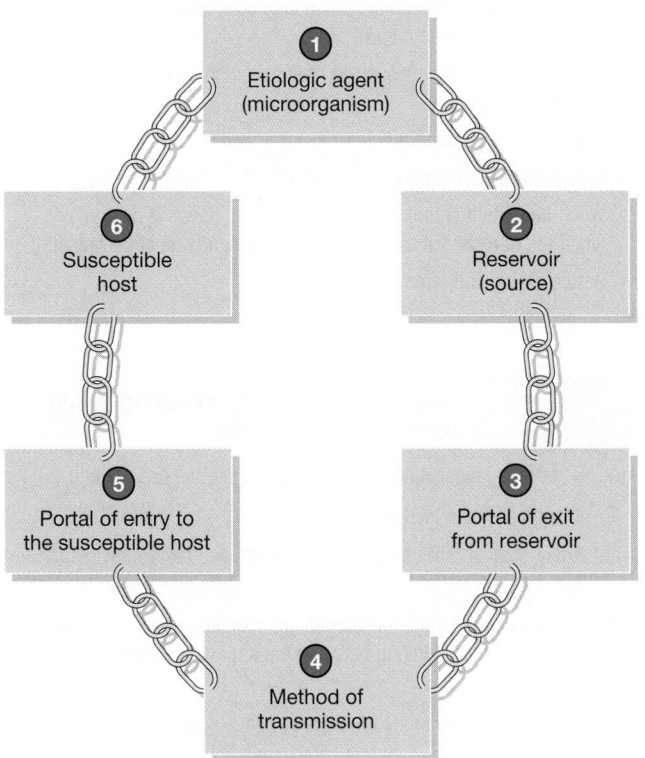

FIGURE 20–2 ■ Chain of infection.

pass by quickly or last for years, but during this time the infected person is contagious. The second stage is the prodromal phase. During the prodromal stage, the symptoms begin to appear. At this point, the symptoms are usually nonspecific such as general malaise, fever, myalgia, and fatigue.

Acute illness occurs during the third stage. During this stage the infective organism is growing and spreading rapidly in the body. The microorganisms produce toxins leading to cell lysis and death. An inflammatory response and immune reaction occur, leading to tissue damage. Along with the vague symptoms, the patient develops more specific symptoms. These include the classic signs of inflammation: swelling, redness, pain, and warmth at the site of infection, along with tachycardia and tachypnea from increased metabolic demands. There are usually other more specific symptoms related to the site of infection and the virulence of the pathogen. As the infection is contained and the pathogen confined by the body's defenses, the individual enters the convalescent stage. During this stage, the damaged tissues begin to heal and symptoms resolve.

An infection can be localized or generalized, acute or chronic. A localized infection affects the host in a small, focal area. Proper care can control the spread of the infection and minimize the illness. Symptoms are localized and may include pain and tenderness at the wound site. A generalized or systemic infection indicates involvement of a large part of the body instead of a single organ or part.

Infections are usually acute, which means that symptoms develop quickly and the body's response is temporary. However, infections can become chronic. In a chronic infection the associated inflammation is covert with the body trying to heal, but with the inflammation flaring up intermittently. It is almost like a battle without either the organism or the body's defenses ever gaining the upper hand.

Infection Control and Prevention

Many actions can be taken to control and prevent infection. Health care facilities are prime targets for the development and transfer of infectious organisms. As discussed earlier, patients in health care facilities generally have weakened defenses and are easy targets for bacteria and other types of infectious organisms. Hospital-acquired infections are as high as 30% in intensive care units (Creedon, 2005).

Hand Hygiene

The single most important action in the control and prevention of infection is hand hygiene. Inadequate hand hygiene is considered the leading cause of health care–associated infections and the spread of multidrug-resistant organisms. Infection associated with the delivery of health care is a topic being addressed by the first Global Patient Safety Challenge. Within that effort is a campaign to promote hand hygiene titled "Clean Hands Are Safer Hands." The simple act of hand washing can decrease the occurrence of infections associated with the delivery of health care (Larson et al., 2006).

The purpose of performing hand hygiene is to remove dirt, organic material, and transient microorganisms, and to prevent the spread of organisms leading to infection. Hands are contaminated daily simply through exposure to skin, patient gowns, bed

linen, bedside furniture, and other objects in the patient's immediate environment that are contaminated with the patient's flora. Simple activities such as lifting a patient, taking a patient's pulse, or touching a hand or shoulder can result in contamination of the hands enough to spread infection to others. It is important to perform hand hygiene before and after patient contact, but there are other indications for hand hygiene as well, as listed in Chart 20–3.

Although hand washing with soap and water may seem like a simple procedure, there are many things to consider when washing hands to prevent spread of infection. It is important to perform the procedure properly in order for it to be effective (Chart 20–4). The compliance of health care workers with hand hygiene recommendations is only about 40% or less (Widmer, Conzelmann, Tomic, Frei, & Stranden, 2007). Health care workers often wash their hands incorrectly and not frequently enough. When using soap and water, the hands should be washed for at least 15 seconds, covering all surfaces of the hands and fingers so that nothing is missed. This allows time for the antimicrobial products to work. The area around and under the fingernails contains higher microbial counts and should be washed thoroughly with debris removed from under the fingernails. The hands are then thoroughly rinsed to remove soap

---

CHART 20–3 Hand Hygiene Requirements

Hand hygiene procedures should be followed in these circumstances:

- When hands are visibly soiled.
- Before and after patient contact.
- After contact with body fluids or excretions, mucous membranes, and wound dressings.
- When hands are moved from a contaminated body site to a clean body site during patient care.
- After contacting objects such as medical equipment in the immediate vicinity of the patient.
- After removing gloves.
- Before invasive procedures are performed.
- When persistent antimicrobial activity on the hands is desired or when the numbers of resident flora on the hands must be reduced.
- Before eating and after using a restroom.

CHART 20–4 Steps in Proper Hand Washing When Using Soap and Water

1. Wet hands under running water using tepid, *not hot,* water.
2. If using antimicrobial soap, use 3 to 5 mL.
3. Apply soap or other hand-washing agent and thoroughly distribute over hands.
4. Vigorously rub hands together for 15 seconds, generating friction on all surfaces including between the fingers and under fingernails.
5. Thoroughly rinse hands to remove residue soap.
6. Dry hands thoroughly using paper towels.
7. Use foot controls or a paper towel to shut off faucet.

residue and then thoroughly dried as well. Microorganisms can be transferred more easily on wet hands than on hands that have been completely dried.

Even when hands are washed and dried correctly, recontamination can occur with the touching of faucet handles that are likely to be contaminated. If the hands are washed correctly and then the faucets are touched to turn them off, the washing is negated. Therefore, faucets should be automatic or controlled by foot, or paper towels should be used for turning them off. When washing the hands for surgical asepsis, the procedure is different, as outlined in Chart 20–5.

Many agents have been tested for use in hand hygiene. The use of plain soap for hand washing is effective in removing dirt, soil, and organic substances; however, plain soap has little antimicrobial activity. The use of antimicrobial hand hygiene products is recommended in any setting where there is a high risk of infection. A 70% ethanol agent effectively reduces microbial counts in less time than other cleansing agents. Alcohol-based agents have been shown to be effective against microorganisms and some viruses and can be more effective than soap in preventing pathogen transmission. The use of an alcohol-based agent results in better adherence to hand hygiene guidelines and saves time for nurses (Somner, Scott, & Gibb, 2007). If using an alcohol-based rub, the product should be applied to the palm of one hand, the hands should be rubbed together, covering all surfaces of the hands and fingers, until the hands are dry.

Some health care facilities have made alcohol-based hand rubs readily available by providing containers to be carried in the nurses' pockets for use at the patient's bedside or close to areas of patient care. Alcohol is not adequate, however, when there is visible dirt or contamination with protein-type materials. Other antiseptic agents used for hand hygiene include chlorhexidine gluconate (CHG), hexachlorophene, and chloroxylenol. These agents work more slowly than alcohol, but have effective residual effects. In addition, agents such as CHG build up an antimicrobial residual, unlike alcohol products.

The wearing of rings and artificial nails can contribute to the spread of infectious organisms (Trick et al., 2003). Rings increase the pathogen counts on the skin, and the more rings that are worn, the greater the contamination (Trick et al., 2003). Therefore, rings should be avoided. Artificial nails are more likely to encourage the growth of microorganisms than are nat-

ural nails and should not be used when caring for patients at high risk for infection. Natural nails should be short enough to allow for thorough cleaning underneath the nail and to prevent tears in gloves. Microorganisms can be found in higher concentrations in subungual areas. Nail polish does not increase the microorganism count, however, chipped nail polish does support the growth of microorganisms on the hands.

Hand hygiene is important regardless of whether gloves are used. However, gloves do provide a protective barrier to the transmission of microbes and prevent heavy contamination of the hands. Some transmission can still occur because gloves may have small defects or be torn during use. The hands can also be contaminated during glove removal. Therefore, hand washing with soap and water or the use of an antiseptic hand rub is recommended after glove removal. Gloves should be changed between patients and between contaminated body sites. Single-use disposable gloves should *not* be reused.

Hand washing can lead to dermatitis from the frequent contact with water and cleansing agents. The cracked, dry skin associated with dermatitis is more readily colonized with pathogens. The tenderness of dry, cracked skin can also lead to the avoidance of hand washing. Therefore, it is important to prevent or correct hand dermatitis. Currently the Occupational Safety and Health Administration (OSHA) recommends avoiding the use of petroleum-based moisturizers because they can lead to a deterioration of latex gloves. The use of an appropriate moisturizer that contains humectants along with fats and oils can increase skin hydration, providing a protective skin barrier without interfering with gloves or antibacterial agents (Larson et al., 2006). The use of tepid water rather than hot water is also recommended to help prevent hand dermatitis and the spread of pathogens.

 **CRITICAL ALERT**   *Hand washing done using the correct procedure and frequency has been shown to be the most important single action in preventing the spread of infection.*

Patient Placement

Placement of a patient with an infection in the hospital setting can be a significant factor in preventing the spread of infection. A private room is the best solution, especially if the infected patient has poor hygiene or cannot assist in implementing precautions to avoid transmission of the microorganisms. If a private room is not available, the infected patient should be placed in a room with the proper roommate. First, consider another patient with the same microorganism as a roommate. If this is not possible, consider the epidemiology and mode of transmission of the infecting pathogen.

Protective Equipment

The use of personal protective equipment (PPE) such as gloves, gowns, and masks plays an important role in the prevention of the spread of pathogens. Protective gowns help prevent the contamination of clothing and protect the skin and clothing of personnel from exposure to blood and body fluids. Gowns can help prevent the transmission of pathogens from patients or equipment in the environment to other patients or equipment. The Healthcare Infection Control Practices Advisory Committee (HICPAC) of the CDC recommends the use of gowns and gloves

---

CHART 20–5   Surgical Hand Antisepsis

1. Hands should be scrubbed before putting on gloves.

2. Remove rings, watches, and bracelets before beginning the scrub.

3. Remove debris from underneath fingernails using a nail cleaner under running water.

4. Using antimicrobial soap or alcohol-based rub, scrub hands and forearms the length of time recommended by the manufacturer, usually 2 to 6 minutes.

5. When using an alcohol-based surgical hand scrub, follow the manufacturer's instructions. Wash hands with non-antimicrobial soap, and dry hands thoroughly before using the alcohol-based scrub.

to prevent nosocomial infections. Gowns need to be impervious to fluids for procedures that may involve fluids. Gowns should *always* be removed before leaving patients' rooms and hand hygiene should be performed.

Masks and face shields or eye shields should be worn by health care personnel when performing procedures that are likely to cause splashing of blood or body fluids. These activities protect the mucous membranes of the eyes, nose, and mouth from exposure to pathogens. When an infected patient leaves his room, a mask is required.

Housekeeping practices should be observed to decrease dust and environmental reservoirs of pathogens. Spills of blood and body fluids must be cleaned up immediately with hospital disinfectant or household bleach and water. Reusable equipment such as blood pressure cuffs and stethoscopes can carry pathogens from patient to patient. Stethoscopes can be disinfected with isopropyl alcohol or disposable covers can be used between patients. Before and after each shift, the bell, diaphragm, and earpieces of stethoscopes need to be wiped down with alcohol. All equipment used on patients in isolation should be left in the room for use only with that patient. If this is not possible, any equipment removed from the room must be disinfected with hospital-grade disinfectant before being used with another patient.

It is important to note that *Clostridium difficile* is a frequent colonizer of the hospital environment. It is a spore former that can live in the environment for very long periods and is able to withstand many normal cleaning procedures.

Disposal of Soiled Equipment

Appropriate disposal of used and/or contaminated equipment is essential in order to protect both health care workers and prevent the spread of disease (Kozier, Erb, Berman, & Snyder, 2004). Linens should be changed so that there is little contact between the dirty linens and the nurse's uniform. Linens are to be carried away from the nurse's body and placed in an appropriate hamper. Throwing dirty linen on the floor or laying it in a chair should be avoided because it could lead to further contamination of the environment. Linens should never be shaken in the air because that creates air currents that spread pathogens. Needles and syringes should be disposed of in a container specifically made for disposal of sharp objects (Figure 20–3 ■). Inadvertent sticks with used sharps can lead to exposure to pathogens.

Contaminated materials need to be placed in plastic bags that are impervious to microorganisms before removing them from an isolated area. The CDC recommends a single bag unless the outside becomes contaminated. The single bag needs to be placed in a second bag if outside contamination occurs (CDC, 1997).

■ Pathogens Causing Infectious Disease

Pathogens must be present in the right quantity in a susceptible host in order to cause infection. The number needed is variable depending on the pathogen and the susceptibility of the host. The severity of the illness depends on the pathogen's pathogenicity or its ability to induce disease. Several factors influence the pathogenicity of an organism, including the pathogen's infectivity or in-

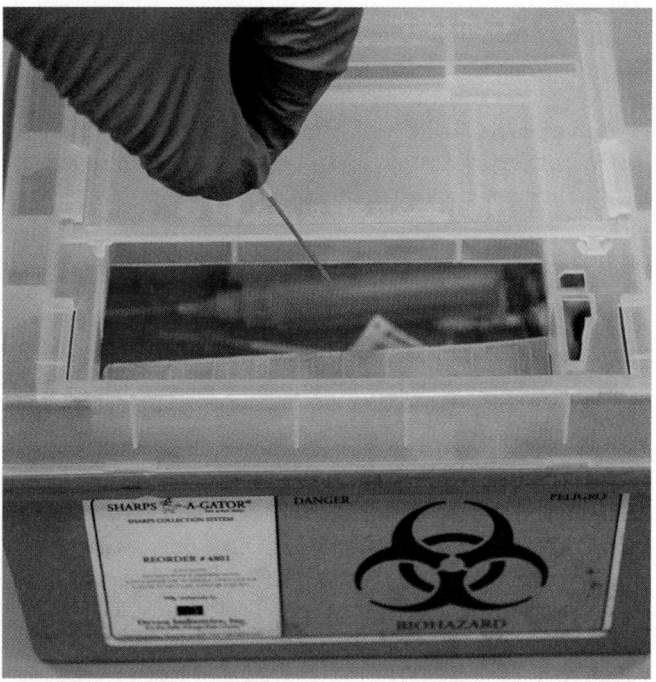

FIGURE 20–3 ■ Sharps container.

vasiveness, virulence, antigenicity, and viability. These terms are defined as follows:

- **Infectivity** or **invasiveness** is the ability of a pathogen to enter the host and then live and grow. Some pathogens are capable of producing toxins or enzymes that help them to invade the host and increase their resistance to the host's defenses.
- **Virulence** is related to the severity of disease a pathogen is capable of causing. Virulence can vary depending on the ability of the host to mount an immune response. It is expressed as the number of cases of infection that are serious or produce a disability in all those infected.
- **Antigenicity** is the ability of the pathogen to elicit an immune defense in the host. It affects the ability of the host to develop long-term immunity.
- **Viability** is the ability of the pathogen to survive outside of the host. Most pathogens cannot live and grow outside the host.

Human pathogens are divided into different categories of disease-causing agents. These include bacteria, viruses, *Mycoplasma*, rickettsiae, fungi, and parasites.

Bacteria

Bacteria are single-celled microorganisms that have a cell membrane that can be penetrated by antibiotics. They are classified in many different ways. They can be round or oval cocci, rod shaped, or spirochetes. Cocci can appear in pairs, called diplococci; or chains, like streptococci; or in clusters, like staphylococci. They can be rod-shaped bacilli, spiral shaped as seen in spirochetes, or curved. Bacteria can be intracellular like *Neisseriae gonorrhoeae* or extracellular like *Staphylococcus*.

Bacteria can be classified according to their need for oxygen. Aerobic bacteria must have oxygen for survival, whereas anaerobic bacteria can survive without oxygen. Bacteria are also classified according to their ability to be stained with crystal violet. Some bacteria have a substance in their outer cell wall that absorbs dye. Gram-positive bacteria stain blue when subjected to crystal violet stain; gram-negative bacteria remain colorless. Yet another classification for bacteria is according to their ability to form protective capsules and spores. See Chart 20–6 for classifications of common bacterial diseases.

Bacteria can cause disease in several ways. Gram-negative bacteria have endotoxins in their outer cell wall. These **endotoxins** are produced by live bacteria and are released when the bacteria are killed. Endotoxins stimulate the immune response, which can lead to changes in coagulation of blood and functions of vital body systems. Endotoxins can stimulate regulatory systems in humans, leading to inflammation, bleeding, hypotension, and fever. **Exotoxins** are proteins released by the bacterial cell during growth and have very specific actions. Exotoxins modify cell enzymes and functions leading to cell death or dysfunction. They are usually named for the site they affect. For example, enterotoxins affect the gastrointestinal tract. Some toxins disrupt cell membranes causing them to lyse, leading to cell death. Examples of bacteria include *Streptococcus, Staphylococcus, Neisseriae gonorrhoeae, Enterococcus,* and *Pseudomonas aeruginosa.*

Viruses

Viruses are the smallest of human pathogens. They occupy the body intracellularly because they require the genetic material of the host cell to replicate. Viruses contain a core made up of either RNA or DNA surrounded by a protein coat that helps the virus attach to the host cell. They cannot live and grow outside of a host cell. Viruses are classified according to the type of genetic material (RNA or DNA), the type of disease they cause (hepatitis, herpes), and how they reproduce (retrovirus) or how they are transmitted (as an enterovirus or sexually).

Viruses attach to receptors on the host cell membrane and penetrate the cell. Once inside the cell, the virus uses the cell's genetic material to replicate itself. The virus then matures and exits the cell ready to invade another host cell. The virus causes disease through the process of entering the cell and replicating, which leads to disruption of the cell's normal functions. The virus evokes an immune response against the host cell as it spreads from cell to cell. Most viruses are self-limiting, but viruses can also cause irreversible and lethal injury in a susceptible host. Examples of diseases caused by a virus include the common cold, acquired immunodeficiency syndrome (AIDS), hepatitis, mononucleosis, and herpes simplex.

CHART 20–6	Common Classifications of Bacterial Disease	
Organism	**Area of the Body**	**Antibiotic Treatment**
Gram-Positive Cocci		
Staphylococcus aureus	Found in nasopharynx, skin, clothing. Common in subcutaneous and cutaneous abscesses, and foreign devices such as IVs. Frequent cause of osteomyelitis, pneumonia.	Penicillin, first-generation cephalosporins, vancomycin, erythromycin
Staphylococcus epidermidis	Found commonly on the skin, nasopharynx, and lower GU tract. Infection occurs with indwelling devices that are inserted through the skin, such as catheters. Can be a contaminant of cultures if area not properly disinfected prior to obtaining the culture.	Penicillins, first-generation cephalosporins, vancomycin
Group A beta-hemolytic streptococci	Found in nose and throat, respiratory secretions, hands. Cause of acute pharyngitis, cutaneous impetigo, and systemic infection.	Penicillin, erythromycin, first-generation cephalosporins, vancomycin
Gram-Positive Bacilli		
Corynebacterium diphtheriae	Present in nasopharyngeal secretions, respiratory infections, and skin infections. Transmitted by airborne droplets and direct contact with exudates from infected lesions.	Erythromycin, penicillin
Gram-Negative Diplococci		
Neisseria meningitidis	Found in the nasopharynx and transported through respiratory tract. Causes meningitis.	Penicillin, third-generation cephalosporins
Gram-Negative Bacilli		
Enterobacteriaceae	Important in nosocomial infections. Can be found in the intestinal tract. Causes lower respiratory tract infections, urinary tract infections, and traveler's diarrhea.	Third-generation cephalosporins, penicillins, imipenem
Pseudomonas	Found in the soil, water, raw fruits and vegetables, plants, animals and man. Causes nosocomial infections. Can affect any body system but frequently seen in moist wounds and upper airways.	Penicillins, aminoglycosides, ciprofloxacin, ceftazidime, imipenem
Anaerobic Bacteria		
Clostridium difficile	Occurs as an overgrowth in the gut of patients during or after antibiotic therapy. Also transmitted on the hands and unsterilized equipment and is a frequent colonizer of the hospital environment. It can live in the environment for long periods and is able to withstand normal cleaning procedures.	Discontinue antibiotics, vancomycin, metronidazole

Mycoplasma

Mycoplasma is a small pathogen that is neither bacteria nor virus. It lives independently and does not require a host cell. It does not have a cell wall but does have a lipid outer membrane (Porth, 2007). This characteristic makes *Mycoplasma* resistant to antibiotics that usually attack cell walls. *Mycoplasma* has the ability to kill cells directly and leads to an autoimmune, antigen–antibody response and inflammation. It usually infects the respiratory tract and leads to many serious respiratory problems such as pneumonia. It also is responsible for pharyngitis, urethritis, and pelvic inflammatory disease (Porth, 2007).

Rickettsiae

Rickettsiae are small, intracellular, gram-negative organisms. They have no cell wall and, therefore, require a host cell to live and multiply. Rickettsiae are transmitted through the bites of arthropods such as ticks, lice, fleas, or mites or through exposure to their waste products. They primarily attack vascular epithelial cells causing vasculitis. Infections related to rickettsiae include Rocky Mountain spotted fever, typhus, and Q fever.

Fungi

Fungi have a nuclear membrane and a nucleus with several chromosomes. They can reproduce sexually or asexually. They are classified as either molds or yeasts. Molds are organisms with hyphae that produce spores for reproduction. Yeasts are single-celled, oval-shaped organisms that reproduce by budding. Fungal disease is also known as mycosis.

Fungi are found most everywhere on earth. They can live in a wide variety of environments and do not necessarily need a host. Temperature is important to the survival of fungi. Some can grow only on cooler surfaces like the skin, whereas others require warmer core body temperatures. Cutaneous mycosis is caused by skin contact. Systemic disease is due to inhalation of the fungi, which is then spread through the lymphatic system. Examples of cutaneous myosis include candidiasis, *tinea pedis,* and *tinea capitis.* Examples of systemic mycosis include cryptococcosis, histoplasmosis, and aspergillosis.

Parasites

Parasites are pathogens that infect and cause disease in other animals. Protozoa and helminths belong to this classification. Protozoa are small, single-celled animals that can be transmitted to the host by direct or indirect contact. They are mainly transmitted through ingested food or water or through an arthropod vector. They reproduce inside the host and are easily mobile in the body. Once inside, they stimulate an inflammatory response or cause disease by ingesting and/or invading human tissue.

Helminths are multicellular parasites. They require intermediate hosts and cannot reproduce inside the human host. Therefore, many exposures are required before a human can be infected. Helminths are transmitted by ingestion of eggs, breaks in the skin, or arthropod vectors. Like protozoa, helminths stimulate an inflammatory response. Infestation by helminths can lead to malnutrition and anemia in the host because they compete with the host for nutrients in the gastrointestinal tract.

New or Reemerging Infection

Infectious diseases are constantly emerging and reemerging. Since 1973, 30 new infections have been identified such as Lyme disease, Ebola virus, West Nile virus, severe acute respiratory syndrome (SARS), and AIDS (CDC, 2004). Diseases that were thought to be under control have reemerged due to antibiotic resistance and the development of new strains of pathogens. Tuberculosis is an example of a reemerging disease.

Biological Warfare

Biological warfare has become a concern since the terrorist attacks of September 11, 2001. The most likely pathogens to be used in biological warfare are the smallpox virus, *Bacillus anthracis* (anthrax), *Clostridium botulinum* (botulism), and viruses that cause hemorrhagic fevers. Smallpox immunizations were stopped in 1972 because the World Health Organization believed the disease had been eradicated. Smallpox is caused by the poxvirus *Variola* and spreads by direct contact or inhalation of respiratory droplets. Symptoms include high fever, headache, malaise, and a vesicular/pustular rash on the face and extremities. It is highly contagious and has a high mortality in unvaccinated people. Anthrax is an acute bacterial infection caused by a gram-positive, spore-producing organism that occurs in inhaled, cutaneous, and gastrointestinal forms. The inhaled form has the highest mortality rate (CDC, 2003). The symptoms are flu-like and include fever, nonproductive cough, headache, and malaise. Eventually the patient develops respiratory failure and hemodynamic collapse that can lead to death in 2 to 3 days.

Health care workers need to be alert to unusual illness patterns that indicate unusual infections. Signs to watch for include an increased incidence in the same geographic area, a disease pattern that is inconsistent with the patient's age, or patient presentation with symptoms of a rare disease. The presence of these indicators should be reported to the public health authorities. Biological warfare is covered in detail in Chapter 72 ⊕.

Isolation Precautions

In 1996, HICPAC developed isolation precautions that were then updated in 2007 (Siegel, Rhinehart, Jackson, Chiarello, & HICPAC, 2007). HICPAC's guidelines follow a two-tiered program. The first tier involves standard precautions. Standard precautions are designed to reduce the risk of transmission of pathogens from blood and body fluids containing blood. Patients with HIV or hepatitis B often have no apparent symptoms but can transmit the disease to others. Therefore, standard precautions apply to all hospitalized patients regardless of their diagnosis. The HICPAC guidelines are designed to control the spread of these diseases, as well as other nosocomial infections. The HICPAC guidelines should be used by all health care workers who have direct or indirect contact with patients or with their body fluids. This includes not only nurses and physicians, but those who empty trash, change linens, or clean the room. Standard precautions apply to blood, body fluids and secretions, nonintact skin, and mucous membranes. The National Guidelines box lists the HICPAC standard precautions.

The second tier is the transmission-based precautions, also outlined in the National Guidelines box. These precautions are

NATIONAL GUIDELINES for Standard and Transmission-Based Precautions

Category	Precaution
Standard Precautions	
Hand hygiene	Perform hand hygiene after touching blood, body fluids, secretions, excretions, and contaminated items whether or not gloves are worn.
Gloves	Wear clean, nonsterile gloves when touching blood, body fluids, secretions, excretions, and contaminated items. Put on clean gloves just before touching mucous membranes and nonintact skin.
Mask, eye protection, face shield	Worn to protect mucous membranes of the eyes, nose, and mouth during procedures and patient care activities that generate splashes or sprays of blood, body fluids, secretions, or excretions.
Gown	Wear a clean, nonsterile gown to protect skin and prevent soiling of clothing during procedures and patient care activities that may generate splashes or sprays of blood, body fluids, secretions, or excretions. Gowns should be impervious to fluids.
Patient care equipment	Handle used patient care equipment soiled with blood, body fluids, secretions, or excretions in a manner that prevents skin and mucous membrane exposure and contamination of clothing, and transfer of microorganisms to other patients and environments.
Environmental control	Adequate procedures should be in place for routine care, cleaning, and disinfection of environmental surfaces.
Linen	Handle soiled linen in a manner that prevents skin and mucous membrane exposure and contamination of clothing.
Occupational health and bloodborne pathogens	Prevent injuries when using and disposing of needles, scalpels, and other sharp instruments or devices. Never recap needles or use any technique that involves pointing the sharp end toward part of the body. Use mouthpieces, resuscitation bags, or other ventilation devices as an alternative to mouth-to-mouth resuscitation.
Patient placement	Place a patient who contaminates the environment in a private room if possible. If not possible, place patients with the same diagnosis in the same room.

Transmission-Based Precautions

Airborne precautions	1. Place patient in private room with N95 respirator, monitored negative air pressure, 6 to 12 air changes per hour, and appropriate discharge of air outdoors. Keep room door closed and patient in room.
	2. Wear respiratory protection when entering room.
	3. If leaving the room, the patient should wear a mask.
	4. Limit the movement and transport of the patient from the room.
Droplet precautions	1. Place patient in private room or in a room with cohort patients with the same disease.
	2. Wear a mask when working within 3 feet of patient.
	3. If leaving the room, the patient should wear a mask.
	4. Limit movement and transport of patient from room.
Contact precautions	1. Place patient in private room or with a very low risk roommate.
	2. Wear gloves when entering room and remove gloves before leaving room. Then perform hand hygiene.
	3. Wear a gown when entering the room and remove gown before leaving room.
	4. Limit the movement and transport of the patient from the room.
	5. Dedicate the use of noncritical patient care equipment to a single patient.

Source: Siegel, J. D., Rhinehart, E., Jackson, M., Chiarello, L., & the Healthcare Infection Control Practices Advisory Committee. (2007, June). *Guideline for isolation precautions: Preventing transmission of infectious agents in healthcare settings 2007.* Retrieved June 6, 2008, from http://www.cdc.gov/ncidod/dhqp/pdf/guidelines/Isolation2007.pdf.

for patients "known or suspected to be infected by highly transmissible or epidemiologically important pathogens" (Siegel et al., 2007). They are used in addition to standard precautions. They are classified into three types: airborne precautions, droplet precautions, and contact precautions (Garner, 1996). These precautions can be used either singularly or in combination for diseases that have multiple routes of transmission.

Airborne precautions are designed to protect against infectious agents that are transmitted through particles that remain suspended in the air and can become inhaled or deposited on a host. These precautions require the use of special ventilation and air handling, such as a room with negative air pressure and an increased number of air changes with the air discharged to the outside and no recirculation of the air in the room. If the air is recirculated, the return air must be filter through a high-efficiency particulate air (HEPA) filter (Schulster & Chinn, 2003). Personal respiratory protection or a mask is indicated for persons entering the room when caring for the patient. Precautions include the use of a National Institute for Occupational Safety and Health (NIOSH)-approved N95 particulate respirator with qualitative fit testing of the respirator required. Use of these engineering controls is needed for TB, varicella (and disseminated varicella-zoster), measles, and smallpox.

Droplet precautions protect against the risk of transmission of infection through droplets in the air. Infected droplets can make contact with the conjunctivae or the mucous membranes of the nose or mouth. They are generated primarily during talking, coughing, or sneezing by someone who is infected with the organism. These droplets do not remain suspended in the air and travel only short distances (usually 3 feet or less), therefore, special air handling is not required. The wearing of masks is important if working closely with a patient, when doing procedures such as suctioning. Droplet precautions may be necessary to use when caring for a patient with meningitis or diphtheria.

Contact precautions reduce the risk of organism transmission by direct or indirect contact. Direct contact occurs when there is skin-to-skin contact such as might occur when turning or bathing a patient or even touching an infected patient's hand. Transmission could also occur from an infected patient to a susceptible patient if the patients shake hands or touch in some way. Indirect contact involves contact of a host with a contaminated intermediate object in the patient's environment. Contact precautions involve wearing gloves and gowns and dedicating the use of equipment to a single patient. This type of precaution would be necessary when caring for a patient with *Clostridium difficile* infection or a major abscess.

Patients who are immunocompromised may be at high risk of developing infections, especially is they are severely neutropenic with an absolute neutrophil count of less than 500 cells/mm^3 (cubic millimeter) (Porth, 2007). This may occur in patients who have had a transplant or have leukemia. These patients must be in a protective environment that minimizes exposures to pathogens. Of course, the standard isolation precautions are observed. The length of time this patient is outside the room for diagnostic procedures or other activities must be limited. If the patient must be outside the room, respiratory protection should be provided. The room should be kept very clean without dust. All visitors and health care workers should perform hand hygiene carefully before entering the room or touching the patient. No one with any type of infection should be allowed to enter the room.

The 2007 expanded and revised isolation guidelines (Siegel et al., 2007) include specific diseases and new terminology and equipment. The National Guidelines box summarizes these 2007 revisions of the 1996 guidelines.

Immunization Programs

Prevention of infection is the best approach, and immunizations help protect children and adults against infections. Infection can be prevented anywhere along the chain of infection. Efforts to prevent infection include anything from eradication of infectious agents, to eliminating the reservoirs for infection, to eliminating a vector that carries the disease. One method used to eliminate the risk for some infections is immunization. Active or passive immunization improves the host's defenses. **Active immunization** involves the introduction of a live, killed, or attenuated toxin of a disease organism into the body. The immune system responds by producing antibodies. Active immunization provides long-term and possibly lifelong immunity. Some vaccines require boosters to maintain the immunity. Examples of active immunizations include those for measles, mumps, hepatitis B, and hepatitis A.

Passive immunization provides immunity for a short period of time, usually around 6 to 12 weeks. This involves the injection of already formed antibodies into the body. The individual may still have the disease, but it will be a less severe case. An example of this type of immunity is immunoglobin injections given to people exposed to hepatitis A. The recommendations regarding immunizations are based on scientific knowledge regarding the principles of active and passive immunization, the epidemiology and burden of disease, the safety of vaccines, and the cost analysis of preventive measures.

Certain benefits and risks are associated with immunizations. No vaccine is completely safe or 100% effective. Benefits include protection against the consequences of disease to the individual and to society as a whole. This protection includes not having to experience the symptoms of the illness, improved quality of life and productivity, and prevention of death. The risks of immunization include common, minor, and local adverse effects and rare, severe, and life-threatening conditions. The recommendations for immunizations represent a balance of the benefits for each person and society against the potential risks and problems associated with vaccinations. A vaccination schedule has been developed based on age-specific risks for disease, age-specific risks for complications, ability of an individual to respond to the vaccine, and potential interference with the immune response by passively transferred maternal antibodies. Studies have demonstrated that recommended ages and intervals between doses of multiple-dose antigens provide optimal protection or have the best evidence of efficacy. The immunization schedule for children is revised annually and published each year in January by the Centers for Disease Control and Prevention (2008). The schedule for adolescents and adults is revised less frequently, except for the influenza vaccine recommendations that are published annually.

Although immunizations are relatively safe, there are some contraindications and certain precautions should be followed. Most are adverse reactions are temporary and the vaccination can be given at a later time. A contraindication is any condition that increases the risk for a serious adverse reaction. The only true contraindication applicable to all vaccines is a history of a severe allergic reaction after a prior dose of vaccine or to a vaccine constituent. For example, a person who has an anaphylactic allergy to egg protein should not receive the influenza vaccine because it could cause serious illness or death in the recipient. A precaution is a condition in a recipient that might increase the risk for a serious adverse reaction or might compromise the ability of the vaccine to produce immunity. Those individuals with mild, acute illness such as diarrhea or upper respiratory tract infection can be safely vaccinated. Individuals with moderate or severe illness should be vaccinated as soon as possible after they have recovered from the acute illness. All vaccines may cause adverse reactions that are local, systemic, or allergic. Local reactions are least severe and mainly involve redness or soreness at the site. Systemic reactions such as fever occur less frequently. Serious allergic reactions such as anaphylaxis are rare.

NATIONAL GUIDELINES Summary of 2007 Revisions to the HICPAC Isolation Guidelines

Standard Precautions: New Elements

Respiratory hygiene/cough etiquette

Use of masks: to insert catheters for injections into spinal or epidural spaces, via lumbar puncture (e.g., myelogram, spinal or epidural anesthesia)

Safe injection practice

Safe Injection Practice: Defined

Use sterile, single-use needles and syringes for each injection given.

Prevent contamination of injection equipment, medication, and spaces used to prepare the injections.

Use single-dose vials whenever possible.

Include these practices in policies and training programs and monitor for adherence.

Empiric Transmission-Based Precautions

These precautions are to be observed in addition to standard precautions, pending confirmation of diagnosis. More than one transmission-based precaution may be used for diseases that have multiple routes of transmission. Some examples follow:

Meningitis

Neisseria meningitides: Use droplet precautions for the first 24 hours of antimicrobial therapy; mask and face protection for intubation. (*Note:* This is the *only type of meningitis* that requires transmission-based precautions.)

Enteroviruses: Use contact precautions for infants and children.

Mycobacterium tuberculosis: Use airborne precautions if pulmonary infiltrate; use airborne plus contact precautions if potentially infectious draining body fluid is present.

Respiratory Infections

In infants and young children, especially bronchiolitis and pneumonia (RSV, parainfluenza, adenovirus, influenza virus, human metapneumonia virus): Use contact plus droplet precautions; droplet may be discontinued when influenza and adenovirus have been ruled out.

Cough/ fever/ upper lobe pulmonary infiltrate (M. tuberculosis, respiratory viruses, Staphylococcus pneumoniae and/or S. aureus (MSSA or MRSA): Use airborne plus contact precautions, or resistant organism (RO) precautions for MRSA.

For HIV-positive patients (or patients at high risk for HIV infection): Use eye/face protection if aerosol-generating procedure performed or contact with respiratory secretions anticipated. Tuberculosis is more likely in an HIV-infected individual than in an HIV-negative individual. If tuberculosis is unlikely and there is no airborne infection isolation room or respirator available, use droplet instead of airborne precautions.

For patients with history of recent travel (10 to 21 days) to countries with active outbreaks of SARS (avian influenza): Use airborne plus contact precautions plus eye protection. If SARS and/or TB are unlikely, use droplet only instead of airborne.

Ambulatory Care

Patient-to-patient transmission of *Burkholderia* species and *Pseudomonas aeruginosa* can occur in outpatient clinics for adults and children with cystic fibrosis. Implement transmission-based precautions. Segregate patients in the waiting room and decontaminate surfaces.

New Terminology

Airborne infection isolation room (AIIR) replaces *negative pressure room.*

Transmission-based precautions replaces *isolation categories.*

New Equipment: Purified Air Particulate Respirator

The purified air particulate respirator (PAPR) is a type of respiratory protection used for rule-out and confirmed TB, SARS, and avian influenza.

The N95 respirators will continue to be used. Annual fit-testing is required for the N95 respirators. N95 respirators have different shapes, sizes, and colors.

Please continue to use surgical masks for standard, droplet, and contact transmission-based precautions.

Source: Centers for Disease Control. (2007a). *Guidelines and recommendations: Infection control guidance for the prevention and control of influenza in acute-care facilities.* Retrieved June 20, 2007, from http://www.cdc.gov.

Healthy People 2010 Guidelines

The *Healthy People 2010* guidelines (DHHS, 2000) are a set of national health objectives designed to serve as a basis for the development of state and community health plans. It allows for diverse groups to work together as teams to improve health for everyone. These objectives were developed by leading federal agencies based on the best scientific knowledge available and designed to measure program outcomes over time. One of the objectives included in the *Healthy People 2010* report is to "[p]revent disease, disability, and death from infectious diseases, including vaccine-preventable diseases" (DHHS, 2000). Infectious diseases remain a major cause of illness, disability, and death in this country and worldwide. Pneumonia, influenza, and septicemia were among the top 10 causes of death in the United States in 2003. Infectious diseases are an economic drain on society, not only in terms of financial costs but also in terms of time lost from work and treatment of disabilities.

Immunizations can prevent infectious diseases and the disabilities caused by the diseases. The vaccines not only protect the person who is vaccinated but also protect society. When the vaccination levels in the community are high, those who have not been vaccinated due to contraindications are not likely to get the disease. Significant progress has been made, with vaccine-preventable diseases at or near record-low levels; however, these efforts need to be continued. The organisms responsible for these diseases have not disappeared—they have merely receded. Therefore, the major strategies identified by *Health People 2010* to protect people from vaccine preventable diseases are as follows:

- Improve the quality and quantity of vaccinated delivery services.
- Minimize financial burdens for needy persons.
- Increase community participation, education, and partnership.

- Improve monitoring of disease and vaccination coverage.
- Develop new or improved vaccines and improve vaccine use.

The National Guidelines box summarizes the *Healthy People 2010* objectives related to immunizations and infectious diseases.

▪ Nursing Management

The nursing management of a patient with an infection requires the assessment of the patient and the development of a specific plan to meet the individual patient's needs. Nursing care should be well planned and adapted as necessary so that the patient receives quality care, further infection is prevented, and infections are not transmitted to others. Nursing assessment is essential to identify potential complications and responses to treatment.

Assessment

When assessing the patient with an infection, the nurse should take into account the signs and symptoms of the infection, the site of the infection, the pathogenicity of the organism, and the body's immune response. A thorough assessment will help identify the infection and/or its complications so that appropriate therapy can be implemented.

Fever

One feature common to most infections is a fever. Fever is defined as a body temperature of more than 38°C (100°F). Fever is an indication of the severity of the inflammatory response in the patient with an intact immune response. As stated earlier in this chapter, fever is induced by mediators known as endogenous pyrogens that act directly on the hypothalamic regulating center that controls the body's temperature. Fever can be beneficial because some microorganisms are very sensitive to changes in temperature and cannot survive when temperatures go up. Fever can also be present when no infectious process is occurring, such as with malignancy or myocardial infarction. In these cases, the injured cells produce endogenous pyrogens, resulting in a fever.

Although a fever can have beneficial effects, a fever of 40°C (104°F) can be harmful. *Hyperpyrexia,* an elevated body temperature, leads to an increased metabolic rate, which increases the demand for oxygen and the need for calories. This is associated with tachycardia and tachypnea. These conditions put an increased workload on the heart and lungs and can lead to impaired cardiac and pulmonary function. The increased need for calories can lead to protein breakdown for energy. With the increase in temperature, diaphoresis increases, which can lead to dehydration. High fevers can also lead to febrile seizures.

NATIONAL GUIDELINES *Healthy People 2010* Objectives Related to Immunization and Infectious Disease

Diseases Preventable Through Universal Vaccination

Reduce or eliminate indigenous cases of vaccine-preventable diseases.

Reduce chronic hepatitis B virus infections in infants and young children.

Reduce hepatitis B.

Reduce bacterial meningitis in young children.

Reduce invasive pneumococcal infections.

Diseases Preventable Through Targeted Vaccination

Reduce hepatitis A.

Reduce meningococcal disease.

Reduce Lyme disease.

Infectious Diseases and Emerging Antimicrobial Resistance

Reduce hepatitis C.

Increase the proportion of persons with chronic hepatitis C infection identified by state and local health departments.

Reduce tuberculosis.

Increase the proportion of all tuberculosis patients who complete curative therapy within 12 months.

Increase the proportion of contacts and other high-risk persons with latent tuberculosis infection who complete a course of treatment.

Reduce the average time for a laboratory to confirm and report tuberculosis cases.

Increase the proportion of international travelers who receive recommended preventive services when traveling in areas of risk for select infectious diseases: hepatitis A, malaria, and typhoid.

Reduce invasive early-onset group B streptococcal disease.

Reduce hospitalizations caused by peptic ulcer disease in the United States.

Reduce the number of courses of antibiotics for ear infections in young children.

Reduce the number of courses of antibiotics prescribed for the sole diagnosis of the common cold.

Reduce hospital-acquired infections in intensive care unit patients.

Reduce antimicrobial use among intensive care unit patients.

Vaccination Coverage and Strategies

Achieve and maintain effective vaccination coverage levels for universally recommended vaccines among young children.

Maintain vaccination coverage levels for children in licensed day care facilities and children in kindergarten through the first grade.

Increase the proportion of young children and adolescents who receive all vaccines that have been recommended for universal administration for at least 5 years.

Increase the proportion of providers who have measured the vaccination coverage levels among children in their practice population within the past 2 years.

Increase the proportion of children who participate in fully operational population-based immunization registries.

Increase routine vaccination coverage levels for adolescents.

Increase hepatitis B vaccine coverage among high-risk groups.

Increase the proportion of adults who are vaccinated annually against influenza and ever vaccinated against pneumococcal disease.

Vaccine Safety

Reduce vaccine-associated adverse events.

Increase the number of persons under active surveillance for vaccine safety via large linked databases.

Source: U.S. Department of Health and Human Services. (2000). *Healthy people 2010: Understanding and improving health.* Retrieved June 5, 2008, from http://www.healthypeople.gov.

The assessment of fever can provide information about the possible cause of the infection. The pattern of fever occurrence should be observed. Fever can be described as intermittent, remittent, sustained, or relapsing. An intermittent fever is defined as a fever that is cyclical. The temperature goes up and then returns to normal at least once in 24 hours. The remittent fever is one in which the fever stays elevated throughout the day but can vary a few degrees. Sustained fever is a continuous fever that has very little variation. A relapsing fever resolves but returns after a period of time in which the infection was thought to be resolved. A fever that lasts 2 weeks or more without identification of the cause is known as a **fever of unknown origin (FUO).**

 A fever of 40.5°C (105°F) can cause or worsen cardiac and pulmonary problems and also cause febrile seizures.

Patient History

When assessing the patient for a risk for infection or the presence of an infection or fever, the first step is to take a history. A thorough history can help identify the cause of the infection and can direct the focus for the physical examination and diagnostic tests. The first part of a patient history is the *history of present illness.* This section should provide an in-depth view of the patient's problem. One way to remember what should be included in the history of present illness is the mnemonic OLD CARTS (Chart 20–7). It is usually beneficial to begin with a general question such as "What brought you here?" Then direct the patient—without putting words in the patient's mouth—so that pertinent information is obtained.

Information pertaining to past medical history is gathered next. This should include information on any previous infectious diseases such as hepatitis, sexually transmitted infections, or TB. History of childhood infections and vaccinations should be included in the inquiry. The patient should be asked about any preexisting conditions that might affect the immune system such as the use of steroids, chemotherapy, transplants, or other chronic illnesses. A travel history should be included. Where has the patient traveled, how long, and what were the living circumstances? Hiking, camping, and caving can increase the risk of infection as well as travel to countries where sanitation is poor. It is important to note what foods were eaten and whether the foods were cooked or raw.

Has the patient been exposed to any infected animals? If the patient has pets, how are the animal feces handled? Has the patient recently experienced any insect bites or been exposed to rodents in the home? Exposure to infected people is also important. The nurse should inquire about sexual history. It is important to know about all sexual partners and whether the sexual activity is high risk. Ask the patient about drug, tobacco, and alcohol use. Drugs and alcohol can lead to exposure to bloodborne pathogens via needles and sexual contact. Smoking increases the risk of respiratory infections due to effects of smoke on cilia that normally protect the airway. Sharing tobacco products, drinks, lip balm, and so forth has been implicated in the transmission of gram-negative diplococci *Neisseria meningitidis,* which may lead to meningococcal disease. Diet history should be obtained related to what is eaten, as well as the sanitation of food, dining out, how food is cooked, and where it is obtained.

Physical Examination

Once the history is completed, the physical examination should focus on the areas identified in the history as being the potential source of infection. A focused physical exam aimed at assessing for an infection should include the following:

- *Vital signs:* Record height and weight, temperature, respiratory rate, pulse rate, and blood pressure.
- *Skin and mucous membranes:* Inspect for breaks in skin integrity, redness, warmth, rash, jaundice, signs of insect bites; check skin turgor and hydration status, drainage from lesions or wounds. Inspect skin folds for candidal skin infections and scabies.
- *Head and neck:* Examine eyes, nose, and ears for redness, drainage, or swelling. Assess visual acuity. Assess pharynx for redness, swelling, the presence of masses, and the presence of discharge or exudates. Inspect the oral mucosa for lesions and the teeth for caries, swelling of the gums, foul smell, or drainage. Palpate over the sinuses for pain or swelling.
- *Lymph nodes:* Palpate all superficial lymph nodes. Check for enlargement and pain. Also note the size of the lymph nodes and whether they are movable or very firm.
- *Lungs:* Auscultate lungs for abnormal breath sounds. Note decreases in breath sounds, the presence of crackles, rhonchi, friction rubs, or wheezes. Note the presence of a cough. Note color and consistency of sputum.
- *Heart:* Auscultate the heart for the rate and rhythm of the heart sounds. Note any abnormal sounds such as murmurs or friction rubs.
- *Abdomen:* Auscultate for the presence of bowel sounds. Palpate for masses, tenderness, and enlarged liver or spleen. If diarrhea is present, note amount, frequency, color, and consistency. Note presence of vomiting including the consistency, color, and amount.
- *Genitourinary tract:* Assess for costovertebral angle tenderness, suprapubic tenderness, fullness over the bladder. Inspect the perineum for redness or drainage.
- *Reproductive system:* Pelvic examination should be completed on women as indicated by the history. Check for discharge, cervical motion tenderness, or masses. The prostate gland should be assessed on men when indicated by history.

CHART 20–7 **History of Present Illness: OLD CARTS**

The OLD CARTS mnemonic can be used to elicit information about a patient's current illness:

Onset

Location

Duration

Character

Aggravating/alleviating factors

Relieving factors

Temporal factors

Severity

Check for size, tenderness, and discharge. Note color, odor, and amount of urine.

- *Nervous system:* Assess for changes in mental status. Note any changes in neurological signs such as weakness, tremors, seizures, or parenthesis.

 CRITICAL ALERT *Frequently assess areas where tubes enter or leave the body for signs of infection such as increasing redness or drainage around the tube.*

Diagnostic Tests

Diagnostic tests are used to confirm the diagnosis, to decide on or see the response to treatment options, or to pinpoint the location and severity of the infection. The Diagnostic Tests box summarizes the tests related to infection. One of the most important diagnostic tests is the complete blood count. The number and variety of leukocytes, or WBCs, can give the nurse some insight into the presence and severity of an infection. The normal count is 5,000 to 10,000 WBC/mm^3. A WBC of more than 10,000

DIAGNOSTIC TESTS Related to Infection

Test and Normal Values	Expected Abnormality	Rationale for Abnormality
WBC count, n = 5,000–10,000 cells/mm^3	Elevated in acute infections, tissue injury, tissue necrosis. Decreased in viral infections, some bacterial infections, bone marrow depression.	WBC count increases in order to phagocytize or kill bacteria or cell debris.
• Neutrophils, n = 50–70% of the total WBC count; band, n = 3–6%	Neutrophils and bands are elevated in acute infections.	Neutrophils are the first WBCs to arrive at the site of infection. They have a short life span and must be continually produced when needed. So the immature neutrophil or band will be elevated quickly.
• Basophils, n = 0.5–1.0% of total WBC count	Elevated with allergic and parasitic responses. Do not respond to bacterial or viral infections.	Involved in phagocytosis of antigen–antibody complexes.
• Eosinophils, n = 1–4% of total WBC count	Elevated in allergic and parasitic reactions.	Respond later in inflammation and help control the inflammatory process.
• Monocytes, n = 2–8% of total WBC count	Elevated with infection, tuberculosis, bacterial endocarditis.	Phagocytic cells that perform like neutrophils but start later and stay longer in the bloodstream.
• Lymphocytes, n = 20–40% of total WBC count	Elevated with some bacterial diseases, infectious mononucleosis, leukemia, some viral diseases.	Function to fight chronic bacterial infection and acute viral infections. Responsible for immune reactions.
Erythrocyte sedimentation rate (ESR): *Males:* up to 15 mm/hr *Females:* up to 20 mm/hr	Elevated with acute and chronic infection, inflammation, cancer, tissue necrosis.	Nonspecific test that measures the rapidity at which red blood cells (RBCs) clump together. This process occurs more rapidly when there is an alteration in blood proteins due to inflammation. Therefore, an elevation indicates the presence of an inflammatory process.
Culture and sensitivity: Normally negative	Positive if pathogens are present in the specimen. The culture will identify the organism and the sensitivity will identify what antibiotic will work best.	If pathogens are present on the substance being tested, they will grow on a special culture medium and can be identified.
Gram stain: None with no organisms present	Differentiates between gram-negative and gram-positive organisms.	Useful for identifying the microorganisms so proper treatment can occur.
Febrile agglutinins: No agglutinins in titers ≤1:80	Increased in infectious diseases such as rickettsial disease, salmonellosis, brucellosis, and tularemia.	A group of tests that helps identify the type of organism responsible for an infection based on antibodies.
Viral antibody tests: None with no organisms present	This is a group of tests for specific viruses. Will be elevated with viral infections.	Used to determine exposure to or existing viral infections that are difficult to culture. Includes several tests, each specific to an organism and antibody reaction. They must be specifically ordered.
Fungal infection: Antibody tests negative	Elevated in the presence of a fungal-induced infection.	Looks for the presence of antibodies related to fungal infections or the presence of parasitic organisms.

WBC/mm³ usually indicates the presence of inflammation and/or infection. The higher the WBC count, the more serious the infection is thought to be. A viral infection can often cause the WBC count to decrease. The differential count of WBCs should also be assessed. There are five types of WBCs; neutrophils, eosinophils, basophils, lymphocytes, and monocytes. Neutrophils are the first type of WBC to arrive at the site of inflammation or infection and their job is to phagocytize or ingest bacteria. This process is described in Chapters 62 and 63 .

Cultures are also very important in diagnosing and treating infections. The nurse is often responsible for collecting the specimen to be cultured. Each institution has its own policy for collecting specimens, however, it is very important to collect the specimen correctly so that the results of the culture are useful. The following guidelines should be followed:

- Sufficient material must be collected to ensure an accurate examination.
- The specimen should be collected where the suspected organism is most likely to be found.
- Observe standard precautions when collecting the specimen.
- Culture only for a specific pathogen and not where there are areas of normal flora.
- Collect the specimen in a sterile container with a tight-fitting lid. Polyester-tipped swabs in a collection system with a transport medium ensure the adequacy of the specimen for 72 hours.
- Place the specimen in a biohazard bag.
- Label the specimen correctly with patient information, the source of the specimen, and the time of collection.
- Make sure the specimen gets to the laboratory as soon as possible. Most specimens can be refrigerated for a few hours if necessary.

CRITICAL ALERT   *Remember to collect specimens for culture before beginning treatment with an antibiotic. This gives a more accurate picture of the original infection.*

Emotional care of the patient is very important. Patients and their families may not know the origin of the infection, and may therefore be apprehensive about the effectiveness of treatments. The use of standard precautions or transmission-based precautions makes visits with family and friends difficult. Hugs and touching are hindered by gloves and masks. The necessary use of protective masks, gloves, and gowns may make the patient feel isolated and rejected. Education about the necessity of isolation procedures is important for the patient and family. The nurse needs to allow the patient to verbalize feelings about the isolation and the concerns about being ostracized.

Nursing Diagnosis

Nursing diagnoses are determined based on an in-depth analysis of the data from the patient history and physical examination. Nursing diagnoses will vary depending on the type and location of the infection or an increased risk for infection. For example, the patient with pneumonia may also be given the nursing diagnosis of *Ineffective Airway Clearance*. Another example might be the patient with a wound infection who has a nursing diagnosis of *Impaired Tissue Integrity*.

When the patient is at risk for an infection the nursing diagnosis is *Risk for Infection*. The etiology or cause may be a break in the body's defense mechanisms, an alteration in secondary defenses such as a low hemoglobin or suppressed inflammatory response, the presence of a chronic disease, malnutrition, or increased environmental exposure. The Nursing Process: Patient Care Plan (p. 474) outlines the nursing management for a patient with an infectious communicable disease.

Health Promotion

Prevention and control of infection is the number one goal of health care no matter what the setting. Health care–associated infections are an increasing problem. The best way to address infection is to prevent it. Prevention requires education of health care professionals and the general public. An educational program related to the prevention of infection has several facets. Everyone should be educated on the importance of proper hand hygiene. Understanding the importance of immunization is an important part of educating the public. Family members must be instructed to check all immunization records and keep them up to date. Community members should understand the disease they are being protected against, why the immunization is necessary, the relative safety of immunizations, and when booster doses are due.

It is important to educate the public on the use of antibiotics. Antibiotics are not effective for all organisms. Many infections will resolve completely without the use of antibiotics. Antibiotic resistance is occurring, in part, because of the misuse of antibiotics. Patients need to have an understanding of when antibiotics are effective and when alternatives may be appropriate. It is important to stress that it is necessary to take all of the medication prescribed. If the full treatment is not taken, this could result in a worse infection due to the development of resistant organisms. The Pharmacology Summary (p. 477) lists medications used to treat infectious disease.

A healthy lifestyle is a deterrent to infection. An individual, who practices good hygiene, eats a well-balanced diet, exercises regularly, and gets an adequate amount of sleep will have a stronger immune system and be better able to resist infection. Although exposure will occur no matter how careful an individual is, it is important to prevent transmission of the organism. To decrease exposure, an individual should do the following:

- Avoid crowds and contact with susceptible persons.
- Use disposable tissues when coughing or sneezing.
- Use appropriate food-handling precautions.
- Practice frequent hand hygiene.
- Clean equipment and eating utensils.
- Avoid contact with or sharing of body fluids through needles or razors.
- Use condoms during sexual activity.

Research has shown that effective strategies for the prevention and control of health care–related infections include proper hand hygiene, utilizing barrier techniques when needed such as wearing gowns and gloves, appropriate care of invasive devices, and cautious use of antibiotics (Larson, 2005; Wiseman, 2006).

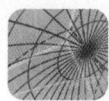

NURSING PROCESS: Patient Care Plan for Infection

Assessment of Pain

Subjective Data:
Do you hurt?
On a scale of 1 to 10 with 10 being the worst possible pain, how bad is the pain?
Where is the pain located?
How would you describe the pain?
Does anything make the pain better or worse?
What have you tried to relieve the pain and has it worked?
How long have you had the pain?

Objective Data:
Heart and respiratory rate may be increased.
Patient demonstrates a facial grimace or gritting of teeth.
Patient guards painful area.
Diaphoresis and pallor may be present.
Presence of nausea and vomiting.
Patient may be crying or moaning.

Nursing Assessment and Diagnoses	Outcomes and Evaluation Parameters	Planning and Interventions with *Rationales*
Nursing Diagnosis: *Acute Pain* related to tissue inflammation and damage	**Outcomes:** Patient reports pain early. Patient reports no adverse effects from pain or medication. Patient verbalizes pain relief and rates the pain lower on the scale of 1 to 10. Pain decreases, requiring less medication. **Evaluation Parameters:** Patient reports that pain is relieved or improved. Heart rate is <100 beats/min. Respiratory rate is <20 breaths/min. Facial muscles are relaxed. Patient is willing to participate in activities and therapies.	**Interventions and *Rationales:*** Instruct the patient to report and describe pain before it becomes unmanageable. Pain should be assessed and medication given before pain gets unbearable. Intervention will be more effective if given before the pain is severe. Describe any adverse effects of unrelieved pain. *Pain may lead to physiological and psychological morbidity factors.* Review patient's chart for frequency of medication administration and overall relief of pain. *Tracking of pain helps the nurse and patient plan ahead and improve pain management.* Support the patient's use of nonpharmacologic measures to control pain such as distraction, imagery, etc. *Some nonpharmacologic strategies can restore the patient's sense of control and help decrease pain.* Plan care activities around periods of greatest comfort. *The presence of pain diminishes the patient's ability to be active.* Assess cultural and religious impact on the patient's responses. *Different cultures and religions respond differently to pain.*

Assessment of Fever

Subjective Data:
Are you feeling unusually warm?
Do you have body aches?
Have you had chills?
Have you taken your temperature and what were the results?

Objective Data:
Temperature >37.2°C (>99°F)
Tachycardia
Respiratory rate of >20 breaths/minute
Decreased alertness
Restlessness
Diaphoresis

Nursing Assessment and Diagnoses	Outcomes and Evaluation Parameters	Planning and Interventions with *Rationales*
Nursing Diagnosis: *Hyperthermia* related to increased metabolic rate from infection	**Outcome:** Normal body temperature **Evaluation Parameters:** Body temperature will be within normal limits. Changes in body temperature will be noted quickly. Patient will remain warm and dry. Patient hydration status will be adequate. Skin will be warm and dry. Alert and oriented without restlessness or malaise. Heart rate <100 beats/min. Respiratory rate <20 beats/min. Resolution of infection.	**Interventions and *Rationales:*** Assess temperature at regular intervals and when the patient complains of chills or myalgia. *Recognize pattern for fever and note when rising or decreasing.* Keep patient comfortable with dry clothing and linens. *Patient in wet clothes and linens will shiver, leading to increased energy needs and possibly increasing fever.* Encourage an intake of eight to ten 8-oz glasses of fluids. *Fluids lost through perspiration need to be replaced.* Administer antipyretics *to decrease temperature.* Administer antibiotics *to treat organism responsible for infection.*

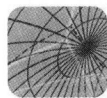

NURSING PROCESS: Patient Care Plan for Infection—*Continued*

Assessment of Fatigue

Subjective Data:
Are you feeling tired?
How much activity makes you tired?
Can you complete activities of daily living?
What makes your fatigue better or worse?

Objective Data:
Inability to stay awake
Unwillingness to participate in activities or therapeutics
Expressionless face.

Nursing Assessment and Diagnoses	Outcomes and Evaluation Parameters	Planning and Interventions with *Rationales*
Nursing Diagnosis: *Fatigue* related to increased energy production	**Outcome:** Increased energy level **Evaluation Parameters:** Patient voices an increase in energy. Patient performs only those essential tasks and asks for help with other activities as energy level increases. Patient takes rest periods throughout the day. Patient eats small frequent meals containing high-energy foods if not contraindicated.	**Interventions and *Rationales:*** Assist the patient with activities of daily living as necessary. *Encourage independence and some activity.* Help the patient identify essential from nonessential tasks *to help conserve energy while providing some independence.* Allow the patient to take rest periods without interruption every couple of hours or more often if needed. *Rest will allow energy to be restored.* Teach the patient strategies for conserving energy. *Some activities can be done sitting instead of standing or in ways that require less energy.*

Assessment of Fluid Volume Status

Subjective Data:
Do you feel thirsty?
How often are you urinating?
Do you feel diaphoretic?

Objective Data:
Skin that is moist and warm
Decreased intake of fluids
Decreased urine output
Poor skin turgor
Dry mucous membranes
Increased urine specific gravity
Tachycardia
Tachypnea

Nursing Assessment and Diagnoses	Outcomes and Evaluation Parameters	Planning and Interventions with *Rationales*
Nursing Diagnosis: *Deficient Fluid Volume* related to increased perspiration and inability to drink	**Outcome:** Fluid balance is maintained. **Evaluation Parameters:** Urine output is equal to or less than intake. Skin is warm and dry. Skin turgor is normal. Mucous membranes are moist.	**Interventions and *Rationales:*** Monitor trends in output related to intake. Note color and specific gravity of urine. *Provides a picture of the patient's hydration status.* Monitor for decreased skin turgor, thirst, dry mucous membranes, dry skin, sunken eyeballs, weakness, and confusion. *These are signs of fluid deficit.* Provide oral hygiene before each meal and at bedtime. *Oral hygiene decreases unpleasant taste, increasing the patient's desire to eat and drink.* Provide fresh water and oral fluids as requested by the patient evenly distributed over 24 hours. *Helps increase oral intake and counter dehydration. When distributed throughout the day, the intake has a greater chance of being retained.*

Assessment of Anxiety Related to Infection

Subjective Data:
What do you know about your infection and/or disease process?
How does this disease affect your daily life?
Do you have family members or friends to provide support?
Do you feel anxious or afraid?

Objective Data:
Presence of restlessness
Withdrawal from activities
Inability to sleep

(continued)

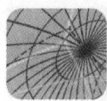

NURSING PROCESS: Patient Care Plan for Infection—*Continued*

Nursing Assessment and Diagnoses	Outcomes and Evaluation Parameters	Planning and Interventions with *Rationales*
Nursing Diagnosis: *Anxiety* related to threat to health status	**Outcome:** Anxiety level is minimal and coping is effective. ***Evaluation Parameters:*** Acknowledges and verbalizes feelings of anxiety. Verbalizes that anxiety is decreased. Verbalizes that physical manifestations of anxiety are decreased or absent. Participates in activities. Able to sleep without restlessness.	**Interventions and *Rationales:*** Monitor patient's level of anxiety and physical reactions. *Signs of anxiety are very individual. Monitoring those reactions helps in the development of a plan to address the anxiety.* Explore coping skills the patient has used in the past for anxiety. *Methods that have been successful in the past are likely to be successful again.* Encourage the patient to use new techniques to reduce anxiety such as imaging, relaxation techniques, or soothing music. *Many techniques will help patients cope with anxiety.* Encourage the patient to express feelings of anxiety. *Recognizing and expressing feelings sometimes helps to relieve them.* Explain all procedures and allow time for mental preparation. *Increased knowledge decreases anxiety related to the unknown.* Explain the disease process and therapies involved in the treatment. *Increased knowledge decreases anxiety related to the unknown.*

Assessment of Knowledge of Disease Process

Subjective Data:
What do you know about your disease?
What do you know about the treatment involved with your infection?
Do you understand how to prevent infection?
Do you know what symptoms to report immediately?

Objective Data:
Assess knowledge of infection, how it occurred, how to prevent it, and how to treat it.

Nursing Assessment and Diagnoses	Outcomes and Evaluation Parameters	Planning and Interventions with *Rationales*
Nursing Diagnosis: *Deficient Knowledge* related to infection and its prevention	**Outcome:** Verbalizes understanding of condition and treatment plan. ***Evaluation Parameters:*** Patient and family verbalize an understanding of the signs of infection and how to prevent an infection. Patient and family verbalize an understanding of the treatment modalities being used. Patient and family verbalize the signs and symptoms to report to the health care provider.	**Interventions and *Rationales:*** Teach patient and family the signs of infection and what to report to the physician *to allow for early recognition and treatment.* Teach the patient and family causes of infection. *Helps the patient to avoid getting an infection.*

Discharge Priorities

With the movement toward decreasing the length of hospital stays and preference to receive care at home, many patients are being cared for in their homes. Infection control has been a concern of hospitals but consideration should now be given to the home environment as well. The prevention of infection in the home is different than in the hospital. Patients being cared for at home are not exposed to other patients and reservoirs of pathogens that would be present in the hospital setting. Home care patients are usually not as ill as hospitalized patients, so their ability to resist infections may be better. However, other environmental resources in the home, such as plumbing, sanitation, and ventilation, typically are more difficult to control than in an institution.

The basic principles of prevention and control still apply. The focus should not be on getting rid of household germs but on using good hygiene measures such as hand washing to prevent exposure to germs and cross infection. Families must be taught infection control principles so that they can develop their own approaches and make knowledgeable decisions related to reducing the chances of infection. Hand hygiene remains a very important part of preventing infection. Other procedures such as care of catheters and wounds can be adapted to the home. Equipment needs to be cleaned in the dishwasher if possible or with regular household cleaning products. Use of gowns, gloves, and masks is only necessary when family members need to be protected from the patient's infection. The Patient Teaching & Discharge Priorities box (p. 479) outlines the teaching needs of a patient who is discharged with an open wound.

There is a requirement that cases or suspected cases of certain diseases or conditions, called **notifiable diseases,** be reported to

PHARMACOLOGY Summary of Medications to Treat Infectious Disease

Medication Category	Action	Application/Indication	Nursing Responsibility
Antibiotics			
Used to treat infections related to bacterial agents	Act by killing bacteria or by inhibiting their growth.	Each type of antibiotic is effective against a different type of organism.	Assess for history of allergies to the medication. Assess the patient's response to the medication in terms of effectiveness and possible side effects. Patient education should include the importance of completing the entire regimen and the medication and reporting any clinical manifestations related to allergies or side effects.
Specific Types of Antibiotics			
Aminoglycosides • Gentamicin • Streptomycin	Act as bactericidal agents by interrupting the bacteria's protein synthesis.	Used against gram-negative bacilli, some aerobic gram-positive organisms, mycobacteria, and some protozoa. May be used to treat nosocomial infections, urinary tract infections, eye infections, and infections of the central nervous system.	Given intravenously because they are poorly absorbed through the GI tract. Assess kidney and hearing function. Check peak and trough levels so that blood levels are maintained in a narrow margin. Watch for drug interactions.
Penicillins • Penicillin G • Ampicillin • Nafcillin	Bactericidal action is through destruction of the cell wall of the bacteria.	Are broad spectrum and act against gram-positive, gram-negative, and anaerobic organisms. Used for upper respiratory tract infections, syphilis, endocarditis.	Assess for adverse reactions and interactions with other medications. Ensure adequate hydration of the patient. Provide small, frequent meals to minimize stomatitis, and sore mouth. If patient of childbearing age, advise her to use a backup method of birth control.
Cephalosporins • Cefazolin • Cefaclor • Ceftazidime	Inhibit bacterial cell-wall synthesis by binding to protein located on the cell membrane.	Act against gram-positive organisms and gram-negative organisms. Used for patients who are allergic to penicillin. Treat respiratory tract infections, skin infections, otitis media, urinary tract infections, septicemia, endocarditis.	Take on an empty stomach. Refrain from drinking alcohol. Maintain adequate hydration.
Tetracyclines • Doxycycline • Minocycline	Bacteriostatic. Inhibit cell growth by inhibiting protein synthesis leading to prevention of cell division.	Used for infections caused by *Rickettsia* species, *Mycoplasma,* and *Chlamydia.* Treats Lyme disease, *Helicobacter pylori,* acne vulgaris, skin infections.	Must use an additional birth control method while taking. Absorption may be decreased if taken with some over-the-counter medications. Take on an empty stomach. Will cause increased sensitivity to the sun.
Macrolides • Erythromycin • Azithromycin • Clarithromycin	Can prevent the cell from dividing or can kill the bacterial cell. Act by inhibiting RNA-dependent protein synthesis.	More effective against gram-positive organisms than gram-negative organisms. Treats *Staphylococcus, Streptococcus, Chlamydia, Mycoplasma.* Used to treat urethral, endocervical, or rectal infections, bronchitis, pharyngitis, skin infections, respiratory infections, pharyngitis, pneumonia.	Monitor the patient's hearing. Medication should be taken 1 hour before or 2 hours after meals.
Vancomycin	Has bacteriocidal activity that inhibits cell-wall synthesis by altering the cell's permeability.	Used to treat bacterial septicemia, endocarditis, bone and joint infections, and *Clostridium difficile* infections. Effective against streptococci and staphylococci.	Monitor hearing and renal function. Monitor fluid status. Assess peak and trough serum levels.
Carbapenems • Ertapenem • Meropenem	Bactericidal. Work by inhibiting cell-wall synthesis.	Have beta-lactam activity for use against anaerobes. Are broad spectrum and effective against gram-positive and gram-negative organisms. Frequently used for serious or life-threatening infections.	Give with caution in patients with head trauma or brain lesions because they can induce seizures.

(continued)

PHARMACOLOGY Summary of Medications to Treat Infectious Disease—*Continued*

Medication Category	Action	Application/Indication	Nursing Responsibility
Monobactams • Aztreonam	Inhibits cell-wall synthesis, leading to cell death.	Effective against gram-negative aerobic organisms such as *Pseudomonas aeruginosa*. Also used to treat urinary tract infections, septicemia, skin, and lower respiratory tract infections.	Given IV or IM. Monitor for signs of thrombophlebitis at the insertion site.
Fluoroquinolones • Ciprofloxacin • Levofloxacin • Ofloxacin	Interrupt DNA synthesis during bacterial replication, interfering with replication.	Used to treat urinary tract infections, respiratory tract infections, skin, bone and joint infections, pneumonia, gynecologic infections, sexually transmitted infections.	Antacids will lead to decreased absorption. Avoid sunlight. Tendon rupture is a potential adverse event and should be assessed.
Sulfonamides • Sulfasalazine	Interferes with synthesis of folic acid needed for DNA synthesis. This prevents reproduction of the bacteria.	Treats urinary tract infections, lower respiratory tract infections, diarrhea, skin, bone and joint infections, gynecologic infections.	Antacids will decrease absorption. Monitor folate deficiency. Monitor fluid intake. Photosensitivity can be a problem. Take on an empty stomach with a full glass of water. Monitor hematologic function.
Nitrofurantoin	Is bacteriostatic by inhibiting the energy production of the bacteria.	Is rapidly excreted in the urine and, therefore, is used only for urinary tract infections.	Monitor for peripheral neuropathy and pulmonary reactions.
Antivirals Used to treat viral infections			
Nucleoside analogues • Acyclovir • Famciclovir	Inhibits viral DNA polymerase, leading to disruption of viral growth.	Treat viral syndromes that occur in immunocompromised patients such as herpes simplex.	Monitor for adverse reactions. Monitor for nephrotoxicity. Is expensive so consider referring patient to social services for financial help.
Influenza A and syncytial virus drugs • Amantadine • Zanamivir	Appear to inhibit viral replication by blocking the uncoating of the virus particle and release of viral RNA into the host cell.	Used to treat influenza A infections and respiratory syncytial virus infections.	Should not be used with central nervous system stimulants such as alcohol.

local, county, or state public health departments. This process helps with disease surveillance efforts so that the health of individuals and families can be protected and the diseases controlled or prevented. The National Guidelines box (p. 480) lists diseases that were designated as reportable at the national level as of 2007. Other additional diseases may be reportable to the state as designated by state law and vary from state to state. The list of diseases designated as reportable changes to reflect the needs of the public at any given time. Annual recommendations for what diseases should be on the list are made by the Council of State and Territorial Epidemiologists (CSTE) and the CDC. The reporting of a disease to a public health authority leads to an immediate response that includes case investigation, contact prophylaxis, and outbreak control. Analysis of the information supplied for the notifiable diseases allows for the establishment of public health priorities and the monitoring of trends.

Collaborative Management

The goals of care are to identify the site of the infection and the causative organism so that a cure can be achieved quickly and

without complications. This will require a collaborative approach to care. The multidisciplinary team may consist of nurses, physicians, occupational therapists, physical therapists, nutritionists, psychologists, and pharmacists. A thorough history and physical examination will help identify the system involved. The physician will order diagnostic tests to help narrow the focus and identify the site and causative agent. It is the nurse's responsibility to continually assess the patient as the presenting signs and symptoms become more defined and to ensure that diagnostic tests are completed and specimens collected correctly.

Once the infecting agent has been identified, therapy can be ordered that is narrowly focused on the patient's problem. A pharmacist will help identify the proper medications and educate the patient on the use and side effects of the medications. A viral infection will often resolve with only supportive care. If antibiotics are administered systemically, it is important to watch for any adverse effects caused by the drugs. It also is the nurse's responsibility to protect the patient from obtaining new infections and decrease the potential for spreading the infection to others.

Nutritionists can help provide the patient with a well-balanced diet to help keep the immune system strong. Physical and occupa-

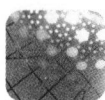

PATIENT TEACHING & DISCHARGE PRIORITIES for Infection

Need	Teaching
Wound care: Patient/family/support system Setting	Perform daily cleansing and dressing changes for open areas.
	Elevate areas where edema formation occurs.
	Avoid scratching the healed areas as this could cause breakdown: • Use liberal amounts of emollient lotions for dryness and flaking. • Use diphenhydramine hydrochloride (Benadryl) for pruritus (itching). • Keep fingernails short and use gloves when sleeping.
	Avoid sunlight because it can cause, among other things, healed wounds to permanently discolor or darken. • Avoid overexposure to sun. • Use sunscreen products when exposed to sunlight. • Use clothing and hats for added protection.
	Avoid exposure to extreme temperatures and harsh chemicals.
	Wear loose-fitting, soft clothing.
	Assess availability, knowledge, and compliance with treatment regimen.
	Assess discharge placement needs for the home, rehabilitation facility, or extended care facility.
	Assess home environment for need for assistive devices.
	Assess for professional home health needs.
	Assess need for follow-up appointments.
Wound infection: Patient/family/support system Setting	Assess for infection of open wounds and healed wound breakdown with each dressing change and report as necessary.
	Signs and symptoms include odor and exudate, fever, increased drainage, swelling, and lack of wound closure.
	Apply antibiotic ointments as prescribed.
	Teach minimization of risk factors for infection.
	Explain signs and symptoms that require medical attention.
	Assess environment for risk factors.
Nutrition: Patient/family/support system Setting	Maintain a high-calorie, high-protein diet.
	Continue taking vitamins and mineral supplements as ordered.
	Observe for appetite and weight loss and food intolerance.
	Taper calorie intake once preinjury or ideal weight has been achieved to prevent excessive weight gain.
	With professional guidance (i.e., physical therapist) institute an exercise program.
	Assess financial resources.
Pain management: Patient/family/support system Setting	Assess pain level and report any increase in pain.
	Assess effectiveness of pharmacologic interventions.
	Wean patient off pain medication when pain lessens.
	Assess environment for safety and promotion of therapeutic needs.
Emotional adjustment: Patient/family/support system Setting	Answer questions honestly.
	Encourage verbalization of frustrations and anger.
	Encourage positive reinforcement from the family.
	Encourage independent functioning as soon as possible.
	Stress that it is not uncommon to feel letdown after discharge.
	Encourage participation in a support group.

tional therapists will be needed to maintain or regain physical functioning. Every member of the health care team along with the patient and the patient's family must be cognizant of the importance of proper hand hygiene and its huge role in the prevention of disease transmission.

Antimicrobials are chosen based on a number of factors. The clinical and diagnostic evaluation is used to decide whether therapy should be instituted as well as what type. If the severity of the infection merits, the physician may decide to begin therapy before the culture results are available. This is known as **empiric**

therapy. Data used to decide on the medication of choice in this instance includes the usual susceptibility of the suspected organism, the capability of medication to penetrate the site of infection, and patient factors such as other illnesses, medication allergies, immune status and pregnancy status. Once the culture results are available, the medication is chosen based on what is most effective against the identified organism, with the least risk of toxicity and fewest adverse effects for the patient. The physician, in consultation with the pharmacist, also considers patient compliance, cost, and dosing schedule.

NATIONAL GUIDELINES Diseases Designated as Notifiable at the National Level During 2007

Acquired immunodeficiency syndrome (AIDS)

Anthrax

Arboviral neuroinvasive and nonneuroinvasive diseases

California serogroup virus disease

Eastern equine encephalitis virus disease

Powassan virus disease

St. Louis encephalitis

West Nile virus disease

Western equine encephalitis virus disease

Botulism

Brucellosis

Chancroid

Chlamydia trachomatis, genital infection

Cholera

Coccidioidomycosis

Cryptosporidiosis

Cyclosporiasis

Diphtheria

Ehrlichiosis

Human granulocytic

Human monocytic

Human, other or unspecified agent

Giardiasis

Gonorrhea

Haemophilus influenzae, invasive disease

Hansen disease

Hantavirus pulmonary syndrome

Hemolytic uremic syndrome, postdiarrheal

Hepatitis A, acute

Hepatitis B, acute

Hepatitis B, perinatal infection

Hepatitis C

Hepatitis viral, chronic B and C

Human immunodeficiency virus (HIV) infection

Adult and pediatric HIV

Influenza-associated pediatric mortality

Legionellosis

Listeriosis

Lyme disease

Malaria

Measles

Meningococcal disease

Mumps

Novel influenza A virus infections

Pertussis

Plague

Poliomyelitis, paralytic

Poliovirus infection, nonparalytic

Psittacosis

Q fever

Rabies, animal

Rabies, human

Rocky Mountain spotted fever

Rubella

Rubella, congenital syndrome

Salmonellosis

Severe acute respiratory syndrome– associated coronavirus (SARS-CoV) disease

Shiga toxin-producing *Escherichia coli* (STEC)

Shigellosis

Smallpox

Streptococcal disease, invasive, group A

Streptococcal toxic-shock syndrome

Streptococcus pneumoniae, drug-resistant, invasive disease

Streptococcus pneumoniae, invasive, in children <5 years old

Syphilis

Syphilis, congenital

Tetanus

Toxic-shock syndrome

Trichinosis

Tuberculosis

Tularemia

Typhoid fever

Vancomycin intermediate-resistant *Staphylococcus aureus* (VISA)

Vancomycin-resistant *Staphylococcus aureus* (VRSA)

Varicella

Varicella deaths

Vibriosis

Yellow fever

Source: Centers for Disease Control and Prevention Morbidly and Mortality Weekly Report. Summary of Notifiable Diseases—-United States, 2007. Retrieved June 12, 2008 from http://www.cdc.gov/mmwr/preview/mmwrhtml/mm5553a1.htm.

 Be sure to assess patient for signs of an allergic reaction or side effects of the medication being given.

The nurse serves as the patient advocate and liaison between the patient and other members of the health care team. The nurse coordinates and facilitates communication between all members of the health care team and the patient. The educational needs and emotional support needs are the responsibility of the nurse.

 Research

There are many research opportunities in nursing related to infection. The goals of research are to identify more effective means of caring for the patient with infection and to prevent infection from occurring. A list of research topics related to infection is provided in the Research Opportunities and Clinical Impact box.

RESEARCH OPPORTUNITIES AND CLINICAL IMPACT RELATED TO INFECTION

Research Area	Clinical Impact
Immunization	
Effects of nursing role on compliance with immunizations	Increases the numbers of people who are immunized so that the numbers exposed to infectious disease can be decreased.
Effects of laws on compliance with immunization	
Adverse effects of vaccines on the outcomes of pregnancy or the unborn child	
Home Care	
Prevention techniques needed in the home	Little is known about the prevalence of infection in the home and the best techniques to prevent it.
The development of surveillance systems for infection in the home	
Prevention of Nosocomial Infections	
The degree and type of organisms related to environmental surface contamination	More information is needed about where the organisms come from and how to prevent their transmission.
Assessment of prevention strategies at specific sites such as ventilator-associated pneumonia	
Compliance of health care personnel with hand hygiene practices	
What agents are most effective for hand hygiene and what time intervals are needed	
Treatment	
Studies related to improved antibiotic usage and management of antibiotic resistance	Although much progress has been made in the treatment of infection, new problems are developing that need to be addressed.

EVIDENCE-BASED PRACTICE

Effects of Infection and Antibiotic-Resistant Bacteria on Wound Healing

Clinical Problem

Antimicrobial resistance occurs when the antibiotics taken to stop the infection do not kill the bacteria that cause the infection. The bacteria resist the effects of the antibiotic, which allows them to continue to survive and grow causing more harm. After repeated exposure to an antibiotic that does not kill them, microorganisms develop the ability to avoid the inhibitory or lethal activity of an antimicrobial agent through several mechanisms. Research has been done to increase understanding about how bacteria protect themselves. Bacteria can become resistant by neutralizing the antibiotic, pumping the antibiotic out, or changing the antibiotic attack site so the function of the bacteria is not affected. Bacteria that were at one time killed by an antibiotic can become resistant through mutation of their genetic material or by acquiring pieces of DNA that code for the resistance properties from other bacteria. The transfer of one piece of DNA may allow the bacteria to become resistant to many antibiotics.

There are several resistant pathogens on the rise. These include penicillin-resistant *Streptococcus pneumoniae* (DRSP), group A streptococci of enhanced virulence, and vancomycin-resistant enterococci. As long as bacteria are able to mutate, the battle against infection will be a struggle. Infection will become more prominent. One of the areas affected by infection and antibiotic-resistant bacteria is that of wound healing. The presence of bacteria in the wound leads to inflammation, delayed healing, and increased scarring.

Research Findings

Ryan (2007) reviewed research on the effects of infection and antibiotic-resistant bacteria on wound healing. As research continues, new mechanisms have been discovered by which bacteria protect themselves. Research has reported that bacteria use a biofilm cover and that bacteria may mutate their genes and horizontally transfer their genes to other bacteria. The ability of bacteria to make adaptations like these causes concerned about prescribing antibiotics. An understanding of these mechanisms will help to identify other ways of attacking the bacteria.

Bacteria in wounds are initially gram positive, but gram-negative bacteria also play a role in the delay of wound healing. In order for the right antibiotic to be prescribed, it is important to identify the right bacteria. Wounds are often contaminated with other materials or may grow different bacteria in different areas of the wound. A good understanding of how to take samples from the wound for culture is important.

Other factors related to wound healing and preventing contamination of the wound should be considered. The healing of the wound and signs of inflammation can be influenced by factors such as the presence of anemia and malnutrition. Medications that the patient may be taking such as steroids or immunosuppressive agents may delay wound healing and make the patient more susceptible to infection. Good nutrition with adequate amounts of vitamins A and C, iron, and zinc is necessary for wound healing. Accurate diagnosis and assessment is important so that antibiotics will be prescribed correctly and only when needed. The traditional implementation of activities thought to be antibacterial is being questioned. Actions such as preoperative bathing and hair removal have been found in some studies to have no effect on the rate of infection. The one activity that has been shown through research to be effective in preventing infection is proper hand hygiene, especially when alcohol is used.

Implications for Nursing Practice

This study demonstrates the need for nurses to help to prevent infections in wounds so that healing can occur. Nurses need to perform hand hygiene before and after caring for the patient. Gloves should be worn to provide wound care. The patient's overall health should be enhanced through a well-balanced diet, proper hydration, good hygiene, and some exercise, if possible, to increase circulation. The proper use of antibiotics can help reduce the development of antibiotic resistance. Patients should be assessed for their response to antibiotic treatment to help decide if the antibiotic is effective. Patient education about the use of antibiotics is also supported in this research. Patients often want an antibiotic when one may not be indicated. Nurses can help the patient and the patient's family understand when the use of an antibiotic is needed and how to take the antibiotic properly.

Critical Thinking Questions

1. Develop a plan for helping the patient prevent a wound infection preoperatively.

2. Describe the proper assessment of a wound when concerned about the possibility of infection.

3. Identify nursing measures that would decrease the chances for infection in a patient wound.

4. Identify interventions that would help decrease resistance to antibiotics.

Answers to Critical Thinking Questions appear in Appendix D.

Reference

Ryan, T. J. (2007). Infection following soft tissue injury: Its role in wound healing. *Current Opinion in Infectious Disease, 20*(2), 124–128.

Clinical Preparation

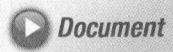 CRITICAL THINKING

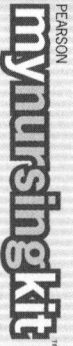

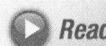 Read

- History of Current Illness
- Past Medical History
- Physical Exam
- Admitting Medical Orders
- Laboratory Study Results

Document

- Summary of Hospitalization
- Pathophysiology Form
- Laboratory Values
- Laboratory Results Explanation

Apply

- List of Potential Nursing Diagnoses
- Concept Map
- Critical Thinking Questions

Log on to MyNursingKit.com to download forms you will need and to complete further steps in the Clinical Preparation assignment.

HISTORY OF PRESENT ILLNESS

Mr. Ralph Newman is a 68-year-old black male admitted with a diagnosis of "infection of right leg wound." Mr. Newman was struck in the right leg with a piece of wood while cutting up firewood. He finished cutting the wood then went in the house and washed off his leg. However, 3 days later the wound began to drain thick greenish, yellow liquid and was painful. He visited his doctor who cleaned the wound and put him on Keflex. However, the wound continued to get worse so he was admitted to the hospital. On the day of admission, Mr. Newman was taken to surgery for a cleaning and debridement of his leg wound.

Medical-Surgical History

Insulin-dependent diabetes mellitus
Myocardial infarction 10 years ago but has been doing well since that time
Allergies: none known
Drug intolerance: none known

Social History

Retired and likes to work outside around his home
Smokes 1 pack of cigarettes per day
Lives with his wife in the country

Physical Exam

Weight: 200 lb; height: 5 ft 8 in.
BP 164/90; P 85; RR 20; T 101°F
HEENT: PERRLA, ears appear normal; pharynx pink with no exudates
Neck: no cervical lymphadenopathy; thyroid nonpalpable
Heart: regular rate and rhythm; no extra heart sounds
Lungs: clear to auscultation
Abdomen: bowel sounds present × 4 quadrants; soft and nondistended; no tenderness or masses; no hepatomegaly
Extremities: left leg 1+ pitting edema; brown discoloration from midcalf down to ankle; toes slightly pink in color
Pedal pulses 1+ left foot
Pulses absent in right foot; toes on right foot pink and cool to touch
Right leg 2+ pitting edema
Open wound on anterior shin approximately 4 inches in diameter. Draining moderate amount of greenish yellow, thick liquid. Necrotic tissue noted in wound bed. Skin around wound red and warm to touch

MS: moves all extremities; full ROM except right ankle due to pain; normal muscle strength
Neuro: sensation slightly diminished in both lower legs. DTRs 2+. CN ii-xii intact

Admitting Medical Orders

Admit to surgical service
Diagnosis: right leg wound infection; status post-incision and drainage of right leg
No known allergies
Vital signs with oxygen saturation q4h
Wet-to-dry dressing with Dakin's solution q4h
Up in chair
Bathroom privileges
ADA diet
Accu-Chek ac and HS
Sequential compression devices (SCD) to lower extremities
Incentive spirometry q hour while awake
IV: saline lock; NS flushes q8h
Intake and output
Call house officer: pulse < 60 & > 110/minute; BP < 90 & > 160 systolic; temperature > 38.5; urine output < 30 mL/hr for 2 hours; respiratory rate > 30/minute: oxygen saturation < 92%; blood sugar < 70 & >130

Scheduled Medications

Insulin 15 units SQ of 70/30 in a.m. and 10 units of 70/30 SQ at HS
Cefoxitin 1 g IV q8h
Aspirin 81 mg po daily
Lipitor 10 mg po daily

PRN Medications

Phenergan 25 mg IV q6h prn nausea
Mylanta 30 mL po q4–6h prn dyspepsia
Triazolam 0.125–0.25 mg po q noc, prn sleep
Ativan 0.5-2 mg IV q6–8h prn anxiety
Milk of Magnesia 30 mL po daily, prn constipation
Tylenol 650 mg po/pr q4h for pain
Vicodin 1-2 tabs po prn q6h for mild to moderate pain
Morphine sulphate 1-8 mg IV q4h prn severe pain

Ordered Laboratory Studies

Wound culture
ESR × 1
Chemistry panel q a.m.
CBC q a.m.

Ordered Diagnostic Studies

Chest x-ray

LABORATORY STUDY RESULTS

Test	Day 1	Day 2	Day 3
Hemoglobin A_1C	9.1%		
Random glucose	160 mg/dL		
Fasting glucose	140 mg/dL	138 mg/dL	142 mg/dL
WBC	12,000/mm³	15,000/mm³	14,000/mm³
Lymphocytes	11%	12%	11%
Monocytes	1%	2%	2%
Bands	12%	18%	17%
Neutrophils	78%	80%	79%
Basophils	10%	10%	9%
RBC	3.08/mm³	3.10/mm³	3.10/mm³
Hemoglobin	9 gl/L	9.5 gl/L	9.7 gl/L
Hematocrit	27%	28%	28%
Wound culture	Staph. aureus		
ESR	48 mm/h		
Chest x-ray	Normal		

CRITICAL THINKING QUESTIONS

1. When Mr. Newman is admitted to the unit there are no private rooms available. The choices are as follows: room 110 with Mr. Jonas, diagnosis: leukemia; room 115 with Mr. Smithson who has a GI bleed; or room 122 with Mr. Kendrick who was admitted for deep venous thrombosis. In which room should Mr. Newman be placed?

2. Should Mr. Newman be placed in isolation. If so, why?

3. What factors does Mr. Newman have that make him susceptible to infection?

4. What nursing diagnoses would be appropriate for Mr. Newman?

Answers to Critical Thinking Questions appear in Appendix D.

NCLEX® REVIEW

1. The nurse is caring for a patient with a wound infection. Which of the following would explain an increase in purulent exudate in the wound?
   1. Response of white blood cells to the cellular injury
   2. Temporary vasoconstriction to avoid blood loss after injury
   3. Vasodilatation to increase blood supply to the area
   4. Leakage of fluid and cells out of capillaries into interstitial spaces

2. The nurse is assessing a patient with an infection. Which of the following assessment findings could indicate the cause for the infection?
   1. Inadequate nutrition
   2. Personality disorder
   3. Age 45 and employed
   4. Urban living

3. A patient is admitted with tuberculosis. The nurse realizes that this patient received this infection through which mode of transmission?
   1. Contact
   2. Airborne
   3. Vehicle
   4. Vector

4. While providing care to patients, the nurse realizes that preventing the control and spread of infection is a priority. Which of the following should the nurse do when washing the hands between patients?
   1. Use water as hot as tolerated.
   2. Clean under artificial nails prior to starting the shift.
   3. Use a petroleum-based lotion for prevention of dryness.
   4. Wash for at least fifteen seconds covering all surfaces.

5. A patient with an indwelling urinary catheter is demonstrating signs of having a urinary tract infection. The nurse realizes this infection is most likely caused by:
   1. Group A beta-hemolytic streptococci.
   2. *Staphylococcus aureus.*
   3. *Neisseria meningitidis.*
   4. *Staphylococcus epidermidis.*

6. A patient is experiencing an infectious disease. The nurse realizes that this is an expected result of passive immunity which is characterized by:
   1. Providing long-term and possibly lifelong immunity.
   2. The introduction of live, killed or attenuated toxin into the body.
   3. Injecting already formed antibodies into the body.
   4. Being immunized for such diseases as measles and mumps.

7. The nurse is admitting a patient with tuberculosis. Which of the following is a *Healthy People 2010* guideline for this disease process?
   1. Eradicate the incidence of tuberculosis in the United States.
   2. Increase the proportion of all tuberculosis clients who complete curative therapy within 12 months.
   3. Increase the percentage of health care workers who are immunized against tuberculosis.
   4. Decrease the communicable spread of tuberculosis among the rural population.

8. The nurse is interviewing a patient for a history of infectious diseases. Which of the following questions would provide the most information about these diseases?
   1. How many hours a week do you work out of the home?
   2. What types of activities do you participate in for recreation?
   3. Have you received chemotherapy for cancer, psoriasis, or rheumatoid arthritis?
   4. Explain your exercise routine.

Answers for review questions appear in Appendix D

KEY TERMS

active immunization *p.468*
antigenicity *p.464*
carrier *p.461*
chain of infection *p.461*
community-acquired infection *p.457*
empiric therapy *p.479*
endotoxins *p.465*

exotoxins *p.465*
fever of unknown origin (FUO) *p.471*
infectivity *p.464*
invasiveness *p.464*
mode of transmission *p.461*
nosocomial infection *p.457*
notifiable disease *p.476*

passive immunization *p.468*
pathogenicity *p.461*
portal of entry *p.461*
portal of exit *p.461*
reservoir *p.461*
viability *p.464*
virulence *p.464*

REFERENCES

Centers for Disease Control and Prevention. (2003). *Anthrax: What you need to know*. Retrieved July 14, 2007, from http://www.bt.cdc.gov/agent/anthrax/needtoknow.asp

Centers for Disease Control and Prevention. (2004). *International conference on new and emerging diseases*. Retrieved July 14, 2007, from http:// www.cdc.gov/iceid/2004/index.htm

Centers for Disease Control. (2008). *2008 Child & Adolescent Immunization Schedules*. Retrieved June 12, 2008 from http://www.cdc.gov/vaccines/recs/schedules/child-schedule.htm

Creedon, S. A. (2005). Healthcare workers' hand decontamination practices: Compliance with recommended guidelines. *Journal of Advanced Nursing, 51*(3), 208–216.

Garner, J. S. (1996). *Guidelines for isolation precautions in hospitals: Hospital Infection Control Advisory Committee*. Atlanta, GA: Centers for Disease Control and Prevention.

Kozier, B., Erb, G., Berman, A., & Snyder, S. (2004). *Fundamentals of nursing: Concepts, process, and practice* (7th ed.). Upper Saddle River, NJ: Pearson Prentice Hall.

Larson, E. L. (2005). State-of-the-science 2004: Time for a "no excuses/no tolerance" (NET) strategy. *American Journal of Infection Control, 33*(9),548–557.

Larson, E. L., Girard, R., Pessoa-Silva, C. L., Boyce, J., Donaldson, L., & Pittet, D. (2006). Skin reactions related to hand hygiene and selection of hand hygiene products. *American Journal of Infection Control, 34*(10), 627–635.

Porth, C. M. (2007). *Essentials of pathophysiology: Concepts of altered health status* (2nd ed.). Philadelphia: Lippincott Williams & Wilkins.

Schulster, L., & Chinn, R. Y. W. (2003). Guidelines for environmental infection control in health-care facilities. *MMWR, 52*(RR10), 1–42.

Siegel, J. D., Rhinehart, E., Jackson, M., Chiarello, L., & the Healthcare Infection Control Practices Advisory Committee. (2007, June). *Guideline for isolation precautions: Preventing transmission of infectious agents in healthcare settings 2007*. Retrieved June 6, 2008, from http://www.cdc.gov/ncidod/dhqp/pdf/guidelines/Isolation2007.pdf

Somner, J.E.A., Scott,K. M. & Gibb, A.P. (2007). What is the Optimum Location of Alcohol-Based Hand Cleanser? *Infect Control Hosp Epidemiol 28*:108–109.

Trick, W. E., Vernon, M. O., Hayes, R. A., Nathan, R., Rice, T. W., Perterson, B. J., et al. (2003). Impact of ring wearing on hand contamination and comparison of hand hygiene agents in a hospital. *Clinical Infectious Diseases, 36*(11), 1383–1390.

U.S. Department of Health and Human Services. (2000). *Healthy people 2010: Understanding and improving health*. Retrieved June 5, 2008, from http://www.healthypeople.gov

Widmer, A. F., Conzelmann, M., Tomic, M., Frei, R., & Stranden, A. M. (2007). Introducing alcohol-based hand rub for hand hygiene: The critical need for training. *Infection Control and Hospital Epidemiology, 28*(1), 50–54.

Wiseman, S. (2006). Prevention and control of healthcare-associated infection. *Nursing Standard, 20*(38), 41–45.

Hypertension

Ann Harley

Outcome-Based Learning Objectives

After studying this chapter, the learner will be able to:

1. Compare and contrast the differences between the types of hypertension: prehypertension, stage 1 hypertension, and stage 2 hypertension.

2. Describe the pathophysiology of hypertension.

3. Discuss the risk factors associated with the development of hypertension.

4. Explain the therapeutic agents used to manage hypertension.

5. Compare and contrast how social and cultural influences affect the plan of care for the hypertensive patient.

6. Develop a nursing plan of care with the hypertensive client.

7. Discuss how multidisciplinary therapeutic interventions are associated with patient outcome.

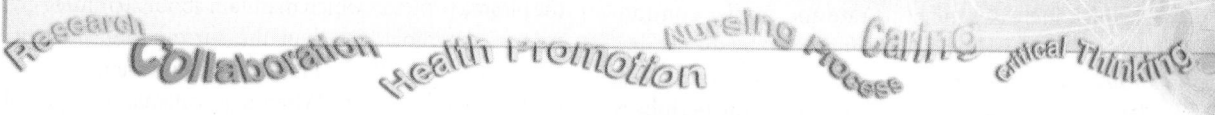

Blood pressure is defined as the pressure created by the circulating blood through the arteries, veins, and the chambers of the heart. Blood pressure readings are classified into four stages: normal tension, prehypertension, stage 1 hypertension, and stage 2 hypertension (National Heart, Lung, and Blood Institute [NHLBI], 2003; Yuan, 2004).

A severe form of hypertension is referred to as malignant hypertension. In the NHLBI's May 2003 publication titled *Seventh Report of the Joint National Committee on Prevention, Detection, Evaluation, and Treatment of High Blood Pressure (JNC 7)*, malignant hypertension is referred to as a hypertensive urgency and emergency that reflects the patient's markedly elevated blood pressure and acute target organ damage requiring immediate hospitalization and parental drug therapy.

The various stages of high blood pressure are discussed throughout this chapter. Nurses should monitor patients for hypertension using the assessment points listed in Chart 21–1.

Regulation of Blood Pressure

Due to the pulsating blood flow created by the contraction and relaxation of the heart, there are two readings associated with blood pressure: the systolic and diastolic. The **systolic** blood pressure is the maximum pressure in the aorta and major arteries. It occurs when the left ventricle contracts and ejects blood into the central vascular system. This systolic reading averages 120 mmHg

CHART 21–1 Clinical Awareness and Monitoring

- Anticipate adherence problems for young men.
- Ask about smoking history:
  - Use of "Smoke Ender" or a similar program
  - History of success in quitting smoking.
- Consider nonadherence as cause of:
  - Failure to reach goal blood pressure
  - Resistant hypertension
  - Sudden loss of control.
- Encourage patients to bring all medications from all physicians and other sources, whether prescription, complementary, or over the counter, to each visit to review and cull out iatrogenic causes of high blood pressure.
- Ask what the patient takes for pain.
- Recognize depression and other psychiatric illnesses, including panic attacks, and manage appropriately.
- Be willing to change unsuccessful regimens and search for those more likely to succeed.

in a healthy adult individual. The **diastolic** blood pressure reflects cardiac relaxation, thus it is the minimum pressure in the arteries, which occurs just prior the next cycle of ventricular ejection of blood. This reading is approximately 80 mmHg in healthy individuals. The difference between the systolic and diastolic pressure is about 40 mmHg and is called the **pulse pressure** (Guyton & Hall, 2005). The pulse pressure is the ratio of stroke volume (amount of blood ejected with each heartbeat) to compliance of the arterial system (systemic vascular resistance) (Guyton & Hall, 2005).

Blood pressure is the product of cardiac output (the amount of blood pumped by the heart each minute) and systemic **peripheral vascular resistance** (the resistance to the flow of blood as determined by the vascular musculature and the diameter of the blood vessels and by influences on the ability of the cardiovascular system to adapt). The homeostatic systems that influence blood pressure changes in accordance with body needs are neural regulation, arterial baroreceptors and chemoreceptors, regulation of fluid volume, and humoral regulation (Guyton & Hall, 2005).

Neural Regulation

The pons and medulla of the brain are the neural control centers for the regulation of blood pressure. These areas are where the autonomic nervous system is integrated and modulated and where the vasomotor control center and cardiovascular control center are located. These control centers transmit parasympathetic impulses through the vagus nerve and sympathetic impulses through the spinal cord and peripheral sympathetic nerves to the heart and blood vessels. The parasympathetic impulse slows the heart rate as opposed to the sympathetic impulse dominance, which increases the heart rate and cardiac contractility. Blood vessels also are selectively innervated by the sympathetic nervous system. When this system is stimulated, vasoconstriction occurs, decreasing blood flow to the periphery and shunting blood to critical organs such as the heart and brain.

Arterial Baroreceptors and Arterial Chemoreceptors

Baroreceptors located in the walls of blood vessels are pressure-sensitive receptors that respond to changes in the stretch of the blood vessels by sending impulses to the brain and heart to adjust the heart rate and smooth muscle tone. These stretch receptors are located in various large vessels throughout the body, such as the carotid sinus and the wall of the left ventricle. They respond to changes in arterial pressure (high or low) and signal the central nervous system (CNS). Signals are then transmitted back through baroreceptors to counteract the abnormal changes in the arterial pressure. If the pressure is elevated, the vagus nerve is stimulated, thereby slowing the heart rate and causing vasodilation, which decreases the pressure in the arteries. This system needs to function effectively to prevent hypertension. When failure occurs in regulating the determinants of blood pressure—cardiac output and the total peripheral resistance—the body needs to reset the baroreceptor and chemoreceptor sensitivity to more adequately respond to the changes in the systemic blood pressure.

The chemoreceptors located in the carotid bodies and the aorta respond to changes in oxygen, carbon dioxide, and hydrogen ion content in the arterial blood. Chemoreceptors regulate ventilation and communicate with the brainstem and cardiovascular centers to cause widespread vasoconstriction.

When the sympathetic nervous system detects an inadequate (low) blood pressure, a lack of oxygen, or a buildup of metabolic end products, the baroreceptors and chemoreceptors are activated. Changes in blood pressure are transmitted back to the CNS. A drop in blood pressure causes parasympathetic system inhibition and cardiac sympathetic nerve activation, resulting in an increased heart rate. In a resting position, the heart rate is under the parasympathetic influence and the heart rate is 60 to 80 beats/minute.

Regulation of Fluid Volume

Fluid volume throughout the body is maintained through multiple homeostatic mechanisms. Normal fluid volume is the result of a dynamic equilibrium between oral fluids and other dietary intakes and fluid output, which occurs through perspiration, urination, and respiration. The cardiovascular, renal, and respiratory areas are involved as are the pituitary gland, parathyroid glands, and adrenal glands.

When changes occur in the osmolarity (i.e., the concentration of the solute), the number of particles in fluid is conserved or eliminated in order to maintain a system homeostatic state. Guyton and Hall (2005) state that 80% of the total osmolarity of the interstitial fluid and plasma is due to sodium and chloride ions. The intracellular fluid is composed of potassium ions, which make up 50% of the osmolarity, and the balance is divided among the other intracellular substances (Guyton & Hall, 2005). The difference between plasma and interstitial fluid is due to the osmotic effects of the plasma proteins, which maintain about 20 mmHg greater pressure in the capillaries than the surrounding interstitial spaces (Guyton & Hall, 2005). Fluid balance is essential to maintaining normal blood pressure. When hypovolemia or hypervolemia occurs, it is reflected in the systemic blood pressure. A loss of fluid or hypovolemia results in a decrease in blood pressure due to the loss of circulating blood volume. With an excess of fluid volume, hypervolemia occurs.

Humoral Regulation

A second mechanism that plays a role in blood pressure regulation is the intrinsic hormones of the body. These include the renin-angiotensin-aldosterone mechanism, vasopressin, and epinephrine and norepinephrine. These hormones are essential in maintaining normal blood pressure on an ongoing basis.

Renin-Angiotensin-Aldosterone System

Renin is an enzyme that is produced and stored by the kidney. It is released with:

- Increased sympathetic nervous system stimulation
- Decreased blood pressure
- Increased extracellular fluid volume
- Increased extracellular sodium concentration.

Once in the bloodstream renin acts as an enzyme to the inactive plasma protein substrate angiotensinogen to convert it to angiotensin I. Angiotensin I travels to the lung and is converted to angiotensin II by the angiotensin-converting enzyme present in the blood vessels of the lungs. Angiotensin II is a potent vasoconstrictor hormone, which increases peripheral vascular resistance, thus increasing blood pressure. A second function of angiotensin II is to stimulate the adrenal glands to release aldosterone. Aldosterone, a steroid, increases sodium and water retention by the kidneys, thereby increasing blood pressure (Figure 21–1 ■).

Vasopressin

Vasopressin, also known as antidiuretic hormone (ADH), is a peptide produced by the posterior pituitary gland. Vasopressin is released in response to decreases in blood volume and blood pressure, as well as when an increase in the osmolality occurs. Its major functions are to increase water reabsorption by the kidneys and cause vasoconstriction, thus increasing blood pressure (Guyton & Hall, 2005). Vasopressin also serves as a neurotransmitter to modify the autonomic nervous system response, as discussed later in this chapter.

Epinephrine and Norepinephrine

The catecholamines, epinephrine and norepinephrine, exert their effects on target cells, which impact blood pressure. The function of the adrenal medulla is to secrete these two catecholamines and depend on the receptor cell designation for their effects. Norepinephrine excites alpha receptors and beta receptors to a lesser degree than does epinephrine. Epinephrine excites both alpha and beta receptors equally. Thus, the effect of norepinephrine and epinephrine differs by the type of receptors in the organs (Guyton & Hall, 2005).

Epinephrine differs from norepinephrine in the following ways: epinephrine stimulates the beta receptors, increasing the effect on cardiac stimulation and weak vasoconstriction (Guyton & Hall, 2005). The heart increases the stroke volume (amount of blood ejected from the ventricle in one systole), the heart rate, and the muscle contractility. Blood vessels are able to constrict and dilate, thus impacting peripheral vascular resistance, which is the resistance to blood flow determined by the tone of the vascular system and the diameter of the blood vessel lumen. Through the action of these catecholamines, blood pressure is maintained. Norepinephrine also increases the heart rate and blood pressure.

■ Epidemiology and Etiology of Hypertension

The National Heart, Lung, and Blood Institute in 2004 reported that 65 million adult Americans—or one-third of the general adult population in the United States—have hypertension (Fields et al., 2004). If high blood pressure remains undiagnosed and untreated, it has a high morbidity and mortality rate.

This universal health dilemma of high blood pressure in the general population is undergoing intense inspection. The health care industry, health insurance groups, pharmaceutical companies, and the federal government are involved in solving this universal problem. The National Guidelines box (p. 490) outlines the *Healthy People 2010* midcourse review objective, target goal, and baseline data for people with hypertension. To make the condition of hypertension more easily understood, the name *hypertension,* a medical term, is gradually being changed to *high blood pressure.* This change is designed to make the term more easily understood in a worldwide multicultural community. The JNC 7 report (NHLBI, 2003b) states that many experts consider high blood pressure a "silent killer." It is a complex syndrome that can occur at any age, involves multiple systems of the body, and requires aggressive treatment.

■ Pathophysiology of Hypertension

Hypertension is diagnosed when the average blood pressure is higher than the accepted norm over a period of time consisting of two or more consecutive office visits. The May 2003 JNC 7 report (NHLBI, 2003b) included revised guidelines for what constitutes hypertension and divided these parameters into three separate classifications for adults over the age of 18 years, as listed in the National Guidelines box (p. 490).

The term **prehypertension,** introduced in the JNC 7 report (NHLBI, 2003b), describes those individuals with a blood pressure finding on two or more office visits of 120–139 mmHg systolic or 80–89 mmHg diastolic. These individuals are at twice the risk of developing hypertension as those with lower values.

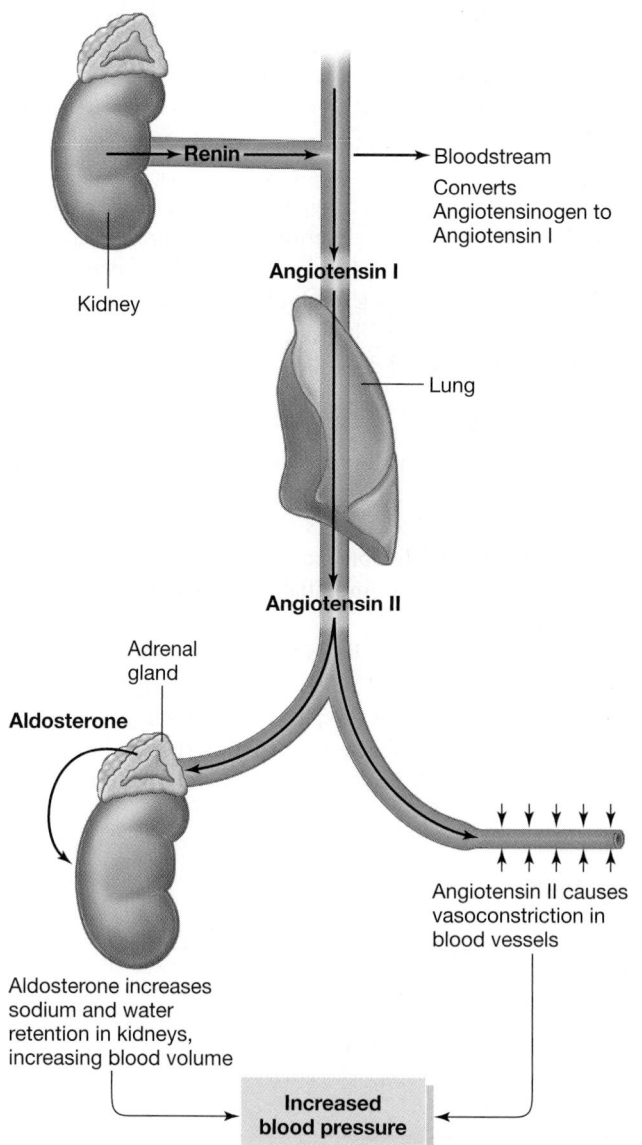

Renin → Bloodstream
Converts Angiotensinogen to Angiotensin I

Angiotensin I

Kidney

Lung

Angiotensin II

Adrenal gland

Aldosterone

Angiotensin II causes vasoconstriction in blood vessels

Aldosterone increases sodium and water retention in kidneys, increasing blood volume

Increased blood pressure

FIGURE 21–1 ■ Renin-angiotensin-aldosterone system.

NATIONAL GUIDELINES *Healthy People 2010* Midcourse Review: Objectives, Target Goals, and Baseline Data

12.9. Reduce the proportion of adults with high blood pressure.
Target: 14 percent
Baseline: 26 percent of adults ages 20 years and older had high blood pressure in 1988–1994 (age adjusted to the year 2000 standard population).

12.10. Increase the proportion of adults with high blood pressure whose blood pressure is under control.
Target: 68 percent
Baseline: 25 percent of adults ages 18 years and older with high blood pressure had it under control in 1988–1994 (age adjusted to the year 2000 standard population).

12.11. Increase the proportion of adults with high blood pressure who are taking action (for example, losing weight, increasing physical activity, or reducing sodium intake) to help control their blood pressure.
Target: 98 percent
Baseline: 84 percent of adults ages 18 years and older with high blood pressure were taking action to control it in 1998 (age adjusted to the year 2000 standard population).

12.12. Increase the proportion of adults who have had their blood pressure measured within the preceding 2 years and can state whether their blood pressure was normal or high.
Target: 95 percent
Baseline: 90 percent of adults ages 18 years and older had their blood pressure measured in the past 2 years and could state whether it was normal or high in 1998 (age adjusted to the year 2000 standard population).

Source: U.S. Department of Health and Human Services. (2006). *Midcourse review: Healthy People 2010: Heart disease and stroke—12.* Retrieved June 9, 2008, from http://www.healthypeople.gov/data/midcourse/html/focusareas/FA12TOC.htm.

MyNursingKit Animation: Stages of Hypertension Table

Prehypertension is the early phase when the relationship between the blood pressure measurement and the need for health education is the primary focus of care. The individual demonstrating prehypertension is at risk for development of stage 1 or stage 2 hypertension. The JNC 7 report emphasizes increasing the awareness of the need to reduce blood pressure levels and prevent the development of high blood pressure in the general population through the education of health care professionals.

Stage 1 hypertension and stage 2 hypertension parameters are outlined in the National Guidelines box. **Stage 1 hypertension** is a blood pressure of 140–159 mmHg systolic or 90–99 mmHg diastolic measured during multiple office visits following the guidelines for accurate blood pressure measurement. Lifestyle changes as well as medications would be part of the therapeutic plan.

Stage 2 hypertension is a systolic blood pressure measured on multiple occasions during an office visit of greater than 160 mmHg or a diastolic pressure of greater than 100 mmHg. The measurement of the blood pressure would follow the guidelines for accuracy (Chart 21–2). Both medications and lifestyle changes would be a part of the therapeutic plan.

In addition, **white coat phenomenon** is an elevated blood pressure when the assessment of the blood pressure is done by a physician or another health care professional. If this phenomenon occurs frequently over time, the patient is responding to a perceived stressful situation and may need early hypertensive treatment. Often the physician will request the patient measure her blood pressure in the home setting and record the findings in order to diagnosis high blood pressure. This process is used to determine if the patient is demonstrating white coat phenomenon.

Hypertension is further categorized by cause. There are two types: essential and secondary hypertension. *Essential hypertension* is defined as a chronic elevation in blood pressure that occurs without the evidence of disease. *Secondary hypertension* is high blood pressure that is a result of some other disorder such as kidney disease. Essential hypertension may be systolic, diastolic, or both systolic and diastolic.

Risk Factors

Certain identifiable contributing elements increase the risk of the development of high blood pressure. These risk factors are classified as modifiable factors and nonmodifiable factors (Chart 21–3). The modifiable factors are those that the patient can control, whereas nonmodifiable factors cannot be controlled by the patient.

A patient evaluation includes determining the risk factors, lifestyle, possible causes of hypertension, and target organs for damage including the heart (e.g., from coronary heart disease). A review of the multiple risk factors contributing to high blood pressure, as listed in the Risk Factors box, can be done while taking the

NATIONAL GUIDELINES JNC 7 Classification of Blood Pressure for Adults

BP Classification	SBP (mmHg)	DBP (mmHg)	Lifestyle Modification Encouraged
Normal	<120	and <90	
Prehypertension	120–139	Or 80–89	Yes
Stage 1 hypertension	140–159	Or 90–99	Yes
Stage 2 hypertension	>160	Or >100	Yes

Note: DBP, diastolic blood pressure; SBP, systolic blood pressure. Treatment determined by highest BP level.
Source: National Heart, Lung, and Blood Institute. (2003, May). *Seventh report of the Joint National Committee on Prevention, Detection, Evaluation, and Treatment of High Blood Pressure (JNC7).* Retrieved June 9, 2008, from http://www.nhlbi.nih.gov/guidelines/hypertension/jnc7full.pdf.

CHART 21–2 Guidelines for Assessing Blood Pressure in Adults

QUESTIONS TO BE ASKED BEFORE A BLOOD PRESSURE ASSESSMENT IS DONE
- Have you drunk any caffeinated beverages within the last hour?
- Have you eaten any chocolate within the last hour?
- Have you smoked within the last 15 minutes?
- Are you using any nasal decongestants? (If yes, assess whether the decongestant contains phenylephrine.)
- Do you use eyedrops for pupillary dilation?
- Does the environment feel cold to you?
- Have you just eaten a meal?
- Do you need to use the restroom?
- Do you exercise? If so, what do you do, for how long and how many times per week?

ENVIRONMENT
- A quiet, warm and comfortable setting.
- Home readings.

EQUIPMENT
- *Cuff size for adult:* The bladder should encircle and cover two-thirds of the length of the arm. If the bladder is too small, a high reading may result.
- *Manometer:* Aneroid gauges should be calibrated every 6 months against a mercury manometer.
- *Infants and children:* Use a Doppler method.

POSTURE
- *Initial assessment:* For patients over age 65 receiving antihypertensive therapy or a diabetic check for postural changes in blood pressure, the first reading is taken after the patient has been supine for 5 minutes and then immediately and 2 minutes after the patient stands.

- *Follow-up:* For a follow-up, a sitting pressure is recommended. The patient should be seated quietly for 5 minutes with the back supported. The arm is then supported at the level of the heart.

TECHNIQUE
- Initially, the blood pressure assessment is taken in both arms. The findings are recorded, identifying the arm and the pressure reading.
- On each occasion, take at least two readings. These are separated by as much time as practical. When readings vary more than 5 mmHg, take additional readings until two readings are close.
- When making the diagnosis of high blood pressure, three sets of readings are obtained at least 1 week apart.
- When the arm pressure is elevated in a patient younger than 30, take the blood pressure in the leg.

PERFORMANCE
- Find the brachial artery.
- Inflate the bladder quickly to a pressure at least 20 mmHg above the systolic pressure. This can be checked by determining that the radial pulse has disappeared.
- Deflate the bladder at about 3 mmHg every second.
- Record the Korotkoff phase V (disappearance) in adults. In children use phase IV (muffling).
- If the Korotkoff sounds are weak, have the patient raise the arm, open and close the hand 5 to 10 times, and then inflate the bladder quickly.
- Recording the findings.
  - Note the pressure obtained.
  - Note which arm was used.
  - Note the patient's position.
  - Note the cuff size.

Example: 140/90, seated, right arm, large adult cuff

Source: This article was published in Cecil essentials of medicine, 6th Ed., Andreoli, T. E., Carpenter, C. C. J., Griggs, R. C. & Loscalzo, J., pp. 38–39 (2004). Cecil essentials of medicine. (6th Ed.) Philadelphia: Saunders, pp. 38–39.

CHART 21–3 Factors Contributing to Hypertension

MODIFIABLE FACTORS
- High sodium dietary intake
- Overweight
- Excessive alcohol consumption
- Low potassium intake
- Smoking

NONMODIFIABLE FACTORS
- Family history
- Age
- Race

Source: National Heart, Lung, and Blood Institute. (2003, May). *Seventh report of the Joint National Committee on Prevention, Detection, Evaluation, and Treatment of High Blood Pressure (JNC7)*. Retrieved June 9, 2008, from http://www.nhlbi.nih.gov/guidelines/hypertension/jnc7full.pdf.

RISK FACTORS for Hypertension

Cigarette smoking

Obesity (BMI > 30 kg/m^2)

Physical inactivity

Dyslipidemia

Diabetes mellitus

Microalbuminuria or estimated GFR < 60 mL/min

Age (older than 55 years for men and 65 years for women)

Family history of premature cardiovascular disease (men under age 55 and women under age 65)

Gender

Sodium intake

Excessive alcohol consumption

Atherosclerosis

Source: Adapted from National Heart, Lung, and Blood Institute. (2003, May). *Seventh report of the Joint National Committee on Prevention, Detection, Evaluation, and Treatment of High Blood Pressure (JNC7)*. Retrieved June 9, 2008, from http://www.nhlbi.nih.gov/guidelines/hypertension/jnc7full.pdf.

patient and family history. The nurse needs to evaluate the patient's stress level in terms of physical and emotional stresses, the reported amount of sodium intake, the patient's weight, the amount of alcohol consumed, the serum potassium level, and use of tobacco. Chart 21–4 outlines the causes of high blood pressure.

Culture, Environment, Race, Genetics, and History

The assessment of an individual's culture, environment, and race is obtained from the patient and family. It is essential for these factors to be assessed during the interview because diversity is well established in the American lifestyle. It is estimated that half of the population in the United States in the year 2050 will be from a minority group (Donnelly, 2000). For example, the health care provider needs to be cognizant that African American individuals have twice as high a possibility of developing high blood pressure than do Caucasian Americans. If the patient lives in the southeastern portion of the United States as opposed to other parts of the country, the incidence of high blood pressure also is higher. In addition, environmental factors such as obesity, cigarette smoking, sedentary lifestyle, use of illegal drugs, and sodium intake have an impact on blood pressure.

The family may contribute medically historic information and report on any therapies the patient may have used. The interview may be both a teaching and learning opportunity, giving the nurse a further opportunity to gather data concerning the lifestyle of the patient and family. The Genetic Considerations box addresses how genetics might affect a patient's propensity for high blood pressure.

Psychosocial Assessment

When the nurse is obtaining a patient's psychosocial data, care must be used when listening to how the patient describes the meaning of the diagnosis of high blood pressure. Life stresses can make the patient's ability to participate in a partnership of care difficult. Areas of stress may be related to job stresses, economic position, losses and/or gains of any kind, and many other issues of life. The activation of the sympathetic nervous system

GENETIC CONSIDERATIONS Related to Hypertension

Despite the advances in medical science, the causes of prehypertension and stage 1 and stage 2 hypertension are not discernible in most cases (Andreoli, Carpenter, Griggs, & Loscalzo, 2004). The genetic profile may assist by providing information about alterations in the genetic coding of angiotensinogen in the hypertensive population. Hypertension is seen most often with persons who have a family history of hypertension, thus implicating a genetic predisposition. If an individual has two or more family members with hypertension before the age of 55 years, there is a 3.8 times greater risk for the development of hypertension (Porth, 2005). A family history of high blood pressure and heart disease may suggest a genetic predisposition for the development of these disorders.

is a significant response to stress. When a patient experiences severe stress, the amount of catecholamines is increased. This is frequently referred to as the "fight-or-flight" response. This response increases the blood pressure.

The assessment of anger and the patient's coping skills need to be incorporated into any care plan. Good patient participation and ownership of the negotiated therapeutic plan are essential to the success of lifestyle changing strategies.

■ Clinical Manifestations

High blood pressure is asymptomatic in the initial period. The patient may be of any age ranging from early childhood to elderly. It is estimated that high blood pressure may be present in some individuals for many years prior to discovery. During this time, the major organs may be slowly damaged.

Clinical signs and symptoms the patient describes may be nonspecific such as a headache or dizziness, sleepiness, nausea and vomiting, irritability, and visual disturbances. More serious complications may occur when a patient remains undiagnosed for years. Myocardial infarction, heart failure, cerebral vascular accidents, and renal failure may all be the result of untreated high blood pressure and occur without further warning.

Assessment

The assessment of a patient includes a review of history, signs, symptoms, prescribed medications, alternative therapies, and over-the-counter (OTC) medicines. The purpose of this assessment is to determine what risk factors are present, what concomitant therapies may have been used, the patient's lifestyle choices, and family history. The nurse records any signs and symptoms such as weakness, muscle cramps, polyuria (possible diabetes mellitus), headache, palpitations, or hyperhidrosis (possible excess of catecholamines). If end-organ involvement is suspected, the history should include symptoms of coronary artery disease, heart failure, cerebral vascular disease, and uremia.

Blood Pressure Measurement

The blood pressure is properly measured using both arms on two or more different occasions, when the patient has been seated for at least 5 minutes prior to measurement. Chart 21–2 (p. 491) includes the guidelines for assessing blood pressure in the adult.

CHART 21–4	Identifiable Causes of Hypertension

Sleep apnea

Drug-induced or -related causes

Chronic kidney disease

Primary aldosteronism

Renovascular disease

Chronic steroid therapy and Cushing's syndrome

Pheochromocytoma

Coarctation of the aorta

Thyroid or parathyroid disease

Cause may be unknown

Source: Adapted from National Heart, Lung, and Blood Institute. (2003, May). *Seventh report of the Joint National Committee on Prevention, Detection, Evaluation, and Treatment of High Blood Pressure (JNC7).* Retrieved June 9, 2008, from http://www.nhlbi.nih.gov/guidelines/hypertension/jnc7full.pdf.

Diagnostic Tests

There are no specific diagnostic tests for hypertension, except the tracking of serial blood pressures. When any stage of hypertension is diagnosed, a complete workup needs to be completed to determine target organ damage. This provides a baseline from which to assess future changes. The Diagnostic Tests box (p. 494) outlines tests that can be used during the initial workup of a newly diagnosed hypertensive patient.

Medical Management

The outcome of the therapeutic plan is to effectively lower and maintain the systemic blood pressure at a normal level. The plan needs to be individualized for each patient. The following factors should be considered when tailoring a plan for a given patient:

- Culture
- Age
- Risk factors
- Degree of blood pressure elevation
- Coexisting diseases
- Cost of prescribed pharmacologic agents
- Family/social support
- Amount and type of follow-up care needed.

A comprehensive plan includes addressing all factors that influence the occurrence of hypertension. This includes dietary restrictions, weight reduction where appropriate, medication regimen, exercise program, and finally stress reduction. Additionally, an evaluation needs to be made to determine if the patient is able to follow through with the lifestyle changes, monitoring of his blood pressure, and maintaining contact with the health care team.

Diet

The Dietary Approaches to Stop Hypertension diet, known as the **DASH** diet, is low in sodium, saturated fat, cholesterol, and total fat. The diet focuses on fruits, vegetables, nuts, and low-fat dairy products. This plan is rich in potassium and calcium. Although, lowering total and saturated fats has no direct effect on controlling blood pressure, it will lower cholesterol and have an effect on the development of coronary artery disease. Therefore, it is an important adjunct to the dietary plan.

There are two versions of the DASH plan in relation to sodium restrictions. Plan 1 limits the patient to 2,400 mg of sodium per day, whereas plan 2 limits the patient to 1,500 mg of sodium per day. The health care provider would assess the stage of hypertension in order to determine the degree of sodium restriction that is necessary. Increasing the intake of potassium-rich foods also is encouraged, due to the side effect of some of the antihypertensive medications and because it is known that a low potassium level is linked to increased blood pressure (Welton, 2003). It is thought that one of the major benefits of a potassium-rich diet is increased elimination of sodium (natriuretic effect) and suppression of the renin-angiotensin system. Note that many processed foods tend to be low in potassium and high in sodium. Thus, patients should be encouraged to consume natural foods and avoid processed foods.

The patient with stage 1 or stage 2 high blood pressure should be encouraged to make the following lifestyle changes: Eat a low-sodium diet (DASH meal plan), reduced-calorie diet (weight re-duction diet), or low-cholesterol diet; decrease the intake of saturated fats; limit the use of alcohol; and stop smoking. The DASH diet plan is considered to be equivalent to a single-drug therapy (NHLBI, 2003b). Chapter 14 🔗 provides an overall description of healthy sensible eating plans, using the Food Guide Pyramid and a description of the DASH diet.

Exercise

Regular physical activities assist in the promotion of cardiovascular fitness and beneficial changes: They lower blood pressure and raise a person's high-density lipoproteins (the good cholesterol). It is essential to have an organized aerobic exercise program, approved by a health care provider, which is completed on a regular basis for 30 to 45 minutes three to five times per week. This plan is begun slowly and stopped if the patient develops shortness of breath, fainting, or chest pain. Physical conditioning has a positive impact on both lowering and maintaining normal blood pressure, as further discussed in the Complementary and Alternative Therapies box (p. 495). Chapter 40 🔗 includes an in-depth discussion of the lipids and the benefit of exercise on the heart.

Light weight training is recommended to lower blood pressure, but heavy lifting is known to raise blood pressure due to the vasovagal response that occurs with intense isometric exercise. Thus, heavy lifting should be avoided in hypertensive individuals.

Weight Control

According to the Centers for Disease Control and Prevention (2008) obesity has risen to epidemic proportions in the past 20 years. A standard measurement for expressing the relationship (or ratio) of weight-to-height is the body mass index (BMI). The BMI is calculated by dividing the body weight in kilograms by the square of height in meters. A person with a BMI of 25 to 29.9 is considered overweight, and individuals with a BMI of 30 or more are considered obese. A BMI of 27 or greater correlates closely with high blood pressure.

A second risk factor for the development of high blood pressure is the presence of excess fat accumulated in the torso that is out of proportion to the rest of the body fat distribution. Men with a waist circumference of 40 inches or more and women with a waist circumference of 35 inches or more are at risk for developing high blood pressure (National Heart, Lung, and Blood Institute, 1998).

For individuals who are 10% or greater above ideal body weight, as little as a 10-pound reduction in weight will lower the blood pressure. Additionally, antihypertensive medication effectiveness is enhanced with weight reduction. During the weight reduction process, the blood pressure needs to be assessed regularly and medications adjusted appropriately.

Stress Reduction

A priority for the nurse is discussion of the issue of stress with both the patient and family. Often individuals are not totally aware of the impact of stress on the development of high blood pressure. Frequently, individuals may feel helpless about how to control their stress levels. It is important for the nurse to explain clearly the impact of stress on the development of high blood pressure. Teaching the patient stress reduction techniques is an essential part of the plan for controlling high blood pressure. Exercise, the use of support systems, and some alternative therapies have all been identified as stress reduction techniques.

DIAGNOSTIC TESTS for Hypertension

Test and Normal Values	Expected Abnormality	Rationale for Abnormality
Aldosterone (blood) *Supine:* 3–20 ng/dL *Upright* (sitting for at least 2 hr): *Males:* 6–22 ng/dL *Females:* 5–30 ng/dL	An increased aldosterone serum level is associated with hypertension and hypokalemia.	Primary aldosteronism may be due to aldosterone-producing adenomas. Aldosterone causes the kidneys to retain salt and excrete potassium, causing the retention of water and, thus, increasing the blood volume and blood pressure (Nicoll, McPhee, & Pignone, 2004, p. 44).
Renin assay, plasma (PRA) (Plasma renin concentration [PRC]) *Adult/Elderly:* *Upright (sodium-restricted diet):* *Age 20–39 years:* 2.9–24 ng/mL/hour *Age >40 years:* 2.9–10.8 ng/mL per hour *Upright (normal sodium diet):* *Age 20–39 years:* 0.1–4.3 ng/mL per hour *Age >40 years:* 0.1–3.0 ng/mL per hour	Increased in some hypertensive states (e.g., renal artery stenosis). Decreased in hyporeninemic hypoaldosteronism, and some hypertensive states: primary aldosteronism, severe preeclampsia.	PRA is helpful in the differential diagnosis of aldosteronism and the evaluation of hypertension. The PRA is increased in dehydration, edematous states due to cirrhosis, nephritic syndrome, heart failure, hypokalemic states, adrenal insufficiency, chronic renal failure, and left ventricular hypertrophy. Test is useful in the evaluation of hypoaldosteronism (low-sodium diet and patient standing) (Nicoll et al., 2004, p. 158).
Glucose (blood) *Adult:* 70–110 mg/dL	The expected finding is an increase in renal damage as a result of hypertension and the acceleration of atherosclerosis, arteriosclerosis, and renal failure.	Prevalence, prematurity, and severity of coronary atherosclerosis are demonstrated among patients with diabetes. When this occurs, the peripheral resistance in the blood vessels increases and the clinical sign is hypertension. Diabetes mellitus may be associated with accelerated arteriosclerosis and primary aldosteronism (Kasper et al., 2005, p. 1469).
Creatinine (blood) *Males:* 0.6–1.2 mg/dL *Females:* 0.5–1.1 mg/dL *Elderly:* decreased values due to decreased muscle mass	Increased in acute renal failure. Decreased when there is a reduced muscle mass.	Nitrogenous end product of protein metabolism. As creatinine and BUN rise, the glomerular filtration rate decreases. With deterioration of renal function occurring, glomerular hypertension occurs within the nephrons.
Sodium (blood) 135–145 mEq/L	Increased sodium levels increases fluid retention, which increases blood pressure. .	Link between sodium intake and high blood pressure is described as increased renal vascular resistance, which reduces renal blood flow and GFR mainly in the cortical collecting tubules (Guyton & Hall, 2005, p. 376).
Cholesterol (serum) *Desirable:* <200 mg/dL *Borderline:* 200–239 mg/dL *High risk:* >240 mg/dL	Increased	Associated with hypertension, predisposition to arteriosclerosis.
Calcium *Total calcium, adult:* 9.0–10.5 mg/dL *Ionized calcium, adult:* 4.5–5.6 mg/dL	Decreased calcium intake is associated with increased blood pressure.	Increased calcium excretion occurs in chronic renal insufficiency. There is a potential link between salt sensitive forms of high blood pressure and calcium (Kasper et al., 2005, p. 1464).
Lipoprotein (HDL [alpha lipoproteins]) *Males:* >45 mg/dL *Females:* >55 mg/dL	HDL is a carrier of cholesterol. It is thought to be the protective cardiac characteristic. Low levels are found with heart disease.	Measurement of the lipoproteins is essential in the therapeutic management of a patient with hypertension because an increase in lipoproteins indicates a risk of atherogenic heart disease and peripheral vascular disease, which may further increase high blood pressure.
LDL (beta lipoproteins) and VLDL (pre-beta-lipoproteins) *LDL:* 60–180 mg/dL *VLDL:* 25–50%	Increased LDL is associated with atherosclerotic heart disease and peripheral vascular disease, which increase the peripheral resistance and blood pressure.	LDL is carried to peripheral tissues and is associated with an increased risk of arteriosclerotic hypertension and peripheral vascular disease.
Urinalysis *Color and appearance:* amber yellow and clear *Odor:* aromatic *pH:* 4.6–8.0 *Protein:* 0–8 mg/dL *Glucose:* none with fresh specimen.	Urine is tested for protein blood and glucose to determine if target organ damage is present.	Part of the screening test for hypertension is to gain information about the potential target organ damage and the etiology of the patient's high blood pressure. Concentration of urine is controlled by secretion of ADH and the renin-angiotensin feedback.

Source: Adapted from National Heart, Lung, and Blood Institute. (2003, May). *Seventh report of the Joint National Committee on Prevention, Detection, Evaluation, and Treatment of High Blood Pressure (JNC7)*. Retrieved June 9, 2008, from http://www.nhlbi.nih.gov/guidelines/hypertension/jnc7full.pdf.

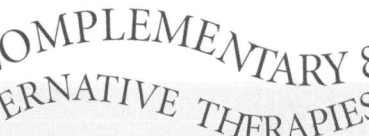

COMPLEMENTARY & ALTERNATIVE THERAPIES

Exercise

Description:

Exercise need not be complex. A patient can create an effective exercise program that is as simple as setting up a treadmill in the bedroom. Other exercise options that are more structured include working with a personal trainer, joining a class, or walking with a group of neighbors. Many organizations offer participatory classes that can promote program adherence and provide instruction in the proper exercise technique. Such organizations include Jazzercise, YMCA, Curves, as well as local gyms.

Research Support:

When the human body is under threat, it exhibits a set of neuroendocrine responses collectively known as the "fight or flight" response. These responses include an increased secretion of glucocorticoids (GCs) and catecholamines from the adrenal gland and the activation of the sympathetic nervous system. These hormones mobilize endogenous substrate and induce a state of insulin resistance in the liver and skeletal muscles. This stress response was essential to survival in ancient times, where the increased metabolic demand was put to immediate use. However, in modern times, one can no longer fight or flee the most common stressors, which often involve emotional, professional, and social stressors. These types of psychological stressors may be protracted and create long-term metabolic disturbances. These metabolic disturbances can lead to a number of comorbidities including central obesity and hypertension. The stress response is a neuroendocrine mechanism that was intended to provide the energy needed for survival-focused physical action. Therefore, physical activity should be the natural means to prevent the comorbid consequences of stress. Indeed, there is a great deal of evidence that documents the beneficial effects of regular exercise in preventing or ameliorating the stress-induced metabolic and psychological comorbidities. It is believed that exercise reduces the body's sensitivity to stress and also the peripheral actions that influence metabolic functions. Of particular importance are the documented effects of exercise on insulin sensitivity and metabolizing calories for fuel rather than storage. It is concluded that when chronic psychosocial stress accompanies physical inactivity, it contributes to our current epidemic of cardiometabolic and emotional disease. Regular exercise provides a way to prevent and combat this burden (Tsatsoulis & Fountoulakis, 2006).

There is evidence that two conditions in particular, hypertension and stroke, are improved with increased physical activity. The following two paragraphs discuss this evidence.

Rates of hypertension and hypertension-related death in older African Americans are very high versus all other American ethnic groups. A lifestyle factor in this population that contributes to their hypertension-related health problems is that they are also one of the most physically inactive groups. Interventions can assist them to increase their exercise activities and thereby gain better hypertension control. Findings of one study by Cromwell and Adams (2006) supported a strong association between physical activity level and exercise self-efficacy in this population. These findings suggest that interventions that address exercise self-efficacy would be helpful for increasing the level of exercise in older African Americans (Cromwell & Adams, 2006).

Stroke is another condition that may be improved through increased physical activity. In order to prevent a first-time stroke, it is vital to identify at-risk patients and control as many risk factors as possible. Some risk factors, such as lifestyle factors, can be eliminated; others, such as hypertension, can be controlled or treated. Exercise provides one way to control the risk of stroke (Sauerbeck, 2006). In the general as well as elderly populations, aerobic exercise is effective for reducing blood pressure (McDonald, Blackwell, & Meurer, 2006). Researchers have found that, when a patient adheres to either supervised or unsupervised moderate-intensity exercise, it is sufficient to reduce short- and long-term blood pressure (Cox, 2006).

References

Cox, K. L. (2006). Exercise and blood pressure: Applying findings from the laboratory to the community setting. *Clinical and Experimental Pharmacology and Physiology, 33*(9), 868–871.

Cromwell, S. L., & Adams, M. M. (2006). Exercise, self-efficacy, and exercise behavior in hypertensive older African-Americans. *Journal of National Black Nurses Association, 17*(1), 17–21.

McDonald, K. C., Blackwell, J. C., & Meurer, L. N. (2006). Clinical inquiries. What lifestyle changes should we recommend for the patient with newly diagnosed hypertension? *Journal of Family Practice, 55*(11), 991–993.

Sauerbeck, L. R. (2006). Primary stroke prevention. *American Journal of Nursing, 106*(11), 40–41, 43–45, 48–50.

Tsatsoulis, A., & Fountoulakis, S. (2006). The protective role of exercise on stress system dysregulation and comorbidities. *Annals of the New York Academy of Sciences, 1083*, 196–213.

Alcohol Consumption

Research indicates that regular consumption of three or more drinks per day increases the risk of hypertension. The systolic blood pressure is more affected by alcohol than the diastolic. The exact mechanism whereby alcohol exerts it effect on blood pressure is unclear, but elevated blood pressure may improve and return to normal when alcohol consumption ceases. Patients tend to understate the amount of alcohol consumed. The nurse needs to realize the amount may be more and tailor the teaching to the possibility of greater consumption.

Pharmacologic Agents Used to Treat Hypertension

The care of the patient with high blood pressure includes the use of pharmacologic agents. These agents have reduced the morbidity and mortality associated with high blood pressure as well as the incidence of cerebrovascular accident. The Pharmacology Summary (p. 497) outlines the eight classifications of medications

used to treat high blood pressure. The summary also includes the nursing responsibilities for patient and family teaching that are necessary for the safe use of these medications. Chart 21–5 (p. 496) outlines herbal therapies for treatment of hypertension.

Complementary and Alternative Therapies

The use of complementary or alternative therapies may be attractive to the patient because of the ease of availability and the lower cost of medicinal herbs as opposed to pharmacologic agents. Eisenhower (2002) reported the finding from the *Descriptive Study of Client Use of Herbal Substances and Over-the-Counter Medications* that 100% of the study subjects took herbs and OTC drugs. In addition, Eisenhower reported (1) that 95% of the subjects mixed herbal and OTC drugs with prescription medications, (2) that the subjects reported they believed these herbal remedies helped 80% of the time, and (3) that 55% of subjects had not told their health care provider of these practices.

Complementary and/or alternative therapies include autogenic therapy, healing, hypnosis, exercise, relaxation and visualization,

CHART 21–5	Selected Herbal Products for Treating Hypertension		
Name	**Action**	**Application/Indications**	**Nursing Responsibility**
Black cohosh	Unknown. Therapeutic effect produced by glycosides isolated from fresh or dried rhizome with attached roots. May decrease symptoms of menopause, including hot flashes, sweating, sleep disturbances, and anxiety.	May potentiate hypertensive drugs and hypertension. Patients need to be warned not to take this drug as a supplement with other antihypertensive drugs without consulting with the health care provider.	Teach patient to monitor blood pressure when taking antihypertensive drugs. Assess for reports of nausea and vomiting, history of seizures, liver disease, and alcohol intake.
Hawthorne	Active compounds are flavonoids and procyanidins that increase coronary blood flow and have positive inotropic and chronotropic effects due to increased permeability to calcium and inhibition of phosphodiesterase. Cardiac output increases; myocardial workload and oxygen consumption decrease. The pharmacokinetics of hawthorne are unknown.	Hawthorne does not cure heart failure but keeps control of symptoms. Do not take hawthorne unless you have the approval of a health care professional. The substance may cause hypertension.	Assess the patient's lung sounds for signs of heart failure. Teach importance of taking daily weights and of taking the pulse for rate and rhythm. Teach symptoms of "heart attack" and heart failure. Instruct therapy may not take effect for 6–8 weeks. Adverse responses to hawthorne may cause drowsiness, profuse sweating, and dehydration leading to severe hypotension. Teach that during hot weather exercise should always be minimized.

Sources: Deglin, J. H., & Vallerand, A. H. (2005). *Davis's drug guide for nurses* (10th ed.) Philadelphia: F. A. Davis Company; Rankin-Box, D. (2001). *The nurse's handbook of complementary therapies* (2nd ed.) London: Bailliere Tindall.

and therapeutic touch. Other therapies include animal-assisted therapy, aromatherapy, biofeedback, herbs (e.g., garlic and hawthorn), message, meditation, qi gong, vitamin C and calcium supplements (if high blood pressure is pregnancy induced), t'ai chi, and yoga. Lily of the valley, an herb containing cardioactive glycosides, would not be prescribed with digitalis because it increases the action of each product (Rankin-Box, 2001). The Complementary and Alternative Therapies box (p. 499) outlines the most common alternative therapies for high blood pressure.

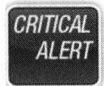 *Assessment of the patient's treatment routine must include the determination of use of herbal and complementary therapies. Nurses are responsible for teaching patients about the use of herbal products and their interactions with prescription drugs.*

■ Nursing Management

A partnership of care with the hypertensive patient involves the process of devising a role for each patient, family member, and the nurse. The nurse is the coordinator of care and provider of information concerning risk reduction, health promotion, disease prevention, and the nursing care plan. The nursing needs of the individual with prehypertension or stage 1 or stage 2 hypertension focus on educating the patient about lifestyle changes and implementing the therapeutic regimen.

The nurse functions with autonomy and creativity in providing the patient with information that the patient/family can use to make informed choices and decisions. Throughout this process, the nurse will use assessment data and technical skills to maintain pri-

vacy, cultural sensitivity, and confidentiality. Jhala (2001) suggested that individuals of a different culture view themselves differently and reflect their own culture in the area of attitudes, beliefs, and values that are embedded in their own world. In addition, language barriers play a large role in the feelings of vulnerability and helplessness (Jhala, 2001). The Cultural Considerations box (p. 499) discusses various cultures' susceptibility to high blood pressure.

As the patient's hypertension moves from one stage to the next, the nursing process provides a framework for assessing, following clinical data, and evaluating the patient outcomes. The nursing care needs of the individual with any classification of high blood pressure are complex and multifaceted. Use of the nursing process will facilitate a comprehensive approach to patient assessment and care. The Nursing Process: Patient Care Plan (p. 500) feature applies the nursing process to the applicable nursing diagnoses and provides a comprehensive care plan for a hypertensive patient.

Health Promotion

Health care providers are beginning to place more responsibility with the individual for healthy lifestyle choices across the life span because, as mentioned earlier, a healthy lifestyle assists in controlling high blood pressure. A healthy lifestyle includes eating three balanced meals per day, eating to maintain a healthy weight, exercise, limited use of alcohol, no smoking, adequate sleeping time (7 to 8 hours per night), and reduction of stress. The individual and family need to be familiar with their current blood pressure measurements. If the findings are higher than 120/80 mmHg, the nondiabetic individual needs to seek medical advice. If an individual has diabetes and her blood pressure is higher than 130/80 mmHg, she too should seek medical advice.

PHARMACOLOGY Summary of Medications to Treat High Blood Pressure

Medication Category	Action	Application/Indication	Nursing Responsibility
Thiazide diuretics: • Chlorothiazide • Hydrochlorothiazide	Prevents sodium and water reabsorption in the distal tubules, thus facilitating excretion of fluid and electrolytes, which decreases the blood volume, thereby decreasing the blood pressure.	Treatment goal is prevention of end-organ damage. Used to lower the blood pressure to the lowest diastolic pressure the patient can tolerate.	Instruct the patient to take this medication at the same time daily. Encourage the intake of foods high in potassium such as bananas and orange juice. Review the frequency of prescription renewal as a measure of compliance. Teach that abrupt withdrawal will cause rebound hypertension.
Potassium-sparing diuretics • Spironolactone • Triamterene	Causes the loss of sodium bicarbonate and calcium while preserving the potassium and hydrogen ions. The fluid follows sodium, facilitating the loss of volume, leading to a decrease in blood pressure while preventing diuretic-induced hypokalemia.	Medication used singly or with another agent to treat hypertension or edema.	Teach to monitor blood pressure daily and report sudden weight gains over a 2-day period to health care provider. Teach regular monitoring of serum electrolytes.
Beta-adrenergic blocking agents • Propranolol • Atenolol • Nadolol	Agents block stimulation of the beta-1 (myocardial) and beta-2 (pulmonary), vascular, and uterine adrenergic receptor sites. This blockage causes vasodilation, decreasing intravascular pressure and blood pressure.	Used in the management of hypertension, heart failure, and angina pectoris. Blocks the stimulation of beta and beta-adrenergic receptor sites.	Teach blood pressure and pulse taking prior to medication. If pulse is below 60, inform the health care provider prior to taking the medication. Medication to be taken at the same time each day. Teach that rapid withdrawal of medication may cause life-threatening dysrhythmias. Instruct patient to report to health care provider any fatigue, difficulty with sexual activity, weakness, or depression. Assess for reported orthostatic hypotension, cough, and shortness of breath.
Calcium channel blockers • Diltiazem hydrochloride • Nifedipine • Verapamil	Agents block the calcium ion from entering the cells of the smooth muscle and myocardium, causing a loss of cell excitation. This results in dilation of the arteries and slowing of the SA node excitation and conduction. These actions decrease both heart rate and blood pressure.	Alone or with other agents for the management of hypertension, angina pectoris, vasospastic angina, supraventricular tachyarrhythmias, and rapid supraventricular rates in atrial flutter and fibrillation.	Instruct that sustained-action capsules or tablets cannot be crushed, broken up, or chewed. Teach monitoring pulse, blood pressure, and weight at regular intervals. Teach that if irregular heartbeats occur, notify the health care provider quickly. Assess the patient's reports of dizziness and use of OTC medications and alcohol unless approved by the health care professional. Teach patient to wear sunscreen to avoid a photosensitive reaction.

(continued)

PHARMACOLOGY Summary of Medications to Treat High Blood Pressure—*Continued*

Medication Category	Action	Application/Indication	Nursing Responsibility
Angiotensin-converting enzyme (ACE) inhibitors • Captopril • Enalapril • Lisinopril	Action blocks the conversion of angiotensin I to vasoconstrictor angiotensin II. Because angiotensin II is a potent vasoconstrictor, the primary vasoactive hormone of the renin-angiotensin-aldosterone system, when it is blocked vasodilation occurs, resulting in a decrease in blood pressure. It also inactivates the vasodilator bradykinin and other vasodilator prostaglandins. ACE inhibitors increase the plasma renin levels and reduce aldosterone levels, causing systemic vasodilation.	Used in the management of hypertension as a single medication or in combination with other agents. It reduces the risk of heart failure following a myocardial infarction.	Encourage the patient to practice good dental hygiene. Instruct patient to contact the health care professional if any of the following occur: irregular heartbeat, chest pain, difficulty breathing, dry cough, sore throat, mouth sores, rash, fever, swelling of the hands and feet and/or face. Teach monitoring of blood pressure daily. Monitoring of renal function tests should be done regularly. Instruct about danger of double medication dosing.
Central alpha agonists • Clonidine	Stimulates the alpha-adrenergic receptors in the CNS, resulting in decreased sympathetic outflow and, hence, inhibition of cardioacceleration and vasoconstriction centers, and also prevents the reuptake of norepinephrine. This results in a drop in blood pressure.	Used in the management of hypertension.	Instruct patient to monitor blood pressure and pulse. Instruct that sudden changes in position may produce dizziness. Instruct that medication is administered at bedtime because of the sedative effect at the beginning of therapy and/or when the dosage is changed. Assess for skin rash when using the transdermal route. Men may have sexual difficulty, which should be reported to the health care professional.
Vasodilators • Hydralazine • Fenoldopam • Nitroprusside	The vasodilator lowers the blood pressure by relaxing the smooth muscle tone of the blood vessel, thus reducing the peripheral resistance.	Short-term hospital management in hypertensive emergencies includes malignant hypertension and end-organ deterioration.	Monitor the blood pressure 2–6 hour after initiating therapy or dosage adjustment. Assess patient for reports of dizziness. Teach that medication should be taken at bedtime to reduce effect of hypotension. If the patient experiences tinnitus, dyspnea, dizziness, headache, and/or blurred vision, these conditions need to be reported to the health care provider.
Angiotensin II receptor blockers • Candesartan • Valsartan	Blocks vasoconstriction and aldosterone-producing effects of angiotensin II at receptor sites, vascular and smooth muscle, and adrenal glands.	Lowers blood pressure and risk of stroke. Decreases hospitalization in patients with heart failure. Used in the management of hypertension.	Teach patient to take medication as directed, not to double dose. Instruct patient to take blood pressure weekly and report any significant changes to the health care provider. Instruct that medication may cause dizziness. Instruct to check with health care provider prior to taking any OTC medications, herbals, cough, cold, or allergy medications. Instruct on the need for follow-up with health care provider. Check for compliance via frequency of refills.

Sources: Deglin, J. H., & Vallerand, A. H. (2007). *Davis's drug guide for nurses* (10th ed.). Philadelphia: F. A. Davis; Rankin-Box, D. (2001). *The nurse's handbook of complementary therapies* (2nd ed.) London: Bailliere Tindall.

COMPLEMENTARY & ALTERNATIVE THERAPIES

Management of High Blood Pressure

Type of Therapy	Purpose	Comments
Healing "is the practice of conscious intentionality to improve health and well-being" (Rankin-Box, 2001, p. 171).	To instill a feeling of relaxation and calm to improve the patient's health and well-being.	*Contraindication:* May cause light-headedness or faintness in some patients. Patient must give informed consent prior to participating in this method of healing when it involves spiritual and/or cultural belief systems.
Relaxation and visualization are "techniques using the imagination to create any desired changes in the individual's life" (Rankin-Box, 2001, p. 276).	Relaxation helps patient feel peaceful and free from anxiety and fear. Visualization creates positive changes in the patient's life.	*Contraindication:* Patient may have difficulty learning the skill, or may be too weak to use the energy to concentrate to elicit a response. A patient with breathing difficulties or cardiac arrhythmias may have increased problems; use should be limited to two to three times per day for 20 minutes because some may experience withdrawal from life, experiencing insomnia or hallucinations. These techniques are to be taught by an individual experienced with these techniques.
Therapeutic touch "is the interaction between energy fields of two or more people with the focus of rebalancing the energy field to enable relaxation and self healing" (Rankin-Box, 2001, p. 276).	To promote relaxation, pain relief, and self-healing through the interaction of people's energy fields, which rebalances or repatterns the energy field.	*Contraindication:* Caution should be used when using the therapy with babies, frail elderly, pregnant women, people with head injuries, emaciated patients, people experiencing psychosis, and patients in shock. The practice of therapeutic touch is taught through course work or home study. Certification as a healing touch practitioner is available through the American Holistic Nurses Association.
Hypnosis is a deliberate use of a trance state to increase the feeling of health and well-being (Rankin-Box, 2001).	To use a trance state to foster a sense of well-being and health.	The therapist must be competent in the technique. Hypnosis gives the patient responsibility for his own healing.
Animal-assisted therapy is the use of selected animals as a treatment modality in health care settings.	To promote human–animal interactions such as bonding, attachment, and to provide cardiovascular and other benefits.	Research supports the value of human–animal interaction in the management of high blood pressure.
Qi gong T'ai chi is a series of postures and exercises developed by the Chinese characterized by relaxed, circular motions.	To foster the generation of energy and conserves their energy to maintain health or to treat illness. As a health discipline, t'ai chi combines physical fitness, meditation, and self-defense. Considered to be the "root of motion."	These are individual personal disciplines. It is best when learning these skills to have an instructor. The teacher is considered to be the only way to advanced skill. Honor and reverence of the teacher is part of the belief system that empowers the disciple.

Sources: Rankin-Box, D. (2001). *The nurse's handbook of complementary therapies* (2nd ed.). London: Bailliere Tindall; Fontaine, K. L. (2004). *Healing practices: Alternative therapies for nursing.* Upper Saddle River, NJ: Pearson Prentice Hall.

CULTURAL CONSIDERATIONS for Hypertension

African Americans have a three to four times higher risk than Caucasians of angioedema and cough attributed to ACE inhibitors. American Indian and Asian populations undergoing Westernization will have significant increases in high blood pressure. Individuals living in the southeastern region (sometimes called the Salt Belt) of the United States have a higher percentage of high blood pressure.

Discharge Priorities

The discharge priorities represent a cooperative effort among the patient, family, and nurse. The focus is to determine if the patient knows the rationale for the prescribed therapy. The pa-

tient should also know how to monitor his blood pressure to maintain it at <120/80 mmHg (or with diabetes mellitus, <130/80 mmHg). In addition, the patient should demonstrate no signs or symptoms of target organ damage. The Patient Teaching & Discharge Priorities box (p. 502) outlines the necessary teaching for discharging a patient with hypertension.

Collaborative Management

The outcome goal of therapy for high blood pressure is to reduce the cardiovascular, cerebral vascular, and renal morbidity and mortality through achieving a systolic blood pressure of <120 mmHg and a diastolic blood pressure of <80 mmHg. However, if the patient has diabetes mellitus, the systolic blood

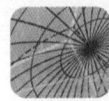

NURSING PROCESS: Patient Care Plan for Hypertension

Assessment of Knowledge Related to Hypertension

Subjective Data:

What did the health care provider tell you about the family member's prognosis?

Do you know the meaning of high blood pressure to the patient?

Do you know if family members understand the diagnosis of high blood pressure?

Nursing Assessment and Diagnoses	Outcomes and Evaluation Parameters	Planning and Interventions with *Rationales*
Nursing Diagnosis: *Deficient Knowledge* related to the relationship between lifestyle choices and the management of hypertension	**Outcome:** The patient/family has a clear understanding of the modification of lifestyle choices. **Outcome:** States understanding of the long-term nature of the partnership between the health care team and the patient. ***Evaluation Parameters:*** The patient/family states an understanding of: Disease process. Modifiable elements of lifestyle. Cultural influences. Blood pressure measurement. Monitoring of condition. Therapeutic plan with its rationale. Signs and symptoms of noncompliance and/or complications. Patient states an understanding of the partnership between the health care team and the patient over the long term. Patient states preferences in modifying lifestyle.	**Interventions and *Rationales*:** Teach patient that health beliefs and practices influence lifestyle choices. *Build a trusting and sharing relationship between the patient and health care team.* Monitor blood pressure in the health care office and home. Monitoring is done by the nurse, patient, and/or family member. *Blood pressure findings may vary dependent on the lifestyle choices, time of day, and degree of stress experienced by the patient.* Monitor exercise and weight patterns. *Weight may be in excess of the body's needs and can lead to potential complications of therapy.* Assess the degree of patient anger. *Self-concept changes when the individual is physiologically and psychologically threatened as reflected by ineffective coping and high blood pressure.* Teach the patient to report to the health care provider the use of herbal products and OTC medications prior to taking them because they frequently change the action of the hypertensive drugs. *Herbal substances are not regulated by the federal Food and Drug Administration and may vary in strength. OTC medicines may interact with prescription medications either by increasing or decreasing the therapeutic effect.* Teach the patient to monitor the amount of alcohol consumed per day/week because many hypertensive drugs labels warn about the consumption of alcohol. *Alcohol consumption elevates arterial blood pressure and adds "empty" calories to the patient's diet.* Teach that smoking cessation is important. *Cigarette, cigar, and pipe smoking affects the cardiovascular system through the action of inhaled nicotine.*

Assessment of Fatigue

Subjective Data:

What symptoms of fatigue do you have?

How many hours of sleep do you require?

Objective Data:

Family reports increasing fatigue.

Patient appears tired.

Nursing Assessment and Diagnoses	Outcomes and Evaluation Parameters	Planning and Interventions with *Rationales*
Nursing Diagnosis: *Fatigue* related to biochemical changes due to chronic disease	**Outcome:** Patient's fatigue level is manageable. ***Evaluation Parameters:*** Patient states an understanding of the use of prescribed therapeutic agents. Patient states the possible side effects of the therapeutic agents.	**Interventions and *Rationales*:** Instruct the patient/family about potential side effects of the prescribed therapeutic agents *to identify any areas of misunderstanding or misinformation concerning the therapeutic plan.* Instruct the patient to read medicine bottle labels and to follow the directions for pulse and blood pressure assessment prior to taking the dose of medication *to promote the therapeutic medication dose levels and the safe physiological levels when administering the pharmaceutical treatment.* Instruct the patient to report and have approved by the health care professional prior to taking any OTC medications, herbal substances, alcohol, diet supplements, or stimulants *to identify any untoward reactions like fatigue between the therapeutic regime and other substances.* Plan rest periods to decrease fatigue level.

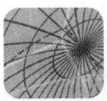

Assessment of Nutrition

Subjective Data:
What diet are you currently following?
What is your weight pattern during the past 6 months?

Objective Data:
What are the following measurements: weight, height, and abdominal girth?

Nursing Assessment and Diagnoses	Outcomes and Evaluation Parameters	Planning and Interventions with *Rationales*
Nursing Diagnosis: *Imbalanced Nutrition: More than Body Requirements* related to excessive caloric intake	**Outcome:** Demonstrates the ability to select a diet to meet nutritional requirements. **Evaluation Parameters:** The patient states an understanding of modifications needed in lifestyle. The health care team verbalizes the importance of cultural influences, the meaning of food, financial concerns, and the patient's choices.	**Interventions and *Rationales*:** Discuss with the patient realistic goals for weight reduction and an exercise program. This plan is age dependent. *Weight is a modifiable cause of high blood pressure. A relationship between saturated fat and cholesterol to weight is well established.*

Assessment of Perfusion

Subjective Data:
Do you have difficulty walking around home, a grocery store, or a shopping mall/center?
Do you have difficulty breathing after exercising?

Objective Data:
Does the patient cough after exercising? Have a flushed face?
Does the patient have edema of the extremities?

Nursing Assessment and Diagnoses	Outcomes and Evaluation Parameters	Planning and Interventions with *Rationales*
Nursing Diagnosis: *Impaired Tissue Perfusion* related to resistance to blood flow	**Outcome:** The patient has a clear understanding of the adequacy of perfusion and pulmonary gas exchange. **Evaluation Parameters:** Patient verbalizes an understanding of the seriousness of adequate systemic perfusion.	**Interventions and *Rationales*:** Teach combination of medications, diet, and exercise for the protection of the target organs. *Knowledge and ownership of the treatment plan by the patient will increase the patient's motivation to modify lifestyle.*

Assessment of Noncompliance

Subjective Data:
Do you have a support system?
Do you consider the treatment plan to be requiring too many lifestyle changes?

Objective Data:
How many missed appointments have been recorded?
Does the patient refill prescriptions promptly?
Does the patient have transportation to the medical office?
Does the patient have financial problems?

Nursing Assessment and Diagnoses	Outcomes and Evaluation Parameters	Planning and Interventions with *Rationales*
Nursing Diagnosis: *Risk of Noncompliance* related to the medical treatment plan	**Outcome:** Demonstrates the ability to make decisions regarding compliance with the therapeutic plan. **Evaluation Parameters:** Partnership between patient and health care team evolves with the patient verbalizing the meaning of the therapeutic plan.	**Interventions and *Rationales*:** Teaches and demonstrates a partnership with the patient/family so that the treatment regimen is understood. Teaches the goals of therapy and the dangerousness of a relapse in the treatment plan. *Compliance is a positive behavior that patients demonstrate when therapeutic goals are mutually agreed on. Compliance is a continuum of coordinated action.*

Assessment of Ineffective Sexual Patterns

Subjective Data:
Have you experienced any changes in sexual performance?
When did these sexual patterns change?

Objective Data:
Observe interactions between family and/or significant other.

Nursing Assessment and Diagnoses	Outcomes and Evaluation Parameters	Planning and Interventions with *Rationales*
Nursing Diagnosis: *Sexual Dysfunction* related to disease and/or therapy	**Outcome:** Verbalizes effective patterns of sexual relationship. **Evaluation Parameters:** Patient verbalizes satisfaction with the quality of life.	**Interventions and *Rationales*:** When assisting with patient discussion of sexuality, teach that it is part of the plan of care and may be discussed at any health care visit. The patient needs reassurance that the information is confidential. *It is important that the health care provider be educated concerning sexual health and sexuality throughout the life span. The health care provider needs to know his or her feelings and beliefs concerning sexuality within the culture. Patients want to know if their feelings are normal versus abnormal concerning this important information.*

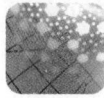

PATIENT TEACHING & DISCHARGE PRIORITIES for Hypertension

Need	Teaching
Prior to discharge the nurse instructs the patient and family on how to measure the blood pressure.	The patient and family will demonstrate to the nurse how to take the blood pressure.
	The interaction may be in a clinic, health provider's office, patient's home, or hospital.
The nurse teaches the patient and family about the medications prescribed. The patient and family know the name of each medication and: 1. Dosage for each medication 2. Time of medication administration 3. Precautions, such as foods to avoid, medication interactions, and the need to take blood pressure and pulse prior to taking the medication 4. Possible side effects 5. What to do if side effects do occur 6. Cautions about using OTC medications, herbals, stimulants, diet supplements, alcohol, and tobacco.	Patient and family need to be knowledgeable about the medications prescribed. Frequently, the nurse may supplement the teaching plan by giving the patient a written guide outlining the medications with a list of do's and don'ts. If the patient has difficulty reading the information, pictures may be used. In addition, tape recording or video recording the teaching session for the patient and family may be very helpful.
The nurse needs to review all of the medications the patient is taking such as vitamins, herbal products, prescribed medications, "cold medicines," stimulants, and diet supplements because these products may cause elevation in the systemic blood pressure. In addition, herbal substances such as black cohosh and hawthorne may lower blood pressure. The patient and family will demonstrate to the nurse how to take the blood pressure.	The nurse has a responsibility to teach the patient and family about the hazards of mixing OTC products, herbal substances, diet substances, stimulants, alcohol, and tobacco with prescription medications.
The nurse demonstrates how menu planning is carried out using a prescribed diet plan such as the DASH diet. Frequently, a referral needs to be made to a therapeutic dietitian for assistance in initiating and maintaining these lifestyle changes. Suggestions for lifestyle changes include: 1. Weight reduction 2. Exercising 3. Stopping smoking 4. Reducing alcohol consumption 5. Reducing stress. The patient may need referrals to support groups for making these lifestyle changes.	Family and patient meet with the nurse and/or the therapeutic dietitian for instruction in how to structure the diet plan. Personal preferences and cultural sensitivity are important because food is an essential part of lifestyle. Family and patient are given the necessary referrals to approved organized groups within their community. With full permission of the patient, involve caring family members or social support (e.g., faith based or community organizations) in the treatment process. Suggest common interest group activities (e.g., walking group) to enhance natural support and motivation.
Reasons for the patient/family to call the health care provider include: 1. Experiencing a headache 2. Fainting 3. Dizziness 4. Need for a follow-up appointment 5. Medication renewal of prescription.	Family and patient need to be aware that there are specific reasons to call the health care provider. These symptoms are potential signs of an elevated blood pressure.
The patient needs to join a community support group.	Family and patient visit and join support group(s) for continuing encouragement and community.

pressure should not be greater than 130 mmHg and the diastolic blood pressure less than 80 mmHg.

The objective of care for the patient with high blood pressure requires a multidisciplinary approach to begin to facilitate the patient and family in making lifestyle changes. The nurse is the coordinator of care, accessing the health team members to facilitate the ongoing care of the patient and family. Ingle (2001) reported from *Factors Assisting with Management of Hypertension* that male subjects stated they cannot trust their body anymore, living with hypertension is dangerous, and it requires learning to live with hypertension on a daily basis. Multiple resources may be needed to support the patient and family during the

management of this chronic illness. The roles of resource individuals for the patient are as follows:

- **Clinical dietitians**—The patient/family will be making a number of lifestyle changes including the selection of food and the amount to be eaten. The patient needs the clinical expertise of a therapeutic dietitian to assist in the modification of diet, menu planning, and modification of recipes. This is viewed as a major lifestyle change with many cultural consequences.

- **Fitness/exercise leader**—The fitness/exercise leader is one employed by a recognized, organized health care system. The leader is able to assess, follow a physician's prescription, and modify the types and kind of activities for the individual with hypertension.

- The pharmacist provides information about the action of the antihypertensive medications as well as precautions and side effects.

Throughout this process, the patient must take ownership and responsibility for maintaining the regimen over the long term.

Complications of High Blood Pressure

The impact of uncontrolled high blood pressure on organs occurs insidiously over an extended period of time throughout the body. The JNC 7 report (NHLBI, 2003b) referred to certain complications of hypertension as target organ damage, with the heart, kidney, brain, peripheral vasculature, and retina considered to be target organs. Prolonged untreated hypertension causes both large and small blood vessels to become sclerotic, tortuous, and weak. These changes cause narrowing of the artery lumen, decreased blood flow to organs, and increased blood pressure. Additionally, the weakened arteries are more prone to rupture. Large arteries tend to occlude or rupture, causing a loss of the blood supply to organs and tissues. Small arteries that are damaged decrease the blood supply to organs, resulting in structural changes. An increased diastolic blood pressure causes injury to the intimal wall of the arteries, resulting in plaque buildup and local inflammation, which in turn results in plaque rupture, platelet aggregation, and subsequent vessel occlusion. The result is a decreased blood supply to organs, leading to progressive loss of function. The organs that are the most affected by these changes are the heart, brain, kidney, and retina. Chart 21–6 outlines the target organs that are most prone to damage.

CHART 21–6 **Target Organ Damage**

Heart
Left ventricular hypertrophy
Angina or prior myocardial infarction
Prior coronary revascularization
Heart failure
Brain
Stroke or transient ischemic attack
Chronic kidney disease
Renal failure
Peripheral arterial disease
Peripheral ischemia
Retinopathy
Vision changes leading to blindness

Source: Adapted from National Heart, Lung, and Blood Institute. (2003, May). *Seventh report of the Joint National Committee on Prevention, Detection, Evaluation, and Treatment of High Blood Pressure (JNC7)*. Retrieved June 9, 2008, from http://www.nhlbi.nih.gov/guidelines/hypertension/jnc7full.pdf.

Ischemic heart disease is the most common site of target organ damage associated with high blood pressure (NHLBI, 2003b). As a result of prolonged hypertension, the coronary arteries are unable to deliver an adequate blood supply to the myocardium. This loss causes the heart muscle to lose its ability to contract sufficiently, resulting in decreased cardiac output. The shearing force of blood flowing with increased pressure over time causes irregularities in the intima of the lumen of the arteries. This causes an increased buildup of plaque, ultimately narrowing the lumen of the artery and decreasing blood flow to the myocardium, resulting in ischemic heart disease.

Heart failure occurs because of the increased cardiac workload due to pumping against an increased afterload, which is the increased pressure created by the narrowed lumen of diseased blood vessels, as the heart attempts to eject its blood supply. Eventually the left ventricle hypertrophies to compensate for increased pressure. Left ventricular hypertrophy increases with age and is most prevalent in persons with blood pressure of 160/95 mmHg (Porth, 2005). Heart failure is a systolic or diastolic ventricular impairment, which can be caused by both ischemic heart disease and long-standing uncontrolled high blood pressure. Heart failure leads to a backup of blood into the pulmonary circulation, causing pulmonary edema and left-sided heart failure. Serous fluid is forced back through the pulmonary capillaries into the alveoli and quickly enters the bronchioles and bronchi. The patient will experience tachypnea, restlessness, apprehensiveness, air hunger or cyanosis, and frothy, blood-tinged sputum. The peripheral and neck veins are engorged and the blood pressure and heart rate are increased. Edema may be present in the extremities and crackles in the lung; respiratory acidosis and profuse diaphoresis may also be present (Andreoli et al., 2004). Ventricular hypertrophy and an increased workload of the heart contribute to approximately 50% of high blood pressure deaths due to myocardial infarction or myocardial failure.

Hypertension leads to nephrosclerosis, which is a common cause of renal insufficiency. This condition is caused by diseased blood vessels that are no longer able to deliver adequate blood supply to the kidneys, resulting in decreased renal function. Additionally, high blood pressure accelerates other types of kidney diseases, particularly in diabetes. The American Diabetic Association recommends that diabetic's maintain a blood pressure of less than 130/80 mmHg (Porth, 2005).

The patient with diabetes may have high levels of circulating cholesterol and other lipids, which impacts the development of atherosclerosis, arteriosclerosis, and severe coronary heart disease, as well as multiple microcirculatory lesions. Due to the complications of diabetes, atherosclerosis increases the probability of developing hypertension, diabetic retinopathy, cataracts, and chronic renal disease (Guyton & Hall, 2005).

Metabolic syndrome is being diagnosed more frequently within the adult obese population. It is estimated that one-fourth of the U.S. population has this syndrome. The characteristics are insulin resistance, hypertension, dyslipidemia, high triglyceride levels, diabetes mellitus, low HDL cholesterol level, and a tendency for the patient to form blood clots (NHLBI, 2003b). Metabolic syndrome is discussed in detail in Chapter 40.

Cerebral vascular disease is caused by arteriosclerotic plaques that occur in the feeder arteries to the brain. When these arteries are damaged by prolonged hypertension, plaque forms and it becomes vulnerable to rupture away from the wall of the artery. Ruptured plaque activates the clotting mechanism and platelets aggregate, causing a clot to form and block the artery, thus leading to an acute loss of brain function in the local area (Guyton & Hall, 2005). High blood pressure may cause the vessel to rupture. Hemorrhage follows, compressing the local brain tissue. Subsequent clotting of the blood vessel leads to blood vessel blockage (Guyton & Hall, 2005).

Hypertensive eye disease includes the retinal arterioles, retinal parenchyma, choroids, and optic nerve. High blood pressure can be detected in the eye by the presence of diffuse arteriolar narrowing, bleeding, cotton wool patches, hard exudates, microaneurysms, zones of nonperfusion, and flame-shaped bleeding at or near the retina (NHLBI, 2003b). All of these conditions are visible through an ophthalmoscope. The ability of the patient to have visual acuity is dependent on the degree of pathology.

Aortic artery disorders are commonly associated with hypertension. An aortic aneurysm is a weakened area in the wall of an artery that bulges out over time. This disorder is associated with vessel wall degeneration and high blood pressure. It is estimated that approximately 50% of the population with aortic aneurysms have high blood pressure (Porth, 2005). Controlling blood pressure will help diminish vessel degeneration.

Hypertensive Emergencies

If left untreated on rare occasions high blood pressure can become a life-threatening emergency. Approximately 90% of the cases of untreated hypertension will lead to death from myocardial infarction, stroke, renal failure, or aortic dissection. The most common emergencies are discussed next.

Hypertensive Crisis

Hypertensive crisis is rare and sometimes has a fatal occurrence characterized by the sudden onset of a diastolic blood pressure of between 120 and 130 mmHg, the clinical manifestation of target organ vascular damage, and the presence of retinal exudates and hemorrhage. A diastolic blood pressure of greater than 120 mmHg causes acute vascular damage, and structural organ changes begin to occur. The release of catecholamines and the activation of the renin-angiotensin mechanism occur, raising the blood pressure even further. The symptoms may include unstable angina, pulmonary edema, myocardial infarction, eclampsia, stroke, life-threatening arterial bleeding, aortic dissection, morning headache, blurred vision and dyspnea, and potential signs of uremia.

The causes of a hypertensive crisis include acute and chronic renal failure, exacerbation of chronic hypertension, sudden withdrawal of antihypertensive medications, and vasculitis. The management of a hypertensive crisis includes immediate hospitalization in a special care area such as a coronary care unit. The goal of management is to bring the blood pressure down within 1 hour of the crisis, without sending the blood pressure too low. Decreasing the blood pressure too severely can cause cerebral and/or myocardial infarcts and renal failure. Intravenous **vasodilator** medications and adrenergic inhibitors are used to treat the hypertension (Yuan, 2004). Sodium nitroprusside has

been the drug of choice in these situations because it has an instantaneous onset and a short half-life. If the blood pressure begins to drop too severely, its effect is short acting.

 *Hypertensive crisis is a medical emergency. Rapid onset: a systolic blood pressure of greater than 240 mmHg and/or a diastolic blood pressure of greater than 130 mmHg.*

Hypertensive Encephalopathy

Hypertensive encephalopathy is a very dangerous state of multifocal cerebral ischemia due to a severely acute or subacute elevated blood pressure. The pathogenesis of hypertensive encephalopathy is the effect of high blood pressure on the brain's arterioles. "If [the] elevated pressure exceeds the upper limits of normal cerebral autoregulation, a combination of multifocal arteriolar vasodilatation and vasoconstriction occurs, producing diffusely distributed small zones of microhemorrhages and ischemia" (Andreoli et al., 2004). The patient with this diagnosis needs urgent and immediate treatment. The decreasing incidence of this emergency is due in part to the use of effective antihypertensive drugs.

Dissecting Aortic Aneurysm

Dissecting aortic aneurysm is a localized dilation of the aorta that has a longitudinal dissection between the outer and middle layers of the vascular wall. A patient demonstrating signs and symptoms of a dissecting aortic aneurysm needs to be admitted to an intensive care unit for hemodynamic monitoring and the monitoring of urinary output.

High blood pressure generally precedes the dissecting aortic aneurysm. Blood penetrates the tear in the aortic intimal lining, forming a false channel with the aortic media. Blood in this false channel may reenter the true aortic channel via a second intimal tear or rupture through the adventitia into the periaortic tissues. Aortic dissection occurs suddenly with severe chest pain, which radiates to the back. The symptoms will vary depending on the location of the dissection (Andreoli et al., 2004). Kasper and colleagues (2005) stated that a type A aneurysm is an ascending aortic dissection that requires emergency surgical repair with a composition graft. A type B aneurysm is described as the compromising of the aortic branches, leading to impending rupture and pain. Transcatheter techniques may be used with stenting of narrow vessels to preserve blood flow to compromised organs. In both cases, long-term therapy includes careful control of hypertension and decrease of cardiac contractility.

Research

Research into the diagnosis, treatment, and prevention of high blood pressure is a universal high priority. The topic is being approached using a variety of methods and by multiple disciplines (see the Evidence-Based Practice feature). Much information is being revised to reflect the need for prevention of high blood pressure by living a healthy lifestyle from birth to old age. Studies about care models to assist patients and families to maintain motivation for a lifetime of health are beginning to be reported in the literature. The reported research indicates that meaningful and positive relationships assist in gaining and nurturing trust between patient and health care provider. There is recognition that diversity of beliefs, culture, and previous experiences within the environment will influence the meaning the patient attributes to the experience with high blood pressure. The patient's ownership of the treatment plan and lifestyle changes is essential. There is gathering evidence that when patient and health care professionals work collaboratively in communicating, exploring, setting goals, and reinforcing them, the patient's management is more successful.

The numbers of therapeutics available to provide protection of the target organs against vascular damage due to high blood pressure are increasing. Teaching aids that use multimedia techniques and information sources need to be devised and made available to the patient and family in their native languages. The Research Opportunities and Clinical Impact box (p. 506) outlines various topics on hypertension that are either under current investigation or in need of investigation.

Impact of Hypertension

Clinical Problem

In the adult practice setting, patients learning to live with hypertension were asked to tell their story concerning what factors have assisted them in managing their hypertension on a daily basis. What do hypertensive adults describe as useful to them in managing their high blood pressure and finding the meaning in their everyday life? Measurement techniques used in a quantitative approach do not reveal a meaningful whole for understanding the hypertensive patient's lived experience. The essence of the hypertensive patient's experience was unveiled through the description of the experiences by the participant using qualitative techniques.

Research Findings

DeWitt and Ploeg (2006) reported that the interpretative phenomenology method should be used to assist in the expression of rigor in the preservation of integrity and legitimacy of nursing research. In a study by Ingle (2001) participants described the everydayness of hypertension, their realization that they were no longer in control of their life, and their learning that life was dangerous. Participants said that individuals with hypertension can no longer take their health for granted. Health becomes a choice made each day by the patient. The therapeutic plan of medication management and care was not part of the patient's narrative. Each patient was describing how they wanted to live in this world.

In a study reported by Peters (2006), the relationship between the factors of perceived racism, emotion-focused stress, and blood pressure were examined within the African American community. This descriptive-correlational, causal modeling study with a convenience sample of 162 community-dwelling adults reported bias, prejudice, and stereotyping by health care providers in conjunction with other racially discriminatory experiences that lead to health care disparities among minorities. Further study is needed to determine the relationship between racism, emotions, psychological factors, and hypertension.

Implications for Nursing Practice

Findings from qualitative and quantitative research studies reveal the need for an increased awareness of the multiple factors that influence the care of patients with hypertension. Assessing the hypertensive patient using narrative interviewing techniques can provide an understanding of the situation. Patients and family were experiencing anger and denial that a problem exists, and that hypertension is perceived as "no big deal." Physical factors were reported to be less significant and did not emerge as a theme (Ingle, 2001). The acronym NURSE is a useful assessment tool.

Acronym	Request	Example
N	Narrative *Assist the patient to understand and state her feelings about hypertension.*	Tell me your story about having high blood pressure.
U	Understanding *Listen with empathy to the situation.*	It is important for me to know what this diagnosis means to you.
R	Reflect *When a patient tells his story, it is difficult to acknowledge it.*	It is difficult to acknowledge and support the various emotions of the story.
S	Silence *During the conversation, pauses will occur.*	Take your time and process both your and the patient's thoughts.
E	Explain *Take time to clarify any misconceptions or to answer any questions.*	I am here to answer any questions.

Critical Thinking Questions

1. After the narrative interview, the patient asks if you would listen to some insights that have become apparent through the process. How would you answer this individual?

2. How will you use silence with the patient?

Answers to Critical Thinking Questions appear in Appendix D.

References

De Witt, L., & Ploeg, J. (2006). Critical appraisal of rigor in interpretive phenomenological nursing research. *Journal of Advanced Nursing, 55*(2), 215–229.

Ingle, E. A. (2001). *Factors assisting with client management of hypertension.* Unpublished master's thesis, Carson-Newman College, Jefferson City, TN.

Peters, R. M. (2006). The relationship of racism, chronic stress emotions, and blood pressure. *Journal of Nursing Scholarship, 38,* 234–240.

EVIDENCE-BASED PRACTICE

RESEARCH OPPORTUNITIES AND CLINICAL IMPACT RELATED TO HYPERTENSION

Research Area	Clinical Impact
How do hypertensive drug actions vary between men versus women?	Selection of gender-specific pharmaceutical packages may decrease target organ injury.
What is the difference between men and women in the description of their symptoms of high blood pressure?	Men and women describe their symptoms differently.
How do childhood obesity and hypertension affect the rate of development of end-organ damage?	Children's physiological response to obesity and hypertension is different than that of adults and the elderly.
What are the roles of heredity and environment in the prevention of hypertension?	Determine the role of genetics and the environment in prevention and treatment of hypertension.
Describe the relationship between aging and hypertension.	Determine the relationship between the aging process and the progression of hypertension.
How does the meaning of living with a diagnosis of hypertension influence the patient's prognosis?	Knowing the meaning and significance of the diagnosis of hypertension to the patient will enhance teaching and learning opportunities.
How does the family cope with the long-term burden of the chronic illness of hypertension?	Knowing the meaning of a chronic illness to a patient will facilitate the partnership care of this individual and the family.
How do the ethics of hypertension, a long-term illness, determine care?	Potential justification of care for patients with chronic long-term illnesses.
How can assessment tools for the measurement of anger be incorporated into adult health assessments?	Such tools could help determine the effect of anger on the blood pressure.
Do hypertensive patients beginning pharmaceutical interventions make self-modifications to maintain sexual performance?	Impact on lifestyle and potential need for intervention.
How does the community function as a long-term support group?	Long-term impact on target organs, body image, and compliance with the therapeutic plan.
How can cultural sensitivity in the care of the patient with hypertension be improved?	Such knowledge would help promote cultural insight surrounding chronic hypertensive care.

Clinical Preparation

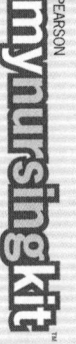

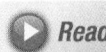 **Read**

- History of Current Illness
- Past Medical History
- Physical Exam
- Admitting Medical Orders
- Laboratory Study Results

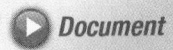 **Document**

- Summary of Hospitalization
- Pathophysiology Form
- Laboratory Values
- Laboratory Results Explanation

 **Apply**

- List of Potential Nursing Diagnoses
- Concept Map
- Critical Thinking Questions

*Log on to MyNursingKit.com to download forms you will need and to complete further steps in the Clinical Preparation assignment.

HISTORY OF PRESENT ILLNESS

Ms. Grace Bell is a 65-year-old Caucasian female with hypertension. She is of German-American heritage. For the past year and a half, she has been experiencing headaches, irritability, anger, and fatigue. She arrived at the nurse practitioner office for an appointment 1 month ago to discuss the recent death of her husband. She also stated "I'm not feeling too great." Her sitting blood pressure in the left arm was 190/92, her height was 5'2" and she weighed 150 pounds. Ms. Bell was asked if she was taking any over-the-counter medications or any alternative or complementary medications. Her response was "No. I'm allergic to everything." At the first appointment she was advised to reduce her intake of cholesterol-rich foods and to reduce her intake of salt by not adding it to food during preparation or at the table. She indicated she had become a "couch potato" and did little exercising. She was given a return appointment for the following week. Ms. Bell's admitting diagnosis to the nurse practitioner's practice was "rule out stage 2 hypertension and white coat hypertension."

Ms. George, FNP, notes that Ms. Bell's voice is loud and her speech fast, she is apparently angry with the office wait, and she reports she has a bad headache. She also wants to know why everyone is so interested in her blood pressure. Ms. Bell states, "It will come down, if you could just let me rest a minute."

Medical–Surgical History

Ms. Bell's medical history includes one vaginal birth of a live female. There is no history of hypertension in the family.

Social History

Ms. Bell reports she has just lost her husband. Her daughter lives nearby and very helpful.

Physical Exam

Weight: 150 lb; height: 5 ft 2 in.
T 98.0; P 120; R 22
Blood pressure: left arm and right arm have a 5-point discrepancy:
    lying 200/100; sitting 190/95; standing 184/90
Capillary refilling times: 3 seconds in both hands

Laboratory Studies

Total cholesterol
HDL
LDL
Glucose
Creatinine
Urinalysis

Scheduled Medications

Atenolol 50 mg once per day
Quinapril 40 mg once per day

PRN Medications

Tylenol 500mg for headache

LABORATORY STUDY RESULTS

Test	Week 1	Week 2	Week 3
Total cholesterol	300 mg/dL	310 mg/dL	295 mg/dL
HDL	50 mg/dL	45 mg/dL	49 mg/dL
LDL	250 mg/dL	275 mg/dL	255 mg/dL
Glucose (fasting)	175 mg/dL	182 mg/dL	170 mg/dL
BUN	25 mg/dL	25 mg/dL	23 mg/dL
Creatinine	2.0 mg/dL	2.0 mg/dL	1.9 mg/dL
Urinalysis	Protein 2+ Glucose 2+	Protein 2+ Glucose 2+	Protein 2+ Glucose 2+

CRITICAL THINKING QUESTIONS

1. Ms. Bell just entered the office for her third appointment and states "I've just become unemployed, I have no health insurance and no income. What shall I do?" What essential recommendations does Ms. Bell need to maintain control of her hypertension? What would you do if Ms. Bell relapses into noncompliant behavior?

2. What process would you use to help Ms. Bell accept responsibility for her own health care?

3. How are you as Ms. Bell's nurse going to listen to her therapeutically?

4. Using the nursing process, develop a plan of care for Ms. Bell related to the impact of chronic illness and ineffective coping with changes in lifestyle.

Answers to Critical Thinking Questions appear in Appendix D.

NCLEX® REVIEW

1. The nurse recognizes that a patient with two consecutive blood pressure readings, a month apart, of 132/80 and 130/88 is considered to have:
   1. Normal blood pressure.
   2. Prehypertension.
   3. Stage 1 hypertension.
   4. Stage 2 hypertension

2. From the list provided, choose the factors having a direct influence on regulation of blood pressure. (Select all that apply.)
   1. Cardiac output
   2. Peripheral vascular resistance
   3. Production of adrenocorticotropic hormone
   4. Baroreceptors
   5. Chemoreceptors
   6. Body fluid volume

3. Which of the following patients represents the highest risk for development of hypertension?
   1. 46-year-old female, African American, recently fired from her job
   2. 46-year-old female, Caucasian, 50 pounds over ideal body weight
   3. 56-year-old male, African American, insulin dependent diabetic
   4. 56-year-old male, Caucasian, excessive alcohol consumption

4. The nurse would teach a patient prescribed nifedipine (procardia XL) to:
   1. Add foods high in potassium such as bananas and orange juice to the diet.
   2. Report the common adverse effect of dry cough to the health care provider.
   3. Not crush, break in half, or chew the extended release form of the drug.
   4. Assess the pulse prior to taking the medication with each dose.

5. The nurse is aware which of the following cultural components play a role with hypertension? Select all that apply.
   1. Asian populations undergoing Westernization will have significant increases in high blood pressure.
   2. Individuals living in southeastern region of the United States have a higher percentage of high blood pressure.
   3. Caucasians adapt more readily to following the DASH diet and starting a routine exercise program.
   4. African Americans tolerate using the ACE inhibitor drug group better than any other ethnicity.

6. A nurse developing a plan of care for an individual with prehypertension would emphasize the need for which of the following? Select all that apply.
   1. A sedentary lifestyle will lower the body's oxygen needs and manage hypertension.
   2. Set a goal to reduce cigarette smoking from two packs, to a half pack a day.
   3. Developing a diet plan that is low in saturated fats and sodium.
   4. Avoid any activities or relationships which are stress-producing.
   5. Target weight loss at five pounds per week until ideal body mass index is obtained.
   6. Eliminating or reducing alcohol consumption to one ounce a day.

7. A priority patient outcome for an individual with long-term Stage 2 hypertension would include:
   1. Avoiding use of generic brands of anti-hypertensive medications.
   2. Verbalizing the warning signs and symptoms of cerebral vascular accident.
   3. Maintaining healthy, supportive relationships among friends and family.
   4. Recording blood pressure measurements once a month with home monitoring.

Answers for review questions appear in Appendix D

KEY TERMS

blood pressure *p.487*
DASH diet *p.493*
diastolic *p.487*
dissecting aortic aneurysm *p.504*
hypertensive crisis *p.504*

hypertensive encephalopathy *p.504*
peripheral vascular resistance *p.488*
prehypertension *p.489*
pulse pressure *p.488*
stage 1 hypertension *p.490*

stage 2 hypertension *p.490*
systolic *p.487*
vasodilator *p.504*
white coat phenomenon *p.490*

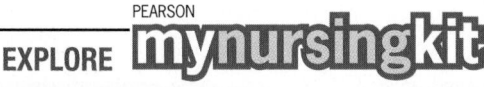

PEARSON

EXPLORE mynursingkit™

MyNursingKit is your one stop for online chapter review materials and resources. Prepare for success with additional NCLEX®-style practice questions, interactive assignments and activities, web links, animations and videos, and more!

Register your access code from the front of your book at
www.mynursingkit.com

REFERENCES

Andreoli, T. E., Carpenter, C. C. J., Griggs, R. C., & Loscalzo, J. (2004). *Cecil essentials of medicine* (6th ed.). Philadelphia: W. B. Saunders.

Centers for Disease Control and Prevention. (2008). *Overweight and Obesity Trends Among Adults.* Retrieved June 13, 2008 from http://www.cdc.gov/nccdphp/dnpa/obesity/trend/

Donnelly, P. (2000). Ethics and cross-cultural nursing. *Journal of Transcultural Nursing, 11,* 119–125.

Eisenhower, J. S. (2002). *Descriptive study of client use of herbal substances and over-the-counter medications.* Unpublished master's thesis, Carson-Newman College, Jefferson City, TN.

Fields, L. E., Burt, V. L., Cutler, J. A., Hughes, J., Roccella, E. J., & Sorlie, P. (2004). The burden of adult hypertension in the United States 1999 to 2000: A rising tide. *Hypertension, 44,* 1–7.

Guyton, A., & Hall, J. E. (2005). *Textbook of medical physiology* (11th ed.). Philadelphia: W. B. Saunders.

Ingle, E. A. (2001). *Factors assisting with client management of hypertension.* Unpublished master's thesis, Carson-Newman College, Jefferson City, TN.

Jhala, S. (2001). *The healthcare needs of Asian Indian females.* Unpublished master's thesis, Carson-Newman College, Jefferson City, TN.

Kasper, D. L., Braunwald, E., Fauci, A. S., Hauser, S. L., Longo, D. L., & Jameson, J. L. (2005). *Harrison's principles of internal medicine* (16th ed.). New York: McGraw-Hill.

National Heart, Lung, and Blood Institute. (1998). *Clinical guidelines on the identification, evaluation, and treatment of overweight and obesity in adults.* Bethesda, MD: Author.

National Heart, Lung, and Blood Institute. (2003, May). *Seventh report of the Joint National Committee on Prevention, Detection, Evaluation, and Treatment of High Blood Pressure (JNC7).* Retrieved June 9,

2008, from http://www.nhlbi.nih.gov/guidelines/hypertension/jnc7full.pdf

Nicoll, D., McPhee, S. J., & Pignone, M. (2004). *Pocket guide to diagnostic tests* (4th ed.). New York: Lange Medical Books/McGraw-Hill.

Porth, C. M. (2005). *Pathophysiology: Concepts of altered health status* (7th ed.). Philadelphia: Lippincott Williams & Wilkins.

Rankin-Box, D. (2001). *The nurse's handbook of complementary therapies* (2nd ed.). Edinburgh: Bailliere Tindall.

Welton, P. K. (2003). Potassium and blood pressure. In J. E. Izzo & H. R. Black (Eds.), *Hypertension primer* (3rd ed., pp. 280–283). Dallas: American Heart Association.

Yuan, S. Y. (2004). *Handbook of diseases* (3rd ed.). Philadelphia: Lippincott Williams & Wilkins.

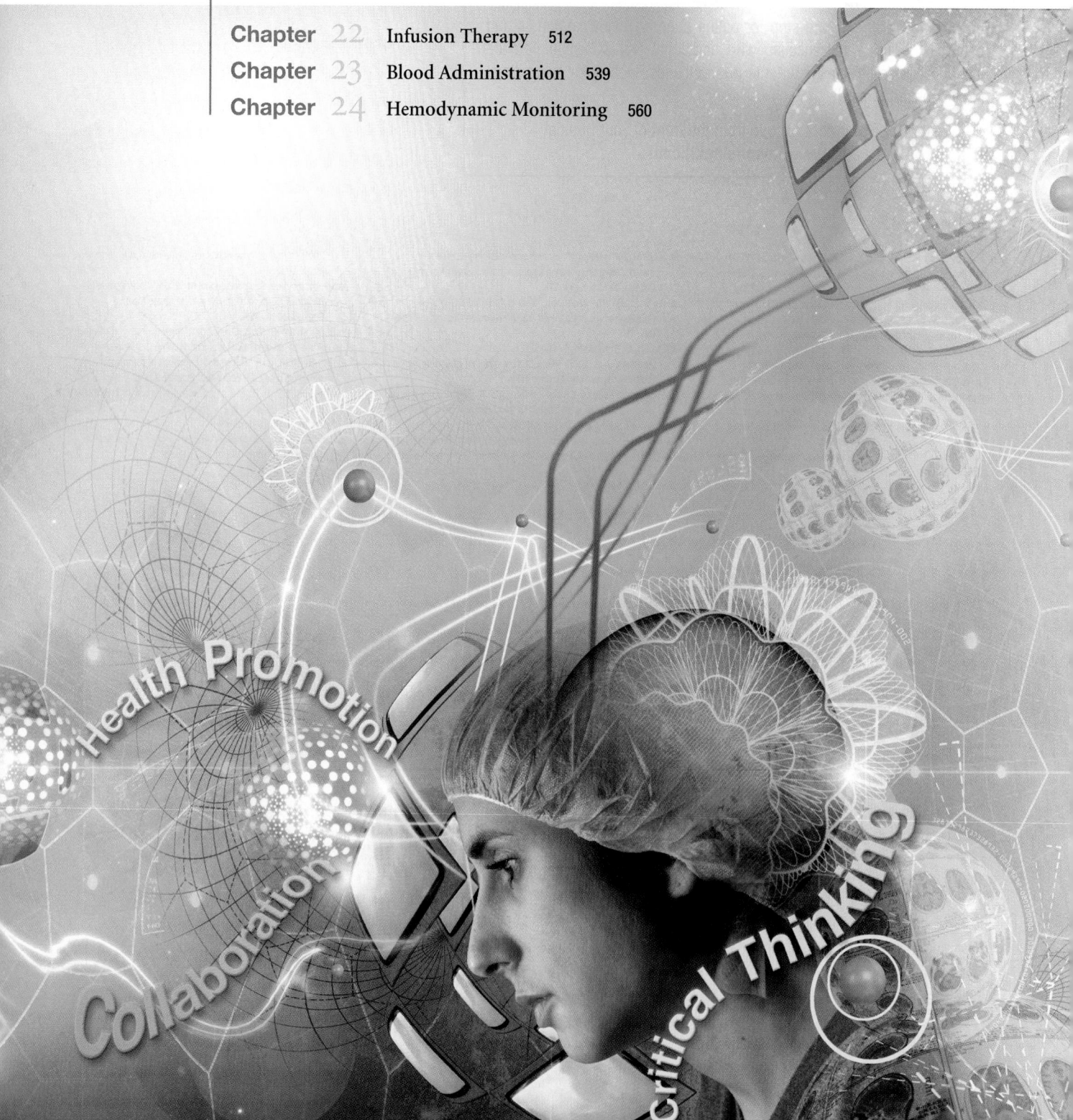

Health Promotion

Collaboration

Critical Thinking

Profiles in Nursing

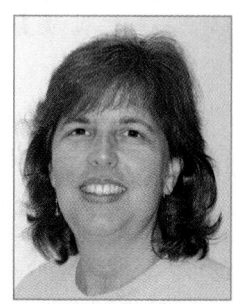

CINDY   My name is Cindy and I am the nurse manager of the Apheresis/Transfusion and Infusion Unit at the Albany Medical Center hospital in Albany, New York. I am also presently comanaging the Surgical Intensive Care Unit (ICU), while a new nurse manager is being recruited and trained. Albany Medical Center is a large 614-bed Level I trauma center with an extremely busy flight program, a medical college involved in educating physicians, and a nationally recognized research program.

I began work at this hospital approximately 28 years ago, in the Burn Unit. This experience provided me with the opportunity to embrace **compassion, commitment,** and **confidence** in my practice as a health care professional. This was when I first began to appreciate the importance of critical thinking skills and clinical reasoning; as a result, I looked for any and all opportunities to float to other critical care areas within the facility to enhance my clinical skills.

I now work full time in the Apheresis Unit as a hands-on manager. I have always lived by the notion that managers should never ask of staff what they themselves are not willing to do. Therefore, I am actively involved in the coordination of care for all of our patients, while ensuring a collaborative team-centered approach to the care. Quality is of the highest priority not only for our patients, but for the staff working in the unit as well. We collaborate on a daily basis with a variety of constituents in order to ensure positive patient outcomes and coordination of care.

Our patient population is as diverse as the age range of the patients that we serve. They have hematologic, immunologic, and oncologic challenges and are in various stages of their disease processes. The goal of the program is to foster an environment that allows patients to spend as much time at home with their families as possible, while addressing their emotional and physical health care needs.

I cherish the memory of a 5-year-old boy whom I had cared for during the last 3 years of his very short life. He had become so riddled with pain that during treatments his mother would lie next to him in bed and rub his tiny spine to make the pain tolerable. During his care one day, the doctors wanted to discuss with the family his next phase of treatment, which meant the parents would have to leave the unit. The child became very distraught at the idea that he would be left and not held. I remember climbing into bed next to him and rubbing his spine as I had watched his mother do. The child immediately calmed; he reached up and started twisting my hair, as he often did with his mother. When his parents arrived back to the unit, the child looked up at me and said "Cinny, I love you." A few days later Michael lost his battle with cancer and when I went to the wake, I was overwhelmed to see that laying there beside him was a picture that his parents had taken of the two of us, lying together in bed. This situation emulates our need to respond not just as health care providers in the clinical sense, but to be able to utilize our compassion in a way that provides for the emotional support that our patient's need.

Most recently we were caring for a patient who had been diagnosed with cancer and required a blood transfusion. To many this process appears quite benign on the surface; I even had an orientee tell me that this "wasn't rocket science." The patient had no indicators that would preclude us from going forward with the plan of care; therefore, the first unit of blood was hung. I remember being only about 10 paces outside of the room when I overheard the patient say "Gee, my lower back hurts." I called for help and immediately stopped the transfusion. Because of the team approach our unit has to nursing, everyone assumed a role: vital signs, oxygen applied, crash cart at bedside, physician called, epinephrine and steroids drawn and ready to administer. Because of their knowledge and expertise, everyone involved recognized that a transfusion reaction was taking place.

You see, what the orientee learned that day was that a mere 2 mL of blood caused this patient to have a true anaphylactic response to blood and that the staff demonstrated how critical thinking, collaboration, and respect could salvage a potentially life-threatening outcome. This patient had an unknown IgA antibody problem and 3 mL of blood would have been enough to cause a lethal situation.

I'd like to conclude by saying that it is the work that we do every day as health care professionals—work that involves thoughtful action, critical thinking, mindfulness, and an ability to understand through reflection and discussion while making sound judgments that lead to justifiable actions—that is true nursing praxis.

> "Quality is of the highest priority not only for our patients, but for the staff working in the unit as well. We collaborate on a daily basis with a variety of constituents in order to ensure positive patient outcomes and coordination of care."

Infusion Therapy

Deborah Benvenuto
Mary Alexander

Outcome-Based Learning Objectives

After studying this chapter, the learner will be able to:

1. Compare and contrast the types and uses of catheters for parenteral administration of solutions and medications.
2. Describe the types and uses of parenteral administration equipment and infusion devices.
3. Evaluate the tenets of infusion nursing practice including competencies, skill validation, and patient assessment.
4. Describe components of infusion-specific documentation.
5. Discuss the recognition and management of infusion-related complications, and strategies to prevent complications for the patient receiving infusion therapy.

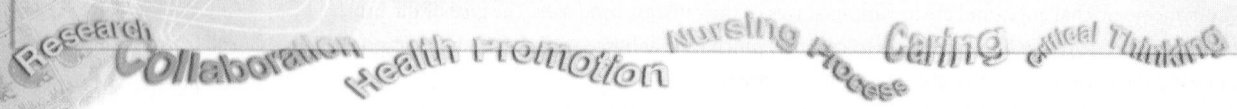

Research Collaboration Health Promotion Nursing Process Caring Critical Thinking

INFUSION THERAPY began in the late 1400s when the vascular system was accessed with crude hollow-bore instruments that consisted of feather quills, animal veins, and bladders. Today, research and technology have produced devices that can be easily inserted into vascular and nonvascular spaces and allowed to **dwell** (remain in place) for periods of several days to many months and sometimes years. These devices are used for delivery of prescribed **infusates** (solutions and medications) over a period of time for specific therapeutic indications or diagnostic evaluations. This method of delivery is referred to as the **parenteral** route, which means that the alimentary canal is bypassed and medications and solutions are instead delivered by subcutaneous, vascular, intramuscular, or nonvascular routes. This chapter discusses these infusion therapies and focuses on the administration of infusates via the subcutaneous, vascular, and nonvascular routes.

Because infusion therapy requires that specific sterile compartments within the body be accessed, standard precautions and sterile technique are to be practiced with all infusion-related procedures. More information about standard precautions is given in Chapter 20 ⊙. Single-use catheters and infusion-specific products are used to promote safety for the patient and health care provider and to prevent and minimize development of infusion-related complications such as infection.

Pathogens associated with infusion therapy causing the greatest health care risk are the hepatitis B and C viruses (HBV and HCV) and the human immunodeficiency virus (HIV). Hollow-bore needles, which are commonly used for obtaining blood samples, administering injections, or accessing vascular and nonvascular structures, are implicated in the transmission of bloodborne diseases because contaminated blood can become lodged within the internal space, or **lumen**, of the device.

■ Vascular Access Devices

A **vascular access device (VAD)** or **catheter** is a device that is introduced through the skin, into the vascular network, for the purpose of infusing parenteral solutions and medications. These devices require the nurse to become proficient in not only insertion techniques for the devices, but patient assessment and monitoring practices, and care and maintenance strategies for these devices.

Peripheral Vascular Access Devices

Vascular access devices that are used primarily for infusion therapies administered via locations found on the upper extremities, or the peripheral vasculature, are addressed in the following sections. These devices are used with parenteral therapies administered in a variety of care settings.

Peripheral-Short Catheters

Peripheral-short catheters are VADs that are less than 7.5 cm (3.0 in.) in length and are placed in the superficial peripheral vasculature of the arms of adult and pediatric patients. In children, VADs also may be inserted in other locations such as the occipital, superficial temporal, posterior auricular, and saphenous veins.

Peripheral short catheters are manufactured with various configurations, lengths, and sizes, and from polyurethane-based and silastic materials. Certain materials such as Teflon (polytetrafluoroethylene) decrease the occurrence of catheter-related phlebitis and thrombogenesis. Another material, Vialon, is considered hemocompatible, and becomes "slick" when moistened. It softens soon after insertion, which minimizes intimal trauma and thrombus formation. Typically, the lengths of peripheral-short catheters vary from 1.5 to 7.5 cm (5/8 to 3.0 in.). Needles range in size, or **gauge**, from a 24-gauge needle, which is the smallest size, to 10- and 12-gauge needles, which are used for large-volume replacement and emergency and trauma care procedures.

During catheter insertion, the stylet is held stationary with the bevel up to prevent vein trauma and facilitate adequate blood flashback. The **bevel** is the slant or angle of the needle that facilitates puncture of the skin and cannulation of the vascular lumen. The **flashback chamber** is a small space in the hub of the stylet that allows for confirmation of the presence of blood and indicates access to the vascular lumen. The nurse must be able to stabilize the stylet assembly during insertion in order to minimize vein trauma and patient discomfort and to prevent accidental exposure to blood or body fluids.

As a result of the Needlestick Safety and Prevention Act of 2000, manufacturers have made great strides in redesigning catheters to afford a measure of safety against accidental blood exposure and possible sharps-related injuries. One type of engineered safety mechanism is identified by the **self-sheathing** stylet, which causes the needle to become encased in a protective chamber upon removal from the inserted catheter. These protective devices require the nurse to purposefully activate the safety mechanism after the needle is withdrawn. Other devices, after withdrawal from the catheter, capture the tip of the exposed stylet with a protective metal casing.

Dwell times for peripheral-short catheters usually range from 72 to 96 hours. Dwell times for winged steel infusion sets (see next section) should be kept under 4 hours and relegated to single-dose therapies due to the increased incidence of complications associated with rigid devices, such as **infiltration** (the inadvertent administration of nonvesicant solutions or medications into surrounding tissues), or for such procedures as phlebotomy procedures.

Removal or discontinuance of the catheter should be accomplished using standard precautions, and aseptic technique must be observed. The dressing materials should be removed from the catheter insertion site followed by gentle retraction of the catheter. Close assessment of the exit site is necessary to detect complications such as phlebitis or drainage, and a dry sterile dressing is applied to the site until hemostasis occurs. The nurse should also inspect the catheter for its condition upon removal. Patients must be educated as to the scope of activities they may engage in and should be instructed to report any drainage or tenderness from the catheter's former site.

The various types of peripheral-short catheters are discussed next. Figure 22–1 ■ shows the most common veins used for intravenous infusions.

Winged Steel Infusion Set

The **winged steel infusion set** is identified by its flexible plastic attachments, or "wings," that extend from either side of the steel needle to facilitate its insertion (Figure 22–2 ■, p. 514). The needle of this device comes in several lengths, from approximately 3/8 to 1.5 inches. Needle gauges vary from 19 to 27. Steel needle gauges are often odd numbered, with the lower number being the larger lumen. Fastened to the winged attachments and needle is plastic tubing generally made of polyvinyl chloride (PVC). This tubing or extension ranges in length from several inches to usually no more than 12 inches. At the distal portion of the extension is an **adapter** to which the administration equipment may be attached. Winged steel infusion sets are now manufactured with safety sheaths that must be activated by the clinician to prevent accidental needlesticks. The winged steel infusion set is biocompatible; therefore, low rates of device-related phlebitis are documented with this infusion product.

Insertion techniques require the nurse to be knowledgeable about vascular anatomy, proficient in desired site selection, and skilled at insertion procedures. Due to the rigidity of the steel

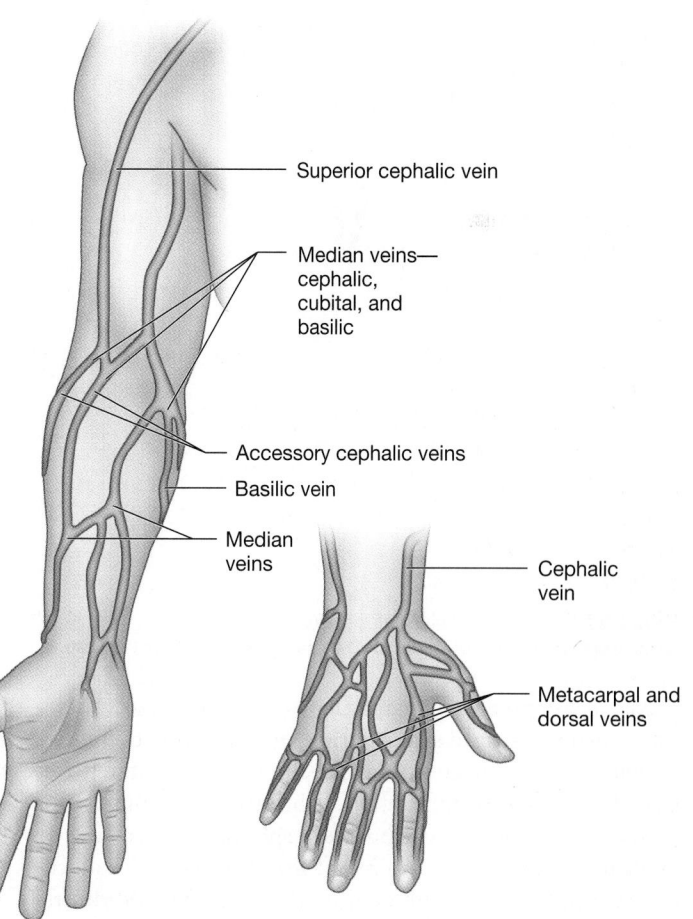

FIGURE 22–1 ■ Common veins used for intravenous therapy.

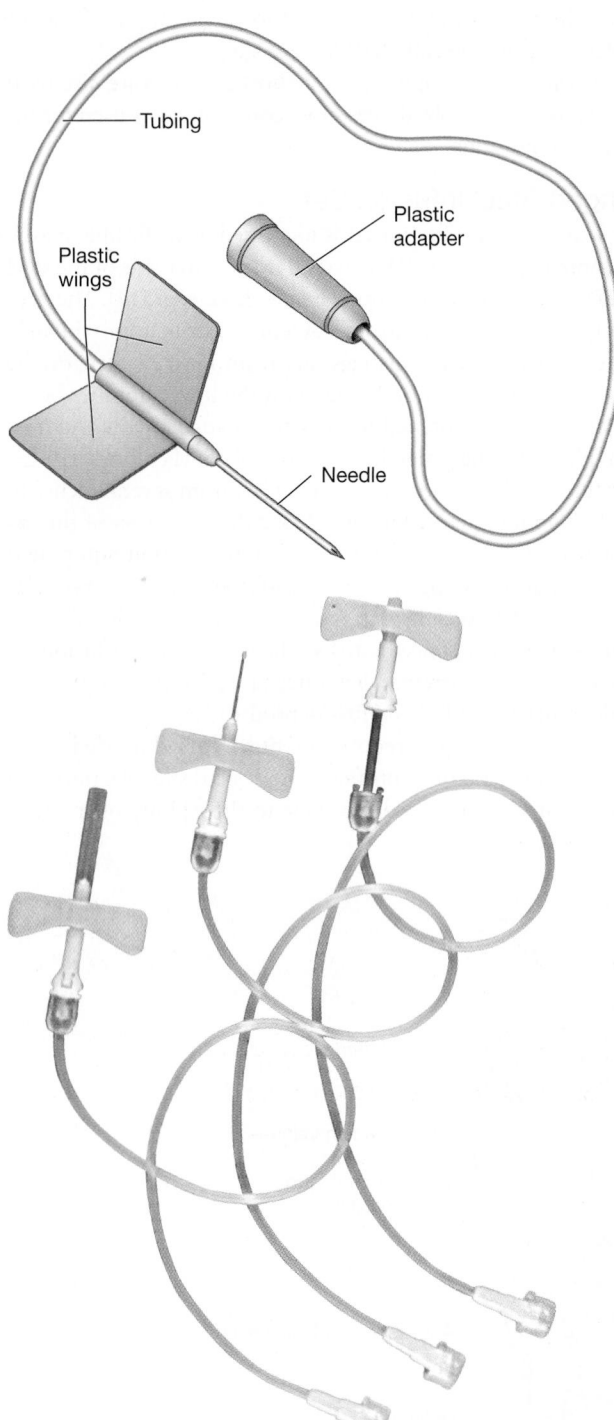

FIGURE 22–2 ■ Winged steel infusion set.
Source: (bottom) Winged safety steel infusion set. Courtesy Exel International Inc., St. Petersburg, FL

needle, development of complications is a serious risk. Therefore, when the winged steel infusion set is used for continuous parenteral administration, the site should be monitored frequently for signs of infiltration or bruising. Temporary supportive devices such as arm boards or splinting surfaces may be applied to assist in preservation of the infusion device's location during short-term therapy. Care should be used during device removal to prevent injury to sensitive or fragile anatomic structures. Adherence to standard precautions and observation of aseptic technique are required. Smooth gentle

retraction on the wings will facilitate device removal. Hemostasis will be achieved with the application of sterile dressing material and gentle pressure applied to the exit wound.

 *Winged steel infusion sets have demonstrated a tendency to infiltrate easily due to rigidity of the steel needle. Observe the patient closely for sudden development of complications such as bruising and infiltration during venipuncture and infusion procedures.*

Over-the-Needle Peripheral-Short Catheters

Over-the-needle peripheral-short catheters (Figure 22–3 ■) are commonly used for short-term infusion therapies. They are less than or equal to 7.5 cm (3.0 in.) in length. They are made of radiopaque materials for ease of x-ray visualization. During the manufacturing process, a hollow-bore metal stylet needle is inserted through the lumen of the flexible catheter. This provides stability to the plastic catheter and facilitates penetration of the skin and vascular or nonvascular structures during device insertion. The presence of blood in the flashback chamber, situated on the posterior aspect of the catheter, indicates when the lumen of the vessel has been accessed. The stylet is then withdrawn as the catheter is moved forward into the vein.

Through-the-Needle Peripheral-Short Catheters

A **through-the-needle peripheral-short catheter** allows passage of the catheter through the lumen of the steel introducer needle, which is the rigid device that allows passage into the vessel. The introducer is withdrawn after successful penetration and positioning within the vessel lumen, leaving the flexible catheter in place. Because the introducer needle cannot be separated from the catheter, it is covered with a protective clip or sleeve to prevent inadvertent catheter shearing or patient injury.

 *When inserting a catheter via this method, be extremely careful **not** to withdraw the catheter back through the steel introducer needle in order to prevent accidental shearing of the catheter. After catheter placement is confirmed, withdraw the introducer needle carefully from the venipuncture site, taking care not to accidentally cut the catheter, and secure with a sterile clip to stabilize the device.*

Midline Catheters

Another example of a peripherally inserted VAD is the midline catheter. Made of materials similar to peripheral-short catheters, the **midline (ML) catheter** is approximately 7.5 to 20 cm (3.1 to

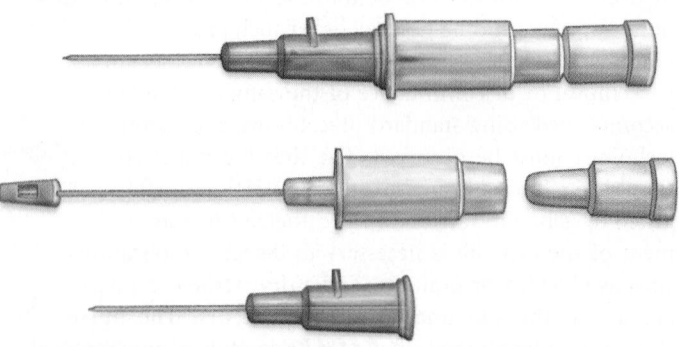

FIGURE 22–3 ■ Introcan safety over-the-needle peripheral-short catheters.

8.0 in.) in length. Dwell periods of these devices are usually recommended not to exceed 4 weeks. Insertion location of the catheter is the antecubital fossa, with alternate sites considered for pediatric patients such as the saphenous, posterior auricular, and superficial temporal veins. The distal tip dwells in the basilic, cephalic, or brachial veins, and is level with the axilla and distal to the shoulder. Because of the extended dwell time, insertion preparations are more extensive than those of the peripheral-short VADs in an effort to minimize development of complications.

ML catheters are generally inserted using an introducer technique, described above. The vein is selected and prepared for venipuncture with appropriate antiseptic agents. An introducer is inserted into the selected vein. The stylet is withdrawn once a positive blood aspirate is confirmed. The ML catheter is then threaded through the introducer. Once the full length of the ML has been inserted, the introducer is withdrawn. Due to its specialized design, the introducer is next peeled apart or separated, allowing its removal from around the ML without disruption to the catheter's location.

A nurse may remove an ML catheter at completion of therapy provided the nurse is educated and skilled in ML catheter removal. It is recommended that antiseptic ointment and an occlusive sterile dressing be applied to the exit wound after removal. This aids hemostasis by occluding the original catheter pathway, and provides a measure of antimicrobial activity due to the extended dwell time of the ML catheter. Due to the length of the device, the catheter must be measured upon removal and be compared to preinsertion documentation.

Therapies infused through a ML catheter are the same as for peripheral-short catheters since the tip of the ML catheter does not pass beyond the peripheral circulatory system. Peripheral infusion prescriptions restricted to ML catheter use are those with pH ranges of 5 to 9, osmolarities of less than 500 mOsm/L, and solutions not to be administered for greater than 4 weeks of therapy.

Central Vascular Access Devices

The **central vascular access device (CVAD)**, defined as a catheter inserted into a centrally located vein with the tip residing in the vena cava, was once relegated to emergent resuscitative procedures and therapies for critically ill patients. Today, their use has evolved to patients in multiple care settings including those outside of the traditional confines of the acute care setting. After insertion, but prior to initiation of therapy, the catheter tip location must be confirmed by radiologic examination.

Nontunneled and Noncuffed CVADs

CVADs are typically divided into three separate and distinct categories for product identification and access configuration purposes. The **nontunneled and noncuffed device** (Figure 22–4 ■) is one that is inserted **percutaneously** via a direct skin puncture with passage of the catheter directly into the vasculature. A catheter inserted using this method is generally not considered a long-term device because it is not tunneled under the skin. A percutaneous catheter may have a single or multiple lumens and is made of polyurethane- or silastic-based materials. A common misnomer is to identify the catheter product by its vascular point of entry such as "subclavian," "jugular," or "femoral" rather than by product name.

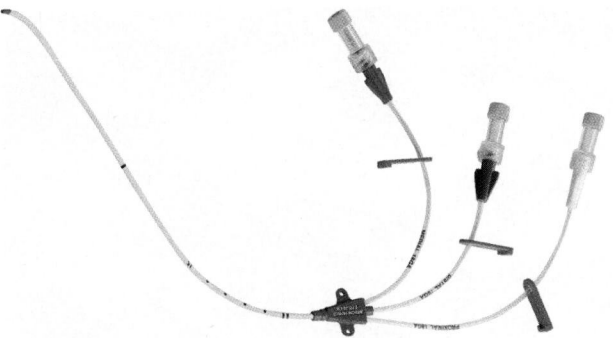

FIGURE 22–4 ■ Triple-lumen noncuffed central catheters.
Source: Reprinted with permission of Arrow International, Inc.

Typically, most CVADs are inserted by physicians or by advanced practice clinicians who are skilled and competent to perform the procedure. Once inserted, the device must be secured, usually with sutures, to prevent inadvertent dislodgment and loss of access. Insertion procedures require sterile technique and maximal barrier precautions.

Removal of nontunneled and noncuffed devices may be done by a nurse skilled and educated in the procedure. Adherence to standard precautions and observation of aseptic technique are required. The patient is placed in a recumbent position and is instructed to perform the Valsalva maneuver, which is to take a deep breath, hold it, and bear down as if to defecate. When the patient bears down, air is prevented from entering the catheter wound and pathway, preventing an **air embolism**, which is caused by the entry of air into the vascular system. While the patient is performing the maneuver, the nurse, having already removed the dressing and released the securement devices, removes the catheter and applies pressure to the catheter exit wound, followed by immediate application of an antiseptic ointment and a sterile occlusive dressing to the site. Then, the nurse instructs the patient to breathe normally and remain inactive and recumbent for approximately 30 minutes, in order to achieve hemostasis and allow monitoring for untoward events related to CVAD removal. The nurse also must inspect the integrity of the device and measure for preinsertion catheter length. This confirms whether the catheter has fractured, leaving a segment in the patient's circulation.

Another type of CVAD that falls into the category of percutaneously inserted nontunneled and noncuffed devices is the **peripherally inserted central catheter (PICC)** (Figure 22–5 ■, p. 516). This is classified as a long-term catheter that is typically inserted at the patient's bedside by nurses educated and skilled in the procedure. Therapies to be infused through a PICC include the following:

- Therapies that require vascular access for several weeks to many months to as long as 1 year
- Therapies with extreme variations in solution pH (>5 and <9) and osmolarity (>600 mOsm/L) and including those solutions with irritant and **vesicant** (causes blistering) properties
- Therapies commonly associated with CVADs such as parenteral nutrition and antineoplastic, anti-infective, and inotropic therapies.

Radiologic confirmation of the catheter tip location prior to therapy initiation is mandatory. Due to the insertion location in

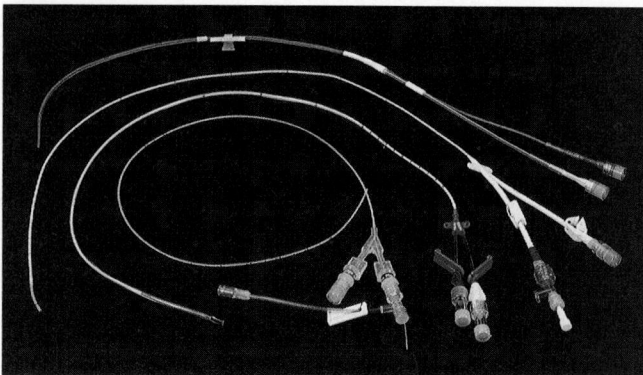

FIGURE 22–5 ■ Peripherally inserted central catheters.
Source: Courtesy of Infusion Nurses Society, PICCC Education Module, 2003

the antecubital region for most PICCs and ML catheters, the ability of the patient to participate in self-care and self-administration practices makes these popular devices among both patients and health care providers.

The PICC is also less commonly associated with development of complications such as site infection, due to the decreased bacterial ecosystem of the antecubital region, and air embolism, because the device does not externally penetrate the thorax during its dwell time. It does lend itself, however, to other complications associated with VADs such as device fracture, tip malposition, device occlusion, and thrombus formation. When removing a PICC, the educated and skilled nurse instructs the patient in the Valsalva maneuver, places the patient in a recumbent position, and performs the removal procedure following the same procedure indicated for removal of other CVADs. Documentation must include measurement of the PICC and preinsertion length comparisons.

Tunneled and Cuffed CVADs

A second category of CVAD is the **tunneled and cuffed device** (Figure 22–6 ■). The cuff is the manufactured piece of the catheter generally made of synthetic materials such as nylon or Dacron. It is attached to the catheter in such a manner that the device is stabilized during its dwell time, and it reduces the risk of catheter-related infection by inhibiting the migration of microorganisms along the catheter track. Some cuffs are impregnated with antimicrobial agents such as a silver-impregnated collagen matrix. The catheter is usually made of silastic-based

materials for its durability and antithrombogenic characteristics. It is configured with either single or multiple lumens. These CVADs are often identified by the physician(s) who developed such clinical devices: Broviac, Hickman, Raaf, and Groshong.

Tunneled and cuffed catheters are typically inserted in the surgical or radiology suite. Tunneling under the skin is the technique used to access the vasculature. An entrance wound is created at a point generally near a large vein, typically the subclavian or femoral vein. The catheter is inserted into the vena cava and radiologic confirmation of tip placement is mandatory prior to initiation of therapy. After tip insertion, the catheter's remaining length is drawn though an exit wound located lower on the chest wall. This technique minimizes the potential for microorganisms gaining access into the body by establishing mechanical barriers (the skin), as well as enabling the cuff to act as a securement device once the tissues heal from the procedure. These CVADs are intended for long-term infusion therapies, with the patient often participating in self-care in the home setting.

Implanted Ports

Implanted ports comprise the third category of central vascular access devices. Implanted ports are indicated for long-term or chronic therapies such as antineoplastic, inotropic, antimicrobial, and blood replacement therapies. An **implanted port** is a chambered device, containing either single or double reservoirs, with an attached silastic catheter (Figure 22–7 ■). The catheter may be a single- or a double-lumen catheter, depending on the configuration of the port. The catheter's tip is directed to dwell in a designated structure, which could be either vascular or nonvascular, depending on the intended infusion prescription.

Implanted ports are in their own category because of their unique physical structure, implantation procedures, clinical indications, and recommended lengths of dwell time. Typically, these devices are surgically placed either in the operating or radiology suite by physicians or advanced practice clinicians. The device is considered long term because it can remain in place for several years. It is inserted, or implanted, under the skin in a surgically designed pocket of skin, and placement of the port or reservoir portion is usually located over a bony surface to enhance port stability and facilitate access. When the port is not in use, it requires very little maintenance.

The port chamber, or reservoir, will have one or two chambers leading to either a single- or double-lumen catheter with the catheter tip located in the vena cava (Figures 22–8 and 22–9 ■).

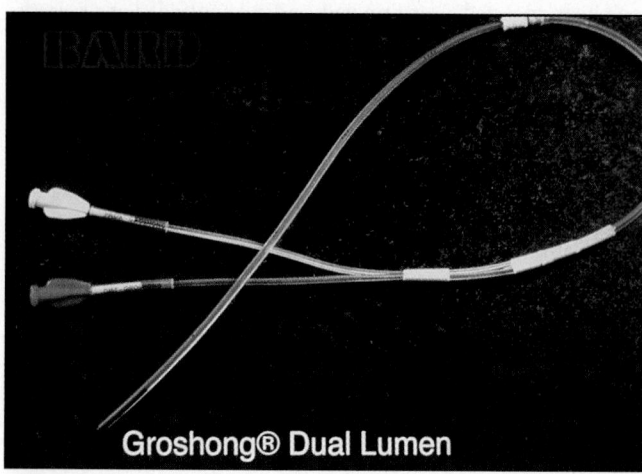

Groshong® Dual Lumen

FIGURE 22–6 ■ Tunneled and cuffed CVAD device.
Source: Courtesy of Bard Access Systems, Salt Lake City, UT

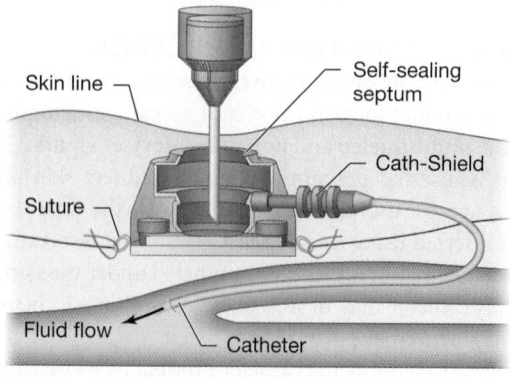

Skin line — Self-sealing septum
Cath-Shield
Suture
Fluid flow — Catheter

FIGURE 22–7 ■ Implanted port.
Source: Courtesy of Infusion Nurses Society, PICC Education Module, 2003.

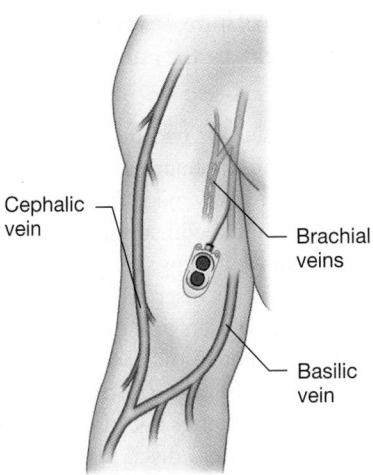

FIGURE 22–8 ■ Double-lumen implanted ports.
Source: Courtesy of Bard Access Systems, Salt Lake City, UT

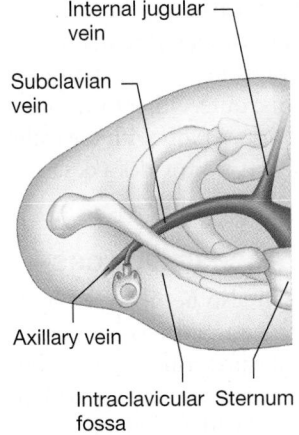

FIGURE 22–9 ■ Single-lumen implanted ports.
Source: Courtesy of Bard Access Systems, Salt Lake City, UT

The port is usually less than 1 inch in height and diameter. There also are low-profile ports that are smaller, less than 1/2 inch in height and width, allowing for placement in children or the inner aspect of the adult's upper arm or ventral surface of the forearm.

The septum is a key factor for optimal functioning of the port. The **septum** is the access point of the port and is usually made of highly compressed silicon. If the septum becomes damaged in any way, then the whole device must be surgically removed and replaced. The septum is designed to accommodate a **noncoring needle** (Figure 22–10 ■). The bevel of the noncoring needle opens on the *side* of the needle, preventing coring of the septum. Damaging the septum would allow leakage of infusate from the septum, placing the patient at potential risk for infiltration and extravasation, air embolism, and infectious processes. It would also cause the patient to face another surgical procedure in order to replace the port.

Removal of tunneled and cuffed catheters and implanted ports and reservoirs is performed by the physician or by advanced practice clinicians who are competent in performing the procedure, and are therefore not included within the scope of practice for most nurses.

In summary, CVADs are indicated for critical care and long-term therapies. These devices are used in all care settings such as hospitals; homes; long-term, rehabilitation, and subacute facilities; ambulatory infusion centers; and physicians' offices. Certain properties of solutions and medications mandate the use of CVADs to avoid damaging the sensitive peripheral vascular structures. Additionally, CVADs are useful for medications, such as inotropics and antineoplastic therapies, that are administered in cycles and over many months. Medications for chronic conditions or illnesses such as immunodeficiency diseases or genetic conditions such as cystic fibrosis are amenable to longer dwell infusion devices.

Specialized Infusion Catheters and Devices

Some VADs are indicated for hemodynamic monitoring in the critical care setting. These types of catheters are used exclusively

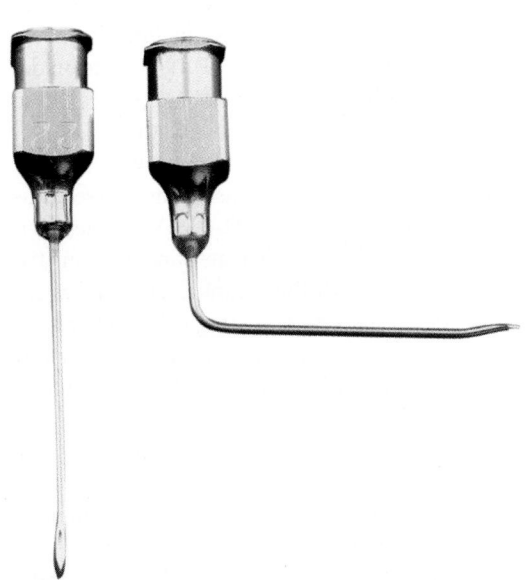

FIGURE 22–10 ■ Noncoring needles.
Source: Courtesy of Bard Access Systems, Salt Lake City, UT

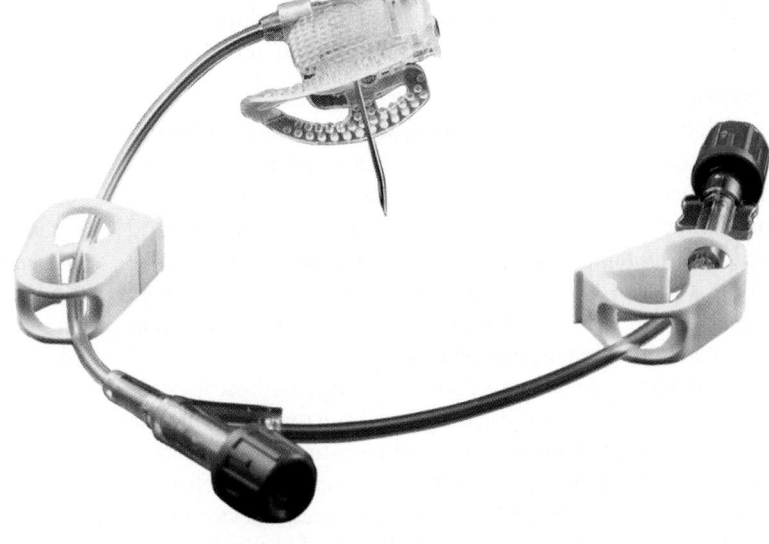

for cardiac monitoring and hemodynamic analyses. They have multiple lumens and are used to measure central venous pressure, pulmonary artery pressure and cardiac output, pulmonary wedge pressure, and temporary heart pacing and for parenteral administrations.

The most common is the pulmonary artery catheter, which is inserted into the pulmonary artery via the right atrium and ventricle. This device is indicated for patients in need of critical monitoring, such as those experiencing acute cardiac and respiratory failures. The brand name is **Swan-Ganz catheter**, named after the two physicians, Drs. Harold James Swan and William Ganz, who developed it. Chapter 24 ⊕ provides a complete description of the many uses and functions of pulmonary artery catheters.

Dialysis and Pheresis Catheters

Dialysis and pheresis catheters are rarely considered for routine infusion administrations. They are instead used for procedures where large volumes of blood need to be treated for specific medical indications. They may be inserted at the bedside or in the radiology or operating suite. The **dialysis catheter** is inserted and used for dialysis until a permanent shunt can be inserted. A **pheresis catheter** may be inserted for plasmapheresis procedures where large volumes of blood are filtered in attempts to remove undesired plasma components. The lumen of the catheter is large enough for blood flow in both directions, thereby facilitating flow through a dialysis or pheresis machine. Dialysis catheters that are inserted for temporary kidney dialysis are reserved for that function only due to the prevalence of high infection rates and problems associated with device occlusion. This also holds true for pheresis catheters. Pheresis and dialysis catheters are known by many brand names, including Quinton, Hohn, Tesio, and Perma-Cath. Pheresis catheters can be used interchangeably for infusions and pheresis procedures, again depending on patient condition, available vascular access, and the infusion prescription.

Both devices are available in silastic and polyurethane materials. The softer silastic devices are reserved for long-term dwell times. These catheters are generally shorter in overall length than typical tunneled and cuffed devices ranging in length from 7.5 to 20 cm (about 3 to 8 in.), and they have larger gauge sizes (12 to 16). The catheter tip resides in the vena cava allowing for high flow rates, which are necessary for fluid and blood volume exchange. Chapter 47 ⊕ provides a description of dialysis.

Arterial-Venous Shunts

Arterial-venous shunts are Gor-Tex or silicone-based devices that are used to anastomose venous and arterial structures, usually located in the arm, such as the radial artery and the cephalic or brachial veins. These shunts are used for specific infusion and exchange therapies and as VADs. When used for dialysis, the shunt is accessed with a large-bore needle. Occasionally these access devices can be used for other infusion therapies such as parenteral nutrition or fluid rehydration.

Assessment for patency is done by placing a stethoscope over the top of the shunt and listening for a bruit, or by placing the fingers of the hand over the site and palpating for a vibration feeling. If present, the shunt is patent. This is necessary when assessing the patient for additional vascular access device placement because no other VADs should be placed in the extremity with an AV shunt for fear of complication development such as infection, compromise and rupture of the shunt, and thrombo-

sis of the peripheral vasculature. If a shunt is damaged, surgical repair and/or replacement are the only options available.

Arterial Catheters

Arterial catheters are used for two primary indications: blood pressure monitoring and vascular access for obtaining blood samples. The catheter is usually made from stiff material such as polyurethane because it must withstand dwell time–limiting effects such as kinking and softening. Peripherally located arterial catheters are most commonly inserted into the radial artery and attached to pressure transducers and monitors. These catheters provide an ongoing assessment of blood pressure as well as access to arterial blood for laboratory testing. No medications are delivered through these catheters because that would cause severe injury to tissues and areas distal to the catheter insertion site. Chapter 24 ⊕ provides a complete description of the use and care of arterial catheters.

Hepatic Artery Catheters

The **hepatic artery catheter**, in contrast to the arterial catheters just discussed, is used to deliver specific, or targeted, antineoplastic therapy. Regionalized antineoplastic therapy is best delivered by this route. Other infusions may be attached to an implanted port or reservoir with the catheter tip positioned arterially. Chapter 46 ⊕ provides a description of the diagnosis and treatment of liver cancer.

Nonvascular Access Devices

Infusion therapy can also be delivered by nonvascular routes such as the subcutaneous, intraosseous, and intraspinal routes. Although many of the prescribed therapies are complicated, the catheter products used in conjunction with these modalities are the same as those used with vascular access.

Subcutaneous Infusion Therapy

Subcutaneous infusion therapy involves the infusion of parenteral solutions and medications via absorption through the subcutaneous tissues. The technique used to infuse a large amount of isotonic solutions in this manner is known as **hypodermoclysis**. Infusing smaller volumes such as medications prescribed for pain control or diabetes mellitus is known as **continuous subcutaneous infusions (CSI)**. The infusion devices are manufactured with extremely small gauge sizes (25 to 27 gauge) and are approximately 1/2 inch in length.

The needle may be positioned at a 90-degree angle and attached to an adhesive disk or may appear as a winged steel infusion set used for vascular access (Figure 22–11 ■). The device is inserted over an area where there is adequate subcutaneous tissue and capillary beds to absorb the infusate. These areas include the abdomen, outer aspects of the thigh and upper arm, and subclavicular and subscapular regions. These areas allow adequate visualization of the infusion site in addition to allowing the patient unfettered mobility.

Even though these are nonvascular insertion procedures, the nurse must prime the administration set and access device with the prescribed parenteral solution prior to initiation of therapy. The intended site is prepared with the appropriate antiseptic agent, allowed to dry, and the device inserted. The device must be aspirated with a syringe to confirm the absence of blood in the area of insertion. If no blood is found, then the device is se-

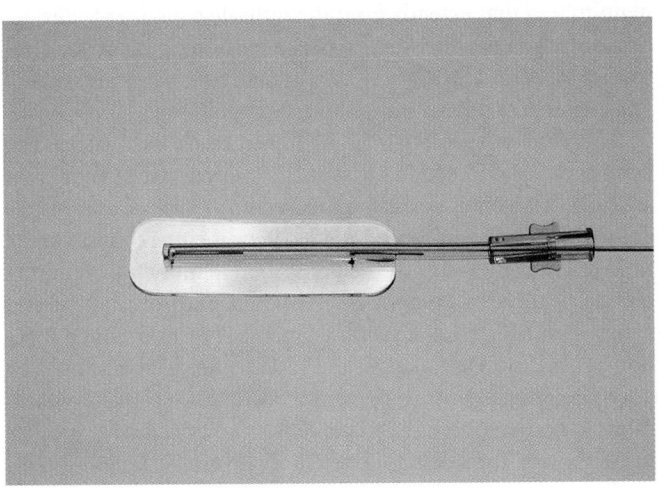

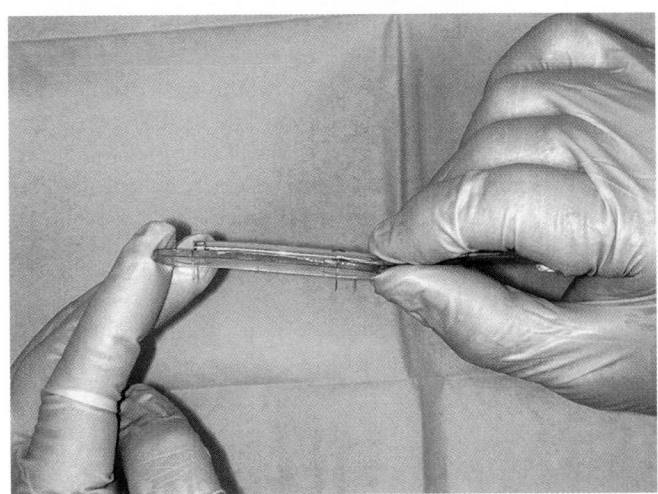

FIGURE 22–11 ■ Clysis infusion set.
Source: Aqua-C Hydration System. Courtesy of Norfolk Medical Products, Inc. Skokie, IL

cured with sterile dressing material and the infusion started. If blood is obtained, the device is removed and another infusion site selected and prepared. A new device is then readied and inserted, once again aspirating to confirm the absence of blood at the insertion site.

Common complications associated with this type of treatment are localized skin irritation including erythema and itching, infection, and dislodgment of the access device. Systemic complications are associated with the medication or solution being infused. Ineffective dosing may require another infusion site or route to be secured. Site rotation usually occurs every 3 to 5 days, depending on the concentration and rate of the fluid or medication being administered.

Hypodermoclysis has been found to be an effective treatment for older patients who require short-term isotonic fluid resuscitation to treat dehydration. Additional criteria for this treatment modality include fluid needs of less than 3 liters per day, no evidence of existing coagulopathies, and intact skin sites.

Intraosseous Therapy

Intraosseous therapy is the insertion of a hollow-bore needle into the bone, with the device tip accessing the marrow space. The tip of the needle is protected by an obturator, which has screw-like threads, facilitating penetration of the bony structure. The long bones of the leg or iliac crest are usually preferred in the pediatric patient, while the sternum has been used equally effectively in adults. Children less than 6 years of age and patients with thermal injuries, trauma, cardiac arrest, or other life-threatening illnesses can be treated in this manner until traditional vascular access can be obtained. Complications include bone fracture, infiltration, osteomyelitis, and cellulitis, in addition to occlusion of the obturator or needle and needle breakage. Emergent access of the bone core allows rapid infusion of large volumes of parenteral fluids and medications until vascular access can be obtained.

Intraspinal Catheters

Intraspinal catheters are located within the spinal spaces such as the epidural and intrathecal spaces. The intraspinal space has been used with great reliability for many procedures such as delivery of anesthesia, diagnostic testing, and infusions. Catheters

used for the intraspinal route have 22- to 26-gauge lumens and vary from 10 to 30 inches in length. They are made of biocompatible materials such as polyurethane and silastic. For temporary placement the catheter is inserted percutaneously into the desired spinal space and secured externally. For more stable long-term placement and as an infection control measure, the catheter can be tunneled to an isolated exit site.

Implanted infusion ports also can be used for intraspinal access. These are usually reserved for those patients with intractable pain who require lifelong pain control and who have a life expectancy of months to a year, or for those patients diagnosed with terminal cancer who require ongoing pain control. The device consists of a catheter whose tip is located in the epidural space. The catheter is attached to an infusion pump that is often implanted under the skin, in the vicinity of the abdominal region or chest wall. A blood return should never be obtained from these devices because the device tip is located in the epidural space where there should not be any blood. Additionally, epidural catheters should have a negative aspirate for spinal fluids because the epidural compartment does not communicate directly with the subarachnoid space, where the spinal cord resides.

Infusates, drugs, and diluents must be preservative free due to the neurotoxic effects of preserving agents. The epidural space can usually accommodate an infusion rate no greater than 15 mL/min due to limitations imposed by physical structures and restrictions of the epidural space. Medications and solutions given via this route have the ability to cross the dura mater, and have direct effects on the central nervous system (CNS). Complications such as infection and catheter malposition must be avoided through skilled manipulation of these infusion systems and observation of sterile technique. Surfactant-free filters on the administration system and alcohol-free skin antiseptic agents are used to prevent potential neurotoxic agents from entering the CNS.

Intrathecal Therapy

Intrathecal therapy involves the administration of medications directly into the cerebrospinal fluid (CSF) via an implanted reservoir system. The most common device, the **Ommaya reservoir**, allows delivery of medications directly into the CSF without relying on diffusion. Unlike epidural catheter systems where medications and solutions enter the CNS by diffusing across the dura mater, medications are injected directly into the CSF, permitting immediate therapy. The catheter attached to the reservoir terminates in the ventricular space of the cerebrum. Not all medications can pass the blood–brain barrier and target specific areas of the brain for treatment. The Ommaya reservoir is very effective for the following therapies:

- Delivering medications such as preservative-free opioids
- Administering selected antineoplastic agents such as methotrexate and cytarabine
- Measuring CSF pressures
- Draining excess CSF
- Obtaining CSF samples for laboratory assay.

The reservoir is surgically placed via a burr hole in the skull and the skin is secured over the device. Care and maintenance practices are dependent on the intended therapy, and standard precautions and sterile technique must be maintained. Complications are the same as those associated with intraspinal devices.

Infusion Delivery Systems

Vascular access devices are just one piece of the entire infusion delivery system. Fluid containers, administration sets, infusion flow control devices, and add-on devices also are integral components to effective therapy delivery.

Fluid Containers

Fluid containers are made of either glass or plastic. Glass containers allow for easy visualization and accurate recording of contents, but are heavy, bulky to store, and may break. Glass containers require a venting mechanism to be inserted into the container in order to facilitate solution delivery. Venting permits movement of air into the fluid container, facilitating flow of parenteral fluid. One such design is an *open airway*, in which a tube is attached to the inside of the bottle stopper. When the bottle is inverted, environmental air moves up the tube and displaces the fluid in the container. A vented administration set is not necessary. The second type of container, a closed system, does require a venting mechanism on the administration set. Air is allowed to access the bottle through a filter attached to the administration set spike.

Plastic containers are the preferred type of container because of easy portability, storage, and reduced manufacturing costs. Due to the flexibility of plastic containers, however, volume and dose administrations may be inaccurate. Plastic containers collapse as the fluid drains, which eliminates the need for vented administration sets. Plastic containers are highly amenable to fluctuations in temperature, which makes freezing of drugs post-admixture advantageous for availability and storage.

Administration Sets

The **administration set** is the tubing that delivers the parenteral fluid from the infusate container to the catheter that is in the patient's vein. *Primary* and *secondary sets* are terms used to describe the function of the set. The **primary set** is typically the main tubing that extends from the infusate container to the access device. It permits fluid passage by using gravity, an electronic infusion device set, or specialized microbore tubing attached to a syringe pump-delivery system.

Any extra equipment such as filters, stopcocks, extensions, connectors, and injection ports or caps added to the primary set are called **add-on devices** (see later section). The use of multiple add-on devices is not recommended because interruption in the fluid pathway increases the risk of system malfunction, inadvertent separation of component elements, and infusion-related complications such as air embolism and infection. All connections to the catheter adapter and for add-on devices should be Luer-Lok attachments to prevent inadvertent separation of administration equipment. A **Luer-Lok** is an attachment mechanism that is threaded to prevent inadvertent separation of equipment.

The **secondary set** is tubing that attaches to the primary set and permits additional infusion administrations. Typically, secondary sets are used to infuse medications and solutions that are administered on an intermittent basis, for example, every 4 hours. The secondary set is attached to a small bag of intravenous solution and then it is "piggybacked" into the primary set and hung up higher than the primary solution so it infuses instead of the primary solution (Figure 22–12 ■). When the bag is empty, the primary solution simply takes over again. Both the primary infusate and the secondary infusate must be compatible in order to prevent complications such as precipitate formation, which can result in occlusion of the fluid pathway.

The drip factor in either set can be described as macrodrip or microdrip, with the set being vented or nonvented. The **drip factor** is the number of drops that will equal 1 milliliter (mL) of infusate. Drip factor sizes vary from 10 to 60 drops/mL. A macrodrip calculation varies from 10 to 20 drops/mL and a microdrip is 60 drops/mL, depending on the manufacturer. This information is critical when calculating the exact amount of solution to be infused. Several formulas are used for fluid delivery calculations and these are dependent on drip factors, prescribed drug, and infusate solutions, as well as other parameters such as body surface area and weight.

Metered-volume chambered sets consist of an administration set topped with a metered, small-volume container that is attached to a fluid container (Figure 22–13 ■). Markings on the chamber vary from 1- to 5-mL increments. The use of this type of administration set is often seen in special patient populations, such as neonate and pediatric groups, in critical care units, and for those older adults with fluid control issues requiring close observation and monitoring. Metered-volume chambered administration sets also are often used with drugs and solutions that require significant control or intermittent delivery, with titrated medications, and for patients with fluid restrictions. Medications can be added to the chamber and diluted with the infusate, thereby not increasing the amount of fluid the patient is receiving.

Clamping mechanisms are features of administration sets that regulate the prescribed infusion rates (Figure 22–14 ■). *Roller clamps*, generally found on primary infusion sets, allow the nurse to regulate the parenteral fluid by either opening or closing the clamp. *Slide and pinch* clamps are not volume controlling, but instead provide an "on–off" feature to the set. These

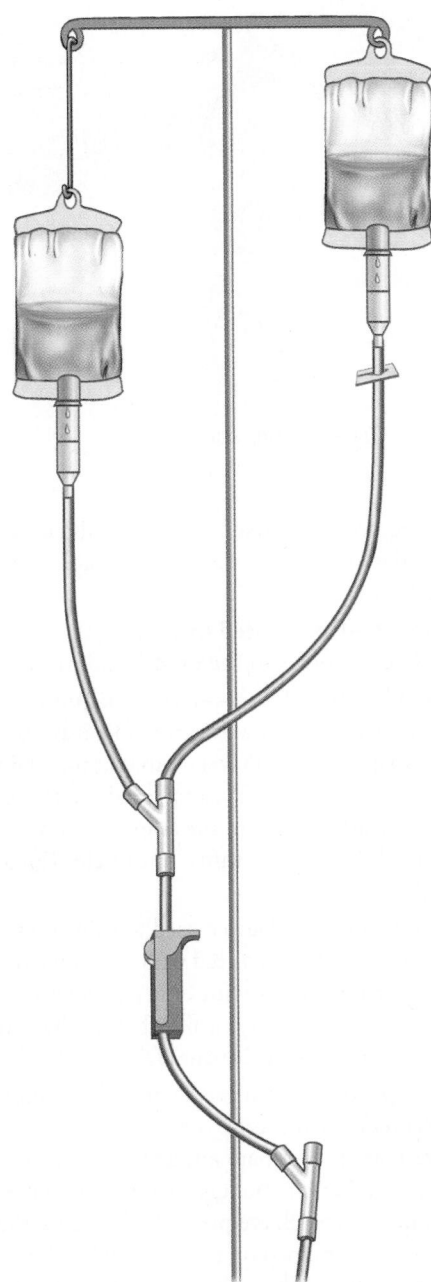

FIGURE 22–12 ■ Piggyback system.

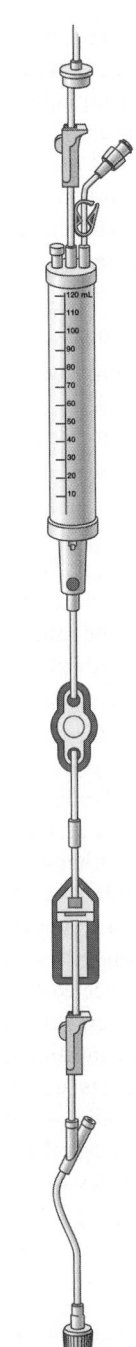

FIGURE 22–13 ■ Metered-volume chambered set.

clamps are seen often on add-on equipment and secondary sets. *Screw* clamps may also be found on administration sets and offer "on–off" and flow regulation functions comparable to those of roller clamps.

Flow Control Device

An add-on device that can be used for regulation of fluid administration is the **flow control device**. This device is added to a gravity infusion system at the point closest to the patient, and used to regulate fluid flow instead of using the clamp provided on the set. (A *gravity* infusion is one in which the infusion is regulated by hand and is affected by the container position above the patient and by patient activities.) At issue is the efficacy of calibrations and effective rate adjustments. Accuracy and consistency of infusion rates are affected by patient activity, height of the fluid container above the patient, and fluid composition and temperature.

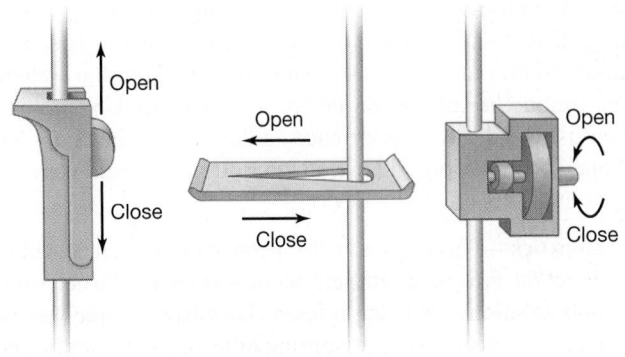

FIGURE 22–14 ■ Administration set clamps.

Once the flow rate is "dialed" or set, it is subject to wide variations in fluid delivery if the patient is ambulatory or the fluid container's height is adjusted. Clamping mechanisms do not negate the effect of close monitoring and fluid regulation by the nurse.

Some infusion products and medications, such as nitroglycerin, lipid emulsions, and blood products, have specific requirements associated with their delivery. Specialized administration sets are manufactured with features that meet these requirements, as discussed here:

- Nitroglycerin is incompatible with standard PVC tubing. Hence, nitroglycerin administration sets are manufactured from non-PVC materials. Also, nitroglycerin is admixed in glass containers for medication delivery to minimize drug loss.

- According to recent controversial reports, lipids are affected by containers and administration sets that contain DEHP (a *plasticizer* in manufacturing of articles made of polyvinyl chloride) (Hankins, Lonsway, Hedrick, & Perdue, 2001). Lipid emulsions are manufactured in glass containers. Due to the limited hang time for the infusion itself, researchers believe the limited contact with plastic tubing does not place the patient at risk (Hankins et al., 2001).

- Blood infusion sets are designed to accommodate the specific properties of blood and its components. Blood administration sets may have Y-shaped tubing and will contain filter systems to remove debris and accumulated by-products that result from blood storage. Other systems require the nurse to attach a separate filter product to a standard administration set. The Y-tubing permits a container of 0.9% sodium chloride to be connected to one access spike of the set and the blood container to be connected to the second access spike. Some sets can be used for gravity infusion while others are compatible with electronic infusion devices. When rapid infusion is indicated, some sets are equipped with an in-line hand pump. These sets should only be used in areas such as emergency departments, surgical suites, and intensive care units. Chapter 23 ⊕ provides a description of the blood administration procedure.

Add-on-Devices

Add-on devices are pieces of equipment that extend the efficacy of the existing administration set. Devices are added to the administration set either proximally at the spike end, or distally at the patient end. Devices can also be added at side ports along the administration set. Add-on devices are used to add length to the administration set, add filter infusates, and increase access to the patient's VAD. Add-on devices should contain a Luer-Lok feature to prevent accidental separation of the infusion system. The routine use of add-on devices is discouraged. Restricting their use will decrease occurrences of fluid contamination, accidental disconnection, and overall infusion supply costs. Here are some examples of add-on devices:

- **Stopcock**—This is a manually operated device that is used to direct the flow of an infusate. Stopcocks are used when multiple solutions are being infused. They have a three-way or four-way mechanism, permitting infusions to be connected at a common aperture, which is located at the VAD's hub. The

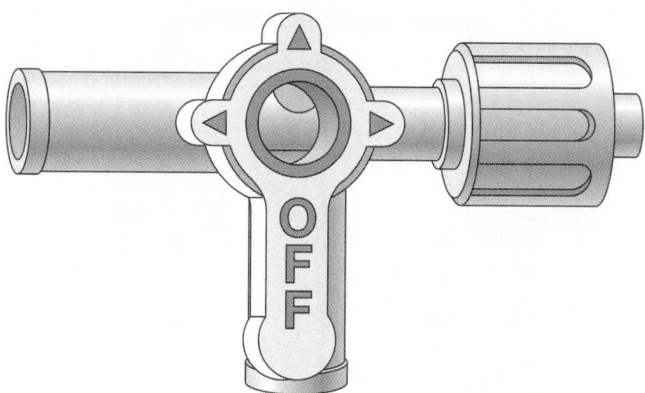

FIGURE 22–15 ■ Three-way stopcock.

stopcock requires the nurse to manually direct the infusion by turning the valve toward a specific infusion in order to initiate fluid flow (Figure 22–15 ■).

- **Extension set**—Device used to add length as well as additional side access ports to the existing administration set.

- **Multiflow adapter** and **Y set**—Devices used for administration of two or more infusates simultaneously. Access to the multiflow adapter is usually via a cap that maintains sterility of the fluid pathway. Each access of the adapter must be primed before attachment to the administration system and prior to attachment to the infusion catheter (Figures 22–16 and 22–17 ■).

- **Injection port or cap**—Device used to gain access to the indwelling catheter. Manufactured with resealable rubber caps, the device permits access with either needles or needleless safety infusion cannulas. Typically, they are lightweight and vary in length from 1/2 to 2 inches (Figure 22–18 ■).

- **Filter**—The purpose of filters is to provide sterility to the infused parenteral medications or solutions. Filters remove particulate matter, eliminate air, and retain or capture microorganisms. Filters are not used when certain medications, such as amphotericin B, are prescribed because the medication may become trapped on the filter bed and not reach the patient. Additionally, filters should not be used in line when administering IV push medications or very small volumes because these medications can also become trapped on the filter bed.

Infusion Delivery Devices

As discussed in the following sections, several methods other than gravity are used to enhance effective delivery of prescribed parenteral solutions. Note, however, that infusion delivery devices should never be used to replace nursing care, but as an adjunct to that care.

Mechanical Infusion Devices

Mechanical infusion devices (MIDs) are devices that do not require the use of an external power source to operate. MIDs are relatively easy to use and monitor, but the nurse should realize that they cannot detect flaws in the administration system such as air in the set, infiltration, or catheter occlusion.

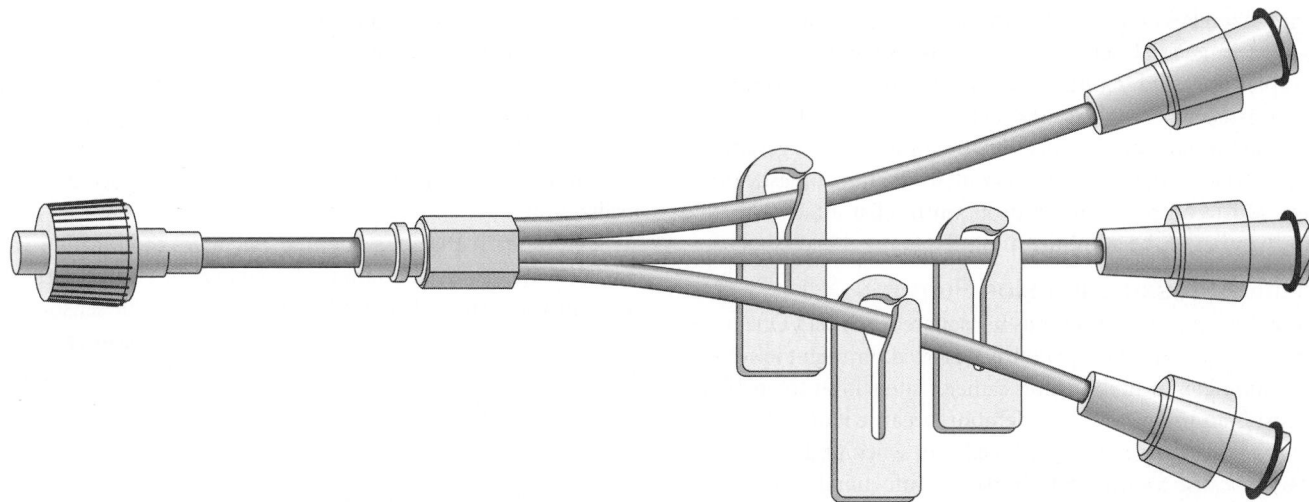

FIGURE 22–16 ■ Three-lumen multiflow adapter.

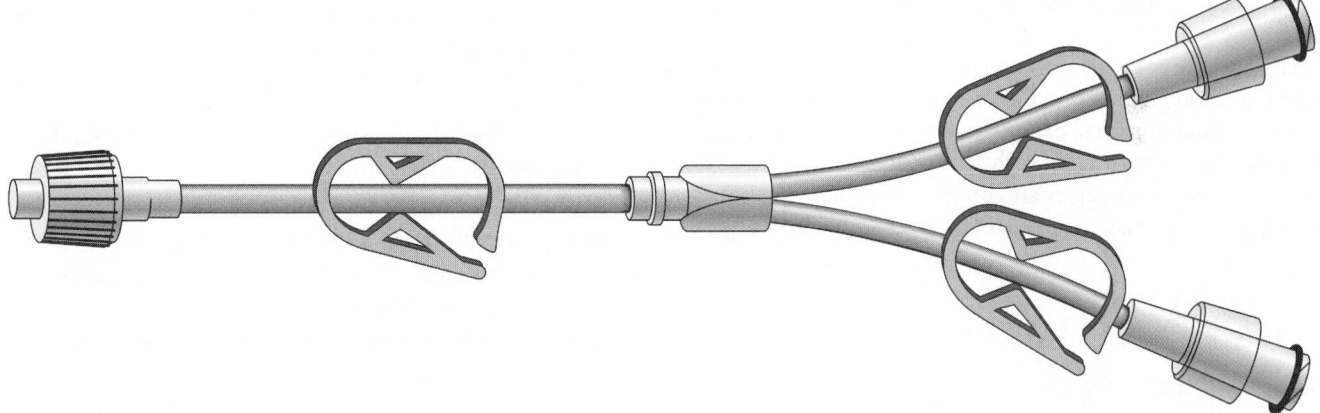

FIGURE 22–17 ■ (A) Two-lumen multiflow adapter.

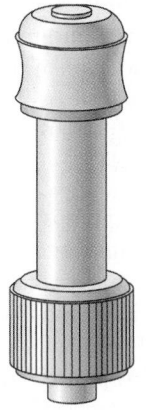

FIGURE 22–18 ■ Injection cap.

Mechanical infusion devices include these types:

- **Elastomeric balloons** are made of soft, expandable material contained within a transparent hard plastic casing. The prescribed medication is contained within the balloon-like container. Microbore tubing is attached to its outlet and, depending on its bore size, delivers the fluid at a corresponding rate over 30 minutes or more, depending on the volume

of the fluid. The small size of the tubing impedes the flow, preventing undue pressure on the patient's catheter. These MIDs are usually reserved for home care situations. These devices tend to be costly because they are a one-time-use product.

- The **spring-coil syringe** acts by powering the plunger of a syringe and delivering the medication to the patient. Once the syringe is empty, a new syringe must be fitted into the locking mechanism. This type of delivery system is more bulky than elastomeric balloons, and its function is relegated to a specific syringe size.

- The **spring-coil container** is a combination of the spring coil and a collapsible disk. The mechanism is activated by applying pressure on the top and bottom disk, causing collapse of the container and allowing its contents to infuse with flow being controlled by microbore tubing. Both the spring-coil syringe and container are used for small-volume parenteral administrations and are seen in acute and home care settings.

Electronic Infusion Devices

Electronic infusion devices (EIDs) can be divided into two categories, pumps and controllers. The *pump* is a device that delivers its solutions via positive pressure, whereas the *controller* is a device that relies on gravity to assist its action. A controller is often seen in general patient populations where uncomplicated therapies are used. Controllers usually do not contribute to infusion-related complications such as infiltration and vascular injury so they are safe for special populations such as geriatrics, neonates, pediatrics, and patients with most antineoplastic therapies. Most controllers use a drop sensor that attaches to the drip chamber of the administration set.

Positive Pressure Infusion Pump

Pressure is expressed in pounds per square inch (psi). One psi is equal to 50 mmHg. This pressure is exerted through the system and culminates at the infusion catheter site within the patient. The psi is an important consideration because it affects the integrity of the entire system and is a factor when undue infusion pressures cause a catheter to burst, an unfortunate and sometimes life-threatening complication of infusion therapy. Gravity-initiated pressures usually average around 2 psi if the infusate container is maintained approximately 60 cm (2 feet) above the patient's head. The higher the container, the greater the pressure exerted.

The **positive pressure infusion pump** creates pressure to infuse the fluid and overcome vascular resistance (Figure 22–19 ■). Pumps have psi parameters somewhere in the vicinity of 10 psi. Pumps are used in high acuity care areas such as critical care where the therapies are complex. Depending on hospital policy, pumps may be used in the general medical–surgical

areas or when medications are being delivered that require strict monitoring, such as anticoagulation, parenteral nutrition, and inotropic therapies. The pump delivers infusate at an accurate prescribed rate and has an alarm system that detects infusion-related errors of delivery such as free flow, air in the line, and changes in vascular resistance such as occlusion or infiltration.

A **volumetric pump** is one that calculates the infusion volume delivered by the amount displaced in a reservoir. Drop sensors can also be included in this pump category. The sensor may be located internally in the pump where the fluid passes through a chamber, but it is usually found externally attached to the drip chamber. Syringe pumps are infusion specific and are limited to small-volume parenterals such as anti-infectives or pain medications. Syringe pumps are unable to detect "no flow" unless significant back pressure is generated from the distal set or indwelling catheter.

Alarms on infusion delivery devices indicate pending disruptions in fluid delivery. Not all devices have comparable alarms or a full array of similar controls. In effect, these systems serve to protect the patient and alert the nurse to evaluate the patient and the patient's infusion system. The following are some alarm features:

- **Air in the line**—Detects the presence of air in the fluid pathway of the set.
- **Occlusion**—Infusion pumps detect disruption of flow above the catheter and resistance to flow occurring below the device.
- **Infusion complete**—This alarm sounds when a preset volume limit has been reached.
- **Free flow**—This alarm is *essential* for preventing the inadvertent bolus dosing of fluid or medications. The administration set, upon its removal from the EID, must have a self-clamping mechanism that prevents free flow of infusate. The alarm detects rapid infusion of fluid as a result of partial disengagement of the pumping mechanism.
- **Other alarms**—Alarms indicating low battery; nonfunctional; not infusing; door open; pressure capabilities; programming capabilities: rate, volume to be infused, and volume infused; ramping; and timed infusion are but a few of the alarms integral to EIDs.

Several types of infusion pumps are designed for very specific care settings or infusions. Ambulatory infusion pumps are lightweight and small enough to be easily carried. They may be attached to the patient's belt, contained within a backpack, or placed on a table top. The power supply is usually a disposable battery. **Patient-controlled analgesia (PCA) pumps** are available in ambulatory, semiportable, or pole-mounted versions. The PCA pump is capable of delivering medication continuously or on patient or clinician demand. **Multichannel** and **dual-channel pumps** are pole-mounted EIDs that can be operated by manufactured housing or channels within a single device. Each channel can be operated independently of each other. Different medications and solutions can be programmed for delivery at assigned times for predetermined doses via a single infusion pathway to the patient.

In addition to the type of VAD, the infusion prescription(s), and care setting, particular features of infusion delivery devices are highly important when selecting the appropriate device.

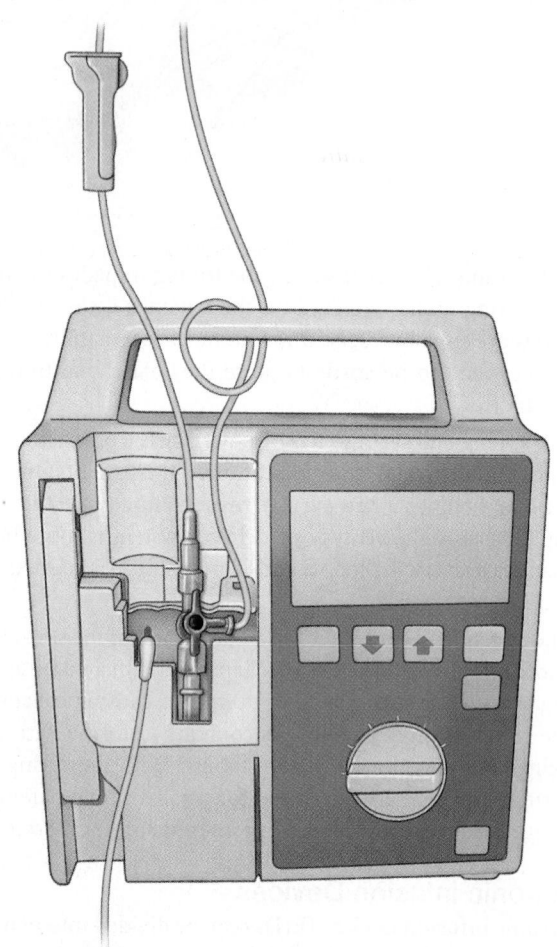

FIGURE 22–19 ■ Positive pressure pump.

Specific controls and alarm systems are integral to the infusion delivery device as safety measures for the patient and they also ensure accurate administration of solutions and medications. Infusion delivery devices are never to be considered a substitute for nursing care, but rather an adjunct. Monitoring and evaluation of response to therapy, in addition to effective care and maintenance strategies for the infusion patient, will provide the foundation for positive outcomes.

Infusion Nursing Practice

Competency and skill validation are required for nurses providing infusion therapy in order to be proficient in its technical aspects, demonstrate competency in clinical judgment, and practice in accordance with their state's nurse practice act. Basic competencies are intended to serve as guidelines and define the knowledge, skill, and abilities necessary to fulfill the expectations of the nurse practicing infusion therapy. Clinical skill validation and competency are vital to health care organizations that participate in annual reviews to ensure that their policies and procedures agree with those of regulatory and nonregulatory agencies (Infusion Nurses Society [INS], 2006b).

Calculations

Infusion therapy is ordered by the health care provider or by a legally authorized prescriber. It is the responsibility of the nurse to be knowledgeable about the drugs' and solutions' properties, intended outcomes, and potential side and adverse effects that may occur. Although many formulations are available for deriving correct dosing volumes and amounts, certain methods are relatively easy to use and are used consistently.

Keep in mind that certain patient conditions and patient populations (i.e., pediatric and geriatric patients and patients receiving antineoplastic or antimicrobial therapies) have specific restrictions and requirements based on body surface area, weight, and age. Medication error reduction and patient safety should remain in the forefront of nursing practice when administering infusion therapies. The nurse should be skilled and knowledgeable about the Joint Commission's approved abbreviations and medication ordering procedures.

Flow rate determination is used to calculate the amount of fluid to be delivered over a specific time period. Flow rates can be ordered as milliliters per hour or minute, total volume over a set period such as multiple hours or a 24-hour period, or number of drops per minute. The nurse must be knowledgeable of the available drop factor of the administration sets on hand and select the most appropriate for the infusion prescription.

One simplified order conversion technique is to divide the milliliter rate per hour by a specific number associated with the drop factor. The formula and an example are given in Chart 22–1. Consistent use and knowledge of the variety of calculations associated with accurate dosing and therapy administration criteria will result in safe nursing practice for the clinician, fewer medication errors, increased patient safety, and positive infusion outcomes.

Infusion Nursing Standards of Practice

Standards of practice enable those outside of a profession to measure a practitioner's performance; thus, standards protect

---

CHART 22–1 **Infusion Rate Calculation Formula**

Example: The flow rate of therapy is ordered at 120 mL per hour via gravity. The administration set on hand has a drip factor of 15 gtts/mL. To calculate drops per minute:

$$\frac{120\ (mL/hr)\ \times\ 15\ (gtt\ factor)}{60\ (time\ in\ minutes)} = 30\ drops\ per\ minute$$

Typically the 30 is divided by 4 and the nurse counts the number of drops in 15 seconds.

---

both patients and practitioners. Standards of practice focus on the provider and define the activities and behavior needed to achieve patient outcomes. They are consistent with valid research findings, national norms, legal guidelines, and complement expectations of regulatory agencies. The goal of the *Infusion Nursing Standards of Practice* is to preserve the patient's right to safe, quality care, and protect the nurse who administers infusion therapy (INS, 2006a). The INS standards define the criteria relative to nursing accountability in the delivery of infusion therapies. They provide a framework to use in evaluating patient outcomes and are used as a mechanism for evaluating the quality of patient care and the competency of the nurse delivering infusion therapy. The INS standards are applicable in all practice settings, such as hospitals, homes, long-term care facilities, and physician offices. Therefore, nurses are accountable for adherence to them regardless of the care setting.

National guidelines are also incorporated into infusion practice. An example related to infusion nursing is the *CDC Guidelines for the Prevention of Intravascular Catheter-Related Infections* (Centers for Disease Control and Prevention [CDC], 2002). This publication provides recommendations that, when incorporated in practice, are designed to reduce infectious complications associated with infusion therapy (see the National Guidelines box).

Required Order and Informed Consent

Before initiation of any type of infusion therapy, the nurse must obtain an order from a health care provider. A medication order needs to include the type of medication or solution, dose of the medication, volume to be infused, duration of therapy, frequency, rate, and route of administration. An order must also be obtained to discontinue infusion therapy. For example, in infusion therapy, informed consent would be obtained prior to inserting a PICC.

NATIONAL GUIDELINES Prevention of Intravascular Catheter-Related Infections

The CDC's guidelines for the prevention of intravascular catheter-related infections were developed for practitioners who insert catheters and for persons responsible for surveillance and control of infections in hospital, outpatient, and home health care settings. A complete copy of the guidelines can be found at http://www.cdc.gov/ncidod/dhqp/gl_intravascular.html.

Source: Centers for Disease Control and Prevention. (2002). *CDC Guidelines for the Prevention of Intravascular Catheter-Related Infections.* Retrieved June 12, 2008, from http://www.cdc.gov/ncidod/dhqp/gl_intravascular.html.

The nurse would provide the patient with accurate and complete information, including a description of the procedure, potential benefits of such a device, possible risks associated with the procedure, and available alternatives. The consent must reflect the patient's voluntary agreement and understanding of the procedure.

Patient Assessment

Patient assessment is an ongoing process to determine the appropriateness of the therapy and ensure desired patient outcomes. The results of the initial assessment identify the baseline for the patient's care and treatment. Ongoing assessment chronicles the patient's response to treatment and provides data to measure outcomes. Pertinent information obtained during assessment and monitoring should be communicated to other health care professionals responsible for the patient's care.

Patient assessment should include the patient's past and present medical history, including diagnosis, medical and surgical histories, age, allergies, vascular access history, and patient preferences regarding VAD types and site locations. Prior to initiation, the prescribed therapy should be assessed for appropriate dose, route, and rate of infusion; potential incompatibilities among infusates, oral medications, and food; and appropriateness of the care setting.

Because infusion therapy is directly related to the patient's fluid volume and electrolyte status, reviewing laboratory data is an important component of the assessment process. Necessary components of the process include, but are not limited to, the patient's electrolytes, serum proteins, blood chemistries, and renal function tests. Clinical assessment of the patient may include height and weight, body surface area, nutritional status, pain threshold, skin turgor, vital signs, intake and output, and vascular access integrity.

The type and frequency of patient monitoring will be determined by the prescribed therapy, access device, patient's condition and age, and care setting. In addition, the nurse must monitor the catheter–skin junction site and surrounding area, flow rate, clinical data, patient response, side effects, and the patient's compliance with the prescribed therapy.

Hand Hygiene

Because of the inherent risks associated with the invasive nature of infusion therapy, knowledge of infection control principles is essential for minimizing and preventing complications from infection. Hand hygiene is a fundamental practice that reduces the transmission of pathogenic microorganisms. Hand hygiene should be done before and after performing patient care procedures, and before donning and after removal of gloves. The use of gloves does not preclude the need to perform hand hygiene. Acceptable products for decontaminating hands include antiseptic soap and water as well as waterless alcohol-based gels and foam (Boyce & Pittet, 2002; O'Grady et al., 2002).

Site Selection

Vein selection for cannulation will need to accommodate the gauge and length of the catheter. Site selection is based on the patient's condition, age, and diagnosis; the vein condition, size, and location; the type and duration of prescribed therapy; and the patient's history. Veins that should be considered for peripheral cannulation are those found on the dorsal and ventral surfaces of the upper extremities including the metacarpal, cephalic, and basilic veins (see Figure 22–1 ■, p. 513). Use of veins of the lower extremities of adults should be avoided due to the risk of embolism and thrombophlebitis formation.

Site selection should be routinely initiated in the distal areas of the upper extremities with subsequent cannulations made proximal to previous cannulated sites. Areas of flexion should be avoided, except when placing a ML catheter or PICC. Also, avoid veins in arms with compromised circulation, postmastectomy or postaxillary node dissection, or fistulated extremities as potential venipuncture sites.

Assess vascular access by applying a tourniquet 10 to 20 cm (4 to 8 in.) proximal to the intended venipuncture site. Palpate the extremity to assess the condition of the vein. An appropriate vein for venipuncture will feel soft and bouncy. A hard, cordlike feeling indicates a sclerosed or compromised vein. Valves can be detected by a hard lump or "knot-like" feeling. Resilient veins that are easily depressed are required for successful venipuncture. Palpation also differentiates arteries from veins, because veins do not pulsate.

Site Preparation

While adhering to standard precautions during site preparation, disinfect the skin with an antiseptic solution before catheter insertion. Apply the agent using friction and allow it to dry thoroughly before making the venipuncture. Fanning, blowing, or blotting the prepared area is contraindicated. Agents recommended for skin preparation include 2% chlorhexidine-based solutions, 1% to 2% tincture of iodine, 10% povidone-iodine, or 70% alcohol as single agents or in combination preparations.

Dressings

Dressings are used to protect the catheter from external environmental contamination. Sterile dressings should be aseptically applied at the initiation of vascular access, when the integrity of the dressing is compromised, and at specified time intervals determined by organizational policy and procedure. Dressings should not be reinforced if they become damp, loose, or visibly soiled, but replaced with new dressing materials. Types of dressings include the following:

- Gauze and tape dressings can be used to cover the venipuncture site. To adequately assess the catheter–skin junction and monitor for development of complications, a gauze dressing needs to be changed according to hospital protocol.

- Transparent semipermeable membrane (TSM) dressings facilitate daily catheter–skin junction inspection without disruption of the therapy, and allow direct observation of the insertion site. For peripheral-short catheter sites, a TSM dressing should be changed at the time of catheter site rotation and immediately if the integrity of the dressing is compromised. For other VADs, the TSM dressing should be changed per protocol or if the dressing has lost its integrity. It is not recommended that topical ointments be placed on the insertion site, because their efficacy at reducing infections is not proven (O'Grady et al., 2002).

Research supporting the choice of dressings is limited, and evidence does not support one choice over the other. In a systematic review of controlled trials that compared the effects of gauze and tape with transparent dressings, there was no evidence of differences in the incidence of infectious complications between dressing types. Because the studies were from small samples, however, the authors recommend the need for more research (Gillies et al., 2003).

Antiseptic dressings, such as the chlorhexidine-impregnated foam dressing, are being used more frequently. A small, round disk is placed around the catheter at the exit site, covered with a transparent dressing. In a meta-analysis published by Ho and Litton in 2006, chlorhexidine-impregnated dressings were found to be effective in reducing bacterial colonization at vascular sites, although they were also identified with a trend toward catheter-related bloodstream infections. As more research becomes available, it will be important that nurses evaluate the technology and incorporate that which will make a positive impact in patient care.

Catheter Securement

Catheters are to be stabilized so as not to interfere with assessment and monitoring of the site or impede delivery of the prescribed therapy. Devices used to secure and stabilize catheters include sterile tapes, sterile surgical strips, and sterile manufactured stabilization devices. Minimizing catheter movement helps prevent mechanical irritation to the vein lining and reduces the risk of phlebitis formation. When feasible, using a manufactured stabilization device is preferred, because it prevents the catheter from telescoping within the vein or becoming dislodged (INS, 2006a).

Flushing

Flushing, which is the infusion of a sterile solution, is performed to ensure and maintain patency of the VAD and to prevent mixing of incompatible medications and solutions. Routine flushing should be performed in the following situations:

- Administration of blood and blood components
- Sampling of blood
- Administration of incompatible medications or solutions
- Intermittent therapy
- Converting the VAD from continuous to intermittent therapies.

Patency flushing is performed at established intervals determined by organizational policy and procedure and the patient's condition. Acceptable flush solutions are saline (preservative-free 0.9% sodium chloride, injection) and heparin in the lowest concentration to achieve patency, while not affecting the patient's clotting factors. Many organizations flush intermittent peripheral devices with 0.9% sodium chloride solution only. Most studies that have compared the use of normal saline versus heparin recommend normal saline for use with peripheral VADs (Hankins et al., 2001). The volume of the flush should be equal to two times the volume capacity of the catheter plus any add-on devices that are attached to the system.

The equipment being used will dictate the correct flushing procedure. If positive pressure is to be exerted to prevent reflux of blood in the catheter lumen, then a forward motion is applied to the syringe plunger as it is removed from the injection port, or the clamping mechanism on the device is activated prior to removal of the syringe.

An occluded or partially occluded catheter should never be forcibly flushed to restore patency because of the potential risk of embolizing the contents into the patient's circulation. The size of the syringe must be considered, because the smaller the syringe, the greater the pressure exerted on the catheter. Excessive pressure may cause the catheter or the vessel to rupture.

Compatibility flushing is accomplished by using 0.9% sodium chloride solution before and after medication administration. Flushing the catheter should prevent incompatible medications and solutions from forming precipitates that can occlude the device. When heparin is used to complete the flushing procedure, *SASH* criteria are used, as outlined in Chart 22–2.

Documentation

Accurate documentation in the patient's medical record objectively describes the care rendered and the patient's response. It also allows for tracking patient outcomes and monitoring care. Chart 22–3 (p. 528) lists the pertinent information that should be documented when an infusion therapy-related procedure has been performed

■ Complications Associated with Infusion Therapy

Due to the invasive nature of infusion therapy, there is a risk for the development of complications that range from minor to severe problems. Complications increase hospital stays, length of therapy, cost of treatment, and nursing responsibilities, and can put the patient at risk for other medical problems. Most infusion-related complications are preventable, but knowledge and understanding of the risks involved with infusion therapy and the use of measures to prevent their occurrence can eliminate many of the problems associated with this treatment. If appropriate interventions are not implemented in a timely manner to treat serious complications, death can result.

Complications associated with infusion therapy are classified by their location. Local complications are generally recognized at the site of venipuncture or occur as a result of mechanical failure. Timely recognition and nursing intervention can often prevent escalation into more serious occurrences. Systemic complications are defined as those that occur within the vascular system distant from the venipuncture site. Although these complications are less common than local complications, they are often more difficult to treat. Prevention of complications is a primary responsibility of the nurse caring for the infusion patient.

CHART 22–2 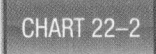 **Intermittent VAD Flushing: The SASH Criteria**

S: Saline

A: Administer medication/solution

S: Saline

H: Heparin (if necessary)

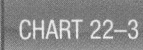

CHART 22–3 Documentation for Insertion and Removal of VADs

- Patient consent and education
- Variations in the procedure such as patient sensitivity or allergy to preparatory agents, latex, or securement adhesives
- Use of anesthetics for preprocedure medications
- Size, length, and type of catheter
- Name of vein used for access and number of insertion attempts (successful and unsuccessful)
- Securement method and dressing
- Administration set, extension equipment, and access caps used
- Flush or infusate initiation
- Patient's response to the procedure
- Name and title of the nurse

Similar documentation should occur when a VAD is removed including:

- Patient consent and education
- Size, length, and type of catheter and condition (e.g., was the catheter intact or fractured upon removal?)
- Condition of the venipuncture site (evidence of erythema, drainage, bleeding, skin tears)
- Dressing materials applied
- Patient's response to the procedure
- Name and title of the nurse

Local Complications

Local complications are usually associated with mechanical failure of the infusion system or traumatic injury to the vasculature. Mechanical difficulties may lead to the inability to deliver or infuse solutions and medications to the patient as prescribed. Trauma to the vasculature may occur with unskilled venipuncture techniques, patient agitation, and noncompliance with infusion therapy. The injured vein will become edematous as a result, which can lead to interruption in the infusion prescription, tissue injury, phlebitis, thrombus formation, and possibly sepsis.

Mechanical Complications

Mechanical complications usually are the result of failure of the infusion administration system to deliver the prescribed therapy, as opposed to the venous access. They are typically the most easy to identify and correct. Areas to be evaluated when determining the causal factors include the patient and the cannulated extremity, the venipuncture site, the catheter, the administration set, and the infusate container and its contents.

The patient's extremity should be checked for constricting clothing, identification bands or bracelets, jewelry, tapes, physical positioning, and restraints. The catheter–skin junction at the venipuncture site and the immediate surrounding area should be assessed for swelling that can impede flow. Verification of catheter placement should be confirmed prior to initiation and periodically throughout the infusion period. A catheter that is inserted so that the tip is against a valve or venous bifurcation may impede the infusion by slowing or stopping the flow. The catheter may become dislodged, bent, or kinked due to patient activity or inadequate device securement.

Placement of a catheter in an area of flexion may adversely affect the infusion rate and the dwell time of the device. If the flow rate slows or increases, the catheter can be stabilized by applying an armboard. The use of restraints and armboards needs to be in accordance with the organization's policies.

Administration sets can easily be pinched, bent, kinked, or crimped. The infusion pathway will be affected and not allow delivery of fluid from the infusion container to the patient. In-line filters or add-on equipment may become clogged due to undissolved medications or precipitate formation from the introduction of incompatible medications into the administration system.

The infusate container and its contents need to be assessed as a contributing factor of mechanical failure. Inadequate height of the fluid container in relation to the patient and catheter insertion site can adversely affect gravity flow, or an empty container can lead to diminished flow or cessation of flow. Rigid containers, such as those made from glass, should be checked for the presence of a venting mechanism. Soft, flexible plastic containers do not need to be vented. The entry port on a container must be completely penetrated in order for the solution to infuse into the patient. Refrigerated solutions need to be brought to room temperature prior to administration. Cold infusates not only cause discomfort for the patient but also may cause venospasm resulting in vasoconstriction and decrease or cessation of flow.

Catheter-Related Complications

Complications related specifically to the vascular access device versus those related to the infusion system and infusate are readily identifiable. Addressing catheter-related complications should begin with the evaluation of the inserter's skill and technique.

Bruising

Bruising (skin discoloration due to infiltration of blood into the subcutaneous tissue) may be attributed to unskilled insertion technique, tourniquet placement (too tight), vigorous device securement and restraining techniques, or preexisting poor skin integrity. For example, patients who are prescribed long-term steroid or anticoagulant therapies are more susceptible to bruising.

Bruising may be particularly notable after multiple attempts at device insertion during a prescribed therapy period. These injuries adversely impact future visualization of intended venipuncture sites. Bruising may predispose the patient to development of cellulitis and other localized infections. The term *ecchymosis* is used to define generalized bleeding into the tissues, whereas *hematoma* describes uncontrolled bleeding at the venipuncture site that usually creates a hard painful lump (Figure 22–20 ■).

Infiltration

Infiltration, as mentioned earlier, is the inadvertent administration of nonvesicant solutions or medications into surrounding tissues. It is manifested by swelling either along the venous pathway or generally located around the venipuncture site (Figure 22–21 ■). The patient may complain of "heaviness" or coldness in the extremity, or may observe generalized swelling. The patient may realize that he cannot remove a ring or other piece of jewelry or cannot close the hand. The extremity will appear enlarged with the skin appearing stretched or shiny. The venipuncture site dressing may appear taut.

The amount of discomfort experienced by the patient is proportional to the type of infusate, rate of infusion, and infusion

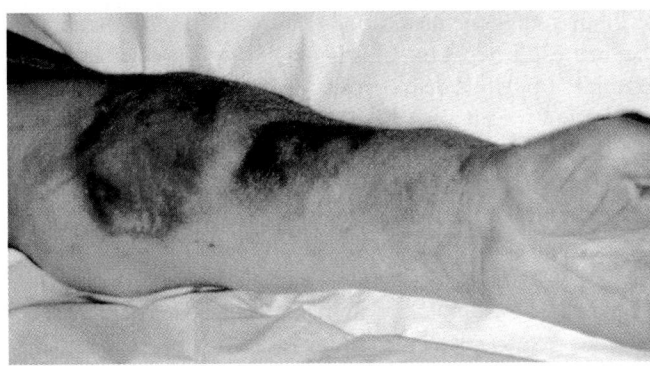

FIGURE 22–20 ■ Hematoma.
Source: Johnson & Johnson—Ethicon Inc.

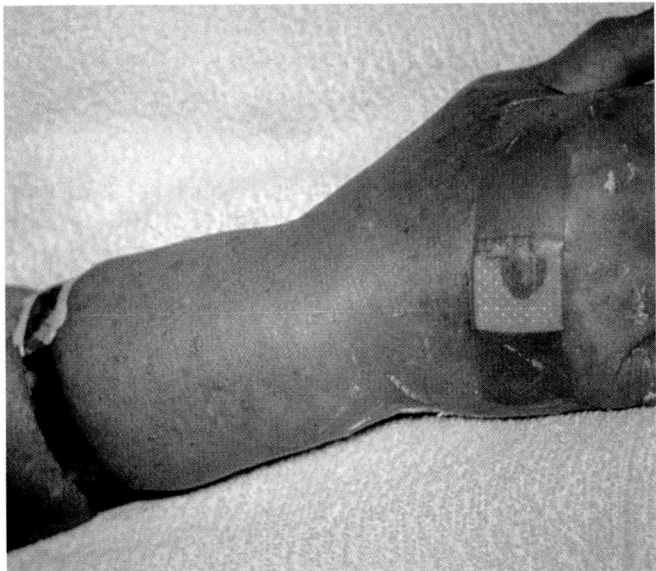

FIGURE 22–21 ■ Intravenous infiltration.
Source: Johnson & Johnson Medical, Inc. 1997. Used by permission of the copyright owner

history. Isotonic solutions generally do not produce much discomfort when an infiltration occurs. Solutions with acidic or alkaline pH or those that are slightly more hypertonic are more irritating and usually cause discomfort (Hankins et al., 2001). If left undetected, infiltration may cause compression of pressure-sensitive tissues such as neurological and arterial structures.

A complete assessment of the patient, the venipuncture site and surrounding area, the involved extremity, and the infusion system may be necessary to determine the presence of an infiltration. The site around the tip of the catheter and the extremity should be inspected for swelling, blanching, stretched skin, firm tissues, and coolness. It may be helpful to compare the site with the same area on the opposite extremity. If both extremities appear edematous, the patient's medical status should be evaluated.

In determining the presence of an infiltration, pressure should be applied to the vein with a finger or tourniquet about 5 cm (2 in.) proximal to the insertion site. If the catheter is in the vein, manual pressure will slow or stop the infusion. If the infusion continues despite venous obstruction, an infiltration has occurred.

If infiltration is noted or suspected, discontinue the infusion immediately and remove the catheter. Elevation of the affected extremity relieves patient discomfort and assists in absorption of excess fluids and improving circulation.

Preventive measures can minimize the severity of the infiltration. When inserting a VAD, areas of flexion should be avoided if possible. The catheter should be secured adequately and the site protected from excessive movement or pressure by use of an armboard or restraint.

 **CRITICAL ALERT** *Be aware that despite the presence of a positive blood aspirate, an infiltration may have occurred. Remove the VAD immediately and restart it, preferably in the opposite extremity.*

Extravasation

Extravasation is the inadvertent administration of a vesicant solution or medication into the surrounding tissues. The solution produces tissue damage by causing blister-like formations with subsequent tissue sloughing (Figure 22–22 ■). Initially the patient may complain of pain or burning along the vein pathway or at the venipuncture site. Fluid can also seep into adjacent tissues as it passes through a previous proximal venipuncture site.

Tissue sloughing may take several weeks to occur as it progresses from edema and erythema to necrosis. Necrosis may involve not only superficial skin layers but may penetrate into basement supporting tissues, muscles, tendons, and bones. The severity of the injury is related to the type, concentration, and volume of the medication or solution infiltrated. This is an adverse condition that could severely impact the future of the patient, resulting in loss of the extremity, prolonged hospitalization, protracted treatments involving surgery and rehabilitation, and potentially loss of life.

When an extravasation is suspected, discontinue the infusion immediately and remove the catheter. Treatment protocols established in written policies and procedures are initiated and a new site is established, preferably in the opposite extremity or in a site above and away from the extravasated site.

Prevention is the key in minimizing extravasation episodes. Only qualified, skilled nurses who have demonstrated proficiency and knowledge in infusion therapy along with knowledge of medications that have the potential for causing injury should be allowed to administer vesicant medications. The venipuncture site must be observed for signs of pending extravasation prior to, during, and after the infusion treatment. Many organizations require

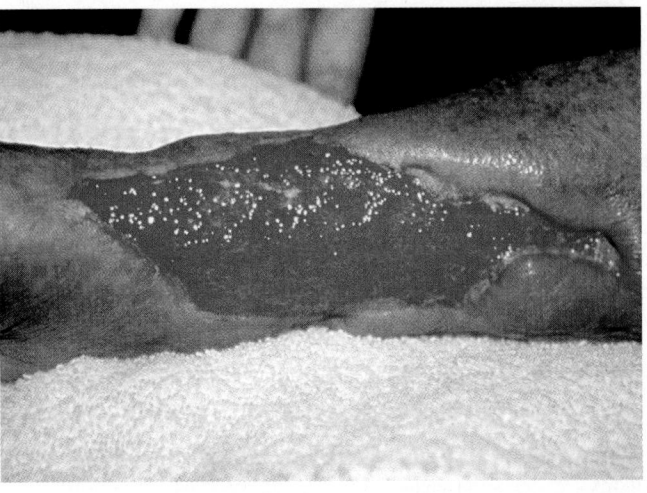

FIGURE 22–22 ■ Extravasation.
Source: Johnson & Johnson Medical, Inc. 1997. Used by permission of the copyright owner

that a new VAD be placed prior to the administration of vesicants in order to avoid questionable patency issues.

If a vesicant medication is delivered directly into a vein via a syringe, the patency of the catheter should be ascertained intermittently throughout the infusion by gently pulling back on the syringe plunger to confirm the presence of a blood return. The catheter should be appropriately secured so as to prevent movement in the vein, while allowing for frequent visualization of the site and venous pathway throughout the administration procedure. Areas of flexion, bony prominences, and the hands should be avoided as access sites for vesicant therapies. Consideration should be given to the possibility of using a CVAD for vesicant therapies given the chronicity of many antimicrobial, inotropic, or antineoplastic therapies.

 CRITICAL ALERT *Continuous observation of the venipuncture site is necessary prior to, during, and after administration of a vesicant. Have knowledge of the protocols needed to treat an extravasation.*

Phlebitis

Phlebitis is defined as an inflammation of the vein's tunica intima (Figure 22–23 ■). It is a common catheter-related complication that is often associated with erythema along the venous pathway, discomfort and tenderness of varying intensities, and inflammation and warmth at the site. Causes of phlebitis include:

- Inappropriate catheter length, gauge, or material
- Inexperience at insertion by the nurse
- Inappropriate site selection
- Prolonged dwell time for the catheter
- Ineffective device securement
- Chemical properties of the infusate(s)
- Patient age, infusion history, compliance, existing disease, or conditions.

Phlebitis can be classified by causative factors: chemical, mechanical, bacterial, and post-infusion phlebitis.

Chemical phlebitis is often associated with infusates with varying ranges of pH values or osmolarities. Improper admixing or dilution of some medications can result in incompatibilities that may cause irritation. Infusion rates may cause irritation. For example, rapid fluid delivery can cause a higher concentration of medication within a localized area, resulting in poor or inadequate hemodilution leading to inflammation. Particulate matter has been demonstrated to cause irritation of the vein wall.

Mechanical phlebitis is primarily associated with the catheter, its insertion, and the selected site. Using areas of flexion and too large a gauge size for the intended vein and prescribed therapy can result in the development of mechanical phlebitis. Poor device securement allows telescoping of the catheter within the vein. Patient noncompliance insofar as unrestricted physical activity will enhance the development of phlebitis. The skill of the nurse inserting the device may contribute to the development of mechanical phlebitis.

Bacterial phlebitis is associated with infectious processes. It is a very serious condition because it may progress to a systemic infection that is potentially life threatening. Hand hygiene and the observance of aseptic techniques throughout the catheter insertion procedure are mandatory for the prevention of catheter- and infusion-related infections. All infusion-related equipment must be inspected prior to use to confirm product integrity and detect any presence of contaminants. Expiration dates, damaged packaging, particulate matter, and presence of color or cloudiness are signs that may indicate compromised products. Appropriate site selection and preparation reduces the opportunity for catheter-related infections to occur. Shaving the intended venipuncture site is not recommended because of the potential to cause microabrasions that would allow for the entry of microorganisms into the circulation. If hair removal is necessary, clipping should be performed.

Postinfusion phlebitis is commonly seen 2 to 4 days after the catheter has been removed. Occurrence is often attributed to the original insertion technique, patient condition, condition of the vein that was cannulated, the properties of the infusate that was delivered, size and length of the catheter, and the dwell time of the device. It is recommended that the identification of phlebitis be standardized and classified according to the phlebitis scale (Chart 22–4) published in the *Infusion Nursing Standards of Practice* (INS, 2006a).

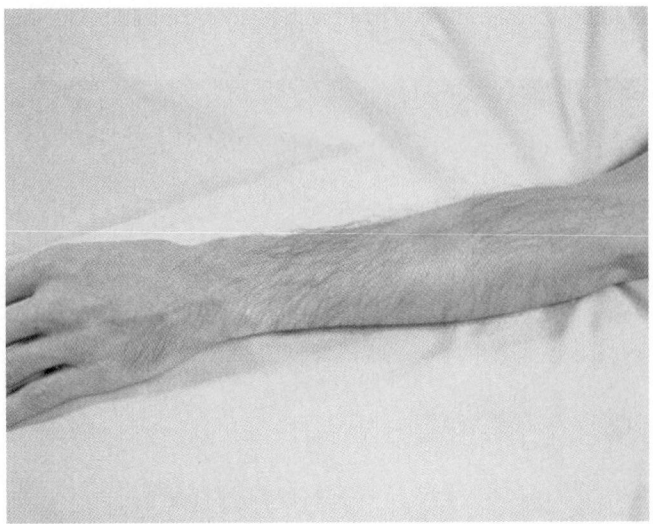

FIGURE 22–23 ■ Phlebitis.
Source: Johnson & Johnson Medical, Inc. 1997. Used by permission of the copyright owner

CHART 22–4	**Phlebitis Scale**
Grade	**Clinical Criteria**
0	No symptoms
1	Erythema at access site with or without pain
2	Pain at access site with erythema and/or edema
3	Pain at access site with erythema and/or edema Streak formation Palpable venous cord
4	Pain at access site with erythema and/or edema Streak formation Palpable venous cord >1 in. in length Purulent drainage

Source: From Infusion Nurses Society. Infusion Nursing Standards of Practice. JIN Supplement. 29 (IS) Standard 53: Phlebitis, p. S59

The most effective treatment for phlebitis is prevention. Venipuncture sites should be assessed frequently. At the first signs of phlebitis, remove and relocate the catheter. Gently palpate the venous pathway at the tip of the catheter to ascertain tenderness while observing for warmth, edema, and induration. If an infection is suspected, remove the catheter and obtain a health care provider order to culture the catheter tip. Establish a new venipuncture site, preferably in the opposite extremity. Document the degree of phlebitis in the patient's medical record and monitor the site frequently at specified intervals.

Thrombosis

Thrombosis is the formation of a blood clot within the vein. It is caused by an injury to the cells lining the vein, usually occurring at the junction where the catheter comes into contact with the tunica intima of the vessel. The causes of thrombus formation are similar to those of phlebitis:

- Poor insertion technique
- Multiple attempts at venipuncture
- Inappropriate catheter gauge and length for the patient and/or prescribed therapy
- Poor circulation
- Administration of incompatible medications and solutions, or those with extreme variations in pH and osmolarity
- Catheter material.

Thrombophlebitis is the combination of thrombus formation in association with inflammation of the vein. Figure 22–23 ■ shows an arm with phlebitis from an intravenous infusion complication. The inflammation may be first detected along the venous pathway, followed by edema, pain, and warmth. The vein will become markedly hardened as the thrombosis progresses.

The patient should be assessed for causative factors that may lead to the development of thrombosis and thrombophlebitis. Slowing or cessation of the infusion may be the first sign that complications are developing. Mechanical problems should be eliminated. If the infusion is being administered via an EID, occlusion alarms may offer an important clue. Patient complaints of discomfort and generalized swelling in the involved extremity are important clinical indications of this pending complication.

The degree of circulatory involvement should be monitored because deprivation of blood flow could seriously impact the functional use of the extremity. Thrombus formation has also been a precursor to systemic infections and embolic events. If thrombosis or thrombophlebitis is detected, remove the catheter and establish a new venipuncture site in the opposite extremity, if possible.

To prevent these complications, skilled insertion techniques are necessary. Avoid cannulation of veins in the lower extremities, particularly in adults, because these veins are very small and allow pooling of blood with subsequent damage to the vein intima and clot formation. Appropriate catheter selection, avoidance of insertions over bony prominences and points of flexion, and proper catheter securement are nursing interventions that have proven to be effective preventive measures against thrombus formation.

Infection

Infection is considered a localized event when it occurs at the insertion site. Evidence of phlebitis may not be apparent. Typical signs of infection such as erythema, tenderness, and drainage will be detected at the catheter–skin junction. The cause of this type of infection is usually due to a faulty insertion technique, such as nonadherence to aseptic technique during catheter insertion, site care, or device removal. The use of contaminated equipment, improper hand hygiene, or patient manipulation may also contribute to the development of an infection. There are instances when infection becomes apparent only after catheter removal.

If an infection is suspected, remove the catheter immediately, obtain a health care provider order to culture the site, and establish a new site. Place a sterile dressing over the site, notify the health care provider, and document appropriately. Topical antimicrobial ointments with sterile dressings may be ordered. Antimicrobial infusions may be required, and surgical intervention may be necessary to treat the infection.

Occlusion

Occlusions are caused by thrombus formation, drug precipitates, or lipid deposits. Slowing of the flow or cessation of the flow from the solution container and an inability to flush the device are signs of possible occlusion. Catheters will become occluded if infusion containers are allowed to "run dry" or when incorrect flushing techniques are used. The administration of incompatible infusates may contribute to the development, causing occlusion of the fluid pathway.

When attempting to restore catheter patency, never forcibly flush the catheter because catheter fracture or embolization of the catheter contents can occur. The occluded catheter must be removed and another site located for the continuation of the prescribed therapy. Containers of solution should be replaced when the contents are nearly empty. Frequent monitoring of the entire infusion system should occur at specified intervals. Establish compatibility of prescribed infusates prior to initiation. Follow policies and procedures for flushing intermittent infusion devices.

 CRITICAL ALERT *Never use force when flushing an occluded VAD. Administer the appropriate flushing solution and technique to maintain VAD patency.*

Systemic Complications

Systemic complications are those complications that occur in the circulation and have the potential to affect the entire body. Although these complications can occur in patients receiving peripheral infusion therapy, they are more frequently seen in those receiving therapies through a CVAD.

Air Embolism

The symptoms of an air embolism, which is caused by entry of air into the vascular system, include chest pain, shortness of breath, shoulder or low back pain, anxiety, cyanosis, hypotension, weak rapid pulse, and loss of consciousness. If left untreated, shock or cardiac arrest may result.

If an air embolism is suspected, the patient should be placed on the left side in the Trendelenburg position. Identify the source of air intake and correct the problem immediately. If the air embolism results from an open or leaking administration system, the administration set should be changed immediately and replaced with a new one flushed with solution.

Measures need to be incorporated to prevent the occurrence of an air embolism.

Administration sets should be clamped when they are being changed. Solution containers should be changed before they are completely empty. Luer-Lok connections should be used to prevent the accidental disconnection of infusion systems. Infusion systems need to be purged of air prior to the initiation of an infusion. Infusions using EIDs with "air-in-line" alarm systems should be used.

 CRITICAL ALERT *Accidental disconnection of the administration set can lead to an air embolism. The nurse must be able to recognize symptoms of an air embolism and be prepared to administer resuscitative measures.*

Catheter Embolism

A **catheter embolism** occurs when a piece of catheter is fractured and enters the circulatory system. The catheter may block a major vein, causing loss of circulation, or may travel to the heart, causing cardiac irritability and cardiac arrest. Catheter fracture is commonly associated with poor insertion technique such as retracting a catheter back through an introducer, partially withdrawing a stylet from a catheter, then reinserting and advancing the now-torn catheter, or forcibly flushing an occluded catheter.

Signs that a peripheral catheter has broken are separation of the catheter and hub or a severed catheter on withdrawal from the venipuncture site. A rupture of a CVAD may not be noted until the device is used and the patient is symptomatic. If a catheter embolism is suspected, the nurse should observe the patient for signs of cyanosis, chest pain, hypotension, increased central venous pressure, tachycardia, fainting, and loss of consciousness.

For a peripheral catheter that has embolized, immediate interventions need to be initiated. Secure a tourniquet on the patient's arm proximal to the venipuncture site, and place the patient on bed rest to minimize the movement of the catheter within the vascular system. If a central venous catheter embolism is suspected, place the patient on bed rest, notify the health care provider, and monitor the patient for signs of shock. Radiographic studies will be ordered to detect the location of the catheter fragment. Medical intervention will depend on the catheter location.

Knowledge of measures to employ to prevent a catheter embolus is important. Inspect catheters for defects before use. Never pull through-the-needle catheters back through the needle once it has been inserted into the patient. Also, never withdraw or reinsert over-the-needle catheters once they have been partially or fully threaded in the vein.

Pulmonary Edema

Pulmonary edema is caused by the presence of excess fluid volume in the circulatory system. If the condition persists, the patient can develop heart failure, shock, and cardiac arrest. This condition is frequently caused by too rapid infusion rates or too much volume infused within a given time period. Patients prone to developing pulmonary edema are pediatric and elderly patients, and those patients with cardiac and renal disease.

Signs of pulmonary edema include shortness of breath, cough, increased pulse, dyspnea, hypertension, moist rales, frothy sputum, and periorbital edema. If pulmonary edema is suspected, the infusion should be slowed immediately to a rate that maintains vascular access, and the patient placed in high Fowler's position. The health care provider should be notified and oxygen administered as ordered. Emergency treatment may include the administration of diuretics, vasodilators, and opiates. Chapter 36 ⊙ includes an in-depth discussion of pulmonary edema.

Before initiating infusion therapy, assess the patient's cardiac and respiratory history, ability to tolerate fluid volume, and any previous problems associated with fluid volume while receiving infusion therapy. Closely monitor patients receiving infusion therapy for tolerance of the amounts of fluids being administered. Maintain infusion rates as ordered and do not increase rates for solutions that are behind schedule. Use volumetric devices and infusion controllers when accurate measurements are required or when the patient's condition warrants management to prevent fluid overload.

Septicemia

Septicemia is caused when pathogenic bacteria enter the bloodstream. Contributing factors placing the patient at risk for septicemia can lead to increasing the patient's susceptibility to infection and allowing microorganisms to enter the infusion system. Risk factors associated with septicemia are outlined in the Risk Factors box.

Early symptoms of septicemia must be evaluated for possible causes. Fever in a patient with a CVAD should be attributed to the device until proven otherwise. Erythema at the insertion site could indicate an infectious process that could lead to sepsis. The health care provider should be notified and cultures of the catheter and the patient's blood may be ordered.

The most effective treatment for septicemia is prevention. Appropriate hand hygiene and strict adherence to aseptic technique should be used when initiating or manipulating an infusion system. All solutions and equipment should be inspected for intact packaging and product integrity. Venipuncture sites should be disinfected with approved antimicrobial agents. Catheter sites are to be rotated, dressings and administration sets changed, and sites

---

RISK FACTORS for the Development of Septicemia

- Patient susceptibility
- Alteration in host defenses
- Presence of other infectious processes
- Contaminated infusion equipment
- Inexperience of the nurse inserting the VAD
- Inadequate site preparation
- Manipulations of the administration delivery system
- Dwell time of the device
- Lack of or improper hand hygiene

monitored according to the *Infusion Nursing Standards of Practice* (INS, 2006a) and organizational policy and procedure.

Allergic Reactions

An allergic reaction is a response to a medication or solution to which the patient is sensitive. The most common reactions are those seen as a result of administering antimicrobial, biologic, and blood products. The patient may experience chills, fever, urticaria, erythema, itching, shortness of breath, or wheezing. Patients should be assessed for a complete allergy history. Use of identification bracelets and special identifying labels on the patient's medical record serve to inform all health care providers about patient allergies.

 CRITICAL ALERT *Be aware of the risk of an allergic reaction occurring when administering antimicrobial, biologic, or blood products. Maintain vascular access and be prepared to treat an anaphylactic event.*

If an allergic reaction is suspected, the infusion should be stopped immediately, the administration set and solution container changed, and vascular access maintained to allow for emergent treatment for possible anaphylactic shock. The health care provider should be notified and the nurse prepared to administer resuscitative measures.

Needlestick Complications

Sharps-related injuries take place at an alarming rate with an estimate of more than 800,000 needlesticks occurring annually among more than 5.6 million health care workers (Perry, Parker, & Jagger, 2003). Unfortunately, it is also estimated that at least one-half of these injuries go unreported. Additionally, of those injured, more than 1,000 reportedly contract a serious infection from the injury (Perry et al., 2003). Data collection for statistical information concentrates on the categories listed in Chart 22–5 for risk of injury with nurses reporting the most percutaneous injuries at 43.6% (Perry et al., 2003). The International Healthcare Worker Safety Center at the University of Virginia Health System provides extensive resources on sharps safety and occupational exposure prevention: tools for conducting exposure surveillance, a list of safety-engineered sharp devices, and statistics.

The Needlestick Safety and Prevention Act was signed into law November 6, 2000, and was incorporated into the revised bloodborne pathogen directive published January 2001 by the Occupational Safety and Health Administration (OSHA). The act changed OSHA's original 1991 *Bloodborne Pathogens Standards* from a directive to law, enforceable in the same manner as any other safety law enforced by OSHA. This legislation, effective on April 18, 2001, with final enforcement and implementation July 17, 2001, clarified OSHA's previous bloodborne standard that required health care workers to use devices that eliminate or minimize chances of exposure or injury by needles and other sharps.

The needlestick act was introduced as a response to two issues: increased concern over inadvertent or accidental needlestick injuries in health care settings, and advancements in technology to prevent health care professionals, patients, and caregivers from sharps-related injuries. The importance of using safety-engineered technologies in an effort to deliver safe infusion therapies is not diminished with the implementation of the act, because it also requires employers currently covered by the *Bloodborne Pathogens Standards* to continually evaluate and use devices that reduce the risk of injuries.

Needleless Infusion Systems

Needlestick injuries can occur as a result of unsafe products or improper use of a product. Factors that contribute to exposure to body fluids include equipment without adequate safety features, failure to observe standard precautions, and actively engaging in hazardous activities such as recapping needles. Needled syringes, winged steel infusion sets, vacuum blood collection tubes, and vascular access devices are often associated with high rates of injury. Other devices or equipment such as infusion connectors and Luer slip tips are considered high risk due to the potential for inadvertent separation of the equipment during a procedure. Needles manufactured as permanent components attached to infusion administration sets are difficult to dispose of without causing injury. Equipment such as blood collection systems may cause inadvertent exposure due to disassembly practices.

Improperly disposing of needles or other sharps often places at risk many employees, patients, and visitors within the health care organization. Expended sharps should never be temporarily placed on food service trays or stuck into bed linens prior to disposal because those procedures greatly increase the risk of injury to others. Procedures that require the use of multiple needles such as flushing intermittent infusion devices are often associated with injury. Needles and syringes should be disposed of immediately after use, and not stored in a uniform pocket to be dropped into the sharps box when next at the medication cart or closet.

Drawing blood poses special risks to the health care worker. Vacuum tubes are frequently associated with higher than normally expected injury rates; recapping needles and removing needles from reusable tube holders for disposal hold risk for personal injury.

Other procedures can pose a risk of exposure to blood or injury. Glass-based tubes may crack and break during phlebotomy procedures or during transport. Administration of infusates and medications presents special risks when piggybacking into primary infusion systems or when connecting to intermittent infusion devices. Equipment with longer lengths of extension tubing can become entangled and expose the clinician and other staff members to sharps-related injury. Injuries may occur when equipment is not properly attached and must be forced apart, or when unfamiliar equipment is not used appropriately. Nurses who are not skilled at certain tasks, such as inserting infusion catheters or performing such procedures on specific patient populations such as pediatrics or confused, combative, or elderly patients, are more susceptible to injury.

CHART 22–5   **Data Collection Categories**

- Injection devices
- Blood-drawing and vascular access devices
- Glass containers
- Surgical instruments

In response to these issues, manufacturers have devised engineered controls for sharps injury protection. Engineered safety products have demonstrated a reduction in needlestick injuries and subsequent exposure to bloodborne pathogens. Needleless systems are examples of engineering controls. A **needleless system** is a device that does not use needles for the collection of body fluids or withdrawal of such fluids after initial access is established or for the administration of medications or fluids or any other procedure involving the potential for occupational exposure to pathogens due to percutaneous injuries from contaminated sharps.

More than 200 needleless products have been approved by the Food and Drug Administration (FDA). These products are classified by the mode of engineered safety incorporated into the device or equipment:

- Elimination of sharps:
  - ✓ Needleless injection system
  - ✓ Presplit septum and blunted cannula
  - ✓ Threaded Luer-Lok adapter.
- Passive (the engineered safety mechanism is a component within the system):
  - ✓ Recessed needles
  - ✓ Self-advancing sheathing syringe
  - ✓ Self-blunting cannula
  - ✓ Vascular access device.
- Active (the safety mechanism must be activated by the nurse):
  - ✓ User-activated needle cover
  - ✓ Sheathing vascular access device, winged steel infusion set, syringe.
- Disposal (safe disposal via nonpermeable, tamper-proof, puncture-resistant containers):
  - ✓ Mailbox or drop-in style.

Using prefilled syringes and other commercially prepared solutions and medications negates the occurrence of injuries during preparation. Needle-free systems using vial adapters can prevent percutaneous injury. Vacuum tubes for laboratory analysis are now available in glass-free materials. Sharps disposal containers should be at eye level and near the patient's bedside. They should also be emptied according to manufacturer's instructions, specifically when the container is three-quarters full. All sharps are to be accounted for at the completion of any procedure. Needles are not to be recapped.

The use of needleless systems does not negate the fact that sterile technique is *always* observed when accessing and manipulating the infusion delivery system. Infection control practices must be adhered to throughout all infusion therapy administrations.

Nursing Management

Infusion therapy is prescribed to deliver many types of solutions and medications to patients in all care settings via vascular and nonvascular routes. Disruptions and variances in accepted standardized care and maintenance practices will adversely impact the patient by jeopardizing the safety, therapy delivery, and prescription compliance. Additionally, ineffective nursing skill and

care competencies will negatively impact intended outcomes. Thus, the nurse must possess a variety of skills and knowledge in order to safely manage patients receiving infusion therapies. These include:

- Knowledge of aseptic technique in order to prevent both local and systemic infections
- Skill in venipuncture
- Knowledge of care and maintenance procedures to preserve vascular access sites and devices
- Knowledge of the impact that solutions and infusion rates have on the body systems, especially in the presence of disease
- Ability to identify and treat catheter-related complications
- Critical thinking skills necessary to troubleshoot equipment problems when they occur
- Knowledge of the impact of medication administration via the intravenous route, including administering more than one medication simultaneously
- Ability to provide emotional support to the patient and family members.

The Nursing Process: Patient Care Plan uses the nursing process to provide a comprehensive plan of care for patients receiving infusion therapy.

Collaborative Management

With emphasis on clinical care and performance competence, collaboration with members of the health care team and the patient and her family will provide the patient with specialized support through education and technical expertise. Members of the health care team, include the primary care physician, the nurse and members of the infusion team, the infection control practitioner, the pharmacist, and the case manager, will collaborate on specific issues such as appropriate VAD selection for the prescribed therapy and home-based infusion services and other indicated support systems as appropriate.

Once the health care provider discusses the purpose of the treatment and orders the patient's therapy, the nurse is responsible for the continued assessment of the patient's infusion needs. The nurse educates the patient about the treatment plan and determines the level of participation the patient can be engaged in. The patient's caregiver is also included in the education process and taught the necessary skills if needed to assist the patient with the infusion care.

Others on the health care team involved with infusion therapy include infection control practitioners and pharmacists. The infection control specialist monitors sharps injuries, infection rates, and disseminated infection control practices. Pharmacists have knowledge of medication and solution concentrations and compatibility issues. The case manager plays an integral role in the care coordination for the patient within the care setting. Knowledge of the intricacies of insurance benefits, availability of health care providers, and logistics coordination activities falls within the purview of the case manager.

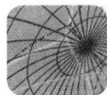

NURSING PROCESS: Patient Care Plan for Infusion Therapy

Assessment of Potential for Injury Secondary to Placement and Dwell Time of VAD and Disruption of the Infusion Delivery System

Subjective Data:

Do you know why you are having infusion therapy, and how long do you expect to have it?

Have you ever had an intravenous catheter? If so, did you ever experience any problems with it?

What "handedness" are you?

Have you ever had a stroke (CVA) or surgery on your arm or chest, such as mastectomy, fracture, vascular surgery, AV fistula or shunt?

Are you sensitive to tape or any antiseptic agents?

Do you use any ambulatory aids?

Objective Data:

Does the patient have a preference for VAD location?

Does the patient have observable physical limitations or conditions that will impact site selection, site preparation, and dwell time of the VAD?

Nursing Assessment and Diagnoses	Outcomes and Evaluation Parameters	Planning and Interventions with *Rationales*
Nursing Diagnosis: *Deficient Knowledge* related to therapeutic infusion management and maintenance practices	**Outcomes:** Patient and/or caregiver will successfully demonstrate VAD care and maintenance practices. Patient and/or caregiver will be educated in disease process and progression, signs and symptoms of distress, and indicated infusion-specific treatment regimen(s). ***Evaluation Parameter:*** Verbalizes understanding of complications associated with infusion therapy.	**Interventions and *Rationales:*** Patient/caregiver will be able to: Explain rationale for VAD placement. Explain rationale for hand hygiene. Describe appropriate condition of VAD location, i.e., intact dressing, clean securement device, intact skin integrity. Describe symptoms of pending complications secondary to VAD dwell, i.e., infiltration, phlebitis, leaking of fluids (bloody drainage, exudates) from catheter–skin junction, pain, and erythema. Describe signs and symptoms of potential infusion-related complications, i.e., air in the line, occlusion, empty infusion container, retrograde blood flow, nonflow of infusate, alarming of infusion assistive device. *Patient and/or caregiver will be able to identify signs and symptoms of possible catheter-related complications through education processes. Patient/caregiver will be able to identify and seek emergency assistance as appropriate.*

Assessment of Knowledge Deficit Related to Infection Control Measures Pertaining to Infusion-Specific Care and Maintenance Practices

Subjective Data:

Have you ever had an infection related to an earlier infusion?

Have you needed an infusion catheter replaced due to an occlusion or infiltration, infection, or catheter malposition?

Have you ever been assessed for a VAD reserved for long-term therapy such as a PICC or implanted port?

Objective Data:

Is the VAD dressing dry and intact?

Is there presence of erythema, swelling, or drainage along the vascular pathway or at the catheter–skin junction?

Is the patient complaining of discomfort or pain along the vascular pathway or at the catheter–skin junction?

Are the EID alarms going off frequently for "occlusion" or "no flow"?

Is there a lack of blood return?

Nursing Assessment and Diagnoses	Outcomes and Evaluation Parameters	Planning and Interventions with *Rationales*
Nursing Diagnoses: Infection, risk for Injury, risk for	**Outcomes:** The VAD will dwell according to established organizational policies and procedures. The VAD will be asymptomatic for the length of dwell time. The patient will achieve intended infusion-related outcomes. ***Evaluation Parameters:*** The patient will be able to verbalize understanding of care and maintenance practices associated with the prescribed infusion therapy and mode of delivery to prevent catheter-related complications.	**Interventions and *Rationales:*** Patient/caregiver will be able to: Explain rationale for hand hygiene. Explain rationale for use of aseptic technique when changing infusion containers and administration sets. Explain rationale for use of antiseptic agent(s) when preparing injection cap/access port for injection. *Patient and/or caregiver will be able to identify signs and symptoms of possible infusion-related complications through education processes. Patient/caregiver will be able to identify and seek emergency assistance as appropriate. Patient and/or caregiver will be able to identify sources for information and nursing support, and will be able to make informed decisions regarding infusion care.*

(continued)

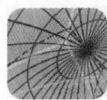

NURSING PROCESS: Patient Care Plan for Infusion Therapy—*Continued*

Assessment of Knowledge Deficit Related to Information Pertaining to Parenteral Medication Use and Administration at Home

Subjective Data:
Do you wear a hearing aid or glasses?
Do you have trouble using your hands due to disease (arthritis) or injury?
Do you have pets?
Do you have someone who can assist you at home?
Do you have running water, refrigeration, electricity, a telephone?
Can you read?
What is the language spoken in your home?
Do you know how long the doctor has prescribed this therapy?

Objective Data:
Do pediatric patients have arrangements for tutoring or for monitoring the infusion in the school setting?

Nursing Assessment and Diagnoses	Outcomes and Evaluation Parameters	Planning and Interventions with *Rationales*
Nursing Diagnosis: *Effective Therapeutic Regiment Management* related to home environment	**Outcome:** Patient and/or caregiver will successfully demonstrate infusion system care and maintenance practices, and safe infusion administration procedures. *Evaluation Parameter:* Patient demonstrates competency related to prescribed infusion therapy.	**Interventions and *Rationales:*** Patient and /or caregiver will be able to: Describe prescribed infusion treatment regimen including anticipated outcomes. Describe expected care and maintenance procedures for prescribed infusion therapy including, but not limited to: 1. Parenteral solution and/or medication use and action. 2. Storage of parenteral medication(s) and solution(s), and equipment. 3. Elements of effective infection control practices including hand hygiene, standard precautions and aseptic technique, and disposal of expended equipment and supplies. 4. Preparation and administration practices for infusion therapy. 5. Signs and symptoms of untoward medication reactions. 6. Use of infusion-specific equipment. *Patient and/or caregiver will successfully describe parenteral infusion treatment protocols and seek interventions and assistance as appropriate.* *Patient and/or caregiver education processes will be documented in the patient's permanent medical record.*

■ Research

Research within the specialty nursing field of infusion therapy is essential in order to advance the practice, but also to identify areas requiring specific data, supporting performance improvement indicators, and identifying concerns and considerations that affect anticipated outcomes and patient safety. Although ongoing assessment is critical for the patient receiving infusion prescriptions, post-therapy assessments and achievement and evaluation of indicators will continue to suggest improved methods of infusion care. Advances in technologies affecting infusion care delivery will need to be addressed in all care settings. Examples of promising areas of research are presented in the Research Opportunities and Clinical Impact box.

■ Summary

Infusion therapy will continue to be practiced in all care settings and administered to patient populations of all ages. Technologic advances affecting insertion, care and maintenance, and research-based practices will continue to shape this nursing specialty. Education and continued competence are necessary to keep nurses abreast of proper techniques and new technology that are essential components of the specialty practice of infusion therapy.

RESEARCH OPPORTUNITIES AND CLINICAL IMPACT RELATED TO INFUSION THERAPY

Research Area	Clinical Impact
Evaluate the process of early patient assessment related to VAD selection.	Timely initiation of therapy
	Appropriate site and VAD selection to preserve sites and minimize the number of venipunctures
	Patient education to promote therapy compliance
Determine the efficacy of saline versus heparin flushes of CVADs in the home care patient.	Prevention of VAD occlusion
	Continuation of therapy without impacting patient's clotting mechanisms
Determine whether a 72- to 96-hour site rotation interval for peripheral-short catheters is appropriate.	Site preservation
	To minimize number of venipunctures
	To decrease risks associated with catheter-related complications

NCLEX® REVIEW

1. A patient, being discharged, will need to receive antibiotic therapy for an additional three weeks. The peripheral vascular access device that would be the best for this patient would be:
   1. A peripheral-short catheter
   2. A winged steel infusion set
   3. A midline catheter
   4. A PICC line

2. A patient receiving parenteral fluids is prescribed an intravenous medication to be infused every 6 hours. Which of the following infusion devices should the nurse use for this medication?
   1. Stop cock
   2. Extension set
   3. Elastomeric balloon
   4. Secondary administration set

3. The staff development department is planning an annual skills review day for the basics of intravenous therapy. If the Infusion Nursing Standards of Practice are being followed, the purpose of this skills day would be to:
   1. Ensure all nurses follow standard precautions.
   2. Preserve the patient's right to safe, quality care and protect the nurse who administers infusion therapy.
   3. Ensure the nurses are in compliance with all regulatory agencies.
   4. Ensure the nurses' skill levels are adequate.

4. A patient is prescribed parenteral fluid therapy. Which of the following should the nurse do first?
   1. Wash hands.
   2. Gather the equipment to insert the peripheral access device.
   3. Prepare the flush to use once the peripheral access device is in place.
   4. Review the procedure with the patient and obtain consent.

5. A patient receiving parenteral fluid therapy complains of the arm "feeling cold" and the dressing "feeling tight." What should the nurse do?
   1. Check for a blood return in the catheter.
   2. Stop the infusion and remove the catheter.
   3. Turn off the infusion, reposition the catheter.
   4. Change the dressing and observe the site.

Answers for review questions appear in Appendix D

KEY TERMS

adapter *p.513*
add-on devices *p.520*
administration set *p.520*
air embolism *p.515*
arterial-venous shunts *p.518*
bacterial phlebitis *p.530*
bevel *p.513*
catheter *p.512*

catheter embolism *p.532*
central vascular access device (CVAD) *p.515*
chemical phlebitis *p.530*
continuous subcutaneous infusion
   (CSI) *p.518*
dialysis catheter *p.518*
drip factor *p.520*
dual-channel pump *p.524*

dwell *p.512*
elastomeric balloon *p.523*
electronic infusion device (EID) *p.523*
extension set *p.522*
extravasation *p.529*
filter *p.522*
flashback chamber *p.513*
flow control device *p.521*

EXPLORE PEARSON **mynursingkit**™

MyNursingKit is your one stop for online chapter review materials and resources. Prepare for success with additional NCLEX®-style practice questions, interactive assignments and activities, web links, animations and videos, and more!

Register your access code from the front of your book at
www.mynursingkit.com

REFERENCES

Boyce, J. M., & Pittet, D. (2002). Guideline for hand hygiene in health-care settings: Recommendations of the Healthcare Infection Control Practices Advisory Committee and the HICPAC/SHEA/APIC/IDSA Hand Hygiene Task Force. *Infection Control and Hospital Epidemiology, 23*(12 Suppl.), S1–S40.

Centers for Disease Control and Prevention. (2002). *CDC Guidelines for the Prevention of Intravascular Catheter-Related Infections.* Retrieved June 12, 2008, from http://www.cdc.gov/ncidod/dhqp/gl_intravascular.html

Gillies, D., O'Riordan, L., Carr, D., Frost, J., Gunning, R., & O'Brien, I. (2003). Gauze and tape and transparent polyurethane dressings for central venous catheters. *Cochrane Database of Systematic Reviews, 4,* CD003827.

Hankins, J., Lonsway, R. A., Hedrick, C., & Perdue, M. (Eds.) (2001). *Infusion therapy in clinical practice.* (2nd ed.). Philadelphia: W. B. Saunders.

Infusion Nurses Society. (2006a). Infusion nursing standards of practice. *Journal of Infusion Nursing, 29*(Suppl.1).

Infusion Nurses Society. (2006b). *Policies and procedures for infusion nursing* (3rd ed.). Norwood, MA: Author.

O'Grady, N. P., Alexander, M., Patchen Dellinger, E., Gerberding, J. L., Heard, S. O., Maki, D. G., et al. (2002, August 9). Guidelines for the prevention of intravascular catheter-related infections. *Morbidity and Mortality Weekly Report, 51*(RR-10), 1–26.

Perry, J., Parker, G., & Jagger, J. (2003). EPINet report: 2001 percutaneous injury rates. *Advances in Exposure Prevention, 6*(3), 32–36.

Blood Administration

Kathleen Osborn

Outcome-Based Learning Objectives

After studying this chapter, the learner will be able to:

1. Describe the rationale for blood donation requirements and restrictions.
2. Describe the advantages of blood component therapy and the therapeutic uses for each component.
3. Compare and contrast the hazards of transfusion therapy and the nursing measures used to assess and prevent them.
4. Using the nursing process, describe the administration procedure for blood administration.
5. Delineate the critical thinking and clinical judgment nursing skills necessary to appropriately treat adverse reactions to blood transfusions.

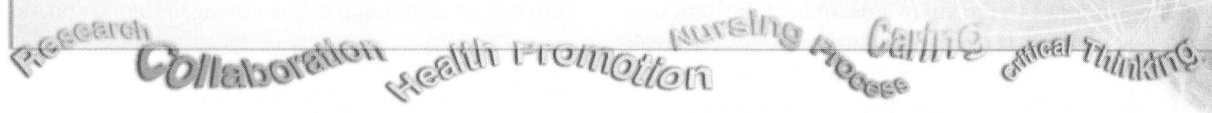

Research Collaboration Health Promotion Nursing Process Caring Critical Thinking

Blood transfusion is defined as the infusion of blood products for the purpose of restoring circulating volume and thereby increasing oxygen carrying capacity. The benefit of a blood transfusion is that it reverses the tissue hypoxia caused by clinically significant anemia and/or blood loss. This reversal can be lifesaving. Blood transfusions are given to approximately 5 million people in the United States annually (Mayo Clinic, 2005). Approximately 14 million units of blood are collected annually in the United States and of these 12 million are transfused (Pearl & Pohlman, 2002). About 60% of the population in the United States is eligible to donate blood; only 5% do (America's Blood Centers, 2006). As the population ages, it is expected that the demand for blood products will increase, perhaps exceeding the supply. The specialty of transfusion medicine is no longer just the practice of storing and administering blood; it now also includes the management of blood resources to ensure the right patients receive transfusions appropriately.

Blood may be administered as either whole blood or blood components. **Whole blood** is obtained from a donor, processed, and infused into a recipient. Whole blood contains red blood cells (RBCs), white blood cells (WBCs), and **platelets**, which are suspended in the **plasma**. Because patients seldom require all of the components of whole blood, in recent years blood component therapy has become the more frequently used method of transfusion. It is more appropriate and economical to separate

blood into its component parts and use only that portion needed by the patient for a specific condition or disease. Two advantages of blood component therapy are (1) conservation of blood resources, because one unit can be used for multiple recipients; and (2) the patient receives only the needed components, thereby decreasing volume overload and reducing side effects and complications.

Blood is fractioned into component parts by either a centrifuge or a cell separator. Each component is then processed and stored appropriately, so as to maximize longevity and cell viability. (See discussion later in the chapter about blood storage.)

Another type of transfusion is **apheresis,** a technique in which blood is withdrawn from a donor, a portion is separated out, and the remainder is returned to the donor. This is useful when a blood donor has been in, say, a malaria-active area of the world. The RBCs from such a donor cannot be used because they may carry the malaria virus, but the plasma portion of the blood can be used.

Donor Considerations

To protect both the donor and the recipient, every potential donor is examined and interviewed. According to the American Red Cross (2005), to be a donor of blood the individual must be healthy, at least 17 years old or 16 years old if allowed by state law, weigh at least 110 pounds, and not have donated blood in the last 8 weeks (56 days). "Healthy" is defined as the ability to perform normal activities. In the presence of a chronic disease such as diabetes or high blood pressure, "healthy" means that the condition is being treated and is under control.

Both the federal Food and Drug Administration (FDA) and the American Association of Blood Banks (AABB) have specific criteria that must be met before a person is accepted for blood donation. The donor must complete a donor history questionnaire. The FDA approved a revised version of a donor history questionnaire developed by the AABB in 2005. A summary of the questions included on the questionnaire are outlined in the National Guidelines box.

Following the history, donors undergo a brief medical examination to evaluate for any obvious signs of illness or conditions that would disqualify them from blood donation. Vital signs are checked and individuals with a fever, high blood pressure, very high or very low pulse rate (with the exception of highly conditioned athletes), and irregular heartbeat are not permitted to donate blood.

Donation Procedure

Blood is obtained from the donor using standard precautions for both donor and phlebotomist. Typically the donor sits in a reclining chair and the antecubital fossa is cleansed with an antiseptic solution. Withdrawal of 450 mL of blood typically takes about 15 minutes. After completion, a firm bandage is applied and the donor is asked to remain in a recumbent position until she feels ready to sit up. If dizziness, light-headedness, or weakness occurs, the donor is asked to remain seated for awhile longer.

Blood banks typically offer donors both food and fluids and ask them to remain for about 15 minutes after standing up. Follow-up donor instructions include (1) leave the dressing in place and avoid heavy lifting for several hours, (2) increase fluid intake for 2 days,

(3) avoid alcoholic beverages for 3 hours, (4) avoid smoking for 1 hour, and (4) eat healthy meals for 2 weeks.

Complications of Donation

Many individuals have the misconception that diseases are transmitted during blood donation. Education of potential donors is necessary to ensure understanding that the equipment is sterile, used once, and that it is a closed system from the beginning to the end of the blood collection process.

Excessive bleeding at the donor venipuncture site is a complication of blood donation. Causes include donor bleeding disorder, laceration of the vein during the puncture, excessive tourniquet pressure, and/or failure to apply adequate pressure after the needle is withdrawn. The phlebotomist must ensure that the bleeding has completely stopped before allowing the donor to leave the blood donation center.

Other complications of blood donation include anginal chest pain in unsuspected individuals with coronary artery disease, and on rare occasions, a blood donation can precipitate a seizure in people with epilepsy. Both of these complications require medical evaluation prior to leaving the blood donation center.

The most common complication of blood donation is fainting, typically due to emotional factors, vasovagal reaction, or inadequate fluid or food intake before donation. Hypotension and syncope also may occur due to loss of blood volume when the donor assumes a standing position. These individuals need to lie down or sit with their head between the knees. The donor needs to be symptom free for 30 minutes before leaving the blood donation center.

■ Blood Supply Safety

The FDA is responsible for ensuring the safety of the blood supply in the United States. Specifically, the Center for Biological Evaluation and Research (CBER) regulates the collection of

---

NATIONAL GUIDELINES for Minimum Requirements for Blood Donation

Oral temperature must be less than 37.5°C (99.6°F).

Regular pulse rate between 50 and 100 beats per minute.

Systolic blood pressure between 90 and 180 mmHg.

Diastolic blood pressure between 50 and 100 mmHg.

Hemoglobin greater than 13.5 g/dL for men and 12.4 g/dL for women.

Body weight must be greater than 50 kg (110 lb) to donate 450 mL. Donors weighing less than 50 kg may donate proportionately less blood.

Age of 17 to 65 years old.

Normal liver function tests.

No blood or plasma donations in the previous 8 weeks.

Medication use (prescription, over the counter, blooding thinners, recent immunization, and illicit).

Exposure to illnesses.

Travel to high-risk areas of the world.

Pregnancy.

Transfusion history.

Surgical history.

Sexual preferences and history (including male-to-male contact even once).

Body piercing and/or tattoos in the last 12 months.

Treatment for syphilis or gonorrhea.

Prison or juvenile hall in the last 12 months.

Residing in the United Kingdom from 1980 to 1996 for greater than 3 months.

Residing in Europe for greater than 5 years.

Lived in Africa or had sex with someone who was born or lived in Africa.

Tested for HIV/AIDS.

History of hepatitis, malaria, Chagas' disease, babesiosis, cancer, leukemia, heart or lung disease, bleeding disorder, Creutzfeldt-Jakob disease.

History of selling illicit drugs.

History of IV drug use.

Source: American Red Cross. (2005). *Blood donation eligibility guidelines.* Retrieved November 7, 2006, from http://www.redcross.org/services/biomed/0,1082,0_557_,00.html#top.

blood and blood components, including manufactured pharmaceuticals derived from blood, such as clotting factors (FDA, 2006a). Additionally, CBER develops and enforces quality standards, inspects blood donation centers, and monitors reports of errors, accidents, and adverse clinical events. This organization also works closely with the federal Public Health Service to identify and respond to potential threats to the blood supply and to develop safety and technical standards to ensure consistent monitoring of the blood supply.

Once blood has been received from the donor it is immediately tested for blood type and infectious diseases. A negative result for the disease testing is required before the blood is used, and each unit is labeled to certify the results.

ABO and Rh Factor Testing

Equally important as disease testing is accurate determination of blood type. Each individual has one of four types of blood: A, B, AB, or O. In a large percentage of the population, two related inherited antigens, A and B, occur on the surface of RBCs and form the basis for the ABO blood typing. Those individuals with A antigen have **type A blood** (41%), those with B antigen have **type B blood** (12%), and those with both A and B have **type AB blood** (3%). If neither A nor B antigens are present, the individual has **type O blood** (44%). Type O blood does not have the genetic information required to make any antigenic formation (Josephson, 2004; Porth, 2005).

Antibodies develop in the serum of people who do not have the corresponding antigen, referred to as anti-A and anti-B. The person with blood type A has B antibodies, someone with type B has A antibodies, someone with type AB has no antibodies, and a person who has type O blood has both antibodies. Therefore, the person with type AB blood can receive any type of blood in an emergency situation and is referred to as the universal recipient. A person with the O blood type is considered a universal donor in an emergency situation. Chart 23–1 outlines each blood type, its antigens and antibodies, and what type of blood a person with each blood type can safely receive. Even though a person is a universal donor or recipient, unless there is an emergency, blood typing should be done to avoid transfusion reactions. ABO incompatibility is an immediate and often fatal cause of transfusion reaction.

 CRITICAL ALERT *In emergency hemorrhage situations, O negative blood can be lifesaving. This is referred to as "uncrossed matched blood," which means that the patient will not react to type O blood because there are no antigens or Rh factor. However, the number of units of O negative blood that can be given is still restricted because of the other antibodies in the blood that can be received. The uncross matched blood places the patient at high risk for transfusion reaction because of these other antibodies.*

The **Rh factor,** also called factor D, is made up of numerous complex antigens. When it is present on the surface of RBCs, the person is Rh positive (Rh⁺); if not present, the person is Rh negative (Rh⁻). The designation of Rh positive or negative is influenced by race, with African Americans being approximately 95% Rh⁺, Native Americans 100% Rh⁺, and about 85% of Caucasians Rh⁺ (Guyton & Hall, 2000). An Rh⁻ person must receive only Rh⁻ blood to avoid antibody formation from Rh⁺ blood. An Rh⁺ person may receive either negative or positive blood. The first time an Rh⁻ person receives Rh⁺ blood, there is usually no reaction. But antibodies will form during the next 2 to 4 weeks and if another transfusion of Rh⁺ blood is given, the antibodies will agglutinate or clump with the Rh antigens of the blood being transfused. Agglutination of cells causes obstruction of the capillaries and blockage of blood flow to the organs. Agglutination and antibody testing are done using the direct Coombs' test (see Chart 23–2, p. 542).

After the blood is taken from the donor, a series of procedures determines both donor and recipient ABO and Rh types. These procedures are referred to as "type and crossmatch" and are listed in Chart 23–2 (p. 542). Typing the blood determines the ABO and Rh factor, whereas crossmatching determines compatibility between donor and recipient blood. To determine blood compatibility, the donor's blood is mixed with the recipient's and observed for agglutination of the cells. If the cells do not agglutinate, and the blood tests negative for diseases, then the blood is compatible and ready to transfuse into the recipient. The blood is stored in a blood bank until needed.

Disease Testing

The blood also is tested for the diseases outlined on Chart 23–3 (p. 542) prior to be being released for patient use. A blood-screening test using nucleic acid technology (NAT) is able to detect minute amounts of the RNA and DNA of specific viruses in blood. Prior to NAT testing, blood could only be tested for antibodies to the virus. There is always a lag time between infection and production of antibodies during which the blood could test negative even though the virus is present. NAT testing markedly reduces this time period, thus making the blood supply safer. NAT testing has been approved by the FDA for hepatitis C, human immunodeficiency virus (HIV), and most recently West Nile virus.

◼ Therapeutic Uses of Blood Products

Major therapeutic uses for blood, as stated earlier, are to restore circulating volume and oxygen carrying capacity. This makes blood transfusions useful to replace blood volume during and after surgery. Many surgeries could not be performed without blood transfusions. Additionally, blood replacement is essential in the treatment of trauma when large amounts of blood have been lost.

CHART 23–1	Blood Types, Antigens and Antibodies, and Transfusion Types	
Blood Type with Antigen	**Antibody Produced**	**Type for Transfusion**
Blood type A Antigen A	Antibody B	Can receive A or O blood
Blood type B Antigen B	Antibody A	Can receive B or O blood
Blood type AB Antigen AB	None	Can receive A, B, or O type blood Universal recipient
Blood type O No antigens	Antibodies A and B	Can receive O type blood only Universal donor

CHART 23–2 **Blood Type and Crossmatch and Antigen Testing**

Name of Test	Purpose of Test	Test Results
Blood type and crossmatch Mandatory test prior to blood transfusion (exception in extreme medical emergency/hemorrhage)	Tests for antigens on the patient's RBCs: ABO antigens on RBCs determine blood type. Rh antigen determines negative or positive Rh factor.	Type A Type B Type AB Type O Rh– Rh+
Indirect Coombs' test Screening prior to blood transfusion	Tests for antibodies present in the patient's serum. Patient's serum is mixed with donor's RBCs. If the patient has antibodies to a specific antigen on the donor RBCs, an antigen–antibody complex is formed and agglutination (clumping) occurs. Blood is tested for more than 40 antibodies.	Normal results: no agglutination; negative for a specific antibody. Abnormal results: agglutination; positive for a specific antibody.
Direct Coombs' test Usually only tested if a transfusion reaction is suspected	Tests for antibodies on the patient's RBCs (not in the serum). Used to detect antibodies from the donor blood that are coating and destroying the patient's RBCs. Patient blood is mixed with Coombs' serum that contains various components of complement and antibodies to IgG to determine antigen–antibody reaction and agglutination.	Normal results: no agglutination; negative for antibodies. Abnormal results: agglutination; positive for antibodies.

Source: Kozier, Barbara J; Erb, Glenora: Berman, Audrey; Snyder, Shirlee. Fundamentals of Nursing: Concepts, Procedures, & Practices, 7th, © 2004. Electronically reproduced by permission of Pearson Education, Inc., Upper Saddle River, New Jersey.

CHART 23–3 **Transmission of Bloodborne Diseases**

Disease	Test	Safety Margin
Hepatitis B	Core antibodies (anti-HBc) and surface antigen (HbsAG) are tested. Not for the virus itself. Research has just begun on the use of NAT (DNA) testing of blood products that will detect the virus itself.	There is still a window from the time an individual is infected to the time the antibodies are produced. Risk of transmission is 1 in 220,000. There is a 7- to 10-day window.
Hepatitis C	NAT testing for the DNA in the virus. Anti- HCV.	If the blood tests positive, it is sent out for confirmatory testing. If it confirmed positive, it is not used. Risk of transmission is 1 in 1.6 million. There is a 7- to 10-day window.
HIV-1	NAT testing for the DNA in the virus. If the test comes out positive, the blood is sent for confirmatory testing.	This test reduces the period of time from infection to detecting the presence of antibodies from 12 weeks to 11 days. Risk of transmission is 1 in 1.8 million.
Human T-lymphocyte virus-1 (retrovirus present with leukemia)	Screened with EIA for HTLV antibodies. If the test comes out positive, the blood is sent for confirmatory testing.	It is possible to have both false positives and negatives. If the blood tests positive, it is sent out for confirmatory testing. If it is confirmed positive, it is not used.
West Nile virus	NAT testing for the DNA in the virus.	If the blood tests positive, it is not used.
Syphilis	PK 7200 with RPR backup. PK 7200: Tests IgM and IgG antibodies for syphilis (*Treponema pallidum*). Immucor Captive CMV: Also tests for IgM and IgG antibodies. RPR test for reagent antibodies. If the test comes out positive, the blood is sent for confirmatory testing.	It is possible to have both false positives and negatives. If the blood tests positive, it is sent out for confirmatory testing. If it is confirmed positive, it is not used.
Malaria	If a donor has been in a malaria-active area of the world in the last 3 years blood is not accepted.	The only exception is if an individual has taken prophylactic medication. Plasma apheresis (using the plasma portion of the blood only) is still possible because malaria is only carried on the RBCs.
Creutzfeldt-Jakob disease (mad cow disease)	If an individual has spent an extended period of time in Great Britain and Europe from 1980 to 1996, the blood is refused.	If the blood tests positive it is not used. No further testing is done. Diagnosis is usually made by autopsy, biopsy, or process of elimination.
Cytomegalovirus	PK 7200 and Immucor Captive CMV as performed as backup.	Transmission risk greater for premature newborns and immunocompromised recipients who are CMV negative. Leukocyte reduction helps reduce transmission of virus. CMV-negative blood is frequently specifically ordered.

Sources: American Association of Blood Banks. (2003). *Testing of donor blood for infectious disease.* Retrieved November 9, 2006, from http://www.aabb.org/Content/About_Blood/ Facts_About_Blood_and_Blood_Banking/fabloodtesting.htm; Josephson, D. (2004). *Intravenous infusion therapy for nurses* (2nd ed.). Clifton Park, NY: Thompson Delmar Learning.

Additional therapeutic uses for blood products are to replace platelets and other clotting factors, which is lifesaving for hemophiliacs. Platelet replacement also is important for cancer patients receiving radiation and chemotherapy. Cancer treatments can cause bone marrow depression and platelet depletion. Blood also can provide protein and other nutrients in severely undernourished patients. Each unit of blood contains approximately 35 grams of protein in the form of plasma proteins, and further sources of protein are found in the cellular elements.

Note that some individuals may refuse blood transfusions for cultural or religious reasons, as discussed in the Cultural Considerations box.

 Types of Blood Products

Administering blood products has become more complex with the advent of blood component therapy. It is essential for the nurse to know the correct blood type, the specific rationale for administration, as well as any special considerations of a given blood product and patient. Chart 23–4 (p. 544) outlines the various types of blood products and their volume, storage, and uses. Chart 23–5 (p. 546) lists the necessary information needed by the nurse to safely administer blood. In addition, the nurse must follow strict institutional guidelines and protocols to ensure safe administration with the fewest number of side effects.

CULTURAL CONSIDERATIONS Related to Refusal of Blood Products

It is not unusual for persons to refuse blood transfusions. Many people are frightened of disease transmission and therefore opt to instead replenish their blood supply with blood alternatives, iron supplements, and diet. Although slower, these treatments are effective unless there has been significant blood loss in a short period of time.

Certain religions ban the use of blood products. For example, Jehovah's Witnesses strictly prohibit receiving blood or agents in which blood is an ingredient in any form. This belief is based on scriptural references and precedents in the history of Christianity (Andrews & Boyle, 2003; Lipson, Dibble, & Minarik, 1996). Jehovah's Witnesses do accept blood volume expanders and vigorously pursue blood alternative therapies as long as they do not contain any derivative of blood. Mechanical devices for circulating blood are acceptable as long as they have not been primed with blood.

Other religions' rules vary with regard to blood transfusion. For example, Christian Scientists generally do not believe in any type of medical interventions except those mandated by law such as immunizations. Thus, they do not accept or donate blood products (Andrews & Boyle, 2003). The Jewish religion prohibits the ingestion of blood (blood sausage, raw meats); however, this belief does not apply to receiving blood products. The following religions have no restrictions on the use of blood or blood products (Andrews & Boyle, 2003):

- Amish
- Baha'i
- Catholic
- Hindu
- Mennonite
- Muslim
- Seventh-Day Adventist
- Unitarian.

Each product has its own special consideration beginning with simple administration of whole blood.

Whole blood contains the normal constituents of blood. After being obtained from a donor, anticoagulants and preservatives are added, and the blood is ready for the recipient. Most of the platelets and WBCs are removed or destroyed during the processing of the blood. **Packed RBCs** have had the plasma portion of the blood removed by a centrifuge process. This is the most common blood product given in the hospital. **Washed RBCs** are indicated when previous transfusion reactions have occurred. The washing process increases the removal of immunoglobulins and proteins that cause reactions. **Frozen RBCs** are coated in glycerol prior to freezing and then washed after thawing to remove the glycerol prior to administration.

Leukocyte-poor RBCs have had most of the WBCs removed as soon as the blood has been taken from the donor (prior to storage). The reason the reduction is done prior to storage is because the storage process causes necrosis of the WBCs, creating by-products that can cause serious adverse signs and symptoms for the recipient of the blood. White blood cells do not contribute to the efficacy of blood transfusions and are generally regarded as contaminants that potentially reduce transfusion safety. Until recently, the use of blood with fewer WBCs has been reserved for patients who are considered a high risk for developing problems from the presence of WBCs. That would include immunocompromised individuals who have cancer or acquired immunodeficiency syndrome (AIDS), and transplant patients. Currently the majority of the blood banks in the United States reduce the WBCs from every unit of blood.

Fresh frozen plasma (FFP) is prepared from whole blood by separating it from the cell portion and freezing it within 4 to 6 hours of taking it from the donor. Platelets are prepared from individual units of whole blood by a centrifuge process. Usually 6 to 10 units are given at one time and the units are usually pooled into one bag for easier administration. **Albumin** is derived from the plasma portion of the blood. It is a commercially prepared product that has no risk of disease transmission and does not require ABO compatibility screening. **Cryoprecipitates** are collected by thawing FFP and collecting the white precipitate that remains (May & Kauder, 2006). This precipitate, which is rich in von Willebrand's factor, **factor VIII,** and fibrinogen are given to treat bleeding associated with hemophilia and disorders that cause a depletion of the clotting factors.

 The platelet count must be assessed within 1 hour following all types of platelet transfusions. This is the best way to accurately assess the therapeutic effect.

Homologous Transfusion

A **homologous transfusion** is one in which blood is collected from a donor for transfusion into other individuals who are in need of blood. The blood may come from volunteers, designated donors, and/or cadavers. Volunteer donors visit a blood bank periodically and donate a unit of blood to be used by an unspecified person. This blood is labeled "volunteer donor." Designated donors are individuals chosen by the intended recipient to donate blood. Cadaver blood is usually collected with the body still on artificial life support. Regardless of which method is used to

CHART 23–4   **Types of Blood Components**

Type of Blood Product	Amount	Action	Uses	Storage	Special Considerations
Whole blood	500 mL.	Increases RBCs to carry the oxygen (O_2) to the tissues. Increases plasma to augment intravascular volume and protein and clotting factors.	Shock, hemorrhage, low hemoglobin, hematocrit, and circulating volume.	For up to 35 days at 0–10°C. Warm for 20–30 minutes prior to administration.	Monitor for volume overload. Give slowly. Use fresh blood when possible to avoid increased amounts of potassium, ammonia, and cellular debris that accumulates in stored blood.
Packed RBCs	250–300 mL. 80% of plasma removed. Hematocrit 70%.	Increases RBCs, hematocrit. Increases O_2 carrying capacity.	Anemia associated with cancer, liver, and cardiac disease, renal disease, and for moderate blood loss. Useful when volume overload is a risk.	Same as whole blood.	More viscous than whole blood; slows transfusion. Most common blood product given.
Washed RBCs	250–300 mL. 80% of plasma removed. Hematocrit 70%.	Increases RBCs, hematocrit. Increases O_2 carrying capacity.	Same as packed RBCs, except previous transfusion reactions have occurred. Decreased fibrinogen coating.	Same as whole blood.	RBCs washed with sterile isotonic saline before transfusion. More viscous than whole blood; slows transfusion.
Frozen RBCs	250–300 mL. 80% of plasma removed. Hematocrit 70%.	Increases RBCs, hematocrit. Increases O_2 carrying capacity.	Storage of rare blood type or frequent transfusion reactions. Storage for autologous future use.	Frozen up to 3 years at −87°C (−188.6°F). Must be used within 24 hours of thawing. Storage in liquid state after 24 hr results in loss of clotting factors.	Relatively free of WBCs and microemboli. Expensive.
Leukocyte-poor RBCs	200–325 mL. 80% of plasma removed. Hematocrit 70%.	Increases RBCs, hematocrit. Increases O_2 carrying capacity.	Previous sensitivity to WBC antigens from prior transfusions or pregnancy.	Same as whole blood.	Decreases transfusion reactions.
Fresh frozen plasma	200–250 mL.	Restores plasma volume in shock without increasing RBCs. Increases factors V, VII, VIII, IX, and X.	Bleeding due to liver disease and hemophilia disseminated intravascular coagulation (DIC), hemorrhage, massive transfusion.	Frozen up to 1 year. Must be used within 24 hours after thawing to prevent deterioration of factors V and VIII.	Effective for rapid volume replacement. Give through a filter. No platelets in FFP.
Platelets	50–70 mL.	Increases platelets and maintains normal blood coagulability. Expected increase of 10,000 mm^3	Bleeding due to thrombocytopenia (<10,000 to 20,000 mm^3) and thrombocytopathy. Bone marrow depression and DIC.	Five days at room temperature depending on type of collection and storage bag.	Can be made packed, washed, or leukocyte poor. Bag needs to be agitated periodically. Failure to increase platelets after administration could be due to fever, sepsis, splenomegaly, and DIC.

CHART 23-4	Types of Blood Components—*Continued*				
Type of Blood Product	**Amount**	**Action**	**Uses**	**Storage**	**Special Considerations**
Albumin (5% or 25% solution)	25-mL, 50-mL, and 100-mL bottles.	Increases plasma colloid osmotic pressure. Increases plasma volume.	Hypovolemic shock and chronic liver failure. Hypoalbuminemia. Burns. Pulmonary and peripheral edema and hypoproteinemia.	Up to 5 years. Check expiration date prior to administration.	No preservatives so each bottle must be used at once. Rapid infusion can cause volume overload. Rate of infusion should not exceed 1 mL/min. Potential capillary leakage in shock due to increased permeability. Often administered with diuretic to prevent fluid overload.
Cryoprecipitate	5–20 mL/unit.	Increases factors VIII and XIII, von Willebrand's factor, and fibrinogen.	Hemophilia, congenital or acquired fibrinogen deficiency, von Willebrand's disease.	Frozen up to 1 year. When thawed must be used within 6 hours.	Multiple units (8–15) typically given depending on reason for administration.
Factor VIII	Number of units is stated on each vial.	Increases factor VIII.	Hemophilia A.	Given either IV push or IV drip.	A factor VIII coagulant level of 30–50% is common end point therapy.
Factor IX	Number of units is stated on each vial.	Increases factor IX.	Hemophilia B or Christmas disease, congenital factor VII or X deficiency.	IV push.	Factor IX levels need to be performed at appropriate intervals to determine response.

Sources: U.S. Department of Health and Human Services, 2000; Josephson, D. (2004). *Intravenous infusion therapy for nurses* (2nd ed.). Clifton Park, NY: Delmar Cengage Learning.

obtain the blood, it must be ABO and Rh typed and tested for all of the diseases outlined earlier in Chart 23–3 (p. 542).

Designated (Directed) Blood

Designated, or directed, blood is collected from a donor designated by the intended recipient. Compatibility testing is required and the blood must meet all of the requirements of homologous blood including being free from transfusion-transmitted diseases. This method of blood donation is controversial due to the risk of a donor whom the recipient knows not disclosing high-risk behaviors.

Autologous Transfusion

Autologous transfusion is the process of collection and reinfusion of the patient's own blood. There are three forms of autologous transfusion; (1) preoperative donation, (2) perioperative blood salvage, and (3) postoperative blood salvage. The advantages to this type of blood replacement are:

- Elimination of infectious disease transmission
- No risk of transfusion reaction
- Provides a source of blood for persons with a rare type or antibodies that make it difficult to find compatible blood.

These blood products require special handling and labeling under strict guidelines by trained personnel before storage and reinfusion; therefore, an autologous transfusion is more expensive than blood obtained from a volunteer donor (Josephson, 2004).

Preoperative Donation

The blood is collected from individuals who are preparing for surgery at a later date. This method is useful for healthy patients who are having elective surgery where the potential need for transfusion is high (e.g., orthopedic surgery). Typically the blood is collected 1 to 6 weeks prior to surgery and stored for reinfusion. The patients are given iron supplements to help build up the RBCs. Occasionally erythropoietin (Procrit, Epogen) is given to stimulate erythropoiesis to maintain the required hematocrit.

CHART 23–5 Blood Administration Procedure

PURPOSE

- To administer blood products safely to patients with altered hematologic function.
- To replace circulating blood volume.
- To restore oxygen carrying capacity.
- To stop and prevent bleeding.

EQUIPMENT

- Y-type blood transfusion tubing (see Figure 23–1 ■, p. 552).
- 250- to 500-mL bag of normal saline (0.9% NaCl).
- Blood product from blood bank.
- Blood administration record for vital sign assessment (Figure 23–2 ■, p. 553).
- Nonsterile gloves.
- Alcohol wipes.
- Tape.
- 18- to 20-gauge IV catheter.
- IV pole.

ASSESSMENT PARAMETERS

- Size of IV catheter (18 to 20 gauge).
- Health care provider's order for type, amount, and rate of blood administration.
- History of blood transfusion reactions.
- Religious or other personal objections to receiving blood products.
- Compatibility of blood product to recipient blood type.
- Circulatory and respiratory status.
- Vital signs before, during, and after transfusion.
- Presence of rash prior to transfusion.

SPECIAL CONSIDERATIONS

- No medications are to be piggybacked into a transfusion.
- The transfusion is never interrupted for medication administration.
- Only 0.9% NaCl is to be infused in the same line as the blood.

PLANNING FOR BLOOD ADMINISTRATION

- Obtain patient transfusion history (previous transfusions, transfusion reactions).
- Ensure the patient understands the need for blood administration and is willing to sign the informed consent. Informed consent is obtained by the health care provider. The blood is not given without the consent.
- Check health care provider's order for type of blood product to be administered.
- Check size and insertion date of the IV catheter:
  - 18- or 20-gauge catheter, depending on the hospital protocol.
  - If the catheter is more than 48 hours old, it should not be used for administration of blood products. (*Note:* Specific agency protocols supersede this procedure.)

NURSING IMPLEMENTATION: ADMINISTRATION PROTOCOL

- Wash hands and assemble appropriate equipment.
- Explain to patient/family the procedure and rationale, length of transfusion, as appropriate. Assess understanding.
- Instruct patient to report *any* unusual symptoms.

- Follow hospital protocol for obtaining blood products from the laboratory.
- Close all three clamps on the Y-type blood tubing with filter and attach the 0.9% NaCl (NS) bag, open the clamp to the NS, and purge the Y-tubing (see Figure 23–1 ■, p. 552).
- Make sure the filter chamber is completely filled with saline.
- Using aseptic technique, connect tubing to IV catheter or to saline lock.
- Check identification of blood product with two (2) *licensed staff nurses* and the patient:
  - Patient name and medical record number (in chart and on the blood product). (*Note:* It is often useful to check the birth date as well.)
  - Blood product type and unit number.
  - Blood ABO group and Rh factor of both donor blood and patient.
  - Expiration date of blood product (may be given up to midnight on expiration day).
  - Both nurse's sign and date blood bank slip that is attached to the blood bag.
- Compare the above patient identification information with the patient's name band.
- Obtain baseline vital signs (TPR, BP) and document on the chart. Follow hospital protocol for frequency of reassessing vital signs.
- Prior to handling any blood products, put on nonsterile gloves and use standard precautions.
  - Connect blood bag to the free arm of the Y-tubing (see Figure 23–1 ■, p. 552) and open the roller clamp on the same arm of the Y.
  - Close the clamp on the NS side of the Y tubing before opening the clamp on the blood side of the Y tubing.
  - Begin infusion of blood product by adjusting the roller clamp closest to the patient's IV site.
  - Take vital signs prior to the infusion of the blood.
  - The nurse must remain with the patient for this 15-minute period and observe the patient for transfusion reactions (Chart 23–6, p. 549). Blood products should be infused very slowly for the first 15 minutes of the transfusion.
  - Vital signs are taken after the first 15 minutes.
  - If there are no indications of a transfusion reaction, increase the infusion rate to the prescribed rate or the standard hospital infusion rate.
- Continue observation for transfusion reactions until the blood product has completely infused.
- Terminating the transfusion:
  - Flush the IV tubing with normal saline by closing the blood product roller clamp and opening the saline roller clamp.
  - Follow hospital protocol for discarding blood product bag and tubing.
  - Flush IV catheter after discontinuing blood tubing.

DOCUMENTATION IN PATIENT RECORD AND BLOOD ADMINISTRATION RECORD (SEE FIGURE 23–2 ■, P. 553)

- Date.
- Time the infusion was started and completed.
- Volume of blood product and normal saline infused (Intake and output record).
- Blood product and number.
- Signature of the two nurses who checked the blood product.
- Baseline and continuing patient assessment.

CHART 23–5   **Blood Administration Procedure—*Continued***

SPECIAL EQUIPMENT USED FOR TRANSFUSION THERAPY

- Blood warmers are used when blood is infused rapidly.
- Infusion pumps are used when blood needs to be given at a very specific rate to prevent fluid overload.

NURSING EVALUATION

- Vital signs before, during, after the transfusion.
- Lung assessment during and after the transfusion.
- Hemoglobin and hematocrit.
- Transfusion reaction.
- Changes in fatigue levels.
- Increased tissue perfusion.
- Clinical manifestations of anemia.

Source: Kozier, Barbara J; Erb, Glenora; Berman, Audrey; Snyder, Shirlee. Fundamentals of Nursing: Concepts, Procedures, & Practices, 7th, © 2004. Electronically reproduced by permission of Pearson Education, Inc., Upper Saddle River, New Jersey.

One unit of blood is typically collected each week, up to 72 hours prior to surgery. The number of needed units varies depending on the surgical procedure. Individual units of blood components also can be collected and stored for future use. The American Red Cross (ARC) requires that autologous blood be given only to the donor. If the blood is not used, it can be stored up to 10 years for future surgeries. It can never be placed in the general donor supply to be used by someone else.

Criteria for donation include a minimum hemoglobin of 11 g/dL, hematocrit of 33%, and no presence of infection. Individuals with unstable angina, acute cardiovascular and cerebrovascular disease, and hypertension may not donate. Cancer patients may donate provided they meet the minimum criteria for donation, as listed earlier in the National Guidelines box (p. 540). Before the transfusion the patient and blood are typed and crossmatched to confirm the ABO and Rh factors and tested for diseases (see Chart 23–3, p. 542) to protect the people handling the blood. The blood is processed and stored in designated blood banks until reinfusion.

Most patients take iron supplementation (ferrous sulfate 325 mg three times per day or ferrous gluconate 325 mg five times daily) starting 1 week before donation and continuing until surgery.

Perioperative Blood Salvage

Perioperative blood salvage is defined as the collection and reinfusion of blood lost during both the intraoperative and early postoperative periods. This is a common procedure employed for major surgeries such as cardiovascular bypass, orthopedic, and vascular surgeries, splenectomy, organ transplantation, and trauma when major blood loss has occurred (Josephson, 2004). The blood is collected under sterile conditions and may be reinfused back into the patient with a standard blood filter and gravity. Suction is used to salvage the blood but it does not traumatize the RBCs. The viability of recovered RBCs is comparable to that obtained with homologous transfusions. This salvage process has all the advantages of an autologous transfusion as outlined earlier, except that the blood has to be given within 12 hours after collection. The amount of blood recovered is usually about 50% of what is lost, so it often precludes the need for a transfusion.

Perioperative blood salvage, however, has a number of disadvantages, the main one being a considerable loss of coagulation factors and platelets. Due to the risk of spreading infection, blood is not used if there is an infection present or if intestinal contents have contaminated the sterile surgical field. Washing and filtering the blood does not eliminate bacteria from the salvaged blood. If malignancy is present, the blood is not used due to risk of causing the cancer to metastasize to other organs.

Postoperative Blood Salvage

Postoperative blood salvage is used following major surgeries, typically cardiovascular, thoracic, and some orthopedic procedures. Blood is obtained from mediastinal and chest tubes and then reinfused. Even though the blood has been diluted with normal saline, it still has viable RBCs, making it useful for increasing tissue perfusion.

Therapeutic Apheresis

As mentioned earlier, apheresis, a Greek word meaning to "separate," is a process in which blood is removed from the donor and passed through an automated cell separation device that removes specific components. The remaining blood is then returned to the donor. Apheresis platelets are collected from a single donor rather than multiple donors, and each unit contains 200 to 400 mL. This is equivalent to six to eight units of platelets obtained from separate donors. Donors can have platelets apheresed about 24 times per year (Kleinman, 2006b).

White blood cells can be obtained in a similar manner, typically after the donor has received growth factors (G-CSF, GM-CSF) to stimulate WBC formation. Growth factors also release stem cells into the circulation that can be harvested over a period of several days and used for a peripheral blood stem cell transplant (Chapter 60 ⊕).

Another use for apheresis is to remove specific components of the blood to treat certain diseases. For example, WBCs and platelets can be removed by a centrifuge process and the remaining blood given back to the patient. When platelets and WBCs are removed, the temporary reduction in the number of these cells decreases immunity, thus allowing time for chemotherapy to have a therapeutic effect. Finally, removal of plasma is typically done so that specific abnormal proteins can be transiently lowered until long-term therapy is initiated. This process is performed for many reasons some of which include autoimmune diseases such as Raynaud's phenomenon (Chapter 43 ⊕), hematologic disorders such as sickle cell anemia (Chapter 65 ⊕), and some neurological conditions including myasthenia gravis and multiple sclerosis (Chapter 31 ⊕) (McLeod, 2000).

Risks Associated with Transfusion Therapy

Transfusion therapy is associated with a variety of risk factors that need to be evaluated prior to and monitored during the transfusion to ensure patient safety. Risks of transfusion therapy include disease transmission, bacterial contamination, acute or delayed transfusion reactions, and circulatory overload. When it is necessary to administer massive transfusions (replacement of greater than one blood volume in 24 hours), the risks include hypothermia, hemodilution, and platelet dysfunction (Rose, 2007). Finally, there is also a somewhat rare risk for the development of a pulmonary reaction to blood administration, referred to as *transfusion-related acute lung injury,* which is discussed in a later section. When informing the recipient about the reason for the transfusion, it is important for the nurse to explain the risks, the benefits, and what to expect during and after the transfusion. Patients must understand that the blood supply is not completely risk free. Each of the risks of transfusion therapy is discussed next. Note also that the nurse must be aware of how blood transfusions can affect the elderly, as discussed in the Gerontological Considerations box.

Disease Transmission

The FDA (2006b) states that the blood supply in the United States is not without risk of transmitting infectious disease, although the blood supply is safer than ever before. Currently tests for the nine diseases outlined earlier in Chart 23–3 (p. 542) are conducted on each unit of blood (AABB, 2003). It remains a nursing responsibility to inform the patient that there are still some risks associated with blood transfusion therapy.

Bacterial Contamination

Bacterial contamination of blood products is very rare, but may occur at any point from procurement to processing and during administration. A unit of contaminated blood product may appear normal or it may have an abnormal color. The refrigeration process helps prevent the growth of bacteria in the donated blood because most bacteria cannot survive the cold temperatures. Platelets are stored at room temperature and therefore are more susceptible to bacterial growth. Besides refrigeration, other

measures that help prevent bacterial contamination and growth include meticulous care in the handling of blood products and following time guidelines when administering the blood. For example, whole blood and RBCs need to be infused within 4 hours because room temperature promotes bacterial growth.

The clinical manifestations of bacterial contamination may not occur until the transfusion is complete, or in some instances several hours later depending on the virulence of the infecting organism. Fever, chills, and hypotension are common initial symptoms. Endotoxic shock and even death will occur if the infection is left untreated (Brown & Whalen, 2000). Fluid replacement, antibiotics, and vasopressors (for blood pressure) are needed immediately to prevent irreversible shock and death.

 As soon as abnormal clinical manifestations occur when transfusing blood, the transfusion is stopped, the doctor is notified, and the blood and tubing are sent to the laboratory for testing and culturing. The nurse may not know the exact reason for the clinical manifestations, but when they occur, the focus is on preventing complications and, at times death.

Transfusion Reactions

With blood administration there is always the risk of having a transfusion reaction occur. It is essential for the nurse to know the signs and symptoms of each type of transfusion reaction and comprehend the importance of immediate treatment in order to prevent potentially fatal complications. During and after the transfusion, it is vital for the nurse to observe the patient for complications of transfusion therapy and know how to carry out the necessary interventions to reverse the reaction, if possible.

Transfusion reactions may be acute or delayed. Acute or immediate reactions can occur as soon as 5 minutes after starting the transfusion, whereas delayed transfusion reactions may occur from 48 hours to 6 months later. There also may be a reaction when a patient receives multiple units of blood products due to preservatives used to store the blood. If possible prior to administering blood, the nurse needs to obtain a health history including allergies and reactions to previous transfusions. Patients with allergies potentially have a higher risk of transfusion reaction and need to be observed closely. Patients who have had previous transfusion reactions or have received multiple transfusions frequently are medicated with antipyretics and/or antihistamines prior to the transfusion due to the presence of antibodies. Chart 23–6 outlines the essential information related to transfusion reactions and the associated nursing care requirements. The Critical Alert discusses the essential nursing actions required during an acute transfusion reaction.

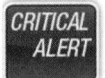 *When a transfusion reaction is occurring and it is necessary to stop the transfusion, it is essential for the nurse to keep the intravenous (IV) line patent. It may be needed to administer emergency medication to treat the presenting signs and symptoms. The line will need to be flushed with normal saline and/or a continuous infusion of fluid initiated by the nurse as soon as the blood transfusion is disconnected from the IV site.*

White Blood Cell Reduction

White blood cells do not contribute to the efficacy of blood transfusions. They are generally regarded as contaminants that

---

GERONTOLOGICAL CONSIDERATIONS for Blood Transfusions

The nurse must possess critical thinking and clinical judgment skills in order to assess the patient's tolerance of a transfusion. Unless the patient is acutely hemorrhaging or is significantly hypovolemic, blood is administered slowly to prevent fluid overload. The nurse needs to know the patient's medical history in order to be aware of the risk for this development. This is especially true for elderly patients with a history of heart failure or renal insufficiency/failure who would be more at risk than a young patient with a healthy heart. Frequent monitoring of high-risk patients will typically prevent complications. Often with elderly patients with previous heart failure problems, the health care provider orders furosemide (diuretic) to be given before or after the transfusion. If the patient is to receive more than one unit, furosemide is often ordered to be given between the two units.

CHART 23–6	Transfusion Reactions		
Class	**Cause**	**Clinical Manifestations**	**Nursing Care**
Allergic reaction	Recipient's sensitivity to foreign plasma proteins. Common in patients with allergies.	Itching, hives, flushing, and chills.	Slow the transfusion. Take vital signs. Notify the health care provider. May be necessary to medicate with antipyretic and/or antihistamine. Then resume the transfusion.
Febrile nonhemolytic reaction	Due to leukocyte or thrombocyte incompatibility (donor's WBCs or platelets react with recipient's antibodies). Usually occurs after multiple transfusions. Accounts for 90% of transfusion reactions. Fever begins about 2 hours after the transfusion. WBC reduced blood helps prevent these reactions.	Increased pulse rate, temperature > 1°C, chills, headache, nausea and vomiting, anxiety, flushing, back pain, muscle aches.	Stop transfusion, but maintain IV site. Give antipyretics as prescribed. Take vital signs. Notify health care provider. Obtain urine and blood sample. Send blood bag, normal saline, and IV tubing to the laboratory. Consider using leukocyte-poor blood.
Delayed hemolytic reaction	May occur up to 14 days after a transfusion when the level of the antibodies has increased to the extent that a reaction occurs.	Fever, anemia, increased bilirubin level, decreased or absent haptoglobin, and jaundice.	Generally not dangerous, but it is important to recognize the reaction because subsequent transfusions may cause a more severe hemolytic reaction. Typically not recognized or treated due to the mild nature of the reaction.
Acute hemolytic reaction	ABO incompatibility of the blood and recipient. May be due to a mistake in labeling by laboratory or blood bank or nursing error. Causes agglutination of cells, which causes obstruction of the capillaries and blockage of blood flow.	Bloody urine and decreased urine output. Petechiae, jaundice, decreased BP, chest tightness, low back pain, nausea, anxiety, and dyspnea. Hypotension, bronchospasm, and vascular collapse may occur. Hemoglobinemia, acute renal failure, shock, cardiac arrest, death. Symptoms typically occur within the first 15 minutes of the transfusion.	Emergent life-threatening situation. Stop transfusion, but maintain IV site and infuse IV colloid solutions to maintain BP. Give diuretics as prescribed to maintain urine flow. Insert urinary catheter to assess output and color. Obtain vital signs. Treat shock. Start CPR if necessary. Give epinephrine. Notify health care provider. Obtain urine and blood sample. Send blood bag, normal saline, and IV tubing to the laboratory.
Hemolytic or anaphylactic reaction	Reaction to donor plasma proteins. Specifically, infusion of IgA proteins to an IgA-deficient recipient who has an IgA antibody.	Wheezing, restlessness, anxiety; progressing to cyanosis, shock, and possibly cardiac arrest.	Stop infusion, but maintain IV site. Give epinephrine per doctor's order. Initiate CPR if necessary. Notify health care provider. Obtain urine and blood sample. Send blood bag, normal saline, and IV tubing to the laboratory.

Sources: Josephson, D. (2004). Intravenous infusion therapy for nurses (2nd ed.). Clifton Park, NY: Delmar Cengage Learning; Porth, C. M. (2005). Pathophysiology: Concepts of altered health status (7th ed.). Philadelphia: Lippincott Williams & Wilkins.

potentially reduce transfusion safety (ARC, 2006). As mentioned earlier, until recently, reducing WBCs has been reserved for patients who are considered high risk for developing problems from the presence of WBCs, including immunocompromised patients. Recent advances in leukocyte reduction technology have contributed to the ease and effectiveness of removing leukocytes from blood and blood products including

whole blood and RBCs (FDA, 2006b). Currently most blood banks reduce WBCs for every recipient. White blood cell reduction reduces the incidence of febrile transfusion reactions (see Chart 23–6) and the transmission of cytomegalovirus (ARC, 2006). The FDA concluded that there are no significant adverse effects with leukocyte reduction. All leukocyte-reduced blood products are specifically labeled "leukocyte reduced."

Noninfectious Serious Hazards of Transfusion Therapy

According to the AABB (2003) there has been a 10,000-fold reduction in transfusion-transmitted infectious diseases in recent decades, but there has been very little progress in reducing the risk of noninfectious serious hazards from transfusions. As a result patients are harmed from noninfectious hazards at a rate of 100-fold to 1,000-fold. The most common noninfectious transfusion-related problems include:

- Mistransfusion and ABO/Rh incompatible transfusion
- Cardiopulmonary toxicity/circulatory overload
- Transfusion-related graft versus host disease
- Transfusion-related acute lung injury
- Metabolic derangements in pediatric and massive transfusion
- Undertransfusion.

Mistransfusion and ABO/Rh Incompatible Transfusion

Transfusion of incompatible blood (see Chart 23–6, p. 549) or mistransfusion is the most common cause of serious morbidity and mortality associated with transfusions (AABB, 2003). Errors may occur at the time of sample collection, within the laboratory, when the blood is issued from the laboratory, or at the bedside. This type of transfusion reaction is typically fatal and the incidence has not significantly decreased. One study by the New York State Department of Health reported that the incidence of these fatal reactions has not decreased significantly in decades in New York State (Linden, Wagner, Voytovich, & Sheehan, 2000).

Circulatory Overload

Circulatory overload can occur with transfusions when the blood is infused too rapidly or in too large a quantity, thus causing hypervolemia. The osmotic makeup of the blood causes fluid to be mobilized from the interstitial space, thereby increasing intravascular volume well beyond that given during the transfusion. High-risk patients include the elderly and those individuals who already have increased circulatory volume or who have a history of heart failure. Clinical manifestations of circulatory overload include dyspnea, tachycardia, distended neck veins, crackles in the lungs, and a rise in blood pressure. If the transfusion is not slowed down or stopped, pulmonary edema will result. A complete description of heart failure and the impact of fluid volume are discussed in Chapter 42 ✆.

If the blood is administered slowly, typically circulatory overload can be prevented. The only time blood is given rapidly is when a patient is hemorrhaging or is severely volume depleted. Packed RBCs are safer than whole blood for high-risk individuals because the plasma portion of the blood has been removed, which decreases the volume of the unit by approximately one-half. Frequently diuretics are administered between units or after the transfusion to high-risk individuals to decrease the circulating volume. If pulmonary edema is present, oxygen, diuretics, morphine, and in severe cases mechanical ventilation may be necessary.

Transfusion Related Graft Versus Host Disease

Graft versus host disease (GVHD) occurs in severely immunocompromised patients when transfused lymphocytes attack host lymphocytes or body tissues. Clinical manifestations include diarrhea, fever, diffuse red skin rash, nausea, vomiting, and hepatitis. The primary prevention is to administer leukocyte-reduced blood products. There is no effective therapy or cure for GVHD, thus nursing care focuses on managing the signs and symptoms. Mortality resulting from acute GVHD is directly related to severity, with overwhelming sepsis being the primary cause of death in patients with acute GVHD (Kuechle, 2005).

Transfusion-Related Acute Lung Injury

See Evidence-Based Practice box for Transfusion of Blood Products (p. 554). **Transfusion-related acute lung injury (TRALI)** is a serious, life-threatening clinical syndrome that is a complication of blood transfusions (Silliman, Ambruso, & Boshkov, 2005). In fact, TRALI is the most commonly reported cause of transfusion-related deaths in the United States, surpassing those caused by ABO incompatibility and bacterial contamination (Silliman et al., 2005). Due to the difficulty of specifically identifying the disorder, it is difficult to calculate the incidence. One group of investigators calculated that it occurs in approximately 1 in every 1,000 to 2,400 units of blood (Finlay, Cassorla, Feiner, & Toy, 2005). No identifiable risk factors have been found.

The exact cause of this complication is not fully understood. One prevailing theory is that TRALI is thought to be caused by the presence of granulocyte antibodies and biologically active lipids in the donor plasma that the recipient reacts to. If antibodies are present in the donor's plasma, they stimulate the WBCs in the recipient's blood. Aggregates of WBCs form and occlude the microvasculature of the lungs (Halpern, Taichman, & Hansen-Flaschen, 2005). Whatever the cause, the end result is increased pulmonary vascular permeability leading to the clinical manifestations described next. All plasma-containing blood components, including RBCs, platelets, FFP, and cryoprecipitates, can be a cause of TRALI.

Clinical manifestations include sudden onset of respiratory distress during or shortly after a transfusion. Hypoxemia, hypotension, severe pulmonary edema, cyanosis, and fever may also occur. Diffuse crackles and decreased breath sounds in the lungs are typically present. In its most severe form, TRALI is indistinguishable from adult respiratory distress syndrome (Chapter 36 ✆). It can occur during the transfusion and as late as 6 hours after a plasma-containing transfusion, but most frequently occurs 1 to 2 hours after the transfusion. The severity of symptoms can range from mild to severe. The symptoms usually last about 96 hours and then begin to resolve. Treatment is supportive and related to the severity of symptoms. Frequently patients need ventilatory support, and diuretics are indicated if pulmonary edema is present (Halpern et al., 2005). Once TRALI has occurred the recipient should not receive any more transfusions from the same donor. Transfusion from other donors poses no increased risk.

Less Common Noninfectious Transfusion-Related Hazards

Other less common noninfectious hazards of transfusion therapy include iron overload and the side effects of multiple and massive transfusions. Repeated exposure to blood transfusion not only carries an increased risk of the transmission of blood-borne diseases but also can cause iron overload.

Iron Overload

Iron overload, referred to as hemochromatosis, may occur in patients who have chronic transfusion requirements. One unit of RBCs contains 250 mg of iron. Patients who receive repeated transfusions acquire more iron than they need and the excess builds up in the tissues. Over time these deposits can cause organ damage, particularly to the pancreas, liver, heart, and testes. Laboratory tests conducted to diagnose hemochromatosis are the total iron binding capacity (TIBC), serum iron (SI), and serum ferritin (SF) tests. These values will all be elevated in iron overload.

The treatment goal is to induce a mild anemia and maintain it until the stored iron is greatly reduced. The SF test value is a measure of stored iron and this number needs to come down to normal range. This is accomplished by bloodletting, that is, therapeutic phlebotomies. Phlebotomy refers to the removal of a full unit of blood from the patient, approximately 500 mL. This should be done in a medical setting. The schedule of this treatment should be twice a week or a minimum of once a week. Chelation therapy that is promptly initiated can prevent end-organ damage from iron toxicity.

Multiple and Massive Transfusion Reactions

A massive transfusion is defined as the replacement by transfusion of more than 50% of a patient's blood volume in 12 to 24 hours. Patients who have repeated exposure to blood products and the preservatives used to store blood products have an increased risk of developing elevated blood ammonia titers, coagulation imbalances, hypocalcemia, acid–base imbalance, and hyperkalemia (Kleinman, 2006a). The ammonia level increases in stored blood due to decomposition of the blood products. Coagulation imbalance occurs due to dilutional thrombocytopenia and decreased platelets that are destroyed in stored blood. Depending on the age of the blood product, it may have few viable clotting factors; therefore, an inability to clot normally may result from multiple transfusions. The longer the blood is stored, the more ineffective the clotting factors become. Replacement of clotting factors, plasma, and platelets is typically necessary (Kleinman, 2006a). The decrease in calcium is due to its binding with the citrate (the preservative), and hyperkalemia occurs when potassium leaks from the stored RBCs. Finally, hypothermia may occur with massive transfusions if refrigerated blood is rapidly transfused. This can be prevented by the use of a blood warming device. It is essential for the nurse to monitor for all of the potential side effects when a patient is receiving repeated transfusions.

Nursing Responsibilities Before, During, and After Transfusions

Nursing care of the patient receiving a blood transfusion requires the nurse to follow strict protocols set forth by the AABB, state licensing boards, individual employers, the Infusion Nurses Society (INS), and the American Nurses Association nurse practice act. The nurse is responsible for all aspects of blood transfusion therapy and must continually assess the patient's response to the transfusion. Knowledge specific to blood transfusions includes blood types, blood component therapy, administration equipment, specific techniques for administering each component, and hazards of transfusion therapy. Critical thinking and clinical judgments skills are necessary because the clinical manifestations of a transfusion reaction are not always "textbook." Therefore, the nurse is responsible for evaluating each situation and being knowledgeable about and able to respond with the appropriate care when problems occur.

Nursing Management

Blood transfusion therapy occurs most frequently in the acute care setting, although under certain circumstances patients will receive blood in other settings. Patients who need chronic transfusions may use free-standing infusion centers, ambulatory care settings, doctor's offices, and even private homes for their transfusions. Nurses need to have the skill and knowledge to adapt to any of these settings when performing a blood transfusion. Use of the nursing process provides the template that enables the nurse to safely perform transfusion therapy in multiple settings. Outlined next are the necessary steps within the nursing process for safe blood administration.

Patients are required to sign a consent form prior to the transfusion. It is the health care provider's responsibility to explain why the transfusion is needed and what risks are associated with the procedure. The nurse's responsibility includes verifying that the patient understands the health care provider's explanation prior to signing the consent form. It is essential for the patient to understand that once the transfusion begins, any unusual signs or symptoms must be reported to the nurse.

Assessment

Prior to beginning a transfusion, the nurse needs to obtain a transfusion history from the patient. This includes information about previous transfusions, allergies, and any transfusion reaction. Information about the type of transfusion reaction, its manifestations, and treatment also is necessary and must be documented in the patient's record. This will alert the nurse about the risk of transfusion reactions and possibly the need for premedication to prevent an allergic reaction.

The physical assessment includes vital signs prior to beginning the transfusion. This provides a baseline for vital sign assessment during the transfusion. An acute rise in the body temperature may indicate a transfusion reaction, thus it is essential to know the baseline temperature. Fluid overload causes changes in both pulse and blood pressure, therefore obtaining baseline vital signs enables the nurse to monitor and assess significant changes. Additionally, lung sounds need a baseline assessment. The development of rales may also indicate fluid overload. Any concurrent health problems relating to cardiac, respiratory, or renal diseases need to be assessed.

 *During a transfusion it is essential for the nurse to assess the patient's vital signs and lungs sounds. The heart rate and respiratory rate increase when fluid overload occurs and rales can be heard in the lungs. Additionally, these patients tend to develop cardiac dysrhythmias. If these changes occur, the nurse needs to slow the transfusion and notify the health care provider.*

Nursing Diagnosis

The nursing diagnoses associated with the need for blood administration include:

1. *Fluid Volume Deficit* related to blood loss.
2. *Gas Exchange Impaired* related to low hemoglobin.
3. *Ineffective Tissue Perfusion* related to hypovolemia.
4. *Fatigue* related to low hemoglobin.
5. *Decreased Cardiac Output* related to hypovolemia.
6. *Risk of Injury* related to complications of blood transfusion.

Planning

In addition to reviewing the patient's medical history, the nurse must plan for and prepare the equipment that will be used during blood administration.

Equipment Preparation

A 16- to 20-gauge catheter is required for RBCs to pass through without being damaged. Using a smaller gauge needle also may slow or stop the transfusion. Special Y-type blood tubing with an in-line filter is always used for the administration of blood products (Figure 23–1 ■). Normal saline (0.9% NaCl) is attached to one of the Y sites and the tubing is primed with normal saline prior to blood administration.

 **CRITICAL ALERT** *Only normal saline can be administered with blood. Dextrose solutions cause hemolysis of the cells. Calcium, which is present in lactated Ringer's solutions, can cause coagulation in citrated (preservative) blood. To increase the rate of the transfusion and decrease the viscosity of the blood, normal saline may run simultaneously to help thin the blood product.*

The purpose of an in-line filter is to trap clots and other debris from all blood components older than 5 days. Some institutions require additional in-line filters to be added to the blood tubing. There are basically two purposes for these additional filters. One type of filter augments the in-line filter in trapping clots and debris, and the other filter removes leukocytes for patients with a history of febrile reactions.

Other optional equipment used for transfusions includes electronic infusion pumps, pressure cuffs, and blood warmers. Electronic pumps regulate the rate or speed of the transfusion and are used when blood needs to be given very rapidly or very slowly. Special blood tubing can be inserted into infusion pumps, and the rate of administration is dialed into the pump. External cuffs may be applied to the outside of the blood bag and the cuffed bag is inflated, which pushes the blood in and therefore increases the rate of infusion. These bags are contraindicated unless large-bore catheters are used. The bag pressure should never exceed 300 mmHg. Blood warmers are used when rapid infusion of blood products is necessary and there is an increased risk of hypothermia. Cold blood may precipitate cardiac dysrhythmias and cardiac arrest associated with rapid, massive infusion of cold blood products. Blood warmers have a preset maximum temperature of 38°C (100.4°F) so as not to damage the RBCs. Blood should never be immersed under hot water or placed in a microwave oven for warming.

Outcome and Evaluation Parameters

The outcome of blood administration is dependent on the reason for the transfusion. For example if it is needed for a low red

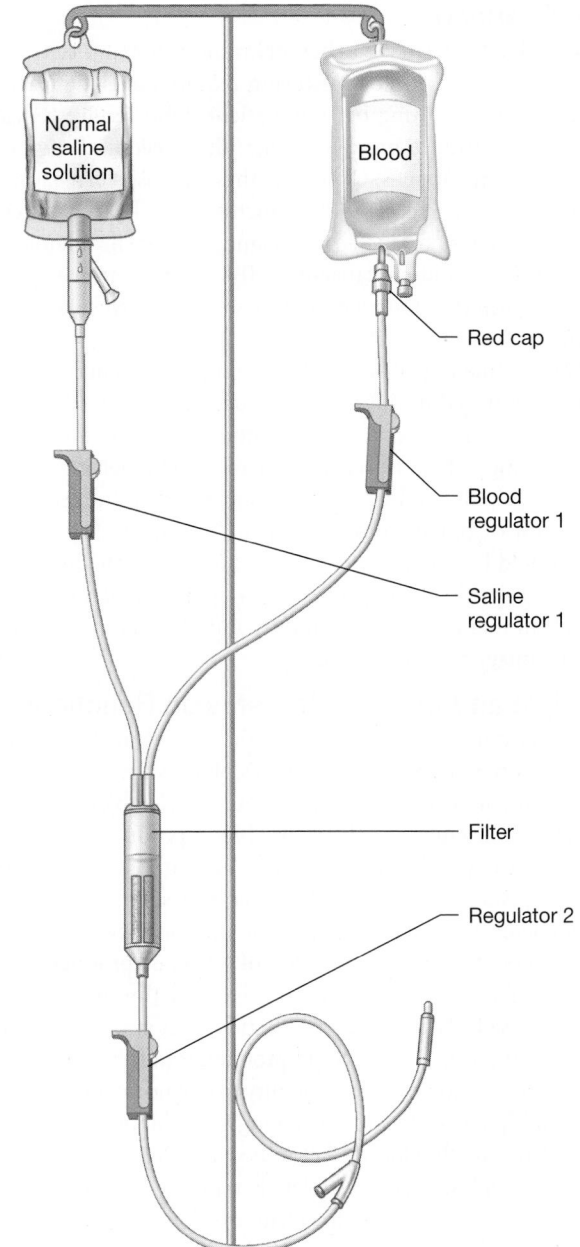

FIGURE 23–1 ■ Y-type blood tubing.

blood cell count, then the outcome is to normalize the value. If the need for the transfusion is due to low platelets resulting in bleeding, the outcome is to normalize the platelet count and stop or prevent blood loss. Since blood administration is just part of a treatment plan, it is imperative that the reason for the abnormality be identified and corrected, if possible. Evaluation parameters include a normal red blood cell count, hemoglobin, hematocrit, platelet count, and clotting factors. Additionally, part of the evaluation would be relief from the clinical manifestations that resulted from the abnormality. These manifestations are the nursing diagnoses listed above.

Interventions and Rationales

Once the blood has been taken from the blood bank, it must be administered within 30 minutes. It cannot be stored in the refrigerator on the nursing unit because a lack of temperature control may damage the blood. When administering a blood product, it is essential to follow institutional policy. The nurse must ensure positive patient identification, appropriateness of blood component, blood product inspection, verification of donor–recipient compatibility, and verification of product expiration date.

Additionally the nurse must have knowledge of the appropriate rate at which to infuse the blood product. Occasionally the health care provider will order a specific rate; otherwise, the institution will identify safe rates of infusion of various blood products in their blood administration policy and procedure. For example, a common infusion rate for a unit of whole blood is 4 hours. Chart 23–5 (p. 546) earlier in the chapter outlines the blood administration procedure, and Figure 23–2 ■ shows a sample blood administration record.

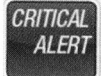 **CRITICAL ALERT** To protect both the patient and the nurse, strict hospital protocols must be followed when checking blood in order to prevent fatal transfusion reactions. It is the nurse's responsibility to know and follow the hospital protocol when checking blood. The protocols vary from institution to institution. Most agencies require that two registered nurses verify the right unit, patient, blood type, and blood product.

Evaluation

During and after the transfusion, the nurse needs to evaluate the patient for response to the transfusion. The nurse must stay with the patient for the first 15 minutes of the transfusion to assess for any clinical manifestations of a transfusion reaction (see Chart 23–5, p. 546). If the patient begins to have clinical manifestations that indicate an abnormal response, the nurse must have knowledge of the appropriate interventions. It is a nursing responsibility to possess the necessary clinical judgment to evaluate a normal versus abnormal response during a blood transfusion. For example, vital signs are monitored at frequencies prescribed by the institution. Both immediate and delayed reactions are manifested by altered vital signs and indicate an abnormal response to the blood. Additionally, the lungs are monitored during and after the transfusion to assess for fluid overload.

The alteration in tissue perfusion that was occurring prior to the transfusion may be assessed by evaluating the hemoglobin and hematocrit. After administration of one unit of packed RBCs in a nonbleeding adult, the hemoglobin increases by 1 g/dL and the hematocrit by 3 percentage points (U.S. Department of Health and Human Services, 2000). The patient should have

UNIVERSITY OF CALIFORNIA DAVIS
MEDICAL CENTER,
SACRAMENTO, CALIFORNIA

Blood Administration Record

PATIENT PROGRESS RECORD

Date	Product Type	Unit#	Blood Type	Time Beg.	Time End	Pre-meds ? Y	Pre-meds ? N	Pre-Infusion T	HR	RR	BP	15 minutes T	HR	RR	BP	30 minutes T	HR	RR	BP	End of Infusion T	HR	RR	BP	Bld Wmr ? Y	Bld Wmr ? N	S/S Reaction? Y	S/S Reaction? N	Signature

RECORD REACTION # IN THE "S/S REACTIONS?" COLUMN

Acute Reactions:
1 = fever
2 = temperature of > 1°C during or immediately following transfusion
3 = chills, mild itching or urticaria, sometimes confluent
4 = pain, sudden onset of dyspnea or complaints of inability to breathe
5 = hypotension
6 = sudden drop of systolic blood pressure 40 mmHg
7 = hemoglobinuria
8 = patient complaining of sense of impending doom (particularly for possible acute hemolytic reaction)
9 = abrupt change in urine color to a deep red/brown color or unexpected, sudden decrease in urine output
10 = unexplained bleeding or unexpected oozing from puncture/incision sites, chest pain, shock, pulminary edema

Delayed Reactions:
11 = unexplained onset of jaundice
12 = unexpected decrease in (or failure to increase) hemoglobin level occurring 5–13 days after transfusion
13 = unexpected elevations in liver function tests
14 = sudden and unexplained appearance of rash or diarrhea occuring 6–10 days

Transfusion Reaction Workup:
1. Send ASAP: 7mL clotted blood, and 10mL urine collected after reaction.
2. Six (6) hours post blood sample is required only for acute hemolytic transfusion reaction (HTR) or requested by Medical Director.
3. Send the remainder of the implicated unit(s) or empty blood bags, attached to administration set, all "Y" tubing with Transfusion Reaction investigation form to the Blood Bank.

FIGURE 23–2 ■ Sample blood administration record.

increased endurance and less fatigue after the transfusion due to the increased oxygen carrying capacity.

Blood Alternatives

Due to the risks associated with blood transfusion, alternative treatments for replacement of hemoglobin are sought. Recombinant technology has provided a means to augment the production of blood cells within functioning bone marrow. Referred to as *blood modifier medications,* these drugs are being used in place of transfused blood in certain groups of patients. These medications have the same biological activity as endogenous human erythropoietin. They induce erythropoiesis by stimulating the division and differentiation of cells in the bone marrow. Indications for their use are the same as for blood transfusions: anemia associated with blood loss, HIV, cancer, and renal failure. These drugs are being used in place of a blood transfusion

---

Transfusion of Blood Products

Clinical Problem

Transfusing blood products is beneficial and often lifesaving, especially in the critically ill population. Blood transfusions are not without risk, however. Anemia is common among patients admitted to intensive care units (ICUs), and studies indicate that more than 40% of patients receive RBC transfusions while in the ICU (Corwin et al., 2004; Walsh et al., 2004). Two life-threatening risks include transfusion-related acute lung injury (TRALI) and fluid overload resulting in pulmonary edema. Nurses need to understand and apply evidence-based findings when administering blood in order to mitigate the occurrence of these complications.

Research Findings

Rena and colleagues (2006) conducted a study to assess the incidence of transfusion-related acute lung injury (TRALI) and transfusion-associated circulatory overload (TACO) in critically ill patients. Patients in four different ICUs who were not on ventilatory support at the time of transfusion were followed by a custom electronic surveillance system that tracked the time of transfusion and onset of respiratory failure. For this study respiratory failure was defined as the need for noninvasive or invasive ventilator support within 6 hours of transfusion.

The study evaluated 8,902 units that were transfused in 1,351 patients. From this sample, 94 patients required new respiratory support within 6 hours of transfusion. For analysis the data were separated into categories of (1) suspected TRALI, (2) possible TRALI, and (3) TACO. The incidence of suspected TRALI was 1 in every 1,271 units transfused; possible TRALI, 1 in 534 per unit transfused; and TACO, 1 in 356 per unit transfused. It was noted that suspected and possible TRALI patients received larger amounts of plasma. The authors concluded first that in the ICU, pulmonary edema frequently occurs after blood transfusion, requiring some form of ventilatory support. Secondly, they concluded that there is an association between infusion of plasma and the development of suspected or possible TRALI, which may have important implications with regard to etiology and prevention of this syndrome.

Implications for Nursing Practice

The impact on nursing practice from the findings of this research is multidimensional and requires critical thinking skills. The nurse must be vigilant of the transfusion infusion rate for a given patient. The patient's age, medical history, current diagnosis, and hemodynamic stability all influence the infusion rate. Except in emergent situations where acute blood loss impacts hemodynamic stability, blood is transfused slowly in order to prevent fluid overload. Monitoring the patient's response to the transfusion also is of critical importance. Vital signs, lung sounds, and oxygen saturation are assessed during and after the transfusion in order to evaluate the patient's tolerance. It is essential for the nurse to report to the health care team the occurrence of abnormal lung sounds and/or a change in the rate and depth of respirations, as well as a decrease in oxygen saturation levels. The nurse needs to understand when ventilatory support is required and facilitate the plan to get it instituted.

The nurse also must be aware of the clinical manifestations of TRALI. Because this complication is often difficult to diagnose and can occur several hours after the transfusion, the nurse must continue ongoing monitoring of the patient subsequent to the transfusion. It is essential for the next shift of nurses to be told that the patient had a transfusion, especially if it was plasma, so that monitoring for side effects will be continued. Typically it is easier to limit the progress of the disorder if it is diagnosed and treated early in its development. Typically it is the nursing staff that picks up the clinical manifestations.

Critical Thinking Questions

1. You are the nurse caring for a patient who received a blood transfusion during the last shift. The nurse reported that the transfusion had occurred without incidence and that the follow-up blood work indicated that there was no need for another transfusion right now. When you assess your patient, you note that the heart respiratory rates are increased and the oxygen saturation has dropped. You suspect that the patient may be experiencing TRALI. Your nursing actions are based on:
   a. Symptoms will last a few minutes and then begin to subside.
   b. The symptoms usually last about 96 hours and then begin to resolve.
   c. Frequently patients need ventilatory support and diuretics.
   d. Since the symptoms are self limiting no medical intervention is needed.
   e. a & d
   f. b & c

2. You are caring for an 86-year-old patient with cardiac problems who is receiving his second unit of packed RBCs. During the transfusion he becomes short of breath and develops wheezes in his lung bases. What are the appropriate nursing actions?

Answers to Critical Thinking Questions appear in Appendix D.

References

Corwin, H. L., Gettinger, A., Pearl, R. G., et al. (2004). The CRIT study: Anemia and blood transfusion in the critically ill—Current clinical practice in the United States. *Critical Care Medicine, 32,* 39.

Rena, R., Fernandez-Perez, E. R., Khan, S. A., Rana, S., Winters, J. L., Lesnick, T. G., et al. (2006). Transfusion-related acute lung injury and pulmonary edema in critically ill patients: A retrospective study. *Transfusion, 46*(9), 1478–1483.

Walsh, T. S., Garrioch, M., Maciver, C., et al. (2004). Red cell requirements for intensive care units adhering to evidenced-based transfusion guidelines. *Transfusion, 44,* 1405.

EVIDENCE-BASED PRACTICE

because they are a safe and effective way to improve oxygen uptake and therefore tissue perfusion (Vernon & Pfeifer, 2003). In cases of massive hemorrhage, blood transfusion is still the treatment of choice due to the acute need for circulating volume and hemoglobin. See Chapter 64 for a complete description of blood modifier therapy.

A second method used to minimize the use of blood products is recombinant factor VIIa. Clotting occurs with the administration of factor VIIa due to the activation of factor X, which causes additional generation of thrombin, resulting in the conversion of fibrinogen to fibrin. It is useful for a variety of clinical situations including (Rose, 2007):

- Massive hemorrhage
- Thrombocytopenia
- Trauma
- Liver failure

- Oral anticoagulant toxicity
- Surgical, intracranial, and obstetrical hemorrhage
- Hemophilia.

Administration of factor VIIa has resulted in cessation of bleeding, reduced blood product use, and an improved coagulation profile (Bliss & Hanley, 2005; Growers & Parr, 2005; Mayo et al., 2004).

Research

Research is essential in order to continue improving the safety and efficacy of blood transfusion therapy. The goal of research is to identify areas where current practice could improve and then evaluate and test methods to improve these areas. The Research Opportunities and Clinical Impact feature provides a list of research topics still under investigation. Electronic databases also are a source for finding specific studies related to these topics.

RESEARCH OPPORTUNITIES AND CLINICAL IMPACT RELATED TO BLOOD ADMINISTRATION

Research Area	Clinical Impact
Prevention of disease transmission.	Ensure a safe blood supply.
Development of a synthetic product that can be used to raise hemoglobin and replace volume quickly in emergent situations and for persons who refuse blood transfusions.	Would provide a safe method for volume and cell replacement when blood products are not available due to the type and crossmatch process. Will provide a safe effective blood replacement for persons who refuse blood transfusions.
Development of a method to prevent ABO incompatibility errors.	Prevent the wrong blood being given to a patient.
A storage process that prevents the loss of viable cells and clotting factors.	Increase the therapeutic effectiveness of blood products.
Evaluate the impact of infusion devices (IV pumps) on cell integrity.	Obtain evidence that supports or negates the use of infusion pumps.
The need for additional in-line blood filters to prevent the infusion of clots and other debris.	Obtain a safer blood product.
Stimulating production of RBCs.	Treat anemia and decrease the need for a blood transfusion.
Measures to prevent or reduce blood transfusion reactions.	Increase safety of blood supply.

Clinical Preparation

CRITICAL THINKING

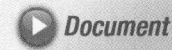 **Read**

- History of Current Illness
- Past Medical History
- Physical Exam
- Admitting Medical Orders
- Laboratory Study Results

 **Document**

- Summary of Hospitalization
- Pathophysiology Form
- Laboratory Values
- Laboratory Results Explanation

Apply

- List of Potential Nursing Diagnoses
- Concept Map
- Critical Thinking Questions

Log on to MyNursingKit.com to download forms you will need and to complete further steps in the Clinical Preparation assignment.

HISTORY OF PRESENT ILLNESS

Mr. B., an 86-year-old male, is admitted to the medical–surgical floor after being seen and evaluated in the emergency department (ED). His chief complaint is abdominal pain, nausea, and vomiting of moderate to large amounts of dark red liquid. Mr. B. has moderate to severe abdominal pain and nausea. He states he has been vomiting for 2 days and taken in very little food or water in 3 days. ED laboratory work: complete blood count (CBC), complete metabolic panel, UA, PTT, PT, and INR; liver function studies; troponin; type and crossmatch for 4 units packed cells. Vital signs in the ED were BP 90/60, HR 118, RR 28, T 37ºC. On admission to the floor, the patient is awake and alert. He states he feels weak and light-headed. Two 500-mL fluid boluses of 0.9% NS were administered in the ED.

You are the nurse caring for Mr. B on his second day of hospitalization. The night nurse reported that there had been no vomiting or bloody stools since his admission. He does continue to complain of abdominal tenderness. After morning report you evaluate the patient's morning laboratory values. All laboratory work except the hemoglobin and hematocrit are normal. When you note that the hemoglobin is 8 g/dL and the hematocrit is 24%, you call the health care provider. Two units of packed RBCs are ordered to be given this a.m. followed by an Hgb & Hct and potassium. An endoscopy is scheduled for today.

Medical–Surgical History

Non-Q wave MI: 1998
Osteoarthritis
No known allergies
Denies a history of syncope
Denies history of gastric ulcers
Denies fever, chills, and night sweats

Home Medications

ASA 81 mg po daily
Lipitor 50 mg po daily
Lopressor 100 po mg bid
Celebrex 200 mg po daily
MVI po daily
Surgeries: appendectomy in 1982

Social History

He lives with his wife; has three grown children who live in the local area

Physical Exam

Elderly male, mild discomfort due to abdominal pain
Oxygen sat 94% on RA
BP: 90/62　HR 118　RR 26
HEENT: normal
Neck: negative JVD, no bruits
Heart: NL S1, S2

Lungs: clear
Abdomen: mildly distended soft, tender, hyperactive bowel sounds
Pulses: present in all extremities; strong throughout; good cap refill
Normal neuro exam
No rash
Poor skin turgor
Osteoarthritis
12-lead EKG showed sinus tachycardia, low voltage, and nonspecific ST wave changes
Chest x-ray is within normal limits

Admitting Medical Orders

Medicine Service
Admit to Telemetry Unit
Admitting diagnosis: GI bleed of unknown etiology
No known allergies
Vital signs and oxygen saturation: q2h
Daily weight
Foley catheter
Strict I&O
NPO
Full code status
Call house officer: BP systolic < 90 > 150 & diastolic > 90; HR > 120 & < 60; RR > 30; < 30 mL of urine per hour × 2 hours; oxygen saturation < 92%

NG: Salem sump lavage until clear and clamp; if vomiting occurs, apply low wall suction

Bed rest: out of bed to bedside commode with assist only

Incentive spirometer q2h

Sequential compression device (SCD) to lower extremities

IV: 0.9 normal saline with 20 mEq of KCl via infusion pump at 125 mL/hr

Keep 2 units of RBCs on hold at all times

GI consult ordered

Scheduled Medications

Protonix 40 mg IV q12h

PRN Medications

Morphine sulfate 2–4 mg IV push q2h prn for pain

Zofran 4 mg IV q8h prn nausea and vomiting

Ordered Laboratory Studies

Amylase and lipase now

Hgb & Hct now and q6h

Chem 7 panel now and in a.m.

Liver function studies now

PT, PTT and INR in a.m.

Potassium after blood

Ordered Diagnostic Studies

Abdominal CT scan

LABORATORY STUDY RESULTS

Test	Pt. Values # 1	Pt. Values #2	Pt. Values #3
Chemistry	Emergency Department	Pre-blood	Post-blood
Sodium	148 mEq/L	143 mEq/L	
Potassium	3.5 mEq/L	3.7 mEq/L	4.2 mEq/L
Chloride	113 mEq/L	110 mEq/L	
Carbon dioxide (CO_2)	25 mEq/L	24 mEq/L	
Blood urea nitrogen (BUN)	40 mg/dL	9 mg/dL	
Creatinine	1.0 mg/dL	1.0 mg/dL	
Blood, glucose	150 mg/dL	136 mg/dL	
Calcium	8.1 mg/dL		
Amylase		60 units/L	
Lipase		82 units/L	
Magnesium	2.2 mEq/L		
Troponin I	0.2 ng/mL		
Albumin	3.9		
Alkaline phosphorus	100 units/L		
GGT (0–65)	56 units/L		
Total bilirubin	1 mg/dL		
CPK total	200 units/L		
CPK MB	2.5%		
LDH	166 units/L		
AST	42 units/L		
ALT	60 units/L		
Hematology			
WBC	8000/mm³	7000/mm³	7000/mm³
Hemoglobin	10.2 g/dL	8 g/dL	10 g/dL
Hematocrit	32%	24%	37.9%
RBC	5/mm³		
Platelets	395/mm³	325/mm³	250/mm³
PTT	24 second		
PT	16.4 second	12 seconds	
INR (<1.19)	1.5	1.19	
Urine analysis	Normal		

CRITICAL THINKING QUESTIONS

1. What might be one cause of the gastric bleeding?

2. What are some possible reasons for the hemoglobin/hematocrit to decrease on the second hospital day?

3. What are critical nursing assessments during blood administrations?

4. What might Mr. B. be at high risk for during blood administration?

5. In the presence of dehydration, why would this patient's heart rate not be more elevated?

6. Compare and contrast the first and second set of labs. What lab data indicate that the patient was dehydrated when he came into the ED?

7. Why is the health care provider ordering an amylase and lipase study?

8. Why is the first PT/INR elevated?

Answers to Critical Thinking Questions appear in Appendix D.

NCLEX® REVIEW

1. A patient is prescribed to receive a transfusion of albumin. The nurse realizes that this transfusion will:
   1. Increase plasma colloidal osmotic pressure and plasma volume.
   2. Increase platelets and increase coagulation.
   3. Increase circulating RBCs.
   4. Increase plasma volume without increasing RBCs.

2. The teenage daughter of a patient asks for information to donate blood for her mother's health care needs. Which of the following should the nurse include in this information?
   1. Family members are discouraged from donating blood for patients.
   2. The youngest age for a blood donor is 17.
   3. A donor's blood pressure has to be greater than 180/90.
   4. A donor's blood count has to be greater than 13.5 mg/dL.

3. The nurse is planning to administer a unit of PRBCs to a patient. Which of the following should be included in this planning?
   1. History of blood transfusion reactions
   2. Circulatory and respiratory status
   3. Assemble appropriate equipment
   4. Patient provides informed consent for the transfusion

4. An elderly patient receiving a blood transfusion begins to cough and has an increase in blood pressure. What should the nurse do to help this patient?
   1. Stop the blood transfusion.
   2. Administer an antipyretic.
   3. Administer epinephrine.
   4. Stop the transfusion, flush the peripheral access device, and resume the transfusion.

5. A patient receiving a unit of PRBCs complains of chest pain within 5 minutes of the start of the transfusion. What should the nurse do?
   1. Slow the transfusion rate.
   2. Stop the transfusion, call for help and begin life-supporting measures.
   3. Administer epinephrine as according to the health care provider's order.
   4. Provide antipyretics.

Answers for review questions appear in Appendix D

KEY TERMS

albumin *p.543*
apheresis *p.539*
autologous transfusion *p.545*
blood transfusion *p.539*
cryoprecipitates *p.543*
factor VIII *p.543*
fresh frozen plasma *p.543*
frozen RBCs *p.543*

homologous transfusion *p.543*
leukocyte-poor RBCs *p.543*
packed RBCs *p.543*
perioperative blood salvage *p.547*
plasma *p.539*
platelets *p.539*
postoperative blood salvage *p.547*
Rh factor *p.541*

transfusion-related acute lung injury (TRALI) *p.550*
type A blood *p.541*
type AB blood *p.541*
type B blood *p.541*
type O blood *p.541*
washed RBCs *p.543*
whole blood *p.539*

REFERENCES

American Association of Blood Banks. (2003). *Testing of donor blood for infectious disease.* Retrieved November 9, 2006, from http://www. aabb.org/Content/About_Blood/Facts_About_Blood_and_Blood_ Banking/fabloodtesting.htm

American Red Cross. (2005). *Blood donation eligibility guidelines.* Retrieved November 7, 2006, from http://www.redcross.org/ services/biomed/0,1082,0_557_,00.html#top

American Red Cross. (2006). *Leukocyte reduction Q&A.* Retrieved November 9, 2006, from http://www.redcross.org/services/biomed/ blood/supply/ulr/qanda.html

America's Blood Centers. (2006). *56 facts about blood.* Retrieved November 7, 2006, from http://www.americasblood.org/ go.cfm?do=Page.View&pid=12

Andrews, M. M., & Boyle, J. S. (2003). *Transcultural concepts in nursing care.* Philadelphia: Lippincott Williams & Wilkins.

Bliss, T., & Hanley, J. (2005). Recombinant activated factor VII (rFVIIa/NovoSeven) in intractable haemorrhage: Use of a clinical scoring system to predict outcome. *Vox Sang, 90,* 45–52.

Brown, M., & Whalen. P. K. (2000). Red blood cell transfusion in critically ill patients. *Critical Care Nurse* (Suppl.).

Finlay, H. E., Cassorla, L., Feiner, J., & Toy, P. (2005). Designing and testing a computer-based screening system for transfusion-related acute lung injury. *American Journal of Clinical Pathology, 124,* 601.

Food and Drug Administration. (2006a). *About CBER.* Retrieved November 8, 2006, from http://www.fda.gov/cber/blood.htm

Food and Drug Administration. (2006b). *Blood.* Retrieved November 9, 2006, from http://www.fda.gov/cber/blood.htm

Growers, C., & Parr, M. (2005). Recombinant activated factor VIIa use in massive transfusion and coagulopathy unresponsive to conventional therapy. *Anesthesia Intensive Care, 33,* 196–200.

Guyton, A., & Hall, J. (2000). *Textbook of medical physiology* (10th ed.). Philadelphia: W. B. Saunders.

Halpern, S. D., Taichman, D. B., & Hansen-Flaschen, J. (2005). *Transfusion-related acute lung injury (pulmonary leukoagglutinin reactions).* Retrieved November 16, 2006, from http://www. uptdol.com

Josephson, D. (2004). *Intravenous infusion therapy for nurses* (2nd ed.). Clifton Park, NY: Thompson Delmar Learning.

Kleinman, S. (2006a). *Massive blood transfusion.* Retrieved November 16, 2006, from http://www.uptdol.com

Kleinman, S. (2006b). *Patient information: Blood donation and transfusion.* Retrieved November 8, 2006, from http://patients. uptodate.com/topic.asp?file=blod_dis/2419

Kuechle, M. (2005). *Graft versus host disease.* Retrieved November 10, 2006, from http://www.emedicine.com/derm/topic478.htm

Linden, J. V., Wagner, K., Voytovich, A. E., & Sheehan, J. (2000). Transfusion errors in New York State: An analysis of 10 years' experience. *Transfusion, 40,* 1207–1213.

Lipson, J. G., Dibble, S. L., & Minarik, P. A. (1996). *Culture and nursing care: A pocket guide.* San Francisco: UCSF Nursing Press.

May, A. K., & Kauder, D. R. (2006). *Use of blood products in the critically ill.* Retrieved November 18, 2006, from http://www.uptodate.com

Mayo, A., Misgav, M., Kluger, Y., et al. (2004). Recombinant activated factor VII (NovoSeven): Addition to replacement therapy in acute, uncontrolled and life-threatening bleeding. *Vox Sang, 87,* 34–40.

Mayo Clinic. (2005). *Blood donation: A life saving gift.* Retrieved November 7, 2006, from http://www.mayoclinic.com/health/blood-donation/GA00039

McLeod, B. C. (2000). Introduction to the third space issue: Clinical applications of therapeutic apheresis. *Journal of Clinical Apheresis, 15*(1/2), 1–5.

Pearl, R. G., & Pohlman, A. S. (2002). Understanding and managing anemia in critically ill patients. *Critical Care Nurse* (Suppl.), 1–14; quiz 15–16.

Porth, C. M. (2005). *Pathophysiology: Concepts of altered health status* (7th ed.). Philadelphia: Lippincott Williams & Wilkins.

Rose, L. (2007). Recombinant factor VIIa. *AACN Advanced Critical Care, 18*(2), 141–148.

Silliman, C., Ambruso, R., & Boshkov, L. (2005). Transfusion-related acute lung injury. *Blood, 105,* 2266–2273.

U.S. Department of Health and Human Services. (2000). *Healthy people 2010: Understanding and improving health.* Retrieved June 11, 2008, from http://www.healthypeople.gov

Vernon, S., & Pfeifer, G. M. (2003). Blood management strategies for critical care patients. *Critical Care Nurse, 23*(6), 34–41.

Hemodynamic Monitoring

Patricia A. Baker

Outcome-Based Learning Objectives

After studying this chapter, the learner will be able to:

1. Explain the concept of hemodynamic monitoring.
2. Identify components of a hemodynamic monitoring system.
3. Compare and contrast arterial, central venous, and pulmonary artery pressure monitoring.
4. Identify adequate central venous and pulmonary artery pressures.
5. Evaluate nursing management of arterial lines and central venous and pulmonary artery catheters.
6. Discuss how alterations in preload, afterload, and contractility affect cardiac output.
7. Compare and contrast how measurements obtained from a central venous catheter differ from the data obtained from a pulmonary artery catheter.

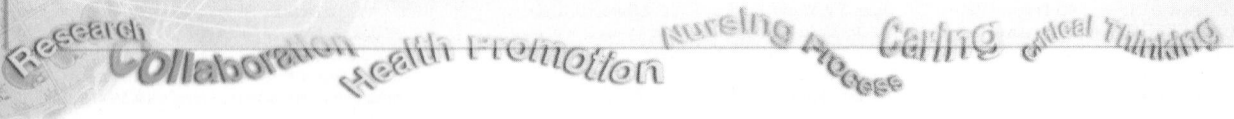

Hemodynamic monitoring is the monitoring of blood flow and pressures within the body. Current technology allows for the monitoring of both the cardiac and neurological systems. This chapter describes invasive and noninvasive hemodynamic monitoring techniques used for the cardiovascular system. The purposes of hemodynamic monitoring are to (1) aid in the diagnosis of various disorders, (2) assist in guiding therapies to minimize or correct dysfunction, and (3) evaluate the patient's response to therapy. For safe operation of hemodynamic monitoring devices, nurses must be familiar with the anatomy and physiology of the system being monitored. Moreover, the nurse must be knowledgeable about therapeutic interventions and their rationales in order to achieve optimal, patient-specific stable outcomes. Nurses must be prepared to provide care based on the findings obtained from the hemodynamic monitoring, to institute interventions, and to report changes to the health care provider when they occur.

Hemodynamic monitoring capability is not restricted to the intensive care unit (ICU). Patients who require hemodynamic assessment are treated in emergency departments, postanesthesia care units, and intermediate care units. The level of intervention differs depending on the patient's diagnosis and hemodynamic stability, but may include monitoring arterial blood pressure, central venous pressure, or intracardiac pressures, all of which are discussed throughout this chapter.

■ Equipment

Both noninvasive and invasive devices are available for hemodynamic monitoring. The required equipment depends on the parameter monitored. Noninvasive monitoring often involves a stethoscope and sphygmomanometer; however, technologies such as ultrasound, and impedance cardiography are also considered noninvasive.

Invasive monitoring necessitates the insertion of a catheter into an artery or vein for direct and ongoing measurement of vascular pressures and volumes. Hemodynamic pressures are transmitted from the intravascular space via this specialized catheter into the monitoring system for the health care team to read and interpret. Invasive monitoring requires informed consent and staff who are knowledgeable about the equipment and techniques for safe use during the procedure. Assembling the equipment and maintaining the system are usually the responsibilities of the bedside nurse.

Informed Consent

Hemodynamic monitoring is not without risk. The physician or licensed provider who will be performing the procedure is responsible for discussing its risks with the patient. The nurse assesses the patient's understanding, reinforces the information as part of ongoing patient and family education, and witnesses a signature on the consent form. Consent in the critical care environment can be implied if a patient experiences an acute, life-threatening event. Chapter 6 discusses informed consent.

CRITICAL ALERT *Analgesics, sedatives, anxiolytics, and hypnotic medications impair judgment and thinking. The elderly are particularly susceptible to adverse reactions (confusion and disorientation) with other classes of medications. Nurses should inform the medical team if there is suspicion of cerebral impairment that would preclude informed consent.*

Components of the Monitoring Equipment

An invasive hemodynamic monitoring system has five basic components: the monitor, flush system, transducer, high-pressure tubing, and catheter (Figure 24–1 ■). The system is referred to as a transducer system and is assembled in an identical fashion whether used for an artery or vein. Chart 24–1 describes the step-by-step process for setting up the hemodynamic monitoring system.

These systems require a constant flow of sterile solution in order to maintain patency and decrease the risk of clot formation. The most common solution used is 0.9% normal saline (NS). Because these catheters are placed into high-pressure systems in the body, a sleeve is placed over the NS bag that is

---

CHART 24–1   Setup of Pressure Transducer System

1. Obtain an intravenous (IV) flush solution of normal saline and a transducer system.
2. Attach the transducer system to the IV flush solution and prime all tubing, ensuring that air bubbles are removed from the system.
3. Replace all vented caps with nonvented (dead-end) sterile caps.
4. Inflate the pressure bag to 300 mmHg.
5. Assist the patient to the supine position with the head of the bed elevated no more than 45 degrees.
6. Accurately measure and mark the patient's phlebostatic axis with an indelible marker.
7. Level the air–fluid interface to the phlebostatic axis.
8. Zero the system.
9. Set alarm limits.

Source: Adapted from American Association of Critical-Care Nurses. (2005). AACN Procedure manual for critical care. (5th Ed). D. J. Lynn-McHale Wiegand & K. K. Carlson. (Eds). Philadelphia: Elsevier, p. 591.

MyNursingKit | Video: Peripheral Vascular: Arterial Pressure Monitoring

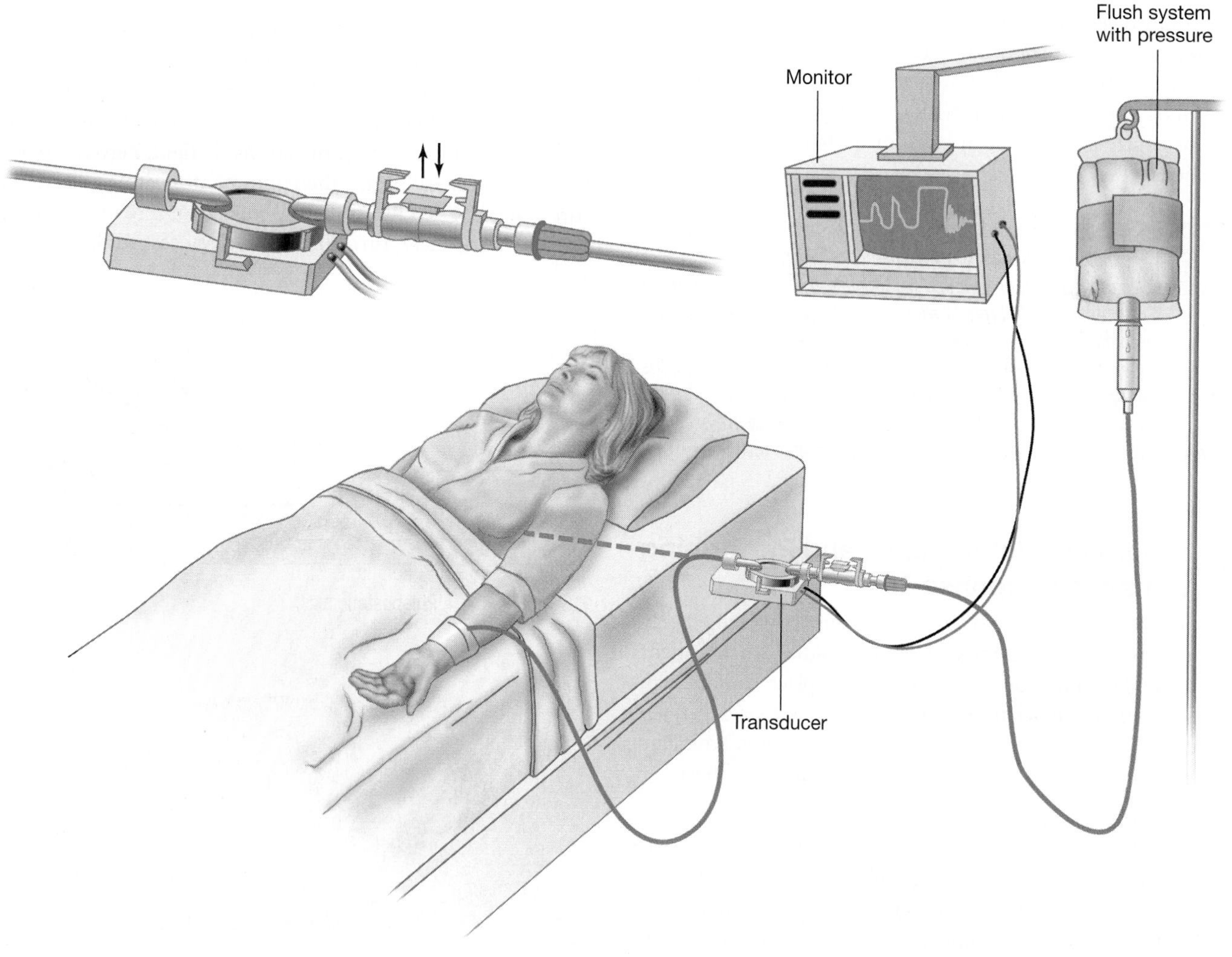

FIGURE 24–1 ■ Components of the hemodynamic monitoring system.

inflated to 300 millimeters of mercury (mmHg) to counteract the pressure in the vessel and allow the solution to flow into the patient. High-pressure tubing instead of flexible intravenous (IV) tubing is necessary to withstand the external pressure exerted by the sleeve and to decrease the distortion of the waveform.

After the transducer system has been assembled and attached to the catheter, the infusion rate is held constant by the transducer system and the pressure sleeve. The information on the transducer package insert will indicate the constant infusion rate, but 1 to 3 mL/hour is common (Lynn-McHale Weigand & Carlson, 2005). The transducer converts pressure detected at the catheter tip into an electrical signal. This signal is displayed on a bedside or portable monitor. Both reusable and disposable transducers are available. Reusable transducers must be disinfected between patients in accordance with institutional policy.

Heparin versus No Heparin Flush Bags

The effect of heparinized versus nonheparinized flush solution on the patency of arterial catheters has been studied. Nursing research has demonstrated that heparin does influence the patency of arterial lines (Urden, Stacy, & Lough, 2006). When heparinized flush solutions were used on arterial lines in place for 72 hours, a greater percentage of arterial lines remained patent; however, heparin in the flush solution did not guarantee patency. Caution should be taken when exposing patients to heparin unnecessarily because the risk of heparin-induced thrombocytopenia increases with every exposure. Some institutions utilize only NS flush bags for all hemodynamic pressure lines.

 Heparin-induced thrombocytopenia occurs 4 to 7 days after exposure to heparin. Any exposure to heparin places the patient at risk of an immune response. The heparin stimulates an antibody that reacts with circulating platelets. This causes platelet aggregation and thrombosis. Diagnosis of heparin-induced thrombocytopenia is made when, during or after reexposure to heparin, the platelet count drops to <50% of baseline or the platelet count is <100,000/μL and other potential causes of thrombocytopenia are excluded. All heparin must be discontinued including heparin-coated invasive catheters.

Leveling, Zero Referencing, and Performing the Dynamic Response Test

Leveling the transducer, zero referencing, and performing the dynamic response test are nursing responsibilities when patients have hemodynamic monitoring catheters in place. Variability in technique among clinicians conducting these operator-dependent procedures influences the accuracy of the hemodynamic data (Urden et al., 2006). Each of these variables is discussed next.

Leveling the Transducer

Leveling the transducer means placing the transducer at the same level as the tip of the catheter sitting in the patient. A reference point on the patient, referred to as the **phlebostatic axis**, is identified to use as a baseline for consistent transducer height placement. To locate the phlebostatic axis, a horizontal line is identified that is halfway between the anterior and posterior di-

ameter of the chest. This horizontal line intersects with a vertical line from the fourth intercostal space (Figure 24–2 ■). Marking this reference point with an indelible marker permits ready identification by others.

The transducer is typically mounted on an IV pole beside the bed and a yardstick with a carpenter level aids the nurse in aligning the transducer with the phlebostatic point. Figure 24–3 ■ illustrates adjustment of the reference point for a patient in a lateral position. Research has shown that when the patient is supine, with the head of the bed elevated up to 45 degrees, the accuracy of pressure readings does not change (Giuliano, Scott, Brown, & Olson, 2003).

The importance of using the same reference point cannot be overstated. Incorrect transducer placement results in invalid pressure readings. Positioning the transducer above the reference point will decrease the pressure reading, and lowering the transducer will increase the reading. This discrepancy can expose a patient to unnecessary or erroneous treatment.

 To ensure accurate pressure readings, it is imperative that when the patient is repositioned, including raising or lowering the head of the bed, the transducer must be zeroed out again at the phlebostatic point. When the transducer is pole mounted and the bed height is raised or lowered, the zeroing out process should be repeated.

Zero Referencing the Transducer

Once the transducer is level with the reference point, the next step is to zero reference the system. Prior to performing this procedure, ensure the transducer system is intact, the tubing is without air bubbles, and connections are tight. **Zero referencing** the transducer calibrates the equipment to atmospheric pressure. Figure 24–4 ■ illustrates the concept of zero referencing. To zero the transducer, turn the stopcock closest to the patient to

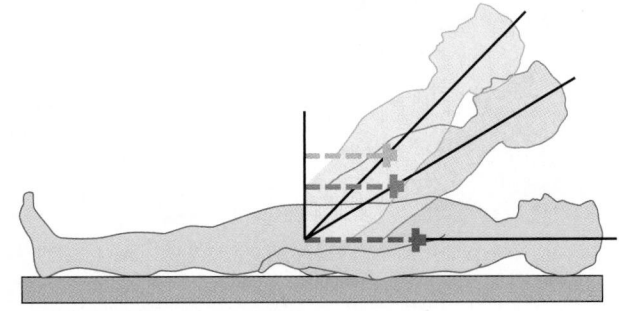

FIGURE 24–2 ■ Phlebostatic axis.

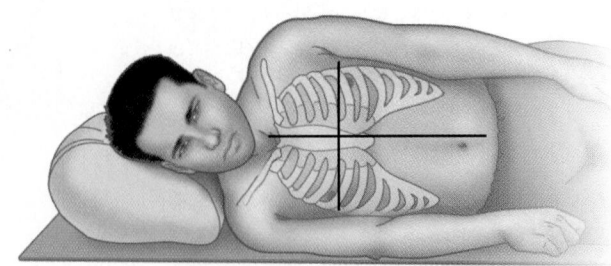

FIGURE 24–3 ■ Identification of phlebostatic axis when patient is in the lateral position.

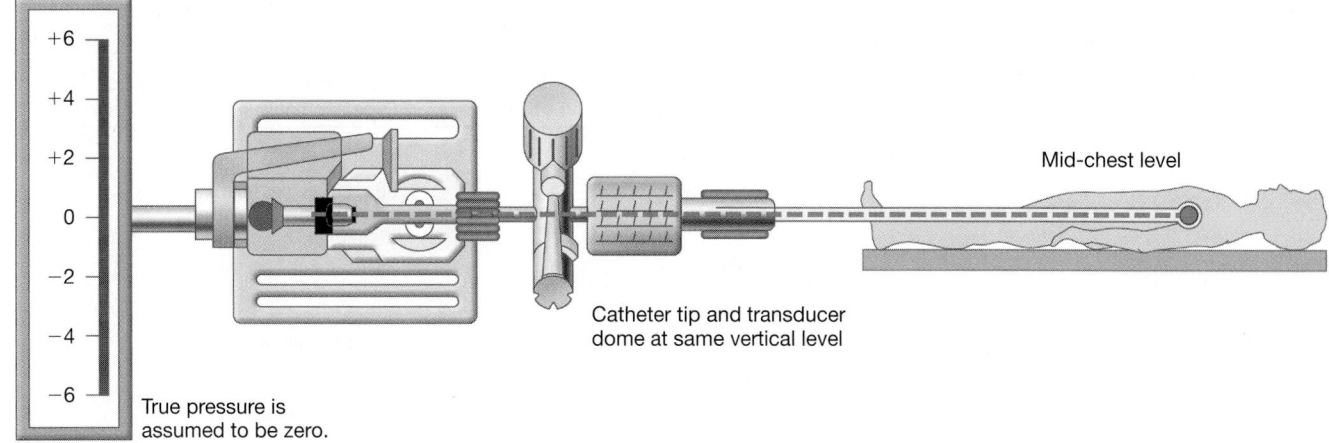

FIGURE 24–4 ■ Leveling and zero referencing the transducer to the phlebostatic axis.

the off position. This turns the transducer off to the patient. Remove the cap from the transducer to allow for equilibration of the transducer with atmospheric pressure. Initiate the zero function on the monitoring system. Wait for the display to read zero then turn the stopcock knob back to the neutral position. The frequency of zeroing the transducer varies between institutions; however, zeroing should be done once per shift, after turning a patient, and whenever pressure readings are questionable (Darovic, 2004).

Dynamic Response Test/Square Wave Test

To test whether the transducer system is accurately transmitting the pressure detected in the vessel, a **dynamic response test** is performed. Poor dynamic response affects readings, making them either appear lower or higher than the actual reading. Dynamic response testing, also called the square wave test, is initiated by using the built-in flush system (pigtail) in the transducer. The nurse quickly pulls the pigtail and releases it, a process that is referred to as "fast flushing" the catheter. This results in a "square wave" in place of the normal waveform. If the test is normal, one or two oscillations will appear below the baseline (Kaplow & Hardin, 2007). The dynamic response test should be performed every 8 to 12 hours, after the system is opened for blood sampling, or whenever the accuracy of readings is questioned (Lynn-McHale Weigand & Carlson, 2005). The waveforms in Figure 24–5 ■ compare an appropriate dynamic response test with abnormal findings.

■ Hemodynamic Terminology

Invasive and noninvasive hemodynamic monitoring provide for close examination of cardiac function. This section explains the terms referred to in hemodynamic monitoring and provides examples to clarify their use. Chart 24–2 (p. 564) summarizes these terms.

Stroke Volume

Stroke volume (SV) is the amount of blood leaving the left ventricle with each contraction. For a healthy heart, the expected SV is 60 to 100 mL per beat. Stroke volume is sensitive to alterations in preload, afterload, and contractility, which are discussed later.

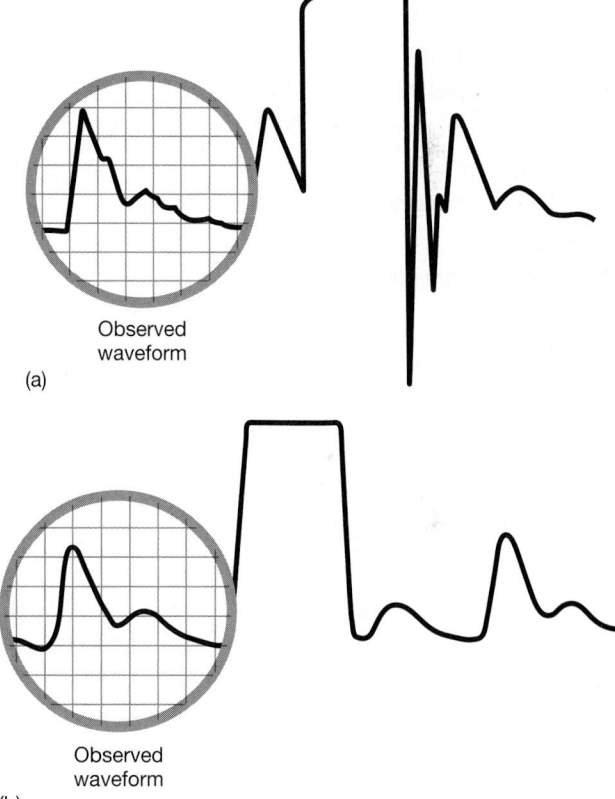

Observed
waveform

(a)

Observed
waveform

(b)

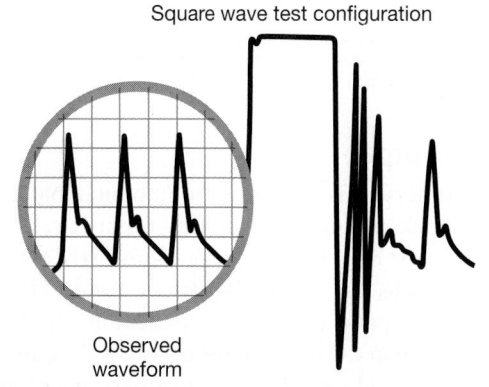

Square wave test configuration

Observed
waveform

FIGURE 24–5 ■ Dynamic response testing: (A) normal response; (B) abnormal response.

CHART 24–2	Hemodynamic Parameters	

Parameters	Calculation	Expected Value
Cardiac Output (CO)		
Stroke volume (SV)	$\dfrac{CO \times 1000}{HR}$	60–100 mL per beat
Stroke volume index (SVI)	$\dfrac{SV}{BSA}$	35–75 mL/m² per beat
Cardiac index (CI)	$\dfrac{CO}{BSA}$	2.8–4.2 L min m^{-2}
Heart rate (HR)		60–100 beats/min
Cardiac output	HR × SV	4–8 liters/min
Preload		
Central venous pressure (CVP)		2–6 mmHg
Right atrial pressure (RAP)		4–6 mmHg
Left atrial pressure (LAP)		4–12 mmHg
Pulmonary artery diastolic pressure (PAD)		5–15 mmHg
Pulmonary artery occlusion pressure (PAOP, PAWP, or PCWP)		4–12 mmHg
Right ventricular end-diastolic pressure (RVEDP)		0–8 mmHg
Left ventricular end-diastolic pressure (LVEDP)		4–10 mmHg
Afterload		
Mean arterial pressure (MAP)	$DBP + \dfrac{(SBP - DBP)}{3}$	
Systemic vascular resistance (SVR)	$\dfrac{MAP - CVP \ (or\ RAP) \times 80}{CO}$	900–1600 dyn sec cm^{-5}
Systemic vascular resistance index (SVRI)	$\dfrac{MAP - CVP \ (or\ RAP) \times 80}{CI}$	1970–2390 dyn sec cm^{-5}
Pulmonary vascular resistance (PVR)	$\dfrac{PAM - PAOP \ (or\ PAWP) \times 80}{CO}$	155–255 dyn sec cm^{-5}
Pulmonary vascular resistance index (PVRI)	$\dfrac{PAM - PAOP \ (or\ PAWP) \times 80}{CI}$	255–285 dyn sec cm^{-5}
Contractility		
Ejection fraction (EF)	$\dfrac{LVEDV \times 100}{SV}$	60–75%
	$\dfrac{RVEDV \times 100}{SV}$	45–50%

Source: Adapted with permission from Whalen, D. A., & Kelleher, R. M. (1998). Cardiovascular patient assessment. In M. R. Kinney et al. (Eds.), *AACN clinical reference for critical care nursing* (4th ed., p. 279). St. Louis: Mosby.

Cardiac Output

Cardiac output (CO) is defined as the amount of blood leaving the left ventricle per minute. Cardiac output is calculated by multiplying heart rate (HR) by stroke volume (HR × SV). With a healthy ventricle, this amount is between 4 and 8 L/min. Adequate cardiac output is essential for circulation and tissue oxygenation. A drop in CO or when the heart is failing and cannot pump effectively reduces the amount of oxygen and nutrients delivered to the tissues.

Cardiac Index

Cardiac index (CI) is a more accurate measurement of circulation than cardiac output. The calculation for cardiac index incorporates the patient's body surface area (BSA). The cardiac index is the CO per square meter of the body. Body surface area can be calculated using the DuBois scale, software in a personal digital assistant (PDA), or by computing it as follows:

$$BSA = (weight\ in\ kg \times 0.425) \times (height\ in\ cm \times 0.725) \times 0.007184$$

If using the DuBois scale, a line is drawn between the patient's height and weight to obtain a BSA.

Whichever method is used to obtain a BSA, the BSA value is then divided into the cardiac output to obtain the cardiac index. An adequate CI is between 2.8 and 4.2 L/min. Most bedside monitors automatically calculate the BSA during a cardiac output measurement, provided the patient's height and weight have been preprogrammed into the monitor. The nurse is responsible for entering the correct height and weight into the bedside monitoring system. Frequently, the patient's admission weight is used. The CO and CI are hemodynamic parameters obtained with a pulmonary artery catheter, discussed later in this chapter.

Ejection Fraction

With each contraction, the left and right ventricles of the heart do not empty completely. The percentage of the total volume that is ejected with each beat is called the **ejection fraction (EF)**. Ejection fraction is a calculation that compares the end-diastolic volume to the stroke volume. It is expressed as a percentage. A normal EF is 65%, meaning that 65% of the blood in the left ventricle is ejected under normal circumstances with each heartbeat and 35% is left for periods of high demand.

The volume of blood remaining in the ventricle is considered a reserve. During periods of stress or exercise, this cardiac reserve, combined with a healthy ventricular contraction, assists in meeting the increased demand for adequate tissue oxygenation. Myocardium with abnormal contractile fibers is unable to pump as effectively as usual; thus, more blood remains in the ventricle with each beat, thereby decreasing the EF. Ejection fraction is an important parameter because a low EF value indicates ventricular dysfunction. An EF of less than 35% indicates serious ventricular failure. In patients with right or left ventricular failure, the administration of volume to improve stroke volume is poorly tolerated and may actually lead to a further decrease in cardiac performance.

Contractility

Contractility is the force generated by the contracting myocardium. The ability of the ventricles to contract or squeeze against resistance is determined by the contractile force of the ventricle. The force of contraction is related to the ability of the ventricular muscle fiber to lengthen or stretch. According to the **Frank-Starling law**, the muscle fibers in healthy ventricles will stretch to accommodate the venous return received during diastole. Generally, if the ventricle receives excess venous blood return during diastole, the ventricular contraction will be more forceful, resulting in an increased stroke volume. A filling pressure between 10 and 12 mmHg is considered optimal (Porth, 2007). When the pressure exceeds 12 mmHg and the myocardial fibers are overstretched, the force of ventricular contraction will decrease, eventually resulting in heart failure.

Contractility is enhanced by circulating catecholamines, sympathetic nervous system stimulation, and certain positive inotropic medications such as digoxin, dopamine, or dobutamine. Contractility is depressed with acidosis, hypoxemia, and beta-adrenergic blocking medications.

Preload

Preload is the volume of blood in the ventricle at the end of diastole. Although reflective of volume, preload is referred to as an end-diastolic pressure (EDP). Right ventricular preload is dependent on total blood volume returning to the heart, cardiac output, and venous vascular resistance (Porth, 2007). **Central venous pressure (CVP)** and right atrial pressure (RAP) are measurements that reflect venous return to the right side of the heart. A central venous pressure of less than 2 mmHg or a RAP of less than 4 mmHg is indicative of hypovolemia. True hypovolemia results from fluid losses such as excess diuretic therapy or the blood losses associated with hemorrhage. Relative hypovolemia occurs with venodilation. Venodilation results in less blood volume being returned to the heart. In patients with increased capillary permeability, as exhibited with sepsis, there is a generalized movement of fluid out of the vascular space and into the transcellular space referred to as "third spacing" of fluid (Porth, 2007). In these patients the CVP or RAP may be an unreliable indicator of preload, but can be monitored for an increasing or decreasing trend.

Hypervolemia, a CVP or RAP of more than 6 mmHg indicates that an increased volume of blood is being returned to the right atrium. Increased preload may be the result of volume overload, renal failure, or cardiac tamponade. Usually the volume of increased preload is the result of intravascular excess. An increase in preload may be noted after a rapid, large-volume IV infusion; however, a patient in renal failure or in heart failure will also exhibit an elevated CVP due to either an inability to excrete fluid or to the buildup of excess pressure in the heart due to poor ventricular function. An elevation in the CVP or RAP also occurs when fluid accumulates in the pericardial sac and exerts external pressure on the heart chambers, as in cardiac tamponade (Chapter 41 👁). Further investigation is required to determine the exact cause. When assessment of preload must be more precise, a pulmonary artery catheter with a lumen in the right ventricle provides measurement of right ventricular volume using the previously described transducer system.

Afterload

Afterload is the pressure or resistance the ventricles must overcome to eject blood during systole. Vascular resistance is the major determinant of afterload. The right ventricle pumps blood into the pulmonary system through the pulmonic valve into the pulmonary artery (Kaplow & Hardin, 2007). Afterload of the pulmonary system is termed pulmonary vascular resistance (PVR). The left ventricle pumps blood into systemic circulation through the aortic valve. Systemic afterload is termed systemic vascular resistance (SVR). Elevations in vascular resistance are the result of vasoconstriction, which has many causes such as hypothermia or hypoxemia. Vascular resistance can also be elevated from mechanical barriers such as aortic or pulmonary artery stenosis. Decreases in vascular resistance are noted in hyperthermia or when vasodilators are administered. Unlike the direct measurement of preload, afterload is a calculated value.

▮ Normal Hemodynamic Pressures

Human physiology relies on a dynamic balance between blood flow, resistance, and pressure. Hemodynamic monitoring provides

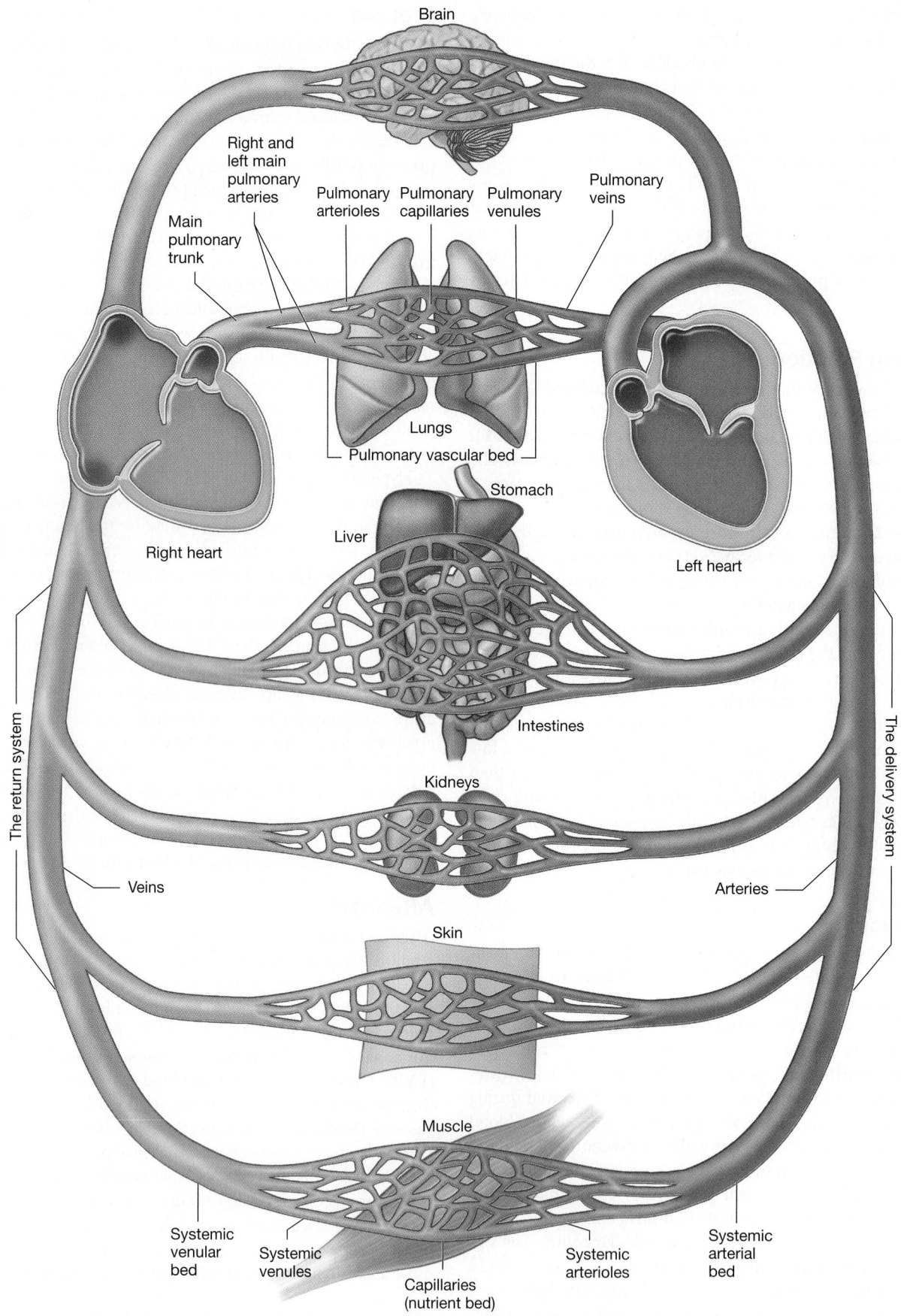

FIGURE 24–6 ■ Vascular circuit.

an overall assessment of this balance with individual components focusing on circulation, perfusion, and tissue oxygenation. This in-depth assessment of these interactions helps health care providers as they diagnose, guide, and evaluate therapies.

The Pump and the Circuit

The closed loop of the cardiovascular system relies on pressure gradients to maintain the normal forward movement of blood flow (Figure 24–6 ■). The low-pressure pulmonary and systemic venous systems deliver blood to their respective atria. Pressure changes in the atria and ventricles are the end result of electrical and mechanical activities. When atrial pressure exceeds ventricular pressure, the tricuspid and mitral valves open and blood passively flows into the ventricle. At the end of this passive flow, when the tricuspid and mitral valves are open, the mean pressure between the atria and the ventricles is equal. When ventricular pressure exceeds pressure in the atria, the tricuspid and mitral valves close. When ventricular pressure exceeds the pressure in the pulmonary artery and aorta, the pulmonic and aortic valves open. Disruption to any segment in the closed loop or cardiac dysfunction can cause an alteration in preload and afterload.

Waveforms and the Cardiac Cycle

When an invasive catheter senses the cardiovascular system's pressures, they are displayed on a monitor as pressure readings. Pressure changes produce positive waves and negative deflections. The waveform correlates with the cardiac cycle, but because the pressures are being transmitted through fluid-filled tubing, there is a slight delay. Simultaneous dual-channel recording of the electrocardiogram (ECG) and pressure waveforms improves the accuracy of the pressure readings, or tracings (Figure 24–7 ■) (Dietz & Smith, 2002). Pressure readings are most accurate at the end of expiration when the effect of intrathoracic pressure is negligible. The location of end expiration on a pressure tracing differs between a spontaneously breathing patient and a patient on positive pressure mechanical ventilation. When a patient is spontaneously breathing, end expiration on a pressure tracing will be higher. With less intrathoracic pressure compressing the great vessels, there is a corresponding increase in preload. Conversely, when a patient is receiving positive pressure ventilation, the intrathoracic pressure is lower during expiration due to the reduction in intrathoracic pressure during exhalation. Figure 24–8 ■ (p. 568) illustrates the differences between the end expiration point in a

spontaneously breathing and a mechanically ventilated patient. Identification of end expiration is important due to its influence on preload, with a falsely elevated preload leading to a falsely elevated cardiac output measurement.

■ Invasive Pressure Monitoring

Invasive hemodynamic monitoring provides a method of direct measurement of vascular pressures. Medical therapies are based on the interpretation of the parameter being assessed. Systemic, central venous, and pulmonary artery monitoring devices are frequently used for this purpose. Each of these is discussed in this section along with information on complications and nursing management.

Intra-arterial Catheters

An **arterial line** is an indwelling catheter inserted into an artery by a physician or an advanced practice nurse in order to monitor blood pressure. These catheters, which are inserted either percutaneously or by a surgical cutdown technique, are recommended for patients whose blood pressure is unstable and therefore require frequent monitoring. These patients include those who are hypotensive, hypertensive, or receiving vasoactive medications requiring titration and careful monitoring. Arterial lines also provide access for obtaining frequent blood specimens.

 CRITICAL ALERT   *An arterial line is* never *used for infusion of IV solutions or medications. Both IV solutions and medications are irritating to the vessel and may compromise tissue perfusion distal to the catheter.*

Insertion of Arterial Catheters

The radial artery is the most common site for arterial catheter placement. Other sites such as the brachial, axillary, femoral, dorsalis pedis, and posterior tibial are possible alternatives. Although the diameter of the radial artery is smaller than that of the ulnar artery, the radial artery is easily accessible because of its proximity to the skin surface, making it the preferred site. An **Allen's test** is performed prior to insertion of the radial arterial catheter to assess ulnar circulation in the hand (Figure 24–9 ■, p. 568). To perform an Allen's test, raise the patient's hand above his head and ask the patient to make a tight fist. While the fist is tight, apply pressure to occlude the radial and ulnar arteries simultaneously. Lower the patient's hand and ask him to release the tight fist. The nurse then releases the pressure over the ulnar

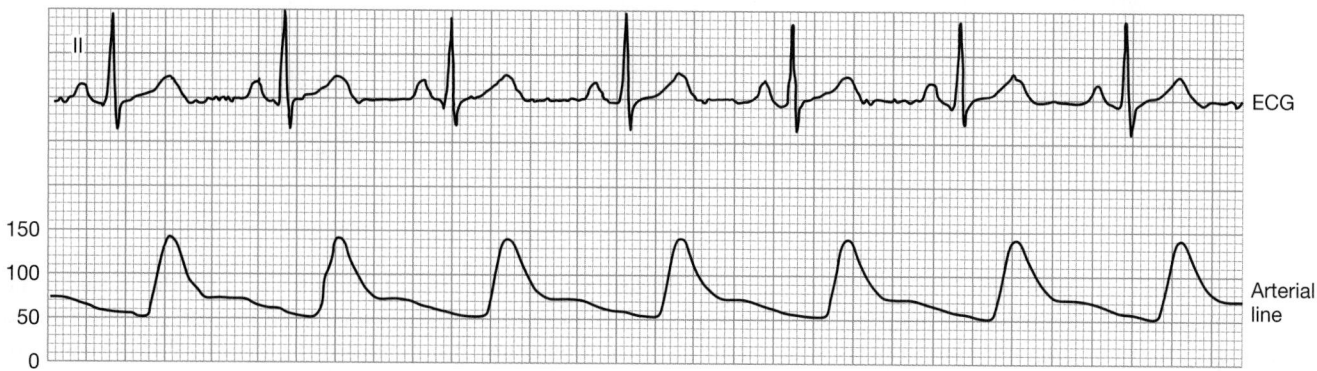

FIGURE 24–7 ■   Single-lead ECG and arterial pressure waveform.

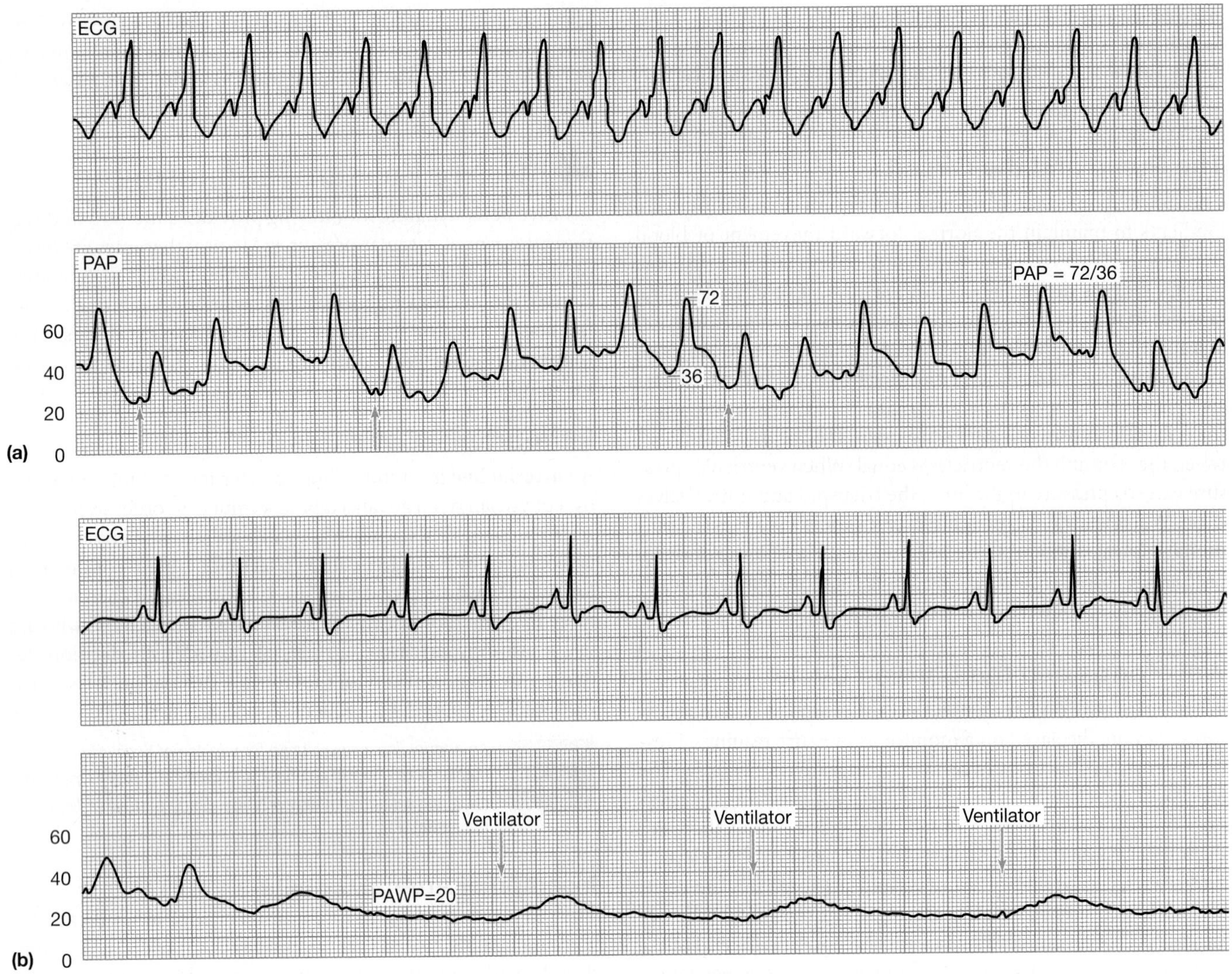

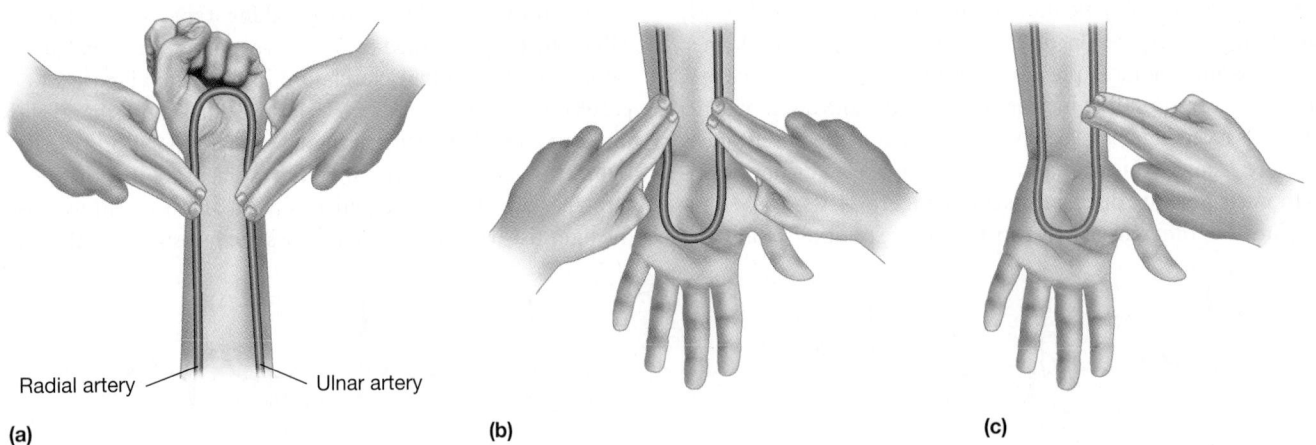

FIGURE 24–8 ■ End expiration: (A) spontaneously breathing patient; (B) mechanically ventilated patient.

Radial artery — — Ulnar artery

(a)

(b)

(c)

FIGURE 24–9 ■ Performing the Allen's test.

artery and observes the return of color to the hand. An Allen's test is positive if the color returns to the hand in 7 seconds or less after release of the ulnar artery. If return time is greater than 7 seconds, the test is inconclusive, but if greater than 15 seconds, the test is negative. If color does not return to the hand after re-

leasing the ulnar artery, the health care provider should be notified prior to an arterial puncture. If the test is negative, the radial artery should not be used for an arterial line because the superficial palmar arch is not intact. This may place the patient at risk for vascular thrombosis and arterial occlusion, which may lead to necrosis and in severe cases amputation of the hand. The nurse must always document that the Allen's test was performed, the results, and any action taken if the test is negative. Ongoing assessment of circulation distal to the insertion site is the responsibility of the bedside nurse.

 *The Allen's test can be performed on an unconscious patient by holding the patient's arm above her head and clenching her hand into a fist. Apply pressure to both ulnar and radial arteries while the arm is overhead. Lower the arm and release the pressure from the radial artery.*

Ensuring the integrity of the monitoring system, preventing infection, and assessing for thrombus formation also are fundamental nursing responsibilities associated with arterial line placement (Urden et al., 2006). Once the catheter is secured, an occlusive dressing is applied. The arterial catheter can be sutured in place prior to the application of the dressing. Also prior to applying the dressing, ensure the arterial catheter is tightly attached to the hub on the pressure tubing. The monitoring system has upper and lower limit alarming capabilities, and it is the responsibility of the nurse to set, adjust, and ensure these alarms are engaged at all times.

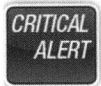 *Always set the patient's alarms based on the patient's baseline hemodynamic pressures and the abnormality being monitored. Never turn the alarms off entirely. To allow alert patients periods of uninterrupted rest, the intensity or volume of the alarm can usually be adjusted on bedside monitors without affecting the alarm signal or message from the central station.*

Arterial Pressure Waveforms

When the pressure transducer system is attached to the arterial catheter, an identifiable arterial waveform appears on the monitor. This waveform represents systolic and diastolic pressures generated by the mechanical activity of the heart (Figure 24–10 ■). The systolic pressure represents maximum left ventricular systolic pressure. The dicrotic notch represents closure of the aortic valve and distinguishes the end of systole and beginning of diastole. The beginning of diastole is a significant cardiac event. Diastolic pressure indicates the pressure in the ventricle at rest and is directly related to blood vessel elasticity (Darovic, 2004).

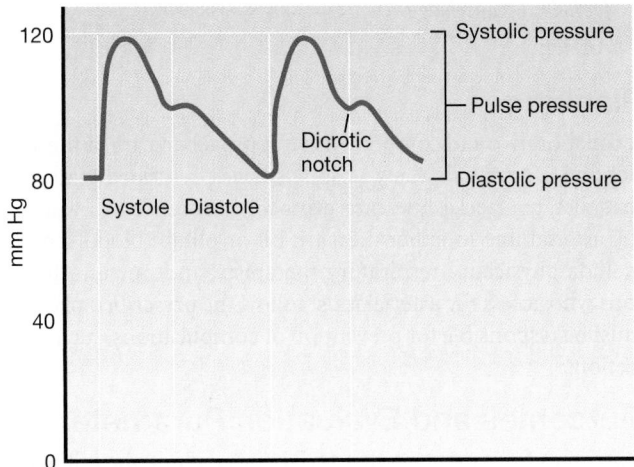

FIGURE 24–10 ■ Analyzing arterial pressure waveform.

Complications of Arterial Blood Pressure Monitoring

Complications of arterial blood pressure monitoring include hemorrhage, emboli, vascular occlusion or spasm, and infection. Occult hemorrhage may occur, particularly after a femoral artery catheter has been inserted. Signs of hypovolemia, lower abdominal firmness, or swelling or bruising at the site should alert the nurse to notify the health care provider immediately. Due to high pressure in arteries, massive blood loss can occur if the catheter dislodges or is disconnected from the patient or if the connections are loosened. Assessment of circulation distal to the insertion site, prior to insertion of the catheter, does not preclude vascular ischemia and necrosis. Arterial clots, fibrin, or air may cause emboli. Risk factors include multiple arterial punctures of the same limb or site, vasoconstriction, low cardiac output, severe peripheral vascular disease, prolonged duration of catheter, and an active infectious process (Darovic, 2004). Vascular occlusion or spasm cannot be predicted and risk factors for spasm are the same as embolic events. Aseptic technique is used for all dressings and sterility is maintained when obtaining blood specimens.

Factors Influencing Arterial Pressure

Alterations in the conduction system of the heart influence arterial pressure. Patients who have irregular cardiac rhythms, such as atrial fibrillation or premature contractions, demonstrate arterial waveforms with varying systolic pressures. These patients experience a decrease in systolic pressure as a result of the decrease in diastolic filling time. Premature contractions prevent complete filling of the ventricle during diastole. With less blood volume filling the heart, there is less volume to eject on the next systole, which results in the lower arterial systolic pressure. Figure 24–11 ■ (p. 570) illustrates this phenomenon. Chapter 38 🖳 provides an in-depth discussion of these dysrhythmias.

As the distance between the heart and the catheter site increases, the shape of the arterial waveform will change: The systolic pressure waveform becomes higher and the diastolic pressure waveform becomes lower. Figure 24–12 ■ (p. 570) illustrates the changes in the shape of an arterial waveform as distance from the heart increases. The mean arterial pressure, however, remains constant irrespective of the arterial catheter site. **Mean arterial pressure (MAP)** is the average pressure in the arteries during one cardiac cycle. When administering vasoactive medications, the MAP is usually specified as the titration parameter. Mean arterial pressure is used in the equation to calculate afterload or SVR.

Pulsus paradoxus refers to a pattern in the arterial waveform in which the systolic pressure decreases by 10 mmHg or more during the inspiratory phase of ventilation. This pattern is the classic sign of cardiac tamponade, but can also be present in any condition that results in compression of the right side of the heart (Urden et al., 2006). In tamponade, fluid or blood has accumulated in the pericardial sac causing compression of the heart. This compression is temporarily relieved during the inspiratory phase of ventilation. During inspiration, a drop in intrathoracic pressure occurs that allows for an increase in venous return. The increased venous return translates into an increase in stroke volume during the next systole. Chapter 41 🖳 describes the causes of pulsus paradoxus and cardiac tamponade.

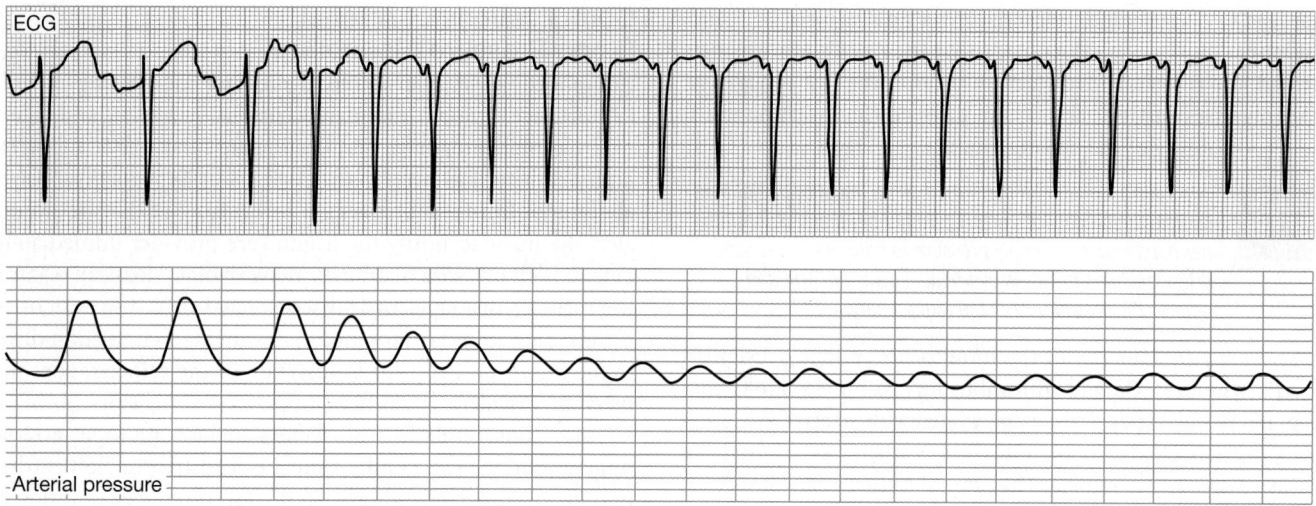

FIGURE 24–11 ■ Effect of atrial tachycardia on arterial pressure.

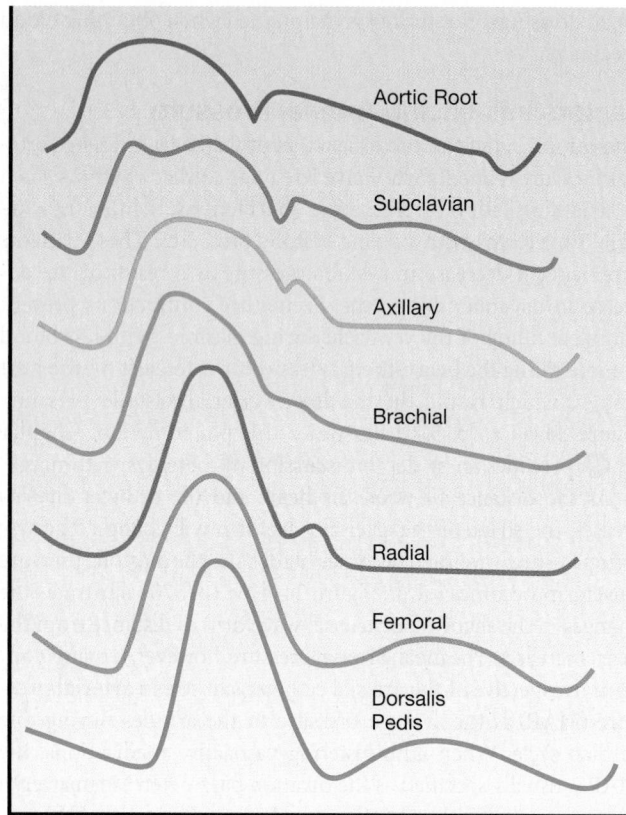

FIGURE 24–12 ■ Changes in arterial pressure waveform.

■ Nursing Management

Explaining the procedure to the patient and family will assist in decreasing their anxiety and elicit their cooperation. Prior to insertion a modified Allen's test must be performed and documented. The bedside nurse can facilitate radial artery cannulation by hyperflexion of the patient's wrist during insertion. After insertion a padded armboard is sometimes necessary after an arterial line is placed to keep the wrist hyperflexed and to optimize the waveform. The nursing process serves as a guideline for nursing management of patients with arterial lines.

Assessment

An in-depth assessment can identify patients at risk, so that actions can be taken to prevent complications from the arterial line. The nurse needs to assess the arterial line insertion site for redness, pain, and swelling, because this is an indication of infection. Assessment of the circulation also is essential to prevent ischemic changes due to compromised circulation. Note the presence and quality of pulses in the extremity. Regularly observe for changes in skin color and assess for motor and sensory changes in the extremity distal to the insertion site. Assessment of the blood pressure (BP) is done on a continuous basis and documented per health care provider orders or unit guidelines. The nurse must note the waveform, and when changes occur the patient should be reassessed and troubleshooting done on the equipment.

Nursing Diagnosis

Nursing diagnoses related to arterial line placement include:

- *Risk for Infection*
- *Impaired Tissue Integrity*
- *Ineffective Tissue Perfusion*
- *Deficient Knowledge*
- *Anxiety.*

Planning

A collaborative and comprehensive approach to care of the arterial line is essential. Many hospitals have prescribed guidelines that dictate arterial line care protocols. Professionals who use the arterial line to either measure BP or obtain blood samples include physicians, respiratory therapists, and nurses. All persons who access the arterial must follow the prescribed plan and must be responsible for prevention of complications, such as infection.

Outcomes and Evaluation Parameters

Outcomes for patients with arterial lines include the following:

- Stabilization of the BP without vasoactive drugs
- No infection at the catheter site or in the bloodstream

- No bleeding from the arterial line site or catheter
- Having the arterial discontinued due to BP stabilization.

Interventions and Rationales

An arterial line can be inserted for the sole purpose of obtaining blood specimens. More commonly, however, a catheter is placed so that blood pressure can be closely monitored. Nursing interventions include monitoring the blood pressure and, if administered, assessing the effectiveness of vasoactive therapy. When a patient is receiving vasoactive medications, which either increase or decrease BP, the bedside nurse is responsible for medication titration to keep the blood pressure within the parameters ordered by the health provider. Frequent assessment of blood pressure (usually at 5- to 10-minute intervals) and documentation of amount of medication infusing are required. When the goal blood pressure is achieved and maintained, then the institutional policy related to documentation is followed.

Each monitor has the ability to notify the nurse that the blood pressure is too high or too low. After the arterial line is inserted, set the high and low alarm limits. These alarms should never be turned off when the nurse leaves the room. When high or low alarms occur, assess the patient for changes. If changes occur in the arterial waveform, *first* assess the patient and take a manual cuff pressure. If the cuff pressure varies from the arterial pressure, it is necessary to troubleshoot the equipment by systematically inspecting and, if necessary, tightening all connections and tubing from insertion site to pressure bag.

Care of an arterial line site includes changing the dressing per unit protocol or whenever the occlusive dressing becomes loose or when contamination is suspected. If infection is suspected, the health care professional should be notified and preparation for a new line instituted. After the dressing is applied, obtain a strip of the arterial line tracing and document the procedure in the patient's record.

Nurses can remove an arterial catheter according to institutional policy and on order by the health care provider. Explain to the patient that the catheter is being removed and pressure will be applied to the site. Prior to removing a radial artery catheter, don goggles and apply nonsterile gloves. Remove the dressing, then remove the suture, if present, with a suture removal kit. With one hand, gently remove the catheter, and apply direct site pressure as soon as the catheter is removed. Continue to apply pressure until hemostasis is achieved, then apply a sterile dressing. The procedure is the same when removing a femoral arterial catheter; however, with the large femoral artery more time is required to achieve hemostasis by direct pressure. Routinely sending catheter tips for culture after removal is not recommended (Centers for Disease Control and Prevention [CDC], 2002). Observe the catheter site regularly for bleeding and/or hematoma formation after the catheter has been removed.

Evaluation

While the arterial line is in place, the nurse should correlate the cuff blood pressure with the arterial line pressure by simultaneously obtaining a reading from the arterial line and a sphygmomanometer. The pressure reading obtained by the arterial line is higher than the cuff pressure because the arterial catheter is a direct measurement rather than an indirect measurement obtained with a sphygmomanometer or by an automated noninvasive

blood pressure machine. Evaluation of the arterial line site should be done every shift and clinical manifestations of infections need to be reported to the health care professional.

Central Venous Catheters

Single- or multiple-lumen catheters are inserted for monitoring central venous pressure, which is the pressure in the right atrium. The subclavian, internal or external jugular, and femoral veins are potential insertion sites. Depending on the selected site and the length of the catheter, the tip transmits pressure from the right atrium, superior vena cava, or inferior vena cava. Specialized central venous catheters with a fiber-optic sensor allow for measurement of systemic central venous oxygen saturation (ScvO$_2$) (Kaplow & Hardin, 2007). The use of central venous oxygen saturation readings for the treatment of severe sepsis is discussed in Chapter 61  .

Insertion of Central Venous Catheters

After obtaining consent, the patient is placed supine. Positioning the patient during line placement is important. If the subclavian or a jugular vein site is selected and if tolerated by the patient, then the nurse may be asked to place the patient in the Trendelenburg position. This position facilitates venous dilation of the central veins and reduces the risk of an air embolus. Also, a rolled-up towel placed between the shoulder blades and parallel with the spine aids in landmark identification and reduces the risk of a pneumothorax. The patient may be asked to turn her head away from the insertion site to minimize contamination of the site. Patients should be informed of the necessity of maintaining a sterile barrier, which for upper torso sites, involves temporarily covering the patient's face with sterile drapes. The health care provider and anyone assisting with catheter insertion wear a cap, mask, sterile gown, and gloves. The nurse and anyone present in the room during the procedure wear a cap and mask. If, at any point during the procedure, the nurse expects to be in contact with the sterile field, then sterile attire is required for the nurse.

When the catheter is secured, the sterile drapes are removed and a sterile dressing is placed over the insertion site. Despite blood return from the central venous catheter port(s) after insertion, the catheter should not be accessed for intravenous infusions or monitoring until a chest x-ray confirms correct placement and a pneumothorax is ruled out. A chest x-ray is not necessary for femoral lines. Reassess the patient and compare the postinsertion findings with the preinsertion assessment.

> **CRITICAL ALERT** *If in doubt as to whether the catheter is in a vein or artery, remove a sample of blood and send or test it for oxygen saturation. This can be included in the line insertion procedure.*

Central Venous Pressure Monitoring

The central venous pressure reflects the blood pressure of the vena cava and the right atrium. CVP monitoring requires the insertion of a catheter into a central vein that is used for monitoring volume status and venous return to the heart. When a central venous catheter is attached to a transducer system, a CVP or RAP waveform can be obtained. The CVP or RAP waveform should be continually displayed on the bedside monitor. A venous pressure of 2 to 6 mmHg is adequate; however, patients may be hemodynamically stable or unstable with lower or higher pressures. Monitoring the trend in CVP, either increasing or decreasing, is of more importance than one observed value. As with other measurements, correlation of findings with patient assessment is essential.

The CVP may be intermittently monitored. When the central venous catheter is the sole IV access and CVP monitoring is required, a stopcock connector may be used in combination with the transducer system. It is important to understand that when the knob on the stopcock is turned so that the CVP can be checked, any IV infusion at the stopcock is stopped until the stopcock is returned to its original position, allowing for infusion therapy to continue.

Central Venous Pressure Waveform

The normal CVP waveform has three positive waves that correspond to atrial cardiac events. The *a* wave correlates with the P wave or atrial contraction (systole). The next positive wave, the *c* wave, may not be visible on the tracing. The *c* wave reflects retrograde swelling of the tricuspid valve into the right atrium, which occurs during ventricular contraction. The *v* wave represents atrial filling (diastole) and the increased pressure against the closed tricuspid valve in early diastole. Figure 24–13 ■ illustrates these relationships.

Complications of Central Venous Pressure Monitoring

Infection can occur any time the catheter is in place, therefore prevention of infection is an important nursing responsibility. The transmission of organisms is preventable when strict aseptic technique is maintained during catheter insertion and dressing changes (see the National Guidelines box about prevention of catheter-related infections). An air embolus is a complication that may occur during insertion or removal of a central catheter, if the IV disconnects from the catheter hub, or when obtaining blood specimens. Assessment findings that may indicate an air embolus include dyspnea, tachypnea, cyanosis, hypotension, and chest pain. A pneumothorax is another risk associated with thoracic central line placement. It can occur when a needle or intro-

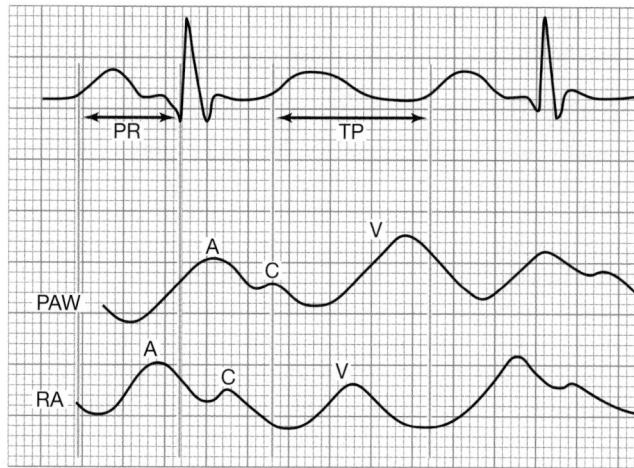

FIGURE 24–13 ■   Correlation of cardiac cycle to CVP and pulmonary artery waveforms.

ducer penetrates the vessel wall, causing air to enter the pleural space. Assessment findings associated with a pneumothorax include those for an air embolus, plus absence of breath sounds on the side of insertion.

■ Nursing Management

Nursing management of central venous catheters focuses on preventing complications, starting with catheter insertion and ending with catheter removal. When compared to arterial catheters and pulmonary artery catheters, the rate of catheter-related infections is highest for central venous catheters (CDC, 2002). The National Guidelines box provides a synopsis of key points from the national guidelines released in 2002 by the CDC.

Further recommendations include replacing all central venous catheters if the patient is hemodynamically unstable and catheter-related bloodstream infection is suspected. In this instance, the bedside nurse alerts the health care team to the catheter replacement need and assists with new central line placement.

NATIONAL GUIDELINES Prevention of Intravascular Catheter-Related Infections

1. Sterile barrier precautions are necessary for all personnel assisting with central venous access insertion.

2. A 2% chlorhexidine preparation is the preferred antiseptic before catheter insertion and during dressing changes.

3. The antiseptic should remain on the insertion site and be allowed to air dry before catheter insertion.

4. Inspect catheter sites visually or manually palpate on a regular basis. Remove dressing to examine if site is tender to palpation.

5. Remove any vascular device that is no longer essential to patient care.

6. Replace disposable transducers, tubing, flush devices, and flush solution at 96-hour intervals.

7. Replace administration sets, including secondary sets and add-on devices, no more frequently than at 72-hour intervals.

8. To prevent infection, avoid routine replacement of central venous catheters.

9. Clean injection port with 70% alcohol or iodophor before accessing.

10. Do not routinely culture catheter tips.

Source: Adapted from Centers for Disease Control and Prevention. (2002). Guidelines for the prevention of intravascular catheter-related infections. *Morbidity and Mortality Weekly Report, 51,* 1–26.

Assessment

Nursing management of a central venous catheter, whether new or *in situ*, involves patient education, assessing the site for infection and leakage, dressing changes, and monitoring of pressures. Prior to insertion of a central venous catheter, the nurse is responsible for assessing the patient for contraindications to the procedure. These include assessing the insertion site, assessing potential difficulties in positioning the patient, and obtaining a baseline physical assessment, including vital signs, pulse oximetry, and heart and breath sounds. Preassessment provides a point of reference for comparison when the procedure is complete. Ensure that external monitoring devices such as ECG wires and electrodes, noninvasive blood pressure cuffs, and pulse oximetry cables are clear of the insertion site. Check the ECG electrodes for good skin contact. If necessary due to the choice of insertion site, relocate ECG electrodes prior to the procedure and before the patient is covered with sterile drapes.

Nursing Diagnosis

Nursing diagnoses related to hemodynamic monitoring include:

- *Anxiety*
- *Risk for Imbalanced Fluid Volume*
- *Ineffective Health Maintenance*
- *Risk for Injury*
- *Deficient Knowledge*
- *Risk for Infection*

Planning

Patient education decreases anxiety and increases patient participation in care. Inform the patient that routine dressing changes and close examination of the insertion site will occur. Before the procedure patients should be informed of the risks of the procedure, the expected duration of the procedure, and that repositioning may be required. Planning for interventions for care for the patient with invasive lines is multifaceted. Each institution has specific procedures for maintaining a sterile occlusive dressing over the line insertion site. The nurse must be knowledgeable of these procedures and carry them out within the required time frames.

Outcomes and Evaluation Parameters

Outcomes associated with central venous catheters include:

- Stabilization of the central venous pressure readings to within normal limits
- No infection at the catheter site or in the bloodstream
- No bleeding from the site or catheter
- Having the central venous catheter discontinued due to patient stabilization.

Interventions and Rationales

Once the central venous catheter is in place, the nurse is responsible for site care and dressing changes. Routine site inspection includes assessing the insertion site and surrounding skin for signs of infection or leakage. Institutional policies vary as to the type of dressing applied; however, hand hygiene and nonsterile gloves are always used to remove the old dressing. If using a prepackaged dressing kit, don the sterile gloves and clean the insertion site and catheter using the disinfectant provided. Allow the disinfectant to air dry. Do not fan the area to speed the drying time because this may lead to site contamination. After the new dressing has been applied, document the procedure, including patient education, date and time of procedure, description of the catheter site, and type of dressing. Some institutions require the date and time of dressing change plus the initials of the person changing the dressing to be placed on the dressing. After assisting with placement of a central venous line, do not access the line until a chest x-ray has confirmed correct placement.

Monitoring the CVP, interpreting the information, and correlating the data collected with the patient's condition are nursing responsibilities. Monitoring the CVP is accomplished with the previously described transducer system. By leveling and zero referencing the transducer and performing the dynamic response test, the nurse can help ensure that the CVP values are accurate.

The CVP reflects preload. Conditions causing an increased CVP include venoconstriction, fluid volume overload, cardiac tamponade, pulmonary hypertension, or depressed cardiac function, especially right ventricular function. Corroborate elevations in CVP with physical assessment findings, which include dependent edema; tachypnea, dyspnea, or orthopnea; anxiety; crackles; and jugular vein distention. Central venous pressures below normal are indicative of venodilation or hypovolemia. Low pressures are frequently seen with major burn injuries, hemorrhage, and spinal cord injuries. Physical findings include postural hypotension, tachycardia, and decreased mean arterial pressure. If continuous monitoring of CVP is not routine, then institutional policy and the health care provider's orders dictate the frequency of obtaining readings. A single CVP value that is less than or more than normal is not as alarming as is a trend in values up or down coupled with a change in the physical assessment findings. Contacting the health care provider is indicated when an abnormal CVP measurement correlates with assessment findings.

Removal of a central venous catheter is done in much the same manner as an arterial line catheter. However, when removing a central venous catheter from the subclavian or jugular site, the removal is timed with the inspiratory phase of the respiratory cycle. When the patient takes a deep breath, the intrathoracic pressure is increased. This maneuver decreases the potential for air embolus. At the peak of inspiration, gently remove the catheter and tell the patient to breathe normally. Continue to hold pressure until hemostasis is achieved and then apply a sterile dressing.

Although CVP and RAP assess preload based on volume status and venous return to the heart, these measurements are often insufficient. When medical therapies depend on accurate evaluation of cardiac output, then measurement of preload, afterload, and contractility is required. Invasive and noninvasive methods are available for this purpose.

Evaluation

Due to the risk of infection, the expected outcome for these patients is stabilization with the intent of getting the invasive catheters removed as soon as possible. Fluid balance as determined by heart rate, BP, and urine output is the evaluation parameter. Not every patient will have normal readings, thus, the goal is to achieve readings that are tolerated by the patient.

Measuring Cardiac Output

Variations in heart rate, preload, afterload, or contractility influence cardiac output. Healthy individuals maintain homeostatic balance through intact compensatory pathways. Athletes, for example, are frequently bradycardic (heart rate below 60 beats/min), but their CO is maintained with above-normal stroke volumes. Critically ill patients either lack reserve or have exhausted their compensatory responses. In other words they are unable to significantly increase contractility to increase the stroke volume. The bedside nurse should be knowledgeable about the components that influence cardiac output, because these factor into determining not only initial therapy, but also evaluation of therapy.

Invasive Methods with Pulmonary Artery Catheters

A **pulmonary artery catheter (PAC)** is a flow-directed, balloon-tipped catheter. The brand name for this catheter is Swan-Ganz, so named for the inventors (Urden et al., 2006). Since the development of the PAC, multiple generations have evolved, although the basic technologies of the catheter remain identical. These catheters allow for assessment of cardiac function, calculation of vascular resistance, measurement of cardiac output, and infusion of IV fluids. The readings obtained with the PAC assist the health care team in diagnosing, treating, and estimating the prognoses of patients who are critically ill. When the PAC was

introduced into critical care, little research existed on its therapeutic use and, yet, the catheter became commonplace in the care of critically ill patients (Adams, 2004). Controversy exists over which patient groups benefit from pulmonary artery catheter guided therapy and if insertion of a PAC decreases mortality rates (Urden et al., 2006).

The American Society of Anesthesiologists (ASA) recommends the use of a PAC for patients undergoing surgical procedures associated with an increased risk of complications from hemodynamic changes (ASA, 2003). Observational studies report mixed results concerning the use of PACs. Chittock and associates (2004) reported that the "mortality rate associated with use of the PAC may be greater if used in a lower severity of illness group but of potential benefit when used in an extremely ill population."

Because controversy still exists over whether the benefits of PACs outweigh the risks, major educational efforts are under way to ensure that patients receive appropriate care based on information derived from the pulmonary artery catheter. The Pulmonary Artery Catheter Education Project is a web-based program for critical care clinicians that focuses on interpretation and application of data obtained from a PA catheter.

Ports and Lumens on a Pulmonary Artery Catheter

The pulmonary artery catheter is a multiple-lumen catheter, with each lumen having a specific purpose (Figure 24–14 ■). The external ports of the catheter correspond to internal lumens that lie either in the right side of the heart or pulmonary artery. There are several types of PACs, some of which have more ports and lumens than others, depending on the intended purpose of the catheter and the manufacturer. Newer multifunction PACs

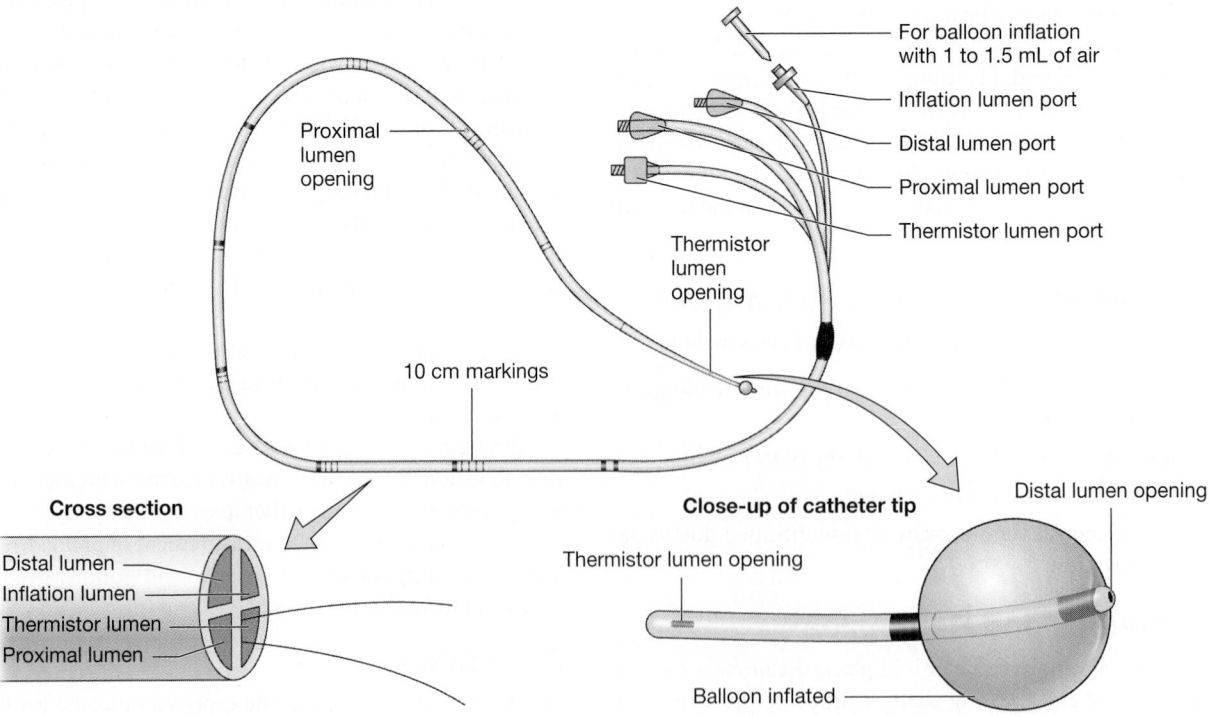

FIGURE 24–14 ■ Ports and lumens of a pulmonary artery catheter.

with additional lumens are used to measure continuous mixed venous oxygen saturation (SvO$_2$), right ventricular volume, continuous cardiac output, or additional ports for insertion of transvenous pacing electrodes. Specialized pulmonary artery catheters are discussed later in the chapter.

The proximal port of the PAC sits in the right atrium and is used to infuse IV fluids and nonvasoactive medications. If a transducer is attached to this port, right atrial pressures can be obtained. The second port, which also sits in the right atrium, is the proximal injectate port, used for measuring cardiac output, which is discussed later. The distal port located at the end of the catheter is positioned in the pulmonary artery. The distal port is connected to the pressure transducer system with the flush solution and used for continuous monitoring of pulmonary artery pressures. The tip of the PAC also contains a thermometer, referred to as a **thermistor**. The thermistor permits measurement of the blood temperature in the pulmonary artery, termed the core temperature. The external thermistor connector is attached to the cardiac output computer.

The final port is the balloon inflation port, which is used to inflate the balloon at the distal end of the catheter. The balloon is inflated during insertion to assist with "floating" the catheter through the heart. The balloon port is also used to obtain pulmonary capillary pressure or the **pulmonary artery occlusion pressure (PAOP)**. The amount of air used to inflate the balloon differs among manufacturers. Usually this volume of air is up to 1.5 mL; however, the capacity of the balloon is limited by the catheter size. Manufacturers of PACs usually indicate the maximum balloon inflation volume on the catheter hub and provide a volume-limiting syringe to prevent accidental overinflation. Overinflation may cause rupture of the balloon or pulmonary artery. Once insertion of the catheter is complete, the balloon *never* remains inflated but rather lies uninflated in the pulmonary artery until it is necessary to obtain the PAOP.

Insertion of the Pulmonary Artery Catheter

For insertion the patient is prepped and draped in a similar manner as for any central venous access because strict sterile technique is required. An introducer is inserted in either the jugular, subclavian, or femoral vein. A protective sheath should be placed over the PAC prior to insertion through the introducer. The sheath is an infection control barrier and allows for repositioning of the PAC after insertion. The PAC is passed through the introducer and advanced into the selected vessel to the right atrium. Once the catheter is in the right atrium, the balloon is inflated to allow it to flow with the blood through the heart chambers. This facilitates passage of the PAC through the tricuspid valve, right ventricle, pulmonic valve, and into the pulmonary artery. The balloon is then deflated and the introducer is sutured in place. Right atrial and right ventricular pressures are measured during the insertion of the catheter.

Hemodynamic pressures and waveforms are generated by myocardial contraction (systole) and relaxation (diastole). When the PAC is advanced through the heart, each chamber has a characteristic waveform (Figure 24–15 ■). As the catheter enters the right atrium, the waveform appears similar to a CVP waveform. The identification of the *a, c,* and *v* waves of the RAP is the same as with a CVP tracing. The normal mean RAP is 4 to

Interpreting hemodynamic waveforms

Right atrium

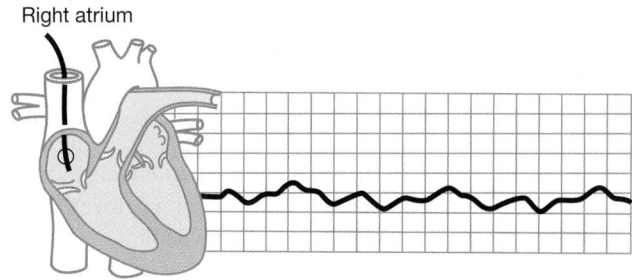

Right ventricle

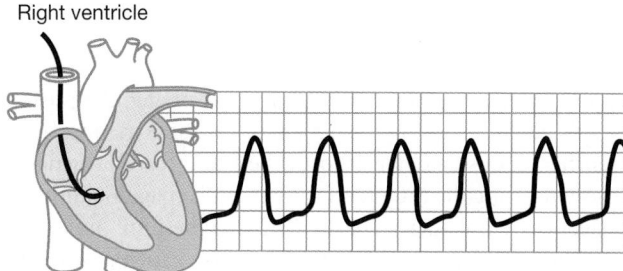

Pulmonary artery

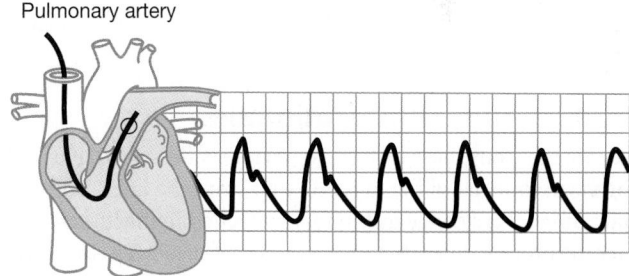

Pulmonary capillary wedge

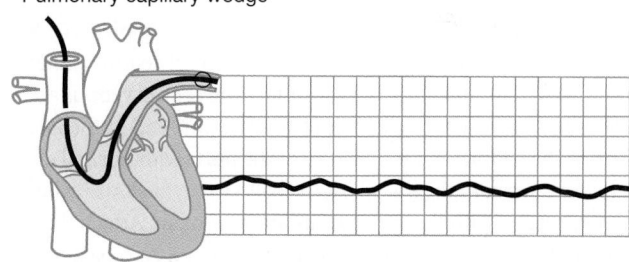

FIGURE 24–15 ■ Cardiac pressures during PAC insertion.

6 mmHg. Normal systolic pressures in the right ventricle (RV) are between 20 and 30 mmHg, and diastolic pressures are between 0 and 8 mmHg (Lynn-McHale Weigand & Carlson, 2005). As the PAC passes through the RV, the tip of the catheter can irritate the ventricle. Monitor the ECG closely for ectopy. Patients may exhibit premature ventricular contractions (PVCs). This ectopy usually ceases when the catheter is advanced into the pulmonary artery or withdrawn from the right ventricle.

As the catheter enters the pulmonary artery, the waveform resembles an arterial pressure waveform with not only systolic and diastolic pressures but also a dicrotic notch. The dicrotic notch represents closure of the pulmonic valve. The normal pulmonary artery systolic (PAS) pressure is 20 to 30 mmHg and the pulmonary artery diastolic (PAD) pressure is 5 to 15 mmHg. Notice that the normal right ventricular systolic pressure and the pulmonary artery systolic pressure are the same

Nursing Management

Nursing management of patients needing pulmonary artery catheters requires critical thinking and clinical judgment. These patients are typically critically ill and hemodynamically compromised. Insertion of a PAC is an intervention that will provide the nurse with advanced assessment parameters as well as a central intravenous line to administer the necessary medications and fluid.

Assessment

Prior to insertion of a pulmonary artery catheter, the nurse is responsible for assessing the patient in the same manner as for a central venous catheter. Inform the health care provider or person inserting the catheter if the patient is coagulopathic, has an electrolyte imbalance (particularly magnesium, potassium, or calcium), or has an acid–base imbalance. Patients with a coagulopathy are more likely to have bleeding complications, and patients with electrolyte or acid–base imbalances are at increased risk for cardiac irritability that may lead to intractable arrhythmias.

Interventions and Rationales

Prepare the transducer system as previously described. Flush all ports with normal saline to remove air from the lines. The normal saline flush syringe may remain attached to the lumen until after the procedure. Attach the distal end of the PAC to the transducer system and zero balance the system. Test the balloon on the PA catheter by inflating the syringe with the appropriate amount of air.

Assist with setup of the sterile field and opening of sterile kits. Sterile barriers identical to those used for central venous catheters are employed for insertion of PACs. Once the central venous access is obtained and the introducer inserted, the port end of the PAC is given to the bedside nurse. Flush all of the ports with normal saline to remove air from the lines. Test the balloon on the PAC by inflating the syringe with the appropriate amount of air. Attach the distal end of the PAC to the transducer system and zero balance the system.

During catheter insertion, watch the monitor for waveform changes as the PAC passes through the chambers of the heart. When the catheter is in the right atrium, the nurse inflates the balloon. This facilitates passage of the catheter through the tricuspid valve. During this time, watch closely for ventricular ectopy.

Note the distance the catheter is inserted. The PAC has thin and wide black lines on the exterior. The thin line represents 10-cm increments and the wide line signifies 50 cm. Document the number of centimeters. This will serve as a reference to others caring for the patient.

Evaluation

After the catheter is placed, secure the site with an occlusive dressing. Reassess the patient to determine tolerance to procedure. Follow through with the health care provider on orders for

a chest x-ray. Once the x-ray confirms proper placement and rules out a pneumothorax, the bedside nurse connects the IV infusions to the remaining ports of the PAC and obtains pulmonary artery occlusion pressures and cardiac output measurements, as discussed in a later section.

Complications of a Pulmonary Artery Catheter

As with central venous catheters, complications from a pulmonary artery catheter include infection, air embolus, and pneumothorax (Urden et al., 2006). However, with a PAC there are additional risks of pulmonary artery rupture, pulmonary infarction, balloon rupture, catheter coiling or displacement, arrhythmias, and conduction defects. Pulmonary artery rupture is a life-threatening complication and, although rare, the mortality rate is 45% to 65% (Weininger, Ginosar, Sprung, & Weiss, 2002). Rupture of the pulmonary artery may occur when the balloon is overfilled or if the tip of the PAC migrates through the pulmonary artery intima. In most cases, hemoptysis is the presenting symptom (Weininger et al., 2002). If a pulmonary artery rupture is suspected, immediately place the patient with the affected side down to prevent blood from leaking into the unaffected lung and notify the health care provider.

Balloon rupture may cause air or balloon pieces to embolize the pulmonary vasculature. The likelihood of balloon rupture increases with catheter duration, because the balloon loses its elasticity over time. If blood is noted in the air inflation port or if no PAOP tracing appears with balloon inflation, then after placing the patient with the affected lung down, notify the health care provider.

Pulmonary infarction can occur if the balloon accidentally remains inflated or if the PA catheter tip occludes a branch of the artery. Continuous monitoring of the PAC waveform noting the contour of the wave and the corresponding numeric values is an important nursing intervention to detect pulmonary infarcts. It is especially important to note the return of the normal pulmonary artery waveform after obtaining the PAOP or wedging of the catheter, which is discussed later. If the nurse suspects that the PAC is remaining wedged despite balloon deflation, then turning the patient side to side or having the patient cough may unwedge the catheter. If these techniques are unsuccessful, the catheter may need repositioning by the health care provider or advanced practice nurse.

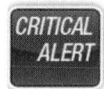 *After obtaining the PAOP, remove the syringe from the balloon inflation port and allow passive deflation of the balloon. Using the syringe to remove the air causes damage to the balloon and may lead to rupture.*

The PAC may coil on itself at any time. Usually the coiling occurs within the right atrium or right ventricle. An x-ray is necessary to detect this complication and requires an invasive procedure to correct. Arrhythmias and conduction defects result when the PAC is touching the endocardium and septal wall. Conduction defects, especially right bundle branch blocks, can occur when the PAC is advanced through the right ventricle. In patients with a preexisting left bundle branch block (LBBB), a new right bundle branch block (RBBB) places the patient at risk for developing a complete bundle branch block. For a patient with a preexisting LBBB, having trans-cutaneous pacing equipment available is advisable. As previously discussed, electrolyte or acid–base imbalances should be corrected prior to PAC insertion in an effort to decrease the likelihood of arrhythmias from these sources.

Pulmonary Artery Occlusion Pressure

The pulmonary artery occlusion pressure (PAOP), also referred to as pulmonary artery wedge pressure (PAWP) and pulmonary capillary wedge pressure (PCWP), is an indirect measurement of left ventricular end-diastolic pressure (LVEDP), or left-sided preload. To obtain this measurement, the balloon of the PAC is inflated, which facilitates forward movement of the catheter until it wedges in the pulmonary capillary (Figure 24–16 ■). The pressure is measured at the tip of the catheter; thus, when the balloon is inflated, blood flow in through the pulmonary artery is temporarily stopped and only pressures in front of the balloon are measurable. Therefore, the PAOP is the most direct bedside measurement of left heart function. A normal PAOP reading is between 4 and 12 mmHg.

Left ventricular (LV) failure and myocardial ischemia, constrictive pericarditis, mitral valve disease, or volume overload are conditions that elevate the PAOP. The diminished contractility and ensuing increase in left ventricular volume seen with LV failure and ischemia are reflected in an increased PAOP. Constrictive pericarditis, like pericardial tamponade, causes an increase in PAOP when the external pressure exerted on the left side of the heart in-creases. Infectious processes, trauma, and uremia secondary to renal disease are examples of conditions causing constrictive pericarditis. Mitral valve disease increases the PAOP when either the mitral valve does not allow for complete emptying of the left atrium due to stenosis (narrowing of the outlet) or when the valve leaflets cannot close completely (insufficiency), causing a reflux of blood into the left atrium during left ventricular contraction. The volume overload of the left heart is usually secondary to LV failure. PAOPs decrease when patients are hypovolemic, in shock, or when receiving vasodilating medications. Vasodilators decrease SVR, making it easier for left ventricular ejection and improvement in ejection fraction (Urden et al., 2006).

Correlating the PAOP Waveform with the Cardiac Cycle

There is a delay in the transmission of pressure changes in the PAOP waveform. Therefore, the *a* wave occurs 0.20 to 0.24 seconds after the P wave, near the end of the QRS complex as illustrated earlier in Figure 24–13 ■ (p. 572). The *v* wave corresponds with the T-P interval. The *c* wave occurs with closure of the tricuspid valve and is found on the *a* to *x* downslope. Identification of the *c* wave is important because prior to the *c* wave occurring, the pressure equilibrates between the atrium and the ventricle. This is the point where the PAOP left ventricular end diastolic volume (LVEDV) is measured. If the *c* wave is indistinguishable, the PAOP is obtained by averaging the *a* and the *x* wave.

Thermodilution Cardiac Output

With the thermodilution method of obtaining a cardiac output reading, a specified amount of solution, typically 5 to 10 mL, is injected through the proximal injectate port of the PAC (see Figure 24–14 ■, p. 574). This process is commonly referred to as "shooting" a cardiac output. The injectate is at room temperature (about 21°C [70°F]) when it enters the right atrium and mixes with blood (about 37°C [98.6°F]). The CO computer calculates the time required for the solution of a different temperature to reach the thermistor, located at the end of the catheter in the pulmonary artery. The change of temperature occurs over time to

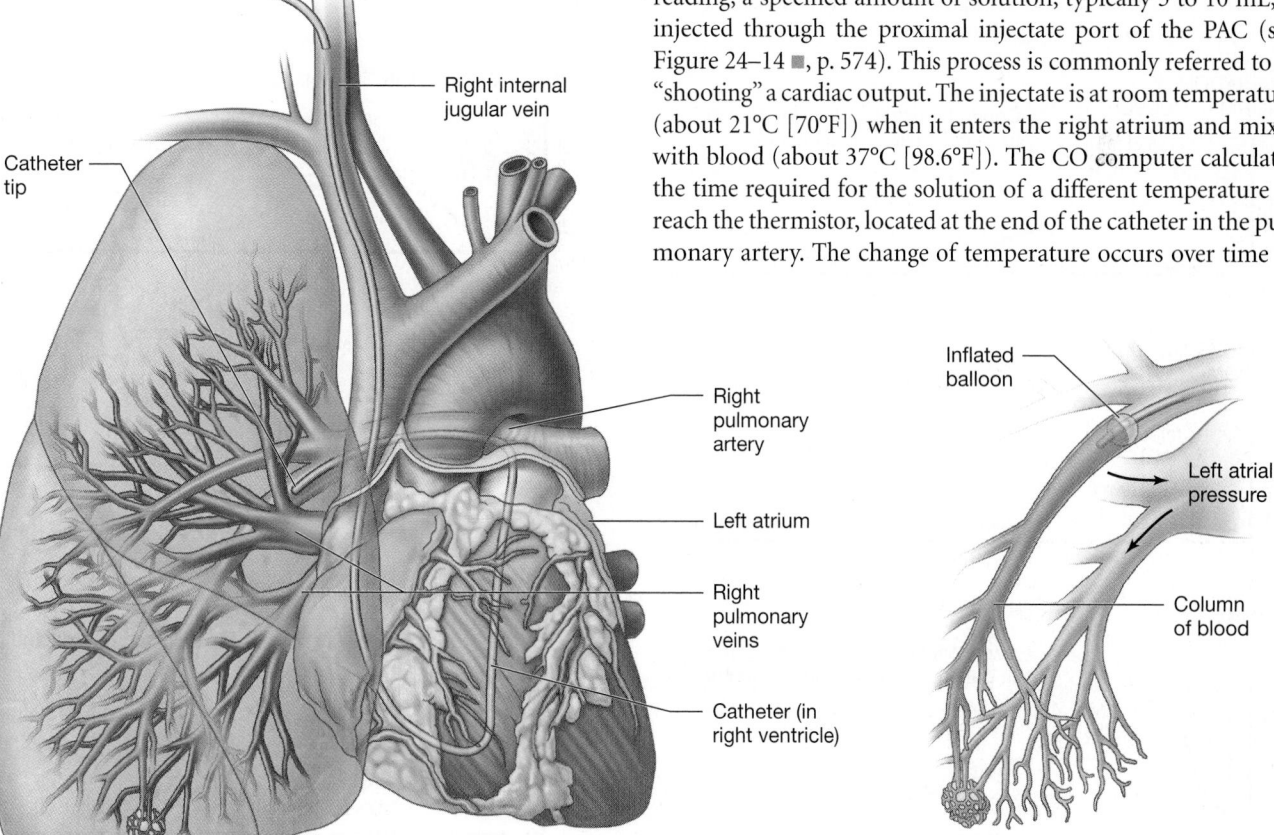

FIGURE 24–16 ■ Position of pulmonary artery catheter during PAOP.

yield a CO curve, as shown in Figure 24–17 ■. The area under the CO curve inversely corresponds to the cardiac output. When the area under the curve is large, the CO is low. Conversely, when the area under the curve is small, the CO is high.

Awareness of what constitutes a normal curve is important. Assessment of the shape of the cardiac output curve is necessary to determine if the CO measurement should be accepted or rejected. A normal CO curve starts at the baseline and has a smooth incline and decline. Hesitation or starting and stopping during a CO injection would yield an invalid curve. The injectate should be injected smoothly and in less than 4 seconds. This prevents prolonged injection times that would yield a lower CO result. Additionally, injecting less than or greater than the recommended amount of injectate invalidates the measurement. Cardiac output measurements are performed 1 to 2 minutes apart with an average of three measurements obtained. Also, the injectate should be timed to the end-expiratory phase of respiration. This will minimize the variation in intrathoracic pressure during respiration. Any CO that is questionable based on the curve or two CO measurements differing by 10% should be discarded (Lynn-McHale Weigand & Carlson, 2005).

Influence of Heart Rate on Cardiac Output

A slow or rapid heart rate affects cardiac output. Heart rates greater than 100 decrease diastolic filling time. For example, a heart rate of 150 beats/min and a reduced stroke volume to 20 mL is detrimental to CO:

$$HR\,(150) \times SV\,(20) = 3,000\ mL\ or\ 3.0\ L/minute$$

Dysrhythmias such as atrial fibrillation and atrial flutter cause not only a decreased diastolic filling time but also a loss of atrial kick, which is responsible for up to 25% of the total cardiac output (Chapter 38).

Bradycardia allows sufficient time for the ventricles to fill and usually is not detrimental to cardiac output because of compensatory mechanisms. However, when patients have lost their compensatory mechanisms, a bradycardic rhythm may not provide sufficient cardiac output. For example, a heart rate of 35 beats/min and a normal stroke volume of 60 mL/beat yields a CO of 2.1 L/min:

$$HR\,(35) \times SV\,(60) = 2,100\ mL\ or\ 2.1\ L/minute$$

Additionally, consider a patient with frequent premature ventricular contractions. If a patient has a heart rate of 80 but every other beat is a PVC, the heart rate is effectively reduced by one-half, due to little or no cardiac output with PVCs.

Influence of Preload on Cardiac Output

Reduced preload (CVP < 2, RAP < 4, PAOP < 4) signals vasodilation or volume loss. Exploration of cause is essential so that appropriate action is taken. Treatment of hypovolemia is the

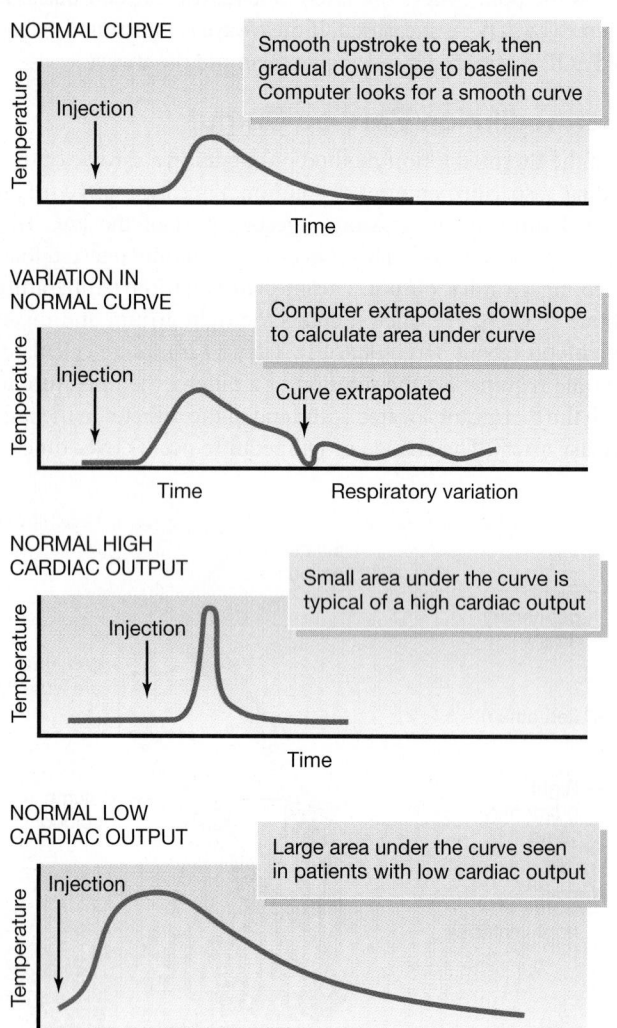

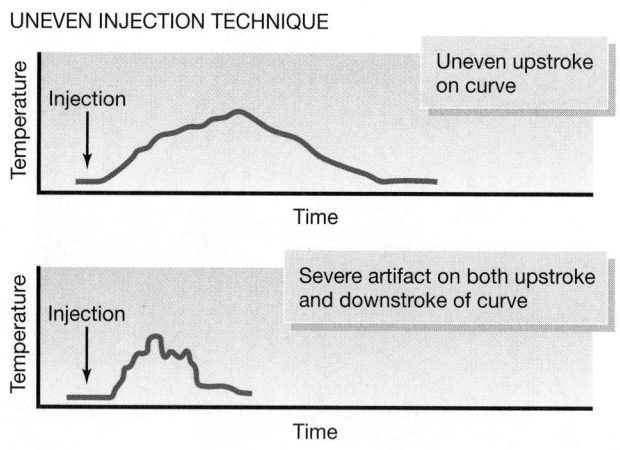

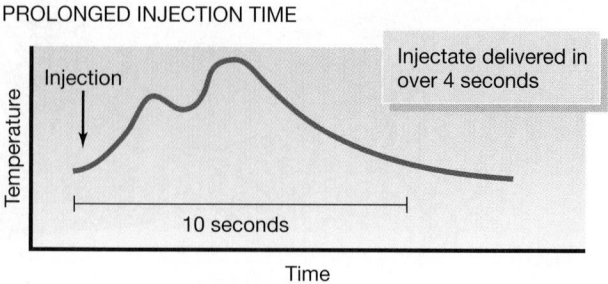

FIGURE 24–17 ■ Normal and abnormal cardiac output curves.

administration of crystalloids, volume expanders, and/or blood products. Examples of obvious fluid losses occur after trauma, during surgery, with diuretic therapy, profuse sweating, or excessive upper or lower gastrointestinal losses. Internal, nonvisible blood loss is an example of insidious hypovolemia and may go undetected unless considered as a suspected cause of preload reduction.

Vasodilation and loss of venous tone demonstrated in neurogenic or anaphylactic shock have a profound effect on preload. In neurogenic shock, the loss of vasomotor tone is secondary to the loss of neural output or from spinal cord damage. This can result from general or spinal anesthesia or, in the case of spinal cord injury, from loss of sympathetic tone. In anaphylactic shock, the antigen–antibody response triggers the release of vasoactive chemicals in the body (histamine, bradykinin), which create massive vasodilation. Shock is discussed in Chapter 61 $\textcircled{\tiny{co}}$.

Excess preload (CVP/RAP > 6, PAOP > 12) may indicate hypervolemia or ventricular failure. Excessive circulating volume strains the heart and compromises adequate tissue oxygenation. Excess preload increases the workload of the heart and increases myocardial oxygen demands. Diuretics and venodilators are ordered if the cause is hypervolemia. If patients do not respond to diuretic therapy or renal failure is diagnosed, then continuous renal replacement therapy utilizing ultrafiltration or dialysis may be considered. If ventricular failure is determined to be the cause, inotropic medications are prescribed.

Influence of Afterload on Cardiac Output

Reduced afterload (PVR < 155, SVR < 900) suggests vasodilation of the pulmonary and systemic vasculature. Decreased afterload lessens the workload on the heart and reduces myocardial oxygen requirements. With reduced resistance to ventricular ejection, an increase in stroke volume occurs as the ventricles empty. For example, patients with sepsis present with hypotension, fever, and vasodilatation, which reduce the SVR. The cardiac output of a patient with sepsis can elevate to as much as 10 L/min.

Excessive afterload (PVR > 255, SVR > 1,600) imposes great strain on the ventricles, increases the myocardial oxygen requirement, and decreases the stroke volume. Conditions that increase pulmonary resistance include hypoxia, acute respiratory distress syndrome, positive end-expiratory pressure, pulmonary embolism, chronic obstructive pulmonary disease (COPD), increased interstitial lung water, and pulmonary fibrosis (Urden et al., 2006). Left ventricular afterload is the resistance to ejection into the systemic circulation. Conditions that increase resistance include aortic valve stenosis, hypertension, and vasoconstriction of the peripheral vasculature.

Influence of Contractility on Cardiac Output

Contractility, the intrinsic ability of the myocardium to contract, occurs independent of changes in preload and afterload. Myocardial damage during an infarction or the presence of cardiomyopathy decreases contractility. Cardiomyopathy is discussed in detail in Chapter 41 $\textcircled{\tiny{co}}$. Positive inotropic medications, such as dobutamine and epinephrine, stimulate the sympathetic nervous system and increase contractility, but these events also increase myocardial oxygen demand. Negative inotropic medications, such as beta-adrenergic blockers, are administered when myocardial work and oxygen consumption are detrimental, such as with a myocardial infarction.

Specialized Pulmonary Artery Catheters

Subsequent to the development of the generic thermodilution catheter, multiple generations evolved. This section explains different PAC models and provides supplemental information. Although presented as separate entities, many of these features are combined on one PAC model. Model variations are usually not available within one institution. The available model is dependent on hospital contracts, health care provider preference, and the patient population needs.

Continuous Cardiac Output PAC

This catheter modifies the thermodilution PAC by adding a thermal filament that slightly warms the blood. This warmed blood is sensed at the thermistor in the catheter tip. The CO result is based on temperature changes at preset intervals, usually every minute (Urden et al., 2006). The updated calculation is then displayed on a CO monitor. The advantages to this system include recognition of CO as a dynamic, fluctuating parameter, the elimination of "shooting" cardiac outputs with the inherent risk of operator variability, plus the elimination of extra fluid a patient receives during that process.

Continuous Mixed Venous Oxygen Saturation

A **mixed venous oxygen saturation** (SvO_2) PAC provides information about the supply of oxygen to the tissues and demand for oxygen by the tissues (Kaplow & Hardin, 2007). This catheter is positioned like a thermodilution catheter with the distal end in the pulmonary artery. These specialized catheters have fiber-optic fibers. One fiber emits a light wave to illuminate red blood cells (RBCs) and the second fiber receives the reflected light signal. The amount of light reflected by the RBCs is determined by their hemoglobin saturation. Because this analysis occurs in the pulmonary artery, it reflects the saturation of all venous blood returned to the right side of the heart. This means that the SvO_2 reflects the consumption of oxygen at the tissue level. The numeric value displayed on the SvO_2 monitor reflects the saturation of mixed venous blood or the amount of deoxygenated blood that returns to the heart. The normal SvO_2 value is 60% to 80%.

Four factors affect mixed venous oxygen saturation: cardiac output, hemoglobin, arterial oxygen saturation, and oxygen consumption. Mixed venous oxygen saturation parallels cardiac output, hemoglobin concentration, and arterial oxygen saturation: A drop in cardiac output, hemoglobin, or oxygen saturation will cause a decrease in SvO_2; an increase in cardiac output, hemoglobin, or oxygen saturation will elevate SvO_2. High tissue extraction of oxygen (low SvO_2) occurs when patients are in pain (high oxygen demand) or when patients are experiencing respiratory failure (low oxygen supply). Low tissue extraction (high SvO_2) occurs when patients are sedate (low oxygen demand) or after blood transfusions (high oxygen supply). Nursing procedures such as patient repositioning and dressing or linen changes are oxygen-consuming activities for the patient and correspondingly lower the SvO_2.

 Use the information offered by the SvO_2 catheter to prioritize and plan nursing interventions. Patients who are compromised do not tolerate turning, suctioning, and dressing changes in a short time interval.

Right Ventricular Ejection Fraction Volumetric Catheter

This catheter provides data on right ventricular systolic and diastolic volumes. Two sensors in the catheter, one in the right ventricle (RV) and one in the pulmonary artery, detect ventricular depolarization, heart rate, and temperature change. Using the information on systolic volume and diastolic volume, the ejection fraction is calculated. Accurate measurement of preload using the right ventricular end-diastolic volume instead of estimation of preload by CVP or PAOP is helpful in assessing the fluid requirement after right ventricular infarction and during high levels of positive end-expiratory pressure (PEEP) on mechanically ventilated patients (Weininger et al., 2002). Accurate calculation of RV systolic and diastolic volumes relies on temperature consistency. Large-volume resuscitations with room temperature IV fluid or cool blood components diminish the accuracy of RV end-diastolic volumes and influence the calculation.

Transpulmonary Thermodilution with Pulse Contour Analysis

Using a special thermistor-tipped catheter inserted in the femoral or brachial artery and a regular central venous catheter, intermittent and continuous cardiac outputs can be evaluated. For an intermittent CO, a preset volume of cold injectate is injected into the central venous catheter. After completion of the vascular circuit, the temperature change is detected by the thermistor in the arterial catheter. As with the previously described thermodilution method, the calculation of CO is based on temperature change over time. For continuous cardiac output monitoring, the value obtained by an intermittent CO is used to calibrate the monitoring equipment. An internal algorithm combines this information with continual analysis of the arterial pressure wave contour to determine CO. Rather than measuring preload, afterload, and stroke volume, this device calculates intrathoracic volume and pulmonary volume by analysis of the CO distribution curve. End-diastolic volumes are automatically calculated. The advantage of measuring end-diastolic volume during fluid resuscitation without a PAC is useful. Nursing care requires knowledge of cardiac and pulmonary physiology plus a shift in thinking from hemodynamic pressure monitoring to hemodynamic volume monitoring (Genahr & McLuckie, 2004).

▉ Nursing Management

The bedside nurse is responsible for management of the pulmonary artery catheter from preinsertion until removal. These responsibilities include patient and family education, assisting with insertion, site care, assessment and interpretation of hemodynamic waveforms and parameters, and titration of vasoactive medications. The nurse should provide information about the PAC and how the measurements obtained will direct therapy. Use of the nursing process facilitates an organized approach for management of patients with invasive catheters.

Assessment

Assessment includes monitoring the insertion site for infection, monitoring of PA pressures, measuring PAOP, and cardiac outputs, and monitoring the patient when changes occur.

Nursing Diagnosis

Nursing diagnoses related to hemodynamic monitoring include:

- *Anxiety*
- *Decreased Cardiac Output*
- *Risk for Imbalanced Fluid Volume*
- *Ineffective Health Maintenance*
- *Risk for Injury*
- *Deficient Knowledge*
- *Risk for Infection.*

Planning

Planning for interventions for care for the patient with invasive lines is multifaceted. Each institution has specific procedures for maintaining a sterile occlusive dressing over the line insertion site. The nurse must be knowledgeable of these procedures and carry them out within the required time frames.

Outcomes and Evaluation Parameters

Outcomes and evaluation parameters associated with pulmonary artery catheters include:

- Stabilization of the pulmonary artery readings to within normal limits
- Normal or stable cardiac output
- No infection at the catheter site or in the bloodstream as evidenced by no fever and a negative blood culture
- No bleeding from the site or catheter
- Having the PAC discontinued due to patient stabilization.

Interventions and Rationales

Appropriate interventions include changing the occlusive dressing if loosened and inspecting the site for redness, swelling, and leakage. The nurse must also possess the knowledge required to operate and troubleshoot the catheter. The transducer system must be inspected for kinks and air bubbles from site to pressure bag. After leveling, zero referencing, and checking the dynamic response, the pulmonary artery systolic, diastolic, and mean pressures are usually documented hourly and after changes in therapies. PAOP and CO readings are obtained when changes occur in the patient's clinical status; with initiation, titration, or discontinuation of vasoactive medications; when significant changes occur in heart rate or rhythm; or when greater than 5 cm of PEEP is applied during mechanical ventilation. Increases in PEEP over 5 cm are associated with increased intrathoracic pressure, which may decrease cardiac output. PEEP is discussed in detail Chapter 36 👁.

Evaluation

The expected outcome for these patients is hemodynamic stabilization with the intent of getting the invasive catheters removed as soon as possible. Not every patient will have normal readings; thus, the goal is for readings that are tolerated by the patient. One gauge of tolerance is the patient's ability to perform activities of daily living.

Health Promotion During Invasive Procedures

Family members should be given the opportunity to stay during invasive procedures, if desired. Based on evaluations conducted in emergency department settings from family presence programs for pediatric patients, family members are grateful and voice their approval (American Heart Association [AHA], 2000). However, there is a lack of evidence related to family presence during adult resuscitations and invasive procedures. Nursing research on family presence is progressing. Initial results indicate that families and patient's favor this practice change (Eichhorn et al., 2001; Meyers et al., 2000). The success of these programs in adult populations is predictable, according to the AHA (2000), when health care workers demonstrate the same level of care and concern seen in pediatric programs.

 **CRITICAL ALERT** *If family members wish to be present during invasive procedures, a staff member should stay with them to answer questions and clarify what is happening.*

Alternative Methods of Determining Cardiac Output

Patients who are coagulopathic or immunosuppressed are at high risk of complications from invasive devices. Additionally, patients who may not tolerate positioning for a pulmonary artery catheter or are clinically unstable may be candidates for noninvasive determination of cardiac output. Minimally invasive and noninvasive monitoring devices estimate hemodynamic pressures in patients who are critically ill and are used in ICUs. Some devices are gaining acceptance in intermediate care units, emergency departments, and outpatient clinics to evaluate and treat patients with congestive heart failure and to optimize pacemaker settings. These devices, the supporting hardware, and monitoring systems are incompatible with the transducer systems used in invasive monitoring. Therefore, separate supporting hardware must be available.

Transesophageal Ultrasound

Transesophageal ultrasound is a minimally invasive method for continuous monitoring of cardiac function. An ultrasound probe is inserted into the esophagus similar to the insertion of a nasogastric tube. When the probe is properly positioned, the ultrasound waves detect red blood cells descending through the aorta. Figure 24–18 ■ illustrates probe position in the aorta. The blood flow and velocity are transmitted to a display monitor where an internal algorithm converts blood flow, velocity, heart rate, and diameter of the aorta into estimations of cardiac output and stroke volume (Turner, 2003). Sedation is recommended before passage of the probe. Nurses assisting with this procedure must have knowledge of conscious sedation protocols.

Thoracic Impedance

Thoracic impedance cardiography is an external, noninvasive method of hemodynamic monitoring. Impedance electrodes are applied to the body, one set at the base of the neck and another set to both sides of the thorax (Figure 24–19 ■, p. 582). These electrodes work in tandem: The outer electrodes inject a

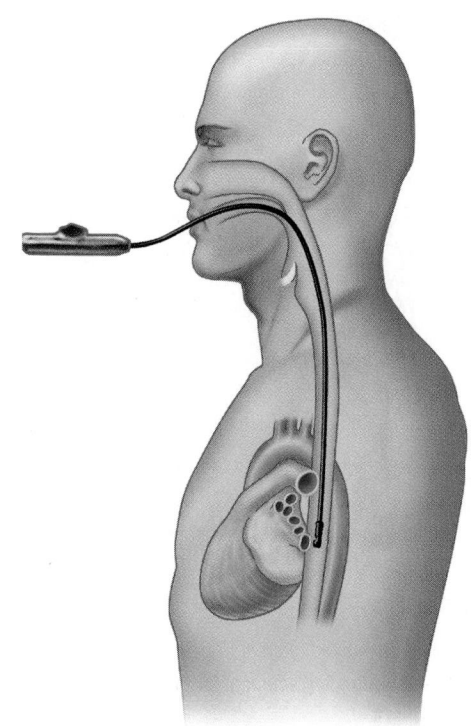

FIGURE 24–18 ■ Transesophageal ultrasound.

low-level electric current (harmless current) and the inner electrodes sense thoracic impedance. Changes in thoracic impedance are associated with changes in aortic blood flow during systole and diastole. Peak blood flow during systole, combined with heart rate analysis from the ECG, is used to compute stroke volume and cardiac output. Unlike invasive monitoring, which hinders patient mobility, when thoracic impedance monitoring is used, patients can be mobilized, including ambulation, by disconnecting the monitoring leads from the system.

The evolution of hemodynamic monitoring does not preclude investigations of current technology. The nursing research discussed in this chapter needs replication, because study replication produces a body of knowledge that enhances nursing science and produces evidence-based practice. All nurses make a contribution in the research process, whether by collecting data or explaining in lay terms the research behind relocating a transducer after turning a patient. Bedside nurses are prime candidates for identification of potential research projects, as outlined in the Research Opportunities and Clinical Impact box (p. 582).

Summary

Exposure to patients who are critically ill and experience with invasive technologies enables the nurse to initiate and actively participate in discussions regarding utilization of invasive devices. As health care team members, nurses' responsibilities include patient advocacy. Nurses are not just accountable for safe care, but also for reasonable care. The nurse should always ask, "What information will be obtained if this catheter is inserted?" and "How will having that information enhance this patient's quality of life?" These questions are not easy to answer, nor is the answer always evident.

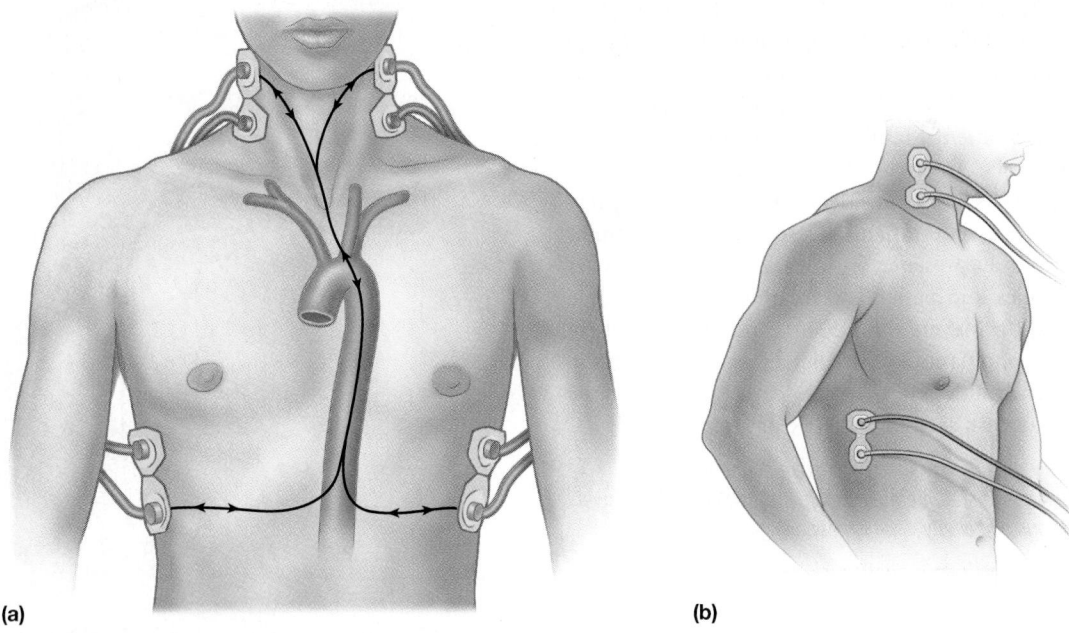

(a)   (b)

FIGURE 24–19 ■ Electrode placement for thoracic impedance cardiography: (A) anterior view; (B) lateral view.

Although hemodynamic monitoring technology has evolved (and will continue to do so), the clinical assessment combined with laboratory data analysis and patient history are equally important in the provision of quality care. Linking a clinical presentation with hemodynamic data requires repeated exposure.

With each experience managing critically ill patients, nursing actions will be become incorporated into daily practice even before an invasive catheter is inserted so that treatment can be initiated quickly.

RESEARCH OPPORTUNITIES AND CLINICAL IMPACT RELATED TO HEMODYNAMIC MONITORING

Research Area	Clinical Impact
Exploration of cultural beliefs about medical decision making	Improves the delivery of care, patient satisfaction, and health care providers' knowledge of other cultures.
Comparison of techniques used to secure arterial catheters	Results in fewer dislodged or accidentally removed arterial catheters, improved patient safety.
Techniques to decrease the infection rates associated with central venous catheters	Prevention of infections will decrease patient morbidity and mortality rates.
Continuous monitoring of left ventricular ejection fraction	Provides immediate information about cardiac function.
Noninvasive methods to accurately measure cardiac output	Decreases exposure to invasive catheters and the associated complications and risks.
Methods of facilitating family presence programs	Recognizes the impact of family systems on patient health and well-being.
The effect of prone positioning on hemodynamic pressures	Provides for accurate hemodynamic assessment during therapeutic proning.

NCLEX® REVIEW

1. A patient is admitted to the ICU in critical condition. The use of hemodynamic monitoring for this patient will be to:
   1. Make measuring the patient's blood pressure more accurate.
   2. Help with diagnosis, treatment, and evaluation of care.
   3. Reduce the amount of nursing time needed to provide care.
   4. Determine when the patient can be transferred to a step-down unit.

2. The nurse is assessing the waveform created after the placement of a hemodynamic monitoring device. The waveform appears distorted. What can the nurse do?
   1. Increase the flow rate through the device.
   2. Reposition the catheter.
   3. Find out if the correct type of tubing was used.
   4. Check the patient and alert the health care provider and begin interventions to improve hemodynamic stability.

3. During the placement of a hemodynamic monitoring device the patient demonstrates premature ventricular contractions upon ECG. Which of the following should be done?

   1. Flush the arterial line with normal saline.

   2. Reposition the CVP monitor.

   3. Zero the transducer.

   4. Advance the catheter into the pulmonary artery.

4. A patient's central venous pressure is 10 mmHg. What should the nurse do?

   1. Report the measurement to the health care provider and prepare for interventions.

   2. Access the algorithm for an elevated CVP and begin the protocol.

   3. Adjust the catheter tip.

   4. Compare the result with other measurements.

5. While shooting a patient's cardiac output, the nurse obtains readings that are inconsistent. What should the nurse do?

   1. Begin again and inject the injectate over 10 seconds.

   2. Eliminate any values that differ by 10%.

   3. Warm the injectate to body temperature.

   4. Use 45 mL of injectate.

6. A patient's central venous pressure reading is 12 mmHg with a right atrial pressure of 14 mmHg. The nurse realizes these pressures reflect:

   1. Fluid volume overload or ventricular failure.

   2. Hypotension.

   3. Vasodilation.

   4. Anaphylactic shock.

7. During the placement of a pulmonary artery catheter a tracing begins to resemble an arterial line tracing but with a dicrotic notch. The nurse realizes that this notch indicates:

   1. Atrial contraction.

   2. Retrograde swelling of the tricuspid valve.

   3. Atrial filling.

   4. Closure of the pulmonic valve.

Answers for review questions appear in Appendix D

KEY TERMS

afterload *p.565*
Allen's test *p.567*
arterial line *p.567*
cardiac index (CI) *p.564*
cardiac output (CO) *p.564*
central venous pressure (CVP) *p.565*
contractility *p.565*
dynamic response test *p.563*

ejection fraction (EF) *p.565*
Frank-Starling law *p.565*
hemodynamic monitoring *p.560*
leveling *p.562*
mean arterial pressure (MAP) *p.569*
mixed venous oxygen saturation *p.579*
phlebostatic axis *p.562*
preload *p.565*

pulmonary artery catheter (PAC) *p.574*
pulmonary artery occlusion pressure (PAOP) *p.575*
stroke volume (SV) *p.563*
thermistor *p.575*
thoracic impedance *p.581*
transesophageal ultrasound *p.581*
zero referencing *p.562*

PEARSON

EXPLORE mynursingkit™

MyNursingKit is your one stop for online chapter review materials and resources. Prepare for success with additional NCLEX®-style practice questions, interactive assignments and activities, web links, animations and videos, and more!

Register your access code from the front of your book at
www.mynursingkit.com

REFERENCES

Adams, K. L. (2004). Hemodynamic assessment: The physiologic basis for turning data into clinical information. *AACN Clinical Issues, 15,* 534–546.

American Heart Association. (2000). Guidelines 2000 for cardiopulmonary resuscitation and emergency cardiovascular care. *Circulation, 102*(8), I-136–I-139.

American Society of Anesthesiologists. (2003). Practice guidelines for pulmonary artery catheterization: An updated report by the American Society of Anesthesiologists Task Force on Pulmonary Artery Catheterization. *Anesthesiology, 99,* 988–1014.

Centers for Disease Control and Prevention. (2002). Guidelines for the prevention of intravascular catheter-related infections. *Morbidity and Mortality Weekly Report, 51.*

Chittock, D. R., Dhingra, V. K., Ronco, J. J., Russell, J. A. Forrest, D. M., Tweeddale, M., et al. (2004). Severity of illness and risk of death associated with pulmonary artery catheter use. *Critical Care Medicine, 32,* 911–915.

Darovic, G. O. (2004). *Handbook of hemodynamic monitoring.* St. Louis, MO: W. B. Saunders.

Dietz, B., & Smith, T. T. (2002). Enhancing the accuracy of hemodynamic monitoring. *Journal of Nursing Care Quality, 17,* 27–34.

Eichhorn, D. J., Meyers, T. A., Guzzetta, C. E., Clark, A. P., Klein, J. D., Taliaferro, E., et al. (2001). Family presence during invasive procedures and resuscitation: Hearing the voice of the patient. *American Journal of Nursing, 101,* 48–55.

Genahr, A., & McLuckie, A. (2004, Spring). Transpulmonary thermodilution in the critically ill. *British Journal of Intensive Care,* 6–10.

Giuliano, K. K., Scott, S. S., Brown, V., & Olson, M. (2003). Backrest angle and cardiac output measurement in critically ill patients. *Nursing Research, 52,* 242–248.

Kaplow, R., & Hardin, S. R. (2007). *Critical care nursing: Synergy for optimal outcomes.* Sudbury, MA: Jones and Bartlett.

Lynn-McHale Weigand, D. J., & Carlson, K. K. (Eds.). (2005). *AACN procedure manual for critical care* (5th ed.). Philadelphia: Elsevier.

Meyers, T. A., Eichhorn, D. J., Guzzetta, C. E., Clark, A. P., Klein, J. D., Taliaferro, E., et al. (2000). Family presence during invasive procedures and resuscitation: The experience of family members, nurses, and physicians. *American Journal of Nursing, 100,* 32–43.

Porth, C. M. (2007). *Essentials of pathophysiology: Concepts of altered health states* (2nd ed., p. 36). Philadelphia: Lippincott Williams & Wilkins.

Turner, M. A. (2003). Doppler-based hemodynamic monitoring. *AACN Clinical Issues, 14,* 220–231.

Urden, L. D., Stacy, K. M., & Lough, M. E. (2006). *Thelan's critical care nursing: Diagnosis and management* (4th ed., pp. 355–359). St. Louis: Mosby.

Weininger, C. F., Ginosar, Y., Sprung, C. L., & Weiss, Y. (2002). Arterial and pulmonary artery catheters. In J. E. Parillo & R. P. Dellinger (Eds.), *Critical care medicine* (2nd ed., pp. 36–63). St. Louis: Mosby.

UNIT

5

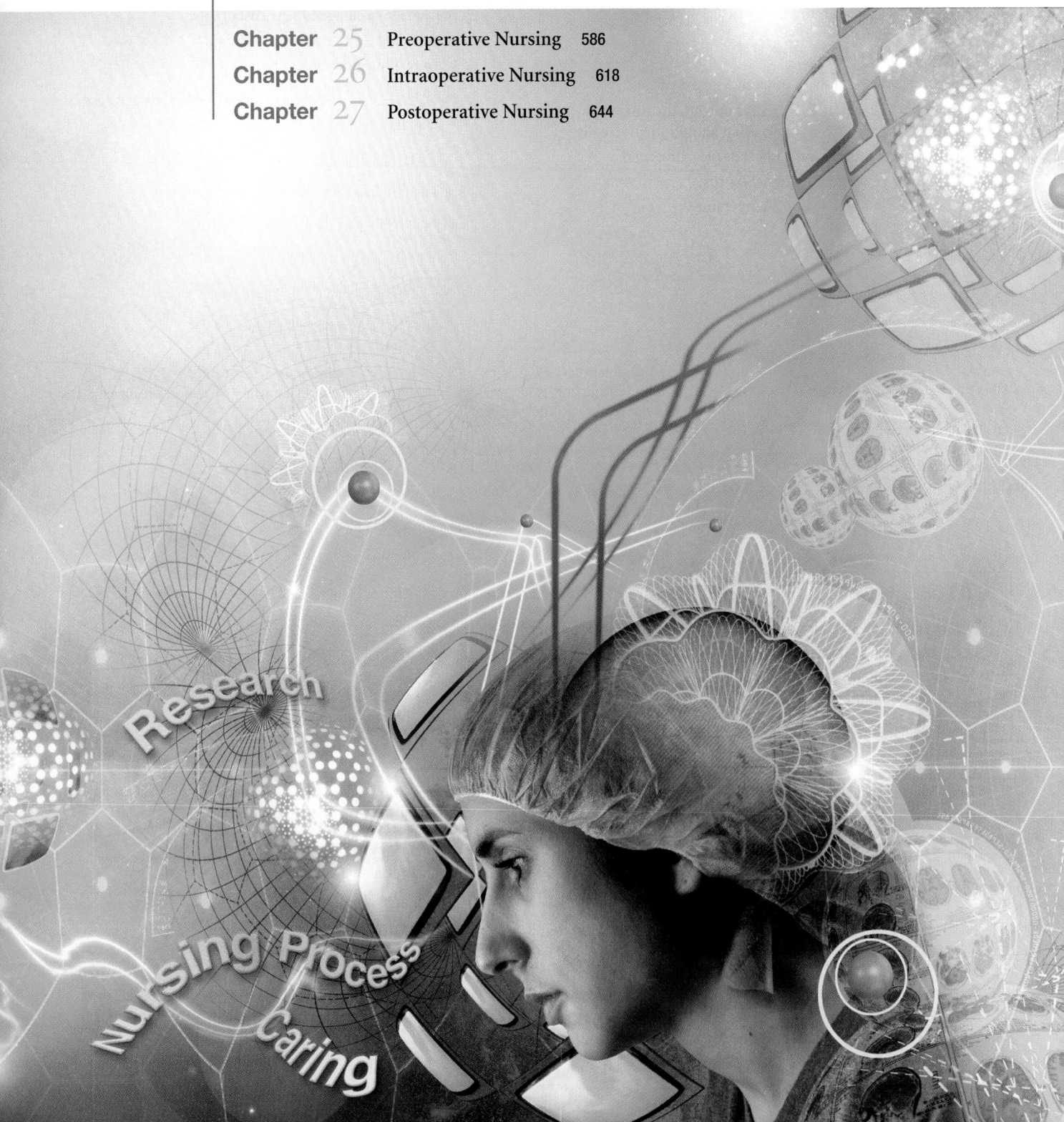

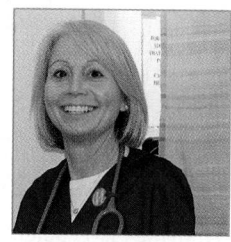

BETTY   My name is Betty and I am a staff nurse in the Ambulatory Surgery Center at Stanford Hospital and Clinics in Stanford, California. Stanford has 600 beds and is the primary teaching hospital for the Stanford University School of Medicine. The Ambulatory Surgery Center has 12 operating rooms, two procedure rooms, and three interventional radiology suites. We care for patients ranging from 1 year old to more than 100 years old. The majority of our patients are admitted for surgery and discharged the same day, but because we are part of Stanford Hospital, our surgery schedule also includes patients who are scheduled to be admitted to the hospital. In a typical day we may have 50 surgeries and procedures scheduled.

At Stanford, I am encouraged to advance in my nursing career. The hospital supports nurses in obtaining advanced degrees or certification in a nursing specialty, or promotion to a management position. I knew I always wanted to remain a "bedside" nurse, but was looking for that next challenge. As the clinical nurse educator for preoperative care and PACU in the Ambulatory Surgery Center, I found a good balance. I coordinate the orientation needs of new staff and provide ongoing education to staff for new procedures in our department. I am also a member of our Nursing Practice Council, led by staff nurses to establish and implement standards of practice for our department. We collaborate with other departments to ensure we give the best care possible. For example, the PACU nurses are currently working on a project with the anesthesiologists to redefine our extubation policy.

I enjoy being a perianesthesia nurse and I appreciate the opportunities it affords me to practice all components of caring. The competence of the preoperative nurse in assessing the patient ensures that the patient meets all of the criteria necessary for a safe and successful surgery. The **commitment** to teaching is evident throughout the perioperative experience. It begins with the preoperative call the night before surgery, then continues in the preoperative area. Questions are answered and learning needs are assessed. Every patient is assessed to make sure he or she has the knowledge and support to ensure successful care once he or she returns home. Each patient and caregiver is given detailed instructions regarding postoperative care before the patient is discharged from our facility.

When a patient first arrives from surgery, many things are done simultaneously. The first priority is to ensure that the airway is unobstructed and the patient is breathing adequately. Monitors are applied and the patient is assessed and appropriate interventions are initiated.

Many patients are confused or frightened when they emerge from anesthesia. One of the most important aspects of our care is to assure patients that their surgery is completed and they are doing well. Patients always remember the **compassion** and comfort care you give—I recall taking care of a patient who had a very unstable course in the PACU, requiring extensive monitoring and critical care. On a subsequent visit to our unit, he did not remember how sick he had been, but he thanked me for giving him the warm blanket after surgery.

Taking care of patients after they have undergone a general anesthetic requires critical thinking skills and clinical reasoning. A patient who is difficult to arouse after anesthesia might be hypercarbic or simply sleeping deeply because he worked the night shift. Pain management can be quite challenging, especially in patients on chronic opiates. It is easy to just give more narcotics, but looking for other reasons and solutions can sometimes be more beneficial. PACU nurses often consult with anesthesiologists about these issues.

Most of the pediatric patients we care for in our PACU are healthy children undergoing tonsillectomies, placement of myringotomy tubes, or hand surgery. It is a frightening experience for the child and the parents. Children often wake up quite agitated, but by **confidently** handling the child and reassuring the parents that this is normal, I can make their surgical experience a positive one.

My **comportment** while charge nurse in the PACU sets the tone for the other members of the PACU team. When critical situations arise, the team pulls together to handle the situation. New staff members are given autonomy in caring for their patients, but always have the backup of a more experienced PACU nurse.

"The competence of the preoperative nurse in assessing the patient ensures that the patient meets all of the criteria necessary for a safe and successful surgery. The **commitment** to teaching is evident throughout the perioperative experience."

Preoperative Nursing

Jane Ashley

Outcome-Based Learning Objectives

After studying this chapter, the learner will be able to:

1. Describe the components and significance of preoperative assessments.
2. Identify critical preoperative assessment findings that require further intervention.
3. Discuss the elements of preoperative preparation.
4. Prioritize nursing interventions for the preoperative patient.
5. Develop a teaching plan for the preoperative patient.
6. Identify and discuss areas of future research relevant to the preoperative patient.

Research   Collaboration   Health Promotion   Nursing Process   Caring   Critical Thinking

ACCORDING TO data from the National Center for Health Statistics, approximately 71 million surgeries were performed in the United States in the year 2004. Of these, 40 million were inpatient procedures and 31 million were outpatient procedures. Surgeries performed on the digestive tract, including endoscopy, colonoscopy, colectomy, appendectomy, and cholecystectomy, are the most common followed by surgeries on the musculoskeletal system, cardiovascular system, and eye. Surgeries are performed in hospital-based inpatient or outpatient settings or in free-standing surgical centers. **Same-day admission,** in which the patient reports from home directly to the reception area of the operating room is becoming standard procedure for many surgeries including complex cardiac procedures.

◼ Categories of Surgery

Surgical procedures are categorized in a variety of ways, and any given procedure will fall into several of the categories. Each of the categorizations provides a small piece of information about the patient who is having surgery. For example, knowing the specific procedure to be performed allows the nurse to begin formulating plans for preoperative teaching. Knowing that a procedure needs to be done emergently gives information about patient acuity. Commonly, procedures are categorized according to the:

- General anatomic location of the surgery (e.g., abdominal, gynecological)
- Specific procedure to be performed (e.g., colectomy, total hip replacement)
- Purpose of the surgery (e.g., diagnostic, cosmetic)
- Urgency of the surgery (e.g., elective, urgent, emergent)
- Degree of risk associated with the surgery (low, moderate, high).

Surgery may also be performed for diagnostic, curative, reconstructive, palliative, or cosmetic purposes. **Diagnostic procedures** are those that are performed for the purpose of making or confirming a medical diagnosis. These procedures frequently require the removal of tissue or cells for analysis. Examples of diagnostic surgeries include procedures such as breast biopsy, arthroscopy, and laparotomy. In some cases, diagnostic surgery is referred to as **exploratory surgery** because the surgeon examines or explores the tissues and structures in order to decide what further procedures or treatments needs to be done.

Curative procedures are those that are done for the purpose of affecting a cure, for example, the successful treatment of a disease or condition. Many surgeries are done for this purpose including cholecystectomy, hernia repair, open reduction of a fracture, and mammoplasty.

Reconstructive surgery is done for the purpose of rebuilding tissues or body structures to achieve a more normal function and appearance. Examples include skin grafting and breast reconstruction following mastectomy.

Palliative procedures are those that are done for the purpose of alleviating symptoms caused by disease or a condition. Palliative surgery does not affect a cure, but it frequently improves quality of life. Examples include tumor debulking, performing a laminectomy to reduce spinal cord compression in a patient with metastatic cancer, and creation of a colostomy in a patient with severe inflammatory bowel disease.

Cosmetic surgery is performed for the primary purpose of improving physical appearance. Examples include liposuction, rhinoplasty, and breast augmentation.

Surgeries are also classified according to the urgency with which the procedure needs to be performed. **Elective procedures** are those that are scheduled in advance for a nonacute condition. Performing a procedure electively is always preferred because the patient will be in better health than he would be during an acute illness, and it allows optimum physiological and psychological preparation of the patient. There also is a technical advantage to elective procedures because the tissues are not distorted by inflammation or infection.

Urgent procedures are those that require prompt attention, within the next 24 to 48 hours, but they describe situations where the patient's condition is not currently life threatening. An appendectomy performed for a ruptured appendix is an example of an urgent procedure. An **emergent** (or emergency) **surgery** is a procedure that must be performed immediately to prevent serious consequences. Failure to perform emergency surgery in a timely manner can result in a patient's death or disability. A fas-ciotomy performed to treat compartment syndrome in a fractured leg is an example of an emergent procedure.

Surgical procedures are accompanied by varying levels of risk. This risk is sometimes characterized using the terms *minor* or *major surgery*. Minor surgery refers to procedures associated with minimal risks. These procedures are often done under local anesthetic and do not require hospitalization. Major surgery describes procedures accompanied by more significant risks. The surgical risk associated with particular procedures can also be described as low, moderate, or high. Low-risk surgeries refer to those that have few complications, and when complications do occur, they are not serious. High-risk surgery describes procedures that are associated with a larger number of and more serious complications. One practice guideline developed by the American College of Cardiology (ACC) and the American Heart Association (AHA), classifies surgical procedures as high, intermediate, or low risk according to how much hemodynamic stress the procedure places on the heart (Eagle et al., 2002). In the guidelines, risk refers specifically to the perioperative development of a myocardial infarction, heart failure, or sudden death. In high-risk surgeries, cardiac events occur more than 5% of the time; in intermediate-risk surgeries, they occur between 1% and 4% of the time; and in low-risk surgeries, they occur less than 1% of the time. The National Guidelines box shows the ACC/AHA surgery-specific classification (Eagle et al., 2002).

Common Surgical Suffixes

There is no standardization for the naming of surgical procedures. Consequently, any given surgical procedure may have several names that are used interchangeably. Knowing the meaning

---

NATIONAL GUIDELINES ACC/AHA Surgery-Specific Classification

High-Risk Surgical Procedures	Emergent operations, particularly in elderly
	Aortic and other major vascular surgery
	Peripheral vascular surgery
	Prolonged surgical procedures, usually longer than 2 hours, associated with large fluid shifts and/or blood loss (e.g., major spinal surgery, pancreas resection)
	Cardiac procedures
Intermediate-Risk Surgical Procedures	Carotid endarterectomy
	Head and neck surgery
	Intraperitoneal and intrathoracic surgery
	Orthopedic surgery
	Prostate surgery
Low-Risk Surgical Procedures	Endoscopic procedures
	Superficial procedures
	Cataract surgery
	Breast surgery
	Cosmetic surgery

Source: Reprinted from ACC/AHA Guideline update for perioperative cardiovascular evaluation for non-cardiac surgery: A report of the American College of Cardiology/American Heart Association Task Force on Practice Guidelines (Committee to Update the 1996 Guidelines on perioperative cardiovascular evaluation for non-cardiac surgery). Eagle, K., Berger, P., Calkins, H., Chaitman, B., Ewy, G., Fleischmann, K., Fleisher, L., Froehlich, J., Gusberg, R., Leppo, J., Ryan, T., Schlant, R., & Winters, W. (2002). Reprinted with permission from Elsevier. American College of Cardiology Web site. Available at http://www.acc.org/clinical/guidelines/perio/dirIndex.htm

of common surgical suffixes, however, provides some help in understanding what type of surgery is to be performed:

- **ectomy**—removal of, surgical excision to remove (e.g., colectomy)
- **ostomy**—surgical creation of permanent opening (e.g., colostomy)
- **otomy**—surgical incision of or cutting into (e.g., thoracotomy)
- **plasty**—surgical repair or reconstruction of (e.g., rhinoplasty)
- **orraphy**—surgical repair or suture of (e.g., herniorrhaphy)
- **scopy**—use of a scope to view an area, looking into (e.g., laparoscopy).

Perioperative Nursing and Perioperative Nursing Practice Standards

The term **perioperative** encompasses the entire surgical experience: preoperative, intraoperative, and postoperative. The nurse's role in a perioperative setting includes preparing the patient for surgery, assisting and observing the patient during the operation, preventing and treating postoperative complications, and preparing the patient for discharge. Practice standards and practice guidelines are the basis for providing consistent, high-level care for the patient who is undergoing surgery. Practice standards developed by professional organizations set the expectations and responsibilities of professional nursing performance.

Standards are subject to ongoing evaluation and refinement so that they reflect current and best practices. The American Nurses Association's (ANA's) *Standards of Clinical Nursing Practice* and the *Code of Ethics for Nurses with Interpretive Statements* describe the roles and responsibilities of nurses regardless of practice setting. These standards are presented in Chapter 1 ☺. Specialty organizations in nursing use the ANA's conceptual framework for developing practice guidelines specific to the specialty. An example of this is the *Standards, Recommended Practices and Guidelines* developed by the Association of peri-Operative Registered Nurses (AORN, 2005). One part of the AORN standards, the *Standards of Perioperative Clinical Practice,* uses the nursing process (assessment, nursing diagnosis, outcome, planning, implementation, and evaluation) to describe how the perioperative nurse provides care to the surgical patient. Another part of the AORN standards, the *Standards of Perioperative Professional Performance,* focuses on professional role activities.

Several critical beliefs underlie AORN's standards. Among these is the belief that quality nursing care:

- Is a partnership between the nurse and the patient
- Is individualized
- Respects the patient's personal, cultural, and religious beliefs
- Respects the patient's autonomy
- Incorporates the patient's goals and preferences
- Focuses on collaboration, education, and advocacy.

Another organization important to perioperative nurses is the American Society of PeriAnesthesia Nurses (ASPAN). This organization develops and publishes standards of practice for care of the patient during recovery from surgery (ASPAN, 2006b).

Perioperative nurses need to be familiar with standards developed by groups interested in promoting quality care. Such groups include the National Council of State Boards of Nursing (NCSBN), the Joint Commission, the Institute for Healthcare Improvement (IHI), and the Medicare Quality Improvement Community. Hospitals also develop policies and procedures for the purpose of defining quality care. Hospital policies need to be rational, reasoned, current, and consistent with state and nationwide clinical and evidence-based practice (Meeker & Rothrock, 1999). Practice guidelines and clinical pathways are used to promote quality care. Clinical pathways are evidence-based and reflect critical activities, interventions, time frames, and desired outcomes for specific surgeries or diseases. It is the responsibility of perioperative nurses to use standards, guidelines, pathways, and policies in conjunction with their expertise and judgment when delivering high-level nursing care.

Collaborative Management

A successful surgical experience includes all members of the health care team. The surgeon and anesthesia care providers assess the patient prior to surgery. Consults from specialty areas such as cardiology, endocrinology, or neurology may be required depending on the patient's past or current medical condition. Some surgeries, such as organ transplantation or the creation of an ostomy, will require the patient to learn a whole new set of health maintenance skills. In these situations, the health care team may include a nurse who works directly with the surgeon and specializes in health care teaching for those surgeries.

A **preoperative health evaluation** is done within 30 days of a planned operation and must be documented in the patient's chart per the Joint Commission requirements (American Society of Anesthesiologists [ASA], 2006a; Institute for Clinical Symptoms Improvement [ICSI], 2006). An internist, surgeon, or anesthesia provider performs the evaluation, and it frequently is done as an outpatient examination. This evaluation is performed specifically to clear the patient for the planned surgical procedure. It provides data for confirming the overall appropriateness of performing the planned surgery (by answering questions such as "Is the patient healthy enough to have surgery?"), and confirms the plan to perform the surgery either as an outpatient, as a same-day admission, or as an inpatient. If abnormal findings are identified during this evaluation, further tests may be required prior to having the surgery. The preoperative evaluation includes a medical history; a focused review of issues pertinent to the planned anesthesia and surgical procedure; an abbreviated physical exam including height, weight, vital signs, cardiac and pulmonary systems; and an assessment of the patient's overall functional ability (ICSI, 2006). The preoperative health evaluation and any recommendations from the evaluation must be sent to the site where the surgery will be conducted.

The anesthesia provider also conducts a preoperative history and physical exam. This preprocedure assessment includes a review of systems with a focus on issues that affect the choice and administration of anesthesia. The patient is asked about any family history of anesthetic problems and any history of motion sickness or anesthesia-related nausea and vomiting. The latter two are risk factors for postoperative nausea and vomiting. The anesthesia assessment includes an examination of the patient's airway, neck (for range of motion), and teeth. Permanent dental prostheses may be documented during the exam. Chart 25–1 lists the ASA guidelines for classifying a patient's physical status and operative risk. Patients are classified in one of six categories, with lower classifications (e.g., I and II) representing those who are healthy or with mild systemic disease and good operative risks, and higher classifications (V and VI) representing patients who have severe disease and who are unlikely to survive surgery (ASA, 2006a).

A newer approach to surgery, accelerated recovery programs, relies on a multidisciplinary team approach with emphasis on collaboration. At the center of accelerated recovery programs, also referred to as fast-track surgery, is the view that patient outcomes are improved by expediting postoperative recovery. Key elements of accelerated programs include the following (Pasero & Belden, 2006):

- Preoperative education to prepare patients to take an active part in their recovery
- Use of anesthetics, analgesics, and surgical techniques that minimize surgical trauma and physiological stress, thereby allowing faster recovery
- Aggressive postoperative rehabilitation including early feeding and intensive ambulation
- Selective and evidence-based use of traditional postoperative practices such as the use of drains, tubes, and monitoring.

In accelerated recovery programs, patient assessment and education are important collaborative roles for nurses working in preoperative care.

■ Nursing Management

Nursing management in the preoperative setting is a cluster of activities (e.g., assessing, planning, teaching, and evaluating) performed by the nurse in anticipation of surgery. The purpose of preoperative care is to evaluate the patient's readiness for surgery, to identify potential risks and hazards of the surgery, to advise the patient about the surgical procedure, to prepare the patient for the postoperative experience, to plan for home care, and to provide emotional support.

Nursing Assessment of the Preoperative Patient

Assessment of the preoperative patient is a nursing responsibility identified in practice standards (AORN, 2005). A complete and thorough preoperative assessment serves several purposes. The assessment identifies risk factors for intraoperative and postoperative problems. The risk of surgery is influenced by several factors including the patient's age, health history, current cardiac and pulmonary status, functional ability, and the type of surgery planned (Eagle et al., 2002). Once risk factors have been identified, the nurse takes steps to correct, minimize, or prevent potential problems. The assessment also provides the data necessary for developing preoperative and postoperative teaching plans. Importantly, the preoperative assessment provides a baseline of physical and functional ability. Nurses caring for the patient postoperatively will use preoperative assessments in deciding if a sign or symptom is a new finding, if the patient is progressing as expected, or if the patient needs specialized care, rehabilitation, or follow-up home services.

The preoperative assessment may be done in a separate appointment before the surgery or on the morning of the surgery. Many hospitals use their own forms for preoperative assessment to ensure completeness and simplicity. Most of these forms will represent an abbreviated version (using checklists for example) of the assessment described next. Figure 25–1 ■ (p. 590) is an example of a nursing assessment form. Preoperative assessment includes a patient history with physical examination and functional assessment. Patient history includes:

- Age
- Allergies
- Current health problem
- Type of surgery planned
- Plans for autologous blood donation
- Family history
- Past medical history
- Past surgical history and experiences with anesthesia
- Current medications
- Current herbal medications and nutritional supplements
- Alcohol, cigarette, social drug use.

Each of the areas listed is discussed in more detail in the following subsections.

Age

Approximately one-third of all surgeries are performed on elderly people. Age alone is not a contraindication for surgery; however, the risks of surgery increase with advancing age. (For more information refer to the Gerontological Considerations section later in this chapter, p. 599.)

CHART 25–1	ASA Physical Status Classification
ASA I	A normal healthy patient
ASA II	A patient with mild systemic disease
ASA III	A patient with severe systemic disease that limits disease but is not incapacitating
ASA IV	A patient with severe systemic disease that is a constant threat to life
ASA V	A moribund patient who is not expected to survive 24 hours without the operation
ASA VI	A patient declared brain dead and whose organs are being removed for transplantation

Source: Adapted from American Society of Anesthesiologists Classification of Physical Status. ASA Relative Value Guide, 2008. http://www.asahq.org/clinical/physicalstatus.htm

PRE PROCEDURE ASSESSMENT

Date: _____ PROCEDURE: _____

Confirmation of Procedure Including Site and Side if Applicable	☐ Outpatient ☐ Inpatient	Height:_____ Weight:_____
☐ Patient procedure confirmed ☐ Patient identified using two identifiers ☐ ID Bracelet on ☐ N/A Patient states: _____ Patient points to: _____ Consent form states: _____	☐ Waive ☐ Telephonic Interview ☐ Consent not available	**PAT ONLY** Arrival Time _____ Start Time _____ End Time _____
☐ **Discrepancy noted, surgeon notified Date __/__/__ Time_____ RN Initials_____**		Visit Level _____

ALLERGIES:

Latex Allergy ☐ No
☐ Yes ☐ O.R. aware Precautions: _____

Review of Systems	☐ Refer to Nursing Assessment in patient's medical record dated: _____ (if within 30 days of procedure)
Cardiovascular & Respiratory	☐ Heart/valve ☐ Hypertension ☐ Angina ☐ Dyspnea ☐ Asthma
GI/Endo/Renal	☐ Diabetes ☐ Digestive/Reflux ☐ Kidney ☐ Liver
Neuromuscular	☐ CVA ☐ Seizures
Other	☐ Anemia ☐ Bleeding/Clotting ☐ Cancer
Habits	Tobacco Use ☐ No ☐ Yes Amount: _____ ETOH ☐ No ☐ Yes Amount: _____ Recreational Drug Use ☐ No ☐ Yes Amount: _____
Surgical History	
Anesthesia History	TMJ/Neck Problems? ☐ No ☐ Yes _____ Past Anesthesia? ☐ No ☐ Yes _____ Problems? ☐ No ☐ Yes _____

MEDICATIONS (Include herbal supplements)

Medication	Dose	Frequency	Medication	Dose	Frequency

Psycho/Social	**Pain**
Lives: ☐ Alone ☐ w/Family ☐ w/Spouse ☐ Other Occupation: _____ Cultural/Religious Preference: _____ Do you feel safe in your relationships? ☐ Yes ☐ No If patient answers no, contact ☐ Safe Transitions (#31389) and/or ☐ Social Work for assistance	Baseline Pain score (0-10): _____ Location: _____ Quality: _____ Daily Narcotic use: ☐ No ☐ Yes Type and daily dosage: _____
Cognitive/Perceptual	**Nutrition/Elimination**
Visual/Hearing Deficit: ☐ No ☐ Yes _____ Primary language other than English: _____ Interpreter: ☐ No ☐ Yes ☐ Requested	Difficulty Swallowing ☐ No ☐ Yes _____ Bladder/Bowel Problems ☐ No ☐ Yes _____ Unintentional Weight Loss > 10lbs: ☐ No ☐ Yes _____
Activity/Mobility	**Patient has Health Care Proxy** ☐ Yes ☐ No
Self ADL ☐ Yes ☐ No _____ Balance ☐ Steady ☐ Unsteady Hx Slips & Falls ☐ No ☐ Yes Judgement ☐ Intact ☐ Impared	If no, Proxy Explained & Patient Advised how to Obtain ☐ No ☐ Yes Name of Proxy: _____ Phone Number: _____ **Advanced Directives** ☐ Yes ☐ No If no, directives explained & patient advised how to obtain

Preoperative teaching completed, patient verbalizes understanding ☐ Yes ☐ PAT Communication Form No ___ Completed and Sent ☐ N/A
Nursing Diagnoses 1-2 Outcomes Met   ☐ Yes   ☐ No
Notes: _____

Signature: _____ RN Printed name: _____ RN Date: ____ / ____ / ____

FIGURE 25–1 ■ Preoperative nursing assessment form.

Source: Courtesy of Beth Israel Deaconess Nursing Department

PREOPERATIVE ASSESSMENT

Allergies: _____   Precautions: _____

ID verified: ☐ Patient identified using two identifiers   ☐ Bracelet on   NPO since: Date _____ Time _____

Last void: Time _____   ☐ Foley cath.   ☐ Other _____

Meds. taken today: _____

V.S.   T _____   P _____   R _____   SpO2 _____   O2 Source _____   B/P in _____   arm: _____

Test results drawn in Holding Area: Hgb. _____   Glucose _____   K _____   T&S _____
Other _____

Consents: ☐ H&P   ☐ Surgical   ☐ General Agreement   ☐ Anesthesia [☐ N/A]

☐ Patient Procedure Confirmed   ☐ No Laterality
☐ No discrepancy, preadmission testing documentation reviewed
OR schedule says _____
Consent form says _____
Patient states & points to _____
Side/site marked is _____

☐ **Discrepancy noted, Surgeon notified**   date ___ /___ /___   time ___ : ___
Surgeon's final side/site directive with surgeon's signature _____   RN Initials _____

Implants: _____

Level of Consciousness: ☐ alert   ☐ unresponsive   ☐ oriented   ☐ disoriented   ☐ somnolent but arousable

Emotional status: ☐ calm   ☐ anxious   ☐ agitated

Pain: ☐ Reviewed baseline pain from pre-procedure assessment. Current baseline pain score (0-10): _____
Location/Quality & pain relief methods in use today: _____

Interpreter: Name _____   ☐ N/A

Escort/Contact: Name _____
Phone number: _____   Location: _____

Nursing Diagnoses 1-4 Outcomes Met: ☐ Yes   ☐ No   Notes: _____
_____
_____   _____ RN Initials

Medication: dose/route/time/by   **Medication:**   dose/route/time/by
1. _____   3. _____
2. _____   4. _____

PATIENT BELONGINGS	Transport	To PACU	w/Patient	w/Escort	PACU Safe	BIDMC Safe	N/A	Locker
Dentures: ☐ upper ☐ lower								
Glasses								
Contact lenses								
Hearing Aid: ☐ right ☐ left								
Prosthesis								
Jewelry:								
Clothing								
Cash ($)								
Credit Cards								
Other:								
Medications brought from home:								

☐ Patient aware of policy, but declines to place valuables in safekeeping.

Signature of Patient/Family _____   **RN Initials** _____   **Signature of Recipient** _____   **RN Initials** _____

1. _____   RN _____   RN _____   ___ /___ /___
       Signature   Printed name   Initials   Date

2. _____   RN _____   RN _____   ___ /___ /___
       Signature   Printed name   Initials   Date

Patient's name _____   Med. Rec. # _____   DOB _____

Allergies

Allergies and allergic reactions to medications, chemicals, and foods must always be identified and prominently displayed on the patient's wristband, in the chart, and in the medication record. Patients with histories of allergic reactions have a greater risk of hypersensitivity to anesthesia, so the type of allergic reaction is very important. They also are much more likely to develop latex allergies. A special operating room setup is required for patients with latex allergy. Latex skin allergy is discussed in detail in Chapter 60 . Patients who are allergic to shellfish or iodine may also be allergic to the solution for surgical preparation, povidone-iodine.

CRITICAL ALERT *Allergic responses to latex range from mild dermatitis to anaphylaxis. If latex allergy is suspected, a blood or skin test can be performed to confirm the allergy. A latex-reduced environment must be created for individuals who are allergic to latex.*

Current Health Problem

The patient's current health problem may influence various aspects of perioperative care. It may affect the type of anesthesia used, the type and amount of fluid replacement given, and the type of intraoperative monitoring performed. It may also determine priorities of postoperative care.

For women, anesthesia should be avoided during the first trimester of pregnancy. It is important to know the date of the last menstrual period. A pregnancy test is done if there is uncertainty about whether or not the patient is pregnant.

Type of Surgery Planned

The surgical procedure planned influences every aspect of perioperative care including the preoperative assessment, preoperative teaching and preparation, the setup of the operating room, the type of anesthesia used, and priorities of postoperative care. The preoperative assessment is a good time for the nurse to review the operative permit (e.g., consent), to evaluate the patient's understanding of the surgical procedure to be performed, and to clarify questions for the patient.

Plans for Autologous Blood Donation

Patients scheduled for elective surgery may make arrangements to donate their own blood in advance of the surgery. To be eligible for preoperative autologous donation, the patient must be in good health, be afebrile, have a hemoglobin of 11 g/dL or higher, and have the approval of her physician or surgeon. Chapter 23 includes a complete description of autologous blood donation and its administration procedures and nursing interventions.

Family History

Family history is important to determine the presence of possible genetic predispositions. It is particularly important to ask about family history of diabetes, heart disease, sudden cardiac death, and malignant hyperthermia (MH). Malignant hyperthermia is a life-threatening condition of sustained muscle contraction precipitated by common agents of anesthesia such as inhalation agents and the muscle relaxant succinylcholine. Malignant hyperthermia is an autosomal dominant trait so that each child of an MH parent has a 50% chance of inheriting the susceptibility. MH is discussed in detail in Chapter 26 .

Past Medical History

Past medical history (PMH) can increase the risk associated with surgery as well as the possibility of postoperative complications. Patients are asked about all previous diseases and conditions. Preexisting disease influences many perioperative decisions including whether or not to proceed with the operation, the type of anesthesia used, the need for additional testing or procedures prior to surgery, and the need for intraoperative and postoperative monitoring. The implications of specific conditions are discussed next.

Neurological conditions assessment includes asking about any history of stroke or transient ischemic attacks (TIAs). If a patient has a history of a stroke, it is important to determine what, if any, deficits remain and whether or not the patient is receiving anticoagulation therapy. Deficits in cognitive functioning may affect the patient's ability to understand preoperative and postoperative instructions. Mobility deficits may place the patient at increased risk for postoperative atelectasis, pneumonia, abdominal distention, constipation, skin breakdown, and deep venous thrombosis (DVT). DVT is discussed in Chapter 43 . Patients who have neuromuscular disorders (myasthenia gravis, multiple sclerosis) or spinal cord injury also may be at a higher risk for postoperative complications associated with limited mobility. Patients who are experiencing transient ischemic attacks (TIA) may need to have a procedure to improve blood flow to the brain (carotid endarterectomy) prior to having any other surgical procedure in order to decrease the risk of a perioperative stroke. Seizure disorder also is a significant surgical factor because some anesthetic agents are known to lower the threshold for seizures.

The *cardiovascular disorders* assessment is important because surgery is a major stress to the heart as a result of the hemodynamic changes that occur with tissue injury and fluid loss. All anesthetic drugs have known cardiovascular affects. Disorders of the cardiovascular system are particularly important in establishing surgical risk for the patient. The highest risk is associated with acute myocardial infarction (AMI) (within 7 days preceding the operation), recent MI (occurred in the month prior to the operation), unstable angina, heart failure, significant arrhythmia, and severe valvular disease (Eagle et al., 2002). It is recommended that patients wait a minimum of 4 to 6 weeks after an MI to have elective surgery to prevent the likelihood of reinfarction. Patients with unstable angina may require stabilization either with medications or coronary revascularization prior to having any other surgical procedures. Patients with heart failure are at increased risk of postoperative pulmonary complications and fluid and electrolyte imbalances (Qaseem et al., 2006). These patients will need to have their fluid status monitored closely during the intraoperative and postoperative periods. Brain natriuretic peptide (BNP) is a chemical that is released when the heart ventricle is stretched. Serum BNP is used preoperatively to screen or monitor heart failure. Postoperatively, it is used to decide whether dyspnea is caused by heart failure or some other condition (Pagana, 2007). Patients with valvular disorders may require antibiotic prophylaxis to reduce the risk of bacterial endocarditis (Chapter 41). Also, these patients must be monitored postoperatively for the development of worsening heart failure.

Patients with a history of dysrhythmias will require postoperative cardiac telemetry. Patients with pacemakers or implantable cardioverter defibrillators (ICDs) present specific concerns during surgery. The presence of a pacemaker affects placement of the electrocautery grounding pad and choice of anesthetic agents. Electrocautery, used in the operating room, can create an electromagnetic interference that may cause pacemaker dysfunction or damage (Rooke, 2007). The use of succinylcholine, a depolarizing muscle relaxant sometimes used during anesthesia, causes muscle fasciculations and postoperative shivering that can suppress pacemaker function (Rooke, 2007). Preoperative information required for patients with pacemakers includes identification of the underlying cardiac rhythm that necessitates pacemaker, and information about the pacemaker itself (e.g., type, device, lead system, availability of technical support). All patients with pacemakers need to have the unit interrogated (i.e., tested to check battery status, and thresholds for sensing and pacing leads) within 3 months of scheduled surgery. Pacemaker interrogation after surgery is also recommended. Patients with ICDs also need to supply information about the device as well as evidence of unit interrogation prior to surgery. It is recommended that the tachyarrhythmia detection of the ICD unit be turned off prior to surgery (Rooke, 2007). Electromagnetic noise from electrocautery can mimic the signal for ventricular tachycardia or ventricular fibrillation, causing the ICD to deliver an unnecessary shock during surgery. A magnet is used to turn off the tachycardia detection feature on the morning of surgery. Postoperatively, the unit must be turned back on.

Patients undergoing cardiac surgery may have a beta-adrenergic blocking medication prescribed preoperatively to reduce the risk of developing atrial fibrillation postoperatively (Bradley et al., 2005) and statin drugs to improve surgical outcomes (Pan et al., 2004). Generally, patients with hypertension will continue to receive antihypertensive medications throughout the perioperative period especially in patients with hard to control hypertension.

Patients with *chronic respiratory conditions* such as chronic obstructive pulmonary disease (COPD) and severe asthma, as well as the elderly and people who smoke cigarettes, have an increased risk of postoperative atelectasis and pneumonia (Qaseem et al., 2006). Preoperative pulmonary function tests may need to be performed on patients with COPD. Patients with an upper respiratory infection may have surgery postponed. Obstructive sleep apnea (OSA) is a serious condition that is evaluated in the preoperative assessment. OSA is associated with airway collapse, hypoventilation, and sensitivity to the respiratory depressant effects of medications such as anesthetics, narcotics, and sedatives (ASA, 2006b).

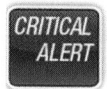 *Notify the anesthesia care provider of patients with suspected or documented OSA. It may be difficult to intubate this patient and he will require continuous monitoring for hypoventilation and hypoxemia during surgery and postoperatively until he is stable.*

Patients with *chronic renal failure* (CRF) will require close monitoring of fluid and electrolyte balance and medication administration. The effectiveness of drugs may be altered because the kidney excretes most drugs. Patients with CRF are at a higher than expected risk of an intraoperative cardiac event (Eagle et al., 2002). Patients with benign prostatic hypertrophy (BPH) should be monitored postoperatively for problems with urinary retention.

Musculoskeletal conditions such as arthritis can have a major impact on the ability to properly position a patient intraoperatively and postoperatively. Care must be taken not to injure arthritic joints. Temporomandibular joint (TMJ) syndrome and limitations of neck mobility can interfere with intubation for general anesthesia. Myotonic dystrophy, a rare form of muscular dystrophy, increases the patient's sensitivity to anesthesia and narcotics.

 Patients with a history of certain neuromuscular disorders, such as myotonic dystrophy, may be highly sensitive to anesthesia and require special precautions when planning surgery. The patient should wear a medical alert bracelet and all health care providers need to be aware of this condition. Monitor the use of narcotics carefully.

Several issues must be considered in caring for the surgical patient with an *endocrine disorder* such as diabetes. Type I diabetes is associated with an increased risk of perioperative cardiac morbidity (Eagle et al., 2002). Poor glucose control is associated with higher rates of surgical site infections (IHI, 2006; Schweon, 2006). Patients with diabetes also experience slower wound healing. The physiological stress of surgery changes the insulin requirement. Careful monitoring of blood sugar is needed to prevent hypoglycemia and ketosis.

Patients who are immunocompromised present a special surgical challenge. Examples of patients at high risk for immune system dysfunction include those with human immunodeficiency virus (HIV) or cancer, those who have undergone chemotherapy, splenectomy, or organ transplantation, those taking immunosuppressive drugs such as prednisone, and those who are malnourished, experience chronic pain, or abuse alcohol (Neil, 2007). Surgery depresses the normal immune system for up to a week, and this effect is heightened in patients already immunocompromised. Immunosuppression increases the surgical risks for hypothermia, infection, and hypoadrenal function. Preoperative assessment for immunosuppressed patients includes weight, blood pressure, a complete blood count, liver and renal function tests, and chest x-ray (Neil, 2007).

Other disorders that may impact surgery include anemia, bleeding or clotting disorders, cancer, and morbid obesity. Skin and tissues that have been irradiated, as a treatment for cancer, are more easily damaged and heal more slowly than other tissues. The effects of chemotherapy depend on the drugs given. Morbid obesity, a body mass index of 40 or greater, is associated with significant comorbidities including diabetes mellitus, hypertension, gastroesophageal reflux disease, and OSA (Owens, 2006). Surgical procedures may also take longer, requiring a longer period of anesthesia (Rogers et al., 2006).

Past Surgical History and Experience with Anesthesia

A patient's previous experience with surgery and anesthesia will influence decisions about the current surgery. A complete surgical history should be obtained, focusing specifically on previous surgeries, dates they were performed, problems with anesthesia, and postoperative complications. Some problems are likely to repeat themselves. If it was difficult to intubate the patient with a previous surgery, it will likely be difficult with the current surgery. Difficulty with intubation needs to be prominently noted in the medical record, and the patient should wear a colored wristband identifying the problem. Other problems with prior surgery may not reoccur because of changes in surgical techniques, improved technologies, better anesthetic agents, or new medications.

CRITICAL ALERT *Alert the anesthesia care provider if the patient reports a history of difficult intubation with a prior surgery. This patient needs an airway examination and specialized airway equipment must be available.*

A preoperative risk assessment for postoperative nausea and vomiting (PONV) needs to be completed. Risk factors for PONV are outlined in the Risk Factors box. The preoperative risk assessment is used to plan for surgery and prophylaxis for postoperative nausea and vomiting. Patients with multiple risk factors may be given different anesthetics (e.g., total intravenous anesthesia or regional blocks) and preoperative medications (ASPAN, 2006a). Patients with moderate to high risk of PONV need a multimodal approach to prevention. Some medications are given to the patient in the presurgical area, whereas others such as a transdermal scopolamine patch are applied by the patient the night before surgery.

Current Medications

Patients are asked to provide a specific and detailed list of regularly taken medications, including over-the-counter (OTC) medications and herbal preparations. The list includes the name of the medication, as well as the amount and how often it is taken. Information on medications is used in numerous ways. Many medications have the potential to either increase or decrease the effect of anesthetic agents. Certain medications may necessitate specific preoperative tests. For example, patients taking digoxin or a diuretic (furosemide, hydrochlorothiazide) may need to have potassium levels tested prior to surgery.

Some medications require dose adjustments prior to surgery. Examples of drugs that may be adjusted prior to surgery include insulin, oral hypoglycemic agents, corticosteroids, and antihypertensive agents. Medications that slow coagulation are frequently discontinued prior to surgery. Examples of these are aspirin, enoxaparin, heparin, vitamin E, and warfarin. Chart 25–2 (p. 595) shows selected medications and the implications for surgery.

RISK FACTORS for Postoperative Nausea and Vomiting

Gender (women more than men)

History of nausea and vomiting with a previous surgery

History of motion sickness

Nonsmoker

Use of certain inhalation anesthetics (volatile anesthetic gases and nitrous oxide)

Use of opioid analgesics

Type of surgery (gynecologic, abdominal, and those on the ear or eye)

Longer surgeries.

Sources: American Society of PeriAnesthesia Nurses. (2006). ASPAN's evidence-based clinical practice guideline for the prevention and/or management of PONV/PDNV. *Journal of PeriAnesthesia Nursing, 21*(4), 230–250; Murphy, M., Hooper, V., Sullivan, E., Clifford, T., & Apfel, C. (2006). Identification of risk factors for postoperative nausea and vomiting in the perianesthesia adult patient. *Journal of PeriAnesthesia Nursing, 21*(6), 377–384.

Current Herbal Medications and Nutritional Supplements

The use of herbal remedies and nutritional supplements is becoming increasingly common in the United States. Studies show that between 40% and 70% of patients do not tell their health care providers or pharmacists about the use of herbal remedies (Bennett & Brown, 2000; Pribitkin & Boger, 2000; Roberts et al., 2005; Vallerand, Fouladbakhsh, & Templin, 2005; Yoon, Horne, & Adams, 2004). Often, patients combine herbs, prescription medications, and OTC products in treating health problems (Roberts et al., 2005; Yoon et al., 2004).

Patients need to be asked specifically about the use of herbs and nutritional supplements in a preoperative assessment. Although herbs are considered relatively safe, they do have pharmacologically active properties that can produce drug interactions or adverse effects. For example, several herbs are known to inhibit platelet function and delay clotting time (Hatcher, 2001). In the United States, herbs are classified as diet supplements; they are not subject to federal regulation and there is no standardization in herb potency. Consequently, it is difficult to know how much of a pharmacologic effect is exerted by any given herbal product. The ASA (1999a) recommends discontinuing all herbal products 2 to 3 weeks prior to surgery.

The use of nutritional supplements can also affect surgery. Fish oil, a popular supplement thought to reduce the effects of atherosclerosis and prevent myocardial infarction and angina, may slow blood clotting. Patients should stop taking fish oil 2 to 3 weeks before surgery. Chart 25–3 (p. 596) lists some common herbs, their uses, and the implications for surgery.

Alcohol, Cigarette, and Drug Use

A careful history of alcohol and illicit drug use is important because excessive and chronic use of these substances can interfere with anesthesia, increase the patient's tolerance to anesthesia, reduce the effectiveness of postoperative pain medication, and cause serious physiological issues such as drug or alcohol withdrawal syndromes. If surgery must be performed on patients who are addicted to alcohol or narcotics, then the careful titration of benzodiazepines (for alcohol) and methadone (for narcotics) may be used to prevent withdrawal symptoms.

CRITICAL ALERT *When the possibility of alcohol withdrawal exists, the nurse and surgical team need to monitor the patient closely. A standardized alcohol withdrawal rating scale, such as the Clinical Institute Withdrawal Assessment (CIWA) scale, helps in identifying serious withdrawal symptoms and in monitoring treatment for alcohol withdrawal syndrome.*

A lifetime history of cigarette smoking is described in pack-years, the number of packs smoked per day multiplied by the number of years smoked. Cigarette smoking increases surgical risk for several reasons. Smoking damages the mucociliary clearance system, resulting in increased secretions and a higher risk of postoperative atelectasis and pneumonia (Barrera et al., 2005). Smoking increases circulating carboxyhemoglobin, which reduces circulating oxygen resulting in less oxygen delivery to body tissues. Smoking causes vasoconstriction, a serious concern for patients undergoing cardiac or vascular surgery. Smoking cessation is thought to reduce sputum production, increase ciliary action and clearance of secretions, and improve small airway function. Patients are asked to stop smoking 6 to 8

CHART 25–2 Medications and Their Implications for Surgery

Drug Classification and Sample Medications	Implications for Surgery
ACE inhibitors Enalapril Lisinopril (Zestril) Quinapril (Accupril)	Inhibit angiotensin-aldosterone system, resulting in decreased peripheral resistance. Can cause hypotension. Monitor blood pressure closely. Surgeon may recommend holding drug on the morning of surgery unless prescribed for heart failure.
Antiarrhythmics Amiodarone Procainamide (Pronestyl) Quinidine	Depress myocardial excitability and contractility and slows heart rate. Some agents can cause hypotension. Can increase the cardiac effects of anesthetic agents.
Anticoagulants Enoxaparin sodium Heparin sodium Warfarin sodium (Coumadin)	Increase the risk of bleeding intraoperatively and postoperatively. Coagulants may be discontinued 24 to 48 hours before surgery. Monitor coagulation studies (PT, INR, aPTT). Watch for signs of bleeding.
Antidepressants Citalopram (Celexa) Paroxetine (Paxil) Sertraline (Zoloft)	Restart the medication as soon as possible once the patient is able to tolerate oral intake.
Antidiabetic agents Glyburide (Glibenclamide) Glipizide (Glucotrol XL) Insulin Metformin (Glucophage)	The physiological stress of surgery increases serum glucose levels and insulin requirements. Hospitals have standard protocols to guide insulin and glucose administration in the perioperative period. Monitor serum glucose levels closely during postoperative period. Expect patients with diabetes to be on regular insulin sliding scale coverage during periods of acute stress and infection. Surgeon may recommend that patient hold the medication at least 8 hours prior to surgery.
Antihypertensives Amlodipine (Norvasc) Atenolol Metoprolol (Lopressor)	Side effects include hypotension and bradycardia. Monitor blood pressure and heart rate. Frequently taken on the morning of surgery especially when hypertension is difficult to manage.
Antiplatelet drugs Clopidogrel (Plavix)	Inhibit platelet aggregation, increasing the risk of bleeding postoperatively. Monitor platelet count. Surgeon may want the drug stopped 2 weeks before surgery.
Antiseizure medications Gabapentin (Neurontin)	Dose may need to be adjusted for surgery. Some anesthetic agents can lower the potential for seizures.
Corticosteroids Dexamethasone (Decadron) Hydrocortisone (Solu-Cortef) Prednisone	Steroids decrease inflammation, delay wound healing, and mask signs of infection. Steroids increase serum glucose levels and insulin requirements. Steroids increase risk of postoperative bleeding. Surgery increases the need for steroids and patients may need to have their steroid dose adjusted.
Diuretics Furosemide (Lasix) Hydrochlorothiazide	Diuretics cause urinary excretion of sodium, chloride, potassium, bicarbonate, magnesium, and calcium. Serum electrolytes should be checked regularly. Monitor intake and output. Surgeon may recommend holding medication on the morning of surgery unless the patient is taking for heart failure.
Gastric acid inhibitors Lansoprazole (Prevacid) Omeprazole (Prilosec)	Proton pump inhibitors also inhibit a liver enzyme needed for the metabolism of other drugs. They can prolong the half-life of some drugs including benzodiazepines. Usually taken on the morning of surgery.
Hormones Levothyroxine (Synthroid)	Should be given intravenously while the patient is NPO.
NSAIDs Aspirin Celecoxib (Celebrex) Ibuprofen	Increase the risk of intraoperative and postoperative bleeding. Aspirin inhibits platelet aggregation and the effect lasts the duration of the thrombocyte life span (7 to 10 days). NSAIDs are stopped 2 weeks before surgery.

weeks prior to surgery. For patients who are unable to quit before surgery, a nicotine patch can be applied postoperatively to prevent nicotine craving and withdrawal.

Physical and Functional Assessment

An important part of the preoperative assessment is the physical examination and functional assessment. During this assessment the nurse documents the patient's baseline physical findings such as vital signs and mental status as well as his baseline functional ability. The components of the assessment remain the same regardless of the type of surgery being performed, but the level of detail provided in certain categories may change by type of surgery. Patients admitted for neurosurgery will have a more thorough reporting of their neurological exam, whereas patients admitted for gastrointestinal surgery will need a more detailed abdominal and nutritional assessment. The patient's past medical

CHART 25–3	Herbs, Their Common Uses, and Implications for Surgery	

Herb	Common Use	Implications for Surgery
Black cohosh	Hot flashes, dysmenorrhea	Unknown
Cayenne	Neuropathy, cluster headaches	Unknown
Echinacea	Cold, sore throat	Unknown
Ephedra	Weight loss	Cardiac stimulation with tachycardia and elevated blood pressure.
Feverfew	To control migraine headache	Impairs platelet function.
Garlic	Cold, flu, hypertension	Interferes with platelet aggregation and prolongs clotting time with risk of bleeding. May decrease blood glucose levels.
Ginger	Nausea, motion sickness	Prolongs clotting time with risk of bleeding.
Ginkgo biloba	Vertigo, tinnitus, intermittent claudication, Alzheimer's disease	Interferes with platelet aggregation. May increase seizure potential.
Ginseng (American)	To strengthen the immune system	May lower serum glucose levels in patients with diabetes.
Ginseng (Asian)	To improve stamina and vitality	Inhibits platelet function.
Guargum	To lower cholesterol	May interfere with gastrointestinal absorption of some antibiotics.
Milk thistle	Liver disease	Unknown
Saw palmetto	Benign prostatic hypertrophy	Increases risk of bleeding.
St. John's wort	Depression, anxiety	Unknown
Valerian	Sedative, anxiety	May potentiate sedative effects of anesthetic agents.

Sources: Flanagan, K. (2001). Preoperative assessment: Safety considerations for patients taking herbal products. *Journal of PeriAnesthesia Nursing, 16*(1), 19–26; Hatcher, T. (2001). The proverbial herb. *American Journal of Nursing, 101*(2), 36–43; Miller, L. (1998). Herbal medicinals: Selected clinical considerations focusing on known or potential drug–herb interactions. *Archives of Internal Medicine, 158*(20), 2200–2211; Pribitkin, E., & Boger, G. (2000). Surgery and herbal therapy: Essential guidelines on bleeding, skin reactions, and wound healing. *Complementary Health Practice Review, 6*(1), 29–40.

history will also direct the nurse's attention toward specific categories of assessment.

Neurological Assessment

The neurological examination includes a baseline mental status examination as well as an assessment of motor and sensory function. An evaluation of mental status includes level of consciousness, judgment, ability to follow commands, appropriateness of behavior, speech, and the ability to express oneself and to understand what is being said. These data are especially helpful in designing pre- and postoperative teaching plans. It is particularly important to document baseline performance for older patients because they are at a higher risk than other adults of experiencing a surgery-related change in mental status. Evaluation of motor function includes strength, movement, balance, and gait. Any physical limitations or impairments such as difficulty with hearing, vision, speech, swallowing, or walking should be noted as well as any history of falls. The risk of falls is associated with many factors, but two factors consistently identified across studies are altered mental status and impaired mobility (Chang et al., 2004; Evans, Hodgkinson, Lambert, & Wood, 2001). During the evaluation, the nurse makes a determination about the patient's fall risk and begins developing a safety plan. A patient's neurological status may affect a patient's ability to carry out activities of daily living (ADLs) independently such as bathing, dressing, toileting, feeding, walking, and transferring.

 CRITICAL ALERT *The reduction of patient falls is a Joint Commission National Patient Safety Goal. A multifactorial falls assessment combined with a fall reduction program is an effective means of reducing falls in the hospital setting.*

The patient is asked about issues of pain and pain tolerance. The location, description, and rating of preoperative pain are noted, and the patient is asked about successful strategies for dealing with pain. This is a good time to discuss postoperative pain, to teach about using a numeric rating scale, and to reassure the patient that pain control is a key concern for health care providers. Patients who are taught preoperatively how to use a pain rating scale are better able to describe their pain postoperatively (Bond et al., 2005). Pain assessment and management is discussed in detail in Chapter 15 🔗.

Cardiovascular Assessment

Baseline vital signs are established for the preoperative patient. It is helpful to know baseline pulse and blood pressure because postoperative problems such as anxiety, pain, hypoxia, and dehydration can manifest via a change in vital signs. The nurse assesses heart rate and rhythm, blood pressure, and peripheral pulses in addition to observing the extremities for color, sensation, capillary refill, and the presence of edema. The physician is made aware of any cardiac-specific abnormalities present on exam such as hypertension, chest pain, dyspnea, pedal edema, or heart rhythm irregularities.

Cardiac abnormalities may need further evaluation prior to surgery to prevent an intraoperative cardiac event (Eagle et al., 2002). Additional evaluation may include an electrocardiogram, echocardiogram, cardiac stress test, and pacemaker or ICD interrogation. In patients with a history of cardiovascular disease, the effect of the disease on the patient's ability to walk, exercise, and participate in ADLs is investigated. It is important to document baseline activity levels for all patients. Research suggests that those who participate in exercise and muscle strengthening activities preoperatively walk greater distances postoperatively and are discharged earlier than those with more sedate lifestyles (Whitney & Parkman, 2002).

Respiratory Assessment

Baseline findings of respiratory rate and depth, quality of respiratory effort, lung sounds, and oxygen saturation level with room air and with oxygen, if the patient requires oxygen, are established. The nurse also asks the patient about any problems breathing, whether or not shortness of breath interferes with ADLs, and about the use of inhalers, oxygen, or continuous positive airway pressure (CPAP) devices at home. Baseline information is important because postoperative atelectasis is a common problem and because the nurse is usually responsible for weaning patients off oxygen in the postoperative period.

Gastrointestinal Assessment

Physical exam includes palpation of the abdomen and auscultation of bowel sounds. Patients are asked about the usual pattern and consistency of bowel movements, the date of the last bowel movement, and what, if any, medications they take for their bowels. Abdominal distention and constipation can occur postoperatively as a result of factors such as anesthesia, limited physical mobility, and the use of narcotics for pain. A patient who has an ostomy is asked about any ostomy-specific issues such as skin care and regularity and about the required supplies during the hospitalization.

Genitourinary Assessment

Patients are asked about their usual pattern of urinary elimination as well as urinary issues such as any difficulty starting a stream, controlling continence of urine, completely emptying the bladder, and dysuria. Patients with chronic renal failure are asked if they are anuric (no urine production) and their usual schedule for dialysis. If a patient is on dialysis, then the arteriovenous (AV) fistula or graft, if present, is documented and checked for patency. The AV fistula or graft is palpated for the presence of a thrill and auscultated for a bruit. Baseline data are important for interpreting postoperative findings and anticipating potential problems. Postoperatively, fluid balance is monitored using urinary output. Urinary retention is a postoperative problem that is associated with certain surgeries, such as gynecologic and genitourinary procedures.

Musculoskeletal Assessment

Musculoskeletal assessment is concerned with patients' ability to move themselves and their extremities. The nurse notes any problems with range of motion, arthritic joints, or mobility restrictions. These data are important to the proper positioning of the patient intraoperatively as well as postoperatively. If a patient uses a prosthetic device, electrocautery grounding pads, which are used in surgery, should be placed away from the site of prosthesis to prevent potential injury to the tissue. Assistive devices (e.g., prostheses, crutches, a walker, a wheelchair) that the patient requires for mobilization need to be available to the patient postoperatively to facilitate early mobilization.

Endocrine Assessment

Patients with diabetes are asked about the frequency of glucose testing and use of oral hypoglycemic agents and insulin. Surgery and anesthesia can affect the regulation of glucose. The physiological and psychological stress of surgery and illness tend to elevate serum glucose levels, whereas factors such as preoperative restriction of food and fluids tend to lower glucose levels. The patient with diabetes should be scheduled for surgery early in the day to limit prolonged fasting. The patient will need frequent monitoring of serum glucose with insulin coverage using a sliding scale. Patients who ordinarily take oral hypoglycemic agents may need the temporary coverage of insulin during periods of stress and illness.

Nutritional Assessment

The nutritional assessment includes a baseline height and weight. The nurse asks specific questions about the patient's appetite, usual diet, food preferences, recent weight loss or gain, and any problems with chewing or swallowing. The nurse notes signs of poor nutrition including brittle nails and dry, flaky, skin. The patient's nutritional status has a profound effect on surgical outcomes. Surgery increases basal metabolic rate and the need for proteins, vitamins, and calories. Patient's who are malnourished with a negative nitrogen balance and deficits of vitamins A, C, and B complex are at risk for experiencing problems with their wound including infection, delayed healing, and dehiscence. A low serum albumin (less than 3.5 mg/dL) or a low or declining prealbumin are markers of poor nutrition and are associated with a higher risk of postoperative pulmonary complications (Qaseem et al., 2006). Prealbumin or a transthyretin test is considered a more sensitive marker of nutrition than albumin and correlates with patient outcomes (Beck & Rosenthal, 2002). Postoperatively, a dropping prealbumin alerts the caregiver to a declining nutritional status.

Patients who are morbidly obese face a number of potential postoperative problems. Access to the operative site is difficult and may prolong the operation and length of time anesthesia is used. Anesthetic agents are absorbed by adipose tissue, prolonging the effects of anesthesia on all body systems. Research shows obesity to be a significant risk factor in the development of postoperative complications (Brooks-Brunn, 2000; Owens, 2006). Wound approximation during surgical closure is difficult and decreased tissue vascularity contributes to slower healing. These factors and others such as insulin resistance increase the potential for wound infection, dehiscence, and evisceration in the obese patient.

Integumentary Assessment

The nurse asks about skin sensitivities and problems, and observes the condition of the skin for moisture, turgor, and color. Any area of injury or breakdown is noted. Many hospitals adopt the use of a tool or scale to measure the risk or likelihood of pressure ulcer development. Chapter 67 ☺ has an example of the Braden Scale as well as other skin breakdown assessment data.

Maintaining skin integrity is a priority of care in the operating room. Surgical cleansing materials, surgical tape, electrodes, and other materials have the potential to cause allergic skin reactions. The grounding pad used with electrocautery can cause a burn if improperly placed. Pressure ulcers can develop within 2 to 3 hours of unrelieved pressure (Heizenroth, 1999). Preoperative risk factors for development of skin breakdown include older age; the presence of comorbidities such as diabetes, hypertension, and vascular disorders; poor nutritional status; and low hemoglobin and hematocrit levels (Price, Whitney, & King, 2005).

Psychosocial Assessment

Surgery is a stressful life event for patients and their significant others. Among the reported sources of anxiety are fears—of the unknown, of death, of mutilation, of disability and loss of independence, of loss of sexuality, of waking up during the surgery, of pain, of separation from family, and of the financial impact. The nurse asks open-ended questions to illicit the patient's concerns about surgery and anesthesia. The nurse also assesses for physiological indicators of stress and anxiety including crying, restlessness, tachycardia, tachypnea, diaphoresis, complaints of inability to sleep, stomach upset, nausea, and diarrhea. Numeric rating scales of anxiety, similar to those used to rate pain, are an effective, easy, and valid way to measure anxiety (Elkins, Staniunas, Rajab, Marcus, & Snyder, 2004). Patients' level of stress will influence their ability to listen and absorb perioperative instruction. It can also affect their response to anesthesia and pain medication and their ability to comply with postoperative care. Patients who are highly anxious about surgery may benefit from receiving premedication with an antianxiety agent. A meta-analysis of 16 studies in which medication for anxiety was used preoperatively showed that using an antianxiety agent did not slow down the time frame for postoperative ambulation or discharge from the postanesthesia care unit (Walker, Smithy, & Pittaway, 2003).

The nurse asks about patients' support systems including family (traditional and nontraditional), friends, and other sources of support such as neighbors and religious affiliations. Patients are also asked if there are spiritual or cultural rituals or traditions that they would like to maintain during their hospitalization. The nurse is sensitive to the view that the hospital culture and its routines and food may be alien to some patients. All cultures hold beliefs about health, illness, and healing. Culturally competent nurses support and build positive cultural health care practices (Spector, 2004). The Cultural Considerations box identifies cultural and ethnic concerns for the perioperative nurse.

Diagnostic Tests

Laboratory tests are not required for routine, non–high-risk surgical procedures unless there is a specific reason for performing the test (ICSI, 2006). Nevertheless, many patients have preoperative laboratory testing as part of a routine examination. Some hospitals require a complete blood count on all patients over a certain age, usually 55 years old. Generally, a hematocrit and hemoglobin as well as a urine pregnancy test are performed on all menstruating females. It is recommended that all patients with diabetes have a hemoglobin A1C level drawn as part of preoperation testing and a fasting blood sugar drawn immediately before the surgical procedure (IHI, 2006). A patient may have a specific indication for performing a laboratory test. A patient taking digoxin (Lanoxin) or a diuretic may need to have a potassium level checked. When laboratory tests are indicated, they should be performed within 30 days of the planned procedure, although many surgeons prefer laboratory tests to be performed within the 1 to 2 weeks prior to surgery. If the need for a blood transfusion is anticipated, the patient will require a blood type and cross-match test to be processed at the facility performing the surgery.

Diagnostic studies performed preoperatively depend on the patient and the surgery to be performed. These studies are de-

CULTURAL CONSIDERATIONS for Perioperative Nurses

Use an interpreter for preoperative teaching. If a patient does not speak English and the nurse does not speak the patient's primary language, schedule an interpreter to assist with the assessment and teaching rather than relying on the patient's family member or significant other. The interpreter should be the same gender as the patient and the nurse should speak directly to the patient regardless of the presence of an interpreter.

Ask the patient about any special needs concerning the scheduling of surgery. In some cultures, the patient may need to consult a religious leader or healer, a special reader, or the zodiac in order to schedule surgery at the most opportune time. In some religions (e.g., Orthodox Jewish, Seventh-Day Adventist, Muslim) Friday evening and Saturday are times of observance and are avoided when scheduling elective surgery.

Consider the patient's view of "time" when scheduling surgery and preoperative appointments. Not all cultures view the concept of time as "clock" time. In some cultures, time is seen in relation to an activity that needs to be completed. The nurse needs to understand that cultures may view time differently and provide an explanation that an appointment time in this culture is an actual time period that is set aside for the patient.

Respect the family structure in getting surgical consent. In some cultures, there is a strict family hierarchy that is based on gender (e.g., the male is head of household) or age (e.g., the oldest member of the family is head of household). Be respectful of family hierarchies when getting consent for surgery and in teaching the patient.

Respect the patient's beliefs. Certain culturally held beliefs will affect preparations for surgery. An amulet may be worn, in some cultures, to ward off evil or bad spirits. When possible, patients should be allowed to wear the amulet into the operating room. If the amulet needs to be removed, remove it after induction of anesthesia and replace it as soon as the surgery is complete. In some cultures or religions (e.g., East Indian, Sikh) there are prohibitions against shaving body hair.

Find out the patient's view of the surgery. Surgery and anesthesia may be viewed as harbingers of death in some cultures (e.g., Roma). Allow family members to stay with the patient as long as possible in the preoperative area, and teach the patient and family about the surgical procedure to reduce anxiety.

Individualize your preoperative teaching. In some cultures, preoperative teaching is not a routine part of preoperative care, therefore, teaching can actually increase the patient's anxiety level. Find out what kind of information and how much information the patient wants and tailor the teaching to meet the patient's needs.

Source: Deyirmenjian, M., Karam, N., & Salameh, P. (2006). Preoperative patient education for open-heart patients: A source of anxiety? *Patient Education and Counseling, 62*(1), 111–117; Galanti, G. A. (2006). Applying cultural competence to perianesthesia nursing. *Journal of PeriAnesthesia Nursing, 21*(2), 97–102; Quinn, D. (2006). How religion, language and ethnicity impact perioperative nursing care. *Nursing Clinics of North America, 41,* 231–248; Spector, R. (2004). *Cultural diversity in health and illness.* Upper Saddle River, NJ: Pearson Prentice Hall.

termined by factors such as the reason the surgery is being done, the patient's overall health, surgeon's preference, and significant past medical history. In addition to any studies performed as part of the work-up of the patient's health problem, a chest x-ray, an electrocardiogram, and pulmonary function tests may be part of the preoperative tests for certain patients. A preoperative chest x-ray is not required for routine, low- to moderate-risk surgery but may be performed on patients who are older or who have a history of respiratory or cardiac disease. Similarly, pulmonary function tests are only done preoperatively if there is a specific indication such as in a patient with severe asthma or chronic obstructive pulmonary disease or a patient scheduled for removal of lung tissue (e.g., lobectomy, pneumonectomy). Electrocardiograms are recommended for all preoperative patients who are 55 years or older or in younger patients with a specific indication (ICSI, 2006). Common preoperative laboratory and diagnostic tests and rationales are presented in the Diagnostic Tests box (p. 600).

Gerontological Considerations

Age is a major consideration in the nursing management of patients scheduled for surgery. Age-related changes to the body make it less able to respond and adapt to the physiological demands of surgery. Older people have less reserve capacity and less of a safety margin during times of higher demand (Muravchick, 2004). Also, older persons are more likely than others to have coexisting illnesses that increase surgical risk. A 2005 profile of older Americans by the Administration on Aging (AOA) notes that most people age 65 or older have one chronic illness and many have more than one. The most common conditions reported are arthritis, hypertension, hearing impairment, heart disease, cataracts, orthopedic impairments, sinusitis, and diabetes (AOA, 2005). Heart disease (i.e., angina, hypertension, heart failure, valve disease, and arrhythmias) is a particular concern because it is a significant predictor of surgical risk (Eagle et al., 2002).

Coexisting disease also is likely to place the older patient in a higher category of the ASA's Physical Status Classification (see Chart 25–1, p. 589) (ASA, 2006a). Patients in higher physical status categories experience greater surgical morbidity and mortality than those in lower categories. Some older adults experience memory impairment and depressive symptoms that can interfere with their ability to learn and comply with perioperative instruction. Other factors that increase the risk of surgery for older persons include preoperative anemia, malnutrition, and dehydration, as well as limitations of mobility. Chart 25–4 (p. 601) presents some of the normal changes associated with aging and the associated potential perioperative problems. Chart 25–5 (p. 602) lists the most common surgeries performed on patients age 65 or older as reported by the CDC, 2008).

Health Promotion: Nursing Diagnoses and Outcomes

Nursing diagnoses will emerge from the preoperative assessment. Common diagnoses in the preoperative patient include:

- *Deficient Knowledge* (*Outcome:* The patient will demonstrate knowledge of the surgery, preoperative preparation, and postoperative exercises.)
- *Anxiety* (Outcome: The patient will verbalize decreased or tolerable levels of anxiety.)

- *Pain Acute* (*Outcome:* The patient will report an acceptable level of pain.)
- *Risk for Perioperative Positioning Injury* (*Outcome:* The patient will remain safe from perioperative injury.)
- *Ineffective Thermoregulation* (*Outcome:* The patient will maintain a normal body temperature throughout surgery.)
- *Impaired Home Maintenance* (*Outcome:* The patient will demonstrate an understanding of discharge instructions.)

Preoperative Instructions

Preoperative teaching is an important role of the perioperative nurse. The overall goal of preoperative teaching is to best prepare the patient for surgery, postoperative care, and discharge, and to protect the patient's safety. Depending on where and how teaching is conducted, teaching serves the purposes of clarifying a patient's preoperative concerns, reducing the patient's anxiety about the perioperative experience, increasing the patient's compliance with perioperative care, decreasing patient-controlled risk factors of postoperative complications, and increasing the patient's satisfaction with nursing and with the surgical experience.

Preoperative education is shown to decrease preoperative anxiety (Guruge & Sidani, 2002; Johansson et al., 2004; Lin & Wang, 2005; and McDonald, Hetrick, & Green, 2006), but it may also create worries perhaps more so in individuals who feel healthy but are scheduled for major elective procedures (Letterstal, Sandstrom, Olofsson, & Forsberg, 2004). This highlights the need to individualize teaching. Preoperative education can improve patient outcomes (Asilioglu & Celik, 2004; Deyirmenjian, Karam, & Salameh, 2006; Hering, Harvan, Dangelo, & Jasinski, 2005; Hulzebos et al., 2006; Yung et al., 2005) although more studies, particularly with experimental designs and those using subjects from various cultural groups, are needed to document which outcomes are most amenable to educational programs (Johansson et al., 2004).

Preoperative teaching and support can be categorized into five dimensions (Bernier, Sanares, Owen, & Newhouse, 2003):

- Situational and procedural information refers to teaching about the surgery and anesthesia.
- Sensation and discomfort information refers to teaching about what the patient can expect to see, hear, or feel.
- Patient role information refers to teaching patients how to participate in their own care.
- Skills training information refers to teaching about specific skills to be used postoperatively such as how to get out of bed with less pain or how to use the incentive spirometer.
- Psychosocial support refers to interactions aimed at alleviating fears and anxieties.

Patient teaching is accomplished in several ways. Many hospitals schedule a preoperative appointment days or weeks prior to the surgery for the purpose of conducting preoperative assessment and patient education. It is increasingly common for patients to receive written instructions either at the time of the appointment or mailed to their home that reinforce important aspects of care. Some hospitals and surgical centers use videotapes that explain the surgical procedure as well as preoperative

DIAGNOSTIC TESTS Commonly Performed Preoperatively

Laboratory Test	Abnormalities Preventing Surgery	Rationale for Performing the Test
COMPLETE BLOOD COUNT		
Red blood cell, hemoglobin, hematocrit	Significantly low hematocrit and hemoglobin.	Check for preoperative anemia; patient may need transfusion before surgery.
White blood cell (WBC)	Significantly elevated WBC. Presence of infection may delay or cancel the procedure. Neutropenia may delay surgery due to an increased risk of infection.	Provides information on the patient's immune status. Check for preoperative infection or inflammation. Preexisting infections, even those distant to the site of the operation, increase the risk of surgical site infection.
ELECTROLYTES AND OTHER TESTS		
Sodium, potassium, chloride, bicarbonate, glucose	Electrolyte imbalances, especially potassium, are corrected prior to surgery.	Check for electrolyte imbalances, metabolic status, and glucose regulation.
Blood urea nitrogen (BUN) and creatinine	Elevated creatinine and BUN are noted prior to surgery because renal function affects selection and dosage of medications. Renal failure patients may need to be dialyzed prior to surgery.	Gives information about renal function. Many drugs are excreted by the kidneys.
Brain natriuretic peptide (BNP)	Elevated levels indicate heart failure.	Rapid, bedside test to identify heart failure. Used in the differential diagnosis of shortness of breath.
Albumin	Marker of nutritional status.	Low serum albumin is associated with higher postoperative pulmonary complications.
Prealbumin or transthyretin test	Marker of nutritional status.	Low prealbumin levels are associated with higher postoperative complications and risk of pressure ulcers.
Hemoglobin A1C	A more stable measure of glucose. Indicates the level of diabetic control over the previous 6 weeks.	Poor glucose control is associated with an increased risk of surgical-site infection.
COAGULATION STUDIES		
International normalized ratio (INR), prothrombin time (PT), partial thromboplastin time (PTT)	Elevated levels may delay or cancel surgery.	Provides information about bleeding tendencies and ability to clot.
Arterial blood gas	May be performed preoperatively in patients with severe lung disease.	Provides information on oxygenation and acid–base status.
Type and crossmatch (T&C) for blood replacement	Performed preoperatively in patients who are bleeding or for surgeries that are expected to have large amounts of blood loss.	Patient's blood type is identified and matched with specific blood units for transfusion. For a T&C to be active, it must be recent (within 48 hours).
Pregnancy test	Surgery is avoided, if possible, during the first trimester of pregnancy.	Performed when there is uncertainty about whether or not the patient is pregnant. May be performed on all menstruating females.
Urinalysis	Abnormal results may require additional follow-up prior to surgery.	Provides screening information about the presence of protein, glucose, blood, and bacteria in the urine. Provides an indication of renal function and urinary tract infection.
Chest x-ray	Surgery may be postponed in patients with pneumonia or who have significant heart failure.	Provides baseline data on pulmonary and cardiac function. Can detect cardiac enlargement, heart failure, infiltrates, pneumonia, pleural effusions.
Electrocardiogram	Indications of cardiac injury (elevated ST segment), ischemia (T wave inversion), or myocardial infarction may delay surgery. Abnormal heart rate and rhythm are corrected preoperatively if possible.	Provides baseline data on cardiac rhythm and cardiac disease. Recommended for all preoperative patients 55 years or older.
Pulmonary function tests	Chronic lung conditions increase the risk of surgery.	Provides preoperative information on lung volumes and condition of airways.

| CHART 25–4 | Normal Changes of Aging, Perioperative Risk, and Nursing Implications |

Normal Changes of Aging	Impact on Perioperative Risk	Implications for Nursing Care
Overall		
Decreased reserve capacity of all body organs, which causes various systems to be overwhelmed during periods of physiological stress	Places the patient at a higher risk for many postoperative problems and complications	Minimize physiological stress as much as possible. Provide adequate oxygen, rest, nutrition, hydration, emotional support, and monitor and correct electrolyte imbalance.
Neurological		
Decreased reserve and increased sensitivity to physiological stressors such as fever and hypoxia Lowered ability to adjust to environmental changes and stimuli Slower reaction times Slower cognitive processes	Potential for acute confusion postoperatively that can take months to resolve Potential for sleep–wake disturbances while in the hospital Potential for knowledge deficit	Assess mental status every shift. Avoid using medications known to cause changes in mental status in the elderly (CNS depressants, H2–receptor antagonists, lidocaine, Dilantin, anticholinergics). Provide for uninterrupted sleep. Avoid unnecessary room or unit changes. Encourage ambulation and participation in activities of daily living (ADLs). If acute confusion develops, look for and treat physiological stressors such as fever, hypoxemia, anemia, pain, and dehydration.
Cardiovascular		
Increased workload of the heart Increased arterial resistance Decreased cardiac output Reduction in the maximum attainable heart rate and cardiac output Decreased peripheral circulation Lowered ability to respond to demands for increased blood, oxygen, and nutrients	Potential for decreased cardiac output Potential for intraoperative cardiac complications Potential for activity intolerance postoperatively	Prevent or treat factors such as anemia that increase cardiac workload. Keep warm to prevent shivering. Apply oxygen to keep oxygen saturation above 93%. Monitor fluid balance to prevent dehydration or fluid overload. Monitor BP, heart rate, oxygen saturation, fatigue, and dyspnea with activity.
Respiratory		
Decreased elasticity of lungs Loss of muscle mass, which weakens muscles of respiration Stiff chest wall, which reduces the ability to expand the lungs Less effective protective mechanisms such as coughing and mucociliary transport	Potential for postoperative pulmonary complications Potential for impaired gas exchange Potential for ineffective airway clearance	Encourage deep breathing postoperatively. Monitor for dyspnea as a sign of ventilatory dysfunction. Control pain but avoid overmedication with narcotics.
Gastrointestinal		
Decreased saliva Loss of teeth and changes in dentition More difficulty with swallowing Decreased peristalsis Decreased blood flow to internal organs	Risk of aspiration Potential for poor nutrition Potential for constipation	Follow aspiration precautions. Make sure dentures are in place when patient is allowed to eat. Encourage mobility postoperatively to prevent abdominal distention and constipation.
Genitourinary		
Decreased renal blood flow Decreased renal function Decreased elasticity of bladder Decreased bladder capacity Enlarged prostate	Risk for impaired renal function postoperatively Risk of fluid and electrolyte imbalances	Monitor intake & output, BUN, and creatinine postoperatively. Ensure adequate hydration. Effects of drugs may be prolonged; choose drugs with short half-lives.
Musculoskeletal		
Loss of bone mass and height Changes in balance and gait Decreased range of motion in joints	Potential for falls	Perform a risk assessment for falls. Assist with ambulation. Use assistive devices as necessary. Physical therapy consult after surgery. Home safety evaluation at discharge.

(continued)

CHART 25–4	Normal Changes of Aging, Perioperative Risk, and Nursing Implications—*Continued*

Normal Changes of Aging	Impact on Perioperative Risk	Implications for Nursing Care
Sensory		
Decreased visual acuity and accommodation	Potential for falls	Make sure that glasses, hearing aids, and dentures are
Decreased ability to adapt to changes in light	Potential for acute confusion	available postoperatively.
Hearing loss and change in taste	Potential for alterations in	Assess pain frequently.
Atypical pain response	communication	
Skin		
Slow replacement of epithelial cells	Potential for tissue injury and	Document preoperative condition of the skin.
Decreased elasticity of skin	pressure ulcers	Keep warm postoperatively.
Loss of subcutaneous tissue	Potential for hypothermia	Encourage adequate nutrition.
Decreased circulation	Delayed wound healing and	Offer nutritional supplements as necessary.
	risk of infection	

CHART 25–5	Common Surgical Procedures in Older Patients

Gender	Common Procedures in Older Patients
Men	Prostatectomy
	Cardiac catheterization
	Coronary bypass
	Pacemaker insertion
	Repair of inguinal hernia
	Digestive system biopsies
	Cataract extraction
Women	Cardiac catheterization
	Reduction of fracture
	Pacemaker insertion
	Digestive system biopsies
	Cholecystectomy
	Cataract extraction

and postoperative care. Telephone interviews also are used for preoperative assessment, teaching, and follow-up after discharge. Depending on circumstances surrounding the surgery, preoperative teaching may be done at the patient's bedside the night before surgery if the patient is an inpatient, or on the morning of the surgery if the patient is an outpatient.

Preoperative teaching is best accomplished in a calm, quiet, and private environment that facilitates discussion and questions, and reduces the patient's anxiety or embarrassment. The nurse needs to be sensitive to the patient's level of anxiety, her ability to understand instructions and express herself, and to cultural issues.

Written instructions are important in reinforcing teaching and serving as a reference. When written instructions are given to patients, they should not use medical jargon, be written at a level that is easy to understand, and be available in various languages. The nurse assesses whether or not a patient is literate in English or in another language before giving written instructions.

General Preoperative Teaching

A preoperative patient needs information about the surgery and surgical routines, home preparation for the surgery, what to ex-

pect postoperatively, and preoperative exercises to prevent postoperative complications. Many operations are scheduled as a same-day procedure, so an easy way to start the teaching is to discuss some of the logistics that surround surgery. Provide the patient with information about transportation to the hospital, where to park a car, the cost of parking, what to wear, when to arrive at the hospital, where to report, where significant others may wait during the procedure, and how hospital personnel will communicate with significant others during and after the surgery. Many hospitals are incorporating surgical liaison programs to facilitate better ongoing communication and support for family members and significant others who are waiting for the patient during the surgical procedure. It has been shown that providing the family with updates on the progress of the patient during surgery and early in the recovery period results in better coping and problem-solving skills and reduced anxiety in family members (Cunningham, Hanson-Heath, & Agre, 2003; Leske, 2000).

Similarly, there is a trend to allow and even encourage family members and significant others to visit the patient in the postanesthesia care unit (PACU), recognizing that this can reduce anxiety for the family and provide comfort and support to the patient. Studies report that the presence of others during the perioperative period provides patients with a sense of comfort, safety, and control (Costa, 2001; Susleck et al., 2007). Hospitals that have adopted PACU visitation often have an information sheet that instructs family and significant others about the experience (e.g., keep the visit short, no cell phones, respect the privacy of other patients, comply with requests to leave) (Smykowski & Rodriguez, 2003).

Patients who will be discharged home rather than admitted to the hospital are not allowed to drive after the procedure and must be transported home by a responsible adult.

Teaching About the Surgery

Patients need to be prepared for how they will feel and how things will progress postoperatively. The patient should receive information about the surgery including what is done during the surgery, what the surgery will accomplish, where the incision(s) will be located, the anticipated length of the procedure, and the expected recovery trajectory. It is important that nurses give patients an honest, realistic view of the surgery without creating heightened anxiety. In one study, 89 subjects who had cardiac surgery were interviewed 6 weeks after discharge from the hospital. Researchers found that these subjects were surprised about the intensity of the surgery and wished that they had received more detailed information about such things as the location of incisions, breathing exercises, and what recovery would be like (Doering, McGuire, & Rourke, 2002). Patients need to know that their initial recovery from anesthesia occurs in a PACU where they will be monitored frequently until they are stable enough to be transferred to a surgical unit, or home in the case of outpatient procedures. If a patient is expected to go to an intensive care unit following the surgical procedure, the patient needs to know the routines of intensive care and the length of the anticipated stay.

It is important to prepare the patient and family for any tubes, drains, devices, or attachments that may be present postoperatively. Some of these devices have alarms that can frighten patients unless they are expecting them. In the PACU, the patient will have an intravenous catheter and intravenous fluid and will be attached to a cardiac monitor, blood pressure cuff, and pulse oximeter. Many patients will also have a Foley catheter to accurately measure postoperative urinary output, and pneumatic compression boots or an alternative device to reduce the

risk of deep venous thrombosis. Depending on the type of surgery performed, the patient may have a nasogastric tube for abdominal decompression, wound drains (e.g., Jackson-Pratt, Anderson sump, Hemovac), other drainage devices (e.g., chest tube, biliary tube, gastrostomy tube), or devices for pain control (e.g., PCA pump or epidural catheter).

If the patient is having orthopedic surgery, he may have equipment such as traction, continuous motion devices, or joint immobilizers. Patients should be prepared for postoperative routines so that they do not become excessively anxious with frequent assessments, measures of vitals signs, and observation and manipulation of the accompanying equipment and devices. Teaching is an important piece of health promotion and must be individualized for the patient and the surgery being performed. Chart 25–6 (p. 604) provides an overview of health promotion teaching content for patients experiencing common surgical procedures. The Evidence-Based Practice box provides information about the benefit of preoperative patient teaching for pain management.

Preoperative Fasting Requirements

Patients are instructed to abstain from food and fluids prior to the operation for the primary purpose of reducing the risk of

---

The Benefit of Preoperative Patient Teaching for Pain

Clinical Problem

Although health care professionals agree that preoperative teaching is important, research studies do not consistently demonstrate a specific benefit (Johansson et al., 2004; McDonald, Hetrick, & Green, 2006). Preoperative education studies often focus on increasing patient knowledge and/or on reducing patient anxiety, with fewer studies looking at the effects of preoperative education on functional outcomes such as pain, nausea, or fatigue (Johansson et al., 2004). Can a preoperative education program improve postoperative outcomes?

Research Findings

A small study conducted by Lin and Wang (2005) set out to determine whether or not a preoperative nursing intervention for pain reduces postoperative pain. This study randomly assigned adult patients scheduled for abdominal surgery to a control group who received routine care comprised of physical preparation and education on postoperative coughing and deep breathing and an experimental group who received routine care as well as a nursing intervention. The nursing intervention was a 20- to 30-minute individual educational session where postoperative pain and pain management were discussed. The session encouraged patients to set a postoperative pain goal and to select a favorite nonpharmacologic method of pain control that could be used in addition to pain medication. The researchers found that the two groups used similar amounts of medication postoperatively, but the experimental group reported significantly lower pain scores after surgery, and reported significantly less pain with activities such as repositioning, coughing, and deep breathing than did the control group. The group that received the nursing intervention got out of bed sooner than the other group. There was no difference between the groups in length of hospital stay.

Implications for Nursing Practice

These findings suggest that a preoperative nursing intervention for pain can decrease postoperative pain and the pain associated with

certain postoperative activities. The intervention can serve as a model for other individualized preoperative teaching strategies. The research findings add to the small, but growing, body of knowledge regarding the functional effects of preoperative teaching. Further, an intervention that speeds up postoperative ambulation and reduces pain associated with deep breathing and coughing could, ultimately, help reduce the incidence of postoperative pulmonary complications.

Critical Thinking Questions

1. This study was conducted in Taiwan, a country that provides national health insurance. What are the implications of this information? What further information would you need to fully answer the first question?

2. In this study, pain was measured using a questionnaire and visual analog scales, measures that are appropriate because pain is a subjective experience. Give examples of objective measures the researchers could include in their study to bolster the findings that the intervention reduced pain or the effects of pain. Provide a rationale for your answers.

Answers to Critical Thinking Questions appear in Appendix D.

References

Johansson, K., Salantera, S., Heikkinen, K., Kuusisto, A., Virtanen, H., & Leino-Kilpi, H. (2004). Surgical patient education: Assessing the interventions and exploring the outcomes from experimental and quasiexperimental studies from 1990 to 2003. *Clinical Effectiveness in Nursing, 8*(2), 81–92.

Lin, L. Y., & Wang, R. (2005). Abdominal surgery, pain and anxiety: Preoperative nursing intervention. *Journal of Advanced Nursing, 51*(3), 252–260.

McDonald, S., Hetrick, S., & Green, S. (2006). Pre-operative education for hip or knee replacement. *The Cochrane Library, 4* (CD003526).

EVIDENCE-BASED PRACTICE

| CHART 25–6 | Health Promotion Teaching for Common Surgical Procedures | | | | | | |

Surgery	Incision Site	Drains	Pain Control	Activity	Diet After Surgery	Special Concerns or Instructions	Length of Stay
Abdominal hysterectomy	Pfannenstiel	Foley is removed first day	Patient-controlled analgesia (PCA)/Intra-muscular (IM)/per oral (po)	Ambulate the evening of surgery	Clear liquids with advance diet as tolerated (ADAT)	Urinary retention sometimes occurs. Risk of DVT.	2–3 days
Appendectomy, open	Lower right quadrant of abdomen	Wound drain if abscess or perforation present	PCA/IM	Ambulate the evening of surgery	Clear liquids first day if no perforation	Wound infection is more likely with perforation of appendix. Hospital stay longer (4 to 7 days) with perforation.	1–2 days if no perforation
Carotid endarterectomy	Right or left neck	None but may have wound drain	PCA/IM/po	Ambulate evening of surgery or first day postop	Clear liquids with ADAT	May overnight in ICU or PACU. Neurological assessment is critical. Check incision for edema or hematoma. Monitor BP.	2–3 days
Cholecystectomy, open	Right upper quadrant of abdomen	T-tube if common bile duct explored, Foley, wound drain, and sometimes a nasogastric tube (NGT)	PCA	Ambulate evening of surgery or first day postop	Nothing per oral (NPO) for 2–3 days.	Risk of atelectasis is increased because of subcostal incision. Encourage deep breathing, ambulation, and pain control.	3–5 days
Colon resection	Abdomen, lower midline, or transverse	Foley, may have NGT, may have temporary colostomy	PCA/PCEA	Ambulate first day postop	NPO for several days	Encourage deep breathing; may have temporary colostomy if bowel perforation present.	5–7 days
Inguinal hernia	Right or left lower quadrant of abdomen	None	po	Ambulate day of surgery	Clear liquids with ADAT	Men may experience swelling of scrotum. Ice applications to decrease swelling.	Outpatient
Lumbar laminectomy	Back, 5–13 cm (2–5 in.) long	Foley, may require wound drain	PCA/PCEA	Ambulate evening of surgery	Clear liquids with ADAT	Back brace may be required when out of bed. Expect involvement of physical therapy. No bending or twisting of the back.	1–4 days
Mastectomy	Right or left chest	1 to 2 Jackson-Pratt drains	PCA/Patient Controlled Epidural Analgesia (PCEA) first day	Ambulate evening of surgery or first day postop	Clear liquids with ADAT	May be discharged with wound drains. Check with MD about arm and shoulder exercises on the affected side. Body image may be concern.	1–2 days
Transurethral resection of the prostate	None	Three-way Foley with continuous bladder irrigation	IV/IM/po	Ambulate evening of surgery	Clear liquids with ADAT	Run bladder irrigant to keep urine clear. Catheter removed day 1 or 2. Bladder spasms common.	1–2 days

pulmonary aspiration of stomach contents associated with anesthesia. Traditionally, patients were told to take nothing by mouth (NPO) after midnight on the night preceding surgery, but 1999 ASA guidelines loosened these requirements because the evidence showed that pulmonary aspiration rarely occurs with modern anesthesia (ASA, 1999b). Current guidelines recommend that patients fast from the intake of solid food (i.e., a light meal) for 6 or more hours before procedures and from clear liquids for 2 or more hours. Fasting is implemented for patients who will have general anesthesia, regional anesthesia, or conscious sedation. Clear liquids (nonparticulate fluids without fat) include water, fruit juices, carbonated drinks, broth, coffee, and tea. Studies show that despite the change in standards, many patients are instructed to fast longer than is necessary, creating feelings of thirst and hunger and sometimes resulting in dehydration, hypovolemia, and hypoglycemia (Crenshaw & Winslow, 2002; Madsen, Brosnan, & Nagy, 1998; Murphy, Ault, Wong, & Szokol, 2000). The new standards allow individualization of fasting instructions so that a patient scheduled for an afternoon procedure is not fasting excessively before the procedure. Patients with known delay in gastric emptying should be assessed on an individual basis and may require longer fasting periods (Soreide & Ljungqvist, 2006). On the day of surgery, patients are asked about the last time that they ate or drank and surgery may need to be delayed or canceled if a patient has not complied with fasting requirements.

 Notify the anesthesia care provider immediately if the patient has not followed the preoperative food or fluid restrictions. This patient will be at a higher risk for aspiration and the surgery may need to be postponed. In some states, patients must sign a document to confirm that they have followed food and fluid restrictions.

Other Home Instructions

Patients may be given other instructions to follow at home prior to the surgery. Patients who smoke cigarettes are instructed to stop smoking. Eight weeks prior to surgery is suggested as the optimal time frame, although research has not established if there is any benefit to a patient who quits smoking days or even a few weeks before surgery (Barrera et al., 2005; Brooks-Brunn, 2000). It is recommended that patients stop taking any herbal remedies 2 to 3 weeks before surgery because of the uncertain effect of herbs on anesthesia and in some cases on blood clotting. Medications that interfere with blood clotting, such as heparin, enoxaparin, warfarin, clopidogrel, aspirin, and vitamin E are usually stopped before surgery although the time frame for stopping will vary according to the drug taken, the reason it is being taken and laboratory tests.

Some experts recommend stopping warfarin 5 to 6 days before surgery depending on the patient's INR, stopping enoxaparin 12 to 18 hours before procedures, and stopping heparin 6 to 8 hours before an operation (Merli, 2000). Time frames for stopping anticoagulation are under investigation. A recent study of 80 patients taking enoxaparin found markedly elevated levels of anti-Xa heparin (a marker of anticoagulation activity) 14 hours after the last dose (O'Donnell et al., 2007). The finding suggests that stopping enoxaparin the evening before surgery may not be long enough to minimize the risk of surgical bleeding. Some patients may need to be admitted to the hospital 2 to

3 days in advance to make a safe transition from warfarin to heparin in the preoperative period.

Usually, it is acceptable for patients to take their regular oral medications with a small amount of water, not more than 150 mL, on the morning of surgery, but patients should check with the surgeon and the anesthesiologist. Patients who take insulin need to check with their doctor about proper preoperative dosage. The ASA established diabetic protocols to guide the administration of insulin and glucose during the perioperative period (Maurer, Borkowski, & Parker, 2004). Usually one-half the usual morning dose is administered on the morning of surgery. Frequent monitoring of blood glucose levels will determine the need for additional sliding scale insulin coverage. Some research suggests that tight glucose control (e.g., maintaining blood glucose levels at 80 to 110 mg/dL) using continuous intravenous insulin during certain surgeries is beneficial to patients (Van den Berghe et al., 2001), but other studies not only challenge these results but also found a deleterious effect with the practice of continuous intravenous insulin (Gandhi et al., 2005, 2007). Clearly more research is needed to determine how best to manage intraoperative glucose levels. Other medications may also need adjustment with surgery. For example, the dose of a corticosteroid might need to be increased depending on the reason it is taken.

 All diabetic medications taken in the 24 hours prior to surgery need to be carefully documented in the patient's record.

Patients will receive surgery-specific instructions to follow at home. For example, patients who are scheduled for colorectal surgery may be asked to follow a special diet, take a laxative, and administer an enema on the night before and morning of surgery to empty the bowel of stool and reduce microorganisms (Nichols, 2001). Some studies question the effectiveness of mechanical bowel preparation (Guenaga, 2002), and in some elective colon resections, patients are allowed a normal diet and require no routine bowel preparation ahead of time (Soreide & Ljungqvist, 2006). The Centers for Disease Control and Prevention (CDC) guidelines recommend that patients take a shower the night before a surgical procedure with an antimicrobial body wash containing 2% chlorhexidine gluconate, although this practice has not yet been shown to reduce surgical-site infections (Schweon, 2006; Seltzer, Horsman, & Korniewicz, 2002).

Preoperative Teaching to Prevent Postoperative Complications

Patients who are scheduled for major surgery that reduces mobility and requires inpatient recovery should be taught breathing exercises, how to splint the incision, coughing (to help clear airways), leg exercises, and the importance of postoperative ambulation. The patient may also benefit from the use of an alternative therapy, such as the mind/body practice of eliciting the relaxation response, as discussed in the Complementary and Alternative Therapies box (p. 606).

Breathing Exercises

Deep breathing is taught as an intervention to decrease the risk of the postoperative pulmonary complications of hypoxemia, atelectasis, and pneumonia. In one small study of patients scheduled for coronary artery bypass graft surgery, patients who received inspiratory muscle training preoperatively were much less likely to develop postoperative pulmonary complications than a comparison group (Hulzebos et al., 2006). To perform deep breathing, the patient breathes out normally then takes a deep breath through the nose or mouth, holds inspiration to the count of three or longer, and slowly releases the breath. Postoperatively, the patient is asked to take 5 to 10 deep breaths every hour.

Research suggests that the effects of deep breathing are not sustained over time and must be performed regularly to achieve physiological outcomes (Orfanos, Ellis, & Johnston, 1999). Deep breathing slows the respiratory rate and produces a sustained maximal inspiration. It is thought that deep breathing increases lung volumes by increasing tidal volume and minute ventilation. It also generates higher flow rates, and stimulates surfactant to help keep alveoli open (Brooks et al., 2001; Orfanos et al., 1999).

Deep breathing can also be used as a technique to reduce pain when moving. Encouraging the patient to focus on taking continuous deep breaths while moving or changing positions may help to prevent the patient from tensing muscles, which tends to worsen postoperative pain. One study found that patients who had received videotape instruction on how to use breathing and

COMPLEMENTARY & ALTERNATIVE THERAPIES — Relaxation Response

Description:

More than 30% of American adults use mind–body practices that elicit the relaxation response (RR). Although the mechanisms that mediate the RR remain unknown, eliciting the RR reduces volumetric oxygen consumption from rest and counteracts the effects of stress (Dusek et al., 2006). RR is an integrated psychophysiological response that originates in the hypothalamus and is the direct operate of the stress response. It leads to a generalized decrease in central nervous system arousal. The RR is a hypometabolic state that can be useful in many situations. The patient who activates the RR can use the body's own innate mechanisms to calm and slow down. The RR can occur through the repetition of a word or short phrase. The patient can return to this gentle repetition whenever distracting thoughts occur. This technique triggers a series of physiological changes (slower breathing, heart rate, blood pressure, etc.) that reduce stress.

The pre- and perioperative areas are excellent settings in which to instruct the patient in various RR techniques, such as how to slow down, focus on breathing techniques, and repeat a simple relaxing phrase. The nurse can utilize this technique at the bedside or in the perioperative area prior to anesthesia. A good place for the nurse to begin is to instruct the patient to breathe in through the nose, out through the mouth, and "focus on my voice." The nurse should practice this technique often to help in its delivery. This technique is also used as a preliminary step in many other CAM therapies.

Research Support:

One study investigated whether brief psychologic interventions to reduce perioperative stress in patients undergoing abdominal surgery would improve the patients' postoperative recovery. Participants involved 60 elderly cancer patients undergoing conventional resection of colorectal carcinoma. Researchers used a randomized, controlled, partially blinded trial to evaluate the differential effectiveness of guided imagery and progressive muscle relaxation on analgesic requirement, pain perception, pulmonary function, duration of postoperative ileus, and fatigue after surgery. Of the 60 patients, 20 used guided imagery, 22 used relaxation, 18 were the control. The effects on analgesic consumption and subjective pain intensity at rest and while coughing did not differ between groups. Pulmonary function recovery, postoperative ileus duration, and subjective postoperative fatigue were also not influenced. Results did not show a clinically relevant influence on the postoperative physiologic course. However, the results showed that imagery and relaxation yielded a very positive patient response. Ninety percent of the patients indicated that they would recommend the techniques to other patients (Haase, Schwenk, Hermann, & Muller, 2005).

Another study investigated whether nitric oxide (NO) mediates RR elicitation. Researchers measured percentage changes in fractional exhaled nitric oxide to evaluate whether depth of RR elicitation was correlated with changes in NO. In this randomized, controlled trial, 46 participants were randomized to either 8 weeks of RR training using audiotapes (n = 34) or 8 weeks of exposure to a control condition in which participants received health education by audiotapes (n = 12). Prior to randomization, participants' volumetric oxygen consumption and fractional exhaled nitric oxide levels were measured while the participants listened to a control audiotape. Eight weeks later, researchers measured participants' volumetric oxygen consumption and fractional exhaled nitric oxide levels while the RR group listened to a RR-eliciting audiotape and the control group listened to a control audiotape. There was no association between volumetric oxygen consumption slope and fractional exhaled nitric oxide prior to the training. However, after training, the results showed an inverse correlation between volumetric oxygen consumption slope and fractional exhaled nitric oxide in the RR group, but not in the control group. Based on these results, the researchers concluded that the depth of RR elicitation was associated with increased concentrations of fractional exhaled nitric oxide after RR training. Their further conclusion was that the RR may be mediated by NO, which helps to explain its clinical effects in stress-related disorders (Dusek et al., 2006).

Another group of investigators conducted a single-blind, 3-arm, randomized controlled trial by evaluating the efficacy of an RR intervention program on the quality of life (QOL) and exercise capacity of CHF patients. Study intervention group patients (n = 95) attended a weekly RR group for 15 weeks and were requested to practice the techniques at home twice a day. An alternative intervention was a 15-week cardiac education (EDU) program. The control group was involved usual care (UC). Researchers administered the QOL questionnaires and a bicycle test at baseline and after intervention (or 15 to 19 weeks). Results were adjusted for baseline scores, time between assessments, age, education, diet, and medication. After these adjustments, results showed that the RR group had significantly better QOL change scores in peace–spiritual scales than did the UC group. However, no significant difference was observed between the EDU and UC groups. Researchers observed a similar trend in emotional QOL. The researchers found no statistically significant intervention effect on physical QOL or exercise capacity (Chang et al., 2005).

References

Chang, B.H., Hendricks, A., Zhao, Y., Rothendler, J. A., LoCastro, J. S., & Slawsky, M. T. (2005). A relaxation response randomized trial on patients with chronic heart failure. *Journal of Cardiopulmonary Rehabilitation, 25*(3), 149–157.

Dusek, J. A., Chang, B. H., Zaki, J., Lazar, S., Deykin, A., Stefano, G. B., et al. (2006). Association between oxygen consumption and nitric oxide production during the relaxation response. *Medical Science Monitor, 12*(1), CR1–10.

Haase, O., Schwenk, W., Hermann, C., & Muller, J. M. (2005). Guided imagery and relaxation in conventional colorectal resections: A randomized, controlled, partially blinded trial. *Diseases of the Colon and Rectum, 48*(10), 1955–1963.

imagery while performing postoperative activities reported significantly less pain, more mobility, and more independent mobility than patients who had not received the instruction (Heye, Foster, Bartlett, & Adkins, 2002).

Incentive Spirometry

The use of incentive spirometry (IS) as a mechanism to encourage deep breathing is widespread. An incentive spirometer is a device that is activated by the inspiratory effort of the patient. Incentive spirometers come in many different models but there are two basic types, flow oriented and volume oriented. To operate the IS, the patient takes a deep breath, which causes a plate or a ball to rise up a calibrated cylinder. The cylinder displays either the inspired volume (a volume-oriented incentive spirometer) or the generated flow (a flow-oriented incentive spirometer) (Weindler & Kiefer, 2001). An incentive spirometer can be helpful postoperatively because it provides a numeric reading of how effectively patients are taking deep breaths, and the use of IS encourages patients to take responsibility for their care, but it is probably not any better than deep breathing in preventing postoperative complications (Overend et al., 2001).

Splinting the Incision

Patients with thoracic or abdominal incisions can be taught preoperatively how to splint the incision to prevent painful stress on the area. The patient can use a small, flat pillow or a small, folded blanket, sometimes referred to as a "cough pillow," to apply gentle, firm pressure over the incision when performing activities that tend to pull the incision such as when getting out of bed, getting up from a chair, or coughing. Splinting the incision is helpful in reducing pain.

Coughing

Postoperative patients have an increase in mucous production and a decreased ability to clear mucus from the airways as a result of anesthesia (Smith & Ellis, 2000). Retained mucus places patients at risk for the development of atelectasis and pneumonia. Coughing can help to clear mucus from the airways and facilitate full expansion of the lungs because it requires an increase in intrathoracic pressure and a rapid expiratory flow (Smith & Ellis, 2000). Coughing can be quite painful for some patients because of the stress it places on the suture line. Splinting the incision will help protect it and reduce some of the pain that occurs with movement of the incisional area. Coughing may be contraindicated after some surgeries because of the stress it puts on the incision (e.g., hernia) or because it increases intracranial pressure (e.g., craniotomy). Generally a health care provider's order will be written to avoid coughing for surgical procedures where it is contraindicated.

Leg Exercises

Guidelines on prevention of venous thromboembolism recommend that a risk assessment be performed on all surgical patients (Blondin, 2006). Most patients receive some form of prophylaxis against the development of DVT (i.e., venous blood clot in the leg) postoperatively. Leg exercises are a simple way of stimulating venous return in the patient with limited mobility. They are used in addition to other devices to prevent venous stasis.

Several types of leg exercises can be performed. The exercises should be done on each leg and should be repeated several times before moving to the next exercise. Descriptions of various leg exercises follow:

- Alternate between flexing the foot and dorsiflexing the foot.
- Lift the foot off the bed and make circles with the ankle several times.
- Bend the knee and lift the leg off of the bed holding the position for a few seconds.
- With knees bent, push the ball of the foot into the bed or floor, contracting the calf and thigh muscles.

Ambulation and Mobility

Early ambulation is beneficial to the postoperative patient for a number of reasons. Ambulation increases heart rate and cardiac output and stimulates circulation to all body systems. The increase in circulation helps to rid the body of the effects of anesthesia. Ambulation increases respiratory rate and minute ventilation, and it helps to mobilize respiratory secretions. Increased circulation to the intestinal tract helps to stimulate peristalsis, and increased blood flow through the kidneys stimulates the production of urine. Blood flow to skin and muscles brings nutrients needed for wound healing. Ambulation stimulates calf muscles and increases venous return. Frequent ambulation, a minimum of three times per day, may help prevent some of the complications associated with immobility. Patients need to understand the importance and emphasis that is placed on walking after an operation and be shown effective ways of getting out of bed postoperatively. In one intervention study, women who were scheduled for abdominal hysterectomy were taught a specific technique for getting out of bed, practiced the technique preoperatively, and were encouraged to use the skill after surgery. The authors reported that the women who received coaching and skill training ambulated for longer periods of time postoperatively than the women who did not receive the training (Oetker-Black et al., 2003). Most patients will be allowed to walk with assistance on the evening of surgery or the first postoperative day. For some surgeries, ambulation is initially restricted. These patients need to turn and reposition every 1 to 2 hours to prevent complications of immobility until they are allowed to ambulate. Older patients have the same informational needs as other adults, but the teaching process may require a different approach, as discussed in the Gerontological Considerations box.

GERONTOLOGICAL CONSIDERATIONS
for Preoperative Teaching

Teaching techniques for older adults who are scheduled for surgery include going over the material more slowly, repeating the material, asking the patient to confirm their understanding of the instruction, and reinforcing verbal instructions with written materials and instructions. Including someone from the elder's social support system in the preoperative teaching session can be helpful as well. Older patients may have more worries about surgery than others because the surgery presents very real threats to their physical function and a potential loss of independence. Older patients having surgery may also worry about the care of an elderly spouse, partner, or sibling during their absence. The nurse must be sensitive to these issues and encourage patients to discuss concerns they may have. A social worker may need to be consulted for assistance in problem solving.

Legal Preparation and Ethical Considerations

The nurse must consider both legal and ethical considerations when preparing a patient for surgery. Patients have a right to be informed about the risks of surgery and anesthesia and to make treatment decisions. They also have the right to decide what course of treatment to follow in the event that they experience a serious postoperative complication.

Informed Consent

The patient must sign an informed consent form prior to surgery. The informed consent protects all parties involved: the patient, the surgeon, and the hospital. In order for the consent to be valid, there must be full disclosure of the treatment to be performed, the patient must sufficiently understand the information provided (i.e., must be competent), and the patient must voluntarily consent to the treatment. Full disclosure includes a description of the condition requiring surgery, the surgical procedure, the possible risks and benefits, alternative treatments, and prognosis. The surgeon is responsible for discussing the procedure with the patient and securing an informed consent. If a patient is unable to sign, an "X" is an acceptable substitute provided there are two witnesses. Consent is voluntary and can be withdrawn at any time. The surgical consent form may include additional consents such as consent for a blood transfusion and for the disposal of body tissues. The nurse's role in the process is to clarify information for the patient and advocate for the patient as needed.

In cases where the patient is unable to participate in informed consent (e.g., an unconscious or incompetent patient), the consent is obtained from the legally responsible person. This person might be the health care proxy, the next of kin, or a court-appointed legal guardian. In emergencies, telephone consent is acceptable. In cases of extreme emergency where the legally responsible person is not available and delaying the operation might result in death or serious impairment, the medical emergency overrides the need for consent and the surgery proceeds without consent. In such circumstances, hospitals have set protocols for documenting in the patient's chart the gravity of the situation and the nature of the emergency.

Frequently, the consent for anesthesia is a separate process performed by the anesthesia care provider. The patient receives information about the type of anesthesia planned and the possible risks associated with it. Figure 25–2 ■ is an example of an informed consent form for surgical treatment. Chapter 4 ⊘ provides a complete description of informed consent.

Resuscitation Orders

It is not unusual for a patient with a do-not-resuscitate (DNR) order to require surgery. Surgery might be done for palliative reasons (e.g., to decrease pain associated with tumor growth) or to facilitate care (e.g., the insertion of a feeding tube) or to improve quality of life. Some older patients who are in reasonably good health request a DNR order in case of an untoward event even though the surgery to be performed is elective. In the past, DNR orders were suspended for the length of the surgery and early postoperative period.

Professional organizations of surgeons, anesthesiologists, and perioperative nurses have challenged the routine suspension of DNR orders (AORN, 1999; ASA, 2001). The position of the AORN is that a patient's autonomy should be respected in the operating room and therefore DNR orders should not be routinely suspended for surgery. Instead, AORN recommends that there be a required reconsideration of the DNR order with the scheduling of surgery. The patient is given the opportunity to consider the consequences of withholding resuscitation efforts during surgery and what, if any, resuscitation efforts she might want performed. The ultimate DNR decision falls with the patient and must be clearly documented in the record. If the patient decides to suspend DNR orders intraoperatively, then the point at which the DNR is to be reinstituted needs to be clearly stated.

Common Routines and Medications

Preoperative care and routines are designed to protect the safety of patients and to minimize the likelihood of postoperative complications. Surgical preparation may include bowel preparation, skin preparation, and hair removal. Bowel preparation is usually ordered for major abdominal surgery of the colon or rectum. The goal of preoperative bowel cleansing is to clear the intestine of feces and to decrease intestinal bacteria. It is thought that this preparation reduces the risk of contamination of the operative site with stool, however, some studies question the necessity and effectiveness of mechanical bowel preparation (Guenaga, 2002). Most surgeons continue to use mechanical bowel preparation prior to colorectal surgery. There are several methods to clear the colon of fecal material. Conventional bowel preparation requires a low-residue diet for several days prior to surgery, administration of laxatives 1 to 2 days before surgery, and the administration of enemas on the evening before surgery (Guenaga, 2002). Bowel preparation also may include the administration of oral antibiotics (e.g., neomycin and erythromycin, or metronidazole). Bowel preparation is a time-consuming and exhausting process, and it can contribute to preoperative dehydration in older patients.

Skin preparation may require the patient to shower the night before surgery or the morning of surgery with an antiseptic solution (i.e., 2% chlorhexidine gluconate). Hair removal prior to surgery is a controversial practice. If hair is to be removed for an operation, the CDC recommends using sterile supplies, clipping rather than shaving, in the direction of hair growth, and performing the procedure as close to the time of operation as possible (Mangram, Horan, Pearson, Silver, & Jarvis, 1999; Niel-Weise, Willie, & van den Broek, 2005; Schweon, 2006). Figure 25–3 ■ (p. 610) shows the areas of skin preparation for common surgical sites.

Preoperative Medications

Preoperative medications refer to those that are given specifically in preparation for surgery. It is increasingly common for preoperative medications to be given in the **holding area** of the surgical suite immediately prior to the operation. The Pharmacology Summary box (p. 611) lists common preoperative medications and the rationale for their administration.

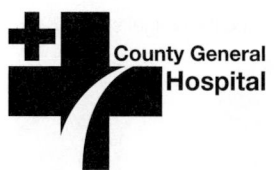

County General
Hospital

Patient's name _____

Med. Rec. # _____

DOB _____

Consent for Medical/Surgical Procedure

_____ has explained that I have a condition called _____ and
(Name of Healthcare Provider)

has recommended a medical or surgical treatment called _____

_____ .

Benefits and Alternatives to Treatment: My doctor has spoken with me about the benefits I may expect from this treatment,

such as _____ but has made no guarantees or promises. My doctor has also spoken about what

could happen if I do not get this treatment, and explained other options for my care including _____

_____ .

Risks:

My doctor has explained that there are some risks to this treatment. The risks include, but are not limited to, allergic reactions, drug reactions, bleeding, blood clots, nerve injury, brain damage, infection, loss of bodily function or life, or the need for more procedures or treatments. My doctor has also explained that there may be other risks or complications. Particular risks include, but are not limited to _____

_____ .

☐ **N/A**   **Blood Transfusion:**

I may also need a blood transfusion. There are risks to this, even when all safety measures are taken. The risks of getting blood transfusion include (but are not limited to) fever; chills; allergic reactions (rashes including hives); heart failure; hemolysis (destruction of the transfused red blood cells) with fever; shock; chest pain; red urine; transmission of infectious agents such as bacteria, hepatitis virus, or HIV (human immunodeficiency virus).

☐ **N/A**   **Disposal of Tissues:**

I give permission to County General Hospital to dispose of any tissue, fluid, or bone that may be removed during my treatment. I understand that this tissue, fluids, or bone may be used, saved, or transferred to others for scientific or teaching purposes.

☐ **N/A**   **Non-Anesthesiologist Delivered Moderate Sedation:**

I understand that I will receive sedation through my intravenous line (IV) in order to help me feel more comfortable during my procedure. This sedation is not general anesthesia and is not administered by an anesthesiologist. With this sedation I may still be aware of what is happening. There are risks to sedation, including (but are not limited to) allergic reactions, drug reactions, bleeding, blood clots, breathing problems that require a breathing tube, nerve injury, brain damage, infection, or loss of bodily function or life.

☐ **N/A**   **Industry Representative:**

I understand that an industry representative(s) will be present during my procedure. My doctor has explained the reasons why the industry representative(s) will be present.

   ☐ **I do not** consent to the presence of an Industry Representative(s).

☐ **N/A**   **Tracking Medical Devices:**

Some surgical treatments include putting in (implanting), or taking out (removing) a medical device. The hospital is asked, by law, to track this device. This means that the hospital is asked to give my name, address, and social security number to the medical device manufacturer, and/or the Food and Drug Administration (FDA). It is my decision whether the hospital can give out this information.

   ☐ **I refuse** to let the hospital give information to the manufacturer and/or FDA.

Trainees & Observers:

County General Hospital is a teaching facility. This means that health care trainees such as resident physicians and students may be involved in or observe my care. All trainees are supervised by professional staff.

Patient Consent:

My questions have been answered. I have read and understood the content of this form. I consent to treatment and medical care.

X_____ or X_____   X __ / __ / __
          Patient   Person authorized to sign for patient and relationship to patient   Date

I have explained the above statements, and answered all the patient's questions.

X_____ or X_____   X __ / __ / __
      Physician/Surgeon/Other Healthcare Provider   Print Name   Date

FIGURE 25–2 ■ Consent for medical–surgical treatment.
Source: Courtesy of Beth Israel Deaconess Nursing Department

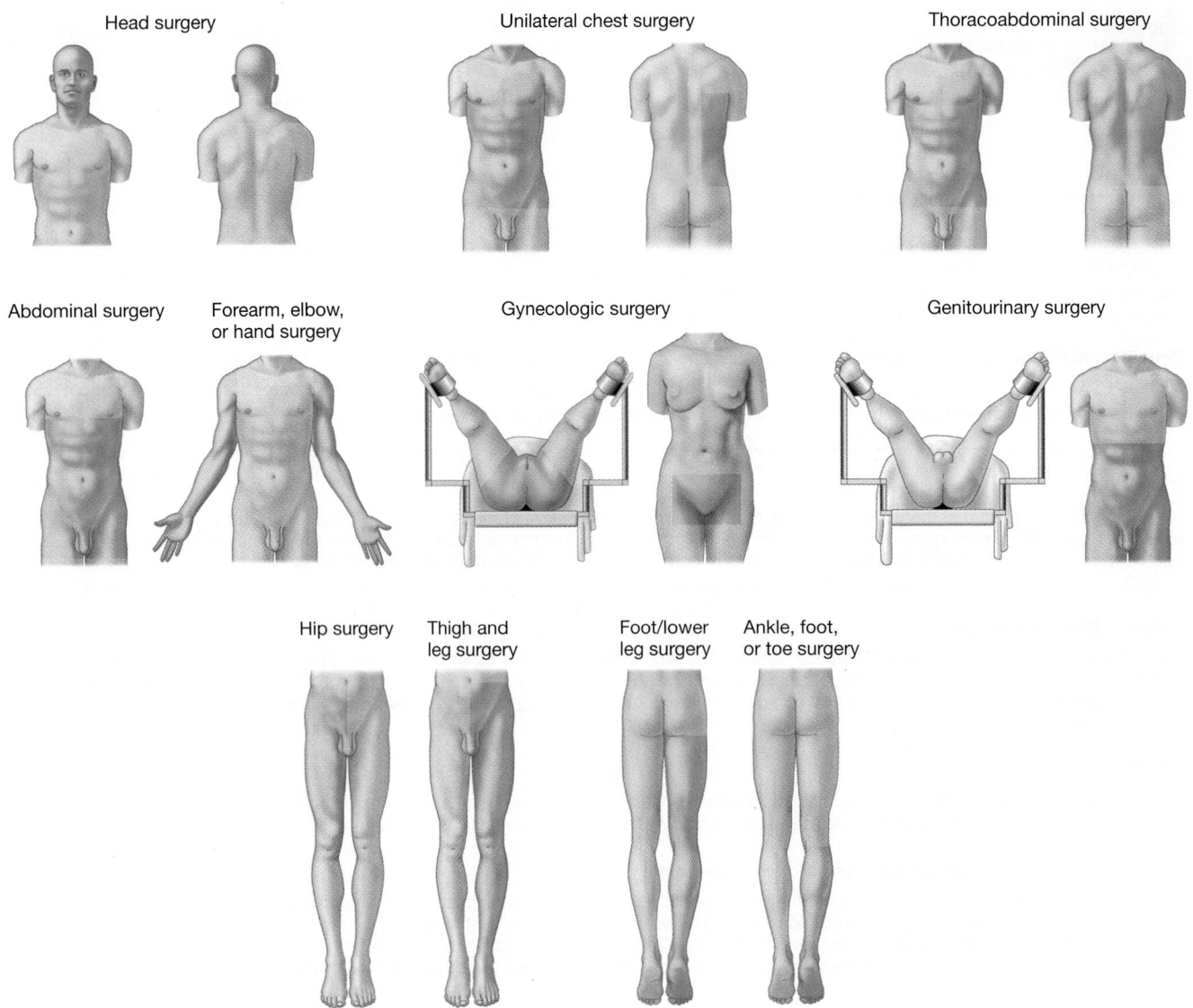

FIGURE 25–3 ■ Skin preparation for common surgical sites.

Antianxiety agents are often given to relax the patient. Prophylactic antibiotics are given in many, but not all, surgical cases. Antibiotics are frequently given intravenously in the surgical holding area or at induction of anesthesia. Research supports the view that the antibiotic must be in the target tissues before bacterial contamination if it is to prevent subsequent infection (Nichols, 2001). Ideally, antibiotics should be given 30 to 60 minutes before an incision is made (Golembiewski, 2004). Cefazolin, a first-generation cephalosporin, is often the drug of choice for surgical prophylaxis, although cefoxitin may be used in colon surgeries. If vancomycin is to be given, it should be started 2 hours before the incision because it takes 60 minutes to administer. In uncomplicated, short, clean surgical cases, one dose of parenteral antibiotic may be sufficient to prevent infection. Additional doses of antibiotics may be given during surgical procedures that last more than 2 to 3 hours or where contamination is suspected (Golembiewski, 2004; Nichols, 2001). Postoperative antibiotic prophylaxis is not recommended beyond 24 hours because studies do not show any benefit and it may contribute to the development of drug resistance (Bratzler & Houck, 2004).

Other preoperative medications that may be given include gastrointestinal stimulants, gastric acid blockers for gastric ulcer prophylaxis, or antiemetics to decrease nausea and vomiting. These medications are not recommended for the purpose of decreasing risk of pulmonary aspiration (ASA, 1999b). Beta-adrenergic blockers are given to patients prior to cardiac surgery to reduce the incidence of postoperative atrial fibrillation. Beta-adrenergic blocker therapy may also be given to high-risk cardiac patients or to those undergoing vascular procedures to reduce the risk of perioperative cardiovascular complications (Fleisher et al., 2006). Currently, it is recommended that beta-adrenergic blocker therapy be started days to weeks before elective surgery although the ideal dose, drug, and timing has not been established.

Preoperative Checklist

Most hospitals use preoperative checklists, like that shown in Figure 25–4 ■ (p. 612), to ensure and document the readiness of the patient for surgery. The admitting nurse completes the preoperative checklist for a patient who is having same-day admission surgery. If the patient is an inpatient, the clinical nurse

PHARMACOLOGY Summary of Common Preoperative Medications

Medication Category	Rationale for Administering Medication to Preoperative Patient
Antibiotics • Cefazolin: recommended for many different types of surgery (e.g., neurosurgical, cardiothoracic, vascular, gastric, biliary tract, urologic, gynecologic, orthopedic procedures) • Erythromycin: may be given orally for surgery on colon and rectum • Neomycin: may be given orally for surgery on colon and rectum • Trimethoprim 160 mg and sulfamethoxazole 800 mg (Bactrim DS) may be given orally to patients having urologic surgery	Antibiotics are given for prophylaxis against infection. Recommendations for the selection of an antibiotic and how it is administered vary according to the surgery and the patient. Prophylactic antibiotics may be given to patients with heart valve abnormalities to prevent bacterial endocarditis. Prophylactic antibiotics are frequently given to patients receiving prostheses (e.g., vascular graft, joint replacement) or transplants (e.g., heart, kidney, pancreas, liver).
Anticholinergics • Atropine • Glycopyrrolate • Scopolamine eyedrops	Given to suppress oral, respiratory, and gastric secretions during surgery. Atropine and glycopyrrolate increase heart rate (prevent bradycardia). Atropine and scopolamine eyedrops may be used in ophthalmic procedures to dilate pupils.
Antiemetics • Droperidol (Inapsine) • Ondansetron (Zofran) • Metoclopramide (Reglan)	Given to reduce nausea and vomiting. Metoclopramide speeds gastric emptying.
Anticoagulants, Low-Dose • Low-dose heparin • Low-molecular-weight heparin (e.g., enoxaparin, dalteparin, ardeparin)	Given to prevent the development of thrombus formation and pulmonary emboli in surgeries or patients who are high risk (e.g., orthopedic procedures). Usually not recommended for patients having neurosurgery, spinal needles, or epidural catheters.
Benzodiazepines • Midazolam (Versed) • Lorazepam (Ativan) • Diazepam (Valium)	Given to reduce anxiety, increase sedation, and smooth induction of anesthesia.
Beta-adrenergic Blocker Therapy • Atenolol • Metoprolol • Propranolol	Given in cardiac surgery to reduce the risk of atrial fibrillation. Given in noncardiac surgery to select patients to reduce the risk of cardiovascular complications.
Gastric Acid Blockers • Proton-pump inhibitor (e.g., Protonix) • H2-receptor antagonist (e.g., famotidine, ranitidine, cimetidine)	Given to decrease gastric acid production as prophylaxis against development of gastric/duodenal ulcer from physiological stress. May be given to raise gastric pH in specific situations where the patient is high risk for pulmonary aspiration. If aspiration occurs the higher pH of gastric secretions does less damage than those that are very acidic.
Narcotics • Fentanyl • Morphine sulfate • Meperidine	Given to reduce pain and discomfort associated with preoperative procedures, and to reduce anesthesia requirements.

Sources: American Society of Anesthesiologists. (1999). Practice guidelines for preoperative fasting and the use of pharmacologic agents to reduce the risk of pulmonary aspiration: Application to healthy patients undergoing elective procedures. A report by the American Society of Anesthesiologists Task Force on Preoperative Fasting. *Anesthesiology, 90*(3), 896–905; American Society of Health System Pharmacists. (1999). ASHP therapeutic guidelines on antimicrobial prophylaxis in surgery. *American Journal of Health System Pharmacists, 56*(18), 1839–1888; Adams, M., Josephson, D., & Holland, L. (2005). *Pharmacology for nurses: A pathophysiological approach.* Upper Saddle River, NJ: Pearson Prentice Hall; Fleisher, L., Beckman, J., Brown, K., Calkins, H., Chaikof, E., Fleischmann, K., Freeman, W., Froehlich, J., Kasper, E., Kersten, J., Riegel, B., & Robb, J. et al. (2006). ACC/AHA 2006 guideline update on perioperative cardiovascular evaluation for noncardiac surgery: Focused update on perioperative beta-blocker therapy. *Journal of the American College of Cardiology, 47*(11).

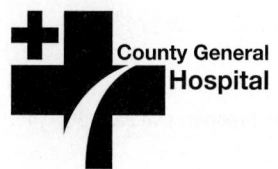

County General
Hospital

PRE-PROCEDURE REPORT

Patient Identification Area

SECTION 1							
PROCEDURE: ☐ Surgical ☐ Cardiac Cath ☐ Angiography ☐ Arteriogram ☐ Tips ☐ Other _____							

CHART PREPARATION	Completed			PHYSICAL PREPARATION	Completed		
	Yes	No	N/A		Yes	No	N/A
Health care Proxy				ID band on			
Surgical/Procedure Consent				Nail polish/hairpins/makeup removed			
Anesthesia Consent				Hospital gown ONLY			
Hemoglobin/Hematocrit				Valuables, jewelry removed			
Interpreted EKG				Prosthesis removed			
Interpreted CXR				Dentures removed			
Addressograph plate				Contact lenses removed			
Medication Adminstration Record				Eyeglasses removed			
Old record				Hearing aide in place L / R			
Insulin record				Preop scrub/prep done			

SECTION 2: PRE-PROCEDURE ASSESSMENT To be completed on the day of surgery/procedure.	
VITAL SIGNS: T_____ BP _____ HR _____ RR _____ O2 SAT_____ ☐ ROOM AIR _____ ☐ NP @ _____ L/M WEIGHT:_____ HEIGHT:_____	**ALLERGIES:** _____ _____ **PRECAUTION STATUS:** _____ **PRIMARY LANGUAGE:** _____

NEURO:
 	
LOC
   ☐ ORIENTED X 3   ☐ CONFUSED
   ☐ SEDATED   ☐ OTHER _____
PAIN
   LOCATION_____
   MEDICATION _____
IMPAIRMENTS: ☐ VISUAL   ☐ HEARING   ☐ COGNITIVE
	MEDICATIONS TAKEN THIS MORNING (ROUTINE):
	_____
	_____
	_____
	_____
	PREOP MEDS:
	_____
	_____
	_____

ENDOCRINE:
   ☐ IDDM   ☐ NIDDM   ☐ AM BS _____
   PRE OP INSULIN (Date, Time)_____
	LOCATION OF FAMILY:
	   CONTACT TO BE CALLED:_____
	   PHONE #:_____
	
	LOCATION OF BELONGINGS:
	_____

GI:
   NPO SINCE _____
GU:
   LAST VOIDED _____ FOLEY_____
   ☐ CRF/LAST DIALYSIS _____
   ACCESS SITE:_____
	TRANSFER NURSE:
	_____ RN
	
	DATE: _____ TIME: _____

COMMENTS: _____ _____ _____	

FIGURE 25–4 ■ Preprocedure report form.

Source: Courtesy of Beth Israel Deaconess Nursing Department

caring for the patient completes the checklist. The patient scheduled for surgery is identified using two indicators (e.g., asking the patient his name and date of birth and checking the wristband). The patient must have a hospital identification wristband in place and allergy band if applicable. Prior to sending the patient to the operating room, the nurse checks to see that signed surgical and anesthesia consents are on file. If consent for surgery or anesthesia is missing, the appropriate physician is contacted. The nurse also checks that the medical record is complete including recent laboratory tests, diagnostic tests, medication records, intake and output sheets, and vital sign graphic records. The nurse records the patient's current level of consciousness and a recent set of vital signs. The nurse notes the medications, routine and preoperative, taken before surgery. Patients should void before going to the operating room.

Commonly cosmetics, including nail polish, are removed preoperatively in order to observe skin color and capillary filling. All jewelry is removed from the patient and locked up with other valuables per hospital policy. It is particularly important to note on the preoperative checklist where valuables are located to prevent loss. Most facilities allow the patient to wear a wedding band that has been taped to the finger to the operating room, but the patient may want to remove the ring if postoperative swelling is expected (e.g., mastectomy with lymph node dissection). Pierced earrings and other body piercings must be removed to prevent accidental burns from electrocautery (Bray, 2006).

All prosthetic devices including dentures, removable bridges, and contact lens are removed prior to surgery. On occasion, the anesthesia care provider may prefer that the patient leave dentures in place to assist in airway maintenance. The presence of dentures in the mouth can assist in creating a tighter seal between the mouth and the oxygen mask (Bray, 2006). When dentures are removed, they must be labeled and stored safely to prevent loss. Patients may want to wear glasses or hearing aids to the holding area, this is acceptable although they will be removed before the surgery. Patients are transported with their medical record, including the medication administration record, to the operating room holding area via gurney.

Additional guidelines for the preoperative phase that deal with pain and comfort are listed in the National Guidelines box (p. 614).

◼ Research

Research is important to improving the care of surgical patients. Advances in technology and changes in surgical technique create the need to research the effects of the change. For example, patients today are sent home earlier after surgery because surgical procedures have become less invasive. What effect does this have on the patient, his or her family, and the home health agency that provides the care that was once provided in the hospital? Research is critical to nurses who want to know that the interventions they perform are based on scientific evidence. The Research Opportunities and Clinical Impact box (p. 615) lists some of the research problems that are important to the care of the preoperative patient. An example of a research study that could have a positive effect on perioperative nursing practice is described in the Evidence-Based Practice feature (p. 603).

NATIONAL GUIDELINES American Society of PeriAnesthesia Nurses Pain and Comfort Clinical Guidelines

Preoperative Phase

Assessment

1. Vital signs including pain and comfort goals (e.g., 0 to 10 scale).

2. Medical history (e.g., neurological status, cardiac and respiratory, instability, allergy to medication, food and objects, use of herbs, motion sickness, sickle cell, fibromyalgia, use of caffeine/substance abuse, fear, and anxiety).

3. Pain history (e.g., preexisting pain, acute, chronic, pain level, pattern, quality, type of source, intensity, location, duration/time, course, pain effect, and effects on personal life).

4. Pain behaviors/expressions or history (e.g., grimacing, frowning, crying, restlessness, tension, and discomfort behaviors, such as shivering, nausea, and vomiting. Note that physical appearance may not necessarily indicate pain/discomfort or its absence.)

5. Analgesic history: type (i.e., opioid, nonopioid, and adjuvant analgesics), dose, frequency, effectiveness, adverse effects, other medications that may influence choice of analgesics (e.g., anticoagulant, antihypertensive, muscle relaxants).

6. Patient's preferences (e.g., for pain relief/comfort measures, expectations, concerns, aggravating and alleviating factors, and clarification of misconceptions).

7. Pain/comfort acceptable levels (e.g., patient and family, as indicated, agree to plan of treatment/interventions postoperatively).

8. Comfort history (i.e., physiological, sociocultural, psychospiritual, and environment, such as spiritual beliefs/symbols, warming measures, music, comfort objects, privacy, positioning, factors related to nausea/vomiting).

9. Educational needs (i.e., consider age or level of education, cognitive and language appropriateness, and barriers to learning).

10. Cultural language preference, identification of personal beliefs, and resulting restrictions.

11. Pertinent laboratory results (e.g., prolonged prothrombin time, partial thromboplastin time, and abnormal international normalized ratio and platelet count to determine risk for epidural hematoma in patients with epidural catheter).

Interventions

1. Identify patient, validate surgeon's order and procedure (i.e., correct name of drug, dose, amount, route, and time), and validate type of surgery and correct surgical site as applicable.

2. Discuss pain and comfort assessment (i.e., presence, location, quality, intensity, age, language, condition, and cognitively appropriate pain rating scale [e.g., a 0 to 10 numerical scale or FACES scale] and comfort scale). Assessment method must be the same for consistency.

3. Discuss with patient and family, as indicated, information about reporting pain intensity using a numerical or FACES rating scales and available pain relief and comfort measures. Include discussion of patient's preference for pain and comfort measures; implement comfort measures (i.e., physiological, sociocultural, spiritual, environmental support as indicated by patient).

4. Discuss and dispel misconceptions about pain and pain management.

5. Encourage patient to take a preventive approach to pain and discomfort by asking for relief measures before pain and discomfort are severe or out of control.

6. Educate purpose of intravenous or epidural patient-controlled analgesia (PCA) as indicated; educate about use of nonpharmacologic methods (e.g., cold therapy, relaxation breathing, music).

7. Discuss potential outcomes of pain and discomfort treatment approaches.

8. Establish pain relief/comfort goals with the patient (e.g., a pain rating of less than 4 on a scale of 0 to 10 to make it easy to cough, deep breathe, and turn). Premedicate patients for sedation, pain relief, and comfort (e.g., nonopioid, opioid, antiemetics as ordered; consider needs of chronic pain patients).

9. Arrange interpreter throughout the continuum of care as indicated.

10. Utilize interventions for patients with sensory impairments (e.g., device to amplify sound, sign language, and interpreters).

11. Report abnormal findings including laboratory values (prolonged PT/PTT and abnormal INR and platelet count among epidural patients).

12. Arrange for parents to be present for children.

Expected Outcomes

1. Patient states understanding of care plan and priority of individualized needs.

2. Patient states understanding of pain intensity scale, comfort scale, and pain relief/comfort goals.

3. Patient establishes realistic and achievable pain relief/comfort goals (e.g., a pain rating of less than 4 on a scale of 0 to 10 to make it easier to cough, deep breathe, and turn upon discharge).

4. Patient states understanding or demonstrates correct use of PCA equipment as indicated.

5. Patient verbalizes understanding of importance of using other nonpharmacologic methods of alleviating pain and discomfort (e.g., cold therapy, relaxation breathing, music).

Source: Reprinted from American Society of PeriAnesthesia Nurses. ASPAN pain and comfort guideline. Journal of PeriAnesthesia Nursing, *18*(4), 232–236, 2003, with permission from Elsevier.

RESEARCH OPPORTUNITIES AND CLINICAL IMPACT RELATED TO CARE OF THE PREOPERATIVE PATIENT

Research Area	Clinical Impact
General Preoperative Teaching	
What is the effect of preoperative education on patients' self-care behaviors postoperatively?	A goal of preoperative education is to increase patients' self-care behaviors and participation in desired postoperative activities.
Is there a difference in knowledge outcomes of preoperative education presented in written versus oral versus video formats?	Provides data for selecting an appropriate format(s) for the presentation of preoperative information.
How does the availability of Internet information on surgical procedures change preoperative education provided by the nurse?	Increased use of the Internet by patients and family members may change the focus of preoperative teaching. It may also affect the type and amount of information desired.
Is there an optimal time for preoperative education?	Provides rationale for scheduling preoperative appointments and for providing written materials to the patient.
What factors (nurse, environment, patient) increase the effectiveness of preoperative education?	Provides background information necessary for understanding the educational process and for creating an effective teaching environment.
Does preoperative education improve patient outcomes postoperatively?	A critical desired outcome of preoperative education programs.
Psychosocial Aspects of Preoperative Care	
How does the timing of preoperative teaching affect patient and family anxiety levels and coping strategies?	Provides information about an optimal time of psychological readiness for preoperative information.
Does family presence in the surgical holding area enhance the well-being of patients and family members?	Provides a rationale for designing a patient/family-friendly environment for surgery.
How do the communication skills of novice nurses in the preoperative area compare to those of experienced nurses?	Provides a basis for understanding the development of therapeutic communication in nurses.
How does a nurse's skill in communication affect preoperative teaching?	Provides a basis for understanding how specific skills affect the teaching–learning process.
What is the effect of an emergency surgery on the informational needs of patients, families, and significant others?	Provides background information for prioritizing information in specific situations.
Culture	
What interventions can be done to support culturally appropriate care preoperatively?	Provides a rationale for developing a range of culture-specific interventions.
What are the differences across cultures regarding the type and amount of preoperative education desired by patients?	Provides information needed for designing culturally sensitive preoperative teaching plans.
Specific Preoperative Instructions	
What is the optimal time frame to quit smoking prior to surgery?	Provides important information about the time frame necessary to achieve positive outcomes.
Does a preoperative shower using antimicrobial soap decrease the risk of surgical-site infection?	Provides rationale for a common preoperative instruction.
What are the physiological effects of a "good nights sleep" before surgery on the preoperative patient?	Provides important psychological and physiological information about the patient going into surgery.
Should gender, ethnicity, and body weight make a difference in the instructions for mechanical bowel preparation for surgery?	Provides information about differences in physiological responses that might support individualizing preoperative preparation.
Does the use of a preoperative risk assessment for venous thromboembolism correlate with reduced incidence of deep vein thrombosis (DVT) postoperatively?	Provides the evidence for a current nursing practice recommendation.
Does specific information about deep vein thrombosis (DVT) prophylaxis increase patients' compliance with leg exercises, ambulation, and use of intermittent pneumatic compression devices postoperatively?	Provides a rationale for preoperative teaching.

NCLEX® REVIEW

1. The nurse asks a preoperative patient about the presence of allergies. The purpose of this information is to:
   1. Reduce allergic reactions to medications or to latex.
   2. Determine the type of anesthesia to be used.
   3. Determine the care area to transfer the patient after the surgical procedure.
   4. Ensure blood products are available for the patient.

2. The nurse is assessing the cardiovascular status of a preoperative patient and learns of the patient's history of valve disease. Which of the following might be indicated for this patient?
   1. Monitor fluid status
   2. Monitor electrolyte status
   3. Antibiotic prophylaxis
   4. BNP level

3. A 40-year-old patient is scheduled for a total knee replacement. Which of the following would be indicated for this patient?
   1. Preoperative arterial blood gas
   2. Stop all NSAIDs two weeks before the scheduled surgery
   3. Recent hemoglobin A1c level
   4. Recent electrocardiogram

4. The nurse is planning preoperative care for an elderly patient. Which of the following should be included to reduce the risk of pulmonary complications?
   1. Encourage deep breathing and coughing
   2. Monitor oxygen saturation
   3. Monitor intake and output
   4. Follow aspiration precautions

5. While providing preoperative instructions in the waiting room, the patient says to the nurse "I don't want to be cauterized." Which of the following should the nurse respond to this patient?
   1. Everyone is cauterized.
   2. Can you explain to me what you mean by cauterized?
   3. The surgeon will cauterize in the operating room if it's necessary.
   4. Who said anything about being cauterized?

6. A preoperative patient tells the nurse that he researched the surgical procedure on the Internet and has no questions at this time. Which of the following should the nurse do?
   1. Document that the patient studied the surgical procedure on the Internet.
   2. Assess the patient's understanding of the procedure to supplement any areas not reviewed through the Internet.
   3. End the preoperative teaching session.
   4. Encourage the patient to use the call light in the event he decides he wants to discuss the procedure.

Answers for review questions appear in Appendix D

KEY TERMS

cosmetic surgery *p.587*
curative procedures *p.586*
diagnostic procedures *p.586*
elective procedures *p.587*
emergent (emergency) surgery *p.587*

exploratory surgery *p.586*
holding area *p.608*
palliative procedures *p.587*
perioperative *p.588*

preoperative health evaluation *p.588*
reconstructive surgery *p.586*
same-day admission *p.586*
urgent procedures *p.587*

REFERENCES

Administration on Aging. (2005). *A profile of older Americans: 2005.* Retrieved on October 21, 2008 from http://www.aoa.gov/prof/Statistics/profile/2005/2005profile.pdf

American Society of Anesthesiologists. (1999a). *Anesthesiologists warn: If you're taking herbal products, tell your doctor before surgery.* Retrieved on October 21, 2008 from http://www.asahq.org/publiceducation/herbal.html

American Society of Anesthesiologists. (1999b). Practice guidelines for preoperative fasting and the use of pharmacologic agents to reduce the risk of pulmonary aspiration: Application to healthy patients undergoing elective procedures. A report by the American Society of Anesthesiologists Task Force on Preoperative Fasting. *Anesthesiology, 90*(3), 896–905.

American Society of Anesthesiologists. (2001). Ethical guidelines for the anesthesia care of patients with do-not-resuscitate orders or other directives that limit treatment. In *ASA standards, guidelines, and statements* (pp.10–11). Park Ridge, IL: Author.

American Society of Anesthesiologists. (2006a). *ASA standards, guidelines, and statements.* Park Ridge, IL: Author.
American Society of Anesthesiologists. (2006b). Practice guidelines for the perioperative management of patients with obstructive sleep apnea: A report by the American Society of Anesthesiologists Task Force on Perioperative Management of Patients with Obstructive Sleep Apnea. *Anesthesiology, 104*(5), 1081–1093.
American Society of PeriAnesthesia Nurses. (2006a). ASPAN's evidence-based clinical practice guideline for the prevention and/or management of PONV/PDNV. *Journal of PeriAnesthesia Nursing, 21*(4), 230–250.
American Society of PeriAnesthesia Nurses. (2006b). *Standards of perianesthesia nursing practice.* New Jersey: Author.
Asilioglu, K., & Celik, S. (2004). The effect of preoperative education on anxiety of open cardiac surgery patients. *Patient Education and Counseling, 1,* 65–70.
Association of periOperative Registered Nurses. (1999). *Perioperative care of patients with do-not-resuscitate (DNR) orders.* Adopted 1995; reaffirmed October 1999. Retrieved from http:// www.aorn.org/about/positions/dnr.htm
Association of periOperative Registered Nurses. (2005). *AORN standards, recommended practices, and guidelines.* Denver: Author.
Barrera, R., Shi, W., Amar, D., Thaler, H., Gabovich, N., Bains, M., et al. (2005). Smoking and timing of cessation: Impact on pulmonary complications after thoracotomy. *Chest, 127,* 1977–1991.
Beck, F., & Rosenthal, T. (2002). Prealbumin: A marker for nutritional evaluation. *American Family Physician, 65,* 1575–1578.
Bennett, J., & Brown, C. (2000). Use of herbal remedies by patients in a health maintenance organization. *Journal of the American Pharmacology Association, 40*(3), 353–358.
Bernier, M., Sanares, D., Owen, S., & Newhouse, P. (2003). Preoperative teaching received and valued in a day surgery setting. *AORN Journal, 77,* 563–582.
Blondin, M. (2006). *Prevention of deep vein thrombosis.* Iowa City, IA: University of Iowa Gerontological Nursing Research Center, Research Dissemination Core.
Bond, L., Flickinger, D., Aytes, L., Bateman, B., Chalk, M. B., & Aysse, P. (2005). Effects of preoperative teaching of the use of a pain scale with patients in the PACU. *Journal of PeriAnesthesia Nursing, 20*(5), 333–340.
Bradley, D., Creswell, L., Hogue, C., Epstein, A., Prystowsky, E., & Daoud, E. (2005). Pharmacologic prophylaxis: American College of Chest Physicians guidelines for the prevention and management of postoperative atrial fibrillation after cardiac surgery. *Chest, 128,* 39S–48S.
Bratzler, D., & Houck, P. (2004). Antimicrobial prophylaxis for surgery: An advisory statement from the National Surgical Infection Prevention Project. *Clinical Infectious Disease, 28*(12), 1706.
Bray, A. (2006). Preoperative nursing assessment of the surgical patient. *Nursing Clinics of North America, 41,* 135–150.
Brooks, D., Crowe, J., Kelsey, C., Lacy, J., Parsons, J., & Solway, S. (2001). A clinical practice guideline on peri-operative cardiorespiratory physical therapy. *Physiotherapy Canada, 53*(1), 9–25.
Brooks-Brunn, J. (2000). Risk factors associated with postoperative pulmonary complications following total abdominal hysterectomy. *Clinical Nursing Research, 9*(1), 25–46.
Centers for Disease Control and Prevention. (2008). *National Center for Health Statistics: Monitoring this nations health.* Retrieved on June 24, 2008 from http://www.cdc.gov/nchs
Chang, J., Morton, S., Rubenstein, L., Mojica, W., Maglione, M., Suttorp, M., et al. (2004). Interventions for the prevention of falls in older adults: Systematic review and meta-analysis of randomized clinical trials. *BMJ, 328*(7441), 653–657.
Costa, M. (2001). The lived perioperative experience of ambulatory surgery patients. *AORN Journal, 74,* 874–881.
Crenshaw, J., & Winslow, E. (2002). Preoperative fasting: Old habits die hard. *American Journal of Nursing, 102*(5), 36–44.
Cunningham, M. F., Hanson-Heath, C., & Agre, P. (2003). A perioperative nurse liaison program: CNS interventions for cancer patients and their families. *Journal of Nursing Care Quality, 18*(1), 16–21.
Deyirmenjian, M., Karam, N., & Salameh, P. (2006). Preoperative patient education for open-heart patients: A source of anxiety? *Patient Education and Counseling, 62*(1), 111–117.
Doering, L., McGuire, A., & Rourke, D. (2002). Recovering from cardiac surgery: What patients want you to know. *American Journal of Critical Care, 11*(4), 333–343.
Eagle, K., Berger, P., Calkins, H., Chaitman, B., Ewy, G., Fleischmann, K., et al. (2002). *ACC/AHA guideline update for perioperative cardiovascular evaluation for non-cardiac surgery: A report of the American College of Cardiology/American Heart Association Task Force on Practice Guidelines (Committee to Update the 1996 Guidelines on perioperative cardiovascular evaluation for non-cardiac surgery).* Retrieved from American College of Cardiology website: http://www.acc.org/clinical/guidelines/perio/dirIndex.htm
Evans, D., Hodgkinson, B., Lambert, L., & Wood, J. (2001). Fall risk factors in the hospital setting: A systematic review. *International Journal of Nursing Practice, 7,* 38–45.
Elkins, G., Staniunas, R., Rajab, H., Marcus, J., & Snyder, T. (2004). Use of a numeric visual analog anxiety scale among patients undergoing colorectal surgery. *Clinical Nursing Research, 13*(3), 237–245.
Fleisher, L., Beckman, J., Brown, K., Calkins, H., Chaikof, E., Fleischmann, K., et al. (2006). ACC/AHA 2006 guideline update on perioperative cardiovascular evaluation for noncardiac surgery: Focused update on perioperative beta-blocker therapy. *Journal of the American College of Cardiology, 47*(11).
Gandhi, G., Nuttall, G., Abel, M., Mullany, C., Schaff, H., O'Brien, P., et al. (2007). Intensive intraoperative insulin therapy versus conventional glucose management during cardiac surgery: A randomized trial. *Annals of Internal Medicine, 146*(4), 233–243, I29–I32.
Gandhi, G., Nuttall, G., Abel, M., Mullany, C., Schaff, H., Williams, A., et al. (2005). Intraoperative hyperglycemia and perioperative outcomes in cardiac surgery patients. *Mayo Clinic Proceedings, 80,* 862–868.
Golembiewski, J. (2004). Antibiotic prophylaxis for preventing surgical site infection. *Journal of PeriAnesthesia Nursing, 19*(2), 111–113.
Guenaga, K. (2002). Preoperative bowel cleansing. *Seminars in Colon & Rectal Surgery, 13*(1), 53–61.
Guruge, S., & Sidani, S. (2002). Effects of demographic characteristics on preoperative teaching outcomes: A meta analysis. *Canadian Journal of Nursing Research, 34*(4), 25–33.
Hatcher, T. (2001). The proverbial herb. *American Journal of Nursing, 101*(2), 36–43.
Heizenroth, P. A. (1999). Positioning the patient for surgery. In M. Meeker & J. Rothrock (Eds.), *Care of the patient in surgery* (pp. 153–172). Philadelphia: Mosby.
Hering, K., Harvan, J., Dangelo, M., & Jasinski, D. (2005). The use of a computer website prior to scheduled surgery: Impact on patient information, acquisition, anxiety level, and overall satisfaction with anesthesia care. *AANA Journal, 73*(1), 29–33.
Heye, M., Foster, L., Bartlett, M. K., & Adkins, S. (2002). A preoperative intervention for pain reduction, improved mobility, and self-efficacy. *Applied Nursing Research, 16*(2), 174–183.
Hulzebos, E., DeBie, R., Favie, N., Helders, J., De La Riviere, A., & Van Meeteren, N. (2006). Preoperative intensive inspiratory muscle training to prevent postoperative pulmonary complications in high-risk patients undergoing CABG surgery: A randomized clinical trial. *JAMA, 296* (15), 1851–1858.
Institute for Clinical Symptoms Improvement. (2006). *Preoperative evaluation.* Retrieved on October 21, 2008 from http://www.icsi.org/preoperative_evaluation/preoperative_evaluation_2328.html. Bloomington, MN: Author.
Institute for Healthcare Improvement. (2006). *Reducing surgical complications.* Retrieved on October 21, 2008 from http://www.ihi.org/IHI/Programs
Johansson, K., Salantera, S., Heikkinen, K., Kuusisto, A., Virtanen, H., & Leino-Kilpi, H. (2004). Surgical patient education: Assessing the interventions and exploring the outcomes from experimental and quasiexperimental studies from 1990 to 2003. *Clinical Effectiveness in Nursing, 8*(2), 81–92.
Leske, J. S. (2000). Family stresses, strengths and outcomes after critical injury. *Critical Care Nursing Clinics of North America, 12*(2), 237–244.
Letterstal, A., Sandstrom, V., Olofsson, P., & Forsberg, C. (2004). Postoperative mobilization of patients with abdominal aortic aneurysm. *Journal of Advanced Nursing, 48*(6), 560–568.
Lin, L. Y., & Wang, R. (2005). Abdominal surgery, pain and anxiety: Preoperative nursing intervention. *Journal of Advanced Nursing, 51*(3), 252–260.
Madsen, M., Brosnan, J., & Nagy, V. (1998). Perioperative thirst: A patient perspective. *Journal of PeriAnesthesia Nursing, 13*(4), 225–228.
Mangram, A., Horan, T., Pearson, M., Silver, L., & Jarvis, W. (1999). Guideline for prevention of surgical site infection. Centers for Disease Control and Prevention, Hospital Infection Control Practices Advisory Committee. *Infection Control and Hospital Epidemiology, 20*(4), 247–280.
Maurer, W., Borkowski, R., & Parker, B. (2004). Quality and resource utilization in managing preoperative evaluation. *Anesthesiology Clinics of North America, 22,* 155–175.
McDonald, S., Hetrick, S., & Green, S. (2006). Pre-operative education for hip or knee replacement. *The Cochrane Library, 4* (CD003526).
Meeker, M., & Rothrock, J. (1999). *Care of the patient in surgery.* Philadelphia: Mosby.
Merli, G. (2000). Prophylaxis for deep venous thrombosis and pulmonary embolism in the surgical patient. *Clinical Cornerstone, 2*(4), 15–25.
Muravchick, S. (2004). *Geriatric anesthesia—Are you ready?* Retrieved April 26, 2004, from ASA Syllabus on Geriatric Anesthesiology, http://www.asahq.org/clinical/geriatrics/geron.htm
Neil, J. (2007). Perioperative care of the immunocompromised patient. *AORN Journal, 85*(3), 544–565.
Nichols, R. L. (2001). Preventing surgical site infections: A surgeon's perspective. *Emerging Infectious Diseases, 7*(2), 220–224.
Niel-Weise, B., Willie, J., & van den Broek, P. (2005). Hair removal policies in clean surgery: Systematic review of randomized, controlled trials. *Infection Control and Hospital Epidemiology, 26*(12), 923–928.
O'Donnell, M., Kearon, C., Johnson, J., Robinson, R., Zondag, M., Turpie, I., et al. (2007). Preoperative anticoagulant activity after bridging low-molecular-weight heparin for temporary interruption of warfarin. *Annals of Internal Medicine, 146*(3), 184–187.
Oetker-Black, S., Jones, S., Estok, P., Ryan, M., Gale, N., & Parker, C. (2003). Preoperative teaching and hysterectomy outcomes. *AORN Journal, 77*(6), 1215–1227.
Orfanos, P., Ellis, E., & Johnston, C. (1999). Effects of deep breathing exercises and ambulation on pattern of ventilation in post-operative patients. *Australian Journal of Physiotherapy, 45*(3), 173–182.
Overend, T., Anderson, C., Lucy, S. D., Bhatia, C., Jonsson, B., & Timmermans, C. (2001). The effect of incentive spirometry on postoperative pulmonary complications. *Chest, 120*(3), 971–978.
Owens, T. (2006). Bariatric surgery risks, benefits, and care of the morbidly obese. *Nursing Clinics of North America, 41,* 249–263.
Pagana, K. (2007). Laboratory and diagnostic testing: A perioperative update. *AORN Journal, 85*(4), 754–762.
Pan, W., Pintar, T., Anton, J., Lee, V., Vaughn, W., & Collard, C. (2004). Statins are associated with a reduced incidence of perioperative mortality after coronary artery bypass graft surgery. *Circulation, 110*(11), S45–S49.
Pasero, C., & Belden, J. (2006). Evidence-based perianesthesia care: Accelerated postoperative recovery programs. *Journal of PeriAnesthesia Nursing, 21*(3), 168–176.
Pribitkin, E., & Boger, G. (2000). Surgery and herbal therapy: Essential guidelines on bleeding, skin reactions, and wound healing. *Complementary Health Practice Review, 6*(1), 29–40.
Price, M., Whitney, J., & King, C. (2005). Development of a risk assessment tool for intraoperative pressure ulcers. *The Journal of Wound, Ostomy and Continence Nursing, 32*(1), 19–30.
Qaseem, A., Snow, V., Fitterman, N., Hornbake, R., Lawrence, V., Smetana, G., et al. (2006). Risk assessment for and strategies to reduce perioperative pulmonary complications for patients undergoing noncardiothoracic surgery: A guideline from the American College of Physicians. *Annals of Internal Medicine, 144*(8), 575–580.
Roberts, C., Baker, F., Hann, D., Runfola, J., Witt, C., McDonald, J., et al. (2005). Patient–physician communication regarding use of complementary therapies during cancer treatment. *Journal of Psychosocial Oncology, 23*(4), 35–60.
Rogers, R., Lebkuchner, U., Kammerer-Doak, D., Thompson, P., Walters, M., & Nygaard, E. (2006). Obesity and retropubic surgery for stress incontinence: Is there really an increased risk of intraoperative complications? *American Journal of Obstetrics and Gynecology, 195*(6), 1794–1798.
Rooke, G. A. (2007). *Pacemakers.* Retrieved August 8, 2007, from Association of Veterans Affairs Anesthesiologists, http://www.vaanes.org/FORUMS/pacer.html
Schweon, S. (2006). Stamping out surgical site infection. *RN, 69*(8), 37–40.
Seltzer, J., Horsman, A., & Korniewicz, D. (2002). Awareness of surgical site infections for advanced practice nurses. *AACN Clinical Issues, 13*(3), 398–409.
Smith, M., & Ellis, E. (2000). Is retained mucus a risk factor for the development of postoperative atelectasis and pneumonia? Implications for the physiotherapist. *Physiotherapy Theory and Practice, 16*(2), 69–80.
Smykowski, L., & Rodriguez, W. (2003). The post anesthesia care unit experience: A family centered approach. *Journal of Nursing Care Quality, 18*(1), 5–15.
Soreide, E., & Ljungqvist, O. (2006). Modern preoperative fasting guidelines: A summary of the present recommendations and remaining questions. *Best Practice & Research Clinical Anaesthesiology, 20*(3), 483–491.
Spector, R. (2004). *Cultural diversity in health and illness.* Upper Saddle River, NJ: Pearson Prentice Hall.
Susleck, D., Willocks, A., Secrest, J., Norwood, B., Holweger, J., Davis, M., et al. (2007). The perianesthesia experience from the patient's perspective. *Journal of PeriAnesthesia Nursing, 22*(1), 10–20.
Vallerand, A., Fouladbakhsh, J., & Templin, T. (2005). Patients' choices for the self-treatment of pain. *Applied Nursing Research, 18*(2), 90–96.
Van den Berghe, G., Wouters, P., Weekers, F., Verwaest, C., Bruyninckx, F., Schetz, M., et al. (2001). Intensive insulin therapy in critically ill patients. *New England Journal of Medicine, 345,* 1359–1367.
Walker, K., Smithy, A., & Pittaway, A. (2003). Premedication for anxiety in adult day surgery. *Cochrane Database of Systematic Reviews, 1* (CD002192).
Weindler, J., & Kiefer, R. (2001). The efficacy of postoperative incentive spirometry is influenced by the device-specific imposed work of breathing. *Chest, 119*(6), 1858–1864.
Whitney, J. A., & Parkman, S. (2002). Preoperative physical activity, anesthesia, and analgesia: Effects on early postoperative walking after total hip replacement. *Applied Nursing Research, 15*(1), 19–27.
Yoon, S., Horne, C., & Adams, C. (2004). Herbal product use by African American older women. *Clinical Nursing Research, 13*(4), 271–289.
Yung, W., Mok, Y., Ling, S., Poon, Y., Wong, K., & Yim, C. (2005). Does preoperative intervention program improve postoperative outcome in high-risk patients undergoing thoracic surgery? *Chest, 128,* 337S–339S.

Intraoperative Nursing

Krista Brecht
Krisna Ogerio
Donna Stanbridge
Danielle Vigeant
Suzanne Watt

With contributions by:
Jane Ashley
Kathleen Osborn

Outcome-Based Learning Objectives

After studying this chapter, the learner will be able to:

1. Discuss the sequence of events for the patient from the beginning of surgery to arrival in the postanesthesia care unit.
2. Differentiate the roles of the surgical team.
3. Describe the interplay between each team member in the success of the surgical intervention.
4. Prioritize nursing interventions to maximize patient safety in the operating room.
5. Evaluate effective nursing measures for patient advocacy in the operating room.
6. Prioritize the nursing care of patients experiencing selected intraoperative complications.
7. Differentiate the role of the certified nurse and the anesthesiologist for the anesthetized patient.

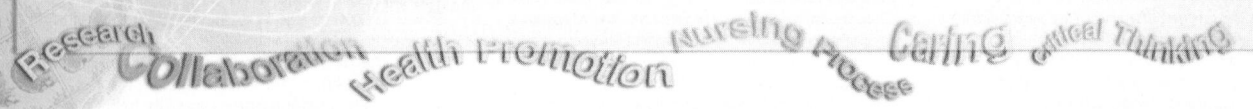

THE GOAL of perioperative or intraoperative nursing practice is to assist patients and their families to achieve a level of wellness equal to or greater than that which they had prior to the procedure (Association of periOperative Registered Nurses [AORN], Perioperative Nursing Data Set (PNDS-2007). The most important role of the perioperative nurse is to be a patient advocate. The essence of the advocacy in the perioperative role is defined as protection, communication (giving a voice), doing, comfort, and caring.

Advocacy is described as an act of informing and supporting the individuals so that they may make the best decisions possible for themselves. It is also speaking up for someone who is unable to speak for himself. Advocacy is a critical issue for surgical patients who are unconscious or sedated and unable to make decisions related to their care. Protecting patients from harm is the essence of the advocacy role of nurses, and it is a critical component for patients whose family members are not readily accessible and whose only possible advocate is the nurse. This is often the case for the patient having surgery. Many perioperative issues involve advocacy. These may include helping patients who are uninformed or have not given adequate consent for surgical procedures, confronting an incompetent colleague, pressing for more analgesia for

a patient in pain, or supporting the patient's view toward prolonging life with extraordinary treatment or technology.

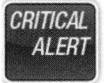 *Surgical patients can be compromised by stress, disease process, and sedation or general anesthesia, and they trust that a perioperative nurse will advocate in their best interest to ensure their privacy, dignity, rights, and safety.*

The nurse must accept accountability for nursing actions that safeguard the rights of the surgical patients. Perioperative nurses act as patient advocates by protecting, and they must be able to quickly and accurately identify advocacy issues and be ready to intervene on behalf of their patients. In recent years, the acceptance of a conceptual model for patient care, published by AORN, has helped to distinguish the relationship of various components of nursing practice and the effect on patient outcomes (Beyea, 2000) (Figure 26–1 ■).

Guidance for Professional Practice

The practice of perioperative nursing is guided by its own professional organization, the Association of periOperative Registered Nurses, as well as the Centers for Disease Control and

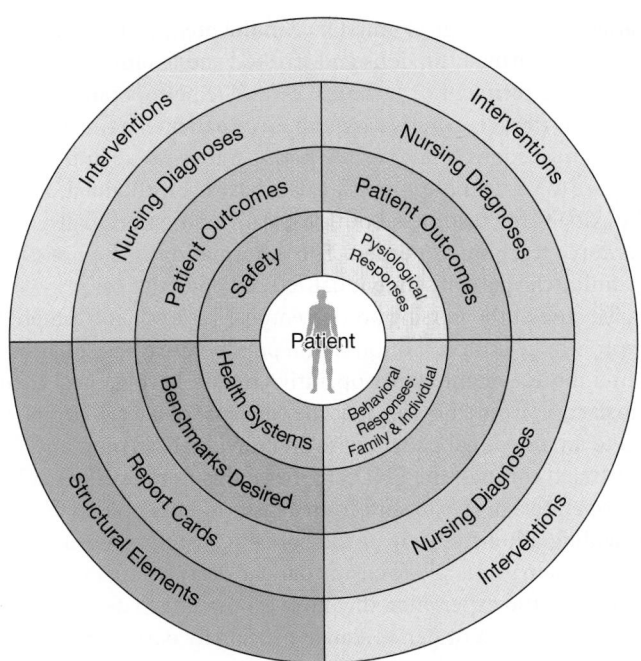

FIGURE 26–1 ■ Perioperative patient-focused model.

Source: Reprinted with permission from "The PNDS model," http://www.aorn.org/PracticeResources/ PNDSAndStandardizedPerioperativeRecord/PNDSModel. Copyright © 2002 AORN, Inc., 2170 South Parker Road, Suite 300, Denver, CO 80231. All rights reserved.

Prevention (CDC) and the Joint Commission. AORN defines its mission as follows: "to promote safety and optimal outcomes for patients undergoing operative and other invasive procedures by providing practice support and professional development opportunities to perioperative nurses." AORN is composed of approximately 41,000 perioperative registered nurses in the United States and abroad who manage, teach, and practice perioperative nursing; who are enrolled in nursing education; and who are engaged in perioperative research (AORN, 2007a). This professional organization has developed a conceptual framework and vocabulary called the Perioperative Nursing Data Set (PNDS). The data set addresses the domains of safety, physiological responses, behavioral responses of the patient and family, and the environment of the perioperative setting within the health system.

The CDC's mission is to promote health and quality of life by preventing and controlling disease, injury, and disability. It also influences perioperative practice. In 1999, the CDC issued guidelines for the prevention of surgical infection. Additionally, it reflected the mission statement of the Joint Commission to continuously improve the safety and quality of care provided to the public through the provision of health care accreditation and related services that support performance improvement in health care organizations (Joint Commission, 2007). The Joint Commission is an independent, not-for-profit organization that is the United States' predominant accrediting body charged with maintaining and improving health care delivery. The Joint Commission's comprehensive accreditation process evaluates an organization's compliance with its standards and other accreditation requirements. Joint Commission accreditation is recognized nationwide as a symbol of quality that reflects an organization's commitment to meeting certain performance standards. To earn and maintain the Joint Commission's Gold Seal of Approval, an organization must undergo an on-site survey by

a Joint Commission survey team at least every 3 years. A complete discussion of the Joint Commission is presented in Chapter 3 .

Surgical Team

Successful surgery relies on the interplay of many individuals working as a team, complementing each other's skills and responsibilities. This multidisciplinary team includes the surgeon and assistants, anesthesiologist and assistants, the nursing team, and support staff. Each of these professionals is responsible for specific functions and plays a role in supporting the other groups. This overlap of responsibilities ensures the safety of patients while they are in a most vulnerable situation of not being able to give any personal input. The roles of each member are described next.

Surgeon

The surgeon heads the surgical team and is responsible for making decisions related to the surgical procedure. Depending on the procedure, an assistant might be required. This assistant could be another surgeon, physician, resident in a university teaching hospital, or the registered nurse first assistant. The surgeon is responsible for performing the procedure and for coordinating the team.

An expanded role for perioperative nurses is that of registered nurse first assistant (RNFA). The RNFA collaborates with the surgeon and performs the role of first assistant during the operation. This role includes handling tissue, providing exposure, using instruments, suturing the wound, and providing hemostasis. The role of an RNFA is highly specialized and demanding. In 2008, AORN approved a policy statement that defines the RNFA role, scope of practice, and qualifications.

Anesthesia Care Provider

The anesthesiologist is a health care provider who specializes in the administration of anesthetic agents and provides care to alleviate pain and promote relaxation. This professional is responsible for maintaining the airway; monitoring and ensuring gas exchanges, respiration, and circulation; estimating and replacing blood and fluid losses; administering medications to maintain hemodynamic stability; managing care in the event of a physiological crisis; and constantly communicating with the surgical and nursing team. The anesthesiologist heads the anesthesia team and might be assisted by a respiratory therapist, anesthesia resident or fellow in a university teaching hospital, or a certified registered nurse anesthetist (CRNA). As Chapter 1 discussed, the CRNA is an advance practice nurse, educated with a master's degree from an accredited nurse anesthesia educational program. CRNAs administer anesthesia and anesthesia-related care in four general categories: (1) preanesthetic preparation and evaluation; (2) anesthesia induction, maintenance, and emergence; (3) postanesthesia care; and (4) perianesthetic and clinical support functions. The CRNA works under the supervision of the anesthesiologist. In a large study examining morbidity associated with anesthesia, researchers found several factors that significantly reduce the risk of anesthesia. Among these are the direct availability of an anesthesiologist during surgery, the presence of a consistent anesthesia care provider throughout the case, and the presence of an anesthetic nurse (Arbous et al., 2005).

Nurses

The perioperative nurse's primary role in the operating room (OR) is that of the circulating nurse. Most states have taken legislative measures in order to ensure the presence of a registered nurse in the circulator role in the OR for every surgical procedure. The circulating nurse's duties are performed outside the sterile field and encompass responsibilities of nursing care management within the OR. The **circulating nurse** observes the surgical team from a broad perspective and assists the team to create and maintain a safe, comfortable environment for surgery. The circulating nurse communicates patient care needs to each member of the surgical team, facilitating a united effort while being the patient advocate whose actions are dedicated to ensuring that the patient's rights and wishes are respected and carried out.

The **scrub nurse** works directly with the surgeon within the sterile field passing instruments, sponges, and other items needed during the surgical procedure. The sterile field is the area closely surrounding the OR table. Surgical team members who work within the sterile field perform a surgical scrub of their hands and arms with special disinfecting solution and, in addition to the regular surgical attire, don a sterile gown and gloves. This role can also be performed by other personnel than an RN, in which case the person is then called a scrub technician. Other roles for RNs are team leader, assistant head nurse, head nurse or nurse manager, nurse educator, and clinical nurse specialist.

As with any specialty, the perioperative nursing assessment is the first step in providing individualized care for perioperative patients. The nursing process serves as a guide to make perioperative nursing assessments comprehensive and holistic in nature. The focus is aimed at promoting and maintaining wellness as well as identifying and preventing illness (Hurley & McAleavy, 2006). These assessments provide valuable information to the entire perioperative team. The nursing care plans that are developed based on the assessment data are utilized to ensure continuity of care during each phase of the individual's perioperative experience. The assessment provides a baseline against which information about the individual's stability can be measured and monitored at any stage of her perioperative experience.

Perioperative Nursing Education

Given that most nursing programs offer limited or no operating room experience in their curricula, nurses initiating a career in the OR get their perioperative education either at the hiring institution or by enrolling in a postgraduate or fellowship perioperative program. It is estimated that a minimum of 3 to 6 months of instruction is required to adequately educate nurses with no previous OR experience depending on the OR's activities (AORN, 2007a). Programs may include the surgical environment, aseptic technique, perioperative assessment, anesthesia, positioning the surgical patient, sterilization and disinfection, surgical instruments, safety considerations, patient teaching, teamwork, scrubbing and circulating, and wound healing and hemostasis (AORN, 2007a). In addition to didactic modules, nurses are often instructed through a cognitive apprenticeship model in the OR in which they take on increasingly complex responsibilities over time.

Health Promotion

Patient teaching for the **intraoperative** patient is usually done in a preadmission testing clinic or the day before the surgery in a patient general surgical unit. Once in the preoperative area, the patient is normally anxious and stressed and assumes a passive role as the recipient of technical care. The perioperative nurse performs the preoperative assessment of patients in the holding area. The responsibilities of the perioperative nurse in this setting are to verify the appropriate data have been obtained, assess the patient for readiness both physically and emotionally, and reinforce teaching as needed. This information is the basis for planning the patient's individualized perioperative care.

The use of the nursing process emphasizes a patient-centered approach; health promotion in the perioperative arena has become more evident as perioperative nurses have gained great satisfaction from knowing that they are part of a team committed to an individual patient with an individualized outcome. As illustrated through the PNDS (p. 624), this framework enables perioperative nurses to shift from a task-oriented role to that of providing a holistic view of the patient. Therefore, even if the nurse's main role is still to ensure patient safety throughout a patient's surgical experience, the nurse is now able to demonstrate the caring aspect of perioperative nursing by participating in a preoperative assessment of the patient.

Surgical Areas

Patients needing surgery go to the operating room for a surgical procedure after having been admitted to the hospital on the same day as surgery, unless an extensive work-up or in-hospital treatments or tests are required prior to surgery. Patients also access the operating room emergently through the emergency department. The practice of same-day admission has become popular for both financial reasons and because evidence suggests that surgical-site infection rates are reduced when the preoperative stay is reduced (Nichols, 2001).

Prior to being admitted to the surgical setting, the patient dons a gown and cap. Surgical-site skin preparation includes a baseline assessment, cleaning of the surgical site and surrounding area, hair removal, and application of an antiseptic agent when required. Traditionally hair removal was extensive and often performed the day prior to surgery. Research studies have revealed that hair removal does not reduce the incidence of surgical-site infections (SSIs). In fact, today, hair removal is instead performed to improve access to surgical site, improve the field of view, or per the institution's policy or surgeon's preference (Evidence-based practice information sheets, 2003; Niel-Weise, Willie, & van den Broek, 2005). Should hair removal be indicated, care needs to be taken to maintain skin integrity and minimize injury. The removal is ideally done outside of the surgical suite as close to the surgery time as possible (AORN, 2007b). There is some evidence that use of hair clippers is superior to use of a razor, but more research is needed (Niel-Weise et al., 2005).

Presurgical or Preoperative Holding Area

The surgical area typically has a presurgical or preoperative holding area next to the operating rooms. The preoperative holding area is a *semirestricted* area usually just inside of the surgical area. This area provides a quiet, calm transition area for the patient to wait immediately before surgery. It provides a shield from the sights and sounds of the busy surgical suite and allows personnel to interview the patient and verify the documentation. Equipment should be readily available in the preoperative holding area for patient care and monitoring. This includes oxygen, suction, electrocardiogram machine, pulse oximetry, and a blood pressure cuff; an emergency medical cart and defibrillator should be nearby (Bailey, McVey, & Pevreal, 2005; Sullivan, 2000).

In the holding area, the nurse must verify that all the relevant documents and studies (films, scans, etc.) are available prior to the start of the procedure, that they have been reviewed and are consistent with each other, and with the patient involved. Team consensus about the intended patient, procedure, and site and as applicable implant is also needed. This verification should occur before the patient leaves the preoperative area and enters the procedure/surgical room.

When the operating room suite is ready to receive the patient, the patient is asked to empty the bladder to prevent incontinence or overdistention because an overly full bladder can hinder access to the surgical site and predispose the patient to inadvertent surgical bladder injury. Urinary catheterization is performed in the OR as necessary (Iorio et al., 2005). The nurse accompanies the patient to the operating room where the patient will be placed on the operating table and prepared for surgery.

Preoperative Operating Room Checklist

The preoperative checklist is a tool for continuing the patient assessment. On it, allergies are documented as per facility policy. Accurate documentation of height and weight is important for proper dosage calculation of the anesthetic agents. The perioperative nurse ensures that the results of all laboratory, radiographic, and diagnostic tests are on the patient's chart.

Any abnormal results are documented and reported to the surgical team as well as any special needs, concerns, or instructions especially with regard to cultural or spiritual beliefs, physical impairments or limitations, and psychosocial conditions. For example, advise the surgical team whether the patient is a member of Jehovah's Witnesses and does not accept blood products or whether the patient is hard of hearing and does not have his hearing aid (Hurley & McAleavy, 2006). Showing respect for patients' spiritual beliefs, psychosocial conditions, and physical limitations facilitates rapport and trust that enable nurses to understand the important role these factors play in how people cope with fear and anxiety related to their perceived perioperative experience.

The perioperative nurse also notes the medical diagnosis, previous surgical experience, patient's physical appearance, visual skin assessment, medical devices accompanying the patient or indwelling medical devices, and any prostheses, jewelry, dentures, and/or capped teeth. The nurse also ensures that prescribed preoperative medications have been taken by the patient and any medications that have been ordered to be given just prior to surgery such as antibiotics are documented on the chart accompanying the patient. The NPO status of the patient is also confirmed by the nurse to assess any potential risk of aspiration. All relevant information is communicated to the surgical team.

Operating Room

Surgery may involve the removal, repair, drainage, replacement, or exploration of body tissue or organs. The operating room or suite is where the surgery will be performed. This room is a *restricted* area where the team of health care professionals wears attire that was donned in the surgery dressing room. This attire, commonly referred to as "scrubs," includes a shirt, trousers, cap, shoe covers, and mask. Those directly involved in the surgical procedure will have scrubbed and will be wearing sterile gowns.

Surgical hand preparation, previously known as a "surgical scrub," is performed prior to participating in a surgical procedure in order to reduce the potential risk of SSI by reducing the number of microorganisms on intact skin of the hands and forearms. Hand preparation considerations include use of a broad-spectrum, fast-acting, nonirritating, FDA-approved antiseptic agent. Traditional scrub techniques with prolonged use of detergent, water, and brushes have contributed to the deterioration of skin, sometimes leading to undesirable changes of hand skin flora and colonization. Additionally, surgical facilities are examining ways to improve the use of physical resources and health care professionals' time. Compared to the traditional surgical scrub, waterless hand preparation boasts a reduction in microbial counts of hands, improved skin health, and reduced use of time and resources (Larson et al., 2001). Below is a list of recommended surgical hand preparation practices (AORN, 2007b), and Chart 26–1 (p. 622) highlights the differences between a surgical scrub and hand rub preparation method:

- Do not wear artificial nails.
- Keep skin free from open lesions and breaks.
- Remove all jewelry from hands and forearms before performing hand hygiene.
- Use only lotions that are approved by infection control staff; lotions must be compatible with the hand antiseptic and gloves, and be stored in disposable, hands-free dispensers.
- Use a standardized hand scrub procedure that follows manufacturer's written guidelines and is approved by the health care facility.

Due to the rapid growth of surgical technologies and innovation during the past decade, many operating rooms have been renovated or reconstructed. This has been done in part to address the abundance of equipment needed in today's operating rooms as well as ergonomic issues. Recent trends in surgery include the move toward less invasive techniques with shorter hospital stays and faster recovery periods. One of the newest trends promising to transform surgery is the *intelligent OR*. The intelligent OR incorporates advanced robotic surgical systems. A speech recognition robot allows the surgeon to control the operating bed, lighting, video displays, and other devices with simple voice commands. A robotic endoscopic camera facilitates optimal views of the surgical field, and the robotic surgical assistant enables the surgeon to control precise technical movements of a robotic arm from a console station. Robotic systems are currently in use for certain cardiac procedures with plans for expansion on the horizon. Surgical robots make it likely that future surgeries could be performed at one facility with the surgeon operating the console from a distant facility. One of the nurse's roles in robotic surgery is to assist the surgeon at the patient's side during the operation.

In addition digital information is becoming the standard format for accessing patient information and images, for communicating with other areas of the hospital or consultants, and for conferring with other health care providers. The operating

CHART 26–1 Traditional and Waterless Surgical Hand Preparation

Traditional Surgical Hand Preparation	**Waterless Surgical Hand Preparation**
1. Wash hands with soap and water.	1. Wash hands with soap and water.
2. Use a disposable nail cleaner to clean nail beds under running water. Discard nail cleaner after use.	2. Use a disposable nail cleaner to clean nail beds under running water. Discard nail cleaner after use.
3. Rinse. Wash hands, then forearms, using antimicrobial-impregnated sponge. Use the counted stroke technique or the recommended amount of time according to the manufacturer's instructions.	3. Rinse and thoroughly dry hands and arms. Apply alcohol-based surgical hand scrub product according to manufacturer's instructions.
4. Rinse.	4. Proceed to operating room.
5. Proceed to operating room.	

Note: Step 2 is performed for the first scrub of the day or as required.

Scrub time for step 3 may vary according to product instructions from 3 to 5 minutes.

Note: Step 2 is performed for the first scrub of the day or as required. Hand preparation time for step 3 generally requires 2 minutes.

room requires convenient real-time access to these digital data and a way to manage the digital information acquired within the operating room. OR design may be categorized into three major areas: physical, information and communication systems, and management.

To accommodate an optimal workflow and facilitate observation of aseptic technique, certain physical considerations need to be taken into account, including the dimensions of the OR suite, positions of exits and entrances, and location of support services. In addition, integration systems are available that permit the control of medical devices, lighting, and the OR bed; access to images; and the routing of all this digital information to any particular monitor for display or to one or more recording devices for archiving, or to pathologists or radiologists via teleconferencing links. Control can be maintained from the surgical field by touch-screen or voice control interfaces, or from a nursing station (Figure 26–2 ■).

Intentional OR design considers the logistics of flow, maintains versatility, optimizes the use of resources, promotes communication, synchronizes services, and adopts technological advances while including all stakeholders in order to promote

successful adoption. The ultimate goal of surgical technology adoption is to enhance patient care and improve patient outcomes.

Surgical table setup is specific to the procedure, facility, and surgeon preference. Scrub tables are often standardized in order to facilitate efficiency and changeover of staff. Instruments vary according to specialty and type of procedure. Figure 26–3 ■ displays the contrast between traditional open surgery and endoscopic instrumentation.

Other perioperative nursing responsibilities include ensuring proper instrument functionality intraoperatively through cleaning and inspection. Inadvertent patient injury may occur due to an instrument malfunction, resulting in an undesirable effect such as tearing tissue, loss of small parts inside the patient, or improper reprocessing leaving a residue of bioburden that can result in postoperative complications. The use of protocols, checklists, and detailed documentation of OR equipment is associated with a significant decrease in perioperative patient injury (Arbous et al., 2005). The majority of surgical instruments are composed of high-grade stainless steel, although advances in surgery such as robotics and minimally invasive surgery (MIS) have resulted in in-

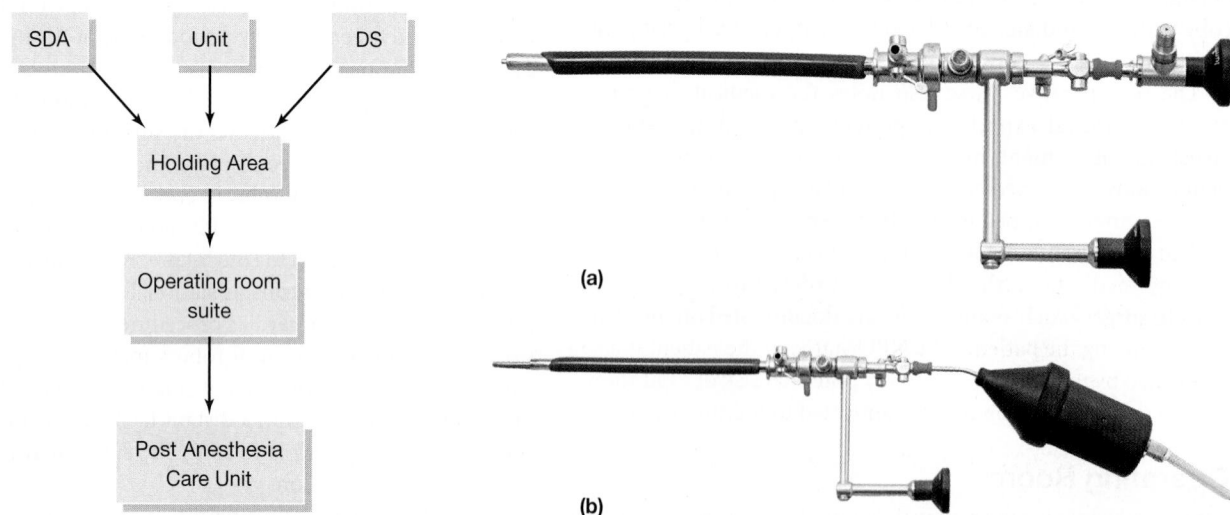

FIGURE 26–2 ■ Layout of a typical surgical unit. (Note: SDA=Same day surgery, DS=day surgery)

FIGURE 26–3 ■ Surgical instruments : (A) traditional versus (B) endoscopic.
Source: © J. Barabe/Custom Medical Stock Photo

novative discoveries of surgical materials and instruments. Surgical instruments are costly and require proper maintenance and care in order to preserve their longevity.

Patient Preparation

Once they enter the surgical suite, patients are cared for by the anesthetist, surgeons, and nurses. Members of the team ask the patient questions, apply electrocardiogram (ECG) leads, remove arms from gown, and so forth. Every effort should be made to limit activity with the patient until she has received a general anesthetic or been given a relaxant if warranted. For example, a patient should have the bladder catheterized following the general anesthetic whenever possible. Also, patients should be kept informed on an ongoing basis. This will prevent and limit anxieties created by the already stressful surgical experience. If regional anesthesia is being used, the patient will remain awake; therefore, a screen is placed in front of the patient's face. Sedatives, hypnotics, or tranquilizers are administered in order to decrease feelings of anxiety and provide sedation.

The perioperative nurse greets the patient on arrival by first asking the patient his name and checks this with the patient's identification bracelet, chart, and hospital card using at least two identifiers, for example, name and date of birth. The nurse reviews the patient's chart, the medical record, and preoperative checklist, and ensures that the consent is signed and that all documentation, preoperative procedures, and orders have been completed. The nurse conducts the preanesthetic assessment by looking at the patient from a holistic viewpoint. This means recognizing the individual person as a dynamic entity made up of components that are continuously interacting with one another. The perioperative nursing assessment is the first step in providing individualized care to the perioperative patient. To harmonize care in all perioperative settings, the Perioperative Nursing Data Set vocabulary can be used as part of the data collection tool (Chart 26–2, p. 624). The PNDS describes the practice of perioperative nursing practice in four domains: safety, physiological responses, behavioral responses, and health care systems. The first three domains reflect phenomena of concern to perioperative nurses and are composed of nursing diagnoses, interventions, and outcomes that surgical patients and their families experience. The fourth domain, the health care system, comprises structural data elements and focuses on clinical processes and outcomes. The model is used to depict the relationship of nursing process components to the achievement of optimal patient outcomes (AORN, 2002).

Comprehensively written nursing care plans have been specifically adapted to the perioperative environment as clinical pathways. Because of the fast-paced environment of the OR, patients' short lengths of stay, and the many routines, some procedures and protocols can be documented on a flow sheet.

Surgical Approaches

Minimally invasive surgery became widespread when the laparoscopic cholecystectomy became a standard of surgical care in the early 1990s. Initial reservations included the limitations of equipment, introduction of new instruments, and the ability of surgeons to adapt and acquire these new surgical skills. Other

concerns included performing surgery on larger patients and the spreading of cancer cells intraoperatively. The latter concerns have been overcome through advances in equipment and instrumentation and adaptive surgical techniques that have enabled the use of laparoscopic gastric bypass surgery for bariatric patients. Study reports confirm MIS to be oncologically safe (Bonjer et al., 2007). The laparoscopic cholecystectomy will be used to illustrate the differences between MIS and open surgery. Open surgery involves an incision under the rib cage on the right side of approximately 15 to 38 cm (6 to 15 in.) in order to allow surgeons access with their hands to perform surgery.

Laparoscopic removal of the gallbladder involves several small incisions, usually four, that are one-quarter to one-half inch in size. Trocars or ports (tubes with valves) are then inserted through these small incisions in order to provide imaging through a telescope attached to a camera for viewing on a monitor while other ports are accessed for instruments used to perform the surgery. To provide space to view and perform surgery, the abdomen is inflated with gas (usually carbon dioxide). Carbon dioxide is used because it is readily accessible, inexpensive, does not support combustion when using surgical energy sources, and is easily absorbed and excreted by the body through the circulatory and respiratory system. In addition, the smaller incisions available with MIS require the use of finer instruments as shown in Figure 26–3b ■ (p. 622) resulting in less surgical trauma and immunosuppression than open surgery (Boo et al., 2007).

Advantages of a laparoscopic surgery over open surgery include less scarring, quicker recovery, shorter hospitalization, faster return to normal activities (work), fewer problems with incisions, less pain, and less use of opioids, which reduces the negative secondary effects associated with opioid use. Often patients undergoing laparoscopic surgery will be discharged the same day as surgery, whereas open surgery procedures can require 3 to 5 days of hospitalization. The intraoperative cost of MIS surgery is often more, but is offset by the reduced hospital stay and quicker recovery (Noblett & Horgan, 2007).

 Many patients complain of discomfort similar to muscle ache in the shoulder area following laparoscopic surgery. This is a referred pain and is due to the distention of the diaphragm, which results from the insufflation of the abdomen with gas that is required for laparoscopic procedures. The discomfort usually subsides within 24 to 48 hours postoperatively.

The Future of Surgery: Natural Orifice Transluminal Endoscopic Surgery

Natural Orifice Transluminal Endoscopic Surgery (NOTES) is the exploration of methods to perform surgery through any of the body's natural orifices (e.g., oral, rectal, urethral, vaginal). NOTES attempts to further minimize the effects of surgery through a totally noninvasive technique.

Anesthesia

Advances in anesthesia, such as improvements in airway devices, use of quickly reversible inhalation agents, and selection of short-acting anesthetic agents, have improved patient outcomes (Arbous et al., 2005; Tarrac, 2006). Anesthesia needs to accomplish several things. It must produce sleep (hypnosis), lack of

| CHART 26–2 | Perioperative Nursing Data Set | | | |

Code	Diagnosis/Intervention/Outcome	Yes	No	Comments
X29	Diagnosis: *Risk of Injury* related to transfer and transport			
I26	Intervention: Confirms identity before the operative or invasive procedure.			
I126	Intervention: Verifies operative procedure.			
I60	Intervention: Identifies baseline tissue perfusion.			
I65	Intervention: Identifies physiological barriers to communication.			
I66	Intervention: Identifies physiological status.			
I59	Intervention: Identifies baseline cardiac function.			
I64	Intervention: Identifies physical alterations that may affect procedure-specific positioning.			
	AORN Outcome: *Patient is free from signs and symptoms of injury related to transfer/transport.*			
X4	Diagnosis: *Risk for Anxiety* related to knowledge deficit and stress of surgery			
I13	Intervention: Assesses coping mechanisms based on psychological status.			
I27	Intervention: Provides continuity of care.			
I30	Intervention: Develops individualized plan of care.			
I57	Intervention: Identifies and reports philosophical, cultural, and spiritual beliefs and values.			
I85	Intervention: Minimizes the length of invasive procedure by planning care.			
I101	Intervention: Provides care to each individual in a manner that preserves and protects the patient's autonomy, dignity, and human rights.			
I106	Intervention: Provides instruction based on age and identified need.			
I56	Intervention: Explains expected sequence of events.			
I50	Intervention: Evaluates response to instructions.			
	AORN Outcome: *Patient participates in decision making affecting the perioperative plan of care.*			
X38	Diagnosis: *Risk for Acute/Chronic Pain*			
I24	Intervention: Collaborates in initiating patient-controlled analgesia.			
I51	Intervention: Evaluates response to medication.			
I61	Intervention: Identifies cultural and value components related to pain.			
I69	Intervention: Implements alternative methods of pain control.			
I71	Intervention: Implements pain guidelines.			
I108	Intervention: Provides pain management instructions.			
I16	Intervention: Assesses pain control.			
I54	Intervention: Evaluates response to pain management interventions.			
	AORN Outcome: *Patient demonstrates and/or reports adequate pain control throughout the perioperative period.*			
X28	Diagnosis: *Risk for Infection*			
I3	Intervention: Administers care to invasive device sites.			
I21	Intervention: Assesses susceptibility for infections.			
I22	Intervention: Classifies surgical wound.			
I94	Intervention: Performs skin preparation.			
I31	Intervention: Dresses wound at completion of procedure.			
	AORN Outcome: *Patient is free from signs and symptoms of infection.*			
X29	Diagnosis: *Risk for Injury*			
I11	Intervention: Applies safety devices.			
I39	Intervention: Evaluates for signs and symptoms of injury to skin and tissue.			
I72	Intervention: Implements protective measures to prevent injury due to electrical sources.			
I73	Intervention: Implements protective measures to prevent injury due to laser sources.			
I77	Intervention: Implements protective measures to prevent skin/tissue injury due to mechanical sources.			
I93	Intervention: Performs required counts.			
I84	Intervention: Manages specimen handling and disposition.			
I112	Intervention: Records devices implanted during the operative or invasive procedure.			
	AORN Outcome: *Patient is free from signs and symptoms of physical injury.*			
X40	Diagnosis: *Risk for Injury: Positioning*			
I38	Intervention: Applies safety devices.			
I39	Intervention: Evaluates for signs and symptoms of injury to skin and tissue.			
I77	Intervention: Implements protective measures to prevent skin/tissue injury due to mechanical devices.			
	AORN Outcome: *Patient is free from signs and symptoms of injury related to positioning.*			

CHART 26–2	Perioperative Nursing Data Set—*Continued*			
Code	**Diagnosis/Intervention/Outcome**	**Yes**	**No**	**Comments**
X30	Diagnosis: *Deficient Knowledge*			
I19	Intervention: Assesses readiness to learn based on physiological status.			
I20	Intervention: Assesses readiness to learn based on psychological status.			
I79	Intervention: Includes family and support persons in the preoperative teaching.			
I103	Intervention: Provides information and explains Patient Self-Determination Act.			
I67	Intervention: Identifies psychological barriers to communication.			
I63	Intervention: Identifies individual values and wishes concerning care.			
I30	Intervention: Develops individualized plan of care.			
I104	Intervention: Provides instruction about prescribed medications.			
I105	Intervention: Provides instruction about wound healing and wound care. *AORN Outcome: Patient demonstrates knowledge of the expected responses to the operative or other invasive procedure.*			

awareness and recall (amnesia), freedom from pain (analgesia), and muscle relaxation. A variety of anesthetic agents can produce these effects. The anesthesia care provider considers the patient and selects the agent or a combination of agents that will produce the best anesthesia with the fewest negative effects for the patient.

Inhalation Agents

Inhalation agents are frequently used for anesthesia because they are fast acting and easily controlled. Anesthetic agents pass through a vaporizer and are mixed with oxygen. The patient inhales the vapors into the lungs. The gas crosses the alveolar membrane, dissolves in the blood, and is carried to body tissues via circulation where it attaches to receptor sites on the cells to produce its effects, primarily depression of the central nervous system (CNS). Frequently, a mixture of gases is used to maintain anesthesia.

A number of theories have been proposed to explain how inhaled anesthetic agents work, but no single theory explains the various effects seen with these agents (Hoffer, 1999). The effects of anesthesia diminish as the gas is washed out of the lungs with 100% oxygen and the remainder is metabolized by the liver. The Pharmacology Summary box (p. 626) lists the advantages, the side effects, and implications of commonly used anesthetic gases.

Intravenous Agents

A variety of intravenous (IV) agents are used to induce and maintain anesthesia. The Pharmacology Summary box (p. 627) lists common intravenous medications used for anesthesia or as adjuncts to anesthesia. Induction of anesthesia may be accomplished with the administration of a sedative hypnotic or anxiolytic drug. Common drugs include barbiturates such as thiopental sodium (Pentothal) and sodium methohexital (Brevital). These drugs cause rapid, short-acting depression of the CNS (sedative hypnotic), but they have limited analgesic effects. A smaller test dose is initially given to make sure the patient tolerates the mediation without reaction. These drugs quickly (within seconds) produce sedation and unconsciousness. Both drugs can cause respiratory and cardiovascular depression.

Nonbarbiturate drugs that depress the CNS may also be used to induce anesthesia. Etomidate (Amidate) produces rapid hypnosis but with less effect on the respiratory and cardiovascular systems than the barbiturate drugs. This makes it an attractive alternative for use with high-risk patients. Etomidate suppresses cortisol secretion causing hypotension. These effects are not significant in short procedures but can be an issue in longer surgeries. Etomidate is used primarily in short procedures. Ketamine hydrochloride (Ketalar) is a fast-acting CNS depressant that causes profound anesthesia but little skeletal muscle relaxation. It is associated with a difficult emergence phase that is characterized by hallucinations and disassociative feelings (feeling separate from the environment). The patient who is recovering from ketamine will do better in a quiet, supportive environment. Propofol (Diprivan) is a rapid-acting hypnotic that causes minimal excitation effects during induction. Risk of the patient's vomiting or thrashing during induction is reduced. A test dose is initially given to test for allergy. Propofol is metabolized rapidly so it does not accumulate in the blood when used to maintain anesthesia. Patients emerge from propofol quite quickly during the recovery period.

Other IV medications used in anesthesia include benzodiazepines and opioid analgesics. Examples of benzodiazepines include midazolam (Versed), lorazepam (Ativan), and diazepam (Valium). The benzodiazepines are antianxiety agents that also have hypnotic, sedative, and muscle relaxant effects. Midazolam is sometimes used to induce anesthesia but these drugs are more commonly used as premedication to reduce the patient's anxiety because they have an amnesic effect. Benzodiazepines are used in combination with other drugs to produce **conscious sedation** or as adjuncts to regional anesthesia to produce sedation and muscle relaxation. Opioids are used in anesthesia for their analgesic effect. Common medications include morphine sulfate, fentanyl citrate (Sublimaze), sufentanil, and alfentanil. Fentanyl is more potent than morphine and is the most commonly used analgesic in anesthesia. The opioid analgesics have good cardiovascular stability but cause respiratory depression.

PHARMACOLOGY Summary of Anesthetic Gases Used During Surgery

Agent	Action and Advantages	Disadvantages and Side Effects	Nursing Responsibility
Desflurane (Suprane)	Maintenance of anesthesia. Very rapid emergence. Good degree of muscle relaxation.	Must be heated to vaporize. Causes increase in heart rate and decrease in blood pressure. Has a strong odor precluding its use for induction of anesthesia. May cause coughing if used for induction.	Monitor for hypotension.
Enflurane (Ethrane)	Maintenance of anesthesia. Good degree of muscle relaxation.	May lower the threshold for seizures. Increases heart rate and decreases blood pressure.	Monitor for hypotension. Contraindicated in patients with seizure disorders.
Halothane (Fluothane)	Maintenance of anesthesia. Rapid induction and emergence but less than that of isoflurane. Low incidence of postoperative nausea and vomiting.	Fair degree of muscle relaxation. Increases heart rate and triggers arrhythmias. Requires a higher degree of liver metabolization than other agents. Causes postoperative shivering.	Can cause hypotension. Monitor for premature ventricular contractions, ventricular tachycardia, and ventricular fibrillation with use of epinephrine. Provide warm blankets during recovery period.
Isoflurane (Forane)	Induction and maintenance of anesthesia. Faster induction and recovery than enflurane or halothane. Minimal metabolization by the liver.	Causes increase in heart rate and hypotension. Hypotension can be unpredictable and severe if concomitant use of antihypertensive agents. Weak stimulation of secretions.	Monitor for hypotension.
Nitrous oxide	Rapid induction and recovery of anesthesia. When used with other inhalants, it reduces the concentration of other agent.	Does not produce muscle relaxation.	
Sevoflurane (Ultane)	Induction and maintenance of anesthesia. Very rapid induction and recovery (3–4 minutes faster than Isoflurane). Minimal metabolization by the liver.		

Sources: Adams, M., Josephson, D., & Holland, L. (2008). *Pharmacology for nurses: A pathophysiological approach.* Upper Saddle River, NJ: Pearson Prentice Hall; Ebert, T. J. (2004). *Physiology of the cardiovascular effects of general anesthesia in the elderly.* Retrieved April 26, 2004, from the ASA Syllabus on Geriatric Anesthesiology website: http://www.asahq.org/clinical/geriatrics/phy. htm; Hoffer, J. L. (1999). Anesthesia. In M. Meeker & J. Rothrock (Eds.), *Care of the patient in surgery* (pp. 203–238). Philadelphia: Mosby; Thompson, A. M. (2002). Anaesthesia. In L. Shields & H. Werder (Eds.), *Perioperative nursing* (pp. 79–105). San Francisco: Greenwich Medical Media.

Muscle Relaxants

Muscle relaxants (neuromuscular blocking agents) primarily affect skeletal muscle and they are used in surgery to facilitate endotracheal intubation and to provide optimal operating conditions. A rapid-acting neuromuscular blocking agent is administered before intubation to paralyze the muscles of the jaw and vocal cords making placement of the endotracheal tube easier. Muscle relaxation is used throughout the surgery to facilitate dissection of tissue. During surgery, the anesthesia care provider monitors the effects of muscle relaxant drugs with a peripheral nerve stimulator. Recovery from neuromuscular blocking agents after surgery is evidenced by the patient's ability to breathe on her own and hold her head upright as well as the presence of a strong hand grasp. There are two types of neuromuscular blocking agents, depolarizing and nondepolarizing.

Succinylcholine is a depolarizing agent and the only one in clinical use. The drug has a strong affinity for acetylcholine receptor sites and once it attaches to the site causes continuous depolarization of the motor end plate. Continuous muscle contractions and fasciculations are followed by flaccid paralysis of the muscles. The onset of paralysis is quick with intravenous administration, 30 to 60 seconds, and the effects last up to 10 minutes. Often succinylcholine is used for intubation because it works very quickly and wears off quickly, but there are disadvantages to the drug. The depolarization of muscle cells causes a transient increase in serum potassium that can produce cardiac dysrhythmia. Muscle fasciculation (twitching) leads the patient to complain of muscle soreness postoperatively. Succinylcholine is known to trigger malignant hyperthermia in susceptible individuals. The drug is broken down by the plasma enzyme cholinesterase. Prolonged paralysis occurs in individuals with insufficient amounts of cholinesterase although this condition is rare.

Nondepolarizing agents work by blocking the depolarizing action of acetylcholine at the motor end plate of the neuromuscular junction, thereby producing muscle paralysis. Muscle fasciculations do not occur with these drugs, eliminating postoperative myalgia. Another advantage is that these agents can be antagonized or reversed with the administration of neostigmine, edrophonium, or pyridostigmine. Use of reversal agents reduces the risk of morbidity associated with anesthesia

PHARMACOLOGY Summary of Intravenous Anesthetic Agents and Other Adjuncts to Anesthesia Used During Surgery

Agent	Action and Advantages	Disadvantages and Side Effects	Nursing Responsibility
Intravenous Anesthetic			
Etomidate (Amidate)	CNS depressant used for induction and maintenance of anesthesia for short procedures. Hypnotic effect but no analgesia. Fewer respiratory and cardiovascular effects than other agents. Onset is 60 seconds with duration of 3–5 minutes.	Suppresses cortisol secretion. Postoperative nausea and vomiting. May cause transient skeletal muscle movements. Metabolized in the liver.	Good anesthetic for patients with asthma or cardiovascular disease. Used in neurosurgery because it causes a slight decrease in intracranial pressure. Monitor cortisol levels and blood pressure.
Diazepam (Valium)	Benzodiazepine with hypnotic and amnesiac properties. Used as adjunct drug in induction of anesthesia and as a preoperative medication to reduce anxiety.	May cause hypotension and tachycardia. Prolonged effect.	Monitor sedation postoperatively.
Ketamine (Ketalar)	CNS depressant used for induction of anesthesia. May supplement nitrous oxide anesthesia. Fewer postoperative nausea and vomiting than other agents.	Increases salivary secretions. Does not produce muscle relaxation. May increase heart rate and blood pressure. Depresses respirations and increases intracranial pressure. Associated with emergence reactions including hallucinations, dissociative feelings, and irrational behavior. Recovery can be prolonged.	Premedicate with anticholinergic agent to reduce secretions. Provide a quiet, calm, reassuring environment for recovery. Monitor heart rate and blood pressure. Monitor airway to prevent aspiration.
Midazolam (Versed)	Benzodiazepine with hypnotic, amnesiac, anxiolytic, and muscle relaxant properties. Used for induction of general anesthesia and for conscious sedation.	Slower induction than with barbiturates. May cause hypotension and tachycardia.	Prepare patient for amnesia. Monitor for respiratory depression.
Propofol (Diprivan)	CSN depressant used for induction and maintenance of anesthesia. Rapid onset with minimal excitation during induction.	Abnormal muscle movement. May cause hypotension.	Monitor blood pressure. Cautious use in patients with allergies to eggs.
Sodium methohexital (Brevital)	Barbiturate used for induction and maintenance of anesthesia. More potent and with a shorter onset and quicker recovery than thiopental.	May cause abnormal muscle movements, coughing, and laryngospasm. Hypotension occurs in some patients. Hiccups may persist postoperatively.	Patient should be recumbent during administration. Monitor blood pressure.
Thiopental sodium (Pentothal)	Barbiturate used for induction and maintenance of anesthesia. Depresses CNS causing sedation and hypnosis. Ultrashort acting with onset in 10–20 seconds and duration of 20–30 minutes.	Depresses respiratory and circulatory function. Can cause anaphylaxis and laryngospasm. Metabolized by the liver.	Test dose given first.
Opioid Analgesics			
Alfentanil (Alfenta)	Narcotic used for induction, analgesia, and balanced anesthesia. Rapid onset and short duration make it a good choice for short surgical procedures.	Causes respiratory depression. Can cause bradycardia and hypotension. Bradycardia is more likely in patients who are taking a beta-blocking drug. Nausea and vomiting common.	Monitor vital signs. Report bradycardia.

(continued)

PHARMACOLOGY   Summary of Intravenous Anesthetic Agents and Other Adjuncts to Anesthesia Used During Surgery—*Continued*

Agent	Action and Advantages	Disadvantages and Side Effects	Nursing Responsibility
Fentanyl (Sublimaze)	Narcotic used as adjunct for induction to anesthesia and for analgesia supplement. The drug of choice for epidural analgesia. Short acting. Causes less nausea and vomiting than morphine.	Causes sedation and respiratory depression. May also cause bradycardia and hypotension.	Monitor vital signs. Watch for signs of respiratory depression.
Morphine sulfate	Narcotic used as premedication and for postoperative analgesia. Long-lasting effect.	Causes respiratory depression. Histamine release causes peripheral vasodilation and hypotension. Nausea and vomiting common.	Monitor vital signs.
Sufentanil (Sufenta)	Narcotic used for analgesic supplement in balanced anesthesia. More potent than fentanyl. Has a quicker onset and shorter recovery than fentanyl. Not associated with histamine release so there is less hypotensive effect.	Prolonged respiratory depression.	Monitor vital signs. Watch for signs of respiratory depression.
Depolarizing Muscle Relaxants			
Succinylcholine	Depolarizing neuroblocking agent with high affinity for acetylcholine receptor sites. Produces muscle relaxation and paralysis. Used to facilitate endotracheal intubation and to produce skeletal muscle relaxation for short surgical procedures. Short-acting agent with onset in 30–60 seconds and duration of several minutes.	Causes muscle fasciculations, bradycardia, and respiratory depression. May precipitate malignant hyperthermia in susceptible individuals.	Monitor vital signs. Maintain airway and clear secretions. Patient may complain of muscle soreness postoperatively.
Nondepolarizing Muscle Relaxants—Intermediate			
Mivacurium (Mivacron)	Intermediate, nondepolarizing muscle relaxant used for endotracheal intubation and to produce relaxation of skeletal muscles for surgery. Effect lasts 15–20 minutes.	Transient hypotension and bradycardia. Metabolized by plasma cholinesterase.	Monitor vital signs.
Vecuronium (Norcuron)	Intermediate, nondepolarizing muscle relaxant used for endotracheal intubation and to produce relaxation of skeletal muscles for surgery. Effect lasts 20–40 minutes.	Metabolized by the liver. Causes respiratory depression. Minimal cardiovascular effects.	Monitor for delay of recovery postoperatively.
Nondepolarizing Muscle Relaxants—Long Acting			
Tubocurarine	Long-acting, nondepolarizing muscle relaxant used for maintenance of relaxation during surgery. Muscle relaxant effects last 30–40 minutes.	Causes histamine release with hypotension. Increases bronchial and salivary secretions.	Monitor blood pressure and airway until full recovery from drug. Observe for residual muscle weakness.
Metocurine (Metubine)	Long-acting, nondepolarizing muscle relaxant used for maintenance of relaxation during surgery. Muscle relaxant effects last 30–90 minutes.	Hypotension, increased salivary secretions, and respiratory depression.	Monitor blood pressure and airway until full recovery. May take several hours for complete neuromuscular recovery.

PHARMACOLOGY   Summary of Intravenous Anesthetic Agents and Other Adjuncts to Anesthesia Used During Surgery—*Continued*

Agent	Action and Advantages	Disadvantages and Side Effects	Nursing Responsibility
Pancuronium (Pavulon)	Long-acting, nondepolarizing muscle relaxant used for maintenance of relaxation during surgery. Muscle relaxant effects last 30–60 minutes.	Tachycardia, hypertension, and premature ventricular contractions.	Monitor vital signs.
Anticholinergics			
Atropine	Anticholinergic agent used to decrease salivary and respiratory secretions, to treat bradycardia and/or hypotension, and to reverse muscle relaxants.	Tachycardia, hypertension, urinary retention, and dry mouth. May cause cardiac arrhythmias.	Monitor heart rate and blood pressure. Heart rate is best indicator of response to the drug.
Glycopyrrolate (Robinul)	Anticholinergic agent used to decrease salivary and respiratory secretions and to reverse neuromuscular block.	Tachycardia, urinary retention, and dry mouth. Fewer problems with cardiac arrhythmias than atropine.	Monitor heart rate.

Sources: Adams, M., Josephson, D., & Holland, L. (2005). *Pharmacology for nurses: A pathophysiological approach.* Upper Saddle River, NJ: Pearson Prentice Hall; Ebert, T. J. (2004). *Physiology of the cardiovascular effects of general anesthesia in the elderly.* Retrieved April 26, 2004, from the ASA Syllabus on Geriatric Anesthesiology website: http://www.asahq.org/clinical/geriatrics/phy. htm; Hoffer, J. L. (1999). Anesthesia. In M. Meeker & J. Rothrock (Eds.), *Care of the patient in surgery* (pp. 203–238). Philadelphia: Mosby; Thompson, A. M. (2002). Anaesthesia. In L. Shields & H. Werder (Eds.), *Perioperative nursing* (pp. 79–105). San Francisco: Greenwich Medical Media.

(Arbous et al., 2005). Reversal drugs cause bradycardia, which is treated with atropine or glycopyrrolate. Nondepolarizing agents are divided into intermediate acting and long acting. Intermediate-acting agents have a quick onset, 60 seconds or less, and last 25 to 40 minutes. Examples of intermediate-acting nondepolarizing agents are vecuronium, atracurium, and mivacurium. Longer acting nondepolarizing muscle relaxants also have a rapid onset but last 45 to 60 minutes. Examples include pancuronium, metocurine, and tubocurarine.

Complications of General Anesthesia

The majority of patients experience **general anesthesia** without problems except for the complaint of a sore throat from the endotracheal tube. Other problems that may occur with intubation are damage to teeth or dental work and trauma to the vocal cords. Complications that arise from general anesthesia include hypoxia, hypotension, hypertension, cardiac dysrhythmia, residual muscle paralysis, hypothermia, and malignant hyperthermia.

A drop in body temperature is common during surgery. Anesthesia interferes with the physiological mechanisms of thermoregulation. This effect combined with environmental factors such as the ambient temperature in the OR, the exposure of body cavities, and the administration of cold solutions (e.g., blood products, IV fluids) or irrigants leads to a reduction in core body temperature. Studies show the most significant drop in body temperature occurs during the first hour of anesthesia (Hasankhani, Mohammadi, Moazzami, Mokhtari, & Naghgizadh, 2007; Sessler & Todd, 2000; Wagner, 2006). Monitoring body temperature and using warming devices during surgery (e.g., blankets, thermal drapes, fluid warmers) is imperative (Hasankhani et al., 2007; Wagner, 2006). Research supports the use of forced-air warming blankets as the most effective method of preventing or treating hypothermia (American Society of PeriAnesthesia Nurses, 2001). Some suggest that using a forced-air warming blanket for 30 minutes prior to surgery helps prevent intraoperative hypothermia and improve patient outcomes (Bitner, Hilde, Hall, & Duvendack, 2007).

Malignant Hyperthermia

Malignant hyperthermia (MH) is a rare but life-threatening complication of anesthesia. The predisposition for MH is genetically transmitted by an autosomal dominant trait. It is thought that MH is triggered by the medications or agents used in general anesthesia with the most common being succinylcholine or one of the inhalant anesthetics. Other factors such as stress, trauma, fatigue, or muscle injury may play a role in increasing susceptibility to the condition or in modifying the patient's response to the condition. Malignant hyperthermia occurs most commonly during induction of anesthesia although it may present anytime during the surgery or early postoperative period.

Malignant hyperthermia is not well understood. With MH, calcium levels within skeletal muscle cells increase, although the reasons for this are not known. The elevation in intracellular calcium activates muscle rigidity and spasm and a hypermetabolic state. The increase in cellular metabolism leads to an increase in carbon dioxide production (hypercarbia) and a metabolic acidosis. As the process continues, the patient becomes hypoxic, hyperthermic, and develops dysrhythmias and hypotension. Muscle breakdown with the release of myoglobins leads to myoglobinuria and an increased risk of renal failure. Damaged muscle cells release intracellular potassium and creatinine phosphokinase (CPK) into the circulation.

The presentation of MH is variable. Early signs are masseter spasm (contracture of jaw), sinus tachycardia, and an increase in expiratory carbon dioxide levels. The anesthesia provider first suspects MH by the rise in the patient's expired CO_2, which is monitored throughout the surgery. An end-tidal carbon dioxide level that is two to three times normal is the earliest and most definitive sign of MH (Redmond, 2001). Other signs are rigor of muscles, hypoxemia evidenced by a drop in oxygen saturation, and tea-colored urine, indicating the presence of myoglobins. Laboratory blood tests results show metabolic acidosis and increases in serum calcium, potassium, and creatinine phosphokinase. Hyperthermia is a late sign and temperature elevations can be extreme with increases of 1 to 2 degrees every few minutes. Other late signs are cardiac dysrhythmia and hypotension.

Malignant hyperthermia can be fatal. The key to treatment is early recognition of the syndrome, immediate discontinuation of the triggering agent, administration of dantrolene sodium to produce muscle relaxation, and providing supportive care. Following emergency treatment, the patient is monitored in the intensive care unit for 24 hours or longer because a small percentage of patients experience a reoccurrence of MH (Redmond, 2001). Chart 26–3 summarizes the management of the patient with malignant hyperthermia.

Other Complications

Other adverse events or complications may occur in the operating room as a result of the surgical procedure. Examples include such things as bleeding with excessive blood loss or inadvertent injury to surrounding organs or tissues. Intraoperative complication rates depend on the surgery, the type of anesthesia, and the patient's physical status. In studies of complications associated with various procedures (e.g., abdominal, spinal, orthopedic, and urologic), 3% to 4% of patients experience intraoperative complications (Rampersaud et al., 2006; Tarrac, 2006).

CHART 26–3 **Management of the Patient with Malignant Hyperthermia**

- Immediately discontinue triggering agent.
- Stop surgery if possible. Otherwise, deepen anesthesia with opioids, sedatives, nondepolarizing muscle relaxants.
- Hyperventilate with 100% oxygen.
- Administer a bolus of dantrolene sodium (Dantrium) 2 to 3 mg/kg intravenously with additional bolus doses up to 10 mg/kg until decreased signs of hypercarbia.
- Administer cooling devices: Apply cooling blanket, use iced normal saline intravenously, lavage open body cavities with iced saline.
- Hydrate with intravenous normal saline.
- Maintain a urine output greater than 2 mL/kg per hour. Administer furosemide and/or mannitol if urine output is less than goal.
- Treat metabolic acidosis with intravenous sodium bicarbonate if it does not self-correct with treatment.
- Treat hyperkalemia with intravenous sodium bicarbonate, 10 units of regular insulin with dextrose intravenously.
- Treat cardiac arrhythmia if it does not self-correct with treatment. Do not use calcium channel blockers.
- Continue to monitor vital signs, oxygen saturation, electrocardiogram, urine output, arterial blood gases, and blood chemistry.
- Transfer to Intensive Care Unit for postoperative care.

Source: Reprinted from Perianesthesia recognition, treatment and care. Redmond, M.C. Copyright 2007, with permission from Elsevier. Retrieved on July 2, 2008 from http://aspan.org/EdCeMalHyper.htm#head 11

Regional Anesthesia

Regional anesthesia is a general classification of anesthesia that includes spinal and epidural anesthesia, peripheral nerve blocks, Bier blocks, and local anesthesia. The common feature of all types of regional anesthesia is the local injection of a medication to block the transmission of sensory impulses from that area to the brain, thus, effectively blocking the sensation of pain. Regional anesthesia has some advantages over general anesthesia. Usually, regional anesthesia does not depress respirations so the patient is at lower risk of postoperative respiratory complications. This makes regional anesthesia a good choice for patients with severe cardiopulmonary disease. Patients who receive a regional anesthetic usually experience less postoperative nausea and vomiting.

Regional anesthesia can be used for any number of surgeries. It is commonly used for repair of inguinal hernia, transurethral resection of the prostate, gynecologic procedures, and arthroscopies and other orthopedic surgeries including repair of hip fractures in the elderly. Typically, patients scheduled for regional anesthesia are premedicated in the holding area with an antianxiety agent to produce mild to moderate sedation. Opioid analgesics may be administered to reduce the pain associated with the insertion of needles and the administration of numbing agents.

Spinal Anesthesia

Spinal anesthesia, also called **intrathecal anesthesia**, is the injection of a local anesthetic into the subarachnoid space and directly into the cerebrospinal fluid (CSF). The anesthetic blocks nerve fibers (i.e., sensory, motor, and sympathetic) at the level of the spinal cord. Spinal anesthesia effectively blocks motor and sensory nerves so that the patient cannot move the affected area (temporary paralysis) or feel pain, touch, temperature, or pressure. The spinal needle is inserted between the 2nd and 3rd lumbar vertebrae (L^2–L^3) or the 3rd and 4th vertebrae (L^3–L^4). For insertion, the patient is placed in a sitting position or in a side-lying position with their head and knees flexed (i.e., fetal position). A spinal needle is inserted in the intervertebral space through the dura mater and into the subarachnoid space. Special spinal needles called *pencil point needles* enter the dura mater by separating the fibers rather than cutting them, reducing the risk of a CSF leak after the needle is removed.

Commonly, spinal anesthesia includes the administration of local anesthetics such as lidocaine, bupivacaine (Marcaine), or chloroprocaine combined with an opioid analgesic such as fentanyl or preservative-free morphine. The medication may be mixed with a dextrose solution to create a hyperbaric solution (i.e., a solution that is heavier than CSF). Once a hyperbaric solution is injected into the CSF, it travels by gravity. The anesthesiologist may have the patient sit for a few minutes to create a block in the lower extremities or place the patient supine with the head tilted slightly downward to create a higher block. After 10 to 15 minutes, the block sets and does not extend further.

Epidural Anesthesia

Epidural anesthesia is the injection of a local anesthetic into the epidural space. The epidural space is located adjacent to the dura mater and contains fat, tissue, and blood vessels. Anesthetic injected into the epidural space affects nerve roots as they leave the spinal cord and some medication diffuses across the dura mater into the subarachnoid space and the CSF. The anesthetic spreads in both directions (i.e., cephalad and caudad) from the site of the injection, and positioning has less effect on movement of the medication than it does with spinal anesthesia.

The same medications used in spinal anesthesia are used in epidural anesthesia, but the concentration of the drugs is greater because they must diffuse across several layers of tissue. The onset of epidural anesthesia is slower than that of spinal anesthesia. A test dose of lidocaine with epinephrine is injected to make sure that the needle is correctly placed in the epidural space and not in the subarachnoid space or in a vein. If the needle is mistakenly in a vein, the test dose produces transient tachycardia; if it is in the subarachnoid space, it produces mild numbness. Frequently, an epidural catheter remains in place after the operation to provide postoperative pain control. Caudal anesthesia is the administration of a local anesthetic into the epidural space, but the approach is through the caudal canal in the sacrum rather than through the lumbar vertebrae.

Complications of Spinal or Epidural Anesthesia Spinal anesthesia may be complicated by the development of headache, hypotension, and meningitis. Spinal headache or post–dural puncture headache (PDPH) is a common postoperative complaint. PDPH is caused by the leaking of CSF through the hole in the dura (e.g., the puncture site). The loss of CSF causes irritation of meningeal nerves and vessels (Hyderally, 2002). Because PDPH develops or worsens when the patient moves to an upright position, patients may be restricted to bed rest for the first 8 to 24 hours postoperatively to reduce the incidence of spinal headache. When headache develops, it is located in the occipital area and resolves in 1 to 3 days. Patients who develop a headache are treated with hydration and analgesics. The patient is placed on bed rest with the head of the bed maintained at less than 30 degrees to reduce CSF leak. PDPH that does not resolve quickly or that produces an intolerable headache may be treated with a "blood patch." The anesthesiologist injects 5 to 10 mL of autologous blood into the epidural space at the site of puncture to seal the leak.

Whereas PDPH occurs postoperatively, hypotension is more likely to occur while anesthesia is still being administered. Hypotension is caused by vasodilation associated with the blocking of sympathetic nerves. When sympathetic nerves are blocked by anesthesia, arteries and veins lose muscle tone and the ability to constrict. This decreases venous return from the extremities and reduces cardiac output. Hypotension can occur with both spinal and epidural anesthesia. Hypotension is avoided with the administration of fluid volume usually normal saline. Medications with strong alpha-adrenergic stimulation effects, such as ephedrine or phenylephrine, are used to prevent or treat hypotension.

Spinal anesthesia is associated with a low risk of aseptic meningitis. When it does occur, signs develop within the first 24 hours after surgery (Hyderally, 2002). The patient presents with the typical signs of meningitis, fever, headache, nuchal rigidity, and photophobia.

Peripheral Nerve Blocks

A **peripheral nerve block** is the injection of a local anesthetic into or around a nerve plexus to produce anesthesia of a selected area. The major advantage of a nerve block is that anesthesia is confined to the area of the surgery and does not have a systemic effect. Long-acting local anesthetics used in the nerve block provide extended control of pain postoperatively. The local anes-

thetic blocks motor, sensory, and sympathetic nerves. Frequently, epinephrine is administered with the local anesthetic. Epinephrine causes vasoconstriction of the area and decreases vascular uptake of the medication, thus prolonging the effect of the local anesthetic. The duration of the block depends on the choice of anesthetic, the volume and concentration of the drug, and the site being injected. Frequently, nerve blocks are administered by anesthesia in the holding area because they may take anywhere from 5 to 30 minutes to take effect.

A nerve block can be performed in a number of different sites. For example, an interscalene or axillary block of the brachial plexus is done for surgeries on the shoulder, forearm, or elbow. Surgery on the lower leg may be accomplished using a femoral or sciatic block. Peripheral nerve blocks are used alone or in combination with general anesthesia. When used with general anesthesia, the amount of general anesthesia can be reduced. Complications that can occur with nerve blocks include hematoma at the site of the block, nerve damage, and toxicity from systemic absorption of local anesthetic. Other, specific complications depend on the site where the block is administered.

Peripheral nerve blocks may be performed as outpatient surgeries. Patients are taught that recovery of motor function occurs first followed by recovery of sensation. Note that while the area is numb, the patient is at risk for inadvertently injuring the area.

A **Bier block** is a specific type of peripheral nerve block that is administered intravenously, but certain techniques are used to trap the anesthetic in the local area. Bier blocks may be used for surgeries on an extremity, usually the arm. An IV catheter is inserted in the extremity at the most distal site possible. A pneumatic tourniquet is applied proximal to the surgical site and inflated higher than the patient's systolic blood pressure. When the local anesthetic (lidocaine) is injected intravenously, the obstruction of blood by the tourniquet prevents it from leaving the surgical area. At the completion of the surgery, the tourniquet is intermittently deflated so that the lidocaine enters the patient's general circulation slowly, preventing a toxic reaction to the anesthetic.

■ Nursing Management

The verification process consists of information gathering and verification, which begins with the determination to do the procedure and continues through all settings and interventions involved in the preoperative preparation of the patient, up to and including the time-out (discussed later) just before the start of the procedure.

Assessment

The nurse asks the patient to confirm the procedure to be completed, the surgical site, and the surgeon. The nurse verifies this information with the surgical consent form, a site verification form per organization policy, and the operating room schedule. In some cases, especially when there is a left or right side involved in the procedure, the correct area for surgery is marked on the patient. Per the AORN (2008) correct site surgery position statement, a comprehensive approach is needed in each health care delivery system to prevent wrong site surgery. In 2003 AORN and the American College of Surgeons developed national guidelines that are to be used with every patient having surgery to eliminate inadvertently operating on the wrong surgical site (see the National Guidelines box, p. 632).

NATIONAL GUIDELINES AORN Guidelines for Eliminating Wrong Site Surgery

The following guidelines are supported by both AORN and the American College of Surgeons.

1. Verify that the correct patient is being taken to the operating room. This verification can be made with the patient or the patient's designated representative if the patient is underage or unable to answer for him/herself.

2. Verify that the correct procedure is on the operating room schedule.

3. Verify with the patient or the patient's designated representative the procedure that is expected to be performed, as well as the location of the operation.

4. Confirm the consent form with the patient or the patient's designated representative.

5. In the case of a bilateral organ, limb, or anatomic site (for example, hernia), the surgeon and patient should agree and the operating surgeon should mark the site prior to giving the patient narcotics, sedation, or anesthesia.

6. If the patient is scheduled for multiple procedures that will be performed by multiple surgeons, all the items on the checklist must be verified for each procedure that is planned to be performed.

7. Conduct a final verification process with members of the surgical team to confirm the correct patient, procedure, and surgical site.

8. Ensure that all relevant records and imaging studies are in the operating room.

9. If any verification process fails to identify the correct site, all activities should be halted until verification is accurate.

10. In the event of a life- or limb-threatening situation, not all of these steps may be followed.

Source: Reprinted from Evolution of Wrong Site Surgery Prevention Strategies. AORN, Carney, B., Volume 83, Issue 5, pp. 1115–1122. Copyright 2006 with permission from Elsevier.

Nursing Diagnoses

The actual and potential nursing diagnoses related to surgery include:

1. *Stress, Overload*
2. *Surgical Recovery Delayed*
3. *Fear*
4. *Infection, Risk for*
5. *Pain, Acute.*

Planning

To provide the safest and least stressful experience for the patient, planning is essential. Planning for the surgical experience typically begins with the admission to the hospital. A comprehensive plan that organizes the care of the patient and family will facilitate the surgical process. The plan includes preoperative, intraoperative, and postoperative management and teaching. Communication is as essential part of executing the plan. Each hospital has specific forms that are used to guide the nurse through the process. Chapter 25 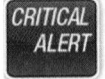 includes an example of a preoperative checklist.

Outcomes and Evaluation Parameters

The desired outcome for patients having surgery is that the patient safely transitions through the entire process. Evaluation parameters include: airway is maintained, oxygen levels are within normal limits, pain is managed and any postoperative complications are effectively mitigated or controlled as much as possible.

Interventions and Rationales

The nurse must communicate pertinent information to the anesthesia team. Information may include allergies, lab/test results, skin condition, NPO status, sensory/mobility impairments, physical particularities, restrictions to jaw and neck range of motion, history of drug use including herbal medication, anticoagulants held for number of days, implanted electronic devices (IEDs), other implants, previous anesthesia/surgery history, artificial or loose teeth, previous surgery, comorbidities, particular patient requests, or any other information deemed crucial to intraoperative patient care. Although this verification takes place in the same-day admission unit or the surgical unit, many ORs have developed a presurgical checklist to ensure that all pertinent information is reviewed and communicated.

Preventing Wrong Site Surgery

When a procedure involves a left/right distinction, multiple structures (such as finger and toes), or multiple levels (such as spinal procedures), the intended site must be marked so that the mark will be visible after the patient has been prepped and draped. The purpose is to identify unambiguously the intended site of incision or insertion. The mark must be made using a marker that is sufficiently permanent to remain visible after the skin preparation. The Joint Commission (2004) recommends that the method and the type of marking should be consistent throughout the organization and that the person doing the marking should be the one doing the procedure. Marking must take place with the patient involved and aware.

CRITICAL ALERT *Exemptions to the marking procedure may include single-organ cases, interventional cases where the point of insertion is not predetermined (such as cardiac catheterization), teeth extractions (although the involved tooth should be documented), and premature infants, for whom the mark may cause a permanent tattoo.*

As the patient's advocate, the perioperative nurse should communicate with all members of the surgical team to verify the correct surgical site. Individual facility policy should clearly delineate the role and responsibility of the health care provider and other team members in marking and verifying the correct surgical site. The 2006 statistics on sentinel events from the Joint Commission identify wrong site surgery as the second most reported sentinel event, accounting for 13% of reported sentinel events (Beyea,

2000). Although it is the surgeon's role to diagnose a patient's need for surgery and to delineate the surgical site, verifying the surgical site at the time of surgery is the responsibility of perioperative nurses and every member of the health care team (AORN, 2008). To this effect, the Joint Commission has issued regulations and is endorsing the Universal Protocol as part of the 2007 National Patient Safety Goals (Joint Commission, 2007).

 The goal of the universal protocol is to prevent wrong site, wrong procedure, and wrong person surgery. The Joint Commission's national guidelines to prevent wrong site surgery are based on the consensus of experts from the relevant clinical specialties and professional disciplines and is endorsed by more than 40 professional medical associations and organizations. The active involvement of the team and the patient or patient's representative and effective communication among all members of the operating room team are important for success.

Surgical Time-Out

Safety initiatives that address communication issues such as the time-out are designed to promote correct site surgery. The time-out checklist has been adopted from the aviation industry model and requires surgical team members to cease all other activities in order to actively, verbally, and mutually verify information such as the correct patient, correct surgery, correct site/side, correct patient position, and possibly additional information such as prophylactic medications being administered at the appropriate time prior to surgery. Figure 26–4 ■ shows a sample of a time-out checklist.

Wrong site surgery may be the result of operating on the wrong patient or performing the wrong procedure, but most commonly it is the result of operating on the wrong site/side; for example, the left hand is operated on instead of the right (Joint Commission, 2007). Although rare, the consequences of wrong site surgery can

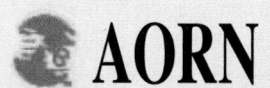

When marking the site
DO NOT USE:
The letter X or the word NO
Do NOT mark the Non-Operative Site

According to AORN standards, the patient is identified by the circulating RN when the patient enters the OR suite. The procedure and surgical site are validated at this time as well.

"TIME OUT"

Takes place in the procedure/OR room, after the patient is prepped and draped and it involves the ENTIRE TEAM.

All team members must verbally verify their agreement on:
- The name of the patient.
- The procedure to be performed.
- The site of the procedure, including laterality, implant to be used and radiologic exams, if applicable.

Validate site mark after draping or confirm ID band with the procedure written on it if used in cases of exemption.

DISCREPANCIES/ISSUES
✓ Procedure does not start until patient verification & missing information is completed and agreed upon by all team members.
✓ If a disagreement is not resolved, follow your facility policy and notify your manager or administrator.
✓ All issues resolved are documented in the medical record.

DOCUMENTATION of "TIME OUT"
Should indicate the following was verified:
- Correct patient.
- Correct site and side.
- Agreement to procedure.
- Correct patient position.
- Implants and/or special equipment or special requirements available.

* Facility determined identifiers should be used.
** Remove the mark at the end of procedure, especially for patients returning for subsequent procedures (e.g., trauma).
*** If operating physician does not mark site, an individual identified by facility policy with knowledge of the patient and planned procedure to be performed may mark the site.

Guidelines for Implementing *JCAHO Universal Protocol* To Promote Correct Site Surgery

PREOPERATIVE VERIFICATION
2 Patient Identifiers Must be Used (for example)*
- Ask patient to state their full name.
- Ask patient to state their date of birth.
- Ask patient to state their planned procedure and document it in the patient's own words.
- The patient's room number is <u>not</u> an acceptable patient identifier:

Confirm and Verify
- Patient's name on their ID band, date of birth, and other documents that correspond with the patient's responses.
- Medical record number.
- Consents.
- Availability of implant if required.
- Availability of blood if ordered.
- Radiologic exams (x-ray, CT scan, MRI, etc.).

PATIENT RESPONSES MUST MATCH:
MARKED SITE * ID BAND * CONSENTS * RADIOLOGIC EXAMS * SCHEDULED PROCEDURE

In the case of pediatric patients and patients unable to verify information for themselves, the RN identifies the patient's legal guardian and verifies with them the following protocol.

SITE MARK:
- Use a permanent marker that is visible after skin is prepped and draped
- Have operating physician/surgeon mark the site with his or her **initials, prior to** patient entering the OR suite. ***
- Mark site(s) with patient participation (e.g., verbal confirmation or visual pointing).
- Use an additional mechanism for identifying site(s) exempt from marking according to facility policy and JCAHO guidelines (For example, an ID band with the procedure written on it is an alternative for site marking. When possible the ID band should be verified during the time out phase similar to the site mark).

FIGURE 26–4 ■ AORN guidelines for verifying the correct surgical site.

AORN SAMPLE Patient Record
(Facility Name and Address)

This record is a sample only. Clinical records should be customized to incorporate data fields that represent the setting, facility, procedure, and patient. Reproductions and variations are encouraged, provided credit is given to AORN.

Addressograph

(Patient Information:
name, age, gender, medical record number, date)

Structural Data:

Operating Room Progress Notes

Room #:	ASA:	Pt. in room:	Anes. start:
Procedure start:	Procedure finish:	Pt. out of room:	Anes. finish:

Anesthesia type:

☐ General   ☐ MAC   ☐ Spinal   ☐ Epidural

☐ Local block, Type: _____   ☐ Other:

Op Dx: _____

Procedure(s): _____

Op Dx: _____

Surgeon 1:	Circulating nurse 1:
Surgeon 2:	Circulating nurse 2:
Assistant 1:	Circ. 1 relief: Time in: ____ Time out: ____
Assistant 2:	Circ. 2 relief: Time in: ____ Time out: ____
Anesthesia care provider 1:	Scrub 1:
Anesthesia care provider 2:	Scrub 2:
Laser operator:	Scrub 1 relief: Time in: ____ Time out: ____
Other authorized personnel:	Scrub 2 relief: Time in: ____ Time out: ____

Nursing Data Elements - Preoperative:

Preoperative checklist reviewed/evaluated

Risk for injury related to transfer and transport (X29):

☐ ID confirmed   ☐ Consent verified   ☐ Site verified
Allergies verified   ☐ Procedure verified
Latex allergy: ☐ Yes   ☐ No   ☐ NPO verified
                                        Time: _____

☐ Alert/oriented   ☐ Drowsy   ☐ Sedated
☐ Asleep   ☐ Unresponsive   ☐ Disoriented
☐ Other: _____

☐ Cool   ☐ Warm   ☐ Intact
☐ Dry   ☐ Moist   ☐ Body jewelry removed
☐ Tattoos: _____

Sensory impairment: ☐ No limitations   ☐ Hearing
                                  ☐ Language barrier   ☐ Sight

Musculoskeletal status: ☐ No limitations   ☐ Paralysis   ☐ Traction

Prosthetics/Assistive devices: ☐ Hearing aid   ☐ Glasses
                                              ☐ AICD
                                              ☐ Prosthetics: _____

Cardiopulmonary status:
Peripheral edema: ☐ Yes Location: _____
                              ☐ No

DVT/PE risk: ☐ High   ☐ Med.   ☐ Low
Respiratory: ☐ Tracheotomy   ☐ Intubated   ☐ Chest tube
                    ☐ Regular   ☐ Labored   ☐ Other findings

Risk for anxiety related to knowledge deficit and stress of surgery (X4):

Psychosocial status:
  ☐ Calm/relaxed   ☐ Anxious   ☐ Talkative
  ☐ Crying   ☐ Restless
  ☐ Other: _____

☐ Provided instruction based on age and identified needs (I106).
☐ Communicated patient concerns to appropriate members of health care team (I128).
☐ Explained sequence of events and preoperative routine (I56).
☐ Evaluated response to instructions (I50).

Risk for acute/chronic pain (X38, X74):

☐ Instructed on use of pain scale
☐ Pain assessment (0-10): _____
   Location: _____

Outcomes:

☐ Verbalizes/indicates decreased anxiety, ability to cope, understanding of procedure and sequence of events. Questions answered.
☐ Demonstrates adequate pain management.
☐ Verbalizes comfort related to transfer/transport.

Transfer to suite via:

☐ Stretcher   ☐ W/C   ☐ Bed
☐ Isolette   ☐ Crib

FIGURE 26–5 ■ Sample of intraoperative nursing documentation.

Source: Reprinted with permission from "AORN sample patient record," in *Perioperative Nursing Data Set,* 2nd edition, pages 212–213; http://www.aorn.org/PracticeResources/PNDSAndStandardizedPerioperative Record/PNDSResources. Copyright © 2002 AORN, Inc., 2170 South Parker Road, Suite 300, Denver, CO 80231. All rights reserved.

Intraoperative Structural Data:

☐ EKG ☐ Oximeter ☐ NIAPB ☐ Temp monitor

Implants/Prosthesis: ☐ Yes ☐ No   Exp. Date:_____

Manufacturer: _____

Type: _____

Size: _____

Lot/Serial #: _____

OR medications: (other than those given by anesthesia care provider)

Time	Medication	Dosage	Route	Initials

Blood products: ☐ Yes ☐ No   Blood band #: _____

Unit #:_____ Start time:_____ Finish time:_____

Unit #:_____ Start time:_____ Finish time:_____

Unit #:_____ Start time:_____ Finish time:_____

Blood recovery: ☐ Yes ☐ No   Unit #:_____

CCs reinfused: _____

Irrigation:

Type: _____

Amount: _____

X-rays: ☐ Yes ☐ No

Site: _____

Type: _____

Protective devices:

☐ Gonadal ☐ Thyroid

Other: _____

Grafts: ☐ Yes ☐ No

Type: _____

Donor site: _____

Recipient site: _____

Pathology specimens:

Routine: ☐ Yes ☐ No
#: _____

Frozen section: ☐ Yes ☐ No
#: _____

Cultures: ☐ Yes ☐ No
#: _____

Comments: _____

Intraoperative Nursing Data:

Risk for infection (X28):

☐ Skin Pre-op intact ☐ Other: _____

☐ Surgical clippers: _____

Area: _____

☐ Skin prep   By: _____

☐ Povidone-iodine ☐ Chlorhexidine
☐ Other: _____

Wound classification:

☐ 1-Clean ☐ 3-Contaminated

☐ 2-Clean/contaminated ☐ 4-Dirty

☐ Urinary catheter:

(size/type/site): _____

OR output: _____ Inserted by: _____

☐ Drains/tubes (size/type/site):_____

OR drainage amount: _____

☐ Packing (size/type/site): _____

☐ Cast (type/site): _____

☐ Dressing (type/site): _____

Risk for hypothermia (X26):

☐ Apply warming blanket #:_____

Temp setting: _____

Applied by: _____

☐ Warm IV fluid

☐ Warm irrigation

☐ Other: _____

Risk for impaired skin integrity (X50):

Position for surgery: ☐ Supine ☐ Prone ☐ Mod. lithotomy ☐ Jackknife

☐ Lt. lateral ☐ Rt. lateral ☐ Other: _____

Positioning devices: ☐ Chest roll ☐ Shoulder roll ☐ Axillary roll

☐ Pillow/wedge ☐ Stirrups ☐ Leg holder

Pad bony prominences: ☐ Elbows ☐ Heels ☐ Arms tucked/padded

☐ Other: _____

Positioned by: _____

Risk for injury (X29):

☐ Apply safety strap to: _____

☐ Apply grounding pad   Site: _____

☐ Electrosurgical unit #: _____ ☐ Bipolar #: _____

Setting: Coag: _____ Cut: _____

☐ Laser Type: _____ Unit #:_____ Settings: _____ Time: _____

☐ Safety measures implemented   Operator:_____

☐ Tourniquet checked & applied #: _____ Site: _____ Applied by: _____

☐ Inflated: _____ ☐ Deflated:_____ Pressure:_____

Sequential stockings: ☐ Yes ☐ No   Other: _____ Unit #:_____

Counts:	Sponge	Needles	Instruments
1st count:	☐ Correct	☐ Correct	☐ Correct
2nd count:	☐ Correct	☐ Correct	☐ Correct
3rd count:	☐ Correct	☐ Correct	☐ Correct
	☐ Unresolved	☐ Unresolved	☐ Unresolved
	☐ N/A	☐ N/A	☐ N/A

☐ Surgeon notified of counts   If counts unresolved, X-ray taken: ☐ Yes ☐ No

Signature: _____   If no, explain: _____

Postprocedure Assessment/Evaluation:

Outcomes: ☐ Patient's surgery performed using aseptic technique and in a manner to prevent cross-contamination (O10).
☐ Skin remains smooth, intact, non-reddened, non-irritated, free of bruising (O5, O2, O8).
☐ Core body temperature remains in expected range (O12).

be devastating and warrant improved systems that promote effective communication such as the time-out initiative.

Intraoperative Patient Record

Most facilities have an intraoperative patient record, like that shown in Figure 26–5 ■, that is used to record intraoperative information. In addition, perioperative nurses may chart information in the nurse's notes when warranted. For example, information may include personnel involved, length of surgery,

position and accessories implemented, wound classification, anesthesia classification, and monitoring devices to name a few.

Protecting the Patient from Infection

Surgical-site infections are the third most frequently reported type of iatrogenic (hospital-acquired) infection (Engemann et al., 2003). Preventing and minimizing associated risks of SSI are fundamental perioperative nursing diagnoses of the surgical patient. According to Nichols (2001), the most critical factor in postoperative infection is the sound judgment and proper practice of the surgical team in addition to the general health and disease state of the patient. It is for this reason that perioperative nurses have become quite expert in the areas of aseptic technique and sterile conscience. Surgical aseptic practice is based on the premise that most infections are caused by exogenous organisms or organisms that are external from the body.

Asepsis is the absence of infectious organisms. In the OR aseptic techniques are practices that minimize contamination due to microorganisms. Frequently aseptic techniques and practices are criticized for being ritualistic in nature and lacking in scientific rigor, but until empiric evidence demonstrates a technique is otherwise unnecessary or ineffective, basic aseptic principles should be observed.

There are no sterilization processes that completely eliminate all microorganisms. The best technologies to date can only limit and reduce the presence of microbial life such as bacteria, viruses, fungi, and spores to an acceptable sterility assurance level. It is for this reason that nurses and surgical team members in the OR need to continually monitor the surgical field and develop strategies to minimize patient risk. An example may include inspecting sterile packaging, delivering items using proper aseptic technique, and ensuring items have been appropriately sterilized.

SSIs may also be predicted based on the surgical wound classification. The CDC publishes norms for SSI rates based on certain indicators, including wound classification (see the National Guidelines box). The CDC data provide benchmarks for health care professionals to evaluate their SSI rates so they can further investigate the problem and implement initiatives should the rates be unusually high.

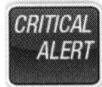 **CRITICAL ALERT** *The purpose of surgical wound classification is to track and learn the cause of infections in order to prevent future incidence. This information is generally recorded on the patient's intraoperative record.*

Over time, surgical team members will in fact develop a surgical conscience. Surgical conscience is defined as "An inner commitment to strictly adhere to aseptic practice, to report any break in aseptic technique, and to correct any violation whether or not anyone else is present or observes the violation. A surgical conscience mandates a commitment to aseptic practice at all times" (Spry, 2005). This allows personnel to function in a more efficient and safe manner.

One of the strategies employed is the creation of the sterile field. The sterile field begins at the surgical site (incision), and extends to the rest of the patient, OR table, surgical team, scrub table, and to a 1-foot parameter around the draped areas (Figure 26–6 ■). This principle is applied to application of prepping solutions, patient draping, room setup, and so forth. It is commonly referred to as the *clean to dirty principle.*

Surgical attire, scrubbing, gowning, and gloving are all functions of OR aseptic technique. Figure 26–7 ■ shows a nurse in

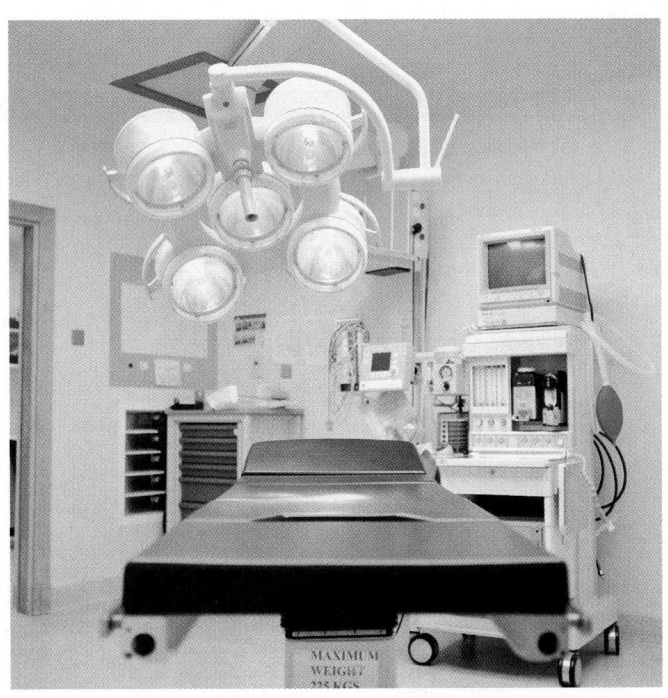

FIGURE 26–6 ■ OR table.
Source: Custom Medical Stock Photo, Inc.

NATIONAL GUIDELINES for Surgical Wound Classification

Clean wounds	An uninfected operative wound in which no inflammation is encountered and the respiratory, alimentary, genital, or uninfected urinary tracts are not entered. In addition, clean wounds are primarily closed and, if necessary, drained with closed drainage. Operative incisional wounds that follow nonpenetrating (blunt) trauma should be included in this category if they meet the criteria.
Clean-contaminated wounds	Operative wounds in which the respiratory, alimentary, genital, or urinary tracts are entered under controlled conditions and without unusual contamination. Specifically, operations involving the biliary tract, appendix, vagina, and oropharynx are included in this category provided no evidence of infection or major break in technique is encountered.
Contaminated wounds	Includes open, fresh, accidental wounds. In addition, operations with major breaks in sterile technique (e.g., open cardiac massage) or gross spillage from the gastrointestinal tract, and incisions in which acute, nonpurulent inflammation is encountered are included in this category.
Dirty or infected wounds	Includes old traumatic wounds with retained or devitalized tissue and those that involve existing clinical infection or perforated viscera. This definition suggests that the organisms causing postoperative infection were present in the operative field before the operation.

Source: Devaney, L., & Rowell K. S. (2004). *Improving surgical wound classification—why it matters.* AORN Journal. Retrieved on July 2, 2008 from http://findarticles.com/p/articles/mi_m0FSL/is_2_80/ai_n6159709.

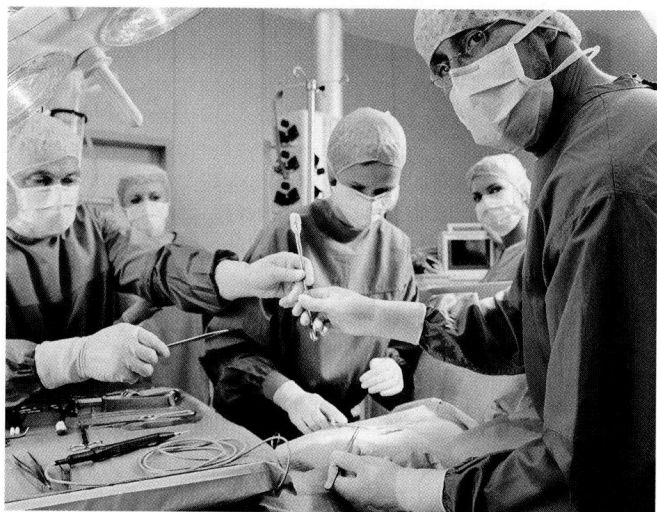

FIGURE 26–7 ■ Correct surgical attire.
Source: Custom Medical Stock Photo, Inc.

proper OR attire and a surgical team member in scrub apparel, highlighting important standards and principles.

Positioning the Patient to Prevent Injury

Patient positioning in the OR is chosen to accommodate surgical access, staff ergonomics, and surgical view while maintaining the patient's skin integrity. It is for this reason that OR tables are narrow (ergonomic for surgeon) and firm (limits movement and allows for CPR). OR tables and accessories are designed to accommodate a wide range of positions in order to allow for the use of gravity to displace organs in order to provide additional working space, surgical access, enhanced ergonomics for professionals, and prevent patient complications.

Complications secondary to positioning include compromised respiratory or circulatory responses, injury to nerves and muscles, and the development of pressure ulcers. Chart 26–4 lists common intraoperative positioning complications and potential causes. Nurses may review patient's intraoperative position via the OR record and assess any relevant patient outcomes. Of these, pressure ulcers have received much attention as a preventable intraoperative complication. The incidence of pressure ulcers in

surgical patients ranges from 4% to a high of 45% depending on the study (Feuchtinger, Halfens, & Dassen, 2005; Price, Whitney, & King, 2005). Researchers report conflicting data on risk factors for the development of pressure ulcers. However, preoperative risk factors commonly cited across studies include age (e.g., older patients); presence of comorbidities particularly diabetes, hypertension, and vascular disorders; and poor nutritional status as measured by low serum albumin and anemia (Feuchtinger et al., 2005; Price et al., 2005). Further research is needed to clarify intraoperative risk factors but those that are suggested include type of surgery (e.g., higher risk with vascular, cardiac, thoracic, and spinal surgery), length of operation (e.g., longer surgeries), care taken during perioperative skin preparation to reduce unnecessary moisture collection under the skin, hypotensive episodes during surgery reducing the blood available to tissues, and the type of anesthetic used. Perioperative nurses need adequate knowledge of anatomy and an understanding of the physiological effects of specific surgical positions. Appropriate positioning accessories and excellent communication between the anesthesia team monitoring physiological responses and the surgical team often requesting position changes is essential in order to prevent patient injury.

 *The primary objective of patient positioning for surgery is to provide maximize exposure while ensuring patient safety. For example, proper positioning can help maintain proper body alignment and access to intravenous and anesthesia support devices.*

Preventing the Retention of Foreign Objects

Surgical counts are the responsibility of perioperative nurses and are performed in order to prevent patient injury due to the high risk of retained foreign body, which can include gauzes, needles, or instruments. Retained foreign objects in patients have resulted in major injuries such as sepsis, bowel perforation, and death. Most facilities follow a legal counting procedure based on the AORN (2007b) recommended standards and practices. The desired patient outcome is a patient free from injury related to extraneous objects. It seems to be a much greater issue than reported, leading to an initiative by health care professional organizations, such as AORN, American College of Surgeons (ACS),

---

CHART 26–4   Intraoperative Positioning Complications

Potential Complications Secondary to Intraoperative Positioning	Potential Intervention
Decreased lung expansion due to supine position resulting in compromised respiratory effects	Position bolsters correctly to minimize compression of thorax, facilitating full lung expansion.
Brachial plexus nerve injury	Position arm correctly to ensure proper arm alignment of less than 90 degrees, supinated, and adequately padded and protected.
Circulatory obstruction due to position resulting in increased risk of postoperative deep vein thrombosis	Apply antiembolic stockings and sequential compression leggings. Use appropriate prophylactic anticoagulant medication administration.
Integumentary injury resulting in pressure ulcers, abrasion, and blistering	Use OR table equipment that will minimize pressure and maximize capillary refill. Appropriate equipment includes gel mattresses. Ensure proper lifting and securing of patient to prevent friction-related injuries.
Dislocation of acetabulum	Ensure proper placement of stirrups and ensure that two health care professionals simultaneously lift, support, and place legs onto stirrups observing correct alignment.

and the Joint Commission, to develop improved methods of accounting for surgical items. One technology that is currently being tested is radio-frequency identification (RFID). This involves RF tags being implanted in surgical sponges (Figure 26–8 ■). This permits the surgical team to pass a wand over the patient following a procedure to verify that no sponges have been left in the patient (Medline, 2006).

The presence of foreign materials in the body can lead to infection, abscess, and other serious problems. Multiple procedures are in place to prevent leaving an instrument or a sponge or other material in the patient when the wound is closed. Sponges, swabs, instruments, and sharps are counted many times during the surgical procedure. Hospitals have written policies describing what is counted, when it is counted, who does the counting, where the counting is documented, and how to resolve a discrepancy in the count. To prevent a foreign object from being left behind:

- All items brought to the operating room are documented.
- No items are removed from the operating room until the final count is complete and verified.
- Sponges, swabs, and other items are counted before surgery, before wound closure begins, and before skin closure begins.
- The circulating nurse and scrub nurse count items in unison.
- The circulating nurse and scrub nurse document the count in the record.

If there is a discrepancy in the count, all personnel try to locate the missing item. If it cannot be found, the patient may be x-rayed. Surgical instruments can be seen by x-ray and soft materials, such as surgical sponges, have a radio-opaque stripe for x-ray identification.

Estimating Blood Loss

The patient is monitored throughout the operation for blood loss. The calculation of blood loss is referred to as the estimation of blood loss (EBL). Blood in suction containers, wound drains, chest tubes, and nasogastric tubes is measured directly at frequent intervals during the surgery. If irrigating fluid is used, it is subtracted from the total amount of drainage to determine the amount of actual blood loss. Blood in sponges can be approximated from their weight with 1 gram of weight being equal to 1 mL of blood. Blood-soaked sponges are collected in a plastic bag and weighed. The weight of the dry sponge(s) and plastic container is subtracted from the total weight to determine blood loss.

Whether or not the patient needs a transfusion during surgery depends on blood loss as well as on other factors such as age, general level of health prior to surgery, history of cardiovascular disease, how well the patient tolerates the blood loss, and the availability of autologous blood. Some religions, such as Christian Science and Jehovah's Witnesses, restrict the administration of blood products.

Adult patients who are generally healthy can tolerate surgical blood loss of up to 500 mL without the need for a transfusion. Blood loss is treated with the administration of packed red blood cells. Chapter 23 ⊘ provides a complete description of blood administration indications and procedures.

Latex Allergy

There has been a significant increase in the number of latex allergies seen in the hospital, including the operating room. Some suggest the increase correlates with the adoption of universal precautions and the increased use of latex gloves. Patients are asked preoperatively about the possibility of latex allergy. A latex sensitivity questionnaire can be used to identify those who have a latex allergy or who are likely to develop the allergy. A high incidence of latex allergy is found in people with spina bifida, patients who have had multiple surgeries, those who work with latex products (health care workers, dental industry workers, rubber workers), and those with a genetic predisposition to allergies (atopy). Patients who report allergies to kiwis, bananas, and avocados are also at an increased risk of latex allergies due to the cross reactivity of the proteins present in these fruits and latex. Blood or skin tests can detect latex-specific IgE antibodies and are performed preoperatively when latex allergy is suspected. Latex allergy is discussed in detail in Chapter 60 ⊘.

It is virtually impossible to create a latex-free environment in the operating room—although it may be possible in the future as more products are being manufactured without latex. For patients with known allergy, a latex-reduced environment is created. Elements of a latex-reduced environment in the operating room include (1) scheduling elective cases as the first cases of the

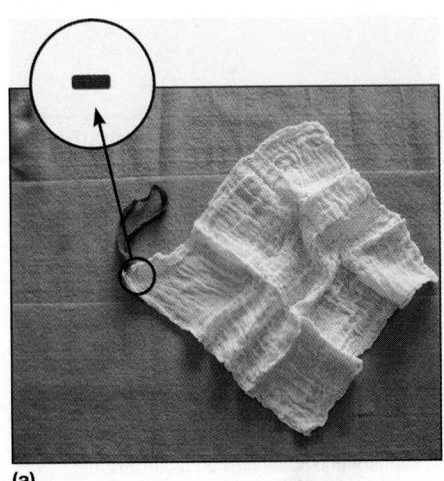
(a)

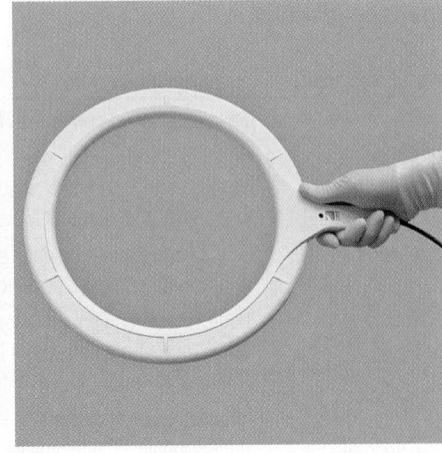
(b)

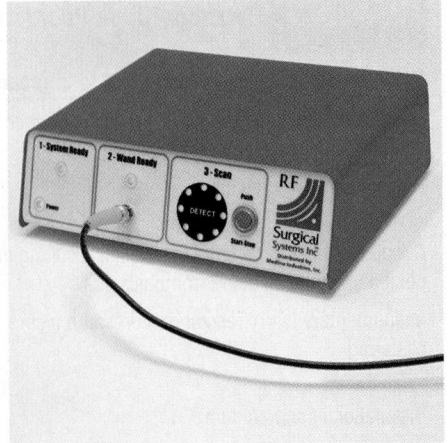
(c)

FIGURE 26–8 ■ RFID technology: (A) RF tag implanted in surgical gauze; (B) wand to detect the RF tag in surgical gauze; (C) surgical RFID detection console.
Source: RF Surgical Systems, Inc. @http://www.rfsurg.com/features.htm

day to minimize contact with aerosolized allergen from latex gloves, (2) using vinyl gloves rather than latex gloves, (3) using powder-free gloves to limit the aerosolization of latex antigens, (4) avoiding latex on the sterile field, (5) using a plastic anesthesia mask, (6) using a stopcock rather than the rubber port for injection of intravenous drugs, (7) removing the rubber cap on medication vials rather than drawing a medication through the cap, (8) using nonlatex equipment such as blood pressure cuff, stethoscope, and electrocardiogram leads, and (9) using nonlatex tape. Premedication of allergic patients with steroids or antihistamines is not recommended.

Allergic responses to latex can range from mild cases of contact dermatitis evidenced by a rash and urticaria to serious cases of anaphylaxis. When a latex allergy is suspected in the operating room, the source of latex in direct contact with the patient is immediately removed. Follow-up treatment includes the administration of 100% oxygen, intravenous fluids to support the blood pressure, and the administration of intravenous epinephrine. Diphenhydramine and steroids may also be given intravenously to attenuate the allergic response.

Postanesthesia Care Unit

Once the surgery is completed, the anesthetist and the nurse will accompany the patient to the postanesthesia care unit (PACU) for further monitoring. Concerns along this route will focus on safety, infection control, medication, communication, positioning, and equipment. The PACU is where the patient will recover from the anaesthetic he has received. This is an unrestricted area where the patient will no longer need to wear a head cover and the nurses will wear regular uniforms. Visitors may be allowed in certain parts of the PACU under certain circumstances.

Poor communication is one of the top contributing factors to medical errors. Therefore, nurses must strive to provide effective and consistent information during patient handoff to a transition unit such as the PACU or Intensive Care Unit (ICU). It is important to give any pertinent information to the unit members where the transfer of responsibility for the surgical patient is occurring and provide an interactive communication that is free of interruptions and includes a systematic process of verification. Figure 26–9 ■ (p. 640) shows a mnemonic that highlights the handoff principles and verification process. PACU is dicussed in detail in Chapter 27 ✿.

Gerontological Considerations

Persons 65 years of age and older, require surgical interventions more often than younger persons because of age-related system changes and comorbid conditions. Degeneration of multiple systems such as the musculoskeletal, nervous, cardiovascular, respiratory, genitourinary, endocrine, and hematopoietic systems and hearing and vision can influence intraoperative and postoperative outcomes. Changes in pharmacokinetics result in changes in drug absorption, distribution, metabolism, and excretion by the body. At this stage of life, both physical and cognitive abilities may vary greatly. Appropriate age-specific interventions should be considered for the geriatric population taking into consideration both physical, cognitive, sensorimotor, and psychosocial factors. The Gerontological Considerations box highlights the special considerations for the gerontological population.

Assess the geriatric patient's history and general health status, in particular medications, previous surgeries, and comorbidities. Promote patient warmth through warming devices and assess range of motion prior to patient being anesthetized in order to ensure correct positioning accessories are available. Additional padding may be necessary due to decreased adipose tissue and circulation, predisposing the patient to the development of pressure ulcers. Efforts should be made to diminish the use of tapes that may lead to denuding of geriatric fragile thinner skin. Ensure adequate time is available to communicate clearly and slowly, keeping in mind possible hearing impairment and need for additional processing and response time.

Hyperglycemia is known to be associated with increased sepsis, suggesting that careful monitoring of glucose levels may be a way to reduce serious postoperative infections. Infections are a major concern for all hospitalized patients, but are especially dangerous for elderly persons. General risk factors for infection in elderly patients are known to include frailty, chronic undernutrition, reduced muscle mass, and poor dentition. Other more general factors common to all age groups are diabetes, aspiration, and the presence of an indwelling urinary catheter.

Patients with postoperative cognitive dysfunction (POCD) experience deterioration in cognitive function that persists for years after the operation. POCD may be related to brain oxygenation during anesthesia, anesthetic agents, and hospital environment (Prough, 2005).

GERONTOLOGICAL CONSIDERATIONS for Elderly Patients Having Surgery

Physical Factors	Cognitive Factors	Sensorimotor Factors	Psychosocial Factors
• Decreased tolerance to heat and cold	• Decline dependent on pregeriatric state and general health and social involvement	• Decreased visual acuity	• Ego integrity important
• Loss of skin tone		• Diminished hearing	• Stressors: end of life, changes in environment, increased cognitive demands
• Declining cardiac/renal function	• Decreased memory, inductive reasoning, and figural relations may occur	• Altered tactile sensation	
• Atrophy of reproductive organs		• Changes in taste and smell	• Death of loved ones
	• Cognitive tasks may require more time to complete	• Diminished response to stress and sensory stimuli	• Concerns for general health increase
• Increased incidence of preexisting health conditions		• Decreased mobility	

Handoff Communications

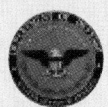

"I PASS THE BATON"

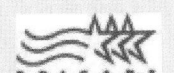

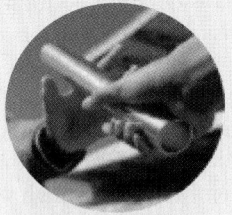

Handoffs and Healthcare Transitions
with opportunities to ask
QUESTIONS, CLARIFY AND CONFIRM

I	Introduction	Introduce yourself and your role/job (include patient)
P	Patient	Name, identifiers, age, sex, location
A	Assessment	Presenting chief complaint, vital signs and symptoms and diagnosis
S	Situation	Current status, medications, circumstances, including code status, level of (un)certainty, recent changes, response to treatment
S	SAFETY Concerns	Critical lab values/reports, socio-economic factors, alllergies, alerts (falls, isolation, etc.)
THE		
B	Background	Co-morbidities, previous episodes, past/home medications, family history
A	Actions	What actions were taken or are required AND provide brief rationale
T	Timing	Level of urgency and explicit timing, prioritization of actions
O	Ownership	Who is responsible (nurse/doctor/team) including patient/family responsibilities
N	Next	What will happen next? Anticipated changes? What is the PLAN? Contingency plans?

FIGURE 26–9 ■ Handoff protocol to improve communication when transferring a patient from the OR to another unit.

Source: Joint Commission (2008). National Patient and Safety Goals. Retrieved July 3, 2008 from http://www.jointcommission.org/NR/rdonlyres/ACA4DBF6-90FD-4400-BE7E-4C6F881E5DCD/0/08_OBS_NPSG_Master.pdf. From the Department of Defense Safety Program.

Prevention of Infection

Clinical Problem

Mild perioperative hypothermia, which is common during major surgery, may promote surgical-wound infection by triggering thermoregulatory vasoconstriction, which decreases subcutaneous oxygen tension. Reduced levels of oxygen in tissue impair oxidative killing by neutrophils and decrease the strength of the healing wound by reducing the deposition of collagen. Hypothermia also directly impairs immune function.

Research Findings

Research was done testing the hypothesis that hypothermia both increases susceptibility to surgical-wound infection and lengthens hospitalization. Good et al. (2006) report that hypothermia itself may delay healing and predispose patients to wound infections. Maintaining normothermia intraoperatively is likely to decrease the incidence of infectious complications in patients undergoing colorectal resection and to shorten their hospitalizations.

Other research was done on prewarming of patients' skin and its influence on core hypothermia (Cooper, 2006; Vanni et al., 2003). Camus et al. (1995) found that a single hour of preoperative skin surface warming reduced the rate at which core hypothermia developed during the first hour of anesthesia.

Antibiotic Administration

Another measure to reduce infection in the operating room is proper timing for antibiotic administration. Antibiotic prophylaxis is being used in a variety of surgical procedures to reduce the incidence of surgical-site infections. Antibiotics should be chosen on the basis of their effectiveness against the pathogens most likely to be encountered. Skin floras (e.g., *Staphylococcus* organisms) are the usual target, so first-generation cephalosporins are most often chosen. Preoperative prophylactic antibiotics should be administered within 60 minutes before the initial incision is made to ensure that antimicrobial levels in the tissue are adequate and maintained for the duration of the procedure (Gordon, 2006; White & Schneider, 2007). To comply with the recommendations of administration within 60 minutes of incision, the holding area was identified as the preferred location (Olin, 2006).

Implications for Nursing Practice

The latest research results have and will influence a change of practice in the perioperative setting based on evidence. In the preoperative setting nurses can use blankets and warming to maintain normothermia. For maintaining normothermia in the OR policies and procedures could be implemented such as use of warming devices under the patient as well as the use of warm solutions. In addition the temperature of the OR suite could be increased.

Nurses also can coordinate the timing of preoperative antibiotic administration. This will necessitate cooperation with both the surgeon and the OR staff to determine the optimal timing of antibiotic administration.

Critical Thinking Questions

1. What nursing interventions will decrease the risk of infection?

Answers to Critical Thinking Questions appear in Appendix D.

References

Camus, Y., Delva, E., Sessler, D., & Lienhart, A. (1995). Pre-induction skin surface warming minimizes intraoperative core hypothermia. *Journal of Clinical Anesthesia, 7,* 384–388.

Cooper, S. (2006). The effect of preoperative warming on patient's postoperative temperatures. *AORN Journal, 83*(5) 1074–1076, 1079–1084.

Good, K. K., Verble, J. A., & Norwood, B. R. (2006). Postoperative hypothermia—The chilling consequences. *AORN Journal, 83*(5), 1055–1066.

Gordon, S. M. (2006). Antibiotic prophylaxis against postoperative wound infections. *Cleveland Clinic Journal of Medicine, 73,* S42–S45.

Olin, J. (2006). Multidisciplinary approach to optimizing antibiotic prophylaxis of surgical site infections. *American Journal of Health-System Pharmacy, 63,* 2312–2314.

Vanni, S. M., Braz, J. R., Modolo, N. S., Amorim, R. B., & Rodrigues, G. R. (2003). Preoperative combined with intraoperative skin surface warming avoids hypothermia caused by general anesthesia and surgery. *Journal of Clinical Anesthesia, 15*(2), 119–125.

White, A., & Schneider, T. (2007). Improving compliance with prophylactic antibiotic administration guidelines. *AORN Journal, 85*(1), 173–180.

EVIDENCE-BASED PRACTICE

NCLEX® REVIEW

1. A preoperative patient is taken into the holding area. The nurse will utilize this time with the patient to do which of the following?
   1. Ensure surgical instruments are operational.
   2. Clean and inspect surgical instruments.
   3. Conduct an interview.
   4. Insert an indwelling urinary catheter if necessary.

2. A registered nurse first assistant is scheduled to assist a surgeon with a surgical procedure. This nurse will be responsible for:
   1. Administering anesthetic agents.
   2. Serving as the patient advocate.
   3. Providing the surgeon with instruments.
   4. Collaborating with the surgeon and suturing the wound closed.

3. During the course of a surgical procedure, the patient's heart rate increases and the blood pressure drops. The care provider who would address these physiological changes to the patient would be the:

1. Surgeon.
2. Anesthesiologist.
3. RNFA.
4. Scrub nurse.

4. While conducting a surgical time-out, the nurse says that the site of surgery is the right knee whereas the left knee was marked as the site of the surgery. Which of the following should be done?

1. Operate on the right knee.
2. Operate on the left knee.
3. Ask a family member which knee is the site of surgery.
4. Stop all preparations until it can be verified which knee is the site of surgery.

5. While an anesthetized patient is being moved to the operating room table, the patient's lower left leg drops and hits the side of the table. Which of the following should the nurse do?

1. Move the leg and place it on the table.
2. Examine the leg for possible or extent of injury and document the event.
3. Nothing because this is considered an acceptable hazard of surgery.
4. Elevate the leg on a pillow.

6. During a surgical procedure the patient begins to demonstrate signs of malignant hyperthermia. Which of the following should be done to support this patient?

1. Administer calcium channel blockers.
2. Stop the surgery or deep the anesthesia.
3. Transfer to the PACU for postsurgical care.
4. Provide 21% oxygen.

7. During a surgical procedure the anesthesiologist directs another care provider to change the oxygen mix being provided to the patient. The care provider most likely to make this oxygen change would be the:

1. RN First Assistant.
2. Scrub nurse.
3. CRNA.
4. Respiratory therapist.

Answers for review questions appear in Appendix D

KEY TERMS

PEARSON
EXPLORE mynursingkit™

MyNursingKit is your one stop for online chapter review materials and resources. Prepare for success with additional NCLEX®-style practice questions, interactive assignments and activities, web links, animations and videos, and more!

Register your access code from the front of your book at
www.mynursingkit.com

REFERENCES

American Society of PeriAnesthesia Nurses. (2001). Clinical guideline for the prevention of unplanned perioperative hypothermia. *Journal of PeriAnesthesia Nursing, 16,* 305–314.

Arbous, M., Meursing, A., van-Kleef, J., de-Lange, J., Spoormans, H., Touw, P., et al. (2005). Impact of anesthesia management characteristics on severe morbidity and mortality. *Anesthesiology, 102*(2), 257–268.

Association of periOperative Registered Nurses. (2002). *PNDS Resources.* AORN. Retrieved June 29, 2008 from http://www.aorn.org/

PracticeResources/PNDSAndStandardizedPerioperativeRecord/PNDSResources/

Association of periOperative Registered Nurses. (2007a). *About AORN.* Retrieved February 16, 2007, from http://www.aorn.org/AboutAORN

Association of periOperative Registered Nurses. (2007b). *Standards, recommended practices and guidelines. Orientation of the registered professional nurse to the perioperative setting.* Denver, CO: Author.

Association of periOperative Registered Nurses. (2008). *RN First Assistant.* AORN. Retrieved on June 29, 2008 from http://www.aorn.org/CareerCenter/CareerDevelopment/RNFirstAssistant/

Bailey, J., McVey, L., & Pevreal, A. (2005). Surveying patients as a start to quality improvement in the surgical suites holding area. *Journal of Nursing Care Quality, 20*(4), 319–326.

Beyea, S. (2000). Preventing surgical site infections—Guiding practice with evidence *AORN Journal.* Retrieved on June 29, 2008 from http:// findarticles.com/p/articles/mi_m0FSL/is_2_72/ai_64424354/pg_3

Bitner, J., Hilde, L., Hall, K., & Duvendack, T. (2007). A team approach to the prevention of unplanned postoperative hypothermia: Clinical report. *AORN Journal, 85*(5), 921–928.

Bonjer, H. J., Hop, W. C., Nelson, H., Sargent, D. J., Lacy, A. M., et al. (2007). Laparoscopically assisted vs open colectomy for colon cancer: A meta-analysis. *Archives of Surgery, 142*(3), 298–303.

Boo, Y. J., Kim, W. B., Kim, J., Song, T. J., Choi, S. Y., et al. (2007). Systemic immune response after open versus laparoscopic cholecystectomy in acute cholecystitis: A prospective randomized study. *Scandinavian Journal of Clinical & Laboratory Investigation, 67*(2), 207–214.

Engemann, J. J., Carmeli, Y., Cosgrove, S. E., Fowler, V. G., Bronstein, M. Z., et al. (2003). Adverse clinical and economic outcomes attributable to methicillin resistance among patients with *Staphylococcus aureus* surgical site infection. *Clinical Infectious Disease, 36,* 592–598.

Evidence based practice information sheets for health professionals. The impact of preoperative hair removal on surgical site infection. (2003). *Best Practice, 7*(2), 1–6.

Feuchtinger, J., Halfens, R., & Dassen, T. (2005). Pressure ulcer risk factors in cardiac surgery: A review of the research literature. *Heart & Lung: The Journal of Acute and Critical Care, 34*(6), 375–385.

Hasankhani, H., Mohammadi, E., Moazzami, F., Mokhtari, M., & Naghgizadh, M. (2007). The effects of intravenous fluid temperature on perioperative hemodynamic situation, post-operative shivering, and recovery in orthopaedic surgery. *Canadian Operating Room Nursing Journal, 25*(1), 20–24, 26–27.

Hoffer, J. L. (1999). Anesthesia. In M. Meeker & J. Rothrock (Eds.), *Care of the patient in surgery* (pp. 203–238). Philadelphia: Mosby.

Hurley, C., & McAleavy, J. (2006) Preoperative assessment and intraoperative care planning. *British Journal of Perioperative Nursing, 16*(1), 187–194.

Hyderally, H. (2002). *Complications of spinal anesthesia.* The Mount Sinai Journal of Medicine. Retrieved June 29, 2008 from http://www.mssm.edu/msjournal/69/v69_1&2_055_056.pdf

Iorio, R., Whang, W., Healy, W. L., Patch, D. A., Najibi, S., & Appleby, D. (2005). The utility of bladder catheterisation in total hip arthroplasty. *Clinical Orthopedics and Related Research, 432,* 148–152.

Joint Commission. (2007). *Facts about the Joint Commission.* Retrieved February 16, 2007, from http://www.jointcommission.org/AboutUs/Fact_Sheets/joint_commission_facts.htm

Larson, E. L., Aiello, A. E., Heilman, J. M., Lyle, C., Cronquist, A., Stahl, A., et al. (2001). Comparison of different regimens for surgical hand preparation. *AORN Journal, 73*(2), 412–432.

Medline. (2006). *RF Surgical Systems, Inc. and Medline Announce Regulatory Clearance to Market RF-Detect, a Breakthrough Surgical Detection System.* Retrieved July 2, 2008 from http://www.medline.com/News/press.asp?ID=39

Nichols, R. L. (2001). Preventing surgical site infections: A surgeon's perspective. *Emerging Infectious Diseases, 7*(2), 220–224.

Niel-Weise, B., Willie, J., & van den Broek, P. (2005). Hair removal policies in clean surgery: Systematic review of randomized, controlled trials. *Infection Control and Hospital Epidemiology, 26*(12), 923–928.

Noblett, S. E., & Horgan, A. F. (2007). A prospective case-matched comparison of clinical and financial outcomes of open versus laparoscopic colorectal resection. *Surgical Endoscopy, 21*(3), 404–408.

Price, M., Whitney, J., & King, C. (2005). Development of a risk assessment tool for intraoperative pressure ulcers. *Journal of Wound, Ostomy and Continence Nursing, 32*(1), 19–30.

Prough, D. S. (2005). Anesthetic pitfalls in the elderly patient. *Journal American College of Surgeons, 200*(5), 784–794.

Rampersaud, Y., Moro, E., Neary, M., White, K., Lewis, S., Massicotte, E., et al. (2006). Intraoperative adverse events and related postoperative complications in spine surgery: Implications for enhancing patient safety founded on evidence-based protocols. *Spine, 31*(13), 1503–1510.

Redmond M. (2001). Malignant hyperthermia: perianesthesia recognition, treatment, and care. *Journal of Perianesthesia Nursing. 16,* 259–270.

Sessler, D., & Todd, M. (2000). Perioperative heat balance. *Anesthesiology, 92*(2), 578–596.

Spry, C. (2005). *Essentials of perioperative nursing* (3rd ed.). Sudbury, MA: Jones & Bartlett.

Sullivan, E. E. (2000). Preoperative holding area, *Journal of PeriAnesthesia Nursing, 15*(5), 353–354.

Tarrac, S. (2006). A description of intraoperative and postanesthesia complication rates. *Journal of PeriAnesthesia Nursing, 21*(2), 88–96.

The Joint Commission (2004). *Procedures Requiring Surgical Site Marking.* Retrieved on July 2, 2008 from http://www.jointcommission.org/AccreditationPrograms/Hospitals/Standards/FAQs/Provsion[plus]of[plus]Care/Operative_HRP_Sed_Anesth/Surgical_Site_Marking.htm

Wagner, D. (2006). Unplanned perioperative hypothermia. *AORN Journal, 83*(2), 470–476.

Postoperative Nursing

Jane Ashley

Outcome-Based Learning Objectives

After studying this chapter, the learner will be able to:

1. Prioritize nursing diagnoses and interventions for the patient in the postanesthesia care unit.
2. Discuss criteria for moving patients through the phases of recovery.
3. Discuss the assessment, prevention, and nursing management of common postoperative problems.
4. Develop a teaching plan for the discharge of a patient after surgery.
5. Identify and discuss areas of future research relevant to the care of the postoperative patient.

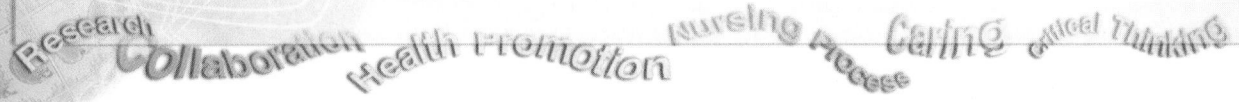

THE POSTOPERATIVE period begins with the completion of surgery and the transfer of the patient to the **postanesthesia care unit** (**PACU**), where the patient recovers from the effects of anesthesia. The PACU, located close to the operating room, is designed to care for patients as they stabilize and recover from surgery and anesthesia. Following surgery, the patient is moved to the PACU accompanied by the circulating nurse and a member of the anesthesia care team. In some circumstances, a surgical patient may be transferred directly to an intensive care unit (ICU) for recovery rather than to the PACU, but most surgical patients stabilize in the PACU before discharge home or transfer to a clinical unit. After discharge from the PACU, postoperative care continues in the home for ambulatory surgical patients, or in the hospital for patients requiring a more monitored recovery.

Nursing Management

Nursing assessment and intervention immediately following surgery focus on patient safety, hemodynamic stability, and the recognition and prevention of postoperative complications. Care in the PACU is organized around postanesthesia phases I and II. Phase I begins with the arrival of the patient and focuses on the recovery of physiological homeostasis and protective mechanisms. During this phase, the patient requires intensive nursing observation and care.

Phase II begins when the patient becomes more alert and functional. The patient requires less intensive nursing and the focus of interventions is on preparing the patient and significant others for the patient's discharge home. As such, phase II refers most specifically to ambulatory surgery. The term **fast-tracking** describes a situation in which the patient is transferred from the operating room to PACU phase II bypassing PACU phase I. Fast-tracking is possible when surgical techniques are minimally invasive and anesthesia is of a short duration. More research is needed to identify which patients are appropriate for fast-tracking, to standardize guidelines and develop protocols used in fast-tracking, and to follow patient outcomes (Ead, 2006).

Nurses should also be aware of certain specifics related to caring for postoperative patients from various cultures, as discussed in the Cultural Considerations box.

Collaborative Management

The PACU nurse works in close collaboration with the anesthesia provider and surgeon. Nurse–physician collaboration in ICUs is linked to better patient outcomes including a reduction in mortality rates (Wheelan, Burchill, & Tilin, 2003). Generally, the anesthesia provider assumes responsibility for coordinating the medical and surgical care of the patient in the PACU. The patient's

CULTURAL CONSIDERATIONS for the Postoperative Patient

- Modesty is extremely important in some cultures and in some religions (e.g., Hispanic, Arab, Muslim). Keep women modestly covered and expose only the body area necessary for examination or treatment. Provide a cover for the head to female patients who desire it. Provide same-gender caretakers when possible.

- Pain assessment may need to be modified for some patients. Numeric rating scales may not be appropriate for all cultures. In some situations, the FACES pain rating scale that uses facial expressions to assess pain may be more useful than numeric rating scales. Some patients may be reluctant to talk about their pain or to take pain medication.

- Pain expression is culturally influenced. In some cultures pain may be openly expressed in words, sounds (e.g., moaning), and physical movement, whereas in other cultures, patients are expected to be stoic about the presence of pain. Nurses need to be aware of and sensitive to cultural expressions of pain.

- Consider cultural beliefs in the selection and use of pain medications. In some cultures, patients may be reluctant to talk about pain and to take pain medication for fear of addition, dependence, or sedation. Explain to patients the importance of treating pain and be sensitive to alternative pain therapies.

- Be aware of and sensitive to treatment restrictions. Some cultures or religions restrict or discourage the use of certain medical treatments such as blood transfusions or organ transplantation.

- Recognize and support the dietary practices in cultures and religions. Many religions (Orthodox Jewish, Muslim, Seventh-Day Adventist, Catholic) have dietary requirements such as vegetarianism or Kosher food preparation, or dietary restrictions such as avoidance of pork, shellfish, or caffeinated products. Hospital kitchens and health care providers need to accommodate these practices. Encourage family members who wish to bring in specially prepared foods to do so. Ask your patient about and be sensitive to special dietary needs.

- Ask about and support the use of alternative healing treatments when possible. Some alternative therapies such as the use of prayer, anointment, healing touch, or communion can be accommodated with little problem. Other therapies such as the use of herbal products to promote healing may need to be evaluated for their effects on wound healing or medications. Talk with patients about what, if any, alternative treatments they believe are important to their recovery.

- Visitors should be encouraged. In some cultures, it is important for family members and extended family members to be present in the hospital with the patient. Consider ways to include family members in the care of the patient.

Sources: Galanti, G. A. (2006). Applying cultural competence to perianesthesia nursing. *Journal of PeriAnesthesia Nursing, 21*(2), 97–102; Lovering, S. (2006). Cultural beliefs about pain. *Journal of Transcultural Nursing, 17*(4), 389–395; McDonald, D. D., McNulty, J., Erickson, K., & Weiskopf, C. (2000). Communicating pain and pain management needs after surgery. *Applied Nursing Research, 13*(2), 70–75; Quinn, D. (2006). How religion, language and ethnicity impact perioperative nursing care. *Nursing Clinics of North America, 41,* 231–248; Spector, R. (2009). *Cultural diversity in health and illness.* Upper Saddle River, NJ: Pearson Prentice Hall.

trajectory in the PACU moves from instability to stability over the course of an hour to several hours (Prowse & Lyne, 2000). Chart 27–1 shows the typical trajectory of a postoperative patient.

Assessment

The PACU nurse ensures patient safety during the transition from the operating room to home or to the clinical unit. The PACU nurse is an intensive care nurse who is prepared to identify and prevent the acute problems and complications associ-

> ### CHART 27–1 Postanesthesia Patient Trajectory
>
> #### Level of Consciousness
> Unconscious → Semiconscious → Conscious
>
> #### Airway
> Unable to maintain airway → Rejects airway support → Supports own airway
>
> #### Cardiovascular
> Cardiovascular instability → Cardiovascular lability → Cardiovascular stable
>
> #### Pain
> No pain perception → Awareness of pain → Adequate pain control
>
> #### Body Temperature
> Hypothermia → Normothermia

Source: Adapted from Prowse, M., & Lyne, P. (2000). Clinical effectiveness in the post-anesthesia care unit: How nursing knowledge contributes to achieving intended patient outcomes. *Journal of Advanced Nursing, 31*(5), 1115–1124.

ated with surgery and anesthesia. The nurse is skilled in the management of situations where the patient's physiological condition is rapidly changing and the nurse is especially attentive to **surveillance** (the systematic and continuous assessment of the patient) and to the recognition and management of potentially catastrophic events (Clarke & Aiken, 2003). The nurse also is prepared to respond to patients' psychological responses to surgery and anesthesia providing reassurance and comfort. Care in the PACU is guided by the *Standards of Perianesthesia Nursing Practice* developed by the American Society of PeriAnesthesia Nurses (ASPAN), the professional organization for PACU nurses (ASPAN, 2006b), the *Standards for Post Anesthesia Care* (ASA, 2004), hospital policies, and clinical guidelines.

The PACU nurse receives a report about the patient's condition from the anesthesia provider. The report provides a description of pertinent medical and surgical history, the condition requiring surgery, the surgical procedure and any complications, the anesthesia, medications given during surgery, any difficulties with intubation, the estimated blood loss from surgery, fluid status of the patient, transfusions, and vital signs. Other pertinent information communicated to the nurse includes the type and location of incisions and drains, intravenous fluids, current medications and medications held prior to surgery, impairments in skin integrity, swallowing, mobility, or communication. The PACU nurse is apprised of concerns the patient expressed preoperatively, any special requirements, and the presence of significant others waiting for the patient.

A complete system assessment of the patient is conducted immediately on arrival to the PACU. The nurse uses the ABCs (i.e., airway–breathing–circulation) to prioritize the initial assessment of the surgical patient starting with observation of the airway for patency. Unless contraindicated, recovering patients are placed in a lateral position to reduce the risk of aspiration. An artificial airway (oral or nasal) prevents the tongue from falling backward and occluding the airway. It may be used until the patient is able to support her airway unassisted. Humidified oxygen is placed via face mask and titrated to keep oxygenation saturation levels above 93% or at a level determined by the health care provider. For the first 2 hours after surgery, the patient may be placed on high levels of oxygen (e.g., FIO_2 greater than 80%) because evidence suggests that this will destroy pathogens and reduce the risk of surgical-site infections (Greif, Akca, Horn, Kurz, & Sessler, 2000; Hopf et al., 2004; Schweon, 2006). The nurse assesses the patient's respiratory rate and depth, breath sounds, and oxygen saturation via a continuous pulse oximeter.

Some patients will remain intubated and on mechanical ventilation following the surgery. In such cases, the nurse performs the respiratory assessments described above and, in addition, checks the endotracheal tube and ventilator settings. A cardiac monitor is attached to the patient as well as a blood pressure cuff. Apical pulse and blood pressure are taken and the patient's heart rhythm is noted. If the patient has a pulmonary artery catheter in place, pulmonary artery pressures and cardiac output are measured and recorded. The nurse assesses peripheral pulses and the patient's color as indices of the adequacy of circulation.

The patient's core body temperature is measured using the monitoring device considered best according to agency policy and the nurse's judgment. Temperature can fluctuate rapidly during recovery. Core body temperature can be measured in the tympanic membrane using a tympanic thermometer. Oral and axillary temperatures provide only an estimate of the core body temperature, and a rectal temperature is considered unreliable in hyperthermic crisis (ASPAN, 2002). A temporal scanner, a device that relies on an infrared scanner to detect the highest temperature of forehead skin, provides a rapid measurement of body temperature, but may not be accurate in recording core body temperatures under some circumstances (Low et al., 2007).

The PACU nurse performs a systematic, head-to-toe assessment of the patient. Figure 27–1 ■ is an example of a PACU assessment form. The following areas are assessed during the head-to-toe examination.

- **Level of consciousness (LOC)**—Is the patient unconscious, arousable, fully awake? LOC is documented every 15 minutes for the first hour, then hourly thereafter. Describe pupil size and response. If awake, is the patient oriented to person, place, and time? Is the patient's speech clear? Intracranial pressure will be measured following selected cranial surgeries.
- **Cardiovascular**—Record the patient's vital signs and cardiac rhythm. If applicable, measure and record cardiac output, pulmonary artery pressures, and central venous pressure. Examine the extremities for color, sensation, motion, and pulses. An ankle-brachial index may be measured in vascular procedures (Chapter 43 🌐).
- **Respiratory**—Describe patient's airway and need for artificial airway, respiratory rate, depth, breath sounds, oxygen

saturation, cough, secretions, arterial blood gases, chest tubes, and need for suctioning, if applicable.

- **Pain management**—Describe the location, quality, and rating of pain. If a spinal or epidural was used, describe the sensory level of numbness and the motor ability of the extremities.
- **Gastrointestinal**—Describe abdominal assessment (Is the abdomen flat and soft or firm and distended? Are bowel sounds present?). If the patient is nauseated, describe whether the nausea is mild, moderate, or severe. Is the patient vomiting?
- **Genitourinary**—Does the patient have a urinary catheter? Describe the amount and color of urine output. If no catheter, is the bladder distended? Has the patient voided? Note when the patient is due to void. If a gynecologic procedure was performed, describe vaginal bleeding.
- **Skin integrity**—Describe skin color, temperature, areas of bruising, redness, or ulceration.
- **Temperature**—Record core body temperature.
- **Incision**—Describe location and condition of incision. Describe any bleeding, wound drainage, or the presence of a hematoma. If the suture line is not visible, describe the condition of the dressing. Describe the type and drainage from any wound drains.
- **Activity/movement**—Is the patient able to hold his head up? Is the patient able to move all extremities? Are movements voluntary or on command? Describe strength of extremities; is it equal on both sides? Does the patient have compression stockings, pneumatic compression boots, or another type of deep venous thrombosis (DVT) prophylaxis device in place?
- **Psychosocial**—If the patient is awake, describe the level of psychosocial comfort. Is the patient calm, relaxed, and sleeping or anxious and distressed?
- **Intravenous fluids**—Describe the location of intravenous catheters, the type of catheter, and the type and rate of intravenous fluid.
- **Drains and other tubes**—Describe the type, location, and drainage of any tubes.
- **Other medical devices**—Describe any other devices the patient may have such as an arterial line, pulmonary artery catheter, or traction.

The American Society of Anesthesiologists (ASA, 2004) recommends using a scoring system as part of the continuous evaluation of PACU patients. Numerical rating systems are endorsed by the Joint Commission and they have several advantages. Scoring systems are easy to use, reliable, and they provide objective data for monitoring how well the patient is progressing. Additionally, data from scoring systems can be used in research studies to compare the postoperative progression associated with particular patient characteristics or specific types of surgeries.

Various numerical rating systems are available but the most commonly used system is the Aldrete Post Anesthesia Recovery Score (PARS) (Figure 27–2 ■, p. 655). In this scoring system, the patient receives a score of 0 to 2 for respirations, oxygen saturation, consciousness, circulation, and activity. Total scores range from 0 to 10 with higher scores indicating a higher level of func-

Patient's name _____

Med. Rec. # _____

DOB _____

POSTOPERATIVE ASSESSMENT

| TIME | | | | | | | | | | | | | | **POST ANESTHETIC SCORE** |

POST ANESTHESIA RECOVERY SCORE

ACTIVITY
Able to move 4 extremities voluntarily or on command ... 2
Able to move 2 extremities voluntarily or on command ... 1
Unable to move extremities voluntarily or on command ... 0

RESPIRATION
Able to breathe deeply and cough freely ... 2
Dyspnea, limited breathing, or tachypnea ... 1
Apneic or on mechanical ventilator ... 0

CIRCULATION
BP plus or minus 20% of preoperative baseline ... 2
BP plus or minus 20%-40% of preanesthetic level ... 1
BP plus or minus 40% of preanesthetic level ... 0

CONSCIOUSNESS
Fully awake ... 2
Arousable on calling ... 1
Not responding ... 0

O2 Saturation
Able to maintain O2 saturation > 92% on room air ... 2
Needs O2 inhalation to maintain O2 saturation > 90% ... 1
O2 saturation <50% even with O2 supplement ... 0

TOTAL PAR SCORE | **TOTAL PAR SCORE**

POST ANESTHESIA DISCHARGE SCORE

VITAL SIGNS
BP and pulse within 20% of preoperative baseline ... 2
BP and pulse 20%-40% of preoperative baseline ... 1
BP and pulse <40% of preoperative baseline ... 0

ACTIVITY LEVEL
Steady gait, no clumsiness, or meets preoperative level ... 2
Requires assistance ... 1
Unable to ambulate ... 0

NAUSEA & VOMITING
Minimal to none ... 2
Moderate ... 1
Severe ... 0

PAIN
Minimal to pain free ... 2
Moderate pain handeled by oral medication ... 1
Severe pain requiring parenternal medication ... 0

SURGICAL BLEEDING
Minimal to none ... 2
Moderate ... 1
Severe ... 0

TOTAL PAD SCORE | **TOTAL PAD SCORE**

LABORATORY RESULTS

	Hematology			Coagulation			Chemistry									Miscellaneous TEST RESULTS
Time	Hct	WBC	Plts	PT	PTT	INR	BS	BUN	Cr	Na	K	Cl	CO$_2$	Mg	iCa	

FIGURE 27–1 ■ Sample PACU assessment form.

tioning. A patient receives a score on admission and every 30 minutes until a score of 8 or higher is achieved. The PARS score is the criterion by which patients progress from phase I PACU recovery to phase II PACU recovery (Ead, 2006).

The frequency of patient assessment in the PACU depends on the stability of the patient. A patient's physiological status can change rapidly during recovery. In acute crisis, patients are con- tinuously monitored (every 1 to 5 minutes) until the situation no longer warrants such close observation. For the person who is stable, vital signs and patient assessment are performed on admission and every 15 minutes for the first hour (i.e., four assessments). This is followed by every 30 minutes for the next 2 hours (i.e., four assessments), then every hour until discharge from the unit. Chart 27–2 (p. 655) lists abnormal findings on assessment

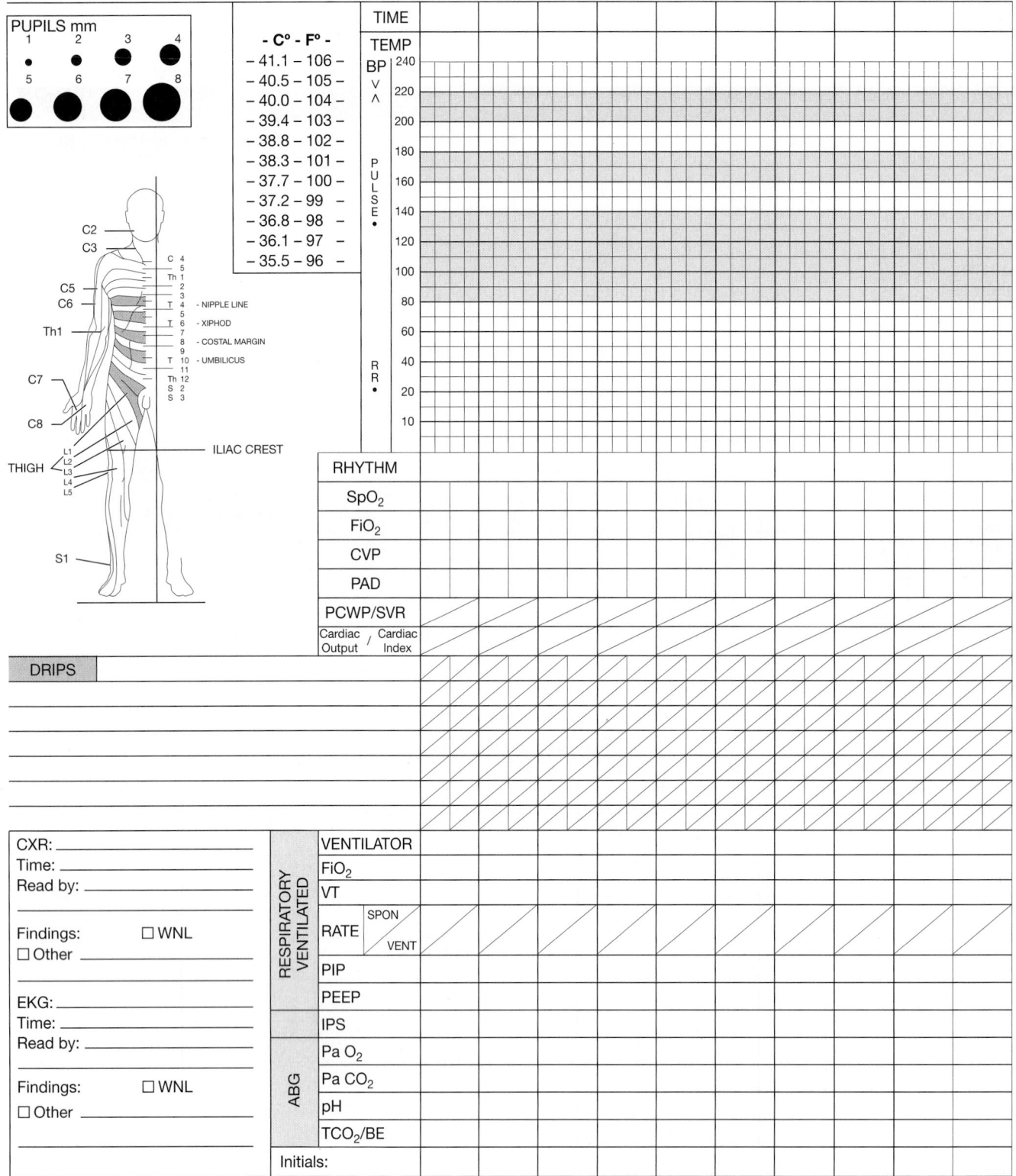

FIGURE 27–1 ■ *Continued*

that suggest the need for closer observation and consultation with the anesthesiologist.

Initially, patients are placed in a lateral position. As they become more awake, they are placed with the head of the bed elevated if not contraindicated by the surgery. Patients are repositioned every 1 to 2 hours or as needed. A patient who is experiencing nausea and vomiting may remain in a lateral position to prevent aspiration.

Nursing Diagnoses and Expected Outcomes

The patient recovering from anesthesia and surgery is at risk for a number of problems. Some of these problems occur early in the course of recovery and are much more likely to be seen in the PACU than elsewhere. Others may occur both in the PACU and on the clinical unit. Some problems occur later in recovery and

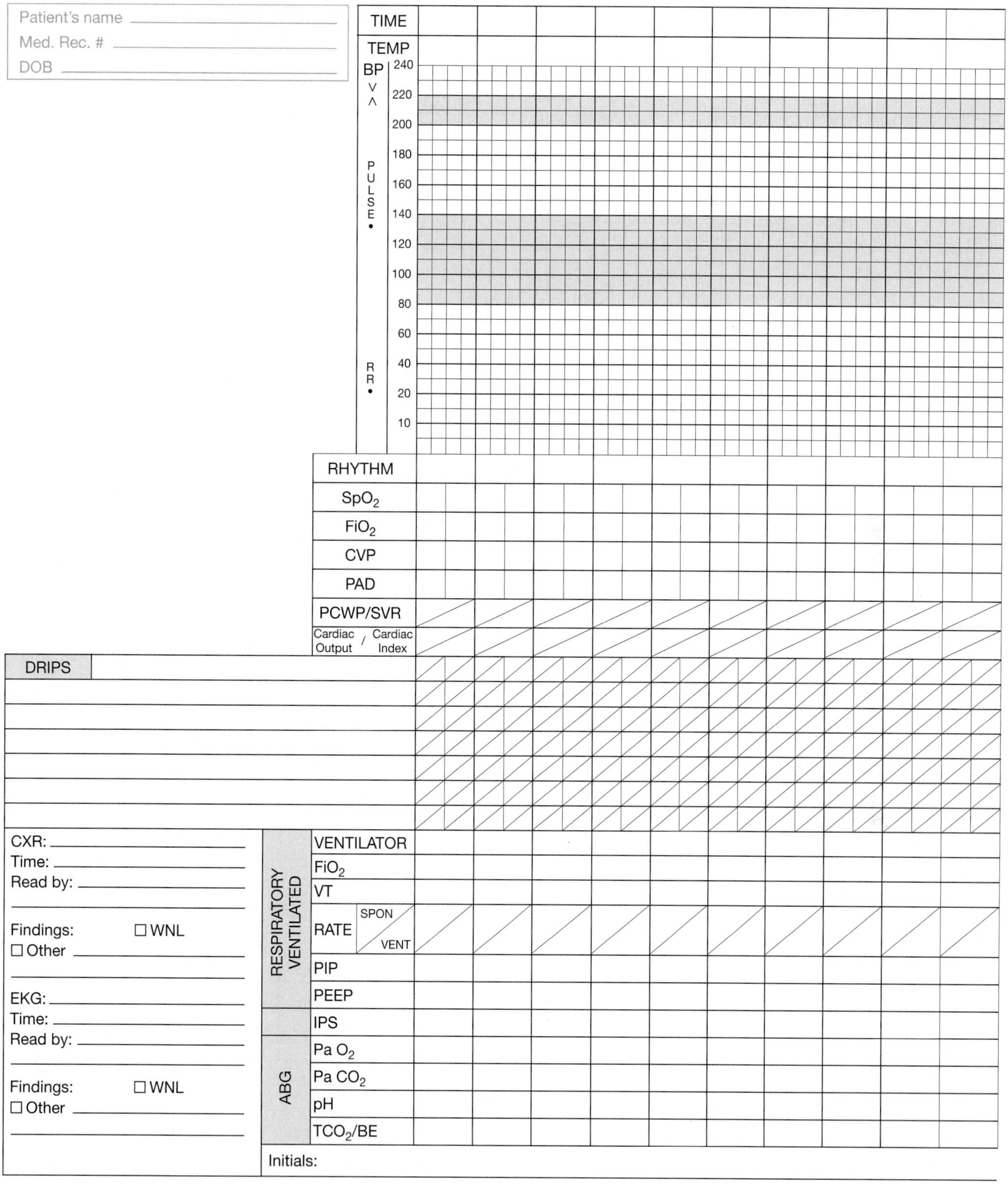

Patient's name _____
Med. Rec. # _____
DOB _____

TIME	
TEMP	
BP	240
V ∧	220
	200
	180
PULSE •	160
	140
	120
	100
	80
	60
R R •	40
	20
	10

RHYTHM	
SpO₂	
FiO₂	
CVP	
PAD	
PCWP/SVR	
Cardiac Output / Cardiac Index	

DRIPS

CXR: _____	VENTILATOR
Time: _____	FiO₂
Read by: _____	VT
	RATE SPON / VENT
Findings: ☐ WNL	
☐ Other _____	PIP
	PEEP
EKG: _____	IPS
Time: _____	Pa O₂
Read by: _____	Pa CO₂
Findings: ☐ WNL	pH
☐ Other _____	TCO₂/BE
	Initials:

RESPIRATORY VENTILATED
ABG

FIGURE 27–1 ■ *Continued*

are more likely to be seen on the clinical unit or at home after discharge. Common nursing diagnoses with expected outcomes in the PACU are as follows:

- *Risk for Impaired Gas Exchange* (airway obstruction, laryngospasm, hypoxia).

  Outcomes: The patient will have an open airway. The patient will have breathing patterns consistent with or improved from baseline. The patient will demonstrate adequate oxygen saturation levels.

- **Risk for Imbalanced Fluid Volume** (bleeding, hypovolemia, fluid overload)

  Outcomes: The patient will achieve adequate hemostasis. The patient will demonstrate normal fluid and electrolyte balance.

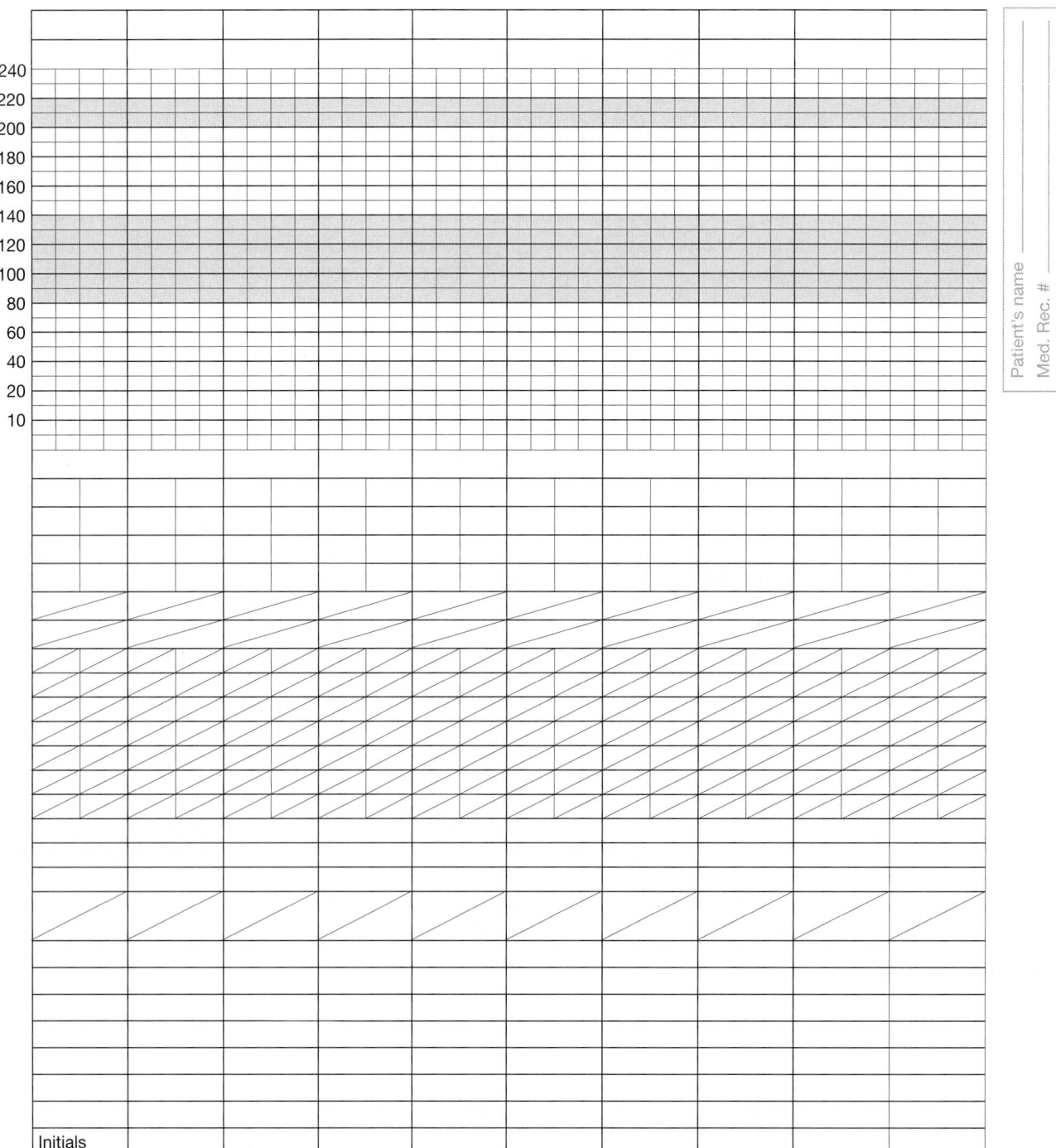

FIGURE 27–1 ■ *Continued*

- **Risk for Decreased Cardiac Output:** (dysrhythmia, hypotension, hypertension).

  Outcomes: The patient will have normal cardiac rhythm. The patient will achieve adequate cardiac output. The patient's blood pressure and heart rate will return to normal or be consistent with baseline values.

- **Risk for Imbalanced Body Temperature:** *Hypothermia*

  Outcome: The patient will demonstrate a normal core body temperature.

- **Readiness for Enhanced Comfort:** *Nausea and Vomiting*

  Outcome: The patient will report adequate relief from nausea and vomiting.

- **Readiness for Enhanced Comfort:** *Pain*

  Outcome: The patient will report an acceptable level of pain control.

- **Anxiety**

  Outcomes: The patient will report diminished anxiety levels. The patient will report an acceptable level of anxiety.

Interventions, Rationales, and Evaluation

The interventions and rationales for the nursing diagnoses often seen with patients in the PACU are discussed next, and additional guidelines for patients in postoperative phase I that deal with pain and comfort are listed in the National Guidelines box (p. 656).

TIME																			
(?) Yes (-) No (*) See Notes (N/A) Not applicable																			
☐ Patient identified using two indicators																			
LEVEL OF CONSCIOUSNESS																			
Fully awake																			
Arousable upon calling																			
Not responding																			
PUPIL SIZE (mm) REACTION R																			
SL = sluggish R = reactive NR = nonreactive L																			
PAIN: Location & Level (0-10) (Quality*)																			
SPEECH CLEAR & APPROPRIATE																			
BREATH SOUNDS																			
SYMMETRICAL																			
COUGH/DEEP BREATHE																			
AIRWAY																			
Patent																			
____ oral ____ nasal D/C ____																			
CPT/IS																			
SUCTIONING																			
EXTREMITIES WARM & WNL																			
PERIPHERAL PULSES R																			
L																			
SEQUENTIAL COMPRESSION DEVICE 45 mmHg																			
POSITION																			
SPINAL/EPIDURAL SENSORY LEVEL R																			
L																			
MOTOR RESPONSE R Arm																			
3 = Lifts & holds L Arm																			
2 = Lifts & falls back R Leg																			
1 = Moves on bed L Leg																			
0 = No movement																			
DRESSING D&I: Site(s)																			
DRAINS PATENT/DRAINAGE																			
1. Type drain/site:																			
1. Type drainage:																			
2. Type drain/site:																			
2. Type drainage:																			
SKIN INTEGRITY:																			
ARTERIAL LINE Dressing D&I																			
CENTRAL LINE Dressing D&I																			
PERIPHERAL IVs:																			
REWARMING DEVICE:																			
VAGINAL FLOW																			
NAUSEA OR VOMITING																			
NGT -> CONTINUOUS SUCTION																			
-> Type drainage																			
ABDOMEN SOFT																			
FOLEY CATHETER PATENT																			
Type drainage																			
BLADDER NOT PALPABLE																			
Voided QS																			
No void. Discharge voiding instructions reviewed.																			
DTV@																			
INITIALS																			

Side label: NURSING OBSERVATIONS AND INTERVENTIONS

FIGURE 27–1 ■ *Continued*

NURSING OBSERVATIONS AND INTERVENTIONS

TIME (?) Yes (-) No (*) See Notes (N/A) Not applicable						
☐Patient identified using two indicators						
LEVEL OF CONSCIOUSNESS						
Fully awake						
Arousable upon calling						
Not responding						
PUPIL SIZE (mm) /REACTION R						
SL = sluggish R = reactive NR = nonreactive L						
PAIN: Location & Level (0-10) (Quality*)						
SPEECH CLEAR & APPROPRIATE						
BREATH SOUNDS						
SYMMETRICAL						
COUGH/DEEP BREATHE						
AIRWAY						
Patent						
____ oral ____ nasal D/C ____						
CPT/IS						
SUCTIONING						
EXTREMITIES WARM & WNL						
PERIPHERAL PULSES R						
L						
SEQUENTIAL COMPRESSION DEVICE 45 mmHg						
POSITION						
SPINAL/EPIDURAL SENSORY LEVEL R						
L						
MOTOR RESPONSE R Arm						
3 = Lifts & holds L Arm						
2 = Lifts & falls back 1 = Moves on bed R Leg						
0 = No movement L Leg						
DRESSING D&I: Site(s)						
DRAINS PATENT/DRAINAGE						
1. Type drain/site:						
1. Type drainage:						
2. Type drain/site:						
2. Type drainage:						
SKIN INTEGRITY:						
ARTERIAL LINE Dressing D&I						
CENTRAL LINE Dressing D&I						
PERIPHERAL IVs:						
REWARMING DEVICE:						
VAGINAL FLOW						
NAUSEA OR VOMITING						
NGT -> CONTINUOUS SUCTION						
-> Type drainage						
ABDOMEN SOFT						
FOLEY CATHETER PATENT						
Type drainage						
BLADDER NOT PALPABLE						
Voided QS						
No void. Discharge voiding instructions reviewed.						
DTV@						
INITIALS						

TIME	NOTES

FIGURE 27–1 ■ *Continued*

MEDICATION	DOSE	ROUTE	TIME			

MEDICATIONS

Patient's name _____

Med. Rec. # _____

DOB _____

MEDICATION	DOSE	ROUTE	TIME			

TIME	NOTES	TIME	NOTES

_____ RN	_____ RN	_____ ___/___/___
Signature	Printed name	Initials Date
_____ RN	_____ RN	_____ ___/___/___
Signature	Printed name	Initials Date
_____ RN	_____ RN	_____ ___/___/___
Signature	Printed name	Initials Date
_____ RN	_____ RN	_____ ___/___/___
Signature	Printed name	Initials Date

FIGURE 27–1 ■ *Continued*

INTAKE & OUTPUT												
ENTERAL		CRYSTALLOID			COLLOID			OUTPUT				
TIME	AMT	TIME	AMT	ABS	TIME	ABS	TIME	IRRIGATION UP / IN	HOURLY URINE / TOTAL	NG/EMESIS	CHEST	HEMOVAC/ JP
O.R. ⟶							EBL=					

DISCHARGE SUMMARY

NURSING DIAGNOSES 1-14 OUTCOMES MET: ☐ Yes ☐ No _____

SURGICAL CRITERIA MET: ☐ Yes ☐ No _____

Time Ready for Discharge: _____ Discharged: _____

☐ Room #: _____ ☐ Transfer Communication Completed _____

Discharge ☐ Home Time: _____ ☐ Valuables Returned to Patient

_____   _____
Signature of Recipient   RN Initials

Discharge teaching completed. Patient verbalizes understanding.

☐ Yes ☐ No (See note)

Prescriptions: _____

Copy of instructions given to patient: ☐ Yes ☐ No

OUTPATIENT POST-OP PHONE CALL

Phone #: _____

Date: _____ Time: _____

Pain: Score (0-10) _____ : Location/Quality _____

Nausea/Vomiting: ☐ No ☐ Yes _____

Voiding: ☐ Yes ☐ No _____

Any problem with procedure site? ☐ No ☐ Yes _____

Any concerns? ☐ No ☐ Yes _____

Did you need to call MD? ☐ No ☐ Yes _____

☐ Voice mail left. Patient to call with questions.

Comments: _____

_____

Signature RN _____   Print Name _____

FIGURE 27–1 ■ *Continued*

Source: Courtesy of Beth Israel Deaconess Nursing Department

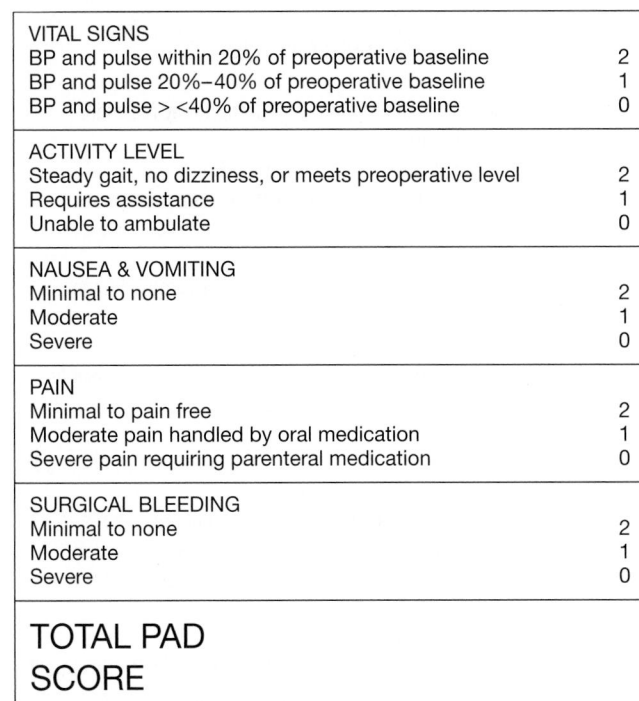

VITAL SIGNS	
BP and pulse within 20% of preoperative baseline	2
BP and pulse 20%–40% of preoperative baseline	1
BP and pulse > <40% of preoperative baseline	0
ACTIVITY LEVEL	
Steady gait, no dizziness, or meets preoperative level	2
Requires assistance	1
Unable to ambulate	0
NAUSEA & VOMITING	
Minimal to none	2
Moderate	1
Severe	0
PAIN	
Minimal to pain free	2
Moderate pain handled by oral medication	1
Severe pain requiring parenteral medication	0
SURGICAL BLEEDING	
Minimal to none	2
Moderate	1
Severe	0
TOTAL PAD SCORE	

FIGURE 27–2 ■ Aldrete Post Anesthesia Recovery Score.
Source: Courtesy of Beth Israel Deaconess Nursing Department

Impaired Gas Exchange

Most patients will arrive in the PACU with supplemental oxygen to prevent **hypoxemia**, insufficient oxygen content in the blood. Common causes of hypoxemia in the early postoperative period include airway obstruction, hypoventilation, and laryngospasm. Respiratory complications, especially the need for upper airway support, are the most frequent postoperative problem in the PACU (McAlister, Bertsch, Man, Bradley, & Jacka, 2005; Tarrac, 2006).

Airway obstruction occurs most often because medications used in anesthesia cause the muscles to relax. When the tongue relaxes, it can fall backward blocking the airway. Signs of an obstructed airway include snoring, stridor, retraction of intercostal muscles, and a fall in oxygen saturation levels. To prevent airway obstruction, patients are positioned on their side and an artificial airway is inserted. An oral airway is effective with the patient who is minimally responsive, but a patient who is more arousable may gag, choke, or spit out the airway. For these patients, a nasal airway may be more effective and comfortable. A patient who is experiencing an acute airway obstruction needs to be stimulated. If a patient is arousable, the problem can often be resolved by speaking to the patient, encouraging her to take deep breaths, and turning up the oxygen level if necessary. Patients who are not arousable may need to have their airway opened. The nurse can perform the chin-tilt/jaw-thrust maneuver used in cardiopulmonary resuscitation to open the airway. An oral airway is inserted to maintain patency. Airway occlusion becomes less of a threat once the patient is more responsive and regains protective mechanisms.

In some patients, a delay in the excretion of neuromuscular blocking agents used in anesthesia can result in weakened respiratory muscles causing *hypoventilation*, insufficient inspiratory

CHART 27–2 Abnormal PACU Assessments That Are Reported to the Anesthesiologist

NEUROLOGICAL FINDINGS

- Prolonged unresponsiveness
- Change in level of consciousness
- Abnormal responses such as slurred speech, asymmetrical smile, weak hand grasps, inability to move all extremities

CARDIOVASCULAR FINDINGS

- Heart rate >120 beats/min
- Hypotension (e.g., systolic blood pressure of less than 90 mmHg)
- New cardiac dysrhythmia
- Hypertension (e.g., systolic blood pressure 20% to 30% higher than baseline)
- Absence of peripheral pulses

RESPIRATORY FINDINGS

- Oxygen saturation < 93%
- Respiratory rate <10 breaths/min
- Indications of respiratory distress and/or hypoventilation such as stridor, retraction of intercostal muscles, minimal respiratory effort

OTHER FINDINGS

- Urine output < 30 mL hour or < 5 mL/kg per hour
- More than the expected amount of bleeding at the incision site
- Enlarging hematoma
- Loss of pulse(s) in a graft site
- Unexpected presence of blood in drainage tubes
- More than the expected amount of drainage from chest tubes or wound drains
- Vomiting associated with possible aspiration

and expiratory effort. This should be suspected in patients who are unable to sustain a head lift or have weak hand grasps although this may be hard to evaluate in a patient who is obtunded. The prolonged effects of anesthetic agents also can produce a slow respiratory rate (i.e., less than 10 per minute) and shallow breathing. The continuous assessment of oxygen saturation helps to identify the patient who is becoming hypoxemic as a result of poor ventilatory effort. The nurse reports to the anesthesiologist a respiratory rate of less than 10 or oxygen saturation rate of less than 93% or less than a health care provider–prescribed value. Some patients experiencing hypoxemia may benefit from the application of continuous positive airway pressure (CPAP) to keep airways open (Squadrone et al., 2005).

Laryngospasm occurs when the muscles of the larynx contract forcefully, causing a closure or partial closure of the airway. It can be caused by irritation from secretions, inhalants, or medications and is an emergency situation because the patient can quickly become hypoxic. Treatment may include opening the airway, suctioning secretions, administering oxygen, administering an aerosolized epinephrine solution, and in severe cases reintubation.

NATIONAL GUIDELINES American Society of PeriAnesthesia Nurses Pain and Comfort Clinical Guidelines

Postanesthesia Phase I

Assessment

1. Refer to preoperative phase assessment, interventions, and outcomes data.

2. Type of surgery and anesthesia technique, anesthetic agents, reversal agents.

3. Analgesics (i.e., nonopioid, opioid, adjuvants given before and during surgery, time and amount at last dose, and regional [e.g., spinal/epidural]).

4. Pain and comfort levels on admission and until transfer to receiving unit or discharge to home. Reassess frequently until pain or discomfort is controlled. During sedation procedure, assess continuously.

5. Assessment parameters:
   A. Functional level and ability to relax.
   B. Pain: type, location, intensity (i.e., using self-report pain rating scale whenever possible [age, language, condition, and cognitive appropriate tools], quality, frequency [continuous or intermittent], and sedation level; patient's method of assessment and reporting need to be the same during the postoperative continuum of care for consistency). Note pain level at rest and during activity.
   C. Self-report of comfort level using numerical scale (0 to 10 scale) or other institutionally approved instruments.
   D. Physical appearance (e.g., pain/discomfort behaviors. [*Note:* Pain behaviors are highly individual and the absence of any specific behavior, e.g., facial expression or body movement, does not mean the absence of pain].)
   E. Other sources of discomfort (e.g., position, nausea and vomiting, shivering, environment such as noise, noxious smell, anxiety).
   F. Achievement of pain relief/comfort treatment goals.

6. Age, cognitive ability, and cognitive learning methods.

7. Status/vital signs:
   A. Airway patency, respiratory status, breath sounds, level of consciousness, and pupil size as indicated and other symptoms related to the effects of medications.
   B. Blood pressure.
   C. Pulse/cardiac monitor rhythm.
   D. Oxygen saturation.
   E. Motor and sensory functions postregional anesthesia technique.

Interventions

1. Identify patient correctly; validate health care provider's order; implement correct drug, dose, amount, route, and time; include type of surgery and surgical site as applicable.

2. Pharmacologic (medicate as ordered).
   A. *Mild to moderate pain:* Use nonopioids and may consider opioid (e.g., acetaminophen, NSAIDs, cyclooxygenase 2 [Cox-2] inhibitors). All of the patient's regular nonopioid prescription medications should be made available unless contraindicated and per institutional approval.
   B. *Moderate to severe pain:* Use multimodal therapy (e.g., combine nonopioid and opioid).

C. Utilize the three analgesic groups appropriately (consider multimodal therapy):
   i. Nonopioids (e.g., acetaminophen, NSAIDs, Cox-2 inhibitors); adjuvants nonopioids (acetaminophen and NSAIDs, such as aspirin, ketorolac, ibuprofen, Cox-2 inhibitors).
   ii. Beta-agonist opioids (e.g., morphine, hydromorphone, fentanyl).
   iii. Adjuvants:
      a. Multipurpose for chronic pain (e.g., anticonvulsants, tricyclic antidepressants, corticosteroids, antianxiety medication).
      b. Multipurpose for moderate to severe acute pain (e.g., local anesthetics, ketamine).
      c. Neuropathic continuous pain (antidepressants, tricyclic antidepressants, oral or local anesthetic).
      d. Neuropathic lancinating pain, e.g., stabbing, knifelike pain (anticonvulsant, baclofen).
      e. Malignant bone pain (corticosteroids, calcitonin).
      f. Post–orthopedic surgery: Consider muscle relaxants if patient experiences muscle spasm.

3. Initiate and adjust IV and regional infusions, i.e., patient controlled analgesia (PCA) as indicated and ordered, and based on hemodynamics status. (Refer to institutional permissive procedure.)

4. Nonpharmacologic intervention use to complement, not replace, pharmacologic interventions.

5. Administer comfort measures as needed:
   A. Physiological (e.g., positioning, pillow, heat and cold therapies, sensory aids [e.g., dentures, eye glasses, hearing aids]; use meperidine [Demerol] for shivering, antiemetics [e.g., Reglan, Zofran] as ordered).
   B. Sociocultural (e.g., family/caregiver, interpreter visit).
   C. Psychospiritual (e.g., chaplain or cleric of choice, religious objects/symbols).
   D. Environmental (e.g., confidentiality, privacy, reasonably quiet room).

6. Cognitive behavioral (e.g., education/instruction, relaxation, imagery, music, distraction, biofeedback).

Expected Outcomes

1. Patient will maintain hemodynamic stability including respiratory/cardiac status and level of consciousness.

2. Patient will state achievement of pain relief/comfort treatments goals (e.g., acceptable pain relief with mobility at time of transfer or discharge).

3. Patient will state he/she feels safe and secure with the instructions (e.g., use of PCA machine).

4. Patient will show effective use of at least one nonpharmacologic method (i.e., breathing relaxation techniques).

5. Patient will show effective use of PCA as indicated and discuss expected results of regional techniques.

6. Patient will verbalize evidence of receding pain level and increased comfort with pharmacologic and nonpharmacologic interventions.

NATIONAL GUIDELINES American Society of PeriAnesthesia Nurses Pain and Comfort Clinical Guidelines—*Continued*

Postanesthesia Phase II/III

Assessment

1. Refer to preoperative phase and phase I assessments, interventions, and outcomes data.

2. Achievement of pain/comfort treatment goals and level of satisfaction with pain relief and comfort management.

3. Pain relief/comfort management plan for discharge and patient agreement.

4. Educational and resource needs, considering age, language, condition, and cognitive appropriateness.

Interventions

1. Identify patient correctly; validate health care provider's order; implement correct drug, dose, amount, route, and time.

2. Pharmacologic interventions (medicate as ordered): nonopioid (e.g., acetaminophen, NSAIDs, Cox-2 inhibitors), beta-agonist opioids (e.g., morphine, hydromorphone, fentanyl), and adjuvant analgesics (e.g., local anesthetics).

3. Continue and/or initiate nonpharmacologic measures from phase I.

4. Educate patient and family/caregiver:
   A. Pain and comfort measures.
   B. Untoward symptoms to observe.
   C. Regional or local anesthetic effects dissipating after discharge (e.g., numbness, motor weakness, or inadequate relief) and potential adjustments as applicable.
   D. Availability of resources as needed.

5. Discuss misconceptions and expectations and implement plan of action satisfactory to patients.

6. Address nausea with pharmacologic interventions or other techniques and discuss expectations.

Expected Outcomes

1. Patient will state acceptable level of pain relief and comfort with movement or activity at time of transfer or discharge to home.

2. Patient will verbalize understanding of discharge instruction plans:
   A. Specific drug to be taken.
   B. Frequency of drug administration.
   C. Potential side effects of medication.
   D. Potential drug interactions.
   E. Specific precaution to follow when taking medication (e.g., physical limitation, dietary restrictions).
   F. Name and telephone number of the health care provider/resource to notify about pain, problems, and other concerns.

3. Patient will state understanding or show effective use of nonpharmacologic methods (e.g., cold/heat therapy, relaxation breathing, imagery, music).

4. Patient will state achievement of pain/comfort treatment goals and level of satisfaction with pain relief and comfort management in the perianesthesia setting.

Source: Reprinted from American Society of PeriAnesthesia Nurses. ASPAN pain and comfort guideline. *Journal of PeriAnesthesia Nursing, 18*(4), 232–236, 2003, with permission from Elsevier.

Risk for Imbalanced Fluid Volume

The patient is monitored postoperatively for evidence of bleeding, hypovolemia, and fluid overload. Bleeding is identified in several ways depending on the specific surgery performed. Bleeding can be seen on surgical wound dressings and in drainage tubes such as a nasogastric tube, a chest tube, a urinary catheter, or a wound drainage tube. The nurse examines the wound and dressing for signs of bleeding every hour or more frequently as needed.

Often, the surgical wound is expected to ooze small to moderate amounts of blood or sanguineous drainage. The nurse does *not* take off the surgical dressing, because it aids in hemostasis. Instead, an area of drainage is marked (e.g., circled in pen) on the dressing, monitored for enlargement, and reported to the surgeon. The sheets under the patient are examined for evidence of bleeding because gravity may cause blood to leak from the dressing and pool underneath the patient. If blood soaks through a dressing, the dressing should be reinforced and the event reported to the surgeon. Drains are monitored with dressing checks. The nurse reports the presence of blood or sudden increased amounts of drainage in a drain as a new finding to the surgeon. Certain tubes, such as chest tubes following a lung resection, a nasogastric tube following a gastrectomy, or wound drainage tubes, might be expected to drain blood initially with the drainage gradually changing from sanguineous to serosanguineous drainage during the next several hours or days. The nurse needs to have a sense of the expected amount and type of drainage from a drainage tube in order to respond promptly to any increases in drainage. The surgeon must be notified of any changes.

Internal bleeding is sometimes seen as distention of tissues or the formation of a bruise or hematoma. A hematoma forms in an area where blood is collecting, and often causes increased pain. Generally this will be in the area surrounding the wound but in some cases, a hematoma may form in what appears to be a distant site. Other signs of internal bleeding are seen when blood loss is large enough to produce a drop in blood pressure, an increase in heart rate, or a decrease in cardiac output (Clancy, McVicar, & Baird, 2002). Initially the heart rate increases in an attempt to maintain a normal cardiac output and blood pressure; thus, it is an early sign of bleeding. Other indications of bleeding include a change in the patient's level of consciousness (anxiety, agitation, and confusion), a decrease in blood pressure (hypotension) with an increase in heart rate (tachycardia) and respiratory rate (tachypnea), and a drop in oxygen saturation. The patient may appear pale, cold and clammy, or cyanotic. Urine output may decrease as a result of poor renal perfusion.

Significant postoperative bleeding is an emergency and is always reported immediately. It may require an operation to explore the surgical site. The patient is monitored continuously until arrangements for the operating room are complete. If needed and not contraindicated, the patient is positioned with the head flat and the legs elevated or in Trendelenburg position (head lowered and feet elevated) to increase venous return and raise the blood pressure. The patient is supported with supplemental oxygen to prevent hypoxemia and the administration of intravenous fluids, blood transfusions, and/or plasma expanders to replace blood volume. Chapter 61 🔗 provides a complete description of nursing care for the patient experiencing shock.

Surgery has a significant effect on a patient's fluid balance and it is unlikely that the patient will have a normal urinary output in the first 24 to 48 hours postoperatively (Clancy et al., 2002). The surgical patient is affected by factors that can lead to dehydration or fluid overload. Factors that contribute to fluid loss and dehydration in the surgical patient include preoperative fasting from foods and fluids, preoperative bowel preparation, hyperventilation from anxiety, blood loss intraoperatively, wound drains, nasogastric drainage, vomiting, evaporative water loss from exposed tissues during the operation, and decisions about intravenous (IV) fluid replacement. Some surgeons prefer a conservative approach to the administration of IV fluids in the operating room because research shows that these patients progress better postoperatively than patients who receive more liberal amounts of IV fluid (Nisanevich et al., 2005). Another factor in fluid balance is that tissue injury can cause a third spacing of fluids that contributes to dehydration initially because the fluid is not in the intravascular space. Postoperatively, fever, hypermetabolism, and sweating can significantly increase insensible water losses from an average of 600 to 800 mL/day to as high as 1,500 mL/day (Arieff, 1999).

Alternatively, certain factors contribute to overhydration and *fluid overload.* The primary factor is the secretion of hormones that occurs with physiological stress. Stress, pain, and anxiety stimulate the release of epinephrine, aldosterone, and antidiuretic hormone (ADH). These hormones affect fluid balance by causing the retention of sodium and water. Fluid overload may also occur as a result of the administration of intravenous fluid. The replacement of fluids during surgery is a clinical approximation of fluid loss, and monitoring is needed to prevent fluid overload.

Although dehydration is more common than fluid overload postoperatively, patients are monitored for signs of overhydration. The risk of overload is highest during the first 24 to 48 hours postoperatively when hormonal influences are at their peak. Most healthy patients can tolerate an overexpansion of fluid volume but the problem can be serious in those with altered physiological reserves. For those patients, the increased cardiac workload associated with fluid overload can precipitate heart failure or pulmonary edema. Patients who are at an increased risk of fluid overload are the elderly and those with preexisting cardiac, pulmonary, or renal disease. Early indicators of fluid retention are heavy, swollen eyelids, edema in the hands and feet, weight gain, and an intake that is greater than output. The patient may complain of headache, apprehension, or dyspnea. Other signs are agitation, distended neck veins, crackles in the lungs, and a drop in urinary output. Vital sign changes include an increase in heart rate, blood pressure, and respiratory rate. Treatment of fluid overload depends on the severity. Continuous close monitoring of weight, intake and output, and lung sounds is paramount, and the administration of IV fluids may be slowed or

discontinued. In some cases, the patient may be given a diuretic, such as furosemide, intravenously to facilitate fluid excretion.

It is more common, however, for a patient to be dehydrated after surgery rather than overhydrated (Clancy et al., 2002). Intake may exceed output for approximately 24 to 48 hours. Fluid balance begins to correct approximately 48 to 72 hours after surgery. At this time, fluid in the interstitial space begins to shift back into the vascular space and the effect of stress hormones decreases, producing a urinary diuresis.

Careful assessment of fluid balance is the key to maintaining adequate hydration and preventing fluid overload. Intravenous fluid is monitored closely. A number of formulas are available for calculating postoperative fluid replacement. As an example, approximately 2,500 mL/day (or 30 to 35 mL/kg body weight per day) is needed for routine fluid replacement with additional amounts, from 500 to 3,000 mL/day, for replacement of losses from third spaced fluid, drains, or other sources (Arieff, 1999). Isotonic solutions (normal saline, Ringer's lactate) are frequently used for routine IV fluid replacement.

In the PACU, urine output is measured hourly. A urine output that is less than 30 mL/hr or 0.5 mL/kg per hour is reported to the health care provider as a significant finding. Frequently, a low urine output in the postoperative patient is the result of depressed renal function from dehydration. Other indications of dehydration include dry mouth, dry tissues, poor skin turgor, and complaints of headache. Tachycardia occurs as a compensatory mechanism for dehydration and the blood pressure tends to decrease as a result of too little blood volume.

A patient with low urine output or other signs of hypovolemia may be given a fluid bolus to expand blood volume and increase renal blood flow. A typical fluid bolus is 250 to 1,000 mL of 9.9% sodium chloride administered over 30 to 60 minutes. The nurse monitors urine output to determine the effectiveness of the fluid bolus. If effective, urine output increases. Vital signs may return to normal although issues other than dehydration (e.g., anxiety, pain) affect vital signs. In some patients, particularly the elderly, a fluid bolus can overwhelm the pumping ability of the heart, resulting in heart failure and pulmonary edema. Older patients need to be monitored during a fluid bolus to ensure that they are able to tolerate the rapid administration of fluid. Crackles (i.e., rales) in the lungs, dyspnea, or a drop in oxygen saturation indicate that the patient is unable to tolerate the fluid.

Risk for Decreased Cardiac Output

Following surgery, patients may have problems with cardiac irregularities, hypotension, or hypertension. Abnormal cardiac rhythms are a frequent finding after surgery. Most abnormal rhythms are a result of expected postoperative issues such as pain or fluid and electrolyte imbalances but an abnormal rhythm can also indicate a more serious problem such as cardiac ischemia. Cardiac telemetry is used to monitor heart rhythms and abnormal beats in the PACU. Telemetry is discontinued when the patient is transferred to a clinical unit, but it will be continued for patients who have signs of myocardial ischemia or abnormal cardiac rhythms or for those who need monitoring for heart or blood pressure medications.

The apical pulse is a more reliable measure than a peripheral pulse of heart rate and rhythm in the postoperative patient. The health care provider usually writes parameters that specify vital signs to report. The nurse relies on these parameters as well as on clinical judgment in reporting changes in the patient's condition. In addition to changes in heart rate, the nurse reports and investigates evidence of new irregularity in the heart rhythm. Irregularity in the heart rhythm may indicate premature ventricular contractions or new-onset atrial fibrillation.

Sinus tachycardia (i.e., a heart rate greater than 100 beats/min) is the most common dysrhythmia and it is caused by fever, anxiety, pain, hypovolemia, anemia, and hypoxia among other reasons. As a rule of thumb, a heart rate greater than 100 beats/min in a postoperative patient is investigated initially to determine the likely cause. If the patient is persistently tachycardic, the nurse must assess for other signs and symptoms (e.g., vertigo, syncope, hypotension, hypoxemia, chest pain) and report heart rates greater than 120 beats/min. The goal is to treat the underlying cause (e.g., give pain medication, fluids, oxygen, or blood transfusion). Although many patients experience tachycardia in the postoperative period, it is important to remember that an increase in heart rate increases the workload of the heart, so in compromised patients decompensation can occur rapidly.

Sinus bradycardia (i.e., a heart rate less than 60 beats/min) occurs postoperatively as a result of anesthetic medications or vagal stimulation. Patients with bradycardia are observed for its effect on cardiac output. If the patient is asymptomatic, further treatment is not usually necessary. Bradycardia that produces hypotension, syncope, or other symptoms may need to be treated with medications such as atropine or with a pacemaker.

Premature ventricular contractions (PVCs) are not unusual after surgery. PVCs may be caused by anxiety, pain, hypoxia, hypovolemia, and electrolyte imbalances particularly hypokalemia or hypomagnesia. Occasional PVCs are often benign and do not require treatment. The nurse reports an increase in the frequency of PVCs, the clustering of PVCs (i.e., couplets, triplets), and episodes of ventricular tachycardia (i.e., four or more PVCs in a row). Treatment is directed toward the underlying cause of the abnormal beats, but an antiarrhythmic drug such as amiodarone may be used to suppress episodes of ventricular tachycardia. It is important to remember that an antiarrhythmic drug given intravenously is also proarrhythmic (i.e., it has the potential to trigger an abnormal rhythm), therefore, these drugs are used cautiously. Chapter 38 ☝ includes a complete discussion of cardiac dysrhythmias.

Hypotension is a systolic blood pressure of less than 90 mmHg or a drop in the patient's systolic blood pressure of more than 20% from baseline. Hypotension can occur for a variety of reasons including bleeding, hypovolemia, depressed myocardial function, abnormal heart rhythm (e.g., atrial fibrillation), pulmonary emboli, and medications. Hypovolemia is the most likely cause of postoperative hypotension. The nurse reports hypotension and monitors the patient for other signs of decreased tissue perfusion. Interventions to treat hypotension depend on the underlying cause, but include placing the patient in Trendelenburg position and administering IV fluids rapidly to increase blood volume.

Hypertension is a systolic blood pressure equal to or greater than 140 mmHg, a diastolic blood pressure equal to or greater than 90 mmHg, or an increase greater than 20% from baseline in the patient's blood pressure. There are many reasons for a postoperative patient to be hypertensive including pain, anxiety, hypothermia, fluid overload, and distention of the bladder. Interventions are focused on treating the cause. If the patient was on antihypertensive medications at home, these are restarted as soon as possible. Patients who are NPO are sometimes allowed to take medications with small sips of water or they may be temporarily switched to an antihypertensive medication that can be given intravenously.

Risk for Imbalanced Body Temperature: Hypothermia

Hypothermia is defined as a core body temperature of less than 36°C (96.8°F) or a condition, regardless of body temperature, in which a person experiences shivering, peripheral vasoconstriction, piloerection, and feeling cold. Hypothermia is a common problem in the PACU, and it can have significant consequences for patients. Hypothermia is linked to patient discomfort, sympathetic stimulation, altered drug metabolism, increased intraoperative blood loss and the need for postoperative transfusions, impaired platelet function and clotting ability, slowed wound healing, increased susceptibility to infection, and untoward cardiac events such as angina (ASPAN, 2002; Scott & Buckland, 2006). Slow drug metabolism means that the hypothermic patient remains anesthetized longer than necessary.

Patients at risk for hypothermia include those with history of vascular and endocrine diseases, those who are immunocompromised, those with open wounds, older patients, and persons who are malnourished with low reserves of body fat. Also, longer surgeries (those lasting more than 1 hour) and the use of cold irrigation solution intraoperatively contribute to the development of postoperative hypothermia. On admission to the PACU, the patient is assessed for evidence of hypothermia and the core body temperature is taken. Clinical guidelines for the prevention of hypothermia recommend maintaining ambient room temperature between 20° and 24°C (68° and 75°F) and using passive insulation such as warm cotton blankets, socks, head coverings, limiting skin exposure, and a circulating water mattress for all patients (ASPAN, 2002; Good, Verble, Secrest, & Norwood, 2006; Wadlund, 2006; Wagner, 2006). Hypothermic patients must be actively rewarmed using a forced-air warming system. These systems help to raise body temperature because they blow warm air through a blanket that covers the patient. Other warming techniques include warming IV fluids and applying warm, humidified oxygen (Hasankhani, Mohammadi, Moazzami, Mokhtari, & Naghgizadh, 2007).

Patients who are hypothermic require more oxygen than they would if they had a normal temperature because shivering increases oxygen demand of the tissues and workload of the heart. Meperidine (Demerol) 12.5 to 25 mg IV is given to treat postoperative shivering, thus reducing oxygen demand. Achieving **normothermia** (i.e., a normal body temperature) reverses the immediate effects of hypothermia (e.g., shivering), but patients who experience perioperative hypothermia develop more cardiac events and wound infections postoperatively than patients who do not experience hypothermia (Scott & Buckland, 2006). Assessment of the patient's comfort and temperature are made every 30 minutes until discharge. The patient must achieve a minimum core body temperature of 36°C (96.8°F) prior to PACU discharge.

Readiness for Enhanced Comfort:
Nausea and Vomiting

Postoperative nausea and vomiting (PONV) is a significant problem that can be more debilitating than the surgical procedure. Despite advances in anesthesia, a large number of patients are affected by nausea and vomiting. Incidence of postoperative nausea and vomiting ranges from 40% to 84% depending on the surgery (Goldman & Ausiello, 2004; Schultz, Andrews, Goran, Mathew, & Sturdevant, 2003). Nausea and vomiting contribute to the development of fluid and electrolyte imbalances, poor nutritional intake, and patient discomfort. Often, patients who experience nausea and vomiting are reluctant or unable to ambulate, increasing the likelihood of other postoperative complications. Predisposing factors for postoperative nausea and vomiting include gender (women more than men), the surgery (there is a higher risk with gynecologic, abdominal, eye, and ear surgeries), longer surgeries (increased risk with surgeries longer than 2 hours), use of opioid analgesics, use of inhalation agents during anesthesia, a history of motion sickness, a history of nausea and vomiting with previous surgery, and a nonsmoking status (ASPAN, 2006a; Gunta, Lewis, & Nuccio, 2000; Murphy, Hooper, Sullivan, Clifford, & Apfel, 2006).

There are three types of PONV. Early postoperative nausea and vomiting occurs quickly, within 2 to 6 hours after the surgery. Late PONV develops 6 to 24 hours after the surgery, and delayed PONV extends beyond the first 24 hours after surgery. The causes of nausea and vomiting are complex and it may be that different types of PONV are caused by different factors and stimuli. PONV occurs as a result of stimulation of the vomiting center in the brain (Goldman & Ausiello, 2004). The vomiting center is activated by pathways from (1) the chemoreceptor trigger zone (CTZ) in the brain, (2) the gastrointestinal (GI) tract and other viscera via the vagus nerve, (3) the vestibular apparatus in the ear, and (4) the cerebral cortex. The CTZ contains serotonin and dopamine receptors that, when stimulated by certain toxins, substances, and drugs, activate nausea and vomiting in the vomiting center. The gastrointestinal (GI) tract also contains receptors—serotonin (5-HT3), dopamine (D2), and histamine (H1)—that when stimulated send messages to the brain via the vagus nerve to trigger nausea and vomiting. Factors such as GI irritation, gastric distention, inflammation, or ischemia can cause nausea and vomiting. For the postoperative patient, anesthesia and medications, especially narcotics, are important triggers of nausea.

Most postoperative nausea and vomiting occur early in the course of recovery and improve over time. One study of 300 postoperative patients found the highest incidence of nausea and vomiting occurred within 2 hours following surgery (Gunta et al., 2000). Interventions to reduce nausea and vomiting begin in the preoperative or intraoperative period with the administration of antiemetic medication. It is thought that early administration of antiemetic drugs (i.e., the drug is administered before emesis is triggered) is more effective than waiting until the patient experiences nausea and vomiting (Clancy et al., 2002). When preventative therapy fails, experts recommend rescue therapy using an agent from a different antiemetic class (ASPAN, 2006a). All patients with PONV need to be well hydrated with IV fluid.

The various antiemetic drugs that are available have different modes of action, and the ideal drug or drug combination has yet to be found. In some cases, a combination of drugs may work more effectively than a single drug (Wallenborn et al., 2006). One large study compared the effectiveness of six different two-drug combinations (e.g., dexamethasone, droperidol, ondansetron) in reducing PONV. The researchers reported that all of the drug combinations reduced PONV by 25% to 30%, but none of the combinations proved superior (Apfel et al., 2004). Not all antiemetics are effective for the nausea and vomiting associated with anesthesia, and all of the drugs have limitations. Some researchers are investigating the antiemetic effects of drugs not generally used for this purpose. In a small trial of patients having laparoscopic surgery, the prophylactic use of gabapentin, an antiseizure drug, decreased PONV (Pandey et al., 2006). The Pharmacology Summary describes common antiemetics used for postoperative nausea and vomiting.

Unfortunately, antiemetic medication does not work for everyone and there are few effective alternatives to the use of drugs. One study found that ginger (1 gram) was better than placebo in decreasing PONV (Chaiyakunapruk, Kitikannakorn, Nathisuwan, Leeprakobboon, & Leelasettagool, 2006), although other studies do not support the finding (Pittler & Eberhart, 2003). Acupuncture, P6 acupoint stimulation bands, aromatherapy, music, and self-hypnosis have limited success in reducing nausea and vomiting (Ezzone, Baker, & Terrepka, 1998; King, 1997; Lee & Done, 2004; Odom-Forren, Fetzer, & Moser, 2006; Phillips & Gill, 1994; Schultz et al., 2003). The nurse provides comfort by allowing the patient periods of uninterrupted rest, offering empathy and support, and encouraging deep breathing. The nurse also offers applications of a cool washcloth, frequent mouth care, and ice chips. Patients frequently report increased nausea with head elevation and movement. Slow position changes may help to prevent this trigger.

Pain

Achieving adequate pain control and comfort are major goals of postoperative care. The physiological effects of pain are well known and include an increase in sympathetic stimulation with an increase in blood pressure, heart rate, respiratory rate, and cardiac workload. The body enters a catabolic state that uses up physiological reserves. From a psychological standpoint, pain contributes to loss of sleep, lack of appetite, depression, anxiety, anger, helplessness, and hopelessness. Postoperative pain is associated with delayed ambulation and diminished functional performance (Horvath, 2003; Morrison, Magaziner, & McLaughlin, 2003). Pain control is necessary in promoting mobility and preventing complications such as atelectasis, ileus, DVT, and poor wound healing. The goal in postoperative pain control is to achieve a level of comfort without producing too much sedation or other side effects. Patients who are sedated will not be able to participate in postoperative breathing exercises or ambulation.

Incisional pain is expected to be highest in the first 24 to 48 hours postoperatively followed by a gradual reduction in pain, but the course of pain varies with the surgery and the individual. In one study, subjects with abdominal surgery reported more pain than those with cardiac surgery, and neither group experienced a reduction in pain 3 days postoperatively as might be expected (Puntillo & Weiss, 2003). Activities and procedures can also alter the course of pain. In a large study of more than

PHARMACOLOGY Summary of Common Drugs Used to Control Postoperative Nausea and Vomiting

Drug	Class and Action	Major Side Effect	Nursing Responsibility
Aprepitant	Neurokinin-1 (NK-1) receptor antagonist. Blocks NK-1 receptors in the central pathway of the vomiting center.	Headache, hypotension, bradycardia, pruritus, constipation.	Used only for prophylaxis. Give as a single dose 3 hours before surgery.
Dexamethasone	Corticosteroid. Augments the antiemetic effect of 5HT3 blockers. May also antagonize prostaglandins or release endorphins that increase mood and well-being.	Headache, gastrointestinal irritation, glucose elevation, retention of sodium and water.	Used in combination with other antiemetics. Watch for GI bleeding.
Diphenhydramine (Benadryl)	Blocks effects of histamine at H1 receptor sites.	Sedation, vertigo, hypotension.	Used more often for nausea associated with motion sickness or chemotherapy. Elderly may be very sensitive to the sedative effects of the drug.
Droperidol (Inapsine)	Blocks dopamine type 2 receptors in the chemoreceptor trigger zone in brain to reduce nausea and vomiting.	Sedation, hypotension, tachycardia, extrapyramidal symptoms (restless, tremor).	Low doses are used for postoperative nausea and vomiting. Watch for sedation and respiratory depression in patients receiving other CNS depressants. Monitor heart rate and blood pressure.
Metoclopramide (Reglan)	Increases gastric emptying and raises threshold for triggering the chemoreceptor trigger zone.	Mild sedation, extrapyramidal symptoms, (dystonia, restless, tremor).	Drug should be discontinued if extrapyramidal symptoms occur. Has not been shown to be effective in prophylactic management of PONV.
Ondansetron (Zofran) Dolasetron Granisetron	Serotonin receptor antagonist. Blocks 5HT3 receptor sites in the CTZ and peripherally to reduce nausea and vomiting.	Headache, diarrhea, or (more commonly) constipation.	Headache may be treated with Tylenol. Give stool softener or laxatives to prevent constipation.
Prochlorperazine (Compazine)	Phenothiazine that depresses CTZ in the brain.	Extrapyramidal symptoms, suppresses cough.	Be alert for development of extrapyramidal symptoms such as motor restlessness and parkinsonism.
Promethazine (Phenergan)	Long-acting phenothiazine derivative that depresses the chemoreceptor trigger zone.	Sedation, dizziness, dry mouth.	Monitor for increased sedation when administered with other CNS depressants. Monitor patient safety.
Scopolamine	Antagonizes muscarinic type 1 receptors in hypothalamus and vomiting center.	Visual disturbances, dry mouth, mydriasis.	Used for prophylaxis of PONV, limited use in rescue because of delayed action.

6,000 subjects, an increase in pain was reported with activities such as turning, drain removal, wound care, and suctioning (Puntillo et al., 2002). Cardiac surgical subjects reported coughing as the most painful activity followed by moving or turning in bed, getting out of bed, and using the incentive spirometer (Milgrom et al., 2004).

Pain may come from sources other than the incision. Residual carbon dioxide, used to inflate the surgical area in laparoscopic procedures, can produce shoulder or back pain. The position used during surgery may cause specific muscle aches. In one research study, 52% of patients placed in the lithotomy position for surgery reported back pain postoperatively (Pietrocola, Riley, Beanland, Kelly, & Radnell, 2004). Studies continue to report the undermedication of pain in postoperative patients (Cheever, 1999; Puntillo & Weiss, 2003; Puntillo et al., 1997, 2002; Sjostrom, Dahlgren, & Haljamae, 2000).

The PACU nurse continuously assesses the patient's level of comfort. The Agency for Health Care Policy and Research (AHCPR; now known as the Agency for Healthcare Research and Quality, AHRQ) developed guidelines for the management of acute pain in 1992. These guidelines recommend the use of a rating scale to measure the patient's self-report of pain. Most hospitals use a numeric rating system where patients report their level of pain on a scale of 0 (no pain) to 10 (the worst pain imaginable) (ASPAN, 2003). Postoperative patients rate their pain at rest and with movement.

Self-report is the best indicator of pain (AHCPR, 1992). Studies suggest that nurses and health care providers consistently underestimate patients' pain (Puntillo et al., 1997; Sjostrom et al., 2000) or have difficulty separating pain from anxiety (Stannard et al., 1996) except in situations where they use a pain scale and listen to the patient's response (Sjostrom et al., 2000). Pain assessment in patients who cannot self-report is more complicated and relies on clinical judgment. The nurse needs to consider the usual pain associated with a particular procedure or surgery and assess the patient for behavioral indicators of pain. Based on these factors, an analgesic trial is used and evaluated for effectiveness (Pasero & McCaffery, 2005).

The American Society of PeriAnesthesia Nurses published pain and comfort guidelines for postoperative patients (ASPAN, 2003). The nurse documents the location and character of the pain. The patient is expected to feel pain at the area of the surgical incision, but pain located in other areas requires further investigation. Pain in other sites may be caused by any number of factors and can be benign. Examples include pain referred from the incision, pain as a result of positioning during the operation, or pain caused by the accumulation of carbon dioxide gas from a laparoscopic procedure. Chest pain not related to an incision can be serious indicating cardiac ischemia and it requires further evaluation.

Postoperative pain should be well controlled with medications and other strategies. Early postoperative pain control is important for patient comfort, but it may also play a role in reducing persistent postsurgical pain, a phenomenon in which pain continues long after the incision heals (Kehlet, Troels, Woolf, & Woolf, 2006). The nurse consults with the health care provider when the patient is not getting acceptable pain relief. Another situation requiring consultation is the report of increased pain when the pain was previously well controlled. This finding suggests the possibility of surgical complications, such as infection or hematoma formation, and requires prompt evaluation.

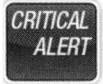 **CRITICAL ALERT** *Uncontrolled postoperative pain or a sudden increase in postoperative pain warrants an immediate investigation. These signs can signal a postoperative complication such as bleeding or leaking of the surgical anastomosis. Report findings to the surgeon immediately.*

Initially, most patients in the PACU receive small doses of intravenous narcotic analgesics for pain control. Common medications include morphine sulfate, hydromorphone, and fentanyl. A typical standing order may be written for morphine sulfate 1 to 5 mg IV every 5 minutes as needed to a maximum total dose of 0.3 mg/kg body weight. Fentanyl also is used in the PACU because it provides comparable analgesia to morphine, but it has a more rapid onset and excretion (Golembiewski, Torrecer, & Katke, 2005). A typical standing order might read: fentanyl 25 mcg IV as needed to a maximum of 100 mcg. The nurse assesses patients' responses to interventions every 15 to 30 minutes or more frequently if appropriate. Patients are monitored for respiratory depression and narcotics are withheld or even reversed if the respiratory rate falls to 10 per minute or less.

 **CRITICAL ALERT** *Patients who require close neurological monitoring need an individualized regimen for pain control. Check with the anesthesiologist for special orders if the patient has major head trauma, increased intracranial pressure, a recent cerebrovascular accident, or recent seizures.*

Patient-controlled analgesia (PCA) or patient-controlled epidural analgesia (PCEA) is commonly used to control postoperative pain. With PCA, a narcotic analgesic can be administered continuously at a basal rate although continuous infusion is not standard because it increases the risk of adverse effects and opioid overdose (Golembiewski et al., 2005). More common is PCA using small boluses when the patient pushes the control button. The PCA delivers a set amount of medication at specified intervals until a maximum amount of medication is reached. The computerized pump keeps a record of how often the patient attempts to access the medication and how many injections the patient receives. The nurse uses this information to determine whether the patient is using the pump effectively. A typical PCA order for a postoperative patient might read: PCA morphine sulfate 1 mg every 6 minutes with a lockout maximum of 10 mg/hour.

Patients receiving PCA are monitored for pain relief and for the untoward effects of the narcotic, including a depressed respiratory rate, sedation, nausea, pruritus, and slowed gastrointestinal function. In a review of studies comparing PCA with nurse-administered analgesics, researchers found consistent evidence that PCA provides better pain control and increased patient satisfaction with very few adverse effects (Hudcova, McNicol, Quah, Lau, & Carr, 2006).

Patient-controlled epidural analgesia delivers medication via a catheter to the epidural space. PCEA, like PCA, can be set to deliver medication continuously, as a bolus, or both. PCEA is used to deliver a local anesthetic such as bupivacaine (0.0625% to 0.125%) or ropivacaine (0.1% to 0.2%) alone or in combination with a narcotic. Fentanyl is used frequently as the narcotic of choice because it is lipid soluble and easily dissolves in epidural fat, but preservative-free morphine also can be given as an epidural medication. It is thought that local anesthetics and opioids work synergistically to provide better pain relief in smaller doses.

The nurse checks the site of the epidural catheter for signs of infection and patency. Infection is uncommon, but the catheter is taped not sutured and displacement can occur. Catheter displacement is suspected by new complaints of pain in a patient who previously had good pain control with the epidural. The nurse monitors the patient for overall pain control and also notes the sensory level of the epidural (i.e., the area of the body where the patient reports diminished sensation). In the PACU, these assessments are made hourly; on the clinical unit, they are made every 4 hours unless the situation warrants more frequent assessments. It is also important to note any areas of motor deficit. The goal of epidural analgesia in the postoperative patient is to reduce sensation and pain without affecting motor ability. If the epidural is affecting motor ability, it will need to be adjusted downward so that the patient will be able to ambulate safely. Other possible side effects include nausea, pruritus, hypotension, and urinary retention. Some health care providers elect to leave a urinary catheter in place while a patient is receiving epidural medication to avoid urinary retention although others believe this practice to be unnecessary.

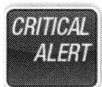

CRITICAL ALERT

If a patient with patient-controlled epidural analgesia is unable to lift his legs off of the bed or describes heaviness in their lower extremities, the health care provider should be consulted. These assessments suggest that the dose of medication is too high, causing motor blockade.

The use of PCA and PCEA is an important advance in control of postoperative pain. Many studies show that PCEA provides better pain control with fewer side effects and better functional outcomes than PCA (Carli et al., 2002; Mann et al., 2000; Mann, Pouzeratte, & Eledjam, 2003; Nishimori, Ballantyne, & Low, 2006; Pasero, 2003a, 2003b, 2005; Schumann et al., 2003). Continuous epidural analgesia with local anesthetics for 24 to 72 hours postoperatively is associated with faster return of GI function, improved respiratory function, and a reduced stress response (Brown, Christo, & Wu, 2004; Holte & Kehlet, 2002). As soon as appropriate, the patient is transitioned away from intravenous or parenteral medications to oral medications.

Experts recommend a multimodal approach (e.g., using multiple agents with different modes of action) for postoperative pain management. When multiple medications are used, pain control can be achieved with smaller doses of narcotics and with fewer adverse effects (Pasero & McCaffery, 2007; Richman, Liu, & Courpas, 2006). For example, infusions of local anesthetics may be used along with intravenous or oral opioids. A continuous wound infusion is the administration of a local anesthetic through a catheter implanted directly into the surgical site. An alternative is the use of continuous perineural infusion. In this type of infusion, a catheter is inserted near the peripheral nerves affected by surgery. An infusion of a short-acting local anesthetic in this area effectively blocks the pain from these nerves (Pasero & McCaffery, 2007).

Nonsteroidal anti-inflammatory drugs (NSAIDs) are used in conjunction with opioids for pain control except where contraindicated. Acetaminophen does not affect postoperative bleeding, so it can be added to most pain control regimens (Kuchta & Golembiewski, 2004). Keterolac (Toradol) is a particularly effective anti-inflammatory agent but its use is often limited to 72 hours because of its deleterious effect on kidney function. The anticonvulsant agents, pregabalin and gabapentin, may be used postoperatively when there is a neuropathic component to pain as is frequently the case with orthopedic conditions (Pasero & McCaffery, 2007).

Other pain control techniques include the application of heat or cold, primarily cold for the postoperative patient, and elevation. Application of ice or a cold pack helps reduce tissue swelling, one factor that contributes to postoperative pain. Ice packs are applied for 20 minutes then removed for 20 minutes and repeated as necessary. The application of cold is seen with various orthopedic procedures as well as some plastic surgeries. Elevation of an affected area above the level of the heart reduces edema and assists with pain control. Elevation is used most often with open reduction of an extremity fracture. Chapter 15 🔗 provides a complete description of pain management techniques.

Nurses use nonpharmacologic interventions to reduce pain, but these interventions should complement medications not replace them. The evidence of the effectiveness of selected nonpharmacologic approaches to pain is inconsistent. In two studies, for example, patients reported that the use of positioning, massage, distraction, and relaxation techniques combined with pain medication is more effective than pain medication alone in providing pain relief and comfort (Smith, Kemp, Hemphill, & Vojir, 2002; VanKooten, 1999). In a systematic review of relaxation interventions, researchers found support for the effectiveness of these techniques in reducing pain in approximately half of the 15 studies they examined (Kwekkeboom & Gretarsdottir, 2006). Similarly, research on the effects of healing touch on postoperative pain control show mixed results (Wardell & Weymouth, 2004). Clearly more studies are needed to establish the efficacy of nonpharmacologic approaches in the management of postoperative pain.

Anxiety

Anxiety is an unpleasant emotional response. Anxiety is associated with increased morbidity and mortality and longer, more complicated hospitalizations in the postoperative patient. Anxiety causes stimulation of the sympathetic nervous system, which can increase blood pressure by 30% to 40% and heart rate by 20% (Frazier et al., 2003). Anxiety depresses the immune system, delays wound healing, and alters blood coagulation. Other reported physiological responses to anxiety include increases in myocardial ischemia, cardiac dysrhythmias, and postoperative pain. The nurse assesses the patient for signs of anxiety, similar to pain assessment. The best indicator of anxiety is patient reports of how anxious they feel. Patients are encouraged to verbalize fears and concerns.

Nurses play a critical role in reducing the anxiety of postoperative patients. The PACU nurse provides frequent reassurance to patients about their condition and how well they are progressing. Reassurance and caring are major factors in reducing anxiety. In one study of critically ill medical and surgical patients, subjects reported an overwhelming need to "feel safe" in their environment, and they identified nurses as the key to either feeling safe or not feeling safe (Hupcey, 2000). The researcher found that nurses who came right away when called, who listened, who expressed genuine interest, and who explained what was happening to the patient were deemed trustworthy and fostered patients' beliefs that they were being "watched over" and therefore safe. Other studies supporting these findings show that nurses' caring behaviors are associated with patients' sense of emotional comfort, well-being, and security, and lead to better functional outcomes (Doering, McGuire, & Rourke, 2002; Meade, Bursell, & Ketelsen, 2006; Swan, 1998; Werner et al., 2002; Williams & Irurita, 2005). Whenever possible, patients should be given choices regarding their care. Regaining a sense of control helps the patient to feel a sense of security (Susleck et al., 2007; Williams & Irurita, 2005).

The nurse individualizes nursing interactions with patients and provides information consistent with the individual's preference for information and personal coping style. Some patients will want and need detailed information about their status, whereas others may become more anxious if the nurse provides too much information or explanations that are too explicit. Nurses should speak slowly and calmly, and maintain a quiet and restful environment. The trend toward allowing significant others to visit with the patient in the PACU is likely to be beneficial in reducing the anxiety of the patient and the significant other. Family and friends are an important source of support and comfort

(Cunningham, Hanson-Heath, & Agre, 2003; Hupcey, 2000; Leske, 2003; Smykowski & Rodriguez, 2003; Susleck et al., 2007).

Other techniques that are helpful in reducing anxiety are sitting with the patient, touch, massage, distraction, meditation, guided imagery, relaxation exercises, and music. It may be very useful to incorporate music into a plan of care. Music therapy is presented in the Complementary and Alternative Therapies box in Chapter 41 🔗. One study found that 20 minutes of music significantly reduced anxiety, heart rate, respiratory rate, and cardiac workload in patients admitted to a coronary care unit (White, 1999).

Despite nonpharmacologic interventions, some patients may require antianxiety agents. A number of antianxiety agents are available. Lorazepam (Ativan) works quickly (1 to 5 minutes) when given intravenously, but can also be administered as an intramuscular (IM) injection or given orally. The dose is titrated to produce desired effects so that oversedation of the patient is avoided. It is important for the nurse to follow up on the effectiveness of interventions to reduce anxiety. In a study of 843 postoperative patients and their nurses, the nurses tended to overrate the amount of anxiety relief that the patient received from interventions (Leinonen, Leino-Kilpi, Stahlberg, & Lertola, 2003).

Discharge from the Postanesthesia Care Unit

Patients are discharged from the PACU to home or to an inpatient unit. PACUs use written criteria and a numeric rating scale to determine the patient's readiness for discharge home or to an inpatient unit. The Aldrete Post Anesthesia Discharge Score (PADS) (Figure 27–3 ■) is one measure of a patient's readiness

for discharge. The PADS assigns a numerical rating of 0 to 2 for each of the following: vital signs, activity level, nausea and vomiting, pain, and surgical bleeding. Patients can be transferred to an inpatient unit with a PADS of between 8 and 10, but a score of 9 or better is required if the patient is being discharged home. If patients have a baseline PADS of less than 8 due to a preexisting condition, the anesthesia provider makes the decision to discharge on an individual basis.

Ambulatory Surgery Discharge

Ambulatory settings require a PADS of 9 or higher for discharge, but other criteria may need to be met before the patient is allowed to go home. Discharge criteria vary depending on the surgery, the patient, and health care provider preference. Additional discharge criteria may include the following:

- Stable vital signs for 1 hour
- Baseline level of consciousness
- Wound is stable with minimal bleeding
- Able to take fluids orally (applicable to selected patients)
- Able to void (applicable to certain surgeries or selected patients)
- Pain is at an acceptable level
- Able to dress and ambulate with assistance
- Adult caretaker available to accompany the patient home.

Patients are no longer required to void or to take oral fluids prior to discharge. Evidence from research studies found that many patients can be safely discharged home without voiding or drinking fluids (Ead, 2006; Mulroy, Salinas, Larkin, & Polissar, 2002). Patients who are considered at low risk for urinary retention may be discharged home without voiding as long as their bladder is not distended. Patients are given explicit instructions to seek medical attention in the emergency room if they have not voided after 8 hours at home. Patients who do not void and who have bladder distention need an ultrasonic bladder scan and may require an intermittent catheterization before discharge. Patients at high risk of postoperative urinary retention are still required to void before discharge. Many patients will be able to drink fluids before discharge, but in most cases, it is not necessary to delay discharge for those who do not tolerate oral fluids. Certain patients, such as those with diabetes, the elderly and the frail, remain under observation until they are able to drink fluids postoperatively.

Patients discharged home need to have complete and concise information about performing self-care. The information is presented verbally as well as in writing using simple language. When home care involves performing a procedure, the nurse demonstrates the technique then asks the patient to return the demonstration (Ross, 2007). The nurse reviews any new medications including the purpose of the drug, the dose, the frequency of administration, and any significant side effects. Pain management is discussed as well as wound care. The nurse reviews any restrictions on bathing, activity, and diet. Patients should be clear about how they are expected to feel after surgery and what symptoms require follow-up with their surgeon. Patients are given instructions about how to contact their health care provider should a problem develop. Information about follow-up appointments is also given to patients. The Patient Teaching & Discharge Priorities box pro-

POST ANESTHETIC SCORE	
ACTIVITY	
Able to move 4 extremities voluntarily or on command	2
Able to move 2 extremities voluntarily or on command	1
Unable to move extremities voluntarily or on command	0
RESPIRATION	
Able to breathe deeply and cough freely	2
Dyspnea, limited breathing or tachypnea	1
Apneic or on mechanical ventilator	0
CIRCULATION	
BP plus or minus 20% of preoperative baseline	2
BP plus or minus 20%–40% of preanesthetic level	1
BP plus or minus 40% of preanesthetic level	0
CONSCIOUSNESS	
Fully awake	2
Arousable on calling	1
Not responding	0
O2 Saturation	
Able to maintain O2 saturation > 92% on room air	2
Needs O2 inhalation to maintain O2 saturation > 90%	1
O2 saturation <90% even with O2 supplement	0
TOTAL PAR SCORE	

FIGURE 27–3 ■ Aldrete Post Anesthesia Discharge Score.
Source: Courtesy of Beth Israel Deaconess Nursing Department

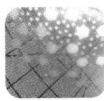

PATIENT TEACHING & DISCHARGE PRIORITIES Following a Breast Biopsy

Need	Teaching
Care of Incision	Your incision is covered with Steri-Strips and a bandage. Leave the bandage in place tonight. Tomorrow, you may remove the bandage (but not the Steri-Strips) and shower. Gently wash the area and pat it dry. Leave the Steri-Strips in place until they fall off by themselves. If you have sutures, they will be removed during your follow-up appointment. It is not unusual to have mild bruising around the area of the incision.
Pain control	You should have very little pain after your biopsy. Your health care provider has given you a prescription for pain medication if you need it. Do not drive while taking the prescription medication. If your pain is mild, you may take acetaminophen (Tylenol) regular or extra strength every 4 to 6 hours as needed instead of the prescription medication. Do *not* take aspirin or ibuprofen because these medications may cause you to bleed.
	Ice will help to reduce swelling and discomfort. An ice pack can be inserted in the bra. Leave the ice pack in place until it gets warm, then remove and replace. Apply ice packs off and on for the remainder of today.
	You should wear a bra for the next 24 to 36 hours to support your breast. This means that you should sleep in the bra tonight. A soft, front-closing bra may be more comfortable for you than other types.
Activity level	Do not drive on the day of your surgery. You should rest and take it easy for the remainder of the day. You received medications during surgery that may make you feel tired. You may return to work when you feel able. For most people, this will be in 1 or 2 days after the procedure. You can begin performing normal activities tomorrow but avoid strenuous exercise until the follow-up appointment with your health care provider.
Possible problems that require attention	You should watch for signs of infection. If your incision becomes red, painful, or develops drainage you should call your health care provider. You should also call if you develop a fever (>38°C [100.4°F]) or if you have pain that is not relieved by pain medication.
Follow-up with the health care provider	The results of your biopsy will be available in 2 or 3 days. Your health care provider will call you at home with the results. If you have sutures, you should make a follow-up appointment for 7 to 10 days after the procedure. If you do not have sutures, you should make a follow-up appointment for 1 month after the procedure.

vides examples of discharge priorities following ambulatory surgery for a breast biopsy.

Many ambulatory surgery centers contact the patient by telephone the day after surgery. The nurse performs the telephone follow-up and inquires about the patient's recovery. The nurse asks questions about pain, nausea and vomiting, voiding, and the surgical site, and gives the patient the opportunity to ask questions. Often, the surgeon or surgical assistant will also contact the patient at home to monitor recovery. Follow-up phone calls help to ensure patient safety. Also, they may be helpful in reducing emotional stress and improving self-care abilities after surgery although more research is needed in this area (Allard, 2007).

Transfer to an Inpatient Unit

The surgeon and anesthesiologist discharge patients from the PACU to an inpatient unit when the patient meets specific discharge criteria including an acceptable PADS. Other criteria for PACU discharge may require the patient to be normothermic, with pain and bleeding controlled, and all tubes, drains, catheters, and IV lines patent and functioning.

Postoperative orders are written before transfer to the nursing unit. The PACU nurse reports to the receiving nurse all pertinent information about the patient. The report includes relevant past history, a description of the surgery and type of anesthesia, any significant postoperative events, estimated blood loss from surgery, recent laboratory data, a summary of OR and PACU fluid status, recent vital signs, a description of the dressing, drains, pain medication, and antiemetics given, and any equipment required postoperatively. Figure 27–4 ■ (p. 666) is an example of a PACU report. The PACU report may be given verbally or in written form.

■ Nursing Management

The nurse on the clinical unit admits the PACU patient and performs a head-to-toe assessment beginning with vital signs and an admitting weight. The elements of the assessment are similar to the PACU admission assessment described earlier. The nurse makes sure that all equipment is set up correctly and functioning well. The safety of the patient is assessed using a fall risk assessment tool. Patients at risk for falls need an individual plan to prevent a fall. Such plans often include simple strategies such as putting the call light within reach, placing the bed in the low position, monitoring the patient frequently, educating the patient and family about falls, and activating the bed alarm if needed (Lyons, 2004; Resnick, 2003).

Postoperative patients are assessed often because their condition can change rapidly. The usual routine on a surgical unit includes a full head-to-toe assessment at the beginning of a shift followed by frequent follow-up assessments as the day progresses. Vital signs with oxygen saturation are taken every 4 hours, although the timing of postoperative observations is

PACU FAX REPORT   RM#

OR PROCEDURE: _____
_____
_____

ANESTHESIA:

☐ General   ☐ Spinal   ☐ Epidural   ☐ MAC   ☐ Other

(ADDRESSOGRAPH)

SIGNIFICANT POST OP EVENTS:

ALLERGIES: _____
_____
_____

HISTORY

CV	☐ WNL	☐ CABG
		☐ VASCULAR BYPASS
		☐ MI
		☐ ANGINA
		☐ HYPERTENSION
		☐ OTHER

I & O   OR/PACU TOTAL

CRYST	COLLOID	EBL	UOP

PULM	☐ WNL	☐ THORACOTOMY
		☐ SMOKING
		☐ OTHER
		☐ PRE-OP O2 SAT

VITAL SIGNS:

T _____ BP_____ HR _____ RHYTHM _____ RR _____
O2 SAT_____   ☐ ROOM AIR   ☐ NP @ _____ L/M

RENAL	☐ WNL	☐ TRANSPLANT
		☐ CRF/DIALYSIS
		☐ OTHER

IV: _____ mL/hr   AMT. REMAINING _____
      ☐ D5 1/2 S   ☐ D5 1/2 + 20Kcl   ☐ LR

OTHER: _____

NEURO	☐ WNL	☐ CVA
		☐ RESIDUAL
		☐ NO RESIDUAL
		☐ OTHER

DRESSING:

☐ D & I   ☐ SM TO MOD SEROSANG
☐ REINFORCED   ☐ CHANGED IN PACU

GI	☐ WNL	☐ GERD
		☐ OTHER

DRAINS:

☐ NG   ☐ FOLEY   ☐ CT X _____   ☐ JP x _____
☐ HEMOVAC   ☐ DAVOL X _____   ☐ OTHER

SUCTION   ☐ WALL   ☐ SELF

ENDOCRINE	☐ WNL	☐ IDDM
		☐ NIDDM
		☐ OTHER

PAIN MEDICATIONS:	ANTI-EMETICS:
MSO4 _____	DROPERIDOL _____
DEMEROL _____	ZOFRAN _____
KETOROLAC _____	REGLAN _____
OTHER _____	OTHER _____
☐ PCA	
☐ EPIDURAL	
APS ☐ YES ☐ NO	

OTHER

EQUIPMENT

☐ IV POLE   ☐ SUCTION
☐ OXYGEN   ☐ BOOT MACHINE
☐ IMED/IVAC
☐ OTHER _____

☐ PLEASE REMOVE BED FROM ROOM
   THANK YOU!

LABS: HCT _____   K+ _____   BS _____
OTHER _____

INSULIN: PRE-OP _____   POST-OP _____

PRIMARY NURSE

_____ RN

FAX TIME _____   ETA TO FLOOR _____

FIGURE 27–4 ■ Sample PACU report.

PACU Report Sheet   Name: _____

Hx: _____

_____

_____

_____

Anes: GA   ETT   Pre-med: _____

        LMA   _____

        Mac   Epidural _____

        Spinal   _____

Intra-op Events of note: _____

_____

_____

_____

Intra-op meds: _____   Antiemetics _____

               _____   _____

               _____   _____

Fluids: Cryst: _____   Colloid: _____

FIGURE 27–4 ■ *Continued*
Source: Courtesy of Beth Israel Deaconess Nursing Department

based on tradition rather than on empirical evidence (Dip, Dip, & McCutcheon, 2006; Zeitz & McCutcheon, 2006). Hospital policy or a health care provider's order may specify parameters for reporting changes in vital signs. Policies do not cover the range of events that can occur in the postoperative period.

The nurse uses clinical judgment in deciding which data require health care provider notification. Chart 27–3 (p. 668) describes findings that are usually reported to the health care provider. Initially, postoperative patients may run a low-grade fever as a result of tissue injury, inflammation, and mild dehydration so mild temperature elevations are not cause for alarm (Vermeulen, Storm-Versloot, Goossens, Speelman, & Legemate, 2005). The nurse reports a fever of 38°C (100.4°F) or higher unless otherwise directed by the health care provider. Atelectasis is often associated with the development of a fever in the first 24 to 48 hours after surgery, so the nurse assesses breath sounds and encourages deep breathing if fever is present. Oxygen saturation is also an important postoperative measurement. Many patients arrive from the PACU with oxygen in place and orders to maintain oxygen saturation above 93%. If the patient's oxygen saturation is acceptable, the nurse begins the process of titrating the oxygen downward.

While performing the head-to-toe assessment, the nurse asks specific questions to assess the patient's level of consciousness, orientation, and cognition. The nurse also asks about the patient's ability to sleep in the hospital. There is a high rate of sleep disturbance in the hospital and sleep is thought to have restorative functions (Redeker, 2000). The nurse asks the patient to rate his pain and assesses the adequacy of pain control measures. If the patient is using PCA for pain control, the nurse checks the

accuracy of the settings on the pump and reviews the history to see how frequently the patient is using the PCA. If the patient has an epidural catheter, the nurse assesses the insertion site on the patient's back for redness, swelling, leaking, or kinking of the tubing. The nurse also reviews the pump settings, and evaluates the level of sensation and the patient's ability to move and use his extremities. The nurse listens to lung sounds, asks about sputum production, and evaluates the patient's ability to perform deep breathing exercises.

The nurse listens to bowel sounds, palpates the abdomen, and asks the patient about nausea, vomiting, passing flatus, and moving of his bowels. General anesthesia and narcotics slow peristalsis but bowel function is expected to return within several hours after surgery unless the patient has had pelvic or abdominal surgery. In these surgeries, peristalsis may be delayed for 24 to 48 hours or longer. Patients are expected to void 6 to 8 hours after surgery and urine output is measured and recorded with each void. If the patient has a urinary catheter in place, urine output is measured frequently and a urine output of less than 30 mL/hr or less than 0.5 mL/kg per hour is reported to the health care provider.

The nurse examines the patient's wound dressing and notes the color and amount of any drainage. The nurse checks the color, sensation, and motion of the extremities and the presence of pedal pulses. The nurse teaches the patient how to perform leg exercises and makes sure that any devices ordered to prevent DVT are in place and functioning properly.

At the conclusion of the assessment, the nurse works with the patient to establish goals for the day and a specific plan to accomplish the goals. One of the most important tasks for the nurse to

CHART 27-3 **Abnormal Postoperative Assessments That Need to Be Reported to the Surgeon**

METABOLIC
- Temperature >38°C (100.4°F)

NEUROLOGICAL FINDINGS
- Change in level of consciousness

CARDIOVASCULAR FINDINGS
- Heart rate < 60 or >120 beats/min
- Hypotension (e.g., systolic blood pressure of less than 90 mmHg)
- New cardiac arrhythmia
- Hypertension (e.g., systolic blood pressure 20% to 30% higher than baseline)
- Chest pain
- Loss of pulses

RESPIRATORY FINDINGS
- Oxygen saturation < 93%
- Respiratory rate < 10 breaths/minute or >24 breaths/minute
- Indications of respiratory distress such as dyspnea, crackles, wheezing

GASTROINTESTINAL
- Abdominal distention
- Vomiting uncontrolled by antiemetics

FLUID BALANCE
- Urine output < 30 mL/hr or < 0.5 mL/kg per hour
- Unable to void in 6 to 8 hours

WOUND
- More than the expected amount of bleeding at the incision site
- More than the expected amount of drainage from chest tubes or wound drains
- Incision with redness, purulent drainage, or opened areas

PAIN
- Pain not adequately controlled

EXTREMITIES
- Absence of peripheral pulses
- Swelling, redness, pain in calf

OTHER
- Unexpected presence of blood in tubes

---

accomplish is to assist the patient with rest and ambulation. It can be difficult to plan uninterrupted periods of rest, given frequent nursing assessments, health care provider visits, blood draws, and consultations by physical therapists, nutritionists, case managers, and social workers among others, visits with family and friends, and the noise level of the clinical unit. Despite these problems, the nurse creates periods where the patient is able to rest because rest is thought to be important in immune function, wound healing, and mental outlook (Redeker, 2000).

Early ambulation is one of the most important interventions that can assist in recovery from anesthesia and surgery. Unless contraindicated, ambulation begins on the evening of surgery or on the first postoperative day. The nurse is present to assist patients with their first attempt at ambulation. Patients may feel dizzy or nauseated when they first move to a sitting or standing position. Splinting the incision, deep breathing, moving slowly, and moving at the patient's pace may help to minimize pain, nausea, and vertigo. Allow patients to sit on the side of the bed for a few minutes before moving to a standing position. Some patients may be inclined to hunch over in a move designed to protect their incisions, but this posture creates muscle tension and distorts balance, so patients are encouraged to relax and assume the correct posture. Patients may be able to ambulate only a short distance initially, but the nurse provides reassurance that the distance will gradually lengthen. Postoperative patients need to ambulate at least three times daily. Early ambulation and physical therapy correlates with faster functional recovery after some surgeries (Kondo et al., 2005; Oldmeadow, McBurney, Robertson, Kimmel, & Elliott, 2004), particularly orthopedic procedures, and early and aggressive ambulation is an important element of accelerated recovery programs (Pasero & Belden, 2006).

Evidence-based demonstration projects are being used to develop models of nursing care delivery (Smith et al., 2002). The Evidence-Based Practice feature describes a model of nursing care delivery that was successful in creating a healing environment for its patients.

Collaborative Management

It is important for the nurse to work closely with the surgeon and other members of the health care team in order to facilitate the patient's rapid recovery from surgery and to prevent complications. Some hospitals are using a collaborative, comanagement approach that teams the surgeon and nurse with a hospitalist in managing postoperative patients. One study of more than 500 patients showed a decrease in minor postoperative complications for patients managed in this type of system (Huddleston et al., 2004).

Other members of the health care team are also closely involved in the patient's care. Clinical nurse specialists provide assistance regarding selected aspects of a patient's recovery such as wound care for more complicated wounds or teaching for a new ostomy or organ transplantation. Physical therapy and occupational therapy provide valuable information about postoperative exercises, ambulation, transfer, and use of assistive devices. A nutritionist may be consulted to make specific recommendations about diet or diet supplementation. Social workers are consulted to provide support and counseling for patients and their families. Case managers help provide a seamless transition from hospital to rehabilitation facility or to home with services. Many patients will be discharged home after surgery without the need for home services. Some postoperative patients, however, will require services at

Impact of Scheduled Nursing Rounds on Use of Call Light

Clinical Problem

Hospital environments, with their noise, restrictions, and loss of personal control, are not generally conducive to patient recovery. Patients report feeling a loss of personal control in the hospital and that this feeling leads to a sense of vulnerability and a poor outlook on their health status. Factors that contribute to the loss of personal control include such things as having to wait for assistance in going to the bathroom or in performing personal care, an inability to reach needed objects, such as a call light, and having to wait to receive a response to requests made (Williams & Irurita, 2005). Can a routine nursing intervention create a more therapeutic environment for patients?

Research Findings

A multisite, quasi-experimental study set out to determine the effect of making "nursing rounds" on patients' use of call lights and on patient satisfaction (Meade, Bursell, & Ketelsen, 2006). In this study, 27 nursing units at 14 hospitals implemented regular nursing rounds for a period of 4 weeks. The nursing units could opt to conduct the rounds every hour from 6 a.m. to 10 p.m. or every 2 hours from 10 p.m. to 6 a.m. A protocol for the rounds was established that included a pain assessment, offers to toilet and reposition patients, placing needed items such as the call light, telephone, and water within patient reach, and concluding the round by asking whether the patient needed anything else and indicating the time of the next scheduled round.

The researchers found that regularly scheduled rounds significantly decreased patients' use of call lights while increasing patient satisfaction. The nursing units that conducted hourly rounds also reported significant reductions in patient falls. Interestingly, even nurses who were initially reluctant to add "nursing rounds" to an already busy day were satisfied with the protocol because it increased their contact with patients in more productive ways. Perhaps most impressive is the finding that 1 year after the study was completed,

85.7% of the nursing units involved in the study continued to use nursing rounds.

Implications for Nursing Practice

This study is important because it takes a cluster of common nursing activities and demonstrates that the performance of these activities in a consistent, caring way has positive patient outcomes. The findings of the study suggest that simple changes in the delivery of nursing care can make a difference to patients—and perhaps to nurses. Understanding how and why this simple intervention worked and testing the intervention with different outcome measures is the next step in the process.

Critical Thinking Questions

1. Explain, using a theory of nursing or of growth and development, why conducting nursing rounds was an effective intervention.

2. An outcome of this study was the reduction of falls on the units that used an hourly nursing rounds protocol. If the study were replicated, what other patient outcomes might be influenced by a nursing rounds protocol?

3. Suggest specific changes in the sample or intervention that might be helpful if the study were replicated.

Answers to Critical Thinking Questions appear in Appendix D.

References

Meade, C., Bursell, A., & Ketelsen, L. (2006). Effects of nursing rounds on patients' call light use, satisfaction, and safety. *American Journal of Nursing, 106*(9), 58–70.

Williams, A., & Irurita, V. (2005). Enhancing the therapeutic potential of hospital environments by increasing the personal control and emotional comfort of hospitalized patients. *Applied Nursing Research, 18*(1), 22–28.

EVIDENCE-BASED PRACTICE

---

home such as physical therapy, speech therapy, intravenous antibiotics, wound and drain checks, or teaching. The surgical nurse collaborates with home health agencies to make sure that the patient's discharge to home is a successful one.

Preventing Postoperative Complications

A significant role of the nurse on a surgical unit is to prevent postoperative complications when possible. Chart 27–4 (p. 670) lists postoperative problems that are common to many surgeries. Common problems that occur after surgery include atelectasis, pneumonia, abdominal distention, constipation, urinary retention, wound infection and venous stasis among others. The Nursing Process: Patient Care Plan (p. 671) feature is for a patient following general surgery. Examples of appropriate nursing diagnoses in the postoperative period are described in the care plan.

Atelectasis and Pneumonia

Atelectasis refers to the collapse of alveoli and the surrounding airways. When alveoli collapse, lung volume is reduced, and mucus accumulates, causing localized airway obstructions from mucous plugs. If atelectasis remains untreated, it leads to fever and hypoxia. Although it is not entirely clear, some theorize that the re-

tention of secretions associated with atelectasis increases the risk of developing pneumonia (Smith & Ellis, 2000). Pneumonia is the inflammation of lung parenchyma caused by a virus, bacteria, or other organism. The invasion of lung tissue by an organism causes an inflammatory response and the alveoli fill with inflammatory exudates. These changes are seen on chest x-ray as new infiltrates. Signs of pneumonia include fever, dyspnea, crackles in the lung fields, purulent sputum, congested cough, hypoxia, and an elevation in the white blood cell count. The incidence of postoperative atelectasis varies according to the surgery performed, but it is estimated to be as high as 84% (Smith & Ellis, 2000). The incidence of postoperative pneumonia is much lower, around 15%, although certain surgeries such as abdominal or thoracic procedures have much higher rates (as high as 40%) (Brooks, 2001).

Atelectasis and pneumonia are referred to collectively as postoperative pulmonary complications. Some researchers also include hypoxia in that description. It can be difficult to distinguish atelectasis from pneumonia initially, and the factors that predispose patients to atelectasis also predispose them to postoperative pneumonia. Older age, preexisting respiratory conditions, heart failure, decreased level of consciousness, poor functional ability, a history of cigarette smoking, and malnutrition predispose the patient to postoperative pulmonary complications (Qaseem et al., 2006).

CHART 27–4 **Common Postoperative Problems**

Problem	Cause/High Risk	Goal	Assessment	Interventions
Pain	Cell injury, muscle spasm, drains, anxiety.	Pain free, rate pain a 3 or less.	Pain rating scale 0–10 Increased HR, BP, RR Guarding, grimacing	Narcotics: PCA or epidural NSAIDS: Tylenol, Toradol Comfort measures
Fluid retention (overload)	Stress response, excess IV fluid, medical diagnosis such as heart failure.	Ensure adequate perfusion without causing overload. (Diuresis is expected by day 3 postop.)	Swelling in hands, feet, eyelids. Weight gain. Decreased urine output of <30 mL/hour or < 0.5 mL/kg per hour. Crackles or rales.	Monitor urine output every 1–4 hours. Check breath sounds. Monitor IV fluid.
Fluid deficit (dehydration)	Excess fluid losses during surgery, from wound, drains; vomiting, fever.	Ensure adequate tissue perfusion.	Dry skin, mucous membranes. Decreased urine output of <30 mL/hour or < 0.5 mL/kg per hour. HR >100, SBP < 90 mmHg, narrow pulse pressure.	Fluid bolus: normal saline (NS) 250–500 mL over 1 hour. Monitor urine output, heart rate, and BP.
Bleeding	High risk for surgery on vascular tissue or on patient with history of clotting disorder, use of anticoagulants, malnourished.	Hemodynamic stability.	Cool, clammy skin. HR >100, SBP < 90 mmHg, narrow pulse pressure. Decreased Hct/Hgb. Decreased urine output of <30 mL/hr or < 0.5 mL/kg per hour. Swelling or distention, oozing from wounds, hematoma, bloody drainage.	Fluid replacement: NS bolus. Transfusion packed red blood cells if active bleeding. Transfusion with fresh frozen plasma (if clotting factors need replacing).
Atelectasis (risk of pneumonia)	Most common problem in first 48–72 hours postop. Primary cause is anesthesia. Risk increases with surgery on chest or abdomen, with uncontrolled pain, decreased mobility, obesity, smoker, chronic obstructive pulmonary disease, asthma.	Patient will demonstrate adequate oxygenation and will not develop postop pneumonia.	Fever is most common sign. Breath sounds diminished or crackles. Increased RR Oxygen (O_2) saturation< 93%. Sputum: increased production and consistency.	Incentive spirometer or turn–cough–deep breathe 10 times per hour. Turn every 1–2 hours. Adequate pain relief. Splint incision during movement. Increase head of bed 30 degrees or higher. Ambulate 3 times per day (tid). Titrate oxygen to maintain O_2 saturation >93%.
Nausea and vomiting (N&V)	Most N&V peaks in 24–36 hours postop. Anesthesia, narcotics, antibiotics, retained gastric secretions.	Will not experience N&V or N&V will be relieved.	Nausea and vomiting. Nausea increases with movement. Abdominal distention.	IV fluid to maintain hydration. Medicate with antiemetic: droperidol, ondansetron, promethazine, metoclopramide. Maintain function of nasogastric tube if needed for comfort. Minimize use of opioids and increase use of nonopioids for pain. Advance diet slowly (ice chips—clear liquids—full liquids—regular diet).
Abdominal distention (postoperative ileus)	Following surgery on the bowel, it will take 3–5 days for return of GI function. Factors that decrease bowel function: anesthesia, surgical trauma, narcotics, decreased mobility.	Return of bowel peristalsis.	Abdomen is distended. No stool or flatus. Nausea and vomiting. No bowel sounds or hypoactive bowel sounds.	NPO until flatus; may be 3–5 days post-gastrointestinal (GI) surgery. NGT to suction for comfort if vomiting. Ambulate tid. Advance diet slowly.

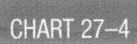

CHART 27–4   **Common Postoperative Problems—*Continued***

Problem	Cause/High Risk	Goal	Assessment	Interventions
Syncope (orthostatic hypotension)	Anesthesia, immobility, dehydration, some medications.	Patient will not experience orthostatic hypotension.	Complaints of dizzy, light-headedness, diaphoresis. Increased symptoms with standing or sitting. Orthostatic (postural) vital sign changes: HR increases at least 10 beats/minute (from lying to standing); BP decreases by at least 10 mmHg (from lying to standing).	Get out of bed slowly; dangle legs before standing. If symptomatic, take orthostatic vital signs. If syncope is from dehydration, give patient a fluid bolus.
Urinary retention	Anesthesia, narcotics, anticholinergics, spasm of abdominal or pelvic muscles.	Patient will void (minimum 200 mL) after surgery or 6–8 hours after removal of Foley catheter.	No voiding or small, frequent voids. Fullness above symphysis pubis.	Ambulate. Avoid use of bedpan. Check intake and output and offer fluids. Bladder scan. Catheterize (per order) if not void in 8–12 hours.
Wound healing: risk of infection Dehiscence Evisceration	Infection usually not evident until 3–7 days after surgery. High risk with obesity, poor circulation, diabetes, malnourishment.	Wound well approximated and without drainage. Wound heals.	Local: redness, swelling, increased pain, edges not approximated, increased drainage from incision. Systemic: fever, elevated white blood cells count.	Adequate nutrition. Limit stress on wound. Prophylactic antibiotic for 24 hours only. Use sterile technique.
Deep venous thrombosis (DVT)	Occurs 5–7 days after surgery and is caused by venous stasis and pressure. DVT can dislodge and become a pulmonary embolus.	Adequate circulation without evidence of venous stasis.	Calf: red, painful, swollen. Positive Homans' sign.	Ambulate tid. Leg exercises. Antiembolism stockings or pneumatic compression boots. Antithrombotic medication. Avoid pressure under the knees.

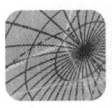

NURSING PROCESS: Patient Care Plan for the Postoperative Patient Following General Surgery

Assessment of Discomfort

Subjective Data:
Ask the patient to describe the pain, its location and intensity.
Ask patient to rate pain from 0–10 on the pain scale.

Objective Data:
Watch for physical signs of pain including guarding, grimacing, crying, increased blood pressure (BP), heart rate (HR), and respiratory rate (RR).

Nursing Assessment and Diagnoses	Outcomes and Evaluation Parameters	Interventions with *Rationales*
Nursing Diagnosis: *Readiness for Enhanced Comfort* related to surgical incision, muscle spasm, positioning in the operating room, the presence of drains, and anxiety	**Outcome:** The patient will be comfortable and rate the pain at a 3 or less. **Evaluation Parameters:** Patient is comfortable. Patient participates in postoperative activities and exercises without discomfort.	**Interventions and *Rationales:*** Use pain scale (0–10) to assess pain every 2–4 hours. *Increases consistency in quantifying pain.* Watch for physical signs of pain including guarding, grimacing, crying, increased BP, HR, and RR. *Some patients are reluctant to ask for pain medication. Different cultures respond to and express pain differently.* Administer pain medication, narcotics and anti-inflammatory agents as prescribed. *Postoperative pain is highest in the first 48 hours after surgery.* Provide teaching about patient controlled analgesia (PCA) or patient controlled epidural analgesia (PCEA) if prescribed. Elevate affected area if appropriate *to decrease tissue swelling.* Apply ice to affected area if appropriate *to decrease tissue swelling.* Teach to splint the incision. *Provides stability to injured area.* Use nonpharmacologic interventions such as massage, distraction, relaxation techniques. *These measures augment other pain control measures.*

(continued)

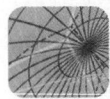

NURSING PROCESS: Patient Care Plan for the Postoperative Patient Following General Surgery—*Continued*

Assessment of Nausea and Vomiting

Subjective Data:
Ask patient about feeling nauseated.

Objective Data:
Patient vomits.
Abdomen is firm, distended with hypoactive bowel sounds.

Nursing Assessment and Diagnoses	Outcomes and Evaluation Parameters	Interventions with *Rationales*
Nursing Diagnosis: *Alteration in Nausea* related to anesthesia, narcotics, antibiotics, slowed peristalsis	**Outcomes:** Patient will get relief from nausea and vomiting. Patient will have a soft abdomen and pass flatus. Patient will have adequate intake of fluids. ***Evaluation Parameters:*** Abdomen soft. Appetite is present. Oral fluid intake is 1,500–2,500 mL in 24 hours. Passing flatus and stool.	**Interventions and *Rationales:*** Assess for nausea, vomiting, abdominal distention, and flatus. *Most nausea and vomiting peaks in 24 to 36 hours after surgery.* Maintain nasogastric tube (NGT) as prescribed for comfort. *An NGT decompresses the stomach and prevents vomiting.* Maintain NPO status until nausea recedes and bowel function returns. *Flatus and passing stool are the best indicators that bowel function has returned.* Advance diet slowly from ice chips to clear liquids to full liquids and regular diet. *Vomiting can occur when the diet is advanced too rapidly.* Medicate with antinausea medication as prescribed. *Early administration of medication is more effective than waiting until the patient experiences nausea and vomiting.* Encourage patient to change positions slowly. *Movement is a trigger for nausea and vomiting.* Provide comfort measures such as rest, a cool washcloth, mouth care, and deep breathing.

Assessment of Fluid Volume

Subjective Data:
Patient reports vertigo.
Are you thirsty?

Objective Data:
Watch for signs of active bleeding including blood on dressing, hematoma, presence of blood in drainage tubes, and decreased hematocrit and hemoglobin.
Watch for signs of dehydration including heart rate (HR) >100, systolic blood pressure (BP) <90, narrow pulse pressure, decreased urine output of <30 mL/hour or <0.5 mL/kg per hour.

Nursing Assessment and Diagnoses	Outcomes and Evaluation Parameters	Interventions with *Rationales*
Nursing Diagnosis: *Deficient Fluid Volume* related to hemorrhage, blood loss with surgery, fluid loss, wound drains, vomiting, or fever	**Outcome:** Patient will have adequate hemostasis and normal intravascular volume. ***Evaluation Parameters:*** Normal vital signs. Urine output >0.5 mL/kg per hour. No evidence of active bleeding.	**Interventions and *Rationales:*** Assess for indications of bleeding and dehydration every 1–4 hours. *There is a higher risk of bleeding if surgery is performed on tissue that is vascular. The patient is most at risk for dehydration in the first 24–48 hours postop.* Report HR >120, systolic blood pressure (SBP) <90, urine output <30 mL/hour or <0.5 mL/kg per hour, or more drainage than expected on dressing or in tubes. *Indicators or risk of imbalanced fluid volume and possible postoperative bleeding.* Check dressing and circle any new drainage with pen *to monitor for bleeding.* Reinforce dressing as needed. *The surgeon changes the primary dressing.* Administer IV fluids as ordered *to replace fluids lost during surgery.* Administer normal saline fluid bolus if required. *Used to expand blood volume and increase urine output.*

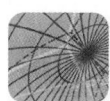

NURSING PROCESS: Patient Care Plan for the Postoperative Patient Following General Surgery—*Continued*

Assessment of Fluid Volume

Subjective Data:
Patient reports dyspnea.

Objective Data:
Swelling in hands, feet, and eyelids, weight gain, urine output < 30 mL/hr or <0.5 mL/kg per hour crackles in the lungs.

Nursing Assessment and Diagnoses	Outcomes and Evaluation Parameters	Interventions with *Rationales*
Nursing Diagnosis: *Risk for Imbalanced Fluid Volume* related to response to stress hormones, excess intravenous fluids, or preexisting medical condition such as congestive heart failure	**Outcome:** Patient will have adequate fluid volume without evidence of overload. **Evaluation Parameters:** Urine output is >30 mL/hr or >0.5 mL/kg per hour. Intake and output (I&O) is balanced. Clear breath sounds. Normal vital signs without tachycardia or tachypnea.	**Interventions and *Rationales:*** Assess for swelling, weight gain, urine output <30 mL/hr or <0.5 mL/kg per hour, crackles in lungs, and dyspnea every 1–4 hours. *The effect of stress hormones is greatest in the first 24–48 hours.* Monitor IV fluid administration carefully. *Fluid given too rapidly can exacerbate fluid overload.*

Assessment of Respiratory Status

Subjective Data:
Patient states it is painful to take deep breaths.

Objective Data:
Watch for fever, diminished breath sounds, crackles in the lungs, sputum production, increased respiratory rate, and decreased oxygen saturation.

Nursing Assessment and Diagnoses	Outcomes and Evaluation Parameters	Interventions with *Rationales*
Nursing Diagnosis: *Ineffective Breathing Pattern* related to anesthesia, surgical pain, location of the surgery, limited mobility, a history of smoking, or preexisting medical condition	**Outcome:** Respiratory status will be stable and within normal limits. **Evaluation Parameters:** Afebrile. Clear lung sounds. Oxygen saturation >93%. Normal respiratory rate. Denies shortness of breath and air hunger.	**Interventions and *Rationales:*** Monitor respiratory rate, depth, breath sounds, and oxygen saturation every 4 hours *to assess for atelectasis.* Encourage deep breathing or use of incentive spirometry 10 times every hour *to increase maximal inspiration and stimulate surfactant.* Encourage patient to cough every hour. Splint incision if appropriate. *Coughing clears mucous secretions.* Elevate head of the bed 30 degrees or higher *to lower the diaphragm and facilitate lung expansion.* Provide adequate pain relief. *Patients consistently give high pain ratings to coughing and deep breathing.* Ambulate three times daily. *Increases RR, minute ventilation, and tidal volume.* Titrate oxygen (O$_2$) to maintain the O$_2$ saturation at or >93%. *Oxygen dries the airways and reduces mucociliary clearance.*

Assessment of Urine Output

Subjective Data:
Patient states he cannot void or is only able to void small amounts.

Objective Data:
Patient does not void or voids only small amounts.
Palpable fullness above symphysis pubis or a bladder scan showing a full bladder.

Nursing Assessment and Diagnoses	Outcomes and Evaluation Parameters	Interventions with *Rationales*
Nursing Diagnosis: *Urinary Retention* related to anesthesia, narcotics, anticholinergic medications, or spasm of abdominal or pelvic muscles	**Outcome:** Patient voids >100–150 mL within 6–8 hours after surgery or after removal of Foley catheter. **Evaluation Parameters:** I&O is balanced. Voids adequate amounts without difficulty.	**Interventions and *Rationales:*** Monitor I&O *to determine adequacy of urine output.* Encourage oral fluids if appropriate. *Inability to void may be due to dehydration.* Ambulate frequently *to stimulate circulation and production of urine.* Perform measures to stimulate voiding reflex (i.e., use commode rather than bedpan; have male patients stand to use urinal; run water; run warm water over perineum; use spirits of peppermints). If patient is unable to void 8 hours after surgery or after Foley catheter is removed, perform a bladder scan and call the surgeon for an order to perform catheterization. *The patient should feel the urge to void when the bladder has 300 mL of urine.*

(continued)

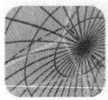

NURSING PROCESS: Patient Care Plan for the Postoperative Patient Following General Surgery—*Continued*

Assessment of Activity Level

Subjective Data:
Patient states he has vertigo, fatigue, or dyspnea with activity.

Objective Data:
Positive orthostatic vital signs with activity or an increased heart rate of >10 beats/minute, increased respiratory rate of >10 beats/minute, decreased oxygen saturation, or labored breathing with activity.

Nursing Assessment and Diagnoses	Outcomes and Evaluation Parameters	Interventions with *Rationales*
Nursing Diagnosis: *Activity Intolerance* related to anesthesia, narcotics, surgery, and limited mobility	**Outcome:** Patient will carry out postoperative activities and activities of daily living without signs of activity intolerance. **Evaluation Parameters:** Ambulates without experiencing symptoms. Completes activities of daily living without experiencing symptoms. Postactivity vital signs and oxygen saturation are within normal limits.	**Interventions and *Rationales:*** Encourage muscle strengthening activities every shift *to increase circulation.* Encourage use of slow changes in position. Dangle legs at bedside before attempting to ambulate. Assist with two people during first attempt at ambulation *to provide for patient safety.* If symptomatic, take orthostatic vital signs and notify surgeon. Anticipate administering a fluid bolus. *Positive orthostatic vital signs are an indication of dehydration.* Ambulate a minimum of three times daily.

Assessment of Wound

Subjective Data:
Patient states that incision feels painful and swollen.

Objective Data:
Incision is red, painful, or swollen. Wound edges are not approximated and the wound has increased drainage.
Elevated white blood cells count (WBC) and fever.

Nursing Assessment and Diagnoses	Outcomes and Evaluation Parameters	Interventions with *Rationales*
Nursing Diagnosis: *Risk for Infection* related to altered skin integrity, and high-risk factors (e.g., diabetes, obesity, diminished arterial circulation, malnutrition)	**Outcomes:** The patient will be free from infection. The wound will heal within appropriately 7–10 days. **Evaluation Parameters:** The patient is afebrile. The wound edges are well approximated without drainage, redness, or swelling.	**Interventions and *Rationales:*** Monitor temperature, WBC count, and serum glucose. *Infection causes a fever and increased WBC and glucose.* Change dressing every shift using sterile technique and monitor for signs of infection. *The inflammatory response in an infected wound will cause redness, pain, swelling, and drainage.* Encourage adequate nutrition that is high in protein and vitamins. *Protein, calories, calcium, iron, zinc, and vitamins A, B_6, B_{12}, and C are needed for wound healing.*

Assessment of Blood Flow to the Extremities

Subjective Data:
Patient complains of pain in calf.

Objective Data:
Calf is red, painful, and swollen. Patient reports a positive Homans' sign.

Nursing Assessment and Diagnoses	Outcomes and Evaluation Parameters	Interventions with *Rationales*
Nursing Diagnosis: *Ineffective Tissue Perfusion, Venous Stasis* related to immobility, surgical procedure, and high-risk factors (e.g., age, use of estrogen, cancer, history of previous deep vein thrombosis [DVT])	**Outcome:** The patient will have adequate peripheral circulation and no evidence of DVT. **Evaluation Parameters:** Palpable dorsal pedis and posterior tibialis pulses. Calf is pain free without evidence of redness or swelling.	**Interventions and *Rationales:*** Assess for signs of DVT. A red, warm, swollen, or painful calf alerts the nurse to the possibility of a venous clot. *Venous thrombosis is most likely to occur 5 to 7 days after surgery.* Administer anticoagulant medication as prescribed *to prevent clot formation.* Measure the circumference of the calf and thigh of each leg and compare them prn. *The leg will increase in size with DVT formation.* Any indication of a clot is reported immediately to the health care provider. *Early treatment will decrease the risk of further clot formation.* The patient is placed on bed rest until the possibility of a clot is evaluated. *There is an increased chance of clot migration with activity.* Encourage ambulation and leg exercises three times daily *to stimulate circulation.* Apply pneumatic compression boots, antiembolism stockings or other antithrombotic devices as ordered *to increase venous return and prevent venous stasis.* Avoid pressure under the knees. *Venous compression contributes to the development of DVT.*

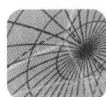

NURSING PROCESS: Patient Care Plan for the Postoperative Patient Following General Surgery—*Continued*

Assessment of Knowledge Regarding Surgery and Postoperative Care

Subjective Data:
Patient states that she needs information on how to care for herself at home.

Objective Data:
Patient is being discharged home following a recent surgery.

Nursing Assessment and Diagnoses	Outcomes and Evaluation Parameters	Interventions with *Rationales*
Nursing Diagnosis: *Deficient Knowledge* related to postoperative care	**Outcomes:** The patient will recover from surgery without complications. The patient is knowledgeable about how to care for herself at home. ***Evaluation Parameters:*** Demonstrates appropriate care of her wound and drains (if applicable). Verbalizes an understanding of pain management. Verbalizes an understanding of activity restrictions and other discharge instructions. Verbalizes an understanding of danger signs and what to do about them.	**Interventions and *Rationales:*** *The specific information taught depends on the surgery (refer to the appropriate disorder chapter in this text for specific information) and the preferences of the surgeon. General areas for teaching are listed below.* Teaching is done in the patient's native language, through an interpreter, if necessary. • General information about recovery • Wound care • Activity • Specific exercises to aid recovery • Diet • Medication • Symptom management: pain, constipation, fatigue • Recognition and prevention of complications • Follow-up appointments • Who to call with questions

There is a higher risk of postoperative atelectasis and pneumonia with surgeries of the chest and abdomen because the incision is located close to the diaphragm, making it painful to take deep breaths, turn, and ambulate. Studies show that vital capacity can decrease by as much as 60% in the first 24 hours following abdominal surgery (Brooks-Brunn, 1998; Shea, Brooks, Dayhoff, & Keck, 2002). Immobility increases risk because the movement of the diaphragm and chest wall are restricted, resulting in diminished lung volumes (Brooks, 2001). Longer surgeries, those that take more than 4 hours, also increase risk as a result of prolonged anesthesia (Smith & Ellis, 2000). Other procedures associated with increased risk of postoperative pulmonary complications are neurosurgery, head and neck surgery, vascular surgery, and emergency surgery (Qaseem et al., 2006).

The nurse assesses the patient's respiratory rate, depth, lung sounds, and oxygen saturation at frequent intervals. Postoperative atelectasis most often occurs in the lower lobes of the lungs. Lung sounds may be diminished as a result of shallow respirations or crackles, which are most noticeable on inspiration and may be heard as collapsed alveoli are forced open. Crackles also occur with pneumonia as air is forced through mucus and fluid in the alveoli. The crackles with pneumonia may be present throughout the respiratory cycle. Atelectasis can clear with repeated deep breathing, so the nurse assesses lung sounds before and after use of incentive spirometry or deep breathing. Fever can be present with either atelectasis or pneumonia and is caused by inflammatory mediators.

A number of interventions are designed to decrease postoperative pulmonary complications. Unless contraindicated, the patient is placed in semi-Fowler's, Fowler's, or high-Fowler's position. Elevating the head of the bed 30 to 90 degrees lowers the diaphragm, thus facilitating chest expansion.

The patient is encouraged to use lung expansion therapies, deep breathing, or incentive spirometry. Deep breathing reverses alveolar collapse by forcing and holding maximal inspiration. Techniques for deep breathing and incentive spirometry are discussed in Chapter 26 ☺. Deep breathing is most effective when maximal inspiration is held for 3 seconds or longer and when the exercises are performed frequently. Patients are encouraged to take 5 to 10 deep breaths every hour, but more is better. Nasal continuous positive airway pressure, a specially designed face mask and pump that forces air into the nasal passages at pressures high enough to keep the airway open, may be helpful to patients who are unable to perform deep breathing (Qaseem et al., 2006).

Forced coughing is used postoperatively to clear secretions. To have an effective cough, the patient must take a deep breath, increase intrathoracic pressure, and produce a high expiratory flow rate. Both volume and force of airflow are required to remove secretions. Coughing can be painful and the incision should be splinted with a pillow or small rolled blanket held firmly across the incision to prevent undue stress. Coughing is usually performed with deep breathing exercises, but the practice is contraindicated in some situations (e.g., cranial surgery, eye surgery) because it can increase intracranial and intraocular pressures and in other circumstances because it places too much stress on the incision (e.g., hernia surgery). Interventions to loosen and remove secretions such as percussion and postural drainage are recommended in specific situations but they are not employed universally after surgery (Brooks et al., 2001).

Ambulation is an important intervention to prevent postoperative pulmonary complications. Ambulation increases respiratory rate, minute ventilation, tidal volume, and inspiratory flow rates (Orfanos, Ellis, & Johnston, 1999). Patients who walk more and who walk longer distances tend to recover quicker and are discharged sooner than patients who are less mobile (Whitney & Parkman, 2002). There are no practice guidelines describing optimal postoperative ambulation. As soon as allowed by the surgeon, patients are encouraged to walk a minimum of three times daily. Patients are encouraged to walk with good posture and to take deep breaths with ambulation. More ambulation is likely to be better, provided that the patient does not overexert. Patients are monitored during ambulation for signs of activity intolerance. Signs include shortness of breath, tachypnea, hypoxia, tachycardia, chest pain, and fatigue. It is also beneficial for patients to get out of bed to a chair several times each day (Markey & Brown, 2002). Sitting facilitates excursion of the diaphragm, and it is associated with improved respirations and lung volumes (Brooks, 2001; Smith & Ellis, 2000).

Pain control is absolutely essential to getting patients to participate in pulmonary exercises and ambulation. Postoperative patients consistently give high pain ratings to turning, movement, coughing, and deep breathing (Puntillo, 2003; Puntillo et al., 2002; Stanik-Hutt, Soeken, Belcher, Fontaine, & Gift, 2001). Higher pain scores are associated with reluctance to walk and to take deep breaths and with higher rates of atelectasis and pneumonia (Edelen & Perlow, 2002; Puntillo & Weiss, 2003; Shea et al., 2002). Patients are medicated prior to periods of mobility and, when possible, the nurse plans to ambulate patients when pain medication is at its peak. Encouraging the use of nonpharmacologic interventions for pain control is also useful. In one study, the use of relaxation techniques 15 minutes before deep breathing exercises was associated with higher inspiratory volumes (Edelen & Perlow, 2002).

The use of nasogastric tubes for patients with nausea and vomiting or symptomatic abdominal distention is shown to reduce the incidence of postoperative atelectasis and pneumonia (Lawrence et al., 2003; Qaseem et al., 2006). Conversely, quick removal of the nasogastric tube when it is no longer necessary may reduce microaspiration and bacterial colonization of the oropharyngeal area, both of which are risk factors for postoperative pneumonia (Brooks, 2001; Smith & Ellis, 2000).

Other interventions may be helpful in reducing atelectasis and pneumonia although the benefit is not established through research. Titrating the patient off of oxygen may be helpful because supplemental oxygen can dry airways and reduce mucociliary clearance (Smith & Ellis, 2000). The Centers for Disease Control and Prevention (CDC, 1997) recommends using sterile water to fill oxygen humidifiers and to rinse medication nebulizers to reduce the introduction of microorganisms to the respiratory tract. Poor nutrition correlates with postoperative pulmonary complications but the routine use of enteral feedings using a gastrostomy, jejunostomy tube, or total parenteral nutrition is not recommended. Enteral feedings pose a risk of aspiration and are discontinued as soon as possible. While feeding tubes are needed, interventions are used to reduce the risk of aspiration including elevating the head of the bed a minimum of 30 degrees and checking tube placement regularly (CDC, 1997). Dental plaque and poor oral care provide a site for bacterial growth and are thought to predispose patients to pneumonia. Good oral hygiene may stimulate salivary flow, reducing the

growth of microorganisms in the mouth. Adequate hydration aids in mucous clearance.

 A fever in the first 48 hours after surgery is commonly related to atelectasis. Encourage the patient to cough, deep breathe, and ambulate, if appropriate. If the fever is accompanied by crackles in the lungs, respiratory congestion, respiratory distress or low oxygen saturations, contact the health care provider because these signs are consistent with pneumonia.

Abdominal Distention, Ileus, and Risk for Constipation

As part of a routine gastrointestinal assessment, the nurse palpates the abdomen for firmness and tenderness and asks about the presence of nausea and vomiting, passing of flatus, and recent bowel movement. Multiple factors place postoperative patients at risk for abdominal distention, a bloated abdomen, and **ileus**, a hypoactive bowel with delay in peristalsis. Surgical trauma, physiological stress, and the inflammatory process stimulate the release of catecholamines, neurotransmitters, and hormones that slow gastrointestinal motility. The inhibitory effects of anesthesia and opioids further reduce peristalsis. Despite these factors, most patients regain bowel function several hours after surgery except in abdominal procedures where the return of bowel function is delayed for several days.

A postoperative ileus (POI) occurs when peristalsis does not return as expected after surgery. An ileus is more likely to occur in patients who have had major abdominal surgery, particularly if inflammation or leakage of an abdominal organ was involved (e.g., leaking appendix or ruptured gallbladder). Other factors such as postoperative fluid and electrolyte imbalance can cause POI. Minimally invasive surgical approaches (laparoscopy), epidural analgesia, and lower doses of opioids are associated with lower rates of POI (Ead, 2006; Saclarides, 2006; Zutshi, Delaney, Senagore, & Fazio, 2004). Indications of an ileus include a hard, firm abdomen, hypoactive or absent bowel sounds, and no passing of flatus or stool. Patients with severe abdominal distention may also experience nausea, vomiting, pain, and hiccups caused by irritation of the diaphragm. Research efforts are focused on preventing postoperative ileus and on speeding resolution of ileus after abdominal surgery. Chart 27–5 lists some of the strategies used to prevent or correct postoperative ileus.

 *The nurse gives priority to performing an abdominal assessment early in the shift on patients who are recovering from abdominal surgery. A hard, distended, painful abdomen can indicate internal bleeding and the surgeon should be notified.*

There are many approaches to treatment of postoperative ileus although not all treatments are evidence based. POI may resolve with time alone or with the correction of dehydration or electrolyte imbalance. In some cases, a nasogastric tube (NGT) or a longer intestinal tube is used to decompress the stomach and/or intestine. Studies show that nasogastric intubation does not improve postoperative ileus (Person & Wexner, 2006; Saclarides, 2006), but it may provide comfort by reducing abdominal bloating and nausea and vomiting. The NGT is attached to suction and the nurse checks that the suction is functioning correctly. NGT drainage is measured every shift. If a disposable

CHART 27–5	Strategies Used to Reduce Postoperative Ileus

Good Evidence that Strategies Are Effective in Reducing POI	Some Evidence that Strategies Might Be Effective in Reducing POI, But Further Research Is Needed
Use of minimally invasive surgical techniques	Use of laxatives postoperatively
Use of epidural analgesia	Chewing gum
NSAIDS for pain control	Early feeding of patient postoperatively
Opioid antagonists for pain control	Sham feeding: allowing patients to chew food without swallowing it
	Alternative therapies: guided imagery, mechanical massage, acupuncture

system is being used, the entire setup is replaced, rather than emptied, once a day or as often as needed. The NGT is taped firmly to the patient's nose to prevent dislodgement. Usually, an NGT can be flushed with 30 mL of normal saline to maintain patency except when contraindicated by the presence of internal sutures. The nurse does not flush an NGT if the patient has had esophageal or gastric surgery except by order of the health care provider because a strong flush could disrupt sutures and stimulate bleeding. Ambulation helps to stimulate peristalsis and return the bowel to normal function. Usually, it is acceptable to clamp an NGT temporarily for the purpose of ambulation or transfer to a chair.

The passing of flatus and stool marks the return of bowel motility and function. The presence of bowel sounds is not a good marker of the return of bowel function in the postoperative patient and is probably an unnecessary assessment (Madsen et al., 2005). The trend in postoperative care is toward early feeding. Most patients (except those with abdominal surgery) will be started on clear fluids the evening of surgery. Traditionally, patients begin on clear liquids and the diet is advanced if the patient tolerates clear liquids without nausea and vomiting, but this practice may be unnecessary. Studies show that many postoperative patients, perhaps 80% to 90%, tolerate oral feedings without problems (Basse, Billesbolle, & Kehlet, 2002; Person & Wexner, 2006; Rimmele et al., 2005; Saclarides, 2006). In a review of 15 research studies, 86% of patients progressed well with early feeding without problems of aspiration, bowel obstruction, anastomotic leak, or pneumonia (Ng & Neill, 2006). Further, early feeding may stimulate gastric emptying, help with tissue repair, and improve patient comfort (Ead, 2006; Saclarides, 2006), but further research is needed to substantiate these benefits.

Many postoperative patients experience constipation. Most patients receive a stool softener such as docusate sodium (Colace). Fluids, ambulation, and bulk laxatives such as Metamucil or MiraLax are also helpful with postoperative bowel regularity. If a patient is unable to move her bowels, she may require a laxative such as milk of magnesia or bisacodyl or an enema, but health care provider approval is necessary.

Urinary Retention

Many patients will have a urinary catheter for the first 12 to 24 hours after surgery. Urine output is observed frequently in patients with a Foley catheter. If urine output falls below 30 mL or .5 mL/kg per hour, the health care provider is notified. The catheter will be removed as soon as possible to avoid the possibil-

ity of a urinary tract infection (UTI). Once the catheter is removed, the patient is at risk for development of urinary retention. Urinary retention is common and occurs as a result of general anesthesia from relaxation of the detrusor muscle, spinal anesthesia from blocking parasympathetic fibers in the sacral region of the spine controlling micturition, certain preoperative medications, and narcotics. Urinary retention is also more likely to occur in surgeries of the lower abdomen, pelvis, and genitourinary tract where manipulation of tissues may cause swelling of or around the urethra.

Once the urinary catheter is discontinued, the patient must void within the next 6 to 8 hours. The time when the patient is due to void (DTV) is noted on the intake and output (I&O) record and in the nursing note. The void must be substantial, a minimum of 100 to 150 mL, to be considered adequate. A patient who only voids small amounts may have urinary retention with overflow or a UTI.

When a patient is unable to void, the nurse palpates the bladder. A bladder scan can be used to estimate the amount of urine in the bladder and to determine the need for catheterization. The I&O record is also reviewed because dehydration may be partially to blame. Techniques to help patients void include running warm water over the perineum, allowing the patient to stand or use the bathroom rather than a bedpan, running water in the bathroom, and allowing the patient to smell spirits of peppermint. These techniques may help, however, their efficacy has not been demonstrated through research.

Patients who do not void within the specified time frame are usually straight catheterized to empty the bladder. The nurse needs a health care provider's order to perform urinary catheterization. Sometimes the catheter is left in place if more than 1,000 mL is drained during the catheterization. The patient is reassured and encouraged to continue to drink fluids. Urinary retention resolves over time, but it may take one or two straight catheterizations before the patient is able to void on his own.

 Urinary retention can place pressure on internal sutures in a patient recovering from some types of urological surgery. Contact the surgeon immediately if a patient is unable to void within the prescribed time period.

Wound Infection

Wound healing begins immediately after tissue injury. In the first stage (days 1 to 4), the inflammatory process is triggered bringing blood, lymph, and fibrin to the area. Fibrin strands form along the area of injury, creating a blood clot that holds the wound edges together. Increased blood flow to the site brings white blood cells (WBCs) that remove damaged tissue and fight off microorganisms. In the second stage (days 5 to 14 or longer), epithelial cells migrate to the area and proliferate, forming a protective barrier at the wound site. While the process of epithelialization is occurring, collagen synthesis is taking place, filling in tissue gaps and giving the wound added strength. Collagen synthesis helps contract the wound, making it smaller than its original size. The last stage of healing begins 2 to 3 weeks after injury and lasts a year or longer as the wound is reshaped. As collagen breaks down and is replaced, the new fibers become more closely packed shrinking the scar and making it less bulky. Until the wound is completely healed, infection is a concern.

Surgical-site infections (SSIs) continue to be a serious postoperative problem. To qualify as a SSI, the infection occurs within 30 days of the operation. In 1992, the CDC classified surgical site infections into those that are incisional (superficial or deep) and those that are in an organ or organ space (Horan, Gaynes, Martone, Jarvis, & Emori, 1992). The CDC has established definitions for each of the classifications, as shown in the National Guidelines box.

The risk of developing a SSI is affected by characteristics of the patient, the operative procedure, and the type of surgery performed. Older patients, smokers, those who are obese, and those who are malnourished are at a higher risk of developing a wound infection. Patients with diabetes or peripheral vascular disease heal more slowly and are at increased risk. Patients who are immunocompromised have insufficient defenses to fight infection and to repair tissues (Neil, 2007). Factors associated with operative procedures that increase the risk of infection include ineffective preoperative skin preparation, breaks in sterile technique, inadequate sterilization of instruments, hypothermia during surgery, failure to administer appropriate antibiotic coverage, and procedures that last significantly longer than expected according to a preestablished standard (Seltzer, Horsman, & Korniewicz, 2002). The type of surgery also affects the risk of SSI. The National Guidelines for Surgical Wound Classification box in Chapter 26 lists the CDC's classifications for surgical wounds. The classification is standardized and documented in the surgical record. The CDC's National Nosocomial Infections Surveillance (NNIS) program uses three criteria to assess risk of SSI: wound classification, duration of the surgical procedure, and the ASA physical status classification (described earlier).

Best practices for preventing SSIs come from the CDC and the American College of Surgeons. The CDC clinical guidelines recommend protecting the surgical wound with a sterile dressing for 24 to 48 hours postoperatively. They also recommend using sterile technique for dressing changes. The question of whether clean technique is as effective as sterile technique in the incidence of wound infection is being researched. At present, there is not enough evidence to recommend clean technique over sterile technique (Horan et al., 1992; St. Clair & Larrabee, 2002). Dressings are used postoperatively for a number of reasons. Dressings act to reduce contamination of the incision by microorganisms (i.e., dry sterile dressing), to reduce bleeding or swelling (i.e., pressure dressing), to cushion the wound and absorb drainage, and in some cases to debride the wound (i.e., wet to dry dressing).

Traditionally, the surgeon performs the first dressing change. Until then, the nurse monitors the surgical site for evidence of bleeding or drainage. Some amount of drainage is normal after surgery. Small to moderate amounts of drainage are circled with a pen directly on the dressing. This allows the nurse to watch for an increase in the amount of drainage. The dressing can also be reinforced. Excessive amounts of bleeding or drainage are reported to the surgeon. After the first dressing change, the wound may be left open to air or covered with a dry sterile dressing according to health care provider preference. Dressing changes are usually performed once or twice a shift using sterile technique. During the dressing change, the nurse notes the condition of the incision. It should be well approximated, slightly pink, and free of purulent drainage. Crusting along the incision is a normal finding. The nurse reports signs of wound infection including pain and tenderness at the site, swelling, redness, purulent drainage, odor, or evidence of dehiscence to the surgeon. Systemic indicators of infection include fever (38°C [100.4°F] or higher), elevated WBC count, and elevated serum glucose. Studies confirm that fever is a nonspecific and insensitive measure of infection. In one study of 284 general surgical patients, 63% of infected patients did not have a fever (Vermeulen et al., 2005).

NATIONAL GUIDELINES CDC Criteria for Defining Surgical Site Infection

Infection Site	Time Frame for Developing Symptoms	Patient Symptoms (Patient Must Have at Least One of These)
Superficial incisional (involves only the skin and subcutaneous tissue)	Infection occurs within 30 days of the surgery.	Purulent drainage from the site. Organisms isolated from a culture of fluid or tissue from the site. One sign and symptom of infection: pain, tenderness, redness, localized swelling and heat.
Deep incisional (involves deep soft tissue such as fascia and muscle layers of incision)	Infection occurs within 30 days of surgery or if an implant is placed within 1 year and the infection appears to be related to operative procedures.	Purulent drainage from the deep incision but not from an organ or body cavity. A deep incision dehisces, or is deliberately opened by the surgeon when the patient presents with at least one of the symptoms of infection: fever, localized pain, or tenderness. Abscess or other evidence of infection involving the deep incision.

Source: Adapted with permission from Mangram, A., Horan, T., Pearson, M., Silver, L., & Jarvis, W. (1999). Guideline for prevention of surgical site infection. Centers for Disease Control and Prevention (CDC), Hospital Infection Control Practices Advisory Committee. *Infection Control and Hospital Epidemiology, 20*(4), 247–280.

Fever that starts or persists after the fifth postoperative day is more likely to be clinically significant for wound infection than is a fever earlier in the postoperative course (Dellinger, 2005).

Parenteral antibiotic prophylaxis may continue for 24 hours after surgery but should not extend beyond this period because it is thought to be unnecessary and may lead to the development of drug resistance (Golembiewski, 2004). Prophylactic antibiotics may be necessary in situations where an organ ruptured or leaked prior to surgery because these wounds are more likely to become infected. Other factors that may aid in wound healing include improving the patient's nutritional status. Protein, calories, calcium, iron, zinc, and vitamins A, B_6, B_{12}, and C are needed for wound healing. Chapter 14 ☺ provides a complete description of adequate nutrition. Chapter 67 ☺ discusses normal and abnormal wound healing.

Wound Dehiscence and Evisceration

Two potential problems of the wound site are wound dehiscence and wound evisceration (Figure 27–5 ■). Wound dehiscence is a partial or complete separation of the wound layers with an opening of the wound. Evisceration is a complete separation of the wound layers and the protrusion of internal organs or viscera. Any wound can dehisce, but it occurs most frequently with abdominal incisions and it occurs most often 5 to 10 days postoperatively. Wound disruption can occur because of poor surgical closure, poor wound healing, or increased stress on the surgical incision.

Risk factors for dehiscence and evisceration are the same (see Rick Factors box). Patients may report "feeling like something popped" and dehiscence is sometimes preceded by a gush of serosanguineous drainage. Wound dehiscence and wound evisceration are emergencies. The nurse calls for help and assists the patient back to bed. The patient is positioned supine with knees bent, and the nurse covers the wound and internal organs with sterile towels or gauze soaked in normal saline. The nurse keeps

RISK FACTORS for Wound Dehiscence and Evisceration
Age (elderly patients)
Diabetes
Obesity
Current wound infection
Preoperative malnutrition
Low serum albumin
Coughing
Vomiting
Straining
Moving

the wound moist and does *not* attempt to replace the organs. The surgeon is called and the patient's vital signs are taken every 5 minutes. Wound dehiscence may be treated medically with dressings or surgically with wound closure. Evisceration is treated with surgical closure.

Wound Drains

Drains are used for a variety of reasons. Wound drains are inserted through an intentional stab wound into an area close to the incision and site of the operation. The purpose of the drain is to remove inflammatory fluid (serum, blood, lymph) that might otherwise accumulate at the operative site causing infection or abscess. The surgeon inserts a closed, suction-type drain such as a Jackson-Pratt or a Hemovac. Applying negative pressure in the drain reservoir creates suction in the drain and speeds the removal of fluid. The nurse empties the drain and records the color and amount of drainage every 8 hours or as often as necessary. The drainage may be sanguineous initially but progresses to serosanguineous and sometimes serous. The nurse reports an increase in the amount of drainage and any unexpected change in the type of drainage. Wound drains are removed when there is minimal drainage (e.g., less than 30 mL in 24 hours). Patients report that the removal of wound drains is quick but very painful (Mimnaugh, Winegar, Mabrey, & Davis, 1999; Puntillo et al., 2002). Patients should be medicated prior to the discontinuation of a drain. Many patients are now discharged to home with wound drains in place. The nurse teaches patients how to empty and measure the drainage so they will be able to continue the care at home.

Other drains and tubes may be inserted during surgery. Chest tubes are used to drain fluid and air from the pleural space and to reestablish a negative intrapleural pressure after thoracotomy. A biliary tube (or T-tube) may be inserted in the common bile duct to prevent biliary obstruction after surgery on the common bile duct. A jejunostomy tube may be inserted during surgery on the pancreas to provide an alternative method of feeding the patient. Chart 27–6 (p. 680) lists common tubes with their purpose and expected drainage. Chapter 67 ☺ further discusses drains and provides pictures.

Venous Thromboembolism

Deep venous thrombosis is the formation of a venous blood clot in a deep vein, usually in the lower leg or pelvis, and it is a serious

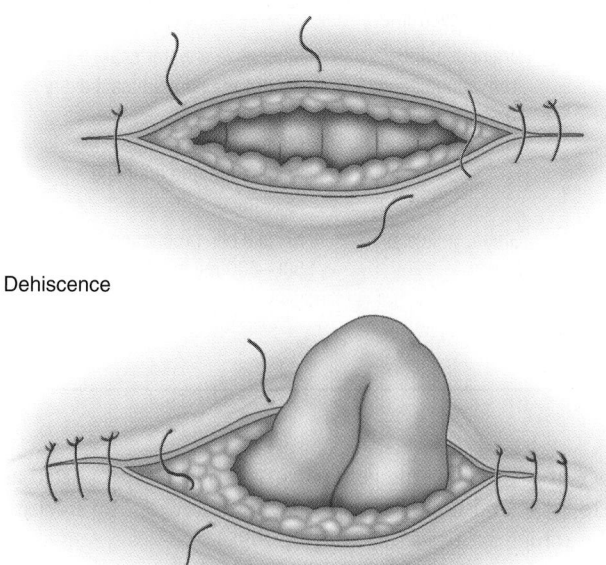

Dehiscence

Evisceration

FIGURE 27–5 ■   (A) Wound dehiscence; (B) wound evisceration.

| CHART 27–6 | Common Tubes and Expected Drainage |

Tube	Purpose	Drainage Amount	Drainage Color	Other
Foley (bladder)	Drains urine and decompresses the bladder.	1,500–2,500 mL in 24 hours or a minimum of 30 mL/hour	Clear, yellow	Report hematuria, or cloudy urine. Report low urine output.
Three-way Foley (bladder) May have a 30-mL balloon rather than a 5- to 10-mL balloon.	Drains urine and is used for continuous bladder irrigation (CBI).	1,500–2,500 mL/24 hour and any irrigating fluid that is instilled	If used for CBI then expect urine to be pink.	Normal saline is used to irrigate. Regulate the CBI to keep the urine clear. Watch for bladder spasms and clots. Careful intake & output (I&O).
Suprapubic tube (bladder)	Drains urine.	1,500–2,500 mL/24 hour or 30 mL/hour	Clear, yellow	Report no urine output. Report dislodgement.
Nephrostomy tube (kidney pelvis)	Drains urine from the kidney.	Amount depends on function of the kidney.	Clear, yellow	Can be gently flushed with 5 to 10 mL of normal saline.
Nasogastric tube (NGT) Salem sump (stomach) Levine tube (stomach)	Decompress the stomach Low, continuous, or intermittent suction is used; intermittent use if the tube does not have an air vent.	Depends on the situation; up to 1,500 mL/24 hour	Usually pale, yellow-green	Expect some blood in the drainage for 8 hours after gastrectomy. NGT can be flushed with 30 mL or more of saline except after gastric or esophageal surgeries.
Gastrostomy tube	Drainage or feeding.	Varies	Green to dark brown, bloody	Flush with normal saline to keep patent.
Jejunostomy tube	Drainage or feeding.	Varies	Green to dark brown, bloody	Flush with normal saline to keep patent.
Blakemore-Sengstaken tube (triple lumen Esophageal balloon, gastric balloon, drainage	Drains stomach and compresses esophageal or stomach varices.	Varies	Green to dark brown, bloody	Measure pressure in esophageal balloon. Balloon is only inflated for a 48-hour period. Periodic release of balloon pressure.
Wound drains, such as Jackson-Pratt, Hemovac	Drains inflammatory fluid from area surrounding incision.	Varies, but the need to empty the drain frequently (e.g., more than every 4 hours) should be cause for concern.	Sanguineous to serosanguineous. Drainage should become more serous over time.	Drains usually removed when drainage is < 30 mL in 24 hours.
Chest tube (pleural space)	Drains fluid or air from pleural space, restores negative intrapleural pressure. Reexpands the lung.	Not more than 100 mL/hour	Drainage varies from sanguineous to serosanguineous to serous.	Must have a water seal. Record drainage at least every 8 hours. Clamp the chest tube *only* prior to changing the drainage system.
T-tube (common bile duct)	Drains bile if the common bile duct (CBD) is obstructed. Maintains patency of CBD after surgery on the bile duct.	Varies from 0 to 500 mL in 24 hours.	Green, yellow, or brown	Normal bile production is 500–800 mL in 24 hours.

postoperative problem. Once the clot forms, there is a danger of detachment and the possibility of a pulmonary embolus (PE), a serious condition in which the clot obstructs an artery in the lungs. Venous thromboembolism (VTE) is the collective term for DVT and PE. It describes the process of blood clot formation and travel through the veins. The overall incidence of DVT is around 9% to 10% but the rate in some surgeries is much higher. The in-

cidence of DVT following general surgery has been reported at 20% to 30%, and the incidence of DVT following hip fracture may be as high as 50% (Clagett et al., 1998).

DVT occurs as a result of vascular stasis (injury to the intimal layer of the vein) and hypercoagulability. The postoperative patient is at risk for DVT because anesthesia vasodilates vessels, leading to stasis and decreased venous return. Longer surgeries cause prolonged immobilization of the patient during the procedure and are associated with a higher risk of blood clot formation. Reduced mobility after surgery contributes to vascular stasis and DVT. Major orthopedic surgery, multiple trauma, and pelvic surgeries are associated with a higher risk of DVT than other procedures (Geerts et al., 2004; Merli, 2000). Other risk factors include age (over age 60), obesity, prolonged immobilization, use of estrogen, cancer, and history of previous DVT.

Prevention of venous thromboembolism is a goal for all postoperative patients and the nurse should discuss prophylaxis with the health care provider if a postoperative patient arrives on the clinical unit without such orders (Blondin, 2006). The American College of Chest Physicians (ACCP) established guidelines for the prevention of DVT and PE at a consensus conference (Geerts et al., 2004). Several methods of DVT prophylaxis are recommended. Chart 27–7 summarizes some of the recommendations for surgical patients.

Antithrombotic drug therapy is frequently used to prevent DVT. Low-dose unfractionated heparin (LDUH) or low-molecular-weight heparin (LMWH) is given subcutaneously in large enough doses to prevent clot formation but the dose is not large enough to produce systemic anticoagulation. LDUH, as a fixed dose, is given as 5,000 units subcutaneously every 8 hours for high-risk patients, or every 12 hours for moderate-risk patients. LMWHs are better absorbed, have longer action, are more effective in producing anticoagulation, and cause bleeding less often than unfractionated heparin, but they are substantially more expensive (Merli, 2000). There are at least six types of LMWH but the most common are enoxaparin, dalteparin, and ardeparin. Enoxaparin is given 30 to 40 mg subcutaneously daily or twice a day. An alternative to LMWH is fondaparinux. This drug inhibits Factor X and has a longer half-life, a more predictable response, and fewer adverse effects than does LMWH (Finnish Medical Society, 2006).

Oral medication, such as warfarin (Coumadin), can also be used for DVT prophylaxis in some situations but the dose must be titrated to achieve a target INR of 2.5 (Geerts et al., 2004). Patients in higher risk categories for venous thromboembolism may need to continue antithrombotic drug therapy for 2 to 4 weeks after hospital discharge. Examples of surgeries that are higher risk for VTE and therefore require extended DVT prophylaxis include hip fracture repair, total hip or knee replacement surgeries, and major gynecologic surgeries.

Some patients should not receive either LDUH or LMWH even in low doses because if bleeding does occur, it could be catastrophic. Patients having cranial surgery (risk of intracranial bleed) or spinal surgery (risk of spinal cord compression from hematoma) might be better served with another form of prophylaxis.

Other ways to decrease the risk of DVT include intermittent pneumatic compression devices (IPCs) or graduated compression stockings (GCSs). There are several manufacturers of **intermittent pneumatic compression devices** and all of them work on the basis of applying intermittent compression of the calf muscle, thereby increasing venous return. The pump is set to apply 45 mmHg of pressure with inflation. Pneumatic compression devices may be applied in the operating room and worn almost continuously (except when ambulating or bathing) for the next several days. Patients sometimes complain that the plastic leg sleeves are hot, cause sweating, or interrupt sleep. Some machines have a switch that cools the airflow through the sleeves. Experts suggest that pneumatic compression devices not be used on patients who are immobilized for 72 hours without prophylaxis. If a clot has formed, the device could dislodge it (Merli, 2000).

Graduated compression stockings are elastic stockings that apply varying degrees of pressure on the lower leg with the greatest exertion of pressure at the ankle and the lowest pressure at the thigh (or knee in shorter stockings). GCSs increase venous return and velocity, thereby reducing venous wall distention and venous stasis (Evans et al., 2001). GCSs have been shown through research to be effective in reducing the incidence of DVT (Amaragiri & Lees, 2006). Pneumatic compression devices and gradient stockings may be used in conjunction with antithrombotic drug therapy or as an alternative to it in patients who should not receive any type of anticoagulation.

CHART 27–7 **Summary of Recommendations for DVT Prophylaxis in the Surgical Patient**

Level of Risk for Venous Thromboembolism	Recommendation
Low risk: minor procedure, age < 40 years, no other risks OR Gynecologic procedures lasting < 30 minutes OR Low-risk urological procedures (TURP)	Early and persistent ambulation
Moderate risk: non–major general surgery, age 40 to 60 years Gynecologic surgery (benign disease)	LDUH 5,000 units bid OR LMWH <3,400 units daily
Higher risk: non–major surgical procedure and age >60 years Extensive gynecologic surgery	LDUH 5,000 units tid OR LMWH >3,400 units daily
Very high risk: major surgery with multiple risk factors	LDUH tid OR LMWH (higher doses) daily AND Graduated compression stockings OR Intermittent pneumatic compression boots
High risk for bleeding	Intermittent pneumatic compression boots OR Graduated compression stockings

Source: Adapted from Geerts, W., Pineo, G., Hit, J., Bergqvist, D., Lassen, M., Colwell, C., et al. (2004). Prevention of venous thromboembolism: The Seventh AACP Conference on Antithrombotic and Thrombolytic Therapy. *Chest, 126*(3 Suppl), 338S–400S.

Early ambulation is important in preventing deep venous thrombosis. Patients are encouraged to ambulate several times a day and to change positions in bed every 1 to 2 hours. Leg exercises can be done while the patient is in a chair or in bed. Chapter 43 contains a complete description of DVT cause and treatment.

Gerontological Considerations

Care of the older adult after surgery is similar to care of younger adult patients with a few exceptions. Older adults have decreased physiological reserves, making them less able or slower to respond to the specific demands of surgery (Mamaril, 2006). It may take older patients 48 hours or longer to fully recover from the effects of anesthesia (Asher, 2004). Also, older adults tend to experience more postoperative complications than younger people because of preexisting illness, nutritional deficits, and altered drug metabolism and, when complications occur, the elderly experience higher death rates (Hamel, Henderson, Khuri, & Daley, 2005). The risk of postoperative complications varies depending on the surgery; however, in a large study (>500,000), 20% of seniors over the age of 80 years developed postoperative complications (Hamel et al., 2005).

The assessment of older patients may show slight variations from those of younger adult patients. For example, older adults tend to run slightly lower body temperatures or oxygen saturation levels (i.e., 93% to 95%) than younger patients, but the nurse needs to use the same parameters of concern for older adults that would be used for others. The nurse also uses the same priorities of postoperative care. The older adult does have special needs (e.g., replace hearing aids, dentures, and glasses as soon as possible) and problems. Major issues to address include pain management, postoperative delirium, medication management, restoring functional ability, and discharge planning. Older patients also have an increased risk for falls, as discussed in the Gerontological Considerations box.

Pain management is a challenge in older adults, and some studies report that postoperative pain is undertreated (Sauaia et al., 2005) or inappropriately treated (Titler et al., 2003). Teaching older patients about communicating their pain may improve pain treatment (McDonald, Thomas, Livingston, & Severson, 2005), and studies show that even elders with mild or moderate cognitive impairments can accurately report pain using a verbal or numeric rating scale (Kaasalainen & Crook, 2004).

The rule of thumb in treating pain in older patients is to start low and go slow (i.e., use the lowest doses first and slowly titrate medications upward) (Mamaril, 2006). Opioids are used to control postoperative pain, but the concurrent use of NSAIDS can decrease the amount of narcotics required. All older patients receiving narcotics should also receive a stool softener to offset the constipating effect of the narcotic (Asher, 2004). Certain narcotics, such as meperidine (Demerol), are avoided in older adults because they produce toxic metabolites that can cause seizures or confusion. Nurses and health care providers need more training in pain management for older adults. In one study of more than 700 patients being treated for hip fracture, pain management was a serious problem. The study reported that acetaminophen, the drug of choice for pain treatment, was administered in subtherapeutic doses; that half of the patients received at least one dose of meperidine, although the drug is not recommended for the elderly; and that only 27% of patients received pain medication around the clock even though this is a suggested practice for postoperative pain control (Titler et al., 2003).

Postoperative delirium, an acute change in cognitive function with decreased ability to focus or sustain attention and altered perceptions, is a serious problem for older adults. Postoperative delirium increases morbidity and mortality for those affected. The incidence of postoperative delirium ranges from 3.8% in low-risk patients (Kalisvaart et al., 2006) to as high as 60% in higher risk patients (Milisen, Lemiengre, Braes, & Foreman, 2005). Postoperative delirium can occur at any time during hospitalization but it is more likely to occur shortly after surgery. In one small study of orthopedic patients, the highest incidence of postoperative confusion occurred on postoperative days 1 and 2 (35% and 37%, respectively) compared with a 12% incidence on postoperative day 4 (Wong, Wong, & Brooks, 2002).

The development of postoperative delirium is multifactorial with the most vulnerable and frail elders being at highest risk. Risk factors include prior cognitive impairment, severity of illness on admission, depression, increased age, sensory deficits, impaired functional ability, and use of certain medications (Kalisvaart et al., 2006; Leung, Sands, Mullen, Wang, & Vaurio, 2005; Milisen et al., 2005; Wong et al., 2002). Patients needing emergency surgery may be more likely to develop acute confusion than those admitted for elective procedures (Kalisvaart et al., 2006).

Programs designed to prevent postoperative delirium have had some success in preventing delirium, reducing the severity of it, or shortening the course (Marcantonio, Flacker, Wright, & Resnick, 2001; Milisen et al., 2001, 2005). Such programs generally include identification of high-risk patients preoperatively, daily consultation with a geriatrician or advanced practice nurse specializing in geriatrics, reducing the use of unnecessary medications, training of bedside nurses in the early recognition of acute confusion, and aggressive correction of factors that may be contributing to confusion (e.g., hypoxia, fluid and electrolyte imbalance, pain). Some have tried to prevent postoperative delirium by administering low doses of haloperidol prophylactically; however, haloperidol does not seem to prevent delirium

GERONTOLOGICAL CONSIDERATIONS Related to Falls

The Joint Commission's 2007 National Patient Safety Goals require hospitals to implement a fall reduction program. Older surgical patients are more likely to fall than younger patients. Risk factors for falls include a prior history of falls, fear of falling, cognitive impairment, bowel and bladder incontinence, and functional impairment (Lyons, 2004; Resnick, 2003). The older postoperative patient will likely have additional risk factors associated with surgery or anesthesia including the use of narcotics for pain control, the attachment of medical equipment (e.g., intravenous lines, urinary catheters) that can limit ambulation, and a temporary functional impairment from the presence of incisions. All postoperative patients are assessed for their risk for falls after surgery and at other times as their condition warrants. The hospital-based fall reduction program must be implemented for all patients who are identified as being at risk.

but it may decrease the severity and duration of it (Kalisvaart et al., 2005).

Older patients experience more adverse effects with medications than do younger adults. Aging causes changes in the absorption, distribution, protein binding, metabolism, and elimination of drugs (Kuchta & Golembiewski, 2004). These changes tend to increase the plasma concentration of some drugs and narrow the therapeutic range. In general, giving smaller doses of drugs or increasing the dosing interval may help reduce adverse effects. Certain drugs should be used sparingly or avoided altogether because of their propensity for causing sedation or confusion in older patients. Examples of these medications include meperidine, cimetidine, long-acting benzodiazepines (e.g., diazepam), and diphenhydramine (Kuchta & Golembiewski, 2004).

It is important to restore functional ability to the older surgical patient as soon as possible. A collaborative effort among health care providers, nurses, physical therapists, and others is required to optimize the elder's recovery. Postoperative imbalances such as dehydration, electrolyte disturbances, or anemia should be corrected. Older patients are not routinely transfused with red blood cells postoperatively, but anemia will impair functional ability. A large study (n = >5,700) of older patients recovering from hip fracture surgery showed that those with higher hemoglobin levels were able to walk further distances postoperatively than those with lower levels (Lawrence et al., 2003).

Early mobilization and muscle strengthening can have positive effects. In one small study, elders who received muscle resistance training after hip surgery showed increased muscle mass, muscle strength, and functional ability over those who did not receive the training (Suetta et al., 2004). Other studies support these findings. A study of 224 patients suffering hip fracture showed that those who began weight bearing and ambulation training early in the postoperative course were more likely to be able to walk independently within a month of hospital discharge (Kondo et al., 2005). Some older patients may be able to be discharged home rather than to rehabilitation when an increased emphasis is placed on muscle strengthening and physical therapy (Oldmeadow et al., 2004).

There are special concerns when discharging an older person home. The nurse needs to ask the patient about the availability of social support, the specifics of the home environment, and any surgery-related needs (Burden, 2004). Specific concerns include the following:

- Is the elder able to perform self-care?
- Who is available to assist the elder in meeting her needs?
- Is the elder a primary caretaker for someone else?
- What is the condition of the home environment (e.g., stairs, location of bedrooms and bathrooms, availability of telephone, presence of a lifeline)?
- Does the home environment need a safety evaluation?
- What supplies, medications, or other equipment (wheelchair, hold bars, raised toilet seat, etc.) does the elder need at home?
- How will the elder get to follow-up appointments?

Another concern for the nurse is the patient's psychological readiness for discharge. Patients need to feel that they will be safe at home. The sense of safety is related to patients; confidence in their ability to care for themselves and in the support they will have from others (Heine, Koch, & Goldie, 2004; Nilsson, Unosson, & Kihlgren, 2006). Nurses need to work closely with patients so that the patient develops the confidence needed to feel safe and ready for discharge.

Health Promotion

Discharge teaching is critical now that the length of hospitalization is shorter. Surgeries that once required a 10-day hospital stay now require a 3- to 4-day stay. Minimally invasive surgical techniques allow some patients to go home on the same day as surgery. It is not unusual to discharge patients home with dressings, drains, and even IV antibiotics or parenteral nutrition. Understandably, patients are concerned about how to care for themselves after discharge. Patients want information about wound care, medications, activities, diet, symptom management, and other aspects of self-care.

Teaching is provided to the patient as well as to others who will be involved in providing care for the patient. It is important to use language the patient understands and to check the patient's understanding of the information. In one study that compared nurses' perceptions of discharge teaching with patients' perceptions, there were significant differences in the understanding of discharge information, with nurses overestimating patients' understanding of the material (Reilly et al., 1996). It is critical to provide written instructions. Research suggests that written information fosters the patient's understanding and compliance with discharge instructions (Holmes & Lenz, 1997; Jacobs, 2000). Also, being able to call the nurse with questions may be especially important to patients in their adjustment after surgery (Burt, Caelli, Moore, & Anderson, 2005; Oermann, Harris, & Dammeyer, 2001; Ross, 2007). The teaching needs of the patient vary according to the surgery and other factors, but general areas to be covered in discharge teaching are discussed next.

Patients need to be advised about the trajectory of recovery. It is theorized that postoperative recovery includes four dimensions: physiological recovery, marked by a return of bodily functions; psychological recovery, a return of well-being; social recovery, a return to social activities and independence; and habitual recovery, a point at which the person returns to a full range of normal activities (Allvin, Berg, Idvall, & Nilsson, 2007). Patients need to know that recovery takes time. One study of patients following cardiac surgery found that patients were surprised to find that recovery took much longer than expected and they felt unprepared for prolonged symptoms such as fatigue (Doering et al., 2002). Uncomplicated surgery often takes 4 to 6 weeks or even longer for recovery. The effects from general anesthesia can linger, wound healing requires energy, it takes weeks to make sufficient red blood cells to replace those lost in surgery, and patients may experience pain or soreness until healing is well on its way. Patients may lack their usual level of energy during recovery. Pain, fatigue, and depression are common symptoms during recovery from major surgery (Hodgson & Given, 2004; Horvath, 2003; Lupien, Schoneboom, & Wren, 2000; Nilsson et al., 2006; Zalon, 2004), but these symptoms will gradually resolve. Social support is important to the psychological well-being of patients as they recover from surgery (Nilsson et al., 2006).

Information on how to care for the wound following discharge is a common need for postsurgical patients. The nurse checks with the surgeon about any special requirements of wound care. Some patients will have a dressing in place that is kept clean and dry until the follow-up appointment with the surgeon. In other situations, incisions are kept covered for the first 24 to 48 hours and then the dressing is removed and the wound left open to the air. These wounds are gently cleaned each day and the dressing replaced if there is risk of contamination. Staples and sutures are often removed 7 to 10 days after the surgery in a follow-up appointment with the nurse or health care provider. If Steri-Strips cover the wound, they are left in place until they fall off naturally. Wound drains are emptied as often as needed and the amount and type of drainage recorded. Any sudden increase in the amount of drainage or a change in the character or color of the drainage needs to be reported to the surgeon.

Information about those activities that are allowed and those that are not allowed after surgery is especially important to provide. Research consistently finds that patients are unclear about what activities are allowed at home and they want specific information on this topic (Doering et al., 2002; Hughes, Hodgson, Muller, Robinson, & McCorkle, 2000; Jacobs, 2000; Reilly et al., 1996). This information also is important because patients may judge their postoperative progress on the activities they are able to perform. Examples of the type of questions that patients' have are as follows:

- When can I bathe or shower?
- When can I exercise? Are there any restrictions on exercising?
- Can I do housework?
- When can I start driving?
- When can I resume sexual activity?
- How much rest should I get?
- When can I return to work?

Usually, patients are encouraged to bathe or shower daily. If a dressing is in place, it is kept clean and dry. For most surgeries, the patient is discouraged from lifting anything heavier than 10 to 15 pounds until the incision has healed in 4 to 6 weeks. Walking at a reasonable pace is encouraged and limited only by pain and fatigue, but heavier aerobic-type workouts are restricted until approved by the surgeon. Similarly, light housework is generally acceptable when the patient feels able but heavier housework may be restricted. Most restrictions on driving are based on the need for road safety rather than potential injury to the wound. Often patients are allowed to drive when their ability to move is no longer restricted by pain or soreness. For some surgeries driving is restricted for several days and for others, it may be several weeks. Once patients are able to drive, they are cautioned not to drive while taking narcotic analgesics. Except with certain gynecologic or genitourinary surgeries, sexual activity after surgery is restricted as a result of pain. Most people will be able to resume sexual activity in 2 to 3 weeks. The time frame for returning to work will depend on the surgery and the type of work performed. For less invasive procedures such as arthroscopy, patients can return to work in 2 to 4 days. Most patients will be out of work for 3 to 6 weeks following major surgery and up to 10 weeks for major abdominal or thoracic resections.

The postoperative diet for most patients emphasizes good nutrition for wound healing. Patients are encouraged to get adequate calories, proteins, and vitamins. Diet restrictions or recommended modifications are made for some surgeries. Examples of these include Nissen's fundoplication, gastrojejunostomy (Bilroth II), pancreatic resection (Whipple), radical neck dissection, and ileostomy.

Research suggests that patients may not feel adequately prepared to manage their medication regimens at home (Cutilli, 2007; Jacobs, 2000; Reilly et al., 1996). Discharge teaching includes a discussion of medications including purpose, how to take the medication, and key side effects. Most postoperative patients will be discharged with an oral narcotic for pain control and some will have antibiotics prescribed. They need to know when to take pain medication, how much medication to take, alternative strategies for pain control such as elevation and ice applications, and how to prevent constipation, a common side effect of narcotics.

Early discharge puts the burden of recognizing and responding to potential complications on the patient. Often, signs of wound infection take several days to develop and may not show up until after the patient is discharged home. Research studies show that patients feel unprepared to identify possible postoperative complications (Hughes et al., 2000; Jacobs, 2000) or to manage expected postoperative problems (Burt et al., 2005). Chart 27–8 lists some of the danger signs that patients should report to their surgeons. Discharge information includes contact phone numbers for emergencies. Most patients will have a follow-up appointment in 7 to 10 days after discharge.

The information needs of surgical patients are complex and it is unrealistic to think that the needs of every patient can be met on discharge from the hospital. Patients need to be carefully evaluated on their ability to provide care for themselves at home, and nurses must make referrals to community services (e.g., visiting nurses association [VNA], physical therapy, hospice) when home assistance is required. Appropriate referrals not only improve patient care but can prevent hospital readmission. Nurses need to develop skills in evaluating patients for discharge.

One study found that nurses and health care providers did not always recognize the needs of their patients on discharge. The study concluded that health care professionals need increased knowledge of the discharge process, of the community services available, training in identifying patients' needs and improved collaboration among themselves with regard to patient discharge (Bowles, Foust, Naylor, & Ware, 2003). Surgical patients may need the services of a VNA or other home health agency to assist

---

CHART 27–8   **Danger Signs That Patients Should Report to Their Health Care Provider**

- Temperature greater than 38°C (100.4°F)
- Fever with chills
- Pain that is increasing or that is not adequately controlled by medication
- Incision that is red, painful, or has drainage
- Difficulty voiding or unable to void
- Painful urination

with their recovery. Services that may be appropriate, particularly for the elderly, include home nursing care for dressing changes, wound checks, antibiotic administration, home safety evaluation, and the coordination of other services such as a home health aide to assist with meeting personal care needs, home physical therapy to assist with rehabilitation, homemaker services for housekeeping, and meal preparation.

Patients are discharged home when the health care provider and health care team determines they no longer need the care and close attention of an acute care hospital and they are safe to care for themselves at home. The nurse has an obligation to speak with the health care provider and advocate for patient safety in situations where the nurse questions the readiness of the patient for discharge. There are no set criteria for determining readiness for discharge; it is a clinical judgment, but the nurse can use indicators to assist in making this judgment. Indicators of stability and readiness for discharge are:

- Stable vital signs; vital signs at patient's baseline
- Baseline level of consciousness
- Wound is stable without bleeding
- Able to take food and fluids orally without nausea and vomiting
- Able to void and move bowels

- Pain is at an acceptable level
- Able to ambulate without assistance
- Able to perform ADLs independently or at baseline
- Home services are adequate to meet the needs of the patient.

Discharge teaching for both the patient and the family/support system is outlined in Patient Teaching & Discharge Priorities box.

Research

Research is changing the way nurses care for postoperative patients. Nurses are looking for evidence to support their practice. It is important to know whether or not nursing interventions are having the desired outcome. A culture of answering practice questions by using the best available research evidence or by designing a research study is evolving. The Research Opportunities and Clinical Impact box (p. 686) lists research problems that are important to the care of the postsurgical patient.

Research is also being used to design structures and nursing care delivery models to create healing environments. Single rooms in hospitals create space for privacy and personal control and provide a place for family to stay overnight. Researchers are examining the effects of single rooms on outcomes such as infection control, pain management, and rest and recovery (Chaudhury, Mahmood, & Valente, 2006).

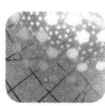 **PATIENT TEACHING & DISCHARGE PRIORITIES for Postoperative Nursing**

Need	Teaching
Incision and drain care	Inspect wound daily.
	Assess for redness, warmth, swelling, increased pain, or drainage. Mild bruising around the wound is often normal.
	Keep wound dry for first 48 hours or as directed by the surgeon.
	After 48 hours, wash gently around the incision site(s) and pat dry.
	If Steri-Strips are in place, allow them to fall off by themselves.
	Sutures are usually removed in 7 to 10 days.
	If drains are in place, empty daily or as often as indicated. Note color and amount of drainage.
	Assess availability, knowledge, and comfort with treatment regimen.
	Report a fever >38°C (>100.4°F) or an incision that becomes red, painful, swollen, or has increased drainage.
	Assess respite needs and resources.
	Assess need for follow-up appointments.
	Assess need for wound checks by health professional.
Pain control	Take pain medication as prescribed.
	Do not drive while taking prescription pain medication.
	Increase fluids and take a stool softener to prevent constipation from prescription pain medication.
	Take acetaminophen (Tylenol) regular or extra strength for mild pain.
	Do *not* take aspirin or ibuprofen unless approved by your surgeon.
	Assess pain level and report any increase in pain.
	Assess environment for safety.
Activity	Expect that the effects of surgery, anesthesia, wound healing, and pain medication will make you feel more tired than usual.
	Fatigue may last several weeks. Plan rest periods and pace your activities.
	Avoid strenuous exercise until the follow-up appointment with the surgeon.
	You will need to check with the health care provider about a time frame for returning to work and normal activities.
	Assess support systems for meal preparation, household chores, child care, or spousal care.
	Assess need for home care services.

RESEARCH OPPORTUNITIES AND CLINICAL IMPACT RELATED TO CARE OF THE SURGICAL PATIENT

Research Area	Clinical Impact
Comparison of deep breathing exercises and incentive spirometry in reducing postoperative pulmonary complications.	Important for evidenced-based practice.
Effectiveness of alternative interventions (e.g., relaxation techniques) in reducing postoperative pulmonary complications.	Provides rationale for common nursing interventions performed after surgery.
Effectiveness of ambulation (distance and frequency) in reducing the incidence of postoperative complications (e.g., pneumonia, abdominal distention, urinary retention).	Provides data to support or refute the use of innovative approaches to common postoperative problems.
Effectiveness of various interventions in treating postoperative urinary retention.	
The effect of early feeding after surgery in stimulating the return of bowel function.	
Factors that increase wound healing postoperatively.	
Comparison of wound dressing technique, clean technique versus sterile technique, in the incidence of postoperative wound infection.	
The effectiveness of interventions in the treatment of postoperative nausea and vomiting.	
Effectiveness of interventions to prevent postoperative confusion in older patients.	
Critical Thinking	
Factors influencing nurses' decisions in weaning patients off of oxygen postoperatively.	Provides a basis for understanding how nurses develop clinical judgment.
Factors influencing nurses' decisions in postoperative pain management.	
Comparison of nursing management to prevent postoperative complications by experienced and novice nurses.	
Comparison of decisions to report abnormal findings to surgeons by experienced and novice nurses.	
Factors influencing the use of "alternative" nursing interventions in the prevention of postoperative complications.	
Strategies used to increase patient compliance with postoperative interventions (e.g., ambulation, coughing, and deep breathing).	
Pain Management	
Effectiveness of nonpharmacologic interventions (e.g., splinting, elevation, application of ice, relaxation techniques) in reducing postoperative pain.	Increased patient comfort.
Evaluation of pain and discomfort associated with common postoperative interventions.	Improve interventions to decrease pain associated with the surgical experience.
Strategies to reduce pain associated with procedures.	
Factors that influence the effectiveness of patient-controlled analgesia in the postoperative patient.	
Factors that reduce persistent postoperative pain.	
Psychosocial Responses	
Predictors of anxiety in surgical patients.	Improve the psychological well-being of postoperative patients.
Factors that influence anxiety levels in the older surgical patient.	
Strategies to reduce anxiety in postoperative patients.	Understand the impact of sleep and rest on postoperative recovery.
Effect of family visits on postoperative anxiety.	
Description of the sleep and rest patterns in postoperative patients.	
Influence of sleep on postoperative recovery.	
Factors important to patients and families in selecting a rehabilitation facility.	
Discharge	
Common problems experienced by the patient following discharge home.	Improve health care professionals' understanding of the issues that patients face following discharge.
Interventions used by patients to manage problems at home (e.g., fatigue, depression, constipation, pain, wound healing).	
Strategies to increase the patient's ability to manage symptoms at home.	Increase patient's competence in managing their own recovery.
Adjustment of discharge teaching to accommodate cultural differences.	

Clinical Preparation

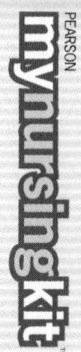

 Read

- History of Current Illness
- Past Medical History
- Physical Exam
- Admitting Medical Orders
- Laboratory Study Results

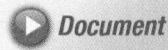 **Document**

- Summary of Hospitalization
- Pathophysiology Form
- Laboratory Values
- Laboratory Results Explanation

 **Apply**

- List of Potential Nursing Diagnoses
- Concept Map
- Critical Thinking Questions

Log on to MyNursingKit.com to download forms you will need and to complete further steps in the Clinical Preparation assignment.

HISTORY OF PRESENT ILLNESS

Ryan Landry is a 67-year-old man who is admitted to the surgical unit following a left hemicolectomy. Mr. Landry was in reasonably good health until 2 months ago when he began to experience cramping abdominal pain that he attributed to constipation and gas. When the abdominal cramping continued and he noticed that his stools were narrower than usual, he made an appointment with his primary health care provider. A routine exam uncovered occult blood in the stool, and Mr. Landry was referred for a colonoscopy.

Several polyps were removed during the colonoscopy and biopsy results revealed adenocarcinoma of the colon. A left hemicolectomy without colostomy was performed. Once the results of lymph node biopsies taken during surgery are available, Mr. Landry will be referred to an oncologist for discussion of follow-up treatment, including possible chemotherapy. Currently Mr. Landry is second day postoperative from the hemicolectomy.

Medical–Surgical History

Patient has hypertension and elevated cholesterol. He smokes 1 pack per day and has done so for the past 40 years. His father died of colon cancer at the age of 70. His hypertension is treated with metoprolol 50 mg daily and the elevated cholesterol levels are treated with atorvastatin 80 mg daily. He has failed many times to quit smoking.

Social History

He lives with his wife and a grown son.

Physical Exam

Vital signs: T 101.4, HR 108, RR 20, BP 142/84

Alert and oriented; reports feeling very anxious; asks frequent questions often repeating them; looks worried and seems overly vigilant any time a health care worker comes into the room

Reports a significant amount of pain, rating it as a 7 at rest and a 10 with movement

Cardiac telemetry: sinus tachycardia with occasional premature ventricular contractions

Taking shallow breaths; crackles in the lung bases bilaterally

Oxygen saturation: 93% on 4 liters of oxygen via nasal cannula; using the incentive spirometer sporadically; weak cough

Abdomen: slightly firm; distended with hypoactive bowel sounds and negative flatus

Nasogastric tube attached to low intermittent suction; draining small amount of green fluid

Complains of being thirsty and having a sore throat; slightly nauseated especially with movement

Foley catheter in place; draining concentrated urine

Urine output in the last 2 hours: 42 mL

Skin: warm and dry

Abdominal incision covered by a primary dressing that is dry and intact

2+ pedal pulses bilaterally and no peripheral edema

Patient requires assistance with ambulation. He complains of severe pain and vertigo when standing. He ambulates a very short distance before requesting to go back to bed. Following activity his respiratory rate was 32 and his heart rate was 118.

Admitting Medical Orders

Surgical service

Admit to Telemetry Unit

No known allergies

Vital signs every 4 hours

Call house officer: pulse < 60 and > 110/minute; BP < 90 and > 160 systolic; temperature > 38.5; urine output < 30 mL/hr for 2 hours; respiratory rate > 30/minute; oxygen saturation > 92%

NPO

Maintain nasogastric tube to low continuous suction

Incentive spirometry 10 times every hour

Foley to gravity drainage

Monitor intake and output

Sequential compression device (SCD) to lower extremities while in bed

Ambulate three times daily

Cardiac telemetry while receiving IV metoprolol

IV: D5½NS with 20 mEq KCl at 125 mL/hr

Scheduled Medications

Heparin 5,000 units subcutaneous twice a day

Nicotine transdermal patch 15 mg daily

PCA morphine sulfate 1 mg/mL incremental dose 1 mg and lock
   out 6 minutes

Metoprolol 5 mg IV every 6 hours while NPO

PRN Medications

Phenergan 25 mg IV q6h prn nausea

Mylanta 30 mL po/NG q4–6h prn dyspepsia

Lorazepam 0.5 to 2 mg IV q6–8h prn anxiety

Tylenol 650 mg po/pr q4h prn pain/fever

Milk of magnesia 30 mL po/NG q4h prn constipation

Ordered Laboratory Studies

Chemistry 20 and CEA on admission

Chemistry 7 with magnesium, phosphorus, and calcium every 48
   hours postoperatively

CBC daily

LABORATORY STUDY RESULTS

Test	Day 1 (Preop)	Day 2 (Postop Day 1)	Day 3 (Postop Day 2)
Sodium	136 mEq/L		142 mEq/L
Potassium	4.1 mEq/L		3.9 mEq/L
Chloride	102 mEq/L		106 mEq/L
Bicarbonate	26 mEq/L		21 mEq/L
Blood urea nitrogen (BUN)	24 mg/dL		33 mg/dL
Creatinine	0.8 mg/dL		1.1 mg/dL
Glucose	113 mg/dL		153 mg/dL
Magnesium	2.2 mEq/L		2.4 mEq/L
Phosphorus	3.2 mg/dL		2.5 mg/dL
Calcium	9.3 mg/dL		10.1 mg/dL
White blood cell (WBC)	7,000/mm^3	11,000/mm^3	13,000/mm^3
Hematocrit	37%	32%	27%
Hemoglobin	13 g/dL	10.6 g/dL	9.2 g/dL
Carcinoembryonic antigen (CEA)	6.0 ng/mL		

CRITICAL THINKING QUESTIONS

1. What five nursing diagnoses are of the highest priority for Mr. Landry today? Why?

2. Review Mr. Landry's current physical examination. What postoperative problems, if any, is Mr. Landry currently experiencing?

3. The following activities need to be performed with or for Mr. Landry: Change the syringe in the PCA pump, empty and record urine output, perform a.m. care, teach use of the incentive spirometer, and call the surgeon for an additional antiemetic order. In which order should the nurse perform these activities? Why?

4. Later in the day, Mr. Landry says to the nurse, "The surgeon told me he's pretty sure he got all of the cancer. I guess I won't need that appointment with the oncologist." What is the nurse's best response to this situation?

Answers to Critical Thinking Questions appear in Appendix D.

NCLEX® REVIEW

1. A postoperative patient in the PACU begins to demonstrate an increased heart rate. The nurse realizes this increase is most likely because of:
   1. Bleeding.
   2. Anxiety.
   3. Nausea.
   4. Pain.

2. The nurse is assessing a postoperative patient in the PACU. Which of the following would indicate the patient is stable enough for transfer to another inpatient care area?
   1. Breathing with an oral airway
   2. Easily arousable and moving all four extremities
   3. Lower extremities without sensation post spinal anesthesia
   4. Moderate amount of vomiting

3. A postoperative patient is demonstrating a distended abdomen with no bowel sounds. Which of the following should the nurse do to help this patient?
   1. Advance to full diet.
   2. Restrict fluids.
   3. Ambulate three times a day.
   4. Administer antiemetic medication.

4. The nurse is instructing a postoperative patient about care needed when at home. Which of the following should the nurse include in these instructions?
   1. Habitual recovery will occur in a short period of time.
   2. Keep the wound open to air and permit the Steri-Strips to fall off on their own.
   3. Return to the doctor's office to have the staples removed in 3 weeks.
   4. Full recovery from surgery will be unexpectedly short.

5. The nurse would like to study how a nurse's critical thinking skills can be improved when working with a postoperative patient. Which of the following research topics would provide information on nurses' critical thinking skills?
   1. Factors that influence anxiety levels in the older surgical patient
   2. Strategies to increase the patient's ability to manage symptoms at home
   3. Nurse's ability to manage post operative pain
   4. Adjustment of discharge teaching to accommodate cultural differences

Answers for review questions appear in Appendix D

KEY TERMS

airway obstruction *p.655*
fast-tracking *p.644*
graduated compression stockings *p.681*
hypothermia *p.659*

hypoxemia *p.655*
ileus *p.676*
intermittent pneumatic compression
   devices *p.681*

laryngospasm *p.655*
normothermia *p.659*
postanesthesia care unit (PACU) *p.644*
surveillance *p.645*

EXPLORE **PEARSON** **mynursingkit**™

MyNursingKit is your one stop for online chapter review materials and resources. Prepare for success with additional NCLEX®-style practice questions, interactive assignments and activities, web links, animations and videos, and more!

Register your access code from the front of your book at
www.mynursingkit.com

REFERENCES

Allard, N. (2007). Day surgery for breast cancer: Effects of a psychoeducational telephone intervention on functional status and emotional distress. *Oncology Nursing Forum, 34*(1), 133–141.

Allvin, R., Berg, K., Idvall, E., & Nilsson, U. (2007). Postoperative recovery: A concept analysis. *Journal of Advanced Nursing, 57*(5), 552–558.

Amaragiri, S., & Lees, T. (2006). Elastic compression stockings for prevention of deep vein thrombosis. *Cochrane Library, 4* (CD001484).

American Society of Anesthesiologists. (2004). *Standard for post anesthesia care.* Park Ridge, IL: Author.

American Society of PeriAnesthesia Nurses. (2002). *Clinical guideline for the prevention of unplanned perioperative hypothermia.* Cherry Hill, NJ: Author.

American Society of PeriAnesthesia Nurses. (2003). ASPAN pain and comfort clinical guideline. *Journal of PeriAnesthesia Nursing, 18*(4), 232–236.

American Society of PeriAnesthesia Nurses. (2006a). ASPAN's evidence-based clinical practice guideline for the prevention and/or management of PONV/PDNV. *Journal of PeriAnesthesia Nursing, 21*(4), 230–250.

American Society of PeriAnesthesia Nurses. (2006b). *Standards of perianesthesia nursing practice.* Cherry Hill, NJ: Author.

Apfel, C., Korttila, K., Abdalla, M., Kerger, H., Turan, A., Vedder, I., Zernak, C., Danner, K., Jokela, R., Pocock, S., Trenkler, S., Kredel, M., Biedler, A., Sessler, D., & Roewer, N., et al. (2004). A factorial trial of six interventions for the prevention of postoperative nausea and vomiting. *New England Journal of Medicine, 350*(24), 2441–2451.

Arieff, A. (1999). Fatal postoperative pulmonary edema. *Chest, 115*(5), 1371–1377.

Asher, M. (2004). Surgical considerations in the elderly. *Journal of PeriAnesthesia Nursing, 19*(6), 406–414.

Basse, L., Billesbolle, P., & Kehlet, H. (2002). Early recovery after abdominal rectopexy with multimodal rehabilitation. *Diseases of the Colon and Rectum, 45*(2), 195–199.

Blondin, M. (2006). *Prevention of deep vein thrombosis.* Iowa City: University of Iowa Gerontological Nursing Research Center, Research Dissemination Core.

Bowles, K., Foust, J., Naylor, M., & Ware, M. (2003). Hospital discharge referral decision making: A multidisciplinary perspective. *Applied Nursing Research, 16*(3), 134–143.

Brooks, D., Crowe, J., Kelsey, C., Lacy, J., Parsons, J., & Solway, Sherra. (2001). A clinical practice guideline on peri-operative cardiorespiratory physical therapy. *Physiotherapy Canada, 53*(1), 9–25.

Brooks, J. (2001). Postoperative nosocomial pneumonia: Nurse-sensitive interventions. *AACN Clinical Issues, 12*(2), 305–323.

Brooks-Brunn, I. (1998). Validation of a predictive model for postoperative pulmonary complications. *Heart & Lung, 27,* 151–158.

Brown, A., Christo, P., & Wu, C. (2004). Strategies for postoperative pain management. *Best Practices & Research. Clinical Anesthesiology, 18,* 703–717.

Burden, N. (2004). Discharge planning for the elderly ambulatory surgical patient. *Journal of PeriAnesthesia Nursing, 19*(6), 401–405.

Burt, J., Caelli, K., Moore, K., & Anderson, M. (2005). Radical prostatectomy: Men's experiences and postoperative needs. *Journal of Clinical Nursing, 14*(7), 883–890.

Carli, F., Mayo, N., Klubien, K., Schricker, T., Trudel, J., & Belliveau, P. (2002). Epidural analgesia enhances functional exercise capacity and health-related quality of life after colonic surgery: Results of a randomized trial. *Anesthesiology, 97*(3), 540–549.

Centers for Disease Control and Prevention. (1997). Guidelines for the prevention of nosocomial pneumonia. *Morbidity and Mortality Weekly Report, 46* (RR-1), 1–79.

Chaiyakunapruk, N., Kitikannakorn, N., Nathisuwan, S., Leeprakobboon, K., & Leelasettagool, C. (2006). The efficacy of ginger for the prevention of postoperative nausea and vomiting: A meta-analysis. *American Journal of Obstetrics and Gynecology, 194*(1), 95–100.

Chaudhury, H., Mahmood, A., & Valente, M. (2006). Nurses' perception of single-occupancy versus multioccupancy rooms in acute care environments: An exploratory comparative assessment. *Applied Nursing Research, 19,* 118–125.

Clagett, G. P., Anderson, F., Geerts, W., Heit, J. A., Knudson, M., Lieberman, J. R., Merli, G. J., & Wheeler, H. B., et al. (1998). Prevention of venous thromboembolism. *Chest, 114*(5, Suppl.), 531S–560S.

Clancy, J., McVicar, A., & Baird, N. (2002). *Perioperative practice: Fundamentals of homeostasis.* New York: Routledge.

Clarke, S., & Aiken, L. (2003). Failure to rescue. *American Journal of Nursing, 103*(1), 42–47.

Cheever, K. (1999). Pain, analgesic use, and morbidity in appendectomy patients. *Clinical Nursing Research 8*(3), 267–282.

Cunningham, M. F., Hanson-Heath, C., & Agre, P. (2003). A perioperative nurse liaison program: CNS interventions for cancer patients and their families. *Journal of Nursing Care Quality, 18*(1), 16–21.

Cutilli, C. (2007). Health literacy in geriatric patients: An integrative review of the literature. *Orthopedic Nursing, 26,* 43–48.

Dellinger, E. (2005). Should we measure body temperature for patients who have recently undergone surgery? *Clinical Infectious Diseases, 40*(10), 1411–1413.

Dip, K., Dip, G., & McCutcheon, H. (2006). Observations and vital signs: Ritual or vital for the postoperative monitoring of postoperative patients? *Applied Nursing Research, 19*(4), 204–211.

Doering, L., McGuire, A., & Rourke, D. (2002). Recovering from cardiac surgery: What patients want you to know. *American Journal of Critical Care, 11*(4), 333–343.

Ead, H. (2006). From Aldrete to PADSS: Reviewing discharge criteria after ambulatory surgery. *Journal of PeriAnesthesia Nursing, 21*(4), 259–267.

Edelen, C., & Perlow, M. (2002). A comparison of the effectiveness of an opioid analgesic and a nonpharmacologic intervention to improve incentive spirometry volumes. *Pain Management Nursing, 3*(1), 36–42.

Evans, D., Read, K., Charles-Barks, C., Edwards, S., Gill, S., Leith, S., Morrison, H., Nelson, J., Sandison, S., & Wilkie, A., et al. (2001). Graduated compression stockings for the prevention of post-operative venous thromboembolism. *Best Practice, 5*(2), 1–5.

Ezzone, S., Baker, R., & Terrepka, E. (1998). Music as an adjunct to antiemetic therapy. *Oncology Nursing Forum, 25,* 1551–1556.

Finnish Medical Society Duodecim. (2006). Prevention of venous thrombosis. In *EMB guidelines: Evidenced-based practice.* Helsinki: Duodecim Medical Publications.

Frazier, S., Moser, D., Daley, L., McKinley, S., Riegel, B., Garvin, B., & An, K., et al. (2003). Critical care nurses' beliefs about and reported management of anxiety. *American Journal of Critical Care, 12*(1), 19–27.

Geerts, W., Pineo, G., Hit, J., Bergqvist, D., Lassen, M., Colwell, C., & Ray, J., et al. (2004). Prevention of venous thromboembolism: The Seventh AACP Conference on Antithrombotic and Thrombolytic Therapy. *Chest, 126*(3 Suppl.), 338S–400S.

Goldman, L., & Ausiello, D. (Eds.). (2004). *Cecil textbook of medicine.* Philadelphia: W. B. Saunders.

Golembiewski, J. (2004). Antibiotic prophylaxis for preventing surgical site infection. *Journal of PeriAnesthesia Nursing, 19*(2), 111–113.

Golembiewski, J., Torrecer, S., & Katke, J. (2005). The use of opioids in the postoperative setting: Focus on morphine, hydromorphone, and fentanyl. *Journal of PeriAnesthesia Nursing, 20*(2), 141–143.

Good, K., Verble, J., Secrest, J., & Norwood, B. (2006). Postoperative hypothermia—The chilling consequences. *AORN Journal, 83*(5), 1054–1069.

Greif, R., Akca, O., Horn, E., Kurz, A., & Sessler, D. (2000). Supplemental perioperative oxygen to reduce the incidence of surgical-wound infection. *New England Journal of Medicine, 342*(3), 161–168.

Gunta, K., Lewis, C., & Nuccio, S. (2000). Prevention and management of postoperative nausea and vomiting. *Orthopaedic Nursing, 19*(2), 39–48.

Hamel, M., Henderson, W., Khuri, S., & Daley, J. (2005). Surgical outcomes for patients aged 80 and older: Morbidity and mortality from major noncardiac surgery. *Journal of the American Geriatrics Society, 53*(3), 424–429.

Hasankhani, H., Mohammadi, E., Moazzami, F., Mokhtari, M., & Naghgizadh, M. (2007). The effects of intravenous fluids temperature on perioperative hemodynamic situation, post-operative shivering, and recovery in orthopaedic surgery. *Canadian Operating Room Nursing Journal, 25*(1), 20–24, 26–27.

Heine, J., Koch, S., & Goldie, P. (2004). Patients' experiences of readiness for discharge following a total hip replacement. *Australian Journal of Physiotherapy, 50*(4), 227–233.

Hodgson, N., & Given, C. (2004). Determinants of functional recovery in older adults surgically treated for cancer. *Cancer Nursing, 27*(1), 10–16.

Holmes, K., & Lenz, E. (1997). Perceived self-care information needs and information-seeking behaviors before and after elective spinal procedures. *Journal of Neuroscience Nursing, 29,* 79–85.

Holte, K., & Kehlet, H. (2002). Epidural anaesthesia and analgesia on perioperative outcome: Effects on surgical stress responses and implications for postoperative nutrition. *Clinical Nutrition, 21,*199–206.

Hopf, H., Hunt, T., Rosen, N., Akca, O., Sessler, D., Greif, R., Sessler, D.I., Harten, J., Anderson, K., Kinsella, J., Lee, J., O'Neill, M., Pryor, K., Fahey, T., Lien, C., & Goldstein, P., et al. (2004). Surgical site infection and the routine use of perioperative hyperoxia in a general surgical population: A randomized controlled trial. *Journal of the American Medical Association, 291*(16), 1956–1965.

Horan, T., Gaynes, R., Martone, W., Jarvis, W., & Emori, T. (1992). CDC definitions of nosocomial surgical site infections. *Infection Control Hospital Epidemiology, 13,* 606–608.

Horvath, K. (2003). Postoperative recovery at home after ambulatory gynecologic laparoscopic surgery. *Journal of PeriAnesthesia Nursing, 18*(5), 324–334.

Hudcova, J., McNicol, E., Quah, C., Lau, J., & Carr, D. (2006). Patient controlled opioid analgesia versus conventional opioid analgesia for postoperative pain. *Cochrane Library, (4)* (CD003348).

Huddleston, J., Long, K., Naessens, J., Vanness, D., Larson, D., Trousdale, R., Plevak, M., Cabanela, M., Ilstrup, D., & Wachter, R., et al. (2004). Improving patient care. Medical and surgical comanagement after elective hip and knee arthroplasty: A randomized, controlled trial. *Annals of Internal Medicine, 141*(1), 28–38.

Hughes, L., Hodgson, N., Muller, P., Robinson, L., & McCorkle, R. (2000). Information needs of elderly postsurgical cancer patients during the transition from hospital to home. *Journal of Nursing Scholarship, 32*(1), 25–30.

Hupcey, J. (2000). Feeling safe: Psychosocial needs of ICU patients. *Journal of Nursing Scholarship, 32*(4), 361–367.

Jacobs, V. (2000). Informational needs of surgical patients following discharge. *Applied Nursing Research, 13*(1), 12–18.

Kaasalainen, S., & Crook, J. (2004). An exploration of seniors' ability to report pain. *Clinical Nursing Research, 13*(3), 199–216.

Kalisvaart, K., de Jonghe, J., Bogaards, M., Vreeswijk, R., Egberts, T., Burger, B., Eikelenboom, P., & van-Gool, W. et al. (2005). Haloperidol prophylaxis for elderly hip-surgery patients at risk for delirium: A randomized placebo-controlled study. *Journal of the American Geriatrics Society, 53*(10), 1658–1666.

Kalisvaart, K., Vreeswijk, R., de Jonghe, J., van der Ploeg, T., van Gool, W., & Eikelenboom, P. (2006). Risk factors and prediction of postoperative delirium in elderly hip-surgery patients: Implementation and validation of a medical risk factor model. *Journal of the American Geriatrics Society, 54*(5), 817–822.

Kehlet, H., Troels, S., Woolf, J., & Woolf, C. (2006). Persistent postsurgical pain: Risk factors and prevention. *Lancet, 367,* 1618–1626.

King, C. (1997). Nonpharmacologic management of chemotherapy-induced nausea and vomiting. *Oncology Nursing Forum, 24*(Suppl.7), 41–47.

Kondo, A., Kanda, K., Isokawa, Y., Nishibayasi, K., Nanpo, S., Kadowaki, R., Anai, K., & Mibu, Y., et al. (2005). The relationship in hip fracture patients of post-operative days to initial rehabilitation activities and their ambulatory ability on postoperative day 20. *Journal of Orthopaedic Nursing, 9*(3), 146–156.

Kuchta, A., & Golembiewski, J. (2004). Medication use in the elderly patient: Focus on the perioperative/perianesthesia setting. *Journal of PeriAnesthesia Nursing, 19*(6), 415–427.

Kwekkeboom, K., & Gretarsdottir, E. (2006). Systematic review of relaxation interventions for pain. *Journal of Nursing Scholarship, 38*(3), 269–277.

Lawrence, V., Silverstein, J., Cornell, J., Pederson, T., Noveck, H., & Carson, J. (2003). Higher Hb level is associated with better early functional recovery after hip repair. *Transfusion, 43*(12), 1717–1722.

Lee, A., & Done, M. (2004). Stimulation of the wrist acupuncture point P6 for preventing postoperative nausea and vomiting. *Cochrane Database of Systematic Reviews, 3* (CD003281).

Leinonen, T., Leino-Kilpi, H., Stahlberg, M., & Lertola, K. (2003). Comparing patient and nurse perceptions of perioperative care quality. *Applied Nursing Research, 16*(1), 29–37.

Leske, J. S. (2003). Comparison of family stresses, strengths, and outcomes after trauma and surgery. *AACN Clinical Issues, 14*(1), 33–41.

Leung, J., Sands, L., Mullen, E., Wang, Y., & Vaurio, L. (2005). Are preoperative depressive symptoms associated with postoperative delirium in geriatric surgical patients? *Journals of Gerontology Series A: Biological Sciences and Medical Sciences, 60A*(12), 1563–1571.

Low, D., Vu, A., Brown, M., Davis, S., Keller, D., Levine, B., & Crandall, C., et al. (2007). Temporal thermometry fails to track body core temperature during heat stress. *Medicine & Science in Sports and Exercise, 39*(7), 1029–1035.

Lupien, A., Schoneboom, B., & Wren, K. (2000). Limitations to self-care in the ambulatory surgical patient. *Journal of PeriAnesthesia Nursing, 15*(2), 102–107.

Lyons, S. (2004). *Fall prevention for older adults.* Iowa City: University of Iowa Gerontological Nursing Interventions Research Center, Research Dissemination Core.

Madsen, D., Tamara, S., Cullen, L., Folkedahl, B., Mueller, T., Richardson, C., & Titler, M., et al. (2005). Listening to bowel sounds: An evidence-based practice project. *American Journal of Nursing, 105*(12), 40–49.

Mamaril, M. (2006). Nursing considerations in the geriatric surgical patient: The perioperative continuum of care. *Nursing Clinics of North America, 41,* 313–328.

Mann, C., Pouzeratte, Y., Boccara, G., Peccoux, C., Vergue, C., Brunat, G., Domergue, J., Millat, B., & Colson, P., et al. (2000). Comparison of intravenous or epidural patient-controlled analgesia in the elderly after major abdominal surgery. *Anesthesiology, 92*(2), 433–441.

Mann, C., Pouzeratte, Y., & Eledjam, J. (2003). Postoperative patient-controlled analgesia in the elderly: Risks and benefits of epidural versus intravenous administration. *Drugs and Aging, 20*(5), 337–345.

Marcantonio, E., Flacker, J., Wright, R., & Resnick, N. (2001). Reducing delirium after hip fracture: A randomized trial. *Journal of the American Geriatrics Society, 49,* 516–522.

Markey, D. W., & Brown, R. J. (2002). An interdisciplinary approach to addressing patient activity and mobility in the medical-surgical patient. *Journal of Nursing Care Quality, 16*(4), 1–12.

McAlister, F., Bertsch, K., Man, J., Bradley, J., & Jacka, M. (2005). Pulmonary complications after noncardiac surgery. *American Journal of Respiratory and Critical Care Medicine, 171*(5), 514–517.

McDonald, D., Thomas, G., Livingston, K., & Severson, J. (2005). Assisting older adults to communicate their postoperative pain. *Clinical Nursing Research, 14*(2), 109–127.

Meade, C., Bursell, A., & Ketelsen, L. (2006). Effects of nursing rounds on patients' call light use, satisfaction, and safety. *American Journal of Nursing, 106*(9), 58–70.

Merli, G. (2000). Prophylaxis for deep venous thrombosis and pulmonary embolism in the surgical patient. *Clinical Cornerstone, 2*(4), 15–25.

Milgrom, L. B., Brooks, J. A., Qi, R., Bunnell, K., Wuestefeld, S., & Beckman, D. (2004). Pain levels experienced with activities after cardiac surgery. *American Journal of Critical Care, 13*(2), 116–125.

Milisen, K., Foreman, M., Abraham, I., deGeest, S., Godderis, J., Vandermeulen, E., Fischler, B., Delooz, H., Spiessens, B., & Broos, P., et al. (2001). A nurse-led interdisciplinary intervention program for delirium in elderly hip-fracture patients. *Journal of the American Geriatrics Society, 49,* 523–532.

Milisen, K., Lemiengre, J., Braes, T., & Foreman, M. (2005). Multicomponent intervention strategies for managing delirium in hospitalized older people: Systematic review. *Journal of Advanced Nursing, 52*(1), 79–90.

Mimnaugh, L., Winegar, M., Mabrey, Y., & Davis, J. (1999). Sensations experienced during removal of tubes in acute postoperative patients. *Applied Nursing Research, 12,* 78–85.

Morrison, R., Magaziner, J., & McLaughlin, M. (2003). The impact of post-operative pain on outcomes following hip fracture. *Pain, 103,* 303–311.

Mulroy, M., Salinas, F., Larkin, K., & Polissar, N. (2002). Ambulatory surgery patients may be discharged before voiding after short-acting spinal and epidural anesthesia. *Anesthesiology, 97*(2), 315–319.

Murphy, M., Hooper, V., Sullivan, E., Clifford, T., & Apfel, C. (2006). Identification of risk factors for postoperative nausea and vomiting in the perianesthesia adult patient. *Journal of PeriAnesthesia Nursing, 21*(6), 377–384.

Neil, J. (2007). Perioperative care of the immunocompromised patient. *AORN Journal, 85*(3), 544–565.

Ng, W., & Neill, J. (2006). Evidence for early oral feeding of patients after elective open colorectal surgery: A literature review. *Journal of Clinical Nursing, 15*(5), 696–709.

Nilsson, U., Unosson, M., & Kihlgren, M. (2006). Experience of postoperative recovery before discharge: Patients' views. *Journal of Advanced Perioperative Care, 2,* 97–106.

Nisanevich, V., Felsenstein, I., Almogy, G., Weissman, C., Einav, S., & Matot, I. (2005). Effect of intraoperative fluid management on outcome after intraabdominal surgery. *Anesthesiology, 103*(1), 25–32.

Nishimori, M., Ballantyne, J., & Low, J. (2006). Epidural pain relief versus systemic opioid-based pain relief for abdominal aortic surgery. *Cochrane Library, (4)* (CD005059).

Odom-Forren, J., Fetzer, S., & Moser, D. (2006). Evidence-based interventions for post discharge nausea and vomiting: A review of the literature. *Journal of PeriAnesthesia Nursing, 21*(6), 411–430.

Oermann, M. H., Harris, C. H., & Dammeyer, J. A. (2001). Teaching by the nurse: How important is it to patients? *Applied Nursing Research, 14*(1), 11–17.

Oldmeadow, L., McBurney, H., Robertson, V., Kimmel, L., & Elliott, B. (2004). Targeted postoperative care improves discharge outcome after hip or knee arthroplasty. *Archives of Physical Medicine and Rehabilitation, 85,* 1424–1427.

Olsson, U., Bergbom, I., & Bosaeus, I. (2002). Patients' experiences of the recovery period 3 months after gastrointestinal cancer surgery. *European Journal of Cancer Care, 11,* 51–60.

Orfanos, P., Ellis, E., & Johnston, C. (1999). Effects of deep breathing exercises and ambulation on pattern of ventilation in post-operative patients. *Australian Journal of Physiotherapy, 45*(3), 173–182.

Overend, T., Anderson, C., Lucy, S. D., Bhatia, C., Jonsson, B., & Timmermans, C. (2001). The effect of incentive spirometry on postoperative pulmonary complications. *Chest, 120*(3), 971–978.

Pandey, C., Priye, S., Ambesh, S., Singh, S., Singh, U., & Singh, P. (2006). Prophylactic gabapentin for prevention of postoperative nausea and vomiting in patients undergoing laparoscopic cholecystectomy: A randomized, double-blind, placebo-controlled study. *Journal of Postgraduate Medicine, 52,* 95–99.

Pasero, C. (2003a). Epidural analgesia for postoperative pain, Part 1. *American Journal of Nursing, 103*(10), 62–64.

Pasero, C. (2003b). Epidural analgesia for postoperative pain, Part 2. *American Journal of Nursing, 103*(11), 43–45.

Pasero, C. (2005). Improving postoperative outcomes with epidural analgesia. *Journal of PeriAnesthesia Nursing, 20*(1), 51–55.

Pasero, C., & Belden, J. (2006). Evidence-based perianesthesia care: Accelerated postoperative recovery programs. *Journal of PeriAnesthesia Nursing, 21*(3), 168–176.

Pasero, C., & McCaffery, M. (2005). No self-report means no pain-intensity rating: Assessing pain in patients who cannot provide a report. *American Journal of Nursing, 105*(10), 50–53.

Pasero, C., & McCaffery, M. (2007). Orthopaedic postoperative pain management. *Journal of PeriAnesthesia Nursing, 22*(3), 160–174.

Person, B., & Wexner, S. (2006). The management of postoperative ileus. *Current Problems in Surgery, 43*(1), 12–65.

Phillips, K., & Gill, L. (1994). The use of simple acupressure bands reduces postoperative nausea. *Complementary Therapies in Medicine, 2,* 158–160.

Pietrocola, P., Riley, R., Beanland, C., Kelly, C., & Radnell, J. (2004). A randomized controlled trial to measure the effectiveness of a sacral wedge in preventing postoperative back pain following trans-uretheral resection of the prostate in lithotomy position. *Journal of Clinical Nursing, 13*(8), 977–985.

Pittler, M., & Eberhart, L. (2003). No effect of *Zingiber officinale* (ginger) on postoperative nausea and vomiting. *Focus on Alternative and Complementary Therapies, 8*(4), 416–418.

Prowse, M., & Lyne, P. (2000). Clinical effectiveness in the post-anaesthesia care unit: How nursing knowledge contributes to achieving intended patient outcomes. *Journal of Advanced Nursing, 31*(5), 1115–1124.

Puntillo, K. (2003). Pain assessment and management in the critically ill: Wizardry or science? *American Journal of Critical Care, 12*(4), 310–316.

Puntillo, K., Miaskowski, C., Kehrle, K., Stannard, D., Gleeson, S., & Nye, P. (1997). The relationship between behavioral and physiological indicators of pain, critical care patients' self reports of pain and opioid administration. *Critical Care Medicine, 5,* 1159–1166.

Puntillo, K., & Weiss, S. J. (2003). Pain: Its mediators and associated morbidity in critically ill cardiovascular surgical patients. *Nursing Research, 43,* 31–36.

Puntillo, K., Wild, L., Morris, A., Stanik-Hutt, J., Thompson, C., & White, C. (2002). Practices and predictors of analgesic interventions for adults undergoing painful procedures. *American Journal of Critical Care, 11*(5), 415–429.

Qaseem, A., Snow, V., Fitterman, N., Hornbake, R., Lawrence, V., Smetana, G., Weiss, K., Owens, D., Aronson, M., Barry, P., Casey, D., Cross, J., Fitterman, N., & Sherif, K., et al. (2006). Risk assessment for and strategies to reduce perioperative pulmonary complications for patients undergoing noncardiothoracic surgery: A guideline from the American College of Physicians. *Annals of Internal Medicine, 144*(8), 575–580.

Redeker, N. (2000). Sleep in acute care settings: An integrative review. *Journal of Nursing Scholarship, 32*(1), 31–38.

Reilly, P., Iezzoni, L., Phillips, R., Davis, R., Tuchin, L., & Calkins, D. (1996). Discharge planning: Comparison of patients' and nurses' perceptions of patients following hospital discharge. *Journal of Nursing Scholarship, 28*(2), 143–147.

Resnick, B. (2003). Preventing falls in acute care. In M. Mezey, T. Fulmer, & A. Zwicker (Eds.), *Geriatric nursing protocols for best practice* (pp. 141–164). New York: Springer.

Richman, J., Liu, S., Courpas, G., et al. (2006). Does continuous peripheral nerve block provide superior pain control to opioids? A meta-analysis. *Anesthesia and Analgesia, 102,* 248–257.

Rimmele, T., Combourieu, E., Wey, P., Boselli, E., Allaouchiche, B., Chassard, D., & Escarment, J., et al. (2005). Immediate postoperative refeeding in orthopedic surgery is safe. *Journal of Anesthesia, 19*(4), 323–325.

Ross, J. (2007). Health literacy and its influence on patient safety. *Journal of PeriAnesthesia Nursing, 22*(3), 220–223.

Saclarides, T. (2006). Current choices—good or bad—for the proactive management of postoperative ileus: A surgeon's view. *Journal of PeriAnesthesia Nursing, 21*(2, Suppl. 1), S7–S15.

Sauaia, A., Min, S., Leber, C., Erbacher, K., Abrams, F., & Fink, R. (2005). Postoperative pain management in elderly patients: Correlation between adherence to treatment guidelines and patient satisfaction. *Journal of the American Geriatrics Society, 53*(2), 272–282.

Schultz, A. A., Andrews, A. L., Goran, S. F., Mathew, T., & Sturdevant, N. (2003). Comparison of acupressure bands and droperidol for reducing post-operative nausea and vomiting in gynecologic surgery patients. *Applied Nursing Research, 16*(4), 256–265.

Schumann, R., Shikora, S., Weiss, J. M., Wurm, H., Strassels, S., & Carr, D. B. (2003). A comparison of multimodal perioperative analgesia to epidural pain management after gastric bypass surgery. *Anesthesia & Analgesia, 96*(2), 469–474.

Schweon, S. (2006). Stamping out surgical site infection. *RN, 69*(8), 37–40.

Scott, E., & Buckland, R. (2006). A systematic review of intraoperative warming to prevent postoperative complications. *AORN Journal, 83*(5), 1090–1112.

Seltzer, J., Horsman, A., & Korniewicz, D. (2002). Awareness of surgical site infections for advanced practice nurses. *AACN Clinical Issues, 13*(3), 398–409.

Shea, R., Brooks, J. A., Dayhoff, N., & Keck, J. (2002). Pain intensity and postoperative pulmonary complications among the elderly after abdominal surgery. *Heart & Lung, 31*(6), 440–449.

Sjostrom, B., Dahlgren, L., & Haljamae, H. (2000). Strategies used in post-operative pain assessment and their clinical accuracy. *Journal of Clinical Nursing, 9,* 111–118.

Smith, M., & Ellis, E. (2000). Is retained mucus a risk factor for the development of postoperative atelectasis and pneumonia? Implications for the physiotherapist. *Physiotherapy Theory and Practice, 16*(2), 69–80.

Smith, M., Kemp, J., Hemphill, L., & Vojir, C. (2002). Outcomes of therapeutic massage for hospitalized cancer patients. *Journal of Nursing Scholarship, 34*(3), 257–262.

Smith, T., White, M., O'Connor, L., Salinas, T., Lucas, J., Bowar-Ferres, S., & Fitzpatrick, J., et al. (2002). Nursing care quality initiative (NCQI) for hospitalized elders and their families: A demonstration and quality improvement model of nursing care. *Applied Nursing Research, 15*(1), 48–51.

Smykowski, L., & Rodriguez, W. (2003). The post anesthesia care unit experience: A family centered approach. *Journal of Nursing Care Quality, 18*(1), 5–15.

Squadrone, V., Coha, M., Cerutti, E., Schellino, M., Biolino, P., Occella, P., Belloni, G., Vilianis, G., Fiore, G., Cavallo, R., & Ranieri, V., et al. (2005). Caring for the critically ill patient. Continuous positive airway pressure for treatment of postoperative hypoxemia: A randomized controlled trial. *Journal of the American Medical Association, 293*(5), 589–595.

Stanik-Hutt, J., Soeken, K., Belcher, A., Fontaine, D., & Gift, A. (2001). Pain experiences of traumatically injured individuals in a critical care setting. *American Journal of Critical Care, 10,* 252–259.

St. Clair, K., & Larrabee, J. (2002). Clean versus sterile gloves: Which to use for postoperative dressing changes? *Outcomes Management, 6*(1), 17–21.

Suetta, C., Magnusson, S., Rosted, A., Aagaard, P., Jakobsen, A., Larsen, L., Duus, B., & Kjaer, M., et al. (2004). Resistance training in the early postoperative phase reduces hospitalization and leads to muscle hypertrophy in elderly hip surgery patients: A controlled, randomized study. *Journal of the American Geriatrics Society, 52*(12), 2016–2022.

Susleck, D., Willocks, A., Secrest, J., Norwood, B., Holweger, J., Davis, M., Myhan, G., & Trimpey, M. et al. (2007). The perianesthesia experience from the patient's perspective. *Journal of PeriAnesthesia Nursing, 22*(1), 10–20.

Swan, B. (1998). Research utilization: Postoperative nursing care contributions to symptom distress and functional status after ambulatory surgery. *Medsurg Nursing, 7,* 148–151, 154–158.

Tarrac, S. (2006). A description of intraoperative and postanesthesia complication rates. *Journal of PeriAnesthesia Nursing, 21*(2), 88–96.

Titler, M., Herr, K., Schilling, M., Marsh, J. L., Xie, X.-J., Ardery, G., Clarke, W., & Everett, L., et al. (2003). Acute pain treatment for older adults hospitalized with hip fracture: Current nursing practices and perceived barriers. *Applied Nursing Research, 16*(4), 211–227.

VanKooten, M. (1999). Non-pharmacologic pain management for postoperative coronary artery bypass graft surgery patients. *Journal of Nursing Scholarship, 31*(2), 157.

Vermeulen, H., Storm-Versloot, M., Goossens, A., Speelman, P., & Legemate, D. (2005). Diagnostic accuracy of routine postoperative body temperature measurements. *Clinical Infectious Disease, 40,* 1404–1414.

Wadlund, D. (2006). Prevention, recognition, and management of nursing complications in the intraoperative and postoperative surgical patients. *Nursing Clinics of North America, 41,* 151–171.

Wagner, D. (2006). Unplanned perioperative hypothermia. *AORN Journal, 83*(2), 470–476.

Wallenborn, J., Gelbrich, G., Bulst, D., Behrends, K., Wallenborn, H., Rohrbach, A., Krause, U., Kuhnast, T., Wiegel, M., & Olthoff, D., et al. (2006). Prevention of postoperative nausea and vomiting by metoclopramide combined with dexamethasone: Randomized double blind multicentre trial. *British Medical Journal, 333,* 324–328.

Wardell, D., & Weymouth, K. (2004). Review of studies of healing touch. *Journal of Nursing Scholarship, 36*(2), 147–160.

Werner, J., Wendler, M., McCormick, J., Paulus-Smith, S., Jackson, C., & Nie, J. (2002). Human response outcomes influenced by nurse caring. *International Journal for Human Caring, 6*(3), 15–23.

Wheelan, S., Burchill, C., & Tilin, F. (2003). The link between teamwork and patients' outcomes in intensive care units. *American Journal of Critical Care, 12*(6), 527–534.

White, J. (1999). Effects of relaxing music on cardiac autonomic balance and anxiety after acute myocardial infarction. *American Journal of Critical Care, 8,* 220–230.

Whitney, J. A., & Parkman, S. (2002). Preoperative physical activity, anesthesia, and analgesia: Effects on early postoperative walking after total hip replacement. *Applied Nursing Research, 15*(1), 19–27.

Williams, A., & Irurita, V. (2005). Enhancing the therapeutic potential of hospital environments by increasing the personal control and emotional comfort of hospitalized patients. *Applied Nursing Research, 18*(1), 22–28.

Wong, J., Wong, S., & Brooks, E. (2002). A study of hospitalized recovery pattern of acutely confused older patients following hip surgery. *Journal of Orthopaedic Nursing, 6*(2), 68–78.

Zalon, M. (2004). Correlates of recovery among older adults after major abdominal surgery. *Nursing Research, 53*(2), 99–106.

Zeitz, K., & McCutcheon, H. (2006). Observations and vital signs: Ritual or vital for the monitoring of postoperative patients. *Applied Nursing Research, 19*(4), 204–211.

Zutshi, M., Delaney, C., Senagore, A., & Fazio, V. (2004). Shorter hospital stay associated with fastrack postoperative care pathways and laparoscopic intestinal resection are not associated with increased physical activity. *Colorectal Disease, 6,* 477–480.

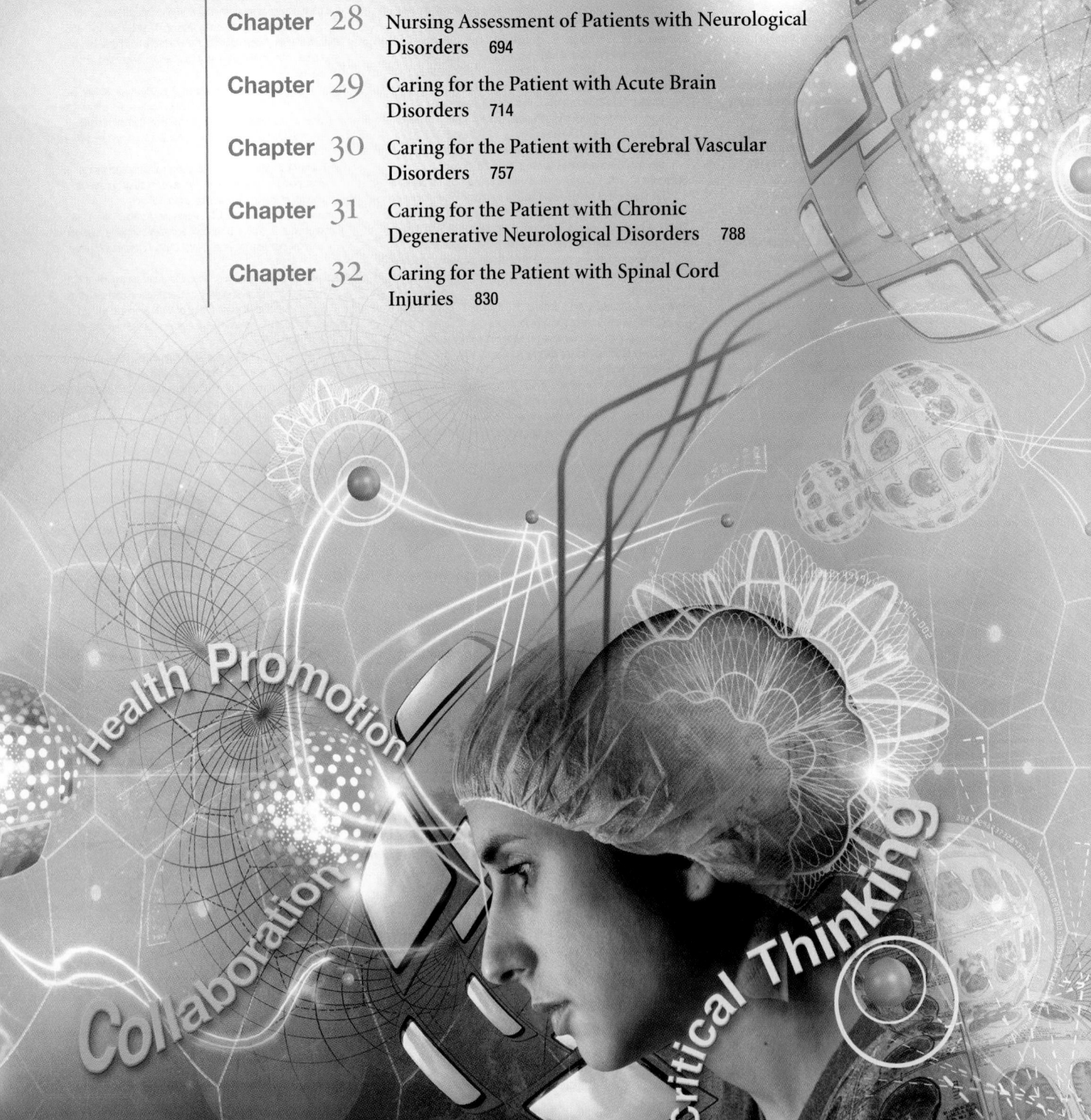

UNIT 6

Nursing Management of Patients with Neurological Disorders

Health Promotion

Collaboration

Critical Thinking

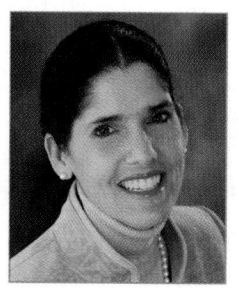

MARY KAY BADER, MSN, CCNS, CNRN, CCRN, FAHA, Neurosurgical Clinical Nurse Specialist, Mission Hospital, I have worked as the neuroscience/critical care clinical nurse specialist (CNS) for 10 years. As the CNS, my position incorporates the multiple roles of clinical expert, educator, leader, change agent, researcher, mentor, and team builder. To be a CNS, I must be master's prepared and clinically competent in the specialty area in which I work.

On a typical day, I conduct clinical rounds in the 12 bed Surgical-Trauma ICU. The purpose of the morning rounds is to assess each patient's clinical status, discuss any issues with the patient's nurse, and talk with family members present about the previous 24 hours. The team in the ICU uses a series of algorithms/clinical guidelines to direct the care of the severe traumatic brain injury (TBI). As the primary developer of these hospital-based guidelines, my role involves educating and collaborating with the nurses, respiratory therapists, and pharmacists on the application of the complex interventions.

I also work with a multidisciplinary vascular team made up of vascular surgeons, interventional radiologists, cardiologists, interventional technologists, and nurses. My role as CNS involves assisting with the development of the IRB research proposal, conducting preprocedure neurological examinations, assisting with the pre- and postprocedure patient/family education, monitoring the neurological status during the procedure, briefing the ICU nursing team on the patient status, following the patient in the hospital, collecting data for the study, and tracking patient visits postprocedure for the year following carotid stent placement.

I have the privilege of following the neurosurgical patients throughout their hospitalization. This helps me build a strong rapport with the patient and family. As I check on patients, I collaborate with the floor nurse and discuss each patient's progress. We advance patients activities and evaluate their responses to therapies.

In the role of CNS, I respond to a "Code Trauma" on all neurological cases, and whenever the team needs an extra hand. I help the trauma nurse with patient care, accompany them to the CT scanner, and await the results. Upon completion of the CT scan I collaborate with the team to develop a plan of care.

The CNS role participates in hospital committees. I attend the Collaborative Practice Council (CPC) meeting. I have been working closely with the CPC as a consultant on the revision of the clinical practice manuals containing procedures, standards of care, patient education plans, and protocols.

In the afternoon I round with the neurosurgeons. I value this time each day as it is an opportunity to engage the team in conversation about the patients. I also participate in the afternoon rehabilitation rounds which is a multidisciplinary team meeting held in the ICU each Wednesday involving nursing members from the various units, therapists, psychiatrist, social worker, and discharge planner. Reviewing the in-house trauma and neurosurgical patients allows the team to anticipate progression of the patients and coordinate timing of referrals.

As an advanced practice nurse, I have the privilege of working with great physicians, nurses, therapists, and other health care providers. I am part of a team in which the whole is greater than the sum of its parts. I consider it an honor to be part of this collaborative team who welcomes the knowledge and skills I can share with them. I would never be able to impact patient care outcomes alone. It takes a synergistic team to save a life when the odds are against them, heal the sick, comfort the dying, and empower families to make tough end-of-life decisions. I am honored and humbled to be part of the nursing profession.

"As the primary developer of these hospital-based guidelines, my role involves educating and collaborating with the nurses, respiratory therapists, and pharmacists on the application of the complex interventions."

CHAPTER 28

Nursing Assessment of Patients with Neurological Disorders

Michele Grigaitis

Outcome-Based Learning Objectives

After studying this chapter, the learner will be able to:

1. Correlate the anatomic and physiological aspects of the nervous system with the neurological examination.
2. Explain the importance of history taking in the neurological assessment.
3. Categorize the cranial nerves with common functional deficits seen in neurological disease.
4. Describe the components of the mental status exam and methods to complete the assessment.
5. Explain the rationale for and methods of measuring and documenting muscle stretch reflexes.
6. Explain the methods of assessing the presence of pathologic reflexes and the method of documentation.
7. Explain the normal age-related differences in the neurological examination of the elderly patient.

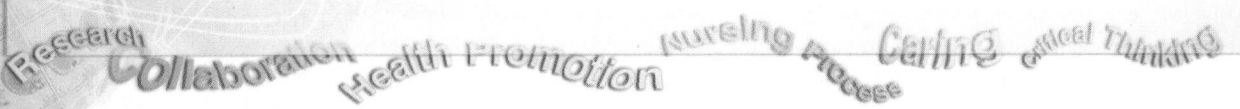

IN THE CARE OF THE PERSON with a known or suspected neurological disorder, the initial neurological assessment becomes the baseline against which all further examination is compared. The need for a thorough and accurate assessment cannot be overemphasized. Patient management is guided by the use of evidence-based medicine, standardized clinical pathways, policies and procedures, or predetermined protocols. The initiation of the management strategy is based on the initial assessment completed by the nurse.

The nursing process is the framework within which the nurse is able to generate a database from the patient's history; construct a list of problems using nursing diagnoses with expected outcomes; design a plan of care; initiate interventions; and evaluate desired patient outcomes. This chapter presents guidelines for the assessment of the adult patient in a variety of clinical settings. The American Nurses Association *Scope and Standards of Neuroscience Nursing Practice* (2002) were used as a framework in determining neurological assessment guidelines.

■ Anatomy and Physiology of the Nervous System

It is necessary for the nurse to correlate knowledge of normal neuroanatomy and physiology with clinical findings to identify clinically significant abnormalities of the nervous system. The nervous system is, to many, the most complex of the body systems. Separated into three areas, the nervous system consists of the central nervous system (CNS), the peripheral nervous system (PNS), and the autonomic nervous system (ANS). Although complex, a basic understanding of the structure and function of the nervous system is critical to the nurse in order to competently assess a patient.

The basic unit of the nervous system is the **neuron.** The primary function of the neuron is to receive information and subsequently transmit this information to other neurons. This information transmission takes place in the **synapse,** the channel between neurons, as shown in Figure 28–1 ■. The size and shape of neurons are different based on the location in the nervous system, but conceptually they are the same. Each neuron is a single cell body. From this body, several branches, or dendrites, extend. These branches communicate through the synapse to other dendrites.

A nerve fiber originating in the body is the axon. The axon can divide into several branches, through which impulses can be distributed to a number of destinations simultaneously. Information transmitted neuronally is dependent on cellular changes in electrical activity. When a neuron is stimulated, the electrical stimulus proceeds down the axon, stimulating vesicles containing chemicals called neurotransmitters. Neurotransmitters act in the synapse, causing the stimulation of the next neuron.

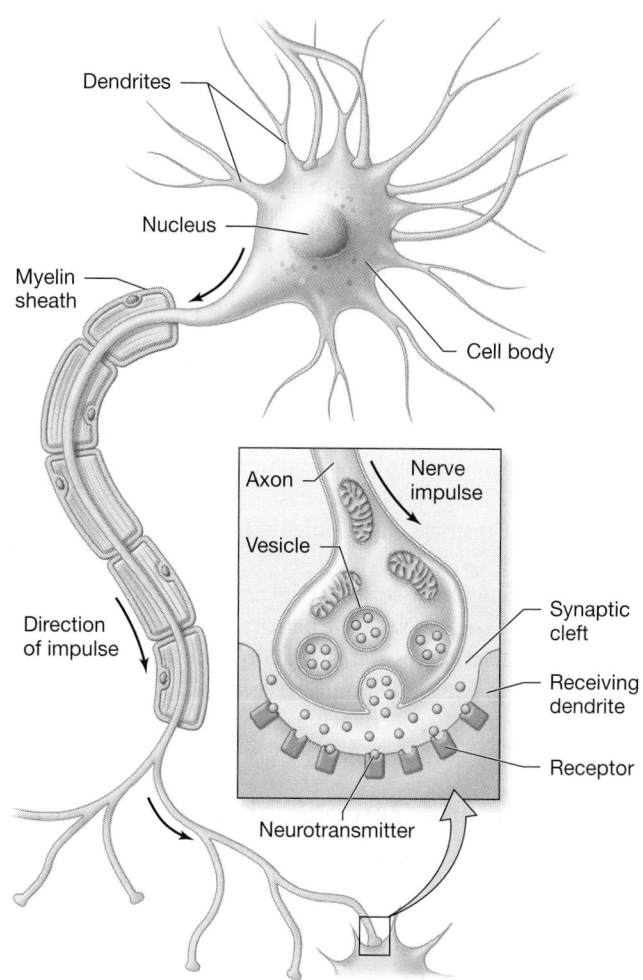

FIGURE 28–1 ■ Two neurons with a synapse between.

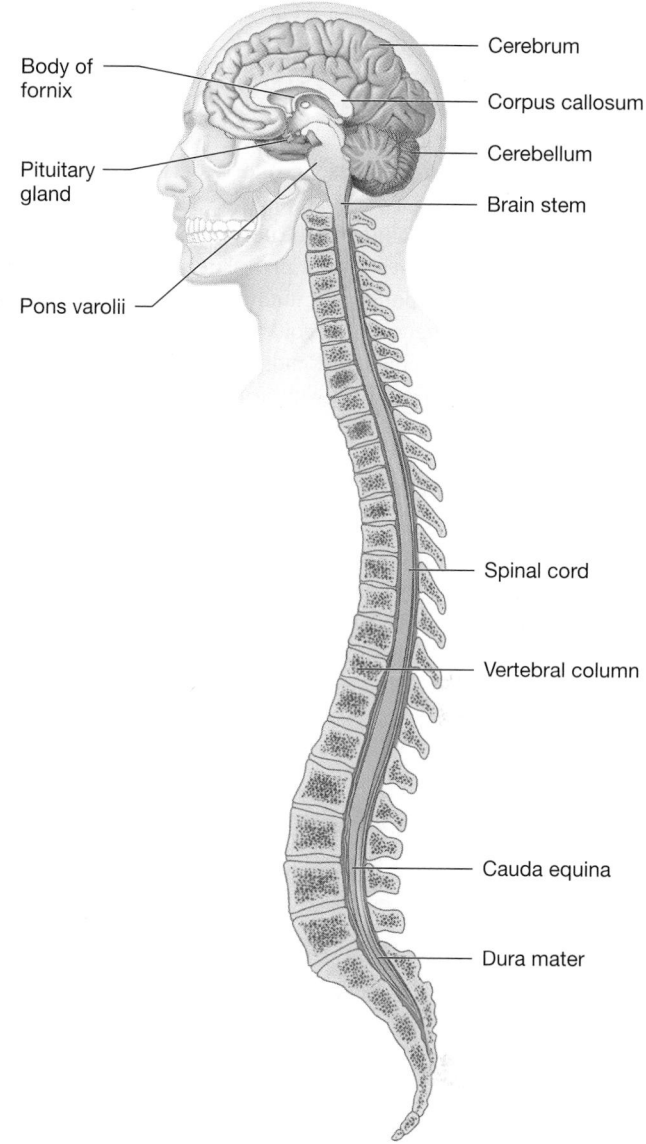

FIGURE 28–2 ■ Brain and spinal cord.

Neuroglia comprise the other major cellular component of the nervous system. Unlike neurons, neuroglia do not directly transmit information. There are three main types of neuroglia: oligodendrocytes, astrocytes, and microglia. Oligodendrocytes form the myelin sheath that covers many neuronal axons. Astrocytes are a key component of the blood–brain barrier, and microglia have a role in removing cellular debris in nervous system damage. Knowledge of the cellular components of the nervous system assists the nurse in understanding the etiology of disease states, such as multiple sclerosis or a primary neoplastic condition. Neurological disorders are discussed in Chapters 29 through 32 ☺ .

Central Nervous System

The central nervous system consists of the brain and spinal cord, as shown in Figure 28–2 ■. It contains the majority of axons and synapses. The CNS is consistent in its apportionment of neurons. Areas with a high density of cell bodies are called gray matter; those primarily containing axons are referred to as white matter. Axons are generally myelinated, which results in a pale color, hence the term *white matter*.

In general, CNS pathways conveying sensory information to the cerebral hemisphere cross over, or decussate, from one side of the CNS to the other. This holds true of descending pathways also. Therefore, each cerebral hemisphere generally perceives sensation from and controls the movement of the contralateral side of the body.

Three protective membranes called the meninges cover the brain and spinal cord. Specifically these membranes are the dura mater, arachnoid mater, and the pia mater. The space between the arachnoid and pia is known as the subarachnoid space. This is the space through which cerebrospinal fluid (CSF) flows. Blood is supplied to the brain through the internal carotid and vertebral arteries.

Peripheral Nervous System

The peripheral nervous system is the link between the CNS and structures of the body from which it receives information and to which it sends information. The PNS consists of nerves joined to the brain and spinal cord, for example, the cranial nerves and spinal nerves. The spinal nerves are shown in Figure 28–3 ■ (p. 696). The spinal nerves branch and combine in areas called plexuses and in groups of cell bodies in structures called ganglia.

The spinal cord lies in the vertebral column, which provides support and protection (Figure 28–3 ■). Vertebrae are bones that are separated by intervertebral disks. These disks act as a cushion to the vertebrae and absorb stress. The spinal cord has 31 pairs of nerves corresponding to the vertebrae they are adjacent to: 8 cervical, 12 thoracic, 5 lumbar, 5 sacral, and 1 coccygeal. Nerves C_1 through C_7 exit over their corresponding vertebrae, but thoracic nerve 1 (T_1) and the remainder of the nerves exit below their correspondingly numbered vertebrae. Cervical nerve 8 (C_8) is unique in that there is no correspondingly numbered vertebra. The spinal cord is shorter than the vertebral column so the spinal roots extend downward. The spinal cord ends at vertebral level L_2, but nerves L_2 through S_5 continue downward as the *cauda equina* or "horse's tail" (see Figure 28–3 ■).

Autonomic Nervous System

Neurons that have the capacity to detect changes in, and control the activity of, the viscera are collectively called the autonomic nervous system. The components of the ANS are found in both the CNS and PNS. The ANS innervates smooth muscle, cardiac muscle, and glands. The primary control of the ANS is the brain and spinal cord. The ANS is separated into two distinct divisions, the sympathetic and parasympathetic nervous systems.

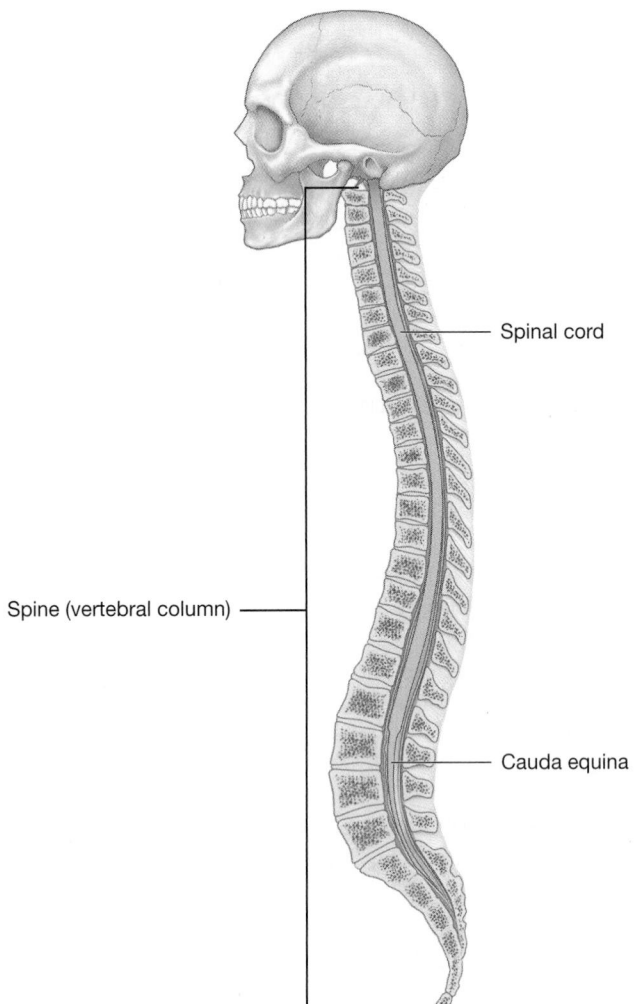

Spinal cord

Spine (vertebral column)

Cauda equina

FIGURE 28–3 ■ Spinal nerves with corresponding vertebrae, to include the cauda equina.

The sympathetic nervous system is the system used to mediate stress. The parasympathetic system, conversely, is associated with conservation and restoring energy. The nurse must have a thorough knowledge of the ANS when dealing with the spinal cord patient. Autonomic dysreflexia (AD) is a hypertensive emergency that can lead to death if untreated.

■ Health History

The traditional health history has several parts, each with its specific purpose. In the patient with neurological symptoms it has been said that the most critical aspect of the assessment is the history (Fuller, 2004). Special care, then, must be taken to ensure the history is comprehensive and accurate. The components of the history include biographic and demographic information, presenting problem, past medical history, family history, social history, environment, and cultural assessment. (See Chapter 9 ⊙.)

The neurological assessment begins with the health care provider's first contact with the patient. Observation of general appearance, facial expression, distractibility, eye contact, and response to verbal stimuli should be assessed. Cognition, emotional expression, speech patterns, and ability to follow directions are noted.

Biographic and Demographic Information

Biographic and demographic data refer to identifying facts. These include age, sex, race, place of birth, current residence, marital status, and religion. These data points serve not only to establish who the patient is but also to give the nurse tentative suggestions as to what areas to further explore. Many neurological conditions occur in specific populations, for example, Alzheimer's disease in the elderly or multiple sclerosis in the young adult. Ethnicity plays a role in cerebral vascular accidents, as epidemiological studies indicate minority populations are at higher risk (Centers for Disease Control and Prevention [CDC], 2007). Current residence is an important piece of information when looking at region-specific diseases such as West Nile virus or cystosarcosis (CDC, 2007).

Presenting Problem

The presenting problem is the reason the individual is seeking care. This reason is best documented in the patient's own words, in quotations. Often, patients with neurological problems have a spouse, family member, or friend present at the time of initial assessment. This should be allowed if possible, because this may provide both support and reassurance to the patient as well as offer validation of the history. In the acute setting, the patient may not be capable of conveying information if the patient is elderly or cognitively impaired or has experienced a traumatic injury; validation of information may be necessary.

History of Presenting Problem

The presenting problem is followed by the history of the presenting problem. The nurse should begin with the initial presentation of the symptom and proceed to the present. If the patient has a single complaint, it is necessary to ascertain when the symptom began and how it evolved over time. If the patient has multiple complaints, a common occurrence in the neurological population, the nurse should explore each symptom individually. One should obtain as full a description as possible. Use of the mnemonic OLD CARTS can be helpful in ensuring all necessary information is obtained. The system of OLD CARTS is designed to assist the health care provider in remembering an assessment order by the use of sequential initials and what they stand for. This tool is shown in Chart 28–1.

When gathering historical information, it is necessary to be very specific. For example, the term *dizziness* can be used to describe vertigo (a sensation of the environment spinning around the patient or spinning of the patient in an immobile environment), light-headedness (a feeling of faintness), momentary visual loss, or overall weakness. The term *weakness* can be used to describe loss of muscle strength, but also imbalance, lack of coordination, or a sensory disturbance. Using the symptom of *headaches* as an example, the questions the nurse would ask include these:

- When did it start?
- What is the location of your headache (frontal, temporal, occipital, global)?
- How long does your headache last?
- How often do the headaches occur (if monthly, related to menses? daily?)? Is the pain throbbing (as with vascular or migraine headaches) or dull (as with chronic daily headaches or rebound headaches)?
- Is a visual disturbance associated with the headache?
- Do the symptoms change with position, for example, are they worse when sitting or standing, and improve with lying flat? (This can indicate increased intracranial pressure caused by, e.g., a tumor, or low-pressure headaches, commonly seen with cerebral spinal fluid leakage.)
- What makes the headache better?
- Has the patient taken any medication, herbal remedy, or supplement to help the headache in the past?
- Rate the pain on a scale of 1 to 10.

 CRITICAL ALERT *When evaluating a patient presenting with headache in the ambulatory setting, difficulty with vision, large palpable temporal arteries, and temporal tenderness are the hallmark of temporal arteritis. This is a neurological emergency and will result in blindness if not treated.*

 CRITICAL ALERT *A patient with the "worst headache of my life" with or without photophobia and meningeal signs could have a subarachnoid hemorrhage. This is a neurological emergency and can result in death if not treated immediately.*

Past Medical History

The past medical history includes major illnesses, which encompass all hospitalizations, surgeries, ambulatory procedures, and illnesses, both acute and chronic. In addition, childhood diseases, immunizations, medications, and allergies are explored.

Childhood Diseases and Immunizations

Many diseases associated with neurological sequelae commonly occur in childhood. Rubella, rubeola, cytomegalovirus, herpes, influenza, and meningitis are examples. It is important to determine vaccination status. Has the patient received adequate vaccination? Vaccines have proven effective against development of certain types of bacterial meningitis. For patients older than 65 years of age, the pneumococcal vaccine should be considered due to the risk of pneumococcal meningitis. Is the patient an immigrant? Many diseases eradicated in the United States occur in other countries. Poliomyelitis, for example, occurs in Africa and South Asia (World Health Organization, 2007).

Major Illness

Several medical conditions are associated with neurological dysfunction. Diabetes mellitus can result in peripheral neuropathy (see Chapter 53 ⊘). Hypertension is a risk factor for cerebrovascular disease (see Chapter 30 ⊘). Infections and neoplastic conditions can result in a myriad of neurological symptoms. Metabolic conditions, such as vitamin deficiency or electrolyte imbalance, can cause neurological symptoms and also exacerbate existing disorders.

A history of trauma is important, as are seizures, stroke, and cranial nerve problems. Important also is the history of surgical procedures. Cognitive impairment has been noted in up to three-quarters of all cardiac surgery patients (Newman, 2007).

Medications

The medication history should include all medications the patient currently is taking or historically has taken. Herbal, over-the-counter, home remedies, and supplements need to be listed as well as prescribed medications. The nurse will need to specifically ask

CHART 28–1	**OLD CARTS Mnemonic for Assessment of Presenting Problem**
Onset of symptom:	When did the symptoms begin?
Location of symptom:	Note the location of the manifestation.
Duration of symptom:	How long has the manifestation been affecting you?
Characteristics:	Describe the characteristics of the manifestation in common language.
Aggravating/**A**ssociated factors:	What factors make the situation worse? What symptoms occur that are associated with the main symptom or manifestation?
Relieving factors:	What factors alleviate the symptoms or make you feel better?
Temporal factors:	Is the onset of the manifestation gradual or sudden? When does it occur? How frequently does it occur? Does it occur in specific settings or environments, e.g., usually after breakfast?
Severity of symptoms:	How severe is the problem? Rate on a scale of 1 to 10 with 10 being the most severe.

if any of these preparations are taken, because many people do not associate them with the term *medication*. This is especially important in the minority and elderly populations. Many ethnic groups commonly use herbs, poultices, tisanes, and teas for medicinal use, both orally and as inhalants. The elderly frequently take "memory-enhancing" supplements. This can be critical information because many of these compounds contain antioxidants, some of which can interfere with prescriptive drugs such as warfarin. When obtaining the medication history, the dose, route, reason for taking, length of time taken, and last dose taken are necessary pieces of information.

Allergies

Many patients believe they have "allergies" to medication, when in fact they are experiencing an adverse drug reaction. Explore the response the patient experienced and list the medication involved. The health care provider should specifically ask about iodine allergies, because many neurological conditions are best ruled in or out with a contrasted imaging study, which uses iodine. All patients should be questioned regarding an allergy to latex.

Family History

A thorough family history includes age, if living, and cause of death if deceased, of all immediate biological family members: parents, grandparents, siblings, and children. Many neurological disorders are inherited. In others, a positive family history represents a risk factor. Examples of inherited disorders are those with autosomal dominant inheritance, such as Huntington disease, or autosomal recessive inheritance, such as Friedreich's ataxia (Victor & Ropper, 2001). An example of a neurological disorder that includes a positive family history as a risk factor is Alzheimer's disease of the late-onset sporadic type (Reyes, Nowak, & Rice, 2006). CADASIL (cerebral autosomal dominant arteriopathy with subcortical infarcts and leukoencephalopathy) is the most common form of hereditary stroke disorder (Joute, Corpechot, & Ducros, 1996). Oftentimes these patients have family members with diagnoses of multiple sclerosis, strokes, and/or dementia. A thorough family history can lead the treating health care provider to these disorders.

Social History

It is important that the social history be obtained in a nonjudgmental fashion. The social history begins with determining the highest level of education the patient has attained, as well as performance in school. The history of current and past employment indicates possible occupational toxin exposure. Marital status and sexual orientation are necessary data points. Drug and alcohol use is critical in the assessment of patients with cognitive impairments. For example, it is necessary to know the answers to these questions: What is the drug/drink of choice? When was it last used? How often is it used? This information will be essential in mediating withdrawal symptoms in the acutely ill hospitalized patient. Tobacco use should be explored as well.

Given the disabling consequences of trauma to the CNS with head and spinal cord injury, the nurse should establish if high-risk factors are present such as drinking and driving, or using recreational drugs and driving. It also is necessary to determine if the patient undertakes high-risk endeavors without appropriate safety equipment, such as not wearing a helmet when riding a motorcycle.

Environment

The home and workplace environment should be assessed for possible exposure to industrial toxins (lead, arsenic, asbestos, benzene, polyvinylchloride, and other carcinogens), as well as the use of any protective safety devices. Potential for falls should be evaluated. Travel or exposure to contagious diseases also should be explored.

Cultural Considerations

Cultural components are present in all patients. Differences, both subtle and obvious, exist. The nurse must take care not to assume that any patient has a prescribed cultural behavior pattern, because this would constitute stereotyping. It is important to explore communication styles, nutrition, family relationships, health beliefs, and religion. This exploration can occur concurrently with the history portion of the assessment. The nurse should ascertain the patient's beliefs regarding the presenting problem. What does the patient believe the cause of the problem is? Being culturally aware is important to the nursing process, as discussed in the Cultural Considerations box.

Physical Examination

The physical examination of the patient with neurological symptoms is conceptually the same as any other system physical examination. The findings of the physical exam are interpreted with the focus on the nervous system.

General Appearance

The physical examination begins when the nurse first encounters the patient. What is the patient's expression? Are there signs of distress, anger, depression, or apathy? Does the patient appear the stated age? The patient's body habitus and nutrition, skin color, amount and distribution of hair, and grooming of hair and nails should be observed. Many chronic illnesses are associated with pallor and weight loss, leading to emaciation.

Vital Signs

Vital signs should be taken by measuring height and weight, and obtaining a temperature. Blood pressure, pulse rate, and respiratory rate also should be obtained. Many cardiovascular anomalies can result in neurological symptoms (see Chapters 40, 42, and 43).

CULTURAL CONSIDERATIONS Related to the Health History

Maintaining cultural awareness indicates a nurse's recognition that patients' attitudes and reactions to illness are reflective of their beliefs as well as practices. Being aware of cultural beliefs and practices enables the nurse to more effectively evaluate and plan appropriate nursing interventions. Medication administration may need to be modified for various cultural groups in order to enhance communication and decrease misconceptions. When patients are evaluated within the context of their cultural orientation and current health care beliefs, improved assessment and planning for interventions are more likely to occur. Chapter 1 ⊕ contains a full discussion of cultural considerations and cultural competence.

Skin

It is necessary to examine the skin of the face, extremities, trunk, and legs, and note the color, temperature, moisture, and dryness in order to detect any signs indicative of a neurological problem. In Parkinson's disease, for example, the face is often oily, a condition called seborrhea (Victor & Ropper, 2001). Sebaceous adenomas following a butterfly area distribution over the bridge of the nose may suggest tuberous sclerosis (Victor & Ropper, 2001).

The nurse also should check for café au lait spots, which can be indicative of neurofibromatosis. Café au lait spots are more or less oval, with the long axis situated along a cutaneous (skin) nerve tract. They are light to medium brown, as reflected by the name, which means "coffee with milk" in French. They usually are present at birth, but may arise later in the first few years of life. They are much more common in black infants. To have a few such spots is totally normal. However, more than six such spots of greater than 1.5 mm in diameter in prepubertal or greater than 5 mm in diameter in postpubertal children will get the doctor's attention, because they are then essentially diagnostic of neurofibromatosis (although other features are required to make the diagnosis and some individuals may have multiple spots without having the disease—a trait that is itself inherited).

The nurse should also pay special attention to the lower lumbar area at the base of the spine. A dimple, with or without a tuft of hair, in that area can signify spina bifida or meningocele (Fuller, 2004).

Head, Neck, and Extremities

The health care provider should observe the responsiveness of the patient's facial expression and look for asymmetry. Parkinson's disease results in a poverty of facial expression, called **masked facies**, and facial asymmetry can be a subtle indication of facial weakness. Other assessment factors include the following:

- Listen to the patient speak to determine whether the speech is clear and fluent or hesitant. Is the patient able to find the correct words to express himself?
- Examine the head to determine whether the skull is abnormally large (**macrocephalic**) or small (**microcephalic**).
- Inspect the scalp for old incisions and palpate the skull to detect deformities that may suggest previous surgery or fractures.
- Palpate the temporal arteries, noting if the patient experiences tenderness.
- Inspect and palpate the neck, looking for thyroid enlargement or cervical lymphadenopathy (disease of the lymph nodes, synonymous with swollen or enlarged lymph nodes).
- Passively flex the neck to detect pain or limitation of movement, which suggests meningeal irritation.

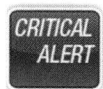 **CRITICAL ALERT** *When examining the neck of the patient, note if the patient has pain on flexion or extension. Brudzinski sign is flexion of the hips when the neck is flexed from a supine position. This is consistent with meningitis, and must be evaluated further.*

- Inspect for **Battle's sign** bruising immediately behind the ears, which refers to ecchymosis on the mastoid bone. **Raccoon sign** (or **eyes**), a darkening around the periorbital area that generates the appearance of a raccoon, refers to periorbital ecchymosis. These signs raise suspicion of basal skull fracture.

- Inspect the hands and fingers to detect deformity. Multiple ungula fibromas are a primary feature of tuberous sclerosis (Victor & Ropper, 2001).
- Inspect the legs to detect abnormally high arches or hammer toe deformity. Friedreich's ataxia, an inherited disease that causes progressive damage to the nervous system resulting in symptoms ranging from gait disturbance and speech problems to heart disease, and some of the hereditary sensor motor neuropathies are associated with high arches and hammer toes (Victor & Ropper, 2001).
- Observe hair distribution over the lower portion of the legs. Loss of hair from these regions occurs with autonomic neuropathies, frequently diabetic neuropathy.
- Use an otoscope to observe the canals and tympanic membrane. Cholesteatoma, or "pearly tumor," though rare, can be seen in the middle ear (Victor & Ropper, 2001). These tumors involve cranial nerve XII (discussed later in the chapter), and are associated with a history of chronic middle ear infections.
- Inspect the lips for cyanosis or pallor, and then look at the gingivae and teeth to detect **gingival hyperplasia**, proliferation of cells causing enlargement, pyorrhea, redness, or erosion. Examine the gums for hyperplasia, which can occur with phenytoin ingestion and ascorbic acid deficiency. Discoloration of the gums can result from heavy metals, notably copper and arsenic, and adrenocorticotrophic hormone.
- Note the color of the tongue and determine whether it is abnormally red, smooth, or fissured. Several vitamin deficiencies, such as niacin, riboflavin and cyanocobalamin are associated with a red, smooth tongue.

Lungs, Cardiac, and Abdomen

The nurse should assess for dyspnea, orthopnea, or shortness of breath. Heart sounds should be auscultated, noting the rate, rhythm, and tone and listening for murmurs. The carotid and subclavian arteries should be auscultated, listening for bruits.

The abdomen should be inspected and palpated to detect tenderness, masses, and abnormal pulsations. The nurse also should listen for bowel sounds. In the hospitalized patient with neurological disorders, bowel function is important to monitor. Ileus, or sluggishness of the bowel, can be common postoperatively.

◼ Neurological Examination

The neurological examination can be divided into five areas: the evaluation of mental status, cranial nerves, motor system, sensation, reflexes, and cerebellar function. In taking the history from the patient, the nurse has developed an impression of the mental status of the patient. However, formal mental status testing must be completed.

Mental Status Examination

Mental status is defined as "the functional state of the mind as judged by the individual's behavior, appearance, responsiveness to stimuli of all kinds, speech, memory, and judgment" (Thomas, 1997). The mental status examination assesses the higher cortical functions of thinking and reasoning as well as level of consciousness, orientation, attention, memory, affect and insight, speech and language, fund of knowledge, and abstraction.

Level of Consciousness

Level of consciousness (LOC) is a critical component of the neurological assessment. Consciousness is a state of awareness and can be a sensitive indicator of cortical function. Consciousness is disrupted easily by neurological damage or disease. Coma is the opposite state to consciousness, and between the two are a variety of altered states of awareness. Arousal is a state of responsiveness to sensory stimulation. Arousal requires both hemispheres and the upper brainstem to be intact (Stewart-Amidei & Bader, 2004). The health care provider should observe the patient's ability to respond to noxious stimuli in an appropriate manner. Awareness is the orientation to person, place, and time, and implies interaction with, and reaction to, environmental stimuli. In documenting the patient's LOC, the health care provider should include both the response and the stimulus that was required to produce the response. Evaluation of the LOC is most accurate when the patient is stimulated to a maximal state of arousal.

The Glasgow Coma Scale (GCS) is the most widely recognized LOC assessment tool (Chart 28–2). It is commonly used in emergency departments, trauma units, and intensive care areas (Teasdale & Jennett, 1974). This tool evaluates three areas: eye opening, verbal response, and best motor response. The highest score that can be attained is 15, and the lowest is 3. In general, a GCS of 8 or lower indicates a coma. When using the GCS for serial assessment, the clinician should note that it is not a sensitive tool for evaluation of altered sensorium. It does not account for aphasia and is not an indicator of lateralization of neurological deterioration. When completing the GCS it is important to score the best response for each category. For the motor response, the upper extremities are scored.

Another validated tool that has been developed more recently than the GCS is the FOUR Score Consciousness Scale (Wijdicks, Bamlet, Maramattom, Manno, & McClelland, 2005). This scale evaluates four components: eye, motor, brainstem, and respiration). Each component has a maximal score of 4. This scale provides greater neurological detail than the GCS. In contrast to the GCS, verbal response is not a component of the FOUR Score Consciousness Scale, making it fully applicable in intubated patients. See Chart 28–3 for a description of the scale.

Orientation

The patient is assessed for orientation to time, place, and person. Time orientation is assessed by evaluating awareness of the year, season, month, day of the week, and date. Place orientation is assessed via awareness of the state the patient is in, followed by city, county, name of the current location (hospital or medical office), and the floor the patient is currently on (or office number).

CHART 28–2 **Scoring for Glasgow Coma Scale**

Eye Opening (E)	Verbal Response (V)	Motor Response (M)
4 = Spontaneous	5 = Normal conversation	6 = Normal
3 = To voice	4 = Disoriented conversation	5 = Localizes to pain
2 = To pain	3 = Words, but not coherent	4 = Withdraws to pain
1 = None	2 = No words; only sounds	3 = Decorticate posture
	1 = None	2 = Decerebrate
		1 = None

Total = E + V + M

With the Glasgow Coma Scale, one determines the best eye opening response, the best verbal response, and the best motor response. The score represents the sum of the numeric scores of each of the categories. There are limitations to its use. If the patient has an endotracheal tube in place, she cannot talk. For this reason, many prefer to document the score by its individual components; so a patient with a Glasgow Coma Scale score of 15 would be documented as follows: E4 V5 M6. An intubated patient would be scored as E4 V intubated M6. Of these individual factors, the best motor response is probably the most significant.

Source: American College of Surgeons Committee on Trauma (2004). Advanced Trauma Life Support for Doctors (7th ed). Chicago: American College of Surgeons.

Time orientation often is impaired early, and many times may be the first sign of neurological change. In the hospitalized patient this may be the result of a sleep disturbance and/or sensory overload. Impaired orientation to place may occur with moderate cerebral dysfunction (Stewart-Amidei & Bader, 2004). Impaired orientation to person is generally the last parameter lost and occurs with severe dysfunction such as delirium or dementia.

Confusion is defined as not being aware of or oriented to, time, place, or self (*Dictionary of Cell and Molecular Biology*, 2008; Thomas, 1997). Confusion may be acute or chronic, and etiologies include metabolic disorders, infections, changes in underlying neurological disorder, and drug or alcohol intoxification. A list of validated tools to assess cognition is shown in Chart 28–4.

Attention and Concentration

Attention refers to the ability to focus on a particular stimulus, task, or situation. Concentration refers to the ability to sustain attention. Alteration in attention and concentration can be early indicators of delirium. To evaluate attention and concentration, the nurse asks the patient to count backwards from 100 by 7 (93, 86, 79, 72, 65). In the patient who is lacking in formal education, the nurse can ask for the days of the week or the months of the year backwards.

CHART 28–3 **FOUR Score Consciousness Scale**

Eye Response	Motor Response	Brainstem Reflexes	Respiration
4 = Eyelids open, tracking or blinking on command	4 = Thumbs up or fist to command	4 = Pupil and corneal reflex present	4 = Not intubated, regular breathing
3 = Eyelids open, not tracking	3 = Localizing to pain	3 = One pupil wide and fixed	3 = Not intubated, Cheyne-Stokes pattern
2 = Eyelids closed, but open to loud noise	2 = Flexion to pain	2 = Pupil **or** corneal reflex absent	2 = Not intubated, irregular pattern
1 = Eyelids closed, but open to pain	1 = Extensor posturing	1 = Pupil **and** corneal reflex absent	1 = Breathes above ventilator rate
0 = Eyelids closed with pain	0 = No response to pain or myoclonus status epilepticus	0 = Absent pupil, corneal, and cough reflex	0 = Breathes at ventilator rate or apnea

CHART 28–4   Cognitive Assessment Tools

Test Name	Evaluation	Scoring
Mini-Mental Status Examination (MMSE)	Evaluates orientation, language, memory, writing, ability to follow commands, calculations, constructional abilities.	30-item examination scored by correct responses: Maximum score = 30 Average score = 27.6 Cognitive impairment = 25 or less.
Short Portable Mental Status Questionnaire (SPMSQ)	Evaluates orientation, language, personal history, awareness and remote memory, and calculational ability.	Ten-item instrument scored by errors. Score of 3 or greater indicates impairment. Able to adjust for educational level. Add one error if person has completed 12th grade. Delete one error if person has not completed 12th grade.
Cognitive Capacity Screening Examination (CCSE)	Evaluates orientation, memory, attention, calculation, and extracting abilities. Most reliable for distinguishing between delirium and dementia.	30-item instrument scored by correct responses. Most reliable for distinguishing between acute and chronic disorders. Maximum score = 30. Score of 20 or below indicates cognitive impairment.

Memory

Memory, the ability to recover information about past events or knowledge, can be subdivided into remote, intermediate, and recent. Most questions related to memory can be asked in the context of obtaining the history.

Remote Memory

Some of the following questions can be asked to evaluate remote memory. The information from the patient can be validated by family or friends.

- Where and when were you born?
- How old are you?
- When did you graduate from high school?
- When were you married?
- What are the names, ages, and birth dates of your children?

Intermediate Memory

Intermediate memory can be evaluated by referring to personal and general events of the previous 5 years; for example, the patient could be asked to give a chronological account of the presenting illness including dates. The nurse could also inquire about common events of the previous 5 years, such as presidential elections.

Recent Memory

Recent memory can be tested in a variety of ways. The nurse could name three objects (i.e., apple, penny, table) and ask the patient to repeat them. Inform the patient you will be asking later for the patient to repeat the names of these objects. Wait 5 minutes, completing other aspects of the assessment, and then ask the patient to recall the three objects named previously. A person without cognitive deficit should be able to correctly recall the three objects. Another method is to ask the patient how she arrived at the place of assessment and with whom, or to name what she had for breakfast that day.

Affect and Insight

Assessment of affect, or display of emotions, begins with observation. **Euthymia** refers to a normal state; that is the patient is calm and appropriate. **Euphoria** is excessively cheerful or inappropriately cheerful. **Apathetic** is used to describe the patient who is flat or dull in appearance. **Dysphoria** is noted as being depressed, despondent, or sad. Validated tools to assess mood or affect are listed in Chart 28–5.

Insight refers to the ability to assess and monitor one's own cognitive, motor, or sensory function. Insight and reality orientation are frequently impaired in neurological diseases. The nurse

CHART 28–5   Affective Assessment Tools

Test Name	Evaluation	Scoring
Beck Depression Inventory (BDI)	Measures manifestations of depression. The BDI takes approximately 10 minutes to complete, although patients require a fifth to sixth grade reading age to adequately understand the questions. Is considered the gold standard for self-rating depression.	21-item self-report scale.
Hamilton Depression Rating Scale	Assesses the severity of depression for clinical purposes in adults of any age.	17-item scale that is rated by semistructured interview with trained interviewer.
Duke Anxiety-Depression Scale (DUKE-AD)	Brief screen for clinical anxiety and depression.	Seven items measured with a score of 5 or above indicates high risk for anxiety or depression.

can assess insight by asking the patient "Why are you being seen today?" or "Why are you in the hospital?"

Speech and Language

Fluency refers to the spontaneity, articulation, hesitancy, and duration of the patient's response. The nurse has evaluated the fluency of speech throughout the assessment. **Aphasia** is a disorder of speech and language due to cerebral dysfunction. The three primary aphasic deficits are in comprehension of spoken language, expressive language, and naming. Aphasic deficits can be localized to the area of dysfunction. Approximately 90% of the U.S. population is right-handed and left hemisphere dominant for language. Among people that are left-handed, two-thirds are thought to have left hemisphere language dominance, while the remainder has varying degrees of mixed or right hemisphere dominance (Fuller, 2004).

Most patients with neurological disorders have some communication function left intact. Carefully evaluating the patient's ability to communicate can aid in localizing a lesion to a specific area of the brain. The various aphasias can be subdivided into categories, and are listed in Chart 28–6 along with the respective areas of involvement.

To assess comprehension, or the ability to understand the spoken word, the patient is first asked to follow a simple instruction, such as "Close your eyes." If the patient is able to do so, increasing complex commands are given, "Touch your right ear with your left index finger." If the patient is able to carry out complex commands, this portion of the communication system appears intact.

- To evaluate the ability to understand the written word, commands of increasing difficulty are written on cards that are shown to the patient, who is asked to follow the instructions. Examples include "Open your mouth," "Stick out your tongue," and "Point to your right ear."
- To assess the ability to express ideas verbally, the patient is asked to identify common objects, such as a pencil or watch. The nurse then proceeds to ask open-ended questions, such as "Tell me about the kind of work you do" or "What types of activities do you enjoy in your free time?" or "Tell me about your illness."
- To test for naming, also called word finding difficulty, the patient is shown common objects such as a pen and watch, and asked to name the object.

CHART 28–6	Aphasias by Location

Aphasia	Location
Auditory receptive aphasia	Lesion at Wernicke's area of the temporal lobe
Visual receptive aphasia	Lesion at parietal-occipital area
Expressive speaking aphasia	Lesion at Broca's area of frontal lobe
Expressive writing aphasia	Lesion at posterior frontal area
Global aphasia (a form of aphasia that involves both expressive and receptive aphasias)	Lesions (extensive) of Broca's area, Wernicke's area, parietal-occipital area, and posterior frontal area

- If there is a question about the inability to express oneself in writing, the patient is given paper and pencil and asked to write his name and address. As with other aphasia evaluations, complexity is increased. The patient could be asked to write an account of a current news event or to describe the weather.

Fund of Knowledge and Abstraction

General fund of knowledge refers to the patient's knowledge base—an understanding of one's natural and social environment. This may be tested by asking questions such as, "How many nickels are in $1.15?" or asking the patient to list the last five presidents of the United States, or to list five major U.S. cities. The higher the number of correct answers, the better the understanding and knowledge base, taking into consideration the individual's educational background and other training.

Abstraction is measured by assessing the patient's ability to determine similarities. For example, one may ask the patient how two items are alike, an apple and an orange or a car and an airplane. The first answer would be good if the patient said "fruit"; it would be poor if the patient said "round." The second answer would be good if the patient said, "modes of transportation." The patient also may be asked the interpretation of proverbial phrases, e.g., what is the meaning of "do not cry over spilt milk?" A good response would be "do not get upset over the little things"; whereas a poor response might be "spilling milk is bad."

Cranial Nerve Examination

The cranial nerves (CNs) are referred to by specific name, as well as an assigned Roman numeral. For documentation purposes, they are referred to by the Roman numeral. They are called cranial nerves because they emerge from the cranium and can have sensory function, motor function, or both ability to recover information about past events or knowledge (Wilson-Pauwels, Akesson, Stewart, & Spacey, 2002). Cranial nerves numbered II through XII arise from the brainstem, as shown in Figure 28–4 ■.

Olfactory Nerve (CN I)

CN I has sensory function only. The sense of smell is tested by occluding one nostril while testing the other. A common odoriferous substance is placed under the unobstructed nostril. Coffee, lemon oil, and peppermint are common substances used. **Anosmia** is the inability to smell. Common neurological causes of anosmia include tumors of the frontal lobe, fractures of the anterior fossa, meningitis, hydrocephalus, and traumatic brain injury. Common nonneurological causes of anosmia include the common cold and inflammation of the nasal cavity. Recently, olfactory deficits have been described early in both Alzheimer's disease and Parkinson's disease (Luzzi, Snowden, Neary, Coccia, Provinciali, & Lambon, 2007). (See Chapters 33, 34, and 69 🕮.)

Optic Nerve (CN II)

CN II has sensory function only. Assessing the optic nerve involves inspecting the globe for cataracts, foreign bodies, or other obvious abnormalities; testing visual acuity; testing visual fields; and completing a funduscopic examination (see Chapter 71 🕮). To assess CN II, each eye is evaluated separately. Visual acuity can be assessed by asking the patient to read from a newspaper, or in the ambulatory setting a Snellen chart is frequently used. A Snellen chart is an eye chart used by eye care professionals and

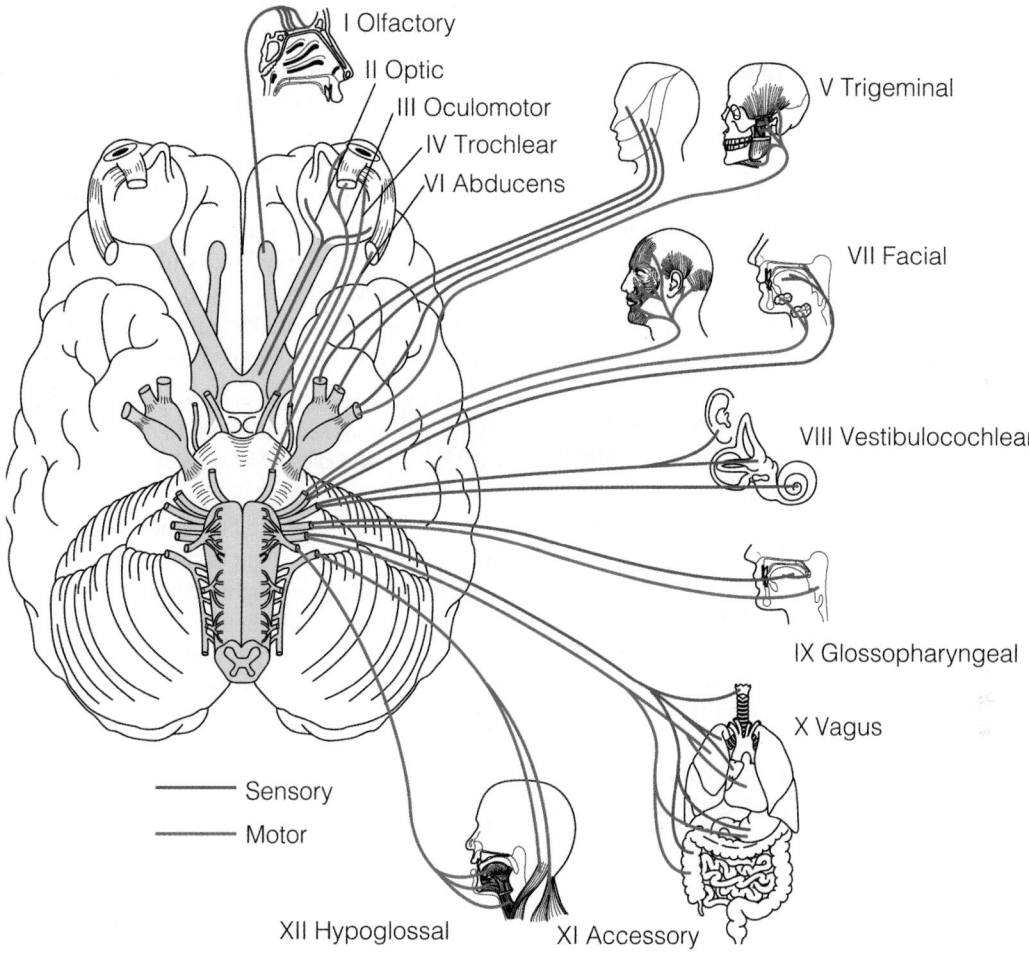

FIGURE 28–4 ■ Dorsal aspect of brain with cranial nerves noted.

others to measure visual acuity. Normal vision is 20/20, which means the patient can read the Snellen chart from a distance of 20 feet. A reading of 20/30 means the patient can read at 30 feet what the normal eye can read at 20 feet.

A visual field extends 60 degrees to the nasal side, 110 degrees to the temporal side, and 130 degrees vertically (Digre & Corbett, 2003). Visual fields are assessed using the confrontation test, whereby the patient and nurse face each other 2 feet apart. The patient is directed to cover one eye and look directly at the nurse. The nurse brings an object, such as a pencil, into each cardinal gaze and the patient indicates when she first sees the object. This test reveals only gross defects. Further testing would be indicated.

The funduscopic examination requires the use of an ophthalmoscope. The ophthalmoscope has a special lens that is used to visualize the inside of the eye by shining light directly into the eye. The room should be dimmed while performing this exam for best results. The nurse examines the patient's right eye by holding the ophthalmoscope in the right hand and using his right eye. The opposite is the case with the left eye. Figure 28–5 ■ illustrates obtaining a pupil response.

The fundus includes the optic disc, macula, and blood vessels on the back wall of the eye. The funduscopic examination is perceived as a difficult task, and is avoided by many nurses. It is essential, however, for the assessment of papilledema, or optic disc swelling, which is a hallmark of increased intracranial pressure.

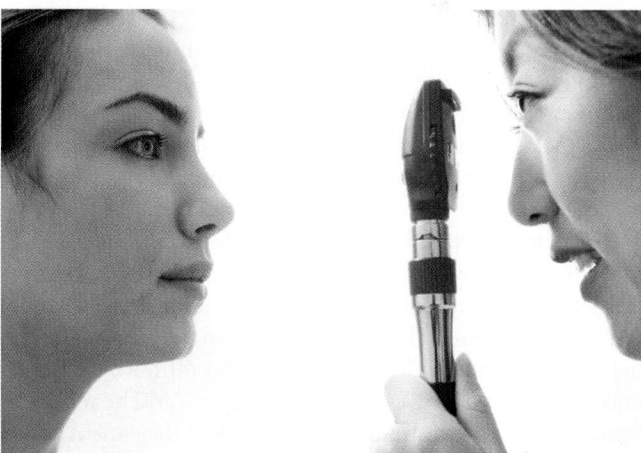

FIGURE 28–5 ■ Obtaining a pupil response.
Source: © Timothy Tadder/CORBIS All Rights Reserved

As with all things, practice increases comfort level, so the nurse is encouraged to practice funduscopic exams when possible. (See Chapter 71 😊).

Oculomotor (CN III), Trochlear (CN IV), and Abducens (CN VI) Nerves

Cranial nerves III, IV, and VI are usually tested together because they supply the various muscles that move the eye, and have motor function only. These three nerves supply the extraocular muscles, pupils, and eyelids. The first step in assessing these nerve functions is to observe the eyes. Note the position of the eyeball within the head. Are the eyes symmetrical? The abnormal protrusion of one or both eyeballs is called **proptosis** or **exophthalmos**. This is commonly seen in hyperthyroidism. Next, note the position of the upper eyelid in relation to the pupil and iris in each eye and compare. **Ptosis** is the term for a drooping upper eyelid, and can be seen in Horner's syndrome and myasthenia gravis.

Extraocular movements are evaluated by asking the patient to follow a finger or pencil through the six cardinal fields of gaze. In the patient without deficits, both eyes move at the same time in the same direction. This is referred to as **conjugate gaze**. If the eye movements are not the same, this is called **dysconjugate gaze**. Double vision may be present if the patient cannot move the eye in a particular direction. The loss of function of the muscles necessary for these movements may be caused by direct damage to the muscle or by injury of the cranial nerve. **Nystagmus** is an involuntary movement of the eyes that may be horizontal, vertical, or mixed in direction. There are multiple types of nystagmus; however, all involve a "jerky" movement of the eyes. Nystagmus is not uncommon in patients taking phenytoin for seizures.

In assessing the unconscious patient, the oculocephalic reflex (doll's eye response) and the oculovestibular reflex (cold calorics) are evaluated for reflex movement of the eye. The **oculocephalic reflex**, or **doll's eyes reflex**, is one in which the eyes move opposite the direction the head is turned, thus maintaining a more or less steady gaze. It is produced by moving the patient's head left to right or up and down. When the reflex is present, the eyes of the patient remain stationary while the head is moved, thus moving in relation to the head. In a normal, alert person, this brainstem reflex is inhibited by gaze control mechanisms. The eyes go wherever the cortex wants them to go. In the comatose patient, this inhibition is lost, and the oculocephalic reflex becomes disinhibited, and clinically demonstrable. Therefore, the eyes deviate in the direction opposite the head turning. This is a positive doll's eyes response. Eyes stay focused on whatever they were looking at before head turning.

The **oculovestibular reflex**, or cold calorics, is a reflex movement that stabilizes images on the retina during head movement by producing an eye movement in the direction opposite to head movement. This can be produced by placing the patient's upper body and head at 30 degrees off horizontal, and injecting 50 to 100 mL of cold water into an ear. The water has the same effect on the semicircular canal as if the patient's head was turned to the opposite side of the injection. Therefore, the patient's eyes will look toward the ear of injection. The eye deviation lasts for a sustained period of time. This is an excellent maneuver to assess extraocular muscles in the comatose patient with possible cervical spine injury. If the oculovestibular reflex is absent, a lesion of the pons, medulla, or less commonly the III, IV, IV, or VIII nerves is present. Unlike the oculocephalic reflex, the oculovestibular reflex is present in patients who are awake. In alert patients, this reflex not only induces eye deviation, it also produces nystagmus in the direction of the noninjected ear. The slow phase is toward the injected ear and the fast phase is away. The presence of these reflexes indicates the brainstem is intact.

To assess the pupils, the patient is directed to look at an object in the room, preferably straight ahead. In the unconscious patient, the pupils are examined as found. Pupils are examined for size, shape, and equality. The normal size of the pupil ranges from 2 to 6 mm. When the pupils are compared to each other, they should be equal; however, approximately 17% of the population has unequal pupil size without the presence of pathology (Wilson-Pauwels et al., 2002). This is called **anisocoria**. The normal pupil is round. Patients who have had cataracts removed will have a "keyhole"-shaped pupil of the affected eye.

 *An ovoid pupil indicates papillary dysfunction, and is seen in early herniation. This is a neurological emergency and must be addressed immediately.*

The pupils are next tested for reaction to light. This is called the direct light reflex. A light is directed into each pupil and then withdrawn. When the light is shone in the eye, the pupil should constrict; conversely, when the light is withdrawn, it should dilate. Additionally, when the light is directed to the eye, the opposite eye should constrict slightly. This is called the consensual light reflex.

 *A unilateral papillary dilation may represent excessive pressure and ultimately herniation of the medial temporal lobe. The nurse must communicate the assessment and observe the patient closely with serial assessments.*

The accommodation reflex is evaluated next. The patient is asked to focus on an object, such as the nurse's finger, that is positioned 2 or 3 feet directly in front of her and asked to follow it with her eyes. The finger is rapidly moved toward the patient's nose. The pupils should constrict when looking at the finger near her face.

In the unconscious patient, the maneuver to assess these nerves is called the doll's eyes maneuver, as previously discussed. To complete, the nurse must first ensure that cervical injury has been ruled out. The nurse then holds the eyelids open and briskly turns the head from side to side. If the eyes lag to the opposite side to which the head is turned, that is considered a positive response. Positive in this instance means the brainstem is intact. If the eyes are fixed, and move with the direction of the head, that is considered a negative response. Negative in this instance means there is a brainstem lesion.

Trigeminal Nerve (CN V)

The trigeminal nerve has both a sensory and motor component. The sensory component is tested with the patient's eyes closed as follows:

- The nurse places warm and cold objects on each side of the face randomly and asks the patient to identify the temperature.
- Touch is evaluated by using a piece of cotton or gauze and lightly touching each side of the face randomly, again asking the patient to identify the sensation.
- Pain is tested by using a sharp object to lightly touch each side of the face.
- The corneal reflex is tested by lightly touching the cornea with cotton, resulting in the patient blinking the stimulated eye.

The motor aspect of the fifth nerve innervates the muscles used for chewing. The patient is asked to tightly clamp the jaw and close the mouth. Palpate the muscles of the jaw, looking for symmetry.

Facial Nerve (VII)

The facial nerve has a sensory and motor function. The seventh nerve innervates the sense of taste in the anterior two-thirds of the tongue. Each side of the tongue is tested separately. The patient is asked to stick out his tongue and identify the taste of sugar. Water is then given and then repeated with a salty or sour substance.

The motor component is tested by observing the face at rest and while completing deliberate movements such as smiling, blowing air into the cheeks, wrinkling the forehead, and raising the eyebrows. If weakness or asymmetry is noted, it is essential to determine if the lesion involved is central or peripheral. Central facial weakness, indicated by weakness below the eyes indicates the cause is in the central nervous system, and can be related to a lesion in the contralateral frontal lobe, such as a patient with a stroke. The patient with central facial weakness is unable to lift the corner of the mouth to smile, but can wrinkle the forehead. If the entire side of the face is involved, the patient has a peripheral facial weakness, involving CN VII, such as Bell's palsy. In this case, the patient may have lost the ability to close the eyelids. The nurse must be aware of this and ensure that the eye is kept moist and protected. During sleep, the use of an "eye bubble" is appropriate. These are clear plastic devices that allow moisture to remain, yet protect the eye from trauma. Use of an eye patch or taping the lid closed while sleeping is appropriate as well.

Vestibulocochlear or Acoustic Nerve (CN VIII)

The acoustic nerve is a pure sensory nerve that is divided into two branches. The cochlear branch deals with hearing, and the vestibular branch is involved with balance. The vestibular branch is not routinely assessed. If the patient identifies symptoms of vertigo, tinnitus, or disturbed balance, more specific testing can be done, generally by the neurologists. These symptoms are common in Ménière's disease and acoustic neuromas (see Chapter 70 ☺).

The cochlear branch is tested by the nurse whispering numbers and the patient repeating them, or by asking the patient to close her eyes while the nurse rubs the thumb and first two fingers together testing each ear separately, and asking the patient to identify on which side they hear the noise. Bone and air conduction tests, using a tuning fork, though not routine, can be done as well. Damage to this nerve can result in impaired hearing, tinnitus, vertigo, nystagmus, and unilateral or bilateral deafness.

Glossopharyngeal (CN IX) and Vagus (CN X) Nerves

The glossopharyngeal and vagus nerves are generally tested together because their innervation overlaps in the pharynx. They have both sensory and motor functions. The glossopharyngeal nerve supplies sensory function to the pharynx, tonsils, and posterior third of the tongue. The motor component elevates the pharynx. To test, the patient is directed to open the mouth and say "aaah." The palate and uvula should move upward. The pharyngeal (gag) reflex is innervated by both the 9th and 10th nerves. To evaluate, the posterior pharynx is stimulated with a tongue blade. The pharynx should elevate and constrict and the tongue should

retract, or "gag." In the unconscious patient, the suction catheter can be used.

The vagus nerve controls swallowing and speaking by innervating the larynx and pharynx. When the patient has the mouth open and is saying "aaah," the uvula should be midline. The quality of the voice is assessed for hoarseness. The patient can be asked to repeat "No ifs, ands, or buts." Damage to this nerve can result in impaired sensation, dysphasia, dysarthria, dysphonia, excessive drooling, and stridor (see Chapter 34 ☺).

Spinal Accessory Nerve (CN XI)

The spinal accessory nerve has motor function only. This nerve innervates the sternocleidomastoid and trapezius muscles. To assess function, the patient is first asked to shrug the shoulders while the nurse uses resistance. The patient is then asked to turn the head to one side and push the chin against the nurse's hand. Damage to this nerve can result in impaired strength in lifting the shoulders or difficulty in turning the head to either side.

Hypoglossal Nerve (CN XII)

The patient is asked to open the mouth and stick out the tongue. The tongue is observed for deviation, atrophy, and **fasciculation,** a small, local involuntary muscle contracting or twitching visible under the skin. Next, the patient is asked to push the tongue against a tongue blade, to each side, to assess strength.

Motor Examination

The motor examination consists of assessing gait, muscle bulk, tone, and strength. The first aspect of the motor examination is the evaluation of the patient's gait. The patient is asked to walk naturally in the examination room. It is necessary to note posture, movement of body parts, and the type of steps taken. See Chart 28–7 for a description of gaits.

Each of the muscles to be evaluated is inspected. Each side of the body is compared against the other. Palpating the muscles can assist with detecting atrophy. Observe for fine or gross involuntary movements such as fasciculations, tremors, or myoclonic jerks. If muscles in an extremity appear asymmetric, each limb should be measured. A difference of 1 cm or less is not significant. As a general rule, loss of muscle bulk may be due to a peripheral nerve dysfunction such as brachial plexus or Guillain-Barré

CHART 28–7	Types of Gait
Gait	**Description**
Steppage	Associated with flaccidity of the leg and foot drop. The patient lifts the thigh and leg high, and the foot slaps against the floor. The patient looks as if he is walking up stairs.
Ataxic	Wide-based, staggering, and uncoordinated. Cannot stand with feet together.
Spastic	Leg extension, and shuffles with the legs stiff without lifting the feet.
Parkinsonian	In this gait, the hallmark is the loss of arm swing while walking. The head and body can be flexed forward and the legs are rigid. The feet shuffle, and the gait is slow.

syndrome. Guillain-Barré syndrome is a disorder in which the body's immune system attacks part of the peripheral nervous system. The first symptoms of this disorder include varying degrees of weakness or tingling sensations in the legs. In many instances the weakness and abnormal sensations spread to the arms and upper body. These symptoms can increase in intensity until certain muscles cannot be used at all and, when severe, the patient is almost totally paralyzed. In these cases the disorder is life threatening—potentially interfering with breathing and, at times, with blood pressure or heart rate—and is considered a medical emergency.

Muscle tone represents muscle resistance to passive movements. Tone is assessed by passive range of motion. Slight resistance on movement is indicative of normal muscle tone. Each extremity should be assessed, and should demonstrate smooth movement without change. Rigidity is a state of resistance that can be intermittent, such as cogwheel rigidity, when small regular jerks are felt. Flaccidity describes decreased muscle tone, or hypotonia. The muscle is weak and flabby.

In the unconscious patient, stimuli may elicit an abnormal motor response. Passive range of motion is done to assess muscle tone in these patients. Additionally response to pain is evaluated. Pain is elicited by means of a sternal rub, squeezing of a nail bed, or pinching of the sternocleidomastoid muscle. When painful stimuli are applied, if the patient demonstrates flexion of the arm, wrist, and fingers while adducting the upper extremity, this is known as **decorticate posturing**, or abnormal flexion. The lower extremities are extended, internally rotated, and plantar flexed. **Decerebrate posturing**, an abnormal body posture that involves rigid extension of the arms and legs, downward pointing of the toes, and backward arching of the head, is seen in the presence of noxious or painful stimuli. The patient clenches his teeth with arm extension in an adducted and hyperpronated fashion. Lower extremities are extended with plantar flexion. Because the lower extremities have similar positions in both motor responses, the upper extremities are used to identify the posturing. It is possible to demonstrate both abnormal responses simultaneously, or each intermittently. Abnormal extension is believed to be the more grave of the two responses (Wilson-Pauwels et al., 2002). It is imperative that the nurse caring for the unconscious patient notify the responsible health care provider treating the patient for immediate intervention.

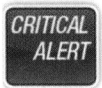 **CRITICAL ALERT** *When caring for the unconscious patient, it is imperative for the nurse to contact the treating clinician when a patient begins to demonstrate abnormal flexion or extension, or if the patient alternates between one and the other.*

Muscle strength is evaluated in both the upper and lower extremities. Each muscle group is assessed by using passive range of motion against gravity followed by active resistance positioned by the nurse and graded based on the ability to move against resistance. Chart 28–8 shows gradations of muscle strength.

To evaluate the upper extremities begin by observing for mild hemiparesis. Direct the patient to close his eyes and place the arms straight out in front of him with the palms up. Observe for 20 to 30 seconds. If one arm lowers slowly, this is referred to as drift. If the hand pronates, this is noted as pronator drift. These are subtle signs of hemiparesis (muscle weakness on one side of the body). Ask the patient to place the arms at the side

CHART 28–8 **Muscle Strength**

Muscle Function Level	Grade	Percentage of Normal
No evidence of contractility	0	0
Slight contractility, no movement	1	10
Muscle able to move with support against gravity	2	25
Muscle able to move without support against gravity	3	50
Muscle able to move without support against gravity with weakness to applied resistance	4	75
Muscle able to move through full range of motion with no weakness to applied resistance	5	100

with elbows flexed and abducted to 90 degrees. Resistance is applied. This assesses the deltoid muscle. The biceps is tested by flexing the elbow and, with the forearm supinated, the patient is directed to pull in against resistance. The patient is then directed to push the arm away against resistance, testing the triceps.

To evaluate the lower extremities, the patient is asked to sit on the examination table, or on the edge of the hospital bed, with the legs dangling freely. The patient is asked to lift the knee up as if walking up a stair. Resistance is then applied, allowing the nurse to assess the iliopsoas muscle. The patient is then asked to pull the lower leg back toward the table, which tests the hamstring group. This is followed by directing the patient to push the lower leg out toward the nurse applying resistance, thereby testing the quadriceps.

Next the feet are examined. The patient is directed to pull the toes up; this dorsiflexion tests the tibialis anterior; the patient then follows up with plantar flexion, which tests the gastrocnemius. These are important in assessing for foot drop. Chart 28–9 indicates major spinal cord segments with the corresponding functional ability and specific muscles to be tested.

Muscle strength assessment is a key factor in determining a diagnosis. Weakness or asymmetry can be seen in neuromuscular disorders such as myasthenia gravis, cerebral vascular accidents, cranial space–occupying lesions, spinal cord lesions or compression, and many others.

Sensory Examination

In the evaluation of sensory function, the patient is tested with the eyes closed. As with muscle testing, each side of the body is

CHART 28–9 **Muscle Innervation**

Reflex	Spinal Level
Biceps	C_5–C_6
Triceps	C_6–C_7
Patellar	L_4
Achilles	S_1

compared to the opposite. The examination is completed in a distal to proximal fashion. Areas for evaluation include hands, forearms, upper arms, trunk, thighs, legs, feet, and perineal and perirectal regions. Primary sensory modalities include light touch, superficial pain, temperature, position sense, and vibratory sense. A dermatome chart is helpful to use as a reference when assessing sensation and the patient's response to testing (Figure 28–6 ■).

Light touch is tested by using a wisp of cotton as the stimulus. The patient is asked to identify when he feels something. The nurse lightly touches the skin with the cotton beginning at the head and moving downward. Light touch can be preserved while other modalities are compromised in lesions of the spinal cord (see Chapter 32 ☺). Superficial pain is assessed in the same manner as light touch; however, the nurse uses a pin or other disposable sharp instrument for the stimulus. Temperature sensation is assessed in the same fashion as pain and touch. Test tubes filled with warm and cold water can be used. Others prefer to run warm and cold water over tuning forks. The disparate temperature objects are used as the stimuli.

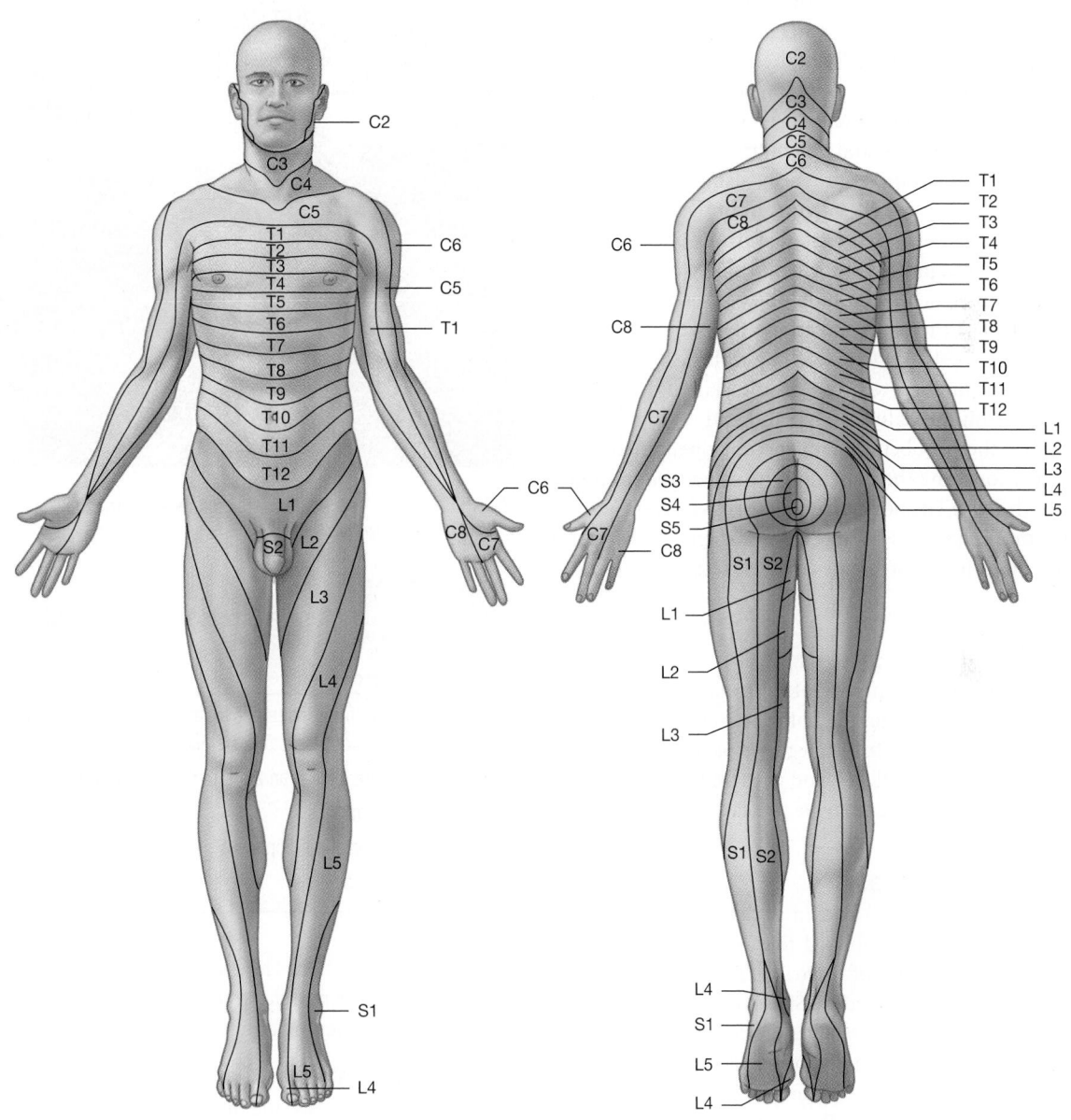

Levels of principal dermatomes

C5	Clavicles
C5, 6, 7	Lateral parts of upper limbs
C8, T1	Medial sides of upper limbs
C6	Thumb
C6, 7, 8	Hand
C8	Ring and little fingers
T4	Level of nipples
T10	Level of umbilicus
T12	Inguinal or groin regions
L1, 2, 3, 4	Anterior and inner surfaces of lower limbs
L4, 5, S1	Foot
L4	Medial side of great toe
S1, 2, L5	Posterior and outer surfaces of lower limbs
S1	Lateral margin of foot and little toe
S2, 3, 4	Perineum

FIGURE 28–6 ■ Dermatome man.

Vibratory sense is tested using a tuning fork. The bony prominences are used, such as the great toe, malleolus, patella, elbow, and wrist. The vibrating tuning fork is placed on these areas and the patient is asked to describe the feeling. Many will use the word "buzzing" to describe the sensation. The patient is then asked to tell the nurse when the feeling stops. Diminished distal vibratory sense is commonly seen in diabetic neuropathy and involves the dorsal columns of the spinal cord (Ziegler, Siekeirka-Kleiser, & Schweers, 2005). (See Chapters 31 and 32 ⊙.)

To assess **proprioception**, the ability to determine spatial body position, the patient again is instructed to close the eyes. The nurse should grasp the great toe by the side of the joint and move the toe in a forward-to-backward manner. This also may be done using the thumb as well. Once the thumb or great toe is pointing in an upward or downward position, the patient is asked to state which direction the digit is pointing. This is repeated using both the upward and downward positions.

Two-point discrimination is tested by using calipers or a compass. The patient is touched with one or both sharp objects at the same time and then asked to state if it was one object or two. Stereognosis (recognition of form and shape of objects by touch) is assessed by placing common objects, such as a pencil or key, in the palm of the hand and asking the patient to identify the object. Graphesthesia (the sense by which a person recognizes figures or numbers written on the skin) is tested by tracing a number on the palm of the hand and asking the patient to identify the number. The extinction phenomenon is tested by lightly touching the patient in the same area simultaneously on both sides. The normal response is to feel both stimuli; an abnormal response is noted if the patient consistently feels only one stimuli. Abnormalities in these tests indicate cortical dysfunction.

Reflex Examination

Evaluating reflexes provides important information on the status of the central nervous system in both the conscious and unconscious patient. There are three categories of reflexes: muscle stretch reflexes, superficial reflexes, and pathologic reflexes. Abnormalities in reflex responses may be the earliest sign of CNS dysfunction.

Muscle Stretch Reflexes

Muscle stretch reflexes are also known as deep tendon reflexes (DTRs). These reflexes are evaluated first, using a percussion hammer at the muscle's point of insertion. The stimulus of the hammer causes the muscle to stretch. Sites commonly tested are the biceps, triceps, patella, and Achilles tendon. The procedure for testing these reflexes is shown in Figure 28–7 ■.

Forearm flexion is the normal response when the brachial tendon is tapped with the hammer. Forearm extension is the response to the triceps stimuli. Stimuli to the area just below the patella results in leg extension, and plantar flexion of the foot is seen when the Achilles is tapped. Muscle stretch reflexes are graded based on the briskness of the response. The grade ranges from zero (no response) to four (hyperactive). Chart 28–10 illustrates muscle stretch reflexes.

Superficial Reflexes

Superficial reflexes are elicited by lightly stroking the skin or mucous membrane of the area tested. Chart 28–11 lists the most

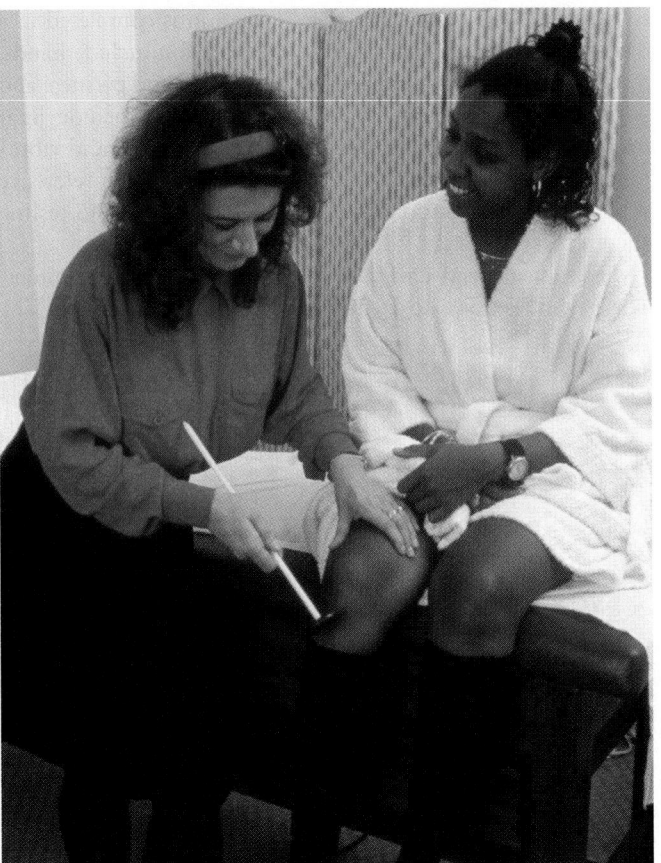

FIGURE 28–7 ■ Procedure for testing muscle stretch reflexes.
Source: © Hattie Young/Photo Researchers, Inc.

CHART 28–10	Muscle Stretch Reflexes and Scoring
Grade	**Description**
4+	Very brisk, hyperactive; muscle contracts multiple times, generally indicative of disease
3+	More brisk than 2+, can be normal for the individual
2+	Normal
1+	Diminished response
0	No response

common reflexes tested. The grading of superficial reflexes is different from that of muscle stretch reflexes. When evaluating superficial reflexes, they are scored as present (+) or absent (−).

Pathologic Reflexes

Pathologic reflexes, as the name implies, are abnormal responses. The extensor plantar response is also known as the Babinski reflex. It is tested by using a moderately sharp object, such as the handle of the percussion hammer, and stroking the lateral aspect of the sole of the foot from the heel to the ball of the foot, curving medially across the ball. Observe the movement of the toes, normally in flexion. Dorsiflexion of the great toe, with fanning of the other toes is seen. Figure 28–8 ■ shows pathologic reflexes.

Additional pathologic reflexes include the grasp reflex, snout reflex, and sucking reflex. These reflexes also are known as prim-

CHART 28–11   Superficial Reflexes

Reflex	Corresponding Spinal Nerve	Description
Abdominal	$T_8, T_9, T_{10}, T_{11}, T_{12}$	Each side of the abdomen is stroked lightly. Each quadrant is tested separately. The umbilicus should move in the direction of the skin stimulated.
Anal	S_3, S_4, S_5	The skin at the side of the anus is scratched with a blunt instrument or pin. There should be puckering of the anus.
Bulbocavernous	S_3, S_4	Direct pressure is applied to the muscle behind the scrotum and pinching the glans penis. The muscle should contract.
Cremasteric	L_1, L_2	The inner aspect of the thigh or lower abdomen is stroked lightly. There should be elevation of the opposite testicle, or both testicles.

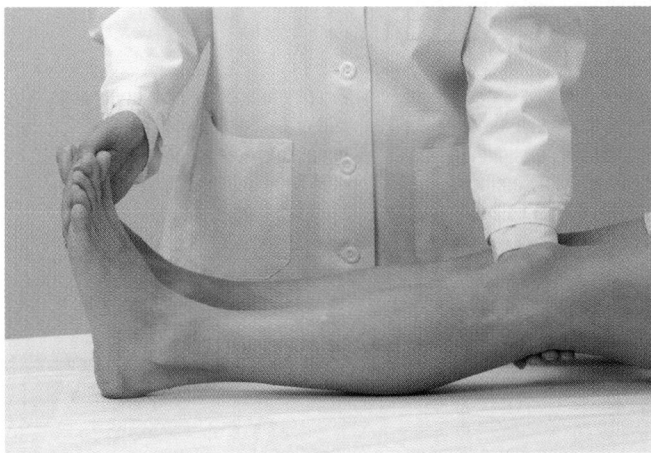

FIGURE 28–8 ■ Procedure for testing pathologic reflexes.

itive reflexes because they are normally seen in early stages of development and disappear. The grasp reflex is elicited by placing two fingers in the palm of the patient's hand. The hand grasps the fingers involuntarily. The snout reflex is seen when the oral region is gently percussed. The response is the puckering of the lips. The sucking reflex is seen when the oral region is stimulated. This may be seen when the patient's mouth is suctioned, or when oral care is done. Pathologic reflexes are graded in the same fashion as the superficial reflexes, in that the reflex is either present or absent. The difference is that in pathologic reflexes, present (+) is abnormal and absent (−) is normal.

Cerebellar Examination

The cerebellar system is important in the coordination of movement. The cerebellum can be separated into two clinically useful divisions: the midline and lateral. The midline aspect of the cerebellum is concerned mainly with head position, maintenance of posture, and oculomotor function. The lateral aspect is involved with limb use and execution of fine coordinated movements. Patients with cerebellar pathology can exhibit dysfunction of both divisions.

Various methods are used to assess balance and coordination. The following are some of the more commonly used methods:

1. Starting with the arms outstretched, the patient is asked to touch her nose. Then the patient is asked to repeat the maneuver with her eyes closed.

2. The nurse, using his index finger, asks the patient to touch the nurse's index finger with the patient's own index finger while the nurse is moving the finger, essentially asking the patient to touch a moving target.

3. In the Romberg test the patient is asked to stand with the feet together, first with the eyes open, and then closed. If the patient can stand with the eyes open, but sways or loses balance with them closed, she is said to have a positive Romberg's test.

 *When performing the Romberg test, it is important for the nurse to stand close to the patient to prevent the patient from falling.*

4. In the patient who is supine, the patient is directed to run the heel of the foot down the shin of the opposite leg. The procedure is repeated on the opposite leg.

A composite list of neurological assessment guidelines is shown in Chart 28–12 (p. 710).

Gerontological Considerations

Neurological disorders are the primary cause of disability in older adults. These disorders account for 50% of disability in those over 65 years of age and greater than 90% of serious dependency (Drachman, Long, & Swearer, 1994; Partners in Research, 2008). The impact of neurological diseases and disorders in the older adult is significant. Whether the older adult is experiencing an acute neurological event or a chronic disabling condition, nurses are pivotal in assessment, treatment, and continuing care. The assessment guidelines are derived from the American Association of Neuroscience Nurses' *Neurological Assessment of the Older Adult: A Guide for Nurses* (2007), a publication in its Clinical Practice Guidelines Series.

History

When obtaining a history from patients over 65 years of age, it is important to use a calm, ordered approach. Due to decreased processing speed, it is helpful to allow adequate time for the patient to respond and for giving verbal instructions (Whitney, Pugh, & Mortimer, 2004). If the patient uses adaptive devices, such as hearing aids, glasses, or walkers, one should attempt to have them in place during the assessment (Pepper, 2006).

CHART 28–12	**Neurological Assessment Guidelines**

Function	Neuroanatomic Correlate	Assessment Strategy	Common Disorders

Mental Status
1. Consciousness
2. Cognition
3. Affect
4. Speech and language
    4a. Dysarthria
    4b. Aphasia
	1. CNS: bilateral hemispheres, reticular activating system
	2. CNS: Bilateral hemispheres, primarily cortical areas
	3. CNS: limbic system, specific cortical areas
	    4a. CNS and PNS: subcortical lesions— brainstem, cerebellar, CN V, VII, IX, X, XII
	    4b. CNS: specific areas of the left frontal, temporal, parietal, and occipital lobes
		Observation: Is the patient alert? Responding to environment? Requiring painful stimuli to respond?
		Assessment: Does the patient know the date? Time? Month? Can he recall how he arrived at the point of care? Is the mood congruent with affect? Does he see things others do not see (hallucinations)? Can he repeat this sentence: "Around a rugged rock the ragged rascal ran"? Is speech free flowing? Can he identify objects correctly?
			Delirium, dementia, coma, accidents, trauma, infection, cerebral vascular accidents, tumors, neurodegenerative disorders

Cranial Nerves 1. Motor 2. Sensory 3. Motor and sensory	PNS 1. CN III, IV, VI supply the extraocular muscles, pupils, and eyelids. CN XI innervates the sternocleidomastoid and trapezius muscles. CN XII innervates the tongue. 2. CN I, II supply the sense of smell, visual acuity, and visual fields. CN VIII supplies hearing and balance. 3. CN V is responsible for facial temperature, touch, pain, and corneal reflex. Jaw muscles are innervated. CN VII innervates taste in the anterior 2/3 of tongue, and facial movements. CN IX, X supply the pharynx including gag reflex. Voice quality, including hoarseness, is involved.	*Examination:* Necessary equipment includes odiferous substance, ophthalmoscope, pen light, Snellen chart (or other acuity method), tongue blade, cotton ball, tuning fork.	Brainstem lesions, pituitary lesions, cerebral vascular accidents, neoplasm, neurodegenerative disorders, Bell's palsy, Ménière's syndrome, acoustic neuromas, schwannoma, local trauma
Motor 1. Gait 2. Bulk 3. Tone 4. Strength	CNS, PNS: Involves the cortical motor strip, pyramidal tracts, cerebellum and spinal cord as well as the innervation of peripheral muscles.	*Observation:* Is there a normal gait? Does she walk straight? Does she need an assistive device? Is her stance wide based? Do her feet leave the floor? Are involuntary movements present? Is muscle tone normal?	Cerebral vascular accidents, spinal cord injury, demyelinating disorders such as multiple sclerosis, transverse myelitis, neurodegenerative-normal pressure hydrocephalus, multisystem atrophy, Parkinson's disease, familial ataxic disorders, neuromuscular disorders such as amyotrophic lateral sclerosis
Sensory/Reflex 1. Light touch 2. Superficial pain 3. Temperature 4. Proprioception 5. Vibratory sense 6. Muscle stretch reflex Superficial reflex Pathologic reflex	CNS, PNS: Involves spinothalamic tracts, postcentral gyrus, parietal lobe, dermatomes.	*Examination:* Necessary equipment includes cotton ball, lancet (or other disposable sharp object), test tubes with disparate temperature liquid, and tuning fork, reflex hammer.	Spinal cord injury, polyneuropathy (B_{12} deficiency, anemias, diabetes), neurodegenerative disorders, cerebral vascular accidents, coma
Elimination 1. Bowel 2. Bladder	CNS, ANS 1. ANS: spinal nerves S_3–S_5, cortical areas 2. ANS: spinal nerves T_9–L_2, S_4, cortical areas	*Examination:* Check for incontinence or impaction, assess muscle tone and sensation, bladder scan for postvoid residual.	Spinal cord injury, cerebral vascular accident

In the geriatric population, the use of anticoagulant mediation is common. The use of an anticoagulant, in the presence of fall risk, can lead to a subdural hematoma if the patient were to fall and strike his head. The nurse must evaluate the fall potential of all older patients who are on anticoagulant medication.

Mental Status Examination

Older patients generally have normal levels of consciousness and are alert. It is an abnormal finding if the patient is not oriented to situation, time, and place (Sirven & Mancall, 2002). Similarly, it is an abnormal finding if the patient has difficulty with calculations or impaired judgment. Remote and recent memory are normal; however, the processing speed and information retrieval capability are slowed (Sirven & Mancall, 2002; Whitney et al., 2004). Therefore, if problems are noted with speech and language, underlying pathology must be considered. Mood and affect should be evaluated. Two questions to ask are "During the past month have you been bothered by feeling sad, depressed, or hopeless?" and "During the past month have you often been bothered by decreased interest or pleasure in doing things?" These questions have 96% sensitivity for detecting major depression, signifying the need for further follow-up (Johnston, Covinsky, & Landefeld, 2005).

Cranial Nerve Assessment of the Elderly

Cranial assessment of the elderly provides a basis for a functional assessment, which provides data regarding possible and potential impairments as well as ability to care for self.

Cranial Nerve	Comment
CN I	Deficits are common with aging (Larner, 2006).
CN II	Presbyopia. Depth, motion perception, and contrast sensitivity decreased (Larner, 2006).
CNs III, IV, VI	Pupils are generally smaller, known as *senile myosis*, and reflexes to light and accommodation become slower. This is due to aging changes in the muscles of the sphincter pupillae and lens, not neurological changes. Restricted upward motion may also result in convergence difficulties (Benassi, D'Alessandro, Gallassi, Morreale, & Lugaresi, 1990; Larner, 2006).
CN V	Decreased lacrimal secretions (Hobdell et al., 2004).
CN VII	Presbycusis (a progressive bilaterally perceptive hearing loss) (Larner, 2006).
CNs VII, IX, X	Decreased taste bud number, but increased perception of salty, sweet, sour, and bitter (Hobdell et al., 2004).
CN XI	Delay in swallowing (Hobdell et al., 2004).

Motor Examination

Muscle tone can alter with age, with increased tone being the most common. Strength is preserved except for a mild reduction in power proximally with advancing age (Sirven & Mancall, 2002). Action tremors often occur; however, they are not a normal aspect of aging. Motor reaction time is decreased with older age (Sirven & Mancall, 2002).

Sensory Examination

The most common expression of aging seen on the neurological examination is in the sensory evaluation. Impairment of loss of vibratory sense in the distal aspect of the lower extremities is a well-known finding. Conversely, proprioception is preserved. Decreases in two-point discrimination and stereognosis have been reported, but are not well characterized (Sirven & Mancall, 2002).

Reflex Examination

Muscle stretch reflexes are generally preserved in the elderly, and absence or asymmetry generally indicates disease. Decreased or absence of ankle jerks are common but thought to be due to Achilles tendon inelasticity versus true neurological change (Sirven & Mancall, 2002). Superficial reflexes may be diminished or absent, likely due to other causes such as pregnancies, history of abdominal surgery, and the like. The snout reflex may return, and is not considered pathologic. However, the suck and grasp reflex are indicative of frontal lobe disease.

Summary

The neurological assessment of a patient begins in the same fashion as any other type of system assessment, and that is with the history. The examination consists of the evaluation of cognition, cranial nerves, motor function, sensation, and reflexes. The techniques described in this chapter will assist the nurse in the incorporation of the nursing process and the development of a problem list and a plan of care.

NCLEX® REVIEW

1. The nurse, providing care to a patient with multiple sclerosis, realizes the patient has a disorder within which of the following areas of the neurological system?

   1. Central nervous system
   2. Peripheral nervous system
   3. Sympathetic nervous system
   4. Autonomic nervous system

2. The nurse is assessing a patient who is demonstrating a neurological disorder. In which area of the health history would the nurse document current medications?

   1. Presenting problem
   2. History of presenting problem
   3. Medication history
   4. Past medical history

3. While assessing a patient's neurological status, the nurse notes the patient is unable to move his head from left to right. This finding could indicate a disorder with which of the following cranial nerves?

   1. Vagus
   2. Hypoglossal
   3. Spinal accessory
   4. Facial

4. While assessing a patient's neurological status, the nurse uses the Glasgow Coma Scale. For which part of the mental status examination is this tool most likely used?

   1. Level of consciousness
   2. Language
   3. Memory
   4. Attention

5. After assessing a patient's patellar reflex, the nurse documents +2 on the patient's medical record. This document indicates the patient's reflex is:

   1. Indicative of disease.
   2. More brisk.
   3. Normal.
   4. Diminished.

6. The nurse is going to assess for the presence of a Babinski reflex. Which of the following will the nurse use to assess this reflex?

   1. Rubber triangle end of the reflex hammer
   2. Handle of the reflex hammer
   3. Safety pin
   4. Cotton swab

7. While assessing an elderly patient's cranial nerves, the nurse notes a sluggish pupilary response to light and accommodation. This finding could be indicative of:

   1. Cranial frontal lobe disease.
   2. Cerebellar disease.
   3. A pending stroke.
   4. Nothing; this can be a normal finding.

Answers for review questions appear in Appendix D

KEY TERMS

anisocoria *p.704*
anosmia *p.702*
apathetic *p.701*
aphasia *p.702*
Battle's sign *p.699*
conjugate gaze *p.704*
decerebrate posturing *p.706*
decorticate posturing *p.706*
doll's eye reflex *p.704*
dysconjugate gaze *p.704*

dysphoria *p.701*
euphoria *p.701*
euthymia *p.701*
exophthalmos *p.704*
fasciculation *p.705*
gingival hyperplasia *p.699*
macrocephalic *p.699*
masked facies *p.699*
microcephalic *p.699*

neuron *p.694*
nystagmus *p.704*
oculocephalic reflex *p.704*
oculovestibular reflex *p.704*
proprioception *p.708*
proptosis *p.704*
ptosis *p.704*
raccoon sign (eyes) *p.699*
synapse *p.694*

REFERENCES

American Association of Neuroscience Nurses. (2007). *Neurological assessment of the older adult: A guide for nurses.* Glenview, IL: Author.

American Nurses' Association. (2002). *Scope and standards of neuroscience nursing practice.* Silver Spring, MD: Author.

Centers for Disease Control and Prevention. (2007). Prevalence of stroke—United States, 2005. *Morbidity and Mortality Weekly Report.* Retrieved April 15, 2008, from http://www.cdc.gov/MMWR/previdw/mmwrhtml/mm5619a2.htm

Dictionary of Cell and Molecular Biology. (2008). Confusion. Retrieved June 24, 2008, from the Centre for Cancer Education, University of Newcastle, website: http://cancerweb.ncl.ac.uk/cgi-bin/omd?confusion

Digre, K. B., & Corbett, J. B. (2003). *Practical viewing of the optic disc.* New York: Butterworth-Heinemann.

Fuller, G. (2004). *Neurological examination made easy* (3rd ed.). Philadelphia, PA: Churchill Livingstone.

Johnston, C. B., Covinsky, K. E., & Landefeld, S. (2005). Geriatric medicine. In L. M. Tierney, Jr., S. J. McPhee, & M. A. Papadakis (Eds.), *Current medical diagnosis and treatment.* New York: Lange.

Joute, A., Corpechot, C., & Ducros, A. (1996). Notch 3 mutations in CADASIL, a hereditary adult-onset condition causing stroke and dementia. *Nature, 383,* 707–710.

Luzzi, S., Snowden, J. S., Neary, D., Coccia, M., Provinciali, L., & Lambon, R. (2007). Distinct patterns of olfactory impairment in Alzheimer's disease, semantic dementia, frontotemporal dementia, and corticobasal degeneration. *Neuropsychologia, 45*(8), 1826–1831.

Newman, M. F. (2007). Open heart surgery and cognitive decline. *Cleveland Clinic Journal of Medicine, 74*(1) 52–55.

Pepper, G. A. (2006). Critical care patient with special needs: Geriatric patients. In J. G. Alspach (Ed.), *Core curriculum for critical care nurses* (6th ed.). Philadelphia: W. B. Saunders.

Reyes, P. F., Nowak, L. A., & Rice, S. G. (2006). Alzheimer's disease: Clinical diagnosis and treatment. *Barrow Quarterly, 22*(1), 9–15.

Sirven, J. I., & Mancall, E. (2002). Neurological examination of the older adult. In J. I. Sirven & B. L. Malamut (Eds.), *Clinical neurology of the older adult.* Philadelphia: Lippincott.

Stewart-Amidei, C. (2006). Why bother with practice guidelines? *Journal of Neuroscience Nursing. 38*:3.

Teasdale, G., & Jennett, B. (1974). Assessment of coma and impaired consciousness: A practical scale. *Lancet, 2,* 81.

Thomas, C. L. (Ed.), (1997). *Taber's cyclopedic medical dictionary.* Philadelphia: F. A. Davis.

Victor, M., & Ropper, A. (2001). *Adams and Victor's principles of neurology* (7th ed.). New York: McGraw-Hill.

Whitney, F., Pugh, D., & Mortimer, D. (2004). Geriatric issues. In M. K. Bader & L. R. Littlejohn (Eds.), *AANN core curriculum for neuroscience nursing* (4th ed.). St. Louis, MO: W. B. Saunders.

Wijdicks, E. F., Bamlet, W. R., Maramattom, B. V., Manno, E. M., & McClelland, R. L. (2005). Validation of a new coma scale: The FOUR Score. *Annals of Neurology, 58*(4), 585–593.

Wilson-Pauwels, L., Akesson, E. J., Stewart, P. A., & Spacey, S. D. (2002). *Cranial nerves in health and disease* (2nd ed.). Hamilton, Ontario: BC Decker.

World Health Organization. (2007). *Weekly epidemiological record.* No. 12, *82,* 93–194.

Ziegler, D., Siekeirka-Kleiser, E., & Schweers, M., (2005). Validation of a novel screening device (NeuroQuick) for quantitative assessment of small nerve fiber dysfunction as an early feature of diabetic polyneuropathy. *Diabetes Care, 28*(5), 1169–1174.

Caring for the Patient with Acute Brain Disorders

Denita Ryan

Outcome-Based Learning Objectives

After studying this chapter, the learner will be able to:

1. Describe basic pathophysiology of increased intracranial pressure as presented in this chapter.
2. List possible signs or symptoms of increased intracranial pressure.
3. Explain rationale of nursing interventions in caring for patients with increased intracranial pressure.
4. Identify various types and causes of head trauma according to level of injury.
5. Compare and contrast differences between bacterial meningitis and viral meningitis, including causes, signs and symptoms, diagnostic evaluation, and treatment.
6. Identify and distinguish between the major types of brain tumors: intra-axial, extra-axial, and metastatic.
7. Explain treatment options for brain tumors.
8. Explain the role of the nurse in family teaching of patients with acute brain disorders.

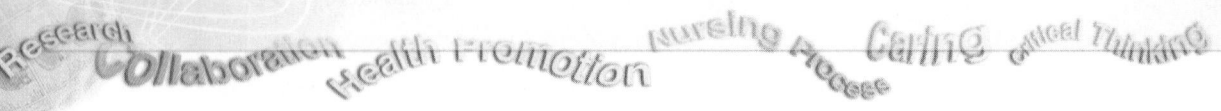

ACUTE BRAIN disorders include a wide range of conditions, such as traumatic injuries, brain tumors, and infectious diseases of the brain. Each of these disorders may affect not just the central nervous system, but every other system of the body as well. The symptoms of the disorders have a tremendous effect on not only the patient, but also on family, friends, and their community.

Intracranial Pressure

An important and underlying physiological concept in the care of any patient with an acute neurological disorder is that of **intracranial pressure (ICP)** or pressure in the head and the mechanisms of its alteration. Any disorder of the brain can cause an increase in intracranial pressure, which may have wide-reaching effects on the patient's neurological status and overall health.

Healers throughout history have known, or at least suspected, that pressure in the head causes harmful outcomes. Trepanations, or the creation of holes in the skull, were apparently performed for thousands of years to relieve pressure in the brain. A historic archeological find in France discovered 120 skulls, 40 of which had been trepanned. The trepanation tools found in Europe were thought to be 4,000 to 5,000 years old. Trepanations have also been attributed to the Incas and a large number of other ancient civilizations throughout the world (Walker, 1967). Hippocrates acknowledged in his early writings on ancient medicine

that relieving pressure in the head must be done to relieve "dropsy of the brain" (Key, Rothrock, & Falk, 1997).

Monro-Kellie Doctrine

Monro wrote in 1783 "brine enclosed in a case of bone ... the substance of the brain ... is nearly incompressible, the quantity of blood in the head must be the same ... those cases only excepted in which water or other matter is effused or secreted from the blood vessels, for in these, a quantity of blood, equal in bulk to the effused matter will be pressed out of the cranium" (cited in Maramou & Beaumont, 2004). This statement became the precursor to the **Monro-Kellie doctrine**, which is the foundation for understanding increased ICP. The Monro-Kellie doctrine has two basic tenets. The first tenet is the relative incompressibility of the intracranial contents, such as the brain tissue, blood, and cerebrospinal fluid (CSF). The second basic tenet is that changes in the volume of one component must cause a reciprocal change in the other components (Maramou, 1996). Once the sutures in the developing cranium become closed, the brain is sealed within a nonexpandable vault.

In some instances brain volume actually decreases. This can occur, for instance, as part of the normal aging process, and it is detected on imaging studies of the brain as cerebral atrophy. The Monro-Kellie doctrine, however, holds true in this condition as well, with the amount of CSF usually increasing to offset the decreasing brain volume.

Pathophysiology

The fixed nature of the skull is the reason that the volume of its contents, brain tissue, blood, and CSF must remain constant. If the volume of any one of the three components of the brain changes, the volume of the other components also may change (be displaced), but the total volume will not change. ICP is the pressure exerted within the skull, in association with the volume of its three components: brain tissue, blood, and CSF. A normal ICP ranges from 0 to 15 mmHg. Brain tissue itself, known as the parenchyma, is a relatively fixed mass. Thus, the presence of a space-occupying lesion, such as a hematoma, tumor, hydrocephalus, or edema, will ultimately cause compression and/or displacement of the two other components, the vasculature and CSF. The body has several compensatory mechanisms that it can access to adapt to changes.

Compensatory Mechanisms

In order for the brain to maintain a normal ICP, attempts are made to compensate for changes in any of the three components within the brain. Initial mechanisms may include changing the volume of CSF by decreasing production or altering absorption. A decrease in brain tissue may be exhibited by the compression of tissue. Alterations in blood volume may occur as a result of local changes in cerebral vasculature, cerebral perfusion pressure, and cerebral blood flow.

Cerebral Blood Flow

Cerebral blood flow (CBF) is the amount of blood that passes through 100 grams of brain tissue in 1 minute. Normal CBF is approximately 50 mL per minute per 100 grams of brain tissue. Because the brain has a high requirement for the oxygen and glucose found in blood, the maintenance of an adequate level is extremely important. The brain utilizes 20% of the body's oxygen, and 25% of its glucose supply. The brain has the ability to alter its blood flow in response to its needs for oxygen and glucose. The process by which this is done is referred to as **autoregulation**. Autoregulation is defined as the process by which the brain is able to alter its vasculature to accommodate changes in ICP.

Cerebral Perfusion Pressure

Cerebral perfusion pressure (CPP) is defined as the pressure gradient that drives cerebral blood flow. It is the amount of pressure needed to provide adequate blood flow to the brain. The purpose of autoregulation is to provide consistent CBF to ensure adequate CPP to meet the metabolic needs of the brain. When the systemic arterial blood pressure is normal, and ICP is normal, there is very little difference between the mean arterial blood pressure (MAP) and the CPP. In the damaged brain however, the compensatory mechanisms that usually preserve CPP are compromised (Feldman & Robertson, 1997). The initial mechanisms used by the various components within the brain to maintain normal ICP begin to fail. Chart 29–1 shows the calculations used to determine CPP.

When the CPP decreases, CBF also decreases due to failure of autoregulation. Normal CPP is 70 to 100. As the CBF and CPP

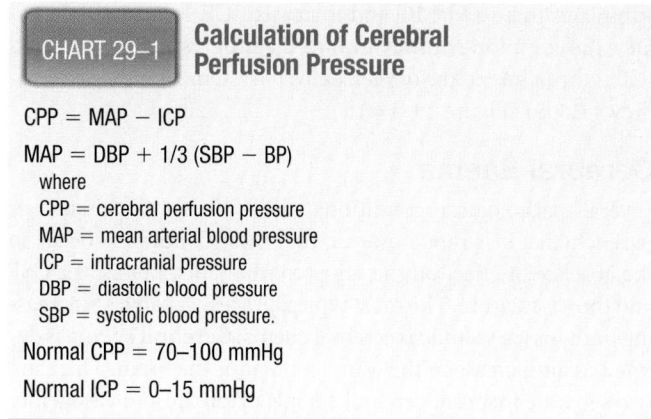

CHART 29–1 Calculation of Cerebral Perfusion Pressure

CPP = MAP − ICP

MAP = DBP + 1/3 (SBP − BP)

where

CPP = cerebral perfusion pressure
MAP = mean arterial blood pressure
ICP = intracranial pressure
DBP = diastolic blood pressure
SBP = systolic blood pressure.

Normal CPP = 70–100 mmHg

Normal ICP = 0–15 mmHg

fall, neuronal ischemia, or lack of oxygen to nerve cells, and death occur. CPP of 50 to 60 mmHg is necessary to adequately perfuse brain tissue. CPP of less than 30 is considered incompatible with neuronal life.

In a normal brain, autoregulation maintains adequate tissue perfusion by adjusting metabolic needs and by altering cerebral vasculature, either by vasoconstriction or vasodilation. These adjustments are made to maintain normal ICPs. When ICP is elevated, it is of utmost importance to maintain an adequate MAP. Though CPP strives to maintain adequate tissue perfusion, this may not be the case in all areas of the brain. The damaged brain may have areas of increased edema, causing a localized area of limited tissue perfusion, resulting in ischemia and further neurological compromise.

Increased Intracranial Pressure

Increased ICP is caused by an increase in the volume of any of the intracranial compartments. Many conditions can cause an increase in ICP (Chart 29–2). Examples of these are craniocerebral trauma (blood), vascular abnormalities, tumors, or edema. ICPs are considered elevated when sustained at greater than 20 mmHg.

At approximately 25 mmHg, increased ICPs become evident by decreased CBF, decreased CPP, and distortion of brain tissue (Geraci & Geraci, 1996). Increased ICPs are associated with increased mortality and morbidity. In the presence of increased ICP, many events take place to perpetuate the process. The **vasodilatory cascade** is a series of events triggered by hypoxia, with the result being increased ICP. Common causes of hypoxia are decreased blood volume and decreased respiratory effort. Hypoxia, from any cause, is a potent vasodilator. Vasodilation

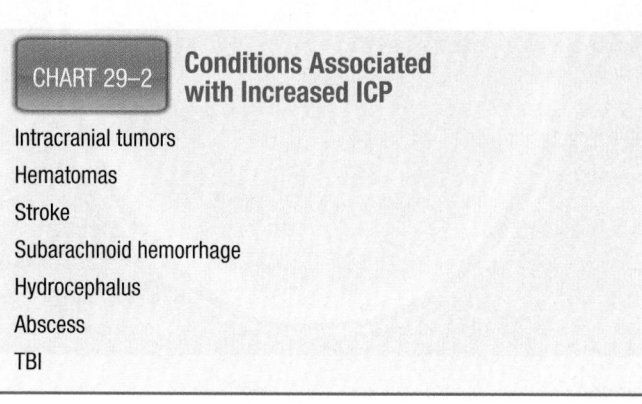

CHART 29–2 Conditions Associated with Increased ICP

Intracranial tumors

Hematomas

Stroke

Subarachnoid hemorrhage

Hydrocephalus

Abscess

TBI

stimulates increased CBF and increased ICP. In acute brain injury, the common pathway toward the progression of increased ICP is the failure of the oxygen delivery system, or ischemia (Andrews, 2005) (Figure 29–1 ■).

Cerebral Edema

Several pathological conditions affect the brain tissue, or parenchyma. It is rare, however, that these conditions occur in the absence of effect on the other components, that is, the CSF and the vasculature. The most typical process capable of increasing brain tissue volume is cerebral edema. **Cerebral edema** is defined as an increase in the water content of the brain. There are two separate forms of cerebral edema: cytotoxic and vasogenic.

Cytotoxic edema is the accumulation of intracellular water. This type of edema occurs as a result of a hypoxic, or possibly toxic event, which damages the cells' ability to pump water out of the intracellular space. Examples include anoxic events such as cardiac arrest or asphyxiation. It is also seen in severe water intoxication due to hyponatremia. This process may or may not be reversible (Farrell & Bower, 2003; Quinn, 2008; Smith & McIntosh, 1996). **Vasogenic edema** represents an alteration in vascular permeability, with disruption of the blood–brain barrier. This results in increased extracellular space. Vasogenic edema frequently is seen in neoplastic diseases, and may be treated with corticosteroids, such as dexamethasone. It also may be treated with osmotic agents such as mannitol.

Cytotoxic edema and vasogenic edema may be seen together. An example of this is a malignant brain tumor in which vasogenic edema exists, causing increased ICP. This in turn decreases tissue perfusion, causing hypoxia to the brain, resulting in cytotoxic edema. Regardless of the process, an increase in brain mass mandates the displacement of other components, which results in increasing ICPs.

Herniation Syndromes

When cerebral edema occurs as a result of a space-occupying lesion, such as a tumor or a hematoma, the pressure exerted on surrounding tissue may not be evenly distributed. The result is a movement of brain mass from an area of high pressure to an area of lower pressure. This movement of brain tissue is referred to as mass effect. The term **herniation** refers to the protrusion of brain structures under pressure into areas causing compression and damage of the brain tissue, with possible catastrophic results. The three most common forms of herniation are cingulate, transtentorial, and uncal and are described by Plum and Posner in their early works and most recent editions (Plum and Posner, 1980; Posner, Saper, Schiff, & Plum, 2007). Herniation syndromes are shown in Figure 29–2 ■.

Cingulate Herniation

Cingulate herniation, also referred to as falcine herniation, is caused by an expanding lesion located in one hemisphere that shifts toward the opposite hemisphere, forcing the cingulate gyrus under the falx cerebri and displacing it to the opposite side. This shift causes displacement of the local blood supply, resulting in compression of the local blood supply, often that of the anterior cerebral artery. Cerebral edema, local cerebral tissue ischemia, and increased ICP follow. Cingulated herniation is common in head trauma and brain tumors; the signs and symptoms are dependent on the specific location affected.

Transtentorial Herniation

Transtentorial herniation, also referred to as central herniation, is caused by lesions that precipitate downward displacement of the cerebral hemispheres, the basal ganglia, the diencephalons, and the brainstem through the tentorial notch (Posner et al., 2007). Cerebral edema, ischemia, and possibly hemorrhage may occur. Signs and symptoms of transtentorial herniation may include decreasing levels of consciousness, altered respiratory patterns, and contralateral motor weakness.

Uncal Herniation

The most common herniation syndrome is uncal herniation. Uncal herniation is caused by an expanding lesion, often located in the temporal lobe. Pressure is exerted across the midline, pushing the medial edge of the uncus into the edge of the tentorium. Brainstem compression may occur. The third cranial nerve (oculomotor nerve) may become compressed, causing ipsilateral pupillary abnormalities, such as a dilated pupil, a common early sign in uncal herniation (Posner et al., 2007).

Often, the first sign of impending uncal herniation is a sluggishly reactive pupil on the ipsilateral side of the lesion (Chart 29–3). This is an early sign, and may be present before any other clinical symptom. Later signs and symptoms of uncal herniation are contralateral hemiparesis, altered levels of consciousness, beginning with restlessness, and progressing through sleepiness, obtundation, and coma. Late signs are altered respiratory patterns, such as Cheyne-Stokes, or pathological positioning, such as decorticate or decerebrate positioning. Very late signs are dilated, fixed pupils.

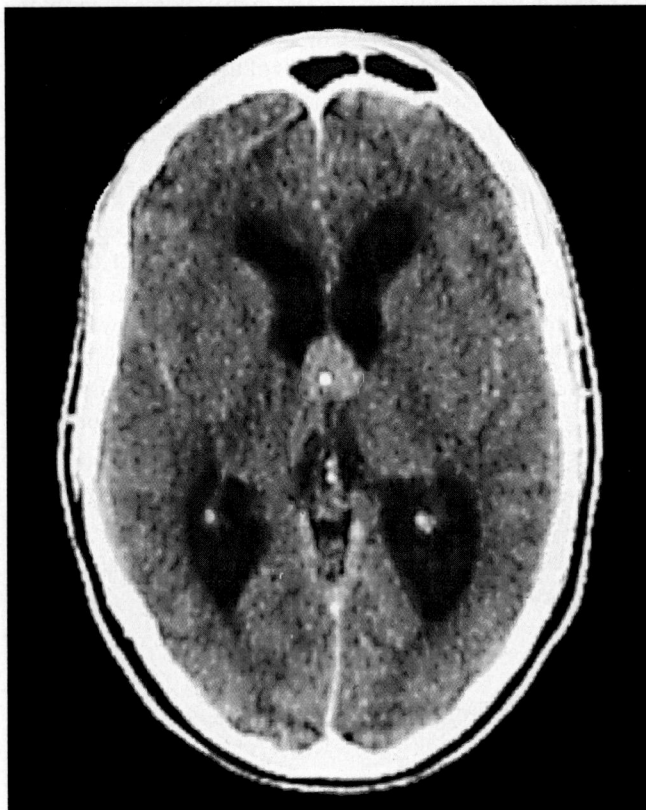

FIGURE 29–1 ■ Progression of increased ICP.
Source: ISM/Phototake NYC

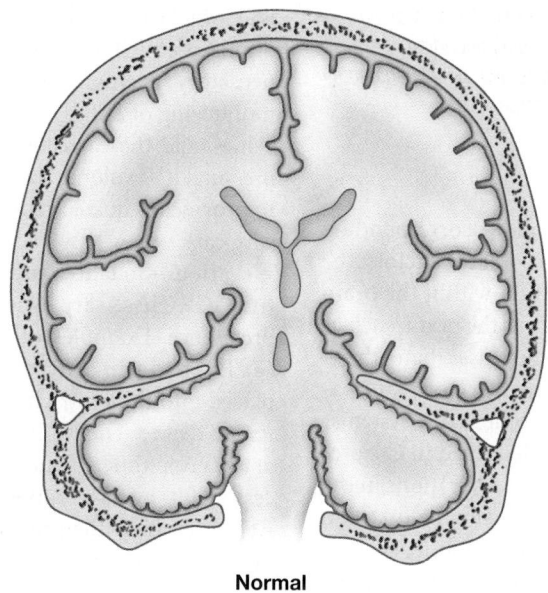

Normal

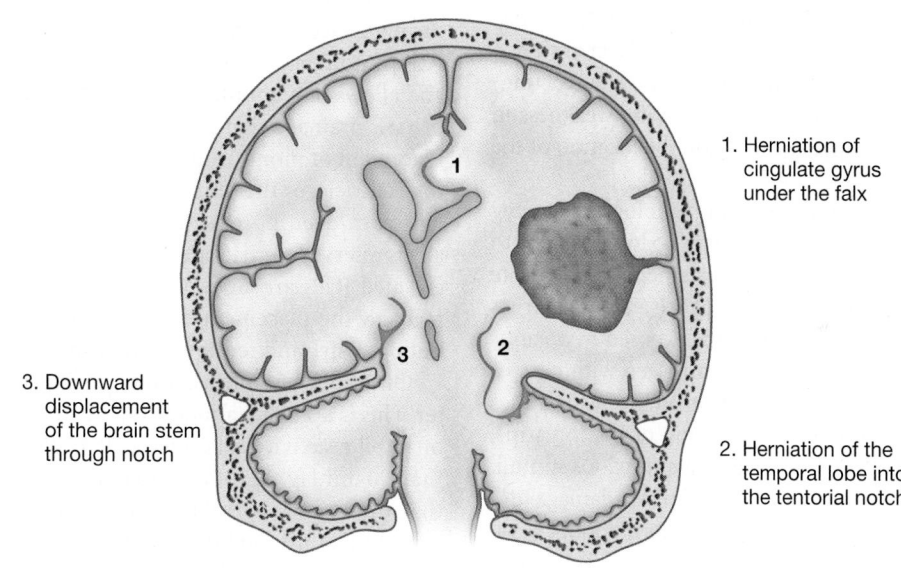

1. Herniation of
   cingulate gyrus
   under the falx

3. Downward
   displacement
   of the brain stem
   through notch

2. Herniation of the
   temporal lobe into
   the tentorial notch

Herniation syndromes

FIGURE 29–2 ■ Herniation syndromes.

| CHART 29–3 | **Pupillary Changes Associated with Herniation** |

Location of Herniation	Pupillary Change
Compression on CN III	Unilateral dilating pupil Sluggishly reactive Usually ipsilateral to lesion
Compression on midbrain to upper pons	Midposition Fixed
Compression on lower pons to upper medullary	Midposition Fixed
Compression on medulla	Dilated Fixed

Urgent surgical intervention to decompress the brain is often the treatment of choice. This may include surgical resection of a mass lesion with or without craniectomy (removal of the bone flap) to allow the brain to swell. Often an intermediate intervention is the placement of a ventriculostomy (catheter placed within the ventricles to drain the CSF) to relieve pressure by allowing CSF to travel another path of less resistance. It also is a valuable tool to measure the ICP. Prior to surgical treatment, hyperosmolar drugs, such as mannitol, can be used to decrease extracellular volume as a temporizing measure.

Herniation syndromes are life-threatening neurological emergencies that, left untreated, can progress rapidly to death. Nursing intervention is aimed at prevention by careful monitoring of neurological status and early recognition of impending problems.

CRITICAL ALERT *New onset of restlessness, agitation, or confusion may be early signs of increased ICP and possible impending herniation. Monitor neurological assessment hourly, and notify MD of any changes in neurological status.*

Clinical Manifestations

The effect of increased ICP on the brain and the corresponding neurological exam is dependent on several common factors: the rate of the pressure increase and the location within the brain that is exerting the pressure. Different parts of the brain, such as the brainstem, are less tolerant of pressure increases than others. The rate and location of pressure increase are reflected in the patient's neurological examination, as well as other body systems.

A complete neurological assessment as described in Chapter 28 🔗 is essential to detecting increasing ICP. Alterations in the patient's level of consciousness (LOC) are usually the first sign of impending changes. These changes may be subtle, such as restlessness or slight confusion. They also may be catastrophic, presenting as coma or even death. The earlier the change is detected and treated, the better the prognosis.

Changes in the cranial nerve exam also may be an early sign of increased ICP. Pressure on the oculomotor nerve (CN III) may result in the impaired ability of the pupil on the affected side to constrict, resulting in a dilated, unreactive (or slow-reacting) pupil. Decrease in motor function with presenting weakness in the extremities also may result, depending on the location of the pressure.

Unrelieved increased ICPs may result in pathologic posturing of the body. These may be seen when a patient no longer is able to follow commands or display purposeful movements. Decorticate (flexor) positioning is described as flexion of the arms and wrists in an adduction posture when the patient is exposed to noxious stimuli, such as pain. A more ominous sign is seen with decerebrate (extensor) posturing. This is seen when all four extremities are in rigid extension, with outward pronation of the forearms, and plantar flexion of the feet, when exposed to noxious stimuli. Both of these postures are indicators of brainstem damage and may indicate more serious conditions, such as herniation.

Other signs, such as headache and vomiting, are less specific. Headaches are generally not a specific indication of ICP problems. Headaches that are "different," such as more severe, unrelenting, and not responsive to modalities that are usually effective, may warrant notification of the health care provider. An example of a "different" headache is one that is "worse in the morning," which may be present with tumors in the posterior fossa. Vomiting, without prior nausea, may be an indication of increased ICP. Vomiting may be without warning, and projectile.

Changes in vital signs may be caused by pressure on the brainstem and/or the hypothalamus. They may be seen as increasing systolic pressure (widening pulse pressure), bradycardia, and/or irregular respiratory patterns. These are known as **Cushing's triad** and are a late indicator of increased ICP. Alterations in respiratory patterns may be a sign of impending neurological decline, especially when associated with a decrease in LOC.

Medical Management

The major goal of medical management of ICP is the prevention of secondary injury due to cerebral edema and increased ICP. This is accomplished by close monitoring of the ICP. The management of increased ICP requires an understanding of the various compensatory systems involved in the regulation of ICP. The goal is the monitoring of ICP dynamics, identifying normal and abnormal values, and the correction of abnormal values. Systemic blood pressure, ICP, volume status, and oxygenation must all be known to provide adequate management. Treatment may be medical or surgical.

Various modalities are available to determine, monitor, and treat ICP. These vary by institution and by health care provider preference. Examples of these are external ventricular drains (EVDs) and parenchymal wires or bolts. An EVD is a catheter placed into the ventricle and connected to a continuous monitoring device. The EVD allows the practitioner to monitor ICP at any given time, including trends. It also allows drainage of excess CSF if necessary to lower the ICP. Another purpose of the EVD is to allow the practitioner to collect CSF for the purpose of sending it to a laboratory for evaluation. The desired range of ICP is 0 to 15 mmHg.

Other monitoring devices also can be used to monitor ICP. In most institutions, the EVD described above is the most commonly used intervention, but it also is possible to place a monitoring device into the brain tissue, or parenchyma, to monitor ICP. Although it is easier to place than an EVD, it is less accurate and allows only monitoring of pressure, without the possibility of CSF drainage that is possible with an EVD (Bader, 2006a). Placement of monitoring devices, such as a catheter or bolt into the ventricle, or the brain parenchyma, usually is done in an intensive care setting, emergency room, or operating room. It usually is reserved for patients with decreased LOC or ones in which elevated ICPs are suspected. Although there are many advantages to the placement of these monitoring devices, they are both invasive and require an intensive level of nursing care.

One type of noninvasive monitoring device is the pupillometer. This is a small, handheld device that measures the dynamics of pupil reactivity. The idea is that patients with ICPs higher than 20 mmHg are thought to have lower constriction velocities than those with normal ICPs. This device is used in limited markets at this time, and data are being collected regarding its use. At this time, the pupillometer is being used in some institutions as a supplemental monitoring device (Bader, 2006b).

Another type of monitoring device is the brain tissue oxygen monitor, which may be used in conjunction with other methods of monitoring. The purpose is to recognize and treat ischemic injuries to the brain. Following an insult to the brain, compensatory mechanisms attempt to maintain autoregulation. The two most frequent causes of secondary injury are hypotension and hypoxia. Therefore, the measurement of oxygenation in brain tissue ($PbtO_2$) leads to valuable information regarding the supply and demand of oxygen within the brain. Measurement of $PbtO_2$ is accomplished by the placement of an oxygen-sensitive probe into the brain tissue. This probe is able to monitor both the level of oxygen and the temperature of the brain tissue. The probe must be placed in healthy tissue, not in area of damage or injury. The measurements are displayed in millimeters of mercury. The type of system used to measure $PbtO_2$ impacts the range of normal levels. However, lower levels of $PbtO_2$ correspond with lower levels of tissue oxygenation, translating to poor neurological outcome.

Jugular bulb venous oxygenation saturation is another method of monitoring cerebral oxygenation. This method consists of a catheter inserted into the jugular bulb of the internal jugular vein. The purpose is to obtain a continuous measurement of jugular venous oxygen saturation (SjO_2). This method provides a measurement of the oxygen saturation of venous blood leaving the brain. The goal of the measurement of SjO_2 is early identification of cerebral hypoxia. A low SjO_2 saturation (less than 54%) is indicative of ischemia (Bader, 2006a). However, measurements are not indicative of specific areas of cerebral tissue oxygenation, but are global readings.

The cerebral microdialysis system is being researched for its effectiveness as a method for measuring extracellular levels of cerebral metabolites. Energy metabolites, such as glucose, pyruvate, lactate, and glycerol, and amino acids, such as aspartate and glutamate, are produced when the brain experiences ischemia (Sarrafzadeh et al., 2002). A tiny microcatheter is inserted into the brain parenchyma, and a dialysate fluid is pumped into the brain. The dialysate fluid is recovered at set intervals and analyzed for levels of chemical metabolites. Changes in the cerebral metabolites indicate the presence of cerebral ischemia, with or without tissue damage. Microdialysis is an emerging technology, but at this point, not widely used. It is an area in which more research is needed (Bader, 2006a).

Various pharmacologic agents may also be used in the management of ICP. Hyperosmotic fluids, such as mannitol or hypertonic saline solutions, can be used to decrease ICP. These are effective in that they move water from cerebral tissue into the circulation. Hemodilution of red blood cells (RBCs) occurs, reducing viscosity and allowing more blood flow to occur within smaller vessels. Vasoconstriction follows, which decreases ICP. It is important to closely monitor the patient's fluid status, including electrolytes and serum osmolality, to avoid negative fluid balance.

Maintenance of adequate vascular volume is of utmost importance in the maintenance of adequate CPP. Central venous catheters and pulmonary artery catheters also may be used to adequately monitor volume status. Also important in the management of CPP is close monitoring of arterial blood pressure with the use of an arterial line. Vasopressors such as phenylephrine and dopamine may be necessary to elevate the systemic arterial blood pressure to support adequate CPP. The goal of treatment is based on the relationship of ICP and CPP.

Patients at risk for neurological deterioration due to ICPs refractory to other methods of treatment may be placed in a barbiturate coma. Patients are given a barbiturate such as pentobarbital, via a loading dose, then a maintenance dose. This method is used in order to decrease LOC, thus decreasing cerebral metabolic needs. The negative aspect of barbiturate coma is that the neurological assessment, including the most basic reflexes, such as gag, swallow, and cough, are lost. The patient in pentobarbital coma must be mechanically ventilated, with intensive nursing care. It also is necessary to monitor patients in pentobarbital coma with continuous electroencephalography (EEG) monitoring. This is done to ensure proper barbiturate dosage. The EEG pattern that is used to regulate appropriate dosing is called burst suppression (BS). The BS pattern is a characteristic signal in the EEG. It is recognized by a period pattern of low voltage of less than 10 μv and a relatively shorter pattern

of higher amplitude complexes. The BS pattern is classified as an EEG abnormality because of its relation to severe encephalopathy. It can be generalized or lateralized. Depending on the initial cause, the state is reversible in some instances (Burst Suppression Tutorial, 2003). The BS pattern may indicate that the barbiturate dose is adequate to suppress brain activity. Continuous monitoring of ICP and hemodynamic and respiratory functions also is vital.

Other, less aggressive means of sedation, such as use of propofol, can be used to keep patients' pain and/or anxiety under control. The goal of sedation is to decrease ICP, CBF, and oxygen demand. Propofol has a short half-life, allowing practitioners to suspend infusion temporarily to accurately assess neurological status.

In some circumstances the best method of treating increased ICP is surgical intervention. In cases of extreme cerebral edema, a hemicraniectomy may be performed. This is a surgical procedure in which a portion of the skull (bone flap) is removed. This method allows room for the swollen brain, lessening the risk for brain tissue damage. The bone flap often is replaced 2 to 4 months later when the patient's condition has stabilized.

Nursing Management

The nursing management of patients with elevated ICP is complex and requires constant vigilance in terms of the neurological exam and trending of monitoring data. An increased ICP affects the brain's overall function and leads to dysfunction in many body systems, including the respiratory, cardiovascular, metabolic, and neurological systems. Therefore, nursing assessment of ICP management must encompass all of these systems.

Assessment

Any patient with neurological compromise must be assessed for adequate respiratory function. Patients with a decreased LOC may have a decreased level of respiratory function. Adequate oxygenation is essential to neurological function. Patients with a Glasgow Coma Scale (GCS) score of 8 or less should be considered for intubation, with possible mechanical ventilation. The GCS is a scale that measures the level of consciousness and is explained in detail in Chapter 28 ☺. Pulse oximetry should be used with supplemental oxygen to maintain oxygen saturations of 95% or greater.

Normocapnia, the normal level of carbon dioxide in the blood, is an important nursing implication. In the past, hypocapnia was the standard of care after head injury. However, recent studies have shown that aggressive hyperventilation and hypocapnia ($PaCO_2 < 30$ mmHg) may actually aggravate secondary brain injury. This occurs through a process where the brain compensates for decreased levels of carbon dioxide, altering the pH of the CSF and initiating autoregulatory responses (Wong, 2000). Ultimately, this leads to increased CBF, increased ICP, decreased CPP, and decreased oxygen to the already ischemic brain tissue (see Figure 29–1 ■, p. 716).

The role of hyperventilation in the management of early brain injury is limited. Prophylactic use of hyperventilation should be avoided. Normocapnia (i.e., PCO_2 values between 35 and 40 mmHg) is recommended to avoid further brain injury. Another important nursing implication is that of monitoring and maintaining the patient in a euglycemic state. Brain trauma induces the increased release of glutamate, which increases cerebral metabolism. This, in turn, increases the metabolic breakdown of glucose, the major energy source for the brain. Decreased CBF results in inadequate oxygen delivery for the increased cerebral demands. This process leads to tissue acidosis, ischemia, and a worsened neurological outcome due to secondary injury.

Hyperglycemia in the setting of an ischemic brain has been shown to be an independent predictor of poor outcome. The goal of nursing is to maintain a normal blood glucose level. Blood levels should be monitored closely, approximately every 4 hours or less. Insulin should be administered to keep the blood levels within parameters associated with normal blood glucose levels, usually between 80 and 120 mg/dL.

Normothermia, the normal body temperature, is another important implication for nursing. Fever is a relatively common finding in neurological patients. It is estimated that between 70% and 100% of patients with traumatic brain injury experience fever during their hospitalization (McIlvoy, 2005). Increases in body temperature may increase metabolic demands, causing an increase in CBF, cerebral blood volume, and ICP. Hyperthermia may lead to ischemia and further brain injury. It is understood that fever in patients with neurological injury is associated with poor outcomes (Thompson, Kirkness, Mitchell, & Webb, 2007). Nursing interventions in maintenance of normal temperature include close monitoring of the patient's temperature. Measuring accurate core temperature is essential, and may require taking rectal temperatures, unless more accurate methods are available. Treatment should be considered as early as a temperature of 37.5°C (99.5°F). Cooling mechanisms may be implemented, if necessary. These include ice packs, cooling blankets, or bathing with tepid water. Care should be taken to prevent the patient from shivering, because this raises temperatures and metabolic demands. Skin integrity also should be monitored closely. Use of acetaminophen is appropriate to lower temperature, if not contraindicated.

The maintenance of normal blood pressure also is an important nursing intervention. To prevent cerebral ischemia, adequate CBF is mandatory. Hypotension in the presence of brain trauma has a strong negative effect on outcome. Patients with hypotension (systolic blood pressure <90 mmHg) in the early phase of brain trauma demonstrate a mortality rate twice as high as those who remain normotensive (Carroll, 1994; Manley et al., 2001; Olson, 2006). Therefore, maintenance of adequate CPP (>60 mmHg) is imperative to prevent further brain injury. Invasive lines, such as arterial lines and Swan-Ganz catheters, may be warranted to adequately monitor blood pressure and hemodynamic status. If necessary, vasopressive or inotropic agents may be necessary to maintain adequate blood pressure. The nursing implications for the management of ICP are summarized in Chart 29–4.

Interventions and Rationales

Many studies have been done to explain the relationship of various nursing activities such as turning, suctioning, and bathing to ICP. Most activities demonstrate only transient increases in ICP; however, this suggests that nurses be aware of such tendencies for increasing ICP and to administer these activities cautiously. Fan (2004) suggests that head positioning in the brain-damaged patient has both positive and negative effects on ICP. The suggestion is that head positioning, both in terms of elevation and rotation, has a definite effect on ICP. Winkleman (2000) studied bed positioning in patients with head injuries and found that elevation of the head of the bed provided optimal CPP and ICP in adults with brain injuries not vascular in

---

CHART 29–4   Nursing Implications and Interventions for Management of ICP

Actual and Potential Problems	Nursing Action	Rationale for Action
Monitoring of ICP	Monitor ICP via EVD or other intracranial pressure device.	Maintenance of normal ICP is essential to prevent further brain injury.
Patient positioning	Keep head of bed at 30°. Maintain head and neck in neutral position.	Decreases resistance to venous return. Prevents pulmonary complications.
Euglycemia	Monitor blood glucose levels. Administer insulin when appropriate.	Prevents increased cerebral metabolic needs and resulting ischemia.
Normocapnia	Maintain PCO$_2$ between 35 and 40 mmHg.	Avoids hyperventilation and potential for rebound increase in ICP.
Normothermia	Monitor body temperature. Use cooling devices if necessary. Administer appropriate antipyretics, if warranted.	Normothermia protects cerebral metabolic needs.
Normotension	Monitor blood pressure, using arterial line, if necessary. Administer vasopressors or inotrope if indicated.	Hypotension increases mortality. Adequate blood pressure is necessary to maintain adequate CPP.
Adequate oxygenation	Monitor oxygen saturations. Maintain adequate oxygenation via pulmonary toilet. Prevent deep vein thrombosis (DVT) through use of sequential compression devices and ambulation as appropriate.	Increased oxygen demands of the brain require adequate oxygenation to prevent further cerebral hypoxia.
Regulate nursing activities	Decrease external stimulation. Coordinate activities, to limit stimulation.	Helps prevent increased ICP.

origin. However, it is recommended that head position be established on an individual basis, with the help of monitoring devices to avoid the possible elevation of ICP.

Traumatic Brain Injury

A damaged skull from the species *Australopithecus africanus*, found in South Africa, provides the first evidence of brain injury, in a murder committed more than 1 million years ago. In this case, the cause of death was probably skull fracture, caused by clubbing (Evans, 1996).

Injuries to the brain have long been considered fatal. In 1682, Younge published a literature review of all recorded medical literature dating from approximately 500 A.D., and found reports of only 100 patients who had survived a brain wound (Evans, 1996). As recently as the 1970s, approximately 90% of all patients with brain injuries died (Senelick & Dougherty, 2001).

Epidemiology and Etiology

Traumatic brain injury (TBI) is and has always been a major health problem globally. In the United States, the Centers for Disease Control and Prevention (CDC) estimate the incidence of patients with closed-head injuries admitted to hospitals is conservatively 1.5 million each year. Approximately 235,000 cases of TBI are admitted to hospitals every year, with approximately 50,000 deaths (CDC, 2007). Although the causes of TBI differ by region, gender, and age group, the largest number of TBI appears to be secondary to motor vehicle crashes, falls, and acts of violence, such as gunshot wounds and assault. Studies have shown that African American men have higher rates of brain injury than other groups. Penetrating head injuries in the United States, such as gunshot wounds and skull fractures, are estimated to be 12 per 100,000, the highest of any developed country in the world (Langlois, Rutland-Brown, & Thomas, 2006). Motor vehicle crashes account for the largest percentage, followed by acts of violence and auto–pedestrian collisions (Burnett et al., 2003). Military personnel in combat zones are most likely to sustain a TBI from a blast (Defense and Veterans Brain Injury Center, 2005). Males are 1.5 times as likely as females to sustain a TBI (Langlois, Rutland-Brown, & Walk, 2006). For some ethnic and socioeconomic groups, risk exposure for TBI is elevated in various ways:

- Increased exposure to physically demanding employment settings (such as construction and manual labor)
- Increased exposure to personal violence
- Increased exposure to older homes and vehicles
- Greater reliance on substandard housing (Evans, 1996; Mayo Clinic Staff, 2008).

The Risk Factors box summarizes the risks for TBI.

The direct and indirect costs of treatment and rehabilitation for TBI patients were estimated at about $60 billion in the United States in 2000 (Finkelstein, Corso, & Miller, 2006). The effect on the lives of the patient, the family, and the entire community is beyond comprehension and is impossible to calculate or predict.

RISK FACTORS for Traumatic Brain Injury

Age 18–25 or over age 70
Alcohol intake
Males (1.5:1)
Military
Participation in certain sports activities

Classification of Acute Head Trauma

Acute head trauma occurs in varying degrees of severity and complexity. It can range from minor scalp lacerations requiring little to no treatment, to severe TBIs resulting in prolonged hospitalization, permanent disabilities, or death.

Superficial Injuries

Injuries to the scalp are relatively common. Although usually minor, they must be carefully assessed and treated diligently. The degree of subsequent treatment is dependent on the extent and depth of the injury. The scalp consists of five layers that cover the skull (Figure 29–3 ■, p. 722). The skin, or dermal, layer contains hair and protects the scalp. The subcutaneous fascia is a fatty, vascular layer, and contains blood vessels that may bleed profusely. The galea aponeurotica is a thick, flexible, and fibrous tissue. The subgaleal space is below the galea, and is a potential space for blood to collect and form cephalohematomas, or "goose eggs." Below the subgaleal space is the periosteum, a thin layer of tissue, covering the skull.

The most common and least severe scalp injury is a simple abrasion. An abrasion is a simple scraping of the skin. It may bleed slightly. A contusion is a bruise of the skin. Treatments for both abrasions and contusions include a thorough cleansing of the wound with possible application of an antibiotic ointment.

Scalp lacerations account for a large number of emergency department visits. The scalp is extremely vascular, and exsanguination has been known to occur in extreme cases. This vascularity is what allows the scalp to heal well in most cases. With any scalp laceration, the possibility of an underlying skull fracture must be addressed. An accurate history of the event surrounding the injury is very important. Based on the mechanism of injury, if there is any reason to suspect a skull fracture, a computerized tomography (CT) scan or, at the very least, a plain x-ray of the skull should be obtained. Once the degree and extent of the scalp injury have been determined, the wound should be carefully cleaned with a standard skin-sterilizing solution, such as a povidone-iodine compound. The wound may require suturing and antibiotic ointment. In addition to a careful history of the event, the immunization history of the patient should be obtained, and a tetanus toxoid should be administered, if appropriate.

Skull Fractures

The skull, or calvarium, is the bony structure that houses the brain. It is composed of the frontal, parietal, temporal, and occipital bones. It also includes the multiple facial bones that make up the facial structure. Of these facial bones, only the mandible is movable. The skull itself is asymmetrical and varies in thickness. The temporal bone is the thinnest; the occipital bone is the thickest. The floor of the skull, known as the

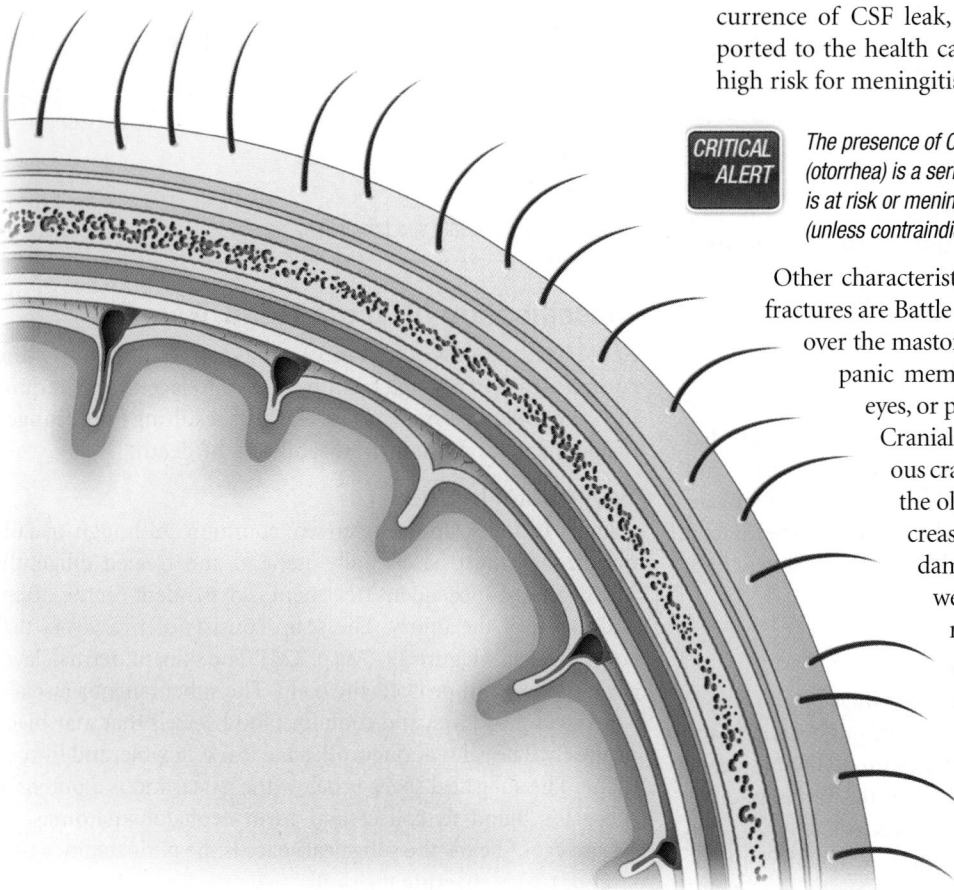

FIGURE 29–3 ■ Cross section of skull.

skull base, is rough and uneven, attributing to an important role in brain injury. Skull fractures are categorized according to type of break and severity of the fracture as listed here:

- **Linear skull fractures** are the most common type of skull fracture. They are simple breaks in the continuity of bone, with no displacement, and most commonly are seen in low-velocity impact situations. Linear fractures of the temporal bone may result in a tear of the middle meningeal artery, resulting in more serious brain injury, such as an epidural hematoma.

- **Comminuted skull fractures** are fragmented interruptions of the skull resulting from multiple linear fractures. An area of bone depression at the point of impact is characteristic of a comminuted fracture.

- **Basal skull fractures** usually are an extension of a linear fracture into the skull base. The mechanism of injury generally is the same as linear skull fractures with a more serious result. The inner aspect of the skull is closely associated with the dura, the thin membrane that covers the brain. The skull base is rough and uneven, and its texture may cause tears to the delicate dura. Consequently, CSF may leak through the tear in the dura. This may result in CSF leaking from the nose or the ear. CSF leaking from the nose is called rhinorrhea. CSF leaking from the ear is called otorrhea. Drainage of CSF may be visualized directly, or may be seen on dressings or bed linens. It is distinguishable by its characteristic halo sign, which appears as blood with a yellow ring around it. The oc-

currence of CSF leak, while not unexpected, must be reported to the health care provider because the patient is at high risk for meningitis.

CRITICAL ALERT *The presence of CSF leaking from the nose (rhinorrhea) or ears (otorrhea) is a serious complication. The patient with CSF leak is at risk or meningitis. Place head of bed at 30 to 45 degrees (unless contraindicated) and call MD.*

Other characteristic signs and symptoms of basal skull fractures are Battle sign, which is ecchymosis, or bruising, over the mastoid bone (Figure 29–4 ■); bulging tympanic membranes; and the presence of raccoon eyes, or periorbital ecchymosis (Figure 29–5 ■). Cranial nerve deficits, due to damage to various cranial nerves, also may occur. Damage to the olfactory nerve (CN I) may result in decreased sense of smell. Visual deficits, due to damage to the optic nerve (CN II), facial weakness, due to damage to the facial nerve (CN VII), and decreased hearing, due to damage to the acoustic nerve (CN VIII), also may be seen.

- **Depressed skull fractures** are the displacement of a comminuted skull fracture (Figure 29–6 ■). They frequently are seen with other injuries to the brain, such as contusions and/or lacerations of the brain. The degree of neurological symptoms depends on the degree and location of brain involvement. Hair, dirt, and other debris may be found within the wound and present risk for infection.

Clinical Manifestations

Skull fractures alone do not cause neurological symptoms, but frequently they are seen in conjunction with other, more serious

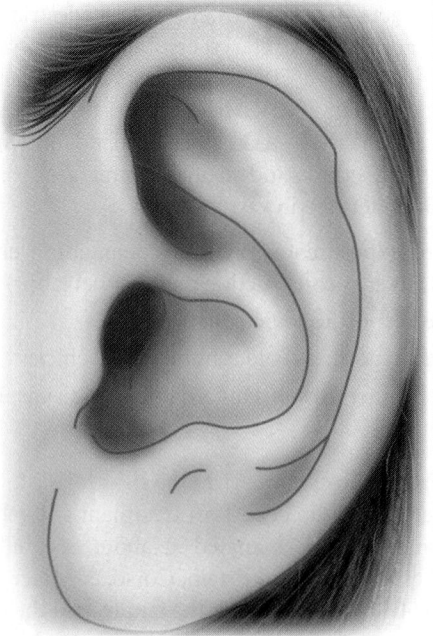

FIGURE 29–4 ■ Battle sign.

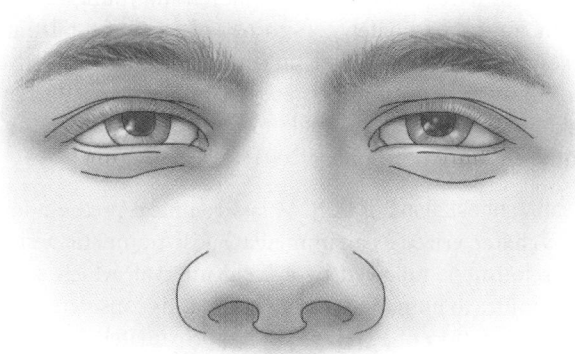

FIGURE 29–5 ◼ Raccoon eyes.

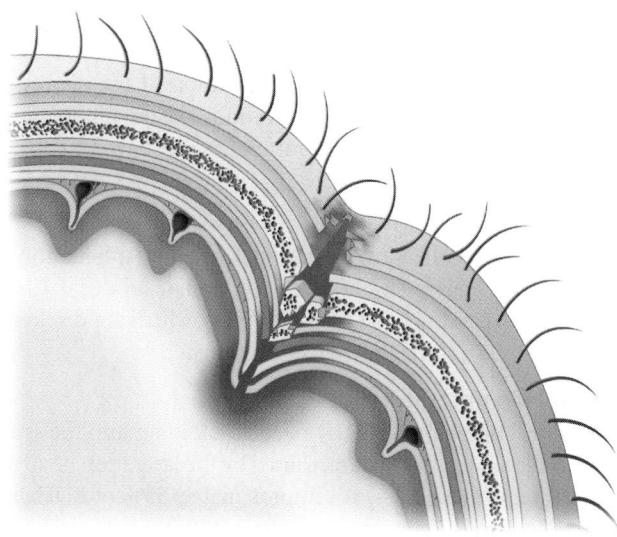

FIGURE 29–6 ◼ Depressed skull fracture.

brain injuries, such as hematomas or contusions. Clinical manifestations then are representative of the other brain injuries that may be present.

Laboratory and Diagnostic Procedures

Diagnosis of skull fractures can be made with plain skull x-rays. However, if a skull fracture is suspected based on the physical assessment and knowledge of the mechanism of injury, a CT scan of the head should be obtained, because the question of underlying brain trauma must be addressed. Fractures of the facial bones and basal skull fractures may be seen best with a thin-cut

CT scan. The Diagnostic Tests box provides more details about appropriate tests for skull fractures.

Medical Management

Treatment depends on the type of fracture. Linear fractures usually do not require treatment, other than close observation of the patient for neurological deterioration. Open or comminuted

DIAGNOSTIC TESTS for Acute Brain Disorders

Test	Expected Abnormality	Rationale for Abnormality
Plain skull films	Fracture lines, linear, basal, depressed, or comminuted	Skull fractures are best seen in plain films.
CT of head	Hematomas (SDH, EDH), contusions, hydrocephalus. Test is time sensitive, as the presence of blood (in SDH) changes characteristics with time	CT scans are best suited to examining presence of blood, edema, CSF.
MRI	DAI (late) tumors	MRI will demonstrate small lesions not seen on CT scan. Best suited to demonstrate heterogeneity of tumors.
Lumbar puncture	Blood in CSF (subarachnoid blood) Abnormalities in fluid chemistry	**Contraindicated** until space-occupying lesions are ruled out—possibility of induced brain herniation. Bacterial or viral pathogens affect glucose, protein, cell counts, RBCs, and WBCs.
Electroencephalogram (EEG)	Seizure activity	Common in head trauma, brain tumors, and infectious process due to altered electrical activity in brain.
Serum electrolytes	Hyponatremia (serum Na+ less than 134 mEq/L) or hypernatremia (Na greater than 145)	Risk factor for increased cerebral edema.
Blood glucose	May be elevated	Indicative of steroid use (dexamethasone).
Complete blood count (CBC)	Elevated WBC count Alteration in hemoglobin/hematocrit	Indicates infection. Also may be present with steroid use. Important for accurate hemodynamic monitoring, especially in patients at risk for vasospasm.
Culture of CSF	Presence of pathogens	Indicated for suspicion of infectious CNS process.
Tissue pathology	Presence of malignancy, pathogen	Indicated for suspicion of tumor or abscess.
Arterial blood gases	Hypoxia, hypercapnia	Depressed neurological state may also indicate depressed respiratory drive. Decreased levels of oxygen and increased levels of CO_2 are a concern for increasing ICPs.

fractures should be considered contaminated, and careful wound debridement with surgical closure often is required. Depressed skull fractures may require elevation of the depressed bone as well as debridement of the wound. The possibility of infection must be considered, and antibiotics are started if considered appropriate.

Hematomas

Hematomas are collections of blood. Intracranial hematomas are defined by their location, either epidural or subdural. Chart 29–5 summarizes the types of hematomas, which are discussed in more detail in the following subsections.

Epidural Hematoma

An **epidural hematoma (EDH)** refers to bleeding into the space between the skull and the dura, caused by the laceration of an artery or a vein (Figure 29–7 ■). Approximately 85% of EDHs are caused by arterial lacerations (Greenberg, 2001), most commonly the middle meningeal artery, with or without fracture of the temporal bone. As bleeding occurs, an enlarging hematoma develops as the dura is stripped away from the inner table of the skull. Pressure is exerted on the brain tissue by the expanding lesion, with resulting neurological compromise.

CHART 29–5	**Types of Hematomas**	
Hematoma	**Onset of Symptoms**	**Characteristic on CT Scan**
Epidural	Immediate loss of consciousness, followed by lucid interval (considered "textbook presentation")	Hyperdense, elliptical
Subdural, acute	Up to 48 hours after injury	Hyperdense
Subdural, subacute	48 hours to 3 weeks	Isodense
Subdural, chronic	3 weeks to several months	Hypodense

EDHs most frequently occur in children and young adults and account for approximately 2% to 6% of intracerebral trauma (Hickey, 2003). It is seen rarely in children younger than 2 years old, or the elderly, possibly because the dura is more adherent to the skull at those ages. The male-to-female ratio of EDH is approximately 4 to 1 (Greenberg, 2001).

Clinical Manifestations of EDH   Classic clinical presentation of EDH is characterized by an immediate post-traumatic period of unconsciousness, followed by a lucid interval, which can last from minutes to hours. The "lucid interval" is considered a textbook presentation of EDH, seen in approximately 85% of patients with EDH. A rapid deterioration in LOC may follow, characterized by sleepiness, confusion, obtundation, coma, and possibly death. Neurological decline is caused by the rapidly increasing pressure, or mass effect, caused by the enlarging hematoma. Other possible signs and symptoms are an enlarging pupil on the same side of the injury (ipsilateral), increasing headache, seizures, motor weakness, and/or pathological positioning (refer to Chapter 28 👁 on assessment).

Subdural Hematoma

Subdural hematoma (SDH) is defined as bleeding between the dura and the arachnoid layers of the meninges (Figure 29–8 ■). Approximately 30% of intracranial traumatic lesions are SDHs (Hickey, 2003). They usually are caused by the tearing of bridging veins located over the surface of the brain. SDHs are divided into three categories based on the amount of time between the initial injury and the presentation of signs and symptoms.

Acute Subdural Hematoma   Acute SDH is characterized by the presentation of neurological signs and symptoms up to 48 hours after injury. On CT of the head, the acute SDH appears as a hyperdense lesion. The most common signs are severe headache with possible gradual deterioration of LOC, starting with drowsiness and progressing through confusion, obtundation, and coma. Pupillary signs also may be present, most commonly an ipsilateral dilation, and sluggish reactivity. Hemiparesis of the contralateral arm and leg also may be present.

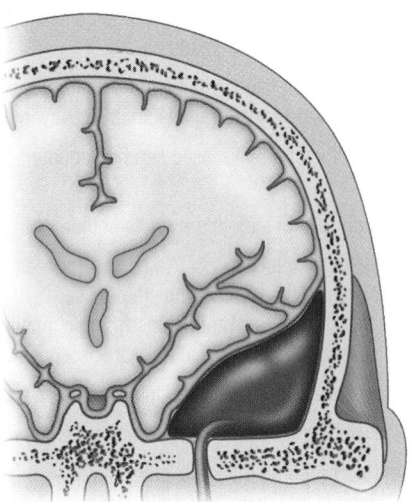

FIGURE 29–7 ■ Epidural hematoma.

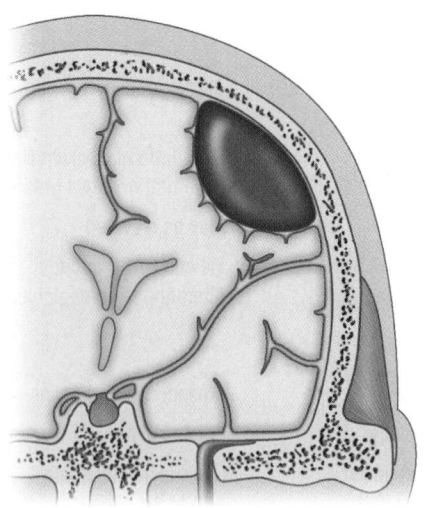

FIGURE 29–8 ■ Subdural hematoma.

Subacute Subdural Hematoma   With subacute subdural hematoma neurological signs and symptoms develop from 48 hours postinjury up to about 3 weeks. They are associated with less serious lesions, perhaps due to bleeding at a much slower rate. The blood in a subacute SDH appears isodense with hyperdense areas and a clear blood–fluid level on a CT scan.

Chronic Subdural Hematoma   With chronic subdural hematoma neurological signs and symptoms develop over 3 weeks to several months. These are associated with minor head injuries, possibly occurring weeks to months prior to the presentation of neurological signs. The SDH increases slowly in size, possibly from repeated small venous bleeds, until a significant mass effect develops and symptoms occur.

Chronic subdural hematomas also are associated with the elderly, who may have atrophic brains that provide more free space to bleed into. Also of significance in the aging brain, bridging veins are stretched as the brain atrophies, which also may cause bleeding into the subdural space. Because there is more room for the clot to expand, the SDH may become quite large before symptoms occur. On CT scan, the chronic SDH appears isodense. However, because chronic SDH may occur from repeated small episodes of subdural bleeding, it is not uncommon to have acute or chronic SDH, as evidenced by areas of varying density demonstrated on CT scan. Chronic SDHs usually do not present with the rapid and dramatic deterioration of neurological function as do acute SDHs. The most common symptom is increasing headache, slowing mentation, confusion, and drowsiness. Seizures are a common presenting symptom.

 Patients with a diagnosis of SDH are at risk for expanding hematoma. Therefore, frequent neurological assessments are required (i.e., hourly until stable, then q2h). A decrease in neurological function, such as increasing confusion or lethargy, increasing motor weakness, or an enlarging pupil is a medical emergency. The doctor should be notified immediately.

Laboratory and Diagnostic Procedures
CT scan of the head remains the most accurate diagnostic tool, along with a thorough and accurate history of the event. EDH is characterized by a high-density elliptical-shaped mass adjacent to the skull. Mass effect also is seen with a shift of the brain from the side with the EDH to the opposite side. CT scan is highly diagnostic for SDH, as well as for the determination of the acute, subacute, or chronic type of hematoma.

Medical Management
The treatment for EDH is almost always surgical. The exception to surgical management is a small lesion that is causing little to no neurological impairment. The patient is hospitalized, possibly in the intensive care unit (ICU), with frequent neurological assessment, and serial CT scans are taken to monitor the size of the hematoma. A decline in the neurological assessment of the patient, with or without radiographic evidence of increased size, warrants emergent surgical evacuation of the hematoma. Mortality rates are dependent on the availability of neurosurgical treatment.

The treatment for SDH is dependent on several factors. Observation with medical management may be appropriate for a small SDH with little to no neurological deterioration, because

a small SDH may reabsorb with time. However, a large SDH, with significant neurological compromise requires immediate surgical evacuation. SDH is commonly associated with therapeutic anticoagulation, and correction of coagulopathy is a critical step in preparing the patient for operative care. It is possible to drain a small liquefied hematoma with twist drill burr holes. Burr holes are small holes made with a twist drill into the skull, over the area of hematoma. Commonly, a drain is left in to drain the hematoma over time. Larger acute, subacute, and chronic SDH may require an open craniotomy for evacuation of the hematoma. Twist drill drainage of chronic SDH may not be possible, because the clotted blood is the consistency of motor oil and may be too gelatinous to be successfully evacuated with burr holes.

Postoperatively, the patient should remain in the ICU, with close monitoring of neurological status. Use of intracranial monitoring is done with caution, because an EVD may cause the SDH to worsen. The patient may require hemodynamic monitoring and/or ventilatory assistance, depending on the size and location of the lesion, as well as the presence of any accompanying injuries.

Because seizures are a common occurrence in SDH, the use of antiepileptic drugs (AEDs) may be warranted. The prophylactic use of AEDs is controversial, because they have many side effects and contraindications. If a patient has a seizure due to a lesion, the patient should be started on an AED such as phenytoin (Dilantin). Seizures and their management are addressed later in the chapter.

Cerebral Contusions
Contusions of the brain are defined as bruising of the brain tissue, often associated with other neurological injuries, such as skull fractures or hematomas. They may occur from blunt trauma, penetrating wounds, or acceleration/deceleration injuries. Causes may include motor vehicle crashes, falls, and assault. The injuries are referred to as coup, in which bruising occurs directly below the point of impact on the skull, or contrecoup, which occurs directly on the opposite point of impact. Contrecoup contusions usually have a coup component, in which case they are referred to as coup-contrecoup contusions. Contrecoup contusions occur as a result of the brain moving with the skull, and bruising itself during acceleration/deceleration movement.

Clinical Manifestations
The clinical presentation of cerebral contusion is highly dependent on the location, size, and the amount of cerebral edema associated with the lesion. For example, a patient with temporal contusions, especially bilateral contusions, may have a significant decrease in LOC with motor and speech deficits. This patient is at high risk for cerebral edema and herniation. A patient with a frontal contusion may be alert, possibly confused, and may be monitored in the hospital for a short period of time with no obvious consequences. However, the patient may experience more obvious neuropsychological deficits such as disinhibition in social situations; therefore, careful observation of the patient's cognitive status is warranted. Patients with neurocognitive deficits often require 24-hour care following discharge for this reason.

Laboratory and Diagnostic Procedures

As with all cerebral traumas, a thorough and accurate history is important. Diagnosis is made by radiographic detection on imaging studies to evaluate for the presence of contusion and possibly edema.

Medical Management

Once the diagnosis of cerebral contusion(s) is made, along with determination of the location and size of the contusion, treatment is dependent on the neurological condition of the patient. Close monitoring of the patient's neurological assessment is important. Monitoring of ICP may be necessary since cerebral edema may be present. Serial CT scans over several days may be warranted to assess the size of the contusion as the brain heals. "Blossoming" or expansion of the contusion may occur at approximately 3 days.

Seizures may be a presenting sign; therefore, use of AEDs may be necessary. Prophylactic use of AEDs is controversial, though some health care providers believe their use is warranted for a limited time (usually 7 days) due to the potential risk of seizures.

Hyponatremia is another common sequelae to TBI, often requiring both salt supplementation and fluid restriction for management.

Concussion

Concussion refers to a recognized collection of symptoms as a result of mild head injury. It is described as a temporary, neurological dysfunction caused by an external force to the head. It is also described as a "shaking of the brain."

Clinical Manifestations

Concussion is associated with a myriad of symptoms, including confusion, possible brief loss of consciousness, headache, intellectual impairment, and memory loss. Concussion is characterized by a nonfocal neurological exam. The American Academy of Neurology Practice has issued a grading scale to define levels of concussion and make recommendations for treatment, as described in the National Guidelines box.

Laboratory and Diagnostic Procedures

An accurate history of the event is essential, including questions such as length of period of loss of consciousness, if any; presence of confusion; and length of time until symptoms subside. No radiographic findings are associated with concussions. However, if the patient has a focal neurological exam, or an extended period of unconsciousness, the patient should be admitted to the hospital, and a CT of the head should be obtained to rule out other, more serious brain trauma.

Medical Management

The management of the concussion is dependent on the grade determined. However, the treatment recommendations are guidelines, and each patient should be assessed individually.

Second-Impact Syndrome

Second-impact syndrome is characterized by a second concussion, in an indeterminate time frame, that occurs before the brain can completely recover from the first concussion. It is caused by a loss of disordered autoregulation of the brain's blood supply as a result of the first injury (Bowen, 2003; Terrell, 2004). Because of poor brain compliance, persistent vascular congestion and increased ICP persist. This condition may persist for an indeterminate length of time. Because second-impact syndrome is the result of a second injury before the brain has recovered from the first injury, the result can be massive cerebral edema and possibly death. The mortality rate is 50% and the morbidity rate is 100% (Proctor & Cantu, 2000). It is for this reason that consideration must be made of the advisability of continuing risk-taking activities after receiving an initial concussion. An example of this is the athlete who continues playing football after receiving one or more concussions and then collapses and dies on the sidelines after an apparent mild injury. For these reasons, well-recognized return-to-play guidelines are now used that progress in a stepwise fashion. The athlete has a period of rest and when symptom free may return to limited noncontact activity and progress each week to full play if no symptoms such as headache or recurrent cognitive problems are experienced. The player must return to repeat the previous step if symptoms recur (Aubry et al., 2001; Terrell, 2004).

Postconcussion Syndrome

Postconcussion syndrome is a condition that follows mild head injury and is characterized by one or more of the following symptoms: headaches, dizziness, vertigo, tinnitus, hearing loss, blurred vision, light and/or noise sensitivity, alteration in smell, anxiety, depression, personality change, sleep disorders, decreased libido, decreased appetite, memory loss, alteration in cognitive function, personality changes, and physical or cognitive decline (Rees & Bellon, 2007). It was once thought that these symptoms were psychological, and the patient perhaps malingering. However, current literature supports a physiological basis for this condition. Symptoms usually subside with time; however, it can take months for total resolution (Mittenberg & Strauman, 2000).

The only treatment for postconcussive syndrome is education and support for the patient and family members. Counseling may be helpful to cope with personal and work-related problems.

Diffuse Axonal Injury

Diffuse axonal injury (DAI) is defined as a primary injury of diffuse white matter that results in tearing or shearing of axons and small blood vessels. Presentation of the patient with DAI is

---

NATIONAL GUIDELINES American Academy of Neurology Practice Parameter Grading System for Concussion

Grade	Type of Concussion
Grade 1	Transient confusion, no loss of consciousness, symptoms of mental status abnormalities on examination resolve in less than 15 minutes.
Grade 2	Transient confusion, no loss of consciousness, symptoms of mental status abnormalities on examination last more than 15 minutes.
Grade 3	Any loss of consciousness, either brief or prolonged.

Source: Kelly, P., & Rosenburg, J. H. (1997). Diagnosis and management of concussion in sports. *Neurology, 483,* 575–580.

MyNursingKit | American Association of Neuroscience Nurses

frequently seen as neurological compromise, possibly coma, with decerebrate or decorticate posturing as described in Chapter 28 . DAI lesions may be microscopic, and not initially detected by CT scan. Magnetic resonance imaging (MRI) is more appropriate for the detection of small DAI lesions. Surgery is not indicated because the injury is diffuse. Treatment is determined by the neurological presentation of the patient and is usually supportive. Support of respiratory and hemodynamic functions may be warranted. DAI is classified as mild, moderate, and severe. Patients with mild DAI may have only mild long-term cognitive disabilities, whereas severe DAIs are associated with significant mortality and long-term disabilities.

Primary/Secondary Injuries

Head injuries can be divided into primary and secondary injuries. **Primary injury** refers to the mechanical injury to the brain. The injury is a direct result of the initial insult to the brain and may be localized, such as occurs with a laceration or contusion, or diffuse, such as with a concussion or DAI.

Secondary injury is a result of the body's response to the primary insult to the brain. It is caused by a flow–metabolism mismatch, which results in **cerebral ischemia**, which then triggers the **ischemia cascade**, which is a series of events that results in changes on the cellular level, which then results in **cerebral infarction** (Goldman & Ausiello, 2004; Porth, 2007). It can be the result of a single event or a series of events. Deficits in cellular metabolism in the brain can cause cell death, leading to death of brain tissue, compromised neurological function, and poor patient outcomes. Causes of secondary injury are many, and include respiratory insufficiency, hypoxia, sepsis, hypotension, metabolic dysfunction, cerebral edema, and increased ICP. It has been estimated that 50% of patients with head trauma succumb to effects of secondary injury (Hilton, 2000; Porth, 2007).

■ Nursing Management

Nursing care of TBI patients has several goals. The first is protection of the patient's neurological function. This is accomplished by a thorough neurological assessment aimed at determining the patient's level of consciousness and possible focal neurological deficits.

Assessment

A good neurological assessment is essential for communication between medical personnel, as well as for a baseline to detect changes. A tool, such as the Glasgow Coma Scale, is helpful to provide standardized information to other medical personnel. The GCS is a widely used scoring system used in quantifying level of consciousness following traumatic brain injury. The scale and its scoring mechanism is discussed in detail in Chapter 28 . Any unfavorable change in a neurological exam, even the most subtle, may indicate deterioration in the patient's condition and is reportable. The National Guidelines box lists the questions used by the CDC to screen for detection of mild TBI.

TBI may be a mild head injury, such as a concussion, or cerebral contusion. TBI also may be a severe, life-threatening situation. It is not uncommon for other serious conditions also to be present,

---

NATIONAL GUIDELINES CDC Screening Instrument for Detection of Mild TBI

Questions

1. At the time of your trauma, did you experience any period of transient confusion, disorientation, or impaired consciousness?

2. At the time of your trauma, did you experience any dysfunction of memory?

3. Did you experience any of the following in relation to your trauma: seizures, headache, dizziness, irritability, fatigue, or poor concentration?

4. At the time of your trauma, did you experience any loss of consciousness lasting 30 minutes or less?

An answer of "yes" on any of these questions indicates mild TBI.

Source: Bay, E., & McLean, S. A. (2007). Mild traumatic brain injury: an update for advanced practice nurses. *American Association of Neuroscience Nurses, 39*(1), 43–51; Centers for Disease Control and Prevention. (2005). *CDCt toolkits.* Retrieved September 25, 2006 from http://www.cdc.govncipe/pub-res/tbi_toolkit/toolkit.htm/.

---

which also may be life threatening. Patients with severe injury or potentially severe conditions are usually admitted to the ICU and monitored carefully. It is imperative to remember the ABCs of patient management with any trauma patient. Assessing and securing an adequate airway are always of primary consideration. Trauma victims frequently have respiratory compromise due to a number of factors, including other injuries. Whether a patient is severely injured and intubated, or awake and talking, maintenance of an adequate airway is essential. Rate and quality of respirations should be assessed initially, and ongoing. A pulse oximeter may be of assistance in early determination of respiratory decline. This is especially important if the patient has an altered LOC. Any patient with a GCS of 8 or less, with 15 being considered normal, should be considered for intubation. Maintenance of adequate oxygenation is an important tenet of ICP management.

 CRITICAL ALERT *Patients with a decreased level of consciousness are at risk for aspiration and respiratory compromise. Monitor respiratory status carefully, suction as needed, and ensure airway protection.*

Assessment of adequate circulation is the last part of the ABCs of life support. Patients with TBI may exhibit alterations in circulatory function, such as bradycardia, hypotension, or hypertension. They may also be hemodynamically unstable due to blood loss secondary to trauma. Therefore, the initial nursing assessment must include a complete set of vital signs and a thorough assessment of the circulatory status of the TBI patient. After the initial ABCs of patient management, the most common concern for nurses caring for patients with TBI is that of ICP. Many patients with TBI require placement of a device to monitor ICP. The nursing management of patients with increased ICP was addressed earlier in this chapter.

Interventions and Rationales

Nursing is in a good position to recognize signs and symptoms, or the potential, of cognitive impairment due to TBI. It is often in the

EVIDENCE-BASED PRACTICE

Traumatic Brain Injury

Clinical Problem

Traumatic brain injury is a major health problem globally. It occurs with varying degrees of severity and disability. It can affect all ages, but the National Institutes of Health (NIH) states that the majority of those with TBI are between the ages of 18 and 25 (NIH Consensus Panel, 1999).

Although the causes of TBI differ by region, gender, and age group, the largest number of TBIs appears to be secondary to motor vehicle crashes, falls, and acts of violence, such as gunshot wounds and assault. In the United States, the incidence of people with closed head injuries admitted to hospitals is conservatively estimated to be 1.5 million each year. Approximately 235,000 cases of TBI are admitted to hospitals every year, with approximately 50,000 deaths (Langlois, Rutland-Brown, & Thomas, 2006).

Mild TBI accounts for approximately 75% of all diagnosed TBI (Bazarian et al., 2005). Persons experiencing mild TBI may enter the health care system through emergency departments; others may present through their primary care health care providers. The signs and symptoms may be mild or even unnoticed. It has been estimated that approximately 25% of those with mild TBI do not seek medical treatment at all (Dawodu, 2007).

The symptoms of mild TBI are frequently cognitive and may consist of memory problems, difficulty with concentration, personality changes, or other alterations in thought processes. These deficits may lead to problems with relationships, education, and/or occupation. For these patients, it is essential that signs and symptoms of mild TBI are recognized early to provide appropriate management. Diagnosis of mild TBI may be obtained through screening procedures, cognitive assessment, and accurate and thorough interviewing and history-taking. A management plan for the patient with mild TBI is based on evidence-based practices.

Research Findings

Management of the patient with mild TBI is based on symptom management. This includes environmental modifications, compensatory strategies, and support and education of the patient and family while gradually returning to work and home responsibilities (Bay & McLean, 2007).

Many of these compensatory strategies are the focus of speech and occupational therapists, either in an acute or outpatient setting. An evidence-based review article published by Cicerone et al. (2005) found evidence to support the use of aids, such as voice organizers and memory journals, to help patients with memory impairment after TBI.

A study by Mittenberg and colleagues (1996) described a printed manual and a 1-hour treatment session regarding symptom management to a small group of patients with mild TBI. They compared this group to a usual treatment group. They compared the two groups 6 months later and found that the first group reported fewer and less severe symptoms. They suggest that even brief educational interventions are beneficial to reducing prolonged symptoms post-TBI.

A review of the literature regarding screening and symptom management of patients with mild TBI suggests that awareness of actual and potential cognitive deficits and subsequent education regarding symptom management are beneficial to reducing prolonged symptoms. There is great need for continued research in the management of mild TBI patients.

Implications for Nursing Practice

Patients with mild TBI may exhibit a vast array of symptoms, including headache, dizziness, and/or subtle symptoms of cognitive impairment. Some of these symptoms include difficulty with concentration, memory, or attention. Personality changes may also be seen. Nurses are in an excellent position to identify signs and symptoms of mild TBI. Screening tools can assist in determining the severity of TBI (see the National Guidelines box titled CDC Screening Instrument for Detection of Mild TBI, p. 727). Nursing staff should also assist patients in obtaining the appropriate therapies, including support and education of patients and their families.

Critical Thinking Questions

1. What patient complaints might be suspicious for signs and symptoms of mild TBI?

2. What part of a patient's history would lead to concern about a possible mild TBI?

3. What would be appropriate management strategies for patients with mild TBI?

Answers to Critical Thinking Questions appear in Appendix D

References

Bazarian, J., McClung, J., Shah, M., Cheng, Y., Flesher, W., & Kraus, J. (2005). Mild traumatic brain injury in the United States, 1998–2000. *Brain Injury, 19*(2), 85–91.

Cicerone, K. D., Dahlberg, C., Malec, J., Langenbahn, D., Felicetti, T., Kneipp, S., et al. (2005). Evidence-based cognitive rehabilitation: Updated review of the literature from 1998 through 2002. *Archives in Physical Medicine Rehabilitation, 86,* 1681–1692.

Dawodu, S.T. (2007). Traumatic brain injury: definition, epidemiology, pathophysiology. *EMedicine.* Retrieved July 14, 2008 from http://www.emedicine.com/pmr/TOPIC212.HTM.

Langlois, J. A., Rutland-Brown, W., & Thomas, K. E. (2006). *Traumatic brain injury in the United States: Emergency department visits, hospitalizations, and deaths.* Atlanta, GA: Centers for Disease Control and Prevention, National Center for Injury Prevention and Control.

Mittenberg, W., Tremont, G., Zielinski, R., Fichera, S., & Rayls, K. (1996). Cognitive-behavioral prevention of post-concussion syndrome. *Archives of Clinical Neuropsychology, 11*(2), 139–145.

National Institutes of Health Consensus Panel. (1999). NIH consensus statement: Rehabilitation of persons with traumatic brain injury. *Journal of the American Medical Association, 282,* 974–983.

Source: From "Mild Traumatic Brain Injury: An Update for Advanced Practice Nurses," E. Bay and S. McLean (2007). *Journal of Neuroscience Nursing, 39*(1), 43–51.

patient's best interest to obtain therapy consults in order to recognize and define possible cognitive problems. Evidence-based practice asserts that early recognition and education regarding possible cognitive deficits may aid in the patient's rehabilitation and recovery (see the Evidence-Based Practice box).

A second goal for the neuroscience nurse is the prevention of complications, many of which are common and known to be complications common to patients with TBI. Examples of these are respiratory failure, development of deep venous thrombosis, and other systemic complications. These complications can be extremely serious and may even be life threatening. Many of these systemic complications are addressed later in this chapter.

TBI is almost always unexpected and usually comes at a time that finds both patients and their families unprepared. The early period of hospitalization requires critical thinking and astute assessment skills. It always requires understanding, empathy, and strong emotional support. Nurses may be equipped with the skills needed to care for TBI patients efficiently, but skills to appropriately care for families of patients with devastating, perhaps potentially fatal injuries also is extremely important. Families of severely injured patients are frequently overwhelmed, often angry, and not uncommonly in denial. The nurse caring for the patient's family members may be their only link for communication, support, and encouragement. It is important to keep them as involved as they want to be in the care of their family member, as informed as possible, and given as much control as is possible. Experienced nurses often relate that the most frequent complaint heard from families is that they "don't know what is going on." It also is important to answer questions honestly, educating the family about the treatment plan and the expected rehabilitation process. It is important to encourage, educate, and offer hope, without misleading. Determining brain death in patients and working with patients' family members are discussed in the Ethical Issues box.

Collaborative Management

The patient with TBI is one with multifaceted challenges. TBI patients require the collaboration of many specialists and ancillary services. Medically, it is not uncommon for a TBI patient to be under the care of several health care providers, such as a pulmonologist to manage respiratory problems, a neurologist to manage seizures, an orthopedic surgeon and/or a trauma surgeon to manage coexisting injuries, and possibly a critical care specialist.

It also is important to have a dietitian involved in the TBI patient's care. Metabolic needs should be determined in order to ensure that caloric needs are met. TBI patients often require enteral feedings, and the type and amount are important to ensure the patient receives the appropriate nutrition for his needs. Nutrition should be started as soon as it is medically possible (see Chapter 14).

Most TBI patients will, at some point in their hospital stay, require therapists. In many hospitals this may consist of physical therapists, occupational therapists, and possibly recreation therapists. Speech pathologists also may be called on to assess swallow function as well as cognitive function. Sometimes a neuropsychologist will be consulted to assess higher cognitive function and to help determine the safety and feasibility of returning home or to a previous occupation. In some hospitals, a psychiatrist, specializing in rehabilitation, may be consulted to facilitate post-hospital therapies. Many TBI patients benefit from a post-hospital stay in a rehabilitation facility to prepare them for return to home and their previous lives.

Social services may be called on to assist in attaining resources the patient and her family may need. Many patients and their families find TBI support groups to be helpful. This is especially important for the families of patients experiencing long-term rehabilitation or those experiencing significant changes in their jobs and/or lifestyles. Nursing support is important in providing and encouraging care for the caregiver.

ETHICAL ISSUES Related to Brain Death

Brain death can be defined as damage to the brain that is irreversible and extensive to the point that there is no potential for recovery. Brain damage can result from numerous causes, including trauma, stroke, or tumor.

Brain death determination is done by a physician and includes the following criteria:

- Absence of brainstem reflexes: fixed pupils, absent corneal reflexes, absent oculovestibular reflexes, absent gag reflex, no spontaneous respirations with apnea challenge
- No response to deep central pain
- Core temperature less than 32.2°C (89.9°F)
- SBP > 90 mmHg.

Determination of brain death is not appropriate in patients with possibility of intoxication, either alcohol or drug.

Consider organ donation for patients in which brain death is a possibility.

Persistent Vegetative State

The term *persistent vegetative state* (PVS) was proposed by Jennett and Plum (1972) to describe the state following coma in some patients who have experienced severe brain injury. This is a state following coma characterized by an awakened state, without cognitive awareness. Patients in a PVS have sleep–wake cycles, with eyes open spontaneously. Normal vital signs, including respiratory function, are maintained. There is no attempt to follow commands, or to communicate. There is no evidence of cognition.

Patients in a PVS may survive many years following a brain injury. This often presents a very difficult situation for family. It is helpful if a living will is available and the patient and family have had discussions regarding the prolongation of life in a situation where quality of life appears minimal at best.

Family conferences with physicians, nursing, therapists, social work, and clergy are frequently helpful in determining prognosis, including quality of life. Discussions involving discontinuance of medical treatment, including nutrition, are difficult at best, and should be done with the patient's living will and/or advance directive. Assuring the family that such decisions are reflections of the patient's own wishes may be comforting and may assuage feelings of guilt or responsibility.

Health Promotion

The most important principle of TBI management is prevention. A vast number of programs in hospitals and communities nationwide are aimed at the prevention of TBI. Community education and public awareness programs are essential in the prevention of TBI. Such programs include the promotion of helmets for bicycle and motorcycle riders and seat-belt laws, which are known to have an effect on the severity of TBI due to motor vehicle collisions.

Infectious Diseases of the Central Nervous System

Many infectious diseases may affect the nervous system. Meningitis, encephalitis, and cerebral abscesses are examples of infections of the central nervous system (CNS) that can be caused by a number of pathogens including common bacteria, fungi, and viruses. Infectious diseases may be acquired or nosocomial. Nosocomial infections are those that are acquired due to hospitalization; they were not present or in the incubation period prior to admission. The nationwide rate of nosocomial infections is about 7% to 10%. It is estimated that approximately 20% of all hospital-acquired infections occur in critical care areas (Smith et al., 2005).

Meningitis

Meningitis is defined as an inflammation of the meninges. **Bacterial meningitis** is an inflammation of the meninges caused by a bacterial pathogen. **Viral meningitis** is an inflammation of the meninges caused by viral pathogens, such as herpes simplex virus, mumps, measles, or any other virus.

Epidemiology

Before the introduction of antibiotics in the 1930s and 1940s, acute bacterial meningitis was fatal in most cases (Koedel, Scheld, & Pfister, 2002). Nowadays, most cases of meningitis are curable, with variable morbidity related to variable pathogens. Bacterial meningitis occurs most often in three patient populations, the very young and the very old, and those with head trauma or surgery. According to the American Association of Neuroscience Nurses (AANN), 70% of all cases of bacterial meningitis occur in children under the age of 5 years old. In adults over age 40, the incidence is 5 to 10 per 100,000. It also has been noted that patients with diabetes mellitus appear to have a higher than average incidence of acquired bacterial meningitis (Huang et al., 2002). Prognosis is good if treated early; however, if left untreated, it has a mortality rate of greater than 70% (Bader & Littlejohns, 2004). Viral meningitis also affects all age groups, including children. Incidence and type of pathogen are highly dependent on geographic locale. An example of a region-specific virus is that which is arthropod-borne, such as the West Nile virus. This virus is more prevalent around water and in humid locales. Viral meningitis may occur as an epidemic or as an isolated occurrence.

Etiology and Pathophysiology

Meningitis involves the layers of the meninges, and the subarachnoid space. Through a complex physiological process, the response of the meningeal tissue causes an alteration in the blood–brain barrier. This process may result in vasogenic edema with an increase in ICP.

Bacteria can enter the meninges by various methods and structures. Bloodborne pathogens are the most common, entering via the bloodstream. Other bacteria enter the body via other structures, such as the sinuses or the inner ear, by dental procedures, or endocarditis. Cerebrospinal fluid is a common route for infection. A dural tear caused by trauma or surgery can create a route for the introduction of pathogens. Patients with skull fractures, for example, may experience rhinorrhea or otorrhea. If a route is available for CSF to leave the body, organisms have a route to enter the body. Unsterile technique during surgical procedures, including lumbar puncture, placement of an EVD, or collection of CSF from an EVD, is a method of introducing organisms into the CSF.

The most common causative agents differ in children and adults. The age of the patient directs suspicion toward the identity of the pathogen. Adults contract bacterial meningitis most frequently from trauma and/or brain surgery. *Staphylococcus aureus, Staphylococcus epidermidis,* and gram-negative bacilli are common causative agents as introduced by neurological procedures, such as surgery or lumbar puncture.

Clinical Manifestations

A common and early sign of bacterial and viral meningitis is that of meningeal irritation, or **meningismus**. Symptoms of meningismus include photophobia, nuchal rigidity, or stiff neck, Kernig's sign, and Brudzinski sign. Kernig's sign is elicited by flexing the patient's hip to approximately 90 degrees, then straightening the leg at the knee. Pain in the hamstring area prevents the straightening of the leg. This is referred to as a positive Kernig's sign, and must be present bilaterally to be considered positive. Brudzinski sign is positive when flexion of the patient's neck elicits flexion of the hips and knees. The discomfort associated with meningismus is caused by inflammation of the meninges.

Headache is another common and early symptom of meningitis. These headaches are usually described as severe and difficult to control. Fever also is common, and is usually high. Altered levels of consciousness, such as lethargy, irritability, and confusion, may occur as the disease progresses. Seizures may be seen at the onset.

Laboratory and Diagnostic Procedures

A thorough and accurate history is very important, focusing on recent illnesses, such as any "flu-like" illness. The presence of systemic viral infections is significant. A history of recent dental procedures, head trauma, and/or brain surgery also is pertinent.

Once meningitis is suspected, lumbar puncture must be done to determine the presence and identity of organisms as well as other diagnostic criteria of CSF. Before a lumbar puncture can be done, however, a CT scan of the head should be done to ascertain that no space-occupying lesion is present to cause mass effect. A lumbar puncture done in the presence of a space-occupying lesion could cause downward shifting of the brain and herniation through the foramen magnum, with neurologically devastating results as described earlier in the chapter (herniation syndromes).

Lumbar puncture can prove with certainty if pathogens are present in the CSF. Also of benefit is examination of the fluid for other diagnostic factors. The CSF may be turbid or cloudy in the presence of bacteria. Other chemical constituents are diagnostic for bacterial meningitis, that is, protein and glucose. The amount of protein in the CSF is usually high, whereas the glucose level is low. Viral meningitis differs in that the glucose count is usually normal, whereas the protein count remains elevated. The CSF appears clear. Intracranial pressure also may be measured via lumbar puncture. Chart 29–6 lists CSF findings under various conditions.

Medical Management

The treatment for bacterial meningitis is antibiotics. They are usually given intravenously, but may be given intrathecally in certain circumstances. The type and route of antibiotics used are determined by the identity of the pathogen. For appropriate antibiotic determination, a CSF Gram stain and culture is very important. It also is important to obtain blood cultures to assist with therapy determination. For an antibiotic to be effective in

CHART 29–6	**CSF Findings in Various Pathologic Conditions**					
Condition	**Opening Pressure (cm H$_2$O)**	**Appearance**	**Cells (per mm^3)**	**Protein (mg %)**	**Glucose (% serum)**	**Cultures**
Normal	7–18	Clear, colorless	0	15–45	50	No organisms
Bacterial meningitis	Frequently increased	Turbid, cloudy	20–50+	100–1,000	Less than 40	Bacterial organisms
Viral meningitis/encephalitis	Normal	Normal, may be cloudy	Few–350	40–100	Normal	No bacterial organisms; viral organisms present on viral cultures only
Subarachnoid hemorrhage	Increased	Bloody	Increased RBCs	50–400	Normal	No organisms

treating meningitis, it must have a bactericidal effect against the causative organism, and it must be able to penetrate the blood–brain barrier. The antibiotic most sensitive to the causative agent is the drug of choice. Because recovery depends on the timeliness of treatment, it usually is important to start treatment as soon as possible, even before the causative agent is identified.

It is important to note that some antibiotics interfere with the metabolism of other drugs, including phenytoin. This is significant because it generally decreases the blood levels of phenytoin, leaving the patient more susceptible to seizure activity.

 CRITICAL ALERT *Seizure precautions must be taken with any patient having seizures or the potential for seizures. While the patient is in bed, the rails should be padded and in the upright position. All patients should be on AEDs, unless contraindicated. Drug levels should be monitored to maintain therapeutic range.*

Because meningitis may cause vasogenic edema, the use of dexamethasone is strongly recommended. Studies also have shown that dexamethasone has been found to decrease mortality when given early (van de Beek et al., 2002). Prognosis also appears to correlate with the causative agent, age, degree of neurological impairment, the presence of underlying disease, such as diabetes, and the general health condition. Mortality and morbidity rates range from 10% to 30%, but if left untreated, the morbidity is greater than 70% (Bader & Littlejohns, 2004). Prognosis depends on many factors: the causative agent, the severity of the infection, the age and general health condition of the patient, and the timeliness of effective treatment.

Treatment of viral meningitis consists mainly of supportive measures. These measures may consist of relief of symptoms, such as fever or pain. A more seriously ill patient may require respiratory and/or circulatory support. AEDs may also be necessary. Frequent monitoring of the patient's neurological status is important, with any decline in the neurological exam reported. Prognosis is dependent on variable factors, similar to those with the bacterial form of meningitis. Occasional neurological impairment has been reported, but full recovery is frequent.

Isolating the patient with a CNS infection usually is not necessary. In the acute phase of meningococcal meningitis, it is possible to spread the infection to others by respiratory droplets. In such a situation, respiratory isolation of these patients may be needed to protect other patients and the nursing staff for a short

period of time. Universal precautions are usually adequate protection from the spread of CNS infections.

Encephalitis

Encephalitis refers to an inflammation of the brain tissue. The cause may be bacterial, viral, fungal, or parasitic. There are many causes of encephalitis worldwide. Like meningitis, the specific pathogen is highly influenced by geographic location. The most common form of encephalitis in the United States is viral. The most common of these viruses is herpes simplex virus (HSV). Other types of viruses include arthropod-borne, such as those carried by mosquitoes. Another cause of viral encephalitis is postviral disease, from measles, mumps, or chickenpox.

HSV exists as type 1 and type 2. HSV-1 is the virus that causes cold sores, and exists in the dormant form in most adults. HSV-1 is the virus that causes HSV encephalitis. It is unknown how or why the virus changes from the dormant phase to the active phase. HSV-2 is the virus that causes genital herpes through sexual transmission.

Pathophysiology

The mechanism by which a virus infects the brain varies with the type of virus. Effects include degenerative changes within the nerve cell. Also seen are localized edema, hemorrhages, and areas of necrosis. HSV has a special affinity for the frontal and temporal lobes. Increased ICP may be present.

Clinical Manifestations

Symptoms are usually more pronounced than those with meningitis. They also are dependent on the type of virus infecting the brain. Symptoms include severe headache, fever, nausea and vomiting, confusion, alterations in LOC, such as lethargy, and focal deficits, such as motor weakness. It is not unusual for patients to have seizures and bizarre behavior. If the virus is causing cerebral edema, the patient will have signs and symptoms of increased ICP, as discussed earlier in this chapter. Death or severe neurological deficits can occur if the condition is left untreated.

Laboratory and Diagnostic Procedures

Diagnosis is made primarily by examination of CSF. Glucose levels are low, protein levels are high, and white blood cells (WBCs) are elevated. Opening pressure is elevated during lumbar puncture. It is important to make a diagnosis as quickly as possible to initiate treatment. A thorough history is important to rule out other causes of the current illness. MRI scan may show early evidence of small localized hemorrhagic lesions. Definitive diagnosis of HSV is accomplished only by brain biopsy.

Medical Management

Treatment is supportive management of symptoms, such as support of respiratory system, and management of increased ICP, nutritional support, and close evaluation of intake and output. Laboratory values, such as a complete blood count (CBC), also should be monitored to assess systemic response to the disease.

Antiviral agents, such as acyclovir or famciclovir, are the standard for treatment of HSV. They are given intravenously and must be started early in the disease process to be effective. Other important medications include dexamethasone to reduce cerebral edema, phenytoin for seizure management, and medication for pain and fever control. Medications used in treatment of seizures are shown in the Pharmacology Summary box. Prognosis is dependent on early diagnosis and treatment. Neurological deficits such as cognitive impairment, motor weakness, seizure disorder, swallowing difficulties, and personality changes are common.

Brain Abscess

A **brain abscess** is a localized infection carried from other sites of the body extending into the cerebral tissue. There are several mechanisms by which an abscess can be introduced into the brain, such as infection, congenital abnormalities, or by penetrating wounds. An abscess may be caused by various agents, including bacteria, fungus, virus, and parasites.

Epidemiology and Etiology

Brain abscesses occur most often in the cerebellum, but can occur in the frontal, parietal, or occipital lobes. They can occur at any age. There is a 2:1 male-to-female ratio in the occurrence of brain abscesses (Greenberg, 2001). Forty percent of all brain abscesses result from the mastoid, or inner ear; 10% come from the sinuses. Penetrating head wounds, such as trauma, or intracranial surgery account for a small number. Almost half of all abscesses are carried through the blood from other infected sources, as with pneumonia or endocarditis (Hickey, 2003). It is believed that in approximately 25% of all brain abscesses, no primary focus is identified (Bader & Littlejohns, 2004). Note, however, that brain abscess in intravenous (IV) drug users carries especially high morbidity and mortality rates (Tunkel & Pradhan, 2002).

Pathophysiology

Brain abscesses begin as an infectious organism that invades the brain from a nearby location, such as the sinuses, mastoid, or inner ear. The initial focus for infection also may be head or facial trauma or a neurosurgical procedure. Bacteremia in IV drug users may seed in the brain tissue or the epidural space. The invading bacteria cause inflammation, cerebral edema, increased ICP, and necrosis. With time, the necrosis liquefies and capsulates. If untreated, it is possible the abscess could rupture, causing more widespread disease.

Clinical Manifestations

Initial symptoms are directly related to the location of the forming abscess. Headache is common, as well as generalized malaise, fever, nausea and vomiting, and chills. Neurological deficits correspond to the location of the lesion, and may include motor weakness, sensory deficits, cranial nerve weakness, speech disturbances, and alterations in LOC, such as confusion and lethargy. The patient may experience seizures.

As the abscess develops, secondary symptoms may occur due to the expansion of the space-occupying lesion. Symptoms are dependent on the location of the lesion. Cerebellar lesions may result in ataxia, nystagmus, or postoccipital headache. Frontal lesions may result in contralateral hemiplegia, aphasia, or personality changes. Headaches may become more severe, and signs of increased ICP may occur. Herniation syndromes may occur if the abscess is left untreated.

Laboratory and Diagnostic Procedures

Diagnosis is made by history and by imaging studies such as CT scan or MRI. Imaging studies show the encapsulated abscesses. CT scan also is helpful in identifying hydrocephalus, mass effect, and cerebral edema. Occasionally abscesses in the brain may appear to be cystic brain tumors. Diffusion-weighted MRI can be used to identify infectious brain lesions and to differentiate between cystic lesions and abscesses (Guzman et al., 2002). Lumbar puncture usually is not performed because abscesses are space-occupying lesions, capable of causing herniation in certain circumstances. If examination of the CSF is possible, the glucose usually would be normal, with an increased protein and WBC count.

Medical Management

Treatment is surgical drainage of the abscess if possible. Medical management consists of administering the appropriate antibiotics, along with steroids. Support of symptoms, such as ICP management, and respiratory and cardiovascular systems is important. Management of fever and pain issues is warranted. Prognosis is excellent if treated early and aggressively. Also significant in determining prognosis is the number of abscesses noted. Patients with single lesions do considerably better than those with multiple lesions. Patients who survive brain abscess have an approximately 30% chance of neurological deficits, seizures being the most common (Hickey, 2003).

◼ Nursing Management

The single most important intervention on the part of nursing and every hospital employee is prevention. The advent of universal precautions has been successful to educate employees in ways to prevent, or at least reduce, the occurrence of infections. The population of patients with neurological disorders appears to have an affinity for infections. One reason for this is the drugs common to patients in this environment. Many patients are given steroids such as dexamethasone, which is an immunosuppressant. Radiation and chemotherapy also act as immunosuppressants. Many patients with neurological disorders have respiratory compromise, requiring intubation and possibly mechanical ventilation. These patients are at high risk for developing nosocomial infections.

Nutritional deficits also are predisposing factors for infection. Many patients enter the hospital in debilitated conditions, in advanced stages of brain tumor, vegetative conditions, or stroke. The widespread use of antibiotics for hospitalized patients plays a role in diminishing the normal flora of a person's

PHARMACOLOGY Summary of Medications to Treat Acute Brain Disorders

Drug	Category	Application/Indication	Nursing Concerns
Dexamethasone	Corticosteroid	Reduce vasogenic edema.	Can cause psychosis, alteration in sleep, GI upset, leukocytosis, hyperglycemia
Mannitol	Osmotic solution	Reduce vasogenic edema.	Monitored unit; monitor serum sodium, osmolality levels
Famotidine (Pepcid) Ranitidine (Zantac) Omeprazole (Prilosec)	H2-blocker	Reduce acid in the stomach.	Thrombocytopenia
Phenytoin (Dilantin) Carbamazepine (Tegretol) Divalproex (Depakote) Gabapentin (Neurontin) Lamotrigine (Lamictal) Phenobarbital Clonazepam (Klonopin) Ethosuximide (Zarontin)	Antiepileptic drug	Prevent seizures.	Thrombocytopenia, gingivitis; allergic reactions can be severe
Diazepam (Valium) Lorazepam (Ativan)	Benzodiazepines	Treatment for seizure cessation, status epilepticus.	Oversedation, respiratory depression
Oxycodone (Percocet, Oxy-IR, OxyContin) Hydromorphone (Dilaudid) Hydrocodone (Vicodin, Lortab) Morphine Fentanyl (Sublimaze, Duragesic)	Opioids	Provide pain control for moderate to severe pain.	Respiratory depression, oversedation, constipation, difficulty with urination
Codeine Tramadol (Ultram)	Opioids	Provide pain control for mild to moderate pain.	Respiratory depression, oversedation
Ketorolac (Toradol) Indomethacin (Indocin) Ibuprofen (Motrin, Advil) Naproxen (Naprosyn)	Nonsteroidal anti-inflammatory drug (NSAID)	Provide pain control and fever reduction.	GI upset
Acetaminophen	Analgesic and anti-inflammatory	Provide pain control and fever reduction.	Liver toxicity
Naloxone (Narcan) Flumazenil (Romazicon)	Opioid antagonist; benzodiazepine antagonist	Reverse opiate effects and benzodiazepine effects.	
Propofol (Diprivan)	Sedative hypnotic	Provide sedation.	Short-acting, reverses quickly, oversedation
Ondansetron (Zofran) Metoclopramide (Reglan) Trimethobenzamide (Tigan) Prochlorperazine (Compazine) Promethazine (Phenergan)	Antiemetics (nonphenothiazines, phenothiazines)	Reduce/prevent nausea.	Psychosis, extrapyramidal symptoms
Carisoprodol (Soma) Cyclobenzaprine (Flexeril) Diazepam (Valium)	Antispasmodics	Muscle relaxants	Oversedation, respiratory depression
Temozolomide (Temodar) Procarbazine Cisplatin/carboplatin Vincristine Methotrexate	Chemotherapy	Treat malignant primary brain tumors.	Thrombocytopenia, neutropenia, anemia, nausea and vomiting

immune system, leaving the patient vulnerable to hospital-acquired infection. Nursing plays a vital role in the prevention of nosocomial infections. The most obvious actions might be the observation of universal precautions, the practice of meticulous hand hygiene, and the monitoring of signs and symptoms of impending infection.

Assessment

Patients with infectious diseases of the brain such as meningitis, encephalitis, or brain abscess initially may appear to be neurologically intact, but systemically ill. They and their families are usually frightened by the intensity of their illness. Often, it is the nurse who identifies that the patient is becoming ill with symptoms such as fever or signs of nuchal (back of neck) rigidity and brings it to the attention of the physician so that diagnostic testing can be done (see the Diagnostic Tests box, p. 723). Meningeal signs, such as nuchal rigidity (neck stiffness that prevents flexion), often are the first symptom. Patients not only experience headache and neck discomfort, they usually are photophobic, complaining of light sensitivity. A careful neurological exam, including testing for nuchal rigidity, Kernig's sign (severe stiffness of the hamstrings), and Brudzinski sign, yields important information.

Interventions and Rationales

The patient with suspected meningitis will need a lumbar puncture for diagnostic purposes. A nurse assisting with this procedure can help alleviate some of the fears of the patients, informing them of the procedure, the purpose of the procedure, and what is expected of them. It also is important for the patient to stay flat for approximately 4 hours after the lumbar puncture to avoid low-pressure spinal headaches. Once the lumbar puncture has been done, the CSF is sent to the laboratory for chemistry tests such as glucose, protein, cell count, and microbiology cultures.

It is important to monitor vital signs closely to watch for fever. The patient should be treated with antipyretics for fever reduction and kept cool and comfortable. Pain management also is important, because headaches may be severe. Use of narcotics to relieve pain must be balanced with the need to preserve the patient's clinical examination. Excessive use of narcotics will result in sedation and an inability to distinguish deterioration from medication effect.

Nursing management of patients with infectious processes of the CNS includes consideration of family members by keeping them involved and informed of their family member's condition. There is a great deal of fear involving diseases such as meningitis, encephalitis, and brain abscesses. There is concern about these conditions being contagious. Sometimes meningitis is contagious, such as in meningococcal meningitis caused by *Neisseria meningitidis*. When cultures are negative for unusual strains passed by contact, family and friends can be reassured that they cannot "catch" these diseases from the patient.

Medications for these disease processes include dexamethasone to decrease cerebral edema, an AED such as phenytoin, for seizure treatment or prophylaxis, antipyretics, and medications for pain control. The use of these medications is described in the Pharmacology Summary box (p. 733). It also is extremely important to start the patient on the appropriate antibiotic as soon as possible to combat the suspected pathogen.

These antibiotics should be started as soon as the CSF has been obtained.

Patients with brain abscess may present with symptoms such as those with any space-occupying lesion in their brain. They may have neurological compromise dependent on the size and location of the lesion. The abscess may cause mass effect and possible cerebral edema. Accurate and thorough neurological assessments are essential to identifying even a slight change in the patient's neurological status. These changes may be caused by an increase in the mass effect caused by an abscess or increased edema.

Evaluation

Brain abscess, once diagnosed, may require removal, with identification of the causative pathogen. Once identified, an aggressive regiment of IV antibiotic therapy is required under the guidance of an infectious disease specialist, if available. Postoperatively, patients will be admitted to the ICU. Though not usually the case, they may require monitoring of ICP and/or hemodynamic monitoring. They certainly will require close monitoring of their neurological status, with frequent, perhaps hourly, neurological assessment, as well as monitoring of their heart rate, blood pressure, respiratory rate, and oxygen saturation. A postoperative MRI is usually done to assess the degree of resection and to look for postoperative changes, such as hemorrhage or edema.

◼ Collaborative Management

Consultation with an infectious disease specialist may be indicated, if available. Commonly, antibiotic courses are 4 to 6 weeks in the duration of the cerebral abscess. Infectious disease health care providers specialize in the management of infections, including method of transmission, appropriate antibiotics, and drug interactions. They also monitor disease trends and outbreaks.

Future Directions

It is important to continue to monitor the epidemiological trends of CNS infections to understand infection dynamics and to develop appropriate medical interventions. Although the mortality rate for meningitis and encephalitis is still significant, it appears that the rate is decreasing. One important trend is that of vaccines for meningococcal infections (Moura, Pablos-Mendez, Layton, & Weiss, 2003).

Another important consideration is that of antimicrobial resistance. The large volume of antibiotics prescribed has contributed to the emergence of highly resistant pathogens, among them vancomycin-resistant enterococci and methicillin-resistant *Staphylococcus aureus*. Some clinicians are very concerned that unless preventive measures are taken and new drugs are developed, at some point in the future, pathogens will appear that are not responsive to antibiotics (Yoshikawa, 2002). It is easy to imagine the high mortality rates we would face if bacterial meningitis could not be treated.

Other studies have demonstrated an inflammatory cascade evident in the tissue destruction in bacterial meningitis. Genetic targeting or pharmacologic blockage of these pathways may be beneficial in developing treatment or vaccines for bacterial pathogens (Koedel et al., 2002).

Brain Tumors

The diagnosis of a brain tumor often brings feelings of fear and uncertainty to the patient and his family. Most patients have little understanding of the concept of brain tumors, and many harbor misconceptions about the cause, treatment, and prognosis of their disease.

Epidemiology

According to the American Cancer Society (ACS), it was estimated that more than 20,000 people in the United States would be diagnosed with a malignant CNS tumor in the year 2007. In the same period approximately 13,000 people will die from brain, spinal cord, or other CNS malignancies (ACS, 2006). Although possible at any age, brain tumors are most commonly seen in children under the age of 10 and in adults from 30 to 50 years old. The average age at onset of all primary brain tumors is 53 years. Age prevalence differs with tumor type (Central Brain Tumor Registry of the United States, 2000). Incidence of gliomas is 40% higher among males; incidence of meningiomas is 80% greater in females (Surawicz, McCarthy, & Kupelian, 1999). Malignant brain tumors account for approximately 1% of all cancers, and 2% of all cancer-related deaths (ACS, 2006).

Etiology

The cause of CNS tumors is not well understood. It is known that brain tumors, like other tumors, are caused by abnormal changes in the genes. DNA, found in all genes, is considered the "building block of life." Genes are inherited from parents, and they literally make people what they are. Abnormal genes are called **gene mutations**, and also are inherited. Mutations can develop into diseases, including tumors. Cancer is believed to develop through an accumulation of genetic mutations or alterations, which allow the cells to grow out of control of normal regulatory mechanisms or to escape destruction by the immune system (see Chapter 64 ☺) (Minn, Wrensch, & Bondy, 2002).

Some inherited diseases, such as neurofibromatosis, are associated with increased risk of developing CNS tumors. It also is known that some gene mutations are not inherited. Research into these mutations has led to experimental laboratory treatments for brain tumors, with further refinement expected in the future (ACS, 2006).

It is not known why some people have gene mutations that cause brain tumors. Much research has been done looking for causes for brain tumors, such as cell phone use or environmental factors. There has been no link confirmed for the development of brain tumors with the use of cellular phones (Inskip, Tarone, & Hatch, 2001). However, children living in the vicinity of electromagnetic fields and having high exposure to them have shown increased risk for brain tumors, as have exposed workers (Meinert & Michaelis, 1996). Environmental factors, such as cigarette smoke, are known to cause lung cancer, which can metastasize to the brain to form metastatic lesions; however, no link has been found for primary disease (Wrensch, Minn, & Bondy, 2000).

Classification of Brain Tumors

The term *benign* can be misleading. Benign refers to microscopic cells that are well differentiated and resemble normal cells, but do not carry out the functions of normal cells. Instead they form slow-growing, space-occupying tumors. Histologically, although a tumor may be benign, if it is in a deep, eloquent area of the brain that is not accessible surgically, the tumor is not resectable. A tumor that is not resectable can continue to grow, producing neurological symptoms and possibly death. Some benign tumors also may progress into more malignant tumors if left untreated. A patient whose benign tumors are surgically resected can be considered cured.

Malignant tumors are those with poorly differentiated cells. Malignant tumors tend to be both aggressive and invasive. Although surgical resection may reduce the tumor, it is not curative. The prognosis for malignant tumors usually is poor.

Brain tumors may be primary or metastatic. **Primary tumors** are those that originate in the brain. These tumors rarely, if ever, travel to other areas of the body, remaining only in the brain. **Metastatic tumors** are those that originate in other areas of the body and travel to the brain. Examples of these are tumors that originate in the lung or breast tissue and metastasize to the brain. Tumors within the brain are classified as intra-axial, extra-axial, or metastatic.

Intra-Axial Tumors

Intra-axial tumors, located in the cerebrum, the brainstem, and the cerebellum, arise from glial cells, astrocytes, primitive brain structures, and ependymal structures. Glial cells are the supportive or nourishing cells of the brain. Any tumor arising from glial cells is referred to as a glioma. There are several types of gliomas: astrocytomas, oligodendrogliomas, and ependymomas. They are named for the type of cells they originate from and are graded for their degree of malignancy. Some tumors exist in a homogeneous form; others exhibit heterogeneous, or mixed, cell types.

Astrocytomas

Astrocytomas arise from the astrocyte cell. They have varying degrees of differentiation and are graded dependent on their degree of malignancy. Astrocytomas range from low grade (grades I and II), to anaplastic astrocytoma (grade III), to the most aggressive form of astrocytoma (grade IV), also known as glioblastoma multiforme. Low-grade astrocytomas, grade I or II, have well-differentiated cells. As the tissues become more malignant, cellularity increases, cell atypia increases, and mitotic activity increases. An astrocytoma with these cellular characteristics is termed anaplastic astrocytoma and is considered to be more malignant.

Astrocytomas account for approximately 50% of all primary brain tumors (Adesina, Leech, & Brumback, 2002). They are seen most commonly in the 30- to 50-year-old population, though they do occur in all age groups. Though astrocytomas may spread into surrounding normal brain tissue, it is rare for them to spread outside the brain and CSF system. Some astrocytomas spread throughout the CNS via CSF pathways.

Survival rates are dependent on many factors. These include grade, age of patient, extent of surgical resection, and response to treatment. The strongest predictor of survival with low-grade gliomas is age. One study reported a mean survival time of 8.5 years for adults less than 40 years of age. This contrasts with 4.9 years for adults 40 years of age and older (Piepmeier, 1987). Though this study is approximately 20 years old, the age factor has remained a strong prognostic factor.

Anaplastic astrocytomas (grade III) are noted to be more aggressive than lower grade astrocytomas. They have a median survival rate of approximately 3 to 5 years (Burton & Prados, 2002). Clinical manifestations are dependent on many factors including location and size of the lesion. They may include a single seizure, behavior changes, headaches, or sensorimotor alterations.

Glioblastoma Multiforme A grade IV astrocytoma also is referred to as a glioblastoma multiforme (GBM). These are the most malignant of the astrocytic tumors. Though they too arise from astrocytes, as do all astrocytomas, they are characterized by much more aggressive and invasive cellularity. They are rapidly growing, sometimes doubling in size in as little as 10 days. The GBM is composed of heterogeneous cells, which demonstrate the transformation of cells within this tumor from a low-grade to a high-grade or more malignant tumor. They are characterized by the presence of necrosis and hemorrhage within the tumor.

GBMs account for approximately 50% of all gliomas, and approximately 35% to 45% of all adult brain tumors. They are found most commonly in adults in their fourth to seventh decade, although they can be seen in young adults. The average age of patients with a GBM is 62 years, and they occur more often in men than women (Cox & Ang, 2003). The clinical history of GBM is relatively short. It frequently is less than 3 months before the patient presents with symptoms. The most common presenting symptoms are seizure, focal symptoms, such as motor weakness or aphasia, or nonfocal symptoms, such as headache or personality changes. The most dangerous aspect of symptomatology is the potential for rapidly increasing ICP caused by the rapid growth potential of this tumor (Kleihues, Davis, Coons, & Burger, 2000).

GBMs are the most malignant of all brain tumors. Despite improvements in surgical techniques, and the advancement of adjunctive therapies such as radiation therapy, chemotherapy, and radiosurgery, the prognosis is grim. The median survival rate is approximately 12 months (Burton & Prados, 2002). Although the prognosis is bleak, there is reason for hope in the treatment of high-grade gliomas. Research is ongoing, and new treatment protocols are being developed to treat this difficult and devastating disease.

Treatment is aimed at prolonging quality of life and may include the following strategies: surgical resection, radiation therapy, stereotactic radiosurgery, and chemotherapy. Despite what appears to be complete gross total resection, it is felt that this group of tumors is highly invasive at a microscopic level. This accounts for tumor recurrence despite resection in most cases. Radiation therapy (RT) is considered adjunctive. The most common form of radiation is focal external beam RT or conformal RT. Gamma knife radiosurgery has been shown to increase survival time in some cases. It can be used as a boost, or at tumor recurrence.

In some institutions, the implantation of radioactive materials, or a localized chemotherapeutic agent is used. This has met with mixed results, extending life by 4 to 10 weeks, but may be associated with seizures and craniotomy wound breakdown requiring additional hospital care. Chemotherapy also is an option for treatment of GBMs. Most treatment decisions are made based on the life expectancy and personal goals of the patient.

Some patients choose biopsy only and decide to spend their remaining time in their home with their family, whereas others prefer to exhaust all treatment measures. Nursing support for the family during their difficult decision process is essential.

Oligodendrogliomas

Tumors originating in brain cells are called oligodendrocytes. They grow and spread in much the same manner as astrocytomas. Specific to oligodendrogliomas is the frequent presence of calcification noted in diagnosed lesions (Adesina et al., 2002). They are slow growing, and can also spread to the CSF pathways, but rarely outside of the brain or spinal cord. Presenting signs and symptoms of oligodendrogliomas are dependent on the size and location of the tumor. Frequently, the initial presenting symptom is seizures. Oligodendrogliomas occur mostly in middle-age adults, but are occasionally seen in children. Treatment is surgical resection and radiation therapy. Prognosis for survival is thought to be approximately 7 years (Shaw, 2002).

Ependymomas

Ependymomas are tumors that originate in the ependymal cells lining the ventricles. They can be found in the brain or spinal cord. They do not spread into normal brain tissue, but they may spread along the CSF pathways. Therefore, there is a much better chance for complete surgical resection of ependymomas, especially from the spinal cord. Because these tumors are found in and around the ventricles and the CSF pathways, they occasionally cause obstruction of CSF flow, and hydrocephalus may occur.

Signs and symptoms are related to the location of the lesion. Seizures, motor weakness, cranial nerve deficits, or alterations in LOC may be present. If hydrocephalus is present, symptoms of increased ICP also may be present. Treatment consists of surgical resection and placement of a shunt if hydrocephalus is present. Radiation may be beneficial. Prognosis is excellent with surgical resection.

Extra-Axial Tumors

Extra-axial tumors are those that originate outside of the brain. The most common extra-axial tumors are meningiomas, schwannomas, and pituitary tumors.

Meningiomas

Meningiomas are the most common type of brain tumor, accounting for approximately 15% of all primary adult brain tumors (Cox & Ang, 2003). They arise from the meninges, the layer of tissue covering the brain and spinal cord. They are firm, encapsulated tumors that are extremely slow growing. Because they grow so slowly, they can grow to become quite large before they start causing symptoms. Meningiomas are most common in the middle-aged and the elderly. The peak occurrence is in the sixth and seventh decade of life. In middle-aged patients, there is a 3:2 female-to-male prevalence (Louis, Scheithauer, Budka, von Deimling, & Kepes, 2000). Presenting signs and symptoms depend on the location and size of the lesion.

Treatment is surgical resection in most cases. Occasionally, a complete resection is not possible because of the size of the lesion and its proximity to vital structures within the brain. In this case, radiation and/or gamma knife radiosurgery may be necessary. It also is necessary to follow these patients closely with yearly MRI scans to monitor the possible growth of the tumor. Tumor recurrence occurs in approximately 50% of patients with subtotal resection (Cox & Ang, 2003). In some cases, a lesion may be considered too small to warrant a surgical procedure. In these cases, monitoring of the lesion may be sufficient. Though considered benign, there is an atypical form and a malignant form of this disease, which may cause recurrence. It also is possible to have multiple meningiomas, which carries a high morbidity. Although the prognosis is extremely favorable with complete resection, it also is highly dependent on the degree of cell differentiation.

Schwannomas

Schwann cells are those that surround cranial nerves and other nerves. **Schwannomas** usually are benign tumors. The most common are schwannomas of the acoustic nerve (CN VIII), also referred to as **acoustic neuromas**. Acoustic neuromas usually are diagnosed when the patient experiences gradual hearing loss. Tinnitus and/or dizziness may also be noted. If left untreated, these lesions can become quite large, causing compression of the facial nerve (CN VII) or the trigeminal nerve (CN V).

For symptomatic lesions, gamma knife radiosurgery is the preferred treatment due to the ease of treatment, the excellent control of tumor growth, and reduction in unfavorable cranial nerve defects. Gamma knife treatment can also be planned to preserve hearing in those patients who still have functional hearing.

Open surgery is more appropriate for lesions that exceed 3 cm (about 1 in.). Surgical resection of acoustic neuromas can cause damage to cranial nerves in proximity to the tumor. In some instances, hearing may be sacrificed in the attempt to remove the tumor. The proximity of the brainstem and cranial nerves may result in damage to these nerves. Acoustic neuromas are located in the cerebropontine angle (CPA) with cranial nerves in proximity. Damage to the facial nerve (CN VII) may be present before surgery or as a result of surgery. Other cranial nerves also may be affected, specifically those involved with swallowing (CN IX, X, and XII). Therefore, a thorough cranial nerve assessment is important, both preoperatively and postoperatively.

If the facial nerve is damaged, it is important to note the degree of facial weakness exhibited. A facial weakness scale, known as the House/Brackmann scale, is used to note the degree of weakness (House & Brackmann, 1985). If significant facial weakness is observed, special care should be taken to protect the eye that does not close adequately. It is important to protect the eye from dryness and even abrasions by keeping it well lubricated with eyedrops. Occasionally, complete resection is not possible due to the size and location of the tumor. Residual tumor may be radiated and/or monitored with serial MRIs. Gamma knife radiosurgery may be a beneficial adjunctive treatment.

Pituitary Adenomas

Tumors of the pituitary gland occur most frequently in the anterior lobe, but both lobes may show symptoms. Tumors are classified by the type of hormone secreted (Chart 29–7, p. 738). Examples of these are prolactin, growth hormone, or ACTH secreting tumors. Pituitary tumors also are classified as functioning, hormone secreting, or nonfunctioning. Functioning pituitary adenomas produce endocrine symptoms, such as acromegaly, hyperprolactinemia, or Cushing's syndrome. Nonfunctioning pituitary adenomas produce symptoms caused by pressure of the tumor on surrounding structures, such as the optic nerve. Frequently, visual loss is the presenting symptom. It may be in the form of decreased acuity, hemianopsia, or scotomas. Headaches frequently accompany visual symptoms. Treatment may be medical and/or surgical. With treatment, prognosis is excellent.

Metastatic Tumors

Metastatic brain tumors originate in another part of the body from another type of cancer and travel to the brain. They are not considered to be cancer of the brain, but rather cancer from another source that has migrated to the brain.

Epidemiology and Etiology

Metastases to the brain come from many sources. The most common sites of primary disease are lung, breast, and skin. Metastatic lesions are probably more common than primary lesions. Males and females are represented equally, most commonly seen between the fifth and seventh decade of life (Sneed, 2002). The method of spread of metastatic lesions varies by the type of primary disease. Lesions most commonly spread from their primary site via the arterial route. They also may spread via the meninges. Occasionally, direct extension of melanoma lesions of the head or neck may lead to melanoma in the brain.

Other characteristics of metastatic lesions vary by primary disease. The number and location of lesions also vary by primary disease. Single lesions are more common, but multiple lesions occur frequently in some types of primary disease, such as lung cancer. The cerebral cortex is the most common site of metastatic disease, with the cerebellum less so.

Clinical Manifestations

Presenting symptoms of metastatic tumors are dependent on the location of the tumors. Most common symptoms are similar to those of primary tumors, and include headache, motor weakness, alteration of mentation, and/or behavioral changes. Seizures are the presenting symptom in many cases.

Laboratory and Diagnostic Procedures

Diagnosis of brain tumors always begins with an accurate and thorough history and physical. Symptom analysis, including duration and frequency of symptoms, is a valuable tool for determining presence and onset of symptoms. It also is important to have an accurate accounting of seizure events, including type, and frequency.

The actual diagnosis of a brain tumor is made by MRI of the suspected region, with and without gadolinium. It is possible with this test to determine the location, size, and characteristics of the lesion, including heterogeneity and presence of necrosis or hemorrhage. MRI also will determine the presence of calcification, cystic qualities, or enhancement. Ventricle size also is seen, as hydrocephalus is a potentially dangerous side effect of the presence of tumor, and the presence of edema and/or mass effect also can be determined. Although it is possible to diagnose a brain tumor with the aid of MRI, it only is possible to assume the type of tumor, not to diagnose the type of tumor. The only positive diagnosis of tumor type is by obtaining tissue for pathology diagnosis.

Medical Management

Once the diagnosis of brain tumor is made, treatment options must be explored. As just stated, the only means for positive

| CHART 29–7 | Classification of Brain Tumors |

Type	Average Age at Onset	Symptoms	Treatment	Prognosis
Meningioma	Age 40–60s	Dependent on location and size Seizures Headaches	Surgery Radiation for residual or recurrence (gamma knife, cyberknife)	Excellent with resection
Astrocytoma	Variable	Dependent on location and size	Surgery Radiation for residual recurrence	3–7 years with treatment, dependent on grade and extent of resection
Glioblastoma multiforme (GBM)	Age 50–60s	Dependent on location and size	Surgery Radiation Chemotherapy	12–18 months with treatment
Oligodendroglioma	Age 40–50s	Dependent on location Seizures	Surgery Radiation Chemotherapy	5–10+ years with treatment
Ependymoma	All ages (60% are children)	Signs and symptoms Increased ICP Hydrocephalus	Surgery Radiation Chemotherapy for recurrence May need shunt	7–8+ years with surgery, less with recurrence
Pituitary adenomas	Variable	Hormone abnormalities dependent on area of pituitary affected Visual disturbances Headaches	Medical Surgical possible Radiation possible	Excellent
Acoustic neuromas	Age 40–50s	Hearing loss	Surgery Radiation for residual (gamma knife)	Excellent
Metastatic tumors	Variable	Dependent on location, size, single or multiple	Surgery if single metastasis or symptomatic Radiation (gamma knife) Chemotherapy	Usually poor, dependent on single or multiple and identification of primary disease

diagnosis is pathologic examination of the tissue. Neurosurgical consultation is imperative if a brain tumor is suspected. In addition to surgical intervention, options of radiation therapy, chemotherapy, and/or radio surgery may be available.

Surgical Excision

The role of surgical excision has several goals. The first is to establish a pathology diagnosis. As previously stated, the only way to obtain a positive diagnosis is to have a pathologist specializing in neuropathology make a positive identification of tumor type. Tumor type and grade, if appropriate, are necessary to establish an appropriate treatment plan. The second goal of surgery is to obtain the maximum tumor debulking possible while maintaining function. In many cases, the success of the treatment—and the prognosis—is based on the amount of tumor resection.

Surgical excision of a brain tumor requires monitoring in an ICU setting initially. Some patients may require ICP monitoring postoperatively. A postoperative MRI usually is done to assess the extent of resection and to assess the presence of hemorrhage, edema, and the status of the ventricles. The National Guidelines box provides the AANN national guidelines for the care of craniotomy patients.

Radiation Therapy

Once a pathologic diagnosis is made, some patients will require a consultation for a radiation oncologist. Brain tumors that cannot be cured by surgery alone may be treated with radiation. Recurrent, intermediate, or high-grade astrocytomas, metastatic tumors, incomplete or subtotal resections, or any other tumor deemed appropriate by the neurosurgeon or the neuro-oncologist may benefit from recommendations from a radiation oncologist. There are many types of radiation, and radiological treatment varies by pathologic diagnosis.

Radiation from an external source focused directly on the tumor is called external beam radiation. These treatments are given over a period of several weeks. Three-dimensional treatments are referred to as conformal radiation. Whole-brain radiation is given over a period of weeks. It generally is reserved for patients with several metastatic lesions for whom other methods of radiation would not be appropriate. Radiation therapy using any of these methods is used after surgical resection. The purpose is to slow growth, or to stabilize the residual tumor. It also may be used to prevent recurrence. The addition of RT to the treatment regimen of brain tumor patients adds to the comfort and quality of life and also increases survival time.

NATIONAL GUIDELINES AANN Guidelines for the Care of Craniotomy Patients for Brain Tumor

Neurological

- Most complications occur within the first 6 hours postoperative
- ICU admission postoperative
- Frequent neurological assessments
  - Ask the neurosurgeon what complications or deficits are expected
- Incision care
  - Monitor incision for drainage
  - Keep incision dry
- Drains
  - Make sure the location of each drain is known; label clearly

Cardiovascular

- Cardiac arrhythmias
- Hypovolemic shock
- Monitor rate and rhythm
- Monitor blood pressure and maintain ordered parameters

Respiratory

- Related to decreased level of consciousness/inability to protect airway
- Especially relevant to surgery near brainstem
- Prevent atelectasis and pneumonia
- Maintain $SaO_2 > 94\%$
- Incentive spirometry unless contraindicated (transsphenoidal surgery)

Gastrointestinal

- Prevention of gastric ulceration (antacids, proton pump inhibitor, H2-blockers)
- Some drugs used in neurological treatment can contribute to gastric irritation (dexamethasone, phenytoin, some antibiotics)

Nutrition

- May require swallow evaluation
- May require enteral feedings

Serum Glucose

- Hyperglycemia may increase cerebral edema
- Hyperglycemia may result from steroid therapy
- Monitor blood glucose as ordered
- Maintain euglycemia

Serum Sodium

- Diabetes insipidus
  - Especially relevant to surgery involving or near the pituitary gland
  - Monitor intake/output and specific gravity
  - Notify health care provider for urine output > 200 mL/hr × 2 consecutive hours
- Syndrome of inappropriate antidiuretic hormone
  - Monitor sodium levels; treat as ordered

Activity

- Population at risk for deep vein thrombosis (DVT)
  - Early ambulation
  - DVT prophylaxis, such as low-molecular-weight heparin, when ordered
  - Therapy consults
- Pain control
  - Assess per hospital protocol
  - Administer pain medication as ordered
  - Offer other techniques for pain management, such as deep breathing or music

Source: Adapted from American Association of Neuroscience Nurses, AANN Reference Series for Clinical Practice. (2006). *Guide to the Care of the Patient with Craniotomy Post-Brain Tumor Resection.* Glenview, IL: American Association of Neuroscience Nurses.

Stereotactic Radiosurgery

Stereotactic radiosurgery is another treatment option. It is a form of radiation therapy that delivers a single, high dose of radiation directly at the tumor or tumor bed. Despite the terminology, it is not a surgical procedure; however, it is meant to provide a highly conformed dose of radiation to the lesion. It may be used as the first preferred treatment or it may be used as a follow-up to other forms of treatment. The goal of radiosurgery is to treat all tumor cells in its path. Two types of radiosurgery most commonly used for treatment of brain tumors are gamma knife and cyber knife radiosurgery.

Gamma knife radiosurgery is a system that uses focused radiation in a single dose. It is used to irradiate very specific areas of tumor, such as the tumor bed of a metastatic lesion. This is a system developed by Lars Leksell that delivers multiple source beams (more than 200) to a specific, small target (Hickey, 2003). The name, however, is misleading because it is not really surgery and it is not really a knife. It may be used as the "first line" of treatment, or it may be used as adjunctive therapy. It may be used to "shrink" the residual tumor when complete resection is not possible. Gamma knife radiosurgery also may be beneficial in treating tumors that are considered inoperable or small enough that a surgical procedure is not necessary.

Cyber knife radiosurgery is a relatively new addition to the radiation arsenal. It is a radiosurgical system that consists of a linear accelerator and a robotic arm. This system can locate tumors using image guidance, and then deliver multiple beams of radiation directly to the tumor site. This system has some important advantages. It minimizes radiation exposure to surrounding tissue and has the capacity to treat tumors up to 6 cm (2.4 in.) in size (Quinn, 2002). It has proven beneficial in treating metastatic brain tumors (Shimamoto et al., 2002).

Brachytherapy is referred to as an internal form of radiation therapy. It is the surgical implantation of radioactive capsules, or "seeds," directly into the tumor bed. These may be temporary or permanent. This procedure is generally reserved for high-grade gliomas.

Radiation is more damaging to cancer cells than to normal tissue, but it can cause damage to normal tissue. Sometimes an area of dead tissue forms at the site of an irradiated tumor. This is referred to as tissue necrosis and can appear as a mass on MRI, making it difficult to differentiate between dead tissue and tumor.

Positron emission tomography (PET) imaging may be used to aide in differentiating tissue necrosis, which has no metabolic activity, from new tumor growth, which has a high metabolic activity. Surgical resection may be necessary to debulk the mass and to differentiate between tumor regrowth and treatment effect. Radiation therapy is not without risk for adverse symptoms. However, the benefits of tumor suppression may outweigh the risks of radiation.

Chemotherapy

The purpose of chemotherapy is to destroy tumor cells, either by destroying the cells themselves or by destroying their capacity to reproduce themselves. Chemotherapy uses anticancer drugs, which are given intravenously or orally. They also may be given intrathecally, usually into an implanted reservoir. The implantation of a wafer soaked in a chemotherapeutic agent is occasionally used in the treatment of GBMs. The types of drugs used, dosage, and route are determined by the tumor type. Special concerns when treating malignant brain tumors with chemotherapeutic agents include the following:

- The location of the tumor in the brain affects choice of treatment.
- Cerebral edema affects drug entry into the brain.
- Brain tissue has a low capacity to remove dead tissue, cell debris, fluid, and drugs because there is no lymphatic drainage in the brain.
- Tumor cell resistance can occur (when tumor cells are no longer susceptible to damage by a particular drug).
- Malignant tumors (GBM) are composed of diverse (heterogeneous) cells, resulting in differences in the chemosensitivity of cells within the tumor.
- Many drugs cannot cross the blood–brain barrier (Shapiro & Shapiro, 1986).

Chemotherapy drugs kill cancer cells, but also can damage normal cells. Some normal tissue, such as bone marrow, the lining of the mouth and intestines, and hair follicles, grow rapidly to replace cells that wear out naturally. These cells are the ones most affected by chemotherapy drugs. Although care is taken to avoid or reduce the side effects of chemotherapy, these patients may experience hair loss, decreased white cell counts, fatigue, mouth sores, decreased appetite, and nausea and vomiting. These side effects are temporary and generally cease once treatment is over.

The survival of patients with brain tumors has improved somewhat with the addition of chemotherapy. However, the most effective drugs or combination of drugs is not yet known. At this point in time, the most common chemotherapeutic drugs are the alkylating agents such as carmustine (BCNU), lomustine (CCNU), procarbazine, vincristine, and temozolomide. They are typically used in combination with other therapies, such as RT. The use of chemotherapy in the treatment of cancer also is discussed in Chapter 64 ☺.

■ Nursing Management

Nursing management of the patient with a brain tumor includes the opportunity to support patients and their families through one of the most difficult experiences they will experience. The patient and her family are presented with a life-altering diagnosis, which will affect every facet of the patient's life and every member of the patient's family. Innumerable factors can affect the patient's needs, both emotional and physical. The response to the diagnosis by the family and the patient is dependent on many factors, including the type of tumor, the location of the tumor, treatment plan, degree of neurological deficits, age of the patient, numerous family dynamics, educational status of the patient and family, and many other factors that change as the course of the disease changes.

Assessment

When the patient is initially diagnosed with a brain tumor, it may be because of an initial event that brought the patient into the emergency room, such as a seizure. Respiratory status must be monitored carefully, especially if the patient is admitted with a decreased level of consciousness. The ABCs of any emergency assessment (airway–breathing–circulation) are equally as important in patients with neurological deterioration. Monitoring of respiratory rate, rhythm, and effort are paramount, with preparations made for emergency intubation should the patient's respiratory status decline.

Usually, however, the patient is not in medical distress or even particularly ill. The patient's first exposure to a hospital setting may be on admission for surgery to remove the brain tumor. It may be unknown as to the patient's level of knowledge regarding his diagnosis or plan. An important nursing intervention is education, both of the surgical experience and what to expect postoperatively. The surgeon will review the planned surgery, surgical approach, projected length of hospital stay, and possible side effects with the patient and family. However, most patients and their families have many other questions that they do not ask their surgeon. Examples of these are: Will I have my head shaved? When will I be able to eat, or get out of bed, or go to the bathroom by myself? Will I be in pain? When can I go back to work? What's going to happen to me when I go home? It is not uncommon for the patient and family to depend on the nurse to provide them with the information that will affect their everyday lives.

Interventions and Rationales

As with other types of acute brain disorders, it is of utmost importance to adhere to the nursing care regimen associated with increased ICP, discussed earlier in this chapter. Certain tumor types are more prone to cause vasogenic edema. This may lead to cerebral edema, and increased ICP causing a variety of neurological deficits (refer to Chart 29–4, p. 720, on the nursing implications and interventions for management of ICP earlier in the chapter). These deficits include personality changes, decreased level of consciousness, aphasia, motor deficits, sensory deficits, visual deficits, and/or cranial nerve deficits. These deficits are dependent on the location and size of the lesion. Cerebral edema can be seen with almost any tumor type, but is most common with GBM, metastatic lesions, and even some "benign" tumors, such as meningiomas. The medical treatment of choice is dexamethasone. It is important that this drug be given exactly as ordered, because an abrupt halt—or even a decrease in dose—can cause an increase in edema and associated neurological symptoms. A patient care plan for patients with acute brain disorders applies to this clinical discussion, as it does with other types of acute brain disorders, and is discussed in the Nursing Process: Patient Care Plan for Acute Brain Disorders.

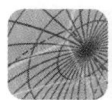

NURSING PROCESS: Patient Care Plan for Acute Brain Disorders

Assessment of Altered Levels of Consciousness

Subjective Data:

Does the patient have any history of health problems, such as hypertension, heart disease, bleeding disorders, renal disease, or cancer?
What were the patient's presenting symptoms/complaints?
How long ago did the first symptoms present?

Objective Data:

Neurological assessment, including mentation, cranial nerve examination, motor and sensory examination.
Imaging studies, including magnetic resonance imaging (MRI), computed tomography scan (CT), and/or lumbar puncture.
Laboratory data, including complete blood count (CBC), cerebral perfusion pressure (CPP), and drug levels.

Nursing Assessment and Diagnoses	Outcomes and Evaluation Parameters	Planning and Interventions with *Rationales*
Nursing Diagnoses: *Actual and Potential Alteration in Level of Consciousness* related to traumatic brain injury (TBI), intracranial tumor, or infectious process	**Outcome:** Improvement to optimum level of function. *Evaluation Parameters:* Stable neurological examination. Glasgow Coma Scale. Laboratory tests, including serum sodium and cultures of blood and cerebrospinal fluid (CSF) if suspicious for infection.	**Interventions and *Rationales:*** Monitor neurological examination hourly, or as directed. *Allows early recognition of pending neurological deterioration.* Monitor lab values, including serum sodium levels and cultures. *Early recognition and treatment of hyponatremia or infection.*
Impaired Physical Mobility related to altered level of consciousness	**Outcome:** Improvement to optimum level of motor function. *Evaluation Parameters:* Neurological motor and sensory examination. Level of participation in therapies and ADLs.	**Interventions and *Rationales:*** Monitor motor strengths and limitations. *Allows early recognition of neurological changes.* Initiate therapies, such as physical and occupational unless contraindicated. *Early initiation of therapies helps to identify deficits and needed areas for improvement.* Initiate activity as tolerated, unless contraindicated. *Physical activity will increase strength and endurance, as well as decrease complications, such as pneumonia or blood clots.*
Ineffective Tissue Perfusion related to immobility	**Outcome:** Adequate tissue perfusion. *Evaluation Parameter:* Absence of deep vein thrombosis (DVTs) or pulmonary embolus.	**Interventions and *Rationales:*** Encourage activity as tolerated, unless contraindicated. *Physical activity will prevent immobility and the formation of blood clots.* Apply thigh-high elastic stockings and sequential compression stockings *to increase venous circulation.* Administer subcutaneous injections of low-molecular-weight heparin, if indicated *to discourage the formation of blood clots.* Monitor lower extremities frequently for signs/symptoms of DVT. *Early recognition and treatment of a DVT may prevent extension of the clot or pulmonary embolus.*
Impaired Verbal Communication related to anatomical defect.	**Outcome:** Maximum level of communication. *Evaluation Parameter:* Ability to adequately communicate with others.	**Interventions and *Rationales:*** Assess type and degree of communication deficit *to determine patient needs and establish a baseline.* Arrange a speech therapy consult. *Early intervention and therapy optimizes results.*
Actual or Potential Alteration in Visual Perception related to TBI or brain tumor	**Outcome:** Maximum level of vision/visual acuity. *Evaluation Parameter:* Formal and informal vision screening including visual fields.	**Interventions and *Rationales:*** Assess vision by informal testing (i.e., counting fingers, reading the clock) *to assess type and degree of visual deficit present.* Institute safety measures, such as placing call light within reach, orienting patient to surroundings, *to prevent accidents/falls.* Obtain occupational therapy evaluation if warranted. *Evaluation of visual deficits and education regarding coping mechanisms.*
Ineffective Cerebral Tissue Perfusion related to electrolyte imbalances in TBI, brain tumors, or infectious process	**Outcome:** Optimum neurological function. *Evaluation Parameters:* Stable neurological examination. Electrolyte levels, specifically sodium.	**Interventions and *Rationales:*** Monitor serum sodium as indicated, at least daily *to assess for hyponatremia.* Conduct neurological assessments frequently *to assess for decreased level of consciousness.* Administer fluids as directed *to maintain adequate fluid balance.* Notify health care providers immediately of abnormal lab values or change in neurological examination. *Such changes may indicate hyponatremia.*

(continued)

NURSING PROCESS: Patient Care Plan for Acute Brain Disorders—*Continued*

Assessment of Airway and Gas Exchange

Subjective Data:
Does the patient have any preexisting medical problems such as emphysema or asthma, or any cardiac diseases?

Objective Data:
Respiratory rate
Oxygen saturation
Arterial blood gases

Vital signs
Lung sounds
Skin/nail bed/lip color

Nursing Assessment and Diagnoses	Outcomes and Evaluation Parameters	Planning and Interventions with *Rationales*
Nursing Diagnoses: *Ineffective Airway Clearance* related to altered level of consciousness	**Outcome:** Adequate respiration status. ***Evaluation Parameters:*** Adequate arterial blood gases. Respiratory rate within normal limits. Normal oxygen saturation levels. Clear lung sounds. Mental status, such as confusion or agitation.	**Interventions and *Rationales:*** Monitor respiratory status (i.e., rate, rhythm, and quality). *Changes in respiratory rates or patterns may indicate pending respiratory failure. It may also indicate neurological change.* Monitor mental status. *Restlessness, agitation, or confusion may indicate hypoxia.* Monitor oxygen saturation *to assess adequacy of gas exchange.* Encourage deep breathing or use of an incentive spirometer *to promote adequate gas exchange.* Position with head in neutral position, head of bed elevated at 30 degrees, unless contraindicated *to promote adequate gas exchange.* Suction as necessary. *Patients with decreased neurological status may be unable to protect their airways.* Report changes in respiratory patterns to MD. *Such changes indicate possible risk for respiratory failure.* If patient not intubated, have necessary intubation equipment available. *Protecting the airway is the priority. Intubation may be necessary to protect airway.*
Risk for Aspiration related to altered level of consciousness	**Outcome:** No aspiration. ***Evaluation Parameters:*** Adequate oxygen saturation. Safe swallowing techniques.	**Interventions and *Rationales:*** Keep NPO until alert and/or swallow reflex is assessed and deemed safe. *Altered level of consciousness may depress the cough and/or swallow reflex.*

Assessment of Hemodynamic Status

Subjective Data:
Does the patient have any preexisting cardiac or respiratory problems?

Objective Data:
Vital signs, including heart rate, blood pressure, respiratory rate, and central venous pressure, if available
Oxygen saturation
Skin, lips, and nail bed color
Lung sounds
Cardiac rhythm strips or ECG

Nursing Assessment and Diagnoses	Outcomes and Evaluation Parameters	Planning and Interventions with *Rationales*
Nursing Diagnoses: *Decreased intracranial adaptive capacity* related to increased intracranial pressure	**Outcome:** Hemodynamic stability. ***Evaluation Parameters:*** Adequate blood pressure to maintain central perfusion pressure (CPP). Stable vital signs, including central venous pressure (CVP), Pulmonary Arterial Pressure (PAP), and intracranial pressure (ICP).	**Interventions and *Rationales:*** Monitor vital signs as directed *to establish a baseline and note changes in vital signs.* Administer fluids and medications as directed *to assist in maintaining blood pressure as ordered to maintain adequate CPP.* Monitor ECG rhythm *to assess for alterations in rhythm or rate.* Monitor intake and output *to assess fluid balance to maintain hemodynamic parameters.* Notify health care provider of hemodynamic changes. *Medical intervention may be necessary to prevent hemodynamic instability leading to neurological decline.* Monitor neurological assessments closely. *Hemodynamic stability is closely related to CPP and ICP changes in neurologically compromised patients.*

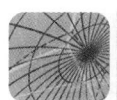

NURSING PROCESS: Patient Care Plan for Acute Brain Disorders—*Continued*

Assessment of Pain

Subjective Data:
Does the patient complain of pain?
Facial expressions (i.e., grimacing).

Objective Data:
Increased heart rate, blood pressure, or respiratory rate?

Nursing Assessment and Diagnoses	Outcomes and Evaluation Parameters	Planning and Interventions with *Rationales*
Nursing Diagnosis: Readiness for enhanced comfort related to brain tumor, head injury, meningitis, or surgical procedure	**Outcome:** Adequate pain control. **Evaluation Parameters:** Vital signs within normal limits. Patient verbalizes pain control.	**Interventions and *Rationales*:** Assess presence of pain or efficacy of pain control frequently *to ensure patient comfort.* Administer pain medications as ordered *to ensure patient comfort.*

Assessment of Coping

Subjective Data:
What are patient's complaints?
What is the patient's understanding of present condition or disease?
What are patient's concerns for the future?

Objective Data:
What is the patient's level of education?
What is the patient's occupation?
What is the patient's family support system?
Does the patient have a religious affiliation?

Nursing Assessment and Diagnoses	Outcomes and Evaluation Parameters	Planning and Interventions with *Rationales*
Nursing Diagnoses: *Ineffective Coping* related to knowledge deficit	**Outcome:** Patient and family will have information needed. **Evaluation Parameter:** Discussions with patient, with verbalization of condition and treatment.	**Interventions and *Rationales*:** Provide information as needed and answer questions honestly and completely. *Information and education are important to the patient.* Involve family as appropriate. *Family support is important for recovery.*
Readiness for Enhanced Family Coping related to neurological deficits	**Outcome:** Family will have improved coping with neurological disability. **Evaluation Parameters:** Discussions with patient and family with verbalization of concerns. Observation of family/patient interactions.	**Interventions and *Rationales*:** Reassure patient and family with honesty and compassion *to provide encouragement and information needed for coping.* Encourage family members to voice concerns *to help with assessment of family needs.* Provide family with support as needed, such as spiritual, therapies, or psychological. *Neurological disability affects the whole family and community.*

These patients usually are started on corticosteroids, such as dexamethasone (Decadron). The most common dose is 4 mg every 6 hours, but it may be necessary to give 10 mg every 6 hours in the presence of cerebral edema. Use of steroids such as dexamethasone usually increases blood glucose levels, possibly requiring treatment. It also raises white blood counts, which may mask underlying infectious processes. Steroids can cause significant alterations in behavior and produce insomnia, elation, and even psychosis. Nursing care should include careful monitoring to detect behavioral changes. Refer to the Pharmacology Summary (p. 733) for more explanation of these medications.

Patients undergoing chemotherapy may experience many side effects. Common side effects of the various chemotherapeutic drugs include fatigue, nausea and vomiting, loss of appetite, rash, neuropathies, myelosuppression, constipation, and immunosuppression. Side effects differ with the agent, and may range from mild to severe. Occasionally treatment cannot be continued due to the severity of the reaction. It is important for nurses to be aware of side effects specific to the treatment of each patient. All side effects should be reported to the health care provider.

Also associated with some brain tumors are seizures. Although seizures may be seen with other acute brain disorders, they are closely associated with certain types of brain tumors. Seizures are the most common presenting symptom of patients with oligodendrogliomas. They also are seen frequently with other tumor types, especially those located in the temporal region, due to the high intensity of seizure focus in that area. These seizures are treated with antiepileptic drugs such as phenytoin. The nursing implications of seizure treatment are discussed later in this chapter.

Patients with newly diagnosed brain tumors may present with overwhelming emotional needs. Nursing intervention comes in the form of education and support. An important discharge intervention may be acquainting patients and their families with available brain tumor support groups. Many patients and families feel that the diagnosis of brain tumor is one without hope. Providing the patient and their family with education and support may be helpful in relieving the fear of the unknown.

Collaborative Management

The diagnosis, treatment, and management of patients with brain tumors require the expertise of multiple disciplines. These include, but are not limited to, nursing, neurosurgery, neuro-oncology, radiation oncology, physical therapy, speech and cognitive therapy, occupational therapy, pathology, rehabilitation specialists, neuropsychologists, research scientists and nurses, dietitians, and support groups. Once the diagnosis of brain tumor is made, the patient should be referred to a neurosurgeon. Postoperatively, the patient may require the services of various therapists, such as physical, occupational, and/or speech therapists. Therapies are important for evaluation, and treatment if necessary. It is also important for discharge recommendations. Dependent on the pathology of the tumor, consultations with neuro-oncology, medical-oncology, and/or radiation oncology may be warranted. These consultations may be for the purpose of recommendations, with or without treatment.

Upon discharge from the hospital, the patient may need further therapy. This may be in the form of outpatient therapies, home health therapy, or an acute inpatient rehabilitation stay. Determination of the patient's need for further therapy is usually made by specialists in rehabilitation medicine. (For more on patient education regarding discharge, see the Patient Teaching & Discharge Priorities box.)

At the center of the brain tumor patient's plan of care is nursing. As stated previously, newly diagnosed brain tumor patients are frequently in a state of confusion and emotional upheaval. Their lives are full of changes: physical, emotional, practical, and possibly financial. They may be facing the loss of a job and fi-

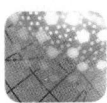

PATIENT TEACHING & DISCHARGE PRIORITIES for Acute Brain Disorders

Need	Teaching

Wound infection:
  Patient
  Family support system
  Setting
	Assess surgical wound for signs/symptoms of infection.
	Signs and symptoms of infection include:
	  Redness
	  Tenderness
	  Exudate and/or odor
	  Swelling
	  Poor healing.
	The presence of fever or any of the above symptoms should be reported.
	Assess family support for needed assistance.

Mobility assistance:
  Patient
  Family support system
  Setting
	Assess motor strengths and ability for ambulation.
	Obtain consults for physical and occupational therapy.
	Assess need for assistive devices, such as wheelchair, walker, or splints.
	Assess availability of family for support with mobility and ADLs.
	Conduct family teaching.
	Assess environment for risk factors.

Pain control:
  Patient
  Family support system
  Setting
	Assess need for pain control.
	Is present medication regimen adequate? Is pain controlled sufficiently to allow patient to participate in ADLs?
	Assess need for family intervention in dispensing pain medication.
	Assess patient/family understanding of medication instructions.

Safety:
  Patient
  Family support system
  Setting
	Assess patient cognitive status:
	  Is patient a fall risk?
	  Assess safety awareness.
	Assess patient understanding of medication schedule and needs.
	Assess patient need for supervision.
	Obtain consults for speech/cognitive evaluation.
	Obtain social service consult.
	Obtain home health consult.
	Assess family involvement in patient's recuperative period.
	Conduct family teaching regarding possible cognitive impairments.
	Conduct family teaching regarding need for supervision.
	Assess environment for safety. May require home health or social service involvement.

Follow-up needs:
  Patient
  Family support system
  Setting
	Assess need for follow-up appointments for needed therapies or interventions:
	  Radiation therapy
	  Outpatient therapies: physical, occupational, speech
	  Physician appointments
	  Laboratory visits for evaluation of drug levels or electrolytes
	  Follow-up x-rays.
	Assess family understanding and need for further explanation.
	Assess availability of resources for follow-up.

nancial security and changes within their family structure (e.g., spouses becoming caregivers). It is important to supply these patients with as much education and support as they require. If support groups are available, it is usually helpful to give this information to the patients and their families.

Health Promotion

Much research has been done to look for causes of brain tumors. These research inquiries include genetic research, environmental factors, dietary factors, and hereditary factors. As mentioned earlier, attention has been given to the use of cellular phones and a possible connection with the development of brain tumors. Use of cellular phones has not been shown to be harmful (Inskip et al., 2003). Studies have been completed to answer the concern about the possibility that exposure to the polio vaccine in the 1950s may have exposed millions to a precursor to the development of brain tumors. No evidence was found to link polio vaccine with the development of brain tumors (Brenner et al., 2002).

Some of the stronger leads concerning potential causes of brain tumors have come from studies of occupation. Suspected occupations of high risk include employment in the petroleum industry, electricity-related jobs, farming, and work involving pesticides, and electric and magnetic fields (DeRoos et al., 2003). Because there are inconsistencies among study results, there is a defined need for further study in certain fields, such as environmental and occupational hazards.

Despite much attention to the potential risk factors of brain tumors, the etiology of brain tumors remains largely unknown. There are some familial genetic cancer syndromes, such as neurofibromatosis and tuberous sclerosis, but these account for a very small number. The only environmental risk factor that is well established is that of ionizing radiation. It is therefore important to continue research to look for factors that may cause brain tumors, and factors that may protect us from brain tumors (Brenner et al., 2002).

Future Directions

A diagnosis of brain tumor is life altering, at best. Even with more than 20 years of clinical trials and new technologies to combat this disease, few improvements in prognosis have been seen, especially in the treatment of high-grade tumors. However, the team of professionals aligned to fight this disease and find a cure, or at very least improved treatment, also is formidable. Neuro-oncologists are facing great challenges in the management of brain tumors. They are joined by radiation oncologists, geneticists, cellular biologists, neurologists, and neurosurgeons.

Pueschel, Ashby, and Shapiro (2003) described the results of clinical trials in the treatment of adult and pediatric CNS tumors published in a single year (2001). These studies described various chemotherapy regimens, delivered with and without adjunctive RT. There is no doubt that these trials will continue examining new and different drug and treatment combinations until one is found that will successfully treat, and, it is hoped, cure brain tumors.

The Radiation Therapy Oncology Group (RTOG) (2008) protocols also are important in identifying optimal RT programs for various tumor types. Radiosurgery has become and will continue to be important in the treatment of various tumor types. Information is being obtained and processed continually to determine the efficacy of various treatment plans.

Research into the genetics of brain tumors is dynamic. Genetic aberrations are being defined for the various glial tumors previously described. It is known that tumors can evolve by different pathways. Genetic aberrations differ from grade of malignancy and the type of tumor. Additional research is needed to continue in this field of brain tumor research to identify causes and look for treatment (Shapiro, 2001). Immunotherapy and gene therapy offer exciting challenges for future investigation of treatment for brain tumors (Pueschel et al., 2003).

■ Hydrocephalus

Cerebrospinal fluid is a clear, colorless fluid produced within the ventricles, in the choroid plexus. Its purpose is to circulate within the subarachnoid space and bathe the brain and spinal cord in fluid to cushion it. A normal adult has approximately 125 to 150 mL of CSF at any one time. It is normally produced at approximately 25 mL an hour. The most common pathologic condition concerning CSF is hydrocephalus. Hydrocephalus is an excessive accumulation of CSF in the intracerebral ventricles. It may be caused by overproduction or inadequate drainage or absorption. Two types of hydrocephalus are communicating and noncommunicating.

Communicating hydrocephalus refers to large ventricles in a system with communication between all of the ventricles and the pathway for CSF. The size of the ventricles is relatively proportional. The cause of communicating hydrocephalus usually is due to blockage or malabsorption of CSF by the arachnoid granulations. Common causes include subarachnoid hemorrhage (SAH) or the presence of infection, such as coccidiomycosis.

Noncommunicating (also referred to as obstructive) hydrocephalus refers to a blockage somewhere within the CSF pathway. One or more of the ventricles may be larger than the other ventricles, depending on the level of the obstruction. The most common cause of noncommunicating hydrocephalus is space-occupying lesions, such as tumors.

The most important concept to understanding hydrocephalus is that of resistance to the absorption of CSF, which can cause hydrocephalus and the increase of ICP. The most common cause of malabsorption of CSF is subarachnoid hemorrhage, in which protein from blood product breakdown clogs the arachnoid granulations, hindering absorption of CSF. In the absence of a lymphatic drainage system in the CNS, open communication between the CSF and the interstitial fluid is necessary for maintenance of homeostasis (Sato, Takei, & Yamada, 1994).

In the presence of cerebral edema, there may be no increase in ventricular size, due to the pressure of the brain tissue (parenchyma) against the ventricular system. Ventricular size is a balance between brain tissue forces attempting to compress the ventricles and intraventricular pressure, attempting to enlarge the ventricles This concept of intracranial pressure was discussed earlier in the chapter. Hydrocephalus is a common occurrence in brain trauma, some brain tumors, subarachnoid hemorrhage, and some encephalopathic conditions, including meningitis, encephalitis, and brain abscess.

Clinical Manifestations

The presentation of increasing ventricular size in adults is dependent on the type of hydrocephalus. Examples of symptoms are similar to those of increased ICP and include papilledema, headache, nausea and vomiting, incontinence, gait changes, difficulty with extraocular movements particularly upgaze, and alterations in LOC.

Laboratory and Diagnostic Procedures

A CT scan of the head, without contrast, is the quickest and most definitive means of diagnosing hydrocephalus. MRI is also an effective diagnostic study, and may be a better choice for imaging when pathology, such as a brain tumor, is suspected. As always, close clinical correlation of the patient's history and presenting symptoms is recommended.

Medical Management

Hydrocephalus is a surgically treated condition. In emergency situations, removal of spinal fluid by means of an external ventricular drain is a temporary solution. However, placement of a shunting device to remove extra spinal fluid is the gold standard for treatment of hydrocephalus. There are several types of shunts; the most common are the ventriculo-peritoneal shunt and the lumbo-peritoneal shunt. Other less commonly used shunts include the ventriculo-atrial shunt, the ventriculo-gallbladder shunt, and the ventriculo-cyst shunt. These are used most commonly when the more common types of shunts are not successful or their use is not possible for some reason.

Disadvantages of shunts are obstruction of the proximal or distal end, infection, or failure due to disconnection. There also is the possibility of overshunting, that is, the drainage of too much CSF, resulting in slit ventricles and headaches for the patient. In extreme cases, subdural hematoma (SDH), caused by tearing of bridging veins, may occur. Undershunting, or too little fluid removal, results in the ventricles remaining large. A CT scan after the placement of a shunt is recommended to document appropriate placement of the shunt and to assess the efficiency of the shunt by checking for decrease in ventricle size.

■ Nursing Management

Nursing management of patients with hydrocephalus consists primarily of accurate neurological assessment. Hydrocephalus can occur with virtually any neurological condition. Decrease in mental status can occur slowly, over days, or rapidly. Any change in neurological status is significant and should be reported. These changes include a decrease in LOC, decrease in ability to speak, decrease in ability to ambulate, and/or incontinence of bowel or bladder. Please refer to the Nursing Process: Patient Care Plan for Acute Brain Disorders (p. 741) for the details of how to care for a patient with hydrocephalus.

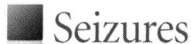

Seizures

Seizures are described as a single, temporary event that consists of uncontrolled, electrical neuronal discharge of the brain that interrupts normal brain function. Seizures may occur as a result of most acute brain disorders: a brain tumor, brain trauma such as a hematoma or concussion, or in conjunction with an infectious process such as meningitis, encephalitis, and abscesses. They also may be seen with other, nonneurological disorders, such as metabolic disorders including severe dehydration, electrolyte imbalances, or withdrawal from alcohol or drugs. Idiopathic seizures also may occur in the absence of underlying abnormalities. Epilepsy is a condition in which seizures occur spontaneously, and they can recur due to an underlying condition or without a known cause.

Epidemiology and Etiology

There are many causes of seizures. These causes are different with age of the patient at onset. In newborns, birth trauma is the most common cause for seizures. In children, fever, trauma, and CNS infections are the most common. Structural abnormalities, such as tumors, strokes, and trauma, are the most common cause in adults. Genetic causes account for approximately 30% of epilepsy in adults and approximately 60% of epilepsy in children (Hirose, Okada, Kaneko, & Mitsudome, 2000).

Clinical Manifestations

The clinical manifestations of seizures are dependent on the location of the seizure focus, or electrical aberrancy. Seizures are divided into two main divisions: generalized and partial (Chart 29–8). Generalized seizures affect the whole brain (Shapiro & Shapiro, 1986). They may be characterized by alterations in mentation, behavior, sensation, or motor tonic–clonic, or grand-mal, seizures. They are characterized by bilateral, symmetric electrical discharges, and are described as a stiffening of the body, with jerking of all extremities (Shapiro & Shapiro, 1986). The patient may become cyanotic, have excessive drooling, and bite the inside of the mouth and/or tongue. Urinary incontinence is common with this type of seizure. The patient loses consciousness and is not communicative or interactive during the event. There may be pupillary changes, with a gaze deviation (away from the side of a structural abnormality, if present). After the seizure, the patient enters the postictal stage, which usually is characterized by extreme lethargy, allowing the patient to sleep. The patient has no memory of the seizure event.

Partial seizures are further divided into simple or complex, with the differentiating factor being consciousness. Simple partial seizures are described as those with specific motor or sensory abnormalities. These would include focal motor seizures or those with somatosensory components, such as the visualization of flashing lights or hearing of noises that are not real. There is no loss of consciousness. Complex partial seizures may begin as a simple partial seizure. They may share many of the same features as simple partial seizures, but consciousness is impaired. They also may progress to a generalized seizure.

Status Epilepticus

Status epilepticus has been described as "either continuous seizures lasting at least five minutes or two or more discrete

| CHART 29–8 | **Types of Seizures** | | | | |

Type of Seizure	Characteristics	Consciousness	Medications	Age Groups
Tonic–clonic Generalized Grand mal Absence	Bilateral Symmetric No warning Stiffening of the body Jerking Cyanosis Tongue-biting Incontinence Abnormal behavior Staring spells	Loss of consciousness for seconds to minutes	Phenytoin (Dilantin) Carbamazepine (Tegretol) Levetiracetam (Keppra) Lamotrigine (Lamictal) Phenobarbital Topiramate (Topamax) Divalproex (Depakote) Klonopin Divalproex (Depakote)	All children
Partial, simple	Focal Motor and/or sensory May progress	No loss of consciousness	Same as above Pregabalin (Lyrica) Gabapentin (Neurontin) Oxcarbazepine (Trileptal)	All
Partial, complex	Focal Motor and/or sensory Automatisms	Altered state of consciousness Clouding or confusion Déjà vu	Same as above	All

seizures between which there is incomplete recovery of consciousness" (Sirven, & Waterhouse, 2003). Status epilepticus is a medical emergency, because continued seizure activity could result in severe neurological injury due to cerebral hypoxia. It also may result in respiratory and/or cardiovascular failure.

Laboratory and Diagnostic Procedures

The diagnosis of seizures is dependent on many factors. First, a detailed account of the event must be available. This includes clinical presentation, medications, and past medical history. A physical examination, with a focus on neurological assessment is essential.

Diagnostic tests include, but are not limited to, imaging studies, such as MRI or CT scan, to rule out structural abnormality as a cause (see the Diagnostic Tests box, p. 723). This does not address whether or not a seizure has occurred, but rather is used to determine if there is an underlying cause present that could potentiate a seizure. EEGs record the electrical potential of the brain. This is done by placing electrodes on the patient's scalp and recording tracings of the electrical activity of the brain. Patients with epilepsy have abnormal electrical tracings. EEGs should be used in conjunction with other diagnostic tests, such as MRI, PET scans, or other tests that determine potential organic causes for seizures, such as a tumor. EEGs are very helpful in recording abnormal electrical activity if a seizure occurs during the tracing. However, these tracings can be normal in the interictal period, between seizure events. Other tests may be used to help determine the exact location of a seizure focus and the area and function of the brain affected. Wada tests, officially known as the intracarotid sodium amobarbital procedure (ISAP), are used to determine which side of the brain controls language function and also how important each side of the brain is with regard to memory function. Functional MRIs also are very helpful to determine where specific functions lie in the brain.

Medical Management

Treatment of seizures begins with treatment of an underlying condition, if present. Medical treatment of seizures should begin immediately, and it depends on the type of seizure. Antiepileptic drugs should be started immediately to prevent further seizures. Many antiepileptic drugs are available, and research is being done to best determine the most efficacious according to seizure types. Antiepileptic drugs are described in the Pharmacology Summary box (p. 733) earlier in the chapter.

In some circumstances, surgical resection of an identifiable seizure focus is warranted. To determine suitability for resection, these patients may be evaluated extensively in a specialized monitoring unit (e.g., the Epilepsy Monitoring Unit) equipped with 24-hour EEG and surveillance monitors to identify the seizure focus. Invasive EEG electrodes may be placed surgically. These data are reviewed along with continuous video surveillance of the patient and all possible seizure activity. This information, along with diagnostic imaging studies, gives useful information to specialists in seizures, called epileptologists. These specialized neurologists work closely with neurosurgeons to determine if surgical resection of a seizure focus would be warranted. This surgery is referred to as a selective amygdalohippocampectomy (SAHC).

Management of status epilepticus consists of two important points. Termination of the seizure is of primary importance. This usually is accomplished with medications, such as short-acting benzodiazepines. Secondly are the ABCs of life support, such as assessment of the patient's respiratory status, with administration of oxygen by mask or nasal cannula and ventilatory support if necessary.

◼ Nursing Management

One of the most important factors in the management of seizures is the reporting of the seizure event. Often, nursing staff are the ones who witness a seizure.

Assessment

Accurate and thorough assessment and reporting of the characteristics of the event is important to the classification of the seizure type and its management. See Chart 29-9 for assessment guidelines.

Interventions and Rationales

Certain tumor types, such as high-grade gliomas and metastatic melanoma to the brain, cause the patient to be at high risk for seizures. All TBI patients are at risk for seizures, as are patients with any type of infectious process in the brain. If the patient is admitted to the hospital after having his first seizure, an important nursing intervention is to prevent further harm to the patient having a seizure. Padding the rails of the bed is one simple nursing action. Administering the necessary antiepileptic drug is another.

 It is important to be aware of precautions and adverse risks concerning the administration of phenytoin. Phenytoin must be administered at a rate of no more than 50 mg/min when given intravenously to avoid pain at the administration site, or hemodynamic compromise, such as bradycardia or hypotension.

Phenytoin may cause drowsiness. When given as routine dosing, it may be necessary to give full daily dose at night to avoid drowsiness during day.

Phenytoin is thought to work by maintaining adequate blood levels of the drug. It is important to monitor drug levels periodically. Most seizures are controlled with a serum level between 10 and 20. Certain drugs interfere with the metabolism of phenytoin, altering the blood levels. It is important to be aware of drugs that interact with phenytoin.

Unexplained rash and/or fever may be attributed to allergy to phenytoin. Report to MD if patient develops rash or fever while on phenytoin.

A common first line AED is phenytoin (Dilantin). Phenytoin is given as a loading dose of 1 gram, or 17 mg/kg intravenously over a period of 30 minutes to 1 hour. The patient is then started on a maintenance dose of 100 mg three times a day. The efficacy of phenytoin is determined by seizure control. Blood testing also is done to measure the serum level of phenytoin. Seizure control is often achieved with a level between 10 and 20, but phenytoin levels are managed based on seizure control and the occurrence of

---

| CHART 29–9 | **Nursing Assessment of Seizure Event** |

- Was the seizure witnessed? If so, by whom?
- Were there precipitating events?
- Where did the seizure start and did it progress to other areas?
- What type of movement of the extremities?
- Were there pupillary changes?
- Was there gaze deviation? If so, which direction?
- Was there incontinence of bowel or bladder?
- What was the patient's mental status (unconscious or awake and talking)?
- How long did the event last?
- After the seizure, what was the patient's mental status?
- Was there any motor weakness after the seizure?
- Did the patient experience an injury from the event?

---

side effects. Occasionally a patient will be started on phenytoin without having had a seizure when health care providers feel that the patient is at risk for seizures. If the patient has a seizure while on phenytoin and while blood levels appear to be in the therapeutic range, a second AED may be necessary.

Phenytoin is not without side effects. It has been known to cause fatigue, which can be alleviated by giving the patient his entire dose at nighttime. Therapeutic drug levels may be achieved with a once daily dose if it is easier for the patient and causes him fewer side effects. Other side effects include nausea, dizziness, gait and balance problems, gingival hyperplasia, and drug-induced fever. Occasionally phenytoin has been associated with severe allergic reactions, ranging from a mild rash to a severe hypersensitivity condition known as Steven-Johnson syndrome (Greenberg, 2001). This condition can be severe and can lead to multisystem failure.

 Confusion, lethargy, and/or seizure may be a sign of hyponatremia. Check recent serum Na+ level, check intake and output, and determine which intravenous fluids are running, if any. Notify health care provider of suspicions of Na+ level less than 135 mEq/L.

Patients with hyponatremia are at risk for seizures. Institute seizure precautions.

Many other AEDs are available. Research is ongoing to determine the most appropriate and efficacious AED for each seizure type. Many patients do not tolerate the first AED prescribed and must switch to another. Some patients require more than one drug to effectively treat their seizures. It should also be recognized that many drugs interact with AEDs. These drugs can increase or decrease the action of AEDs, particularly phenytoin. They include many antibiotics, warfarin, hormones such as estrogen, antihistamines, and various cardiac drugs. It is important that a thorough record be made of all medications taken by any patient taking AEDs.

Protecting the patient from secondary injury is an important concern regarding patients with seizures. It is imperative that the patient not be left alone while having a seizure. It is also important never to force anything into the patient's mouth, such as a "bite stick." Occasionally, a patient may stop breathing after a seizure, especially if the patient is in status epilepticus. This is a medical emergency, and CPR should be started immediately. Oxygen should be administered by nasal cannula or face mask. The ABCs of life support may be instituted. The health care provider should always be notified in the case of seizure. (See also the Nursing Process: Patient Care Plan for Acute Brain Disorders, p. 741.)

▇ Collaborative Management

Seizure management, specifically AED management, is a specialty area in some institutions. If epileptologists or neurologists specializing in seizure management are available, consulting this service may be helpful, especially if seizure management proves to be difficult. Phenytoin dosing services are available in some institutions, and are a welcome addition to management of this drug, dosing in accordance to laboratory drug levels.

Pharmacists also may be of assistance with the many drug interactions associated with AEDs. Many common drugs, as well as foods, can interact with and potentiate or diminish the effects of AEDs. It is important for the patient and family to be aware of these common foods and drugs and the effect they may have on seizure management.

Systemic Response to Acute Brain Disorders

Although the primary nursing focus for patients with acute brain disorders is the neurological status, other systems also must be considered to ensure the best possible outcome for the patient. Insults to the brain affect many other major organ systems and must be carefully evaluated and monitored.

Respiratory Effect

Patients with decreased neurological status frequently have compromised respiratory status. Protecting the patient's airway must be of paramount importance. The patient with decreased level of consciousness is at risk for aspiration, ineffective airway clearance, and respiratory failure. Injuries to the brainstem can cause altered respiratory patterns, which can increase the risk of cerebral hypoxia, extending the neurological damage. The nurse must carefully assess respiratory status by monitoring respiratory patterns, effectiveness of respiration, O_2 saturation, respiratory rates, and arterial blood gases. The possibility of intubation and mechanical ventilation must be considered, especially for patients with GCS ≤ 8.

Neurogenic pulmonary edema is a phenomenon associated with head injury. This is due to a systemic response of the body to shunt blood away from the brain and to the lungs as a result of brain trauma. Treatment is supportive, with possible mechanical ventilation, management of increased ICP, and the use of pharmacologic agents such as dobutamine (Pyeron, 2001).

Pneumonia is a frequent complication of brain injury. The patient is at risk for more than one type of pneumonia, whether it is from bacteria introduced to an already compromised patient, nosocomial from the hospital environment, or aspiration, from a compromised swallow reflex. Ventilator-acquired pneumonia (VAP) is a specific risk for patients in this population. For this reason it is imperative that nursing staff take specific precautions when treating neurologically compromised patients requiring mechanical ventilation.

Of utmost importance is the monitoring of respiratory parameters, such as rate, rhythm, and breath sounds. Accurate monitoring of arterial blood gases is important to recognize patterns of abnormal ventilation. One of the most important nursing functions in supporting respiratory status is turning the patient frequently, if not contraindicated (such as a patient with a potential neck injury). Encouraging the patient to move as much as her condition warrants is helpful to avoid pneumonia.

Mechanically ventilated patients are especially at risk for developing VAP. Intubated patients may require suctioning of their endotracheal or tracheal tubes to clear out excess secretions. Also of importance in reducing VAP is aggressive oral care. Patients with a decreased LOC are at an increased risk for aspiration. This may be due to impairment of the swallow reflex or because of extreme lethargy. The potential for aspiration and/or pneumonia due to an unprotected airway mandates close observation of respiratory status and immediate reporting to the health care provider of any changes. A nurse caring for a patient with an acute brain disorder should be prepared for sudden changes, and the possibility of intubation to protect the airway. (See also the Nursing Process: Patient Care Plan for Acute Brain Disorders, p. 741.)

Cardiovascular Effect

It is common for patients with TBI to experience alterations in cardiovascular function. Arrhythmias are seen, some potentially lethal, such as premature ventricular beats. Bradycardia and tachycardia also are seen. Most common, however, is hypertension. This may indicate increasing intracranial pressure. Hypotension is not frequently associated with head injury, but may be seen in conjunction with an associated injury, such as bleeding. As discussed in the section on ICP management, prevention of hypotension is essential to maintenance of adequate CPP.

Nurses caring for TBI patients, especially in the acute phase, must carefully monitor vital signs, including heart rate and rhythm and blood pressure. Close monitoring of electrocardiograph (ECG) patterns also are essential, including changes in pattern. Acute changes in vital signs may be signs of increasing ICP or changes in nonneurological systems. This is especially important in trauma patients and should be reported without delay.

Monitoring of hemodynamic functions frequently is warranted. To adequately assess cardiovascular function, the placement of invasive lines is common. Arterial lines may be inserted to continually monitor blood pressure. Central venous pressure (CVP) and Swan-Ganz catheters allow practitioners to closely monitor cardiovascular parameters, such as volume, which is essential to the maintenance of adequate CPP. Alterations in blood pressure pose a frequent problem for nurses caring for this population. It is important to know the patient's previous medical history including medications. A trauma patient may experience hypotension due to blood loss from injuries. As observed in the section on ICP management earlier in the chapter, hypotension has a strongly negative effect on CPP and ICP. The use of vasopressors, blood transfusions, and/or fluid challenges may be warranted. Hypertension also may be seen and treated as appropriate. Laboratory values such as serial hemoglobin and hematocrit levels should be monitored closely. (See also the Nursing Process: Patient Care Plan for Acute Brain Disorders, p. 741.)

Gastrointestinal Effect

The most common gastrointestinal (GI) problem is stomach ulcers (Cushing's ulcer). In the initial stage of head injury, GI bleeding may be common due to an increase in gastric acid production. Use of H2-blockers that work to reduce acid in the stomach, such as famotidine, is recommended early in the hospital course to avoid this unnecessary complication. Another potential complication involving the GI system is that of constipation. Patients may be receiving an alternate form of nutrition, such as enteral feedings. Coupled with medications, such as narcotics, and relative immobility, constipation is a constant possibility.

If not closely monitored, constipation may progress to bowel obstruction, a serious (and preventable) complication. Nursing should be aware of elimination patterns and in the event of constipation, stool softeners and laxatives should be given as ordered.

Support of nutritional needs also is of paramount importance to the patient with neurological disease or trauma. It is especially important for the neurologically compromised patient.

A complete nutritional assessment should be done and nutrition should be started as early as possible. Often this means the placement of a feeding tube to provide enteral nutrition. If available, a dietitian can assist in determining caloric needs and optimal nutritional options. If the patient is able to take oral nutrition, it may be necessary to do a calorie count to ensure the patient's caloric support. For more on nutrition, see Chapter 14  . (See also the Nursing Process: Patient Care Plan for Acute Brain Disorders, p. 741.)

Metabolic Effect

The occurrence of brain injury may cause alterations to electrolyte balance. Of primary concern is the maintenance of appropriate sodium levels. Hyponatremia, low serum sodium, is relatively common in head injury. Syndrome of inappropriate antidiuretic hormone (SIADH), an electrolyte imbalance caused by excessive ADH release from the pituitary, must be considered and sodium levels monitored. Hyponatremia is associated with cerebral edema, manifesting symptoms such as lethargy, confusion, seizures, and neurological decline. Diabetes insipidus also must be considered, although it is much less common. Diabetes insipidus is characterized by hypernatremia and low urine specific gravities and is seen with pituitary tumors (see Chapter 18).

Normal levels of serum sodium are between 135 and 145 mEq/L in most institutions. Close monitoring of serum sodium levels and serum osmolality is important because low levels of serum sodium, especially less than 130 mEq/L, can facilitate cerebral edema, causing decreased levels of consciousness, confusion, seizures, and even death.

Fluid restriction, especially of free water, is the treatment of choice of SIADH, while administration of salt tablets, and hyperosmolar saline is the preferred treatment for cerebral salt wasting. Sodium levels should be checked every 6 hours if there is concern for SIADH, or if the patient is receiving treatment for SIADH to prevent overcorrecting. Accurate intake and output is an important nursing function. (See also the Nursing Process: Patient Care Plan for Acute Brain Disorders, p. 741.)

Hematologic Effect

Occasionally patients with an acute brain disorder may develop clotting abnormalities. The most devastating of these is disseminated intravascular coagulopathy (DIC). This is caused by the release of large amounts of thromboplastin by the injured brain. Treatment is the normalization of clotting factors and the maintenance of adequate blood volume.

The development of deep venous thrombosis (DVT) is another potentially dangerous hematologic complication. The cause of DVT usually is immobility; it is, therefore, usually preventable. DVT can lead to the potentially fatal development of a pulmonary embolus. Some brain tumors, especially high-grade gliomas, seem to be a risk factor for the development of DVT and/or pulmonary embolus. Diagnosis is made by ultrasound of the lower extremities.

> **CRITICAL ALERT** *Patients with acute brain disorders, especially those with lower extremity weakness, are prone to formation of DVT. Activity is extremely important. Patients should get out of bed and into a chair or ambulate with assistance, unless contraindicated.*
>
> *All patients who are not ambulating independently should wear antiembolism stockings and compression stockings. Subcutaneous injection of low-molecular-weight heparin or enoxaparin should be considered. Notify health care provider for any signs of DVT (i.e., calf pain).*

If the patient is experiencing motor weakness postoperatively, great care must be taken to avoid DVT due to immobility. Prevention is the ideal treatment.

The use of antiembolism hose or pneumonic stockings is highly recommended and should be applied as soon as possible, even before the patient goes to surgery. Frequent turning of the patient and early mobilization, with health care provider approval, is of utmost importance. Prophylactic use of subcutaneous enoxaparin also is recommended in instances of motor deficits that cause immobility of the limb and when it is not otherwise contraindicated. Early mobilization is a key preventive strategy in avoiding DVT; however, patients must be able to ambulate a minimum of 150 feet per day to discontinue adjunctive prevention treatment.

Any patient with an acute brain disorder, especially one associated with immobility, should be assessed frequently for DVT. Pain in the lower extremity, especially the calf, is a frequent complaint in the presence of DVT. However, many patients in this population may be unaware of, or unable to complain of, this discomfort. Therefore, it is important for nursing to include an examination of the patient's lower extremities in the routine assessment of patients with any neurological disorder. This includes observation for the presence of edema, redness, warmth of calf, and/or pain in the lower extremity. Any abnormality, including patient complaint, should be reported. (See also the Nursing Process: Patient Care Plan for Acute Brain Disorders, p. 741.)

■ Gerontological Considerations for Acute Brain Disorders

Acute brain disorders, such as traumatic brain injury, brain tumors, or infectious diseases, can cause substantial injury to patients across the age continuum. TBI in the elderly, however, has some specific considerations. The incidence of TBI in the elderly may be influenced by age-related changes, such as decreased vision, decreased mobility, decreased muscle and bone mass, and decreased physical agility. Adding to the increased fall risk of the elderly is the fact that many elderly patients live alone.

TBI in the elderly carries a higher percentage of mortality and morbidity than other age groups. Ritchie and colleagues (2000) found that overall mortality of TBI in the elderly is approximately 33.5%, with overall poor functional outcomes. Less favorable outcomes may be due to several factors including chronic, preexisting comorbidities, such as pulmonary or cardiovascular problems. Preexisting cognitive impairment is another factor influencing outcome. Medication, specifically anticoagulation, also plays a significant role in outcome.

According to the U.S. Census Bureau (2000), the number of people age 65 or older approximated 13% of the total population. Those over the age of 85 are projected to be the fastest growing age group in America, with a projected population of more than 8.5 million by the year 2030. Mild or moderate TBI is associated with 2.3% and 4.5%, respectively, increased risk over Alzheimer's disease in the elderly (Langlois, Rutland-Brown, & Walk, 2006). These numbers support the importance of recognizing the specific considerations of TBI in the gerontological population.

Other acute brain disorders, such as brain tumors also may have age-specific characteristics. As noted, brain tumors affect all ages, but certain tumor types are more common in the elderly. Meningiomas are found most commonly in the sixth or seventh decade.

Rehabilitation

During the patient's hospitalization, the patient's nurse may be the one he sees the most often, and the one who is looked to for support and encouragement. Often, the realization that life may be changed, perhaps drastically, is overwhelming. Patients need to know that there is support and resources available to help them and their family through whatever the future holds.

At the time of discharge, it may be necessary to transfer the patient to another facility for rehabilitation, or perhaps to arrange for rehabilitation as an outpatient. For patients with brain tumors, this may be coordinated with radiation therapy and possibly chemotherapy. It is helpful to be able to provide the patient and family with information about the benefits of rehabilitation, and what is available to that patient. In many cases, rehabilitation is very important to allow the patient to return home with optimum independence. According to a study done by Mukand and colleagues (2001), impaired cognition, motor weakness, and visual-perceptual deficits were the most common problems in the population studies. Their study supports the benefits of a comprehensive and interdisciplinary rehabilitation program for patients with primary or metastatic brain tumors.

For patients with altered level of consciousness or deficits, rehabilitation also is necessary to provide the patient with the opportunity to maximize functional abilities. The goal for all rehabilitation is to return patients to their optimum level of independence. According to Jennett and Teasdale (1981) in their classic work on level of consciousness, the six aspects of living must be addressed for rehabilitation purposes: activities of daily living (ADLs), mobility and life organization, social relationships, work or leisure activities, present satisfaction, and future prospects. These factors cannot be measured quantitatively, although several outcome measurement scales are available that can be used to address outcomes. The Glasgow Outcome Scale (Jennett & Bond, 1975) and the Karnofsky Performance Status Scale (Karnofsky & Burchenal, 1949) are two such examples.

RESEARCH OPPORTUNITIES AND CLINICAL IMPACT RELATED TO ACUTE BRAIN DISORDERS

Research Area	Clinical Impact
Examine the advantage of various modalities to prevent venous stasis in patients with TBI and brain tumors, such as antiembolism stockings, early ambulation, and the use of low-molecular-weight heparin.	DVTs and pulmonary embolisms are a worrisome complication of head injury and are fairly common in patients with brain tumors. Identifying and implementing DVT prophylaxis may reduce the rate of thromboembolic events, such as DVTs and pulmonary embolisms.
Examine various treatment modalities for hyponatremia (i.e., hypertonic saline, salt tablets, fluid restriction, or other medications) and their impact on the treatment of hyponatremia in the presence of brain tumors.	Hyponatremia is relatively common in the presence of brain tumors and head injury, and it also is associated with cerebral edema. The appropriate treatment of hyponatremia may be significant to a positive patient outcome.
Examine the outcome of patients with TBI or brain tumor who are provided with rehabilitation services versus patients who receive no rehabilitation after discharge (retrospective study).	Define the benefits of therapies and rehabilitation to patients with brain injury due to TBI or tumor.
Examine different monitoring devices for the maintenance of adequate brain oxygenation.	Maintenance of adequate brain oxygenation, with the reduction of neurological injury.
Examine various administration routes (oral, enteral, IV) for the administration of phenytoin and any possible differences in maintenance of adequate blood levels of the drug.	Maintenance of adequate blood levels of phenytoin, possibly reducing the risk of seizures.

Clinical Preparation

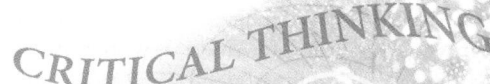

CRITICAL THINKING

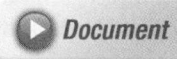

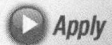

▶ **Read**

- History of Current Illness
- Past Medical History
- Physical Exam
- Admitting Medical Orders
- Laboratory Study Results

▶ **Document**

- Summary of Hospitalization
- Pathophysiology Form
- Laboratory Values
- Laboratory Results Explanation

▶ **Apply**

- List of Potential Nursing Diagnoses
- Concept Map
- Critical Thinking Questions

Log on to MyNursingKit.com to download forms you will need and to complete further steps in the Clinical Preparation assignment.

HISTORY OF PRESENT ILLNESS

As a nurse in the neuroscience ICU of a large metropolitan teaching hospital, you receive a phone call from the charge nurse of the emergency department (ED). The nurse is calling to give a report on a new patient being admitted to your unit. The patient is a 32-year-old Hispanic male brought to the ED by his brother, who found him wandering outside their home, confused and disoriented. He also noted that his brother had trouble opening the car door with his right hand. He stated that his brother had come home from his job stocking supplies in a grocery warehouse complaining of a headache. Coworkers told his brother that they had seen several boxes that had fallen, but were unaware that any had actually struck the patient.

On admission to the ED, a CT scan was done and a moderate-sized subdural hematoma was noted in the left temporal area. A skull fracture was ruled out. The patient is now being admitted to the neuroscience ICU for close monitoring of his neurological status. A craniotomy for evacuation of the left temporal subdural hematoma is planned for early the following morning. The ED nurse tells you that the patient is on his way, and his family is accompanying him. His family consists of several siblings, his wife, his parents, and two small children. They are very concerned and do not speak English.

Medical–Surgical History

This history was obtained from multiple family members: On examination of the patient's records, you note that the patient, whose name is Jose R., has no past medical history and has, in fact, never been in the hospital for any reason. He has no allergies and takes no medication. Illnesses: none, with the exception of "usual" childhood illnesses, per parents

Social History

His social history, according to his family, includes a wife, two small children, and multiple family members. His wife denies any drug or alcohol use; however, his brother relates moderate alcohol consumption "on the weekends." He works in a warehouse stocking groceries and supplies. He has completed high school. He has lived in this country for many years and is a citizen of this country. He has not traveled outside of the country since he was a young child.

Physical Exam

His emergency department assessment and orders are as follows:
Young Hispanic male, resting quietly, appears in no distress
Vital signs: afebrile; HR 62 regular, RR 16, BP 134/74
HEENT: normocephalic, with small tender, bruised area near L temple
Heart: rhythm and rate regular, S_1S_2 heard, no abnormal murmurs, good capillary refill, pulses 2+ all extremities, no pitting edema
Lungs: clear to auscultation bilaterally

O_2 sat at 97% on room air
Abdomen: soft, nontender, bowel sounds heard all quadrants

Neurological Exam

GCS = E4 M6 V4 = 14; oriented to name only, confused to date and surroundings
Pleasant, cooperative, and attentive
Speech clear and fluent
Cranial nerves: CN II–XII intact bilaterally
Motor:
  Right upper extremity 5/5
  Right lower extremity 5/5
  RUE pronator drift
  Left upper extremity 5/5
  Left lower extremity 5/5
Sensory: grossly intact to light touch bilaterally

Imaging Studies

Head CT scan done in the ED reveals an acute left-sided subdural hematoma
Chest x-ray: negative for abnormal pathology

Admitting Medical Orders

Admit to Neuroscience ICU
Diagnosis: acute left subdural hematoma
Condition: guarded
Allergies: none known
Vital signs and neuro assessment: q1h

Bed rest

Diet: NPO

Notify resident on call: any change in neurological status; increase in severity of headache or nausea, temperature > 38°C, HR < 60 or > 120, systolic BP < 100 or > 160, RR < 10 or > 30, O_2 sat less 92%, urine output < 30 mL/hr × 2

Sequential compression devices (SCDs) to lower extremities prior to surgery

IV: D5/0.45NS @ 75 mL/hr

Continuous ECG, pulse oximetry

Foley catheter

Intake and output q2h

Consent for craniotomy for evacuation of left subdural hematoma by Dr. XYZ

Scheduled Medications

Pepcid 20 mg IV q12h

PRN Medications

Acetaminophen 650 mg po/PR q4h for pain or fever

Morphine sulfate 2–4 mg IV q2h for pain

Promethazine 25–50 mg po/IV/PR q4h for nausea

Ordered Laboratory Studies

ABG × 1 now

Serum and urine osmolality × 1 now

CBC now and q a.m.

PTT, INR. Chem 7 panel, magnesium, phosphorous, and ionized CA now and q12h

Urinalysis now

Ordered Diagnostic Studies

Preoperative ECG

After Jose is settled in your unit, you examine the patient. His vital signs and neurological assessment are unchanged from the admitting assessment. (Refer to Chapter 28 🌐 for a review of neurological assessment.)

Jose is resting comfortably, talking with the nursing staff, and is quite pleasant and cooperative. He is complaining of a headache and is medicated with intravenous morphine. He has an IV line running. He is denying nausea at this time, but is not hungry. He is in the ICU for close monitoring. He is considered to be stable, and safe to wait the few hours until morning to evacuate his hematoma.

About 2 hours after Jose is admitted, he requests more pain medication, because his headache is worse. Before you can bring his medication, he attempts to crawl over the side rails of his bed. He is clearly agitated, worried about his family, and wants to go home. You convince him to return to bed. Within minutes, he has projectile emesis, and now is clearly confused. He is unable to tell you his name or where he is. His vital signs are essentially unchanged, although his heart and respiratory rate are slightly elevated. His neurological examination is as follows: He is alert, restless, and agitated. He is clearly confused, unable to state name or where he is. His pupils are equal, but his left pupil is slow to react. His right pronator drift is still present, but does not appear to be any worse. The neurosurgical resident you call wants another CT scan, but states that he may go straight to surgery after his scan. As you are preparing to take the patient to radiology, you look up his labs, and check his paperwork to make sure the surgical consent is in the chart. As the patient is receiving his scan, you go to the waiting room to speak to the family and keep them aware of events.

LABORATORY STUDY RESULTS

Test	On Admission
pH	7.36
$PaCO_2$	40 mmHg
PaO_2	80 mmHg
SO2	96%
HCO_3	24 mEq/L
Sodium	140 mEq/L
Potassium	3.6 mEq/L
Chloride	92 mEq/L
Carbon dioxide	23 mEq/L
Blood urea nitrogen (BUN)	26 mg/dL
Creatinine	1.4 mg/dL
Blood glucose	93 mg/dL
Blood alcohol	NA, 00.0%
White blood cells	9200 /µL
Hemoglobin	14.2 g/dL
Hematocrit	39.8%
Platelets	312,000 µL
Protime (PT)	11.8 seconds
International normalized ratio (INR)	0.9 INR
Partial thromboplastin time (PTT)	34 seconds
Serum osmolality	280 mOsm/kg
Urine osmolality	600 mOsm/kg H_2O

CRITICAL THINKING QUESTIONS

1. What neurological findings might you expect in a patient with an injury to the left temporal area?

2. At what point did Jose's neurological status change?

3. What is the significance of Jose's change in mental status?

4. Based on the change in Jose's condition, what might the nurse expect Jose's CT scan to show?

5. What other clinical findings might support the nurse's concern about rising ICPs?

Answers to Critical Thinking Questions appear in Appendix D.

NCLEX® REVIEW

1. The encased structure of the adult brain is the reason that the relationship between brain mass, cerebrospinal fluid (CSF), and blood must remain constant. Initial mechanisms to compensate for pressure changes in any of these components include which of the following?

   1. Increasing production of CSF
   2. Expansion of brain tissue
   3. Blocking the auto-regulation of cerebral blood flow
   4. Increasing absorption of CSF

2. A patient is admitted with a gradual increase in intracranial pressure due to an enlarging tumor. Early signs of increased intracranial pressure may include which of the following?

   1. Changes in the optic nerve (CN VIII) may result in ringing in the ears
   2. Decorticate movement observable in the arms
   3. Complaints of a 'different' headache and projectile vomiting
   4. Cushing's triad

3. The nursing management for the patient with increased intracranial pressure involves assessment of respiratory, cardiovascular, metabolic, and neurological processes. Desired parameters to avoid complications include which of the following? Select all that apply.

   1. Pulse oximetry should be used with supplemental oxygen to maintain saturations of 90% or greater
   2. Normocapnia levels (PaCO$_2$ levels of 35–40mm Hg)
   3. Euglycemic levels of 80–120 mg/dL
   4. Normothermia and interventions for body temperatures >99.5°F rectally

4. A 50-year-old patient is admitted to the ED with a scalp laceration that was bleeding profusely and was bandaged at the scene by emergency personnel. The patient is currently stable. The nurse is aware that before wound closure is initiated, which of the following activities is a priority?

   1. A complete neurological assessment to rule out cerebral contusion
   2. A CAT scan of the head to rule out skull fracture
   3. A cerebral arteriogram to identify which vessel has been ruptured
   4. A skull series to determine the presence of hematomas

5. The presenting signs and symptoms for bacterial and viral meningitis are the same. It is important, therefore, for the nurse to utilize laboratory data to differentiate between these acute processes. Which of the following is true concerning bacterial meningitis?

   1. In the spinal fluid, protein levels will be high and glucose levels will be low.
   2. In the spinal fluid, the color will be clear.
   3. In the spinal fluid, the protein and glucose levels will be low.
   4. The spinal fluid will be bloody.

6. Brain tumors are a threat to life whether they are benign or malignant. Which of the following statements reflects the characteristics of benign tumors of the brain?

   1. These tumors are nonmalignant and are easily removed by surgery.
   2. The tumors are self-limiting and do not influence the function of surrounding tissues.
   3. Benign tumors may be surgically difficult to remove and may compress vital structures.
   4. These tumors do not progress into malignant tumors.

7. Chemotherapy in the treatment of brain tumors may be administered intrathecally, intravenously, or orally. Special concerns with the use of chemotherapy for brain tumors include:

   1. Brain tissue, due to increase lymph flow, has an improved mechanism to remove cellular debris.
   2. Chemotherapy is the treatment of choice because all of these drugs readily cross the blood–brain barrier.
   3. Malignant cells are homogenous and are consistent in their sensitivity to chemotherapeutic agents.
   4. A flexible approach due to the changing resistance patterns to specific drugs.

8. The role of the nurse in family teaching of patients with acute brain disorders is:

   1. Limited to teaching the early detection of cognitive impairment.
   2. Different than other long term-care patients because of the early implementation of rehabilitative therapies.
   3. Provide answers to questions honestly as they arise, educate them about the treatment plan, and involve them in discussions of the rehabilitation process.
   4. Geared to offering the family a realistic perspective of the limited abilities of the patient.

Answers for review questions appear in Appendix D

KEY TERMS

acoustic neuromas *p.737*
autoregulation *p.715*
bacterial meningitis *p.730*
basal skull fracture *p.722*
brain abscess *p.732*
cerebral blood flow (CBF) *p.715*
cerebral edema *p.716*
cerebral infarction *p.727*
cerebral ischemia *p.727*
cerebral perfusion pressure (CPP) *p.715*
comminuted skull fracture *p.722*
concussion *p.726*
contusions *p.725*
Cushing's triad *p.718*

cytotoxic edema *p.716*
depressed skull fracture *p.722*
diffuse axonal injury (DAI) *p.726*
encephalitis *p.731*
ependymomas *p.736*
epidural hematoma (EDH) *p.724*
extra-axial tumors *p.736*
gene mutations *p.735*
herniation *p.716*
intra-axial tumors *p.735*
intracranial pressure (ICP) *p.714*
ischemia cascade *p.727*
linear skull fracture *p.722*
meningiomas *p.736*

meningismus *p.730*
metastatic tumors *p.735*
Monro-Kellie doctrine *p.714*
postconcussion syndrome *p.726*
primary injury *p.727*
primary tumors *p.735*
schwannomas *p.737*
second-impact syndrome *p.726*
secondary injury *p.727*
subdural hematoma (SDH) *p.724*
traumatic brain injury (TBI) *p.721*
vasodilatory cascade *p.715*
vasogenic edema *p.716*
viral meningitis *p.730*

EXPLORE PEARSON **mynursingkit**™

MyNursingKit is your one stop for online chapter review materials and resources. Prepare for success with additional NCLEX®-style practice questions, interactive assignments and activities, web links, animations and videos, and more!

Register your access code from the front of your book at
www.mynursingkit.com

REFERENCES

Adesina, A. M., Leech, R. W., & Brumback, R. A. (2002). Histopathology of primary tumors of the central nervous system. In M. Prados (Ed.), *Brain cancer* (pp. 16–45). London: B. C. Decker.

American Cancer Society. (2006). Detailed guide: brain/cnss tumors in adults. What are the key statistics for brain and spinal cord tumors in adults. *Cancer Reference Information*. Retrieved July 13, 2008 from http://www.cancer.org/docroot/CRI/content/CRI_2_4_1X_What_are_the_key_statistics_fo…

Andrews, P.J.D. (2005). Cerebral perfusion pressure and brain ischemia: Can one size fit all? *Critical Care, 9,* 638–639.

Aubry, M., Cantu, R. C., Dvorak, J., Graf-Baumann, T., Johnston, K., & Kelly, J. (2001). *Concussion in sport group: Summary and agreement statement of the First International Concussion in Sport.* Vienna, Austria.

Bader, M. K. (2006a). Gizmos and gadgets for the neuroscience intensive care unit. *Journal of Neuroscience Nursing, 38*(4), 248–260.

Bader, M. K. (2006b). Recognizing and treating ischemic insults to the brain: The role of brain tissue oxygen monitoring. *Critical Care Nursing Clinics of North America, 18,* 243–256.

Bader, M. K., & Littlejohns, L. (Eds.). (2004). *Core curriculum for neuroscience nursing* (4th ed.). Chicago: American Association of Neuroscience Nurses.

Bay, E., & McLean, S. A. (2007). Mild traumatic brain injury: An update for advanced practice nurses. *Journal of Neuroscience Nursing, 39*(1), 43–51.

Bowen, A. P. (2003). Secondary impact syndrome. *Journal of Emergency Nursing, 29*(3): 287–289.

Brenner, A. V., Linet, M. S., Fine, H. A., Shapiro, W. R., Selker, R. G., Black, P. M., et al. (2002). History of allergies and autoimmune diseases and risk of brain tumors in adults. *International Journal of Cancer, 99,* 252–259.

Burnett, D. M., Kolawkowky-Hayner, S. A., Slater, D., Stringer, A., Bushnik, T., Zafonte, R., et al. (2003). Ethnographic analysis of traumatic brain injury patients in the National Model Systems Database. *Archives of Physical Medicine and Rehabilitation, 84*(2), 263–267.

Burst suppression tutorial. (2003, December). Reykjavik, Iceland: Taugagreininghf.

Burton, E., & Prados, M. (2002). Management of primary malignant brain tumors in adults. In Prado, M. (Ed.), *Brain cancer* (pp. 262–277). London: B. C. Decker.

Carroll, S. (1994). Secondary brain injury and the role of neuroprotective agents. *Journal of Neuroscience Nursing, 26,* 251–254.

Centers for Disease Control and Prevention. (2007). *Brain injuries and mass casualty events.* Retrieved June 25, 2007, from http://www.bt.cdc.gov/masscasualties/braininjuriespro.asp

Central Brain Tumor Registry of the United States. (2000). *Statistical report: Primary brain tumors in the United States, 1992–1997.* Chicago: Author.

Cox, J. D., & Ang, K. K. (2003). *Radiation oncology* (pp. 801–806). St. Louis: Mosby.

Defense and Veterans Brain Injury Center. (2005). *Living with Brain Injury,* Brain Injury Association of America, Washington, DC: Walter Reed Army Medical Center.

DeRoos, A. J., Stewart, P. A., Linet, M. S., Heineman, E. F., Dosemeci, M., Wilcosky, T., et al. (2003). Occupation and the risk of adult glioma in the United States. *Cancer Causes and Control, 14,* 139–150.

Evans, R. W. (1996). *Neurology and trauma.* Philadelphia: W. B. Saunders.

Fan, J. (2004). Effect of backrest position on intracranial pressure and cerebral perfusion pressure in individuals with brain injury: A systematic review. *Journal of Neuroscience Nursing, 36*(5), 278–288.

Farrell, D. J., & Bower, L. (2003). Fatal water intoxication. *Journal of Clinical Pathology, 56*(10), 803–804.

Feldman, Z., & Robertson, C. S. (1997). Monitoring of cerebral hemodynamics with jugular bulb catheters. *Critical Care Clinics, 13*(1): 55–77.

Finkelstein, E., Corso, P., & Miller, T. (2006). *The incidence and economic burden of injuries in the United States.* Oxford University Press: New York.

Geraci, E. B., & Geraci, T. A. (1996). A look at recent hyperventilation studies: Outcomes and recommendations for early use in the head injured patient. *Journal of Neuroscience Nursing, 28*(4), 222–233.

Goldman, L., & Ausiello, D. (2004). *Cecil textbook of medicine* (22nd ed.). Philadelphia, PA: W. B. Saunders.

Greenberg, M. S. (2001). *Handbook of neurosurgery* (5th ed.). New York: Thieme.

Guzman, R., Barth, A., Lovblad, K. O., El-Koussy, M., Weis, J., Schroth, G., et al (2002). Use of diffusion-weighted magnetic resonance imaging in differentiating purulent brain processes from cystic brain tumors. *Journal of Neurosurgery, 97*(5), 1101–1107.

Hickey, J. (2003). *The clinical practice of neurological and neurosurgical nursing* (5th ed.). Philadelphia: Lippincott.

Hilton, G. (2000). Cerebral oxygenation in the traumatically brain-injured pateint: Are ICP and CPP enough? *Journal of Neuroscience Nursing, 32*(5): 278–281.

Hirose, S., Okada, O., Kaneko, S., & Mitsudome, A. (2000). Are some idiopathic epilepsies disorders of ion channels? A working hypothesis. *Epilepsy Research, 41,* 191–204.

House, J. W., & Brackmann, D. E. (1985). Facial nerve grading scale. *Otolaryngology, 93*(2), 146–147.

Huang, C. R., Lu, C. H., Chang, H. W., Lee, P. Y., Lin, M. W., & Chang, W. N. (2002). Community-acquired spontaneous bacterial meningitis in adult diabetic patients: An analysis of clinical characteristics and prognostic factors. *Infection,30*(6), 346–350.

Inskip, P. D., Tarone, R. E., & Hatch, E. E. (2001). Cellular-telephone use and brain tumors. *New England Journal of Medicine, 344,* 79–86.

Inskip, P. D., Tarone, R. E., Hatch, E. E., Wilcosky, T. C., Selker, R. G., Fine, H. A., et al. (2003). Laterality of brain tumors. *Neuroepidemiology, 22*(3): 130–138.

Jennett, B., & Teasdale, G. (1981). *Management of head injuries.* Philadelphia: F. A. Davis.

Jennett, W. B., & Bond, M. (1975). Assessment of outcome after severe brain damage: A practical scale. *Lancet,* 480–484.

Jennett, W. B., & Plum, F. (1972). The persistent vegetative state: A syndrome in search of a name. *Lancet, 1,* 734–737.

Karnofsky, D. A., & Burchenal, J. H. (1949). In C. M. Macleod (Ed.), *Evaluation of chemotherapeutic agents* (pp. 191–205). New York: Columbia University Press.

Key, C. B., Rothrock, S. G., & Falk, J. L. (1997). Cerebrospinal fluid shunt complications: An emergency medicine prospective. *Pediatric Emergency Care, 11*(5), 265–272.

Kleihues, P., Davis, R. L., Coons, S. W., & Burger, P. C. (2000). Anaplastic astrocytoma. In P. Kleihues & W. K. Cavenee (Eds.), *Pathology & genetics of tumours of the nervous system* (pp. 27–28). Lyon, France: IARC Press.

Koedel, U., Scheld, W. M., & Pfister, H. W. (2002). Pathogenesis and pathophysiology of pneumococcal meningitis. *Lancet Infectious Disease, 2*(12), 721–736.

Langlois, J. A., Rutland-Brown, W., & Thomas, K. E. (2006). *Traumatic brain injury in the United States: Emergency department visits, hospitalizations, and deaths.* Atlanta, GA: Centers for Disease Control and Prevention, National Center for Injury Prevention and Control.

Langlois, J., Rutland-Brown, W., & Walk, M. (2006). The epidemiology and impact of traumatic brain injury: A brief overview. *Journal of Head Trauma Rehabilitation, 21*(5), 375–378.

Louis, D. N., Scheithauer, B. W., Budka, H., von Deimling, A., & Kepes, J. J. (2000). Meningiomas. In P. Kleihues & W. K. Cavenee (Eds.), *Pathology & genetics of tumours of the nervous system* (pp. 176–184). Lyon, France: IARC Press.

Manley, G., Knudson, M. M., Morabito, D., Damron, S., Erickson, V., & Pitts, L. (2001). Hypotension, hypoxia, and head injury. *Archives of Surgery, 136*(10): 1118–1123.

Maramou, A. (1996). Physiology of intracranial pressure. In R. K. Narayan, J. E. Wilberger, & J. T. Povlishock (Eds.), *Neurotrauma.* New York: McGraw-Hill.

Maramou, A., & Beaumont, A. (2004). Physiology of the cerebrospinal fluid and intracranial pressure. In M. Kliot (Ed.), *Youman's neurological surgery* (5th ed., pp. 175-194). Philadelphia: W. B. Saunders.

Mayo Clinic Staff. (2008). *Traumatic Brain Injury.* Retrieved July 13, 2008 from http://www.mayoclinic.com/health/traumatic-brain-injury/DS00552/DSECTION=risk-fact...

McIlvoy, L. (2005). The effect of hypothermia and hyperthermia on acute brain injury. *AACN Clinical Issues, 16,* 488–500.

Meinert, R., & Michaelis, J. (1996). Meta-analyses of studies on the association between electromagnetic fields and childhood cancer. *Radiation & Environmental Biophysics, 35,* 11–18.

Minn, Y., Wrensch, M., & Bondy, M. L. (2002). Epidemiology of primary brain tumors. In M. Prados (Ed.), *Brain cancer.* London: B. C. Decker.

Mittenberg, W., & Strauman, S. (2000). Diagnosis of mild head injury and the postconcussion syndrome. *Head Trauma Rehabilitation, 15*(2), 783–791.

Moura, A. S., Pablos-Mendez, A., Layton, M., & Weiss, D. (2003). Epidemiology of meningococcal disease, New York City, 1989–2002. *Emerging Infectious Disease, 9*(3), 355–361.

Mukand, J. A., Blackinton, D. D., Crincoli, M. G., Lee, J. J., & Santos, B. B. (2001). Incidence of neurologic deficits and rehabilitation of patients with brain tumors. *American Journal of Physical Medicine and Rehabilitation 80*(5), 346–350.

Olson, D. A. (2006). Head injury. *EMedicine.* Retrieved July 13, 2008 from http://www.emedicine.com/neuro/TOPIC143.HTM

Piepmeier, J. M. (1987). Observations on the current treatment of low-grade astrocytic tumors of the cerebral hemispheres. *Journal of Neurosurgery, 67,* 177–181.

Plum, F., & Posner, J. (1980). *Diagnosis of stupor and coma* (3rd ed., Contemporary Neurology Series). Philadelphia: F. A. Davis.

Porth, C. M. (2007). *Essentials of pathophysiology: Concepts of altered health states.* (2nd Ed.). Philadelphia: Lippincott Williams & Wilkins..

Posner, J. B., Saper, C. B., Schiff, N., & Plum, F. (2007). *Plum and Posner's diagnosis of stupor and coma* (4th ed.). New York: Oxford University Press.

Proctor, M. R., & Cantu, R. C. (2000). Head and neck injuries in young athletes. *Clinics of Sports Medicine, 19*(4).

Pueschel, J. K., Ashby, L. S., & Shapiro, W. R. (2003). Brain tumors. In G. Giaccone, R. Schilsky, & P. Sondel (Eds.), *Cancer chemotherapy and biological response modifiers* (Annual 21). New York: Elsevier Science.

Pyeron, A. M. (2001). Respiratory failure in the neurological patient: The diagnosis of neurogenic pulmonary edema. *Journal of Neuroscience Nursing, 33*(4), 203–207.

Quinn, A. M. (2002). CyberKnife: A robotic radiosurgery system. *Clinical Journal of Oncology Nursing, 6*(3), 149–156.

Quinn, E. (2008). Water intoxication—hyponatremia. *Sports Medicine.* Retrieved March 30, 2008, from http://sportsmedicine.about.com/od/hydrationandfluid/a/Hyponatremia.htm

Radiation Therapy Oncology Group (RTOG). (2008). *Brain tumor protocols.* Retrieved July 14, 2008 from http://www.rrtog.org/summaries/brain.html

Rees, R. J., & Bellon, M. L. (2007). Post concussion syndrome ebb and flow: Longitudinal effects and management. *NeuroRehabilitation, 22*(3), 229–242.

Ritchie, P. D., Cameron, P. A., Ugoni, A. M., & Kaye, A. H. (2000). A study of the functional outcome and mortality in elderly patients with head injuries. *Journal of Clinical Neuroscience, 7*(4), 301–304.

Sarrafzadeh, A. S., Sakowitz, O. W., Kiening, K. I., Benndorf, G., Lanksch, W. R., & Unterberg, A. W. (2002). Bedside microdialysis: A tool to monitor cerebral metabolism in subarachnoid hemmorrhage patients? *Critical Care Medicine, 30,* 1062–1070.

Sato, O., Takei, F., & Yamada, S. (1994). Hydrocephalus: Is impaired cerebrospinal fluid circulation only one problem involved? *Child's Nervous System, 10*(3), 151–154.

Senelick, R., & Dougherty, K. (2001). *Living with brain injury: A guide for families* (2nd ed., p. 3). Birmingham, AL: Healthsouth Press.

Shapiro, J. R. (2001). Genetics of nervous system tumors. *Hematology/Oncology Clinics of North America, 15*(6), 961–977.

Shapiro, W. R., & Shapiro, J. R. (1986). Principles of brain tumor therapy. *Seminars in Oncology, 13*(1), 56–69.

Shaw, E. G. (2002). Management of low-grade gliomas in adults. In M. Prados (Ed.), *Brain cancer.* London: B. C. Decker.

Shimamoto, S., Inoue, T., Shiomi, H., Sumida, I., Yamada, Y., & Tanaka, E. (2002). CyberKnife stereotactic irradiation for metastatic brain tumors. *Radiation Medicine, 20*(6), 299–304.

Sirven, J. I., & Waterhouse, E. (2003). Management of status epilepticus. *American Family Physician, 68*(3), 469–476.

Smith, D. H., & McIntosh, T. K. (1996). Traumatic brain injury and excitatory amino acids. In R. K. Naryan, J. E. Wilberger, & J. T. Povlishock (Eds.), *Neurotrauma.* New York: McGraw-Hill.

Smith, D. L., Levin, S. A., & Laxminarayan, R. (2005). Strategic interactions in multi-institutional epidemics of antibiotic resistance. *Proceedings. National Academy of Sciences. USA 102,* 3153–3158.

Sneed, P. K. (2002). Metastatic brain tumors. In M. Prados (Ed.), *Brain cancer.* London: B. C. Decker.

Surawicz, T. S., McCarthy, B. J., & Kupelian, V. (1999). Descriptive epidemiology of primary brain and CNS tumors: Results from the Central Brain Tumor Registry of the United States, 1990–1994. *Neurooncology 1999, 1,* 14–25.

Terrell, T. R. (2004). Concussion in athletes. *Southern Medical Journal, 97*(9), 837–842.

Thompson, H. J., Kirkness, C. J., Mitchell, P. H., & Webb, D. J. (2007). Fever management practices of neuroscience nurses: National and regional perspectives. *Journal of Neuroscience Nursing, 39*(3), 151–161.

Tunkel, A. R., & Pradhan, S. K. (2002). Central nervous system infections in injection drug users. *Infectious Disease Clinics of North America 16*(3): 589–605.

U.S. Bureau of the Census. (2000). *United States census 2000: Your gateway to census 2000.* Retrieved October 20, 2008. http://www.census.gov/main/www/cen2000.html

van de Beek, D., Schmand, B., de Gans, J., Weisfelt, M., Vaessen, H., & Vermeulen, M. (2002). Cognitive impairment in adults with good recovery after bacterial meningitis. *Journal of Infectious Disease, 186*(7), 1047–1052.

Walker, J. T. (1967). *History of neurological surgery.* New York: McGraw-Hill.

Winkleman, C. (2000). Effect of backrest position on intracranial and cerebral perfusion pressures in traumatically brain-injured adults. *American Journal of Critical Care, 9*(6), 373–380.

Wong, F. W. H. (2000). Prevention of secondary brain injury. *Critical Care Nurse, 20*(5), 18–27.

Wrensch, M., Minn, Y., & Bondy, M. L. (2000). Epidemiology. In M. Bernstein & M. Berger (Eds.), *Essential neuro-oncology* (pp. 1–17). New York: Thieme.

Yoshikawa, T. T. (2002). Antimicrobial resistance and aging: Beginning of the end of the antibiotic era? *Journal of American Geriatric Society, 50*(7), 226–229.

Caring for the Patient with Cerebral Vascular Disorders

Denita Ryan

Outcome-Based Learning Objectives

After studying this chapter, the learner will be able to:

1. Identify and distinguish between the different types of stroke and their reported impact on rehabilitation and recovery to a functional status.
2. Describe the basic pathophysiology of each type of identified stroke.
3. Explain the events of the ischemic cascade as it relates to the pathophysiology of stroke.
4. Compare and contrast the different medical management options for the treatment of ruptured aneurysms.
5. Explain nursing interventions associated with management of vasospasm.

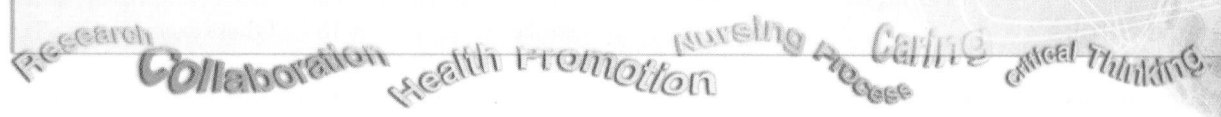

THE CEREBRAL VASCULAR disorders discussed in this chapter consist of stroke and arterial venous malformations. Both represent major disorders that cause an assault on the brain, and in many ways they manifest symptoms similar to the disorders discussed in Chapter 29 🔗 on acute brain disorders. The prevalence, current modes of diagnosis and treatment, and nursing management of these disorders are discussed, as are the societal implications.

▋ Stroke

Stroke is brain attack. This strong statement is indicative of the new definition for stroke. "Time is brain" is another strong statement exclaiming the importance of timely treatment before neurological deterioration. Hickey (2003) defines stroke as "a heterogeneous, neurological syndrome characterized by the gradual, or rapid, nonconvulsive onset of neurological deficits that fit a known vascular territory and that last for 24 hours or more."

A stroke, or brain attack, occurs in one of two ways. A blood vessel or artery is clogged or obstructed, which interrupts blood flow to a certain area of the brain. The second method of stroke is when the vessel or artery hemorrhages, with the blood itself interrupting blood flow to a certain area of the brain. Both methods cause ischemia, or a lack of oxygen to the brain cells. Cells that are deprived of oxygen for an undetermined amount of time begin to die; this area of dead tissue is called an **infarction**.

As certain areas of the brain become damaged or infarcted, the control of various bodily functions may become affected. These functions include motor function, sensory function, speech, memory, and other cognitive mechanisms. The type and extent of neurological disabilities are dependent on the location of the stroke. Strokes are divided into two categories: ischemic stroke and hemorrhagic stroke. Ischemic strokes are further divided by mechanism, embolic, arteriosclerotic cerebrovascular disease, or lacunar infarct. A lacunar infarct is a thrombosis of a small penetrating artery that results in tissue death. The outcome is a small cavity in the deep white matter of the brain, referred to as a *lacuna*.

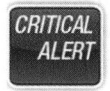 **CRITICAL ALERT** *The onset of neurological symptoms indicating stroke is a medical emergency. Notify health care provider immediately for any new symptoms indicating possibility of a stroke. Stroke protocols must be initiated immediately.*

Public awareness has changed the outlook for stroke. No longer is stroke viewed as fatal or devastating. Education has broadened public knowledge about stroke and clarified some misconceptions. The term *cerebrovascular accident*, or *CVA*, implies that stroke is an isolated event, somehow unexpected and random. Stroke actually is a vascular event that results from an actual disease of the blood vessels (Adams, del Zoppo, & von Kummer, 2006). Education has taught the public that they have some control over their own health. Research has brought public new sets of guidelines and recommendations for the prevention and management of brain attack.

Epidemiology

Stroke is a leading cause of death and disability in many developed nations. In the United States, it is the third leading cause of death, after heart disease and cancer (American Heart Association [AHA], 2005a). There are approximately 750,000 cases of stroke each year (American Heart Association [AHA], 2004), of which 160,000 are fatal (AHA, 2008a).

Approximately 4 million people in the United States have survived a brain attack and are living with the aftereffects. Although stroke is considered a condition of the elderly, stroke can happen to anyone—28% of its victims are under the age of 65 (AHA, 2008a). The annual cost of ischemic stroke is approximately $71.8 billion (Matchar & Samsa, 2000; Rosamond et al., 2007). The prevalence for stroke is almost twice as high for African Americans than Caucasians, and more men than women experience stroke. However, women account for approximately 60% of all stroke deaths (AHA, 2005b). Stroke kills almost twice as many women as breast cancer (Adams et al., 2006).

Etiology and Classification

As mentioned earlier, strokes generally are classified according to two main categories, ischemic and hemorrhagic, contingent on the pathology of the lesion or infarct that develops. Each category of stroke is further broken down into specific types.

Ischemic Stroke

Ischemic strokes are the most common form of stroke, accounting for approximately 400,000 cases or 80% (Rosamond et al., 2007). Ischemic strokes are further divided into several subtypes, including atherosclerotic thrombotic strokes, cardioembolic strokes, and lacunar strokes. A small percentage of ischemic strokes are caused by other vascular conditions.

Thrombotic Strokes

Thrombotic strokes occur most commonly in older individuals with underlying atherosclerosis (Alberts, 1999; Rosamond et al., 2007). Atherosclerosis is a condition in which the large arteries, both extracranial and intracranial, are subject to a buildup of "plaque," which narrows the lumen of the artery. Narrowing of the arteries is referred to as stenosis. Blood clots may form on an atherosclerotic vessel, further narrowing the lumen of the artery and causing severe stenosis. Large arteries, such as the internal carotid artery or the vertebral artery, can become stenotic, as can small, deep intracerebral vessels. Hypercoagulable states, conditions which promote platelet aggregation and clotting, also contribute to stenotic arteries.

Embolic Strokes

Embolism results when a clot breaks off and travels to an area of decreased circulation, blocking off blood flow. The tissue may then become hypoxic and finally infarcted, or dead. This embolism could be made of plaque from within the arterial lumen, or a blood clot from a faulty heart valve. Embolisms from cardiac sources are referred to as **cardiogenic embolisms**. The most common cause is atrial fibrillation, which accounts for almost 20% of all ischemic strokes (Hickey, 2003). Any condition that can cause a reduction in systemic blood flow can cause an ischemic event.

Examples of this are shock, hypotension, or cardiac arrest. Extremely low rates of blood flow may be responsible for the lack of cerebral oxygenation, resulting in ischemia and infarction.

Lacunar Strokes

Lacunar strokes also are known as small artery occlusive disease, or penetrating artery strokes. As mentioned earlier, the term *lacuna* refers to a small cavity that remains in brain tissue after dead tissue that results from an infarct has sloughed away. Lacunar strokes occur primarily in the deep areas of the brain, such as the basal ganglia or the thalamus. Although lacunar strokes usually are small, they are usually in eloquent, or highly functional, areas of the brain and can cause significant deficits. Hypertension is the predominant risk factor.

Transient Ischemic Attacks

Transient ischemic attacks (TIAs) are episodes of neurological deficit resulting from ischemia that is temporary and resolves in minutes to hours. This ischemia is a result of vascular disease and is specific to a defined vascular territory. Neurological deficits are a result of ischemia in a specific vascular territory. Examples of focal neurological deficits are weakness or sensory loss to one side of the body, unilateral visual deficits, loss of speech, and/or facial droop. Global deficits, such as confusion or lethargy, are not indicative of TIAs.

Onset is usually rapid. Resolution of accompanying neurological deficits occurs in less than 24 hours, often in less than 1 hour. Waxing and waning symptoms are not common with TIAs. Many patients have TIAs before having a large-vessel stroke. Approximately 10% of those experiencing a TIA will experience a major stroke within a year. The risk for stroke is greatest within the first 48 hours after a TIA (Howard et al., 2006; Johnson, Gress, Browner, & Sidney, 2000). TIAs are an important warning sign of impending stroke.

Hemorrhagic Strokes

Hemorrhagic strokes also are referred to as intracerebral or intraparenchymal hemorrhages. Approximately 20% of all strokes are hemorrhagic. The most common causes of intracerebral hemorrhage are hypertension or amyloid angiopathy. Intracerebral hemorrhage is seen most often in the elderly, although it is seen in the younger population with certain high-risk factors. Trauma, such as motor vehicle crashes, assaults, and falls, also accounts for intracerebral hemorrhage. When intracerebral hemorrhage is seen in a young adult, and trauma is ruled out as the cause, drug use should be suspected, specifically cocaine or amphetamines.

Another type of hemorrhagic stroke is subarachnoid hemorrhage (SAH). Rupture of an intracerebral aneurysm, with hemorrhage into the subarachnoid space, is the most common case of SAH. SAH and cerebral aneurysms are discussed later in the chapter.

Pathophysiology

The pathophysiology of stroke varies contingent on the different types of strokes. Factors that need to be considered include predisposing factors, including risk factors, comorbidities, duration of symptoms, and age (Stanford School of Medicine, 2008).

Ischemic Strokes

Atherosclerosis is the strongest contributing factor to ischemic stroke. The term **atherogenesis** refers to the development of the condition of atherosclerosis. The most fundamental lesion of atherosclerosis is a fatty streak, located in the intimal layer of large arteries. Fatty streaks may be in existence for many years, possibly starting in the early adult years. As years pass, the fatty streak becomes a fatty plaque. The growth and enlargement of the plaque occurs over years and decades. The patient is unaware of the presence of plaque until the plaque starts to invade the diameter of the artery and interfere with blood flow. The plaque disrupts the integrity of the arterial lining, causing blood to enter the plaque, which in turn causes thrombus (Hickey, 2003).

Smaller arteries are probably affected by a different process. It is thought that the smaller vessels become coated with a lipid compound in a process called lipohyalinosis. **Lipohyalinosis** is indicative of a vascular abnormality due to hypertension (Greenberg, 2001). This lipid coating causes the vessel walls to gradually become thicker, until the lumen becomes extremely narrow and blood flow is obstructed. Lipohyalinosis is believed to be the mechanism behind lacunar strokes.

Regardless of the mechanism involved—plaque, embolus, or thrombus—the result is the same. As the vessel becomes obstructed, blood flow becomes inadequate to perfuse brain tissue, and ischemia results. If this ischemia is left untreated, the tissue dies, which is referred to as cerebral infarction. Dead tissue is referred to as necrotic.

Ischemia causes injury at the cellular level because of lack of blood flow. The brain is extremely sensitive to lack of blood flow, and ischemic injury can occur within minutes. Further (secondary) injuries are due to the effects of the molecular changes due to ischemia. In cerebral infarction, an area of dead, necrotic tissue exists at the core of the damage. Around the necrotic core, there exists an area referred to as the penumbra. The cells within the penumbra are damaged, but not destroyed, and may be salvaged if blood flow is restored. The ischemic penumbra was described for the first time in 1970 as the hypoperfused zone surrounding an area of infarction. It is referred to as functionally silent tissue that is able to regain its function if promptly reperfused (Pestalozza, DiLegge, Calabresi, & Lenzi, 2002).

The ischemic penumbra that surrounds the necrotic core is comprised of edematous, oxygen-starved brain cells. A process known as the ischemic cascade refers to a series of events that occur in response to cellular hypoxia. This process induces intracellular swelling, further propagating cerebral edema, cerebral ischemia, and, finally, cerebral infarction and cell death. This further extends the area of infarction, or the necrotic core. Chart 30–1 depicts the ischemic cascade. The concept that cells within the ischemic penumbra are viable and can be saved if blood flow is returned quickly cannot be overstated. Time *is* indeed brain.

Reperfusion injury refers to injury to cells due to released oxygen free radicals that occurs after the blood supply has been reestablished to the ischemic area. Reperfusion injury results in further injury to already damaged tissue that is compromised, but viable (Ayata & Ropper, 2002; Clark, 2007). Reperfusion injury is seen most often with thrombolytic therapy.

Hemorrhagic Stroke

The pathology of hemorrhagic stroke is associated with increased intracranial pressure (ICP). This event triggers a series of conditions, such as increased mass effect, decreased cerebral blood flow, and cerebral edema. It may further increase ICP and possibly lead

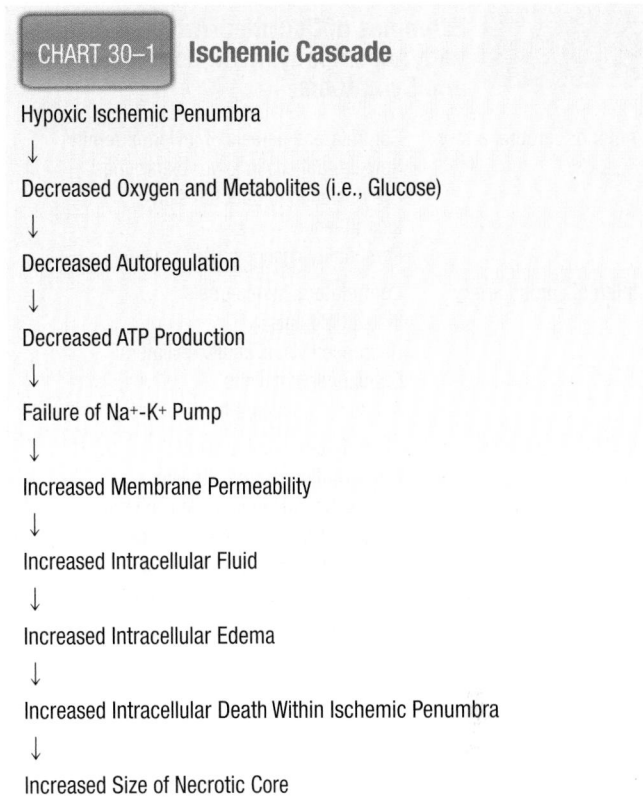

CHART 30–1   **Ischemic Cascade**

Hypoxic Ischemic Penumbra

↓

Decreased Oxygen and Metabolites (i.e., Glucose)

↓

Decreased Autoregulation

↓

Decreased ATP Production

↓

Failure of Na$^+$-K$^+$ Pump

↓

Increased Membrane Permeability

↓

Increased Intracellular Fluid

↓

Increased Intracellular Edema

↓

Increased Intracellular Death Within Ischemic Penumbra

↓

Increased Size of Necrotic Core

to herniation. The events associated with hemorrhagic stroke are closely related to the pathophysiology of increased ICP and herniation syndromes (see Chapter 29 🌐 for a review of herniation syndromes).

Clinical Manifestations

The signs and symptoms of ischemic stroke vary widely, and are dependent on the location of the vessel involved and the extent of the occlusion. Examples of occluded arteries and their associated signs and symptoms are found in Chart 30–2 (p. 760).

In hemorrhagic strokes, intracerebral bleeds happen quickly. Therefore, the presenting signs and symptoms occur rapidly. There may be little to no warning. Severe headache is a common sign. The other signs and symptoms are dependent on the region of the brain affected and the size of the hemorrhage. The most common areas for hemorrhagic stroke are the putamen and the surrounding internal capsule. These are the very deep structures, and account for approximately 50% of all hemorrhagic strokes due to hypertension (Hickey, 2003). Other areas in which hemorrhages frequently are found are the thalamus, the cerebellum, the brainstem, and the white matter of the frontal, temporal, and the parietal lobes.

As stated, hemorrhagic strokes occur rapidly. Often, there is no warning sign, and the patient presents with loss of consciousness and severe neurological impairment, possibly death. The area of hemorrhage may represent a large volume, which gathers quickly, causing rapid displacement of brain tissue. The presenting signs and symptoms of hemorrhagic stroke may be focal signs associated with the specific location of the hemorrhage, but also may be those of increased ICP and herniation syndromes.

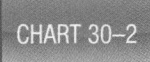

CHART 30–2

Examples of Occluded/Affected Arteries with Accompanying Signs and Symptoms

Anterior cerebral artery	Contralateral paresis of lower extremity
	Sensory deficits in lower extremities
	Eye deviation to affected side
	Incontinence
	Personality changes
Internal carotid artery	Contralateral hemiparesis
	Visual field cuts
	Decreased visual acuity ipsilateral
	Cranial nerve deficits
	Aphasia if dominant hemisphere
Middle cerebral artery	Contralateral hemiparesis
	Eye deviation to opposite site
	Dysphagia if dominant hemisphere
	Aphasia if dominant hemisphere
	Contralateral sensory impairment
	Apraxia if nondominant hemisphere
Vertebral/basilar arteries (posterior circulation)	Visual field deficits
	Ataxia
	Cranial nerve deficits:
	Eye movement disorders
	Dysphagia
	Dysarthria
	Quadriparesis
	Vertigo
	Sensory deficits
	Mutism

RISK FACTORS for Stroke

Hypertension
Family history
Atrial fibrillation
Hyperlipidemia
Diabetes mellitus
Stress
Excessive alcohol use
Sedentary lifestyle
Obesity
Smoking
Valvular disease
Coronary artery disease

Laboratory and Diagnostic Procedures

Diagnosis of stroke is made by a careful and accurate history of events, and presentation of symptoms. It also is important to determine a patient's risk factors for stroke (see the Risk Factors for Stroke box). A noncontrast computerized tomography (CT) scan of the head should be obtained as soon as possible to rule out hemorrhagic stroke. This is especially important if any condition exists that may predispose the patient to hemorrhage. Examples of these conditions are anticoagulation, known presence of lesions such as brain tumors, or a rapid deterioration of neurological status. It is important to rule out hemorrhage in order to provide the patient with the optimum treatment plan.

Once hemorrhage has been ruled out, diagnosis of ischemic stroke is made by cerebral angiography. Angiography provides details of the vasculature, which artery is occluded, and the extent of occlusion. Note that a CT scan does not immediately show infarcted tissue, and the patient may have a normal CT scan, yet have an occluded artery.

Another important imaging tool for the diagnosis of carotid stenosis is duplex sonography with Doppler imaging. Koga and colleagues (2001) studied diagnostic tools for imaging of carotid arteries and asserted that carotid ultrasound was an effective tool for the diagnosis of carotid stenosis.

Medical Management of Ischemic Stroke

Both medical and surgical approaches are used to treat ischemic stroke. The medical treatment for ischemic stroke is antiplatelet

and antithrombotic therapy. **Antiplatelet therapy** inhibits platelet adhesion and aggregation and is the cornerstone of therapy for occlusive artery disease. For more than 100 years, the only antiplatelet drug available was aspirin (Lubbe & Berger, 2002). Recently, the addition of a second-line drug, clopidogrel (Plavix), a thienopyridine, has added benefits to the patient at risk for progression of a stroke or the possibility of another stroke. Dual antiplatelet drug therapy, with the addition of clopidogrel (Plavix), has significantly improved clinical outcomes in reducing ischemic events. One limitation of dual antiplatelet therapy is an increased risk of bleeding (Lubbe & Berger, 2002).

Another class of drug that has gained much attention is the glycoprotein receptor antagonist, abciximab (ReoPro). Abciximab inhibits platelet aggregation and leukocyte adhesion. When used with aspirin and heparin, it has been shown to reduce the risk of ischemic complications for patients undergoing endovascular intervention. Abciximab appears to be particularly beneficial to high-risk patients, including those with diabetes mellitus (Ibbotson, McGavin, & Goa, 2003). In clinical trials, abciximab has been shown to dissolve intravascular thrombi and to improve neurological outcomes after stroke and endovascular intervention (Winkley & Adams, 2000). It appears that the use of antiplatelet drugs, such as aspirin, clopidogrel, and glycoprotein inhibitors, provides strategies that block multiple platelet activation pathways, providing increased safety for patients with vascular disease (Brinkman, Terramani, Najibi, & Chaikof, 2002).

Recent studies of angiotensin-converting enzyme (ACE) inhibitors have identified an important role for the secondary prevention of stroke, even in patients who are not hypertensive (MacWalter & Shirley, 2002). Lipid-lowering drugs, such as the statins, also have an important role in the prevention of stroke. These drugs also have a role in the reduction of risk factors of those patients who are at risk for stroke or who have already had a stroke.

The term **neuroprotection** refers to therapies, both pharmacologic and nonpharmacologic, that are used to arrest the sequence of events that occur during the ischemic cascade (Hinkle & Bowman, 2003). During an ischemic stroke, the cerebral blood flow (CBF) decreases, causing ischemic tissue to become infarcted, with an ischemic penumbra around it. At this point, it is important to restore blood flow to the ischemic tissue that still has potential for revitalization. Currently, the only available treatment is tissue plasminogen activator (t-PA), which lyses the clot and restores blood flow to the ischemic penumbra (Alberts, 1999). See the Evidenced-Based Practice box which presents the latest research on treating ICH (p. 782).

Administration of t-PA is approved by the U.S. Food and Drug Administration (FDA) and must be administered within 3 hours of onset of symptoms. Note that the administration of t-PA does not affect the infarcted, necrotic core, but may revitalize the penumbra and limit the extent of damage caused by ischemic stroke (National Institute of Neurological Disorders and Stroke t-PA Study Group, 1995). t-PA is given intravenously, although it also may be given via an intra-arterial route. The advantage of the intra-arterial route is that the agent can be given directly into the clot. It also may be given within a longer time frame, 6 hours, rather than 3 hours for the intravenous (IV) route. The disadvantages to both administration routes are the risk of intracerebral hemorrhage (Saver, 2001).

Anticoagulation with IV infusion of heparin for several days during the acute care management of a patient with ischemic stroke is common. Some institutions are using low-molecular-weight heparin (LMWH) subcutaneously instead of intravenous heparin. It also may be administered at the onset of warfarin therapy until prothrombin time and International Normalized Ratio (INR) levels are therapeutic. The advantage of this method is a shorter length of hospitalization. Warfarin therapy is commonly used for patients with cardioembolic strokes due to atrial fibrillation.

Anticoagulation is one type of treatment for ischemic stroke due to an embolus. Patients receiving heparin therapy must have partial prothromboplastin times done every 6 hours, with the rate of heparin adjusted appropriately in order to reach the target goal. Patients on warfarin or enoxaparin must have daily prothrombin times taken to ensure therapeutic levels.

Neuroprotective agents are defined as those that protect the brain from further injury. Thrombolytic drugs (that cause the break-up of a blood clot), such as t-PA, are considered neuroprotective. Much research has been done to look for other drugs that can protect the brain from further stroke. Very few have been shown to improve outcome. Glutamate antagonists, calcium channel blockers, gamma-aminobutyric acid (GABA) agonists, and free-radical scavengers are neuroprotective drugs that currently are under investigation for the treatment of ischemic stroke. These drugs interact during the ischemic cascade, and have shown promise in animal studies (Hinkle & Bowman, 2003).

Another neuroprotective strategy is mild hypothermia. Studies have shown that mild hypothermia, even when delayed by as much as 2 hours, decreased inflammatory responses in stroke (Deng, Han, Cheng, Sun, & Yenari, 2003). It is thought that hypothermia may limit the extent of ischemic injury.

Other drugs used in the treatment of strokes and other cerebrovascular disorders are listed in the Pharmacology Summary box (p. 762).

Surgical Management of Ischemic Strokes

Patients with atherosclerotic disease in selected vessels may be candidates for surgical intervention. The diseased vessels can be either intracranial or extracranial. The goal of treatment is to prevent further strokes or TIAs. Surgical intervention may consist of a carotid endarterectomy, percutaneous angioplasty with or without intervascular stenting, or possibly an extracranial to intracranial bypass procedure. A **carotid endarterectomy (CEA)** is a surgical procedure to correct carotid stenosis. Surgical options are dependent on several variables: the location of the stenotic or occluded vessel, the extent of occlusion, and the accessibility of the appropriate facilities and surgical expertise available.

Neurovascular procedures such as CEA, stenting, and bypass procedures are highly specialized. The risks of all three procedures are significant and potentially devastating to the patient. The major risks of CEA are wound hematoma, stroke, or hemorrhage. The risks of percutaneous angioplasty with or without stenting are hemorrhage of the vessel, extravasation of contrast material, or stroke. Bypass procedures carry significant risk to the patient, such as hemorrhage of the vessel, stroke due to clot in the graft, blood pressure instability, or stroke due to a variety of other factors. All surgical procedures carry risks of infection and alteration in wound healing.

Carotid Endarterectomy

Carotid endarterectomy has been proven to be superior to medical treatment alone for the prevention of stroke by the North American Symptomatic Carotid Endarterectomy Trial (NASCET, 1991). The practice of CEA has not always met with favor. In the 1980s, the practice of CEA was controversial. It was not apparent that CEA was performed for appropriate conditions. Since then, several clinical trials have supported the classic study conducted by the NASCET by demonstrating that under appropriate conditions, CEA is the most beneficial treatment for carotid stenosis (Barnett, Taylor, & Eliasziw, 1998). In 1999, more than 130,000 CEAs were performed in the United States alone (Gross, Steiner, Bass, & Powe, 2000). Patients with a greater than 70% stenosis of the internal carotid artery have a greater than 60% risk reduction with CEA, assuming they have no major surgical risk factors. CEA is not recommended for patients with a less than 50% stenosis of the internal carotid artery. These patients are usually placed on antiplatelet therapy (NASCET, 1991).

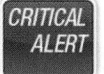

Patients who have had a carotid endarterectomy are at risk for hematoma at the incision. Monitor the incision at least every 2 hours for the first 24 hours. If hematoma occurs, measure the neck circumference, noting the presence of tracheal deviation, or respiratory distress. Notify health care provider immediately.

Endovascular Procedures

Endovascular procedures have been a tremendous asset to the treatment of stenotic disease and the prevention of stroke. Endovascular procedures include intravascular stenting and **percutaneous angioplasty**. These are interventional radiological procedures done by endovascular neurosurgeons or interventional radiologists. Angioplasty and stenting may be appropriate alternatives for patients who are at high risk for CEA. Percutaneous angioplasty is a form of catheterization with microcatheters. These catheters are floated into a large vessel, such as the carotids, middle cerebrals, vertebrals, or the basilar

PHARMACOLOGY Summary of Medications to Treat Cerebrovascular Disorders

Drug	Category	Application/Indication	Nursing Concerns
Dopamine Dobutamine (Dobutrex) Phenylephrine (Neo-Synephrine) Norepinephrine (Levophed) Epinephrine	Vasopressors	Increase blood pressure.	Monitored unit Hypertension
Labetalol hydralazine Nitroglycerine (NTG) Nitroprusside (Nipride) Enalapril Metoprolol	Vasodilators	Reduce blood pressure.	May raise ICP Monitored unit for IV use Possible hypotension
Nimodipine (Nimotop) Nicardipine (Cardene)	Calcium channel blockers Triple-H therapy	Reduce blood pressure. Reduce vasospasm.	Hypotension
Clopidogrel (Plavix) Aspirin Warfarin (Coumadin) Heparin	Antithrombotic agents	Reduce platelet aggregation. Provide anticoagulation.	Monitor for bleeding Monitor protime/INR Monitor PTT Family teaching for home care
t-PA Streptokinase	Antithrombotic agents	Recanalize occluded arteries. Restore oxygenation and cerebral blood flow.	Must meet eligibility criteria Increased risk for bleeding or reperfusion injury Monitored unit
Mannitol	Osmotic solution	Reduce vasogenic edema.	Monitored unit Monitor serum sodium, osmolality levels
Famotidine (Pepcid) Ranitidine (Zantac) Omeprazole (Prilosec)	H2-blockers	Reduce acid in the stomach.	Thrombocytopenia
Phenytoin (Dilantin) Carbamazepine (Tegretol) Divalproex (Depakote) Gabapentin (Neurontin) Lamotrigine (Lamictal) Phenobarbital Clonazepam (Klonopin) Ethosuximide (Zarontin)	Antiepileptic drugs	Prevent seizures.	Thrombocytopenia Allergic reactions can be severe Gingivitis Monitor blood levels when appropriate Possible drug interactions
Diazepam (Valium) Lorazepam (Ativan)	Benzodiazepines	Used as treatment for seizure cessation, status epilepticus.	Oversedation Respiratory depression
Oxycodone (Percocet, Oxy-IR, Roxicet, OxyContin) Hydromorphone (Dilaudid) Hydrocodone (Vicodin, Lortab) Morphine Fentanyl (Sublimaze, Duragesic)	Opioids	Control moderate to severe pain.	Respiratory depression Oversedation Constipation Difficulty with urination
Codeine Tramadol (Ultram)	Opioids	Control mild to moderate pain.	Respiratory depression Oversedation
Ketorolac (Toradol) Indomethacin (Indocin) Ibuprofen (Motrin, Advil) Naproxen (Naprosyn)	Nonsteroidal anti-inflammatory drugs	Control pain. Reduce fever.	GI upset, GI bleed
Acetaminophen	Analgesic and anti-inflammatory	Control pain. Reduce fever.	Liver toxicity
Naloxone (Narcan) Flumazenil (Romazicon)	Opioid antagonists Benzodiazepine antagonists	Reverse opiate action. Reverse benzodiazepine action.	
Ondansetron (Zofran) Metoclopramide (Reglan) Trimethobenzamide (Tigan) Prochlorperazine (Compazine) Promethazine (Phenergan)	Antiemetics, nonphenothiazines Antiemetics, phenothiazines	Reduce/prevent nausea.	Psychosis Extrapyramidal symptoms

artery. The catheter then enters the stenosed, or narrowed, vessel, and the atherosclerotic plaque is broken apart by inflation of a balloon within the catheter. The patency of the vessel may be preserved by the use of a **stent**, which is an open-ended tube. The stent supports the vessel wall and widens the lumen of the vessel.

Revascularization

Bypass procedures are highly controversial. These procedures are extracranial to intracranial (EC-IC) anastomosis and, frequently, the superficial temporal artery to the middle cerebral artery (STA-MCA). This is a microsurgical procedure done to improve circulation to the area of the brain served by a specific artery, often the MCA. This procedure was initially looked on as unfavorable because of the negative results reported in the EC-IC Bypass Trial (Barnett et al., 1987). This study was unable to prove that this procedure reduced the risk of stroke (Martin, Kureshi, & Coiteiro, 2004). However, this procedure offers favorable results when done by surgeons who are highly specialized in neurovascular techniques. It is used most often as a refined revascularization technique in the treatment of aneurysms.

Medical Management of Hemorrhagic Stroke

Treatment of hemorrhagic stroke is dependent on the location of the hemorrhage, the extent of the hemorrhage, and the neurological condition of the patient. Management is frequently both medical and surgical. After an initial neurological examination, the patient must be monitored closely in the intensive care unit (ICU), with frequent neurological assessment. The patient's symptoms are usually as a result of increased ICP and mass effect due to a hematoma. Placement of an external ventricular drain (EVD) may be necessary to monitor ICP and to treat elevation of ICP by drainage of cerebrospinal fluid (CSF). Medical support of blood pressure and respiratory effort also may be necessary. If the hemorrhage is large enough to cause a shift due to mass effect, a craniotomy may be done to evacuate the hematoma to relieve mass effect.

◼ Cerebrovascular Malformations

Cerebrovascular malformations are congenital lesions composed of a complex tangle of arteries and veins connected by one or more fistulae. They represent several types of complex disorders whose exact etiology is not known, but which typically produce neurological deficits (Schumacher & Marshall, 2006).

Cerebral Aneurysms

The word *aneurysm* comes from the Greek word *aneurysma*, which means "widening" (Khurana & Spetzler, 2006). A **cerebral aneurysm** is defined as a "saccular outpouching of a cerebral artery" (Hickey, 2003). Though aneurysms may consist of varied shapes, the saccular, or **berry aneurysm**, is by far the most common, accounting for approximately 85% to 95% of all intracerebral aneurysms. These aneurysms are generally located on a major artery at the site of maximum hemodynamic stress, and they have a neck (Figure 30–1 ◼). Common locations are the middle cerebral artery, the anterior communicating artery, the anterior cerebral artery, and the internal carotid artery. Saccular aneurysms also are located in the posterior circulation, on the vertebral or basilar arteries, although this placement is not as common. Fre-

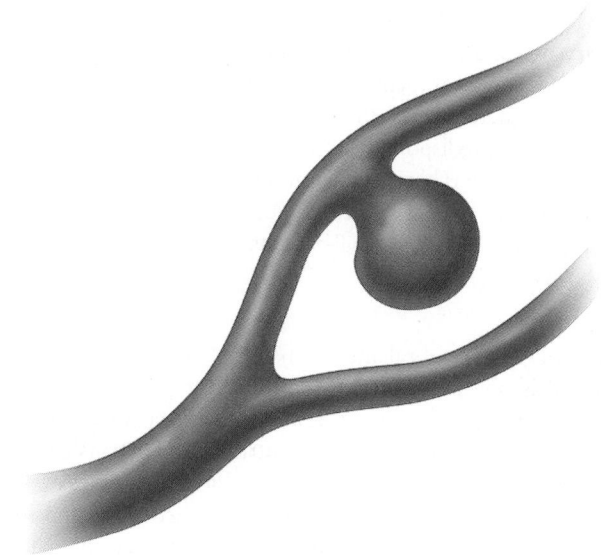

FIGURE 30–1 ◼ Intracerebral saccular aneurysm.

quently seen in the posterior circulation are **fusiform aneurysms**, which are elliptical in shape. Intracerebral aneurysms may occur singularly or in multiples. **Familial intracranial aneurysms** are defined as two or more family members with documented cerebral aneurysms.

Rupture of an intracerebral aneurysm results in **subarachnoid hemorrhage (SAH)**. SAH is defined simply as bleeding into the subarachnoid space. Though SAH can occur from other causes, such as trauma, or be idiopathic, SAH most often occurs from aneurysm rupture. This is referred to as aneurysmal SAH.

Epidemiology

Each year in the United States there are approximately 30,000 new cases of aneurysmal SAH (Schumacher & Marshall, 2006). Autopsy studies demonstrate an incidence of approximately 5% of the population (Khurana & Spetzler, 2006). The morbidity and mortality of SAH is relatively high. Despite vast improvements in medical technology and surgical techniques, outcome of SAH is still poor, with a fatality rate of approximately 40% to 50% (Juvela, 2003). Survivors of SAH may have significant neurological, physical, and/or cognitive deficits (Ballard et al., 2003). The incidence of SAH increases with age, the mean age being approximately 50 years, and is higher in women than in men (Kaminogo, Yonekura, & Shibata, 2003). Literature indicates that African Americans are at higher risk than Caucasians (Sacco et al., 1998). In one study, the author found that heterogeneity, based on ethnicity, was a risk factor for SAH (Kim, 2007). Kim concluded that the ethnic groups involved in the study had a higher propensity for smoking versus the nonethnic participants, and that the harmful health effects of smoking may be one cause for the higher incidence of SAH. The Stanford Stroke Center also identified race as a risk factor; however, they did not elaborate on or describe an interpretation of this factor (Stanford School of Medicine, 2008).

Familial Aneurysms

Familial intracranial aneurysms are defined as the presence of two or more family members among first- and second-degree relatives with proven aneurysms, either ruptured or incidental (Hickey, 2003). Multiple studies have been done regarding familial aneurysms, and they have determined that the incidence is between 7% and 20% (Schievink, 2004). Because family members may have different risk factors and show no signs of other disorders that may predispose them to intracranial aneurysms, it is believed that there is a genetic component to familial intracranial aneurysms (Wills et al., 2003). Multiple aneurysms occur in approximately 10% to 20% of all patients with SAH (Brown & Piepgras, 2004).

Etiology

The etiology of cerebral aneurysms is not clear. Genetic predisposition is one possibility. It is probable that genetic factors, combined with various intrinsic and extrinsic factors, may be an explanation. There are also many intrinsic and extrinsic factors that affect the integrity of the vascular system. Examples of these factors are hypertension and smoking. A genetic predisposition for weakened vasculature, coupled with hypertension and/or smoking that may exacerbate the weakened vessel, could cause rupture (see Risk Factors for Aneurysms).

As stated earlier, the saccular aneurysm, also known as the berry aneurysm, is the most common type of aneurysm. It is formed by a ballooning of the vessel at the weakened portion of the artery. In contrast, fusiform aneurysms are elliptically shaped. They do not have a neck. They look like "swollen" areas of the artery, and are associated with fatty plaque buildup in the artery. Although they do not usually rupture, they may cause neurological compromise due to pressure exerted on surrounding brain. Most fusiform aneurysms are located in the posterior circulation.

The etiology of cerebral aneurysms remains an area where research is warranted; however, the cause for some aneurysms is well understood. Some aneurysms are caused by bacterial or fungal infections, resulting in mycotic aneurysms. These aneurysms do not result in SAH.

Location and Classification of Aneurysms

The location of cerebral aneurysms, their size, and whether or not they have ruptured are the most important factors in determining signs and symptoms of the patient. Four main arteries enter the brain. The two internal carotid arteries enter in the front of the brain. Two vertebral arteries enter from the back. These four arteries form a ring that circles the underside of the brain. This ring is referred to as the circle of Willis. Many smaller arteries branch off from the larger arteries (Figure 30–2 ■). The arteries at the top of the ring are in the **anterior circulation**; the arteries at the lower portion of the ring are in the **posterior circulation**.

RISK FACTORS for Aneurysms

Smoking
Hypertension
Previous aneurysms
Family history of aneurysms
Connective tissue disorder
Age greater than 40 years
Female
Blood vessel injury or dissection

Aneurysms also are classified by their size, with small aneurysms being the most common (Chart 30–3). Small and large aneurysms are more prone to rupture. Although giant aneurysms occasionally rupture, most often giant aneurysms cause patients to be symptomatic due to compression on surrounding brain tissue (Khurana & Spetzler, 2006).

Pathophysiology

The occurrence, natural history, and eventual rupture of intracerebral aneurysms appear to occur as a result of several factors. The formation of an aneurysm seems be precipitated by the integrity of the vasculature. Weakening of the vascular wall may occur due to structural limitations of the vessel. Hemodynamic stressors further influence the formation and growth of aneurysms. Intrinsic and extrinsic factors, such as hypertension, smoking, and various autoimmune diseases, further affect the history of aneurysms.

Once an aneurysm ruptures, the arterial pressure forces blood into the subarachnoid space, creating an SAH. Pressure in the brain tissue stops the bleeding. The blood irritates brain tissue, causing an inflammatory response, which may further cause cerebral edema. The circulating blood in the CSF is an irritant that may inhibit CSF absorption, causing hydrocephalus. The presence of SAH causes hemodynamic changes, with a resultant increase in ICP. The pathophysiology of increased ICP is discussed in Chapter 29 .

Clinical Manifestations

Patients with aneurysms of the anterior circulation have different symptoms than those with aneurysms of the posterior circulation. Those patients who experience SAH also have more severe neurological compromise than those without SAH. Clinical manifestations are dependent on the location and size of the hemorrhage. See Chart 30–2 (p. 760) for specific arteries that are occluded or somehow compromised due to stroke and the accompanying symptoms that may be present.

Ruptured Aneurysms

In patients with SAH, the most frequent presenting sign is headache, then progressively deteriorating neurological status. The headaches are described as the "worst headache of my life," almost without exception. Neurological deterioration usually follows, with focal signs dependent on location and the size of the hemorrhage. Seizures are not uncommon. Not infrequently, the presenting sign is death.

SAH in the posterior circulation also produces severe headaches. If the patient is conscious, extreme vertigo and nausea and vomiting usually are present. Neurological deterioration may also be present in posterior circulation aneurysms.

Unruptured Aneurysms

Although most patients are completely asymptomatic until rupture occurs, some aneurysms produce warning signs. They are frequently attributed to other causes and ignored. Occasionally, an aneurysm is found incidentally, when the patient has imaging studies for another purpose. When an aneurysm becomes large enough to cause symptoms, the most frequent symptom appears to be localized headache and/or cranial nerve signs. The most common cranial nerve deficits are dilated pupil, decreased mobility of the eye, or ptosis (drooping of the eyelid), all due to pressure on cranial nerve (CN) III (oculomotor nerve). The aneurysm be-

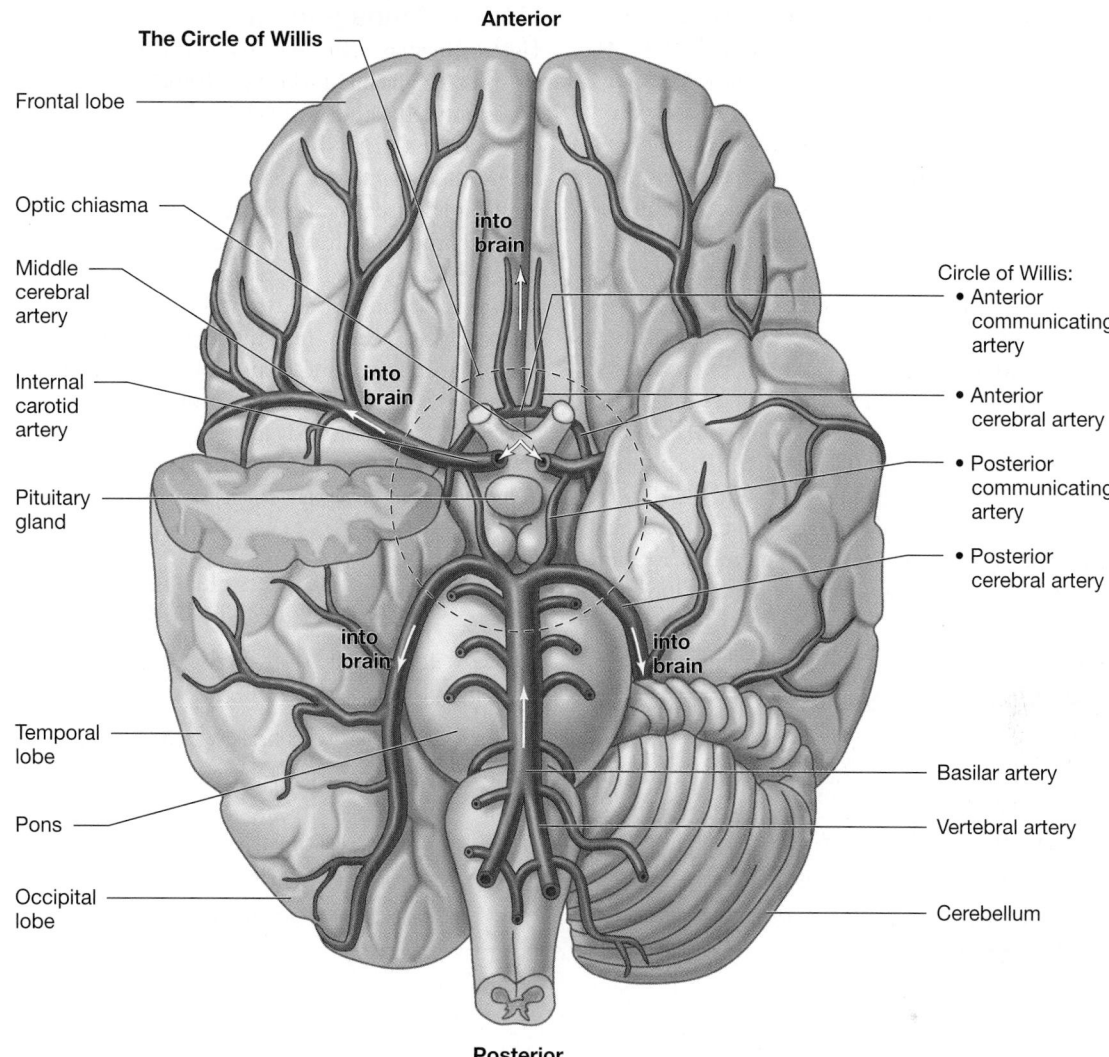

FIGURE 30–2 ■ Circle of Willis.

CHART 30–3 **Classification of Aneurysm Size**

Classification	Size
Small	Up to 10 mm
Medium	10–15 mm
Large	15–25 mm
Giant	>25 mm

comes a space-occupying lesion, causing symptoms dependent on the location and size of the aneurysm. Clinical manifestations of unruptured aneurysms of the posterior circulation are those of dizziness and balance difficulties. The symptoms are caused by the size of the aneurysms exhibiting mass effect.

Risk Factors for Subarachnoid Hemorrhage (SAH)

Risk factors for SAH have been shown to be age, gender, and race, as described earlier. As with other types of stroke, smoking is a strong risk factor for SAH, especially in women (Anderson et al., 2004). In the past, the use of oral contraceptives was felt to be a strong risk factor, but with the change in the estrogen composition of these drugs, the risk appears significant for thrombotic stroke, but not SAH (Chan et al., 2004). Drug abuse has been associated with SAH, especially use of stimulants, such as cocaine and amphetamines. It appears that while the use of cocaine or amphetamines may not actually cause a hemorrhage, the vasoactive properties of the drugs appear to worsen an already weakened vasculature. There is evidence that the patients who indulged in cocaine use prior to SAH have a greater incidence of vasospasm (Conway & Tamargo, 2001). Smoking, drug use, and hypertension are all modifiable risk factors.

Once an aneurysm ruptures, risk factors differ slightly. Once SAH has occurred, factors such as the patient's initial clinical condition, the amount of subarachnoid blood, and the continued presence of hypertension are strong negative prognostic factors. Cigarette smoking also appears to be a strong risk factor for poor outcome (Juvela, 2003). It is believed that approximately 60% to 70% of all SAH patients are smokers (Juvela, 2000).

Laboratory and Diagnostic Procedures

The patient who comes into the emergency department in a neurologically compromised condition should always receive a CT scan of the head immediately. The CT scan will demonstrate blood in the ventricles and subarachnoid space. The patient is assigned a grade based on the **Fisher grading scale** (Chart 30–4). This scale is used to determine the amount of blood demonstrated on CT scan. It also is used as a predictor for vasospasm. Once SAH is diagnosed, the patient should have a cerebral angiogram to ascertain the location of the ruptured aneurysm. Lumbar puncture no longer is the definitive examination because, even though it will show blood in the CSF, it will not determine the location of the aneurysm or even whether it is caused by aneurysmal rupture. The Diagnostic Tests box provides more information about tests used for determining whether an aneurysm or other cerebral vascular disorder exists.

Once aneurysmal rupture is diagnosed, a grading scale is used to assign an SAH classification to the patient. This SAH grading scale is the **Hunt-Hess classification** (Chart 30–5). The purpose of this grading scale is to determine the severity of the SAH, and possibly assist with treatment options. It also is a common language that health care professionals use to communicate with when discussing the patient and the severity of his condition.

Medical Management

The treatment of aneurysms is highly dependent on many factors, the most important of which is whether the aneurysm is ruptured or unruptured. Other factors include the generalized medical condition of the patient, the Hunt-Hess grade, and the facilities available to the patient. Patients with SAH due to ruptured aneurysm should be transported to facilities with the capabilities and training to appropriately treat patients with ruptured aneurysms. A national study looked at surgery of unruptured aneurysm nationwide, and found that for patients with unruptured aneurysms treated in the United States between 1996 and 2000, surgery at high-volume institutions performed by high-volume surgeons was associated with significantly lower morbidity and mortality (Carter, Amin-Hanjani, Butler, Ogilvy, & Barker, 2003).

Historically, the treatment of choice has been surgical. For years, the neurovascular surgeon treated the aneurysm, both

CHART 30–4 Fisher Grading Scale

Group	Blood on CT Scan
1	No blood detected
2	Diffuse or vertical layers less than 1 mm thick
3	Localized clot and/or vertical layer greater than 1 mm thick
4	Intracerebral or intraventricular clot with diffuse or no SAH

CHART 30–5 Hunt-Hess Classification of Subarachnoid Hemorrhages

Grade	Description
0	Unruptured
I	Asymptomatic, or mild headache and slight nuchal rigidity
II	Cranial nerve palsy, moderate to severe headache, nuchal rigidity
III	Mild focal deficit, lethargy, or confusion
IV	Stupor, moderate to severe hemiparesis, decerebrate rigidity
V	Deep coma, decerebrate rigidity, moribund

DIAGNOSTIC TESTS for Cerebrovascular Disorders

Test	Expected Abnormality	Rationale for Abnormality
CT of head	Hematomas, SAH, hydrocephalus	CT scans are best suited to examine presence of blood, edema, CSF.
Cerebral angiogram	Vascular abnormalities, i.e., cerebral aneurysms, arteriovenous malformations.	Angiogram is gold standard for visualization of the arterial system.
Magnetic resonance angiography (MRA)	Vascular abnormalities	Demonstrates the vascular system, best when large aneurysms are present (>0.5 cm).
MRI, including diffusion-weighted images (DWI)	Ischemic abnormalities, cavernous malformations	MRI will demonstrate small lesions not seen on CT scan. Best suited to demonstrate ischemic areas of stroke.
Lumbar puncture	Blood in CSF (subarachnoid blood) Time-sensitive blood in CSF presents as yellow with passage of time	Contraindicated until space-occupying lesions are ruled out; possibility of induced brain herniation.
Electroencephalogram (EEG)	Seizure activity	Common in head trauma, SAH, vascular malformations due to altered electrical activity in brain.
Serum electrolytes	Hyponatremia (serum Na+ less than 134 mEq/L)	Risk factor for increased cerebral edema. Significant in the presence of SAH and vasospasm.
Blood glucose	May be elevated	Indicative of steroid use (dexamethasone). Hyperglycemia a significant risk for ischemic brain.
Complete blood count (CBC)	Elevated white blood cell count	Indicates infection. Also may be present with steroid use.
Arterial blood gases	Hypoxia, hypercapnia	Depressed neurological state may also indicate depressed respiratory drive. Decreased levels of oxygen and increased levels of CO_2 raise concerns about increasing ICP.

ruptured and unruptured, by placing a surgical clip across the neck of the aneurysm to completely obliterate it (Figure 30–3 ▪). Improvement in outcomes came with the improvement of the clips themselves and with the development of more efficient methods of approaching the aneurysm. Again, the institutions doing a high volume of aneurysm clippings by surgeons doing the highest volume of surgeries were associated with more favorable outcomes than lower volume institutions.

Regardless of the expertise of the surgeons, or the volume of surgery done at various institutions, some aneurysms still were felt to be inoperable. This challenge has led to the innovative use of techniques devised by cardiac surgeons to perform cardiac bypass surgeries. In a limited number of institutions, certain aneurysms are being clipped under cardiac standstill, cooling the body of the patient and stopping blood circulation. Large basilar artery aneurysms that previously were not amenable to being surgically clipped can now at least be considered for treatment in the hands of surgeons skilled in this highly technical procedure. Although the number of institutions that have the capability to perform this intervention is relatively small, it is exciting to realize the possibilities that exist and are constantly being revised.

The advent of endovascular procedures has presented nonsurgical options, such as coiling or stenting. The goal of any treatment is to prevent rebleeding by obliterating the aneurysm with either a surgical clip or a coil.

Unruptured Aneurysms

In 1998, a group of researchers nationwide collaborated to study unruptured aneurysms to determine the most advantageous treatment plan. The International Study of Unruptured Intracranial Aneurysms (ISUIA) studied 1,449 patients with 1,937 unruptured aneurysms from 53 participating centers. In studies published on clipping of unruptured aneurysms, the mortality rate was reported at 2.6%, and the morbidity at 10.9%. The mortality rate for SAH was 66%. The high mortality associated with rupture of aneurysms suggests that preventive surgery for the obliteration of unruptured aneurysms is a good therapeutic option (Raaymakers, Rinkel, Limburg, & Algra, 1998).

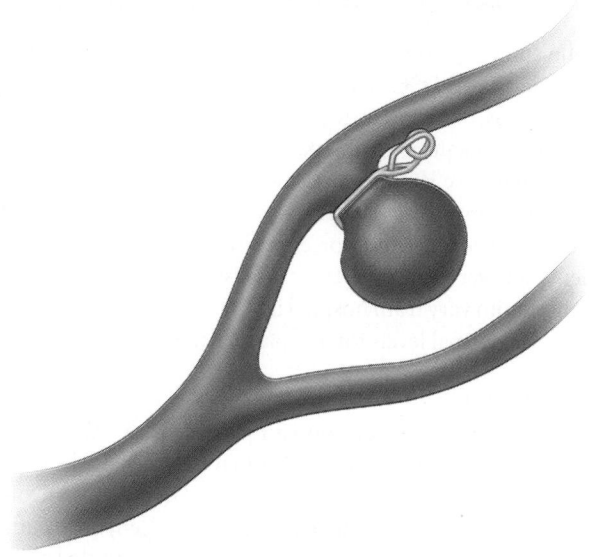

FIGURE 30–3 ▪ Aneurysm with clip applied.

Ruptured Aneurysms

Patients with ruptured intracranial aneurysms should be treated as soon as possible after the hemorrhage. The purpose of treatment is to prevent rebleeding. It also is important to aggressively manage medical complications associated with SAH, such as **vasospasm**. The choice of treatment—endovascular or surgical—is a source of ongoing debate. The choice of treatment should be based on the angiographic demonstration of the aneurysm. According to the International Subarachnoid Aneurysm Trial [ISAT] Collaborative Group (2002), if the aneurysm is suitable for coiling, that is the preferred method (van den Berg, Rinkel, & Vandertop, 2003). Preferably, treatment would occur at a hospital with neurosurgeons specially trained in the clipping of aneurysms, and interventional neuroradiologists.

The ISAT Collaborative Group (2002) found that in patients with ruptured intracranial aneurysm, for which endovascular coiling and neurosurgical clipping are both options, the outcome for survival free of disability at 1 year is significantly higher with endovascular coiling (Molyneux et al., 2002). Although not a factor in the decision-making process of clip versus coil, both treatment options have financial implications. Bairstow and colleagues (2002) reported that the expense of endovascular coiling was actually higher than that of surgical clipping, but the expense was more than compensated for by the decreased hospital length of stay and the patient's earlier return to work and normal activities of daily living (ADLs).

Complications of Subarachnoid Hemorrhage

The complications of aneurysmal SAH are varied and potentially life threatening. The major risks are rebleeding, vasospasm, hyponatremia, seizures, and hydrocephalus.

Rebleeding

The risk of rebleeding is highest in the first 2 weeks after the initial bleed. Aneurysms rebleed because the area of weakened vasculature is even weaker after it bleeds. Rebleeding is also possible if the risks, such as hypertension, remain. The hemodynamic forces that aided the rupture of an aneurysm will continue to weaken the vessel, causing it to bleed again. The highest incidence of rebleeding is in the first 24 to 48 hours. Seventy percent of patients whose aneurysms rebleed will die (LeRoux & Winn, 2004). Historically, the preferred treatment option is to treat as early as possible to prevent rebleeding.

Cerebral Vasospasm

Cerebral vasospasm is defined as narrowing of the arterial lumen due to overcontraction of the vessel wall (Khurana & Spetzler, 2006). Vasospasm occurs in approximately 30% of all patients with SAH. Vasospasm decreases CBF to the area supplied by the vessel in question, causing signs and symptoms of cerebral ischemia, and infarction if left untreated. In patients already compromised by the SAH itself, vasospasm may introduce additional signs of neurological deterioration (Chart 30–6, p. 768). The peak incidence of vasospasm is from 3 to 14 days from the incidence of SAH, although it may occur up to 21 days after the bleed occurs.

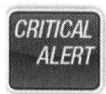 *Patients with SAH are at significant risk for vasospasm. Monitor fluid intake and output carefully. DO NOT discontinue IV fluids even if patient has adequate oral intake. Check with health care provider before discontinuing IV fluids. Monitor blood pressure at least hourly. Do not administer antihypertensive medications without parameters for administration.*

Clinical Presentation of Cerebral Vasospasm

- Confusion
- Impaired level of consciousness
- Focal neurological impairment, such as hemiplegia, aphasia
- Fever
- Neck stiffness

Diagnosis of vasospasm is made in several ways. The easiest way is through transcranial Doppler studies (TCDs). TCDs monitor the CBF through the cerebral arteries in question and can clearly demonstrate impaired flow. Cerebral angiography shows the artery in vasospasm as a narrowed vessel. Obviously cerebral angiograms are more invasive and take more time than TCDs, but are more definitive about the vessel itself. TCDs can be performed at the bedside and may be ordered routinely on patients with SAH.

It is not uncommon for patients to demonstrate vasospasm by angiogram or TCDs, while being completely asymptomatic. It is estimated that up to 50% of patients with vasospasm are asymptomatic. Usually, however, vasospasm is characterized by a neurological decline distinguished by the specific territory supplied by the vessel in spasm. Patients may experience a decrease in the level of consciousness (LOC), but may also exhibit a focal neurological impairment. Examples of these are motor weakness, aphasia, confusion, and/or cranial nerve deficits.

Treatment of vasospasm is a medical triad of therapies referred to as **triple-H therapy**. Triple-H therapy consists of hypertension, hemodilution, and hypervolemia. The goal of triple-H therapy is to increase cerebral perfusion pressure and CBF, therefore, reducing the risk for further neurological deficits.

Hypertension is one form of therapy to treat vasospasm in the presence of a clipped or coiled aneurysm. Systolic blood pressure should be kept at no less than 160 mmHg, and may be kept as high as 180 to 200 mmHg in patients with vasospasm that does not respond to standard treatment. If necessary, hypertension may be induced with vasopressors, such as dopamine, phenylephrine, or dobutamine. It is also common to use hypervolemia as a method of maintaining blood pressure. Patients must be in a monitored ICU, with a central venous catheter, and a pulmonary artery catheter for hemodynamic monitoring.

Hemodilution increases CBF. The balance of viscosity and oxygen-carrying capability is maintained at a hematocrit of 32% to 35% (Hickey, 2003). To maintain the hematocrit at this range, the infusion of volume expanders, such as albumin, may be used.

Calcium channel blockers, such as nimodipine, have been shown to reduce ischemic neurological deficits after aneurysmal SAH (Rinkel, Feigin, Algra, Vermeulen, & van Gijn, 2002). It also has been shown to increase CBF. In many institutions, nimodipine is given routinely to patients with SAH. Nimodipine has antihypertensive properties, however, that might limit its effectiveness for some patients.

Another neuroprotective strategy for the treatment of vasospasm is hypothermia. The use of mild hypothermia is controversial; however, there is some support for its use for treatment of cerebral ischemia due to vasospasm (Nagao et al., 2003).

Vasospasm is a dangerous complication of SAH, often causing secondary neurological declines. Thirteen percent of patients with SAH die or have serious neurological impairments due to vasospasms (Oyama & Criddle, 2004). However, the treatment for vasospasm is not without risk. Patients with underlying pulmonary or heart disease are at risk for complications from triple-H therapy. Nurses play a critical role in assessment and treatment of vasospasms. Nurses must be aware of pulmonary compromise and congestive heart failure caused by hypervolemic therapy in patients with preexisting pulmonary or heart conditions or those who are at risk due to age or other predisposing factors (Friedman et al., 2003).

Hyponatremia

Hyponatremia is another common complication of SAH. Hyponatremia occurs in approximately one-third of all SAH cases (MacDonald & Weir, 2004). Hyponatremia in SAH is caused by either syndrome of inappropriate antidiuretic hormone (SIADH) or **cerebral salt wasting**. It is very important for the cause of hyponatremia to be determined, because the treatment strategies for SIADH and cerebral salt wasting are very different. The treatment for SIADH is fluid restriction, and the treatment for cerebral salt wasting is the addition of salt. This is an important clinical differentiation, because two of the risk factors for SAH are low volume and hyponatremia. Fluid restriction for patients with SAH can be catastrophic, attributing to increased vasospasm. Generally, the treatment for hyponatremia in SAH is hypertonic saline, with oral salt supplements, if possible. This is in addition to IV fluids, usually normal saline, administered at 100 to 150 mL/hr for the prevention of vasospasm. It is very important for the patient's serum sodium levels to be monitored frequently, every 6 hours if the patient is receiving hypertonic saline. It also is important for the patient's fluid intake and output to be carefully monitored. As stated earlier, hemodynamic monitoring also may be warranted. An important feature of hyponatremia in the presence of SAH is that it frequently accompanies vasospasm, so very careful nursing monitoring of this patient is extremely important.

 *Patients with SAH are at significant risk for hyponatremia. Monitor serum Na^+ levels at least daily. Levels at or below normal should be treated. Standard treatment is the administration of salt, both as oral tablets and as IV hypertonic saline. Fluid restriction in this setting is absolutely CONTRAINDICATED.*

The clinical picture of patients with hyponatremia usually is that of decreased LOC. This patient may become suddenly confused, restless, or lethargic. It is not uncommon for hyponatremia to become evident when the patient has a seizure. Patients with SAH should have sodium levels done at least daily, even if their levels are normal. Those with levels at baseline or slightly below should be treated to avoid worsening hyponatremia because these patients are very sensitive to vasospasm. The normal levels of serum sodium vary from hospital laboratories, and it is important to note the normal levels for any particular institution.

Seizures

Seizures also are not uncommon for patients with SAH. They can occur immediately after the bleed or may be delayed. The seizures may be generalized or focal, depending on the area involved. Treatment for seizures usually consists of phenytoin initially; however, other drugs may be added as needed. Prophylactic use of antiepileptic drugs is controversial.

Hydrocephalus

Hydrocephalus is a common complication of SAH. As the blood products in the CSF break down, the high protein levels actually "clog" the absorption of CSF, causing communicating hydrocephalus (refer to Chapter 29 ©). Symptoms of hydrocephalus include lethargy, confusion, or other focal neurological deficits. Hydrocephalus is diagnosed by a CT scan. Many patients have serial CT scans while hospitalized to monitor ventricle size. The treatment for hydrocephalus is placement of a shunt, usually a ventriculo-peritoneal shunt. Hydrocephalus in SAH patients frequently occurs while the patient is still hospitalized, but it is not uncommon for delayed hydrocephalus to occur weeks after the initial bleed.

Arteriovenous Malformations

Malformations of the cerebrovascular system are believed to be developmental anomalies that result from failure of the embryonic vasculature to develop properly (National Institute of Neurological Disorders and Stroke, 2007a; Tatter & Ogilvy, 1995). The two most common types of cerebrovascular malformations are arteriovenous malformations and **cavernous malformations**.

Arteriovenous malformations (AVMs) are a mass of abnormal blood vessels in which arterial blood flows directly into the venous system. AVMs contain blood vessels that are thin walled and do not have normal characteristics of blood vessels. AVMs appear as a tangled mass of vessels (Figure 30–4 ■). There is no normal brain tissue within the AVM. Because arterial blood is flowing into the venous system, this is a medium- to high-flow system. Therefore, bleeding is often the first symptom.

Epidemiology and Etiology

AVMs account for approximately 8.6% of all SAH. The incidence is approximately 1 per 100,000 person/year. There is a slight male prevalence, with the most common age at diagnosis being between 20 and 40 years old (Soderman, Andersson, Karlsson, Wallace, & Edner, 2003). About half of AVMs are diagnosed with hemorrhage being the presenting symptom. AVMs are congenital, which implies a lifelong risk of hemorrhage (Greenberg, 2001).

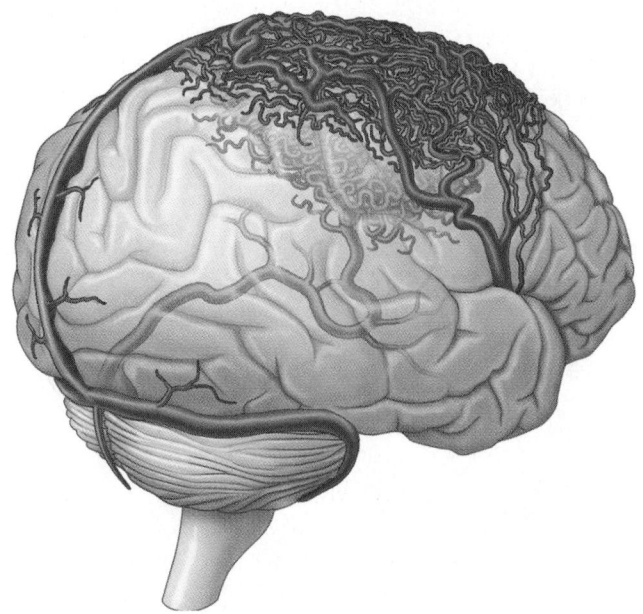

FIGURE 30–4 ■ Arteriovenous malformation.

Pathophysiology

There are several important points to consider regarding AVMs. One is that an AVM is actually a mass, which displaces normal tissue as it grows in size. Therefore, the presence of mass effect is possible, even in cases where hemorrhage has not occurred. The result may be increased ICP, as discussed in Chapter 29 ©. AVMs are considered to be errors in the developing vasculature of the brain that are associated with abnormal connectivity between the venous and the arterial system. The largest concentration of abnormal vessels is located in the center of the AVM, referred to as the **nidus**. The nidus is composed of these abnormal vessels that are a cross between veins and arteries. These AVMs are supplied by one or more arteries and drained by one or more draining veins.

Normal effects of blood flow lead to an atypical shunting of arterial blood into the venous system (Soderman et al., 2003). This results in an elevated intravascular pressure and possible rupture and hemorrhage of vessels. It also is possible for aneurysms to form on the artery that supplies the AVM. These aneurysms are prone to rupture due to high intravascular pressure. Approximately 6% to 7% of patients with AVMs have associated aneurysms (Khurana & Spetzler, 2006). Neurological deterioration may be rapid in the presence of hemorrhage. Diversion of arterial blood to the AVM may increase intravascular pressure, thus decreasing cerebral perfusion pressure. The brain tissue surrounding the AVM may become ischemic. Neurological deficits may progress slowly without the presence of hemorrhage.

Classification of AVMs

AVMs have three distinguishing characteristics: the size of the nidus, the eloquence of the surrounding tissue, and the presence/pattern of draining veins. The presence of aneurysms also is an important diagnostic factor. Nidus refers to the size of the focus of the AVM. Eloquence refers to the location and to the "value" of identifiable neurological function. Eloquent areas are those in which speech, sensory and motor, and vision functions are located. The pattern of venous drainage refers to the characteristics of draining veins, whether they are superficial or located in deep subcortical tissue.

To assist in decision making regarding treatment of a lesion, and to aid in consistency in referring to these lesions, a grading scale has been determined, and each AVM is given a grade based on a standardized scale. Spetzler and Martin (1986) devised a scale based on the degree of surgical difficulty in resecting these lesions. The **Spetzler-Martin AVM grading scale** rates AVMs by assigning points for size, eloquence, and the presence of draining veins (Chart 30–7, p. 770). Lower grade AVMs have a low morbidity and mortality with treatment; higher grade AVMs have a high morbidity and mortality, and treatment is usually restricted to medical management and observation.

Clinical Manifestations

Signs and symptoms of AVMs are dependent on several variables. The most important are size, the location, and the presence of hemorrhage. As previously stated, the AVM is itself a mass lesion. The symptoms exhibited by a patient with an unruptured AVM might be related to the location of the lesion and to the function of the brain it is displacing. This lesion is generally slow growing, and neurological symptoms may be slow in progressing.

CHART 30–7	Spetzler-Martin Grading Scale for Arteriovenous Malformations				
Size of AVM*		**Eloquence of Adjacent Brain†**		**Pattern of Venous Drainage‡**	
Small (<3 cm)	I	Noneloquent	0	Superficial only	0
Medium (3–6 cm)	II	Eloquent	I	Deep component	I
Large (>6 cm)	III	. . .		. . .	

*Measure the largest diameter of the nidus of the lesion on angiography.
† Eloquent areas include sensorimotor, language, visual, thalamus, hypothalamus, internal capsule, brainstem, cerebellar peduncles, and deep cerebellar nuclei.
‡ The lesion is considered superficial only if all drainage is via the cortical drainage system.

If the AVM has hemorrhaged, the symptoms may be considerably more drastic. For many patients with AVM rupture, severe neurological compromise, even coma or death, are the presenting symptoms. The severity of the neurological deficits depends on the size of hemorrhage and the eloquence of the brain affected. Seizures are not uncommon with AVM hemorrhage.

Laboratory and Diagnostic Procedures

Diagnosis of the presence of an AVM, with or without hemorrhage, is usually by CT scan or MRI. Once the diagnosis of AVM has been made, cerebral angiography is warranted for determination of involvement of cerebral vasculature, including the presence of associated aneurysms.

Medical Management

The treatment options for AVMs are surgical resection, endovascular embolization, radiosurgery, or conservative treatment, such as management of symptoms and observation. The determination of a treatment plan for patients with cerebral AVMs is dependent on the Spetzler-Martin grade given to the AVM. Grades I and II have favorable results with surgical resection in a setting where a large number of neurovascular procedures are routinely done. Grade III may warrant resection, depending on the individual analysis of the case. Grades IV and V, which are not shown on the chart, usually call for alternate treatment, because surgical resection has high morbidity and mortality even in the hands of the most experienced neurovascular surgeon.

Higher grade AVMs may benefit from endovascular treatment, such as **coiling** or **embolization**. Both coiling and embolization are a highly developed specialty of neurosurgery or interventional neuroradiology. The use of flow-directed microcatheters has made the navigation of the arterial system much safer, and a viable option to conventional surgery. In embolization, selected arteries, including aneurysms, may be obliterated with material such as glue.

The coiling of intra-AVM aneurysms with a Guglielmi detachable coil (GDC), such as those used in coiling of other intracerebral aneurysms, also has allowed some AVMs to be surgically resected that may otherwise not be amenable to surgical resection. The goal of embolization or coiling is to occlude aneurysms and other high-flow areas within the AVM. It may be used exclusively or as adjunctive therapy before surgical resection.

Gamma knife radiosurgery is another option. This treatment modality is used to treat surgically inaccessible lesions. It also is used to treat larger lesions in conjunction with other forms of treatment, usually surgical.

Conservative treatment is usually reserved for those AVMs that are a higher grade (grades III through V) and are felt to be unsafe to treat. Patients with these types of AVMs should be watched with serial magnetic resonance images (MRIs) and/or cerebral angiograms (see the Diagnostic Tests box, p. 766). Managing symptoms, such as headaches or seizures, is appropriate.

Cavernous Malformations

Another type of vascular malformation is the cavernous malformation. Historically, cavernous malformations have been called cavernous angiomas, cavernous hemangiomas, capillary hemangiomas, and cavernomas (National Institute of Neurological Disorders and Stroke, 2007a; Zabramski, Henn, & Coons, 1999). Cavernous malformations are composed of clusters of enlarged capillary channels, separated by dense fibrous tissue, with little to no intervening normal brain tissue. These lesions have a characteristic "grape-cluster" type of appearance (Figure 30–5 ■). Unfortunately, cavernous malformations usually are not diagnosed until they bleed, causing neurological deficits specific to the location of lesion. There are two types of cavernous malformations: sporadic and hereditary (or familial).

Epidemiology and Etiology

Cavernous malformations are believed to affect approximately 0.4% of the population (Passacantilli, Zabramski, Lanzino, & Spetzler, 2002). They comprise approximately 5% to 10% of all cerebral vascular malformations (Zabramski & Han, 2004). There is no gender bias and they may be found in all age groups.

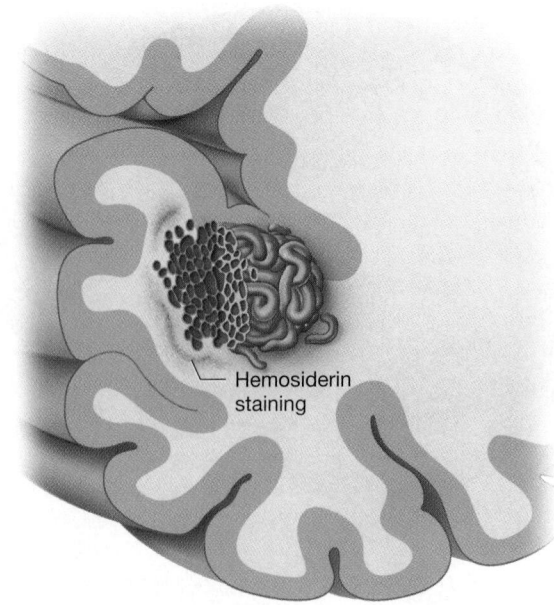
Hemosiderin staining

FIGURE 30–5 ■ Cavernous malformation.

Familial Form of Cavernous Malformations

Genetics appears to play a part in the familial form of cavernous malformations. It is an autosomal dominant inheritance and is characterized by the presence of multiple lesions, often presenting with seizures (Passacantilli et al., 2002). It appears to be more prevalent in Mexican American families (Zabramski et al., 1994). Approximately 50% of documented cavernous malformations are felt to be familial (Johnson, Marchuk, & Zabramski, 2004). A gene contributing to cavernous malformations, both sporadic and hereditary, has been identified (Laurans et al., 2003). (See Chapter 11 🔗 for more information on genetics.)

Pathophysiology

Cavernous malformations are clusters of enlarged capillary channels separated by dense fibrous tissue with little to no intervening brain tissue. These malformations grow and increase in size as a result of recurrent bleeding and thrombosis. Gradual buildup of iron and other blood breakdown products occurs as a result of recurrent hemorrhages. There is an abundant amount of hemosiderin, a blood breakdown product, in virtually every cavernous malformation.

Clinical Manifestations

Clinical manifestations of cavernous malformations are dependent on several factors, including location, size of the lesion, and whether the lesion has bled. A cavernous malformation may produce neurological symptoms because it is a space-occupying lesion. It is not uncommon for the patient to be unaware of the cavernous malformation until it bleeds, causing deficits based on its location. The most common presenting symptom of cavernous malformation is seizures. Other symptoms include headaches and/or focal neurological deficits, such as motor and/or sensory deficits or cranial nerve deficits. Repeated hemorrhages usually worsen the neurological deficits, especially if the lesion is in the brainstem (Wang, Liu, Zhang, Sun, & Zhao, 2003). It is not uncommon for the patient to recover from neurological deficits, but rarely does he completely return to baseline.

Laboratory and Diagnostic Procedures

Because cavernous malformations are low-flow lesions, angiography is not diagnostic. Diagnosis is made via an MRI scan. A CT scan may be helpful to determine the presence of a lesion, but is not specific to the type of lesion. CT scans may be falsely negative in 30% to 50% of studies. (See the Diagnostic Tests box, p. 766.)

Medical Management

Treatment almost always is surgical resection if the lesions are in accessible areas. In the hands of an experienced neurovascular surgeon, these lesions are curable if a complete resection is possible (Nakaji, 2004). Indications for surgery include refractory or worsening seizures, or neurological deterioration due to repeated hemorrhages and/or mass effect. Surgery may not be warranted if the lesion(s) are felt to be small and/or not threatening. These lesions are watched with serial MRIs. Gamma knife radiosurgery is not indicated, because these vascular lesions are not radiosensitive.

As seizures are commonly seen with cavernous malformations, the use of antiepileptic drugs may be appropriate. Steroids are not a common treatment for cavernous malformations. (See the Pharmacology Summary box, p. 762.)

◼ Nursing Management

Nursing management of patients with acute brain disorders was discussed in Chapter 29 🔗. Many of the management implications of patients with brain insults, such as tumors, or trauma are identical to those with stroke. All are caused by insults to the brain, whether the mechanism is trauma or stroke. All insults to the brain can cause neurological deterioration due to cerebral edema and increased ICP. Nursing management of ICP is discussed in Chapter 29 🔗. Nursing management that is specific to stroke and cerebrovascular malformations, such as aneurysms, AVMs, and cavernous malformations, is discussed in this chapter.

Nursing management of patients who have had a stroke, either ischemic or hemorrhagic, is a multifaceted endeavor. Strokes may also be seen in the form of an SAH from a ruptured intracerebral aneurysm or AVM. Nursing management requires comprehensive knowledge of the neurological assessment as well as virtually every system of the body (Chart 30–8).

Assessment

Neurological evaluation is important throughout the patient's course. Ischemic stroke may be an ongoing process, with stepwise changes in a patient's neurological condition. Hemorrhagic stroke may be sudden, with subtle or catastrophic results, such as those seen in SAH. In either case, the neurological consequences may be subtle and/or transient, or extreme and life changing. The nurse taking care of patients with cerebrovascular disease must be able to recognize subtle changes in the neurological exam and act appropriately. The patient's course may begin with emergent measures to stabilize both the neurological system, as well as systemic measures. It continues throughout the patient's hospital stay, through the rehabilitation process and beyond.

At the onset of stroke symptoms, the patient should be admitted to the hospital, usually through the emergency department, and ultimately to the ICU. Initially, patients present to the emergency department with symptoms of stroke, the type of which is unknown. It is imperative that nurses do complete and frequent neurological assessments. Any change, regardless of how insignificant it may appear, should be reported. At the very onset, the patient must be assessed for the basic ABCs: airway, breathing, and circulation.

Patients with cavernous malformations require careful neurological assessment in order to determine the full extent of their deficits. It is helpful for the nurse to be aware of the location of the cavernous malformation and what deficits would be expected in that location. It is imperative to know the patient's

---

CHART 30–8	**Nursing Implications in Treatment of Stroke**

- Blood pressure
- Fever
- Blood glucose
- Immobility
- Respiratory compromise
- Cardiac arrhythmias
- Seizures
- ICP management
- Identification and modification of risk factors

history, including the number of hemorrhages the patient may have had, and surgical history, if any. It would also be helpful to know if the patient has family members who have also experienced a hemorrhage from a cavernous malformation.

Planning

Once neurological deficits have been determined, it is important to ensure that the patient is receiving any and all therapy evaluations that might be helpful. For example, a patient with a brainstem cavernous malformation is at risk for swallowing difficulties. These may not be readily apparent, allowing the patient to experience "silent aspiration" with potentially serious consequences. A swallow evaluation by a speech therapist trained in dysphagia is helpful to determine if a patient is able to swallow safely or if alternate forms of nutrition are required.

As stated, patients admitted with stroke should be assessed for airway and breathing. Nursing management of patients with respiratory compromise due to increased ICP or head trauma was discussed in Chapter 29 ☻. As with other types of brain insult, patients with hemorrhagic stroke, including SAH, may present with severely compromised LOC. These patients may require intubation and mechanical ventilation. They also may require frequent suctioning to keep their airway clear. Patients with stroke in the brainstem, either hemorrhagic or ischemic, may experience nausea and vomiting, possibly requiring airway protection.

Interventions and Rationales

Management of blood pressure is a very important nursing consideration in patients with stroke. It may be managed differently depending on the type of stroke. Patients with aneurysms also are treated differently, dependent on whether the aneurysm is ruptured or unruptured, or clipped or unclipped. Occasionally, patients with ischemic stroke may have elevated blood pressure. Many clinicians will not only allow the patient to have an elevated blood pressure, but may actually give the patient vasopressors to raise it. It is sometimes felt that the patient's blood pressure needs to be elevated in order to perfuse the ischemic brain. Measures to lower blood pressure could worsen the neurological condition, perhaps increasing the area of stroke.

Hemorrhagic stroke may be treated differently. As stated, the most common cause of hemorrhagic stroke is hypertension. It is important to know any medications the patient was prescribed prior to admission. It also is important to determine if the patient was compliant and took the medication as prescribed. Any other medications, including herbals, may be significant and should be noted, as should any retrievable information regarding the use of any illegal drugs, such as cocaine or methamphetamines, which are known to raise blood pressure.

Management of blood pressure may be treated differently in the presence of an aneurysm. A patient with a ruptured aneurysm may require an elevated blood pressure to ensure adequate cerebral perfusion after the aneurysm has been clipped. It is possible that hypertension may be induced via fluids and/or vasopressors. In the presence of an unruptured aneurysm, or a ruptured, but unclipped aneurysm, blood pressure is usually well controlled.

Cardiac arrhythmias may be present with stroke, especially cardioembolic stroke. It is possible that a cardiac arrhythmia such as atrial fibrillation may not be diagnosed until the patient experiences an embolic stroke due to small clots sent off to the brain as a result of atrial fibrillation. These patients require diligent cardiac monitoring, with cardiac drugs designed to treat and stabilize atrial arrhythmias. Cardiac arrhythmias are not uncommon in the presence of SAH.

The presence of fever is uncommon at the initial onset of stroke. However, it is associated with decreased levels of neurological function over time. Patients with decreased levels of consciousness are prone to aspiration pneumonia due to their inability to protect the airway. Pneumonia due to immobility is a possibility and is another reason to promote early activity.

Central fever also is a possibility for patients with hemorrhage in thermoregulatory centers of the brain. In some cases, fever may be attributed to certain drugs, such as phenytoin. However, it is important to look for the source of fever for appropriate treatment. Efforts to treat fever should be aggressive. The use of antipyretics, such as acetaminophen, and cooling devices is encouraged. Several studies support the idea that the presence of fever promotes undesirable outcomes (Jorgensen et al., 1999). The presence of fever is known to increase the metabolic demands of the brain; thus, every effort should be made to determine the cause of fever.

Other nursing considerations include close monitoring and control of blood glucose levels, and observation of other laboratory values, such as sodium. These implications are addressed in Chapter 29 ☻.

Immobility is a strong nursing implication, as previously discussed. The initiation of early activity and therapy evaluations is extremely important to the prevention of deep venous thrombosis (DVT) and pulmonary embolus. These complications are frequently preventable and require appropriate nursing interventions to prevent this potentially serious, even fatal, complication.

If the patient has a new diagnosis of seizure, education regarding antiepileptic drugs is important. Nurses should educate patients and/or their families regarding the administration, side effects, and drug interactions of their medications. They also should be instructed if blood testing is required for evaluation of efficacy. (Refer to the section on the nursing management of seizures in Chapter 29 ☻.)

Another important aspect of nursing management is the identification and modification of risk factors. Smoking cessation is an obvious area in which nursing can assist the patient in identifying strategies to quit. Other modifiable risk factors include diet and exercise. Education of the patient and family is an invaluable service to help avoid future stroke.

As part of every discharge plan, the nurse should evaluate the type and extent of family and patient teaching required. Some patients with cavernous malformations, particularly in the brainstem, may have significant neurological deficits. Some deficits may require the patient and/or family member to learn adaptive measures, such as administering enteral feedings. Nursing plays an integral role in teaching and also assessing the need for further education and support.

The nursing care of patients with cerebrovascular disorders is exciting and challenging. This patient has needs that often are complex and multisystemic. Nursing care should address multiple body systems, with many actual and potential problems. Nursing diagnoses are included in the Nursing Process: Patient Care Plan feature. This plan addresses many of the nursing diagnoses, with an appropriate care plan for the patient with a

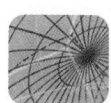

Assessment for Level of Consciousness
Subjective Data:

Do you have any history of hypertension, heart disease, bleeding disorders, renal disease, or cancer?
What day is it and where are you?
Squeeze my hands.
Push your feet against my hands.
Have you noticed any facial droop?
Do you have any memory loss that you are aware of?
How long ago did the first symptoms present?

Objective Data:

Glasgow Coma Scale number.
Neurological assessment, including mentation, cranial nerve examination, motor and sensory function.
Imaging studies, including MRI, CT, and/or lumbar puncture.
Laboratory data, including CBC, Complete Metabolic Panel CMP, and drug levels.

Nursing Assessment and Diagnoses	Outcomes and Evaluation Parameters	Planning and Interventions with *Rationales*
Nursing Diagnosis: *Decreased Intracranial Adaptive Capacity* related to SAH, stroke, or intracerebral hemorrhage	**Outcome:** Improvement to optimum level of neurological function ***Evaluation Parameters:*** Improved level of consciousness. Intracranial pressure readings within normal limits. Normal or stable Glasgow coma scale score. Oriented to time, place, person, and circumstances. Pupils equal and reactive to light. Normal ICP < 10 mmHg. Normal P_2 ICP wave form. Normal serum sodium level. Vital signs, especially the blood pressure and temperature remain within normal limits.	**Interventions and *Rationales:*** Monitor neurological assessment using the Glasgow Coma Scale hourly, or as ordered by the health care provider. Assess pupil size and reactivity. *To assess changes in motor and sensory function, and orientation to time, place, person, and circumstances. To assess changes in pupil function that reflect an increase in intracranial pressure.* Monitor ICP reading. *To assess changes in intracranial pressure that may be life threatening. To ascertain when medical intervention is necessary to decrease the pressure. To identify which interventions raise or lower the pressure.* Monitor lab values (serum Na+). *To maintain a normal range to prevent fluid retention that would raise intracranial pressure.* Monitor vital signs as ordered by the health care provider and report changes when abnormalities occur. *To prevent a rise in the blood pressure that would increase intracranial pressure. To report any increase in temperature that may indicate an infection.*

Assessment of Airway and Gas Exchange
Subjective Data:

Do you have a history of emphysema or asthma, or any cardiac diseases?
Do you become short of breath with exertion?
How far are you able to walk before having to rest?
How active are you on a daily basis?
Have you ever experienced chest pain or fainting?

Objective Data:

Respiratory rate.
Oxygen saturation.
Arterial blood gases.
Vital signs.

Lung sounds.
Skin, lips, and nail bed color.
Cough reflex and ability to clear secretions.

Nursing Assessment and Diagnoses	Outcomes and Evaluation Parameters	Planning and Interventions with *Rationales*
Nursing Diagnoses: *Ineffective Airway Clearance and Gas Exchange Impaired* related to SAH, stroke, intracerebral hemorrhage, or increased intracranial pressure *Actual or Risk for Aspiration* related to altered neurological status *Actual or Risk for Ineffective Airway Clearance* related to immobility and ineffective cough reflex	**Outcomes:** Respiratory function within normal limits and stable. Gas exchange within normal limits. ***Evaluation Parameters:*** Respiratory rate within normal limits. Airway clear of secretions. Patient will be able to manage secretions. Stable or improved ABGs. No shortness of breath. Patient able to eat without aspiration occurring.	**Nursing Intervention and *Rationales:*** Monitor respiratory status, i.e., rate, rhythm, quality. *To determine changes due to altered cerebral function.* Suction as necessary. *To maintain a clear airway.* Monitor oxygen saturation as ordered and when clinical manifestations such as increased respiratory rate occur. *To determine need for interventions such as oxygen or endotracheal intubation.* Provide respiratory therapy treatments as ordered. Position patient with neck in neutral position. Elevate head to 30 degrees unless contraindicated. If patient is not intubated, have supplies ready for possible intubation. If patient is intubated, suction as necessary, but limit to 10 seconds to avoid increased ICP. Administer oxygen as needed. Monitor ABG results. Notify health care provider if change in respiratory status occurs. *To improve and stabilize oxygen exchange and promote patient comfort.* Keep patient NPO until alert and/or swallow function is assessed and deemed safe. Conduct swallows evaluation *to assess safety.* Initiate aspiration precautions. *To prevent aspiration and allow normal oral intake.*

(continued)

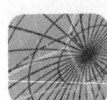

NURSING PROCESS: Patient Care Plan for Cerebral Vascular Disorders—*Continued*

Assessment of Hemodynamic Status

Subjective Data:
Do you have any preexisting cardiac or respiratory problems?
Do you ever experience chest pain?
Do you have high blood pressure?
Are you taking any cardiac or blood pressure medications—if so, what are they?

Objective Data:
Vital signs, including heart rate,
blood pressure, respiratory rate, and central venous pressure, if available.
Oxygen saturation.
Skin, lips, and nail bed color.
Lung sounds.
Cardiac rhythm strips or ECG.

Nursing Assessment and Diagnoses	Outcomes and Evaluation Parameters	Planning and Interventions with *Rationales*
Nursing Diagnoses: *Cardiac Output, Decreased* related to arrhythmias, hemodynamic instability, and hypotension/hypertension *Actual or risk for Ineffective Tissue Perfusion* related to decreased cardiac output	**Outcomes:** Cardiac output within normal limits. Adequate tissue perfusion maintained. ***Evaluation Parameters:*** Stable rate and rhythm Blood pressure maintenance within established parameters Patient able to perform activities of daily living comfortably and independently.	**Nursing Intervention and *Rationales:*** Monitor ECG continuously. Notify health care provider of changes in rate or rhythm. Administer cardiac and hypertension medications as ordered and monitor for effectiveness. *To assess and treat cardiac dysrhythmia that affect cardiac output.* Monitor vital signs. Measure cardiac output with Swan-Ganz catheter, if in place. Notify health care provider of changes in blood pressure. *To determine cardiac output and tissue perfusion and treat if necessary. To assess for heart failure.*

Assessment of Motor and Sensory Status

Subjective Data:
Can you move your arms and legs?
Where am I touching you?

Objective Data:
Bilateral motor and sensory function.
Orientation and ability to follow directions.
Family member who can assist the patient with mobility and adherence to directions for safe care, verbally and graphically.

Nursing Assessment and Diagnoses	Outcomes and Evaluation Parameters	Planning and Interventions with *Rationales*
Nursing Diagnoses: *Self Care Deficit* related to altered motor and sensory function from neuro deficit. *Actual or Risk for Impaired Physical Mobility* related to decreased strength and endurance *Risk for Injury* related to fall risk. Risk for Tissue Injury related to immobility	**Outcomes:** Patient will attain maximum motor function. Patient will be free from injury. Family/significant other who is able to assist with care. Adequate tissue perfusion. ***Evaluation Parameters:*** Patient will be safe. Able to progress with ambulation and complete self-care. No deep vein thrombosis (DVT) or pulmonary embolism.	**Nursing Intervention and *Rationales:*** Monitor strengths and limitations. Initiate physical therapy consultation. Initiate activity as tolerated, unless contraindicated. Obtain occupational therapy consult to assist with activities of daily living. *To regain and increase strength on affected side and promote independence.* Encourage family involvement in patient care and mobility. Educate patient and family regarding safety measures. *To promote family involvement and prepare for discharge.* Institute safety measures, i.e., place call light within reach, ask patient to call nurse before getting out of bed. Apply restraints as ordered. Keep bed rails in high position at all times. *To promote safety and prevent falling.* Apply thigh-high elastic stockings. Apply sequential compression stockings. Administer subcutaneous injections of LMWH if indicated. Monitor lower extremities frequently for signs/symptoms of DVT. Notify health care provider for signs/symptoms of DVT. *To prevent, assess for, and treat deep vein thrombosis.*

Skin Assessment

Subjective Data:
Are you having pain on your skin in any area of your body?
Are you able to turn yourself in bed?
Are you able to get out of bed?

Objective Data:
Skin breakdown.
Patient's ability to move.
Patient's activity level.

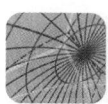

NURSING PROCESS: Patient Care Plan for Cerebral Vascular Disorders—*Continued*

Nursing Assessment and Diagnoses	Outcomes and Evaluation Parameters	Planning and Interventions with *Rationales*
Nursing Diagnosis: Risk for Impaired Skin Integrity *related to immobility*	**Outcome:** Skin intact and healthy, without evidence of breakdown. **Evaluation Parameters:** Patient will maintain skin integrity. Understands importance of changing positions and is able to do it.	**Nursing Intervention and *Rationales:*** Turn and reposition every 2 hours, unless contraindicated. *To take the pressure off bony prominences and promote tissue perfusion.* Provide skin care frequently, keeping skin clean and dry. *To prevent breakdown.* Monitor skin for redness and possible skin breakdown. Do not position patient on areas of redness. *To detect areas that may be beginning to break down and treat them to prevent further deterioration.* Assess need for air mattress or other pressure relief bed. *To prevent break down.* Assess need for nutrition consult. *To provide the necessary nutrients to promote healing.* Monitor vital signs. *To assess for the presence of infection.*

Nutrition Assessment

Subjective Data:
How is your appetite?
Do you have sores in your mouth?
What kinds of foods are you eating?
What kinds of foods do you like or dislike?
Are there any cultural practices that would influence your diet?
Does any type of food make you choke?
Have you noticed a change in your ability to swallow?

Objective Data:
Assess nutritional status.
Assess 24-hour food intake.
Assess for ability to swallow.

Nursing Assessment and Diagnoses	Outcomes and Evaluation Parameters	Planning and Interventions with *Rationales*
Nursing Diagnosis: *Actual or Risk for Imbalanced Nutrition:* Less than Body Requirements related to neuro deficit	**Outcomes:** Stable weight. Adequate nutritional intake. No aspiration. **Evaluation Parameters:** Patient will maintain current body weight. Patient will maintain or improve albumin levels. Patient will tolerate diet or tube feedings.	**Nursing Intervention and *Rationales:*** Monitor food intake. *Food intake needs to be adequate for healing.* Serve small amounts of high calorie, high protein food every 2 hours. *Patient is more likely to eat small amounts more frequently than large amounts less often.* Provide a well-balanced diet with foods the patient likes. *Patient will be more likely to eat.* Consult with a dietician. Assess the need for parenteral or enteral feedings. *If the patient is unable to eat enough food orally to keep up with the body's demands, other avenues may need to be explored and utilized.* Keep calorie count. *To assess adequacy of intake.* Assess ability to swallow. Assess which foods make the patient choke—if any. *To prevent aspiration.*

Assessment of Pain

Subjective Data:
Are you in pain, if so where?
What makes the pain better or worse?
Does it radiate anywhere on your body?

Objective Data:
Increased heart rate, blood pressure, or respiratory rate.
Facial expressions, i.e., grimacing.
Use pain scale (0–10) to quantify pain level.
Assess cultural or religious impact on the patient's response. Assess location, duration, and onset of pain.

(continued)

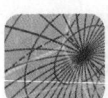

NURSING PROCESS: Patient Care Plan for Cerebral Vascular Disorders—*Continued*

Nursing Assessment and Diagnoses	Outcomes and Evaluation Parameters	Planning and Interventions with *Rationales*
Nursing Diagnoses: *Pain, Acute* related to Impaired Physical Mobility and motor deficits	**Outcome:** Able to ambulate safely with little to no pain. ***Evaluation Parameters:*** Patient expresses pain control. Attains maximum motor function.	**Nursing Intervention and *Rationales:*** Administer pain medications as ordered. Use pain scale (0–10) to quantify pain level. *Quantifying pain increases consistency.* Instruct patient to inform nurse if pain is not relieved. *Indicates need to change pain management plan.* Assess cultural and religious impact on patient's responses. *Different cultures and religions respond differently to pain.* Correct misconceptions about risk of addiction and overdose. *To decrease anxiety related to medication addiction.* Explain, prepare, and medicate patient for painful procedures (physical therapy) and anticipated discomforts. *To control increased pain level related to procedure.* Provide a supportive environment where patient is able to express pain level. *Opens communication and facilitates pain management.* Use pain control measures before it becomes severe. *This increases comfort and decreases need for medication.* Teach nonpharmacologic method of control, i.e., guided imagery and massage, and breathing exercises. *These measures augment pain relief.* Plan diversional activities. *To augment pain relief measures.*

Assessment of Communication Ability
Subjective Data:
Are you able to speak?
Has it become more difficult?

Objective Data:
Speech clarity.
Is there any slurring?
Does the mouth droop?

Nursing Assessment and Diagnoses	Outcomes and Evaluation Parameters	Planning and Interventions with *Rationales*
Nursing Diagnosis: *Actual or Risk for Impaired Verbal Communication*	**Outcome:** Patient is able to communicate needs and preferences verbally. ***Evaluation Parameters:*** Patient attains maximum communication. Speech skills begin to return.	**Nursing Intervention and *Rationales:*** Assess type and degree of communication deficit. *To identify the appropriate therapy.* Initiate speech therapy consultation. *To begin speech rehabilitation.* Provide communication board for intubated patient. *To facilitate communication.*

Assessment of Coping
Subjective Data:
What are your complaints?
What is your understanding of present condition or disease?
What are patient's concerns for the future?

Objective Data:
What is the patient's level of education?
What is the patient's occupation?
What is the patient's family support system?
Does the patient have a religious affiliation?
Facial expressions.
Mood.
Verbalization of fear regarding illness, impact on family, and future.

Nursing Assessment and Diagnoses	Outcomes and Evaluation Parameters	Planning and Interventions with *Rationales*
Nursing Diagnoses: *Ineffective Coping* related to sudden change in physiological status *Anxiety related to apprehension regarding potential outcome*	**Outcomes:** Patient/family is coping with illness in a positive manner. Patient displays reduced anxiety.	**Nursing Intervention and *Rationales:*** Provide factual information concerning diagnosis, treatment, disfigurement, disabilities, and prognosis. *Truthful explanations increase trust and potentially decrease anxiety and may increase coping.* Encourage family involvement. *To assist all members to learn to cope by decreasing fear.* Provide spiritual support as needed, if desired.

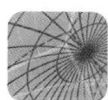

NURSING PROCESS: Patient Care Plan for Cerebral Vascular Disorders—*Continued*

Nursing Assessment and Diagnoses	Outcomes and Evaluation Parameters	Planning and Interventions with *Rationales*
	Evaluation Parameters: Manifests coping mechanisms with what is happening, verbally if possible, and by facial expression. Appears calm; discusses possible outcomes. Maintains self-composure when discussing the future. Verbalizes what relieves anxiety. Verbalizes absence of sensory perceptual disorders. Verbalizes absence of physical manifestations of anxiety.	Assess and document level of anxiety. *To track trends in anxiety levels.* Explore with the patient/family techniques to reduce anxiety. *This gives the patient a sense of control and opens communication about the subject.* Explain all procedures and allow time for mental preparation. *This decreases fear and anxiety of the unknown.* Explore with patient effective ways to minimize anxiety. *This gives the patient a sense of control.* Instruct patient on use of relaxation techniques. *To relieve anxiety.* Assess need for and administer antianxiety and pain medication. *If alternative measures are not effective, may need antianxiety agents.* Assist patient/family in setting realistic long-term goals for progress. *Indicates effectiveness of emotional adjustment.* Consider psychiatric counseling for patients/families who exhibit inability to accept situation. *Provide an ongoing plan and interventions to promote long-term relief of anxiety.*

Assessment of Knowledge of Disease Condition

Subjective Data:
What do you understand about your illness?
Do you have questions about the treatment program?
What would you like me to tell you about your illness?

Objective Data:
Patient/family verbalizes questions about the seriousness of illness and prognosis.

Nursing Assessment and Diagnoses	Outcomes and Evaluation Parameters	Planning and Interventions with *Rationales*
Nursing Diagnosis: *Deficient Knowledge* related to **diagnosis**.	**Outcome:** Patient and family knowledgeable about condition and long-term ramifications. **Evaluation Parameter:** Patient and family or significant others verbalize understanding of condition and rehabilitative education provided.	**Nursing Intervention and *Rationales*:** Provide patient with information as needed. Provide patient and family education. Provide patient with resources as needed. *To increase their knowledge about all phases of illness and the necessary treatments.*

cerebrovascular disorder, such as stroke, subarachnoid hemorrhage due to aneurysm rupture, arteriovenous malformation, or cavernous malformation.

Collaborative Management

Patients who experience cerebrovascular insults—whether an ischemic stroke or an intracerebral hemorrhage due to a ruptured aneurysm, arteriovenous malformation, or a cavernous malformation—present a complex, multifaceted situation. There is virtually no system within the body that is unaffected. In addition, every aspect of patients' lives is affected, as well as that of their families and the community.

Because the treatment goal of each patient is to maintain an optimum level of function, a team of practitioners typically is required to aid the patient in this endeavor. In addition to nurses, multiple health care providers of various specialties are part of the team: specialists in neurosurgery, neurology, internal medicine or critical care medicine, endovascular surgeons, and rehabilitation specialists, among others. Also playing an integral part of this multidisciplinary team are the therapists (i.e., physical

therapy, occupational therapy, and speech therapy). Other specialists, such as dietitians, radiologists, and pharmacists, may be involved. Once a patient is admitted to the hospital with a diagnosis of a cerebral vascular disorder, the decision regarding treatment is made with the help of the appropriate specialists, usually neurosurgery and/or endovascular surgeons.

During the patient's hospitalization, it is common to use the help of internal medicine or critical care physicians to manage possible medical complications, such as respiratory failure, pneumonia, hypertension, electrolyte imbalances, and other preexisting conditions. After the initial treatment, the patient will require the entire team of nurses, specialists, and therapists to evaluate and assess for possible therapy needs. It is not unusual for patients with cerebral vascular disorders to need physical therapy and occupational therapy to evaluate and treat motor and functional deficits. It also is frequently beneficial for speech therapy to assess for cognitive deficits, some of which may not be readily apparent. Speech therapy also is of great benefit to assess and treat functional speech abnormalities, as well as swallow evaluations. Once the patient is medically stable, the need for further rehabilitation, frequently in an inpatient facility, may be addressed. See the Complementary and Alternative Therapies box for other options for patient treatments.

The patient with cerebrovascular disorder usually experiences a complicated, multisystem disorder. These patients require the expertise of many modalities. Nursing is the center and coordinator of each patient's care. Collaborative care, involving many of the other disciplines mentioned above, may be required to help each patient return to their optimum level of function.

Rehabilitation

Once a diagnosis has been made, and treatment options have been explored and implemented, the promotion of optimum health is centered on rehabilitation. Rehabilitation for patients with brain injury, whether it be a result of stroke, tumor, or trauma, is discussed in Chapter 29 ☺. The patient who has had a stroke as a result of a ruptured aneurysm, an intracerebral hemorrhage, or an ischemic infarction may have residual neurological deficits.

 **CRITICAL ALERT** *Patients with cerebral vascular disorders may have residual neurological deficits. These deficits may be subtle cognitive deficits that may hinder the patient's return to school or work. Obtain consults as soon as possible for therapies: physical, occupational, speech, and possibly neuropsychology. Consults for rehabilitation, either in an acute or outpatient setting, may be warranted.*

These deficits may be motor, sensory, learning, or cognitive. It is important that physical, occupational, or speech therapists be consulted and their recommendations initiated early in the patient's hospitalization. It also is important for nursing staff to be diligent in assessing the needs of stroke patients. The nurse is the first line in identifying and assessing deficits and in the education of the patient and family. Several outcome measurement scales that are helpful in determining the type and degree of deficits are available. One such scale from the National Institutes of Health is shown in the National Guidelines box, and another is shown in Chart 30–9.

It is in the patient's best interest to obtain a rehabilitation consult for either inpatient or outpatient therapy. It also is important to obtain information about the patient's home environment

COMPLEMENTARY & ALTERNATIVE THERAPIES — Biofeedback

Description:
Biofeedback employs a way of monitoring changes in one's own body with the aid of sensitive machines. The patient consciously visualizes, relaxes, or imagines while feedback is provided through light, sound, or specialized feedback. This feedback allows the patient to learn to make subtle adjustments to move toward a more balanced internal state. Through repeated practice, a patient can use biofeedback as a self-training therapy to control physical conditions and psychological states. Tension-causing conditions such as hypertension, insomnia, and headaches are also improved by biofeedback.

Research Support:
Many hypertensive patients try CAM therapies, including biofeedback, for blood pressure control (Ernst, 2005). More than 100 randomized controlled trials indicate that behavioral treatments can modestly reduce blood pressure (BP). This reduction in BP is greater than that produced by wait-list or other inactive controls. Greater BP reductions are experienced with multicomponent, individualized psychological treatments than with single-component treatments. There are many types of biofeedback treatments, and two of them—thermal feedback and electrodermal activity feedback—perform better than EMG or direct BP feedback, which tend to produce no effect (Linden & Moseley, 2006).

In one study by Yucha and colleagues (2005), 54 adults with stage 1 or 2 hypertension (78% of which were taking BP medications), researchers administered 8 weeks of relaxation training in addition to thermal, electromyographic, and respiratory sinus arrhythmia biofeedback. Researchers measured blood pressure in the clinic and over 24 hours using an ambulatory BP monitor pretraining and post-training. Results showed that systolic BP dropped from 135.0 +/− 9.8 mmHg pretraining to 132.2 +/− 10.5 mmHg post-training. In addition, diastolic BP dropped from 80.4 +/− 8.1 mmHg pretraining to 78.5 +/− 10.0 mmHg post-training. Researchers developed a prediction model using data from 37 participants with baseline BP of 130/85 mmHg or greater. In this model, regression showed that those who were able to lower their systolic BP 5 mmHg or more:

1. Were not taking antihypertensive medication;

2. Had the lowest starting finger temperature;

3. Had the smallest standard deviation in daytime mean arterial pressure; and

4. Had the lowest score on the Multidimensional Health Locus of Control-internal scale. Researchers concluded that, since these types of persons are most likely to benefit from biofeedback-assisted relaxation (BFAR), they should be offered BFAR prior to starting hypertensive medications (Yucha, Tsai. Calderon, & Tian, 2005).

Another set of researchers, Nakao and colleagues (2003), classified biofeedback interventions into two types: simple biofeedback and relaxation-assisted biofeedback. They found that only the relaxation-assisted biofeedback significantly decreased both systolic and diastolic blood pressures compared with those in sham or nonspecific behavioral intervention controls. These results suggest that biofeedback is more effective in reducing blood pressure in patients with essential hypertension than no intervention. It is important to note, however, that the treatment was only found to be superior to sham or nonspecific behavioral intervention when combined with other relaxation techniques (Nakao, Yano, Nomura, & Kuboki, 2003). Another study concluded that, according to research conducted to date, biofeedback can be a useful alternative or adjunct to conventional forms of treatment (Kranitz & Lehrer, 2004).

References
Ernst, E. (2005). Complementary/alternative medicine for hypertension: A mini-review. *Wiener Medizinische Wochenschrift, 155*(17–18), 386–91.

Kranitz, L., & Lehrer, P. (2004). Biofeedback applications in the treatment of cardiovascular diseases. *Cardiology Review, 12*(3), 177–181.

Linden, W., & Moseley, J. V. (2006). The efficacy of behavioral treatments for hypertension. *Applied Psychophysiology and Biofeedback, 31*(1), 51–63.

Nakao, M., Yano, E., Nomura, S., & Kuboki, T. (2003). Blood pressure-lowering effects of biofeedback treatment in hypertension: A meta-analysis of randomized controlled trials. *Hypertension Research, 26*(1), 37–46.

Yucha, C. B., Tsai, P. S., Calderon, K. S., & Tian, L. (2005). Biofeedback-assisted relaxation training for essential hypertension: Who is most likely to benefit? *Journal of Cardiovascular Nursing, 20*(3), 198–205.

NATIONAL GUIDELINES Outcome Grading Scales: The Modified National Institutes of Health Stroke Scale

Item	Name	Response
1A	Level of consciousness	0 = Alert 1 = Not alert, but arouses easily 2 = Not alert, obtunded 3 = Unresponsive
1B	Questions	0 = Answers both questions correctly 1 = Answers one correctly 2 = Answers neither correctly
1C	Commands	0 = Performs both tasks correctly 1 = Performs one task correctly 2 = Performs neither task correctly
2	Gaze	0 = Normal 1 = Partial gaze palsy 2 = Total gaze palsy
3	Visual fields	0 = No visual loss 1 = Partial hemianopsia 2 = Complete hemianopsia 3 = Bilateral hemianopsia
4	Facial palsy	0 = Normal 1 = Minor paralysis 2 = Partial paralysis 3 = Complete paralysis
5	Motor arm a. left b. right	0 = No drift 1 = Drift before 10 seconds 2 = Falls before 10 seconds 3 = No effort against gravity 4 = No movement
6	Motor leg a. left b. right	0 = No drift 1 = Drift before 5 seconds 2 = Falls before 5 seconds 3 = No effort against gravity 4 = No movement
7	Ataxia	0 = Absent 1 = One limb 2 = Two limbs
8	Sensory	0 = Normal 1 = Mild loss 2 = Severe loss
9	Language	0 = Normal 1 = Mild aphasia 2 = Severe aphasia 3 = Mute or global aphasia
10	Dysarthria	0 = Normal 1 = Mild 2 = Severe
11	Extinction	0 = Normal 1 = Mild 2 = Severe

CHART 30–9   The Barthel Index

1. **Feeding**
   - 10 = Independent; able to apply any necessary device; feeds in reasonable time
   - 5 = Needs help (i.e., for cutting food)
   - 0 = Inferior performance

2. **Bathing**
   - 5 = Performs without assistance
   - 0 = Inferior performance

3. **Personal grooming**
   - 5 = Washes face, combs hair, brushes teeth
   - 0 = Inferior performance

4. **Dressing**
   - 10 = Independent; ties shoes, fastens fasteners, applies braces
   - 5 = Needs help but does at least half of tasks within reasonable time
   - 0 = Inferior performance

5. **Bowel control**
   - 10 = No accidents
   - 5 = Occasional accidents
   - 0 = Inferior performance

6. **Bladder control**
   - 10 = No accidents
   - 5 = Occasional accidents
   - 0 = Inferior performance

7. **Toilet transfers**
   - 10 = Independent with toilet or bedpan
   - 5 = Needs help for balance, handling clothes or toilet paper
   - 0 = Inferior performance

8. **Chair/bed transfers**
   - 15 = Independent
   - 10 = Minimum assistance
   - 5 = Able to sit, but needs maximum assistance to transfer
   - 0 = Inferior performance

9. **Ambulation**
   - 15 = Independent for 50 yards; may use assistive devices except for rolling walker
   - 10 = With help for 50 yards
   - 5 = Independent with wheelchair for 50 yards
   - 0 = Inferior performance

10. **Stair climbing**
    - 10 = Independent
    - 5 = Needs help or supervision
    - 0 = Inferior performance

and the resources available at home. Whether or not the patient has someone available to provide 24-hour supervision may make the difference between discharge to the home with family supervision and admission to a skilled nursing facility for therapies. Knowledge of a patient's occupation and level of responsibility on discharge also is important. It may be necessary for a patient to have neuropsychological testing prior to returning to the work environment.

It is important to teach the patient and family what to expect on discharge. Patients need to be encouraged with the understanding that there will be disappointments and setbacks, as well as improvement. Encourage questions and give honest answers. It usually is helpful to provide home health visits on discharge to support the family and patient and answer any further questions or concerns they may have. It also is helpful to provide lists of resources for further support. The Patient Teaching & Discharge Priorities box (p. 780) lists some teaching suggestions for patients who have had strokes.

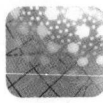

PATIENT TEACHING & DISCHARGE PRIORITIES for Stroke

Need	Teaching
Risk factors: Patient Family Setting	Assess presence of risk factors for patients with atherosclerotic cerebral vascular disease, i.e., smoking, hypertension. Educate patient and family regarding risk factors, and the appropriate interventions. Assess family support and resources.
Wound infection: Patient/family support system Setting	Assess surgical wound for signs/symptoms of infection. Signs and symptoms of infection include: Redness Tenderness Exudate and/or odor Swelling Poor healing. The presence of fever or any of above symptoms should be reported. Assess family support for needed assistance.
Pain control: Patient Family Setting	Assess need for pain control. Is present medication regimen adequate? Is pain controlled sufficiently to allow patient to participate in ADLs. Assess need for family intervention in dispensing pain medication. Assess patient/family understanding of medication instructions.
Safety: Patient Family Setting	Assess patient cognitive status: Is patient a fall risk? Assess safety awareness. Assess patient understanding of medication schedule and needs. Assess patient need for supervision. Obtain consults for speech/cognitive evaluation. Obtain social service consult. Obtain home health consult. Assess family involvement in patient's recuperative period. Provide family teaching regarding possible cognitive impairments. Provide family teaching regarding need for supervision. Assess environment for safety. May require home health or social service involvement.
Anticoagulation: Patient/family support system Setting	If patient requires anticoagulation following an embolic stroke: Assess follow-up plans. How will blood draws be obtained? Which health care provider will be monitoring the lab tests and managing the medication? Assess patient/family understanding of the medication ordered and the reason for the anticoagulation. Assess risk factors concerning anticoagulation: Is patient a fall risk? Will patient be compliant with medication and blood draws? Assess family support. Assess resources. Assess patient ability to follow instructions.
Follow-up needs Patient Family Setting	Assess need for follow-up appointments for needed therapies or interventions: Radiation therapy Outpatient therapies: physical, occupational, speech Health care provider appointments Laboratory visits for evaluation of drug levels, or electrolytes Follow-up x-rays Assess family understanding and need for further explanation. Assess availability of resources for follow-up.

Health Promotion

Stroke is the third leading cause of death in the United States (AHA, 2008b). Many of the risk factors for stroke are preventable. One of the most important defenses against stroke is education. Public awareness of stroke and its risk factors is increasing because of a massive education of not only the public, but health professionals, who are learning that "time is brain." Stroke protocols are being set up in hospitals and in prehospital settings, saving precious time in the treatment of stroke.

Many of the risk factors are genetic and, therefore, unalterable. However, many risk factors are manageable, even preventable. The National Stroke Association's Prevention Advisory Board released its Stroke Prevention Guidelines, a set of recommendations on what the public can do to prevent stroke (NSA, 2008). The guidelines are presented in the accompanying National Guidelines box.

For the majority of patients with diagnosis of vascular malformations and abnormalities, such as aneurysms, arteriovenous malformations, and cavernous malformations, there is no prevention and no warning signs. Patients are unaware of the presence of these lesions until they become symptomatic.

■ Future Directions

With rapidly growing public awareness regarding stroke, the future direction of stroke treatment is education and prevention. As stated earlier in this chapter, many of the risk factors for stroke are preventable. There is hope that with education about the risk factors of stroke, the number of strokes will decrease. Education about the signs and symptoms of stroke will facilitate quicker treatment. Stroke centers are being developed in communities throughout the United States, with protocols for speedy treatment

---

NATIONAL GUIDELINES National Stroke Association Prevention Advisory Board's 1997 Stroke Prevention Guidelines

Guidelines	What You Can Do
1. Know your blood pressure.	Have your blood pressure checked annually.
	If your doctor recommends antihypertensive medication, compliance is critical.
	A diet of low salt and low fat will help lower your blood pressure.
	Start and maintain an exercise program.
	Hypertension is the leading cause of stroke. Fifty million Americans have elevated blood pressure, or are taking antihypertensive medications, yet most do not have their blood pressure adequately controlled. The Systolic Hypertension in the Elderly Program demonstrated that the treatment of systolic hypertension decreased stroke by 36%. A prospective meta-analysis of observational studies showed that a decrease of 10 mmHg in diastolic blood pressure reduced strokes by 50% (NSA, 2008). Compliance with antihypertensive therapy is critical.
2. Find out if you have atrial fibrillation.	Atrial fibrillation is an irregular heartbeat that alters heart function and allows blood to collect in the lower chambers of the heart. Blood clots may form and be pumped into the bloodstream, and into the arterial system, causing embolic stroke. If atrial fibrillation is diagnosed, warfarin or aspirin may be prescribed to thin the blood, making blood less likely to clot and cause stroke. Atrial fibrillation can be diagnosed with a simple electrocardiogram (ECG).
3. If you smoke, STOP.	Smoking doubles the risk for stroke. Cessation of smoking immediately decreases the chance for stroke. Smoking is a completely preventable risk factor for stroke.
4. If you drink, do so in moderation.	If you drink, drink no more than two drinks daily.
	Studies show that drinking one or two alcoholic beverages daily may actually reduce the chance for stroke. However, more than two drinks a day increases the risk for stroke by two to three times. Alcohol also interacts with the actions of many medications, including warfarin.
	If you don't drink, don't start.
5. Know your cholesterol level.	High cholesterol levels, especially of low-density lipoproteins, increase your risk for stroke. High cholesterol can be controlled with diet in most cases. Some people may require cholesterol-lowering medication.
6. If you have diabetes, control it.	Diabetes puts people at increased risk for stroke. By controlling diabetes, via medication or lifestyle modification, patients with diabetes can lower their risk for stroke.
	Maintain an exercise program.
7. Exercise.	Sedentary lifestyle is another preventable risk factor.
8. Reduce salt and fat in the diet.	Increased sodium is associated with hypertension. The role of fat as a stroke risk factor is uncertain, but it may increase the risk of stroke.
9. Develop awareness of circulation problems.	See your doctor if you experience circulatory symptoms, or if you have a history of anemia or sickle cell anemia.
10. Know the symptoms.	Know the signs and symptoms of stroke.
	Call 911 immediately.

that will minimize neurological deficits. These protocols incorporate not only hospitals, but prehospital personnel and the public.

The area of neurovascular surgery also is growing rapidly. Studies such as the International Subarachnoid Aneurysm Trial, the North American Symptomatic Carotid Endarterectomy Trial Group, the International Study of Unruptured Intracranial Aneurysm, and the Carotid Revascularization Endarterectomy versus Stenting Trial have examined the alternative methods of treatments for aneurysms, and are being reviewed constantly to offer patients the best treatment option. Other trials are in progress to study the differences between coiling and clipping of intracerebral aneurysms and make recommendations for the best possible treatment.

Endovascular neurosurgery is a relatively new field of neurosurgery that is committed to developing new treatment strategies for the treatment of endovascular disease. Intravascular stenting and percutaneous angioplasty are just beginning to be explored as treatment methods for cerebrovascular disease.

Revascularization techniques also are an area in which much research is being committed. The extracranial–intracranial arterial bypass is a procedure that has given patients hope for optimum neurological function that would otherwise have little chance for a functional future. These are procedures that are done by a select group of neurovascular surgeons who are committed to teaching these procedures to surgeons who will continue to expand the capabilities of research and surgery.

EVIDENCE-BASED PRACTICE

Intracerebral Hemorrhage

Clinical Problem

Intracerebral hemorrhage (ICH) is defined as bleeding into brain tissue. Also referred to as hemorrhagic stroke, it accounts for approximately 15% of all strokes. It is a potentially devastating type of stroke, associated with significant mortality and morbidity. The mortality rate in the first 30 days is approximately 35% to 50% (Hickey, 2003). In the United States, an estimated 37,000 to 52,000 people will be affected annually by ICH (Qureshi et al., 2001). Though seen mostly in the elderly, it can also affect people who are middle aged. African Americans and Asians (particularly Japanese) are most often affected (Broderick et al., 1999). It is most commonly associated with uncontrolled hypertension. It is also associated with the use of anticoagulation agents, such as Coumadin.

Clinical manifestations of ICH are usually of sudden onset. Signs and symptoms are dependent on location and size of the hemorrhage. Most common symptoms include severe headache, weakness or numbness on either side of the body, difficulty with speech or understanding speech, or visual disturbances. It is suggested that the size of the hematoma is one of the most important factors in determining outcome for patients with ICH. The use of recombinant-activated Factor VII is a therapy used as medical management of patients with ICH. Nurses caring for patients with ICH must be familiar with this treatment.

Research Findings

It has been suggested that arresting expansion of the hematoma may improve outcome for patients with ICH. The administration of Factor VII to patients with acute ICH may promote coagulation at the site of the hemorrhage and prevent expansion of the clot.

In a Phase IIb randomized, double-blind, placebo controlled trial of 400 patients, Factor VII was administered according to a patient's weight. Single intravenous injections were given within 4 hours of hemorrhage. Treatment with Factor VII was found to decrease the size of the hematoma. A confirmatory, Phase III trial will follow (Mayer et al., 2005).

Implications for Nursing Practice

Nursing responsibilities while caring for the patient with ICH are multiple and varied. As with any medical emergency, the ABCs (airway–breathing–circulation) are of primary concern. Close monitoring of neurological status is critical. Any decline in the patient's neurological status could suggest a worsening condition. This possible decrease in neurological status warrants an emergent CT scan to assess for an increase in the size of the hematoma. Early recognition of neurological decline is necessary to obtain imaging studies, such as CT scans, to alert the medical team of an expanding hematoma. This would allow the patient to be treated with Factor VIIa, if eligible, and hopefully avoiding further neurological deficits.

Other important nursing responsibilities include careful monitoring of blood pressure parameters, optimizing treatment. This would include titration of vasoactive medications. Other neuroprotective mechanisms must be undertaken, if warranted. These include cooling mechanisms, closely controlling blood glucose and other electrolytes, fever management, seizure management, and any other monitoring of physiological processes.

Nurses are in a position to recognize and communicate changes in neurological assessment, sometimes gradual and/or subtle. Nurses skilled in neurological assessment play an important role in the care of patients with ICH, and may prevent further decline due to expanding hematoma.

Critical Thinking Questions

1. What types of patients are at risk for intracerebral hemorrhage?

2. What patient complaints or admitting signs and symptoms are worrisome for ICH?

3. What are appropriate nursing responsibilities for a patient with ICH?

Answers to Critical Thinking Questions are in Appendix D.

References

Broderick, J. P., Harold, A. P., Barsan, W., Feinberg, W., Feldmann, E., & Grotta, J. (1999). Guidelines for the management of spontaneous intracerebral hemorrhage: A statement for healthcare professionals from a special writing group of the Stroke Council, American Heart Association. *Stroke, 30,* 905–915.

Hickey, J. (2003). *The clinical practice of neurological and neurosurgical nursing.* (5th ed.). Philadelphia: Lippincott: Philadelphia.

Mayer, S. A., Brun, N. C., Broderick, J., Davis, S., Diringer, M. N., & Skolnick, B. E. (2005). Safety and feasibility of recombinant Factor VIIa for acute intracerebral hemorrhage. *Stroke, 36,* 74–79.

Presciutti, M. (2006). Nursing priorities in caring for patients with intracerebral hemorrhage. *Journal of Neuroscience Nursing, 38*(4), 296–299.

Qureshi, A. I., Tuhrim, S., Broderick, J. P., Batjer, H. H., Hondo, H., & Hanley, D. (2001). Spontaneous intracerebral hemorrhage. *New England Journal of Medicine, 344,* 1450–1460.

Source: From "Nursing priorities in caring for patients with intracerebral hemorrhage," M. Presciutti (2006). *Journal of Neuroscience Nursing, 38*(4), 296–299.

The role of nursing in the care of patients with cerebral vascular disorders is one of exciting challenges for the future. Nursing has the responsibility and the challenge to explore opportunities to improve the care and possibly the outcome of patients experiencing cerebral vascular insult. There are many opportunities for nursing research, including the treatment of vasospasm, postoperative pain control, and the effect of nursing interventions on ICP (see the Research Opportunities box). Patients who have experienced stroke offer the nurse many opportunities to explore and research treatment modalities to improve patients' quality of life.

RESEARCH OPPORTUNITIES AND CLINICAL IMPACT RELATED TO CEREBRAL VASCULAR DISORDERS

Research Area	Clinical Impact
Examine the various treatment modalities for hyponatremia, such as hypertonic saline, oral salt supplements, diet, or other medicines, and their impact on treating hyponatremia in the presence of subarachnoid hemorrhage.	Hyponatremia in the presence of subarachnoid hemorrhage is common. It is also associated with vasospasm, which is extremely significant to patient outcomes. Evaluation of hyponatremia treatments may be significant to successfully treating vasospasm and having a positive patient outcome.
Examine the differences in postoperative pain in patients who have had a craniotomy for clipping of an aneurysm versus patients who have had aneurysms coiled endovascularly.	Decreased postoperative pain.
Examine the advantages of early ambulation and therapies in patients with stroke.	Earliest possible return to previous level of function.
Examine the impact of ruptured aneurysms in specific arterial locations and the potential for return to previous cognitive function. For example, study the rupture of anterior communicating aneurysms and the long-term cognitive impact.	Identifying cognitive risk factors associated with specific aneurysm locations may lead to early testing and intervention, resulting in improved cognitive function and quality of life.

Clinical Preparation

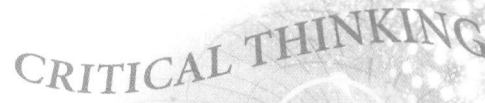

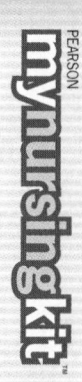

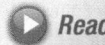 **Read**

- History of Current Illness
- Past Medical History
- Physical Exam
- Admitting Medical Orders
- Laboratory Study Results

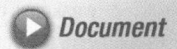 **Document**

- Summary of Hospitalization
- Pathophysiology Form
- Laboratory Values
- Laboratory Results Explanation

 **Apply**

- List of Potential Nursing Diagnoses
- Concept Map
- Critical Thinking Questions

Log on to MyNursingKit.com to download forms you will need and to complete further steps in the Clinical Preparation assignment.

HISTORY OF PRESENT ILLNESS

Mrs. J.M. is a 42-year-old woman admitted to the ICU in a major metropolitan hospital. She was brought into the emergency department (ED) by paramedics who responded to a frantic call from her husband. He reports that she has always been in perfect health until about 3 hours prior to admission. They were about to sit down to dinner with friends when she gasped, grabbed her forehead, and complained of the "worst headache of her life." She then lost consciousness and slid to the floor.

When paramedics arrived, they found Mrs. J.M. moaning and localizing to pain with her left side. She had no obvious movement on her right side. Her respirations were labored, blood pressure 192/110. She was immediately transported to the hospital.

On arrival at the ED, her respirations became labored, and she required intubation to protect her airway. She was placed on a ventilator, and a neurosurgical consult was requested.

She was immediately sent for a CT scan of her head that revealed a subarachnoid hemorrhage (SAH). The neurosurgical resident immediately sent her for cerebral angiography, which revealed a ruptured aneurysm of the left middle cerebral artery. The surgeon discussed the findings with the patient's husband and obtained permission for the patient to go to surgery for a clipping of the left middle cerebral artery aneurysm. While the surgical team assembles, the patient is admitted to the ICU, where you assume care of her.

Medical–Surgical History

Obtained from husband

No known allergies

Medications: regular insulin, per sliding scale; occasional over-the-counter medications, such as acetaminophen

No past surgical history

Social History

No tobacco use; rare social alcohol use

Married, with two daughters, ages 8 and 10

Works as a hotel manager

Physical Exam

Young woman, appearing stated age, sedated, appears in no distress

Vital signs: temp 37.0°C degrees rectally, heart rate 62, respiratory rate 12 (assisted), blood pressure 174/80

HEENT: rhythm and rate regular, S_1S_2 heard, no abnormal murmurs, good capillary refill, pulses 2+ all extremities, no pitting edema

Lungs: clear to auscultation bilaterally

Abdomen: soft, nontender; bowel sounds heard in all quadrants

Neurological Exam

GCS = E3 M4 VT1 = 8T (eyes open to speech only, withdraws her left side to pain, no verbal response, intubated)

Cranial nerves: CN II–XII intact bilaterally

Motor:

Left upper extremity: withdraws to pain

Left lower extremity: withdraws to pain

Right upper extremity: no response to pain

Right lower extremity: no response to pain

Sensory: Unable to examine

Cerebellar: Unable to examine

Imaging Studies

CT scan done in the ED reveals subarachnoid blood

Cerebral angiogram reveals the presence of a left middle cerebral aneurysm

Chest x-ray: no abnormal pathology

ECG: normal

Admitting Medical Orders

Admit to Neuroscience ICU

Diagnosis: subarachnoid hemorrhage; status postinsertion EVD

Condition: critical

Allergies: none known

Vital signs and neuro assessment q1h

Bed rest

NPO

NG tube to low intermittent suction

Foley catheter

Intake and output: q1h

Continuous ECG, arterial pressure, ICP monitoring

Keep EVD (external ventricular drain) at the level of the EAC (external auditory canal) open to drain for ICP > 20 until ICP is less than 20; then resume monitoring

Call resident on call: any change in neurological status; any change in vital signs: HR < 60 or > 120; systolic blood pressure < 100 or > 140; RR < 12 or > 30; temperature > 38°C; O_2 saturation < 92%; ICP > 20; CPP < 80 or > 100; glucose < 70 or > 120 mg/dL

IV: NS with 20 mEq KCl @ 75 mL/hr

Ventilatory settings: O_2: 40%, TV: 600, IMV: 12

Consent for: craniotomy for clipping of left middle cerebral artery aneurysm by Dr. XYZ

Sequential compression stockings (SCDs) to lower extremities prior to surgery

Internal medicine consult for management of diabetes

Scheduled Medications

Sliding scale regular Insulin, dosage to be determined by internist

Pepcid 20 mg IV bid

PRN Medications

Acetaminophen 650 mg rectal q4h prn fever

Morphine sulfate 2–6 mg IV q1h prn pain

Ativan 0.5–2 mg IV q2h prn agitation

Zofran 4 mg IV q8 prn nausea

Ordered Laboratory Studies

CBC, Chem 7 panel, PTT, PT, INR on admission and q a.m.

Accu-Chek q6h

Ordered Diagnostic Studies

Head CT scan in the morning postoperatively

Head CT scan stat prn if neuro signs change and notify physician

Trans cranial Doppler study every other day

An external ventricular drain (EVD) is placed to monitor and assist with controlling her ICP. Her opening pressure is 26 and her cerebrospinal fluid (CSF) is grossly bloody. A central line is placed to assist with hemodynamic monitoring. An arterial line is also being placed to assist with blood pressure monitoring. Laboratory tests, including coagulation studies done in the ED, are reviewed and are unremarkable. Mrs. J.M. is sent to surgery.

Postoperatively, when Mrs. J.M. returns to the ICU, she is still sedated, but waking up. She opens her eyes and moves her left side purposefully. She does not move the right arm or leg. She remains intubated and ventilated with her EVD in place.

Mrs. J.M. is extubated on postop day 3. She is no longer sedated. Her neurological exam is as follows: GCS = E4 M6 V3. Her pupils are equal and reactive, and her gaze is conjugate. Her face shows some weakness on the right side. She follows commands by showing two fingers on the left side. She is unable to move the right arm or leg. Her speech consists of barely intelligible words. Her EVD is closed to drainage and a follow-up CT scan the following morning shows no increase in ventricular size with the EVD closed, so it is removed.

Transcranial Doppler studies are being performed every other day to monitor blood flow in the affected arteries, and to assess for vasospasm. Her laboratory values are stable, her sodium level is 136 mEq/L. Medications include nimodipine 30 mg sublingual every 2 hours; Pepcid 20 mg orally bid; salt supplements, 2 grams three times a day with food; sliding scale insulin; and prn medications for pain, nausea, and fever. Her vital signs have been stable: afebrile, heart rate in the 70s, blood pressure 140/82–150/90, respirations stable at 16. She does not require supplemental oxygen. She is eating a pureed diet (due to impaired swallow reflex), and nursing is getting her out of bed to sit in a chair. Her IV is running at 100 mL/hr with a solution of NS.

She is transferred to general floor care on postop day 4. She has orders to increase her activity as tolerated and to attempt to eat solid foods. Her IV has been discontinued. Physical therapy and occupational therapy are ordered to assist with mobility and ambulation. Speech therapy is consulted to assist with the evaluation of her swallowing and to assist with her severe aphasia.

On postop day 5, the nurse notes that she is slightly agitated. On questioning her, it is noted that her speech has deteriorated to moans only. Her vital signs are unchanged with the exception of a blood pressure of 100/62. The rest of her exam is unchanged. Laboratory values reveal a sodium level of 130 mg/L. The MD is called, and the patient is sent for a stat angiogram. The angiogram results prove that Mrs. J.M. has vasospasm of her left middle cerebral artery. She is placed on hy-

pertonic saline for her hyponatremia. She is transferred back to the ICU and her triple-H therapy (for hypervolemia, hypertension, and hemodilution) is resumed.

LABORATORY STUDY RESULTS

Test	Day 1	Day 2	Day 3
Sodium	142 mEq/L	138 mEq/L	135mEq/L
Potassium	3.8 mEq/L	3.5 mEq/L	3.6 mEq/L
Chloride	98 mEq/L	97 mEq/L	98 mEq/L
Carbon dioxide	22 mEq/L	22 mEq/L	23 mEq/L
Blood urea nitrogen (BUN)	22 mg/dL	21 mg/dL	22 mg/dL
Creatinine	1.2 mg/dL	1.2 mg/dL	1.2 mg/dL
Blood glucose	290 mg/dL	240 mg/dL	180 mg/dL
White blood cells	8200 µL	8100 µL	8200 µL
Hemoglobin	12.3 g/dL	12.2 g/dL	12.4 g/dL
Hematocrit	35.4%	33%	34%
Platelets	210,000 µL	200,000 µL	205,000 µL
Protime (PT)	10.6 seconds	10.5 seconds	10.5 seconds
International Normalized Ration (INR)	0.8 INR	0.8 INR	0.75 INR
Partial thromboplastin time (PTT)	33 seconds	34 seconds	32 seconds

CRITICAL THINKING QUESTIONS

1. What is the significance of Mrs. J.M. complaining of "the worst headache of her life"?

2. What symptoms did Mrs. J.M. experience that specified the location of the affected artery?

3. What symptoms of vasospasm did Mrs. J.M. exhibit?

4. What interventions could be expected to treat vasospasm?

Answers to Critical Thinking Questions appear in Appendix D.

NCLEX® REVIEW

1. Of the 500,000 strokes that occur annually, 80% of them are ischemic strokes. Which of the following accurately reflects this type of stroke?

1. The strokes are hemorrhagic in nature.
2. The signs and symptoms, though acute, resolve without permanent disability.
3. The strokes are commonly caused by artherosclerosis.
4. Patients experiencing this type of stroke are usually younger.

2. The pathophysiology of a stroke differs according to its underlying process. In the following selections, identify those processes that can cause a brain attack. Select all that apply.

1. Plaque formation that alters the internal diameter of a cerebral artery
2. Embolus that separated from a deep venous thrombosis in the left leg
3. Thrombus formation as a result of plaque formation
4. Lipohyalinosis, a vascular abnormality, caused by hypertension

3. The ischemic cascade is a response to cellular hypoxia and may result in additional cell damage. In describing this process, the nurse understands that:
   1. Tissues that surround the necrotic area have themselves undergone anoxia.
   2. Ischemic cascade further extends the area of infarction.
   3. This tissue may be reperfused, but its ability to function has been permanently impaired.
   4. The penumbra of a stroke is the necrotic core.

4. Nurses play a crucial role in the management of patient with vasospasm associated with subarachnoid hemorrhage treated with Triple–H therapy. The nurse must continuously assess for the complications. Assessment parameters include:
   1. Assessing renal output to detect the onset of cerebral salt wasting.
   2. Assessing lung and heart sounds to detect fluid overload.
   3. Detection of the nidus which can warn of impending seizure onset.
   4. Monitoring for focal seizure onset as these warn of a dire complication.

5. There are two major medical management options for the treatment of ruptured aneurysm. When diagnostic testing has found that both endovascular coiling and neurosurgical clipping are treatment options, the choice is based upon which of the following factors?
   1. Endovascular coiling is associated with a longer length of hospital stay.
   2. Neurosurgical clipping is associated with a higher survival and lower morbidity rates one year after procedure.
   3. Endovascular coiling is associated with the patients being able to return to their activities of normal living and work earlier than patients who had undergone neurosurgical clipping.
   4. There is little difference in either treatment option other than the availability of an interventional neuroradiologist.

Answers for review questions appear in Appendix D

KEY TERMS

anterior circulation *p.764*
antiplatelet therapy *p.760*
arteriovenous malformation (AVM) *p.769*
atherogenesis *p.758*
berry aneurysm *p.763*
cardiogenic embolism *p.758*
carotid endarterectomy (CEA) *p.761*
cavernous malformation *p.769*
cerebral aneurysm *p.763*
cerebral salt wasting *p.768*
coiling *p.770*

embolization *p.770*
familial intracranial aneurysms *p.763*
Fisher grading scale *p.766*
fusiform aneurysms *p.763*
Hunt-Hess classification *p.766*
infarction *p.757*
lacunar stroke *p.758*
lipohyalinosis *p.759*
neuroprotection *p.760*
nidus *p.769*

percutaneous angioplasty *p.761*
posterior circulation *p.764*
reperfusion injury *p.759*
Spetzler-Martin AVM grading scale *p.769*
stent *p.763*
stroke *p.757*
subarachnoid hemorrhage (SAH) *p.763*
transient ischemic attack (TIA) *p.758*
triple-H therapy *p.768*
vasospasm *p.767*

REFERENCES

Adams, H. P., del Zoppo, G. J., & von Kummer, R. (2006). *Management of stroke: A practical guide for the prevention, evaluation, and treatment of acute stroke* (3rd ed.). West Islip, NY: Professional Communications.

Alberts, M. J. (1999). Diagnosis and treatment of ischemic stroke. *American Journal of Medicine, 106,* 211–221.

American Heart Association. (2004). *Heart disease and stroke statistics—2004 update.* Dallas, TX: Author.

American Heart Association. (2005a). *Heart disease and stroke statistics.—2005 update.* Dallas: Author.

American Heart Association. (2005b). American Heart Association and American Stroke Association national survey of stroke risk awareness among women. *Circulation, 111,* 1321–1326.

American Heart Association. (2008a). *Heart disease and stroke statistics: 2008 update at-a-glance.* Dallas, Texas: American Heart Association.

American Heart Association. (2008b). Heart disease and stroke statistics—2008 update. *Circulation, 117,* e25–e146.

Anderson, C. S., Feigin, V., Bennett, D., Lin, R. B., Hankey, G., & Jamrozik, K., et al. (2004). Active and passive smoking and the risk of subarachnoid hemorrhage: An international population-based case-controlled study. *Stroke, 35*(3), 633–637.

Ayata, C., & Ropper, A. H. (2002). Ischaemic brain oedema. *Journal of Clinical Neuroscience, 9*(2), 113–124.

Bairstow, P., Dodgson, A., Linto, J., & Khangure, M. (2002). Comparison of cost and outcome of endovascular and neurosurgical procedures

in the treatment of ruptured intracranial aneurysms. *Australian Radiology, 46*(3), 249–251.

Ballard, J., Kreiter, K. T., Claassen, J., Kowalski, R. G., Connolly, E. S., & Mayer, S. A. (2003). Risk factors for continued cigarette use after subarachnoid hemmorrage. *Stroke, 34,* 1859–1863.

Barnett, H. J. M., Sackett, D., Taylor, D. W., Haynes, B., Peerless, S. J., Meissner, I., et al. (1987). Are the results of the extracranial–intracranial bypass trial generalizable? *New England Journal of Medicine, 316*(13), 800–824.

Barnett, H. J., Taylor, D. W., & Eliasziw, M. (1998). Benefit of carotid endarterectomy in patients with symptomatic moderate or severe stenosis: North American Symptomatic Carotid Endarterectomy Trial Collaborators. *New England Journal of Medicine, 339,* 1415–1425.

Brinkman, W. T., Terramani, T. T., Najibi, S., & Chaikof, E. L. (2002). Platelets: Is aspirin sufficient or must we know how to pronounce abciximab? *Seminars in Vascular Surgery, 15*(4), 245–255.

Brown, R. D., & Piepgras, D. G. (2004). Screening for intracranial aneurysms after subarachnoid hemorrhage: do our patients benefit? *Neurology, 62,* 354–356.

Carter, B. S., Amin-Hanjani, S., Butler, W. E., Ogilvy, C. S., & Barker, F. G. (2003, February). *In-hospital mortality and morbidity after surgical treatment of unruptured intracranial aneurysms in the United States from 1996 to 2000: The effect of hospital and surgeon volume.* Oral abstract presentation at the Sixth Joint Meeting of the AANS/CNS Section on Cerebrovascular Surgery and the American Society of Interventional & Therapeutic Neuroradiology, Phoenix, AZ.

Chan, W. S., Ray, J., Wai, E. K., Ginsburg, S., Hannah, M. E., Corey, P. N., et al. (2004). Risk of stroke in women exposed to low-dose oral contraceptives: A critical evaluation of the evidence. *Archives of Internal Medicine, 164*(7), 741–747.

Clark, W. M. (2007). Reperfusion injury in stroke. *eMedicine.* Retrieved April 2, 2008, from http://www.emedicine.com/neuro/topic602.htm

Conway, J. E., & Tamargo R. J. (2001). Cocaine use is an independent risk factor for cerebral vasospasm in aneurysmal subarachnoid hemorrhage. *Stroke, 32*(10), 2338–2343.

Deng, H., Han, H. S., Cheng, D., Sun, G. H., & Yenari, M. A. (2003). Mild hypothermia inhibits inflammation after experimental stroke and brain inflammation. *Stroke 34,* 2495–2501.

Friedman, J. A., Pichelmann, M. A., Piepgras, D. G., McIver, J. I., Toussaint, L. G., McClelland, R. L., et al. (2003). Pulmonary complications of aneurysmal subarachnoid hemorrhage. *Neurosurgery, 52*(5), 1025–1031.

Greenberg, M. S. (2001). *Handbook of neurosurgery* (5th ed.). New York: Thieme.

Gross, C. P., Steiner, C. A., Bass, E. B., & Powe, N. R. (2000). Relation between prepublication release of clinical trial results and the practice of carotid endarterectomy. *Journal of the American Medical Association, 284,* 2886–2893.

Hickey, J. (2003). *The clinical practice of neurological and neurosurgical nursing* (5th ed.). Philadelphia: Lippincott.

Hinkle, J. L., & Bowman, L. (2003). Neuroprotection for ischemic stroke. *Journal of Neuroscience Nursing, 35*(2), 114–118.

Howard, V. J., McClure, L. A., Meschia, J. F., Pulley, L., Orr, S. C., & Friday, G. H. (2006). High prevalence of stroke symptoms among persons without a diagnosis of stroke or transient ischemic attack in a general population: The Reasons for Geographic And Racial Differences in Stroke (REGARDS) study. *Archives of Internal Medicine, 166*(18), 1952–1958.

Ibbotson, T., McGavin, J. K., & Goa, K. L. (2003). Abciximab: An updated review of its therapeutic use in patients with ischaemic heart disease undergoing percutaneous coronary revascularization. *Drugs, 63*(11), 1121–1163.

International Subarachnoid Aneurysm Trial Collaborative Group. (2002). International Subarachnoid Aneurysm Trial (ISAT) of neurosurgical clipping versus endovascular coiling in 2143 patients with ruptured intracranial aneurysms: A randomized trial. *Lancet, 360,* 1267–1274.

Johnson, E. W., Marchuk, D. A., & Zabramski, J. M. (2004). The genetics of cerebral cavernous malformations. In R. F. Spetzler & F. B. Meyer (Eds.), *Youman's neurological surgery* (5th ed., pp. 2299–2303). Philadelphia: W. B. Saunders.

Johnson, S. C., Gress, D. R., Browner, W. S., & Sidney, S. (2000). Short-term prognosis after emergency department diagnosis of TIA. *Journal of American Medical Association, 284,* 2901–2906.

Jorgensen, H. S., Reith, J., Nakayama, H., Kammersgard, L. P., Raaschous, H. O., & Olsen, T. S. (1999). What determines good recovery in patients with the most severe strokes? The Copenhagen Stroke Study. *Stroke, 30,* 2009–2012.

Juvela, S. (2000). Risk factors for multiple intracranial aneurysms. *Stroke, 31,* 392–397.

Juvela, S. (2003). Prehemorrhage risk factors for fatal intracranial aneurysm rupture. *Stroke, 34,* 1852–1858.

Kaminogo, M., Yonekura, M., & Shibata, S. (2003). Incidence and outcome of multiple intracranial aneurysms in a defined population. *Stroke, 34*(1), 16–21.

Khurana, V. G., & Spetzler, R. F. (2006). *The brain aneurysm: A comprehensive resource for brain aneurysm patients, their families, and physicians.* Bloomington, IN: AuthorHouse.

Kim, K. V. (2007). Ethnic differences in risk factors for subarachnoid hemorrhage. *Neurosurgery, 107*(3), 522–529.

Koga, M., Kimura, K., Minematsu, K., & Yamaguchi, T. (2001). Diagnosis of internal carotid artery stenosis greater than 70% with power Doppler duplex sonography. *American Journal of Neuroradiology, 22*(2), 413–417.

Laurans, M. S., DiLuna, M. L., Shin, D., Niazi, F., Voorhees, J. R., Nelson-Williams, M., et al. (2003). Mutational analysis of 206 families with cavernous malformations. *Journal of Neurosurgery, 99*(1), 38–43.

LeRoux, P. D., & Winn, H. R. (2004). Surgical decision making for the treatment of cerebral aneurysms. In R. F. Spetzler & F. B. Meyer (Eds.), *Youman's neurological surgery* (5th ed., pp. 1793–1809). Philadelphia: W. B. Saunders.

Lubbe, D. F., & Berger, P. B. (2002). The thienopyridines. *Journal of Interventional Cardiology., 15*(1), 85–93.

MacDonald, R. L., & Weir, B. (2004). Perioperative management of subarachnoid hemorrhage. In R. F. Spetzler & F. B. Meyer (Eds.), *Youman's neurological surgery* (5th ed., pp. 1813–1835). Philadelphia: W. B. Saunders.

MacWalter, R. S., & Shirley, C. P. (2002). A benefit-risk assessment of agents used in the secondary prevention of stroke. *Drug Safety, 25*(13), 943–963.

Martin, N. A., Kureshi, I., & Coiteiro, D. (2004). Revascularization techniques for complex aneurysms and skull base tumors. In R. F. Spetzler & F. B. Meyer (Eds.), *Youman's neurological surgery* (5th ed., pp. 2107–2119). Philadelphia: W. B. Saunders.

Matchar, D. B., & Samsa, G. P. (2000). *Secondary and tertiary prevention of stroke: Patient Outcomes Research Team (PORT) final report phase 1.* (AHRQ Pub. No. 00-N001). Rockville, MD: Agency for Healthcare Research and Quality.

Molyneux, A., Kerr, R., Stratton, I., Sandercock, P., Clarke, M., Shrimpton, J., et al. (2002). International Subarachnoid Aneurysm Trial (ISAT) of neurosurgical clipping versus endovascular coiling in 2143 patients with ruptured intracranial aneurysms: A randomised trial. *Lancet, 360*(9342), 1267–1274.

Nagao, S., Irie, K., Kawai, N., Nakamura, T., Kunishio, K., & Matsumoto, Y. (2003). The use of mild hypothermia for patients with severe vasospasm: A preliminary report. *Journal of Clinical Neuroscience, 10*(2), 208–212.

Nakaji, P. (2004). Management of brainstem cavernous malformations. For the Proceedings of the 29th Stroke Conference of the Japan Stroke Society. Submitted for publishing.

National Institute of Neurological Disorders and Stroke. (2007a). *NINDS arteriovenous malformation information page.* Retrieved April 3, 2008, from http://www.ninds.nih.gov/disorders/avms/avms.htm

National Institute of Neurological Disorders and Stroke t-PA Study Group. (1995). Tissue plasminogen activator for acute ischemic stroke. *New England Journal of Medicine, 333,* 1581–1587.

National Stroke Association. (2008). *Stroke risk factors.* Retrieved April 5, 2008, from http://www.stroke.org/site.PageSeravcer?pagename=RISKN

North American Symptomatic Carotid Endarterectomy Trial Collaborators. (1991). Beneficial effect of carotid endarterectomy in symptomatic patients with high-grade stenosis. *New England Journal of Medicine, 325*(7), 445–453.

Oyama, K., & Criddle, L. (2004). Vasospasm after aneurysmal subarachnoid hemorrhage. *Critical Care Nurse, 24*(5), 58–60.

Passacantilli, E., Zabramski, J., Lanzino, G., & Spetzler, R. F. (2002). Cavernous malformations: Genetic, molecular biology, and familial forms. *Operative Techniques in Neurosurgery, 5(3),* 145–149.

Pestalozza, I. F., DiLegge, S., Calabresi, M., & Lenzi, G. L. (2002). Ischaemic penumbra: Highlights. *Clinical Experience with Hypertension, 24*(7–8), 517–529.

Raaymakers, T. W. M., Rinkel, G. J. E., Limburg, M., & Algra, A. (1998). Mortality and morbidity of surgery for unruptured intracranial aneurysms: A meta-analysis. *Stroke, 29,* 1531–1538.

Rinkel, G. J., Feigin, V. L., Algra, A., Vermeulen, M., & van Gijn, J. (2002). Calcium antagonists for aneurysmal subarachnoid hemorrhage. *Cochran Database System.*

Rosamond, W., Flegal, K., Friday, G., Furie, K., et al. (2007). Heart disease and stroke statistics—2007 update: A report from the American Heart Association Statistics Committee and Stroke Statistics Subcommittee. *Circulation, 115*(5), e69–e171.

Sacco, R. L., Boden-Albala, B., Gan, R., Chen, X., Kargman, D. E., Shea, S., et al. (1998). Stroke incidence among white, black, and Hispanic residents of urban community: The Northern Manhattan Stroke Study. *American Journal of Epidemiology, 147*(3), 259–268.

Saver, J. (2001). Intra-arterial thrombolysis. *Neurology, 57,* 58–60.

Schievink, W. I. (2004). Genetics of intracranial aneurysms. In R. F. Spetzler & F. B. Meyer (Eds.), *Youman's neurological surgery* (5th ed., pp. 1769–1777). Philadelphia: W. B. Saunders.

Schumacher, H. C., & Marshall, R. S. (2006). Arteriovenous malformations. *eMedicine.* Retrieved April 2, 2008, from http://www.emedicine.com/NEURO/topic21.htm

Soderman, M., Andersson, T., Karlsson, B., Wallace, M. C., & Edner, G. (2003). Management of patients with brain arteriovenous malformation. *European Journal of Radiology, 46*(3), 195–205.

Spetzler, R. F., & Martin, N. A. (1986). A grading system for arteriovenous malformations. *Journal of Neurosurgery, 65,* 476–483.

Stanford School of Medicine. (2008). Stroke prevention. Retrieved April 2, 2008, from Stanford Stroke Center website: http://strokecenter. stanford.edu/guide/prevention.html

Tatter, S. B., & Ogilvy, C. S. (1995). Vascular malformations: General considerations. In C. W. Mitchell (Ed.), *Surgical management of neurovascular disease.* Baltimore: Williams & Wilkins.

Van den Berg, R., Rinkel, G. J., & Vandertop, W. P. (2003). Treatment of ruptured intracranial aneurysms: Implications of the ISAT on clipping versus coiling. *European Journal of Radiology, 46*(3), 172–177.

Wang, C. C., Liu, A., Zhang, J. T., Sun, B., & Zhao, Y. L. (2003). Surgical management of brain-stem cavernous malformations: Report of 137 cases. *Surgical Neurology, 59*(6), 444–454.

Wills, S., Ronkainen, A., van der Voet, M., Kuiuvaniemi, H., Helin, K., Leinonen, E., et al. (2003). Familial intracranial aneurysms: An analysis of 346 multiplex Finnish families. *Stroke, 34,* 1370–1374.

Winkley, J. M., & Adams, H. P. (2000). Potential role of abciximab in ischemic cerebrovascular disease. *American Journal of Cardiology, 85,* 47C–51C.

Zabramski, J. M., & Han, P. P. (2004). Epidemiology and natural history of cavernous malformations. In R. F. Spetzler & F. B. Meyer (Eds.), *Youman's neurological surgery* (5th ed., pp. 2292–2298). Philadelphia: W. B. Saunders.

Zabramski, J. M., Henn, J. S., & Coons, S. (1999). Pathology of cerebral vascular malformations. *Neurosurgery Clinics of North America, 10,* 395–410.

Zabramski, J. M., Spetzler, R. F., Johnson, B., Golfinos, J., Drayer, B. P., Brown, B., et al. (1994). The natural history of familial cavernous malformations: Results of an ongoing study. *Journal of Neurosurgery, 80,* 422–432.

Caring for the Patient with Chronic Neurological Disorders

Gale Kittle

Outcome-Based Learning Objectives

After studying this chapter, the learner will be able to:

1. Distinguish among the neurodegenerative disorders of Alzheimer's disease, Parkinson's disease, multiple sclerosis, amyotrophic lateral sclerosis, and myasthenia gravis by describing the etiology and pathophysiology of each disorder.
2. Compare and contrast the presenting signs and symptoms of each of the neurodegenerative disorders discussed in the chapter.
3. Develop a generalized plan of care for each of the neurodegenerative disorders discussed.
4. Develop a comprehensive discharge teaching plan for each of the neurodegenerative disorders discussed.
5. Describe generalized health promotion needs for each neurodegenerative disorder discussed.
6. Explain gerontological implications for each neurodegenerative disorder discussed.
7. Evaluate research implications for nursing practice when caring for persons with a neurodegenerative disorder.

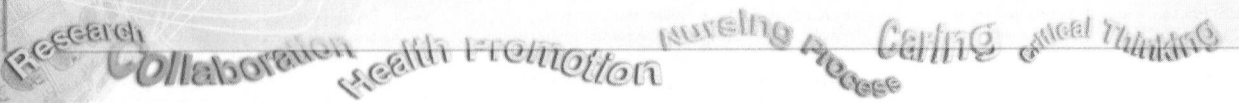
Research   Collaboration   Health Promotion   Nursing Process   Caring   Critical Thinking

CARING for patients with the neurodegenerative disorders of Alzheimer's disease, Parkinson's disease, multiple sclerosis, amyotrophic lateral sclerosis, and myasthenia gravis challenges the nurse's ability to manage diverse conditions. Characterized by neuronal loss in specific areas of the central nervous system (CNS), neurodegenerative disorders are chronic, progressive, and without cure. Although these disorders manifest with differing signs and distinctive symptoms, they share many common aspects that contribute to the complexity of diagnosing and treating them.

In many cases, a diagnosis cannot be confirmed without autopsy. Clinically, neurodegenerative diseases often have a variable course. Families face a future of uncertain prognosis—other than the knowledge that symptoms will worsen. Complicated treatment strategies only compound the difficulty of these cases. As patients' mental and/or physical symptoms progress and as they lose more and more of their ability to care for themselves, these patients begin to rely on a spouse, a close family member, or another lay caregiver. The ongoing and long-term care of a person with a degenerative disorder is labor intensive and can carry over to threaten the physical and mental well-being of the patient's family.

Nurses caring for patients with neurodegenerative disorders find themselves in a dual role of caring for both the patient and the caregiver, often becoming a vital link among the patient, caregiver, and health care system in a variety of environments.

Because of the prolonged, chronic nature of these diseases, the common settings in which one finds these patients are the home, outpatient clinic, or long-term care facility. Patients may be hospitalized during the initial diagnostic phase or for complications associated with their condition. The wide range of care for those with neurodegenerative disorders creates a unique opportunity for a nurse to have a profound impact on the patient and family response to a seemingly hopeless condition.

Alzheimer's Disease and Related Dementias

Dementia is a general term for brain dysfunction characterized by deterioration of memory and cognition (Desai & Grossberg, 2005). Although other forms of dementia are addressed, this chapter focuses primarily on the most common form of dementia, Alzheimer's disease. **Alzheimer's disease (AD)** is a chronic, progressive, irreversible brain disorder. Long-term care of AD patients is as likely to take place in the home as it is in a nursing facility. Obviously, nurses who specialize in treatment of neurological disorders most often are the providers of ongoing, clinical care in these settings; however, hospital nurses working in other specialties may see AD patients with concurrent health issues.

Epidemiology and Etiology

Alzheimer's disease is found most frequently in adults ages 65 and older (Desai & Grossberg, 2005). The onset of AD begins with subtle lapses of memory, which gradually and progressively develop into a chronic loss of personality, recognition, reasoning, and independence. Neurologists estimate that approximately 4 million Americans have this disease. As the general population grows, the projected number is expected to double by the year 2030 and nearly quadruple by 2050. AD is now emerging as a major public health crisis based on the projected number of people expected to be affected (Leifer, 2003). The causes of dementia are numerous and are listed in Chart 31–1.

Pathophysiology

The pathology of AD is marked by the profusion of amyloid plaques and neurofibrillary tangles, which form in the hippocampus and other parts of the brain critical to memory (Figure 31–1 ■). While normal aging of the brain can cause plaques and tangles, they develop at a much greater rate and mass in those affected with AD (National Institute on Aging [NIA], 2007).

Neurofibrillary tangles were one of the initial discoveries that first described hallmark pathology in AD. The findings revealed a specialized protein known as **tau**. A key component of tangles, tau normally helps maintain the health of neurons. In AD, mutations in tau cause it to distort and twist, creating tangled threads of the protein within neurons (NIA, 2007; Porth, 2007). These neurofibrillary tangles eventually lead to cell death, neuronal degeneration, and the symptoms associated with AD (DeKosky, 2003). Figure 31–2 ■ (p. 790) depicts this process.

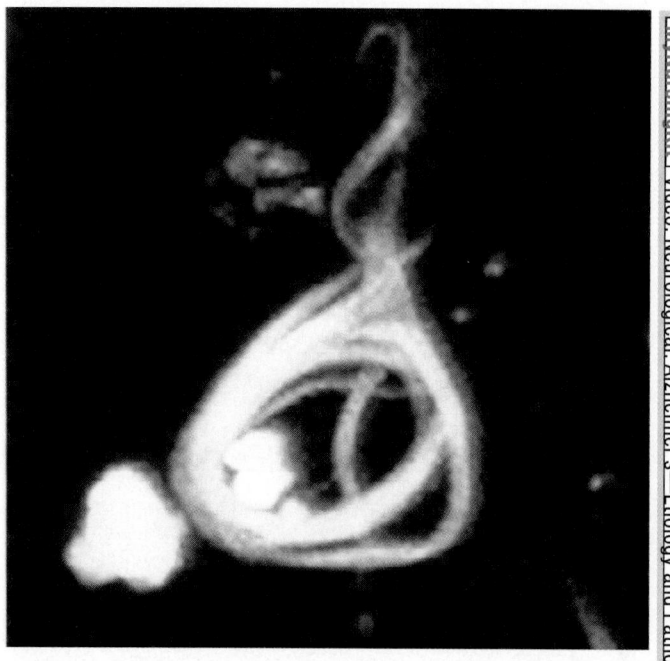

FIGURE 31–1 ■   An AD neurofibrillary tangle.
Source: Photo from Alzheimer's Disease: Unraveling the Mystery, U.S. National Institute on Aging, 2002

Most recently, researchers have focused on the impact amyloid plaques have on determining other pathologic characteristics of AD. Composed of the protein beta-amyloid and clipped from the larger amyloid precursor protein, these thick, insoluble plaques form around neurons, causing oxidative stress and inflammatory changes. Cholesterol also may play a part in the formation of amyloid plaques, and it has become suspect in the development of AD (DeKosky, 2003). It is not known whether amyloid plaques cause AD or if they are a product of the disease process. Research continues to focus on oxidative stress, inflammation, and cholesterol and their relationship to the formation and presence of amyloid plaques in AD (NIA, 2007). The accompanying Risk Factors and Genetic Considerations boxes (p. 790) provide more information about Alzheimer's disease.

Clinical Manifestations

Slow and insidious in onset and ranging over a course of 3 to 20 years, AD progressively degrades cognitive function (Feldman & Woodward, 2005). While the span of the disease varies in length and severity from patient to patient, its symptoms develop in stages corresponding to the area of the brain where degeneration is present (NIA, 2007). Typically, neuronal degeneration starts in the hippocampus, an area of the brain critical to short- and long-term memory. From there, it spreads to other regions that control cognition, judgment, behavior, and physical movement. General descriptions of each of the four basic stages of AD are given below (NIA, 2002).

Preclinical AD

Researchers suspect that the damaging effects of AD on the brain start 10 to 20 years before signs of the disease begin to show. Initially, the degeneration originates in the entorhinal cortex, an area adjacent to the hippocampus (Figure 31–3 ■, p. 791). The first symptom is likely to be an elusive, difficult-to-distinguish

---

CHART 31–1   **Causes of Dementia**

Alzheimer's disease

Vascular dementia

Diffuse Lewy body dementia

Frontotemporal atrophy/Pick's disease

Parkinson's disease

Huntington's disease

Postcortical or post-thalamic stroke

Postanoxic encephalopathy

Hydrocephalus

Brain tumors

Infectious disorders: meningitis, Creutzfeldt–Jakob disease, HIV, neurosyphilis

Toxins: drugs, alcohol, heavy metals

Delirium

Depression

Vitamin B_{12} deficiency

Polypharmacy

Sources: Desai, A. K., & Grossberg, G. T. (2005). Diagnosis and treatment of Alzheimer's disease. *Neurology, 64*(Suppl. 3), S34–S39; Leifer, B. P. (2003). Early diagnosis of Alzheimer's disease: Clinical and economic benefits. *Journal of the American Geriatrics Society, 51,* S281–S288.

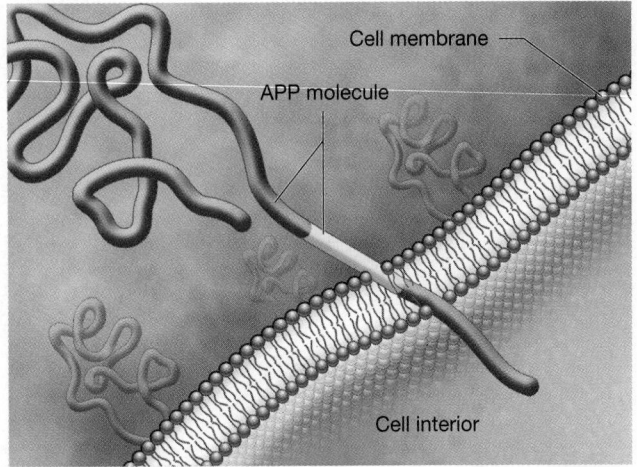

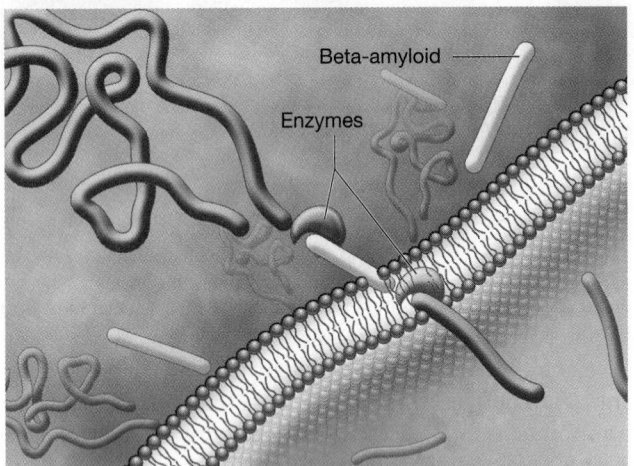

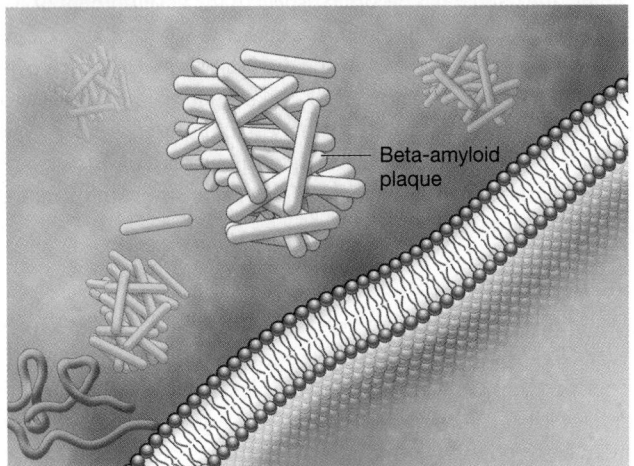

FIGURE 31–2 ■ From amyloid precursor protein (APP) to beta-amyloid and formation of amyloid plaque.

loss of memory. If the patient's memory loss appears to be greater than might be expected for his or her age, while other functions of cognition remain intact, then a diagnosis of **mild cognitive impairment (MCI)** may be rendered. In cases of MCI, the patient's experience of cognitive impairment may be uncorroborated by friends or family who do not notice the subtle behavior changes and memory anomalies of which the patient complains. The relationship between MCI and AD is not fully understood; however, MCI is sometimes considered a precursor to AD.

Mild AD

Once the degeneration of neurons spreads to the cerebral cortex (Figure 31–4 ■), the escalating problems with memory and cognitive function become obvious. Friends and family who do recognize the patient's transitory condition corroborate these difficulties. Clinical testing will reveal the following signs of mild AD:

- Confusion about the location of familiar places
- Slow to accomplish simple tasks
- Difficulty handling money matters
- Loss of spontaneity and sense of initiative
- Mood swings and personality changes.

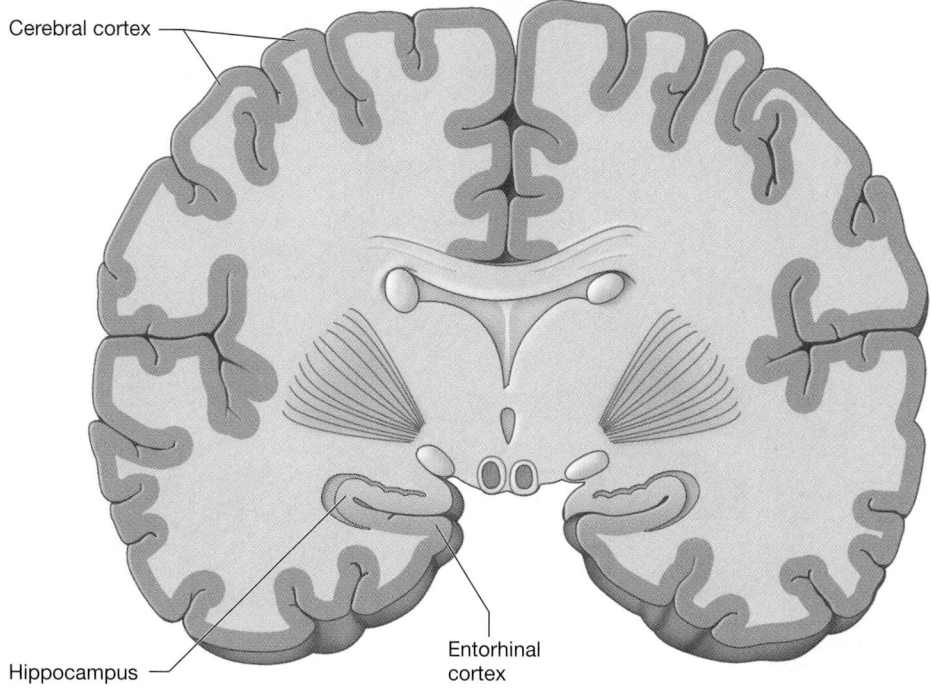

FIGURE 31–3 ■ Preclinical AD.

Moderate AD

At this stage of the disease, neuronal degeneration expands to areas that control language and reasoning. The symptoms worsen as atrophy continues to spread. The patient may have a bout of wandering and can be easily agitated by the routines of daily living. The following symptoms are indicators of moderate AD:

- Progressive memory loss and confusion
- Unable to recognize friends and family
- Language difficulties

- Difficulties with reading, writing, and simple math
- Problems learning new material, aligning thoughts, and thinking logically
- Hallucinations, delusions, paranoia.

Severe AD

In the most advanced phase of AD, plaques and tangles have spread throughout the brain, causing generalized atrophy (Figure 31–5 ■, p. 792). The patient becomes completely dependent and

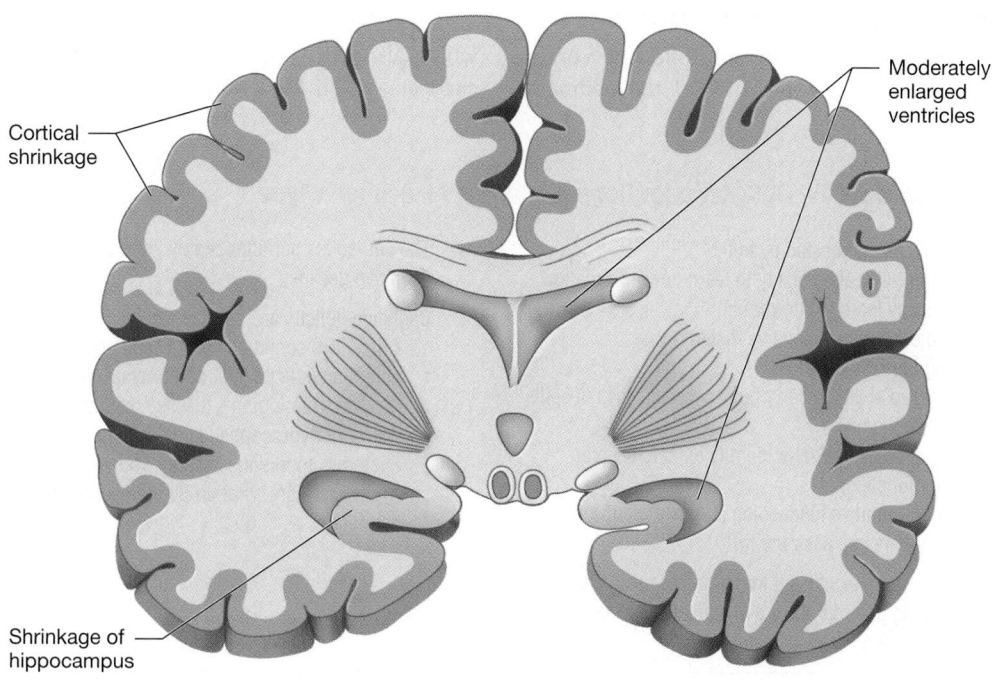

FIGURE 31–4 ■ Mild AD.

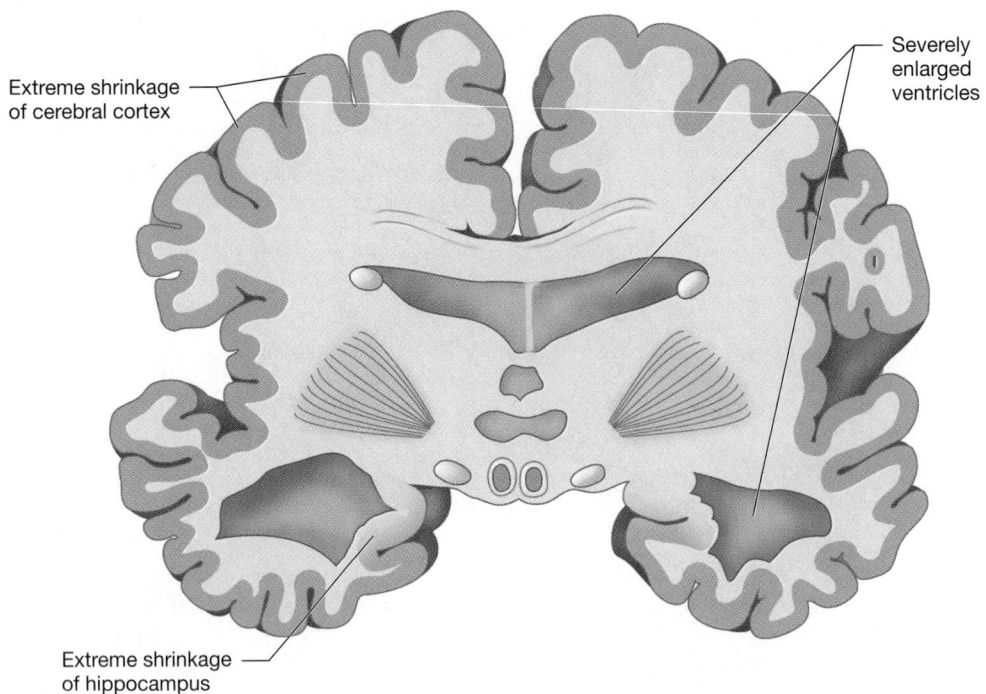

Extreme shrinkage of cerebral cortex

Severely enlarged ventricles

Extreme shrinkage of hippocampus

FIGURE 31–5 ■ Severe AD.

is not able to recognize loved ones. Other characteristics of advanced AD include:

- Inability to communicate
- Weight loss secondary to difficulty eating and swallowing
- Bowel and bladder incontinence
- Increased sleeping.

Death usually occurs as a result of aspiration pneumonia or from other concurrent health conditions.

Laboratory and Diagnostic Procedures

A definitive diagnosis of AD can be made only following a brain autopsy, which can determine the presence of the hallmark plaques and tangles. However, diagnostic tools are available that can assist in a preliminary diagnosis of AD (Leifer, 2003). The *Diagnostic and Statistical Manual of Mental Disorders, Fourth Edition,* Text Revision (*DSM-IV-TR*; American Psychiatric Society, 2000) outlines the criteria used to diagnose Alzheimer's dementia (see the National Guidelines box).

Routine laboratory and radiological tests are used to rule out other causes of dementia. These other causes can include metabolic imbalances, vitamin B_{12} deficiency, stroke, and brain tumor. Magnetic resonance imagining (MRI) of the brain is performed primarily to rule out other conditions such as normal pressure hydrocephalus or subdural hematoma, which also can cause dementia symptoms (Leifer, 2003). In early stages, an MRI may show atrophy in the hippocampal

---

NATIONAL GUIDELINES DSM-IV-TR Criteria for Dementia of the Alzheimer's Type

A. Multiple cognitive deficits manifested by both:
1. Memory impairment (impaired ability to learn new information or to recall previously learned information)
2. One or more of the following cognitive disturbances:
   a. Aphasia (language disturbance)
   b. Apraxia (impaired ability to carry out motor activities despite intact motor function)
   c. Agnosia (failure to recognize or identify objects despite intact sensory function)
   d. Disturbance in executive functioning (i.e., planning, organizing, sequencing, abstracting).

B. The cognitive deficits cause significant impairment in social or occupational functioning and represent a significant decline from a previous level of functioning.

C. The course is characterized by general onset and continuing cognitive decline.

D. Cognitive deficits are not due to:
1. Other CNS conditions that cause progressive memory and cognition deficits (i.e., cerebrovascular disease, Parkinson's disease, Huntington's disease, subdural hematoma, normal pressure hydrocephalus, brain tumor).
2. Systemic conditions that are known to cause dementia (e.g., hypothyroidism, vitamin B_{12} deficiency, neurosyphilis, HIV infection).

Source: Adapted from American Psychiatric Association. (2000). *Diagnostic and statistical manual of mental disorders* (4th ed.). Washington, DC: Author.

area, while later stages will show generalized atrophy (Desai & Grossberg, 2005). Positron emission tomography (PET) has been shown to detect significant alterations in brain metabolism produced by AD and is increasingly being used as a diagnostic tool, especially in cases where a diagnosis of dementia remains uncertain despite a thorough evaluation (Desai & Grossberg, 2005; Silverman, et al., 2001). Functional MRI (fMRI) is used primarily for research purposes to measure changes in brain function and structure, although it has future potential as a diagnostic and monitoring tool (NIA, 2007). In addition to the test results and patient assessment, interviewing a close relative or associate is considered to be another important diagnostic tool. Other tests are listed in the Diagnostic Tests box.

The diagnostic process includes a detailed medical history, physical examination, and neurological assessment, paying particular attention to the duration and progression of the patient's memory loss. Complete and accurate charting of former and current medical conditions, medications, and behavioral symptoms are necessary considerations when prescribing treatments.

Whenever the patient has cognitive and memory difficulties, interviewing the primary caregiver and/or other family members can help to supplement the history. Cognitive status is often evaluated using the Folstein Mini-Mental Status Exam (MMSE). The MMSE is an 11-question measure that tests five areas of cognitive function: orientation, registration, attention and calculation, recall, and language. The maximum score is 30. A score of 23 or lower is indicative of cognitive impairment. The MMSE takes only 5 to 10 minutes to administer and is, therefore, practical to use repeatedly and routinely. The MMSE is considered to be a national standard as a screening device to identify patients with cognitive impairment from those without it in both clinical practice and research (Kurlowicz & Wallace, 1999).

For a detailed evaluation of cognitive functioning, a neuropsychological evaluation of language, memory, problem-solving skills, and visuospatial skills provides a cognitive baseline and measures performance in comparison with an age-matched cohort. The diagnostic work-up concludes with an evaluation of the patient's ability to perform self-care and function normally in daily living (Cummings, Frank, Cherry, Kohatsu, & Kemp, 2002a, 2002b).

After the initial diagnosis, biannual follow-up assessments are recommended. These ongoing examinations are necessary to evaluate response to medications, concurrent medical conditions, and progression of memory impairment (Cummings et al., 2002a, 2002b). When monitoring MMSE results in cases of AD, scores drop at an average rate of 4 points per year (Leifer, 2003).

The presence of depression can complicate the diagnosis of dementia or AD. Depression is the most common form of psychiatric illness in the elderly. Symptoms common to both AD and depression include behavioral slowing, complaints of cognitive difficulties, fatigue, and changes in sleep and appetite. Depression also can occur concurrently with AD, making it critical to separate the diagnosis of AD and depression before appropriate treatments can be implemented (Cummings et al., 2002a, 2002b).

Delirium also could manifest symptoms similar to dementia. Delirium is a transient and potentially reversible condition with fluctuating levels of awareness, hallucinations, and cognitive impairment (Gleason, 2003). Delirium also is discussed in Chapter 10 as relevant to the aging patient.

The critical difference between dementia and delirium is that delirium is transient and caused by an underlying medical condition, whereas dementia is progressive and irreversible. Common causes of delirium include renal or liver failure, vitamin B_{12} deficiencies, trauma such as hip fractures and head injuries, and medications.

Other Forms of Dementia

Besides AD, other primary dementias include vascular dementia, Lewy body dementia, and frontotemporal dementia. While

---

DIAGNOSTIC TESTS for Alzheimer's Disease

Test	Expected Result	Rationale
Complete blood count (CBC), electrolytes, blood urea nitrogen (BUN), creatinine, random blood glucose, calcium	Within normal limits (WNL)	Rule out metabolic abnormalities.
TSH	WNL	Rule out hypothyroidism.
Vitamin B_{12}	WNL	Rule out vitamin B_{12} deficiency.
Syphilis serology*	Negative	Rule out syphilis.
HIV*	Negative	Rule out HIV.
Heavy metals*	Negative	
MRI or CT scan	WNL for age; in early stages, mild atrophy may be present in hippocampal regions; in moderate to severe stages, atrophy may be more generalized	Rule out stroke, brain tumor, hydrocephalus, or other structural abnormalities.

*If history indicates.

Sources: Adapted from Alzheimer's Association. (2003). *Provider checklist for treating a confused elder*. Retrieved April 30, 2008, from http://alzla.org/medical/Checklisthtml.html; Farlow, M. R. (2005).The search for disease modification in moderate to severe Alzheimer's disease. *Neurology, 65* (Suppl. 3), S25–S30; Knopman, D. S., DeKosky, S. T., Cummings, J. L., Chui, H., Corey-Bloom, J., Relkin, N., et al. (2001). Practice parameter: Diagnosis of dementia (an evidence-based review). *Neurology, 56*, 1143–1153; Leifer, B. P. (2003). Early diagnosis of Alzheimer's disease: Clinical and economic benefits. *Journal of the American Geriatrics Society, 51*, S281–S288.

CHART 31–2	**Overview of Other Common Types of Dementia**	
Type	**Characteristics**	**Pathology**
Vascular dementia	Most common form of dementia after AD Abrupt onset with stepwise deterioration Focal neurological symptoms; signs or history of stroke	Multiple infarcts on MRI
Lewy body dementia (LBD)	Gradual onset Fluctuating cognitive deficits Parkinsonian symptoms (rigidity, bradykinesia) not responsive to levodopa Visual hallucinations	Lewy bodies (identified on brain autopsy) present in cytoplasm of cortical neurons
Frontotemporal dementia (FTD)	Insidious onset Slowly progressive Psychiatric symptoms include disinhibition, delusions, and social inappropriateness Neglect of hygiene/grooming Incontinence	Atrophy of frontal lobes and anterior temporal lobes Neuronal loss Tau tangles Gliosis

Sources: Leifer, B. P. (2003). Early diagnosis of Alzheimer's disease: Clinical and economic benefits. *Journal of the American Geriatrics Society, 51*, S281–S288; National Institute on Aging, U.S. Nation Institutes of Health. (2007). Frontotemporal dementia connections reprint. Retrieved July 18, 2008 from http://www.nia.nih.gov/Alzheimers/Publications/FTDreprint.htm.

the diagnostic work-up for any form of dementia is the same, treatments for some types will make symptoms worse in other types, thereby making it important to distinguish the type of dementia afflicting the patient. The unique clinical and pathologic characteristics of various forms are summarized in Chart 31–2.

Medical Management

A handful of medications are available to treat AD. At best, these drugs only temporarily slow cognitive and functional loss. As AD continues to progress, treatment increasingly focuses on non-pharmacologic approaches to managing behavioral symptoms.

Drug Therapy

The goals of pharmacologic treatment for AD are to preserve cognitive and functional abilities, minimize behavioral disturbances, and slow the progression of the disease (Geldmacher, 2003). With AD, levels of **acetylcholine**, a neurotransmitter critical in the process of memory formation and especially important to neurons in the hippocampus and cerebral cortex, are lowered as neuronal degeneration occurs. The resulting decreases of acetylcholine and cholinergic activity in general are associated with memory impairment. Increasing available acetylcholine can potentially improve memory symptoms. The only medications approved by the Food and Drug Administration (FDA) for the treatment of mild to moderate AD are acetylcholinesterase inhibitors (AChEIs), which increase cholinergic activity and can improve cognitive symptoms of AD (DeKosky, 2003). Although these medications do not reverse or prevent cell death (Geldmacher, 2003), there is evidence that they may improve cognitive functioning and decrease behavioral symptoms, at least in the mild to moderate stages (Cummings et al., 2002a, 2002b). Three FDA-approved AChEIs, donepezil (Aricept), rivastigmine (Exelon), and galantamine (Reminyl), are currently used in the treatment of AD. See the Pharmacology Summary for a description of these medications, including common dosages and side effects.

Late in 2003, the FDA approved the first *N*-methyl-D-aspartate (NMDA) receptor antagonist, memantine (Namenda), for the treatment of moderate to severe AD. Memantine is thought to block the action of **glutamate**, an excitatory neurotransmitter. Glutamate activates NMDA receptors, which modulate the chemical environment necessary for memory. An excess of glutamate overstimulates NMDA receptors, which can lead to cell death. Memantine may protect cells from excess glutamate by partially blocking NMDA receptors (Alzheimer's Association, 2004). While memantine and AChEIs may help symptoms of AD, it does not prevent or slow the neurological degeneration associated with it (FDA, 2003).

Treating Behavioral Symptoms

Behavioral symptoms that present with the disease often are the most difficult for caregivers to manage (Cummings et al., 2002a, 2002b). Restlessness, agitation, anger, anxiety, wandering, or psychotic symptoms may require treatment with psychotropic medications (Geldmacher, 2003). Nonpharmacologic approaches to managing behavioral symptoms center on reducing environmental stimuli, establishing predictable routines, simplifying tasks, and using distraction and redirection (Cummings et al., 2002a, 2002b). See the Pharmacology Summary for a list of drugs used to treat behavioral symptoms of AD.

Before implementing psychotropic medications, other conditions that may contribute to behavioral symptoms should be disqualified. These include, but are not limited to, delirium, pain, infection, or other acute medical conditions (Cummings et al., 2002a, 2002b).

Potential Treatments Undergoing Research

Several agents are undergoing research as potential treatments or preventive therapies for AD. Cholesterol has been associated with ApoE, beta-amyloid, and vascular damage. Studies have shown a decreased AD prevalence and risk reduction in those patients taking statin drugs. Prospective research trials are in process to further delineate the potential role of cholesterol in the prevention of AD (DeKosky, 2003). Because inflammatory changes are associated with the disease process, anti-inflammatory medications may have a role in preventing AD. Large-scale studies examining

PHARMACOLOGY Summary of Medications to Treat Alzheimer's Disease

Medication Category	Action	Application/Indication	Nursing Responsibility
Acetylcholinesterase Inhibitors			
• Galantamine (Reminyl) • Rivastigmine (Exelon) • Donepezil (Aricept)	Increase acetylcholine levels in the brain.	Treatment of mild to moderate disease	Monitor for nausea, vomiting, diarrhea, weight loss.
NMDA Receptor Antagonist			
• Memantine (Namenda)	Blocks action of glutamate, decreasing activation of NMDA receptors.	Treatment of moderate to severe disease	Monitor for headache, constipation, confusion, dizziness.
Behavioral Symptoms of Alzheimer's Disease **Atypical Antipsychotics**			
• Olanzapine (Zyprexa) • Quetiapine (Seroquel)	Act as antagonists of dopamine and serotonin.	Delusions, hallucinations, agitation, combativeness	Monitor mental status and response to drug therapy. Monitor for orthostatic hypotension, somnolence.
Selective Serotonin-Reuptake Inhibitors			
• Sertraline (Zoloft) • Citalopram (Celexa)	Inhibit uptake of the neurotransmitter serotonin in CNS, potentiating the effects of serotonin. Has little or no effect on other neurotransmitters.	Depression, irritability	Monitor for mood changes, somnolence, and insomnia.

anti-inflammatory drugs and their potential use as a treatment are being conducted now (DeKosky, 2003).

Researchers also are looking at folate. Deficiencies of folate have been associated with increased levels of homocysteine, which is another possible risk factor for developing AD (DeKosky, 2003). Estrogen also could be a possible preventive therapy. Studies suggest that it may protect against AD. More research is needed and in process (DeKosky, 2003). Antioxidants vitamins C and E are believed to be neurologically protective against oxidative damage, again present in AD. Clinical trials to evaluate the role of vitamin E in slowing disease progression are under way. The herbal supplement gingko biloba also has been considered as a treatment, as discussed in the Complementary and Alternative Therapies box.

Gerontological Considerations

Because dementia affects primarily the elderly, its signs are often characterized as naturally occurring senility common to old age. This misunderstanding could confuse the signs of dementia and AD with normal aging. This not only perpetuates fallacies of aging, it runs the risk of delaying early, accurate diagnosis and prompt treatment.

With the highest prevalence rates in the oldest segment of the population, nurses will need to recognize the factors that influence an elderly person's response to drugs prescribed for AD. Inevitably, the aging patient likely may have concurrent medical conditions that require multiple medications, presenting the potential for drug interactions and adverse effects. Slowed renal clearance and hepatic metabolism may influence medication

COMPLEMENTARY & ALTERNATIVE THERAPIES   Ginkgo Biloba

Ginkgo biloba has undergone research as a potential treatment for AD. It is thought to have antioxidant and possibly anti-inflammatory and antiplatelet activity (DeKosky, 2003). It is commonly used in Germany to treat AD; however, insufficient studies preclude recommended use in the United States. Results are pending from the Ginkgo Evaluation of Memory Study, sponsored by the National Center for Complementary Medicine, the National Institute on Aging, and the National Heart, Lung, and Blood Institute. This interventional study will help determine the effect of ginkgo biloba in decreasing the incidence of AD and slowing cognitive decline and functional disability (Alzheimer's Disease Education and Referral Center, 2003). Ginkgo biloba should only be taken under the direction of a health care provider, as the risk of spontaneous bleeding increased when it is taken

with non-steroidal anti-inflammatory drugs (NSAIDS) and anticoagulants such as heparin or warfarin (De Smet, 2002).

References

Alzheimer's Disease Education and Referral Center. (2003). *Gingko biloba fact sheet.* Retrieved April 14, 2008, from http://www.alzheimers.org.

De Smet, P. (2002). Herbal remedies. *New England Journal of Medicine, 347*(25), 2046–2076.

DeKosky, S. T. (2003). Pathology and pathways of Alzheimer's disease with an update in new developments in treatment. *Journal of the American Geriatrics Society, 51,* S314–S320.

tolerance. Drugs that cause sedation have an adverse effect on cognition.

The crippling effect AD has on those who develop it also comes with significant psychosocial ramifications. Often it will impact an elderly spouse or adult children who are called on to provide care and support. Research has demonstrated that the implications of the elderly caring for the elderly in terms of stress and burden on an older caregiver's physical, mental, and financial well-being are substantive.

Special nursing interventions for this population include a complete medical history with special attention to concurrent medical problems and to polypharmacy. Caregiver burden and stress should be periodically assessed, with assistance to develop coping mechanisms. Referrals should be made to appropriate community resources for example, the local area agency on aging.

■ Nursing Management

Use of the nursing process will facilitate a comprehensive approach to patient and caregiver support throughout the course of the disease (see the Nursing Process: Patient Care Plan for Alzheimer's Disease feature). Protecting the patient from injury, managing dysfunctional behaviors, and supporting the patient and caregiver in activities of daily living (ADLs) are the primary focus of nursing care. Nurses must be prepared to assist family caregivers in dealing with denial, anger, guilt, grief, or clinical depression as the patient progresses, with the goal of helping the caregiver adjust and adapt to the changes associated with the progressive stages (Volcifer & McKee, 2001). See the Cultural Considerations box for a discussion related to the care of the patient and family with AD.

■ Collaborative Management

Throughout the disease process, a multidisciplinary approach facilitates optimal disease management. In the early and mid-stages of the disease, periodic outpatient visits to the neurologist will be required for medication management. Neuropsychologists play critical roles in the periodic evaluation of cognitive function. Geriatric psychiatrists may become involved either at the time of diagnosis or as the behavioral symptoms increase.

CULTURAL CONSIDERATIONS Related to Alzheimer's Disease

Throughout the nursing process, cultural sensitivity is imperative. The meaning of dementia, how families care for elders, and help-seeking methods can all vary depending on ethnicity. Recent studies suggest that ethnically diverse older people frequently subscribe to folk beliefs to explain dementia, rather than the biomedical explanation of a physical disease or condition. Such folk explanations might include that AD is caused by psychosocial stress or that it is a normal part of aging (Hinton, Franz, Yeo, & Levkoff, 2005). Nurses need to consider the patient's and family's perspective of dementia, and approach the provision of care in a way that considers those views and values.

Sources: Ackley, B. J., & Ludwig, G. B. (Eds.). (2003). *Nursing diagnosis handbook: A guide to planning care* (6th ed.). St. Louis: Mosby; Doenges, M. E., & Moorhouse, M. F. (2003). *Application of nursing process and diagnosis: An interactive text for diagnostic reasoning* (4th ed.). Philadelphia: F. A. Davis.

Physical therapy may be needed as mobility becomes affected and to counteract contractures in the end stages. Occupational therapy will help the patient and caregiver accomplish ADLs. A psychologist, social worker, or mental health professional is needed to help the family work through altered dynamics and to plan for long-term care.

Discharge Priorities

Discharge plans for the patient with AD, as discussed in the Patient Teaching & Discharge Priorities box (p. 799), are extremely important to maintaining functional goals.

Health Promotion

The physical and mental health of the primary family caregiver is critical to the care of the Alzheimer's patient. Caregivers suffer from higher rates of depression and physical illness than persons not functioning in a caregiver role (Schultz, O'Brien, Bookwala, & Fleissner, 1995). Nurses can optimize both patient and caregiver health by (Cummings et al., 2002a, 2002b):

- Providing pertinent information, both written and verbal, about AD

- Referring to organizations for assistance with finding community resources, support groups, financial and legal advice, respite, and long-term care options

- Encouraging discussion about advance directives for management of advanced stages of AD

- Assisting the primary caregiver in managing stress and developing coping mechanisms through psychoeducational interventions and individual and/or group therapy.

In its attempt to produce excellence in the care of Alzheimer's patients, the Alzheimer's Foundation of America (AFA) has developed a nationwide standard of excellence for settings that provide care to individuals with Alzheimer's disease or related dementias. This new initiative, called Excellence in Care, involves on-site evaluations of dementia care settings and assistance in meeting the comprehensive set of standards. The standards reflect what AFA believes to be essential components of any quality dementia care program. Areas of evaluation include the physical environment, safety procedures, program activities, staff–client interaction, and training of staff and families (AFA, 2006).

■ Parkinson's Disease

Parkinson's disease (PD) is second to Alzheimer's disease as the most common of the neurological degenerative disorders (Nussbaum & Ellis, 2003). It is recognized as the most common movement disorder (Dawson & Dawson, 2003).

Epidemiology and Etiology

With the cardinal symptoms of tremor, rigidity, bradykinesia, and postural instability, PD is estimated to afflict about 1,000,000 Americans (Nutt & Wooten, 2005), with a lifetime risk of 1 in 40 to 50 (Schapira, 2006). Incidence increases with age, rising sharply after age 60; about 4% of the cases occur before age 50 (Van Den Eeden et al., 2003).

Although the cause of idiopathic PD is not known, both genetic and environmental factors have been implicated (Schapira,

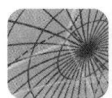

NURSING PROCESS: Patient Care Plan for Alzheimer's Disease

Assessment of Safety and Self-Care Ability

Subjective Data:
(Involve family members.)
Does the patient fall frequently?
Has the patient been hurt as a result of falling?
Does the patient wander?
Does the patient wear glasses or a hearing aid?
Does the patient use a walker?

Objective Data:
Neurological status, including orientation, memory, sensory, gait judgment, insight
Wandering behavior

Nursing Assessment and Diagnoses	Outcomes and Evaluation Parameters	Planning and Interventions with *Rationales*
Nursing Diagnosis: *High Risk for Injury* related to poor memory, insight, judgment, and self-control; unstable gait	**Outcome:** Patient remains injury free. *Evaluation Parameters:* Patient uses sensory aids and assistive devices. Family identifies potential environmental hazards. Patient does not fall. Patient does not wander.	**Interventions and *Rationales*:** Encourage use of eyeglasses, hearing aids, and assistive devices such as a walker. *Optimal eyesight and hearing will help patient with environmental awareness; assistive devices will stabilize gait.* Remove potential hazards from environment such as sharp objects and medications *to prevent patient from harming self.* Ensure that patient has identification bracelet. Encourage family to register patient with Safe Return program of the Alzheimer's Association. *Patient may wander and cause harm to self or others.*

Assessment of Cognition and Thought Processes

Subjective Data:
(Involve family members.)
Does the patient hear voices or see things that are not there?
Is the patient easily agitated?
Does the patient act impulsively?

Objective Data:
Neurological status, including orientation, memory, sensory, gait judgment, insight
Ability to follow instructions
Agitation/restlessness
Paranoia

Nursing Assessment and Diagnoses	Outcomes and Evaluation Parameters	Planning and Interventions with *Rationales*
Nursing Diagnosis: *Disturbed Thought Processes* (inappropriate reactions, dysfunctional behavior, delusions and paranoia) related to cognitive decline	**Outcome:** Remains oriented to extent possible given stage of disease. *Evaluation Parameter:* Demonstrates fewer episodes of agitation, delusions, paranoia, or other dysfunctional behavior.	**Interventions and *Rationales*:** When communicating with patient: Approach patient in a gentle, calm manner *to prevent patient from being startled or frightened.* Communicate using short, simple sentences, yes/no questions. *Negative feedback leads to increased confusion and agitation.* Break directions down into short, simple steps. *Unable to follow complex directions; decreases frustration.* Redirect conversation without contradicting or criticizing the patient's statements *to decrease anxiety, frustration.* Maintain consistent daily schedule *to decrease anxiety; situational anxiety due to change can lead to agitation.* Monitor for nonverbal behaviors such as grimacing or increased restlessness. *May indicate pain or discomfort, which may increase agitation.* Create calming environment. Eliminate noise and clutter. *Sensory overload can contribute to disruptive behavior and agitation.* Provide cues to orientation including verbal cues, clocks, and calendars. *Reorients patient to reality as much as possible.* Display pictures, mementos, and encourage reminiscence. *Can comfort patient and trigger memories.*

(continued)

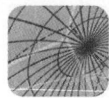

NURSING PROCESS: Patient Care Plan for Alzheimer's Disease—*Continued*

Assessment of

Subjective Data:

(Involve family members.)

Does the patient bathe, groom, and dress independently?

Are these activities accomplished appropriately?

Does the patient become agitated during these activities?

Does the patient require assistance with self-care activities?

Do you have an established schedule for these activities?

Objective Data:

Neurological status, including orientation, memory, sensory, gait judgment, insight, apraxia, agnosia

Appearance

Ability to draw bath or start shower, brush teeth, select and put on clothing

Ability to follow instructions

Nursing Assessment and Diagnoses	Outcomes and Evaluation Parameters	Planning and Interventions with *Rationales*
Nursing Diagnosis: *Self-Care Deficits* (bathing, hygiene, dressing, grooming) related to cognitive losses, impaired judgment	**Outcome:** Self-care needs are met. **Evaluation Parameters:** Performs self-care independently to the extent possible given disease progression. Daily routine of bathing, hygiene, dressing, and grooming is established with patient and family. Staff and family assist with self-care needs.	**Interventions and *Rationales:*** Assist patient to perform self-care such as bathing, dressing, and toileting *to obtain a baseline assessment of ability.* Keep instructions short, simple, and repeat frequently *to allow patient to perform activities; complicated directions can lead to frustration and agitation.* Avoid distractions during bathing, toileting, and dressing. *Sensory overload contributes to agitation and confusion.* Allow sufficient time to perform activities. *Rushing the patient may lead to agitation.* Provide privacy during self-care activities *to demonstrate respect for patient.* Maintain consistent schedule for bathing, dressing, and toileting. *Establishing routine may help decrease agitation during self-care tasks.* Provide care that patient is not able to do *to ensure that all care tasks are completed.*

Sources: Jankovic, J. (2006). Therapeutic strategies in Parkinson's disease. *Geriatrics, 61,* 3–7; Schapira, A. H. V. (2006). Etiology of Parkinson's disease. *Neurology, 66* (Suppl. 4).

2006). It is thought that the resulting disease process results from a complex interaction between genetic and environmental factors that differ from one individual to another (Jankovic, 2006) (see the Genetic Considerations and Risk Factors boxes, p. 800).

Pathophysiology

PD is a disease of the basal ganglia, a structure deep in the brain that includes the corpus striatum and globus pallidus (Figures 31–6 and 31–7 ■, p. 800). These structures are critical to the system of connections that joins the cerebral cortex and the thalamus and allows for ease of movement. The origin of PD pathology lies in the **substantia nigra**, a structure located in the midbrain, beneath the basal ganglia. Neurons in the substantia nigra produce **dopamine**, a neurotransmitter that is necessary for smooth, voluntary movement. Through the connections of the nigral striatal pathway, dopamine is transmitted from the substantia nigra to the striatum. This cycle allows for the smoothness and ease of normal, voluntary movement. In PD, the neurons of the substantia nigra inexplicably begin to degenerate and die. The resulting lack of dopamine production leads to difficulty with movement, tremor, rigidity, and difficulty maintaining posture.

When approximately 70% of the neurons in the substantia nigra have degenerated and/or died, the symptoms of PD begin to appear. Acetylcholine, another neurotransmitter, also is believed to be involved in the pathology. The lack of dopamine upsets the delicate balance between these two neurotransmitters. The defining pathologic feature of PD is the presence of Lewy bodies and neuronal loss in the substantia nigra (Schapira, 2006). Lewy bodies are detected only at brain autopsy, which is required for a definitive diagnosis of PD.

Several medications can cause parkinsonian symptoms, although they do not cause the idiopathic form of PD. These symptoms are often called drug-induced parkinsonism, or pseudo-parkinsonism. Drugs that can cause symptoms of PD include neuroleptics, such as haloperidol and risperidone, and antiemetics, such as Compazine and metoclopramide. Withdrawal from the offending agents will reverse the parkinsonian symptoms, although it may take weeks and possibly months. These medications should be avoided in patients with PD (Nutt & Wooten, 2005).

 Common drugs contraindicated in Parkinson's disease include:

Antiemetics

Prochlorperazine (Compazine)

Metoclopramide (Reglan)

Neuroleptics

Chlorpromazine (Thorazine)

Haloperidol (Haldol)

Nutt & Wooten (2005)

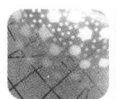

PATIENT TEACHING & DISCHARGE PRIORITIES for Alzheimer's Disease

Need	Teaching
Medication management: Patient/family	Adhere to medication schedule. Monitor response to medication. Monitor and report side effects.
Disease process: Patient/family	Describe diagnostic tests and need for brain autopsy for confirmation. Describe pathophysiology; cause not known. State signs, symptoms, and stages of disease progression. Describe possible treatments.
Activities of daily living: Family Setting	Use wall calendar to mark events and activities to aid orientation and mark passage of time. Place clocks prominently around house. Keep belongings consistently in one place. Use automatic dialing phone. Keep bathing and dressing routines consistent.
Safety: Family Setting	Remove potential hazards: • Cover electrical outlets to prevent shock. • Put locks on cabinets that contain potentially hazardous materials such as medications, cleaning agents, kitchen appliances, knives, or razor blades. • Store firearms in locked area. • Lower water heater temperature to avoid burns. • Remove furniture with sharp corners or pad the corners. • Serve food on plastic plates to prevent breakage. • Use professionally installed safety rails in bathroom and stairway. Hide car keys if necessary. Use signaling device if wandering is a problem. Enroll in Alzheimer Association's Safe Return program.
Managing wandering, aggression, agitation: Family	Reduce stressful situations. Establish daily routines. Simplify surroundings. Look for signs of pain or illness. Encourage light exercise, walking if possible.
Communication: Family	Listen and communicate patiently and in calm, relaxed manner. Replace contradicting with listening and questioning in caring manner. Use words or pictures to cue memories.
Community resources: Family	Contact the Alzheimer's Association (1-800-272-3900) and its local chapter for information about disease process, managing symptoms, and local support groups. Enroll in Alzheimer Association's Safe Return if wandering is a problem. Contact local area agency on aging for home care, respite, or adult day care referrals.
End-of-life issues: Patient/family	Establish advance directive, living will. Explore option of using hospice services.
Caregiver issues: Family	State signs/symptoms of increasing stress and burnout. Get adequate rest. Eat balanced meals and nutritious foods. Exercise. Use relaxation techniques such as deep breathing or meditation. Use community resources for assistance and respite. Attend caregiver support groups.

Sources: Fischer Center for Alzheimer's Research Foundation. Alzheimer's Research Foundation. (2002–2008). Alzheimer's Disease Cause, Care, & Cure. Retrieved July 18, 2008 from http://www.alzinfo.org.

GENETIC CONSIDERATIONS Related to Parkinson's Disease

Several recent studies confirm that PD is more common in relatives of PD patients than in those without relatives affected with PD. Studies of PD in twins have concluded that genetic factors do not play a significant role in cases of those with onset commencing at over age 50; however, genetic factors may be at work in earlier onset cases. While genetic research has linked mutations in the alpha-synuclein and parkin genes to PD, only about 1% of cases are clearly genetic (Schapira, 2006; Tanner et al., 1999).

RISK FACTORS for Parkinson's Disease

Without a known cause of idiopathic PD, definitive risk factors are not clear. However, certain factors have been linked with PD, including the following:

Family history

Pesticide exposure

Rural living

Farming as an occupation

Drinking well water

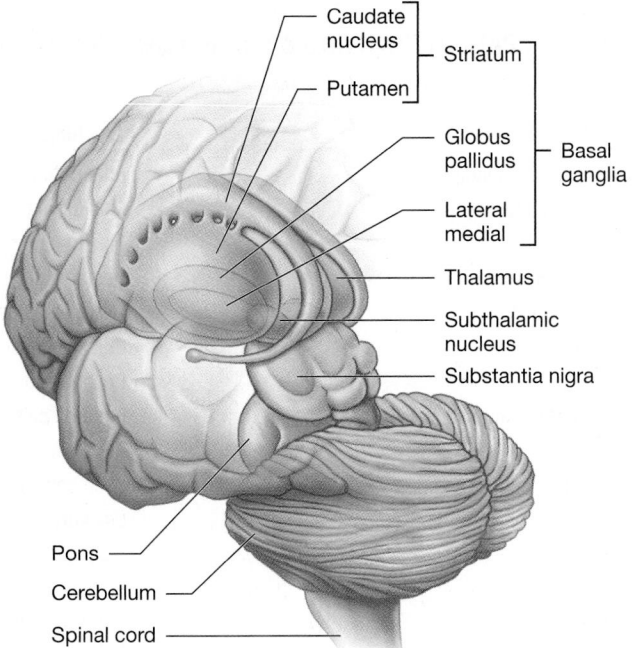

FIGURE 31–7 ■ Main connections of the basal ganglia.

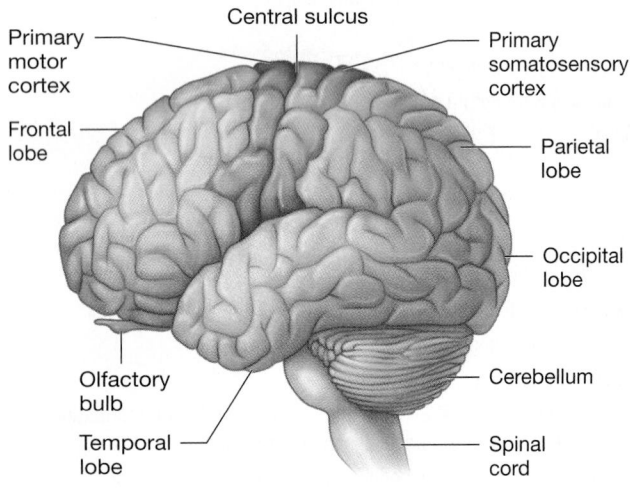

FIGURE 31–6 ■ Cerebral hemispheres and brainstem.

Clinical Manifestations

PD is characterized by four primary symptoms: resting tremor, rigidity, bradykinesia, and postural instability. Secondary and autonomic symptoms also may be present. Secondary symptoms often result from combinations of the primary symptoms.

Primary Symptoms

A parkinsonian tremor characteristically occurs at rest and manifests as involuntary shaking in the hand and wrist or feet while the muscles are relaxed. The tremor may decrease with activity. Although a resting tremor is commonly the first symptom, about 20% of patients do not exhibit this symptom (Nutt & Wooten, 2005). The tremor usually is present only on one side of the body in the early stages of PD, but may spread to the other side as the disease progresses. A "pill-rolling" tremor is particularly characteristic and appears as though a person is rolling a pill between his thumb and forefinger (National Institute of Neurological Disorders and Stroke [NINDS], 2006).

Rigidity, or muscle stiffness, may be felt throughout any given range of movement. Typically, Parkinsonian rigidity is characterized as hypertonicity of muscles resulting in stiffness of motion and is often associated with aching and discomfort (Nutt & Wooten, 2005).

Bradykinesia, one of the more disabling symptoms of PD, refers to slowness of movement. Bradykinesia is often the most prominent and disabling symptom, causing difficulty with walking, changing positions, and speaking and swallowing (NINDS, 2006).

Postural instability refers to the balancing difficulties that result from the diminishing of the reflexes that allow a person to maintain her balance (NINDS, 2006). The patient will have difficulty staying balanced and may even fall when changing positions.

Secondary Symptoms

Secondary symptoms usually are the result of the overarching, primary symptoms. Rigid facial muscles combined with bradykinesia lead to **hypomimia**, or decreased facial expression, resulting in the characteristic "masked" face of a PD patient. The decrease in facial expression often conveys lack of emotion, or a depressed affect, which may or may not actually be present. Muscle rigidity, bradykinesia, and postural instability may combine to produce gait abnormalities, like a shuffled walk, difficulty turning while walking, and stooped posture. Face and neck muscles used for talking may be affected as well. Voice changes associated with PD are known as **hypokinetic dysarthria**. They include **hypophonia**, or a soft, muffled speech. Similarly, the muscles used for swallowing become rigid, leading to dysphagia, or difficulty swallowing. **Micrographia**, or small, cramped handwriting, results from rigidity and bradykinesia in the hands (Jankovic, 2006).

Autonomic Symptoms

PD affects the autonomic nervous system, which can lead to symptoms not related to movement. Constipation is common and PD medications may exacerbate it. Orthostatic hypotension, sexual dysfunction, excessive sweating, and urinary incontinence are other common symptoms (Jankovic, 2006).

Neuropsychiatric Symptoms

Neuropsychiatric changes and cognitive impairments including dementia are estimated to occur in 30% of patients. Up to 60% of people with PD may suffer from depression. Depression in this population may be difficult to detect, since many of the symptoms are similar to PD, such as loss of facial expression, motor and mental slowing, and cognitive difficulties (Calne, 2003).

Disease Progression

As PD progresses, motor complications develop. **Dyskinesias**—involuntary, writhing motions that may involve the limbs, trunk, face, and neck—are a side effect of dopaminergic medications and result from overstimulation of dopamine receptors. Drug therapy regimes can create fluctuations in movement ability, known as **on–off phenomena**. When "on," the patient is experiencing a positive response to medication, but the effects may suddenly wear off, rendering the patient barely able to move, or "off." These reactions are related to building a tolerance to or having an unpredictable response to levodopa (Pahwa et al., 2006). Dyskinesia and the associated motor fluctuations can cause a great diversity and range of physical capacity and disability during the course of an average day. The unpredictable nature of these fluctuations interferes greatly with the patient's ability to plan for and perform routine activities.

As motor function worsens, so can other PD symptoms. Dysphagia often worsens over time and a feeding tube may be required to prevent the aspiration of food. Worsening orthostatic hypotension and postural instability increase the risk of injuries resulting from a fall (Bunting-Perry, 2006). Although PD is not considered a fatal disease, the degrading effect it has on the patient's ability to carry out basic daily functions can cause susceptibility to more threatening conditions such as pneumonia or traumatic injury.

Laboratory and Diagnostic Procedures

There is no definitive laboratory or radiological test to diagnose PD. Diagnosis is based on a neurological exam and clinical history. Laboratory tests and MRI are used to rule out other possible causes of the presenting symptoms. The positive response to dopaminergic medications reassures the PD diagnosis. Diagnostic criteria include the following (Pahwa, Lyons, & Wilkinson, 2003):

- Bradykinesia and either resting tremor or rigidity
- Positive response to levodopa
- Other causes ruled out, such as drugs, stroke, or metabolic abnormalities
- Definite diagnosis only by autopsy.

PD is commonly staged using the Hoehn and Yahr scale (1967):

- **Stage I**—Unilateral disease
- **Stage II**—Bilateral disease with preservation of postural reflexes

- **Stage III**—Bilateral disease with impaired postural reflexes; able to ambulate
- **Stage IV**—Severe disease requiring assistance
- **Stage V**—End-stage disease, confined to bed or chair.

Medical Management

An effective treatment for protecting against the loss of dopamine-producing neurons remains to be discovered. Because PD involves the loss of dopamine-producing neurons and the subsequent diminished supply of dopamine in the striatum, dopaminergic drugs that can increase dopamine levels are the first line of treatment. Novel new surgical procedures also can provide relief in advanced cases. Treatment of the secondary symptoms such as hypotension and constipation also is included in a broad approach to increase mobility, decrease symptoms, and improve quality of life, as the underlying disease progresses despite all treatments.

Also noted are the new guidelines published by the American Academy of Neurology regarding the treatment of Parkinson's disease. The guidelines tend to be more proscriptive than prescriptive (Susman, 2006). The guidelines inform the health care provider, as well as patients, that there is no neuroprotective therapy that has shown any proven value. The guidelines demonstrate that nutritional supplementation, for example, does not work. They do note 20 specific recommendations that are categorized under four broad areas:

- Diagnosis and prognosis of new-onset disease
- Neuroprotective treatments and alternative therapies
- Management of Parkinson's disease with motor fluctuations and dyskinesias
- Depression, psychosis, and dementia that are associated with Parkinson's disease (American Academy of Neurology, 2006; Susman, 2006).

Dopaminergic Drugs

Often referred to as dopaminergic drugs, these medications enhance the levels of dopamine naturally produced in the brain. Levodopa was the first breakthrough in treatment for PD in the 1960s, and it is still considered the most effective drug for PD (Jankovic, 2006; Nutt & Wooten, 2005). Dopamine itself cannot cross the blood–brain barrier (Ahlskog, 2001). **Levodopa** is the amino acid precursor of dopamine, and it can cross the blood–brain barrier. Once in the brain, levodopa is converted to dopamine (Ahlskog, 2001). However, a portion of levodopa is converted into dopamine by dopa-decarboxylase prior to entering the brain, leaving dopamine in the circulating system and causing severe nausea and vomiting.

Levodopa is given with carbidopa, a dopa-decarboxylase inhibitor, which blocks premature conversion of dopa into dopamine and minimizes nausea and vomiting (Jankovic, 2006; Nutt & Wooten, 2005). A combination of carbidopa/levodopa is available in tablet form and it varies in dosage combinations. For example, carbidopa/levodopa 25/100 tablets contain 25 mg of carbidopa and 100 mg of levodopa. The first number indicates milligrams of carbidopa, and the second indicates milligrams of levodopa.

Levodopa therapy effectively manages motor PD symptoms in most patients for 4 to 6 years; after that time, nearly half of the patients will develop motor fluctuations and/or dyskinesia (Ahlskog, 2001). Common side effects that may manifest at initiation of therapy include nausea, vomiting, loss of appetite, hypotension, confusion, and hallucinations (Nutt & Wooten, 2005). The motor complications resulting from levodopa therapy have a lower likelihood of occurring with dopamine agonist therapy (Ahlskog, 2001).

Although slightly less effective than levodopa, dopamine agonists are an alternative to levodopa for initial treatment of PD (Nutt & Wooten, 2005). Dopamine agonists approved for the treatment of PD include bromocriptine (Parlodel), pergolide (Permax), pramipexole (Mirapex), ropinirole (Requip), and apomorphine hydrochloride (Apokyn). While levodopa is converted into dopamine within the brain, dopamine agonists act on dopamine receptors within the brain and essentially mimic the effect of dopamine. The side effects of dopamine agonists are similar to those of levodopa. Dopamine agonists are prescribed initially in very low doses and slowly titrated upward to therapeutic amounts (Nutt & Wooten, 2005).

The older dopamine agonists pergolide and bromocriptine are seldom used nowadays because of adverse effects on the heart and lung (Jankovic, 2006), including pleural fibrosis and thickening of cardiac valves (Nutt & Wooten, 2005). Apomorphine hydrochloride differs from the other dopamine agonists in that it is injectable, and it is used as a rapid "rescue" for the PD patient who is undermedicated or "frozen." Symptoms abate 4 to 8 minutes after injection, although the benefit only lasts for 45

to 60 minutes. This drug can cause hypotension and severe nausea and, hence, must be taken with specific antiemetics (Mylan Bertek Pharmaceuticals, 2004).

 CRITICAL ALERT *Patients receiving apomorphine injectable should be monitored closely for the following side effects (Bowron, 2004; Mylan Bertek Pharmaceuticals, 2004):*

Severe nausea: *This side effect may decrease with continued use. Assess patient for previous use of apomorphine with concomitant nausea and vomiting. If antiemetic is needed, it should be administered prior to injection. Trimethobenzamide is the recommended antiemetic. Phenothiazines such as prochlorperazine and 5HT3 antagonists such as odansetron should NOT be given for nausea.*

Orthostatic hypotension: *Blood pressure should be monitored in supine and standing position. Health care provider notified of drop in systolic BP of > 20 mmHg.*

Dyskinesia: *Notify health care provider of onset of involuntary writhing movements of limbs, face, or trunk.*

Anticholinergic Drugs

Anticholinergics are the oldest class of medications used to treat PD. They were commonly used before the discovery of levodopa. These medications are used primarily to treat tremor (Pahwa et al., 2003). Side effects such as dry mouth, blurred vision, constipation, oversedation, urinary retention, and confusion deter their long-term use. The most commonly prescribed medications in this category are trihexyphenidyl (Artane) and benztropine (Cogentin) (Nutt & Wooten, 2005).

PHARMACOLOGY Summary of Medications to Treat Parkinson's Disease

Medication Category	Action	Application/Indication	Nursing Responsibility
Carbidopa/Levodopa • Immediate release • Controlled release • Carbidopa/levodopa/entacapone (Stalevo)	Levodopa is converted to dopamine in the basal ganglia, increasing dopamine concentration within the brain. Carbidopa blocks the peripheral decarboxylation of levodopa, making more levodopa available to the brain.	Symptomatic treatment of idiopathic Parkinson's disease; may be given alone or in combination with other anti-Parkinsonian drugs	Monitor for nausea, hypotension, confusion, hallucinations, motor fluctuations, dyskinesia.
Dopamine Agonists • Bromocriptine (Parlodel) • Pergolide (Permax) • Pramipexole (Mirapex) • Ropinirole (Requip) • Apomorphine hydrochloride (Apokyn) • Rotigotine	Stimulate dopamine receptors in the brain.	May be given as initial treatment or adjunctively with levodopa in advanced cases	Monitor for postural hypotension, nausea, confusion, hallucinations.
Anticholinergics • Benztropine (Cogentin) • Trihexyphenidyl (Artane)	Block cholinergic activity in CNS.	Tremor	Monitor for dry mouth, constipation, urinary retention, blurred vision, hallucinations, confusion.
Antiviral • Amantadine (Symmetrel)	Exact action not clear; likely potentiates dopaminergic transmission in CNS.	Motor fluctuations, dyskinesia	Monitor for lower extremity edema, livedo reticularis, urinary retention, hallucinations.

PHARMACOLOGY Summary of Medications to Treat Parkinson's Disease—*Continued*

Medication Category	Action	Application/Indication	Nursing Responsibility
MAO-B Inhibitors • Seleginine (Eldepryl) • Rasagiline	Exact action not clear; believed to enhance dopaminergic activity in substantia nigra by blocking the enzyme MAO-B.	Sometimes given as monotherapy for initial treatment for PD; usually given adjunctively	Monitor for agitation, insomnia, vivid dreams, hallucinations, orthostatic hypotension.
COMT Inhibitors • Entacapone • Tolcapone	Blocks COMT, an enzyme that metabolizes levodopa; enhances available dopamine.	Given adjunctively with levodopa/carbidopa	Same as for levodopa.

Management of Selected Nonmotor Symptoms of Parkinson's Disease

Medication Category	Action	Application/Indication	Nursing Responsibility
Tricyclic Antidepressants • Amitriptyline (Elavil) **Selective Serotonin Reuptake Inhibitors (SSRIs)** • Fluoxetine (Prozac) • Sertraline (Zoloft) • Paroxetine (Paxil) • Citalopram (Celexa)	Potentiates serotonin and norepinephrine in CNS. Inhibits uptake of neurotransmitter serotonin in CNS, potentiating the effects of serotonin. Has little or no effect on other neurotransmitters.	Depression	*Tricyclics:* Monitor for cognitive changes. May improve insomnia, drooling. Monitor for constipation. *SSRIs:* Monitor for restlessness or agitation. *All:* May take several weeks to reach therapeutic dose. Should not be discontinued suddenly. Assess suicide risk. Encourage concomitant counseling.
Atypical Antipsychotics • Clozapine (Clozaril) • Quetiapine (Seroquel)	Likely act as antagonists of dopamine and serotonin.	Hallucinations	Assess anti-Parkinsonian medication schedule for timing and dosage changes. Assess all current medications for possible cause of hallucinations. Assess for infection. Assess for dehydration or constipation. *Clozapine:* Monitor for agranulocytosis.
Glucocorticoid • Fludrocortisone (Florinef)	Acts on distal renal tubule to promote sodium reabsorption and water retention.	Severe, chronic postural hypotension	Assess medication regime for antihypertensives. Monitor blood pressure sitting and standing. Monitor fluid balance and salt intake. Monitor for signs of fluid retention.
Vasopressor • Midodrine (ProAmatine)	Stimulates alpha$_1$-adrenergic receptors, increasing total peripheral resistance, resulting in increased systolic and diastolic blood pressure.	Severe, chronic postural hypotension	Assess medication regime for antihypertensives. Monitor blood pressure sitting and standing. Monitor fluid balance and salt intake.
Genitourinary Antispasmodic • Oxybutynin (Ditropan) • Tolterodine tartrate (Detrol)	Exert a direct spasmolytic action and an antimuscarinic action on smooth muscle, relaxing bladder smooth muscle.	Urinary symptoms of overactive bladder	Monitor for urinary frequency and urgency. Monitor fluid balance. Monitor for signs of urinary tract infection.

Sources: Alzheimer's Association. (2003). *Provider checklist for treating a confused elder.* Retrieved April 30, 2008, from http://alzla.org/medical/Checklisthtml.html; American Society of Health-System Pharmacists. (2006). *AHFS drug information.* Bethesda, MD: Author; Calne, S. M. (2003). The psychosocial impact of late-stage Parkinson's disease. *Journal of Neuroscience Nursing, 35*(6), 306–313; Calne, S. M., & Kumar, A. (2003). Nursing care of patients with late-stage Parkinson's disease. *Journal of Neuroscience Nursing, 35*, 5, 242–251; Jankovic, J. (2006). Therapeutic strategies in Parkinson's disease. Pahwa, R., Lyons, K., & Wilkinson, B. (2003). *Deep brain stimulation for Parkinson's disease: An update.* Retrieved January 23, 2004, from http://www.medscape.com/viewprogram/2274_pnt.

COMT Inhibitors

Catechol-*O*-methyltransferase (COMT) is an enzyme that metabolizes levodopa and dopamine. Inhibiting COMT decreases levodopa metabolism so that more is available to cross the blood–brain barrier (Pahwa et al., 2003). Because they increase the effective duration of the levodopa dosage, COMT inhibitors are effective only when taken in conjunction with levodopa. They are used most often to counteract wearing-off responses (Jankovic, 2006). Approved COMT inhibitors are tolcapone (Tasmar) and entacapone (Comtan). Tolcapone is used less often because of the risk of liver toxicity. Stalevo combines both levodopa/carbidopa and entacapone into one tablet.

Other Medications

Amantadine, an antiviral drug, has proven to provide modest improvement for PD symptoms. It is particularly useful for treating dyskinesias. Side effects include fatigue, agitation, the red or purple skin blotches of livedo reticularis, and edema of the lower extremities (Nutt & Wooten, 2005).

Inhibition of the enzyme monoamine oxidase type B (MAO-B) interferes with the metabolism of dopamine. Although the MAO-B inhibitor selegiline was thought to prevent degeneration of dopamine-producing neurons and delay the progression of PD, studies have not successfully confirmed this. Nonetheless, selegiline reduces the metabolism of dopamine, does improve PD symptoms, and can reduce total levodopa dosage by 10% to 25% in some patients. Unlike other MAO-B inhibitors, selegiline has no dietary restrictions at the recommended dose of 10 mg/day. Because of its stimulating effects, it should be taken in the morning and not later than noon to avoid disruption of sleep. There is potential for serious and possibly fatal drug interactions when taken concurrently with meperidine (Demerol), and therefore should be discontinued at least 2 weeks before surgery (Jankovic, 2006; Nutt & Wooten, 2005). Other medications can be used to treat secondary symptoms of PD including depression, cognitive changes, sleep problems, and genitourinary issues. The Pharmacology Summary box (p. 802) provides more information about medications for Parkinson's disease.

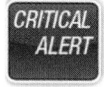 **CRITICAL ALERT** *Meperidine should not be given to patients taking selegiline due to risk of fatal drug interaction (Nutt & Wooten, 2005).*

Surgical Approaches

Neurosurgical intervention is an option reserved for certain carefully selected patients with advanced PD. Surgical treatments include ablative procedures, deep brain stimulation (DBS; Figure 31–8 ■), and cell transplantation. Ablative procedures include thalamotomy and pallidotomy, which is the surgical placement of a permanent lesion in the thalamus or the globus pallidus, respectively. Ablative procedures are older procedures and rarely used today.

Recently, DBS became another viable option. DBS involves surgically placing electrodes in targeted areas of the brain. As with ablative procedures, the most common targets are specific areas within the subthalamic nucleus or globus pallidus. The electrodes are attached to an external pacemaker-like device that is implanted underneath the collarbone. High-frequency stimulation provides effects similar to ablative surgery (Pahwa et al., 2003). Like PD drug treatments, surgical interventions do not cure the disease.

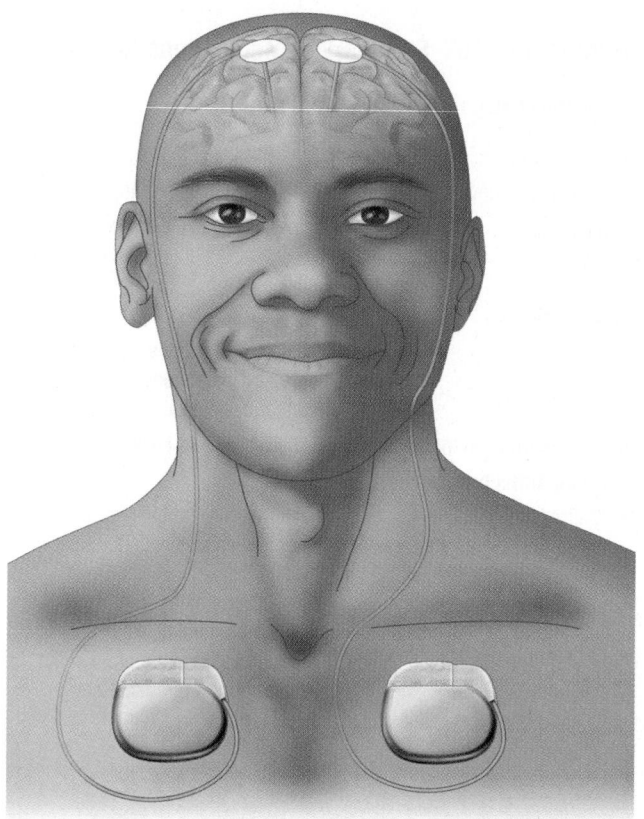

FIGURE 31–8 ■ Parkinson's control therapy: deep brain stimulation.

Transplantation therapy involves transplanting stem cells, in an effort to replace lost substantia nigra cells. Currently, these controversial procedures are experimental and the ongoing focus of research (Pahwa et al., 2003).

Complementary and alternative therapies also may be used to treat PD. One such alternative, t'ai chi, is discussed in the Complementary and Alternative Therapies box.

Gerontological Considerations

People with PD ages 65 and older account for 17% of neurology outpatient visits. After Alzheimer's disease, it is the second most common neurological condition requiring home health care (Pahwa et al., 2003). PD imposes socioeconomic burdens as well. Research studies indicate that the individual costs of PD are estimated as to be as high as $24,000 per year, with the cost of medications alone over $2,000 (Pahwa et al., 2003). Medication expense for patients beyond their productive years can be particularly burdensome.

People can live with PD for many years. The chronic and progressive nature of PD can significantly impact older, spousal caregivers, who may not have the physical strength to handle the weight of a patient with limited mobility. Caregiver stress and burden have been shown to increase as the disease progresses (Carter et al., 1998).

■ Nursing Management

Application of the nursing process will facilitate a comprehensive approach to patient care throughout the disease process. Relevant nursing diagnoses, assessment, outcomes, and interventions are

COMPLEMENTARY & ALTERNATIVE THERAPIES   T'ai Chi

Description:

T'AI CHI is an Asian exercise technique that consists of a series of flowing, graceful movements conducted in a specific pattern. Unlike many other forms of exercise, breathing and balance are central to t'ai chi. There are many different t'ai chi styles throughout the world and it is becoming increasingly used as a part of many preventative and restorative health regimens.

Research Support:

One of the diseases that research has shown t'ai chi to improve is Parkinson's disease. The primary effects associated with Parkinson's disease occur in tandem with the secondary, often preventable, effects of immobility (Kluding & McGinnis, 2006). The majority of studies on t'ai chi show that the method may lead to improved balance, reduced fear of falling, increased strength, increased functional mobility, greater flexibility, and increased psychological well-being for patients with Parkinson's disease (Kuramoto, 2006).

One small study examined the effects of 3 months of various physical activities on two 66-year-old males in early or middle stages of Parkinson's disease. The men participated in balance classes twice weekly during the first month, joined a fitness center and self-directed their exercise program during the second month, and participated in group t'ai chi classes twice weekly during the third month. The results of the 3-month program showed improvements in functional reach for both participants, and both demonstrated improvement in their balance test performance over a 3-month period (Kluding & McGinnis, 2006). Once the program ended, participants were given suggestions for continued physical fitness activities, and both participants continued to exercise regularly for at least 8 months following the program.

Another small study described the effects of an 8-week t'ai chi class on two participants: one with Parkinson's disease, the other with multiple system atrophy. The results showed that both participants demonstrated improved scores on the Activities-specific Balance Confidence Scale and the Functional Reach Test. Both participants also reported subjective improvements in balance and balance awareness. Based on these results, researchers concluded that t'ai chi may be a viable option for improving balance in patients with mild Parkinsonism (Venglar, 2005).

Another larger study involved 15 participants who received 12 weeks of weekly t'ai chi instruction in 45-minute sessions at a community facility. After the participants completed the program, researchers evaluated their results by administering a survey questionnaire, analyzing themes of a focus group discussion, assessing instructor reflections, and reviewing attendance records. Participants perceived benefits in physical, psychological, and social domains. The results showed that improved balance was reported most frequently. In addition, instructor observations and participant testimony suggest that performing t'ai chi may improve movement capability for individuals with Parkinson's (Klein & Rivers, 2006).

References

Klein, P. J., & Rivers, L. (2006). T'ai chi for individuals with Parkinson disease and their support partners: A program evaluation. *Journal of Neurologic Physical Therapy, 30*(1), 22–27.

Kluding, P., & McGinnis, P. Q. (2006). Multidimensional exercise for people with Parkinson's disease: A case report. *Physiotherapy Theory and Practice, 22*(3), 153–162.

Kuramoto, A. M. (2006). Therapeutic benefits of T'ai Chi exercise: Research review. *Wisconsin Medical Journal, 105*(7), 42–46.

Venglar, M. (2005). Case report: T'ai Chi and parkinsonism. *Physiotherapy Research International, 10*(2), 116–121.

---

all part of the nursing process, as outlined in the Nursing Process: Patient Care Plan for Parkinson's Disease feature (p. 806).

Collaborative Management

With the goal of maintaining independence and quality of life, a multidisciplinary plan will help to effectively manage the symptoms and complications of PD. Physical, speech, and occupational therapy can counteract effects of progressive movement and speech complications. Dietary consultation can address nutritional concerns. In the later stages of PD, a multidisciplinary approach will best address the goals of symptom relief, prevention of complications, maintaining patient dignity, and supporting the family caregivers (Thomas & MacMahon, 2004).

Discharge Priorities

Discharge priorities for the patient with PD involve both the patient and the patient's family, or caretakers (see the Patient Teaching & Discharge Priorities box, p. 807).

Health Promotion

In addition to medicines and treatment specifically designed to alleviate symptoms, a complete care plan for the PD patient will include diet, exercise, and mental health needs of the patient and caregiver. People with PD are at risk for dehydration, weight loss, and constipation. A dietitian or nutritionist who is familiar with dysphagia can assess nutritional needs (see Chapter 14 ⊙) and recommend adequate amounts of fluids and proper foods for such conditions (Holden, 2003).

Cardiovascular exercise, strength training, and muscle stretching routines can help combat losses of balance, dexterity, and normal movement. Exercise also will improve the strength, endurance, and compensatory qualities of the unaffected parts of the body. Patients should know that physical exercise may help them improve function (Suchowersky, Gronseth, Perlmutter, Reich, & Zesiewicz, 2006).

Parkinson's support organizations offer understanding and hope for both the patients and their families. Local and national support groups provide information, educational programs, and social activities tailored especially for people with PD. Some PD patients choose to participate in clinical research studies as a way of advancing science while keenly managing their condition with the latest, most promising treatments.

Multiple Sclerosis

A chronic and progressive neuroimmunologic disease, **multiple sclerosis (MS)** is characterized by multiple areas of demyelination in the white matter of the brain and spinal cord. The demyelination leaves sclerotic areas, also known as plaques, and subsequent scarring leading to a variety of neurological symptoms including weakness, spasticity, visual difficulties, and **paresthesias**.

Epidemiology and Etiology

In the United States, an estimated 350,000 cases affect almost twice as many women as men. Typically, symptoms first appear

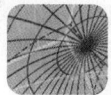

Assessment for Independent Activity

Subjective Data:

Do you have stiffness and slowness of movement?

Do these symptoms interfere with your daily activities?

Do you have trouble with balance?

Have you ever fallen?

Do you need assistance when you walk?

Do you use a cane or walker?

Does your medication regimen help your symptoms?

Do you have times during the day when you function better than at other times?

Objective Data:

Neurological status, including motor status (coordination, gait, balance, tremor, rigidity, bradykinesia)

Nursing Assessment and Diagnoses	Outcomes and Evaluation Parameters	Planning and Interventions with *Rationales*
Nursing Diagnosis: *Impaired Physical Mobility* related to rigidity, bradykinesia, postural instability, altered gait	**Outcomes:** Patient demonstrates maximum independent physical function. Patient is free of immobility complications. **Evaluation Parameters:** Patient maintains as much independent mobility as possible given degree of disease progression. Patient uses assistive devices to maximize mobility. ADLs and therapy schedule coincide with medication peak effectiveness.	**Interventions and *Rationales*:** Assist patient to ambulate and perform ADLs *to provide assessment of abilities.* Consult with patient regarding medication schedule. *Medication schedule may be complex and may not fit traditional medication timelines.* Schedule therapies and ADLs to coincide with optimum medication benefit. *Movement will be easier when medications are working at peak effectiveness.* Instruct patient to stand as straight as possible and walk with a wide-based gait while swinging arms *to help maintain balance and momentum.* Perform range of motion to all joints *to counteract the effects of rigidity.* Encourage use of walker or other assistive device *to increase mobility by stabilizing gait.* Use side rails or overhead trapeze on bed. *Both act as grab bars and assist with turning over in bed.* Instruct patient to use straight-back chairs with firm seats and arm rests when possible. *It is difficult for patients to get up from low, soft surfaces such as easy chairs or sofas.* Consult with physical therapist. *Can prescribe and tailor appropriate gait assistive devices and also exercises to counteract stiffness and rigidity.* Consult with occupational therapist. *Can assess need for adaptive aids for ADLs such as specialized eating utensils or button hook for dressing.*

Assessment for Ability to Communicate

Subjective Data:

Do people ask you to repeat things?

Do you frequently feel misunderstood?

Do you get frustrated when trying to converse?

Objective Data:

Difficulty understanding patient

Lack of facial expression

Nursing Assessment and Diagnoses	Outcomes and Evaluation Parameters	Planning and Interventions with *Rationales*
Nursing Diagnosis: *Impaired Verbal Communication* related to voice and speech changes and decreased facial expression	**Outcome:** Patient is able to converse and communicate needs. **Evaluation Parameters:** Staff and family members are able to understand verbalizations. Patient and family members verbalize disease process and effect on speech and expression.	**Nursing Interventions and *Rationales*:** Assess and monitor for decreased voice volume, slurred or mumbled speech, difficulties initiating speech. *Common symptoms of PD.* Observe ability of patient to communicate needs and converse with family members. *Provides information about impact of speech changes on family dynamics and assesses need for education.* Consult with speech-language pathologist. *Can evaluate speech difficulties and develop treatment program, including assistive devices.* Eliminate background noise (TV, radio) while patient is speaking. *Decreases environmental interference when listening to patient.* Allow ample time for patient to speak and communicate. *Communicating takes longer for patient; allowing ample time decreases stress and anxiety, which may improve speech.*

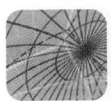

NURSING PROCESS: Patient Care Plan for Parkinson's Disease—*Continued*

Assessment for Orientation to Time, Place, and Person
Subjective Data:
States name when asked.

Objective Data:
Neurological status including level of consciousness, orientation, MMSE
Agitation
Visual hallucinations
Medication regimen
Signs of infection: fever
Hydration status, including intake and output
Laboratory studies including blood chemistry and CBCs

Nursing Assessment and Diagnoses	Outcomes and Evaluation Parameters	Planning and Interventions with *Rationales*
Nursing Diagnosis: *Disturbed Thought Processes* (confusion, hallucinations and delusions) related to cognitive changes, medication regimen, and/or infection	**Outcome:** Patient remains oriented. ***Evaluation Parameters:*** Patient does not exhibit evidence of having delusions or hallucinations. Patient is oriented. Family remains calm in event of visual hallucinations.	**Interventions and *Rationales:*** Assess and monitor patient's level of cognitive functioning using rating scale such as MMSE. *Provides a basis of planning care.* Assess changes in medication dosage and/or schedule and monitor for increased or decreased confusion or hallucinations and physical mobility. *Dopaminergic drugs can stimulate hallucinations or cause confusion and may need to be adjusted; these side effects may preclude a dosage high enough to improve mobility.* Assess for treatable causes of confusion such as infection, recent general anesthesia, dehydration. *Can be sources of delirium or increased confusion.* Assess and monitor response to antipsychotic drugs. *May be prescribed to counteract hallucination and delusions.* Reassure patient and family during hallucinations. *Patient may or may not become frightened during hallucinations; hallucinations can be distressing to family.* Minimize environmental hazards *to decrease risk of injury due to confusion.*

Sources: Ackley, B. J., & Ludwig, G. B. (Eds.). (2003). *Nursing diagnosis handbook: A guide to planning care* (6th ed.). St. Louis: Mosby; Calne, S. M. (2003). The psychosocial impact of late-stage Parkinson's disease. *Journal of Neuroscience Nursing, 35*(6), 306–313; Calne, S. M., & Kumar, A. (2003). Nursing care of patients with late-stage Parkinson's disease. *Journal of Neuroscience Nursing, 35,* 5, 242–251; Doenges, M. E., & Moorhouse, M. F. (2003). *Application of nursing process and diagnosis: An interactive text for diagnostic reasoning* (4th ed.). Philadelphia: F. A. Davis; Holloway, N. (2003). *Medical-surgical care planning* (4th ed.). Philadelphia: Lippincott Wilkins & Williams.

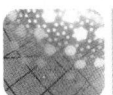

PATIENT TEACHING & DISCHARGE PRIORITIES for Parkinson's Disease

Need	Teaching
Disease process: Patient/family	Assess knowledge of disease process: • PD is chronic and slowly progressive. • No clear cause or cure is known. • General progression through stages but progression varies from person to person. • Treatment approaches.
Educational resources: Patient/family	National Parkinson Foundation (1-800-327-4545) Parkinson Disease Foundation (1-800-457-6676) American Parkinson's Disease Association (1-800-223-2732) Local PD clinical and research centers Local support groups Internet resources

MyNursingKit | Parkinson Disease Foundation

MyNursingKit | American Parkinson's Disease Association

MyNursingKit | National Parkinson Foundation

(continued)

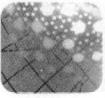

PATIENT TEACHING & DISCHARGE PRIORITIES for Parkinson's Disease—*Continued*

Need	Teaching
Dopaminergic medications: Patient/family	Side effects of dopaminergic medications: • Nausea/vomiting • Light-headedness • Drowsiness • Confusion • Hallucinations. Take as directed, usually starting with low dose and titrating upward. Allow time to reach dosage required for symptom improvement. Take carbidopa/levodopa 30 to 60 minutes before a meal or 1 to 2 hours after a meal for optimal absorption. Do not abruptly stop medications unless directed by health care provider. Use medication diary to track schedule, dosage, and side-effects. Need to work closely with health care provider to arrive at optimal, individualized dosage.
Fall prevention: Family Setting	Remove throw rugs. Move electrical cords out of walkways. Create clear, uncluttered walking paths. Rearrange furniture so that it is easy to get around. Install railings along hallways and on stairways. Minimize sharp edges or corners on furniture, wet floors, and hot surfaces. Install grab bars in shower and next to commode. Do not use towel racks as grab bars.
Nutrition: Patient/family	Hydration is important to counteract low blood pressure, constipation, and for general health. Fiber helps to counteract constipation. Calcium is important for maintaining bone density and decreasing the risk of fracture from falls. Protein may interfere with levodopa absorption in a small percentage of patients. Take levodopa at least 30 minutes before eating or 1 hour after eating. Consult with dietitian for weight loss.
Exercise: Patient/family Setting (home/clinic)	Stress importance of the following in accordance with patient's physical ability: • Resistance training to strengthen muscles and bones • Mild aerobic conditioning for cardiovascular health • Stretching to counteract stiffness and rigidity.
Constipation: Patient/family Setting (home/clinic/hospital)	Part of disease process and worsened by medications. Avoid use of laxatives. May use stool softeners and bulking agents such as psyllium on daily basis. Increase dietary fluid and fiber.
Urinary problems: Patient/family Setting (home/clinic/hospital)	Urinary frequency and/or urgency is common. Signs/symptoms of urinary tract infection (UTI): • Foul-smelling urine • Painful urination. Call health care provider if signs/symptoms of UTI develop. Consult with health care provider regarding urinary problems.
Orthostatic hypotension: Patient/family Setting (home/clinic/hospital)	Signs of low blood pressure include light-headedness, dizziness, fainting. Part of disease process, medications also contribute. Change position slowly when rising from a lying or seated position. Increase fluids and salt if not contraindicated by other conditions. Use support stockings and elevate legs throughout the day. Remain seated for 20 to 30 minutes after a large meal or dose of medication. Sit down to towel after hot bath or shower.

Sources: Calne, S. M., & Kumar, A. (2003). Nursing care of patients with late-stage Parkinson's disease. *Journal of Neuroscience Nursing, 35,* 5, 242–251; Cianci, H. (2004). *Fitness counts* (2nd ed.). Brochure. Miami, FL: National Parkinson Foundation; Holden, K. (2003). *Parkinson's disease: Guidelines for medical nutritional therapy for use by nutrition professionals.* Miami, FL: Five Star Living; Marjama-Lyons, J. & Shomon, M. J. (2003). *What your doctor may not tell you about Parkinson's disease: a holistic program for optimal wellness.* New York, NY: Warner Books, Inc.

RISK FACTORS for Multiple Sclerosis

Research has shown that people who spend their first 15 years of life in temperate climates, at a distance from the equator, are more at risk than those who spend the same time in tropical regions closer to the equator (Schapiro, 2003).

There is evidence that a genetic link may influence susceptibility to MS. Generally, a person's chance of developing MS is about one-tenth of 1%; however, if there is a first-degree relative with MS, the risk jumps up to 3%. In identical twins, the chance that the second twin will develop MS if the first twin does is 30%; in fraternal twins, the risk is decreased to 4%. Many researchers hypothesize that MS is not caused by a single gene, virus, or environmental factor, but is the result of a combination of factors (NINDS, 2002).

between 20 and 40 years of age. Onset of the disease may have a geographical component (Schapiro, 2003). Risk for MS increases geographically from southern to northern latitudes. The highest frequency areas of North America include the northern United States and southern Canada. There is also evidence that migration to and from higher frequency areas in early life influences the risk of developing MS (Franklin & Nelson, 2003).

Pathophysiology

MS is a neuroimmunologic disease that attacks **myelin**, the protective sheath surrounding nerve fibers. Demyelinating lesions or plaques form along nerve fibers in the brain and spinal cord, producing symptoms related to the location of damage. The breakdown of myelin interferes with normal nerve conduction in the affected areas (Schapiro, 2003). Demyelination results from an inflammatory process and also leads to irreversible axonal injury and permanent loss of nerve function (Holland, 2003; O'Connor & Canadian Multiple Sclerosis Working Group, 2002). This process may be triggered by a virus or other environmental stimulus that activates T cells specific for the production of myelin basic protein (MBP). The T cells cross the blood–brain barrier into the CNS, where they release cytokines, initiating an immune response that ultimately damages the myelin sheath and axons (O'Connor et al., 2002). Although viruses and environmental factors are suspect for their role in MS, the cause is still unknown (see the Risk Factors box).

Clinical Manifestations

Because MS can damage different parts of the CNS, symptoms vary, not only from patient to patient, but within the same patient over time. The most common initial signs include fatigue, nystagmus, vertigo, gait disturbances, sensory loss, lower extremity weakness, spasticity, bladder disturbance, and optic neuritis. Other symptoms that may present at any time during the course of the disease include cognitive changes such as euphoria or depression, and physical conditions such as muscle cramping and sexual dysfunction (Holland, 2003).

The symptoms of MS are listed in four categories: sensory, motor, cerebellar, and miscellaneous. The symptoms correspond specifically with the area in the brain or spinal cord that is damaged. Sensory symptoms include numbness, paresthesias, loss of proprioception, and **L'Hermite's sign**, or a shocklike pain that results from flexion of the neck. Motor symptoms include weak-

ness, particularly in the lower extremities, and spasticity. Cerebellar symptoms include **ataxia**, or loss of balance and coordination, as well as speech difficulties including dysarthria or slurred and scanning speech. Other symptoms such as fatigue and loss of vision associated with a central scotoma often are an early sign of the disease. Vertigo, sometimes accompanied by vomiting and nystagmus, affects some patients while bowel and bladder problems beset others. Emotional disturbances and cognitive impairment may be present as well.

As with the wide range of symptoms, the course any particular case might take is varied. The four main types of MS are listed here (O'Connor et al., 2002):

- *Relapsing-remitting MS* is the most common type. It is known for its acute attacks followed by complete or partial remission. It makes up about 85% of initial diagnoses.
- *Primary-progressive MS* progresses without remission, although plateaus or minor improvements can happen. Approximately 10% to 15% of the diagnoses are for this form of the disease.
- *Secondary progressive MS* begins as relapsing-remitting, but then it develops into the primary-progressive course.
- *Progressive-relapsing MS* intersperses the progression of the disease with acute attacks.

Both age and duration of the disease have the greatest influence on the rate of relapse.

Laboratory and Diagnostic Procedures

In addition to a comprehensive medical history and neurological exam, diagnostics for MS include MRI, cerebrospinal fluid (CSF) tests, and visual evoked potentials (VEP) (Chaudhuri & Behan, 2004; Holland, 2003). Lesions that represent inflammation or demyelination often are referred to as plaques and are easily detected with T_2-weighted and flair MRI tests. Enhancing lesions, or those enhanced by the contrast agent gadolinium, are considered new. They may appear and then disappear. Nonenhancing lesions can be seen without gadolinium, and reflect older, permanent damage. CSF studies look for inflammatory proteins and oligoclonal bands. The VEP test is done to measure transmission of impulses across nerve fibers, which are slowed in areas of demyelination (Holland, 2003). Other diagnostics are listed in the Diagnostic Tests box (p. 810).

Medical Management

Treating MS relies on drug therapy, relapse management, and symptom management. The nurse plays a critical role in education and health management in all of these areas (Costello, Halper, Harris, & Kennedy, 2003).

Disease-Modifying Drugs

Disease-modifying drugs reduce the frequency of relapses and potentially delay progression. Interferon beta-1b (Betaseron) is used to treat ambulatory patients with relapsing-remitting MS and secondary-progressive MS. Interferon beta-1a (Avonex) helps relapsing forms of MS as well as the initial MS attack. Another interferon beta-1a (Rebif) treats relapsing forms of MS.

These medications are injected either subcutaneously or intramuscularly. Side effects resulting from these treatments range from flu-like symptoms that subside over time and injection-site

DIAGNOSTIC TESTS for Multiple Sclerosis

Test	Expected Result	Rationale
MRI	White matter lesion(s) identified	Rule out other conditions; look for white matter lesions (plaques).
CSF studies	Elevated IgG index or synthesis rate Presence of oligoclonal bands	Uncovers signs of inflammation and myelin breakdown.
VEP	Slowed conduction	Identifies lesions in sensory pathway; may help identify lesion not easily visualized by MRI; for example, optic nerve.

Sources: Chaudhuri, A., & Behan, P.O. (2004). Multiple sclerosis is not an autoimmune disease. *Archives of Neurology, 61,* 1610–1612; NMSS (2008); Holland, N. (2003). *Urinary dysfunction in multiple sclerosis.* Retrieved May 2, 2008, from http://www.nationalmssociety.org;pdf/forpros/Bladder.pdf.

reactions such as erythema to pain, menstrual irregularities, and nausea (Costello et al., 2003). Depression also is a possible side effect. Flu-like symptoms can be minimized by slowly increasing the dose and use of antipyretics. Teaching correct technique and applying ice to the site can manage injection-site reactions. Blood chemistry and hematology should be checked regularly because, even though abnormalities are rare, they do occur. Particular attention should be given to monitoring liver function tests (Costello et al., 2003).

Glatiramer acetate (Copaxone) is not an interferon; nevertheless, it is a disease-modifying drug used to treat relapsing-remitting MS. Like interferons, glatiramer acetate is injected. Localized site reactions are common and can be minimized in the same way as interferon site reactions. Systemic reactions occur rarely. Although not dangerous, they may invoke tachycardia, sweating, anxiety, dyspnea, faintness, flushing, and nausea. Educating patients about the possibility of a postinjection reaction will help to minimize anxiety (Costello et al., 2003).

Traditionally used as a treatment for cancer, mitoxantrone (Novantrone), an antineoplastic drug, suppresses the activity of T cells, B cells, and macrophages. It is used to treat the secondary progressive, progressive-relapsing, and worsening relapsing-remitting forms of MS (National Multiple Sclerosis Society [NMSS], 2008). The therapy calls for its intravenous administration every 3 months. The blue-colored fluid may cause a bluish tinge in urine and bluing in the whites of the eyes. Use of mitoxantrone for more than 2.5 years increases the risk of cardiac toxicity (Schapiro, 2003).

 **CRITICAL ALERT** *Cardiac output should be recorded prior to starting mitoxantrone drug therapy and periodically thereafter (NMSS, 2008).*

In 2006, the FDA approved natalizumab (Tysabri) for the treatment of relapsing MS. A laboratory-produced monoclonal antibody, this drug inhibits the movement of damaging immune cells across the blood–brain barrier and into the brain and spinal cord. Due to the increased risk of progressive multifocal leukoencephalopathy, an opportunistic viral brain infection, it is available only through a restricted distribution program (FDA, 2006).

The Pharmacology Summary box provides more information about drugs used for the treatment of multiple sclerosis.

Relapse Management

A relapse is a new sign or a worsening of neurological symptoms with a duration that is greater than 24 hours. Recovery from relapse is variable. After onset of neurological deterioration, symptoms plateau and patients recover over weeks or months. Symptoms gradually resolve and patients fully or partially recover. Several conditions are known to precipitate symptoms or relapses. These include, but are not limited to, excessive exertion, extreme temperatures, infections, hot baths, fever, emotional stress, and pregnancy (Costello et al., 2003).

Relapses often are treated with an orally or intravenously administered glucocorticoid, such as methylprednisolone. Common side effects from the use of these types of drugs include weight gain, a metallic taste in the mouth, insomnia, hyperglycemia, and gastrointestinal ulceration and upset. Less common side effects include psychosis and blurred vision (Costello et al., 2003).

Detailing the history of relapse and the consequential symptoms becomes the basis of care and treatment of the MS patient. The record should show when the relapse began, the severity of symptoms, and the impact on the patient's daily activities. The patient care plan should address the patient's understanding of factors that can contribute to the worsening of symptoms, common diagnostic evaluations, and a review of common medical therapy.

Symptom Management

Fatigue is a common symptom in patients diagnosed with MS, and it is the most disabling symptom (Schapiro, 2003). MS fatigue may have sudden onset and interfere with normal function. When managing fatigue, the patient's sleep habits, current and former medications, experiences of depression, and applied coping strategies all need to be collectively, as well as individually, taken into consideration. Patients should understand that a hot ambient temperature can trigger the onset of fatigue and symptoms. Countermeasures such as air conditioning, cool drinks, and ice packs can help to restore a patient's strength. Occupational therapists can teach energy conservation strategies that can help the patient accomplish ADLs. The practices of light exercise, scheduling rest times between activities, and using labor-saving tools and appliances often become part of the therapy. Medications prescribed to combat fatigue include amantadine, pemoline, modafinil, and low-dose antidepressants (Lisak, 2001; Schapiro, 2003).

Muscle spasticity also is common. Infection, disease relapse, incorrect body positioning, and a full bowel and/or bladder all can contribute to spasticity. The nurse should obtain a detailed history of the time, place, and circumstances associated with spasticity. Stretching and breathing exercises, cool-water therapy, and relaxation techniques may be incorporated into strategies

PHARMACOLOGY Summary of Medications to Treat Multiple Sclerosis

Medication Category	Action	Application/Indication	Nursing Responsibility
Immunomodulator/Interferons • Interferon beta-1a (Avonex) • Interferon beta-1b (Betaseron) • Interferon beta-1a (Rebif)	Although action is not clear, thought to inhibit proliferation of leukocytes and antigens; modulate production of anti-inflammatory cytokines; inhibit T-cell migration across blood–brain barrier.	Relapsing forms of MS	Assess frequency of exacerbations. Monitor hemoglobin, WBC, platelets, blood chemistries. Instruct patient on correct injection technique.
Immunomodulator • Glatiramer acetate (Copaxone)	Although action is not clear, thought to modulate T cells to promote production of anti-inflammatory cytokines.	Relapsing-remitting forms	Assess frequency of exacerbations. After injection, assess for flushing, chest pain, palpitations, and dyspnea. Instruct patient on correct injection technique.
Antineoplastic/Immunosuppressive • Mitoxantrone (Novantrone)	Inhibits DNA synthesis.	Rapidly worsening relapsing-remitting, progressive-relapsing, secondary-progressive	Assess frequency of exacerbations. Monitor for cardiotoxicity, fatigue, nausea, immunosuppression.
Monoclonal Antibody • Natalizumab (Tysabri)	May hamper the movement of immune cells across the blood–brain barrier.	Relapsing forms in patients who have inadequate response or who cannot tolerate other disease-modifying treatment	Due to risk of progressive multifocal leukoencephalopathy, a serious viral infection of the brain, this drug is only available at select authorized infusion sites requiring mandatory patient registration and follow-up.
Management of Selected Symptoms of Multiple Sclerosis **CNS Stimulants** • Pemoline • Modafinil	Produce CNS stimulation.	Fatigue	Monitor for restlessness or sleep disturbances. Counsel patient regarding dosing schedule and titration.
Genitourinary Antispasmodics • Oxybutynin (Ditropan) • Tolterodine tartrate (Detrol)	Exert a direct spasmolytic action and an antimuscarinic action on smooth muscle, relaxing bladder smooth muscle.	Bladder dysfunction	Assess for urinary tract infection. Monitor for urinary retention. Monitor intake and output. Monitor overall elimination pattern.
Skeletal Muscle Relaxant • Oral or intrathecal baclofen	Acts at spinal cord level to decrease frequency and amplitude of muscle spasms.	Spasticity	Time doses to maintain therapeutic blood levels. Titrate doses up. Monitor for sedation or cognitive symptoms. Intrathecal baclofen requires surgical insertion of programmable pump; monitor closely during titration.
Benzodiazepines • Diazepam • Clonazepam	Inhibit polysynaptic afferent pathways.	Spasticity	Assess spasticity. Monitor vital signs during therapy. Assess risk of falls and implement fall prevention strategies. Monitor for psychological/physical dependence during long-term therapy.

Sources: Costello, K., Halper, J., Harris, C., & Kennedy, P. (2003). Multiple sclerosis treatment and the importance of early intervention [online]. *International Journal of MS Care.* Retrieved from http://www.mscare.org/cmsc/Journal-of-MS-Care.html; Food and Drug Administration. (2006). *Natalizumab (marketed as Tysabri) information.* Retrieved April 30, 2008, from http://www.fda.gov/cder/drug/infopage/natalizumab; Forest Pharmaceuticals. (2003). *Namenda (memanatine HCL)* [Package insert]. St. Louis: Author; Rizvi, S. A., & Agius, M. A. (2004). Current approved options for treating patients with multiple sclerosis. *Neurology, 63* (Suppl. 6), S8–S14.

designed to minimize these symptoms. In some cases, orthotic devices are used to prevent contractures and maintain proper body posture and alignment. Medications used to treat spasticity include baclofen, tizanidine, clonazepam, gabapentin, and diazepam (Lisak, 2001; Schapiro, 2003). In some cases, injections of botulinum toxin or implantation of an intrathecal baclofen pump may be necessary (Costello et al., 2003).

Bowel and bladder problems are common in MS. Bladder dysfunction can be classified as failure to store, failure to empty, or a combination of both conditions. Urinary tract infections, urinary urgency, incontinence, and dribbling are typical symptoms (Lisak, 2001; Schapiro, 2003). Medication management includes oxybutynin HCL (Ditropan), propantheline (Pro-Banthine), tolterodine (Detrol), and terazosin (Hytrin). Patients should be encouraged to avoid caffeine, alcohol, and other diuretics. Teaching the Kegel technique of contracting and holding the pubococcygeal muscle and the Credé technique of applying pressure to the lower abdomen to express urine may help patients adjust to retention and elimination anomalies. In cases of urinary retention, intermittent catheterization may be necessary. Patients should be instructed on correct straight catheterization technique and care. In some cases, a Foley or suprapubic catheter may be required (Lisak, 2001; Schapiro, 2003). The management of constipation and bowel incontinence is best served with the help of a dietitian familiar with the needs of the MS patient. Stressing a diet and hydration appropriate for the condition (see Chapter 14) along with moderate exercise is helpful (Lisak, 2001).

About half of the people with MS suffer from some form of cognitive impairment as a result of the disease. Although the symptoms vary, they are most likely to manifest as short-term memory deficits and attention difficulties. At times, the person's mental condition may worsen when tired, stressed, or exposed to hot weather. Many patients turn to list making, calendar keeping, and tape recording to aid them with memory lapses (Schapiro, 2003). As discussed in the Complementary and Alternative Therapies box, some therapies related to temperature control may be useful in relieving some of the symptoms of MS.

Gerontological Considerations

MS most often strikes young adults. There are comparatively few occurrences in older people. Those who have MS can expect to live an average life span (Schapiro, 2003).

■ Nursing Management

Nursing care needs of the patient with MS are multifaceted and complex, encompassing both inpatient and outpatient care. Symptom management is a major area of focus, with nursing care concentrating on nonpharmacologic management, patient education, and support. The nursing process can effectively help develop a plan of care, as outlined in the Nursing Process: Patient Care Plan for Multiple Sclerosis. Relevant nursing assessments, diagnoses, outcomes, and interventions in the care of the MS patient must be addressed.

■ Collaborative Management

The MS patient presents with a range of needs that are best addressed by a multidisciplinary team approach. Complicated medication regimens to prevent or treat relapses are managed by the neurology team including a neurologist, neuroscience nurses, and rehabilitation services. Physical therapists often participate in the rehabilitation efforts following relapse. They play a critical role in determining the need for mobility aids and design exercise regimes to combat fatigue and spasticity. Occupational therapy is important for developing energy conservation plans. Neuropsychologists may be called on to evaluate cognitive changes. Urologists may be consulted to manage bladder dysfunction common to MS. Issues related to self-esteem, body image, and interpersonal communication may be referred to a psychologist. Gynecologists or sexual therapists may be needed to address sexual dysfunction.

Discharge Priorities

Discharge priorities for patients with MS focus on adaptive strategies for them and their caretakers in the outpatient or home environment, as addressed in the Patient Teaching & Discharge Priorities box (p. 815).

Health Promotion

Like other chronic, degenerative, neurological conditions, physical and emotional stress can exacerbate the symptoms of MS. Patients should be instructed to avoid extreme temperatures and exposure to infections. Techniques to manage emotional stress should be emphasized.

Patients should be encouraged to engage in a regular exercise program and practice healthy eating habits. Exercise may help manage fatigue, spasticity, and bowel and bladder problems. Good nutrition can aid in resistance to infection. Increasing fluids and fiber is particularly useful for bladder problems and constipation (Lisak, 2001). A low-fat, high-fiber diet (see Chapter 14) should be recommended (NMSS, 2008).

The majority of MS cases occur in women of childbearing age, and the disease does not affect a women's ability to conceive or bear children (Giesser, 2003). However, symptoms such as

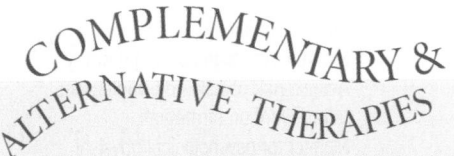

COMPLEMENTARY & ALTERNATIVE THERAPIES for Multiple Sclerosis

Heat is known to exacerbate symptoms of MS. A recent study showed that cooling suits may help improve fatigue, strength, and cognition when worn on a daily basis over a month (NASA/MS Study Group, 2003). Cooling suits, which cover the trunk and extremities, work by circulating a cooling liquid throughout the garment, which lowers body temperature and may improve conduction of nerve impulses in people with MS. Studies have not addressed the potential benefits of using passive cooling systems, such as ice packs (Rocky Mountain MS Center, 2003).

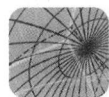
NURSING PROCESS: Patient Care Plan for Multiple Sclerosis

Assessment for Self-Care and Safety

Subjective Data:
Have you ever fallen?
Do you have double vision?
Do you have trouble sensing the temperature of water?

Objective Data:
Neurological status including muscle tone, gait, balance, vision, sensory perception

Nursing Assessment and Diagnoses	Outcomes and Evaluation Parameters	Planning and Interventions with *Rationales*
Nursing Diagnosis: *Risk of Injury* related to muscle weakness, ataxia, decreased sensory perception	**Outcome:** Patient remains free of injury. **Evaluation Parameters:** Demonstrates correct use of mobility aids. Practices safety measures to compensate for sensory losses.	**Interventions and *Rationales:*** Ambulate patient *to evaluate gait, ataxia, potential for falling.* Consult with physical therapist. *Can evaluate need for mobility assistive equipment.* Instruct on use of mobility aids such as cane, walker, or wheelchair *to help prevent injury, provide security, and increase independent movement.* Consult with occupational therapist. *Can provide instruction to compensate for sensory deficits while accomplishing ADLs.* Teach patient and caregivers safety measures to compensate for sensory loss, such as the use of a thermometer to test water temperature or the wearing of an eye patch to alleviate visual disturbance such as double vision. *Impaired sensory perception increases risk of injury.*

Assessment for Energy and Ability to Perform Own ADLs

Subjective Data:
How many hours per night do you sleep? Do you nap and if so, how often?
How many times do you get up during the night?
Are you or have you been feeling depressed?
Are you able to accomplish your usual activities during the course of a day?
Do you exercise?
Do you notice that you become very tired in hot temperatures?

Objective Data:
Neurological status including gait, coordination, and spasticity
Nutritional status including appetite and weight
Activity level including exercise/therapy
Medications

Nursing Assessment and Diagnoses	Outcomes and Evaluation Parameters	Planning and Interventions with *Rationales*
Nursing Diagnosis: *Fatigue* related to disease process	**Expected Outcomes:** Patient verbalizes increased energy. Patient is able to accomplish daily routines. **Evaluation Parameters:** Patient verbalizes understanding that fatigue is part of disease process. Patient practices prescribed energy conservation strategies. Patient uses prescribed assistive devices to accomplish ADLs. Patient verbalizes understanding that hot ambient temperatures worsen fatigue.	**Interventions and *Rationales:*** Discuss relationship of fatigue and disease process with patient and family; allow both to verbalize coping mechanisms. *Educates patient and family and assesses needs and coping strategies.* Provide rest periods between physical activity and activities of daily living *to minimize fatigue and conserve energy.* Teach patient and caregivers to avoid prolonged exposure to hot ambient temperatures, hot baths or showers. *Can trigger onset of fatigue.* Consult occupational therapist. *Can develop energy conservation plan, and assess need for and prescribe adaptive equipment to assist with ADLs, which helps to minimize fatigue.* Consult physical therapist. *Can develop light exercise regime, which may increase endurance and minimize fatigue.*

Assessment for Ability to Void Normally

Subjective Data:
How many times per day do you void?
Do you feel like your bladder empties completely?
Are there times when you cannot make it to the bathroom in time?
Do you have sudden urges to void?
Do you dribble in between voiding?
Is it hard to get started when voiding?
Do you have burning when you void?

Objective Data:
Intake and output
Voiding pattern
Bladder distention
Postvoid residual
Urine appearance/odor
Urinalysis, culture, sensitivity

(continued)

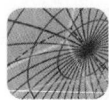

NURSING PROCESS: Patient Care Plan for Multiple Sclerosis—*Continued*

Nursing Assessment and Diagnoses	Outcomes and Evaluation Parameters	Planning and Interventions with *Rationales*
Nursing Diagnosis: *Impaired Urinary Elimination* related to spastic or flaccid bladder	**Outcomes:** Patient empties bladder completely by voiding and/or catheterizing. Patient remains free of urinary tract infection. ***Evaluation Parameters:*** Patient demonstrates correct techniques for bladder emptying. Patient is able to verbalize signs and symptoms of UTI.	**Nursing Interventions and *Rationales:*** Discuss voiding patterns with patient. Encourage patient to verbalize concerns. *Provides opportunity for patient to verbalize coping strategies and assesses voiding patterns.* Monitor voiding patterns *to establish baseline voiding patterns.* Assist patient to use the bathroom *to assess patient mobility status and ability to get to and from bathroom.* Assess for signs of urine retention including bladder distention, and urine overflow and intake greater than output. *Signs of retention.* Assess for signs of urinary tract infection. *Urinary retention and catheterization increase risk of infection.* Teach patient Credé maneuver. *Fully expresses urine from bladder for failure-to-empty difficulties, which decreases risk of infection.* Teach patient Kegel exercises. *Contracting and holding pubococcygeal muscle strengthens it, which helps improve failure-to-store problems.* Teach correct technique for prescribed bladder elimination: intermittent catheterization, suprapubic or indwelling catheter care. *Decreases risk of infection and ensures emptying of bladder.* Monitor medications for therapeutic and side effects *to aid in early detection of side effects or adverse reactions.*

Sources: Holloway, N. (2003). *Medical-surgical care planning* (4th ed.). Philadelphia: Lippincott Wilkins & Williams; Schapiro, R. (2003). *Managing the symptoms of multiple sclerosis* (4th ed.). New York: Demos.

urinary urgency and fatigue may flare during pregnancy and may require special management. The use of disease-modifying agents before and during pregnancy is an issue (Giesser, 2003), and patients will need education and counseling regarding treatment choices and recommendations during this time.

Amyotrophic Lateral Sclerosis

Amyotrophic lateral sclerosis (ALS) is a degenerative disease involving upper and lower motor neurons. Degeneration of motor neurons in the spinal cord, brainstem, and cerebral cortex leads to the characteristic symptoms of weakness, muscular atrophy, and spasticity. ALS, also known as Lou Gehrig's disease, is progressive, incurable, and fatal (Charles & Swash, 2001).

Epidemiology and Etiology

Approximately 20,000 Americans have ALS. Another 5,000 diagnoses are made each year (NINDS, 2008a). In the 1930s Lou Gehrig, a baseball player for the New York Yankees, was diagnosed with ALS, thus explaining why the disease is identified by his name in the United States. His celebrity has brought recognition to this disease in the way of public awareness and research funding. Estimates of prevalence rates range from 3 to 7 cases per 100,000 worldwide, making it one of the most common neuromuscular disorders (Borasio, Voltz, & Miller, 2001; Charles & Swash, 2001). The onset of ALS typically occurs between 40 and 60 years of age; however, it can affect younger and older people. It strikes men more often than women (NINDS, 2003a).

The cause of ALS is unknown. The excitatory neurotransmitter glutamate is believed to have a part in motor neuron degeneration (Charles & Swash, 2001). Other investigations have focused on autoimmune responses, environmental toxins, and infectious agents. Still, there is insufficient evidence to implicate any of these factors as causes of ALS (NINDS, 2003a). A genetic link to ALS is possible, as discussed in the Genetic Considerations box.

Pathophysiology

In ALS, degenerative changes occur in the anterior horn cells of the spinal cord, the motor nuclei of the brainstem, and the corticospinal tracts. Upper motor neuron degeneration leads to spasticity and reduced muscle strength, while lower motor neuron degeneration causes flaccid muscles, paralysis, and atrophy. Cognition, sensory function, vision, and hearing are spared. The bowel and bladder functions are not affected until the later stages of the disease (Borasio et al., 2001).

Clinical Manifestations

Subtle at the onset and slow in progression, the symptoms of ALS include painless muscle weakness and wasting, spasticity, cramping, fatigue, **fasciculation** (involuntary twitching) of the limb and tongue muscles, dysarthria, dysphagia, and dyspnea (Charles & Swash, 2001). Symptoms in an arm first present in roughly half of the cases, with about 20% of the occurrences affecting a leg. Initial complaints range from difficulty walking and problems with tripping and stumbling to trouble performing fine tasks

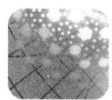

PATIENT TEACHING & DISCHARGE PRIORITIES for Multiple Sclerosis

Need	Teaching
Disease information:	Contact the National Multiple Sclerosis Society (1-800-FIGHTMS).
Patient/family	Disease progression is variable; some patients never become incapacitated.
	MS is rarely direct cause of death; expect fairly normal life span.
Medication information:	Purpose, dosage, administration schedule.
Patient/family	Correct technique for administering injectable medications.
	Administer on schedule.
	Expected side effects.
Exacerbating factors:	Mild fever worsens symptoms; take acetaminophen promptly for any fever-associated illness.
Patient/family	Prevent infections; use hand hygiene, avoid exposure to infection; get flu shot.
Setting	Avoid emotional stress, undue fatigue, and exertion.
	Avoid exposure to heat, include home temperature, hot baths, or showers.
	Use air conditioning in warm months.
Bladder management:	Correct technique for:
Patient/family	• Catheterization, if warranted
	• Credé maneuver
	• Kegel exercises.
	Call health care provider if signs/symptoms of UTI arise.
Relapse management:	Report new or worsening symptoms to health care provider.
Patient/family	
Safety:	Use thermometer to track water temperature for bathing.
Patient/family	
Health promotion:	Mild exercise is beneficial, but do not exercise to point of fatigue.
Patient/family	Consume high-fiber, low-fat diet.
	Adequate hydration.
Mobility:	Correct use of mobility aids.
Patient/family	Ambulation and transfer techniques.
Setting	Home evaluation for adaptive equipment needs.

Sources: Chaudhuri, A., & Behan, P.O. (2004). Multiple sclerosis is not an autoimmune disease. *Archives of Neurology, 61,* 1610–1612; Holloway, N. (2003). *Medical-surgical care planning* (4th ed.). Philadelphia: Lippincott Wilkins & Williams.

GENETIC CONSIDERATIONS Related to Amyotrophic Lateral Sclerosis

Genetic research has discovered a defect occurring on the gene responsible for the production of the enzyme superoxide dismutase 1 (SODI1) that may be linked to ALS. SODI1 is a powerful antioxidant that protects against free radicals, which are thought to play a role in cell degeneration. The role of the SODI1 gene mutation in motor neuron degeneration is unclear. The theory is that the malfunctioning gene allows for an excessive accumulation of free radicals.

Ninety to 95% of ALS cases are sporadic, while 5% to 10% are classified as familial. The SODI1 gene mutation accounts for approximately 20% of familial cases. Other familial forms involve mutations on the ALS2 gene, which also is implicated in the death of motor neurons.

Sources: Mitchell, J. D., & Borasio, G. D. (2007). Amyotrophic lateral sclerosis. *Lancet, 369,* 2031–2040; National Institutes of Health. (2003). *Genetics home reference: Amyotrophic lateral sclerosis.* Retrieved April 30, 2008, from http://ghr.nlm.nih.gov/condition=amyotrophiclateralsclerosis; National Institute of Neurological Disorders and Stroke. (2003a). *Amyotrophic lateral sclerosis fact sheet.* Retrieved April 2, 2008, from http://www.ninds.nih.gov/disorders/amyotrophiclateralsclerosis/detail_amyotrophiclateralsclerosis.htm.

such as buttoning clothing and writing (Charles & Swash, 2001; NINDS, 2003a).

As the disease progresses, weakness and atrophy extend throughout the muscles. The arms and legs become severely impaired. Muscles involved with speech and swallowing progressively deteriorate to the point of severe dysarthria and dysphagia (Borasio et al., 2001; Charles & Swash, 2001). Swallowing becomes difficult and increases the risk of aspirating food or saliva into the airway. Difficulties eating lead to weight loss. Because cognitive functions remain intact, patients are highly aware of the disease and its progression. Anxiety or depression is likely to complicate the condition (NINDS, 2003a). In the final stage, speaking is nearly impossible if at all. Acute dyspnea sets in and, eventually, a ventilator is required for breathing. Aspiration, infection, and respiratory failure are usually the ultimate causes of death. Average disease duration is 3 to 4 years (Borasio et al., 2001).

Laboratory and Diagnostic Procedures

Like other neurodegenerative diseases, there is no definitive test that will confirm the presence of ALS. Diagnosis is based on medical history, neurological examination, symptoms, and laboratory tests that rule out other metabolic conditions (NINDS, 2003a). Electromyography (EMG) may distinguish characteristic fibrillations that result from denervation, muscle wasting, and atrophy (Borasio et al., 2001). Brain and spinal MRI can detect structural lesions, herniated disks, or cervical spondylosis in the process of eliminating other conditions that mimic ALS symptoms. In the same manner, nerve conduction velocity (NCV) tests can discount peripheral neuropathy and myopathy (NINDS, 2003a). Several different tests are commonly used to aid in the diagnosis of ALS, as presented in the Diagnostic Tests box.

Medical Management

Like other neurodegenerative diseases, there is no cure for ALS. Medical treatment focuses on slowing the progression and on symptom management. Riluzole (Rilutek), a benzothiazole, is the only drug known to slow the progression of ALS (Mitchell & Borasio, 2007). The drug is thought to protect motor neurons by inhibiting glutamate production. Patients who respond well to riluzole delay the need for ventilatory support and lengthen their life expectancies by an average of 3 months (Mitchell & Borasio, 2007). While generally well tolerated, riluzole should be administered with strict monitoring of liver function. Dizziness, vertigo, and somnolence may result from taking the drug. Medications for symptom management may include diazepam or dantrolene for spasticity and quinine sulfate or baclofen for muscle cramping, as discussed in the Pharmacology Summary box for ALS, p. 817.

 **CRITICAL ALERT** *Patients taking riluzole should have periodic liver function tests to monitor for elevation of liver enzymes (American Society of Health-System Pharmacists, 2006).*

Nursing Management

A home health care plan is critical for patients and families who will be in particular need of ongoing support and assistance in coping with a progressive and fatal illness. They will be faced with making difficult decisions regarding artificial feeding and ventilation. It is important that the choices be made prior to a crisis so that the individual's wishes regarding end of life are honored. Throughout this process, it is critical to respect cultural differences in the meaning of death and dying. Pertinent nursing assessments, diagnoses, assessment, outcomes, and interventions are all part of the nursing process, as outlined in the Nursing Process: Patient Care Plan for Amyotrophic Lateral Sclerosis (p. 818).

Collaborative Management

Management of ALS requires a multidisciplinary approach to meet the needs of both the patient and family (Charles & Swash, 2001; Van den Berg, Kalmijn, Lindeman, Veldink, & de Visser, 2005). Treatment goals should focus on providing symptom relief and on preserving comfort and dignity, because disease progression renders the patient to a completely dependent state. In addition to the previously mentioned drug therapy, supportive care depends on a multidisciplinary approach as depicted below (Borasio et al., 2001; Charles & Swash, 2001):

- Physical therapists can conduct range-of-motion exercises that are used to combat spasticity. They also can recommend the use of orthopedic equipment such as walkers, wheelchairs, splints, and braces.
- Occupational therapists can suggest devices for performing the routine activities of eating, dressing, and bathing. Specialized eating utensils, shower chairs, and case-specific tools assist the patient in prolonging self-sufficiency. These therapists also teach energy conservation, which helps manage fatigue.
- Speech therapists can teach adaptive strategies and techniques to cope with the effects of dysarthria. They may adapt a computer-based communication system to compensate for loss of speech. In addition, these therapists can evaluate and, more importantly, monitor the patient's ability to swallow.
- Dietitians and nutritionists can assess dietary needs and modify the patient's meals to maintain nutrition and prevent aspiration. Inevitably, as the patient's condition deteriorates, the use of a gastrostomy tube will become an issue for both the patient and family.
- Respiratory therapists manage assistive ventilation based on periodic assessment of the patient's respiratory function. Respiratory therapy can be applied as intermittent positive pressure ventilation (IPPV) or bilevel positive airway pressure (BiPAP). The option of whether or not to apply mechanical ventilation will be a growing concern of both the patient and family.
- Social workers can assist with the social, emotional, and financial ramifications of ALS. Support groups, powers of attorney, living wills, financial assistance, and hospice services are areas where expertise in social services can help patients adjust to extremely difficult concerns.
- Spiritual counselors consistent with patient and family beliefs can help the patient and family accept and cope with inevitable death.

DIAGNOSTIC TESTS for Amyotrophic Lateral Sclerosis

Test	Expected Result	Rationale
Electromyogram (EMG)	Fibrillations	May show signs of denervation, muscle wasting, and atrophy.
CPK level	May be elevated	Indicates breakdown of muscle tissue.
MRI brain and spine	Normal	Rule out conditions that could mimic symptoms of ALS.

Sources: Borasio, G. D., & Miller, R. G. (2001). Clinical characteristics and management of ALS. *Seminars in Neurology, 21,* 155–166; Muscular Dystrophy Association. (2003). *Facts about ALS.* Retrieved April 30, 2008, from http://www.als-mda.org/publications/fa-als.html; National Institute of Neurological Disorders and Stroke. (2003). *Multiple sclerosis: Hope through research.* Retrieved April 30, 2008, from http://www.ninds.nih.gov.

Discharge Priorities

The Patient Teaching & Discharge Priorities box (p. 819) covers a wide range of topics that apply to the patient with ALS.

PHARMACOLOGY Summary of Medications to Treat ALS

Medication Category	Action	Application/ Indication	Nursing Responsibilities
Anti-ALS			
riluzole (Rilutek)	Slows progression of ALS by protecting motor neurons through inhibition of glutamate production.	Treatment of ALS	• Monitor for adverse effects: muscular weakness, dizziness, somnolence, nausea, diarrhea, decreased lung function. • Monitor liver function and blood count. • Be aware of multiple drug interactions; (theophylline, barbiturates, aminoglycosides and others). Monitor riluzole plasma levels and observe for hepatotoxicity. • Warn patient caffeine, cigarette smoking, high fat diet, and charcoal-broiled food affect riluzole level. • Give on an empty stomach.
Skeletal Muscle Relaxants			
centrally acting diazepam (Valium) baclofen (Kemstro, Lioresal)*	Relaxes skeletal muscle most likely by depressing afferent reflex activity at the level of the spinal cord.	Spasticity, muscle spasms	• Monitor for adverse effects: drowsiness, dizziness, weakness, confusion, hypotension, nausea, constipation. • Monitor for psychiatric disturbances, especially in elderly. • Monitor liver and kidney function, especially in elderly or if renal or hepatic disease present. • Warn patient to avoid alcohol and other CNS depressants. • Be aware abruptly stopping drug may result in adverse reactions. • Monitor diabetics for hyperglycemia.*
Peripherally Acting			
dantrolene (Dantrium)	Relaxes skeletal muscle by interfering with calcium ion release within muscle.	Spasticity	• Monitor for adverse effects: muscle weakness, slurred speech, fatigue, diarrhea, constipation. • Monitor blood count, liver and renal function. • Monitor for signs of pleural effusion and pericarditis in patients with cardiac disease, respiratory depression in patients with pulmonary dysfunction. • Warn patient not to use alcohol, check with health care provider before using OTC medications. • Warn patient about possible photosensitivity and need for sun block. • Teach patient symptoms of hepatitis. Notify health care provider if present.
Antimalarial			
quinine sulfate (Quinamm, Quiphile)	Reduces muscle cramping by direct action at the neuromuscular junction.	Muscle cramping	• Monitor for adverse effects: headache, sweating, tinnitus, vertigo, visual disturbances, vomiting, diarrhea, abdominal pain, cardiac arrhythmias. • Be aware of multiple drug interactions; monitor for toxicity or decreased drug efficacy (digoxin, antacids, warfarin, anticonvulsants, and others). • Give with food or milk.

Sources: Geriatrics, 61, 3–7; Mylan Bertek Pharmaceuticals. (2004). Apokyn [Package insert]; National Institutes of Health. (2003). *Genetics home reference: Amyotrophic lateral sclerosis.* Retrieved April 30, 2008, from http://ghr.nlm.nih.gov/condition=amyotrophiclateralsclerosis.

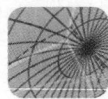

NURSING PROCESS: Patient Care Plan for Amyotrophic Lateral Sclerosis

Assessment for Comfort in Breathing

Subjective Data:
Do you feel comfortable?
Do you have a headache?
Do you feel tired?

Objective Data:
Neurological status including level of consciousness, cognition
Vital signs
Respiratory status, including respiration rate, pattern, lung sounds, accessory muscles, pulmonary function studies
Skin and nail bed color
Restlessness

Nursing Assessment and Diagnoses	Outcomes and Evaluation Parameters	Planning and Interventions with *Rationales*
Nursing Diagnosis: *Ineffective Breathing Pattern* related to neuromuscular dysfunction	**Outcome:** Patient receives ventilatory assistance to extent desired. ***Evaluation Parameter:*** Patient reports minimal respiratory discomfort.	**Interventions and *Rationales:*** Discuss wishes with patient and family. Consult with spiritual care. Record advance directives/patient wishes for ventilatory assistance in medical record. *Ensures that patient's wishes are met.* Assess respiratory rate and lung sounds q4h *to assess for respiratory distress.* Monitor pulmonary function studies and arterial blood gases as ordered *to assess adequacy of gas exchange.* Assess for morning headaches, restlessness, nightmares, or poor quality of sleep. *Indicates poor gas exchange with resultant brain hypoxia.* Assess skin and nail bed color. *Indicator of poor gas exchange with resultant tissue hypoxia.* Consult with respiratory therapist for noninvasive ventilatory device. *May be recommended if vital capacity is < 70%.*

Assessment for Ability to Swallow Foods and Liquids

Subjective Data:
Do you feel like you have trouble swallowing food or liquids?
Are you afraid of choking?

Objective Data:
Neurological assessment including swallowing and gag reflex
Vital signs
Respiratory status including rate and lung sounds
Choking on food or liquids
Tube feedings
Swallowing studies

Nursing Assessment and Diagnoses	Outcomes and Evaluation Parameters	Planning and Interventions with *Rationales*
Nursing Diagnosis: *High Risk for Aspiration* related to impaired swallowing muscles	**Outcome:** Patient does not show signs of aspiration. ***Evaluation Parameters:*** Patient is able to swallow food without choking or aspirating. Patient does not aspirate oral secretions. Lung sounds clear. No signs of infection.	**Interventions and *Rationales:*** Monitor for persistent coughing after swallowing liquids. *May indicate aspiration.* Consult with speech-language pathologist. *Can evaluate swallowing ability.* Consult with dietitian. *Can develop diet consistent with patient's swallowing abilities.* Administer and evaluate response to medications. *Medications may be given to dry oral secretions.* Discuss wishes regarding tube feedings with patient and family. Consult with spiritual care if needed. Record advance. directives/patient wishes for nutritional support in medical record *to ensure that patient's wishes are met.*

Assessment for Psychological and Spiritual Comfort

Subjective Data:
Do you have a spiritual counselor?
Has your family ever experienced loss and/or death?

Objective Data:
Patient/family interactions
Patient/family cultural background and religious preferences
Use of spiritual resources

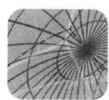

NURSING PROCESS: Patient Care Plan for Amyotrophic Lateral Sclerosis—*Continued*

Nursing Assessment and Diagnoses	Outcomes and Evaluation Parameters	Planning and Interventions with *Rationales*
Nursing Diagnosis: *Anticipatory Grieving*, patient and family, related to fatal illness	**Outcome:** Patient and family move through the grieving process and come to terms with fatal illness. *Evaluation Parameters:* Patient and family use culturally appropriate coping mechanisms to deal with loss. Patient and family utilize spiritual resources to cope with pending death. Patient and family verbalize the grieving process and how it relates to their situation. Patient and family express feelings related to fatal illness. Patient and family attend support group. Patient and family formulate advance directives.	**Interventions and *Rationales:*** Discuss cultural beliefs with patient and family. *Provides knowledge of cultural beliefs that may influence the grieving process.* Provide patient and family opportunity to verbalize feelings related to prognosis *to help facilitate acceptance.* Encourage patient/family to consult with spiritual counselor consistent with culture and beliefs. *Can help facilitate acceptance and coping.* Encourage patient and family to attend appropriate support groups. *Such groups provide safe environment to express feelings.* Help patient and family become familiar with the grieving process *to help facilitate acceptance and coping.* Encourage patient and family to formulate advance directives. *Provides a sense of control and ensures that patient's wishes are met.*

Sources: Borasio, G. D., Voltz, R., & Miller, R. G. (2001). Palliative care in amyotrophic lateral sclerosis. *Neurologic Clinics, 19*(4), 829–845; Carter, G., & Miller, R. (1998). Comprehensive management of amyotrophic lateral sclerosis. *Physical Medicine and Rehabilitation Clinics of North America, 9*(1), 271–283; Charles, T., & Swash, M. (2001). Amyotrophic lateral sclerosis: Current understanding. *Journal of Neuroscience Nursing, 33*, 245–253.

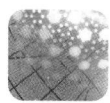

PATIENT TEACHING & DISCHARGE PRIORITIES for Amyotrophic Lateral Sclerosis

Need	Teaching
Disease process: Patient/family	Disease symptoms and progression; fatal illness.
	Notify health care professional of increasing weakness, difficulty swallowing.
	Cognition is generally not affected by disease process.
	Contact the Muscular Dystrophy Association (1-800-572-1717; http://www.mdausa.org) or the ALS Association (1-800-782-4747; http://www.alsa.org) for educational materials.
Psychosocial: Patient/family	Encourage consultation with mental health professional.
	Encourage participation in support group.
Respiratory care: Patient/family	Correct use of respiratory equipment such as oxygen therapy, noninvasive ventilatory devices, and suction equipment.
	Guidelines for breathing: • Don't lie down after eating. • Avoid eating large meals. • Sleep with head elevated 15 to 30 degrees.
Communication: Patient/family	Develop alternative methods to communicate, such as blinking, if not able to speak.
Diet and oral care: Patient/family	Clean corners of mouth after eating.
	Soft diet as tolerated.
	Pureed foods should be placed on posterior tongue.
	Solid foods should be eaten slowly, in small pieces, and swallowed after every bite.
	Correct care of feeding tube if utilized.
Activity: Patient/family	Balance activity with rest periods.
	Mild low-impact aerobic exercise OK if able; do not exercise to exhaustion; stop if experiencing muscle cramping, heaviness in extremities, prolonged shortness of breath.
	Correct use of braces, splints, or other orthotic devices.
	Correct positioning and transfer techniques.
End-of-life issues: Patient/family	Need to make proactive decisions regarding mechanical ventilation, artificial hydration, and nutrition.
	Hospice services can help ensure comfortable death at home in accordance with patient and family wishes.
	Encourage spiritual guidance in accordance with patient, family, and cultural beliefs.

Sources: Borasio, G. D., Voltz, R., & Miller, R. G. (2001). Palliative care in amyotrophic lateral sclerosis. *Neurologic Clinics, 19*(4), 829–845; Carter, G., & Miller, R. (1998). Comprehensive management of amyotrophic lateral sclerosis. *Physical Medicine and Rehabilitation Clinics of North America, 9*(1), 271–283; Charles, T., & Swash, M. (2001). Amyotrophic lateral sclerosis: Current understanding. *Journal of Neuroscience Nursing, 33*, 245–253.

Health Promotion

People with ALS do maintain careers and interests. They are encouraged to remain active for as long as possible. Referral for psychological and/or spiritual counseling may help the patient and family come to terms with the disease and its prognosis. Many find support groups their most valuable asset in the struggle against the condition. Internet organizations also connect individuals who wish to communicate about the disease.

◼ Myasthenia Gravis

Myasthenia gravis (MG) is a chronic, autoimmune neuromuscular disorder in which acetylcholine receptors at the neuromuscular junction are destroyed. The two major clinical forms of MG are ocular and generalized (Awwad & Maluf, 2007). The hallmark feature is fluctuating weakness and fatigability of voluntary muscles.

Epidemiology and Etiology

MG is a relatively uncommon disorder, with an annual incidence of 2 new cases per million people in the United States (Awwad & Maluf, 2007). It occurs at any age, although the age of onset is commonly either at 20 to 40 years of age for women or 60 to 80 years of age for men. Overall, the disorder is more common in women than in men, with a female-to-male ratio of 3:2 (Phillips, 2004).

Although the primary etiology remains speculative, there is increasing evidence that the thymus might play an important role. Histological studies have shown prominent germinal centers (Awwad & Maluf, 2007). Epithelial myoid cells normally present in the thymus do resemble skeletal muscle cells and possess acetylcholine receptor (AChR) on their surface membrane; therefore, it is hypothesized that they may become antigenic and set free an autoimmune attack of the muscular end plate AChR by molecular mimicry. Note also that the majority of people affected by MG also have thymus gland abnormalities. It remains unclear why the disease afflicts first and predominantly the extraocular muscles.

Pathophysiology

Muscle weakness in MG is the result of dysfunction at the neuromuscular junction. Acetylcholine (ACh) is a neurotransmitter vital for the transmission of nerve impulses to skeletal muscles, and it is produced in motor nerve endings. In MG, antibodies generated by an autoimmune response bind to AChRs, blocking the transmission of nerve impulses. This inefficient neuromuscular transmission together with the normally present presynaptic rundown phenomenon results in a decremental amount of nerve fibers being activated by successive nerve fiber impulses. This, then, accounts for the fatigability and characteristic muscular weakness of those with the disease (Augustus, 2000; Awwad & Maluf, 2007).

Clinical Manifestations

Usually the initial complaint is a specific muscle weakness rather than generalized muscle weakness. The severity of the weakness typically fluctuates over hours being least severe in the morning and worsening as the day progresses. It also varies over the course of weeks or months, with exacerbations and remissions. Exposure to sunlight, viral illness, surgery, immunization, emotional stress, menstruation, and physical factors might trigger or worsen exacerbations (Awwad & Maluf, 2007). As MG progresses, symptom-free periods decrease, and muscle weakness fluctuates from mild to severe (Keesey, 2004).

Symptoms are classified by some as ophthalmic and nonophthalmic. A majority of the patients initially complain of ocular disturbance, mainly ptosis and diplopia. Ptosis may be unilateral or bilateral and it may shift from eye to eye. Eventually 90% of patients with MG develop ocular symptoms. About 50% of patients present solely with ocular symptoms, and about 50% to 60% progress to develop generalized disease. Of the nonophthalmic symptoms, oropharyngeal muscle disturbances come second in presentation, with approximately 15% of patients first experiencing difficulty in swallowing, talking, and chewing (Awwad & Maluf, 2007).

MG can affect any skeletal muscle group, with 10% of patients initially complaining of limb and trunk weakness. Weakness in the bulbar muscles produces dysarthria and dysphagia, and a nasal quality to the voice. If facial muscles are involved, the patient may appear expressionless or impart a snarling expression when attempting to smile. Involvement of respiratory muscles may lead to symptoms of respiratory insufficiency, and even respiratory failure, an emergency known as **myasthenic crisis**. Patients also demonstrate incremental weakness upon repeating the motor power test over and over.

Patients with MG are at risk for two life-threatening situations with a similar clinical picture: myasthenic crisis and cholinergic crisis. The patient will present with extreme weakness and respiratory insufficiency. Myasthenic crisis is caused by undermedication (lack of acetylcholine) or stressors such as infection, surgery, or incompatible medications. The less common **cholinergic crisis** results from overmedication (excess acetylcholine). Both conditions are medical emergencies because they require mechanical ventilation (Augustus, 2000).

Laboratory and Diagnostic Procedures

MG is initially diagnosed through a detailed history and physical assessment, including a neurological examination. The Tensilon test may be administered, in which 2 mg of edrophonium chloride (Tensilon), a cholinesterase inhibitor with rapid onset and short duration of action, is administered intravenously at 30- to 60-second intervals up to a total of 10 mg. Patients with MG will demonstrate a distinct increase in muscle strength within 30 to 60 seconds. Administration of cholinergic drugs, however, may precipitate a cholinergic crisis, which is a life-threatening situation. Symptoms of cholinergic crisis include muscle weakness, cramps, difficulty talking, difficulty swallowing, bradycardia, bronchospasm, excessive salivation, vomiting, diarrhea and excessive sweating. A Tensilon test should not be administered without the ready availability of intravenous atropine, an antidote for edrophonium (Augustus, 2000; Hood, 1999).

Though not definitive, EMG may contribute to a diagnosis of MG. Repetitive nerve stimulation may be used to evaluate the decremental response in compound action potentials on EMG. A computerized tomography (CT) or MRI scan may be performed to evaluate the thymus gland and to rule out mass lesions compressing cranial nerves. Laboratory studies will include immunologic assays to detect AChR antibodies (Augustus, 2000). Thyroid function tests are indicated to rule out associated Graves' disease or hyperthyroidism. This is particularly essential in patients with ocular MG where the concomitant hyperthyroidism is most frequent.

Recently, the ice pack test (i.e., placing ice over the eyelid) has gained interest among ophthalmologists to assess improvement in ptosis and diplopia in ocular MG, the rationale being that cooling might improve neuromuscular transmission. This remains questionable by some (Awwad & Maluf, 2007; Larner, 2004), as they have demonstrated that patients with ocular MG actually improve on the ice, heat, and modified sleep tests. Hence, rest might be the cause of the improvement in ocular signs. Benatar & Kaminski, (2007) has countered that both the ice test and the rest test are sensitive and specific in ocular MG.

Medical Management

A wide range of treatments may be used for patients with MG. There is not, however, a consensus about which to start first or which to combine. According to Awwad and Maluf (2007), there is general agreement that medical treatment is administered best by a neurologist, and an ophthalmologist should follow up on the ophthalmic symptoms, such as diplopia and ptosis. Ptosis, when it becomes bothersome, is treated best by lid crutches; surgery is contraindicated because of the fluctuation of the disease. Diplopia is treated with the use of Fresnel prisms unless the deviation is large and variable, in which case an opaque lens over the affected eye is preferred.

Surgical treatment includes thymectomy, strabismus surgery, and blepharoptosis. Thymectomy may be performed in the absence of a thymoma. Approximately 85% of patients experience improvement, and 35% of these patients achieve drug-free remission. Patients often experience some transient worsening of symptoms early in the postoperative period, and improvement usually is delayed for months or years. Strabismus surgery may be used for selected patients with a stable course of MG. If a patient has stable ptosis, which has failed to respond to medical therapy, blepharoptosis may be performed.

Drug Therapy

The neurologist tends to coordinate the pharmacologic treatment. Cholinesterase inhibitors (neostigmine, pyridostigmine, or ambenonium) are used to treat the symptoms of MG by preventing the breakdown of acetylcholine at the neuromuscular junction. Pyridostigmine is the most commonly prescribed cholinesterase inhibitor, because it tends to have the least severe muscarinic side effects, including abdominal cramping, diarrhea, increased peristalsis, increased salivation, bradycardia, and blurred vision. Dosage is adjusted to manage the patient's symptoms (Augustus, 2000).

Patients with MG who remain symptomatic on cholinesterase inhibitors may require immunotherapy. Commonly prescribed immunotherapeutic drugs include corticosteroids, azathioprine, and cyclosporine (Saperstein & Barohn, 2004). Although administration of corticosteroids leads to marked improvement in the majority of patients, there may be an initial worsening of symptoms. For this reason, initiation of corticosteroids is reserved for hospitalized patients (Augustus, 2000).

The Pharmacology Summary discusses other drug therapies for myasthenia gravis (p. 822).

Plasmapheresis

Plasmapheresis may be used when a patient is in crisis or not adequately responding to other therapy. Circulating AChR antibodies are removed from the patient's circulation by removing whole blood, extracting the plasma from it, and returning the blood along with fresh or frozen plasma to the patient. The outpatient procedure is repeated three to four times over a period of 8 to10 days (Augustus, 2000).

Intravenous Immunoglobulin Therapy

Intravenous immunoglobulin (IVIG) therapy is an alternative to plasmapheresis for treating the patient with MG who is experiencing increasing weakness. It may be used as preoperative treatment before thymectomy. Monthly courses of IVIG therapy may be administered until the slower immunotherapy approaches, such as corticosteroids, take effect. The mechanism of action for IVIG therapy is not certain (Saperstein & Barohn, 2004).

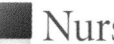 # Nursing Management

Application of the nursing process will facilitate a comprehensive approach to patient care throughout the disease process. Relevant nursing diagnoses, assessment, outcomes, and interventions are all part of the nursing process.

Assessment

Nursing diagnoses for the patient with MG will depend on the muscles affected for each individual. A thorough history of disease onset and progression should be reviewed. Baseline data for respiratory function, bulbar function, and fatigue should be established, including (Augustus, 2000):

- Vital signs, with special attention to respiratory rate
- Breath sounds and breathing pattern
- Lung vital capacity
- Integrity of gag/swallow reflex
- Ability to chew and swallow
- Ability to see correctly without diplopia, ocular motility disturbance, or ptosis
- Ability to perform self-care activities.

Nursing Diagnoses

Possible diagnoses include (Augustus, 2000):

- *Ineffective Breathing Pattern* related to neuromuscular weakness
- *Alteration in Vision Acuity* related to ocular muscle involvement and ptosis
- *Imbalanced Nutrition: Less Than Body Requirements* related to dysphagia, bulbar weakness
- *Self-Care Deficit* related to weakness
- *Deficient Knowledge* related to disease process, medications, and/or energy conservation.

PHARMACOLOGY Summary of Medications to Treat Myasthenia Gravis

Medication Category	Action	Application/Indication	Nursing Responsibility
Cholinesterase Inhibitors			
neostigmine (Prostigmin) pyridostigmine (Mestinon) ambenonium (Mytelase) edrophonium chloride (Tensilon)	Increases strength of muscle contraction by preventing the breakdown of acetylcholine at the neuromuscular junction.	Symptomatic treatment of myasthenia gravis diagnosis of myasthenia gravis, differentiation between cholinergic and myasthenic crises (not recommended for maintenance therapy due to short duration of action)	• Monitor for adverse effects: abdominal cramping, nausea, vomiting, diarrhea, diaphoresis, blurred vision, bradycardia, hypotension, bronchospasm. • Monitor for cholinergic crisis. Assess vital signs, respiratory and neuromuscular function. Have atropine and resuscitation equipment immediately available for treatment. • Be aware of drug interactions (corticosteroids, aminoglycoside, antibiotics, and others).
Immunosuppressants			
azathioprine (Imuran) cyclosporine (Sandimmune, Neoral)	Suppresses immune response by inhibiting lymphocyte replication or disrupting helper T cells.	Treatment of myasthenia gravis	• Monitor for adverse effects: hirsutism, hypertension, nausea, vomiting, infection. • Observe for signs of toxicity: tremors, seizures, altered mental status, visual disturbances. • Monitor CBC, liver and renal function tests, *magnesium, *potassium, *blood sugar. • Be aware of multiple drug interactions (digoxin, NSAIDS, erythromycin, verapamil, cimetidine, and others with cyclosporine; allopurinal, ace inhibitors, warfarin, and others with azathioprine). Monitor for altered drug levels, nephrotoxicity, or leukopenia.
Corticosteroid			
prednisone	Reduces acetylcholine receptor antibody levels, may enhance neuromuscular transmission.	Myasthenia gravis immunosuppression	• Monitor for adverse effects: mood swings, anxiety, insomnia, nausea, vomiting, weight gain, acne, delayed wound healing. • Monitor clinical response to guide incremental dosing. • Observe for transient steroid induced exacerbation of MG with initiation of drug. • Monitor blood count, glucose, and electrolytes. • Be aware of drug interactions (theophylline, warfarin, and others). Monitor for toxicity or decreased efficacy. • Warn patient of potential need for dose adjustment if ill or stress increases and to not abruptly stop drug.

Planning

The overall goals of nursing care for the patient with MG are to minimize symptoms and to detect early signs of myasthenic or cholinergic crisis.

Outcomes and Evaluation Parameters

The outcomes and evaluation parameters are as follows (Augustus, 2000):

- Respiratory rate of 16 to 20 breaths per minute
- Vital capacity 4,600 mL
- Total lung capacity 5,800 mL
- Intact gag/cough reflex
- Able to read and establish visual field
- Heart rate of 60 to 100 beats per minute
- Weight maintained at baseline
- Patient/family verbalizes understanding of disease process, treatments, and signs of myasthenic or cholinergic crises.

In terms of evaluation parameters, the patient with MG will not show evidence of respiratory insufficiency. Weight will be at baseline. The patient will be able to independently complete ADLs and will verbalize an understanding of the disease process, treatment, and signs of myasthenic or cholinergic crisis.

Interventions and Rationales

Because respiratory muscles are often affected, the patient with MG should be monitored closely for signs of respiratory insufficiency that could indicate impending myasthenic crisis. MG often affects the bulbar muscles involved with chewing and swallowing, so ability to chew and swallow should be monitored closely. Other nutritional parameters such as weight, intake and output, electrolytes, and serum albumin should be monitored. The patient should be educated on energy conservation techniques, such as taking frequent rests when completing ADLs. Assistance with bathing and dressing may be needed.

Discharge Priorities

The importance of taking medications on time and as ordered should be emphasized. If bulbar muscles are affected, the patient should be instructed to eat and chew slowly and to match food consistency to the ability to swallow. Nutritional counseling may be necessary if optimal weight cannot be maintained. Caregivers should be instructed on the Heimlich maneuver technique. Patients should be taught measures to prevent respiratory infection, and to contact their health care provider immediately if signs or symptoms occur. Energy conservation strategies such as undertaking physical activities early in the day, and alternating activity with frequent rest periods should be emphasized. It is critical for the patient to know the signs and symptoms of crisis and to seek immediate help should they occur. The patient should also wear a medic alert bracelet and carry a card stating diagnosis, medication dose, and medication schedule (Augustus, 2000).

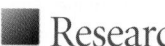 Research

Neurodegenerative conditions offer a plethora of opportunities for nursing research. These are summarized in the Research Opportunities feature.

EVIDENCE-BASED PRACTICE

Family Caregiver Assistance

Clinical Problem

It is estimated that there are more than 44 million family caregivers in the United States who provide 80% of home care to chronically ill older adults (Habermann & Davis, 2005; National Alliance for Caregiving, 2005). Family caregivers may provide a multitude of tasks in the daily care of their loved ones, from assisting with ADLs, to tasks requiring problem-solving skills and clinical judgment, such as managing symptoms and carrying out treatments as in medication regimes. In addition, family caregivers are often responsible for coordinating health care and social services (Schumacher, Beck, & Marren, 2006). Decades of research has confirmed that providing care to an older, chronically ill family member is stressful and can negatively affect family caregivers' physical and mental health (Schumacher et al., 2006).

While much of the current knowledge of family caregiving has been learned from studies of caregivers to individuals with AD (Habermann & Davis, 2005), further studies suggest that caregivers of individuals with other illnesses have similar negative physical and mental health outcomes. Nurses, particularly those who care for patients with neurodegenerative diseases, will encounter family caregivers in a variety of health care settings, and are often the primary source for family caregivers to learn how to provide care (Schumacher et al., 2006; Shyu, 2000).

Research Findings

Habermann and Davis (2005) conducted a study to compare the assistance needs of family caregivers for individuals with Alzheimer's disease and Parkinson's disease, with the overarching goal of exploring whether there is a core set of caregiver needs across illness groups. The authors opted to study the needs of caregivers of family members with the neurodegenerative diseases AD and PD. These conditions were selected because, although they have a similar downhill disease trajectory, each condition presents unique challenges for the family caregiver. Forty caregivers took part in the study; twenty of whom cared for a family member with AD, and twenty who cared for a family member with PD. The study participants participated in a semistructured, interview which included a self-scored caregiver needs assessment tool as well as open-ended questions addressing the challenges and satisfaction of caregiving. The caregiver needs assessment tool addressed needs in the following areas: (1) caregiving knowledge and skills, (2) finding and using community resources, and (3) accessing personal assistance. This sample of two groups of family caregivers agreed on 75% of these assistance needs. There was additional agreement between the two groups on the challenges of caregiving.

Implications for Nursing Practice

Although further research needs to be conducted regarding specific interventions to increase knowledge, skills, and self-care for caregivers, nurses should be cognizant that there may be common family caregiver needs and challenges across the span of neurodegenerative disorders. Specifically, family caregivers for individuals with AD and PD identified high needs for information about the illness as well as the need for practical training on how to provide care. When providing education and support to individuals with these conditions, nurses need to identify and include the family caregiver. Furthermore, caregivers need information about self-care for their own health promotion, and encouragement to pursue activities to support their own health and well-being.

Critical Thinking Questions

1. What are the important points that would be included in an education plan for patients and families with a neurodegenerative disorder such as AD or PD?

2. How might a nurse determine that a family caregiver understands education and information that has been provided in the plan of care?

3. What measures could nurses recommend to family caregivers to encourage self-care?

Answers to Critical Thinking Questions appear in Appendix D

References

Habermann, B., & Davis, L. L. (2005). Caring for family with Alzheimer's and Parkinson's disease: Needs, challenges and satisfactions. *Journal of Gerontological Nursing, 31,* 49–54.

National Alliance for Caregiving. (2005). *Caregiving in the U.S.* Bethesda, MD: Author.

Schumacher, K., Beck, C. A., & Marren, J. M. (2006). Family caregivers: Caring for older adults, working with their families. *American Journal of Nursing, 106,* 40–49.

Shyu, Y. L. (2000). Role tuning between caregiver and care receiver during discharge transition: an illustration of role function mode in Roy's adaptation theory. *Nursing Research Quarterly, 13*(4), 323–331.

RESEARCH OPPORTUNITIES AND CLINICAL IMPACT RELATED TO NEURODEGENERATIVE DISEASES

Research Area	Clinical Impact
Quality-of-Life (QOL) Research	Established domains of QOL.
• Assessing domains of QOL.	
• Impact of disease progression on QOL.	Improve interventions that enhance QOL in face of degenerative disease.
• Factors that mediate QOL.	
• Interventions that improve QOL.	
• Cultural implications for QOL.	
Patient/Family Education Research	Proven interventions for effective patient/family education.
• Assessing the changing learning needs of patient/family throughout disease trajectory.	
• Efficacy of interventions to educate patient/family throughout disease trajectory.	
• Literacy levels of educational materials versus literacy levels of patient/family.	
• Use of multimedia educational interventions.	
• Use of Internet as patient/family education tool.	
• Factors influencing patient/family learning.	
• Cultural implications for patient/family education.	
Caregiver Research	Maintain family caregiver health.
• Changing education and support needs throughout disease trajectory.	
• Skill-building educational interventions.	
• Anticipatory grief.	
• Factors influencing positive and negative caregiver experience.	
• Barriers to accessing community resources.	
• Cultural implications of family caregiving.	
Emotional and Psychological Research	Adaptation to progressing disability.
• Ambiguous loss.	
• Impact of role change.	
• Sexuality and intimacy issues.	
• Successful coping.	
• Factors that influence patients/families to seek mental health services.	
Complementary/Alternative Approach	Impact of complementary approaches on disease management and experience.
• Impact of meditation and prayer on disease management and experience.	
• Factors influencing patients and family members to seek alternative treatments.	

Clinical Preparation

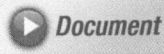 **Read**

- History of Current Illness
- Past Medical History
- Physical Exam
- Admitting Medical Orders
- Laboratory Study Results

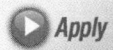 **Document**

- Summary of Hospitalization
- Pathophysiology Form
- Laboratory Values
- Laboratory Results Explanation

Apply

- List of Potential Nursing Diagnoses
- Concept Map
- Critical Thinking Questions

*Log on to MyNursingKit.com to download forms you will need and to complete further steps in the Clinical Preparation assignment.

HISTORY OF PRESENT ILLNESS

You are the on-coming nurse receiving report on Mr. X, a 65-year-old male admitted with a diagnosis of Parkinson's disease (PD). Today he underwent surgery for unilateral deep brain stimulation (DBS) therapy. His surgery lasted approximately 5 hours. Mr. X was awake for the surgery that involved placement of the DBS lead, so he did not have general anesthesia. There were no complications during surgery. The implantable pulse generator (also called the battery or pacemaker) will be placed in 1 week in outpatient surgery. Thus, the leads are not yet generating electrical stimulation.

Medical–Surgical History

Mr. X has been diagnosed with PD for 10 years. His case of PD is staged as Hoehn and Yahr Stage III. He has had peak-dose dyskinesia for the past 3 years, as well as unpredictable on–off fluctuations. His medical and surgical history is negative otherwise. His medications include ropinirole, carbidopa/levodopa LA 50/200, amantadine, citalopram, and apomorphine injections prn. His medical history is significant for an appendectomy at 21 years of age.

Social History

Mr. X is a retired bank manager. He is married and has two adult children.

Physical Exam

Mr. X is sleepy but easily aroused and oriented to person, place, and time. His pupils are equal, round, and reactive to light at 4 mm. His speech is low and muffled, and slightly slurred. He is able to move all four extremities equally although movement is slow and stiff. He denies numbness and tingling in his extremities. He has pronounced tremor in his upper extremities. He denies nausea, and has been sipping on clear liquids with assistance. His abdomen is soft, with bowel sounds present in four quadrants. His lungs are clear. He has voided in a urinal standing at the bedside. He has not had a bowel movement. He has a heparin lock in his right forearm. Mr. X has a 1-cm wound at the top of the cranium. He took his anti-PD medications last evening, but has not had any today. Mr. X needs assistance to sit at the bedside, and is able to turn himself over in bed.

Admitting Medical Orders

Admit to Neurosurgical Floor, Neurosurgery Service
Diagnosis: Parkinson's disease, scheduled DBS surgery
Allergies: none noted
VS q4h
Neuro checks q1h × 4, then q2h × 2, then q4h
Ambulate with assistance
Bathroom privileges
I/O q shift
Diet: advance diet as tolerated
Call house officer: HR < 50 or > 120, systolic BP < 90 or > 160, temperature >38.5°C, RR < 10 or > 30, change in neuro status, urinary output < 240 mL in 8 hours, O₂ saturation < 92%
Saline lock with NS flushes q8h
Wound care: dry sterile dressing to scalp wound daily and prn; if drainage present, notify health care provider

Scheduled Medications

Ropinirole 4 mg po tid
Carbidopa/levodopa CR 50/200 po tid
Amantadine 100 mg po bid
Citalopram 40 mg po daily

PRN Medications

Apomorphine 0.2–0.4 ml sq q4h prn for muscle stiffness or lack of muscle control
Darvocet N-100 i-ii po q6h prn for pain, maximum 8 tabs/day

Ordered Laboratory Studies

CBC, Chem 7 panel, PT, PTT, and INR daily

Laboratory Findings

On admission, all lab values were WNL, including CBC, chemistry panel, and bleeding times.

LABORATORY STUDY RESULTS

Test	On Admission	Postop Day 1	Postop Day 2
Sodium	135 mEq/L	137 mEq/L	140 mEq/L
Potassium	3.5 mEq/L	3.7 mEq/L	3.7 mEq/L
Chloride	97 mEq/L	100 mEq/L	101 mEq/L
Carbon dioxide	22 mEq/L	23 mEq/L	24 mEq/L
Blood urea nitrogen (BUN)	22 mg/dL	23 mg/dL	25 mg/dL
Creatinine	1.3 mg/dL	1.3 mg/dL	1.2 mg/dL
Blood glucose	90 mg/dL	94 mg/dL	100 mg/dL
White blood cells	8000 µL	8200 µL	8200 µL
Hemoglobin	140 g/dL	13.5 g/dL	13.6 g/dL
Hematocrit	50%	53%	50%
Platelets	200,000 µL	210,000 µL	220,000 µL
Protime (PT)	12 seconds	12 seconds	13 seconds
Partial thromboplastin time (PTT)	60 seconds	62 seconds	65 seconds
International Normalized Ratio (INR)	2.0 INR	2.0 INR	2.5 INR

CRITICAL THINKING QUESTIONS

1. What are potential postop complications for which you would want to carefully assess?

2. As Mr. X restarts his oral anti-PD meds postop, what aspects of his neuro check would you carefully assess?

3. What are some of the psychosocial issues that you would assess Mr. X for?

4. If Mr. X requests an injection of Apomorphine, what would you assess before the injection?

Answers to Critical Thinking Questions appear in Appendix D.

NCLEX® REVIEW

1. A patient is demonstrating agnosia. The nurse realizes this impairment is characteristic of which of the following disorders?
   1. Multiple sclerosis
   2. Alzheimer's disease
   3. Parkinson's disease
   4. Myasthenia gravis

2. A patient is experiencing a disorder that is caused by demyelinating nerve fibers and plaque formation. The nurse realizes this patient is experiencing:
   1. Alzheimer's disease.
   2. Myasthenia gravis.
   3. Multiple sclerosis.
   4. Parkinson's disease.

3. The nurse is devising a plan of care for a patient with multiple sclerosis. Which of the following interventions should the nurse include to help reduce the incidence and frequency of fatigue?
   1. Discuss voiding patterns.
   2. Plan for a daily hot shower.
   3. Minimize the use of assistive devices.
   4. Instruct to avoid prolonged exposure to hot temperatures including showers, baths, and environmental temperatures.

4. The nurse is preparing a discharge plan of care for a patient with Parkinson's disease. Which of the following should be included to help the patient with constipation?
   1. Restrict fluids.
   2. Increase dietary fiber.
   3. Take a laxative every evening.
   4. Limit protein intake.

5. A patient with Alzheimer's disease is being cared for at home by her adult daughter. Which of the following should the nurse instruct the daughter to support health promotion needs?
   1. Discuss advance directives for management of advanced stages of the disease.
   2. Encourage getting involved in clinical research studies.
   3. Instruct to avoid extreme temperatures and exposure to infections.
   4. Refer for psychological and spiritual counseling.

6. A patient with Parkinson's disease tells the nurse that she's worried about her 80-year-old husband's ability to care for her as she gets older. Which of the following would be an appropriate response for the nurse to make to this patient?

   1. That's not something that you should be worried about.

   2. You are so healthy now that I'm sure you won't be a burden to your husband.

   3. Would you like to talk about things that can help you and your husband?

   4. I'll get the doctor for you so you can talk with him about your concerns.

7. The nurse is interested in research that focuses on complementary approaches to neurodegenerative diseases. Which of the following topics would the nurse find the most interesting?

   1. Interventions that improve quality of life

   2. Literacy levels of educational materials versus literacy levels of patient/family

   3. Anticipatory grief

   4. Impact of meditation and prayer on disease management and experience

Answers for review questions appear in Appendix D

KEY TERMS

acetylcholine *p.794*
Alzheimer's disease (AD) *p.788*
amyotrophic lateral sclerosis (ALS) *p.814*
ataxia *p.809*
bradykinesia *p.800*
cholinergic crisis *p.820*
dementia *p.788*
dopamine *p.798*
dyskinesia *p.801*
fasciculation *p.814*

glutamate *p.794*
hypokinetic dysarthria *p.800*
hypomimia *p.800*
hypophonia *p.800*
levodopa *p.801*
L'Hermite's sign *p.809*
micrographia *p.800*
mild cognitive impairment (MCI) *p.790*
multiple sclerosis (MS) *p.805*
myasthenia gravis *p.820*

myasthenic crisis *p.820*
myelin *p.809*
on–off phenomena *p.801*
paresthesias *p.805*
Parkinson's disease (PD) *p.796*
postural instability *p.800*
rigidity *p.800*
substantia nigra *p.798*
tau *p.788*

PEARSON
EXPLORE **mynursingkit**™

MyNursingKit is your one stop for online chapter review materials and resources. Prepare for success with additional NCLEX®-style practice questions, interactive assignments and activities, web links, animations and videos, and more!

Register your access code from the front of your book at
www.mynursingkit.com

REFERENCES

Ahlskog, J. E. (2001). Parkinson's disease: Medical and surgical treatment. *Neurologic Clinics, 19*(3), 579–604.

Alzheimer's Association. (2004). *Fact sheet: Memantine (Namenda).* Chicago: Author.

Alzheimer's Foundation of America. (2006, November 17). Alzheimer's Foundation of America sets standard of excellence for dementia settings. *Medical News Today.* Retrieved April 14, 2008, from http://www.medicalnewstoday.com/articles/56912.php

American Academy of Neurology. (2006). Practice parameters: Parkinson disease diagnosis and treatment. *Journal Watch, 66,* 968–975.

American Psychiatric Association (1994). *Diagnostic and statistical manual of mental disorders.* (4th Ed.). Washington, DC: Author.

American Society of Health-System Pharmacists (2006). *AHFS drug information.* Bethesda, MD: Author.

Augustus, L. (2000). Crisis: Myasthenia gravis. *American Journal of Nursing, 100,* 24AA–24HH.

Awwad, S., & Maluf, R. (2007). *Myasthenia gravis.* Retrieved April 11, 2008, from Emedicine website: http://www.emedicine.com/oph/topic263.htm

Benatar M., & Kaminski H. J. (2007). Evidence report: the medical treatment of ocular myasthenia (an evidence-based review): report of the Quality Standards Subcommittee of the American Academy of Neurology. *Neurology. 68*(24):2144–2149.

Borasio, G. D., Voltz, R., & Miller, R. G. (2001). Palliative care in amyotrophic lateral sclerosis. *Neurologic Clinics, 19*(4), 829–845.

Bowron, A. (2004). Practical considerations in the use of apomorphine injectable. *Neurology, 62*(Suppl. 4), S32–S36.

Bunting-Perry, L. (2006). Palliative care in Parkinson's disease: Implications for neuroscience nursing. *Journal of Neuroscience Nursing, 38,* 106–114.

Calne, S. M. (2003). The psychosocial impact of late-stage Parkinson's disease. *Journal of Neuroscience Nursing, 35*(6), 306–313.

Carter, J. H., Stewart, B. J., Archbold, P. G., Inoue, I., Jaglin, J., Lannon, M., et al. (1998). Living with a person who has Parkinson's disease: The spouse's perspective by stage of disease. *Movement Disorders, 13*(1), 20–28.

Charles, T., & Swash, M. (2001). Amyotrophic lateral sclerosis: Current understanding. *Journal of Neuroscience Nursing, 33,* 245–253.

Chaudhuri, A., & Behan, P. O. (2004). Multiple sclerosis is not an autoimmune disease. *Archives of Neurology, 61,* 1610–1612.

Costello, K., Halper, J., Harris, C., & Kennedy, P. (2003). Multiple sclerosis treatment and the importance of early intervention [online]. *International Journal of MS Care.* Retrieved from http://www.mscare.org/cmsc/Journal-of-MS-Care.html

Cummings, J. L., Frank, J. C., Cherry, D., Kohatsu, N. D., & Kemp, B. (2002a). Guidelines for managing Alzheimer's disease. Part I: Assessment. *American Family Physician, 65*(11), 2263–2272.

Cummings, J. L, Frank, J. C., Cherry, D., Kohatsu, N. D., & Kemp, B. (2002b). Guidelines for managing Alzheimer's disease. Part II: Treatment. *American Family Physician, 65*(11), 2263–2272.

Dawson, T. M., & Dawson, V. L. (2003). Molecular pathways of neurodegeneration in Parkinson's disease. *Science, 302,* 819–821.

DeKosky, S. T. (2003). Pathology and pathways of Alzheimer's disease with an update in new developments in treatment. *Journal of the American Geriatrics Society, 51,* S314–S320.

Desai, A. K., & Grossberg, G. T. (2005). Diagnosis and treatment of Alzheimer's disease. *Neurology, 64*(Suppl. 3), S34–S39.

Feldman, H. H., & Woodward, M. (2005). The staging and assessment of moderate to severe Alzheimer's disease. *Neurology, 65*(Suppl. 3), S10–S17.

Food and Drug Administration. (2003). *FDA approves memantine (Namenda) for Alzheimer's disease.* Retrieved April 30, 2008, from http://www.fda.gov/bbs/topics/NEWS/2003/NEW00961.html

Food and Drug Administration. (2006). *Natalizumab (marketed as Tysabri) information.* Retrieved April 30, 2008, from http://www.fda.gov/cder/drug/infopage/natalizumab/

Franklin, G. M., & Nelson, L. (2003). Environmental risk factors in multiple sclerosis: Causes, triggers and patient autonomy. *Neurology, 61,* 1032–1034.

Geldmacher, D. S. (2003). Alzheimer's disease: Current pharmacotherapy in the context of patient and family needs. *Journal of the American Geriatrics Society, 51,* S289–S295.

Giesser, B. (2003). *Reproductive issues in persons with multiple sclerosis.* Retrieved from http://www.nationalmssociety.org/download.aspx?id=168

Gleason, O. C. (2003). Delirium. *American Family Physician, 67,5,* 1027–34.

Hinton, L., Franz, C. E., Yeo, G., & Levkoff, S. E. (2005). Conceptions of dementia in a multiethnic sample of family caregivers. *Journal of the American Geriatrics Society, 53,* 1405–1409.

Holden, K. (2003). *Parkinson's disease: Guidelines for medical nutritional therapy for use by nutrition professionals.* Miami, FL: Five Star Living.

Holland, N. (2003). *Urinary dysfunction in multiple sclerosis.* Retrieved May 2, 2008, from http://www.nationalmssociety.org;pdf/forpros/Bladder.pdf

Hood, L. (1999). The Tensilon test. *American Journal of Nursing, 99*(5), 24HH, 24JJ– 24KK.

Jankovic, J. (2006). Therapeutic strategies in Parkinson's disease. *Geriatrics, 61,* 3–7.

Keesey, J. C. (2004). Clinical evaluation and management of myasthenia gravis. *Muscle Nerve, 29,* 2004.

Kurlowicz, L., & Wallace, M. (1999). The mini mental state examination (MMSE). *Best Practices in Nursing Care to Older Adults, 3.*

Larner, A. J. (2004). Case report: The place of the ice pack test in the diagnosis of myasthenia gravis. *International Journal of Clinical Practice, 58*(9), 887–888.

Leifer, B. P. (2003). Early diagnosis of Alzheimer's disease: Clinical and economic benefits. *Journal of the American Geriatrics Society, 51,* S281–S288.

Lisak, D. (2001). Overview of symptomatic management of multiple sclerosis. *Journal of Neuroscience Nursing, 33*(5), 224–230.

Mitchell, J. D., & Borasio, G. D. (2007). Amyotrophic lateral sclerosis. *Lancet, 369,* 2031–2040.

Mylan Bertek Pharmaceuticals. (2004). *Apokyn.* Package insert.

NASA/MS Cooling Study Group. (2003). A randomized, controlled study of acute and chronic effects of cooling therapy for MS. *Neurology, 60,* 12: 1955–1960.

National Institute on Aging, U.S. Nation Institutes of Health. (2007). Frontotemporal dementia connections reprint. Retrieved July 18, 2008 from http://www.nia.nih.gov/Alzheimers/Publications/FTDreprint.htm

National Institute of Neurological Disorders and Stroke. (2003). *Amyotrophic lateral sclerosis fact sheet.* Retrieved April 2, 2008, from http://www.ninds.nih.gov/disorders/amyotrophiclateralsclerosis/detail_amyotrophiclateralsclerosis.htm

National Institute of Neurological Disorders and Stroke. (2004). *The dementias: Hope through research.* Bethesda, MD: National Instutututes of Health.

National Institute of Neurological Disorders and Stroke. (2006). *Parkinson's disease: Hope through research.* Bethesda, MD: National Institutes of Health.

National Institute of Neurological Disorders and Stroke. (2008). *NINDS amyotrophic lateral sclerosis information page.* Retrieved May 7, 2008, from http://www.ninds.nih.gov/disorders/amyotrophiclateralsclerosis/amyotrophiclateralsclerosis.htm

National Institute of Neurological Disorders and Stroke. (2008). *Multiple sclerosis: hope through research.* Retrieved July 18, 2008 from http://www.ninds.gov/disorders/mikltiple_scleerosis/detail_multiple_sclerosis.htm?css=…

National Multiple Sclerosis Society. (2008). *Just the facts 2006–2007.* Washington, DC: Author.

Nussbaum, R. L., & Ellis, C. E. (2003). Alzheimer's disease and Parkinson's disease. *New England Journal of Medicine, 348*(14), 1356–1364.

Nutt, J. G., & Wooten, G. F. (2005). Diagnosis and initial management of Parkinson's disease. *New England Journal of Medicine, 353,* 1021–1027.

O'Connor, P., & Canadian Multiple Sclerosis Working Group. (2002). Key issues in the diagnosis and treatment of multiple sclerosis: An overview. *Neurology, 59*(6), S1–S33.

Pahwa, R., Lyons, K., & Wilkinson, B. (2003). *Deep brain stimulation for Parkinson's disease: An update.* Retrieved January 23, 2004, from http://www.medscape.com/viewprogram/2274_pnt

Pahwa, R. A., Factor, S. E., Lyons, K. E., et al. (2006). Practice parameter: Treatment of Parkinson disease with motor fluctuations and dyskinesia (an evidence-based review). *Neurology, 66,* 983–1005.

Phillips, L. H. (2004). The epidemiology of myasthenia gravis. *Seminars in Neurology, 24,* 17.

Porth, C. M. P. (2007). *Essentials of pathophysiology: concepts of altered health status.* Philadelphia: Lippincott Williams & Wilkins.

Rocky Mountain MS Center (2003). *Cooling.* Retrieved April 30, 2008, from http://www.ms-cam.org

Saperstein, D. S., & Barohn, R. J. (2004). Management of myasthenia gravis. *Seminars in Neurology, 24*(1), 41–48.

Schapira, A. H. V. (2006). Etiology of Parkinson's disease. *Neurology, 66*(Suppl. 4).

Schapiro, R. (2003). *Managing the symptoms of multiple sclerosis* (4th ed.). New York: Demos.

Schultz, R., O'Brien, A. T., Bookwala, J., & Fleissner, K. (1995). Psychiatric and physical morbidity effects of dementia caregiving: Prevalence, correlates, and causes. *Gerontologist, 35,* 771–791.

Silverman, D. H., Small, G. W., Chang, C. Y., Lu, C. S., Kung de Aburto, M. A., et al. (2001). Positron emission tomography in evaluation of dementia: Regional brain metabolism and long-term outcome. *Journal of the American Medical Association, 286*(17), 2110–2127.

Suchowersky, O., Gronseth, G., Perlmutter, J., Reich, S., & Zesiewicz, T. (2006). Practice parameter: Neuroprotective strategies and alternative therapies for Parkinson disease (an evidence-based review). *Neurology, 66,* 976–982.

Susman, E. (2006). *AAN: New Parkinson's disease treatment guidelines issued.* Retrieved April 14, 2008, from http://www.medpagetoday.com/Neurology/ParkinsonsDisease/tb/3025

Tanner, C. M., Ottman, R., Goldman, S. M., Ellenberg, J., Chan, P., Mayeux, R., et al. (1999). Parkinson's disease in twins: An etiologic study. *Journal of the American Medical Association, 281*(4), 341–346.

Thomas, S., & MacMahon, D. (2004). Parkinson's disease, palliative care and older people: Part 1. *Nursing Older People, 16*(1), 22–27.

Van den Berg, J. P., Kalmijn, S., Lindeman, E., Veldink, J. H., & de Visser, M. (2005). Multidisciplinary ALS care improves quality of life in patients with ALS. *Neurology, 65,* 1264–1267.

Van Den Eeden, S. K., Tanner, C. M., Bernstein, A. L., Fross, R. D., Leimpeter, A., Bloch, D. A., et al. (2003). Incidence of Parkinson's disease: Variation by age, gender, and race/ethnicity. *American Journal of Epidemiology, 157*(11), 1015–1022.

Volcifer, L., & McKee, A. (2001). Dementia. *Neurologic Clinics, 19*(4), 867–883.

Caring for the Patient with Spinal Cord Injuries

Laurie Baker

Outcome-Based Learning Objectives

After studying this chapter, the learner will be able to:

1. Compare and contrast the most common causes of acute spinal cord injury in persons under the age of 65 as opposed to persons over the age of 65.
2. Differentiate between a complete and an incomplete spinal cord injury.
3. Explain three complications of spinal cord injury and strategies to prevent these complications.
4. Discuss the psychosocial impact of spinal cord injury on the patient and family.
5. Identify rehabilitative needs and goals for discharge for the patient who has experienced a spinal cord injury.
6. Select three nursing diagnoses and apply the nursing process in the care of the patient who has experienced a spinal cord injury.

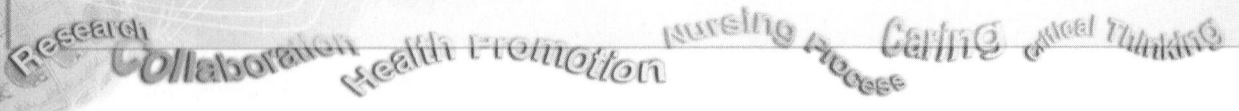

Research Collaboration Health Promotion Nursing Process Caring Critical Thinking

SPINAL CORD injury may be caused by trauma, neoplasm, hemorrhage, infection, and even degenerative changes of the spine. Regardless of its etiology, spinal cord injury is a cause of major morbidity and disability. Treatment of this injury and its associated complications is very costly and is estimated to be in the billions of dollars in the United States (National Center for Injury Prevention and Control [NCIPC], 2006). People who have had a spinal cord injury not only experience the physical effects of this injury, but also face significant psychosocial impacts. Patients with spinal cord injury often are faced with major life changes including loss of lifestyle, independence, economic security, and body image.

Patients who have experienced a spinal cord injury can pose a significant challenge to nurses. There may be a profound physiological response as a result of this injury, which can affect all major body systems. The recovery from this injury is variable and can range from no discernible deficit to permanent, severe disability. Nurses caring for this population must have an understanding of the mechanisms of injury and subsequent sequelae, be able to perform an accurate neurological assessment, and institute appropriate interventions to optimize neurological function and avoid potential complications.

Spinal cord injury (SCI) occurs when a mechanical force is applied to the spinal cord, causing either a temporary or permanent loss of sensory, motor, or autonomic function below the level of injury. The majority of SCIs occur because of trauma to the spinal column. Other traumatic injuries also may be present and can influence outcomes after this injury. Morbidity and mortality after SCI is generally affected by age at the time of injury as well as the level and severity of the injury. Persons of advanced age and those with severe injuries high in the spinal cord generally have higher mortality rates (McIlvoy, Meyer, & McQuillan, 2004).

Epidemiology

It is estimated that more than 200,000 persons are currently living with a SCI in the United States, and approximately 11,000 new cases of SCI occur each year. Young adults are primarily affected, with the majority of SCIs (approximately 78%) occurring among males. The average age at injury currently is 38 years and has been gradually increasing since the 1970s. The percentage of people over the age of 60 who have experienced a SCI has also increased from approximately 5% of the total number of cases in 1980 to 12% in 2000 (National Spinal Cord Injury Statistical Center [NSCISC], 2006). More than 50% of all SCIs occur in the cervical spine. The thoracolumbar juncture is the second most common site for injury because of the relative mobility of the spine at this level (Sekhon & Fehlings, 2001).

The average length of stay for those who are hospitalized in an acute care system that has expertise in treating SCIs is less than 3 weeks. The majority of these patients also will spend an average of 39 days in a rehabilitation facility. Persons with the most severe injuries will have longer lengths of stay. Most people will be discharged eventually to a home environment. The life expectancy for persons who survive at least 1 year after injury is dependent on age and severity of injury, but is steadily increasing. Younger patients with less severe injuries have the best survival rate, whereas older patients, those with severe injuries located high in the spinal cord, and those who are ventilator dependent have the least favorable survival rates (NSCISC, 2006).

Etiology

The vast majority of SCIs are the result of a traumatic event. The most common cause of SCIs in persons under the age of 65 is motor vehicle crashes. Falls rank as the most common cause of SCI in people over the age of 65. Sports and recreation-related SCIs are more likely to occur in people under the age of 30. Spinal cord injuries due to nontraumatic causes are more likely to occur in persons older than 40 years of age (NCIPC, 2006; Spinal Cord Injury Information Network [SCIIN], 2006).

Spinal Tumors

Less than 10% of SCIs are due to medical reasons such as neoplasm or hemorrhage from a vascular abnormality (NCIPC, 2006; SCIIN, 2006). Spinal tumors are broadly classified according to their location within the spine. More specific tumor classifications are based on histology. Intramedullary lesions describe neoplasms that arise from within the spinal cord itself. These types of tumors can cause dilation and distortion of the central portion of the spinal cord or they can infiltrate normal spinal cord tissue. The most common forms of intramedullary spinal cord tumors include ependymoma in adults and astrocytoma in children. Ependymomas are most commonly seen in the conus medullaris and cauda equina. Astrocytomas are most frequently seen in the cervical and thoracic regions of the spinal cord (Bloomer, Ackerman, & Bhatia, 2006; Henson, 2001).

Intradural/extramedullary lesions describe neoplasms that arise between the dura and the spinal cord. These lesions tend to cause compression but do not invade the neural tissue. Schwannoma and meningioma are the most common intradural/extramedullary spinal tumors. Schwannomas can be found anywhere in the spine, but there is a slightly higher incidence in the thoracic spine. Meningiomas are seen most frequently in females after the age of 40 and have a higher incidence of occurring in the thoracic spine (Bloomer et al., 2006).

Extradural lesions, or neoplasms that occur outside of the dural covering of the spinal cord, are the most common form of spinal tumors. The majority of these tumors involve the bony structures of the spine, such as the vertebral bodies, and are metastatic in nature. These tumors cause destruction and weakening of the bone, resulting in spinal instability and collapse. Mass effect from the tumor also may cause compression of the spinal cord. Lung cancer is the most common spinal metastatic lesion followed by breast cancer. Other cancers that commonly metastasize to the spine include myeloma, prostate, and lymphoma (Bloomer et al., 2006).

Pathophysiology

To fully understand the pathophysiology associated with spinal cord injury, it is critical to understand the anatomy and physiology related to the spinal cord. The spinal cord extends from the first cervical vertebra to approximately the first lumbar vertebra in the adult. The spinal nerves exit the spinal cord in pairs. Each nerve has two roots, an anterior or ventral root and a posterior or dorsal root. The anterior root connects to the anterior portion of the spinal cord and contains **efferent** motor fibers, which carry motor information from the brain to the body. The posterior nerve root attaches to the posterior spinal cord and contains **afferent** sensory fibers, which carry sensory information from the body to the spinal cord (Figure 32–1 ■). The spinal cord then transmits this information to the brain (Hickey, 2003a; Mulnard, 2001).

The spinal cord is divided into segments according to region and groups of nerves (Figure 32–2 ■, p. 832). The segments are numbered according to the level of the vertebral column. For example, C_3 denotes the third cervical pair of nerves and the third cervical segment of the spinal column. The spinal cord tapers as it passes through the thoracic region and ends at the conus medullaris at approximately the first lumbar vertebra. Below this is the cauda equina. The cauda equina is comprised of the lumbar and sacral nerve roots as they arise from the conus medullaris (Mulnard, 2001).

A cross section of the spinal cord reveals the gray matter, shaped like an "H" or butterfly, in the center of the cord surrounded by white matter (Figure 32–3 ■, p. 832). The gray matter of the spinal cord contains unmyelinated cells such as the axons and dendrites. It is divided into the anterior (ventral), the posterior (dorsal), and the lateral columns or horns. The lateral columns of the gray matter extend only from T_1 to L_2 or L_3. The motor fibers of the anterior nerve roots originate in the ventral and lateral columns of the gray matter. The posterior columns of the gray matter receive sensory input from the dorsal nerve roots (Hickey, 2003a; Mulnard, 2001).

The white matter serves to link the separate segments of the spinal cord and to link the spinal cord to the brain. It is comprised of ascending and descending tracts that contain mostly myelinated nerve fibers. These tracts are organized into anterior, posterior, and lateral columns. The ascending tracts contain primarily sensory fibers, whereas the descending tracts contain

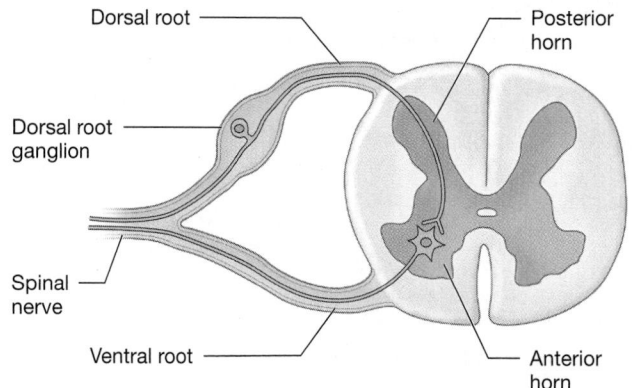

FIGURE 32–1 ■ Ventral and dorsal nerve roots.
Source: Lindsay, K. W. & Bone, I. (2004). Localised neurological disease and its management: peripheral nerves and muscles. In *Neurology and Neurosurgery Illustrated,* 4th Edition

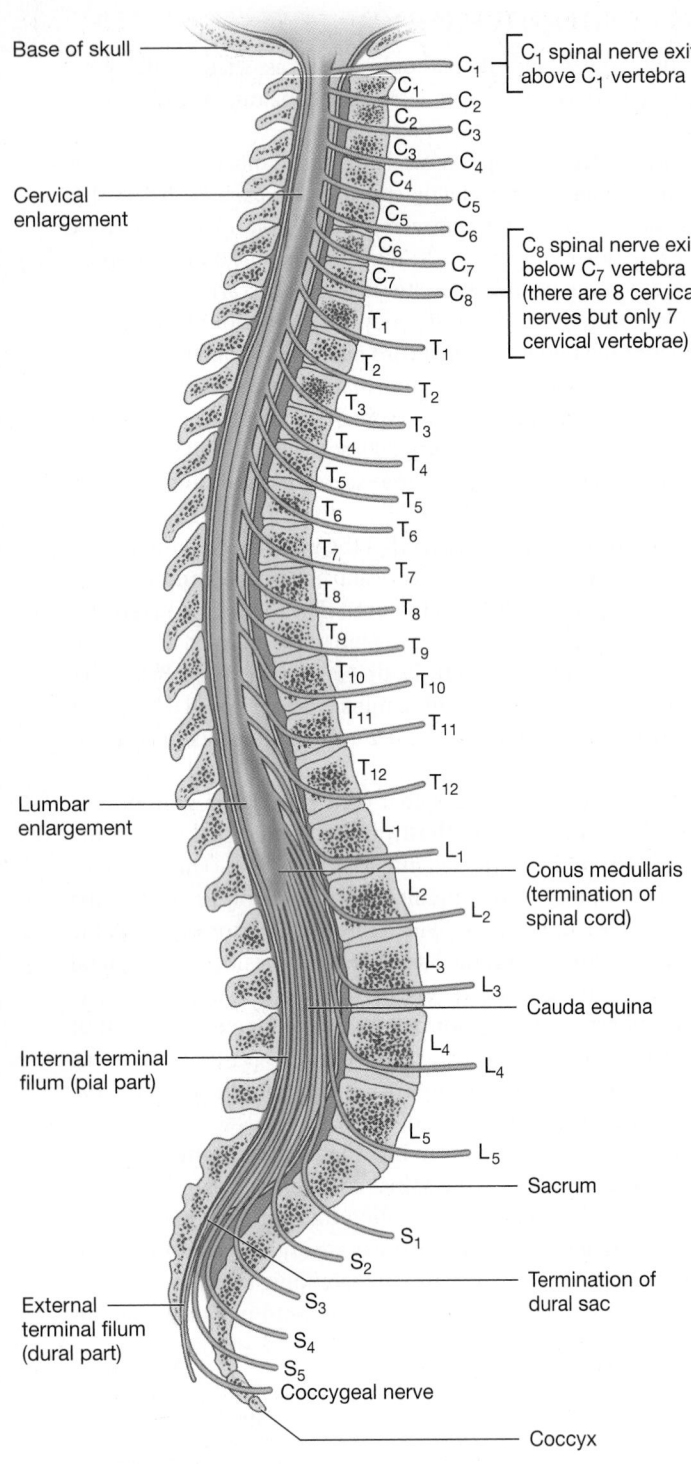

Base of skull

Cervical enlargement

C_1 spinal nerve exits above C_1 vertebra

C_8 spinal nerve exits below C_7 vertebra (there are 8 cervical nerves but only 7 cervical vertebrae)

Lumbar enlargement

Conus medullaris (termination of spinal cord)

Internal terminal filum (pial part)

Cauda equina

Sacrum

External terminal filum (dural part)

Termination of dural sac

Coccygeal nerve

Coccyx

FIGURE 32–2 ■ Spinal column.

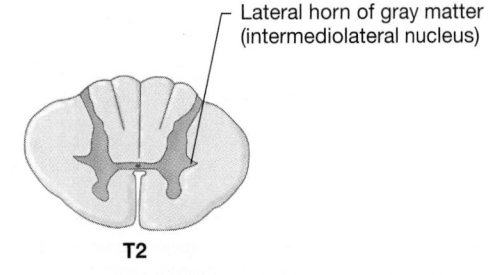

Lateral horn of gray matter (intermediolateral nucleus)

T2

FIGURE 32–3 ■ Cross section of the thoracic spinal cord.

primarily motor fibers. The ascending tracts in the anterolateral columns of the white matter are responsible for the conveyance of pain and temperature sensations to the brain. Afferent impulses enter the spinal cord from the dorsal nerve roots. These impulses then cross the midline of the spinal cord to the contralateral side. From here, the impulses travel up the spinal cord to the thalamus. Injury involving the anterolateral columns will result in loss of pain and temperature sensation on the opposite side of the body below the level of the injury. Proprioception includes the sense of position and movement. The ascending tracts responsible for the conveyance of proprioception lie in the dorsal columns of the white matter. These tracts do not cross the spinal cord, but ascend on the same or ipsilateral side to the medulla. Injury involving the ascending tracts in the dorsal column will result in loss of proprioception below the level of injury on the same side. The descending tracts are responsible for motor function and are located in the anterior columns of the white matter. These tracts do not cross in the spinal cord (Connelly, 2001).

The main vessels that provide the blood supply to the spinal cord include the anterior and posterior spinal arteries. These arteries run along the length of the spinal cord and have several vascular feeders. The anterior spinal artery arises from the vertebral arteries and lies along the midline of the anterior surface of the spinal cord. This vessel perfuses the anterior two-thirds of the spinal cord including the anterior and part of the posterior portions of the gray matter. It has a relatively poor collateral blood supply and is therefore susceptible to vascular disease or injury. The posterior spinal arteries are paired arteries that are located laterally on each side of the posterior aspect of the spinal cord. These arteries form a plexus on the posterior aspect of the spinal cord and have a rich collateral blood supply. As a result, the posterior aspect of the spinal cord is less susceptible to vascular disease or injury. The upper cervical spinal cord also is perfused by a plexus of vessels formed by the vertebral and subclavian vessels. The blood supply of the midthoracic region of the spinal cord is augmented by branches of the intercostal artery. The lower portion of the thoracic spinal cord and the conus medullaris receive additional perfusion from the artery of Adamkiewicz. The sacral arteries supply perfusion to the sacrum and cauda equina (Lindsay & Bone, 2004).

Classification

Spinal cord injuries are classified according to the degree of loss of motor and sensory function below the level of injury. Rehabilitation goals and degree of independence after recovery are dependent on the type of SCI.

Complete Spinal Cord Injury

A **complete spinal cord injury** indicates complete loss of voluntary motor and sensory functions below the level of injury. Injuries involving the cervical spinal cord will result in **tetraplegia** (a Greek term; **quadriplegia** is the Latin term) or loss of motor and sensory function involving both upper extremities, both lower extremities, bowel, and bladder. Injuries involving the thoracic or lumbar spinal cord will result in **paraplegia** or loss of motor and sensory function in both of the lower extremities, bowel, and bladder (Chart 32–1). The damage to the spinal cord in this type of injury is irreversible.

| CHART 32–1 | **Functional Loss After Complete Spinal Cord Injury** |

Level of Injury	Motor Function	Deep Tendon Reflexes	Sensory Function	Bowel and Bladder Function
C_1–C_4	Tetraplegia (quadriplegia) *Lost:* All motor function below the neck	All reflexes lost	*Lost:* All sensation from the neck down	Lost
C_5	Tetraplegia (quadriplegia) *Lost:* All function below the shoulders *Intact:* Sternocleidomastoid Cervical paraspinal muscles Trapezius	C_5, C_6 Biceps	*Lost:* Sensation below the clavicles Most of the arms Hands Chest Abdomen Lower extremities *Intact:* Sensation to head Shoulders Deltoid Clavicle Lateral aspect of the forearm	Lost
C_6	Tetraplegia (quadriplegia) *Lost:* All function below the shoulders and upper arms *Intact:* Deltoid Biceps Rotator muscles of the shoulder	C_5, C_6 Brachioradialis	*Lost:* Sensation below the clavicles Chest Abdomen Lower extremities *Intact:* Sensation to the head Shoulders Arms Palms of hands Thumbs	Lost
C_7	Tetraplegia (quadriplegia) *Lost:* Function in portions of the hands and arms *Intact:* Shoulder depressors Shoulder abductors Shoulder internal rotators Radial wrist extensors	C_7, C_8 Triceps	*Lost:* Sensation below the clavicles Chest Abdomen Lower extremities *Intact:* Sensation to the head Shoulders Most of the arms and hands	Lost
C_8	Tetraplegia (quadriplegia) *Lost:* Function in portions of the hands and arms *Intact:* Elbow extensors Wrist Finger extensors and flexors		*Lost:* Sensation below the chest Portions of the hands *Intact:* Sensation to the head Shoulders Part of the upper chest	Lost
T_1–T_6	Paraplegia *Lost:* Function below the midchest including the muscles of the trunk *Intact:* Shoulders Upper chest Arms Hands		*Lost:* Sensation below the midchest *Intact:* Everything above the midchest T_1, T_2 provide sensation to the inner arm T_4 provides sensation to the nipple area	Lost

(continued)

CHART 32–1	Functional Loss After Complete Spinal Cord Injury—*Continued*			
Level of Injury	Motor Function	Deep Tendon Reflexes	Sensory Function	Bowel and Bladder Function
T_6–T_{12}	Paraplegia *Lost:* Function below the waist *Intact:* Shoulders Arms Hands Long trunk muscles		*Lost:* Sensation below the waist *Intact:* Shoulders Arms Hands T_{10} provides sensation to the umbilicus T_{12} provides sensation to the groin	Lost
L_1–L_3	Paraplegia *Lost:* Most control of the legs and pelvis *Intact:* Shoulders Arms Hands Torso Hip rotation	L_2–L_4 Knee jerk	*Lost:* Lower abdomen Legs *Intact:* Some sensation to the inner and anterior thigh L_3 supplies the knee	Lost
L_3–L_4	Paraplegia *Lost:* Portions of the lower legs Ankles Feet *Intact:* Increased knee extension		*Lost:* Sensation to portions of the lower legs Ankles Feet *Intact:* Sensation to the upper legs	Lost
L_4–S_5	Incomplete paraplegia *L_4–S_1:* Abduction and internal rotation of the hip Ankle dorsiflexion Foot inversion *L5–S_1:* Foot inversion *L_4–S_2:* Foot eversion *S_1–S_2:* Plantar flexion *S_2–S_5:* Bowel and bladder control	S_1–S_2 Ankle jerk	*L_5:* Medial aspect of the foot *S_1:* Lateral aspect of the foot *S_2:* Posterior aspect of the thigh/calf *Lower sacral nerves:* Perineum	Possibly spared *S_2–S_4:* Urinary control *S_3–S_5:* Bowel control

Source: Adapted from Hickey, J. V. (Ed.). (2003). *The clinical practice of neurological and neurosurgical nursing* (5th ed., pp. 424–425). Philadelphia: Lippincott Williams & Wilkins.

Incomplete Spinal Cord Injury

Patients who have experienced an **incomplete spinal cord injury** will have some preservation of sensory and/or motor function below the level of injury. In these patients, there is sparing of some of the spinal cord tracts, which allows neurotransmission to occur. Five main syndromes are associated with incomplete SCI, each classified according to the portion of the spinal cord damaged and the preservation of function below the level of injury (Figure 32–4 ▪) (McIlvoy et al., 2004).

Central Cord Syndrome

Central cord syndrome is the most common incomplete SCI. This injury can occur at any age, but is seen most frequently in older patients who have degenerative bony changes in the cervical spine resulting in narrowing of the overall diameter of the spinal canal (Kirschblum & O'Connor, 2000). It most often is

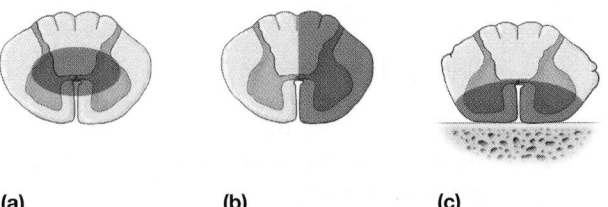

FIGURE 32–4 ▪ Incomplete spinal cord injury. a) Central cord syndrome b) Anterior cord syndrome c) Brown & Sequard syndrome.
Source: Hickey, J. (2003). Vertebral and spinal cord injuries. In J. Hickey, *The Clinical Practice of Neurological and Neurosurgical Nursing,* 5th edition, p. 419. Philadelphia, PA: Lippincott/Williams and Wilkins. p. 427. Philadelphia, Pa: Elsevier

caused by a hyperextension injury resulting in damage to the center of the spinal cord. The spinal tracts in the cervical spinal cord are arranged so that the fibers leading to the upper extremities are more centrally located, whereas the fibers leading to the lower extremities are located more laterally. Therefore, there is greater loss of motor and sensory function in the upper extremities than in the lower extremities. Bladder dysfunction is variable (Hickey, 2003b). The overall prognosis for recovery from this injury is generally favorable; however, patients older than 50 years of age have the least favorable prognosis (McIlvoy et al., 2004). The typical pattern of recovery is return of lower extremity function first followed by return of bladder function. Recovery of hand intrinsic function is variable and often the last to return (Kirschblum & O'Connor, 2000).

Anterior Cord Syndrome

Anterior cord syndrome is caused by direct injury to the anterior portion of the spinal cord or disruption of the anterior spinal artery resulting in ischemia and infarction of the anterior two-thirds of the spinal cord (McIlvoy et al., 2004). This is often due to compression from either an acute disk herniation or from a hyperextension injury resulting in fracture-dislocation of the vertebra. Paralysis and loss of pain and temperature sensation are evident below the level of injury. Light touch, vibration, and proprioception are preserved because these tracts are located in the dorsal columns of the spinal cord, which are perfused by the posterior spinal arteries. The prognosis for recovery from this injury is variable, although generally not favorable (Hickey, 2003a; Kirschblum & O'Connor, 2000).

Brown-Séquard Syndrome

Brown-Séquard syndrome occurs usually as a result of a penetrating injury causing transverse hemisection of the spinal cord. This injury accounts for less than 4% of all spinal cord injuries and is rarely seen in its pure form (McIlvoy et al., 2004). Paralysis and loss of proprioception are seen on the ipsilateral side of the injury, and pain and temperature sensation are lost on the contralateral side. The spinal tracts responsible for motor and proprioception do not cross the spinal cord as they travel to the brain; however, the spinal tracts responsible for the conveyance of pain and temperature do cross to the opposite side of the cord (Hickey, 2003a). Functional recovery from this type of injury is variable, although it can be quite favorable (Kirschblum & O'Connor, 2000).

Cauda Equina Syndrome

Compression of the lumbar nerve roots below the level of L_1 can result in **cauda equina syndrome**. This is most commonly seen with large disk herniations at the L_4/L_5 level that cause mass effect on the nerve roots as they descend through the spinal canal. The deficits related to this syndrome are variable depending on specific nerve root involvement, but can involve motor and sensory functions of the pelvic organs and lower extremities. Weakness, sensory deficits, loss of the Achilles reflex, and bowel and bladder dysfunction including bowel incontinence, urinary retention, and overflow urinary incontinence can be seen. Recovery is variable (Hickey, 2003b; McIlvoy et al., 2004).

Spinal Cord Injury Without Radiographic Abnormality

Spinal cord injury without radiographic abnormality (SCIWORA) is defined as spinal cord injury following a traumatic event without signs of fracture, dislocation, or ligamentous injury on plain radiographs, computed tomography (CT), or myelography. This phenomenon was first described in older patients with spondylitic changes of the cervical spine who developed central cord injury or acute **myelopathy** resulting in changes in sensory, motor, and reflex functions after experiencing a hyperextension injury. These patients had no evidence of spinal fracture or dislocation on radiographic evaluation, but were noted to have significantly narrowed spinal canals due to the degenerative changes of the spinal column common in **spondylitic disease** (Kothari, Freeman, Grevitt, & Kerslak, 2000).

This injury pattern also has been described in patients under the age of 16 years. Anatomic and biomechanical characteristics of the immature pediatric spinal column allow it to be hypermobile, increasing the stress on the spinal cord, predisposing it to injury particularly in flexion-extension type mechanisms (Pang & Wilberger, 1982). Magnetic resonance imaging (MRI) provides good imaging of the soft tissue structures of the spinal column including the intervertebral disks, ligaments, and spinal cord itself. Patients who have experienced a SCIWORA type injury often will demonstrate abnormality of the soft tissue structures or spinal cord on MRI that is not evident on standard radiography (Hendy, Wolfson, Mower, & Hoffman, 2002).

Primary Mechanisms of Injury

Regardless of the etiology of SCI, there are five common primary mechanisms of injury including hyperflexion, hyperextension, rotation, compression, and penetrating injury. Each of these mechanisms of injury is related to the type of mechanical force that is applied to the spinal column.

- **Hyperflexion injuries** occur when there is a sudden deceleration in motion such as can occur in a head-on motor vehicle collision or diving accident. As a result, the head and neck are flexed forward in an exaggerated motion. This can result in fracture of the anterior portion of the vertebral body as well as fracture and dislocation of the facets in the posterior aspect of the spinal column. The posterior spinal ligament and the intervertebral disk also may be disrupted (Figure 32–5 ■). The facet joints and the ligaments are important structures in maintaining the stability of the spine. If

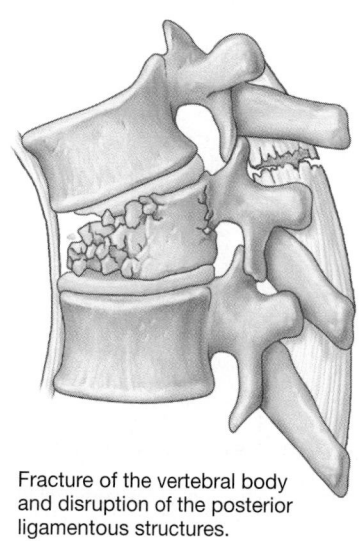

Fracture of the vertebral body and disruption of the posterior ligamentous structures.

FIGURE 32–5 ■ Flexion injury.

these structures are compromised, the spine will be unstable and surgical stabilization of the spine may be required. The presence of fracture and dislocation of the facet joints increases the probability of injury to the spinal cord.

- Hyperextension injuries occur when the spine is extended backward as can occur in rear-impact collisions when the head and neck are forcefully extended back, or in forward falls in which the chin or forehead is struck. The spinal cord can be stretched and degenerative changes of the spinal column including the presence of bone spurs and hypertrophy of the ligaments can cause excessive compression of the spinal cord resulting in a SCI. Injury to the ligaments may not be evident and dislocations are relatively uncommon. Fractures involving the posterior elements of the spinal column including the spinous processes may be present (Figure 32–6 ■).

- **Rotational injuries** occur when there is extreme lateral flexion or rotation and flexion of the spine (Figure 32–7 ■). This injury occurs most commonly in the neck because of the relative mobility of the spine in this region. The posterior ligaments may rupture and fracture and dislocation of the facets may occur, resulting in spinal instability. If the facets on both sides of the spine are affected, the incidence of SCI is in-

creased. The fracture and dislocation may need to be reduced with application of traction, and the spine will need to be surgically stabilized.

- **Compression injuries** occur because of axial pressure or loading of the spine. A vertical force is applied to the spine causing fracture of the vertebral body (Figure 32–8 ■). These injuries typically occur as a result of landing on the feet or buttocks after a fall from a significant height or from extreme flexion of the spine (Figure 32–9 ■). A compression fracture also can occur because of weakening of the vertebral body due to infection, malignancy, or osteoporosis. Bone fragments from the fracture can cause compression or mass effect on the spinal cord. These injuries may require decompression of the spinal canal and stabilization of the spine.

- Penetrating injuries occur as a result of a projectile such as a bullet or sharp object entering the spinal column. The spinal

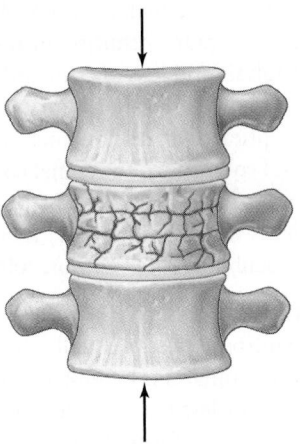

Compression fracture of vertebral body by axial loading forces.

FIGURE 32–8 ■ Compression fracture.

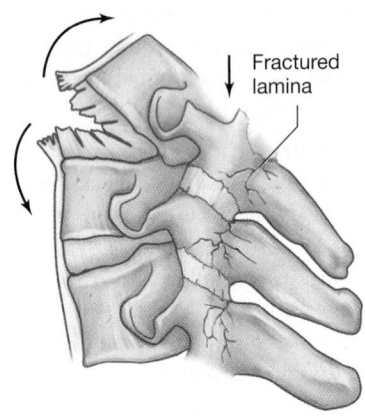

Intervertebral disc and fracturing of the lamina caused by distraction/compression forces.

FIGURE 32–6 ■ Hyperextension injury.

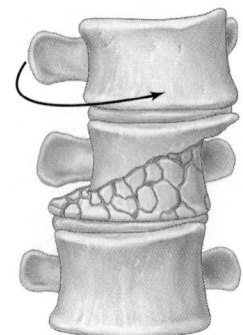

Comminuted fracture of the vertebral body.

FIGURE 32–7 ■ Rotational injury.

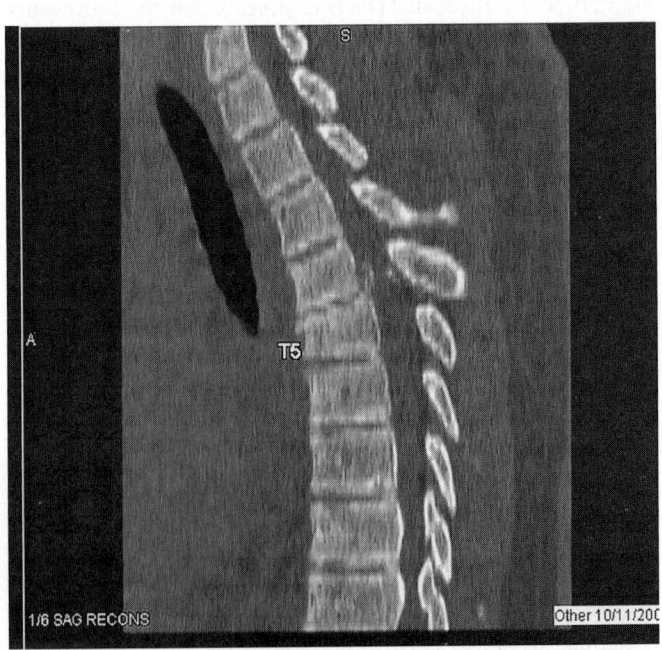

FIGURE 32–9 ■ CT scan of thoracic spine compression fracture.
Source: Laurie Baker

cord can suffer a **contusion** (bruising) or even a partial or complete **transection** (severing of the cord). Damage to the bony structures of the spine can also occur resulting in bone fragments in the spinal canal, which can cause additional compression of the spinal cord. The degree of injury to the spinal cord is related to the velocity of the object as it enters the spinal canal.

Types of Injury

The spinal cord may sustain one or a combination of several types of injuries as a result of the above mechanisms of injury:

- **Concussion**—Usually occurs as a result of a blow to the spinal column. The spinal cord is jarred or shaken. A temporary loss of function can be seen for a period of hours or days.

- **Contusion**—Often caused by fracture, dislocation, or direct trauma to the spinal cord. The spinal cord is bruised, resulting in hemorrhage and edema into the cord. Necrosis of spinal cord tissue may occur because of compression from bleeding or edema or because of direct damage of neural tissue. The degree of neurological dysfunction is dependent on the severity of the contusion.

- **Compression**—Occurs as a result of squeezing or pressure on the spinal cord. The pressure can last momentarily as in a hyperextension injury or can be prolonged because of mass effect from bone fragments, neoplasm, hemorrhage, or disk herniation (Figure 32–10 ■). The spinal cord may also suffer contusion, concussion, laceration, or transection as a result.

- **Laceration**—A tear or cut in the spinal cord. Neurological deficits resulting from this type of injury are permanent.

- **Transection**—Severing of the spinal cord.

- **Hemorrhage**—Bleeding that can occur either within the spinal cord or the surrounding tissues. This can result in compression on the spinal cord or irritation to the neural tissues.

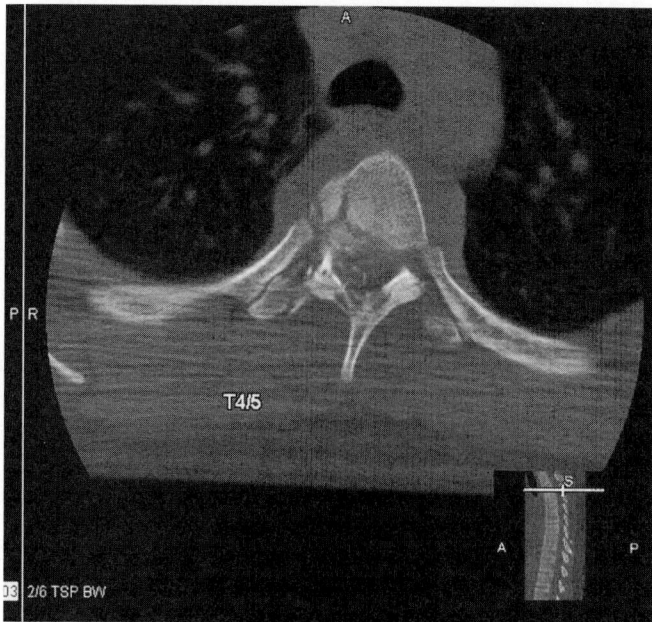

FIGURE 32–10 ■ CT axial view of thoracic spine fracture with bone fragments in the canal.
Source: Laurie Baker

- **Infarction**—Ischemia of the spinal cord as a result of interruption of blood flow. This type of injury can occur because of compression or injury to the vessels that perfuse the cord.

Primary Injury

The initial insult to the spinal cord at the time of trauma is known as the primary injury. The spinal cord suffers physical damage as a result of this insult. The degree of damage to the spinal cord is dependent on the amount of force applied to the cord at the time of the initial injury and may range from mild cord concussion resulting in a transient loss of function to severe injury resulting in complete and permanent loss of function. As a result of the initial trauma, the neural elements of the spinal cord, including nerve cells and the ascending and descending spinal tracks, will be disrupted at the level of the injury. The vasculature of the spinal cord also can be affected, resulting in hemorrhage and ischemia of the spinal cord (Kwon, Tetzlaff, Grauer, Beiner, & Vaccaro, 2004; McIlvoy et al., 2004).

Spinal shock is a state of **areflexia** in which there is a loss of all motor, sensory, and reflex activity at the level of the injury and below. Spinal shock occurs as a result of the primary injury. The duration of spinal shock is quite variable, lasting as little as a few hours or as long as several weeks after injury. During this state, it is impossible to determine the extent of the SCI. As spinal shock abates, signs of muscle spasticity and **hyperreflexia** (exaggeration of the deep tendon reflexes) become evident. The return of the perianal reflexes indicates the resolution of spinal shock (Hickey, 2003a; McIlvoy et al., 2004).

Secondary Injury

The initial or primary SCI sets forth a cascade of complex events that can worsen the extent of the injury by causing damage to the adjoining neural tissues. The exact mechanism of this injury is not entirely understood, but many of the current treatment strategies for SCI are directed at reducing the damage caused by this secondary process. The secondary process begins almost immediately after the initial trauma to the spinal cord. Ischemia within the spinal cord at the time of the primary injury leads to additional vascular changes, which worsen the disruption of the normal perfusion of the spinal cord (Kwon et al., 2004). As a result of these vascular changes, cell membrane permeability is affected due to dysfunction of the cellular sodium-potassium pump (see Chapter 18 ☺). Intracellular potassium is depleted and sodium and calcium ions enter into the cell, resulting in cellular edema and subsequent cell death. The increased intracellular calcium triggers the release of enzymes and free radicals, which worsens cellular necrosis and leads to additional tissue damage. An inflammatory response is triggered, resulting in increased vascular permeability, edema, and macrophage activity leading to additional tissue damage and glial scarring (Hickey, 2003a; McIlvoy et al., 2004).

Disruption of autonomic regulation occurs as a result of SCI and can lead to **neurogenic shock**. This is a phenomenon most commonly seen in patients who have had a SCI at T_6 or above and should be differentiated from spinal shock. Spinal shock results in the loss of sensorimotor control and loss of the muscle stretch and cutaneous reflexes below the level of the injury. Neurogenic shock results in the disruption of the sympathetic nervous system. The sympathetic nervous system originates in the thoracolumbar region of the spinal cord and is responsible for elevations in heart rate and blood pressure and for vasoconstriction of the peripheral vascular system during stress situations. Neurogenic shock occurs when the normal impulses from the brainstem, which contribute to the reflexive control of heart rate and blood pressure, are disrupted, resulting in interruption of normal sympathetic outflow. Vagal tone is, therefore, left unopposed (Hickey, 2003a). As a result, bradycardia, peripheral vasodilation below the level of injury resulting in decreased systemic vascular resistance, hypotension, and decreased cardiac output are evident. The resulting hypotension and diminished cardiac output are thought to contribute to ischemia of the spinal cord at the site of injury.

The trauma patient who also is suspected of having a SCI may also experience hypovolemic shock. It is important to distinguish between neurogenic shock and hypovolemic shock in order to ensure that appropriate treatment strategies are implemented. Hypotension is a hallmark sign for both neurogenic shock and hypovolemic shock. The patient experiencing neurogenic shock will exhibit bradycardia with a heart rate of 50 to 70 beats per minute and will often require vasopressor support for treatment. The patient's skin also will be warm and hyperemic. The patient who has hypovolemia will exhibit tachycardia and will usually respond to volume replacement (McIlvoy et al., 2004).

Autonomic Hyperreflexia

Autonomic hyperreflexia occurs as a result of a noxious stimulus below the level of the SCI. Common causes include urinary tract abnormalities such as a distended bladder, abnormalities of the lower intestinal tract such as constipation or fecal impaction, and pressure ulcers. As a result of the noxious stimulus, a sympathetic response is triggered, resulting in vasoconstriction below the level of the SCI. Blood volume is shifted from the vasculature below the SCI to the vasculature above the injury, causing elevation of blood pressure. The baroreceptors in the carotid body and the aortic arch stimulate the vasomotor center of the medulla, which in turn triggers slowing of the heart and vasodilation. The vasculature above the level of injury responds, resulting in flushing of the skin, piloerection, and nasal congestion; however, these impulses are blocked at the level of the SCI and vasoconstriction continues unchecked below the level of injury. This response will continue until the noxious stimulus is removed (Hickey, 2003a; Krassioukov, 2004; McIlvoy et al., 2004; National Guideline Clearinghouse, 2001).

 **CRITICAL ALERT** *It is easy to confuse neurogenic shock and hypovolemic shock in the trauma patient with SCI. Both conditions may be present concomitantly and will manifest with hypotension, but an important distinction is bradycardia. Patients experiencing neurogenic shock will exhibit bradycardia, whereas tachycardia is most often associated with hypovolemia. Patients with neurogenic shock will also exhibit warm, hyperemic skin due to vasodilation. Atropine to increase the heart rate and vasopressor support will be necessary to treat the patient in neurogenic shock.*

■ Clinical Manifestations

The clinical manifestations of spinal cord injury assume a systemic effect. The injury can affect the function of multiple organ systems depending on the level and severity of the injury. It is vital that nurses caring for this population understand the systemic effects of SCI so that appropriate assessment and interventions can be undertaken to avoid potential medical complications.

Cardiovascular

Neurogenic shock resulting in cardiovascular compromise is most evident in the patient who has sustained a SCI at T_6 or above. Sympathetic innervation is lost leaving vagal tone unopposed. Bradycardia, peripheral vasodilation below the level of injury, decreased systemic vascular resistance, and hypotension are seen. Cardiac preload and afterload subsequently are decreased resulting in decreased cardiac output (see Chapters 37 and 42). The use of atropine to increase the heart rate and vasopressors such as dopamine or dobutamine may be required to increase the heart rate, promote vasoconstriction, and increase cardiac output (Hickey, 2003a; McIlvoy et al., 2004).

Orthostatic hypotension also may be problematic for this patient population. The loss of sympathetic vascular tone results in blood pooling in the abdomen and lower extremities and a loss of arteriole vasomotor control. Prolonged immobility and decreased intravascular volume also are contributing factors. The patient experiences a drop in blood pressure when placed in an upright position and may complain of dizziness, light-headedness, visual disturbance, or syncope because of diminished blood supply to the brain, a phenomenon referred to as orthostatic hypotension. If this phenomenon if left unchecked, cerebral ischemia is possible (Hickey, 2003a; McIlvoy et al., 2004).

Pooling of blood in the peripheral vascular system, flaccidity of the extremities, and immobility predispose the patient with SCI to the development of venous thrombosis. This condition, if left untreated, could lead to the more serious complication of pulmonary embolus. The risk of development of deep venous thrombosis (DVT) seems to be highest in the first 2 to 3 months after injury (Apuzzo, 2002b). Patients may initially be asymptomatic unless they have some preservation of sensation. Signs of DVT include the presence of low-grade fever, edema in the affected limb, or change in temperature of the affected limb. If patients have sensory sparing, they may complain of pain and tenderness of the site (Hickey, 2003b; McIlvoy et al., 2004).

If signs of DVT are identified, additional testing is required. Venography is the "gold standard" for diagnosing DVT, but it is an invasive procedure and has associated risks, therefore it is rarely used. Duplex Doppler ultrasound screening is most frequently used to evaluate for DVT. This test has a high sensitivity for detecting DVT and carries a low risk to the patient. If a DVT is diagnosed, treatment with anticoagulant therapy should be instituted. Placement of an intravascular filter to prevent migration of the blood clot to the lungs also may be warranted. National guidelines for prevention of thromboembolism after spinal cord injury have been established (see the National Guidelines box).

Pulmonary embolus (PE) is a potentially life-threatening condition. A decline in oxygen saturation may be the only sign of PE; however, other symptoms may include chest pain or dyspnea. If any of these signs are evident and a PE is suspected, additional evaluation such as helical CT scan of the chest should be obtained immediately. Once diagnosed, treatment of PE is supportive with the administration of oxygen therapy and anticoagulation (Apuzzo, 2002c; National Guideline Clearinghouse, 2005b).

NATIONAL GUIDELINES for Prevention of Thromboembolism After Spinal Cord Injury

Risk Factor	Guideline
DVT	**Assessment:**
	Obtain history that could add to the increased risk of DVT after spinal cord injury:
	• Age over 40
	• Obesity
	• Estrogen therapy
	• Malignancy
	• Congestive heart failure
	• History of tobacco use
	• Concomitant injuries, specifically fractures of the lower limb
	• Previous history of DVT.
	Perform physical assessment twice daily and inspect all extremities for signs of DVT:
	• Increased circumference of calf or thigh
	• Pain, tenderness of the affected extremity
	• Low-grade fever of unknown origin
	• Erythema of the extremity.
	Prophylaxis:
	Prophylactic measures should be instituted within 72 hours of injury unless there is a medical contraindication. If application of mechanical prophylactic devices is delayed for >72 hours, the presence of lower extremity DVT should be ruled out prior to employing the following devices:
	• Compression stockings
	• External pneumatic compression devices
	• Anticoagulation with either low-molecular-weight heparin or unfractionated heparin
	• Initiation of early mobilization or passive range-of-motion exercises once the patient is medically and surgically stable.
	If DVT Is Suspected:
	Duplex ultrasound should be obtained of the affected extremity.
	Placement of vena cava filter to decrease the risk of development of PE.

Source: National Guideline Clearinghouse. (2005). *Prevention of thromboembolism in spinal cord injury.* Washington, DC: Consortium for Spinal Cord Medicine, Paralyzed Veterans of America. Retrieved April 29, 2008, from http://www.guideline.gov/summary/summary.aspx?doc_id=2965&nbr=002191&string=spinal+AND+cord+AND+injury.

 CRITICAL ALERT *Pulmonary embolus is a life-threatening disorder that can result in death if not recognized and treated promptly. Common signs and symptoms include decrease in oxygen saturation, shortness of breath, and chest pain. If the patient exhibits any of these symptoms, the managing medical team should be notified immediately.*

Pulmonary

Patients who have sustained a SCI above T_{12} have potential for impairment of respiratory function. The degree of this impairment is dependent on the level of injury. Generally, higher level injuries have more significant impairment (McIlvoy et al., 2004). Atelectasis and pneumonia are common complications after SCI regardless of the involved spinal level and also can contribute to decompensation in respiratory function.

The diaphragm receives innervation from the phrenic nerve, which arises above C_5. The diaphragm is responsible for inspiration and deep breathing as well as the initiation of an effective cough. Injuries at C_4 or higher will cause paralysis of the diaphragm, necessitating intubation and ventilation (Hickey, 2003b). Patients who have experienced injuries involving the lower cervical spine, thoracic spine, or lumbar spine usually will

not require immediate intubation, but warrant close monitoring for signs of respiratory decompensation because of loss of use of the respiratory accessory muscles. The intercostal and abdominal muscles that aid inspiration, forced expiration, and cough are innervated by the T_1–T_{12} nerves. Loss of use of these accessory muscles will result in a decrease of about 70% of forced vital capacity and maximal inspiratory force in the acute period following SCI (Ball, 2001; McIlvoy et al., 2004).

Gastrointestinal

Gastrointestinal effects of spinal shock include gastroparesis, loss of intestinal peristalsis, and ileus. The resulting abdominal distention places the patient at risk for vomiting and aspiration and also may interfere with respiratory function. Placement of a nasogastric or oral gastric tube will be necessary in the acute phase of SCI for decompression of the stomach and minimization of these risks (Prendergast & Sullivan, 2000).

Patients with SCI also are at risk for gastric stress ulceration. Loss of sensation to the visceral organs, especially in patients with high-level injuries, may interfere with the ability of these patients to feel gastric pain. This may delay early identification of gastric ulceration, which, in turn, will delay appropriate treatment and increase the risk of gastric hemorrhage. A prophylactic medication regimen should be instituted in all SCI patients (Prendergast & Sullivan, 2000).

Patients with SCI will experience abnormalities in both sensory and motor function of the bowel due to disruption of the spinal tracts responsible for bowel control. Generally, patients with injury above T_{12} will experience decreased intestinal peristalsis, absent rectal sensation, and an increase in anal sphincter tone. Anal reflex activity may be preserved. These patients are prone to chronic constipation. Patients with injury at or below L_1 will experience loss of tone throughout the colon and rectal sphincters. These patients are more likely to experience bowel incontinence (Enck, Greving, Klosterhalfen, & Wietek, 2006; Hickey, 2003a).

Genitourinary

The spinal tracts responsible for bladder control also are disrupted in SCI, resulting in loss of the normal bladder reflexes and control of urination. As a result, the bladder becomes atonic and the patient experiences urinary retention and bladder distention. Urinary incontinence may occur as the result of overflow of urine from a distended bladder into the urethra. Overdistension of the bladder can cause impairment of the blood supply to the bladder and reflux of urine into the ureters and kidney because of the increased bladder pressures. These patients are at risk for complications such as urinary tract infection (UTI), hydronephrosis, decline in renal function, and the development of renal calculi. In some cases of incomplete SCI, bladder function may return after recovery of spinal shock. It is important to assess postvoid residuals in these patients to ensure adequate bladder emptying (Hickey, 2003a; Pataki, Woodhouse, Hamid, Shah, & Craggs, 2006).

Integumentary

Patients with SCI are at high risk for development of pressure ulcers because of impairment in sensory and motor functions as well as impairment of tissue perfusion due to hypotension and pooling of blood in the lower extremities. Once these wounds develop, they can be very difficult to heal and can increase the risk of infection. Factors that contribute to the development of pressure ulcers in this population also include fever, infection, poor nutrition, and prolonged immobilization on the firm spinal board used to maintain optimal spinal alignment during transport to the hospital. Prevention is the best strategy to deal with pressure ulcers.

 *Autonomic hyperreflexia is a medical emergency that could lead to serious complications if left untreated. When the patient exhibits symptoms of autonomic hyperreflexia, it is important to institute measures to treat the blood pressure and to identify and correct the cause.*

◼ General Evaluation and Management

Evaluation and management of SCI begins at the scene of the trauma and is carried throughout the acute care hospitalization and rehabilitation phases. Early assessment and management are vital for determining the extent of injury and minimization of secondary injury to the spinal cord. Acute care assessment and management are directed toward optimizing neurological function and avoidance of early complications. Rehabilitative management and evaluation focus on adaptation and avoidance of long-term complications.

Prehospital

Expert evaluation and management of the trauma victim at the scene can make a difference in the victim's ultimate neurological outcome. Improper mobilization of the trauma victim with an unrecognized, unstable spinal fracture can worsen or even cause injury to the spinal cord. Impairment of respiratory and circulatory function also can worsen SCI. First responders follow the general principles of trauma management including rapid assessment of the victim, evaluation and management of the ABCs (airway–breathing–circulation), stabilization and control of life-threatening injuries, and rapid transport to an appropriate facility for continuation of care.

Spinal precautions are methods of immobilizing the spine and moving patients to prevent or avoid additional spinal injury. Spinal precautions are initiated at the scene of the trauma and are carried out until spinal injury has been ruled out or appropriate treatment strategies have been implemented. Immobilization of the entire spine is necessary because 20% of patients with a spinal injury have injuries at more than one spinal level (Apuzzo, 2002a). Spinal precautions usually are implemented in any trauma patient; however, determination of the mechanism of injury at the scene can prove invaluable in helping to identify potential injuries. Victims of a traumatic event with a significant mechanism of injury have a greater risk for multiple organ injuries and neurological injuries. First responders should have a high suspicion of spinal injury in any victim with multiple injuries, complaint of spinal pain, spinal deformity, or abnormality on sensory and/or motor examination. Also, those victims who have sustained head injury, experienced loss of consciousness, have an altered mental status, have complaint of motor or sensory disturbance at the scene, or are under the influence of drugs or alcohol warrant careful handling until a spinal injury can be definitively ruled out (Apuzzo, 2002a; Hickey, 2003a).

Spinal precautions can be initiated with the patient in an upright position if necessary until extrication and movement to a long back board is possible. A rigid cervical collar is applied and the patient is log rolled onto a back board in the supine position with the spine in a neutral position. Sandbags or blocks are placed on both sides of the head to prevent lateral rotation of the neck. The head is then secured to the back board utilizing tape or straps across the forehead to limit neck flexion. The patient also will be secured to the board utilizing appropriately placed straps.

Pediatric patients pose a special challenge in positioning because of their relatively large sized head. These patients require padding under the torso in order to prevent flexion of the neck. Elderly patients also may also warrant special consideration with positioning due to arthritic changes of the spine affecting spinal alignment. All patients require vigilant monitoring of airway and respiratory function. Immobilization on a back board can contribute to respiratory impairment because forced vital capacity is decreased by 20%. If respiratory function deteriorates and the patient requires ventilatory support, care must be taken to ensure spinal alignment is maintained (Apuzzo, 2002c; Bernbeck & Delamarter, 2000).

Emergency Department

Once the patient arrives in the emergency department, a complete survey of injuries and continued stabilization of the patient will continue while spinal precautions are maintained. A baseline assessment of the patient's physical and neurological status as well as information pertaining to the trauma and the patient's past medical history will be obtained. Efforts should be made to expedite diagnostic testing to facilitate early identification of spinal cord compression or spinal instability so that appropriate surgical measures can be taken if needed or restrictive protective equipment can be removed if not required. After the initial assessment and diagnostic evaluation is complete and the treatment plan established, the patient should be removed from the back board to avoid additional complications related to prolonged immobilization.

Initial Assessment

Evaluation of pulmonary and circulatory function will take precedence in the trauma patient. The patient should be assessed and monitored for adequacy of respiratory efforts and ventilatory function. All patients should receive supplemental oxygen and have oxygenation monitored continuously with pulse oximetry. A baseline arterial blood gas (ABG) should be obtained. Lung sounds should be assessed on admission and repeated periodically. The patient with SCI may initially present with adequate respiratory function but can quickly deteriorate. Apnea, stridorous respirations, use of accessory muscles, rapid, shallow respirations, and decline of oxygen saturation are indicative of inadequate respiratory efforts. Ventilatory support should be considered if the patient exhibits signs of inadequate respiratory function. If intubation is necessary, care should be taken to ensure the spine remains in alignment and extension or flexion of the neck is avoided (Ball, 2001; Hickey, 2003a; Prendergast & Sullivan, 2000).

Circulatory function including heart rate, rhythm, and blood pressure also should be closely monitored. The patient with SCI may be bradycardic and hypotensive on presentation to the emergency department due to disruption in vagal tone because of neurogenic shock. Blood pressure may be further compromised by hypovolemia. Central venous pressure monitoring can be helpful in determining volume status and distinguishing between neurogenic and hypovolemic shock (Hadley, 2002).

Patients with SCI due to trauma also are at risk for other organ injuries. These patients may not be able to experience visceral pain because of the SCI. Therefore, it is vital that emergency department providers be vigilant in assessing for signs of other organ injury during their initial assessment.

A careful baseline neurological examination is crucial in the initial assessment of the patient suspected of having a spinal injury. This assessment will be the basis for management of the patient as well as for determination of change in neurological status. This assessment should take place before the patient receives pain medication, sedatives, or paralytics if possible. These medications can interfere with the ability to obtain an accurate neurological assessment.

The overall level of consciousness should be assessed in all trauma patients utilizing a Glasgow Coma Scale (GCS) score because there is a possibility of concomitant brain injury (Chart 32–2). The GCS score is the sum of scores for the patient's best eye opening, verbal, and motor responses. This score provides a

---

CHART 32–2	Glasgow Coma Scale

Eye Opening (E)	Verbal Response (V)	Motor Response (M)
4 = Spontaneous	5 = Normal conversation	6 = Normal
3 = To voice	4 = Disoriented conversation	5 = Localizes to pain
2 = To pain	3 = Words, but not coherent	4 = Withdraws to pain
1 = None	2 = No words; only sounds	3 = Decorticate posture
	1 = None	2 = Decerebrate
		1 = None

Total = E + V + M

With the Glasgow Coma Scale, one determines the best eye opening response, the best verbal response, and the best motor response. The score represents the sum of the numeric scores of each of the categories. There are limitations to its use. If the patient has an endotracheal tube in place, she cannot talk. For this reason, many prefer to document the score by its individual components; so a patient with a Glasgow Coma Scale score of 15 would be documented as follows: E4 V5 M6. An intubated patient would be scored as E4 V intubated M6. Of these individual factors, the best motor response is probably the most significant.

Source: American College of Surgeons Committee on Trauma (2004). Advanced Trauma Life Support for Doctors (7th ed.). Chicago: American College of Surgeons

---

means for monitoring changes in the patient's mental status and predicting a prognosis from the time of injury in patients who have sustained a traumatic brain injury. A score of 15 is the maximum score and indicates a normal level of consciousness; a score of 3 is the lowest score and is indicative of a poor prognosis.

A detailed assessment of motor function of all major muscle groups in both the upper and lower extremities will be obtained as part of the initial assessment and repeated hourly as part of the routine monitoring of vital signs for the first 48 to 72 hours. The strength of each major muscle group is tested individually and compared with the corresponding muscle group on the contralateral side. The muscle strength is graded on a scale of 0 to 5 with 0 indicating no motor function and 5 indicating normal strength (Chart 32–3). Each muscle group is innervated by a corresponding spinal nerve (Chart 32–4, p. 842). Abnormalities in motor function can help with approximating the level of the SCI.

 *Frequent monitoring of vital signs and neurological function is necessary for the first 48 to 72 hours after SCI to assess for any change in status. The managing medical team should be notified immediately if any decline in status is noted so that prompt intervention can be initiated to preserve existing function.*

CHART 32–3	Grading of Muscle Strength

Grade	Strength
0	No contraction
1	Trace or flicker contraction
2	Movement with gravity eliminated
3	Movement against gravity
4	Movement against resistance
5	Normal strength

CHART 32–4	**Major Muscle Group Innervation and Function**	
Spinal Nerve	**Muscle**	**Function**
C_5	Deltoid	Abduct arm
C_6	Biceps	Bend elbow
C_6, C_7	Extensor carpi radialis	Extend wrist
C_7	Triceps	Straighten elbow
C_8, T_1	Hand intrinsics	Spread fingers
L_1, L_2	Iliopsoas	Raise knee to chest
L_3, L_4	Quadriceps	Extend knee
L_5	Tibialis anterior	Dorsiflex the foot
S_1	Extensor hallucis longus	Extend the great toe
	Hamstring	Flex knee
	Gastrocnemius	Plantar flex the foot

A sensory examination also is performed assessing the patient's response to pinprick in all dermatomes using a sequential side-to-side manner. Abnormalities in sensation are documented according to the corresponding dermatome. An anatomical dermatome chart is a helpful resource in determining the specific level of sensory abnormality (see Figure 28–6 ■, p. 707 in Chapter 28 🌐).

Evaluation of the deep tendon reflexes (DTRs) and rectal sphincter tone also will take place as part of the initial assessment. Each reflex is innervated by a corresponding spinal nerve (Chart 32–5). Reflex activity is lost below the level of injury when spinal shock is present. As spinal shock abates, reflexes will generally return. The DTRs usually are not tested on a routine basis after the initial assessment; however, sphincter tone and sensation can be monitored during the routine bowel regimen (McIlvoy et al., 2004).

In addition to the neurological assessment, the entire spine should be palpated as part of the initial evaluation. Bony deformity, alteration in alignment, pain, and focal tenderness should be noted because these signs may be indicative of spinal fracture or dislocation.

Acute Care Hospital

Once the extent of injury has been determined, the patient has been stabilized, and the treatment plan established, the patient will be admitted to the intensive care unit (ICU) where close monitoring and support of neurological, respiratory, and circulatory functions will take place. The patient will be transferred to the general care floor once those functions have stabilized. The treatment plan will then be expanded from physiological

CHART 32–5	**Spinal Reflexes**
Spinal Level	**Reflex**
C_5–C_6	Biceps
C_7	Triceps
L_4	Patellar
S_1	Achilles

support and minimization of secondary injury to prevention of complications, education of the patient and family, and optimization of existing function.

Laboratory and Diagnostic Procedures

All patients who are suspected of having a spinal injury will undergo radiographic evaluation of the spine. Initially, plain x-rays will be obtained of the entire spinal axis to assess spinal alignment and the integrity of the spinal elements. Anterior-posterior (AP) and lateral views will be obtained. The **odontoid process**, the tooth-like projection of C_2 that sits behind the anterior portion of C_1, is difficult to visualize on standard x-ray views; therefore, an x-ray through the patient's open mouth will be necessary for visualization of the odontoid process and the C_1–C_2 junction.

The cervicothoracic junction can also be difficult to visualize with plain radiographs because of interference of the shoulder joint. Visualization of this area of the spine often requires pulling downward on the patient's shoulders or obtaining a lateral swimmer's view with the patient's arm fully abducted. This type of positioning may not be possible if the victim has sustained trauma to the upper extremities.

A CT scan provides detailed imaging of the bony structures of the spine and is very helpful in identifying fractures that may be missed on plain radiographs (Figure 32–11 ■). An MRI may be obtained to provide imaging of the soft tissue structures including the spinal cord, intervertebral disks, and ligaments; however, an MRI is not indicated for all patients (Figure 32–12 ■). Patients who are morbidly obese or have ex-

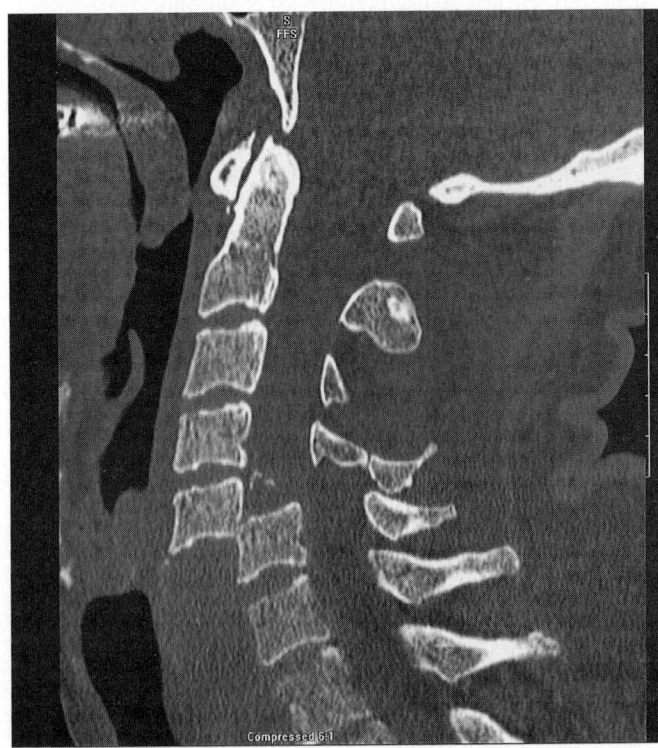

FIGURE 32–11 ■ CT of C_5–C_6 fracture and subluxation.
Source: Laurie Baker

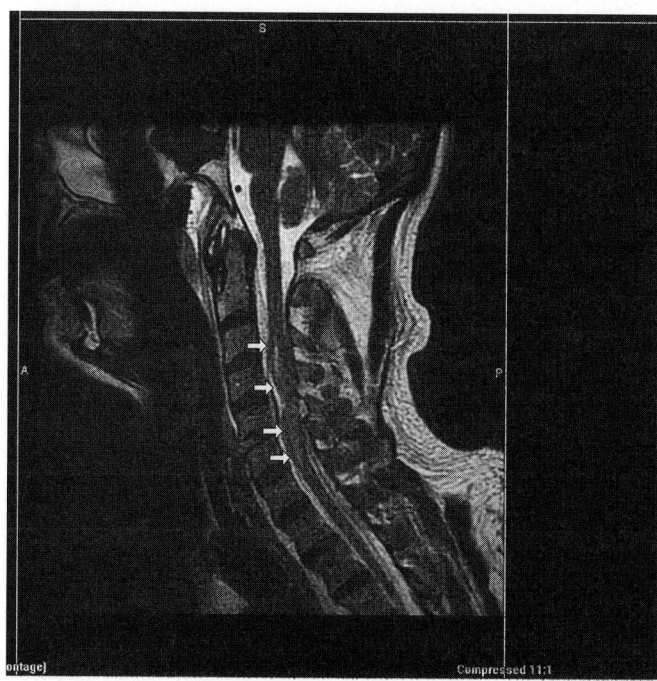

FIGURE 32–12 ■ MRI of the cervical spine.
Source: Laurie Baker

treme claustrophobia will not be able to undergo an MRI scan. Also, patients with implanted medical devices such as pacemakers or those with retained metal from shrapnel injuries will not be candidates for this test. Another disadvantage of an MRI scan is the length of time it takes to perform this test. A spinal axis MRI can take up to 60 to 90 minutes to

complete. Patients who are medically unstable may be unsuitable for this type of imaging (Apuzzo, 2002e; France, Bono, & Vaccaro, 2005; Hickey, 2003a; National Guideline Clearinghouse, 2005c). See the Diagnostic Tests box for a listing of tests for acute SCI.

■ Medical Management

Decisions regarding treatment strategies for the patient with SCI are guided by the patient's presentation and results of the imaging studies. The ultimate goals of treatment are to stabilize the spine at the level of injury, optimize neurological outcome, and prevent neurological deterioration. Early medical management of the patient with SCI is geared toward stabilization of the spine and lessening of the secondary injury processes.

If stability of the vertebral column or ligaments is in question, immobilization of the spine utilizing an orthotic device will be necessary. Most of these devices are noninvasive and each device is designed to maintain alignment and stability of a particular spinal region. Rigid cervical collars are commonly used to provide stability to the cervical spine (Figure 32–13 ■, p. 844). A halo brace also may be used to stabilize cervical fractures, especially if a collar does not provide adequate stability (Figure 32–14 ■, p. 844). The application of cervical traction with such devices as Gardner-Wells tongs may be necessary to reestablish alignment of the cervical spine or to reduce cervical fractures before surgical stabilization (Figure 32–15 ■, p. 844).

Injuries in the cervicothoracic juncture or high thoracic spine require the use of a device that provides stabilization to both the lower cervical and upper thoracic regions such as a

DIAGNOSTIC TESTS for Acute Spinal Cord Injury

Test and *Normal Values*	Expected Abnormality	Rationale for Abnormality
Spinal x-rays: AP & Lat views Cervical spine x-rays should also include open mouth views and swimmer's view *Normal spinal alignment* *Bony elements of the spine are intact without evidence of fracture*	Subluxation of the vertebral bodies Compression or abnormal shape of the vertebral body Crush deformity of the vertebral body Widening or collapse of the intervertebral space	Injuries to the spinal ligaments or fracture of the stabilizing structures of the spine allow the vertebral body to slip out of alignment. Compression fracture of the vertebra will result in crushing of the vertebral body, altering its normal shape. Disruption of the intervertebral disk will cause changes in the space between the vertebral bodies.
CT scan of the spine *Normal spinal alignment* *Normal configuration of the bony elements of the spine* *No evidence of fracture* *No bone fragments within the canal*	Abnormal alignment of the spine Fracture of the bony elements of the spinal column Bone fragments within the spinal canal	Fracture or ligamentous injuries allow the spine to become unstable and the vertebral bodies to move out of place. Bone fragments from spinal fractures can be propelled or migrate into the canal, causing compression of the spinal cord or nerves.
MRI of the spine *Spinal alignment maintained* *Intervertebral disks intact* *Spinal cord is surrounded by cerebrospinal fluid without evidence of compression or abnormality in signal intensity* *Normal signal intensity of the surrounding ligaments and tissue*	Abnormal alignment of the spine Protrusion of the intervertebral disk into the canal, causing compression of the spinal cord Narrowing of the spinal canal with compression of the spinal cord Hyperintensity within the spinal cord Hyperintensity of the surrounding ligaments and tissues	Brightness or hyperintense signal within the spinal cord or surrounding tissue indicates the presence of swelling or edema due to the inflammatory response of injury. If present only in the surrounding tissue and not the spinal cord, this could be indicative of ligamentous injury, which increases the risk of spinal instability.

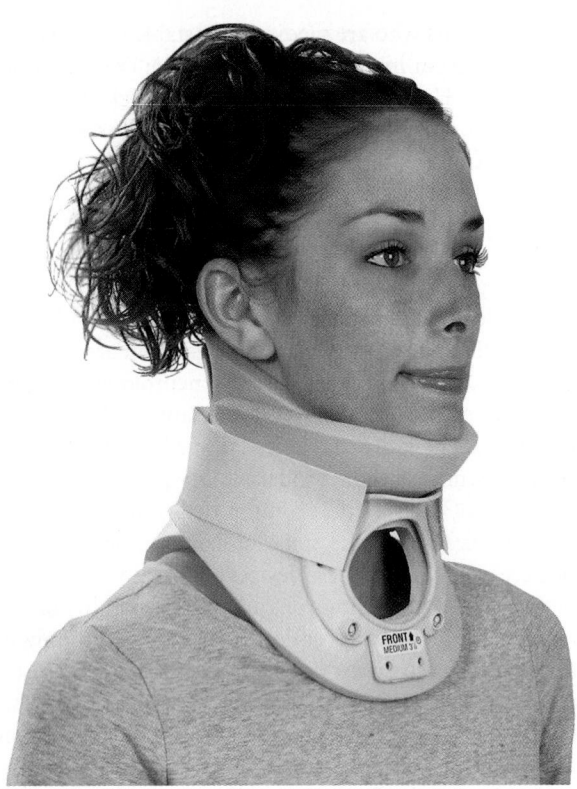

FIGURE 32–13 ■ Philly collar.
Source: Courtesy of Ossur

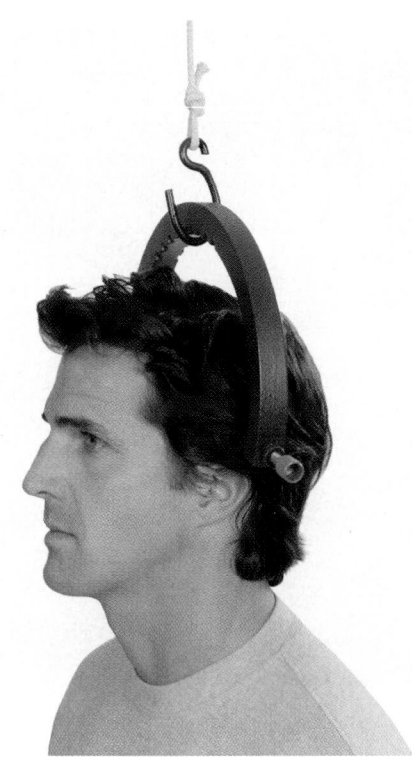

FIGURE 32–15 ■ J tongs.
Source: Courtesy of Ossur

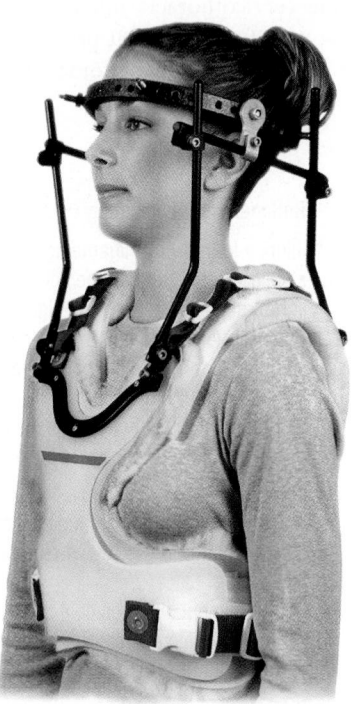

FIGURE 32–14 ■ ReSolve Halo.
Source: Courtesy of Ossur

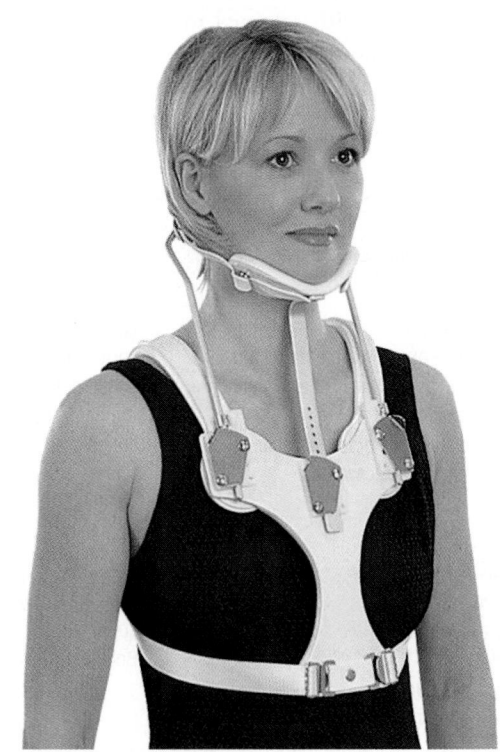

FIGURE 32–16 ■ SOMI brace.
Source: Courtesy of Trulife

SOMI brace (Figure 32–16 ■). A thoracolumbosacral orthosis will be required to stabilize the thoracic and lumbar regions. This orthotic consists of a fiberglass or rigid plastic vest fitted specifically to the patient.

Methylprednisolone administration in acute SCI has become a standard of care in many treatment centers; however, there is

much controversy in the literature regarding the effectiveness of this treatment strategy. Methylprednisolone is thought to provide protection to the neural tissues and lessen the effects of the secondary processes that contribute to the decline in neurological function in the early postinjury period (Hurlbert, 2006). Early studies indicated improvement of both motor and sensory function after administration of high-dose methylprednisolone; however, these results have not been duplicated in subsequent trials. Also, administration of high-dose steroids have associated risks including sepsis, pneumonia, blood sugar elevation, and delayed wound healing (Sayer, Kronvall, & Nilsson, 2006; Walker & Criddle, 2001). Despite the criticism in the literature, it remains a treatment option. The current standardized regimen for the treatment of acute SCI is methylprednisolone 30 mg/kg intravenously

(IV) over 15 minutes followed by a continuous infusion of methylprednisolone 5.4 mg · kg^{-1} · hr^{-1} for 23 hours if the patient is seen within 3 hours following injury. For patients who are seen between 3 and 8 hours following injury, the recommendation is to administer 30 mg/kg IV over 15 minutes, then 5.4 mg · kg^{-1} · hr^{-1} for 48 hours (Apuzzo, 2002d, Hickey, 2003b; McIlvoy et al., 2004; Prendergast & Sullivan, 2000). The Pharmacology Summary box lists medication used for treatment of spinal cord injuries.

PHARMACOLOGY Summary of Medications Used in Early Spinal Cord Injury

Medication Category	Action	Application/Indication	Nursing Responsibility
Steroid: • Methylprednisolone	Stabilizes cell membrane permeability. Decreases immune response.	Decreases secondary injury due to inflammatory response.	Assess for side effects including mental status and mood changes. Monitor blood glucose levels. Monitor for symptoms of infection.
Cardiac: • Atropine • Dopamine/dobutamine	Alter autonomic activity of the heart. Act to increase the heart rate. Sympathomimetic. Increases blood pressure and cardiac output.	Bradycardia. Hypotension due to neurogenic shock.	Monitor heart rate and rhythm. Monitor blood pressure. Titrate dosage to keep systolic BP > 90 mmHg and MAP > 85 mmHg.
Anticoagulant: • Low-molecular-weight heparin • Warfarin sodium	Inhibit blood clot formation.	Prevention or treatment of DVT.	Monitor patient for signs and symptoms of DVT formation. Monitor coagulation factors PT, PTT, INR. Assess patient for signs of too much anticoagulation, such as excessive bleeding, bruising, or signs of GI bleed.
Gastrointestinal: *Proton pump inhibitors:* • Lansoprazole • Omeprazole • Pantoprazole *Stool softeners:* • Colace • Peri-Colace • Senokot *Bowel stimulants:* • Dulcolax suppository • Therevac *Osmotic laxative:* • MiraLax *Psychological:* Anxiolytics: • Diazepam • Alprazolam • Lorazepam Antidepressants: • Venlafaxine • Fluoxetine • Duloxetine • Sertraline • Paroxetine	Inhibit gastric acid secretion. Maintain water content of feces. Stimulate bowel activity. Promote water retention in the stool producing a laxative effect. Depress the central nervous system. Inhibit the reuptake of serotonin.	Prevent gastric stress ulceration. Prevent constipation. Encourage regular emptying of the colon. Prevent constipation. Reduces anxiety related to hospitalization, injury, and loss of control over patient's own environment. Mood stabilizers help the patient cope with the injury and focus on rehabilitative goals.	Monitor patient for development of stress ulcer: c/o abdominal pain, signs of GI bleeding. Monitor frequency and quality of bowel movements. Institute bowel program as soon as patient's medical condition warrants. Assess the patient's response to the medication. Monitor patient for alteration in mood.

Current treatment strategies for medical management of acute SCI stress the importance of maintaining adequate oxygenation and blood pressure to ensure perfusion of the spinal cord. Hypotension is thought to be a contributor to worsening spinal cord injury by worsening spinal cord ischemia. Systolic blood pressure should be maintained above 90 mmHg with mean arterial blood pressure targeted above 85 mmHg to ensure adequate spinal cord perfusion (Apuzzo, 2002c; Hadley, 2002; Hickey, 2003a; Hurlbert, 2006; McIlvoy et al., 2004; Prendergast & Sullivan, 2000).

Surgical Management

Surgical management of spinal cord injuries will be considered in patients who have fractures of the spinal column that are unstable and in those patients who have compression of the spinal cord as a result of bone fragments, disk herniation, tumor, or hematoma. There is some controversy among surgeons surrounding the optimal timing for surgical intervention. Advocates for early surgical treatment point to the benefits of early decompression of the spinal cord. These benefits include improvement of spinal cord perfusion, resulting in preservation or possibly even improvement of spinal cord function by decreasing spinal cord ischemia particularly in patients with incomplete injuries. Early stabilization of an unstable spinal column also will allow for earlier mobilization of the patient, resulting in improved pulmonary function and decreased risk of development of DVT and pressure ulcers (Apuzzo, 2002a; Hickey, 2003a).

Surgery often will consist of decompression of the spinal canal and/or fusion to provide structural stability for spine fractures or dislocations. A laminectomy is the surgical procedure of choice for decompression of the spinal canal. This procedure is performed through a posterior approach and consists of removing the ligament and lamina from the back of the spinal column. Bone fragments, disc fragments, tumor, or hematoma resulting in compression of the spinal cord also will be removed when indicated. If the spine is unstable due to fracture, dislocation, or ligamentous injury, spinal instrumentation with fusion will be performed to restore spinal alignment and stability. Spinal fusion with instrumentation consists of placement of a combination of titanium screws, plates, wires, rods, or intervertebral cages and bone from either the bone bank or the patient's iliac crest to bridge fractured, unstable spinal segments with healthy, well-aligned bone. Fusion can be performed through either an anterior, posterior, or lateral approach to the spinal column (Figures 32–17 ■ and 32–18 ■).

Nursing Management

The focus of nursing care for the patient with an SCI is accurate, ongoing assessment of the patient and prevention of complications. Evaluation of the physiological response to the injury and corresponding treatment as well as the patient's emotional response to the injury are important aspects of the nursing assessment. The nursing assessment also is vital in determining the effectiveness of the treatment plan as well as prevention of potential complications and deterioration of the patient's status by allowing for early identification of problems and prompt intervention. The nursing plan of care will reflect the needs of the pa-

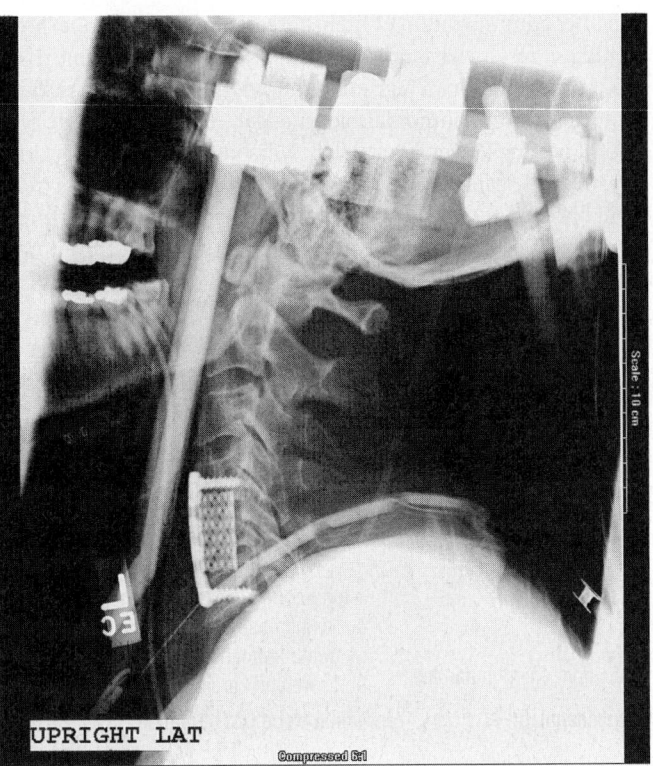

FIGURE 32–17 ■ Lateral cervical spine x-ray of C_4–C_6 fusion.
Source: Laurie Baker

tient and family and employ strategies to prevent complications and optimize the patient's function (see the Nursing Process: Patient Care Plan feature, p. 848).

Assessment
Physical Assessment and Interventions

Nursing assessment of the patient with an SCI includes routine assessment of all major organ systems. Neurological assessment includes evaluation of the patient's mental status and motor and sensory functions. Any decline in status warrants additional investigation and should be reported immediately. Range-of-motion exercises and devices such as specialized splints to prevent contracture formation from disuse should be instituted for the affected joints as soon as the patient is stable enough to tolerate these activities.

Routine cardiovascular assessment will include monitoring of blood pressure, heart rate and rhythm, and peripheral circulation including assessment of peripheral pulses and temperature of the extremities. Patients in the ICU may have a pulmonary artery catheter in place to allow for monitoring of the central pressures and cardiac output. The use of vasopressors, cardiotropic medications, and volume replacement should be instituted as ordered to maintain adequate cardiac output and mean arterial blood pressure (MAP). Intake and output should be monitored to evaluate fluid status. Once patients have clearance for mobilization, they should be monitored closely for signs of orthostatic hypotension when upright. If orthostatic hypotension is problematic, measures to prevent blood pooling in the peripheral vascular system and increase venous return to the heart should be instituted. These measures include the use of compression stockings and an abdominal binder. Expansion of intravascular volume also may be helpful. The use of devices such as a tilt table or a reclining

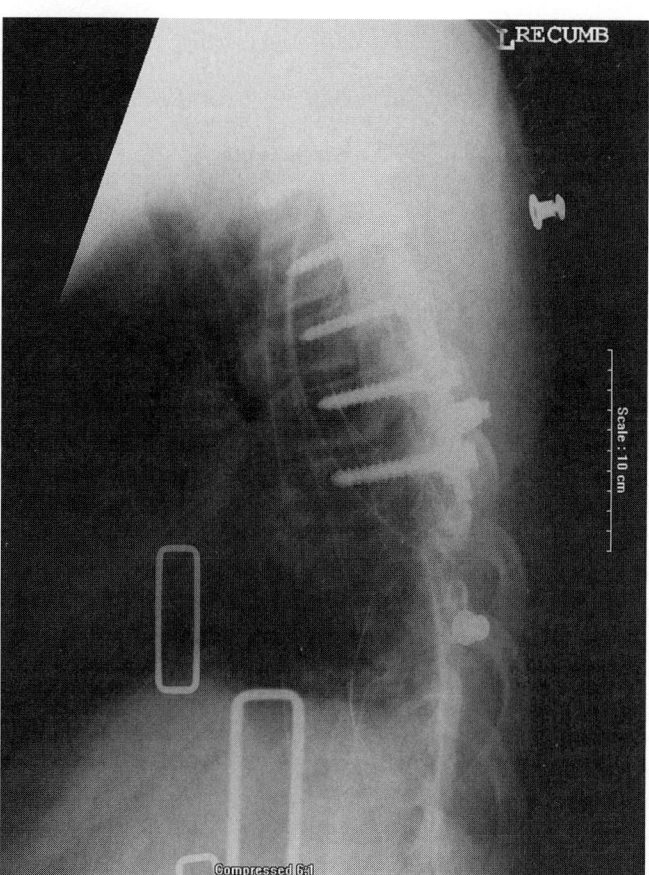

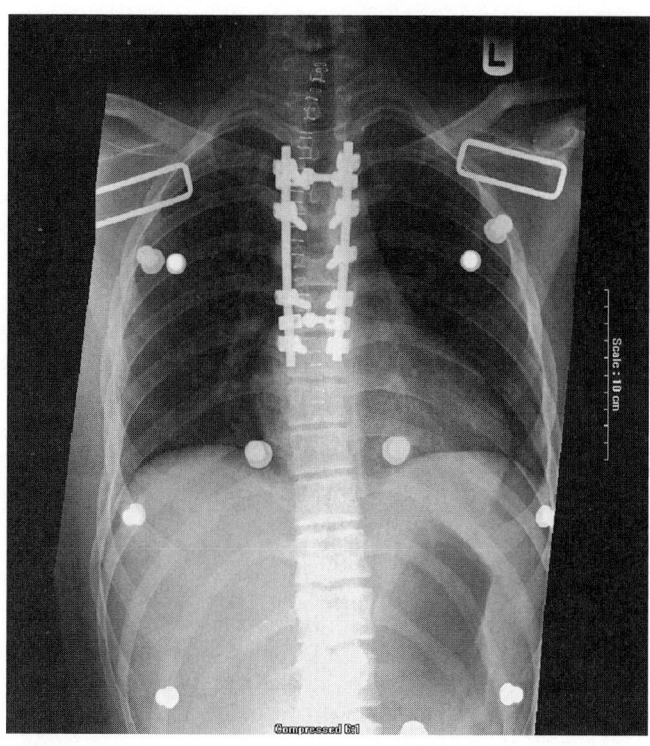

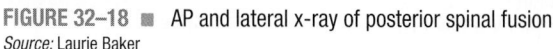

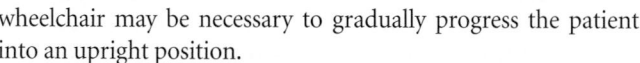

FIGURE 32–18 ■ AP and lateral x-ray of posterior spinal fusion.
Source: Laurie Baker

wheelchair may be necessary to gradually progress the patient into an upright position.

Prophylactic measures to prevent DVT formation, including the use of antiembolic hose and sequential compression boots, should be instituted once the patient is admitted to the hospital. Anticoagulant therapy and mobilization may be initiated after clearance from the surgical team. It is imperative that the nurse be vigilant in assessing for objective signs of DVT including the presence of low-grade fever, change in temperature in an extremity, swelling of an extremity, or loss of a peripheral pulse. All four extremities should be assessed because a DVT can occur in an upper extremity as well as in a lower extremity. If a DVT is suspected, the medical team should be notified immediately so that the appropriate diagnostic study can be performed and treatment initiated.

All patients with SCI should be monitored closely for signs of respiratory impairment. These signs include fever, tachypnea, tachycardia, shortness of breath, use of accessory muscles, increased volume and change in characteristic of secretions, and mental status change including increased anxiety or decrease in mental alertness. Assessment of lung sounds noting the presence of adventitious sounds indicative of pneumonia or atelectasis should be performed routinely and if any change in respiratory function is detected. Respiratory rate and use of accessory muscles in respiration also is to be noted. Pulse oximetry should be monitored on a routine basis and ABGs should be obtained to monitor for the development of hypoxemia in the patient who is at high risk for respiratory decompensation and if a decline in respiratory function or change in mental status not explained by

other means is noted. Assessment of respiratory parameters including tidal volume, vital capacity, and negative inspiratory force can be helpful in determining the need for ventilatory assistance. A chest x-ray should be obtained if alteration in respiratory function is noted (see Chapter 33 @).

The patient should be instructed on pulmonary hygiene measures including coughing and deep breathing exercises and the use of an incentive spirometer. Suctioning may be necessary if the patient is unable to clear her own secretions. Assisted coughing techniques may be beneficial as well as chest physiotherapy especially in patients with high-level injuries. The use of continuous positive airway pressure (CPAP) or bilevel positive airway pressure (BiPAP) may also be instituted to assist with reexpansion of lung tissue (Hickey, 2003a; McIlvoy et al., 2004; National Guideline Clearinghouse, 2005c). The National Guidelines box (p. 851) lists guidelines that have been established for respiratory management after spinal cord injury.

Bowel activity should be monitored with routine assessment of bowel sounds and inspection of the abdomen for distention and tenderness. The patient should be monitored for complaints of nausea and/or vomiting. If abdominal distention is present and bowel sounds are absent, an abdominal x-ray may be warranted to evaluate for an ileus. It may be necessary to insert a nasogastric tube for decompression of the stomach if ileus is present. If a drop in hematocrit occurs that is not explained by other means, evaluation for gastrointestinal hemorrhage should be performed by testing for occult blood in the stool. The nurse will need to ensure that a stress ulcer prophylactic regimen has

NURSING PROCESS: Patient Care Plan for Spinal Cord Injury

Assessment of Neurological Status

Subjective Data:
Are you able to move your arms, hand, legs, feet?
Do you have numbness or tingling anywhere?

Objective Data:

Motor strength	Deep tendon reflexes
Sensory level	Sphincter tone

Nursing Assessment and Diagnoses	Outcomes and Evaluation Parameters	Planning and Interventions with *Rationales*
Nursing Diagnoses: *Risk for Constipation* related to spinal cord injury *Disturbed Sensory Perception* related to spinal cord injury *Risk for Injury* due to spinal instability	**Outcomes:** Stabilization or improvement of neurological function. Maintenance of spinal alignment. **Evaluation Parameters:** Existing neurological function is preserved. Spine is immobilized with the appropriate orthotic device and mobility restrictions.	**Interventions and *Rationales:*** Spinal precautions maintained as ordered by the treating health care provider. *Measures to limit additional mechanical injury to the spinal cord.* Administer methylprednisolone per hospital protocol. *May limit inflammatory response and secondary injury to the spinal cord.* Maintain adequate oxygenation and mean arterial pressure (MAP) above 85 mmHg and systolic BP above 90 mmHg *to prevent secondary injury due to hypoxia and hypotension.* Monitor motor and sensory function *to assess for change in neurological function allowing for prompt medical attention if needed.*

Assessment of Pulmonary Function

Subjective Data:
Do you feel short of breath?
Do you feel like you are unable to clear your secretions?

Objective Data:

Lung sounds	Adequacy of cough
Monitor respiratory rate	Monitor pulse oximetry
Use of accessory muscles for breathing	Monitor arterial blood gases
Amount and character of secretions	Change in mental status (i.e., anxiety, confusion, increased lethargy)

Nursing Assessment and Diagnoses	Outcomes and Evaluation Parameters	Planning and Interventions with *Rationales*
Nursing Diagnoses: *Ineffective Breathing Pattern* related to pulmonary complications of spinal cord injury *Ineffective Airway Clearance* related to the loss of spinal innervation of the respiratory muscles	**Outcome:** Adequate gas exchange. **Evaluation Parameters:** Adequate oxygenation is achieved as evidenced by normal blood gases and pulse oximetry. Patient is able to clear airway secretions. Patient is without complaint of dyspnea. Lung sounds remain clear. Patient remains alert and oriented without anxiety or restlessness.	**Interventions and *Rationales:*** Monitor respiratory status. *Evaluate for change indicative of declining respiratory function including increased use of accessory muscles, inability to clear secretions, drop in oxygen saturation, change in mental status, change in respiratory parameters (tidal volume, vital capacity, negative inspiratory force).* Institute pulmonary hygiene, including cough and deep breathing exercises, chest physiotherapy, assisted cough techniques, suctioning *to promote gas exchange and airway clearance.* Administer humidified oxygen as ordered *to increase oxygenation.* Report decline in respiratory function to the medical team. *Medical management including mechanical ventilatory support may be necessary.*

Assessment of Cardiovascular Status

Subjective Data:
Are you dizzy or light-headed?

Objective Data:

Heart rate and rhythm	Blood pressure	Urine output

Nursing Assessment and Diagnoses	Outcomes and Evaluation Parameters	Planning and Interventions with *Rationales*
Nursing Diagnosis: *Risk for Ineffective Tissue Perfusion* related to cardiovascular effects of neurogenic shock	**Outcomes:** Patient maintains hemodynamic stability. Patient is able to tolerate being in an upright position. **Evaluation Parameters:** MAP > 85 mmHg SBP > 90 mmHg HR > 50–60 Patient does not complain of dizziness or light-headedness.	**Interventions and *Rationales:*** Monitor hemodynamic status *to assess for change to allow for prompt medical intervention.* Administer vasoactive agents and atropine as ordered *to ensure adequate blood pressure, heart rate, and cardiac output.* Monitor intake and output and replace intravascular volume *to ensure adequate fluid status. Hypovolemia can contribute to hemodynamic instability.* Utilize abdominal binder and thigh-high compression stockings *to increase venous return to the heart and limit blood pooling in abdomen and lower extremities due to vasodilation.* Transition patient slowly into an upright position *to avoid orthostatic hypotension.*

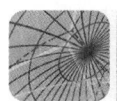

NURSING PROCESS: Patient Care Plan for Spinal Cord Injury—*Continued*

Assessment of Peripheral Tissue Perfusion

Subjective Data:
Do you have any pain or pressure in your extremities?
Have you noticed any abnormal swelling or redness in your extremities?
Have you noticed change in temperature in one or more extremity?

Objective Data:
Peripheral pulses
Temperature and color of the extremities
Unilateral swelling in the extremities

Nursing Assessment and Diagnoses	Outcomes and Evaluation Parameters	Planning and Interventions with *Rationales*
Nursing Diagnosis: *Risk of Ineffective Peripheral Tissue Perfusion* related to deep venous thrombosis (DVT)	**Outcome:** Patient does not develop DVT. **Evaluation Parameters:** The patient does not exhibit signs of DVT: redness, edema, change in temperature of extremity. Patient does not complain of pain or tenderness. Peripheral pulses remain intact.	**Interventions and *Rationales:*** Utilize antiembolic hose and sequential compression boots *to limit blood pooling in the lower extremities.* Administer prophylactic dose of anticoagulant as ordered once cleared by the surgical team *to prevent formation of peripheral DVT.* Begin mobilization of patient including range-of-motion exercises as soon as cleared by the surgical team *to limit the effects of prolonged immobility.* Assess color, temperature, and size of extremities and check peripheral pulses. Report abnormalities to the medical team *to enable early detection and prompt treatment.*

Assessment of Gastrointestinal Function

Subjective Data:
Are you nauseous?
Do you have any abdominal pain?
When was your last bowel movement?

Objective Data:
Abdominal pain
Abdominal distention
Bowel sounds
Frequency of bowel movements
Guaiac stools
Hematocrit
Dietary intake

Nursing Assessment and Diagnoses	Outcomes and Evaluation Parameters	Planning and Interventions with *Rationales*
Nursing Diagnoses: *Risk for constipation* related to impaired gastric motility due to spinal cord injury *Potential for Gastric Ulceration* related to stress of critical injury *Readiness for Enhanced Nutrition* related to increased metabolic need and inadequate caloric intake	**Outcomes:** Gastrointestinal function will be maintained. Patient will be without evidence of gastric stress ulceration. A regular pattern of bowel movements will be established. Patient will receive adequate nutrition to meet caloric requirements. **Evaluation Parameters:** Abdomen will remain soft, nontender, and nondistended. Patient will be without complaints of nausea, vomiting, constipation, or epigastric pain. Hematocrit will remain stable. Nutrition will be implemented.	**Interventions and *Rationales:*** Assess abdomen for tenderness and distention. Auscultate bowel sounds. *Evaluation of gastrointestinal function.* Monitor hematocrit and check stool for occult blood if drop in hematocrit noted without other explanation (i.e., surgery) *to assess for GI bleed due to gastric stress ulceration.* Use nasogastric tube if ileus is present *to provide for decompression of the stomach.* Administer stress ulcer prophylactic regimen as ordered by the medical team. Institute bowel regimen of stool softener, chemical stimulation such as a suppository, and mechanical (digital) stimulation *to establish a regular bowel elimination pattern.* Institute parenteral nutrition until patient is able to tolerate enteral feedings. Call for dietary consult *to determine patient's caloric needs.*

Assessment of Urinary Elimination

Subjective Data:
Are you able to urinate?
Do you feel like your bladder is full?
Have you had any incontinence of urine?

Objective Data:
Urinary output
Bladder scan to assess for urinary retention

(continued)

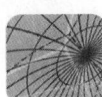

NURSING PROCESS: Patient Care Plan for Spinal Cord Injury—*Continued*

Nursing Assessment and Diagnoses	Outcomes and Evaluation Parameters	Planning and Interventions with *Rationales*
Nursing Diagnoses: Impaired Urinary Elimination due to neurogenic bladder *Risk for Autonomic Dysreflexia* related to autonomic dysfunction as a result of spinal cord injury	**Outcomes:** The patient will establish a normal pattern of urinary elimination. The patient will be able to recognize the signs of autonomic hyperreflexia, identify potential causes, and describe treatment of hyperreflexia. **Evaluation Parameters:** The patient or caregiver is able to perform clean intermittent catherization (CIC). The patient and caregiver can verbalize common causes of hyperreflexia, common symptoms of hyperreflexia, and actions to take should hyperreflexia occur.	**Interventions and *Rationales:*** Use indwelling catheter during the acute period *to allow for complete bladder emptying and accurate measurement of urinary output.* Check postvoid residuals by either intermittent catheterization or bladder scan *to assess for urinary retention.* Teach CIC to patient and caregiver *to encourage a consistent manner of bladder emptying.* Instruct patient and caregiver on common causes and signs of autonomic hyperreflexia and interventions to institute when these signs occur.

Assessment of Pain

Subjective Data:
Are you having pain?
Where do you hurt?

Objective Data:

Facial grimacing	Elevated blood pressure
Crying	Elevated heart rate
Increased spasticity	

Nursing Assessment and Diagnoses	Outcomes and Evaluation Parameters	Planning and Interventions with *Rationales*
Nursing Diagnosis: Readiness for enhanced comfort due to injury and/or surgical procedure	**Outcome:** Effective control of pain. **Evaluation Parameters:** The patient will report improvement of pain. The patient is able to participate in therapies.	**Interventions and *Rationales:*** Assess pain utilizing a pain scale *to provide a method of measuring degree of pain and response to pain control measures.* Administer analgesics as ordered *to provide pharmacologic treatment of pain.* Utilize distraction and repositioning techniques *to augment pharmacologic treatment of pain.*

Assessment of Psychosocial State

Subjective Data:
Are you feeling sad, depressed?
How have you dealt with stress in the past?
Who is your support person?

Objective Data:

Refusal to communicate	Anger
Refusal to participate in activities	Crying
Avoidance of eye contact	Expressing feelings of hopelessness

Nursing Assessment and Diagnoses	Outcomes and Evaluation Parameters	Planning and Interventions with *Rationales*
Nursing Diagnoses: *Ineffective Coping* related to loss of control over environment and uncertainty of the future	**Outcomes:** Patient will exhibit appropriate coping strategies. Patient will exhibit less anxiety. **Evaluation Parameters:** Patient reports improved mood. Patient participates in care. Patient is able to express feelings.	**Interventions and *Rationales:*** Encourage the patient to express her feelings *to provide for self-expression and identification of feelings.* Allow patient to participate in decisions *so the patient regains some control over self and the environment.* Request psychiatric consultation. *Assist with crisis counseling and to help the patient to identify appropriate coping strategies.* Administer antianxiolytics and antidepressants as prescribed.

Assessment of Adaptation

Subjective Data:
What are you able to do for yourself?
What adaptive equipment do you have available and what will be needed?

Objective Data:
Functional assessment based on preserved motor function
Patient/caregiver knowledge of use of equipment
Patient/caregiver knowledge of available resources

Nursing Assessment and Diagnoses	Outcomes and Evaluation Parameters	Planning and Interventions with *Rationales*
Nursing Diagnoses: *Self-Care Deficit* related to spinal cord injury *Deficient Knowledge* regarding adaptation strategies and resources	**Outcome:** Patient will implement self-care strategies utilizing the appropriate adaptive devices within the limitations of his injury. **Evaluation Parameters:** The patient participates in his own care. The patient will be able to identify available resources to help him to be independent within the limitations of his injury.	**Interventions and *Rationales:*** Schedule nursing care around PT/OT sessions *to ensure patient is able to participate in rehabilitative activities.* Have adaptive equipment readily available and encourage patient to use the equipment in self-care activities. *Encourages self-care strategies and reinforces education on the use of the equipment.* Assist the patient in identifying available community resources *to assist in independent living.*

NATIONAL GUIDELINES for Respiratory Management Following Spinal Cord Injury

Risk Factor	**Guideline**
Respiratory failure	Assessment:
	History:
	• Relevant past medical history
	• Prior history of pulmonary disease
	• Medications
	• History of substance abuse
	• Neurological impairment
	• Coexisting injuries
	Examination:
	• Physical exam of the respiratory system including lung sounds, respiratory rate, use of accessory muscles
	• Respiratory complaints
	• Oxygen saturation with continuous pulse oximetry
	• Chest x-ray
	• Measurement of vital capacity, maximal negative inspiratory pressure, forced expiratory volume in 1 second
	• Neurological level and extent of impairment
	• Assess risk for aspiration
	Initial laboratory and radiographic evaluation:
	• Arterial blood gases
	• CBC, chemistry panel, coagulation profile, cardiac enzymes, urinalysis, toxicology
	• Chest x-ray
	• EKG
	Intubation Parameters:
	• Intractable respiratory failure
	• High risk for aspiration plus respiratory compromise
Atelectasis and pneumonia	Assessment:
	Monitor indicators for the development of pneumonia or atelectasis:
	• Rising temperature
	• Change in respiratory rate
	• Increasing heart rate
	• Increasing anxiety
	• Increased volume and change in character of secretions
	• Decline in vital capacity
	• Decline in peak expiratory flow
	Obtain chest x-ray. If atelectasis or pneumonia present on x-ray, monitor serial x-rays.
	Prevention and Treatment:
	Incentive spirometry and coughing and deep breathing exercises
	Chest physiotherapy
	Assisted coughing techniques
	Intermittent positive pressure breathing
	CPAP or BiPAP
	Turning and alternative positioning when patient is medically and surgically stable
	Mobilization once patient is medically and surgically stable
	Prevent aspiration
	Antibiotic therapy as indicated by sputum culture

Source: National Guideline Clearinghouse. (2005). *Respiratory management following spinal cord injury: A clinical practice guideline for health-care professionals.* Washington, DC: Consortium for Spinal Cord Medicine, Paralyzed Veterans of America. Retrieved April 29, 2008, from http://www.guideline.gov/summary/summary.aspx?doc_id=7198&nbr=004301&string=spinal+AND+cord+AND+injury.

been implemented as part of the medical treatment plan. Nutritional intake should be initiated as soon as possible. A dietary consult may be necessary to ensure adequate caloric intake to meet the patient's metabolic needs.

Regardless of the level of injury, all patients with SCI should have a regular bowel management regimen instituted as part of their ongoing care once the patient's condition allows. This program should be based on the patient's preinjury elimination patterns and provide for a consistent schedule of elimination to avoid such problems as bowel impaction or incontinence. This regimen should include the use of stool softeners, chemical stimulants such as suppositories, and mechanical stimulants such as digital stimulation of the bowel. The patient's bowel elimination pattern should be monitored closely to ensure adequate bowel evacuation. Dietary recommendations to aid in bowel evacuation include ensuring a minimum of 15 grams of dietary fiber per day as well as adequate fluid intake (Enck et al., 2006; Hickey, 2003b; National Guideline Clearinghouse, 2005a).

All patients who have had a SCI will require the use of an indwelling urinary catheter in the acute phase following injury. The catheter allows for bladder decompression and adequate monitoring of intake and output. A catheter can increase the risk of UTI. Urine that is cloudy or has a foul odor may indicate the presence of a UTI and urinalysis and culture should be obtained.

As the patient progresses through the recovery period, the indwelling catheter should be removed. The patient will need to be monitored for signs of urinary retention. Postvoid residuals should be checked either with intermittent catheterization or bladder scan. Urinary incontinence may be due to overflow of urine from a distended bladder. If the patient is unable to void or has high postvoid residual volumes, an alternative method of urinary elimination to allow for complete emptying of the bladder should be implemented. The most common means of urinary management after SCI is the use of clean intermittent catheterization (CIC). Intermittent catheterization should be taught to the patient if there is adequate preservation of hand function or to the patient's primary caregiver if the patient is unable to perform this task.

It is vital that the nurse maintain excellent skin care for the patient with a SCI in order to maintain skin integrity. Patients should be removed from the firm spinal board as soon as the initial trauma assessment is complete and it is deemed safe to move the patient. Routine assessment of the skin particularly in areas over bony prominences and under orthotic devices should be performed a minimum of twice daily. Redness and/or blanching of the skin are early signs of pressure ulcer formation. Areas most vulnerable to pressure ulcer formation include the trochanters, ischial tuberosities, sacrum, coccyx, heels, and occiput. Pressure ulcers can also occur on the elbows and scapula. The patient should be turned every 2 hours with careful attention paid to positioning the patient to avoid pressure over bony prominences and avoidance of shearing forces when moving the patient. The skin, clothing, and sheets should be kept dry and wrinkle free. Devices such as air flotation mattresses, pillows, and wheelchair cushions designed to unload pressure sites should be instituted. Patients also should be instructed in repositioning techniques to unload pressure sites while sitting in the wheelchair.

If the patient requires the use of an orthotic brace for immobilization, the skin under the brace should be routinely in-

spected. Rigid braces such as cervical collars and thoracic lumbar braces can be removed and the skin underneath can be inspected while the patient is supine in bed. Patients who are immobilized with a halo brace or other traction devices should have the cranial pin sites cleaned with normal saline and inspected for signs of infection twice daily. The vest plates of the halo vest can be removed by an experienced orthotist while the patient is supine, and skin care to the thoracic area can be performed at that time. Incisions and abrasions should be inspected regularly for signs of infection. Nutritional measures should be instituted as soon as possible to ensure the patient receives adequate calories, protein, and micronutrients (Hickey, 2003b; Paralyzed Veterans of America, 2001).

If the patient experiences symptoms of autonomic hyperreflexia, he should be placed in an upright position with the lower extremities dependent to lower the blood pressure. The causative factor should be identified and removed. If hypertension persists, administration of a quick-acting antihypertensive agent may be necessary. The best strategy for managing autonomic hyperreflexia is avoidance of the precipitating stimulus. The patient and family will need to be educated on the signs and symptoms of autonomic hyperreflexia, strategies to avoid this condition, and actions to take should this condition occur (Hickey, 2003b; Krassioukov, 2004; McIlvoy et al., 2004; National Guideline Clearinghouse, 2001). National guidelines for acute management of autonomic hyperreflexia have been established.

Psychosocial Assessment and Intervention

Patients who have experienced a SCI are not only faced with the physical challenges associated with this injury, but also with a significant psychosocial impact. These patients are faced with changes related to loss of body image, loss of independence, loss of control over their immediate environment, loss of economic security, and lifestyle changes. This injury also can place a significant stress and strain on existing relationships. The patient may exhibit a wide range of emotions including denial, grief, anger, hopelessness, and depression.

The nurse should monitor the patient for signs of inadequate coping including withdrawal from social interactions, avoidance of eye contact, and refusal to participate in activities. The patient should be encouraged to discuss her feelings and be allowed to participate in decision making whenever possible. The patient's family members also will need support and ongoing education to help them deal with the stress of having a critically ill loved one and the role changes associated with becoming a primary caregiver. In some cases, consultation with a chaplain, social worker, or psychiatrist may be necessary. Healing touch may also be helpful to patients with SCI, as discussed in the Complementary and Alternative Therapies box (p. 854).

Rehabilitation

Rehabilitation for patients with SCI will consist of a comprehensive, interdisciplinary program designed to help patients adapt to the limitations of their injury, reach the highest level of independence possible, and reintegrate into the home environment and community. During the rehabilitation period, the patient will undergo extensive inpatient physical and occupational

NATIONAL GUIDELINES for Acute Management of Autonomic Hyperreflexia

Risk Factor	Guideline
Autonomic hyperreflexia	Patient's with SCI at or above T_6 are at risk for autonomic hyperreflexia.

Recognize the signs and symptoms of autonomic hyperreflexia:

- Elevated blood pressure: a sudden, significant increase (20–40 mmHg) in both diastolic and systolic blood pressures above the patient's usual level
- Pounding headache
- Bradycardia: may be within normal range but relative slowing compared to the patient's normal heat rate
- Profuse sweating above the level of the lesion, especially the face, neck, and shoulders
- Piloerection above and possibly below the level of injury
- Cardiac dysrhythmias including atrial fibrillation, premature ventricular contractions, and atrioventricular conduction abnormalities
- Flushing of the skin above the level of injury, especially the face, neck, and shoulders
- Patient complaint of visual disturbance such as blurred vision or spots in the visual field
- Nasal congestion
- Feelings of apprehension or anxiety
- Symptoms may be absent or minimal despite significantly elevated blood pressure (silent autonomic hyperreflexia)

Treatment:

- If the person is supine, immediately sit the patient up and lower the legs if possible. This allows the blood to pool in the lower extremities and may lower the blood pressure.
- Loosen any clothing or constricting devices.
- Monitor the blood pressure and pulse frequently. Blood pressure can fluctuate rapidly due to impaired autonomic regulation.
- Quickly assess the patient for the instigating cause and remove it as quickly as possible.
  - The most common cause of autonomic hyperreflexia is bladder distention:
    - Check indwelling catheter for patency and proper placement.
    - If the catheter is blocked, gently irrigate with 10 to 15 mL normal saline at body temperature.
    - Avoid compressing or tapping on the bladder.
    - If the catheter does not drain, remove and replace the catheter.
  - If no catheter is in place, catheterize the patient:
    - Instill 2% lidocaine jelly into urethra and wait 2 minutes if time allows before inserting the catheter to decrease sensory input and relax the urinary sphincter.
  - The second most common cause of autonomic hyperreflexia is fecal impaction:
    - If systolic blood pressure is >150 mmHg, consider pharmacologic treatment to reduce blood pressure without causing hypotension prior to checking for fecal impaction.
    - If systolic blood pressure is <150 mmHg, check for fecal impaction:
      - Instill 2% lidocaine jelly into the rectum.
      - Wait 2 minutes.
      - Insert gloved, lubricated finger into the rectum and check for the presence of stool.
      - If stool is present, gently remove.
      - If autonomic hyperreflexia worsens, stop the manual evacuation, instill additional topical anesthetic, and recheck the rectum after approximately 20 minutes.
  - If urinary and fecal causes of autonomic hyperreflexia have been eliminated and symptoms persist, assess for other instigating causes and treat accordingly:
    - Pressure ulcerations
    - Abdominal pathology
    - Ingrown toenails
    - Long bone fractures
    - Infection

Education:

- Educate the patient and family about common causes of autonomic hyperreflexia and appropriate treatment strategies.

Source: National Guideline Clearinghouse. (2001). *Acute management of autonomic dysreflexia: Individuals with spinal cord injury presenting to a health-care facility.* Washington, DC: Consortium for Spinal Cord Medicine, Paralyzed Veterans of America. Retrieved November 14, 2006, from http://www.guideline.gov/summary/summary.aspx?doc_id=2964&nbr=002190&string=Autonomic+ AND+dysreflexia.

therapy to strengthen functioning muscles and optimize functionality. The patient and family will receive instruction regarding strategies for self-care and performance of activities of daily living (ADLs) including proper transfer and mobility techniques. Patients and families also will receive advice regarding appropriate modifications to the home to accommodate the patient's disability and adaptive equipment.

A social worker and psychologist will work with patients and their families to assist with psychosocial issues related to lifestyle including sexuality and recreation. Patients will receive advice on maintaining an active lifestyle within the limitations of their injury. They also will receive instruction specific to sexual activity early in the acute rehabilitative period and this information will be frequently reinforced. It is important that these patients

COMPLEMENTARY & ALTERNATIVE THERAPIES — Healing Touch and Spirituality

Description:

Healing touch is a form of energy-based therapy in which the practitioner's hands move to realign energy that resides just outside the physical body. While it is still a new and somewhat controversial technique, many nurses practice healing touch, and many advocate its use. There are also many anecdotal reports that confirm its beneficial effects. This feature will discuss healing touch as it specifically applies to spinal cord injuries. Many patients with spinal cord injuries experience spiritual crisis during their journey to recovery and a new way of living. Therefore, anything that shows a benefit should be tried to help those suffering this trauma.

Research Support:

A pilot study assessed how healing touch (HT) modulates chronic neuropathic pain and the associated psychological distress from post–spinal cord injury. During six weekly home visits, 12 veterans were assigned to either HT or guided progressive relaxation. Researchers then measured the participants' progress using several instruments: the Brief Pain Inventory, the Profile of Moods, and the Diener Satisfaction with Life Scale. Although there was a large variation among the groups, the instruments did show sensitivity. The composite of interference on the Brief Pain Inventory showed a significant difference. In the fatigue subscale of the Profile of Moods, the mean score decreased (ns) in the HT group, and in the subscale of confusion the mean score remained stable in the control group. The Diener Satisfaction with Life Scale showed increased well-being in the HT group and no change in the control group. Researchers concluded that HT sessions may have benefit in the complex response to chronic pain (Wardell, Rintala, Duan, & Tan, 2006).

A national U.S. sample of insured adults with physical disabilities were examined to estimate the prevalence of CAM practitioner use, assess the reasons for use, and determine the symptoms for which CAM practitioners were consulted. Data for this study were obtained from a longitudinal survey conducted in 2000 and 2001 on a national sample of 830 adults with health insurance. These adults had one of four disabling conditions: multiple sclerosis, cerebral palsy, spinal cord injury, and arthritis. A cross-sectional analysis of the 2001 survey data was used to estimate annual prevalence and reasons and symptoms for which CAM practitioners were consulted. The 2000 survey was used to assess prior use of CAM. Nineteen percent of the sample population consulted CAM practitioners, which is a rate similar to, or higher than, the general population. Results showed that CAM use was more prevalent among women than men (24% versus 10%); in the Western United States (30%) compared to the Midwest (20%), Northeast (14%), and South (10%); and among prior users (62%) compared to nonusers (8%). Results showed no significant differences in CAM use by condition, although individuals with spinal cord injury reported the lowest CAM use (14%). Common symptoms treated included pain (80%), decreased functioning (43%), and lack of energy (24%). Common reasons for using CAM practitioners included lifestyle choice (67%) and because they are perceived to be more effective than conventional medicine (44%). This evidence suggests that a significant proportion of people with physical disabilities consult CAM prac-

titioners. Researchers noted that many of those who use CAM do so because it fits their lifestyle and because they perceive it to be more effective than conventional medicine for treating common symptoms including pain and decreased functioning (Carlson & Krahn, 2006).

An essential component in providing holistic care to patients is spiritual care. Although nursing education often lacks practical guidelines on how to provide culturally competent spiritual care, all nurses are required to provide spiritual care. Rehabilitation patients often face a lengthy recovery time and have special needs; therefore, rehabilitation nurses, in particular, are challenged to be competent in this area (Rieg, Mason, & Preston, 2006).

Nurses must be competent to provide care on a physical, mental, social, and spiritual level in order to deliver spiritual care. In one study, three main nursing competencies associated with the role of the nurse as a professional and as an individual person were identified: delivery of spiritual care by the nursing process; nurses' communication with patients, interdisciplinary team, and clinical/educational organizations; and safeguarding ethical issues in care. Spiritual care is complex, and the Nursing Code of Ethics recommends that nurses increase their awareness of each patient's individual uniqueness and the connection between mind, body, and spirit, and to assess the spiritual status of patients during illness and the implementation of holistic care (Baldacchino, 2006).

Another study investigated the relationship of spirituality and life satisfaction among persons with spinal cord injury. The study involved a nationwide sample of 230 persons with long-term spinal cord injury. These participants completed the Satisfaction with Life Scale (SWLS), the Quality of Life Index (QLI), and a demographic data form. Results indicated a significant positive correlation between life satisfaction and psychological/spiritual factors of the QLI instrument.

The International Council of Nurses, the Joint Commission on Accreditation of Healthcare Organizations, and the Patient's Bill of Rights mandate nurses to provide spiritual care for clients. Rehabilitation nurses, in particular, have the opportunity to support spirituality and life satisfaction when assisting clients with disabilities to redefine their lives and explore new life opportunities (Brillhart, 2005).

References

Baldacchino, D. R. (2006). Nursing competencies for spiritual care. *Journal of Clinical Nursing, 15*(7), 885–96.

Brillhart, B. (2005). A study of spirituality and life satisfaction among persons with spinal cord injury. *Rehabilitation Nursing, 30*(1), 31–4.

Carlson, M. J., & Krahn, G. (2006). Use of complementary and alternative medicine practitioners by people with physical disabilities: Estimates from a national U.S. survey. *Disability and Rehabilitation, 28*(8), 505–13.

Rieg, L. S., Mason, C. H., & Preston, K. (2006). Spiritual care: Practical guidelines for rehabilitation nurses. *Rehabilitation Nursing, 31*(6), 249–56.

Wardell, D. W., Rintala, D. H., Duan, Z., & Tan, G. (2006). A pilot study of healing touch and progressive relaxation for chronic neuropathic pain in persons with spinal cord injury. *Journal of Holistic Nursing, 24*(4), 231–240.

understand they can continue to be active both sexually and recreationally despite their injury. It is even possible for them to have children in the future if they so desire. The ongoing support of a urologist or gynecologist after discharge from the rehabilitation facility will be important in maintaining sexual health.

Once the patient is ready for discharge, identification of community resources for continued support to the patient and family and to assist with reintegration into the home environment and community is beneficial. Other patient teaching priorities are listed in the Patient Teaching & Discharge Priorities box.

Collaborative Management

The patient with a SCI will require a multidisciplinary team approach to treatment throughout the continuum of care. The medical team will often consist of members of the trauma team and surgical team until stabilization of injuries is accomplished. Health care providers specializing in critical care medicine are helpful in management of cardiopulmonary issues in the acute phase after injury. A respiratory therapist will assist with pulmonary management including suctioning and cough and deep breathing strategies. Dietary consultation is helpful to ensure the patient's nutritional requirements are met.

Once the patient has been stabilized, physical and occupational therapy evaluation and treatment are necessary to assist with optimization of function through range-of-motion exercises, strengthening exercises, and instruction regarding mobility and use of adaptive equipment. Involvement of a social worker with expertise in SCI is vital to assist with issues related to lifestyle changes and loss of income as well as identification of resources to assist with transition into the community. The assistance of a

mental health expert, such as a psychologist, will be helpful to assist with issues of depression and adjustment to lifestyle changes related to the injury. Once the acute care issues of hemodynamic and spinal stability have been addressed, involvement of a physiatrist to direct rehabilitation efforts will be necessary.

Nurses are an integral part of the multidisciplinary team, providing a common link for all team members as well as providing education and support to the patient and family through all phases of treatment.

Gerontological Considerations

The number of patients over the age of 60 who have sustained an SCI has gradually increased during the last decade. Falls account for the leading cause of injury in this population. The elderly are at increased risk of injury to the spinal cord because of degenerative changes in the spinal column including ossification and hypertrophy of the spinal ligaments and development of bone spurs within the spinal column leading to narrowing of the spinal canal. Weakening of the bone due to osteoporosis also increases the risk of spinal fracture in these patients. This patient population presents an added challenge to the management of acute SCI because of preexisting medical problems such as diabetes and heart disease, as well as the normal physiological effects of aging (Chart 32–6, p. 856). These factors may affect overall outcomes in this age group (NSCISC, 2006; Villanueva, 2000).

Health Promotion

The majority of SCIs occur as a result of trauma and many of these injuries are preventable. The key to reducing the incidence of these injuries is to decrease high-risk behaviors such as driving while under the influence of drugs or alcohol, lack of seat belt use, and diving into shallow water. Several educational programs geared to both adults and children have been designed to increase

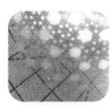

PATIENT TEACHING & DISCHARGE PRIORITIES for Spinal Cord Injury

Need	Teaching
Understanding of bowel/bladder regimen	The patient and family are taught how to perform CIC and how to perform bowel care including insertion of a suppository, digital stimulation of the bowel, and disimpaction of stool.
Prevention of complications	The patient and family are taught strategies such as frequent position changes and skin care to avoid the formation of pressure ulcers.
	The patient and family will understand the importance of maintaining a regular bowel and bladder regimen to avoid complications of UTI and bowel impaction.
Safety	Proper instruction on the use of adaptive equipment and transfer strategies will be given to the patient and family.
	The patient and family will be instructed on the signs and symptoms of autonomic hyperreflexia, common causes of hyperreflexia, and strategies to implement if autonomic hyperreflexia occurs.
Emotional adjustment of patient and family to psychosocial impact of SCI	The patient and family are encouraged to discuss their feelings openly.
	The patient and family will be able to identify supportive resources to help them cope with both the physical and psychosocial changes due to SCI.
Adaptation of environment	The patient and family will be provided instruction on necessary adaptation to the home environment and resources to assist with completion of environmental changes necessary to accommodate the patient's deficits and adaptive equipment.
	If the patient is unable to be discharged to a home environment, arrangements for an assisted living environment will be made.

CHART 32–6	**Changes Associated with Aging**

System	Associated Changes
Cardiovascular	↓ Contractile strength of the myocardium ↓ Cardiac output and stroke volume ↓ Vessel elasticity
Pulmonary	↓ Vital capacity ↓ Functional residual capacity ↑ Residual volume
Gastrointestinal	↓ Peristalsis ↓ Gastric acid secretion
Integument	↓ Subcutaneous tissue ↑ Thinning of epidermal layer
Musculoskeletal	↑ Osteoarthritic, degenerative joint changes ↓ Muscle mass, tone, and strength

Source: Adapted from Villanueva, N. E. (2000). Spinal cord injury in the elderly. *Critical Care Nurse Clinics of North America, 12,* 509–519.

awareness of those high-risk behaviors as well as to educate the public on simple strategies to decrease the risk of sustaining a SCI. These programs have been implemented in schools, workplaces, and communities, and often are comprised of a team of volunteers including a person who has sustained a permanent SCI and a health care provider who has experience in treating SCIs.

Prevention of complications is important to the maintenance of optimal health for the person with an SCI. Early detection and prompt treatment of problems such as alteration in skin integrity and UTIs are keys in preventing more serious complications such as sepsis and osteomyelitis. The person with an SCI should also be encouraged to obtain regular health maintenance evaluations for screening and treatment of chronic health problems including diabetes and heart disease. Counseling regarding smoking cessation and drug and alcohol use should not be overlooked in this patient population. Many people who have had an SCI are eventually able to return to active productive lives with the appropriate adaptive strategies and optimal health maintenance.

Research

Current spinal cord injury research continues to focus on ways to improve outcomes for patients with SCI as well as improving functional ability (see the Research Opportunities and Clinical Impact box). Much of this research is focused on limiting the secondary effects of spinal cord injury as well as restoration of function.

RESEARCH OPPORTUNITIES AND CLINICAL IMPACT RELATED TO SPINAL CORD INJURIES

Research Area	Clinical Impact
Administration of methylprednisolone or GM-1 ganglioside	Reduce secondary effects of spinal cord injury
Early versus delayed surgical decompression	
Cell transplantation into the spinal cord	Repair of spinal cord damage
Restorative therapy techniques	Improvement and restoration of function
Electrical stimulation of muscles below the level of injury	

Respiratory Complications Related to Spinal Cord Injury

Clinical Problem

Respiratory complications account for the most common cause of death in patients who have sustained a spinal cord injury. Patients with injury in the cervical spine are at the highest risk for morbidity and mortality related to respiratory issues due in large part to disruption of innervation to the diaphragm and respiratory accessory muscles; however, aspiration also contributes to pulmonary-related complications (Neville et al., 2005). Patients who have sustained a cervical spinal cord injury are at increased risk for aspiration not only because they are not able to adequately protect their airways due to ineffective protective measures such as cough, but also because these patients experience abnormality in swallowing.

Research Findings

Neville and colleagues (2005) conducted an evaluation of esophageal function in patients who had sustained traumatic cervical spinal cord injury. These authors hypothesized that patients with cervical spinal cord injury had abnormality of esophageal function that put them at risk for aspiration. The study sample consisted of 18 patients who had sustained traumatic cervical spinal cord injury. A control group for comparison was comprised of five patients who had sustained spinal cord injury at T_1 or below. Patients were excluded if they had associated head injury, known history of gastroesophageal reflux disease, previous gastric surgery, or previous antireflux surgery. All patients were subjected to measurement of esophageal pressures utilizing a manometric catheter inserted transnasally into the esophagus. Pressures were obtained at both the upper esophageal sphincter and lower esophageal sphincter. Measurement of peristaltic activity along the length of the esophagus during swallow was also obtained.

All patients in the study group had abnormally elevated pressures of the upper esophageal sphincter on swallow. This was not reflected in the control group. No abnormality of lower esophageal pressures or esophageal peristaltic activity was present for either the study or control group. The authors concluded that patients with cervical spinal cord injury have abnormal pressures of the upper esophageal sphincter necessitating increased force to move secretions or food from the oral pharynx into the esophagus during swallow and increasing the patient's risk for aspiration.

The effect of cervical bracing on swallow also has been evaluated. Stambolis et al. (2003) performed radiographic observation of swallow in 17 normal adults utilizing both solids and liquids without a cervical orthosis and in a rigid cervical collar, a SOMI brace, and in a halo brace. None of the subjects had previous history of swallowing abnormalities. Swallowing abnormalities were apparent in all bracing conditions and were most evident with liquid boluses. The investigators observed changes in the point of initiation of swallow, increased laryngeal penetration, increased residue in the pharynx, and reduced hyoid bone movement. They determined that cervical bracing placed the subjects in an unnatural eating position and limited the use of compensatory swallowing mechanisms. Many people slightly flex their necks when swallowing. This action was limited by the orthoses.

Also, most orthoses placed the subjects in a 90° head position, which caused narrowing of the oropharynx in some of subjects.

Morishima, Ohota, and Miura (2005) also evaluated the effect of halo brace fixation on swallow. Their study sample was comprised of six neurologically intact, healthy volunteers. Radiographic evaluation of swallow with thin liquids was obtained with the subjects in a neutral position without the brace and with the subjects in the halo brace with the head in a neutral position and in a hyperextended position. Activity of the muscles associated with swallow also was observed with electromyography. The investigators demonstrated changes in the activation of the muscles associated with swallow as well as prolonged transit of the liquids in the pharyngeal phase of swallow with the subjects in the halo brace with the head hyperextended. Penetration of liquid into the larynx and aspiration during swallow was also evident.

Implications for Nursing Practice

Based on these studies, the risk of aspiration due to swallowing abnormalities in the patient with cervical spinal cord injury is clearly present. These patients not only have abnormalities in the mechanics of swallow, but treatment modalities such as cervical bracing also contribute to swallowing dysfunction. It is important for nurses caring for this population to be aware of this risk so that appropriate assessment and prevention strategies can be instituted as part of the nursing plan of care. The patient and family also will need to be educated on the risk for aspiration as well as precautions to take to prevent it. If the patient exhibits signs of aspiration such as a wet quality to the voice, coughing with oral intake, or difficulty managing oral secretions, a referral for formal swallow evaluation is warranted. Prevention of aspiration is one of the key strategies in decreasing the risk of pulmonary complications.

Critical Thinking Questions

1. What are the risks for aspiration in the patient with cervical spinal cord injury?

2. What signs may indicate aspiration?

3. What precautions should be taken to avoid aspiration?

Answers to Critical Thinking Questions appear in Appendix D.

References

Morishima, N., Ohota, K., & Miura, Y. (2005). The influences of halo-vest fixation and cervical hyperextension on swallowing in healthy volunteers. *Spine, 30,* E179–E182.

Neville, A., Crookes, P., Velmahos, G., Vlahos, A., Theodorou, D., & Lucas, C. (2005). Esophageal dysfunction in cervical spinal cord injury: A potentially important mechanism of aspiration. *Journal of Trauma, 59,* 905–911.

Stambolis, V., Brady, S., Klos, D., Wesling, M., Fatianov, T., & Hildner, C. (2003). The effects of cervical bracing upon swallowing in young, normal, healthy volunteers. *Dysphagia, 18,* 39–45.

EVIDENCE-BASED PRACTICE

Clinical Preparation

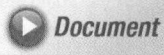 **Read**

- History of Current Illness
- Past Medical History
- Physical Exam
- Admitting Medical Orders
- Laboratory Study Results

 **Document**

- Summary of Hospitalization
- Pathophysiology Form
- Laboratory Values
- Laboratory Results Explanation

Apply

- List of Potential Nursing Diagnoses
- Concept Map
- Critical Thinking Questions

Log on to MyNursingKit.com to download forms you will need and to complete further steps in the Clinical Preparation assignment.

HISTORY OF PRESENT ILLNESS

You are the nurse assigned to Mr. H., a 24-year-old male who sustained a spinal cord injury (SCI) 3 days ago. He dove into a pool from the roof of a house while attending a party. When his friends noted he did not surface, they jumped into the pool and brought him out of the water. They estimated he was submerged for 1 to 2 minutes. Once out of the water, Mr. H. was noted to only shrug his shoulders. He was unable to move his arms or legs and complained of feeling "numb" and short of breath. His friends called 911 and Mr. H. was transported to the hospital where he was diagnosed with a compression fracture of C_6, spinal cord contusion at C_6, and a complete SCI. There was no evidence of continued spinal cord compression from bone fragments within the canal, therefore, Mr. H. was placed in a halo brace.

Medical–Surgical History

Mr. H. denies significant past medical or surgical history.

Social History

Mr. H. is single. He lives alone and his parents are out of state. He smokes approximately 1.5 packs of cigarettes per day and drinks 24 to 48 cans of beer on the weekends. He denies recreational drug use.

Physical Exam

Mr. H. has a halo brace in place and the pin sites are clean. He has a triple-lumen, subclavian central line with normal saline infusing at 75 mL/hr in one port, and dopamine infusing at

15 mcg kg^{-1} min^{-1} into a second port to maintain a systolic blood pressure greater than 90 mmHg and O_2 saturation at 90%. He is receiving 50% oxygen via face mask. A nasogastric tube is in place and connected to low intermittent wall suction. An indwelling urinary catheter is draining yellow urine.

Mr. H. is awake, but does not open his eyes to answer questions or acknowledge staff. He is oriented to person, place, time, and current events. He denies complaint of pain, but does report feeling short of breath. Cranial nerve testing is normal. Motor exam reveals 5/5 strength with shoulder shrug and deltoid function bilaterally. Bicep strength is graded as 4/5 bilaterally. He has 0/5 motor function in the triceps, wrist extension, and hand intrinsics bilaterally. His lower extremities are flaccid.

He denies sensation to pinprick below the clavicle including the chest, abdomen, and lower extremities. He has intact sensation in the neck, shoulders, and palmar aspect of the hands. Deep tendon reflexes are 1+ in the biceps, but otherwise absent. Rectal tone is absent. Lung sounds are diminished in the bases. The patient is tachypneic and respirations are shallow. His abdomen is soft, nontender, with hypoactive bowel sounds. He has not had a bowel movement since admission. His extremities are warm without erythema or edema. Peripheral pulses are intact.

Vital signs reveal a temperature of 37°C (98.6°F). Blood pressure is 90/46. Heart rate is 50 beats per minute, sinus bradycardia. Respiratory rate is 38 and shallow.

Admitting Medical Orders

Service: Neurosurgical
Admit to Neurosurgical ICU
Diagnosis: compression fracture of C_6, spinal cord contusion at C_6, and complete SCI
Allergies: none reported
Vital signs: q1h
Bed rest
Diet: NPO
Nasogastric tube to low intermittent suction
Call house officer: HR < 50 or <120, systolic blood pressure < 90 or > 160, RR < 12 or > 30, temperature < 38.5°C, urinary output less than 30 mL/hr × 2, O_2 saturation < 92%

Respiratory care: incentive spirometer q1h when awake, IPPB respiratory treatment q4h
CVP monitoring q4hours, notify health care provider if < 8 or > 20
Foley catheter
Maintain I&O
Pin site care with 0.5% H_2O_2 and normal saline bid
IVs: Normal saline at 75 mL/hr

Scheduled Medications

Famotidine 20 mg per NG bid
Senokot liquid 15 mL per NG bid
Dopamine titrated to keep the systolic BP above 90 mmHg

PRN Medications

Atropine 0.5–1 mg IV every 3–5 minutes prn heart rate less than 45 beats per minute, and call physician

Ordered Laboratory Studies

Daily ABGs, Chem 7, CBC, and albumin weekly

LABORATORY STUDY RESULTS

Test	Day 1	Day 2	Day 3
ABGs			
PO_2	90 mmHg	88 mmHg	72 mmHg
PCO_2	36 mmHg	38 mmHg	48 mmHg
pH	7.35	7.34	7.31
Chemistry			
Sodium	141 mEq/L	145 mEq/L	142 mEq/L
Potassium	3.8 mEq/L	4.0 mEq/L	4.0 mEq/L
Chloride	95 mEq/L	102 mEq/L	103 mEq/L
CO_2	23 mEq/L	21 mEq/L	21 mEq/L
Glucose	134 mg/dL	121 mg/dL	118 mg/dL
Blood urea nitrogen (BUN)	8 mg/dL	12 mg/dL	16 mg/dL
Creatinine	0.8 mg/dL	1.1 mg/dL	1.0 mg/dL
CBC			
WBC	10.5 µ/L	11.3 µ/L	15.1 µ/L
Hgb	14.7 g/dL	13.8 g/dL	13.0 g/dL
Hct	40.6 ml/dL	39.6 ml/dL	39.8 ml/dL
Platelets	300,000 µL	350,000 µL	300,000 µL
Albumin	2.6 g/dL		

CRITICAL THINKING QUESTIONS

1. What are the indicators in the assessment that should alert the nurse about potential for and/or actual decline in pulmonary status?

2. What measures should be instituted for DVT prophylaxis?

3. What are the possible GI complications for this patient?

4. What are the indicators Mr. H. may be experiencing depression?

5. What are common signs for autonomic hyperreflexia and what are measures to take should this occur?

Answers to Critical Thinking Questions appear in Appendix D.

NCLEX® REVIEW

1. The nurse is teaching a group of nursing students about the causes of spinal cord injury. Which of the following statements made by one of the students indicates a clear understanding of the topic?

1. "Forward falls in which the chin or forehead strikes the ground might produce compression spinal cord injuries."

2. "When axial pressure is loaded on the spine, the resultant rotational injuries might include fracture of the vertebral body."

3. "Hyperextension injuries can cause anterior vertebral body fractures and posterior spinal column facet fracture and dislocation."

4. "A sudden deceleration injury, such as a head-on motor vehicle collision, is frequently the cause of hyperflexion injuries."

2. The patient was involved in a motor vehicle collision with rear impact and is now experiencing severe neck pain and decreased upper extremity motor function, but there is normal motor function in the lower extremities. The patient complains of parasthesias in both the upper and lower extremities but greater in the arms. Based on these findings you suspect the patient may have which of the following types of injuries?

1. Anterior cord syndrome

2. Central cord syndrome

3. Cauda equina syndrome

4. Brown-Séquard syndrome

3. Which of the following statements best describes appropriate prophylaxis for some of the most common complications following spinal cord injury?

   1. Use of an abdominal binder and compression stockings to decrease the peripheral venous pooling that can cause neurogenic shock
   2. Use of a Duplex Doppler ultrasound to dissolve deep vein thromboembolisms and reduce the likelihood of pulmonary embolus
   3. Use of a reclining wheelchair to gradually progress the patient into an upright position so as not to cause orthostatic hypotension
   4. Use of sound nutritional measures such as an increased caloric, protein, and micronutrient intake to promote bowel evacuation

4. When planning educational opportunities related to the psychosocial impact of spinal cord injury, the nurse understands that:

   1. The patient's family will need ongoing education to help deal with the stress of any role changes associated with the injury.
   2. The patient may exhibit any number of negative emotions about physical challenges, including elation and jubilation.
   3. The patient should be encouraged to discuss his feelings openly and to support the decisions made for him by the health care provider.
   4. The patient is usually so preoccupied with the physical challenges faced after a spinal cord injury that psychosocial problems rarely occur.

5. The nurse understands that the needs of the patient with a spinal cord injury (SCI) are unique. When planning the discharge of the patient with SCI, the nurse should include which of the following?

   1. Information regarding support systems that can help the patient and his family adjust to the changes in lifestyle and roles
   2. Referral to a rehabilitation program that uses a single, specialized discipline to help the patient adapt to his injury limitations
   3. Strategies such as infrequent position changes that avoid shearing and will help in the prevention of pressure ulcer formation
   4. Instruction on the importance of avoiding use of suppository medication or other bowel stimulation so as to prevent hyperreflexia

6. When planning care for the patient with spinal cord injury, which nursing diagnosis has the highest priority?

   1. Risk for imbalanced nutrition less than body requirements related to increased metabolic need and inadequate caloric intake
   2. Anxiety related to loss of independence, loss of control over environment and uncertainty of the future
   3. Risk for ineffective peripheral tissue perfusion related to the formation of deep venous thrombosis
   4. Ineffective airway clearance related to the loss of spinal innervation of the respiratory and accessory muscles

Answers for review questions appear in Appendix D

KEY TERMS

afferent *p.831*
areflexia *p.837*
autonomic hyperreflexia *p.838*
cauda equina syndrome *p.835*
complete spinal cord injury *p.832*
compression injuries *p.836*
contusion *p.837*
efferent *p.831*

hyperflexion injuries *p.835*
hyperreflexia *p.837*
incomplete spinal cord injury *p.834*
myelopathy *p.835*
neurogenic shock *p.837*
odontoid process *p.842*
paraplegia *p.832*
quadriplegia (*Latin*) *p.832*

rotational injuries *p.836*
spinal cord injury (SCI) *p.830*
spinal precautions *p.840*
spinal shock *p.837*
spondylitic disease *p.835*
tetraplegia (*Greek*) *p.832*
transection *p.837*

REFERENCES

Apuzzo, M. L. (Ed.) (2002a). Cervical spine immobilization before admission to the hospital. Guidelines for the management of acute spine and spinal cord injuries. *Neurosurgery, 50*(Suppl.), S7–S17.

Apuzzo, M. L. (Ed.) (2002b). Deep venous thrombosis and thromboembolism in patients with cervical spinal cord injuries. Guidelines for the management of acute spine and spinal cord injuries. *Neurosurgery, 50*(Suppl.), S73–S80.

Apuzzo, M. L. (Ed.) (2002c). Management of acute central cervical spinal cord injuries. Guidelines for the management of acute spine and spinal cord injuries. *Neurosurgery, 50*(Suppl.), S166–S171.

Apuzzo, M. L. (Ed.) (2002d). Pharmacologic therapy after acute cervical spinal cord injury. Guidelines for the management of acute spine and spinal cord injuries. *Neurosurgery, 50*(Suppl.), S63–S72.

Apuzzo, M. L. (Ed.) (2002e). Radiographic assessment of the cervical spine in symptomatic trauma patients. Guidelines for the management of acute spine and spinal cord injuries. *Neurosurgery, 50*(Suppl.), S36–S43.

Ball, P. A. (2001). Critical care of spinal cord injury. *Spine, 15*(Suppl.), S27–S30.

Bernbeck, J., & Delamarter, R. B. (2000). Pathophysiology and initial treatment of acute spinal cord injuries. In J. M. Cotler, J. M. Simpson, H. S. An, & C. P. Silveri (Eds.), *Surgery of spinal trauma* (pp. 45–60). Philadelphia: Lippincott Williams & Wilkins.

Bloomer, C., Ackerman, A., & Bhatia, R. (2006). Imaging for spine tumors and new applications. *Topics in Magnetic Resonance Imaging, 17,* 69–87.

Connelly, C. (2001). Alterations in affiliative relationships. In C. Stewart-Amidei & J. A. Kunkel (Eds.), *AANN's neuroscience nursing: Human responses to neurologic dysfunction* (2nd ed., pp. 391–405). Philadelphia: W. B. Saunders.

Enck, P., Greving, I., Klosterhalfen, S., & Wietek, B. (2006). Upper and lower gastrointestinal motor and sensory dysfunction after spinal cord injury. *Progress in Brain Research, 152,* 373–384.

France, J. C., Bono, C. M., & Vaccaro, A. R. (2005). Initial evaluation of the spine after trauma: When, what, where, and how to image the acutely traumatized spine. *Journal of Orthopaedic Trauma, 19,* 640–649.

Hadley, M. (2002). Blood pressure management after acute spinal cord injury. *Neurosurgery, 50*(Suppl.), S58–S62.

Hendy, G. W., Wolfson, A. B., Mower, W. R., & Hoffman, J. R. (2002). Spinal cord injury without radiographic abnormality: Results of the national emergency x-radiography utilization study in blunt cervical trauma. *Journal of Trauma, Injury, Infection and Critical Care, 53,* 1–4

Henson, J. W. (2001). Spinal cord gliomas. *Current Opinion in Neurology, 14,* 679–682.

Hickey, J. V. (2003a). Overview of neuroanatomy and neurophysiology. In J. V. Hickey (Ed.), *The clinical practice of neurological and neurosurgical nursing* (5th ed., pp. 45–92). Philadelphia: Lippincott Williams & Wilkins

Hickey, J. V. (2003b). Vertebral and spinal cord injuries. In J. V. Hickey (Ed.), *The clinical practice of neurological and neurosurgical nursing* (5th ed., pp. 407–450). Philadelphia: Lippincott Williams & Wilkins.

Hurlbert, J. R. (2006). Strategies of medical intervention in the management of acute spinal cord injury. *Spine, 31*(Suppl.), S16–S21.

Kirschblum, S. C., & O'Connor, K. C. (2000). Levels of spinal cord injury and predictors of neurologic recovery. *Physical Medicine and Rehabilitation Clinics of North America, 11,* 1–27.

Kothari, P., Freeman, B., Grevitt, M., & Kerslak, R. (2000). Injury to the spinal cord without radiologic abnormality (SCIWORA) in adults. *Journal of Bone and Joint Surgery, 82-B,* 1034–1037.

Krassioukov, A. (2004). Autonomic dysreflexia in acute spinal cord injury: Injury, mechanisms, and management. *SCI Nursing, 21,* 215–216.

Kwon, B. K., Tetzlaff, W., Grauer, J. N., Beiner, J., & Vaccaro, A. R. (2004). Pathophysiology and pharmacologic treatment of acute spinal cord injury. *Spine Journal, 4,* 451–464.

Lindsay, K. W., & Bone, I. (Eds.) (2004). Localized neurologic disease and its management: B. Spinal cord and roots. In *Neurology and neurosurgery illustrated* (4th ed., pp. 385–423). London: Churchill Livingston.

McIlvoy, L., Meyer, K., & McQuillan, K. A. (2004). Traumatic spine injuries. In M. K. Bader & L. R. Littlejohns (Eds.), *AANN core curriculum for neuroscience nursing* (4th ed., pp. 335–402). St. Louis: W. B. Saunders.

Mulnard, R. A. (2001). Sensation: An overview. In C. Stewart-Amidei & J. A. Kunkel (Eds.), *AANN's neuroscience nursing: Human responses to neurologic dysfunction* (2nd ed., pp. 533–556). Philadelphia: W. B. Saunders.

National Center for Injury Prevention and Control (2006). *Spinal cord injury (SCI): Fact sheet.* Retrieved April 28, 2008, from http://www.cdc.gov/ncipc/factsheets/scifacts.htm

National Guideline Clearinghouse. (2001). *Acute management of autonomic dysreflexia: Individuals with spinal cord injury presenting to a health-care facility.* Washington, DC: Consortium for Spinal Cord Medicine, Paralyzed Veterans of America. Retrieved November 14, 2006, from http://www.guideline.gov/summary/ summary.aspx?doc_id=2964&nbr=002190&string=Autonomic+ AND+dysreflexia

National Guideline Clearinghouse. (2005a). *Neurogenic bowel management in adults with spinal cord injury.* Washington, DC:

Consortium for Spinal Cord Medicine, Paralyzed Veterans of America. Retrieved November 14, 2006, from http://www.guideline.gov/summary/summary.aspx?doc_id=850&n br=000394&string=spinal+AND+cord+AND+injury

National Guideline Clearinghouse. (2005b). *Prevention of thromboembolism in spinal cord injury.* Washington, DC: Consortium for Spinal Cord Medicine, Paralyzed Veterans of America. Retrieved April 29, 2008, from http://www.guideline.gov/ summary/summary.aspx?doc_id=2965&nbr=002191&string= spinal+AND+cord+AND+Injury.

National Guideline Clearinghouse. (2005c). *Respiratory management following spinal cord injury: A clinical practice guideline for health-care professionals.* Washington, DC: Consortium for Spinal Cord Medicine, Paralyzed Veterans of America. Retrieved April 29, 2008, from http://www. guideline.gov/summary/summary.aspx?doc_id= 7198&nbr=004301&string=spinal+AND+cord+AND+injury

National Spinal Cord Injury Statistical Center. (2006). *Spinal cord injury: Facts and figures at a glance.* Retrieved November 14, 2006, from http://www.spinalcord.uab.edu

Pang, D., & Wilberger, J. E. (1982). Spinal cord injuries without radiographic abnormalities in children. *Journal of Neurosurgery, 57,* 114–129.

Paralyzed Veterans of America. (2001). Pressure ulcer prevention and treatment following spinal cord injury: A clinical practice guideline for health-care professionals. *Journal of Spinal Cord Medicine, 24*(Suppl. 1), S40–S101.

Pataki, P., Woodhouse, J., Hamid, R., Shah, J., & Craggs, M. (2006). Lower urinary tract dysfunction in ambulatory patients with incomplete spinal cord injury. *Journal of Urology, 175,* 1784–1787.

Prendergast, V., & Sullivan, C. (2000). Acute spinal cord injury: Nursing considerations for the first 72 hours. *Critical Care Nursing Clinics of North America, 12,* 499–508.

Sayer, F. T., Kronvall, E., & Nilsson, O. G. (2006). Methylprednisolone treatment in acute spinal cord injury: The myth challenged through a structures analysis of the published literature. *Spine Journal, 6,* 335–343.

Sekhon, L., & Fehlings, M. (2001). Epidemiology, demographics, and pathophysiology of acute spinal cord injury. *Spine, 26*(24 Suppl.), S2–S12.

Spinal Cord Injury Information Network. (2006). *Etiology of SCI since 1990.* Retrieved November 22, 2006, from http://www.spinalcord .uab.edu/show.asp?durki=25426.

Villanueva, N. E. (2000). Spinal cord injury in the elderly. *Critical Care Nurse Clinics of North America, 12,* 509–519.

Walker, J., & Criddle, L. M. (2001). Methylprednisolone in acute spinal cord injury: Fact or fantasy? *Journal of Emergency Nursing, 27,* 401–403.

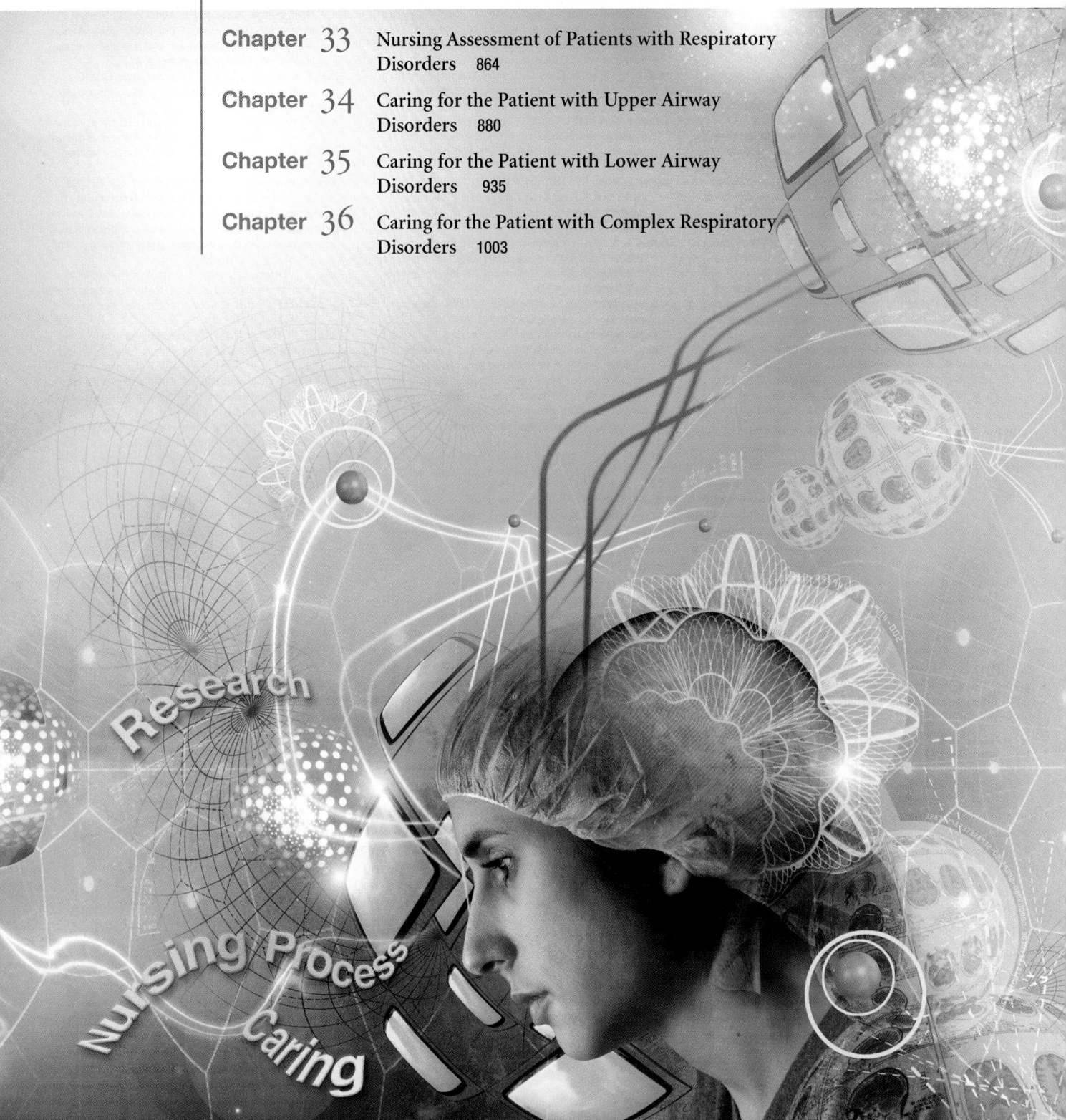

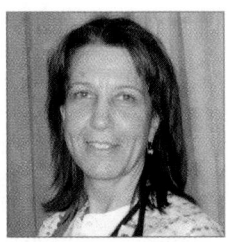

LINDA My name is Linda and I am a clinical resource nurse (CN III) in the Trauma/Surgical ICU (SICU-I) at a 540-bed teaching hospital in Northern California. The hospital is a Level I trauma center associated with the University of California Davis, School of Medicine. In my unit we care for the sickest of the adult trauma patients. Although I mainly care for trauma victims, anyone needing intensive monitoring and critical care is a potential patient. In addition to patient care, I also precept new nurses and I am one of a six-member clinical resource team responsible for contributing to the continuing education of all nursing staff in our 12-bed unit.

In the course of performing as a patient-care advocate, six important characteristics of caring have become evident. These characteristics are an integral part of my role as a professional nurse and are incorporated into the daily care of my patients. For example, I cared for a female patient who had been injured in a car crash months ago but whose poor health, chronic back pain, and anxiety were prolonging weaning from the ventilator. She had a tracheostomy and required numerous doses of prn analgesics and frequent repositioning throughout the day to treat her pain. **Compassion** for what I thought was inadequate pain and anxiety control prompted me to obtain an order for a Pharmacy Pain Service consultation. My **conscience** would not allow me to simply give more doses of sedatives without attempting to find a better solution. The pharmacist evaluated her history, spoke with the patient, and developed a plan that added three new medications and cancelled one. The results were impressive. Her need for prn medication in a 24-hour period went from 17 doses of two narcotics down to 6 doses of one narcotic. She appeared much more comfortable and started smiling more. I cannot express how pleased I was to be a part of easing her discomfort after witnessing her previous misery.

Another patient I vividly remember was an elderly Korean pedestrian who had been hit by a car. Her injuries included multiple fractures and a small liver laceration. She had been recently extubated following surgery but still required oxygen at 4 L/min, and her arterial blood gas (ABG) results were of concern because she had documented pneumonia. She had nearly absent breath sounds on the right side. She spoke Korean and was confused and therefore unable to cooperate with incentive spirometry or deep breathing and coughing exercises. There were new physician orders to feed her. After performing an initial morning assessment, I was reluctant to feed her due to concern about her respiratory status and possible compromised swallowing ability. My concern was that if she aspirated her food that she would further compromise her already tenuous respiratory status. I expressed my concerns to the resident who had written the orders to feed her, and he disagreed and wanted her fed.

The patient's daughter was in the room and asking questions about her mother. In answering her, I gave her physiological reasons for my concerns but also let her know about my many years of experience and that of the physicians, to ease her mind. In situations like this, my **comportment** can make a difference in how family members respond to what is happening to their loved ones.

I subsequently verbalized my concerns to the attending physician who put eating on hold until he could view the morning chest x-ray results. **Confidence** in my experience and abilities allows me to pursue patient-care issues like this despite the disagreement with the resident. As it turned out, the x-ray showed a large right pleural effusion. The patient then needed a CT scan of the chest. Taking any critically ill patient to the radiology department involves planning for the worst and hoping for the best. Preparing for any emergency is part of my responsibility as a **competent** critical care nurse. In this case, I took all the emergency equipment and drugs to the radiology department, but fortunately none of it was needed. Although, based on the CT scan a chest tube was placed, which drained a liter of blood. Needless to say, she didn't eat that day.

Being an ICU nurse isn't only about the drama of car crashes, gunshot wounds, and saving lives. It is also about my role as patient advocate and protector. There is no doubt this can be challenging and frustrating, but the rewards include pride in my contribution to helping others and tremendous satisfaction that what I do has value to individuals and to society in general. I also must confess to appreciating the intermittent adrenaline rush and sense of camaraderie that results from working together to save a life. I feel fortunate to have a career for which I continue to have passion.

> The internal **commitment** I have made as a nurse is to do as much as I can for my patients on each shift, which includes anything from washing the bloody, glass-riddled hair of an accident victim to doing CPR on a cardiac patient.

CHAPTER 33

Nursing Assessment of Patients with Respiratory Disorders

Karen Cooper

Outcome-Based Learning Objectives

After studying this chapter, the learner will be able to:

1. Compare and contrast normal and adventitious breath sounds.
2. Defend the importance of obtaining information on recent travel as a component of the patient history.
3. Describe the relationship of data obtained from the review of a patient's social and occupational history with risk for pulmonary disease.
4. Describe the essential components of a physical assessment of the pulmonary system.
5. Compare and contrast adjuncts used during physical assessment of the pulmonary system.

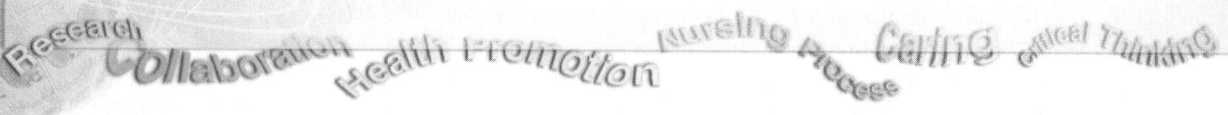

Research   Collaboration   Health Promotion   Nursing Process   Caring   Critical Thinking

NURSES IN ALL health care settings require an in-depth knowledge of the pulmonary system and pulmonary skills to be able to rapidly assess the respiratory status of their patients. Breathing and oxygenation are essential to life. The nursing history and physical examination can uncover valuable clues to the origin of actual or potential problems limiting the patient's ability to breathe effectively. Many pathologic conditions can interfere with the body's ability to exchange oxygen and carbon dioxide both within the pulmonary system as well as on a cellular level in all body structures. Nursing assessment of a patient's respiratory status encompasses all of the senses and accurate and appropriate use of a stethoscope as well as information obtained from review of laboratory tests, pulmonary function tests, chest x-rays, and pulse oximetry. Nurses need to be able to recognize normal assessment findings and identify subtle deviations from normal that signal worsening of the patient's condition. Rapid intervention based on assessment findings is crucial to prevent adverse outcomes.

Ventilation is the movement of air into and out of the lungs. As the lung tissue expands, it increases the surfaces available for exchange of oxygen and carbon dioxide. The levels of oxygen in the pulmonary tree set up a gradient forcing the exchange of oxygen on the pulmonary side with carbon dioxide from the vascular side. The act of breathing is regulated by the respiratory centers in the brainstem, voluntary muscle activity, and stimula-

tion of chemoreceptors by changes in pH and oxygen levels in the blood. The respiratory rate and depth are also influenced by these mechanisms. Disease states as well as emotions can also influence these mechanisms. The nurse must utilize knowledge of the patient's history and perform a comprehensive physical assessment to assist in determining the causes of changes in respiratory patterns and findings.

■ Anatomy and Physiology of the Pulmonary System

Ventilation consists of the movement of air from the environment into the pulmonary system. Respiration consists of the diffusion of oxygen across the alveolar–capillary membrane into the pulmonary circulation, which includes oxygen molecule attachment to hemoglobin molecules and the release of carbon dioxide molecules from hemoglobin across the alveolar–capillary membranes and through the airways out to the environment.

Conducting airways such as the trachea and bronchi do not participate in oxygen–carbon dioxide exchange, but allow passage of these molecules and gases from the bloodstream in and out of the environment. If the conducting airways are blocked by secretions or other conditions causing obstruction, they are unable to permit adequate movement of air and oxygen to the alveoli for gas exchange.

Ventilation is dependent on neurological and musculoskeletal integrity. The central nervous system (CNS) responds to changes in the carbon dioxide and oxygen levels in the blood to influence increases or decreases in the rate and depth of respiration. The medulla and pons respond to changes in respiratory rate and depth as well as changes in the oxygen and carbon dioxide levels in the blood to increase or decrease the rate and depth of respiration. Musculoskeletal structures influencing respiration include the intercostal muscles, diaphragm, abdominal muscles, and thoracic muscles such as the scalene, sternomastoid, and trapezius.

Inspiration and expiration are also influenced by intrapleural pressures. When the pressure of air in the lungs during inspiration reaches capacity, expiration occurs. Inspiration is an active procedure related to neuromuscular activities, but expiration is essentially passive, related to reaching the maximum elastic stretch of the respiratory muscles and the recoil of these muscles. The movement of air in one breath is the tidal volume. The movement of air over 1 minute is the minute ventilation. Tidal volume is usually about 500 mL during normal ventilation, but can increase if more is demanded by the body, as can occur during exercise or times of stress.

The alveoli are the structures where exchange of oxygen and carbon dioxide occurs. For adequate exchange of these gases, the alveoli must be adequately expanded by air and have adequate contact with hemoglobin molecules in the capillaries. If the alveoli are fully expanded but unable to exchange oxygen with the capillaries due to edema or secretions lining the alveoli, a ventilation/perfusion mismatch occurs and the patient will exhibit signs and symptoms of hypoxia. If the alveoli are not able to distend adequately, despite adequate blood flow (perfusion), ventilation/perfusion mismatch will again occur and the patient will exhibit signs and symptoms of hypoxia.

Perfusion, the movement of oxygen across the alveolar–capillary membrane, is dependent on gravity, oxygen concentrations on the alveolar and capillary sides, and the availability of hemoglobin molecules for oxygen binding. Patients who are anemic will have fewer hemoglobin binding sites for oxygen. Also, if a patient's circulation is compromised by conditions such as shock or heart failure, the patient will not be able to exchange oxygen and carbon dioxide because blood flow is diverted from the alveoli and will not allow the exchange of gases to occur.

The nurse must be knowledgeable of the physiology of the pulmonary system and the physical integrity of the patient to be able to determine the ability of the patient to adequately exchange oxygen and carbon dioxide. Physical examination findings, diagnostic testing, and diagnostic criteria are described in this chapter for the nurse to assess the patient's current status and determine if current therapies are effective.

■ History

Components of the patient history include both objective and subjective data. Effective interviewing skills are necessary to elicit pertinent data regarding the symptoms and the effect the symptoms have on the patient's ability to carry out life functions. Biographic and demographic data assist the interviewer in determining if any cultural or educational factors figure importantly into the manner and style of the interview process.

The health history should begin with the complaint that caused the patient to seek care (the chief complaint), and what the patient thinks may have initiated the problem. The past medical history may provide clues as to the nature of the current problem. For example, a patient with a prior history of breast or testicular cancer may present with shortness of breath related to metastases from the primary site. The social history not only gives valuable clues regarding the availability of potential caregivers, but also may indicate potential occupational sources of the current patient problems.

One of the issues facing nurses caring for patients with respiratory disease is shortness of breath. Patients may not be able to verbally complete the health history due to **dyspnea**, the subjective feeling of shortness of breath or difficulty breathing. Therefore, it may be necessary for the nurse to obtain information from family members or the available medical record regarding the basic history, and limit the history obtained from the patient to focused responses and information not available from other sources. The nurse may need to focus on allowing the patient to rest and limit all forms of exertion during the history. Use of yes and no questions or allowing the patient to write or use a communication board may be useful. The nurse may need to provide supplemental oxygen for the patient to relieve distress and, in doing so, the nurse should follow established facility protocols. Patients with chronic respiratory diseases may respond adversely to increased oxygen levels, which can suppress their respiratory drive. Normally, hypoxia will cause an increase in respiratory drive. Patients with chronic hypoxia, such as that seen in chronic obstructive pulmonary disease (COPD), may no longer respond to hypoxia, and instead will respond to elevated carbon dioxide levels to stimulate breathing. Use of high-flow oxygen in this group may result in respiratory arrest.

Biographic and Demographic Data

Assessment of biographic and demographic data includes information regarding age, race, gender, and culture that can influence the patient's understanding, preconceptions, and susceptibility to some pulmonary disorders. In some instances, knowledge of the patient's place of birth or current address may give clues to the origin of the current complaints. For example, patients with a productive cough and night sweats who were born in or recently relocated from areas where tuberculosis (TB) is common should be isolated and appropriate precautions taken both during the interview and during discussions with the patient, family members, and continued care providers. If TB is suspected, testing measures such as sputum testing, chest x-ray, and/or intradermal tuberculin placement (PPD) testing must take place. Places of residence may also include areas with poor air quality or the presence of allergens and irritants that affect the respiratory system.

Gender no longer appears to be a factor in the development of pulmonary disease. Lung cancer, COPD, and emphysema occur only slightly more frequently in men than in women. Lymphangiomyomatosis is a disease affecting young women in their 20s and 30s that may have a genetic or hormonal component that causes changes in the smooth muscle tissue of the lung and cyst development. The symptoms and treatment of this disease are similar to those for emphysema. Normal aging may also play a part in activity-related shortness of breath. The nurse must utilize knowledge of age-related changes in the pulmonary vessels and tissue when performing a respiratory assessment.

Chief Complaint

The chief complaint is the patient's impression of what caused him to seek care. It should be recorded in the patient's own words. Often, by asking what exactly caused him to seek care, the patient will give information on both the symptoms and the impact the symptoms have had on his lifestyle and functional abilities. The chief complaint should direct a focused assessment of the patient's perception of the problem and the presenting symptoms.

Presenting Symptoms

A review of symptoms explores the patient's symptoms in a systematic fashion. The nurse may use any of a number of guidelines for this exploration. The PQRST (Dillon, 2003) or the COLDSA (Weber & Kelley, 2003) method may be helpful in performing a systematic analysis of symptoms. Each of these methods is used to describe a specific symptom in terms of location, onset, duration, quality, severity, aggravating and relieving factors, and related symptoms (Chart 33–1). The patient should be asked specifically when the symptoms began and how the symptoms progressed. Aggravating and relieving factors must be explored, as well as the timing at which the symptoms occur. For example, if shortness of breath occurs at night or with activity, the nurse must explore the possibility of a cardiovascular component to the presenting symptom.

Dyspnea, difficulty breathing, is a very common chief complaint for patients with respiratory illness. Because dyspnea is considered a subjective finding, current research is attempting to validate specific dyspnea scales so that they can be utilized in a manner similar to the analog and Wong-Baker pain scales. Orthopnea is shortness of breath that occurs in the supine position. Orthopnea may be related to gastrointestinal reflux, heart failure, or pulmonary disease. Exploration of symptoms with specific questions will aid the nurse in pinpointing the origin of the dysfunction. Presenting symptoms associated with pulmonary disease that should be explored with the patient include cough, sputum production, shortness of breath, chest, back or thoracic pain, activity intolerance, hemoptysis (bloody sputum), sleep disorders, and "noisy" respirations.

Past Medical History

The past medical history gives insight into the effect that prior illnesses and conditions may have on the current presenting symptom. For example, a prior history of prolonged intubation associated with cardiac surgery may indicate the risk of either cardiovascular system associated complications or preexisting pulmonary problems that can impact the patient's current condition. If the patient has received treatment for cardiac dysrhythmias, the nurse can explore the potential for medication-related pulmonary fibrosis such as occurs with the use of amiodarone. A history of thyroid disease may implicate myxedema or thyrotoxicosis as precipitating factors in the development of shortness of breath (see Chapter 52).

Childhood Diseases and Immunizations

Premature birth, childhood diseases, congenital pulmonary disease, and immunization (or lack thereof) are important to include in the history portion of the respiratory assessment. Current immunization status for influenza and pneumococcal pneumonia should also be assessed. Today, a number of adults present to health care systems with cystic fibrosis, often considered a childhood disease state. Asthma symptoms are frequently first seen during childhood. Cystic fibrosis and asthma are discussed in detail in Chapter 35 . Finally, the patient should be asked if she had frequent colds, episodes of wheezing, or shortness of breath during childhood.

Patients born prematurely who were mechanically ventilated for long periods in neonatal intensive care units (NICUs) may suffer from primary or secondary pulmonary disease. Pulmonary disease in this population may be related to lung injury such as barotrauma from ventilation pressures, to prolonged use of high oxygen levels, to primary pulmonary disease such as pulmonary atresia, to pulmonary hypertension, or to primary congenital heart disease or valvular dysfunction. Neonatal respiratory distress syndrome is caused by a lack of surfactant in the immature lungs of premature babies. Although synthetic exogenous surfactant is available today to treat this complication of preterm birth, adults currently presenting with pulmonary problems may not have had treatment with the medication and are at risk for long-term or chronic complications.

The nurse should also ask the patient if he suffered any childhood trauma. Swimming accidents during childhood could result in aspiration of water and resultant lung injury. Likewise, aspiration of foreign bodies in childhood may cause structural damage to airways.

Adults who work in areas where they will be exposed to flu, such as health care workers, the elderly, and patients with chronic conditions such as asthma and COPD, should receive yearly flu vaccination. The elderly and patients with chronic diseases should also receive pneumococcal vaccine to prevent pneumococcal pneumonia.

CHART 33–1	**Symptom Assessment Mnemonics**

PQRST EVALUATION OF SYMPTOMS

P	Palliative and/or Provocative
Q	Quality and Quantity
R	Radiation and location
S	Severity
T	Time of day and duration

COLDSA EVALUATION OF SYMPTOMS

C	Character
O	Onset
L	Location
D	Duration
S	Severity
A	Associated factors

Previous Illnesses and Hospitalizations

The frequency of previous episodes of pneumonia, asthma exacerbations, and respiratory distress should be elicited from the patient as well as any hospitalizations associated with these conditions. This will give insight into the potential severity of the patient's condition or to the progression of the disease process. Treatment modalities, such as tracheostomy, chest tube insertion, intubation, and use of oxygen, should also be elicited. Information regarding hospitalizations and illnesses not necessarily related to the pulmonary system are also important. For example, a patient hospitalized with a bowel obstruction may have suffered aspiration related to reflux of gastric contents. Cardiac disease frequently has an adverse impact on the pulmonary system. Heart failure is a classic example of cardiac disease causing pulmonary symptoms and may result in residual pulmonary problems. Heart failure is discussed in detail in Chapter 42 . Mitral valve disease, or papillary muscle rupture associated with myocardial infarction may cause pulmonary congestion. Mitral valve abnormalities are discussed in Chapter 41 .

Treatment for thyroid disease may include local radiation therapy that could result in narrowing of the trachea due to goiter compression or tissue damage and edema from therapy. Patients who have been diagnosed with cancer may have metastases to the lung or a treatment that affects the pulmonary system. Thoracic trauma causing a rib fracture may impair the patient's ability to deep breathe and expectorate secretions. The patient with rib fractures is at risk for hypoventilation and pneumonia. Liver failure associated with alpha$_1$-antitrypsin (AAT) deficiency is also associated with the development of emphysema and pulmonary disease.

The patient's response to hospitalization and previous illness gives the nurse valuable information regarding prior experience with invasive and noninvasive testing and treatment. The analysis of previous illnesses and hospitalization also provides knowledge of comorbid conditions that may complicate diagnosis and care.

Diagnostic Procedures or Surgeries

The results of diagnostic procedures performed and the surgical history should be obtained by the nurse performing a respiratory assessment. Prior thoracic surgery, lung biopsy, or bronchoscopy indicates prior pulmonary dysfunction. Pulmonary function tests can give insight into the extent or nature of pulmonary disease. Chest x-rays give valuable information regarding the condition of pleural tissue, presence of rib fractures, pneumothorax, hemothorax, pulmonary edema, pneumonia, interstitial disease, and lung lesions. Electrocardiography (ECG) may indicate a cardiac component to the patient's condition or demonstrate changes related to pulmonary embolism. The ventilation and perfusion (V/Q) scan is the gold standard for diagnosis of pulmonary embolus determining lung perfusion status. Deep venous thrombosis (DVT), a precursor to pulmonary embolism, may be diagnosed from Doppler studies or suggested by a positive D-dimer blood test. Patient's who have had immobilizing illnesses and surgery of the abdomen or lower extremities are at risk for the development of DVT.

Arterial blood gas (ABG) analysis is utilized to determine oxygen and carbon dioxide levels and oxygen saturation. Laboratory tests such as the complete blood count (CBC) may give insight into an infectious process or anemia causing shortness of breath.

Carboxyhemoglobin levels should be obtained on patients exposed to smoke or fire, particularly if the exposure was in an enclosed space, or patients exposed to excessive automobile exhaust fumes. Sputum cultures are utilized to determine organisms causing pneumonia. In addition acid-fast bacilli testing of sputum cultures is utilized to determine if the patient has tuberculosis. Tuberculin skin testing is also used to determine exposure to tuberculosis. The AAT blood test is utilized to diagnose AAT deficiency, which is related to the development of pulmonary and liver disease in susceptible individuals. Allergy testing may be performed in patients exhibiting frequent occurrences of wheezing, pulmonary congestion, or chronic cough.

Medications

The patient should be encouraged to carry a list of all current medications. If possible, the medical record can also be explored for the use of medications prior to the present time. When discussing current medications with the patient, the nurse should inquire about dosage, frequency, and the last time the medication was taken. This is especially relevant if the patient is prescribed bronchodilators, anticholinergics, and steroids. Increased use of these medications may indicate that the patient's condition is worsening. Failure to take medications as directed may also increase pulmonary symptoms. The correct order in which to take inhaled medications is to take bronchodilators first to open the airways. Steroids should be taken after bronchodilators to improve absorption when the airways are dilated (open). Over-the-counter (OTC) medications such as cough suppressants, expectorants, antihistamines, or herbal supplements may be overlooked by patients in their report of medications taken. The nurse should specifically ask about OTC medication use.

If the patient is currently prescribed medications to treat tuberculosis, or antibiotics to treat pneumonia, the nurse should ensure that the patient is taking the medications as prescribed. Patients will frequently stop taking medications when they feel well. It should come as no surprise that symptoms return when patients fail to take medications as prescribed. When patients fail to complete a course of antibiotic therapy, the organism may develop a resistance and the antibiotic will no longer be effective in its treatment. Use of medications other than those prescribed for pulmonary disease may cause pulmonary symptoms. For example, angiotensin converting enzyme (ACE) inhibitors may cause cough, and amiodarone may cause pulmonary fibrosis. Respiratory medications are discussed in detail in Chapters 35 and 36 .

Patients who use inhalers should be requested to demonstrate their technique. If they are using metered-dose inhalers or spacers, the nurse should ensure that they are used correctly. Patients may assume that it is correct to use a spacer with all inhaled medications, when this is not true. For example, Advair, a combination inhaler, is not supposed to be taken with a spacer. Patients should be encouraged to bring all inhalers to their assessment. If patients bring inhalers that are no longer part of the prescribed regimen, they should be discarded to prevent the patient from potential overmedication with one of the inhaler components.

Allergies

Allergies frequently cause pulmonary symptoms ranging from simple congestion, coughing, and wheezing to anaphylactic reactions and airway obstruction. Patients should be instructed to report allergies to plant products, foods, medications, dusts, molds, and animal sources. Knowledge of *all* allergies is important to the nurse because patients frequently do not realize that the contents of some medications or OTC supplements may contain allergens to which they are susceptible. For example, Atrovent and Combivent (combination) inhalers should not be used in patients who are allergic to soy or nuts. Patients may recognize that they are allergic to certain plants or pollens, but not understand that most herbal supplements are made from plants and that they should carefully read the ingredients and understand the components of the supplement prior to taking them.

Use of Oxygen or Ventilatory Assist Devices

Outpatient oxygen therapy indicates that the patient has extensive or chronic pulmonary disease. Increased shortness of breath despite use of oxygen or ventilatory assistive devices should send up a red warning flag about the potential for imminent decompensation. The nurse should immediately assess the patient and determine if the health care provider needs to be notified or the patient requires immediate intervention such as airway suction. Prior need for oxygen therapy or assistive devices such as tracheostomy or mechanical ventilation may also indicate the existence of previous pulmonary problems.

Cough and Sputum Production

Coughing is a symptom associated with pulmonary congestion as well as reactive airway disease. It is a protective mechanism to rid the lungs of mucus in airways or to prevent inhalation of irritants. The nurse must evaluate the symptom of coughing in relation to its timing, frequency, duration, and the nature of sputum produced. Chronic cough is a classic warning sign of lung cancer. Patients who smoke may cough upon awakening. Cough at night may be related to heart failure, postnasal drip, or esophageal reflux, which occurs when supine. If decongestants and cough suppressants are utilized, the cough may have a specific pattern related to the timing of the dosage. Persistent or continuous coughing may be related to smoking, pneumonia, cancer, or chronic irritation.

The character and nature of sputum production gives valuable clues as to the potential cause of the cough. Hemoptysis may indicate a ruptured pulmonary blood vessel, pulmonary embolus, or cancer. Sputum that is thick is usually related to pneumonia. The color of the sputum also gives insight as to the cause or causative organism. Pink, frothy sputum is the hallmark of pulmonary edema. Bronchitis and pneumonia are associated with yellow, tan, green, or gray colored mucus. The color of the sputum does not indicate a particular organism nor should it influence the decision to obtain sputum cultures. Black or carbonaceous sputum may be related to burn trauma. A nonproductive cough may be related to ACE inhibitor use or irritation from dust or fumes. The amount of sputum production should be quantified as well.

Pain associated with cough may be related to musculoskeletal strain, pleurisy, or pneumothorax.

Family Health History

The family history gives information on potential genetic relationships associated with disease development as well as environmental and behavior-related risks for disease development. The family health history should include investigation of the presence of family members who smoke(d), and if any family members had pulmonary disease, lung cancer, or cardiovascular disease. Lung cancer and cardiovascular disease tend to run in families. The familial risk of lung cancer is likely related to the presence of cigarette smoke in the household. The occurrence of childhood asthma and preterm birth is greater in instances where the mother smoked. See Chapter 37 ⊙ for cardiovascular risk factors.

Risk Factors

Cigarette smoking, inactivity, cardiovascular disease, obesity, substance abuse, and trauma are some of the more common risk factors that contribute to the development of respiratory disorders. The *Healthy People 2010* initiative sites physical activity, obesity, tobacco use, and substance abuse as leading health indicators. The goal under respiratory diseases is to "Promote respiratory health through better prevention, detection, treatment, and education efforts" (U.S. Department of Health and Human Services, 2000).

Cigarette Smoking

The primary risk factor for the development of pulmonary disease is cigarette smoking. All patients should receive counseling on smoking cessation. The number of cigarettes smoked per day and the time in years a patient has smoked should be elicited from the patient (pack-years). Patients may be reluctant to accurately describe their smoking history to the nurse. After all, they know that it causes COPD, emphysema, and lung cancer. The risk for these three disorders increases with the number of cigarettes smoked and the length of time a patient has been a smoker. Patients ages 50 or older who have smoked a pack of cigarettes (20) per day are at highest risk of pulmonary complications (Dillon, 2003).

Inactivity

Patients who are physically inactive are at higher risk for DVT and pulmonary embolism. Immobility causes decreased venous return, venous stasis, and hypercoagulability. The longer the patient is inactive, the greater the risk for development of DVT. Patients with pulmonary disease may become short of breath with activity and become physically inactive to prevent development of shortness of breath. This starts a vicious cycle that further predisposes them to deconditioning, inactivity, and the potential for the development of thromboembolic disease. Recent weight loss unrelated to specific diet may indicate risk for tuberculosis or lung cancer.

Cardiovascular Disease

Patients with cardiovascular disease experience pulmonary complications related to the inability of the heart to effectively pump blood to the lungs due to pulmonary hypertension, or to the periphery due to hypertension, aortic disease, or diseases of the myocardium and valves. Frequently this results in a failure to adequately oxygenate or circulate oxygenated arterial blood to supply body tissues to meet metabolic demands. The result is activity intolerance, hypoxemia, and tachycardia, which further increase the myocardial oxygen demand and the potential for inadequate oxygen to supply these needs. A history of cardiovascular disease should alert the nurse to the potential for heart failure and pulmonary edema.

Obesity

Obesity is associated with a number of respiratory-related dysfunctions. There is hypoventilation related to restriction of thoracic expansion by excess adipose tissue. Upper airway changes related to fat deposits in the neck and poor muscle tone in the upper airway cause intermittent partial and complete airway obstruction (Jubber, 2004). In many obese patients, obstructive sleep apnea interrupts effective sleep patterns.

Patients with obstructive sleep apnea may wake up at night short of breath or may be unaware of breathing difficulties during sleep. A classic symptom is snoring, which is a form of partial airway obstruction (Merritt & Berger, 2004) Classically, the patient wakes up when the airway is completely obstructed, or when hypoxic or hypercapnic reflexes cause them to resume breathing. Obese patients with obstructive sleep apnea are also more prone to associated conditions such as diabetes, heart failure, dysrhythmias, hypercoagulability, coronary artery disease, and stroke (Shamsuzzaman, Gersh, & Somers, 2003).

Substance Abuse

Patients who abuse intravenous (IV) medications are at risk for a multitude of complications affecting almost every organ system. IV drug abusers are at high risk for pneumonia, pulmonary emboli, and pulmonary edema (Gotway et al., 2002). Inhaled drugs may cause pulmonary injury or pulmonary hemorrhage. CNS depression from alcohol or drugs can contribute to aspiration pneumonia, chemical pneumonitis, and respiratory arrest (Wilson & Saukkonen, 2004).

Trauma

Thoracic and abdominal traumatic injuries predispose patients to the development of pneumonias, hypoventilation, and atelectasis. Fractures of long bones are most closely associated with fat emboli, although they also can occur with other invasive fat-related procedures such as liposuction and lipid infusions. The clinical picture of the patient with fat emboli includes dyspnea, tachypnea, tachycardia, cyanosis, and petechiae (Harris, 2004). ABG analysis is very important in the patient with actual or potential fat emboli because the actual degree of hypoxemia may not be apparent until the patient decompensates (Peltier, 2004).

Both blunt and penetrating trauma may cause pneumothorax and/or hemothorax. Pneumothorax may be described as either open or closed. With an open pneumothorax, as a patient inhales, air enters the pleura, causing positive pressure and resultant lung collapse. In a closed pneumothorax, there is nowhere for the air to escape to, causing a rapid buildup of positive pressure and lung collapse, which can shift the trachea and mediastinal contents toward the uninjured lung side. This results in cardiovascular collapse if untreated. Treatment for pneumothorax may include high-flow oxygen if the pneumothorax is small or less than 10% of the lung. Large and symptomatic pneumothoraces are treated with needle thoracostomy, chest tube, or thoracic vent insertion. A hemothorax is treated with chest tube insertion.

Burn injury can occur in the pulmonary tree from inhalation of heated gases (see Chapter 68). The damaged lung tissue becomes edematous and the patient develops acute respiratory distress. Edema of the airways can cause upper airway obstruction. ABG studies are valuable in the early burn period because pulse oximetry values may be unreliable. The pulse oximeter is unable to recognize the difference between oxygenated hemoglobin and carboxyhemoglobin. The normal value for carboxyhemoglobin in a nonsmoking patient is <2.5%. A person who smokes may have a normal carboxyhemoglobin level of 4% to 5%; a heavy smoker 5% to 12% (Kee, 2005).

Trauma to the brain and spinal cord may also affect the respiratory system and assessment findings (see Chapters 29 and 32). The medulla and pons control respiratory rate and depth in response to changes in oxygen levels in the blood. Chemoreceptors relay information on blood pH to the cardiorespiratory centers in the brainstem. Spinal cord injuries above cervical level 3 will paralyze the muscles normally used in ventilation, including the diaphragm. Below cervical spine level 4, intercostal muscle paralysis may occur.

Social History

The social history includes information about patients' lifestyles and habits that may be relevant to their current state of health. For example, patients who smoke have increased risk for pulmonary disease, and patients who have allergies and engage in outdoor social activities such as golfing may have exacerbations of symptoms after participating in these activities. If patients frequent social events in which they are exposed to people with upper respiratory infections or poor hygienic conditions, they may be predisposed to the development of pulmonary infections.

Occupation

Many occupations are associated with exposure to airborne particles, vapors, and irritants. These occupational irritants can result in acute or chronic respiratory disease in susceptible individuals. The Occupational Safety and Health Administration (OSHA) sets and enforces standards in the work environment in the United States to ensure a safe work environment; however, it is impossible in many circumstances to prevent airborne or inhalation exposure, particularly in the out-of-doors. Farmers may be exposed to pesticides, and construction workers and masons may be exposed to cement dust. Even when personal protective equipment is available and recommended, it is each person's own decision to utilize precautions and the equipment.

Asbestos inhalation is associated with the development of pleurisy and pleural effusion up to 20 years after exposure. Mesothelioma is a rare form of asbestos-related malignancy in which symptoms may not appear for 40 years after exposure (Corbridge, Kamp, & Richlin, 2004). Patients at risk for asbestos-related pulmonary disease worked in naval shipyards, construction, and insulation prior to the 1970s. Today, firemen and demolition workers are at risk of asbestos-related pulmonary disease because older buildings still contain significant amounts of asbestos. Asbestos is also present in vehicle brake linings, placing auto mechanics at risk.

Occupational asthma may occur in many settings. Persons who work around animals are exposed to dander, hair, and allergens picked up from the environment. In the food industry, dust, proteins, and fumes may cause asthmatic reactions. Any occupation in which workers come into contact with fumes or vapors may provoke occupational asthma. This includes cleaning solvents that are utilized in work environments as well as the home. Symptoms associated with work-related asthma include wheezing, shortness of breath, and coughing when the worker is exposed to the allergen. The disease is progressive with each exposure. Initially the person may have symptoms only while at work, but as the airways become more reactive, symptoms occur in any setting.

Early recognition, diagnosis, and treatment of occupational asthma can prevent pulmonary complications.

Culture

Culture plays an important role in acceptance of diagnostic testing and treatment of respiratory symptoms (see the Cultural Considerations box). Cultural indoctrination may also influence the patient's responses to attempts to obtain the patient's history and to perform the physical examination. The nurse needs to have an understanding of cultural considerations specific to the patient's frame of reference. For example, East Indian patients may feel that eye contact is rude. The nurse must make allowances for this conception and not conclude that the lack of eye contact indicates deception or abuse.

Cultural practices such as the wearing of protective amulets may interfere with planned diagnostic testing. The nurse must respect the patient's belief and perhaps suggest an alternate placement of the amulet so that interference with diagnostic testing does not occur. For example, if an amulet is worn around the neck and would interfere with a chest x-ray, the nurse may suggest that the patient continue to wear the amulet but wrap it around the wrist during the diagnostic test. Refugees from countries that have been involved in civil conflict may have experienced traumatic injuries or toxic exposures.

Physical assessment of the patient may reveal cultural practices such as coining and cupping. Southeast Asian people may feel that respiratory illness is due to "wind illness" and traditionally treat the symptoms with "cupping." Cupping involves utilizing a cup applied to the skin to draw out the disease. This practice leaves circular marks on the skin. This traditional therapy is also practiced by people in Greece. "Coining" involves scraping the skin of the thorax with a coin or a spoon and is practiced in Southeast Asia, Italy, and Russia. Both coining and cupping may result in skin lesions or burns that may be mistaken as signs of abuse or cause complications that require medical treatment. Prior to coining or cupping, the skin may be treated with an herbal lotion or ointment (Kose, Karabagli, & Cetin, 2005; Snyder & Miska, 2003; Yoo & Tausk, 2004).

If the patient is experiencing respiratory symptoms, some cultures feel that the patient should avoid water or bathing because these may contribute to illness. Many cultures have herbal remedies for respiratory illness. A Native American herbal treatment for respiratory illness felt to boost the immune system is echinacea. Current research seems to vacillate regarding the effectiveness of this remedy. Among the Hmong (from Laos), opium is used as an analgesic. Smoking opium causes respiratory complications, and lung disease may be considered by the Hmong as an accepted part of life.

Environment

The nurse should explore the home and work environment for potential allergens or contributing factors for the development of pulmonary symptoms. If the environment contains allergens, they should be removed. Pets and mold allergens are easily removed. Patients with asthma should have allergy tests prior to suggestions that specific allergens and triggers be removed from the home environment. House dust mites are a common trigger for allergy and asthma symptoms. Weekly vacuuming and removal of stuffed products such as toys and pillows may help remove dust mites. Cockroach allergens may be removed with commercial cockroach insecticides as well as preventive measures such as disposing of trash daily to an area outside of the home. Although little can be done regarding workplace allergen containment, the workplace should be reviewed regarding patient triggers and accommodations made prior to specific activities such as painting, insecticide treatment, and use of specific cleansers. For persons with reactive airway disease who work outdoors, environmental agents such as cement dust and specific fumes that affect the patient may be avoided with appropriate communication.

Habits

Cigarette smoking is the most specific habit that should be avoided. Patients should be counseled regarding avoidance of situations in which cigarette smoking is present to prevent exposure to secondhand smoke. Personal hygiene habits should also be explored with the patient. Good oral hygiene can help prevent pulmonary disease. Oral infections can travel to the pulmonary tree to cause abscess formation or pneumonia. Hand hygiene is also important. Patients should be counseled to wash their hands frequently and always before eating and drinking. Proper clothing for the weather should be encouraged.

Exercise

Exercise tolerance is often decreased in patients with pulmonary disease. The nurse should obtain specific information regarding

---

CULTURAL CONSIDERATIONS Cultural Practices Related to Respiratory Disorders

Cultural Practice	Nursing Considerations
Use of amulets (many cultures)	May interfere with diagnostic testing such as x-rays, MRI, ultrasound. Suggest alternate placement of amulet for test duration or placement of amulet within eye contact but not in MRI.
Cupping (Southeast Asia, Greece)	May be mistaken for signs of abuse; may delay medical treatment. Burns or skin infections may occur and necessitate medical treatment.
Coining (Southeast Asia, Italy, and Russia)	May be mistaken for signs of abuse; may delay medical treatment. Burns or skin infections may occur and necessitate medical treatment.
Herbal remedies (used in many cultures)	Herbal remedies may be related to allergies because they are derived from plants that are associated with allergens. Herbal remedies may also interfere with the actions of medications and antibiotics or increase bleeding tendencies.

the distance that the patient can walk on a flat surface as well as specific activities that cause shortness of breath. Frequently, the distance a patient can ambulate independently will affect the level of care necessary for the patient on discharge from the hospital. For example, if the patient cannot ambulate 50 feet unassisted or without shortness of breath, she may need to be discharged to a skilled nursing facility. A specific plan for progressive exercise should be developed for the patient. Goals to be set for the patient on a daily basis require knowledge of the patient's baseline activity and exercise status.

Some forms of recreation and exercise predispose to pulmonary symptoms. Water sports such as wake boarding expose the rider to carbon monoxide fumes. Water sports that involve riding a ski or board in the exhaust path are the most frequent cause of carbon monoxide poisoning.

Nutrition

Frequently patients with shortness of breath have poor nutritional status. Obtaining, preparing, and consuming meals requires energy. Shortness of breath can interfere with the patient's abilities to shop for, prepare, and consume food. A typical body type is associated with pulmonary disease. The patient with chronic bronchitis or emphysema may be thin with muscle wasting. Inadequate nutrition places the patient at risk for infection. Nutrition is discussed in detail in Chapter 14 .

Travel and Area of Residence

Area of recent travel may become an important aspect of the history in diagnosing potential respiratory problems. In 2003, a severe acute respiratory syndrome (SARS) outbreak demonstrated to the world that viral pulmonary disease could be traced to a specific location. Although there have been no subsequent episodes of SARS, recent travel and area of residence have been demonstrated to be an important factor in the history of respiratory symptoms and should be included in the interview process.

High-altitude pulmonary edema (HAPE) can occur in persons who are not acclimated and travel to altitudes greater than 5,000 feet. As altitude increases, atmospheric pressure decreases and the oxygen available in air also decreases. Persons with pre-existing illness may develop rapid onset of hypoxemia related to the decreased oxygen levels. Compensatory increases in respiratory rate to compensate for the decreased available oxygen may contribute to fatigue and further respiratory insufficiency. Compensatory mechanisms cause initial pulmonary vascular vasoconstriction. Later, inflammatory mediators cause vasodilation. The alveolar–capillary membrane becomes more permeable in response to these mediators and engorges with fluid, causing pulmonary edema. HAPE is discussed in detail in Chapter 36 .

Physical Examination

The physical examination of the patient begins with the first contact. All of the nurse's senses are utilized. Whether the patient is ambulating into a clinic or is a patient on a ventilator in the ICU, the nurse begins collecting data. The nurse may hear audible wheezes or stridor from a distance. When speaking with the patient, the nurse notes the amount of words in each sentence and if there is foul odor to the breath. Foul odor on the breath may be a sign of pulmonary infection or abscess. The

general appearance of the patient, the skin color, the presence of oxygen or assistive devices all provide data for the nurse in the assessment of the patient.

The assessment of any patient should be systematic and proceed from noninvasive data collection to invasive data collection. All available information should be elicited. If medical records are available, they should be obtained and included in data collection. Comparison of previous assessments should be applied to the patient's current physical status. If findings indicate new symptoms or an increase in symptoms of pathology, the nurse must document findings and take appropriate steps to ensure that the patient receives appropriate care. The nurse must pursue appropriate and complete evaluation of all physical findings and symptoms of respiratory dysfunction to assist in the determination of the cause and to prevent further compromise of the patient's ability to carry out activities essential to health and satisfaction with lifestyle.

Inspection

Inspection is the initial activity for any assessment of the patient. It involves observation of obvious physical characteristics that may indicate potential health problems or characteristics that indicate a need for more in-depth evaluation. Evaluation of the respiratory rate, pattern, and patient's ease of breathing should occur continually throughout the assessment of the patient.

General Appearance

The nurse should evaluate the patient's general appearance. Does the patient appear to have the physical capability to take care of himself? Does he appear comfortable or assume a tripod position to breathe easily? Is the patient in obvious distress?

The facial appearance may indicate that the patient is anxious, a symptom of hypoxia. Patients with COPD may exhibit facial flushing related to the effort of breathing. Pursed lip breathing during exhalation prolongs the expiratory phase of respiration. This maintains the smaller airways in an open position so that there is a longer period for exchange of oxygen and carbon dioxide and prevents collapse of the alveoli. Normal expiration time is twice the duration of inspiration. Nasal flaring may also be evident in the patient with pulmonary disease. Nasal flaring indicates that the patient is making a voluntary effort to inhale through the nostrils, which is a sign of increased work in breathing.

Patients may assume a posture that eases the work of breathing. The "tripod" position, in which the patient leans forward resting on both arms, allows expansion of the thorax and eases breathing. Sitting upright with the legs dependent may ease breathing in the patient with heart failure by decreasing venous return to the heart from the legs and allowing thoracic expansion.

Mentation

The brain relies on oxygen for function. Hypoxia causes changes in mental status including agitation, poor judgment, poor memory, and attention deficits. Symptoms of elevated carbon dioxide in the blood include lethargy, headache, and decreased level of consciousness. The nurse must assess the patient for orientation to person, place, and time as part of the assessment process.

 *The nurse should first rule out hypoxia as the cause for changes in metal status in patients with changes in behavior or level of consciousness.*

Rate, Depth, and Rhythm of Respirations

Respiratory rate should be counted for a full minute in patients with an irregular respiratory rhythm, and for 30 seconds in patients with a regular rhythm. The normal respiratory rate is 12 to 20 per minute. **Tachypnea** is considered to be a respiratory rate greater than 20 breaths per minute. A respiratory rate greater than 24 indicates respiratory distress. **Bradypnea** is considered to be a respiratory rate less than 12 breaths per minute. Bradypnea may be related to neurological disease or oversedation. Increased respiratory rate may be seen with fever, anxiety, and exercise. In general, for each increase in temperature of one degree, the heart rate will increase four beats per minute and the respiratory rate increase one breath per minute.

Hyperpnea refers to both increased rate and depth of respiration and is associated with metabolic acidosis. It is sometimes referred to as Kussmaul's breathing. Cheyne–Stokes breathing is a pattern of breathing in which the patient breathes rapidly then has a period of apnea. During deep inspiration, the lungs move downward to the 8th to 10th intercostal space anteriorly and the 10th to 12th space posteriorly. At the end of expiration, the lungs move upward to the 5th intercostal space anteriorly and the 9th to 10th intercostal space posteriorly. Shallow respirations may be seen with sedation, pneumonia, pain, or hypercalcemia. The respiratory pattern is normally rhythmic. Breathing patterns that are not rhythmic signal neurological dysfunction.

Thoracic Size and Shape

The thoracic size and shape provide important clues about risk for pulmonary disease. Structural abnormalities such as pectus excavatum (sternal depression) or pigeon chest (pectus carinatum), an outward bowing of the sternum, may indicate underlying structural abnormalities in the heart. Pectus excavatum may cause compression of the heart or great vessels. Barrel chest, an increased anterior-posterior diameter of the thorax, may indicate emphysema. Scoliosis and kyphoscoliosis (hunching and curvature of the spine) may prevent full expansion of the affected lung. These structural changes also prevent full lung expansion. Lung expansion is integral for oxygen and carbon dioxide exchange and for clearance of secretions. Cough may be ineffective to clear secretions in patients with structural deformities. This increases the risk of pneumonia.

Thoracic Expansion and Symmetry

During normal inspiration the diaphragm flattens and the lower rib cage expands. Although the lungs are paired, the right lung has three lobes and the left lung has two lobes. The liver causes the diaphragm on the right side to be higher than the left. In terms of overall expansion of the rib cage during inspiration, a 5 to 13 cm (2 to 5 in.) increase in diameter can be observed. In patients with COPD, the chest diameter during inspiration is decreased. Expansion is symmetrical, except when pneumothorax, structural abnormality, or pneumonia is present. Paradoxical movement may be present in flail chest. Flail chest occurs when two or more adjacent ribs are fractured in two or more places.

Use of Accessory Muscles

During normal inspiration the diaphragm and intercostal muscles contract, expanding the thorax and moving it upward. Patients with pulmonary disease may have difficulty with inspiration or ex-piration. **Accessory muscles** of inspiration include the trapezius, sternomastoid, and scalenus. During inspiration they may become pronounced in a patient with pulmonary dysfunction. Abdominal muscles may also be used in patients with pulmonary disease to force expiration.

Color and Appearance of Skin and Extremities

The color and appearance of the skin and extremities may give clues to the presence of hypoxia or anemia. Physical characteristics such as clubbing of the fingers may also indicate chronic hypoxia. Cardiovascular causes of pallor or skin changes must be explored as well. The nurse should corroborate findings of the physical examination with the patient to determine if they are familial characteristics or changes related to disease progression.

Pallor

Pallor can be related to vasoconstriction from cold ambient temperatures, melanin deficiencies, and heredity. It may also indicate that the patient is anemic. The nurse should check the mucous membranes and conjunctiva if pallor is suspected to be due to anemia. Ninety-eight percent of oxygen in the blood is bound to hemoglobin. In anemia there is a decrease in hemoglobin and a resultant decrease in the oxygen-carrying capacity. Patients with anemia tend to compensate for the decrease in oxygen-carrying capacity by increasing the heart rate. The hemoglobin moves through the vascular tree more rapidly, to the lungs to be oxygenated, to the body where it exchanges oxygen for carbon dioxide. Anemic patients are generally exercise intolerant because they cannot tolerate further increases in heart rate.

Cyanosis

Cyanosis is a very nonspecific and somewhat subjective sign. It is a bluish discoloration of the skin that occurs when oxygen levels are low in the presence of sufficient hemoglobin levels. It may also be seen in some patients with normal oxygen levels, polycythemia, and peripheral vascular disease. Ability to evaluate the presence of cyanosis also depends on available lighting and the eyesight and color discrimination of the person evaluating the patient's skin. Newborns may exhibit peripheral cyanosis when cold or agitated. Central cyanosis occurs when the mucous membranes, mouth, and lips are blue tinged. In the adult, central cyanosis indicates hypoxia.

The nail beds should be examined for the presence of cyanosis. Normally the nail beds are pink. Widening of the tips of the fingers and nail beds with loss of the normal angle, may indicate chronic hypoxia. This finding is known as clubbing.

Neck Inspection

The neck should be examined for tracheal deviation or the presence of goiter or lesions, which may cause upper airway obstruction and jugular venous distention. The trapezius, scalenus, and sternomastoid muscles may be enlarged in patients with COPD. **Tracheal deviation** occurs in pneumothorax and hemothorax. Deviation is usually away from the affected lung. Neck vein distention, or jugular venous distention, may be related to right heart failure. Right heart failure decreases flow of blood to the pulmonary tree for oxygenation. Jugular venous filling during expiration may be seen in COPD due to hyperinflation of the lungs.

Palpation of Skin and Extremities

Palpation of the thorax and dependent extremities helps determine if changes are due to cardiac, vascular, or pulmonary causes. Edema of the lower extremities points to heart failure as the cause for edema. Palpation of the thorax may uncover subcutaneous emphysema, step-off defects caused by rib fractures, and vibrations caused by respirations. Tactile **fremitus** is the palpation of vibrations in the thorax related to vocal speech. Capillary refill time can indicate a cardiovascular cause for dyspnea.

Edema

Edema of the lower extremities is generally related to right heart or heart failure. Right heart failure or combined left- and right-sided failure is common in patients with COPD. Right-sided failure is caused by pulmonary hypertension. Chronic distention of the lower airways makes forward blood flow more difficult. Over time, the right heart hypertrophies in an attempt to increase the force of blood through the pulmonary tree. Eventually the right heart fails, and fluid that cannot be accommodated is sequestered in dependent interstitial spaces (usually the lower extremities and coccyx) and causes edema. Edema is classified as pitting or nonpitting, and graded according to depth. Using one finger, the skin is depressed for 5 seconds and then released. If the nurse is able to depress the tissue up to 8 mm, the patient has 4+ edema; 6 mm, the patient has 3+ edema; 4 mm, 2+ edema; and 1+ edema measures 2 mm.

Skin Temperature and Moisture

The skin temperature and moisture status can give the nurse information on the patient's hydration, breathing effort, and temperature. Patients with COPD and asthma exacerbations may have very dry skin due to the loss of moisture through the respiratory tract. Shortness of breath with asthma and COPD exacerbations may prevent the patient from replacing fluids lost through rapid respiration, thus causing dehydration. Fever from pulmonary infections may increase skin temperature and moisture or cause cool, dry skin. Warm, moist skin may also be related to increased effort of breathing.

Clinical Reference Points

Although certain visible reference points, such as the trachea, nipple line, and sternum, are utilized in respiratory assessment, it is important to palpate and count ribs and interspaces for accuracy (Figure 33–1 ■). Landmarks utilized in the cardiorespiratory assessment include the anterior axillary line, the midaxillary line, and the midclavicular line. If a lesion is seen or adventitious breath sounds heard along one of these lines, it is then described further by its vertical location as delineated by the rib number or intercostal space.

Chest Excursion

Chest excursion is measured by placing the hands on the patient's back, equidistant from the spine or the center of the back, at the level of the 10th rib. When the patient takes a deep breath, the examiner's hands should move an equal distance laterally. This examination may also be performed on the anterior chest. The normal chest excursion (i.e., the distance between the thumbs with inspiration) should be 5 to 10 cm (2 to 4 in.). Elderly patients

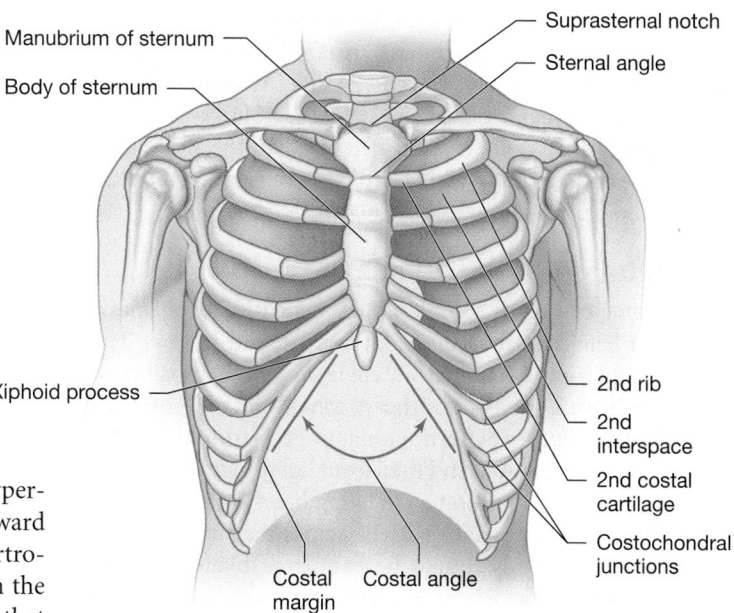

FIGURE 33–1 ■ In a respiratory assessment, it is important to palpate and count ribs and interspaces to accurately record the location of lesions or adventitious breath sounds.

may have decreased chest excursion as a normal finding. COPD patients may have decreased chest excursion due to anatomic flattening of the diaphragm from hyperinflation at the base of the lungs. Patients with rib fractures, pneumothorax, hemothorax, or pneumonia may also have decreased chest excursion.

Tactile Fremitus

Tactile fremitus is palpated over the thorax by having the patient vocalize the word "ninety-nine." Voice vibrations from the large airways are transmitted to the surface skin of the thorax. Start palpating with the ulnar side of the hand from the scapulae on the back and clavicles on the anterior chest, and move down bilaterally on each side of the thorax while the patient repeats "ninety-nine." The vibrations should be strongest over the large airways on the upper thorax and decrease in strength as you move down the thorax. Compare each side for symmetry. Unequal fremitus may be due to unilateral airway obstruction, pneumothorax, or pleural effusion causing a decrease in fremitus on the side with the defect. Increased fremitus is seen with consolidation or pneumonia and an increase in fremitus is felt over these areas.

Tenderness

Point tenderness may be seen in muscle strain or rib fracture. Excessive coughing may strain intercostals and thoracic muscles. Pneumonia and consolidation may also cause tenderness with deep inspiration. To avoid tenderness from any of these conditions, the patient may limit chest excursion and breathe shallowly. Shallow respirations promote atelectasis and may contribute to hypoxia.

Crepitus

Crepitus is also called **subcutaneous emphysema**. It is caused by air that escapes into the subcutaneous tissue. Crepitus may occur with rupture of pulmonary bullae, pneumothorax, or around chest tube insertion sites. Because air rises, crepitus is not generally seen in dependent areas. If noted, the nurse should mark the outline of crepitus so that increases in air escape can be evaluated. Excessive increases of crepitus may cause upper airway obstruction if located in the neck area. Crepitus feels like tiny packing bubble wrap under the skin and is often painless.

Auscultation of the Lungs

Auscultation of breath sounds is performed in a systematic manner utilizing a stethoscope (Figures 33–2 and 33–3 ■). The nurse should ensure as quiet an environment as possible to auscultate breath sounds and heart tones. On the posterior chest, the auscultatory pattern should progress from the apices located above the scapula and then from left to right across the back in a downward fashion to the lung bases. Breath sounds should follow a left-to-right pattern across the anterior chest as well. Breath sounds should be compared bilaterally. The breath sounds on the left posterior chest are generally heard about 2.5 cm (1 in.) lower than on the right side due to the location of the liver and increased height of the right diaphragm.

The diaphragm of the stethoscope is utilized to listen to breath sounds. Breath sounds are best auscultated with the pa-

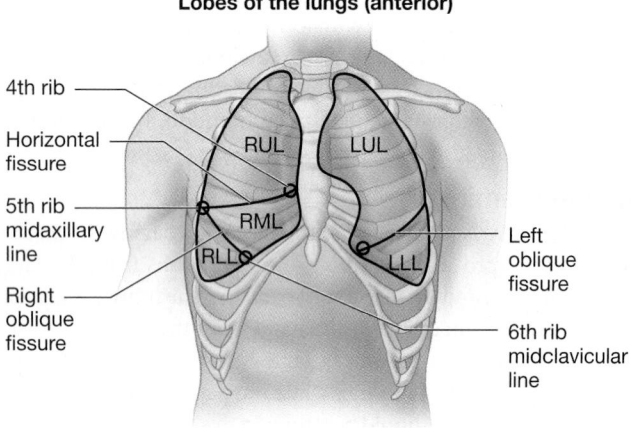

Lobes of the lungs (anterior)

4th rib
Horizontal fissure
5th rib midaxillary line
Right oblique fissure

RUL   LUL
RML
RLL   LLL

Left oblique fissure
6th rib midclavicular line

FIGURE 33–2 ■ Lobes of the lung—anterior.

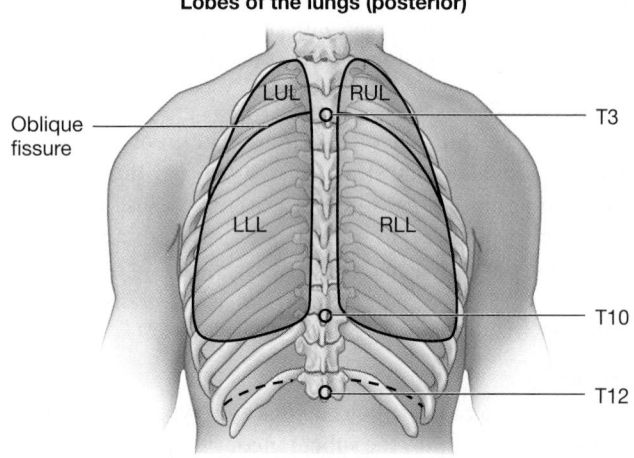

Lobes of the lungs (posterior)

Oblique fissure

LUL   RUL — T3
LLL   RLL
— T10
— T12

FIGURE 33–3 ■ Lobes of the lung—posterior.

tient in an upright position. Do not listen to breath sounds over clothing or hospital gowns. The movement of clothing causes rustling that will interfere with accurate auscultation of breath sounds.

Normal Breath Sounds

When listening for normal breath sounds, the patient should be upright so that the breath sounds can be auscultated bilaterally without interference and so that expansion is not restricted. Most texts advocate auscultating from the superior thorax at the level of C_7 posteriorly and anteriorly from above the clavicles. The diaphragm of the stethoscope should be used. The nurse should then move systematically from right to left and move steadily downward right to left toward the lung bases. Each site should be auscultated through both inspiration and expiration.

When the patient is obese, excess subcutaneous tissue may make it difficult to hear breath sounds because of the increased distance they must travel through the chest wall. Sometimes, having the patient stand so that gravity pulls subcutaneous tissue downward can aid in the auscultation of breath sounds in the obese person.

In the bedbound patient, the dependent areas are restricted from fully expanding by the pressure of the mattress. If the patient must remain supine, it is best to listen to the dependent areas before the superior areas because fluid and exudates will migrate to dependent areas with gravity. When the patient is turned so that these areas are no longer dependent, evidence of consolidation or fluid may disappear.

Tracheal Breath Sounds

Breath sounds auscultated over the trachea are called **tracheal breath sounds,** and they are loud and high pitched. The sounds heard in this location are caused by turbulent airflow through the tubular trachea. Because this is the largest airway, these sounds are also the loudest. As the airways become smaller, there is less turbulence and the sounds become softer and fainter. The duration of time that tracheal breath sounds are heard is equal during inspiration and expiration. They are best heard over the neck and trachea. Tracheal breath sounds should be auscultated if upper airway obstruction is suspected.

Bronchial Breath Sounds

Bronchial breath sounds are heard over the anterior chest on either side of the sternum, over the right and left main stem bronchus from the second to fourth intercostal spaces. On the back, they are best heard lateral to the spine between the third and sixth intercostal spaces. They are loud in pitch, harsh, less turbulent, and lower in frequency than tracheal breath sounds. A gap is heard between inspiration and expiration, and expiration is heard for a longer time than inspiration. The sounds over smaller airways are low pitched and softer.

Bronchovesicular Breath Sounds

Bronchovesicular breath sounds are heard during inspiration and expiration. They are midway in pitch and loudness between vesicular and bronchial breath sounds. They are best heard in the 1st and 2nd intercostal spaces of the anterior chest and between the scapulae of the posterior chest. Bronchovesicular breath sounds represent air movement in the moderate airways between the bronchi and the smaller airways.

Vesicular Breath Sounds

Vesicular breath sounds are heard over most of the thorax. The sounds are soft and low pitched, like a rustling, from air moving through small airways. Vesicular breath sounds are heard longer during expiration, because expiration generally lasts twice as long as inspiration.

Adventitious Breath Sounds

Abnormal breath sounds are decreased or absent sounds where normal breath sounds would normally occur. Diminished breath sounds indicate atelectasis, shallow respirations, pneumothorax, or decreased respiratory effort. These findings should be correlated with the patient's clinical condition and diagnoses. For example, a patient with myasthenia gravis who has diminished breath sounds should be assessed for respiratory muscle fatigue or paralysis. If the patient had a central venous line placed and develops diminished breath sounds, a pneumothorax should be suspected. Diminished breath sounds demonstrate decreased airflow and potentially decreased oxygen exchange. It is also abnormal for some breath sounds to occur where they should not be located. For example, bronchial breath sounds may be heard over consolidated areas or areas of pulmonary fibrosis because of increased tissue density.

Adventitious breath sounds are extra, abnormal sounds not normally heard during auscultation of breath sounds (Chart 33–2). They represent pathologic conditions of the heart or lungs, and indicate the presence of airway spasm, fluid, or secretions that disrupt airflow.

 Bronchial breath sounds over the large airways and diminished or absent breath sounds over smaller airways may indicate airway obstruction or pneumothorax.

Crackles

Crackles are sounds caused by fluid in the airways. They are described as intermittent or discontinuous, nonmusical, or popping sounds. They are caused by fluid, inflammation, infection, or secretions. (Note that the term *rales* is no longer used to describe fluid effects in the airways.) Crackles are described as either fine or coarse. Crackles occur when closed airways snap open during inspiration. Crackles may also be described as to timing, such as early inspiratory crackles or late inspiratory crackles. Sound is also produced when the airways close, but this sound is generally softer than heard on inspiration.

Wheezes

Wheezes are heard equally during inspiration and expiration. They are high-pitched musical sounds caused by air flowing across strands of mucus or swollen pulmonary tissue that narrows the airway or from bronchospasm. (Note that the term *rhonchi* is no longer used to describe harsh sounds caused by secretions in the airways.) Wheezes may be heard without a stethoscope. When auscultated, wheezes should be described as inspiratory or expiratory, continuous or discontinuous, and mild, moderate, or severe. Wheezing is typically heard in patients with asthma, allergic or reactive airway reactions, or after exercise. In patients who are experiencing acute asthma exacerbations, the absence of wheezing may indicate lack of airflow and is an ominous sign heralding respiratory arrest. Notify the health care provider or arrange for emergency care (911) immediately.

 Absence of wheezing in a patient with asthma exacerbation indicates lack of airflow and impending respiratory arrest. Notify the health care provider immediately.

Stridor

Stridor is heard only during inspiration, as air attempts to flow across an obstruction. Stridor may be heard without a stethoscope as a high-pitched, crowing sound. With a stethoscope it is heard best over the large airways, such as the trachea or bronchus. Stridor must be reported to the health care provider immediately and should alert the nurse to the presence of airway obstruction and the need for interventions to relieve the mechanical obstruction. Bronchoscopy may be necessary to remove the obstruction.

Pleural Friction Rub

Pleural friction rubs are low-pitched, creaking or squeaking sounds that occur when inflamed pleural surfaces rub together during respiration. They are most easily heard on inspiration. The pitch of the sound usually increases with chest expansion. To determine if the sound is due to pleural or pericardial friction, have the patient hold her breath. The pericardial friction rub will continue with each heartbeat, whereas the pleural friction rub will not occur when the patient is not actively breathing.

Percussion

Percussion is a skill rarely performed by nurses. Percussion is considered to be ultrasound without the technology, and helps

CHART 33–2	**Adventitious Breath Sounds**			
Breath Sound	**Inspiration**	**Expiration**	**Sound Description**	**Significance**
Crackles	Louder	Softer	Discontinuous, nonmusical	Fluid in the pleural tissue, asthma, bronchitis, consolidation, pneumonia, congestive heart failure, pulmonary edema, fibrosis
Wheeze	Yes	Yes	High-pitched, continuous musical sound	Bronchospasm, secretions, airway inflammation
Stridor	Yes	No	High-pitched crowing	Airway obstruction
Pleural friction rub	Yes	No	Rubbing or grating sound	Pleural inflammation

assess whether the underlying tissues are air filled, fluid filled, or solid. Sounds produced by percussion are described as flat, dull, resonant, hyperresonant, or tympanic. The lungs are approximately 99% air filled; therefore, percussion over the lungs produces resonance. Decreased sounds indicate a lack of air.

Resonance should be heard throughout most lung fields during inspiration while they are air filled. **Resonance** is a low-pitched, clear sound that is heard over normal lung tissue.

Abnormal percussion sounds include hyperresonance and dullness. Tympany is not heard over lung tissue but may be heard over an air-filled cheek or abdomen. Hyperresonance is very loud, with a lower pitch and a longer sound than resonance and indicates hyperinflation of the airways, or an excess of air in the absence of lung tissue. Hyperinflation is seen and heard in emphysema. Pneumothorax causes the collapse of lung tissue and excess air in the pleural space.

Dullness is a percussive tone that is heard over solid tissue. Dullness occurs over the lungs when air is absent. This is heard over the lower thorax during expiration, when consolidation is present as in pneumonia, pleural effusion, hemothorax, or the presence of solid tumors. The sound elicited is a dull thumping sound without vibration.

Pain

Pain associated with breathing may be related to pulmonary embolism, pleural disease, pneumothorax, musculoskeletal injury, pericarditis, or pneumonia. Sudden onset of shortness of breath or pain may be related to pulmonary embolism or pneumothorax. Progressive development of pain may be related to heart failure, pneumonia, asthma, or conditions that cause coughing. Pain with respiration will decrease inspired tidal volumes and promote atelectasis. Pain medication should be provided to patients so that they can participate in pulmonary rehabilitation activities and breathe deeply to prevent pneumonia and atelectasis. Cough suppressants should be used with caution because the primary purpose of the cough is to remove secretions that block the airways.

Genetic Considerations

Cystic fibrosis is an autosomal recessive genetic disorder that produces multiple problems and pulmonary complications. Most patients with cystic fibrosis are diagnosed in childhood. Pulmonary complications are the primary cause of death in patients with cystic fibrosis. In the past, children with cystic fibrosis did not survive to adulthood. Today, approximately 60% of children with cystic fibrosis will reach adulthood (Crosier & Wise, 2001). They have ineffective airway clearance related to thick mucus. The thickness of the mucus is related to a defect in the cystic fibrosis transmembrane regulator (CFTR). CFTR affects the movement of sodium and water across epithelial tissues, producing thick mucus. Thick mucus is difficult to expectorate from the airways and promotes colonization of bacteria. The most common bacteria infection seen is *Pseudomonas aeruginosa.*

The patient with cystic fibrosis suffers from exacerbations of respiratory infection. Chest physical therapy and devices that support airway clearance may be used by both child and adult patients with cystic fibrosis. Rarely, cystic fibrosis has been diagnosed in adulthood. Children who survive to adulthood with cystic fibro-

sis may be unable to maintain employment and may have other physical and emotional challenges. Social isolation is not uncommon. In addition, as adult patients with cystic fibrosis leave their pediatricians and cystic fibrosis clinics, there are few adult health care providers who are as knowledgeable as the pediatricians about the problems associated with cystic fibrosis.

Gerontological Considerations

Respiratory function decreases with advancing age for a variety of reasons. Skeletal changes from osteoporosis may cause stooped posture and decreased rib expansion. The rib cage becomes more rigid and the anterior-posterior diameter increases. The alveolar surface area decreases with age. In addition, lung tissue becomes less elastic and reduced tidal volume and decreased exchange of oxygen and carbon dioxide result in lowered arterial oxygen values.

Geriatric patients are at higher risk for pneumonia because of ineffective coughing related to the aforementioned physiological changes and due to risk of disease states that increase risk for aspiration. Decreased subcutaneous fat may make the geriatric patient more susceptible to cool room temperatures during respiratory physical assessment, so care must be taken to provide heat or warmed blankets or sheets to promote comfort during the examination.

Health Promotion

Avoidance of cigarette smoking is a primary avenue to prevent the development of pulmonary disease. Adolescents and adults who do not smoke should not start and if they do smoke, should stop. Nurses in all realms of practice should offer smoking cessation information and support for patients to stop smoking.

Hand hygiene is recognized in health care settings as an important means to prevent the spread of infection. Frequent hand washing or the use of alcohol degermers in school settings and public places may prevent the spread of bacteria and decrease the spread of cold, flu, and pneumonia.

Flu vaccines and pneumococcal vaccines should be available to patients in high-risk populations. Frequently these frail patients are physically unable to go to local centers or wait in lines to obtain the vaccination. Insurance and health care providers should develop and execute plans to get the vaccines to the patients, instead of forcing these patients to "come to the vaccine."

Governmental agencies have been active in promoting healthy and safe workplaces. In occupations that commonly encounter environmental irritants and allergens, education in the use of personal protective equipment (PPE) should be provided in an ongoing basis. Although PPE may be uncomfortable at first, consistent insistence on its use should be provided. Construction workers have gotten used to hard hats; it is time for them to get used to respirator masks. Reduction of the effects of environmental allergens and irritants will prevent the development of chronic disease in this population.

■ Respiratory Monitoring

Whether the patient is on the medical–surgical ward, ICU, or postanesthesia recovery unit, respiratory monitoring includes observation, physical assessment, and the use of electronic monitoring devices. The nurse must be knowledgeable about the oxygen delivery method and the expected outcomes for the patient. If a patient is receiving supplemental oxygen, the nurse should expect that the patient will be able to maintain appropriate arterial oxygen levels. These are assessed using ABGs, physical assessment, and pulse oximetry. In a normal patient, with normal lungs, the nurse can expect that the FiO_2 delivered to the patient will increase the PaO_2 four times. That is why the PaO_2 in a normal patient inspiring room air that has an FiO_2 of approximately 24% is approximately 95%.

The standard of care for patients with cardiac and respiratory illness now includes continuous or intermittent observation of the patient's oxygen saturation and end-tidal carbon dioxide levels. The peak flow is utilized to trend treatment effectiveness in patients with asthma.

Pulse Oximetry

Pulse oximeters provide a digital readout of the percentage that the hemoglobin is saturated with oxygen (Figure 33–4 ■). Pulse oximeters use infrared light technology or reflectance photometry to reflect light off the hemoglobin molecules. The computer in the pulse oximeter then measures the absorption of light by hemoglobin during pulsatile arterial waves.

The oxygen saturation measured by infrared technology does not necessarily provide the same values obtained from the calculated oxygen saturation obtained from an ABG. Normal infrared oxygen saturation (SPO_2) and ABG saturations range from 95% to 100%. Nail polish color may interfere with the ability of the machine to read infrared pulsations. Pulse oximetry probes should not be placed on extremities with automated blood pressure cuffs, hemodialysis fistulas, or arterial lines, because these interfere with blood flow (Grap, 2002). Shock and hypovolemia also cause low-flow states that contribute to inaccurate pulse oximetry readings. Patient movement, ambient light, and venous pulsations may also cause inaccurate readings. The accuracy of the readout should be suspect if the waveform does not match the patient's pulse rate and amplitude. If ambient light is interfering with readings (producing results higher than suspected), cover the probe with a towel to see if the result is different.

Pulse oximetry does not distinguish methemoglobin or carboxyhemoglobin from oxygen-saturated hemoglobin. Fifty percent carboxyhemoglobin reads as 95% SpO_2 (Ford, 2002). Patients who have suspected thiocyanate toxicity or inhalation injury should have an ABG analysis to determine respiratory status and oxygen saturation.

Peak Flow

Peak flow meters are utilized to determine trends in a patient's condition or to evaluate air movement to determine severity of asthma exacerbation (Figure 33–5 ■). Many different types of meters and results graphs are available. Some peak flow meters are computerized so that the patient can provide a diary of results to the health care provider.

Peak flow meters measure the peak expiratory flow rate. Normal values for peak flow measurements are based on age and body size. Many peak flow meters utilize a red, yellow, and green zone to determine the severity of decrease in peak flow. Green is the "good zone," meaning that the patient meets at least 80% of normal. The yellow zone is a caution zone. Values in this area are below normal. The red zone means that the patient is in danger of respiratory complications and has a peak flow of less than 50% of the normal value. As a general rule, values of less than 400 L/min indicate poor airflow. The peak flow measures the peak expiratory flow rate, the amount of air the patient can exhale.

Arterial Blood Gas

ABG studies are utilized to provide information on arterial oxygen and carbon dioxide levels. The oxygen saturation, bicarbonate, and blood pH are also calculated. The carbon dioxide level is utilized as the major determinant for diagnosing respiratory alkalosis and respiratory acidosis. The bicarbonate level is the determinant of metabolic acidosis and alkalosis.

Low oxygen levels in the arterial blood may be due to a variety of pathologies. Oxygen travels in the arterial blood attached to hemoglobin. If the hemoglobin levels are decreased as in anemia, there are fewer sites to which oxygen can bind. Hemoglobin affinity for oxygen is affected by the blood pH. If the pH is elevated (alkalosis), less oxygen is delivered to tissues.

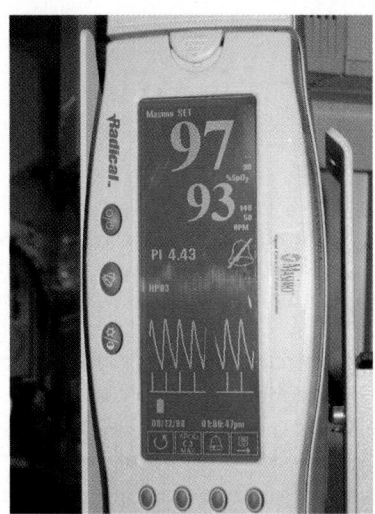

FIGURE 33–4 ■ Pulse oximetry monitor.
Source: Cheryl Wraa

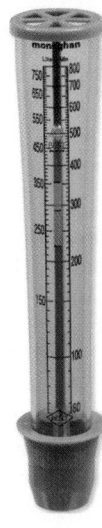

FIGURE 33–5 ■ Peak flow meter.
Source: Courtesy of Monaghan Medical Corporation

CHART 33–3 Acute ABG Analysis

ABG	Normal	Respiratory Acidosis	Respiratory Alkalosis	Metabolic Acidosis	Metabolic Alkalosis
pH	7.35–7.45	<7.35	>7.45	<7.35	>7.45
PaO_2	80–100 mmHg	Normal or decreased	Normal	Normal	Normal
$PaCO_2$	35–45 mmHg	>45 mmHg	<35 mmHg	Normal	Normal
HCO_3^-	22–26 mEq/L	Decreased	Normal	Decreased	Increased

There is an increased affinity of hemoglobin for oxygen. In acidotic states, the affinity of hemoglobin for oxygen is decreased and it is readily released to tissues. Chart 33–3 outlines normal ABGs and the changes seen with acute respiratory and metabolic acidosis and alkalosis.

Capnography

Capnography is the measurement of exhaled carbon dioxide (Figure 33–6 ■). Small disposable capnographers are utilized to test endotracheal tube placement utilizing treated paper that changes color in the presence of an acid such as carbon dioxide. Some machines also measure amounts of carbon dioxide in exhaled breath through spectography. These analyzers also provide waveform readings corresponding to the patient's inspiratory and expiratory cycles. Capnography waveforms and CO_2 values are useful in determining the patient's ventilatory status and readiness for extubation or pulmonary vessel perfusion in patients with pulmonary embolus.

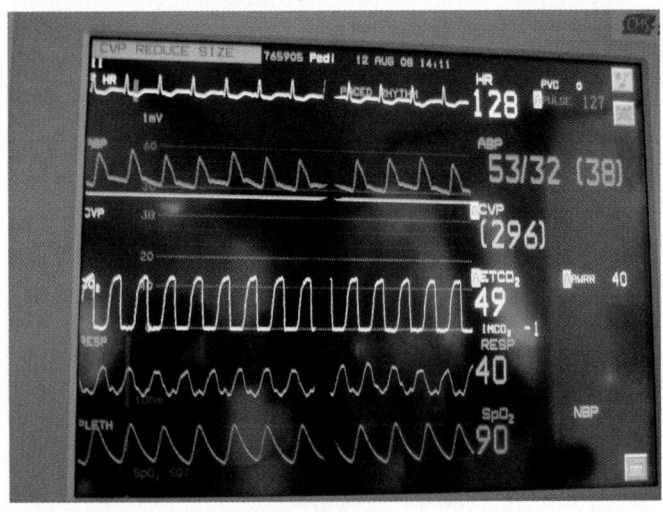

FIGURE 33–6 ■ End-tidal CO_2 monitoring.
Source: Cheryl Wraa

■ Summary

All nurses must be skilled in respiratory assessment because breathing is essential to life. The respiratory assessment must include pertinent data regarding the patient's history and current complaints. Acute changes in respiratory status must be acted on quickly to prevent patient compromise. Patients with chronic pulmonary disease will have abnormal physical findings, but the patients' usual and customary status must be ascertained by the nurse so that the progression of symptoms and the current status of the patient can be determined. This knowledge is also valuable in planning care for the patients. Data obtained from the respiratory assessment will determine if the current plan of care is adequate for a patient's needs. Is the patient getting better or worse? Utilizing the objective data from the respiratory assessment, the nurse can advocate for the patient with the health care provider to ensure an appropriate plan of care. Early recognition of symptoms by the nurse is important to provide education in risk reduction and to assist in determining possible environmental irritants and allergens that can then be eliminated and thus prevent chronic disease.

NCLEX® REVIEW

1. While auscultating a patient's lungs, the nurse hears intermittent popping sounds. The nurse would document this assessment finding as:
   1. Rales.
   2. Crackles.
   3. Wheezes.
   4. Rhonchi.

2. A patient tells the nurse that he just returned from visiting Asia and has had an upper respiratory infection for 2 weeks. Why is this information beneficial to aid in the care of this patient?
   1. It will help determine the patient's socioeconomic status.
   2. It will help determine the patient's occupation.
   3. It might help to know if there are any recent outbreaks of pulmonary disorders in the area of travel.
   4. It might help determine the patient's immunological status.

3. A patient, who is a nonsmoker, comes into the clinic with symptoms of a respiratory disorder. Which of the following should the nurse include regarding this patient's social history while conducting the assessment?

1. Do you have any heart problems?

2. Have you been to any activities or functions around other people with respiratory problems?

3. Do you have any family members with known respiratory problems?

4. Do you remember which immunizations you received as a child?

4. During the assessment of a patient with a respiratory disorder, the nurse observes lower extremity edema. This finding is important in respiratory disorders because:

1. It will indicate the patient's ability to ambulate.

2. Edema indicates the amount of fluid the patient can tolerate.

3. Edema indicates heart failure, a common finding in a patient with COPD.

4. It aids in determining if the patient will need assistance with activities of daily living.

5. A patient in the burn unit has a pulse oximetry reading of 98%. Which of the following should the nurse do about this reading?

1. Cover the probe to see if the reading is different.

2. Move the probe to another extremity.

3. Have an arterial blood gas analysis done to compare the readings.

4. Ask the patient to not move while doing another reading.

Answers for review questions appear in Appendix D

KEY TERMS

accessory muscles *p.872*
adventitious breath sounds *p.875*
bradypnea *p.872*
bronchial breath sounds *p.874*
bronchovesicular breath sounds *p.874*
capnography *p.878*
crackles *p.875*

crepitus *p.873*
dyspnea *p.865*
fremitus *p.873*
hypernea *p.872*
pleural friction rubs *p.875*
resonance *p.876*

subcutaneous emphysema *p.873*
tachypnea *p.872*
tracheal breath sounds *p.874*
tracheal deviation *p.872*
vesicular breath sounds *p.875*
wheezes *p.875*

REFERENCES

Corbridge, S. J., Kamp, D. W., & Richlin, D. (2004). Asbestos related pulmonary diseases. *AAOHN Journal, 52,* 49–51.

Crosier, J., & Wise, L. C. (2001). Coming of age: Cystic fibrosis once a childhood disease makes its way to adulthood. *Nursing Management, 33*(11), 30–31.

Dillon, P. M. (2003). *Nursing health assessment: A critical thinking, case studies approach.* Philadelphia: F. A. Davis.

Ford, S. (2002). Common errors in clinical measurement. *Anesthesia and Intensive Care Medicine, 3*(12), 464–467.

Gotway, M. B., Marder, S. R., Hanks, D. K., Leung, J. W., Dawn, S. K., Gean, A. D., et al. (2002). Thoracic complications of illicit drug use: An organ system approach. *Radiographics, 22,* S119–S135.

Grap, M. (2002). Protocols for practice: Pulse oximetry. *Critical Care Nurse, 22*(3), 69–76.

Harris, H. (2004). Action stat fat embolism. *Nursing 2004, 34,* 96.

Jubber, A. S. (2004). Respiratory complications of obesity. *International Journal of Clinical Practice, 58,* 573–580.

Kee, J. L. (2005). *Handbook of laboratory & diagnostic tests* (5th ed.). Upper Saddle River, NJ: Pearson Prentice Hall.

Kose, A. A., Karabagli, Y., & Cetin, C. (2005). An unusual cause of burns due to cupping: Complications of a folk medicine remedy. *Burns, 33,* 126–127.

Merritt, S. L., & Berger, B. E. (2004). Obstructive sleep apnea-hypopnea syndrome. *AJN, 104,* 49–52.

Peltier, L. F. (2004). Fat embolism. *Clinical Orthopedics and Related Research, 422,* 148–153.

Shamsuzzaman, A. S., Gersh, B. J., & Somers, V. K. (2003). Obstructive sleep apnea implications for cardiac and vascular disease. *Journal of the American Medical Association, 290,* 1906–1914.

Snyder, M., & Miska, K. (2003). Cultural related complementary therapies: Their use in critical care units. *Critical Care Clinics of North America, 15,* 341–346.

U.S. Department of Health and Human Services. (2000). *Healthy people 2010: Understanding and improving health.* Washington, DC: Author.

Weber, J., & Kelley, J. (2003). *Health assessment in nursing* (2nd ed.). Philadelphia: Lippincott Williams & Wilkins.

Wilson, K. C., & Saukkonen, J. J. (2004). Acute respiratory failure from abused substances. *Journal of Intensive Care Medicine, 19,* 183–193.

Yoo, S. S., & Tausk, F. (2004). Cupping: East meets West. *International Journal of Dermatology, 43,* 664–665.

34

Caring for the Patient with Upper Airway Disorders

Ann Sievers

With contributions by:
Kathleen Osborn
Annita Watson

Outcome-Based Learning Objectives

After studying this chapter, the learner will be able to:

1. Compare and contrast nursing management of the most common facial fractures.
2. Explain nursing care for a patient with sinus disease.
3. Differentiate the essential components for developing a teaching plan for patients with infections of the upper airway.
4. Discuss the implications of the loss of the senses of smell, sight, and taste in patients with upper airway disorders and disfigurement.
5. Compare and contrast the nursing management of patients with partial versus total airway obstruction.
6. Identify the risk factors of head and neck cancer.
7. Explain the nursing management of a patient with head and neck cancer in the acute care setting related to airway, wounds, pain, and nutrition.

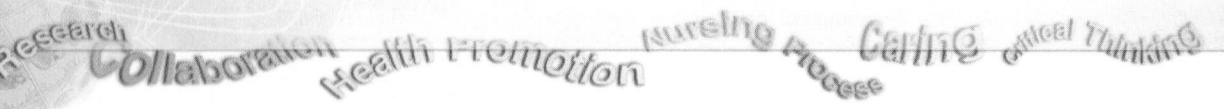

Otolaryngology, also called **otorhinolaryngology**, is the study of disorders of the head and neck, including the ears, nose, and throat. Disease and trauma that affect these structures impact a person's outlook on the world. They can change the way a person smells, tastes, breathes, sees, hears, and touches, and how a person is perceived by others.

Disorders of the head and neck area can not only be disfiguring, but also can involve vital tissues that function to meet the basic human needs of intake of air, fluids, and food. These tissues serve to assess the environment via the special senses of sight, hearing, taste, and smell. Speech also may be affected, as in the case of cancer and subsequent treatment. Any interference with facial appearance, basic human needs, or ability to communicate can be a devastating experience for the patient and family and is a meaningful component of caring for patients of this type. Nurses must be aware of the immense impact of otolaryngology disease and respond to their patients' needs accordingly. It is important for nurses to understand the physiological care needs of their patients and also to be sensitive to the impact on the patient's quality of life. Assisting and teaching patients how to cope with otolaryngologic illnesses and life changes is an essential part of the healing process.

This chapter focuses on disorders of the head and neck and is presented in discrete sections, each describing a specific type of disorder of the head and neck related to structure, function, and disease entities.

Structural, Traumatic, and Deformity Disorders of the Nose and Facial Structures

The facial skeleton serves to protect the brain, house and protect the sense organs of smell, sight, and taste, and provide a frame for the soft tissues of the face. It also helps to facilitate eating, facial expression, breathing, and speech. The primary bones of the face are the nasal bones, mandible, maxilla, zygoma, temporal bone, and frontal bone. Numerous types of deformities affect the facial structures of the head and neck, many of which deal with fractures. The head is the most frequently injured part of the body. Head injuries occur in approximately 75% of all motor vehicle crashes, with approximately 30% of head traumas resulting in skull fractures (Connell & Belafsky, 2005). The ear is the most frequently damaged sense organ.

Nasal Fractures

The skeletal structure of the nose is composed of paired nasal bones, the nasal process of the frontal bone and the maxilla, which form a framework to support the cartilaginous skeleton of the nose. The nasal bones rigidly support the upper portion of the nose between the eyes. The cartilages are flexible supports that maintain the shape of the rest of the nose. The septum divides the nostrils and is also made of both cartilage and bone. Figure 34–1 ■ shows the anatomical relationship between the nasal bones, cartilage, and septum. Underlying the framework of the nose are soft tissues, mucous glands, and nerves responsible for sensation and function of the nose. A "broken nose" may have injured bone, cartilage, nerves, skin, and/or mucosa (the nasal lining). Because the nose is the most prominent anterior feature of the face, nasal fractures account for approximately 40% of bone injuries (Bermant, 2007). According to Smith and Perez (2004), fracture of the nasal bones is the most common site-specific bone injury of the facial skeleton in the United States.

Epidemiology and Etiology

Nasal fractures typically are caused by a traumatic injury to the bone or cartilage of the nose. Although most of the nasal structure is made up of cartilage, the nasal bones usually are fractured in injury. Fights and sports injuries account for most nasal fractures in adults, followed by falls and vehicle crashes. Play and sports account foremost for nasal fractures in children. When nasal fractures are seen in children and women, physical abuse should be considered and appropriately ruled out (Smith & Perez, 2004). Nasal fractures occur more frequently in males than females (>2:1), with the incidence increasing in patients ages 15 to 30 years (Smith & Perez, 2004).

Laboratory and Diagnostic Procedures

Nasal fractures may be diagnosed by facial x-rays. If it is suspected that the ethmoid bone also is damaged due to its proximity to the nasal bones, neurological tests are indicated to assess cognition and response. The ethmoid bone lies posterior to the nasal bones and can be damaged from a direct trauma to the nose. A patient with this type of injury will have a profound headache and may have a cerebrospinal fluid (CSF) leak. Any clear fluid draining from the nose is highly suspect for CSF. Diagnosis is confirmed by allowing the fluid to drain on a clean white dressing. If a halo of red-tinged fluid is demonstrated (halo test), then a CSF leak is present.

Clinical Manifestations

Patients with a nasal fracture usually present with some combination of deformity, tenderness, hemorrhage, edema, ecchymoses, instability, or crepitation. Nasal fractures can occur and not be displaced. In this case, no surgical treatment is indicated. Edema can mask underlying nasal bone displacement, which, if untreated, can result both in unfavorable appearance and function.

Air traveling through the nose normally is controlled by the position of the bones and cartilages and, if displaced, obstruction of the nose can occur. Mucosal swelling and clotted blood also will limit airflow. An injured nose can bleed from lacerations of the skin or from the mucosa inside the nose. These cuts may need to be evaluated and repaired. A septal hematoma can injure or thicken the septal structures, impairing airflow through the nose. Bruises often migrate around the eyes and eventually down the cheeks. Repositioning or moving fractured bones and cartilage typically results in additional swelling. The upper airway passages may be at risk for considerable edema and bruising.

Medical Management

With an uncomplicated (nondisplaced) acute nasal fracture, it is appropriate to prescribe pain medication and release the patient with instructions to rest, apply ice, and maintain head elevation. Follow-up evaluation and management can safely be scheduled after the swelling resolves, usually within 3 to 5 days. If there is displacement of the nasal bones, reduction should be accomplished between the 5th and 10th day after the injury, before the nasal bones start to fixate. Septal hematomas should be drained if possible to prevent nasal obstruction.

Most acute nasal fractures are able to be reduced in the primary care setting. However, for some fractures, open reduction in an operating room is necessary to obtain proper alignment of the nasal bones. Sometimes the aesthetic outcomes of closed-reduction techniques are less than optimal, and patients should be counseled that nasal reconstruction might eventually be necessary. A combination of medications inside the nose and injections around the nose lessens the discomfort of the reduction.

■ Nursing Management

Assessment is a key function of the nurse in caring for patients with a fractured nose. It is imperative that the nurse evaluate the patient for type and severity of injury, bleeding, swelling, patency of airway, skin discoloration, and pain. The immediate goals are to control bleeding, reduce swelling with application of ice, and provide pain control. The nurse will need to assess for further injury by testing the patient for facial numbness or tingling. The presence of tingling needs to be reported to the health care provider. An isolated nasal fracture does not require hospitalization.

Septal Deviation

The nasal septum is the wall dividing the nasal cavity into halves; it is composed of a central supporting skeleton covered on each side by mucous membrane. The front portion of this natural partition is a firm but bendable structure made mostly of cartilage and is covered by skin that has a substantial supply of blood vessels. The ideal nasal septum is exactly midline, separating the left and right sides of the nose into passageways of equal size. A septal deviation occurs when the septum is severely shifted away

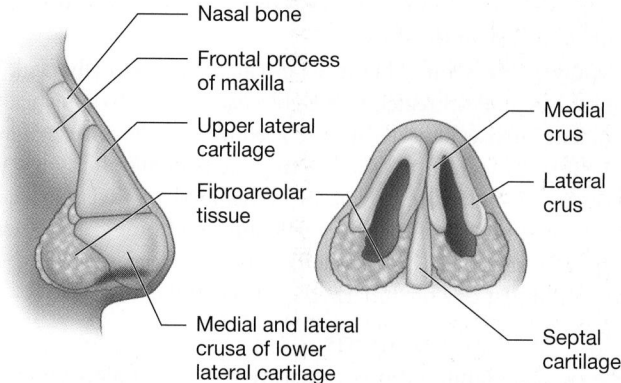

FIGURE 34–1 ■ Anatomical relationship between nasal bones, cartilage, and septum.

Nasal bone
Frontal process of maxilla
Upper lateral cartilage
Fibroareolar tissue
Medial and lateral crusa of lower lateral cartilage
Medial crus
Lateral crus
Septal cartilage

from the midline. Diagnosed septal deviations are a common occurrence in individuals, reportedly as high as 75%. Note, however, that the American Academy of Otolaryngology–Head and Neck Surgery (2007) has reported that 80% of all nasal septums are somewhat off-centered. The majority of diagnosed septal deviations that cause pathophysiological symptoms to patients are caused by trauma to the nose.

Epidemiology and Etiology

Deviations of the nasal septum may develop during growth or by trauma due to a fall, a blow to the nose, or surgery that further exaggerates the deviation. These deviations are common and, for the most part, cause no symptoms and require no treatment. However, the septal deviation may be severe enough to obstruct the passage of air through the nostrils. This obstruction predisposes the patient to sinusitis, infection, and epistaxis.

Pathophysiology and Clinical Manifestations

Although septal deviations usually present no problem for the individual, they may cause one or more of the following: blockage of one or both nostrils; nasal congestion, sometimes one sided; frequent nosebleeds; frequent sinus infections; at times, facial pain; headaches, postnasal drip; and noisy breathing during sleep, particularly in infants and young children.

In some cases, a person with a mildly deviated septum has symptoms only when an upper respiratory tract infection is also present. In these individuals, the respiratory infection triggers nasal inflammation that temporarily amplifies any mild airflow problems related to the deviated septum. Once the infection resolves, and the nasal inflammation subsides, symptoms of a deviated septum often also resolve.

Medical Management

It is easy to diagnose that a septum is deviated; it is more difficult to determine if that deviation needs correcting. A patient's complaint that she can breathe through only one nostril is the usual determinant of treatment. Decongestants, such as pseudoephedrine or phenylpropanolamine, will shrink the members and thereby enlarge the passages. Antihistamines, nasal cortisone spray, and other allergy treatments also may be temporarily beneficial. Normal saline drops and sprays are very helpful in loosening mucus in the obstructed side and preventing drying in the other side, where all of the air blows. These therapies are useful to take care of symptoms, but do not correct the problem.

If the patient complains of obstruction or has cosmetic complaints, a septoplasty, or surgical repositioning of the septum, may be performed. It is performed with a local anesthetic and conscious sedation. Some health care providers insert nasal splints and suture them into place as a temporary structural support. The splints are removed a few days after surgery. Surgical repair is curative and carries little risk. A nasospecific procedure in which a deflated balloon is inserted in the nostril and inflated to a large enough degree to adjust the septal deviation, can be an alternative to surgery. A practitioner trained in this nasospecific procedure is necessary.

■ Nursing Management

Nursing management focuses on maintaining a clear air passage, detecting signs of infection, and maintaining patient comfort. The nurse is instrumental in teaching the patient how to instill nose drops and sprays and perform a saline lavage. In the event of a surgical repair, the nurse provides routine postoperative care and is alert for bleeding, swelling, and pain.

Epistaxis

Epistaxis is defined as any bleeding from the nostril, nasal cavity, or nasopharynx. Epistaxis is common due to the highly vascular linings of the nose. One of the primary causes of nosebleeds is traumatic nose injuries, although they may occur for other reasons. Air moving through the nose can dry and irritate the membranes lining the inside of the nose, forming crusts. These crusts bleed when irritated by rubbing, picking, or blowing the nose.

Epidemiology and Etiology

As noted, nosebleeds are very common. They tend to occur more frequently in the winter when viruses are common and heated indoor air dries out the nostrils. Common etiologies include injuries such as trauma; systemic problems, such as coagulation disorders or hypertension; environmental problems, such as dry air; irritation from nose picking; use of drugs and medications; or postoperatively with any nasal or sinus surgery. A foreign object in the nose or direct impact to the nose also can cause a nosebleed. A deviated septum also may make a person prone to nosebleeds.

The elderly are susceptible to nosebleeds for several reasons. As a person ages, the skin becomes more friable and retains less turgor. The same is true of the lining in the nose. Any mechanical irritation, such as nose picking or excessive rubbing, may cause a bleed. Individuals who use any type of inhaled drug also are at risk of damaging the nasal tissues and are highly prone to nosebleeds.

Pathophysiology

There are two areas within the nasal passage where a plexus of anastomotic vessels can be found. The anterior area is referred to as Kiesselbach's plexus (or Little's area), and the posterior area is known as Woodruff's plexus (Kucik, 2005). These areas often are implicated in nosebleeds. Anterior bleeds from Kiesselbach's plexus are the most common. They account for approximately 90% of nosebleeds. The bleeding erupts when the relatively thin nasal mucosa overlying a dilated septal vessel dries, scabs, and falls (or is picked) off. Posterior bleeds originating from Woodruff's plexus, which is located over the posterior middle turbinate, are less common. In these cases the site of bleeding is higher and deeper within the nose and the blood flows primarily down the back of the throat.

Only rarely is a nosebleed life threatening or actually fatal. In most cases of life-threatening nosebleeds, some underlying health problem, such as hypertension, a bleeding disorder, or use of anticoagulant medication, is impacting the patient's ability to clot (Pope & Hobbs, 2005). Hereditary hemorrhagic telangiectasia (also called HHT or Osler-Weber-Rendu syndrome) may be evidenced by nosebleeds. This is a disorder involving a blood vessel growth similar to a birthmark in the back of the nose.

Clinical Manifestations

The clinical manifestation of epistaxis consists of bleeding from the nose. There may be slight or profuse bleeding dependent on the cause of the nosebleed. If the bleeding does not stop after 20 minutes, it is imperative that the patient seek emergency care. If the nosebleed occurs after an injury to the head, this may indicate a skull fracture. It could also indicate a broken nose and x-rays should be taken no matter how trivial the blow seems to be at the time. Skull fractures are discussed in Chapter 29 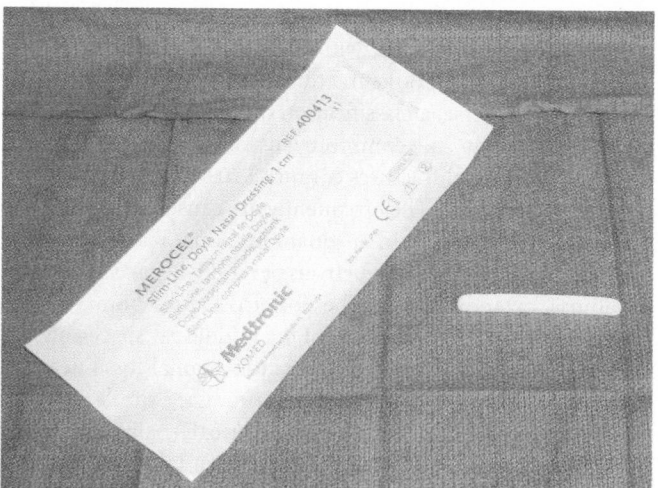.

Laboratory and Diagnostic Procedures and Medical Management

Laboratory and diagnostic tests that may need to be performed include a complete blood count (CBC), partial thromboplastin time measurements, prothrombin (PT) measurements, and x-rays of the skull. Nasal endoscopy (examination of the nose using a camera) also may be called for.

Anterior bleeds generally resolve on their own by pinching the nares together and leaning forward for several minutes. The health care provider should apply cold packs to the face and have the patient lean forward or to the side to protect the airway and prevent swallowing of blood. This maneuver may prevent emesis. Electrocautery, chemical cautery, or anterior or posterior nasal packing may be used for any bleeding that does not quickly resolve (Figure 34–2 ■). Cryotherapy, laser therapy, embolization, or surgery may be used to ligate bleeding vessels (Pope & Hobbs, 2005).

Instruction for any patient recovering from a nosebleed should include refraining from picking or blowing of the nose, no heavy lifting, and no straining for 2 days to 2 weeks, as recommended by the health care provider. Stool softeners, pain medications, nasal emollients, or nasal saline spray may be prescribed.

■ Nursing Management

For patients with anterior epistaxis and anterior packing, a feeling of airway obstruction can arise. The nurse will need to take special note of the patient's concerns and provide reassurance as needed. The head of the bed should be elevated, and a face mask should be provided for humidity. In the event of surgery, routine postoperative care protocols should be followed. Pain medications should be provided as needed. The patient with posterior epistaxis, requiring posterior packing, should be observed in an intensive care unit (ICU). These patients are at risk

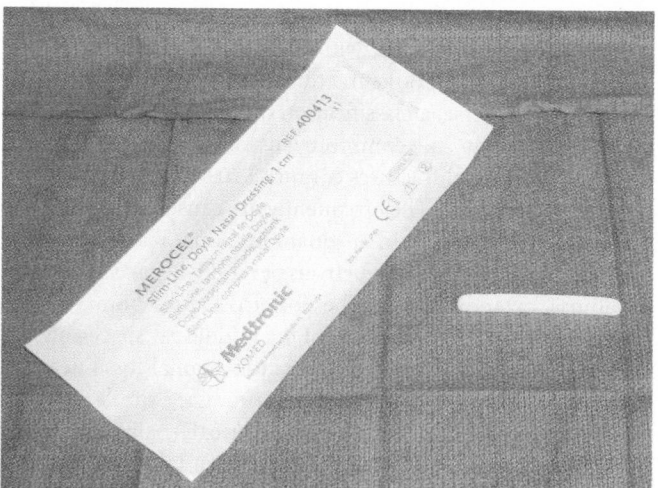

FIGURE 34–2 ■ Nasal tampon for the treatment of anterior epistaxis. This is placed in the anterior nasal cavity, impregnated with normal saline, and left in place for at least 5 days. Most nasal packing is bilateral to provide pressure support on either side of the nasal septum.
Source: University of California, Davis Medical Center

for airway obstruction if the packs slip. They also are at risk for developing bradycardia and hypercarbia due to the nasopulmonary reflex. Therefore, cardiac monitoring and pulse oximetry are mandatory.

The nurse also should advise patients of risk factors for nosebleeds, including a hot, dry climate, colds and allergies, a deviated septum, exposure to irritating chemicals, medical conditions, heavy alcohol use, and medications that interfere with blood clotting. Patient education should include advice on preventive measures that can be taken. These include not picking the nose, gently blowing the nose one nostril at a time, keeping mouth open when sneezing, not smoking, using a humidifier if indoor climate is dry, applying a dab of butter/petroleum jelly to the inside of the nostrils before bedtime, and avoiding aspirin and other medications that prolong the bleeding time.

Facial Fractures

Facial fractures refer to any injuries that result in a broken bone or bones of the face. Because nose fractures were discussed earlier, this discussion is restricted to the mandible, maxilla, zygoma, temporal bones, and the frontal bone. Multiple facial fractures may occur simultaneously, typically resulting from an injury to the face. Many situations can cause facial fractures. Motor vehicle crashes, sporting injuries, falls, and assault account for the majority, although injuries from gunshot wounds and stabbings occur as well. When dealing with facial fractures, the nurse should always be concerned that other injuries may exist. Other parts of the body may be injured, for example, if the patient has facial injuries caused by a motor vehicle crash.

Mandible Fractures

The mandible is a U-shaped bone; together with the maxilla, the mandible is the largest and strongest bone of the face. It forms the lower jaw and holds the lower teeth in place. The mandible consists of a curved, horizontal portion, referred to as the *body*; two perpendicular portions, the *rami*, which unite with the ends of the body nearly at right angles; the alveolar process; the tooth-bearing area of the mandible (upper part of the body of the mandible), the condyle; superior (upper) and posterior projection from the ramus, which makes the temporomandibular joint with the temporal bone; and the coronoid process, superior and anterior projection from the ramus, which provides attachment to the temporalis muscle.

The inferior alveolar nerve, a branch of the mandibular division of the trigeminal (V) nerve, enters the mandibular foramen and runs forward in the mandibular canal, supplying sensation to the teeth. At the mental foramen the nerve divides into two terminal branches: incisive and mental nerves. The incisive nerve runs forward in the mandible and supplies the anterior teeth. The mental nerve exits the mental foramen and supplies sensation to the lower lip (Babak & Blackwell, 2005). The mandible articulates with the two temporal bones at the temporomandibular joints. It is the only mobile bone of the facial skeleton, and since it houses the lower teeth, its motion is essential for mastication. Mandibular fractures often are accompanied by a "twin fracture" on the contralateral (opposite) side. The mandible may be dislocated anteriorly (to the front) and inferiorly (downward) but very rarely posteriorly (backward).

Maxilla Fractures

The maxilla forms the largest component of the middle third of the facial skeleton, and is a fusion of two bones along the palatal fissure that forms the upper jaw. This is similar to the mandible, which also is a fusion of two halves at the mental symphysis. The alveolar process of the maxilla holds the upper teeth and is referred to as the maxillary arch. The maxilla attaches laterally to the zygomatic bones (cheekbones) and assists in forming the boundaries of three cavities: the roof of the mouth, the floor and lateral side of the nasal antrum, and the floor of the orbit. The maxilla also enters into the formation of two fossae: the infratemporal and pterygopalatine, and two fissures, the inferior orbital and pterygomaxillary. The maxilla articulates with nine bones: two of the cranium (frontal and ethmoid) and seven of the face (nasal, zygomatic, lacrimal, inferior nasal, concha, palatine, vomer) and the adjacent fused maxillary bone. Sometimes it articulates with the orbital surface, and sometimes with the lateral pterygoid plate of the sphenoid. The maxilla is a key bone in the midface that is closely associated with adjacent bones providing structural support between the cranial base and the occlusal plane.

Fractures of the maxilla occur less frequently than those of the mandible or nose due to the strong structural support of this bone. The midface consists of alternating thick and thin sections of bone that are capable of resisting significant force. This structurally strong bone provides protection for the globes and brain, projection of the midface, and support for occlusion. Reestablishing the continuity of these buttresses is the foundation on which maxillary fracture treatment is based.

Le Fort Classification of Fractures

René Le Fort provided the earliest classification system of maxillary fractures in 1901. His model, which is still generally used, described "great lines of weakness in the face" using low-velocity impact forces directed against cadaver skulls. The categorization and assessment of Le Fort fractures are discussed next.

Le Fort I Fracture

Le Fort I fractures (horizontal) may result from a force of injury directed low on the maxillary alveolar rim in a downward direction. The Le Fort I fracture, or transverse fracture, extends through the base of the maxillary sinuses above the teeth, essentially separating the alveolar processes, palate, and pterygoid processes from the facial structures above. This transverse fracture across the entire lower maxilla separates the alveolus as a mobile unit from the rest of the midface. Fracture dislocations of segments of the alveolus may be associated with this fracture. With high-energy injuries, the palate may be split in the midline in addition to the Le Fort I fracture.

Le Forte II Fracture

Le Fort II fractures (pyramidal) may result from a blow to the lower or midmaxilla. A pyramidal fracture of the maxilla is synonymous with a Le Fort II fracture. This fracture pattern begins laterally, similar to a Le Fort I, but medially diverges in a superior direction to include part of the medial orbit as well as the nose. The fracture extending across the nose may be variable, involving only the nasal cartilage or being so extensive that the nasofrontal suture is separated. The fracture extends diagonally from the pterygoid plates through the maxilla to the inferior orbital rim and up the medial wall of the orbit to the nose. This separates the maxillary alveolus, the medial wall of the orbit and nose, as a separate piece.

Le Fort III Fracture

Le Fort III fractures (transverse) may result from impact to the nasal bridge or upper maxilla. A Le Fort III fracture, also referred to as a craniofacial disjunction, denotes a complete separation of the midface or facial bones from the cranium. This fracture transverses the zygomaticofrontal suture, continues through the floor of the orbit, and finally through the nasofrontal suture. The bones of the orbit are separated through the lateral wall, floor, and medial wall. It is unusual to have this fracture as a single segment of bone; more commonly, it comminutes with varying combinations of zygomatic, nasoethmoid, and orbital fractures. The fractures may not be symmetric on both sides and minimal mobility may be present.

Zygoma Fractures

The zygomatic bone (malar bone) is a paired bone of the human skull. It articulates with the maxilla, the temporal bone, the sphenoid bone, and the frontal bone. It forms part of the orbit, the lateral portion of the interior orbital rim, as well as the lateral rim and lateral wall of the orbit, and is commonly referred to as the cheekbone. It is situated at the upper and lateral part of the face, forming the prominence of the cheek, part of the lateral wall and floor of the orbit, and parts of the temporal and infratemporal fossae. This bone presents a malar and a temporal surface; four processes, the frontosphenoidal, orbital, maxillary, and temporal; and four borders.

Additionally, it forms the anterior zygomatic arch. The zygomatic arch is made up of three bone components: the zygomatic bone, coming off the zygomatic prominence of the maxilla, and the zygomatic process of the temporal bone. The masseter muscle also is suspended from the zygomatic arch. The masseter muscle acts to close the mandible for mastication and speech.

Temporal Bone Fractures

The temporal bones are situated at the sides and base of the skull. The temporal bone supports that part of the face known as the temple. It is considered by many to be the most complex bone in the human body (Connell & Belafsky, 2005). The temporal bone houses many vital structures, including the cochlear and vestibular end organs and the facial nerve, carotid artery, and jugular vein. It is possible that an involvement of all or some of the structures may occur with a temporal bone fracture.

Typically temporal bone fractures are classified into longitudinal and transverse, a classification originally set forth by Ullrich in 1926, but still commonly used (Connell & Belafsky, 2005). Longitudinal fractures comprise 70% to 90% of all temporal bone fractures. They frequently are caused by a blunt lateral force over the mastoid or squamous bone. The fracture line parallels the long axis of the petrous pyramid. It starts in the pars squamosa, extends through the posterosuperior bony external canal, continues across the roof of the middle ear space anterior to the labyrinth, and ends in the middle cranial fossa near the foramen spinosum. Oblique fractures produce a similar fracture line in the middle cranial fossa but differ externally. They cross the petrotympanic fissure, and longitudinal fractures are contained within it (Connell & Belafsky, 2005).

Frontal Bone Fractures

The frontal bone is the large bone that makes up the forehead and supplies the upper edge and roof of the orbit (eye socket). It resembles a cockle-shell in shape, and forms the anterior portion of the cranium. This bone consists of two portions: a vertical portion known as the squama frontalis, corresponding with the region of the forehead, and an orbital or horizontal portion, the pars orbitalis, which enters into the formation of the roofs of the orbital and nasal cavities (Babak & Blackwell, 2005). It articulates with a number of other bones including the parietal, nasal, ethmoid, maxillary, and zygomatic bones. The frontal sinus is a pyramid, air-filled cavity that lies between the lamina of the frontal bone. The anterior wall generally is considered the strongest of the tables. The posterior wall is much thinner and weaker, and separates the sinus from the dura of the frontal lobe of the anterior facial fossa. The eyebrows and the buttress of the supraorbital rim demarcate the lower anterior border of the frontal sinus. The sinus floor consists of membranous bone that is the thinnest of the sinus boundaries and the most vulnerable to injury. The floor also forms two-thirds of the medial orbital roof. The primary purpose of the frontal sinus is to serve as a mechanical barrier to protect the brain from trauma. The frontal sinuses are positioned more anteriorly than the other paranasal sinuses and are situated to absorb anterior cranial facial trauma.

Epidemiology and Etiology

All facial fractures usually occur as a result of an injury or trauma to the face. These injuries often are induced by motor vehicle crashes, motorcycle crashes, or from direct blows to the face.

A mandibular fracture generally is caused by trauma such as a direct blow or lateral blow to the face as a result of a motor vehicle crash, assault, fall, or contact sports. As with mandibular fractures, maxillary fractures also are often the result of motor vehicle crashes. The bones that make up the zygomatic arch frequently are fractured in collisions and as a result of blunt trauma. These high-velocity injuries many times produce fracture patterns not classified by the standard Le Fort system, but are described simply by the anatomic structure fractured and the degree of comminution present.

Temporal bone trauma usually is the sequelae of blunt head injury. Damage to the temporal bone typically requires the application of great force and may cause fracture, hemorrhage, nerve trauma, vascular damage, or disruption of the middle or inner ear structures. Associated intracranial injuries, such as extra-axial hemorrhage, shear (or diffuse axonal injury), and brain contusion, are common (Woodcock, 2007). Temporal bone injuries reportedly occur in 14% to 22% of all skull fractures, with motor vehicle crashes causing approximately 31% of temporal bone fractures (Connell & Belafsky, 2005).

Other causes, in descending order of frequency, are physical assaults, falls, motorcycle crashes, pedestrian injuries, bicycle crashes, and gunshot wounds. Males ages 21 to 40 years old comprise the most commonly involved group. Transverse temporal fractures are less common, comprising 10% to 30% of all temporal bone fractures. They usually are caused by a frontal or parietal blow, but may result from an occipital blow, producing a profound sensorineural hearing loss and severe ablative vertigo. Fractures may extend through the internal auditory canal and injure the nerves directly. Cochlear and vestibular structures usually are destroyed

Fractures involving the frontal region represent some of the least common injuries that affect the facial skeleton. The incidence is 5% to 15% of all facial fractures (Piccolino et al., 2007).

For purposes of initial evaluation, frontal sinus fractures should be regarded as head injuries. The majority of these patients are victims of automobile collisions with multiple injuries requiring a multiple-specialty team approach and complete evaluation. Skull fractures are discussed in detail in Chapter 29 🔗.

Laboratory and Diagnostic Procedures

The clinical exam, facial x-ray, or computed tomography (CT) scan is used to make the diagnosis of most facial fractures. The exact location and extent of injury for the majority of facial fractures determines the type of x-ray to be used. For example, the diagnosis of a mandibular fracture is by panorex, or CT scan, accompanied by presenting dental malocclusion, pain, and a history of trauma to the area.

As noted earlier, maxillary facial fractures are described by using the Le Fort categories. These fractures almost always require surgical repair and CT scans, and the more recent development of three-dimensional (3D) reconstructions has aided greatly in the diagnosis, classification, and preoperative planning of complex maxillary fractures.

A zygomatic fracture is diagnosed with a combination of a CT scan, a history of the trauma, and from the presenting signs and symptoms. In the case of temporal and frontal fractures high-resolution CT (HRCT) of the bones is useful in assessing injuries complicated by CSF leak or facial paralysis. If transient or persistent neurological deficits are present in a patient with basilar skull fracture, HRCT or temporal bone with CT angiography is indicated to evaluate for petrous carotid injury. With fractures of the temporal bones, it is necessary to test for hearing loss.

Clinical Manifestations

With most facial bone fractures there is some overt sign of the deformity, which may include bleeding, swelling, bruising, a change in the facial shape, and pain. With mandibular fractures, patients will have difficulty opening their mouths and chewing (masticating). A patient with a mandibular fracture will have pain and difficulty with talking and chewing. Paresthesia and numbness also may be present on the affected side due to swelling at the site of injury. With maxillary fractures, the face seems to be sunken in and, on palpation, irregularities and boney stepoffs, or misalignments, demonstrate free movement. Because of considerable and extensive facial edema, the nurse may not fully appreciate these assessments. Patients will have pain, difficulty on opening the mouth and chewing, and sometimes difficulty talking. They also may have paresthesia or numbness or a sensation of "pins and needles" on the affected side due to the proximity of the swelling to the trigeminal (CN V) and facial (CN VII) nerves. Of the three fracture types, the most extensive and life threatening is the Le Forte III. With this type of fracture, airway obstruction and severe bleeding are likely. The airway usually is supported with a temporary tracheotomy. A **tracheotomy** is a surgical airway. A **tracheostomy** is the opening created by the surgical procedure. In this chapter these terms are used interchangeably.

In zygomatic and orbital fractures, the orbital contents can become entrapped by bony fragments from the floor of the orbit. The patient will experience pain, diplopia, difficulty with eye movement, and sometimes blindness. Global entrapment must be surgically corrected very early on to prevent further visual damage. Swelling to the area may mask the fracture. Patients will have pain, difficulty on opening the mouth and chewing, and sometimes difficulty talking.

The two kinds of temporal bone fractures produce different findings. A longitudinal fracture runs vertically, usually causing injury to the tympanic membrane and ossicles. This produces conductive hearing loss (negative Rinne test, lateralization with Weber test), otorrhea of either blood or CSF, and, occasionally, facial nerve paralysis. Rinne and Weber tests evaluate hearing. The Rinne test distinguishes between conductive and sensorineural hearing loss and the Weber test evaluates bone conduction; both use a tuning fork. Other findings include headache, nystagmus, or vertigo. Some temporal bone fractures are difficult to see on x-ray. All clinical findings may not be present at the time of injury, but may develop later. Hearing impairment is discussed in detail in Chapter 70 🔗.

Medical Management

Medical management of all facial fractures includes airway support, pain control, and closed reduction or surgical repair depending on the type and severity of the fracture. The patient's airway should be assessed for patency because hemorrhage or edema can cause airway obstruction. Treatment generally consists of realigning the fractured pieces of bone with wires or repairing the break with metal plates and fine screws. If fragments of bone have pierced the skin or if teeth were lost or loosened, an antibiotic generally is ordered to reduce the risk of infection.

Maxillary fractures are treated by reduction and immobilization. Surgical repair of the fractures involves plating the bones together to stabilize the bony facial structure (Figure 34–3 ■). The maxilla and mandible also may be wired together for further stabilization. Establishment of preinjury occlusion and midface buttress alignment provides the foundation for this treatment.

The goals of treatment of Le Fort fractures are to reestablish preinjury occlusion with normal height and projection of the face. To accomplish this, the structural buttress of the maxilla must be aligned and stabilized to provide the necessary support and contour to the midface. The proper occlusal relationship between the dental arches is established with intermaxillary fixation (IMF), or more appropriately termed maxillomandibular fixation. Early placement of the patient in IMF can eliminate some of the secondary deformities caused by Le Fort fractures. IMF is established by securing arch bars to the upper and lower dental arches with individual wire ligatures around the teeth. The appropriate occlusion is then determined by wear facets, and the maxillary and mandibular arch bar are secured together. This is one of the simplest and most effective forms of treatment. However, IMF is more commonly used in conjunction with other immobilization and stabilization techniques.

Recent advances in the treatment of maxillary fractures include the use of extended open-reduction techniques with rigid plate and screw fixation of the facial buttresses. Bone grafts have been used to replace missing or comminuted bone with early treatment of these injuries. This more aggressive surgical approach has dramatically improved the aesthetic results now obtainable with fewer secondary deformities.

Zygomatic and mandibular fractures are usually treated surgically. Fractures are reduced by using screws, bars, wires, and plates. Following open-reduction internal fixation (ORIF) of the

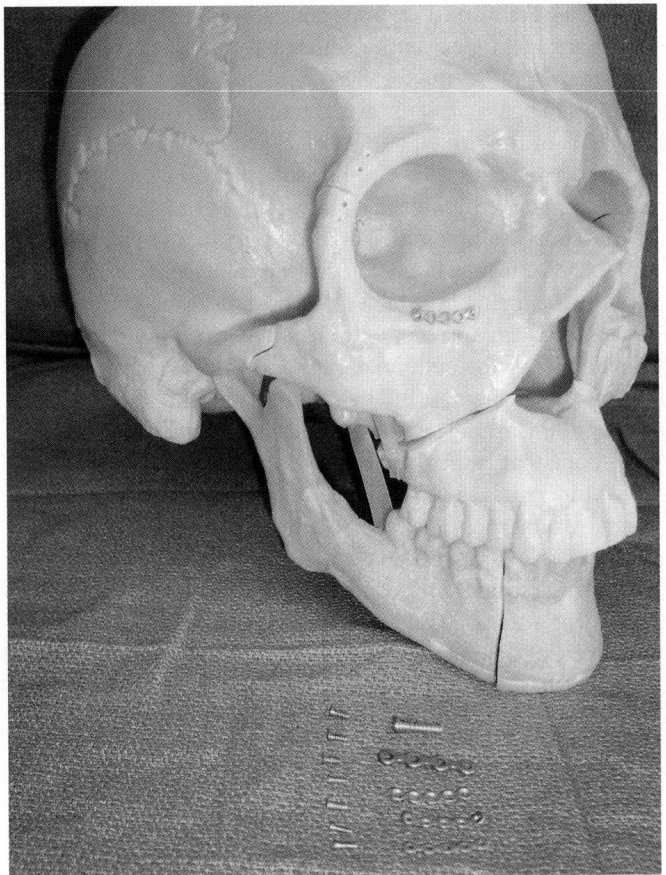

FIGURE 34–3 ■ Plating facial fractures is the current method of internal fixation. Facial plates remain in place (or can be removed at a future surgery) for at least 6 to 8 weeks until the fractures heal. This plate demonstrates the fixation of an orbital rim fracture.
Source: University of California, Davis Medical Center

fractures, the jaws can be wired shut with or without plating of the fractures. Intermaxillary-mandibular fractures (IMMFs) are repaired with wires and bands, which are similar to braces, to maintain alignment during healing.

Management of temporal bone fractures generally is conservative. If the facial nerve (CN VII) is lacerated or impacted, the patient must undergo surgical facial nerve decompression. If a dural leak is suspected, systemic antibiotics are given to prevent meningitis. Transverse fractures across the middle ear produce pain, blood behind the eardrum (hemotympanum), and a sensorineural hearing loss resulting in a positive Rinne test, and showing lateralization in the Weber test due to vestibulocochlear (CN VIII) damage. Facial nerve (CN VII) injury or paralysis produces a facial droop, loss of a blink reflex, and paresthesia. The care of a patient with a temporal bone fracture and/or a temporal bone resection is similar; the focus is on care of the eye after facial nerve resection, cable grafting, or repair. Eye protection adding lubrication prevents corneal abrasions.

The long-range goals of treatment of frontal sinus fractures are cosmetic restoration and prevention of early and late complications including acute and chronic sinusitis, mucocele formation, brain abscess, and osteomyelitis. The first step, however, is to evaluate and manage more serious life-threatening injuries. Thus, in the case of frontal fractures, the standard trauma protocol must be followed with emphasis on ensuring an adequate airway, breathing, circulation, central nervous system (CNS) status, and C-spine. Frontal sinus fractures do not require immediate surgical attention unless they are associated with a neurosurgical or ophthalmologic emergency. The choice of treatment usually is dictated by the site and extent of the damage (Piccolino et al., 2007).

There are no uniform treatment guidelines for patients with fractures of the frontal sinus. Controversies exist regarding timing and indications for surgical intervention as well as the best types of surgical ablative materials to use. For anterior table fractures, displaced fractures require treatment to correct aesthetic deformity. With injury to the nasofrontal duct, an anterior table fracture is treated with duct occlusion and frontal sinus obliteration. Treatment of posterior table fractures is fraught with controversy. Some authors advocate sinus obliteration whenever there is a posterior table fracture in order to avoid complications with undetected nasofrontal duct injury or CSF leak. Other authors recommend treatment based on displacement, or the presence of CSF leak or nasofrontal duct injury. For nondisplaced fractures, surgical treatment is not required. For displaced fractures, sinus obliteration is only recommended if there is simultaneous injury to the nasofrontal duct and/or the presence of a CSF leak (Corey, 2006).

■ Nursing Management

With mandibular fractures, the patient's nutritional requirements and knowledge deficits should be determined regarding the planned procedure and self-care after discharge. Oral nutrition with a liquid diet high in protein and calories is essential. Weight loss should be avoided if possible to ensure nutritional adequacy for healing. A feeding nasogastric or oral gastric tube may be required for nutritional support for the patient with extensive facial swelling.

Assessment

For all patients with these types of fractures, it is critical for the nurse to observe for nausea and vomiting and to intervene to prevent aspiration when necessary.

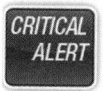

Postoperatively give nausea medication to reduce the chances of vomiting. If, following surgery, the patient vomits and is unable to maintain his airway, the nurse, or family if at home, should cut the wires to open the mouth to protect the airway. The patient must then have the wires resecured to reestablish the fracture repair.

Planning

Effective oral care is essential for healthy healing and prevention of dental complications. Patient education includes use of the water pick for mouth and teeth cleaning and dietary requirements. A nutritional consult can assess the patient's nutrition and home requirements for enteral feeding or an oral soft or liquid diet. Dental follow-up is important during and following the 6-week healing process. Chapter 14 ☉ includes a discussion of enteral feedings and their importance for maintaining nutritional balance.

Interventions and Rationales

Management of temporal bone fractures usually is conservative. The nurse must continually assess for nerve damage and hear-

ing loss. It is essential to test for any otorrhea (inflammation of the ear with purulent discharge), which may indicate a CSF leak. The nurse needs to institute CSF leak precautions which include the following:

- Keep the head of the patient's bed at 30 to 45 degrees at all times.
- Teach the patient not to bend over, strain, or lift heavy objects.
- Provide instruction about not straining during a bowel movement because this may prevent a CSF leak from healing or make it worse.

A lumbar drain is inserted to lessen the increased intracranial pressure at the site of injury and allow it to heal. If facial nerve injury is present, the nurse should provide eye care including artificial tears every 2 hours, ointment at night, and use of an eye shield to protect the eye from drying and corneal abrasion.

Patients who present with a frontal facial fracture have generally experienced other severe injuries as well. The nurse must be alert to patency of airway, bleeding, swelling, pain, and possible other injuries.

■ Inflammation, Infection, and Obstruction of the Nose and Paranasal Sinuses

Disorders affecting the nose and paranasal sinuses include inflammation, infection, and obstruction. The effect of these phenomena leads individuals to feel ill, tired, and irritable. Common disorders that fall within these categories are discussed following a review of the anatomy and physiology of the paranasal sinuses.

Anatomy and Physiology of the Paranasal Sinuses

The paranasal sinuses are the eight cavities in the skull that connect with the nasal cavity. They are arranged bilaterally in four pairs. The pairs are the maxillary sinuses in the maxillae, the frontal sinuses in the frontal bone, the sphenoid sinuses in the sphenoid bone behind the nasal cavity, and the ethmoid cells (sinuses) in the ethmoid bone behind and below the frontal sinuses. The exact function of the sinuses is not certain. They are believed to help the nose in circulating, warming, and moistening air as it is inhaled, thereby lessening the effect of cold, dry air to the lungs. They also are thought to have a role as resonating chambers for the voice (Miller-Keene & O'Toole, 2003). The anatomy of the sinuses varies tremendously from person to person. In some individuals, anatomical differences may affect breathing and block the normal nasal drainage.

The upper aerodigestive tract mucous membrane in the nose and sinuses acts to condition inhaled air. It warms, moisturizes, and filters the air. The mucous membrane creates clear, wet, slightly sticky mucus that gathers any dust, smoke, bacteria, or virus particles that may have been in the air. Tiny hairs along the membrane called cilia rotate to move the mucus along through the sinuses and out the nose. The mucous membrane also is one the body's frontline defense systems. It releases chemicals that help to destroy bacteria and viruses. If a virus, bacteria, allergen, or other irritant is strong enough to prevent the mucous membrane and cilia from functioning, an infectious obstruction can occur in any of the pairs of sinus.

Rhinitis

Rhinitis is an inflammation of the nasal mucous membrane and typically is classified as allergic or nonallergic (Quillen & Feller, 2006). Associated clinical symptoms of rhinitis include excessive mucous production, congestion, sneezing paroxysm, watery eyes, and nasal and ocular pruritus. Although the symptoms of both types of rhinitis may be similar, the etiology and treatment may vary, thus requiring a differential diagnosis.

Allergic rhinitis is considered a systemic illness and may be associated with generalized symptoms such as fatigue, malaise, and headache. It also may be a comorbidity in patients with asthma, eczema, or chronic sinusitis (Quillen & Feller, 2006). The three types of allergic rhinitis are (1) seasonal, which occurs particularly during pollen season, (2) perennial, which occurs throughout the year, and (3) occupational, which is triggered by exposure to irritants and allergens.

Nonallergic rhinitis usually is the result of a viral or bacterial infection. It resembles allergic rhinitis in symptoms and clinical manifestations, but not in etiology.

Epidemiology and Etiology

Rhinitis is common among individuals, affecting approximately 40 million people in the United States. Recent U.S. figures suggest a 20% cumulative prevalence rate (Sheikh, 2007). Allergic rhinitis occurs in persons of all races. A prevalence of allergic rhinitis seems to vary among different populations and cultures, which may be due to genetic differences, geographic factors, environmental differences, and/or other population-based factors. The prevalence of rhinitis is approximately equal between men and women in adulthood. The onset of rhinitis is common in childhood, adolescence, and early adulthood, with a mean age of onset of 8 to 11 years. However, allergic rhinitis may occur in persons of any age, with 80% of cases developing by age 20. In the geriatric population, rhinitis is less commonly allergic in nature (Sheikh, 2007).

Nonallergic rhinitis affects 5% to 10% of the population, and approximately half of these individuals seek treatment for relief of the symptoms (Ramakrishnan & Meyers, 2006). Nonallergic rhinitis has seven basic subclassifications: (1) infectious rhinitis, (2) vasomotor rhinitis, (3) occupational rhinitis, (4) hormonal rhinitis, (5) drug-induced rhinitis, (6) gustatory rhinitis, and (7) nonallergic rhinitis with eosinophilia syndrome (Ramakrishnan & Meyers, 2006).

- *Infectious rhinitis* is usually caused by an upper respiratory tract infection of viral origin. The most common causes are infections due to rhinovirus, coronavirus, adenovirus, parainfluenza virus, respiratory syncytial virus, or enterovirus. They are generally self-limiting, lasting between 7 and 10 days.

- *Vasomotor rhinitis* is believed to result from disturbed regulation of the parasympathetic and sympathetic systems in which the parasympathetic system dominates, resulting in vasodilatation and edema of the nasal vasculature. Resulting symptoms of rhinorrhea are sneezing and congestion. Cold air, strong odors, stress, or inhaled irritants may exacerbate symptoms.

- *Occupational rhinitis* causes patients to have symptoms only in the workplace. These symptoms usually are due to an inhaled irritant, for example, metal salts, animal dander, latex, wood dusts, chemicals. Patients with occupational rhinitis frequently present with concurrent occupational asthma (Quillen & Feller, 2006).

- *Hormonal rhinitis* occurs during periods of hormonal imbalance. Estrogens are known to affect the autonomic nervous system by means of several mechanisms. Central parasympathetic activity, acetylcholine content, and activity of acetylcholine transferase are increased. The most common causes of hormonal rhinitis are pregnancy, menstruation, puberty, use of exogenous estrogen, and hypothyroidism.

- *Drug-induced rhinitis* is precipitated by several medications: angiotensin-converting enzyme inhibitors, reserpine, guanethidine, phentolamine, methyldopa, beta-blockers, chlorpromazine, gabapentin, penicillamine, aspirin, nonsteroidal anti-inflammatory drugs, inhaled cocaine, exogenous estrogens, and oral contraceptives. Rhinitis medicamentosa represents a different etiology. This is a drug-induced rhinitis resulting from prolonged use of nasal sympathomimetics.

- *Gustatory rhinitis* occurs after eating, particularly hot and spicy foods. The end results are profuse watery rhinorrhea secondary to nasal vasodilation that is vagally mediated and generally occurs within a few hours of oral ingestion. Symptoms of rhinitis rarely are secondary to ingestion of specific preservatives or dyes in food.

- *Nonallergic rhinitis with eosinophilia syndrome* (NARES) accounts for as many as 20% of the rhinitis diagnoses. Abnormal prostaglandin metabolism has been implicated as a cause of NARES. Eosinophil counts are elevated in approximately 20% of nasal smears in the general population; however, not everyone with eosinophilia has symptoms of rhinitis. A distinguishing feature of NARES is the presence of eosinophils, usually 10% to 20% on nasal smears. In general, patients with NARES present with nasal congestion, sneezing, rhinorrhea, nasal pruritus, and hyposmia.

Pathophysiology

An allergy is actually an inappropriate immune response to a substance in the environment that is normally harmless. When a person with allergies breathes in an allergen, histamine and other chemicals are released as part of the immune response, causing itching and swelling, mucous production, and in serious cases, hives and rashes, as well as other symptoms.

Allergic rhinitis involves inflammation of the mucous membranes of the nose, eyes, eustachian tubes, middle ear, sinuses, and pharynx. It is a reaction that occurs when airborne irritants (allergens) trigger the release of immune mediators. The mediators that are immediately released include histamine, tryptase, chymase, kinins, and heparin. These mediators act via various interactions and ultimately lead to the symptoms of rhinorrhea. Mucous glands are stimulated, leading to increased secretions.

Vascular permeability is increased, leading to plasma exudation. Vasodilation occurs, leading to congestion and pressure. Sensory nerves are stimulated, leading to sneezing and itching. Histamine causes inflammation and fluid production in the fragile linings of nasal passages, sinuses, and eyelids. All of these events can occur in minutes; hence, this reaction is called the early, or immediate, phase of the reaction.

Over 4 to 8 hours, these mediators, through a complex interplay of events, lead to the recruitment of other inflammatory cells to the mucosa, such as neutrophils, eosinophils, lymphocytes, and macrophages. This results in continued inflammation, termed the late-phase response. The symptoms of the late-phase response are similar to those of the early phase, but usually with less sneezing and itching, and more congestion and mucous production tend to occur. The late phase may persist for hours or days (Sheikh, 2007).

Nonallergic rhinitis follows the same path of symptom development as allergic rhinitis; however, autonomic stimuli have a greater effect on patients with nonallergic rhinitis than with those with allergic rhinitis. Autonomic imbalance favoring the parasympathetic system increases nasal blood flow, edema, and secretions, creating an overall presentation of rhinitis and nasal obstruction. Changes in body posture from erect to supine can increase nasal airway resistance. In the supine position pressure is lower in the right nostril than in the left nostril when the patient lies on the right side. Temperature also can affect nasal blood flow and compliance, both of which decrease in cold environments (Ramakrishnan & Meyers, 2006).

Clinical Manifestations

Patients with allergic rhinitis typically present with rhinorrhea, sneezing, pruritus, and conjunctivitis. Physical examination may demonstrate the "allergic shiner" (dark circles under the eyes that resemble bruises from a black eye) (Ramakrishnan & Meyers, 2006). Clinical manifestations of nonallergic rhinitis mimic those of allergic rhinitis (Chart 34–1). The usual symptoms of acute viral rhinitis include an initial profuse, clear, watery rhinorrhea (which often turns cloudy later in the course of the illness), nasal obstruction, postnasal discharge, and fever. Obstruction of the sinuses and/or eustachian tube causes referred facial pain or ear fullness. Many symptoms emanate from

the edema of the mucosal membranes. Rhinitis usually causes self-limiting, but annoying, symptoms that resolve in 7 to 10 days. The patient also may express feelings of fatigue, malaise, and headache (Quillen & Feller, 2006).

Laboratory and Diagnostic Procedures

The most common diagnostic tests for allergic rhinitis are the percutaneous skin test and the allergen-specific immunoglobulin E (IgE) antibody test. Less common diagnostic tools include nasal provocation testing, nasal cytology (e.g., blown secretions, scraping, lavage, and biopsy), nasolaryngoscopy, and intradermal skin testing. Skin testing involves introducing controlled amounts of allergen and control substances into the skin. Percutaneous testing is the most common type of skin testing and is preferred in primary care. It is conventional, safe, and widely accepted. Occasionally, intradermal testing is used because it is more sensitive, but less specific than percutaneous testing.

Allergic rhinitis can have an immediate or delayed response. Skin testing elicits both types of responses; however, the primary goal of skin testing is to detect the immediate allergic response caused by the release of mast cells or basophil IgE-specific mediators, which create the classic wheal and flare reaction after 15 minutes. The delayed response occurs 4 to 8 hours after exposure to the sensitizing allergen and is less useful in clinical diagnosis.

Other tests that may be used include, rhinoscopy, and imaging studies may include radiography, CT scanning, and magnetic resonance imaging (MRI). These latter studies are helpful in establishing possible structural abnormalities or for helping detect complications of comorbid conditions, such as sinusitis or adenoid hypertrophy. Imaging is particularly helpful in establishing obstruction of the ostiomeatal complex, and in delineating polyps, turbinate swelling, and septal and bony abnormalities, such as concha bullosa.

Medical Management

A wide variety of etiologies are involved in nonallergic rhinitis. Therefore, treatment options should not be implemented randomly. Instead, they should be aimed primarily at resolving the underlying causative physiology. The health care provider also must differentiate between acute and chronic rhinitis as well as allergic versus nonallergic rhinitis before a treatment method is chosen. Rhinitis is not a disease; it is simply a term used to describe the symptoms produced by nasal irritation or inflammation: a runny, itchy, or stuffy nose. If the rhinitis lasts less than 6 weeks, it is called acute rhinitis, which usually is caused by infections or chemical irritation and probably is classified as nonallergic rhinitis. If symptoms linger for longer than 6 weeks, the symptoms would be called chronic rhinitis. Chronic rhinitis may be caused by allergy or a variety of other factors.

It often is confusing to differentiate among the types of rhinitis, thus, a thorough and comprehensive history usually suggests the correct diagnosis. Health care providers should focus on symptoms (i.e., duration, exposures, magnitude of reaction, patterns, and chronicity) and triggers. The symptoms can be similar to allergic rhinitis, but with a less prominent nasal itch and conjunctiva irritation. Symptoms also tend to be consonant with seasonal variation, environmental influences, allergies, medical history (i.e., trauma, family and treatment histories) and current treatments. An acute onset of 1 week or less has a

---

| CHART 34–1 | **Symptoms of Allergic Rhinitis** |

Coughing

Headache

Itching (nose, mouth, eyes, palate, throat)

Runny nose

Impaired sense of smell

Sneezing

Stuffy nose (nasal congestion)

Sore throat

Tearing eyes

Wheezing

limited differential and usually suggests a viral etiology; an acute exacerbation of allergic rhinitis; or, less commonly, a foreign body, particularly when symptoms are unilateral with purulent discharge.

The goal of treatment is to reduce the allergy symptoms caused by the inflammation of affected tissues. The best "treatment" is to avoid what causes the allergic symptoms. It may be impossible to completely avoid all allergens that produce the sensitivity, but one can often take over-the-counter (nonprescription) medications, which relieve mild to moderate symptoms but tend to cause drowsiness. Longer acting antihistamines that require prescriptions and nasal corticosteroid sprays and decongestants are useful in relieving symptoms. Each individual must find the correct combination of medications to treat his specific symptoms. The use of antihistamines that have a rapid onset and a long duration of action with the least amount of side effects, especially drowsiness, is effective in maintaining a quality of life in people with seasonal allergic rhinitis (Hampel et al., 2003; Howarth, Stern, Roi, Reynolds, & Bousquet, 1999).

 **CRITICAL ALERT** *Sedating antihistamines may impair driving performance as seriously as alcohol. The first-generation antihistamine diphenhydramine may have an even greater impact than does alcohol on the complex task of operating an automobile (Weiler et al., 2000).*

In some cases people may outgrow an allergy as the immune system becomes less sensitive to the allergen. As a general rule, however, once a substance causes allergies for an individual, it can continue to affect the person over the long term. More severe cases of allergic rhinitis require immunotherapy (allergy shots) or removal of tissue in the nose (e.g., nasal polyps) or sinuses.

With allergy injections patients generally receive small amounts of diluted allergy products once or twice a week. Gradually the dose is increased to a maintenance concentration, which takes about 5 to 6 months. When at dose maintenance, the timing can be increased to every 2 weeks, then 3 weeks, and then to a maximum of 4 weeks. If an injection is missed, it may be repeated at the same dosage or the patient may need to back up a few doses. Most people notice improvement after they reach a maintenance dose. Patients may receive allergy injections for 3 to 5 years, predicated on symptoms.

To prevent complications, the health care provider should review a standard series of allergy questions with the patient prior to each injection. These questions include previous injection reactions, any new medications, any changes in health status, any increase in allergy/asthma (seasonal response), and determining if the patient has taken an antihistamine that day. Following the injection, the patient is monitored for reactions (Chart 34–2). After the injection is given, the patient is required to wait for 30 minutes. The risk for reaction is reduced by selecting low-risk patients and by educating patients about warning signs. Medical personnel are aware of symptoms and treatment and should educate patients about them (Hallet, 2006). Fatalities occur in less than 1 per million injections, but they do occur.

Treatment, dependent on etiology, generally consists of anticholinergics, nasal corticosteroids, antihistamines, sympathomimetics, capsaicin, and bacterially derived immunostimulants. Elderly patients typically are treated with antihistamines (e.g., fexofenadine, cetirizine, and loratadine) to avoid unwanted adverse effects such as loss of bladder control. One alternative therapy that may be helpful to patients with upper respiratory mucus and swelling is inhalation of peppermint oil, as discussed in the Complementary and Alternative Therapies box.

Patients also should be advised to take measures to stay away from any allergens that they know may trigger a reaction. These measures include:

- Reducing outdoor exposure during the season in which a particular type of pollen is present
- Limiting outdoor exposure by keeping the windows and doors of the house and car closed as much as possible during the pollen season

CHART 34–2 Allergy Reactions and Treatments

Reaction	Symptoms	Treatment	Medications
Local reaction	Erythema arm swelling of 2–3 cm, itchy eyes, slight body itching, transient local itching	Ice elevation. Observe closely until reaction resolves. Fill out anaphylaxis treatment record in patient chart.	Antihistamines, steroids Claritin, Zyrtec, Benadryl
Systemic reaction, anaphylaxis	Conjunctivitis, urticaria, chest tightness, problems breathing, syncope, wheezing, difficulty swallowing, shortness of breath, dyspneic hives, decrease in blood pressure	Maintain airway O_2 at 5 L/min. Place venous tourniquet above injection site. Check vital signs, peak flow, pulse ox every 5–10 min. Start two (14–16) IVs bolus 250–500 mL normal saline (NS). Repeat prn for BP stability. Continue to check vital signs every 5 min until reaction is resolved. Call 911 and transport to ED. Fill out anaphylaxis treatment record in patient chart.	1:1000 epinephrine up to 0.3–0.5 mL IM Chlorpheniramine 4 mg po or diphenhydramine 25–50 mg po or IM Albuterol 2.5 mg nebulizer or 8 puffs metered-dose inhaler if wheezing Prednisone 60 mg po or Solu-Medrol 125 mg IV Zantac 50 mg IV/Pepcid 20 mg IV Glucagon 1 mg (especially if on beta-blockers)

- Covering mattress and pillow with impermeable covers to reduce exposure to dust mites, washing linens every 2 weeks, and treating carpets and rugs as appropriate
- Reducing excessive humidity and removing standing water
- Practicing environmental controls for dust mites to help reduce mold spores
- Eliminating exposure to smoke, strong perfumes and scents, fumes, rapid changes in temperature, and outdoor pollution for patients with nonspecific triggers.

For animal allergies, complete avoidance is the best option. Confining the animal to a noncarpeted room and keeping it entirely out of the bedroom can be of some benefit. For occupational allergens, as with animal allergens, avoidance is the best measure. When this is not possible, using a mask or respirator might be helpful.

Patients with intermittent symptoms often are treated adequately with oral antihistamines, decongestants, or both as needed. Regular use of an intranasal steroid spray may be more appropriate for patients with chronic symptoms. Daily use of an antihistamine, decongestant, or both can be considered either instead of or in addition to nasal steroids. The newer second-generation (i.e., nonsedating) antihistamine drops usually are preferable to avoid sedation and other adverse effects associated with the older first-generation antihistamines. The second-generation oral antihistamines currently available in the United States are cetirizine, desloratadine, fexofenadine, and loratadine (Sheikh, 2007).

Nursing Management

Nursing management of patients with rhinitis is very similar to medical management. It is essential that during the assessment phase, the nurse secure a thorough history from the patient by asking questions such as these: What are the symptoms? When did they start? How long have they been occurring? Do you know what triggered the symptoms? Have they occurred before; if so, when and for how long? Is there a pattern that can be recognized?

If allergy medications are to be administered, this is typically the nurse's responsibility. The nurse should advise the patient of what the medication involves, and stay with the patient after the administration of the medication to determine any adverse effects.

Another major component of the nurse's role is education, helping the patient identify the known allergen and how to avoid subsequent allergic reactions. In many situations this is difficult because patients are being asked to change their lifestyles or elements within their life that are very important to them (e.g., pets). In these instances the nurse acts as a support

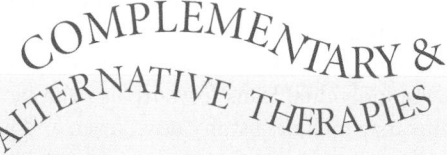

COMPLEMENTARY & ALTERNATIVE THERAPIES   Peppermint Oil Inhalation

Description:

The congestion caused by upper respiratory mucus and swelling is uncomfortable, and many seek relief from this discomfort. One CAM technique is the use of peppermint oil inhalation. This is an old Chinese healing technique in which a bowl is filled with steaming hot water. A few drops of peppermint oil are placed into the water. The patient immediately places a large towel over his or her head and leans over the vessel. The towel should cover both the head and the bowl, allowing the steam to rise directly into the nostrils. The patient then takes deep breaths through the nose, with the eyes and mouth closed. The menthol steam opens nasal passageways and loosens mucus. This is a safe technique, but the person should be careful to not make the water so hot that the steam burns. Although this technique is poorly documented in Western scientific literature, anecdotal evidence shows that it is an effective technique.

Research Support:

The peppermint (*Mentha piperita L.*) plant is one of the most widely used ingredients in herbal teas. Both peppermint tea, which is brewed from the plant leaves, and the essential oil of peppermint are used in traditional medicines. The acidic compounds (phenols) of the leaves include rosmarinic acid and several flavonoids, primarily eriocitrin, luteolin, and hesperidin. In the essential oil, the main volatile components are menthol and menthone. In vitro studies of peppermint show significant antimicrobial and antiviral properties, strong antioxidant and antitumor properties, and some antiallergenic properties. Animal model studies demonstrate that peppermint exerts a relaxation effect on gastrointestinal (GI) tissue, analgesic and anesthetic effects on the central and peripheral nervous system, immunomodulating properties, and chemopreventive properties. Human studies are limited; however, several clinical trials have been conducted that examine the effects of peppermint oil on irritable bowel syndrome (IBS) symptoms. No human studies have been conducted on peppermint tea. No

adverse reactions to peppermint tea have been reported. However, patients with GI reflux, hiatal hernia, or kidney stones should use peppermint oil with caution (McKay & Blumberg, 2006).

A literature review was performed to determine which herbs are most commonly used as CAM treatments for asthma, allergies, and immunologic conditions. Searches were conducted on the PubMed and OVID databases using the keywords that combined asthma, allergy, and CAM, plus the following herb names: echinacea (*Echinacea angustifolia, Echinacea pallida, and Echinacea purpurea*); garlic (*Allium*); angelica; chamomile; ephedra; gingko; grape seed extract; licorice root (*Glycyrrhiza*); St. John's wort (*Hypericum*); kava kava (*Piper*); peppermint oil and leaf (*Mentha*); stinging nettle (*Urtica*); and ginseng (*Panax*). The results showed that echinacea is one of the most common herbs used to treat symptoms of the "common cold" and upper respiratory tract allergies. Garlic is primarily used for cardiovascular health and relief of cough, colds, and rhinitis. Other herbs, including angelica, German chamomile flower, ephedra, gingko, grape seed extract, licorice root, St. John's wort, kava kava rhizome, peppermint, stinging nettle, and ginseng were also mentioned. The goal of this review was to alert practitioners of possible adverse effects, as the allergy and immunology fields have seen the second largest increase in CAM use (second only to practitioners who treat lower back pain). The most common adverse effect is in the form of a hypersensitivity reaction (Bielory, 2004).

References

Bielory, L. (2004). Complementary and alternative interventions in asthma, allergy, and immunology. *Annals of Allergy, Asthma, & Immunology, 93*(2 Suppl 1), S45–S54.

McKay, D. L., & Blumberg, J. B. (2006). A review of the bioactivity and potential health benefits of peppermint tea (Mentha piperita L.). *Phytotherapy Research, 20*(8), 619–633.

person to the patient. A person can prevent the symptoms of allergic rhinitis by avoiding known allergens. During the target season, people should remain indoors in an air-conditioned atmosphere whenever possible. It also is incumbent on the nurse to advise the patient of warning signs of an allergic reaction, and when and how to seek medical advice.

Sinusitis

Sinusitis is the inflammation of one or more of the paranasal and frontal sinuses, and occurs with obstruction of the normal drainage mechanism. It is traditionally subdivided into acute (symptoms lasting less than 3 weeks), subacute (symptoms lasting 3 weeks to 3 months), and chronic (symptoms lasting more than 3 months) (Kennedy, 2007).

Epidemiology and Etiology

More than 30 million patients in the United States are estimated to have sinus disease (Kennedy, 2007). A viral infection associated with the common cold is the most frequent etiology of acute sinusitis. Only a small percentage of viral sinusitis cases is complicated by bacterial sinusitis. The challenge is to differentiate a simple upper respiratory infection and allergic rhinitis from sinusitis.

Sinusitis can be caused by bacterial, viral, and fungal infections. Although the majority of community-acquired respiratory tract infections are viral in origin, bacteriologic causes are common (Chart 34–3). They include *Streptococcus pneumoniae*, *Haemophilus influenzae*, and *Moraxella catarrhalis* (File, 2005). Sinusitis may occur during an upper respiratory tract infection when infection in the nose spreads to the sinuses. It is sometimes encouraged by excessively strong blowing of the nose, thereby, disseminating bacteria. It also can occur as a complication of tooth infection, allergy, or certain infectious diseases such as pneumonia and measles. Basically, anything that causes swelling in the sinuses or keeps the cilia from moving mucus can cause sinusitis. Contributing factors, not causative, are air pollution, diving and underwater swimming, sudden extremes of temperature, and structural defects of the nose that interfere with normal breathing, such as a deviated septum (O'Toole, 2003).

Pathophysiology

The paranasal sinuses, a part of the upper respiratory tract, are in direct communication with the nasopharynx. Because of the proximity to nasopharyngeal flora, obstruction can cause bacterial infection. When sinusitis is caused by a bacterial or viral infection, a person develops a sinus infection.

Diseases that obstruct drainage can result in a reduced ability of the paranasal sinuses to function normally. For example, sinus and nasal tumors can block critical drainage pathways. When tumors, polyps, trauma, or benign growths occur near the sinus openings (ostia), the sinuses can become obstructed. When the ostia are obstructed, the normal flow of air into the sinuses and mucous drainage out of the sinuses is impeded. The mucociliary transport system becomes impaired, leading to more stagnation of secretion and epithelial damage, followed by decreased oxygen tension and subsequent bacterial growth. The reduced flow of air and mucus allows mucus to become stagnant, which, in turn, contributes to the growth of bacteria and infection. Once a bacterial infection is present, it causes inflammation and swelling, which leads to an increase in mucous production. The cycle continues and ultimately leads to sinusitis. Figure 34–4 ■ shows a picture of the sinuses that house sinusitis.

Clinical Manifestations

Symptoms of sinusitis can include fever, weakness, fatigue, cough, and congestion. Nasal congestion and discharge come first. The discharge typically is pus that is yellowish to yellow-green. There also may be mucous drainage in the back of the throat, called postnasal drip. A respiratory infection such as the common cold that starts to get better and then gets worse may be a sign of acute sinusitis. Pain or pressure in some areas of the face (forehead, cheeks, maxilla, or between the eyes) often is a sign of acute sinusitis. Pain in one's forehead that starts or becomes worse when the individual leans forward also can be a sign. Other symptoms may include a stuffy nose, fever, and an ache in the upper teeth, as well as increased fatigue.

Recurrent acute, chronic, and subacute sinusitis tend to take the following course. Symptoms are more vague and generalized than with acute sinusitis, and they last longer than 4 weeks. Subacute sinusitis lasts longer than 4 weeks but less than 8 weeks. Chronic sinusitis lasts 8 weeks or longer. Symptoms occur throughout the year, even during nonallergy seasons. Site-

---

> **CHART 34–3**   **Common Causes of Sinus Disease**
>
> Rhinoviruses
> Influenza
> Parainfluenza
> Respiratory syncytial virus
> Adenoviruses

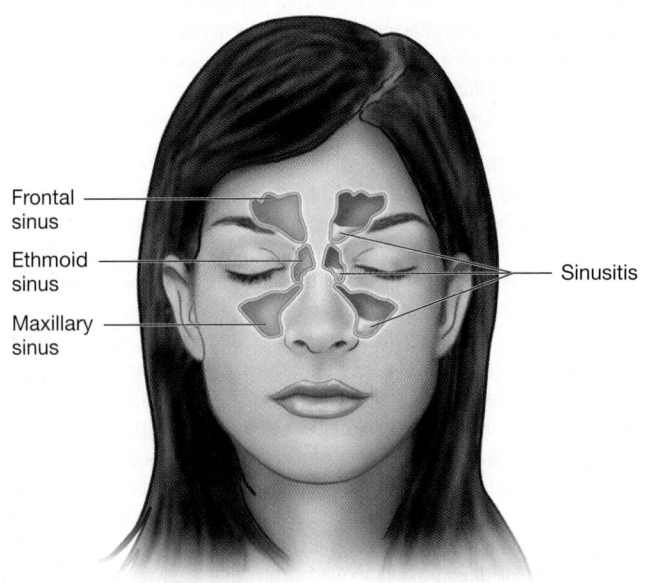

FIGURE 34–4 ■ Sites of sinusitis.

specific symptoms also may occur depending on the location of the infection:

- Frontal sinusitis causes pain across the lower forehead.
- Pain from maxillary sinusitis occurs over the cheeks and may travel to the teeth, and the hard palate in the mouth sometimes becomes swollen.
- Ethmoid sinusitis causes pain behind the eyes and sometimes redness and tenderness in the area across the top of the nose.
- Sphenoid sinusitis rarely occurs by itself; when it does, the pain may be experienced behind the eyes, across the forehead, or in the face (University of Maryland Medical Center, 2006).

Laboratory and Diagnostic Procedures

Diagnosis of chronic sinusitis may be extremely difficult because patients commonly have vague symptoms. Unless sinusitis is suspected as a possible cause of symptoms, it may go undiagnosed. CT scans are commonly performed for the diagnosis of chronic sinusitis. In some cases, plain sinus films are adequate to make the diagnosis of acute sinusitis in the maxillary and sphenoid sinuses. A limited coronal CT scan allows visualization of all of the sinuses and potentially the ostiomeatal unit. It is also possible to visualize thickening of the lining of the sinuses, indicative of inflammation, on the CT scan (Kennedy, 2007).

Laboratory tests are sometimes useful. For example, a nasal smear may show polymorphonuclear leukocytes, which are suggestive of infection, versus eosinophils, which are suggestive of allergic rhinitis. Patients with chronic sinusitis that cannot be adequately controlled warrant immunologic testing for an immunodeficiency. Such testing should include immunoglobulin levels, IgG subtypes, antibody response to common bacterial antigens, and allergy testing by an allergist/immunologist.

Medical Management

Unlike a viral cold or an allergy, acute bacterial sinusitis requires antibiotic treatment to cure the infection. If sinus symptoms do not improve after 5 to 7 days, it becomes more likely that the infection is caused by bacteria and will respond to an antibiotic. The hallmark of any bacterial infection is fever and production of pus. However, about half of all bacterial sinus infections will resolve without antibiotics.

Chronic sinusitis symptoms can be difficult to treat, in part because treatment may require the coordinated efforts of several specialists to address all of the aspects of the disease. However, in general, treating chronic sinusitis is similar to treating acute sinusitis. If antibiotic treatment fails, allergy testing, desensitization, and or surgery may be recommended. Depending on the severity and duration of the sinusitis infection, there are five main treatments a health care provider may consider: oral antibiotics, nebulized antibiotics, topical rinses, intravenous antibiotics, and sinus surgery (Strong & Senders, 2003).

Functional Endoscopic Sinus Surgery

Currently, functional endoscopic sinus surgery (FESS) is the most common corrective surgery for chronic sinus inflammation (Strong, 2006). Performed under the magnification of a small telescopic endoscope, FESS is precise enough to remove diseased tissue and bone, open the sinuses, and help to restore the nose

and sinus to health. FESS is much less invasive than older conventional surgical methods. The extent of sinus disease varies from person to person, and surgery may be a relatively minimal procedure or an extensive and prolonged operation. Endoscopic sinus surgery can correct chronic or severe blockages in one or more of the maxillary, ethmoid, frontal, or sphenoid sinuses.

With FESS the patient experiences very little postoperative discomfort and has an excellent chance of improvement in symptoms. Ongoing medical therapy controls the underlying causes of inflammation. After surgery severe chronic inflammation may take months or even years to disappear completely. Serious complications, such as blindness, are very rare, but because of the proximity of sinus structures to the eyes and the brain, risks are present. During the preoperative informed surgical consent meeting, the potential complication of blindness should be discussed.

Image-Guided Surgery

Image-guided surgery is surgery guided by CT registered guidance (Strong, 2006). Traditional sinus surgery is a complex procedure. The proximity of the sinuses to the brain, the eye, and major arteries can make the surgery risky. In addition the surgery can be disfiguring and painful because it involves making incisions in the mouth and face. Image-guided surgery, also known as stealth surgery, allows the surgeon to minimize the chances of sinus surgery complications, operate more thoroughly, and perform more difficult procedures.

A CT scan of the patient's head creates a "road map" of the patient's skull; the surgeon can then correlate the registered CT image with the position of the probe (Figure 34–5 ■). During the procedure, the surgeon places a handheld probe in the patient's nose while correlating the 3D position with the scan on a computer screen. This 3D image guidance system shows the location of the probe tip so the surgeon can safely navigate through trouble spots. Stealth technology is particularly useful if a patient's

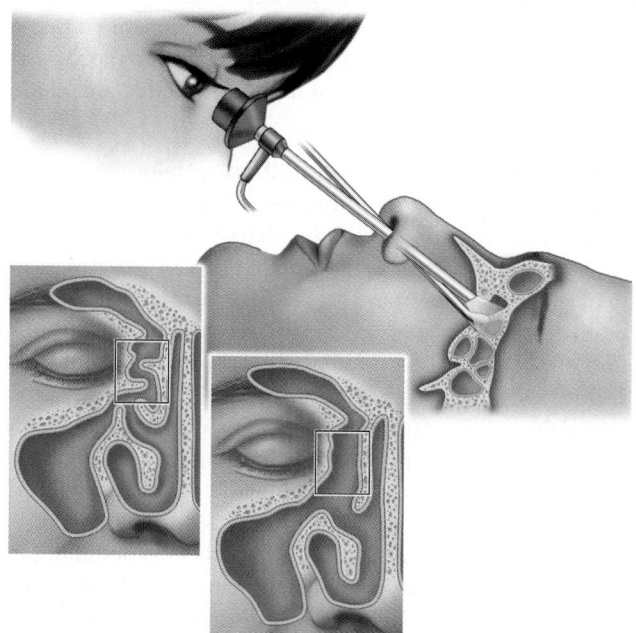

FIGURE 34–5 ■ CT registered with probe for sinus surgery.

sinus anatomy is unusual, or for "revision" surgeries, when a patient has already had one or more sinus procedures.

Nursing Management

Nursing care of the patient relies heavily on assessment of signs and symptoms, which, in turn, is dependent on obtaining a thorough patient history. The history must include the onset and duration of the symptoms including site of pain or discomfort, redness of eyes, flushing of face across the nose, fever, weakness or fatigue, cough, congestion, sore throat, muscle ache, and sore teeth. It also is important to know if any particular event or incident triggered the patient's symptoms.

If the patient is experiencing acute sinusitis requiring surgical intervention, postoperative care becomes important. This care includes educating the patient about the signs and symptoms of potential complications contingent on the type of surgery that was performed. Patient education also includes information about the cause of the sinusitis and how to avoid the triggers: air pollution, diving, underwater swimming, and known allergens and irritants.

Nasal Obstruction

Nasal obstruction may be broadly described as any occurrence that blocks the flow of air in the nose. This feeling of blockage can result from many nasal disorders previously discussed in this chapter. These include those that cause a deformity of the cartilaginous or bony structures that make up the framework of the nose (e.g., fractures, a deviated nasal septum) and those that cause swelling and infections of the nasal lining and the turbinate bones (rhinitis and sinusitis). Two other common causes of nasal obstruction are nasal polyps and foreign bodies.

Nasal Polyps

Nasal polyps are small, saclike growths consisting of inflamed nasal mucosa and sinus linings. The nasal examination reveals a grayish, grapelike mass within the nasal cavity. Nasal polyps are smooth, pear-shaped growths of nasal mucosa that are gelatin-like, semitranslucent, and pale.

Epidemiology, Etiology, and Pathophysiology

Polyps are benign, can occur on one or both sides of the nose, and are more commonly seen in adults than in children. The polyps may originate near the ethmoid sinuses (located at the top of the nose) and grow into the sinus cavities. Large polyps can obstruct this part of the upper airway. The most common cause of polyps is allergy, followed by chronic sinus infection (Rosin, 1998). Aside from causing nasal blockage, polyps may plug up the normal sinus opening (ostia) and contribute to the development of sinus infection. Although nasal polyps in children are unusual, their occurrence before age 16 may indicate cystic fibrosis.

Nasal polyps are associated with a number of conditions, including asthma, hay fever, and sinus infections. In some patients, there is an association between asthma, nasal polyps, and aspirin intolerance known as Samter's triad (McClay, 2007; Rosin, 1998; Zitt, 2003). Almost one out of four patients with nasal polyps is intolerant to aspirin. In these individuals ingestion of aspirin is followed by wheezing, excessive watery nasal discharge, and swelling of the throat, which can be fatal if not treated immediately.

Medical Management

The initial treatment of polyps usually is medical. Polyps shrink after a course of cortisone (or other steroids). If there is significant shrinkage following cortisone, then an extended course of a cortisone-containing nasal spray may keep the nasal passages clear and prevent reformation of polyps. Cortisone-containing sprays have rare, minor side effects, so they can be used safely in most people for many months under a doctor's supervision. They do not cause rebound congestion as is seen with nonprescription decongestant sprays.

Despite appropriate medication, many polyp patients require surgery to remove polyps and open the nasal passages. Surgical polyp removal, or polypectomy, can be performed in an office or outpatient setting. Although, most polyps are not cancerous, once removed, they should be sent for pathologic examination to ensure that there is no malignancy present. Very infrequently these tissues may demonstrate abnormal growth patterns called inverting papillomas (adults) or juvenile angio neurofibromas (male teenagers) (Donald, Enepikedes, & Boggan, 2004).

Although most patients notice marked improvement in their breathing after removal of polyps, they should be aware that polyps often recur. If they start to grow back in a matter of months, then a more thorough search for the cause should be undertaken. This usually includes an allergy work-up and CT scan x-ray if they have not already been done. One way to prevent polyp regrowth after removal is to stay on topical steroid sprays for an extended period of time.

Nursing Management

Nurses assist in the examination of patients for polyps by assessing and documenting symptoms, including history, length of "stuffy nose" syndrome, and other related allergy symptoms. If surgical intervention is required, nurses are responsible for pre- and postoperative care of the patient. A major focus of nursing intervention and evaluation is education for the patient as to symptoms to look for, reasons to seek medical care, and relief of pain and difficulty breathing. It also is important to complete a health history to determine allergic patterns and any signs of genetic implications.

Foreign Bodies

The term *foreign bodies* refers to any foreign objects inserted into the nose. Common objects found in children include beads, buttons, crayons, small plastic toys, peanuts, raisins, popcorn, and pencil erasers. These objects, if allowed to remain in the nose, may lead to irritation, infection, and difficulty breathing. The symptoms are foul-smelling or bloody nasal discharge, difficulty breathing through the affected nostril, irritation, or a sensation of something in the nostril. It is important not to probe the nose with cotton swabs or other instruments. Doing so may push the object farther into the nose. The nurse should have the patient breathe through the mouth and avoid breathing in forcefully, which may force the object further inward.

Once it is determined which nostril is affected, the nurse should have the patient gently press the other nostril closed and have the patient gently blow through the affected nostril. Avoid blowing the nose too hard or repeatedly. Local or general anesthesia may be used for examination and object removal if conservative measures fail.

Anosmia

Anosmia is the loss or impairment of the sense of smell. To many people, the ability to sense thousands of different odors is a normal occurrence and something that may be taken for granted. However, to a minority, this natural skill is lost due to a disorder of the olfactory system. Odors bring both enhancement and improvement of life to an individual, whether it is the smell of food, fragrances, or a scent associated with a particular event or person. More than this, smell has other functions. Taste is to a great extent determined by smell, so a loss of smell often leads to a loss of taste.

Epidemiology, Etiology, and Pathophysiology

It has been estimated that 2 million Americans have smell and taste disorders and about 200,000 visit a doctor each year (Jafek, Murrow, & Linschoten, 2000). The loss of smell usually is the result of nasal congestion, a cold, or an obstruction, but sometimes it can indicate a neurological disorder. Loss of the sense of smell may be idiopathic (without any identifiable cause). Some diminution of smell occurs normally with aging, and in most cases, there are no obvious or immediate causes and there is no treatment (Medline Plus, 2006).

Temporary anosmia is common with colds and nasal allergies such as hay fever. It may occur following a viral illness. The sense of smell also is lost with disorders that prevent air from reaching the part of the nose where smell receptors are located (the cribriform plate located high in the nose). These disorders may include nasal polyps, nasal septal deformities, and nasal tumors. Other disorders that may cause anosmia include tumors of the head or brain, head trauma, endocrine and nutritional disorders, and neurological disorders.

Many medications may change or decrease the ability to detect odors. Most people who lose the sense of smell are unable to differentiate between salty, sweet, sour, and bitter tastes that are sensed on the ventral tongue. Individuals with such a disorder may not be able to distinguish other flavors. Some spices such as pepper may stimulate cranial nerves, but may be sensed rather than smelled. The olfactory nerve (CN I) is responsible for the sense of smell. This sensory organ is located in the roof of the nasal cavity.

Clinical Manifestations

There are many definitions of the various categories of smell dysfunction. The following definitions come from Seiden (1997):

- **Anosmia**—a complete loss of smell
- **Hyposmia**—a partial loss of smell
- **Hyperosmia**—enhanced smell sensitivity
- **Dysosmia**—distortion in odor perception (includes parosmia (distorted sense of smell) and phantosmia
- **Parosmia**—distortion of perception of external stimulus
- **Phantosmia**—smell perception with no external stimulus.

In all of the categories enumerated above, the patient experiences a change in the sense of smell. Changes in the sense of smell range from a lack of smell to smelling a perceived foul odor that no one else can smell; hence, the use of the word *phantom* as in *phantosmia*. It is necessary to determine, upon assessment, what the patient is experiencing.

Medical and Nursing Management

Several methods of diagnosis are used by primary care providers with respect to olfaction disorders. A thorough patient history and physical evaluation are essential for establishing the cause of the disorder (Jafek et al., 2000). In particular, when investigating the patient's history, identifying the time that the loss occurred and whether any other conditions may have contributed are fundamental for a diagnosis. It is important to distinguish between a smell-related disorder and a taste-related disorder because commonly they are misidentified or misunderstood.

It is important to identify events that occurred prior to the onset of the disorder. Some of the questions asked to do so are the length of time of olfactory loss and whether it is an intermittent or continuous olfactory loss. Fluctuation usually is a sign of conductive loss and hence may indicate a nasal or sinus disorder (Seiden, 1997).

A complete head and neck examination is essential to determine the cause of anosmia. The examination should focus on the nose to determine whether it is a conductive or sensorineural loss. An endoscope is used to provide reliable observations. Chemosensory testing and a neuroradiologic evaluation also are used to detect the type of dysfunction a patient is experiencing.

Treatment of underlying disorders may correct the loss of sense of smell. This includes antihistamines (if the condition is related to allergy), surgical correction of physical blockages, treatment of other disorders, and changes in medication. If loss of the sense of smell is permanent, dietary counseling may include use of highly seasoned foods and stimulation of taste sensations that remain. Caution should be taken to ensure safety around the home. Smoke detectors and electric appliances rather than gas appliances should be used as should technologies that detect the presence of gas fumes in the home. The health care provider is responsible for educating patients about these cautions.

Nurses are responsible for assessing the patient's symptoms, documenting and reporting them to the primary health care provider, and providing supportive care to the patient. Education as to the cause and alleviation of symptoms is primary for the nurse. The nurse also plays a key role in assessing and evaluating the patient's response to treatment and communicating this to the primary care provider.

Mucormycosis

Mucormycosis is a rare but often fatal disease caused by certain fungi. It is sometimes called zygomycosis or phycomycosis (Beers & Berkow, 2004). Mucormycosis is an opportunistic infection that typically develops in patients with weakened immune systems, diabetes, kidney failure, organ transplants, or chemotherapy for cancer. It also may develop in patients receiving an iron chelating drug called desferrioxamine (Desferal) as treatment for acute iron poisoning.

Epidemiology and Etiology

In the United States mucormycosis mostly occurs in patients who are immunocompromised, though cases in immunocompetent patients also are reported (Baugh & Earhart, 2006). It also is most likely that patients in the United States will develop mucormycosis in the nasal areas or in the lungs; however, it also may develop on the skin or in the digestive tract. Gastrointestinal disease usually develops only in severely malnourished patients. Cutaneous mucormycosis is most likely to develop under occlusive surgical dressings. Although occlusive dressings are intended to keep the air out of incisions and wounds, they also trap body heat and moisture.

Common fungi, frequently found in the soil among vegetation, cause mucormycosis. These fungi are prevalent in nature, but may be more prone to cause infection in moist, temperate climates (Baugh & Earhart, 2006). Most individuals are exposed to these fungi on a daily basis, but people with immune disorders or diabetes are at a higher risk for developing this rare infection. Aside from these, environmental spore exposure (from exposure to construction activities) also has led to clinical cases of mucormycosis. Other cases have been reported in patients with traumatic skin injury (as with the use of non-sterile adhesive tape or with the use of tongue depressors as splints in neonates). Exposure to voriconazole, which is not active against mucormycosis, is noted to be a risk factor in patients with cancer (Varman & Whaley, 2006). The incidence of the disease is difficult to evaluate because it is very rare; however, there is some indication that it is increasing (Beers & Berkow, 2004) (see the Risk Factors for Mucormycosis box).

Pathophysiology and Clinical Manifestations

Mucormycosis is caused by fungi of several different species, including *Mucor, Rhizopus, Absidia,* and *Rhizomucor.* The fungus gains entry into the body through the nasopharynx. It can be inhaled into the lungs, or it can extend to the sinuses, orbit, and brain, with mucormycosis development dependent on host immunity. Upon gaining access to the mucous membranes of the patient's nose or lungs, the organisms multiply rapidly and invade the nearby blood vessels. The fungi destroy soft tissue and bone, as well as the walls of blood vessels. Regardless of the anatomic site involved, characteristic histopathologic findings include angioinvasion with subsequent tissue infarction and necrosis leading to tissue destruction.

- With rhinocerebral mucormycosis, the fungus destroys the tissue of the nasal passages, sinuses, or hard palate, producing a black or pus-filled discharge and visible patches of dying tissue. The overt symptoms of rhinocerebral mucormycosis include acute sinusitis, fever, eye swelling and protrusion of the orbit (proptosis), dark nasal eschar (scabbing), and redness progressing to ecchymoses of the overlying skin. General symptoms also may include headache, nausea, and lethargy. Visual loss secondary to thrombosis of retinal artery or direct fungal invasion may occur. The fungus then invades the tissues around the socket and eventually the brain. At that point the patient may have convulsions or paralysis on one side of the body.

- Most patients with pulmonary mucormycosis are being treated for leukemia and are immunocompromised. The fungus enters the patient's lungs, where it eventually invades a major blood vessel, causing the patient to cough up blood or hemorrhage into the lungs. Early symptoms of pulmonary

RISK FACTORS for Mucormycosis	
Diabetes mellitus	A risk factor particularly with poor glycemic control and acidosis as it relates to cellular immune dysfunction.
Iron overload	May be a risk factor as observed with hemochromatosis and deferoxamine treatment in patients receiving dialysis. Iron enhances fungal growth and leads to increased host susceptibility.
Burn patients	In burn patients, *Mucor* generally involves the skin and only rarely causes the rhinocerebral form.
Leukemia	Researchers estimate that the incidence in hematologic malignancy is approximately 1%.
Lymphoma	May result from immunosuppressions.
Transplantation	Infection may occur after solid organ (liver, kidney) and bone marrow transplants and in association with graft versus host disease (GvHD), severe neutropenia, or steroid therapy.
Immunosuppression	Those who are immunosuppressed are more susceptible to the fungal infection.
Prolonged neutropenia	The lowering of white blood cell count compromises immunity.
Chemotherapy	Neutropenia and immunosuppressions may result from administration of chemotherapeutic drugs.
High-dose steroids	Steroids affect metabolism and promote immunosuppressions thus facilitating the spread of mycormycosis.
Following donor leukocyte infusions	Infection may occur after donor infusions die to transfer of mucor fungi.
Acquired immunodeficiency syndrome (AIDS)	Immunosupression contributes to susceptibility of the fungal infection.
Intravenous drug use (embolic to brain)	Mucor hyphae, obtained from contaminated equipment, may invade the blood vessels and cause necrosis.

Source: Baugh, W. P., & Earhart, K. C. (2006). Rhinocerebral mucormycosis. *eMedicine.* Retrieved September 2, 2007, from the eMedicine website: http://www.emedicine.com/med/topic2026.htm.

mucormycosis include fever and difficulty breathing, with eventual bleeding from the lungs.

- The symptoms of gastrointestinal mucormycosis are not unique to the disease, which may complicate diagnosis. Patients typically complain of pressure or pain in the abdomen and nausea and vomiting.

Mucormycosis is a feared complication associated with diabetes. Diabetic ketoacidosis helps to potentiate the growth of mucormycosis. Patients with type II diabetes can present in ketoacidosis (Eledrisi, Alshanti, Shah, Brolosy, & Jaha, 2006; Linfoot & Bergstrom, 2005). The site of involvement is typically the nasopharyngeal region, but the infection can spread to involve soft tissues and bones of the face, orbit, skull, and brain. Rhinocerebral infection may start as a sinus infection and progress rapidly over hours to complete obtundation and coma. The disease may progress to involve inflammation of cranial nerves and blood vessels, causing blood clots that block blood supply to the surrounding tissue and brain (thrombosis). There is an increased incidence of cavernous sinus thrombosis and carotid involvement with rhinocerebral mucormycosis.

 *Any patient who presents in diabetic ketoacidosis with findings of orbital cellulitis and vision changes must be evaluated immediately for mucormycosis. The progression of the disease occurs very quickly over a few hours. The time lapse between making an accurate diagnosis and instituting therapy is critical.*

Laboratory and Diagnostic Procedures

Diagnosis usually is based on a combination of the patient's medical history and a visual examination of the nose, throat, and eyes. Once mucormycosis is suspected, obtaining tissue for culture is vital. Specimens should be obtained from areas such as suggestive skin lesions, black eschars found in the nasopharynx, and nasal discharge that may appear like clotted blood. The tissue specimen reveals *Mucor* fungi and the species is oryzae. Serial CT scans and MRI scans are used to identify the extent of the disorder, the destruction of soft tissue of bone in patients with advanced disease. Chest x-rays sometimes reveal a cavity in the lung or an area filled with tissue fluid if the patient has pulmonary mucormycosis.

Medical Management

Treatment usually is begun without waiting for laboratory reports because of the rapid spread and high mortality rate of the disease (Beers & Berkow, 2004). The mainstay of treatment for mucormycosis is early aggressive surgical intervention to remove all dead and infected tissue along with intravenous and possibly intrathecal antifungal therapy of amphotericin and liposomal amphotericin. Surgery is disfiguring for rhinocerebral mucormycosis because it may involve the removal of the palate, nasal, and orbital structures. Reconstructive surgery is inevitable for those who have disfigurement due to severe rhinocerebral mucormycosis. Hyperbaric oxygenation (HBO) may be indicated and has proven to be very helpful in conjunction with long-term therapy with antifungal drugs. In addition, underlying comorbidities such as hyperglycemia, acidosis in diabetic patients, nutritional problems, neutropenia, lymphopenia, and immunosuppressions must be addressed.

■ Nursing Management

The nurse is responsible for assessing the patient for clinical manifestations of mucormycosis on the first interview with the patient. Obtaining an accurate and complete patient history is essential. Following diagnosis and treatment, the nurse assumes postoperative care of the patient. During this phase the nurse should be particularly sensitive to the fear and anxiety related to possible/potential disfigurement and high mortality rate of the disease. Follow-up care includes educating patients about the signs of recurrent mucormycosis, particularly facial swelling and a black discharge from the nose, and advising them to see a health care provider at once if they notice these symptoms.

Prevention also is critical to caring for patients with mucormycosis. It depends on protecting high-risk patients from contact with sugary foods, decaying plants, moldy bread, manure, and other breeding grounds for fungi. In addition, when caring for patients in the hospital, the nurse should be careful to change occlusive dressings frequently and check the underlying skin for any signs of possible fungal infection.

■ Disorders of the Pharynx and Oral Cavity

The oral cavity, tongue, and pharynx are the anatomic conduits to the esophagus and airway. The pharynx assists in speech and swallowing and begins the division of the airway from the esophagus. The oral cavity, which includes the tongue, is responsible for ingestion, taste, and other sensory responses to food, chewing, swallowing, speech, and respiration. The tongue is an articulator for speech, a propulsion device for swallowing, and a sensor for taste. These organs are susceptible to disease, which may affect an individual's ability to communicate and take in nutrition. Disorders specific to the pharynx and oral cavity are discussed in the following sections.

Sleep Apnea

Sleep apnea is a disorder in which a person stops breathing for more than 10 seconds, typically more than 20 to 30 times in an hour. The three main types of sleep apnea are central, obstructive, and a combination of central and obstructive.

Etiology, Epidemiology, Pathophysiology, and Clinical Manifestations

The cause of *central sleep apnea* is impairment in the respiratory center drive such that the brain fails to send the appropriate signal to the breathing muscles to initiate respirations. This is the less common form of sleep apnea. *Obstructive sleep apnea* (OSA) is caused by physical obstruction from tissues in the upper airway. Air cannot flow into or out of the person's mouth, despite continued efforts to breathe. Approximately 12 million Americans have obstructive sleep apnea. More than half the people who have sleep apnea are overweight or obese (National Heart, Lung, and Blood Institute [NHLBI], 2006). OSA is usually marked by recurrent sleep interruptions, loud snoring, choking and gasping spells on awakening, daytime drowsiness, loss of memory, and concentration caused by the lack of normal sleep. Alcohol consumption makes OSA worse. Patients usually wake up not feeling rested or refreshed. Individuals at risk for sleep apnea include those who:

- Are overweight.
- Have high blood pressure.
- Have a decreased airway size in the nose, throat, or mouth. This can be caused by the shape of these structures or by medical conditions causing congestion in these areas, such as hay fever or other allergies.
- Have a family history of sleep apnea (NHLBI, 2006).

Combination sleep apnea, also called *mixed*, starts as central sleep apnea, quickly followed by thoracoabdominal movements

MyNursingKit | Video: Respiratory: Sleep Apnea—Etiology and Pathophysiology and upper airway obstruction. Mixed apnea occurs more often than central, but less often than OSA, and is treated the same way as OSA (Beers & Berkow, 2004).

Diagnostic Studies

For a formal diagnosis a patient should undergo a full ear, nose, and throat (ENT) examination and history, and a physical examination with fiber-optic endoscopy. An x-ray or CT scan of the head and neck is very helpful in identifying obstructive structures and checking the position of the tongue in relation to the jaw. The majority of patients with obstructive sleep apnea experience upper airway obstruction at the level of the soft palate (nasopharynx) or the level of the tongue and base of the tongue (oropharynx).

If a routine examination is inconclusive, the patient may require a formal sleep study or polysomnography. Although usually done in a controlled setting such as a sleep center, home sleep studies are being evaluated for their reliability. During a sleep study, several objective measurements are collected. These include oxygen saturation levels, electrocardiography (ECG) monitoring, air movement including chest wall and abdominal movements, electrical activity of the brain, eye movements, and airflow. These measures are evaluated for frequency of occurrence and physiological effect. These tests are used both to diagnose sleep apnea and to determine its severity.

Medical Management

Treatment for OSA varies depending on the degree of sleep apnea and the willingness and compliance of the patient. Behavioral changes such as weight loss are an important part of the treatment program. The individual should avoid the use of alcohol, tobacco, and sleeping pills. In some patients with mild sleep apnea, breathing pauses occur only when they sleep on their backs. In such cases, the use of pillows and other devices that help them sleep in a side-lying position is often helpful. In cases of mild sleep apnea, some patients may obtain relief from the use of a dental device that moves the tongue or mandible forward.

Severe symptoms of OSA need more aggressive treatment. **Continuous positive airway pressure (CPAP)** opens the airway and prevents airway collapse. It involves blowing air into the respiratory tract with just enough pressure to prevent the tissue collapse during sleep, reducing the number and severity of apneic episodes and significant oxygen desaturation. Although, CPAP is an effective treatment, many patients find it difficult to keep the device in place, especially if they are claustrophobic. The most common side effects of CPAP are dry mouth, rhinitis, and sinus congestion. Humidification and antihistamines effectively treat these side effects.

Patients also have several surgical options. Surgical intervention is available for those patients for whom CPAP has failed or those who are unable to comply with the rigors of home CPAP. An uvulovelopalatopharyngoplasty (UVPPP) is a surgical procedure in which a resection of the uvula and soft palate is done. This shortens and stiffens the palate. It is effective in about 40% of patients (Young et al., 2004). Another surgical approach involves the advancement of the tongue and maxillary/mandibular bone complex. This brings the pharynx forward and out of the airway path.

Tracheotomy

Tracheotomy, the surgical placement of an artificial airway, provides definitive correction because it bypasses the obstructive OSA. This still does not correct central apnea, but allows unrestricted airflow. All patients benefit from such a procedure, but it does cause significant changes in the lifestyle and quality of life of the OSA patient. Some patients require a tracheotomy to live, and extensive counseling is necessary before and after the procedure. A complete discussion of managing patients with a tracheostomy is provided later in the chapter.

■ Nursing Management

The nursing process guides the management of patients with sleep apnea. Nursing management of the patient with OSA after UVPPP focuses on airway patency. The outcome objective is to have normal airway function and relief of symptoms. Patients who undergo surgical intervention are placed on a pulse oximeter to monitor oxygen saturation level, and lung sounds are assessed for adventitious sounds. Patients who have had obstructive sleep apnea for an extended period of time develop higher pulmonary pressures due to the obstruction. Once the obstruction has been modified, the positive end-expiratory pulmonary (PEEP) pressures decrease. This can result in a condition called flash pulmonary edema, which is potentially life threatening. This change can happen very quickly; therefore, the patient is monitored closely for the first 24 hours after surgery. The integrity of the surgical site in the posterior pharynx and tonsillar pillars is monitored by direct observation with a tongue blade and flashlight. As with most oropharyngeal surgery, use of straws is prohibited so as not to disrupt clot formation with higher intraoral pressures.

Oral Cavity Disorders

Disorders of the oral cavity involve the teeth, tongue, and floor of the mouth, the maxilla, and tonsils. These affect chewing, taste, nutrition, and speech articulation. Nursing care should be directed toward maintaining the patient's oral health, nutrition, and control of pain.

Etiology and Clinical Manifestations of Hairy Tongue

Hairy tongue is a condition in which the tongue is covered with hairlike papilla due to the overgrowth of the fungus *Candida albicans* or *Aspergillus niger*. It usually is the result of antibiotic therapy that inhibits the growth of normal flora in the mouth. Antifungal agents, such as Diflucan, are used to treat the condition.

Etiology and Clinical Manifestations of Dental Caries

Dental caries are the result of the destruction of tooth enamel caused by dental plaque. Plaque, a substance formed by the interaction of saliva and food proteins, coats the teeth. Plaque breaks down tooth enamel. Deep crevasses in teeth, poor quality enamel, lack of fluoridated water, and poor dental hygiene also contribute to dental caries. Left untreated, dental caries can lead to a dental abscess and eventually loss of the affected tooth.

Etiology, Pathophysiology, Clinical Manifestations, and Medical Management of Ludwig's Angina

Ludwig's angina is a dental abscess that develops in the floor of the mouth. It is a deep neck infection involving the sublingual, submandibular, and submental spaces. Pus collects above the mylohyoid muscle in the sublingual space, pushing the tongue up and back. Posterior, superior displacement of the tongue results in obstruction of the oropharyngeal airway. This infection typically spreads rapidly through the anterior deep neck spaces. Immediate surgical intervention and tracheotomy often are necessary to maintain an airway. A neck incision is made, and surgical drains allow for external drainage of the abscess. Postoperatively, the wound is irrigated and packed with gauze to promote healing. Extraction of any abscessed teeth is important to control the infection.

Dental Abscess

A dental abscess (dentoalveolar abscess) is an acute lesion bacterial infection characterized by localization of pus in the structures that surround the teeth. Milder cases of a dental abscess result in painful swelling of the gums adjacent to the tooth in question. The tooth or, in some cases, multiple teeth have a large cavity or mandible fracture that infects the dental pulp (Schneider & Segal, 2006). Mandibular dental abscesses can progress to the floor of mouth, causing infection if not treated appropriately.

Pathophysiology

The term *dentoalveolar abscess* denotes three distinct processes as follows:

* A periapical abscess that originates in the dental pulp and usually is secondary to dental caries is the most common dental abscess in children. Dental caries erode the protective layers of the tooth (i.e., enamel, dentin) and allow bacteria to invade the pulp, producing a pulpitis. Pulpitis can progress to necrosis with bacterial invasion of the alveolar bone, causing an abscess.
* A periodontal abscess involves the supporting structures of the teeth (periodontal ligaments, alveolar bone). This is the most common dental abscess in adults but may occur in children with impaction of a foreign body in the gingiva.
* Pericoronitis describes the infection of the gum that overlies a partially erupted third molar.

Odontogenic infections are polymicrobial, with an average of four to six different causative bacteria. The dominant isolates are strictly anaerobic gram-negative rods and gram-positive cocci, in addition to facultative and microaerophilic streptococci. Anaerobic bacteria outnumber aerobes 2:1 to 3:1. In general, strictly anaerobic gram-negative rods are more pathogenic than facultative or strictly anaerobic gram-positive cocci (Schneider & Segal, 2006).

Epidemiology and Etiology

There are few epidemiological and etiological factors that are predictive of a dental abscess. No race predilection exists, nor is there a sex predilection. Dental abscesses are rare in infants because abscesses do not form until teeth erupt. In children, as noted, a periapical abscess is the most common type of dental abscess. This is because of the combination of poor hygiene, thinner enamel, and the primary dentition having a more abundant blood supply, which allows for an increased inflammatory response. In adults, periodontal abscess is more common than periapical abscess.

Laboratory and Diagnostic Procedures

An uncomplicated (i.e., simple) abscess does not require any laboratory or imaging studies, although x-rays may be taken. With a complicated abscess a CBC may reveal leukocytosis with neutrophil predominance. A blood culture may be taken to determine the bacteria before initiating parenteral antibiotics. A needle aspirate also may be done and is indicated for Gram stain and culture. There also are several levels of imaging, which may be completed for a complex abscess:

* Plain radiography represents the first level of investigation.
* Lateral and anterior-posterior neck views may be used to reveal a neck mass.
* A panoramic radiograph may be helpful to indicate whether bone or teeth are involved.

Clinical Manifestations

The main symptom of a tooth abscess is a severe, persistent, throbbing toothache. Initially, the tooth may be sensitive to heat and pressure with chewing or biting. Dependent on the age of the abscess, a patient also may have a fever, swelling in the face or cheek, and tender, swollen lymph nodes under the jaw or in the neck. If the abscess ruptures, the patient will experience a sudden rush of foul-smelling and foul-tasting fluid in the mouth.

Medical Management

A dental abscess is treated with antibiotics. If the abscess responds to treatment, no further intervention is needed. In larger abscesses surgical incision and drainage are done. General anesthesia may be necessary due to the size of the incision and the number of teeth involved or to be extracted. Intravenous (IV) antibiotic treatment continues postoperatively. Dental abscess infections have been known to spread upward to the face or distally into the neck and chest causing swelling, redness, drainage collection, and airway obstruction. These patients will require extensive surgery with wound debridement, a tracheotomy, aggressive frequent dressing changes, and antibiotic therapy. Management of an abscess also includes pain medicine to control the pain. Additional pain medication is given with antianxiety medicines during an incision and drainage of a larger abscess.

■ Nursing Management

Nursing assessment of the patient with a dental abscess is primarily focused on pain determination and observation of the wound, if present. Interventions include frequent oral dressing changes and oral packing after incision and drainage. The nurse must assess the patient for pain and administer medications as necessary or teach the patient when and how to take analgesics. Interventions include a strong educational component. It is necessary to teach the patient the importance of oral care especially after surgery. Prevention also is instrumental in patient education. The patient should be advised of how to recognize symptoms early and to seek treatment early before the abscess has a chance to become a major health problem.

Etiology, Pathophysiology, and Clinical Manifestations of Tonsillitis

The tonsils are masses of lymphoid tissue found in the root of the tongue (lingual tonsil), on both sides of the oropharynx (palatine tonsil, anterior and posterior), and on the superior wall of the nasopharynx (pharyngeal tonsil). **Tonsillitis** is an inflammation of the tonsils, most commonly caused by a virus, and occurs mainly in children. Symptoms are sore throat, red, swollen tonsils, dysphagia, odynophagia, fever, and enlarged, tender lymph nodes in the neck. Tonsillitis usually is self-limiting and treated symptomatically. However, if a throat culture reveals the cause as group A beta-hemolytic streptococci, then an antibiotic such as penicillin will be prescribed. Complications such as sinusitis, mastoiditis, rheumatic fever, or peritonsillar abscess may occur with tonsillitis. Surgery to remove the tonsils (tonsillectomy) may be necessary for individuals with repeated infections.

Etiology and Clinical Manifestations of Peritonsillar Abscess

Peritonsillar abscess, also known as Quinsy tonsillitis, is a rare complication of tonsillitis in which infection spreads to the tissue around the tonsillar capsule. Symptoms are severe throat pain, mouth breathing, drooling, and muffled voice. Physical examination reveals a large unilateral fullness of the affected tonsillar pillar and soft palate, and deviation of the uvula to the unaffected side. A peritonsillar abscess is treated with incision and drainage of the abscess and use of antibiotics. Four to 6 weeks after recovery a tonsillectomy may be necessary. This prevents recurrent infection and removes scar tissue from the tonsillar area. Nursing care should focus on antibiotic therapy, pain control, hydration, nutrition, and airway protection, during the acute episode.

Etiology of Pharyngitis

Pharyngitis is an inflammation of the pharynx, which results in a sore throat. Upper respiratory infections such as the common cold or flu may lead to pharyngitis. It occurs most frequently in the winter months and usually resolves on its own. For symptomatic comfort the patient should increase fluid intake, take analgesics, and gargle with warm saltwater. Pharyngitis from a *Streptococcus* infection requires antibiotics.

Etiology, Clinical Manifestations, and Medical Management of Epiglottitis

The epiglottis is a flap of tissue and cartilage that covers the opening of the trachea during swallowing. **Epiglottitis** is a life-threatening bacterial illness that may lead to airway obstruction. Epiglottitis is seen more frequently in children, but also occurs in adults. The cause of the infection usually is *Haemophilus influenzae* group B. The infection and inflammation affects the epiglottis and surrounding supraglottic structures. Symptoms are a cherry red epiglottis, drooling, inspiratory stridor, dyspnea, and high fever. **Stridor** is the raspy noise heard in the upper airway as the result of air attempting to move through a narrowed opening. Initial treatment focuses on maintaining a patent airway with conservative measures of oxygen, humidification, and inhaled respiratory therapy. Corticosteroids are given to reduce edema, antibiotics are prescribed to thwart the infection, and IV fluids are given for hydration. Only if the airway is in immediate jeopardy is a tracheotomy or endotracheal tube inserted. If a patient is suspected of having epiglottitis, avoid the use of a tongue blade or oral thermometer because either may cause further edema or laryngeal spasm and can obstruct the airway.

■ Disorders Related to the Larynx and Trachea

Caring for a patient with a disorder of breathing requires expert nursing care. Knowledge of airway anatomy and physiology is critical in the delivery of safe care. Nurses must advocate for these patients who often are unable to speak and breathe without assistance. Specific disorders related to the larynx and trachea are discussed below.

Anatomy and Physiology of the Larynx

The glottic structures include the larynx, epiglottis, the arytenoids, and the true and false vocal folds. The larynx and trachea are two major structures of the upper airway. The larynx is composed of four anatomic units: mucosa, skeleton, intrinsic muscles, and extrinsic muscles (Sataloff et al., 1998). The larynx, which connects the oropharynx to the trachea, is supported by firm cartilaginous structures that prevent collapse during inspiration. The larynx functions to protect the lungs from foreign substances and is needed for normal speech.

The epiglottis, which is located above the larynx, moves downward acting like a sphincter during swallowing to cover the larynx, thus, preventing food and fluid from entering the lungs. This same sphincter-type function is what allows for coughing, completion of a Valsalva maneuver, and vocalization. Closing of the glottis (vocal folds) creates a brief increase in intrathoracic pressure and intra-abdominal pressure. Rapid opening of the glottic opening allows quick upward movement of the air and produces a cough, or a bolus of air, that can be transformed into speech.

The cavity of the larynx is divided into two pairs of folds: upper vestibular folds and lower vocal folds. The vestibular folds function as protection, and the vocal folds vibrate to make vocal sounds (Porth, 2005). The vocal fold itself is composed of five layers: the epithelium, the superficial layer, the intermediate layer, the deep layers of the lamina propria, and the vocalis muscle (Figure 34–6 ■). The larynx, also referred to as the glottis, transmits air to and from the upper airway or the oropharynx

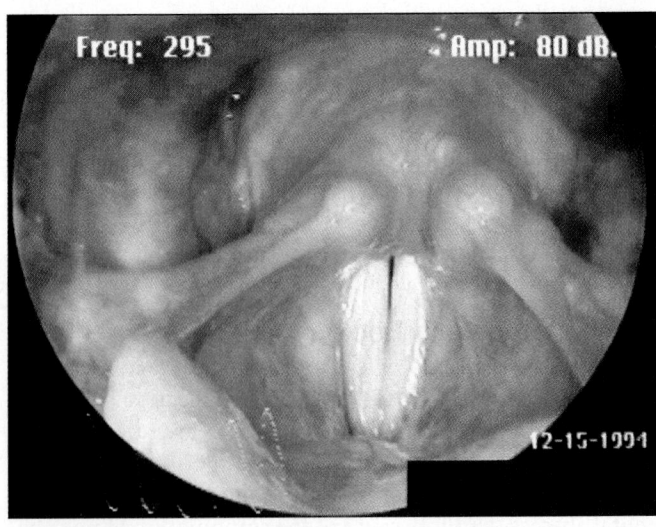

FIGURE 34–6 ■ Normal vocal cords in resting position.
Source: University of California, Davis Medical Center

and trachea and lungs. The vocal cords produce sound and the oral cavity, the palate, tongue, and lips function as articulators as the air passes through the oropharynx and mouth.

There are two synovial joints in the larynx that are of importance, the cricothyroid joint and the cricoarytenoid joint. The cricothyroid joint allows movement of the cords by changing the length of the vocal cords; thereby, controlling vocal pitch. The cricoarytenoid joint allows for the adduction (movement toward the midline) and abduction (movement away from the midline of the vocal cords during breathing, eating, and speaking. At the onset of inspiration, the recurrent laryngeal nerve is stimulated, which causes the vocal cords to abduct or open just before air is taken into the lungs.

These structures are vulnerable to trauma, disease, infection, inflammation, edema, and damage to the structures or to the nerves innervating these structures. This type of damage can result in respiratory, swallowing, and speaking disorders. The larynx is evaluated with fiber-optic laryngoscopy (Figure 34–7 ■), stroboscopy, and voice evaluation (Leonard & Kendall, 2001).

The 10th cranial nerve (CN X), the vagus nerve, innervates the larynx. The superior laryngeal branch and the recurrent laryngeal branch are responsible for both motor and sensation to the larynx. The superior laryngeal nerve supplies sensation to the larynx above the vocal folds, and motor function to the cricothyroid muscle, which helps to control vocal pitch by lengthening the cords. The recurrent laryngeal nerve provides sensory innervation to the larynx below the vocal folds, and motor innervation to the posterior cricoarytenoid muscle, which shortens and opens the vocal cords, the lateral cricoarytenoid muscle, which shortens and closes the vocal cords; and the thyroarytenoid muscle, which helps to create tension or resistance to airflow.

Damage to either one of these nerves can have a great impact on the quality of life for the patient. The location of these nerves makes them very vulnerable to damage by surgery or trauma to the neck and chest. Surgery of the larynx, thyroid, carotid, cardiac, or anterior cervical spine surgery and trauma to the chest or root of the neck may precipitate damage to these tissues. A patient with damage to the superior laryngeal nerve is at high risk for aspiration, because the loss of sensation above the vocal cords does not allow sensation of saliva, foods, or fluids as they are swallowed and drop into the airway. This is termed *silent aspiration* because patients may not be aware of aspirating until they develop pneumonia. Without the sensory innervation of the superior laryngeal nerve, the patient does not experience the typical reaction to aspiration, which is coughing while eating or drinking.

 *Any patient after laryngeal or thyroid surgery or anterior chest or neck trauma must be observed for airway and voice changes. The implication is a temporary or permanent injury to the larynx. These patients should also be observed eating and drinking and assessed for any difficulty with swallowing. This can include coughing, struggling while eating, or experiencing a foreign body sensation.*

Etiology, Epidemiology, Pathophysiology

Vocal cord paralysis is a disorder that occurs when one or both of the vocal cords (or vocal folds) do not open or close properly. This paralysis results in difficulty swallowing and coughing. Food or liquids slip into the trachea and lungs because the paralyzed cord or cords remain open, leaving the airway passage and the lungs unprotected.

Vocal Cord Paralysis

Vocal cord paralysis is a common disorder, and symptoms can range from mild to life threatening (National Institute on Deafness and other Communication Disorders, 2002).

Vocal cord/fold paralysis may occur at any age from birth to advanced age. It occurs equally in males and females from a variety of causes. It can be the result of an infectious process, trauma to the neck or chest area, neurological disorders, and cancer; however, transection of the recurrent laryngeal nerve during thyroidectomy remains a common cause (Bailey, Johnson, Newlands, Calhoun, & Deskin, 2006).

In total thyroidectomy surgery with dissection on both sides of the neck, there is a risk of damage to both recurrent laryngeal nerves, which could lead to bilateral vocal cord paralysis. Often the damage is apparent in the immediate postoperative period when the patient is extubated. The patient experiences respiratory difficulties and may require reintubation or a tracheostomy.

Due to the lengthy pathway of the vagus nerve to the recurrent laryngeal nerve, any surgery or injury involving the neck and chest area potentially can lead to vocal cord paralysis. The left recurrent laryngeal nerve is more susceptible to injury because of the course and location of the nerve through the chest. In addition to post-thyroid surgery, those patients having carotid endarterectomy, cervical spine surgery, surgery in the mediastinum, skull base surgery, or thoracic surgery are at high

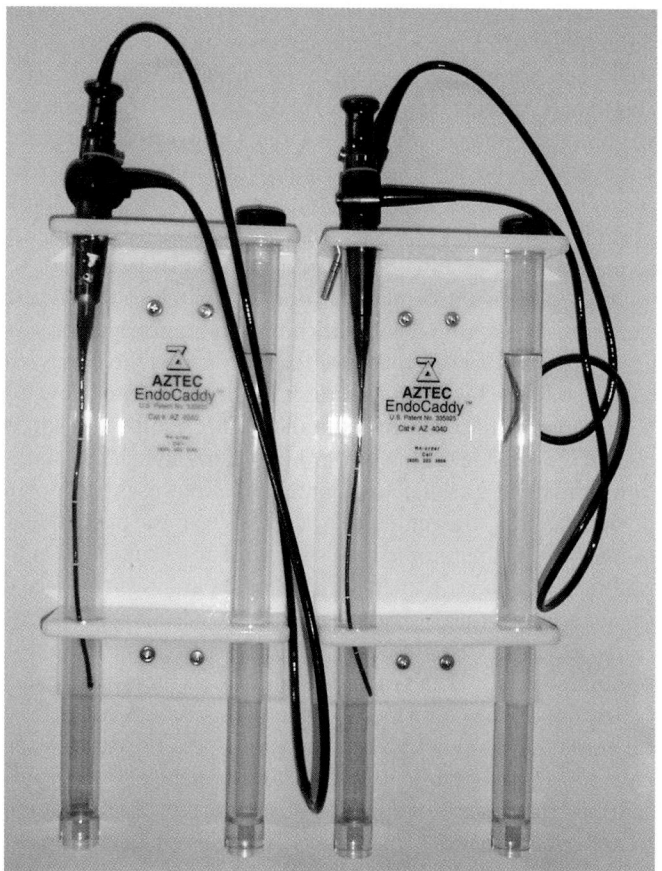

FIGURE 34–7 ■ Fiber-optic scopes for upper airway endoscopy.
Source: University of California, Davis Medical Center

risk of vocal cord paralysis if the vagus or the recurrent laryngeal branch is damaged during the procedure. If the nerve is completely severed, there is little hope of regaining motion to the affected cord. However, if the nerve is stretched or bruised during the procedure, there may be slow return of vocal cord function over a period of up to 12 months. Airway obstruction usually is not a problem with unilateral vocal cord paresis, but voice changes and possible aspiration remain a concern.

Clinical Manifestations

The primary clinical manifestation of vocal cord paralysis is a change in the voice. It may become hoarse (croaky or rough); breathy, as though the individual is exhaling excessive air when speaking; and weakened. Other clinical manifestations include:

- Shortness of breath
- Noisy breathing
- Choking or coughing while swallowing food, drink, or saliva
- The need to take frequent breaths while speaking
- Inability to speak loudly
- Inability to "bear down" while lifting (Mayo Clinic, 2006).

If a patient indicates that she is breathing normally, but is unable to speak or is **aphonic** (without a voice), suspect bilateral vocal cord paralysis in the abducted (AB) or open position. Without cord closure, the patient will not be able to speak, produce an effective cough, or perform a Valsalva maneuver when lifting or straining for a bowel movement. If the patient has paralysis to only one of the vocal cords, the nurse can expect to hear a soft breathy or hoarse voice and minimal to no difficulty breathing. When the paralyzed cord is fixed in the lateral position, the mobile cord cannot meet with the other cord, and the air escaping through the cords when the patient talks creates the breathy sound. The severity of the patient's symptoms (breathy voice, ineffective cough, and dysphagia) is dependent on the position of the paralyzed cord, the degree of injury to the cord (paresis versus paralysis), and the ability of the opposite cord to compensate.

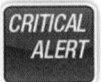 *If the patient is able to speak and appears to be in respiratory distress, suspect vocal cord paralysis. With the cords closed together in the midline, it is difficult for the patient to move air in and out of the airway. These patients may require intubation or emergency tracheotomy to establish a safe airway. If the patient is able to breathe but not speak, suspect vocal cord paralysis. The airway is open for respiration, but the vocal cords are unable to move together to produce sound.*

Damage to the vagus nerve and its branches can have a significant impact on the patient's quality of life. Because the vocal cords have an integral role in the protection of the airway from aspiration, damage here can affect the patient's ability to eat and drink. This damage also may alter the sensation of the larynx, making the individual unable to sense the insults of aspiration. Persistent aspiration can be significant enough that the patient will not be able to eat orally. The larynx and the vocal cords must be able to close completely to prevent food and fluids from entering the airway and to allow the patient to build up sufficient intrathoracic and intra-abdominal resistance to be able to produce an effective cough. Additionally, the patient's ability to communicate is affected because this nerve is necessary to allow the opening, closing, and vibration of the vocal cords as air moves up from the lungs. Without this ability the voice may be hoarse, weak, or nonexistent. Alteration in communication, method of eating, and body image are significant changes for any patient.

Laboratory and Diagnostic Procedures

Direct visualization of the vocal cord is done by endoscopy. The endoscope is a thin flexible tube with a light and camera that can be passed down the patient's throat for direct visualization of the cords to determine if one or both cords are affected. Additionally, laryngeal electromyography (LEMG) is a test that measures the electric currents in the cords. This will determine the degree of paralysis and what types of treatment may be most effective. During this test, the health care provider inserts small needles into the vocal cord muscles to measure the electric currents to the muscles.

Because other disorders can cause damage to the cords, additional tests may be needed to identify the cause of the paralysis. Tests may include blood work, x-rays, CT scans, or MRI of the head, neck, and chest. Referral to a neurologist may be necessary to rule out damage to nerves other than those of the vocal cords (Mayo Clinic, 2006).

Medical Management

Treatment alternatives to profound uncontrolled aspiration are a permanent enteral feeding option with placement of a gastrostomy tube and usually a tracheostomy. A gastrostomy or jejunostomy tube directs feeding through the anterior wall of the abdomen directly into the stomach or jejunum. Nutrition is taken as liquid supplements. However, if aspiration of oral secretions alone is causing recurrent pneumonias, this option is not realistic to prevent the problem as the insult to the larynx is not eliminated. Another alternative is to completely separate the larynx and the esophagus, similar to a total **laryngectomy**, the total removal of the larynx. This surgery provides the patient with the ability to eat without aspiration, but removes the ability to speak normally. Alternative speech is taught by speech pathologists trained in alaryngeal (without a larynx) speech.

In the patient with unilateral vocal cord paralysis with severe symptoms of aspiration and difficulty communicating, the surgeon may perform a procedure that medializes the paralyzed cord so that the two cords can meet in the midline to allow for vocalization and to prevent aspiration. The mobile cord still is able to move aside during breathing to allow adequate respiration. Different types of materials are used with this procedure to push the cord to the center. Silastic or fat from the patient's abdomen is used to plump up the vocal cord and bring it closer to midline. Patients with bilateral vocal cord paralysis may need a tracheostomy if the cords are adducted and a feeding tube if the cords are abducted, in the immediate period after injury, trauma, or surgery. Later in the healing process there may be surgeries that can be performed to open the space between the vocal cords (glottis) enough to allow air to pass through, so the patient will not require a tracheostomy, and without significantly affecting the voice quality. It is important for the patient to understand that the voice and airway will not return to normal with this procedure, but the goal is to communicate verbally and to breathe without a tracheostomy.

Nursing Management

The nursing process guides the management of patients with vocal cord paralysis.

Assessment

It is essential for the assessment to begin with identifying the patient's risk for aspiration.

Outcomes and Evaluation Parameters

The expected outcome is prevention of aspiration and the evaluation parameters include the following:

- Lungs are clear to auscultation.
- Oxygen saturation is greater than 95% or within normal range.
- There is no increase in respiration or work of breathing.
- The patient denies feeling short of breath.

These parameters need to be assessed regularly and after each oral intake.

Interventions and Rationales

Nursing interventions to prevent aspiration include having the patient sit upright in a chair to eat and staying with the patient to observe for coughing or frequent throat clearing after swallowing. If the patient appears to be having significant problems with fluids or foods, the tray should be taken away and the patient's response to eating should be reported to the health care provider and documented.

Evaluation

A formal evaluation by a health care provider and a trained speech pathologist should be done with fiber-optic laryngoscopy, and a dynamic swallow study should be completed to determine the safest and most appropriate diet for the patient. Liquid nutrition is discussed in detail in Chapter 14 . Patients with unilateral vocal cord paralysis are likely to have trouble with swallowing thin liquids safely. Solid foods, thickened fluids, or foods with a custard-like consistency seem to be less of a problem because the patient has more control of the food bolus, which stimulates sensation when swallowing thus decreasing the risk of aspiration.

For some patients their voice is their livelihood and damage to their vocal cords can create psychological as well as physical changes. Singers, teachers, preachers, and politicians who depend on their voices may be unable to return to their chosen profession.

The patient should be observed for signs and symptoms of depression and these should be discussed with the health care provider. Working with a speech therapist and learning how to maximize the remaining function of the vocal cords can help the patient physically by decreasing the risk of aspiration and mentally by increasing the patient's communication skills.

Etiology, Epidemiology, and Pathophysiology of Laryngeal Disorders

Hoarseness of the voice occurs because of the disruption of the normal vibration of the vocal cord. **Hoarseness** is defined as having difficulty producing sound when trying to speak. The voice may have a change in the pitch or quality and may sound weak, excessively breathy, scratchy, or husky (Medline Plus, 2005a). The causes are lesions on the vocal cords, lesions along the cranial nerves, vocal trauma, stiffness of the vocal cords, and a change in the mass of the cords due to swelling or growths or changes in the normal coordination of vocal cord movement.

A major cause of hoarseness is smoking and, hence, tobacco cessation is of the upmost priority (Rudy, 2006). Other common causes are acute and chronic laryngitis (Baitha, Raizada, Kennedy-Singh, Puttewar, & Chaturvedi, 2002). Any of these changes will affect the quality of the voice. Patients with hoarseness for more than 2 weeks should have a complete head and neck exam because this could be the presenting symptoms of vocal nodules or an early vocal cord cancer. Hoarseness in elderly patients is discussed in the Gerontological Considerations box.

Etiology, Pathophysiology, and Medical Management of Acute Laryngitis

Laryngitis is an inflammation of the larynx and vocal cords or just the larynx. The most common cause of acute laryngitis is a viral upper respiratory tract infection or acute vocal strain. When laryngitis occurs as part of an upper respiratory infection, the patient also may experience coughing, rhinorrhea, and a mild sore throat. The infection causes edema and inflammation of the vocal cords, which prevents them from vibrating properly.

The vocal cords may show submucosal hemorrhage and edema with any vocal strain such as after loud cheering for a sports team or trying to carry on a conversation over the dance music at a club. Any edema or changes to the surface of the vocal cords can disrupt the motion of the vocal cords and cause hoarseness.

Acute laryngitis secondary to a viral infection usually is self-limiting and does not require medical treatment. Antibiotics rarely are necessary unless there is evidence of a coexistent bacterial infection. Humidification, hydration, and voice rest usually are sufficient to allow the edema to resolve and the voice to return to normal. Symptomatic relief of sore throat, fever, and cough is appropriate.

Etiology, Pathophysiology, and Clinical Manifestations of Chronic Laryngitis

Chronic laryngitis is a result of long-standing inflammation to the larynx and vocal folds. Examination of the larynx usually

---

GERONTOLOGICAL CONSIDERATIONS for Hoarseness

In the elderly patient hoarseness can be a result of changes in the texture or shape of the vocal cords. It also can be the result of dehydration from poor nutritional intake and or medications. Bowing may occur which does not allow the cords to meet fully in the middle and stiffness decreases the normal vibratory action of the cords, resulting in a coarse and breathy voice. Arthritic changes in the cricoarytenoid joints can decrease the motion of the vocal cords. How the patient is affected by these changes depends on the severity of the decreased motion and how it manifests in the patient.

reveals redness of the true vocal cords and possibly edema. Causes include frequent inhalation of smoke, chemicals, and pollens, and exposure to gastric acids in patients with reflux disease, or mechanical irritation from frequent coughing or throat clearing, whether due to any of the just-mentioned exposures to irritants or simply as a bad habit.

Chronic irritation can lead to a chronic inflammatory state clinically presenting as a hoarse voice and a barking cough. Individuals who overuse and abuse their voices such as loud screaming sports fans or singers, teachers, preachers, and politicians who use their voice for long periods at a time day after day may develop forms of chronic irritation and inflammation to their vocal cords. Speech therapy is indicated for the person to learn to speak and project their voices in a nontraumatic method through education in the techniques of voice control.

Medical Management

The health care provider should obtain a thorough medical history from any patient presenting with a hoarse voice. This includes observing specific qualities of the voice such as coarse, raspy, breathy, or a quivering quality. Assessment of the patient's troublesome or stridorous breathing should be completed. It is essential to determine and report the use of any accessory muscles of respiration, because this indicates respiratory distress.

It is important to ask the patient how much difficulty he is having breathing and whether this has been a rapid or slow-onset change. The health care provider should attempt to elicit any potentially triggering events leading up to the change in voice. This is accomplished by inquiring if the patient has had a viral or bacterial illness or if this is a result of voice abuse or trauma. Assess smoking and secondhand smoke exposure and work history. Document the patient's environmental exposure to paint, chemicals, fertilizers, pets, or cleaning solutions. Answers to questions about these topics can assist in focusing in on the cause of hoarseness. Hoarseness is treated with voice rest, hydration, humidification, changes in voicing practices, or removal of the known inhaled irritant. Referral to a speech pathologist trained in voice is important.

Health Promotion

Instructions regarding voice rest must be reinforced for patients with laryngitis. Instruct the patients that if she must speak in an emergency to use a regular speaking voice and not whisper. Whispering is more strenuous on the vocal cords than speaking in a normal voice and, thus, can exacerbate the problem. The patient should be instructed to carry a notepad and pen or a handheld communication device. If the patient is in the hospital for any condition that requires strict voice rest, a sign should be placed above the patient's bed indicating "Patient Is on Voice Rest." This alerts the staff and visitors entering the room that the patient is not to speak. If clerks at the nurses' station answering the call light understand that the patient is on voice rest, they can say "I know you cannot speak, therefore I am paging your nurse to come to your room now" to reassure patients that their call has been acknowledged.

Patients should be instructed to avoid inhaling irritants if this is the cause of the chronic inflammation. It also is important to stress the importance of smoking cessation (Rudy, 2006). Refer the patient to a smoking cessation program and instruct

to avoid exposure to secondhand smoke (Wynd, 2006). It may be necessary to wear a mask in the workplace if there are irritating substances in the environment. Encourage the patient to work with the occupational health nurse at the worksite and to find protective equipment to prevent further exposure to those substances.

Etiology and Clinical Manifestations of Edema of the Larynx

Laryngeal edema is defined as swelling in any region of the larynx. There are a variety of causes including allergic reactions, gastroesophageal reflux disease, laryngopharyngeal reflux disease, and endotracheal intubation. Allergic reaction is a common inflammatory response that potentially can lead rapidly to airway obstruction. Laryngeal edema usually is of sudden onset and results from exposure to a specific allergen. Common precipitators are bee stings, foods, or medicines. The edema may be mild at first, causing hoarseness and a scratchy sensation in the throat. Rapid progression to airway obstruction can develop if the patient is particularly sensitive to the allergen or has a significant exposure to a target food or medication. When airway obstruction occurs, it becomes a medical emergency.

Medical and Nursing Management

The priority for nursing management of edema to the larynx is to summon medical assistance and support the patient's airway until expert assistance arrives. The nurse should place a tracheostomy insertion tray at the bedside, elevate the head of the bed, monitor oxygen saturations, and provide supplemental oxygen. An IV line should be inserted to administer medications, which may include IV steroids and antihistamines. Epinephrine given subcutaneously or in aerosolized form via nebulizer treatments typically is effective. If the obstruction is severe and the patient does not respond rapidly enough to medications, a tracheotomy can establish an airway until the edema resolves.

Patients with allergies to medication should be given information on how to obtain a medic alert bracelet indicating the medication to which they are allergic. If they are taken ill and are unable to speak, the alert tag can speak for them. A patient with a bee sting allergy should, in addition to the medic alert information, be given an EpiPen auto-injector with instructions. An EpiPen is a dose of epinephrine that the patient or family injects into the subcutaneous tissue to help decrease the histamine release initiated by exposure to the allergen. The patient may feel better after the injection, but should still get medical help for follow-up treatment. EpiPen use is discussed in detail in Chapter 60 .

Etiology, Pathophysiology, Clinical Manifestations, and Medical Management of Vocal Cord Pathology

Vocal cord nodules, also called "singer's" or "screamer's" nodes, are a result of chronic microtrauma from vocal strain, and generally can be thought of as scars or calluses on the vocal cords (Figure 34–8 ■). The nodules develop initially from submucosal hemorrhages resulting from an impact injury between the cords. The nodule may appear as a red edematous area on the cord, but

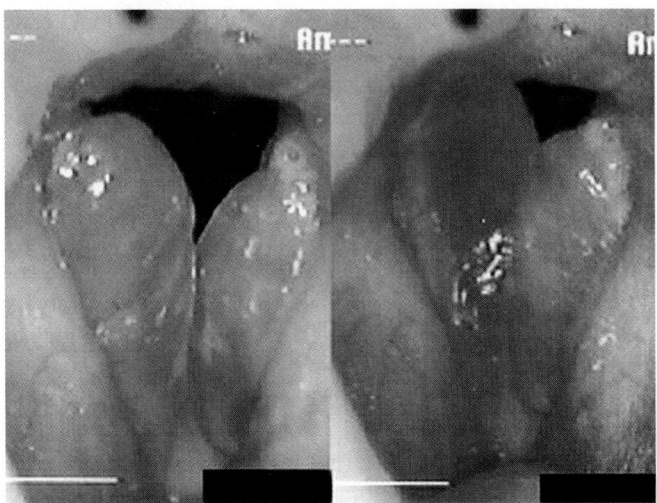

FIGURE 34–8 ■ Vocal cord nodules/vocal hemorrhage/abuse.
Source: University of California, Davis Medical Center

with continued trauma to the area, it becomes thick and fibrosed. Vocal cord nodules typically occur in individuals who abuse their voices such as cheerleaders, singers, teachers, bartenders, coaches, and politicians. These nodules, though painless, produce persistent hoarseness as they inhibit normal vibration and closure of the vocal cords. The patient will present with complaints of painless hoarseness, inability to sing in the higher ranges, inability to speak for a long period of time, or always have a breathy voice. Typically the nodules will resolve with humidification, hydration, voice rest, and treatment by a speech therapist to correct the underlying abuse issues. Some patients require surgical removal of the nodules.

Etiology, Pathophysiology, Clinical Manifestations, and Medical Management of Vocal Cord Polyps

A vocal cord polyp is a growth that typically occurs only on one side of the vocal cord, in a variety of shapes and sizes. Vocal cord polyps are a result of long-term vocal abuse or chronic irritation. The main causative factors include smoking, voice strain, and gastric reflux. What begins as microhemorrhages on the vocal folds turns into polyps, cystlike growths filled with a gelatinous material. Indirect laryngoscopy demonstrates significant vocal cord edema but no redness. Hoarseness occurs due to the disruption of the vibration of the cord, and breathiness develops due to incomplete closure of the cords due to the polyp. Treatment for polyps is voice therapy and often surgery with microlaryngoscopy to remove the polyp.

Because polyps may return after surgical removal if the same predisposing conditions exist, postoperative treatment must include treatment of the underlying etiologic factors to help prevent recurrence and speech therapy. Smoking cessation is encouraged; the patient must be offered information on programs and support groups at the health care facility or in the community.

Individuals who have polyps resulting from chronic vocal abuse should be instructed that humidification, hydration, and voice rest are necessary. These patients will benefit from an evaluation by a speech therapist, which serves to direct treatment at correcting the underlying causes for vocal strain. Patients who develop polyps as a result of laryngopharyngeal reflux, discussed later, require changes in diet and lifestyle, weight reduction, medical management, or surgical management.

Etiology, Epidemiology, Pathophysiology, and Medical Management of Laryngeal Papillomas

Laryngeal papillomas are benign laryngeal growths associated with the human papilloma virus. Although, laryngeal papillomas can affect any age group, it is children who seem to have the most aggressive form in terms of recurrence, spread, and requirements for frequent intervention. As the child approaches puberty, sometimes the severity and recurrences of the disease slow down.

The papillomas can be widespread, and patients present with hoarseness and, if severe, progressive respiratory distress. Treatment of this disorder involves carbon dioxide (CO_2) laser ablation of the papillomas during laryngoscopy. Despite frequent surgical interventions the papillomas may recur or spread. It is important to keep the papillomas from becoming large enough to cause airway obstruction. Placing a tracheostomy tube in a patient with laryngeal papillomas should be avoided to prevent spreading of the disease to the trachea. If the papillomas spread to the trachea, bronchial tree, and lungs, the disease usually is fatal.

Etiology, Pathophysiology, Clinical Manifestations, and Medical Management of Laryngeal Spasm

Laryngeal spasm is an abnormal reflexive response to a laryngeal insult. The laryngeal glottis reflexively closes with a swallow to protect the airway from aspiration of food or fluids. Laryngospasm is an abnormal response to this reflex. It may occur spontaneously or be triggered by certain foods, inhalants, or by reflux at night. After extubation of a laryngeal tube, patients also may experience laryngospasm. Although the episodes usually are transient (lasting several seconds to several minutes), this period of respiratory distress is quite disturbing to the patient. Although the patient may be stridorous and unable to speak (aphonic), these episodes usually are not associated with severe hypoxia or loss of consciousness.

Effective interventions include keeping the offending food or environmental stimulants (chemicals, cleaners, or perfumes) away from the patient in order to avoid triggering a spasm. If the laryngeal spasm occurs at night as a result of reflux, educate the patient regarding diet and lifestyle changes as discussed later in the section on laryngopharyngeal reflux disease.

Etiology and Clinical Manifestations of Laryngeal Injury

Laryngeal injury usually is the result of blunt trauma to the neck. Scenarios include a patient arriving in the emergency room after a motor vehicle crash, a child who has been thrown over and hits the handle bars of his bike, a softball player getting hit in the neck by a ball, a patient attempting suicide via hanging, or assault victims with strangulation injuries. The patient's symptoms and physical findings on examination may initially seem benign, and if the clinician is not aware of the potential complications of a direct blow to the larynx, a patient could conceivably be seen in the emergency department, discharged home, and then develop significant and life-threatening airway obstruction after discharge.

 CRITICAL ALERT *Symptoms that have developed over a period of hours may progress to full obstruction very quickly.*

Initially patients presenting with no acute airway obstruction may develop obstruction hours later as the edema increases. In a stable patient with an adequate airway on admission, the initial evaluation includes a transnasal fiber-optic laryngoscopy to assess for fractures of the cartilage of the anterior neck and larynx, the functioning of the vocal cords, and any other internal damage from the trauma. Additional work-up may include a CT scan, a barium swallow, and an endoscopy.

If the blow is severe and the patient develops laryngeal edema rapidly, there may be a complaint of pain with swallowing, and a notable change in voice quality. The patient's breathing may be labored and sound stridorous, and the patient may complain of neck pain or coughing of blood (hemoptysis). On physical exam the thyroid cartilage notch or "Adam's apple" may not be visible and may be tender on palpation. Subcutaneous crepitus in the neck indicates leakage of air from the aerodigestive tract into the tissue of the neck, often due to a tear in the laryngeal mucosa. Hemoptysis is an ominous sign of mucosal tears and needs to be reported to the health care provider.

Swelling may come on slowly and progression to airway compromise or obstruction may be subtle. If a cartilage fracture of the larynx penetrates into or obstructs the airway or swelling occurs rapidly, the patient will immediately demonstrate signs of airway distress. Securing and maintaining an airway at this point is of utmost importance. When there is a strong suspicion of a fracture to the larynx, the nurse should prepare to assist with placement of a tracheostomy tube. Patients with suspected laryngeal injury should not be intubated because this may create further damage to the fragments of laryngeal cartilage or be difficult due to the vocal cord edema. It is critical to establish an effective airway first, then examine the larynx more thoroughly and stabilize the fracture for repair.

Laboratory and Diagnostic Procedures and Medical Management

Due to the vital structures and function in the anterior neck, any laryngeal injury must be fully investigated. The patient's ability to protect the airway must be determined as well as the ability to take in nutrition. The Diagnostic Tests for Laryngeal Injury and Disease box outlines the tests needed to determine injury and function.

A speech therapist trained in dysphagia can determine the type of diet, position for eating, and safety while eating. Examples of strategies include double swallowing, holding the breath while swallowing, coughing after each swallow, and positioning the head to the unaffected side to best protect the airway from aspiration. Sometimes just changing the thickness of the liquids the patient drinks can decrease the risk of aspiration. With thicker fluids, the patient has more control of the liquid as it is swallowed, thus helping to reduce the incidence of aspiration.

Although the majority of patients presenting to the emergency department (ED) with laryngeal trauma have experienced blunt trauma to the neck, patients may arrive in the ED with laryngeal injury secondary to intentional or accidental ingestion of caustic chemicals (lye, ammonia, bleach, Lysol), thermal burns from ingestion of hot food or liquids, or inhalation of hot air or gases. Patients should *not* be encouraged to vomit because aspiration of a caustic substance can lead to further damage to healthy airway tissues. Laryngeal injury after radiation treatment also can occur because radiation weakens the tissue and causes irritation; inflammation and stenosis also can occur as a result of the radiation therapy. Airway stabilization is the first priority in these patients because the most common

DIAGNOSTIC TESTS for Laryngeal Injury and Disease

Test	Expected Abnormality/Findings	Rationale for Abnormality
Flex scope	Revealed fixation of the left vocal cord in the open or abducted position. Decreased sensation throughout the left side of the larynx as evidenced by no response to touch with the scope.	Any injury to the anterior neck demands an inspection of the larynx.
Videostroboscopy	Decreased movement on the right side and no movement on the left side of the larynx. No mucosal wave.	Evaluate movement of the vocal folds. Test is done at postinjury day 14 to allow for swelling to dissipate and have a more accurate exam.
Dynamic swallow study	Timing delayed to 2.0 seconds (WNL 1.0 seconds). Oropharynx and oral cavity: normal transition of bolus to pharynx. Obvious pooling in the vallecula and pyriform sinus on the L side of the larynx and pharynx.	Objectively evaluate the patient's ability to protect her airway and ability to safely take oral nutrition. Establish safe methods of compensation and rehabilitation.
CT Scan	Injury to the structural support of the larynx, fracture of the thyroid cartilage. Significant soft tissue damage.	Evaluate the structure of the larynx used predominantly for soft tissue.
MRI scan	Injury to the structural support of the larynx. Fracture of the thyroid cartilage.	Evaluate the structure of the larynx used predominantly for bony structural and organ definition.

cause of severe respiratory distress in patients with caustic ingestion is supraglottic swelling (Calhoun, Eibling, & Wax, 2001). Endotracheal intubation with direct visualization by the oral route is preferred. The procedure of nasotracheal intubation is contraindicated because of the high risk of tracheal, pharyngeal, and esophageal perforation (Calhoun et al., 2001).

Endotracheal (ET) tube intubation may cause laryngeal trauma (Maktabi, Smith, & Todd, 2003). The placement of an ET tube may induce laryngeal swelling, which is a cause of upper airway obstruction after extubation (Tanaka, Isono, Ishikawa, Sato, & Nishino, 2003). Endotracheal intubation can result in laryngeal injury either at the time of insertion, or secondary to prolonged intubation or intubation with an inappropriately sized endotracheal tube. The acute complications include perforation or laceration of the trachea or esophagus, bleeding, and arytenoid dislocation. The arytenoid cartilages are attached to the upper edge of the cricoid cartilage and to the posterior cricoarytenoid muscles that are responsible for abducting, or opening, the vocal cords. Damage here can lead to speech and swallowing problems.

Routine tracheal intubation also produces mucosal changes in the airway (Tanaka et al., 2003). The long-term complications associated with endotracheal intubation include laryngeal, subglottic, and tracheal stenosis as well as vocal cord paralysis. Irritation and inflammation to the subglottic and upper tracheal mucosa most often are caused by the cuff on the ET tube. Before the advent of low-pressure endotracheal and tracheal cuffs, tracheal stenosis and tracheal esophageal fistulas were not uncommon in patients requiring long-term intubation. A **fistula** is a communication between two specific areas such as the oral cavity and the skin, or trachea and esophagus. Today, damage secondary to high cuff pressure is less of a problem than irritation and inflammation from the cuff on an improperly secured ET tube. This inflammation can cause subsequent scarring and subglottic stenosis.

To prevent any or all of the long-term complications of intubation, it is important that all health professionals who perform direct care of patients with ET tubes ensure the tube remains properly positioned and secured in place. Unnecessary movement of the tube can irritate and inflame the laryngeal tissue. Sedation of the patient may be necessary if the patient is restless due to withdrawal from alcohol or drugs or as a result of anxiety, pain, or head trauma. The risk of laryngeal or tracheal long-term complications can be reduced by changing the patient to a tracheostomy tube if intubation is anticipated to be necessary for longer than 7 to 14 days (Harris & Huntoon, 2007). Tracheostomy is an effective method of establishing an airway and has fewer complications than long-term endotracheal intubation.

Laryngopharyngeal Reflux Disease

Etiology, Pathophysiology, and Clinical Manifestations

The etiology of **laryngopharyngeal reflux disease (LPRD)** is reflux of gastric acid into the larynx. The reflux occurs when there is intermittent relaxation of the lower esophageal sphincter (LES). Patients with this problem most often seek medical care because of hoarseness and throat irritation rather than heartburn symptoms. Upon further questioning the patient may say,

"It feels like something is in my throat and I seem to be clearing my throat a lot." Typical clinical manifestations include:

- Hoarseness
- Chronic (ongoing) cough
- Frequent throat clearing
- Pain or sensation in throat
- Feeling of a lump in throat
- Problems while swallowing
- Bad/bitter taste in mouth (especially in morning)
- Asthma-like symptoms
- Referred ear pain
- Postnasal drip
- Difficulty with high notes when singing.

Laboratory and Diagnostic Procedures

Usually the diagnosis of LPRD is based on the patient's symptom history and examination of the larynx. Twenty-four-hour pharyngoesophageal pH monitoring is the gold standard for monitoring reflux events associated with LPRD (Belafsky, 2006). A tube with dual pH probes monitors the pH in the patient's esophagus. The pH monitor records values just below the upper esophageal sphincter and just above the LES. Patients are instructed to eat and drink normally and include foods that they know cause symptoms of indigestion. The patient wears the monitor for 24 hours and records any incidence of discomfort, throat irritation, or heartburn, and the time of occurrence. The recordings are reviewed to determine how many reflux episodes reached the upper pH monitor and how long and how acidic those exposures were.

If a patient complains of persistent hoarseness, a transnasal fiber-optic laryngoscopy or indirect laryngoscopy is used to assess the condition of the larynx. The vocal cords and arytenoids appear edematous and red on patients with this disease. During the fiber-optic exam, the health care provider or a specially trained speech pathologist can show the patient evidence of the irritation the gastric acid is having on her larynx. A videotape of the exam is an excellent teaching model.

Medical Management

The three major methods of treating LPRD are (1) behavioral and lifestyle changes, (2) medication, and (3) surgical intervention. It is necessary to teach the patient dietary and lifestyle changes that can decrease the incidence of laryngopharyngeal reflux. These include teaching the patient not to eat for 3 hours before bedtime and to avoid:

- Eating aggravating foods such as chocolate and peppermint (which are known to relax the LES)
- Fatty foods
- Substances that tend to increase the production of gastric acid such as caffeine, alcohol, milk, and nicotine
- Spicy, acidic, and tomato-based foods such as Mexican or Italian food
- Acidic fruit juices such as orange juice, grapefruit juice, or cranberry juice.

Elevating the head of the bed by 6 inches has been shown to decrease the incidence of reflux episodes and increase acid clearance (Belafsky, 2006). Using extra pillows to elevate the head actually may worsen the reflux by increasing intra-abdominal pressure. If the person is overweight, weight loss is imperative, and clothes that fit tightly around the waist should be avoided because this increases intra-abdominal pressure and, therefore, increases the incidence and severity of gastric acid reflux.

When diet and lifestyle changes are ineffective or when the edema and irritation are significant on physical exam, medications that neutralize the gastric acid, increase gastric emptying, or decrease the secretion of gastric acids help lessen the exposure of caustic acids to the sensitive tissues of the larynx. Medical management for LPRD is necessary for much longer than for gastroesophageal reflux disease because the tissues of the larynx are much more sensitive to the gastric acid and, therefore, take longer to respond to therapy and heal completely.

A surgical option is available for patients who fail dietary, lifestyle changes, and medical management, and who have a weak lower esophageal sphincter on esophageal manometry. Laparoscopic Nissen fundoplication tightens the LES, making it more difficult for the gastric acid to reflux into the esophagus and larynx. Combined medical and surgical treatment is curative for LPRD. The cessation of acid reflux into the larynx is the definitive goal of therapy.

Nursing Management

Nursing management of patients with laryngopharyngeal reflux disease depends on the severity of the disorder and the patient's general state of health. The nursing process guides the management of these patients.

Assessment

The nurse begins with an in-depth assessment of the patient with airway being the first priority. Any difficulty with breathing and gas exchange must be addressed immediately. Nursing assessment of the airway includes gathering both objective and subjective data. Objective data include lungs sounds, oxygen saturation levels, and respiratory rate and depth. Subjective data include a report of increasing difficulty breathing or shortness of breath.

Outcomes and Evaluation Parameters

Outcomes for these patients should be a treatment plan that allows for a resolution of the symptoms of laryngopharyngeal reflux disease. The patient should be experiencing clear lung sounds, respiratory rate and depth within normal limits, and O_2 sats within the normal range.

Evaluation

In the case of patients with intentional ingestion of caustic substances, it is imperative that plans for a psychiatric evaluation and follow-up be in place before patient discharge. It is essential for the patient to be allowed to communicate fears and concerns and for the nurse to provide comfort and reassurance as appropriate. Encourage patience when communication is difficult or not immediately understood, and share that this can be a frustrating experience for family and friends as well.

Nutritional evaluation by the dietician is important for the patient with LPRD. Patients with severe dysphagia or unhealed esophageal burns and erosions will need nutritional supplementation through a gastrostomy tube to allow the damaged tissue to heal and the patient to receive adequate nutrition to aid the healing process.

Health Promotion

Patients with LPRD have a difficult time understanding how they can have irritation in the throat without experiencing irritation in the esophagus. It needs to be explained that the tissue of the larynx is much more sensitive to the acids from the stomach than the esophagus; therefore, it does not take as much exposure to create irritation in the throat as it does in the esophagus. It is important for the patient to understand the correlation between reflux disease and hoarseness. If the patient does not understand this connection, there may be reluctance to initiate the medication and dietary and lifestyle modifications required to treat this disease.

Airway Obstruction

Airway obstruction is a potentially life-threatening event that requires immediate and skilled intervention. It is imperative to determine the cause of the obstruction in order to intervene and prevent a worsening of the obstruction. The obstruction could be caused by a variety of situations, such as a foreign object, allergy, lesions, stenosis, and swelling.

Etiology and Clinical Manifestations

Specific causes include viral and bacterial infections; fire or inhalation burns; allergic responses to foods, medications, or bee stings; and infections after dental extraction that have a large amount of swelling. Other causes include laryngeal trauma secondary to a motor vehicle crash, strangulation, nerve damage to the vocal cords during a surgical procedure or intubation, or a cancerous tumor large enough to press on the nerves or structures of the larynx or trachea or to physically narrow the airway opening. Aspiration of food material also is a cause of airway obstruction. Large boluses as well as small pieces of food, such as peanuts, can partially or totally obstruct the airway. In patients who have altered sensation or anatomy, talking while eating may cause aspiration. This can present acutely or as a chronic cough or infection.

The one clinical manifestation that is present in nearly all patients with partial airway obstruction is stridor. The patient's ability to speak must be determined. Ability to speak helps determine if the obstruction is partial or complete. With a complete obstruction, the patient is unable to speak. Labored respirations and use of accessory muscles is a common finding with airway obstruction. Mild obstruction may result in air hunger, whereas more severe obstruction can lead to cyanosis. Confusion and unconsciousness indicate a progression in the severity of the obstruction. If not treated a partial obstruction can lead to a complete obstruction, rapid suffocation, and death (Medline Plus, 2005b).

Diagnosis and Medical Management

If the patient is not in extreme distress as with a partial airway obstruction, obtain a medical and surgical history from the patient or the family regarding the onset and progression of the respiratory difficulty. Inquire about recent symptoms of an infection (sore throat, runny nose, fever, cough, dysphagia, or odynophagia), head and neck trauma, new medications, foreign body ingestion, or recent dental extractions. Ask the patient if he or she has recently been diagnosed and/or treated for a cancer of the head and neck, and determine whether the patient has had any prior experience with respiratory difficulty. Often patients presenting with partial obstruction secondary to a head or neck malignancy will relate recent weight loss, difficulty eating, coughing with meals, hoarseness, difficult or painful swallowing, or shortness of breath with minimal activity for a time before this more acute respiratory episode was significant enough for them to seek medical attention.

Surgical scars to the neck should be noted and the patient questioned about those past surgeries. It is necessary to determine if the patient had a thyroidectomy, carotid endarterectomy, goiter removal, tracheostomy, or cervical spine surgery with an anterior neck approach. This information can help the health care provider focus on possible causes of the airway distress.

It is imperative to keep the patient safe and provide oxygen. The patient should be placed in an upright position so as to straighten the airway and help alleviate the obstruction. Extending the patient's head and pulling the mandible forward to displace the tongue base away from the pharyngeal wall also may be helpful. This will straighten the airway and may improve air exchange until help arrives.

An IV line should be placed for medication and fluid administration, and oxygen and humidification are indicated. Administration of IV steroids to decrease swelling in the airway may be ordered by the health care provider. Even a small increase in the diameter of the airway can make a significant improvement in the patient's symptoms. Antibiotic therapy is indicated if the cause is a bacterial infection.

Patients with complete airway obstruction require immediate attention with endotracheal intubation, cricothyroidotomy, or tracheostomy to establish an airway. In the case of a full respiratory arrest secondary to airway obstruction, ventilating with a resuscitation bag will be futile. Therefore, it is critical to secure an emergency surgical airway.

◼ Nursing Management of Airway Obstruction

The nursing process guides the management of patients with a partial or complete airway obstruction.

Assessment

The initial assessment of objective and subjective data includes:

- Presence of spontaneous breathing
- Rate, depth, and effort of respirations
- Presence of grunting or wheezing
- Use of accessory muscles of respiration
- Symmetry of chest expansion (determined through palpation) (Galler, Skinner, & Ng, 2005)
- Vital signs

- Oxygen saturation level
- Quality of the voice, such as hoarse, raspy, weak, muffled, normal, or nonexistent
- Stridor or any type of noisy breathing
- Patient complaint of "not getting enough air."

The patient's orientation, mentation, and general demeanor should be monitored on an ongoing basis. The patient may be cooperative and able to answer questions appropriately on arrival to the unit, but as the obstruction increases the patient may begin to appear anxious and agitated or confused. The patient who was cooperative initially may become disoriented and unable to follow directions. If the obstruction has been progressing gradually, the patient may not report as much discomfort breathing as his appearance belies.

Assessment also should include the patient's ability to handle oral secretions, and whether the patient is having pain with speaking or swallowing. Any frequent drooling or productive coughing to clear the airway should be noted. Drooling is an ominous sign that signifies an inability to swallow oral secretions, indicating near complete obstruction. It is essential to determine how long it has been since the patient has noticed voice or respiratory changes. Symptoms that have developed over a period of days may indicate a slower progressing airway problem.

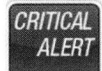 Hoarseness and early respiratory distress are signs that must not be overlooked or discounted on initial exam. Patients with blunt neck trauma should be carefully assessed for hoarseness, respiratory distress, hemoptysis (bloody sputum), and dysphagia because these symptoms indicate airway injury and respiratory compromise.

Planning

A patient with complete airway obstruction appears very anxious, agitated, and apprehensive, and progresses quickly to cyanosis and respiratory arrest. The chest wall may be moving in and out as the individual tries to breathe, but there will be no air exchange. As the patient becomes more hypoxic, agitation, combativeness, and loss of consciousness may ensue. There is no cough and the patient will be cyanotic and unable to speak. If the patient is unable to speak, a Heimlich maneuver should be performed in case the obstruction is from a foreign object or food or more information). Anticipation is the key to saving patients with a complete airway obstruction. Supplies should be kept at the bedside for creating an immediate artificial airway, such as tracheostomy insertion, cricothyroidotomy, or endotracheal intubation equipment. Resuscitation equipment should be brought to the bedside in case there is a subsequent cardiac arrest.

Outcomes and Evaluation Parameters

The outcome is relief of the obstruction and return of normal oxygenation. Evaluation parameters include an alert oriented patient who has normal oxygen saturation levels, respiratory rate and depth, and vital signs. It is necessary to continuously monitor vital signs and pulse oxygen saturations. It is the overall assessment of respiratory effort, stridor, body positioning, restlessness, agitation, cyanosis, and decreasing level of consciousness that will provide the true picture of how the patient is doing.

Tracheotomy

Patients with severe facial injuries, edema in the head and neck area, infection, surgery, large obstructive tumors, or neurological changes to the larynx may require an altered airway. A tracheotomy can be performed to provide an artificial airway.

Placement of a tracheostomy tube usually is temporary to support the patient through the initial period of obstructive swelling or to provide an airway in a patient with airway obstruction. Most health care providers recommend a tracheostomy for patients whom they expect to be intubated for longer than 7 to 10 days. This decreases the risk of permanent injury to the vocal cords or tissues in the larynx or upper airway. Patients with severe lung disease, as in chronic obstructive pulmonary disease (COPD), may have a tracheostomy to provide direct access to the lungs for vigorous pulmonary toilet. Another indication for tracheostomy is obstructive sleep apnea for those who have failed conservative therapy. Patients with short thick necks and large tonsils or a large amount of soft tissue in the posterior pharynx may have their airways obstructed as they relax to sleep. The tracheostomy allows the patient unobstructed breathing while sleeping.

The tracheostomy incision is below the prominent thyroid cartilage (Adam's apple) and below the cricoid cartilage, usually between the second and third, or third and fourth tracheal cartilages, and continues on through the anterior tracheal wall. The tracheostomy tube is placed into the tracheal stoma to keep the airway open. It is initially sutured into place to prevent inadvertent dislodgement. In addition, ties are placed through the faceplate of the tracheostomy tube and around the neck to further secure the tube. The tube remains sutured in place until the tract from the anterior neck into the trachea becomes well established. A post-tracheostomy tray is kept at the bedside or on the nursing unit; in it are instruments to help with reinsertion in the event of early accidental decannulation or early tube obstruction (Figure 34–9 ■). **Decannulation**, a term used to refer to the process of weaning toward the goal of removing the tracheostomy tube, is discussed later.

The tracheostomy tubes are usually made of silicone, plastic, stainless steel, or silver. The tube consists of an outer tube and a removable inner cannula. Remove the inner cannula for cleaning if it is a reusable one, or discard it if it is disposable. The inner cannula serves as a safety device. Remove the cannula if it becomes obstructed with crusts or thick secretions and the patient still has an adequate airway. The patient should always have an inner cannula in place except when cleaning it or when the tube is capped during weaning.

Tracheostomy tubes with a cuff are used for patients on mechanical ventilation to seal the airway around the tube (Figure 34–10 ■). The cuff is *not* intended to hold the tube in place. At best, it keeps the tube centered in the airway. Cuffed tubes may be used to minimize aspiration, although dependence on the cuff to prevent aspiration is not always successful (Tolentino-DelosReyes, Ruppert, & Shiao, 2007). The trachea expands during inhalation and often secretions can fall from around the cuff into the main stem bronchus. Sometimes special tubes must be used or customized to fit the patient appropriately. In patients with thick necks, the regular length tube

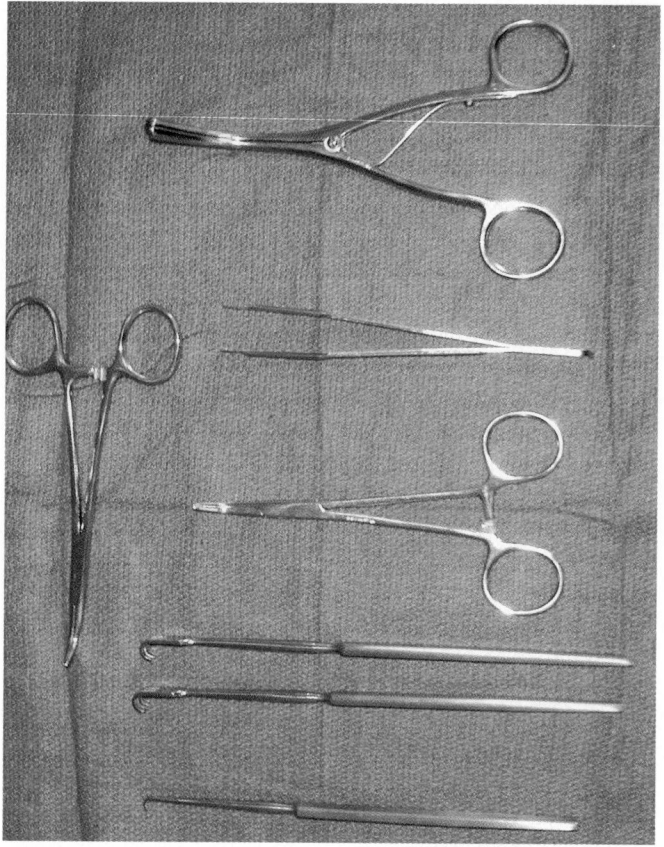

FIGURE 34–9 ■ Post-tracheotomy tray instruments are kept near the new tracheotomy patient for surgical access in the event of accidental decannulation.
Source: University of California, Davis Medical Center

may not be long enough to reach into the trachea, so a tube with a longer shaft must be used (Figure 34–11 ■).

■ Nursing Management of an Artificial Airway

The nursing process is used to guide the care of the patient with an artificial airway.

Assessment

Nursing assessment of the patient with a new tracheostomy includes auscultation of the lungs, monitoring of oxygen saturation, and assessment for any increase in amounts of blood in the sputum, subcutaneous emphysema in the neck, respiratory distress, and patency of the tracheostomy tube itself.

Most patients with a new tracheostomy will have some blood in their sputum and around the tracheostomy tube insertion site. If bleeding in and around the tracheotomy site is continuous and beyond mild oozing, the health care provider needs to be notified. The neck and thyroid area is rich with blood vessels, so trauma to this area during placement of the tracheotomy can lead to postoperative bleeding and may require some local cauterization or packing for control. Bleeding in the early postoperative period is usually from the thyroid vessels that are ligated during the proce-

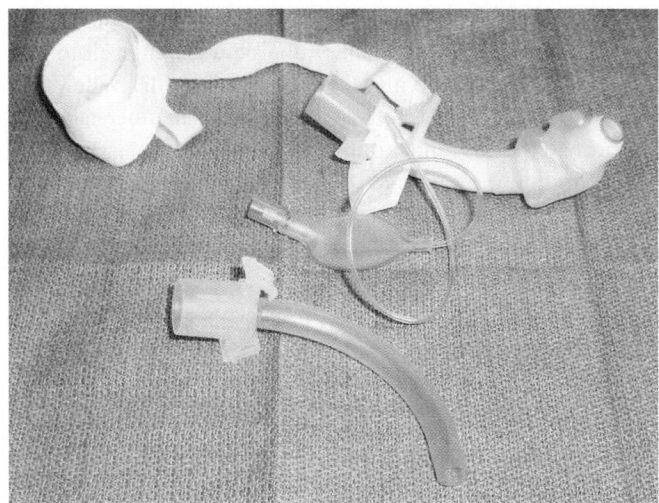

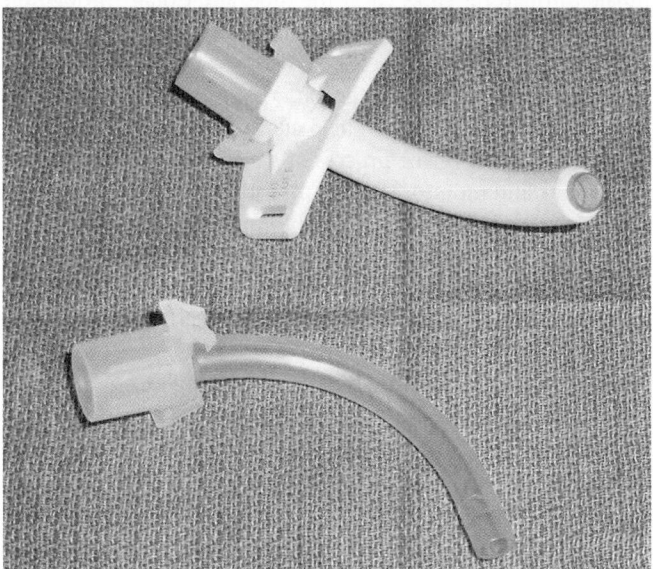

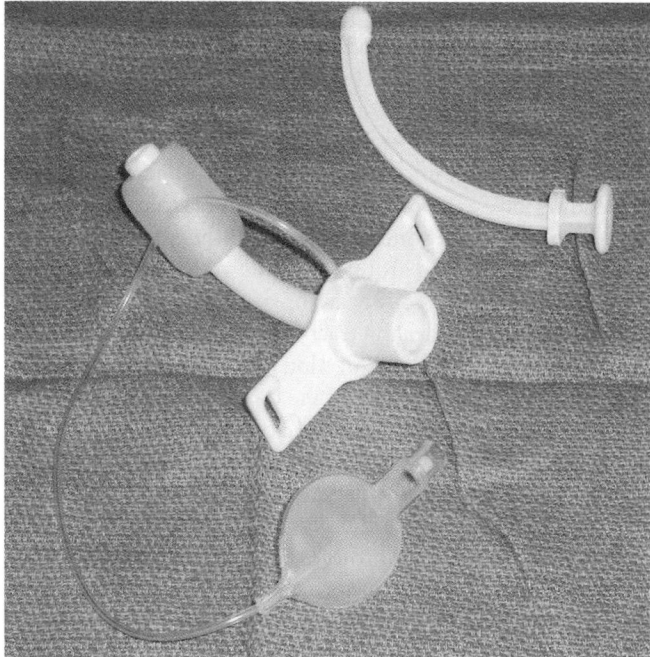

FIGURE 34–11 ■ Shiley single-cannula tracheotomy tube used for patients who require an extra length to span the skin to trachea distance, or those who require a lower cuff placement. A single-cannula tube requires more aggressive nursing care to keep the single cannula free from lumen obstruction.
Source: University of California, Davis Medical Center

FIGURE 34–10 ■ Shiley (A) cuffed and (B) uncuffed tracheotomy tube with disposable inner cannula.
Source: University of California, Davis Medical Center

dure. Ligatures slip or the effect of local lidocaine and epinephrine is reversed. Hemorrhage seen very late in the postoperative period can be caused by erosion of the innominate artery by the tracheostomy tube through the anterior tracheal wall.

 CRITICAL ALERT *In all cases of bleeding, suction the tracheotomy tube to maintain patency of the patient's airway. Inflate the cuff if one is present. Request help to control a potentially very dangerous circumstance.*

If the patient has had a long-standing obstruction preoperatively, careful assessment of the lungs in the postoperative period is necessary. After placement of a tracheostomy, postobstructive pulmonary edema can occur in a patient with significant preoperative obstruction. Negative pressure is thought to be transmitted to the pulmonary interstitium, reducing the hydrostatic pressure around the pulmonary vessels and resulting in an increased hydrostatic pressure and interstitial water accumulation. This is referred to as postobstructive pulmonary edema (POPE) (Fidrose & Elamin, 2004). Signs and symptoms are frothy spu-

tum and moist rales on auscultation of the lungs. This condition is treated with a diuretic and ventilatory support if indicated by respiratory failure.

Interventions and Rationales

The patient should be encouraged to cough, deep breathe, and be suctioned as necessary. If the patient is able to take five to six deep breaths to maintain oxygenation, it is preferable to have the patient cough to clear secretions. The amount of tracheal suctioning should be limited, because excessive suctioning leads to irritation to the tracheal mucosa below the level of the tube. If necessary, give the patient supplemental oxygen and use a resuscitation bag prior to suctioning to prevent oxygen desaturation. The bagging should be timed to coincide with the patient's own inspiratory effort. The suction catheter should be inserted into the tube with the suction off and limited to 5 to 10 seconds, or as long as one can hold one's breath comfortably. Care should be exercised not to use suction greater than 100 mmHg pressure to prevent trauma to the tracheal mucosa. If the patient's oxygen saturation decreases after suctioning, the nurse can use the resuscitation bag with oxygen for a two- to six-breath interval to increase the patient's oxygen level, and further suctioning requires preoxygenation. If the patient is restless or agitated due to alcohol or drug withdrawal, upper extremity restraints may be necessary to keep the patient from removing the tube. When suctioning, the nurse must be careful not to injure the carina by inserting the suction catheter too far into the trachea. Suctioning a patient with a tracheostomy tube requires using only a small percentage of the suction catheter. The catheter may touch the delicate membrane of the carina and cause the patient to cough, but the catheter should not be inserted into the trachea and forcibly collide with the carina. Suctioning technique is discussed in detail in Chapter 36 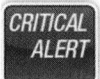.

Ensuring that the inner cannula is changed routinely to prevent occlusion is an important component of the nursing care. Depending on secretions the inner cannula can be changed every 8 to 12 hours or once a day. Care of the tracheostomy site itself involves cleaning around the tube with half-strength hydrogen peroxide on cotton swabs and rinsing with normal saline. Secretions under the tracheostomy plate can cause skin breakdown and can lead to infection if not cleaned regularly. Assess the area under the edges of the tracheostomy face plate for signs of skin breakdown. Keep the face plate flush with the skin of the neck.

Occasionally, due to the patient's anatomy, the lower edge of the plate puts pressure on the skin and can lead to skin breakdown if not assessed and protected. A split gauze dressing provides some padding, or some form of manufactured skin barrier such as DuoDerm or a stoma wafer can be used to protect the skin. The nurse needs to assess frequently for secretions undermining the barrier and change the barrier as necessary.

Outcomes and Evaluation Parameters

Outcomes for the patient with an artificial airway include lack of complications and normal oxygenation. Airway complication can occur from a variety of causes including bleeding, tube obstruction or dislodgement, and displacement into the subcutaneous tissue of the neck. Most complications of tracheotomies can be avoided by securing the tube well. Check the ties frequently and change them if they become wet or soiled. Cotton ties work well but do stretch as they become wet. The ties should be tied tightly enough so that only one finger can be placed between the skin and the ties.

The nurse should monitor the patient's oxygen and respiratory status and take note of changes in the patient's behavior. Increasing restlessness or agitation or changes in mentation (decreasing level of consciousness or increasing confusion) could indicate that the patient is not oxygenating well. If these symptoms occur remove the inner cannula and make sure the tracheostomy tube is clear; then suction the patient. If unable to pass a suction catheter down the tracheostomy tube, the tube may have become dislodged. If the tube becomes displaced or dislodged, the nursing priority is to stay with the patient and to position the patient with her head up and slightly extended. A health care provider who is able to reinsert the airway tube needs to be summoned, and the patient needs reassurance that help is on the way. If necessary the patient may need to be ventilated with a resuscitation bag until the airway is replaced. Acute respiratory distress is very frightening for the patient; therefore it is essential for the nurse to reassure the patient that everything is being done to rectify the situation. It is important to assemble the necessary equipment for reintubation or replacement of the tracheostomy tube. The obturator, which is used to guide the tracheostomy tube during insertion, should always be kept with the patient.

Decannulation

Decannulation, or removal of the tube, occurs with the resolution of the initial airway problem. This process typically begins by downsizing the size of the tracheostomy tube and/or capping the tracheostomy tube. A smaller tube allows enough air to pass around the tube and up into the natural larynx. This allows the patient to breathe in the normal physiological manner, taking in air through the nose and mouth and into the upper airway. Oxygen saturation is monitored continuously during and after this change. If the patient tolerates the downsizing, the tube is again downsized and a cap is placed over the end of the tracheostomy tube (Figure 34–12 ■).

CRITICAL ALERT *If at any time the patient experiences respiratory distress during weaning, remove the cap and encourage the patient to cough. Suction if necessary, and recap the tube if the patient is able to tolerate.*

Teach the patient to occlude the end of the tracheostomy tube with a finger and to speak on exhalation. Instruct the patient to inhale through the tube, cover the tube, and exhale through the natural airway. Regaining communication can be very rewarding for the patient.

It also is critical to teach the patient how to uncap or remove the cap of the tube. This can help allay fears that may be associated with capping or the process of decannulation. Cap the patient's tube and monitor saturations for an extended period and while the patient is sleeping, before completely removing the tracheostomy. If the patient tolerates the capping throughout the night without episodes of oxygen desaturation, the health care provider removes the tracheostomy tube and places a dry sterile occlusive dressing over the site. Explain to the patient the importance of putting pressure on the site when coughing or talking to prevent air from passing through the stoma. The more consistent the patient is with this, the sooner the stomal incision will close. The incision is never closed with sutures. It is important for the wound to heal from the inside out. Closure of the skin edges before the tracheal incision itself closes can lead to subcutaneous emphysema in the neck. The dressing is changed as

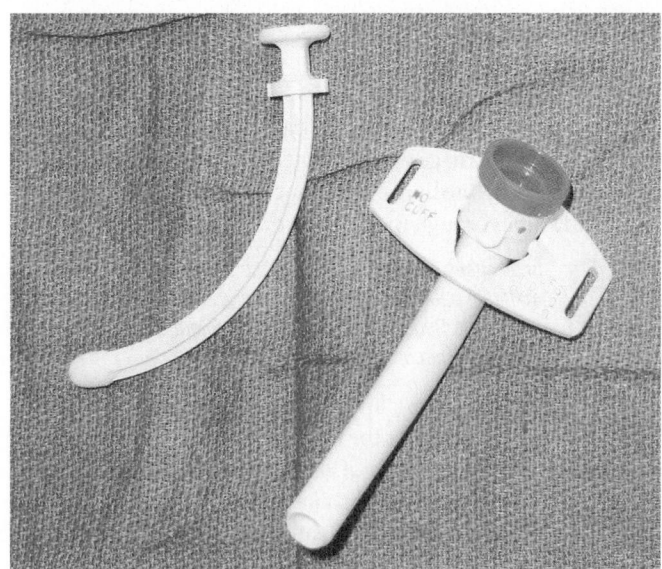

FIGURE 34–12 ■ Shiley tracheotomy tube with red cap for weaning and eventual decannulation. If possible, the patient should be taught to uncap the tube if distress occurs. The nurse in the hospital must be vigilant for subtle and overt signs of distress during this process.
Source: University of California, Davis Medical Center

needed until there is no evidence of air passage through the incision and the skin edges are approximated. Wound care to the healing site is typically ordered twice a day and as needed, with half- or full-strength hydrogen peroxide and rinsing with normal saline before applying a dry dressing.

Oral communication is very important. If the patient cannot be decannulated for reasons such as vocal cord dysfunction, then the use of a speaking valve may help. These valves are one-way valves that allow the patient to breathe in through the valve; the valve then shuts and the patient then breathes out through his natural airway (Figure 34–13 ■). This flutter valve is very simple but very effective. Some types can be used inline and assist ventilator-dependent patients to speak.

Discharge Priorities for Patients with Tracheostomy

If a patient is to go home with a tracheostomy, the goal is for the patient to be safe at home, resume normal activities, and have an acceptable quality of life. Safety with an artificial airway is the priority for teaching. The patient and family must demonstrate safe care before discharge. This should include suctioning, saline instillation, wound care, inner cannula care, tracheostomy change, and emergency measures. Encourage the patient and family to participate in care early in the hospitalization to increase their confidence.

Total Laryngectomy Permanent Airway

Removal of the larynx or laryngectomy necessitates a permanent tracheal artificial airway. (Refer to the section on head and neck cancer for more information on causes for removal and management of patients who have had a laryngectomy.) A similar surgery called laryngotracheal separation is done for patients with severe aspiration resulting in repeated, frequent hospitalizations for aspiration pneumonia. In both surgeries the trachea is transected, and the distal portion of the trachea is brought to the skin surface in the anterior neck and sewn into

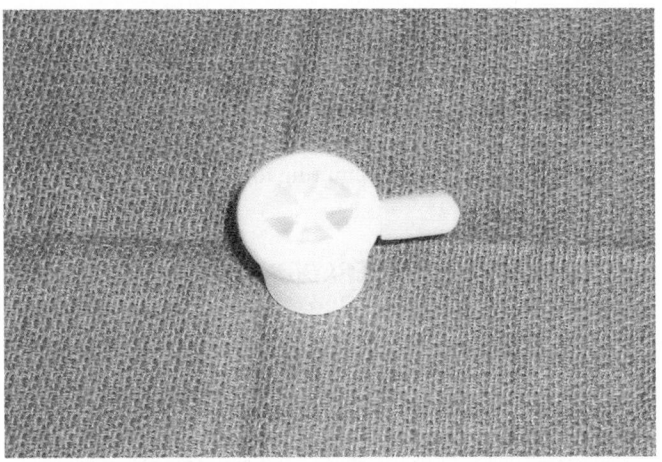

FIGURE 34–13 ■ The Shiley speaking valve with oxygen port is a one-way valve that allows airflow on exhalation upward into the larynx, thereby supporting speech. These valves are fragile and any secretions interfere with their operation.
Source: University of California, Davis Medical Center

place. This surgery completely separates the trachea from the esophagus and thus prevents problems with aspiration. However, because air no longer passes through the structures of the larynx, such as the vocal cords, the patient will not be able to speak in the normal way.

The loss of the ability to communicate verbally can be very frightening to the patient. Few things are as disabling as the impairment resulting from total loss of laryngeal speech. The impact of the total removal of the larynx is so dramatic that it may impact the patient's decision regarding treatment. Even though the total surgical removal of the larynx may provide the greatest chance of successfully controlling a malignancy, it is not unusual for a patient to knowingly compromise a chance for cure by choosing another form of treatment that would result in preservation of the larynx and the ability to speak (Bailey et al., 2006). Much time and care must be taken with these patients and their families during the diagnostic and preoperative phases. It is important for the health care provider to explain to the patient and family all of the risks and benefits of each form of treatment. It is equally important that the patient feel support in whatever decision is made—even though it might not seem the best choice for complete removal of the disease. Some patients opt for other treatments first, radiation or a combination of radiation and chemotherapy, or only a partial laryngectomy in order to preserve their voice. If cancer recurs or there is a significant problem with aspiration, then the patient may subsequently consent to a total laryngectomy.

■ Nursing Management

The nursing process guides the management of the postoperative laryngectomy patient. As always the airway is the first priority.

Interventions and Rationales

The laryngectomy stoma must be kept clean and free of crusts. It is a *life-threatening* situation if the laryngectomy stoma becomes obstructed with mucus or crusts. The outcomes for these patients are a patent airway and normal oxygenation as evidenced by normal oxygen saturation levels, lungs that are clear to auscultation, and unlabored respirations. Crusts of secretions and blood form when there is not enough humidity. The lungs are accustomed to heated, humidified, and filtered inspired air by the nose and upper airway. With the trachea positioned directly out to the neck now, this process is bypassed. It is important, therefore, to provide warm humidified mist to the patient's stoma to keep the airway moist. Occasionally the placement of a stoma button can keep the skin edges from contracting (Figure 34–14 ■, p. 914). Stoma buttons also can be used if a dressing around the stoma endangers the lumen of the airway.

Until the internal incision lines in the pharynx heal, the patient will not be able to eat orally. This typically takes 5 to 7 days postlaryngectomy. For this reason, a nasogastric feeding tube is placed intraoperatively. Before the patient resumes an oral diet, a barium swallow is completed to evaluate the internal suture lines of the pharynx, thereby ensuring that the suture lines are intact and there is no leak of barium through the incisions, referred to as internal dehiscence. Aspiration *cannot* be a problem for these patients because the esophagus and airway are

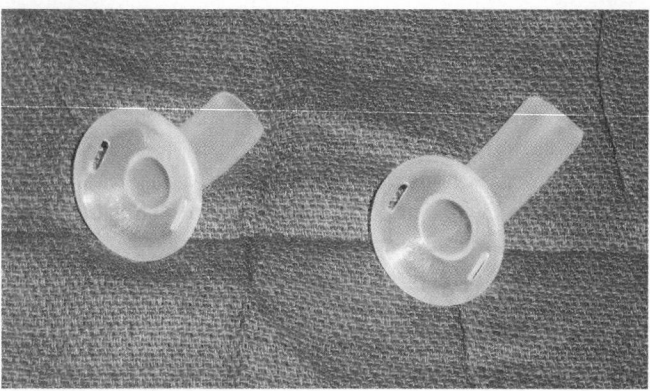

FIGURE 34–14 ■ Bivona stoma buttons for laryngectomy are placed into the laryngectomy stoma to prevent cicatricule (or circular) scarring and maintain the patient's only airway.
Source: University of California, Davis Medical Center

completely separated. There may be some swallowing issues initially as the patient learns to control food and fluids in the reconstructed esophagus.

Meticulous wound care includes cleaning incision lines with hydrogen peroxide and rinsing with normal saline to decrease infection and promote wound healing. Many times patients undergoing this surgery are poorly nourished. Difficulties eating and drinking due to tumor size and location lead to weight loss and malnourishment preoperatively. Patients with poor nutrition or patients with prior radiation to the area tend to take longer to heal and are at higher risk for complications, such as infection.

In the event an infection causing an abscess, called an oropharyngeal fistula, does develop, the health care provider may open the area widely to drain purulence, and begin wound packing with saline–soaked, wet-to-dry dressings. This allows the wound to heal from the inside outward to the skin.

 **CRITICAL ALERT** *Notify the heath care provider if the temperature increases or there is swelling, pain, or redness at the suture line. Separation of the suture lines may be indicative of a wound infection or potential fistula formation.*

As with the patient with a tracheostomy or someone on voice rest, it is important to be patient with the new laryngectomy patient as he or she tries to communicate. This can be an extremely frustrating time for the patient and for the nurse if care is not taken to establish a workable form of communication. It is important to acknowledge the patient's frustration and to explain to her that writing and pantomiming, though tedious, are very effective communication tools. Some patients articulate well enough to read lips and use gestures so that writing may not be necessary all the time. For others, writing is the only way to communicate. Pen and paper or a dry erase board should be provided for this purpose.

Some individuals may not be able to write to communicate, which increases the frustration. Thus, the nurse should assess the patient's ability to read and write prior to surgery and establish a suitable form of communication. Remember that almost 50% of Americans are functionally illiterate, and it is difficult for low-literacy patients to read and understand such routine health information as dosage instructions on medication bottles, poi-

son warnings, appointment slips and consent forms, and written patient education information (Kutner, Greenberg, Jun, & Paulsen, 2006). Answering call lights promptly is extremely important for patients who cannot speak.

Health Promotion

Nursing assessment in the preoperative setting must include assessment of the patient's support systems. It is important to determine if the patient and spouse or other primary support person are able to read and write. Initially this will be the most used form of communication for the patient to express his needs and concerns. The Cultural Considerations box addresses the needs of patients who may not understand English.

It is important for the patient to understand that various options are available for vocal restoration procedures. Meeting with a speech therapist preoperatively and discussing these options may help the patient realize that having a total laryngectomy does not necessarily mean the end to communication with some form of speech. It may be helpful to have someone who has had the same procedure and has been trained to work with patients who have had laryngectomies visit with the patient to show him how to speak after surgery and how the voice sounds.

Tracheoesophageal puncture (TEP) is a procedure that can be done at the time of the original surgery or at a later date when healing is completed. This procedure provides voice restoration to patients who have had a total laryngectomy. A puncture is made through the posterior wall of the trachea into the anterior wall of the esophagus. A feeding tube is threaded through this puncture and used to help form a tract by acting as a stent. It also is used to feed the patient enterally while the surgical site heals. After the tract heals and matures, a one-way prosthetic valve is inserted into this tract for purposes of speech (Figure 34–15 ■). The purpose of the valve is to allow the patient to shunt air from the trachea into the esophagus, but not allow food and fluid from the esophagus to enter the trachea. The airflow through the one-way valve causes vibration in the upper esophagus when the stoma is occluded, and the mouth, tongue, and lips articulate the sound to produce speech.

Gerontological Considerations

One of the more common and difficult problems with the older patient is postoperative delirium. Family members become concerned when they see their loved ones picking and pulling at tubes, removing IV lines, attempting to get out of bed alone de-

 CULTURAL CONSIDERATIONS for Patients with Total Laryngectomy

For patients with a total laryngectomy who speak a language other than English, communication can be even more difficult. It is helpful to have the family assist by making signs with words both in English and the patient's native language for things such as "pain," "bathroom," and "difficulty breathing." This allows the patient to just point to the appropriate sign. If no one in the family speaks English, use interpreting services. If a staff member speaks the patient's native language, assign her as one of the primary nurses. This can ease the patient's fears of not being understood.

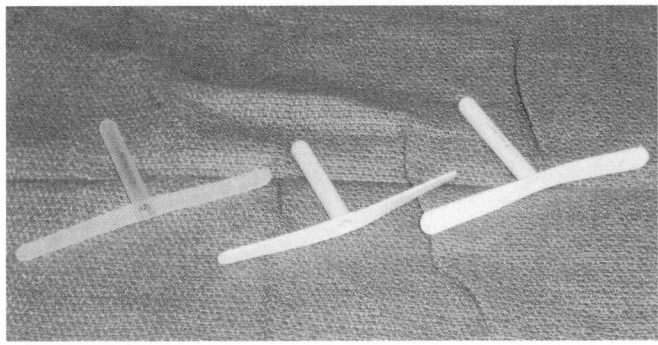

FIGURE 34–15 ■ Bivona tracheoesophageal puncture speech prosthesis. This speech prosthesis is placed into the TEP to shunt air from the stoma (lungs) into the esophagus to produce speech after total laryngectomy.
Source: University of California, Davis Medical Center

spite frequent reminders to call for help, and generally behaving in an uncharacteristic manner (Jett, 2007). According to Kagan (personal communication, 2004), it is estimated that as many as 50% of hospitalized patients over the age of 65 experience some level of delirium during the course of their hospital stay.

Causes for the delirium include anesthesia, medications, stress, and/or an unfamiliar place with unfamiliar faces. It is important not to restrain the elderly physically or pharmacologically, unless absolutely necessary for safety. One-to-one supervision to prevent restraining the patient can help to decrease the length of the period of delirium. If possible, the number of new medications added to the patient's home regimen should be limited.

It is prudent to request a psychological evaluation to assess the patient and to perform the Mini-Mental State (State) Examination (MMSE) (Brannon, 2006). The MMSE is a nationally recognized tool that can be used to systematically and thoroughly assess mental status and separate patients with cognitive impairment from those without it. If used repeatedly the instrument is able to measure changes in cognitive status that may benefit from intervention. The MMSE is considered to be a standard diagnostic instrument by the American Psychiatric Association and, as such, is used in a variety of settings. Chart 34–4 (p. 916) provides more information about the MMSE. When used, the health care provider can assess orientation, memory attention, calculation, language, writing, and drawing. Preoperative cognitive function is an invaluable piece of information. If the delirium is not cleared by discharge, it is important to assess whether or not the family will be able to manage their loved one at home, or whether a temporary stay in a skilled nursing facility might be necessary until the patient clears mentally and can return safely to the home environment. Most likely if the patient is older, the spouse or primary caregiver also is elderly, so it is important to be realistic about how much he or she can do. Patient safety is the first priority.

Other issues with the older patient may be limited mobility, decreased manual dexterity, and decreased vision and hearing. Changing tracheostomy ties, managing tube feedings, and performing wound care can be difficult for someone with limited mobility and limited vision. Patients going home post-tracheostomy or with vocal cord paralysis may have decreased volume with their voice and if their spouse has impaired hearing, communication can be difficult.

Head and Neck Cancer

Head and neck cancer is one of the more uncommon cancers; however, the challenges the patient, family, and health care team face during diagnosis, treatment, and recovery are intense and persistent. Ablative surgery often is used to treat this type of cancer, leaving the patient with facial disfigurement and functional impairment. The use of an interdisciplinary team (early in diagnosis) will provide the patient with the clinical expertise that will optimize the patient's recovery potential and improve his quality of life.

If detected early head and neck cancer is treatable and curable. It is, however, an insidious disease and may not present itself until the patient has a large tumor burden. Discussions with family and significant others often help to explain the consequences of head and neck cancer and its treatment. Unfortunately, if not treated, this type of cancer is very disfiguring and alters the normal functions of breathing, eating, smelling, tasting, and facial attributes and expressions. Decisions regarding treatment must be informed decisions that include the outcome without treatment and the implications, risks, and benefits of surgery and radiation therapy.

Etiology

A variety of risk factors are associated with head and neck cancer, although some patients do not have any of the known risk factors, so it is not possible to know for sure how much they contributed to causing the cancer (American Cancer Society [ACS], 2006). The Risk Factors box (p. 917) lists the most common risk factors associated with head and neck cancer.

People of Asian heritage, predominantly first generation, can develop nasopharyngeal cancer from the Epstein–Barr virus. It seems that their culture-based risk factor for nasopharyngeal cancer from the consumption of salt-preserved fish decreases with each generation (Chang & Adami, 2006). The cessation of tobacco product (cigarettes, cigars, chewing tobacco, snuff) use and the limitation of alcohol in combination with tobacco is a goal for health promotion (Rudy, 2006).

Pathophysiology

The predominant cell type in head and neck cancer is squamous cell cancer. There are many other types, but in far less frequent occurrence. Squamous cells or epithelial cells line the aerodigestive tract and are irritated and altered by the environmental agents outlined earlier. Cells change from the normal fast growing and dividing cells into altered cells that grow along tissue planes and into adjacent structures. Chapter 64 ☺ includes a complete discussion of the pathogenesis of cancer.

Laboratory and Diagnostic Procedures

Diagnosing head and neck cancer involves the accurate assessment of health history, physical condition, social factors, and presence of support systems. When a patient presents to an otolaryngologist, a thorough history is taken with emphasis on specific symptoms in the head and neck. Length of time each symptom has been present and sequence of symptom development also is documented. The 12 cranial nerves are evaluated carefully because they provide important clues to the invasion

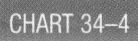 CHART 34–4 **The Mini-Mental State Examination**

The MMSE is an 11-question measure that tests five areas of cognitive function: orientation, registration, retention and calculation, recall, and language. The maximum score is 30. A score of 23 or lower is indicative of cognitive impairment. The MMSE takes only 5 to 10 minutes to administer and is, therefore, practical to use repeatedly and routinely.

The MMSE is effective as a screening tool for cognitive impairment with older, community dwelling, hospitalized, or institutionalized adults. Assessment of an older adult's cognitive function is best achieved when it is done routinely, systematically, and thoroughly. Examples of questions included in the Mini-Mental State Examination are shown below.

MMSE Sample Items

Orientation to Time

"What is the date?"

Registration

"Listen carefully. I am going to say three words. You say them back after I stop.

Ready? Here they are...

APPLE (pause), PENNY (pause), TABLE (pause). Now repeat those words back to me."

[Repeat up to 5 times, but score only the first trial.]

Naming

"What is this?" [Point to a pencil or pen.]

Reading

"Please read this and do what it says." [Show examinee the words on the stimulus form.]

CLOSE YOUR EYES

Source: Reproduced by special permission of the Publisher, Psychological Assessment Resources, Inc., 16204 North Florida Avenue, Lutz, Florida 33549, from the Mini Mental State Examination, by Marshal Folstein and Susan Folstein, Copyright 1975, 1998, 2001 by Mini Mental LLC, Inc. Published 2001 by Psychological Assessment Resources, Inc. Further reproduction is prohibited without permission of PAR, Inc. The MMSE can be purchased from PAR, Inc. by calling (813) 968-3003

RISK FACTORS for Head and Neck Cancer

- *Tobacco Use*—Approximately 90% of people with oral cavity and oropharyngeal cancers use tobacco; risk is correlated with the length and amount smoked or chewed.
  - Tobacco smoke from cigarettes, cigars, or pipes can cause cancers anywhere in the mouth or throat, as well as causing cancers of the larynx (voice box).
  - Pipe smoking has a particularly significant risk for cancers in the area of the lips that touch the pipe stem.
  - Oral tobacco products (snuff or chewing tobacco) are associated with cancers of the cheek, gums, and inner surface of the lips. Long time snuff use poses an especially high risk.
- *Heavy Drinking*—Drinking alcohol strongly increases a smoker's risk of developing oral cavity and oropharyngeal cancers. Particularly heavy, non-smokers and alcohol drinkers also have a high risk of these cancers; however, the combination of drinking and smoking is the most dangerous.
- *Gender*—Oral and oropharyngeal cancers are about twice as common in men as in women, possibly due to the fact that men are more likely to use tobacco and alcohol, though this trend is changing.
- *Ultraviolet Light*—Cancers of the lip are more common in people who have prolonged exposure to sunlight.
- *Poor Nutrition*—A diet low in fruits and vegetables is linked with an increased risk of cancers of the oral cavity and oropharynx.
- *Human Papilloma Virus Infection*—HPV infection may contribute to oral and oropharyngeal cancers, 20–30% of such cancers.
- *Lichen Planus*—A severe case may slightly increase the risk of oral cancer in middle aged people.
- *Uncertain, Unproven or Controversial Risk Factors*
  - *Mouthwash*—Some studies have suggested that mouthwash with high alcohol content might be linked to a higher risk of oral and oropharyngeal cancers.
  - *Irritation From Dentures*—It has been suggested that long-term irritation of the lining of the mouth caused by poorly fitting dentures may be a risk factor for oral cancer.

Source: American Cancer Society. (2006). *Detailed guide: Oral cavity and oropharyngeal cancer. What are the risk factors for oral cavity and oropharyngeal cancer?* Retrieved August 23, 2007, from http://www.cancer.org/docroot/CRI/content/CRI_2_4_2X_What_are_the_risk_factors_for_oral_cavity_and_oropharyngeal_cancer_60.asp?rnav=cri

and location of the cancer. This information helps the health care provider better understand the patient's disease and recovery potential.

Integral to the complete evaluation of the patient and before a final decision for treatment is complete, the patient usually undergoes a panendoscopy. **Panendoscopy** includes tumor mapping and biopsy to confirm histologic diagnosis; it includes bronchoscope, esophagoscopy, nasal endoscopy, examination of the oral cavity, and anatomical mapping of the cancer. This tumor mapping directs the therapy that is recommended to the patient. From a surgical perspective this allows the surgeon to determine what must be removed and what can be saved during a surgical resection, and the method of reconstruction. The Diagnostic Tests box (p. 918) outlines specific tests for head and neck cancer.

Clinical Manifestations

Clinical manifestations of head and neck cancer include sore throat without fever, unilateral earache, change in voice or articulation, dental changes, and weight loss. Most symptoms are related directly to the location and invasion of the cancer, such as change in articulation with an oral tongue cancer, or hoarseness and dysphagia (difficulty swallowing) with a base of tongue or laryngeal cancer. Many people first recognize a mass in the neck, and may not even be aware of the site of the primary tumor. This neck mass represents nodal extent of the disease and the investigation must be done to locate the primary tumor.

◼ Collaborative Management

A multidisciplinary team of experts including otolaryngologists, medical oncologists, radiation oncologists, social service providers, clinical nurse specialists, speech pathologists, nurses, and dentists or maxillofacial prosthodontists provides a collaborative approach to providing care for patients with head and neck cancer. This panel of experts reviews the patient's history, findings from the physical exam, and results of radiologic studies. This panel also examines the patient. The team develops a consensus opinion for the best chance for cure and develops a plan of therapy. Then, in a private session the plan is presented to patients so they can make their decisions. The nursing role is to participate as a team member, to act as an advocate for the patient, and to help interpret medical terms into lay terms for the patient and family.

The patient and family require assistance in understanding the choices and plan of care because many choices and decisions regarding treatment are available. Patients must understand that they may choose no treatment. Although unusual, some individuals elect no therapy as their option, with the ultimate outcome being death. When such a choice is made, it is important for the patient, family, friends, and significant others to understand that therapy is available for symptoms and palliative care (Meyers & Linder, 2003). Aggressive symptom control can be very powerful in life-threatening illnesses. Patients also must understand the process that lies ahead and the resources that are available to help. Aggressive palliative care and hospice can be an integral part of this process (Meyers, 1999).

Staging System

Head and neck cancer is defined by the organ or origins of the tumor, for example, the larynx, tongue, tonsil, and sinus, with subdefinitions within parts of that organ. Once a diagnosis is made, staging or evaluation is done to determine the size and extent of the solid tumor, using the American Joint Committee on Cancer guide (Greene et al., 2002). *Tumor staging* is an internationally recognized method of comparison of types, sizes, and locations of cancers (Greene et al., 2002). With this staging system, tumors are described by the acronym TNM. The *T* stands for tumor, which includes the size. The *N* represents the presence or absence of nodal extension, particularly into the cervical nodal system in the necks. The *M* represents metastatic disease to other organ systems, as described by clinical, laboratory, and radiographic investigations. Each section (TNM) has many subdivisions that further elucidate the extent of the tumor involvement. This staging system allows each health care practitioner to

DIAGNOSTIC TESTS for Head and Neck Cancer

Test	Expected Abnormality	Rationale for Abnormality
Fine-needle biopsy	Fine-needle aspirate of tumor or neck nodes. Taken with a very small needle, so as not to invade tissue planes.	To extract cells for microscopic evaluation, To determine cell type of tumors.
Fiber-optic laryngoscopy	Uses fiber-optic light bundle channel to transmit light. Local or no anesthesia required.	To look into the upper aerodigestive tract without using general anesthesia.
Panendoscopy	Includes laryngoscopy, nasopharyngoscopy, and esophagoscopy, examination of the oral cavity, tumor mapping, and biopsy. Conducted under general anesthesia.	To completely evaluate the upper aerodigestive tract with the patient asleep. Define the organ of origin. Map the extent or regions of the tumor and biopsy the tumor for pathologic conformation.
Blood tests	Chemistry 20. Complete blood count. Liver function tests.	To evaluate for alterations in liver function that may indicate metastatic disease and or liver failure.
CT head and neck	Computerized tomography.	To evaluate the extent of tumor involvement focusing on tissue.
CT chest	Computerized tomography.	To evaluate the lungs for metastatic disease or primary lung cancer.
MRI	Magnetic resonance imaging.	To evaluate the extent of tumor involvement and bony structures.
BTO	Balloon test occlusion.	To evaluate the carotid artery and assess the ability of the contralateral carotid artery to crossfill if the artery is resected.
SPECT scan	Single photon emission computerized tomography.	To evaluate brain activity before and after BTO. To assess for brain activity after carotid artery resection.
PET scan	Proton emission scan based on the uptake of glucose in tissues. Hypermetabolic tissues can be identified.	To measure the biological and metabolic changes associated with disease.
Doppler	This test uses Doppler technology to evaluate the blood flow in an artery or vein.	To assess the competency of an artery or vein for use in microvascular free flap reconstruction.

compare treatment results and survival with those of similar patients around the world. Chapter 64 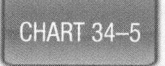 includes a complete description of the TNM staging system.

Medical Management

Traditionally head and neck cancer has been treated with radiation alone, surgery alone, or the combination of surgery followed by radiation. Currently there also is the option of radiation with chemotherapy used to make the tumor more sensitive to the radiation therapy (Vokes & Stenson, 2003). The location and size of the tumor, patient choices, and the patient's general medical condition dictate most treatment recommendations (Forastiere et al., 2003). Ultimately, the choice is the patient's own. Chart 34–5 outlines the options for treatment of head and neck cancer.

Radiation is used not only as an attempt to cure, but also to save organ function and avoid debilitating surgery. Radiation has its own inherent side effects of permanent dry mouth, loss of taste or smell, and problems swallowing. Gene therapy is a very experimental, but promising, therapy and researchers hope it will be a viable frontline choice in the future (Merritt, Roth, & Logothetis, 2001; Nettelbeck & Curiel, 2003). Gene transfer is a new treatment modality that introduces new genes into a cancerous cell or the surrounding tissue to cause cell death or slow

CHART 34–5
Treatment Options for Head and Neck Cancer

Surgery, conventional or laser resection

Surgery and postoperative radiation therapy

Radiation therapy

Radiation and sensitizing chemotherapy

Radiation and conventional chemotherapy

Chemotherapy

Gene therapy

Combination of any of the above

Alternative therapies

No therapy; just palliative care and/or hospice

the growth of the cancer. This therapy technique is very flexible, and a wide range of genes and vectors are being evaluated in clinical trials (Cross & Burmester, 2006).

Early stage disease (stage I or II) typically is treated with either surgery or radiation therapy. In moderately advanced disease (stage III), those cases deemed resectable are treated with surgery plus postoperative radiation therapy; or radiation therapy with or without surgery, as feasible. Chemoradiation therapy is considered in select cases, based on the patient's choice and general medical condition. Advanced, unresectable disease is treated with chemoradiation therapy or definitive radiation therapy. The patient should be informed of all aspects of therapy including the pros and cons of each treatment. Chapter 64 🌐 includes a complete description of radiation and chemotherapy.

Surgical Resection

There are six general types of surgical resection: oral cavity resection, laryngectomy (partial or total), temporal bone resection, maxillary (with or without orbital exenteration) or bimaxillary resection, skull base resection, and the combination of each. Each surgery has its own subgroups based on the site of origin of the tumor. Each surgical resection presents with unique requirements because of the location of the tumor. Essentially all of the surgical approaches have similar needs in relation to airway, wound care, nutrition, self-image, self-care education, and recovery.

Neck dissection may accompany tumor resections. A neck dissection is necessary for metastatic disease in the lymph nodes of the neck or when there is a very high suspicion of tumor because of the behavior or tumor bulk at the primary site. A **neck dissection** includes lymph tissue, the jugular vein, the spinal accessory nerve, and the sternocleidomastoid muscle (SCM). Chart 34–6 outlines the various surgical approaches for head and neck cancer.

Reconstruction Flaps and Grafts

In otolaryngology cancer surgery, after the tumor is resected, the goal is to reconstruct the patient for optimum function and cosmetics. The surgical site can be primarily closed or left open to granulate by secondary intention. Frequently flaps and composite grafts of muscle, bone, and tissue are used for reconstruction. A **myocutaneous flap**, composed of muscle and skin, is used to reconstruct the defect caused by the tumor resection. A flap from the pectoralis major is commonly used for reconstruction. This rotation flap is supplied by its native blood supply, but rotated into the surgical defect. Free flaps that are harvested from a distant site also can be used for reconstruction. Common sites include the radial forearm, fibula, scapula, lateral arm, or lateral thigh. These flaps can include tissue, bone, and muscle as well as the artery and vein for the microvascular anastomosis (Figure 34–16 ■, p. 920).

A dermis graft may be harvested using the dermis layer of skin to cover the carotid artery or the bed of the resection. It acts as a watertight second layer seal. This allows the tissue to adhere and heal to the wound bed.

When assessing a reconstruction flap, myocutaneous or free, it should be pink and warm with brisk capillary refill (<2 seconds). A flap that is *blue* or cyanotic is a sign of venous congestion, *white* indicates no arterial supply, and *deep red* is a sign of partial venous congestion with a vigorous arterial supply. Tracheostomy and cupola ties should be positioned away from the graft to prevent pressure on the area, which may lead to impaired or decreased blood flow to the tissue and loss of the graft. The head position should be maintained straight or toward the operative side to prevent pressure or tension on the flap. The head of the bed is elevated to at least 30 degrees to facilitate drainage of fluid and to prevent edema of the head and neck area.

CHART 34–6   **Otolaryngology Surgical Resections for Head and Neck Cancer**

Type of Surgery	Major Areas Resected *(Predicated on primary tumor location)*	Major Implications
Oral cavity resection	Tongue, buccal mucosa, mandible	Speech, articulation, chewing, swallowing, facial cosmesis
Oropharyngeal resections, bimaxillary resection	Tongue, base of tongue, tonsil, maxilla, mandible	Swallowing, speech, aspiration Facial cosmesis
Laryngectomy, partial (often called hemi or vertical hemi laryngectomy)	Larynx, partial	Speech, swallowing Aspiration (partial laryngectomy only) Cosmesis
Laryngectomy, total	Larynx, total	Speech, cosmesis *Complete* separation of airway and esophagus
Temporal bone resection	Temporal bone, parotid, maxilla, mandible	Hearing, balance Cosmesis Facial nerve impairment or paralysis Eye protection concerns
Maxillary, with or without orbital exenteration	Maxilla, orbit	Speech, swallowing, chewing, sight Cosmesis
Skull base resection (anterior, middle, posterior, or combination)	Skull base carotid artery	Cognition, speech, swallowing, balance Cosmesis
Neck dissection (radical, modified, *paired* with the above surgeries for lymph node involvement)	Lymph nodes, SCM, jugular vein, spinal accessory nerve CN XI	Impaired lymph drainage Trapezius muscle paralysis Facial edema (especially if bilateral neck dissections are performed at the same time) Cerebral edema with bilateral neck dissection
Combination of any of the above surgical resections	Any anatomical *combination* as required by tumor invasion for oncologic purposes	*All of the above* predicated on location of tumor and invasion

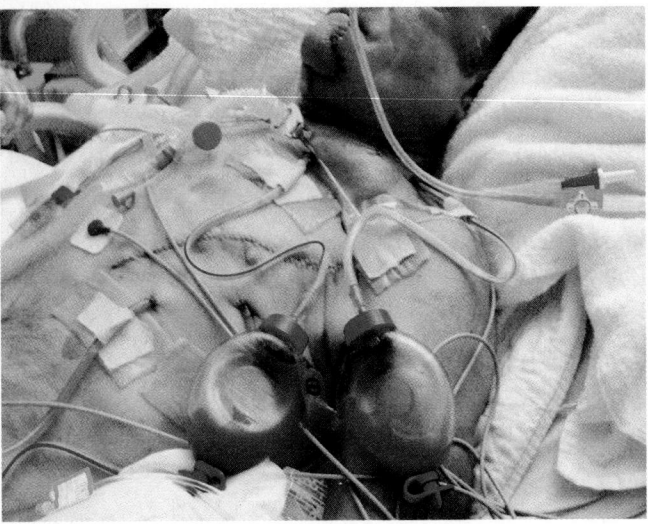

FIGURE 34–16 ■ Pectoralis major myocutaneous reconstruction flap.
Source: University of California, Davis Medical Center

The free flap is assessed for a pulse by Doppler per the surgeon's order, typically every 2 hours (Figure 34–17 ■). It also is important in the immediate postoperative period to maintain an adequate blood pressure with a mean arterial pressure (MAP) of at least 60 to ensure tissue perfusion to the graft.

■ Nursing Management

Nursing care management priorities for patients with head and neck cancer are airway maintenance, pain management, and nutrition. If surgery was done, these patients have special needs and consideration including wound management, drain assessment and care, oral care, wound complications, and carotid artery exposure assessment and management. There are also special nursing management priorities related to reconstruction flaps. The Nursing Process: Patient Care Plan outlines the care for a patient who has had an orbital exenteration and maxillectomy.

Airway Management

As always the patient's airway is the first priority. The outcome for these patients is to maintain a patent airway and normal gas

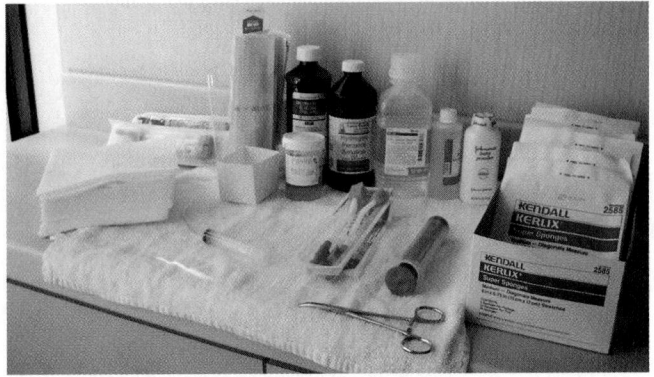

FIGURE 34–17 ■ Nursing care equipment for Doppler monitoring for arterial patency following microvascular free flap reconstruction.
Source: University of California, Davis Medical Center

exchange. Critical symptoms that need to be assessed on an ongoing basis are shortness of breath, stridor, blood-tinged sputum, and infection. Some blood may be present in the sputum, especially within the first 24 hours of having surgery and/or placement of a tracheostomy tube. Clinical manifestations of airway obstruction are increased work of breathing and increased use of accessory muscles, especially facial musculature that uses a higher amount of oxygen. There also may be an increased heart rate and decreased oxygen saturation levels. Nursing assessment of the airway needs to include the type of airway that is being used. There are many types and varieties of tracheotomy and endotracheal tubes. It is important for the nurse to become familiar with the different types and their uses. A complete discussion of airway assessment and management was presented earlier in this chapter.

Nursing interventions include securing the airway with the appropriate ties in order to prevent the possibility of the tube being dislodged or accidentally removed. The tracheostomy tube ties should be secured to the chest laterally with suspended ties. Circumferential ties can place pressure on the incision lines or reconstruction flaps or grafts. The ties should be changed every day or when soiled to decrease the possibility of infection. The tracheostomy site should be cleaned on a regular basis such as every 8 hours and more frequently as needed to remove crusts and secretions that could obstruct the airway. If the tracheostomy tube has an inner cannula, it should be changed if disposable or cleaned when every tie tracheostomy care is done. This will prevent the buildup of secretions in the tube and the possibility of airway obstruction. Frequent assessment is essential to patient safety when there are large amounts of secretions. (See earlier section for a complete description of the care of a patient with a tracheostomy tube.) If the patient is unable to clear the secretions from the airway independently, suctioning is indicated.

All patients who have an artificial airway require humidification to the airway because the normal upper airway passages that humidify sections are bypassed. This is done by tracheotomy cupola or collar. Many times in the early postoperative period, a patient is unable to clear her own secretions and may require bagging and deep suctioning. This procedure will mobilize mucous plugs, stimulate a cough, and clear the airway.

Patients who have had long surgical cases, large amounts of sedation, or have underlying lung conditions may require mechanical ventilation during the early postoperative period. Patients with head and neck cancer often have long histories of smoking with related chronic lung disease. Because their thorax or abdomen is not interrupted and their ventilation is not compromised, they usually wean early and easily from the ventilator. These patients need to be carefully but aggressively weaned as soon as they are awake and spontaneously breathing. Close monitoring is indicated including, pulse oximetry, arterial blood gases (ABGs), and respiratory rate and effort. The cuff of the tracheotomy tube should be deflated when the patient is off positive pressure ventilation. This will prevent serious complications that may include airway scarring and stenosis at the cuff site.

Other measures to improve airway and gas exchange include turning, coughing, and deep breathing, respiratory treatments with bronchodilators, and chest physiotherapy. Although very time consuming and labor intensive, early mobilization and

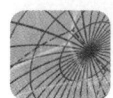

NURSING PROCESS: Patient Care Plan for Head and Neck Cancer

Assessment of Gas Exchange

Subjective Data:

Do you feel like you are getting enough air?

Are you short of breath?

Do you have any preexisting health problems such as heart, lung, or kidney disease?

Do you smoke? If so, for how long?

Objective Data:

Oxygen saturation

Work of breathing (e.g., gasping, increased rate, loudness)

Heart rate

Nail bed and skin color

Use of accessory respiratory muscles

Cough present, type of secretions

Level of consciousness and orientation

Lung sounds

Arterial blood gases

Nursing Assessment and Diagnoses	Outcomes and Evaluation Parameters	Planning and Interventions with *Rationales*
Nursing Diagnosis: *Risk for Impaired Gas Exchange*	**Outcome:** Adequate gas exchange. *Evaluation Parameters:* Free of dyspnea: unlabored respirations < 24/min. Alert and oriented. Clear breath sounds. No restlessness, cyanosis, or fatigue. Oxygen saturation and ABGs are within normal limits.	**Interventions and *Rationales:*** Assess for adventitious or diminished breath sounds. *Indicates decreased gas exchange.* Note presence of cough and amount, color, and consistency of sputum *to assess for inhalation injury.* Monitor ABGs and oxygen saturation *to assess adequacy of gas exchange and level of shock state.* Monitor respiratory rate and depth *to assess for respiratory distress.* Monitor restlessness and confusion. *Indicators of inadequate gas exchange with resultant brain hypoxia.* Observe for cyanosis, especially in the mucous membranes. *Indicators of inadequate gas exchange with resultant tissue hypoxia.* Turn, cough, deep breathe, elevate head of bed, instruct on use of incentive spirometry. *Measures to promote gas exchange.* Administer humidified oxygen as prescribed *to loosen secretions and promote airway clearance.* Report respiratory distress to the health care provider. *Medical intervention may be indicated to prevent respiratory failure.* Assess need for suctioning and/or endotracheal intubation *to maintain adequate gas exchange.* **Tracheostomy:** <ul><li>Cuff inflated while on ventilator</li><li>Always check cuff pressures</li><li>Cuff deflated at all other times</li><li>Position by securing from shoulders (not chest) Stomahesive and Elastoplast</li><li>Wound care</li><li>Remove crusts over suture lines</li><li>Spare tube at bedside (Bivona or similar stoma button if stoma contracts).</li></ul> *To maintain a patent airway.*

Assessment of Knowledge Regarding Diagnosis and Treatment

Subjective Data:

What do you understand about your diagnosis and treatment plan?

Do you have questions about the treatment program?

What would you like me to tell you about your diagnosis?

Objective Data:

Facial expressions

Verbalization of questions by patient and family

(continued)

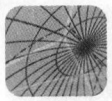
Nursing Assessment and Diagnoses	Outcomes and Evaluation Parameters	Planning and Interventions with *Rationales*
Nursing Diagnosis: *Deficient Knowledge* related to diagnosis and treatment	**Outcome:** Adequate knowledge of treatment regimen. ***Evaluation Parameter:*** Patient and family will verbalize understanding of treatments and care.	**Interventions and *Rationales:*** Assess patient/family's readiness and ability to learn and individual learning needs. *The person must be psychologically ready to learn.* Determine level of existing knowledge. *Begin the teaching where existing knowledge ends.* Instruct patient and significant other about anatomic changes related to nasal and paranasal sinus surgery. *Preoperative education empowers the patient and decreases anxiety.* Provide factual information about diagnosis, treatments, and prognosis *to increase knowledge and understanding.* Explain all procedures in simple, concise language and allow for questions *to increase understanding.* Encourage questions. *Keeps open communication and augments understanding.* Provide ongoing education about treatment plan and rationale. *Ongoing education is necessary as situations and conditions change.* Document response to teaching *to assist health care team when implementing a teaching plan.*

Assessment of Cerebrospinal Fluid (CSF) Leak Related to Repair of Dural Defect

Subjective Data:
Do you have a headache or blurred vision?
Do you feel drowsy?

Objective Data:
Nasal drainage for presence of CSF

Nursing Assessment and Diagnoses	Outcomes and Evaluation Parameters	Planning and Interventions with *Rationales*
Nursing Diagnosis: *Risk for Injury* related to CSF leak	**Outcome:** Orbital graft site will heal without complications. ***Evaluation Parameter:*** No evidence of CSF leak.	**Interventions and *Rationales:*** Observe all nasal drainage for CSF leak with a halo test. CSF on a clean dressing demonstrates a halo of clear encircled with a red–tinged halo. Notify the surgeon when leak occurs. *This indicates an abnormal leak.* Instruct patient not to strain and to avoid excessive coughing *to minimize increased intracranial pressure.*

Assessment of Perioperative Anxiety Related to Diagnosis, Hospitalization, and Surgery

Subjective Data:
Tell me what you are feeling about your diagnosis and treatment plan?
Who are the people in your life that are your support system?
How have you handled fearful situations in the past?

Objective Data:
Facial expressions
Mood
Verbalization of fear regarding injury, impact on family, and future

Nursing Assessment and Diagnoses	Outcomes and Evaluation Parameters	Planning and Interventions with *Rationales*
Nursing Diagnosis: *Anxiety* related to changes in health status/role functioning; situational crisis	**Outcomes:** Patient will verbalize fears and concerns. Accurate preoperative teaching will help decrease patient's fear of the unknown. ***Evaluation Parameter:*** Patient states she is comfortable with care and interventions.	**Interventions and *Rationales:*** Assess and document level of anxiety *to track trends in anxiety levels.* Explore with the patient/family techniques to reduce anxiety. *This gives the patient a sense of control and opens communication about the subject.* Provide factual information concerning diagnosis, treatment, disfigurement, disabilities, and prognosis. *Truthful explanations increase trust and potentially decrease anxiety.* Explain all procedures and allow time for mental preparation. *This decreases fear and anxiety of the unknown.* Explore with patient effective ways to minimize anxiety. *This gives the patient a sense of control.* Instruct patient on use of relaxation techniques *to relieve anxiety.* Assess need for and administer antianxiety and pain medication. *If alternative measures are not effective, the patient may need antianxiety agents.* Assist patient/family in setting realistic goals for progress. *Indicates effectiveness of emotional adjustment.* Consider psychiatric counseling for patients/families who exhibit inability to accept situation. *Provide an ongoing plan and interventions to promote long-term relief of anxiety.*

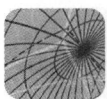

NURSING PROCESS: Patient Care Plan for Head and Neck Cancer—*Continued*

Assessment of Impaired Skin Integrity Related to Surgery

Subjective Data:
Where are you hurting?

Objective Data:
Color, blanching, odor, bleeding from graft donor and surgical site
Size and depth of wound

Nursing Assessment and Diagnoses	Outcomes and Evaluation Parameters	Planning and Interventions with *Rationales*
Nursing Diagnosis: *Impaired Skin Integrity* related to surgery	**Outcome:** Suture lines will heal normally, without complications. **Evaluation Parameters:** On inspection of the graft, no areas of dehiscence are seen. Continuous airway maintenance. Gas exchange within normal limits.	**Interventions and *Rationales:*** Assess wound and incisions. Cleanse incisions and initiate oral care per surgeon's order. Assess nutritional intake. No tracheostomy ties over reconstruction flaps or grafts. *Preventing infection and promotion of wound healing.* Provide orocutaneous, pharyngocutaneous care: • Wet-to-dry dressing that is packed carefully into the wound per surgeon's order. Protect airway at all times *to prevent infection and maintain airway.* **Free Flap Care** • Do not change dressings. • Check neurovascular status. *Radial forearm free flap:* assess the fingers. *Fibular free flap:* assess the toes. *Assessment of blood supply distal to the flap site.* **Drain Care** Secure with Stomahesive and Elastoplast. • Strip to prevent clots. • Strict output recording. • Call surgeon if sudden increase or decrease in output or air leaks from the drains. Pressure dressing 24 hours after drain removal. **Internal Carotid Artery** Exposed external or intraoral: • Wet-to-wet dressing to keep carotid in a wet and clean environment. • Hespan at bedside. • Type and cross (or hold) two units of blood. • Two large–bore IV lines in place. • Alert operating room that the patient is on precautions. • If bleed occurs, apply DIRECT pressure do not remove. • Call surgeon and operating department emergently and prepare patient for transfer.

Assessment for Infection

Subjective Data:
Is your pain increasing in the surgical areas?
Do you feel weaker?

Objective Data:
Previously healed wounds are breaking down
Open wounds not healing
Partial thickness injuries/donor sites converting to full-thickness injuries
Increased odor and drainage from wound sites
Wound cultures positive for organisms
Fever
Increased WBC

(continued)

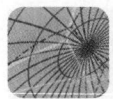

NURSING PROCESS: Patient Care Plan for Head and Neck Cancer—*Continued*

Nursing Assessment and Diagnoses	Outcomes and Evaluation Parameters	Planning and Interventions with *Rationales*
Nursing Diagnoses: *High Risk for Infection* related to loss of skin integrity and impaired healing	**Outcome:** Effective infection prevention. ***Evaluation Parameters:*** Surgical sites will not be colonized by organisms. Healing and reepithelialization will occur as noted by wound closure. Skin integrity will be restored.	**Interventions and *Rationales:*** Cleanse wounds per protocol *to prevent contamination.* Assess for infection and document with each dressing change *to prevent spread of infection.* Assess for drainage: exudate, color, odor, and amount. *These factors indicate infection.* Assess for undermining or sinus tract formation. *Indicates infection.* Use strict aseptic technique *to prevent infection.* Notify health care provider of presence of infection or wound enlargement *to facilitate medical intervention.* Monitor serum WBC daily. *Increased WBC indicates presence of infection.* Maintain nutritional therapies. *Malnutrition increases the risk of infection.* Monitor and record temperature. *Indicates infection.* Culture wounds and body secretions per protocol *to assess for infection.* Observe donor site for drainage, odor, and an increase in wound depth. Observe and document bolster orbital dressing for foul smell or purulence. *Indicates presence of infection.*

Assessment of Patient Safety

Subjective Data:
Do you feel safe when up walking?
How are you adapting to seeing out of only one eye?
What adjustments have been necessary?

Objective Data:
Is the patient able to navigate safely?
What assistive devices are necessary?

Nursing Assessment and Diagnoses	Outcomes and Evaluation Parameters	Planning and Interventions with *Rationales*
Nursing Diagnosis: *Risk for Falls*	**Outcome:** Patient will adapt safely to monocular vision. ***Evaluation Parameter:*** Patient is able to navigate safely in hospital and home environment.	**Interventions and *Rationales:*** Explain anatomic changes and discuss implications for decreased vision. Discuss the implications of monocular vision and safety implications. *Patient has knowledge of limitations.* Encourage patient to wear glasses as soon as possible. *Helps improve vision.* Arrange for home evaluation to make needed adjustments to ensure fall prevention. *Improve the safety of the environment.*

Assessment of Psychological Adjustment to Facial Disfigurement

Subjective Data:
What impact does the change in your physical appearance have on your life?
How do you plan to cope with these changes?

Objective Data:
Does patient look at the changes in the mirror?
Does patient ask questions about the wounds?
Are the patient and family members willing to learn and participate in the required care after hospital discharge?
Is patient's perception realistic regarding body image changes?

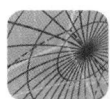

NURSING PROCESS: Patient Care Plan for Head and Neck Cancer—*Continued*

Nursing Assessment and Diagnoses	Outcomes and Evaluation Parameters	Planning and Interventions with *Rationales*
Nursing Diagnoses: *Disturbed Body Image* related to facial disfigurement and formation and functional loss. *Anticipatory Grieving* related to body image change, risk of family role change, and possible occupational change	**Outcomes:** Acceptance of body image changes. Patient is safe and competent in wound care. Patient and family will cope with deficit. ***Evaluation Parameters:*** Patient will return to activities of daily living and social interactions. Patient verbalizes understanding of body changes.	**Interventions and *Rationales:*** Teaching will have begun preoperatively with patient education and informed consent. Teach patient and family about the anatomy, reconstruction, and prosthetic rehabilitation. Begin teaching wound care, orbital packing, and obturator care as soon as possible after packing removal. *To increase knowledge and potentially decrease anxiety of the unknown.* Have patient complete dressing with nurse's support, instruction, and understanding of the visual implications of self-image changes. *Begins the adjustment process and increases independence and autonomy.* Use eye patch (flesh tones) until orbital prosthesis is made. *More aesthetic and less visible.* Consider psychiatry or social service consults as needed. *May be necessary if patient is not adjusting to change in body image.* Arrange for home health nursing consult at discharge *to assist in the transition from hospital to home environment.* Assess patient's ability to participate in self-care of the orbital cavity. Assess need for psychiatric liaison support by consultation with social service, colleagues, and health care provider.

Assessment of Nutritional Intake

Subjective Data:	Objective Data:
Does your stomach feel full? Are you experiencing any nausea?	Bowel sounds Lung sounds Residual volume

Nursing Assessment and Diagnoses	Outcomes and Evaluation Parameters	Planning and Interventions with *Rationales*
Nursing Diagnosis: *Risk for Imbalanced Nutrition; Less Than Body Requirements* related to surgery	**Outcomes:** Patient will have sufficient nutrition to heal. Home nutritional care plan is instituted as needed. ***Evaluation Parameters:*** No weight loss. Nutritional parameters at normal levels. Intake and output within normal limits. Prealbumin levels normal. No aspiration.	**Interventions and *Rationales:*** Observe ability to oral nourish self safely without aspiration. Arrange for nutrition consult for calorie and protein requirements and intake. Measure intake and output with calorie counts. *Nutrition is essential for wound healing.* Institute enteral nutrition by nasogastric (NG) or gastrostomy (GT) tube feeding as necessary. • If chyle leak, feed only no-fat formula (Vivonex TEN or similar). • Do not move NG tube. • Secure with Stomahesive and tape to nares. • Do not remove nasal stitch. • Do not attempt to replace NG without health care provider order. • Aspirate NG/GT tube at regular intervals to check residual volumes. Hold tube feeding if greater than amount specified by health care provider. *Safe administration of nasogastric feedings will prevent aspiration and not disturb suture lines.*

(continued)

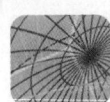

NURSING PROCESS: Patient Care Plan for Head and Neck Cancer—*Continued*

Assessment of Pain

Subjective Data:

What is your pain level, using the 1 to 10 scale? (A 1 is very little pain; a 10 is the worst imaginable pain.)

What is your experience with pain?

Do you routinely take pain medications at home; if so, what for and what kind?

Are you allergic to any pain medication?

Do you have any cultural or religious beliefs that impact your pain control?

Objective Data:

Grimacing upon movement

Restlessness and irritability

Taut facial expression

Nursing Assessment and Diagnoses	Outcomes and Evaluation Parameters	Planning and Interventions with *Rationales*
Nursing Diagnosis: *Pain* related to surgery	**Outcome:** Comfort level maintained. **Evaluation Parameters:** Able to communicate pain level and therapies that help alleviate it. Pain reduced and/or absent as evidenced by patient report and no pain behaviors (i.e., no grimacing). Nonpharmacologic method of control is effective as evidenced by patient report and no pain behaviors. Reports satisfaction with pain management program.	**Interventions and *Rationales:*** Use pain scale (0–10) to quantify pain level. *Quantifying pain increases consistency.* Instruct patient to inform nurse if pain is not relieved. *Indicates need to change pain management plan.* Assess cultural and religious impact on patient's responses. *Different cultures and religions respond differently to pain.* Correct misconceptions about risk of addiction and overdose *to decrease anxiety related to medication addiction.* Explain, prepare, and medicate patient for painful procedures (dressing change) and anticipated discomforts *to control increased pain level related to procedure.* Provide a supportive environment where patient is able to express pain level. *Opens communication and facilitates pain management.* Use pain control measures before pain becomes severe. *This increases comfort and decreases need for medication.* Teach nonpharmacologic method of control (i.e., guided imagery, massage, breathing exercises). *These measures augment pain relief.* Cover wounds. *Covering areas where there is no skin decreases the pain.* Provide rest periods between procedures to assist with coping with ongoing pain. *Decreases the fatigue related to long-term pain.* Revise pain management plan as wounds heal and pain decreases *to prevent overmedication.* Plan diversional activities *to augment pain relief measures.*

Source: Adapted from Mulgrew and Dropkin, Memorial Sloan-Kettering Cancer Center. Mulgrew, B., & Dropkin, M. J. (1991). Coping with craniofacial resection: A case study. *ORL–Head and Neck Nursing,* 9(3), 8–18.

ambulation of the patient will greatly improve the respiratory status by stimulating coughing, encouraging greater lung expansion, recruiting lung fields, and mobilizing secretions. Early ambulation also benefits circulation and increasing muscle strength. The routine standards of turn, cough, and deep breathing are extremely important in this population.

Laryngectomy Stoma Care

Patients who have undergone surgery for cancer of the larynx and have had a total laryngectomy have a permanent change in their airway and their ability to speak naturally. These patients breathe *only* from their stoma because the aerodigestive tract has been separated and the trachea is sutured to the anterior neck. Care of the permanently reconstructed airway is similar to that of the patient with a temporary tracheostomy tube in place. Careful cleaning of the stoma should be done at least every 8

hours and as needed to prevent the buildup of secretions and debris around the suture line and to prevent scarring and narrowing of the airway. If edema causes narrowing of the airway, a stoma button can be inserted to open the airway and improve ease of breathing.

The patient's head should be positioned in a neutral position or slightly extended position so as not to occlude the airway and compromise breathing. Humidification must be provided and used after discharge from the hospital until the airway becomes used to unfiltered unwarmed air. Patients usually carry small spray bottles of normal saline to mist their stomas. A simple bedside humidification device is used at night.

Pain Management

One of the greatest fears for any patient undergoing cancer surgery is the fear of pain, and with patients with head and neck cancer their fear is augmented by their inability to communicate orally. Therefore, one of the highest nursing priorities and outcomes of care is to alleviate pain and anxiety related to pain. The pain of the cancer and the pain of the procedure must be defined and each treated together (Miaskowski, 2002). For many head and neck cancer patients, pain may have been the issue that brought them in to see the doctor in the first place. They may have been taking pain medications prior to the surgery. This is a key detail to ascertain, because normal pain relief measures may be ineffective for this type of patient.

It is important to do a very careful and exact assessment of the type and location of the pain. Have the patient set a goal pain level, using a pain rating scale, and use this scale to evaluate the effectiveness of the medication and intervention. This is a useful tool to use for a patient who is awake and alert and able to cooperate with the nurse. For patients who are uncooperative and unable to communicate, more subjective signs such as diaphoresis; restlessness; agitation; increased blood pressure, heart, and respiratory rates; facial grimacing; and lack of interaction may be clues to the need for pain medication. These signs also are useful for patients who are stoic and are not asking for pain medication.

The patient should be taught not to wait until the pain is unbearable to request pain medication because, once the pain sets in, it will take longer and require more medication to achieve relief. Nursing intervention for pain relief needs to occur early and frequently in the immediate postoperative period. The patient should receive small frequent doses of analgesia. Initially, the patient's pain is managed by morphine sulfate intravenously, the commonly preferred drug of choice. Increasing the dosage as the patient's respiratory status tolerates the higher doses may achieve the goal of pain relief. The use of patient-controlled analgesia (PCA) for alert cooperative patients can be considered. Transition to oral medications is predicated on the patient's ability to swallow safely and in sufficient quantity to sustain nutrition and medication. If a feeding tube is in place, as soon as tube feedings are tolerated the patient should start on acetaminophen with codeine or hydrocodone because the enteral route has a longer effect than the IV route.

Because head and neck oncology surgeries are very long, often exceeding 15 hours, many patients complain of joint pain. Particularly in the elderly, pain from immobility often is severe and not very responsive to opioids (White & Cohen, 2006). It is not appropriate to begin nonsteroidal medications in the early postoperative period because of the complication of bleeding. An excellent method of treating this pain is with mobility, frequent ambulation, or turning in bed, even as early as postoperative day 1.

Older adults may choose not to take pain medications, but instead opt for immobility as their treatment. They then have inadequate pain control and add the risk of immobility (Kemper, 2002). Patients should know that following surgical resection the cancer pain will be eliminated. The pain of surgical resection can be controlled by multiple methods. In-depth communication, ongoing evaluation, and documentation with the health care provider should be established (Miaskowski, 2001). Pain management is discussed in detail in Chapter 15 🔗 .

Nutrition Management

Many patients with head and neck cancer present with inadequate nutrition caused by the tumor burden, cancer cachexia, or the mechanical difficulty of eating because of tumor impingement into the aerodigestive tract. Early recognition of nutritional inadequacy and nutritional intervention is critical to ensure a positive nitrogen balance with enough calories and protein to heal following surgery and radiation therapy (van Bokhorst-de van der Schueren et al., 2000).

The preoperative evaluation will identify those patients who are at risk for malnutrition and outline interventions. Those at risk are patients presenting with significant weight loss (>10%) in the past few months and those presenting with low prealbumin levels. Body height and weight are included to calculate body mass index (BMI). BMI is a method of calculating a person's height-to-weight ratio (body mass index kg/m^2). Rapid turnover proteins are the most practical window for viewing catabolic state and nitrogen loss despite the varying effects of kidney and liver failure and of steroids. The best test is serum prealbumin, transthyretin, or thyroxin-binding prealbumin (TBPA). Prealbumin is the laboratory measure of choice for assessing visceral protein status and should replace routine use of both albumin and transferrin for this purpose. Prealbumin is essential for monitoring nutrition status and nutritional therapy (Beck & Rosenthal, 2002; Bernstein et al., 1995).

The inclusion of a nutritionist in the multidisciplinary team is mandatory. Following cancer resection or during radiation therapy, nutrition consults are very helpful in targeting maintenance and replenishment goals. In the postoperative period a nutritional goal for caloric intake is estimated at 35 kcal/kg with specific attention to an increased need for hydration due to insensible water loss. Normal water loss per day is about 400 mL. In a patient with an artificial airway, water loss is about 500 to 600 mL insensible volume with an additional 600 to 700 mL per day with suctioning. Replacement requirements need to be carefully calculated in order to ensure proper hydration. The choice of feeding method, whether oral or enteral, is dependent on the patient's level of consciousness and ability to swallow. Feeding can proceed by an oral route, nasogastric route, gastrostomy, jejunostomy, or any combination thereof. Nutrition replacement must begin early and be continuous throughout the therapy for cancer. Most feeding can begin on postoperative day 1 and be advanced to goals as quickly as tolerated.

Dysphagia is a common issue that needs to be dealt with in patients with head and neck cancer. Swallowing is difficult because of tumor burden, invasion of the aerodigestive tract, and pain. Aspiration is a significant concern with patients who are unable to maintain their airway protection (Metheny, 2002; Metheny, Aud, & Wunderlich, 1999). See the Risk Factors for Aspiration box (p. 928).

Beginning as early as 1989, Logeman greatly advanced dysphagia research by directing the medical community to more accurately and objectively assess the amount, type, cause, and directed therapy for the treatment of swallowing problems and aspiration. Leonard and Kendall (1997) described an objective method of radiographic identification and quantification of aspiration. These more precise evaluations direct the process of intervention and swallow rehabilitation (Leonard & Kendall, 2007).

Enteral feeding routes are used because most patients with head and neck cancer have intact and functioning gastrointestinal systems. Once the patient is able to take oral food, the process needs to begin slowly with careful monitoring of tolerance and

RISK FACTORS for Aspiration

Documented previous episodes of aspiration

Decreased level of consciousness (sedation, increased intracranial pressure, coma)

Structural abnormalities of the aerodigestive tract (post head and neck cancer resection)

Neuromuscular disease

Endotracheal intubation

Vomiting

Persistently high gastric residual volumes

Need for prolonged supine position

Additional Factors

Presence of a nasoenteric tube

Noncontinuous or intermittent feeding

Abdominal/thoracic surgery or trauma

Delayed gastric emptying

Diabetes, hyperglycemia independent of diabetes, electrolyte abnormalities, drugs known to reduce gastroenteritis

Poor oral care

Age

Inadequate nursing staff

Large size or diameter of feeding tube

Malpositioned feeding tube

Transport

Source: McClave, S. A. et al. (2002). North American Summit of Aspiration in the Critically Ill Patient: Consensus statement. *Journal of Parenteral and Enteral Nutrition, 26* (6 Suppl.), S80–S85.

risk for aspiration. Sievers, Leonard, and McKenzie (1992) described a safe method for oral rehabilitation using an adaptive device (Figure 34–18 ■). All of these methods of nutritional support can and should be used to assist the patient with head and neck cancer to attain successful nutrition.

Wound Care

Gentle wound care is done with hydrogen peroxide to remove crusts, and normal saline is used to cleanse the skin wound and incisions. The surgeon dictates the frequency, but generally rou-

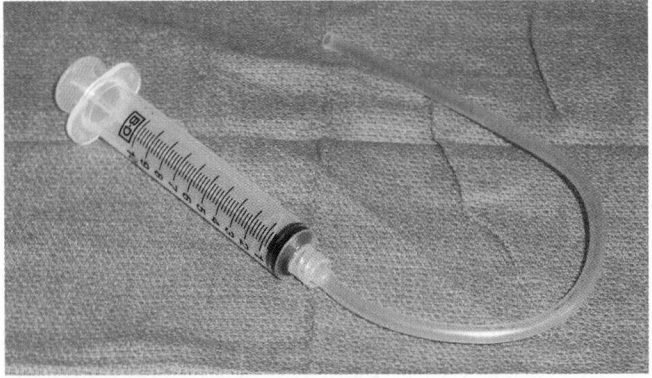

FIGURE 34–18 ■ Syringe with catheter for feeding placement for accurate placement of oral nutrition in the patient with oral tongue resections. Safe oral placement is critical to prevent aspiration.
Source: University of California, Davis Medical Center

tine care is considered to be every 4 hours and as needed (prn) to keep the wound clean and free from crusts. Depending on surgeon preference, the cleaning should be followed by the application of a thin layer of antibiotic ointment for the first 48 hours. This will help keep the incision clean and free from drainage and will aid in sealing the wound. Care of the suture lines also includes assessment for drainage, redness, odor, or other signs of infection. Any surgical incisions that are not well approximated or are draining pus, bile, saliva, or tube feedings must be reported to the health care provider at once because they indicate serious changes in the integrity of the surgical site. Oral care is included in wound care because many of the patients have intraoral incisions. The inside of the mouth should be very carefully cleaned on the side away from the internal suture lines using very soft toothbrushes and rinsing well.

The purpose of the placement of drains in the surgical site is to evaluate blood and other fluids from the surgical site. The assessment of the postoperative patient includes observing the drains for patency and the amount and type of drainage. Each drain is individually labeled and firmly secured, so the drain will not accidentally become dislodged or pulled out by the patient. Every drain is numbered, labeled, and documented precisely for position on the neck and chest. Document the color, type, and amount of output, and record each drain individually in the intake and output section of the nursing documentation record. The health care provider determines when the drain should be removed; typically this is done when there is less than 30 mL of drainage in a 24-hour period. A dressing is placed over the site for 24 hours following removal.

Wound Complications

A number of postoperative complications can occur in the patient with head and neck cancer. Patients who have a history of radiation therapy or have a poor nutritional status are at greater risk for alterations in wound healing and possible complications. Any type of excessive drainage may indicate a problem and, if caught early, treatment will mitigate complications. For example, a large amount of milky colored fluid (possibly up to 1 liter in 24 hours) is referred to as a chyle leak. A **chyle leak** is a disruption in the lymph system that causes lymphatic fluid to leak from the thoracic duct on the left side and the lymphatic duct on the right side. This condition should be reported to the health care provider immediately because it can result in serious fluid and electrolyte imbalances. Shifts in potassium, sodium, calcium, and magnesium can be life threatening with serious cardiac manifestations. The affected drain is placed to gravity drainage and a zero-fat diet is implemented. A decrease in fat in the diet will result in a decreased production of lymph. This is done with the hope that the leak will seal itself given the decrease in production of lymphatic fluid. The nurse must monitor fluid and electrolytes.

Bright red, excessive clots or large amounts of drainage indicate abnormal bleeding. Monitoring the patient's hematocrit (HCT) and hemoglobin (HBG) and carefully assessing vital signs are essential when bleeding occurs. A decrease in the HCT and HGB and/or an increase in the pulse rate and decrease in the blood pressure are reported to the surgeon. Each drain is milked or stripped according to the surgeon's orders to ensure patency. Stripping will remove excess fluid, drainage, and clots from the surgical area and tubing that may lead to problems of congestion, flap failure, and hematoma at the surgical site. The tube is stripped by first lubricating it with lotion or water-soluble jelly, then pinching the tube between two fingers and pulling down the length of the tubing, creating suction. Great care must be taken not to dislodge the tube from its position in the body. Any suspected problems with drain function should be reported to the surgeon for immediate intervention.

Other possible postoperative complications include the accumulation of fluid (seroma) or blood (hematoma) in the bed of the surgical wound, infection, fistulas, carotid artery exposure, and flap failure. As discussed earlier, fistulas are dehiscent wounds that traverse between two different tissue planes. In the head and neck, a fistula that occurs between the pharynx and the skin is termed a pharyngocutaneous fistula (Figure 34–19 ■).

A serious, potentially life-threatening complication is carotid artery exposure and potential rupture. This can occur in the patient who has problems with wound healing, fistula formation, poor nutrition, and/or a history of radiation therapy to the area. A tumor that has been removed close to the carotid artery leaves the artery in jeopardy of rupture, and if the tumor recurs or a fistula forms, the risk further increases. If the primary closure of the surgical incision fails and the artery is exposed to air, it can lead to drying and weakening of the arterial wall. If this occurs, place the patient on special alert for what is referred to as *carotid blowout* precautions. The patient should be in sight of a nurse at all times and specific supplies are placed in the patient's room that will be needed in the event of a rupture. A "herald" bleed (massive bleed), or prerupture sign, indicating an imminent bleed, can occur 24 to 48 hours prior to a major carotid bleed. If a rupture occurs, direct digital pressure should be placed on the vessel and the airway maintained with suctioning and positioning. The patient is transported to the operating room immediately to undergo carotid resection. Never release direct pressure until surgical intervention has been secured. Chart 34–7 outlines typical health care provider orders for carotid artery precautions.

Physical Therapy

As the patient progresses through the hospital stay, it is important to include physical therapy in the plan of care. If the patient has had a neck dissection with the resection of CN XI, he will be unable to fully move the shoulder due to the enervation of the trapezius muscle. Physical therapy exercises help the patient to regain mobility, prevent a frozen shoulder, and improve general reconditioning. These exercises should be continued after hospital discharge either in the home or as an outpatient. Written instructions with pictures are very helpful for the patient and family to follow. This also gives the home health nurse and outpatient physical therapist goals for home therapy.

Discharge Priorities

Discharge priorities for patients with head and neck cancer are related to safety at home, airway maintenance, nutrition, wound care, follow-up therapy, compliance with the treatment regimen, and adaptation to illness (see Patient Teaching & Discharge Priorities box, p. 930). As these patients finish their hospital stay, it is the nurse's responsibility to become part of the team to help the patient transition from hospital to home. With the clinical nurse specialist, dietitian, speech therapist, discharge planner, physician, physical therapist, and social services providers, all efforts must be directed toward adaptation and safety. The most important part of the discharge process is to remember that discharge planning begins at the time of diagnosis.

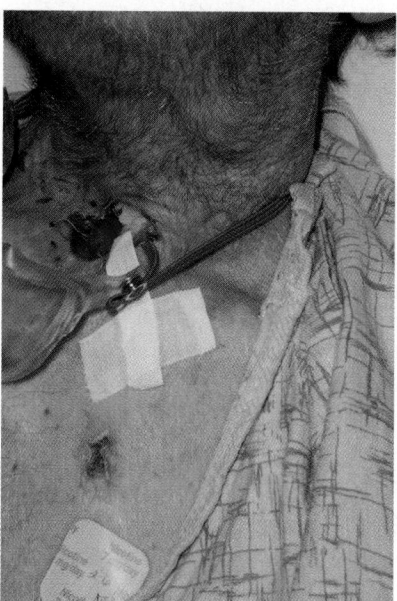

FIGURE 34–19 ■ This post-laryngectomy patient developed a fistula on his left side just lateral to his laryngectomy stoma. Packing in place is changed four times a day to encourage healing and prevent saliva from entering his stoma.
Source: University of California, Davis Medical Center

CHART 34–7   Carotid Artery Precautions

1. Carotid tray at bedside
2. Four packages fluffs at bedside
3. Dual-suction machines with large oral suction at bedside
4. Portable suction on unit for transport
5. One-liter lactated Ringer's solution at bedside with connecting tubing
6. Two large-bore IVs at all times
7. Blood administration set at bedside
8. Type and antibody screen every 48 hours (1 adult clot tube) or per hospital protocol
9. Two units Hespan (or similar) at bedside
10. *Wound care:* saline-soaked dressings (Wet to wet every 2 hours. When stable and healing, advance to every 2 hours while awake and every 4 hours at night, with wetting of the dressing with normal saline every 2 hours.)
11. Frequent observation of patient for "herald" bleed (prerupture bleed), dry or dark area of artery or aneurysm formation
12. Call House Officer or Primary Care Provider immediately if any of the above occur.
13. Assess for higher level of care if other compounding problems are present.
14. Alert OR and blood bank that patient is on carotid precautions.

RESEARCH OPPORTUNITIES AND CLINICAL IMPACT RELATED TO UPPER AIRWAY DISORDERS

Research Area	Clinical Impact
What is the effect of anterior and posterior nasal packing on oxygenation and CO_2?	Currently patients who have anterior and/or posterior packing require cardiac monitoring and therefore advanced nursing care. What is the appropriate level of care required for these patients?
What is the effect of weight loss on the life of OSA patients?	Improved quality of life with OSA.
	Decreased hospitalizations and medical costs.
	Education of patients about the importance of weight control and OSA.
Insensible water loss with a tracheotomy.	Improved method of caring for patients with an artificial airway.
Use of normal saline in the ambulatory patient with an artificial airway.	Better hydration and fluid replacement techniques.
	Decreased frequency of dehydration.
Perceptions of patients with head and neck cancer.	Better adapted and better prepared patients.
Quality of life with patients and caregivers of those with head and neck cancer.	Improved quality of life.
What is safe staffing for an otolaryngology unit or clinic given the fragility of patients with artificial and at-risk airways?	Ability to define the appropriate staffing mix for an ENT nursing unit or clinic based on nursing decisions, patient education, and interventions.

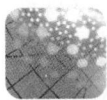

PATIENT TEACHING & DISCHARGE PRIORITIES for Head and Neck Cancer Patients

Need	Teaching
Knowledge of home and self-care following surgery for head and neck cancer	Health care needs include verbal and written instructions for treatment plan and follow-up care.
	Assess patient and family understanding of disease process, surgical procedure performed, and health maintenance needs in the home setting.
Maintenance of airway	Patient and family or significant others are taught how to maintain an open airway by: • Providing verbal and written instructions on self-care needs, equipment usage, and indicators for emergency assistance. • Providing instructions on self-suctioning, wound care, change of tracheostomy tube, and safety precautions.
Nutrition	Patient and family are taught about nutritional needs by: • Instructing patient/family on nutritional needs, calories needed per day, and how to use enteral feedings. • Providing consultation from a dietitian as necessary.
Wound care	Ascertain patient/family's ability to care for the wound using aseptic technique: • Instruct patient/family on wound care and evaluate ability to complete by ensuring a return demonstration. • Providing all necessary supplies for wound care and ask patient/family to keep track of availability of necessary supplies.
Physical therapy	Assess patient's need for transportation to appointments.
	Determine patient's ability to perform exercises as directed by demonstrating exercises.
Speech therapy	Assess patient's need for transportation to appointments.
	Establish means of communication; practice speech.
	Instruct patient to keep track of therapy appointments and observe compliance to prescribed therapy.
Safety	Stress importance of safety precautions by: • Instructing to keep emergency numbers by phone. • Instructing to keep written instructions for self-care easily accessible. • Reinforcing instructions for airway maintenance. • Identifying ways to detect gas alerts if patient/family unable to smell.
Family/significant other support system	Assess availability, knowledge, and compliance with treatment regimen.
	Assess for need for professional home health needs.
	Establish a plan for caretaker rest and support.
	Establish a plan for assurance of meeting patient's rest needs.
	Discuss with patient and family independence goals and establish markers for advancement toward independence.
Follow-up therapy	Instruct patient on criticality of follow-up therapy.
	Assist patient in establishing a calendar of appointments with expected outcome that patient will keep appointments.
Compliance	Evaluate patient for knowledge of compliance needs in self-care with potential outcome of patient maintaining ongoing appointments as scheduled.
Adaptation to illness	Assess patient's coping needs and methods of coping.
	Encourage open discussion of feelings and concerns.
	Provide psychological counseling as needed.

Clinical Preparation

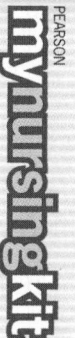

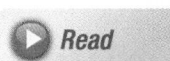 **Read**

- History of Current Illness
- Past Medical History
- Physical Exam
- Admitting Medical Orders
- Laboratory Study Results

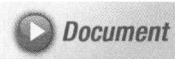 **Document**

- Summary of Hospitalization
- Pathophysiology Form
- Laboratory Values
- Laboratory Results Explanation

 **Apply**

- List of Potential Nursing Diagnoses
- Concept Map
- Critical Thinking Questions

Log on to MyNursingKit.com to download forms you will need and to complete further steps in the Clinical Preparation assignment.

HISTORY OF PRESENT ILLNESS

A 23-year-old female was brought in by ambulance to the emergency department (ED). She was transported because of an injury to her anterior neck after being hit by a softball during practice. The patient was responsive sitting in an upright forward position. She was initially evaluated by the ED physician. Otolaryngology was urgently consulted because the patient's airway distress was increasing as her neck swelling increased. There was too much swelling to safely view the vocal cords for intubation. With fluid resuscitation and stabilization, the patient was taken to the operating room where a tracheotomy was performed.

Following recovery from anesthesia, she was alert, cognitively intact, and could write to the staff. After 2 days in the ICU to rule out any other injuries such as closed head injury, the patient was stable and transferred to an acute care unit where you assumed care of her. The patient's tracheotomy was downsized from a cuffed #8 to an uncuffed #6 tracheotomy tube. The patient was taught to speak by covering the tube with finger occlusion. The patient's voice was very hoarse, and she coughed while drinking liquids. Aspiration precautions were initiated and otolaryngology speech therapy was called in to assess the patient's voice and swallowing. Otolaryngology continued to evaluate the patient's hoarse, breathy voice and dysphagia. On fiber-optic examination it was apparent that she was not able to medialize her right vocal cord and her larynx was insensate, thus the hoarseness and inability to protect the airway during eating. The patient did not appear to be experiencing any further respiratory difficulties and her vital signs and oxygen (O_2) saturations were all within normal limits. She had a low-grade temperature (38°C), which was presumed to be a result of atelectasis from prolonged bed rest.

A dynamic swallow study was done in the speech lab to further assess the degree of difficulty the patient had protecting her airway while eating and to evaluate the patient's vocal cord status. The speech therapist worked with the patient with different types of food textures to determine which ones the patient could safely handle. It was determined that pureed food with thick liquids would be the safest diet for this patient.

Dietary was notified of the change in diet and a request was put in to have the diet tray left on the cart to be delivered to the patient by the nurse. That way, it was certain that the patient would be positioned properly in a chair or with the head of the bed at 90 degrees and that she would be observed for aspiration throughout the meal. Suction was available at the bedside for use as needed.

Medical–Surgical History

Appendectomy and tonsillectomy as a child

Social History

Married no children; attends graduate school

Travels frequently in the United States with her softball team

Physical Exam

Head: normocephalic, nontraumatic, no lacerations or bruising

Eyes: normal EOM bilaterally, PERL

Ears: WNL no hemotympanum or trauma

Nose: WNL

Mouth: WNL no evidences of trauma, tongue not swollen, occasional coughing of blood

Neck: Significant bruising was noted in the anterior of the neck; attributed to the direct injury of the softball

Cranial nerves: CN I not tested; CN X impairment on the L side; others WNL

Admitting Medical Orders

Otolaryngology Service

Admit to Medical–Surgical floor

Admitting diagnosis: 23-year-old woman admitted status postinjury to the neck by a softball; tracheotomy

Allergies: none known
Up ad lib with bathroom privileges
Head of bed at 90 degrees or up in chair for meals
Diet: pureed food with thick liquids
Vital signs and oxygen saturation q4h
Neuro assessment q4h
I&O
IV D51/2 NS at 75 mL/hr until tolerating fluids; then convert to saline lock: flush q8h with NS
Aspiration precautions
Routine tracheostomy care
Suction prn
O_2 per humidified trach collar to keep oxygen saturation > 92%
Call house officer: pulse < 60 and > 130/minute; BP < 90 and > 160 systolic; temperature > 38.5; urine output < 30 mL/hr for 2 hours; respiratory rate > 30/minute; oxygen saturation < 92%
Sequential compression devices (SCDs) to lower extremities while in bed

Scheduled Medications

Morphine sulfate PCA: 1 mg incremental dose q10min. If pain not well controlled, give morphine sulfate bolus 1–5 mg IV × 1

PRN Medications

Temazepam 15–30 mg po qhs prn insomnia
Droperidol 1.25–2.5 mg IV q6h prn nausea
Ativan 1 mg IV q6h prn anxiety
Milk of Magnesia 30 mL daily prn constipation
Tylenol 650 mg po/PR q4h prn for pain

Ordered Laboratory Studies

Chemistry 7 panel, CBC, ABGs, and magnesium daily
INR × 1

Ordered Diagnostic Studies

Flexible fiber-optic laryngoscopy
Videostroboscopy
Dynamic swallow study

LABORATORY STUDY RESULTS

Test	Day 1	Day 2	Day 3
Sodium	137 mEq/L	136 mEq/L	139 mEq/L
Potassium	3.8 mEq/L	3.8 mEq/L	3.7 mEq/L
Chloride	106 mEq/L	103 mEq/L	11 mEq/L
Blood urea nitrogen (BUN)	4 mg/dL	4 mg/dL	6 mg/dL
Creatinine	1.1 mg/dL	0.9 m/dL	0.7 m/dL
Blood glucose	143 mg/dL	120 m/dL	98 m/dL
Calcium	7.9 mEq/L	7.8 mEq/L	9.1 mEq/L
Total protein	6.3 g/dL	6.0 g/dL	5.8 mg/dL
Magnesium	2.1 mEq/L	1.9 mEq/L	2.4 mEq/L
White blood count	12,600 µL	19.1 µL	13.4 µL
Hemoglobin	9.8 g/dL	10.6 g/dL	12.5 g/dL
Hematocrit	28.1%	29.6%	31.5%
Red blood cells	3.35 million/ µL	3.26 million/µL	3.67 million/µL
Platelets	195,000 µL	189,000 µL	241,000 µL
INR	1.00 INR		
ABGs			
PaO_2	98 mmHg	112 mmHg	96 mmHg
O_2 sat	96	99	97
pH	7.44	7.46	7.56
$PaCO_2$	36 mmHg	35 mmHg	24 mmHg
HCO_3	25 mEq/L	25 mEq/L	20 mEq/L

CRITICAL THINKING QUESTIONS

1. Explain what the nurse's responsibility is to a patient who is unable to communicate by natural voice. What are the alternatives and what are the nurse's professional responsibilities?

2. Discuss the implications of nursing interventions used with a patient in airway obstruction following traumatic injury. How can the nurse help the patient adapt to a new airway?

3. Think of the quality-of-life implications for a 23-year-old athlete who has a tracheostomy and airway injury. Discuss the role of compassion and comportment in the nursing care of such a patient.

Answers to Critical Thinking Questions appear in Appendix D

NCLEX® REVIEW

1. The nurse is caring for a pediatric patient recovering from a fractured mandible. Which of the following should be included in this patient's plan of care?
   1. Provide system antibiotics to prevent meningitis.
   2. Once stable, instruct in the use of a water pik.
   3. Provide eye protection.
   4. Assess for facial droop every 2 hours.

2. Which of the following should the nurse include in a plan of care for a patient with acute sinusitis?
   1. Restrict fluids
   2. Administer antibiotics as prescribed
   3. Maintain on bedrest
   4. Dental consultation for gum and tooth pain

3. The nurse is planning instruction for a patient with seasonal allergic rhinitis. Which of the following should be included in this instruction?
   1. Expect to have allergy injections for 6 months.
   2. Spend time outdoors to increase immunity to the allergen.
   3. Boil a pan of water on the stove every day to increase environmental humidity.
   4. Avoid exposure to strong perfumes, smoke, and rapid changes in temperature.

4. During an assessment, an elderly patient tells the nurse that he "just doesn't smell things the way he used to." Which of the following should the nurse include in this patient's assessment?
   1. Presence of smoke detectors in the home and the type of cooking appliances used
   2. Mobility of head and neck
   3. Appetite
   4. Respiratory rate

5. A patient with obstructive sleep apnea is having difficulty using the CPAP device at home. Which of the following can the nurse instruct this patient?
   1. Only wear the device for a few hours every night.
   2. Assess the type of difficulty and provide recommendations accordingly.
   3. Sleep propped up with pillows instead of using the device.
   4. Use a dental device instead.

6. A patient diagnosed with neck cancer says he's never smoked and wants to know what caused the disease. Which of the following should the nurse respond to this patient?
   1. Most people deny a smoking history.
   2. Smoking is only one cause for the disease. Others include chronic mouth lesions and poor nutrition.
   3. You would be surprised to hear what can cause this type of cancer.
   4. It's because you drink alcohol.

7. The nurse is providing care to a patient with a tracheostomy because of neck cancer. Which of the following should be included in this patient's plan of care?
   1. Provide tracheostomy care every 24 hours.
   2. Change tracheostomy ties every 4 hours.
   3. Provide inner cannula care every day.
   4. Secure the tube ties laterally to the chest with suspended ties.

Answers for review questions appear in Appendix D

KEY TERMS

anosmia *p.895*
aphonic *p.902*
chyle leak *p.928*
continuous positive airway pressure
   (CPAP) *p.878*
decannulation *p.910*
epiglottitis *p.900*
epistaxis *p.882*
fistula *p.907*
hairy tongue *p.898*
hoarseness *p.903*

laryngeal spasm *p.905*
laryngectomy *p.902*
laryngitis *p.903*
laryngopharyngeal reflux disease
   (LPRD) *p.907*
Ludwig's angina *p.899*
mucormycosis *p.895*
myocutaneous flap *p.919*
nasal polyps *p.894*
neck dissection *p.919*
otolaryngology (otorhinolaryngology) *p.880*

panendoscopy *p.917*
peritonsillar abscess *p.900*
pharyngitis *p.900*
rhinitis *p.888*
sinusitis *p.892*
sleep apnea *p.897*
stridor *p.900*
tonsillitis *p.900*
tracheostomy *p.885*
tracheotomy *p.885*

REFERENCES

American Academy of Otolaryngology–Head and Neck Surgery. (2007). *Fact sheet: Deviated septum.* Retrieved May 19, 2008, from http://www.entnet.org/HealthInformation/deviatedSeptum.cfm

American Cancer Society. (2006). *Detailed guide: Oral cavity and oropharyngeal cancer. What are the risk factors for oral cavity and oropharyngeal cancer?* Retrieved August 23, 2007, from http://www. cancer.org/docroot/CRI/content/CRI_2_4_2X_What_are_the_risk_factors_for_oral_cavity_and_oropharyngeal_cancer_60.asp?rnav=cri

Babak, J., & Blackwell, K. (2005). *Facial bone anatomy.* Retrieved July 14, 2007, from http://www.emedicine.com/ent/topic9.htm

Bailey, B. J., Johnson, J. T., Newlands, S. D., Calhoun, K. H., & Deskin, R. W. (2006). *Head and neck surgery—otolaryngology.* Philadelphia: Lippincott Williams & Wilkins.

Baitha, S., Raizada, R. M., Kennedy-Singh, A. K., Puttewar, M. P., & Chaturvedi, V. N. (2002). Clinical profile of hoarseness of voice. *Indian Journal of Otolaryngology and Head and Neck Surgery, 54*(1), 554–558.

Baugh, W. P., & Earhart, K. C. (2006). *Rhinocerebral mucormycosis.* Retrieved September 2, 2007, from the eMedicine website: http://www.emedicine.com/med/topic2026.htm

Beck, F. K., & Rosenthal, T. C. (2002). Pre-albumin: A marker for nutritional evaluation. *American Family Physician, 65,* 1575–1578.

Beers, M. (Ed.). (2004). Neurological disorders. Section 14: Sleep disorders. In *The Merck manual of health and aging* (central ed.). West Point, PA: Merck Research Laboratories.

Beers, M. H. & Berkow, R. (2004). Mucormycosis. Section 13 Chapter 158. In *the merck manual of diagnoses and therapy.* Whitehouse Station, NJ: Merck Research Laboratories.

Belafsky, P. C. (2006). Empiric treatment with PPI's is not appropriate without testing. *American Journal of Gastroenterology, 101*(1), 6–8.

Bermant, M. (2007). *Nasal fractures.* Retrieved July 15, 2007, from http://www.plasticsurgery4u.com/procedure_folder/nasal_fx.html

Bernstein, L., et al. (1995). Measurement of visceral protein status in assessing protein and energy malnutrition: Standard of care prealbumin in nutritional care consensus group. *Nutrition, 11*(2), 169–171.

Brannon, G. E. (2006). *History and mental status examination.* Retrieved September 8, 2007, from http://www.emedicine.com/med/topic3358.htm

Calhoun, K., Eibling, D. E., & Wax, M. K. (Eds.). (2001). *Expert guide to otolaryngology.* Philadelphia: American College of Physicians and American Society of Internal Medicine.

Chang, E., & Adami, H. O. (2006). The enigmatic epidemiology of nasopharyngeal carcinoma. *Cancer Epidemiology, Biomarkers and Prevention, 15,* 1765–1777.

Connell, S., & Belafsky, P. C. (2005). *Temporal bone fractures.* Retrieved July 23, 2007, from http://www.emedicine.com/ent/topic477.htm

Corey, C. L. (2006). *Frontal sinus fractures.* Houston: Baylor College of Medicine, Bobby R. Alford Department of Otolaryngology–Head and Neck Surgery, Grand Round Archive.

Cross, D., & Burmester, J. (2006), Gene therapy for cancer treatment: Past, present and future. *Clinical Medicine & Research, 4*(3), 218–227.

Donald, P. J., Enepikedes, D., & Boggan, J. (2004). Giant juvenile nasopharyngeal angiofibroma: Management by skull-base surgery. *Archives of Otolaryngology—Head & Neck Surgery, 130,* 882–886.

Eledrisi, M. S., Alshanti, M. S., Shah, M. F., Brolosy, B., & Jaha, N. (2006). Overview of the diagnosis and management of diabetic ketoacidosis. *American Journal of the Medical Sciences, 331*(5), 243–251.

Fidrose, R., & Elamin, E. (2004). Pulmonary edema secondary to dynamic tracheal collapse. *Journal of Bronchology, 11*(2), 118–121.

File, T. M. (2005). Telithromycin new product overview. *Journal of Allergy and Clinical Immunology, 115*(2), S1–S13.

Forastiere, A. A., Goepfert, H., Maor, M., Pajak, T., Webers, R., Morrison, W., et al. (2003). Concurrent chemotherapy and radiotherapy for organ preservation in advanced laryngeal cancer. *New England Journal of Medicine, 349* (22), 2091–2098, and Correction, *350*(10),1049.

Galler, D., Skinner, A., & Ng, A. (2005). *Critical care considerations in trauma.* Retrieved January 25, 2006, from http://www.emedicine.com/med/topic3218.htm#section-neurotrauma

Greene, F. L., Page, D. L., Fleming, I. D., Fritz, A. G., Balch, C. M., Haller, D. G., et al. (Eds.). (2002). *AJCC cancer staging manual* (6th ed.). New York: Springer.

Hallet, R. (2006, October). *Allergy and immunology management.* Lecture given at the University of California Davis Medical Center.

Hampel, F., Ratner, P., Mansfield, L., Meeves, S., Liao, Y., & Georges, G. (2003, October). Fexofenadine hydrochloride exhibits equivalent efficacy to cetirizine with less drowsiness in patients with moderate-to-severe seasonal allergic rhinitis. *Annals of Allergy, Asthma and Immunology, 91*(4), 354–361.

Harris, L., & Huntoon, M. (Eds.). (2007). *Core curriculum for otorhinolaryngology head–neck nursing* (2nd ed.). New Smyrna Beach, FL: Society of Otorhinolaryngology and Head-Neck Nurses.

Howarth, P., Stern, M., Roi, L., Reynolds, R., & Bousquet, J. (1999). Double-blind, placebo-controlled study comparing the efficacy and safety of fexofenadine hydrochloride and cetirizine in seasonal allergic rhinitis. *Journal of Allergy and Clinical Immunology, 104*(5), 927–933.

Jafek, B. W., Murrow, B., & Linschoten, M. (2000). Evaluation and treatment of anosmia. *Current Opinion Otolaryngology & Head & Neck Surgery, 8,* 63–67.

Jett, K. F. (2007). Dementia, delirium and depression. *Advance for Nurses, 4*(6), 15–19.

Kemper, J. A. (2002). Pain management of older adults after discharge from outpatient surgery. *Pain Management Nursing, 3* (4), 141–153.

Kennedy, E. S. (2007). *Sinusitis.* Retrieved August 30, 2007, from http://www.emedicine.com/EMERG/topic536.htm

Kucik, C. J. (2005). Management of epistaxis. *American Family Physician, 71*(2), 305–311.

Kutner, M., Greenberg, E., Jun, Y., & Paulsen, C. (2006). *The health literacy of America's adults: Results from the 2003 National Assessment of Adult Literacy.* Washington, DC: National Center for Education Statistics, U.S. Department of Education.

Leonard, R., & Kendall, K. (Eds.). (1997). *Dysphagia assessment and treatment planning: A team approach.* San Diego: Singular Publishing.

Leonard, R., & Kendall, K. (2001). Phonoscopy: A valuable tool for otolaryngologists and speech language pathologists in the management of dysphonic patients. *Laryngoscope, 111*(10), 1760–1766.

Leonard, R., & Kendall, K. (Eds.). (2007). *Dysphagia assessment and treatment planning: A team approach.* San Diego: Singular Publishing.

Linfoot, P., & Bergstrom, C. (2005). Pathophysiology of ketoacidosis in Type 2 diabetes mellitus. *Diabetic Medicine, 22*(10), 1414–1419.

Maktabi, M., Smith, R., & Todd, M. (2003). Editorial views: Is routine endotracheal intubation as safe as we think or wish? *Anesthesiology, 99*(2), 247–248.

Mayo Clinic. (2006). *Nervous system: Vocal cord paralysis.* Retrieved August 28, 2007, from http://www.mayoclinic.com/health/vocal-cord-paralysis/DS00670/DSECTION=2

McClay, J. E. (2007). *Nasal polyps.* Retrieved May 29, 2008, from http://www.emedicine.com/PED/topic1550.htm

Medline Plus. (2005a). *Hoarseness or changing voice.* Retrieved August 28, 2007, from http://www.nlm.nih.gov/medlineplus/ency/article/003054.htm#Definition

Medline Plus. (2005b). *Upper airway obstruction.* Retrieved August 16, 2007, from http://www.nlm.nih.gov/medlineplus/ency/article/000067.htm

Medline Plus. (2006). *Smell—impaired.* Retrieved September 3, 2007, from http://www.nlm.nih.gov/medlineplus/ency/article/003053.htm

Merritt, J., Roth, J., & Logothetis, C. (2001). Clinical evaluation of adenoviral-mediated gene transfer: Review on INGN 201 studies. *Seminars in Oncology, 28* (5 Suppl. 16), 105–114.

Metheny, N. A. (2002). Risk factors for aspiration. *Journal of Parenteral and Enteral Nutrition,* S26–S31, and Discussion, S32–S3.

Metheny, N. A., Aud, M. A., & Wunderlich, R. J. (1999). A survey of bedside methods used to detect pulmonary aspiration of enteral formula in intubated tube-fed patients. *American Journal of Critical Care, 8,* 160–169.

Meyers, F. (1999). Perspectives on palliative care: A chair of medicine viewpoint. *Journal of Palliative Medicine, 2,* 371–375.

Meyers, F., & Linder, J. (2003). Simultaneous care: Disease treatment and palliative care. *Journal of Clinical Oncology, 21*(7), 1412–1415.

Miaskowski, C. (2001). Words with new meanings [Editorial]. *Pain Management Nursing, 2*(3), 73.

Miaskowski, C. (2002). The need to assess multiple symptoms [Editorial]. *Pain Management Nursing, 3*(4), 115.

National Heart, Lung, and Blood Institute. (2006). *Obstructive sleep apnea.* Retrieved August 16, 2007, from http://www.nhlbi.nih.gov/health/dci/Diseases/SleepApnea/SleepApnea_WhatIs.html

National Institute on Deafness and Other Communication Disorders. (2002). *Vocal cord paralysis.* Retrieved August 16, 2007, from http://www.nidcd.nih.gov/health/voice/vocalparal.htm

Nettelbeck, D., & Curiel, D. (2003, October). Tumor-busting viruses. *Scientific American,* 68–75.

O'Toole, M. T. (Ed). (2003). *Miller-Keane encyclopedia and dictionary of medicine, nursing, and allied health* (7th ed.). Philadelphia: W. B. Saunders.

Piccolino, P., Vetrano, S., Mundula, P., Di Lella, G., Tedaldi, M., & Poladas, G. (2007). Frontal bone fractures: A new technique of closed reduction. Technical strategies. *Journal of Craniofacial Surgery, 18*(3), 695–698.

Pope, L. E. R., & Hobbs, C. G. L. (2005). Epistaxis: An update on current management. *Postgraduate Medical Journal, 81,* 309–314.

Porth, C. M. (2005) *Pathophysiology: Concepts of altered health status* (7th ed.). Philadelphia: Lippincott Williams & Wilkins.

Quillen, D. M., & Feller, D. B. (2006). Diagnosing rhinitis: Allergic vs. nonallergic. *American Family Physician, 73*(9), 1583–1590.

Ramakrishnan, V. R., & Meyers, A. D. (2006). *Nonallergic rhinitis.* Retrieved August 19, 2007, from http://www.emedicine.com/ent/topic402.htm

Rosin, D. (1998). Nasal obstruction. *The sinus source book.* Los Angeles: Lowell House.

Rudy, S. F. (2006). Staying motivated in providing tobacco cessation advice and counseling. *ORL–Head and Neck Nursing, 24*(4), 6–9.

Sataloff, R., et al. (1998). *Performing arts medicine.* San Diego: Singular Publishing.

Schneider, K., & Segal, G. (2006). *Dental abscess.* Retrieved July 29, 2007, from http://www.emedicine.com/ped/topic2675.htm

Seiden, A. M. (1997). *Taste and smell disorders.* New York: Thieme.

Sheikh, H. (2007). *Rhinitis, allergic.* Retrieved August 25, 2007, from http://emedicine.com/med/topic104.htm

Sievers, A., Leonard, R., & McKenzie, S. (1992). The safe use of an adaptative early feeding device for impaired patients. *ORL–Head and Neck Nursing, 10,* 17–19.

Smith, J. E., & Perez, C. L. (2004). *Nasal fractures.* Retrieved August 15, 2007, from http://www.emedicine.com/radio/topic468.htm

Strong, B. (2006). Image-guided functional endoscopic sinus surgery. *Current Opinion in Otolaryngology Head and Neck Surgery, 8*(1), 3–6.

Strong, E. B., & Senders, C. W. (2003). Surgery for severe rhinosinusitis. *Clinical Reviews in Allergy and Immunology, 2*(25),165–176.

Tanaka, A., Isono, S., Ishikawa, T., Sato, J., & Nishino, T. (2003). Laryngeal resistance before and after minor surgery. *Anesthesiology, 99*(2), 252–258.

Tolentino-DelosReyes, A. F., Ruppert, S. D., & Shiao, S.-Y. P. K. (2007). Evidence-based practice: Use of the ventilator bundle to prevent ventilator-associated pneumonia. *American Journal of Critical Care, 16*(1), 20–28.

University of Maryland Medical Center. (2006). *Sinusitis.* Retrieved August 30, 2007, from http://www.umm.edu/patiened/articles/what_ symptoms_of_sinusitis_000062_4.htm

van Bokhorst-de van der Schueren M., et al. (2000).The impact of nutritional status on the prognoses of patients with advanced head and neck cancer. *Cancer, 86*(3), 519–527.

Varman, M., & Whaley, D. (2006). *Mucormycosis.* Retrieved September 2, 2007, from http://www.emedicine.com/ped/topic1488.htm

Vokes, E., & Stenson, K. (2003). Therapeutic options for laryngeal cancer. *New England Journal of Medicine, 349,* 2087–2089.

Weiler, J. M., Bloomfield, J. R., Woodworth, G. G., Grant, A. R., Layton, T. A., Brown, T. L., et al. (2000). Effects of fexofenadine, diphenhydramine, and alcohol on driving performance: A randomized, placebo controlled trial in the Iowa Driving Simulator. *Annals of Internal Medicine, 132* (5), 354–363.

White, H. K., & Cohen, H. J. (2006). The older cancer patient. *Medical Clinics of North America, 90*(5), 967–982.

Woodcock, R. (2007). *Temporal bone: Fractures.* Retrieved July 29, 2007, from http://www.emedicine.com/radio/topic678.htm

Wynd, C. A. (2006), Smoking patterns, beliefs, and the practice of healthy behaviors in abstinent, relapsed and recalcitrant smokers. *Applied Nursing Research, 19*(4), 197–203.

Young, T., Skatrud, J., & Peppard, P. E. (2004). Risk factors for obstructive sleep apnea in adults. *Journal of the American Medical Association, 291,* 2013–2016.

Zitt, M. J. (2003, November). *New developments in the medical management of rhinosinusitis. Current concepts in rhinosinusitis.* Program and abstracts of the American College of Allergy, Asthma & Immunology 2003 Annual Meeting, New Orleans, LA.

Caring for the Patient
with Lower Airway Disorders

Ellen DeLuca
Kathleen Osborn

Annita Watson

Outcome-Based Learning Objectives

After studying this chapter, the learner will be able to:

1. Differentiate between restrictive and obstructive lung diseases.

2. Compare and contrast the etiology, pathophysiology, clinical manifestations, nursing management, and prevention of the various pulmonary infections and inflammatory disorders.

3. Explain the etiology, pathophysiology, and nursing management of COPD, chronic bronchitis, asthma, cystic fibrosis, pulmonary embolism, and cor pulmonale.

4. Compare and contrast the etiology and nursing management for patients with a variety of chest trauma and thoracic injuries.

5. Discuss the etiology, pathophysiology, and nursing management for patients with lung cancer and lung transplant.

6. Discuss the etiology, pathophysiology, and nursing management of occupational lung diseases.

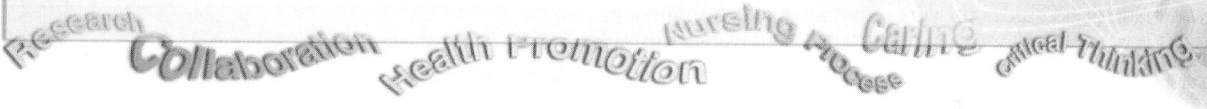

A VARIETY of pathologies can affect the respiratory system. These respiratory alterations include infections, obstructive diseases, occupational diseases, chest trauma, restrictive disorders, and pleural, vascular, and malignant disruptions. This chapter provides in-depth backgrounds for the common respiratory problems faced by individuals and families and also a thorough plan of care for nurses who are members of health teams that care for people with respiratory disorders.

◼ Infections and Inflammatory Disorders

Respiratory infections are a common occurrence among Americans. For example, most individuals will experience symptoms of influenza during their lifetime. However, infections of the respiratory tract are potentially life threatening and a significant cause of morbidly and mortality (Esmond, 2000). The increasing number of resistant organisms enhances the complexity of treatments. The nurse's awareness of assessment, treatment, and prevention of respiratory infections is essential to nursing practice.

Acute Bronchitis

Acute bronchitis is defined as the sudden inflammation of the tracheobronchial tree, which comprises the trachea and the bronchi. Bronchitis can be acute or chronic (a discussion of chronic bronchitis occurs later in this chapter). Acute bronchitis is one of the most common conditions treated by primary care physicians.

Etiology and Epidemiology

Acute bronchitis is most prevalent in children and older adults, and its incidence is highest in the winter. Individuals who suffer from allergies, other respiratory illnesses such as chronic obstructive pulmonary disease (COPD), chronic sinusitis, chronic tonsillitis, or infected adenoids and smokers are at a higher risk (McCance & Huether, 2007; Pulmonology Channel, 2002). Chart 35–1 (p. 936) lists triggers of acute bronchitis.

Pathophysiology

When airways are assaulted by chemical agents or microorganisms, the result is an inflammation of the lower bronchial mucous membranes. Acute bronchitis commonly follows a respiratory viral illness and is usually self-limiting. Most often, its cause is viral; however, a wide variety of agents can produce acute bronchitis including viruses, bacteria, yeast, and fungi and noninfectious triggers (Knutson & Braun, 2002). In adult patients, the most common viral triggers include adenovirus, influenza virus, and respiratory syncytial virus (RSV). Parainfluenza virus, enterovirus, and rhinovirus infections most

- Viruses (e.g., adenovirus, rhinovirus, and influenza types A and B)
- Bacterias (e.g., *Streptococcus pneumoniae, Haemophilus influenzae*)
- Yeast and fungi (e.g., *Candida albicans*)
- Pollutants (e.g., asthma, air pollutants, ammonia, and tobacco)

commonly occur in the fall, whereas RSV and coronavirus occur in winter and spring. Other causes of acute bronchitis are pollutants, such as ammonia and tobacco. Common bacterial causes are *Streptococcus pneumoniae, Haemophilus influenzae*, and *Bordetella pertussis* (Knutson & Braun, 2002).

Clinical Manifestations

Many of the clinical manifestations (i.e., fever, cough, chills, and malaise) mimic pneumonia, but the physical exam and chest x-ray often are normal. Bacterial cultures are of limited use. The cough typically gets steadily worse for 10 to 12 days, is more profound at night, and becomes increasing loose over time. Most patients have a cough for less than 2 weeks; however, for some individuals, a cough may last for 6 to 8 weeks (Knutson & Braun, 2002). Shortness of breath and wheezing also are common manifestations.

Nursing Management

The nursing process guides the care of patients with pulmonary infections. Diagnosis of acute bronchitis is based on symptom history.

Assessment

Assessment findings reveal a cough as the most commonly observed symptom in acute bronchitis. Individuals with viral bronchitis have a nonproductive cough. The cough often occurs in paroxysms and is aggravated by cold, dry, or dusty air (McCance & Huether, 2007). Patients with a bacterial bronchitis have a productive cough, and fever and pain behind the sternum that is aggravated by coughing.

Nursing Diagnoses

Priority nursing diagnoses for the patient with bacterial bronchitis include *Ineffective Airway Clearance, Impaired Gas Exchange*, and *Activity Intolerance*.

Outcomes

The outcomes of nursing management include relief of the clinical manifestations and a return to the previous level of functioning.

Interventions and Rationales

Nursing interventions focus on assisting patients with prescribed therapies. These include use of antitussives, analgesics, and bronchodilator medications; encouraging fluids; and teaching patients to cough effectively and avoid infections. Because viruses are the most common cause of acute bronchitis, treatment in this case is focused on preventing the cough with antitussive therapy such as codeine or dextromethorphan or on making the cough more effective with protussive therapy. Terbutaline (Brethine), amiloride (Midamor), and hypertonic saline aerosols have been shown to be the most effective of these (Knutson & Braun, 2002).

In addition to administering these treatments, the nurse encourages an increase in fluid intake to 2 to 3 L/day for thinning secretions and offers mild analgesics such as aspirin or acetaminophen (Tylenol) for discomfort. Deep breathing exercises and use of an incentive spirometer help maintain oxygen and carbon dioxide exchange. For the patient who is wheezing or demonstrating asthmatic symptoms, bronchodilators such as albuterol are administered by the nurse. Antibiotics have not been shown to be effective with acute bronchitis except in patients with COPD (Hunter & King, 2001; Knutson & Braun, 2002). The American Thoracic Society (ATS) has recommended strategies for managing acute exacerbations of chronic bronchitis and emphysema (Voelkel & Tuder, 2000). These strategies include beta-2 agonists, the addition of anticholinergics, antibiotic therapy (when indicated), and the intravenous administration of corticosteroids or methylxanthines such as aminophylline.

Evaluation

Nursing evaluation of a patient with bronchitis includes relief of the respiratory symptoms, e.g., cough, wheezing, and shortness of breath. The patient needs teaching regarding prevention and avoidance of risk factors.

Influenza

Influenza, also known as the *flu*, is a contagious disease that is caused by the influenza virus. Most people recover from influenza in 2 weeks, but some develop life-threatening complications such as pneumonia. About 10% to 20% of people in the United States get influenza yearly. An average of 36,000 people per year die from influenza in the United States. People ages 65 years old and older and people of any age with chronic medical conditions are likely to have complications from the flu (Centers for Disease Control and Prevention [CDC], 2004b).

Epidemiology

Epidemics of influenza occur typically during winter months. Influenza A and B are the two types of influenza viruses that cause epidemic human disease. Influenza virus type C has not been classified and usually does not induce illness. Antigenic variations in influenza type A and B account for the yearly epidemics. These minor variations account for the yearly updating of vaccine strains to be employed (Fishman et al., 2002).

Yearly epidemics of influenza begin abruptly and last 5 to 6 weeks. Epidemics occur from December to April in the Northern Hemisphere. Immunocompromised individuals initially experience illness from influenza; this is the first indication of an impending epidemic followed by increasing numbers of febrile respiratory illnesses in children (Fishman et al., 2002). Worldwide pandemics occur when a new virus emerges for which there is no immunity. Three of the pandemics of the 20th century (1957, 1968, and 1977) began in China. One hypothesis for this geographic source is that influenza viruses can be isolated throughout the year in China and other parts of Asia where the proximity of birds, swine, and humans increases the opportunity for recombination of animal and human influenza viruses, leading to new antigenic shifts (Fishman et al., 2002).

Pathophysiology

Transmission of influenza occurs by small-particle aerosols. Viruses deposited in the lower respiratory tract attach to and infect epithelial cells (Fishman et al., 2002). This can happen when an infected person coughs or sneezes and droplets are propelled through the air and deposited on the mouth or nose of people nearby. Though a less frequent means of transmission, viruses also can be spread when a person touches respiratory droplets on another person or an object and then touches his own mouth or nose before washing his hands (CDC, 2006).

Clinical Manifestations

Typically, influenza has an abrupt onset and is characterized by fever, chills, headache, fatigue, dry, nonproductive cough, sore throat, nasal congestion, and myalgia. The cough may be associated with chest pain. Fever usually persists for 3 to 4 days and occasionally 1 week, at which point systemic symptoms abate. Lung sounds are usually normal, although the most common complication is pneumonia, which may be primary influenza pneumonia or a secondary bacterial pneumonia. The elderly and patients with COPD are at an increased risk for this complication (Fishman et al., 2002).

■ Nursing Management

The primary care goals are relief of symptoms and prevention of secondary infection. Patients are advised to rest, drink plenty of fluids, avoid using alcohol and tobacco, and take aspirin or acetaminophen (Tylenol) for symptom relief.

Medical Management and Health Promotion

The nurse works with the health care provider to ensure that medications are taken appropriately. Three antiviral drugs, amantadine, rimantadine, and oseltamivir, have been approved by the federal government and are commercially available for preventing flu. They are 70% to 90% effective for preventing illness in healthy adults (CDC, 2004b). Four antiviral drugs have been approved for treatment of the flu: amantadine, rimantadine, zanamivir, and oseltamivir. If taken within 2 days of getting sick, these drugs can reduce the symptoms of flu and shorten the time of illness by 1 or 2 days. Antiviral drugs most often are used to control flu outbreaks in institutions such as nursing homes or hospital wards where people are at high risk for complications (CDC, 2004b).

Pneumonia

Pneumonia is an inflammatory process that results in edema of the parenchymal lung tissue, such as alveoli and bronchioles. It also includes extravasation of fluid into the alveoli, thus causing hypoxemia. It is a condition that affects the terminal gas-exchanging portions of the lung primarily. Although at one time pneumonia was a major cause of death, antibiotics have reduced mortality significantly.

Epidemiology

Pneumonia is the sixth leading cause of death in the United States and the number one cause of death from an infectious disease (Niederman et al., 2001; Porth, 2007). The death rates from pneumonia and influenza increased by 59% in the 25-year period prior to 1994, perhaps reflecting an increased population of older Americans (Schultz, 2003). The incidence and mortality of pneumonia are highest in the elderly. Risk factors for pneumonia include advanced age, a compromised immune system, underlying lung disease, alcoholism, altered consciousness, smoking, endotracheal intubation, malnutrition, and immobilization (see the Risk Factors for Community-Acquired Pneumonia box). In general, nosocomial infections and those affecting immunocompromised individuals have a higher mortality rate than community-acquired pneumonias (McCance & Huether, 2007).

Pneumonia was a major cause of death in the 19th and early 20th centuries. The discovery of antibiotics has reduced mortality significantly. The most recent challenge in the treatment of pneumonia is the development of a variety of resistant strain organisms. This has occurred because of overuse and misuse of antibiotics, global transmission of resistant bacteria as a result of poverty and poor medical infection control practices in both developing countries and in the United States, increased world travel, and the increasing costs of developing new antibiotics (Wooten & Salkind, 2003).

Aspiration of oropharyngeal secretions is the most common route of lower respiratory infection. The nasopharynx and oropharynx constitute the first line of defense for most infectious agents. Another route of infection is through the inhalation of microorganisms that have been released into the air when an infected individual coughs, sneezes, or talks, or from aerosolized water, such as that from infected respiratory equipment. Pneumonia also can occur when bacteria are spread to the lungs in the blood from bacteremia, which can result from infection elsewhere in the body or from intravenous (IV) drug abuse (McCance & Huether, 2007).

Etiology

Pneumonia is an acute inflammation of lung tissue caused by inhalation of bacteria, viruses, fungi, protozoa, or parasites to the lung or transportation of these agents via the bloodstream. Other causes are radiation therapy; aspiration of water, food, fluid, and vomitus; and inhalation of toxic gases, chemicals, and smoke (McCance & Huether, 2007).

RISK FACTORS for Community-Acquired Pneumonia

- Advanced age
- Immunocompromised state
- Underlying lung disease
- Chronic disease
- Alcoholism
- Smoking
- Immobility
- Malnutrition
- Crowded living conditions
- Exposure to day care

Pneumonias are classified according to the type of agent causing the infection, the distribution of the infection (lobar or bronchopneumonia), and the setting (community or hospital). The causative microorganism influences the signs and symptoms with which the patient presents, the treatment methods to be used, and the prognosis. For example, bacterial pneumonia causes exudate to fill the alveoli, thereby interfering with oxygen and carbon dioxide exchange and resulting in more severe symptoms than viral and mycoplasmal infections, which involve the tissue surrounding the alveoli (Porth, 2007).

Acute bacterial pneumonias are further subdivided into their anatomic locations. Lobar pneumonia refers to consolidation of a part or all of a lung lobe, whereas bronchopneumonia indicates a patchy consolidation of more than one lobe. Pneumonias also are being classified according to the setting where they were acquired. Community-acquired pneumonia tends to be caused by different microorganisms than those infections acquired in the hospital (nosocomial) (McCance & Huether, 2007). Legionnaire's disease is a common community-acquired bronchopneumonia that is caused by a gram-negative rod, *Legionella pneumophila*. The organism is frequently found in warm standing water. Hospital-acquired pneumonia is defined as a lower respiratory infection that was not present or incubating on admission to the hospital (Porth, 2007).

Pathophysiology

In healthy individuals pathogens that reach the lungs are expelled. However, if a microorganism gets past the upper cough reflex and mucociliary clearance, the next line of defense is the alveolar macrophage. If the organism is virulent and overwhelms the macrophage, there is a full-scale activation of the body's defense mechanisms including the release of multiple inflammatory mediators, cellular infiltration, and immune activation. The end result is that bronchial mucous membranes become damaged, causing the acini and terminal bronchioles to fill with infectious debris and exudates. The accumulation of exudates leads to dyspnea, ventilation/perfusion mismatching, and hypoxemia (McCance & Huether, 2007).

Community-Acquired Pneumonia

Community-acquired pneumonia (CAP), which can be bacterial or viral, is defined as an infection that begins outside the hospital or is diagnosed within 48 hours after admission to a hospital in a person who has not resided in a long-term facility (Porth, 2007). The incidence of CAP is highest in winter months with smoking being an important risk factor (ATS, 2001).

In the outpatient setting, the mortality rate for pneumonia is low. Another feature associated with CAP is that drug resistance has been identified with increasing frequency among *Streptococcus pneumoniae, Haemophilus influenzae, Moraxella catarrhalis*, and a number of enteric gram-negative bacteria (Niederman et al., 2001). In general, CAP patients will be managed on an outpatient basis, but hospitalization may be necessary for persons who are acutely ill or for those at special risk for complications, such as the elderly (Schultz, 2003).

Types of Community-Acquired Pneumonias The most common community-acquired pneumonia is caused by *Streptococcus pneumoniae* (also known as pneumococcus), which has a low mortality rate, though higher in the elderly. *Mycoplasma pneu-*

moniae is a common cause of pneumonia in young people, especially those living in group dormitories or army barracks. Influenza is the most common viral CAP in adults.

Pseudomonas aeruginosa, other gram-negative organisms, and *Staphylococcus aureus* are the most common causes of nosocomial or hospital-acquired pneumonia. Immunocompromised individuals are especially susceptible to *Pneumocystis carinii*, mycobacterial infections, and fungal infections of the respiratory tract (Chart 35–2). In the compromised host, these infections can be difficult to treat and have a high mortality rate (McCance & Huether, 2007). Among patients with CAP who require hospitalization, the mortality rate averages 12% (Niederman et al., 2001). This is related to predisposing factors that include general debility, malnutrition, endotracheal intubation, and contaminated respiratory therapy equipment.

Hospital-Acquired Pneumonia

Pneumonia that occurs more than 48 hours after hospital admission is considered to be a hospital-acquired pneumonia (HAP) and has a mortality rate of 20% to 50% (Barnes, 2000). Ninety percent of the infections are bacterial, and individuals with compromised immune systems, chronic lung disease, and those requiring intubation and mechanical ventilation are at higher risk (Porth, 2007). See the Risk Factors for Hospital-Acquired Pneumonia box. Ventilator-associated pneumonia is discussed in detail in Chapter 36 🌐. Some common microorganisms that cause HAP are *Pseudomonas aeruginosa, Staphylococcus aureus, Klebsiella pneumoniae*, and *Escherichia coli* (McCance & Huether, 2007).

Clinical Manifestations

Symptoms suggestive of pneumonia include fever, chills, increased respiratory rates, rusty, bloody sputum, crackles, and x-ray abnormalities. Patients who are immunocompromised,

---

CHART 35–2 | **Microorganisms Associated with Pneumonia**

Community Acquired	Hospital Acquired
Streptococcus pneumoniae	*Pseudomonas aeruginosa*
Mycoplasma pneumoniae	Staphylococcal pneumonia
Haemophilus influenzae	*Klebsiella* pneumoniae
Oral anaerobic bacteria	
Influenza virus	
Legionella pneumophila	
Chlamydial pneumonia	

RISK FACTORS for Hospital-Acquired Pneumonia

- General debility and malnutrition
- Treatment in an ICU
- Depressed level of consciousness
- Endotracheal intubation
- Contaminated respiratory therapy equipment
- Mechanical ventilation
- Immunosuppressed state

hypothermic, or elderly may not have a fever, and in general 20% of all patients presenting with pneumonia are afebrile. Nonrespiratory symptoms include headache, abdominal pain, nausea and vomiting, diarrhea, and muscle aches. In general, elderly persons complain of fewer symptoms (Fishman et al., 2002). Chart 35–3 summarizes the clinical manifestations of pneumonia.

Laboratory and Diagnostic Procedures

Unfortunately, relatively few diagnostic tests can help the clinician clearly differentiate the pathogen specific to the diagnosis of pneumonia. See the Diagnostic Tests for Pneumonia box.

Medical Management

Antibiotics are the primary treatment for CAP. The fluoroquinolones have been very effective in the treatment of pneumonia. Currently available agents in addition to the quinolones ciprofloxacin and ofloxacin include levofloxacin, sparfloxacin, gatifloxacin, and moxifloxacin (Niederman et al., 2001). Use of the antipneumococcal fluoroquinolones is the recommended choice of treatment by the ATS (2001) for CAP because they are likely to be effective with both gram-negative and gram-positive pathogens. Resistance has been noted with both penicillin and ciprofloxacin (ATS, 2001). Other first-line antibiotics include doxycycline and the macrolides. Antibiotic therapy should be started while identifying the pathogen. When the causative organism is identified, drug therapy can be tailored to the specific pathogen (Schultz, 2003).

Therapy for HAP is empiric and uses combinations of broad-spectrum antibiotics. In some patients methicillin-resistant *Staphylococcus aureus* (MRSA) also is a consideration and vancomycin may be added to the combination antibiotic therapy (Fishman et al., 2002). Bronchodilators may be given via an aerosol route or with **metered-dose inhalers (MDIs)** when there is a significant degree of bronchospasm. A spacer is a device that may be added to the MDI to deliver medication more safely and efficiently. Figures 35–1 ■ and 35–2 ■ (p. 940) show various MDIs and how to use them.

The patient's oxygenation should be monitored so that the saturation is maintained at 93% unless otherwise specified by the health care provider. Pulse oximetry is the least invasive assessment tool, but arterial blood gas (ABG) studies should be done if the patient is suspected of being more severely hypoxemic. This may require that the patient be given supplemental oxygen via a nasal cannula or mask (Figure 35–3 ■, p. 940). In addition, the nurse monitors the patient for signs of hypoxemia.

MyNursingKit | Video: Respiratory: Asthma—Using Inhaler

CHART 35–3 Clinical Manifestations of Pneumonia

- Fever, chills, or hypothermia
- Respiratory rate greater than 20
- Heart rate greater than 100
- Crackles heard on auscultation
- Chest discomfort
- Dyspnea
- Rusty-colored sputum
- Cough
- Fatigue, muscle aches, headache, nausea

DIAGNOSTIC TESTS for Pneumonia

Test	Expected Abnormality	Rationale for Abnormality
Chest x-ray	Whiting out of areas of involvement.	Leukocytosis is present with a bacterial infection.
Sputum Gram stain and culture	Presence of pathogen.	Pathogens are present, and will be evident on the Gram stain.
Transtracheal aspiration	Presence of specific pathogen.	A single pathogen present on the Gram stain is indicative of pneumonia; mixed flora may indicate oral contamination of anaerobic infections.
Bronchoscopy with bronchoalveolar lavage	Presence of a specific pathogen or abnormalities of the trachea and bronchioles.	Bronchial washings specimens can be obtained. Protected brush and bronchoalveolar lavage can be performed for quantitative cultures.
CBC	Presence of leukocytosis.	Leukocytosis is present in pneumonia and infectious processes.
ABG study	Evidence of hypoxemia or hypercarbia, acid–base abnormalities.	Decreased oxygenation may be present if pneumonia is present.
Thoracentesis with pleural fluid sample	Presence of abnormal cells and bacteria.	Obtaining fluid from the pleural space for laboratory analysis allows for the differentiation between simple and complicated effusions. This is used to guide therapeutic intervention.
Urine sample	Hematuria, pyuria, or the presence of protein.	A urinary antigen test for pneumococcus is useful in determining the presence of Legionella serogroup 1.
Serum electrolytes, BUN, creatinine, liver function studies	Abnormal laboratory values in elderly individuals and in persons who are chronically ill for whom pneumonia is a secondary problem.	Serology is essential in the diagnosis of unusual causes of pneumonia such as Q fever and brucellosis.

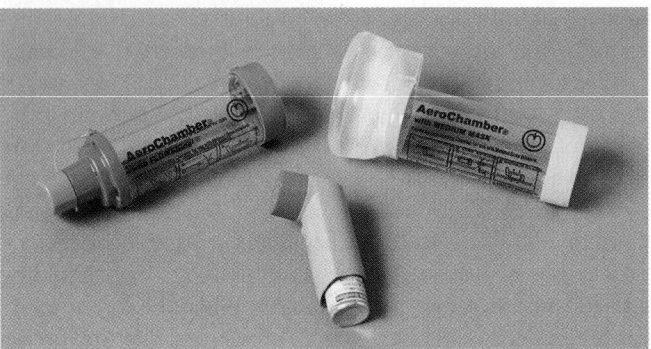

FIGURE 35–1 ■ A variety of inhalers and their use.

Restlessness or increased pulse may be the first signs of hypoxia. Breathlessness and cyanosis are later signs.

Nursing Management

Priority nursing measures for the patient with pneumonia include airway maintenance oxygen saturation above 93% or the level specified by the health care provider. *Readiness for Enhanced Comfort* and *Readiness for Enhanced Nutrition* also are common nursing diagnoses. The nurse promotes nutrition and hydration as a component of care since patients may be anorexic because of the disease process. Small, frequent, high-carbohydrate and high-

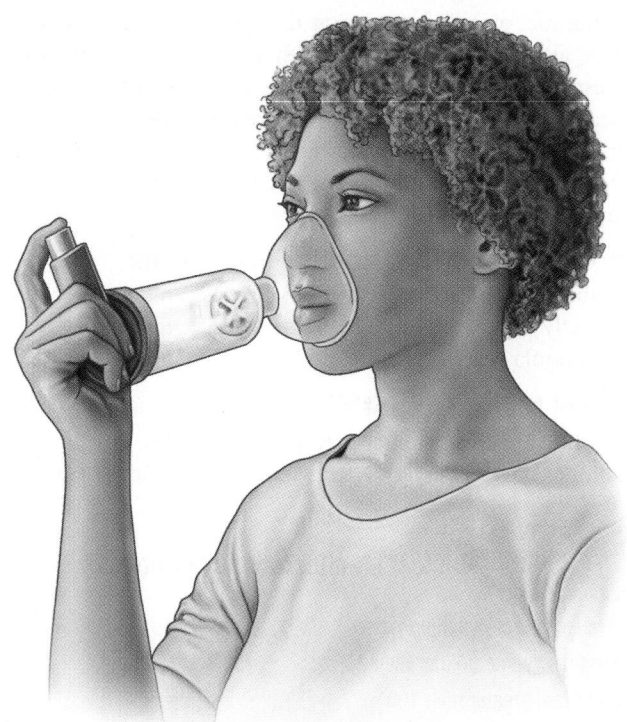

FIGURE 35–2 ■ How to use a metered-dose inhaler.

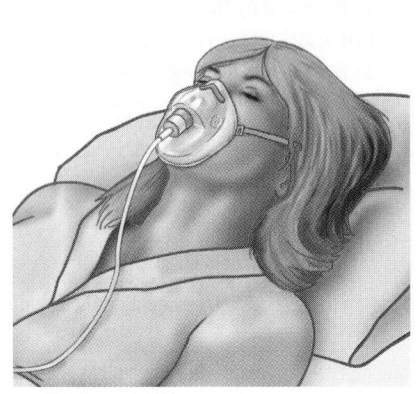

(a) Simple face mask

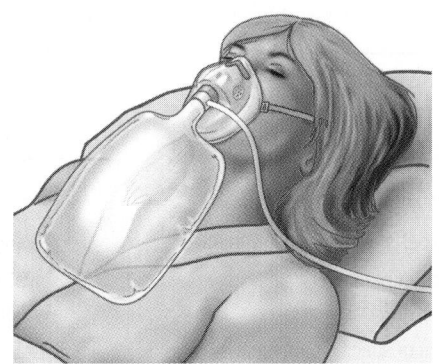

(b) Plastic face mask with reservoir bag

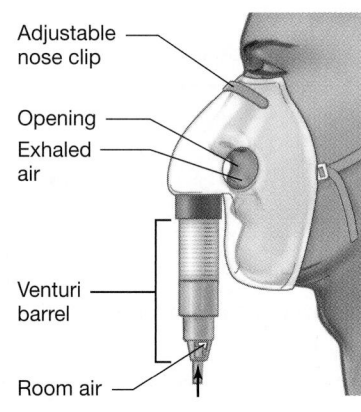

Adjustable nose clip

Opening

Exhaled air

Venturi barrel

Room air

(c) Venturi mask

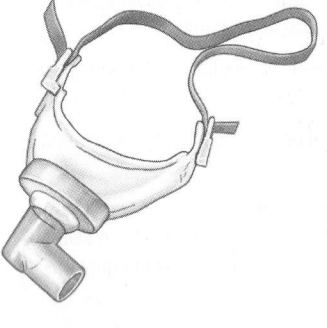

(d) Tracheostomy mask

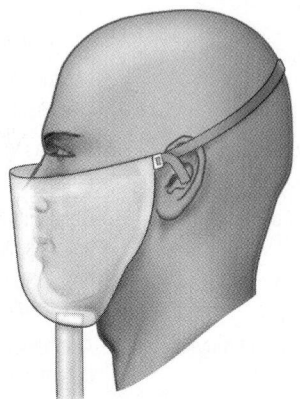

(e) Face tent

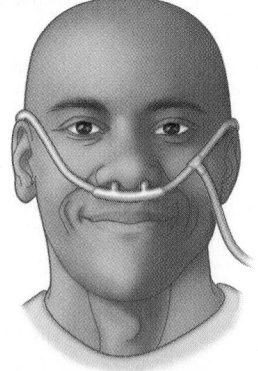
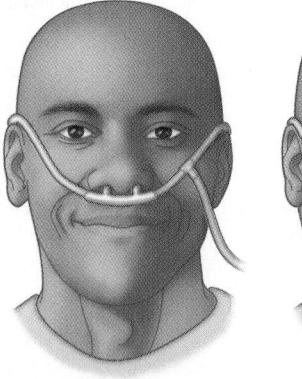

(f) Standard nasal cannulas

FIGURE 35–3 ■ Use of an oxygen mask.

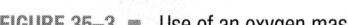

protein meals are provided and fluid intake is monitored closely. Oral hygiene is essential before and after meals. Promoting comfort also is a nursing role. The patient is monitored for chest pain and the character and location are noted. This may occur because of excessive coughing. Usually patients are most comfortable with the head of the bed elevated 45 to 90 degrees. Mild analgesics such as codeine, aspirin, and acetaminophen (Tylenol) are prescribed. Managing these patients is outlined in detail in the Nursing Process: Patient Care Plan for Pneumonia.

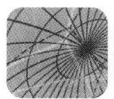

NURSING PROCESS: Patient Care Plan for Pneumonia

Assessment for Pneumonia

Subjective Data:

Do you have a cough, chills, or chest pain?

Describe the sputum you are coughing if any.

How are you treating the symptoms?

What seems to be most helpful?

Do you have any history of exposure to respiratory infections or pulmonary irritants?

Have you recently taken antibiotics?

Do you feel short of breath?

What triggers your discomfort?

Describe your sleeping pattern.

Objective Data:

Lung sounds

Vital signs

Sputum cultures

Chest x-ray

Spirometry

ABGs

Oxygen saturation

Nursing Assessment and Diagnoses	Outcomes and Evaluation Parameters	Planning and Interventions with *Rationales*
Nursing Diagnosis: *Ineffective Breathing Pattern* related to an infectious process in the lungs	**Outcomes:** The patient demonstrates effective coughing and breathing techniques. The patient drinks 3 liters of fluid per day. ***Evaluation Parameters:*** The patient's vital signs and temperature are within normal range. Upon auscultation, lung sounds in all fields are clear. The health care team, patient, and significant other(s) report that patient is drinking fluids as instructed. Sputum is easily expectorated and liquefied. Urine is clear light yellow.	**Interventions and *Rationales:*** Complete a physical assessment that includes vital signs, temperature, assessment of fever and or chills, tachycardia, and tachypnea *to detect early signs of infection and or exacerbation of infection.* Inspect for accessory muscle retraction, cyanosis, grunting on expiration, and restricted chest movement. In addition, auscultate for bronchial breath sounds, inspiratory crackles, decreased vocal fremitus due to pleural effusion, and egophony due to consolidation. *These clinical signs are associated with hypoxemia, atelectasis, and pulmonary congestion. A baseline assessment is performed to ascertain the degree of pulmonary congestion and hypoxemia.* Assist the patient to perform controlled coughing and deep breathing, and place the patient in an upright position to do this. A small pillow used to splint the chest may facilitate coughing and increase comfort. When not sitting in a chair, the patient's position should be changed frequently. *This assists with mobilizing secretions.* Give mild analgesics for chest pain that the patient may experience *due to muscular fatigue as the result of frequent paroxysms of coughing. Coughing allows for expectoration of secretions and clearance of airways. A pillow supports the diaphragm and allows for deeper breaths.* Provide prescribed medications and teach the patient about the purpose of each. This may include the use of an MDI. Prior to discharge the patient should demonstrate accurate use of the MDI, inhalers, or other oxygen equipment, and state the purpose of each medication. In addition to bronchodilators the patient may be placed on antibiotic therapy. The nurse reviews the therapy regime with the patient and ascertains that he is able to take the medications correctly at home. *The patient is placed on bronchodilator medications as well as antibiotics to open airways and clear secretions. Providing teaching about medication and assessing the patient's ability ascertains that the patient will receive the prescribed dose at home.* Encourage fluids to 3 liters/day *to liquefy tenacious secretions and allow for easy expectoration.*

(continued)

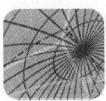

NURSING PROCESS: Patient Care Plan for Pneumonia—*Continued*

Assessment of Oxygen Status

Subjective Data:
Do you have a cough, chills, or chest pain?
Describe the sputum you are coughing if any.
Do you have any history of exposure to respiratory infections or pulmonary irritants?
Have you recently taken antibiotics?
Do you feel short of breath?
Do you feel like you are getting enough air?
If not, what triggers your discomfort?

Objective Data:
Lung sounds
Vital signs
Sputum cultures
Chest x-ray
Spirometry
ABGs
Oxygen saturation

Nursing Assessment and Diagnoses	Outcomes and Evaluation Parameters	Planning and Interventions with *Rationales*
Nursing Diagnosis: *Impaired Gas Exchange* related to infectious process in the lungs	**Outcome:** The patient states she can breathe easily without distress. **Evaluation Parameter:** Pulse oximetry and or blood gas results are within normal range for the patient.	**Interventions and *Rationales:*** Assess the patient's dyspnea at rest, with exertion, and during sleep. Administer oxygen as ordered, usually via nasal cannula or mask, and position the patient in an upright position or with the head up at night. Explain the rationale for oxygen to patient and family members. *Perfusion abnormalities related to pulmonary congestion cause hypoxemia and dyspnea. Supplemental oxygen with a nasal cannula or a mask provides relief. Ventilation is improved in the upright position because it allows for maximal expansion of the lungs.*

Assessment of Ability to Perform ADLs

Subjective Data:
Can you perform the normal activities of daily living (ADL)?
What activities lead to fatigue?
How much activity can you do before needing to stop and rest? How is this different from your usual endurance?

Objective Data:
Exercise tolerance: How much activity can the patient tolerate before developing clinical manifestations?

Nursing Assessment and Diagnoses	Outcomes and Evaluation Parameters	Planning and Interventions with *Rationales*
Nursing Diagnosis: *Activity Intolerance* related to an infectious process in the lungs	**Outcome:** Patient is able to assist with ADLs and initiate short walks of one-quarter to one-half block without dyspnea. **Evaluation Parameter:** Patient's oxygen saturation remains normal during and after performance of ADLs and ambulation.	**Interventions and *Rationales:*** Assess the patient's ability to perform ADLs. Administering oxygen as necessary, encourage the patient to do partial completion of ADLs and assist to a chair position followed by ambulation at short distances until the goal is reached. *Dyspnea indicates increased work of breathing. In the hypoxemic patient, exercise should not be attempted without oxygen. Oxygen allows the patient to perform optimally by providing adequate oxygenation to the muscles and decreasing the work of breathing.*

Assessment of Patient/Family Knowledge

Subjective Data:
Tell me what you know about your health problems.
Do you have questions about your health care?

Objective Data:
Verbalizes education needs.
Identifies mode of receiving educational material.
Participates in education discussion.

Nursing Assessment and Diagnoses	Outcomes and Evaluation Parameters	Planning and Interventions with *Rationales*
Nursing Diagnosis: *Deficient Knowledge* related to disease process	**Outcomes:** Patient avoids risk factors related to pneumonia. Patient complies with follow-up care. **Evaluation Parameter:** Patient verbalizes understanding of health needs and importance of prevention.	**Interventions and *Rationales:*** Assess the patient's and family's learning needs, readiness to learn, and preferred method of education (verbal, written, audiovisual) to present information at a time and in a manner the patient and family can understand. The patient's understanding of the treatment measures decreases anxiety and promotes compliance. Instruct patient to seek immediate medical attention for return of clinical manifestations *to promote seeking early medical treatment of potential life-threatening illness.*

Discharge Priorities

Before discharging the patient recovering from pneumonia, the nurse emphasizes the importance of rest and a gradual increase in activity to avoid fatigue. Patients are instructed to maintain resistance to infection with proper nutrition and adequate fluid intake. They also are warned to avoid chilling and exposure to others with upper respiratory tract infections or viruses.

Health Promotion

The patient and family are made aware of the fact that one episode of pneumonia increases susceptibility to recurrent infections. The patient is taught about all medications that will be continued at home. The nurse provides written instructions as necessary. Patients should be reminded that they should continue deep breathing and coughing exercises 4 times a day for 6 to 8 weeks. They also are instructed to notify the health care provider if experiencing chills, fever, dyspnea, hemoptysis, increasing fatigue, or other respiratory complications.

Pulmonary Fungal Infections

The incidence of fungal infections of the lung has increased dramatically since the 1960s, particularly in immunocompromised patients (Haque, 1992; Mandanas, 2007). Fungal infections of the lung can be divided into those that occur in generally healthy individuals and those that occur in opportunistically immunosuppressed patients (Chart 35–4). Both types are acquired by inhalation of contaminated soil resulting in pulmonary infections.

Etiology and Epidemiology

Fungal lung infections occur more frequently in areas where there are endemic fungi, which include the valleys of the Mississippi and Ohio rivers (histoplasmosis and blastomycosis), the southwestern United States, the San Joaquin valley in California, and northern Mexico (coccidioidomycosis), and Central and South America (paracoccidioidomycosis). The organisms grow in soil that has been enriched with bird excreta: old chicken coops, barns, pigeon nesting areas, and tress where birds roost (Porth, 2007). These infections affect men (75% to 95%) more often than women; estrogen-mediated inhibition of mycelium-to-yeast transformation may be responsible for the male predominance. Estrogen seems to have a protective effect against cryptococcal infection. Cryptococcosis has a male-to-female ratio of 2 to 3:1 (Mandanas, 2007). Known risk factors for the development of the fungal lung diseases include:

- Travel to an area where fungal pneumonia pathogens are endemic

---

CHART 35–4 Fungal Infections of the Lung

FUNGAL INFECTIONS OCCURRING IN IMMUNE COMPETENT INDIVIDUALS	FUNGAL INFECTIONS OCCURRING IN IMMUNE INCOMPETENT INDIVIDUALS
- Histoplasmosis	- Aspergillosis
- Coccidioidomycosis	- Candidiasis
- Blastomycosis	- Mucormycosis

- Regular exposure to bird, bat, or rodent droppings in endemic areas
- Immunocompromised patients who have an increased risk for opportunistic infections, such as cancer and human immunodeficiency virus (HIV)
- Males.

Endemic pneumonias are generally self-limiting in healthy patients. *Coccidioides immitis*, which causes coccidioidomycosis, is the most virulent, yet 90% of patients recover without treatment. However, in patients with acquired immunodeficiency syndrome (AIDS), the mortality rate is as high as 70%. Fungi that affect immunosuppressed individuals include *Aspergillus* and *Candida*, as well as *Cryptococcus neoformans* and fungi of the order *Mucorales* called mucormycosis. In patients with limited defense mechanisms these organisms can produce widespread systemic disease leading to death. A fungal etiology always should be considered in immunosuppressed patients with radiologic abnormalities (Amersham Health, 2004). Aspergillosis in patients who are neutropenic (from either leukemia chemotherapy or bone marrow transplantation) has a mortality rate of 50% to 85% (Mandanas, 2007).

Pathophysiology

Fungi can cause lung disease through direct infection of pulmonary tissue, through infection of pulmonary air spaces/lung cavities, or through their ability to trigger an immunologic reaction when fungal material is inhaled. Once in the lungs, the fungi elicit tissue responses ranging from acute exudative reactions to a prolonged chronic course, and disseminating to other organs and causing systemic infections. Additionally, individuals with fungal pneumonias may develop chronic pulmonary (e.g., cavitation, pleural effusions, bronchopleural fistulas) or extrapulmonary complications.

Clinical Manifestations

Clinical manifestations of fungal lung infections frequently resemble those of tuberculosis. The disease can take any of three forms depending on the host's resistance and immunocompetence:

- An acute primary disease
- A chronic (cavitary) pulmonary disease
- A disseminated infection.

The primary pulmonary lesions present with nodules containing macrophages that have engulfed microorganisms. These nodules may also be in the lymph nodes. Other clinical manifestations include a mild self-limiting flu-like syndrome (Porth, 2007).

When the individual is immunocompromised, chronic cavitary lesions develop, along with a productive cough, fever, night sweats, and weight loss. A disseminated fulminating infection most often occurs in the very young and very elderly who have compromised immune function. These patients present with a high fever, generalized lymph node enlargement, hepatosplenomegaly, muscle wasting, anemia, high white blood cell counts, and thrombocytopenia. Ulcerations of the tongue and mouth and voice hoarseness, nausea, vomiting, diarrhea, and abdominal pain may also occur. Frequently meningitis becomes the most pronounced manifestation (Porth, 2007).

Laboratory and Diagnostic Procedures

The diagnosis of a fungal infection depends on the demonstration of the organisms by culture or histology (Mandanas, 2007). The most characteristic chest x-ray presentation involves one or more nodular infiltrates that progress rapidly, cavitate, and cross lung fissures. Lung scans may demonstrate perfusion defects consistent with fungal disease. However, the patient may be symptomatic without radiologic findings. Skin tests similar to the tuberculin test are used to detect *Histoplasma* and *Coccidioides*.

Medical Management

Amphotericin B is the drug most commonly used in treating serious systemic fungal infections. It is given intravenously and considered a toxic drug with many possible side effects including fever, chills, malaise, nausea and vomiting, thrombophlebitis at the injection site, and renal dysfunction. Recent advances in amphotericin B include the development of lipid formulations, which demonstrate reduced nephrotoxicity when compared with the parent compound (American Lung Association, 2004; Crawford, 2004). Total treatment with the drug may last from 4 to 12 weeks. Many of the side effects can be avoided by premedication with hydrocortisone, an anti-inflammatory, or Benadryl. Renal function is monitored closely, and ensuring adequate hydration is essential. In addition to amphotericin, the oral agents currently available for treatment include the imidazoles, the triazoles, and the echocardins. More details on these agents are given in the Pharmacology Summary feature (p. 981).

■ Nursing Management

Presenting symptoms are often dyspnea, nonproductive cough, and pleuritic chest pain. Fever and chills also may be present (Morrison & Lew, 2001).

Assessment

The nurse assesses the patient's breathing pattern, lung sounds, and presence of cough, sputum production, and pleuritic chest pain. Lung sounds can mimic those of bacterial pneumonia including signs of pulmonary consolidation, such as crackles, bronchial breath sounds, and increased fremitus. The nurse needs to monitor oxygen saturations and ABGs for evidence of respiratory failure. Fever and chills also may be present. Symptoms may range from mild to severe, including respiratory failure; therefore, the assessment must be done on an ongoing basis to monitor for trends in the clinical manifestations.

Outcomes and Evaluation Parameters

Outcomes and evaluation parameters for these patients include an absence of symptoms and an ability to perform activities of daily living (ADLs).

Interventions and Rationales

Nursing interventions depend on the clinical manifestations. The patient may just need to be encouraged and reminded to deep breathe and cough. Supplemental oxygen therapy and in some instances mechanical ventilation may be necessary. Administration of medications and patient education is a priority.

Pulmonary Tuberculosis

Pulmonary tuberculosis (TB) is a contagious bacterial infection caused by *Mycobacterium tuberculosis (M. tuberculosis)*. The lungs are primarily involved but the disease can spread to other organs. The disease can develop after inhaling droplets sprayed into the air from a cough or sneeze by someone infected with *M. tuberculosis*. The disease is characterized by the development of granulomas (granular tumors) in the infected tissues.

Epidemiology

In 1900, tuberculosis (TB) was the leading cause of death in the United States and Europe. In 2005, the total number of new cases of tuberculosis in the United States was 14,093. The annual decrease in tuberculosis cases has slowed from an average of 7.1% in the 1993–2000 period to the current average of 3.8% for the 2001–2005 period. In addition to those with active TB, an estimated 10 to 15 million people in the United States have latent tuberculosis. About 10% of these individuals will develop active TB at some time in their lives. Transmission of TB is rampant in crowded shelters and prisons where people weakened by poor nutrition, drug addiction, and alcoholism are exposed to *Mycobacterium tuberculosis* (Schoenstadt, 2006).

Noncompliance is a major cause of drug-resistant TB. Tuberculosis patients who do not complete drug treatment can stay infectious for longer periods of time and therefore can spread TB to more people. These treatment failures result in TB strains that are resistant to one or more of the standard medicines given to TB patients (Schoenstadt, 2006).

Many elderly people whose general health has declined develop active TB from TB infection that they had much earlier in life. Other elderly people, especially those with weak immune systems, become newly infected with *M. tuberculosis* and can develop active TB rapidly.

Cases of multidrug-resistant TB have declined sharply in the United States during the past decade. In 2003, the most recent year for which there is resistance rate reporting, 114 individuals were reported with multidrug-resistant TB—a 76.5% decline since 1993. Of these individuals, 28 were born in the United States, and 86 were born in other nations (Schoenstadt, 2006).

Etiology

The organism *Mycobacterium tuberculosis* is nonmotile, nonsporulating, and an acid-fast rod that secretes niacin. The tubercle bacillus is transmitted via aerosolization (i.e., an airborne route). Individuals who are most commonly infected are those having repeated close contact with an infected person who has not yet been diagnosed with TB.

TB also is one of the opportunistic infections common to persons with HIV/AIDS. According to the World Health Organization (WHO) (2003) the AIDS epidemic is considered a major factor in the increase of TB cases. The suppression of the immune system caused by HIV both opens the door to new active infection and permits activation of latent disease. One-third of the increase in global TB cases during the last five years can be attributed to HIV (WHO, 2003). Continuous assessment and intervention to prevent the spread of the disease must continue.

The newest form of TB is multidrug-resistant tuberculosis (MDR TB). It is resistant to two or more of the primary drugs (isoniazid and rifampin) used for the treatment of tuberculosis. Extensively drug-resistant TB (XDR TB) is TB resistant to isoniazid and rifampin among the first-line anti-TB drugs; and among the second-line drugs, it is resistant to any fluoroquinolone and at least one of three injectable drugs (Raviglione & Smith, 2007). Resistance occurs when bacteria develop the ability to withstand antibiotic attack and relay that ability to newly produced bacteria. Because that entire strain of bacteria inherits this capacity, resistance can spread from one person to another. Inadequate treatment of TB and/or improper use of antituberculosis medications is an important cause of drug-resistant tuberculosis. Drug-resistant TB is difficult and costly to treat and can be fatal (Raviglione & Smith, 2007).

Pathophysiology

TB is a highly communicable disease that is transmitted via aerosolization. When an infected person laughs, sneezes, or sings, droplet nuclei are produced and may be inhaled by others. When the tubercle reaches a suitable site (bronchi or alveoli), it multiplies freely. An exudative response occurs, causing a nonspecific pneumonitis. With the development of acquired immunity, further multiplication of bacilli is controlled in the majority of initial lesions. The lesions typically resolve and leave very little or no residual. A small percentage of those who are initially infected develop the disease (5% to 15%). Cell-mediated or type IV immunity develops 2 to 10 weeks after infection and is manifested by a significant reaction to a tuberculin test. A primary infection may be microscopic in size and may never appear on x-ray film.

The process of infection appears in the following way. The granulomatous inflammation created by the tubercle bacillus becomes surrounded by collagen, fibroblasts, and lymphocytes. In the center of the lesion (Ghon's tubercle), necrosis, which is called caseation necrosis, occurs. After this development, areas of caseation localize and undergo resorption, hyaline degeneration, and fibrosis. These necrotic areas may calcify (calcification) or liquefy (liquefaction). If the latter occurs, the liquid material then empties into a bronchus, and the evacuated area becomes a cavity (cavitation). Bacilli continue to proliferate in the necrotic cavity wall. The evacuated material leads to endobronchial spread of disease into new areas of the lung; this process can be a recurring one. A lesion also may progress by direct extension if bacilli multiply rapidly and there is marked exudative response. These lesions may extend into the pleura, which results in tuberculosis pleural effusion with a small number of organisms. Similarly, pericardial effusions may occur. Initial infection is seen more often in the middle or lower lobes of the lung. If a large number of organisms enter the bloodstream, disseminated disease, which is called miliary tuberculosis, occurs. Typically, many tiny discrete nodules scattered throughout the lung are visualized on x-ray film. If disseminated disease occurs through bloodborne foci, the brain, meninges, liver, kidney, and bone marrow are commonly involved.

Clinical Manifestations

The nurse inquires about presenting signs and symptoms such as dyspnea, weight loss, cough, sputum production, sleep disturbances, night sweats, and fatigue. The signs and symptoms of pulmonary TB are insidious and many patients do not become aware of symptoms until the disease is well advanced. Typically, the patient presents with lethargy, exhaustive fatigue, activity intolerance, nausea, irregular menses, and low-grade fever, which may have occurred for weeks or months. Fever also may be accompanied by night sweats. The patient finally notices a cough and the production of mucoid and mucopurulent sputum, which is occasionally streaked with blood. A dull aching chest pain may accompany the cough. The physical examination of the chest does not provide conclusive evidence of tuberculosis. The nurse may hear dullness with percussion over involved parenchymal areas, bronchial breath sounds, and increased transmission of spoken or whispered sounds. Wheezing related to obstruction may also be heard.

Laboratory and Diagnostic Procedures

The tuberculin skin test, chest x-ray, acid-fast bacillus smear, and sputum culture are used to diagnose TB. If the patient has had the bacille Calmette-Guérin (BCG) vaccine containing attenuated tubercle bacilli, which is used routinely in foreign countries to produce resistance to TB, she will have a positive skin test and should be evaluated via chest x-ray. See the Diagnostic Tests for Tuberculosis box (p. 946) for specific details.

Medical Management

Early detection of TB depends on subjective data rather than presentation of symptoms. Possible exposure and travel to foreign countries in which there is a high incidence of TB need to be determined. It is important to note whether the patient has had any prior tests for TB and what they were. There is a difference between being infected with TB and having TB disease. Someone who is infected with TB has the TB bacteria in his body and his body's defenses are protecting him from the bacteria and therefore the person is not sick. Someone with TB disease is sick and, if not properly treated, can spread the disease to other people. A person with symptoms of TB disease or evidence of infection needs to be seen by a health care provider.

Most patients are treated on an outpatient basis, and with effective drug therapy many individuals continue to work and lead normal lives. Medical management for TB centers on drug therapy (see the Pharmacology Summary, p. 981). Drug therapy is used for those who have clinical manifestations and for individuals who are infected. The patient receives instructions for the chemotherapy regime from the health care provider who follows up for at least a year during active treatment. The diagnosis also is reported to the local health department, which follows up on patient progress through treatment and provides resources.

The hospitalized patient with active TB or suspected active TB is placed in a negative pressure room with respiratory airborne isolation and use of standard precautions. Negative pressure is effective in moving airborne bacilli out into the atmosphere. The patient should remain in isolation until three consecutive sputum cultures have tested negative. Until the sputum cultures return negative, there is no certainty that an individual is not infectious.

Possible complications of TB include multidrug resistance, hemorrhage, and pleurisy; any of these complications may

DIAGNOSTIC TESTS for Tuberculosis

Test	Expected Results	Rationale
Mantoux test for TB (PPD)	A reaction at the injection site occurs 48–72 hours after injection of a small amount of intermediate strength purified protein derivative (PPD) given intradermally into the forearm. A reaction includes induration and erythema. The diameter of induration is measured at its widest part. An induration of 5 mm or greater may be significant for individuals at risk such as HIV patients. An induration of 10 mm or greater is significant in individuals with normal or mildly impaired immunity.	An individual with a positive PPD test has been exposed to TB and has developed antibodies. Also individuals who have received the BCG vaccine used routinely in Europe and South America to provide resistance to TB develop antibodies.
Chest x-ray	Visualizes tuberculosis lesions, cavities, and inflammation.	Visualizes the extent of lung involvement but does not confirm diagnosis. Used to assess patients with a positive PPD.
Sputum for acid–fast bacilli	Three sputum samples are positive on an acid-fast smear.	Confirms TB diagnosis.

indicate recurrence of tuberculosis activity, and the patient and family should be made aware of these complications.

■ Nursing Management

Nursing care for the TB patient focuses on preventing the spread of the infection, assisting the patient and family to manage the environment, and prescribed chemotherapy. The nurse addresses patient anxiety related to the disease and issues such as poor nutrition, pain, and fatigue (see Nursing Process: Patient Care Plan for Tuberculosis).

Health Promotion

The main focus of TB management is prevention of the spread of the infection. Most TB can be cured with drugs, but a patient must continually take the prescribed medication, usually for 9 months. Some patients require a year or more for successful treatment. If the drug is stopped before completion, the TB may come back more resilient than before. Surviving bacteria may become resistant to the drugs used to treat TB, causing MDR TB (ATS, CDC, and Infectious Disease Society of America, 2003). Finally, all persons who live with or have been in close contact with the infected individual must be tested and treated if necessary.

Atypical Mycobacterium

Atypical mycobacteria are a group of bacteria that are widely distributed in nature. They are found in water, soil, animals, and man, and usually do not produce disease. These are *Mycobacterium avium, M. intracellulare, M. kansasii, M. xenopi*, and *M. fortuitum*. Usually infections from these organisms are caused by exposure to infected water, soil, dust, or aerosols (Medical College of Wisconsin Healthlink, 2008).

Epidemiology and Etiology

The largest numbers of *M. avium* or mycobacterium avium complex (MAC) encounters have been among persons who were immunocompromised with HIV disease and other forms of immune compromise (Fishman et al., 2002). MAC disease is the second most commonly diagnosed opportunistic infection second to *Pneumocystis carinii*, commonly experienced by persons with HIV.

Clinical Manifestations

MAC and *Mycobacterium scrofulaceum* are associated with lymphadenitis in immunocompetent children. All nodes in the cervical chain can be affected, but the nodes of the submandibular region appear to be the most commonly involved. Disseminated infections are usually associated with HIV infection. Host immunity seems to play a major role because a low CD4+ lymphocyte count (fewer than 100 cells/μL for adults and age-appropriate decreases in children) is associated with an increased frequency of disseminated MAC disease (Dieudonne, 2008). Patients present with cough, increased sputum production, fever, weakness, and weight loss. A chest x-ray is likely to show abnormalities, and blood cultures or cultures of body fluids are likely to confirm the diagnosis.

Medical Management

Medical management involves administration of prescribed antibiotics and assessment of pulmonary status and oxygen saturation. Usually the patient is on two antibiotics. Common antibiotics include Zithromax, Biaxin, ciprofloxacin, and Mefoxin. Oxygen therapy is administered if the patient experiences dyspnea and low oxygen saturations. Family members and significant others are taught that there is no concern for person-to-person spread of these organisms so isolation is not necessary (Medical College of Wisconsin Healthlink, 2008). If the patient experiences weight loss or wasting syndrome, the nutritionist becomes very involved with meal planning. Patients may require follow-up with a home care nurse, respiratory therapist, and nutritionist upon discharge. Arrangements are also made for any respiratory therapy equipment or oxygen to be delivered and managed in the home setting.

Lung Abscess

A **lung abscess** is a localized area of lung destruction caused by liquefaction necrosis usually related to pyogenic bacteria.

Epidemiology and Etiology

The incidence of lung abscess is not well known due to it not occurring in isolation. It may be solitary or may occur in multiple discrete lesions. Most often such an abscess is secondary to anaerobic and aerobic organisms that colonize the upper respiratory tract and may be associated with periodontal disease (Fishman et al., 2002). Patients who present with this problem often have a history of pneumonia, possibly complicated by aspiration of oropharyngeal contents. Other causes of lung abscess include bacteremia seeding in the lungs, tricuspid endocarditis leading to septic pulmonary embolus, extension of hepatic abscess, associated with bronchial carcinoma, and bronchial obstruction (Patient UK, 2007). For example, an obstruction of a bronchus may cause a necrotizing process in the distal lung that eventually becomes an abscess. Formation of multiple abscesses and cavities occurs commonly in patients with TB or fungal infections of the lung.

Clinical Manifestations

Clinical manifestations are often insidious, although more acute if a lung abscess follows pneumonia. Typically the patient experiences spiking temperature with rigors and night sweats; a cough with sputum that is often foul tasting, foul smelling, and blood stained; pleuritic chest pain; tachycardia; and shortness of breath. Lung sounds are diminished and there is a dullness on percussion over the abscess. Depending on the size, oxygen saturation may be decreased.

Laboratory and Diagnostic Procedures

A CT scan is used if there is a question of cavitation not clearly seen. Pleural fluid and blood cultures may be obtained. Bronchoscopy may be used in the case of delayed drainage or suspected malignancy. If the health care provider is unable to obtain sputum, transtracheal aspiration via suction may be done to obtain a sample so that sputum can be cultured and appropriate organisms identified. The patient needs to be evaluated for signs of severe periodontal disease and infective endocarditis, as a possible cause of the lung abscess.

Medical Management

The type of organism isolated on sputum culture and the findings of the history, physical exam, and diagnostic work-up will determine the treatment required. Adequate drainage of the lung abscess can be achieved through postural drainage and chest physiotherapy. The patient should be assessed for adequate cough. Some patients may benefit from a percutaneous chest catheter placed for drainage of the abscess (Sharma, 2004). Intravenous antibiotic therapy with penicillin G or clindamycin is the pharmacologic therapy of choice followed by penicillin with metronidazole. The dose is continued until there is evidence of symptom improvement. Long-term therapy with oral antibiotics prevents relapse (Sharma, 2004). In addition, a diet high in protein is provided. Supportive care and emotional support for the long-term nature of this problem is necessary.

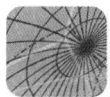

NURSING PROCESS: Patient Care Plan for Tuberculosis

Assessment of Airway and Gas Exchange

Subjective Data:
Have you been exposed to TB?
Have you had recent travel to foreign countries in which there is a high incidence of TB?
Have you had any prior tests for TB?
If so what were they?
Have you had the BCG vaccine?
Have you had dyspnea, weight loss, cough, sputum production, sleep disturbances, night sweats, or fatigue?

Objective Data:
Lung sounds
Vital signs
Sputum culture for acid-fast bacilli
Chest x-ray
Work of breathing
Oxygen saturation

Nursing Assessment and Diagnoses	Outcomes and Evaluation Parameters	Planning and Interventions with *Rationales*
Nursing Diagnosis: *Ineffective Airway Clearance* related to tracheobronchial secretions as evidenced by copious sputum production	**Outcome:** Upon auscultation of lung fields by the nurse, breath sounds are clear or with fewer adventitious sounds. **Evaluation Parameter:** Upon assessment by the nurse, vital signs are within normal range and the patient is afebrile.	**Interventions and *Rationales:*** Instruct the patient on methods to facilitate airway clearance. Teach proper coughing and deep breathing and postural drainage techniques. Encourage hydration with 2–3 liters of fluid daily. *Effective coughing and deep breathing techniques and good hydration promote liquefication of secretions and facilitate expectoration.* Assess respiratory status for changes, also observing for temperature spikes or recurrence of symptoms. The patient who is progressing well should show a remission of symptoms. *A temperature spike or changes in respiratory status may indicate a complication or drug resistance.*

(continued)

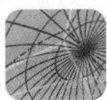

NURSING PROCESS: Patient Care Plan for Tuberculosis—*Continued*

Assessment of Patient/Family Knowledge of Disease

Subjective Data:
What is your understanding of TB?
Do you know who you got it from?
Do you know how it is spread?
Can you list your medications and how to take them and what precautions are necessary?
Do you understand the treatment of TB and how you can help clear your lungs?

Objective Data:
Can you give examples of when you would call your health care provider?
What are the best methods for preventing the spread of TB?

Nursing Assessment and Diagnoses	Outcomes and Evaluation Parameters	Planning and Interventions with *Rationales*
Nursing Diagnosis: *Deficient Knowledge about treatment regimen and preventive health measures* related to TB management as evidenced by inability to plan care without assistance	**Outcomes:** Patient demonstrates to the nurse accurate coughing and deep breathing techniques, positioning and postural drainage techniques, and proper use of humidification and hydration to facilitate airway clearance. ***Evaluation Parameters:*** Demonstrates an adequate level of knowledge with regard to the medication regime, side effects, and indications for contacting the health care provider. Describes methods for preventing the spread of TB. Describes methods for minimizing drug side effects such as regular checkups, laboratory evaluation, supplemental vitamins, and avoidance of alcohol and foods containing tyramine and histamine.	**Interventions and *Rationales:*** Review the necessary information regarding coughing and breathing techniques and drug therapy and provide written information and instructions. Information is repeated as needed, enlisting the support of family members. If the patient is not English speaking, an interpreter is sought as well as patient education materials in the appropriate language. The importance of scheduled laboratory evaluation of renal and liver function is stressed. Teach the patient that rifampin causes urine to become darker in color. In addition, rifampin can increase the metabolism of other medications, making them less effective. These include beta-blockers, oral anticoagulants, corticosteroids, digoxin, quinidine, oral hypoglycemic agents, oral contraceptives, theophylline, and verapamil. Patients taking isoniazid (also called isonicotinyl hydrazine or INH) are taught to avoid foods containing tyramine and histamine. These are tuna, aged cheese, red wine, soy sauce, and yeast extracts. Eating these foods while on INH causes headaches, flushing, hypotension, light-headedness, palpitations, and diaphoresis. Medications should be taken 1 hour before meals or on an empty stomach since food interferes with absorption. The patient is instructed to cover his or her mouth and nose when coughing and sneezing. The patient should alert the health care provider regarding any fever or recurrence of symptoms. He should avoid exposure to silicone or dust because these substances cause further lung damage. The patient also must understand that taking medications is the most effective method of preventing transmission. *The major reason treatment fails is that patients do not take medications regularly and for the prescribed duration. Adherence to the therapeutic regime is essential to recovery. Patients who are not compliant with medication regimes are likely to remain infectious, and also prone to developing resistant strains of TB that are much more difficult to treat.*

Assessment of Ability to Perform Activities of Daily Living (ADL)

Subjective Data:
What daily activities can you accomplish without assistance?
Describe your activity schedule.
Describe any physical symptoms you have while exercising or performing ADLs.

Objective Data:
Observation of physical status during exercise
Oxygen saturation pre- and postactivity
Lung sounds pre- and postactivity
Vital signs pre- and postactivity

Nursing Assessment and Diagnoses	Outcomes and Evaluation Parameters	Planning and Interventions with *Rationales*
Nursing Diagnosis: *Activity Intolerance* related to fatigue as evidenced by inability to engage in normal activities without dyspnea or fatigue	**Outcome:** Maintains an activity schedule without fatigue or dyspnea. ***Evaluation Parameters:*** Walks one-half block without experiencing dyspnea or fatigue. Completes ADLs independently and without dyspnea. Oxygen saturation is within normal range at rest and after completion of ADLs.	**Interventions and *Rationales:*** Plan a gradual progression of activity *to increase exercise tolerance and muscle strength.*

Nursing Management

The nursing management of patients with lung abscess focuses on assessment, treatment, and evaluation. It is critical that the nurse assess the patient's recent past medical history, and plan interventions based on the patient's knowledge base and understanding. The nurse also must take into consideration the patient's support system and ability to care for self.

Assessment

It is important for the nurse to assess the patient's recent history of influenza, pneumonia, febrile illness cough, and sputum production. Physical assessment of the patient often reveals a febrile patient who appears pale and fatigued. The patient may complain of pleuritic chest pain, which is stabbing in nature when taking a deep breath. Auscultation of breath sounds may reveal decreased sounds in the involved area of the lung. Bronchial breath sounds and fine crackles are heard over the site of the lesion.

Nursing Diagnoses

Nursing diagnoses include *Impaired Gas Exchange* and *Ineffective Tissue Perfusion*, both of which are related to diminished gas exchange in the area of the abscess.

Outcomes

The nursing outcomes for the patient with a lung abscess include a relief of clinical manifestations and a return to the previous level of function.

Interventions and Rationales

Nursing interventions include management of the patient's clinical manifestations. Management of the oxygen status needs constant monitoring. The nurse assesses the oxygen saturation, the respiratory and heart rate, and the work of breathing. Nursing interventions also include administration of antipyretic, antibiotic, and pain medications, with a follow-up assessment of effectiveness. Physical care such as bathing needs to be spaced to allow for periods of rest between activities. If a catheter has been placed to drain the abscess, the amount and a description of the color, odor, and viscosity need to be assessed and documented.

Evaluation

Evaluation focuses on the ability or status of the patient in meeting the outcome parameters. If the desired outcomes are not met, an analysis of the reason why must be undertaken and different interventions must be considered.

Subdiaphragmatic Abscess

A subdiaphragmatic abscess is a collection of pus located in the left or right diaphragmatic space. The usual cause is infected fluid ascending from the pelvis. This movement is facilitated by the negative pressure caused by the movement of the right diaphragm.

Etiology, Clinical Manifestations, and Medical Management

A subdiaphragmatic abscess occurs more commonly on the right side where the right paracolic space provides an easy pathway for infected fluid. Changes in the level and configuration of the diaphragm and signs of pleural effusion or basal lung opacities on the side of the suspected abscesses are indirect signs observed on chest x-rays. Computed tomography (CT) scanning may be used to visualize the abscess. Drainage of the abscess may be accomplished percutaneously using an image-guided radiologic procedure. Nursing management is much the same as for a lung abscess.

Collaborative Management for Pulmonary Infections

To optimize the patient care, the nurse collaborates with the health care provider for monitoring and adjusting medications, treatments, patient education, and the overall plan of care. The pharmacist is consulted regarding medication effectiveness and side effects, and the respiratory therapist assists with administration of the pulmonary toilet, including breathing and coughing techniques that allow for clearing pulmonary secretions.

The physical therapist may assist with ambulation and some physical rehabilitation if the patient is in a weakened state. The nurse provides adequate pain relief in advance of physical therapy. If anorexia is present, which is common with infections, especially with TB, the nutritionist plans for small frequent meals and nutritional supplements as needed. The treatment of anorexia is discussed in Chapter 14 ☞. If monitoring is required after discharge, a social worker and home care nurse are enlisted. A community health nurse is likely to provide continuity of care.

Health Promotion for Pulmonary Infections

Patients should be taught principles of prevention. These include washing hands frequently, especially after using the bathroom, before meals, and after blowing the nose. Influenza vaccination is the primary method for preventing influenza and its severe complications. As indicated in a report from the Advisory Committee on Immunization Practices (ACIP) (MMWR, 2004 of the CDC), an annual influenza vaccination is now recommended for persons at high risk for influenza-related complications and severe disease, including children ages 6 to 59 months, pregnant women, persons 50 years or older, persons of any age with certain chronic medical conditions, and persons who live with or care for persons at high risk, including household contacts who have frequent contact with persons at high risk and who can transmit influenza to those persons at high risk, and health care workers who also have frequent contact with persons at high risk (CDC, 2006). A flu shot can be 70% to 90% effective in preventing the flu.

Elderly persons and those with chronic diseases such COPD and diabetes are at high risk for pneumonia and should avoid smoking (see the Gerontological Considerations box, p. 950). Exposure to environmental smoke, pollutants, and crowds also can be risk factors for these individuals. Those at risk should be inoculated with the influenza and pneumococcus vaccines. Individuals older than 65 years and younger patients who have chronic illnesses or are immunocompromised should also receive the pneumococcal vaccine, which is 60% effective in preventing bacterial pneumococcal infections in adults (Schultz, 2003). Gerontological considerations also are discussed at length in Chapter 10 ☞.

CRITICAL ALERT *Patients older than 50 years with a chronic disease, respiratory disease, or those who are immunocompromised should get a flu shot yearly and should be inoculated with the pneumococcal vaccine.*

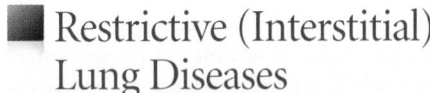

Restrictive (Interstitial) Lung Diseases

Restrictive lung diseases (also known as interstitial lung diseases) are those that result in reduced lung volumes, either because of an alteration in lung parenchyma or because of a disease of the pleura, chest wall, or neuromuscular apparatus. They are characterized by reduced total lung capacity, vital capacity, or resting lung volume. Accompanying characteristics are preserved airflow and normal airway resistance, which are measured as the functional residual capacity. If caused by parenchymal lung disease, restrictive lung disorders are accompanied by reduced gas transfer, which may be marked clinically by desaturation after exercise. The many disorders that cause reduction or restriction of lung volumes may be divided into two groups based on anatomic structures (Sharma, 2006b). These groups are classified as intrinsic lung diseases and extrinsic lung diseases.

Intrinsic lung diseases are diseases of the lung parenchyma. These diseases cause inflammation or scarring of the lung tissue (interstitial lung disease) or result in filling of the air spaces with exudate and debris (pneumonitis). These diseases can be characterized according to etiologic factors. They include idiopathic fibrotic diseases, connective tissue diseases, drug-induced lung disease, and primary diseases of the lungs (including sarcoidosis). Idiopathic pulmonary fibrosis and sarcoidosis are discussed independently in this chapter. Others are discussed throughout the text in Chapters 36 and 58 🔄.

Extrinsic lung diseases are also called extraparenchymal diseases. Diseases of the chest wall, pleura, and respiratory muscles result in lung restriction, impaired ventilatory function, and respiratory failure (e.g., nonmuscular diseases of the chest wall and neuromuscular disorders).

Epidemiology and Etiology

For intrinsic lung diseases, studies cite an overall prevalence of 3 to 6 cases per 100,000 persons, with a prevalence of idiopathic pulmonary fibrosis (IPF) of 27 to 29 cases per 100,000 persons (Sharma, 2006b). The prevalence for adults ages 35 to 44 years is 2.7 cases per 100,000 persons. Prevalence exceeded 175 cases per 100,000 persons among patients older than 75 years. Exposure to dust, metals, or organic solvents and agricultural employment are associated with increased risk.

- In North America, the prevalence of sarcoidosis is 10 to 40 cases per 100,000 persons.
- The incidence of chronic interstitial lung diseases in persons with collagen vascular diseases is variable, but it is increasing for most diseases.
- Kyphoscoliosis is a common extrinsic disorder associated with an incidence of mild deformities amounting to 1 case per 1,000 persons, with severe deformity occurring in 1 case per 10,000 persons.
- Other nonmuscular and neuromuscular disorders are rare, and their incidence and prevalence are not well known.

The mortality and morbidity from various causes of restrictive lung disease are dependent on the underlying etiology of the disease process. For example, the median survival time for patients with IPF is less than 3 years. Factors that predict poor outcome include older age, male gender, severe dyspnea, history of cigarette smoking, severe loss of lung function, appearance and severity of fibrosis on radiologic studies, a lack of response to therapy, and prominent fibroblastic foci on histopathologic evaluation.

Although a familial variant of IPF exists, a genetic predisposition is not documented (Diaz & Quellette, 2008). U.S. prevalence of sarcoidosis is estimated to be 10 to 17 times higher among African Americans compared to Caucasian Americans (Diaz & Quellette, 2008). Lymphangioleiomyomatosis (LAM) and lung involvement in tuberous sclerosis occur exclusively in premenopausal women. Men are more likely to have pneumoconiosis because of occupational exposure, IPF, and collagen vascular diseases (e.g., rheumatoid lung). Worldwide, sarcoidosis is slightly more common in women (Sharma, 2006a).

Relative to age, IPF is rare in children. Some intrinsic lung diseases present in patients ages 20 to 40 years. These include sarcoidosis, collagen vascular–associated diseases, and histiocytosis X. Most patients with IPF are older than 50 years (Sharma, 2007).

Pathophysiology

Most restrictive (interstitial) lung diseases, regardless of the cause, have a common pathogenesis. It is thought that these disorders are initiated by some type of injury to the alveolar epithelium, followed by an inflammatory process that involves the alveoli and interstitium of the lung. As the inflammatory and immune cells accumulate, damage continues to develop and fibrous scar tissue replaces functioning lung tissue (Porth, 2007). Normally, air flows to and from the alveoli as lungs inflate and deflate during each respiratory cycle. Lung inflation is accomplished by a contraction of respiratory, diaphragmatic, and external intercostal muscles, whereas deflation is passive. Functional residual capacity (FRC) is the volume of air in the lungs when the respiratory muscles are fully relaxed and no airflow is present. The volume of FRC is determined by the balance of the inward elastic recoil of the lungs and the outward elastic recoil of the chest wall. Restrictive lung diseases are characterized by a reduction in FRC and other lung volumes because of pathology in lungs, pleura, or the structures of the thoracic cage.

The distensibility of the respiratory system is called compliance, the volume change produced by a change in the distending pressure. Lung compliance is independent of the thoracic cage, which is a semirigid container. The compliance of an intact respiratory system is an algebraic sum of the compliances of both of these structures; therefore, it is influenced by any disease of the lungs, pleura, or chest wall.

In cases of intrinsic lung disease, the physiological effects of diffuse parenchymal disorders reduce all lung volumes by the excessive elastic recoil of the lungs, in comparison to the outward recoil forces of the chest wall. Expiratory airflow is reduced in proportion to lung volume. Arterial hypoxemia in these disorders is primarily caused by ventilation/perfusion mismatching, with further contribution from an intrapulmonary shunt. The diffusion of oxygen is impaired, which contributes a little toward hypoxemia at rest, but is primarily the mechanism of exercise-induced desaturation. Hyperventilation at rest and exercise is caused by the reflexes arising from the lungs and the need to maintain minute ventilation by reducing tidal volume and increasing respiratory frequency.

In cases of extrinsic disorders of the pleura and thoracic cage, the total compliance by the respiratory system is reduced and, hence, lung volumes are reduced. As a result of atelectasis, gas distribution becomes nonuniform, resulting in ventilation/perfusion mismatch and hypoxemia. In kyphoscoliosis, lateral curvature, anteroposterior angulation, kyphosis, or several of these conditions are present. The Cobb angle, an angle formed by two limbs of a convex prime curvature of the spine, is an indication of the severity of disease. An angle greater than 100 degrees is usually associated with respiratory failure.

Neuromuscular disorders affect an integral part of the respiratory system, a vital pump. The respiratory pump can be impaired at the level of the central nervous system (CNS), spinal cord, peripheral nervous system, neuromuscular junction, or respiratory muscle. The pattern of ventilatory impairment is highly dependent on the specific neuromuscular disease.

Clinical Manifestations

Restrictive lung diseases may be acute or insidious in onset, depending on the causes. Symptoms of intrinsic diseases include progressive exertional dyspnea, which is the predominant symptom; a dry cough (a productive cough is an unusual sign in most patients); and hemoptysis or grossly bloody sputum, which occurs in patients with diffuse alveolar hemorrhage syndromes and vasculitis. Wheezing is an uncommon manifestation but can occur in patients with lymphangitic carcinomatosis, chronic eosinophilic pneumonia, and respiratory bronchiolitis. Chest pain also is uncommon, but pleuritic chest pain may occur in patients with rheumatoid arthritis, systemic lupus erythematosus, and some drug-induced disorders.

Symptoms of extrinsic disorders tend to occur in middle-aged patients who develop dyspnea, decreased exercise tolerance, and respiratory infections. The cause of respiratory failure is multifactorial and is secondary to spinal deformity, muscle weakness, disordered ventilatory control, sleep disordered breathing, and airway disease. As neuromuscular disorders occur and progress, the respiratory muscle weakness progresses. Patients develop dyspnea upon exertion, followed by dyspnea at rest, with their condition ultimately advancing to respiratory failure. Also, patients with neuromuscular diseases develop significant respiratory muscle weakness and may demonstrate fatigue, dyspnea, impaired control of secretions, and recurrent lower respiratory tract infections. Acute and chronic respiratory failure, pulmonary hypertension, and cor pulmonale eventually ensue (Sharma, 2006c).

From a physical examination perspective, patients with intrinsic lung disorders may exhibit distinguishing findings. Those with chest wall disorders:

- Show obvious massive obesity and an abnormal configuration of the thoracic cage.
- Have alveolar crackles.
- Have inspiratory squeaks or scattered, late, inspiratory high-pitched rhonchi.
- Demonstrate cyanosis at rest as a late manifestation of advanced disease.
- Have digital clubbing (in those with IPF) (Sharma, 2006a).

With extrinsic disorders, severe kyphoscoliosis and massive obesity easily are recognizable. The pleural disorders are associated with decreased tactile fremitus, dullness upon percussion, and decreased intensity of breath sounds. In cases of neuromuscular diseases, the physical examination findings may indicate accessory muscle usage, rapid shallow breathing, paradoxical breathing, and other features of systemic involvement (Sharma, 2006c).

Laboratory and Diagnostic Procedures

Routine laboratory evaluations are completed to reveal positive findings in intrinsic lung diseases. Though they often fail to reveal positive findings, anemia can indicate vasculitis, and polycythemia can indicate hypoxemia in advanced disease. Leukocytosis can suggest acute hypersensitivity pneumonitis. Additional tests should be directed by the findings of the clinical assessment. Extrinsic disorders rely on an elevated creatinine kinase level that may indicate myositis, which, in turn, may cause muscle weakness and restrictive lung disease.

Imaging studies consist of chest radiography and computed tomography of the chest to diagnose intrinsic disorders, whereas fluoroscopy often is used to diagnose extrinsic disorders. Other tests include pulmonary function testing and tests for extrinsic lung disorders, such as bronchoalveolar lavage, lung biopsy, and surgical lung biopsy.

Medical Management

Medical management depends on the specific diagnosis, which is based on findings from the clinical evaluation, imaging studies, and lung biopsy. Corticosteroids, immunosuppressive agents, and cytotoxic agents are the mainstay of therapy for many of the interstitial lung diseases. Ancillary therapies include supplemental oxygen therapy, which alleviates exercise-induced hypoxemia and improves performance. The treatment regime also may include antifibrotic therapies.

Relative to the treatment of extrinsic lung disorders, it is imperative that the cause of muscle weakness be identified. Preventive therapies are used to minimize the impact of impaired secretion clearance and the prevention and prompt treatment of respiratory infections. Patients who develop respiratory failure or have severe gas exchange abnormalities during sleep may be treated with non-invasive positive pressure ventilation via a nasal or oronasal mask. Patients in whom these devices fail may require a permanent tracheotomy and ventilator assistance with a portable ventilator.

Treatment for massive obesity consists of weight loss, which causes dramatic improvement in pulmonary function test findings but is harder to achieve. These patients require polysomnographic study because of the high incidence of nocturnal hypoventilation or upper airway obstructions. Either continuous positive airway pressure or noninvasive pressure ventilation helps correct hypoventilation and upper airway obstruction (Sharma, 2006c).

In advanced disease, when respiratory failure develops, patients are treated with mechanical ventilation. If they have copious secretions, cannot control their upper airway, or are not cooperative, invasive ventilation with a tracheotomy tube is indicated. If patients have good airway control and minimal secretions, noninvasive ventilation is used, initially nocturnally and then intermittently.

◼ Nursing Management of Restrictive (Interstitial) Airway Diseases

Nursing management of patients with restrictive (interstitial) lung disease follows the protocols of patients with any type of lung disease. It is imperative that the nurse use the nursing process in determining what the patient's individual needs are and implement nursing interventions to ensure that the patient can meet individual health potential in carrying out normal daily activities without respiratory distress. Specific examples of nursing diagnoses, desired outcomes, and interventions are consistent with those for patients with obstructive pulmonary disease when airflow is lessened or restricted and are shown in the Nursing Process: Patient Care Plan for Chronic Obstructive Pulmonary Disease later in this chapter (p. 962).

◼ Idiopathic Pulmonary Fibrosis

Idiopathic pulmonary fibrosis is a chronic, progressive, fibrosing interstitial lung disease of unknown etiology characterized by a poor prognosis and no proven effective treatment. Its pathogenesis remains unknown, but disordered fibroproliferation and alveolar epithelial cell function have been identified (Diaz & Quellette, 2008). The most common histologic pattern found in surgical lung biopsy specimens from patients with IPF is called usual interstitial pneumonia (UIP), making IPF and UIP interchangeable terms in most patients.

Epidemiology and Etiology

Idiopathic pulmonary fibrosis is a disease with unknown cause with a very severe prognosis. Typically, when detected, IPF is already in an advanced stage. Patients who have IPF cannot develop normally with pulmonary gas exchange and have a much reduced quality of life. Because of lack of an effective treatment, they rarely survive 5 years after being diagnosed. Idiopathic pulmonary fibrosis affects 13 out of 100,000 men and 7 out of 100,000 women,

normally over 40 years of age. Approximately 80,000 cases of IPF have been identified in the United States, with an estimated 30,000 new cases developing each year. England and Wales report a prevalence of 6 cases per 100,000 people.

The course of IPF is variable and unpredictable. Some patients exhibit a rapidly progressive fatal course over several months, whereas others demonstrate deterioration in lung function over a longer period. The median survival is 3 to 5 years from the onset of symptoms. IPF has no racial predilection (Patel, 2008).

More males than females have been reported to have IPF. Patients with IPF are often middle aged, usually between 40 and 70 years of age. Approximately two-thirds of patients with IPF are over the age of 60 years at the time of presentation, with a mean age at diagnosis of 66 years (Diaz & Quellette, 2008). The incidence of the disease increases with older age.

IPF has no distinct geographic distribution. It is reported worldwide in both rural and urban settings with no predilection by race or ethnicity. However, the age-adjusted mortality rates appear higher among Caucasians and lower among African Americans. The reason for this finding is unclear and likely relates to inadequate reporting rather than to differences in the disease course in Caucasians compared with African Americans (Diaz & Quellette, 2008). There is geographic variation in the age-adjusted mortality from pulmonary fibrosis. This variation may reflect differences in occupational or environmental exposures. In the United States, age-adjusted mortality rates due to pulmonary fibrosis are lowest in the Midwest and Northeast, and highest in the West and Southeast. In the United Kingdom, the highest rates of mortality secondary to IPF occur in the industrialized central areas of England and Wales (Antoniou et al., 2008).

It is documented that deaths from pulmonary fibrosis increase with increasing age (Verma & Slutsky, 2007). The mortality rate for IPF per 100,000 population is estimated to be 3.3 in men and 2.5 in women, with an overall rate of 3.0 in both sexes in Japan. A summary of various studies reports that the mean length of survival from the time of diagnosis of IPF varies between 3.2 and 5 years (Diaz & Quellette, 2008).

Potential risk factors for IPF include:

- Cigarette smoking
- Exposure to commonly prescribed drugs, such as antidepressants
- Chronic aspiration
- Environmental factors, such as metal dust and wood dust, solvents
- Infectious agents, such as Epstein–Barr virus, influenza, cytomegalovirus, hepatitis C, and HIV
- Genetic predisposition, based on familial cases of IPF, meaning at least two members of a primary biologic family (parent, child, sibling) (Dauber, 2006).

Pathophysiology

The pathogenesis of IPF remains unknown. It was once thought that intra-alveolar inflammation played a big role; however, anti-inflammatory agents and immune modulators have proved to be only minimally effective in the treatment of IPF. IPF is characterized by diffuse interstitial fibrosis with only mild inflammation, honeycomb cysts, and fibroblastic foci (areas of accumulation of fibroblasts and connective tissue). A disruption in the homeostasis of alveolar epithelial cells caused by unknown endogenous or environmental stimuli is thought to occur. This disruption in the homeostasis results in diffuse epithelial cell activation and aberrant epithelial repair, in which cytokines and dysfunctional apoptosis are involved (Verma & Slutsky, 2007).

Clinical Manifestations

Clinical manifestations of IPF consist of progressive dyspnea upon exertion, interstitial infiltrates on chest radiographs, and abnormal pulmonary function test results indicating restrictive disease (Patel, 2008). Symptoms depend on the extent of lung damage. Initially, patients present with shortness of breath on exertion, cough, and diminished stamina. Weight loss and fatigue are common. Complications include lung infections and cor pulmonale as the disease progresses (Merck, 2008). The definitive diagnosis should be made only after clinical, radiologic, and pathologic evaluations of the patient and only after excluding other causes of interstitial lung disease.

Laboratory and Diagnostic Procedures

Blood test results are not specific for IPF; however, some abnormal values can be related to the pathophysiology of IPF. For example, an elevated hemoglobin value may reflect chronic hypoxemia secondary to IPF. The erythrocyte sedimentation rate is elevated in 50% of patients. Serologic test results are nonspecific; however, high titers should raise the possibility of connective-tissue disorders.

Imaging studies may be used but are not specific to IPF. At the time of diagnosis of IPF, almost all patients have abnormal chest radiography findings of bilateral diffuse reticular or reticulonodular infiltrates at the periphery and the bases of the lungs.

Pulmonary function tests are conducted with a typical finding of a restrictive ventilatory defect. The most common abnormality found in patients with IPF is a decreased diffusing capacity. Bronchoalveolar lavage, echocardiography, and bronchoscopy also may be done to isolate or confirm diagnosis.

Lung biopsy of patients with IPF may be done. During the period of accelerated IPF, lung biopsy typically shows a combination of UIP with superimposed diffuse alveolar damage, characterized by fibroblast proliferation of the alveoli septa, hyperplasia of type 2 pneumocytes, and hyaline membrane remnants (Diaz & Quellette, 2008).

Medical Management

Medical management of IPF focuses on preserving as much lung function as possible, and enabling the patient to engage in normal activities as long as possible. In this regard, oxygen therapy should be prescribed for patients with documented hypoxemia; thereby, improving exercise tolerance. A pulmonary specialist generally is consulted to mange the patient with corticosteroids and cytotoxic or antifibrotic agents. Patients with acute respiratory failure may require mechanical ventilation, with consultation from a critical care specialist.

Maintaining adequate nutritional intake and immunizations is important for quality of life. Participation in a pulmonary rehabilitation should be encouraged in order to maintain functionality and address psychosocial aspects of this disease.

Patients with pneumothorax should be admitted to inpatient care as should patients with severe hypoxemia. Further outpatient care focuses on closely monitoring the patient for adverse drug effects and complications, maintaining functionality through pulmonary rehabilitation, encouraging smoking cessation, and recommending vaccines as appropriate.

Referral to a lung transplantation center should be instituted early in patients with histologic or radiographic evidence of UIP. Lung transplantation also should be considered, and a referral to an appropriate transplantation center may be appropriate. Referrals to a specialized center for any ongoing clinical trials for new treatments that may offer new hope for patients with IPF also should be considered.

■ Nursing Management

Nursing management of patients with IPF is based on the principles of caring for any patient with lung or respiratory disorders. The main focus is on assisting the patient to remain functional and to maintain as much self-care and life management as possible. The nurse works with the interdisciplinary health care team in carrying out treatment goals: identifying and removing the injurious agent, suppressing the inflammatory response, preventing progression of the disease, and providing supportive therapy for persons with advanced disease. The Nursing Process: Patient Care Plan for Chronic Obstructive Pulmonary Disease (p. 962) contains an approach to implementing the nursing process for IPF.

IPF does not have a positive prognosis, and the nurse must be aware of the psychosocial needs of the patient and family. These may become paramount in planning the care of the patient and in instituting discharge priorities. As noted under medical management, the nurse may assist the patient in referrals to transplant programs as well as pulmonary rehabilitation programs.

■ Sarcoidosis

Sarcoidosis is an inflammatory immune system disorder that affects multiple organ systems. It is characterized by noncaseating granulomas (small inflammatory nodules) that most often occur in the lungs or lymph nodes. They can clump together and form larger clumps that attack other organs including the skin, liver, eyes, spleen, bone marrow, kidneys, salivary glands, heart, endocrine system, and gastrointestinal system (Barreiro, DeMarco, Gemmel, & Schaub, 2005; Gould, 2006; Yakobi, 2007). Some people have signs and symptoms related to a specific organ, such as shortness of breath from lung problems, but others may have only a vague feeling of illness or no signs or symptoms at all.

Epidemiology, Etiology, and Pathophysiology

Although anyone can develop sarcoidosis, the disease mainly affects adults between the ages of 20 and 40. People of Scandinavian descent and African Americans are particularly at risk. African Americans also are more likely to have severe, chronic symptoms than are Caucasians. The annual incidence of sarcoidosis in the United States is approximately 10 cases in 100,000 among Caucasians, and 36 cases per 100,000 in the African American population. It is most commonly seen in the Mid-Atlantic States and in the South, rarely in the Southwest.

The disease does seem to run in families, particularly African Americans who present with a more aggressive course (Barreiro et. al., 2005).

Although the exact cause of sarcoidosis is unknown, it is believed to occur when a person's immune system overreacts to an unknown toxin, drug, or pathogen that enters the body through the airways (Mayo Clinic, 2008). Normally, a person's immune system helps protect the person's body from foreign substances and invading microorganisms, such as bacteria and viruses. But in sarcoidosis, T-helper lymphocytes—white blood cells that play a key role in the body's immune response—seem to respond too strongly to a perceived threat. This triggers small areas of inflammation called granulomas.

As the disease progresses, granulomas and scarring (fibrosis) may occur in the tissue between the air sacs, stiffening the lungs and reducing the amount of air the lungs can hold. Some experts speculate that the causative agent may be a nontuberculous mycobacterium, a noncontagious member of the family of bacteria that causes tuberculosis. In a small portion of people, sarcoidosis may have a genetic component. Studies are ongoing to investigate the genetic and environmental components of this disease (Gould, 2006).

Clinical Manifestations

Patients with symptoms of sarcoidosis most commonly present in winter and early spring, which suggests a possible environmental trigger. They may have no symptoms, having been diagnosed by chest x-ray, or they may have fever, night sweats, malaise, fatigue, weight loss, dry cough, wheezing, and dyspnea.

Sometimes sarcoidosis develops gradually and produces signs and symptoms that last for years. Or it may appear suddenly and then disappear just as quickly. In either case, signs and symptoms can vary, depending on which organs are affected and how long the individual has had the disease (American Lung Association, 2007). Ninety percent of patients present with pulmonary involvement, but if this is not the case they are likely to experience remission within 2 years or experience a milder disease presentation. Additional signs and symptoms of sarcoidosis that should be considered include small red bumps on the face, arms, or buttocks, a condition more common in African Americans than in Caucasians, and red, watery eyes. Arthritis in the ankles, elbows, wrists, and hands commonly is associated with bumps in the skin over a person's shins (erythema nodosum) (Gould, 2006; Yakobi, 2007).

Laboratory and Diagnostic Procedures

Chest x-rays are performed, but usually are nonspecific; CT scans and magnetic resonance imaging (MRI) are more helpful in confirming a diagnosis. Pulmonary function is assessed with pulmonary function studies, ABGs, and oxygen saturation. A fiber-optic bronchoscopy with transbronchial biopsies including culturing is helpful. A total chemistry and hematologic work-up is performed including liver function tests, and a TB skin test is administered to rule out TB (Barreiro et al., 2005).

Medical Management

Medical management of sarcoidosis is individualized, with the need for medical therapy varying based on the symptoms and organ systems involved in each patient. Many patients require no

treatment; symptoms usually are not disabling and tend to disappear spontaneously. Because sarcoidosis can disappear even without therapy, health care providers may disagree on when to start treatment, what medication and dose to prescribe, and how long to continue the medicine. When therapy is recommended, the main goal is to keep the lungs and other affected body organs working and to relieve symptoms. The disease is considered inactive once the symptoms fade. The decision to initiate drug therapy depends on the organ system involved and how far the inflammation has progressed. If the disease appears to be severe, especially in the lungs, eyes, heart, nervous system, spleen, or kidneys, the doctor may prescribe medications.

Currently, corticosteroid drugs are the primary treatment for inflammation and granuloma formation. Prednisone probably is the corticosteroid most often prescribed today (Gould, 2006). Corticosteroid treatment usually results in improvement. However, symptoms often start up again when it is stopped. Treatment, therefore, may be necessary for several years. At present, there is no treatment to reverse the lung scarring (fibrosis) that might be present in advanced sarcoidosis.

Note also that more than one test is needed to diagnose sarcoidosis. Diagnostic tests also can determine if patients with sarcoidosis are getting better. Occasionally, a blood test will show a high blood level of calcium accompanying sarcoidosis. The reasons for this are not clear. When it does occur, the patient may be advised to avoid calcium-rich foods, vitamin D, or sunlight, or to take prednisone, as indicated earlier. Frequent checkups are important so that the health care provider can monitor the illness and, if necessary, adjust the treatment.

For example, corticosteroids can have side effects: mood swings, swelling, and weight gain because the treatment tends to make the body hold on to water; high blood pressure; high blood sugar; and a craving for food. Long-term use can affect the stomach, skin, and bones. This situation can bring on stomach pain, an ulcer, or acne or cause the loss of calcium from bones. However, if the corticosteroid is taken in carefully prescribed low doses, the benefits from the treatment usually are far greater than the problems.

◼ Nursing Management

If the patient presents with pulmonary symptoms, the nurse monitors respiratory status frequently including oxygen saturation and lung sounds. Oxygen is administered if the patient is dyspneic or oxygen saturation falls below 90%. A total physical assessment is performed and may reveal abnormalities in vital signs, heart rhythm, skin, and eyes; cranial nerve damage may affect the gag reflex, causing swallowing difficulties, facial numbness, or unilateral drooping. If dyspnea is severe the patient may be started on prednisone 60 mg daily and gradually reduced to smaller doses of 10 to 30 mg as symptoms subside. The nurse educates the patient and family regarding administration of prednisone, the dangers associated with abrupt stoppage, and side effects such as weight gain, mood changes, hypokalemia, and muscle weakness.

Second-line drugs used include methotrexate and azathioprine (Imuran) for which patients are also educated. Persons with cardiac involvement may be on medications for dysrhythmias, hypertension, and congestive heart failure. Topical med-

CHART 35–5 Research on Assessment of Dyspnea

Researchers Kendrick, Baxi, and Smith (2000, pp. 2–3) wished to answer the following questions: (1) Can patients with acute bronchospastic asthma or COPD adequately communicate their level of dyspnea using the modified Borg scale (MBS)? (2) Does subjective improvement in the patient's dyspnea using the MBS correlate with improvements in pulmonary functions as measured by the peak flow meter and cutaneous oxygen saturation (SaO_2)?

Four hundred male veterans ages 24 to 87 presented with a chief complaint of dyspnea. The assessing health care provider identified 102 of these patients as having acute bronchospasm, 42 were diagnosed with asthma, and 60 were diagnosed as COPD. All study patients were able to use the MBS to rate their perception of the severity of dyspnea. As the peak flow measurements increased, the MBS scores of difficulty breathing decreased. Researchers concluded that the MBS is a valid and reliable assessment tool for dyspnea. The emergency department triage and primary care nursing staff rated the MBS as highly satisfactory along with the patients. Respiratory assessment in the triage notes was streamlined to consistently include three measures: peak flow, MBS, and SaO_2. Long respiratory narratives were found to be unnecessary in many cases.

Source: This article was published in *Journal of Emergency Nursing 26*(3). Kendrick, K., Baxi, S., & Smith, R. Usefulness of the modified 0–10 Borg scale in assessing the degree of dyspnea in patients with COPD and asthma. pp. 216–222. Copyright Elsevier, 2000.

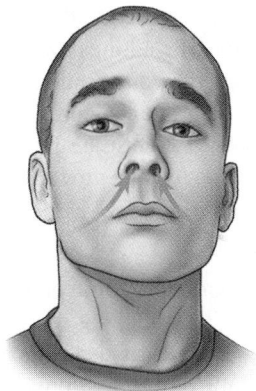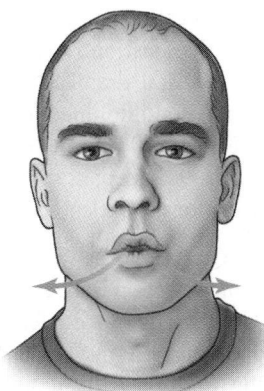

FIGURE 35–7 ■ Patient doing pursed lip breathing.

symptoms. The nurse monitors ABG results to determine the patient's status and make clinical decisions regarding treatment. The nurse assists the patient to manage the anxiety that often accompanies dyspnea related to asthmatic attacks or complications of chronic bronchitis and emphysema.

A major role of the nurse is patient and family education with the often complex therapies associated with chronic COPD. This may be in the form of a structured program or may incorporate

COMPLEMENTARY & ALTERNATIVE THERAPIES   Inhalation of Herbal Preparations

Description:
CAM use is increasingly popular for respiratory conditions, and is particularly well documented in German research. The aromatic components of herbal preparations are commonly used in a number of proprietary products to improve lung mucus clearance in patients with chronic airway obstruction.

Aromatics from nasturtium, horseradish root, ivy leaf, thyme, aniseed, and marshmallow and primrose root are used in many herbal products to improve mucus clearance.

Research Support:
A study conducted in the United Kingdom investigated the efficacy of inhaled aromatics on lung clearance. Twelve patients with chronic bronchitis were studied in a randomized, single-blind, placebo-controlled crossover trial. The mean age of the participants was 67. Relative to a baseline, airway mucus clearance observed during the first hour of testing was significantly correlated with the concentration level of aromatics (Hasani, Pavia, Toms, Dilworth, & Agnew, 2003).

A prospective cohort study was conducted in 251 German medical centers that involved 536 participants with acute sinusitis, bronchitis, or urinary tract infections (UTI) for 4 years or more. The participants were treated either with the herbal drug Angocin Anti-Infekt N (containing nasturtium and horseradish root) or with standard antibiotic therapy. The physician determined the treatment, dosage, and duration according to the patient's needs. Standard antibiotic therapy was found to be comparable to therapy with the herbal drug in treating acute sinusitis, acute bronchitis and acute urinary tract infection. In addition, the group treated with the herbal drug needed less supportive procedures and administration of concurrent medication, leading the investigators to conclude that there is a clear advantageous safety profile compared to the group treated with standard antibiotics (Goos, Albrecht, & Schneider, 2006).

A clinical trial involving 62 participants with common cold, bronchitis, or respiratory tract disease evaluated changes in the symptoms of cough

and tolerability after treatment with a combined herbal cough syrup preparation containing dry ivy leaf extract as the main active ingredient, decoctions of thyme and aniseed, and mucilage of marshmallow root (Weleda Hustenelixier, new formulation). At the end of the trial, there was an improvement in all symptom scores as compared to baseline, as well as good tolerability (Buechi, Vogelin, von Eiff, Ramos, & Melzer, 2005).

Another study of 150 outpatients with bronchitis evaluated the efficacy of a fixed combination of thyme fluid extract and primrose root tincture. The results showed a clinically relevant and more pronounced decrease of bronchitis symptoms (the primary outcome criterion) and a shortened duration of acute bronchitis (the secondary outcome criterion) when compared to placebo (Gruenwald, Graubaum, & Busch, 2005).

References
Buechi, S., Vogelin, R., von Eiff, M. M., Ramos, M., & Melzer, J. (2005). Open trial to assess aspects of safety and efficacy of a combined herbal cough syrup with ivy and thyme. *Forschende Komplementarmedizin und Klassiche Naturheilkunde, 12*(6), 328–332.

Goos, K. H., Albrecht, U., & Schneider, B. (2006). Efficacy and safety profile of a herbal drug containing nasturtium herb and horseradish root in acute sinusitis, acute bronchitis and acute urinary tract infection in comparison with other treatments in the daily practice/results of a prospective cohort study. *Arzneimittelforschung, 56*(3), 249–257.

Gruenwald, J., Graubaum, H. J., & Busch, R. (2005). Efficacy and tolerability of a fixed combination of thyme and primrose root in patients with acute bronchitis. A double-blind, randomized, placebo-controlled clinical trial. *Arzneimittelforschung, 55*(11), 669–676.

Hasani, A., Pavia, D., Toms, N., Dilworth, P., & Agnew, J. E. (2003). Effect of aromatics on lung mucociliary clearance in patients with chronic airways obstruction. *Journal of Alternative & Complementary Medicine, 9*(2), 243–249.

patient education and practice opportunities offered by the nurse, physical therapist, and respiratory therapist. Breathing retraining, use of postural drainage techniques, energy conservation, and physical reconditioning are the foci of education (Figures 35–8, 35–9, and 35–10 ■). The Nursing Process: Patient Care Plan for COPD (p. 962) depicts specific steps of the nursing process used in caring for the patient with COPD.

Health Promotion

Smoking cessation is the single most important factor in preventing COPD. The nurse refers the patient to a smoking cessation program or assists in a personal plan. Even for the patient who has COPD, quitting is likely to prevent future complications. The nurse educates the patient regarding the hazards of smoking and provides counseling opportunities as needed. In addition, it is important to teach the patient some of the subtle changes that may occur, such as fatigue, dyspnea, and change in sputum color, consistency, or amount, indicate a respiratory infection. To prevent infection, the nurse cautions patients to avoid extremes of temperature, exposure to crowds, poor air quality, or high pollen counts. These conditions may cause bronchospasm.

 CRITICAL ALERT   *Subtle changes indicating a respiratory infection are fatigue, dyspnea, and change in sputum color, consistency, or amount. To prevent infection, the nurse cautions patients to avoid extremes of temperature, exposure to crowds, poor air quality, or high pollen counts. These conditions may cause bronchospasm.*

■ Collaborative Management

Individuals with COPD will receive treatment from a team of professionals including nurses, respiratory therapists, physical therapists, social workers, pharmacists, and other health care

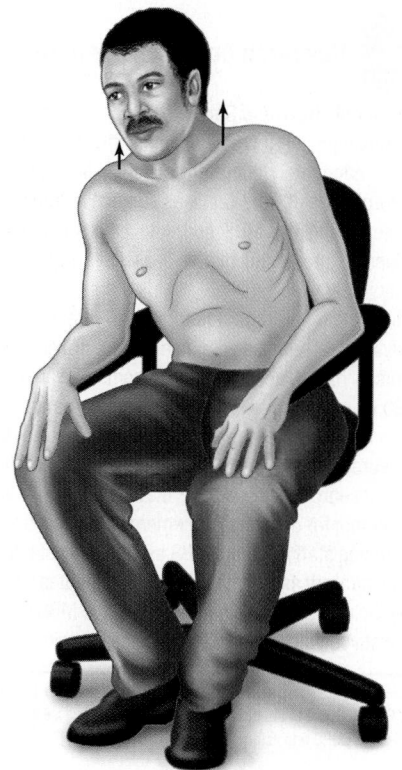

FIGURE 35–9 ■ Typical posture of patient with COPD.

providers. A social worker and or a psychologist also may assist with financial issues and vocational concerns.

It is likely that the COPD patient may require follow-up in a rehabilitation setting following discharge from an acute care setting. Follow-up with a home care nurse also is likely. Many patients and caregivers benefit from a formal or informal pulmonary rehabilitation program provided in the outpatient setting. Aside from assisting the patient with physical and respiratory rehabilitation and muscle strengthening, patients receive emotional support from staff and other participants. The Nursing Process: Patient Care Plan for COPD (p. 962) details nursing care priorities.

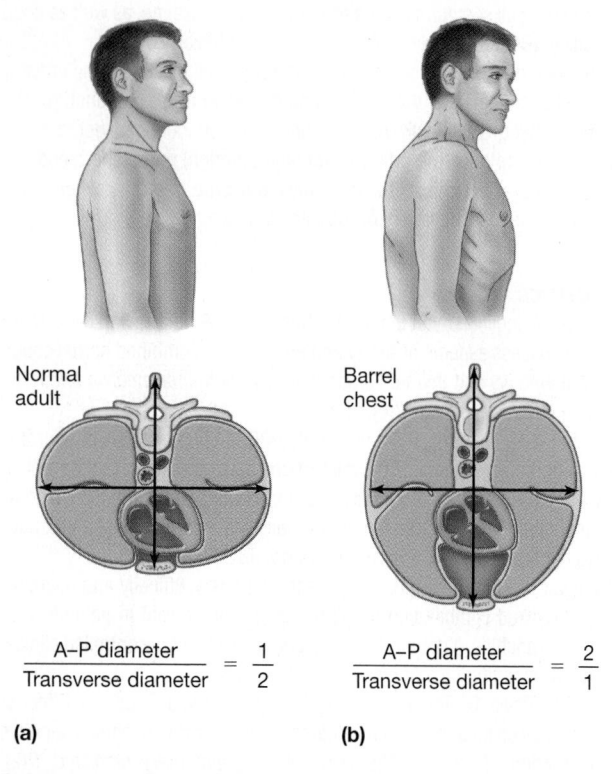

Normal adult

Barrel chest

$$\frac{\text{A–P diameter}}{\text{Transverse diameter}} = \frac{1}{2}$$

$$\frac{\text{A–P diameter}}{\text{Transverse diameter}} = \frac{2}{1}$$

(a)   **(b)**

FIGURE 35–8 ■ Barrel chest.

■ Asthma

Asthma is a chronic hyperreactive disorder of the airways (bronchioles) that is characterized by episodic reversible airflow obstruction and airway inflammation, persistent airway hyperreactivity, and airway remodeling (changes in wall structure) (Morris, 2007; Porth, 2007). The National Heart, Lung, and Blood Institute's (NHLBI's) Second Expert Panel on Management of Asthma defined bronchial asthma as "a chronic inflammatory disorder of the airways in which many cells and cellular elements play a role, in particular, mast cells, eosinophils, T lymphocytes, and epithelial cells" (NHLBI, 1997/2002). Morris (2007) notes that it is one of the most common chronic diseases worldwide and is the most common cause of hospitalization for children in the United States. This inflammatory process causes recurrent episodes of wheezing, breathlessness, chest tightness, and coughing, particularly at night or in the early morning, in

MyNursingKit | Video: Respiratory: Asthma—Etiology and Pathophysiology

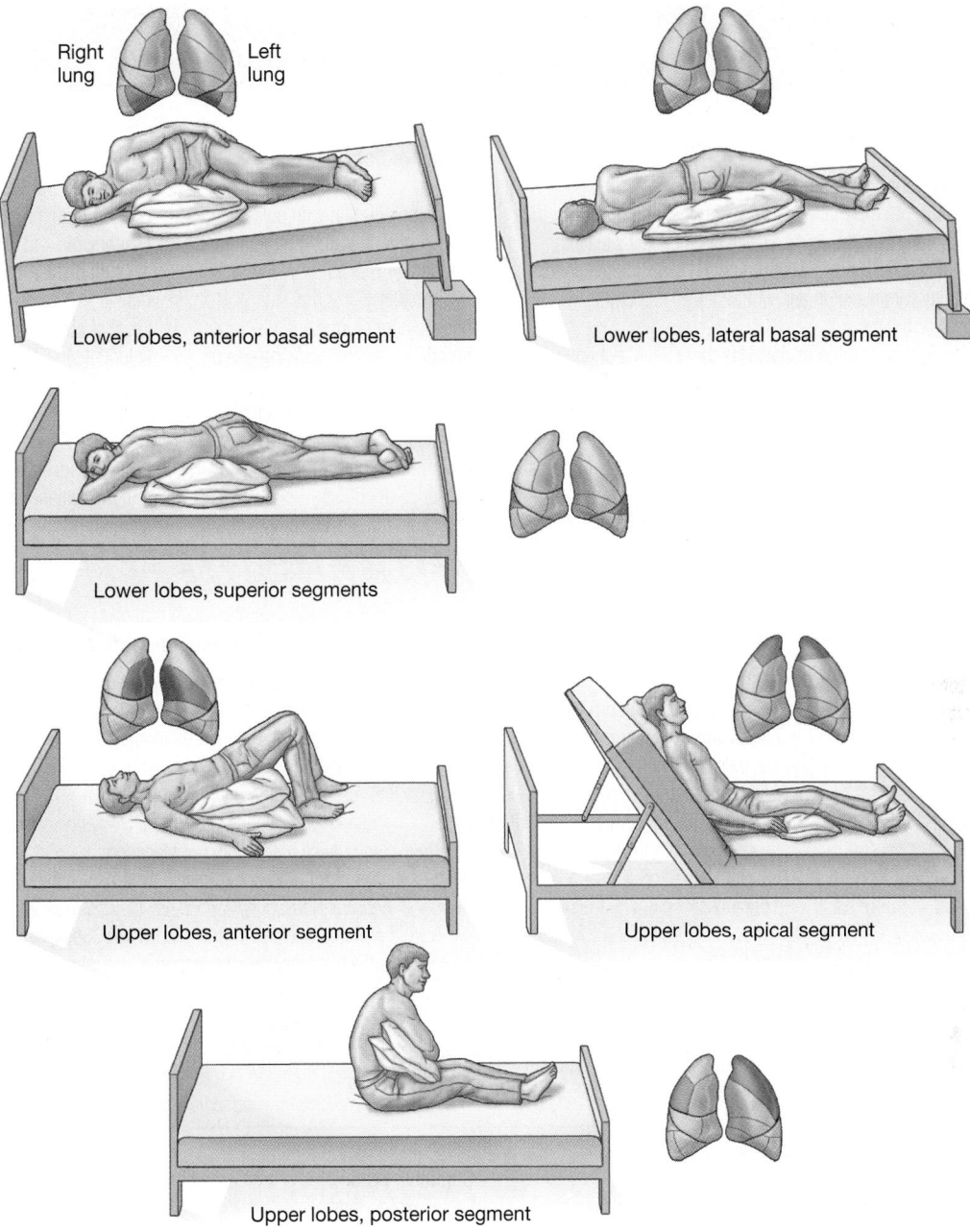

Right lung   Left lung

Lower lobes, anterior basal segment

Lower lobes, lateral basal segment

Lower lobes, superior segments

Upper lobes, anterior segment

Upper lobes, apical segment

Upper lobes, posterior segment

FIGURE 35–10 ■ Postural drainage positions.

susceptible individuals. These episodes are usually associated with widespread but variable airflow obstruction that is often reversible either spontaneously or with treatment. The inflammation also causes an associated increase in the existing bronchial responsiveness to a variety of stimuli.

Sometimes asthma is classified as intrinsic or extrinsic. Intrinsic asthma, also referred to as nonallergic asthma, is triggered by diverse nonimmune mechanisms, including respiratory tract infections, exercise, ingestion of aspirin, emotional upset, and exposure to bronchial irritants such as cigarette smoke, dust, chemicals, and fumes.

Extrinsic, or atopic, asthma is initiated by a type 1 hypersensitivity response to an extrinsic antigen, such as pollens and allergens. Although this distinction is considered helpful from a pathophysiological perspective, it is less helpful from a clinical view because many people with asthma manifest overlapping characteristics of both extrinsic an intrinsic asthma (Porth, 2007). Note, however, that treatment of allergic asthma should include avoiding the primarily indoor and sometimes outdoor allergens to which the patient has become sensitized, and treatment of intrinsic asthma is aimed at avoiding respiratory infections (viral infections, colds, influenza, and all contact with smoke and fumes).

Epidemiology and Etiology

The prevalence of asthma appears to have increased continuously since the 1970s, and asthma now affects an estimated 4% to 7% of people worldwide (NHLBI, 2007). As the prevalence has increased, so has the mortality and morbidity. Although asthma occurs across races worldwide, in the United States,

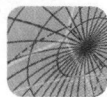

NURSING PROCESS: Patient Care Plan for Chronic Obstructive Pulmonary Disease

Assessment of the COPD Patient

Subjective Data:

Do you experience cough, shortness of breath, or wheezing?

Describe the type of cough you experience. Is it dry hacking, productive, and/or triggered by smoking or other environmental, social, or emotional situations?

Is sputum clear or colored and how much would you say is expectorated per day?

Do you have any difficulty with sleeping and what position is most comfortable for you?

What is your current weight and eating habits? Has there been a change during the last month or year?

Do you or have you ever smoked any type of tobacco? If so, describe your smoking history.

Describe your medications and breathing treatments.

Do you use supplemental oxygen? If so, please describe.

Describe your activity tolerance. Has this changed during the last month or year?

If you experience wheezing or chest tightness, what situations seem to trigger this?

Objective Data:

Vital signs

Oxygen saturation with pulse oximetry

Spirometry results (FEV_1/FVC)

ABG results

Assessment of lung sounds and breathing pattern including use of accessory muscles

Presence or absence of clubbing

Presence or absence of barrel chest

Color of face, lips, and nail beds

Presence of cough

Color and amount of sputum production

Exercise tolerance

Oxygen requirements

Hemoglobin and hematocrit

Sputum culture and sensitivity results

Level of consciousness

Orientation

Note whether the patient responds with lucid answers and states them in compete sentences.

Breathlessness may be so severe that the patient can only respond with one- or two-word answers.

Nursing Assessment and Diagnoses	Outcomes and Evaluation Parameters	Planning and Interventions with *Rationales*
Nursing Diagnosis: *Ineffective Airway Clearance* related to inadequate cough and excessive mucous production	**Outcome:** Patient will demonstrate controlled cough and postural drainage. **Evaluation Parameters:** After completion of pulmonary toilet, lung sounds are clear or significantly improved upon auscultation. Oxygen saturation after pulmonary toilet is within normal range. Patient expectorates secretions effectively upon assessment by the nurse.	**Interventions and *Rationales:*** Assess the patient's ability to mobilize secretions. If unable to do so, suction as necessary to remove secretions *to clear the airway.* Teach use of postural drainage and chest physiotherapy or refer to respiratory therapist. Note characteristics of sputum. *Secretions can obstruct airways and cause respiratory complications.* Assess for presence of adventitious lung sounds every 4–8 hours. *Auscultation of lung sounds provides information on respiratory status.* Administer expectorants as ordered. Observe the patient for drug effectiveness. *Airway dilation is the result of medications.* Provide hydration of at least 2 L/day if not medically contraindicated. Administer vaporization therapy and perform physical therapy and postural drainage as ordered at least 1 hour before meals. *Hydration and vaporization help to liquefy secretions.*

Assessment of Anxiety and Coping with Disease

Subjective Data:

How do you think you are coping with episodes of dyspnea or chest tightness?

What are triggers for increasing anxiety?

Objective Data:

Facial expressions

Mood

Verbalization of fear regarding illness and its impact on family and the future

Nursing Assessment and Diagnoses	Outcomes and Evaluation Parameters	Planning and Interventions with *Rationales*
Nursing Diagnosis: *Anxiety* related to dyspneic episodes or asthmatic attacks	**Outcome:** Patient is able to identify activities that tend to decrease anxious behaviors. **Evaluation Parameters:** Demonstrates the ability to initiate purse-lipped breathing at the onset of dyspnea related to anxiety. Verbalizes anxious feelings and thoughts. Anxiety is relieved by consistently demonstrating aggression and anxiety control, coping, impulse control, self-mutilation restraint, and substantially effective social interaction skills. Verbalizes absence of sensory perceptual disorders. Verbalizes absence of physical manifestations of anxiety. Behavioral manifestations of anxiety absent.	**Interventions and *Rationales:*** Ask the patient to identify in writing various factors that elicit an anxious response. *Clarifying thoughts gives the patient control and may decrease anxiety.* Help the patient formulate a plan for coping with dyspneic and or wheezing episodes. *A plan allows the patient to prepare.* Encourage verbalization of feelings *to decrease anxiety.* Teach patient interventions for coping such as relaxation techniques and biofeedback. *These types of interventions decrease stress and anxiety.*

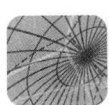

NURSING PROCESS: Patient Care Plan for Chronic Obstructive Pulmonary Disease—*Continued*

Assessment of Patient/Family Knowledge

Subjective Data:
Describe your disease history and the progression of symptoms. For example, has the shortness of breath worsened over time?

Objective Data:
Able to verbalize prevention techniques

Nursing Assessment and Diagnoses	Outcomes and Evaluation Parameters	Planning and Interventions with *Rationales*
Nursing Diagnosis: *Deficient Knowledge* related to COPD	**Outcome:** Patient and significant others describe breathing exercises and energy conservation techniques prior to discharge. ***Evaluation Parameters:*** Patient demonstrates breathing exercises and energy conservation techniques prior to discharge. Patient and family members describe the treatment regime with rationale prior to discharge. Patient discusses emotional reactions to lifestyle changes prior to discharge. Prior to discharge, the patient and caregiver verbalize issues that constitute an emergency and what actions they should take. Patient and caregiver describe the appropriate contacts to make in the case of an emergency.	**Interventions and *Rationales:*** Instruct the patient on prevention of infection. Discuss stress with the patient: avoidance of crowded rooms or contact with known cases of colds or flu, avoidance of irritants such as tobacco smoke, importance of receiving pneumococcal and influenza vaccines, importance of recognizing changes in sputum color and density. *These measures prevent complications of COPD.* The nurse, along with the respiratory therapist, physical therapist, and occupational therapist, teaches breathing techniques including breathing exercises and energy conservation strategies. Treadmills, weights, and bicycles may be used to improve muscle strength and endurance. Patients can incorporate use of portable oxygen systems into this exercise routine as needed. Inspiratory muscle training may be prescribed to strengthen muscles used in breathing. This requires that the patient breathe against resistance for 10–15 minutes a day, *thus conditioning muscles and increasing activity tolerance and ventilatory competence. Breathing exercises and physical reconditioning decrease the work of breathing and improve physical stamina.* Review the patient's treatment regime including medications, oxygen, breathing exercises, postural drainage, physical conditioning, and nutritional support. Attention to psychosocial issues is very important *since the patient with end-stage COPD is often discouraged because of immobility, and can easily become angry, depressed, and demanding. Making the necessary lifestyle changes requires that patients talk about the emotions associated with these changes.* Enlist family support and at the same time support caregivers who face these difficult issues daily. Attain resources for patient education from the American Lung Association, the American Association of Cardiovascular and Pulmonary Rehabilitation, the American Thoracic Society, and the American Association for Respiratory Therapy. The nurse plays a major role in educating the patient regarding the disease process and the medical regimen. *Enhancing the knowledge base of the patient and family is likely to facilitate health maintenance and prevention of complications.* Review what issues constitute an emergency and describes what action patients should take in a simulated situation offered by the nurse. The health care team arranges for oxygen, if ordered, to be available in the home setting. Plans for transfer to home should be made in consideration of oxygen needs. Instructions should be given in writing. Arrangements are made with the home oxygen distributor to provide specific education regarding home oxygen and respiratory equipment. *Discharge is a time of transition and anxiety. Repetition of information and visual cues such as written information reinforces what has been taught.* Give contact numbers for nursing and other care providers to the patient and caregiver. The patient and caregiver are instructed to place these near the phone for easy access in case of an emergency.

asthma prevalence, especially morbidity and mortality, is higher in African Americans than in Caucasians. Although genetic factors are of major importance in determining a predisposition to the development of asthma, environmental factors play a greater role than racial factors in the onset of the disease (Morris, 2007). Asthma occurs at all ages, but half of the cases occur during childhood and another third before age 40 (NHLBI, 2006).

During childhood, asthma predominantly occurs in boys with a male-to-female ratio of 2:1 until puberty, when the male-to-female ratio becomes 1:1. After puberty, the prevalence in females is greater, and the majority of adult-onset cases diagnosed in persons older than 40 years occurs in females. Boys are more likely than girls to experience a decrease in symptoms by late adolescence (Morris, 2007). Five percent of adults and 7% to 10% of children in the United States have asthma. It ranks among the most common chronic conditions in the United States, affecting an estimated 14.9 million persons in 1995 and causing 1.5 million emergency department visits (NHLBI, 2006).

The hygiene hypothesis also should be considered when discussing the increase in asthma diagnoses. This is a theory about the cause of asthma and other allergic disease that is supported by epidemiologic data for asthma. For example, asthma prevalence has been increasing in developed countries along with increased use of antibiotics, cesarean sections, and cleaning products (Martinez, 2007). All of these things may negatively affect exposure to beneficial bacteria and other immune system modulators that are important during development and, thus, may cause increased risk for asthma and allergy.

Asthma is caused by a complex interaction of genetic and environmental factors that is not yet fully understood (Martinez, 2007). These factors also can influence how severe a person's asthma is and how well one responds to medication (Choudhry et al., 2007). As with other complex diseases, many genetic and environmental factors have been suggested as causes of asthma, but not all of them have been replicated. In addition, as researchers detangle the complex causes of asthma, it is becoming more evident that certain environmental and genetic factors may only affect asthma when combined. It is likely that genes are inherited for increased interleukin-4 (IL-4) and immunoglobulin E (IgE). These cause responses to allergens and bronchial hyperresponsiveness. Environmental factors also increase the risk of asthma. In many individuals the symptoms of asthma are reversible, but fibrosis of the lung may occur in some patients with asthma and these changes cause abnormalities of lung function. This decreases lung compliance and initiates a restrictive component to the lung disease (McCance & Huether, 2007). See Risk Factors and Precipitating Factors for Asthma.

Pathophysiology

The pathophysiology of asthma involves the following components: (1) airway inflammation, (2) intermittent airflow obstruction, and (3) bronchial hyperresponsiveness (Figure 35–11 ■). The mechanism of inflammation in asthma may be acute, subacute, or chronic, and the presence of airway edema and mucous secretion also contributes to airflow obstruction and bronchial reactivity. Varying degrees of mononuclear cell and eosinophil infiltration, mucous hypersecretion, desquamation of the epithelium, smooth muscle hyperplasia, and airway remodeling are present (Morris, 2007; Porth, 2007).

RISK FACTORS and Precipitating Factors for Asthma

Allergens
- Animal dander (from the skin, hair, or feathers of animals)
- Dust mites (contained in house dust)
- Cockroaches
- Pollen from trees and grass
- Mold (indoor and outdoor)

Irritants
- Cigarette smoke
- Air pollution
- Cold air or changes in weather
- Strong odors from painting or cooking
- Scented products
- Strong emotional expression (including crying or laughing hard) and stress
- Living in large urban area

Others
- Medicines such as aspirin and beta-blockers
- Sulfites in food (dried fruit) or beverages (wine)
- Gastroesophageal reflux disease that causes heartburn and can worsen asthma symptoms, especially at night
- Irritants or allergens at your work, such as special chemicals or dusts
- Infections
- Having one or both parents with asthma
- Obesity

Sources: American Lung Association. (2008). *What is asthma?* Retrieved May 4, 2008 from http://www.lungusa.org/site/apps/s/content.asp?c=dv:IL900E&b=4061173& ct=5314727; Morris, M. J. (2007). Asthma. *eMedicine.* Retrieved July 29, 2008, from http://www.emedicine.com/med/topic177.htm.

Some of the principal cells identified in airway inflammation include mast cells, eosinophils, epithelial cells, macrophages, and activated T lymphocytes. T lymphocytes play an important role in the regulation of airway inflammation through the release of numerous cytokines. Other constituent airway cells, such as fibroblasts, endothelial cells, and epithelial cells, contribute to the chronicity of the disease. Factors such as adhesion molecules (e.g., selectins, integrins) are critical in directing the inflammatory changes in the airway. Finally, cell-derived mediators influence smooth muscle tone and produce structural changes and remodeling of the airway.

The presence of airway hyperresponsiveness or bronchial hyperreactivity in asthma is an exaggerated response to numerous exogenous and endogenous stimuli. The mechanisms involved include direct stimulation of airway smooth muscle and indirect stimulation by pharmacologically active substances from mediator-secreting cells such as mast cells or nonmyelinated sensory neurons. The degree of airway hyperresponsiveness generally correlates with the clinical severity of asthma.

Airflow obstruction can be caused by a variety of changes, including acute bronchoconstriction, airway edema, chronic mucous plug formation, and airway remodeling. Acute bronchoconstriction is the consequence of IgE-dependent mediator release upon exposure to aeroallergens and is the primary component of the early asthmatic response. Airway edema occurs 6 to 24

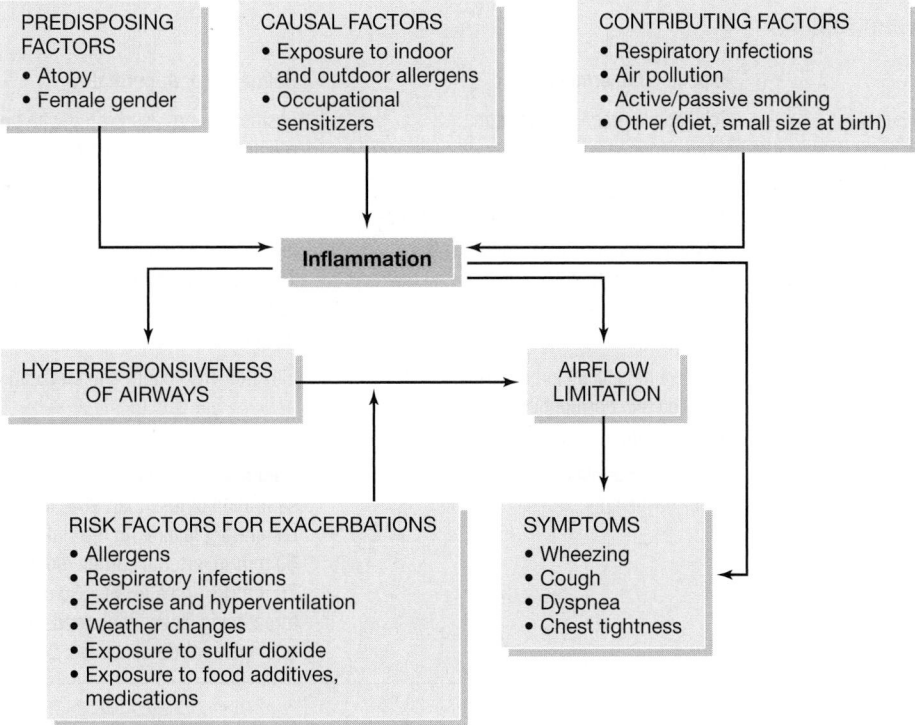

FIGURE 35–11 ■ Pathophysiology of asthma.

hours following an allergen challenge and is referred to as the late asthmatic response. Chronic mucous plug formation consists of an exudate of serum proteins and cell debris that may take weeks to resolve. Airway remodeling is associated with structural changes due to long-standing inflammation and may profoundly affect the extent of reversibility of airway obstruction.

The pathogenesis of exercise-induced asthma (EIA) is controversial. The disease may be mediated by water loss from the airway, heat loss from the airway, or a combination of both. The upper airway is designed to keep inspired air at 100% humidity and body temperature at 37°C (98.6°F). The nose is unable to condition the increased amount of air required for exercise, particularly in athletes who breathe through their mouths. The abnormal heat and water fluxes in the bronchial tree result in bronchoconstriction, occurring within minutes of completing exercise. Results from bronchoalveolar lavage studies have not demonstrated an increase in inflammatory mediators. These patients generally develop a refractory period, during which a second exercise challenge does not cause a significant degree of bronchoconstriction (Morris, 2007; Porth, 2007).

Clinical Manifestations

Persons with asthma exhibit a wide range of signs and symptoms, from episodic wheezing and feelings of chest tightness to acute immobilizing attacks. Attacks vary from person to person, with many people being symptom free between attacks. The physical signs of bronchial asthma vary with the severity of the attacks. A mild attack may produce a felling of chest tightness, a slight increase in respiratory rate with prolonged expiration, and mild wheezing. A cough also may be present.

As attacks become more severe, the individual may exhibit signs of using accessory muscles for breathing, distant breath sounds caused by air trapping, and loud wheezing. Fatigue develops as the attack progresses, with the skin becoming moist and anxiety and apprehension becoming obvious. Dyspnea may be severe, and often the person is able to speak only one or two words at a time before taking a breath. At the point at which airflow is markedly decreased, breath sounds become inaudible with diminished wheezing, and the cough becomes ineffective despite being repetitive and hacking (NHLBI, 1997/2002; Porth 2007). Symptom patterns may vary according to:

- Perennial versus seasonal
- Continual versus episodic
- Duration, severity, and frequency
- Diurnal variations, for example, nocturnal and early-morning awakenings (Morris, 2007).

Despite variations in symptom patterns, clinical manifestations typically include cough, wheezing, shortness of breath, chest tightness, sputum production, and decreased exercise tolerance.

Laboratory and Diagnostic Procedures

The patient undergoes a detailed history to determine causes of airflow limitation in the environment as well as foods and stressful conditions. See Diagnostic Tests for Asthma (p. 966).

Medical Management

The goals for successful management of asthma as outlined in the NHLBI's 2002 Second Expert Panel report (NHLBI, 1997/2002) include the following:

- Achieve and maintain control of symptoms.
- Prevent asthma exacerbations.

DIAGNOSTIC TESTS for Asthma

Test	Expected Abnormality	Rationale for Abnormality
Sputum Gram stain and culture	Eosinophils present in sputum.	Eosinophils are associated with antigen–antibody reactions that occur commonly in allergic reactions and asthma.
FEV_1 (volume of air that the patient can forcibly exhale in 1 second) to FVC (forced vital capacity)	With obstruction, the patient has difficulty exhaling from the lungs, reducing the FEV_1/FVC ratio to 70% or less.	The FEV_1/FVC ratio is usually markedly decreased during an attack and improves with bronchodilator therapy. These spirometric results are expressed as an absolute volume and percent based on normal values for age, height, and weight.
CBC	WBC count is likely to be elevated with infection and eosinophils elevated with allergic response.	Elevated WBC count and elevated eosinophils.
ABG study	Shows hypoxemia or hypercarbia, acid–base abnormalities.	Arterial oxygen of less than 60 mmHg or an oxygen saturation of less than 90% on room air indicates respiratory failure. An arterial oxygen of less than 50 mmHg, arterial carbon dioxide of greater than 70 mmHg, and a pH of 7.30 or less indicates life-threatening illness that needs intensive care management (Chojinowski, 2003).

- Maintain pulmonary function as close to normal levels as possible.
- Maintain normal activity levels, including exercise.
- Avoid adverse effects from asthma medications.
- Prevent the development of irreversible airflow limitations.
- Prevent asthma mortality.

The long-term outpatient management of asthma is based on the Global Initiative for Asthma guidelines (2007). According to these guidelines, medical management should incorporate four treatment components: (1) objective measures of lung function, (2) environmental control measures and avoidance of risk factors, (3) compressive pharmacologic therapy, and (4) patient education. Two additional strategies include management of exacerbations and regular follow-up care (Morris, 2007). The severity of asthma should be classified based on symptom prevalence and measurement of lung function before therapy is initiated. Classification of severity and treatment options are listed here:

Step 1.   Intermittent
- Intermittent symptoms occurring less than once a week
- Brief exacerbations
- Nocturnal symptoms occurring less than twice a month
- Asymptomatic with normal lung function between exacerbations
- No daily medication needed
- FEV_1 or Peak Expiratory Flow (PEF rate of greater than 80%, with less than 20% variability).

Step 2.   Mild Persistent
- Symptoms occurring more than once a week, but less than once a day
- Exacerbations affect activity and sleep
- Nocturnal symptoms occurring more than twice a month

- Inhaled steroid (low dose), cromolyn (adult: 2 to 4 puffs tid/qid; child: 1 to 2 puffs tid/qid), or nedocromil (adult: 2 to 4 puffs bid/qid; child: 1 to 2 puffs bid/qid) (Children usually begin with a trial of cromolyn or nedocromil.)
- FEV_1 or PEF rate of greater than 80% predicted, with variability of 20% to 30%.

Step 3.   Moderate Persistent
- Daily symptoms
- Exacerbations affect activity and sleep
- Nocturnal symptoms occurring more than once a week
- Anti-inflammatory, inhaled steroid (medium dose), or inhaled steroid (low-to-medium dose) and long-acting bronchodilator, especially for nighttime symptoms (either long-acting inhaled beta-2 agonist [adult: 2 puffs q12h, child: 1 to 2 puffs q12h], sustained-release theophylline, or long-acting beta-2 agonist tablets; if needed, give inhaled steroids in a medium-to-high dose)
- FEV_1 or PEF rate of 60% to 80% of predicted, with variability greater than 30%.

Step 4.   Severe Persistent
- Continuous symptoms
- Frequent exacerbations
- Frequent nocturnal asthma symptoms
- Physical activities limited by asthma symptoms
- Anti-inflammatory or inhaled steroid (high dose) and long-acting bronchodilator (either long-acting inhaled beta-2 agonist [adult: 2 puffs q12h, child: 1 to 2 puffs q12h] and sustained-release theophylline or long-acting beta-2 agonist tablets and steroid tablets or syrup long term; make repeated attempts to reduce systemic steroid and maintain control with high-dose inhaled steroid)
- FEV_1 or PEF rate of less than 60%, with variability greater than 30% (Morris, 2007).

Medications usually are divided into two categories, quick relief and long-term control. Quick relief medications are used to relieve acute asthma exacerbations and to prevent EIA symptoms. These medications include short-acting beta agonists, anticholinergics (used for severe exacerbations), and systemic corticosteroids, which speed recovery from acute exacerbations. Long-term control inhaled medications include inhaled corticosteroids, cromolyn sodium, nedocromil, long-acting beta agonists, methylxanthines, and leukotriene antagonists. Use of these medications by the stepwise approach is outlined above in the four steps. Also, drug categories used in the treatment of asthma are described in the Pharmacology Summary table (p. 981).

Medical management also includes consultations, diet control, and activity control. It frequently is necessary to consult with a pulmonologist or allergist to ensure proper stepwise management of asthma, or referral for further evaluation to help rule out other diagnoses. Patients also may be referred to an otolaryngologist for treatment of nasal obstruction from polyps, sinusitis, or allergic rhinitis, or for the diagnosis of upper airway disorders.

The patient's diet also must be considered, because recent studies have suggested that there is an association between asthma and obesity. Patients with an elevated body mass index (BMI) have an increased risk for developing asthma (Morris, 2007). Activity generally is limited by patients' ability to exercise and their response to medications. No specific limitations are recommended for patients with asthma; however, they should avoid exposure to agents that may exacerbate their disease. A significant number of patients with asthma also have EIA, and baseline control of their disease should be adequate to prevent exertional symptoms. The ability of patients with EIA to exercise is based on their level of exertion, degree of fitness, and environment in which they exercise. Many patients have fewer problems when exercising indoors or in a warm, humid environment compared with outdoors or in a cold, dry environment (Morris, 2007).

Nursing Management

Nursing management of patients with asthma relies on a holistic approach to care through the nursing process. Immediate nursing care of patients with asthma depends on the severity of the symptoms and whether they are being treated as outpatients or inpatients. A major emphasis of all nursing care is patient and family education about the prevention of asthma attacks. Throughout the course of the illness, nurses also provide emotional support to the patient and family, who may be frightened and anxious because of the patient's dyspnea.

Assessment

Nursing responsibilities include a thorough assessment of symptoms and history of attacks, coordinating the plan of care as set forth by the health care provider. The nurse assesses the patient's respiratory status by monitoring the severity of symptoms, breath sounds, peak flow, pulse oximetry, and vital signs.

Interventions and Rationales

Administration of medications as ordered is inherent in the nursing role, having first obtained a history of any allergic responses to medications. Patient education is paramount in assisting the patient with taking medications. For example, regular use of anti-inflammatory medications via an MDI controls the symptoms of asthma (see Figures 35–1 and 35–2 ■, p. 940).

Corticosteroids are effective in improving symptoms and normalizing the FEV_1. The patient should use a spacer with this medication and rinse the mouth afterwards to prevent thrush. A spacer is a device that is attached to the inhaler, allowing medication to accumulate as the patient inhales and preventing medication from escaping outside of the patient's mouth. These are particularly helpful for elderly patients or patients with poor dexterity.

Other specific nursing responsibilities include fluid administration if the patient is dehydrated and performance of critical care procedures, such as assisting with intubation, if the patient is hospitalized.

As part of the educational approach to care, the patient should be encouraged to keep a diary regarding responses to triggers, in order to avoid known triggers as much as possible. The nurse teaches the patient to monitor peak flow measurements with a diary (Plaut, 2001).

See the Nursing Process: Patient Care Plan for Asthma feature (p. 968) for details on the nursing process for caring for asthma patients. The importance of patient education cannot be overemphasized. Patients do better the more they know about asthma—what triggers an attack, what drug to use when, proper inhaler technique, how to use a spacer with an MDI, and the importance of early use of corticosteroids in exacerbations. Every patient should have a written action plan for day-to-day management, especially for management of acute attacks that is based on the patient's best personal peak flow rather than on predicted normal value. Such a plan leads to much better asthma control, largely attributable to improved adherence to therapies.

Discharge Priorities

The nurse ensures that the patient is comfortable with the plan of care and is able to follow written instructions for medications and follow-up visits. When possible, the patients are taught to do their own peak flow measurements and can discuss plans for possible emergencies at home or work.

Health Promotion

Educating the public regarding the symptoms and dangers of asthma contributes to community well-being. This includes the role of environmental pollutants, smoking, allergens, chemicals, and inhalants. When the patient is diagnosed the nurse assists in preventing exacerbations by helping the patient and family to develop a health maintenance routine that includes regular checkups, regular assessment of peak flow rates and use of a peak flow meter (Figure 35–12 ■, p. 969), and awareness of individual triggers that cause bronchospasm or exacerbations.

Collaborative Management

In the care of the asthmatic patient, the nurse collaborates with the health care provider and the respiratory therapist, and patient and family education is essential. If there are financial issues related to maintenance care and equipment, the social worker becomes involved. Referral to the home care nurse is instituted if the patient is not able to manage outpatient clinic or office visits.

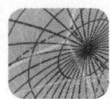

NURSING PROCESS: Patient Care Plan for Asthma

Assessment for Asthma

Subjective Data:

Do you have shortness of breath?

Do you have chest tightness?

Are you able to speak without effort?

Do you have a cough?

Do you produce sputum?

Could you describe the sputum?

At what times of day are your symptoms most evident?

Are there particular exposures that start the symptoms such as smoke, dust, or pollen?

Are there particular times of the year when you have symptoms?

Do any particular activities make you ill?

How long is it between attacks or is it continuous?

Do any family members have asthma?

Objective Data:

Lung sounds

ABGs

FVC and FEV_1

PERF

Vital signs

Chest x-ray

Work of breathing

Oxygen saturation

Observation of physical status during exercise

Oxygen saturation pre- and postactivity

Lung sounds pre- and postactivity

Vital signs pre- and postactivity

Nursing Assessment and Diagnoses	Outcomes and Evaluation Parameters	Planning and Interventions with *Rationales*
Nursing Diagnosis: *Impaired Gas Exchange* related to bronchoconstriction	**Outcome:** Patient will experience relief of chest tightness and dyspnea and will be able to exercise preventive strategies that alleviate frequency of symptoms. **Evaluation Parameters:** Patient will describe breathing as comfortable. Lung sounds will be clear upon auscultation. Pulse oximetry readings will show normal oxygen saturation. Patient or family member will describe the use of the PERF meter at home. Patient or family member will describe the purpose and administration of bronchodilators and anti-inflammatory drugs. Patient or family member will describe environmental or situational triggers she needs to avoid. Patient or family member will describe activities that will decrease stress, anxiety, and onset of symptoms. Patient or family member will describe symptoms that require immediate emergency care.	**Interventions and *Rationales:*** In the acute phase, monitor vital signs, lung sounds, oxygen saturation, and blood gases, noting improvement in air exchange. Later, the nurse plays a major role in prevention by doing patient and family education. After testing to determine triggers, encourage the patient to keep a diary regarding responses to triggers. *He should avoid known triggers as much as possible to prevent episodes of bronchospasm.* If symptoms persist for more than 2 days per week, revise the treatment plan. Teach the patient to monitor peak flow measurements with a diary PERF (Plaut, 2001). *Analysis of peak flow allows for evaluation of bronchoconstriction; a lowered peak flow indicates bronchoconstriction.* Regular use of anti-inflammatory medications via an MDI controls the symptoms of asthma. *Corticosteroids are effective in improving symptoms and normalizing the FEV_1.* The patient should use a spacer with this medication and rinse the mouth afterwards to prevent thrush. *A spacer is a device that is attached to the inhaler, allowing medication to accumulate as the patient inhales and preventing medication from escaping outside of the patient's mouth. These are particularly helpful for elderly patients or patients with poor dexterity. Corticosteroids can also be given orally to treat exacerbations. Cromolyn sodium is an anti-inflammatory agent used commonly in children but may be prescribed for adults. Long-acting beta-adrenergic agonists are used with anti-inflammatory agents to control symptoms* (Fishman et al., 2002; Wilson, Shannon, & Stang, 2006).

Cystic Fibrosis

Cystic fibrosis (CF) is the most common fatal recessive genetic disease among Caucasians (Sharma, 2006b). It affects mainly the exocrine (mucous) glands of the lungs, liver, pancreas, and intestines, causing progressive disability due to multiple-system failure. It is the most common fatal recessive genetic disease among Caucasians (Rowe, Miller, & Sorscher, 2005).

Epidemiology and Etiology

A person is born with CF, and it affects boys more than girls. It affects Caucasians five times more often than it does African Amer-

icans, and it is rare in Asian American children. Predictably, this disease affects 1 in 3,300 live births among Caucasians in the United States. In African Americans it affects 1 in 15,300. The frequency of unaffected carriers of Northern European ancestry is 1 in 25 (Fishman et al., 2002; Murray & Brown, 2007).

CF is caused by a mutation in a single gene, the cystic fibrosis transmembrane conductive regulator (CFTR). This gene controls the production of a protein that regulates how salt is carried across the membranes that separate cells. The gene disturbance leads to production of unusually thick mucus that blocks bodily passages, particularly in the digestive and respiratory systems. The disorder affects all exocrine glands. The pancreatic channel

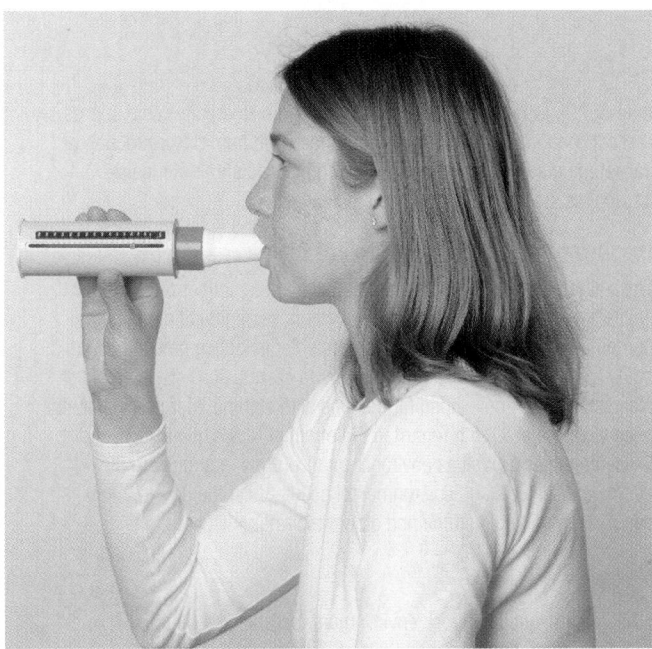

FIGURE 35–12 ■ Use of a peak flow meter.
Source: © Dorling Kindersley

will be affected by sticky fluid, which may result in fibrosis and destruction of the gland. Pancreatic insufficiency may lead to malabsorption and diabetes. People with one copy of the defective gene carry it, but have no symptoms, which is the case for more than 10 million Americans. However, those who receive a copy of the defective gene from both parents will develop cystic fibrosis. The Risk Factors for Cystic Fibrosis box lists common risk factors.

Pathophysiology

The typical features of CF lung disease are mucous plugging, chronic inflammation, and infection. These lead to microabscess formation, bronchiectasis, patchy consolidation and pneumonia, peribronchial fibrosis, and cyst formation. These progressive changes cause gradual destruction of functional lung tissue. Peripheral bullae or blebs may develop because of obstruction and airway wall weakening. This occurs more frequently in older patients and often leads to the occurrence of

---

RISK FACTORS for Cystic Fibrosis

- About 30,000 people in the United States have cystic fibrosis (CF).
- About 1 in every 3,000 babies born in the United States has CF.
- It affects both males and females.
- It affects people from all racial and ethnic groups but is most common among Caucasians whose ancestors came from northern Europe. CF is one of the most common inherited diseases among Caucasians.
- CF also is common in Latinos and Native Americans, especially the Pueblo and Zuni.
- CF is much less common among African Americans and Asian Americans.
- About 12 million Americans are carriers of an abnormal CF gene. Many of them do not know that they are CF carriers.

---

pneumothorax. **Hemoptysis** (bloody sputum) may occur because of enlarged bronchial arteries that develop in response to the inflammation associated with bronchiectasis. Over a long period of time, localized hypoxia and arteriolar vasoconstriction cause pulmonary hypertension. This often leads to the development of cor pulmonale (McCance & Huether, 2007). Local factors in the CF airway environment favor bacterial colonization. *Staphylococcus aureus* is common and *Pseudomonas aeruginosa* ultimately colonizes in 75% of persons with CF. *Pseudomonas* acquisition has been linked with more rapid decline (McCance & Huether, 2007).

Clinical Manifestations

The most common symptoms are respiratory and gastrointestinal. Respiratory symptoms include persistent cough or wheeze and recurrent and severe pneumonia (McCance & Huether, 2007). In CF patients *S. aureus* and *P. aeruginosa* are rarely eradicated even with prolonged use of antibiotics. They often occur together in sputum samples (Fishman et al., 2002). An acute exacerbation is characterized by increasing breathlessness; change in sputum volume, color, and viscosity; tiredness; loss of appetite; and weight loss (Esmond, 2000). Physical signs developing over time include barrel chest (see Figure 35–8 ■, p. 960) and digital clubbing (McCance & Huether, 2007). Gastrointestinal manifestations in young adults include malabsorptive symptoms such as frequent loose and oily stools and abdominal cramping. About 10% of CF patients have no gastrointestinal symptoms or pancreatic abnormalities.

Endocrine function of the pancreas is usually preserved in children, but approximately 50% of adults are overtly diabetic by the age of 30. They experience signs and symptoms of diabetes including abnormal glucose tolerance, polydipsia, polyuria, and polyphagia (Fishman et al., 2002; Porth, 2007). Subtle manifestations of CF include chronic sinusitis, nasal polyps, and rectal prolapse (McCance & Huether, 2007). Infertility is common in males due to maldevelopment of the vas deferens. Women are fertile but frequently face a higher risk of complications with pregnancy. The trajectory of the disease varies among individuals, but death is usually caused by respiratory failure secondary to progressive lung involvement (Sharma, 2006b). Chart 35–6 (p. 971) lists additional clinical manifestations of CF.

Laboratory and Diagnostic Procedures

The standard method of diagnosis for CF is the sweat test, which will reveal a sodium chloride concentration in excess of 60 mEq/L. Other diagnostic studies include chest x-ray, pulmonary function studies, fecal analysis of fat, pancreatic enzyme studies, liver function studies, and semen analysis to determine infertility in males (see Diagnostic Tests for Cystic Fibrosis, p. 971). Genetic analysis can be used to confirm the diagnosis of CF (Fishman et al., 2002).

Medical Management

Early diagnosis and treatment are important in delaying the onset and severity of chronic illness in children with CF. CF has a remarkably variable clinical course, depending on the severity of the genetic mutation, the types of infections acquired, and the organs other than the lung that are affected. For all patients with CF, the median survival has risen steadily during the past four decades and is now approaching the age of 35.1 (Porth, 2007).

Environmental Causes of Asthma

Clinical Problem

It is known that people spend 90% of their time indoors in an increasingly technological environment. There has also been a major increase in respiratory illness in the past 40 years. The indoor environment, particularly the home, has been recognized as a major source of exposure to allergens and toxic chemicals that are associated with the development and exacerbation of asthma and other respiratory diseases (Richardson, Eick, & Jones, 2005). Therefore, Richardson and colleagues (2005) reviewed the literature to identify the factors in the environment that have an evidenced-based link to the development or exacerbation of asthma and to outline measures that health care professionals can use to reduce exposure to risk factors in the home.

Research Findings

The researchers concluded their meta-analysis by stating that there is currently evidence of a link between a small number of indoor environmental factors and the development and or exacerbation of asthma. They also concluded that there are measures to alleviate asthma that could be promoted by health care professionals, but the clinical evidence of symptom alleviation, with the exception of measures to isolate dust mites for atopic asthma in children, does not exist.

Variables associated with strong evidence for a causal relationship with exacerbation and development of asthma included house dust mites and environmental tobacco smoke. Cat allergen and cockroach antigen were associated with strong evidence of a causal relationship with exacerbation only and there is limited evidence regarding an association with exacerbation related to dog allergen. Regarding molds, there is sufficient evidence of an association with exacerbation but more data are needed in this area. Regarding nitrogen dioxide, carbon monoxide, general allergens, and formaldehyde, there is strong evidence of an association and strong evidence of low risk. Regarding pesticides, polycyclic aromatic hydrocarbons, endotoxins, and volatile organic compounds, there is insufficient evidence of an association.

Researchers found that most of the environmental controls that have been recommended lack clinical evidence of success via reduced risk of sensitization. The one exception is the use of mattress encasements with impermeable material such as polyurethane. This was shown to be effective with children, but ineffective with adults.

Other environmental controls include elimination of tobacco smoke, elimination of pets, particularly cats, use of feather-filled versus foam pillows, washing bedding regularly in hot water greater than 55°C, use of a filtered ventilation system to reduce mold spores, use of a dehumidifier to reduce dampness and humidity, reduction of carpeted spaces, and restructuring of homes to eliminate leaks, dampness, and cold.

Implications for Nursing Practice

The results of this study indicate that there are a number of environmental controls individuals with asthma might initiate in their homes. Health professionals might review the evidence presented in this study as the basis for recommendations to clients. Consistent teaching standards can be developed for persons with asthma. More clinical trials need to be initiated with regard to the effect of molds, pesticides, and toxic chemicals as well as environmental controls that mitigate the effects of allergens and environmental pollutants in the development and exacerbation of asthma and other respiratory diseases.

Critical Thinking Questions

1. A good-quality indoor environment is important because
   a. most people spend 90% of time indoors.
   b. most people spend 50% of time indoors.
   c. molds are positively associated with asthma development.
   d. pesticides are positively associated with asthma exacerbations.

2. An implication of this study related to the development of asthma is
   a. tobacco smoke must be eliminated from the indoor environment.
   b. most houses need a total rehabilitation in order to be safe for persons with asthma.
   c. all rugs should be removed in order to prevent dust mites.
   d. pesticide use should be avoided.

3. There is currently not enough evidence to prove that
   a. reducing the exposure to indoor allergens and pollutants will reduce exacerbation of respiratory illness.
   b. reducing exposure to dust mites in children reduces symptoms.
   c. certain allergens are triggers for asthma and respiratory illness.
   d. molds are associated with dampness and humidity.

Answers to Critical Thinking Questions appear in Appendix D.

Source: From "How Is the Indoor Environment Related to Asthma?: Literature Review" by G. Richardson, S. Eick, and R. Jones, 2005, *Journal of Advanced Nursing, 52*(3), 328–339.

Diagnosis typically is based on the presence of respiratory and gastrointestinal manifestations typical of CF, a history of CF in a sibling, or a positive newborn screening test. Confirming laboratory tests are performed, the most common being the sweat test, as mentioned earlier (Murray & Brown, 2007).

At present, there are no approved treatments for correcting the genetic defects in CF or reversing the ion transport abnormalities associated with the dysfunctional CFTR. Thus, treatment measures are directed toward slowing the progression of secondary organ dysfunction and sequelae such as chronic lung infection and pancreatic insufficiency. Aggressive medical treatment is initiated prior to consideration of surgical interventions.

Medical treatments include the use of antibiotics to prevent and manage infections, the use of chest physical therapy (chest percussion and postural drainage) and mucolytic agents to prevent airway obstruction; and pancreatic enzyme replacement and nutritional therapy (Murray & Brown, 2007; Porth, 2007).

It is vital for patients to employ strategies to clear pulmonary secretions to prevent complications arising from airway plugging by viscous secretions. Chest physical therapy includes percussion and postural drainage performed regularly. Patients with CF should maintain a twice-daily routine of chest physical therapy. During periods of exacerbation, the regimen should be performed more frequently.

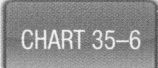

CHART 35–6 Clinical Manifestations of Cystic Fibrosis

PULMONARY SIGNS AND SYMPTOMS IN YOUNG ADULTS

- Persistent cough or wheeze
- *Pseudomonas aeruginosa* and/or *Staphylococcus aureus* in the sputum
- Hyperinflated lungs on chest x-ray
- Barrel chest and digital clubbing
- Chronic sinusitis
- Nasal polyps
- Recurrent episodes of pneumonia
- Chronic bronchitis

GASTROINTESTINAL MANIFESTATIONS

- Frequent loose and oily stools
- Pancreatic abnormalities
- Cramps and abdominal pain
- Rectal prolapse
- Malnutrition and weight loss

ENDOCRINE MANIFESTATIONS

- Glucose intolerance
- Polydipsia, polyuria, polyphasia

REPRODUCTIVE

- Infertility in males
- High risk of complications with pregnancy
- Delayed sexual development

Medical treatments are started whenever patients experience a subjective increase in nasal obstruction, cough, or drainage (Murray & Brown, 2007):

- **Antibiotic choices**—The bacteriology of sinonasal disease in patients with CF differs from that in patients without CF. This difference affects antibiotic choices. The most notable difference is the nearly consistent presence of *Pseudomonas* species in patients with CF.
- **Nasal toilet**—Because mucociliary clearance is chronically impaired, irrigations are critical and should be a daily routine as patients begin to develop condensed symptoms. Nasal saline irrigations serve to decrease bacterial colonization, wash away condensed secretions that lead to obstruction, and temporarily aid in ameliorating vasoconstriction. Irrigation is also required after any surgical intervention because surgery enlarges sinus ostia but does not address underlying defects in mucociliary clearance.
- **Irrigations**—Irrigations with antipseudomonal antibiotics such as tobramycin may be recommended.

The medication regime is a mainstay of treatment. Antibiotics can be used both prophylactically and for treatment of acute exacerbations. Other medications include bronchodilators and pancreatic enzymes. A detailed list can be found in the Pharmacology Summary (p. 981). Pancreatic enzymes are prescribed for patients with pancreatic insufficiency. These must be taken prior to meals and snacks. Fat-soluble vitamins (A, D, E, and K) must be supplemented. The Pharmacology Summary (p. 981) includes all the medications for CF.

Surgical care may be initiated if medical therapy is ineffective. However, surgical interventions for patients with CF must be carefully considered, because CF patients often are at risk for developing severe mucous plugging during general anesthesia,

DIAGNOSTIC TESTS for Cystic Fibrosis

Test	Expected Abnormality	Rationale for Abnormality
Sweat test	Sodium chloride concentration in excess of 60 mEq/L.	Mucous plugging of the sweat duct causes malabsorption of sodium chloride. This is a diagnostic indicator of CF.
Chest x-ray	Shows densities or whiteout in areas of consolidation.	This is a diagnostic indicator of CF.
Fecal fat	Fecal fat concentration is elevated.	Pancreatic enzymes such as amylase, lipase, and trypsinogen do not reach the intestine to digest ingested nutrients. There is malabsorption of fat, protein, and fat-soluble vitamins. This results in steatorrhea (fatty stool).
Pancreatic enzymes	Decreased.	Mucous plugging of the pancreatic duct results in fibrosis of the acinar glands of the pancreas. The exocrine function of the pancreas is altered and may be lost completely.
Pulmonary function studies	Show abnormal findings.	Tidal volume, vital capacity, and other functions are below normal related to the disease process.
Serum glucose	Elevated.	Diabetes mellitus may occur because the islets of Langerhans become fibrotic. CF-related diabetes affects 15% of patients with CF.
Semen analysis	Sperm count abnormally low.	Confirms infertility in males. CF causes maldevelopment of the vas deferens.
Genetic analysis	Positive for CF.	Confirms diagnosis.
Liver enzymes	Elevated.	Mucous plugging causes biliary cirrhosis late in the disease.

and this risk increases with duration of intubation. Indications for surgical intervention include the following:

- Persistent nasal obstruction associated with nasal polyposis and/or medial bowing of the lateral nasal wall following intensive medical management
- Medialization of the lateral nasal wall, as demonstrated by endoscopy or CT scanning
- Pulmonary exacerbations that appear to correlate with sinonasal disease exacerbations, worsening of pulmonary status, or diminished activity level, despite appropriate medical management
- Facial pain or headaches that have no other apparent cause and that adversely affect quality of life
- Desire for improvement in symptom profile beyond what medical management has achieved in a patient with significant nasal cavity and paranasal sinus symptoms (Murray & Brown, 2007).

According to Porth (2007), "up to 90% of patients with CF have complete loss of exocrine pancreas function and inadequate digestion of fats and proteins. They require diet adjustment, pancreatic enzyme replacement, and supplemental vitamins and minerals. Pancreatic enzyme dosage and product are individualized for each patient" (p. 508).

Nursing Management

Nursing management for the CF patient focuses on assisting the patient to maintain adequate airway clearance, reduce risk factors associated with infections, perform ADLs, prevent complications, and involve the patient and family in planning and implementing the therapeutic regimen.

Assessment

Objective and subjective data should be obtained from the patient and family. Subjective data includes obtaining a past health history of recurrent respiratory and sinus infection and persistent cough with excessive sputum production; use of and compliance with corticosteroids, bronchodilators, and antibiotics; functional health patterns, such as family history, diagnosis of cystic fibrosis in childhood; nutritional and metabolic needs and symptoms; elimination; activity patterns; cognitive perceptions of pain; and reproductive symptoms, such as menstrual irregularities.

Objective data includes assessment of general impression, such as mood, anxiety, depression, restlessness, failure to thrive; cyanosis of skin and nail beds; persistent runny nose, diminished breath sounds, sputum characteristics; tachycardia; protuberant abdomen, abdominal distention, foul and fatty stools; the possibility of abnormal ABGs and pulmonary function tests; and an abnormal sweat chloride test, chest x-ray, and fecal fat analysis. Determination of medications being used also is part of the assessment process.

Nursing Diagnoses

Nursing diagnoses may include:

- *Ineffective Airway Clearance* related to thick and abundant mucus, weakness, and fatigue

- *Ineffective Breathing Pattern* related to bronchoconstriction, anxiety, and airway obstruction
- *Impaired Gas Exchange* related to lung infections
- *Imbalanced Nutrition* related to dietary intolerances, intestinal gas, and altered pancreatic enzyme production.

Planning

Planning goals are focused on the patient having adequate airway clearance, reduced risk factors associated with respiratory infections and the ability to perform ADLs, freedom from complications from CF, and active participation in planning and implementing a restorative regime.

Outcomes and Evaluation Parameters

Outcomes and evaluation parameters include the following:

- The patient and family will show evidence of understanding the disease process, methods of maintaining a clear airway, and the ADL performance regime.
- The patient and family will demonstrate an understanding of a nutritional plan and a plan of continuous evaluation of the condition.

Interventions and Rationales

The goal of nursing implementations is to assist patients in gaining and maintaining independence by assuming responsibility for their own care. Active interventions include relief of bronchoconstriction, airway obstruction, and airflow limitation. The nurse is responsible for administering medications as ordered by the health care provider providing oxygen therapy, and instructing the patient and family on nutrition and exercise. Home care instruction consists of postural drainage techniques, aerosol-nebulation therapy, and breathing retraining. The patient also should be taught controlled coughing techniques, deep breathing exercises, and progressive exercise conditioning.

Psychosocial support regarding the financial and emotional burden of the disease should be provided to the patient and family.

Discharge Priorities

Fatigue and weakness related to an exacerbation of cystic fibrosis may render a young adult who was formerly an active and independent participant in care incapable of performing the treatment regime independently. Upon discharge he may need assistance with the treatment regime. Therefore, the family should be included in all patient education and discharge planning. This includes instruction regarding the chest physical therapy regime, oral or IV medications, and aerosols and breathing treatments.

Health Promotion

Because the adult with CF is extremely vulnerable to infection, the nurse should emphasize to the patient and family that the environment be kept as free from infection as possible. The patient is encouraged to wash her hands frequently, especially after coughing. Frequent mouth care is encouraged, especially after the chest physical therapy regime. Patients should avoid exposure to persons who are ill especially with upper respiratory infections. Patients with CF should be screened for

Mycobacterium tuberculosis infection with yearly PPD skin tests and treated prophylactically with the same regimen used for non-CF patients (Fishman et al., 2002).

Collaborative Management

Comprehensive multidisciplinary CF treatment programs have led to a dramatic increase in the median age of survival for those affected patients (Fishman et al., 2002). Care is managed by a multidisciplinary team including the health care provider, nurse, respiratory therapist, physical therapist, and nutritionist. The patient and family members work closely with the team to develop a regimen that is successful. Involvement of the patient is critical. Treatment depends on the severity of both the exacerbation and the underlying lung disease. The aim of treatment is to maintain lung function, which can be achieved by a regular regimen of chest physical therapy, early and effective antibiotic treatment of acute exacerbations, optimal bronchodilation, and attention to optimal nutrition (Esmond, 2000).

The dietitian can manage the caloric needs, which are high especially with advancing disease. High-calorie feedings or even gastrostomy feedings may be required (McCance & Huether, 2007). See Chapter 14 🌐 for details on nutritional management.

Lung transplant has emerged as an option for patients with end-stage CF. The outcome for those with CF who undergo lung transplantation is among the best reported with an average survival rate of 4 years in 50% of cases. Nutritional issues complicate post-transplantation management because 50% of those over age 30 are overtly diabetic, and the treatment with corticosteroids induces diabetes in another 10%. Patients are not considered for transplant unless their weight is greater than 75% of ideal (Fishman et al., 2002). Lung transplant is discussed later in the chapter.

Psychosocial Support

Careful attention should be paid to the social, emotional, and financial needs of the patient with CF and his or her family. Education regarding management of the disease should be ongoing and counseling resources should be available to the patient and family. Active participation in the therapeutic regimen is essential for the well-being of persons with CF. Other issues for young adults include building self-esteem, self-confidence, and meaningful friendships and relationships. The decision to have children should be considered carefully. The nurse might suggest genetic counseling because many men with CF are sterile and women may have difficulty with pregnancy (WHO, 1996). Any children produced will be carriers or have the disease. Britto et al. (2004) found in a study of adolescents with CF that the interpersonal aspects of nursing care were rated as very important and highly valued.

Pulmonary Embolism

Pulmonary embolism (PE) results when a thrombus breaks loose from an attachment and blocks a branch of the pulmonary artery. This produces widespread pulmonary vasoconstriction, which impairs ventilation and perfusion and, thus, produces life-threatening hypoxemia and the potential for ischemia and pulmonary infarction.

Epidemiology

In the United States, there are approximately 650,000 cases annually of PE, and as many as 50,000 patients die each year as a result of PE (Kavita, 2005; Wrong Diagnosis, 2008). PE is predominantly a disease of older individuals, and the highest incidence of recognized PE occurs in hospitalized patients. The incidence of venous thromboembolic events in the elderly is more common among men than women. In patients younger than 55 years, the incidence of PE is higher in females. Patients who survive an acute PE are at high risk for recurrent PE and the development of pulmonary hypertension or chronic cor pulmonale. Subtle population differences may exist in the incidence of deep venous thrombosis (DVT) and PE but the incidence is high in all racial groups. Although, the frequency of PE increases with age, age is not an independent risk factor (Feied & Handler, 2002).

Etiology

Pulmonary embolism is a complication of a DVT, which is a common occurrence after surgery or trauma, childbirth, stroke, heart failure, myocardial infarction, atrial fibrillation, cancer, and prolonged immobilization. Most emboli arise from thrombi in proximal deep veins. They also can originate from the pelvis, particularly with pregnant women and with pelvic fractures. Symptomatic pulmonary embolism occurs in 30% of cases of untreated DVT (McCance & Huether, 2007).

The most common risk factors for PE are a prior history of DVT or PE, recent surgery or pregnancy, prolonged immobilization, or underlying malignancy. Risks for PE include situations in which there is venous stasis or in which there is increased hypercoagulability or a clotting tendency of the blood. Aside from prolonged bed rest, inactivity may include long trips in planes, cars, and trains. Other causes are oral contraceptive use, surgery especially involving the pelvic area, massive trauma, burns, cancer, stroke, myocardial infarction, and fractures of the hips or femur (Fishman et al., 2002). Having an indwelling central venous catheter also increases risk (Morris, Morrison, & Yetsko, 2002). Genetic risk factors include mutations in Factor V, antithrombin III deficiency, protein C or protein S deficiency, and fibrinolysis defects (Kavita, 2005).

Pathophysiology

A pulmonary occlusion occurs when a bloodborne substance occludes a branch of the pulmonary artery and obstructs blood flow to the area that the artery feeds. The embolism can be a thrombus, air accidentally injected through an IV catheter, fat from bone marrow after a fracture, or amniotic fluid that has entered the mother's bloodstream after rupture of the membranes at birth (Porth, 2007). Pulmonary emboli can occur in a variety of ways: (1) a massive occlusion of the pulmonary circulation, (2) an embolus that is large enough to cause infarction of a portion of lung tissue, (3) an embolus without infarction, and (4) multiple pulmonary emboli that may be chronic or recurrent.

Depending on the pattern of occurrence and severity, the pulmonary embolism causes varying degrees of bronchoconstriction in the affected area of the lung, resulting in impaired gas exchange and loss of alveolar surfactant. Pulmonary edema and right heart failure may develop with massive vasoconstriction. **Atelectasis** (collapse of lung) and release of neurohumoral substances such as histamine, serotonin, and thromboxane also may occur. The embolus also may cause systemic hypotension, decreased cardiac output, and pulmonary hypertension, which when severe, results in acute right ventricular failure and death. If the clot does not cause infarction, it is dissolved by the fibrinolytic system (McCance & Huether, 2007).

Clinical Manifestations

The clinical manifestations of PE depend on its size, location, and the amount of obstruction. The classic triad of symptoms of PE is hemoptysis, dyspnea, and chest pain but they occur in fewer than 20% of patients. Many patients with PE are completely asymptomatic, and most of those who do have symptoms have an atypical presentation. Patients may present with pleuritic chest pain, chest wall tenderness, a pulmonary friction rub, or hypotension related to acute cor pulmonale, or they may have a completely normal physical exam. After 24 hours, loss of pulmonary surfactant causes atelectasis and alveolar infiltrates that are indistinguishable from pneumonia on x-ray. In addition, patients with massive PE may have tachypnea, crackles, an accentuated second heart sound, tachycardia, fever, diaphoresis, S_3 or S_4 gallop, thrombophlebitis, lower extremity edema, cardiac murmur, and cyanosis (Feied & Handler, 2002).

Small emboli may be asymptomatic initially; however, repeated small emboli result in a gradual reduction in the pulmonary bed, ultimately resulting in pulmonary hypertension. Massive PEs typically present with sudden crushing substernal chest pain, shock, and loss of consciousness, and they are usually fatal (Porth, 2007).

Diagnostic Studies

Diagnosis of PE is particularly difficult because many of the diagnostic studies used to evaluate lung function may be normal in the patient with PE. See the Diagnostic Tests for Pulmonary Embolism box for details.

DIAGNOSTIC TESTS for Pulmonary Embolism

Test	Expected Abnormality	Rationale for Abnormality
ABGs	Abnormal in some cases.	Altered gas exchange secondary to PE.
Pulse oximetry	Abnormal in some cases, normal in most cases.	Altered oxygen saturation secondary to PE.
CBC	White blood cell count may be normal or elevated.	Atelectasis and infiltrates occur, causing elevated white count.
ECG	Specific abnormalities with PE are tachycardia, tall, peaked P waves in lead 2, right axis deviation, and right bundle branch block. Most significant finding is tachycardia.	Hypoxemia secondary to PE causes cardiac abnormalities.
Chest x-rays	Usually normal initially. Within 24–72 hours atelectasis or infiltrates may be apparent as well as a small pleural effusion.	Altered perfusion pattern not visible via chest x-ray. In massive embolus dilation of the pulmonary vasculature near the embolus may be seen. Infiltrates and pleural effusions are visible later.
D-Dimer test	Positive.	The D-dimer test is a degradation product of cross-linked fibrin generated by plasmin cleavage. When levels are above 500 mg/L, the test is positive. This indicates activation of the fibrolytic pathway, meaning the body is trying to break down clots. Therefore the D-dimer test will be elevated in any condition such as disseminated intravascular coagulation (DIC), PE, DVT, and myocardial infarction where clots are formed. If the D-dimer is positive and the patient also has tachycardia, crackles, dyspnea, pleuritic chest pain, and cough, a PE diagnosis can be confirmed (Woodruff, 1999).
V/Q scan	Diagnostic of abnormal perfusion pattern, or may be normal.	Perfusion pattern is altered by PE, but even if positive, this is not an acceptable end point in the diagnostic process.
Pulmonary angiogram	Positive.	Provides 100% certainty that an obstruction to pulmonary arterial blood flow does exist. A negative angiogram provides greater than 90% certainty in the exclusion of PE. This is still the most reliable diagnostic test for PE.
Ultrasonography and plethysmography	May detect presence of lower extremity DVT. Echocardiography reflects findings of right-sided heart failure.	Detection of lower extremity DVT helps confirm diagnosis of PE, but often cannot be visualized. Findings of right-sided heart failure consistent with PE (Porth, 2007).
Spiral CT scan	Positive.	This is a relatively new noninvasive diagnostic test that provides additional slices of the area visualized. In many patients a spiral or helical CT with intravenous contrast can visualize pulmonary vessels so well that an angiogram is not necessary.

Medical Management

Oxygen should be administered to any patient who is suspected of having a PE even if the arterial PO_2 is normal. Increased alveolar oxygen may help to promote pulmonary vascular dilation. Insertion of a pulmonary artery catheter is helpful to determine the condition of the heart and its ability to manage the circulating fluid volume. This catheter is inserted by a health care provider through the subclavian vein into the chambers of the heart and into the pulmonary artery. Readings are obtained regarding the patient's cardiac output and pressures within the right and left ventricles and within the pulmonary artery. Some pulmonary catheters can be manipulated to obtain sophisticated determinations such as the right ventricular ejection fraction and continuous cardiac output monitoring (Morton, Fontaine, Hudak, & Gallo, 2005). Pulmonary artery catheters are discussed in detail in Chapter 24 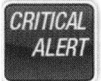. In the case of a cardiac arrest, CPR is not helpful since obstruction of the pulmonary circuit prevents oxygenated blood from reaching the peripheral and cerebral circulation. The only management approaches that are useful in these situations are an emergency cardiopulmonary bypass or emergency thoracotomy. If cardiopulmonary bypass with extracorporeal oxygenation is available, it may be lifesaving for patients with massive PE in whom cardiac arrest has occurred or appears imminent (Feied & Handler, 2002).

Compression stockings that provide a 30 to 40 mmHg compression gradient should be used, because they are a safe and effective adjunctive treatment that can limit or prevent extension of thrombus. Antiembolic or "Ted hose" produce a maximum compression of 18 mmHg, and because of this they have no value in the treatment of DVT or PE (Feied & Handler, 2002).

Fibrinolytic therapy has been the standard of care for patients with massive or unstable PE since the 1970s. Unless overwhelming contradictions are evident, a rapidly acting fibrinolytic agent should be administered immediately to any patient who has suffered any degree of hypotension or is significantly hypoxemic from PE (Feied & Handler, 2002). Fibrinolysis also should be considered in patients with PE who have any evidence of right heart strain and in all patients without contraindications to therapy because research studies have demonstrated that mortality rate, morbidity, and recurrence are reduced with its use (Feied & Handler, 2002). This should be followed immediately by treatment with heparin. Fibrinolytic medications are discussed in the Pharmacology Summary table in Chapter 40 (p. 1191) 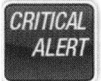.

Heparin is still the most effective treatment for PE because it slows or prevents clot progression and reduces the risk of further embolism. Early heparin anticoagulation should be started as soon as the diagnosis of pulmonary thromboembolism is considered seriously. Long-term anticoagulation is essential for patients who survive an initial DVT or PE. At least 6 months of anticoagulation is associated with significant reduction in recurrences and a net positive benefit (Feied & Handler, 2002). See the Pharmacology Summary table in Chapter 43 (p. 1349) 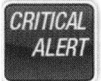 for a complete description of heparin.

Surgical Therapy

Pulmonary embolectomy was the first definitive therapy for PE. This consists of an emergency thoracotomy; then while occluding the pulmonary artery and aorta, the emboli are removed through an incision into the pulmonary artery. When first discovered in 1908 it was considered an extreme therapy with very little hope of success. Two technical advances in the 1960s, cardiopulmonary bypass and pulmonary angiography, made pulmonary embolectomy a more feasible procedure. In spite of this it is only considered in patients with massive PE complicated by shock (Dalen, 2002).

Inferior vena cava (IVC) filters commonly are used in patients with venous thromboembolism who are concomitantly unable to tolerate anticoagulants. They also are indicated for patients who have recurrent PE in spite of anticoagulation. They may be used as an adjunctive therapy in patients undergoing embolectomy or with massive PE. Anticoagulant medications used for PE are outlined in the Pharmacology Summary table in Chapter 43 (p. 1349) 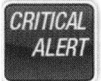.

◼ Nursing Management

The nursing process guides the nursing care for patients with a PE.

Assessment

Nursing assessment must include an evaluation of risk factors on admission and throughout the patient's hospital stay. Although patients initially may be on bed rest, nurses should encourage maximal mobility, including range of motion and walking where appropriate while also staying alert to symptoms of DVT and PE (Morris et al., 2002).

Nursing Diagnoses

Nursing diagnoses related to PE include *Ineffective Tissue Perfusion* and *Impaired Gas Exchange*. Other nursing diagnoses are directly related to the specific clinical manifestations described earlier.

Outcomes and Evaluation Parameters

Nursing outcomes include supporting the patient through the acute period and resolution of the clinical manifestations. Evaluation parameters include normal vital signs, therapeutic blood levels for anticoagulation, and the absence of clinical manifestations.

Interventions and Rationales

Nursing interventions are aimed at assisting the patient to maintain the therapeutic regime during the acute period. Anticoagulant medication should be given at the same time each day. The nurse monitors hemoglobin, hematocrit, platelet, and the international normalized ratio (INR) levels, and other clotting studies as needed to assess the effectiveness of anticoagulants.

CRITICAL ALERT *Anticoagulant medication should be given on time and at the same time each day. The nurse monitors hemoglobin, hematocrit, platelet, INR levels, and other clotting studies as needed to assess the effectiveness of anticoagulants.*

The nurse assesses for symptoms of bleeding and heparin-induced thrombocytopenia and teaches patients to do the same. Monitoring liver function is particularly important in elderly and critically ill patients receiving anticoagulants. The nurse has a major role in the prevention of DVT and PE. This is discussed further in the Health Promotion section below.

Discharge Priorities

Discharge priorities include educating the patient and family about risk factors and treatment regimes. The medication regimen is reviewed carefully with attention to the side effects of anticoagulation such as bleeding. Outpatient appointments for laboratory tests such as INR, clotting studies, and liver function studies should be stressed.

Health Promotion

Nurses should assess patients on admission for risks of PE and DVT. These can occur in young people as well as middle-aged people and the elderly. This assessment continues throughout the hospital stay. Orders for DVT prophylaxis should be obtained in patients with risk factors such as recent surgery, orthopedic surgery, injury, childbirth, stroke, cancer, heart failure and prolonged immobilization, indwelling central venous catheters, and older age. Patients who have had spinal cord injuries and spinal fractures are at increased risk often related to their postinjury status and immobilization (Kennedy, Zolot, & Sofer, 2001; Morris et al., 2002).

A number of deaths from pulmonary embolism caused by DVT have been attributed to long-distance airplane travel. Preventive strategies the nurse can stress for inpatients and outpatients include avoiding alcohol and caffeine before and during the flight, avoiding constrictive clothing, avoiding leg crossing, changing positions frequently while seated, not ingesting sleeping pills, not smoking, requesting bulkhead seating so as to stretch legs, staying well hydrated with water, noncaffeinated drinks, soft drinks, or juices, taking only short naps unless a normal sleeping position can be attained, and wearing compression stockings (Ball, 2003).

■ Pulmonary Hypertension

Pulmonary artery hypertension (PH) is a progressive disorder characterized by abnormally high blood pressure (hypertension) in the pulmonary artery. Hypertension develops when most of the very small arteries throughout the lungs narrow in diameter, thereby increasing the resistance to blood flow through the lungs. The increased pressure causes abnormally high and sustainable blood pressure elevations in the pulmonary arteries.

There are two types of PH: primary, also referred to as idiopathic, and secondary, that is, secondary to some other cause. Primary pulmonary artery hypertension (PPH) may be inherited (familial) or may occur for no known reason (idiopathic). Secondary pulmonary hypertension (SPH) is caused by or occurs either because of another condition, including chronic heart or lung disease or blood clots in the lungs, or a disease such as scleroderma (Porth, 2007).

Pulmonary artery hypertension is not curable, but it is treatable. Prognosis is compromised if the cause of SPH is not found and treated. Currently, many new treatments are being investigated that may help improve the quality of life for those patients experiencing PH (NHLBI, 2006).

Epidemiology and Etiology

Normal pulmonary circulation is a high-flow, low-resistance circuit capable of accommodating the entire right ventricular output at one-fifth the pressure of the systemic circulation level. The thin-walled right ventricle functions primarily as a flow-generator pump, and it is particularly sensitive to increases in its afterload. Increased pulmonary artery pressure and pulmonary vascular resistance characterize pulmonary hypertension. Pulmonary arterial hypertension is a mean pulmonary arterial pressure of greater than 25 mmHg at rest or greater than 35 mmHg during exercise (Merck, 2005b; Morton et al., 2005; Porth, 2007).

In accordance with the distinction between primary and secondary pulmonary arterial hypertension, the epidemiology and etiology of each is different. Idiopathic or primary pulmonary hypertension is the rarer of the two types, with an incidence of about 2 to 3 per million per year and a prevalence of about 15 per million (CDC, 2006). About 300 new cases of PPH are diagnosed in the United States each year, with a mean age of 35 to 37, but it can occur as late as age 60. SPH is much more common (NHLBI, 2006). Women are almost three times as likely to present with PPH as men (Sharma, 2006c). Although anyone can develop either type of pulmonary hypertension, older adults are more likely to have secondary pulmonary hypertension and young people are more likely to have idiopathic (primary) pulmonary hypertension.

PPH can be familial, meaning inherited or clustered, or sporadic. Most cases are sporadic, with approximately 10% being familial (Jassal & Sharma, 2004). In PPH, the precise etiology is unknown. However, presumed mechanisms include the following:

- **Endothelial dysfunction**—With impaired production of both prostacyclin and nitrous oxide, endothelium is overproduced. This overproduction results in vasoconstriction and remodeling of the pulmonary vasculature.
- **Voltage-gated K channel**—A defect in this ion channel changes the resting membrane potential, increasing intracellular calcium and leading to pulmonary vasoconstriction.
- **Thrombosis in situ**—Injury to the endothelial lining of the vessel wall, abnormal fibrinolysis, and platelet abnormalities may all contribute to thrombus formation (Sharma, 2006c, p. 1)

The etiologies and risk factors of PPH include the following:

- Use of appetite suppressants such as fenfluramine and dexfenfluramine; Fen-Phen produced an annual incidence of 25 to 50 per million per year.
- Genetic factors, for example, inheritance as an autosomal dominant trait, could play a role.
- Cocaine or amphetamine ingestion may be a contributing factor.

The specific genetic factors related to primary pulmonary hypertension are listed in the Genetic Considerations box.

Secondary pulmonary hypertension often is caused by several interactive disease processes. These causes may be categorized as pulmonary venous hypertension, chronic hypoxia

GENETIC CONSIDERATIONS Related to Primary Pulmonary Hypertension

Genetic factors, such as defects within the bone morphogenetic protein receptor type II gene, coding for a receptor member of the transforming growth factor-beta family, underlie familial primary pulmonary hypertension (Humbert & Trembath, 2002). About 20% of sporadic cases also have *BMPR2* mutations. Many people with PPH have increased levels of angiopoietin-1, which appears to downregulate *BMPR1A*, a sister receptor to *BMPR2*, and may stimulate serotonin production and endothelial smooth muscle proliferation.

Other possible contributing factors include abnormalities in serotonin transport and previous infection with human herpesvirus 8 (Humbert & Trembath; 2002; Merck, 2005b). Although achievements in determining the impact of genomic approaches on pulmonary hypertension have been made, additional research is indicated to identify specific molecular determinants for this disorder.

with secondary vasoconstriction of the pulmonary vasculature, pulmonary artery obstruction, and left-to-right shunts. Pulmonary venous hypertension is the most common form of pulmonary hypertension and usually due to left-sided heart disease. Pulmonary hypertension develops as a result of the obstruction of blood flow downstream from the pulmonary vein. Causes of pulmonary venous hypertension from distal to proximal of the pulmonary vasculature include coarctation of the aorta, aortic stenosis, aortic regurgitation, hypertrophic cardiomyopathy, constrictive pericarditis, restrictive cardiomyopathy, dilated cardiomyopathy, mitral stenosis, mitral regurgitation, and left atrial myxoma (Jassal & Sharma, 2004; Porth, 2007).

Chronic hypoxia with secondary vasoconstriction of the pulmonary vasculature induces vasoconstriction of the pulmonary vascular bed, causing high pulmonary resistance and hypertension with right ventricular failure. Causes include restrictive lung disease (obesity, pneumoconiosis, neuromuscular disorders) and obstructive lung diseases (asthma, COPD, bronchiectasis).

Concerning pulmonary artery obstruction, chronic major thromboembolic vessel disease is a treatable cause of pulmonary hypertension that results in anatomic obstruction of the arteries. Thrombotic disorders include sickle cell disease and other coagulation disorders. Embolic disease includes chronic thromboemboli, connective tissue disease, lupus, and schistosomiasis.

Individuals with pulmonary hypertension due to left-to-right shunts have high blood flow to the pulmonary vessels, which leads to increased pulmonary vascular resistance over time with reversal of the shunt (Eisenmenger complex). Extracardiac shunts include patent ductus arteriosus, and intracardiac shunts include ventricular and atrial septal defects.

Pathophysiology

Three predominant pathophysiological mechanisms may be involved in the development of SPH: (1) hypoxic vasoconstriction, (2) decreased area of the pulmonary vascular bed, and (3) volume/pressure overload (Sharma, 2006c). Chronic hypoxemia causes pulmonary vasoconstriction by a variety of actions on pulmonary artery endothelium and smooth muscle cells, including downregulation of endothelial nitric oxide synthetase and reduced production of the voltage-gated potassium channel alpha subunit. Chronic hypoxemia leading to pulmonary hypertension can occur in patients with COPD, high-altitude disorders, and hypoventilation disorders (e.g., obstructive sleep apnea). COPD is the most common cause of SPH. These patients have worse than 5-year survival rates, more severe ventilation/perfusion mismatch than other diseases causing SPH, and nocturnal or exercise-induced hypoxemia. Other disorders, such as obstructive sleep apnea, neuromuscular disorders, and disorders of the chest wall, may lead to hypoxic pulmonary vasoconstriction and eventually SPH.

A variety of causes may decrease the cross-sectional area of the pulmonary vascular bed, primarily due to disease of the lung parenchyma. The pulmonary arterial pressure rises only when the loss of the pulmonary vessels exceeds 60% of the total pulmonary vasculature. Patients with collagen vascular diseases have a high incidence of SPH, particularly patients with systemic scleroderma or CREST (calcinosis cutis, Raynaud phenomenon, esophageal motility disorder, sclerodactyly, and telangiectasia) syndrome. A mild-to-moderate elevation in mean pulmonary artery pressure occurs secondary to acute pulmonary embolism. The peak systolic pressures usually do not rise above 50 mmHg, and they generally normalize following appropriate therapy. Chronic pulmonary emboli can result in progressive PH. HIV infection and several drugs and toxins are also known to cause PH.

Disorders of the left heart may cause SPH, resulting from volume and pressure overload. Pulmonary blood volume overload is caused by left-to-right intracardiac shunts, such as in patients with atrial or ventricular septal defects. Left atrial hypertension causes a passive rise in pulmonary arterial systolic pressure in order to maintain a driving force across the vasculature. Over time, persistent pulmonary hypertension accompanied by vasculopathy occurs. This may occur secondary to left ventricular dysfunction, mitral valvular disease, constrictive pericarditis, aortic stenosis, and cardiomyopathy.

Pulmonary venous obstruction is a rare cause of pulmonary hypertension. This may develop secondary to mediastinal fibrosis, anomalous pulmonary venous drainage, or pulmonary veno-occlusive disease.

Clinical Manifestations

Symptoms of pulmonary hypertension may develop very gradually and often are nonspecific. Thus, patients may delay seeing a health care provider for years, and when seen their disorder may be misdiagnosed and treated for more common conditions (Hegewald, Markewitz, & Elliott, 2007). Also, the clinical manifestations of SPH frequently are masked by the underlying etiology. Typically, the interval between the onset of symptoms of PH to diagnosis is about 2 years. The most common presenting symptoms are:

- Exertional dyspnea
- Fatigue and lethargy
- Angina
- Syncope
- Raynaud's disease
- Edema (Jassal & Sharma, 2004).

Less common symptoms include cough, hemoptysis, and hoarseness (due to compression of the recurrent laryngeal nerve by the distended pulmonary artery, i.e., Ortner's syndrome). In advanced disease, signs may include right ventricular heave; widely split second heart sound (S_2); accentuated, pulmonic component of $S_2(P_2)$; pulmonary ejection click; right ventricular third heart sound (S_3); and jugular venous distention. Liver congestion and peripheral edema are common late manifestations (Sharma, 2006c).

Laboratory and Diagnostic Procedures

The diagnosis of PPH is suspected in patients with significant exertional dyspnea who are otherwise relatively healthy and have no signs of other diseases known to cause pulmonary hypertension. Patients usually undergo chest x-ray, spirometry, and electrocardiography (ECG) to identify more common causes of dyspnea, followed by Doppler ECG to assess right ventricular and pulmonary artery pressures as well as to detect structural heart disease causing secondary pulmonary hypertension.

The most common x-ray result in PPH is enlarged hilar vessels that rapidly prune into the periphery. Spirometry and lung volumes may be normal or show mild restriction, but diffusing capacity for carbon monoxide (DLco) is usually reduced. Common ECG findings include right axis deviation, $R > S$ in V_1, $S_1Q_3T_3$, and peaked P waves.

Additional tests are obtained as indicated to diagnose secondary causes not apparent clinically. These include ventilation/perfusion scanning to detect thromboembolic disease, pulmonary function tests to identify obstructive or restrictive lung disease, and serum serologic tests to gather evidence for or against rheumatologic disease. Chronic thromboembolic pulmonary hypertension is suggested by CT or lung scan and is diagnosed by arteriography. Other tests, such as HIV testing, liver function tests, and polysomnography, are performed in the appropriate clinical context.

When initial evaluation reveals no conditions associated with secondary pulmonary hypertension, pulmonary artery catheterization is necessary to measure right atrial and ventricular, pulmonary artery, and pulmonary capillary wedge pressures and cardiac output. Right-sided O_2 saturation should be measured to exclude atrial septal defect. A mean pulmonary arterial pressure greater than 25 mmHg in the absence of an underlying cause defines PPH. However, most patients with PPH present with significantly higher pressure (e.g., 60 mmHg). Vasodilating drugs (e.g., inhaled nitric oxide, IV epoprostenol) often are administered during the procedure; a decrease in right-sided pressures in response to these drugs helps in the selection of drugs for treatment. Biopsy, once widely performed, is neither needed nor recommended because of high morbidity and mortality (Hegewald et al., 2007; Merck, 2005b; Sharma, 2006c).

Once PPH is diagnosed, the patient's family history is reviewed to detect possible genetic transmission, which is suggested by premature deaths in otherwise healthy members of the extended family. In familial PPH, genetic counseling is needed to advise family members of the risk of disease (about 20%) and to advocate serial screening with echocardiograms. Testing for mutations in the *BMPR2* gene in familial PPH may play a future role.

Medical Management

The treatment of SPH is primarily directed at treatment of the underlying disease. Effective therapy should be instituted in the early stages, before irreversible changes in pulmonary vasculature occur. Once the cause of SPH has been established, the management consists of specific interventional therapy, specific medical therapy, or general supportive therapy. Specific interventional and medical therapies are instituted for conditions such as atrial septal defects, mitral stenosis, sleep apnea, and chronic pulmonary thromboembolic disease. General supportive therapy is provided to patients who have right ventricular failure or to those patients in whom the cause cannot be addressed directly. General oxygen has a proven benefit in reducing patient mortality in selected patients with PH. Long-term oxygen is prescribed for those patients who have PaO_2 of less than 55 mmHg at rest from any cause and those who have decreased oxygen saturation during exercise.

Treatment of PPH is rapidly evolving. Oral calcium (Ca) channel blockers sustain reductions in pulmonary artery pressure or pulmonary vascular resistance in about 10% to 15% of patients and are the first drugs used. No differences in efficacy exist by Ca channel blocker type, although most specialists avoid verapamil because of its negative inotropic effects. Response to Ca channel blockers is a favorable prognostic sign, and patients who respond should continue this treatment. Those who do not respond are given other drugs. IV epoprostenol, a prostacyclin analog, improves function and lengthens survival even in patients who are unresponsive to a vasodilator during catheterization. Disadvantages are the need for continuous central catheter infusion and significant adverse effects, including flushing, diarrhea, and bacteremia due to the indwelling central catheter. Inhaled iloprost, oral beraprost, and subcutaneous prostacyclin analogs are under study as alternatives.

Other pharmacologic therapies for treating both primary and secondary pulmonary hypertension include anticoagulants, antidiuretics, anticoagulants, and digoxin. Anticoagulants are used regularly in patients with PPH because they help reduce symptoms and may provide a survival benefit. The role of anticoagulation has not been established in patients with SPH. Nonetheless, anticoagulation with warfarin is indicated in patients with chronic pulmonary emboli, pulmonary veno-occlusive disease, and atrial fibrillation induced by left or right heart failure. Furthermore, long-term anticoagulation therapy should be considered in patients who are at high risk for developing venous thromboembolism (e.g., those with cor pulmonale and patients with immobility secondary to severe dyspnea).

Fluid removal with diuretics reduces hepatic congestion and pulmonary edema. It should, however, be instituted with caution to avoid hypokalemia, metabolic alkalosis, and a decrease in cardiac output. Phlebotomy should be considered if the patient's hematocrit value is greater than 60%. Digoxin has been shown to be beneficial for patients with supraventricular tachycardia or associated left ventricular dysfunction multifocal atrial tachycardia, but verapamil has been proven to be better than digoxin for controlling the heart rate.

Surgical Management

Lung transplantation offers the only hope of cure for PPH (Merck, 2005b). It is reserved for patients with New York Heart Association Class IV disease (defined as dyspnea associated with minimal activity, leading to bed to chair limitations) who have not been helped by prostacyclin analogs. Transplant surgery has a high morbidity due to the problems of rejection and infection and a 60% 5-year survival rate related to bronchiolitis obliterans (Sharma, 2006c).

Patients with an atrial septal defect, mitral stenosis, or chronic pulmonary thromboembolic disease should be considered for surgical management. PH resolves following successful surgical procedures, unless it is too far advanced. Although lung transplantation is reserved for patients with severe PPH, a subset of patients with SPH has undergone successful transplantation at several centers. These patients had SPH due to collagen vascular disease, drug-induced PAH, or pulmonary venous obstruction. Stability of the underlying causative disorder and the patient's ability to tolerate an extensive surgical procedure are prerequisites. Heart-lung transplantation has been performed in patients with SPH due to congenital cardiac disease or severe left ventricular dysfunction (Sharma, 2006c).

Nursing Management

The primary goal of nursing management is to identify those patients subject to or at high risk for pulmonary hypertension. There are numerous conditions, but primary diseases include cystic fibrosis, COPD, hypoventilation syndromes, pulmonary fibrosis, congenital heart disease, pulmonary emboli, mitral valve disease, and connective tissue diseases. See the Risk Factors for Secondary Pulmonary Hypertension for more details.

The nurse also must be alert to the foremost signs and symptoms of pulmonary hypertension: exertional dyspnea, fatigue and lethargy, angina, syncope, Raynaud's disease, and edema of ankles and legs. Nurses also are responsible for oxygen administration and medication administration as ordered. Patient education as to risk factors, activity tolerance, the use of oxygen, and discharge priorities is critical to the care of the patient. The remainder of the nursing management for pulmonary hypertension is covered under nursing management of restrictive pulmonary diseases.

RISK FACTORS for Secondary Pulmonary Hypertension

- Chronic high-altitude exposure
- Obstructive sleep apnea
- Vasculitis
- Infectious diseases
- HIV
- Drugs and toxins
- Amphetamines
- Anorexigens
- Cocaine
- Toxic rapeseed oil ingestion

Discharge Priorities

Discharge priorities are multifaceted and focus on self-care, education regarding medications and home equipment, and emergency needs. Fatigue and weakness related to the disease itself may render the patient dependent on others for self-care. Patients and families need to be advised about an activity regimen that the patient can safely assume. The physical environment also should be configured in order to provide easy and safe navigation, ambulatory or via a wheelchair. Precise instructions as to how and when to take medications should be given to the patient and family, and the patient should be instructed to keep the list in an easily accessible location along with emergency phone numbers to use if needed. Family members also should know the placement of these documents. Return medical appointments should be given to the patient, and the patient should indicate where these are recorded. If the patient is going to be on oxygen therapy at home, instruction should be provided as to how to use the equipment and how to secure replacement as necessary.

Psychological adjustment to the patient's illness also must be considered. The diagnosis carries with it an uncertain and historically very bleak prognosis. Although new oral and chronic parenteral (IV and subcutaneous) treatments have had a significant positive medical impact on the physical functioning of individuals with PAH, patients often struggle with new short- and long-term psychosocial challenges (Wryobeck, Lippo, McLaughlin, Riba, & Rubenfire, 2007).

Health Promotion

With regard to health promotion, patients with pulmonary hypertension should be made aware of risk factors that may exacerbate their disease, and cautioned to avoid them. Patients also may be on a variety of medications, including anticoagulants. They should be advised to avoid situations that would put them at risk for experiencing side effects of the medications. Counseling also is advised to help people cope with the serious and potentially life-threatening outcomes of their disease. Referral to a support group, locally or online, also may assist the patient in the coping process.

Collaborative Management

The health care provider, nurse, and social worker are involved in the care of the patient. They initiate the plan of care and assume responsibility for continuity. Various diagnostic tests, as previously described, are performed. These are essential to determine the cause of secondary hypertension. They also are essential to interrupting the self-perpetuation cycle responsible for the progress of this disease. Although there is no cure for PPH, treatment as prescribed by the health care provider can relieve symptoms, increase quality of life, and prolong life. The nurse is responsible for implementing and evaluating the plan of care. The social worker, occupational therapist, and dietitian may be called on to assist the patient in making appropriate plans for discharge, physical set-up of house that deters overexertion, self-care help, and dietary plans that reduce physiological stress.

Cor Pulmonale: Etiology, Epidemiology, and Pathophysiology

Cor pulmonale is defined as an alteration in the structure and function of the right ventricle caused by a primary disorder of the respiratory system. Pulmonary hypertension is the common link between lung dysfunction and the heart in cor pulmonale. Right ventricular disease caused by a primary abnormality of the left side of the heart or congenital heart disease is not considered cor pulmonale, but it can develop secondary to many cardiopulmonary diseases (Yunis & Crausman, 2006).

Cor pulmonale develops as a result of lung disorders such as chronic lung disease, pulmonary embolism, interstitial lung disease, idiopathic primary pulmonary hypertension, and blood disorders such as polycythemia vera, sickle cell disease, and macrohemoglobinemia (Yunis & Crausman, 2006). Blood disorders are discussed in detail in Chapter 63 ⊚ . Cor pulmonale is estimated to account for 6% to 7% of all types of adult heart disease in the United States with COPD the causative factor in more than 50% of cases (Yunis & Crausman, 2006).

A variety of pathophysiological mechanisms lead to pulmonary hypertension and consequently, cor pulmonale. These include (1) pulmonary vasoconstriction due to alveolar hypoxia, (2) anatomic compromise of the pulmonary vascular bed, (3) increased blood viscosity secondary to blood disorders such as polycythemia vera and sickle cell disease, and (4) idiopathic primary pulmonary hypertension (Yunis & Crausman, 2006).

There are two forms of cor pulmonale, acute and chronic. Acute cor pulmonale usually results from a massive pulmonary embolus or from injury due to mechanical ventilation for acute respiratory distress syndrome. Chronic cor pulmonale is usually caused by COPD (chronic bronchitis, emphysema) and less often by extensive loss of lung tissue due to surgery or trauma, chronic unresolved pulmonary emboli, pulmonary veno-occlusive disease, scleroderma, pulmonary interstitial fibrosis, kyphoscoliosis, obesity with alveolar hypoventilation, neuromuscular disorders involving respiratory muscles, or idiopathic alveolar hypoventilation. In patients with COPD, an acute exacerbation or pulmonary infection may trigger right ventricular overload (Merck, 2005a).

Laboratory and Diagnostic Procedures

Diagnosis is based on the clinical manifestations and diagnostic tests such as echocardiography, which will give information about the size of the heart. Chest x-rays and computed axial tomography CAT scan of the chest are also used for this reason. Pulmonary function tests that evaluate ventilation/perfusion mismatch (Chapters 33 and 36 ⊚) provide information about problems with gas exchange. ABG tests also help identify gas exchange and the presence of acidosis and alkalosis.

Clinical Manifestations

Cor pulmonale is asymptomatic initially, although patients usually have significant clinical manifestations related to underlying lung disorder (e.g., dyspnea, exertional fatigue). Later, as right ventricular (RV) pressures increase, physical signs commonly include a left parasternal systolic lift, a loud pulmonic component of the second heart sound (S_2), and murmurs of functional tricuspid and pulmonic insufficiency. Later, an RV gallop rhythm (third [S_3] and fourth [S_4] heart sounds) augmented during inspiration, distended jugular veins, hepatomegaly, and lower extremity edema may occur. The patient also may complain of fatigue, dyspnea or chest pain on exertion, and cough. In advanced stages hepatic congestion leads to anorexia, right upper quadrant abdominal discomfort, and jaundice (Yunis & Crausman, 2006).

Medical Management

Treatment is directed at the underlying illness. Oxygen therapy is a mainstay for patients with cor pulmonale because it relieves hypoxemic pulmonary vasoconstriction. Because the partial pressure of oxygen or PO_2 is likely to fall with exercise and sleep, oxygen is recommended during these times or continuously (Yunis & Crausman, 2006). Diuretics are used, particularly when the right ventricular filling volume is markedly elevated; however, they are used cautiously to prevent hypokalemia, metabolic acidosis, and a decline in cardiac output.

In addition to diuretics, vasodilator drugs including calcium channel blockers such as oral sustained-release nifedipine and diltiazem are effective. Theophylline has a weak inotropic effect and may improve right ventricular ejection as well as decrease pulmonary vascular resistance. Finally, anticoagulation with warfarin is recommended in patients who are high risk for thromboembolism (Yunis & Crausman, 2006). Phlebotomy is recommended for patients with severe polycythemia, which is defined as a hematocrit of over 65 (Yunis & Crausman, 2006). Cardiac medications are discussed in Chapter 40 ⊚ and anticoagulants in Chapter 43 ⊚ .

Nursing Management

Physical assessment findings include an increased chest diameter, labored respirations with retractions of the chest wall and use of accessory muscles, hyperresonance to percussion, diminished breath sounds, wheezing, and, rarely, cyanosis (Yunis & Crausman, 2006). Auscultation of the heart may reveal a split second heart sound, a systolic ejection murmur with a sharp ejection click over the pulmonary artery, along with a diastolic regurgitation murmur (Yunis & Crausman, 2006). There may be a third ventricular heart sound secondary to systemic venous congestion. This also may be reflected by distended neck veins (Yunis & Crausman, 2006). See the Diagnostic Tests for Cor Pulmonale box (p. 985) for relevant diagnostic studies.

The primary role of the nurse is managing dyspnea by administration of oxygen and medications to treat right ventricular hypertrophy and pulmonary hypertension. This includes medications that treat the underlying disease.

Patient education is another major role of the nurse. The nurse teaches the patient and caregiver to be comfortable managing oxygen equipment and medications. Referrals to home health and pulmonary rehabilitation are usually needed to ensure safe care in the home setting. A plan for regular assessment of oxygen needs and medications should be in place before discharge. The single most preventive measure is to encourage individuals to stop smoking and to avoid exposure to secondhand smoke and respiratory pollutants.

PHARMACOLOGY Summary of Medications to Treat Lower Airway Disorders

Medication Category	Action	Application/Indication	Nursing Responsibility
Mucolytics • Dornase alpha (Pulmozyme) • Acetylcysteine* (Mucomyst) • Amiloride**	Liquefies bronchial secretions by altering the structure of mucous molecule.	Cystic fibrosis, acute and chronic bronchitis, pneumonia, TB.	Monitor for adverse effects: nausea, vomiting. Observe for possible bronchospasm. Establish a routine for elimination of secretions post-treatment. Use with caution in patients with compromised ability to cough.
Decongestants • Sympathomimetics • Ephedrine (Efedron) • Oxymetazoline (Afrin 12 hour, Neo-Synephrine 12 hour) • Phenylephrine (Afrin 4–6 hour, Neo-Synephrine 4–6 hour) • Pseudoephedrine (Chlor-Trimeton, Drixoral, Sudafed) **Anticholinergic** • Intranasal ipratropium (Atrovent, Combivent)	Decreases nasal membrane edema by constricting nasal arterioles. Decreases rhinorrhea by blocking muscarinic receptors in nasal passages.	Common cold, sinusitis, allergic rhinitis, nasal congestion.	Monitor for adverse effects: insomnia, tremors, weakness, anxiety, hypertension, tachycardia, palpitations, arrhythmias. Observe for rebound nasal congestion with intranasal administration, CNS stimulation with oral administration. Monitor for severe reactions: hallucinations, convulsions. Be aware of drug interactions (MAOIs, methyldopa, tricyclic antidepressants and others).
Antitussives • Nonopioid dextromethorphan* (Benylin, Robitussin, Delsym) **Opioid** • Codeine** • Hydrocodone bitartrate (Hycodan, Mycodone)	Suppresses cough by direct action on the cough center in the medulla.	Nonproductive or hyperactive cough.	Monitor for adverse effects: drowsiness, sedation (especially patients on CNS depressants), nausea, vomiting, constipation, dizziness, **pruritus. *Be aware of drug interaction with MAOIs. Monitor for CNS stimulation, hypotension, hyperpyrexia.
Antibiotics • Fluoroquinolones/quinolones • Ciprofloxacin (Cipro) • Ofloxacin (Floxin) • Levofloxacin (Levaquin) • Moxifloxacin (Avelox)	Exerts bacteriocidal effect by disrupting synthesis of gram-negative and gram-positive bacterial DNA.	Acute exacerbation of chronic bronchitis, community-acquired pneumonia, sinusitis.	Monitor for adverse effects: nausea, headache, diarrhea, some may cause dysrhythmias or liver failure. Monitor WBC count, liver and renal function. Monitor for signs of CNS toxicity especially if given in presence of epilepsy, cerebral artery disease, alcoholism. Be aware of drug interactions (warfarin, NSAIDs, theophylline, antacids, caffeine). Monitor for altered efficacy or toxicity. Do not give with antacids or vitamins containing calcium, magnesium, iron, or zinc.
Tetracyclines • Doxycycline (Vibramycin) • Tetracycline (Sumycin)	Exerts bacteriostatic effect by inhibiting bacterial protein synthesis in gram-positive and gram-negative bacteria. May be bactericidal at higher doses.	Respiratory tract infections, *Chlamydia*, gonorrhea, tetanus, *Helicobacter pylori*, Lyme disease.	Monitor for adverse effects: nausea, vomiting, diarrhea, signs of superinfection. Be aware of drug interactions (iron, calcium, magnesium, antacids, lipid lowering drugs, oral anticoagulants, oral contraceptives). Observe for decreased drug efficacy or toxicity. Do not give with milk products, iron, magnesium laxatives, or antacids. Warn patient of photosensitivity and need for sun block.

(continued)

PHARMACOLOGY Summary of Medications to Treat Lower Airway Disorders—*Continued*

Medication Category	Action	Application/Indication	Nursing Responsibility
Macrolides • Clarithromycin* (Biaxin) • Erythromycin (Erythrocin) • Azithromycin (Zithromax)	Exerts bacteriostatic effect by inhibiting bacterial protein synthesis in gram-positive and gram-negative organisms. May be bactericidal at higher doses.	Legionnaire disease, *Mycoplasma pneumoniae* pneumonia, diphtheria, chlamydial infections.	Monitor for adverse effects: urticaria, nausea, vomiting, diarrhea, abdominal cramping, *Clostridium* overgrowth. Observe for exacerbation of existing heart disease or, if given IV, torsades de pointes. Monitor hepatic function. Be aware of multiple drug interactions (warfarin, anticonvulsants, theophylline, and others). Monitor for toxicity or altered drug efficacy. Warn patient not to take OTC drugs without contacting physician. Do not give with fruit juice.
Aminoglycosides • Tobramycin (Nebcin) • Amikacin (Amikin) • Gentamicin (Garamycin)	Exerts bacteriocidal effect on gram-negative organisms and staphylococcus by altering bacterial protein synthesis.	TB, serious respiratory infections, sepsis, meningitis, osteomyelitis.	Monitor for adverse effects: signs of ototoxicity (dizziness, loss of balance, tinnitus, headache), superinfection. *Note:* Hearing loss is usually irreversible. Be aware of increased risk of nephrotoxicity and/or ototoxicity if given concurrently with amphotericin B, furosemide, acetylsalicylic, and others. Monitor renal function for signs of nephrotoxicity.
Sulfonamides • Trimethoprim-sulfamethoxazole (SMZ-TMP) (Bactrim, Septra)	Exerts bacteriostatic activity by inhibiting bacterial folic acid synthesis needed for cell growth.	Exacerbation of chronic bronchitis, pneumonia, traveler's diarrhea, urinary tract infections, otitis media.	Monitor for adverse effects: nausea, vomiting, urticaria. Be aware of drug interactions (warfarin, digoxin, phenytoin, and others). Observe for drug toxicity. Monitor CBC, renal function, urinalysis (crystalluria can occur). Increase fluid intake unless contraindicated.
Miscellaneous Antibiotics • Chloramphenicol (Chloromycetin)	Exerts broad-spectrum bacteriostatic activity by interfering with bacterial protein synthesis. May be bacteriocidal in some organisms.	Serious infections, cystic fibrosis regimes, bacteremia, meningitis, typhoid fever.	Monitor for adverse effects: nausea, vomiting, headache, fungal overgrowth. Monitor blood studies regularly. May cause blood dyscrasias and irreversible bone marrow depression. Increase monitoring of blood glucose in patients on oral antidiabetic agents. Monitor serum drug levels, especially in the presence of renal or hepatic impairment.

PHARMACOLOGY Summary of Medications to Treat Lower Airway Disorders—*Continued*

Medication Category	Action	Application/Indication	Nursing Responsibility
Antifungals • Polyene • Amphotericin B (Fungizone)	Causes fungal cell death by altering fungal cell membrane.	Progressive or potentially fatal systemic fungal or protozoal infections.	Monitor for anorexia, nausea, vomiting. May require premedication with antiemetic. During IV infusion, monitor vital signs, observe for infusion reaction: headache, fever, chills, nausea, vomiting, hypotension, bronchospasm (premedication with diphenhydramine and acetaminophen may reduce infusion reactions). Monitor input and output (I&O), renal function, appearance of urine, CBC, electrolytes, hepatic function. Monitor IV site for extravasation, thrombophlebitis. Be aware of multiple drug incompatibilities when given IV.
Azoles • Fluconazole (Diflucan) • Itraconazole (Sporanox)	Exerts fungistatic effect by interrupting fungal cell membrane function. May be fungicidal at higher concentrations.	Systemic candidiasis, pneumonia, esophageal candidiasis.	Monitor for adverse effects: headache, nausea, abdominal pain, diarrhea. Monitor liver function. Be aware of multiple drug interactions (oral hypoglycemics, Coumadin, phenytoin, theophylline, and others). Monitor for decreased drug efficacy or toxicity. Monitor for hypoglycemia in diabetic patients. Be aware of multiple drug incompatibilities when given IV.
Echocardins • Anidulafungin (Eraxis)	Exerts antifungal effect by inhibiting synthesis of major component of fungal cell wall.	Esophageal candidiasis, candidemia.	Monitor for adverse effects: nausea, vomiting, diarrhea, hypokalemia, rash. Monitor liver function.
Antiviral • Amantadine (Symmetrel) Rimantadine (Flumadine) • Oseltamivir* (Tamiflu) • Zanamivir* (Relenza)	Thought to exert antiviral effect by inhibiting early viral replication.	Prevention and treatment of influenza A. *Treatment of influenza A and B.	Monitor for adverse effects: dizziness, light-headedness, insomnia, nausea. Observe for increased seizure activity in presence of seizure disorder.

(continued)

PHARMACOLOGY Summary of Medications to Treat Lower Airway Disorders—*Continued*

Medication Category	Action	Application/Indication	Nursing Responsibility
Anti–TB • Isoniazid* (INH, Nydrazid, Laniazid) • Rifapentine** (Priftin) • Rifampin** (Rifadin)	Exerts bacteriostatic or bacteriocidal effects by disrupting synthesis of bacterial cell wall or impairing cell metabolism.	Prevention and treatment of pulmonary TB.	Monitor for adverse effects: visual disturbances, orthostatic hypotension*, signs of hepatotoxicity (anorexia, fatigue, nausea, malaise), signs of peripheral neuropathy (burning, tingling, pain, numbness). Monitor hepatic function, CBC. Monitor for hyperglycemia in presence of diabetes. **Be aware of multiple drug interactions (phenytoin, warfarin, diazepam, theophylline and others). Monitor for altered drug efficacy. **Warn patient on oral contraceptives to use alternate birth control method. *Instruct patient to restrict alcohol and intake of foods rich in tyramine (dairy, beef, chicken, bananas, caffeine, and others) and histamine (tuna, yeast extract, brine).
Digestive Enzyme • Pancrelipase (Viokase)	Breaks down fats, proteins, and starches in the final stage of digestion for easier absorption.	Steatorrhea from malabsorption syndrome in cystic fibrosis.	Monitor for adverse effects: nausea, abdominal cramps, diarrhea. Assess for improved nutritional status and decreased steatorrhea. Be aware of religious considerations; drug is pork based.
Bronchodilators • Corticosteroids			

*Acetaminophen toxicity, prevention of contrast-induced renal complications.
**A diuretic that reduces mucous viscosity by altering sputum electrolytes.
*Binds with hepatotoxic metabolite of acetaminophen, protects liver and renal cells from damage.

Pleural Effusion

A **pleural effusion**, which affects 1.3 million people annually in the United States, is defined as the presence of fluid in the pleural space (Figure 35–13 ■) (Abrahamian, 2008). This usually occurs secondary to other diseases. The source of the fluid usually is blood vessels or lymphatic vessels lying beneath either pleura. Occasionally, the source is an abscess or other lesion that drains into the pleural space.

Epidemiology and Etiology

Other common causes of pleural effusion include heart failure, TB, pneumonia, pulmonary infections, nephrotic syndrome, connective tissue disease, pulmonary embolism, fungal lung infections, and neoplastic tumors.

Pathophysiology

The pleura is a thin, transparent, serous permeable membrane that lines the thoracic cavity and encases the lungs. There are two layers: The parietal pleura lies adjacent to the chest wall, and the visceral pleura adheres to the outer surfaces of the lung. The small amount of serous fluid normally present between these two surfaces acts as a lubricant, thereby allowing the chest wall and lung to glide during inspiration and expiration. Fluids that accumulate in the lung can cross into the pleural space, causing a plural effusion (McCance & Huether, 2007). A pleural effusion can cause compression atelectasis and displacement of mediastinal contents. Because there is no communication between the pleural space and environmental air, pressure in the pleural space remains negative, and atelectasis is caused solely by pressure exerted by the effusion.

The effusion can be composed of a relatively clear fluid or it can be bloody or purulent. An effusion may be a transudate or an exudate. Transudates are clear in color, have a low protein content, and are secondary to underlying diseases. Some of these are caused by heart failure, cirrhosis, nephrotic syndrome, and/or medical disorders leading to hypoalbuminemia. Exudates have higher protein content and usually are caused by infection. Typ-

DIAGNOSTIC TESTS for Cor Pulmonale

Test	Expected Abnormality	Rationale
Chest x-ray	Enlargement of central pulmonary arteries; increased transverse diameter of the heart.	Changes in heart and pulmonary vessels are caused by pulmonary hypertension secondary to hypoxemia.
Echocardiography	Shows signs of chronic right ventricular pressure overload.	The right ventricle is strained by pulmonary hypertension.
ECG	Incomplete right bundle branch block, low-voltage QRS, signs of right ventricular hypertrophy, and atrial and junctional dysrhythmias.	ECG changes are secondary to right atrial enlargement and hypoxemia.
Cardiac catheterization	Assesses degree of pulmonary hypertension and differentiates cor pulmonale from occult left ventricular dysfunction.	Chronic hypoxemia causes pulmonary hypertension.
Hematocrit	Abnormally elevated.	Polycythemia developed secondary to hypoxemia.
Serum Alpha 1-antitrypsin	Decreased.	Deficiency of AAT causes COPD symptomatology and leads to cor pulmonale.

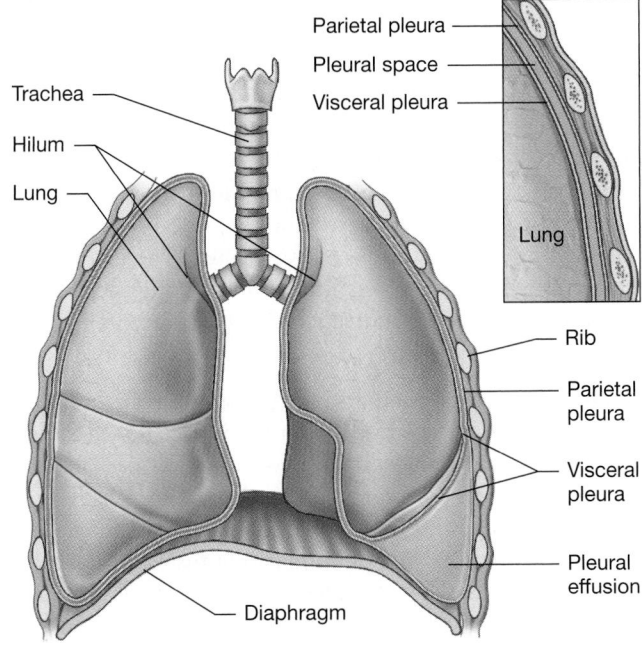

FIGURE 35–13 ■ Pleural effusion.

ically, they are deeper in color with a turbid appearance (Fishman et al., 2002). Causes are malignancy, collagen vascular disease, pneumonia, pancreatitis, or pulmonary embolism (Porth, 2007).

Clinical Manifestations

The symptoms of pleural effusion depend largely on the underlying disease and the size of the effusion. The patient may be asymptomatic if the effusion is small. However, if the effusion is large, clinical manifestations include severe breathlessness, pain, or both. Breath sounds are reduced on the affected side and the percussion note is dull. A pleural friction rub, which is described as a rubbing, grating, harsh, dry, and scratchy sound, may be present and best heard over the area of pleural inflammation. It will disappear with breath holding. There will be asymmetric ex-

pansion of the thoracic cage, with lagging expansion on the affected side. Mediastinal shift is seen only with massive effusions (usually >1,000 mL) and is noted on x-ray as displacement of the trachea and mediastinum to the contralateral side of the pleural effusion. Other important findings that provide clues to the cause of the pleural effusion are anasarca, distended neck veins, S_3 gallop rhythm, clubbing of the fingers, and breast nodule or intra-abdominal mass (Abrahamian, 2008).

Laboratory and Diagnostic Procedures

If more than 200 to 500 mL of fluid is present in the pleural space, the chest x-ray may show blunting of the costophrenic angle. As the volume of fluid increases, the hemidiaphragm becomes obscured as well. A lateral decubitus film may be helpful for showing fluid shifts. A CT scan, ultrasound, or thoracentesis also may be employed to make the final diagnosis. A sample of pleural fluid is obtained for biochemical, microbiologic, and cytologic analysis. Analysis of pleural fluid includes protein and glucose concentration, pH, and bacteria, including acid-fast bacilli and cell content. Cytologic testing reveals a malignant effusion about 80% of the time. Closed-needle biopsy is performed to identify tuberculosis and malignancies (Peek et al., 2000).

Medical Management

As with any other life-threatening condition, airway stabilization with adequate oxygenation and ventilation is the first priority. Administer supplemental oxygen to all unstable patients. Generally, any patient who requires thoracentesis is admitted to the hospital. A thoracentesis is a procedure to remove fluid from the space between the lungs and the chest wall called the pleural space. It is done with a needle (and sometimes a plastic catheter) inserted through the chest wall. This pleural fluid may be sent to a lab to determine what may be causing the fluid to accumulate in the pleural space.

Treatment of transudative effusions most commonly caused by heart failure differs from treatment of exudative effusions caused by infection and malignancy. In the case of a patient presenting with pleural effusion associated with congestive heart failure (CHF), the treatment involves controlling the patient's heart failure before considering thoracentesis (Coding Edge Archives, 2000).

Other treatment options include chemotherapy, radiation, intrapleural instillation of sclerosing agents, indwelling pleural catheters with intermittent drainage, chest tube drainage using the water seal system, pleuroperitoneal shunts, and pleurectomy. If thoracentesis provides relief, intermittent thoracenteses can be scheduled or a chest tube can be inserted to completely evacuate the pleural space. This is usually followed by pleurodesis or instillation of a sclerosing agent into the pleural cavity via the chest tube (Kvale, Simoff, & Prakash, 2003; Taubert, 2001).

When pleural effusion is related to a malignant cause, it may reaccumulate rapidly. Therefore, thoracentesis is done at frequent intervals to provide comfort and relieve dyspnea. The fluid is protein rich and hypoalbuminemia may result. Use of oral diuretics such as spironolactone has been suggested (Nevidjion & Sowers, 2000).

Nursing Management

Nursing assessment includes regular evaluation of the lung sounds. Pulse oximetry is used to assess oxygen saturation. The nurse provides symptomatic relief of dyspnea and pain. If a chest tube is placed, the nurse positions the patient and offers support during the thoracentesis procedure. Pain management is a priority, and the nurse assists the patient to assume positions of comfort and offers analgesics as needed. The nurse continues to assess levels of dyspnea and provides supplemental oxygen, bronchodilators, and opioid analgesics such as morphine for relief of dyspnea (Kvale et al., 2003). This procedure prevents reaccumulation of pleural fluid in the pleural space (Taubert, 2001).

If a chest tube and water seal system are used, the nurse monitors the system function and records the amount of drainage at frequent intervals. The patient is encouraged to turn frequently and ambulate to facilitate chest drainage. Care of the patient with a chest tube is discussed later in this chapter. The nurse also monitors electrolytes for imbalances and intake and output as indicated (see Chapter 18 ⊘).

Discharge Priorities

Patients may be discharged with a pleural catheter for drainage. The nurse is responsible for educating the patient and family regarding management and care of the catheter and drainage system. Another important issue for patient education is pain management. The patient and family should be given concrete instructions on medications to be taken for pain and what to do for breakthrough pain. Patients and families should be instructed to call the health care provider or health care team if dyspnea and discomfort are not relieved by the regimen suggested for discharge.

Chest Trauma and Thoracic Injuries

Chest trauma is the cause of nearly 16,000 deaths in the United States each year and the cause of death in

25% of all trauma patients. Chapter 73 ⊘ discusses chest trauma. Increased hand gun use has contributed to the rise in the number of penetrating injuries (Reeder & Danis, 2001). These injuries impair airway patency, breathing, and circulation so the role of the nurse in maintaining an excellent standard of care in these situations is paramount.

Rib and Sternal Fractures

Rib fractures are the most common blunt thoracic injury in adults. These are frequently associated with other injuries such as flail chest, pulmonary contusion, and pneumothorax.

Epidemiology and Etiology

Rib fractures usually are caused by a direct blow to the ribs. Another mechanism of injury may be due to a forceful compression of the rib cage, as can happen in a "pileup" during a football game (Cerro Coso Coyote Athletics [CCCA], 2004). The most important cause of significant blunt chest trauma is motor vehicle crashes (MVCs). MVCs account for 70% to 80% of such injuries (Sawyer, 2006).

Sternal fractures are most common in MVCs that result in a direct blow to the sternum via the steering wheel, and are most common in female patients over age 50 and those using shoulder restraints (Owens, Chaudry, Eggerstedt, & Smith, 2000). A fracture occurs because the pressure of an injury interrupts the bony integrity of the rib or the sternum. Ribs tend to break just in front of the angle, which is its weakest point. Ribs 4 through 9 are the most likely to be injured by direct blows because they are not protected by the shoulder girdle (CCCA, 2004). The incidence of fractured ribs in patients presenting to the operating department for emergency surgery is more than 60% (CCCA, 2004).

Flail Chest

A **flail chest** occurs when an injury causes a segment of the thoracic cage to be separated from the rest of the chest wall. This usually occurs when at least two fractures per rib occur (producing a free segment), in at least two ribs (Figure 35–14 ■). The significance of a flail chest is that it indicates the presence of an underlying pulmonary contusion, as described in a later section. The separated segment is unable to con-

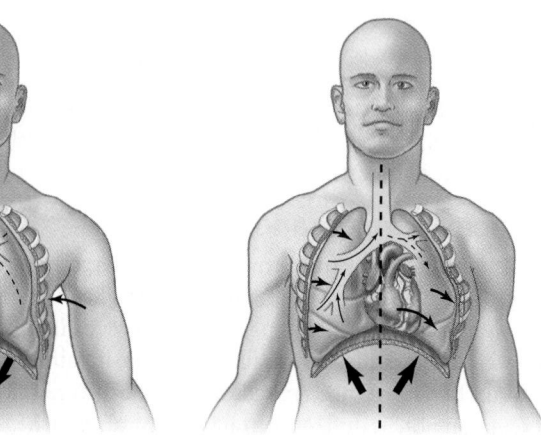

(a) Inspiration **(b) Expiration**

FIGURE 35–14 ■ Flail chest.

tribute to lung expansion; in fact, during spontaneous ventilation the floating segment moves in the opposite direction or paradoxically to the chest wall. Large flail segments will involve a much greater proportion of the chest wall and may extend bilaterally or involve the sternum. In most cases, the severity and extent of the lung injury determine the clinical course and requirement for mechanical ventilation. Thus, the management of flail chest consists of standard management of the rib fractures and of the pulmonary contusions underneath (Trauma.org, 2004).

Laboratory and Diagnostic Procedures

Chest radiography should be obtained to detect rib fractures, but also to look for associated injuries such as pneumothorax, hemothorax, or pulmonary contusion (Devitt, 1995). The patient with a sternal fracture is evaluated closely for underlying cardiac injuries. An ECG should be done and the oxygenation should be monitored with pulse oximetry and ABGs.

No single condition confirms the diagnosis of flail chest. Chest x-ray and ABG measurements along with the patient's description of the pain along the ribs contributes to the diagnostic information. A CT scan also may be useful (Bjerke, 2002).

Clinical Manifestations

The clinical manifestations associated with rib fractures include severe localized pain, which is usually increased on movement of the ribs, deep breathing, coughing, or sneezing. An individual with a rib fracture usually will refrain from breathing deeply by taking shallow breaths, and may also hold the injured side in an attempt to restrict painful movement of the chest. Palpation of the ribs with gentle compression will indicate pain at the fracture site. If the fracture is displaced, there may be a palpable defect and crepitation on movement or coughing. Complications of a rib fracture also can occur with a puncture of the thoracic or visceral structures (Sawyer, 2006; Shahani, 2006). The signs and symptoms of a sternal fracture are similar to a rib fracture except that tenderness exists along the sternum (CCCA, 2004). There also may be anterior chest pain, tenderness, ecchymosis, swelling, and the potential for a chest wall deformity. If there are cardiac complications, crepitus may be detected upon auscultation and subcutaneous emphysema may be palpated.

The patient with flail chest engages in splinting with each breath because of pain, and intrusion of the flail segment on the contusion leads to increased work of breathing and pulmonary shunting with hypoxia (Devitt, 1995). As a result, the patient experiences severe respiratory distress.

Medical Management

The aim of medical management with a chest wall injury is directed toward protecting the underlying lung and allowing adequate oxygenation, ventilation, and pulmonary toilet. This approach will help prevent the most common complication, pneumonia. This is a particular concern in the elderly patient who is at a higher risk for the development of pneumonia and respiratory failure if not appropriately managed. Most commonly patients initially are placed on 100% oxygen via a nonrebreather face mask (Trauma.org, 2004). Oxygen saturation and ABGs are monitored regularly and when changes occur.

Analgesia is a crucial component in the management of rib fractures. Although strapping the chest to splint rib fractures may help with pain, the strapping impedes chest wall movement and prevents adequate inspiration and clearance of secretions. Sedation and pain management allow the patient to begin deep breathing and coughing in order to prevent the development of atelectasis, pneumonitis, and hypoxemia. Opioid analgesics are useful, but must be monitored carefully for respiratory depression, especially in the elderly. Patient-controlled administration of an opioid infusion is an effective method for cooperative patients. Chapter 15 ⊙ includes a complete discussion of patient-controlled analgesia (PCA) for pain management.

The addition of a nonsteroidal anti-inflammatory drug (NSAID) may provide adequate relief, but these should be withheld until other injuries have been excluded (e.g., traumatic brain injury) and used with caution in the elderly. Epidural analgesia for a severe chest wall injury is effective because it provides complete analgesia, allowing normal inspiration and coughing without the risks of respiratory depression. Alternative pain management strategies include intercostal nerve block, ice over the site, epidural analgesia, PCA, and nonopioid analgesia. The pain usually diminishes by the fifth to the seventh day, and healing occurs in 3 to 6 weeks.

Intubation and mechanical ventilation are rarely indicated for chest wall injury alone. Where ventilation is necessary, it is usually for hypoxia due to flail chest and underlying pulmonary contusions. Ventilation is usually necessary only until the resolution of the pulmonary contusion. Positive pressure ventilation may be required for severe chest wall instability that results in inadequate spontaneous ventilation. The patient also is evaluated for any injuries that are associated with the rib fractures. Surgical fixation usually is not necessary unless fragments pose a potential for further injury.

▮ Nursing Management

Nursing management in the emergency setting for patients with rib fractures involves astute assessment for respiratory complications and diligent patient monitoring for dyspnea, hypoxemia, and pain. The nurse emphasizes pain management and gives specific instructions regarding medications for pain until the pain diminishes. The nurse administers pain medication and assesses for pain relief. The nurse assists the patient with coughing and deep breathing techniques, monitors patient response, and auscultates lung fields regularly for adventitious sounds. If the patient is receiving a narcotic and is using PCA, the nurse assesses the rate of breathing, level of alertness, and the presence of hypoxemia hourly. Research shows that patients with flail chest often continue to experience chronic pain, dyspnea, and disability for 6 months.

Discharge Priorities

The patient should be given written instructions regarding the plan of care. Patients and caregivers should be encouraged to call members of the health team for persistent problems such as pain or dyspnea. Patients may be reluctant to ask for more pain medication when it is needed, so the nurse stresses that healing will not occur unless the patient feels comfortable breathing and coughing. The patient should be well versed in situations that would constitute an emergency visit to the hospital and be given resources for handling problem situations. Patients should be aware of emergency contacts in case of increasing dyspnea and pain.

Pulmonary Contusion

A **pulmonary contusion** is an injury to the lung parenchyma, leading to edema and blood collecting in alveolar spaces and loss of normal lung structure and function.

This blunt injury develops over 24 hours, leading to poor gas exchange, increased pulmonary vascular resistance, and decreased lung compliance. There also is a significant inflammatory reaction to blood components in the lung, and 50% to 60% of patients with significant contusions develop bilateral acute respiratory distress syndrome (ARDS) (Wanek & Mayberry, 2004).

Epidemiology and Etiology

The most common cause of pulmonary contusion is trauma. It occurs in 20% of blunt trauma patients with significant injuries. The mortality ranges from 10% to 25%, and 40% to 60% for patients who require mechanical ventilation.

Clinical Manifestations

There are few clinical signs of contusion. Crackles may be heard on auscultation but are rarely heard in the emergency setting on admission. Rib fractures, flail chest, or bruising on the chest indicates the possibility of contusion. Frequently, if the patient has significant chest wall injury, pain will affect the ability to ventilate and clear secretions.

Laboratory and Diagnostic Procedures

Pulmonary contusions are rarely diagnosed on physical examination. Most significant contusions are diagnosed by chest x-ray; however, an x-ray will often underestimate the size of the contusion and lags behind the clinical picture. The true extent of injury may not be present on chest x-ray for 24 to 48 hours (Wanek & Mayberry, 2004). CT scan is very sensitive for identification of pulmonary contusion and may allow for differentiation from areas of atelectasis and or aspiration (2004). ABGs and/or pulse oximetry may be used to assess for hypoxemia and gas exchange.

Medical Management

The patient is monitored closely for hypoxemia. Supplemental oxygen is delivered as needed. If the patient has extreme difficulty with ventilation and clearing of secretions because of pain, intubation and mechanical ventilation are necessary. Patient management involves fluid restriction in order to prevent pulmonary edema and increasing respiratory insufficiency. Usually pulmonary contusions resolve in 3 to 5 days. The main complications are ARDS and pneumonia (Wanek & Mayberry 2004). (ARDS is discussed in Chapter 36 .) Careful discharge planning should allow for maximal supervision in the first few weeks af-

ter discharge. To accomplish patient care goals, the nurse collaborates with the health care provider and respiratory therapist. A referral to a home health nurse may be necessary if the patient is alone or without a supportive environment.

■ Nursing Management

The nurse focuses on assessment for hypoxemia and worsening pain or atelectasis. Management of pain is essential for pulmonary toilet. If fluid restrictions are in place, the nurse monitors fluids closely and frequently assesses the patient's respiratory status.

Pneumothorax

Under normal circumstances the pleural cavity is free of air. When air or gas enters the pleural space, it is referred to as a **pneumothorax**, which results in a partial or complete collapse of the lung on the affected side. It is caused by a rupture in the visceral pleura or the parietal pleura and chest wall. As air separates the pleura, it destroys the negative pressure of the pleural space, disrupting the normal state of equilibrium. Because it is no longer held in check by the recoil forces of the chest wall, the lung recoils and collapses toward the hilus (McCance & Huether, 2007). This may occur spontaneously or without obvious cause or as a result of trauma. Figure 35–15 ■ shows a tension pneumothorax.

Spontaneous Pneumothorax: Epidemiology, Etiology, and Pathophysiology

This anomaly occurs unexpectedly in healthy individuals between the ages of 20 and 40; therefore, it is referred to as spontaneous pneumothorax. It occurs more commonly in men who tend to be taller and thinner than most individuals (Fishman et al., 2002). Smoking also is a risk factor, due to disease it causes in the small airways. The cause of the pneumothorax is a ruptured, air-filled bleb or blister on the lung surface. Bleb rupture allows

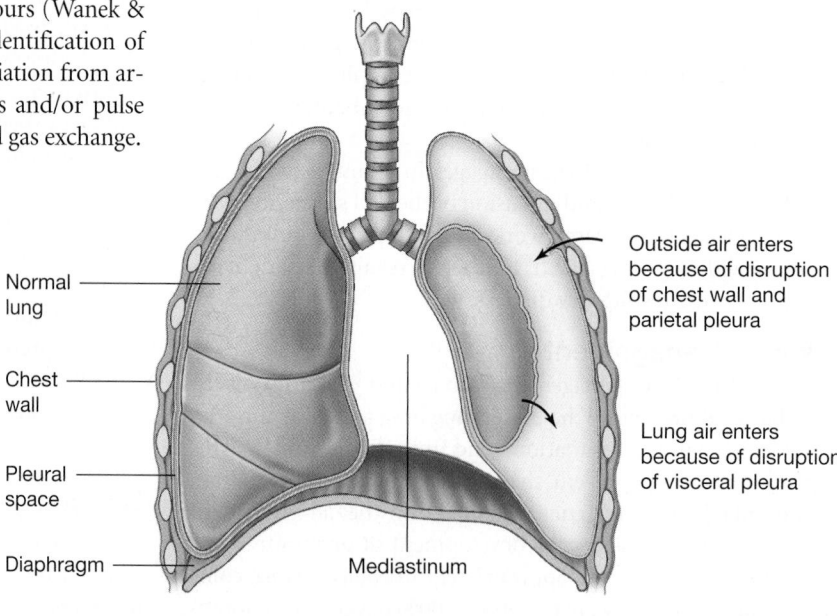

Normal lung

Chest wall

Pleural space

Diaphragm

Mediastinum

Outside air enters because of disruption of chest wall and parietal pleura

Lung air enters because of disruption of visceral pleura

FIGURE 35–15 ■ Tension pneumothorax.

atmospheric air to enter the pleural cavity, resulting in a loss of negative pressure and collapse of the lung (Porth, 2007). How the bleb ruptures is not fully understood but 80% of patients have emphysema-like changes in the lung whether they smoke or do not have blebs (McCance & Huether, 2007). Blebs on the visceral pleura rupture during sleep, rest, or exercise. These blebs usually are located on the apexes of the lung. Tension pneumothorax can develop with this rupture (McCance & Huether, 2007).

Traumatic Pneumothorax: Etiology

The most common causes of traumatic pneumothoraxes are penetrating chest injures such as bullets or stab wounds, and fractured ribs that penetrate the pleura. Hemothorax is frequently associated with these injuries. A traumatic pneumothorax may also occur with fracture of the trachea, bronchus, or esophagus (Porth, 2007).

Aside from trauma, tension pneumothorax can be caused by central venous catheterization and mechanical ventilation in which peak inspiratory pressure rises when the patient fights the ventilator. This more commonly occurs in patients with COPD receiving positive end-expiratory pressure (PEEP) during mechanical ventilation (Fishman et al., 2002).

Tension Pneumothorax: Epidemiology, Etiology, and Pathophysiology

A tension pneumothorax is one of the rapidly developing complications of blunt chest trauma and occurs as a result of an air leak in the lung or chest wall. It often is caused by blunt chest trauma in which the parenchymal injury has failed to seal and causes complete collapse of the lung. The air that enters the pleural space during expiration does not exit during inspiration due to the damaged tissue acting as a one-way valve. In addition to this mechanism, the positive pressure used with mechanical ventilation therapy can cause air trapping and increased intrapleural pressure. This increased pressure pushes the heart and mediastinal structures to the contralateral side. The mediastinum impinges on and compresses the contralateral lung. Hypoxia results as the collapsed lung on the affected side and the compressed lung on the contralateral side are compromised resulting in a diminished ability to effectively exchange gas. This hypoxia and decreased venous return caused by compression of the relatively thin walls of the atria impair cardiac function, thereby decreasing cardiac output and resulting in hypotension and, ultimately, hemodynamic collapse and death if untreated (Bowman, 2006).

Hemothorax: Epidemiology, Etiology, and Pathophysiology

Hemothorax is one of the most common problems encountered following blunt chest trauma. A simple hemothorax is defined as blood loss of less than 2,000 mL into the thoracic cavity. The absence of breath sounds over the lung and dullness to percussion are characteristic signs of a hemothorax (Fishman et al., 2002). Bleeding is caused by injuries to the lung parenchyma, such as pulmonary contusions and lacerations, which often are associated with rib and sternal fractures. Massive intrathoracic bleeding in blunt chest trauma usually stems from the heart, great vessels, or major systemic arteries. Chest surgery may

cause what is classified as a traumatic pneumothorax as a result of air and fluid seeping into the pleural space. It also may emerge as a result of a malignancy that damages blood vessels. As air and blood separate the pleurae, it destroys the negative pressure of the pleural space disrupting the normal state of equilibrium. The lung recoils and collapses toward the hilus (McCance & Huether, 2007).

Pneumothorax and Hemothorax: Clinical Manifestations

Patients with pneumothorax or hemothorax present with pleuritic pain or breathlessness, or both, which can be life threatening. Respiratory distress, which can lead to respiratory arrest if untreated, is also present. The specific manifestations depend on the size of the pneumothorax. Patients may experience increasing levels of agitation especially if this is a sudden event. If cardiac output is affected blood pressure will drop and the patient will be tachycardic (Woodruff, 1999). Upon auscultation, breath sounds are unilaterally decreased or absent and the percussion note is hyperresonant or very loud. Hyperresonance and tracheal deviation are late findings (Woodruff, 1999). Hypotension is typically considered a key sign of a tension pneumothorax and typically occurs immediately before cardiovascular collapse (Bowman, 2006).

Laboratory and Diagnostic Procedures

Plain chest radiography is done and shows lung collapse and air in the pleural space (Ross, 2003). With hemothorax, chest radiography shows fluid accumulation in the pleural space or may show haziness if the quantity of blood in the chest is small. CT scanning is used after the individual is stabilized to determine the risk of recurrence. A CT scan is more sensitive than a chest radiograph in the evaluation of small pneumothoraxes. ABG analysis may be useful in evaluating for hypoxia, hypercarbia, and respiratory acidosis (Bowman, 2006).

Medical Management

The patient with a pneumothorax is experiencing dyspnea and anxiety. Pulse oximetry is used to document oxygen saturation. Based on this and the degree of dyspnea experienced by the patient, supplemental oxygen is given to treat hypoxemia. If a tension pneumothorax is present, the patient may experience severe air hunger and may require higher concentrations of supplemental oxygen. Lung reexpansion is accomplished by inserting a chest tube or chest drainage device. The patient may require mechanical ventilation.

Needle aspiration is a less invasive way of treating pneumothorax. A needle is inserted into the pleural space and air is withdrawn. This approach is not as successful as a chest tube, but it is less painful (Woodruff, 1999). Another approach to correcting a pneumothorax is to use a Heimlich valve, which is typically used as a stopgap measure until a tube can be placed. The valve attaches to a chest tube and is inserted into the chest. As the patient exhales, air and fluid drain through the valve into a plastic bag. When the patient inhales, the flexible tubing in the valve collapses, preventing secretions and air from reentering the pleura (Woodruff, 1999).

■ Nursing Management

The nurse must act promptly to assess pulmonary status quickly and to mobilize the health team to provide reexpansion of the lung via a chest tube. The nurse focuses on relieving dyspnea and supporting oxygenation. The patient may need supplemental oxygen and possibly mechanical ventilation.

Assessment, Interventions, and Rationales

Oxygen saturation and ABGs are monitored to assess the oxygen status. Equipment is prepared for insertion of a chest tube. The nurse explains the rationale for all treatments in advance and often assists with its preparation. Insertion of a chest tube is painful for the patient, so the nurse assists in providing a local anesthetic, IV pain medication, and a sedative (Woodruff, 1999).

The chest tube is attached to a water-controlled device, and usually suction is applied to 20 mmHg pressure. There should be gentle bubbling in the suction control chamber, the water column in the water seal should rise and fall unless air is escaping from the chest cavity, and there should be no kinks or dependent loops in the tubing (see Chapter 36 ✏). Bubbling in the water seal should occur during the initial reexpansion of the lung, but should then subside. In the case of a hemothorax, the nurse assesses vital signs regularly in order to establish blood loss and replenish blood and fluids. The nurse assesses for an excessive amount of bloody drainage in a short period and a repeat chest x-ray should be done in a few hours (Fishman et al., 2002).

Discharge Priorities

The patient should be given written instructions regarding the plan of care. Patients and caregivers should be encouraged to call members of the health team for persistent problems such as pain, dyspnea, congestion, or increasing sputum production. Patients may be reluctant to ask for more pain medication when it is needed, so the nurse needs to stress that healing will not occur unless the patient feels comfortable breathing and coughing. The patient should be made aware of symptoms that are emergency situations and receive resources for handling them.

Health Promotion

Once a patient has experienced a pneumothorax, he needs to understand that it could occur again. The nurse must stress that if the clinical manifestations reappear the patient must seek immediate medical help. The nurse reviews signs and symptoms of breathlessness and anxiety for which the patient and caregiver should seek emergency treatment. When a patient is admitted with a spontaneous pneumothorax, the individual should receive guidance from a pulmonary specialist regarding follow-up treatment and risk factors. The patient should be given information regarding the cause of the pneumothorax. If the health care provider believes pulmonary changes are related to genetic causes, the individual should be counseled regarding follow-up genetic testing and necessary lifestyle changes. The patient who smokes should be guided to quit smoking.

■ Nursing Management of a Patient with a Chest Tube

Many patients who are mechanically ventilated have chest tubes, and part of the nursing management is ensuring that the chest drainage system is intact and functioning properly. There are two types of chest tubes: pleural tubes and mediastinal tubes. A pleural tube is inserted in the pleural space in order to evacuate the air or blood and allow the lung to reexpand. The pleural tube re-creates the normal negative pressure in the chest that has been violated by trauma or surgery. Indications for insertion of a pleural tube include all the conditions listed in Chart 35–7.

A mediastinal tube is placed in the mediastinum after this area has been opened during cardiac or thoracic surgery. Mediastinal tubes prevent fluid and blood from collecting in the mediastinum and exerting pressure on the heart. These tubes do not look any different from pleural tubes. Usually they are inserted in the subxiphoid area, but only the surgeon or the operative report can alert the nurse to the difference in the two types of chest tubes.

Assessment

Pleural tubes are connected to underwater seal drainage or connected to a one-way valve. These devices, either the underwater seal or one-way valve, allow air to exit the chest but prevent air from entering the chest. Pleural tubes exhibit a characteristic called tidaling. With inspiration, the fluid in the tube can be seen moving with respiration. If there is no fluid in the tube, many chest drainage systems have a fluid diagnostic chamber. In this chamber the tidaling can be seen. It is important to assess this fluid movement either in the tube or in the diagnostic fluid chamber to ensure that the chest tube is in the thoracic cavity and there is no blockage.

Mediastinal tubes exhibit no tidaling because they are located in the mediastinal space and not the pleural space. Mediastinal tubes usually drain blood or other fluid. An important intervention with these tubes is to ensure that they are patent and draining freely. Most chest tube systems have available an autotransfusion unit attachment so that blood can be reinfused.

CHART 35–7 | **Indications for Insertion of a Chest Tube**

INDICATIONS FOR A PLEURAL TUBE

- Hemothorax
- Pneumothorax
- Hemopneumothorax
- Pleural effusion
- Drainage of pus (empyema), bile (cholothorax), or chyle (chylothorax) from the pleural cavity
- Postoperative thoracostomy

INDICATIONS FOR A MEDIASTINAL TUBE

- Drainage of the mediastinal space after surgical procedure
- Cardiac surgery
- Pericardial window

Initially chest tubes are connected to suction to increase the drainage and to assist the lungs in reexpansion. The suction is most commonly set at 20 cm of water pressure. Though not recommended, disconnecting the chest tube from suction does not allow air to enter the chest but only stops the suction. As the drainage diminishes and the lung reexpands frequently, the heath care provider will discontinue the suction for a few hours prior to removal.

No chest tube should ever be clamped except under direct observation prior to removal. Clamping a chest tube can allow a tension pneumothorax to develop. The risk of a tension pneumothorax is increased when a patient is receiving positive pressure ventilation.

 Never clamp a chest tube except under direct observation prior to removing the tube.

Insertion of a Chest Tube

The equipment needed for insertion of a chest tube is listed in Chart 35–8. Pleural tubes commonly are inserted at the bedside, whereas mediastinal tubes are inserted in the operating room during surgery. The location on the chest of the tube is related to the reason for the chest tube insertion. If a chest tube is inserted to decompress a pneumothorax, it usually is inserted anteriorly, whereas a chest tube that is inserted to drain fluid or blood from the chest is inserted in a more posterior location on the chest wall. Air rises to the anterior surface of the chest when a patient is supine; therefore, placement of a chest tube is anterior if insertion is required because of a pneumothorax. However, if there is blood in the pleural space, a chest tube will be

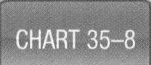 **Necessary Equipment for Insertion of a Chest Tube**

Chest tube insertion tray

Tube (size specified by health care provider)

Scalpel with size 11 blade

Several dissecting, such as curved Kelly clamps or artery forceps

A 10-mL syringe and a 20-ml syringe

One small-gauge needle (size 25)

A needle driver

Local anesthetic (Xylocaine)

Betadine (or other antiseptic)

Scissors

One packet of strong, non-absorbable, curved sutures of size 1.0 or larger, made from silk or nylon

Sterile gloves

4 × 4's

Suction setup

Suction tubing

Chest tube collection system

Vaseline gauze

Silk tape

Source: This article was published in *The AACN Procedure Manual,* 4th ed., p. 110, Lynn-McHale, D. & Carlson, K. Copyright W. B. Sanders, Philadelphia, 2001.

placed posteriorly because the blood will settle in the posterior of the chest cavity. Many different types of chest tube drainage systems are commercially available. Figure 35–16 ■ (p. 992) shows an example of one of those devices.

Near Drowning

Near drowning connotes an immersion episode of sufficient severity that it could lead to morbidity and death and, hence, warrants medical attention (Shepherd, 2003). To be categorized as a near drowning the patient must survive for at least 24 hours after submersion. Immersion in water causes laryngospasm and pulmonary injury resulting in hypoxemia and its effects on the brain and other organs.

Epidemiology and Etiology

Young adults typically drown in lakes, ponds, rivers, and oceans. Diving accidents are a common cause, and alcohol and recreational drugs have been implicated in many cases. Research shows that 30% to 50% of older adolescents and adults who drowned in boating accidents were inebriated (Shepherd, 2003). In the United States drowning deaths number more than 6,500 per year. The highest numbers are in toddlers and adolescent males. Drowning is second only to motor vehicle crashes as the most common cause of injury in children ages 1 month to 14 years. The true incidence of near drowning has yet to be reported, but it is estimated in the range of 20 to 500 times the rate of drowning (Shepherd, 2003).

Pathophysiology

After initial gasping, and possible aspiration, immersion stimulates hyperventilation, followed by involuntary apnea and laryngospasm leading to hypoxemia. The patient is likely to develop cardiac arrest and CNS ischemia. Asphyxia leads to relaxation of the airway, which permits the lungs to fill with water in many individuals (wet drowning). Approximately 10% to 20% of individuals maintain tight laryngospasm until cardiac arrest occurs. Inhalation of water causes pulmonary vasoconstriction, hypertension, destruction of surfactant, alveolar instability, and atelectasis (Shepherd, 2003).

Laboratory and Diagnostic Procedures

ABG analysis is the most reliable clinical parameter to assess level of hypoxia. In addition a complete blood count (CBC), electrolytes, and a coagulation profile are done. Lymphocytosis is commonly seen as well as elevated serum creatinine due to acute renal failure. A chest x-ray is done to determine evidence of aspiration, pulmonary edema, or atelectasis (Shepherd, 2003).

Medical and Nursing Management

Victims of submersion are classified into one of four groups:

1. Asymptomatic
2. Symptomatic
3. Cardiopulmonary arrest
4. Obviously dead.

Symptoms associated with near drowning are hypothermia, tachycardia, bradycardia, anxious appearance, tachypnea, dyspnea or hypoxia, metabolic acidosis, and altered level of consciousness.

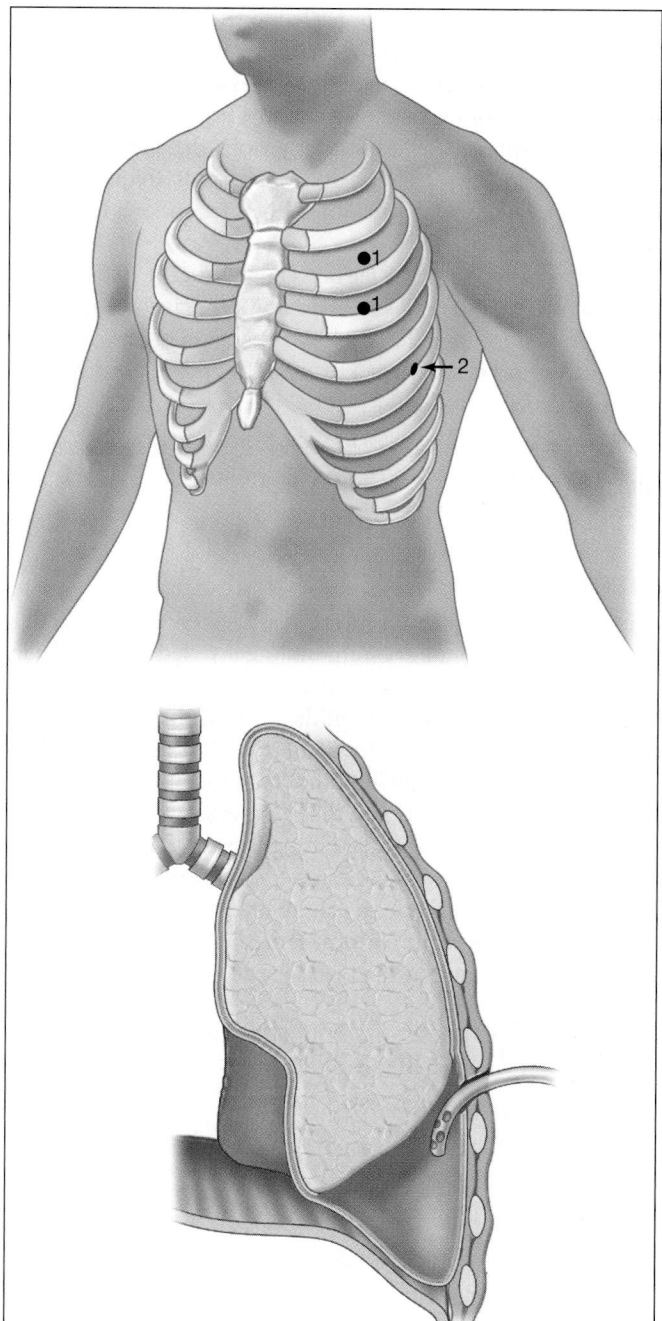

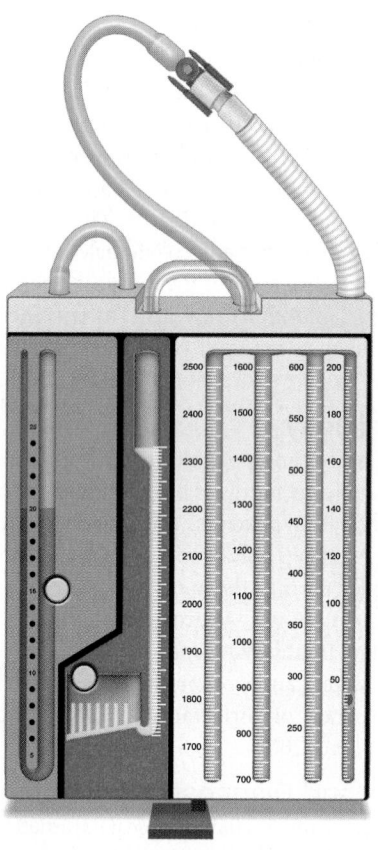

FIGURE 35–16 ■ Chest tube drainage.

In the emergency department phase of treatment, the patient in respiratory failure is intubated, mechanically ventilated, and rewarmed to 30°C (86°F). A nasogastric tube is inserted to decompress the stomach and prevent aspiration. The patient is treated for electrolyte imbalances, seizures, bronchospasm, atelectasis, dysrhythmias, and hypotension as necessary. Resuscitation efforts are not abandoned until the patient is rewarmed. Patients who are alert and oriented are observed in the emergency department until the ABGs become normal and there is an absence of dysrhythmias. If hypoxemia or other complications do not resolve, patients are admitted for observation and treatment (Shepherd, 2003). Possible complications are acute renal failure, ischemic cerebral injury, ARDS, pulmonary damage secondary to the drowning episode, and cardiac arrest.

Key health team members that the nurse collaborates with are the health care provider and respiratory therapist. If a social worker or liaison person is available to keep family members abreast of the patient situation, this is very helpful. The nurse obtains a history from the patient and family members to determine the cause of drowning and the type of water. The nurse assists the emergency department team in stabilizing the patient and communicates the patient status to family members. The major focus of nursing care is assessment and treatment of hypoxemia.

Carbon Monoxide Poisoning

Carbon monoxide poisoning occurs when an individual breathes carbon monoxide fumes that have built up in an enclosed space (CDC, 2004a). Carbon monoxide or CO is an odorless, colorless gas that can cause sudden illness or death. It is found in combustion fumes such as those produced by cars and trucks, small gasoline engines, stoves, lanterns, burning charcoal and wood, and gas ranges and heating systems. Persons who attempt suicide or are victims of smoke inhalation are poisoned with carbon monoxide (Fishman et al., 2002).

Epidemiology, Etiology, and Pathophysiology

Each year more than 500 Americans die from unintentional carbon monoxide poisoning and 2,000 commit suicide by intentionally poisoning themselves (CDC, 2004a). The ultimate injury that carbon monoxide produces is caused by hypoxia. Normally oxygen is carried to the tissues via the hemoglobin in red blood cells. Because carbon monoxide's affinity for hemoglobin is 300 times greater than that of oxygen, it quickly binds with hemoglobin, preventing oxygen molecules from doing so (McCance & Huether, 2007).

Laboratory and Diagnostic Procedures, Clinical Manifestations, and Medical and Nursing Management

Diagnostic tests are not as reliable as clinical assessment in the case of CO poisoning. Pulse oximetry is not valid because the hemoglobin is well saturated. ABG studies often are done to assess oxygen content as well as a chest x-ray to visualize the lung fields. Carboxyhemoglobin blood levels provide guidelines for treatment. Levels of greater than 40% are considered severe (Fishman et al., 2002). Symptoms related to CO poisoning include headache, giddiness, tinnitus, nausea, weakness, and vomiting. Persons at risk are smokers, coal miners, firefighters, unborn babies, and persons with chronic heart disease.

The nursing role is to participate with the emergency department team in stabilizing the patient and to communicate the patient status to family members. The major focus of nursing care is assessment and treatment of hypoxemia and management of mental status changes. The prognosis in carbon monoxide poisoning depends on the level of carbon monoxide inhaled. All persons who are victims of significant smoke inhalation should be resuscitated and transported on 100% oxygen. Hyperbaric oxygen therapy is the treatment of choice; this hastens clearance of carbon monoxide and decreases neurotoxicities, which include hallucinations, ataxia, visual disturbances, headaches, and psychoses (Fishman et al., 2002). The alternative treatment is treatment with 100% oxygen. This usually requires intubation and mechanical ventilation. Oxygen should be administered until the carbon monoxide level is less than 5%. In spite of this, mental status changes may persist and may be a sign of permanent brain damage.

Health Promotion

Educating the public regarding the dangers of smoking and the dangers of allowing exhaust fumes to be present in small enclosed places are preventive activities that increase awareness of the dangers of carbon monoxide. Advocating for the presence of smoke alarms and maintenance of fire safety regulations in all public and private buildings is another preventive strategy to promote community awareness of the problem. Nurses in home care and public health should make fire safety and the possibility of carbon monoxide escape a topic for environmental assessments. When unintentional carbon monoxide poisoning occurs,

the health department should be contacted. Upon discharge, patients and families should be instructed to seek assistance if they experience dyspnea, confusion, altered levels of consciousness, hallucinations, weakness, or nausea.

■ Lung Cancer

Globally, lung cancer is the most common form of cancer; however, in the United States it is the second most common occurring malignancy (Parkin, Bray, & Ferlay, 2005). This disease accounts for the majority of cancer deaths among men since the 1950s and women since 1987 (ACS, 2006). In recent years the seriousness of lung cancer gained the public's attention as many Americans mourned the deaths of news anchorman Peter Jennings and Dana Reeve, wife of *Superman* star Christopher Reeve.

Epidemiology and Etiology

Efforts to combat the prevalence of lung cancer have been targeted at preventing exposure to known risk factors. Cellular genetic destruction results from repeated exposure to carcinogens such as tobacco smoke, radon, and asbestos. Smoking accounts for 87% of all lung cancer deaths (ACS, 2006); approximately 3,000 of these cases are due to environmental tobacco smoke (ETS) commonly referred to as "secondhand smoke." Exposure to radon, a colorless, odorless, radioactive gas, occurs in places where there is reduced air turnover and ventilation, as in underground mines.

Asbestos can still be found in products such as gaskets and roofing and friction items. Exposure occurs not only during the mining and manufacturing of these products but when we are at home, at the office, and in school (National Cancer Institute [NCI], 2005a). Other risk factors such as occupational hazards, air pollution, genetics, dietary factors, advancing age, and race are continuously being studied in an effort to determine more effective strategies to reduce mortality due to exposure. Chapter 64 ☺ presents detailed information regarding cancer risk factors and recommended prevention programs.

Prevention of lung cancer has been primarily aimed at reducing the incidence of smoking. Persons who quit smoking reduce the risk of developing lung cancer over time. Those who refrain from smoking for approximately 10 years will reduce their risk of dying from this disease by 30% to 50% (NCI, 2005b). Multiple resources are now available for nurses and other clinicians as they develop programs designed to help patients and their families understand the importance of smoking cessation.

Pathophysiology

The World Health Organization has identified four major histologic types of lung cancer. These include small cell carcinoma, squamous cell carcinoma, adenocarcinoma, and large cell carcinoma. In the United States 85% of all lung cancers are non–small cell lung cancer (NSCLC) and 15% account for small cell lung cancer (SCLC) (National Comprehensive Cancer Network [NCCN], 2007). SCLC behaves differently from other cell types. Its unique ability to spread and be widely disseminated by the time of diagnosis leads to a poor prognosis, often survival ranging from only 2 to 4 months.

NSCLCs, including squamous cell carcinoma, adenocarcinoma, and large cell carcinoma, all have unique patterns of growth and clinical appearance. Squamous cell tumors typically originate in the proximal bronchi and account for 30% of all lung cancers (Hoffman & Gift, 2007). These malignancies have a tendency to be slow growing, such that a visible mass may not be detected for 3 to 4 years.

Adenocarcinoma is the most common form of lung cancer and the most common cell type in nonsmokers. Cancer cells can be found in the periphery of the lung and are known to present with fewer pulmonary symptoms than those that originate in the central portion of the lung parenchyma. Progression is slow; however, adenocarcinoma invades the lymphatic and blood vessels early in the disease, resulting in a worse prognosis compared to that for SCLCs. Large cell lung cancer commonly is located in the periphery of the lung, often times spreading to the subsegmental bronchi or larger airways. Because this cell type is poorly differentiated and possesses neuroendocrine features, the prognosis is often times very poor. Common metastatic sites for all types of lung cancer include liver, bone, adrenal glands, and the brain. For a more detailed discussion of the pathophysiology of cancer, refer to Chapter 64 🔗.

Clinical Manifestations

Persons with lung cancer access the health care system when they have begun to experience multiple serious symptoms. This makes it very difficult for the patient to function physically, psychologically, and socially. A comprehensive history and physical includes obtaining an accurate history of risk factors. This information combined with the physical symptoms paints a more complete picture indicative of lung cancer. Respiratory symptoms include cough, dyspnea, sputum production, wheezing, hemoptysis, and chest pain. These symptoms need to be explored further so their origin can be identified. Additional manifestations include dysphagia, hoarseness, pain, fatigue, weakness, nausea, disturbed sleep, memory impairments, anorexia, and night sweats.

Lung cancers can produce complications that require the nurse to use sharp assessment skills and to have the ability to recognize manifestations that need immediate interventions. Examples of these complications include superior vena cava syndrome and paraneoplastic syndromes. Superior vena cava syndrome is an oncologic emergency that occurs when a tumor obstructs the superior vena cava, resulting in facial swelling, hands, arm, and neck swelling, distended neck veins, cyanosis of the upper torso, and dyspnea (Aurora, Milite, & Vander Els, 2000). Paraneoplastic syndromes (Cushing's syndrome, syndrome of inappropriate antidiuretic hormone [SIADH], and hypercalcemia) are considered metabolic emergencies that disrupt the homeostasis of vital body functions.

Laboratory and Diagnostic Procedures

Early diagnosis of lung cancer is difficult because most patients do not experience symptoms until the disease has begun metastasize. For those patients who have a localized malignancy without metastasis the likelihood of a 5-year survival rate is 50% (ACS, 2006). Initially, noninvasive tests are done to confirm the type of tumor, clinical stage, and additional information related to any preexisting conditions that may impact the recommended treatment plan (NCCN, 2007). Blood sampling for CBC, liver enzymes, and chemistries provides the clinician with information related to existing comorbidities, possible metasta-

tic disease, and complications commonly found with lung cancer (e.g., paraneoplastic syndromes).

An ECG and pulmonary function tests may be ordered to determine baseline pulmonary and cardiac function, especially if radiation therapy will be part of the treatment plan. Chest x-rays and chest CT scans are commonly used to assess the primary tumor, lymph node involvement, and the possible spread to other organs. Although MRI is infrequently done, it is helpful if there is suspected involvement of the CNS or spinal cord.

Invasive diagnostic tests are done to obtain tissue samples, which are used to diagnose the presence of lung cancer, determine the presence of cancer spread, and confirm whether lymph nodes are malignant or benign (Hoffman & Gift, 2007). Sputum cytology is useful to identify cancerous cells in those patients who experience hemoptysis. Direct tissue sampling is done via bronchoscopy. This test provides the clinician with information related to cell type and ultimately formalizing the diagnosis of lung cancer. Occasionally, transthoracic needle aspiration (TTNA) is necessary to confirm a diagnosis in those patients with peripheral lung masses that are not easily reached by the bronchoscope (Rivera, Detterbeck, & Mehta, 2003).

Medical Management

The medical management of lung cancer differs based on the cell type. Those patients with SCLC will likely receive chemotherapy, radiation therapy, or a combination of the two. Surgical intervention is saved for patients with a rare subset of SCLCs. Patients with NSCLC may receive surgery, chemotherapy, or radiation therapy. Depending on the staging of the disease, treatment options may be prescribed singly or in combination (Hoffman & Gift, 2007). For a better understanding of these three treatment options and the associated nursing responsibilities, refer to Chapter 64 🔗.

◼ Nursing Management

Nursing management of patients with lung cancer is challenging and complex. The nurse must possess an appreciation of the care required for patients who have undergone surgical resection, those who receive chemotherapeutic agents, and those who receive radiation therapy.

Assessment

The surgical patient will need close postoperative observation for cardiac and pulmonary complications such as dyspnea, atelectasis, and atrial dysrhythmias due to surgical irritation of the vagus nerve (Quinn, 2003). Dyspnea is the most common postoperative symptom and can be attributed to decreased lung capacity and a thoracotomy incision. Effective pain management is crucial so the patient will be able to participate in progressive mobilization that, over time, will lead to decreased dyspnea.

Interventions and Rationales

Nurses who care for patients receiving chemotherapy and radiation therapy receive additional specialized training and certification. Regardless of the type of therapy prescribed, the patient may experience some common side effects (e.g., fatigue, nausea and vomiting, compromised immune function, pain, skin breakdown) that can severely impact their quality of life. Refer to Chapter 64 🔗 for a detailed discussion of the nursing care of the cancer patient.

Caring for patients with lung cancer often means caring for the older adult. Since the incidence of developing lung cancer increases with age, in the future, nursing will be faced with caring for more patients diagnosed with lung cancers. It is important for nurses to understand the effects of aging related to treatments and offer education and advocacy to patients and their families.

Lung Transplant

Lung transplantation has evolved as a viable alternative for patients with advanced pulmonary disease. Indications include AAT deficiency, bronchiectasis, cystic fibrosis, emphysema, idiopathic pulmonary fibrosis, interstitial lung disease, and pulmonary hypertension. The selection of patients is central to the success of the transplant and postoperative management. Persons more than 65 years of age are not recommended for a single lung transplant, and for bilateral lung transplants 60 is the recommended age based on international guidelines. These guidelines are more relaxed with pulmonary fibrosis because there is no pharmacologic treatment. The general guidelines for candidate selection for lung transplantation are shown in the International Guidelines box.

For patients with this terminal diagnosis, single lung transplants may be available to those over 65 years of age and double lung transplants for those over 60 years of age (Egan, 2004). Other circumstances that could jeopardize selection for this option are (1) colonization with antibiotic-resistant organisms, (2) noncompliance with medical regime, (3) inability to walk 600 feet (Egan, 2004), (4) diagnosis of a malignancy within 2 years, (5) renal or liver insufficiency, and (6) positive for HIV. Patients undergo an extensive evaluation for lung transplant and wait an average of 1 year for this procedure. The patient and family undergo psychological treatment to ensure that they can cope with a postoperative regimen that requires strict adherence to immunosuppressive therapy and continuous monitoring.

Infection postoperatively is the leading cause of morbidity and mortality. Viral infection with cytomegalovirus (CMV) and herpes simplex occurs frequently. The use of bronchodilator drugs and respiratory therapies to provide clearance of secretions is continued as a component of the patient routine. Acute rejection may occur as soon as 5 to 7 days after the transplant in spite of the patient's faithfulness to the regime. Symptoms of rejection include fever, chills, flu-like aches, shortness of breath, decreased urine output, and pain over the transplanted lung (ChestNet, 2004). Accurate diagnosis is by transtracheal biopsy and treatment is with corticosteroids. The body's response to organ transplant is discussed in detail in Chapter 60 and cardiac transplantation is discussed in Chapter 42.

Occupational Lung Disorders: Pneumoconiosis

Exposure to toxic dust and particulate matter may cause a variety of respiratory disorders. Depending on the degree of intensity of exposure, smoking history, and underlying pulmonary disease, individuals may experience irreversible effects of chronic pulmonary disease after long-term exposures. The dusts of silica, asbestos, and coal are the most common causes of pneumoconiosis. Others include talc, fiberglass, clays, mica, cement, cadmium, beryllium tungsten, cobalt, aluminum, and iron. The dust deposits are permanent. Treatment is palliative and focuses on preventing further exposure and improving workplace safety (McCance & Huether, 2007).

GUIDELINES for the Selection of Lung Transplant Candidates

Evaluation of patients for lung transplantation should include ensuring that patients have, or are receiving, optimal medical therapy for their disease, but are experiencing a decline in function. Candidates generally should have chronic disease for which no further medical or surgical therapy is available and survival is limited, or end-stage lung disease. Those who are acutely critically ill are seldom candidates for lung transplantation. Routine preventive medicinal measures, including mammograms, Pap smears, and colon cancer screening, should be completed where appropriate, and comorbid medical conditions should be optimally treated as appropriate.

Older patients tend to have a significantly worse survival rate than younger patients.

There is no firm age restriction; people from birth to beyond 60 years have benefited from lung transplantation. The general age consideration is 70 years or younger. The International Guidelines for the selection of lung transplantation candidates suggest the following:

Age Limits
- Heart-lung transplants: ~55 years
- Single lung transplants: ~65 years
- Bilateral lung transplants: ~60 years.

Other general medical conditions may affect eligibility for lung transplantation. These include chronic ventricular dependence, current use of corticosteroids, significant chest wall deformity, cardiovascular abnormalities such as irreversible right ventricular dysfunctions, viral diseases, cancer, systemic hypertension, connective tissue disease, nutritional issues, substance abuse, psychological problems, and requirement for invasive ventilation.

Current contraindications for transplantation include the following:

- Dysfunction of major organs other than the lung
- Infection with HIV
- Hepatitis B antigen positivity
- Hepatitis C with biopsy-proven histologic evidence of liver disease.

Lung transplant is not contraindicated per se in patients with systemic disease (e.g., collagen vascular processes, diabetes mellitus). Each potential candidate is considered on an individual basis, with particular attention paid to the presence of any target organ damage outside the lung that might affect long-term outcome. This would constitute a relative or absolute contraindication.

Sources: American Thoracic Society. (1998). *International guidelines for the selection of lung transplant candidates.* Retrieved March 18, 2007, from http://patuents.uptodate.com/print.asp?print=&file=ats_guid/18053; Cedars-Sinai. (2000–2008). *Relative and absolute contraindications for lung transplantation.* Retrieved February 10, 2009, from http://www.csmc.edu/1247.html; Fallon Community Health Plan. (2003). *Lung transplant.* Retrieved February 10, 2009, from lungtransplant update.doc; Mayo Clinic. (2001–2009). *Lung transplant: criteria for lung transplant at Mayo Clinic.* Retrieved February 10, 2009, from http://www.mayoclinic.org/lung-transplant-criteria.html; Meyers, B.G., & Patterson, G.A. (1999). Lung transplantation-current issues and evolving concepts. *Seminar in Respiratory Critical Care Medicine.* 20(5), 429–436; Saint Barnabas Health Care System. (2009). Criteria for lung transplant. Retrieved February 10, 2009, from http://www.saintbarnabas.com/services/lungtransplant/criteria/index.html.

Occupational asthma can result from exposure to particulate matter in the workplace. Occupational asthma affects about 15% of the cases of adult asthma (American Lung Association [ALA], 2004). It is difficult to recognize because the patient continues to experience symptoms when away from the source of exposure. Symptoms experienced by the patient are dyspnea, wheezing, and chest tightness, which can occur within 12 hours of exposure or continue when the patient exercises, has a respiratory infection, and/or is undergoing emotional stress. Chemical irritants used in industry enzymes in food processing, detergents, pharmaceutical agents, and textile fibers may cause these symptoms. Exposure to workplace chemicals, gases, cereal grains, or irritants causes inflammation and edema of any portion of the respiratory tract, resulting in bronchospasm, hypersecretion of mucus from the bronchial mucosa, dyspnea, and wheezing. Nursing and medical management of occupational asthma is discussed under asthma.

Silicosis is a type of pneumoconiosis resulting from the inhalation of free silica and silica-containing compounds. It causes acute fibrosis of the lung tissue as well as fibrous nodules within the lung. Individuals are frequently asymptomatic. Between 1979 and 1995, 2,594 deaths were attributed to silicosis (McCance & Huether, 2007). Each year 200 people die of silicosis, a rate that has been stable since the 1990s. About 1.6 million workers are believed to have been exposed to silica dust and almost 60,000 are expected to suffer from some degree of silicosis. This occurs in coal mining and other industries involved in the extraction and processing of ore, preparation and use of sand, and manufacture of pipe building and roofing materials (McCance & Huether, 2007). Nursing management of silicosis is discussed under pulmonary fibrosis.

Coal miner pneumoconiosis (also called black lung or coal miner's lung) is caused by coal dust deposits in the lung. Its mild form is without symptoms except for chronic bronchitis. The disease affects about 4.5% of coal miners; about 2% have lung scarring causing restrictive disease. Between 1990 and 1999 there were more than 10,000 deaths and annual death counts increase by one-third. Its severe form consists of pulmonary fibrosis with dyspnea and wheezing often occurring. There is no specific treatment for the disease, and in complex cases patients may develop nodular lesions throughout the lungs. These enlarge and coalesce. Dense masses form in the upper portions of the lung, resulting in the loss of pulmonary volume. Patients experience a restrictive disease in which they cannot fully expand their lungs as well as an obstructive disease from secondary emphysema. Nursing management of restrictive lung disease is discussed in above sections of this chapter.

Asbestosis is a progressive lung disease caused by exposure to microscopic fibers of asbestos and resulting in a diffuse interstitial fibrosis with diaphragmatic calcification. Fibrous tissue eventually obliterates the alveoli. Between 1980 and 2002, 6,343 deaths were due to asbestosis (ALA, 2004). There is a considerable latency period between exposure and the development of symptomatology from about 10 to 20 years. Those at high risk for this disease are asbestos miners, millers, and those employed in building trades and shipyards, such as loggers, insulation workers, pipe fitters and steamfitters, sheet metal workers, and welders. Pulmonary function studies usually reveal a restrictive ventilatory defect and restricted lung volume as with silicosis. The patient experiences dyspnea and hypoxemia. The chances of arresting the disease are best in its early stages. Removal of the individual from the asbestos exposure is essential (Fishman et al., 2002).

Clinical Manifestations

Crackles of a dry quality can be auscultated in 70% to 90% of patients with diffuse interstitial fibrosis. Clubbing also is present frequently. Chronic cough and sputum production, similar to acute bronchitis, are often presenting signs. Shrinkage of the lung, which occurs with fibrotic changes, can cause a reduced vital capacity (Ross, 2003). Sputum is expectorated in large amounts and often contains varying amounts of black fluid, particularly with smokers. Eventually, respiratory failure and cor pulmonale result. There is no medical treatment for occupational lung diseases.

◼ Nursing Management

The nurse provides supportive care and education to assist the patient and caregiver. Issues to be addressed are dyspnea, fatigue, and activity tolerance. Physical conditioning and breathing exercises are helpful. The oxygen prescription provides relief from dyspnea. Medications, including bronchodilators, glucocorticoids, and antibiotics, may be prescribed for the relief of bronchospasm and treatment of exacerbations. Fluids should be taken liberally to allow for liquefaction of sputum. The nurse addresses emotional issues such as depression, anxiety, and anger as the patient deteriorates in the end stage.

Discharge Priorities

Before the patient is discharged after an acute episode, she should have received education about all aspects of the treatment regime. Contact numbers for nursing and other care providers should be given to the patient and caregiver. The patient and caregiver should be able to verbalize issues that constitute an emergency. Oxygen, if ordered, should be available in the home setting. Plans for transfer to home should be made in consideration of oxygen needs and instructions should be given in writing.

Health Promotion

Workers who are exposed to these toxic agents must be fitted with appropriate safety equipment. In the industrial setting, the occupational health nurse advocates for the use of safety measures and reduced exposure to dust. The Occupational Safety and Health Administration (OSHA) issues regulations regarding dust control and ventilation that must be followed in the workplace. The nurse must be apprised of these regulations to advocate for workers. Environmental checks must be initiated as required by OSHA. Ongoing educational programs should be provided for workers so that they can be accountable for their own health. Refraining from smoking and receiving a yearly influenza vaccination contribute to pulmonary health.

Collaborative Management

Because there is no definitive treatment for the pulmonary fibrotic changes caused by occupational lung diseases, the health care team's focus is on the provision of supportive care and relief of dyspnea. The social worker often collaborates with the team to provide satisfactory care at home or in the community. Depending on the severity of disease, the patient may be discharged to a pulmonary rehabilitation program, home care, or hospice in the end stages of the disease. The health care provider collaborates with the nurse, physical therapist, and respiratory therapist on the plan of care after discharge. The physical therapist and a home care nurse may see the patient on an outpatient basis. Oxygen equipment along with patient and family education is provided by the medical equipment company.

Gerontological Considerations with Pulmonary Diseases

In the acute care setting, the nurse recognizes that elderly individuals may demonstrate confusion as well as agitation and breathlessness in the face of hypoxemia. This confusion is more likely to occur at night when the environment seems more unfamiliar. Elders also are at a higher risk for PE related to tendencies toward immobilization. They may be less tolerant of anticoagulants. Assessment for bleeding tendencies should be stressed and discharge planning should emphasize patient safety in this regard. Caution should be taken with positioning elders because of the possibility of osteoporosis and arthritis. Attention should be paid to alleviating pain during painful procedures such as the insertion of a chest tube. Attention also should be given to drug interactions and other systemic problems when pain medication is given to maintain the patient's comfort. Elderly individuals may require a lower dosage of medication. Upon ambulation with chest tubes or other equipment, an elderly person should be monitored closely because age and poor mobility constitute a risk for falls.

On discharge from the acute setting, elders benefit from an environmental assessment by a nurse. Hazards that could potentiate symptoms are wood-burning stoves, dust, or the presence of smoking or chemical fumes in the immediate environment. The nurse enlists the assistance of family or significant others to promote safety. Air conditioning in the summer and efficient heating in the winter will facilitate easy breathing for elders. Elderly patients with COPD and asthma should receive the influenza vaccine and the pneumococcal vaccine yearly. Refraining from smoking and staying indoors during extremes of temperatures is important. Written instructions are helpful for the elder person being discharged as is follow-up by a home health nurse to assist with the development of an individualized care plan and an emergency protocol.

Research

The treatment of lower airway disorders is aided by ongoing research on the topic, as outlined in the Research Opportunities and Clinical Impact box (p. 998). The research opportunities enumerated tend to focus on the use of complimentary and alternative medicine, stimulation of positive health behaviors in older adults, enhancement of nursing knowledge, and student nursing learning gaps in caring for asthmatic patients.

RESEARCH OPPORTUNITIES AND CLINICAL IMPACT RELATED TO LOWER AIRWAY DISORDERS

Research Area	Clinical Impact
What complementary therapies are used by asthma sufferers, and are they effective?	A study by Ernst (1999) referenced by Guthrie and Tingen (2002) stated that 60% of asthma sufferers use complementary therapies. Specific data on complementary therapies would add to the knowledge base about asthma treatment and could provide useful information for patient education. For example, "Which complementary modalities such as homeopathy, herbal remedies, and acupuncture, as examples, have been most useful?" Other research questions are: • Do persons who use complementary therapies have fewer exacerbations? • Is there a relationship between anxiety and use of complementary therapies?
Are students in university settings receiving adequate asthma care? (Knowledge base about asthma among college students and interventions for college students with asthma by the student health center)	McClennon, Holcroft, Faul, and Nicolosi (2002) stated that there is a research gap related to health behavior of college students with asthma and there is a need for better ways for a college health center to provide interventions and education for students. Questions that could be studied further are: • How do students' treatment regimes relate to the current asthma guidelines? • What is the relationship of stress and anxiety in the college environment to students' asthma exacerbations? • What is the relationship between the student with asthma and the college health center? Data obtained regarding these topics would add to the clinical nursing research on asthma in young adults and provide useful strategies for asthma management in college and university health centers.
Assessment of dyspnea (Dyspnea scales are currently being developed and tested.)	Kendrick and colleagues (2000) proposed use of a tool to measure dyspnea in patients by use of the Borg scale. Questions that could be studied further include: • How do nurses measure dyspnea in clinical settings? • What objective and subjective data are used by nurses to assess and evaluate severity of dyspnea? • How is the patient involved in assessing his own level of dyspnea? Obtaining survey and interview data regarding general nursing knowledge could be instrumental in framing clinical nursing education curricula and continuing education programs regarding standards of care for patients experiencing dyspnea. It could also provide guidelines for the formulation of dyspnea assessment tools that are practical for the clinical setting. Care algorithms may be developed based on dyspnea scores.
The effect of cues to promote positive health behaviors in older adults regarding obtaining flu shots.	McCall, Johnson, and Rothman (2002) tested the effectiveness of a variety of "cues to actions" or messages for elders regarding importance and availability of flu shots in North Dakota counties. This is an area for future research. Knowledge about effective cues that promote positive health behaviors among elders provides useful information for community health centers. Replication of the McCall et al. (2002) study would be useful since elders in rural settings such as North Dakota might respond to different "cues to action" than elders in other localities. Research regarding "cues to action" that are effective for diverse and poverty-laden populations of risk would be extremely useful as well. Aside from obtaining flu shots, "cues to action" for other positive health behaviors could also be established such as safe sex, weight loss, exercise, and quitting smoking.
Nursing knowledge base about chest drains.	According to Carroll (2000) chest drainage options are expanding and nurses need to know what is out there and when to use each type. Data could be collected regarding nursing knowledge about chest drains among cardiovascular nurses or emergency department nurses. These data could then be used as a basis for continuing education programs and training materials for nurses.
What is the effectiveness of various methods of smoking cessation?	Promotion of the most effective means of smoking cessation should aid patients in successful smoking cessation.
What is the effect of education on smoke avoidance in grade school on the rate of smoking in adolescence?	Early avoidance of primary and secondhand smoke should decrease the development of emphysema and COPD.

Clinical Preparation

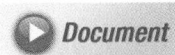

CRITICAL THINKING

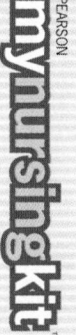

 **Read**

- History of Current Illness
- Past Medical History
- Physical Exam
- Admitting Medical Orders
- Laboratory Study Results

 **Document**

- Summary of Hospitalization
- Pathophysiology Form
- Laboratory Values
- Laboratory Results Explanation

Apply

- List of Potential Nursing Diagnoses
- Concept Map
- Critical Thinking Questions

Log on to MyNursingKit.com to download forms you will need and to complete further steps in the Clinical Preparation assignment.

HISTORY OF PRESENT ILLNESS

Mr. H is a 70-year-old man admitted to the emergency department with complaints of intermittent chest tightness and dyspnea, which he states have gotten progressively worse in the past week. He states he is coughing up large amounts of thick, yellowish sputum and experiences muscle fatigue and dyspnea after bouts of coughing. Mr. H also indicates that he feels winded after a short walk to the bathroom of his apartment.

The patient is started on intravenous (IV) fluids equaling 3 liters per day. He is started on IV Solu-Medrol 200 mg every 6 hours, and he is continued on his captopril orally. The nurse maintains a record of intake and output. A respiratory physical therapist assists him with postural drainage and breathing and coughing exercises. He is maintained on 2 liters of nasal oxygen. He is also started on albuterol nebulization treatments four times a day. The physical therapist and nursing staff ambulate him in the hallway four times a day with oxygen. Because his glucose is controlled, his glipizide is discontinued and he is placed on glucometer checks four times a day. He is placed on an 1,800-calorie diabetic diet, which he tolerates well.

Medical–Surgical History

Mr. H has a history of chronic bronchitis, hypertension, and colon cancer. He has had two to three hospital admissions per year

for exacerbations of chronic bronchitis. Past surgical procedures include a hernia repair at age 50 and a colon resection for colon cancer at age 65. He underwent chemotherapy at that time and is currently in remission. He sees an oncologist every 6 months for follow-up. He is also a non–insulin-dependent diabetic. Current medications include glipizide, captopril, and Atrovent three times a day.

Social History

Mr. H is married and lives with his wife. They have two children who live nearby in the same community. He has a history of smoking, but has quit within the last 5 years.

Physical Examination

Auscultation of lung sounds reveals crackles and a few expiratory wheezes throughout all lung fields. His breath sounds are decreased in the bases. He uses his accessory sternocleidomastoid muscles for breathing. While at rest, his respiratory rate is 30. His vital signs are as follows: blood pressure 160/100, pulse 100 beats per minute, and temp 100.6°F orally. Auscultation of the heart reveals he is tachycardic with an S_3. He seems most comfortable sitting forward in a chair and appears to have a barrel chest.

Admitting Medical Orders

Service: Medical floor
Diagnosis: dyspnea and shortness of breath
Allergies: none noted
Vital signs and O_2 sats q2h
Ambulate in hall with assistance and with oxygen four times daily
Diet: 1,800-calorie diabetic diet
Call house officer: HR < 60 or > 120, systolic blood pressure <100 or > 140, RR < 12 or > 30, temperature > 38°C, O_2 saturation < 92%, glucose < 70 or > 150 mg/dL
IV fluids: 0.45 normal saline at 125 mL/hr
I&O q shift
Respiratory care: maintain on 2 liters of nasal oxygen; postural drainage and breathing and coughing exercises by physical therapist q4h

Scheduled Medications

Albuterol nebulization treatments four times a day
IV Solu-Medrol 200 mg q6h
Captopril 50 mg PO twice daily, 1 hour before meals

PRN Medications

None noted

Ordered Laboratory Studies

Sputum culture × 1
ABGs, CBC, and Chem 7 panel daily
Accu-Chek q ac and hs

Ordered Diagnostic Studies

Anterior/posterior and lateral chest x-ray

Nursing Care Day 2

On day 2 Mr. H is started on a broad-spectrum antibiotic given intravenously in addition to the other therapies. His sliding scale insulin is discontinued and he is placed on oral glipizide. His dyspnea has eased and he is expectorating sputum more easily. Mr. H is tolerating ambulation and an increase in activity. His IV is changed to a saline lock through which he receives his antibiotic. His wife visits at his bedside regularly and is encouraged to assist with coughing and deep breathing exercises as well as a fluid intake of 8 glasses of water per day. Mr. H's vital signs are as follows: BP 130/70, HR 92, respiratory rate 24, and temperature 99.5°F.

LABORATORY STUDY RESULTS

Test	Day 1	Day 2	Day 3
O_2 saturation on room air	88%		
O_2 saturation on 2 L nasal O_2	92%	94%	94%
ABGs			
pH	7.40	7.40	7.40
PO_2	85 mmHg	90 mmHg	92 mmHg
PCO_2	50 mmHg	49 mmHg	49 mmHg
HCO_3	36 mEq/L	35 mEq/L	35 mEq/L
Hct	54%	50%	49%
Hgb	17 g/100 mL	16 g/100 mL	15 g/100 mL
Platelets	200,000 µL	210,000 µL	225,000 µL
RBCs	$4.6 \times 10^6/µL$	$5.0 \times 10^6/µL$	$5.2 \times 10^6/µL$
Sodium	148 mEq/L	128 mEq/L	139 mEq/L
Potassium	4.0 mEq/L	4.2 mEq/L	4.5 mEq/L
Chloride	105 mEq/L	100 mEq/L	100 mEq/L
HCO_3^-	35 mEq/L	35 mEq/L	32 mEq/L
Glucose	150 mg/dL	145 mg/dL	148 mg/dL
Sputum culture		*Staphylococcus aureus*	

CRITICAL THINKING QUESTIONS

1. As the nurse on the unit where Mr. H is admitted, what further assessment data do you plan to collect?

2. Your initial impression is that Mr. H has a barrel chest. How do you verify this with objective data? What is the etiology of a barrel chest in the patient with COPD?

3. Mr. H is placed on IV Solu-Medrol 200 mg every 6 hours. How will this drug alleviate Mr. H's symptoms? What are some potential side effects?

4. After 3 days Mr. H is to be discharged on 2 L nasal oxygen, which is to be administered continuously. His medications include glipizide, captopril, oral prednisone, an oral antibiotic to be taken for 3 more days, albuterol, and steroid inhalers to be taken three times a day. What patient education do you provide and what assessment do you want to make prior to discharge? Describe patient education strategies and use of visual aids.

5. What are some nutritional considerations for Mr. H?

6. What benefits will continuous oxygen therapy afford Mr. H in terms of quality of life?

Answers to Critical Thinking Questions appear in Appendix D.

NCLEX® REVIEW

1. A patient is seen in the emergency department with acute shortness of breath and chest tightness which started after exposure to a carpet cleaning agent in her home. The nurse realizes this patient is most likely experiencing:
   1. The flu.
   2. An acute asthma attack.
   3. COPD.
   4. Cystic fibrosis.

2. A patient with community acquired pneumonia is being discharged. Which of the following should the nurse include in this patient's discharge plan of care?
   1. Take the prescribed antibiotics until the coughing stops.
   2. Limit fluid intake to reduce secretions.
   3. Avoid smoking or environments with smoke.
   4. Resume normal activity level.

3. The nurse is providing care to a patient with chronic obstructive pulmonary disease. Which of the following should the nurse be prepared to administer to the patient?

1. Pancreatic enzymes

2. Ibuprofen

3. Magnesium sulfate

4. Pulmozyme

4. A patient is admitted with rib fractures after falling from a ladder while on the job. Which of the following is a priority for the care of this patient?

1. Pain management

2. Safety precautions

3. Employment counseling

4. Rehabilitation therapy

5. A patient with lung cancer is complaining of increasing arm pain. The nurse realizes the patient could be experiencing:

1. Superior vena cava syndrome.

2. Hypoxia.

3. Hypercalcemia.

4. Pain associated with the primary diagnosis.

6. A patient is admitted with asbestosis. Which of the following should be included in the assessment of this patient?

1. Location of home and surrounding industrial community

2. Current place of employment

3. Place of employment 10 to 20 years prior to current admission

4. Employment with roofing materials

Answers for review questions appear in Appendix D

KEY TERMS

acute bronchitis *p.935*
asbestosis *p.996*
asthma *p.960*
atelectasis *p.973*
carbon monoxide poisoning *p.992*
chronic bronchitis *p.955*
chronic obstructive pulmonary disease
   (COPD) *p.955*
coal miner pneumoconiosis *p.996*

cor pulmonale *p.980*
cystic fibrosis (CF) *p.968*
emphysema *p.955*
flail chest *p.986*
hemoptysis *p.969*
hemothorax *p.989*
influenza *p.936*
lung abscess *p.947*
metered-dose inhaler (MDI) *p.939*

near drowning *p.991*
occupational asthma *p.996*
pleural effusion *p.984*
pneumonia *p.937*
pneumothorax *p.988*
polycythemia vera *p.958*
pulmonary contusion *p.988*
pulmonary embolism (PE) *p.973*
silicosis *p.996*

EXPLORE PEARSON **mynursingkit**™

MyNursingKit is your one stop for online chapter review materials and resources. Prepare for success with additional NCLEX®-style practice questions, interactive assignments and activities, web links, animations and videos, and more!

Register your access code from the front of your book at
www.mynursingkit.com

REFERENCES

Abrahamian, F. M. (2008). *Pleural effusion.* Retrieved April 22, 2008, from http://www.emedicine.com/emerg/topic462.htm

American Cancer Society. (2006). *Cigarette smoking.* Retrieved from http://www.cancer.org

American Lung Association. (2004). *Fact sheet: Occupational lung disease.* Retrieved February 9, 2008, from http://www.lungusa.org/diseases/occupational_factsheet.html

American Lung Association. (2007). *Sarcoidosis.* Retrieved May 10, 2008, from http://www. lungusa.org/site/c.dvLUK900E/b.4061173/apps/s/content.asp?ct=5176723

American Thoracic Society. (2001). *Guidelines for the management of adults with community-acquired pneumonia.* Retrieved February 24, 2007, from http://ajrccm.atsjournals.org/cgi/content/full/163/7/1730

American Thoracic Society, Centers for Disease Control, and Infectious Diseases Society of America. (2003). Treatment of tuberculosis. *Morbidity and Mortality Weekly Report, 52*(RR-11), 1–77.

Amersham Health. (2004). *Pulmonary fungal infection.* Retrieved February 9, 2008, from http://www.amershamhealth.com/medcyclopeaedia/…/FUNGAL%20INFECTION%20PULMONARY.as

Antoniou, K. M., Hansell, D. M., Rubens, M. G., Marten, K., Desal, S. R., Siafakas, N. M., et al. (2008). Idiopathic pulmonary fibrosis:

Outcome in relation to smoking status. *American Journal of Respiratory Critical Care Medicine, 177*(2), 190–194.

Aurora, R., Milite, F., & Vender Els, N. J. (2000). Respiratory emergencies. Seminars in Oncology, *27*(3).

Ball, K. (2003). Deep vein thrombosis and airline travel: The deadly duo. *AORN Journal, 77*(2), 346, 348–349, 351–352, 354, 357–358.

Barnes, P. J. (2000). Chronic obstructive pulmonary disease. *New England Journal of Medicine, 343,* 269–280.

Barreiro, T. J., DeMarco, R., Gemmel, D. J., & Schaub, C. R. (2005, October). Sarcoidosis: An enigmatic disease calls for a measured workup. *Patient Care for the Nurse Practitioner,* pp. 1–10.

Bjerke, S. (2002). *Flail chest.* Retrieved August 22, 2004, from http://www.emedicine.com/emerg/topic2813.htm

Bowman, J. G. (2006). *Pneumothorax, tension and traumatic.* Retrieved April 23, 2008, from http://www.emedicine.com/emerg/TOPIC470.HTM

Britto, M. T., DeVellis, R. F., Hornung, R. W., DeFriese, G. H., Atherton, H. D., & Slap, G. B. (2004). Health care preferences and priorities of adolescents with chronic illnesses. *Pediatrics, 114*(5), 1272–1280.

Carroll, P. (2000). Exploring chest drain options. *RN 63* (10), 50–54, 56.

Centers for Disease Control and Prevention. (2004a). *Carbon monoxide poisoning fact sheet.* Retrieved August 22, 2004, from http://www.cdc.gov/nceh/airpollution/carbonmonoxide/cofaq.htm

Centers for Disease Control and Prevention. (2004b). *Influenza: The disease.* Retrieved from http://www.cdc.gov/flu/about/disease.htm

Centers for Disease Control. (2006). Trends in tuberculosis—United States, 2005. *Morbidly and Mortality Weekly Report, 55*(11), 305.

Cerro Coso Coyote Athletics. (2004). *Chest injuries.* Retrieved May 12, 2008, from http://athletics.cerrocoso.edu/sportsmedicine/chest_injuries.htm

ChestNet. (2004). *A guide to lung transplantation.* Retrieved August 22, 2004, from http://www.chestnet.org/education/patient/guides/transplantation/p6.php

Chojinowski, D. (2003). "Gold" standards for acute exacerbation in COPD. *Nurse Practitioner, 28*(5), 26–39.

Choudhry, S., Seibold, M. A., Borrell, L. N., et al. (2007). Dissecting complex diseases in complex populations: Asthma in Latino Americans. *Proceedings of the American Thoracic Society, 4*(3), 326–333.

Coding Edge Archives. (2000). *Congestive heart failure and related cardiopulmonary conditions.* Retrieved June 5, 2005, from http://www.lagunamedsys.com/EdgeArchive/feature121500.htm

Crawford, S. (2004). *Current anti-fungal treatment in the ICU.* Retrieved February 9, 2008, from http://www.hospital_consult_pda.com?PDAcca44.htm

Dalen, J. (2002). Pulmonary embolism: What have we learned since Virchow? Treatment and prevention. *Chest, 122*(5), 1801–1818.

Dauber, J. H. (2006). *Risk factors for idiopathic pulmonary fibrosis.* Retrieved May 17, 2008, from University of Pittsburgh website: http://www.simmonsfund.pitt.edu/rishfactors.html

Devitt, H. (1995). *Blunt thoracic trauma: Assessment, management and anesthesia.* Retrieved August 22, 2004, from http://www.anesthesia.org/winterlude/w195_4.html

Diaz, J. I., & Quellette, R. R. (2008). *Pulmonary fibrosis, idiopathic.* Retrieved April 20, 2008, from http://www.emedicine.com/med/TOPOC1960.HTM

Dieudonne, A. (2008). *Atypical mycobacterial infection.* Retrieved February 12, 2008, from http://www.medicine.com/ped/TOPIC3034.HTM

Egan, J. (2004). The clinical practice of lung transplantation in America. *Chest, 125*(4), 1183–1184.

Ernst, E. (1999). Complementary/alternative medicine for asthma: We do not know what we need to. *Chest (American College of Chest Physicians), 115,* 1–3.

Esmond, G. (2000). *Respiratory nursing.* London: Harcourt Health.

Feied, C., & Handler, J. (2002). Pulmonary embolism. Retrieved February 28, 2008, from http://www.emedicine.com/EMERG/topic490.htm

Fishman, A. P., Elias, J. A., Fishman, J. A., Grippi, M. A., Kaiser, L. R., & Senior, R. M. (2002). *Fishman's manual of pulmonary diseases and disorders.* New York: McGraw-Hill.

Global Initiative for Asthma. (2007). *Global strategy for asthma management and prevention.* Retrieved July 29, 2008, from http://www.ginasthma.org

Gould, K. P. (2006). Sarcoidosis. *eMedicine.* Retrieved May 20, 2008, from http://www.emedicine.com/DERM/topic281.htm

Guthrie, C., & Tingen, M. S. (2002). Asthma: A case study. Review of pathophysiology and management strategies. *Journal of the American Academy of Nurse Practitioners, 14*(10), 457–462.

Haque, A. K. (1992). Pathology of common pulmonary fungal infections. *Journal of Thoracic Imaging, 4,* 1–11.

Hegewald, M. J., Markewitz, B., & Elliott, C. G. (2007). Pulmonary hypertension: Clinical manifestations, classification and diagnosis. *International Journal of Clinical Practice, 61*(Suppl. 156), 5–14.

Hoffman, A., & Gift, A. (2007). Lung cancer. In M. Langerhorne, J. Fulton, & S. Otto (Eds.), *Oncology nursing* (5th ed.). St. Louis: Mosby.

Humbert, M. and Trembath, R. C. (2002). Genetics of pulmonary hypertension: from bench to bedside. *European Respiratory Journal,* 20, 741–749.

Hunter, M., & King, D. (2001). COPD: Management of acute exacerbations and chronic stable disease. *American Family Physician, 64,* 603–612, 621–622. Retrieved February 24, 2007, from http://www.aafp.org/afp/20010815/603.html

Jassal, D., & Sharma, S. (2004). *Pulmonary hypertension.* Retrieved May 31, 2008, from http://www.emedicine.com/Radio/topic583.htm

Kaplan, V., Clermont, G., Griffin, M. F., Kasal, J., et al. (2003). Pneumonia: Still the old man's friend? *Archives of Internal Medicine, 163*(3), 317–324.

Kavita, G. (2005). Acute pulmonary embolism (helical CT). Retrieved April 21, 2008, from http://www.emedicine.com/RADIO/topic582.htm

Kendrick, K., Baxi, S., & Smith, R. (2000). Usefulness of the Borg scale in assessing the degree of dyspnea in patients with COPD and asthma. *Journal of Emergency Nursing, 26*(3), 216–222.

Kennedy, M., Zolot, J., & Sofer, D. (2001). Preventing thromboembolism after injury. *AJN, 101*(2), 18–19.

Kleinschmidt, P. (2004, June). *Chronic obstructive pulmonary disease and emphysema.* Retrieved August 1, 2004, from http://www.emedicine.com/emerg/topic99.htm

Knutson, D., & Braun, C. (2002). Diagnosis and management of acute bronchitis. *American Family Physician, 65*(10), 2039–2045.

Kvale, P. A., Simoff, M., & Prakash, U. B. (2003). Palliative care. *Chest, 123*(1), 284S–311S.

Mandanas, R. A. (2007). *Pneumonia, fungal.* Retrieved April 17, 2008, from http://www.emedicine.com/med/topic1853.htm

Martinez, F. D. (2007). Genes, environments, development and asthma: A reappraisal. *European Respiratory Journal, 29*(1), 179–184.

Mayo Clinic. (2008). *Sarcoidosis.* Retrieved May 10, 2008, from http://www.mayoclinic.com/health/sarcoidosis/DS00251

McCall, K., Johnson, R., & Rothman, A. (2002). The effects of framing and action instructions on whether older adults obtain flu shots. *Health Psychology, 21*(6), 624–628.

McCance, K., & Heuther, S. (2007). *Pathophysiology: The biological basis for disease in adults and children* (5th ed.). St. Louis: Mosby.

McClennon, S. R., Holcroft, C., Faul, N. Q., & Nicolosi, R. (2002). A look at asthma care in a university setting. *Nurse Practitioner, 27*(12), 35–42.

Medical College of Wisconsin Healthlink. (2008). *Atypical mycobacteria.* Retrieved February 12, 2008, from http://healthlink.mcw.edu/article/954973743

Merck. (2005a). *Cor pulmonale.* Retrieved April 24, 2008, from http://www.merck.com/mmpe/sec07/ch074/ch074c.html

Merck. (2005b). *Pulmonary hypertension.* Retrieved April 24, 2008, from http://www.merck.com/mmpe/sec05/ch058/ch058a.html

Merck. (2008). *Idiopathic pulmonary fibrosis.* Retrieved February 9, 2008, from http://www.merck.com/mmhe/sec04/ch050b.html

Morbidity and Mortality Weekly Report (MMWR): Recommendations and Reports, CDC. (2004). Prevention and control of influenza: recommendations of the advisory committee on immunization priorities (ACIP). Retrieved August 3, 2008 from http://www.cdc.gov/mmrw/preview/mmwrhtml/rr5306al.htm

Morris, B., Morrison, R. B., & Yetsko, C. (2002). Venous thromboembolism. *RN Magazine, 65*(10), 1–8.

Morris, M. J. (2007). Asthma. *eMedicine.* Retrieved July 29, 2008, from http://www.emedicine.com/med/topic177.htm

Morrison, C., & Lew, E. (2001). Aspergillosis. *AJN, 101*(8), 40–48.

Morton, P. G., Fontaine, D. K., Hudak, C. M., & Gallo, B. M. (2005). *Critical care nursing.* Philadelphia: Lippincott William & Wilkins.

Murray, L. N., & Brown, K. R. (2007). *Cystic fibrosis.* Retrieved May 6, 2008, from http://www.emedicine.com/ent/topic515.htm

National Cancer Institute. (2005a). *Asbestos exposure: Questions and answers.* Retrieved from http://cis.nci.nih.gov

National Cancer Institute. (2005b). *Small cell lung cancer.* Retrieved from http://cis.nci.nih.gov

National Center for Health Statistics. (2006). *Summary health statistics for U.S. adults: National health interview survey, 2006, Tables 3 and 4.* Retrieved May 16, 2008 from http://www.cdc.gov/nchs/fastats/copd.htm

National Comprehensive Cancer Network. (2007). *National comprehensive cancer network practice guidelines: Small cell lung cancer.* http://www.nccn.org

National Heart, Lung, and Blood Institute. (1997/2002). *Expert panel report 2: Guidelines for the diagnosis and management of asthma* and *Update on selected topics 2002.* Bethesda, MD: Author. Retrieved July 29, 2008, from http://www.nhlbi.nih.gov/guidelines/archives/epr-2/index.htm

National Heart Lung and Blood Institute (NHLBI). (2006). *What is pulmonary arterial hypertension?* Retrieved April 24, 2008, from http://www.nhlbi.nih.gov/health/dci/Diseases/pah/pah_what.html

National Heart Lung and Blood Institute. (2007). *Expert panel report 3: Guidelines for the diagnosis and management of asthma* (NIH Publication No. 09-5846). Retrieved from http://www.nhlbi.nih.gov/guidelines/asthma

National Institutes of Health. (2001). *Global initiative for chronic obstructive lung disease: Global strategy for the diagnosis, management and prevention of chronic obstructive lung disease* (NIH Publication No. 2701B). Bethesda, MD: Author.

Nevidjion, B., & Sowers, K. (2000). *A nurse's guide to cancer care.* Philadelphia: Lippincott Williams & Wilkins.

Niederman, M. S., Mandell, L. A., Anzueto, A., Bass, J. B., Broughton, W. A., Campbell, G. D., et al. (2001). Guidelines for management of adults with community-acquired pneumonia: Diagnosis, assessment of severity, antimicrobial therapy and prevention. *American Journal of Respiratory Critical Care Medicine, 163*(7), 1730–1754.

Owens, M., Chaudry, M. S., Eggerstedt, J. M., & Smith, L. M. (2000). In R. George, M. Light, M. Mathay, & R. Mathay (Eds.), *Chest medicine: Essentials of pulmonary and critical care medicine.* Philadelphia: Lippincott Williams & Wilkins.

Parkin, D., Bray, F., & Ferlay, J. (2005). Global cancer statistics 2002. *CA: A Cancer Journal for Physicians,* 55.

Patel, R. J. (2008). *Idiopathic pulmonary fibrosis.* Retrieved from http://www.emedicine.com.med/topic1960.htm

Patient UK. (2007). *Lung abscess.* Retrieved April 21, 2008, from http://www.patient.co.uk/showdoc/40000608/

Peek, G., Morocos, G., & Cooper, T. (2000). The pleural cavity. *British Medical Journal, 320,* 1318–1330.

Plaut, T. F. (2001). Lack of knowledge leads to poor asthma care. *Advance for Managers of Respiratory Care, 10*(3), 38, 40–41.

Porth, C. M. (2007). *Essentials of concepts of altered health states* (2nd ed.). Philadelphia: Lippincott Williams & Wilkins.

Pulmonology Channel. (2002). *Bronchitis: Overview, causes and risk factors.* Retrieved April 19, 2008, from http://www.pulmonologychannel.com/bronchitis/index.shtml

Quinn, K. (2003). Managing patients through thoracic surgery. In M. Hass (Ed.), *Contemporary issues in lung cancer: A nursing perspective* (1st ed.). Boston: Jones & Bartlett.

Raviglione, M., & Smith, I. (2007). XDR tuberculosis—Implications for global public health. *New England Journal of Medicine, 356*(7), 24–36.

Reeder, J., & Danis, D. (2001). Penetrating chest trauma: With careful assessment, rapid diagnosis, and relatively simple interventions, most patients with penetrating chest trauma will recover. *AJN, 101*(Suppl.), 15–18.

Rivera, M., Detterbeck, F., & Mehta, A. (2003). Diagnosis of lung cancer: The guidelines. *Chest, 123*(1 Suppl.).

Ross, R. (2003). The clinical diagnosis of asbestosis in this century requires more than a chest radiograph. *Chest, 124*(3), 1120–1129.

Rowe, S. M., Miller, S., & Sorscher, E. J. (2005). Cystic fibrosis. *New England Journal of Medicine, 352,* 1992–2001.

Sawyer, M. (2006). *Blunt chest trauma.* Retrieved May 12, 2008, from http://www.emedicine.com/med/TOPICS3658.HTM

Schoenstadt, A. (2006). *Tuberculosis statistics in the United States.* Retrieved May 13, 2008, from http://tuberculosis.emedtv.com/tuberculoosis-statistics-in-the-united-states.html

Schultz, P. (2003, September–October). Community-acquired pneumonia: Hunting the elusive respiratory infection. *Nursing 2003,* pp. 29–34.

Shahani, R. (2006). *Penetrating chest trauma.* Retrieved May 12, 2008, from http://www.emedicine.com/MED/topic2916.htm

Sharma, S. (2004). *Lung abscess.* Retrieved October 28, 2004, from http://www.emedicine.com/med/topic1332htm

Sharma, S. (2006a). Chronic obstructive pulmonary disease. *eMedicine.* Retrieved May 21, 2008, from http://www.emedicine.com/med/TOPIC373.HTM

Sharma, S. (2006b). Cystic fibrosis. *eMedicine.* Retrieved May 12, 2008, from http://www.emedicine.com/ped/topics535,html

Sharma, S. (2006c). Pulmonary hypertension secondary. *eMedicine.* Retrieved April 26, 2008, from http://www.emedicine.com/MEd/topic2946.htm

Sharma, S. (2007). Chronic bronchitis. *eMedicine.* Retrieved May 16, 2008, from http://www.emedicine.com/med/TOPIC367.HTM

Shepherd, S. (2003). *Submersion injury: Near drowning.* Retrieved August 28, 2004, from http://www.emedicine.com/EMERG/topic744.htm

Taubert, J. (2001). Management of malignant pleural effusion. *Nursing Clinics of North America, 36*(4), 665–683.

Trauma.org. (2004). *Chest trauma rib fractures and flail chest.* Retrieved from http://www.trauma.org/archive/thoracic/CHESTflail.html

Verma, S., & Slutsky, A. S. (2007). Idiopathic pulmonary fibrosis—New insights. *New England Journal of Medicine, 356*(13), 1370–1372.

Voelkel, N. F., & Tuder, R. (2000). COPD: Exacerbation. *Chest, 117,* S376–S379.

Wanek, S. & Mayberry, J. C. (2004). Blunt thoracic trauma: flail chest, pulmonary contusion, and blast injury. *Critical Care Clinic, 20*(1), 71–81.

Wilson, B. A., Shannon, M., & Stang, C. L. (2006). *Nurse's drug guide.* Philadelphia: Pearson Prentice Hall.

World Health Organization. (1996). *Guidelines for the diagnosis and management of cystic fibrosis.* Retrieved February 24, 2007, from http://www.cf.org/WHO/guidelines

World Health Organization. (2003). *Global TB control report.* Retrieved from http://www.cf.org/WHO

Woodruff, D. (1999). Pneumothorax. *RN, 62*(9), 62–66.

Wooten, J., & Salkind, A. (2003). Superbugs: Unmasking the threat. *RN Magazine, 66*(3), 37–44.

Wrong Diagnosis. (2008). *Prevalence and incidence of pulmonary embolism.* Retrieved April 21, 2008, from http://www.wrongdiagnosis.com/p/pulmonary_embolism/prevalence.htm

Wryobeck, J. M., Lippo, G., McLaughlin, V., Riba, M., & Rubenfire, M. (2007). Psychosocial aspects of pulmonary hypertension: A review. *Psychosomatics, 28,* 457–475.

Yakobi, R. (2007). *Sarcoidosis.* Retrieved from http:// www.emedicine.com/emerg/TOPIC516.HTM

Yunis, N. A., & Crausman, R. S. (2006). Cor pulmonale. *eMedicine.* Retrieved May 20, 2008 from http://www.emedicine.com/med/topic449.htm

Caring for the Patient with Complex Respiratory Disorders

Nancy Ames

With contributions by:
Kathleen Osborn

Outcome-Based Learning Objectives

After studying this chapter, the learner will be able to:

1. Describe the etiology, incidence, and types of acute respiratory failure as seen by nurses in acute care settings.

2. Define pulmonary edema and state three of the common etiologies of pulmonary edema that are seen in practice.

3. Differentiate between non-cardiogenic pulmonary edema and cardiogenic pulmonary edema, as it relates to patient symptomology.

4. Distinguish between acute respiratory distress syndrome (ARDS) and acute lung injury (ALI) in patients presenting in an acute care setting.

5. Identify the common ventilator modes and important nursing implications for each mode.

6. Define PEEP and state two complications of this therapy.

7. List the equipment needed for intubation, and explain how the equipment is used with a patient.

8. Review the procedure for suctioning and state two important nursing implications related to conducting this procedure.

9. State two indications for insertion of a chest tube in a patient in an acute care setting.

Research   Collaboration   Health Promotion   Nursing Process   Caring   Critical Thinking

ONE OF THE most challenging groups of patients that nurses will likely care for are those patients who cannot breathe. These patients can be agitated and confused or unconscious and apneic. They might require emergency arterial blood gases (ABGs) or an immediate lifesaving intervention, such as intubation. Patients may need ventilator support and require immediate suctioning for a mucous plug or develop a tension pneumothorax that necessitates emergent placement of a chest tube.

This chapter addresses the different types of complex respiratory disorders that result in an alteration in oxygen perfusion to the tissues. Basic pulmonary physiology is important to understand in order to care for patients with these complex respiratory disorders. The relationship between oxygen and hemoglobin, ventilation/perfusion mismatching producing hypoxemia, and the role of the alveolar-capillary membrane in respiratory failure are reviewed. The reader is referred to other chapters to review such topics as ABG interpretation and other pertinent pulmonary physiology.

Before reviewing the pathophysiology of complex respiratory disorders, the reader is encouraged to review the chapter on acute coronary syndromes and other cardiac pathologies (Chapter 40 ☻). It is important to understand that the heart and lungs are inextricably linked and what affects one system eventually affects the other. An appreciation of this association between the heart and the lungs will aid in understanding complex disorders of the respiratory system. Respiratory complications are frequently a result of a primary disorder somewhere else in the body. Therefore, determining the primary organ system failure and focusing on the treatment of this pathology are the goals for many of the complex respiratory disorders. The nursing management of patients with complex respiratory disorders focuses on airway management and maintaining oxygen for tissue perfusion. A description of the complex respiratory disorders follows. The nursing management for these disorders is similar; therefore, a discussion of nursing management is presented after the description of the disorders.

Respiratory Physiology

The *alveolar-capillary (A-C) membrane* is the central component of gas exchange in the lungs. The A-C membrane consists of many tissue layers through which gas diffuses. West (1998) describes the lungs as "a collection of 300 million bubbles, each 0.3 mm in diameter." (*Note:* One millimeter is equal to approximately 0.04 inch and 0.3 mm equals 0.0118 inch.) Figure 36–1 ■ (p. 1004) presents a section of the lung showing many alveoli. Visualize many of these clusters of alveoli arranged as groups around the terminal bronchioles in the lungs. These groups or

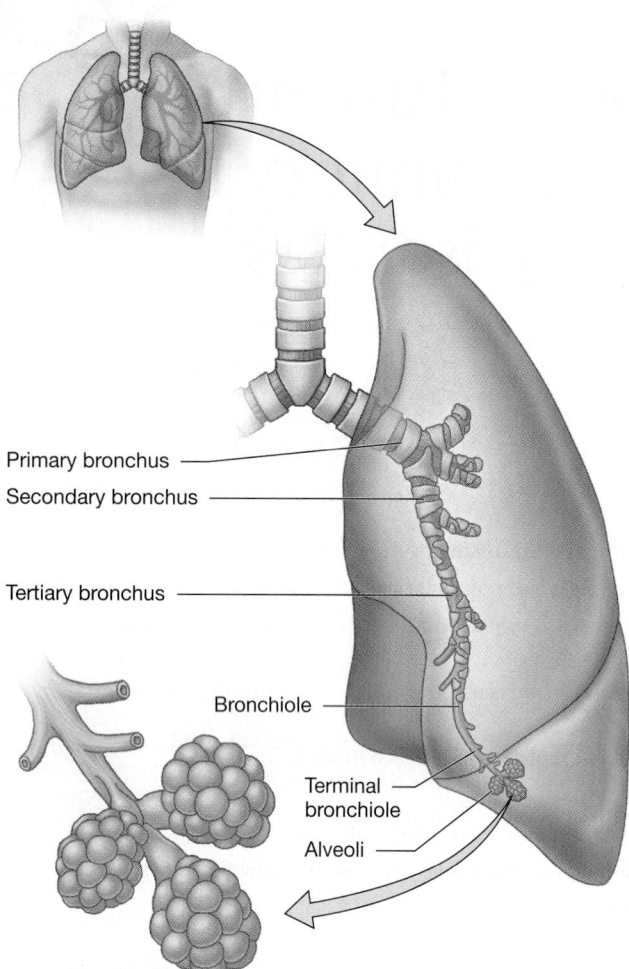

FIGURE 36–1 ■ Alveoli with bronchioles.

Labels in figure: Primary bronchus; Secondary bronchus; Tertiary bronchus; Bronchiole; Terminal bronchiole; Alveoli; **Aveoli enlarged**

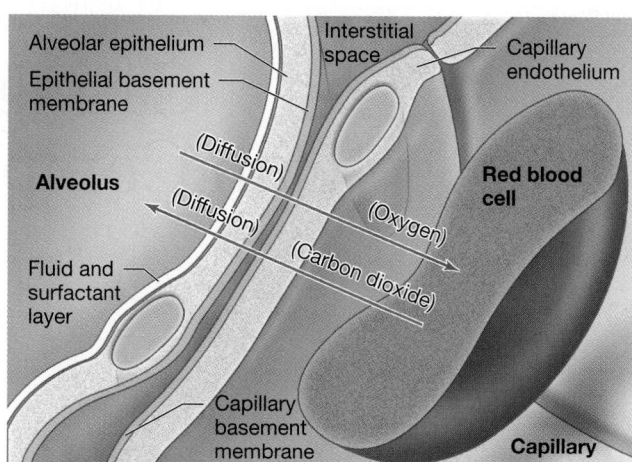

FIGURE 36–2 ■ Alveolar-capillary membrane.

Labels in figure: Alveolar epithelium; Epithelial basement membrane; Interstitial space; Capillary endothelium; (Diffusion); (Diffusion); **Alveolus**; (Oxygen); (Carbon dioxide); **Red blood cell**; Fluid and surfactant layer; Capillary basement membrane; **Capillary**

acini permit 300 million alveoli to fit into the human thorax. The *acinus* is the functional unit of gas exchange and is the terminal respiratory unit of the lung. It is composed of all structures from the respiratory bronchiole to the alveolus, including alveolar ducts, alveolar sacs, and alveoli. This type of formation of the alveoli increases the surface area available for gas exchange in the lungs and makes the pulmonary organ system very efficient.

The 300 million "bubbles" or alveoli are uniquely structured to prevent fluid from filling their air-filled spaces. The distance between the alveolus and the capillary is less than 0.3 micron (a micron is one millionth of a meter). Oxygen diffuses from the alveolus into the pulmonary capillary, and carbon dioxide travels in the opposite direction because the partial pressure of CO_2 is higher in the pulmonary capillaries than it is in the alveoli. This multilayer lamination of tissues begins with the alveolar epithelium that lines the alveoli.

The alveolar epithelium is coated with a thin fluid layer. An important component of this fluid layer is surfactant. **Surfactant** is a surface-active agent that promotes alveolar stability and reduces the likelihood of alveolar collapse. Type II alveolar cells that line the alveoli and the small bronchioles produce surfactant. The alveolus basement membrane provides structure for the alveolus. The next structure, in the middle of the membranes that separate the alveoli from the pulmonary capillary, is a poten-

tial space, called the interstitial space (Figure 36–2 ■). In the normal A-C membrane, the interstitial space contains little or no fluid. In addition to the interstitial space, the pulmonary capillary is composed of a basement membrane and a capillary endothelium through which the gases diffuse. The oxygen diffuses into the red blood cells and attaches to hemoglobin. What is not shown in Figure 36–2 ■ is the lymphatic system in the lungs, which allows transudated fluid to drain from the lungs into the lymph system. Normal flow of this fluid in the lungs is approximately 20 mL/hr at rest (West, 1998). Normally, pressures exerted by water (hydrostatic) and proteins (oncotic) prevent fluid in the pulmonary capillaries and the lymphatics from entering the alveoli. Chart 36–1 describes the normal pressures present in the pulmonary capillaries that cause a net outward movement of a small amount of fluid from the pulmonary capillaries into the interstitial space where it is cleared by the lymphatics.

Oxyhemoglobin Dissociation Curve

The oxyhemoglobin dissociation curve is a commonly used tool for understanding how blood carries and releases oxygen

---

CHART 36–1   Mechanisms of Pulmonary Edema

Forces causing movement of fluid OUT of pulmonary capillaries into pulmonary interstitial space:

Pulmonary capillary hydrostatic pressure	7
Pulmonary interstitial colloid osmotic pressure (oncotic)	14
Negative pulmonary interstitial hydrostatic pressure	8
Total outward force	29

Forces causing adsorption of fluids INTO the pulmonary capillaries:

Pulmonary capillary colloid osmotic pressure	−28
Net outward flow	+ 1

As a result, flow is outward from the pulmonary capillaries into the interstitial space and is pumped away by the lymphatics.

Note: All pressures are in mmHg.

Source: This article was published in *Human Physiology and Mechanism of Disease.* Guyton, A. C., & Hall, J. E. (5 ed., p. 292). Copyright Elsevier 1992.

(Figure 36–3 ■). Specifically, the oxyhemoglobin dissociation curve shows the percentage of oxygen saturation (SO_2) at different oxygen pressures (PaO_2). This is determined by what is called "hemoglobin's affinity for oxygen," that is, how readily hemoglobin acquires and releases oxygen molecules from its surrounding tissue. Oxygen saturation does not change significantly with the higher PaO_2 (flat portion of the curve), but once 60 mmHg is reached, then, very little change in PaO_2 causes a rapid decline in oxygen saturation (steep portion of the curve). The curve can move to either the right or the left. When the curve shifts to the right, the hemoglobin has less affinity for oxygen and O_2 is released easily to the cells. Increased carbon dioxide, decreased pH, and hyperthermia are three conditions that cause a shift to the right. A shift to the left means that it is more difficult for hemoglobin to release oxygen to the tissues. Such a shift is caused by an increased pH, decreased carbon dioxide, and hypothermia (Kaplow & Hardin, 2007). A clear understanding of the association between oxygen and hemoglobin is important to understand the respiratory system pathophysiology. This curve will be referred to throughout this chapter.

Shunts and the Oxyhemoglobin Dissociation Curve

A **shunt** is a passage through which blood may pass or a connection between two locations. In pulmonary physiology, a shunt is present when deoxygenated blood passes through the pulmonary capillary without exchanging oxygen (Guyton & Hall, 2005). There are two types of shunts, physiological shunts and pathologic shunts. A physiological shunt occurs when a portion of the cardiac output goes through the regular pulmonary vasculature without becoming oxygenated in the alveolar sac. There is no abnormal connection between the blood vessels; rather, there is a severe redistribution of pulmonary blood flow due to some pathology. Physiological shunting is often seen in conditions such as pulmonary edema, pneumonia, and lobar atelectasis.

This physiological shunt prevents the SaO_2 (arterial saturation of oxygen) from ever reaching 100% and, for the same reason, prevents the upper arterial plateau of the oxyhemoglobin dissociation curve from reaching 100% saturation (see Figure 36–3).

The other type of shunt is a pathologic shunt. An example of this type of shunt could be a right-to-left septal defect, where deoxygenated blood passes from the right ventricle and flows directly into the left ventricle in a patient with this type of structural cardiac defect. Venous blood from the right heart mixes with oxygenated blood from the left. Breathing 100% oxygen cannot correct a shunt. This is an important diagnostic clue that assists the health care professional in determining the cause of the hypoxemia. Most patients with shunts do not have increased CO_2 levels in the blood because their respiratory center is responding to the hypoxemia by increasing the respiratory rate, therefore maintaining a near normal or low level of CO_2.

Ventilation/Perfusion Mismatching

Ventilation is the movement of air between the atmosphere and the alveoli that is accomplished by respirations, whereas **perfusion** is the movement of blood carrying oxygen and assisting in removing carbon dioxide. Usually there is a near equal relationship of ventilation (V) to perfusion in the lungs. The formula V/Q where ventilation is 4 L/min and perfusion is 5 L/min, explains this relationship. Normal ventilation to perfusion equals 4/5 or 0.8 (Porth, 2007; Shapiro, Peruzzi, & Templin, 1994). Figure 36–4A ■ shows an example of a unit where the perfusion is normal and the ventilation is also normal; that is, V/Q is equal to 0.8. Shapiro's classical example of ventilation and perfusion mismatching explains this principle. There exists a mismatch of ventilation and perfusion when this formula is not equal to 0.8. In Figure 36–4B ■ there is ventilation but no perfusion; note the air sac or alveoli without blood flow, hence no perfusion. This phenomenon is referred to as a dead space unit because there is ventilation and little if

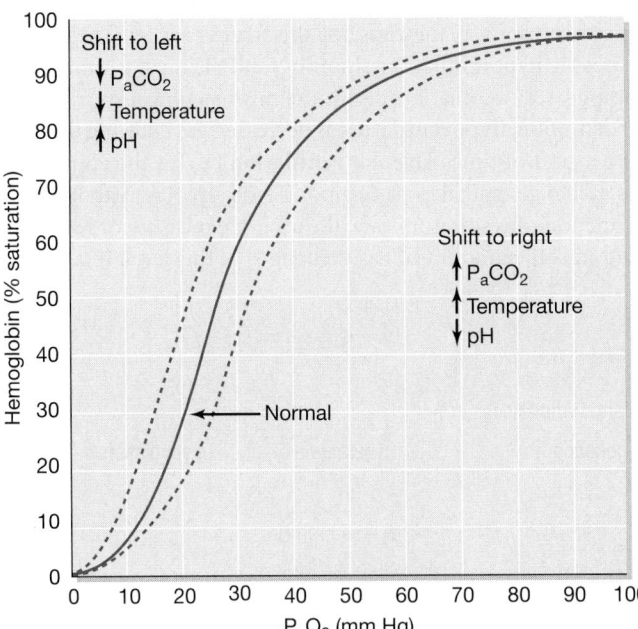

FIGURE 36–3 ■ Oxyhemoglobin dissociation curve.

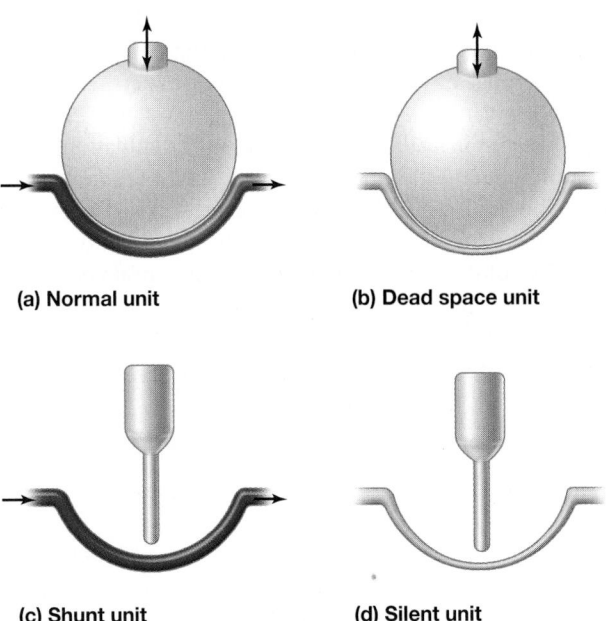

FIGURE 36–4 ■ Ventilation/perfusion relationships: (A) normal unit; (B) dead space unit; (C) shunt unit; (D) silent unit.

any perfusion: V/Q > 0.8. Examples of diseases that are related to an increase in the ventilation-to-perfusion ratio are pulmonary emboli and cardiogenic shock. There is no abnormality in ventilation and the lungs may be normal, but tissues would become hypoxic because of lack of perfusion.

Figure 36–4C ■ (p. 1005) shows a shunt unit where V/Q < 0.8. There is perfusion but little or no ventilation—note that the air sac is collapsed. This occurs in pulmonary edema, pneumonia, and many other causes of respiratory failure. Figure 36–4D ■ (p. 1005) demonstrates both abnormalities producing neither ventilation nor perfusion. Increasing the oxygen concentration can correct some types of V/Q mismatch especially when V/Q < 0.8, but it will not correct other abnormalities caused by shunts. Shunting of blood across collapsed alveoli can cause a type of ventilation/perfusion mismatching that may produce hypoxemia. This "shunt effect" is a type of **ventilation/perfusion mismatch**. It should not be confused with the other main cause of hypoxemia, which was explained previously, even though the same term shunt is used to explain both conditions. Ventilation/perfusion mismatching is a common cause of acute respiratory failure.

■ Acute Respiratory Failure

Acute respiratory failure (ARF) is a condition defined as a failure of gas exchange (Hemmila & Napolitano, 2006). The lungs no longer meet the physiological needs of the body due to a failure of the heart, lungs, or both. The hallmark of ARF is respiratory difficulty with abnormal ABGs.

Epidemiology and Etiology

The purpose of the pulmonary system is to provide oxygen to the cells of the body and remove carbon dioxide and other waste products of metabolism. The inability of the respiratory system to accomplish this function is termed respiratory failure. The epidemiology of acute respiratory failure has recently been reported in four different European countries: Germany, Sweden, Iceland, and Norway (Lewandowski, 2003). The researchers found very similar incidences of ARF among the four countries, namely, a range of 77.6 to 88.6 and 77.6 cases per 100,000 population per year.

ARF results in a failure of oxygenation or ventilation or both (Fink, Abraham, Vincent, & Kochanek, 2005). Respiratory failure can be divided into three main categories, based on etiology: hypoxemic respiratory failure, hypercapneic respiratory failure, and failure of the respiratory centers in the central nervous system. The Diagnostic Tests box lists the normal values for ABGs and compares these normal values to ABGs representative of hypoxemic and hypercapneic respiratory failure.

A failure of oxygenation produces **hypoxemia**, which is defined as an arterial oxygen tension or pressure (PaO_2) that is below normal range. The normal range of PaO_2 is between 80 and 100 mmHg. Therefore, a PaO_2 of less than 60 mmHg and an arterial saturation of oxygen (SaO_2) of less than 90% while breathing room air is representative of hypoxemic respiratory failure. This value of 60 mmHg is located on the steep part of the oxyhemoglobin dissociation curve (see Figure 36–3 ■, p. 1005).

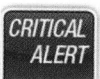

The nurse should assess the patient carefully when:

PaO_2 < 60 mmHg from ABGs
SpO_2 < 90%.

Notify health care provider and increase oxygen delivery.

A failure of the respiratory system to ventilate produces the clinical sign of hypercapnia. Hypercapnia is an abnormal concentration of carbon dioxide ($PaCO_2$) in the blood above normal range. The normal range of $PaCO_2$ is between 35 and 45 mmHg. A $PaCO_2$ of greater than 50 mmHg represents hypercapneic respiratory failure with a pH of less than 7.3. Acute respiratory failure happens quickly, over hours to days, and is not characterized by a gradual worsening of symptoms that would portray chronic respiratory failure. Acute respiratory failure presents with no time for compensation by the renal system. The central and peripheral nervous systems are involved in the control and regulation of respiration. If these systems fail respiratory failure occurs. Chart 36–2 lists the major etiologies causing respiratory failure. This chart is divided into hypoxemic respiratory failure, hypercapneic respiratory failure, and a failure of the respiratory centers in the central nervous system (CNS). These three categories represent the three principal causes of acute respiratory failure.

Pathophysiology

Acute respiratory failure can be traced to three main pathophysiological reasons as the cause of this acute process. These three causes are hypoventilation, shunting, and the most common and complicated, ventilation/perfusion mismatching (West, 1998). By definition, **hypoventilation** is decreased gas entering the alveoli per unit of time. **Alveolar ventilation (V_A)** is the cumulative gas exchange that takes place among each alveolus. Although it is a function of respiratory rate, the accurate measure of hypoventilation is the amount of gas exchanged at this level. It is *not* the

DIAGNOSTIC TESTS for Hypoxemia and Hypercapneic Respiratory Failure

Test		Expected Abnormalities and Rationale	
ABGs	Normal	Hypoxemic-failure of oxygenation	Hypercapneic-failure of ventilation
pH	7.35–7.45	7.35–7.45	< 7.30
PaO_2	80–100 mmHg	< 60 mmHg	80–100 mmHg
$PaCO_2$	35–45 mmHg	35–45 mmHg	> 50–55 mmHg
HCO_3	22–27 mmHg	22–27 mmHg	Can be < 22 mmHg
SaO_2	95–99	< 90 %	> 90 %

CHART 36–2   Etiology of Acute Respiratory Failure

Type of Respiratory Failure	Diagnosis/Disease
Hypoxemic respiratory failure	Acute lung injury Acute respiratory distress syndrome Pneumothorax
Hypercapneic respiratory failure	Oversedation Obesity Diaphragmatic fatigue
Nervous system causes of respiratory failure	Cervical spinal cord injury Guillain-Barré syndrome Myasthenia gravis

CHART 36–3   Clinical Manifestations of Acute Respiratory Failure

System	Signs/Symptoms
Respiratory	Dyspnea Tachypnea Shortness of breath (SOB) Use of accessory muscles for breathing Adventitious lung sounds (crackles, rhonchi, wheezes) Decreased breath sounds Inspiratory/expiratory stridor Cough Increased secretions Orthopnea
Neurological	Agitation Confusion Disorientation Difficult to arouse, sleepiness (hypercarbic respiratory failure) Muscle twitching
Cardiac	Tachycardia Dysrhythmias (ventricular ectopy) Diaphoresis Hypertension or hypotension
Radiologic	Pulmonary infiltrates Atelectasis Pneumothorax Normal

quantity of gas that enters the large airways because the large airways, the trachea, and the bronchi down to the terminal bronchioles have no role in gas exchange. Their role is to transport ambient air beyond the terminal bronchioles where oxygen first meets the alveoli. These transporting airways compose the **anatomic dead space** because no gas exchange occurs. Ventilation of this anatomic region is defined as **dead space ventilation (V_D).**

With hypoventilation, the level of CO_2 in the blood must rise because CO_2 is not exhaled adequately. Some common causes of hypoventilation are drugs that depress the respiratory center, such as morphine and barbiturates. Guillain-Barré syndrome, an immune-mediated disease that affects the peripheral nervous system and eventually causes respiratory depression and failure, respiratory paralysis from a spinal cord injury, and myasthenia gravis that affects the neuromuscular junction are all examples of diseases for which hypoventilation can be the major cause of respiratory failure (Hughes & Cornblath, 2005). Trauma with flail chest or multiple rib fractures, central and obstructive sleep apnea, and morbid obesity also can cause hypoventilation with increased CO_2 retention. Chapter 35 😊 discusses flail chest, Chapter 34 😊 discusses obstructive sleep apnea, and Chapter 19 😊 discusses acid–base disturbances.

Hypoxemia is not a problem with pure hypoventilation and can be easily corrected by increasing the **fraction of inspired oxygen (FiO_2)** concentration. Oxygenation is defined as adding oxygen to any system. In the human body, hemoglobin increases the efficiency of this addition by associating with oxygen at the arterial level and releasing oxygen at the tissue level.

Clinical Manifestations

The presenting symptom in acute respiratory failure is shortness of breath, dyspnea, and increased work of breathing (WOB) with hypoxemia. Dyspnea is difficulty breathing and a subjective symptom (Wang, FitzGerald, Schulzer, Mak, & Ayas, 2005). In addition, the patient may be tachypneic, tachycardic, agitated, confused, and disoriented. There may be increased secretions with a productive cough. Chart 36–3 compares hypoxemic respiratory failure with hypercapneic respiratory failure. Many of the signs and symptoms are shared by both disorders. The central cyanosis of hypoxemic respiratory failure and the muscle twitching caused by the acidosis in hypercapneic respiratory failure are unique for each condition and provide some useful

clues for the nurse. The patient with hypoxemic respiratory failure will rarely become sleepy and usually will not have difficulty being aroused, but the patient who has high CO_2 levels commonly presents with somnolence and a decreased level of consciousness. This is an important diagnostic finding.

Laboratory and Diagnostic Procedures and Monitoring

A chest x-ray assists in determining the primary disorder that is contributing to the respiratory failure, but ABG levels are the most common test for assessing respiratory failure and are useful in predicting the type of respiratory failure the patient may be experiencing (see the Diagnostic Tests box earlier in the chapter for normal ABG values). In acute respiratory failure, no compensation in pH is seen because it takes the kidneys hours to days to compensate for altered pH. See Chapter 19 😊 for a discussion of acid–base imbalance.

Medical Management

Correcting and treating the hypoxemia is the primary goal of treatment of acute respiratory failure. The secondary goal is to discover the cause. Supplemental oxygen devices should be used until treatment can reverse the hypoxemia. Chart 36–4 (p. 1008) outlines the common oxygen delivery devices and percentage of oxygen that they deliver.

 *To treat life-threatening hypoxemia that does not respond to supplemental oxygen, endotracheal intubation is necessary. The nurse must be able to assist with this procedure.*

CHART 36–4	**Common Oxygen Delivery Devices, FiO$_2$, and Flow Rates**	
Device	**FiO$_2$ (%)**	**Flow Rate (L/min)**
Nasal cannula	24	1
	28	2
	32	3
	36	4
	40	5
	44	6
Simple face mask	35–55	5–10
Venturi mask	24	3
	26	3
	28	6
	31	6
	35	9
	40	12
	50	15
Nonrebreather mask	60–80	10–15

Note: FiO$_2$ = fraction of inspired oxygen. These are only approximations, not absolute FiO$_2$ values, because the delivery is via a mask or cannula.

If these devices fail to correct the hypoxemia, intubation and institution of mechanical ventilation are considered. Besides intubation, another intervention that is being used for more causes of acute respiratory failure is **noninvasive positive pressure ventilation (NPPV)**. This intervention uses a ventilator and mask attachment, either a nasal or full-face mask, to deliver the oxygen without requiring the use of an endotracheal tube and intubation. This intervention is discussed in more detail later in the chapter.

Gerontological Considerations

As the population of elderly patients increases, the potential exists for an increase in the incidence of acute respiratory failure. Nurses who care for the elderly must be aware of the important differences between the elderly patient with respiratory failure and those who are younger. There are some significant differences in the elderly person's respiratory system that predispose the elderly to developing respiratory failure. These differences have to do with the physiological effects of aging. Chart 36–5 outlines the physiological effects of aging on the pulmonary system.

A decrease in the forced expiratory volume in one second (FEV$_1$) begins after age 30 and is further pronounced if the patient smokes. The other criteria listed in Chart 36–5 include many important physiological parameters that are accentuated as the person ages and the muscles become deconditioned. Once the elderly patient has respiratory failure and is intubated and placed on mechanical ventilation, her outcome is not that different than that from of her younger counterparts. A recent study determined that the highest risks of death among patients who were 70 years or older were not related to age but to coexistent acute renal failure, shock, and limited functional status (Estebam et al., 2004). These predictors of death were more important than age. Age alone should not be a criterion for anticipating the success or failure of mechanical ventilation. However, age has a complex relationship with the most severe type of respiratory failure: acute respiratory distress disorder (ARDS). In a study of ARDS in trauma patients, patients 60 to 69 years of age showed increasingly higher risks for

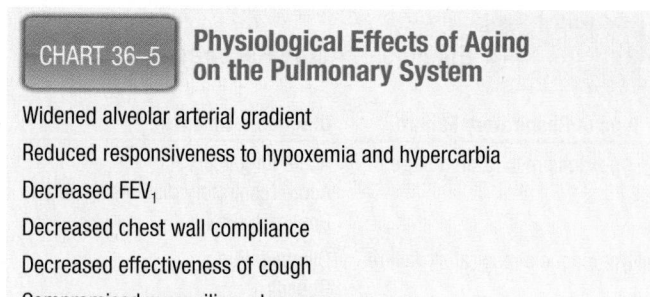

CHART 36–5	**Physiological Effects of Aging on the Pulmonary System**

Widened alveolar arterial gradient

Reduced responsiveness to hypoxemia and hypercarbia

Decreased FEV$_1$

Decreased chest wall compliance

Decreased effectiveness of cough

Compromised mucociliary clearance

ARDS development (Johnston, Rubenfeld, & Hudson, 2003). Patients who were older had a decreased risk of ARDS. Although these results may be confusing, this study further emphasizes the importance of not predicting outcome by using age alone.

■ Acute Pulmonary Edema

Acute pulmonary edema is an abnormal accumulation of fluid in the lungs. This fluid accumulates because of a dysfunction with the lungs and/or the heart. Acute pulmonary edema may be attributed to many different etiologies and types of pulmonary edema, which are discussed below. These etiologies have different names but all can be traced back to a failure of the heart, lungs, or both. Heart failure is discussed in detail in Chapter 42 ⊚.

Epidemiology

Acute pulmonary edema is a common medical problem. Epidemiologic data on heart failure, which is the primary cause of cardiogenic acute pulmonary edema, demonstrates an incidence of 10 per 1,000 in persons more than 65 years old in the United States (Jessup & Brozena, 2003). Most patients with heart failure are admitted to the emergency department for life-saving treatment (Collins, Lindsell, Storrow, & Abraham, 2006). However, there is evidence that the number of patients who present with heart failure is declining because of improved hospital management (Fox et al., 2007). Heart failure, a chronic disease, affects about 5 million people in the United States with an incidence of 550,000 cases annually (Onwuanyi & Taylor, 2007). See Chapter 42 ⊚ for a complete discussion of heart failure.

Etiologies

Acute pulmonary edema refers to the time frame during which the fluid accumulation develops. In acute pulmonary edema, this occurs quickly over minutes to hours. Some clinicians use the term *flash pulmonary edema* to define pulmonary edema that occurs within minutes of a precipitating event. Reported causes of flash pulmonary edema include the classic cardiac pathologies of left ventricular dysfunction as a result of a massive myocardial infarction or valve dysfunction with or without papillary muscle rupture. When the pulmonary capillary pressure rises quickly and reaches two to three times the normal pressures in the pulmonary arteries, edema fluid floods the interstitial space and the alveoli. The pulmonary lymphatic system and other vessels have no time to compensate, unlike in chronic pulmonary edema in which the pressure in the pulmonary arteries can be higher but the lungs have time to compensate. The etiology of pulmonary edema is divided into cardiogenic and noncardiogenic categories.

Cardiogenic pulmonary edema (CPE) is pulmonary edema that results from increased hydrostatic pressures in the pulmonary capillary bed secondary to increased pulmonary venous pressure due to heart failure (Jessup & Brozena, 2003). This pulmonary hypertension is related to many factors, the most common of which is cardiac dysfunction. But fluid overload and chronic hypoxemia also can contribute to this type of pulmonary edema. Pulmonary hypertension is a compensatory mechanism that develops as a result of hypoxemia and can lead to remodeling of the pulmonary vasculature. Pulmonary hypertension is discussed in detail in Chapter 35 .

Heart failure can be from cardiac muscle dysfunction or valvular problems. Dysrhythmias, especially tachydysrhythmias, such as supraventricular and ventricular tachycardias, can precipitate pulmonary edema (see Chapter 38). Constrictive pericarditis is present when a thickened, fibrotic, and adherent pericardium restricts diastolic filling of the heart. It usually begins with an initial episode of acute pericarditis. Dressler's syndrome is a common type of pericarditis that occurs after an acute myocardial infarction. A large majority of cases of constrictive pericarditis are idiopathic or without a known cause (Talreja et al., 2003).

Noncardiogenic pulmonary edema (NCPE) is related to injury of the A-C membrane from numerous causes. Among the most important causes are sepsis, inflammation, inhaled toxins, and drugs. In NCPE usually there is no primary cardiac dysfunction. Chart 36–6 lists typical etiologies of pulmonary edema comparing the cardiac and noncardiac causes. Both types of pulmonary edema, cardiogenic and noncardiogenic, produce, as an end result, excess fluid in the lungs. This excess fluid in the alveoli decreases the number of alveoli available for gas exchange; however, the mechanism is very different. The initial insult in noncardiogenic pulmonary edema is caused by a change in the permeability of the A-C membrane caused by direct injury or as result of inflammation, whereas the initial insult in cardiogenic pulmonary edema is caused by heart failure.

One of the syndromes that is listed as a cause of NCPE is ARDS. Because of its prevalence and high mortality, this disease is discussed in more detail later in this chapter. Cardiogenic pulmonary edema, caused by an increased pressure in the pulmonary capillaries due to heart failure, is the major focus of this section. The next section discusses some common causes of noncardiogenic pulmonary edema other than ARDS.

Neurogenic Pulmonary Edema

Neurogenic pulmonary edema (NPE) is associated with direct insult to the CNS. Seizures, cerebral hemorrhage, and head injury are common precipitating factors to the development of pulmonary edema. The pathophysiology of the edema formation is not clear, but it might be related to disruption in sympathetic tone related to increased venous pressure and hypertension. The presenting symptom for these patients is dyspnea, but the other signs and symptoms of pulmonary edema— crackles, shortness of breath, and pink frothy sputum—also can be seen. Treatment includes treating the underlying events as well as supportive care (Fontes et al., 2003).

Negative Pressure Pulmonary Edema

Negative pressure pulmonary edema (NPPE) is caused by attempting to ventilate with an apparent airway obstruction. *Postobstruction pulmonary edema* and *airway obstruction pul-*

CHART 36–6	Common Causes of Acute Pulmonary Edema
Type of Acute Pulmonary Edema	**Disease/Condition**
Cardiogenic	Myocardial infarction
	Myocardial ischemia
	Hypertension
	Cardiomyopathies
	Viral myocarditis
	Acute dysrhythmias
	Valvular dysfunction
	Atrial myxomas
	Papillary muscle rupture
	Pericarditis
	Cardiac tamponade
Noncardiogenic	Acute lung injury (ALI)
	Acute respiratory distress syndrome (ARDS)
	Neurogenic pulmonary edema
	Excessive intravenous fluid administration
	Postoperative pulmonary edema
	Acute renal failure
	Pneumonia
	Drowning
Population or disease specific	High-altitude pulmonary edema
	Heroin-related pulmonary edema
	Transfusion-related acute lung injury
	Hyperbaric oxygen therapy
	Postanesthesia
	Postcardiopulmonary bypass
	Diving-related pulmonary edema
	Malaria
	Eclampsia
	Negative pressure pulmonary edema
Medication or chemical inhalant related	Certain chemotherapeutic agents
	Smoke and burn injuries
	Biowarfare agents (e.g., anthrax)
	Allergic reaction to IV contrast

monary edema are other names for the same disorder. This type of pulmonary edema develops because of the extreme pressures that are used to attempt to ventilate during the obstruction. These high pressures are transmitted to the pulmonary system, increasing transpulmonary pressures as well as pleural pressures. Once the airway obstruction is relieved, hydrostatic pressure forces fluid into the alveoli and pulmonary edema develops.

The most common cause of NPPE is laryngospasm during intubation or after extubation (Fremont, Kallet, Matthay, & Ware, 2007). NPPE has also been associated with oropharyngeal surgery and patients who have had head and neck surgeries. Symptoms of this type of pulmonary edema mimic other types of pulmonary edema with production of pink frothy sputum, difficulty breathing, tachypnea, and tachycardia. Treatment consists of positive pressure ventilation with positive end-expiratory pressure (PEEP). In some circumstances diuretics can be used. Hemodynamic monitoring will assist the health care provider in differentiating this type of noncardiogenic pulmonary edema from cardiogenic pulmonary edema (Tarrac, 2003).

High-Altitude Pulmonary Edema

High-altitude pulmonary edema (HAPE) is listed as a cause of pulmonary edema in a specific population: skiers and climbers. This type of pulmonary edema develops in persons who rapidly ascend to heights greater than 2,500 to 3,000 meters (8,202 to 9,842 feet). The pathogenesis of the formation of pulmonary edema is debated. The hypothesis is that a pulmonary vasoconstriction causes a relative hypoxemia. This increases the pressure in the pulmonary capillaries, thus forcing fluid into the interstitial space and the alveoli. A direct injury pattern from inflammatory mediators and oxygen free radicals also are believed to be responsible for some of the pulmonary capillary direct injury. Oxygen free radicals are components of oxygen that have an unpaired electron on an oxygen atom. These free radicals are believed to cause tissue injury at the cellular level. An example of an oxygen free radical is the one-electron reduction of O_2, which produces the superoxide radical, O_2. The most important treatment is removal from high altitudes. If this is done, the pulmonary edema should resolve. Other treatment measures include steroids and oxygen therapy (Gabry, Ledoux, Mozziconacci, & Martin, 2003).

Heroin-Related Pulmonary Edema

Another example of population-specific pulmonary edema is *heroin-related pulmonary edema* (HRPE). Heroin is one of the most commonly abused narcotics in the United States (Habal, 2006). This type of edema develops within 24 hours of the administration of heroin and has been reported in users of cocaine and methadone. One review reported that clinical symptoms appear immediately or within 4 hours of the administered dose of heroin and that 39% of patients who develop this type of pulmonary edema require mechanical ventilation (Frishman, Del Vecchio, Sanal, & Ismail, 2003).

Excessive Intravenous Fluid Administration

Any patient who has a continuous intravenous infusion and receives a large amount of fluid over a short period of time can develop pulmonary edema. If the patient has any comorbidities such as cardiac, pulmonary, or renal disease the risk of developing pulmonary edema increases. The pathophysiology of this type of pulmonary edema is very clear. Increased venous return of the excessive fluid contributes to increased pulmonary pressures that cause fluid to leak into interstitial spaces and then into the alveoli. A patient population that is at increased risk for this type of pulmonary edema is the dialysis-dependent patient. Fluid management for the patient who is in renal failure presents a challenge because underresuscitation of hypotension can be as harmful as overresuscitation. Failure of the dialysis-dependent patient to follow dietary restrictions (e.g., salt intake) predisposes this patient population to pulmonary edema.

The patient who is dialysis dependent is at risk for the development of pulmonary edema after excessive fluid administrative (Arieff, 1999; Fleischmann, Goldman, Young, & Lee, 2003). In Arieff's study 13 patients who died of postoperative pulmonary edema were analyzed for predictive factors. In the 13 patients each had retained greater than $67 \text{ mL} \cdot \text{kg}^{-1} \cdot \text{day}^{-1}$ and there was no presenting sign. However, cardiorespiratory arrest was the most frequent clinical presentation.

Transfusion-Related Lung Injury

Patients who receive any type of transfusion are at risk for *transfusion-related acute lung injury* (TRALI), which can cause noncardiogenic pulmonary edema. Transfusions that can cause this syndrome include packed red blood cells, platelets, granulocytes, and fresh frozen plasma (Looney, Gropper, & Matthay, 2004). This syndrome has also been reported following allogeneic stem cell transplantation. The classic symptoms of dyspnea, hypoxemia, and bilateral pulmonary edema occur within 4 to 6 hours of administration of blood products. A large percentage of the patients require support with either intubation or noninvasive ventilation. An impressive feature of this type of NCPE is the speed of development and onset of pulmonary edema. The patient who has no respiratory problem receives a transfusion and within 4 to 6 hours requires maximal ventilation support in order to ventilate and oxygenate. TRALI is discussed in detail in Chapter 23 🔗.

Hyperbaric Oxygen Therapy and Diving-Related Pulmonary Edema

Hyperbaric oxygen therapy and SCUBA (self-contained underwater breathing apparatus) diving can predispose this special population to pulmonary edema related to the increased pressure of oxygen used in both hyperbaric treatment and recreationally for SCUBA diving. Removal from the increased pressure resolves symptoms (Halpern, Gefen, Sorkine, & Elad, 2003).

Inhalation of Toxic Substances Related to Bioterrorism or Accidental Exposure

No discussion of the etiologies of noncardiogenic pulmonary edema would be complete without discussing the causes of NCPE related to inhalation of a toxic chemical or a bioterrorism agent. These agents can be bacteria, viruses, or biotoxins that are naturally occurring compounds, such as ricin, that are released for the purpose of inflicting harm or inciting terror. Many of the agents that are listed by the Centers for Disease Control and Prevention (CDC) as Category A agents cause death by attacking the lung parenchyma either directly or as a result of an inflammatory process. The CDC categorizes agents as A, B, and C based on their ability to inflict harm (CDC, 2007). Category A agents are those that can inflict the greatest harm and pose the greatest threat to the public. The Category A bioterrorism agents are listed in Chart 36–7. Anthrax and plague are discussed next because of their presenting symptoms and as examples of Category A agents. More information on these types of agents is given in Chapter 72 🔗.

Bacillus anthracis is a gram-positive bacillus that is present in nature. Humans contract anthrax when they come in contact with animals or animal products. Three different sources of anthrax infections are known: gastrointestinal, cutaneous, and inhalation. Cutaneous anthrax is the most common type. Lesions on the skin develop a black eschar. With appropriate treatment deaths from cutaneous anthrax are rare (Inglesby et al., 2002). Gastrointestinal anthrax is uncommon. However, inhalation of the bacillus anthrax spores is the most deadly source of the types of anthrax. The various defense mechanisms of the respiratory system assist in activating the anthrax spores. As the spores are inhaled, the natural defense mechanism of the alveoli breaks down the spores. The alveolar macrophages destroy some of the inhaled spores, but others are transported in the lymph system to the mediastinal lymph nodes where they germinate. What causes this germination is not fully understood and the time range for activation of the spores can range in time from 2 to 43 days (Inglesby et al., 2002). Once the spores have germinated, clinical

CHART 36–7	**Category A Bioterrorism Agents**
Agent	**Brief Description**
Anthrax	Caused by *Bacillus anthracis*. Most severe form is inhalational anthrax, which produces fever, chills, malaise, widened mediastinum, pulmonary infiltrates, pleural effusion, and pulmonary edema (Ingelsby et al., 2002).
Plague	Caused by *Yersinia pestis*. Three types of plague: bubonic, septicemic, and pneumonic. Pneumonic plague is characterized by sudden-onset cough, fever, and chest pain (Cobbs & Chansolme, 2004).
Smallpox	Caused by *Variola* virus and is highly infectious. Produces a rash, fever, and chills. Contagious and because of vaccine has been eradicated as a natural occurring disease (Lupatkin, Lupatkin, & Rosenberg, 2004).
Botulism	Caused by *Clostridium botulinum*. Present in contaminated foods, but botulinum toxin can be used as an aerosolized agent in a bioterrorism attack. Bacillus produces neurotoxins that cause paralysis (Karwa et al., 2005).
Viral hemorrhagic fever	Caused by a diverse group of RNA viruses. Produces complex clinical syndrome of fever, chills, disturbances in regional circulation, and bleeding. Marburg and Ebola viruses are in this category (Karwa et al., 2005).
Tularemia	Caused by *Francisella tularensis*, a gram-negative bacterium. Patients present with fever, chills, and generalized weakness. Predisposes patients to pneumonia and ARDS (Karwa et al., 2005).

symptoms appear. Theses symptoms include fever, chills, and sweating with a nonproductive or minimally productive cough. Dyspnea and tachycardia are two other presenting symptoms.

At the presenting stage of the disease, the clinical symptoms for a case of acute febrile respiratory infection and inhalational anthrax are very similar. But as the disease progresses, pleural effusion, a widened mediastinum, and the presence of the bacillus in blood and other fluid cultures help the clinician differentiate the symptoms. The patient's clinical course deteriorates quickly with development of severe hypoxemia, ARDS, and shock. If recognized and treated early with antibiotics, mortality can be as low as 45% (Karwa, Currie, & Kvetan, 2005). Inhalational anthrax is not contagious. Normal universal precautions are all that is required for protection. A vaccine (Biothrax) is available but recommendations for its use are for the military and laboratory workers who are engaged in studying the bacillus (Karwa et al., 2005).

The "Black Death" or plague is really three diseases or clinical entities, namely, bubonic plague, septicemic plague, and pneumonic plague. All three diseases are caused by the bacterial pathogen *Yersinia pestis*. The disease is spread from the bite of a flea or direct contact with an animal that is infected. Two to 8 days after the contact, the person develops symptoms. The symptoms include fever, chills, and weakness. The other classic findings of bubonic plague are swollen and painful lymph glands. These are called buboes and are usually located in the

lymph node closest to where the contact occurred. These buboes appear as nonmovable masses. With antibiotic treatment the mortality is approximately 50% (Cobbs & Chansolme, 2004). Pneumonic plague is spread from infected droplets coughed by patients who are already infected. In this disease the microorganisms develop in the lung and spread systemically. Symptoms include cough, fever, chills, and chest pain. Pneumonia and lung consolidation occur rapidly. Without treatment with appropriate antibiotics, mortality is 100%. This type of plague is highly contagious and is spread from person-to-person contact through the aerosolized droplet. Because of the contagious properties and the mortality rate, pneumonic plague makes an excellent choice as an agent for bioterrorism.

Besides the viruses and bacteria that have been discussed, other agents such as chemicals can cause severe swelling of the respiratory tract, upper airways, and lungs. The subsequent pulmonary edema that develops from the injury caused by these agents produces dyspnea, shortness of breath, and death if the inhalation is severe. Chemical agents include ammonia, bromine, chlorine, hydrogen chlorine, phosgene, phosphine, and phosphorus. They can be inhaled as a result of an accidental exposure or because of bioterrorism. All of these agents produce an injury to the lung tissue and, if severe enough, death. Together these agents are termed pulmonary edemagens (Baker, 2005).

Two chemical agents, chlorine and phosgene, have similar injury patterns. Chlorine is one of the most common chemicals produced by man. It has many uses in bleaching and cleaning. If inhaled, chlorine gas is corrosive to the throat, lungs, eyes, and skin. When chlorine gas comes in contact with water, it forms hypochlorous acid and hydrochloric acid. These acids can cause damage to skin, eyes, and lung tissue. Therefore, water substantially enhances chlorine's oxidizing and corrosive effects. If exposed, washing and flushing of exposed mucous membranes is recommended. The symptoms depend on the amount of gas inhaled. Treatment is supportive.

Phosgene is a liquid and a vapor that is formed by the natural decomposition of chlorinated hydrocarbons. During World War I both sides used phosgene gas as a military weapon. Exposure to this gas causes pulmonary edema. The gas attacks the alveoli and the type I and II pneumocytes. Phosgene gas destroys the alveolar macrophages. The parenchymal lung injury produces platelet aggregation and vasoconstriction with increased capillary permeability. Treatment of phosgene gas inhalation includes supportive care and mechanical ventilation if the injury is severe. There is some information that supports steroid use in toxic gas inhalation (Baker, 2005).

The final category of substances that can be harmful if ingested or inhaled are those listed by the CDC as biotoxins. These naturally occurring proteins include ricin. Ricin is a glucoprotein that is extracted from the castor bean (*Ricinus communis*). Castor beans have been used for centuries all over the world for the oil that is used as a laxative and for lubricating. Ricin is produced from the mash of the castor bean after the oil is extracted. Ricin can be easily manufactured from a substance that is readily available, which makes it an excellent agent for bioterrorism. Ricin works by inhibiting protein synthesis in all cells with which it comes in contact. The toxin binds to the cell membrane and then is incorporated into the cell by a process termed receptor-mediated endocytosis (Doan, 2004). This process eventually destroys the cell. The liver and spleen are susceptible. There is a significant lag time between exposure and symptoms because of this process. Inhalation of ricin is rare but pulmonary symptoms would include increased permeability, pulmonary edema, shock, and death within 35 to 72 hours (Marks, 2004). Usually ingestion of the beans or parenteral injection of ricin is the method of contact. Symptoms include nausea, vomiting, diarrhea, and abdominal cramps with subsequent dehydration. Fever can be present. Treatment is supportive and a vaccine is under development (Doan, 2004).

Pathophysiology

The pathophysiology of acute pulmonary edema and the signs and symptoms of this dysfunction are related to the accumulation of fluid preventing adequate gas exchange across the alveolar-capillary membrane. This fluid accumulates in the interstitial space and floods the alveoli, thereby interfering with gas exchange. The three causes include (1) too much fluid being delivered to the delicate pulmonary capillaries; (2) increased pressure in the capillaries due to constriction, to such an extent that fluid is forced across the capillary into the alveolus; and (3) capillary injury, which causes a leaking of fluid, even if it is a normal amount.

Pathophysiology of Cardiogenic Pulmonary Edema

In cardiogenic pulmonary edema fluid enters the alveoli and prevents the diffusion of oxygen and carbon dioxide across the A-C membrane into the pulmonary capillaries. In CPE, this space is one of the first to fill with transudated fluid that is "pushed out" of the pulmonary capillaries. Transudated fluid is fluid that has decreased protein and cellular elements as compared to normal serum. This fluid shift occurs due to changes in the dynamics of the A-C membrane that are caused by increased pulmonary capillary pressure.

The fluid accumulates because of a primary cardiac etiology that causes the increased pulmonary capillary pressure. The interstitial edema occurs before the alveolar edema. Acute pulmonary edema develops when the pulmonary capillary pressure exceeds the pulmonary oncotic pressure. The increased pressure in the pulmonary capillary forces fluid into the interstitial space and the alveoli. The fluid that enters the interstitial space decreases the interstitial oncotic pressure. Increased fluid overwhelms the lymphatic drainage. Normally the pulmonary capillary oncotic pressure prevents fluid from flowing out of the pulmonary vessels, but this oncotic pressure is now lower than the pulmonary capillary pressure and fluid is forced to exit the pulmonary capillaries. The only place that this fluid can flow is into the interstitial space and then into the alveoli, producing pulmonary edema. Increased pulmonary capillary pressure, above the plasma oncotic pressure, is the central physiological event that causes fluid to follow this pathologic route. This interstitial edema is the first sign of pulmonary edema. As the fluid accumulates, it leaks into the spaces around the bronchi (peribronchial) and, finally, into the alveolus, preventing gas exchange. Eventually, if treatment is not instituted, more alveoli become flooded with fluid and collapse. Surfactant is washed out and deactivated. Lung compliance falls and the work of breathing increases as more and more of the lung becomes un-

available for gas exchange. Chart 36–8 lists the stages of cardiogenic pulmonary edema.

Systolic Dysfunction

Failure of the left ventricle to effectively propel blood into the aorta during systole is one the most common causes of pulmonary edema (Sanderson & Fraser, 2006). There are numerous causes of left ventricular dysfunction including acute myocardial infarction, valvular dysfunction, and viral cardiomyopathies. Chapter 42 ⊘ reviews the pathophysiology of heart failure. Severe heart failure always produces pulmonary edema related to increased pressures in the pulmonary circuit. To compensate for decreased cardiac contractility and decreased ejection fraction, the left ventricle dilates and the pressures in the left ventricle at end diastole increase. This produces increased pressure in the left atrium and in the pulmonary circulation. This pressure is higher than the pulmonary oncotic pressure. The end result is that fluid develops in the interstitial space and then flows into the alveoli.

Diastolic Dysfunction

Another cause of heart failure is diastolic dysfunction (Brutsaert & De Keulenaer, 2006). Diastolic dysfunction produces slowed or decreased ventricular relaxation. This can be initiated by decreased venous return or preload and/or decreased compliance of the ventricle. The result of diastolic dysfunction is an increase in the pulmonary pressure and development of pulmonary edema (Andrew, 2003). Patients who develop acute hypertensive crisis

CHART 36–8	Stages of Cardiogenic Pulmonary Edema
Stages of Pulmonary Edema	**Physiological Abnormality**
Stage I	Fluid and colloids move into the lungs' interstitial space from the pulmonary capillaries. The lymphatics are able to increase flow and remove the fluid. Blood gas exchange does not deteriorate, or it may even be slightly improved.
Stage II	The lymphatics become overwhelmed with fluid and the efficient pump fails. The lung interstitial space becomes flooded. The interstitial space in the lungs is located around the bronchioles, arterioles, and venules in the dependent regions. The accumulation of liquid in the interstitium may compromise the small airways, leading to mild hypoxemia.
Stage III	Fluid continues to flow into the interstitial space. A large amount of fluid can be sequestered in this space in the lungs. With increasing fluid comes increasing pressure and fluid flows across the alveolar epithelium into the alveoli preventing gas exchange. The interstitial space can contain up to 500 mL of fluid. With further accumulations, the fluid crosses the alveolar epithelium into the alveoli, leading to alveolar flooding. This results in abnormalities in gas exchange and vital capacity, respiratory volumes are substantially reduced, and hypoxemia becomes more severe.

Source: Adapted from Sovari, A. A. (2008). Pulmonary edema: Cardiogenic. *eMedicine.* Retrieved June 4, 2008, from http://www.emedicine.com/med/topic1955.htm#.

can have diastolic dysfunction. Increased heart rate is the most common cause of decreased cardiac filling time. In the borderline cardiac patient, increasing the heart rate from 60 to 120 beats/min decreases diastolic filling time by approximately one-half the time the heart has to fill, resulting in cardiac diastolic dysfunction.

Other Cardiac Pathophysiological Causes

Pericardial tamponade from trauma or neoplasms produces increased fluid in the pericardium (Sagrista-Sauleda et al., 2006). This increased pressure around the heart prevents the heart from filling and contracting appropriately and can result in pulmonary edema. The force of the fluid in the pericardium produces increased pressures in the most distensible chambers of the heart, the atria. Again, this increased pressure results in pulmonary artery hypertension and, if not treated, pulmonary edema. This mechanical obstruction to the contraction of the heart usually is easily treated by removal of the fluid.

Valvular dysfunction, whether in a mitral or aortic valve, can cause pulmonary edema. See Chapter 41 ⊙ for a discussion of the pathophysiology of valve dysfunction.

Another cause of pulmonary edema is atrial myxomas. Atrial myxoma usually is a benign primary tumor of the heart that develops either in the right or left atria. Seventy-five to 80% develop in the left atrium (Percell, Henning, & Siddique Patel, 2003). The myxoma is attached to the atrial wall by a stemlike structure. Myxomas can interfere with atrial function and produce pulmonary edema. If the myxoma becomes detached from the wall and occludes the atria, sudden death occurs. Treatment involves cardiac surgery for removal of the tumor.

Pathophysiology of Noncardiogenic Pulmonary Edema

In noncardiogenic pulmonary edema the fluid fills the alveoli because of direct injury to the membrane itself, not because of increased hydrostatic pressure as a primary event. When excess fluid collects in the interstitial space, special receptors are stimulated to help with clearing this fluid. These juxtacapillary receptors, or J receptors, increase respiratory rate and assist in increasing lymphatic drainage from the lungs.

Clinical Manifestations

The primary presenting clinical signs and symptoms of pulmonary edema are those of respiratory distress progressing to respiratory failure. The clinical manifestations include rapidly worsening dyspnea, shortness of breath, tachypnea, agitation, and adventitious lung sounds (Ware & Matthay, 2005). The other clinical signs are hypertension, tachycardia, and possibly S_3 or S_4 heart sounds. The chest x-ray demonstrates increased pulmonary infiltrates. ABGs are significant for hypoxemia and hypercarbia with a respiratory acidosis. Auscultation of the lungs provides the key assessment clue to the diagnosis of pulmonary edema. Crackles in the bases of the lungs bilaterally usually are an early sign of pulmonary edema. The crackles could advance to fill the entire lung field. Other adventitious lung sounds, such as wheezes and rhonchi, heard over the large airways also could be present. Cough and production of pink frothy sputum are the classic presenting signs of pulmonary edema. Central cyanosis and circumoral pallor, that is, a bluish tinge to the lips and mucous membranes, re-

flects worsening hypoxemia. Pulse oximetry (SpO_2) or the percent of saturation of oxygen demonstrates the hypoxemia with readings in the high 80s to low 90s, and ABGs could reflect a respiratory acidosis with increased carbon dioxide levels.

Chart 36–9 contrasts the assessment of cardiogenic pulmonary edema to noncardiogenic pulmonary edema. Notice that the respiratory assessment clues are identical for both types of pulmonary edema. In the cardiac assessment, some very subtle changes might assist the nurse in differentiating the two types of pulmonary edema. Tachycardia with hypotension and cool diaphoretic skin would be prognostic of a cardiogenic pathology, whereas tachycardia with hypertension bounding pulses and dry skin would be more predictive of a noncardiogenic cause. Jugular venous distention (JVD) occurs if there is right heart failure with a present hepatojugular reflex. JVD is a much more common finding in cardiogenic pulmonary edema than noncardiogenic. If a pulmonary artery catheter were placed, a pulmonary artery catheter wedge pressure (PCWP), or pulmonary artery occlusion pressure (PAOP) of greater than 18 mmHg would confirm a cardiogenic cause of the pulmonary edema. See Chapter 24 ⊙ for a complete discussion of pulmonary artery catheters. Agitation and confusion are common symptoms of hypoxemia and sometimes are the first symptoms. The nurse should be alert to not discounting these important symptoms when assessing a patient with any type of respiratory distress.

Laboratory and Diagnostic Procedures

Increased interstitial markings on a chest x-ray can be a diagnostic finding of pulmonary edema. The chest x-ray also may reveal

CHART 36–9	Comparison of Cardiogenic Pulmonary Edema and Noncardiogenic Pulmonary Edema	
Assessment Parameters	**CPE**	**NCPE**
Cardiovascular	Tachycardia	Tachycardia
	Hypotension (LV failure)	Hypertension
	Murmurs (valve dysfunction)	Bounding pulses
	Extra heart sounds present (S_3, S_4)	PCWP < 18 mmHg
	PCWP > 18 mmHg	
	Jugular venous distention	
Pulmonary	Dyspnea, orthopnea, shortness of breath	
	Crackles bilaterally	
	Wheezes and rhonchi	
	SpO_2 and ABGs = hypoxemia and hypercapnia	
	Central cyanosis	
	Cough	
	Pink frothy sputum	
Neurological	Agitation	
	Confusion and disorientation	
	If CO_2 high, difficult to arouse	
Skin	Cool and diaphoretic	Warm and dry
	Pallor or mottling	
Chest x-ray	Diffuse bilateral or alveolar infiltrates	

Note: PCWP = pulmonary capillary wedge pressure; SpO_2 = saturation of oxygen obtained from plethysmograph signal amplitudes.

an enlarged heart. ABGs should be monitored at regular intervals for respiratory acidosis with increased carbon dioxide levels. An echocardiogram is indicated to detect a weak heart muscle, leaky or narrow heart valves, or fluid surrounding the heart. Serum testing for B-type natriuretic peptide has improved diagnostic accuracy (Mattu, Martinez, & Kelly, 2005).

Medical Management of Acute Pulmonary Edema

The most important treatment of pulmonary edema is to provide supplemental oxygen and, if necessary, intubation with mechanical ventilation to relieve the symptoms of hypoxemia. Recently, noninvasive positive pressure ventilation (NPPV) using full or partial masks has been used to treat acute pulmonary edema (Liesching, Kwok, & Hill, 2003). This mode of treatment removes the risks of intubation. Supplemental oxygen should be titrated to increase the SpO_2 and relieve air hunger. This treatment is the first line until the cause of the pulmonary edema is determined. Treatment also includes a short-acting diuretic such as furosemide. Medications to strengthen the heart muscle or to relieve the pressure on the heart may also be given. Specific medications are discussed next.

Medical Management of Cardiogenic Pulmonary Edema

After airway management, diuretics and vasodilators are the mainstay for treatment of cardiogenic pulmonary edema. Treatment should focus on aggressive preload and afterload reduction, not just diuretics. Intravenous (IV) furosemide is the diuretic of choice. Furosemide decreases venous return, reduces blood pressure, and decreases afterload. Diuresis should occur within 30 minutes of an intravenous dose. Morphine sulfate titrated to blood pressure relieves anxiety and decreases venous return, although, in higher doses, it can cause respiratory depression. Administering small doses of morphine sulfate, 2 to 4 mg IV, and titrating to blood pressure can prevent this side effect (Brunton, Lazo, & Parker, 2005). Continuous IV vasodilators, such as nitroglycerin, are useful in decreasing preload. In acute pulmonary edema, the IV route is preferred because of rapid onset of action and ability to relieve symptoms. The intravenous infusion can be discontinued and the effects of the drug are quickly reversed.

The safety and efficacy of the angiotensin-converting enzyme inhibitor (ACEI) enalapril were established in a randomized clinical trial to treat pulmonary edema (Annane et al., 1996). In this landmark study, 20 patients received either enalapril or placebo. Enalapril decreased PCWP, systemic blood pressure, and pulmonary shunt in these patients. Chapter 42 ⊙ includes a summary of the medications used for the treatment of pulmonary edema.

Medical Management of Noncardiogenic Pulmonary Edema

Noncardiogenic pulmonary edema is a wide spectrum of diseases that is caused by either direct or indirect injury of the pulmonary capillary membrane that allows fluids to leak into the interstitial space and then into the alveoli. Another name for NCPE is nonhydrostatic pulmonary edema. This term emphasizes the etiology of this type of acute pulmonary edema, which results from permeability changes in the pulmonary capillaries, not increased hydrostatic pressure in the pulmonary capillaries.

Chart 36–6 (p. 1009) lists some common disease syndromes that are associated with noncardiogenic pulmonary edema (Martin et al., 2005). The first two causes, ALI and ARDS, are covered in the next section. However, some of the other diseases listed in Chart 36–6 (p. 1009) deserve a few words of explanation now. The medical management of these types of NCPE is mentioned if it relates to the etiology and is unique to that type of NCPE.

▪ Acute Respiratory Distress Syndrome and Acute Lung Injury

Acute respiratory distress syndrome (ARDS) is a progressive form of respiratory failure that leads to alveolar capillary inflammation and damage. The term **acute lung injury (ALI)** is sometimes used when referring to ARDS, but ALI is less severe (Kaplow & Hardin, 2007). In 1994, the North American-European Consensus Conference outlined criteria for ALI and ARDS (Bernard et al., 1994). Chart 36–10 lists the criteria for both diseases. Both are reflections of the same mechanisms of lung injury, inflammation and pulmonary edema that results in hypoxemia (Wheeler & Bernard, 2007).

Epidemiology

The incidence of ARDS is difficult to predict because of the lack of a definitive diagnosis of the disease in most cases. Since 1994 when the definition for ARDS began to be used, most experts believe that ARDS is a major health problem (Ware, 2005). A large study group examining the disease noted its incidence as 64 per 100,000 population or approximately 150,000 cases per year (Goss, Brower, Hudson, & Rubenfeld, 2003). ARDS has a mortality rate of 40%, which is significantly decreased from previous years (Howard, Courtney-Shapiro, Kelso, Goltz, & Morris, 2004). Patients usually die from multiple-organ failure complications rather than from the respiratory failure. The lower mortality usually is seen in centers that are accustomed to treating patients with ARDS where the multidisciplinary team has a clear understanding of the goals of treatment and predicted outcomes. Some diseases and conditions increase the mortality of patients who acquire ARDS, as outlined in the Risk Factors box.

CHART 36–10	Criteria That Define Acute Lung Injury and Acute Respiratory Distress Syndrome
Type of Acute Lung Injury	**Criteria**
Acute lung injury	$PaO_2/FiO_2 < 300$ mmHg (regardless of PEEP level) Bilateral patchy infiltrates on chest x-ray PCWP < 18 mmHg or no evidence of left atrial hypertension
Acute respiratory distress syndrome	$PaO_2/FiO_2 < 200$ mmHg (regardless of PEEP level) Bilateral patchy infiltrates on chest x-ray PCWP < 18 mmHg or no evidence of left atrial hypertension

Source: Bernard, G. R., Artigas, A., Brigham, K. L., Carlet, J., Falke, K., Hudson, L., et al. (1994). The American-European Consensus Conference on ARDS. Definitions, mechanisms, relevant outcomes, and clinical trial coordination. *American Journal of Respiratory and Critical Care Medicine, 149* (3 Part 1), 818–824.

RISK FACTORS Predictive of Increased Mortality in Patients with ALI/ARDS

- Liver dysfunction
- Sepsis
- Nonpulmonary organ dysfunction
- Age
- Organ transplantation
- HIV infection
- Active malignancy
- Length of mechanical ventilation prior to ARDS
- Oxygenation index
- Mean airway pressure $\times$ FiO$_2$ $\times$ 100/PaO$_2$
- Mechanism of lung injury
- Right ventricular dysfunction
- PaO$_2$/FiO$_2$ ratio < 100
- Chronic alcoholism

Source: Adapted from TenHoor, T., Mannino, D.M., & Moss, M. (2001). Risk factors for ARDS in the United States: Analysis of the 1993 national mortality followback study. *Chest,* 119, 1179–1184.

Etiology

Acute injury to the lungs can be caused by many factors. Usually, these factors are divided into direct and indirect injury to the lungs. Chest trauma with lung contusions, aspiration, and infectious causes, such as pneumonia, are in the direct injury category. In fact, aspiration of gastric secretions is one of the most common causes of ALI (Murray & Nadel, 2005). These entities can cause direct injury to the airways and parenchyma of the lung. In the indirect category are many nonpulmonary etiologies that result in acute respiratory failure. These indirect causes of ALI require the action of intermediary substances that cause the lung injury. These intermediary substances are host defenses that are released when tissue is injured and when inflammation occurs. They include some of the substances listed in Chart 36–11. Their role is to protect the body from infection and disease, but in the case of ALI and ARDS these substances become "overactivated" and become part of the problem instead of the solution.

Systemic inflammatory response syndrome (SIRS) describes the syndrome when these substances of inflammation are activated. When SIRS is caused by infection, it is called sepsis, and with significant hypotension, septic shock as discussed in Chapter 61 . If other organ systems are involved such as the renal or cardiovascular system, then multiple-organ dysfunction syndrome (MODS) might develop. Severe sepsis with septic shock, acute pancreatitis, and even cardiopulmonary bypass can result in ALI, and if the injury is severe enough ARDS can develop. Acute lung injury associated with pancreatitis is referred to as *pancreatitis-associated acute lung injury* (Pastor, Matthay, & Frossard, 2003). There is a proposed link between sepsis and lung injury. ALI develops in 10% to 45% of patients who develop severe sepsis syndrome (Murray & Nadel, 2005). Chart 36–12 (p. 1016) lists some causes of ALI. This list is not all inclusive and, although it is varied and involves many different disease entities, it is important to realize that almost any disease process that generates a large-scale inflammation and injury pattern in the human body can cause ALI and ARDS. Apprecia-

CHART 36–11 | **Immune Cells and Cytokines Associated with ALI and ARDS**

Type	Definition
Neutrophils or PMNs	White blood cells (WBCs) are part of the nonspecific rapid response to infection or inflammation.
Activated nuclear factor-kappa B in alveolar macrophages	Nuclear factor-kappa B/Rel transcription factors play an important role in the regulation of a variety of genes involved in the inflammatory responses of cells. Alveolar macrophages are monocytes that are located in the alveoli. These cells help the lungs fight infections.
Interleukins (ILs)	Cytokines or cell messengers; inter = between; leukins = white cells.
IL-1-beta	IL-1-beta, also known as lymphocyte activating factor (LAF), activates T-cell lymphocytes, which secrete IL-2, released primarily from macrophages, monocytes, and other cells.
IL-6	A protein that is directly involved in the responses that occur after infection and injury and is called the acute phase response. IL-6 is produced by fibroblasts, activated T cells, activated monocytes or macrophages, and endothelial cells.
IL-8	IL-8, formerly called monocyte-derived neutrophil chemotactic factor. Attracts WBCs.
Tumor necrosis factor-alpha	Tumor necrosis factor-alpha is a serum glycoprotein produced by activated macrophages and monocytes. It has the ability to destroy tumor cell lines and increases the ability to reject tumor transplants. Released early in sepsis, trauma, and other diseases.

Sources: Didier, D., Jean-Damien, R., & Georges, S. (2003). On the physiological and clinical relevance of lung-borne cytokines during ventilator-induced lung injury. *American Journal of Respiratory and Critical Care Medicine, 167,* 1467–1471; Roitt, I., & Delves, P. (2001). *Roitt's essential immunology* (10th ed.). London: Blackwell Scientific.

tion of this concept allows the nurse to recognize a worsening respiratory condition with a potential development of ALI and initiate treatment quickly to prevent further hypoxemia.

There is no cure for ALI/ARDS or treatment that prevents the patient from developing this disease (Vincent, Sakr, & Ranieri, 2003; Ware & Matthay, 2005).

Pathophysiology

ARDS is caused by injury to the alveolar-capillary membrane that allows fluids, proteins, and cell products to flow into the alveoli. Inflammation in the lungs adds to the damage. As alveoli collapse, the lungs become heavy and stiff and difficult to ventilate. Hypoxemia, low lung compliance, and increased **minute ventilation** (V_E) (volume of gas ventilated in 1 minute) are the classic features of respiratory failure caused by ARDS. ARDS is similar to the pathophysiology of pulmonary edema with injury to the A-C membrane. The injury to the A-C

CHART 36–12 Causes of Acute Lung Injury

Types of Disorders	Diagnoses/Clinical Causes

Infectious causes	Gram-negative sepsis or gram-positive sepsis:
	   Bacterial pneumonia
	   Viral pneumonia
	   Mycoplasmal pneumonia
	   Fungal pneumonia
	   Parasitic infections
	   Mycobacterial disease

Aspiration	Gastric acid:
	   Food and other particulate matter
	   Fresh or sea water (near drowning)
	   Hydrocarbon fluids

Trauma	Lung contusion:
	   Fat emboli
	   Nonthoracic trauma
	   Overdistention (mechanical ventilation)
	   Blast injury (explosion, lightning)
	   Thermal injury (burns)
	   Inhaled gases (phosgene, ammonia)

Hemodynamic disturbances	Shock of any etiology:
	   Anaphylaxis
	   High-altitude pulmonary edema
	   Reperfusion
	   Air embolism
	   Amniotic fluid embolism

Drugs	Suicide gesture (aspiration):
	   Heroin
	   Methadone
	   Propoxyphene
	   Naloxone
	   Cocaine
	   Barbiturates
	   Colchicine
	   Salicylates
	   Ethchlorvynol
	   Interleukin-2
	   Protamine
	   Hydrochlorothiazide
	   Obstruction or its release
	   Disseminated intravascular coagulation:
	     Incompatible blood transfusion
	     Rh incompatibility
	     Antileukocyte antibodies
	   Leukoagglutinin reactions
	   Postcardiopulmonary bypass pump
	   oxygenator

Metabolic disorders	Pancreatitis Uremia Diabetic ketoacidosis
Neurological disorders	Head trauma Grand mal seizures Increased intracranial pressure (any cause) Subarachnoid or intracerebral hemorrhage
Miscellaneous disorders	Lung reexpansion Upper airway obstruction

Source: From Murray, J., & Nadel, J. (Eds.). (2005). *Textbook of respiratory medicine* (4th ed., p. 1511, Table 51-4). Philadelphia: W. B. Saunders. Used with permission.

membrane occurs when pro-inflammatory mediators, oxygen free radicals, and other cytokines are activated in response to injury. The injury is multifactorial and can be related to other diseases or can be related to increased pressures or volumes caused by mechanical ventilation. Injury from the ventilator is termed *ventilator-associated lung injury* or *ventilator-induced lung injury* (MacIntyre, 2005). The complexity, interrelatedness, and mechanism of action of these host defense mediators are reasons why no cure for ARDS has been found since the disease was first recognized as a syndrome.

Three phases have been identified in ARDS: the acute exudative phase, the proliferative phase, and a final fibrotic stage (Castro, 2006). Although theses phases may assist in categorizing and explaining the complex pattern of pathophysiological changes seen in ARDS, many researchers do not use them to explain the characteristics of this disease (Matthay et al., 2003).

Acute Exudative Phase

The acute exudative phase occurs within the first 7 to 10 days after injury. During this phase, extensive edema is produced in response to the lung injury. This edema fluid is high in protein content and floods the interstitial space, collapses alveoli, and causes hemorrhage. Further damage is done to alveolar ducts and other supporting structures of the alveoli. This diffuse alveolar damage is indicative of the early phase of ARDS.

The functional residual capacity (FRC) is the amount of gas in the lungs after a normal expiration. The FRC of the lungs decreases because the alveoli are no longer filled with air, but are filled with fluid instead. FRC is an important lung volume that can be measured as part of a pulmonary function test (PFT). It also can be measured in some diseases such as ARDS. It is a higher value in men than women (West, 1998).

In ARDS, because the lung is stiff and not as compliant and because alveoli have collapsed or are flooded with fluid, on expiration, the lung recoils to a smaller volume. More fluid and less air in the lungs decreases the ability of the lungs to exchange oxygen and carbon dioxide. One goal in the treatment of ARDS is to increase FRC. Because the lung is now filled with water, there is less room for air. Not every alveolus is collapsed or injured in this phase of ARDS, giving the disease one of its defining characteristics, heterogeneity (Marini & Gattinoni, 2004). That is, some alveoli remain normal in function and structure. If high pressures are used in an attempt to ventilate the patient, these pressures are transmitted to the "normal" alveoli injuring them.

Increased numbers of polymorphonuclear neutrophils (PMNs) also are found in the capillaries, in the interstitial spaces and in the alveoli, adding to the disruption of gas exchange at the A-C membrane (see Chart 36–11, p. 1015). Neutrophils are the body's nonspecific first responders to infection, injury, or inflammation. Once activated by lung injury, neutrophils produce pro-inflammatory cytokines such as interleukin-1-beta and tumor necrosis factor-alpha. PMNs also attract macrophages by producing specific chemical agents or chemokines that signal macrophages. The neutrophils cause damage by blocking the air spaces, and in their mission to destroy bacteria and limit inflammation, they destroy alveolar endothelial cells in the process (Abraham, 2003).

Neutrophils are not the only initiator of ARDS because this syndrome can occur without neutrophils. Patients who are neutropenic can still develop ARDS (Ognibene et al., 1986). As the disease progresses, the alveolar epithelium is swollen and lifted off the basement membrane. A hyaline membrane that is composed of plasma proteins, fibrin, and other cellular debris coats this basement membrane. This hyaline membrane is another mechanism that prevents normal gas exchange. The hyaline membrane is a collection of cells, proteinaceous materials, and necrotic epithelium that line the respiratory bronchioles, alveolar ducts, and unopened alveoli. In Chart 36–13 alveolar ducts (AD) are lined with hyaline membrane (HM). This hyaline membrane occurs because of decreased surfactant and increased lung injury, further compromising gas exchange at the alveolar-capillary membrane. The dense tissue surrounding this alveolar duct is collapsed alveoli.

Pulmonary hypertension can be another symptom that is seen in this phase caused by refractory hypoxemia and excretion of endothelin-1, a powerful vasoconstrictor (Moloney & Evans, 2003). Surfactant production by type II alveolar cells also is affected. Increased lung edema dilutes the surfactant in the alveoli, and the inflammation and damage to the type II cells produces a decrease in the amount of surfactant that is synthesized and recirculated. There also is some evidence that surfactant composition in patients with ARDS is structurally and chemically altered, preventing normal functioning of this essential ingredient of lung physiology.

Proliferative Phase

The next phase of ARDS begins approximately 7 to 10 days postinjury. It is difficult to distinguish between disease progression and pathophysiological abnormalities that occur because of the high ventilator pressures and oxygen toxicity that must be used at times to treat ARDS at this stage of the disease. The air spaces that have been filled with fluid are now narrowed and filled with fibroblasts, specialized cells that attempt to restructure the alveoli. Type I alveolar cells have been replaced by type II cells in the alveolar epithelium. The A-C membrane is thick and not efficient in gas exchange. This phase is marked by proliferation of these fibroblasts. Fibroblasts now are present in the interstitial spaces and even in the air spaces that continue to collapse at an alarming rate. The compliance of the lung is decreased now, and high pressures are needed to ventilate through narrowed air spaces and collapsed alveoli.

Fibrotic Phase

The final phase of ARDS is marked by fibrotic changes of the alveolar ducts, alveoli, and interstitial space (Hudson & Hough, 2006). This phase can begin as early as 10 days after initial insult. These stiff fibrotic structures can be seen on chest x-ray and their "honeycombed" appearance is a classic finding. This structure is a result of the body's attempt at repair. These pathologic changes still can be reversed if the patient's condition improves and the initial insult has been treated. Frequently, patients in this phase require long-term ventilator support until the lung damaged is repaired. Because of these fibrotic changes in the lungs, increased CO_2 retention can be seen at this phase of the disease. CO_2 retention usually is not present until this final stage of the disease.

Clinical Manifestations

The patient presents with all the symptoms of respiratory failure usually after a precipitating event. An early sign of respiratory failure is hyperventilation with a corresponding respiratory alkalosis. At this stage of ARDS, the chest x-ray may appear normal and this rapid respiratory rate is the only clinical sign that is present. As the hypoxemia increases, dyspnea, shortness of breath, and tachypnea with use of accessory muscles is a frequent finding. The skin may appear cyanotic or mottled, which does not improve with oxygen administration. Respirations are rapid, shallow, with intercostal and suprasternal retractions on inspiration only (Kaplow & Hardin, 2007).

In auscultating the lung fields, the nurse may hear bilateral crackles. These are heard in the bases or throughout the lung fields. Coarse rhonchi and wheezes, depending on the severity of the fluid that is flowing into the alveoli, also are heard. In some cases, the pink frothy sputum of classic pulmonary edema is seen. The hypoxemia quickly becomes refractory to standard oxygen therapies, and the patient requires intubation and mechanical ventilation to maintain oxygenation and ventilation. The ABGs frequently demonstrate a respiratory alkalosis in the early stage and respiratory acidosis in the advanced stage. The chest x-ray exhibits the bilateral patchy infiltrates that are characteristic of the disease. This "whiteout" can cover the entire lung field as the disease progresses. Finally, late findings include hypotension and decreased cardiac output.

Laboratory and Diagnostic Procedures

Once a patient is suspected of having ARDS, ABG values are used to detect and document hypoxemia and pH imbalances.

CHART 36–13 **Hyaline Membrane Disease of the Newborn**

Hyaline membrane disease of the newborn was the name given to the acute respiratory failure of infants who now are classified as having ARDS. The *A* in ARDS had previously been defined as *adult* but was recently changed to stand for *acute*.

The hyaline membrane is a collection of cells, proteinaceous materials, and necrotic epithelium that can line the respiratory bronchioles, alveolar ducts, and unopened alveoli. In the depiction here, the alveolus is lined with this hyaline membrane (arrow pointing to hyaline membrane). This hyaline membrane occurs because of decreased surfactant and increased lung injury. The hyaline membrane further compromises gas exchange at the alveolar-capillary membrane.

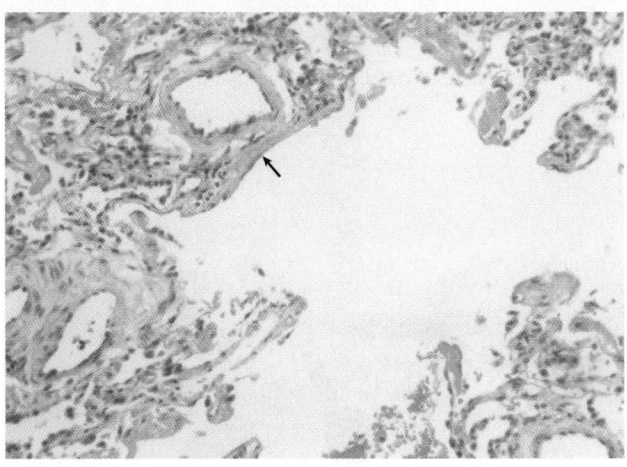

Source: Ware, L. B., & Matthay, M. A. (2005). Clinical practice: Acute pulmonary edema. *New England Journal of Medicine, 353*(26), 2788–2796. Photo © OJ Staats. MD/ Custom Medical Stock Photo.

Hypocapnia is a typical finding early in ARDS, but hypercapnia can be seen later as ventilatory failure progresses. A PaO_2 of less than 50 mmHg is a typical finding. Sputum should be collected for Gram stain and cultures (e.g., bacterial, fungal, viral) if a pulmonary infection is present. Other laboratory studies are non-specific and are obtained as indicated by the underlying or predisposing conditions.

The chest radiograph reveals characteristic diffuse alveolar-interstitial infiltrates in all lung fields, although in early cases, the radiographic findings may not be fully developed. Chest CT may be helpful in advanced cases but is not necessary for diagnosis. Echocardiography may be helpful to exclude a cardiogenic etiology for pulmonary edema.

Medical Management

Because there is no cure for ARDS, treatment is organized into specific therapy to treat the underlying cause of the precipitating event and supportive treatment. Supportive treatment includes administration of oxygen, mechanical ventilation, and fluid management. Newer ventilation therapies for the treatment of ARDS are discussed later in the mechanical ventilation section.

Optimum fluid management in patients with ARDS is centered on attempting to restrict fluids in order to limit the lung edema and at the same time prevent hypotension and renal failure. Vasopressor drugs are used to prevent hypotension and tissue hypoxia and increase cardiac output when the patient is in shock and has been fluid resuscitated without a clinical response. If the patient requires vasopressors, no one drug is superior in the patient who presents with ARDS.

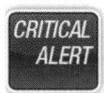 *Vasopressors should be used if the patient remains hypotensive after fluid resuscitation. Vasopressors include dopamine and norepinephrine and other agents that increase blood pressure.*

To promote healing and prevent complications in patients who are seriously ill, adequate nutrition either enterally or parenterally is essential. If the patient can tolerate enteral feeding, this is the preferred route. Recent literature suggests that enteral nutrition is associated with lower septic morbidity rates (Martin, Doig, Heyland, Morrison, & Sibbald, 2004). There are no proven preferred enteral feeding formulas for the patient who has ARDS. It is important to consult a nutritionist in order to calculate caloric goals and prevent overfeeding. See Chapter 14 ⊙ for more information on nutrition.

Mechanical Ventilation

Life-threatening hypoxemia from respiratory failure is treated with intubation and institution of mechanical ventilation. Most patients who develop ARDS cannot be treated with supplemental oxygen alone. There is very little information and weak evidence that patients with ARDS can be successfully treated with noninvasive positive pressure ventilation (Liesching et al., 2003). However, a recent study demonstrated that some patients with ARDS might be candidates for this therapy (Antonelli et al., 2007). Mechanical ventilation instituted early to prevent aspiration and increased work of breathing allows the underlying initiating event to be treated and the lung to begin to heal. No mode of ventilation has been proven superior in treating ARDS (Esteban et al., 2000). Positive end-expiratory pressure has been used since the disease was

recognized as a syndrome and improves oxygenation by numerous mechanisms. For example, PEEP helps maintain FiO_2 at less than 50% and prevents the hazards of oxygen toxicity (Brower, Ware, Berthiaume, & Matthay, 2001). Decreased lung compliance is the classic presenting symptom of ARDS. An important goal of ventilator management is preventing further lung damage of intact alveoli. In a large randomized clinical trial supported by the NIH, the ARDS Network study group ventilated patients with small tidal volume (6 mL/kg) and low (<30 cm H_2O) plateau pressures. These maneuvers were shown to be efficacious in this disease (Acute Respiratory Distress Syndrome Network, 2000).

Two unique modes of ventilation can be employed for the patient with ARDS and very noncompliant lungs. These modes employ very high respiratory rates and small tidal volumes to prevent further lung injury. One ventilator uses a piston to deliver the gas in an oscillating wave; this type of ventilator is called an oscillator and the mode is termed high-frequency oscillatory ventilation (HFOV). The other uses a jet to deliver the gas and this mode is called high-frequency jet ventilation (HFJV). Both of these modes have been used in the neonatal and pediatric population and, with the approval of an adult oscillator in 2001, are currently being used in adults (Figure 36–5 ■) (Chan & Stewart, 2005). HFOV does not use the high pressures that sometimes are needed to ventilate patients with ARDS who have very noncompliant lungs. The oscillating wave, produced by a piston that is the central feature of the ventilator, obliterates lung sounds, but keeps the alveoli open by using extremely high respiratory rates.

HFJV is also used in patients with noncompliant lungs. Another indication for HFJV is presence of an air leak that has failed conventional mechanical ventilation. A special triple-lumen endotracheal tube can be used to deliver the jet ventilation. The

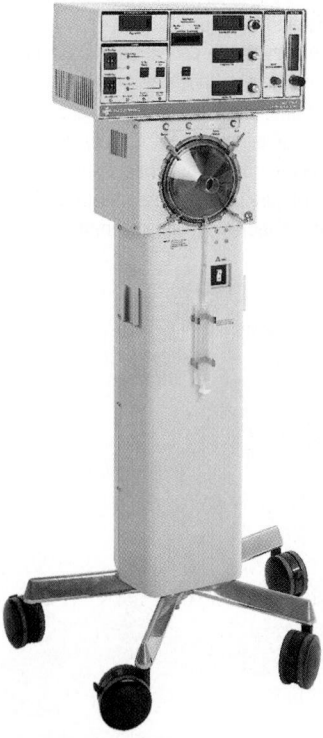

FIGURE 36–5 ■ Sensormedics 3100 B ventilator.
Source: Courtesy of Cardinal Health

three lumens of this "jet tube" are necessary in order to provide the jet ventilation, monitor airway pressures, and provide a connection for a conventional ventilator. As with HFOV, rates with jet ventilation are extremely rapid: from 240 to 660 breaths/min. HFJV is used in neonates and during surgical procedures that require immobilization of the chest (MacIntyre, 2005).

Experimental Medical Therapies

Many new and potential exciting therapies are being studied to determine if they are efficacious for treating patients with ARDS. Genetic susceptibility to ARDS is being studied by a group of researchers who have discovered a difference in the surfactant protein gene (Gong et al., 2004). Administration of surfactant to patients with ARDS has been attempted in the past with inconsistent results. Timing of the administration of surfactant is one facet of this therapy that is critical for success (Lewis & Brackenbury, 2003).

Extracorporeal gas exchange, either with total support, which is called *extracorporeal membrane oxygenation* (ECMO), or limited support, with just removal of CO_2, which is called *extracorporeal carbon dioxide removal* ($EC_{CO2}R$), remains a very invasive, expensive therapy that has a high mortality, but is used in some cases of ARDS. It is capable of supporting the patients until their lungs heal. Data from the ECMO Registry of the Extracorporeal Life Support Organization (ELSO) reported for the 1980–1995 period a total of 197 adult patients with a 41% survival rate. The neonatal cases number more than 10,000. Failure to respond to maximal ventilatory management was the most common indication for adult ECMO (ELSO Registry Information, 2008).

Fluorocarbon liquid–assisted gas exchange has been studied for many years. Fluorocarbon liquid–assisted gas exchange involves breathing an organic fluorocarbon liquid, which can dissolve 17 times more oxygen than water. This therapy potentially represents a way to oxygenate the lungs of a patient with ARDS without causing further damage to alveoli (Kaisers, Kelly, & Busch, 2003).

Research continues with medical therapies that are attempting to limit the inflammation and the activation of neutrophils and monocytes in ARDS. Exogenous surfactant, corticosteroids, and phosphodiesterase are examples of new medical therapies that could be administered to patients with ARDS to stop this cycle of inflammation (Calfee & Matthay, 2007).

Nursing Management of Acute Respiratory Failure and ARDS

The nursing process guides the care of patients who are experiencing acute respiratory failure. It is imperative that the nurse be knowledgeable about the pathophysiology of the disease that caused the acute respiratory failure. The nurse also must recognize that the treatment for acute respiratory failure is based on supporting the patient until the underlying disease can be resolved. Prevention of the complications of hypoxemia is a primary goal.

Assessment

The nursing assessment begins with airway and oxygenation status. This includes both subjective and objective findings. The patient must be questioned about whether he is feeling short of breath. For example, ask the patient if he feels he is getting enough air. Objective assessment includes the respiratory rate, the work of breathing, oxygen saturation, and vital signs. Anxiety is frequently present with respiratory distress and must be evaluated in conjunction with the rest of the clinical manifestations. The skin and nail beds need to be assessed for cyanosis and pallor. Lung assessment is critical when evaluating for respiratory failure. Because respiratory status changes rapidly, it is imperative for the nurse to perform frequent and ongoing assessments. Specific clinical manifestations were discussed earlier in the chapter.

Nursing Diagnoses

Nursing diagnoses that apply to patients with respiratory compromise include:

- *Impaired Gas Exchange*
- *Ineffective Tissue Perfusion: Cardiopulmonary* and *Peripheral*
- *Deficient Knowledge* related to the disease process
- *Self-Care Deficit*
- *Ineffective Airway Clearance*
- *Ineffective Breathing Pattern.*

Outcomes and Evaluation Parameters

Outcomes include stable oxygen status and prevention of or resolution of respiratory failure. Evaluation parameters include vital signs and oxygen saturation within normal limits on room air. Lung sounds are clear and the patient denies shortness of breath or air hunger.

Interventions and Rationales

Nursing interventions include deep breathing and coughing, use of an incentive spirometer if ordered, and reporting to the health care provider when changes occur that may indicate a need for oxygen therapy and/or mechanical ventilation. Frequent turning and repositioning of patients has always been a standard component of the nursing care of the patient who is immobilized. In the patient with ARDS, turning is an important part of their care. The nurse should note if oxygen desaturation is correlated with turning from one side to the other or if desaturation is sustained if the patient is placed on a certain side. Patients with ARDS frequently have little respiratory reserve and develop hypoxemia when turned, suctioned, or bathed. Sometimes this desaturation is related to turning on a certain side or after an activity. The nurse can mitigate this hypoxemia by documenting this effect of the activity, so it is not repeated. Paying careful attention to preoxygenation prior to suctioning or to the grouping of nursing activities can prevent decreased SpO_2 and allow turning and other care activities.

Intubation and mechanical ventilation are two major interventions. Successful intubation is an important procedure that demands that the nurse know how to assist the health care provider, administer medications, demonstrate skill with suctioning and use of the **air-mask-bag unit** (**AMBU**) (a device used to deliver oxygen via a mask when a patient is not adequately ventilating or oxygenating), and document the event in the record.

The nursing care of the ventilated patient involves not only understanding the purpose of mechanical ventilation, its basic operation and common modes, but also the complications of mechanical ventilation. NPPV is being used to treat acute respiratory failure, especially with patients who have chronic obstructive pulmonary diseases and emphysema. Many of the complications of having an endotracheal tube in the airway are avoided with this type of ventilation. This type of mechanical ventilation support is becoming more available to patients who previously were intubated because of technological advances in ventilator design as well as the positive results of controlled studies.

Nursing Priorities During Endotracheal Intubation

The indications for intubation include inability of the respiratory system to maintain oxygenation and/or ventilation. Other indications for intubation include airway protection and elective surgery. Assisting with intubation requires that the nurse know what equipment is necessary and the proper operation of that equipment. It also requires that the nurse anticipate the needs of the health care professional who is performing the procedure. Prior to the procedure, the nurse should explain the procedure to the patient and the family. The patient is positioned on his or her back with a small blanket under the shoulder blades to hyperextend the neck and open the airway. The nurse also confirms that the equipment is working properly. Using an MRB and mask, the nurse preoxygenates the patient. During the procedure, the nurse provides suction as necessary and monitors the patient's SaO_2 by pulse oximetry, as well as the patient's heart rate and blood pressure. Orienting the patient to the need for the endotracheal tube and providing reassurance to the patient are primary nursing interventions.

Documentation of the intubation should include the size of the **endotracheal tube** (a tube used to deliver oxygen that is placed in the trachea) and where the tube is located in the airway. This is determined by the number of centimeters on the tube that is located at the teeth or gum line. The nurse should also document medication administered and how the patient tolerated the procedure. Chart 36–14 includes a list of equipment necessary for intubation.

Oral Endotracheal Intubation

An endotracheal tube located in the mouth produces many of the complications of patients with respiratory failure who require intubation. These complications can be reviewed by referring to Figure 36–6 ■ (Lanken, 2006). If the patient is not properly sedated, the patient can occlude the tube with teeth or gums (1 on the diagram) or remove the tube with her tongue (2). The tongue is a powerful muscle and it is not uncommon for a patient to "tongue-out" the endotracheal tube. The tube can cause pressure ulcers and erode the lips. The endotracheal tube can become kinked in the back of the throat (3).

The cuff of the endotracheal tube is important because it prevents most secretions from being aspirated into the lungs and prevents air from the ventilator from escaping from around the endotracheal tube into the upper airways instead of ventilating the lungs (4). The tube also can be too high in the trachea, which places the cuff in the vocal cords. This apparent herniation of the cuff can prevent the patient from being venti-

---

CHART 36–14 ■ Equipment for Endotracheal Intubation

Personal protective equipment

Endotracheal tubes with intact cuff and 15-mm connectors
Adult female: 7.5- to 8.0-mm tube
Adult male: 8.0- to 9.0-mm tube

Laryngoscope handle with fresh batteries

Laryngoscope blades (straight or curved)

Spare bulbs for laryngoscope blades

Flexible stylet

Self-inflating resuscitation bag with mask connected to 100% oxygen

Oxygen source and connecting tubes

Swivel adapter

Nonsterile gloves

Luer-Lok 10-mL syringe for cuff inflation

Water-soluble lubricant

Rigid pharyngeal suction tip catheter (Yankauer)

Suction apparatus (wall or portable)

Suction catheters

Bite block or oropharyngeal airways

Endotracheal tube securing apparatus or tape

Stethoscope

Anesthetic spray or jelly (for nasal approach)

Sedating or paralyzing medication

Magill forceps

Ventilator

Source: This article was published in *The AACN procedure manual.* Lynn-McHale, D., & Carlson, K. (Eds.). (4th ed., p. 11). Copyright Elsevier 2001.

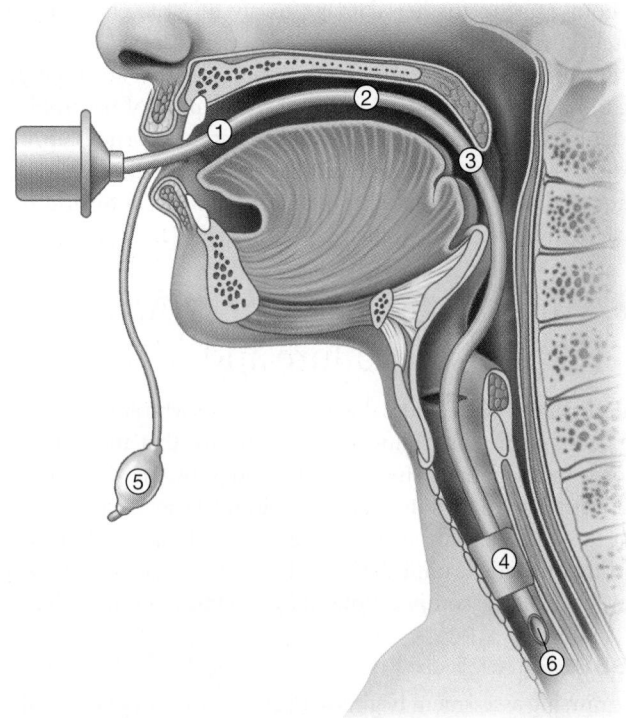

FIGURE 36–6 ■ Endotracheal tube.

lated properly. The pilot balloon (5) can leak and cause insufficient volumes to be delivered to the patient. Finally, the tip of the tube (6) itself can be blocked with secretions, bacteria, or blood that prevent delivery of adequate tidal volumes (Lanken, 2006).

There is increasing evidence that a biofilm develops on endotracheal tubes that are in place for any length of time. This biofilm is a complex matrix of bacteria that has been associated with ventilator-associated pneumonia (Rello et al., 2006).

Mechanical Ventilation

Indications for providing mechanical ventilation to the patient with acute respiratory failure include treating hypoxemia, hypercarbia, or both. Modern ventilators are termed positive pressure ventilators because they provide an increased pressure on inspiration to the lungs. This is the most common type of ventilator used in the acute care setting. There are devices, such as the chest cuirass and iron lung, that create a negative pressure around the chest and assist with exhalation. These devices are sometimes used in the home. Finally, a combined type of ventilator using negative and positive pressure to deliver the gas is used in some situations. The high-frequency oscillator used in pediatric and adult patients with decreased lung compliance produces an oscillating wave of pressures to deliver the gas. This type of ventilator was discussed earlier in the ARDS treatment section.

Figure 36–7 ■ displays the common components of a typical ventilator, and Chart 36–15 outlines common terms associated with ventilators. The ventilator circuit is connected to the patient and consists of a single plastic tube that fits directly onto the endotracheal tube or tracheostomy. The circuit divides at the wye into an inspiratory and expiratory circuit that connects directly to the ventilator. An important component of this system is humidification. Oxygen delivered without humidification can cause drying of the airways and solidification of secretions. Numerous types of humidification are available commercially.

The ventilator monitors rates, pressures, and volumes, and delivers the set volumes or pressures or a combination of the two to the patient during the inspiratory cycle. The ventilator accomplishes this monitoring and delivery of gas by using microprocessors to synchronize and detect when the patient inspires and expires and to time the delivery of machine support. Another necessary component of the ventilator is the compressor. In hospitals without compressed gas that is available piped in from the wall, a compressor is attached to the ventilator. The compressor provides the compressed air that is mixed with the percent of oxygen to deliver the ordered FiO_2. Some ventilators are equipped with the ability to monitor respiratory waveforms. These waveforms allow the health care team to assess the lung mechanics and

CHART 36–15	Common Respiratory Terms
Term	**Definition**
Fraction of inspired oxygen (FiO_2)	Amount of oxygen in the delivered gas; expressed as a percent or decimal
Minute ventilation (V_E)	Total ventilation per minute: Respiratory rate $\times V_T = V_E$
Tidal volume (V_T)	Amount of gas inspired with each breath
Functional Residual Capacity (FRC)	Total amount of gas left in the lungs after a normal expiration
Residual volume (RV)	Amount of gas remaining in the lungs after a maximal expiration
Rapid shallow breathing index (RSBI)	Parameter used for determining weaning success: Respiratory rate/spontaneous tidal volume

better adjust the ventilator to the patient's needs. The respiratory waveforms are monitored on a screen above the ventilator.

Providing nursing care to the patient on a ventilator has become increasingly complicated for two reasons. First, the complexities of ventilators in use today have increased dramatically with more and more of the functions becoming automatic within user-defined limits. Second, the variety and type of ventilators that are available have increased. The nurse who works on a pulmonary unit might have to learn the unique features of five to six different ventilators. Each ventilator manufacturer also uses many different terms to describe modes and ventilator operations.

In the next section, the most common ventilators and the modes they deliver as well as the implications for nursing care are reviewed. A discussion of specific ventilators and their modes is beyond the scope of this chapter. Many fine references and Internet resources are available that describe particular ventilators (Cairo & Pilbeam, 2004). The major resource for the nurse is the respiratory therapist who is responsible for the ventilator and for ensuring that the ventilator is meeting the respiratory needs of the patient. The nurse is responsible for knowing how the ventilator functions and the meaning of different modes to ensure that the patient receives an integrative approach and the best possible outcome. To ensure optimum care of a patient on a ventilator, the entire health care team must share a common goal, that is, to liberate the patient from the ventilator. But the respiratory therapist and the nurse have an added responsibility to work together in the care of the ventilated patient. The nurse and the therapist must ensure that they are communicating with each other with regard to changes in modes, sedation levels, and daily plans for weaning.

The ventilator decreases the work of breathing (WOB) for the patient. If the ventilator does all the work of breathing, that breath is called a mandatory breath. The ventilator starts the breath, controls inspiratory gas delivery, and determines the end of inspiration. Assisted breaths are those breaths that the patient initiates, but the ventilator controls the inspiratory gas delivery and time. If the ventilator provides any type of support during inspiration or expiration, that breath is defined as an assisted breath.

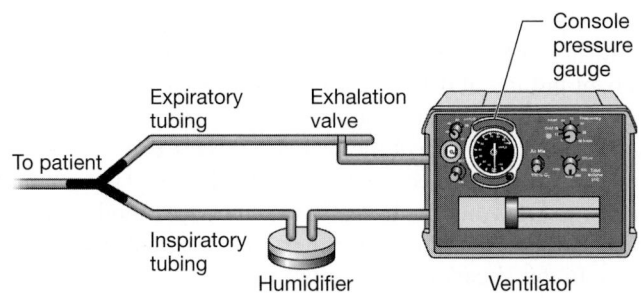

FIGURE 36–7 ■ Model of volume-cycled ventilator.

To patient

Expiratory tubing

Exhalation valve

Inspiratory tubing

Humidifier

Console pressure gauge

Ventilator

If the patient initiates the breath, the trigger or event that begins inspiration is termed patient triggered. If the trigger is not patient triggered, it is usually time triggered. For a respiratory rate of 12 times a minute, the ventilator triggers a breath every 6 seconds. This time-triggered breath also is called control ventilation because the breath is mandatory and the machine is controlling the rate and volume or pressure. Spontaneous breaths are those breaths for which the patient controls the change from inspiration to expiration. Another aspect of this breath delivery is related to the clinician controlling the volume delivered. This is called volume-targeted or volume ventilation. If the clinician wants to limit the pressure, it is called pressure-targeted or pressure ventilation. A debate about which mode is better or more comfortable for the patient began when the ventilator manufactures first gave the clinician a choice between volume ventilation and pressure ventilation. This debate continues today. The nurse should understand the difference between a volume and pressure mode. In volume ventilation, the clinician sets the volume and the pressure varies within certain parameters. In pressure ventilation, the pressure is set and the volume varies. The flow, or the way that the gas is delivered, is different between these two modes.

Nursing Management of the Ventilated Patient and Basic Modes of Ventilation

A mode describes the pattern of the breath delivery (Cairo & Pilbeam, 2004). The health care provider orders the mode that best meets the patient's needs. The mode is selected on the ventilator control panel. Figure 36–8 ■ shows a common ventilator used in critical care units and an enlarged drawing of the control panel, demonstrating the complexity of today's ventilators.

There is no common terminology used in naming the different modes. Different ventilator manufacturers use different names for the modes. Chart 36–16 (p. 1024) compares the modes, key features, and important nursing implications that are reviewed in this chapter.

Assist Control Mode and Nursing Implications

The definition of an assist control mode is one in which the patient can trigger a breath or the breath can be time triggered. Regardless of how the breath is initiated, the preset volume or preset pressure is delivered to the patient each time a breath is initiated. Each breath is a mandatory breath. Some ventilator manufacturers use the term CMV or controlled mandatory ventilation to define this mode. This is a common mode used in caring for the patient who requires ventilatory management. It typically is used with a preset volume instead of a set pressure. It is used in the postoperative patient who is recovering from anesthesia and is still heavily sedated.

Assist control mode allows the ventilator to deliver a set tidal volume for each breath. As the patient awakes and the level of sedation and analgesia decrease, the patient begins initiating breaths. The ventilator attempts to deliver the set tidal volume at a faster rate. Eventually as the rate increases, the ventilator can-

not deliver the set tidal volume and a high-pressure alarm occurs. The patient continues to attempt to initiate a breath because the patient is becoming hypoxemic and anxious because the ventilator continues to alarm without delivering the set tidal volume. There is no time for the full volume to be delivered. This phenomenon is called "stacking" and the high pressures that result from this can cause ventilated-associated lung injury. A simple solution to stacking is to change to a mode that allows the patient to breathe at a comfortable rate and set his own tidal volume. Synchronized mandatory ventilation mode, discussed next, would be one solution. The other option is to increase the level of sedation or analgesia that the patient is receiving.

The nurse who is caring for this patient should be able to assess the situation and intervene to ensure that the patient and the ventilator are working together to prevent patient–ventilator dyssynchrony. Respiratory alkalosis is not uncommon with assist control ventilation because of the patient's ability to increase his minute ventilation (V_E).

Synchronized Intermittent Mandatory Ventilation and Nursing Implications

The definition of synchronized intermittent mandatory ventilation (SIMV) is a mode of ventilation with a set rate during which the ventilator will deliver a set volume or pressure. This is the mandatory rate. Otherwise, patients can breathe between the set rates and receive whatever volume is determined by their effort. These spontaneous breaths also can be pressure supported. The synchronization means that the ventilator will wait for the patient to initiate a breath and then deliver the set mandatory breath in concert with the patient. If the patient does not inspire, the ventilator will initiate the breath.

SIMV is one of the most common modes used in the United States for patients on ventilators. Respiratory alkalosis is not much of a problem unless the set rate is too high. The nurse should record the set rate as well as the patient's rate to determine if the patient is breathing over the ventilator. Most health care providers want the patient to breathe over the set rate in order to use their respiratory muscles. If the patient does not breathe over the set SIMV rate, the team should evaluate the level of sedation and analgesia and consider decreasing it. Also, the set SIMV rate may be set too high. Decreasing the set rate will allow more opportunity for the patient to initiate a breath.

Pressure Support Ventilation and Nursing Implications

Pressure support ventilation (PSV) is an assisted form of ventilation. The patient must have a reliable respiratory effort because there is no set rate nor set tidal volume delivered by the ventilator. If the ventilator senses a negative pressure when the patient inspires, it delivers a set pressure, usually 5 to 10 cm of H_2O to assist with inspiration. Pressure support overcomes some of the resistance of the artificial airways, that is, an endotracheal tube or tracheostomy. It commonly is used in combination with SIMV but can be used as a stand-alone mode in stable ventilator patients who are weaning and have stable respiratory rates. In this situation, the pressure support decreases the work of breathing or at higher levels of pressure support (10 to 20 cm H_2O), the ventilator can assume much of the WOB.

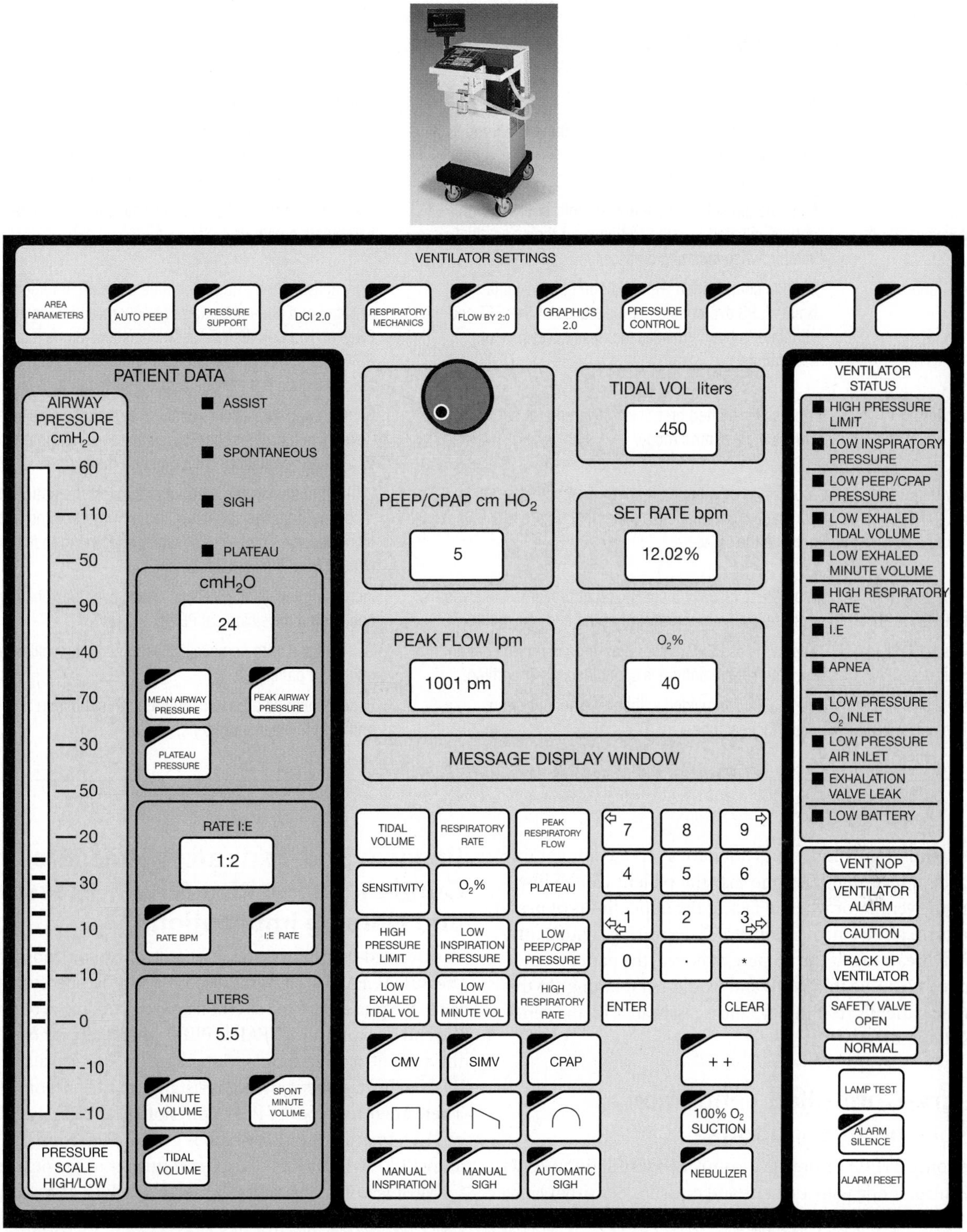

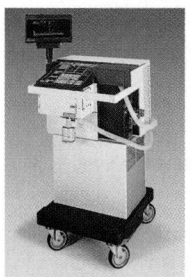

VENTILATOR SETTINGS										
AREA PARAMETERS	AUTO PEEP	PRESSURE SUPPORT	DCI 2.0	RESPIRATORY MECHANICS	FLOW BY 2:0	GRAPHICS 2.0	PRESSURE CONTROL			

PATIENT DATA

AIRWAY PRESSURE cmH₂O

- ASSIST
- SPONTANEOUS
- SIGH
- PLATEAU

cmH₂O
24

MEAN AIRWAY PRESSURE   PEAK AIRWAY PRESSURE

PLATEAU PRESSURE

RATE I:E
1:2

RATE BPM   I:E RATE

LITERS
5.5

MINUTE VOLUME   SPONT MINUTE VOLUME

PRESSURE SCALE HIGH/LOW   TIDAL VOLUME

Airway pressure scale: 60, 110, 50, 90, 40, 70, 30, 50, 20, 30, 10, 10, 0, -10, -10

TIDAL VOL liters
.450

PEEP/CPAP cm HO₂
5

SET RATE bpm
12.02%

PEAK FLOW lpm
1001 pm

O₂%
40

MESSAGE DISPLAY WINDOW

TIDAL VOLUME	RESPIRATORY RATE	PEAK RESPIRATORY FLOW
SENSITIVITY	O₂%	PLATEAU
HIGH PRESSURE LIMIT	LOW INSPIRATION PRESSURE	LOW PEEP/CPAP PRESSURE
LOW EXHALED TIDAL VOL	LOW EXHALED MINUTE VOL	HIGH RESPIRATORY RATE

7	8	9
4	5	6
1	2	3
0	.	*
ENTER		CLEAR

CMV   SIMV   CPAP   ++

MANUAL INSPIRATION   MANUAL SIGH   AUTOMATIC SIGH

100% O₂ SUCTION

NEBULIZER

VENTILATOR STATUS

- HIGH PRESSURE LIMIT
- LOW INSPIRATORY PRESSURE
- LOW PEEP/CPAP PRESSURE
- LOW EXHALED TIDAL VOLUME
- LOW EXHALED MINUTE VOLUME
- HIGH RESPIRATORY RATE
- I.E
- APNEA
- LOW PRESSURE O₂ INLET
- LOW PRESSURE AIR INLET
- EXHALATION VALVE LEAK
- LOW BATTERY

VENT NOP

VENTILATOR ALARM

CAUTION

BACK UP VENTILATOR

SAFETY VALVE OPEN

NORMAL

LAMP TEST

ALARM SILENCE

ALARM RESET

Third-generation control panel for the 7200 ventilator displays potential patient settings. If the mean airway pressure button is selected, the cmH₂O could be 24. In the next section the inspiratory to expiratory ratio is 1:2. If the rate in breaths/minute is selected that will be displayed in this window. The center panel illustrates 5 ventilator settings. In the example the PEEP is 5 cm H₂O, the tidal volumne is .450 liters, and the rate is 12 with a peak flow of 100 liters and an oxygen concentration of 40%.

FIGURE 36–8 ■ Puritan-Bennett 7200 ventilator and control panel.

Source: Photo reprinted by permission from Nellcor Puritan Bennett LLC, Boulder Colorado, part of Corider. Photo Christelle Montichard.

PSV is commonly used in combination with SIMV. If the patient does not breathe over the set rate in the SIMV mode and has a set pressure support of 5 cm of H₂O, the patient does not receive any benefit from the pressure support (PS). Only when the patient initiates a breath does the PS, in this case 5 cm of H₂O, assist the patient in inspiration. The nurse should assess the patient and talk to the team regarding the fact that the patient is not breathing over the set rate and determine a course of action.

Another important factor with PS is assessing how much ventilator support the patient is requiring. Because PSV, when

CHART 36–16	Common Ventilator Modes	

Ventilator Mode	Key Features	Nursing Implications
Assist control (AC)	Each breath, whether patient or machine triggered, is a full pressure or volume breath.	You get "what you set." Patients can become tachypneic and the ventilator has no time to deliver a full breath. "Stacking breaths" can be a complication of this mode.
Synchronized mandatory ventilation (SIMV)	Machine (preset rate) breaths are interspersed with patient-initiated breaths. Patients set their own tidal volume when initiating breaths.	Standard mode used in most critical care units. Used in combination with PS.
Pressure support (PS)	Used in combination with SIMV on patient-initiated breaths. PS overcomes the resistance of the ETT and the ventilator tubing. Provides increased pressure on inspiration.	Only active when patient initiates a breath. If patient is too sedated and does not attempt to overbreathe the set rate, no PS is active. Can also be used in a stand-alone mode called PSV. Patient must have a reliable respiratory rate. The machine does not provide a rate.
Pressure control	A pressure-limited breath is delivered at a certain rate. This is a full control mode.	Usually used for patients who have restrictive disease and worsening lung function. This mode does not guarantee a set V_E (minute ventilation). This must be monitored.
Mandatory minute ventilation (MMV)	A pressure or volume breath that provides a minimum ventilation if the patient's spontaneous breaths do not achieve the set V_E.	Difficult to assess the amount of support the patient is receiving from the ventilator and how much effort is their own. Becomes problematic when attempting to liberate the patient from the ventilator.
Positive end-expiratory pressure (PEEP)	A pressure (usually 5 cm H_2O) that prevents the alveoli from returning to 0 pressure at the end of exhalation.	Increasing levels of PEEP can cause hypotension. All patients need some physiological PEEP.
Continuous positive airway pressure (CPAP)	The same as PEEP except that there is no rate set on the ventilator—the patient is spontaneously breathing.	Can be used with noninvasive ventilation as well as with an intubated patient.
Noninvasive positive pressure ventilation (NPPV)	Ventilation is provided without the benefit of an endotracheal tube.	Patient must be able to cooperate; must be alert and oriented and able to clear secretions.

used as a stand-alone mode, does not have a set rate nor volume delivery, the nurse might assume that the patient can be liberated from the ventilator when in fact, at the upper limits of pressure support, e.g., 20 cm, the ventilator is decreasing significantly the work of breathing. If the PS were removed, the patient would not be able to assume this WOB and would fail weaning. At this point in the patient's respiratory failure, assistance by the ventilator is still required.

Pressure-Controlled Ventilation and Nursing Implications

Pressure control (PC) or pressure-controlled ventilation (PCV) is a full control mode with a set rate and pressure. Sensitivity also is set that allows the patient to trigger a breath. Inspiratory time or the time the patient spends in inspiration is set. The tidal volume (V_T) varies from breath to breath. When the breath is triggered, a rapid flow of gas is delivered to reach the set pressure and then the flow is decelerated. This pattern of flow delivery is an important distinction between PCV and volume ventilation.

In most settings, the PCV is reserved for patients with noncompliant lungs whom it is difficult to ventilate and oxygenate. A patient in acute respiratory failure with ARDS is the perfect example. The nurse should trend the V_E and the expiratory volume over time. If the volume is decreasing, the lungs could be less compliant and the pressure would have to be changed to achieve the same volume.

Positive End-Expiratory Pressure and Continuous Positive Airway Pressure and Nursing Implications

Positive end-expiratory pressure and continuous positive airway pressure (CPAP) are not modes but a ventilator setting that prevents the pressure in the circuit from returning to zero pressure at the end of expiration. CPAP is PEEP when there is no set rate and the patient is breathing spontaneously. The ventilator accomplishes this task by applying resistance at the end of exhalation. There are three types of PEEP: physiological PEEP, which is 5 cm of H_2O; treatment PEEP, which is greater than 5 cm of H_2O; and auto-PEEP, which will be discussed further in the next section.

Most ventilated patients should have PEEP of at least 5 cm of H_2O to prevent the pressure in the alveoli from dropping to zero at the end of expiration. Without physiological PEEP there is a greater chance of alveoli collapsing and not opening again on the next tidal breath. To understand PEEP, it helps to think of pursed-lip breathing. When most people are short of breath, a compensatory mechanism is to breathe through pursed lips. Athletes do this forcibly and older adults use this technique to increase oxygenation after exertion. Obviously, when a patient is intubated the ability to purse-lip breathe is removed. PEEP is a method of allowing the ventilated patient to increase oxygenation. The use of PEEP and increasing the FiO_2 are two methods of increasing oxygenation. The complications of PEEP, that is, PEEP greater than 5 cm of H_2O, are decreased cardiac output, and at higher levels of PEEP, pneumothorax. These complications usually are not seen at PEEP set at 5 cm of H$_2$O. The nurse should be aware of the level of PEEP.

Prior to extubation, a common practice is to place the patient in CPAP alone on the ventilator. This means that the patient is not receiving any support from the ventilator except at the end of exhalation when the ventilator prevents the pressure from returning to zero.

Auto-PEEP, residual PEEP, or intrinsic PEEP is PEEP that is present in the ventilatory system at the end of expiration. This increased pressure is over and above the set PEEP that is ordered for the patient.

Auto-PEEP can be caused by increased respiratory rate where the patient has no time to expire before the next breath is delivered. This is common in patients with asthma who because of their increased airway resistance require long expiration times. With an increased respiratory rate, the ventilator is attempting to deliver a higher volume than is possible in a shortened respiratory cycle. Other pulmonary pathologies such as ARDS can cause the presence of auto-PEEP because of noncompliant lungs and gas trapping. The higher the set rate on the ventilator, the greater the potential for the development of auto-PEEP. The respiratory therapist can assess the level of auto-PEEP by a maneuver called an expiratory hold.

Finally, the clinician can cause auto-PEEP through the over-aggressive use of an AMBU. The patient is removed from the ventilator for transport or for suctioning. Rapid AMBU rates are used to bag the patient instead of the rate that was set on the ventilator. Treatment would involve disconnecting the patient from the AMBU or ventilator for a few seconds; this would allow the excess pressure to dissipate.

The modes that have been discussed can be seen on the ventilator panel in Figure 36–8 ■ (p. 1023). Note that the CMV mode on this particular ventilator is really Assist/Control as explained. This manufacture elected to call it CMV instead of A/C. There is no standard classification of terms used by manufacturers of ventilators when describing modes. This may create confusion and is especially difficult when the novice is attempting to understand the different modes and their implications for patient care.

Complications of Mechanical Ventilation and Nursing Implication

As soon as a patient is intubated and mechanical ventilation is initiated, the next moment is when the nurse should be activating a plan to liberate the patient from the ventilator. An endotracheal tube and positive pressure ventilation expose the patient to an increased risk of morbidity and mortality. The ventilator and endotracheal tube are necessary interventions to treat acute respiratory failure and other diseases where the patient's own pulmonary or cardiovascular system cannot support exchange of oxygen and removal of carbon dioxide. The ventilator provides this support but not without some risk. One way in which the nurse can prevent the occurrence of this increased risk is to coordinate the care of the patient who is ventilated to ensure timely extubation. Another way that the nurse can impact the care of the patient who is mechanically ventilated is to prevent the complications that can occur. The nurse caring for a patient on a ventilator must recognize the possible complications and work diligently to prevent them if at all possible. The important complications of mechanical ventilation are presented next and are organized by organ systems. This

is not an exhaustive list nor does it deal with some of the complications of long-term mechanical ventilation. Chatila and Criner (2002) present an excellent review of these complications. Nursing implications and prevention strategies also are discussed.

Cardiovascular Complications

Cardiovascular complications of mechanical ventilation are variable and depend on the amount of pressure used to ventilate the lungs, the amount of PEEP, and the underlying heart and lung dynamics. The heart and lungs are a system and what affects one component of that system will usually affect the other. In the setting of cardiac failure, mechanical ventilation can unload some of the stress exerted on the heart by decreasing preload and afterload. This assistance by the ventilator remains invisible until the patient is weaned, and then chest pain and other symptoms of heart failure may develop.

One of the most common complications of mechanical ventilation is hypotension. This can occur immediately after intubation and initiation of positive pressure ventilation or anytime during the course of treatment. This hypotension is related to decreased cardiac output, hypovolemia, and positive pressure delivered by the ventilator. This positive pressure changes the pressure in the thorax. Positive pressure ventilation can reduce ventricular filling by decreasing the amount of blood that flows into the atria (preload) and, therefore, decreasing filling during ventricular diastole. This decreased preload produces the hypotension. Compression of the pulmonary vessels can reduce blood flow into the left atrium or impede the ejection of blood from the right heart. The increased pressure in the chest produced by mechanical ventilation also can affect the dispensability of the chambers of the heart especially during diastole. The increased pleural pressure from the chest can be transmitted to the heart and prevent filling.

Assessment of heart failure and intervening with appropriate treatment in the patient on the ventilator is the primary role of the nurse in preventing cardiovascular complications. If hypotension is the presenting symptom without other indications of cardiac failure, fluid boluses can be ordered that usually correct hypovolemia and reverse the hypotension. The nurse should be prepared to intervene, report to the health care provider, and institute treatment for this common complication. The importance of recognizing the hypotension as potentially being related to the mechanical ventilation is important. The premedications used prior to intubation also can cause hypotension, but will respond to increasing intravascular volume. In some situations vasoactive medications, such as dopamine, might be required to support the blood pressure. Increased levels of PEEP, whether it is set PEEP or auto-PEEP, also can cause hypotension. Decreasing set PEEP levels if hypotension is a direct result of increased PEEP is an important intervention. Preventing auto-PEEP, by allowing time for the patient to exhale or preventing stacking of breaths by adequately sedating the patient or selecting the correct mode, also can prevent hypotension. In some patients, decreased cardiac output and decreased pH can predispose the patient to cardiac dysrhythmias. Careful attention to fluid and electrolyte replacement can help prevent this complication from occurring. Chapter 38 ⊕ includes a complete description of cardiac dysrhythmias.

Gastrointestinal Complications

Abdominal distention is a common complication of mechanical ventilation. Gastric distention as a result of swallowed air from pressure ventilation necessitates the routine use of a nasal or oral gastric tube to decompress the stomach. Stress ulcer prevention is another important intervention to prevent gastrointestinal bleeding. Gastric ulcer formation is discussed in Chapter 45 ⊙.

Psychological Complications

Agitation, anxiety, and confusion are all complications of mechanical ventilation. It is very uncomfortable for a patient to be attached to a machine to breathe and unable to communicate simple wishes. In addition, lack of adequate sleep and use of analgesics and sedatives also may contribute to this state.

Providing periods of uninterrupted sleep is important in preventing agitation in the patient on a ventilator. Use of a speaking board, lip reading, or a special endotracheal tube that forces air through the vocal cords are all means that can assist the patient in communicating. Sedating appropriately using a sedation scale and individualizing sedation for each patient is key to providing good nursing care.

Pulmonary Complications

Barotrauma is defined as alveoli damage caused by increased pressure resulting from the ventilator. These high pressures are necessary in order to oxygenate the relatively noncompliant lungs of patients who are receiving mechanical ventilation. **Volutrauma** is similar but the lung damage is caused by increased volume that causes overdistention of alveoli. Generally, this lung injury is termed ventilator-induced lung injury (VILI) or ventilated-associated lung injury (VALI) (Suter, 2006). Alveolar damage and capillary leak can occur in the lungs from positive pressure ventilation and are recognized complications of using high pressures to ventilate. Besides the damage that these high pressures inflict on the alveoli, increased pressure can lead to pneumothorax, pneumomediastinum, or subcutaneous emphysema. Atelectasis or collapse of a segment of the lung can occur because of a mucous plug that obstructs the airway. It also can be the result of tidal volumes that are too low to ventilate the entire lung.

Severe airway injury can occur with high pressures, long-term ventilation, or with a predisposing abnormality. The endotracheal tube, the tape, or other devices used to secure the tube can cause nasopharyngeal injury. Ulcerations of the lips, nose, and mouth are too common in patients who have endotracheal tubes and can be prevented in most instances. Sinusitis is a common infection produced by the increase in secretions and the inability of drainage because of the location of the tube in the upper airway. Tracheal damage and tracheoesophageal fistulas have become less common with the universal use of low-pressure, high-volume cuffed endotracheal tubes. Trachea-innominate artery rupture, although almost always fatal, is a unique and rare complication of tracheostomies (Sue & Susanto, 2003).

Oxygen toxicity is another complication of mechanical ventilation that can occur with FiO_2 levels greater than 50% for long periods of time. Most health care providers who are managing patients on ventilators will attempt to reduce the FiO_2 to below 50% initially before decreasing other parameters (Pilbeam & Cairo, 2006).

In patients with severe ARDS, ventilating with high pressures is necessary to prevent hypoxemia. Plateau pressures should be less than 35 cm H_2O (Acute Respiratory Distress Syndrome Network, 2000). Plateau pressure is the true pressure that is transmitted to the alveoli that can cause lung damage. Plateau pressures are obtained by a maneuver that is performed by a respiratory thera-

pist called an inspiratory hold. Monitoring plateau pressures can alert the team to the increased risk of barotraumas. Keeping the plateau pressure to less than 35 cm H_2O can prevent barotrauma (Acute Respiratory Distress Syndrome Network, 2000). The ARDS Network, as previously described, correlated low tidal volumes (6 mL/kg) with improved outcomes versus higher tidal volumes in patients with ARDS. Note, however, that ventilating all patients with this low tidal volume is not adequate to prevent atelectasis. Adequate tidal volumes are necessary to ensure that the entire lung receives enough volume to prevent collapse.

Prevention of soft tissue injury of the lips, nares, and oral mucosal from the endotracheal tube and its attachment can be accomplished by paying careful attention to how the tube is secured. Many different types of tube holders are available besides the standard cloth tape used to secure the tube. Frequent changes of the device and assessment of underlying soft tissue is important. The nurse and the respiratory therapist working together can prevent the patient from acquiring an injury that is preventable.

Humidification of the entire ventilator circuit prevents excessive mucous plugging. There are many methods of humidification, such as heat and moisture exchanger (HME) and heater-humidifiers. Providing humidification is an important intervention when using any type of artificial airway that bypasses the natural humidification provided by the nose and upper airway. If this is not done, mucous plugging can be a common complication of mechanical ventilation.

Finally, prevention of oxygen toxicity can be accomplished by careful monitoring of ABGs and keeping the PaO_2 to less than 50 mmHg whenever possible.

Ventilated-Associated Pneumonia

Ventilated-associated pneumonia (VAP) has been the second most common hospital-associated infection after that of the urinary tract (CDC, 2005). The primary risk factor for the development of hospital-associated bacterial pneumonia is mechanical ventilation (with its requisite endotracheal intubation). Morbidity and mortality increase when an endotracheal tube is placed in a patient's airway. This is one of the most serious consequences of initiation of mechanical ventilation. This mortality ranges from 24% to 50% and, in the case of some high-risk pathogens, the mortality for VAP can be as high as 76% (Klompas, 2007). The rate of pneumonia for intubated patients is 3- to 10-fold that of patients who are not intubated. Along with the increased rates of pneumonia in intubated patients, the cost per admission is greater in patients who are intubated and the length of stay of these patients is significantly increased (Shorr & Kollef, 2005). The CDC (2003a) has published guidelines that are targeted toward medical and nursing staff for preventing VAP, as listed in the National Guidelines feature.

The most common etiology for a VAP is aspiration of contaminated oropharyngeal secretions. Microaspiration occurs commonly in everyone. A small amount of saliva is aspirated into the lungs but this saliva is not contaminated with the amount of bacteria that is common in the saliva of patients who are critically ill. In patients who require intubation, the saliva is commonly contaminated with pathogens that are not normally present in the mouth. The reason that the saliva is contaminated is multifactorial. Lack of appropriate mouth care, the immune-compromised state that accompanies critical illness, and relative xerostomia (dry mouth) are some of the important factors that

NATIONAL GUIDELINES for the Prevention of Health Care–Associated Bacterial Pneumonia

I. Staff Education and Involvement in Infection Prevention
Educate health care workers about the epidemiology of, and infection control procedures for, preventing health care–associated bacterial pneumonia.

II. **Infection and Microbiologic Surveillance**
   A. Conduct surveillance for bacterial pneumonia in intensive care unit (ICU) patients who are at high risk for health-care–related bacterial pneumonia (e.g., patients with mechanically assisted ventilation or selected postoperative patients) to determine trends and help identify outbreaks and other potential infection-control problems. The use of the new National Nosocomial Infection Surveillance (NNIS) system's surveillance definition of pneumonia is recommended. Include data on the causative microorganisms and their antimicrobial susceptibility patterns. Express data as rates (e.g., number of infected patients or infections per 100 ICU days or per 1,000 ventilator days) to facilitate intrahospital comparisons and trend determination. Link monitored rates and prevention efforts and return data to appropriate health-care personnel.
   B. In the absence of specific clinical, epidemiologic, or infection-control objectives, do not routinely perform surveillance cultures of patients or of equipment or devices used for respiratory therapy, pulmonary-function testing, or delivery of inhalation anesthesia.

III. Prevention of Transmission of Microorganisms
   A. Sterilization or Disinfection and Maintenance of Equipment and Devices
      1. Thoroughly clean all equipment and devices to be sterilized or disinfected.
      2. Mechanical ventilators:
         • Do not routinely sterilize or disinfect the internal machinery of mechanical ventilators.
      3. Breathing circuits, humidifiers, and heat-and-moisture exchangers (HMEs):
         • Do not change routinely, on the basis of duration of use, the breathing circuit (i.e., ventilator tubing and exhalation valve and the attached humidifier) that is in use on an individual patient. Change the circuit when it is visibly soiled or mechanically malfunctioning.
         • Periodically drain and discard any condensate that collects in the tubing of a mechanical ventilator, taking precautions not to allow condensate to drain toward the patient.
         • Wear gloves to perform the previous procedure and/or when handling the fluid. Decontaminate hands with soap and water (if hands are visibly soiled) or with an alcohol-based hand rub after performing the procedure or handling the fluid.
      4. Humidifier fluids:
         • Use sterile (not distilled, nonsterile) water to fill bubbling humidifiers.
         • Ventilator breathing circuits with HMEs.
      5. Changing an HME:
         • Change an HME that is in use on a patient when it malfunctions mechanically or becomes visibly soiled.
         • Do not routinely change more frequently than every 48 hours an HME that is in use on a patient.
         • Do not change routinely (in the absence of gross contamination or malfunction) the breathing circuit attached to an HME while it is in use on a patient.
      6. Oxygen humidifiers:
         • Follow manufacturers' instructions for use of oxygen humidifiers.
         • Change the humidifier-tubing (including any nasal prongs or mask) that is in use when it malfunctions or becomes visibly contaminated.
      7. Small-volume medication nebulizers: in-line and handheld nebulizers:
         • Between treatments on the same patient, clean, disinfect, and rinse with sterile water.
         • Use only sterile fluid for nebulization, and dispense the fluid into the nebulizer aseptically.
         • Whenever possible, use aerosolized medications in single-dose vials. If multidose medication vials are used, follow manufacturers' instructions for handling, storing, and dispensing the medications.
      8. Other devices used in association with respiratory therapy:
         • *Respirometer and ventilator thermometer:* Between their uses on different patients, sterilize or subject to high-level disinfection portable respirometers and ventilator thermometers.
         • *Resuscitation bags:* Between their uses on different patients, sterilize or subject to high-level disinfection reusable hand-powered resuscitation bags.
   B. Prevention of Person-to-Person Transmission of Bacteria
      1. Standard Precautions
         • *Hand hygiene:* Decontaminate hands by washing them with either antimicrobial soap and water or with nonantimicrobial soap and water (if hands are visibly dirty or contaminated with proteinaceous material or are soiled with blood or body fluids) or by using an alcohol-based waterless antiseptic agent (e.g., hand rub) if hands are not visibly soiled after contact with mucous membranes, respiratory secretions, or objects contaminated with respiratory secretions, whether or not gloves are worn. Decontaminate hands as described previously before and after contact with a patient who has an endotracheal or tracheostomy tube in place, and before and after contact with any respiratory device that is used on the patient, whether or not gloves are worn.
         • *Gloving:* Wear gloves for handling respiratory secretions or objects contaminated with respiratory secretions of any patient.
         • Change gloves and decontaminate hands between contacts with different patients; after handling respiratory secretions or objects contaminated with secretions from one patient and before contact with another patient, object, or environmental surface; and between contacts with a contaminated body site and the respiratory tract of, or respiratory device on, the same patient.
         • When soiling with respiratory secretions from a patient is anticipated, wear a gown and change it after soiling occurs and before providing care to another patient.

(continued)

NATIONAL GUIDELINES for the Prevention of Health Care–Associated Bacterial Pneumonia—*Continued*

  2. Care of patients with tracheostomy:
- Perform tracheostomy under aseptic conditions.
- When changing a tracheostomy tube, wear a gown, use aseptic technique, and replace the tube with one that has undergone sterilization or high-level disinfection.

  3. Suctioning of respiratory tract secretions:
- If the open-system suction is employed, use a sterile, single-use catheter.
- Use only sterile fluid to remove secretions from the suction catheter if the catheter is to be used for reentry into the patient's lower respiratory tract.

IV. Modifying Host Risk for Infection
- A. Increasing Host Defense Against Infection: Administration of Immune Modulators
  1. *Pneumococcal vaccination:* Vaccinate patients at high risk for severe pneumococcal infections.
- B. Precautions for Prevention of Aspiration
  1. As soon as the clinical indications for their use are resolved, remove devices such as endotracheal, tracheostomy, and/or enteral tubes.
  2. Prevention of aspiration associated with endotracheal intubation:
     - Use noninvasive ventilation (NIV) to reduce the need for and duration of endotracheal intubation.
     - When feasible and not medically contraindicated, use noninvasive positive pressure ventilation delivered continuously by face or nose mask, instead of performing endotracheal intubation in patients who are in respiratory failure yet do not need immediate intubation (e.g., those who are in hypercapneic respiratory failure secondary to acute exacerbation of COPD or cardiogenic pulmonary edema).
     - When feasible and not medically contraindicated, use NIV as part of the weaning process (from mechanically assisted ventilation) to shorten the period of endotracheal intubation.
     - As much as possible, avoid repeat endotracheal intubation in patients who have received mechanically assisted ventilation.
     - Unless contraindicated by the patient's condition, perform orotracheal rather than nasotracheal intubation on patients.
     - If feasible, use an endotracheal tube with a dorsal lumen above the endotracheal cuff to allow drainage (by continuous or frequent intermittent suctioning) of tracheal secretions that accumulate in the patient's subglottic area.
     - Before deflating the cuff of an endotracheal tube in preparation for tube removal, or before moving the tube, ensure that secretions are cleared from above the tube cuff.
  3. Prevention of aspiration associated with enteral feeding:
     - In the absence of medical contraindication(s), elevate at an angle of 30 to 45 degrees the head of the bed of a patient at high risk for aspiration (e.g., a person receiving mechanically assisted ventilation and/or who has an enteral tube in place).
     - Routinely verify appropriate placement of the feeding tube.
  4. Prevention or modulation of oropharyngeal colonization:
     - *Oropharyngeal cleaning and decontamination with an antiseptic agent:* Develop and implement a comprehensive oral hygiene program (which might include the use of an antiseptic agent) for patients in acute care settings or residents in long-term care facilities who are at high risk for health care–associated pneumonia.
     - *Chlorhexidine oral rinse:* Use an oral chlorhexidine gluconate (0.12%) rinse during the perioperative period on adult patients who undergo cardiac surgery.
     - Oral decontamination with topical antimicrobial agents.
- C. Prevention of Postoperative Pneumonia
  1. Instruct preoperative patients, especially those at high risk for contracting pneumonia, about taking deep breaths and ambulating as soon as medically indicated in the postoperative period.
  2. Encourage all postoperative patients to take deep breaths, move about the bed, and ambulate unless medically contraindicated.
  3. Use incentive spirometry on postoperative patients at high risk for pneumonia.

Source: Centers for Disease Control and Prevention. (2003). *Prevention of health care–associated bacterial pneumonia.* Retrieved May 9, 2008, from http://www.cdc.gov/mmwr/preview/mmwrhtml/rr5303a1.htm.

predispose these patients to developing contaminated saliva that eventually is responsible for VAP (Safdar, Crnich, & Maki, 2005).

Prevention of Ventilated-Associated Pneumonia

What can a nurse do to prevent VAP? A device that has been shown to decrease the risk of VAP is a type of endotracheal tube that has an extra port that allows continuous suctioning of secretions from above the cuff. Secretions collect here and, because of a lack of complete seal between the endotracheal tube cuff and the trachea, drain into the lungs. This aspiration of subglottic secretions prevents the sputum from entering the lungs (O'Neal, Munro, Grap, & Rausch, 2007). The newest endotracheal tube is a silver-coated endotracheal tube that has been scientifically proven as a VAP-preventive device for patients at risk of intubation for 24 hours or longer that minimizes user dependence. In a multicenter clinical trial comparing the silver-coated device to an uncoated tube, the percentage of patients who developed microbiologically confirmed VAP was reduced by 36% for those who received the silver-coated endotracheal tube (Bard, 2008).

Some recommendations by the CDC (2003a) include:

- Hand hygiene using an alcohol-based antiseptic decreased the incidence of hand-transmitted infections.
- Gloving helps prevent cross-contamination. Personnel should use gloves properly and decontaminate their hands after gloves are removed.

- Proper cleaning and sterilization or disinfection of reusable devices used for respiratory therapy, pulmonary diagnostic tests, or delivery of anesthesia helps prevent infection transmission.

The other important intervention is providing oral care to patients who cannot perform their own oral care. Decontamination of the oral cavity either with toothbrushing or use of other interventions has shown a decrease in the rate of VAP in two recent studies (Koeman et al., 2006; Mori et al., 2006). The American Association of Critical Care Nurses (2006) recommends developing and implementing a comprehensive oral hygiene program for patients in critical care and acute care settings who are at high risk for health care–associated pneumonia. Interventions include:

- Brush teeth, gums, and tongue at least twice a day using a soft pediatric or adult toothbrush.
- Provide oral moisturizing to oral mucosa and lips every 2 to 4 hours.
- Use an oral chlorhexidine gluconate (0.12%) rinse twice a day during the perioperative period for adult patients who undergo cardiac surgery. Routine use in other populations is not recommended at this time.

The Complementary and Alternative Therapies box discusses some supportive measures, including the use of vitamin C, that patients can use at home when their pneumonia is not severe enough to warrant hospitalization.

COMPLEMENTARY & ALTERNATIVE THERAPIES

Supportive Measures Plus Vitamin C and Zinc for Pneumonia

Description:

PNEUMONIA is a significant problem in the elderly population. However, it is a condition that is particularly responsive to supportive care. If the patient's condition does not require hospitalization, there are a number of things the patient can do to improve symptoms. Heat is one method of supportive care. When applied in the form of a wrapped hot water bottle to the chest, it can loosen phlegm. Inhaling vapors is another method that can be beneficial in all respiratory conditions, both upper and lower. In addition, postural drainage moves phlegm from within the pulmonary lobes. The older method of postural drainage, cupping, involves a caregiver using a cupped hand patted on the patient's chest also works well. The caregiver should never perform postural drainage soon after the patient has eaten or if the patient has nausea or vomiting.

Vitamin C and zinc are also popular pneumonia treatment and prevention measures. Vitamin C is an antioxidant that protects cells against reactive oxygen species generated during the respiratory burst and in the inflammatory response. Likewise, zinc supports cellular mediators of immunity such as phagocytosis, natural killer cell activity, and the generation of oxidative burst. Both nutrients play important roles in immune function and resistance to infectious agents.

Research Support:

The prophylactic and therapeutic effects of vitamin C on pneumonia was assessed through a Cochrane database search. Researchers identified three prophylactic trials that recorded 37 cases of pneumonia in 2,335 people. In each of these trials, the participants who took vitamin C showed a statistically significant (80% or greater) reduction in pneumonia incidence. Based on these findings, investigators concluded that the prophylactic use of vitamin C to prevent pneumonia should be further studied in populations who have high incidence of pneumonia. This is particularly true for patients whose dietary vitamin C intake is low and who have low plasma vitamin C levels. In the general population, the current evidence is too weak to advocate widespread prophylactic use of vitamin C to prevent pneumonia. However, vitamin C is a low-cost and low-risk supplement, so therapeutic vitamin C supplementation may be reasonable for pneumonia patients who have low vitamin C plasma levels (Hemila & Louhiala, 2007).

A case study in the Netherlands described a 43-year-old male patient with acute sinistral pleuropneumonia and a pronounced thoracic pain syndrome. The patient refused antibiotic treatment, despite his painful ailments. The patient was treated with a complementary therapy comprised of physiotherapy, hydrotherapy, herbal therapy, vitamin C, cupping, and qi gong. A cantharidin blister was applied topically to the left thorax treat the pain syndrome. This combination of CAM treatments resulted in a rapid clinical and x-ray resolution of pneumonia. The cantharidin treatment effectively relieved pain (Rampp & Michalsen, 2006).

A Swiss study evaluated the effect of supplementation with vitamin C and zinc on human immune system function. The study found that vitamin C supplementation improved antimicrobial and natural killer cell activities, lymphocyte proliferation, chemotaxis, and delayed-type hypersensitivity. A large number of randomized controlled trials used intakes of up to 1 g of vitamin C and up to 30 mg of zinc. These trials show that adequate intakes of vitamin C and zinc ameliorate symptoms and shorten the duration of respiratory tract infections including the common cold. They also show that vitamin C and zinc reduce the incidence and improve the outcome of pneumonia (Wintergerst, Maggini, & Hornig, 2006).

A Finnish review evaluated the effect of vitamin C supplementation on respiratory infections in military personnel and other subjects living under conditions comparable to those of military recruits. Seven of the trials involved military personnel, three trials involved students in crowded lodgings, and two trials involved marathon runners. Eight of these trials were double blind and placebo controlled and seven were randomized. In five short, small trials with participants who were under heavy exertion, there was a statistically significant 45% to 91% reduction in common cold incidence. Three other trials found a statistically significant 80% to 100% reduction in the incidence of pneumonia in the vitamin C group (Hemila, 2004).

References

Hemila, H. (2004). Vitamin C supplementation and respiratory infections: A systematic review. *Military Medicine, 169*(11), 920–925.

Hemila, H., & Louhiala, P. (2007). Vitamin C for preventing and treating pneumonia. *Cochrane Database of Systematic Reviews, 24*(1), CD005532.

Rampp, T., & Michalsen, A. (2006). Complementary treatment of pneumonia with pleural effusion. *Forschende Komplementarmedizin und Klassiche Naturheilkunde, 13*(2), 116–118.

Wintergerst, E. S., Maggini, S., & Hornig, D. H. (2006). Immune-enhancing role of vitamin C and zinc and effect on clinical conditions. *Annals of Nutrition and Metabolism, 50*(2), 85–94.

Assessment and Care of the Ventilated Patient

Many of the interventions that are provided by nurses in caring for a patient on a ventilator determine the success of weaning and the prevention of complications. The attention to details and basic nursing care in this population affect the outcome of patients who require ventilators. Among the most important of these interventions is an accurate and detailed assessment. This section reviews the priorities of assessment and care of the patient on ventilation and will include a discussion of suctioning and weaning.

Inspection

Observing the patient and the patient–ventilator interactions is a highly underrated task. To observe the patient on a ventilator, the nurse stands at the foot of the bed and observes how the patient is breathing. The nurse should use a standardized method of observation. A head-to-toe method is one option. The nurse starts at the head of the patient and observes important structures in an organized manner. The endotracheal tube is checked for size and depth of insertion. The method of securing the tube is assessed. A tube that is loose can cause pressure ulcers or, worse, accidental extubation. Presence of an oral airway is noted. Oral airways usually are placed to prevent the patient from biting the tube, but an oral airway can cause significant oral trauma and prevent mouth care. The ventilator circuit is inspected to ensure that it is not pulling on the endotracheal tube or creating tension on the tube. The ventilator circuit should be free of fluid. If fluid is in the tubing, this fluid can lavage the trachea.

The amount and color of secretions in the endotracheal tube and the mouth and nose are noted. Position of the head is assessed. Some patients develop torsion of the neck muscles because they always keep their heads turned toward the side of the bed where the ventilator is situated. Agitation is assessed. Hypoxemia should be ruled out as a cause of agitation and restlessness, especially before administering medication for sedation and analgesia. Cyanosis present around the mouth and mucous membranes suggests central cyanosis and hypoxemia.

Observation of the chest wall for an adequate and symmetrical breathing pattern is crucial in assessing the patient on a ventilator. Assess for asymmetry between the right and left side of the chest. Observe for unusual movements. A tension pneumothorax or pleural effusion can change the size of the affected lung making it appear larger, or the side where an atelectatic segment is located can appear smaller. Both right and left sides of the chest should be symmetrical and rise equally with inspiration and fall with expiration. Paradoxical breathing can occur with trauma to the chest but also with muscle fatigue of the diaphragm. On inspiration the chest rises and the abdomen is drawn in because the fatigued diaphragm cannot descend on inspiration, as it should.

Look for use of accessory muscles of ventilation. Is the patient's WOB increased because of the ventilator mode or size of the endotracheal tube? Phrenic nerve injury or paralysis can affect the diaphragm and can be present on only one side of the chest, producing asymmetry in inspiration or paradoxical movement of the diaphragm, which is another etiology of paradoxical breathing that is described. Is the abdomen distended and protruding into the chest, preventing adequate ventilation? Are the upper extremities more swollen than the feet? Often, patients who have been on a ventilator for a significant period accumulate peripheral edema more in the upper extremities than in the feet. Is mottling present in the extremities? Is the patient shivering? Finally, is there any noise of escaping air heard on expiration that could be caused by too low a volume in the endotracheal tube cuff?

Palpation

Deviation of the trachea is seen in many defects such as tension pneumothorax, flail chest, and in patients who have had pneumonectomies. The nurse begins by palpating the trachea, checking for position as well as mobility. The chest wall is next, feeling for any abnormalities, bulging, or depressions. The point of maximal impulse (PMI) is palpated. Palpating for fremitus is another important component of the assessment. Pleural friction fremitus is a palpable vibration produced when the swollen, inflamed pleural surfaces come in contact with each other. Pleural friction fremitus can be felt during expiration and inspiration but sometimes is felt only during inspiration. Rhonchial fremitus is vibration produced when air is forced through thick secretions.

The chest wall and extremities also are checked for subcutaneous emphysema that is produced by air being forced into the tissue from a pneumothorax or other communication with the airway. Subcutaneous emphysema prompts the team to check for this apparent pathology but usually resolves without treatment. Subcutaneous emphysema is produced when small pockets of air are trapped under the skin.

Auscultation

Auscultation is the most significant component of the assessment in the patient who is ventilated. The frequency of assessment is patient specific and based on other assessment parameters. For example, if the pulse oximetry reading falls to 88% from 99%, after ensuring that the patient is receiving oxygen and ventilation from the ventilator, the nurse should immediately assess lung sounds. For example, absent lung sounds on the left could signal a pneumothorax. The endotracheal tube being advanced down the right main stem bronchus preventing air from entering the left lung also could cause the absence of lung sounds on the left.

The nurse should listen posteriorly as well as anteriorly, starting at the top of the thorax and moving down. It is important for the nurse to listen posteriorly. The importance of this exam cannot be overemphasized. When listening, the nurse should compare right against left lung and never listen through clothing or other material. The clinician should listen laterally in order to appreciate certain lung segments that can be heard in this position. For example, on the right side by listening laterally the nurse can auscultate the anterior basal segment of the right lower lobe. Assessing lung sounds in a ventilated patient can be assisted by performing manual breaths with the ventilator or removing the patient from the ventilator and having someone bag the patient while the other practitioner listens. Normal lung sounds heard in abnormal locations can alert the nurse to certain abnormalities. Bronchial or bronchovesicular sounds heard over the periphery can be indicative of consolidation caused by pneumonia. This sound can also be a result of atelectasis.

Adventitious or abnormal sounds are assessed to ascertain the apparent cause of the abnormality. Crackles occur first in the bases and without the posterior exam the majority of the lung fields cannot be assessed. Inspiratory or expiratory wheezes could be the result of a constriction of the bronchi. Initiation of a bronchodilatory treatment administered as a nebulization through the ventilator circuit might be indicated. Gurgles or rhonchi are low-pitched continuous sounds that are heard over the large airways and sometimes are so loud that the sound is transmitted throughout the lung field. This sound should prompt the nurse to assess the need for suctioning the endotracheal tube. Almost certainly there are secretions that need to be removed. Diminished lung sounds in the ventilated patient can be indicative of pleural fluid accumulation, pneumothorax, or obesity.

Usually, in the ventilated patient, when abnormal or absent sounds are observed, a portable chest x-ray is ordered. The reliance on the chest x-ray should not preclude an excellent clinical exam and an important component of this exam is auscultation of the lungs. Depending on the facility, portable chest x-rays can take minutes to take and even longer to produce the film. Some disorders such as tension pneumothorax can produce a fatal outcome in a few minutes. The nurse at the bedside must be able to quickly assess the change in the lung exam and alert the health care provider.

 Tension pneumothorax is more common in patients who are receiving positive pressure ventilation. Air enters the pleural space through a defect in the lung parenchyma and is trapped in the pleural space. As the pressure in the pleural space increases from the trapped air, the lung collapses and the pressure displaces the trachea and great vessels to the opposite side. If not relieved, the remaining lung collapses. This can occur very rapidly. Successful treatment is a needle thoracostomy and placement of a chest tube.

Nutrition

Preventing malnutrition but at the same time not overfeeding and producing excess CO_2 in the patient who is mechanically ventilated is another important concern for care. Enteral feeding via a nasogastric or oral gastric feeding tube is the preferred method. Small lumen feeding tubes are being used more often than larger bore feeding tubes because of increased patient comfort. Aspiration and other complications including malposition can be prevented by instituting standard protocols and by monitoring problems associated with these tubes at the unit level (Metheny, Meert, & Clouse, 2007). Careful assessment of abdominal distention and bowel frequency can decrease the risk of aspiration. Most patients who are enterally fed in critical care units do not meet their nutritional needs for multiple reasons such as excessive residuals, stopping feeding because of procedures, and loss of access. Interventions to prevent aspiration include keeping the head of the bed elevated and administering medications to assist with gastric motility. Instillation of blue food coloring in the enteral feeding is not recommended because of possible contamination of the tube feeding. A complete description of enteral feedings is presented in Chapter 14 .

Communication and Sleep

One of the important needs of all patients is to be able to communicate their needs to the people who are caring for them. Inability to communicate because of mechanical ventilation is a concern for the patient and should be recognized by the nurse. Many devices are now available to assist with allowing the patient to communicate. Some are sophisticated such as a speak-

ing tracheostomy tube that allows a patient on a ventilator to communicate. This special tracheostomy tube has a port that can be connected directly to another oxygen source. The port exits near the vocal cords and with some training, the patient can learn to speak. Simple devices that allow patients to communicate include a message board with an alphabet or symbols that they can point to if they are unable to write. The concept is to provide some method for communication.

Lack of sleep is another concern for the patients who are receiving mechanical ventilation. Periods of rest and interrupted sleep should be addressed in the plan of care for the patient. Hospitalized patients typically receive very little uninterrupted sleep and patients who are in critical care units or in other specialty units receiving mechanical ventilation are more likely to be suffering from lack of sleep. Noise level also is a concern (Freedman, Gazendam, Levan, Pack, & Schwab, 2001). One unique intervention for dealing with this issue was a "quiet time" introduced by nurses in a neurocritical care unit. This quiet time was instituted to ensure that patients had some time during the 24-hour period during which the noise level was at a minimum and patients were allowed to rest (Reishtein, 2005).

Weaning from Mechanical Ventilation

Difficulty in discontinuation of mechanical ventilation is associated with critical illness, long-term mechanical ventilation, and lung disease. Patients who have been critically ill or "chronically critically ill" and required prolonged mechanical ventilation have difficulty being liberated from the ventilator (Ely et al., 2001). *Weaning* is the process of discontinuation of a patient from the ventilator. The best process of weaning patients from the ventilator is not known. Some researchers believe that weaning is a process that is provided by a multidisciplinary team of health care providers, nurses, respiratory therapists, dieticians, physical therapists, and others who coordinate the process based on a detailed care pathway in order to be successful (Burns et al., 2003). Other researchers and clinicians believe that health care provider directed–weaning with structured rounds and high availability of health care providers is what is needed (Krishnan, Moore, Robeson, Rand, & Fessler, 2004).

How does the nurse know that a patient is ready to be discontinued from the ventilator? There are two tests that have some ability to predict weaning and extubation success. They are the rapid shallow breathing index (RSBI) and the CROP index (Agency for Healthcare Research and Quality [AHRQ], 2000). The CROP index is an integrated scale that includes a thoracic **C**ompliance **R**espiratory rate, **O**xygenation, and maximal inspiratory **P**ressure. This scale is much more involved and difficult to obtain than the RSBI. Chart 36–17 (p. 1032) illustrates the RSBI scale and gives a clinical example.

Other more multidisciplinary screens such as the Burns' Weaning Assessment Tool (Figure 36–9 ■, p. 1032) have been developed that include other patient characteristics such as fever, strength, endurance, and other nonpulmonary system criteria.

Once the decision to wean the patient has been made, there are many different ways to attempt to wean. The use of pressure support with CPAP on the ventilator is one method. If the endotracheal tube is large enough (i.e., if it has a greater than 7-mm internal diameter), another method is to place the patient on a

| CHART 36–17 | **Rapid Shallow Breathing Index** |

Definition	Clinical Example
Ratio of respiratory frequency f (breaths/minute) to V_T (liters). If $f/V_T < 105$, successful weaning is likely.	Calculate the RSBI for a patient whose respiratory rate is 28 breaths per minute and V_T is 250 mL or 0.25 liters: $28/0.25 = 112$ This patient is probably not ready to wean.

Source: Yang, K., & Tobin, M. (1991). A prospective study of indexes predicting the outcome of trials of weaning from mechanical ventilation. *New England Journal of Medicine, 324*(21),1445–1450.

T-piece with oxygen for 1 hour and then extubate if the patient tolerates the procedure (Krishnan et al., 2004). In a classic study by Esteban and colleagues (1995), four different methods of weaning were compared. A once-daily trial of spontaneous breathing accomplished weaning faster than the other three methods. In fact, this method of weaning is supported as a best practice that is recommended by the Agency for Healthcare Research and Quality (AHRQ, 2000). Use of NPPV in some patients with COPD to facilitate weaning was reviewed in five studies. The results were that NPPV might be associated with some clinical benefit (Burns et al., 2003).

When actively weaning the patient, the nurse should monitor SpO_2, respiratory rate, heart rate, and blood pressure closely and be able to return the patient to the ventilator if the patient is in acute distress.

BURNS' WEAN ASSESSMENT PROGRAM (BWAP)
Copyright Burns 1990

Patient Name _____   Patient History Number _____

Patient Weight _____ kg

I. GENERAL ASSESSMENT

YES	NO	NOT ASSESSED	
____	____		1. Hemodynamically stable? (Pulse rate, cardiac output)
____	____		2. Free from factors that increase or decrease metabolic rate (seizures, temperature, sepsis, bacteremia, hypo/hyperthyroid)?
____	____		3. Hematocrit > 25% (or baseline)?
____	____		4. Systematically hydrated? (weight at or near baseline, balanced intake and output)?
____	____		5. Nourished? (albumin > 2.5, parenteral/enteral feedings maximized) If albumin is low and anasarca or third spacing is present, score for hydration should be "no."
____	____		6. Electrolytes within normal limits? (including Ca++, Mg+, PO_4). Correct Ca++ for albumin level.
____	____		7. Pain controlled? (subjective determination)
____	____		8. Adequate sleep/rest? (subjective determination)
____	____		9. Appropriate level of anxiety and nervousness? (subjective determination)
____	____		10. Absence of bowel problems (diarrhea, constipation, ileus)?
____	____		11. Improved general body strength/endurance? (i.e., out of bed in chair, progressive activity program)?
____	____		12. Chest x-ray improving or returned to baseline?

Figure 2. Burns Wean Assessment Program (BWAP), RR respiratory rate; ETT, endotracheal tube; ID, inner diameter; NIP, negative inspiratory pressure; PEP, positive expiratory pressure; STV, spontaneous tidal volume; VC, vital capacity: MV, mechanical ventilation.

FIGURE 36–9 ■ Burns' Weaning Assessment Tool.

II. RESPIRATORY ASSESSMENT

Gas Flow and Work of Breathing

YES NO NOT ASSESSED

13. Eupnic respiratory rate and pattern (spontaneous RR <25, without dyspnea, absence of accessory muscle use).
    *This is assessed off the ventilator while measuring #20–23.
    RR = _____

14. Absence of adventitious breath sounds? (rhonchi, rales, wheezing)

15. Secretions thin and minimal?

16. Absence of neuromuscular disease/deformity?

17. Absence of abdominal distention/obesity/ascites?

18. Oral ETT > #7.5 or trach > #6.0 (I.D.)

Airway Clearance

19. Cough and swallow reflexes adequate?

Strength

20. NIP <−20 (negative inspiratory pressure)
    NIP = _____

21. PEP >+30 (positive expiratory pressure)
    PEP = _____

Endurance

22. STV . 5 ml/kg (spontaneous tidal volume)?
    Spont VNT = _____ STV/BW in kg =

23. VC > 10–15 ml/kg (vital capacity)?
    VC =

ABCs

24. pH 7.30–7.45

25. $PaCO_2$ - 40 mmHg (or baseline) with M.V. <10 L/min
    * This is evaluated while on ventilator.
    $PaCO_2$ - _____ MV =

26. PaO_2 >60 on FiO_2 <40%

Figure 2. Continued.

FIGURE 36–9 ■ Burns' Weaning Assessment Tool—*Continued.*
Source: From Burns, S., Earven, S., Fisher, C., Lewis, R., Merrell, P., Schubart, J., Trawit, J., Bleck, T., University of Virginia Long Term Mechanical Ventillation Team. (2003). Implementation of an institutional program to improve clinical and financial outcomes of mechanically ventilated patients: One-year outcomes and lessons learned. *Critical Care Medicine, 31*(12): 2752–2763.

 CRITICAL ALERT *During weaning, if the patient exhibits any adverse symptoms, the nurse should request that the patient be returned to the ventilator and to the settings that the patient had been on before weaning. Symptoms that might prompt the nurse to terminate weaning include:*

Increase in respiratory rate and complaints of dyspnea

Increase in blood pressure

Increase in heart rate

Decrease in SpO_2.

Other symptoms might include diaphoresis, nausea, and increased anxiety.

Chart 36–18 (p. 1034) is an example of a weaning plan from a recent study that lists criteria for terminating weaning (Krishnan et al., 2004).

Successful weaning is important to patients in order to ensure continued recovery from their respiratory failure whatever the etiology. The nurse can assist with this process by being knowledgeable regarding the factors that are involved in weaning even though the "best practice" regarding weaning has not been fully clarified. As always, the most important nursing action is assessment of the patient's tolerance to ventilator changes and ultimately being off mechanical ventilation. Vital signs,

CHART 36–18	**Example of Weaning Plan**

RAPID SHALLOW BREATHING TEST (RSBT) SCREENING

f/V_T where f = frequency and V_T = tidal volume.

Patient is not advanced to f/V_T measurement if any of the following are present:

- Known or suspected increased intracranial pressure
- Unstable coronary artery disease
- Heart rate > 140
- Wean screen prohibited by health care provider
- SpO_2 < 92%
- PEEP > 5 cm H_2O
- FiO_2 > 0.5
- Receiving paralytics
- Absent cough and gag reflex
- Unresponsive to noxious stimuli

RSBT PERFORMED AND F/V_T <105

Patient is returned to ventilator if, within 1 hour of initiating spontaneous breathing trial (SBT), any of the following occurs:

- Heart rate > 20 beats per minute above rate before initiating SBT, persisting > 5 minutes.
- Systolic blood pressure < 90 torr (12 kPa) or > 30 torr (4 kPa) change after initiating SBT, persisting > 5 minutes.
- Chest pain or ECG changes (ischemia or new arrhythmia).
- SpO_2 < 88% or PaO_2 < 60 torr (8 kPa), persisting > 5 minutes.
- Marked distress or agitation.

Source: From Krishnan, J. A., Moore, D., Robeson, C., Rand, C. S., & Fessler, H. (2004). A prospective, controlled trial of a protocol-based strategy to discontinue mechanical ventilation. *American Journal of Respiratory and Critical Care Medicine, 169,* 673–678.

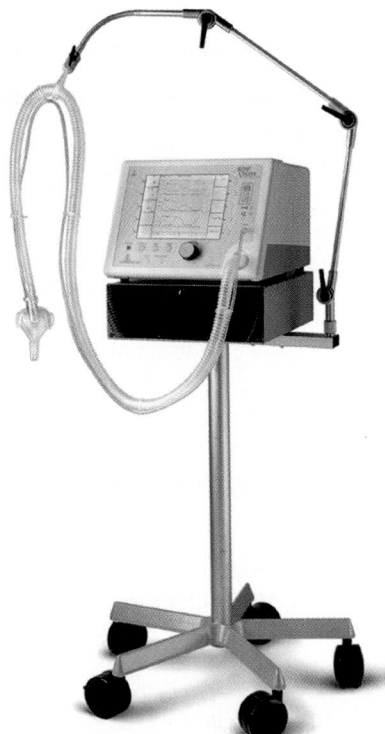

FIGURE 36–10 ■ Example of NPPV: BiPAP.
Source: Image courtesy of Respironics, Inc., Murrysville, PA

ABGs, and oxygen saturation levels are measured continuously. The patient may tire after being off the ventilator for an extended period of time and therefore need to be placed back on it to rest. Typically when the patient tires while on the ventilator, the heart and respiratory rate increase, while the blood pressure and oxygen saturation decrease. It is essential for the nurse to intervene when changes occur in order to prevent complications such as a myocardial infarction due to the physiological stress of trying to maintain oxygenation.

Noninvasive Positive Pressure Ventilation

Noninvasive positive pressure ventilation is the administration of pressure support and PEEP delivered via a face mask or nasal mask (Liesching et al., 2003). Ventilators designed to deliver NPPV can perform many options. Figure 36–10 ■ shows an example of a ventilator used for NPPV. The patient can have just CPAP without any set respiratory rate or the patient can have a combination of pressure support and CPAP. In patients without a stable respiratory drive or who require more support to maintain oxygenation and ventilation, it is possible to set a rate and two levels of CPAP. This mode of ventilation is referred to as **BiPAP**, an inspiratory

level, which is called IPAP or inspiratory positive airway pressure and EPAP or expiratory airway pressure, is set.

The potential benefits of NPPV are that many of the complications of mechanical ventilation with placement of an endotracheal tube are avoided. Among these complications are infections, upper airway trauma, sinusitis, and increased ventilator days related to weaning. It is important to remember that the longer the patient is intubated, the greater the chance of complications related to the endotracheal tube. Psychosocial issues that are avoided by administering NPPV instead of administering ventilator support with an endotracheal tube are another important aspect of this therapy. Patients who are on NPPV can communicate, eat, and require very little, if any, sedation. Figure 36–11 ■ illustrates one type of interface, an oronasal mask that is used to initiate NPPV.

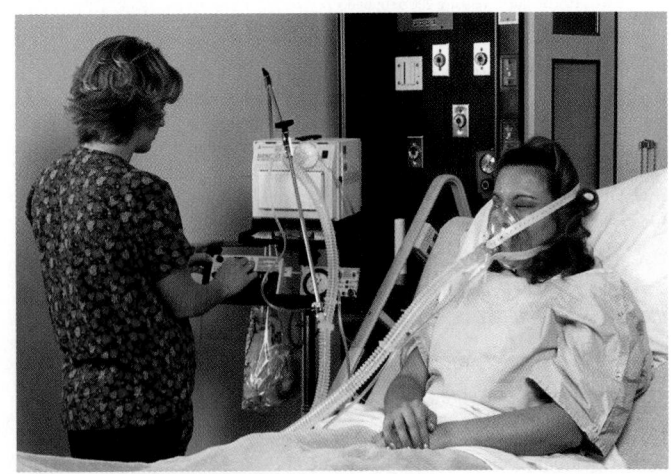

FIGURE 36–11 ■ Oronasal mask.

■ Nursing Management of the Patient with NPPV

Noninvasive positive pressure ventilation is a mode of supporting the patient with acute respiratory failure by using a mask and ventilator instead of an endotracheal tube. NPPV is an intervention that can be successful in preventing intubation but only when a comprehensive approach to the patient is followed. Patients receiving NPPV require many of the continuous monitoring devices that patients who are intubated require. The nurse should be aware that the most serious potentially fatal complication of NPPV is aspiration. Because the airway is not protected as in the patient who is intubated, patients receiving NPPV typically require more frequent assessments. Continuous heart rate, pulse oximetry (SpO_2), and especially trained nurses and respiratory therapists who are experienced with NPPV are essential for these patients. Two other common complications of NPPV include facial trauma related to the tight-fitting mask and abdominal distention. Chart 36–19 outlines the contraindications for NPPV.

A comprehensive approach to the patient who is a candidate for NPPV is outlined in the Nursing Process: Patient Care Plan for the Patient Receiving Noninvasive Positive Pressure Ventilation (p. 1037). This care plan applies the nursing process beginning with a diagnosis of altered respiratory status. Key interventions with rationales are listed for selection, initiation, and assessment of the patient on NPPV.

Discharge Priorities for Patients with Respiratory Failure/ARDS

Quality-of-life research has helped to focus the discharge priorities for patients with ARDS and respiratory failure who spend weeks to months in hospitals receiving mechanical ventilation. Quality of life is an important but elusive outcome measure in many diseases especially after critical illness. It is elusive because it is difficult to define and measure. Quality of life means many different things to patients. Quality of life has important implications for the nurses who care for patients as they recover from ARDS. It is important for the nurse who discharges these patients home or to a rehabilitation facility to understand how this quality-of-life issue affects this group of patients.

What is life like for the patient after surviving ARDS? Studies have suggested that quality of life after ARDS is reduced. Some researchers (Orme et al., 2003) believe that patients' decreased quality of life is related to physical functioning caused by the chronic lung injury after recovering from the acute disease. Others believe that the emotional component, depression or a syndrome not unlike post-traumatic stress, decreases the quality of life. One study has followed these patients for 2 years following ARDS and found significant neurocognitive and emotional impairment besides decreased quality of life (Hopkins et al., 2005).

The nurse should be aware of the following implications for rehabilitation in patients recovering from respiratory failure:

- Recognize that depression, anxiety, and post-traumatic stress syndrome may occur after ARDS and obtain treatment and follow-up with appropriate resources, such as psychiatric consults.
- Inform the patient that crying and depression after recovering from ARDS are common reactions.
- Provide pulmonary rehabilitation for the patients after ARDS with a goal of improving lung function.
- Ensure adequate follow-up of patients with their family health care providers or pulmonologists after discharge from the hospital.

The Discharge Priorities chart summarizes the discharge needs of patients who have had ARDS and respiratory failure.

Health Promotion

Teaching the patient how to remove the ventilator mask and what the different alarms on the ventilator mean helps decrease patient anxiety. The nurse and therapist work closely together to accomplish this patient teaching. It is important to determine if the patient and spouse or primary support person are knowledgeable about the reason for the mask and the limitations the patient will experience while wearing it.

After removal of the mask, the patient is reminded that she should continue deep breathing and coughing exercises at least every 2 hours. Before discharging the patient, the nurse emphasizes the importance of rest and a gradual increase in activity to avoid fatigue. Patients are instructed to maintain resistance to infection with proper nutrition and adequate fluid intake. They also are warned to avoid exposure to others with upper respiratory tract infections or viruses. The patient is taught about all medications that will be continued at home. The nurse provides written instructions as necessary.

■ Collaborative Care

One of the primary examples of collaborative care is the multidisciplinary team of health care providers, nurses, and respiratory therapists who work together to successfully initiate NPPV for a patient.

The health care provider's role is to assess the patient and make the decision that NPPV is an option for the patient. There are many contraindications for NPPV. Timing in initiation of NPPV is crucial. This therapy must be started before the patient

---

CHART 36–19 Contraindications to Noninvasive Positive Pressure Ventilation

- Cardiac or respiratory arrest
- Nonrespiratory organ failure
- Severe encephalopathy (e.g., GCS < 10)
- Severe upper gastrointestinal bleeding
- Hemodynamic instability or unstable cardiac arrhythmia
- Facial surgery, trauma, or deformity
- Upper airway obstruction
- Inability to cooperate/protect the airway
- Inability to clear respiratory secretions
- High risk for aspiration

Source: International Consensus Conferences in Intensive Care Medicine: Noninvasive Positive Pressure Ventilation in Acute Respiratory Failure. Organized jointly by the American Thoracic Society, the European Respiratory Society, the European Society of Intensive Care Medicine, and the Societé de Reanimation de Langue Française, and approved by ATS Board of Directors, December 2000. *American Journal of Respiratory and Critical Care Medicine, 163*(1), 288.

Noninvasive Positive Pressure Ventilation

Clinical Problem

Who should receive noninvasive positive pressure ventilation? There are some patient characteristics and some absolutes with regards to patient selection. These absolute contraindications to NPPV are listed in Chart 36–19 (p. 1035). They were established by an international consensus conference on NPPV (Evans, 2001).

But how does the health care provider, nurse, or respiratory therapist decide who would be a good candidate for NPPV? It is difficult to predict which patient will tolerate NPPV. Some patients who are agitated and anxious when placed on NPPV become calm and relaxed. These patients relax because the cause of the agitation was hypoxemia that was resolved by application of the NPPV. If the patient does have any potential contraindications to NPPV, attempting a trial of this therapy is probably the best course for deciding if the patient will tolerate NPPV. However, there is some research that could assist the team in this regard.

Research Findings

Increased use of NPPV in the past 10 years has positively affected the outcome for many patients who present with acute respiratory failure (Hess & Fessler, 2007). Two surveys conducted in this country and in Canada reported that the most common reason for utilizing NPPV is for patients with COPD and congestive heart failure (Burns et al., 2005; Carlucci, Richard, Wysocki, Lepage, & Brochard, 2001). In fact, two meta-analyses demonstrated a survival benefit in patients who were place on NPPV with COPD (Keenan, Sinuff, Cook, & Hill, 2003; Lightowler, Wedzicha, Elliott, & Ram, 2003). Another meta-analysis of 15 trials compared NPPV or CPAP to conventional oxygen therapy in patients with acute cardiogenic pulmonary edema (Masip et al., 2005). This meta-analysis demonstrated a reduced mortality rate of close to 45% for those who received NPPV support. Another population that has benefited from NPPV are patients who present with acute hypoxemic respiratory failure and are immunocompromised (Antonelli et al., 2000; Hilbert et al., 2001). This therapy provides a bridge to prevent intubation in this high–risk, infection-prone population. Two studies have shown a positive benefit and decreased mortality in the NPPV group.

Some evidence supports NPPV as a tool to wean patients early from invasive ventilation. In other words, patients are extubated to NPPV before being transitioned to standard oxygen therapy. Five studies supported using NPPV to promote early weaning from invasive ventilation (Ferrer et al., 2003, 2006; Girault et al., 1999; Nava et al., 1998, 2005). Finally, in patients who have do-not-intubate orders, this method of ventilator support does not violate the patients' wishes, however, this approach is controversial (Curtis et al., 2007). In one study by Levy and others, they evaluated the outcome of 114 patients who had do-not-intubate orders. Forty-nine of these patients, or 43%, survived to hospital discharge (Levy et al., 2004).

Where is the best place to manage a patient on NPPV? Some experts have questioned the use of NPPV in the intensive care unit only (Kacmarek, 2006). One study demonstrated safe care of this patient population on a medical–surgical unit (Farha, Ghamra, Hoisington, Butler, & Stoller, 2006).

Implications for Nursing Practice

In the final analysis, if the patient does not meet any of the absolute contraindications and is cooperative, a trial of NPPV might be warranted if the clinical team feels that the patient might benefit from this therapy. The clinical judgment of health care providers, nurses,

and respiratory therapists is a key step toward ensuring a successful intervention. The research has provided evidence that patients with COPD, those with cardiogenic pulmonary edema failure, and immunocompromised patients might benefit from this therapy.

Critical Thinking Questions

1. An absolute contraindication to initiating NPPV is
   a. do-not-intubate orders.
   b. age greater than 75 years old.
   c. confused and not able to cooperate.
   d. There are no absolute contraindication to NPPV.

2. A common patient population that research has shown benefits from NPPV and that according to utilization surveys NPPV is used in most frequently is
   a. patients with acute asthma.
   b. patients with COPD.
   c. immunocompromised patients.
   d. None of the above.

Answers to Critical Thinking Questions appear in Appendix D.

References

Antonelli, M., Conti, G., Bufi, M., Costa, M. G., Lappa, A., Rocco, M., et al. (2000). Noninvasive ventilation for treatment of acute respiratory failure in patients undergoing solid organ transplantation: A randomized trial. *Journal of the American Medical Association, 283*(2), 235–241.

Burns, K. E., Sinuff, T., Adhikari, N. K., Meade, M. O., Heels-Ansdell, D., Martin, C. M., et al. (2005). Bilevel noninvasive positive pressure ventilation for acute respiratory failure: Survey of Ontario practice. *Critical Care Medicine, 33*(7), 1477–1483.

Carlucci, A., Richard, J. C., Wysocki, M., Lepage, E., & Brochard, L. (2001). Noninvasive versus conventional mechanical ventilation. An epidemiologic survey. *American Journal of Respiratory and Critical Care Medicine, 163*(4), 874–880.

Curtis, J. R., Cook, D. J., Sinuff, T., White, D. B., Hill, N., Keenan, S. P., et al. (2007). Noninvasive positive pressure ventilation in critical and palliative care settings: Understanding the goals of therapy. *Critical Care Medicine, 35*(3), 932–939.

Evans, T. W. (2001). International Consensus Conferences in Intensive Care Medicine: Non-invasive positive pressure ventilation in acute respiratory failure. *Intensive Care Medicine, 27*(1), 166–178.

Farha, S., Ghamra, Z. W., Hoisington, E. R., Butler, R. S., & Stoller, J. K. (2006). Use of noninvasive positive-pressure ventilation on the regular hospital ward: Experience and correlates of success. *Respiratory Care, 51*(11), 1237–1243.

Ferrer, M., Esquinas, A., Arancibia, F., Bauer, T. T., Gonzalez, G., Carrillo, A., et al. (2003). Noninvasive ventilation during persistent weaning failure: A randomized controlled trial. *American Journal of Respiratory and Critical Care Medicine, 168*(1), 70–76.

Ferrer, M., Valencia, M., Nicolas, J. M., Bernadich, O., Badia, J. R., & Torres, A. (2006). Early noninvasive ventilation averts extubation failure in patients at risk: A randomized trial. *American Journal of Respiratory and Critical Care Medicine, 173*(2), 164–170.

Girault, C., Daudenthun, I., Chevron, V., Tamion, F., Leroy, J., & Bonmarchand, G. (1999). Noninvasive ventilation as a systematic extubation and weaning technique in acute-on-chronic respiratory failure: A prospective, randomized controlled study. *American Journal of Respiratory and Critical Care Medicine, 160*(1), 86–92.

Hess, D. R., & Fessler, H. E. (2007). Should noninvasive positive-pressure ventilation be used in all forms of acute respiratory failure? *Respiratory Care, 52*(5), 568–581.

Hilbert, G., Gruson, D., Vargas, F., Valentino, R., Gbikpi-Benissan, G., Dupon, M., et al. (2001). Noninvasive ventilation in immunosuppressed patients with pulmonary infiltrates, fever, and acute respiratory failure. *New England Journal of Medicine, 344*(7), 481–487.

Kacmarek, R. M. (2006). NPPV in acute respiratory failure: Is it time to reconsider where it may be applied? *Respiratory Care, 51*(11), 1226–1227.

Keenan, S. P., Sinuff, T., Cook, D. J., & Hill, N. S. (2003). Which patients with acute exacerbation of chronic obstructive pulmonary disease benefit from noninvasive positive-pressure ventilation? A systematic review of the literature. *Annals of Internal Medicine, 138*(11), 861–870.

Levy, M., Tanios, M. A., Nelson, D., Short, K., Senechia, A., Vespia, J., et al. (2004). Outcomes of patients with do-not-intubate orders treated with noninvasive ventilation. *Critical Care Medicine, 32*(10), 2002–2007.

Lightowler, J. V., Wedzicha, J. A., Elliott, M. W., & Ram, F. S. (2003). Noninvasive positive pressure ventilation to treat respiratory failure resulting from exacerbations of chronic obstructive pulmonary disease: Cochrane systematic review and meta-analysis. *BMJ, 326*(7382), 185.

Masip, J., Roque, M., Sanchez, B., Fernandez, R., Subirana, M., & Exposito, J. A. (2005). Noninvasive ventilation in acute cardiogenic pulmonary edema: Systematic review and meta-analysis. *Journal of the American Medical Association, 294*(24), 3124–3130.

Nava, S., Ambrosino, N., Clini, E., Prato, M., Orlando, G., Vitacca, M., et al. (1998). Noninvasive mechanical ventilation in the weaning of patients with respiratory failure due to chronic obstructive pulmonary disease. A randomized, controlled trial. *Annals of Internal Medicine, 128*(9), 721–728.

Nava, S., Gregoretti, C., Fanfulla, F., Squadrone, E., Grassi, M., Carlucci, A., et al. (2005). Noninvasive ventilation to prevent respiratory failure after extubation in high-risk patients. *Critical Care Medicine, 33*(11), 2465–2470.

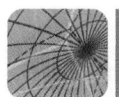

NURSING PROCESS: Patient Care Plan for Patient Receiving Noninvasive Positive Pressure Ventilation

Assessment for Selection, Initiation, and Assessment of Patient on NPPV

Subjective Data:
Do you think you could attempt a trial of NPPV?
Which interface would you prefer?
Are you experiencing any episodes of nausea or vomiting?
Have you ever had problems with claustrophobia?

Objective Data:
Level of consciousness
Hemodynamic stability
Ventilation
Work of breathing
Oxygen saturation
Abdominal and genitourinary assessment
Vital signs
ABGs

Nursing Assessment and Diagnoses	Outcomes and Evaluation Parameters	Planning and Interventions with *Rationales*
Nursing Diagnosis: *Ineffective Breathing Pattern* that can be treated with noninvasive pulmonary pressure ventilation (NPPV) related to *Impaired Gas Exchange, Ineffective Airway Clearance,* and *Ineffective Breathing Pattern*	**Outcomes:** Patient is candidate for NPPV. Improved gas exchange on NPPV. **Evaluation Parameters:** Arterial blood gases improved within 3 hours of NPPV. Decreased work of breathing as exhibited by the patient. Alert and oriented.	**Interventions and *Rationales:*** Assess level of consciousness and ability to follow commands and cooperate *to determine the presence of cerebral hypoxia.* Assess compliance with keeping the mask in place *to determine if the treatment is being tolerated.* Assess level of sedation *to determine if more or less is needed to keep the patient comfortable.*

Assessment for Level of Consciousness and Patient's Ability to Communicate and Procedural Tolerance

Subjective Data:
What is your name, where are you, what is the date, and why are you here?

Objective Data:
Glasgow Coma Scale
Follows commands

Nursing Assessment and Diagnoses	Outcomes and Evaluation Parameters	Planning and Interventions with *Rationales*
Nursing Diagnosis: *Tissue Perfusion Ineffective: Cerebral* related to decreased oxygenation and increased CO_2 levels	**Outcome:** Tolerance of NPPV until it is not needed. **Evaluation Parameters:** Able to follow commands. Responds correctly to questions of time and place. *Glasgow Coma Scale (GCS) < 10 and/or inability to follow commands would disqualify patient from receiving NPPV.*	**Interventions and *Rationales:*** Assess neurological status frequently after initiating NPPV. Increasing confusion related to increased CO_2 levels would signify failure of NPPV.

(continued)

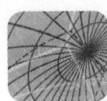

NURSING PROCESS: Patient Care Plan for Patient Receiving Noninvasive Positive Pressure Ventilation—*Continued*

Assessment of Level of Comfort

Subjective Data:

What is your pain level at, using the 1–10 scale? A 1 is very little pain and a 10 is the worst imaginable pain.

What is your experience with pain?

Do you routinely take pain medications at home; if so, what for and what kind?

Are you allergic to any pain medication?

Do you have any cultural or religious beliefs that impact your pain control?

Does the pain get worse with deep inspiration?

Describe the pain: burning, sharp, aching, or any other term that is descriptive of it.

Objective Data:

Grimacing on movement

Restlessness and irritability

Taut facial expression

Nursing Assessment and Diagnoses	Outcomes and Evaluation Parameters	Planning and Interventions with *Rationales*
Nursing Diagnosis: *Pain* related to ventilation or other preexisting conditions	**Outcomes:** Pain controlled with analgesia. Level of sedation is adequate. **Evaluation Parameters:** Appears relaxed. Expresses relief of pain.	**Interventions and *Rationales:*** Assess pain and sedation level. *Increasing levels of pain would require increased analgesics that might decrease respiratory drive.* Provide adequate sedation. *Increasing anxiety would prevent patient from tolerating NPPV. Too much sedation could decrease respiratory rate and prevent ability to cooperate.*

Assessment of Hemodynamic Stability

Subjective Data:

Do you become light-headed or pass out?

Do palpitations or light-headedness occur at the same time?

Do your feet swell and, if so, under what circumstances.

Objective Data:

Vital signs: BP and HR

Oxygen saturation

Level of consciousness

ECG

Lab values: electrolytes and measures of acidosis

Cardiac output

Lung/cardiac

Urine output

Nursing Assessment and Diagnoses	Outcomes and Evaluation Parameters	Planning and Interventions with *Rationales*
Nursing Diagnosis: *Decreased Cardiac Output* related to heart failure and hypotension	**Outcome:** Hemodynamically stable. **Evaluation Parameters:** Adequate blood pressure. Heart rate less than 100 beats per minute. Respiratory rate less than 18 breaths per minute while resting. Urine output minimum of 30 mL/hr. Lungs clear to auscultation. Intake and output within normal limits.	**Interventions and *Rationales:*** Monitor blood pressure and heart rate. *Hemodynamic instability, severe tachycardia, and/or hypotension (shock) would exclude patient. Uncontrolled ischemia or arrhythmias would also disqualify patient.* Auscultate heart sounds. Palpate pulses. Assess cardiac rhythm if patient is on monitor. Obtain 12-lead ECG to *further evaluate rhythm.* Administer antiarrhythmic and or beta-blockers as prescribed. Assess extremities for edema. Assess fluid status and JVD. Weigh patient. Administer diuretics. Monitor intake and output. *Fluid overload can prevent adequate gas exchange.*

Assessment of Respiratory Effort

Subjective Data:

Do you feel short of breath?

Is it becoming worse or better?

How long have you been experiencing shortness of breath?

Do you have it at rest or just with activities?

Objective Data:

Oxygen saturation

ABGs

Skin color and temperature

Respiratory rate

Lung sounds

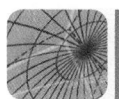

NURSING PROCESS: Patient Care Plan for Patient Receiving Noninvasive Positive Pressure Ventilation—*Continued*

Nursing Assessment and Diagnoses	Outcomes and Evaluation Parameters	Planning and Interventions with *Rationales*
Nursing Diagnoses: *Ineffective Breathing Pattern,* related to lung constriction, lung collapse, low tidal volumes	**Outcome:** Improved ventilation after application of NPPV. ***Evaluation Parameters:*** Decrease in respiratory rate, decreased use of accessory muscles, and decreased dyspnea. Oxygen saturation and ABGs within normal limits. Patient denies increased work of breathing.	**Interventions and *Rationales:*** Assess respiratory status for appropriateness of application of NPPV. *The following respiratory parameters would prompt the provider to **not** attempt NPPV:* *Inability to clear secretion* *Excessive secretions* *No cough or gag* *Impaired swallowing* *Respiratory arrest or unreliable respiratory drive.* Assess facial trauma or anatomic abnormalities that would prevent adequate mask fit. Assess breathing pattern, rate, and depth. Monitor respiratory rate and quality *to assess improvement in ventilation with NPPV.* Assess chest expansion. Note paradoxical respirations. Assess cough and ability to clear secretions. Assess use of accessory muscles during inspiration or prolonged expiratory phase. Assess nasal flaring or pursed-lip breathing.

Assessment for Sufficient Oxygen Saturation Related to Altered Blood Gas

Subjective Data:
Do you have any preexisting health problems such as heart or lung disease?

Objective Data:
Lung sounds
Oxygen saturation
Work of breathing, e.g., gasping, increased rate, loudness
Vital signs
Skin and nail bed color
ABGs
Oxygen saturation

Nursing Assessment and Diagnoses	Outcomes and Evaluation Parameters	Planning and Interventions with *Rationales*
Nursing Diagnosis: *Impaired Gas Exchange* related to pulmonary disease/infection	**Outcome:** Improved oxygen saturation after application of NPPV. ***Evaluation Parameters:*** $SpO_2 > 92\%$ on room air. No increased work of breathing. Lungs sounds clear.	**Interventions and *Rationales:*** Review ABGs and monitor SpO_2. *Ensure that initial ABG/SpO_2 value does not require immediate intervention such as endotracheal intubation.* *Severe acidosis (pH < 7.2) and hypoxemia ($PaO_2 < 60$) would require invasive intubation.* Auscultate breath sounds. Note any adventitious sounds such as wheezes or crackles in the bases. Assess pulse oximetry for absolute value as well as adequacy of waveform. *Waveform should always be monitored with SpO_2 to ensure that SpO_2 is accurate. Dampened waveform can reflect probe displacement.* Maintain $SpO_2 > 92\%$ *to provide appropriate level of oxygen therapy via mask.* Obtain chest x-ray as ordered. Compare film to previous studies *to assess lungs.* Administer bronchodilators if appropriate to increase ventilation.

Assessment of Patient's Coping Abilities

Subjective Data:
How are you feeling about your health and illness?
Tell me what you are feeling about your illness and being on NPPV.
Who are the people in your life that are your support system?
How have you handled fearful situations in the past?

Objective Data:
Facial expressions
Mood
Verbalization of fear regarding injury, impact on family, and future

(continued)

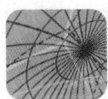

NURSING PROCESS: Patient Care Plan for Patient Receiving Noninvasive Positive Pressure Ventilation—*Continued*

Nursing Diagnosis: *Anxiety* related to discomfort, inability to communicate, lack of adequate sleep, and use of analgesics and sedatives	**Outcome:** Reduced anxiety and confusion. *Evaluation Parameters:* Calm demeanor; acceptance of therapy. Patient can communicate and eat. Mask fits appropriately.	**Interventions and *Rationales:*** Provide constant observation and coaching of patient once NPPV therapy is instituted. *Explaining procedure to patient and coaching will decrease anxiety and promote acceptance of therapy.* Select appropriate mask for patient. Examine patient and note face size. Discuss interfaces and plan for initiation with patient and team (health care provider, respiratory therapist, and patient). *Use of an oronasal or full-face mask with gel mask improves compliance and is more efficient for gas exchange and allows mouth breathing.* Transition to nasal mask if appropriate as patient improves.

Assessment of Soft Tissue Injury of Skin, Nose, Mouth, and Nasopharynx

Subjective Data:
Are you experiencing any pain around, under, or near the mask?

Objective Data:
Skin breakdown near and under mask

Nursing Assessment and Diagnoses	Outcomes and Evaluation Parameters	Planning and Interventions with *Rationales*
Nursing Diagnosis: Risk for impaired skin integrity of face and nose related to poor fitting mask	**Outcome:** Absence of soft tissue injury. *Evaluation Parameters:* No tissue breakdown noted. Skin and soft tissue clear and intact.	**Interventions and *Rationales:*** Apply protective device on bridge of nose *to prevent skin breakdown*. Provide frequent oral care *to prevent mouth dryness and to prevent increase in plaque*. Keep dentures in place *to assist with mask fit.*

Assessment for Abdominal Pain

Subjective Data:
Are you having any abdominal pain?
Do you feel like you are swallowing air?
Are you nauseated?

Objective Data:
Abdominal girth   Vomiting
Oxygen saturation   Bowel sounds

Nursing Assessment and Diagnoses	Outcomes and Evaluation Parameters	Planning and Interventions with *Rationales*
Nursing Diagnosis: *Risk for Injury and Abdominal Distention* related to high pressures, long-term ventilation, and predisposing abnormality	**Outcome:** No abnormal abdominal distention noted. *Evaluation Parameters:* Abdomen soft and nontender. Bowel sounds present. Patient free of nausea and vomiting.	**Interventions and *Rationales:*** Assess abdomen for distention, pain, or tenderness. Assess presence of bowel sounds in all four quadrants. *Persistent nausea and vomiting would be a contraindication to NPPV. Lack of bowel sounds and/or a distended abdomen might increase risk of aspiration with NPPV* If abdomen is distended, consider obtaining order for placement of nasogastric tube *to decompress stomach*. Stop all feeding and oral intake until patient is stable on NPPV. Position patient with head of bed > 30 degrees.

Assessment for Aspiration Related to Insecure Airway

Subjective Data:
Are you feeling like you are getting enough air?
Do you feel more short of breath?

Objective Data:
Lung sounds   Increased work of breathing
Oxygen saturation   Bowel sounds
Vital signs   Abdominal distention

Nursing Assessment and Diagnoses	Outcomes and Evaluation Parameters	Planning and Interventions with *Rationales*
Nursing Diagnosis: *Risk for Aspiration*	**Outcome:** Free of aspiration. *Evaluation Parameters:* Clear lungs. Oxygen saturation within normal limits.	**Interventions and *Rationales:*** Instruct patient how to remove mask if vomiting occurs. *Aspiration is a significant risk for patients with NPPV.*

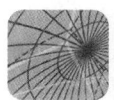

NURSING PROCESS: Patient Care Plan for Patient Receiving Noninvasive Positive Pressure Ventilation—*Continued*

Assessment of Knowledge Deficit

Subjective Data:

What are your concerns about the diagnosis of respiratory disease in terms of prognosis, changes in lifestyle, and progression of disease?

Do you understand how to take medications and their potential side effects?

Do you understand what symptoms you might have and how to monitor them at home and when to contact the health care provider?

Objective Data:

Patients may be anxious, confused, and need repeated information.

Nursing Assessment and Diagnoses	Outcomes and Evaluation Parameters	Planning and Interventions with *Rationales*
Nursing Diagnosis: *Deficient Knowledge* related to the diagnosis, treatments, and long-term management	**Outcomes:** Patient/family understand: The diagnosis of respiratory disease. Their prognosis and treatments. Lifestyle changes. Symptoms to monitor. ***Evaluation Parameters:*** Patient/family will: Ask appropriate questions. Follow appropriate medication regimen. Call when their symptoms worsen for urgent evaluation when needed.	**Interventions and *Rationales:*** Discuss with patient/family the cause and prevention of respiratory disease. *This will enhance their understanding of risk factors and prevention.* Discuss how the NPPV works and how to prevent complications. *This will provide the fundamental treatment strategies and should increase compliance.* Discuss the common symptoms of respiratory disease with the patient and family, describing shortness of breath, cough, fatigue, activity intolerance, weight gain/edema, palpitations, chest tightness, and poor concentration. *This will enable patients to recognize their symptoms and reinforce calling early when their symptoms worsen, so they can be seen and have adjustments made in their medications, preempting an urgent hospitalization.*

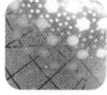

PATIENT TEACHING & DISCHARGE PRIORITIES for a Patient with ARDS

Need	Teaching
Respiratory care: Patient/family Family support/system Setting	Provide supplemental oxygen if appropriate. Instruct use of oxygen therapy and safety measures when using oxygen tanks. Provide pulse oximetry in order to assess oxygenation. Use values for SpO₂ that are individualized for patient. Document these parameters. Provide incentive spirometer if appropriate. Document frequency per day. Respiratory medication administration: • Have patient/family demonstrate use of inhalers. • Document frequency for administration of meds. Ensure that when to notify health care provider is clear. Schedule appointment with pulmonologist and other health care providers. Assess availability and knowledge with treatment regime. Assess respite needs. Assess discharge placement needs: home, rehabilitation, or extended facility.
Emotional and psychological needs, quality of life: Patient/family Setting	Encourage verbalization of frustration with inability to increase activity because of decreased lung function. Encourage increase in independent activity as appropriate. Stress that depression is common after a serious illness. Assess need for psychological counseling. Encourage participation in support groups.
Nutritional: Patient/family	Maintain a diet that is balanced. Continue vitamins or supplements as appropriate. Observe for weight loss and/or loss of appetite. Prevent weight gain. Institute an exercise program with professional consultation.
Pain management: Patient/family Setting	Assess pain level and report any increase in pain. Instruct about the timing and frequency of analgesia medications. Assess environment for safety.

Source: Reprinted from *Clinics in Geriatric Medicine,* 19(1), Sevransky, J. E. & Haponik, D. F., Respiratory failure in elderly patients, 205–294. Copyright 2003, with permission from Elsevier.

is exhausted and unable to sustain a reliable respiratory effort. The respiratory therapist and nurse work hand in hand to select the appropriate interface or mask that will fit the patient and prevent large air leaks. The mask needs to be comfortable but tight enough to allow a flow of air to the patient. Coaching the patient and explaining the goal of NPPV is another important role of the nurse and therapist. Nutrition is an important aspect of care and can be maintained with the help of a registered dietitian.

Nursing Management of the Patient with a Tracheostomy and Chest Tubes

Nursing care of patients with acute respiratory failure involves not only care of the ventilated patient but also care of patients with a tracheostomy. Suctioning is a major intervention that is necessary to perform appropriately to prevent airway injury and cause minimal discomfort. Insertion of chest tubes and assessment of the patient with a chest tube is another skill the nurse must master to care for patients with respiratory compromise. Finally, certain medications that affect the pulmonary system and delivery of these medications are another facet of the care of patients with acute respiratory failure.

Interventions and Rationales
Tracheostomy Tube
There is very little information of when is the optimum time for performing a tracheostomy on a patient who is mechanically ventilated. A tracheostomy is an elective surgical procedure. The surgeon creates a small incision in the skin and opens the lower trachea in order to place a small tube, called a tracheostomy tube. This tube is more stable and secure and has less dead space than an endotracheal tube. Some experts suggest 2 weeks on mechanical ventilation as the optimum time before this surgical procedure is performed (Engoren, Arslanian-Engoren, & Fenn-Buderer, 2004). The benefits to the patient include patient comfort, a secure airway, effective airway suctioning, decreased airway resistance and dead space, better patient mobility, increased opportunities for communication, and the ability to eat.

On the other side, the patient faces some risks with this procedure. The major risks of tracheostomy include bleeding, inappropriate incision location, thyroid injury, pneumothorax, tracheoesophageal fistula, hypoxemia, and infection (Sue & Susanto, 2003). The ability to insert a tracheostomy tube at the bedside percutaneously also has increased the potential frequency of tracheostomies (Polderman et al., 2003).

As the patient improves and is liberated from the ventilator, the tracheostomy tube may be changed and decreased in size until the patient can be decannulated. The first tracheostomy tube change should not be performed until 7 to 10 days after the procedure in order to allow the stoma and tracheostomy tract to mature. In some clinical situations, a fenestrated tracheostomy tube is used (see Figure 36–12 ■). This allows the patient to breathe around

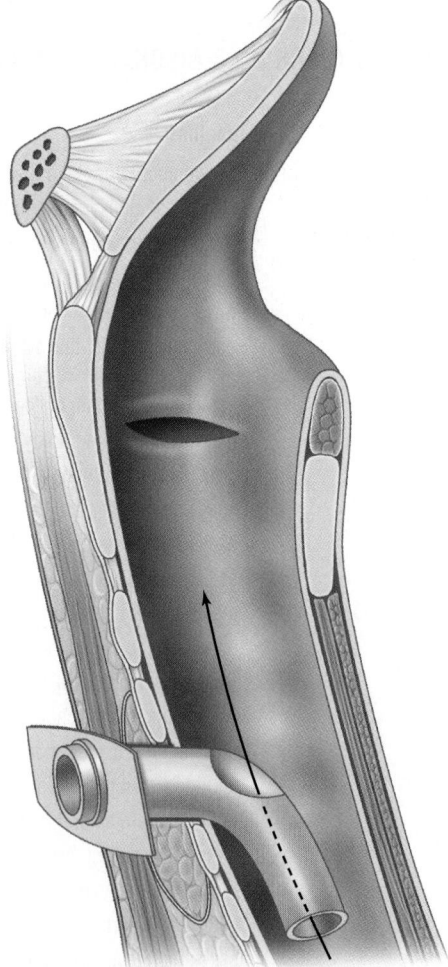

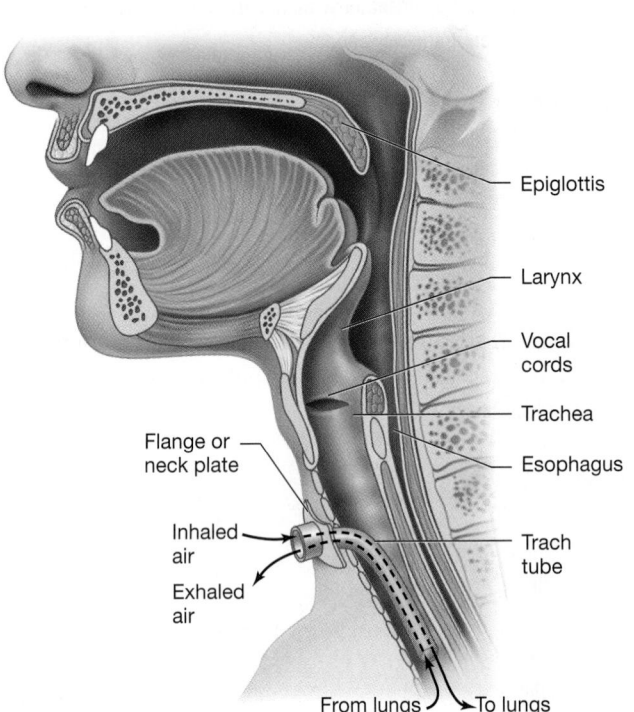

Epiglottis

Larynx

Vocal cords

Trachea

Flange or neck plate

Esophagus

Inhaled air

Exhaled air

Trach tube

From lungs To lungs

FIGURE 36–12 ■ Tracheostomy tube with inner cannula and fenestrated outer cannula.

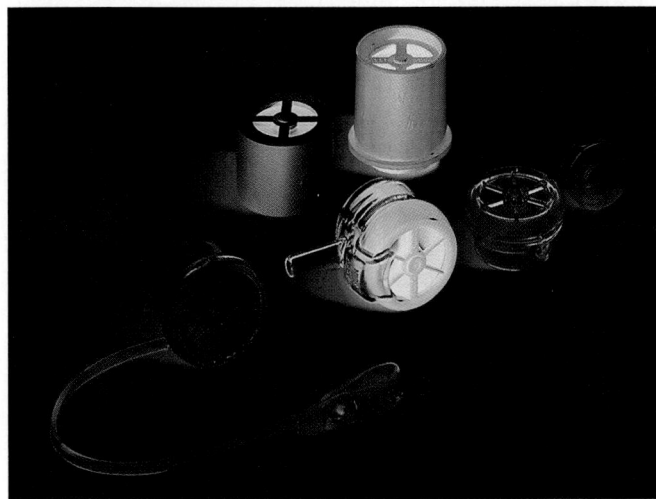

FIGURE 36–13 ■ Passey Muir valve used on end of tracheostomy tube.
Source: Courtesy of Passy-Muir, Inc.

the tube more easily when the cuff is deflated. With the addition of a one-way valve on the end of the tracheostomy tube, the patient can inspire from the tracheostomy tube and expire, forcing air into the larynx around the vocal cord to produce audible sounds. Two devices that are available are the Passey-Muir valve (Figure 36–13 ■) or Olympic Trach-Talk one-way valve. This is a great advantage for the patient who feels elated that he can now communicate directly with the staff. Nursing management of the tracheostomy tube is discussed in detail in Chapter 34 ☺ .

Suctioning

Another important component of the care of the patient who is ventilated is assessing the need for suctioning and performing this procedure appropriately. Chart 36–20 (p. 1044) reviews the suctioning procedure. Some key points of this procedure need to be emphasized:

- Suctioning is only performed based on clinical assessment; it is never ordered routinely.
- Complications of suctioning include hypoxemia, bronchospasms, cardiac arrhythmias, tissue injury, and increased risk of infection.
- Hyperoxygenation prior to and after suctioning is essential to limit hypoxemia.
- Normal saline should *not* be instilled routinely into the airway prior to suctioning.
- Closed suctioning systems (Figure 36–14 ■) should be used in patients with high PEEP and/or FiO_2 and patients who cannot tolerate suctioning with an open system or have an infectious disease that could be spread by aerosolization of secretions.

■ Administration of Common Respiratory Medications

A variety of respiratory medications are delivered through the aerosolized route using many different types of devices. Two of the most common devices are metered-dose inhalers (MDIs) with and without spacers and small-volume nebulizers (SVN).

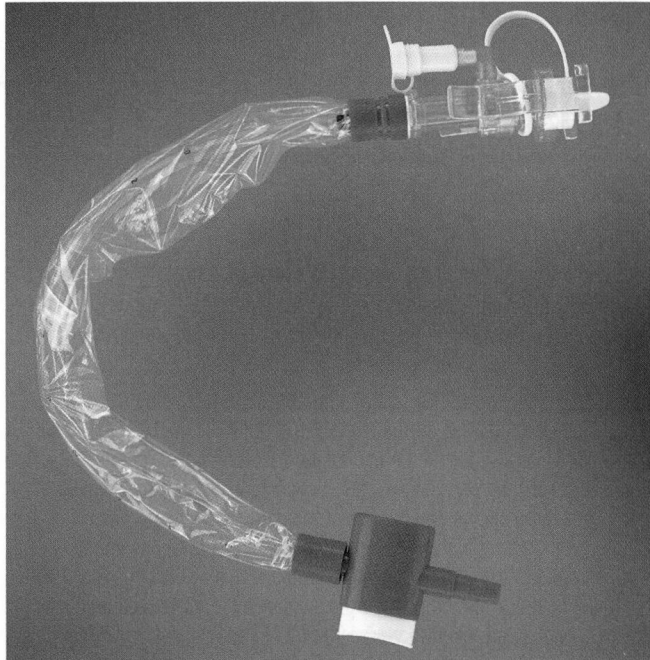

FIGURE 36–14 ■ Ballard catheter.
Source: © 2007 Kimberly-Clark Worldwide Inc. Used with permission.

The nurse should be knowledgeable about the medication that is being administered and the important side effects. The nurse should understand how to administer an MDI and how to teach patients to administer their medication appropriately.

Medication is administered via the aerosolized route for many reasons. Because the medication is not given systemically, the ratio of dose to effect is high. Medication given via this route can be dosed at a lower level because the medication is delivered directly to the lungs. Because of the lower dose, fewer side effects will occur. Delivering medication directly to the lungs also is convenient and less expensive than other routes (Karwa et al., 2005).

Health Promotion

Teaching patients about the proper use and side effects of medication is a basic nursing function. The importance of this teaching is emphasized in teaching patients about respiratory medications. Improper timing and overuse of respiratory medications can prevent the medications from working properly and in a worst case scenario cause increasing symptoms and respiratory failure. For example, one of the most common devices that is used to deliver bronchodilators is the MDI. However, this device must be used correctly and patients must be taught how to use it.

One of the most effective methods of teaching patients about MDIs is for a member of the health care team to demonstrate use of the device and then to ask the patient to perform a return demonstration. This teaching can be accomplished in an acute care setting and usually takes less than 10 minutes. A recent study examined teaching time in an emergency setting and found that the mean teaching time was 6.5 minutes (Numata, Bourbeau, Ernst, Duquette, & Schwartzman, 2002). The majority of the patients in this study reported satisfaction with the teaching and treatment. To teach the patient correctly, the nurse must follow the steps described in Chart 36–21 (p. 1045).

CHART 36–20 | **Suctioning Procedure**

EQUIPMENT

Sterile suction catheter

Sterile gloves

Sterile normal saline for irrigation, when indicated

Sterile disposable container

TECHNIQUE

1. Perform routine procedures before suction. Administer medication, assemble equipment, explain the procedure to the patient, adjust bed to comfortable working position, prepare suction pressure, wash hands, and don gloves.

2. Hyperoxygenate the patient with 100% oxygen, using a manual resuscitation bag (MRB) or the ventilator. If the ventilator method is used, preoxygenation must last at least 3 minutes. Return to the previous oxygen setting after suctioning is completed. (Clinical research shows that the use of the patient's ventilator for preoxygenation delivers higher oxygen concentrations and lower peak pressures than those generated with an MRB (Doering, 1993). In patients who do not tolerate suction with hyperoxygenation, a positive end-expiratory pressure (PEEP) attachment should be on the MRB at the appropriate setting, or in-line suctioning should be used to avoid loss of PEEP and desaturation.

3. Quickly, but gently, insert the catheter as far as possible into the artificial airway without application of suction.

4. Withdraw the catheter 1–2 cm, and apply intermittent suction while rotating and removing the catheter. Limit suction pressure to −80 to −120 mm Hg. Aspiration should not exceed 10 to 15 seconds. (Prolonged aspiration can lead to severe hypoxia, hemodynamic instability, and ultimately, cardiac arrest.

5. Hyperoxygenate the patient before and after each subsequent pass of the catheter for at least 30 seconds, and before reconnection to the ventilator.

6. Monitor heart rate and rhythm and pulse oximetry during and after suctioning.
   Discontinue the procedure if the patient does not tolerate it as evidenced by dysrhythmias, bradycardia, or a drop in SaO_2.

7. Remove equipment.

8. Perform oral hygiene.

9. Clean suction tubing.

10. Wash your hands.

11. Document procedure.

Source: Doering, L. V. (1993). The effect of positioning on hemodynamics and gas exchange in the critically ill: a review. *American Journal of Critical Care, 2,* 208–216. Used with permission; Morton, P. G., Fontaine, D. K., Hudak, C. M., & Gallo, B. M. 8th ed. *Critical care nursing. A holistic approach.* (2005) Philadelphia, Lippincott, Williams & Wilkins.

RESEARCH OPPORTUNITIES AND CLINICAL IMPACT RELATED TO COMPLEX RESPIRATORY DISORDERS

Research Area	Clinical Impact
ARDS and proning in adults	Improving oxygenation and preventing further lung injury
Ventilator management for the treatment of ARDS: Ventilator settings Mode selection Pressure versus volume Noninvasive ventilation in the treatment of ARDS HFOV	
Liquid ventilation	
ECMO for the treatment of ARDS	
Fluid management in ARDS	
Use of hemodynamic monitoring in the patient with ARDS	
Ventilated-associated pneumonia	Preventing VAP
Role of mouth care in decreasing pathogenic organisms in the oral plaque biofilm	
Other methods of preventing VAP: Patient positioning Use of subglottic endotracheal tube Antibiotic-coated endotracheal tube	
Quality of life in patients with lung disease	Improving quality of life after discharge Appropriate discharge criteria
Use of NPPV and weaning	Improving weaning
Incorporate this mode of weaning into weaning strategies	
NPPV and indications for instituting this mode of ventilation in cardiac failure and respiratory failure	Wider use of NPPV for many types of cardiac and respiratory failure
NPPV interfaces: Improved masks Improved ventilators that compensate for leaks	Improved interfaces that will improve patient compliance

CHART 36–21 Steps for Teaching a Patient How to Use a Metered-Dose Inhaler

The nurse should demonstrate this technique and then evaluate the patient's technique using the following checklist:

1. Removes cap from the MDI device.
2. Shakes the MDI.
3. Correctly inserts the MDI into the chamber.
4. Exhales prior to actuation.
5. Places chamber into mouth and closes lips around chamber.
6. Properly times actuation by beginning actuation and inhaling dose.
7. Holds breath for more than 5–10 seconds after dose.
8. Waits at least 30 seconds before administering next dose.

Sources: Numata, Y., Bourbeau, J., Ernst, P., Duquette, G., & Schwartzman, K. (2002). Teaching time for metered-dose inhalers in the emergency setting. *Chest, 122*(2), 498–504; Resnick, D. J., Gold, R. L., Lee-Wong, M., Feldman, B. R., Ramakrishnan, R., & Davis, W. J. (1996). Physicians' metered dose inhaler technique after a single teaching session. *Annals of Allergy and Asthma Immunology, 76*(2), 145–148.

▮ Research

Research on complex respiratory disorders has led to tremendous advances in diagnosis and treatment, ultimately saving lives and improving the quality of life. The treatments outlined earlier in the chapter represent evidenced-based practice that resulted from ongoing research. There continue to be unanswered questions related to all aspects of complex respiratory disease. Therefore, research continues to strive to answer these questions in order to decrease the morbidity and mortality associated with these life-threatening disorders. The Research Opportunities feature outlines future directions in research studies related to complex respiratory diseases.

Clinical Preparation

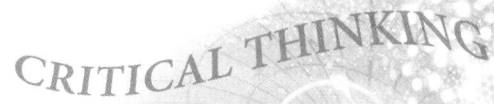
CRITICAL THINKING

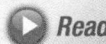 **Read**

- History of Current Illness
- Past Medical History
- Physical Exam
- Admitting Medical Orders
- Laboratory Study Results

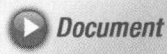 **Document**

- Summary of Hospitalization
- Pathophysiology Form
- Laboratory Values
- Laboratory Results Explanation

 **Apply**

- List of Potential Nursing Diagnoses
- Concept Map
- Critical Thinking Questions

Log on to MyNursingKit.com to download forms you will need and to complete further steps in the Clinical Preparation assignment.

PEARSON **mynursingKit**™

HISTORY OF PRESENT ILLNESS

M r. A is a 52-year-old man admitted to your unit with a diagnosis of pneumonia with increasing shortness of breath during the past several days. He is admitted from the emergency department receiving oxygen via nasal cannula at 6 L/min. Three days ago Mr. A stated that he "didn't feel right" and stayed home from work. He thought he had a cold and was congested and sneezing. He reported not being able to sleep lying flat. Last night he was awakened by an episode of severe shortness of breath. He called 911 and was transported to the hospital. On admission to the emergency department he was febrile at 39.4°C (102.9°F) with a pulse oximeter of 88% on room air. Oxygen via nasal cannula was instituted, which increased the pulse oximetry reading to 92%. A portable chest x-ray demonstrated consolidation of the right middle and lower lobe. Blood, sputum, and urine cultures were obtained and antibiotics were initiated. The patient was admitted to the special respiratory unit for further treatment. Continuous pulse oximetry, coughing and deep breathing encouragement, and Tylenol for fever are the nursing priorities for Mr. A on admission. Careful attention to the timing of his antibiotic doses also is a priority.

Medical–Surgical History

He has never been hospitalized before, but has a history of hypertension that is being treated with the angiotensin-converting enzyme inhibitor irbesartan (Avapro), 150 mg, and hydrochlorothiazide, 12.5 mg, each once a day.

Social History

Mr. A is a sedentary business executive who is 76 inches tall and weighs 250 pounds. He lives by himself, and has no close relatives locally.

Physical Examination

On physical exam, Mr. A is alert and oriented but anxious. His cardiac exam reveals bounding pulses with normal heart sounds and no jugular venous distention. He denies any chest pain or any type of pain except discomfort related to breathing and shortness of breath. His respiratory rate is rapid but his chest excursion is equal bilaterally. He is using accessory muscles for respiration and is sitting straight up in bed. On auscultation, he has decreased breath sounds on the right side with wet crackles heard posteriorly over the entire right lung field. His cough is productive for sputum that is thick, yellow, and tenacious. His blood pressure is 150/90; heart rate is 100 beats per minute with a respiratory rate of 34 to 36 per minute, and pulse oximetry fluctuating between 90% and 92% on 6 liters nasal cannula. His temperature is running 38° to 40°C (100.4° to 104°F). Abdomen is large but soft and nontender. He denies any problems with urination or defecation. His last bowel movement was yesterday. Skin is warm and dry with no areas of breakdown noted. An intravenous infusion is present in his left forearm with antibiotics infusing.

Admitting Medical Orders

Admit to MIC
Service: MICU
Condition: guarded
Admitting diagnosis: pneumonia
Allergies: no known drug allergies
Vital signs and O_2 sats q1h
Activity: bed rest
Diet: regular
Daily weight
Continuous cardiac monitor
Continuous pulse oximetry
Call house officer: HR < 60 or >120, systolic blood pressure < 90 or > 160, RR < 12 or > 30, temperature > 38.5°C, urinary output less than 30 mL/hr × 2, O_2 sat < 92%
IV: D5½ NS @ 50 mL/hr
Strict I/O q1h
Oxygen: via 6 liters nasal cannula; maintain oxygen saturation > 92%
Respiratory Care: Incentive Spirometer q1 hours when awake
Sequential compression stockings to lower extremities while in bed

Scheduled Medications

Irbesartan (Avapro) 150 mg PO once a day
Hydrochlorothiazide 12.5 mg PO once a day
Ceftazidime 2 grams every 8 hours IV

PRN Medications

Tylenol 650 mg po q4h for fever
Morphine 0.3–5 mg IV q4h prn pain
Temazepam 15–30 mg po at bedtime prn insomnia
Droperidol 1.25–2.5 mg IV q4–6h prn nausea

Ordered Laboratory Studies

CPK-MB q8h × 3
Chemistry panel, CBC, and magnesium daily
ABGs daily and prn for respiratory distress

Ordered Diagnostic Studies

Chest x-ray q a.m.

Nursing Priorities

Six hours later, the nurse is called to Mr. A's room. His dinner tray is on his bedside stand. He is cyanotic with pulse oximetry reading in the 70s. He is coughing sporadically with a respiratory rate in the high 40s. Lung sounds are decreased but bronchial sounds are heard throughout the lung fields except for the right side, which is very decreased. The health care provider is called and an emergency chest x-ray is ordered. Oxygen is changed to a face mask, 100% nonrebreather. His pulse oximetry increases to 85%. ABGs are obtained. (The ABGs are listed below with the laboratory results.)

The chest x-ray reveals a new infiltrate in the posterior segment of the left upper lobe and an increasing pattern of consolidation in the right lung. A presumptive diagnosis of worsening pneumonia with possible aspiration pneumonia is considered. On questioning, Mr. A. states that he had difficulty swallowing his dinner and after drinking some of the milk remembers that his coughing increased and he vomited. Presently he can barely talk because he is so short of breath and is increasingly anxious with nasal flaring. Respiratory rate has increased to 45 breaths/min, heart rate has increased to the120s, and the blood pressure is 150/100. Other laboratory tests are ordered with electrolytes and troponin to rule out any cardiac involvement.

Mr. A's status is deteriorating. His respiratory rate is increasing and he is complaining of becoming tired. A repeat ABG is drawn (see below) and shows increasing hypoxemia. The health care provider recommends a trial of noninvasive positive pressure ventilation (NPPV). Mr. A is placed on an NPO regimen and fitted for a mask. A noninvasive ventilator is brought into the room. The mode selected was BiPAP (two levels of CPAP) with an inspiratory pressure or IPAP of 15 cm of H_2O and an expiratory pressure or EPAP of 5 cm of H_2O.

An hour after being placed on the NPPV, Mr. A is less anxious. His respiratory rate is 24 to 26. An ABG examination demonstrates improvement in his hypoxemia. The nurse continues to monitor his progress.

LABORATORY FINDINGS

Test	Day 1	Day 2	Day 3
Sodium	135 mEq/L	136 mEq/L	135 mEq/L
Potassium	4.1 mEq/L	4.0 mEq/L	4.0 mEq/L
Chloride	103 mEq/L	104 mEq/L	95 mEq/L
Carbon dioxide	26 mEq/L	25 mEq/L	25 mEq/L
Blood urea nitrogen (BUN)	16 mg/dL	15 mg/dL	14 mg/dL
Creatinine	1.2 mg/dL	1.3 mg/dL	1.2 mg/dL
Glucose	134 mg/dL	123 mg/dL	120 mg/dL
Phosphorus	2.2 mg/dL	3.4 mg/dL	3.8 mg/dL
Calcium	9.1 mg/dL	8.7 mg/dL	9.1 mg/dL
Albumin	3.7 g/dL	3.7 g/dL	3.5 g/dL
Alkaline phosphatase (ALP)	70 units/L	76 units/L	77 units/L
Bilirubin	0.8 mg/dL	1.0 mg/dL	1.0 mg/dL
Alanine transaminase (ALT)	15 units/L	20 units/L	30 units/L
Magnesium	2.0 mg/dL	1.9 mg/dL	1.9 mg/dL
Creatine kinase	64 units/L	67 units/L	62 units/L

Test	Day 1	Day 2	Day 3
CK-MB	0 ng/mL by immunoassay	0 ng/mL by immunoassay	0 ng/mL by immunoassay
Troponin I	0 mcg/mL	0.2 mcg/mL	0.1 mcg/mL
Troponin T	0 mcg/mL	0.1 mcg/mL	0.1 mcg/mL
WBC	4500/µL	5000/µL	8000/µL
RBC	4.89×10^6/µL	5.09×10^6/µL	4.92×10^6/µL
Hemoglobin	15.9 g/dL	16.5 g/dL	15.9 g/dL
Hematocrit	45.5%	47.8%	45.6%
Platelets	295,000/µL	256,000/µL	300,000/µL
ABGs	Admission	After Aspiration	After NPPV
pH	7.35	7.30	7.35
PaO_2	70 mmHg	53 mmHg	76 mmHg
$PaCO_2$	47 mmHg	50 mmHg	39 mmHg
HCO_3	26 mmHg	25 mmHg	24 mmHg
SpO_2	93%	86%	92%
Oxygen delivery	6 liters nasal cannula	100% FiO_2 via nonrebreather mask	NPPV with BIPAP; IPAP of 15 and EPAP of 5

CRITICAL THINKING QUESTIONS

1. What are the risks of placing Mr. A on NPPV versus intubating him and placing him on conventional ventilation?

2. What types of devices are available for administering NPPV and what are the benefits of each?

3. What are the nursing priorities involved with monitoring Mr. A?

Answers to Critical Thinking Questions appear in Appendix D.

NCLEX® REVIEW

1. A patient with acute respiratory failure is complaining of shortness of breath. Which of the following would be most effective to help this patient?

1. Administer oxygen 2 liters nasal cannula.
2. Maintain oxygen saturation above 85%.
3. Administer a cholinergic medication.
4. Educate to avoid crowds and poor air quality.

2. A patient comes into the emergency department with new onset of dyspnea, SOB, tachypnea, and increased anxiety. The nurse notes increased crackles, coarse rhonchi and pink frothy sputum. Which of the following should the nurse suspect this patient is experiencing?

1. Heroin–related pulmonary edema (HRPE)
2. Neurogenic pulmonary edema
3. Pulmonary edema
4. High altitude pulmonary edema (HAPE)

3. The nurse is caring for a patient with non-cardiogenic pulmonary edema. The nurse should notify the physician if the patient develops which of the following?

1. Heart rate 124 bpm
2. 3+ pulses in the lower extremities
3. B/P 152/88
4. PCWP > 30 mmHg

4. A patient, admitted with respiratory failure, develops ARDS and requires intubation. Which of the following clinical manifestations are usually consistent with this stage of ARDS?

1. Chest x-ray showing absence of infiltrates
2. Temperature of 99°F
3. Arterial blood gases showing respiratory acidosis
4. B/P 124/76 Pulse 86 Respiratory rate 18

5. While caring for a patient on a ventilator, the nurse notes that the patient is experiencing acute distress with a decrease in oxygen saturation to 82%. The nurse's initial intervention would be to:

1. Call the respiratory therapist stat to assess the problem.
2. Remove the patient from the ventilator and use the AMBU bag with 100% oxygen.
3. Call the physician stat regarding the patient's drop in oxygen saturation.
4. Administer a sedative per physician's orders to reduce the patient's anxiety.

6. A patient on a ventilator with 5 cm of H_2O PEEP develops severe hypotension when disconnected from the ventilator. The nurse realizes that:

1. The patient cannot be removed from the ventilator when PEEP is used.
2. The patient is hypovolemic as a result of the PEEP setting.
3. The patient is anxious about being removed from the ventilator.
4. When the patient is removed from the ventilator and the AMBU is used it causes over inflation from the AMBU aggressive rates.

7. A patient with severe respiratory failure has just been intubated. Which of the following should the nurse do first after the intubation?

   1. Auscultate lungs for bilateral breath sounds.

   2. Obtain a pulse oximeter reading to assess oxygenation.

   3. Call for a portable chest x-ray to verify placement.

   4. Secure the ET tube to maintain the patency of the ET tube.

8. The nurse has instructed a family on how to perform tracheostomy suctioning. Which of the following would indicate that the family needs more instruction on the procedure?

   1. Donning sterile gloves in preparation for suctioning

   2. Hyperoxygenating the patient with 100% oxygen prior to suctioning

   3. Placing the head of the bed in a semi-Fowlers position prior to suctioning

   4. Applying suction when passing the catheter into the patient's tracheostomy

9. The nurse has received a change of shift report. Which of the following patients would be of the highest priority for the nurse to assess first?

   1. A patient with oxygen at 2 liters N/C with an oxygen saturation of 96%

   2. A patient with a chest tube on the right side with bubbling in the water seal chamber

   3. A patient who is to receive postural drainage every four hours

   4. A patient being discharged and needs education on how to use a metered-dose inhaler

Answers for review questions appear in Appendix D

KEY TERMS

acute lung injury (ALI) *p.1014*
acute pulmonary edema *p.1008*
acute respiratory distress syndrome (ARDS) *p.1014*
acute respiratory failure (ARF) *p.1006*
air-mask-bag unit (AMBU) *p.1019*
alveolar ventilation (V_A) *p.1006*
anatomic dead space *p.1006*
barotrauma *p.1026*
BiPAP *p.1034*
cardiogenic pulmonary edema (CPE) *p.1009*
dead space ventilation (V_D) *p.1006*

endotracheal tube *p.1020*
fraction of inspired oxygen (FiO_2) *p.1007*
high-altitude pulmonary edema (HAPE) *p.1010*
hypoventilation *p.1006*
hypoxemia *p.1006*
minute ventilation (V_E) *p.1015*
negative pressure pulmonary edema (NPPE) *p.1009*
neurogenic pulmonary edema (NPE) *p.1009*
noncardiogenic pulmonary edema (NCPE) *p.1009*

noninvasive positive pressure ventilation (NPPV) *p.1008*
perfusion *p.1005*
shunt *p.1005*
surfactant *p.1004*
ventilated-associated pneumonia (VAP) *p.1026*
ventilation *p.1005*
ventilation/perfusion mismatching (V/Q) *p.1006*
volutrauma *p.1026*

EXPLORE PEARSON mynursingkit™

MyNursingKit is your one stop for online chapter review materials and resources. Prepare for success with additional NCLEX®-style practice questions, interactive assignments and activities, web links, animations and videos, and more!

Register your access code from the front of your book at
www.mynursingkit.com

REFERENCES

Abraham, E. (2003). Neutrophils and acute lung injury. *Critical Care Medicine, 31*(4 Suppl.), S195–S199.

Acute Respiratory Distress Syndrome Network. (2000). Ventilation with lower tidal volumes as compared with traditional tidal volumes for acute lung injury and the acute respiratory distress syndrome. *New England Journal of Medicine, 342,* 1301–1308.

Agency for Healthcare Research and Quality. (2000, June). *Criteria for weaning from mechanical ventilation. Summary, evidence report/technology assessment: Number 23* (AHRQ Publication No. 00-E028). Retrieved January 10, 2004, from http://www.ahrq.gov/clinic/epcsums/mechsumm.htm

American Association of Critical Care Nurses. (2006). *Practice alert: Oral care in the critically ill.* Retrieved May 6, 2008, from http://www.aacn.org/AACN/practiceAlert.nsf/Files/ORAL%20CARE/$file/Oral%20Care%20in%20the%20Critically%20Ill%208-2006.pdf

Andrew, P. (2003). Diastolic heart failure demystified. *Chest, 124*(2), 744–753.

Annane, D., Bellissant, E., Pussard, E., Asmar, R., Lacombe, F., Lanata, E., et al. (1996). Placebo-controlled, randomized, double-blind study of intravenous enalaprilat efficacy and safety in acute cardiogenic pulmonary edema. *Circulation, 94*(6), 1316–1324.

Antonelli, M., Conti, G., Esquinas, A., Montini, L., Maggiore, S. M., Bello, G., et al. (2007). A multiple-center survey on the use in clinical practice of noninvasive ventilation as a first-line intervention for acute respiratory distress syndrome. *Critical Care Medicine, 35*(1), 18–25.

Arieff, A. I. (1999). Fatal postoperative pulmonary edema: Pathogenesis and literature review. *Chest, 115*(5), 1371–1377.

Baker, D. J. (2005). Critical care requirements after mass toxic agent release. *Critical Care Medicine, 33*(1 Suppl.), S66–S74.

Bard, (2008). Agento I.C. endotracheal tube. Retrieved May 6, 2008, from http://www.bardmedical.com/products/loadProduct.aspx? prodID=391

Bernard, G. R., Artigas, A., Brigham, K. L., Carlet, J., Falke, K., Hudson, L., et al. (1994). The American-European Consensus Conference on ARDS. Definitions, mechanisms, relevant outcomes, and clinical

trial coordination. *American Journal of Respiratory and Critical Care Medicine, 149*(3 Part 1), 818–824.

Brower, R. G., Ware, L. B., Berthiaume, Y., & Matthay, M. A. (2001). Treatment of ARDS. *Chest, 120*(4), 1347–1367.

Brunton, L. B., Lazo, J. S., & Parker, K. L. (Eds.). (2005). *Goodman Gilman's pharmacological basis of therapeutics* (11th ed.). New York: McGraw-Hill.

Brutsaert, D. L., & De Keulenaer, G. W. (2006). Diastolic heart failure: A myth. *Current Opinions in Cardiology, 21*(3), 240–248.

Burns, S. M., Earven, S., Fisher, C., Lewis, R., Merrell, P., Schubart, J. R., et al. (2003). Implementation of an institutional program to improve clinical and financial outcomes of mechanically ventilated patients: One-year outcomes and lessons learned. *Critical Care Medicine, 31*(12), 2752–2763.

Cairo, J. M., & Pilbeam, S. P., I. (2004). *Mosby's respiratory care equipment.* St. Louis: Mosby.

Calfee, C. S., & Matthay, M. A. (2007). Nonventilatory treatments for acute lung injury and ARDS. *Chest, 131*(3), 913–920.

Castro, C. Y. (2006). ARDS and diffuse alveolar damage: A pathologist's perspective. *Seminars in Thoracic and Cardiovascular Surgery, 18*(1), 13–19.

Centers for Disease Control and Prevention. (2003a). *Prevention and control of ventilator-associated pneumonia guidelines.* Retrieved May 6, 2008, from http://www.cdc.gov/ncidod/dhqp/dpac_ventilate_pc.html

Centers for Disease Control and Prevention. (2005). *An overview of ventilator-associated pneumonia.* Retrieved June 4, 2008, from http://www.cdc.gov/ncidod/dhqp/dpac_ventilate.html

Centers for Disease Control and Prevention. (2007). *Bioterrorism overview.* Retrieved June 4, 2008, from http://emergency.cdc.gov/bioterrorism/overview.asp

Chan, K. P., & Stewart, T. E. (2005). Clinical use of high-frequency oscillatory ventilation in adult patients with acute respiratory distress syndrome. *Critical Care Medicine, 33*(3 Suppl.), S170–S174.

Chatila, W. M., & Criner, G. J. (2002). Complications of long-term mechanical ventilation. *Respiratory Care Clinics of North America, 8*(4), 631–647.

Cobbs, C. G., & Chansolme, D. H. (2004). Plague. *Dermatologic Clinics, 22*(3), 303–312, vi.

Collins, S. P., Lindsell, C. J., Storrow, A. B., & Abraham, W. T. (2006). Prevalence of negative chest radiography results in the emergency department patient with decompensated heart failure. *Annals of Emergency Medicine, 47*(1), 13–18.

Doan, L. G. (2004). Ricin: mechanism of toxicity, clinical manifestations, and vaccine development. A review. *Journal of Toxicology–Clinical Toxicology, 42*(2), 201–208.

ELSO Registry Information. (2008). Retrieved August 9, 2008 from http:/ /www.elso.med.umich.edu/Registry.htm

Ely, E. W., Meade, M. O., Haponik, E. F., Kollef, M. H., Cook, D. J., Guyatt, G. H., et al. (2001). Mechanical ventilator weaning protocols driven by nonphysician health-care professionals: Evidence-based clinical practice guidelines. *Chest, 120*(6 Suppl.), 454S–463S.

Engoren, M., Arslanian-Engoren, C., & Fenn-Buderer, N. (2004). Hospital and long-term outcome after tracheostomy for respiratory failure. *Chest, 125*(1), 220–227.

Esteban, A., Alia, I., Gordo, F., de Pablo, R., Suarez, J., Gonzalez, G., et al. (2000). Prospective randomized trial comparing pressure-controlled ventilation and volume-controlled ventilation in ARDS. *Chest, 117*(6), 1690–1696.

Estebam, A., Anzueto, A., Frutos-Vivar, F., Alia, I., Ely, E. W., Brochard, L., et al. (2004). Outcome of older patients receiving mechanical ventilation. *Intensive Care Medicine, 30* (4), 639–646.

Esteban, A., Frutos, F., Tobin, M. J., Alia, I., Solsona, J. F., Valverdu, I., et al. (1995). A comparison of four methods of weaning patients from mechanical ventilation. *New England Journal of Medicine, 332*(6), 345–350.

Fink, M. P., Abraham, E., Vincent, J., & Kochanek, P. (2005). Acute respiratory failure. In *Textbook of critical care* (Chap. 9). Philadelphia: W. B. Saunders.

Fleischmann, K. E., Goldman, L., Young, B., & Lee, T. H. (2003). Association between cardiac and noncardiac complications in patients undergoing noncardiac surgery: Outcomes and effects on length of stay. *American Journal of Medicine, 115*(7), 515–520.

Fontes, R. B., Aguiar, P. H., Zanetti, M. V., Andrade, F., Mandel, M., & Teixeira, M. J. (2003). Acute neurogenic pulmonary edema: Case reports and literature review. *Journal of Neurosurgical Anesthesiology, 15*(2), 144–150.

Fox, K. A., Steg, P. G., Eagle, K. A., Goodman, S. G., Anderson, F. A., Jr., Granger, C. B., et al. (2007). Decline in rates of death and heart failure in acute coronary syndromes, 1999–2006. *Journal of the American Medical Association, 297*(17), 1892–1900.

Freedman, N. S., Gazendam, J., Levan, L., Pack, A. I., & Schwab, R. J. (2001). Abnormal sleep/wake cycles and the effect of environmental noise on sleep disruption in the intensive care unit. *American Journal of Respiratory and Critical Care Medicine, 163*(2), 451–457.

Fremont, R. D., Kallet, R. H., Matthay, M. A., & Ware, L. B. (2007). Post-obstructive pulmonary edema: A case for hydrostatic mechanisms. *Chest, 131,* 1742–1746.

Frishman, W. H., Del Vecchio, A., Sanal, S., & Ismail, A. (2003). Cardiovascular manifestations of substance abuse. Part 2: Alcohol, amphetamines, heroin, cannabis, and caffeine. *Heart Disease, 5*(4), 253–271.

Gabry, A. L., Ledoux, X., Mozziconacci, M., & Martin, C. (2003). High-altitude pulmonary edema at moderate altitude (< 2,400 m; 7,870 feet): A series of 52 patients. *Chest, 123*(1), 49–53.

Gong, M. N., Wei, Z., Xu, L. L., Miller, D. P., Thompson, B. T., & Christiani, D. C. (2004). Polymorphism in the surfactant protein-B gene, gender, and the risk of direct pulmonary injury and ARDS. *Chest, 125*(1), 203–211.

Goss, C. H., Brower, R. G., Hudson, L. D., & Rubenfeld, G. D. (2003). Incidence of acute lung injury in the United States. *Critical Care Medicine, 31*(6), 1607–1611.

Guyton, A., & Hall, J. (2005). *Textbook of Medical Physiology* (11th ed.). Philadelphia: W. B. Saunders.

Habal, R. (2006). *Toxicity, heroin.* EMedicine. Retrieved August 13, 2008 from http://www.emedicine.com/med/TOPIC1003.HTM

Halpern, P., Gefen, A., Sorkine, P., & Elad, D. (2003). Pulmonary oedema in SCUBA divers: Pathophysiology and computed risk analysis. *European Journal of Emergency Medicine, 10*(1), 35–41.

Hemmila, M. R., & Napolitano, L. M. (2006). Severe respiratory failure: Advanced treatment options. *Critical Care Medicine, 34*(9 Suppl.), S278–S290.

Hopkins, R. O., Weaver, L. K., Collingridge, D., Parkinson, R. B., Chan, K. J., & Orme, J. F., Jr. (2005). Two-year cognitive, emotional, and quality-of-life outcomes in acute respiratory distress syndrome. *American Journal of Respiratory and Critical Care Medicine, 171*(4), 340–347.

Howard, A., Courtney-Shapiro, C., Kelso, L., Goltz, M., & Morris, P. (2004). Comparison of three methods of detecting acute respiratory distress syndrome: Clinical screening, chart review and diagnosis coding. *American Journal of Nursing, 13,* 59–64.

Hudson, L. D., & Hough, C. L. (2006). Therapy for late-phase acute respiratory distress syndrome. *Clinics in Chest Medicine, 27*(4), 671–677; abstract, ix–x.

Hughes, R. A., & Cornblath, D. R. (2005). Guillain-Barre syndrome. *Lancet, 366*(9497), 1653–1666.

Inglesby, T. V., O'Toole, T., Henderson, D. A., Bartlett, J. G., Ascher, M. S., Eitzen, E., et al. (2002). Anthrax as a biological weapon, 2002: Updated recommendations for management. *Journal of the American Medical Association, 287*(17), 2236–2252.

Jessup, M., & Brozena, S. (2003). Heart failure. *New England Journal of Medicine, 348*(20), 2007–2018.

Johnston, C. J., Rubenfeld, G. D., & Hudson, L. D. (2003). Effect of age on the development of ARDS in trauma patients. *Chest, 124*(2), 653–659.

Kaisers, U., Kelly, K. P., & Busch, T. (2003). Liquid ventilation. *British Journal of Anaesthesia, 91*(1), 143–151.

Kaplow, R., & Hardin, S. R. (2007). *Critical care nursing: Synergy and optimal outcomes.* Boston: Jones & Bartlett.

Karwa, M., Currie, B., & Kvetan, V. (2005). Bioterrorism: Preparing for the impossible or the improbable. *Critical Care Medicine, 33*(1 Suppl.), S75–S95.

Klompas, M. (2007). Does this patient have ventilator-associated pneumonia? *Journal of the American Medical Association, 297*(14), 1583–1593.

Koeman, M., van der Ven, A. J., Hak, E., Joore, H. C., Kaasjager, K., de Smet, A. G., et al. (2006). Oral decontamination with chlorhexidine reduces the incidence of ventilator-associated pneumonia. *American Journal of Respiratory and Critical Care Medicine, 173*(12), 1348–1355.

Krishnan, J. A., Moore, D., Robeson, C., Rand, C. S., & Fessler, H. E. (2004). A prospective, controlled trial of a protocol-based strategy to discontinue mechanical ventilation. *American Journal of Respiratory and Critical Care Medicine, 169*(6), 673–678.

Lanken, P. N., Ed. (2006). *The intensive care unit manual* (3rd ed.). Philadelphia: W. B. Saunders.

Lewandowski, K. (2003). Contributions to the epidemiology of acute respiratory failure. *Critical Care, 7*(4), 288–290.

Lewis, J. F., & Brackenbury, A. (2003). Role of exogenous surfactant in acute lung injury. *Critical Care Medicine, 31*(4 Suppl.), S324–S328.

Liesching, T., Kwok, H., & Hill, N. S. (2003). Acute applications of noninvasive positive pressure ventilation. *Chest, 124*(2), 699–713.

Looney, M. R., Gropper, M. A., & Matthay, M. A. (2004). Transfusion-related acute lung injury: A review. *Chest, 126* (1), 249–258.

Lupatkin, H., Lupatkin, J., & Rosenberg, A. (2004). Smallpox in the 21st century. *Anesthesiology Clinics of North America, 22* (3), 541–561.

MacIntyre, N. R. (2005). Current issues in mechanical ventilation for respiratory failure. *Chest, 128*(5 Suppl. 2), 561S–567S.

Marini, J. J., & Gattinoni, L. (2004). Ventilatory management of acute respiratory distress syndrome: A consensus of two. *Critical Care Medicine, 32*(1), 250–255.

Marks, J. D. (2004). Medical aspects of biologic toxins. *Anesthesiology Clinics of North America, 22*(3), 509–532, vii.

Martin, C. M., Doig, G. S., Heyland, D. K., Morrison, T., & Sibbald, W. J. (2004). Multicentre, cluster-randomized clinical trial of algorithms for critical-care enteral and parenteral therapy (ACCEPT). *CMAJ, 170*(2), 197–204.

Martin, M., Salim, A., Murray, J., Demetriades, D., Belzberg, H., & Rhee, P. (2005). The decreasing incidence and mortality of acute respiratory distress syndrome after injury: A 5-year observational study. *Journal of Trauma, 59*(5), 1107–1113.

Matthay, M. A., Zimmerman, G. A., Esmon, C., Bhattacharya, J., Coller, B., Doerschuk, C. M., et al. (2003). Future research directions in acute lung injury: Summary of a National Heart, Lung, and Blood Institute working group. *American Journal of Respiratory and Critical Care Medicine, 167*(7), 1027–1035.

Mattu, A., Martinez, J. P., & Kelly, B. S. (2005). Modern management of cardiogenic pulmonary edema. *Emergency Medical Clinics of North America, 23*(4), 1105–1125.

Metheny, N. A., Meert, K. L., & Clouse, R. E. (2007). Complications related to feeding tube placement. *Current Opinions in Gastroenterology, 23*(2), 178–182.

Moloney, E. D., & Evans, T. W. (2003). Pathophysiology and pharmacological treatment of pulmonary hypertension in acute respiratory distress syndrome. *European Respiratory Journal, 21*(4), 720–727.

Mori, H., Hirasawa, H., Oda, S., Shiga, H., Matsuda, K., & Nakamura, M. (2006). Oral care reduces incidence of ventilator-associated pneumonia in ICU populations. *Intensive Care Medicine, 32*(2), 230–236.

Murray, J., & Nadel, J. (Eds.). (2005). *Textbook of respiratory medicine* (4th ed.). Philadelphia: W. B. Saunders.

Numata, Y., Bourbeau, J., Ernst, P., Duquette, G., & Schwartzman, K. (2002). Teaching time for metered-dose inhalers in the emergency setting. *Chest, 122*(2), 498–504.

O'Neal, P. V., Munro, C. L., Grap, M. J., & Rausch, S. M. (2007). Subglottic secretion viscosity and evacuation efficiency. *Biological Research for Nursing, 8*(3), 202–209.

Ognibene, F. P., Martin, S. E., Parker, M. M., Schlesinger, T., Roach, P., Burch, C., et al. (1986). Adult respiratory distress syndrome in patients with severe neutropenia. *New England Journal of Medicine, 315*(9), 547–551.

Onwuanyi, A., & Taylor, M. (2007). Acute decompensated heart failure: Pathophysiology and treatment. *American Journal of Cardiology, 99*(6B), 25D–30D.

Orme, J., Jr., Romney, J. S., Hopkins, R. O., Pope, D., Chan, K. J., Thomsen, G., et al. (2003). Pulmonary function and health-related quality of life in survivors of acute respiratory distress syndrome. *American Journal of Respiratory and Critical Care Medicine, 167*(5), 690–694.

Pastor, C. M., Matthay, M. A., & Frossard, J. L. (2003). Pancreatitis-associated acute lung injury: New insights. *Chest, 124*(6), 2341–2351.

Percell, R. L., Jr., Henning, R. J., & Siddique Patel, M. (2003). Atrial myxoma: Case report and a review of the literature. *Heart Disease, 5*(3), 224–230.

Pilbeam, S. P. & Cairo, J. M. (2006). *Mechanical ventilation: Physiological and clinical applications* (4th ed.). Philadelphia: Mosby.

Polderman, K. H., Spijkstra, J. J., de Bree, R., Christiaans, H. M., Gelissen, H. P., Wester, J. P., et al. (2003). Percutaneous dilatational tracheostomy in the ICU: Optimal organization, low complication rates, and description of a new complication. *Chest, 123*(5), 1595–1602.

Porth, C. (2007). *Essential of Pathophysiology* (2nd ed.). St. Louis: Lippincott Williams & Wilkins.

Reishtein, J. L. (2005). Sleep in mechanically ventilated patients. *Critical Care Nursing Clinics of North America, 17*(3), 251–255.

Rello, J., Kollef, M., Diaz, E., Sandiumenge, A., del Castillo, Y., Corbella, X., et al. (2006). Reduced burden of bacterial airway colonization with a novel silver-coated endotracheal tube in a randomized multiple-center feasibility study. *Critical Care Medicine, 34*(11), 2766–2772.

Safdar, N., Crnich, C. J., & Maki, D. G. (2005). The pathogenesis of ventilator-associated pneumonia: Its relevance to developing effective strategies for prevention. *Respiratory Care, 50*(6), 725–739; discussion, 739–741.

Sagrista-Sauleda, J., Angel, J., Sambola, A., Alguersuari, J., Permanyer-Miralda, G., & Soler-Soler, J. (2006). Low-pressure cardiac tamponade: Clinical and hemodynamic profile. *Circulation, 114*(9), 945–952.

Sanderson, J. E., & Fraser, A. G. (2006). Systolic dysfunction in heart failure with a normal ejection fraction: Echo-Doppler measurements. *Progress in Cardiovascular Disease, 49*(3), 196–206.

Shapiro, B., Peruzzi, W., & Templin, R. (Eds.). (1994). *Clinical applications of blood gases.* St. Louis: Mosby.

Shorr, A. F., & Kollef, M. H. (2005). Ventilator-associated pneumonia: Insights from recent clinical trials. *Chest, 128*(5 Suppl. 2), 583S–591S.

Sue, R. D., & Susanto, I. (2003). Long-term complications of artificial airways. *Clinics in Chest Medicine, 24*(3), 457–471.

Suter, P. M. (2006). Reducing ventilator-induced lung injury and other organ injury by the prone position. *Critical Care, 10*(2), 139.

Talreja, D. R., Edwards, W. D., Danielson, G. K., Schaff, H. V., Tajik, A. J., Tazelaar, H. D., et al. (2003). Constrictive pericarditis in 26 patients with histologically normal pericardial thickness. *Circulation, 108*(15), 1852–1857.

Tarrac, S. E. (2003). Negative pressure pulmonary edema—a postanesthesia emergency. *Journal of Perianesthesia Nursing, 18*(5), 317–323.

Vincent, J. L., Sakr, Y., & Ranieri, V. M. (2003). Epidemiology and outcome of acute respiratory failure in intensive care unit patients. *Critical Care Medicine, 31*(4 Suppl.), S296–S299.

Wang, C. S., FitzGerald, J. M., Schulzer, M., Mak, E., & Ayas, N. T. (2005). Does this dyspneic patient in the emergency department have congestive heart failure? *Journal of the American Medical Association, 294*(15), 1944–1956.

Ware, L. B. (2005). Prognostic determinants of acute respiratory distress syndrome in adults: Impact on clinical trial design. *Critical Care Medicine, 33*(3 Suppl.), S217–S222.

Ware, L. B., & Matthay, M. A. (2005). Clinical practice: Acute pulmonary edema. *New England Journal of Medicine, 353*(26), 2788–2796.

West, J. B. (1998). *Pulmonary pathophysiology: The essentials* (5th ed.). Baltimore: Williams & Wilkins.

Wheeler, A. P., & Bernard, G. R. (2007). Acute lung injury and the acute respiratory distress syndrome: A clinical review. *Lancet, 369*(9572), 1553–1564.

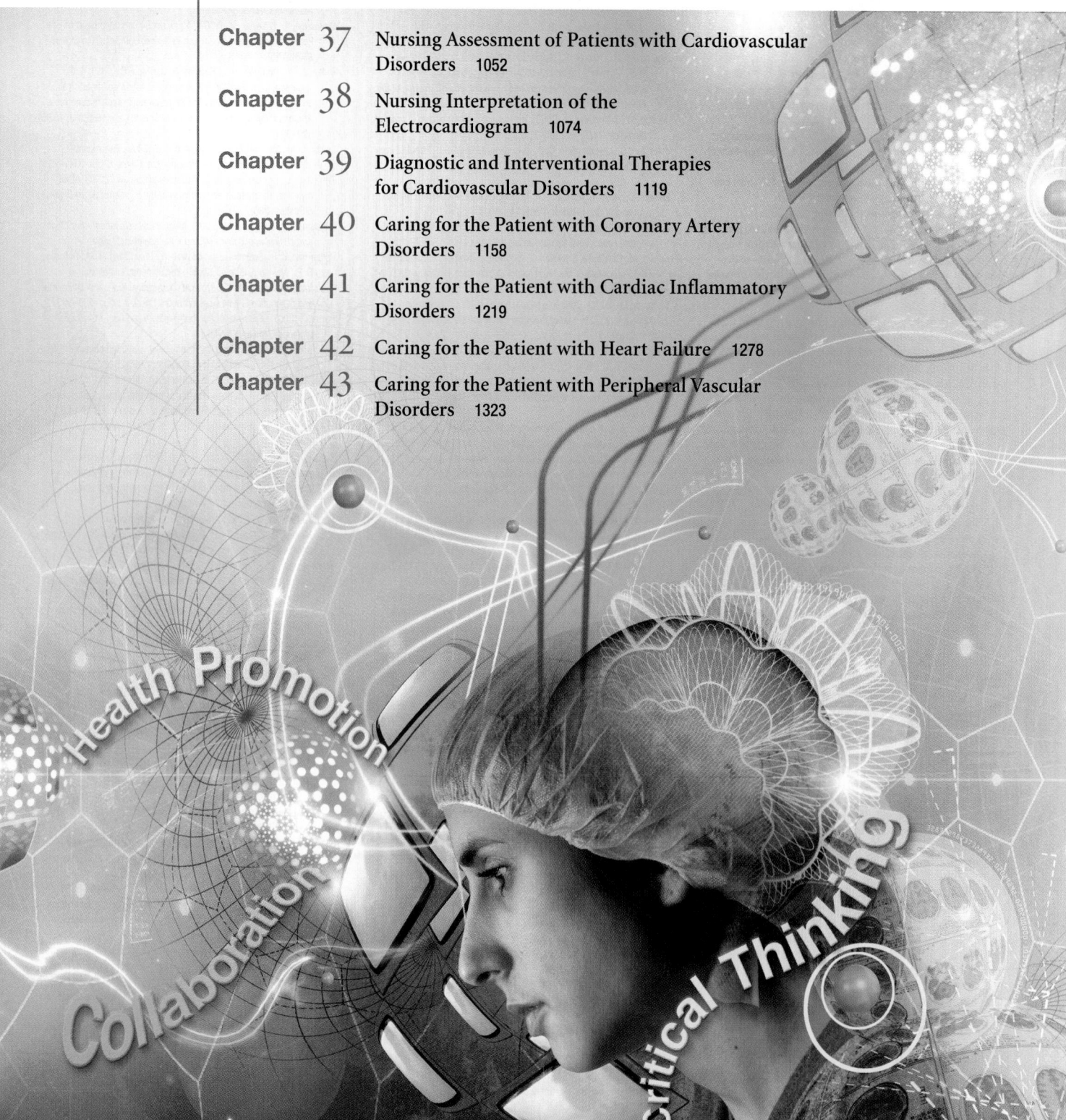

UNIT

8 | Nursing Management of Patients with Cardiovascular Disorders

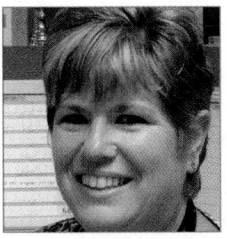

JACKIE My name is Jackie and I am a registered nurse on the Cardiothoracic Progressive Care Unit at UC Davis Medical Center. Our typical patients are postoperative and have had coronary artery bypass graft surgery (CABG), valve replacements, and thoracotomies. We also have a wide variety of patients who are experiencing respiratory failure, alcohol withdrawal, and multiple system failures—all of which require telemetry monitoring. To be competent, all nurses on the unit are required to complete Advanced Cardiac Life Support (ACLS) certification and ECG monitor training.

On a typical day I have three patients. I will obtain report, research each patient's laboratory results, and check their telemetry, making sure that each patient is hemodynamically stable. I will then introduce myself to my patients, assess them and, with confidence, report anything pertinent to the health care team. I listen with compassion to any needs or concerns the patient and family may have. Postoperative patients can have many concerns and questions regarding their future health status. I answer their questions and let them know that I will help them in any way that I am able. As the day progresses, I will educate my patients about their disease process, wound care management, and any discharge needs. It is particularly important to have cardiac patients understand the disease process. The surgery may have reestablished blood flow to the heart muscle, but unless the patient makes lifestyle changes such as a healthy diet and exercise, the arteries can occlude again. It is important to have patients and their family participate in their care early to allay any fears they may have about being able to care for themselves after discharge from the hospital. I also watch for any changes in my patients and their telemetry monitoring. Are they having increased ectopy? Are their electrolytes within normal limits? Is the patient having an increase in pain or chest tube output? These are just a few things that I continually monitor. As the primary nurse I spend the most time with the patient and may be the first to observe subtle changes in their condition. Early recognition of complications can keep them from becoming severe.

Nursing is a rewarding career. Remember to be happy and keep humor in your daily routine—patients like a happy nurse who comports herself well. Always be kind, caring, and compassionate, and treat patients the way you would want your loved ones to be treated.

> "It is important to have patients and their family participate in their care early to allay any fears they may have about being able to care for themselves after discharge from the hospital."

Nursing Assessment of Patients with Cardiovascular Disorders

Kristine L'Ecuyer
With contributions by:
Kathleen Osborn

Outcome-Based Learning Objectives

After studying this chapter, the learner will be able to:

1. Compare and contrast the significance of cardiovascular assessment findings.
2. Evaluate the relationship of current health status and the presence of cardiac risk factors.
3. Describe the relationship of clinical manifestations to data obtained from the review of a patient's social history.
4. Describe the essential components of a cardiovascular physical assessment.

Research Collaboration Health Promotion Nursing Process Caring Critical Thinking

NURSES NEED in-depth knowledge and skills in order to assess the cardiovascular status of their patients rapidly. Although the cardiovascular system is complex, its purpose is simple: to deliver oxygen and nutrients to the tissues and cells of the body. An understanding of cardiovascular anatomy and physiology is essential for cardiovascular assessment. Additionally, it is important to gather data about the patient's medical history as well as the presenting symptoms, because they can provide clues to cardiac status. The relationship between the existence of risk factors and the patient's susceptibility for disease is an important concept this chapter presents.

A thorough physical examination, including inspection, palpation, and auscultation, helps to define an individual's ability to carry out the physiological function of the cardiovascular system. Nurses should be able to recognize normal assessment findings and, more importantly, to identify subtle abnormalities or deviations from normal that might indicate worsening of the patient's condition. Accuracy in monitoring and reporting of data is essential, and nurses have access to a wide variety of non-invasive and invasive technological devices that assist in cardiovascular monitoring and assessment.

Anatomy and Physiology of the Cardiovascular System

An in-depth cardiovascular assessment requires knowledge of cardiovascular anatomy and physiology, and an ability to integrate that knowledge into the current condition of each patient. As seen in Figure 37–1 ■, the heart is housed directly behind the central section of the thorax referred to as the mediastinum. Two-thirds of the heart lies to the left of the midline. The apex lies just above the diaphragm and the base of the heart lies approximately at the level of the third rib. The exact size of the heart varies among individuals, but on the average it is approximately 5 inches long and about 3 inches wide, resembling the size of a closed fist.

The heart is a four-chambered muscular organ composed of two separate pumps, each having one atrium and one ventricle. The upper chambers (atria) of the heart are separated by the interatrial septum, and the ventricles are separated by the interventricular septum. The two atria are located at the base or top of the heart, and the lower chambers are located at the bottom or apex of the heart. The upper chambers are thin walled and re-

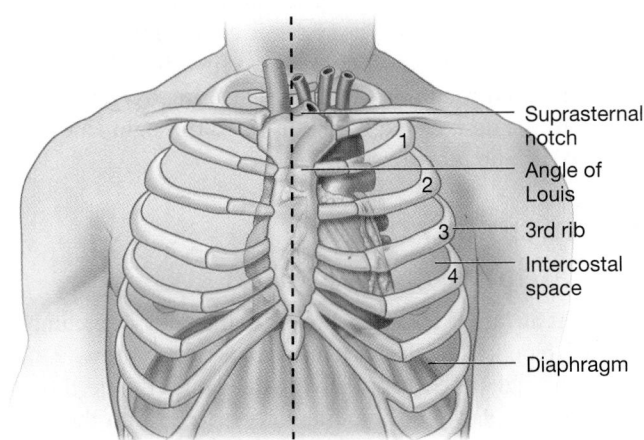

FIGURE 37–1 ■ Diagram of heart in chest.

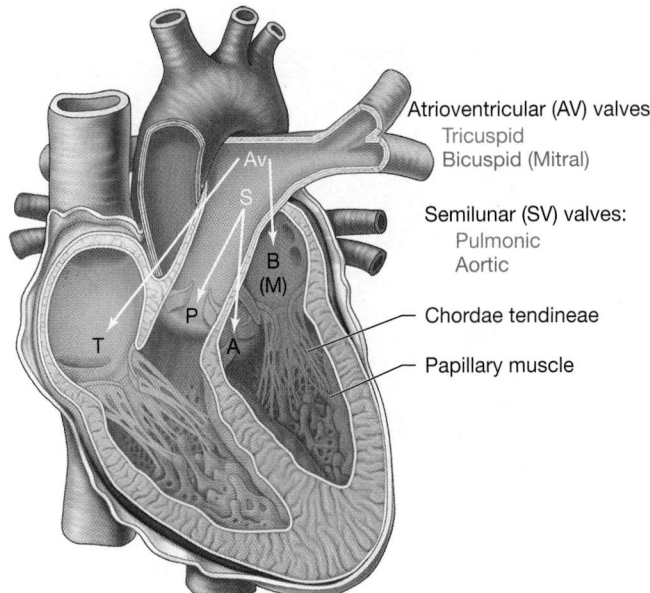

FIGURE 37–2 ■ Cross section of heart.

ceive blood as it returns to the heart. The right atrium receives blood from the systemic venous circulation, while the left atrium receives blood from the pulmonary circulation. The lower chambers have thicker walls and pump blood out of the heart. The right ventricle pumps blood into the pulmonary circulation, while the left ventricle pumps blood into the systemic circulation. Although each ventricle pumps the same volume of blood, the left ventricle has a larger, stronger muscle. This increased strength is needed because the left ventricle has to pump blood into the systemic circulation, which has five times greater pressure than the pulmonic circulation. The heart wall is composed of the three layers:

1. The epicardium: the smooth outer serous layer.

2. The myocardium: the middle muscular layer, which is the thickest of the three layers and is responsible for the heart's ability to contract.

3. The endocardium: the inner lining of the heart, which is composed of thin connective tissue. This smooth inner surface and the valves allow blood to flow more easily throughout the heart.

Cardiac Valves

There are four valves in the heart (Figure 37–2 ■). The purpose of the valves is to ensure that blood travels in only one direction as it passes through the heart. The valve opens to fill a chamber and then closes when the pressure in the chamber builds, thereby allowing blood to continue to flow in one direction. The atrioventricular (AV) valves are located between the atria and the ventricles (see Figure 37–2 ■). These valves are referred to as the tricuspid valve and the bicuspid or mitral valve. The tricuspid valve lies between the right atrium and the right ventricle and is so named because it has three cusps. The mitral or bicuspid valve has only two cusps and is located between the left atrium and the left ventricle. The cusps of both the mitral and the tricuspid extend into the ventricles where they attach to the chordae tendineae. Chordae tendineae are cords of dense connective tissue that attach to the papillary muscles (see Figure 37–2 ■). The chordae tendineae and the papillary muscle work

together to prevent the valve cusps from fluttering back into the atrium and thereby interrupting forward blood flow. The semilunar valves are the pulmonic and the aortic valves. Each semilunar valve contains moon-shaped cusps (semilunar). The pulmonic valve is located between the right ventricle and the pulmonary artery. The aortic valve is located between the left ventricle and the trunk of the aorta.

As blood is filling the ventricular chamber, pressure is rising. The ventricular muscle fibers respond to an increase in blood volume by stretching to allow more fluid into the chamber (Starling law). As pressure in the ventricles increases, the ventricular muscles stretch. When the pressure in the right ventricle is greater than the pressure in the pulmonary system, and likewise, when the pressure in the left ventricle is greater than the pressure in the aorta, the AV valves (tricuspid and mitral) snap together to close as the semilunar valves (pulmonic and aortic) open. The ventricular muscles contract, and blood is ejected through the open pulmonic valve to the pulmonary artery and the pulmonary circuit, and through the open aortic valve to the aorta and the systemic circulation.

Surrounding the heart is a two-layered sac referred to as the pericardial sac (Figure 37–3 ■, p. 1054). The outer layer, called the parietal pericardium, is in direct contact with the pleura (lung). This layer consists of a tough, nonelastic, fibrous connective tissue and serves to prevent overdistention of the heart. The thin, serous inner layer of the pericardium, called the visceral pericardium, lays directly on the epicardium or outer layer of the heart. There is a small amount of fluid between the heart wall and the pericardial sac (approximately 10 mL). This fluid acts as a lubricant to prevent friction during contractions.

Cardiac Circulatory System

The heart has its own circulatory system allowing for constant nourishment of blood to the cardiac muscle. The heart's circulatory system consists of coronary arteries and veins

Transverse section of the heart

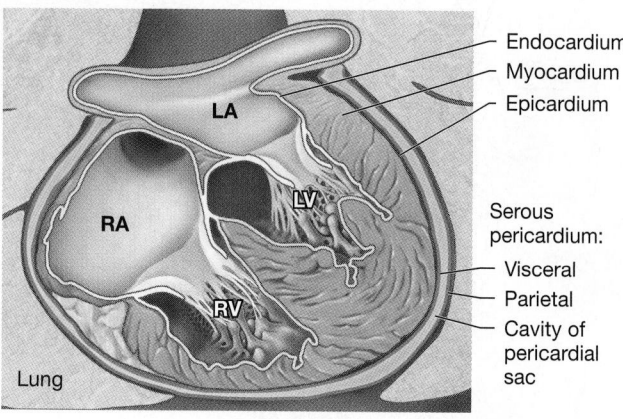

FIGURE 37–3 ■ Layers of heart.

(Figure 37–4 ■). The sinuses or openings into the coronary arteries lie at the base of the aorta, just above the aortic valve. As blood leaves the heart with each beat, it travels through the coronary sinus to supply the cardiac muscle. The two main arteries are the right and left coronary arteries. The right coronary artery and its branches normally supply the right atrium and ventricle and a portion of the posterior wall of the left ventricle. The left coronary artery branches into the left anterior descending and the circumflex arteries, both of which feed the left atrium and the massive walls of the left ventricle. The left coronary artery carries 85% of the blood flow to the myocardium. The left anterior descending (LAD) artery feeds the anterior wall of the left ventricle and the interventricular septum. The circumflex artery feeds the lateral and posterior portions of the left ventricle.

The pulmonary circulation consists of blood flow between the heart and lungs. Blood leaves the right ventricle, enters the

pulmonary artery and lungs, picks up oxygen, and travels to the left side of the heart. The systemic circulation consists of a network of arteries, capillaries, and veins. Blood leaves the heart, travels through these vessels delivering oxygen and nutrients to the tissues, and then returns to the right side of the heart to pick up more oxygen.

■ Physiology of the Cardiovascular System

The right atrium is the central point in the body where unoxygenated blood from the systemic circulation returns. It then travels through the tricuspid valve to the right ventricle, through the pulmonic valve to the pulmonary arteries into the lungs, through the pulmonary alveolar-capillary network into the pulmonary veins, into the left atrium, through the mitral valve into the left ventricle, and finally out the aortic valve to the systemic circulation.

Freshly oxygenated blood, traveling through the aortic valve, also enters into the coronary arteries to supply the myocardium with oxygen. Normally the myocardium extracts 75% of the available oxygen from the coronary arteries. This is more than is extracted from any other tissue in the body; the rest of the body extracts about 40%. If oxygen needs are not met from this near maximal extraction, then blood flow must be increased. With a healthy heart, blood flow is increased in two ways. First, the arteries are able to dilate, thereby increasing their capacity, and second, the myocardial muscle increases the force of the contraction, pumping more blood into the arteries. These two mechanisms result in an increase in the cardiac output and blood flow to the myocardium.

Cardiac Cycle

The pumping action of the heart consists of contraction and relaxation of the myocardial layer of the heart wall. Each contraction and relaxation is one cardiac cycle. During relaxation or diastole blood flows into the ventricles and the contraction that follows, termed systole, propels blood out of the heart. The heart functions as a unit because both atria contract simultaneously, and then both ventricles contract. When both atria contract the ventricles are filled to capacity, and then the ventricles contract and blood is ejected into both the pulmonary and the systemic circulation. At the time of ventricular contraction, the mitral and tricuspid valves are closed by the pressure from the contraction while the pulmonic and aortic valves are opened. The cardiac cycle represents the actual time sequence between ventricular contraction and ventricular relaxation.

Autonomic Nervous System

The autonomic nervous system is a built-in control center for the body. Its purpose is to regulate functions of the body that are not under conscious control. There are two major divisions: the sympathetic and the parasympathetic nervous systems. Most of the organs of the body are innervated with both systems, although the blood vessels are innervated with only the sympathetic nervous system. The sympathetic nervous system (SNS) prepares the body for activity (flight or fight), whereas the

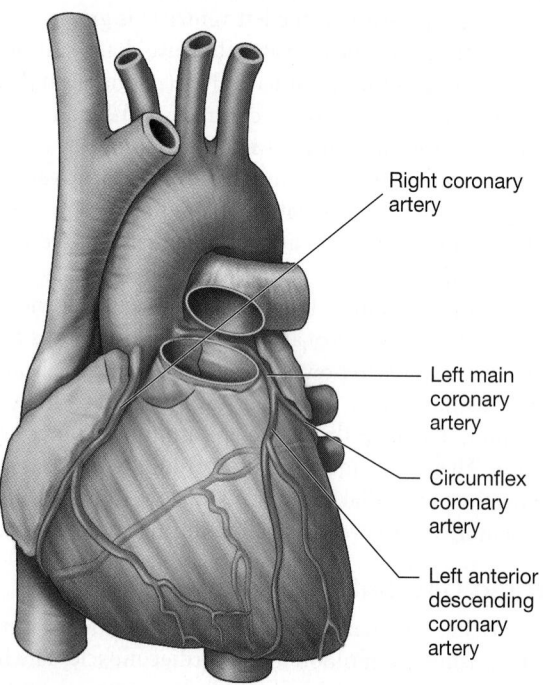

FIGURE 37–4 ■ Coronary arteries.

Right coronary artery

Left main coronary artery

Circumflex coronary artery

Left anterior descending coronary artery

parasympathetic nervous system (PSNS) regulates the calmer (rest and digest) functions. Because the sympathetic nervous system (SNS) and the parasympathetic nervous system (PSNS) innervate the heart, neural impulses are not needed to maintain the cardiac cycle. In other words, the heart will beat in the absence of any nervous system connection. The SNS and the PSNS affect only the speed of the cardiac cycles and the diameter of the coronary arteries. It is said that these nervous systems only "fine-tune" the cardiac cycle.

Receptors and Neurotransmitters

The nerve endings of both the SNS and the PSNS secrete neurotransmitters. The SNS has two types of receptors at the nerve endings, the alpha- and the beta-receptors. These nerve endings are called adrenergic. The neurotransmitter for the SNS is norepinephrine, which causes an increase in heart rate and contractile force of the cardiac fibers. The PSNS nerve endings are known as cholinergic, and the neurotransmitter is acetylcholine, which causes the heart rate and blood pressure to go down.

History

A thorough history will help the nurse identify cardiovascular symptoms as well as current or potential problems that may affect cardiovascular function. Information learned from a thorough history and physical exam could help prevent undesirable responses to current therapies and treatment plans. The essential assessment data included in the cardiovascular history are outlined in this section.

Biographic and Demographic Data

Assessment of biographic and demographic data includes information regarding age, race, gender, and ethnicity, which can impact the susceptibility to some cardiovascular disorders. For example, African Americans have a higher incidence of hypertension than Caucasians (American Heart Association, 2006), and premenopausal women have a lower incidence of atherosclerotic coronary artery disease than men (American Heart Association, 2008b). Additionally, the presenting symptoms of cardiovascular diseases in women are often atypical, which may either delay diagnosis or make diagnosis more difficult. For example, women more frequently present with shortness of breath.

Chief Complaint

During the assessment process the nurse obtains a complete description of the present illness, paying particular attention to the chief complaint, or the reason the patient is seeking health care. The chief complaint focuses the history-taking process and prioritizes treatment regimens. For example, if the patient is complaining of chest pain, then the history should include information regarding the nature of the pain, associated symptoms, exacerbating and alleviating factors, as well as radiation of the pain and intensity of the pain. It also is important to determine what brings the pain and what relieves it.

Presenting Symptoms

Symptomatology is the review of symptoms the patient is experiencing. A review of symptoms helps define the current functional status of the patient. The nurse needs to ask questions about the date and mode of onset of the symptoms to find out when and how the symptoms first began. For example, has the shortness of breath been a problem for many weeks, or is it a new occurrence? Have the symptoms changed in intensity or duration? Additionally, questions about the exacerbations, or what causes the symptoms to worsen, and alleviating factors are important.

Specific Cardiovascular Clinical Manifestations

Patients with cardiovascular disease often present to the health care professional with typical or common cardiovascular symptoms. Knowledge of these common symptoms, their usual presentation, and their etiology can help focus and guide the exam process.

1. *Nurses should be particularly aware of the following common cardiovascular symptoms: chest pain, palpitations, dyspnea, orthopnea, cough, and nocturia.*
2. *The most severe symptoms should be assessed in greater depth and reported to the health care provider, if indicated.*

The most life-threatening symptoms should be addressed first. If the patient is complaining of shortness of breath, it needs to be assessed immediately. Airway management and oxygen status must be stabilized before the remainder of the assessment is completed. The management of airway is discussed in Chapters 34, 35, and 36 ⊙. Next, the patient is asked about the presence, site, and intensity of pain. The primary cardiovascular concern is pain associated with cardiac muscle ischemia, referred to as angina pectoris. The clinical manifestations of angina vary among patients; therefore, specific questions must be asked during the assessment in order to ascertain the cause of the pain. Pain may be described as indigestion, burning, numbness, tightness, or pressure in the midchest, or as epigastric or substernal pain, which can radiate to the shoulder, neck, arms, jaw, or back. It is essential that the nurse inquires about what brings the "pain on" and what makes it go away. An in-depth discussion of angina-type chest pain, the assessment data, and treatment is included in Chapter 40 ⊙. Patients might deny the presence of chest pain but admit to sensations of chest discomfort; therefore, it is important to allow patients to present their symptoms in their own words prior to analyzing their symptoms.

Palpitations are typically described by the patient as sensations of a racing heartbeat, irregular beats, or skipped beats. These sensations may be normal, or they may signify cardiac rhythm disturbances. The presence of **dyspnea**, or shortness of breath, may indicate an imbalance of arterial oxygen supply and demand. **Orthopnea**, the presence of dyspnea when the patient lies flat, is frequently a manifestation of cardiac disease. Often the degree of orthopnea is measured by the number of pillows (for example, 2- to 3-pillow orthopnea) necessary for the patient to use to breathe comfortably while sleeping. A cough may suggest pulmonary congestion resulting from fluid accumulation in the lungs due to either cardiac pump failure or fluid overload. If the patient has **nocturia,** the need to urinate often at night, it may indicate heart failure, although there are other disorders that cause frequent urination, such as an enlarged prostate. During the day as a patient is up and moving, fluid shifts to extremities and extravascular spaces, which serves to decrease fluid workload on a decompensated heart. At night, however, when the patient lies flat, fluid is returned to the central intravascular column, thereby increasing the amount of fluid to the kidneys. Patients with heart failure may report paroxysmal nocturnal dyspnea, which is acute dyspnea caused by lung congestion and edema that occurs suddenly at night, usually an hour or two after falling asleep.

Edema, or fluid accumulation in the extravascular spaces of the body, may be due to decreases in venous return. Fluid retention is manifested by weight gain, a feeling of being bloated, or clothes or shoes that no longer fit comfortably. Changes in weight should be specifically addressed. Large, sudden weight gains correlate with volume overload. Dizziness, **syncope** (fainting), or light-headedness may be experienced with sudden changes of position, and all are related to decreased cardiac output, which decreases blood to the brain.

Fatigue is a common complaint with cardiovascular patients. Fatigue is due to a decreased supply of oxygen to the tissues. Metabolic demands are higher in chronic cardiovascular conditions; however, due to a lowered cardiac output, demands are not met and the result is fatigue. The fatigue is usually progressive over time, and the patient may report decreased ability to complete usual activities of daily living. Additionally, patients may report a lack of energy or the need for more rest than usual. Medications such as diuretics, beta-adrenergic blockers, calcium channel blockers, digoxin, and antihypertensives have long been thought to contribute to fatigue. For example, beta-adrenergic blockers block the response from the beta nerve receptors, which serves to slow down the heart rate and lower the blood pressure. This desired physiological change, which decreases the myocardial oxygen demand, also may cause an undesired side effect of fatigue. Interestingly, clinical trials have not supported the notion that beta-adrenergic blocker therapy is associated with substantial risks of side effects. In a quantitative review of randomized trials that tested beta-adrenergic blockers in myocardial infarction, heart failure, and hypertension, the authors found no significant increased risk of depressive symptoms and only small increased risks of fatigue and sexual dysfunction (Ko et al., 2002). Therefore, the risks of adverse effects (fatigue) should be considered in context with the well-documented benefits of medications such as beta-adrenergic blockers.

Problems with the peripheral vascular system are frequently manifested with intermittent claudication. The patient reports pain in the muscles of the lower extremities associated with activity, which may be due to arterial insufficiency. Chapter 43 includes a complete discussion of both venous and arterial peripheral vascular disorders.

Past Medical History

Past medical history should be reviewed because many past illnesses or disorders of other systems of the body can affect the cardiovascular system directly or indirectly. Additionally, the clinical manifestations of other diseases may mistakenly be attributed to cardiovascular disorders. For example, it is important to determine the presence of respiratory disorders to assess a patient's complaint of dyspnea properly, or a history of rheumatic heart disease may have damaged the heart valves. Unit 7 discusses respiratory management, and Chapter 41 discusses rheumatic fever and valve disorders.

Childhood Illnesses and Immunizations

Childhood illnesses, congenital heart diseases, history of murmurs, cyanosis, streptococcal infections, anemia, and rheumatic fever should all be assessed. They can either exacerbate current cardiovascular conditions or contribute to the development of additional cardiovascular problems and disease states. Nurses should question the status of immunizations and make sure they are up-to-date.

Previous Illnesses and Hospitalizations

Heart failure, coronary artery disease (CAD), stroke, heart valve disease, mitral valve prolapse, previous myocardial infarction (MI), peripheral vascular disease (PVD), diabetes mellitus (DM), hypertension (HTN), hyperlipidemia, dysrhythmias, murmurs, endocarditis, psychiatric illnesses, thrombophlebitis, deep vein thrombosis (DVT), and systemic or pulmonary emboli are all important components of or contributors to cardiovascular disease. Their presence, or a history of their presence, and the potential impact on the present health state must be assessed.

Diagnostic/Interventional Cardiac Procedures or Surgeries

Data from previous diagnostic tests, particularly for cardiovascular symptoms, should be obtained. The patient should be asked whether he had any cardiac studies or interventions in the past such as cardiac catheterizations, cardiac ultrasounds, electrocardiograms (ECGs), exercise tolerance tests (stress tests), or myocardial imaging. Previous chest x-rays or ECGs may be helpful to view for baseline data.

Past surgeries, treatments, or hospital admissions should be explored. Assess for a history of previous percutaneous transluminal coronary angioplasty (PTCA), atherectomy stent placement, or valvuloplasty. See Chapter 39 for more information on diagnostic and interventional therapies for heart disease.

Medications

The patient's current and past medications should be reviewed. This includes over-the-counter (OTC) and any prescription medications. A medication list with the name and dose of each medication and the patient's understanding of its purpose is helpful. The consumption of herbal remedies or dietary supplements should be specifically assessed because some cardiovascular complications have been linked to these substances. Consideration is made of other common medications and their potential side effects on cardiovascular status. Chart 37–1 outlines common medications and their side effects that affect the cardiovascular system.

Cultural Considerations

Health and well-being of a culturally diverse population can be promoted by incorporating the therapies that patients have traditionally used. The basis for many complementary therapies is to promote harmony, promote health, reduce anxiety, and increase comfort (Snyder & Miska, 2003). During the assessment phase, nurses must be able to gather information on the use of all therapies being used by a patient, including complementary and nontraditional therapies, as discussed in the Complementary and Alternative Therapies box, in order to plan care that is safe and comfortable.

CHART 37–1 Common Medications and Side Effects That Affect Cardiovascular Status

Medication	Side Effect
Anabolic steroids	Increased total cholesterol, decreased HDL, hypertrophy
Antihistamines	Dysrhythmias, syncope
Aspirin	Prolonged blood clotting time
Corticosteroids	Sodium and fluid retention
Decongestants	Hypertension and arrhythmias
Doxorubicin (Adriamycin)	Cardiomyopathy
Lithium	Dysrhythmias
Oral contraceptives	Thrombophlebitis
Phenothiazines	Dysrhythmias, hypotension
Recreational or abused drugs	Tachycardia, dysrhythmias
Theophylline preparations	Tachycardia, arrhythmias
Tricyclic antidepressants	Dysrhythmias

Allergies

Certain diagnostic tests to evaluate heart disease use contrast media and medications, so the presence of any allergies, especially to radiographic contrast agents or iodine, should be assessed. Drug interactions or intolerance should also be noted. Information as to the nature of allergic reactions, such as rash, anaphylaxis, or dyspnea, is essential.

Family History

The link between familial history of cardiovascular disease and the risk for similar events is well established (Williams et al., 2001). Specifically, the patient should be asked whether blood relatives have suffered from any of the following: coronary artery

disease (CAD) at or under age 55, myocardial infarction, hypertension, stroke, diabetes mellitus, and/or lipid disorders. Collagen vascular diseases such as lupus or scleroderma may be important, because they are linked to the development of cardiac disease or pericarditis. Additionally, a family health history of noncardiac conditions such as asthma, renal disease, and obesity should be noted due to their impact on cardiovascular function.

Risk Factors

It is necessary to assess for the presence of risk factors to anticipate the likelihood of the development of cardiovascular disorders. Risk factors can be classified as either nonmodifiable or modifiable. Nonmodifiable risk factors are not subject to interventions to decrease their significance yet play an important role in the development of cardiovascular diseases. Nonmodifiable risk factors include such things as age, gender, family history, and race. Modifiable risk factors are those that can be treated with interventions to decrease their impact on the development of the disorder. Modifiable risk factors include cigarette smoking, hypertension (HTN), hypercholesterolemia, physical inactivity, diabetes, stress, and obesity. Chapter 40 includes a complete description of cardiac risk factors. Additionally, recent dental work or infection may put the patient at risk for development of cardiac complications such as endocarditis. Another risk factor associated with cardiovascular disorders is metabolic syndrome, as discussed in the Risk Factors box (p. 1058).

Social History

An assessment of social history is important because of the relationship between social history and the development of, acceleration of, and response to cardiovascular diseases. Risk factor assessment and history taking are done simultaneously. While taking a social history, nurses can gain valuable information from the patient about the presence of risk factors. Nurses then

MyNursingKit | Center for Disease Control

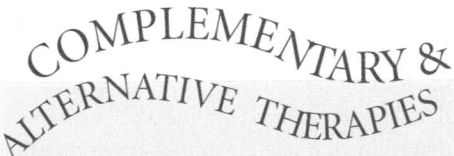

COMPLEMENTARY & ALTERNATIVE THERAPIES Herbal Products

ONE OF THE MOST important complementary therapies that should be addressed during assessment is the use of herbal products. There is a known risk of interaction between herbal products and conventional medications.

Research Support:
A study by Yoon and Claydell (2001) explored the use of herbal products for medicinal purposes and compared differences in demographic characteristics and health status of herbal product users and nonusers among community-dwelling older women. In 1998, a random sample of 86 women aged 65 years and older who lived independently in a north central Florida county was selected. Questionnaires were completed for the 86 subjects. Findings indicated that herbal products had been used by 45% of the sample in the previous 12 months. The average number of herbal products used by the 45% was 2.5. Herbal products were used to prevent health problems (41%), to treat illness (23%), and for both prevention and treatment (36%). The three most commonly used herbal products were ginkgo biloba or ginkgo biloba with other combinations, garlic tablets and cloves, and glu-

cosamine with chondroitin. The women reported using an average of 3.2 prescribed medicines and 3.8 nonprescribed medicines. The most frequently used nonprescribed medicines taken regularly were multivitamins, calcium, vitamin E, vitamin C, and aspirin. Interestingly, there were no differences in demographic characteristics and health status for users and nonusers of herbal products except that herbal product users were more concerned with memory problems than were nonusers (Yoon & Claydell, 2001). The implications for nurses are that it is important for health care providers to be knowledgeable about the use of herbal products to provide comprehensive health care. In order to make these needed adaptations of care, nurses must be knowledgeable and committed to provide culturally competent care.

References
Yoon, S., & Claydell, H. (2001). Herbal products and conventional medicines used by community-residing older women. *Journal of Advanced Nursing, 33*(1), 51–59.

RISK FACTORS Related to Metabolic Syndrome

The metabolic syndrome describes a cluster of risk factors that significantly increases the incidence of an acute cardiac event and other diseases related to plaque buildup in artery walls (e.g., stroke and peripheral vascular disease) and type II diabetes. The metabolic syndrome has become increasingly common in the United States. It is estimated that over 50 million Americans have it (American Heart Association [AHA], 2008a). The *Third Report of the National Cholesterol Education Program Expert Panel on Detection, Evaluation, and Treatment of High Blood Cholesterol in Adults (Adult Treatment Panel III)* (ATP III) defines and describes the importance of metabolic syndrome. Individuals having three or more of the following criteria are defined as having the metabolic syndrome (National Institutes of Health, 2001; AHA, 2006):

- Abdominal obesity: waist circumference > 102 cm in men and > 88 cm in women
- Hypertriglyceridemia: > 150 mg/dL (1.69 mmol/L)
- Low high-density lipoprotein (HDL) cholesterol: < 40 mg/dL (1.04 mmol/L) in men and < 50 mg/dL (1.29 mmol/L) in women
- High blood pressure: > 130/85 mmHg
- High fasting glucose: > 110 mg/dL (>6.1 mmol/L)
- Prothrombotic state (e.g., high fibrinogen or plasminogen activator inhibitor–1 in the blood)
- Proinflammatory state (e.g., elevated C-reactive protein in the blood).

Abdominal obesity, elevated triglycerides, and insulin resistance (a metabolic disorder in which the body is unable to use insulin efficiently) are major features in metabolic syndrome and have a complex relationship. Fat accumulation in the lower body (pear-shaped) is subcutaneous, whereas fat accumulation in the abdominal area (apple-shaped) is largely visceral fat. Excess abdominal fat disrupts the normal balance and functioning of several hormones, including lipids and insulin. Abdominal fat and circulating triglycerides both increase with age, and recent studies have confirmed their relationship as major metabolic risk factors (Kahn & Valdez, 2003). Therefore, waist circumference measurement, as a measure of abdominal fat, is a useful tool in physical assessment and is a reliable, inexpensive indicator that helps identify those at risk for lipid accumulation. While assessing risk factors, nurses should be aware that individuals with metabolic syndrome are at a greater risk for developing cardiovascular disease than are individuals without metabolic syndrome (Kahn, Buse, Ferrannini, & Stern, 2005). Other conditions commonly associated with metabolic syndrome include physical inactivity, aging, hormonal imbalance, and genetic predisposition. Metabolic syndrome is discussed in depth in Chapter 40 ⌐.

---

have an important role in assisting patients to recognize unhealthy habits that require education in order to modify or change to prevent the progression and complications associated with the development of cardiovascular disorders. As nurses develop relationships with patients, they are in a unique position to offer assistance in risk factor analysis and lifestyle modification. The identification of the presence of modifiable risk factors, as well as the patient's ability and interest in adopting lifestyle changes, forms a framework for the nursing discharge teaching plan discussed in the subsequent cardiac disorder chapters.

Occupation

Job stress is a common condition that promotes the occurrence of cardiovascular events. Previous and recent job-related stres-sors should be explored. Stress and tension regardless of their etiology cause vasoconstriction, which increases afterload, oxygen consumption, and release of catecholamines, which in turn can contribute to the development of cardiac symptoms. Another occupational hazard that should be considered is exposure to noxious or harmful substances, and the potential effect of them on the cardiovascular system.

Culture

Nurses should be prepared to care for a diverse group of people, because the numbers of patients from other cultures in the health care system have increased. There is a great deal of variation in cultural consistency of different demographic areas. Beliefs and values related to health, illness, and death, as well as daily habits, nutritional preferences, and health practices, may exist that are culturally important to the patient, but conflict with the health care environment or even the function of the cardiovascular status. Nurses may need to ask questions about upcoming religious celebrations or rituals that might affect dietary patterns or preferences (Smith-Stoner, 2006). For example, the patient should be asked about the salt content in the food, because an increased amount may precipitate an episode of heart failure and/or high blood pressure. As nurses are caring for more diverse populations, they need to be knowledgeable about the health practices of other cultures and religions.

Environment

Environment and lifestyle issues are also strongly correlated with the risk for cardiovascular disease. Environmental conditions such as living conditions and the presence of any cardiovascular toxins may need to be addressed. It is understood that heart disease develops as a result of complex interactions between genes and the environment in which we live (Bhatnagar, 2006). Environmental risk factors are not limited to the better known risk factors of smoking, poor diet, and lack of exercise, but also include exposure to pollutants and chemicals. Similarly to the response to secondhand smoke, cardiovascular tissues are extremely sensitive to environmental chemicals and pollutants; therefore, environmental exposures should be routinely considered during cardiovascular assessment. Specifically, nurses should assess for exposure to particulate matter, arsenic, or metals. Further research is needed to determine the relationship of environmental chemicals and cardiovascular toxicity (Bhatnagar, 2006).

Habits

Lifestyle habits and dietary habits such as the use of tea, coffee, alcohol, recreational drugs, over-the-counter drugs, and smoking should be discussed and documented. If the patient smokes, the number of pack years of smoking (packs smoked per day multiplied by the years smoked) should be calculated. The patient's attitude about smoking and any attempts to stop smoking should be documented. The presence of secondhand smoke also must be assessed. Alcohol use, including type of beverages, amount, frequency, and any change in the reaction to it should be assessed. The use of habit-forming drugs and recreational drugs should be noted.

Exercise

The practice of engaging in physical activity has long been known to reduce the risk of cardiovascular events. Low levels of physical activity as well as consumption of excess calories, combined with inherited genes, cause obesity. Obesity, especially abdominal obesity, is a predisposing factor for the development of cardiovascular disease as well as hypertension and type II diabetes mellitus. The physical activity patterns of a patient, including the type of exercise, the duration and frequency of the exercise, and the presence of any cardiovascular symptoms, should be documented. Any decrease in previous abilities or changes in the response to physical activity should be noted, because they may be indications of the advent or progression of heart disease.

In 1996 with revisions in 1999, the Surgeon General of the United States Public Health Service published a report on physical activity and health. This report contains a comprehensive review of scientific evidence about the relationship between physical activity and health status in an attempt to heighten America's awareness of this important public health issue. The report makes it clear that current levels of physical activity among Americans remain low; however, the emphasis is that people can benefit from even moderate levels of physical activity, and that even greater health benefits can be achieved by increasing the amount (duration, frequency, or intensity) of physical activity (Centers for Disease Control and Prevention [CDC], 2008). The report suggests that adults should strive to meet either of the following physical activity recommendations.

- Adults should engage in moderate-intensity physical activities for at least 30 minutes on 5 or more days of the week (Centers for Disease Control and Prevention, 2008).

OR

- Adults should engage in vigorous-intensity physical activity 3 or more days per week for 20 or more minutes per occasion (U.S. Department of Health and Human Services [DHHS], 2004).

Nutrition

It is important to assess the patient's weight and diet history. An assessment of weight in comparison to height and build must be completed. Being overweight or underweight either may be related to certain cardiovascular disorders or may put the patient at risk for developing certain cardiac problems. Usual dietary intake including amounts of salt, saturated fats, triglycerides, and fluids should be determined. It may be important to identify which dietary habits are related to cultural preferences and which habits are the results of the environment or social situations. For example, an executive may consume many meals at restaurants while out with clients, and a construction worker might eat many meals at fast-food restaurants. In addition, the patient's attitudes and plans in relation to diet should be discussed. Food intake patterns should be accountable to exercise patterns and should be complementary.

The National Guidelines box outlines the dietary guidelines for Americans released by the American Heart Association in 2000. Choosing healthy foods can help to prevent the three major risk factors for heart attack—high blood cholesterol, high blood pressure, and excess body weight. Because heart disease and high blood pressure are major risk factors for stroke, these dietary guidelines also help prevent stroke (American Heart Association, 2006).

Personal Factors

Baseline cognitive functioning, recent life changes especially within the last 12 months, sleep-rest patterns, and relationship

---

NATIONAL GUIDELINES for Diet

American Heart Association 2006 Diet and Lifestyle Recommendations

Achieve an Overall Healthy Eating Pattern

- Choose an overall balanced diet with foods from all major food groups, emphasizing fruits, vegetables, and grains.
- Consume a variety of fruits, vegetables, and grain products.
- Eat at least 5 daily servings of fruits and vegetables.
- Eat at least 6 daily servings of grain products, including whole grains.
- Include fat-free and low-fat dairy products, fish, legumes, poultry, and lean meats.
- Eat at least 2 servings of fish per week.

Achieve a Healthy Body Weight

- Maintain a level of physical activity that achieves fitness and balances energy expenditure with caloric intake; for weight reduction, expenditure should exceed intake.
- Limit foods that are high in calories and/or low in nutritional quality, including those with a high amount of added sugar.

Achieve a Desirable Cholesterol Level

- Limit foods with a high content of saturated fat and cholesterol. Substitute with grains and unsaturated fat from vegetables, fish, legumes, and nuts.
- Limit cholesterol to 300 milligrams (mg) a day for the general population and 200 milligrams a day for those with heart disease or its risk factors.
- Limit *trans* fatty acids. Trans fatty acids are found in foods containing partially hydrogenated vegetable oils such as packaged cookies, crackers, and other baked goods; commercially prepared fried foods; and some margarines.

Achieve a Desirable Blood Pressure Level

- Limit salt intake to less than 6 grams (2,400 milligrams sodium) per day, slightly more than 1 teaspoon a day.
- If you drink, limit alcohol consumption to no more than one drink per day for women and two drinks per day for men.

Source: American Heart Association. (2006). *Dietary guidelines: At-a-glance.* Retrieved January 21, 2008, from http://www.americanheart.org/presenter.jhtml?identifier=851.

---

issues should all be considered. Emotional state, such as the evidence of psychological stress, anger, anxiety, or depression, causes the release of catecholamines, which results in vasoconstriction, thereby increasing cardiac workload and potentially resulting in a decreased cardiac output. Perception of illness and its meaning for the future should also be noted.

Personality type may also be a consideration for cardiovascular assessment. Type A personality behavior has been associated with increased incidence of cardiovascular disease. Researchers have found conflicting evidence to support or refute this notion. Gallacher, Sweetman, Yarnell, Elwood, and Stansfeld (2003) suggest that increased exposure to circumstances that induce extreme cardiovascular activity, as seen in type A personality behavior, may be a "trigger" that precipitates coronary events rather than affecting the process of atherosclerosis. The role of stress and the manner in which an individual deals with life stressors may also have an important role. Individuals with type

A personality may respond to stress with hostility or aggression, which may exaggerate sympathetic and hemodynamic responses leading to greater cardiovascular reactivity (Schroeder et al., 2000).

Physical Examination

A thorough physical examination is the foundation for accurate assessment of the cardiovascular system and encompasses skills of inspection, palpation, and auscultation. Percussion is not utilized for assessment of the cardiovascular system.

Inspection of Skin and Extremities

A great deal of information can be obtained about the status of the cardiovascular system by simply observing and touching the patient. An experienced nurse is able to assess general appearance quickly, including facial expressions, body posture and mentation, as well as color and temperature, and clubbing of the nail beds. Then it is necessary to relate the findings to the patient's current cardiovascular status.

General Appearance

General appearance includes a brief visual inspection of a patient's physical appearance. Observations of a patient who looks unwell, lethargic, exhausted, or breathless are important findings and may indicate reduced cardiac output or heart failure. An obese person who has fat evenly distributed over the body is vulnerable for serious cardiovascular health consequences. Additionally, an accumulation of abdominal (visceral) fat, measured by waist circumference, is a known risk factor for cardiovascular and other diseases.

Interestingly, recent studies suggest that variances in fat distributions (abdominal vs. peripheral) may exhibit different influences on lipid metabolism. Laszlo et al. (2004) studied 1,356 women aged 60 to 85 years and found that abdominal fat mass promoted atherogenesis, whereas peripheral fat deposits actually counteracted atherogenesis. The women with peripheral fat deposits rather than central fat deposits showed a negative correlation with glucose and lipid metabolites. The authors concluded that the localization or distribution of the fat mass is an important consideration in obese patients and should be considered during any risk appraisal.

Observation of facial expression may indicate important findings, such as the assessment of apprehension, pain, or fear. Body posture may indicate the amount of effort it takes to breathe. For example, a patient in acute heart failure may need to sit upright, whereas a patient with pericarditis may lean forward in order to breathe comfortably (Urden, Lough, & Stacy, 2006).

Mentation

Adequate functioning of all subsystems of the body indicates the individual organ is receiving adequate cardiac output. For example, normal neurological function indicates adequate cerebral perfusion. A quick and easy method to estimate baseline cognitive function is to assess the patient's orientation to person, place and time, and situation. Confusion could indicate hypotension or low cardiac output.

Color and Appearance of Skin and Extremities

The skin and mucous membranes are inspected for color and temperature. Extremities should be assessed bilaterally for equal temperature and appearance. The extremities are inspected for signs of peripheral arterial or venous vascular disorders. Arterial vascular disease is suspected when the skin is pale, shiny, with sparse hair growth. Venous vascular diseases cause an edematous limb with deep red rubor, brown discoloration, and leg ulcerations (Urden, Lough, & Stacy, 2006). Chapter 43 includes an in-depth description of peripheral vascular disease.

Cyanosis

Cyanosis is a bluish tinge to the skin due to deoxygenated hemoglobin in the blood vessels close to the skin surface; it can be either central or peripheral. Central cyanosis, which is noted on the lips or tongue, is often characteristic of impaired gas exchange. Central cyanosis may result from a cardiac right-to-left shunt due to septal defects, in which deoxygenated venous blood mixes with blood from the left heart and is ejected into the systemic circulation. In heart failure with significant pulmonary congestion, oxygenation of blood in the pulmonary vascular bed can be impaired, which leads to deoxygenated blood returning to the left heart and being pumped out into the systemic circulation. Peripheral cyanosis, which occurs in the extremities or under the nail beds, may indicate poor circulation. The room where the examination is taking place must have a comfortable temperature because nail beds can become cyanotic with cold temperatures.

Pallor

Pallor suggests poor perfusion, which may be related to peripheral vascular disease (a narrowing in the blood vessels outside the heart); a release of catecholamines and subsequent vasoconstriction; or a low hemoglobin and hematocrit. All of these conditions should be thoroughly assessed. Additionally, temperature changes such as generalized warmth or coolness may indicate altered peripheral perfusion.

Nail Beds

Clubbing of nail beds is easily assessed and appears as swelling of the subcutaneous tissue over the base of the nail and absence of the normal angle between the nail and the nail base. The presence of clubbing indicates long-term oxygen deficiencies such as congenital heart defects or pulmonary diseases with hypoxemia.

Neck Veins

The right external and internal jugular veins (Figure 37–5 ■) are used to assess for jugular venous distention (JVD) and **jugular venous pressure (JVP)** or pulse. Although these terms are often used interchangeably, there is a physiological significance in distinguishing between JVD and JVP. Anatomically, the right jugular veins drain blood from the head into the right atrium of the heart. Both veins reflect activity on the right side of the heart. The internal jugular vein lies in a straight path to the right atrium, but because it is buried beneath the sternomastoid muscle, it is difficult to visualize. The external jugular vein curves a few times before entering the right atrium, and because it is located closer to the skin it is easier to visualize. Findings from neck vein assessment are helpful in confirming suspicions of heart failure; however, the information must be put in context of the presenting symptoms and current health status. The importance of volume status and cardiovascular function is an important hemodynamic concept. Chapter 42 includes an in-depth discussion of the significance of distended neck veins with heart failure.

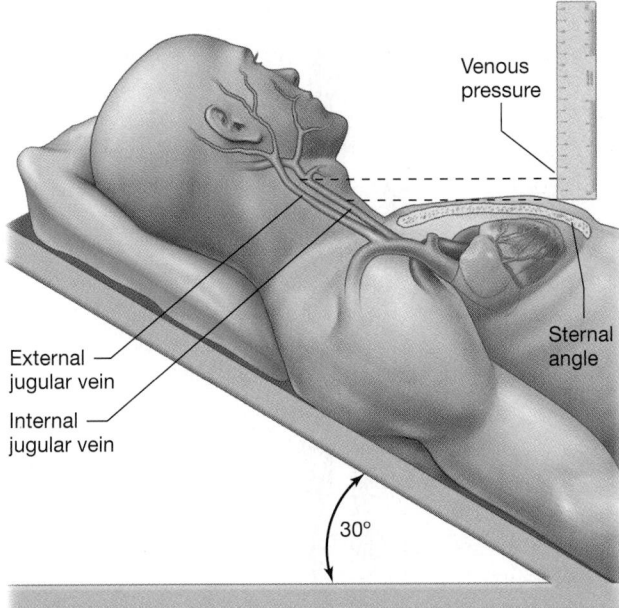

FIGURE 37–5 ■ Jugular veins.

Jugular Venous Distention

Jugular venous distention (JVD) is assessed by visually observing the right external jugular (REJ) vein. Generally noting that this vein is full or overdistended is sufficient for the nursing assessment and provides useful information pertaining to hemodynamic volume status of the cardiovascular system. The REJ vein is always distended when the patient is lying flat and is eliminated as the patient becomes more upright. From a flat position, slowly elevate the head of the bed and observe the right external jugular vein, noting the degree of elevation at which the distention is eliminated (30, 45, 60, or 90 degrees). The finding is reported by noting the highest height of the head of the bed (HOB) when JVD was appreciated; for example, "presence of JVD was noted with HOB elevated to 45 degrees" (Urden et al., 2006).

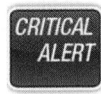
The finding of JVD during inspection of the neck veins can contribute to diagnosis of right heart failure. Treatment to reduce volume, such as diuretics or vasodilators, may be needed. The finding of JVD may also help to explain other findings noted during the exam, such as shortness of breath (SOB), diaphoresis, or confusion.

Jugular Venous Pressure

The right internal jugular (RIJ) vein is used to assess jugular venous pulses and jugular venous pressure. The RIJ lies deep in skin and soft tissues, and its pulsations are transmitted to the overlying tissues. These pulsations are produced by the right atrial and right ventricular activity (Garg & Garg, 2000). Changes in pulsations can be a diagnostic tool for the skilled practitioner. Assessment of RIJ for jugular venous pressure (JVP) provides valuable information as well; and it is a more reliable indicator of central venous pressure (CVP), or the pressure that exists in the central venous system, than is the right external vein assessment. To examine the JVP, stand on the patient's right side, and turn the patient's head slightly to the left. The neck muscles should be relaxed. The head of the bed should be elevated high enough to visualize the top of the

column of blood in the internal jugular vein. Observe the highest point of pulsation during exhalation. The vertical difference between this location and the sternal angle (see Figure 37–5 ■) is measured in centimeters. The normal measurement should be 4 centimeters or less. A measurement of more than 4 centimeters suggests increased JVP, an increase in pressure in the right heart, and therefore an increased CVP. Because the distance between the sternal angle and the mid-right atrium is approximately 5 centimeters, to measure CVP, 5 centimeters is added to the measurement of JVP. The upper limit of normal is a CVP measurement of 9 centimeters (JVP of 4 plus 5 centimeters) (Garg & Garg, 2000). An example of how this finding is reported is "JVP estimated at 9 centimeters with the head of the bed elevated to 45 degrees."

Abdominojugular Reflux

The assessment of the abdominojugular reflux (sometimes called hepatojugular reflux) can also be used as a noninvasive technique to assess cardiovascular volume status. In heart failure, or volume overload, blood volume that normally is pumped proficiently by the heart begins to be displaced throughout the body as a mechanism to minimize cardiac workload. Volume may be displaced in the abdomen, particularly the hepatic system, which has a large capacity to hold fluid. The technique to observe **abdominojugular reflux** is done by compressing the right upper abdomen for 15 to 30 seconds. Observe for JVD before, during, and after abdominal compression. This pressure causes volume in the abdomen to be pushed back to the right atrium. The failing heart will not be able to accommodate this increase in volume, and the pressure will be reflected in the jugular veins. Sustained JVD (longer than 10 seconds) with abdominal compression is another indicator that aids the diagnosis of cardiac failure (Urden et al., 2006).

Palpation of Skin and Extremities

Palpation of the skin and extremities during a cardiovascular assessment includes an assessment of edema, skin turgor, capillary refill, and the arterial pulses for abnormalities associated with cardiovascular disorders.

Edema

Edema is defined as an increase in interstitial fluid that is clinically evident. Although there are many types of edema, cardiovascular patients typically experience edema associated with the accumulation of fluid in the extracellular spaces, particularly the skin of the extremities, as seen earlier. Edema of the skin can be painful, and it interferes with normal blood circulation. Edema is an important assessment finding because it is indicative of an underlying disease process and requires treatment.

Normally two-thirds of the body's water is in the cells (intracellular), while one-third is outside the cells (extracellular). Extracellular fluid consists of water in the plasma and in the tissues (interstitial). Fluid exchange between these compartments is governed by a balance of hydraulic and oncotic pressures as well as the permeability of the capillary wall that separates them. When any of the factors are altered, excess fluid may be moved into the plasma and interstitial spaces. Changes in capillary hydraulic pressure can occur with heart failure. Capillary permeability can be increased as a consequence of the inflammatory process, which can be initiated as a response to numerous events including exposure to allergens. The kidneys play an important role in body fluid distribution as the kidneys respond to changes in blood pressure and volume by adjusting retention of sodium. Therefore, sodium balance is of utmost importance in cardiovascular disease processes involving the development or potential development of edema.

The skin can feel puffy and tight. Edema can be localized in one area of the body or can be generalized throughout. Dependent edema occurs when there is an increase in extracellular fluid volume in a dependent limb or area. Edema is assessed by firmly placing a thumb against a dependent area of the body (arms, hands, legs, feet, ankles). When the pressure is released, an indentation on the skin may be observed. When the indentation remains on the skin after releasing pressure, it is referred to as pitting edema. The degree of pitting edema can be rated on a 4-point scale (Chart 37–2).

Skin Turgor

Palpation of the skin **turgor**, or elasticity, reflects the skin's state of hydration. A small section of the patient's skin (anterior chest, under clavicle, or abdomen) is pinched between the examiner's thumb and forefinger. As the skin is slowly released, the speed at which the skin returns to its original contour is observed. It should return to normal rapidly. If there is poor skin turgor, the skin returns to its original contour very slowly. Dehydration, scleroderma, or aging can decrease skin turgor.

Capillary Refill

Capillary refill, the rate at which blood refills empty capillaries, is a quick method of assessing blood flow to the peripheral microcirculation. The tip of the finger is compressed until blanching of the nail bed is noted. When pressure is released, a return of color should be noted within 2 to 3 seconds. A delayed return of color is a sign of vasoconstriction or poor peripheral perfusion. A delayed capillary refill may be observed in heart failure, peripheral vascular disease (PVD), or shock.

Arterial Pulses

Palpation of the pulses in the neck and extremities provides information about arterial blood flow, particularly volume and pressure within the vessels. Arterial pulses are palpated bilaterally to compare characteristics of the arteries on the right and left sides of the body (Figure 37–6 ■). The volume of the pulsations is judged and recorded as normal, bounding, thready, or absent. Additionally, a common scale can be used for documentation of pulses. A score of 0 indicates an absent pulse. A score of 1+ indicates a pulse is present, but it is weak and thready. A score of 2+ indicates a pulse is present and normal in amplitude. A score of 3+ indicates a full and bounding pulsation. A normal

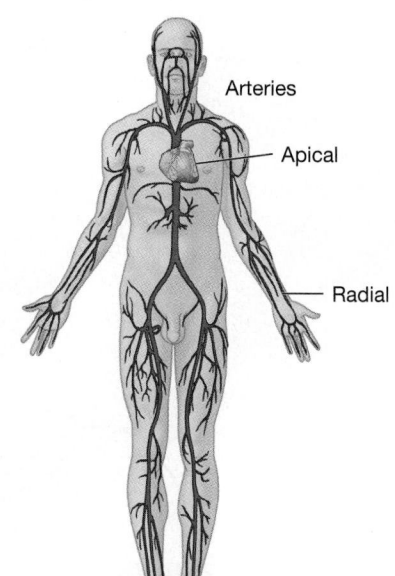

Systemic Circulation

Arteries

Apical

Radial

Pedal

Posterior tibal

FIGURE 37–6 ■ Arterial pulses.

pulse feels like a tap, whereas a vessel that is narrowed or bulging will vibrate. The rate and rhythm of arterial pulses are palpated. The examiner counts the number of pulsations in a minute to determine the heart rate. At the same time, a judgment is made as to the regularity of the pattern of pulses and the intervals between pulses. Pulses can be normal or abnormal. Abnormalities in rate and rhythm of arterial pulses may indicate inadequate cardiac output or cardiac dysrhythmias.

Inspection and Palpation of the Precordium

Inspection and palpation of the bony structures of the thorax, including the sternoclavicular joints, the manubrium, and the upper part of the sternum, are performed using clinical reference points. The precordium is assessed for pulsations, heaves, and thrills described on page 1063, which may indicate vessel abnormalities.

Clinical Reference Points

The normal clinical reference points or landmarks of the chest wall, as well as specific auscultatory areas, should be noted on every patient during cardiovascular assessment in a consistent manner. Experience enhances the ability to identify abnormalities and their significance to cardiovascular disorders (Figures 37–7 ■ and 37–8 ■).

Point of Maximal Impulse (PMI)

The mitral valve area of the thorax is palpated for the point of maximal impulse (PMI). This pulsation is normally located at the left fifth intercostal space (ICS) at the midclavicular line (MCL) (see Figure 37–7 ■). With the patient in a sitting position, the nurse uses fingertips to identify the PMI. Sometimes having the patient lean slightly forward enhances the PMI. The

---

CHART 37–2	**Scale for Rating Edema**

+0″	No pitting
+1	0″–¼″ pitting (mild)
+2	¼″–½″ pitting (moderate)
+3	½″–1″ pitting (severe)
+4	Greater than 1″ pitting (severe)

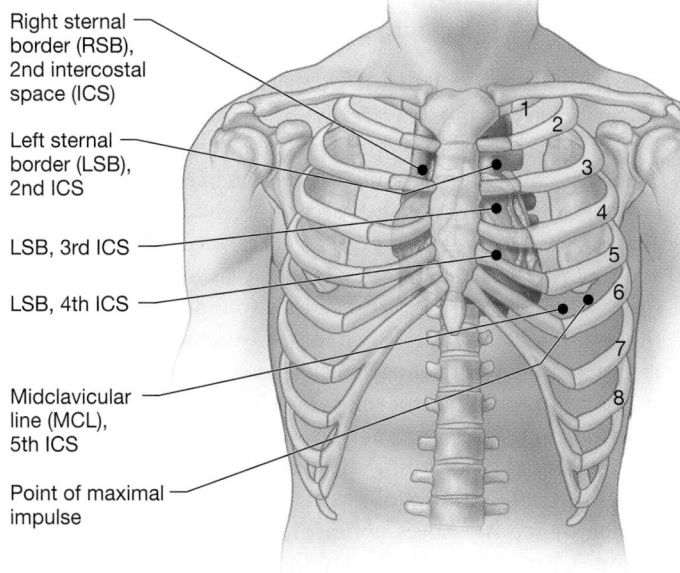

Right sternal border (RSB), 2nd intercostal space (ICS)

Left sternal border (LSB), 2nd ICS

LSB, 3rd ICS

LSB, 4th ICS

Midclavicular line (MCL), 5th ICS

Point of maximal impulse

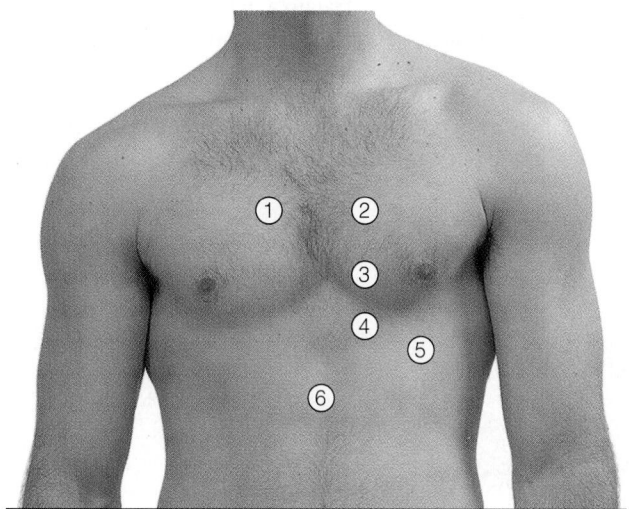

FIGURE 37–7 ■ Clinical reference points for palpation.

PMI is normally felt as a single pulsation or light tap, and is 1 to 2 centimeters in diameter. The position and the diameter of the PMI should be recorded in relation to the MCL and ICSs. If the patient has an enlarged heart (cardiomegaly) due to heart failure, ventricular hypertrophy, or pregnancy, the PMI may be enlarged or displaced laterally and downward. The PMI may also be visualized as a pulsation on the chest in a patient with cardiovascular disease.

Heaves and Thrills

The precordium is inspected for pulsations, heaves, and thrills. Although rare, pulsations may be visualized on the chest wall, particularly in thin patients, and may be caused by pulmonary hypertension or a significant aneurysm. **Heaves** or lifts, which are normally not seen or felt over the precordium, are sustained lifts of the chest wall in the precordial area due to forceful cardiac contractions that cause a slight to vigorous movement of the sternum and ribs. Heaves may be caused by ventricular enlargement or hypertrophy. A **thrill** describes a palpable vibra-

tory sensation from turbulent blood flow across cardiac valves. Thrills are typically described as the throat of a purring cat.

Findings in various clinical reference points may indicate specific cardiac disorders. The respiratory system is observed simultaneously, because the purpose of the cardiovascular system is to deliver oxygen to the tissues that was received from the respiratory system. Alterations in rate and depth of respirations may indicate cardiovascular, respiratory, or neurological disorders.

Auscultation of the Precordium

Auscultation involves listening to the sounds produced by different body areas. Cardiac auscultation is an efficient, noninvasive manner to assess both normal and abnormal heart sounds. Although the technique is simply performed with only a stethoscope, a great deal of practice and expertise is required to appreciate and differentiate cardiac abnormalities associated with valvular alterations. The art of auscultation includes the ability to discriminate subtle differences in intensity, pitch, location, radiation, duration, timing, and intervals of heart sounds (O'Connor, 1998). Generally, nurses should be able to perform the technique proficiently, be able to recognize normal auscultatory sounds, and most importantly be alert to variations from normal that can provide valuable clinical clues and may indicate a change or deterioration in cardiac status.

The skill of auscultation begins with good technique and a quiet environment. The stethoscope should be of good quality with a bell, a diaphragm, and comfortable earpieces. The stethoscope must be applied directly to the skin; listening over clothing will obscure the sound. The patient should be in a comfortable position and asked to lie still and not talk. Imagine the position of the heart and the cardiac valves under the chest wall (see Figure 37–8 ■). Find the angle of Louis, felt as a ridge just below the suprasternal notch (see Figure 37–1 ■, p. 1053). Feel the ribs on each side of this angle and the intercostal space below each rib. Using the bell and the diaphragm of the stethoscope, listen to heart sounds at each auscultatory area (see Figure 37–8 ■), first with the diaphragm for high-pitched sounds and then with the bell with very light pressure for low-pitched sounds at each auscultatory

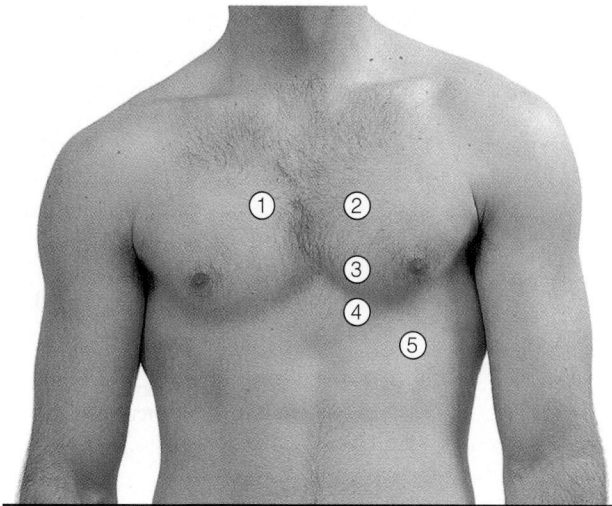

FIGURE 37–8 ■ Auscultatory areas.

site. Listen for the normal S_1 and S_2 heart sounds at each site, and note the intensity, the presence of split sounds, and the effect of the respiratory cycle on the regularity of the sounds. Also note the time between the S_1 and S_2 for regularity. Listen for extra heart sounds and abnormal heart sounds at each site. If abnormal sounds are heard, note the timing, pitch, loudness, duration, and location on the chest wall. If a murmur is heard, note where it can be heard best and whether it is a low-, medium-, or high-pitched sound. The presence of any pericardial friction rubs should also be noted.

Requirements for Auscultation

In order to understand cardiac auscultation, nurses need to have knowledge of the physiology of the cardiac cycle, the normal landmarks of the chest (see Figure 37–7 ■, p. 1063), and the auscultatory sites on the chest wall that correspond to specific valve sounds (see Figure 37–8 ■, p. 1063). When listening to dynamic blood flow across cardiac valves, the sounds associated with the closure of the valves are not heard directly over that valve area, but rather in the direction of the flow of blood. It is helpful to imagine the physical position of the heart under the chest wall, as well as the path or direction of blood flow (Figure 37–9 ■). Because sound is not transmitted through bone, the best auscultatory area of a particular valve would be the nearest tissue area in line with the path of blood flow. The key to a good auscultatory exam is to listen to one sound at a time in each auscultatory

area. The nurse should be in the habit of listening to all the auscultatory areas with the diaphragm and then again with the bell.

Normal Heart Sounds: S_1 and S_2

Normal heart sounds are created by the turbulence of blood flow as the cardiac valves open and close during the cardiac cycle. As the valves move, some turbulence in blood flow is created. (See the Cardiac Valves section at the beginning of the chapter.) Two heart sounds can be heard with each cardiac cycle. The first heart sound is referred to as S_1 and the second heart sound, S_2. S_1 is a called a systolic sound because it signals the beginning of systole. When the pressures in the pulmonary artery and the right ventricle begin to equalize, and the pressures in the aorta and the left ventricle begin to equalize, systolic ejection tapers off and the semilunar valves snap shut. This signals the beginning of diastole, which allows the AV valves to open and diastolic ventricular filling to begin. The closing of the AV valves is heard as the S_2, or second heart sound (Chart 37–3). The S_1 and the S_2 are both high-pitched sounds heard best with the diaphragm. The S_1 is normally loudest over the apex or mitral area, while the S_2 is best heard over the base of the heart, or the aortic area.

Distinguishing S_1 from S_2

It is helpful during auscultation to differentiate the S_1 from the S_2. When there is an abnormality, it must be described as a sys-

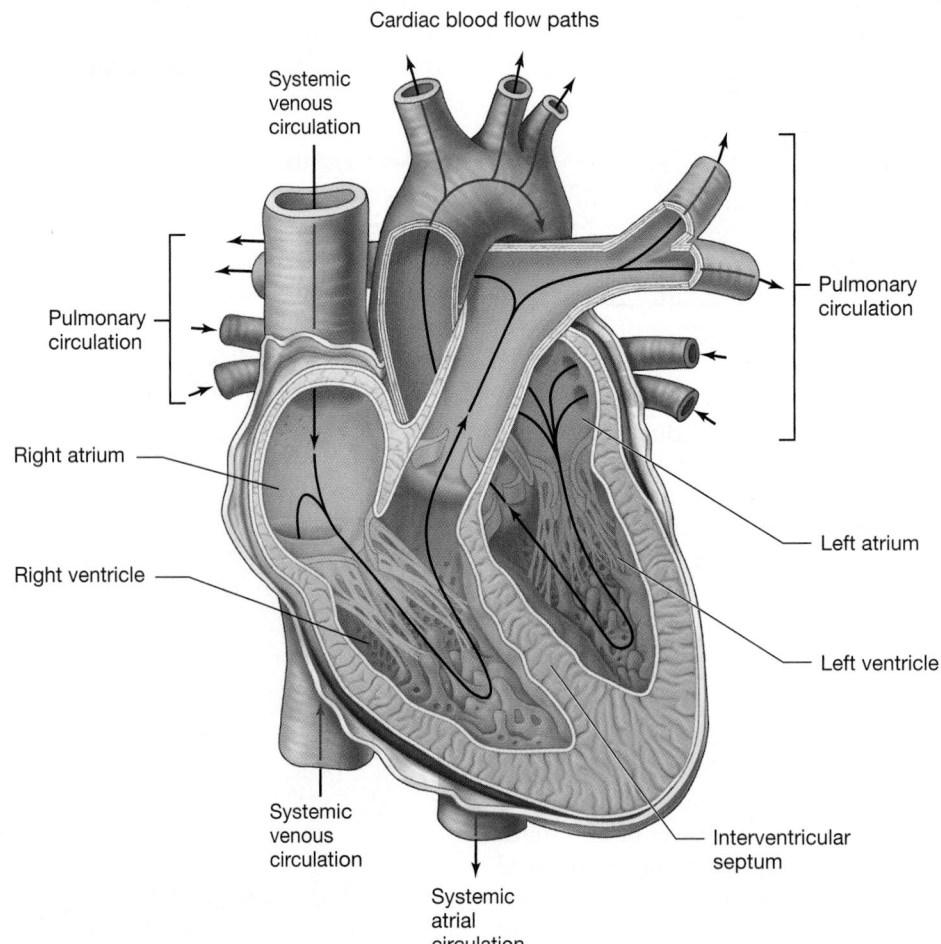

Cardiac blood flow paths

Systemic venous circulation

Pulmonary circulation

Pulmonary circulation

Right atrium

Left atrium

Right ventricle

Left ventricle

Interventricular septum

Systemic venous circulation

Systemic atrial circulation

FIGURE 37–9 ■ Cardiac blood flow path.

CHART 37–3 Summary of Heart Sounds

Heart Sounds		Cardiac Cycle Timing	Ausculation Site	Position	Pitch
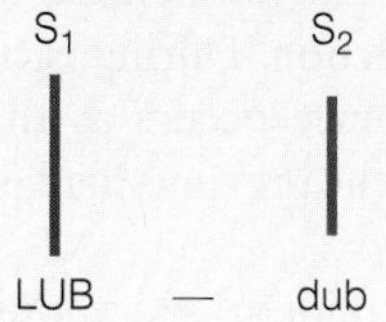 S_1 / S_2 (LUB — dub)	S_1	Start of systole	Best at apex with diaphragm	Position does not affect the sound	High
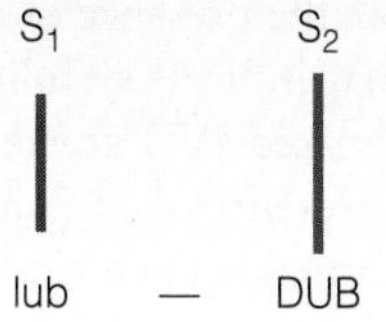 S_1 / S_2 (lub — DUB)	S_2	End of systole	Both at 2nd intercostal space (ICS); pulmonary component best at left sternal border (LSB); aortic component best at RBS with diaphragm	Sitting or supine	High
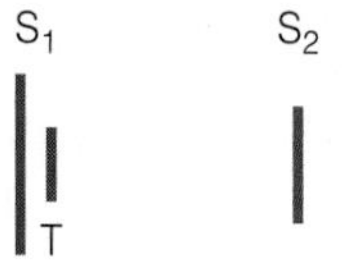 S_1 (T) / S_2	Split S_1	Beginning of systole	If normal, at 2nd ICS, LSB abnormal if heard at apex	Better heard in the supine position	High
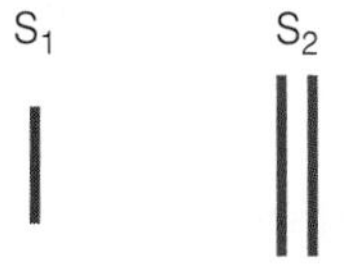 S_1 / S_2	Fixed Split S_2	End of systole	Both at 2nd ICS: pulmonary component best at LSB; aortic component best at right sternal border (RSB) with diaphragm	Better heard in the supine position	High
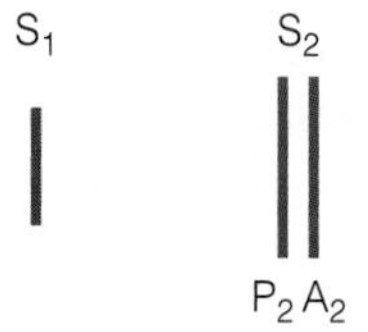 S_1 / S_2 ($P_2 A_2$)	Paradoxial Split S_2	End of systole	Both at 2nd ICS; pulmonary component best at LSB; aortic component best at RSB with diaphragm	Better heard in the supine position	High
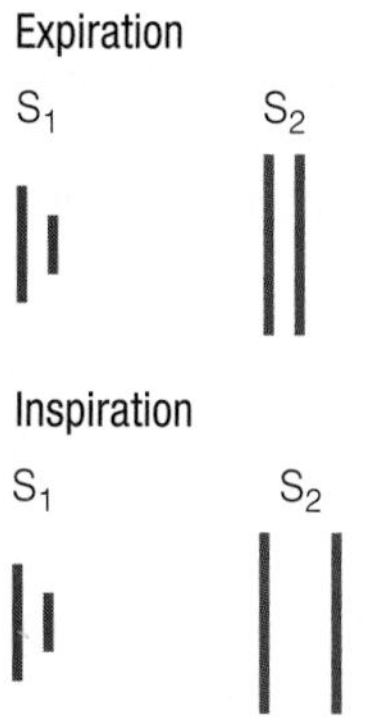 Expiration S_1 / S_2 ; Inspiration S_1 / S_2	Wide Split S_2	End of systole	Both at 2nd ICS; pulmonary component best at LSB; aortic component best at RSB with diaphragm	Better heard in the supine position	High
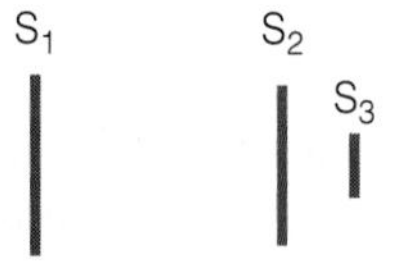 S_1 / S_2 S_3	S_3	Early diastole right after S_2	Apex with the bell	Auscultated better in left lateral position or supine	Low
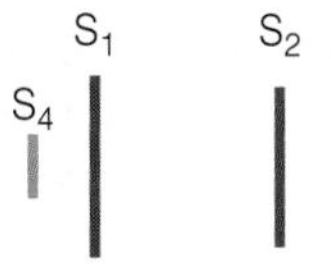 S_4 S_1 / S_2	S_4	Late diastole right before S_1	Apex with the bell	Auscultated better in left lateral position or supine	Low

tolic sound (occurring with or after the S_1) or a diastolic sound (occurring with or after the S_2). By determining where in the cardiac cycle the abnormality occurs, the listener can better estimate which cardiac valve is affected. For example, if the nurse hears an abnormality of the S_1 sound, she would know there is an alteration in either the mitral or the tricuspid valve. The S_1 and the S_2 sounds can be differentiated by three methods. The first is timing. During the cardiac cycle, the amount of time spent in diastole is longer than the amount of time spent in systole. Therefore, there should be a pause between the S_2 and the next S_1 (Chart 37–3, p. 1065). Of course this method is accurate only when the heart rate is slow enough to appreciate the diastolic pause. If, however, the heart rate is accelerated, the S_1 can be identified by palpating either the PMI (point of maximal impulse) or the carotid arterial pulsation. As the practitioner is listening with the stethoscope on the chest wall to the heart sound, she should be palpating these pulsation points. When the pulsation is felt, the S_1 is heard. Pulse points, further downstream, such as the radial artery should not be used to establish correlation, because they are too far away from the heart and are not likely to correspond with the S_1.

Split Heart Sounds: Split S_1 and Split S_2

Because the right and left heart are two separate pumps that function simultaneously, it is normal to hear the closure of two valves, the right and left AV valves, and the right and left semilunar valves, as one sound. Many conditions can alter the timing of the cardiac cycle on the right or left side of the heart causing one valve to close slightly later than normal. When this happens, the sounds of S_1 (closure of the tricuspid and mitral valves) or the sounds of S_2 (closure of the pulmonic and aortic valves) are heard separately, referred to as a split heart sound.

The S_1 is normally heard as a single sound, although there might be a slight split between the mitral component (M_1) and the tricuspid component (T_1) of the S_1. The S_2 exhibits a normal split on inspiration. This is called a *physiological split*, because it is associated with a normal physiological pattern. This physiological split S_2, heard best over the pulmonic area, is a result of asymmetry with the closure of the aortic (A_2) and pulmonic (P_2) valve sounds that make up the S_2 (A_2P_2). On inspiration, there is an increase in intrathoracic pressure that causes an increase in venous return to the right heart. The increased volume causes a delay in ventricular emptying, and thus the pulmonic valve closure (P_2) is slightly delayed. This effect is removed, however, during expiration; the A_2 and P_2 should be closer in synchrony, and the two components of the second heart sound are heard as one. Numerous other conditions, such as ventricular septal defects (VSDs), bundle branch blocks, and ventricular failure, can cause abnormal splitting of the S_2.

Extra Heart Sounds

Extra heart sounds are classified in relation to their timing in the cardiac cycle. Although the presence of an S_3 or S_4 can be normal, these extra heart sounds often signify cardiac disorders. Therefore, nurses should be knowledgeable about these sounds, as well as their significance in relation to heart disease, in order to detect and report their presence. Third and fourth heart sounds, if present, are both heard during diastole. S_3 and S_4 are low-frequency soft sounds, which are best heard by applying the stethoscope softly on the skin or just firmly enough to create a skin seal. It is easier to detect the S_3 or the S_4 by positioning the patient in the left lateral position, which brings the heart closer to the heart wall. S_3s and S_4s are not affected by respirations and are heard as single sounds.

S_3

S_3 is heard early in diastole just after the S_2 and is heard best in the apex (see Chart 37–3, p. 1065). One cardiac cycle (S_1, S_2, S_3,

sounds like lub-dub-dee or "Ken-tuc'-ky." S_3s are heard early in diastole because they are associated with abnormalities of ventricular filling, and they are sometimes called ventricular gallops. S_3s are markers of systolic dysfunction. When there is ventricular systolic dysfunction, the ventricle is not able to empty sufficiently with each systolic contraction. During each consecutive diastolic filling period, turbulence occurs as the "new" load of blood attempts to enter when the previous load of blood has not completely left the ventricle.

An S_3 heard over the left ventricle in children and young adults is normal, although after ages 35 to 40, the presence of a third heart sound is usually abnormal and may indicate systolic dysfunction. An S_3 and the presence of increased JVD are regarded as specific signs of heart failure. The presence of an S_3 in an older person may be the only clue to abnormal left ventricular function (O'Connor, 1998).

S_4

S_4 occurs late in diastole just before the S_1 and is heard best in the apex (Chart 37–3, p. 1065). One cardiac cycle (S_4, S_1, S_2) sounds like dee-lub-dub or "Ten-nes-see." S_4s are heard late in diastole because they are associated with the atrial kick component of diastole, and they are sometimes called atrial gallops. S_4s are markers of diastolic dysfunction. An S_4 occurs when the atria attempt to pump blood into a stiff, noncompliant ventricle that is resistant to further volume expansion.

Diastolic dysfunction may occur with ventricular hypertrophy associated with hypertension, with aortic stenosis, or with altered ventricular compliance associated with ischemia. Normal fourth heart sounds are common in older adults and are associated with an age-related decrease in left ventricular compliance (O'Connor, 1998). A fourth heart sound is almost always abnormal in children and may contribute to a decrease in ventricular compliance. An S_4 cannot be heard during atrial fibrillation, because S_4s are associated with atrial contraction against a noncompliant ventricle.

Summation Gallop

Summation gallops occur when both an S_3 and an S_4 are heard (S_4, S_1, S_2, S_3) (Chart 37–3, p. 1065); in other words, there is a combined ventricular and atrial gallop. A summation gallop is associated with advanced heart failure. The S_3 and S_4 may be heard as two distinct sounds in diastole or, in the case of tachycardia, as a single mid-diastolic sound. Summation gallops are sometimes described as galloping hooves.

Pericardial Friction Rubs

Pericardial friction rubs are due to inflammation of the pericardial sac surrounding the heart in conditions such as pericarditis. Pericarditis is described in detail in Chapter 41 ☺. Pericardial friction rubs are a transient high-pitched sound heard best at the left sternal border. The sound that is produced is a squeaky, rubbing, muffled sound. Pericardial friction rubs are heard best with the patient leaning forward or lying on the left side. Pericardial friction rubs may be a transient assessment finding.

Abnormal Heart Sounds: Murmurs

Murmurs are audible vibrations heard over the heart and great vessels. Murmurs are caused by turbulent blood flow across a diseased valve (stenosis or regurgitation), turbulence caused by increased blood flow through normal structures, or blood flow into a dilated chamber (Chart 37–4). Whereas murmurs are aus-

CHART 37–4	**Classification of Murmurs**
TIMING	• Timing within the cardiac cycle. • Systolic or diastolic (early, mid, late, continuous). • Systolic murmurs are often benign. • Diastolic murmurs are never benign.
LOCATION	Auscultatory area the murmur is best heard. • Aortic, pulmonic, mitral, tricuspid. • Presence of murmurs at specific valve sites leads to the identification of the affected valve.
FREQUENCY	• High-pitched or low-pitched sound. • Low-pitched murmurs are caused by a low velocity of blood flow. • High-pitched murmurs are caused by a rapid velocity of blood flow.
QUALITY	• Descriptive quality of the sound. • Harsh, rumbling, musical, soft, blowing, gurgling. • Quality may indicate regurgitation or stenosis.
PATTERN	• Configuration of sound if one were to draw it. • Crescendo, decrescendo, diamond shaped.
RADIATION	• Sounds may be radiated to the neck, back, shoulders, sternal border, jaw, arm, or left axilla. • Some murmurs radiate in the direction of the bloodstream, by which they are produced.
INTENSITY	Grading scale of loudness • I/VI Very soft, barely audible. • II/VI Soft, but loud enough to be appreciated. • III/VI Loud, easily heard, no thrills or vibrations. • IV/VI Loud, soft palpable thrill. • V/VI Loud, heard with stethoscope barely touching chest wall; palpable thrill. • VI/VI Very loud, can be heard with stethoscope fully off chest wall, pronounced palpable thrill.

cultatory sounds caused by vibrations or turbulence in the heart and great vessels, **bruits** are auscultatory sounds associated with vibrations or turbulence in a blood vessel outside the heart.

Murmur Etiology

Murmurs are due to valve abnormalities of stenosis or regurgitation. Many different physiological conditions can lead to these alterations. A stenotic valve is one whose valve leaflets are hardened, calcified, or narrowed. Blood flow is obstructed as it is forced through a narrowed, stenotic valve orifice. Valve regurgitation occurs when the valve leaflets fail to close completely. This causes valve insufficiency, and a portion of the systolic blood volume is allowed to flow backward. Causes of abnormal valves are discussed in Chapter 41 ☺. As blood flows through these two different types of valve alterations, the sounds generated are very distinct. For example, blood flowing through a stenotic valve would sound very harsh because blood is being forced through a narrow opening, whereas blood flowing through a regurgitant valve would sound softer and have more of a gurgling quality. The sounds associated with particular valve disorders

would be best heard at the corresponding valve's auscultatory site (Chart 37–5). When a murmur is auscultated, the etiology can be suggested by understanding the physiology of the cardiac cycle and heart sounds. For example, during systole the aortic valve is open, allowing blood to flow from the left ventricle through the aortic valve to the aorta, and the mitral valve is closed, preventing blood from flowing back into the left atrium. If the aortic valve were stenotic, the sound would be a harsh murmur during systole over the aortic valve area. Likewise, if the mitral valve were regurgitant, one would typically hear a gurgling sound over the mitral valve area. During the assessment the nurse should evaluate for head bobbing up and down in synchrony with the heartbeat, because this is characteristic of severe aortic regurgitation (D'Amico & Barbarito, 2007).

Systolic murmurs, heard during systole, include mitral regurgitation, tricuspid regurgitation, aortic stenosis, and pulmonic stenosis. Diastolic murmurs, heard during diastole, include mitral stenosis, tricuspid stenosis, aortic regurgitation, and pulmonic regurgitation.

Innocent Murmurs

Some murmurs may be classified as innocent or functional murmurs. An innocent murmur is a sound made by the blood circulating in the heart chambers or valves, or through the blood vessels near the heart. Innocent murmurs are often soft and may vary or disappear with position changes, whereas pathologic murmurs are generally louder and seldom disappear with position changes. Innocent murmurs are harmless, asymptomatic, and are commonly heard in children. Further diagnostic tests may be performed to rule out other conditions.

When a murmur is heard, it is important to describe the sound properly. Murmurs should be described in terms of their timing in the cardiac cycle, the auscultatory location they are heard best, frequency, intensity, radiation, and quality. A summary of murmurs associated with valve disorders is presented in Chart 37–6 (p. 1068).

Gender Implications/Gender Differences

Before the 1980s, it was believed that cardiovascular disease (CVD) affected primarily men. This was due in large part to the fact that most research studies involved men. It is now well known that women respond uniquely to CVD as well as to other diseases. Women experience the signs and symptoms associated with CVD differently than men. More women have asymptomatic and undiagnosed CVD. It is difficult to apply preventive cardiovascular care to women who have not been identified as having CVD. Mortality

CHART 37–5	**Valve Opening and Closing with Cardiac Cycle**		
	Open	**Closed**	**Abnormality**
SYSTOLE	Pulmonic Aortic (stenosis)	Tricuspid Mitral (regurgitation)	Regurgitation is unable to completely close
DIASTOLE	Tricuspid Mitral (stenosis)	Pulmonic Aortic (regurgitation)	Stenosis is unable to completely open

MyNursingKit | Animation: Health and Physical Assessment: Cardiac/Cardiovascular—Heart Sounds: Irregular

| CHART 37–6 | **Summary of Murmurs Associated with Valve Disorders** |

AORTIC STENOSIS

1. Midsystolic, crescendo-decrescendo
2. Harsh
3. Usually heard best in the aortic area
4. Often heard widely over the chest
5. Often radiates to the carotid arteries
6. Loudness unrelated to severity

AORTIC REGURGITATION

1. Present in early diastole
2. Decrescendo configuration
3. High-pitched blowing
4. Heard best with the patient leaning forward; often faint
5. Loudness along Left Lower Sternal Border (LLSB)

MITRAL STENOSIS

1. Long, rumbling diastolic murmur
2. Low pitched
3. Heard best with bell
4. Localized to mitral area (apex)
5. Often accompanied by a diastolic thrill in the area
6. Crescendo occurs in late diastole

MITRAL REGURGITATION

1. Pansystolic
2. Loudest in mitral area (apex)
3. Radiates to left axilla
4. Usually blowing in quality
5. Systolic thrill usually present in mitral area

INNOCENT MURMUR

1. Short, soft, systolic
2. Normal S_1 and S_2
3. Normal ECG and chest x-ray
4. Crescendo-decrescendo
5. Heard in primary aortic area

rates of CVD, particularly from sudden death, are currently higher in women than in men (D'Amore and Mora, 2006). D'Amore and Mora (2006) suggest that women previously deemed at intermediate risk for the development of CVD from standard available guidelines, but who have concerning features in their medical history such as a strong family history, may benefit from stress testing, which may provide further gender-specific prognostic information. Further studies are needed to identify gender-specific predictors of cardiac disease, and more comprehensive approaches to CVD prevention and treatment are needed for women. Although, many of the gender-specific differences in CVD are not well explained, it is well understood that postmenopausal women are at greater risk of developing CVD than are premenopausal women.

This is due to the cardioprotective effect of estrogen in premenopausal women. (Genetic predispositions to cardiovascular disease are discussed in the Genetic Considerations box.)

Gerontological Considerations

The number of elderly people over age 65 in the population of the United States has been steadily increasing. Therefore, it stands to reason that the number of elderly patients cared for in health care settings will also increase. The gerontological population has unique considerations, which are important in cardiovascular assessment. Physiological changes associated with aging include myocardial hypertrophy; an increase in collagen and scarring; a decrease in elasticity; fibrotic and sclerotic changes of the atria and ventricles; calcification, sclerosis, or fibrosis of the cardiac valves; and rigidity and fibrosis of the vessels of the arterial system. These changes can lead to a drop in cardiac output, systolic or diastolic murmurs, increased frequency of dysrhythmias, and altered blood flow dynamics, all of which affect tissue perfusion. For example, elderly persons may have elevations in systolic or diastolic blood pressures. Additionally, in the response to injury or shock, the heart becomes less able to respond or initiate the stimulation of catecholamines needed to increase heart rate and contractility (Whetstone & Boswell, 2002). It is not uncommon to hear an S_4 in an elderly person due to decreased compliance of the left ventricle or a systolic murmur due to aortic or mitral valve abnormalities. Thickened myocardial fibers can also affect the conduction system of the heart and cause cardiac irritability and dysrhythmias. Diseases affecting other body systems can

GENETIC CONSIDERATIONS for Cardiovascular Disease

A great deal is known about the independent risk factors for the development of cardiovascular disease. Advances made in the area of genetics since the Human Genome Project in 1988 have helped scientists understand the genetic causes of cardiovascular disease. It has become clear that most cardiovascular diseases result from various genetic causes (Allen, 2000). Gene mutations and the interaction of genes and the environment are currently being examined. For example, polygenic disorders, such as hypertension, are caused by the combined effect of more than one mutated gene. Interestingly, the nature and severity of polygenic disorders vary significantly and are unpredictable in nature (Allen, 2000).

Coronary artery disease is an example of a multifactorial disorder. Multifactorial disorders may have a genetic component, but the presentation is largely affected by environmental factors. For example, multifactorial disorders may include an interaction of genetic factors (genetic abnormalities that result in lipid disorders, hypertension, and obesity) with nongenetic factors such as smoking, increasing age, and physical activity.

Through a thorough cardiovascular assessment, and potentially future genetic testing, inherited cardiovascular diseases or the susceptibility to diseases can be identified. The hope is that early detection and diagnosis will identify individuals at risk. Then prevention or modulation of the effects can be undertaken by the implementation of a treatment plan, education, and counseling. The goal of genetic testing would be to save lives through preventive treatment and therapeutic interventions. Nurses can complete family history assessments and initiate appropriate referrals for genetic counseling.

affect the heart and blood vessels. Diabetes mellitus is one example of a disease that can have damaging effects on the peripheral vasculature, and another is chronic obstructive lung disease, which contributes to right-sided heart failure.

Normal physiological changes in the elderly can contribute to the significance of cardiovascular signs and symptoms. For example, loss of muscle mass is a normal physiological change but can contribute to symptoms of weakness of fatigue. It is essential to encourage a healthy diet and regular exercise program. The gerontological population is more susceptible to cognitive impairments that make them more vulnerable to the effects of cardiac diseases and their treatments (Garrett, 1997). Dementia and delerium are common cognitive impairments found in the geriatric population. Cognitive losses of dementia affect the overall ability of an individual to interact successfully with the environment. The way the individual responds to stimuli from touch or stimuli from the environment may vary among individuals and should be considered prior to the exam (Garrett, 1997). The nurse needs to understand that there may be limitations in the patient's abilities to learn and apply new knowledge. It will be much more difficult for the individual who is cognitively impaired to manage the complexities of his cardiovascular disease and its treatment. Changes in cerebral perfusion due to atherosclerosis may also be present. When cognitive impairments such as dementia or delerium are suspected, the ability to provide accurate information for the health history will be altered (Garrett, 1997).

Critical Thinking Related to Cardiovascular Assessment

Critical thinking is essential in order to prioritize the most significant clinical manifestations that need further investigation. Cardiovascular clinical manifestations can range from conditions as benign as an innocent murmur to life-threatening disorders such as heart failure. It is imperative that the nurse be able to distinguish normal from abnormal, benign from serious. The nurse must rely on critical thinking skills in interpreting the patient's symptoms and assessment findings to determine possible and potential patient diagnoses and to consider the appropriate actions to take. Analysis of these data allows the nurse to make a diagnosis and then follow up with an intervention. It is imperative that the nurse communicate and collaborate with other members of the health care team in developing and implementing a plan of care.

Because cardiac disease manifestations can mimic other abnormalities such as pulmonary disease, the nurse must question each symptom and then compare and contrast symptoms. For example, when the patient reports a sudden onset of chest pain, the nurse must possess knowledge of the difference in manifestations between the causes of cardiac versus pulmonary chest pain and assess the patient for each of them. Making an assumption that the pain is cardiac in nature would be inappropriate and shortsighted. Effective critical thinking skills include being curious and not making any assumptions. Regardless of the health problem, each symptom identified should be thoroughly described in order for the nurse to gain a full understanding. The nurse can say to the patient, "Tell me more about the problem," or "How did it start?" The patient usually proceeds with a discourse about the symptoms. The nurse uses skillful interview techniques to explore and investigate each symptom further. Any symptom analysis would be incomplete without a thorough description of its characteristics.

Implications for Health Promotion

A good time to discuss the concept of health promotion with a patient is during a cardiovascular exam. Assessment can be a time to review current health status, examine problem areas, identify risk factors that need to be modified, identify possible health goals, discuss options, and potentially develop a plan of care. During a health assessment nurses need to provide health education and supply the patient with educational materials. Nurses are in a unique position to help patients recognize health problems or potential health problems. When abnormalities or positive findings are discovered during the health history process, an opportunity exists to discuss the issue in greater detail. Nurses should also recognize their role in promoting healthy lifestyles and their abilities to empower a patient and her family to make needed changes in their lives. Be aware that certain health topics are very personal, and some nurses have difficulty discussing these sensitive issues with patients.

As the populations that are served in health care settings continue to change and nurses are caring for more diverse populations, they need to be knowledgeable about the health practices of other cultures. Integrating culturally competent care includes incorporation of complementary therapies into the plan of care that will ultimately help nurses accomplish the goal of health promotion for all patients.

Cardiovascular Monitoring

Cardiovascular monitoring is an integral part of nursing management and includes many technologies used to augment the physical exam. Monitoring devices range from simple noninvasive monitoring, including assessment of heart rate, blood pressure, and pulse oximetry, to more invasive monitoring, such as hemodynamic monitoring using indwelling pulmonary artery catheters and arterial catheters. Chapter 24 🔗 includes a complete discussion of invasive hemodynamic monitoring. The goal of cardiovascular monitoring is to obtain the data needed to complete the cardiovascular assessment in a timely fashion, in the safest, most cost-efficient manner.

Assessment of Heart Rate

Counting the number of pulsations of the heart per minute determines heart rate. Assessment of heart rate should be performed when the patient is at rest in a calm environment. Many factors can alter the heart rate. For example, exercise, pain, and anxiety can cause an increase in circulating catecholamines, which may elevate heart rate and blood pressure. Endocrine and metabolic conditions can also affect the heart rate. The heart normally beats 60 to 100 times per minute. Heart rates less than 60 beats per minute (bradycardia) may be caused by hypoxia, parasympathetic stimulation, or beta-adrenergic blocker medication (Docherty, 2002a), although many well-conditioned athletes have resting heart rates well below 60 beats per minute. Bradycardia may not be clinically significant, unless accompanied by systolic blood pressure of less than 90 mmHg, which would indicate that the slow rate is compromising cardiovascular function (Docherty, 2002b).

Heart rates over 100 beats per minute are termed *tachycardia*, and some causes are exercise, pyrexia, hypovolemia, anxiety, and pain. Other clinical conditions that increase oxygen demand, such as myocardial ischemia or respiratory distress, may also cause tachycardia (Docherty, 2002a). Tachycardia can compromise cardiovascular status by decreasing diastolic filling time and increasing oxygen consumption, which may cause a reduction in stroke volume and eventually a drop in cardiac output. The regularity of the pulse should also be assessed. Irregularities suggest an alteration in cardiac conduction and should be further evaluated. Electrocardiogram (ECG) monitoring is a noninvasive method used to assess the heart rate and rhythm, and is commonly utilized in acute care settings. Interpretation and analysis of the ECG is discussed in Chapter 38 🌐.

Assessment of Blood Pressure

Arterial blood pressure (BP) is a measure of the pressure exerted by blood against the walls of the arterial system as it is ejected from the left ventricle. Blood pressure is a dynamic, multidimensional indicator of a person's cardiovascular state (Thomas, Liehr, DeKeyser, Frazier, & Friedmann, 2002). Assessment of blood pressure reflects the events of the pulsatile cardiac cycle and is expressed as systolic/diastolic. The systolic blood pressure (SBP) is the peak pressure exerted against the arteries when the heart ventricles contract during systole. The diastolic blood pressure (DBP) is the residual pressure existing in the arterial system at the end of diastole when the ventricles are relaxed and are filling with blood from the atria.

The recording of blood pressure can provide important information about blood volume, cardiac output, and peripheral resistance. It is a critical component of vital signs and therefore is a basic parameter for nurses' physical assessments (Thomas et al., 2002). When the systolic and diastolic blood pressures are elevated, so is the risk of developing cardiovascular disorders. High blood pressure causes the heart to work harder and directly damages the smooth muscle that lines the cardiovascular system (see Chapter 21 and Chapter 40 🌐). Hypertension must be treated promptly to prevent complications such as the development of atherosclerotic cardiovascular disease, myocardial infarction, and stroke.

Blood pressure can be measured in several ways: either indirectly by use of auscultatory methods such as mercury column or aneroid (clock-face) sphygmomanometers or by use of oscillatory methods such as the electronic automatic blood pressure cuffs that produce a digital readout, or directly by use of invasive monitoring devices.

In many clinic and hospital settings the most common way to obtain blood pressure recordings is by auscultation with the use of an indirect sphygmomanometer. Pressure is exerted on the main artery of the arm by the inflated blood pressure cuff. The stethoscope is used to listen for Korotkoff's sounds, which change in tone and volume as the cuff is deflated and blood flow is gradually restarted. The first sound heard is the systolic blood pressure, which represents the highest blood pressure that occurs each time the heart beats. The second recording is the diastolic blood pressure, which represents the lowest blood pressure that occurs when the heart relaxes between beats.

Accuracy in the measurement of BP is imperative because these data often guide medical and nursing practice. Many ther-

apeutic decisions are made based on BP recordings. Although the skill of measuring blood pressure appears simple, there are many possible causes of errors and inaccuracies (Chart 37–7). Inaccuracies in BP assessment can lead to underestimation or overestimation of blood pressure, causing errors in the diagnosis and treatment of cardiovascular conditions. The American Heart Association has published standard recommendations and a step-by-step protocol for the indirect measurement of blood pressure (Chart 37–8). Guidelines provide a consistent, uniform technique for measuring blood pressure. However, nurses should be periodically retrained in determination of blood pressure. Retraining of blood pressure observers has been shown to reduce variability of blood pressure due to human error (Jones, Apperl, Sheps, Roccella, & Lenfant, 2003).

It is important for nurses to understand that the BP in an artery is a dynamic number and changes throughout the day. It is the lowest during sleep. It rises on waking and can rise with excitation, nervousness, or activity. Therefore, a single reading of high blood pressure is not used to make a diagnosis of hypertension. Treatment of hypertension includes lifestyle management including dietary changes and exercise as well as a variety of medications (angiotensin converting enzyme inhibitors, angiotensin receptor blockers, beta-blockers, calcium channel blockers). Chapter 21 🌐 contains an in-depth discussion of hypertension guidelines and treatment.

Classification of Blood Pressure

The National Heart, Lung, and Blood Institute (NHLBI) has classified two levels of high blood pressure. A blood pressure reading below 120/80 mmHg is considered normal. Blood pressures under 140/90 mmHg are classified as either normal or prehypertension. Prehypertension is systolic blood pressures between 120 and 137, or diastolic readings between 80 and 89. Hypertension is considered when the blood pressure reading is 140/90 mmHg. These clas-

---

CHART 37–7 | **Inaccuracies in Measurement of Blood Pressure**

Inaccuracies in measurement of blood pressure are common clinical problems and can occur due to human error or device error for numerous reasons:

Inappropriately sized cuffs (too wide or too narrow)

Incorrect cuff positioning

Incorrect cuff wrapping (too loose or uneven)

Failure to allow a rest period before measurement

Deflating the cuff too quickly or too slowly

Inaccurate inflation level

Not measuring in both arms

Failure to palpate maximal systolic pressure before auscultation

Improper position of the arm (above or below heart level)

Poor observer concentration

Lack of repeated measurements

Poorly fitting stethoscope.

Sources: Jones, D. W., Apperl, L. J., Sheps, S. G., Roccella, E. J., & Lenfant, C. (2003). Measuring blood pressure accurately: New and persistent challenges. *JAMA, 289*(8), 1027–1030; McAlister, F. A., & Straus, S. E. (2001). Measurement of blood pressure: An evidenced based review. *British Medical Journal, 322*(7291), 908–911.

CHART 37–8 Technique for Measurement of Blood Pressure

The intent and purpose of the measurement should be explained to the subject in a reassuring manner, and every effort should be made to put the subject at ease.

The sequential steps for measuring the blood pressure in the upper extremity, as for routine screening and monitoring purposes, should include the following:

1. Have paper and pen at hand for immediate recording of the pressure.

2. Seat the subject in a quiet, calm environment with her bared arm resting on a standard table or other support so the midpoint of the upper arm is at the level of the heart.

3. Estimate by inspection or measure with a tape the circumference of the bare upper arm at the midpoint between the acromion and olecranon process (between the shoulder and elbow), and select an appropriately sized cuff. The bladder inside the cuff should encircle 80% of the arm in adults and 100% of the arm in children under 13 years old. If in doubt, use a larger cuff. If the available cuff is too small, this should be noted.

4. Palpate the brachial artery and place the cuff so that the midline of the bladder is over the arterial pulsation; then wrap and secure the cuff snugly around the subject's bare upper arm. Avoid rolling up the sleeve in such a manner that it forms a tight tourniquet around the upper arm. Loose application of the cuff results in overestimation of the pressure. The lower edge of the cuff should be 1 inch (2 centimeters) above the antecubital fossa (bend of the elbow), where the head of the stethoscope is to be placed.

5. Place the manometer so that the center of the mercury column or aneroid dial is at eye level and easily visible to the observer, and the tubing from the cuff is unobstructed.

6. Inflate the cuff rapidly to 70 mmHg, and increase by 10 mmHg increments while palpating the radial pulse. Note the level of pressure at which the pulse disappears and subsequently reappears during deflation. This procedure, the *palpatory method*, provides a necessary preliminary approximation of the systolic blood pressure to ensure an adequate level of inflation when the actual, auscultatory measurement is made. The palpatory method is particularly useful to avoid underinflation of the cuff in patients with an auscultatory gap and overinflation in those with very low blood pressure.

7. Place the earpieces of the stethoscope into the ear canals, angled forward to fit snugly. Switch the stethoscope head to the low-frequency position (bell). The setting can be confirmed by listening as the stethoscope head is tapped gently.

8. Place the head of the stethoscope over the brachial artery pulsation, just above and medial to the antecubital fossa but below the lower edge of the cuff, and hold it firmly in place, making sure that the head makes contact with the skin around its entire circumference. Wedging the head of the stethoscope under the edge of the cuff may free up one hand but results in considerable extraneous noise.

9. Inflate the bladder rapidly and steadily to a pressure 20 to 30 mmHg above the level previously determined by palpation, and then partially unscrew (open) the valve and deflate the bladder at 2 mm/s while listening for the appearance of the Korotkoff's sounds.

10. As the pressure in the bladder falls, note the level of the pressure on the manometer at the first appearance of repetitive sounds (Phase I), at the muffling of these sounds (Phase IV), and when they disappear (Phase V). During the period the Korotkoff's sounds are audible, the rate of deflation should be no more than 2 millimeters per pulse beat, thereby compensating for both rapid and slow heart rates.

11. After the last Korotkoff's sound is heard, the cuff should be deflated slowly for at least another 10 mmHg, to ensure that no further sounds are audible, and then rapidly and completely deflated. The subject should be allowed to rest for at least 30 seconds.

12. The systolic (Phase I) and diastolic (Phase V) pressures should be immediately recorded, rounded off (upward) to the nearest 2 mmHg. In children, and when sounds are heard nearly to a level of 0 mmHg, the Phase IV pressure should also be recorded. All values should be recorded together with the name of the subject, the date and time of the measurement, the arm on which the measurement was made, the subject's position, and the cuff size (when a nonstandard size is used).

13. The measurement should be repeated after at least 30 seconds, and the two readings averaged. In clinical situations additional measurements can be made in the same or opposite arm, and in the same or an alternative position.

Source: Perloff, D., Grim, C., Flack, J., Frohlich, E., Hill, M., McDonald, M., et al. (Writing Group). (1993). *Human blood pressure determination by sphygmomanometry* (American Heart Association, Product Code: 2460-2467). Dallas, TX: American Heart Association.

sifications are for adults over age 18 who are not on medicine for high blood pressure, are not having a short-term serious illness, and do not have other conditions such as diabetes or kidney disease. An exception to this classification is that a blood pressure of 130/80 mmHg or higher is considered high blood pressure in persons with diabetes and chronic kidney disease (NHLBI, 2008). Classifications, prevention, and management of hypertension are discussed in detail in Chapter 21 ⊙.

Health Promotion: Preventing Hypertension

The National High Blood Pressure Education Program (NHBPEP), established in 1972, is a cooperative effort among professional and voluntary health agencies, state health departments, and many community groups. The NHBPEP is administered and coordinated by the National Heart, Lung, and Blood Institute (NHLBI). The goal of the NHBPEP is to reduce death and disability related to high blood pressure through programs of professional, patient, and public education. Another goal of the NHBPEP is to achieve the *Healthy People 2010* heart disease and stroke objectives for the nation (DHHS, 2004). Strategies to meet the program's goal include developing and disseminating science-based-educational materials and developing partnerships among the program participants.

Assessment of Oxygen Delivery

Pulse oximetry allows noninvasive estimation of hemoglobin oxygen saturation, or SpO_2, which is the amount of hemoglobin saturated with oxygen (Figure 37–10 ■). These devices work by using a light sensor containing two sources of light (red and infrared) that are absorbed by hemoglobin and then transmitted through the tissue to a photodetector. The amount of light transmitted through the tissue is converted to a digital value, which represents the percentage of hemoglobin saturated with oxygen (Lynn-McHale & Carlson, 2005).

Normal oxygen saturation values are 97% to 99% in a healthy individual, but a value of 95% is clinically acceptable in a patient with a normal hemoglobin level (Lynn-McHale & Carlson, 2005). It should be reinforced that tissue oxygenation is not reflected by oxygen saturation because the affinity of hemoglobin to oxygen may actually either impair or enhance the way oxygen is released at the tissue level. Additionally, oxygen saturation does not reflect a patient's ability to ventilate, and thus its clinical use is limited in patients with obstructive pulmonary disease (Lynn-McHale & Carlson, 2005). SpO_2 values, however, are often monitored to allow for observations of trends and changes over time. For example, in a patient with emphysema, an SpO_2 of 93% might be considered a normal baseline. If however, he had an exacerbation of symptoms and his SpO_2 dropped to 90% or lower, the finding would be significant and reportable.

Oxygen saturation can be measured from several sites, including fingers, toes, and earlobes. It is important to remember that some situations—such as low perfusion, low temperature, anemia, discoloration of the nail bed, and even carbon monoxide poisoning,—will affect the ability of the sensor to estimate venous oxygen saturation accurately. The device should not be used on the same extremity as a blood pressure cuff, which may interrupt blood supply (Docherty, 2002b). The accuracy of the measurement is dependent on peripheral circulation, which may be compromised in a critically ill adult. Pulse oximetry, as a simple, noninvasive monitoring device, can be used continuously to assess adequacy of oxygen delivery. It may also be employed as a substitute for frequent arterial blood gas analysis, which involves needlesticks to obtain arterial blood (Docherty, 2002b). Therefore, pulse oximetry is efficient in that it can save nursing time, cost, and patient discomfort.

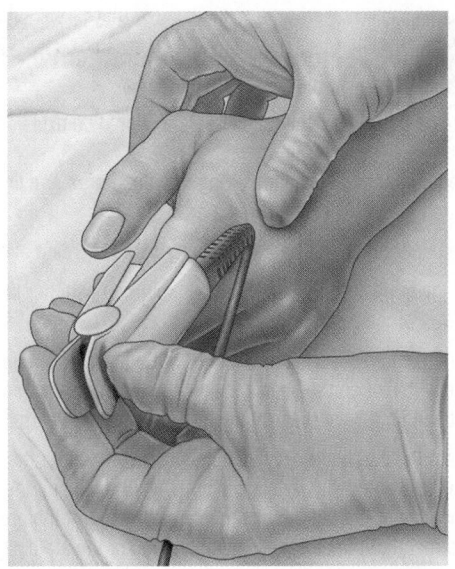

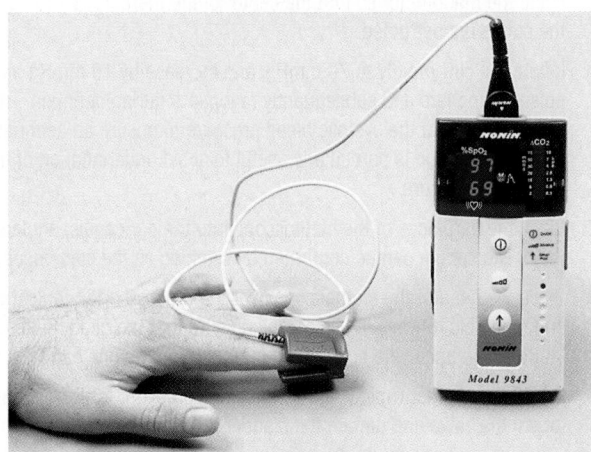

FIGURE 37–10 ■ Pulse oximeter.

■ Summary

A thorough and accurate cardiovascular assessment is an important nursing tool. Findings from cardiovascular assessments can lead to early identification of potentially life-threatening conditions and provide an opportunity for timely application of preventative measures and treatment modalities. Cardiovascular assessment skills are mandatory in acute care as well as in many other nursing settings. Experience with cardiovascular assessment allows a nurse to validate and interpret findings in order to implement appropriate therapeutic interventions. Nurses may implement preventative strategies, initiate treatment plans, or provide education or counseling.

NCLEX® REVIEW

1. The nurse determines a male patient with hypertension and hypertriglyceridemia meets the criteria for metabolic syndrome when the cardiovascular assessment demonstrates which finding?
   1. Random blood sugar is 150 mg/dL.
   2. Waist circumference is 110 cm.
   3. High density lipids, HDLs, are 52 mg/dL.
   4. Fasting blood sugar is 100 mg/dL.

2. When assessing the medication history of a patient with heart disease the nurse would be most concerned when the patient reports frequent use of which medication?
   1. Proton pump inhibitor
   2. Antacids
   3. Bulk forming laxatives
   4. Decongestants

3. A patient reports having difficulty sleeping at night secondary to becoming short of breath when lying down. In order to further assess the degree of orthopnea, the nurse should ask which question.

1. "How often do you wake up at night?"

2. "How many pillows do you sleep on?"

3. "Do you experience palpitations that awaken you?"

4. "How often do you get up to urinate during the night?"

4. When auscultating heart sounds the nurse hears a third heart sound and recognizes the patient has which condition?

1. Diastolic dysfunction

2. Systolic dysfunction

3. Conduction defect of the SA node

4. Dysfunctional mitral valve

Answers for review questions appear in Appendix D

KEY TERMS

abdominojugular reflux *p.1061*
auscultation *p.1063*
bruits *p.1067*
cyanosis *p.1060*
dyspnea *p.1055*

edema *p.1056*
heaves *p.1063*
jugular venous pressure (JVP) *p.1060*
murmurs *p.1066*
nocturia *p.1055*

orthopnea *p.1055*
palpitations *p.1055*
syncope *p.1056*
thrills *p.1063*
turgor *p.1062*

EXPLORE PEARSON mynursingkit™

MyNursingKit is your one stop for online chapter review materials and resources. Prepare for success with additional NCLEX®-style practice questions, interactive assignments and activities, web links, animations and videos, and more!

Register your access code from the front of your book at
www.mynursingkit.com

REFERENCES

Allen, J. K. (2000). Genetics and cardiovascular disease. *Nursing Clinics of North America, 35*(3), 653–661.

American Heart Association. (2006). *Our 2006 Diet and Lifestyle Recommendations.* Retrieved July 2, 2008, from http://www.americanheart.org/presenter.jhtml?identifier=851

American Heart Association. (2008a). *Metabolic syndrome.* Retrieved January 22, 2008, from http://www.americanheart.org/presenter.jhtml?identifier=4756

American Heart Association. (2008b). *Women and coronary artery disease.* Retrieved February 22, 2008, from http://www.americanheart.org/presenter.jhtml?identifier=2859

Bhatnagar, A. (2006). Environmental cardiology: Studying mechanistic links between pollution and heart disease. *Circulation Research, 99*, 692–705.

Centers for Disease Control and Prevention. (2008). *Physical activity for everyone.* Retrieved July 2, 2008 from http://www.cdc.gov/nccdphp/dnpa/physical/everyone/index.htm

D'Amico, D., & Barbarito C. (2007). *Health and physical assessment in nursing.* Upper Saddle River, NJ: Pearson Prentice Hall.

D'Amore, S., & Mora, S. (2006). Gender-specific prediction of cardiac disease: Importance of risk factors and exercise variables. *Cardiology in Review, 14*(6), 281–285.

Docherty, B. (2002a). Cardiorespiratory physical assessment for the acutely ill: 1. *British Journal of Nursing, 11*(11), 750–758.

Docherty, B. (2002b). Cardiorespiratory physical assessment for the acutely ill: 2. *British Journal of Nursing, 11*(12), 800–807.

Gallacher, J. E., Sweetman, P. M., Yarnell, J. W., Elwood, P. C., & Stansfeld, S. A. (2003). Is type A behavior really a trigger for coronary heart disease events? *Psychosomatic Medicine, 65*, 339–346.

Garg, N., & Garg, N. (2000). Jugular venous pulse: An appraisal. *Journal of Indian Academy of Clinical Medicine, 1*(3), 260–269.

Garrett, A. P. (1997). Assessing cardiovascular status in the older adult with cognitive impairments. *Journal of Cardiovascular Nursing, 11*(4), 1–11.

Jones, D. W., Apperl, L. J., Sheps, S. G., Roccella, E. J., & Lenfant, C. (2003). Measuring blood pressure accurately: New and persistent challenges. *JAMA, 289*(8):1027–1030.

Kahn, H. S., & Valdez, R. (2003). Metabolic risks identified by the combination of enlarged waist and elevated triacylglycerol concentration. *American Journal of Clinical Nutrition, 78*(5), 928–934.

Kahn, R., Buse, J., Ferrannini, E., & Stern, M. (2005). The metabolic syndrome: Time for a critical appraisal. *Diabetes Care, 28*(9), 2289–2304.

Ko, D. T., Hebert, P. R., Coffey, C. S., Sedrakyan, A., Curtis, J. P., & Krumholz, H. M. (2002). B-Blocker therapy and symptoms of depression, fatigue, and sexual dysfunction. *JAMA, 288*(3), 351–357.

Laszlo, B. et al. (2004). Novel Associations Between Bioavailable Estradiol and Adipokines in Elderly Women with Different Phenotypes of Obesity: Implications for Atherogenesis. *Circulation. 110:*2246–2252.

Lynn-McHale, D. J., & Carlson, K. K. (2005). *AACN procedure manual for critical care* (5th ed.). Philadelphia: W. B. Saunders.

National Heart, Lung, and Blood Institute. (2008). What Is High Blood Pressure? Retrieved January 25, 2008 from http://www.nhlbi.nih.gov

National Institutes of Health. (2001). *Third Report of the National Cholesterol Education Program Expert Panel on Detection, Evaluation, and Treatment of High Blood Cholesterol in Adults (Adult Treatment Panel III)* (NIH Publication 01-3670). Bethesda, MD: Author.

O'Connor, D. L. (1998). The art of auscultation. *Patient Care, 32*(20), 35–36, 38, 41–2.

Schroeder, K. E., Narkiewicz, K., Kato, M., Pesek, C., Phillips, B., Davison, D., et al. (2000). Personality type and neural circulatory control. *Hypertension, 36*, 830–833.

Smith-Stoner, M. (2006). Caring for patients of diverse religious traditions; Considerations for Buddhist clients in home care. *Home Healthcare Nurse, 24*(7), 459–466.

Snyder, M., & Miska, K. (2003). Snyder related complementary therapies: Their use in critical care units. *Critical Care Clinics of North America, 15*, 341–346.

Thomas, S. A., Liehr, P., DeKeyser, F., Frazier, L., & Friedmann, E. (2002). A review of nursing research on blood pressure. *Journal of Nursing Scholarship, 34*(4), 313–321.

Urden, L. D., Lough, M. E., & Stacy, K. M. (2006). *Thelan's critical care nursing: Diagnosis and management* (4th ed.). St. Louis: Mosby.

U.S. Department of Health and Human Services. (2004). *Healthy People 2010.* Retrieved on July 10, 2006, from http://www.health.gov/healthypeople/document/

Whetstone, G., & Boswell, S. (2002). The geriatric heart: Nurses need to be aware of how aging and disease affect the myocardium. *American Journal of Nursing, 102*(Suppl.), 22–24.

Williams, R. R., Hunt, S. C., Heiss, G., Province, M. A., Bensen, J. T., Higgins, M., et al. (2001). Usefulness of cardiovascular family history data for population-based preventive medicine and medical research. (The Health Family Tree Study and the NHLBI Family Heart Study). *American Journal of Cardiology, 87*(2), 129–135.

CHAPTER 38

Nursing Interpretation of the Electrocardiogram

Kathleen Osborn
Annita Watson

Outcome-Based Learning Objectives

After studying this chapter, the learner will be able to:

1. Describe the configuration of the normal electrocardiogram (ECG).

2. Identify and calculate heart rate, rhythm, PR interval, QRS complex, and QT interval for normal and abnormal cardiac rhythms.

3. Discuss the etiology and significant ECG features of the following dysrhythmia classifications: sinus, atrial, junctional, block, ventricular, and asystole.

4. Interpret the significance of each of the dysrhythmias and formulate nursing responsibilities for each dysrhythmia.

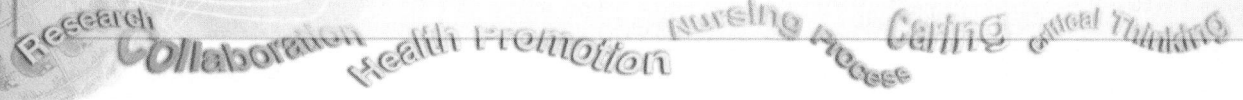

Research   Collaboration   Health Promotion   Nursing Process   Caring   Critical Thinking

THE ELECTROCARDIOGRAM (ECG) is the most important and definitive noninvasive diagnostic procedure that shows a graphic depiction of the electrical activity of the heart. It is used to assist the health care team in diagnosing and monitoring cardiac electrical system function. The ECG was first used less than a century ago, in the early 1900s. Initially the equipment was large and cumbersome and had limited use. As equipment improved, ECG bedside monitoring became possible in the 1960s. Today, due to increased patient acuity levels, the use of ECGs has become widespread, moving outside the traditional critical and emergent care settings. Thus, so has the expectation for nurses to have the knowledge and understanding of ECG interpretation. Nurses are expected to read and interpret ECGs when planning, providing, and evaluating patient care (Holtschneider, McBroom, & Patterson, 2006). In order to orient the learner to the cardiac conduction system, this chapter provides a brief overview of the anatomy and electrophysiology of the heart. This review is followed by information on how to obtain the graphic representation of the electrical activity of the heart, the ECG (also referred to as EKG). The equipment and skills needed to obtain an ECG are described. The learner is guided in the necessary steps for interpretation of both normal and abnormal cardiac rhythms. This is followed by a description of the appropriate nursing interventions and evaluation criteria.

◼ Anatomy of the Heart

Recognition of common cardiac rhythms measured by an electrocardiogram requires a basic understanding of cardiac anatomy and physiology. A complete description of the cardiac anatomy is outlined in Chapter 37 ☺. Knowledge of the cardiac conduction system needed for ECG interpretation is presented here.

Cardiac Conduction System

The heart contains its own **cardiac conduction system** composed of specialized cell fibers called either **nodes** or **bundles.** These fibers enable the heart to generate and transmit action potentials without stimulation from the body's nervous systems. The heart's conduction system is responsible for the electrical activity that controls each normal heartbeat. The special cells and fibers called nodes or bundles are located beneath the endocardium, or inner lining of the heart, in the cardiac conduction system. These are referred to as the sinoatrial (SA) node, the atrioventricular (AV) node, and the Purkinje network (Figure 38–1 ◼). Although the sympathetic nervous system (SNS) and the parasympathetic nervous system (PSNS) innervate the heart, these external neural impulses are not needed to maintain the cardiac cycle. The pacemaker cells are capable of initiating electrical activity automatically and act as a pacemaker; there-

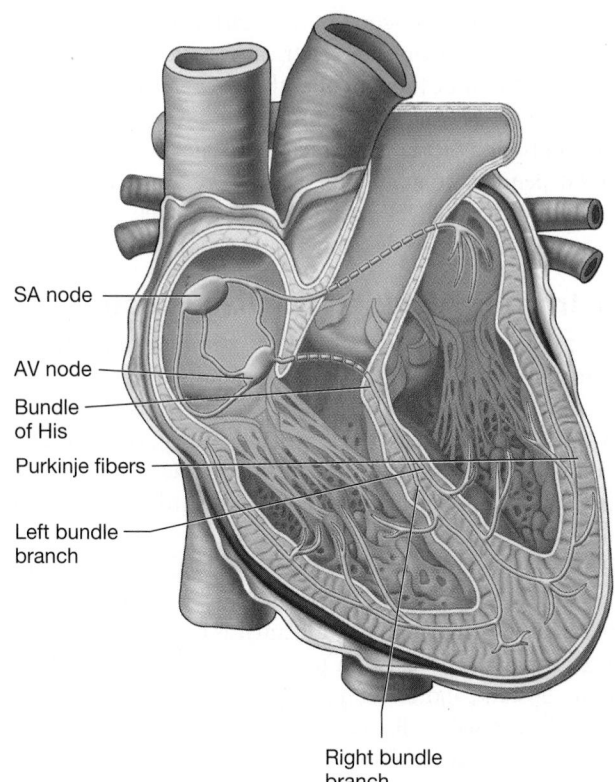

FIGURE 38–1 ■ Electrical conduction system of the heart.

fore, the heart will beat in the absence of any nervous system connection. The SNS and the PSNS affect only the speed of the cardiac cycles and the diameter of the coronary arteries. It is essential to understand the heart's electrical conduction system in order to be able to understand an ECG strip interpretation. Each component of the system follows.

Sinoatrial (SA) Node

The **sinoatrial (SA) node** is located in the upper posterior portion of the right atrial wall, near the opening of the superior vena cava. The node is made up of hundreds of cells that compose a knot of modified heart muscle. The SA node is capable of generating impulses that travel throughout the muscle fibers of both atria, resulting in atrial depolarization. The SA node is commonly called the primary pacemaker of the heart because under normal conditions it depolarizes more consistently, frequently, and reliably than other normal pacemaker cells. The normal firing rate of the SA node is 60 to 100 beats per minute. Depolarization of the atria occurs as the impulse leaves the SA node and travels in a downward or waterfall fashion through the conduction pathways. If the SA node (pacemaker) fails to fire due to some abnormality, other pacemaker cells are able to take over, that is, the AV node or the Purkinje network. The emergence of a pacemaker that is lower in the heart, which sustains a heart rate when the SA node fails, is referred to as an **escape** mechanism or rhythm. During an escape rhythm, the heart rate is slower than the dominant pacemaker. If the rhythm originates in the junctional tissue, it is referred to as a junctional escape rhythm. If the rhythm originates in the ventricle, it is referred to as a ventricular escape rhythm.

Intra-Atrial Pathways

The **intra-atrial pathways,** located in the atria, transport impulses from the SA node to the AV node. There are three pathways: the anterior, middle, and posterior intranodal or intra-atrial pathways, and Bachmann bundle. **Bachmann bundle,** which is a part of the anterior pathway, is a group of fibers contained in the left atrium. All of the intranodal pathways and Bachmann bundle receive electrical impulses as they exit the SA node, distribute these impulses throughout the atria, and transmit them to the AV node (Beasley, 2003).

Atrioventricular (AV) Node and AV Junction

The **atrioventricular (AV) node** is located on the floor of the right atrium just above the tricuspid valve. Electrical activity at the AV node is delayed approximately 0.05 second to allow for atrial contraction, which increases the amount of blood reaching the ventricles. Atrial contraction, commonly referred to as **atrial kick,** augments the blood supply going to the ventricles and ultimately cardiac output. This delay also serves to stop the transmission for a very rapid succession of impulses that can occur under abnormal conditions. These abnormalities, called atrial flutter/fibrillation, are discussed later in the chapter.

The AV junction contains fibers that can polarize spontaneously, forming an impulse that can spread through the heart chambers. This means that if the SA node fails or falls below its normal range, the AV node can take over, thus assuming the role of a secondary pacemaker. Under normal conditions the AV junction is the only pathway for the conduction of atrial impulses to the ventricles.

Bundle of His and Bundle Branches

The **bundle of His** is approximately 15 millimeters long and lies on top of the interventricular septum, between the right and left ventricles. This area, also referred to as the common bundle, contains pacemaker cells that have the ability to self-initiate electrical activity at a rate of 38 to 60 beats per minute. At the top of the interventricular septum, the bundle of His divides into two bundle branches, the right and left bundles. The right bundle, a long, thin structure that lies beneath the endocardium, runs down the right side of the interventricular septum and terminates at the papillary muscles in the right atrium. The left bundle is shorter than the right bundle and divides into pathways that spread from the left side of the interventricular septum throughout the left ventricle. The two pathways of the left bundle branch are called **fascicles,** one being anterior and the other posterior. The anterior fascicle carries electrical impulses to the anterior wall of the left ventricle. The posterior fascicle spreads electrical impulses to the posterior ventricular wall. The bundle branches continue to divide until they finally terminate in the Purkinje network fibers.

Purkinje Network Fibers

Purkinje network fibers consist of a network of fibers that carry impulses directly to the ventricles. The rapid spread of the electrical impulse through the left and right bundle branches, the Purkinje network fibers, and the ventricular muscle initiates ventricular contraction. Purkinje fibers also may be pacemaker cells; they fire at an intrinsic rate of 20 to 40 beats per minute.

Cardiac Cells

There are two basic cardiac cell groups: the myocardial working cells and the specialized pacemaker cells of the electrical conduction system. The atria and the ventricles are constructed of myocardial working cells, which have an abundance of contractile filaments needed to generate cardiac muscle contraction. The cardiac muscle contraction is what actually pumps the blood through and out of the heart into the pulmonic and the systemic circulation. The myocardial working cells have the ability to contract in response to chemical, electrical, or mechanical stimuli.

The second type of cardiac cell is the specialized **pacemaker cell** whose primary function is to generate and conduct electrical impulses (stimuli). These cells found in the heart wall and septum (membrane dividing the right and left sides of the heart) control the heart rate and rhythm by coordinating regular cardiac muscle depolarization (contraction) (see Figure 38–1 ■, p. 1075). The myocardial contractions pump the blood through and out of the heart.

The term **threshold** refers to the point at which an electrical stimulus produces a cell response. When a stimulus is strong enough for cardiac cells to reach this threshold, all of the cells will respond to the stimulus and cause a muscle contraction. This is called the "all-or-none phenomenon"; in other words, either all the cells respond, or none of the cells respond. This principle allows for a coordinated muscle contraction and greater efficiency in pumping blood. Cardiac cells possess four primary characteristics: automaticity, excitability, conductivity, and contractility. These characteristics are described next.

Automaticity

Automaticity is the ability of the pacemaker cells to generate their own electrical impulses without depending on nervous system stimulation external to the heart. This spontaneous activity is what produces regular depolarization of the cardiac muscle. This characteristic is specific to only certain pacemaker cell sites within the conduction system. These cell sites are the sinoatrial (SA) node, the atrioventricular (AV) node, and the Purkinje network fibers.

Excitability

Excitability is the ability of the electrical cell to respond to a stimulus. This ability also is referred to as irritability, and all electrical cardiac cells possess this property. When cardiac cells are highly irritable, a cell other than the normal pacemaker may cause a contraction. Cell irritability can be caused by a number of problems, including cardiac muscle ischemia due to hypoxia, or a lack of oxygen. This is the most common cause of cardiac dysrhythmias, the abnormal rhythms of the heart.

Conductivity

Conductivity is the ability of the cardiac cell to accept and then transmit a stimulus to other cardiac cells. All cardiac cells share this characteristic, thereby portraying the all-or-none property of the heart muscle; the cardiac cells function as a unit.

Contractility

Contractility is the ability of the cardiac cells to shorten and cause the muscle to contract in response to an electrical stimulus. This ability also is referred to as rhythmicity. Contractility is

the only mechanical function of the heart. Excitability, conductivity, and automaticity are electrical functions of the heart. Contractility may be thought of as the mechanical coordination of cardiac muscle contractions producing a heartbeat.

In addition to these cell characteristics, normal cardiac function is dependent on maintaining electrolyte concentrations inside and outside the cell membrane. Specific electrolytes and their relationship to cardiac function are described next.

Electrolytes Affecting Cardiac Function

An electrolyte is a substance or compound whose molecules dissociate into charged components, or **ions,** when placed in water, producing positively and negatively charged ions. A positively charged ion is called a **cation**. A negatively charged ion is called an **anion**. Myocardial cells are bathed in electrolyte solutions; thus, both the mechanical and the electrical cardiac functions are influenced by electrolytes.

The major cations that affect cardiac function are potassium (K), sodium (Na), and calcium (Ca). Magnesium (Mg) also is an important cation, but is not as influential as K, Na, and Ca with regard to stimulating the action potential discussed here. Magnesium, potassium, and calcium are intracellular cations, meaning they reside within the cell; whereas Na is an extracellular cation, residing outside the cell. Chloride (Cl) is a major anion in electrocardiac function. Chloride provides electroneutrality in relation to Na. Transport of chloride is passive and follows the active transport of sodium (Na).

Abnormally high or low levels of electrolytes, especially K, can potentiate very serious, life-threatening ventricular dysrhythmias. Therefore, monitoring and maintaining normal electrolyte values is essential. Nurses have a responsibility to report immediately any significant abnormal values to the health care provider.

 Assessing laboratory values is an essential nursing responsibility. Each time laboratory results are completed on a patient the nurse needs to compare the new results with reference normal values and previous findings, if applicable, and report significant changes and/or trends.

Cardiac Depolarization and Repolarization

When impulses travel through the myocardial muscle, they cause changes in the muscle fibers referred to as depolarization and repolarization. **Cardiac depolarization** refers to cardiac muscle contraction resulting from an electrolyte exchange in the cardiac cells, which then changes the electrical charge. As with all cells of the body, cardiac cells are electrically charged, with the inside of the cell more negative than the outside. To move Na and K across the cell membrane requires active transport by a mechanism referred to as the sodium-potassium adenosine triphosphatase (ATP) pump (Na-K pump). The Na-K pump is an energy-driven mechanism by which 3 Na ions are pumped out for every 2 K ions. Two enzymes, adenosine triphosphate (ATP) and adenosine triphosphatase (ATPase), are involved in the energy production for the pump (Porth, 2004).

Prior to depolarization the cells must be in a resting state, referred to as the **resting membrane potential.** In this state the myocardial cell is negatively charged to −90 millivolts (mV). This negative state is maintained until depolarization occurs.

When a muscle cell receives a stimulus due to the Na-K pump exchange, a rapid change occurs in the resting membrane potential, known as the **action potential,** which is measured in **millivolts** (a unit of electrical voltage or potential difference equal to one-thousandth of a volt). Once the action potential occurs, the cell moves toward a positive charge. The four phases (0–4) of the action potential are shown in Figure 38–2 ■. Phase 0 is rapid depolarization, phase 1 is rapid repolarization, phase 2 is the plateau, phase 3 is final repolarization, and phase 4 is the resting state. To generate this action potential and the resulting muscle depolarization, the threshold potential must be reached, which is phase 0. To initiate phase 0, Na enters the cell causing a sharp positively charged rise of the intracellular ions. The cell moves from −90 millivolts (mV) in its resting state to a positive 15 to 30 millivolts, causing myocardial depolarization to occur. When the threshold is reached, the cell will continue to depolarize with no further stimulation; this phenomenon is referred to as automaticity. During phase 1, the depolarized stage, the interior of the cell has a net positive charge. In this effort to continue to make the inside of the cell more positive, Ca enters; this is phase 2, the plateau phase. During phase 3 the calcium channels close, and Na is pulled from the cell by the Na-K pump; thus the cell is returning to its polarized negative resting membrane potential state (phase 4) (Figure 38–3 ■). The first area of the cardiac muscle to be depolarized is the first area that is repolarized. For example, after the atria depolarize they repolarize while the ventricles are depolarizing. Thus, when the SA node fires again, the muscle will be ready to respond with a new action potential.

Cardiac repolarization is the process whereby the depolarized cell is polarized, causing a return to the resting membrane potential (see Figure 38–2 ■). Repolarization also is referred to as the recovery phase that every cardiac cell must go through in order to be ready to accept another stimulus. It is a slower process than that of depolarization. During repolarization the

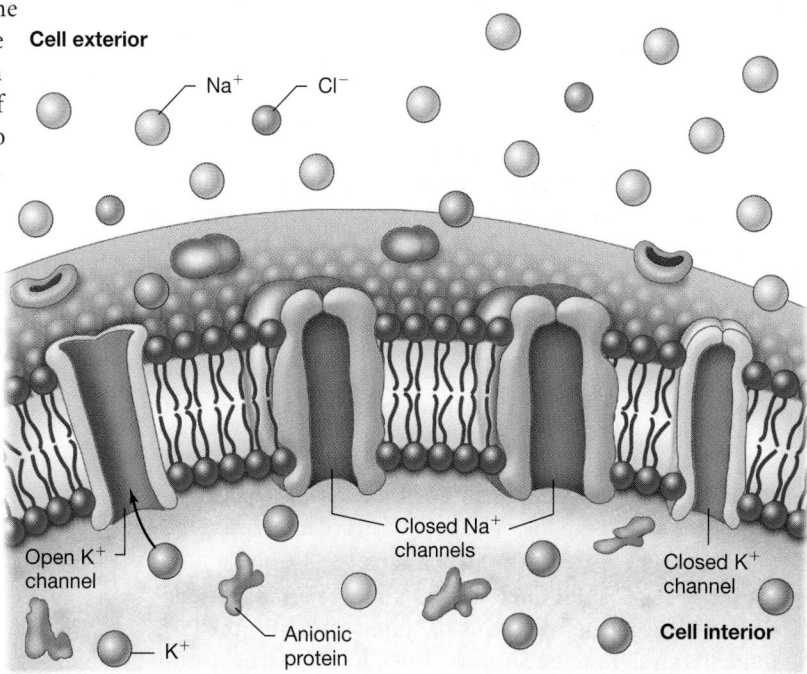

Cell exterior

Na⁺   Cl⁻

Open K⁺ channel

Closed Na⁺ channels

Closed K⁺ channel

Cell interior

K⁺   Anionic protein

FIGURE 38–3 ■ Electrolyte movement during an action potential.

muscle is *refractory* (resistant) to stimulation. This **refractory period** consists of two stages; the absolute and the relative refractory periods. During the **absolute refractory period,** which is the majority of time for repolarization, the cardiac cell is unable to respond to any stimulus and thus cannot spontaneously depolarize (see Figure 38–2 ■).

The **relative refractory period** is a period when repolarization is almost complete (see Figure 38–2 ■). This period is known as the vulnerable period of cardiac cell repolarization. If a stimulus is strong enough, it can cause depolarization that can be life threatening. These situations are discussed later in this chapter. The refractory periods play a major role in either causing or preventing cardiac dysrhythmias. Further discussion of their role is explained regarding the various dysrhythmias and throughout the chapter.

Summary of the Cardiac Conduction System

The electrical impulse begins in the SA node located in the upper right atrium, causing atrial contraction. The impulse then travels through the atria along intra-atrial pathways to the AV node located near the center of the heart. After leaving the AV node the impulse moves down into the bundle of His, through the right and left bundle branches, and into the Purkinje network fibers, causing ventricular contraction followed by repolarization (see Figure 38–1 ■, p. 1075). Then the cycle begins again.

When caring for patients with actual or potential cardiac conduction abnormalities, it is essential that the nurse understand how the cardiac conduction system described here is graphically depicted on an electrocardiogram. Recognizing and interpreting these electrical impulses and their relationship to heart disease is an essential nursing responsibility. A discussion of how the electrical conduction system is depicted in an ECG follows.

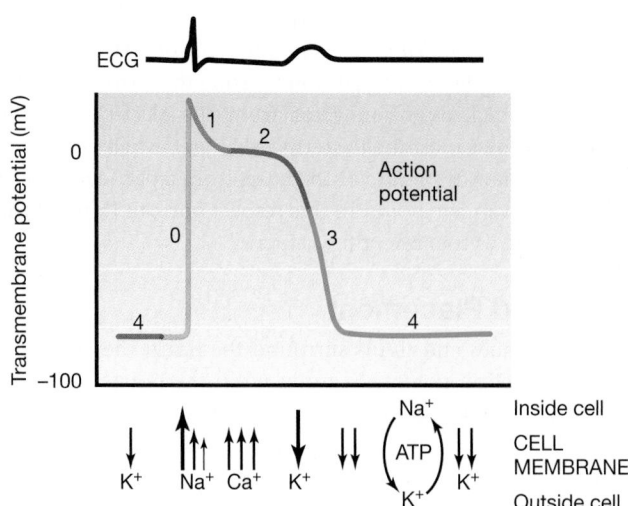

FIGURE 38–2 ■ Action potential.

Cardiac Waveform and Time Intervals Measured on ECG

When the electrical impulse leaves the SA node, a graphical representation of the signal referred to as a waveform is produced and recorded with monitoring equipment. As the electrical impulse travels through the cardiac conduction system, waveforms characteristic of a given anatomical location are recorded. These waveforms are referred to as P, Q, R, S, and T. Additionally, time intervals, which represent the time it takes for the impulse to travel from one anatomical location in the heart to another, are recorded. These time intervals are called PR, QRS, and QT. One complete cardiac cycle has five to six waveforms and time intervals. These are described here and depicted in Figure 38–4 ■.

- **P wave**—The **P wave** represents contraction or depolarization of the atria. Both the right and left atria depolarize at the same time.
- **PR interval**—The **PR interval,** sometimes referred to as the PRI or PR segment, represents the time it takes for the impulse to travel from the SA node down the intra-atrial pathways to the ventricles. In other words, it represents the beginning of the atrial contraction to the beginning of the ventricular contraction.
- **QRS complex**—The **QRS complex** consists of the Q, R, and S waves, and represents the conduction of electrical impulses from the bundle of His near the AV junction to the Purkinje network fibers located in the ventricles, causing them to depolarize.
- **J point**—The point at which the QRS meets the ST segment is called the J point.
- **ST segment**—The **ST segment** is a line extending from the S wave that gradually curves upward to the T wave, represented on the ECG as an almost isoelectric line. The ST segment signifies ventricular repolarization.
- **T wave**—The **T wave** is ventricular recovery or repolarization. This is often referred to as the resting phase of the cardiac cycle. Both the absolute and the relative refractory periods are in place during the T wave.
- **U wave**—The **U wave** is present only on some people's ECG. It follows the T wave. Its etiology is unknown, but it is frequently seen in exercise, in drug toxicity, and most frequently with low potassium levels.

Changes in the configuration of the waveforms or lengthening and/or shortening of time intervals may indicate an abnormality in the heart. These abnormalities are discussed in detail in Chapters 40, 41, 42, and 43 ☍. The following sections discuss the method used to evaluate waveforms and time intervals.

■ ECG Monitoring Equipment

Electrocardiography detects cardiac electrical impulses at various points on the surface of the body. The graphical depiction of these impulses, waveforms, and time intervals is obtained either with an electrocardiograph (ECG machine) or on a bedside cardiac monitor. To obtain an ECG tracing, specific equipment is needed including an electrode, lead wire, and monitor or oscilloscope. An **electrode** is most commonly a round adhesive pad that is impregnated with conducting gel in the center and is attached to a lead wire. Electrodes are sensing devices that detect the electrical activity of the heart and conduct the electrical impulses from the skin surface back to the ECG machine, where they are converted into waveforms. An electrode is much like a camera in that it takes pictures of the electrical activity in the heart. The electrodes are connected to a cardiac monitor by lead wires. Typically, these wires are color coded according to machine manufacturer, and these colors assist the provider in attaching the lead wires to the appropriate electrode. The cardiac monitor records the electrical impulses and provides a real-time visual tracing of the waveforms on the screen and/or a printed version on specialized ECG graph paper, described next. The printed version is called a rhythm strip or ECG strip. The rhythm strip gives the health care provider information about where the pathological processes are occurring in the heart. Figure 38–5 ■ shows the electrodes, lead wire, and cardiac monitor.

The term *lead* is used in different contexts when discussing ECGs. In addition to using the term as just described, as a connector from the electrode to the cardiac monitor, the term also is used when discussing a view or picture of the heart from a particular angle or vantage point. In this respect one can think of the lead as the "eye of the camera."

Lead Placement

Body tissues and fluids surround the heart; therefore, the electrical action potentials produced in the heart are widely conducted throughout the body via these tissues and fluids. The impulses or action potentials can be detected from any point in the body. Electrodes must be placed in certain positions on the body in order to obtain a clear picture of the electrical impulses in the heart, and there must always be a positive, a negative, and a ground electrode/lead. The ground lead minimizes outside

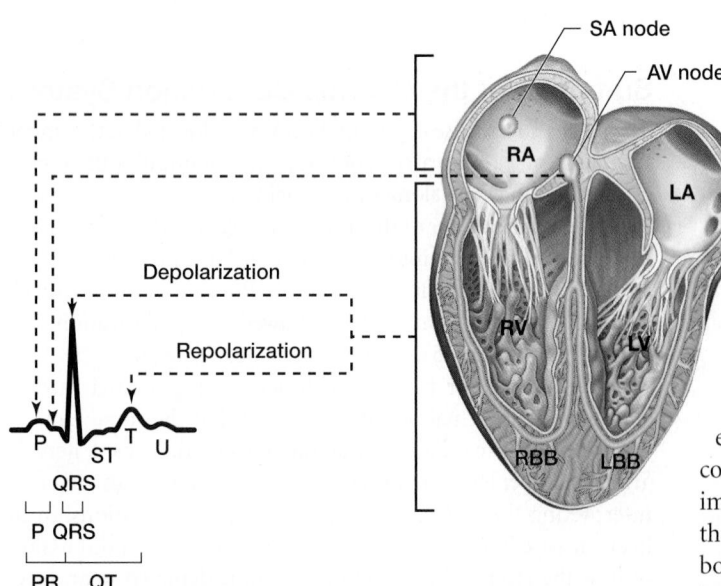

FIGURE 38–4 ■ Waveform relationship to cardiac conduction system.

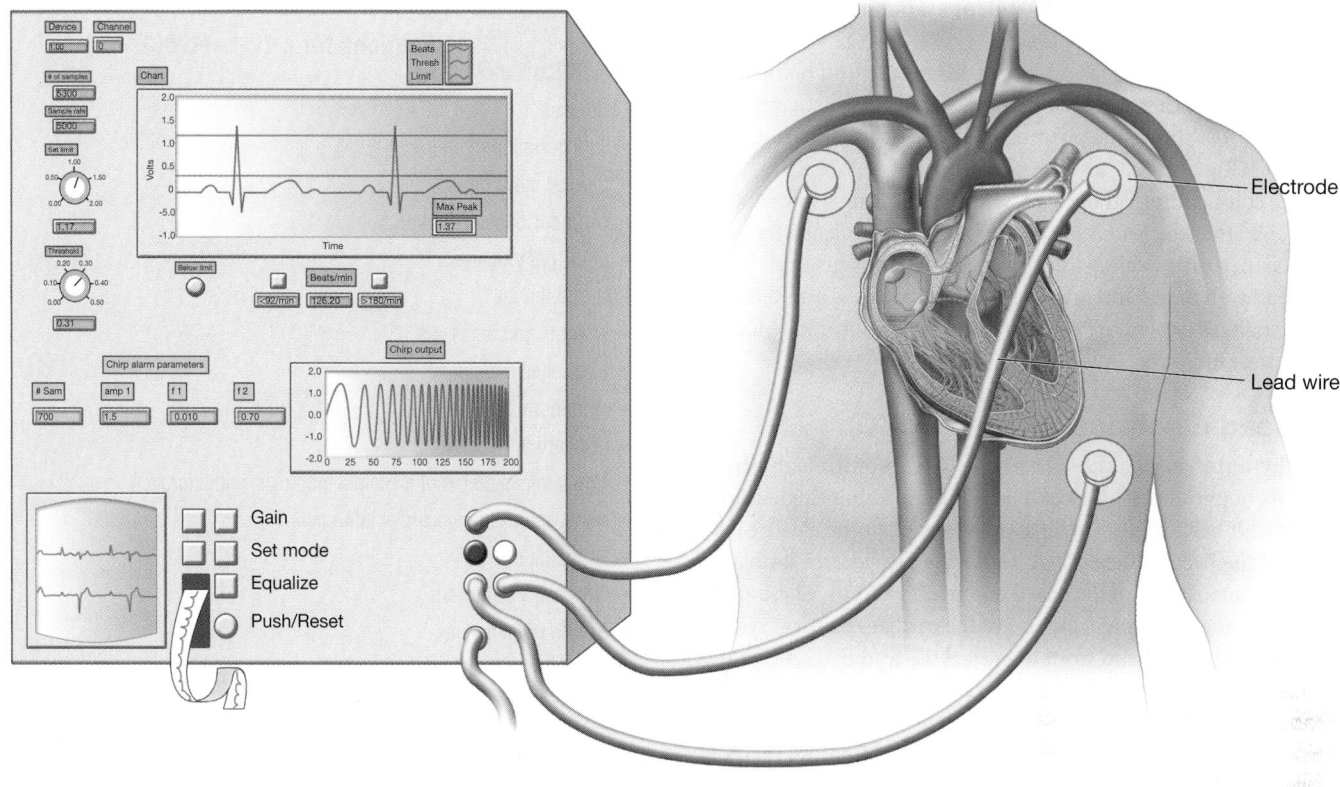

FIGURE 38–5 ■ Electrodes, lead wire, and cardiac monitor.

electrical interference. Each electrode senses the flow of current in the heart in relation to the lead axis. The **lead axis** refers to the imaginary line drawn between the positive and negative electrodes. If the axis is directed toward the positive lead, there is an upward or **positive deflection** on the ECG tracing (above the isoelectric line). If the axis is directed toward the negative lead, there is a **negative deflection** on the ECG tracing (below the iso-electric line) Figure 38–6 ■. Multiple leads, as seen with a **12-lead ECG,** view cardiac electrical conduction from different perspectives. Think of the heart on a pedestal that one is able to move around while a camera takes pictures from various angles. This gives the provider 12 different views of the cardiac electrical activity.

For bedside monitoring it is not practical or necessary to have a 12-lead ECG or 12 continuous views of the heart. Therefore, 1 or 2 of the 12 possible leads from the entire 12-lead ECG are chosen for constant bedside monitoring because they give a clear view of cardiac activity and abnormalities. To obtain a single bedside ECG rhythm strip, a minimum of three electrodes is required: one positive, one negative, and one ground. Either lead II or modified chest lead$_1$ (MCL$_1$) is commonly used for three-electrode bedside monitoring. The MCL$_1$ is one of the V leads from the 12-lead ECG that is modified for bedside monitoring. The lead chosen is dependent on the unit policy and nurse and/or health care provider preference. The specific dysrhythmia being monitored or anticipated may dictate the type of lead chosen.

No single monitoring lead is ideal for every patient. Therefore, if more than one lead or picture of the heart is required, five electrodes are placed to increase the monitor's capability beyond the three-electrode monitoring system. The five-electrode monitoring system has an exploring chest electrode that allows one to obtain the same 12 views as a 12-lead ECG when needed. However, at the bedside typically only two simultaneous leads are used to view the heart with the five-electrode system. Commonly the two leads that are run simultaneously are lead II and MCL$_1$. However, the lead or leads chosen depend on the desired view of the heart. Figure 38–6 ■ shows a cardiac rhythm strip that has simultaneous lead II and MCL$_1$ ECG views.

These two leads provide different perspectives of the various normal and abnormal ECG configurations. For example, lead II produces easily identifiable upright P waves and clear QRS

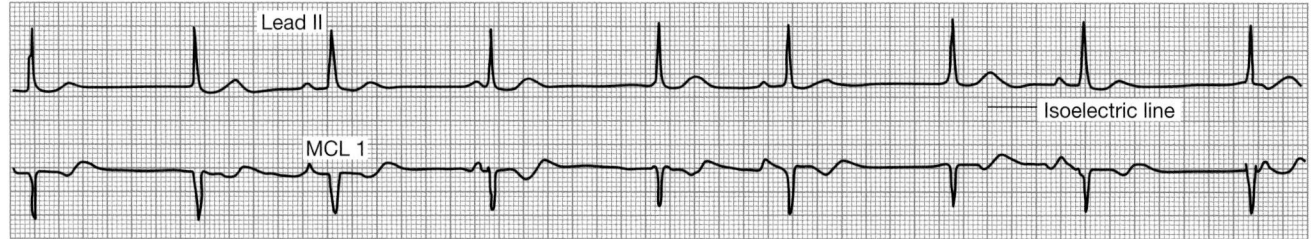

FIGURE 38–6 ■ Lead II and MCL$_1$ ECG configurations.

complexes. An MCL₁ lead is useful for evaluating abnormalities in the ventricles.

Placement of the electrodes depends on the lead being monitored and whether a three- or five-lead system is being used. Figure 38–7 ■ shows the position of the electrodes for both lead II and MCL₁.

The color coding on the lead wire gives the nurse information about whether the lead is positive or negative. Typically the color black is negative, white is positive, and green is ground. In the five-lead system red and brown colors also are used and their polarity changes depending on the lead being monitored (Morton, Fontaine, Hudak, & Gallo, 2005).

12-Lead Electrocardiogram (ECG)

The rhythm strips that have been used to demonstrate dysrhythmias throughout this chapter have all been from a single lead. A single-lead ECG rhythm strip gives one view of the electrical activity of the heart, whereas a 12-lead ECG provides 12 individual views or "snapshots" of the heart's electrical patterns. These added views provide a complete picture of the cardiac electrical system, both top to bottom and front to back. A 12-lead ECG is useful in evaluating not only the presence of damage but also the location in the heart where that damage occurred. Frequently, to assess damage accurately requires viewing the area with more than one lead. Chart 38–1 provides the indications for a 12-lead ECG.

There are 3 bipolar and 9 unipolar leads in a 12-lead ECG. A **bipolar lead** has electrodes with opposite polarity, one positive and one negative. A **unipolar lead** has only a positive polarity (Walraven, 2006). Both bipolar and unipolar leads provide information in one direction only—between two points. The two

CHART 38–1   **Indications for a 12-Lead ECG**

Evaluation of:

- Axis deviation
- Cardiac valve disease
- Chamber dilation or hypertrophy
- Chest pain/angina
- Dysrhythmias
- Effect of cardiac drugs
- Electrolyte imbalance
- Hypothermia
- Myocardial ischemia
- Myocardial patterns of ischemia, necrosis, and infarction
- New versus old myocardial infarction
- Pericarditis
- Pulmonary embolism
- Bundle branch block

dimensions on the chest in which leads can be placed are the frontal plane (up and down) and the horizontal plane (around the chest). Figure 38–8 ■ shows the horizontal plane and frontal plane views.

The axis of a lead is the imaginary line drawn between the positive and the negative electrode in a bipolar lead and between the positive electrode and the zero reference point in a unipolar lead. Thus, depending on where a given lead is placed, it provides

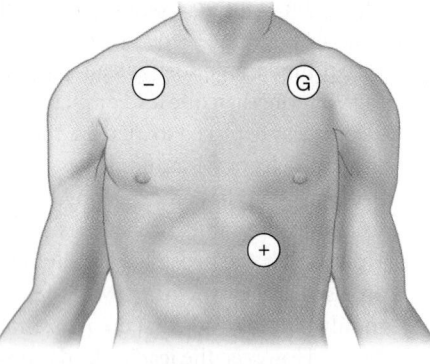

Lead II: Positive electrode left abdomen
Negative electrode right shoulder
Ground electrode left shoulder

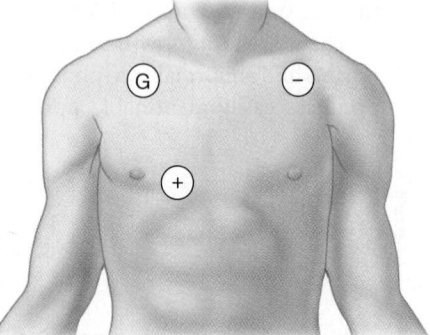

MCL₁: Positive electrode 4th ICS RSB
Negative electrode left shoulder
Ground electrode right shoulder

MCL₁ is modified chest lead 1. It's like V₁.

FIGURE 38–7 ■ Electrode placement for bedside cardiac monitoring.

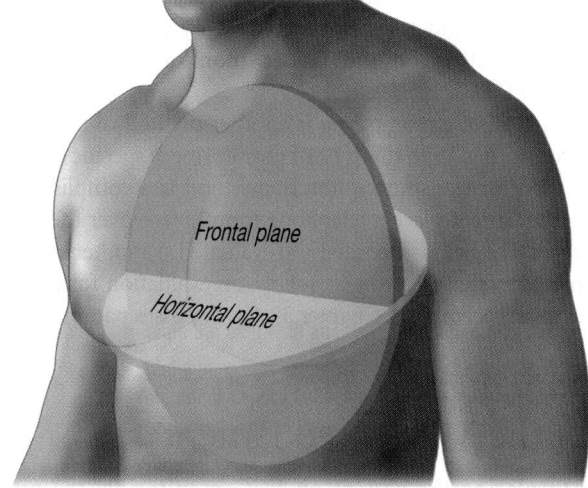

FIGURE 38–8 ■ Horizontal and frontal planes.

a picture of the electrical activity from that vantage point within the heart. Electrical current flowing toward a positive electrode creates a positive deflection on the ECG paper, whereas electrical current flowing toward a negative electrode creates a negative deflection on the ECG paper (Walraven, 2006).

The standard bipolar limb leads—I, II, III—are applied to the right arm (RA), left arm (LA), and left leg (LL). Each lead records the following electrical conduction pattern:

- Lead I records conduction from RA to LA.
- Lead II records conduction from RA to LL.
- Lead III records conduction from LA to LL.

The right leg electrode acts as a grounding electrode.

Three more frontal plane, unipolar augmented limb leads can be created by using a central terminal. Augmented leads are

so named because they generate such small waveforms that the ECG machine must augment, or increase, their size so they will show up on the ECG paper (Ellis, 2002a). These leads are aVR, aVL, and aVF. Each lead records the following electrical conduction pattern:

- aVR: central terminal to right arm
- aVL: central terminal to left arm
- aVF: central terminal to left leg.

The standard bipolar leads and the augmented limb leads provide the 6 frontal plane leads of the 12-lead ECG, whereas the 6 chest (precordial) unipolar leads, V1—V6, evaluate the horizontal plane of the heart. The positive electrode is placed on 6 different sites across the chest as shown in the diagram in Figure 39–1 ■ (p. 1121). These chest leads provide the 6 horizontal leads of the 12-lead ECG. Chart 38–2 describes the procedure for obtaining a 12-lead ECG.

For example, lead V1 evaluates the right ventricle; leads V2 and V3 span the interventricular septum; lead V4 is over the cardiac apex; and leads V5 and V6 evaluate the lateral wall. The Q wave, T wave, and ST segment are used to evaluate the presence of damage, and the lead placement is used to identify the area of damage. Chapter 40 🌐 discusses the myocardial damage associated with changes in the Q wave, T wave, and ST segment.

When performing an ECG, the nurse must have knowledge of the lead placement for each of the 12 leads. Improper placement may result in inaccurate information and treatment. The electrodes must have firm, unbroken contact with the skin. The limb leads are placed on the flat surfaces just above the wrists and ankles. If there is an amputation, the lead is placed on the remaining stump. Chest hair may interfere with skin contact and, if so, should be shaved. The type and sophistication of ECG machines varies; some can record only one lead at a time, whereas others can record 3, 6, or all 12 leads simultaneously.

CHART 38–2	12-Lead ECG Procedure
Electrode Placement	• Bring the portable ECG machine to the patient's bedside in any type of patient care setting.
	• Use 10 electrodes for the standard 12-lead ECG: 6 on the chest and 4 on the limbs. Figure 39–1 ■ (p. 1121) shows the correct placement of the electrodes.
	• Place limb electrodes away from bony prominences and areas of significant muscle movement to prevent interference of other muscle activity.
	• Palpate the intercostal spaces along the sternal border, until the fourth one is reached, for placement of the first chest electrode.
Cable Connection and Machine Operation	• Connect the cable that is attached to each of the electrodes to the ECG machine.
	• Adjust the ECG machine to obtain a clear picture of the cardiac electrical activity.
	• After completing the ECG, remove electrodes and clean the skin as necessary.
	• Leave the electrodes in place if the patient is going to have serial ECGs to ensure consistency of multiple readings.
Patient Instructions	• Explain the procedure and the rationale for the test prior to performing an ECG.
	• Advise the patient to lie still, breathe normally, and refrain from speaking while obtaining the ECG.
Documentation	• Document patient's height, weight, and use of cardiac medications.
	• Document current clinical manifestations if present and chief complaint.
	• Document reason for the ECG.
	• Record patient's response to procedure, if any.

The ECG graph paper is arranged as a series of horizontal and vertical lines. This paper is standardized to allow for consistency in ECG measurement and strip analysis. Both the amplitude and the voltage may be measured on the paper. The vertical axis measures the amplitude and is stated in millivolts (mV). Two large squares on this axis equal 1 millivolt. This measurement is rarely used because the size of the picture or millivolts can be adjusted at the monitoring station, thereby reducing the consistency of this measurement.

The horizontal axis is divided into small squares. The squares on the ECG paper are used to measure the length of time required for the electrical impulse to traverse a specific part of the heart. Figure 38–9 ■ shows an example of ECG graph paper.

These squares are used to measure time intervals as follows:

- The smallest square is 1 millimeter (mm) in length and represents 0.04 second in time.
- The large square is 5 mm in length and represents 0.20 second in time.
- The large square equals 5 small squares.
- Five large squares represent 1 second.

■ ECG Measurements

When assessing either a rhythm strip or a 12-lead ECG, both the individual PQRST complexes need to be evaluated as well as the relationship of each individual complex to the overall rhythm. The assessment of an ECG configuration includes the following:

- **P wave**—There should be one P wave for every QRS complex.
- **PR interval**—This is measured from the beginning of the P wave to the beginning of the QRS complex. The normal PR interval is from 0.12 to 0.20 second or 3 small boxes to 1 large box.
- **QRS complex**—The QRS complex is measured from the beginning of the Q wave to the end of the S wave. The normal range is from 0.06 to 0.12 second or 1.5 boxes to 3 boxes. The shape of the QRS complex varies from individual to in-

dividual and also depends on the ECG lead being used. For example, QRS complexes are mostly positive in the lead II and mostly negative in the MCL₁ lead (see Figure 38–6 ■, p. 1079). Not everyone has a discernable Q wave.

- **QT interval**—This is measured from the Q wave to the end of the T wave. The normal QT interval is 0.34 to 0.43 second or 8.5 to 11 boxes.
- **Heart rate**—This is measured by using the very top of the ECG paper, which is marked off in 3-second intervals with tick marks. The tick mark is a small straight line or hash mark above the tracing. Count up the number of PQRST complexes that occur in 6 seconds and multiply that number by 10. This method provides a general estimate of the heart rate. A more accurate method for measuring heart rate is to count the number of small squares between two R waves and divide the total into 1,500. The normal HR is 60 to 100 beats per minute.
- **Heart rhythm**—This is determined by measuring the distance between P waves for atrial rate and two R waves for ventricular rate and then measuring each subsequent R wave to ensure it is the same distance apart as the previous ones. With a regular rhythm, the distance between R waves is equal.

Calipers (Figure 38–10 ■) are the instrument used to take all these measurements. Figure 38–11 ■ demonstrates where each measurement begins and ends.

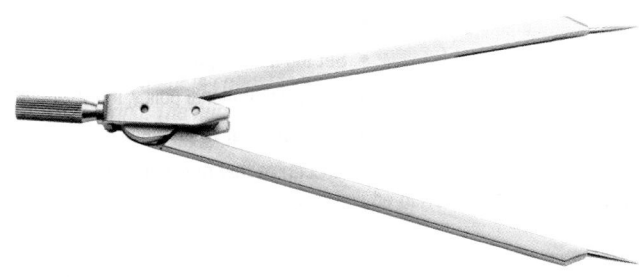

FIGURE 38–10 ■ Calipers.

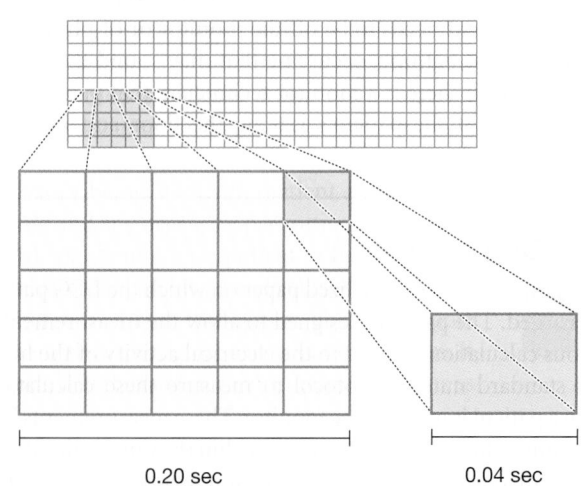

FIGURE 38–9 ■ ECG graph paper.

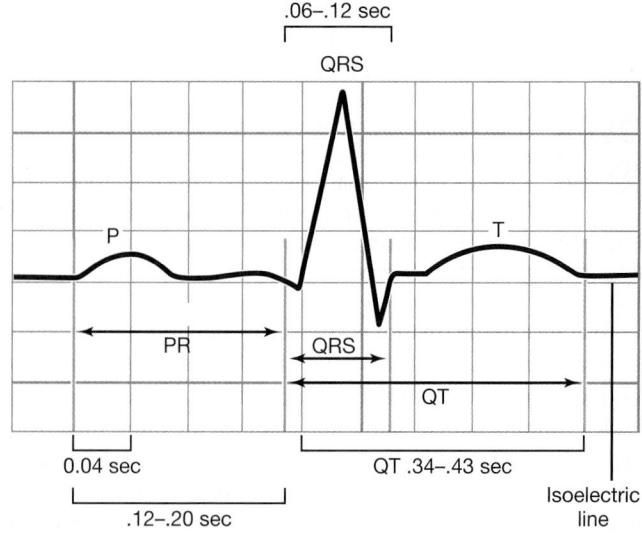

FIGURE 38–11 ■ ECG measurement.

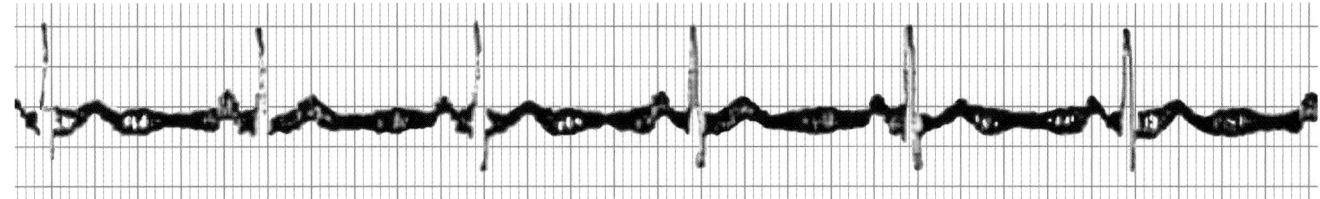

FIGURE 38–12 ■ Artifact.

Isoelectric Line

The **isoelectric line** marks the beginning and ending point of all waves. When the SA node fires, the **ECG waveform** (the actual tracing on the graph paper) begins and moves away from the isoelectric line (see Figure 38–12 ■). Any wave that has an upward deflection, which is above the isoelectric line, is referred to as a positive deflection, and any waveform that goes below the line is referred to as a negative deflection. Depending on the lead, certain waves normally are positive and certain ones are negative. In a lead II the normal P wave has a positive deflection, the PR interval is isoelectric, the Q wave is the first negative deflection, the R wave is positive, the S wave is negative, the ST segment is isoelectric, and the T wave is positive.

Artifact

Artifact is defined as an ECG pattern caused by sources outside the heart creating a false and abnormal pattern on the ECG graph paper. This interference is due to several causes:

- Malfunction of electrodes possibly due to dry conductive gel, clammy skin, or dense chest hair
- Patient movement, which precipitates a fluctuating isoelectric line that corrects itself when the patient lies still
- Improper grounding, which occurs when a patient is in contact with an outside source of electricity, such as poorly grounded beds and/or IV infusion pumps
- Equipment failures, such as broken wires or cables on the ECG equipment, which need to be exchanged for new equipment.

Because of this interference or artifact, the baseline or isoelectric line becomes fuzzy. When artifact is present, it is difficult to diagnose cardiac abnormalities, making it is necessary to correct the cause of the artifact. Figure 38–12 ■ depicts artifact.

Ectopic Focus

Ectopic focus is a heartbeat originating from a site other than the primary cardiac pacemaker tissue. Ectopic foci may affect cardiac output and must be assessed and documented carefully for their impact on the hemodynamic stability of the patient. The terms *dysrhythmia, arrhythmia,* and *ectopic focus* all mean the same thing and are used interchangeably.

ECG Rhythm Strip Evaluation and Documentation

When evaluating an ECG rhythm strip, using a simple stepwise process provides a consistent method for rhythm strip evaluation. This is shown in Chart 38–4. If the rhythm strip falls out of the normal parameters, then there is a high probability of an ab-

CHART 38–4	Stepwise Process for ECG Strip Evaluation
P Waves	Are the P waves regular? Is there one P wave for every QRS and one QRS for every P wave? Is the P wave in front of the QRS or behind it? Is the P wave normal and upright in lead II? Do all the P waves look alike? Are the abnormal P waves associated with ectopic beats?
PR Interval	Are all the PR intervals constant? Is the PR interval measurement within normal range (0.12 to 0.20 second)? If the PR interval varies, is there a pattern to the changing measurements?
QRS Complex	Are all the QRS complexes of equal duration? What is the measurement of the QRS complex size? Is the QRS complex measurement within normal limits (0.06 to 0.12 second)? Do all the QRS complexes look alike? Are the unusual QRS complexes associated with ectopic beats?
QT Interval	What is the length of the QT interval? Is it normal or prolonged? Is the patient on a treatment that prolongs the interval?
Rate	Atrial: how many P waves in 6 seconds times 10. Ventricular: how many R waves in 6 seconds times 10. A second method is to count the number of large boxes between two R waves and divide by 1500. Both methods work best when the rhythm is normal. What is the heart rate?
Regularity (also called rhythm)	Is it regular? Is it irregular? Are there any patterns to the irregularity? Are there any ectopic beats; if so, are they early or late?
Ectopic Beats	Are they present? What are they? How is the patient tolerating them? Do they require treatment?

normality occurring in the conduction system. These abnormalities are discussed at length throughout the remainder of the chapter.

Normal Sinus Rhythm

Normal sinus rhythm (NSR) is a cardiac rhythm initiated from the SA or sinus node that has all the normal waveforms (PQRST) and normal time intervals (PR, QRS, QT) (Figure 38–13 ■).

The following criteria must be present to be NSR:

- P wave has a normal and consistent shape and appears before every QRS complex.
- There is a 1:1 ratio of P wave to QRS complex.
- PR interval is between 0.12 and 0.20 second.
- QRS complex is between 0.06 and 0.12 second.
- QT interval is between 0.34 and 0.43 second.
- Atrial and ventricular rate is between 60 and 100 beats per minute (beats/minute).
- Atrial and ventricular rhythm is regular.

Nursing Management

When the patient is on a cardiac monitor, it is the nurse's responsibility to measure, assess, and document the patient's rhythm strip at least every shift and more frequently depending on the patient's condition and agency protocol. Whenever changes occur in the heart rhythm, the nurse must begin the same process again: measure, assess, and document the rhythm strip. The nurse needs to understand when it is appropriate to report a change in the ECG to the health care provider.

Nursing Documentation

When documenting the heart rhythm in the patient's record, most institutions require that a rhythm strip is attached to the patient's chart once every shift and/or when a change in the rhythm occurs. The patient's name, the date and time of rhythm strip collection, and the ECG lead used for the rhythm strip should be documented. Additionally, the electrical features of the rhythm should be documented including the presence of a P wave, the PR interval, the width of the QRS complex, the QT interval, the heart rate, and rhythm (regular verses irregular), and the presence of ectopy (ectopic focus). Corresponding clinical manifestations associated with a given rhythm also need to be documented in the record. For exam-

ple, change in blood pressure, pulse, level of consciousness, and urine output.

Dysrhythmias

When the cardiac muscle does not receive enough blood, it becomes ischemic and irritable, causing cardiac dysrhythmias to occur. A **dysrhythmia** is an abnormal disturbance of the electrical conduction system of the heart. There are a number of dysrhythmias, which originate in different parts of the heart. This chapter addresses dysrhythmias according to location in the heart, beginning at the top with the atrial dysrhythmias. As the dysrhythmias occur anatomically lower in the heart, the severity is greater due to their impact on cardiac output. The cardiac output decreases as the severity of the dysrhythmia increases.

Heart rhythms are categorized according to the cardiac structure in which they begin, or their site of origin. The most common dysrhythmias begin at the top of the heart with the SA node. These types of dysrhythmias are called sinus dysrhythmias due to their origin in the SA, or sinus, node. The next area in the heart where dysrhythmias may occur is in the intra-atrial pathways, referred to as atrial dysrhythmias. Moving anatomically down to the next area of the conduction system, the AV node or junction is where junctional dysrhythmias occur. The final area of the heart where dysrhythmias may occur is in the ventricles. These ventricular dysrhythmias are considered to be the most dangerous because they precipitate the most profound decrease in the cardiac output.

When observing, assessing, and treating dysrhythmias, it is critical for the nurse to remember that it is the patient being treated, not the dysrhythmia. Treatment is always based on the hemodynamic impact of the dysrhythmia.

Sinus Dysrhythmias

The four common dysrhythmias associated with the sinus area of the heart are sinus bradycardia, sinus tachycardia, sinus arrhythmia/dysrhythmia, and sinus arrest.

Sinus Bradycardia

Sinus bradycardia, often called "sinus brady," occurs when the SA node is firing at a rate of less than 60 beats per minute. Sinus means the rhythm originated in the SA node; therefore, P waves are present. The only difference between sinus bradycardia and normal sinus rhythm (NSR) is the heart rate, but because of this variable, sinus bradycardia is not normal. Sinus bradycardia may result in decreased cardiac output, because while there is adequate time for the heart to fill up with blood, there are not enough contractions per minute to pump the amount of blood needed for normal cardiac output. Significant slowing of the heart rate predisposes the patient to an ectopic focus assuming the role of pacemaker in order to generate sufficient cardiac output. This condition may lead to serious dysrhythmias and warrants careful monitoring. An ECG strip showing sinus bradycardia is in Figure 38–14 ■.

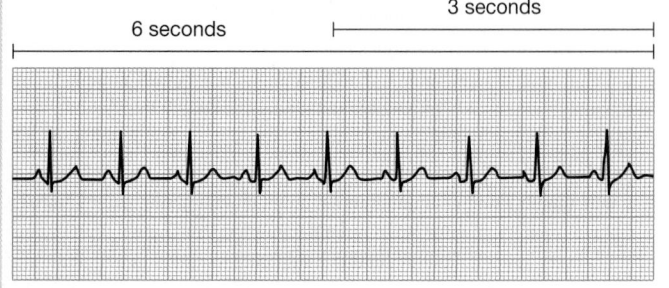

P Wave: Present 1 P wave/QRS complex; PR Interval: 0.18 second; QRS Complex: 0.06 second; QT Interval 0.36 second; Heart Rate: Atrial: 90 beats per minute (bpm); Ventricular: 90 bpm; Rhythm: Regular, Ectopic Beats: None

FIGURE 38–13 ■ Normal sinus rhythm.

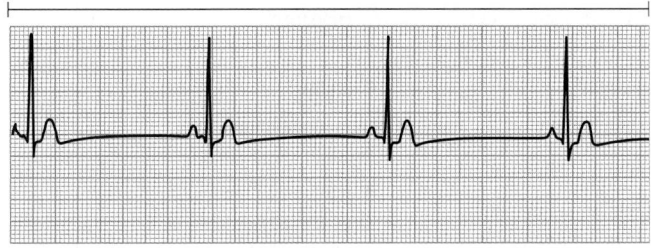

P Wave: Present, 1 P wave/QRS Complex; PR Interval: .16 second; QRS Complex: 0.08 second; QT Interval: 0.32 second; Heart Rate: Atrial: 40 bpm; Ventricular: 40 bpm; Rhythm: Regular; Ectopic Beats: None

FIGURE 38–14 ■ Sinus bradycardia.

Significant ECG features of sinus bradycardia include:

- Both atrial and ventricular rates are less than 60 beats per minute.
- The QT interval tends to lengthen.

The etiology, physical assessment findings, and treatment for sinus bradycardia are outlined in Chart 38–5.

Sinus Tachycardia

Sinus tachycardia is defined as a firing of the (SA) node at a rate greater than 100 beats per minute. It is called *sinus* tachycardia because there is a P wave present, although it may be related to an abnormality of the SA node itself. For example, an acute myocardial infarction (AMI) may cause a decrease in the blood supply to the SA node, resulting in an abnormal response such as tachycardia.

Sinus tachycardia results in increased oxygen consumption, increased workload of the heart, and decreased cardiac output. Whenever the heart rate increases, more oxygen is required to nourish the muscle, resulting in increased work of the heart and increased oxygen consumption. Decreased cardiac output occurs when the heart rate is fast enough to lose the period of time needed for blood to enter the heart, referred to as **fill time.** An ECG strip showing sinus tachycardia is in Figure 38–15 ■ (p. 1089). Significant ECG features of sinus tachycardia include:

- Atrial and ventricular heart rates are over 100 beats per minute.
- As the sinus rate accelerates, both the PR interval and the QT interval tend to shorten slightly.
- The rhythm may be slightly irregular as the rate begins to accelerate, but then becomes a rapid regular rhythm.

The etiology, physical assessment findings, and treatment for sinus tachycardia are outlined in Chart 38–5.

Sinus Arrhythmia/Dysrhythmia

Sinus arrhythmia/dysrhythmia resembles normal sinus rhythm, except for the slight irregularity in the heart rhythm. The rate of impulse formation and conduction varies with the respiratory cycle; thus, the P to P and R to R intervals change with respiration. The heart rate increases during inspiration and decreases with expiration. This dysrhythmia is common in young children and tends to disappear as they grow older (Garcia & Miller, 2004). Additionally, it tends to disappear when the heart increases, for example, with exercise. Typically there is no clinical significance with this dysrhythmia; it is considered a variant of normal. However, the cyclic decreased heart rate may make the heart muscle

CHART 38–5	Sinus Dysrhythmias: Etiology, Physical Assessment, and Treatment		
Dysrhythmia	**Etiology**	**Physical Assessment**	**Treatment**
Sinus bradycardia	Decreased sympathetic tone, or anatomic changes Hypothermia Drugs, such as morphine, digoxin, verapamil, and some sedatives Toxins Vagal stimulation, as with vomiting or Valsalva maneuver Hypothyroidism Infectious diseases Acidosis Hypovolemia Hypo/hyperkalemia Hypoglycemia Cardiac tamponade Tension pneumothorax Thrombosis: coronary and/or pulmonary Trauma Increased intracranial pressure Normal conditions: sleeping and a well-conditioned athlete's heart	Pulse: Less than 60 beats per minute and typically regular. Blood pressure (BP): Lower than usual if for pathological conditions. If cardiac output is decreased, the following clinical manifestations may occur: • Angina • Syncope • Generalized weakness • Dizziness • Shortness of breath. Altered mental state may be present, although rare.	Treat *only* if symptomatic. Treatment is typically instituted when syncope and/or alteration in consciousness occurs. If symptomatic, it means there is a significant drop in cardiac output. Attempt to identify and treat the cause. Assess for changes in vital signs. Observe for other dysrhythmias. With poor perfusion, typical treatment includes: • Oxygen • IV access • Drug therapy (atropine) • Epinephrine or dopamine • Pacemaker evaluation.

(continued)

CHART 38–5	**Sinus Dysrhythmias: Etiology, Physical Assessment, and Treatment—*Continued***

Dysrhythmia	Etiology	Physical Assessment	Treatment
Sinus tachycardia	Exercise Smoking Alcohol Caffeine Cocaine Fever Blood loss/anemia Hypovolemia Early sepsis Hypermetabolic state, e.g., burn injury Heart failure Allergic reactions Emotions Anxiety Pain Decreased PSNS Increased SNS stimulation Drug side effect of many over-the-counter cold drugs and drugs used to treat asthma and sinus conditions Compensatory response to a decreased cardiac output	Pulse: Greater than 100 beats per minute. BP: Lower than normal. If cardiac output is decreased, the following clinical manifestations may occur: • Angina • Syncope • Generalized weakness • Dizziness • Shortness of breath. Altered mental state may be present, although rare.	Treat *only* if symptomatic. Attempt to identify and treat the cause. Treatment may include: • Drug therapy, such as beta-adrenergic blockers, adenosine, diltiazem, and digoxin • Carotid massage/vagal maneuvers • Cardioversion • Anxiety medications • Fluid replacement. If causes are identified and managed, generally the rhythm converts back to NSR.
Sinus arrhythmia/ dysrhythmia	Common and normal finding, especially in children and young adults Pathological causes include underlying cardiac disease, such as sick sinus syndrome and myocardial infarction Digoxin Factors that cause heart rate variability including exercise, mental stress, and circadian rhythms	Pulse: irregular.	Not treated unless the bradycardic phase causes clinical manifestations described under bradycardia. Atropine for bradycardia. Provide reassurance that this rhythm is not dangerous, but it needs to be evaluated to rule out more serious dysrhythmias.
Sinus arrest	Hypoxemia Cardiac muscle ischemia Damage to the SA node Digoxin Aspirin Abnormal potassium levels Myocardial infarction Vagal dominance Hypersensitive carotid sinus reflex, e.g., tight shirt collar	Pulse: irregular. BP: Lower than normal depending on number of pauses per minute. If cardiac output is decreased, the following clinical manifestations may occur: • Angina • Syncope • Generalized weakness • Dizziness • Shortness of breath. Altered mental state may be present, although rare.	Treat *only* if patient is symptomatic and/or condition is complicated by other dysrhythmias. Ascertain and treat cause, if possible. Typical treatment may include permanent or temporary artificial pacemaker for repeated episodes, depending on the prognosis, age, and presence of clinical manifestations.

Source: Adapted from American Heart Association. (2006). *Handbook of emergency cardiovascular care for healthcare providers.* Dallas, TX: Author.

more susceptible to other dysrhythmias. Figure 38–16 ■ shows an ECG strip of sinus arrhythmia/dysrhythmia. Significant ECG features of sinus arrhythmia/dysrhythmia include:

• PR interval may change slightly as the heart rate changes.
• QT interval changes with the heart rate, becoming longer during the slow phase of the rhythm.
• Heart rate is 60 to 100 beats per minute; however, the slow phase may drop below 60 beats per minute.

• Heart rhythm is regularly irregular, with a variance of more than 0.08 second in the acceleration and deceleration phases.
• Ectopic beats may occur during the slow phase of the rhythm.

The etiology, physical assessment findings, and treatment for sinus arrhythmia/dysrhythmia are outlined in Chart 38–5.

Sinus Arrest

Sinus arrest is a momentary cessation of sinus impulse formation (SA node failure), causing a pause in the cardiac rhythm

6 seconds

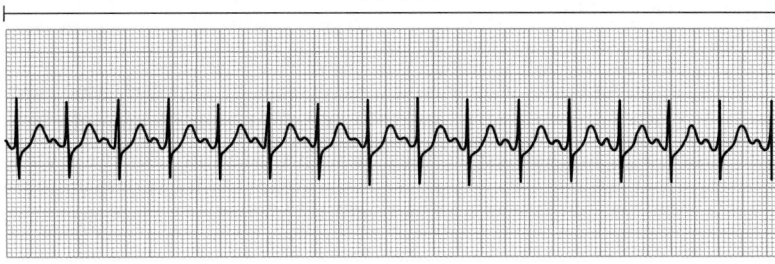

P Wave: Present, 1/QRS Complex; PR Interval: 0.14 second; QRS Complex: 0.08 second; QT Interval: 0.36 second; Heart Rate: Atrial: 140 bpm, Ventricular: 140 bpm; Rhythm: Regular; Ectopic Beats None

FIGURE 38–15 ■ Sinus tachycardia.

6 seconds

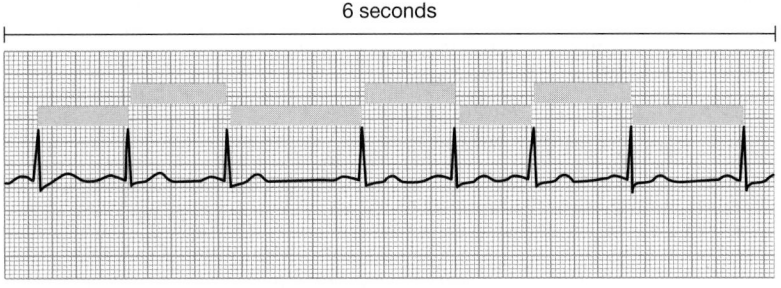

P Wave: Present 1/QRS Complex; PR Interval: 0.18 second; QRS Complex: 0.08 second; QT Interval: 0.40 second; Heart Rate: Atrial: 80 bpm, Ventricular: 80 bpm; Rhythm: Irregular; Ectopic Beats: None

FIGURE 38–16 ■ Sinus arrhythmia/dysrhythmia.

followed by spontaneous resumption of electrical activity. Sinus arrest also is called sinus pause. With a sinus pause there will be an absence of the PQRST complex on the ECG strip and a loss of cardiac output. Figure 38–17 ■ shows an ECG strip of sinus arrest (pause). Significant ECG features of sinus arrest include:

- There is an absence of one entire PQRST complex.
- QT interval changes with the heart rate, becoming longer during the slow phase of the rhythm.
- There may be marked bradycardia due to long sinus pauses.
- Underlying heart rhythm is regular except when the pauses occur.

The etiology, physical assessment findings, and treatment for sinus arrest are outlined in Chart 38–5.

■ Nursing Management for Sinus Dysrhythmias

The nurse should first evaluate the patient's response to and tolerance of any dysrhythmia. Depending on the type of dysrhythmia, the patient may or may not be symptomatic. However, if the abnormal rhythm results in a decreased cardiac output, it is important to assess for the changes outlined on Chart 38–6 (p. 1090).

The psychological impact of having a dysrhythmia also must be addressed. It is frightening to most patients when they experience the clinical manifestations of cardiac dysrhythmias, such as angina, dizziness, syncope, diaphoresis, and disorientation. The nurse should reassure the patient that all appropriate treatment is being provided and offer comfort

Pause

6 seconds

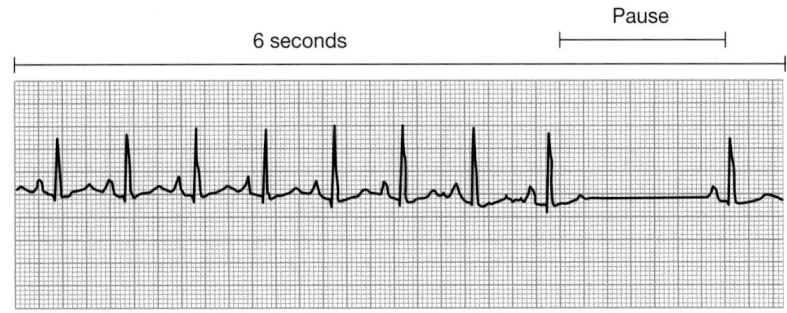

P Wave: Present 1/QRS Complex; PR Interval: 0.20 second; QRS Complex: 0.10 second; QT Interval: 0.40 second; Heart Rate: Atrial: 90 bpm, Ventricular: 90 bpm; Rhythm: Regular except for the pause; Ectopic Beats: None
Conclusion: Sinus arrest (pause)

FIGURE 38–17 ■ Sinus arrest (pause).

CHART 38–6	Clinical Manifestations of Decreased Cardiac Output
Lower than usual blood pressure	Exercise intolerance
Decreased or increased heart rate	Dizziness
Syncope	Alteration in consciousness
Generalized weakness	Angina

Note: Clinical manifestations depend on the degree of decreased cardiac output.

measures. Supply the patient with a quiet environment and treatments to alleviate clinical manifestations. Also provide support by actively listening to the patient's concerns and including family in the plan of care.

The cause of the dysrhythmia, as outlined in Chart 38–5 (p. 1087), must be evaluated and corrected, if possible. Typically the patient is treated only if he becomes symptomatic and/or the condition is complicated by other more serious dysrhythmias. When a dysrhythmia occurs, the nurse needs to do an in-depth assessment of the patient to determine the clinical manifestations. A dysrhythmia may not always occur due to an abnormality in the heart, but may be due to a variety of reasons not associated with a cardiac abnormality. For example, pain and anxiety are two noncardiac causes of tachycardia. Therefore, treatment may consist of pain medications or, if the patient is anxious, providing support, such as talking with the patient. If the patient is hemodynamically unstable, the health care provider should be notified. Chart 38–5 (p. 1087) outlines the standard treatments for each of the sinus dysrhythmias.

Atrial Dysrhythmias

Atrial dysrhythmias usually result from an irritable focus in the atria that initiates an electrical impulse before the SA node has fired in a normal fashion. Because the electrical impulse does not come from the SA node, the P wave configuration of the ECG is different. However, the QRS complex is normal because the electrical impulse travels down the normal pathway from the AV node through the ventricle. Seven different atrial dysrhythmias are discussed next: premature atrial contraction, atrial flutter, atrial fibrillation, supraventricular tachycardia, Wolff-Parkinson-White syndrome, wandering atrial pacemaker, and sick sinus syndrome.

Premature Atrial Contraction

Premature atrial contraction (PAC) is an ectopic focus in the atria that occurs early, before the next expected SA node impulse, causing depolarization and contraction of the cardiac muscle. This electrical impulse originates outside the SA node. It frequently occurs when the underlying rhythm is normal sinus rhythm (NSR), and the only abnormality is the PAC. When there are more than 5 to 6 PACs per minute, they are termed frequent and have more clinical significance. Whenever beats are premature, there is a loss of the time needed for blood to flow into the heart (fill time), which decreases the amount of blood pumped out of the heart, the cardiac output. Thus, if the beats occur frequently cardiac output is decreased. An increase in the frequency of the dysrhythmia also indicates irritability of the atrial muscle and becomes a cause for concern as it tends to increase the risk for other dysrhythmias occurring. Figure 38–18 ■ is a rhythm strip showing premature atrial contractions. Significant ECG features of PACs include:

- P wave is present and is premature.
- P wave configuration (shape) may look different because electrical impulses do not come from the SA node.
- PR interval may be shorter or longer than regular beats.
- PACs are premature, making the rhythm irregular.
- P wave after the PAC falls earlier than expected because of the early electrical discharge, which then resets the SA node rhythm, referred to as a noncompensatory pause.
- Heart rate and rhythm are typically within normal limits, except when the PAC occurs.

The etiology, physical assessment findings, and treatment of PACs are outlined in Chart 38–7.

Atrial Flutter

Atrial flutter is a rapid, regular, atrial rhythm with an *atrial* rate of 200 to 400 beats per minute (Garcia & Miller, 2004). There is loss of SA node dominance, which is the preferential pacemaker. Only a fraction of the atrial impulses are conducted through the AV node to the ventricle. Most of the atrial beats fall during the AV node refractory period when the cardiac cell is unable to respond to any stimulus, thus preventing conduction of the impulse. This makes the AV node the "gatekeeper" for the ventricles by prohibiting all of the atrial impulses from reaching the ventricles, thereby limiting ventricular rate. Atrial flutter also causes a decreased cardiac output due to the loss of the atrial kick or

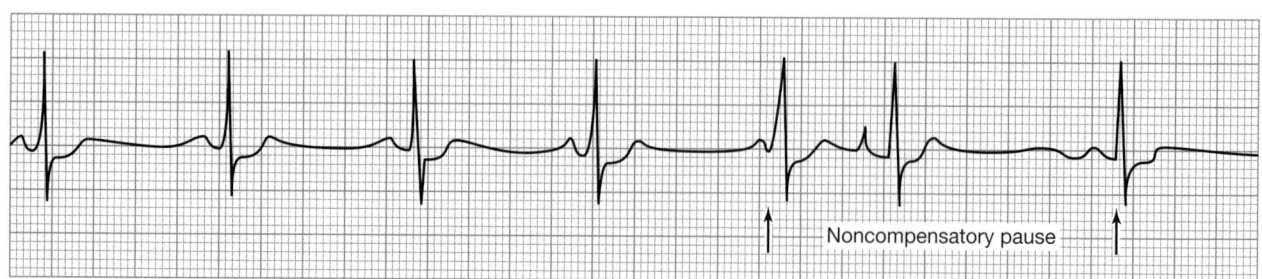

Noncompensatory pause

P Wave: Premature; PR Interval: 0.16 second; QRS Complex: 0.10 second; QT interval: 0.40 second; Heart Rate: Atrial: 70 bpm; Ventricular: 70 bpm; Rhythm: Regular except for premature beats. Ectopic Beat PAC. Conclusion: One premature atrial contraction.

FIGURE 38–18 ■   Premature atrial contraction.

CHART 38–7   Atrial Dysrhythmias: Etiology, Physical Assessment, and Treatment

Dysrhythmia	Etiology	Physical Assessment	Treatment
Premature atrial contraction	Mitral stenosis Mitral valve prolapse Cor pulmonale Underlying cardiovascular disease including ischemia and myocardial infarction Hypoxia Infectious diseases Electrolyte imbalance Increased sympathetic tone Stimulants Drug toxicity, e.g., digoxin Stress Anxiety	Pulse: Irregular BP: If frequent PACs, may be decreased. If cardiac output is decreased the following clinical manifestations may occur: Angina Syncope Generalized weakness Dizziness Shortness of breath Altered mental state may be present, although rare.	Observe the frequency of the PACs, and observe for decreased cardiac output (Chart 38–6). Treat the underlying cause, e.g., stress, anxiety, electrolyte imbalance. Frequent PAC's or those that cause sustained tachycardia may require treatment with drugs that prolong atrial refractoriness, such as digoxin, verapamil, or propranolol.
Atrial flutter	Coronary atherosclerosis Valvular disease; Cor pulmonale Pulmonary edema Myocardial infarction SA node disease Pulmonary embolism Digitalis toxicity ETOH abuse Postsurgical complication: one of the common dysrhythmias following open heart surgery. On rare occasions it may occur with normal healthy hearts.	Pulse: May be regular or irregular BP: Lower than normal if cardiac output is decreased. If cardiac output is decreased the following clinical manifestations may occur: Angina Syncope Generalized weakness Dizziness Shortness of breath Altered mental state may be present, although rare.	Cardioversion is a common intervention. Drug therapy is used to reduce AV conduction: digitalis, propranolol, diltiazem. If a chronic situation the patient may be placed on anticoagulants like warfarin.
Atrial fibrillation	Acute myocardial infarction Left atrial stretch due to mitral stenosis and mitral regurgitation May be a chronic rhythm associated with heart failure Transient after open-heart surgery Long-standing hypertension Digoxin toxicity Alcohol intake, chronic or acute, moderate to heavy Idiopathic	Pulse: Irregular (hallmark feature) BP: Lower than normal If cardiac output is decreased the following clinical manifestations may occur: Angina Syncope Generalized weakness Dizziness Shortness of breath Altered mental state may be present, depending on the ventricular rate.	Control the ventricular response, i.e., heart rate. If a rapid ventricular response control with drugs: digoxin is still the drug of choice; beta-blockers (propranolol) and calcium channel blockers (verapamil, diltiazem). Calcium channel blockers work the fastest, and are the drug of choice when medically unstable. Prevent thromboembolic events with anticoagulant therapy, e.g., warfarin, Cardioversion: Is used if new onset, especially when hemodynamic instability is present. If successful, digoxin is used to prevent reoccurrence.
Supraventricular tachycardia includes paroxysmal Atrioventricular node reentry tachycardia AVNRT Atrial tachycardia	Heart disease Rheumatic heart disease Coronary artery disease (CAD) Hypoxia May be precipitated by a premature atrial contraction (PAC) May occur in healthy adults from a variety of causes: Overexertion Stress Excessive use of stimulants Smoking Hypokalemia	Pulse: Very fast. BP: Decreased if drop in cardiac output. If cardiac output is decreased the following clinical manifestations may occur: Angina Syncope Generalized weakness Dizziness Shortness of breath Altered mental state may be present, although rare.	It is necessary to find and treat the cause, e.g., stress, hypokalemia. Vagal maneuvers, i.e., bearing down, coughing, and carotid artery massage. Specific treatment may include: oxygen therapy and cardioversion. Drug therapy: adenosine is used to briefly terminate the rhythm for differential diagnosis. Verapamil is a calcium channel blocker; decreases heart rate. Cardioversion is performed if drug therapy and vagal maneuvers are unsuccessful.

(continued)

CHART 38-7	Atrial Dysrhythmias: Etiology, Physical Assessment, and Treatment—*Continued*		
Dysrhythmia	**Etiology**	**Physical Assessment**	**Treatment**
Wolff-Parkinson-White (WPW) syndrome	Congenital in origin: twice as common in males, and occurs in 0.1 to 0.3% of the general population.	Pulse: Rapid. Frequent episodes of palpitations. BP: May be decreased due to fast heart rate. If cardiac output is decreased the following clinical manifestations may occur: Angina Syncope Generalized weakness Dizziness Shortness of breath Altered mental state may be present, although rare.	Same as that for supraventricular tachycardia. Radiofrequency ablation to terminate the accessory pathway.
Wandering atrial pacemaker	Frequently seen in normal individuals and is of no consequence. Digoxin toxicity	Pulse: 40–60 bpm BP: Lower than normal If cardiac output is decreased the following clinical manifestations may occur: Angina Syncope Generalized weakness Dizziness Shortness of breath Altered mental state may be present, although rare.	Treat only if symptomatic. Treatment typically is instituted when syncope and/or alteration in consciousness occurs. Attempt to identify and treat the cause. Administer oxygen. Establish IV access Drug therapy: Atropine Evaluate for transcutaneous or permanent pacemaker depending on impact on cardiac output
Sick sinus syndrome	Coronary artery disease Drugs: Cardiac glycoside, Antihypertensive agents, Calcium channel blockers Frequently, intermittent and unpredictable, may occur in the absence of heart disease Myocardial infarction Inflammatory or degenerative processes	Pulse: Bradycardia that alternates with tachycardia, referred to as brady-tachy syndrome. BP: May decrease due to decreased cardiac output. If cardiac output is decreased the following clinical manifestations may occur: Angina Syncope Generalized weakness Dizziness Shortness of breath Altered mental state may be present, although rare.	Clinical manifestations and ECG findings determine treatment. Anticoagulants are used because of blood stasis if atrial flutter/fibrillation is present. The only definitive treatment is a permanent pacemaker to replace the SA node.

normal atrial contraction. Atrial kick forces more blood into the ventricle, which augments cardiac output. With atrial flutter the atria are just fluttering instead of contracting, resulting in a decreased cardiac output by as much as 30% (Shade & Wesley, 2007). Additionally, with the loss of the atrial contraction, blood stasis and pooling occur, leading to an increased incidence of clot formation. Finally, due to the rapid atrial rate myocardial oxygen consumption increases, which eventually leads to the development of hypoxia of the myocardial muscle and predisposes the left ventricular to fail. Figure 38–19 ■ is a rhythm strip showing atrial flutter. Significant ECG features of atrial flutter include:

- P waves are not identifiable; instead there are flutter waves (F waves), creating a "sawtooth" baseline on the ECG strip.

- PR intervals are not measurable.

- QT interval is not measurable because the T waves are buried in the F waves.

- Atrial and ventricular rhythms typically are regular, but they may be irregular depending on how often the AV node allows impulses to travel to the ventricle.

The etiology, physical assessment findings, and treatment of atrial flutter are outlined in Chart 38–7.

Atrial Fibrillation

Atrial fibrillation, also referred to as "atrial fib" or "a-fib," is a common dysrhythmia. The Evidence-Based Practice box outlines the genetic considerations of atrial fibrillation.

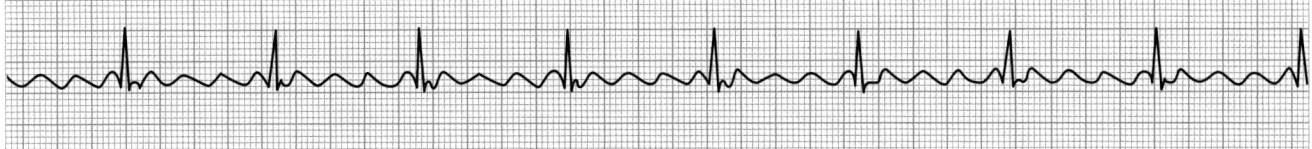

P Wave: None, flutter waves; PR interval: None; QRS Complex: 0.08 second; QT Interval: unable to obtain; Heart Rate: Atrial: about 300 bpm, Ventricular: 90 bpm; Rhythm: Regular; Ectopic Beats: Flutter waves.

FIGURE 38–19 ■ Atrial flutter.

It is characterized by a disorganized, very rapid, and irregular atrial rhythm resulting in an irregular ventricular rhythm, the hallmark feature. Rapid or slow ventricular heart rate, referred to as the ventricular response, depends on the rate that the AV node allows impulses to be conducted to the ventricles. The cells in the atria have an increased irritability typically due to cardiac muscle hypoxia, which causes many sites in the atria to become pacemakers and initiate electrical impulses. The firing of these multiple sites causes the atria simply to quiver instead of contracting effectively. Atrial fibrillation causes three significant clinical manifestations: (1) loss of SA node pacemaker dominance, which is the most reliable pacemaker; (2) decreased cardiac output due to loss

of atrial kick; and (3) increased myocardial oxygen consumption. The immediate concern for atrial fibrillation is the ventricular response because it determines cardiac output. A heart rate that is too slow or too fast impacts cardiac output.

With the loss of the atrial kick, blood stasis and pooling occur, leading to an increased incidence of clot formation. Therefore, those individuals with atrial fibrillation are at high risk for a cardiovascular accident (CVA) and/or pulmonary emboli. The rapid atrial firing also increases the workload on the heart, eventually causing hypoxia of the myocardial muscle. Long-term hypoxia predisposes to left ventricular failure. Figure 38–20 ■ (p. 1096) is a rhythm strip showing atrial fibrillation.

Genetic Considerations

Clinical Problem

A conservative estimate of the number of people who are affected by atrial fibrillation (AF) is approximately 2 million. It is the most common dysrhythmia that causes an irregular heart rate, palpitations, unexplained rapid heart rate, and a sensation of "missed" beats. The incidence of AF increases with age, with less than 1% of the population experiencing it before age 60 years, while it is present in 1 in 10 individuals at age 80 years and over. Elderly white men compose the largest group that is affected by AF.

Research Findings

A new study conducted by the National Heart, Lung, and Blood Institute (2004) assessed the prevalence of AF in individuals who had it in their family history. The study evaluated 2,243 individuals whose parents were in the original Framingham Heart Study. The participants were at least 30 years of age and had no history of AF. Seventy of the subjects developed AF within four years. If individual participants had a history of one parent with AF they were twice as likely to develop the dysrhythmia as subjects who had no family history of AF. If both parents had AF before 75 years of age, the risk tripled. Further research continues to determine which genes are involved and what steps are necessary to enhance early diagnosis and treatment.

Implications for Nursing Practice

Implications for nursing practice begin with the nursing assessment. It is important to specifically question the family history for the presence of AF. This is especially essential if the patient has clinical manifestations and new onset irregular pulse. It needs to be documented in the patient's record that there is a family history of the disease. The nurse also must assess the presence of other risk factors for the development of AF including:

Cardiomyopathy

Hypertension

Heart failure

Excessive alcohol consumption

Previous myocardial infarction

Diabetes

Rheumatic heart disease

Mitral valve disorders such as prolapse, regurgitation, and annular calcification

Smoking

Caffeine

The need for patient/family counseling about the increased risk for the development of AF is necessary along with instructions about the need for medical attention if clinical manifestations described above occur. A major emphasis needs to be placed on increasing public awareness of AF and its many causative factors. Patients with a family history require more frequent and diligent testing. Treatment for AF is outlined on Chart 38–7 (p. 1091).

Critical Thinking Questions

1. When assessing a patient with new onset atrial fibrillation, what types of questions would assist the nurse to determine if there is a risk for a genetic predisposition?

2. When teaching a newly diagnosed patient how to live with AF, in order of priority what must be included in the teaching plan?

Answers to Critical Thinking Questions appear in Appendix D.

Sources: Fox, C. S., Parise, H., D'Agostino, R.B., et al. (2004). Parental atrial fibrillation as a risk factor for atrial fibrillation in offspring. *JAMA: 291*(23): 2852-2856; Pavlovich-Dannis, S.J. (2005). Mom's eyes and dad's atrial fibrillation. *Nurse Week:* 23–24. National Heart, Lung, and Blood Institute (NHLBI), National Institutes of Health. (2004). Parental atrial fibrillation increases risk in offspring, finds NHLBI's Framingham Heart Study. *NIH News.* Retrieved August 8, 2008 from http://www.nhlbi.nih.gov/new/press04-06-15.htm

EVIDENCE-BASED PRACTICE

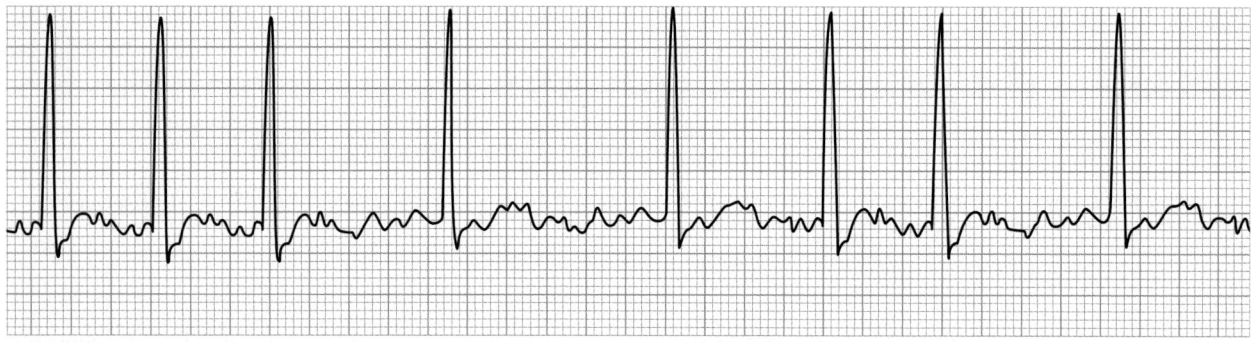

P Wave: None; PR Interval: None; QRS Complex: 0.10 second; QT Interval: unable to obtain; Heart Rate: Ventricular: 80 bpm; Rhythm: Irregular; Ectopic Beats: f waves.

FIGURE 38–20 ■ Atrial fibrillation.

Significant ECG features of atrial fibrillation include:

- P waves are not identifiable due to the atrial quivering, referred to as "f" waves, occurring at 350 to 750 beats per minute.
- PR intervals are not measurable.
- QT interval is not obtainable because the T waves are buried in the f waves.
- Irregularly irregular rhythm occurs, meaning that there is no pattern to the irregularity.
- f waves are ectopic beats.

The etiology, physical assessment findings, and treatment of atrial fibrillation are outlined in Chart 38–7 (p. 1091).

Supraventricular Tachycardia

Supraventricular tachycardia (SVT) is a tachycardia that is generated somewhere above the ventricles. This general term encompasses all fast (tachy) rhythms with normal QRS complexes and heart rates greater than 100 beats per minute. Rhythms included under the SVT umbrella include sinus tachycardia, paroxysmal atrial tachycardia (PAT), and paroxysmal junctional tachycardia (PJT). Clinicians use the term *supraventricular tachycardia* when it is impossible to identify the source of the tachycardia.

Usually this rhythm is benign and is self-limiting when the cause is removed. If sustained, loss of blood *fill time* (diastole) causes a drop in cardiac output. Prolonged episodes of supraventricular tachycardia increase myocardial oxygen demand and also

may result in a conversion to atrial flutter or fibrillation. Eventually, signs and symptoms of congestive heart failure will be present. Figure 38–21 ■ is a rhythm strip showing supraventricular tachycardia (SVT).

Significant ECG features of supraventricular tachycardia include:

- Heart rate is 100 to 250 beats per minute.
- P wave is not seen; it is buried in the QRS complex.
- PR interval is not discernable.
- QRS complex is within normal limits unless distorted by the buried P waves.
- QT interval is not obtainable because the T waves are buried.
- Heart rhythm may be regular or irregular due to varying conduction rates through the AV node.
- Ectopic beats may or may not be present, depending on the pacemaker site.

The etiology, physical assessment findings, and treatment of supraventricular tachycardia are outlined in Chart 38–7 (p. 1091).

Atrioventricular Nodal Reentry Tachycardia

One phenomenon that can cause supraventricular tachycardia is atrioventricular nodal reentry tachycardia (AVNRT). Normally people are born with only a single electrical pathway at the base of the right atrium where impulses travel to the AV node. However, some individuals are born with two separate electrical pathways leading to the AV node, each with its own respective

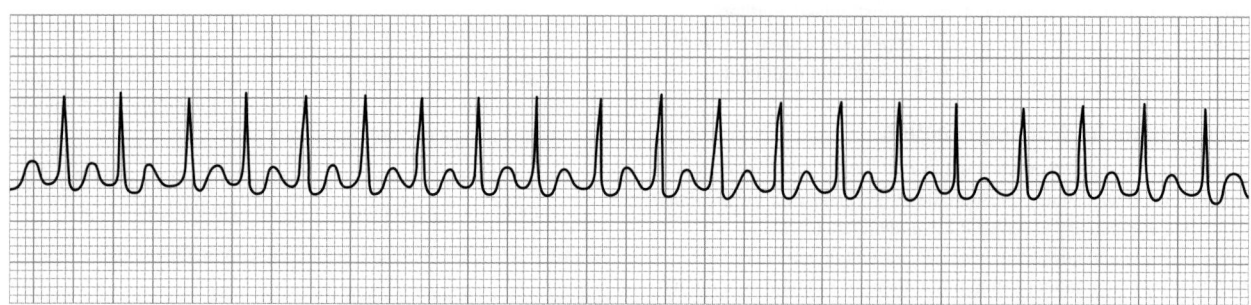

P Wave: None; PR Interval: None; QRS Complex: 0.10 second; QT Interval: unable to obtain; Heart Rate: ⟶ Atrial rate rapid, Ventricular: 200 bpm; Rhythm: Regular; Ectopic Beats: Depends on pacemaker site.

FIGURE 38–21 ■ Supraventricular tachycardia (SVT).

properties. Each pathway has its own refractory period, one fast (beta) and one slow (alpha). The fast track has a long refractory period, and the slow track has a fast refractory period. Impulses travel the two separate pathways simultaneously. When the impulse begins down these two pathways, because of its speed, the one in the fast track stimulates the AV node and bundle of His, causing ventricular depolarization and a normal-width QRS complex. The fast track impulse also travels retrograde (backward transmission) back through the slow track, meeting the impulse coming down the slow track. When the two impulses meet, 99.9% of the time, they cancel each other out and the rhythm is normal. If for any reason, such as the presence of a refractory period in the fast track, the fast track will be unable to transmit the impulse, then the slow track transmits the impulse, causing depolarization of the ventricles. The QRS complex would still be within normal limits, but the PR interval would be longer than the ones coming from the fast track. This creates rhythm strips

that have identical QRS complexes but two different PR interval lengths. These beats still are considered to be sinus complexes, as opposed to coming from another atrial ectopic focus. The PR interval length differences are a result of the conduction alternating intermittently between the two functioning tracks.

The AVNRT phenomenon occurs when a reentrant circuit or loop is created along the two pathways and the AV node (Figure 38–22 ■). An early impulse such as a PAC hits the two pathways; the fast track is in refractory and therefore cannot accept the impulse, but the slow track can. The impulse travels from the slow track, to the AV node, and then retrograde up the fast track because this track has recovered, is no longer in a refractory state, and can accept the impulse. The impulses are now able to continue to cycle the circuit or loop and initiate ventricular depolarization at a fast rate; this is referred to as AVNRT (Garcia & Miller, 2004).

It is estimated that AVNRT occurs in 60% of patients presenting with paroxysmal (sudden onset) SVT and occurs in

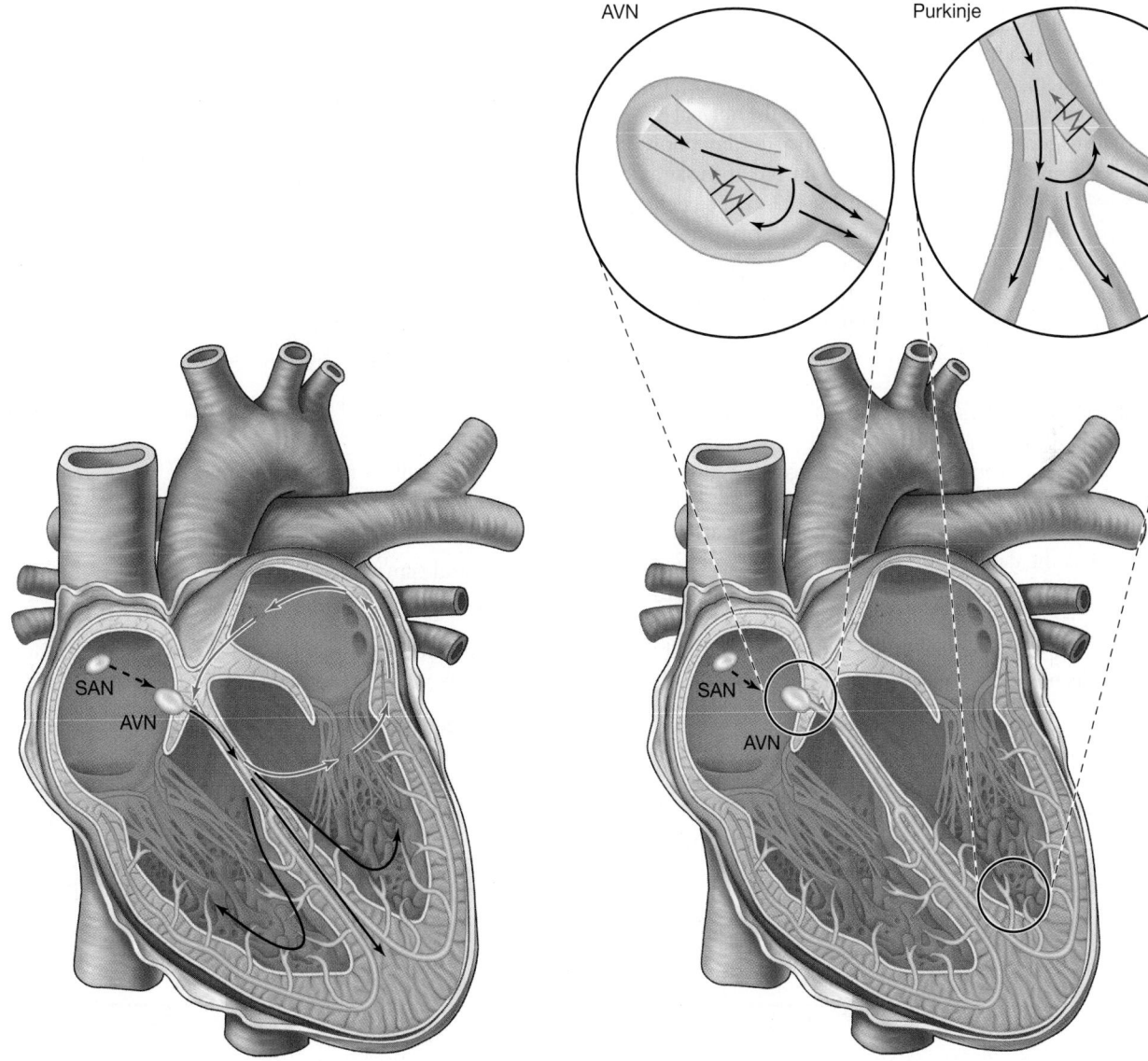

(a) **Macro re-entry circut: antegrade through AV node and retrograde across an assessory pathway.**

(b) **Micro re-entry at the cellular level in the AV node and Purkinje fibers.**

FIGURE 38–22 ■ Reentrant circuit.

approximately several cases per thousand persons worldwide. It is more predominant in women, may occur with individuals of any age, and is common in young adults. AVNRT is usually well tolerated; it often occurs in patients with no structural heart disease. Clinical manifestations are the same as with any tachy dysrhythmia, although AVNRT may cause angina or myocardial infarction in patients with coronary artery disease. Prognosis for patients without heart disease is usually good (Olshansky et al., 2006). Treatment is aimed at breaking the reentrant cycle with the use of vagal maneuvers such as breath holding, stimulating gag reflex, and carotid sinus massage.

Wolff-Parkinson-White Syndrome

Wolff-Parkinson-White syndrome (WPW) is a genetic AV conduction disorder characterized by the presence of two AV conduction pathways, one normal and one abnormal. An impulse leaving the atrium may travel down one or the other pathway without any specific pattern. The abnormal pathway, called the Kent bundle, is composed of an extra muscle bundle made up of working myocardial tissue. This extra muscle bundle forms a connection between the atria and the ventricles outside the normal conduction system, referred to as an accessory pathway. This allows impulses coming from the atrium to bypass the normal AV connection. The hallmark feature on the ECG strip for the abnormal pathway is the presence of a delta wave, a slurred upstroke at the beginning of the QRS complex (Figure 38–23 ■). The delta wave occurs when the impulse travels via the accessory pathway to the ventricles. Because the conduction is outside the normal conduction system, it takes longer for the impulse to travel through the ventricles, thus creating an abnormally wide, bizarre QRS complex (Garcia & Miller, 2004).

Atrial flutter, atrial fibrillation, and supraventricular tachycardia that results in heart rates of greater than 250 beats per minute, are common dysrhythmias in patients with WPW. The increased heart rate increases the workload and oxygen consumption of the heart, predisposing to heart failure, and therefore could cause sudden cardiac death. When the patient does not exhibit any dysrhythmias, but has the delta wave, this is called WPW pattern. When the patient becomes symptomatic or develops dysrhythmias, then the correct terminology is WPW syndrome. Figure 38–23 ■ is a rhythm strip showing Wolff-Parkinson-White dysrhythmia. Significant ECG features of Wolff-Parkinson-White syndrome include:

- PR interval shortens to less than 0.12 second because the AV node is bypassed and delta waves appear just prior to the beginning of the R wave.

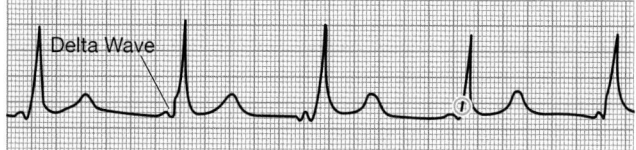

P Wave: Present and irregular; PR Interval: 0.12 second; QRS Complex: 0.16 second. QT Interval 0.52 second, 40-50 bpm, Ventricular: 40-50 bpm; Rhythm: Regular Ectopic Beats: None.

FIGURE 38–23 ■ Wolff-Parkinson-White syndrome.

- QRS complex is greater than 0.12 second due to the delta waves.
- QT interval shortens if tachycardia occurs and lengthens with bradycardia.
- Heart rate frequently tachycardic.
- Heart rhythm is regular, except during heart rate changes.

The etiology, physical assessment findings, and treatment of WPW syndrome are outlined in Chart 38–7 (p. 1091).

Wandering Atrial Pacemaker

Wandering atrial pacemaker is a pacemaker from at least three different sites above the bundle of His acting as the heart's pacemaker. These pacemaker sites may include the SA node, the AV junction, an atrial ectopic site, and/or any combination of these areas. This abnormality occurs because of SA node slowing, which permits an atrial ectopic focus and junctional escape rhythms to "jump in" as atrial pacemakers. Figure 38–24 ■ is a rhythm strip showing wandering atrial pacemaker. Significant ECG features of wandering atrial pacemaker include:

- P waves have multiple shapes, due to multiple atrial sites initiating the conduction.
- QT interval usually is normal, but may be prolonged due to a slow heart rate.
- Heart rhythm is irregular due to changing pacemakers.
- Atrial rate and ventricular heart rate typically are slow.
- Ectopic beats may be present due to the slow rhythm.

The etiology, physical assessment findings, and treatment of wandering atrial pacemaker are outlined in Chart 38–7 (p. 1091).

Sick Sinus Syndrome

Sick sinus syndrome (SSS) encompasses a broad range of abnormalities, including disorders of impulse generation and conduction, failure of pacemakers, and a susceptibility to paroxysmal or

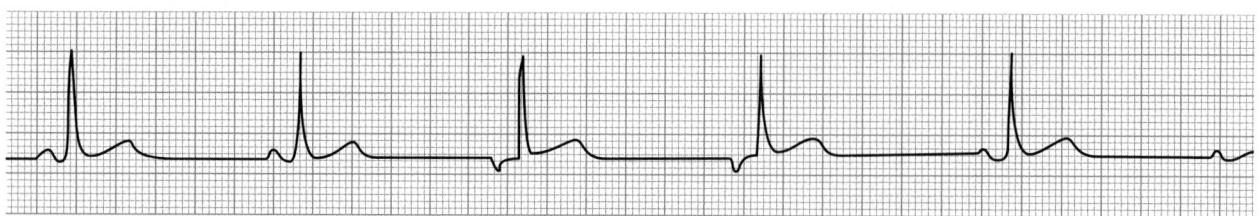

P Wave: Multifocal; PR Interval: 0.16 second; QRS Complex: 0.06 second; QT Interval: 0.04 second; Heart Rate: Atrial: Approximately 60 bpm; Ventricular: 50 bpm; Rhythm: Irregular; Ectopic Beats; Multifocal P waves.

FIGURE 38–24 ■ Wandering atrial pacemaker.

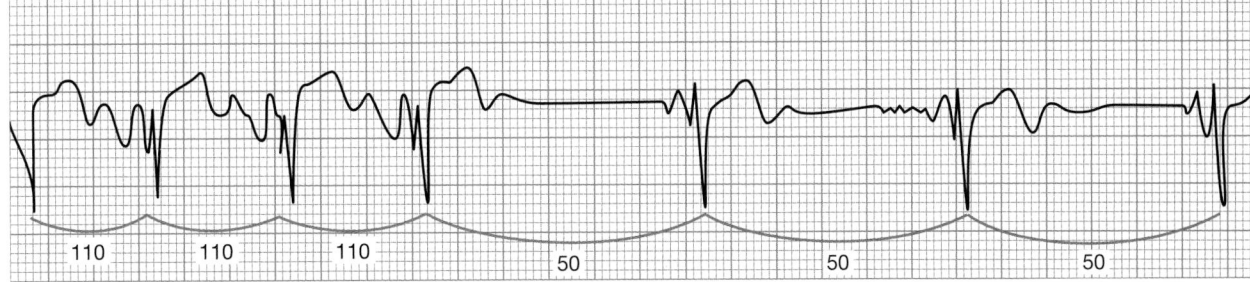

P Wave: Present, but variable configuration; PR Interval: 0.14 second; QRS Complex: 0.08 second; QT Interval: 0.40 second;
Heart Rate: Atrial: 60 bpm, Ventricular: 60 bpm; Rhythm: Irregular; Ectopic Beats: May occur with slow rate.

FIGURE 38–25 ■ Sick sinus syndrome.

chronic atrial tachycardia. This disorder also is referred to as sinoatrial disease and sinoatrial dysfunction. The cause is a severely depressed nonreliable SA node due to heart disease or the side effect of certain cardiac drugs, such as cardiac glycosides, sympatholytic antihypertensive agents, beta-adrenergic blockers, calcium channel blockers, and membrane active antiarrhythmic agents. When the tachycardia occurs with SSS there is increased oxygen consumption and workload for the myocardium. Profound sinus bradycardia with SSS may progress to sinus pauses or arrest, thereby decreasing cardiac output. Figure 38–25 ■ is a rhythm strip showing sick sinus syndrome. Significant ECG features of sick sinus syndrome include:

- P waves may be present or absent depending on which dysrhythmia is occurring.
- PR interval varies due to changing P wave sites.
- QT interval varies due to rate changes.
- Heart rate may be rapid or slow, or a combination of both.
- Heart rhythm is irregular and highly variable.
- Ectopic beats may be present when a slow rate occurs.

The etiology, physical assessment findings, and treatment of sick sinus syndrome are outlined in Chart 38–7 (p. 1091).

■ Nursing Management for Responsibilities for Atrial Dysrhythmias

Nursing responsibility when any dysrhythmia occurs is to assess the patient's response to the rhythm. This is especially true if it is a new onset dysrhythmia and/or if the dysrhythmia causes a drop in the cardiac output. The atrial dysrhythmias do not have the impact on cardiac output that the more serious ventricular dysrhythmias do, but any change in cardiac output may cause clinical manifestations, and therefore, requires an in-depth assessment. The patient is evaluated for the clinical manifestations of reduced cardiac output as outlined in Chart 38–6 (p. 1090). Vital signs and clinical manifestations must be monitored frequently to assess tolerance of the rhythm, especially if it is sustained. The health care provider needs to be notified, especially if this is a new rhythm, because medical intervention must be initiated to convert the rhythm back to normal sinus rhythm.

Atrial flutter and fibrillation may occur as a transient dysrhythmia in healthy young individuals. If these conditions are chronic they are typically associated with heart disease including atrial muscle disease or atrial distention with disease of the sinus node. Atrial fibrillation also is seen in congenital heart disease. If the atrial flutter and/or atrial fibrillation are chronic conditions, and normal sinus rhythm cannot be reestablished, the patient often is placed on an anticoagulant, such as warfarin. This treatment is indicated because a fluttering/fibrillating atrium creates blood stasis, which increases the risk of clot formation. If these clots travel out of the atrium they tend to lodge in the brain, and, on rare occasions in the lung, causing an alteration in normal function in these areas.

Treatment of atrial fibrillation/flutter may include cardioversion, which is the delivery of electrical voltage in order to stop unwanted electrical activity and allow the SA node to resume the heart's pacemaker. Cardioversion is discussed in detail in Chapter 39 ∞. This treatment increases risk for myocardial infarction, cerebral vascular accident (CVA), and pulmonary embolus. The nurse needs to assess the patient post-cardioversion for clinical manifestations of these disorders. Myocardial infarction is discussed in detail in Chapter 40 ∞. Cardiovascular accident (CVA) is discussed in Chapter 30 ∞, and pulmonary embolus is discussed in Chapters 35 and 36 ∞.

Besides heart disease frequently there are other causes for atrial cardiac dysrhythmias that must be evaluated and treated, e.g., stress, pain, and anxiety. The treatment may be narcotics for pain relief or an antianxiety medication for stress and increased anxiety. The nurse may need only to sit and listen to the patient and provide emotional support.

Junctional Dysrhythmias

Junctional dysrhythmias also referred to as nodal rhythms result from either an irritable focus in the junctional tissue that discharges before the SA node has had a chance to or because the SA node has failed to fire and the junctional node becomes the secondary pacemaker. AV junctional dysrhythmias may occur if the impulse from the SA node is blocked as it exits the SA node or if it is not conducted through the atria. AV junctional dysrhythmias have a distinctive pattern on ECG tracings because the impulse is not initiated in the SA node. The impulse is initiated in the AV junctional tissue and must travel in a backward (retrograde) direction to activate the atria. Therefore, the P wave is inverted or negatively deflected, due to this retrograde conduction, and may occur before, after, or buried in, the QRS complex. Retrograde conduction means that the impulse originates in the AV junction so it stimulates the atria from the bottom up instead of the top down. The impulse simultaneously initiates both atrial and ventricular contractions. The location of the P wave is, therefore, dependent on the speed with which the impulses travel in both chambers. The QRS complex configuration is normal in appearance because the impulse travels the normal pathway from the AV junctional node through the ventricles. AV junctional dysrhythmias are not considered lethal or life threatening, but as always, the most important indicator of the clinical significance of any dysrhythmia is the patient's response to or tolerance of the rhythm. The three AV junctional dysrhythmias discussed in this chapter are: junctional escape rhythm, premature junctional contractions, and paroxysmal junctional tachycardia.

Junctional Escape Rhythm

Junctional escape rhythm occurs when there is a problem with normal SA node function, either fails to produce an impulse, or when the SA node's rate of firing falls below the intrinsic rate of the AV node. At this time the AV node will assume the role of the pacemaker. The ability of the AV node to assume this role is a safety measure in that it becomes the pacemaker for the heart when the SA node fails to do so. When an isolated beat from the AV junction occurs it is called a junctional escape beat or complex, as compared to a series of beats that then is called a junctional rhythm. When a rhythm is generated from the junction, the rate is between 40 and 60 beats per minute. If the rate is greater than 60 but less than 100 it is referred to as an accelerated junctional rhythm. If the rate is greater than 100 typically it is called junctional tachycardia.

Figures 38–26 ■ and 38–27 ■ are ECG rhythm strips that show junctional escape rhythm and accelerated junctional rhythm, respectively. Significant ECG features of junctional escape rhythms include:

- P wave is inverted, negatively deflected, due to retrograde conduction, and either occurs before, after, or buried in the QRS complex.
- PR interval is dependent on the location of P wave; thus, the PR interval may or may not be present or normal.
- QRS complex is normal in duration and shape, unless distorted by a buried P wave.
- QT interval is within normal range, unless impacted by the heart rate. It is prolonged with slow heart rate or shortened with increased heart rate.
- Heart rate is usually within normal range for a rhythm generated from the AV junction and is 40 to 60 beats per minute. For an accelerated junctional rhythm the rate is 60 to 100 beats per minute and for junctional tachycardia the heart rate is greater than 100 bpm.
- Heart rhythm is typically regular.
- Entire rhythm is composed of ectopic beats because they all come from the AV junction instead of the SA node. Other ectopic beats may occur with slow heart rate.

The etiology, physical assessment findings, and treatment of junctional escape rhythms are outlined in Chart 38–8.

Premature Junctional Contraction

A **premature junctional contraction (PJC)** originates as an ectopic beat that is initiated in the atrioventricular (AV) junction. It discharges before the next expected SA node impulse causing simultaneous atrial and ventricular contraction to occur. This is not a dangerous dysrhythmia, although it does indicate that some degree of cardiac ischemia is occurring. Figure 38–28 ■ (p. 1100) is

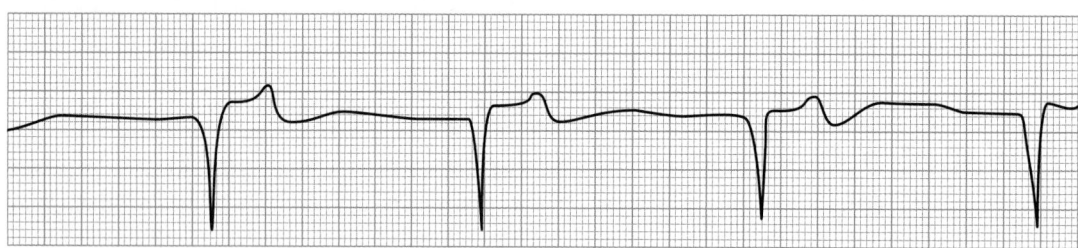

P Wave: None, or buried in QRS Complex; PR Interval: Not measurable; QRS Complex: 0.10 second; QT Interval: 0.40 second; Heart Rate: Atrial: Not measurable, Ventricular: 40 bpm; Rhythm: Regular; Ectopic Beats: None.

FIGURE 38–26 ■ Junctional escape rhythm.

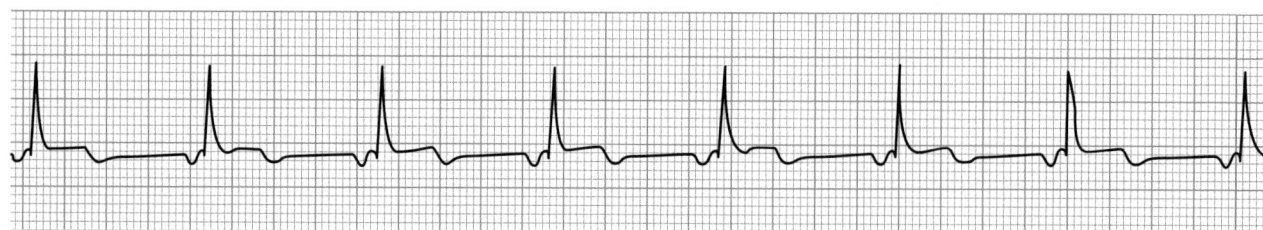

P Wave: Inverted and regular; PR Interval: 0.14–0.16 second; QRS Complex: 0.08 second: QT Interval: 0.44 second; Heart Rate: Atrial: 80 bpm, Ventricular: 80 bpm; Rhythm: Regular: Ectopic Beats: none.

FIGURE 38–27 ■ Accelerated junctional rhythm.

| CHART 38–8 | **Junctional Dysrhythmias: Etiology, Physical Assessment, and Treatment** | | |

Dysrhythmia	Etiology	Physical Assessment	Treatment
Junctional escape rhythm	SA node disease Myocardial infarction Hypoxia and ischemia Heart failure Increased vagal tone Certain cardiac drugs: such as digoxin, beta adrenergic blockers, and calcium channel blockers Sinus bradycardia Digoxin toxicity Hyperkalemia Valve disease	Pulse: rhythm is regular with a usual rate of 40 – 60 bpm unless it is an accelerated rhythm of > 100 bpm If cardiac output is decreased the following clinical manifestations may occur: Angina Syncope Generalized weakness Dizziness Shortness of breath Altered mental state may be present, although rare.	Observe for other dysrhthmias if a slow rate is present. Generally this condition is asymptomatic; however, if symptomatic, typical treatment includes: Oxygen Drug therapy: (atropine, dopamine) Pacemaker Cardioversion
Premature junctional contraction (PJC)	Irritability of the AV junctional tissue caused by: SA node disease Myocardial infarction Sinus bradycardia Mitral stenosis Mitral valve prolapse Cor pulmonale Hypoxia Ischemia Infectious diseases Increased vagal tone Increased sympathetic tone Electrolyte imbalances Digoxin Stimulants Stress Anxiety May precede AV block	Pulse: Irregular BP: Normal unless PJCs occur frequently enough to decrease cardiac output.	Rarely causes symptoms, thus typically not treated. Find and treat the underlying cause, if possible. If it initiates a more serious dysrhythmia, such as tachycardia, therapy becomes more aggressive, contingent on the type of dysrhythmia. If occurring frequently, more than 5 times per minute, they can drop cardiac output, and predispose the patient to other dysrhythmias. Oxygen Drugs such as stimulants, sympathomimetics, and digitalis may be discontinued.
Paroxysmal junctional tachycardia (PJT)	May occur at any age with no prior history of underlying heart disease. Digoxin toxicity (most common cause) Inferior wall myocardial infarction Myocarditis Ischemia Untoward response to open heart surgery Frequent ingestion of stimulants Anxiety Increased catecholamine secretion	Pulse: Rapid, with patient experiencing a fluttering sensation. BP: Lower than usual due to decreased cardiac output. If cardiac output is decreased the following clinical manifestations may occur: Angina Syncope Generalized weakness Dizziness Shortness of breath Altered mental state may be present, although rare.	Find and treat the cause as PJTs may be a predisposition to lethal dysrhythmias, heart failure, and shock. Vagal maneuvers may be applied. Oxygen Drug therapy initiated: includes: amiodarone or beta-adrenergic blockers. Cardioversion may be initiated if necessary.

a rhythm strip showing premature junctional contraction. Significant ECG features of premature junction contractions include:

- P wave is inverted and occurs before, after, or buried in the QRS complex.
- PR interval is dependent on the location of P wave; thus, the PR interval may or may not be present or normal.
- QRS complex is normal in duration and shape, unless distorted by a buried P wave.

- QT interval also is normal unless impacted by the heart rate.
- Heart rate is that of the underlying rhythm.
- Heart rhythm is irregular when PJCs are present; or it may be described as regular with premature beats.
- Ectopic beat is the PJC.

The etiology, physical assessment findings, and treatment of PJCs are outlined in Chart 38–8.

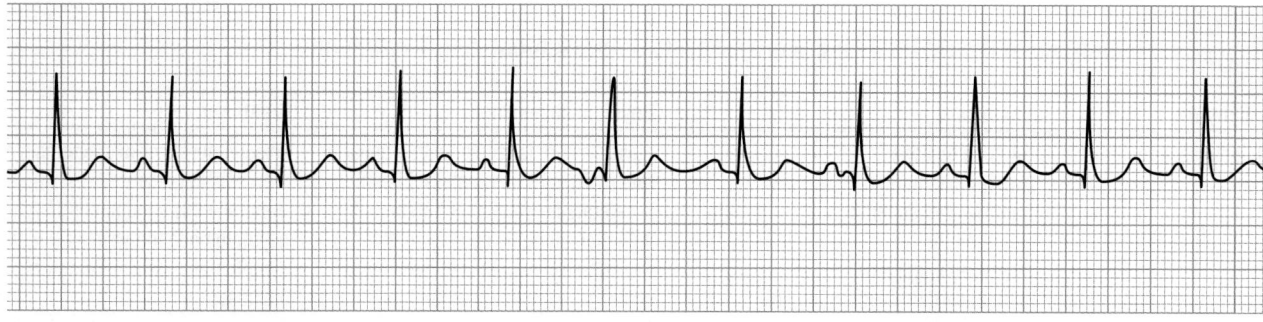

P Wave: Present and regular except for premature beat; PR Interval: 0.16 second; QRS Complex: 0.08 second; second; Heart Rate: Atrial: 110 bpm, Ventricular: 110 bpm; Rhythm: Regular except for premature beats: Ectopic Beats: none

FIGURE 38–28 ■ Premature junctional contraction (PJC).

Paroxysmal Junctional Tachycardia

The **paroxysmal junctional tachycardia (PJT)** rhythm is defined as an irritable focus in the AV junction that assumes the pacemaker role by discharging impulses more rapidly than the SA node. It begins and ends abruptly, which is why it is called paroxysmal. If it is a sustained rhythm, and greater than 60 beats per minute, it may be referred to as junctional tachycardia. The term *junctional tachycardia* sometimes is used interchangeably with the term accelerated junctional rhythm, which was discussed previously. This rhythm produces a junctional rate of over 60 beats per minute. Figure 38–29 ■ is a rhythm strip showing paroxysmal junctional tachycardia. Significant ECG features of paroxysmal junctional tachycardia include:

- Heart rate usually is 160 to 240 beats per minute and constant. It may, however, be as low as 110 beats per minute or exceed 240 beats per minute.
- P wave is inverted and occurs before, after, or buried in the QRS complex.
- PR interval is dependent on the location of P wave; thus, the PR interval may or may not be present or normal.
- QRS complex is normal in duration and shape, unless distorted by a buried P wave.
- QT interval shortens due to increased heart rate.
- Heart rhythm is essentially regular. It may become irregular as the rate increases.
- Entire rhythm is composed of ectopic beats because they all come from the AV junction instead of the SA node.

The etiology, physical assessment findings, and treatment of PJTs are outlined in Chart 38–8 (p. 1099).

■ Nursing Management for Junctional Dysrhythmias

Like atrial dysrhythmias, junctional dysrhythmias generally are not life threatening. However, the decreased and/or increased heart rate does have an impact on cardiac output. This is especially true in the presence of heart disease when the heart is unable to significantly increase the force of the muscle contraction to compensate for the rate changes. Therefore, the nurse must evaluate the patient for clinical manifestations of decreased cardiac output (Chart 38–6, p. 1090). When rhythm is slow other ectopic foci may attempt to become the heart's pacemaker, therefore, the nurse must assess the rhythm for other aberrancies. The health care provider needs to be notified, especially if it is a new onset dysrhythmia in order to determine cause and treatment. It is essential that the nurse assist the health care provider in determining the cause and treatment of dysrhythmias. Since some prescribed medications, e.g., digoxin, cause significant dysrhythmias, the patient's medical history should be reviewed to determine if the dysrhythmia is medication related. Serum drug levels should be ordered as indicated. For symptomatic junctional tachycardia, treatment also may include applying vagal maneuvers, initiating drug therapy, and completing cardioversion if necessary. As always any significant rhythm change or the appearance of new onset dysrhythmias needs to be reported to the health care provider.

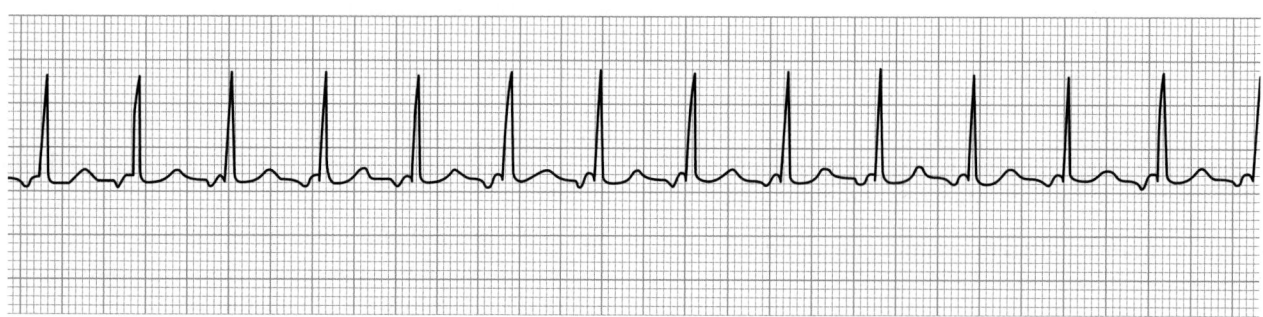

P Wave: Inverted and regular; PR Interval: 0.08 second; QRS Complex: 0.06 second; QT Interval: 0.32 second; Heart Rate: Atrial: 130 bpm, Ventricular: 130 bpm. Rhythm: Regular; Ectopic Beats: None.

FIGURE 38–29 ■ Paroxysmal junctional tachycardia.

Due to the clinical manifestations of these dysrhythmias, the patient and family may experience anxiety. Thus, the nurse also must assess and treat the anxiety by use of supportive measures, such as listening to the patient's concerns, offering reassurance, providing a calm environment, and medicating for anxiety and pain relief as appropriate.

Conduction Block Dysrhythmias

Cardiac conduction block dysrhythmias occur due to an interruption in the continuity of the cardiac electrical conduction system. This discontinuity is caused by a loss of blood supply to the conduction system as a result of ischemic heart disease or coronary artery disease. Heart blocks are classified according to the degree of the block, either partial or complete obstruction of the electrical conduction pathway. These disorders may be either permanent or transient, and minor or significant. The clinical significance of an AV block depends on the degree (severity) of the block, the rate of the escape pacemaker (junctional vs. ventricular), and the patient's response to that ventricular rate. There are four types of heart block dysrhythmias discussed next: first-degree AV block; Mobitz I/Wenckebach/ Type I second-degree heart block; Mobitz II second-degree block; and third-degree AV block (complete).

First-Degree AV Block

First-degree AV block represents a conduction disturbance in which electrical impulses flow normally from the SA node through the atria, but are delayed at the AV node. There is a prolongation or slowing of conduction rather than an actual block. Because of this consistent delay the PR interval is greater than 0.20 second, making it abnormal. First-degree AV block is not actually a dysrhythmia. Its presence only indicates a delay at the AV node, rather than a definite block. Figure 38–30 ■ is a rhythm strip showing first-degree AV block. Significant ECG features of first-degree AV block include:

- P waves are present and normal in size and shape.
- PR interval is prolonged, greater than 0.20 second, but constant.
- QRS duration usually is normal.
- QT interval is normal unless there is an abnormal rate.
- Heart rate is usually within normal range.
- Heart rhythm is regular.

The etiology, physical assessment findings, and treatment of first-degree AV blocks are outlined in Chart 38–9 (p. 1102).

Mobitz I/Wenckebach/Type I Second-Degree Heart Block

The terms Mobitz I/Wenckebach/Type 1 second-degree heart block, are used interchangeably to refer to the same abnormality. This abnormality is depicted as a progressive prolongation of the electrical impulse delay in the AV node until there is a complete loss of the QRS complex, and thus, no ventricular contraction. This dysrhythmia is characterized by progressive lengthening of the PR interval until a QRS complex fails to appear after a P wave (Beasley, 2003). **Mobitz I/Wenckebach** is one of the two types of second-degree block that occurs in the AV node. Figure 38–31 ■ (p. 1104) is a rhythm strip showing Mobitz I/Wenckebach dysrhythmia. Significant ECG features of Mobitz I/Wenckebach dysrhythmia include:

- P waves are present, and they precede the QRS complexes.
- PR interval progressively prolongs until there is a dropped QRS complex and then the progressive prolongation begins again.
- QRS complexes are normal in shape and duration.
- QT interval is within normal limits, unless no QRS complex occurs.
- Atrial heart rate is normal and regular; ventricular heart rate is less than that of the atrial rate.
- Atrial rhythm is regular; the ventricular rhythm is irregular.

The etiology, physical assessment findings, and treatment of Mobitz I/Wenckebach/Type I second-degree heart block are outlined in Chart 38–9 (p. 1102).

Mobitz II Second-Degree Block

Mobitz II second-degree block results from an intermittent block of the AV node, the bundle of His, or bundle branches. This dysrhythmia occurs when this block causes an intermittent interruption in the electrical conduction system near or below the AV node, which prevents the sinus or atrial impulses from getting to the ventricles. On the ECG strip the P wave (atrial contraction) is present at regular intervals because the SA node is generating impulses in a normal manner; however when the block occurs, the P wave is not followed by a QRS complex. An AV conduction ratio of 2 Ps for every 1 QRS; 3Ps for every 1 QRS, or greater is common, with or without a bundle branch block

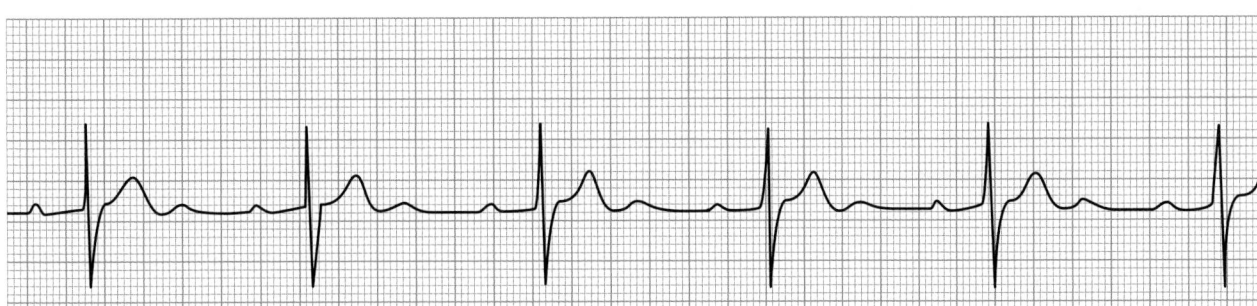

P Wave: Present and regular; PR Interval: 0.24 second; QRS Complex: 0.06 second; QT Interval: 0.40 second; Heart Rate: Atrial: 60 bpm, Ventricular: 60 bpm; Rhythm: Regular; Ectopic Beats: None.

FIGURE 38–30 ■ First-degree AV block.

CHART 38–9	AV Block Dysrhythmias: Etiology, Physical Assessment, and Treatment		
Dysrhythmia	**Etiology**	**Physical Assessment**	**Treatment**
First-degree AV block	May occur without any underlying heart disease May occur in athletes Occurs in about 13% of the population Drug reactions to digoxin, beta-blockers, and CA channel blockers Cardiac related causes include: Ischemia Myocardial infarction Rheumatic heart disease Coronary artery disease	Pulse: Within normal limits BP: Within normal limits	This is not a dangerous rhythm in itself and usually is asymptomatic. May progress to a more advanced heart block, especially in the presence of a myocardial infarction. Observe closely and place on an ECG monitor to detect additional signs and symptoms.
Mobitz I / Wenckebach/ Type I second-degree heart block	Conduction delay within the AV node Most commonly associated with AV nodal ischemia secondary to occlusion of the right coronary artery Other causes may be: Myocardial infarction Inferior/right ventricular structural heart disease or an anatomical abnormality Myocarditis Transient side effect of open heart surgery Increased vagal activity Drug toxicity, e.g., digoxin	Pulse: Irregular BP: May be decreased with frequently dropped beats due to decreased cardiac output. If cardiac output is decreased the following clinical manifestations may occur: Angina Syncope Generalized weakness Dizziness Shortness of breath Altered mental state may be present, although rare.	This is often a transient rhythm and will revert to normal rhythm without treatment. Usually asymptomatic because the ventricular rate often remains nearly normal and cardiac output is not significantly affected. If symptomatic, and is a result of medications, they should be withheld. If the heart rate is slow and serious clinical manifestations such as low BP, angina, shortness of breath, occur, atropine or temporary pacing is considered. When occurs in conjunction with acute myocardial infarction, observe for increasing AV block.
Mobitz II second-degree AV block	Septal wall necrosis Acute inferior or right ventricular MI Myocarditis Advanced coronary artery disease (general ischemia) Electrolyte imbalance Digitalis toxicity Reaction to amiodarone, beta-blockers, or calcium channel blockers	Pulse: slow and typically irregular, depending on ventricular response BP: Decreased due to low cardiac output If cardiac output is decreased the following clinical manifestations may occur: Angina Syncope Generalized weakness Dizziness Shortness of breath Altered mental state may be present.	Often considered an emergent situation. The health care provider should be notified at once. May progress to a third-degree AV block and ventricular asystole, thus, a standby cardiac pacemaker is indicated for asymptomatic patients, and temporary cardiac pacing is required for symptomatic patients. For sustained permanent block, a permanent pacemaker is inserted.
Third-degree AV block (complete)	Ischemic damage Septal wall necrosis Acute inferior or right ventricular MI due to the effect of vagal tone and ischemia on the AV node Acute anterior MI Myocarditis Coronary artery disease Cardiomyopathies Cardiac muscle diseases Rheumatic heart disease Drug toxicity, reaction to amiodarone, beta-blockers, or calcium channel blockers Electrolyte imbalance Rheumatic heart disease Congenital condition usually located at the level of the AV junction	Pulse: Slow and usually irregular BP: Lower than usual If cardiac output is decreased the following clinical manifestations may occur: Angina Syncope Generalized weakness Dizziness Shortness of breath Altered mental state may be present.	Treatment is essential as third-degree block is potentially lethal. If an AV junctional or ventricular escape pacemaker does not take over following a sudden onset of third-degree AV block, asystole will occur. Clinical manifestations depend on the ventricular heart rate, especially for slow rates. If the QRS is narrow and the patient is symptomatic, initial management is atropine and/or transcutaneous pacing. If the QRS is wide and the patient is symptomatic, transcutaneous pacing is started. A temporary pacemaker is inserted, and may be followed by a permanent pacemaker.

CHART 38–9 **AV Block Dysrhythmias: Etiology, Physical Assessment, and Treatment—*Continued***

Dysrhythmia	Etiology	Physical Assessment	Treatment
Bundle branch block (BBB)	Causes vary depending on whether it is the right or left BBB Right BBB may be present in healthy individuals with apparently normal hearts without any apparent underlying cause Common pathological causes include: Coronary artery disease Cardiac tumors Cardiomyopathy Myocarditis Atrial septal defect Cardiac surgery Congenital RBBB Acute anterioseptal MI Acute pulmonary embolism or infarction Acute heart failure Unlike RBBB, LBBB always indicates a diseased heart and generally is more common in individuals with diseased hearts Common causes include: Hypertensive heart disease Cardiomyopathy Myocarditis Syphilitic, rheumatic, and congenital heart disease Cardiac tumors Idiopathic degenerative disease of the electrical conduction system Aberrant ventricular conduction associated with supraventricular premature contractions and tachycardia	Pulse: Within normal limits BP: Within normal limits	Specific treatment usually is not indicated if it is present alone and is not the result of an acute MI. Temporary cardiac pacing is indicated for the treatment of a right or left bundle branch block under the following conditions: results from an acute MI is complicated by a first- or second-degree AV block, or both, especially in the setting of an acute MI if the block progresses to a complete AV block.

(Beasley, 2003). In other words there are 2, 3, or 4 P waves for every QRS complex. Thus, with this dysrhythmia there may be enough dropped QRSs to significantly impact cardiac output. Therefore, Mobitz II is a more serious dysrhythmia than either first-degree AV block or Mobitz I (Wenckebach/ Type I second-degree heart block) because of the impact on the cardiac output and an increased risk of progression to third-degree block or complete heart block. Figure 38–32 ■ (p. 1104) is a rhythm strip showing Mobitz II/second-degree block. Significant ECG features of Mobitz II/second-degree block include:

- QRS complexes are intermittently absent; they may be normal to prolonged when present; and they are usually prolonged due to bundle branch block.
- P waves are present and regular.
- PR intervals are constant with conducted beats.
- QT intervals are within normal limits.
- Atrial heart rate is usually normal; ventricular heart rate is less than the atrial rate.

- Atrial rhythm is regular; ventricular rhythm may be regular or irregular. The ventricular rhythm is irregular when the AV block is intermittent; thereby, causing a varying AV conduction ratio.
- Ectopic beats may be present due to the slow heart rate.

The etiology, physical assessment findings, and treatment of Mobitz II heart block are outlined in Chart 38–9.

Third-Degree AV Block (Complete)

Third-degree AV block, or **complete block,** is the independent excitation and contraction of the atria and ventricles due to the inability of any atrial impulses to reach the ventricles. In other words, the top and bottom of the heart are not communicating; they are beating independently. This dysrhythmia also is referred to as **AV dissociation** because of the independent function of the atria and the ventricles. The SA node fires at regular intervals, producing P waves at a normal rate of 60 to 100 beats per minute; whereas, the ventricles are paced by either a pacemaker site in the ventricles themselves or in the junctional

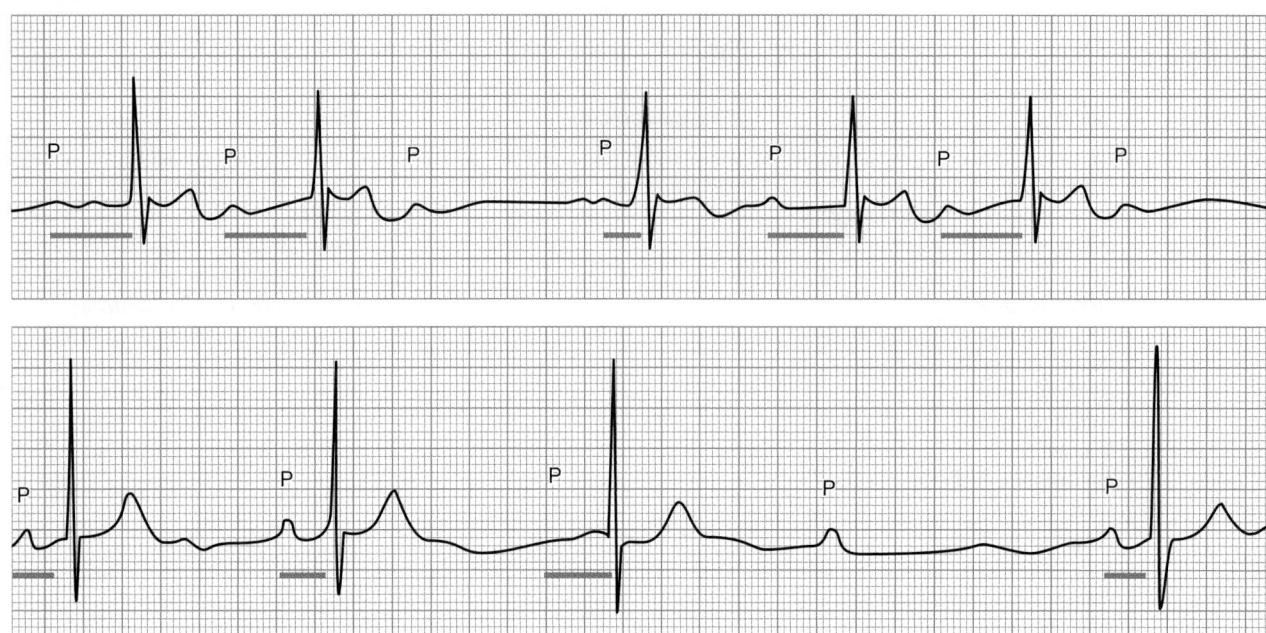

P Waves: Present and regular; PR Interval: Progressively prolonged until one P wave is not conducted and the sequence begins again; QRS Complex: 0.10 second; QT Interval: 0.42–0.60 second; Heart Rate: Atrial: 70 bpm, Ventricular 50 bpm; Rhythm: Atrial: Regular, Ventricular: Irregular due to dropped beat; Ectopic Beats: None. Conclusion: Mobitz I/Wenckeback Second-Degree Heart Block.

FIGURE 38–31 ■ Mobitz I/Wenckebach/second-degree heart block.

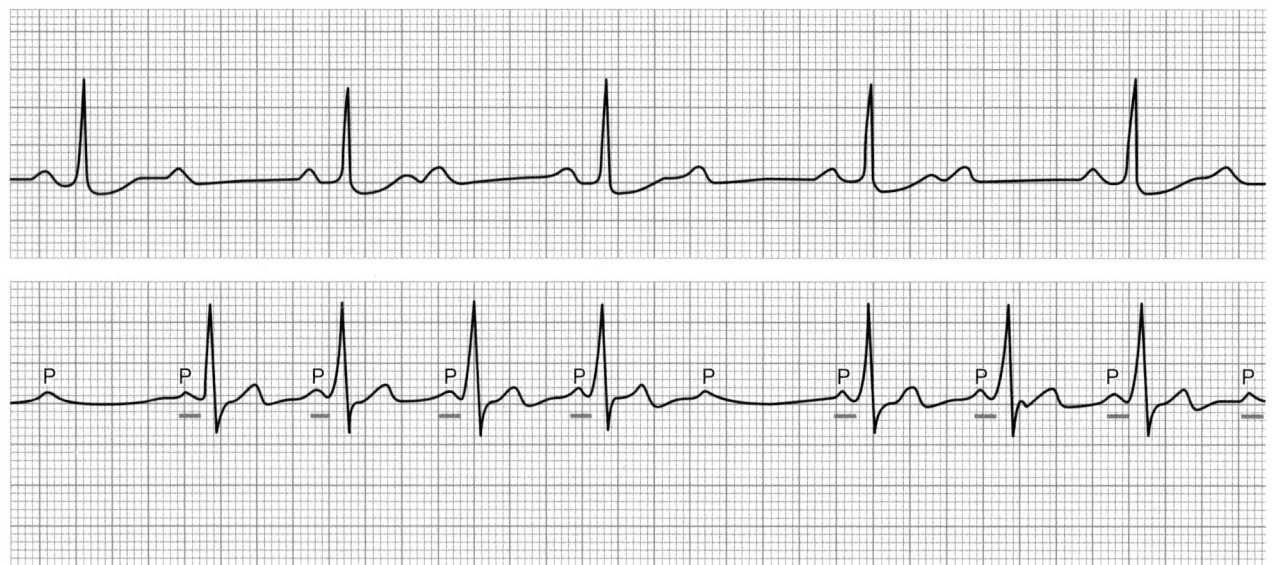

P Waves: Present and regular; PR Interval: 0.24 second; QRS Complex: 0.06 second; QT Interval: 0.48 second; Heart Rate: Atrial: 100 bpm, Ventricular 50 bpm; Rhythm: Atrial: Regular, Ventricular: Irregular due to dropped beat; Ectopic Beats: None.

FIGURE 38–32 ■ Mobitz II/second-degree heart block.

tissue. If the QRS complex is narrow the pacemaker is in the junctional tissue with a rate of 40 to 60 beats per minute. However, if the QRS complex is wide the pacemaker is in the Purkinje network and the heart rate ranges from 20 to 40 beats per minute; this is referred to as an idioventricular rhythm. Complete AV block associated with an inferior myocardial infarction is thought to be a block in the bundle of His, and often occurs after progression from first-degree AV block or second-degree AV

block, type I. Third-degree heart block is the most serious type of heart block because it may progress to asystole (a complete cessation of electrical activity), and the slow ventricular heart rate results in decreased cardiac output. Since the ventricular rhythm may not be able to sustain adequate cardiac output, third-degree heart block is referred to as a lethal dysrhythmia. Figure 38–33 ■ is a rhythm strip showing third-degree or complete heart block. Significant ECG features of third-degree heart block include:

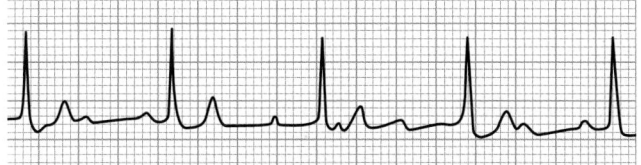

P Waves: Present and regular; PR Interval: None; QRS Complex: 0.12 second; QT Interval: 0.38 second; Heart Rate: Atrial: 90 bpm, Ventricular: 40–50 bpm; Rhythm: Regular; Ectopic Beats: None.

FIGURE 38–33 ■ Third-degree (complete) heart block.

- Atrial and ventricular rhythms are independent of one another (dissociated). Atrial rhythm usually is regular, depending on underlying sinus, atrial, or junctional rhythm. Ventricular rhythm may be regular or irregular.

- P waves are present and regular; however there is no relationship to QRS complexes.

- PR interval is absent.

- QRS complex may be narrow with a junctional rhythm, or wide with an idioventricular rhythm.

- QT interval may change with the rate change, but is not directly affected.

- Atrial heart rate is regular, 60 to 100 beats per minute; nodal rate is 40 to 60 beats per minute; and ventricular rate is 20 to 40 beats per minute.

- Atrial and ventricular rhythms are independent of one another (dissociated). Atrial rhythm usually is regular, depending on underlying sinus, atrial, or junctional rhythm. Ventricular rhythm may be regular or irregular.

- Ectopic beats usually are present due to slow rate.

The etiology, physical assessment findings, and treatment of Mobitz II heart block are outlined in Chart 38–9 (p. 1102).

Bundle Branch Block

Bundle branch block, also referred to as intraventricular conduction defect, is a discontinuity of conduction, complete or incomplete, in one branch of the bundle of His, which affects normal transmission of the impulse through the ventricles. When one bundle is blocked, the ventricles depolarize asynchronously. Bundle branch block is characterized by a delay of excitation to one ventricle; therefore, an abnormal spread of electrical activity through the ventricles occurs. This delayed conduction causes a widening of the QRS complex to more than 0.12 second. When measuring the QRS complex, it is necessary to observe the axis of the complex to determine whether it is right or left bundle branch block. Figure 38–34 ■ is a rhythm strip showing a bundle branch block. Significant ECG features of bundle branch block include:

- QRS complex is more than 0.12 second if a complete bundle branch block is present. P waves are present and regular.

- PR interval is 0.12 to 0.20 second.

- QRS measuring 0.10 to 0.12 second is called an incomplete right or left bundle branch block.

- QT interval is within normal limits.

- Heart rate is 60 to 100 beats per minute.

- Heart rhythm is regular.

The etiology, physical assessment findings, and treatment of bundle branch block are outlined in Chart 38–9 (p. 1102).

■ Nursing Management for Conduction Block Dysrhythmias

The type of heart block determines the severity of the dysrhythmia, and therefore, nursing responsibilities. As with any dysrhythmia the patient's tolerance to the rhythm must be evaluated when heart block develops. First-degree heart block and bundle branch block in isolation, do not impact cardiac output, therefore, patients are not symptomatic. With first-degree heart block, the nurse must observe the cardiac monitor for any changes in the rhythm indicating a progression to a more severe type of heart block.

Mobitz I/Wenckebach often does not require treatment, however, the ECG monitoring and patient assessment are necessary because this type of block may lead to a more serious Mobitz II or complete heart block. It is necessary, therefore, that the nurse frequently checks the monitor to identify potential changes. As with any new dysrhythmia, Mobitz I/Wenckebach needs to be reported to the health care provider.

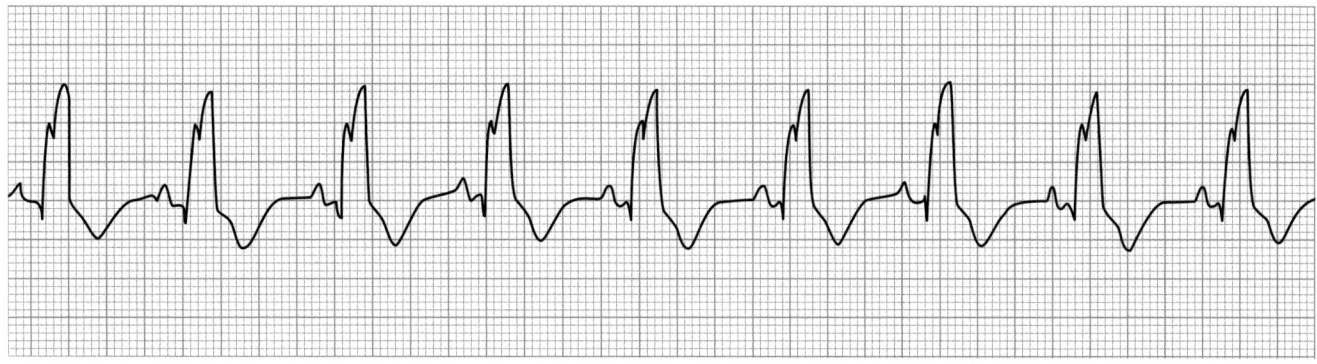

P Wave: Normal sinus rhythm; PR Interval: 0.16 second; QRS Complex: 0.20 second; QT Interval: 0.40 second. Heart Rate: Atrial: 90 bpm, Ventricular: 90 bpm; Rhythm: Atrial: Regular, Ventricular: Regular; Ectopic Beats: None.

FIGURE 38–34 ■ Bundle branch block.

The onset of Mobitz II and complete heart block are emergent situations that require immediate intervention. Mobitz II is described as a "treacherous and unpredictable" rhythm that can deteriorate to become a complete heart block. If untreated, these rhythms may progress to cardiac asystole and sudden death. At any indication of rhythm changes indicative of Mobitz II or complete heart block, the health care provider should be notified at once. The nurse should prepare for a temporary pacemaker insertion (Chapter 39), which generally is indicated for these types of dysrhythmias. A permanent pacemaker may be necessary if the block persists. It is the nurse's responsibility when working with monitored patients to be familiar with equipment location and operation.

CRITICAL ALERT *Signs and symptoms of third-degree AV block are the same as those in symptomatic sinus bradycardia. AV block can be more ominous, especially when associated with wide and bizarre QRS complexes. If an AV junctional or ventricular escape pacemaker does not take over the pacing of the heart following a sudden onset of third-degree AV block or ventricular asystole will occur. Temporary cardiac pacemaker is required immediately for treatment of symptomatic third-degree block with wide QRS complexes. The nurse must report this rhythm immediately to the health care provider in order to initiate treatment before a significant drop in cardiac output occurs.*

Ventricular Dysrhythmias

Ventricular dysrhythmias are caused by ectopic or irritable foci in the walls of the ventricles. The pacemaker cells in the ventricles may, in certain circumstances, serve as the heart's pacemaker. When the SA node fails or the impulse does not get through the AV node, the ventricles take over the pacing role. In this situation, an electrical impulse may be instigated from both the bundle of His and the Purkinje network. The intrinsic ventricular rate is only 20 to 40 beats per minute; therefore, cardiac output is severely compromised. Also, if the atrium is not contracting there is no atrial kick, causing further decrease in cardiac output. Because the rhythm originates in the ventricle there is no P wave, and because it is an abnormal conduction pathway the QRS is wide and distorted. Ventricular dysrhythmias are considered to be very serious dysrhythmias mainly due to their im-

pact on cardiac output. The various types of ventricular dysrhythmias are discussed next: premature ventricular contraction, ventricular tachycardia, torsade de pointes, ventricular fibrillation, pulseless electrical activity, and asystole.

Premature Ventricular Contraction

A **premature ventricular contraction (PVC)** is caused by an irritable focus within the ventricle that discharges before the next sinus impulse, stimulating the ventricle directly, and causing a contraction. PVCs are more likely to occur during bradycardia when there is more time for them to emerge. Premature ventricular contractions (PVCs) are individual beats, one ectopic beat, not a rhythm. PVCs have a wide and bizarre QRS complex that is more than 0.12 second in length. Because the activation begins outside the normal conduction system, it takes longer to travel the ventricular conduction pathways, thereby prolonging the QRS length. PVCs are followed by a full compensatory pause, meaning the SA node rate and rhythm are unaffected by the PVC. In other words, the rate prior to the PVC resumes, following the PVC. A compensatory pause is measured by:

- Measuring the two beats preceding the PVC
- Moving the calipers along, and marking where the next beat should have fallen
- Then placing the calipers on the spot where the beat should have occurred, measure the distance to the next beat, there should not be a change in the cadence of the rhythm.

The full compensatory pause is one of the factors used when evaluating and diagnosing PVCs. To distinguish PVCs from atrial and junctional ectopic beats, the full compensatory pause is present. Typically, atrial and junctional ectopic beats do not have a full compensatory pause, they are said to be non-compensatory or partially compensatory, meaning that there is a rhythm change following these dysrhythmias. Figure 38–35 ■ is a rhythm strip showing premature ventricular contractions (PVCs) with a full compensatory pause.

Unifocal and Multifocal PVCs

Premature ventricular contractions (PVCs) occur in various patterns. Each pattern differs in its severity and prognosis. First, if the PVC configuration (size and shape) remains the same

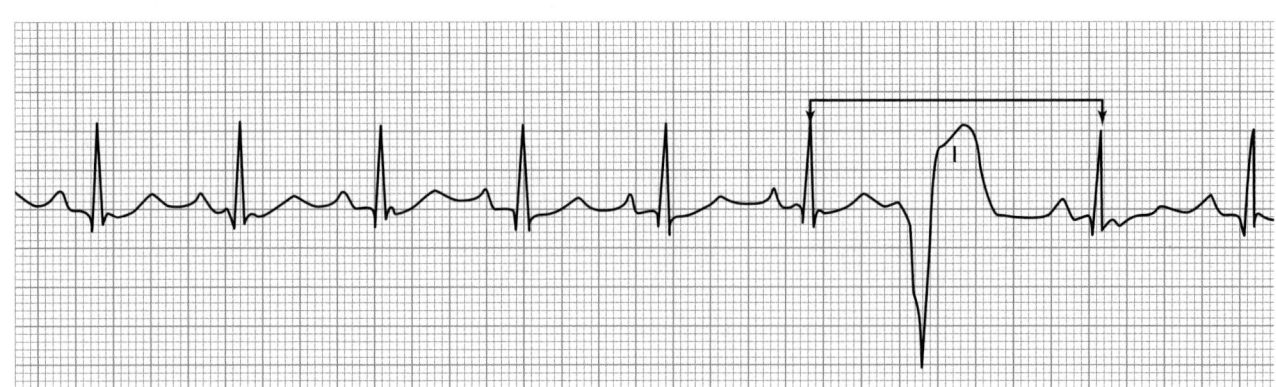

P Wave: Present and regular, except where absent (PVC); PR Interval: 0.20 second; QRS Complex: 0.08 second; QT Interval: 0.42 second; Heart Rate: Atrial: 70 bpm, Ventricular: 80 bpm; Rhythm: Atrial: Regular, Ventricular: Regular except for premature beat; Ectopic Beats: One PVC.

FIGURE 38–35 ■ Premature ventricular contractions (PVCs).

consistently, the dysrhythmia is coming from one irritable focus in the ventricle. These are referred to as unifocal PVCs. If PVCs occur with every other beat the rhythm is referred to as **bigeminy.** If PVCs occur every third beat, the rhythm is called **trigeminy,** and occurrence every fourth beat is **quadrigeminy.** The more often the PVC occurs, the greater the drop in cardiac output, and therefore, the more serious the dysrhythmia. The drop in cardiac output is due to the premature occurrence of the rhythm which does not allow for sufficient diastole or ventricle filling time. As cardiac muscle ischemia increases the muscle becomes more irritable, causing PVCs to be initiated in more than one place in the ventricle. This is referred to as multifocal PVCs. When multifocal, the morphology (shape) of the QRSs varies. Multifocal PVCs are more serious than unifocal PVCs because they indicate that there is more ischemia occurring in the myocardium.

PVC Patterns

When PVCs occur for two or more consecutive beats this is referred to as paired salvos. When there are three or more consecutive PVCs salvos, it is defined as ventricular tachycardia. Ventricular tachycardia may be life threatening due to the severe drop in cardiac output.

The most serious or dangerous time for a PVC to occur is during the relative refractory period, which is the top of the T wave on the ECG. This is referred to as an R on T phenomenon, and this occurrence may precipitate a run of ventricular tachycardia. Significant ECG features with PVCs include:

- QRS complex is premature, 0.12 second or greater in width, complexes are larger than the normal beats, with the T wave always occurring on the opposite side of the isoelectric line from the R wave.
- P waves are not present or are buried in the PVCs.
- PR interval-none.
- QT interval is prolonged for the ectopic beat only.
- PVC occurs prematurely.
- Heart rate usually is within normal range, but depends on underlying rhythm.
- Heart rhythm is irregular because the PVCs are premature.
- Ectopic beats are the PVCs.

The etiology, physical assessment findings, and treatment of premature ventricular contractions are outlined in Chart 38–10 (p. 1108).

Ventricular Tachycardia

Ventricular tachycardia (VT), often referred to as v-tach is a life threatening ventricular rhythm arising from an excitable ventricular focus in the tissue distal to the bifurcation of the bundle of His. In general, ventricular tachycardia affects the diseased heart, although it has been described in patients with apparently normal hearts. It is a rhythm that discharges repetitively, acting as the dominant pacemaker. It is present when three or more PVCs occur in a row at a rate of greater than 100 beats per minute (American Heart Association, 2006a). This dysrhythmia frequently begins rapidly, and is initiated by a PVC which then becomes the heart's pacemaker. A sustained ventricular tachycardia is a rhythm that lasts longer than 30 seconds and usually requires ter-

mination by antiarrhythmic drugs, antitachycardia pacing techniques, or electrical cardioversion. If the rhythm lasts less than 30 seconds it is a non-sustained rhythm or simply a run of ventricular tachycardia (three beats or longer) that terminates spontaneously. Ventricular tachycardia is an emergent situation, requiring urgent evaluation to assess cardiac output and the presence or absence of the pulse. Treatment is guided by published advanced cardiac support (ACLS) guidelines and varies based on the presence of a pulse. Ventricular tachycardia when sustained but hemodynamically stable (with pulse) is treated with pharmacologic agents such as lidocaine, procainamide or amiodarone (AHA, 2006a). Ventricular tachycardia that is hemodynamically unstable and pulseless is treated using the ACLS guidelines for pulseless cardiac arrest (AHA, 2006b). These guidelines dictate that the nurse assess the patient for a pulse, if none is present, cardiopulmonary resuscitation (CPR) is initiated and help is requested. Oxygen is administered and the patient is placed on a monitor/defibrillator when available. The nurse must be prepared to shock the patient per AHA guideline joules, CPR is resumed for 5 cycles, and then rhythm is checked. The patient is re-shocked if VT persists. Vasopressors are administered when intravenous access has been established. CPR and defibrillation cycles are repeated per ACLS guidelines until a viable rhythm is established or death occurs. Figure 38–36 ■ (p. 1110). Significant ECG features of ventricular tachycardia and ventricular fibrillation include:

- QRS complexes are uniform in appearance, usually wide and bizarre, measuring 0.12 second or greater, with the T wave occurring on the opposite side of the isoelectric line from the R wave.
- P waves in rapid VT are usually not recognizable. At slower ventricular rates, P waves may be recognized and may represent normal sinus node depolarization at a rate slower than VT, but the electrical activities do not affect one another.
- PR interval is not discernable.
- QT interval is not measurable.
- Heart rate is greater than 100 beats per minute and usually not faster than 200 beats per minute.
- Heart rhythm is essentially regular but may be irregular.
- Entire rhythm is ectopic beats.

The etiology, physical assessment findings, and treatment of ventricular tachycardia are outlined in Chart 38–10 (p. 1108).

Torsade de Pointes

Torsade de pointes, frequently referred to as "torsades," is a form of ventricular tachycardia that is usually accompanied by prolongation of the QT interval. The QT interval usually is more than 0.50 second in the beats preceding the onset of the rhythm. Once the rhythm has occurred the QRS complexes have varying morphology or shape and width that usually begin after a pause in the rhythm or bradycardia. The name, torsade de pointes, is derived from the French term that signifies the "twisting of the points." The name characterizes the rhythm in that it resembles a turning about or twisting motion along the baseline or isoelectric line. This form of VT, which is rare, is due to age, gender, drug toxicity, or an idiosyncratic reaction to certain cardiac drugs such as

| CHART 38–10 | **Ventricular Dysrhythmias: Etiology, Physical Assessment, and Treatment** |

Dysrhythmia	Etiology	Physical Assessment	Treatment
Premature ventricular contraction (PVC)	Organic heart disease Coronary artery disease Myocardial ischemia/irritability and infarction Cardiac valve disease Mitral valve prolapse Heart failure Primary electrical instability Fever Fluid volume deficit Electrolyte imbalance, e.g., hypokalemia, hypercalcemia, hypomagnesemia Acid/base imbalance Drug excess: e.g. Tricyclic antidepressants; digitalis, sympathomimetic amines, and antiarrhythmic agents Moderate to excessive alcohol intake Increase in catecholamine release and sympathetic tone as in emotional stress Sarcoidosis Change in posture Exercise Emotional excitement Vagal stimulation Normal variation that increases with age	Pulse: May be irregular due to asynchronous firing of the ventricles. The corresponding QRS complex may be detected on the monitor while contractions are felt as a peripheral pulse. BP: Normal or lower than usual due to decreased cardiac output leading to decreased perfusion. Thumping sensation in chest/throat Palpitations If cardiac output is decreased the following clinical manifestations may occur: Angina Syncope Generalized weakness Dizziness Shortness of breath Altered mental state may be present.	PVCs may be isolated when there is no underlying heart condition. Usually, then, they have no significance and require no treatment. Treatment depends on the cause and clinical manifestations. It is essential to identify and treat the underlying cause. When provoked by fast or slow heart rate, correcting the rate can abolish PVCs. Treatment usually is not required. Treatment is directed at uncovering the etiology and providing adequate oxygenation, pain relief, and rapid identification of causes. Antidysrhythmic drugs such as amiodarone and lidocaine should be administered as ordered per frequency of occurrence.
Ventricular tachycardia (VT)	Precipitated by the same conditions as premature ventricular contractions (see above)	Pulse: Rapid and weak BP: Hypotensive Cardiac output is decreased therefore the following clinical manifestations occur: Angina Syncope Generalized weakness Dizziness Shortness of breath Changes in mental status, starting with confusion and restlessness, leading to unconsciousness. Conscious sensation of ineffective cardiac activity often accompanied by anxiety. Presence and severity of the signs and symptoms depends on rhythm duration.	Initial treatment is based on the presence or absence of a palpable pulse. If hemodynamically stable, with a pulse, drug intervention is appropriate e.g., procainamide, amiodarone, lidocaine. If hemodynamically unstable (pulseless) defibrillation and cardiopulmonary resuscitation (CPR) is indicated. After initial stabilization other treatments which may be considered include: Implantable cardioverter defibrillator Electrophysiology Studies (EPS): ventricles are stimulated to produce VT: then antiarrhythmic drugs are administered, followed by a second attempt to produce the VT. If unable to reproduce the dysrhythmia, the drug is considered effective and continuous therapy is instituted. Drugs used include: procainamide, amiodarone, and lidocaiane. Radio-frequency ablation, burning the area or focus in the ventricle where the VT is coming from may also be considered. Chapter 39 ⊕ has a complete description of EPS and ablation.

CHART 38–10	Ventricular Dysrhythmias: Etiology, Physical Assessment, and Treatment—*Continued*		
Dysrhythmia	**Etiology**	**Physical Assessment**	**Treatment**
Torsade de pointes (TdP)	Prolonged QT interval, which may be congenital or acquired Severe bradycardia Electrolyte imbalance, e.g., hypokalemia, hypomagnesemia Central nervous system lesions Tricyclic antidepressants Antidysrhythmic drugs, e.g., quinidine, procainamide, amiodarone Antihistamines, e.g., seldane Antibiotics, e.g., erythromycin Diuretics Liquid protein diets Starvation Or any combination of the above	Pulse: Rapid, palpitations felt, often the first symptom BP: Low due to decreased cardiac output If cardiac output is decreased the following clinical manifestations may occur: Angina Syncope Generalized weakness Dizziness Shortness of breath Changes in mental status, starting with confusion and restlessness, leading to unconsciousness. Seizures may be present with a prolonged rhythm. Clinical manifestations are related to the decreased cardiac output caused by the dysrhythmia.	Assessment of QT interval for prolongation. Magnesium is the treatment of choice to shorten the QT interval. If unsuccessful, overdrive ventricular pacing to keep the heart rate up and the QT interval within normal limits. Stress testing and Valsalva will prolong QT interval and can be used to diagnose congenital prolonged QT interval. All agents that cause torsade de pointe are immediately discontinued. Administer potassium intravenously if QT interval is abnormal. Cardioversion and overdrive pacing are used to terminate torsades, but only may be temporary. Drugs are modified or discontinued if QT interval is prolonged.
Ventricular fibrillation (VF)	Severe myocardial ischemia Coronary heart disease Myocardial infarction Advanced heart block Abnormal repolarization Vagal stimulation Drug toxicity, e.g., psychotropics, digoxin Metabolic abnormalities, e.g., hypokalemia, hypomagnesemia Hypoxia Trauma Terminal event in many disease states Electrical shock	Pulse: None palpable and heart sounds usually absent BP: None Unconscious Seizures Apnea Death, if untreated	Initiate CPR and defibrillation per ACLS guidelines.
Pulseless electrical activity	Profound hypovolemia Massive myocardial damage Excessive vagal tone due to loss of sympathetic tone Obstruction of blood flow to or from the heart, e.g., severe pulmonary embolism Pericardial tamponade Myocardial rupture Massive cardiac trauma resulting in cardiac tamponade and/or tension pneumothorax Severe acidosis Hyperkalemia Hypothermia Drug overdose, e.g., tricyclics, beta-blockers, calcium channel blockers, digoxin	Pulse: None palpable BP: None Unconscious Seizures may occur Death, if untreated	Assess for pulse and blood pressure; initiate CPR protocol per ACLS guidelines. Find cause and treat.
Asystole	Cardiac standstill from massive cardiac muscle damage	Pulse: None palpable BP: None Unconscious Death, if untreated	Check the rhythm in two leads in order to rule out the possibility of fine ventricular fibrillation. Also, check the lead placement to make sure it has not fallen off. Initiate CPR and ACLS protocols. Administer drugs per ACLS guidelines, agency protocol or health care provider's orders.

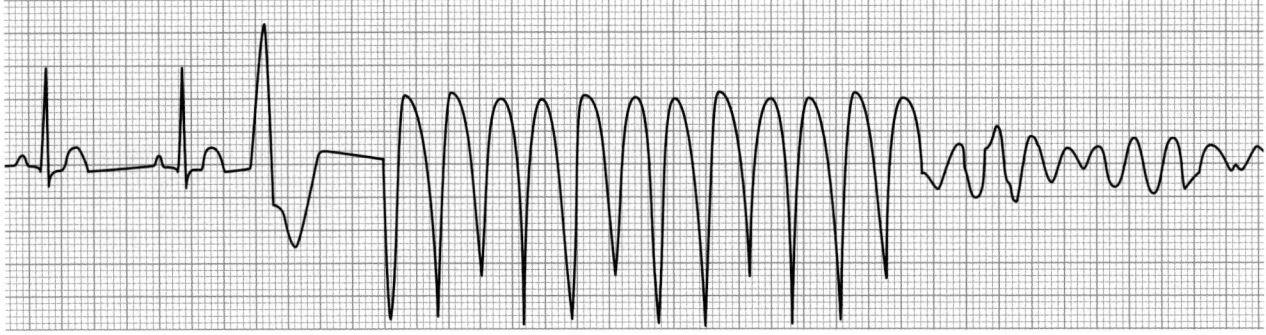

P Wave: Two normal P waves present; PR Interval: Not discernable during dysrhythmia; QRS Complex: Wide and distorted during dysrhythmia; QT Interval: Not discernable during dysrhythmia; Heart Rate: Atrial: Not discernable, Ventricular: Rapid; Rhythm: Both regular and irregular; Ectopic Beats: PVCs, ventricular tachycardia/fibrillation.

FIGURE 38–36 ■ Ventricular tachycardia.

quinidine, procainamide, disopyramide, or other agents that prolong the QT interval. Electrolyte imbalance such as hypokalemia and hypomagnesemia also can initiate torsade de pointes (Garcia & Miller, 2004).

In addition to being a life-threatening dysrhythmia, torsade de pointes tends to recur repeatedly. It is, therefore, essential to find and treat the underlying cause. Figure 38–37 ■ is a rhythm strip showing torsade de pointes. Significant ECG features of torsade de pointes include:

- QRS complex height varies and undulates.
- P waves are not discernable.
- PR interval is not measurable.
- QT is not measurable.
- Heart rate varies; approximately 200 to 250 beats per minute.
- Heart rhythm may be regular or irregular.
- Entire rhythm is ectopy.

The etiology, physical assessment findings, and treatment of torsade de pointes are outlined in Chart 38–10 (p. 1108).

Ventricular Fibrillation

Ventricular fibrillation (VF), often referred to as v-fib, is a dysrhythmia marked by rapid, disorganized depolarization of the ventricles. There are no organized electrical impulses, and therefore, no coordinated atrial or ventricular contraction or palpable pulse. The myocardial cells appear to quiver rather than depolarize normally. With this dysrhythmia multiple ventricular sites initiate electrical impulses that are not transmit-

ted through the normal conduction pathway. There are no waveforms apparent on the ECG strip. The rhythm appears disorganized, rapid, and irregular with waves whose morphology varies greatly. Ventricular fibrillation may be classified further as coarse and fine, just like atrial fibrillation. Coarse waveforms are more easily visible and are greater than 3 mm; those that are less than 3 mm frequently are referred to as fine VF. Coarse VF responds better to treatment than does fine VF. Also, coarse VF typically progresses to fine VF unless treatment is initiated in a timely manner. Fine VF indicates that the rhythm has been present for an extended period of time. Figure 38–38 ■ is a rhythm strip showing ventricular fibrillation.

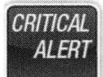 *Ventricular fibrillation (VF) is an ineffective quivering of the heart muscle that results in no blood delivery to tissues, thus, VF must be treated immediately. Detection of VF on a monitor requires immediate patient evaluation by the nurse to begin prompt treatment and to rule out equipment malfunctions that mimic VF such as ECG artifacts produced by loose or dry electrodes, broken ECG leads, or patient movements or muscle tremors.*

Significant ECG features of ventricular fibrillation include:

- P waves, PR intervals, QRS complexes, and QT intervals are all absent.
- Heart rate is not discernable because there are no waves or complexes to measure.
- Heart rhythm is irregular.
- Entire rhythm is ectopy.

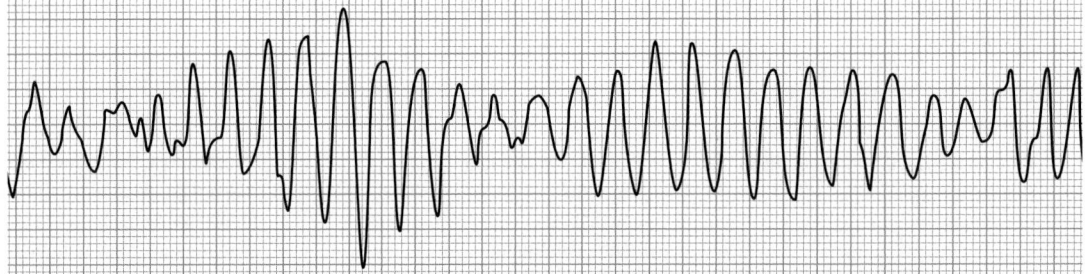

P Waves: Not discernable; PR Interval: Not discernable; QRS Complex: Wide, distorted, and varying heights; QT Interval: not discernable; Rate: Rapid; Rhythm: Both regular and irregular; Ectopic Beats: All.

FIGURE 38–37 ■ Torsade de pointes.

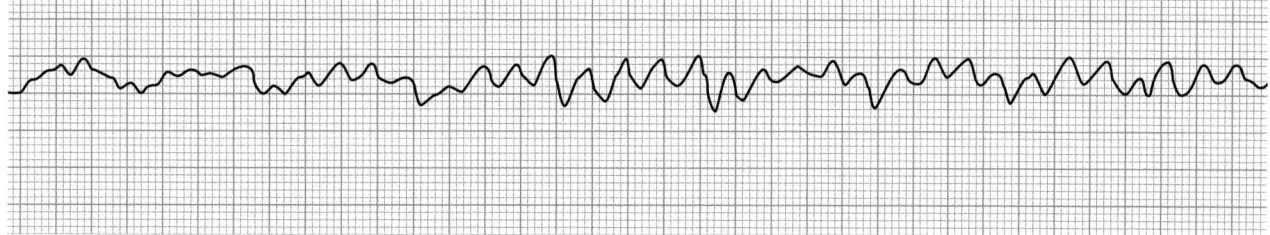

P Waves: Not discernable; PR Interval: Not discernable; QRS Complex: Wide, distorted, and varying heights; QT Interval not discernable; Heart Rate: Not discernable; Ectopic Beats: All.

FIGURE 38–38 ■ Ventricular fibrillation.

The etiology, physical assessment findings, and treatment of ventricular fibrillation are outlined in Chart 38–10 (p. 1108).

Pulseless Electrical Activity

Pulseless electrical activity (PEA) is a clinical phenomenon that occurs when the heart muscle loses its ability to contract even though cardiac electrical activity is present. Cardiac electrical activity is seen on the monitor, but the patient has no detectable pulse or blood pressure. Though the electrical activity is represented as an organized rhythm (other than VT or VF) on the cardiac monitor, (e.g., bradycardia, heart block), the heart muscle is unable to respond to the electrical stimuli. Due to a variety of cardiac and noncardiac disorders such as acidosis, electrolyte imbalance, trauma, and cardiac rupture, the muscle is unable to respond to the stimuli, causing cardiac output and tissue perfusion to cease, and clinical death to occur. When PEA occurs biological death follows within minutes unless the cause is identified and treated (Beasley, 2003). Formerly, pulseless electrical activity was called electromechanical dissociation (EMD). The clinical outcome usually is poor despite aggressive life support measures. Significant ECG features of pulseless electrical activity include:

- P waves may or may not be present dependent on rhythm.
- PR intervals may or may not have a relationship to QRS complexes.

- QRS complex may be narrow or wide.
- QT interval is variable.
- Heart rate and rhythm are variable, usually bradycardia.
- Ectopic beats may be present.

The etiology, physical assessment findings, and treatment of pulseless electrical activity are outlined in Chart 38–10 (p. 1108).

Asystole

Asystole is a complete termination of all cardiac electrical activity. Without an electrical impulse, the atria and ventricles do not contract causing immediate loss of oxygen supply to the brain and tissues. In hospital settings efforts are usually made to reestablish cardiac activity but, often are futile. Figure 38–39 ■ is a rhythm strip showing asystole. In asystole, no measurable electrical activity exists and the rhythm strip appears as a straight line on the ECG monitor. The etiology, physical assessment findings, and treatment of asystole are outlined in Chart 38–10 (p. 1108).

■ Nursing Management for Ventricular Dysrhythmias

As with any dysrhythmia, the first nursing responsibility for ventricular dysrhythmias is to assess the patient's response to

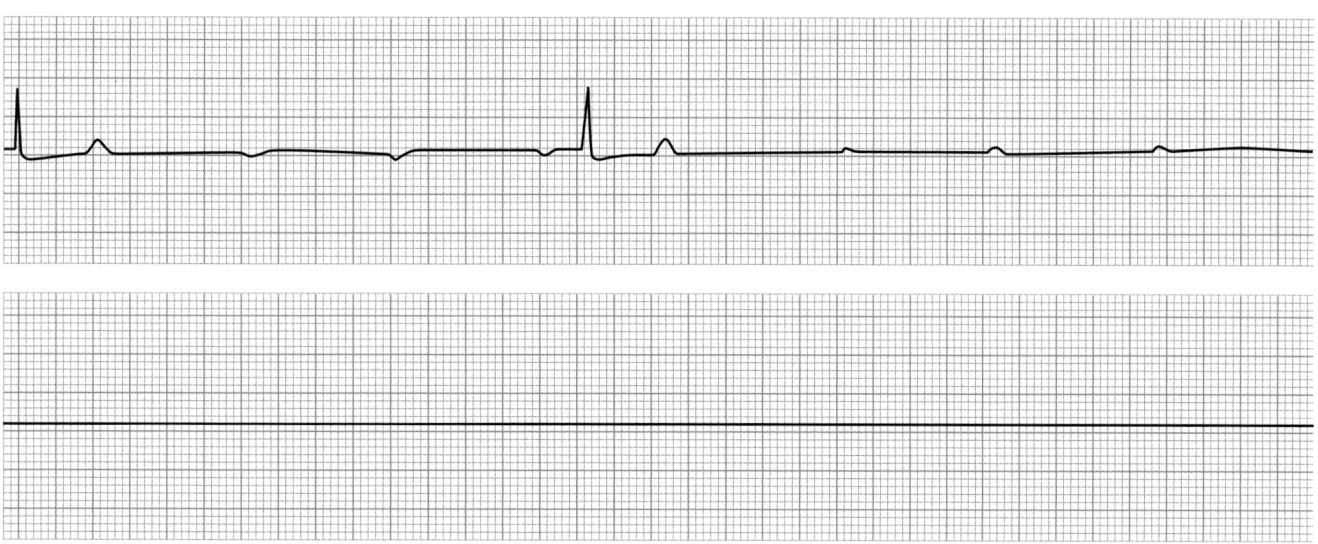

No measurable electrical activity

FIGURE 38–39 ■ Asystole.

the specific abnormality. Nurses need to complete a health history to assess the risk factors related to the occurrence of ventricular dysrhythmias that are outlined in Chart 38–10 (p. 1108). Cultural awareness of populations that are at increased risk for ventricular dysrhythmias is discussed in the Cultural Considerations box.

Ventricular dysrhythmias have the greatest impact on cardiac output and are, therefore, the most serious. Depending on the variation in configuration and the frequency of occurrence, ventricular dysrhythmias require a variety of interventions from simple observation, to drug intervention, to advanced life support treatments. Generally, in monitoring units the health care providers provide protocols or "standing orders" for treating each type of ventricular dysrhythmia. The nurse must be knowledgeable of the treatment regimens required for each of the ventricular dysrhythmias based on the standing orders, basic cardiac life support (BCLS), advanced cardiac life support (ACLS), and agency specific protocols. When reporting ventricular dysrhythmias, the nurse needs to give a detailed description of the dysrhythmia pattern and the patient's clinical response to the health care provider, so treatment is tailored to the specific dysrhythmia. The seriousness and treatment of ventricular dysrhythmias depend on the duration and the impact on hemodynamic stability (blood pressure and cardiac output).

If the resuscitation efforts are initiated it is imperative that family and significant others be kept informed and be allowed to participate in the decision-making process. Research in the United States and the United Kingdom revealed that most family members wished to be present during the attempted resuscitation of a loved one (Boyd, 2000). The research concluded that even family members with no medical background found it comforting to be with their loved one during the final moments of life. It is imperative that the health care team offer this opportunity and be sensitive to the family during this crisis period. If possible, it is optimal to have a health care team member be assigned to the family to answer questions, clarify information, and provide comfort (AHA 2005a). Since the nurse is at the bedside it typically becomes a nursing responsibility to keep the family informed, act as a liaison, and advocate for the patient. Chapter 17 🔗 includes a complete description of end of life issues.

National Guidelines for Cardiopulmonary Resuscitation and Emergency Cardiovascular Care

Since 1974 the American Heart Association has been publishing guidelines for cardiopulmonary resuscitation and emergency cardiovascular care. The guidelines were most recently updated in 2005 and are based on evidenced evaluation from the 2005 International Consensus Conference on Cardiopulmonary Resuscitation and Emergency Cardiovascular Care with Treatment Recommendations (International Liaison Committee on Resuscitation, 2005). These 2005 guidelines supersede the published 2000 guidelines for cardiovascular resuscitation and emergency cardiovascular care. The current guidelines contain recommendations designed to improve survival from sudden cardiac arrest and acute life-threatening cardiopulmonary disorders. These guidelines are based on the most extensive evidence review of CPR yet published. They confirm the safety and effectiveness of many treatments and recommend new treatments that have undergone evidence evaluation. Given that the guidelines do not apply to all situations, the leader of the resuscitation attempt may need to adapt application of the guidelines to unique circumstances. Finally, the guidelines also have streamlined the amount of information that rescuers need to learn and remember, and have clarified the most important skills that rescuers need to perform (American Heart Association, 2006b). Future goals of the AHA are to continue to improve the guidelines based on new and evolving research and practice evidence. Foci will be placed on CPR education, and improving the effectiveness and efficiency of instruction, skill retention, and a reduction in barriers to action for basic and advanced life support providers (Chamberlain & Hazinski, 2003). Continuous quality improvement issues focus on reducing time to CPR and shock delivery and improving the quality of CPR provided (Jacobs et al, 2004; Peberdy et al, 2003). The National Guidelines box outlines the 2005 AHA national guidelines for selected CPR and emergency cardiovascular care.

Nursing Management of Patients with Dysrhythmias

Nursing responsibilities when caring for patients experiencing cardiac dysrhythmias have been discussed throughout this chapter. To assist the learner, the patient care plan outlines a systematic approach to assessing and providing nursing care for

---

CULTURAL CONSIDERATIONS Brugada Syndrome

The term *Brugada sign* is an abnormal finding on an electrocardiogram (ECG) that refers to distance of at least 0.10 second from the onset of the QRS complex or the bottom of the S wave. Its presence may indicate Brugada syndrome which is an abnormality in the heart's electrical system that causes life-threatening heart rhythm disturbances such as ventricular fibrillation. It occurs in patients with a structurally normal heart, and few or no coronary artery disease risk factors, and a family history of sudden cardiac death. It's possible to have a Brugada sign without having Brugada syndrome. This syndrome occurs most often in young adults. It also occurs with increased frequency in Asians. The cause isn't clear, but it appears to be inherited in some cases.

Nursing implications are to assess young patients and patients of Asian decent who are having ventricular dysrhythmias with little to no risk of heart disease, for a family history of sudden cardiac death. Those considered at risk have:

- A family history of sudden cardiac death in young relatives
- A personal history of serious heart rhythm problems
- A personal history of severe fainting spells

Immediate treatment for ventricular fibrillation is outlined in the American Heart Association ACLS guidelines for 2005. Long-term treatment includes antidysrhythmic medication therapy and an implantable defibrillator.

Source: Adapted from: *Brugada Syndrome* (2005). MayoClinic.com. http://www.mayoclinic.com/health/brugada-syndrome/AN00551. Retrieved July 13, 2006.

NATIONAL GUIDELINES for Cardiopulmonary Resuscitation and Emergency Cardiovascular Care

Adult basic life support

Advanced cardiac life support

Electrical therapies

CPR techniques and devices

Adjuncts for airway control and ventilation

Management of cardiac arrest

Management of symptomatic bradycardia and tachycardia

Monitoring and medications

Post-resuscitation support

Stabilizing of the patient with acute coronary syndromes

Source: Adapted from American Heart Association. (2006). *2005 international consensus on CPR and ECC science with treatment recommendations.* Retrieved June 30, 2006, from http://www.americanheart.org/presenter.jhtml?identifier=3022512.

these patients. Beginning with the assessment the nurse needs to identify what type of information is necessary to help find the risk factors and causes that precipitate the occurrence or progression of cardiac dysrhythmias. The nursing diagnosis is generated from the assessment data and guides the nurse toward desired patient outcomes and an intervention plan (see Nursing Process: Patient Care Plan for Dysrhythmias).

To assist the nurse in the comprehensive assessment and interpretation of cardiac dysrhythmias, Chart 38–11 (p. 1114) summarizes the characteristics of each type of dysrhythmia.

Health Promotion

As with any disorder the primary focus is on prevention of the onset and progression of the disease. Health teaching about risk factors and life style habits that cause the disorders that underlie the occurrence of cardiac dysrhythmias is essential for prevention. Once an individual has been diagnosed with heart disease the best way to prevent dysrhythmias is to have the patient closely follow a treatment plan and make the necessary life style habit changes. Life style habits most closely associated with heart disease and the occurrence of dysrhythmias include:

- Smoking
- Alcohol use
- Caffeine intake
- Sedentary life style
- Stress
- Overweight/obesity
- Diet.

The nurse needs to develop a teaching plan that will effectively assist the patient in reducing or eliminating these risk factors. Additionally, the patient needs to be told to note if there is a pattern as to when the dysrhythmias occur, what brings them on and what makes them go away. For example, does it take a long time for the heart rate to return to normal after exercise or exertion? Instruct the patient to identify high-stress situations that bring on the dysrhythmias and examine with the patient how to diminish or avoid them as much as possible. All aspects of life including professional as well as personal relationships need to be examined.

Since the Human Genome Project ongoing research has focused on gaining a better understanding of how genetic disorders can predispose to dysrhythmias. For example, a mutation of gene ankyrin-B is now known to cause cardiac arrhythmia syndrome (Hamby, Mittal, & Stein, 2006). The goal is to use gene-based therapies in the future to better treat dysrhythmias as well as identifying those individuals who are susceptible to dysrhythmias. Nurses will assist in identifying whether or not the patient has a family history of dysrhythmias. This in turn will aid in the early diagnosis, treatment, or prevention of the occurrence of life-threatening dysrhythmias.

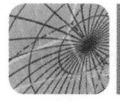

NURSING PROCESS: Patient Care Plan for Dysrhythmias

Assessment	Nursing Diagnosis	Expected Outcomes/Evaluation	Interventions
Health history	*Alteration in Tissue Perfusion*	Maintain adequate cardiac output	Monitoring and managing the dysrhythmia
Social Habits	*Altered Cardiac Output*	Free of clinical manifestations	Finding the cause
Psychosocial assessment	*Anxiety* related to fear of the unknown	Reduced anxiety	Reducing risk factors through
Physical assessment	*Knowledge Deficit* related to dysrhythmias	Verbalizes understanding of	patient teaching
Coexisting conditions:	and their treatment	disorder and treatments	Controlling incidence
Heart disease			Minimizing anxiety
Chronic obstructive			Promoting home and community-
pulmonary disease			based care
Prescription and over-the-			
counter medications			
Clinical manifestations:			
Syncope			
Dizziness			
Fatigue			
Chest discomfort			

| CHART 38–11 | **ECG Measurements for Cardiac Rhythms** |

ECG Rhythm	P Wave	PR Interval	QRS	QT Interval	Rate	Rhythm	Ectopic Beats
Normal Sinus Rhythm	Present and Regular	0.12–0.21	0.06–0.12	0.34–0.43	60–100 bpm	Regular	None
Sinus Bradycardia	Present and Regular	Normal limits	Normal	Lengthens to greater than normal	40–60 bpm	Regular	None
Sinus Tachycardia	Present and Regular	As the sinus rate accelerates, the PR interval tends to shorten slightly.	Normal	Usually shortens	100–180 bpm	May be slightly irregular as rate accelerates; then becomes a rapid regular rate.	None
Sinus Arrhythmia	Present and Irregular	Normal limits	Normal limits	Changes with the heart rate, becoming longer during the slow phase of the rhythm	60–100 bpm	Regularly irregular, with a variance of more than 0.08 seconds in the acceleration and deceleration phases.	May occur during the slow phase of the rhythm
Sinus Arrest (Pause)	Present and Irregular	May be the same before and after sinus pauses.	Normal limits	Changes with the heart rate, becoming longer during the slow phase of the rhythm.	There may be marked bradycardia due to long sinus pauses.	Underlying regular rhythm except where the sinus pauses occur.	Possible during sinus pauses
Premature Atrial Contraction (PAC)	Present and Irregular when PAC occurs.	Normal limits. May change with PAC only.	Normal limits	Normal if rate is normal.	60–100 bpm	Regular except for premature PAC which may reset rhythm.	PAC
Atrial Flutter	No P wave f waves	None	Normal limits	Unable to obtain as T waves are buried in F waves	Depends on the AV conduction ratio. There may be a slow ventricular response, or there may be a fast ventricular response.	Atrial rate regular. Ventricular rate may be regular or irregular.	Flutter waves
Atrial Fibrillation	No P wave f waves	None	Normal limits	Unable to obtain because the T waves are buried in the f waves.	T waves are buried in the f waves.	Irregular	Fibrillation waves
Supraventricular Tachycardia (SVT)	Not seen –buried in QRS complex	Not discernable	Within normal limits, unless distorted by buried P waves.	Unable to obtain as T waves are buried.	100–250 bpm	Regular or irregular due to varying conduction through the AV node.	Rapid ectopic focus takes over rhythm
Paroxysmal Atrial Tachycardia (PAT)	At onset of rhythm, shape of P waves different from sinus P waves.	Varies with rhythm change	Within normal limits, unless distorted by buried P waves.	T waves buried, so unable to obtain with fast rhythm.	100–250 beats/minute dependent on reference source.	Irregular due to varying heart rates.	Ectopic focus at onset of rapid rhythm

CHART 38–11	ECG Measurements for Cardiac Rhythms—*Continued*

ECG Rhythm	P Wave	PR Interval	QRS	QT Interval	Rate	Rhythm	Ectopic Beats
Wolff-Parkinson White Syndrome	Present and Regular	Less than 0.12 second because the AV node is bypassed and contains presence of delta wave	Greater than 0.10 seconds due to delta waves created by the abnormal conduction pathway	Shortens with tachycardia and lengthens with bradycardia	High incidence of tachy-dysrthrymias	Regular, except during heart rate changes	Delta waves: Occur just prior to R wave
Wandering Atrial Pacemaker	Present and Irregular Multiform	Usually normal	Normal limits	Normal. May be prolonged due to slow heart rate	Atrial: Slow, bradycardic Ventricular: Slow, bradycardic	Irregular due to changing pacemakers	May be present due to the slow rhythm
Sick Sinus Syndrome	Present or absent depending on which dysrhythmia is occurring	Variable depending on the rhythm	Normal limits	Variable due to rate change	Bradycardia to tachycardia	Atrial: Irregular Ventricular: Irregular	May be present with slow rate
Junctional Escape Rhythm	May occur before, after, or buried in, the QRS complex	Less than 0.12 second if the P wave occurs before the QRS complex	Normal unless distorted by P wave	Normal unless impacted by rate	Usually 40–60 (normal intrinsic rate for junctional tissue)	Regular	May occur with slow rates
Premature Junctional Contraction (PJC)	May occur before, after, or buried in, the QRS complex	Less than 0.12 second if P wave occurs before QRS complex for the ectopic beat All others normal	Normal unless distorted by P wave for the ectopic beat All others normal	Normal	That of underlying rhythm	Regular except for the premature beat	PJC
Junctional Tachycardia	May occur before, after, or buried in, the QRS complex	Less than 0.12 second if P wave occurs before QRS complex for the ectopic beat	Normal unless distorted by P wave for the ectopic beat	No specific change unless it is heart rate related	Greater than 100 beats per minute	Appears regular, but may increase its rate	May occur due to muscle irritability
First Degree AV Block	Present and Regular	Greater than 0.20 second	Normal	Normal	Variable	Regular	None
Mobitz I/Wenckeback	Sinus P waves	Progressively prolonged until one P wave is not conducted and the sequence begins	Within normal limits	Within normal limits	Atrial rate within normal limits; ventricular rate slower than atrial	Atrial rhythm is regular; ventricular rhythm is irregular	Usually none unless they occur during period when no QRS has occurred and there is a long pause
Mobitz II/Second-Degree Block	Present Not always followed by QRS	Constant with conducted beats	Intermitttently absent; may be normal (AV node) or prolonged when present	Within normal limits	Atrial rate is regular; ventricular rate irregular and bradycardic	Atrial is regular; ventricular is irregular	May occur due to slow rate

(continued)

CHART 38–11	ECG Measurements for Cardiac Rhythms—*Continued*

ECG Rhythm	P Wave	PR Interval	QRS	QT Interval	Rate	Rhythm	Ectopic Beats
Third-Degree (Complete) Heart Block	Present and Regular	P wave has no relationship to QRS complexes; therefore no PR interval is present.	May be narrow (junctional rhythm), or wide (idioventricular rhythm)	May be rate related, but not directly affected.	Atrial rate is regular, 60–100 bpm; nodal rate is 40–60 bpm; ventricular rate is 20–40 bpm.	Atrial is regular; ventricular may be regular or irregular.	May occur due to slow rate.
Bundle Branch Block	Present and Regular sinus P waves	0.12–0.20 second.	Greater than 0.12 second. If notch higher on right, indicates right bundle branch block; if notch higher on left, indicates left bundle branch block.	Within normal limits.	60–100 beats/minute.	Regular	None
Premature Ventricular Contraction (PVC)	None with PVC.	None with PVC.	Broad and premature and has increased amplitude. R and T waves opposite sides of isoelectric line.	Prolonged with PVC.	Underlying rate may be normal or abnormal.	Irregular because PVCs are premature.	PVC more likely to occur during bradycardia when there is more time to emerge.
Ventricular Tachycardia	None visible	Not discernible	Wide and bizarre, measuring > 0.12 seconds. R and T waves opposite sides of isoelectric line	Not discernible.	100–250 beats/minute.	Essentially regular.	All waves are ectopy
Torsade de Pointes	Not discernible	Not discernible	Height undulates	Usually > 0.50 seconds in the beats preceding the onset of the rhythm	Rates vary 200–250 beats/minute.	Typically regular.	All waves are ectopy
Ventricular Fibrillation	None	None	None	None	Atrial: Absent Ventricular: Absent	Irregular	All waves are ectopy
Pulseless Electrical Activity	May or may not be present.	May or may not have a relationship to QRS complexes	May be narrow or wide complex.	Variable.	Variable, depends on rhythm; usually bradycardic.	Variable depends on rate.	May be present but none of the beats perfuse
Asystole	None	None	None	None	None	None	None

Source: Megan Redeen, (2007). California State University, Sacramento.

NCLEX® REVIEW

1. After reviewing the electrocardiogram of a patient, the nurse believes the tracing is normal. Which of the following did the nurse assess on this patient's ECG?

    1. PR interval less than 0.8 second

    2. QRS complex 0.10 second

    3. Absent PR interval

    4. QT interval greater than 0.50 seconds

2. The nurse is assessing the QRS complexes on a patient's electrocardiogram. The complex spans 3 small boxes on the ECG paper. The nurse would identify this patient's QRS complex to be:

    1. 0.03 second

    2. 0.06 second

    3. 0.12 second

    4. 0.15 second

3. A patient comes into the emergency department to be seen for chest pain that started after learning that his brother was killed in an accident. The electrocardiogram shows a normal heart rate with shorter PR intervals. Which of the following should be included in this patient's plan of care?

    1. Plan for cardioversion.

    2. Observe and treat the patient for anxiety.

    3. Medicate with calcium channel blockers.

    4. Provide carotid artery massage.

4. A patient is diagnosed with a junctional dysrhythmia. Which of the following should be included in this patient's plan of care?

    1. Have a serum digoxin level drawn.

    2. Implement ACLS protocols.

    3. Prepare to administer magnesium.

    4. Prepare to administer lidocaine.

Answers for review questions appear in Appendix D

KEY TERMS

absolute refractory period *p.1077*
action potential *p.1077*
anion *p.1076*
artifact *p.1085*
asystole *p.1111*
atrial dysrhythmia *p.1090*
atrial fibrillation *p.1092*
atrial flutter *p.1096*
atrial kick *p.1075*
atrioventricular (AV) node *p.1075*
automaticity *p.1076*
AV dissociation *p.1103*
Bachmann bundle *p.1075*
bigeminy *p.1107*
bipolar lead *p.1080*
bundle branch block *p.1105*
bundle of His *p.1075*
bundles *p.1074*
cardiac conduction system *p.1073*
cardiac depolarization *p.1076*
cardiac repolarization *p.1077*
cation *p.1076*
conductivity *p.1076*
contractility *p.1076*
dysrhythmia *p.1086*
ECG waveform *p.1085*
ectopic focus *p.1085*
electrode *p.1078*
escape *p.1075*
excitability *p.1076*

fascicles *p.1075*
fill time *p.1087*
first-degree AV block *p.1101*
graph paper *p.1083*
intra-atrial pathways *p.1075*
ion *p.1076*
isoelectric line *p.1085*
J point *p.1078*
junctional dysrhythmia *p.1097*
junctional escape rhythm *p.1098*
lead axis *p.1079*
millivolts *p.1077*
Mobitz I/Wenckebach *p.1101*
Mobitz II/second-degree block *p.1101*
negative deflection *p.1079*
nodes (bundles) *p.1074*
normal sinus rhythm (NSR) *p.1086*
P wave *p.1078*
pacemaker cell *p.1076*
paroxysmal junctional tachycardia (PJT) *p.1100*
positive deflection *p.1079*
PR interval *p.1078*
premature atrial contraction (PAC) *p.1090*
premature junctional contraction (PJC) *p.1098*
premature ventricular contraction (PVC) *p.1106*
pulseless electrical activity (PEA) *p.1111*
Purkinje network fibers *p.1075*

QRS complex *p.1078*
QT interval *p.1084*
quadrigeminy *p.1107*
refractory period *p.1077*
relative refractory period *p.1077*
resting membrane potential *p.1076*
sick sinus syndrome (SSS) *p.1096*
sinoatrial (SA) node *p.1075*
sinus arrest *p.1088*
sinus arrhythmia/dysrhythmia *p.1087*
sinus bradycardia *p.1086*
sinus tachycardia *p.1087*
ST segment *p.1078*
supraventricular tachycardia (SVT) *p.1094*
T wave *p.1078*
third-degree AV block (complete block) *p.1103*
threshold *p.1071*
torsade de pointes *p.1107*
trigeminy *p.1107*
12-lead ECG *p.1079*
U wave *p.1078*
unipolar lead *p.1080*
ventricular dysrhythmia *p.1106*
ventricular fibrillation (VF) *p.1110*
ventricular tachycardia (VT) *p.1107*
wandering atrial pacemaker *p.1096*
Wolff-Parkinson-White syndrome (WPW) *p.1096*

REFERENCES

American Heart Association. (2005a). *Handbook of emergency cardiovascular care for healthcare providers.* Dallas, TX: Author.

American Heart Association. (2005b). Part 5: Electrical therapies: Automated external defibrillators, defibrillation, cardioversion, and pacing. *Supplement to Circulation: Journal of the American Heart Association, 112*(24), IV-35–IV-46.

American Heart Association. (2005c). 2005 American Heart Association guidelines for cardiopulmonary resuscitation and emergency cardiovascular care: Part 2. Ethical issues. *Circulation, 112,* IV-6–IV-11.

American Heart Association. (2006a). *BLS guidelines for healthcare providers.* Dallas, TX: Author.

American Heart Association. (2006b). *2005 International Consensus on CPR and ECC Science with Treatment Recommendations.* Retrieved June 30, 2006, from http://www.americanheart.org/presenter .jhtml?identifier=3022512

Beasley, B. M. (2003). *Understanding EKGs: A practical approach* (2nd ed.). Upper Saddle River, NJ: Prentice Hall.

Boyd, R. (2000). Witnessed resuscitation by relatives. *Resuscitation, 43,* 171–176.

Chamberlain, D. A., & Hazinski, M. F. (2003). Education in resuscitation: An ILCOR symposium: Utstein Abbey: Stavanger, Norway: June 22–24, 2001. *Circulation,* 108, 2575–2594.

Ellis, K. M. (2002a). *EKG plain and simple: From rhythm strips to 12-leads.* Upper Saddle River, NJ: Prentice Hall Health.

Ellis, K. M. (2002b). *Q & A review of EKG.* Upper Saddle River, NJ: Prentice Hall Health.

Garcia, T. B., & Miller G. T. (2004). *Arrhythmia recognition: The art of interruption.* Sudbury, MA: Jones and Bartlett.

Hamby, R. L., Mittal, S., & Stein, K. M. (2006). *Arrhythmia.* Retrieved July 17, 2006, from http:// heart.healthcentersonline.com/ arrhythmia/arrhythmia8.cfm

Holtschneider, M. E., McBroom, K. G., & Patterson, A. (2006). ECG everywhere. *Advance for Nurses, 3*(13), 20.

International Liaison Committee on Resuscitation. (2005). International consensus on cardiopulmonary resuscitation and emergency cardiovascular care with treatment recommendations. *Circulation,* 2005, 112: III-I-III-136.

Jacobs, I., et al. (2004). Cardiac arrest and cardiopulmonary resuscitation outcome reports: Update and simplification of the Utstein templates resuscitation registries. A statement for health care professionals from a task force of the international liaison committee on resuscitation (AHA, European Resuscitation Council, Australian Resuscitation Council, New Zealand Resuscitation Council, Heart and Stroke Foundation of Canada, interAmerican Heart Foundation, Resuscitation Council of Southern Africa). *Resuscitation, 63,* 233–249.

Morton, P. G., Fontaine, D. K., Hudak, C.M. & Gallo, B. M. (2005). *Critical care nursing: A holistic approach* (8th ed.). Philadelphia: Lippincott Williams & Wilkins.

Olshansky, B. et al. (2006). Atrioventricular nodal reentry tachycardia (AVNRT). *eMedicine from WebMD.* Retrieved July 13, 2006, from http://www.emedicine.com/med/topic2955.htm

Peberdy, M. A. et al. (2003). Cardiopulmonary resuscitation of adult in the hospital: A report of 14720 cardiac arrests from the National Registry of Cardiopulmonary Resuscitation. *Resuscitation, 58,* 297–308.

Porth, C. M. (2004). *Essentials of pathophysiology: Concepts of altered health states.* Philadelphia: Lippincott Williams & Wilkins.

Shade, B., & Wesley, K. (2007). *Fast and easy ECGs: A self-paced learning program.* Boston: McGraw-Hill.

Walraven, G. (2006). *Basic arrhythmias* (6th ed.). Upper Saddle River, NJ: Prentice Hall Health.

Diagnostic and Interventional Therapies for Cardiovascular Disorders

Sue Apple
Joseph Lindsay, Jr.

Outcome-Based Learning Objectives

After studying this chapter, the learner will be able to:

1. Define sensitivity and specificity as they relate to diagnostic testing.
2. Describe the major noninvasive and invasive diagnostic tests to detect coronary disease.
3. Identify the appropriate screening test and associated nursing management for a given patient population.
4. Compare and contrast major advantages and limitations for each test.
5. Prioritize the nursing management for patients receiving percutaneous coronary interventional procedures.

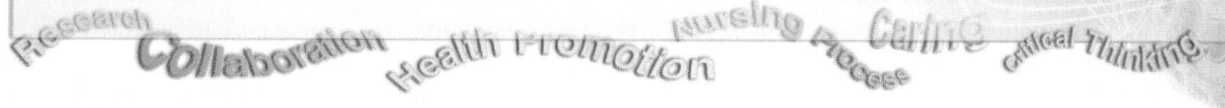

Research   Collaboration   Health Promotion   Nursing Process   Caring   Critical Thinking

ALTHOUGH MUCH information is gained at the bedside by a detailed history and physical examination, health care providers also need results from both noninvasive and invasive diagnostic tests to determine the presence or absence of heart disease in their patients. For persons with known disease, such as the patient who has had a myocardial infarction, these tests provide the basis for determining functional status, treatment, and long-term prognosis.

The heart can be evaluated using x-rays (radiography, angiography, computed tomography [CT]), gamma rays (radionuclide imaging), sound waves (echocardiography), and magnetic properties of the body (magnetic resonance imaging [MRI]) (Thomas, 2002). Given the ever-widening array of tests, choosing the most appropriate test for an individual can be challenging. To be most beneficial, it is important to consider the cost, safety, accuracy, and availability of the particular test.

Certain basic concepts apply to nearly all cardiovascular testing. Each test may be assessed for its *sensitivity* against a known standard. In the case of coronary heart disease the "gold standard" is usually the detection of atherosclerotic plaque by coronary angiography (Baim & Grossman, 2000b). For practical purposes, if the standard is a valid one (and not "fool's gold") and as long as the criteria for discriminating a positive from a negative test remain constant, sensitivity will be constant. It may be defined by means of population testing. **Sensitivity** describes the ability of a test to identify patients with disease (Greenland & Gaziano, 2003). It may be calculated by dividing the number of true positive tests by the sum of true positives plus false negatives. For example, positive tests in subjects with coronary disease are "true positives" whereas negative tests in subjects with disease are "false negatives." Similarly, negative tests in patients who are free of disease are "true negatives" and positive tests in patients without disease are "false positives." **Specificity** is calculated by dividing the number of true negatives in the population by the sum of true negatives plus false positives. Thus, specificity describes the frequency with which the test is normal in subjects who are free of disease (Kadish et al., 2001).

An understanding of test characteristics is only part of the information necessary for the clinician who will apply the test result in an individual subject. The clinician needs to know how often the *single* result reflects accurately the presence or absence of disease. For this interpretation he must understand an additional concept, **predictive accuracy** of a positive and of a negative test; that is, how well the results of the test predict the presence or absence of disease.

The sensitivity and specificity of most diagnostic tests are known for a given disease in a specific population. What is not always known is the **pretest probability**, which is the likelihood

CHART 39–1	Improving Reliability of Test Results

Two patients—a 70-year-old man with symptoms of typical angina and a 35-year-old woman with atypical chest pain—undergo stress electro-cardiography and have positive test results. Who is more likely to have ischemic heart disease? Remember, the predictive value of a positive test result is dependent on the prevalence of the disease in the population being studied, not just the sensitivity and specificity of the test.

that disease is present in the patient before testing. Therefore, choosing the appropriate test requires knowledge of the test, including indications, advantages, and disadvantages, combined with clinical knowledge of the disease and the individual patient (Chart 39–1).

To be useful a positive test should substantially increase the **post-test probability** (likelihood that disease is present), and a negative test should lower the post-test probability.

This chapter will provide an overview of current diagnostic tests used to screen patients for the presence of heart disease as well as determine functional status, treatment outcomes, and long-term prognosis. A brief overview of cardiac pacemakers and percutaneous coronary interventions also will be provided.

Diagnostic Procedures

The choice of diagnostic procedure depends on several factors, including the clinical question, the availability of the test, the cost, and the ability to interpret the results correctly. The most frequently used tests are described next, including the rationale and normal versus abnormal results.

Electrocardiogram

The **electrocardiogram** (ECG) is a body surface recording of the electrical activity of the heart. Introduced in 1902 by Willem Einthoven, the ECG not only is the oldest but also remains the most frequently performed cardiac diagnostic test (Kadish et al., 2001; Rosen, 2002). The standard 12-lead ECG derives its name from the 12 leads that provide 12 different "views" of the electrical activity as it traverses the myocardium. These views are derived from the four limb and six precordial (chest) electrodes attached to the patient (Figure 39–1 ■).

Examining the electrical signals from the heart in different leads provides the clinician with accurate information about a variety of cardiac conditions (Chart 39–2, p. 1122). An in-depth discussion of electrocardiography is covered in Chapter 38 ⊜.

Drew (2002) noted that the ECG continues to be the gold standard for the detection and evaluation of cardiac dysrhythmias and ischemia. Because it is useful in many clinical situations and relatively easy to perform, the nurse at the bedside is frequently expected to obtain the 12-lead ECG. To improve the accuracy of the test, care must be taken to ensure correct positioning of the leads and firm contact with the skin (Drew & Ide, 1999; Kadish et al., 2001). Patient factors that can negatively influence the quality of the tracing include motion artifact, morbid obesity, and chronic obstructive lung disease. Motion artifact distorts the baseline, introducing error into the interpre-

tation. Morbid obesity and obstructive lung disease interfere with transmission of the electrical activity of the heart.

Although the ECG alone gives the clinician much valuable information, the tracing must always be interpreted at the bedside. That is, the ECG should be interpreted in the context of the patient's symptoms, laboratory values, and likely diagnosis.

Echocardiography

If the ECG is the most frequently performed diagnostic test, the echocardiogram (echo) is a close second (Smith & Thomas, 2002). This is not surprising because the echo exam provides a rapid, safe, and relatively inexpensive detailed examination of the heart. **Echocardiography** refers to the noninvasive assessment of the structures and function of the heart and great vessels utilizing high-frequency (ultrasound) sound waves. The first application of ultrasound, or sonar technology, to the clinical arena occurred almost 100 years ago in Sweden, where Edler and Hertz published their work on the utility of ultrasound to record the movements of the heart (Weyman, 2004). Since that time the definition of echocardiography has broadened to include not only traditional M-mode echocardiography but also two-dimensional transthoracic echocardiography, Doppler analysis and transesophageal echocardiography are explained later (Cheitlin et al., 2003).

Echocardiographic imaging relies on the generation of ultrasound waves (Armstrong & Feigenbaum, 2001; Hall, 2005). These waves are emitted from a transducer placed in standard positions on the chest wall. As the waves encounter an interface between solid (muscle) and liquid (blood), a portion of the ultrasound waves are bounced back to the transducer. Interfaces perpendicular to the ultrasound beam reflect echoes much more effectively than those that are not perpendicular. Because the speed of sound traveling in the body is known, the time it takes for the echo to return to the transducer allows determination of the depth of the structure. The fast rate of travel of the ultrasound waves allows for almost instantaneous or real-time recording of the cardiac structures in motion. The three noninvasive types of echocardiography are M-mode, two-dimensional, and Doppler ultrasound.

M-mode (motion) echocardiography was the earliest form of clinical ultrasound. Images are transmitted from a single narrow line of ultrasound and recorded as moving lines that do not resemble cardiac structures, and therefore can be difficult to interpret. M-mode provides information about the distance of each object (valve leaflet, pericardium, etc.) from the transducer and can be used to assess valvular motion and chamber wall thickness and motion.

Two-dimensional (2D) echocardiography came into use in the 1970s. 2D echo provides an anatomically recognizable image of the heart by sending out pulsed ultrasound waves in a fan or arc-shaped configuration, and today the transthoracic 2D echo is considered the mainstay of the echo evaluation (Armstrong & Feigenbaum, 2001).

Doppler ultrasound relies on analysis of frequency shifts as the beam encounters moving targets. In the heart, sound waves are reflected off moving red blood cells. The Doppler effect shifts the sound frequency as the cells move toward or away from the transducer; these shifts are viewed as color changes.

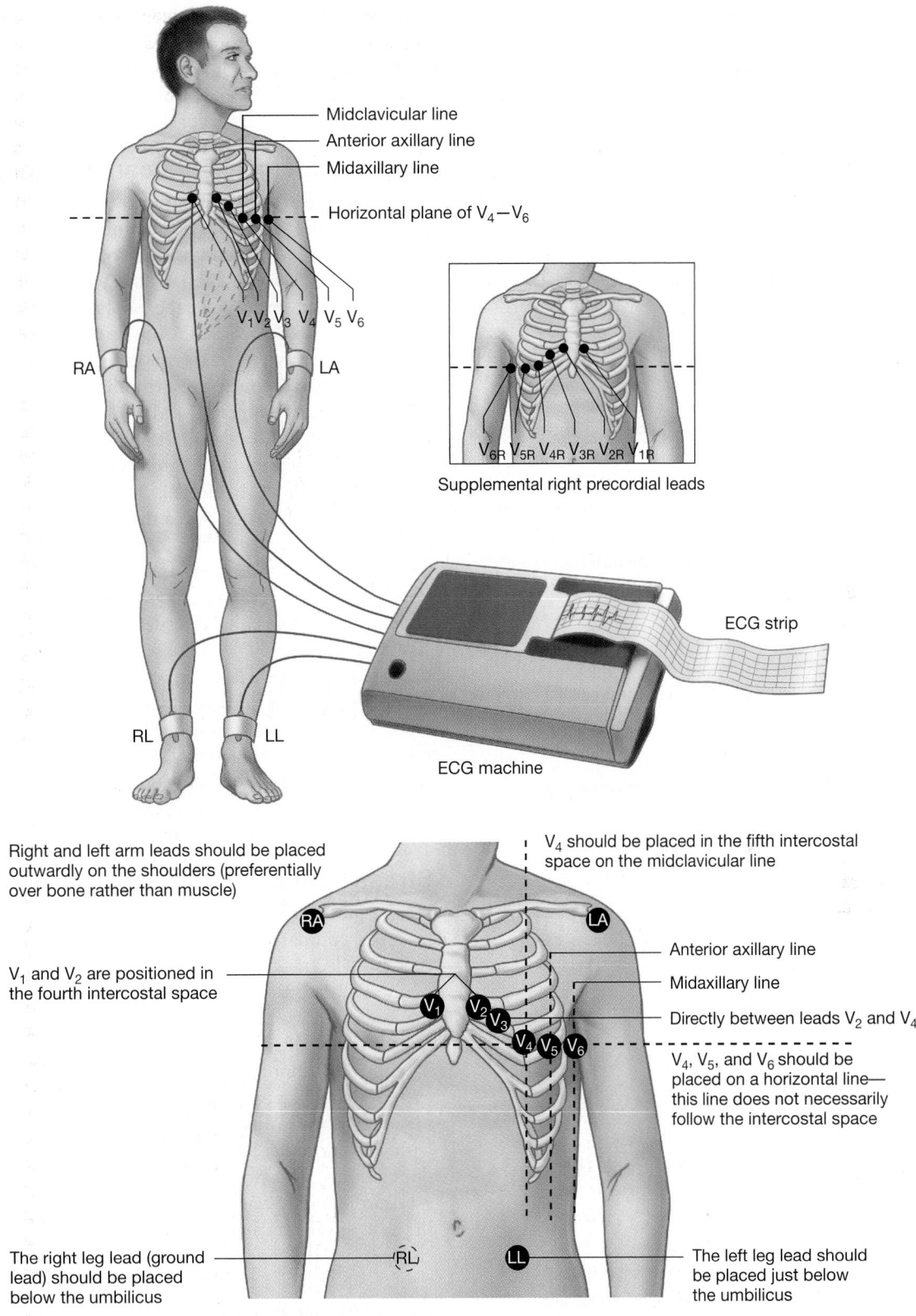

Right and left arm leads should be placed outwardly on the shoulders (preferentially over bone rather than muscle)

V_1 and V_2 are positioned in the fourth intercostal space

The right leg lead (ground lead) should be placed below the umbilicus

V_4 should be placed in the fifth intercostal space on the midclavicular line

Anterior axillary line

Midaxillary line

Directly between leads V_2 and V_4

V_4, V_5, and V_6 should be placed on a horizontal line—this line does not necessarily follow the intercostal space

The left leg lead should be placed just below the umbilicus

Midclavicular line
Anterior axillary line
Midaxillary line
Horizontal plane of V_4–V_6

Supplemental right precordial leads

ECG strip

ECG machine

FIGURE 39–1 ■ Position of the electrodes in the 12-lead electrocardiogram.

This ability to measure blood flow through the heart and great vessels provides hemodynamic data to supplement the anatomic information obtained from M-mode and 2D echo. Hemodynamic data include the amount and speed of blood flow through the valves, enabling the noninvasive detection and follow-up of stenotic or regurgitant heart valves, and measure-

ment of intracardiac pressures, which can be used to detect abnormal flow states such as shunts across the atrial or ventricular septum.

The echocardiogram can also assess the pumping action of the cardiac muscle. This measure is known as an ejection fraction, or EF. A normal EF is around 55% to 65%. Numbers below

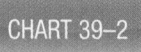

CHART 39–2 **Clinical Conditions Detectable from the 12-Lead Electrocardiogram**

1. Myocardial ischemia, injury, and infarction
2. Cardiac dysrhythmias
3. Electrical conduction abnormalities
4. Cardiac hypertrophy
5. Medication effects (i.e., digitalis toxicity)
6. Electrolyte abnormalities

45% usually represent some decrease in the pumping strength of the heart, whereas numbers below 30% to 35% are representative of an important decrease.

Currently a complete echocardiography exam incorporates all three modalities: M-mode, 2D, and Doppler (Cheitlin et al., 2003). Together they provide the clinician with detailed information about the structure and function of the heart and great vessels (Chart 39–3).

In certain populations the standard transthoracic examination (TTE) has limitations that require the use of further tests to establish the diagnosis or determine the therapeutic course of action. Because ultrasound waves cannot travel through air, echocardiography performed on patients who have chronic obstructive lung disease or who are on mechanical ventilators may

CHART 39–3 **Indications for Echocardiography**

ASSESSMENT OF THE HEART AND GREAT VESSELS

1. Size of the cardiac chambers
2. Size of the cardiac walls
3. Structure and function of the valves
4. Location and quantification of cardiac shunts (i.e., patent foramen ovale or a ventricular septal defect)
5. Cardiac tumors
6. Estimates of left ventricular functioning

ESTABLISHMENT OF CLINICAL DIAGNOSES

1. Aortic dissection
2. Location and quantification of pericardial effusions
3. Cardiac tamponade
4. Endocarditis
5. Murmurs
6. Stroke: identification of intracardiac sources of embolization

TIMING OF THERAPEUTIC INTERVENTIONS

1. When to repair/replace defective cardiac valves
2. Rule out intra-atrial thrombus before cardioversion for atrial fibrillation
3. Intraoperative TEE guidance
4. Ischemic heart disease

result in suboptimal or even inadequate images. Likewise, ultrasound cannot image through bone or heavily calcified structures. In the adult this limits the transducer placement to the intercostal and subxiphoid positions. Finally, excess adipose tissue can make visualization of the borders of the heart difficult.

Transesophageal Echocardiography

Transesophageal echocardiography (TEE) can overcome some of the limitations of TTE (Armstrong & Feigenbaum, 2001; Milani, Lavie, Gilliland, Cassidy, & Bernal, 2003; Peterson, Brickner, & Reimold, 2003). During TEE, the miniaturized transducer is advanced down the esophagus. Because the esophagus passes directly behind the posterior surface of the heart, it affords excellent views of the posterior structures of the heart and great vessels. Because TEE is minimally invasive and usually performed using conscious sedation, it is associated with a slight risk (<0.02%) of complications such as trauma to the structures of the mouth or throat or adverse reactions to the conscious sedation (Milani et al., 2003). Current guidelines recommend using TEE only when the information cannot be obtained from a standard TTE (Quiñones et al., 2003). TEE is frequently used to detect and assess endocarditis, aortic dissection, intracardiac masses such as thrombi or tumors, valvular pathology, and congenital disorders in both children and adults (Quiñones et al., 2003). TEE also is helpful in critically ill patients requiring ventilator support because the posterior images are not distorted by the constant motion of the lungs as the ventilator cycles. Finally, the role of TEE intraoperatively is expanding as evidence mounts that TEE guidance during procedures such as valvular repair improves clinical outcomes (improved valve function after surgery, less need for valve replacement or reoperation) (Cheitlin et al., 2003).

Stress Echocardiography

Stress echocardiography refers to the use of echocardiography to detect coronary artery disease (Marwick, 2002). Although exercise electrocardiography is the standard noninvasive method of detecting CAD, in some settings this test is of limited value because of incomplete data or difficulty in interpreting the test results. These instances include patients who have baseline ECG abnormalities or who are unable or unwilling to exercise to their peak heart rate. The standard treadmill test may also be more difficult to interpret in women and patients with left ventricular hypertrophy (ECG is least reliable in these populations) (Marwick, 2003). In these instances stress echocardiography can be used to make the diagnosis because the test results are based on echo images and not on ECG changes. Stress echocardiography is also used to evaluate patients with known coronary or valvular heart disease, populations who often cannot exercise to their peak heart rate and/or have baseline ECG abnormalities (Quiñones et al., 2003).

Stress echocardiography can be performed using standard forms of exercise (treadmill or bicycle) or a pharmacologic agent such as dobutamine, to increase the heart rate (Quiñones et al., 2003). The normal response to exercise is an increase in heart rate and contractility. The development of a new myocardial wall motion abnormality (failure to contract normally in one or more segments of the heart) or failure of the heart to increase strength of contraction during the test is a positive indication of reversible ischemia.

Contrast agents have been explored as a method of improving visualization of the left ventricle during echocardiography (Mulvagh et al., 2000; Smith & Thomas, 2002; Stewart, 2003). Agitated saline, created by forcefully mixing normal saline with air, is the simplest contrast agent and still the standard by which to detect intracardiac shunts (Armstrong & Feigenbaum, 2001). Because agitated saline results in microbubbles too large to pass through the pulmonary circulation, the visualization of bubbles in the left side of the heart after intravenous injection is considered positive proof of a cardiac shunt (abnormal opening in the atrial or ventricular septum).

Newer contrast agents that possess smaller, more stable bubbles are under investigation (Mulvagh et al., 2000). These agents improve endocardial border detection and thus improve the ability of echocardiography to detect ischemic disease and possibly evaluate **myocardial perfusion** (blood flow to the heart muscle) (Mulvagh et al., 2000; Quiñones et al., 2003; Stewart, 2003).

Finally, the development of three-dimensional echocardiography (3D) allows the clinician to view the structures and valves of the heart in a three-dimensional view noninvasively. This technology, combined with other advances in echocardiography, is bringing diagnostic cardiology closer to having an all-inclusive noninvasive assessment of the anatomy and physiology of the heart.

The advantages of echocardiography—the amount of information obtained with a noninvasive test, its portability and safety, and its relative low cost—can also lead to overuse of this technology. Clinical guidelines for the use of echocardiography are published and should be used to identify appropriate indications for testing (Cheitlin et al., 2003). Another well-known limitation of echocardiography is operator variability in performing and interpreting the results (Armstrong & Feigenbaum, 2001; Smith & Thomas, 2002). Again, standards are published for the performance and interpretation of echocardiography (Quiñones et al., 2003). Adherence to these standards improves the reliability and validity of the test results.

Exercise Testing

Exercise testing is a "cardiovascular stress test that uses treadmill or bicycle exercise and electrocardiographic and blood pressure monitoring" (Gibbons et al., 2002, p. 2). It is the most common noninvasive test used to evaluate patients with suspected ischemic heart disease (Gibbons et al., 2002; Grech, 2003).

Indications

Exercise testing is useful in many situations and populations (Chart 39–4). It is a relatively inexpensive test that can be safely performed in the hospital or in an outpatient setting. As with other diagnostic tests, the value of the information obtained from the test is directly related to the expertise and experience of all the staff performing and interpreting the results. Standards have been established for the performance and interpretation of exercise tests (Fletcher et al., 2001; Gibbons et al., 2002).

In persons with normal cardiac function, upright exercise such as walking on a treadmill results in an increased heart rate that is largely responsible for the increased cardiac output. Sys-

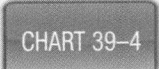

CHART 39–4 Indications and Contraindications for Exercise Testing

INDICATIONS

1. Evaluation of chest pain
2. Evaluation of severity of myocardial disease
3. Risk stratification, especially after a myocardial infarction
4. Prognosis in patients with known or suspected heart disease
5. Detection of exercise-related symptoms, such as syncope due to dysrhythmias
6. Evaluation after revascularization procedures, such as percutaneous coronary interventions or coronary artery bypass surgeries
7. Evaluation for cardiac rehabilitation
8. Patient reassurance

CONTRAINDICATIONS

1. Myocardial infarction within 2 days
2. Unstable angina
3. Aortic stenosis
4. Uncontrolled dysrhythmias
5. Symptomatic heart failure
6. Active endocarditis
7. Uncontrolled hypertension
8. Any acute disorder that may affect exercise (infection, renal failure)
9. Inability to obtain informed consent

Sources: Adapted from Fletcher, G. F., Balady, G. J., Amsterdam, E. A., Chaitman, B., Eckel, R., Fleg, J., et al. (2001). Exercise standards for testing and training. *Circulation, 104,* 1694–1740; Grech, E. D. (2003). ABC of interventional cardiology: Pathophysiology and investigation of coronary artery disease. *British Medical Journal, 326,* 1027–1030; and Myers, J. (2005). Exercise testing. In S. L. Woods, E. S. S. Froelicher, S. A. Motzer, & E. J. Bridges (Eds.), *Cardiac nursing* (5th ed., pp. 439–458). Philadelphia: Lippincott Williams & Wilkins.

tolic blood pressure increases as work increases, but there is minimal or no change in diastolic blood pressure (Fletcher et al., 2001; Myers, 2005).

During exercise there is an increase in heart rate along with increased myocardial oxygen need and thereby a demand for increased coronary blood flow (Myers, 2005). The maximal heart rate that a person can attain at peak exercise declines with age and can be roughly calculated from this formula: $220 -$ age (years) (Chaitman, 2001). Oxygen uptake is usually expressed in **metabolic equivalents (MET),** whereby 1 MET is a unit of sitting/resting oxygen uptake (≈ 3.5 milliliters of O_2 per kilogram of body weight per minute). Maximal oxygen consumption, the greatest amount of oxygen a person can take in while exercising at maximum capacity, is considered the best measure of a person's exercise capacity (Fletcher et al., 2001).

Factors that influence a person's ability to exercise include age, gender, physical conditioning, heredity, and cardiovascular status (Fletcher et al., 2001). Cardiovascular disease causes maximal heart rate and systolic blood pressure, as well as maximal exercise capacity, to be reduced.

Protocols and Patient Preparation

Exercise tests are conducted according to established protocols that usually include a warm-up phase, progressive exercise to a maximal heart rate or prespecified end points, and a recovery phase. Several different exercise protocols are available. Selection of protocol will depend on the purpose of the test, the physical condition of the patient, and of course the equipment and personnel available. The most suitable protocols for clinical testing last 6 to 12 minutes (Fletcher at al., 2001; Myers, 2005).

Patients are usually asked not to eat or smoke for 3 hours before the exam. They should also be instructed about their medications; most centers do not stop cardiac medications before the test. During the test, heart rate, blood pressure, electrocardiographic changes, exercise capacity, and patient symptoms are monitored. The electrocardiogram is the cornerstone of the exercise test; therefore, skin preparation and lead placement are extremely important in order to obtain high-quality results.

Interpretation

The test is usually continued until the patient achieves a maximal level of exertion or displays clinical indications for stopping (Chart 39–5).

The results of the exercise test include both objective and subjective data. Objective information includes blood pressure measurements, heart rate, and exercise capacity reported in METs, or exercise stage achieved, and ECG findings. Failure to achieve 85% of the predicted heart rate is associated with an increased risk of mortality in patients with previously diagnosed coronary artery disease (CAD) (Chaitman, 2001; Fletcher et al., 2001). Numerous ECG criteria are used to diagnose CAD. Patients with exercise- or dobutamine-induced myocardial ischemia often develop ST segment depression. In patients with a normal baseline ECG, the traditional criteria include the development of 1 millimeter or greater ST segment depression (horizontal or downsloping) occurring for at least 60 to 80 milliseconds after the J point—the point on the ECG where the QRS complex ends and the ST segment begins (Fletcher et al., 2001; Myers, 2005) (Figure 39–2 ■). ECG abnormalities at baseline make interpretation of the stress tracing difficult or impossible.

> **CHART 39–5** **Selected Indications for Stopping Exercise Testing**
>
> 1. Target heart rate achieved (>85% of maximum predicted heart rate)
> 2. ST segment elevation (>1.0 millimeter) in leads without Q waves (except leads V_1 and aVR)
> 3. Decrease in systolic blood pressure (>10 mmHg) accompanied by other evidence of ischemia
> 4. Moderate to severe angina
> 5. Dizziness or near syncope
> 6. Sustained ventricular tachycardia
>
> *Sources:* Adapted from Fletcher, G. F., Balady, G. J., Amsterdam, E. A., Chaitman, B., Eckel, R., Fleg, J., et al. (2001). Exercise standards for testing and training. *Circulation, 104,* 1694–1740; Grech, E. D. (2003). ABC of interventional cardiology: Pathophysiology and investigation of coronary artery disease. *British Medical Journal, 326,* 1027–1030; and Myers, J. (2005). Exercise testing. In S. L. Woods, E. S. S. Froelicher, S. A. Motzer, & E. J. Bridges (Eds.), *Cardiac nursing* (5th ed., pp. 439–458). Philadelphia: Lippincott Williams & Wilkins.

Subjective measurements include the development of any chest pain, excessive fatigue, general appearance, and perceived exertion, that is, shortness of breath. Classic symptoms of angina as a result of the test are predictive of coronary artery disease, especially when associated with ST segment depression (Fletcher et al., 2001).

The probability that a patient with a positive exercise test actually has significant coronary artery disease depends in part on the sensitivity and specificity of the test. Sensitivity, or the ability of the test to detect patients with CAD, is relatively low, ranging from 50% to 75%. Specificity in patients who do not have CAD is much higher; that is, the test will be negative in 77% to 90% of cases. The relatively high specificity is the real value of the exercise test in diagnosing CAD (Gibbons et al., 2002; Grech, 2003; Myers, 2005). However, remember that the most important factor affecting the results is the estimation of pretest probability of the patient actually having CAD. Tables are available that estimate the likelihood of CAD based on gender, age, and symptoms (Gibbons et al., 2002); nonetheless, the history and physical examination, as well as the experience of the health care provider, are critically important in deciding who is an appropriate candidate for exercise testing.

Radionuclide Imaging

Nuclear clinical cardiology is a relatively recent field, beginning in the early 1970s with the introduction of the scintillation camera and radioactive potassium to image the heart and great vessels (Iskandrian & Verani, 2002). Today nuclear cardiology techniques are used to establish the diagnosis, assess the severity of disease, calculate risk assessment, and evaluate outcomes of therapy in patients with acute and chronic coronary syndromes and heart failure (Klocke et al., 2003).

Perfusion Imaging

Exercise **myocardial perfusion imaging (MPI)** is the most common application of nuclear imaging techniques. In patients who do not have a normal baseline ECG, or who for other reasons such as physical limitations are not suitable candidates for a standard exercise test, imaging techniques combined with a basic stress test improve the ability to detect significant CAD (Fletcher et al., 2001; Klocke et al., 2003; Wackers, Soufer, & Zaret, 2001). In addition, imaging provides information regarding the location of ischemic myocardium, as well as an estimation of the amount of myocardium at risk. MPI is most useful in patients who have an intermediate risk of CAD (Greenland & Gaziano, 2003; Klocke et al., 2003).

During MPI a radioactive tracer is administered intravenously and given time to circulate in the bloodstream. Areas of the myocardium with normal coronary blood flow (normal perfusion) will absorb relatively large amounts of the tracer, whereas areas with compromised blood flow will absorb less. A gamma camera is placed over the precordium to record the amount of radioactive tracer emissions. Because most significant coronary plaques are associated with normal blood flow at rest, it is necessary to image the heart during a period of maximal exercise. A perfusion defect imaged only during exercise, termed a reversible defect, denotes an area of viable (functioning) but ischemic myocardium. If a defect is present during both exercise and rest, it is termed a fixed defect and probably indicates

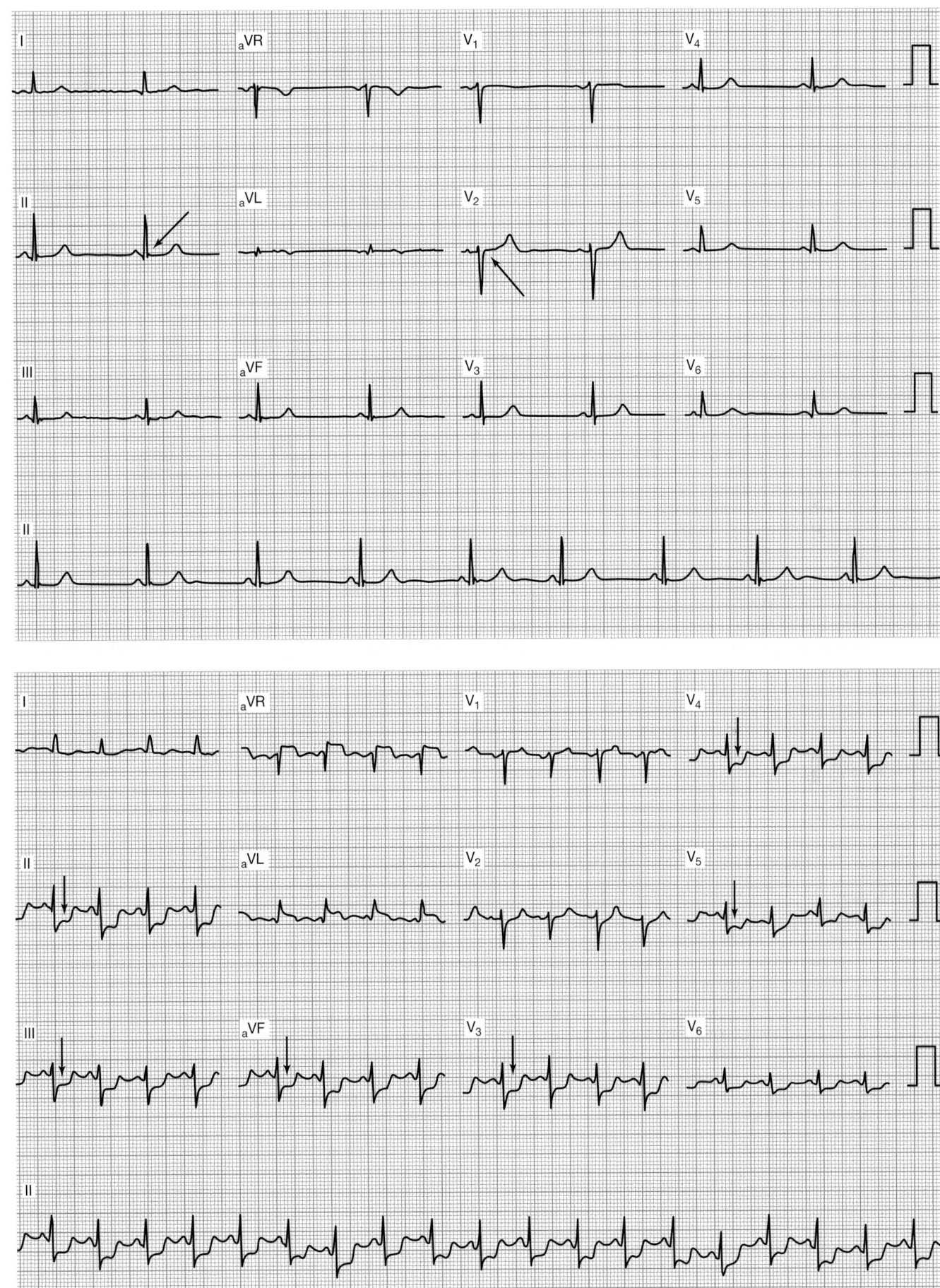

FIGURE 39–2 ■ Positive electrocardiographic ischemic response to exercise.

an area of infarction (defect is not reversible). If the patient is unable to exercise to maximum capacity, pharmacologic agents such as dipyridamole or adenosine can be used to invoke a physiological response in coronary blood flow similar to physical exercise. The results obtained with these methods appear to be as accurate as the results obtained with traditional stress tests (Klocke et al., 2003).

Three perfusion tracers are currently approved for routine clinical use: thallium 201 (t. 201), technetium (Tc) 99m sestamibi, and Tc 99m tetrofosmin (Chart 39–6).

Although t. 201 was the first commercially available tracer and has been the standard for diagnosing CAD, it does appear that any of the three tracers can be used to diagnose CAD accurately (Klocke et al., 2003).

ECG single photon emission computed tomography (SPECT), performed in 80% to 90% of perfusion imaging studies, is considered state of the art (Klocke et al., 2003; Wackers et al., 2001). **Tomography** is the display of images within a single plane (slice) of the heart. SPECT images are obtained with a rotating gamma camera that stops at preset angles to record images. The results are displayed as views of the heart on three different axes (Figure 39–3 ■). SPECT images offer better resolution and better separation of overlapping myocardial segments than do traditional planar images.

SPECT images are often obtained by a technique referred to as **gating,** in which image acquisition is timed to the ECG. The cardiac cycle is divided into segments that, when viewed in cine mode, allow the clinician to evaluate wall motion and systolic thickening in all areas of the left ventricle (Iskandrian & Verani, 2002). This technique allows for more accurate interpretation because the perfusion image can be correlated with the gated image of ventricular contraction.

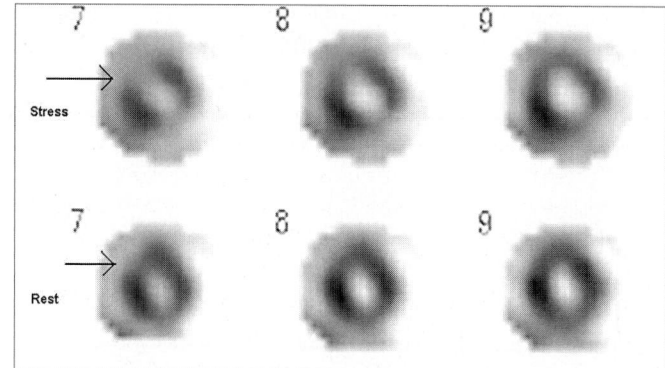

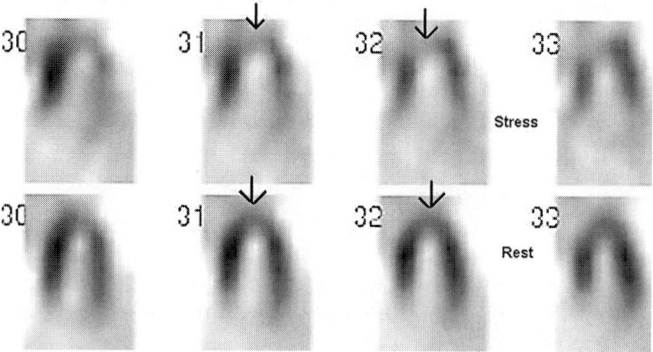

FIGURE 39–3 ■ Exercise–rest myocardial perfusion images.
Source: Courtesy of Dr. Guy Weingold, Director of Cardiac CT, Washington Hospital Center, Washington, DC

Cardiac Magnetic Resonance Imaging

Magnetic resonance imaging (MRI) uses radiofrequency pulses from a large, powerful magnet to disrupt the normal spin of certain atoms within the body temporarily. When the pulses are stopped, the atoms emit small amounts of energy while returning to their original spin; this energy can be imaged and recorded as high-resolution images. These images allow detailed noninvasive assessment of both cardiac anatomy and physiology (Choudhury, Fuster, Badimon, Fisher, & Fayad, 2002; Schvartzman & White, 2002).

MRI can be used to evaluate patients with presumed congenital heart diseases, such as coarctation of the aorta or atrial septal defects (Pohost, Hung, & Doyle, 2003). It also is used to image structures of the heart such as the valves and the pericardium, and assessment of **myocardial viability.** This provides information about areas of the myocardium that appear to have normal functioning as well as areas that appear to be dysfunctional and may improve with revascularization.

Introduced in the late 1970s, the term *hibernating myocardium* defined areas of the heart that initially appeared dysfunctional but after restoration of blood flow (revascularization) were noted to have improved contractility (Wu & Lima, 2003). Similar improvements in function were noted in patients who had undergone successful thrombolytic therapy. Chapter 40 ☺ includes a complete discussion of thrombolytic therapy.

These areas were referred to as "stunned" myocardium by the sudden occlusion of the coronary artery during a myocardial infarction. An in-depth discussion of the pathophysiology of acute myocardial infarction is presented in Chapter 40 ☺.

Whether hibernating and stunned myocardium are different manifestations of the same process or distinct entities remains unknown (Kloner, Bolli, Marbán, Reinlib, & Braunwald, 1998).

CHART 39–6 **Radionuclide Tracers**

THALLIUM 201 (t. 201)

- Uptake similar to potassium in living cells; after injection rapidly taken up by myocardial tissue in proportion to myocardial blood flow
- Half-life 74 hours; only small amounts can be administered
- Need for immediate imaging after injection because it redistributes in the myocardium over time (images obtained late do not reflect blood flow at time of injection)
- Not useful in evaluating chest pain in the emergency department
- Usual imaging protocol involves immediate imaging after injection during exercise; followed in 2 to 4 hours by imaging at rest to evaluate reversibility of any defects

TECHNETIUM 99m (Tc 99m) SESTAMIBI AND TETROFOSMIN

- Tracer trapped in myocardium and does not redistribute
- Less radiation exposure than thallium
- Sestamibi half-life 6 hours; larger doses can be administered
- Useful for imaging acute (emergency department) patients
- Useful for diagnosing coronary artery disease

Usual imaging protocol with sestamibi involves obtaining rest images first; after waiting 60 minutes after injection to allow for uptake and clearance from the liver, a second dose of sestamibi is administered during peak exercise.

However, the importance of identifying areas of the heart that could benefit from revascularization is self-evident.

MRI can identify viable myocardium through the use of low-dose dobutamine, with a sensitivity and specificity to identify functional recovery similar to echo (Wu & Lima, 2003). However, delayed hyperenhancement is rapidly challenging the conventional methods for assessing viability. Using gadolinium (Gd) based contrast agents increases the MRI signal of tissues, allowing characterization of specific areas of the myocardium. Gd is mainly an extracellular, interstitial agent. This property enables it to accumulate near acute infarcts where necrosis results in cell membrane rupture and interstitial edema. Gd also is increased in areas of chronic infarction. Compared to normal myocardium, areas of irreversibly damaged heart muscle appear hyperenhanced, allowing accurate quantification of the amount and location of nonviable myocardium (Higgins, 2002; Pohost et al., 2003; Wu & Lima, 2003).

The clinical uses of MRI are rapidly expanding. The application of this technology is limited by the size and expense of the magnet, the lack of dedicated cardiovascular MRI facilities, and the difficulty in imaging acutely ill patients (the nurse cannot remain with the patient during imaging). Additionally, patients with implanted metal devices such as pacemakers or defibrillators cannot be placed in the magnet (Chart 39–7) (Schvartzman & White, 2002).

Positron-Emission Tomography

Positron-emission tomography (PET) utilizes tracers that emit positrons (positively charged particles). When introduced into the body, these tracers travel only a short distance before interacting with electrons, which results in destruction of both particles and the release of a pair of high-energy photons. These photons travel in opposite directions, always 180 degrees apart. Two detectors positioned on opposite sides are programmed to recognize only simultaneous high-energy photons. Destruction of the tracer is assumed to have occurred somewhere along the straight line connecting the two detectors (Wackers et al., 2001).

The main advantage of PET scanning is the ability to label and image biologically active compounds such as glucose or drugs,

---

CHART 39–7 **Advantages and Disadvantages of Cardiac Magnetic Resonance Imaging**

ADVANTAGES

- Noninvasive
- No exposure to radiation
- Can be repeated serially
- Provides high-resolution images of coronary artery vessel walls and lumen, allowing characterization of atherosclerotic plaque
- Allows noninvasive evaluation of acquired and congenital diseases affecting the heart, pericardium, and great arteries and veins of the thorax

DISADVANTAGES

- Relatively expensive
- Not portable
- Difficulty monitoring acutely ill patients during imaging
- Cannot be used for patients who have metal implants, such as pacemakers or implantable defibrillators

---

which allows quantification of metabolic processes. PET scan is the current gold standard for assessment of myocardial viability. Cardiac metabolism is measured by uptake of tracers, which are analogues of glucose; viable heart muscle has normal or increased glucose uptake (Goldin, Ratib, & Aberle, 2000; Soine & Hanrahan, 2005; Wu & Lima, 2003). However, this technology has limited clinical availability because of the need for expensive equipment as well as the availability of other means of assessing viability.

Electron Beam Computed Tomography

Calcium deposits inside coronary arteries are part of the development of atherosclerosis; these deposits are not found in normal coronary arteries (O'Rourke et al., 2000). Thus the ability to quantify the amount of intracoronary artery calcium may identify asymptomatic individuals at risk for coronary events (Detrano & Carr, 2002; Fuseini, Goodwin, Ferris, & Mehta, 2003).

Computed tomography is very sensitive in detecting calcium, due to the increased absorption of x-rays by elements with high atomic numbers such as calcium. With the development of **electron beam computed tomography (EBCT),** which uses an electron gun and a stationary tungsten target to acquire rapidly (≈ 90 seconds) multiple images of the heart during a single breath hold, detection and quantification of intracoronary calcium are now a clinical reality. Since the 1990s EBCT has become the accepted gold standard for assessing calcified plaques (Detrano & Carr, 2002; Fayad, Fuster, Nikolaou, & Becker, 2002; Greenland & Gaziano, 2003; O'Rourke et al., 2000).

The amount of calcium identified by EBCT is usually reported as a total calcium score (Agatson et al., 1990). A calcium score of zero is normal. There is no currently accepted standard for a high score, but values over 100 are usually considered to indicate high risk for the presence of CAD.

Many issues surround the measuring and reporting of calcium scores. First is the acknowledged low reproducibility rates; scores are influenced by the laboratory and the method of scoring (Detrano & Carr, 2002; Greenland & Gaziano, 2003; O'Rourke et al., 2000). Second, scores must be adjusted for age and gender (O'Rourke et al., 2000). Third, is the fact that a high calcium score is a sensitive but not specific marker for CAD. Sensitivity to detect CAD ranges from 80% to 90%, but specificity has been reported between 40% and 50% (Greenland & Gaziano, 2003; O'Rourke et al., 2000). Lack of data from controlled clinical trials makes it unclear at this time whether calcium scores have true incremental prognostic value.

In addition to lack of a standard reporting system for calcium scores, there is also uncertainty concerning the role of EBCT in detecting and evaluating CAD. Much of the controversy surrounding EBCT is attributable to the fact that, unlike most screening tests, EBCT is available to the public without a health care provider's order, and it has been aggressively marketed directly to consumers as a rapid, inexpensive screening tool to detect CAD (Lee & Brennan, 2002; O'Rourke et al., 2000). EBCT is a promising technology that needs clinical trials in order to assume its place as an important noninvasive, relatively inexpensive, rapid tool in the management of CAD.

Multislice Helical Computed Tomography

More recently, **multislice helical CT** has emerged as an exceptionally promising tool for visualization of general cardiac structures, the great vessels, and especially the coronary arteries (Figure 39–4 ■) (Detrano & Carr, 2002; Fayad et al., 2002; Nikolaou, Poon, Sirol, Becker, & Fayad, 2003; Schoepf, Becker, Hofmann, & Yucel, 2003).

Using 16-slice helical scanners, accompanied by ECG gating and the administration of 80 to 120 milliliters of iodinated contrast, it is possible to scan the entire volume of the heart, the proximal great vessels, and the coronary arteries with a single 25-second breath hold (Figure 39–5 ■). The spatial resolution of multislice helical CT is much higher than that of EBCT, allowing visualization of fine details of the coronary anatomy (Figure 39–6 ■), such as small side branches and atherosclerotic plaques, including "noncalcified" plaques. In addition, multislice helical CT can also detect coronary calcification using a noncontrast, low-radiation-dose scan.

The real advantage of multislice helical CT, however, is its ability to visualize the lumen of the coronary artery with high detail, allowing the interpreter to measure the degree of luminal stenosis, something that EBCT cannot do. In addition, some research suggests that identification of noncalcified plaque may be more significant as a marker of future coronary events, because calcified plaques may represent a more chronic and stable form of CAD (Choudhury et al., 2002).

Multiple-Gated Acquisition Scan (MUGA)

The MUGA scan is a useful noninvasive tool for assessing the function of the heart. The moving images of the beating heart that can be obtained provide important information about the motion of the ventricles. If muscle damage has occurred, as with a myocardial infarction, the MUGA scan can localize the portion of the heart muscle that has sustained damage and can assess the degree of damage. But more importantly, the MUGA scan is able to measure the ejection fraction of the cardiac ventricles. The left ventricular ejection fraction (LVEF), which is the proportion of blood

that is expelled from the ventricle with each heartbeat, is a commonly used measure of overall cardiac function (Fogorus, 2006).

A MUGA scan is performed by attaching a radioactive substance, technetium 99, to red blood cells and then injecting the red blood cells into the patient's bloodstream. The patient is

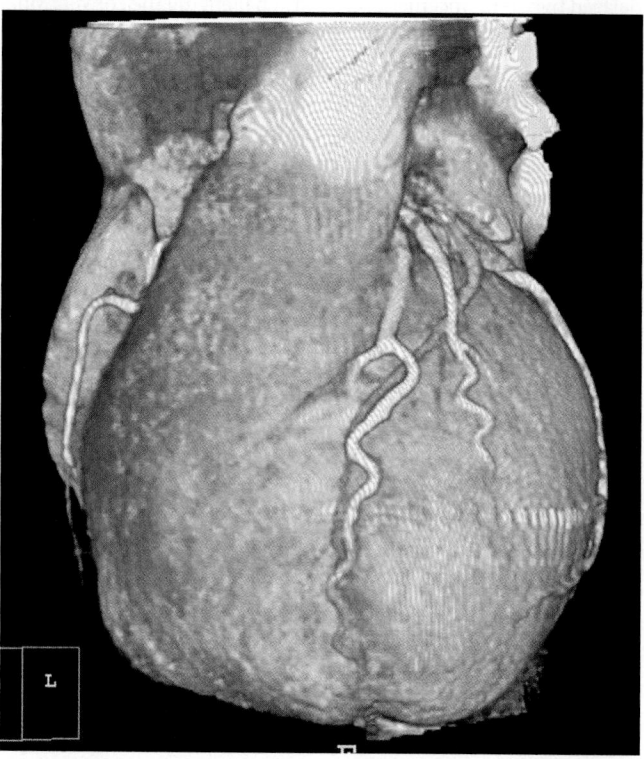

FIGURE 39–5 ■ Multislice helical computed tomography (CT) image of the heart.
Source: Courtesy of Dr. Guy Weingold, Director of Cardiac CT, Washington Hospital Center, Washington, DC

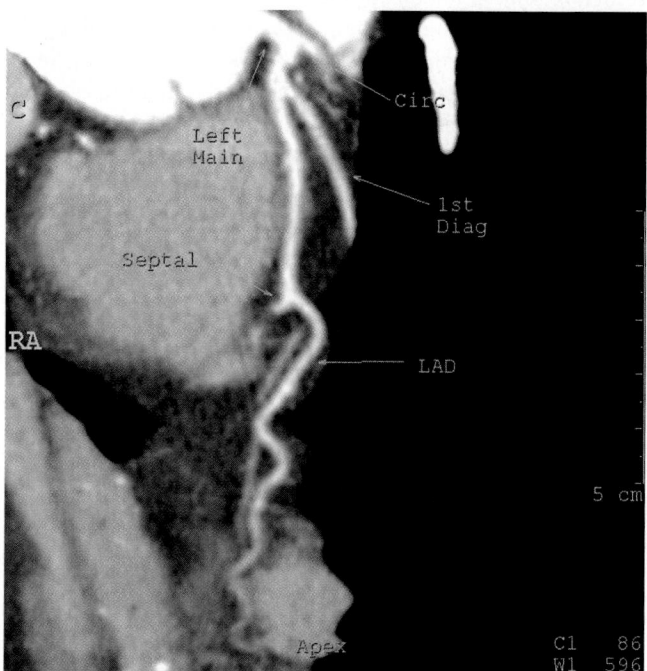

FIGURE 39–4 ■ Multislice helical computed tomography (CT) image of the heart.
Source: Courtesy of Dr. Guy Weingold, Director of Cardiac CT, Washington Hospital Center, Washington, DC

FIGURE 39–6 ■ Multislice helical computed tomography (CT) image of coronary arteries.
Source: Courtesy of Dr. Guy Weingold, Director of Cardiac CT, Washington Hospital Center, Washington, DC

then placed under a gamma camera, which is able to detect the technetium-labeled red cells. The image produced by the gamma camera is essentially an outline of those chambers, and after computer manipulation, the final product is a movie of the heart beating (Fogorus, 2006).

Nursing Management

Undergoing an evaluation for coronary artery disease, whether to detect new disease or to assess the progression or regression of a known clinical problem, can be stressful for the patient and her family. In order to provide optimum care during all phases of testing, the nurse must be knowledgeable about the particular test, including why it is ordered, what information is obtained, and how it is done. Explaining the procedure beforehand helps to calm the patient and may affect the results by improving patient compliance.

In many instances the nurse will actually perform the entire procedure, such as obtaining an ECG. In other situations the nurse may assist during portions of the test, such as monitoring the patient receiving conscious sedation during a TEE. Regardless, the nurse can play a critical role in ensuring a complete and accurate diagnostic exam.

Once the results are obtained, the nurse should be prepared to answer any further questions the patient or family may have regarding the outcome. This will be easier if the nurse if familiar with the standard report forms in her area of practice.

Many imaging techniques are currently available to health care professionals to identify and quantify CAD in their patients (Chart 39–8). There often is more than one appropriate test; factors such as the clinical assessment of the patient, the availability, the cost, and the experience of the professional with the current technology will all influence the choice of test.

Cardiac Catheterization

Cardiac catheterization is a procedure that is done in a special laboratory under sterile conditions. It consists of the insertion of a radiopaque catheter into the left or right side of the heart to provide anatomic and hemodynamic information about the heart and great vessels. This information is then utilized to assess the presence and severity of cardiac disease and assists to determine potential therapy and prognosis. Coronary angiography refers specifically to the use of radiopaque contrast media to image the coronary arteries. The first documented cardiac catheterization was done on a horse by Claude Bernard in 1844. The first human catheterization was performed by Werner Forssmann on himself in 1929. In 1959 Mason Sones accidentally cannulized the right coronary artery, thereby becoming the first person to perform coronary angiography on a human. In 2001 cardiac catheterizations were performed on over 1 million people, making it the second most frequent in-hospital procedure performed in the United States (American Heart Association, 2003; Deelstra & Jacobson, 2005; Grossman, 2000a; Scanlon et al., 1999).

Cardiac catheterization is indicated in a wide variety of clinical situations. Specifically it can provide information about:

- Hemodynamic pressures, which is used to evaluate cardiac and pulmonary function

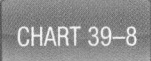

CHART 39–8 **Choosing the Appropriate Diagnostic Test**

Screening can be defined as the identification of previously unrecognized disease. How do you choose the most appropriate procedure?

1. Is the procedure rapid and accessible?
2. Can the results favorably alter the patient's quality or quantity of life?
3. Will the results of any intervention outweigh any potential adverse effects?
4. Does the disease have a clinically asymptomatic period during which the outcome of the disease can be altered?
5. Are acceptable treatments available?
6. Does the prevalence and seriousness of the disease justify the cost of the intervention?
7. Is the screening procedure relatively easy and inexpensive?
8. Are sufficient resources available?

- Heart chambers and the great vessels, which helps determine structural abnormalities
- Pressure gradients across valves to evaluate the extent of stenosis or regurgitation
- The patency of coronary arteries, which is used to evaluate the extent of coronary artery disease.

Chart 39–9 outlines the specific indications for cardiac catheterization.

Exact indications will vary depending on the aggressiveness of the institution in treating CAD (acute, chronic, or congenital). In addition, advances in other technologies such as cardiac MRI and multislice helical CT allow information previously available only by catheterization to be obtained in a noninvasive manner.

Right Heart Catheterization

Catheterization of the right atrium was first reported in the early 1940s. To access the right side of the heart, a catheter is advanced through a major vein into the right atrium (Figure 39–7a ■, p. 1130).

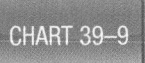

CHART 39–9 **Indications for Cardiac Catheterization**

- Identify coronary artery disease and assess its extent and severity.
- Determine the treatment strategy in patients with acute coronary syndrome.
- Assess the consequences of coronary artery disease (CAD):
  - Ischemic mitral regurgitation
  - Left ventricular dysfunction
  - Ventricular aneurysm.
- In patients with known CAD:
  - Correlate symptoms with extent of CAD.
  - Evaluate response to acute pharmacologic intervention.
  - Assess left ventricular dysfunction in cardiomyopathy.
- Evaluate and determine the treatment strategy in patients with congenital heart disease.
- Obtain hemodynamic information such as shunt size or pulmonary vascular resistance.

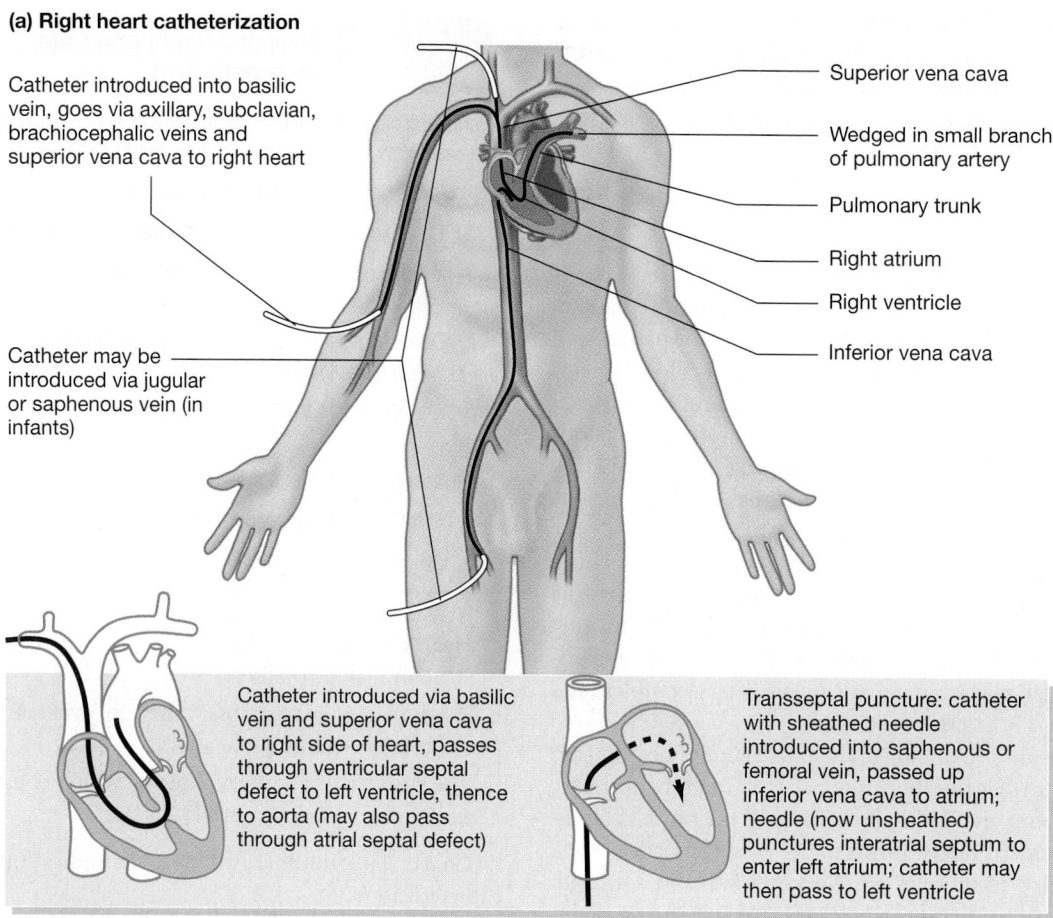

(a) Right heart catheterization

Catheter introduced into basilic vein, goes via axillary, subclavian, brachiocephalic veins and superior vena cava to right heart

Catheter may be introduced via jugular or saphenous vein (in infants)

Superior vena cava

Wedged in small branch of pulmonary artery

Pulmonary trunk

Right atrium

Right ventricle

Inferior vena cava

Catheter introduced via basilic vein and superior vena cava to right side of heart, passes through ventricular septal defect to left ventricle, thence to aorta (may also pass through atrial septal defect)

Transseptal puncture: catheter with sheathed needle introduced into saphenous or femoral vein, passed up inferior vena cava to atrium; needle (now unsheathed) punctures interatrial septum to enter left atrium; catheter may then pass to left ventricle

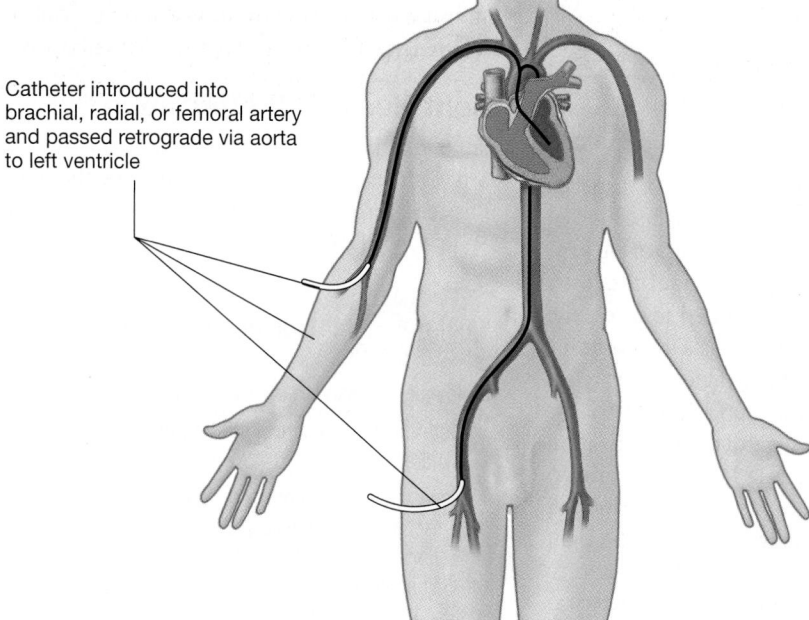

(b) Left heart catheterization

Catheter introduced into brachial, radial, or femoral artery and passed retrograde via aorta to left ventricle

FIGURE 39–7 ■ Heart catheterization.

Right heart catheterization allows for measurement and analysis of right heart pressures and oxygen saturations, pulmonary artery pressures including pulmonary capillary wedge pressures, screening for intracardiac shunts, and temporary ventricular pacing (Baim, 2000; Davidson & Bonow, 2001). Refer to

Chapter 24 🔗 for more detail regarding hemodynamic measurements. Shunts, abnormal blood flow through an opening in the atrial or ventricular septum, can be detected by measuring oxygen saturation levels in the right heart. Clinically significant (needing closure) left-to-right shunts will be evident by a notable increase in the oxygen saturation levels in the right heart, as oxygenated blood from the left side of the heart crosses through the shunt and mixes with the desaturated blood in the right side (Grossman, 2000a).

Right heart catheterization is not a routine part of the evaluation of patients with CAD. In the 1990s several professional groups ruled that necessary information can be obtained with a left heart catheterization alone; since that time the number of right heart catheterizations has steadily declined (Baim, 2000).

Left Heart Catheterization

Left heart catheterization was first reported in the early 1950s. Today left heart catheterization is usually performed by accessing the femoral artery using the Judkins technique, named for Melvin Judkins, who perfected this percutaneous approach in the 1960s (Grossman, 2000). The catheter is inserted into a major artery, usually the femoral, and passed retrograde (opposite direction) to blood flow up the aorta to the openings of the coronary arteries at the base of the aorta, or it crosses the aortic valve to enter the left heart (see Figure 39–7b ■). Left heart catheterization allows for the direct measurement of left heart pressures and pressures on both sides of the aortic valve, ventriculography to measure cardiac output, and evaluation of both left ventricular function as well as the severity of any mitral or aortic valvular disease.

Coronary Angiography

Coronary cine-angiography remains the gold standard to detect significant coronary artery disease. Specialized catheters are inserted into the coronary arteries using the left heart catheterization just described. Then radiographic dye is injected into the arteries. The entire coronary vasculature (tree) is imaged, including any surgically placed saphenous vein or internal mammary artery grafts. Where plaque buildup has occurred, the lumen of the artery appears narrowed (Figure 39–8 ■) (Baim & Grossman, 2000a). See Chapter 40 ⊜ for more information regarding coronary artery disease and coronary artery bypass surgery.

In addition to evaluating the extent of CAD, angiography also is used to define therapeutic options to treat CAD and to evaluate serial changes in the coronary lumen after revascularization or acute pharmacologic therapy (Baim & Grossman, 2000a; Deelstra & Jacobson, 2005; Popma & Bittl, 2001).

Percutaneous Coronary Interventions

Percutaneous transluminal coronary angioplasty (PTCA) refers to treatment of CAD using expandable balloons to crack (tear or rupture) atherosclerotic plaque, thereby enlarging the lumen of the coronary artery (Popma & Kuntz, 2001). The era of PTCA began with the first balloon angioplasty performed in a human by Andreas Grüntzig in 1977 (Grüntzig, 1978). During PTCA, a fluoroscopy-guided catheter with an expandable balloon mounted on the tip is passed into the coronary artery until it traverses the stenotic (narrowed by disease) area. The balloon is then inflated for several seconds, deflated, and then withdrawn. The procedure can be repeated until there is an increase in the diameter of the artery resulting in improved blood flow to the myocardium. Grüntzig's procedure marked the beginning of a period of rapid development in the percutaneous treatment of CAD, which continues even today (Kent, 2000;

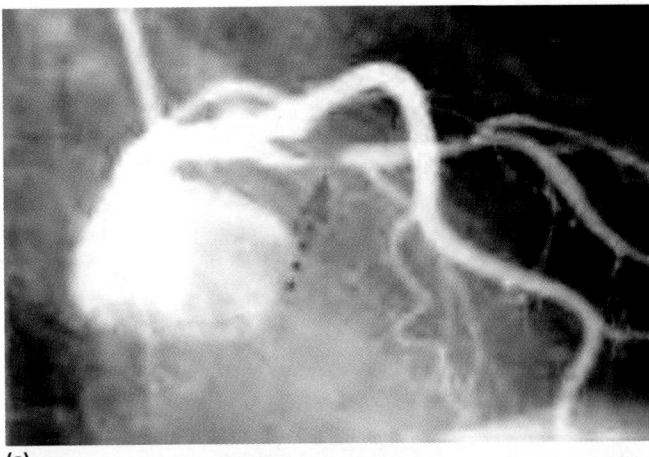

(a)

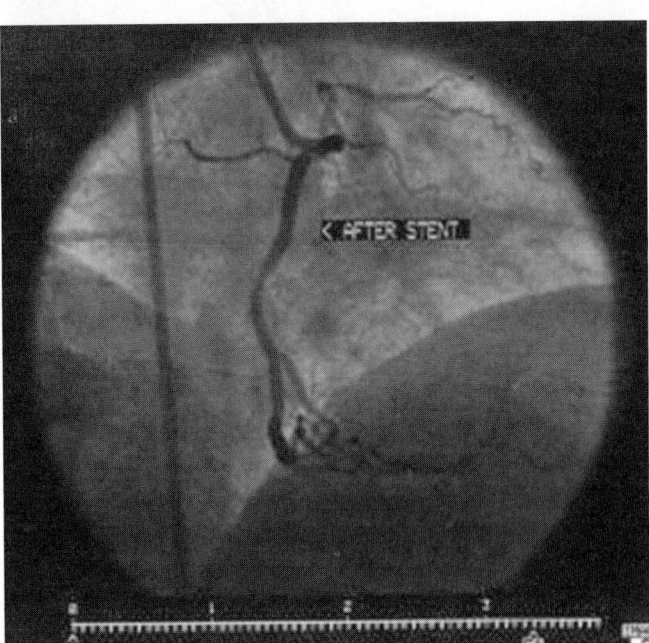

(b)

FIGURE 39–8 ■ Coronary artery with contrast media: (A) before stent placement and (B) after stent placement.
Source: Dr. Walt Marquardt, Mercy Hospital

O'Neill & Dixon, 2004). Figure 39–9 ■ (p. 1132) shows a balloon-tipped catheter that is used to perform a PTCA.

Percutaneous coronary intervention (PCI) includes not only PTCA but also all other devices used either to remove plaque or to alter its morphology in the catheterization laboratory. Such devices include intracoronary lasers, which can be used to open totally occluded coronary arteries; intracoronary stents; and atherectomy devices, which shave the plaque and remove it. Coronary artery **stents,** first approved for elective angioplasty in 1993, are metallic mesh-like structures that are inserted permanently inside the coronary artery, compressing plaque and providing structural support of the vessel (Figure 39–10 ■, p. 1130).

Stents, either alone or in combination with PTCA, are the most frequently used device, with at least one coronary stent placed in over 70% of PCI procedures (Smith et al., 2001) (see Figure 39–8 ■). Currently over 500,000 PCIs are performed annually in the United States; worldwide the figure is estimated at over 1 million procedures (American Heart Association, 2003).

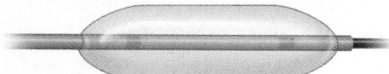

FIGURE 39–9 ■ Balloon-tipped catheter for PTCA.

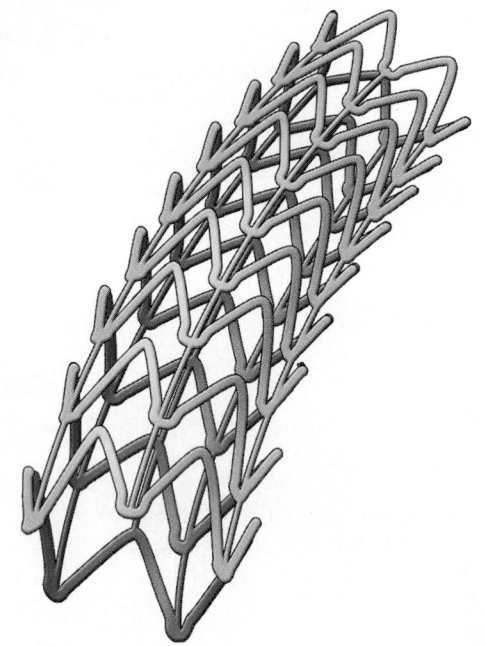

FIGURE 39–10 ■ Intracoronary stent.

Indications for PCI are numerous and depend on the clinical history of the patient, the extent of coronary disease, the presence of any comorbidity, the left ventricular (LV) function, and the institution where the procedure is performed. Comorbidities such as diabetes, hyperlipidemia, renal failure, or hypertension are associated with higher morbidity and mortality rates during PCI. The same applies to patients with poor left ventricular (LV) function. See the National Guidelines for Class I Indications for Percutaneous Coronary Intervention (PCI) box.

Outcomes are measured in terms of success of the procedure and complications. A successful PCI procedure is usually defined as an angiographic success (minimal residual narrowing in the artery at the completion of the procedure) without any in-hospital major adverse cardiovascular event (MACE). A MACE is generally considered death, emergency bypass surgery, or myocardial infarction (MI), with MI defined as a significant elevation in cardiac enzymes even in the absence of new Q waves. Refer to Chapter 40 for more information regarding MI. Clinical success includes angiographic and procedural success, as well as relief of any signs or symptoms of ischemia after the patient recovers from the procedure (short-term success) and ideally for more than 6 months after the procedure (long-term success) (Smith et al., 2001). Although outcomes are constantly changing in response to new technologies, improved operator skills, and changes in adjunct pharmacology, in general PCI angiographic success ranges from 96% to 99%, with MACE event rates from 0.2% to 3%, depending on the event measured. Long-term outcomes (5 to 10 years) are more difficult to measure, due to continuous changes in technology such as improved coronary stents, as well as clinical factors such as an increase in the number of elderly patients with poor left ventricular function undergoing PCI (Lindsay & Pinnow, 2000).

Restenosis, typically defined as a greater than 50% diameter stenosis at follow-up catheterization, has always been the Achilles' heel of PCI (Cannon, 2002; Smith et al., 2001; Waksman, 2000). Restenosis is an accumulation of smooth muscle cells at the site of the original procedure that occurs because of the artery's response to the injury from the PCI. Before the advent of stents, restenosis rates ranged from 30% to 50% within 6 to 12 months after the procedure.

Intracoronary stents marked a dramatic improvement in the incidence of restenosis, primarily by "tacking up" dissections and intimal tears as well as preventing the arterial recoil (tendency of the vessel wall to return to its original size weeks after the procedure) that commonly occurred with PCI. However, stents could not stop the smooth muscle cell proliferation that also occurred. Restenosis was occurring within the metal struts of the stent (in-stent restenosis) as well as near the ends of the device (Cannon, 2002; Carrozza & Baim, 2000; Waksman, 2000).

NATIONAL GUIDELINES for Class I Indications for Percutaneous Coronary Intervention (PCI)

1. Asymptomatic to mild angina
   a. Patients who do not have treated diabetes with one or more significant lesions in one or more coronary arteries and a high likelihood of successful PCI. The artery to be dilated must perfuse a large area of viable myocardium.

2. Moderate to severe symptoms, unstable angina, or non–ST segment elevation myocardial infarction
   a. Patients with one or more significant lesions in one or more coronary arteries suitable for PCI and a high likelihood of success. The artery to be dilated must perfuse a moderate or large area of viable myocardium.

3. Acute myocardial infarction (AMI)
   a. As an alternative to thrombolytic therapy in patients with ST segment elevation AMI or new left bundle branch block, if the

patient can undergo PCI ≤ 12 hours from the onset of ischemic symptoms or > 12 hours if symptoms persist and PCI can be performed quickly in a laboratory with experienced personnel and adequate equipment.
   b. In patients who are within 36 hours of an ST elevation AMI who develop cardiogenic shock, who are ≤ 75 years old, and revascularization can be completed within 18 hours of the onset of shock in a laboratory with experienced personnel and adequate equipment.

4. Prior coronary artery bypass surgery
   a. Patients with ischemia within 30 days of surgery

Note: Class I indications are "Conditions for which there is evidence and/or general agreement that the procedure or treatment is useful and effective."

Source: Adapted from ACC/AHA guidelines for percutaneous coronary intervention," by S. C. Smith, Jr., et al., 2001, *Journal of the American College of Cardiology, 39*, p. iii

Intracoronary **brachytherapy,** the use of localized radiation within the coronary artery, was the next development to treat in-stent restenosis (Teirstein & Kuntz, 2001; Weinberger, Lincoff, & Popma, 2002). The basis of this therapy is the assumption that restenosis is a benign process of smooth muscle cell proliferation, and locally delivered radiation can halt or even prevent this process. Intracoronary brachytherapy has been approved in the United States for the treatment of in-stent restenosis, but its use in the future of PCI is questionable due to advances in coronary stents (Teirstein & Kuntz, 2001a).

Drug eluting stents (DESs) may have the potential to eliminate or at least dramatically reduce the problem of in-stent restenosis (O'Neill & Dixon, 2004; Sousa, Serruys, & Costa, 2003). DESs are bare metal stents coated with immunosuppressive agents such as sirolimus or paclitaxel that are eluted over a period of weeks to months to inhibit smooth muscle cell proliferation. Early clinical trials reported results that were almost too good: 0% restenosis. Although later trials in more complex patients failed to duplicate the initial success, restenosis rates of less than 5% are common with the current DES. The result is that, despite the lack of long-term results, DES has captured the PCI market and become the standard of care worldwide (O'Neill & Dixon, 2004; Sousa et al., 2003; Squires, 2003).

Intravascular Ultrasound

Coronary angiography provides only a two-dimensional image of the coronary artery lumen (a "luminogram") and provides no information regarding the arterial wall. Intravascular ultrasound (IVUS) fills that void. To obtain these images a small ultrasound catheter is threaded into a coronary artery. From it ultrasound images that provide 360-degree cross-sectional images of the artery can be obtained. Important information can be gathered regarding not only the coronary lumen but also the intima, media, and adventitia of the vessel wall. Peter Yock and colleagues recorded the first ultrasound images of human coronary arteries in 1988 (Chou, Fitzgerald, & Yock, 2000; Mintz & Walsh, 2000; Popma & Bittl, 2001).

IVUS can be used to detect vessel wall pathology, to help determine the choice of PCI, as well as to evaluate the results of the intervention, especially intracoronary stenting. IVUS is safe, rapid, and reproducible (results are consistent when performed by different clinicians). However, its use is not universal, owing to its steep "learning curve," additional cost of the equipment, and limited information linking IVUS to improved patient outcomes (Mintz & Walsh, 2000; Popma & Bittl, 2001). In addition, advances in technology such as multislice helical CT will allow similar information to be obtained noninvasively.

■ Nursing Management

Patients undergoing PCI range from the stable person having an elective first procedure to the patient with an acute myocardial infarction (AMI) who is hemodynamically unstable, requiring ventilatory and inotropic support during the procedure. The clinical status of the patient and the planned procedure will dictate the exact patient management.

Before the procedure the nurse should perform a complete assessment, with special attention to the cardiovascular and peripheral vascular system. The patient and family should be questioned about any medications taken today, including warfarin, metformin, diuretics, or insulin. Warfarin, an oral anticoagulant, could lead to increased bleeding during and after the procedure. Metformin, a biguanide indicated in the treatment of non–insulin-dependent diabetes, has been associated with an increased risk of lactic acidosis after PCI. Diuretics in combination with the patient's NPO status can lead to hypovolemia during or after the procedure. Baseline laboratory values include serum chemistries, coagulation factors, and a complete blood count. Finally, the nurse should review the patient and family's understanding of the planned procedure, including postprocedure care. Explaining the purpose of the vascular access devices and monitoring equipment will help to decrease anxiety for everyone during the procedure.

Patients undergoing catheterization are told to have nothing to eat or drink for at least 6 hours before the test. There are a few contraindications to the procedure, which are outlined in Chart 39–10.

Patients with preexisting renal failure and a history of anaphylactic reaction to contrast dye must be pretreated before the catheterization (Scanlon et al., 1999). Pretreatment for the patient with a history of anaphylactic reaction to contrast dye includes antihistamines and steroids. In the laboratory the patient will usually be given a mild sedative. Patients with renal failure (serum creatinine ≥ 1.5 mg/dL) should receive intravenous normal saline for several hours before the procedure.

The length of the procedure will vary depending on the information needed; coronary angiography alone takes about 15 minutes. The patient should be warned that during injection of any contrast medium he may feel hot and flushed; this will pass quickly. After the procedure the patient will have to remain on bed rest for a few hours unless a vascular closure device has been inserted.

Prior to the procedure the patient is given a mild sedative, but remains awake throughout the procedure. The nurse's role during PCI usually includes close monitoring of the patient to ensure a safe environment for the procedure. The nurse must pay particular attention to the patient's airway and respiratory status during the administration of conscious sedation. Continuous assessment of the cardiovascular system, including vital signs and ECG, is also necessary to avoid complications. ECG changes such as ST segment elevation indicating myocardial injury may occur before the patient experiences chest pain. The nurse must always be alert for signs and symptoms of any allergic reaction, such as hypotension or difficulty breathing. Rapid identification of any potential problems is necessary to initiate treatment and to provide optimal care for the patient.

Adjunctive pharmacology is required for every patient undergoing PCI to maintain patency of the coronary artery. These

---

CHART 39-10 **Relative Contraindications for Cardiac Catheterization**

- Severe congestive heart failure
- Severe electrolyte abnormalities
- Bleeding diathesis
- Serum creatinine ≥ 1.5 mg/dL
- Poor patient cooperation

drugs include antiplatelet agents, usually aspirin, and an adenosine diphosphate inhibitor (clopidogrel or ticlopidine). Intravenous antiplatelet drugs include the glycoprotein IIb/IIIa receptor inhibitors, abciximab, eptifibatide, or tirofiban. The dose and time of therapy will depend on the exact clinical status of the patient. Anticoagulants include either unfractionated heparin or low molecular weight heparin. Direct thrombin inhibitors such as bivalirudin or argatroban are increasingly used in place of heparins because of their more reliable anticoagulant effects, shorter half-lives, and lesser rates of complications (Smith et al., 2001). The drug, dose, and time of therapy will depend on the exact clinical status of the patient.

After the catheterization, patients are routinely observed in a holding area or observational unit for several hours, depending on the type of procedure, any anticoagulation administered, and the size of the sheath used for vascular access. The sheaths that are inserted to facilitate the passage of the catheters are usually removed immediately at the conclusion of the procedure. Hemostasis is obtained by manual compression; some institutions are utilizing compression or closure devices in an attempt to speed ambulation and decrease time to discharge (Koreny, Riedmuller, Nikfardjam, Siostrzonek, & Mullner, 2004). Regardless, all patients must have a complete nursing assessment, with special emphasis on the cardiovascular system including peripheral pulses and the vascular access site. This assessment, includes vital signs, ECG monitoring, and assessment of the vascular access site and pulses distal to the puncture site, should be done frequently until the patient is stable and ready for discharge. Evaluation of the access site includes inspection for any signs of bleeding or swelling and palpation for any tenderness. The arterial and venous sheaths (catheters through which the PCI devices are entered into the vascular system) may be removed in the catheterization laboratory or left in until the clotting times return to normal. Hemostasis at the access site can be achieved by manual compression or by a variety of external compression devices or patches. Patients are monitored for any complications such as hematoma, arteriovenous fistula, or retroperitoneal bleed (Apple, 2000).

Diagnosis of suspected arterial injuries is made through a careful physical assessment and confirmed through noninvasive vascular studies or arteriography. Physical examination of the femoral site is performed, assessing for the presence of localized tenderness, bruits, or a pulsatile mass. Hematomas are identified by swelling at the site of the arterial puncture. Large hematomas may need to be assessed by ultrasound to rule out the presence of pseudoaneurysms or arteriovenous fistulas.

A femoral pseudoaneurysm is an extravascular cavity communicating with the femoral artery by a channel or neck at the needle puncture site. Examination will reveal localized tenderness and a palpable, pulsatile mass, often associated with a bruit. Although rare, large pseudoaneurysms can compress the adjacent nerves causing significant discomfort for the patient. Diagnosis is confirmed through ultrasound with Doppler imaging that demonstrates a cavity communicating with the femoral artery as well as to-and-fro flow of blood through the neck. Treatment depends on the size of the pseudoaneurysm and the clinical assessment of the patient. Asymptomatic patients with a well-defined pseudoaneurysm (lumen < 2 centimeters in diameter) can initially be managed conservatively. External compression guided by ultrasound is the standard of treatment for

femoral artery pseudoaneurysms greater than 2 centimeters. Pseudoaneurysms associated with a rapidly expanding hematoma should be considered for urgent operative repair, because they can lead to rupture of the pseudoaneurysm or compression neuropathy.

An arteriovenous (AV) fistula is a direct communication between the artery and vein, resulting in a high-velocity jet from the artery into the vein. Fistulae are identified by the presence of a bruit over the access site. Diagnosis is confirmed by Doppler ultrasound. An AV fistula that is detected in clinically asymptomatic patients without evidence of expansion may be followed conservatively. If treatment is indicated, ultrasound-guided compression is usually attempted first. If this fails to close the fistulae, or there is evidence of clinical deterioration, the patient is referred for surgical repair.

Retroperitoneal hematomas are a rare but potentially fatal complication that accounts for significant morbidity, involving the need for blood transfusions and surgical repair. Bleeding into the retroperitoneal space can be difficult to detect until there has been significant blood loss. Early symptoms include flank or back pain, as well as nausea and vomiting, often associated with a vagal reaction (hypotension and bradycardia). Diagnosis is confirmed through abdominal CT scan. Small retroperitoneal hematomas in stable patients may be managed conservatively. However, surgical repair is indicated at the first sign of expansion of or deterioration in the patient's condition.

Infections at the access site are related to the length of sheath insertion, the need for repeat PCI, and the need for surgical repair. Organisms are typically gram-positive cocci, usually *Staphylococcus aureus*. Treatment may require several weeks of appropriate antibiotic therapy.

Contrast-induced nephropathy is a rare complication after PCI but remains the major cause of hospital-acquired renal failure (Apple, 2000; Smith et al., 2001). Patients with preexisting renal dysfunction and diabetes are at particular risk. Although the creatinine usually returns to baseline within a few days and hemodialysis is rarely required, nephropathy after PCI is a marker for the development of long-term adverse events (Lindsay et al., 2003). Complications from a catheterization are rare; the risk of major complications is less than 2% (Chart 39–11) (Baim & Grossman, 2000a; Scanlon et al., 1999).

Discharge criteria vary, but typically include stable vital signs, tolerating food and fluids, no evidence of complications at the access site, ability to ambulate without assistance, and void-

---

CHART 39–11 | **Potential Complications of Cardiac Catheterization**

- Death
- Myocardial infarction
- Neurological events
- Emergency surgery
- Cardiac perforation
- Dysrhythmias
- Vascular problems
- Vasovagal reactions
- Allergic reactions

ing without difficulty. Discharge instructions to patients and family members should include management of the access site; when to shower, drive, and return to work; and what to do if the patient develops chest pain.

In summary, the nursing management of patients with coronary artery disease who have undergone a PCI is challenging. The nurse must have an understanding of the procedure, including any complications that may arise and the typical medications that are crucial to optimum outcomes. Details of the nursing management of patients after PCI are given in the Nursing Process: Patient Care Plan After Percutaneous Coronary Intervention (p. 1136) feature. The following section will apply the nursing process to care of patients with coronary artery disease treated by PCI.

Collaborative Management

Care of patients with CAD undergoing urgent PCI requires a collaborative approach among all members of the health care team in different areas of the hospital, such as the emergency department, the cardiac critical care unit, the pharmacy, the catheterization laboratory, the cardiovascular operating room, and the step-down units. Staff in the emergency department must be aware of the need for urgent identification and treatment of any patient presenting with AMI. Medications including antiplatelet and antithrombotic agents need to be started as soon as the diagnosis is confirmed. The patient needs to be transported to the appropriate area for treatment (catheterization laboratory, operating room, or nursing unit) without delay. Catheterization laboratory personnel, including invasive cardiovascular professionals, health care providers, and nurses, must be prepared to treat AMI patients quickly, whether it is during the middle of a busy day or in the middle of the night. All health care team members must cooperate in order to meet the goal of restoring blood flow to the occluded artery as quickly as possible. Once the PCI is completed, the patient and family will require intensive education from the health care team regarding identification and management of all cardiac risk factors. For many patients, this procedure represents their first invasive cardiac procedure and usually requires significant changes in lifestyle. Because patients undergoing successful PCI may remain in the hospital for only a few days, this process should be started as soon as possible, because changes in lifestyle affect not only the patient but also the entire family.

Discharge Priorities

Patients are able to leave the hospital 24 to 36 hours after an uncomplicated PCI. Serum laboratory values are checked before discharge to verify that hemoglobin, hematocrit, and creatinine levels are within acceptable range and that there has been no abnormal elevation of cardiac enzymes. Physical examination includes a complete cardiovascular assessment, as well as auscultation and palpation of the vascular access site. If any tenderness, large hematoma, or bruit is noted, discharge must be postponed until the access site is stable.

Patients should be given written instructions regarding care of the access site, as well as what to do if they experience chest pain or other symptoms of CAD. All cardiac medications should be reviewed, with emphasis on the importance of not stopping any

medicine (especially antiplatelet and adenosine diphosphate inhibitor drugs) without first discussing this with the cardiologist. Finally, patients should be reminded of the need for careful follow-up with their health care provider. Comprehensive instructions are presented in the Patient Teaching & Discharge Priorities box (p. 1137).

Health Promotion

Patients should be discharged with instructions regarding risk factor modification and appropriate medical therapy. See Chapter 40 for a more detailed discussion of risk factors and medical therapy.

Depending on the patient's risk factors and clinical history, secondary prevention should include:

- Aspirin therapy
- Control of high blood pressure
- Control of diabetes
- Aggressive control of lipids
- Smoking cessation, if indicated
- Control of weight
- Physical exercise
- Angiotensin-converting enzyme (ACE) inhibitor therapy for patients with poor left ventricular function (ejection fraction < 40%).

The National Heart, Lung, and Blood Institute, the American Heart Association, the American College of Cardiology, and the National Cholesterol Education Program (NCEP) Expert Panel have jointly published national guidelines for the management of cardiovascular risk factors (Grundy et al., 2004). The importance of these guidelines is presented in the National Guidelines for the Management of Risk Factors for Cardiovascular Disease box (p. 1138).

Complementary and Alternative Therapies

Discharge teaching for patients with CAD is not complete without addressing complementary and alternative medicine (CAM). According the National Institutes of Health National Center for Complementary and Alternative Medicine, CAM is "a group of diverse medical and health care systems, practices, and products that are not presently considered to be part of conventional medicine" (National Institutes of Health, 2008). *Complementary* refers to therapies used together with conventional medicine; alternative therapies are used in place of conventional medicine. Estimates of the prevalence of CAM in patients with CAD range from 9% to over 60%; the wide variation is due in part to what exactly is considered CAM and the population surveyed (Bond & Heitkemper, 2005; Gold & Farnsworth, 2002).

Summary

Between 1987 and 2001 the number of PCI procedures in the United States increased by 266% (American Heart Association, 2003). Between the current epidemic of metabolic syndrome (type II diabetes mellitus, obesity, and hyperlipidemia), the aging of the population, and continued advances in technology, this

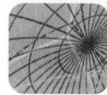

NURSING PROCESS: Patient Care Plan After Percutaneous Coronary Intervention

Assessment of Chest Pain

Subjective Data:
When did the pain start?
Is this pain like your typical angina?

Objective Data:
Vital signs including oxygen saturation.
12-lead electrocardiogram (ECG).

Heart and lung sounds.
Skin.
Peripheral pulses.

Nursing Assessment and Diagnoses	Outcomes and Evaluation Parameters	Planning and Interventions with *Rationales*
Nursing Diagnosis: *Acute Pain* related to transmission and perception of cutaneous, visceral, muscular, or ischemic impulses	**Outcome:** Management of chest pain and rapid initiation of appropriate treatment. *Evaluation Parameters:* 12-lead ECG— no change from previous ECG. Oxygen saturation within normal levels. Patient reports relief or lessening of chest pain. Laboratory values within normal levels. Patient/family are able to verbalize feelings.	**Interventions and *Rationales:*** Obtain 12-lead ECG. *To evaluate ischemic changes.* Administer oxygen as ordered; monitor oxygen saturation. *To assess adequacy of gas exchange.* Administer nitrates as ordered. Monitor vital signs and assess level of pain. *To assess relief of ischemia and prevent side effects, such as hypotension.* Administer analgesia as ordered. Monitor vital signs, and level of consciousness. *To assess relief of ischemia and prevent side effects such as respiratory depression.* Monitor laboratory values, especially cardiac enzymes and hematology. *Elevated cardiac enzymes after PCI may indicate reocclusion of the infarcted artery. A low hemoglobin/hematocrit may precipitate ischemic chest pain.* Assess level of anxiety of patient and family members. *Anxiety related to the procedure and diagnosis of AMI can precipitate nonischemic pain.*

Assessment of Cardiac Risk Factors

Subjective Data:
What are your risk factors for heart disease?
What medications are you taking?
Are you overweight?
How much physical exercise do you do in a typical week?
What type of food do you like to eat?

Objective Data:
Patient's body mass index (BMI) (weight/height^2, ideal < 25).
Blood pressure.
Lipid levels.

Smoking history.
Current medications.
Dietary habits.
Physical exercise.

Nursing Assessment and Diagnoses	Outcomes and Evaluation Parameters	Planning and Interventions with *Rationales*
Nursing Diagnosis: *Deficient Knowledge* related to current management of cardiac risk factors	**Outcome:** All appropriate cardiac risk factors are identified and patient/family verbalize understanding of discharge instructions. *Evaluation Parameters:* 1. Patient/family verbalize understanding of: Diet changes Regular exercise Weight control Medications	**Interventions and *Rationales:*** Measure patient's height and weight to calculate BMI. Evaluate results according to the American Heart Association guidelines. *People underestimate how much they weigh.* Evaluate multiple blood pressure readings after PCI. Evaluate results according to the American Heart Association guidelines. *Current guidelines indicate aggressive treatment of high blood pressure is necessary to decrease the risk of cardiac events. Family members may also need to be screened based upon the results.* Evaluate results of lipid profile with patient and family. *Treatment will depend on values and other risk factors. Family members may also need to be tested based on the results.* Assess patient's willingness to stop smoking, if this is indicated. *Goal for all people is no smoking. Include family members in this discussion in order to enhance compliance.* Assess current medications to ensure appropriate treatment of risk factors. *Patients often need written instructions at the appropriate reading level to enhance compliance.* Assess current dietary habits. Nutritional counseling may be indicated. *People frequently underestimate the amount of fat and calories consumed in an average meal.* Assess level of current physical exercise. *Before starting an exercise program, the patient will need to be cleared by her health care provider.*

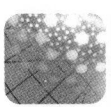
Need	Teaching

Vascular Access Site
 	
Patient
 	
Family
 	
Setting
	Assess the site daily. Some amount of bruising and firmness/tenderness at the site is normal. Patient should call her health care provider if the area of firmness gets bigger instead of smaller. The bruising should resolve by 4 to 6 weeks.
	• Shower or bathe as usual.
	• No special dressing is needed.
	• Take Tylenol for any discomfort at the site.
	
	If the access site was in groin, avoid bending over or straining for the first 48 hours. Avoid heavy lifting for the first week.
	• If patient experiences any of the following in her leg, toes, or foot, she should call her health care provider immediately:
	  • Numbness
	  • Tingling
	  • Coolness.
	
	If patient experiences bright-red bleeding from the site, she should lie down and have someone apply firm pressure just above the site for 20 minutes and then gently release the pressure. If the bleeding cannot be controlled, call 911.
	
	If the access site was sealed using a special closure device, the patient will have received special instructions regarding the device. Usually no special care is required, but patient needs to keep these instructions containing the name of the device in case she or her health care provider has questions or concerns about the site.
	
	Assess availability, knowledge, and compliance with treatment regimen.
	
	Validate follow-up appointment with local health care provider.
	
	Assess availability of emergency health care.

Activity Patient	Patient should not resume or start an exercise program until he has been evaluated by his doctor. Regular exercise is a key component in maintaining a heart-healthy lifestyle. Patient must notify his health care provider immediately if he experiences any of the following during exercise: • Chest pain, especially pain similar to typical angina • Nausea, vomiting, or cool, clammy skin • Extreme or persistent fatigue not relieved by a short rest period • Shortness of breath, especially if it makes talking difficult • A change in heart rhythm. If patient has had a heart attack, he should be able to resume sexual relations in 4 weeks. Again, this should be discussed with his health care provider. Patient should notify his health care provider if he experiences any of the following: • Rapid heartbeat, palpitations, or shortness of breath persisting for 15 minutes after intercourse • Chest pain during or after intercourse • Extreme fatigue. Patient should be able to return to work very quickly. Discuss this with the health care provider.
Knowledge of Disease Process and Prognosis/Risk Factor Modification Patient Family Setting	It is critically important to obtain regular follow-up from one's health care provider. A heart-healthy lifestyle includes: • Weight control • Regular exercise • Smoking cessation • Diet high in fruits and vegetables and low in fat. Medications that may be prescribed include: • Aspirin therapy • Hypertensive control • Diabetes management • Lipid lowering agent. Other medications may be indicated, depending on the health of the patient's heart. Assess availability, knowledge, and compliance with treatment regimen. Assess need for lifestyle modification for all family members. Assess need for cardiac rehabilitation. Assess ability to obtain necessary medications after discharge.
Emotional Adjustment of Patient/Family Due to Chronic Nature of the Disease Patient Family Setting	Assess patient's understanding of need for lifelong medications and potential change in lifestyle. Assess family's ability to support necessary changes. Assess need for referrals to support therapeutic lifestyle changes.

NATIONAL GUIDELINES for the Management of Risk Factors for Cardiovascular Disease

In 2002 the Third Report of the National Cholesterol Education Program (NCEP) Expert Panel on Detection, Evaluation, and Treatment of High Blood Cholesterol in Adults released its final report. This document contained guidelines for the management of risk factors for cardiovascular disease in adults. Since that time, further evidence from clinical trials has indicated that a more aggressive approach to lowering blood lipids is necessary. All nurses, regardless of their specialty, should be familiar with these documents and keep abreast of current changes by visiting the website of the American Heart Association or the National Heart, Lung, and Blood Institute.

Note: American Heart Association, http://americanheart.org; National Heart, Lung, and Blood Institute, http://www.nhlbi.nih.gov/guidelines/cholesterol/

number will certainly continue to increase. All members of the health care team will be challenged to keep up with the latest developments in order to continue to deliver the expert care required of all patients.

■ Evaluating and Treating Dysrhythmias

Cardiac dysrhythmias range from clinically insignificant (occasional premature atrial beats) to potentially lethal (ventricular fibrillation). An in-depth discussion of dysrhythmias is covered in Chapter 38 🔄. The significance of the dysrhythmia also depends on the clinical diagnosis; patients with severe coronary disease or valvular obstructions often cannot tolerate even minor dysrhythmias and require aggressive management. As always, the health care professional should begin with a careful history and physical examination before deciding which diagnostic test to utilize (Fenton, 2001; Miller & Zipes, 2001).

Ambulatory Electrocardiogram Monitoring

Ambulatory ECG monitoring, frequently called **Holter monitoring** after its inventor Norman Holter, was developed in the 1960s and first used clinically to detect ventricular dysrhythmias in patients recovering from acute myocardial infarction (Fenton, 2001; Holter, 1961). Today there are many indications for Holter monitoring, as it has become a valuable noninvasive tool with numerous clinical applications (Chart 39–12) (Crawford et al., 1999; Kadish et al., 2001).

| CHART 39–12 | **Indications for Holter Monitoring** |

1. Assess symptoms that may be related to a dysrhythmia, such as syncope or palpitations.
2. Assess therapy response such as cardiac medications.
3. Monitor the rate of atrial fibrillation.
4. Analyze pacemakers or implantable cardioverter defibrillators.
5. Detect silent myocardial ischemia.
6. Assess heart rate variability.

Holter's original monitor was a 75-pound backpack that could record only a single ECG lead (Helena Cardiology Clinic, n.d.). Current Holter monitoring systems consist of leads placed on the chest that are connected to a small recording device, which can be worn around the waist or on a strap over the patient's shoulder. Typically two or three leads of ECG data are recorded, either continuously for 24 to 48 hours or when activated by the patient during periods of symptoms such as palpitations or dizziness. In general continuous recordings are indicated for assessment of frequent (at least once a day) symptoms that may be related to a dysrhythmia, syncope or near syncope, and unexplained palpitations (Kadish et al., 2001). If the symptoms occur very infrequently and other diagnostic tests have failed to provide a diagnosis, an implantable loop recorder can be utilized. Typically placed subcutaneously in the left subclavian or parasternal areas, these devices can be left in place for months or even years, increasing the probability of capturing the ECG during the time of the clinical event (Fenton, 2001; Futterman & Lemberg, 2002).

Holter monitoring is safe and relatively inexpensive. Because the electrodes must remain in place for 1 to 2 days, skin preparation is very important to ensure tracings free of artifact. Patients should be instructed not to pull at the electrodes, and to go about their normal daily activities. Frequently they are asked to keep a diary to record their activities and the occurrence of any symptoms during monitoring.

Electrophysiology Study

The **electrophysiology study (EPS)** is an invasive procedure that involves placing multiple multipolar catheter electrodes into the venous and sometimes the arterial side of the heart. These electrodes are positioned at various locations inside of the heart and they have two purposes: to record the electrical signal within the heart and to deliver an electrical stimulus at precisely timed intervals (programmed stimulation).

Developed in the 1960s, EPS originally recorded only intracardiac electrical activity during spontaneously occurring dysrhythmias in order to identify the location of the dysrhythmia, thereby determining treatment options. Currently EPS is the standard test for reproducing dysrhythmias in a controlled environment in order to diagnose and treat the disorder. EPS can include delivering programmed electrical stimulation in order to provoke dysrhythmias (a major indication for EPS), as well as pacing protocols to assess AV nodal function. During EPS catheters with several electrodes are advanced percutaneously and positioned within the heart; the exact location depends on the source of the dysrhythmia. Detailed recordings of the electrical activity of the heart are obtained, including interval measurements (time for the electrical activity to travel from one area of the conduction system to another) as well as the direction of conduction. Programmed electrical stimulation involves use of the catheters to deliver programmed stimulus in order to initiate the dysrhythmia. A series of impulses is delivered to the myocardium in an attempt to cause a tachyarrhythmia. If successful, the dysrhythmia is termed inducible. Treatment is instituted and the same procedure is repeated; if the tachy-arrhythmia cannot be induced, the treatment is successful. Medications to increase the heart rate such as epinephrine or isoproterenol also may be utilized to assess the conduction system (Blancher, 2005).

In addition, EPS can assess the function of SA and AV nodes and assess the effectiveness of specific antiarrhythmic medications. When assessing the cardiac conduction, the rate is turned up faster than the intrinsic rate, allowing the catheter to be the cardiac pacemaker. Then the stimulus is shut off and the time it takes for the SA node to take control is assessed. If the time is prolonged, the SA node is diseased.

During the 1980s EPS moved from strictly a diagnostic procedure to include multiple therapeutic and treatment regimens, such as radiofrequency catheter ablation, as permanent treatment for several dysrhythmias (Chart 39–13) (Blancher, 2005; Janosik, Quattromani, & Schiller, 2003; Miller & Zipes, 2001; Tracy, Akhtar, DiMarco, Packer, & Weitz, 2000). **Ablation** refers to destruction of an area of the myocardium through localized delivery of chemicals or electrical energy. Radiofrequency catheter ablation is one of the major advances in the treatment of supraventricular tachycardia (SVT). See Chapter 38 🔗 for more detail about SVT. Prior to the development of radiofrequency catheter ablation, most patients required open-heart surgery to treat SVT. In the late 1980s catheters were developed that allowed the application of safe radiofrequency energy to heat the myocardium in very specific locations, thus destroying tissue responsible for dysrhythmia formation and propagation.

Patient preparation for EPS is similar to that for cardiac catheterization. The length of the procedure will vary greatly, depending on the indication for the test. The patient must be clear of severe infection before EPS and must be able to tolerate lying flat and relatively still for an extended period of time. Complications are very rare, but can include death (usually from intractable ventricular dysrhythmias), myocardial perforation (a risk any time catheters are introduced inside the heart), and thrombosis. The need for anticoagulation will depend on the length of the procedure and the position of the catheters. Conscious sedation may be required for long procedures.

Nursing management postprocedure includes a complete cardiovascular assessment, with special emphasis on the ECG as well as the access site. Specific parameters will depend on the type of procedure. Patients are usually discharged the same day after a diagnostic EPS. Discharge instructions include care of the access site, bathing, driving, and return to work. Specific instructions regarding the results of the EPS will depend on the indication for the test.

▮ Electrical Treatment of Cardiac Dysrhythmias

Diagnosis and treatment of cardiac dysrhythmias are discussed in detail in Chapter 38 🔗. Cardioversion and defibrillation are common additional procedures used to treat cardiac dysrhythmias. Both of these procedures use a defibrillator that delivers a preset level of electrical voltage to the heart for the purpose of terminating an unwanted dysrhythmia. The electrical current depolarizes the myocardial cells, which is then followed by repolarization. During repolarization the sinus node usually is able to take over its role as the heart's natural pacemaker. Three major factors are assessed when deciding to do cardioversion versus defibrillation: timing of the delivery of the electrical current, rationale for use, and amount of voltage used. Cardioversion and defibrillation are discussed next. Chart 39–14 outlines safety rules when using a defibrillator.

Cardioversion

Cardioversion is defined as the delivery of electrical voltage in order to stop unwanted electrical activity and allow the SA node to

---

CHART 39–13   **Selected Indications for Electrophysiology Studies**

DIAGNOSTIC

Evaluate sinus and atrioventricular (AV) nodal function.

Confirm the mechanism of ventricular tachycardia.

Relate symptoms to potential dysrhythmias, such as bradycardia.

THERAPEUTIC

Evaluate and determine whether dysrhythmias are suitable for drug, device, or ablation therapy.

Assess effects of pharmacologic therapy.

INTERVENTIONAL

Ablation of AV node.

Ablation of atrial flutter or atrial tachycardias.

Ablation of accessory pathways such as found in Wolff-Parkinson-White.

Ablation of ventricular tachycardias.

PROGNOSTIC

Assess future risk of serious cardiac events.

Assess patient's predisposition to spontaneously occurring dysrhythmias.

Source: Adapted from O'Rourke, R. A., et al. (2000). American College of Cardiology/American Heart Association expert consensus document on electron-beam computed tomography for the diagnosis and prognosis of coronary artery disease. *Circulation, 102,* 126–140.

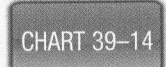

CHART 39–14   **Safety Criteria When Using a Defibrillator**

Use designated conductor pads or paddles.

Use designated conductor medium; gel, pastes, sheet.

Place pads or paddles so they are not in contact with the patient's clothes, bed linen, or near medication patches and monitor leads.

Do not place pads or paddles near a direct oxygen source to prevent a fire hazard.

For cardioversion, defibrillator must be set in a synchronous mode.

For defibrillation, defibrillator must be set in an asynchronous mode.

For cardioversion, make sure the monitor leads are attached to the patient.

Do not charge the defibrillator until ready to shock, and keep fingers off discharge buttons until ready to discharge voltage.

Exert enough pressure on the paddles to ensure adequate contact prior to discharging the voltage.

Call for everyone to clear the area prior to discharging the defibrillator.

Document entire procedure and effectiveness of the intervention.

Inspect skin for burns after the procedure, and report and treat per health care provider's orders.

resume as the heart's pacemaker. It is used for the treatment of tachyarrhythmias: atrial tachycardia, rapid atrial fibrillation, atrial flutter, and junctional tachycardia. The procedure typically is performed at the bedside in an area of the hospital where cardiac monitoring is available. The cardiac defibrillator is set on the synchronous mode, meaning it will discharge only on the down slope of the R wave or with the S wave of the QRS complex. Therefore, the electrical voltage will not discharge during the vulnerable period of ventricular repolarization (T wave), which could precipitate ventricular tachycardia and ventricular fibrillation; referred to as the R on T phenomenon. The patient is instructed not to eat or drink for at least 6 hours prior to the procedure, and digoxin is withheld for 48 hours prior to the procedure to ensure resumption of sinoatrial (SA) node activity and normal conduction to the atrioventricular (AV) node. The patient is sedated intravenously prior to the procedure and full resuscitation equipment is available, if necessary. The voltage on the defibrillator begins at 10 to 20 joules (J). If unsuccessful it is increased to 50 joules and increased at intervals to a maximum of 360 joules. The lower the joules, the less the chance of complications such as cardiac necrosis. Success is measured by conversion to normal sinus rhythm, with a normal heart rate and blood pressure. Nursing responsibilities include recording the postcardioversion rhythm, cardiac output, and vital signs for 2 to 3 hours after the procedure. Vital signs, level of consciousness, and oxygen saturation are measured until the patient recovers from the sedation. If the patient converts back to the unwanted rhythm, this must be reported to the health care provider immediately.

Defibrillation

Defibrillation is basically the same as cardioversion in that electrical voltage is delivered to the myocardium to terminate unwanted rhythms, except defibrillation is done in an emergency situation for life-threatening dysrhythmias. It is indicated for patients in ventricular tachycardia and ventricular fibrillation when they have lost consciousness and cardiopulmonary resuscitation is in progress. The defibrillator is usually set in an asynchronous mode unless there are discernable T waves. The voltage on the defibrillator is set at 360 joules. After each defibrillation, the rhythm is evaluated and voltage delivery is repeated as necessary until there is a viable rhythm or resuscitation is stopped. Between each defibrillation, cardiopulmonary resuscitation (CPR) is done to maintain oxygenation. Medications such as lidocaine, amiodarone, epinephrine, and vasopressin typically are administered during resuscitation to assist in conversion to normal sinus rhythm.

During both cardioversion and defibrillation, paddles or conductor pads are applied to the patient's chest and attached to the defibrillator. Figure 39–11 ■ demonstrates normal paddle placement using both the standard and anteroposterior placement.

Whichever type of pad is used, it must have a conducting medium to prevent burning the patient's skin.

Monophasic Versus Biphasic Defibrillation

Monophasic defibrillation is the traditional means by which electric voltage is delivered to patients in ventricular tachycardia

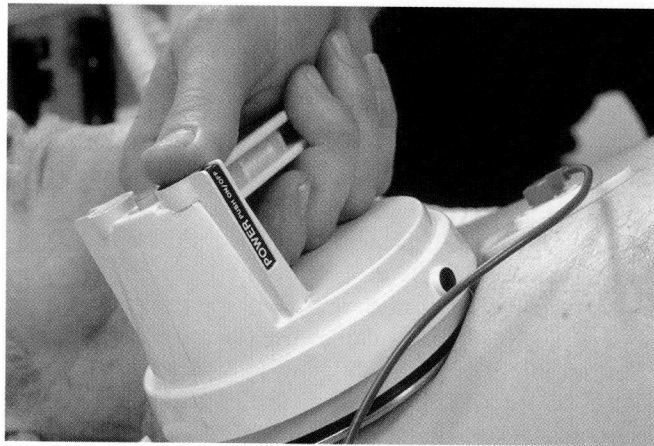

FIGURE 39–11 ■ Defibrillator paddle.

and fibrillation. These high-energy defibrillators deliver an electrical charge in one direction only. Side effects of monophasic defibrillation are the risks of burning the skin on the chest where the site of the voltage is delivered and postshock myocardial dysfunction manifested by prolonged ischemic ST segment changes. Having no other choice, clinicians historically believed that the benefits of monophasic defibrillation outweighed the side effects. In an attempt to reduce or eliminate side effects, researchers in the 1990s began evaluating low-energy biphasic defibrillation. **Biphasic defibrillation** delivers a charge in one direction for half of the shock and in the opposite direction for the second half. Biphasic shocks appear to achieve the same defibrillation success rates (most often defined as termination of ventricular fibrillation [VF] for at least 3 to 5 seconds) as monophasic waveforms, but with significantly lower energy levels (Amato-Vealey & Colonies, 2005). Therefore, fewer side effects such as burned skin and myocardial dysfunction have been noted.

Defibrillator manufacturers are able to achieve some technological advantages from these lower-energy devices in that they can be made smaller, lighter, less expensive, and less demanding of batteries, with fewer maintenance requirements.

Automated External Defibrillator

An **automated external defibrillator (AED)** is a small, lightweight device that can recognize and treat ventricular fibrillation (VF), also known as "sudden cardiac arrest" (SCA). The AED is designed for use by lay rescuers or "first responders" (Hallstrom, Ornato, Weisfeldt, Travers, 2004). If SCA is present, an AED will talk the responder through the very simple steps to defibrillate. These devices have been shown to decrease mortality when used in conjunction with cardiopulmonary resuscitation (CPR) (Federal Occupational Health, 2008). Once the domain of only highly trained emergency professionals, these technologically advanced defibrillators are now available on board airlines, on cruise ships, and in other public places. These defibrillators are appropriate for use with infants and children, as well as adults, as long as the appropriate pads are used. Typically, children over 55 pounds (25 kilograms) or 8 years of age are defibrillated as adults. Precautions when using AEDs include:

- Ensure pulseless criteria are met before AED is applied.
- Withhold unit analysis of the rhythm during cardiopulmonary resuscitation (CPR).

- Withhold unit analysis of the rhythm if the patient is seizing.
- Use caution with rhythm analysis in a moving vehicle.
- Stop frequently for rhythm analysis during transport.
- Place electrodes without shaving chest; not required for effective placement.
- Ensure skin is dry and free of nicks and cuts for effective electrode placement.
- Perform regular maintenance and battery placement according to manufacturer's recommendations.

Implantable Cardioverter Defibrillator

An **implantable cardioverter defibrillator (ICD)** is a device that can automatically terminate potentially lethal dysrhythmias of ventricular tachycardia and ventricular fibrillation. Developed by Dr. Michael Mirowski, the first ICD implanted in humans in 1980 was nonprogrammable and capable of defibrillating only the heart (Mirowski, 1985). Since that time ICDs, like all pacemakers, have become smaller, are programmable, and can combine a variety of therapies in one device, including:

- Tiered electrical therapy—the ability to deliver low-voltage cardioversion or high-voltage defibrillation
- Antitachycardia pacing—the ability to pace the heart at a faster rate than a tachycardia (supraventricular or ventricular), enabling the device to capture (control) the intrinsic heart rate and gradually slow it down to a normal heart rate
- Programmable ventricular or atrial pacing.

Current ICDs have been referred to as "an electrophysiology study (EPS) in a can" for their ability to analyze the ECG and deliver appropriate therapy, and then store this extensive information for later retrieval. Thus far these devices have effectively proven their lifesaving value, resulting in expanded indications for their use (Chart 39–15).

ICD System

The ICD system is similar to traditional pacemakers in that it consists of a pulse generator and defibrillation leads for both dysrhythmia detection and delivery of therapy (Jacobson & Gerity, 2005). Unlike early devices that required open thoracotomy, current ICDs are usually implanted transvenously with generator placement under the chest wall. Depending on the programmed functions of the ICD, the patient may have one, two, or three leads. A single-chamber ICD requires only one lead in the right ventricle. Combining ICD with biventricular pacing requires leads in the right atrium, in the right ventricle, and behind the left ventricle in a coronary vein. The ventricular leads are similar to pacemaker leads in their ability to sense and pace the heart; the difference is the large electrical surface area needed to deliver the shock.

Complications Potential complications of ICD include those related to traditional pacemaker therapy, such as lead dislodgment or fracture and infection. Long-term potential complications unique to ICD include electromagnetic interference (electrocautery during surgery, radiofrequency transmitters, high-powered electromagnetic fields, etc.) that can result in inappropriate shocks or inhibition of the device (Jacobson & Gerity, 2005; Stone & McPherson, 2004).

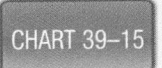

CHART 39–15 **Selected Indications for Implantable Cardioverter Defibrillators**

CLASS I

1. Cardiac arrest due to ventricular tachycardia or ventricular fibrillation not due to a transient or reversible cause

2. Spontaneous sustained ventricular tachycardia associated with structural heart disease

3. Syncope of undetermined etiology associated with clinically significant ventricular tachycardia or ventricular fibrillation, and pharmacologic therapy is ineffective, not tolerated, or not preferred

4. Nonsustained ventricular tachycardia in patients with coronary artery disease, prior myocardial infarction, left ventricular dysfunction, and inducible ventricular fibrillation or sustained ventricular tachycardia during an electrophysiology study that is not suppressed by an appropriate antiarrhythmic medication

5. Spontaneous sustained ventricular tachycardia in patients without structural heart disease not amenable to other therapies

CLASS IIA

1. Patients with a left ventricular ejection fraction ≤ 30% at least 1 month after a myocardial infarction or 3 months after coronary artery bypass surgery

Note: According to the American Heart Association/American College of Cardiology, Class I indications are conditions for which there is evidence and/or general agreement that a given procedure or treatment is beneficial, useful, and effective. Class IIa indications are conditions for which conflicting evidence or a divergence of opinion exists, but the weight of the evidence/opinion favors its usefulness/efficacy.

Source: G. Gregoratos et al. (2002). ACC/AHA/NASPE 2002 guideline update for implantation of cardiac pacemakers and antiarrhythmia devices. Circulation, 106, 2145–2161+

If the patient requires external defibrillation, care must be taken not to position the paddles on or near the generator. In any event, the ICD must be thoroughly evaluated after any episode of external defibrillation.

◼ Nursing Management

Nursing management of the patient immediately after ICD implantation is similar to care of the patient with a permanent pacemaker. However, most patients and their families need additional support in dealing with the emotional response to ICD implantation (White, 2002). The shock delivered by the ICD is lifesaving, but at the same time it is unpredictable and painful. Patients typically equate a shock to being kicked in the chest or being slammed to the ground. If the shock is delivered when the patient is at work or out in public, she may report feeling embarrassed at her reaction to the shock as well as her loss of control during the episode. Some patients report "phantom shocks," or reporting that a shock has been delivered when in fact the ICD has no record of delivering a shock. In addition, anyone touching the patient during an ICD firing will also feel the shock. The result is not fatal but can be painful. Continued emotional support for the ICD patient and her family before the device is implanted and during follow-up can promote acceptance of the technology and lead to improvement in quality of life.

Cardiac Pacemakers

Although the use of electricity to treat cardiac dysrhythmias dates back to the 16th century, it was not until the 1950s that electricity was successfully applied to clinical practice (Lüderitz, 1995). Following seminal publications by Zoll and others, Zoll successfully resuscitated a patient in full cardiac arrest using electrodes placed on the patient's chest to pace the heart (Zoll, 1952). By 1958 the first implantable cardiac pacemaker was placed by Elmquist and Senning. In 1960 the first battery-powered pacemaker with a myocardial lead was safely implanted by Chardack, and the modern era of cardiac pacemakers had begun. This section will review the basic principles of temporary and permanent artificial cardiac pacemakers.

A **cardiac pacemaker** is an electronic device that is capable of delivering an electrical stimulus to the heart. These devices are used to augment or replace the natural cardiac pacemaker when there is either a congenital abnormality or a disease of the cardiac conduction system. The earliest pacemakers stimulated one ventricle and were used to treat symptomatic bradycardia (heart rate of less than 60 beats per minute). Today pacemakers are capable of delivering impulses to multiple chambers of the heart in order to treat not only bradycardias but also tachydysrhythmias (greater than 100 beats per minute) originating from either the atria or the ventricles (Gregoratos et al., 2002; Obias-Manno, 2001). Current pacemakers also are able to vary the heart rate in accordance with a change in the patient's metabolic demand or activity level.

Pacemaker Components

A pacing system is composed of a generator and lead(s). The type of generator and type and number of leads will depend on the reason for implementing pacemaker therapy. There are basically two types of pacemakers, temporary and permanent, both of which are discussed below. Single-chambered devices pace a single chamber of the heart, such as the right ventricle. Dual-chambered pacemakers pace at least two chambers of the heart, such as the right atrium and the right ventricle, or both ventricles. A single-chambered right ventricular and a dual-chambered right atrium and right ventricular are shown in Figure 39–12 ■.

Generator

The generator contains the electronic circuitry and the power source, and is synonymous with the term *pacemaker* (Figure 39–13 ■).

Permanent pacemakers are small and usually implanted in the pectoral area. The generators of permanent pacemakers are typically composed of titanium and are hermetically (airtight) sealed to prevent erosion from contact with bodily fluids. Lithium-iodine batteries are contained within the generator, as well as the microprocessors that control the various functions of the pacemaker. Implanted generators last between 7 and 10 years, depending on multiple factors such as the amount of time the heart is actually paced (Jacobson & Gerity, 2005; Reynolds & Apple, 2001).

Generators of temporary pacing systems are connected to the pacemaker lead(s) but remain outside the body. They are powered by ordinary batteries and are manually programmed as needed (Figure 39–17 ■, p. 1146).

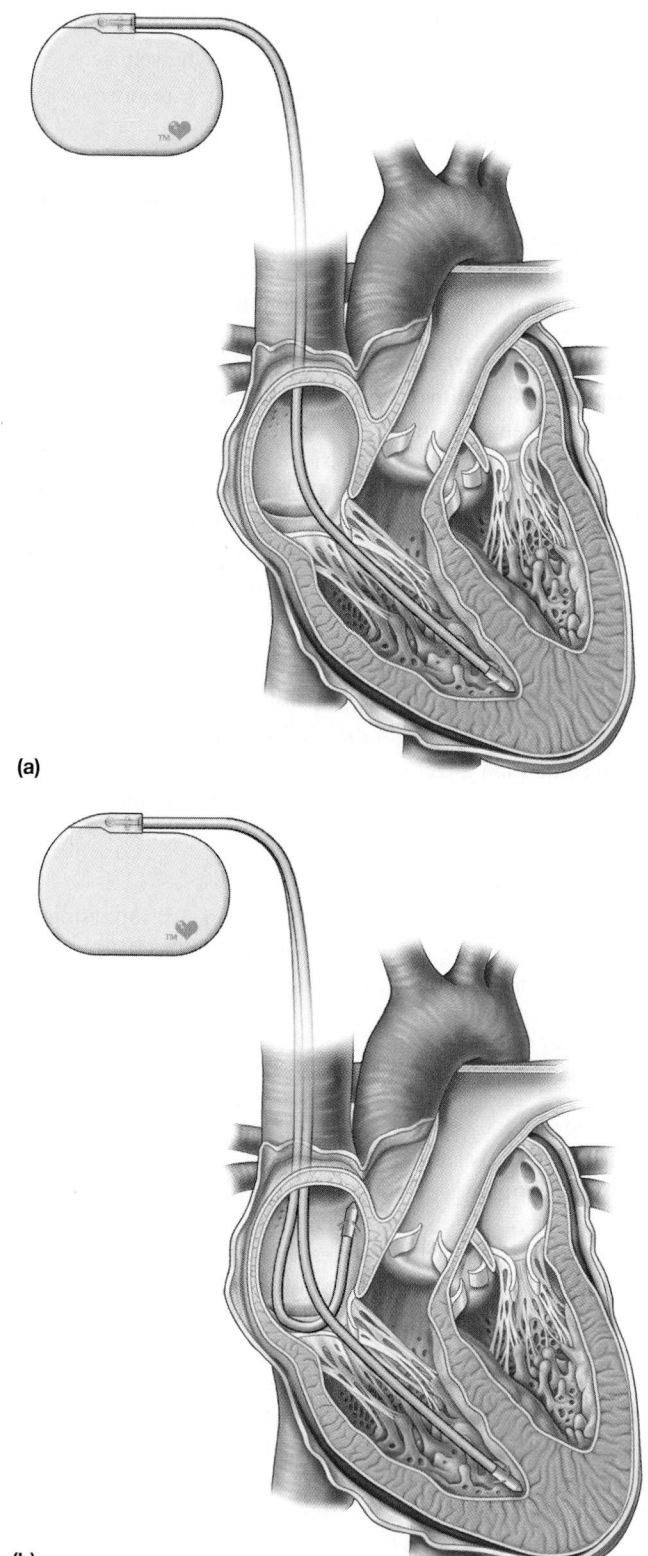

(a)

(b)

FIGURE 39–12 ■ (A) Single- and (B) dual-chambered pacemakers.

Leads

The pacemaker lead is the connection between the generator and the myocardium (Figure 39–13 ■). Permanent pacemaker leads may be placed inside the cardiac chambers (most common) or on the surface of the heart (epicardial leads). Leads contain tip electrodes, conductor, and insulation (Figure 39–14 ■).

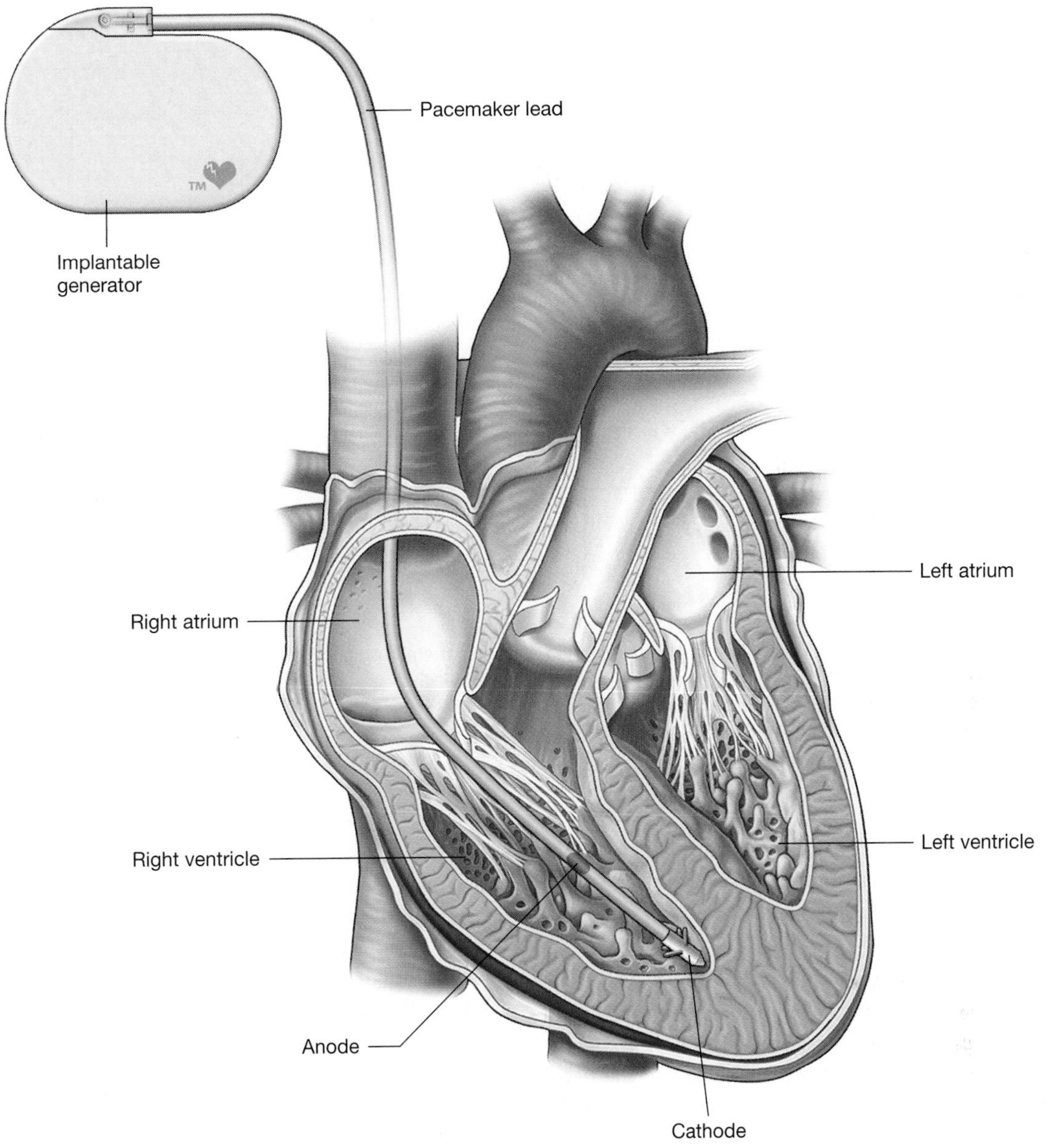

Pacemaker lead

Implantable
generator

Left atrium

Right atrium

Left ventricle

Right ventricle

Anode

Cathode

FIGURE 39–13 ■ Pacemaker components.

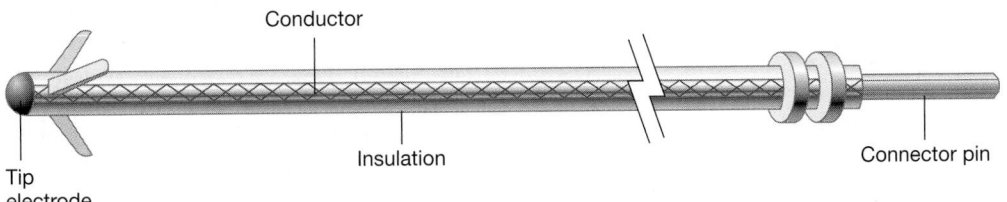

Conductor

Insulation

Connector pin

Tip
electrode

FIGURE 39–14 ■ Pacemaker lead components.

The tip electrode is embedded directly into the cardiac tissue. The lead conducts the electrical stimulus between the negative and positive electrodes (poles). Electrical current flows between two metal poles. In a unipolar system, the tip of the electrode contains only the negative (cathode) electrode; the positive (anode) electrode is located in the generator. Most lead systems today are bipolar, meaning the distal tip of the electrode contains the negative pole; the positive pole is an exposed metal ring located a few

millimeters from the tip (see Figure 39–13 ■). The advantage of a bipolar system is that both electrodes are contained within the heart, making it less susceptible to sensing extraneous electrical activity. In addition, less battery power is needed with the bipolar system, thereby increasing the battery life.

Electrical impulses are carried from the generator to the tip electrode (Figure 39–14 ■) across a very thin wire conductor. The conductor also returns sensed intracardiac intrinsic electrical activity

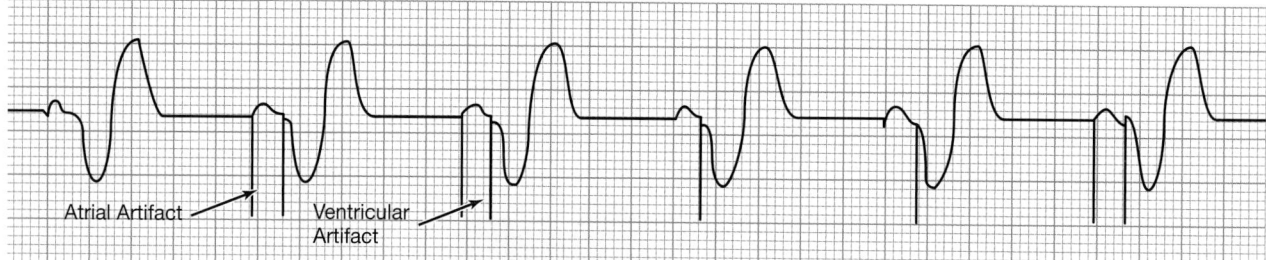

DDD (Dual: Paces both atria and ventricle, Dual: Senses both atria and ventricle: Dual: Can be programmed to be inhibited or triggered in response to intrinsic activity) pacemaker with evidence of 1:1 atrial and ventricular capture. Every pacing artifact is followed by depolarization. Note that pacemaker sensing can not be evaluated from this ECG because there is no intrinsic rhythm.

(a)

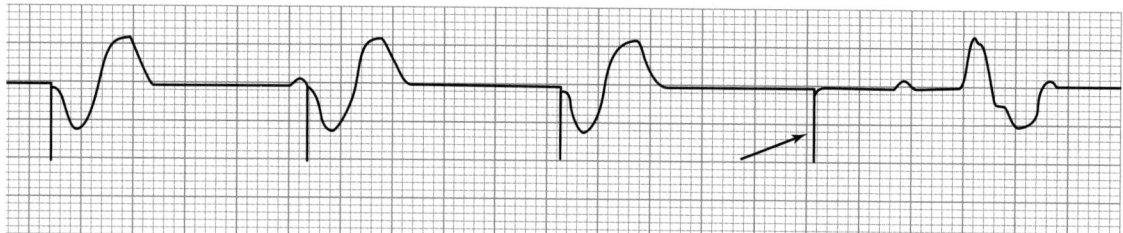

The first three beats exhibit 1:1 capture. After the 4th pacer artifact (arrow), there is no corresponding paced beat. The last QRS complex is an escape beat representing intrinsic ventricular activity.

(b)

FIGURE 39–15 ■ Pacemaker capture: (A) and (B) loss of ventricular capture.

to the generator. This conductor is covered with insulation, silicone or polyurethane, to prevent corrosion of the lead and to prevent current leaking into surrounding body tissues.

Assessment of Pacemaker Function

Information obtained from the ECG must be combined with knowledge of the specific type of pacemaker as well as a complete assessment of the patient in order to evaluate the pacemaker completely. The nurse should review the reason for the pacemaker, the date of insertion, the program settings, and the patient's intrinsic rate, if present.

The ECG should be examined in a systematic fashion regardless of the type of pacemaker (Chart 39–16).

CHART 39–16	**ECG Assessment of the Patient with a Pacemaker**

1. Assess for any intrinsic electrical activity (the patient's own rhythm). Look for intrinsic P waves or QRS complexes.

2. Assess for pacing spikes (pacer artifact). Pacemakers with bipolar pacing leads (most common) have smaller pacing artifacts than those with unipolar leads. Examine the ECG in more than one lead for evidence of pacing activity.

3. Determine the relationship between the P wave and the QRS complex, if any.

4. Look for capture beats (paced beats) with each pacemaker artifact (1:1 capture).

5. Calculate the heart rate. What is the pacemaker's programmed rate?

Pacemaker Capture

Capture is the depolarization of cardiac muscle after a paced electrical stimulus that results in myocardial contraction (Figure 39–15 ■). Loss of capture is noted when pacing artifact is present without depolarization, and is seen on the ECG as pacing artifact with no paced beat (see Figure 39–15 ■). Loss of capture can be continuous or intermittent.

Once loss of capture is identified, it is important to assess the patient because loss of capture can result in profound bradycardia and hypotension (Reynolds & Apple, 2001). Etiology for loss of capture in a temporary pacemaker includes lead dislodgment (most common), lead fracture, battery failure, altered pacemaker thresholds, perforation of the myocardium by the lead wire, and generator failure. Altered thresholds are the result of local inflammation at the site of the pacemaker wire, which interrupts the transmission of pacemaker signals. Typically, threshold levels will increase over several days after pacemaker insertion, sometimes increasing as much as three times the original level. The use of pacemaker wires containing small amounts of steroids that elute over a period of time, thereby suppressing inflammation, has greatly reduced this potential problem.

Pacemaker Sensitivity

Pacemaker sensitivity is the ability of the pacemaker to detect or "hear" intrinsic electrical activity and respond appropriately. Electrical activity also is generated by normal skeletal muscle activity. In order for the pacemaker to function properly, it must be programmed to detect only normal *cardiac* electrical activity. The sensitivity is usually set at two to three times higher than the threshold level (Chart 39–17).

Threshold levels increase during the first few days after implantation due to inflammation at the tip site. Threshold levels

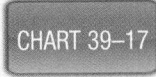

CHART 39–17 **Programming Temporary Pacemaker's Sensing**

1. Set pacemaker programmed rate at least 10 beats per minute (beats/min) above the patient's intrinsic heart rate. Check that there is 1:1 capture; that is, every pacemaker spike is followed by a QRS complex and results in a palpable pulse.

2. Slowly decrease the programmed output (energy in milliamperes) until there is loss of capture.

3. Slowly increase the programmed output until there is 1:1 capture. This is the threshold value.

4. Set the programmed output to two to three times higher than the threshold value.

5. Slowly return pacemaker rate to original programmed value.

are usually checked daily while the temporary pacemaker remains in place (Jacobson & Gerity, 2005; Reynolds & Apple, 2001).

In order to evaluate sensing, there must be intrinsic beats on the ECG and the nurse must know the current pacemaker program. *Undersensing* occurs when the pacemaker fails to detect ("hear") intrinsic electrical cardiac activity and delivers inappropriate pacing artifacts (Figure 39–16A ■). Possible causes of undersensing include lead displacement or fracture, loose connections, or generator failure.

Oversensing (Figure 39–16B ■) occurs when the pacemaker is inhibited by inappropriate electrical artifact, such as extraneous muscle activity, or by the T wave on the ECG. A common cause of oversensing is airport security systems. The patient must be instructed not to go through airport security because the pacemaker will interpret the "electrical noise" as cardiac activity and inhibit itself. Depending on the length of exposure, the patient could experience a drop in cardiac output.

Temporary Pacemakers

Temporary pacing can be performed using transvenous, epicardial, or transcutaneous methods. The system used will depend on factors such as the clinical diagnosis and stability of the patient (elective or emergency situation). Temporary pacing is indicated in a variety of conditions (Chart 39–18).

Temporary Transvenous Pacing

Temporary transvenous pacing involves insertion of the lead through a major vein, such as the internal jugular, subclavian, or femoral. The pacing lead is threaded into the right side of the heart; the proximal end is sutured outside the body and connected to an external generator. If an epicardial lead is used, the lead is attached to the outside of the heart (typically during cardiac surgery) and is introduced through the chest wall. Temporary pacemakers can be either single chambered (lead in the ventricle only) or dual chambered (leads in both the atrium and the ventricle). Dual-chambered temporary pacemakers are not widely used at this time.

CHART 39–18 **Indications for Temporary Pacemakers**

Symptomatic sick sinus syndrome

Symptomatic second- or third-degree heart block

Drug refractory dysrhythmias

Prophylactic after cardiovascular surgery

Prior to insertion of a permanent cardiac pacemaker

Development of significant conduction disturbances after acute myocardial infarction

Overdrive tachydysrhythmias

During cardiac resuscitation

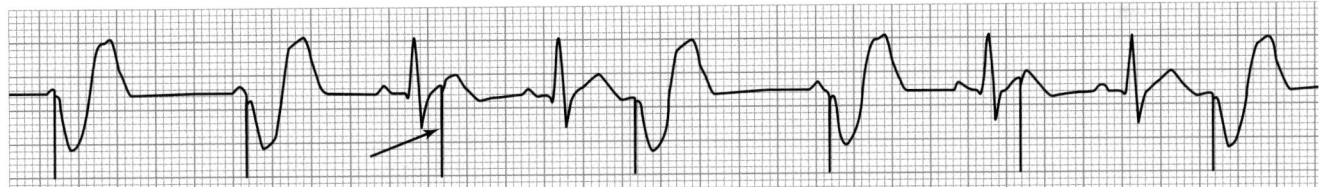

Undersensing. VVI pacemaker programmed at a rate of 60. Pacemaker fails to sense (hear) the intrinsic beat and delivers a pacing artifact into the ST segment of the intrinsic beat (arrow). Pacemaker artifact in this location has been noted to initiate a run of ventricular fibrillation (R on T phenomenon).

(a)

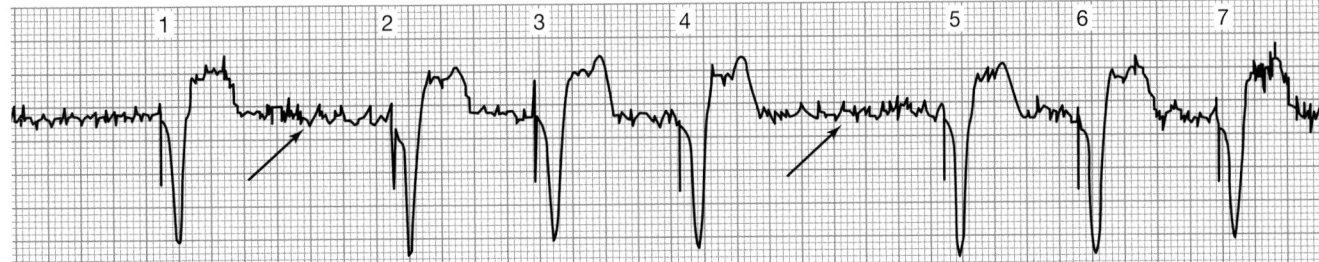

Oversensing. VVI pacemaker programmed at a rate of 60. Pacemaker is inhibited by extraneous electrical activity (arrows). When the pacemaker does fire, there is 1:1 capture.

Note: ECGs from Medtronics, Inc.

(b)

FIGURE 39–16 ■ Pacemaker sensing: (A) undersensing and (B) oversensing.

Programming the External Generator

Once the leads are connected to the generator, the system must be programmed. At a minimum this consists of setting the rate at which the pacemaker will fire, the amount of energy delivered with each paced beat (output), and the sensitivity (Figure 39–17 ■).

The programmed rate determines the patient's minimum heart rate. For example, a single-chamber temporary transvenous pacemaker (VVI) set at 60 beats per minute (beats/min) will deliver an electrical stimulus to the ventricle only when the patient's rate drops below 60. If the patient generates his own heartbeat faster than 60 beats per minute, the pacemaker will be inhibited (Figure 39–18 ■). This is referred to as a demand pacemaker.

The programmed output, the amount of energy delivered by the generator with each paced beat, is measured in milliamperes (ma). The amount of energy must be sufficient to cause capture, which means that a myocardial contraction has occurred.

Pacemaker sensitivity, the amount of electrical activity the pacemaker will sense or "hear," is measured in millivolts (mV).

A sensitivity of 2 millivolts is more sensitive than that of 5 millivolts, because the pacemaker will be able to hear smaller amounts of electrical activity. If the sensitivity is increased to the maximum, the pacemaker becomes asynchronous; that is, the pacemaker cannot sense any intrinsic electrical activity and will pace continuously at its programmed rate. A single-chamber ventricular pacemaker set to asynchronous would be designated VOO (paces the right ventricle, no chamber sensed, and no response to intrinsic beats). The sensitivity is usually set at two to three times higher than *threshold*, which is the minimum amount of current necessary for electrical capture and myocardial contraction (see Chart 39–17, p. 1145).

■ Nursing Management

Care of the patient with an external transvenous pacemaker includes a complete cardiovascular assessment, with special attention to the heart rate. The nurse needs to evaluate the

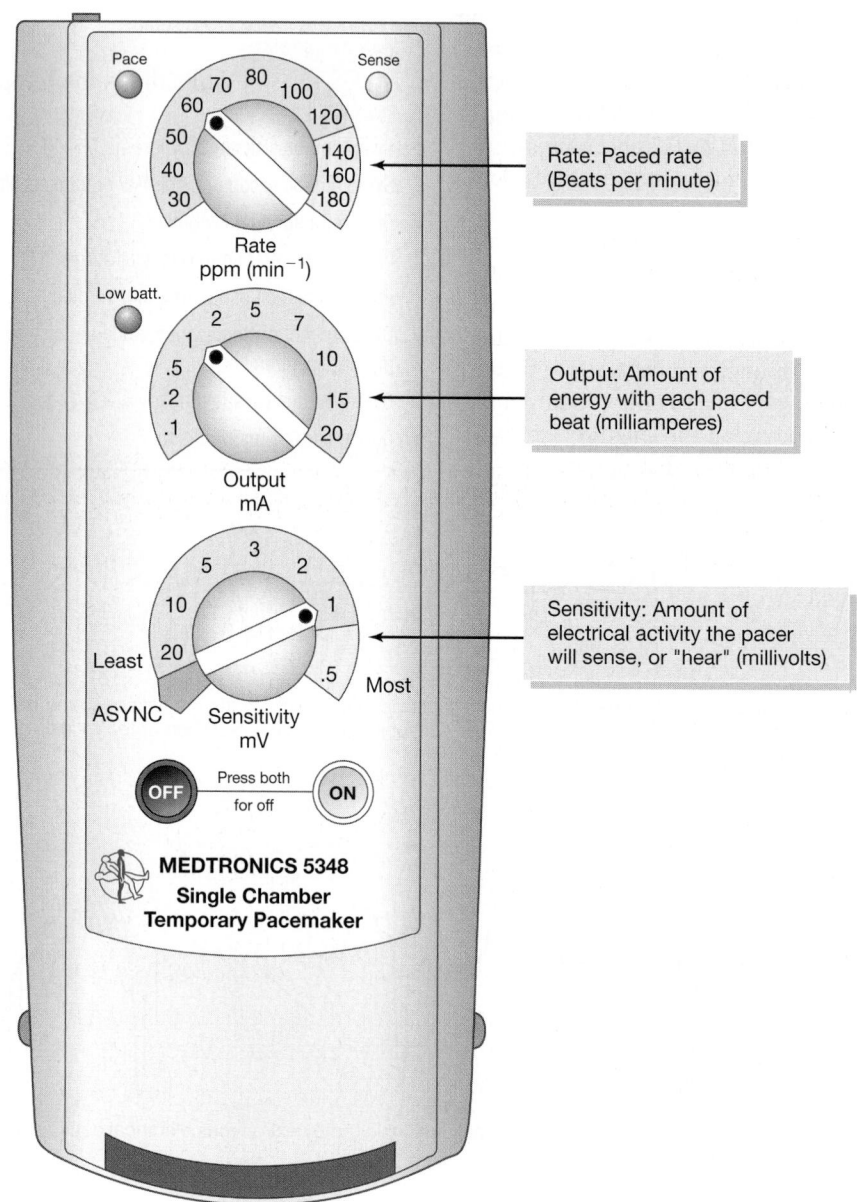

FIGURE 39–17 ■ Temporary pacemaker generator.

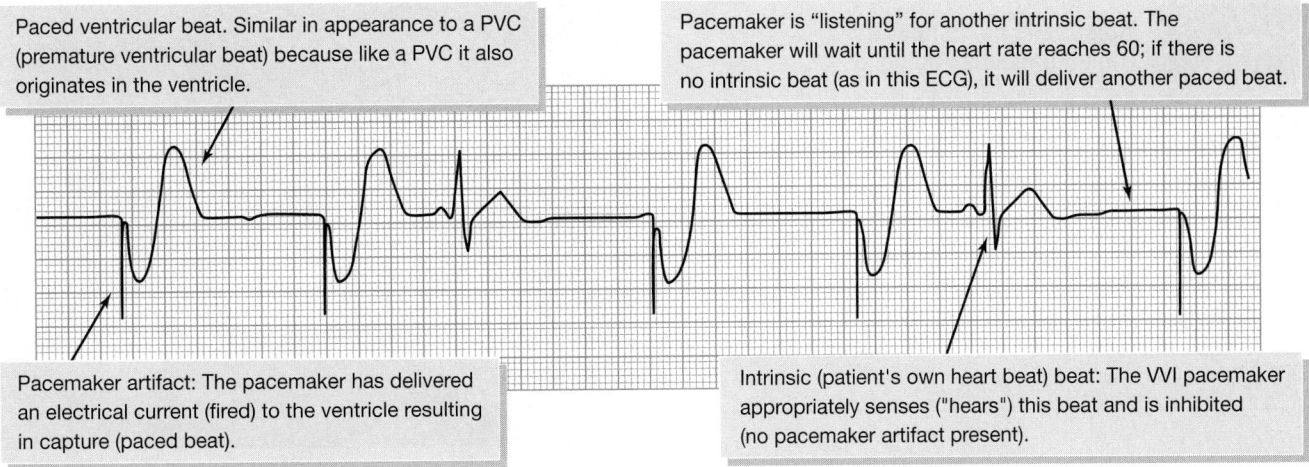

Paced ventricular beat. Similar in appearance to a PVC (premature ventricular beat) because like a PVC it also originates in the ventricle.

Pacemaker is "listening" for another intrinsic beat. The pacemaker will wait until the heart rate reaches 60; if there is no intrinsic beat (as in this ECG), it will deliver another paced beat.

Pacemaker artifact: The pacemaker has delivered an electrical current (fired) to the ventricle resulting in capture (paced beat).

Intrinsic (patient's own heart beat) beat: The VVI pacemaker appropriately senses ("hears") this beat and is inhibited (no pacemaker artifact present).

VVI Pacemaker: (Paces the ventricle; Senses the ventricle; Inhibited when it senses intrinsic electrical activity. This VVI pacemaker is set at a rate of 60.

FIGURE 39–18 ■ VVI pacemaker.

rhythm strip to determine whether capture is occurring appropriately. Thus, the nurse questions: If it is a single-chambered pacemaker, is there a QRS after each pacemaker spike, and if it is dual-chambered pacemaker, is there a P wave after the atrial spike and a QRS after the ventricular spike? Additionally, the nurse needs to assess for normal sensing. For example, does the pacemaker inhibit itself when there is intrinsic cardiac activity? Does the patient's heart rate and blood pressure indicate that the pacemaker rate is appropriate? Another important assessment is how often the pacemaker is pacing the heart. It typically is expressed in percentages and usually is a close approximation; for example, the patient is being paced 50% of the time. With a temporary pacemaker this will assist in determining the need for a permanent pacemaker.

In addition, electrical safety practices are critically important, because the leads are capable of carrying electrical current directly into the heart (Jacobson & Gerity, 2005; Overbay & Criddle, 2004).

1. *Always wear gloves when handling the pacemaker leads or connecting cables.*
2. *Verify that all connections are securely fastened.*
3. *Verify that all equipment in the room is electrically grounded.*
4. *If they are not connected to an external generator, keep epicardial leads covered in a disposable glove or a small tube.*
5. *Do not touch any of the pacemaker components on first entering the patient's room to avoid static electricity.*

Nurses should always wear gloves when handling any component of the pacemaker to avoid microshocks. The generator should be securely attached in order to avoid accidental dislodgment of the leads. Care of the access site should incorporate standards of care for any vascular access site.

Temporary Transcutaneous Pacing

Transcutaneous pacing (TCP) is accomplished by delivering the electrical stimulus directly through the chest wall. A variety

of devices is currently available; most portable defibrillators are now equipped with optional external pacing capabilities (Figure 39–19 ■).

Technological advances have resulted in TCP systems that are more reliable and safer to use, resulting in expanded indications for TCP (Chart 39–19, p. 1148).

Large-surface adhesive electrodes, similar to defibrillation electrodes, are placed on the anterior and posterior chest wall over the heart (Figure 39–20 ■, p. 1148).

If this is not feasible, the pads may be placed on the anterior chest wall on the right shoulder and over the left apex. Skin preparation is critical to optimize capture. If there is time the

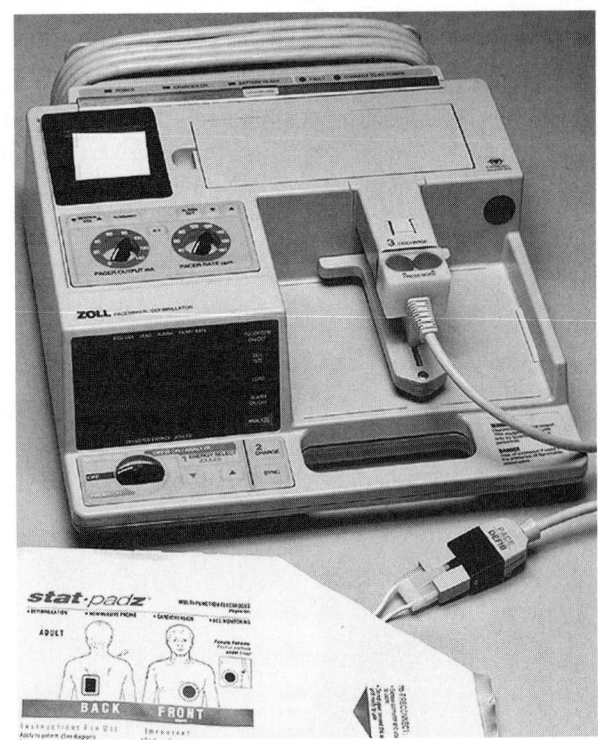

FIGURE 39–19 ■ Temporary transcutaneous pacemaker.
Source: Courtesy of ZOLL Medical Corporation

Indications for Temporary Transcutaneous Pacing

1. Hemodynamically significant (resulting in symptoms such as dizziness or syncope) bradycardia unresponsive to atropine

2. Bradycardia with escape rhythms

3. Pacing for patients in cardiac arrest with profound bradycardia or pulseless electrical activity secondary to drug overdose, acidosis, or electrolyte imbalance

4. Standby pacing in anticipation of clinical deterioration, such as development of bifascicular block in acute myocardial infarction or transport of critically ill patients

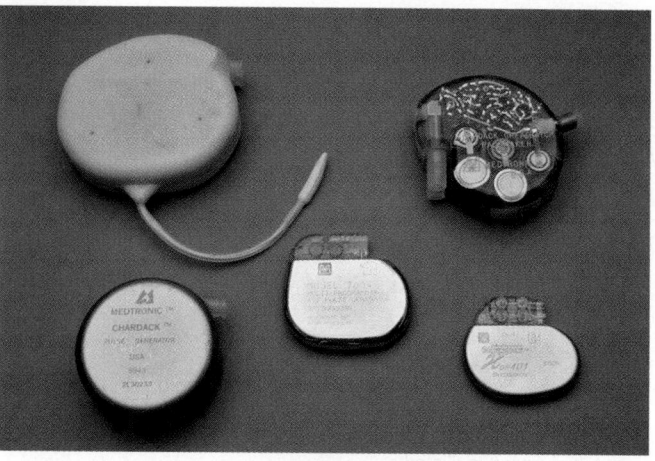

FIGURE 39–21 ■ Permanent pacemakers.
Source: Reproduced with permission of Medtronic, Inc.

nurse should wash the skin with soap and water and thoroughly dry the chest, and avoid alcohol or benzoin. If there is significant body hair it may be trimmed carefully; shaving is avoided because this can leave small cuts, making TCP painful. The electrodes are placed firmly on the chest, avoiding the diaphragm and any metal on the patient, including permanent pacemakers. After the electrodes are applied, the programmed rate is set and the output increased until there is capture. Because TCP results in skeletal muscle movement, it is important to verify capture through palpation of a major vessel, preferably the femoral artery. Problems encountered with TCP include failure to capture, failure to sense, and painful stimulation of the chest wall. Newer systems have overcome many of these limitations.

Permanent Cardiac Pacemakers

The earliest pacemakers were implanted to treat symptomatic bradycardia; that is, "a documented bradydysrhythmia that is directly responsible for the development of the clinical manifestations of frank syncope or near syncope, transient dizziness or lightheadedness, and confusional states resulting from cerebral hypoperfusion attributable to slow heart rate" (Gregoratos et al., 2002, p. 4). Figure 39–21 ■ shows various pacemakers from the very first larger units to the current small, compact unit.

Although correcting symptomatic bradycardia remains the cornerstone of permanent pacemaker therapy, indications for

implantation have greatly expanded. Technological advances have expanded the ability of pacemakers to detect and treat a variety of dysrhythmias as well as structural abnormalities such as cardiomyopathy (Gregoratos et al., 2002; Obias-Manno, 2001) (Chart 39–20).

Device Selection

Once the decision has been made to implant a permanent pacemaker, the clinician and patient are faced with a wide variety of choices (Chart 39–21).

Published guidelines exist to aid in the choice of the most appropriate therapy (Gregoratos et al., 2002). The nurse must be aware that there is frequently more than one treatment option. The choice of pacemaker will depend on the indication(s) for pacing, health care provider and patient preference, and availability and cost of the device.

Permanent Pacemaker Vocabulary

In order to understand pacemakers, the nurse must be familiar with basic pacemaker terminology and functions, which are outlined in Charts 39–22 and 39–23 (p. 1150).

In addition, a standard pacemaker code was originally developed in 1974 by the Inter-Society Commission for Heart Disease (ICHD) to describe the properties of any pacemaker. The original code contained three letters; however, with the advent of the more complex dual-chambered pacemakers, the code was expanded to five letters in 1987 (Chart 39–24, p. 1150).

It is not always necessary to use all five categories to identify clinically significant information. Two of the most commonly used pacing modes include VVI and DDD. The VVI pacemaker has the ability to pace the right ventricle (V), sense the intrinsic electrical activity in the right ventricle (V), and inhibit itself (does not deliver an electrical stimulus) when sensing intrinsic activity (I). The DDD pacemaker (also referred to as a dual-chambered or physiological pacemaker) has leads in both the right atrium and the right ventricle. The first D (dual) in the code indicates that these pacemakers can deliver atrial or ventricular paced beats, or both, depending on the settings. The second D indicates the ability to sense intrinsic electrical activity in both the right atrium and right ventricle. The third D indicates the ability of the

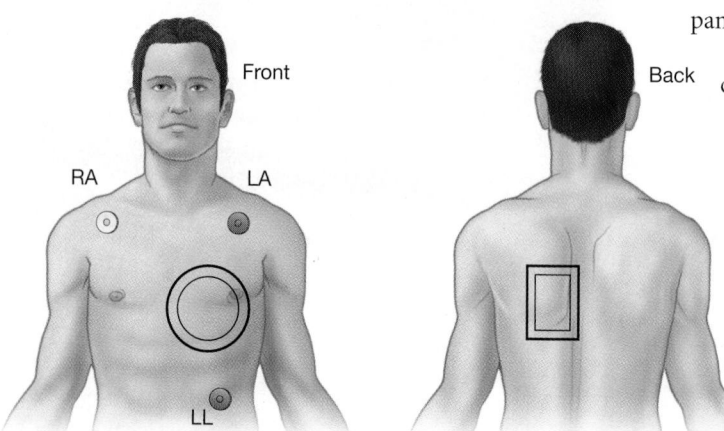

Front   Back

RA   LA

LL

FIGURE 39–20 ■ Transcutaneous conductor pad placement.

CHART 39–20 **Indications for Permanent Cardiac Pacemaker**

1. Acquired atrioventricular block in adults
2. Chronic bifascicular and trifascicular block
3. Atrioventricular block associated with acute myocardial infarction
4. Sinus node dysfunction
5. Prevention and termination of tachydysrhythmias
6. Hypersensitive carotid sinus and neurocardiogenic syncope
7. Patients with congenital heart disease
8. In certain conditions:
   a. Hypertrophic obstructive cardiomyopathy
   b. Idiopathic dilated cardiomyopathy
   c. Cardiac transplantation.

Treatment of the preceding indications does not always require pacemaker implantation, and in many instances acceptable alternative therapies are available.

Source: "ACC/AHA/NASPE 2002 guideline update for implantation of cardiac pacemakers and antidysrhythmia devices." G. Gregortos et al., 2002, Circulation, 106: 2145–2161.

CHART 39–21 **Selection of Pacemaker Device**

GENERATOR

1. Single chamber versus dual chamber (Pace the atria, or ventricle, or both?)
2. Unipolar versus bipolar
3. Rate response; type of sensor for rate response (Pacer will have the ability to adapt to changing physiological needs, such as sleep or exercise.)
4. Advanced features
5. Battery capacity
6. Size of the generator
7. Cost

LEAD

1. Single or dual lead(s)
2. Polarity (bipolar or unipolar)
3. Type of insulation (silicone rubber or polyurethane)
4. Active or passive fixation (active fixation leads are permanently attached, usually by means of a small screw at the tip)
5. Steroid eluting tip (can result in lower thresholds for pacing and thus prolong battery life)

OTHER

1. Programming capabilities
2. Availability of technical support
3. Frequency and type of clinical follow-up required (clinic visits or transtelephonic monitoring)

CHART 39–22 **Basic Pacemaker Vocabulary**

Term	Definition
Anode	Positive electrode
Cathode	Negative electrode
Current	Volume of flow of the energy, measured in milliamperes (ma)
Voltage	Force of electrical energy from the generator through the lead to the electrode tip
Resistance	Function of lead integrity at the electrode and myocardial interface; opposes the flow of current; measured in ohms
Programmer	External device used to communicate with pacemaker for information stored in the pacer memory; enables the clinician to check settings and make changes
Rate modulation	Ability of pacemaker to vary its pacing rate automatically to adapt to physiological needs, such as exercise or sleep (also known as rate response)
Crosstalk	Inappropriate sensing of one lead or chamber activity by another
Tracking	Ventricular pacing in a 1:1 response to sensed atrial activity; that is, the ventricular rate will match the atrial rate

---

pacemaker to be either inhibited or triggered in response to a sensed activity. DDD pacemakers are commonly referred to as physiological pacemakers because of their ability to maintain atrial contraction followed by ventricular contraction, which most closely mimics normal intrinsic cardiac activity. The fourth letter of the code indicates programmability and rate modulation. In the United States, the overwhelming majority of modern permanent pacemakers have rate modulation, the ability to adjust the pacing rate automatically, as a programmable feature (Lamas, Ellenbogen, Hennekens, & Montanez, 2004).

Cardiac Resynchronization Therapy

Cardiac resynchronization therapy (CRT) refers to atrial-synchronized biventricular pacemakers (Abraham & Hayes, 2003; Auricchio & Abraham, 2004; Jacobson & Gerity, 2005; Leclercq & Hare, 2004; Legge & Leeper, 2002). The three leads necessary for this system are a right atrial lead, a right ventricular lead, and a left ventricular lead. The right leads are positioned inside the cardiac chambers; the left ventricular lead is usually placed in a left lateral vein via the coronary sinus.

Normally the right and left ventricles are activated almost simultaneously, resulting in synchronous systole and diastole. In patients with systolic heart failure, approximately 30% have a prolonged QRS complex (>120 milliseconds). A prolonged QRS results in a significant delay in the electrical activation of the left ventricle, resulting in ventricular dyssynchrony (left ventricular systole occurs after right ventricular systole). This dyssynchrony between the right and left ventricles results in a paradoxical motion of the interventricular septum; that is, instead of contracting with the left ventricle, the septal wall moves toward the right ventricle. Ventricular dyssynchrony forces a mechanical disadvantage

---

CHART 39-23 **Basic Pacemaker Functions**

Function	Definition
AV interval	The pacemaker's PR interval; the interval between the programmed or sensed P wave and the programmed or sensed QRS.
Capture	Myocardial contraction in response to the pacemaker firing; a palpable pulse is felt with every paced beat.
Hysteresis	The ability of a pacemaker to wait until a lower heart rate than the pacing rate before initiating pacing. For example, the pacemaker may be programmed to pace at a rate of 80, but the pacemaker will not start pacing until the patient's heart rate has dropped to 65.
Magnet rate	Rate of a pacer that is produced when a magnet is applied to the generator. The ability of the pacemaker to generate a magnet rate is a function of the battery and is useful in determining time to generator replacement.
Program	The parameters of the pacemaker; also refers to the ability to change or set the pacemaker's parameters noninvasively.
Pulse amplitude	Output voltage needed to stimulate the heart, measured in volts (V); how much current is needed to have capture.
Pulse width	The duration of the output, measured in milliseconds (ms); how long the electrical current is delivered to the heart.
Sensitivity	Pacemaker's ability to sense intrinsic cardiac activity (the patient's own heartbeat), measured in millivolts (mV).
Stimulation threshold	Minimum amount of energy required to capture the heartbeat consistently.

---

on an already failing heart (Jacobson & Gerity, 2005; Leclercq & Hare, 2004). This mechanical disadvantage results in a further drop in cardiac output and heart failure.

Biventricular pacemakers were first implanted in the early 1990s. However, the early systems required open-heart surgery and were plagued with high failure rates. Since that time technological advances have resulted in CRT systems that can be inserted percutaneously with a high rate of success. These devices are used for patients with severe systolic heart failure who have a prolonged QRS and remain symptomatic despite optimal medical management; these patients experience improved cardiac function with CRT. This therapy increases cardiac output and decreases ventricular filling pressures. In addition, CRT results in a decrease in heart failure symptoms and improved quality of life. In 2001 CRT was approved by the U.S. Food and Drug Administration (FDA) for use in this population (Abraham & Hayes, 2003; Leclercq & Hare, 2004). The latest advances in CRT devices include combining cardioverter/defibrillation capabilities with biventricular pacing, eliminating the need for a separate ICD in certain patients. In the fall of 2004, these combination devices were approved by the FDA for placement in patients who meet the criteria for CRT, regardless of whether they currently require an ICD. CRT is discussed in Chapter 42 as it relates to heart failure.

Nursing Management

Care of the patient with a new permanent pacemaker is similar to care of a patient with a temporary pacemaker. The nurse should be familiar with the type of pacemaker and current program settings. The patient should be assessed frequently for signs and symptoms of inadequate cardiac output that could be related to the pacemaker, such as hypotension, dizziness, or sudden syncope.

Discharge Teaching

Discharge instructions include care of the access site as well as providing the patient with the pacemaker information card provided by all pacemaker manufacturers. The patient should carry this information with her at all times. In addition, a letter from her health care provider and a medic alert bracelet will aid travel through systems such as airports that require screening by metal detectors. Finally, even though current technology has rendered pacemakers relatively easy to implant and maintenance free, careful long-term follow-up is necessary to avoid potential problems. The complexity of modern pacemakers makes it difficult to evaluate pacemaker function fully with only the ECG. Pacemaker device questioning by a trained professional is necessary to evaluate pacemaker function and settings completely (Jacobson & Gerity, 2005). This may occur in the office or by telephone.

CHART 39-24 **Pacemaker Code**

Chamber Paced	Chamber Sensed	Response of Sensing	Programmability	Antitachycardia Pacing Functions
0 = None	0 = None	0 = None	0 = None	0 = None
A = Atrium	A = Atrium	T = Triggered	P = Simple programmable	P = Antitachycardia pacing
V = Ventricle	V = Ventricle	I = Inhibited	M = Multiprogrammable	S = Shock
D = Dual (A and V)	D = A and V	D = Trigger and inhibited	C = Communicating	D = P and S
			R = Rate Modulation	

Sources: Code adapted from Parsonnet, V., Furman, S., & Smyth, N. P. D. (1974). Implantable cardiac pacemakers: Status report and resource guideline. *Circulation, 50,* 21A–35A; and Berstein, A. D., Camm, A. J., Fletcher, R. D., Gold, R. D., Rickards, A. F., Smyth, N. P., et al. (1987). The NASPE/BPEG generic pacemaker code for antibradycardia and adaptive-rate pacing and antitachyarrhythmia devices. *Pacing and Clinical Electrophysiology, 10,* 794–799.

Gerontological Considerations

Over 80% of pacemakers are implanted in patients over the age of 64 (Gregoratos et al., 2002). Because elderly patients already are at increased risk for falls due to a variety of natural physiological changes, health care professionals must be aggressive in providing careful pacemaker follow-up in order to prevent potential complications in this vulnerable population. The timing of follow-up evaluation depends on several factors, including clinical status of the patient, age of the pacemaker, and geographic location of the patient to a health care facility. Family members may need to be enlisted to ensure that patients adhere to their appointments. Telephone follow-up may be an option if patients have difficulty traveling.

Summary

Advances in pacemaker technologies have led to more complicated but reliable devices that have moved well beyond the ability of the first pacemakers to pace only the right ventricle at a fixed predetermined rate. Modern pacemakers are programmable, have the ability to modulate their rate in response to a variety of triggers, and are indicated not only for the treatment of dysrhythmias but also for clinical conditions such as heart failure. However, the decision to implant a pacemaker does not mean that the patient will not require long-term follow-up or be freed from medications. The pacemaker is just one component, albeit an important one, of comprehensive care for the cardiac patient and his family.

■ Research Opportunities Related to PCI

As with much of medicine and nursing, there is still a great deal to be learned in order to improve patient care and the quality of life for cardiac patients. Cardiac care is an ever-evolving science that requires continued research. The Research Opportunities and Clinical Impact box outlines areas of research that are still under investigation or need future trials.

RESEARCH OPPORTUNITIES AND CLINICAL IMPACT RELATED TO PERCUTANEOUS CORONARY INTERVENTION

Research Area	Clinical Impact
Physiological Research	
Long-term impact of drug eluting stents on restenosis.	Restenosis is the major cause of repeat revascularization procedures.
Vascular management techniques.	Potential to reduce length of stay and improve patient comfort and safety after PCI.
Length of time to continue antiplatelet agents after PCI.	Reduce complications associated with these medications.
Emotional and Psychological Research	
Denial of signs and symptoms of acute myocardial infarction.	Delaying treatment results in increased morbidity and mortality.
Risk factor modification.	Reduce incidence of CAD, as well as improve outcomes after PCI.
Use of alternative therapies such as guided imagery to reduce anxiety during PCI.	Lower stress during PCI while reducing need for sedatives/analgesics.
Effective teaching methods for discharge instructions.	Knowledge alone does not improve patient/family compliance.

Clinical Preparation

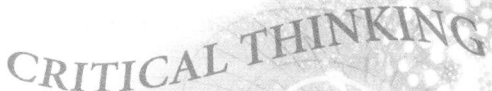

CRITICAL THINKING

PEARSON **mynursingkit**™

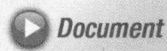 **Read**

- History of Current Illness
- Past Medical History
- Physical Exam
- Admitting Medical Orders
- Laboratory Study Results

 **Document**

- Summary of Hospitalization
- Pathophysiology Form
- Laboratory Values
- Laboratory Results Explanation

Apply

- List of Potential Nursing Diagnoses
- Concept Map
- Critical Thinking Questions

Log on to MyNursingKit.com to download forms you will need and to complete further steps in the Clinical Preparation assignment.

HISTORY OF PRESENT ILLNESS

You are a nurse in a large hospital that is the referral center for cardiac patients needing urgent percutaneous coronary interventional (PCI) procedures or coronary artery bypass surgery. You have just received a report about Mr. W, a 52-year-old engineer who is having an acute myocardial infarction and is being transported to your hospital for urgent PCI. Mr. W went to work this morning despite not feeling well. After several episodes of nausea and chest pain, Mr. W's coworkers called 911. His wife and three children also were so notified and are on their way to your hospital.

Medical–Surgical History

Mr. W has a past medical history of hypertension, non–insulin-dependent diabetes, and hyperlipidemia. He states he is not currently under a doctor's care and is taking no medicines. He has had no prior surgeries. No known allergies.

Social History

Mr. W. lives with his wife and three young children. He works about 60 to 70 hours per week. He coaches his son's baseball team in the evening and weekends. He smokes 1 to 2 packs per day and drinks two to three beers every evening.

Physical Exam

When Mr. W arrives at the hospital, he is restless but able to answer questions appropriately, very anxious, and complaining of chest pain radiating down his left arm. He is diaphoretic and appears short of breath. Vital signs are temperature, 99.6°F; pulse, 118 beats per minute and regular; respiratory rate, 28 per minute; blood pressure, 90/50 mmHg; and his oxygen saturation is 92% on room air. He is 5'9" and weighs 220 pounds.

A 55-year-old man with 4 hours of "crushing" chest pain

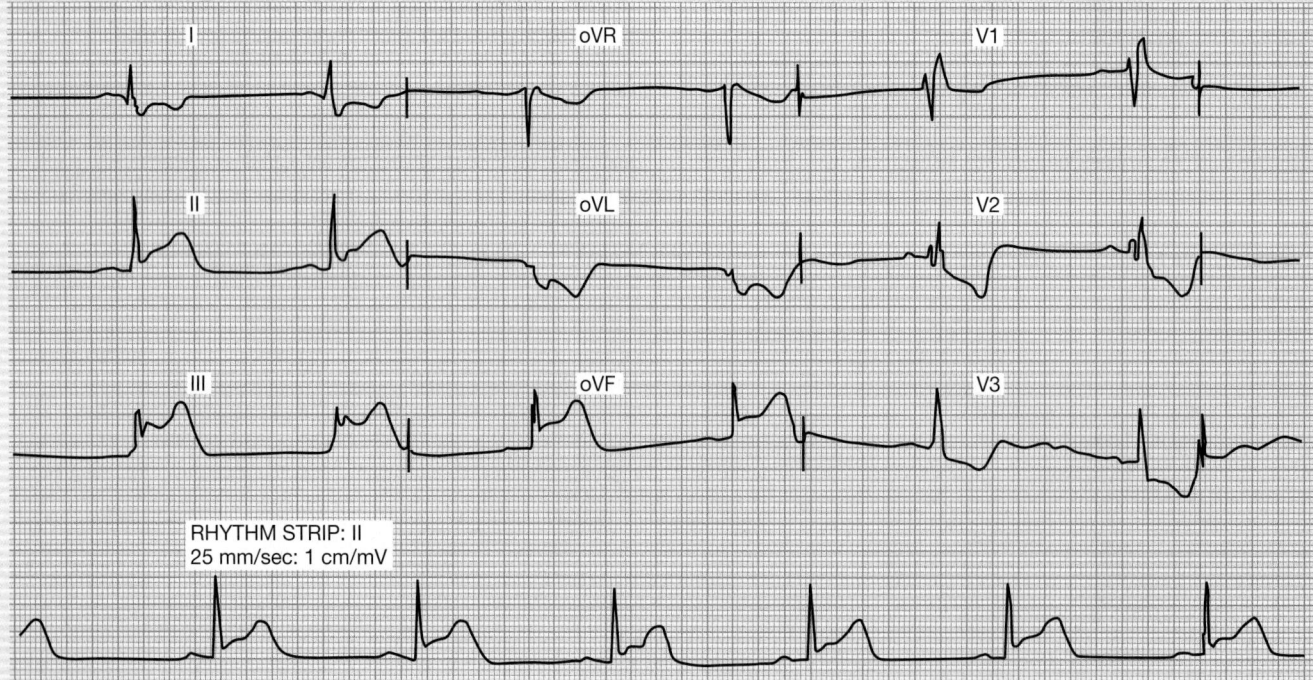

FIGURE V–1 ■ Admission 12-lead ECG. ST segment elevation is present in leads II, III, and aVF, indicating acute inferior myocardial infarction. Note the ST segment depression in the posterior lead V₂, indicating possible posterior involvement. There is also ST segment depression in the lateral (I, and avL) leads. These are probably secondary changes related to the size of the infarct.

Mr. W has bilateral rales in both lung bases. He has a loud third heart sound, but no murmurs or rubs. Extremities are cool; all pulses are present and normal. His abdomen is soft and nontender with active bowel sounds. A Foley catheter has been placed; there is 90 milliliters of clear yellow urine in the bag. Mr. W has one peripheral line in his right arm; normal saline is infusing at 100 mL/hr. He has been given one adult aspirin and one dose of low-molecular-weight heparin. You accompany Mr. W as he is urgently transferred to the catheterization laboratory. Mr. W's admitting ECG indicates that he is experiencing an acute inferior/posterior myocardial infarction (Figure V–1 ■). This is usually related to a significant occlusion in the right coronary artery (RCA).

Mr. W's initial cardiac angiography revealed a total occlusion of the proximal RCA (Figure V–2 ■). After balloon angioplasty there was no blood flow to the artery, and significant thrombus (clot) had now formed in the distal portions of the artery (Figures V–3 ■ and V–4 ■). Despite the placement of multiple coronary stents, the artery remained blocked with thrombus. Eventually the decision was made to remove the thrombus directly with a mechanical thrombectomy device, in this case the AngioJet. This device creates suction at its tip that aspirates and then breaks up a clot, allowing it to be removed with almost no damage to the wall of the coronary artery. The final result was a patent RCA (Figure V–5 ■).

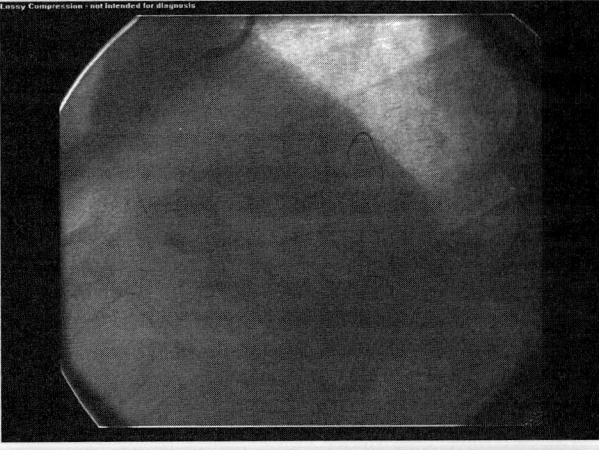

FIGURE V–4 ■ Angiogram after attempted balloon angioplasty. There is no blood flow and significant thrombus (clot) in the distal portions of the artery (arrows).

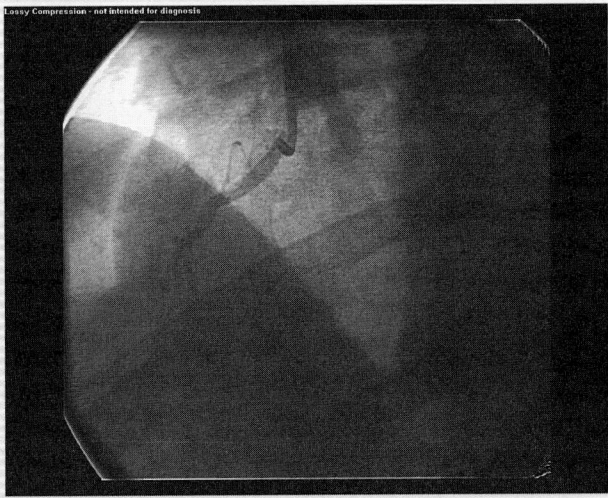

FIGURE V–2 ■ Cardiac angiography indicating a total occlusion in the midportion of the right coronary artery (arrow).

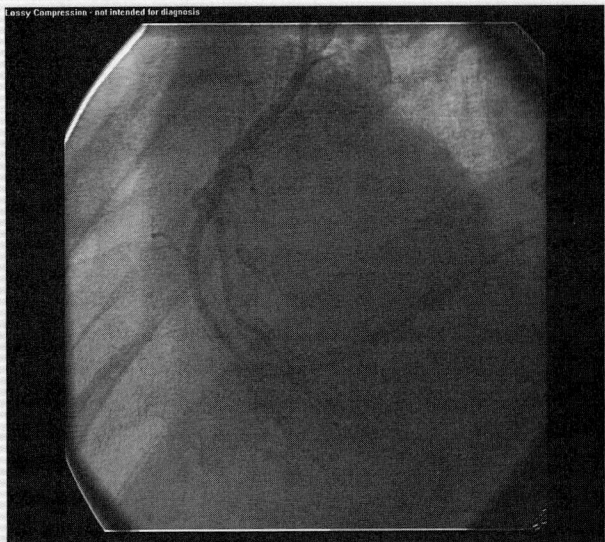

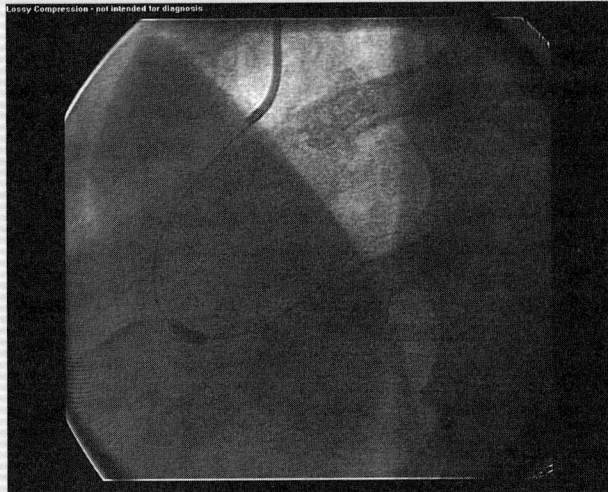

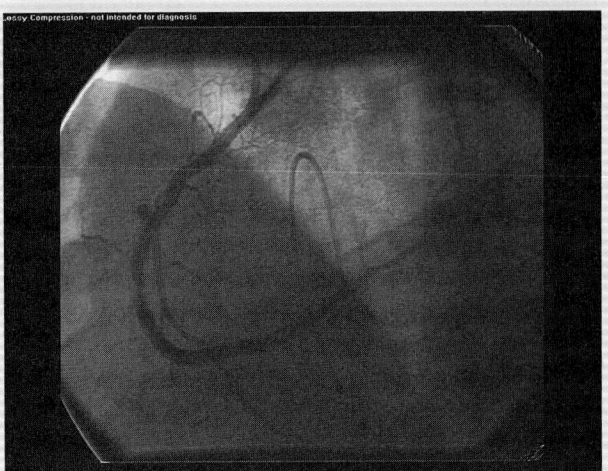

FIGURE V–5 ■ The patient eventually required the placement of multiple coronary stents, as well as direct removal of the clot by a mechanical thrombectomy device. The AngioJet catheter creates a vacuum at its tip that aspirates and removes thrombus and other material from within the artery. The final result is a widely patent RCA with excellent blood flow throughout.
Source: All catheterization images courtesy of Boston Scientific

FIGURE V–3 ■ Balloon angioplasty of the occlusion in the RCA.

Medications Before PCI

Aspirin 325 mg po daily (first dose at least 2 hours before the procedure)

Clopidogrel 300 mg po as a one-time loading dose, then 75 mg daily

Unfractionated heparin 70 international units/kg bolus IV, then 17 international units/kg per hour titrated to clotting time

Nitroglycerin, IV, titrated to maintain systolic blood pressure > 90 mmHg

Morphine, 3–5 mg IV q1h prn pain

Admitting Medical Orders

Admit to cardiology service, coronary care unit

Condition guarded

No known allergies

Diagnosis: acute inferior/posterior myocardial infarction; status postangioplasty, stent placement and thrombectomy

Vital signs and oxygen saturation q1h

Bed rest

Call house officer: pulse < 60 and > 110/minute; BP < 90 and > 160 systolic; temperature > 38.5; urine output < 30 mL/hr for 2 hours; respiratory rate > 30/minute; oxygen saturation < 92%

Diet: cardiac

Daily weight

Continuous cardiac monitor

Sequential compression devices (SCDs) to lower extremities

Strict in/out

Oxygen to 2 liters nasal cannula, maintain oxygen sat > 92%

IV: D51/2 NS @ 75 mL/hr

Scheduled Medications

Aspirin 81 mg po daily

Clopidogrel 75 mg po daily

Lipitor 10 mg po daily

ReoPro gtt @ 0.125 mcg/kg/minute for 12 hours

Lisinopril 10 mg po daily

Rosiglitazone 4 mg po daily

Metoprolol 25 mg po bid

PRN Medications

Nitroglycerin, IV, titrated to maintain systolic blood pressure > 90 mmHg

Morphine, 3–5 mg IV q1h prn pain

Temazepam 15–30 mg po qhs prn insomnia

Droperidol 1.25–2.5 mg IV q6h prn nausea

Ordered Laboratory Studies

Troponin I q8h × 3

CPK–MB q8h × 3

Chemistry panel 7 q a.m.

CBC q a.m.

Magnesium q a.m.

Lipid panel in a.m.

Ordered Diagnostic Studies

ECG q a.m.

Echocardiogram in a.m.

LABORATORY STUDY RESULTS

Test	Before PCI	Day 1 After PCI	Day 2 After PCI
WBC	5,000/mm^3	8,000/mm^3	5,000/mm^3
RBC	4.89/mm^3	4.69/mm^3	4.38/mm^3
Hemoglobin	13 g/dL	11 g/dL	11 g/dL
Hematocrit	35%	30%	29%
Platelets	120,000/mm^3	100,000/mm^3	130,000/mm^3
Prothrombin time	10 seconds	10 seconds	10 seconds
Activated partial thromboplastin time	25 seconds	65 seconds (on heparin)	100 seconds (on heparin)
Glucose	156 mg/dL	130 mg/dL	130 mg/dL
BUN	10 mg/dL	15 mg/dL	10 mg/dL
Creatinine	0.5 mg/dL	0.9 mg/dL	0.7 mg/dL
Sodium	139 mEq/L	137 mEq/L	140 mEq/L
Potassium	3.8 mEq/L	4.9 mEq/L	4.9 mEq/L
Chloride	100 mEq/L	100 mEq/L	100 mEq/L
CO_2	25 mEq/L	25 mEq/L	25 mEq/L
Calcium	9.5 mg/dL	9.5 mg/dL	9 mg/dL
Magnesium	2.2mEq/L	2.0 mEq/L	2.0 mEq/L
Troponin I	0.8 ng/mL	30 ng/mL	25 ng/mL
CPK-MB	>250.00%	>300.00%	259.7%
Cholesterol	260 mg/dL		
High-density lipoproteins (HDL)	34 mg/dL		
Low-density lipoproteins (LDL)	190 mg/dL		
Very low-density lipoproteins (VLDL)	62%		
Apolipoproteins	161 mg/dL		
Triglycerides	200 mg/dL		

CRITICAL THINKING QUESTIONS

1. What factors in Mr. W's past medical history place him at high risk for complications from the planned PCI?

2. What is the rationale for taking Mr. W directly to the catheterization laboratory?

3. Why was Mr. W given an aspirin?

4. Mr. W is restless, tachycardic, with low blood pressure and urine output. What is the most likely cause of these findings?

Answers to Critical Thinking Questions appear in Appendix D

NCLEX® REVIEW

1. A patient with asthma is being treated with a glucocorticoid and has been told that his blood glucose level could increase, creating the picture that he has diabetes. The nurse has instructed the patient on which of the following types of sensitivity to tests?
   1. True positive
   2. False negative
   3. True negative
   4. False positive

2. A patient is demonstrating signs of cardiac valve stenosis. The nurse should be prepared to discuss which of the following diagnostic tests with this patient?
   1. PET scan
   2. MRI
   3. TEE
   4. Echocardiogram

3. A patient with a serum creatinine level of 2.8 mg/dL is scheduled for a cardiac catheterization. Which of the following should be done to assist this patient?
   1. Provide an antihistamine prior to the procedure.
   2. Provide intravenous normal saline prior to the procedure.
   3. Provide an injection of steroids prior to the procedure.
   4. Provide intravenous dextrose prior to the procedure.

4. A patient experienced an acute myocardial infarction the previous day. Of the following diagnostic tests planned for this patient, which of the following would be contraindicated at this time?
   1. ECG
   2. Echocardiogram
   3. PCI
   4. Stress test

5. While assessing a patient recovering from a cardiac catheterization, the nurse is unable to assess the pedal pulse on the limb used for the procedure. Which of the following should the nurse do?
   1. Readjust the patient's foot.
   2. Apply warm blankets to the patient's feet.
   3. Assess the femoral site.
   4. Ask the patient to move the foot.

Answers for review questions appear in Appendix D

KEY TERMS

REFERENCES

Abraham, W. T., & Hayes, D. L. (2003). Cardiac resynchronization therapy for heart failure. *Circulation,108*, 2596–2603.

Agatson, A. S., Janowitz, W. R., Hildner, F. J., Zusmer, N. R., Viamonte, M., Jr., & Detrano, R. (1990). Quantification of coronary artery calcium using ultrafast computed tomography. *Journal of the American College of Cardiology, 15*, 827–832.

Amato-Vealey, E., & Colonies, P. A. (2005). Demystifying biphasic defibrillation. *Nursing2005, 35*(8, Suppl.), ED Insider, 6–11.

American Heart Association. (2003). *Heart disease and stroke statistics—2004 update.* Dallas, TX: Author.

Apple, S. (2000). Interdisciplinary management of the interventional patient. In S. Apple & J. Lindsay, Jr. (Eds.), *Principles and practice of interventional cardiology* (pp. 229–263). Philadelphia: Lippincott Williams & Wilkins.

Armstrong, W. F., & Feigenbaum, H. (2001). Echocardiography. In E. Braunwald, D. P. Zipes, & P. Libby (Eds.), *Heart disease* (6th ed., pp. 160–236). Philadelphia: W. B. Saunders.

Auricchio, A., & Abraham, W. T. (2004). Cardiac resynchronization therapy: Current state of the art cost versus benefit. *Circulation, 109*, 300–307.

Baim, D. S. (2000). Percutaneous approach, including transseptal and apical puncture. In D. S. Baim & W. Grossman (Eds.), *Grossman's cardiac catheterization, angiography, and intervention* (6th ed., pp. 69–100). Philadelphia: Lippincott Williams & Wilkins.

Baim, D. S., & Grossman, W. (2000a). Complications of cardiac catheterization. In D. S. Baim & W. Grossman (Eds.), *Grossman's cardiac catheterization, angiography, and intervention* (6th ed., pp. 35–65). Philadelphia: Lippincott Williams & Wilkins.

Baim, D. S., & Grossman, W. (2000b). Coronary angiography. In D. S. Baim & W. Grossman (Eds.), *Grossman's cardiac catheterization, angiography, and intervention* (6th ed., pp. 211–256). Philadelphia: Lippincott Williams & Wilkins.

Blancher, S. (2005). Cardiac electrophysiology procedures. In S. L. Woods, E. S. S. Froelicher, S. A. Motzer, & E. J. Bridges (Eds.), *Cardiac nursing* (5th ed., pp. 425–438). Philadelphia: Lippincott Williams & Wilkins.

Bond, E. F., & Heitkemper, M. M. (2005). Complementary and alternative medicine in cardiac and vascular disease. In S. L. Woods, E. S. S. Froelicher, S. A. Motzer, & E. J. Bridges (Eds.), *Cardiac nursing* (5th ed., pp. 974–985). Philadelphia: Lippincott Williams & Wilkins.

Cannon, R. O. (2002). Restenosis after angioplasty. *New England Journal of Medicine, 346*, 1182–1183.

Carrozza, J. P., Jr., & Baim, D. S. (2000). Coronary stenting. In D. S. Baim & W. Grossman (Eds.), *Grossman's cardiac catheterization, angiography, and intervention* (6th ed., pp. 639–666). Philadelphia: Lippincott Williams & Wilkins.

Chaitman, B. R. (2001). Exercise testing. In E. Braunwald, D. P. Zipes, & P. Libby (Eds.), *Heart disease* (6th ed., pp. 129–159). Philadelphia: W. B. Saunders.

Cheitlin, M. D., Armstrong, W. F., Aurigemma, G. P., Beller, G. A., Bierman, F. Z., Davis, J. L., et al. (2003). ACC/AHA/ASE 2003 guideline update for the clinical application of echocardiography—Summary article: A report of the American College of Cardiology/American Heart Association Task Force on Practice Guidelines. *Circulation, 108*, 1146–1162.

Chou, T. M., Fitzgerald, P. J., & Yock, P. G. (2000). Intravascular ultrasound. In D. S. Baim & W. Grossman (Eds.), *Grossman's cardiac catheterization, angiography, and intervention* (6th ed., pp. 423–444). Philadelphia: Lippincott Williams & Wilkins.

Choudhury, R. P., Fuster, V., Badimon, J. J., Fisher, E. A., & Fayad, Z. A. (2002). MRI and characterization of atherosclerotic plaque: Emerging application and molecular imaging. *Arteriosclerosis, Thrombosis, and Vascular Biology, 22*, 1065–1074.

Crawford, M. H., Berstein, S. J., Deedwania, P. C., DiMarco, J. P., Ferrick, K. J., Garson, A., Jr., et al. (1999). ACC/AHA guidelines for ambulatory electrocardiography—Executive summary and recommendations: A report of the American College of

Cardiology/American Heart Association Task Force on Practice Guidelines. *Circulation, 100*, 886–893.

Davidson, C. J., & Bonow, R. O. (2001). Cardiac catheterization. In E. Braunwald, D. P. Zipes, & P. Libby (Eds.), *Heart disease* (6th ed., pp. 359–386). Philadelphia: W. B. Saunders.

Deelstra, M. S., & Jacobson, C. (2005). Cardiac catheterization. In S. L. Woods, E. S. S. Froelicher, S. A. Motzer, & E. J. Bridges (Eds.), *Cardiac nursing* (5th ed., pp. 459–477). Philadelphia: Lippincott Williams & Wilkins.

Detrano, R., & Carr, J. J. (2002). Computed tomography of the heart. In E. J. Topol (Ed.), *Textbook of cardiovascular medicine* (2nd ed., pp. 1281–1296). Philadelphia: Lippincott Williams & Wilkins.

Drew, B. J. (2002). Celebrating the 100th birthday of the electrocardiogram: Lessons learned from research in cardiac monitoring. *American Journal of Critical Care, 11*, 387–389.

Drew, B. J., & Ide, B. (1999). Could inaccurate lead placement cause misdiagnosis of the culprit artery in patients with acute myocardial infarction? *Progress in Cardiovascular Nursing, 14*, 33–34.

Fayad, Z. A., Fuster, V., Nikolaou, K., & Becker, C. (2002). Computed tomography and magnetic resonance imaging for noninvasive coronary angiography and plaque imaging: Current and potential future concepts. *Circulation, 106*, 2026–2034.

Federal Occupational Health. (2008). *Automated external defibrillator program.* Retrieved February 24, 2008, from http://www.foh.dhhs.gov/Public/ProductFocus/Apr2006/AED.asp

Fenton, J. M. (2001). The clinician's approach to evaluating patients with dysrhythmias. *AACN Clinical Issues, 12*, 72–86.

Fletcher, G. F., Balady, G. J., Amsterdam, E. A., Chaitman, B., Eckel, R., Fleg, J., et al. (2001). Exercise standards for testing and training. *Circulation, 104*, 1694–1740.

Forgoros, R. N. (2006). *The MUGA scan. About heart disease.* Retrieved May 20, 2007, from http://heartdisease.about.com/cs/cardiactests/a/muga.htm

Fuseini, M., Goodwin, W. J., Ferris, E. J., & Mehta, J. L. (2003). Does electron beam computer tomography provide added value in the diagnosis of coronary artery disease? *Current Opinion in Cardiology, 18*, 385–393.

Futterman, L. G., & Lemberg, L. (2002). Ambulatory electrocardiographic monitoring: Use of the implantable loop recorder in the evaluation of syncope. *Journal of Cardiovascular Nursing, 16*, 24–33.

Gibbons, R. J., Balady, G. J., Bricker, J. T., Chaitman, B. R., Fletcher, G. F., Froelicher, V. F., et al. (2002). ACC/AHA 2002 guideline update for exercise testing: A report of the American College of Cardiology/American Heart Association Task Force on Practice Guidelines (Committee on Exercise Testing). Retrieved, May 10, 2008 from http://linkinghub.elsevier.com/retrieve/pii/S0735109702021642

Gold, M. E., & Farnsworth, N. (2002). Alternative medicines for cardiovascular diseases. *Journal of Cardiovascular Nursing, 16*, v–viii.

Goldin, J. G., Ratib, O., & Aberle, D. R. (2000). Contemporary cardiac imaging. *Journal of Thoracic Imaging, 15*, 218–229.

Grech, E. D. (2003). ABC of interventional cardiology: Pathophysiology and investigation of coronary artery disease. *British Medical Journal, 326*, 1027–1030.

Greenland, P., & Gaziano, J. M. (2003). Selecting asymptomatic patients for coronary computed tomography or electrocardiographic exercise testing. *New England Journal of Medicine, 349*, 465–473.

Gregoratos, G., Abrams, J., Epstein, A. E., Freedman, R. A., Hayes, D. L., Hlatky, M. A., et al. (2002). ACC/AHA/NASPE 2002 guideline update for implantation of cardiac pacemakers and antiarrhythmia devices—Summary article: A report of the American College of Cardiology/American Heart Association Task Force on Practice Guidelines (ACC/AHA/NASPE Committee to Update the 1998 Pacemaker Guidelines). *Circulation, 106*, 2145–2161.

Grossman, W. (2000a). Historical perspective and present practice of cardiac catheterization. In D. S. Baim & W. Grossman (Eds.), *Grossman's cardiac catheterization, angiography, and intervention* (6th ed., pp. 3–14). Philadelphia: Lippincott Williams & Wilkins.

Grossman, W. (2000b). Shunt detection and quantification. In D. S. Baim & W. Grossman (Eds.), *Grossman's cardiac catheterization, angiography, and intervention* (6th ed., pp. 179–191). Philadelphia: Lippincott Williams & Wilkins.

Grundy, S. M., Cleeman, J. I., Merz, C. N. B., Brewer, H. B., Jr., Clark, L. T., Hunninghake, D. B., et al. (2004). Implications of recent clinical trials for the National Cholesterol Education program Adult Treatment Panel III guidelines. *Circulation, 110*, 227–239.

Grüntzig, A. (1978). Transluminal dilation of coronary-artery stenosis. *Lancet, 1*, 263.

Hall, M. L. (2005). Echocardiography. In S. L. Woods, E. S. S. Froelicher, S. A. Motzer, & E. J. Bridges (Eds.), *Cardiac nursing* (5th ed., pp. 307–318). Philadelphia: Lippincott Williams & Wilkins.

Hallstrom, A. P., Ornato, J. P., Weisfeldt, M., & Travers, J. (2004). Public-access defibrillation and survival after out-of-hospital cardiac arrest: The public access defibrillation trial investigators. *New England Journal of Medicine, 351*(7), 637–646.

Helena Cardiology Clinic. (n.d.). *Holter monitoring.* Retrieved March 26, 2004, from http://www.helenacardiology.com/holtermonitor.htm

Higgins, C. B. (2002). Newer cardiac imaging modalities: Magnetic resonance imaging and computed tomography. In E. Braunwald, D. P. Zipes, & P. Libby (Eds.), *Heart disease* (6th ed., pp. 324–358). Philadelphia: W. B. Saunders.

Holter, N. J. (1961). New method for heart studies: Continuous electrocardiography of active subjects is now practical. *Science, 34*, 1214–1219.

Iskandrian, A. E., & Verani, M. S. (2002). Nuclear imaging techniques. In E. J. Topol (Ed.), *Textbook of cardiovascular medicine* (2nd ed., pp. 1192–1211). Philadelphia: Lippincott Williams & Wilkins.

Jacobson, C., & Gerity, D. (2005). Pacemakers and implantable defibrillators. In S. L. Woods, E. S. S. Froelicher, S. A. Motzer, & E. J. Bridges (Eds.), *Cardiac nursing* (5th ed., pp. 709–755). Philadelphia: Lippincott Williams & Wilkins.

Janosik, D. L., Quattromani, A., & Schiller, L. (2003). Electrophysiologic studies and ablation techniques. In M. J. Kern (Ed.), *The cardiac catheterization handbook* (4th ed., pp. 326–398). Philadelphia: Mosby.

Kadish, A. H., Buxton, A. E., Kennedy, H. L., Knight, B. P., Mason, J. W., Schuger, C. D., et al. (2001). ACC/AHA clinical competence statement on electrocardiography and ambulatory electrocardiography: A report of the American College of Cardiology/American Heart Association/American College of Physicians/American Society of Internal Medicine Task Force on Clinical Competence (ACC/AHA Committee to Develop a Clinical Competence Statement on Electrocardiography and Ambulatory Electrocardiography). *Circulation, 104*, 3169–3178.

Kent, K. M. (2000). Development of interventional cardiology. In S. Apple & J. Lindsay, Jr. (Eds.), *Principles and practice of interventional cardiology* (pp. 1–12). Philadelphia: Lippincott Williams & Wilkins.

Klocke, F. J., Baird, M. G., Bateman, T. M., Berman, D. S., Carabello, B. A., Cerqueria, M. D., et al. (2003). ACC/AHA/ASNC guidelines for the clinical use of cardiac radionuclide imaging: A report of the American College of Cardiology/American Heart Association Task Force on Practice Guidelines (ACC/AHA/ASNC Committee to Revise the 1995 Guidelines for the Clinical Use of Radionuclide Imaging). Retrieved March 4, 2004, from http://www.ncbi.nlm.nih.gov/pubmed/12975245

Kloner, R. A., Bolli, R., Marbán, E., Reinlib, L., & Braunwald, E. (1998). Medical and cellular implications of stunning, hibernation, and preconditioning: An NHLBI workshop. *Circulation, 97*, 1848–1867.

Koreny, M., Riedmuller, E., Nikfardjam, M., Siostrzonek, P., & Mullner, M. (2004). Arterial puncture closing devices compared with standard manual compression after cardiac catheterization: Systematic review and meta-analysis. *Journal of the American Medical Association, 291*, 350–357.

Lamas, G. A., Ellenbogen, K. A., with the assistance of Hennekens, C. H., & Montanez, A. (2004). Evidence base for pacemaker mode selection: From physiology to randomized trials. *Circulation, 109,* 443–451.

Leclercq, C., & Hare, J. M. (2004). Ventricular resynchronization: Current state of the art. *Circulation, 109,* 296–299.

Lee, T. H., & Brennan, T. A. (2002). Direct-to-consumer marketing of high-technology screening tests. *New England Journal of Medicine, 346,* 529–531.

Legge, D., & Leeper, B. (2002). Resynchronization therapy for the management of heart failure. *Critical Care Nursing Clinics of North America, 15*(4), 467–475.

Lindsay, J., Jr., Apple, S., Pinnow, E. E., Gevorkian, N., Gruberg, L., Satler, L. F., et al. (2003). Percutaneous coronary intervention–associated nephropathy foreshadows increased risk of late adverse events in patients with normal baseline serum creatinine. *Catheterization and Cardiovascular Interventions, 59,* 338–343.

Lindsay, J., Jr., & Pinnow, E. E. (2000). Outcomes of percutaneous transluminal coronary revascularization. In S. Apple & J. Lindsay, Jr. (Eds.), *Principles and practice of interventional cardiology* (pp. 277–286). Philadelphia: Lippincott Williams & Wilkins.

Lüderitz, B. (1995). *History of the disorders of cardiac rhythm* (2nd ed.). Armonk, NY: Futura.

Marwick, T. H. (2002). Stress echocardiography. In E. J. Topol (Ed.), *Textbook of cardiovascular medicine* (2nd ed., pp. 1115–1142). Philadelphia: Lippincott Williams & Wilkins.

Marwick, T. H. (2003). Stress echocardiography. *Heart, 89,* 113–118.

Milani, R. V., Lavie, C. J., Gilliland, Y. E., Cassidy, M. M., & Bernal, J. A. (2003). Overview of transesophageal echocardiography for the chest physician. *Chest, 124,* 1081–1089.

Miller, J. M., & Zipes, D. P. (2001). Management of the patient with cardiac dysrhythmias. In E. Braunwald, D. P. Zipes, & P. Libby (Eds.), *Heart disease* (6th ed., pp. 700–774). Philadelphia: W. B. Saunders.

Mintz, G. S., & Walsh, C. (2000). Intravascular ultrasound imaging. In S. Apple & J. Lindsay, Jr. (Eds.), *Principles and practice of interventional cardiology* (pp. 161–183). Philadelphia: Lippincott Williams & Wilkins.

Mirowski, M. (1985). The automatic implantable cardioverter-defibrillator. *American Journal of Cardiology, 6,* 461–466.

Mulvagh, S. L., DeMaria, A. N., Feinstein, S. B., Burns, P. N., Kaul, S., Miller, J. G., et al. (2000). Contrast echocardiography: Current and future applications. *Journal of the American Society of Echocardiography, 13,* 331–342.

Myers, J. (2005). Exercise testing. In S. L. Woods, E. S. S. Froelicher, S. A. Motzer, & E. J. Bridges (Eds.), *Cardiac nursing* (5th ed., pp. 439–458). Philadelphia: Lippincott Williams & Wilkins.

National Institutes of Health National Center for Complementary and Alternative Medicine. (2008). The use of complementary and alternative medicine in the United States. Retrieved August 20, 2008, from http://nccam.nih.gov

Nikolaou, K., Poon, M., Sirol, M., Becker, C. R., & Fayad, Z. A. (2003). Complementary results of computed tomography and magnetic resonance imaging of the heart and coronary arteries: A review and future outlook. *Cardiology Clinics, 21,* 639–655.

Obias-Manno, D. (2001). Unconventional applications in pacemaker therapy. *AACN Clinical Issues, 12,* 127–139.

O'Neill, W. W., & Dixon, S. R. (2004). The year in interventional cardiology. *Journal of the American College of Cardiology, 43,* 875–890.

O'Rourke, R. A., Brundage, B. H., Froelicher, V. F., Greenland, P., Grundy, S. M., Hachamovitch, R., et al. (2000). American College of Cardiology/American Heart Association expert consensus document on electron-beam computed tomography for the diagnosis and prognosis of coronary artery disease. *Circulation, 102,* 126–140.

Overbay, D., & Criddle, L. (2004). Mastering temporary invasive cardiac pacing. *Critical Care Nurse, 24,* 25–32.

Peterson, G. E., Brickner, E., & Reimold, S. C. (2003). Transesophageal echocardiography: Clinical indications and applications. *Circulation, 107,* 2398–2402.

Pohost, G. M., Hung, L., & Doyle, M. (2003). Clinical use of cardiovascular magnetic resonance. *Circulation, 108,* 647–653.

Popma, J. J., & Bittl, J. (2001). Coronary angiography and intravascular ultrasonography. In E. Braunwald, D. P. Zipes, & P. Libby (Eds.), *Heart disease* (6th ed., pp. 387–421). Philadelphia: W. B. Saunders.

Popma, J. J., & Kuntz, R. E. (2001). Percutaneous coronary and valvular intervention. In E. Braunwald, D. P. Zipes, & P. Libby (Eds.), *Heart disease* (6th ed., pp. 1364–1405). Philadelphia: W. B. Saunders.

Quiñones, M. A., Douglas, P. S., Foster, E., Gorcsan, J., III, Lewis, J. F., Pearlman, A. S., et al. (2003). American College of Cardiology/American Heart Association clinical competence statement of echocardiography: A report of the American College of Cardiology/American Heart Association/American College of Physicians/American Society of Internal Medicine Task Force on Clinical Competence. *Circulation, 107,* 1068–1089.

Reynolds, J., & Apple, S. (2001). A systematic approach to pacemaker assessment. *AACN Clinical Issues, 12,* 114–126.

Rosen, M. R. (2002). The electrocardiogram 100 years later: Electrical insights into molecular messages. *Circulation, 106,* 2173–2179.

Scanlon, P. J., Faxon, D. P., Audet, A., Carabello, B., Dehmer, G. J., Eagle, K. A., et al. (1999). ACC/AHA guidelines for coronary angiography: Executive summary and recommendations. *Circulation, 99,* 2345–2357.

Schoepf, U. J., Becker, C. R., Hofmann, L. K., & Yucel, E. K. (2003). Multidetector-row CT of the heart. *Radiologic Clinics of North America, 41,* 491–505.

Schvartzman, P. R., & White, R. D. (2002). Magnetic resonance imaging. In E. J. Topol (Ed.), *Textbook of cardiovascular medicine* (2nd ed., pp. 1213–1256). Philadelphia: Lippincott Williams & Wilkins.

Smith, R. L., & Thomas, J. D. (2002). Transthoracic echocardiography. In E. J. Topol (Ed.), *Textbook of cardiovascular medicine* (2nd ed., pp. 1091–1113). Philadelphia: Lippincott Williams & Wilkins.

Smith, S. C., Jr., Dove, J. T., Jacobs, A. K., Kennedy, J. W., Kereiakes, D., Kern, M. J., et al. (2001). ACC/AHA guidelines for percutaneous coronary intervention. *Circulation.* 2001;103:3019.

Soine, L., & Hanrahan, M. (2005). Nuclear and other imaging studies. In S. L. Woods, E. S. S. Froelicher, S. A. Motzer, & E. J. Bridges (Eds.), *Cardiac nursing* (5th ed., pp. 319–325). Philadelphia: Lippincott Williams & Wilkins.

Sousa, J. E., Serruys, P. W., & Costa, M. A. (2003). New frontiers in cardiology: Drug eluting stents. *Circulation, 107,* Part I, pp. 2274–2279, Part II, pp. 2383–2389.

Squires, S. (2003, September 16). The selling of the stent. *The Washington Post,* pp. F1, F5.

Stewart, M. J. (2003). Contrast echocardiography. *Heart, 89,* 342–348.

Stone, K. R., & McPherson, C. A. (2004). Assessment and management of patients with pacemakers and implantable cardioverter defibrillators. *Critical Care Medicine, 32,* S155–S165.

Teirstein, P. S., & Kuntz, R. E. (2001). New frontiers in interventional cardiology: Intravascular radiation to prevent restenosis. *Circulation, 104,* 2620–2626.

Thomas, J. D. (2002). Principles of imaging. In E. J. Topol (Ed.), *Textbook of cardiovascular medicine* (2nd ed., pp. 1031–1045). Philadelphia: Lippincott Williams & Wilkins.

Tracy, C. M., Akhtar, M., DiMarco, J. P., Packer, D. L., & Weitz, H. H. (2000). American College of Cardiology/American Heart Association clinical competence statement on invasive electrophysiology studies, catheter ablation, and cardioversion. *Circulation, 102,* 2309–2320.

Wackers, F. J. T., Soufer, R., & Zaret, B. L. (2001). Nuclear cardiology. In E. Braunwald, D. P. Zipes, & P. Libby (Eds.), *Heart disease* (6th ed., pp. 273–323). Philadelphia: W. B. Saunders.

Waksman, R. (2000). Restenosis. In S. Apple & J. Lindsay, Jr. (Eds.), *Principles and practice of interventional cardiology* (pp. 213–228). Philadelphia: Lippincott Williams & Wilkins.

Weinberger, J., Lincoff, A. M., & Popma, J. J. (2002). New techniques in interventional cardiology: Radiation, emboli protection, and therapeutic angiogenesis. In E. J. Topol (Ed.), *Textbook of cardiovascular medicine* (2nd ed., pp. 1677–1714). Philadelphia: Lippincott Williams & Wilkins.

Weyman, A. E. (2004). The year in echocardiography. *Journal of the American College of Cardiology, 43,* 140–148.

White, M. M. (2002). Psychosocial impact of the implantable cardioverter defibrillator: Nursing implications. *Journal of Cardiovascular Nursing, 16,* 53–61.

Wu, K. C., & Lima, J. A. C. (2003). Noninvasive imaging of myocardial viability: Current techniques and future developments. *Circulation Research, 93,* 1146–1158.

Zoll, P. M. (1952). Resuscitation of the heart in ventricular standstill by external electrical stimulation. *New England Journal of Medicine, 247,* 768–771.

CHAPTER 40

Caring for the Patient with Coronary Artery Disease

Kori Harder
Kathleen Osborn
James Stotts

With Contribution By:
Gina Flaharty, Coronary Artery Bypass Graft
Surgery Section

Outcome-Based Learning Objectives

After studying this chapter, the learner will be able to:

1. Discuss the epidemiological factors of coronary artery disease (CAD) and define the risk factors.

2. Define and identify the etiology and pathophysiology of CAD/ischemic heart disease and explain the nursing assessment data and interventions used when evaluating a patient with angina pectoris.

3. Differentiate the three criteria used to evaluate ischemic heart disease and identify the pathologic significance of each criterion.

4. Compare and contrast the pathogenesis of unstable angina, a non Q wave, subendocardial, non–ST segment elevation myocardial infarction (MI), and a Q wave, transmural, ST segment elevation (MI).

5. Identify the complications of an MI and discuss the variables that affect the prognosis of the patient with an MI.

6. Identify which clinical manifestations and diagnostic finding are an indication for coronary artery bypass graft surgery (CABG).

7. Identify three possible complications of CABG and discuss nursing interventions that potentially reduce the incidence of these complications.

A NEIGHBOR comes frantically knocking on the door saying that her husband is having chest pain and has just passed out. She is asking for help. A postoperative orthopedic patient is complaining of chest pressure. She has a history of myocardial infarction (MI), commonly referred to as a heart attack. A postoperative cholecystectomy patient shows dramatic ST segment elevation on the cardiac monitor. A 33-year-old with peripartum myocarditis complains of shortness of breath and palpitations. Each of these scenarios represents manifestations of coronary artery disease (CAD). The differences in settings highlight the fact that CAD is not gender, age, or specialty specific. Despite where one works the chances of caring for a patient, neighbor, or family member with CAD are high. This chapter discusses the clinical relevance to the prevalence, presentation, diagnostic work-up, and care guidelines for patients with manifestations of CAD.

Coronary Artery Anatomy

Coronary arteries are comprised of three concentric layers of differentiated cells separated by elastic membranes (Figure 40–1 ■). The **tunica intima** consists of endothelial cells, connective tissue, and smooth muscle cells. Once considered simply as a diffusing

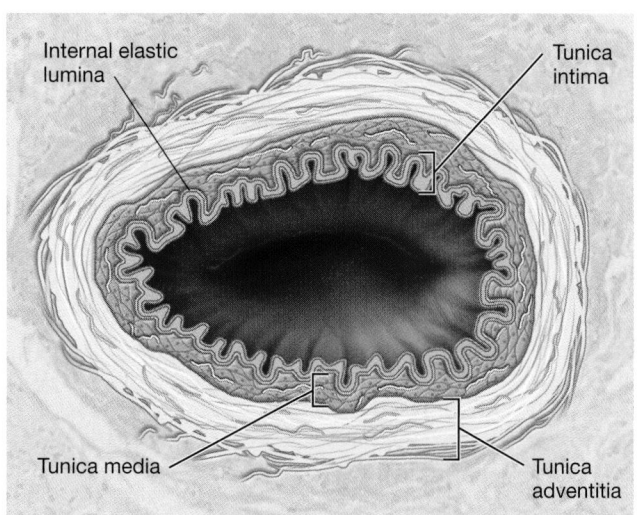

FIGURE 40–1 ■ Normal artery layers.

barrier between blood and the subintimal, it is now recognized that the endothelium regulates vasomotor tone, pro- and anticoagulant stimulation, mediation of inflammatory and growth factors, and the adhesion and entry of inflammatory cells and lipids into the vessel wall. Adjacent to the intima is the internal elastic membrane (internal elastic lumina), a fenestrated sheet of elastic tissue that separates the intima from the medial layer.

The **tunica media**, the middle layer of the artery, consists of multiple layers of smooth muscle cells and connective tissue made up of elastic fibers, collagen, and proteoglycans (Figure 40–1 ■). The external elastic membrane (external elastic lumina) separates the medial layer from the adventitia. The external elastic membrane, comprised of interrupted layers of elastin, is thinner than the internal elastic membrane.

The **tunica adventitia,** the outer layer of the artery, is a flexible stratum consisting of fibrous tissue made of collagen and elastic fibers surrounded by collagen bundles (Figure 40–1 ■). The loose structure of the adventitia and the adjoining collagen bundles facilitates coronary vessel diameter changes during vasodilation and constriction. The adventitia also contains nerve fibers and, in larger vessels, the vasa vasorum, which is a network of arteries and veins that provide blood supply to the vessel wall.

Epidemiology of Coronary Artery Disease

Coronary artery disease (CAD) is defined as a progressive atherosclerotic disorder of the coronary arteries that results in narrowing or complete occlusion of the vessel lumen. This disease claims more lives each year in the United States than the next five leading causes of death combined (American Heart Association [AHA], 2006d). Coronary artery disease is responsible for approximately 50% of cardiovascular events in both men and women under the age of 75 (AHA, 2006d). CAD causes one-fifth of all deaths in the United States, making it the single largest killer of the American population. It is the leading cause of death in both males and females of white, African American, Hispanic, American Indian, and Asian Pacific Island ethnicities (AHA, 2006d). The overall risk of CAD is greater in men than in women, until menopause when it becomes more equal (AHA, 2006d).

The economic impact of CAD is significant. It is the leading cause of early, permanent disability in the U.S. labor force, with 22% of those over age 65 unable to return to work following a myocardial infarction (MI) (AHA, 2006d). Medical costs are significant with diagnostic testing of nearly 6 million patient visits to the emergency department annually for symptoms suspected of CAD and 2 million hospital discharges at an annual cost of $133 billion (AHA, 2006d). CAD is the leading cause of death, afflicts all ethnic groups and ages, and consumes the greatest portion of our national health dollars. The magnitude and pervasiveness of CAD provide sound rationale for advocating a greater allocation of research funds toward the prevention and treatment of CAD. Care providers, regardless of health care setting, are very likely to find that they are responsible for managing the care of a patient with CAD.

Etiology of Coronary Artery Disease

Coronary artery disease (CAD) is not an acute process but one that progresses over time and can begin as early in life as infancy. The rate of progression is related to risk factors such as genetic predisposition, gender, diet, sedentary lifestyle, and smoking.

Atherosclerosis affects the medium-size arteries perfusing the heart, brain, and kidneys and the large arteries branching off the aorta. Men predate women by about 10 years for CAD and 20 years for serious cardiac events such as an acute MI or sudden cardiac death. Because women present with CAD at an older age, they have a greater risk of overall mortality and developing serious complications that will be discussed throughout the chapter. Cardiovascular disease is the number-one killer of women over 40 years of age. According to the American Heart Association (AHA, 2008c), about 500,000 women die each year from heart disease. Recent national guidelines (AHA, 2006a) specifically target treating heart disease in women. The National Guidelines for Treating Women with Heart Disease box outlines these treatments.

Pathophysiology of Coronary Artery Disease

Coronary artery disease includes abnormal conditions such as arteriosclerosis, atherosclerosis, and arteritis of the coronary arteries, all of which result in reduced flow of oxygen and nutrients to the myocardium. **Arteriosclerosis** is characterized by thickening, reduced elasticity, and calcification of the arterial wall. **Atherosclerosis**, a type of arteriosclerosis, is the most common etiologic process that causes reduced myocardial blood flow. Atherosclerosis is coronary artery luminal obstruction caused by plaque buildup of cholesterol, lipids, and cellular debris infiltrating the intimal lining of the arterial wall, causing a reduced blood flow to the myocardium. Reductions in myocardial blood supply, especially in times of increased demand, are the cause of coronary syndromes,

---

NATIONAL GUIDELINES for Treating Women with Heart Disease

- Prevention should be tailored to a woman's level of risk.
- Quitting smoking, regular exercise, diet, and weight maintenance are strong priorities for all women.
- Aspirin is recommended as a preventive measure for all high-risk women; aspirin is not recommended for low-risk women. For intermediate-risk women, aspirin can be considered as long as blood pressure is controlled and the benefits outweigh the risk of side effects.
- Blood pressure–lowering drugs are recommended when blood pressure is greater than or equal to 140/90 mmHg. Blood pressure should be maintained at less than 130/80 mmHg for women with diabetes or with damage to target end organs related to blood pressure.
- Hormone therapy and antioxidant vitamin supplements are not recommended for heart disease prevention for women at any level of risk.
- Women with heart disease should be evaluated for depression and treated or referred for treatment when indicated.
- In addition to a heart-healthy diet, supplementation with omega-3 fatty acids and folic acid may be considered in some high-risk women.
- ACE inhibitors and beta-blockers are recommended for all high-risk women.

Source: American Heart Association. (2008c). Women and Coronary Heart Disease. Retrieved on July 18, 2008 from http://www.americanheart.org/presenter.jhtml?identifier=2859.

which include stable angina, unstable angina (UA), myocardial infarction (MI), and sudden cardiac death (SCD). These conditions depict a continuum of progressively worsening imbalances between the amount of oxygenated blood delivered and that which is required by myocardial tissues.

Normally the myocardium extracts 75% of the available oxygen from the coronary arteries, which is more than is extracted from any other tissue in the body (the rest of body extracts about 40% of available oxygen). If the oxygen needs are not met from this near maximal extraction, then myocardial blood flow must be increased. Normal coronary arteries are able to dilate, and normal hearts are able to increase the force of contraction, resulting in increased blood being delivered to the cardiac muscle and cardiac output. With CAD the arteries are unable to dilate because of the plaque buildup and subsequent calcification. In addition, because of the decrease in blood supply, the heart muscle has significant difficulty increasing the force of the contraction in order to increase the cardiac output. The result of all of the unmet oxygen needs is the shift to anaerobic metabolism and myocardial tissue hypoxia, which results in angina. The term myocardial **ischemia** or tissue hypoxia is a result of this oxygen imbalance. Ischemic heart disease, which is considered reversible, is insidious with prodromal anginal or chest pain symptoms present in only 20% of patients with MI and less than 50% of patients who suffer sudden cardiac death (SCD).

Certain factors, whether experienced internally or environmentally, such as stress or physical activity cause the heart to work harder and therefore increase oxygen demand. Whereas CAD decreases the blood supply to the myocardium, both abnormal demand and supply issues can cause angina to occur. Chart 40–1 outlines the most common factors that impact supply and demand.

The pathophysiology of plaque generation, development, composition, and injury provides the basis on which medical therapies for prevention of coronary artery disease and management of its sequelae have developed. The process of atherosclerotic development is described next.

Atherogenesis

An **atheroma** is an accumulation of plaque in the inner lining of an artery made up of cholesterol and other constituents. The cause of plaque generation is still unclear to researchers. One theory proposes that plaque pathogenesis is a response to injury to the vessel wall. Potential causes of injury include mechanical, chemical, immunologic, viral, bacterial, and subendothelial stressors. Some of these stressors as well as additional stressors are included in Chart 40–2. Once the endothelial lining has been injured, it undergoes a number of structural and functional changes. There is a disruption in cell-to-cell contact or cell to underlying connective tissue contact such that the once relatively impermeable endothelial monolayer can no longer protect or regulate the exposure of subendothelial constituents from elements in the circulating bloodstream. One effect of subendothelial cells coming in contact with blood is that there is a loss of endothelial vasodilatory control, as demonstrated by a decrease in focal endothelial-derived relaxing factor (EDRF) or nitric oxide (NO) synthesis and release, and increased sensitivity to catecholamines. Thus, rather than stimulating compensatory vasodilation, ischemia causes vasoconstriction in areas of vessel disruption. Endothelial injury also causes

CHART 40–1	**Common Factors That Increase Oxygen Demand and Decrease Oxygen Supply**
Increased Oxygen Demand	**Rationale**
Exercise	Increases the heart rate, which increases the workload of the heart, and diseased coronary arteries are unable to deliver an increased amount of oxygen to the heart muscle.
Eating	During digestion after a heavy meal, the blood is diverted to the gastrointestinal system, causing low blood flow to the coronary arteries.
Emotions	Stimulate the sympathetic nervous system and increase the workload of the heart by increasing heart rate and blood pressure.
Exposure to cold	Constricts blood vessels and increases metabolism, both of which put an extra workload on the heart.
Hypertension	Because the heart has to pump against greater pressure (afterload), it increases the workload and oxygen demands.
Sexual activity	Increases sympathetic nervous system stimulation, which increases the workload on the heart.
Decreased Oxygen Supply	**Rationale**
Coronary artery spasm	Causes a decrease in the size of the lumen of the artery, which decreases blood flow to the tissues. When combined with CAD, it markedly decreases blood flow to the tissues.
Coronary artery disease	Decreases vessel lumen, which decreases blood supply to the myocardium.
Hypotension	Decreases cardiac output.
Dysrhythmias	Decreases cardiac output if occurring in significant numbers and areas of the myocardium (ventricle).
Anemia	Decreases the oxygen-carrying capacity of the blood, which decreases oxygen to the myocardium.
Smoking	Causes vasoconstriction, which increases afterload and the workload of the heart.

stimulation of internal mechanisms that result in the smooth muscle extending into the inner layer of the vessel, thereby decreasing in the lumen of the artery and a loss of elasticity. Additionally, this process causes external recruitment of inflammatory and procoagulant cells (platelets, and coagulation factors), causing them to aggregate and further decrease the size of the lumen.

Stage I Lesion

Lesions in the coronary arteries develop in stages. In early atherosclerosis, stage I lesion has grossly visible yellow lesions, known as fatty streaks, in the intimal layer. This earliest form of plaque has been found in the aortas of newborns as well as in both the young and old. These streaks cause little or no obstruction to coronary blood flow; thus, the individuals are not symptomatic. Early fatty streaks consist primarily of macrophages, foam cells, and T lymphocytes, suggesting that plaque genesis may be a response to inflammation. The lesion develops with the migration of smooth muscle cells and the accumulation of macrophages, T lymphocytes, lipids, and foam cells. In response to injury, circulating monocytes

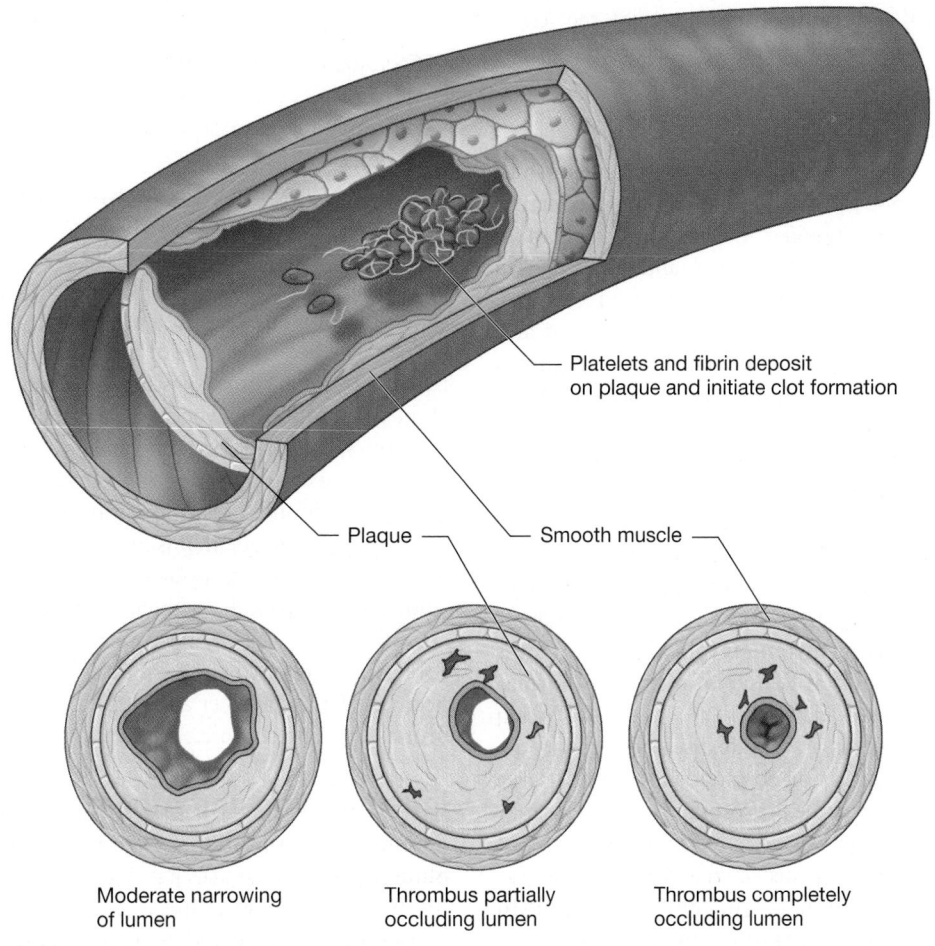

CHART 40–2	**Causes of Intimal Vessel Wall Injury**
Stressor	**Source and Effect**
Mechanical	Sheer stress from blood flow at vessel branches/bifurcation due to HTN; injury secondary to PCI procedures
Chemical	Hypercholesterolemia; homocystinemia; hydrocarbons, nicotine, and carbon monoxide from cigarettes; free fatty acids, oxygen radicals, angiotensin, hormones; oxidized lipids; oxidant stress caused by cigarette smoking, hypertension, and advanced glycation end products in diabetes mellitus; estrogen deficiency; vasoactive amines
Immunologic	Exposure to antigen–antibody complexes; virally induced injuries; exposure to bacteria; activated macrophages; infectious microorganisms such as herpesviruses, *Chlamydia pneumoniae*
Genetic	Alterations
Biologic	Advancing age

and platelets adhere to the damaged segment of endothelium. Activated platelets release their contents, and this release recruits and promotes adhesion of other platelets to the endothelium. This process then causes the release of growth factors, which inhibits cell proliferation and stimulates connective tissue formation, all of which cause a decrease in lumen size. Activated macrophages bind with lipoproteins to form foam cells. Macrophages and foam cells produce cytokines, growth factors, and other chemicals that induce and regulate the accumulation of lipids; the proliferation and migration of monocytes, T lymphocytes, possibly mast cells into the arterial wall, and smooth muscle cells from the media into the intima; and the synthesis of matrix components (Figure 40–2 ■).

Stage II Lesion

Over time, perhaps as a result of repeated injury, plaque lesions may mature with the organization of a lipid core and the formation of a fibrous cap (Figure 40–3 ■, p. 1162). This progression of the disease is referred to as a stage II lesion. During this stage the medial smooth muscle cells invade the intimal lesion, leading to a further buildup of plaque that obstructs luminal blood flow. These lesions contain an accumulation of smooth muscle cells, macrophages, T lymphocytes, intra- and extracellular lipids, foam cells, cellular debris from focal necrosis and foam cell apoptosis, and other blood components such as fibrin, fibrinogen, albumin, and white cells. The smooth muscle cells secrete collagen, elastin, and glycosaminoglycans that form a dense connective tissue matrix called the **fibrous cap**. Stage II lesions are grossly white in appearance and most frequently develop where arteries bifurcate. Figure 40–3 ■ (p. 1162) shows the fibrous cap. If the atheroma grows to occlude 40% to 45% of the vessel lumen, arterial remodeling occurs to maintain luminal diameter (Burke et al., 2002). *Remodeling* is a term used to describe how cells, tissue,

Platelets and fibrin deposit on plaque and initiate clot formation

Plaque — Smooth muscle

Moderate narrowing of lumen

Thrombus partially occluding lumen

Thrombus completely occluding lumen

FIGURE 40–2 ■ Stage of atheroma development in a coronary artery.

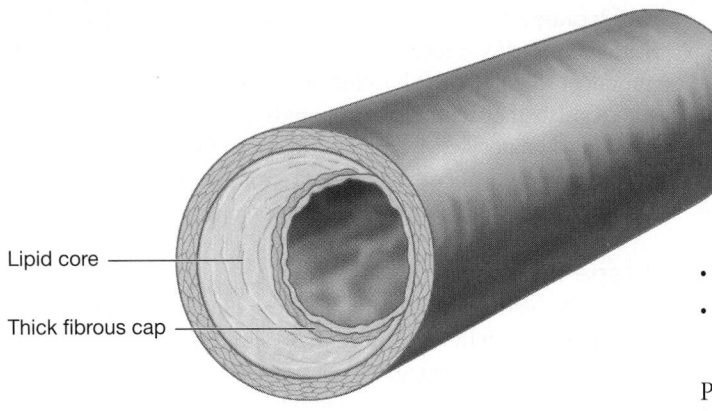

Lipid core

Thick fibrous cap

FIGURE 40–3 ■ Fibrous cap.

or organs react or change in response to injury that either serves to maintain function or structure (positive remodeling) or results in further disruption of normal processes (negative remodeling). With positive remodeling, despite increasing atheroma size within the intima, the vessel accommodates through expansion or stretching of the external elastic lumina. Over time, with continued plaque growth, negative remodeling occurs, which refers to shrinking or constriction of the external elastic lumina, resulting in increasing stenosis of the vessel lumen (Schoenhagen et al., 2002) (see Figure 40–3 ■). Once arterial diameter is reduced by 70%, whether due to plaque size or thrombosis, the patient develops symptoms of CAD such as angina. Coronary artery stenosis is described as either **eccentric,** meaning that the lesion occupies part of the vessel wall circumference, or **concentric**, whereby the lesion occupies the whole circumference.

Stage III Lesion

Advanced or stage III lesions are plaque with a well-established fibrous cap and lipid core. Further development and calcification of the fibrous matrix and lipid core, ulceration and hemorrhage of the fibrous cap and intimal surface, and increased risk of transluminal thrombosis characterize an advanced lesion.

In some lesions the fibrous cap becomes vascularized and grows in size; others calcify and become hardened; still others may be thin and poorly developed. Vessel segments with hardened fibrous caps are less responsive to ischemia-related vasodilatory compensatory mechanisms, which results in the vessel not dilating during periods of increased need for oxygen. In complicated lesions the lipid-rich core increases in size, may become calcified, and fills with necrotic cellular debris. As the atheroma enlarges, the intimal surface may develop fissures or cracks, referred to as plaque rupture, which exposes the subendothelial matrix and initiating **thrombus** (blood clot that forms in a blood vessel and remains at the site of formation) formation, described earlier (see Figure 40–2 ■, p. 1161). When thrombus formation occurs in an already diseased coronary artery, it causes further obstruction to blood flow, and if large enough it may completely occlude the coronary artery. This may stop all blood flow to the tissues being fed by the artery, thus leading to tissue ischemia and, if sustained, cell death.

Plaque anatomy and defining plaque that is vulnerable to rupture have received a great deal of attention. Studies have identified certain characteristics that suggest plaque instabil-

ity, which increases the risk for rupture (Pasterkamp, Fitzgerald, & de Kleijn, 2002). Plaque "prone to rupture" is associated with the following factors:

- Positive remodeling
- A thin fibrous cap
- A core rich in lipids, calcium deposits, macrophages, T lymphocytes, and mast cells
- A paucity of collagen and smooth muscle cells
- Of a size large enough to cause mild to moderate luminal obstruction (Pasterkamp et al., 2002).

Plaque injury occurs in lesions that are predominantly yellow in color with ragged edges. Unstable lesions are associated with areas of plaque hemorrhage and neovascularization (blood supply) within the fibrous cap. They are also associated with points of endothelial disruption or ulceration overlying the fibrous cap; sites where the fibrous cap is thinnest, typically at the shoulder where it attaches to the vessel; and sites where there is a dense concentration of matrix metalloproteinases (MMPs). Matrix metalloproteinases are proinflammatory substances that contribute to the breakdown of the fibrous cap. It is thought that MMPs play a role in plaque vulnerability. These lesions may be difficult to identify. Often there is not a flow-limiting stenosis and the patient is asymptomatic. Normal detection with conventional methods such as stress testing and angiography may be inconclusive.

Unstable angina (UA), non–ST segment elevation MI (NSTEMI), and ST segment elevation MI (STEMI) are the three syndromes that collectively describe **acute coronary syndrome (ACS)**. Acute coronary syndrome, which is discussed later in the chapter, results when the plaque buildup in the artery becomes significant enough to cause ischemia that result in clinical manifestations.

A recent consensus paper suggests that when unstable plaque is conjoined with conditions of blood and myocardial maladies, the risk for ACS increases (Naghavi et al., 2003b). Blood abnormalities include abnormal platelet function or structure, hypercoagulable states, and/or reduced anticoagulation factors. Blood that is prone to coagulate because of one of these blood disorders increases the risk of thrombus formation when combined with plaque development or disruption. Myocardial maladies can be caused by dysrhythmias, reduced or abnormal ventricular function, and reduced myocardial perfusion. These patients are at higher risk of death from chronic and acute coronary artery occlusion.

In contrast, plaque that is more stable is associated with negative remodeling, a smooth surface with a predominant white color and no thrombi, a thick calcified fibrous cap with little smooth muscle cell or macrophage content, a smaller plaque core consisting of collagen, smooth muscle cells, and apoptotic necrosis (Pasterkamp et al., 2002). Lesions of this type are less prone to plaque rupture.

Inflammation and Atherogenesis

Recently the association between atherogenesis and the immune complex response has been described in the literature. Immune complex response is described in Chapter 60 ☺. At every stage of plaque development, leukocytes act as instigators and regulators of many processes that are associated with plaque development, such as endothelial dysfunction, procoagulant activity, subendothelial macrophage and smooth muscle cell activity, fibrous cap matrix formation and degradation, and enhanced lipoprotein transfer in the vessel wall. Research studies have suggested that certain infectious organisms may stimulate an immune response that results in plaque disruption, plaque growth, or thrombosis in areas of existing atheroma (Higuchi et al., 2003; Pieniazek et al., 2001). Increased titers of antibodies to certain organisms such as cytomegalovirus, herpesvirus, *Chlamydia pneumoniae,* and *Helicobacter pylori* have been identified as possible predictors of elevated risk for coronary artery occlusions (Higuchi et al., 2003; Pieniazek et al., 2001). It is unclear what effect these organisms have on the cells of the vessel lining; however, these organisms have been found in atheromatous lesions and organs either at autopsy or from atheroma samples. In addition, patients with ACS demonstrate elevated levels of serum markers of inflammation, activated leukocytosis, and their by-products of cytokine, growth factor, and smooth muscle cell activation, which indicate a heightened inflammatory response (Aggarwal et al., 2004; Nomoto et al., 2003). These findings strongly suggest a role of inflammation in either propagating or promoting atherogenesis, or that inflammatory markers are signs that plaque disruption is ongoing and thus are considered markers of increased risk for future sentinel cardiac events (Porth, 2005; Rosenson & Koenig, 2003). Several serum markers of inflammation have been identified, including C-reactive protein (CRP).

Pathophysiology of Myocardial Injury and Death

Myocardial injury from ischemia begins in the subendocardium and progresses to the epicardium (Figure 40–4 ■). If blood flow is not restored within 20 minutes, cell death ensues, autodigestion of cells begins, and the inflammatory response is initiated. Rupture of the intracellular lysosomes is the final event signaling irreversible cell injury, cell death, and loss of muscle function. At this point the intracellular enzymes are released into the bloodstream. The dead nonfunctional tissue is referred to as the area of infarction, which has a central core comprised of nonfunctional cells with disorganized structures, which are surrounded by peripheral cells with varying amounts of disruption (Figure 40–5 ■, p. 1164). Within hours neutrophils infiltrate infarcted tissue, causing further endothelial damage, contraction of smooth muscles, and an increase in vascular permeability. Enzymes released by macrophages may lead to breakdown of connective tissue and cardiac muscle aneurysm formation or rupture, leaking of fluid into the pericardial space, and/or pericardial inflammation. Necrotic tissue is replaced by granulation tissue in 2 to 3 weeks, which can induce myocardial wall thinning and dilation. Fibroblasts eventually appear and synthesize a collagen matrix that provides the substrate for fibrous tissue and the formation of a mature scar in 2 to 3 months. Scarred or fibrotic myocardium becomes stiff and loses its ability to contract and relax, in other words, to function normally. Over time the myocardium may thin. Muscle cells around scarred tissue enlarge or hypertrophy. Myocardial stiffening, thinning, and hypertrophy also can cause contraction abnormalities. In addition myocardial scarring can cause abnormal conduction of cardiac impulses

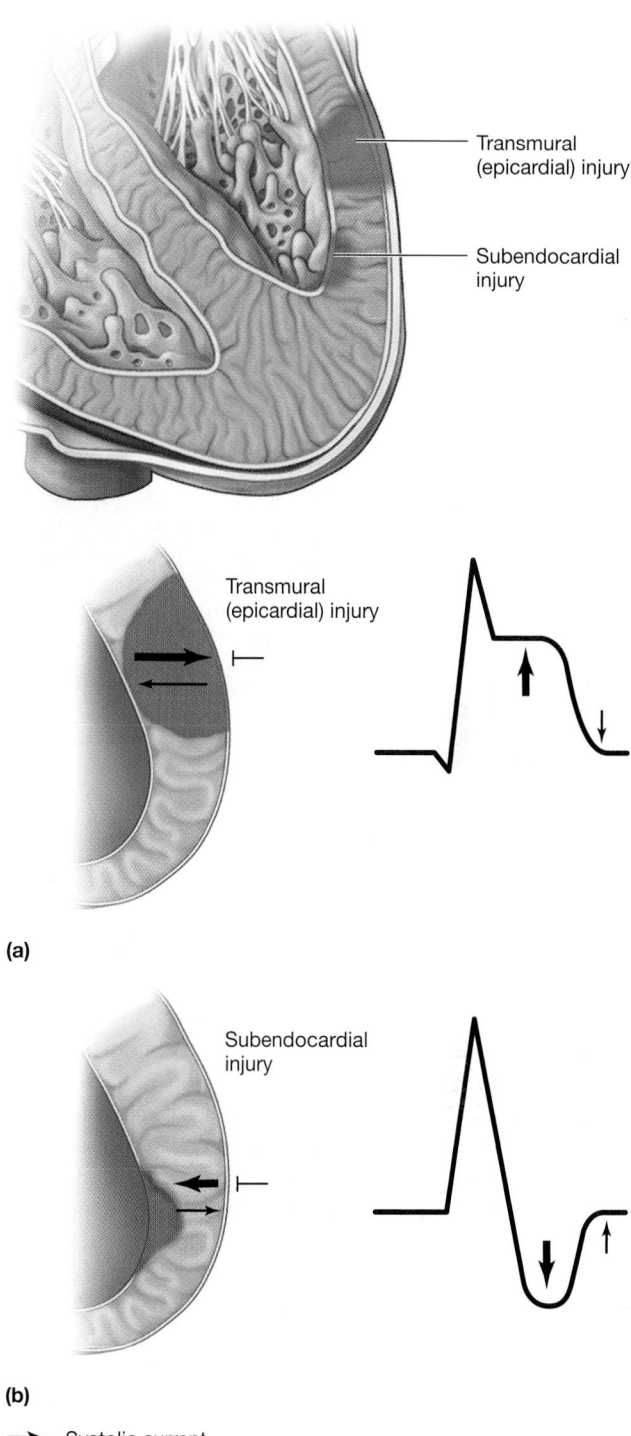

(a)

(b)

➡ Systolic current

→ Diastolic current

⊢ Electrode

FIGURE 40–4 ■ Subendocardial versus transmural damage.

from the sinoatrial (SA) node to the ventricles (Porth, 2005). The cardiac conduction system is discussed in Chapter 38 ⊘.

Surrounding the area of infarction is the zone of injury and the zone of ischemia (see Figure 40–5 ■, p. 1164). These zones are made of potentially viable tissues. They can become necrotic and die, or be reperfused and remain functional. The goal of treatment for an AMI is to establish reperfusion as early as possible to prevent necrosis and salvage the myocardium.

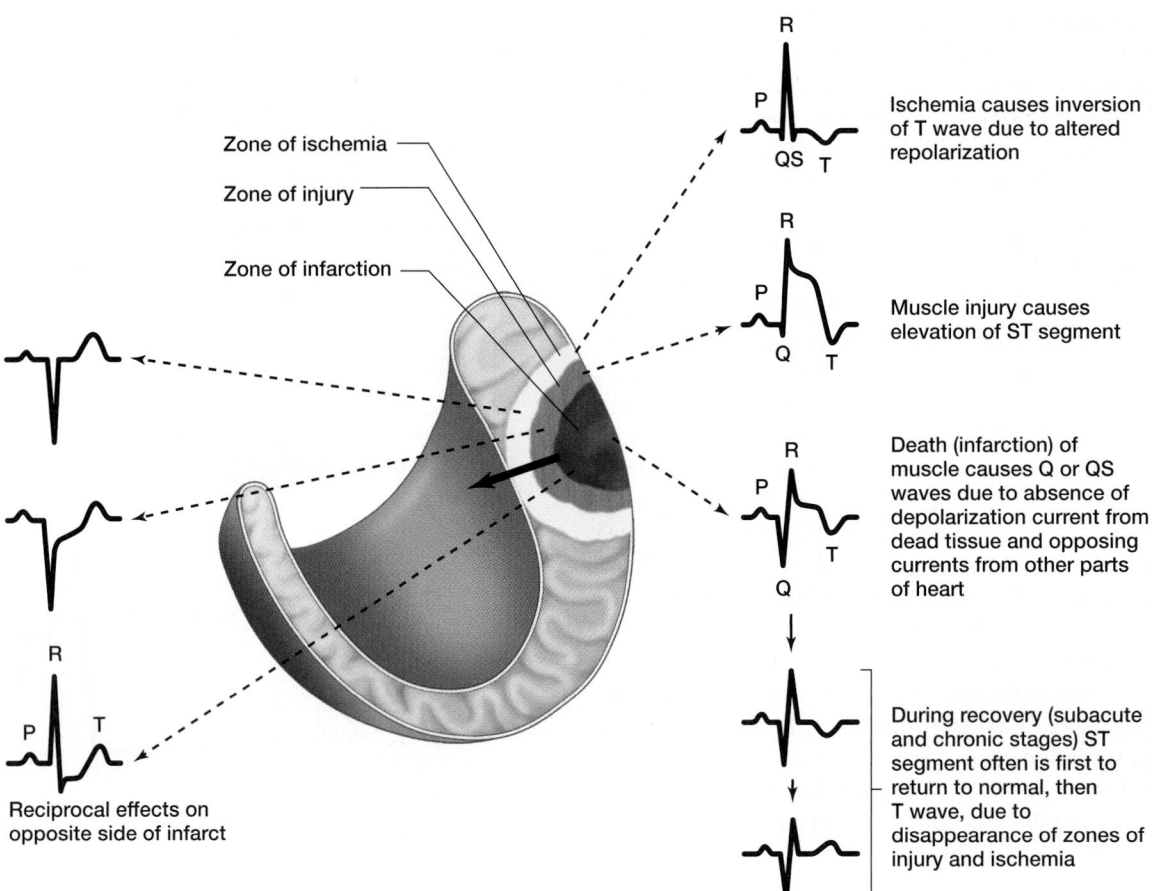

Zone of ischemia
Zone of injury
Zone of infarction

Ischemia causes inversion of T wave due to altered repolarization

Muscle injury causes elevation of ST segment

Death (infarction) of muscle causes Q or QS waves due to absence of depolarization current from dead tissue and opposing currents from other parts of heart

During recovery (subacute and chronic stages) ST segment often is first to return to normal, then T wave, due to disappearance of zones of injury and ischemia

Reciprocal effects on opposite side of infarct

FIGURE 40–5 ■ Zones of infarction and reciprocal ECG changes.

Prevention of cell death, reversing cell injury, limiting infarct size or extension, and preventing myocardial remodeling are all dependent on a number of adaptive responses to acute and chronic ischemia. These include the timing of reperfusion, the presence of ischemic preconditioning, the extent of collateral circulation, myocardial stunning and hibernation, and cellular apoptosis and oncosis (Henning & Olsson, 2001). Reperfusion within 20 minutes will abort cell death. Fibrinolytic, or clot-dissolving, agents (see the Pharmacology Summary of Medications to Treat Coronary Artery Disease box, p. 1199) have a window of less than 12 hours from symptom onset to achieve myocardial salvage. Vessels with chronic subacute thrombosis lasting a few minutes, precondition the tissue for periods of longer ischemia, protecting it from infarction. Chronic, progressive coronary obstruction also stimulates the development of coronary collateral vessels. It is unclear whether these vessels are indigenous and simply recruited in times of coronary insufficiency, or if collaterals represent neovascular development. Neovascular development can occur by angiogenesis, which is the growth of new microvessels budding from arteries in areas of healing infarcted tissue. Myocardial tissue stunning and hibernation are conditions of reversible muscle contractile dysfunction thought to be adaptive responses to chronic coronary occlusion. **Myocardial stunning** is a temporary dysfunction that occurs in response to artery occlusion of short duration or transient global hypoperfusion during a limited low flow state such as shock. The end result is that the myocardial muscle tem-

porarily has a limited ability to contract, whereas with **myocardial hibernation** the tissue actually undergoes cellular structural changes and progressive apoptosis (cell death) in response to prolonged ischemia (Henning & Olsson, 2001). Hibernating tissue is thought to recover contractile function fully once perfusion is reestablished (Brown, 2001).

Oncosis and apoptosis are two processes of cell death. **Oncosis** is cell swelling as a result of changes in membrane permeability. Apoptosis is a genetically derived and substrate controlled process of programmed cell death. Oncosis and apoptosis may contribute to the overall magnitude of ischemic necrosis and myocardial remodeling. Recent studies have identified apoptotic cells and myocyte proliferation in areas around the site of infarction (Barandon et al., 2004). Various hypotheses are the subject of ongoing research as to whether cells can be reprogrammed to limit apoptosis and/or enhance angiogenesis and myocyte regeneration as a means of altering the process of myocardial remodeling.

■ Cardiac Risk Factors

Cardiac risk factors are habits, lifestyles, and/or genetic factors that predispose an individual to the development of coronary artery disease. Risk factors have various categories, which are typically referred to as modifiable versus nonmodifiable, and contributing factors. The risk factors for coronary artery disease are outlined in the Risk Factors box. Modifiable risk factors are ones that an individual has some control over, such as physical

RISK FACTORS for Coronary Artery Disease

Modifiable Factors	Nonmodifiable Factors	Contributing Factors
Elevated low density lipoprotein cholesterol (LDL-C)	Increasing age	High-fat diet
Low high density lipoprotein cholesterol (HDL-C)	Heredity	Alcohol consumption
Triglycerides	Male gender	Increased stress
Elevated total cholesterol		Increased homocysteine level
Hypertension		Increased C-reactive protein
Tobacco smoke		Hormone replacement therapy
Diabetes		
Physical inactivity		
Overweight and obesity*		

Normal weight = 18.5–24.9 kg/m²; overweight = 25–29 kg/m²; obesity = > 30.0 kg/m²; abdominal obesity is defined as waist circumference (men) > 102 centimeters (40 inches); (women) > 88 centimeters (35 inches)

activity, stress, and cigarette smoking, whereas nonmodifiable risk factors are not controllable. Nonmodifiable risk factors include advancing age, male sex, and heredity. The American Heart Association (2006c) recommends that all adults with or without established CAD be assessed for risk beginning at the age of 20. A review of lifestyle and predisposing factors at every annual physical evaluation or at least every 2 years should occur (AHA 2006c).

Since 1948 a longitudinal study has been conducted in Framingham, Massachusetts (Futterman & Lemberg, 2000). This study has been evaluating lifestyles and habits of the city's inhabitants. The results of this study have allowed researchers to identify factors that increase a person's risk for the development of CAD. The study is still going on and it is now evaluating the third and fourth generation of subjects. It continues to provide important information about the development of heart disease. Additionally, an abundance of other research continues to refine and add to the body of knowledge about the development of CAD. The modifiable risk factors include elevated serum total cholesterol, increased low density lipoprotein cholesterol (LDL-C), low levels of high density lipoprotein cholesterol (HDL-C), elevated blood pressure, tobacco smoke, physical inactivity, diabetes mellitus, and obesity/overweight (AHA, 2006c). Of these factors, high cholesterol, high LDL-C, high blood pressure, and smoking are most closely linked to development of atherosclerosis. Each of these factors is an independent predictor of CAD.

Research data from the last few decades have shown conclusively that it is possible to alter the natural history of atherosclerosis by either regression or stabilization of plaque with aggressive risk factor reduction (Naghavi et al., 2003a, 2003b). Risk factor reduction efforts focus on factors that are modifiable, specifically lifestyle changes aimed at promoting smoking cessation, blood pressure control, exercise, weight reduction, low-fat diets, and pharmacologic therapies that control dyslipidemia.

Modifiable Risk Factors

Modifiable risk factor identification is important for both assessment of risk and targets for intervention. The modifiable risk factors include hyperlipidemia, hypertension, tobacco smoke, diabetes, physical inactivity, and obesity/overweight.

 CRITICAL ALERT *When educating patients about CAD, the nurse must stress that if the patient has nonmodifiable risk factors, it is essential to control the modifiable factors in order to prevent or slow the progression of CAD.*

Hyperlipidemia

Hyperlipidemia, is defined as elevated cholesterol and/or triglyceride levels. These are lipids that permeate the arterial wall causing a narrowed lumen that ultimately decreases blood flow to the cardiac muscle. **Hypercholesterolemia** is defined as increased cholesterol level in the blood. **Cholesterol** is a steroid molecule produced primarily by the liver that is essential for the formation and maintenance of cell membranes. Cholesterol also is a building block for sex hormones; it aids in the production of digestive bile salts and enables the conversion of vitamin D in the skin. The serum cholesterol level is a potent indicator of risk for CAD. Approximately 85% of cholesterol in the blood is produced by the body. The other 15% is consumed through the diet. For a person with no cardiac history or risk factors, a total cholesterol level less than 200 mg/dL is considered low risk for the development of CAD. A total cholesterol level of 200 to 250 mg/dL is moderate risk, and levels greater than 250 mg/dL are considered high risk. For patients with known CAD or risk factors, the desired serum levels are lower (Chart 40–3).

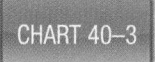 **CHART 40–3 Laboratory Test Parameters That Prevent CAD**

Patient teaching needs to stress that the following blood levels are the goal for prevention of CAD:

Total cholesterol/HDL-C ratio < 4

Total cholesterol < 200 mg/dL

LDL-C < 100 mg/dL

HDL-C > 40 mg/dL

Triglycerides < 150 mg/dL

Hs-C-reactive protein < 0.7 mg/dL = low risk

Homocysteine 4 to 14.

Source: Corbett, J. V. (2004). *Laboratory and diagnostic procedures with nursing diagnoses.* Upper Saddle River, NJ: Prentice Hall Health. Electronically reproduced by permission of Pearson Education, Inc., Upper Saddle River, New Jersey.

Hypercholesterolemia may be inherited as a genetic defect that leads to excessive production of low density lipoproteins or a decreased capacity for their removal. It also can be acquired through diet and lifestyle. Familial hypercholesterolemia is discussed in the Genetic Considerations box. Cultural variations on cholesterol levels have been noted as well. The Cultural Considerations box discusses cultural groups that have a lower rate of CAD. Cholesterol levels tend to increase with age. One correlation is resoundingly clear: The higher the elevated level of cholesterol, the greater the risk of future and acute cardiovascular adverse events. A 1% decrease in cholesterol results in a 2% to 3% decrease in the risk of MI (Castelli, 2001).

Cholesterol is carried in the blood via small proteins. When these carrier proteins join with cholesterol, they are called lipoproteins. The weight or density of lipoproteins depends on the amount of protein in the molecule. Total serum cholesterol is a composite value comprised of all the types of cholesterol carrying lipoproteins. The lipoproteins that alter one's risk for CAD are the low density lipoproteins, the high density lipoproteins, and possibly lipoprotein A. The American Heart Association (AHA) recommends that total cholesterol levels be drawn every 5 years. For men over 45 years, women over 55 years, and patients with elevated cholesterol, or low high density lipoprotein cholesterol (HDL-C), cholesterol levels should be drawn more often.

 CRITICAL ALERT *Patients need to be instructed that cholesterol and lipid panels should be drawn after a person has fasted overnight, including no alcohol.*

Low density lipoprotein cholesterol (LDL-C), the so-called "bad cholesterol," is the major cholesterol carrier in the blood. When circulating LDL-C becomes oxidized, it is modified such that it attaches to and migrates through the cell membrane into the intimal lining of the vessel. Once inside the cell membrane, LDL-C attracts immune complexes from the blood into the intimae. Smooth muscle cells from the medial layer of the vessel wall migrate into the intima, thus creating the substrate for plaque development. Oxidized LDL-C also causes endothelial dysfunction by inhibiting the release of endothelial nitric oxide, a compound that not only prevents LDL-C oxidation but also is necessary for vasodilation. Thus, vessel segments damaged by plaque do not vasodilate in response to local hypoxia caused from vessel occlusion the way undamaged vessel segments do. The optimal target goal for LDL-C is less than 100 mg/dL. Target ranges vary depending on the presence of CAD and the risk factor profile outlined in Chart 40–4.

GENETIC CONSIDERATIONS
for Hypercholesterolemia

Familial hypercholesterolemia (FH) is a dominantly inherited genetic disease that results in markedly elevated low density lipoproteins (LDL), the bad cholesterol, beginning at birth. This leads to premature coronary atherosclerosis, which increases the risk of suffering an acute myocardial infarction (AMI) or stroke at an early age. Men are more commonly affected, having their first AMI in their 40s to 50s, with 85% of them having an AMI by age 60. Women have an increased incidence of AMI, but it is delayed by 10 years.

Hypercholesterolemia has several alternative names including type II hyperlipoproteinemia, hypercholesterolemic xanthomatosis, and low density lipoprotein receptor mutation.

An individual can inherit two genes for this disorder, which magnifies the severity of the condition. The cholesterol level may exceed 600 mg/dL; and waxy plaques (xanthomas) of cholesterol develop beneath the skin over elbows, knees, and buttocks; in tendons; and around the cornea of the eye. Atherosclerosis begins before puberty, and AMI and death may occur before age 30.

Patient teaching for individuals with a strong family history includes stressing the risk of early AMI, and these patients should be evaluated with a lipid screen regularly. Proper diet, exercise, and the use of lipid lowering drugs to bring the cholesterol down to safer levels are also recommended.

Source: Leren, T. P. (2004). Cascade genetic screening for familial hypercholesterolemia. *Clinical Genetics: An International Journal of Genetics and Molecular Medicine. 66* (6). 483–487. Reproduced with permission of Blackwell Publishing Ltd.

CULTURAL CONSIDERATIONS for CAD
Development

Cultures vary in their tendency for high cholesterol levels and the development of CAD. This is dramatized by the fact that rural residents in the developing nations of Asia, Africa, and Latin America typically have low total cholesterol levels, in the range of 125 to 140 mg/dL, and they do not develop CAD (Castelli, 2001).

CHART 40–4	Factors That Affect the Lipid Profile	
HDL-C	Factors that ↑ HDL-C	Smoking cessation by 10% Exercise Weight reduction
	Factors that ↓ HDL-C	Smoking Trans fatty acids Sedentary Obesity Low-fat/high carbohydrate diet
LDL-C	Factors that ↑ LDL-C	Trans fatty acids Saturated fats Cholesterol
	Factors that ↓ LDL-C	Polyunsaturated fatty acids Monounsaturated fatty acids Soluble fiber Soy protein Weight reduction
Triglycerides	Factors that ↑ triglycerides	Excess body weight Reduced physical activity Increased intake of sugar and refined carbohydrates, particularly in the setting of insulin resistance and glucose intolerance Increased alcohol intake
	Factors that ↓ triglycerides	Exercise Weight reduction Reduced carbohydrate consumption

High density lipoprotein cholesterol (HDL-C) is heavier lipoproteins that bind to cholesterol, transporting it back to the liver, and may actually remove excess cholesterol from plaque in the arteries. High levels of HDL-C are thought to be cardioprotective. Levels greater than 40 mg/dL in men and greater than 50 mg/dL in women with no CAD and no risk factors are desirable. Even if one's HDL-C level is elevated above the target level, this does not negate the need to lower one's LDL-C level to target levels. The cardioprotection from HDL-C does not insulate one from the atherogenic effects of LDL-C. When determining one's risk of CAD, clinicians also use a comparison between the total cholesterol level and the HDL-C level. A total cholesterol/HDL-C ratio of 3.5:1 or less is optimal (AHA, 2006c). Methods used to alter lipid levels include dietary and lifestyle modifications, and/or pharmacologic intervention (Chart 40–5).

 When teaching patients about dietary control of cholesterol and lipids, it is important for the nurse to inquire about food preferences and cultural factors. The teaching needs to be tailored to include these preferences and cultural considerations in order to increase compliance with the restrictions.

Triglycerides are a form of fat derived from fats in food and produced by the body from other sources such as carbohydrates. Triglycerides are used as a partial building block for plasma lipids found in cell membranes. Elevated triglyceride levels are associated with high total cholesterol, high LDL-C, low HDL-C, heart disease, obesity, and diabetes (AHA, 2006e). Lowering levels to less than 150 mg/dL has become a part of risk prevention. Levels of 150 to 199 mg/dL are considered borderline high, levels of 200 to 499 mg/dL borderline high to high, and levels greater than 500 mg/dL very high (AHA, 2006e).

CHART 40–5   Therapeutic Lifestyle Dietary Changes

Nutrient	Recommended Intake
Saturated fat	Less than 7% of total calories
Polyunsaturated fat	Up to 10% of total calories
Monounsaturated fat—oils from olives, avocados, nuts	Up to 20% total calories
Total fat	25–35% of total calories
Carbohydrate—predominantly derived from foods rich in complex carbohydrates including grains, whole grains, fruits, and vegetables	50–60% of total calories, if > 60% of diet can cause reduced high density lipoproteins (HDL) and increased triglycerides
Fiber	20–30 grams/day
Protein	Approximately 15% of total calories
Cholesterol	Less than 200 milligrams/day
Total calories (energy)	Balance energy intake and expenditure to maintain desirable body weight/prevent weight gain

Source: Berra, K., & Klieman, L. (2003). National cholesterol education program. Adult treatment panel III—New recommendations for lifestyle and medical management of dyslipidemia. *Journal of Cardiovascular Nursing, 18*(2), 85–92.

Triglycerides are carried to tissues by many types of proteins such as very low density lipoprotein cholesterol (VLDL-C) and chylomicra. VLDL is converted to LDL-C after delivering triglycerides to the muscles and adipose or fat tissue. Chylomicra have the heaviest mass and richest triglyceride content of any lipid-containing particle. Chylomicra are metabolized or broken down into partial fragments or remnants by enzymes called apoproteins, such as lipoprotein A and apoprotein E. Elevated levels of VLDL, chylomicra and cylomicron remnants, and apoproteins have each been suggested as having an associated risk of atherogenesis (Nash, 2004).

Lipid Lowering Therapy

Lipid lowering drugs include hepatic hydroxymethyl glutaryl coenzyme A reductase inhibitors (HMG-CoA reductase inhibitors), also referred to as statins, and the newest generation, which are a combination of these drugs. The Pharmacology Summary (p. 1199) outlines the lipid lowering medications. Lipid lowering agents are considered in patients with CAD and fewer than two risk factors if their LDL-C is ≥ 190 mg/dL, in patients without CAD with two or more risk factors with an LDL-C ≥ 160 mg/dL, or in patients with known CAD with an LDL-C ≥ 130 mg/dL. Drug therapy is delayed in men under age 35 and premenopausal women with LDL-C of 190 to 219 mg/dL, except in high-risk patient groups such as patients with diabetes or patients who are obese or with hypertension. Patients with CAD and LDL-C between 100 and 129 mg/dL may still benefit from lipid lowering therapy. Additionally, lipid lowering therapy is indicated for familial dyslipidemia.

Hypertension

Maintaining a blood pressure within the recommended normal range reduces the mortality from CAD. Every 1 mmHg decrease in diastolic blood pressure results in a 2% to 3% decrease in the incidence of an MI (Diop & Aghababian, 2001). Research has demonstrated that with each age category well into the 80s there was significant reduction in risk of death from CAD or stroke with blood pressure lowering by 20 mmHg, even down to pressures as low as 115/75 mmHg (Lewington et al., 2002). African Americans have the highest overall mortality rate from CAD of all ethnic groups in the United States, which is attributed to the higher prevalence of certain coronary risk factors, among them hypertension and type II diabetes (Clark et al., 2001). A complete description of the cause, incidence, and treatment of high blood pressure is included in Chapter 21 ⊘.

Nonpharmacologic interventions aimed at lowering blood pressure focus on exercise, weight control, reduced salt intake, limited alcohol consumption, and a diet that emphasizes fruits, vegetables, and low-fat dairy products. Reducing sodium intake by 1.8 grams a day is associated with a 4 mmHg drop in systolic and a 2 mmHg drop in diastolic pressure in hypertensive patients. Salt intake should be limited to 2,400 milligrams a day, which is equivalent to a diet that includes no added salt and watching added salts in prepared foods. A weight reduction of 1.6 kilograms has shown to drop pressure by 1.1 mmHg averaged for both systolic and diastolic pressures. The American Heart Association advocates the use of antihypertensive medications if the following blood pressure targets cannot be reached after a 6- to 12-month trial of nonpharmacologic measures: blood pressure < 140/90 mmHg;

< 130/85 mmHg if the patient has heart failure or renal insufficiency; or < 130/80 mmHg if the patient has diabetes (Pearson et al., 2002). Age differences are an important consideration in the treatment of hypertension. According to new research published in the *Journal of the American Medical Association,* people age 60 and older should seek treatment when their systolic blood pressure rises above 160, even if the diastolic reading is less than 90. The researchers found "strong evidence" that treating systolic high blood pressure can decrease the likelihood of developing heart disease or having a stroke. High systolic blood pressure in people age 60 and over is a much more important heart disease risk factor than is high diastolic blood pressure (Sarwat, Krumholz, & Foody, 2004).

Tobacco Smoke

Tobacco smokers have a 50% greater chance of developing CAD with a 70% greater mortality than nonsmokers (Diop & Aghababian, 2001). Women who use oral contraceptives and smoke are at a greater risk of heart disease and stroke than are nonsmoking women who use oral contraceptives (Diop & Aghababian, 2001). Cardiovascular adverse effects are attributed to carbon monoxide and nicotine. Carbon monoxide displaces oxygen on the hemoglobin molecule, thus, reducing the blood's oxygen-carrying capacity. Carbon monoxide also may promote atherogenesis by causing endothelial damage. Nicotine increases myocardial oxygen demand by increasing blood pressure and heart rate, and is thought to promote thrombogenesis through platelet aggregation. Nicotine also causes vasospasm and endothelial dysfunction. The risk of cardiovascular adverse events in male and female smokers who successfully quit dramatically decreases. In fact their risk level approaches that of nonsmokers within 2 to 3 years of smoking cessation. HDL-C levels increase by 10% soon after smoking cessation.

Hospitalization presents a unique opportunity of social support for patients who want to stop smoking. A plan for assisting patients in smoking cessation should include the following: (1) Know that repeated attempts at cessation are often necessary; (2) encouragement by all of the patient's health care providers enhances success; (3) the greater the intensity of tobacco-dependence counseling, the higher the quit rate; (4) participation in a smoking cessation program encourages patients to be conscious of triggers for smoking, to develop diversional activities for cravings and rewards for successes, and to establish person–person contact via individual, group, or telephone support; and (5) pharmacotherapies including nicotine replacement with nicotine gum, patch, inhaler, and nasal spray as well as bupropion SR, clonidine, or nortriptyline may be necessary (Haskell, 2003). Useful contacts for more information on smoking cessation include the Agency for Healthcare Research and Quality and the American Lung Association.

Secondhand smoke, often also referred to as environmental tobacco smoke, is a mixture of the smoke given off by the burning end of a cigarette, pipe, or cigar and the smoke exhaled from the lungs of smokers (American Lung Association, 2006a). The residual smoke lingers in the air for hours, even after the tobacco has been extinguished and is involuntarily inhaled by nonsmokers, causing a wide range of adverse health effects, including cancer, respiratory infections, and asthma. Nonsmokers exposed to environmental smoke were 25% more likely to have coronary

heart diseases as compared to nonsmokers not exposed to smoke (American Lung Association, 2006a). In 2005, 9 smoke-free states prohibited smoking in almost all workplaces, restaurants, and bars (American Lung Association, 2006a). Additionally, in 2006, 20 years after the first U.S. Surgeon General's report on the dangers of secondhand smoke, the Surgeon General reported that there is no safe level of exposure to secondhand smoke (American Lung Association, 2006b; United States Department of Health and Human Services, 2006a). The new report confirms that secondhand smoke is a cause of lung cancer and heart disease and has immediate adverse effects on the cardiovascular system. The report recommends eliminating smoking in all indoor spaces.

Diabetes

Various micro- and macrovascular changes are thought to be responsible for an overall higher rate of cardiovascular morbidity and mortality found in patients with diabetes. Women have twice the risk of men of developing cardiovascular events associated with diabetes (AHA, 2008b &c). These vascular changes are thought to be mediated through intimal proliferation and other pathologies of endothelial function. As a consequence, those with diabetes are at risk for developing the following conditions related to coronary artery disease:

- Cardiac autonomic neuropathy, resulting in a decreased perception of ischemic pain
- Arterial occlusion in the heart and peripheral vascular circulation
- Dyslipidemias
- Hypertension
- Increased platelet aggregation
- Elevated coagulation factors.

Heart failure because of myocyte hypertrophy, interstitial fibrosis, cardiomyopathy (Chapter 42 ⊙), and disease of the microcirculation called microangiopathy are other consequences of diabetes.

Reducing risk of CAD for patients with diabetes goes beyond controlling known cardiac risk factors. Even without additional risk factors those with diabetes are at greater risk for CAD (AHA, 2006c). Risk factor reduction focuses on aggressive treatment for diabetes including glycemic control (blood sugar) and lifestyle changes. Moderate changes in diet, exercise, and weight reduction can decrease the development of diabetes (National Guidelines and Tools for Cardiovascular Risk Reduction, 2006). Glycemic control has been shown to have an impact on decreasing overall CAD morbidity and mortality and reduces long-term mortality following an acute MI.

Physical Inactivity

Obesity, sedentary lifestyle, and lack of physical activity are mutually supporting cardiac risk factors that are the by-product of Western industrialized societies. Modern society is increasingly dependent on laborsaving technologies that once provided physical exercise or activity for the average person. These include transportation, work, computer- and video-based recreational outlets, and food products of supersized portions with flavor enhanced through fats, sugar, and salt.

Regular exercise ($\geq$ 5 times/week lasting $\geq$ 30 minutes) of moderate intensity (brisk walking) decreases heart attack risk by 10% to 50% in both men and women. Cardioprotection from exercise is attributed to improved functional work capacity, decreased heart rate, decreased platelet adhesiveness, enhanced fibrinolysis, attenuation of the sympathetic stress response, weight loss, lowered triglyceride levels, and increased HDL-C levels. The AHA recommends an exercise routine that totals 2.5 hours a week of any combination of days and hours per day. The recommended routine also includes resistance training of 8 to 10 different exercises, 1 to 2 sets per exercise, 10 to 15 repetitions per set, flexibility training, and habits that increase daily activity (AHA, 2006g). Exercise also may prevent obesity and insulin resistance.

Obesity and Overweight

Obesity has become a social stigma associated with Western civilizations and is destined to cause as much disease and preventable deaths as cigarette smoking. In fact obesity is second only to smoking in modifiable risk factors for all causes of death in the United States (National Guidelines for Treatment and Prevention of Obesity, p. 1170). Chronic obesity increases the risk of CAD in men and women and is antithetical to risk reduction in other areas. Obesity is attributed to increases in blood pressure, abnormal lipoprotein levels, insulin resistance, and platelet aggregation. The two units of measure associated with cardiovascular risk are body mass index (BMI) and abdominal circumference. BMI is a person's weight in kilograms divided by the square of one's height in meters, giving a measure of kg/m². Obesity is defined as a body mass index (BMI) > 30, whereas 25.0 to 29.9 is overweight, and 18.5 to 24.9 is normal weight. Abdominal obesity is defined as a waist circumference of > 40 inches (102 centimeters) in men and > 35 inches (88 centimeters) in women. Fat accumulation in the upper body, giving the body an appearance of an "apple," has been linked to a greater risk of CAD as opposed to a "pear" shape with body fat accumulation in the gluteofemoral region. Abdominal obesity is associated with elevated levels of cholesterol and greater risk for CAD.

Obesity is a product of overeating in relation to energy expenditure. General guidelines recommend that total energy intake match overall energy needs, and that activity level matches or exceeds energy intake. The Surgeon General has developed an action plan with specific activities as national priorities for immediate action for individuals, families, communities, schools, work sites, health care, media, industry, organizations, and government to take action to prevent and decrease overweight and obesity. These activities are presented in the National Guidelines for Treatment and Prevention of Obesity box (p. 1170).

 *When counseling a patient in weight reduction, a multidisciplinary approach is typically most effective. In order to achieve lifetime changes in eating habits and adherence to an exercise program, the patient needs counseling from nutritionists, health care providers, nurses, physical therapists, and psychological counselors. Many cities have obesity clinics that provide these services.*

Nonmodifiable Risk Factors

Nonmodifiable risk factors are those present that cannot be modified through lifestyle and habit changes. Meticulous attention in controlling the modifiable risk factors is recommended to mitigate the effects of the nonmodifiable risk factors. The nonmodifiable risk factors of increasing age, heredity, and male gender are discussed next.

Increasing Age

Cardiac aging results in stiffening of myofibrils, which cause a reduced ability of the muscle to relax, stretch, and contract. The number of myocytes decreases with age, cells enlarge or hypertrophy, they become less responsive to stimulation, and the rate of cellular apoptosis or death increases. As mentioned earlier, with advanced age cholesterol and triglyceride levels increase. Aging causes large arterial vessel walls to dilate and thicken, smooth muscle tone to increase, and increased vessel stiffness as elastic and collagen are replaced with fibrotic tissue. The consequences of these changes are an elevated systolic blood pressure, arteriosclerosis, atherosclerosis, and a decrease in cardiac performance. Age is an independent risk factor for CAD and should be a part of every risk assessment.

Heredity

A familial history of CAD dramatically increases the risk that aggregate family members will have cardiac disease as well. Adult offspring of parents with a CAD history also are more likely to have multiple risk factors for CAD and have greater likelihood of an acute cardiac event, even after correcting for other disease risk factors. First-degree relatives (children, parents, and siblings), families with greater prevalence meaning more than one person in the family have CAD, and families with early onset CAD are at greater risk. Reasons for this familial connection are not known. Possible mediators may be environmental or social factors, or genetic predisposition. Research in the area of genetic mapping is beginning to uncover links between the presence of specific genes or genetic mutations and CAD. For example, a gene called ABCC6 plays a role in keeping elastic fibers healthy. A mutation in this gene has been found to be associated with an increased risk of early CAD (Gene Analysis Service, 2005). Also, inherited variations in gene pairing of a gene that controls how beta-2 (β_2) adrenergic receptors influence blood flow may lower the risk of having a heart attack and dying from heart disease.

Health care personnel need to be mindful of the fact that family members are not always aware that others in their family have or are predisposed to heart disease, especially with regard to less obvious risk factors such as hypertension and hyperlipidemia. The good news is that family members predisposed to CAD who modify their risk in other ways, such as getting regular physical activity at a moderate level, have lower odds of developing CAD than those family members who do not modify their risk factors.

Race is also included under the category of heredity. African Americans have a higher overall CAD prevalence and mortality rate than do Caucasians in the United States (AHA, 2006c). Additionally, they also present with a disproportionate number of CAD risk factors such as hypertension, type II diabetes, metabolic syndrome, abdominal obesity, stress, and inactivity. Reasons for these disparities are unclear; however, ethnic, cultural, and physiological differences exist. Studies have highlighted that African Americans (1) perceive cardiac pain differently and often ascribe symptoms to other noncardiac causes; (2) less often seek, ask for, receive, and respond differently to appropriate preventive, diagnostic, and

NATIONAL GUIDELINES for Treatment and Prevention of Obesity

Overweight and Obesity: A Vision of the Future

The Surgeon General identifies specific activities as national priorities for immediate action. Individuals, families, communities, schools, work sites, health care, media, industry, organizations, and government must determine their role and take action to prevent and decrease overweight and obesity.

Communication

The Nation must take an informed, sensitive approach to communicate with and educate the American people about health issues related to overweight and obesity. Everyone must work together to:

Change the perception of overweight and obesity at all ages. The primary concern should be one of health and not appearance.

Educate all expectant parents about the many benefits of breastfeeding.

Breastfed infants may be less likely to become overweight as they grow older.

Mothers who breastfeed may return to prepregnancy weight more quickly.

Educate health care providers and health profession students in the prevention and treatment of overweight and obesity across the life span.

Provide culturally appropriate education in schools and communities about healthy eating habits and regular physical activity, based on the Dietary Guidelines for Americans, for people of all ages. Emphasize the consumer's role in making wise food and physical activity choices.

Action

The Nation must take action to assist Americans in balancing healthful eating with regular physical activity. Individuals and groups across all settings must work in concert to:

Ensure daily, quality physical education in all school grades. Such education can develop the knowledge, attitudes, skills, behaviors, and confidence needed to be physically active for life.

Reduce time spent watching television and in other similar sedentary behaviors.

Build physical activity into regular routines and playtime for children and their families. Ensure that adults get at least 30 minutes of moderate physical activity on most days of the week. Children should aim for at least 60 minutes.

Create more opportunities for physical activity at work sites. Encourage all employers to make facilities and opportunities available for physical activity for all employees.

Make community facilities available and accessible for physical activity for all people, including the elderly.

Promote healthier food choices, including at least 5 servings of fruits and vegetables each day, and reasonable portion sizes at home, in schools, at work sites, and in communities.

Ensure that schools provide healthful foods and beverages on school campuses and at school events by:

Enforcing existing U.S. Department of Agriculture regulations that prohibit serving foods of minimal nutritional value during mealtimes in school food service areas, including in vending machines.

Adopting policies specifying that all foods and beverages available at school contribute toward eating patterns that are consistent with the Dietary Guidelines for Americans.

Providing more food options that are low in fat, calories, and added sugars such as fruits, vegetables, whole grains, and low-fat or nonfat dairy foods.

Reducing access to foods high in fat, calories, and added sugars and to excessive portion sizes.

Create mechanisms for appropriate reimbursement for the prevention and treatment of overweight and obesity.

Research and Evaluation

The Nation must invest in research that improves our understanding of the causes, prevention, and treatment of overweight and obesity. A concerted effort should be made to:

Increase research on behavioral and environmental causes of overweight and obesity.

Increase research and evaluation on prevention and treatment interventions for overweight and obesity and develop and disseminate best practice guidelines.

Increase research on disparities in the prevalence of overweight and obesity among racial and ethnic, gender, socioeconomic, and age groups and use this research to identify effective and culturally appropriate interventions.

Source: United States Department of Health and Human Services. (2006). *Overweight and obesity: A vision for the future.* Retrieved September 17, 2006, from http://www.surgeongeneral.gov/topics/obesity/calltoaction/fact_vision.htm.

---

interventional therapy for CAD; (3) may be financially disenfranchised, which limits access to health care; (4) may experience psychosocial stress, racism, and frustration leading to suboptimal interactions with the health care system; and (5) may have genetic predisposition to vascular disease and atherosclerosis (Venkat, Hekstra, & Lindsell, 2003).

According to the AHA (2006c), CAD is also higher in Mexican Americans, American Indians, native Hawaiians, and some Asian Americans. This is thought to be due in part to higher rates of obesity and diabetes in these populations.

Male Gender

The literature is replete with references to how gender affects cardiovascular health and disease. Prevalence and mortality rates are higher in men than in women, especially men 45 to 70 years of age, surpassed by women only in older age (AHA,

2006c). Even when women's death rate from heart disease increases after menopause, it is not as great as that of men. Men are more likely to seek and receive diagnostic and therapeutic intervention related to differences in pain perception, treatment bias, and social roles. Men also respond differently to therapy with often separate prescription and guideline recommendations. As women achieve advanced financial and social status, there may be a change in CAD disease prevalence and mortality demographics.

 The American Heart Association has created a free online toolkit designed to educate women about cardiovascular disease. It was developed as part of the association's Go Red For Women campaign, which calls attention to the devastating effects of heart disease in women. Access this and other campaign resources through the American Heart Association's website.

Contributing Risk Factors

Contributing risk factors include those factors that one may have a tendency or likelihood to have because of genetics, gender, habits, or other related causes. They are preventable risk factors that usually require self-discipline and motivation in order to avert. Contributing risk factors include high-fat diet, alcohol consumption, stress, homocysteine level, C-reactive protein, and hormone replacement therapy, all of which are discussed next.

High-Fat Diet

The term *heart-healthy diet* has undergone a metamorphosis over the years with on and off restrictive or liberal carbohydrate, protein, or fat portions. The cornerstone of cardiac nutrition stresses a diet low in calories; low in total fat (saturated fats, trans fatty acids, and cholesterol); moderate in protein; and high in fruits, vegetables, and other complex carbohydrates (see Chart 40–5, p. 1167). Limiting caloric intake aids in weight reduction and improves insulin resistance. Diets high in total fats are associated with excess body weight and elevated levels of circulating cholesterol and lipoproteins that are known to be atherogenic. Chapter 14 provides a complete description of heart-healthy diets.

Alcohol Consumption

In observational studies, alcohol consumption of 3 or more alcoholic drinks a day has been associated with elevated blood pressure, heart failure, and stroke (AHA, 2006c). Heavy use of alcohol also has been linked to CAD and related risk factors such as obesity, limited physical activity, diabetes, and malnutrition. Guidelines recommend limiting alcohol intake to no more than 2 drinks a day for men and 1 drink a day for women (AHA, 2006c). Within these limitations, reductions of 20% to 60% in risk have been observed (Diop & Aghababian, 2001). Alcohol in the form of red wine and dark beer may actually protect the heart in ways that have been recently discovered. Flavonals in red wine and dark beer, which are not as plentiful in other forms of alcohol or white wine, are thought to increase HDL-C, improve endothelial function, and reduce platelet aggregation (Goldfinger, 2003). However, drinking in excess of 1 glass of alcohol per day for women and 2 glasses for men, even red wine, is discouraged.

Stress

A number of psychosocial stressors appear to increase one's risk for CAD and morbidity and mortality following an acute MI. Anger, hostility, cynicism, anxiety, depression, lack of social support, type A personality, lack of spiritual support, and lack of financial resources have all been associated with increased risk of and morbidity and mortality from cardiovascular disease. Stress in general enhances autonomic stimulation. Sympathetic stimulation increases myocardial work, blood pressure, heart rate, dysrhythmia generation, and enhances platelet aggregation. Parasympathetic stimulation also predisposes one to dysrhythmias. Depression and lack of social support may affect autonomic impulses and may result in poor adherence to risk modification therapy. Spirituality includes a system of beliefs an individual has about the world and herself. People with greater spiritual awareness appear to display less distress, anxiety, and depression during times of personal turmoil, which may have a direct and indirect effect on CVD risk. The association between psychosocial stressors and CAD is based only on epidemiologic studies thus far. There is a complete discussion of the impact of stress on maladaptive or disease processes in Chapter 12 .

Homocysteine Level

Homocysteine is an amino acid that is a by-product of the enzyme reactions from meat, dairy products, vitamin, and mineral metabolism (Coffey, Crowder, & Cheek, 2003). Homocysteine causes endothelial ulceration and scarring, and increases procoagulant properties of blood, all leading to an increase in the risk of thrombus formation. Elevated levels of homocysteine (Hyc > 15 μmol/L) are associated with an increased risk of CAD, as well as peripheral vascular disease, stroke, and venous thrombosis. A normal homocysteine level is 4 to 14 μmol/L. Vitamins B_6, B_{12}, and folic acid decrease the levels of homocysteine, which can be supplemented by either vitamins or foods such as fruits, vegetables, cereals, and legumes (Coffey, Crowder, & Cheek, 2003). Vitamin therapy including dosing is included in Chapter 14 .

C-Reactive Protein

Inflammation as described earlier is thought to contribute to ACS, whether as a precursor to acute events because of plaque rupture, or as representative of ongoing endothelial and cell membrane damage. A serum marker of inflammation is C-reactive protein (CRP). C-reactive protein is produced and released by liver cells stimulated by activated macrophages. It is called an "acute phase" protein, meaning that within 24 to 48 hours after an inflammatory stimulus, as may occur during an acute coronary event, protein levels increase a thousandfold. CRP is a predictor of increased risk for heart attacks, strokes, and peripheral vascular disease, and is being used as a screening test for atherosclerosis for middle-aged and older people (AHA, 2006d). Elevated levels are present in patients with unstable angina and acute myocardial infarction (AMI) and appear to be predictive of higher risk for short- and long-term cardiovascular morbidity and mortality. A normal CRP value is < 0.9 mg/dL with levels > 1.6 mg/dL denoting risk and possibly a need for medical intervention such as coronary revascularization.

The standard CRP is not sensitive enough to detect small changes in the level of inflammation that occur in the cardiovascular system of individuals who appear free of CAD. A high-sensitivity CRP (hs-CRP) has been developed that can detect low-grade inflammatory activity within the cardiovascular system. An hs-CRP of < 0.7 mg/dL denotes low risk, 0.7 to 1.1 mg/dL mild risk, 1.2 to 1.9 mg/dL moderate risk, 2.0 to 3.8 mg/dL high risk, and 3.9 to 15 mg/dL very high risk. Aspirin, some forms of vitamin E, statin therapy, and weight loss have been shown to reduce CRP levels (AHA, 2006d).

Hormone Replacement Therapy

Recent studies have changed the thinking related to the benefits and risks of hormone replacement therapy (HRT) in women (AHA, 2006d). Menopause is associated with significant elevations in serum dyslipidemias and a threefold increase in risk of CAD. This is thought to be related to a decrease in the level of estrogen. However, studies have been inconclusive with regard to HRT conferring cardiac protection, and in fact it may increase the risk of CAD. Current recommendations dissuade the use of HRT as a CAD risk reduction strategy and suggest that women contact their health care provider to decide whether the therapeutic benefits of HRT outweigh the risks (AHA, 2006d). However, further research is needed to confirm or deny the more recent findings.

Metabolic Syndrome

Recently a cluster of cardiovascular risk factors, referred to as **metabolic syndrome**, has been defined as having three out of the five following conditions: (1) abdominal obesity, (2) high triglycerides, (3) low HDL-C, (4) high blood pressure, and (5) fasting glucose ($\geq$ 100 mg/dL). This cluster of conditions correlates with a higher risk for CAD and type 2 diabetes onset (Nash, 2004). Management of metabolic syndrome consists of targeting each abnormality with modification of corresponding risk factors, especially weight reduction and increased physical activity, and use of direct therapeutic interventions to lower blood pressure, serum glucose, and serum lipids. The American Heart Association recommends that adults over age 40 or those with two or more risk factors have a multirisk assessment score completed every 10 years.

■ Clinical Manifestations of Coronary Artery Disease

Coronary artery disease presents as clinical conditions of angina pectoris, unstable angina pectoris, myocardial infarction, and sudden cardiac death. These conditions depict a continuum of progressively worsening imbalances between the amount of oxygen delivered to and required by myocardial tissues. The underlying pathophysiology of each disorder is the same, atherosclerosis, as described earlier. However, as vessel stenosis intensifies, distinctions in the manifestations of signs and symptoms occur that are important for appropriate disease management. The clinical manifestations of ischemia are described next.

Electrocardiogram (ECG) Changes

When the heart muscle becomes ischemic, injured, or infarcted, depolarization and repolarization of cardiac cells are altered, causing changes in the ECG tracing. Figure 40–6 ■ depicts a normal ECG tracing. The ECG changes are manifested in three specific ways: ST segment elevation or depression, T wave extenuation or inversion, and QRS changes as in the development of pathologic Q waves (Figures 40–7 ■, 40–8 ■, 40–9 ■, p. 1174, 40–10 ■, p. 1175). A bundle branch block and cardiac dysrhythmias may also occur. The ECG is useful in identifying areas of injury or infarction, the infarct-related artery, in determining reperfusion following intervention, and in monitoring for cardiac dysrhythmias associated with myocardial damage. The ECG should be completed within the first 10 minutes of admission to the emergency department per national guidelines of the American College of Cardiology/American Heart Association (ACC/AHA) (Antman, Anbe, Armstrong, Bates, Green, Hand, et al. 2004).

ST Segment Changes

The ST segment begins at the end of the QRS complex and ends at the beginning of the T wave (see Figure 40–6 ■). The point marking the end of the QRS complex is referred to as the *J point* (see Figure 40–7 ■). Normally isoelectric, the ST segment represents the time during which the ventricles have been completely depolarized and are beginning to repolarize. When cardiac tissue

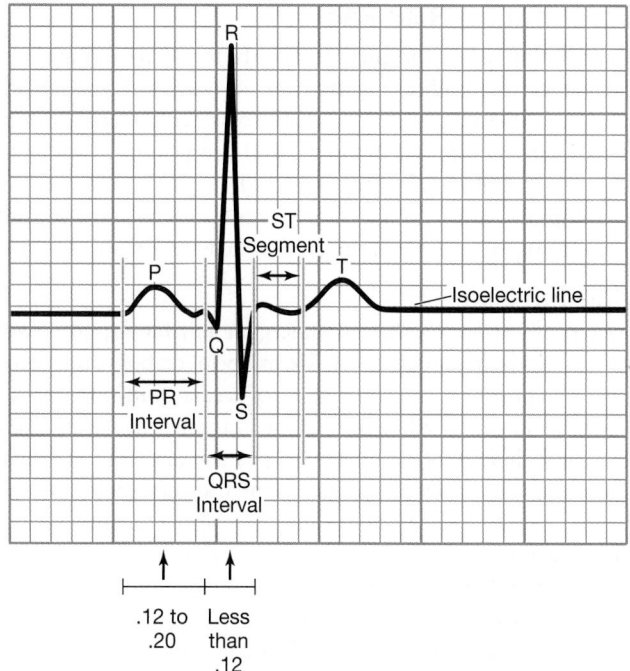

FIGURE 40–6 ■ Normal ECG waveforms.

becomes ischemic, the ST segment becomes abnormal and indicates a total reduction in localized blood flow. When the muscle ischemia involves only a portion of the heart wall, it is referred to as subendocardial injury, and ST segment depression occurs (see Figure 40–8 ■). When the ischemia traverses the entire width of the cardiac muscle, referred to as transmural ischemia, the ST segment becomes elevated (see Figure 40–7 ■). Prolonged, persistent ST segment elevation indicates acute ischemia and injury/infarction, and is associated with elevated cardiac blood markers. The greater the displacement of the ST segment and the more leads involved on the 12-lead ECG, the greater the amount of tissue damage (Morton, Fontaine, Hudak, & Gallo, 2005). The morphology (shape) of ST segment elevation is dependent on the lead. Figure 40–7 ■ depicts the various morphologies of ST segment elevation.

With transmural injury, the ST segment begins to rise almost immediately and can remain elevated for several hours to several days, as long as the ischemia continues. As the ischemia/injury subsides, the ST segment returns to the baseline. Once the ST segment has returned to the baseline, one of the main indicators of the acute MI is lost. Thus, obtaining a 12-lead ECG while the abnormality is present or the patient is having chest pain, is essential prior to treatment so that a diagnosis of a cardiac event can be made.

ST segment elevation greater than 1 millimeter or 1 small box on the ECG graph paper, or ST segment depression greater than 0.5 millimeter or one-half a small box, as determined on a 12-lead ECG, is considered a significant change. ST segment changes seen on continuous cardiac monitoring should be verified by obtaining a 12-lead ECG. The waveforms of continuous monitors are not calibrated and may be artificially enhanced by changes in the signal gain. Patients also may have a slight ST depression or elevation as a result of chronic cardiac disease, which can mimic an acute ECG change.

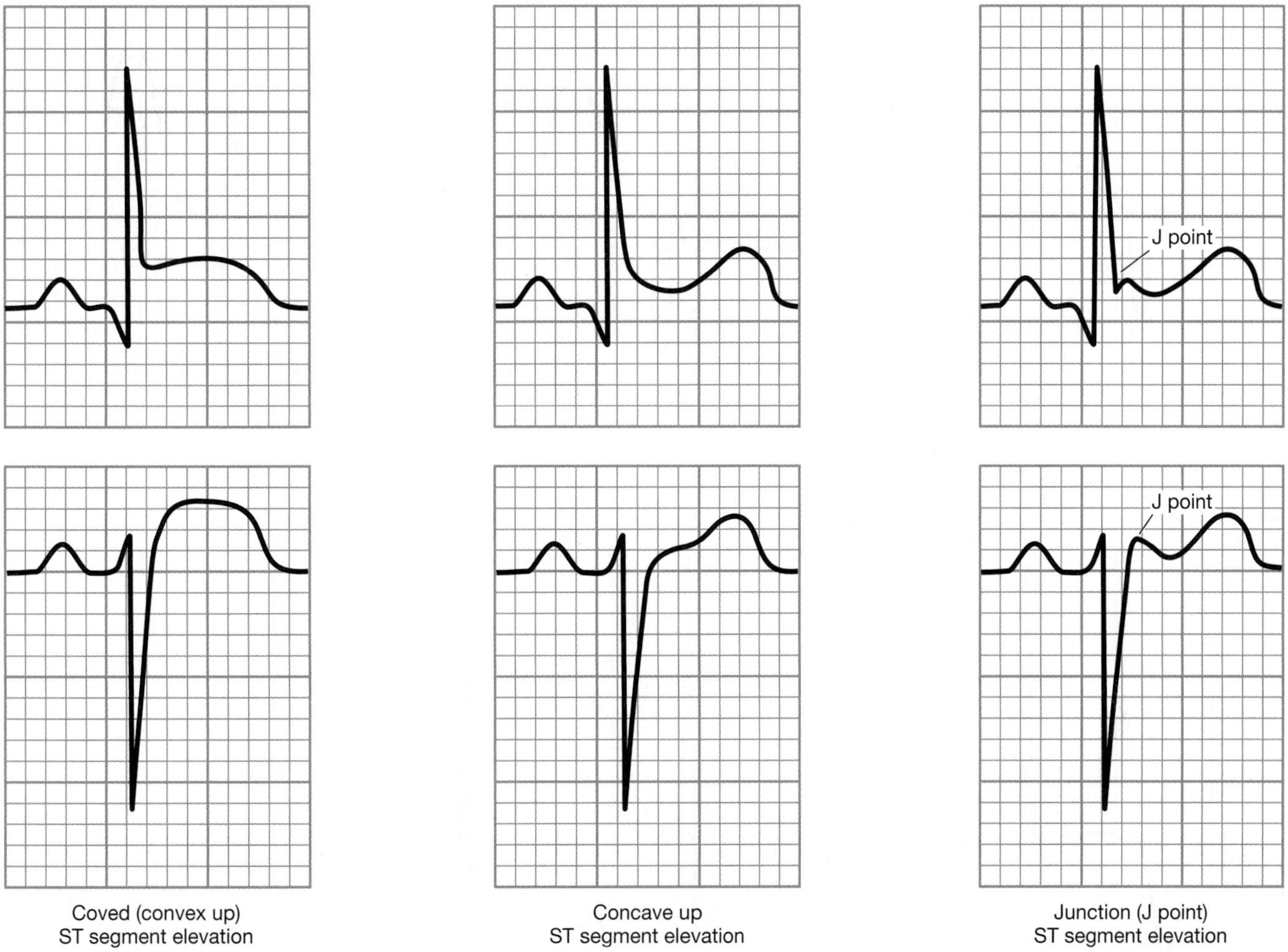

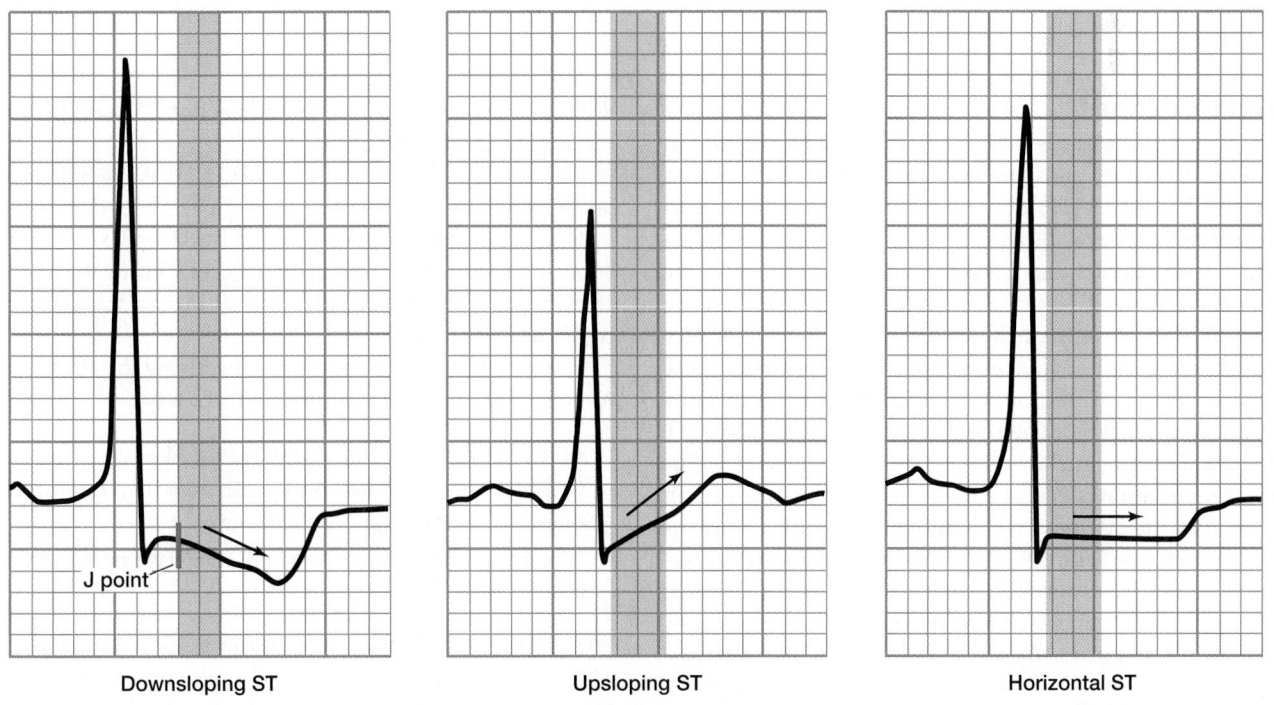

J point
J point
Coved (convex up)
ST segment elevation
Concave up
ST segment elevation
Junction (J point)
ST segment elevation

FIGURE 40–7 ■ ST segment elevation morphology differences.

J point
Downsloping ST
Upsloping ST
Horizontal ST
ST Segment Depression
The J point occurs at the end of the QRS complexes.
The ST segment begins at the J point and extends to a user defined interval.

FIGURE 40–8 ■ ST segment depression.

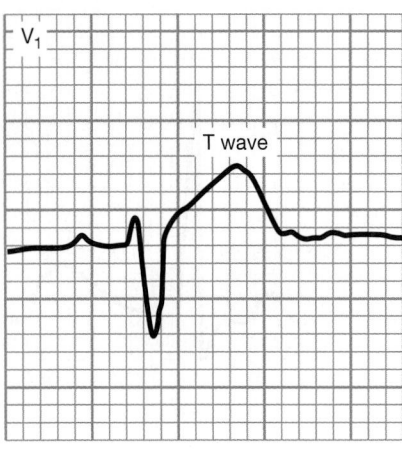
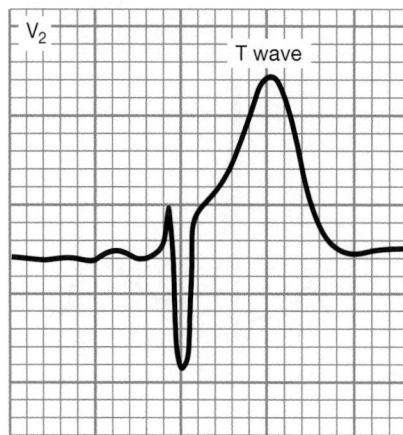
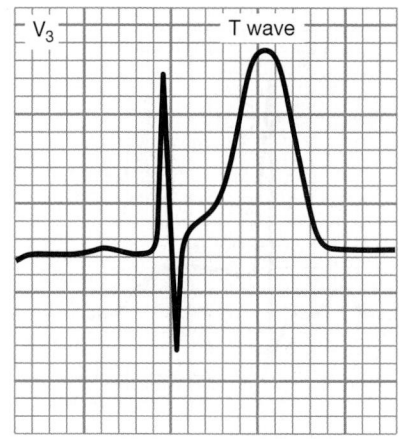

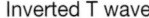

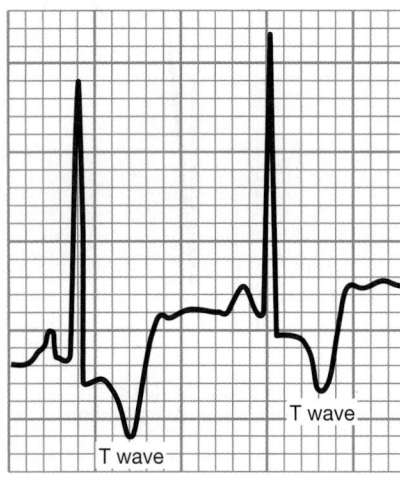
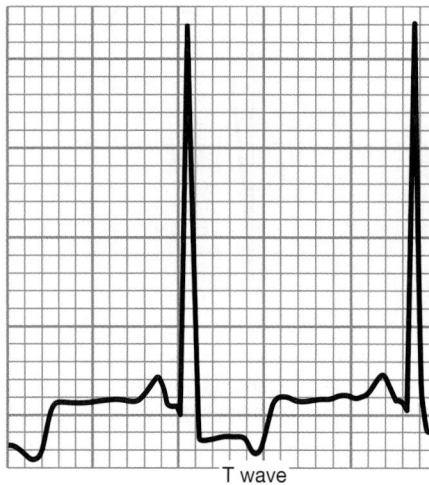

FIGURE 40–9 ■ Abnormal hyperacute and inverted T wave.

T Wave Changes

The T wave begins at the isoelectric line, gently slopes upward in a positive deflection, and represents ventricular repolarization (see Figure 40–6 ■, p. 1172). Abnormal T wave changes occur with ischemia/injury, thus, assisting with the diagnosis of ACS. When ischemia/injury occurs, the T wave inverts (flips over) in some leads and becomes tall or peaked in other leads. Marked T wave peaking and an increase in their width may be present in the very early stages of an acute MI. These are referred to as hyperacute T waves (see Figure 40–9 ■). Even patients with unstable angina have marked T wave peaking and increased width. Peaked T waves, like ST segment elevations, are indicative of acute occlusion. If the occlusion is total and unrelieved, it will evolve into an AMI. Within 5 to 30 minutes of occlusion/ ischemia, T wave inversion occurs (see Figure 40–9 ■). The inverted T wave is symmetrical in shape, relatively narrow, and somewhat pointed. Unlike the ST segment, which returns to normal rather quickly, the T wave can stay inverted for weeks after the ischemic event.

Q Wave Changes

The Q wave is the first component of the ventricular complex, and under normal conditions it is a negatively deflected wave (below the isoelectric line). It is small in size, is less than 0.04 second in duration, and is less than 25% of the amplitude of the R wave (see Figure 40–10 ■). The absence of Q waves is a normal variant of some people's ECG.

The development of an abnormal Q wave is a definitive diagnostic sign of myocardial necrosis. It appears later in time on the ECG than ischemia or injury evident by ST or T wave changes, because necrosis takes the longest to occur. During the first 24 to 48 hours after the AMI as the necrosis occurs, the Q wave becomes deeper and wider (see Figure 40–10 ■).

Q waves will develop in the leads overlying the affected area. Abnormal Q waves are identified in three ways:

- An increase in duration of > 0.04 second
- Greater than 4 millimeters in depth or > than one-fourth to one-third of the height of the R wave
- When they appear in leads where they have previously been absent.

The deep Q wave change seen on the ECG is due to necrosis, which is not reversible; therefore, Q wave changes on the ECGs are permanent, making previous MIs identifiable. The diagnosis of an "old" MI is made when there is a Q wave present in the absence of any ST segment elevation, patient symptoms, and positive blood markers. The ECG cannot determine how long ago the MI occurred; it could have been 2 weeks or 20 years.

Normal

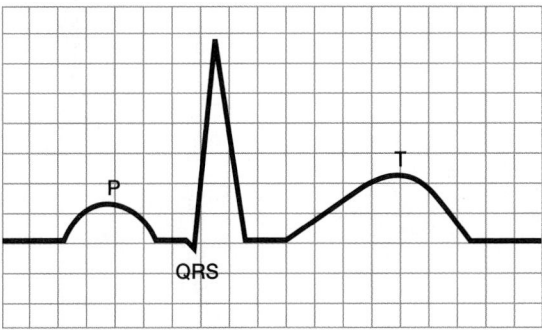

Abnormal Q wave

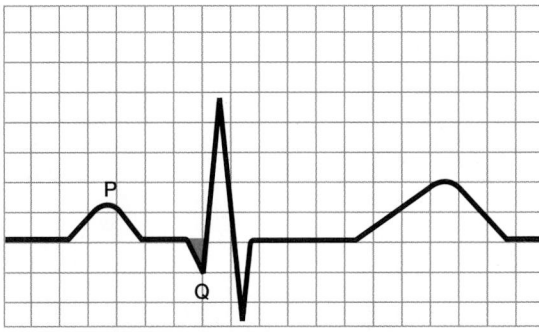

FIGURE 40–10 ■ Normal and abnormal Q wave.

Angina Pectoris

Angina pectoris is defined as transient chest pain due to myocardial ischemia, caused by an inadequate supply of oxygen and nutrients for the myocardium. CAD is the most common cause of a decreased blood supply to the myocardium. In the United States approximately 6,400,000 people suffer from angina. The estimated age-adjusted prevalences of angina in women age 20 and older were 3.5 percent for non-Hispanic white women, 4.7 percent for non-Hispanic black women, and 2.2 percent for Mexican American women. Rates for men in these three groups were 4.5, 3.1, and 2.4 percent, respectively (AHA, 2006b). Angina accounts for 29% of all medical emergency department admissions, at the cost of billions of health care dollars, and has the highest risk for adverse events and death (Libby, Bonow, Zipes, & Mann, 2008). Angina typically appears in middle age, whereas the average age for first heart attacks is 65 years in men and 70 in women. Though considered mostly a white man's disease, incidence rates of angina have increased in Mexican American men and women, and African American women most significantly (AHA, 2006f).

Angina also can occur in people with normal coronary arteries without obstruction, as a result of vasospasm, endothelial dysfunction, valvular heart disease, hypertrophic cardiomyopathy, uncontrolled hypertension, exacerbations of heart failure, and noncardiac conditions of the esophagus, chest wall, or lungs. Angina in the presence of heart disease is a *warning sign* and needs to be treated emergently in an attempt to prevent an acute cardiac event, such as a myocardial infarction.

Clinical Manifestations of Angina

The clinical manifestations of angina pectoris include a sudden onset of discomfort in the chest, jaw, shoulder, back, or arm, aggravated by exertion or emotional stress, and relieved with rest or nitroglycerin (Figure 40–11 ■, p. 1176). Terms such as *burning, crushing, suffocating,* and *pressure* are typical descriptors of chest pain from myocardial ischemia, often with pain radiating to other areas of the upper torso. Cardiac chest pain usually is neither described as sharp nor localized to a defined spot.

Symptoms of chest pain alone are poor predictors of the presence of CAD and the severity of myocardial damage. In nearly one-third to one-half of individuals with myocardial ischemia, symptoms are not present at all. The clinician is faced with comparing data abstracted from the patient to a set of characteristics associated with diseases that have common presenting signs and symptoms. Charts 40–6 (p. 1177) and 40–7 (p. 1178) outline the presentation of patients with diseases that mimic chest pain associated with CAD.

Women, patients with diabetes, and elderly patients may not experience pain with myocardial ischemia. In addition, the characterization of pain by women may be different from that of men, with women expressing pain in less severe terms, if at all, and often ascribing the pain to causes other than cardiac issues.

Types of Angina Pectoris

There are several accepted classifications for angina pectoris that are based on what triggers the occurrence, how long it lasts, when it occurs, what makes it go away, and its seriousness. Angina is classified as either typical or atypical, depending on signs and symptoms and/or by its severity using the Canadian Cardiovascular Society's angina classification scale. It also is assigned various terms that describe its timing, location, and position. Chart 40–8 (p. 1180) outlines the classifications and descriptors of angina.

Two general categories or classifications include stable and unstable angina. Stable angina, the less serious type, is triggered by a predictable degree of exertion or emotions, and there is a pattern in relation to what brings it on, its duration, its intensity of symptoms, and how to relieve it. Stable angina subsides by taking away the precipitating factors and using sublingual nitroglycerin. Stable angina is differentiated from unstable angina pathologically by the absence of plaque disruption and thrombus formation in the lumen of the artery. Unstable angina is discussed in the next section under acute coronary syndrome.

Variant, Prinzmetal, or Vasospastic Angina   is the most serious type of angina. It occurs when single or multiple sites in major coronary arteries and their large branches have vasospasm. Most often the right coronary artery is involved. Sites of vasospasm generally occur over eccentric lesions. Causes of vasospasm are unknown but may be related to an imbalance of vasoactive agents derived from damaged coronary endothelial tissue, vessel segment hypersensitivity to sympathetic stimulation, allergy, or hypomagnesemia. Symptoms are usually episodic, may last several minutes, are often associated with exercise, and can occur frequently at night.

Medical Management of Angina Pectoris

The majority of patients with stable angina achieve symptom control by medical management alone. When patients with symptoms of angina present to a clinician's office or an emergency

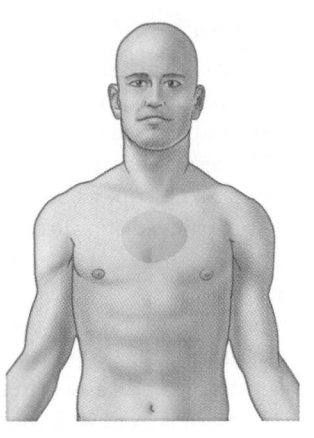

(a) Upper chest

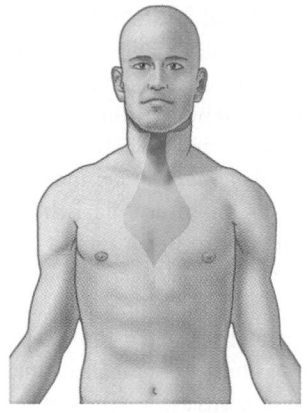

(b) Substernal radiating to neck and jaw

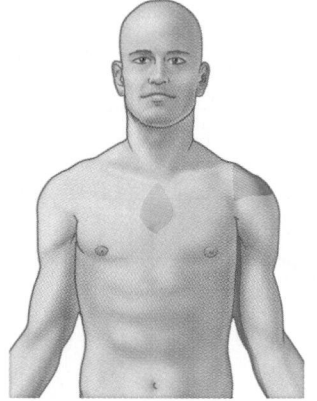

(c) Substernal radiating down left arm

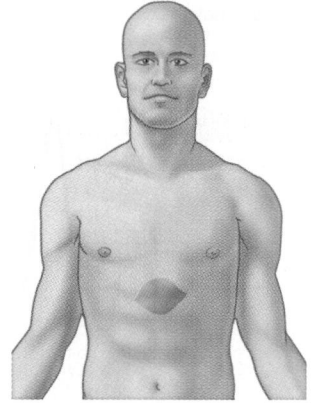

(d) Epigastric

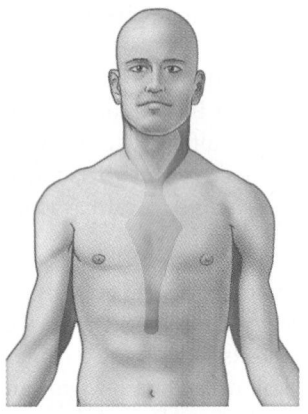

(e) Epigastric radiating to neck, jaw, and arms

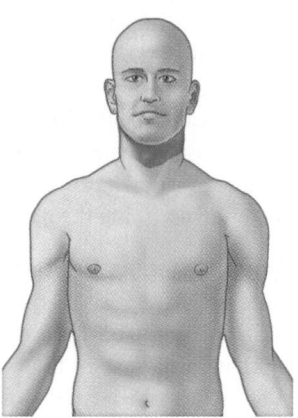

(f) Neck and jaw

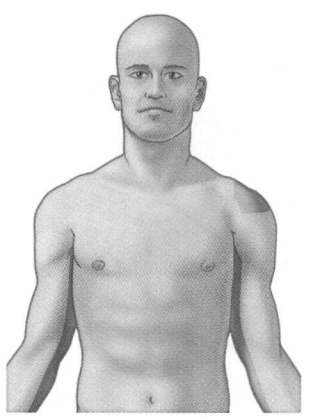

(g) Left shoulder and down both arms

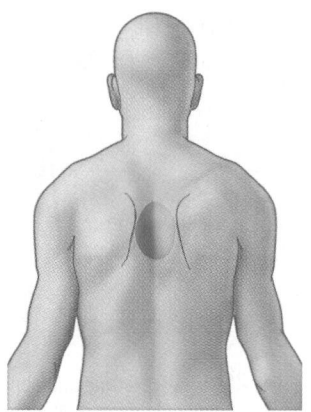

(h) Intrascapular

FIGURE 40–11 ■ Location of anginal pain.

department, they must be taken seriously and evaluated thoroughly by the health care team. Routine evaluations of patients who complain of chest pain include a review of their symptoms, their medical/social history for associated diseases and risk factors, an assessment for physical signs, and diagnostic tests. Emergency department (ED) personnel use guidelines set forth by the American College of Cardiology and the American Heart Association (Antman et al., 2004) that dictate the patients' treatment. (See the Medical Management of Complications of Acute Myocardial Infarction section, p. 1198.)

Predictors of higher risk for complications generally include angina that has increased in duration, frequency, or at rest; associated ST segment or T wave changes on the ECG; and accompanying signs of heart failure such as the following: new or worsening mitral regurgitation murmur; skin changes such as cool, pale, or clammy; pulmonary edema or presence of an S_3 or S_4 heart sound; tachycardia; and hypotension. Patients classified at lower risk are generally treated on an outpatient basis. Goals for outpatient management include treating conditions that exacerbate angina such as anemia, thyrotoxicosis, dysrhythmias, and eliminating or suppressing symptoms through behavioral changes and prescribing antianginal agents.

Pharmacologic management for angina rests primarily on three classes of drugs: calcium channel blockers, nitrates, and beta-adrenergic blocking agents. Symptom characteristics, exer-

cise tolerance, and comorbid conditions dictate which antianginal agent to use. To date no one drug category has proven more effective at improving prognosis for patients treated for angina pectoris. Antianginal medications are outlined in the Pharmacology Summary (p. 1199). In addition to antianginal agents, management of angina includes ASA in daily doses of 81 to 325 milligrams.

Activity restriction and removing the precipitating factors also will help relieve angina due to decreasing the oxygen demand on the heart. Supplemental oxygen is frequently ordered during periods of pain.

■ Nursing Management

Nursing management of a patient who is experiencing angina requires critical thinking and decision-making skills. Angina pectoris is a warning that the myocardium is not getting enough oxygen, and increased perfusion of oxygen and nutrients is needed to prevent permanent myocardial muscle damage. The nursing process serves as the platform to manage the patients experiencing angina pectoris.

Assessment

The patient needs an in-depth nursing assessment of the pain, including the type of sensation, the location and transmission,

CHART 40–6	**Differential Diagnosis of Chest Pain: Common Etiologies**

Pain Description	Associated Findings	History
Angina/Myocardial Infarction		

• Usually retrosternal
• Can originate or radiate at the back, anterior chest, epigastric area, jaw, shoulder, elbow, forearm, wrist
• May be relieved with rest, lasts < 30 minutes
	• Tachycardia
	• Tachypnea, dyspnea
	• Weak heart sounds
	• Rhonchi
	• Diaphoresis
	• Abnormal precordial impulses
	• Evidence of dysrhythmias
		• Cardiac risk factors
		  • Smoking
		  • Male gender
		  • African American
		  • Sedentary lifestyle
		  • Social stressors
		  • High-fat diet.

• Heaviness, burning, tight pressure, aching, indigestion
• Is not relieved with position change
• May increase while supine
• Is not aggravated by deep breathing
	• Fever, elevated white blood count (WBC) count, elevated sedimentation rate
	• Anxiety, sense of impending doom
	• Nausea/vomiting
		• Cardiovascular disease
		  • Heart failure
		  • Dysrhythmias
		  • PVD
		  • Heart valve disease
		  • Angina, unstable angina, myocardial infarction (MI) cardiac interventions
		  • Cardiac surgery
		  • Catheter-based interventions.

Pulmonary Embolism		
• Sudden onset • Sharp • Pleuritic • Lateral chest • Increases on deep inspiration	• Shock • Syncope • Dyspnea, shortness of breath (SOB), cyanosis • Tachycardia • Hemoptysis • Pleural friction rub • Expiratory wheeze • Fever	• Hypercoaguable state • Immobility • Surgery • Trauma • DVT
Gastrointestinal Disorders		
• Burning, squeezing, gripping • Retrosternal without radiation • Lasts many hours or days, constant in nature • Precipitated by bending over, drinking very hot/cold liquids, meals • Relieved with food or beverage	• Reflux • Dysphagia • Dyspepsia	• GERD • Esophageal motility disorders • Esophageal malignancy
Costochondritis		
• Usually superficial and localized • Described as tender, ache, sharp • Can be in any location • Duration variable • Aggravated/provoked by movement or touch	• Sudden movement • Tachypnea, shallow breathing • Tachycardia • Elevated blood pressure	• Falls or trauma • Immobility • Chest tubes newly removed
Acute Anxiety		
• Dull, stabbing	• Breathlessness, hyperventilation	• Acute stress, phobia • Inability to cope

< = less than; PVD = peripheral vascular disease; DVT = deep vein thrombosis; GERD = gastroesophageal reflux disease; w/ = with; w/o = without; SOB = shortness of breath; MI = myocardial infarction; WBC = white blood count

Sources: Williams, J. L. (2003). Gastroesophageal reflux disease: Clinical manifestations. *Gastroenterology Nursing, 26*(5), 195–200; Zoorob, R. J., & Campbell, J. S. (2003). Acute dyspnea in the office. *American Family Physician, 68,* 1803–1810; Lissin, L. W., & Vagelos, R. (2002). Acute aortic syndrome: A case presentation and review of the literature. *Vascular Medicine, 7*(4), 281–287; Pope, J. H., & Selker, H. P. (2002). Diagnosis of acute cardiac ischemia. *Emergency Medical Clinics of North America, 21*(1), 27–59; and Kontos, M. C. (2001). Evaluation of the emergency department chest pain patient. *Cardiology Review, 9*(5), 266–275.

CHART 40–7	Differential Diagnosis of Chest Pain: Less Common Etiologies	

Pain Description	Associated Findings	History
Pericarditis		
• Sudden, sharp	• Pulsus paradoxsus	• AMI
• Dull, aching	• Dyspnea	• Dressler's syndrome
• Stabbing, knife-like	• Low-grade erratic fever	• Tamponade
• Retrosternum or precordial	• Pericardial friction rub	• Pericardial effusion
• Can radiate to neck, left shoulder and arm, back, epigastrium	• Elevated neck veins	• Constrictive pericarditis
	• Tachycardia	• Myocardial/pericardial injury
	• Hiccups	• Connective tissue disease
• Aggravated by deep inspiration, cough, rotation of the chest	• Nausea/vomiting	• Infection
	• Dizziness	• Radiation therapy
	• Generalized malaise	• Neoplasm
• Alleviated by sitting up and forward	• Hoarseness	
	• Abdominal pain	
Dissecting Aortic Aneurysm		
• Acute sharp onset w/o warning	• Syncope	• Hypertension
	• Diaphoresis	• Congenital heart defects
• Tearing, ripping	• Tachycardia	• Syphilitic aortitis
• In synch w/heartbeat	• Hyper/hypotension	• Blunt trauma
• Lasts for hours or days	• Confusion	• Males > 50–70 years
• Upper back, anterior chest, epigastric, shoulders, retrosternal	• Fever	• Third trimester of pregnancy
	• Blood pressure different in each arm	
• Radiates to hips, groin, lower extremity, neck, shoulders, costovertebral area, epigastric area, jaw	• Absent or diminished pulses uni/bilateral	
	• Decreased level of consciousness	
• Settles in lower back	• Melena, hematemesis, nausea, vomiting	
Spontaneous Pneumothorax		
• Sudden	• Dyspnea	• Severe underlying lung disease
• Severe	• Tachycardia	• Necrotizing pneumonia
• Over lateral thorax	• Blood pressure difference in each arm	• ARDS
	• Hyperresonance and decreased breath sounds	• High airway pressures while on mechanical ventilation
		• Common ages 16–25 years
	• Tracheal deviation toward affected side	• COPD
		• Cystic fibrosis
	• Decreased respiratory excursion	• Blebs
	• Bulging intercostal muscles	
Cholecystitis		
• Severe abdominal pain	• Nausea/vomiting	
• Epigastric area	• Fever	
• Tenderness in abdomen, right upper quadrant	• Jaundice	
	• Changes in bowel habit	
• May radiate to back and scapula	• Intolerance to fatty foods	
Pancreatitis		
• Extreme epigastric pain, alternating with dull aching sensation	• Hypotension	
	• Fever	
	• Change in bowel habit	
• Radiates to back, flank	• Weight loss, malnutrition	

AMI = acute myocardial infarction; w/o = without; w/ = with; ARDS = acute respiratory distress syndrome; COPD = chronic obstructive pulmonary disease

Sources: Williams, J. L. (2003). Gastroesophageal reflux disease: Clinical manifestations. *Gastroenterology Nursing, 26*(5), 195–200. Zoorob, R. J., & Campbell, J. S. (2003). Acute dyspnea in the office. *American Family Physician, 68,* 1803–1810; Lissin, L. W., & Vagelos, R. (2002). Acute aortic syndrome: A case presentation and review of the literature. *Vascular Medicine, 7*(4), 281–287; Pope, J. H., & Selker, H. P. (2002). Diagnosis of acute cardiac ischemia. *Emergency Medical Clinics of North America, 21*(1), 27–59; and Kontos, M. C. (2001). Evaluation of the emergency department chest pain patient. *Cardiology Review, 9*(5), 266–275.

Coronary Heart Disease in Women

Clinical Problem

Coronary heart disease (CHD), resulting in an acute myocardial infarction, is the leading cause of death for American women. Many women believe that cancer is more of a threat, but nearly twice as many women in the United States die of heart disease and stroke as from all forms of cancer, including breast cancer. Heart disease and stroke claim more female lives than the next five causes of death combined (AHA, 2006a). Additionally, women have an overall poorer prognosis once they have had an acute myocardial infarction (AMI). According to the American Heart Association (2006a), 38% of women, as compared with 25% of men, will die within 1 year after a heart attack.

Diagnosing CHD in women is challenging, and yet few studies have focused on the scope of women's prodromal and acute CHD symptoms. For example, chest pain, a hallmark symptom of ischemia in men, is often not of significant prognostic value in women. No clear picture has emerged on women's typical prodromal symptoms and how they relate to the onset of an AMI. Currently, the description of typical cardiac symptoms is based primarily on what occurs in white, middle-class men. For nurses to improve patient teaching about prevention and occurrence of an AMI in women, it is imperative to identify prodromal and acute symptoms.

Research Findings

McSweeney et al. (2003) studied 515 women who were diagnosed with an AMI. These women were surveyed 4 to 6 months after hospital discharge. The research questionnaire targeted symptoms, comorbidities, and demographic characteristics. The results indicated that 95% of the women knew their symptoms were new or different a month or more before their AMI. The most common symptoms prior to the AMI were:

- Unusual fatigue (70%)
- Sleep disturbance (48%)
- Shortness of breath (42%)
- Indigestion (39%)
- Anxiety (35%).

Major symptoms during the AMI include:

- Unusual fatigue (43%)
- Weakness (55%)
- Shortness of breath (58%)
- Cold sweat (39%)
- Dizziness (39%).

Approximately 78% of women reported experiencing at least one prodromal symptom for more than 1 month either daily or several times a week before their AMI. Only 29.7% reported chest discomfort, which they described as aching (33%), tightness (33%), pressure (32%), sharpness (23%), burning (21%), fullness (18%), and tingling (18%) (McSweeney et al., 2003, p. 2).

Implications for Nursing Practice

This study indicates that there is still much to learn about women versus men experiencing AMIs. Education about heart disease in

women began in 1997. To extend the effort that began in 1997, in 2004 the American Heart Association and other organizations began a series of national awareness campaigns to educate women about heart disease. At this time the American Heart Association launched its *Go Red For Women* movement to raise women's awareness of their risk for heart disease and to help them take action to reduce their risk. Today the association continues to play a leading role in educating women by providing them with heart-healthy tools through Go Red For Women (AHA, 2008b & c).

It is imperative that nurses educate women about the symptoms of heart disease at every opportunity. A study by Mosca et al. (2006) indicated that women's awareness of the risk of heart disease as the leading killer has risen from 30% in 1997 to 55% in 2006. The study also concluded that due to this awareness women are taking action to improve their own and their family's heart health. These changes in awareness and lifestyles can come about only through education. Nurses play a "key" role in this education process due to their close proximity to patients.

The downside of the study's results (Mosca et al., 2006) is that while 62% of white women surveyed were aware that heart disease was the leading cause of death, only 38% of African Americans and 34% of Hispanics had the same level of awareness. Given these statistics, efforts need to focus on educating the culturally diverse populations.

Teaching needs to include the risk for heart disease and well as the prodromal symptoms. Increasing awareness will ensure that women know whether they have healthy levels of risk factors and what their personal risk is. Mosca's study indicated that women's awareness of heart disease can positively influence their family. Therefore educational efforts for women can have a far-reaching impact.

Critical Thinking Questions

1. How can nurses adapt teaching materials and techniques for patients with limited or no English language skills?

2. When assessing a female patient suspected of having CHD, what types of questions would the nurse ask to help determine the presence of fatigue?

3. What facts would a nurse include in an education program to help increase the awareness of heart disease in women?

Answers to Critical Thinking Questions appear in Appendix D.

References

American Heart Association (2006a). *Facts about women and cardiovascular diseases.* Retrieved August 7, 2006, from http://www.americanheart.org/presenter.jhtml?identifier=2876.

American Heart Association. (2008). *Women and Coronary Heart Disease.* Retrieved July 18, 2008, from http://www.americanheart.org/presenter.jhtml?identifier=2859.

McSweeney, J., Cody, M., O'Sullivan, P., Elberson, K., Moser, D., & Garvin, B. (2003). Women's early warning symptoms of acute myocardial infarction. *Circulation, 108* (21), 2619–2623.

Mosca, L., Mochari, H., Christian, A., Berra, K., Taubert, K., Mills, T., et al. (2006). National study of women's awareness, preventive action, and barriers to cardiovascular health. *Circulation, 113,* 525–534.

EVIDENCE-BASED PRACTICE

| CHART 40–8 | Angina Classifications and Descriptors |

Term	Descriptor(s)/Definitions
Typical angina, three key characteristics	1. Central/substernal chest or left arm pain, discomfort, pressure, tightness, heaviness 2. Provoked by exertion or emotional stress 3. Relieved by nitroglycerin
Atypical angina or ischemic equivalents, any two of the characteristics for typical angina	1. Jaw, neck, ear, arm, back 2. Weakness, dizziness, light-headedness, loss of consciousness, unexplained fatigue, diaphoresis 3. New or worsening dyspnea on exertion 4. Nausea/vomiting unexplained indigestion, belching, epigastric pain or discomfort 5. Burning, aching, cramping
Nocturnal angina	Occurs at night usually during sleep. May be relieved by sitting upright. Commonly associated with left ventricular dysfunction.
Decubitus angina	Angina while lying down.
Preinfarction, postinfarction angina	Prior to or after infarction. Preinfarction angina may precondition the heart for episodes of subsequent infarction, resulting in a reduction in infarct size. Postinfarction angina denotes increased risk for death or recurrent myocardial infarction (MI).
Recurring/stuttering angina	Angina that comes and goes. Denotes instability, thrombus formation, and dissolution.
Canadian Cardiovascular Society Classification for Angina Pectoris	
Class I angina	Angina produced only with strenuous, rapid, or prolonged exertion. Patient is able to engage in ordinary physical activity such as walking and climbing stairs.
Class II angina	Angina that occurs with mild exertion such as climbing stairs rapidly; walking uphill, in the cold, against the wind; walking or stair-climbing after a meal. Angina that occurs under emotional stress or in the first few hours after awakening. Results in slight limitation of ordinary activity.
Class III angina	Angina that occurs during ordinary physical activities such as walking at a normal pace 1–2 blocks on level ground or climbing a flight of stairs under normal conditions. Results in marked limitation of ordinary physical activity.
Class IV angina	Angina at rest. Results in inability to carry on any physical activity without discomfort.

Source: Braunwald, E., Antman, E. M., Beasley, J. W., et al. (2002). ACC/AHA 2002 guideline update for the management of patients with unstable angina and non-ST-segment elevation myocardial infarction: A report of the American College of Cardiology/American Heart Association Task Force on Practice Guidelines (Committee on the Management of Patient with Unstable Angina). *Journal of the American College of Cardiology, 40,* 1366–1370. Retrieved July 15, 2008, from http://www.acc.org/clinical/guidelines/unstable/unstable.pdf. Retrieved July 15, 2008, from http://www.acc.org/qualityandscience/clinical/guidelines/unstable/appendix2.htm.

the duration, what brings it on, and what makes it go away. The nurse must inquire whether this is new onset pain or whether there is a history of anginal chest pain. If this pain has occurred before, is there a change in the pattern or intensity? For example, stable angina is predictable in what causes it, makes it go away, and its intensity, whereas unstable angina is more intense and less predictable in its pattern. The subjective and objective findings during an anginal attack may include tachycardia, increased or decreased blood pressure (BP), cardiac dysrhythmias, apprehension/anxiety, diaphoresis, and pallor. The nurse must assess vital signs, the ECG monitor, and the associated clinical manifestations. Typically the ECG is obtained during pain because the ischemic changes will resolve with treatment. It is also common to have cardiac dysrhythmias occur during angina, due to muscle irritability from the ischemia. Assessment for heart failure also is essential. Lung sounds, peripheral edema, increasing shortness of breath, and respiratory rate must be evaluated. Physical findings between periods of angina are usually normal and therefore not diagnostic.

Outcomes and Evaluation Parameters

The desired nursing outcome is to prevent the progression of ischemia to the myocardium, which would result in permanent cardiac muscle damage and worsening symptoms. The primary evaluation parameter is complete relief of the anginal pain, because this indicates that there is adequate blood supply to the myocardium. Associated outcome parameters include vital signs, cardiac output, activity tolerance, lungs, and mental orientation. The nurse must monitor the patient's vital signs both as the pain is beginning to subside and when it is totally relieved. The goal is for the heart rate and blood pressure to return to the patient's baseline. Normal ECG, absent or decreased dysrhythmias, and normal mentation also are outcomes that indicate an adequate blood supply to the myocardium. Absence of heart failure is an essential outcome because it is a serious long-term complication. Finally, once the pain is relieved, the patient will verbalize less fear and anxiety.

Planning and Interventions with Rationales

Nursing interventions must be instituted including prescribed antianginal medications, described under medical management, that dilate the coronary arteries, thereby increasing blood flow to the ischemic myocardium. Whatever activity was occurring that precipitated the pain must be stopped. The heart is unable to meet the oxygen needs, and stopping activity will decrease the need.

Supplemental oxygen is applied per health care provider orders, and vital signs and oxygen saturation levels are observed. The effectiveness of these interventions is assessed continuously until the patient is pain free and the heart rate and blood pressure are within normal range. If this is not achieved, it may indicate that there is a more serious problem, and the health care provider must be notified to order further interventions and testing.

 The nurse must stay with the patient who is experiencing angina and continue an ongoing assessment until the pain is gone or it is determined that the interventions are not effective and the health care provider needs to be notified.

Health Promotion

Because angina pectoris is an indicator of decreased cardiac reserve, it is imperative that a comprehensive education program be initiated on onset of the symptoms. The best prevention program would be instituted before the clinical manifestations, but often the patient is not seen prior to admittance to an emergency department (ED). The nurse is in an ideal position to begin education about lifestyle changes that will reduce or prevent a progression of the disease. The education needs to include risk factor management (see Charts 40–4, p. 1166 and 40–5, p. 1167), medication instructions, and avoidance of precipitating factors. The nurse must assess the patient/family's ability to understand and be receptive to education. There may be language or cultural barriers, and/or the anxiety level may interfere with the patient/family's ability to absorb the information. It is imperative that the teaching plan includes a review of medication regimens, side effects, symptoms of ischemia, and teaching about self-treatment and handling potentially emergent situations. The patients receiving beta-adrenergic blocking agents and calcium channel blockers need to be taught how to count their pulse and what rate must be reported to the health care provider. If taking nitrates, patients should be taught about safe storage, handling, and side effects of different nitrate preparations as well as how to take sublingual nitrates (see the Pharmacology Summary, p. 1199). Patients should also receive coaching on adaptation to and compliance with risk factor modification activities and be encouraged to seek assistance if therapy becomes a financial burden or creates conflicts within their support group. Families or significant others may need teaching about how to cope or help the patient deal with lifestyle and behavioral change, or referral to community services to learn bystander cardiopulmonary resuscitation.

Acute Coronary Syndrome

Patients who present to the health care provider's office or the ED with a change in their previous pattern of angina or new onset angina, are evaluated for the likelihood that their symptoms represent an ACS secondary to CAD. They are evaluated for the presence of myocardial infarction, myocardial ischemia, and infarction-related complications, as well as a general state of hemodynamic stability. Disposition of patients to either outpatient management or admission to an inpatient unit, selection of therapy, and decisions about revascularization are based on these assessment data.

Categories of Acute Coronary Syndrome

Included under the umbrella of acute coronary syndrome (ACS) are the diagnoses of unstable angina (UA), non–ST segment elevation myocardial infarction (MI) (NSTEMI), and ST segment elevation MI (STEMI). *ACS* is a recent term that has emerged as research into the pathophysiology and optimal management of ischemic heart disease has progressed. Being admitted with a diagnosis of ACS just means there is a cardiac event going on, and after admission and further testing, a more definitive diagnosis is made. Pathogenesis of ACS involves fibrous plaque disruption and thrombosis formation, and can result in either a partial or a total occlusion of the lumen of the coronary artery. This process will either markedly decrease or completely cut off blood flow to the myocardium.

Unstable Angina Pectoris

Anginal symptoms controlled by rest or medical management are considered stable, as described earlier. **Unstable angina** depicts a transitory syndrome falling between stable angina and acute myocardial infarction (AMI) wherein thrombus forms in an area of arterial stenosis but is subsequently fully or partially lysed by endogenous antithrombotic mechanisms. Symptoms worsen such that the patient presents with the development of new onset exertion angina, angina present at rest for longer than 20 minutes, or symptoms that have accelerated in frequency, duration, or intensity (Diop & Aghababian, 2001). When the vessels are assessed with cardiac angiography (Chapter 39), these patients most often show the presence of stenotic eccentric lesions, collateral circulation, and the absence of a totally occluded coronary artery. Blood markers indicating myocardial damage are normal, and ECG changes, if present, are transitory and will return to normal. Based on the assessment and physical findings, patients are categorized as low, intermediate, or high risk and triaged appropriately (Chart 40–9, p. 1182).

Non–ST Segment Myocardial Infarction

The term **myocardial infarction** (**MI**) denotes a loss of myocytes or myocardial cell death as a result of prolonged muscle ischemia. Cell death results in a permanent loss of myocardial muscle function. **NSTEMI** is a correlate syndrome to UA with a common pathogenesis and clinical presentation. Both usually occur as a result of transient subtotal occlusion of a coronary artery with reduced coronary blood flow resulting from plaque disruption and ensuing pathophysiological processes. The presence of serum blood markers and persistent ECG changes distinguishes a more severe myocardial injury associated with NSTEMI and thus a higher risk of death and MI, versus no blood marker release and transitory or no ECG changes seen with UA. See Figure 40–6 ■ (p. 1172), which shows normal ECG waveforms, and compare it to Figure 40–8 ■ (p. 1173) and to Figure 40–12 ■ (p. 1183); the middle figure shows ECG changes associated with the partial obstruction seen with NSTEMI.

ST Segment Elevation Myocardial Infarction

ST segment elevation myocardial infarction (**STEMI**) refers to myocardial injury associated with ST segment elevation on the ECG (see Figure 40–7 ■, p. 1173 & 40–12 ■, p. 1183). Besides the ST segment, STEMI compares differently to NSTEMI in a number of ways. The presence of ST segment elevation means that myocardial tissue is undergoing severe anoxia and cellular damage. In

| CHART 40–9 | Short-Term Risk of Death or Nonfatal MI in Patients With UA/NSTEMI*£ | | |

Feature	Low Risk (No High or Intermediate risk features but may have any of the following)	Intermediate Risk (No High risk features, must have 1 of the following)	High Risk (At least 1 of the following features must be present)
History		Prior diagnosis of arterio-occlusive disease such as MI, PVD, CVD, or CABG; prior aspirin use	Accelerating tempo (increased frequency, severity, or duration) of ischemic symptoms over last 48 hours
Pain Characteristics	Increased frequency, severity, or duration of angina Angina provoked at a lower threshold New onset angina with onset 2 weeks to 2 months prior to presentation	Prolonged (> 20 minutes) rest angina, resolved at presentation, with likelihood of CAD Prolonged (> 20 minutes) angina relieved with rest or sublingual NTG Nocturnal angina New onset or progressive limitation of activity (walking 1–2 blocks, climbing 1–2 flights of stairs, pain with any physical exertion, angina at rest) in past 2 weeks without prolonged (> 20 minutes) rest pain but with likelihood of CAD.	Prolonged (> 20 minutes) ongoing at rest
Clinical Findings		Age > 70 years	Presence of any one of the following: pulmonary edema likely due to ischemia; new or worsening mitral regurgitation; S_3 or new/worsening rales; hypotension, bradycardia, tachycardia Age > 75 years
ECG	Normal or unchanged ECG	T wave changes Pathologic Qs or resting ST-segment depression > 1 mm in multiple lead groups (anterior, inferior, lateral)	Angina at rest with transient ST-segment changes > 0.5 mm BBB new or presumed new Sustained VT
Cardiac Markers	Normal	Slightly elevated TnT, TnI, or CK-MB	Elevated cardiac TnT, TnI, or CK-MB

Note: BBB-bundle branch block; CABG-coronary artery bypass graft surgery; CAD-coronary artery disease; CK-MB-creatine kinase, MB fraction; CVD-cerebral vascular disease; ECG-electrocardiogram; MI-myocardial infarction; NTG- nitroglycerin; PVD-peripheral vascular disease; TnI-troponin I; TnT- troponin T; UA/NSTEMI-unstable angina/non–ST-elevation myocardial infarction; VT-ventricular tachycardia.

*Estimation of risk for adverse events should be done with patients who present with a history and/or signs and symptoms of cardiac ischemia and considered in patient treatment.

£Adapted from Table 7 page e17 of Anderson et. al, ACC/AHA 2007 Guidelines for the Management of Patients With Unstable Angina/Non-ST-Elevation Myocardial Infarction: A Report of the American College of Cardiology/American Heart Association Task Force on Practice Guidelines. Content is meant to illustrate general guidelines and should not be used as practice algorithms.

most cases this is a result of complete coronary artery blockage from thrombotic occlusion over an underlying plaque lesion (Libby, Bonow, Zipes, & Mann, 2008). Unlike NSTEMI, the blockage is sustained. If blood flow is not reestablished in 20 minutes, cell death occurs. Ischemic damage traverses the myocardium vertically outward, starting with the subendocardial layer through to the epicardium (see Figure 40–4 ■, p. 1163). Prior to the current age of rapid revascularization therapies, ST segment elevation was usually associated with transmural myocardial infarction and the appearance of Q waves on the ECG days later. The Q wave changes indicate cell death and permanent loss of muscle function in the affected area. If the occlusion is treated early, a patient presenting with STEMI may suffer only subendocardial cell damage without subsequent Q waves.

Classifications of Myocardial Infarction

Both STEMI and NSTEMI are classified according to the coronary artery involved. Occlusion of the left anterior descending

(LAD) artery is referred to as an anterior wall infarct. The LAD feeds the anterior left ventricle, anterior septum, papillary muscle, apex, bundle of His, and bundle branches. All or some of the function of these tissues is lost with an infarct to the LAD. Most infarcts affect the left ventricle.

Occlusion of the right coronary artery (RCA) results in an inferior wall MI. The RCA supplies the inferior left ventricle, inferior septum, papillary muscle, and right ventricle (the SA node in 60% of the population and the AV node in 90%). Occlusion of the circumflex artery results in a lateral wall infarct because it supplies the lateral wall of the left ventricle (the SA node in 40% of the population and the AV node in 10%).

Occlusion of the left main coronary (LMC) artery results in what is referred to as a massive MI because LMC supplies blood to over 70% of the left ventricle. Myocardial infarctions involving the LMC, often referred to as "widow makers," typically are associated with complications such as heart failure. Figure 40–13 ■ shows a thrombosis in the coronary arteries.

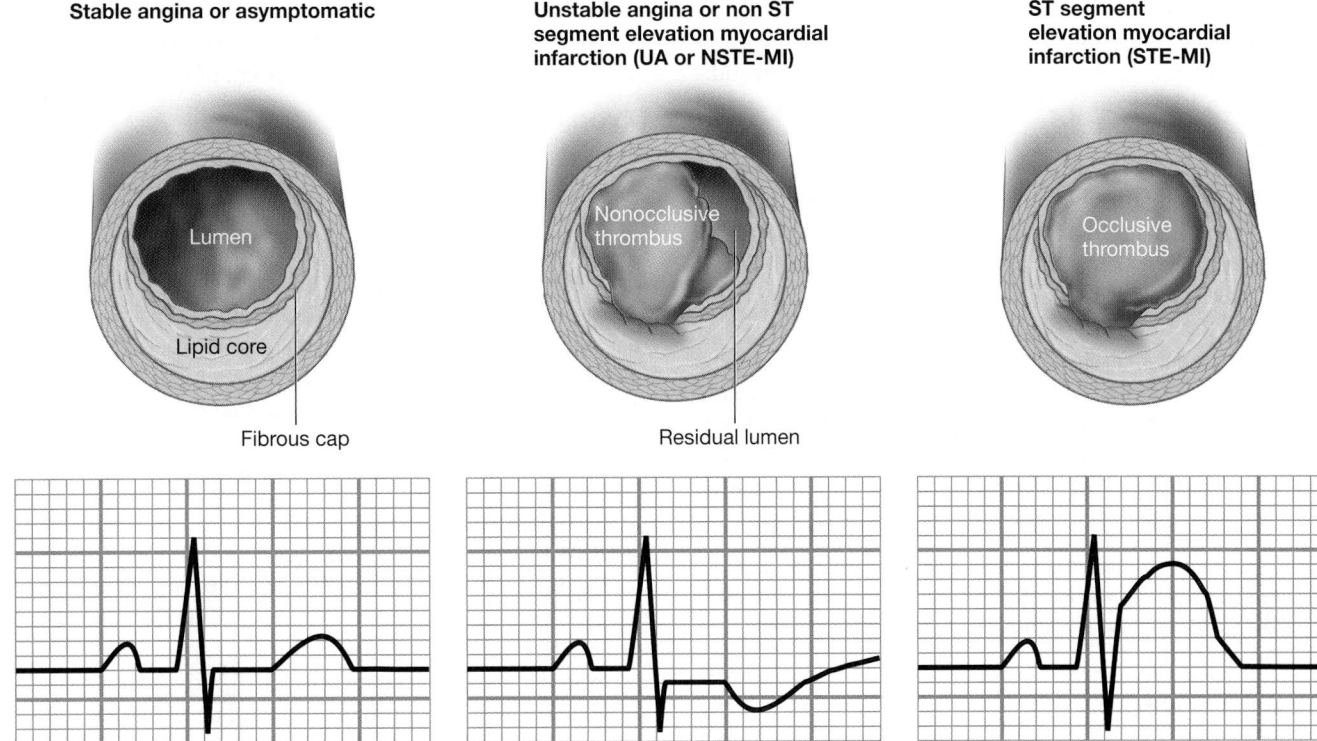

Stable angina or asymptomatic

Unstable angina or non ST segment elevation myocardial infarction (UA or NSTE-MI)

ST segment elevation myocardial infarction (STE-MI)

FIGURE 40–12 ■ Clot formation and ST segment ECG changes associated with ACS.

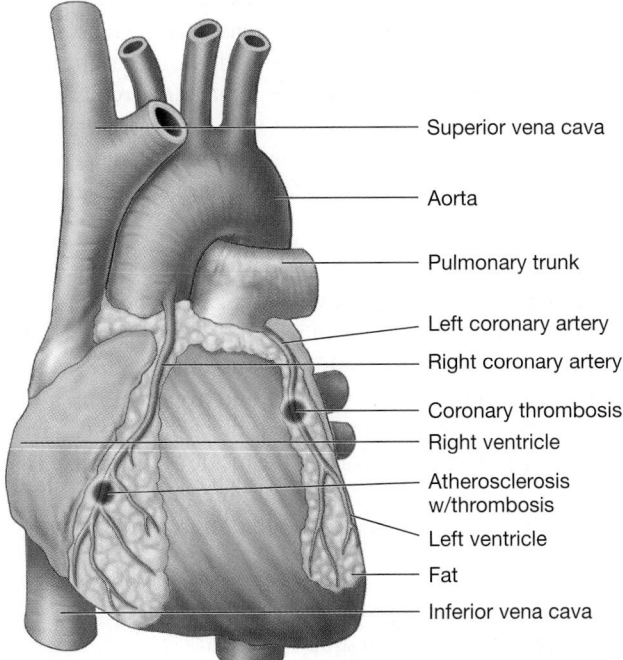

FIGURE 40–13 ■ Thrombosis in a coronary artery.

Silent Ischemia

Nearly 70% to 90% of daily life ischemic episodes are asymptomatic, and 25% of patients who experience an AMI have either no or atypical symptoms (Cohn, Fox, & Daly, 2003). The presence of silent ischemia predicts greater risk of adverse outcomes in patients with stable and unstable angina, and in patients following an AMI or revascularization therapies. Silent ischemia is more prevalent in the elderly, women, patients with diabetes, and patients with three-vessel disease. The lack of symptoms has been attributed to altered pain regulation or perception, higher pain tolerance, higher levels of circulating endorphins, or altered sensory secondary to pain pathway impairment (Cohn et al., 2003).

Sudden Cardiac Death

Sudden cardiac death (SCD) is cardiac arrest most often associated with abrupt coronary artery occlusion from plaque disruption over severely stenotic lesions in the setting of poorly developed collateral circulation. The abrupt occlusion triggers pulseless ventricular tachycardia, ventricular fibrillation, or asystole, which if not treated immediately is almost always fatal. Chapter 38 ⚭ includes an in-depth discussion of these dysrhythmias.

Clinical Manifestations of Acute Coronary Syndrome

Presenting signs and symptoms vary greatly from person to person experiencing acute coronary syndrome (ACS). Typical symptoms include chest pain, diaphoresis, shortness of breath, and generalized weakness. Patients describe the pain from an acute myocardial infarction (AMI) in the same terms as the pain from angina pectoris only usually more intense and longer in duration. If the chest pain lasts longer than 20 minutes, there is a concern that cardiac damage is occurring. The pain from an AMI is not relieved by rest and requires treatment with medications or interventions to open the occluded coronary artery.

Most frequently patients report that the anginal pain occurs in the mid to lower sternal areas of the chest. It also may radiate to the left arm, right arm, neck, jaw, and back areas. Atypical angina occurs in the stomach and back. Due to the close proximity to the epigastric region, many people mistake it for indigestion. Men having an AMI report the mid to lower sternal chest pain more often than women. Women who are having an AMI more typically report shortness of breath (57.9%), weakness (54.8%), and fatigue (40.9%); prodromal symptoms experienced 1 month prior to AMI include unusual fatigue (70.7%), sleep disturbance (47.8%), and shortness of breath (40.1%) (AHA, 2008c McSweeney et al., 2003). Figure 40–11 ■ (p. 1176) outlines the locations where angina occurs.

Other frequent signs and symptoms associated with AMI include nausea, vomiting, dyspnea, syncope, anxiety, and a feeling of impending doom. Approximately one-third of patients experiencing an AMI do not experience chest pain and initially exhibit other symptoms of decreased cardiac output such as shortness of breath and changes in sensorium, or syncope.

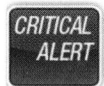 **CRITICAL ALERT** *Some patients are able to sense when a major cardiac event is occurring; and therefore, it is essential that the nurse pay close attention to patients who report impending doom.*

The physical assessment findings of a patient experiencing acute coronary syndrome are also variable. The blood pressure may be low due to a decreased cardiac output, or it may be elevated due to catecholamine release, fear, and anxiety. The heart rate may be bradycardic or tachycardic, depending on where in the heart the damage is occurring and the patient's anxiety level. There may be an S_3 or S_4 present and new systolic murmurs. Chapter 37 🔗 includes a description of S_3 and S_4. The lung sounds may be clear unless there is associated heart failure, in which case rales or crackles, and/or wheezes may be heard with an associated decrease in arterial oxygen saturation. Heart failure is described in Chapter 42 🔗 .

■ Laboratory and Diagnostic Procedures to Diagnose Acute Coronary Syndrome

The clinical manifestations of CAD typically bring the patient to the ED or health care provider's office. The second indicators of acute coronary insufficiency are the laboratory tests and ECG changes that indicate the presence and extent of myocardial damage. As soon as the patient is admitted to the ED, laboratory tests are done to assist in determining the diagnosis. Many of the laboratory values are "time" sensitive, so it is essential that the blood is drawn immediately after admission. The initial laboratory and diagnostic workup includes blood serum markers and a 12-lead ECG. Chart 40–10 outlines normal laboratory values.

Blood (Serum) Markers of Myocardial Ischemia

Laboratory tests include myoglobin, cardiac enzymes (CK total, CK-MB), troponin (T or I), and possibly a C-reactive protein level. A rise in cardiac blood markers occurs when the myocardial cells become damaged from a lack of blood supply that occurs with myocardial injury and death. The cell membrane loses its integrity and intracellular enzymes are released. The extent of en-

zyme release is relative to the amount of tissue damage and, thus, the size of the infarct. Therefore, blood marker levels are useful to help confirm the diagnosis and the extent of tissue injury.

Myoglobin

Myoglobin is a heme-containing, oxygen-binding protein that is exclusive to striated and nonstriated muscle. Because of its very small molecular weight, it is released into the interstitial fluid as early as 2 hours following damage to muscle tissue. Unlike CK-MB, the presence of an elevated myoglobin level is not a specific indicator of just heart damage. Rather it is a sensitive indicator that muscle damage has occurred. For example, if a patient falls or has any type of muscle injury, the myoglobin will rise. In other words, if a patient has had an acute cardiac event, he will have an elevated myoglobin; however, the diagnosis cannot be made on myoglobin alone because of its lack of specificity.

Creatine Kinase

Creatine kinase (CK) is an enzyme found in high concentrations in the heart and skeletal muscle and in smaller concentrations in the brain. Laboratory studies are able to subdivide and analyze the total CK level into its three isoforms: CK-MM coming from damaged skeletal muscle, CK-BB from damaged brain tissue, and CK-MB from damaged cardiac tissue. Of the isoforms, only CK-MB, along with CK total and percentage of CK-MB of CK total, is relevant for determining cardiac ischemia and infarction. Other enzymes have been used in the past such as serum glutamic-oxaloacetic transaminase (SGOT), aspartate transaminase (AST), and lactic dehydrogenase (LDH) along with CK's isoforms. In the last 2 to 3 decades, CK and specifically CK-MB have proven to be more time-efficient, sensitive, and specific indicators of cardiac muscle damage. Currently, newer tests are providing even faster results with the same accuracy as the cardiac enzymes, which include troponin T and I. Chart 40–10 outlines the normal values for the cardiac markers.

Troponin

Troponin is a protein complex that is found in cardiac and skeletal muscle. There are three isotypes—**troponin T**, troponin C, and **troponin I**—all of which help regulate the force and speed of muscle contractions by modulating the interaction of actin and myosin. Troponin T and troponin I are found in cardiac muscle, and during periods of cardiac ischemia, intracellular troponin will leak from the inside of the cell because of changes in myocardial cell membrane permeability. Troponin levels can be detected soon after an ischemic event be-

CHART 40–10	Normal Cardiac Markers' Laboratory Normal Values	
Laboratory Test	**Normal Range**
Creatine kinase (CPK)	0–250 U/L
CPK-MB	<8.0 mcg/mL
CPK-MB relative index	<3.2%
Troponin I (cTnI)	0–.06 ng/mL
Troponin T (cTnT)	0–.05 ng/mL
Myoglobin	17–106 ng/mL

CHART 40–11	**Cardiac Laboratory Markers' Pattern Consistent with Acute Myocardial Infarction**			
Laboratory Test	**Time to Elevation**	**Mean Time to Peak Elevation**	**Time to Return to Normal**	
Myoglobin	1–3 hours	6–7 hours	24 hours	
Troponin I	3–12 hours	24 hours	5–10 days	
Troponin T	3–12 hours	12 hours–2 days	5–14 days	
CK-MB	3–12 hours	24 hours	48–72 hours	
C-reactive protein	24 hours	2–3 days	2 weeks	

Source: This article was published in *Heart Disease: A textbook in Cardiovascular Medicine,* 5th ed., Antman E. M., Braunwald E. In: Braunwald E., ed., p. 1202. Copyright 1997, Philadelphia, PA: WB Saunders.

cause these proteins are very small and therefore leak out quickly. Normal and abnormal troponin T and troponin I laboratory markers are outlined in Chart 40–11.

ECG Changes
12-Lead ECG Changes with Acute Myocardial Infarction

The 12-lead ECG provides 12 different views of the electrical activity in the heart. When evaluating a 12-lead ECG, the Q wave, T wave, and ST segment are used to determine the presence of damage. Changes in specific leads reflect the specific location in the heart where the damage has occurred and which vessel(s) contain the culprit lesions. As the ischemia and injury evolve, so

do the ECG changes. Figure 40–12 ▪ (p. 1183) demonstrates the ECG changes that occur with a transmural AMI.

The ST segment is the major focus when evaluating ischemic injury to the myocardium. As discussed earlier, the location of the AMI is identified by the involved coronary artery. Abnormal changes on the ECG correlate with the area in the myocardium where damage has occurred and, thus, identify the artery involved. Chart 40–12 outlines the artery, the associated 12-lead ECG changes, and complications.

For ST segment and T wave changes to be considered diagnostic, they must appear in two or more contiguous leads. This means that changes must be present in two or more leads that correspond to a given area of myocardium damage. For example,

CHART 40–12	**ECG Changes During an MI, Correlated with Coronary Anatomy**		
	Areas and Structures Supplied	**Type of MI and Leads Involved**	**Associated Symptoms and Complications**
Right Coronary Artery (RCA)	SA node (55%), AV node (90%) Bundle of His Right atrium and ventricle Inferior surface of left ventricle Posterior 1/3 of septum Left bundle branch Posterior/inferior division of right bundle branch	**INFERIOR MI (RCA)** II, III, aVF Reciprocal changes in I, aVL	Vagal symptoms: nausea and bradycardia AV blocks: most common = 1st degree and 2nd degree type I (Wenckebach); 3rd degree possible Usually transient; treat only if symptomatic
Left Anterior Descending (LAD)	Anterior wall of left ventricle Anterior 2/3 of septum Right bundle branch Anterior/superior division of left bundle branch	**ANTERIOR MI (LAD)** $V_1 - V_4$ Reciprocal changes in II, III, aVF **ANTEROLATERAL (LAD/CIRC)** $V_1 - V_4$ I, aVL, V_5, V_6 Reciprocal changes in II, III, aVF	Often associated with loss of large muscle mass If large myocardial infarction (MI), prone to develop diminished left ventricular branch function, signs and symptoms of heart failure (HF), cardiogenic shock Rhythm disturbances: atrial and ventricular dysrhythmias, bundle branch blocks, AV blocks with 2nd degree type II most common; may progress to 3rd-degree block (complete heart block)
Left Circumflex Artery (CIRC, CX)	SA node (45%), AV node (10%) Inferior surface of left ventricle Lateral wall of left ventricle Left atrium Posterior/inferior division of left bundle branch	**LATERAL MI (CIRC/LAD)** I, aVL, V_5, V_6 Reciprocal changes in V_1, V_3 **ANTEROLATERAL MI (LAD/CX)** I, aVL, V_5, V_6 $V_1 - V_4$ Reciprocal changes in II, III, aVF **POSTERIOR MI (RCA, CIRC)** Reciprocal changes only in V_1, V_2 unless 18-lead EKG is done	Frequently seen with large anterior MIs Occasionally seen with inferior MIs Least likely to alter hemodynamics or cause dysrhythmias Uncommon; involves both right coronary artery (RCA) and circumflex (CIRC) Hard to diagnose on traditional 12-lead; researchers developing 18-lead EKG Bradycardia with possible AV block; usually transient

in order for the ECG criteria to be met for an inferior wall MI, a patient would have to have ST segment elevation of 1 millimeter or greater in two of these three leads: II, III, and aVF.

Reciprocal ST Segment Abnormalities

When ST segment changes occur during an AMI, they are present in the leads on the 12-lead ECG that face the damaged myocardium and/or infarction, and are referred to as the indicative leads. Reciprocal (electrically opposite) leads are distant from the injury and reflect in an upside-down, mirror image of the changes or damage seen in the indicative leads. Reciprocal ST segment changes present as horizontal or downsloping of the ST segment. Other reciprocal changes include the absence of a Q wave, an increased height of the R wave in the QRS complex, and a tall, upright T wave. It is generally thought that the presence of reciprocal changes indicates more extensive damage and a worse prognosis. When looking at a 12-lead ECG for indicative and reciprocal changes, one has to keep in mind that ST segment depression interpreted as reciprocal changes may in fact reflect injury rising from a culprit lesion in another vessel (Morton et al., 2005).

Bundle branch block (BBB) is defined as a discontinuity of conduction (complete or incomplete) in one branch of the His bundle, which affects normal transmission of the impulse through the ventricles. The QRS is wider than the normal 0.12 second with BBB. When one bundle is blocked the ventricles depolarize asynchronously, which is characterized by a delay of excitation to one ventricle; therefore, an abnormal spread of electrical activity through the ventricles occurs. Spontaneous left bundle branch block or right ventricular pacing–induced left bundle branch pattern obscures the electrocardiographic diagnosis of an AMI.

ECG Signs of Reperfusion

The goal for the management of AMI is rapid restoration of blood flow to the infarct-related artery (IRA). The lack of reperfusion is an important predictor of cardiac morbidity and mortality following AMI. The amount of time to restoration of blood flow directly correlates to the morbidity and mortality associated with AMI. The resolution of ST segment deviation should occur within 90 minutes following revascularization for the therapy to be considered successful. "Time is muscle"; thus, immediate reperfusion must occur in order to salvage myocardium. Other markers of reperfusion include newly acquired T wave inversion within 4 hours after AMI, accelerated idioventricular rhythms of rates between 60 and 120 beats per minute, isolated premature ventricular contractions, and nonsustained asymptomatic runs of ventricular tachycardia. The emergence of polymorphic ventricular tachycardia and ventricular fibrillation is rare and more often represents reocclusion of the IRA. Chapter 38  has a complete description of ventricular tachycardia and ventricular fibrillation.

Cardiac Dysrhythmias Associated with Acute Myocardial Infarction

Premature atrial and ventricular contractions, conduction abnormalities, tachycardia, and bradycardia can all be seen with myocardial ischemia and infarction. Premature beats and tachycardias occur because of acute tissue hypoxemia and irritability, and derangement of electrical membrane potentials. Tachycar-

dia also is a by-product of elevated levels of circulating catecholamines due to the stress response. Atrial fibrillation may result from myocardial infarction because of enhanced vagal tone, increased atrial pressure, atrial infarction, or pericarditis. Conduction delays and bradycardia relate to the location of the infarct and the mass of involved myocardium.

In summary, although a significant number of patients do not have ECG changes indicative of AMI on admission, they are still considered an important diagnostic indicator when used in conjunction with the patient's history, presenting signs and symptoms, and blood markers indicative of cardiac ischemia.

> **CRITICAL ALERT** *Because the dysrhythmias that accompany an MI are common and varied, it is essential that the nurse understand the impact of each type on the cardiac output and the necessary interventions to terminate the abnormal rhythm.*

■ Medical Management of Coronary Artery Disease

The following case example represents the difficulty in evaluating the cause of a patient's complaint of chest pain:

> A 42-year-old white female with no history of cardiac disease presents to the emergency department (ED) with substernal chest pain she has had for 10 hours. She describes her pain as feeling "like a weight" with nausea, dizziness, left arm numbness, and accompanied by dyspnea. Her medical history is positive for 10 pack/years of smoking, epigastric pain, gastric reflux disease, and black tarry stool. She has a negative family history for heart disease and no history of hypertension, diabetes, or hyperlipidemia. The patient is convinced her pain is epigastric, as she has had this same sensation before. She is given a GI cocktail consisting of Donnatal, viscous Lidocaine, and Maalox, which relieves her symptoms. Her initial set of cardiac markers were negative; her ECG showed ST depression of < 1 millimeter in leads II, III, and aVF.

Routine evaluation of patients who present with symptoms that may represent exacerbations of CAD includes a review of their symptoms, their medical/social history for associated diseases and risk factors, an assessment for physical signs, and diagnostic tests. In this case, the patient's description, history, physical signs, and initial diagnostic workup of her suspected anginal symptoms are compounded with those that are classic for gastric ulcer disease. Subsequent testing demonstrated that she was indeed having an AMI, but she could have easily been treated with antacids and sent home joining the cohort patients admitted to the emergency department with a nondiagnostic workup for CAD, discharged only to return later with ACS.

Tools used to determine the extent of myocardial perfusion depend on six indexes: the presence of physical signs and symptoms representative of tissue hypoxemia or heart failure, abnormal levels of blood serum markers indicating myocardial cell membrane damage, ECG changes consistent with myocardial injury and muscle death, the lack of uptake of substances by cardiac tissue, vessel patency as seen with angiography, and assessments of global intracardiac structure and function (Chapter 38 ). Signs and symptoms, blood markers, and ECG changes are completed expeditiously when a patient is admitted for suspected acute coronary ischemia. ECG testing is done either at rest during an acute event such as the presence of angina, or during exercise to determine the extent of stress on the heart during work. Angiography is used to confirm or define areas of critical stenosis or obstruction, referred to as culprit lesions, as well as for hemodynamic measurements. Viability studies employ the infusion of a radioactive indicator, typically technetium, that is taken up by tissue with good perfusion and is later "washed out" as perfusing blood dilutes the concentration of the isotope over time. Ventricular radiography done during coronary angiography identifies areas of abnormal heart contractility such as **dyskinesia** (impaired muscle movement), **akinesia** (severe loss or no muscle movement), and **hypokinesia** (hypoactive muscle movement) that can result from poor coronary perfusion. Echocardiography uses sonography to assess any damage to valve structure or chamber contractility at rest or during exercise that may result from chronic or acute myocardial ischemia. The studies discussed earlier are described in detail in Chapter 38 ⊙. The Diagnostic Tests box (p. 1188) summarizes the laboratory studies that are used to diagnose the presence and extent of CAD.

Physical findings associated with CAD are not specific to just coronary artery disease but also may be associated with other diseases such as systemic arterial hypertension, hyperlipidemia, valvular heart disease, heart failure, diabetes, or peripheral atherosclerosis. Thus, findings such as the following are not diagnostic for CAD specifically: elevated blood pressure; presence of an S_3, S_4, or paradoxically split S_2; diminished peripheral pulses; murmurs of aortic stenosis or mitral insufficiency; enlarged cardiac silhouette; changes in pulse cadence and rate because of ventricular or atrial ectopic beats; and presence of crackles. However, they may represent exacerbations of associated diseases that result in coronary insufficiency or vice versa. The absence or presence of these findings also provides a baseline in the advent of complications, assists in excluding other conditions, and assists in stratifying risk for appropriate triage of patients who present with the clinical manifestations of CAD.

Pain is most effectively assessed using a systematic approach to help ensure that all aspects are assessed such as the following: aggravating and alleviating factors; timing related to frequency, duration, time of day, and relation to activity or rest; qualitative characteristics such as description, location, intensity, and radiation; and any other associated symptoms.

Medical Management of Acute Coronary Syndrome

Patients with unstable symptoms are at a greater risk and therefore warrant hospital admission for diagnostic workup and treatment. An estimated 5 million or more adults present each year to emergency departments with a primary complaint of chest pain (Libby, Bonow, Zipes, & Mann, 2008). More than 1.4 million Americans patients are subsequently hospitalized, of which one-third are found to have symptoms of cardiac disease (AHA, 2006f).

Patients with suspected cardiac ischemia but with nondefinitive results from the cardiac workup may be triaged to a cardiac observation unit located as part of an emergency department or inpatient unit. Observation units, also referred to as chest pain units, provide space for patients to be "ruled out" for ischemia

using specific protocols. These protocols involve serial ECGs, cardiac blood marker determinations, and possibly stress testing, echocardiography, or perfusion tests. These patients are not admitted to the hospital unless ischemia is "ruled in" or still suspected after 24 hours.

Patients with acute coronary syndrome should be evaluated in an environment where aggressive therapy can be initiated quickly, such as a hospital emergency department, which has advanced life support backup and personnel to provide continuous monitoring. On admission to the emergency department or critical care unit, patients are made NPO, put on bed rest, given supplemental oxygen, and undergo continuous cardiac and oxygen saturation monitoring. Blood chemistries including cardiac markers are drawn, a 12-lead ECG is obtained, and the patient is placed on a cardiac monitor.

The mnemonic **MONA**, cited in the Advanced Cardiac Life Support (ACLS) guidelines, describes a protocol for treatment of patients with suspected myocardial infarction. The mnemonic stands for morphine, oxygen, nitroglycerin, and aspirin. MONA does not, however, imply a correct sequencing of treatment. The platelet-inhibiting action of chewable aspirin in doses of 81 to 325 milligrams decreases platelet aggregation, and supplemental oxygen treatments are intended to increase oxygen supply to ischemic tissue. Nitroglycerin (NTG) dilates the large coronary arteries, thus increasing the blood supply to ischemic tissue. Initially NTG is administered sublingually, as spray, and with persistent symptoms it may be given intravenously. Intravenous morphine sulfate, a potent analgesic, is used to relieve angina, although it is also effective in reducing anxiety. Morphine along with nitroglycerin can cause the veins to dilate, resulting in a decrease in the amount of blood returning to the heart (preload). This reduced preload helps to decrease myocardial oxygen demand. Short-acting nitroglycerin and morphine can precipitate hypotension, especially in patients with a right ventricular infarction. Therefore, both drugs must be titrated cautiously to relieve pain without causing hypotension. For persistent symptoms of ischemia, IV or oral beta-blockers and heparin will be administered. Glycoprotein (GP) IIb/IIIa inhibitors may be added for unrelenting symptoms. A thrombolytic agent (see Pharmacology Summary, p. 1199) may be administered, or the patient is prepared for emergent percutaneous coronary intervention (PCI) (Chapter 39 ⊙), as soon as the ECG and/or cardiac markers indicate the presence of STEMI. Thrombolytic medications are contraindicated in patients with unstable angina (UA) and non–ST segment elevation myocardial infarction (NSTEMI), because studies demonstrate a higher risk of bleeding and lower beneficial results compared to patients with MI (Libby, Bonow, Zipes, & Mann, 2008). Figure 40–14 ■ (p. 1189) is an algorithm for emergent management for patients with acute coronary syndromes.

Once medically stable (without recurrent ischemia, electrical instability [ECG], signs of heart failure, or other serious complications), patients with UA can be transferred to a non–critical care environment where oral nitrates, β-adrenergic blocker, or calcium channel blocker, and possibly low molecular weight heparin (LMWH) (i.e., Lovenox), therapy will be initiated or adjusted to maintain symptom control and hemodynamic stability. If minimal or no episodes of angina occur while the patient is transitioned off oxygen and to a normal activity level, discharge

DIAGNOSTIC TESTS for Coronary Artery Disease

Diagnostic Test and Normal Values	Expected Abnormality	Rationale for Abnormality
ECG: No ST segment elevation or depression. No T wave inversion. No Q waves.	ST segment elevation. ST segment depression. Q waves.	Identify ST segment or T wave abnormalities; and the presence of pathologic Q waves indicates myocardial ischemia, injury, and necrosis, which assists in the diagnosis of an AMI.
Stress test (exercise treadmill or bicycle): Induces abnormal ECG changes, which occur when myocardial oxygen demand increases due to exercise.	ST segment or T wave changes during stress.	Certain changes occur only when the heart is stressed due to the heart's inability to increase cardiac output during periods of high demand.
Nuclear myocardial perfusion imaging: Pharmacologic agent used to induce stress for those patients who cannot exercise.	ST segment or T wave changes during stress.	Identify both functional and nonfunctional myocardium when oxygen demand is increased.
Dobutamine stress echocardiography: Pharmacologic agent used to induce stress for those patients who cannot exercise.	ST segment or T wave changes during stress. Changes in ejection fraction.	Identify both functional and nonfunctional myocardium when oxygen demand is increased.
Electron beam computed tomography (EBCT)/multislice CT: Detect and quantify coronary artery calcification.	Calcium score is age dependent.	Coronary calcium is part of the development of atherosclerosis. It occurs exclusively in atherosclerotic arteries and is absent in the normal vessel wall. The presence of calcification in the coronary arteries indicates the presence of coronary atherosclerosis.
MRI: Identifies plaque size and composition.	Coronary artery stenosis.	Identifies area of plaque buildup from the presence and progression of coronary artery disease (CAD).
Cardiac catheterization: Confirms patency of coronary arteries, determines blood flow in chambers and great vessels, evaluates pressures across valves.	Coronary artery stenosis, valve damage, decreased ventricular function.	Identifies area of plaque buildup from the presence and progression of CAD.
Intravascular ultrasound:	Coronary artery stenosis	Quantify plaque burden and composition from the presence and progression of coronary artery disease.
Chest x-ray (CXR): Evaluate heart size. Identify congestion or effusions. Identify tumors or masses.	Enlarged heart and lung congestion. Pulmonary edema, congestive heart failure. Presence of lung tumor or mass.	Heart failure, cardiomyopathy, and coronary artery disease.
Echocardiogram, transthoracic or transesophageal.	Valvular damage; insufficiency, regurgitation, stenosis, or vegetation. Enlarged chamber size such as ventricular hypertrophy. Abnormal pressure gradients. Decreased ventricular function.	Measures diameters of the cardiac chambers, evaluates structural abnormalities, and identifies valvular vegetation and pressure gradients.
Hs-C-reactive protein: < 10 mg/L	>10 mg/L	Acute phase reactant protein used to indicate an inflammatory process.
Cardiac enzymes:	See Chart 40–10 (p. 1184)	See Chart 40–10 (p. 1184)
Magnesium: 1.3–2.1 mg/dL	<1.5 mg/dL >2.1 mg/dL	Electrolyte balance; decreases ventricular irritability.
Potassium: 3.5–5.0 mEq/L	<3.5 mEq/L >5.0 mEq/L	Electrolyte balance; decreases ventricular irritability.

can be expected in 1 to 3 days. For recurrent chest pain the patient should receive an immediate (stat) 12-lead ECG to document ischemia during pain, followed by sublingual NTG and IV NTG if pain persists. Noninvasive stress testing, perfusion scans, and/or cardiac catheterization may be scheduled to occur while in the hospital or as a follow-up procedure postdischarge. Discharge preparation includes teaching about cardiac risk factors, signs and symptoms of myocardial ischemia, how and when to access emergency medical services, and medication regimes. Patients diagnosed as having an AMI will receive either thrombolytic

CLINICAL PATHWAYS FOR EMERGENCY MANAGEMENT OF URGENT CHEST PAIN

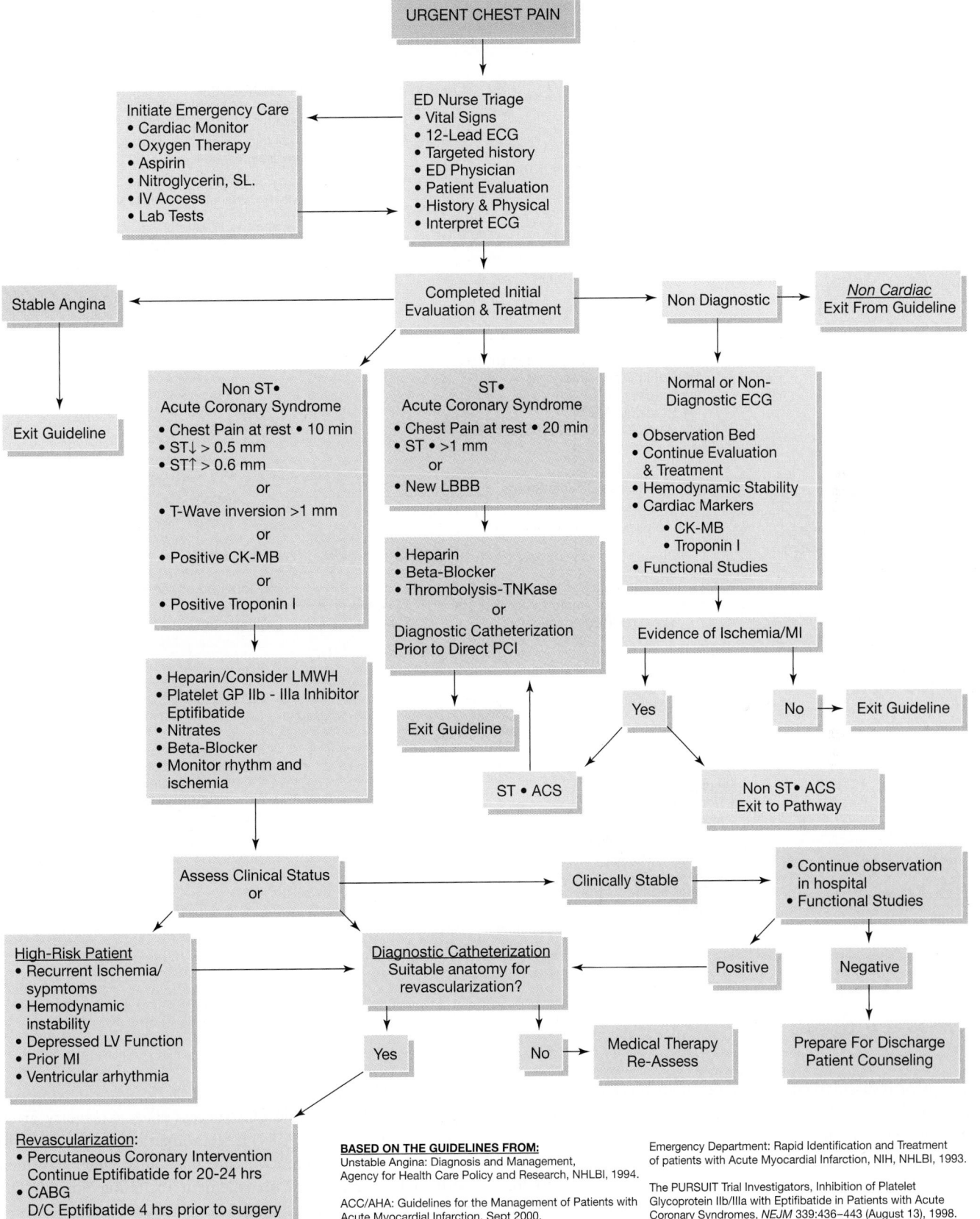

FIGURE 40–14 ■ Algorithm for emergent management of patients with acute coronary syndrome.

CLINICAL PATHWAYS FOR MANAGEMENT OF ACUTE CORONARY SYNDROMES

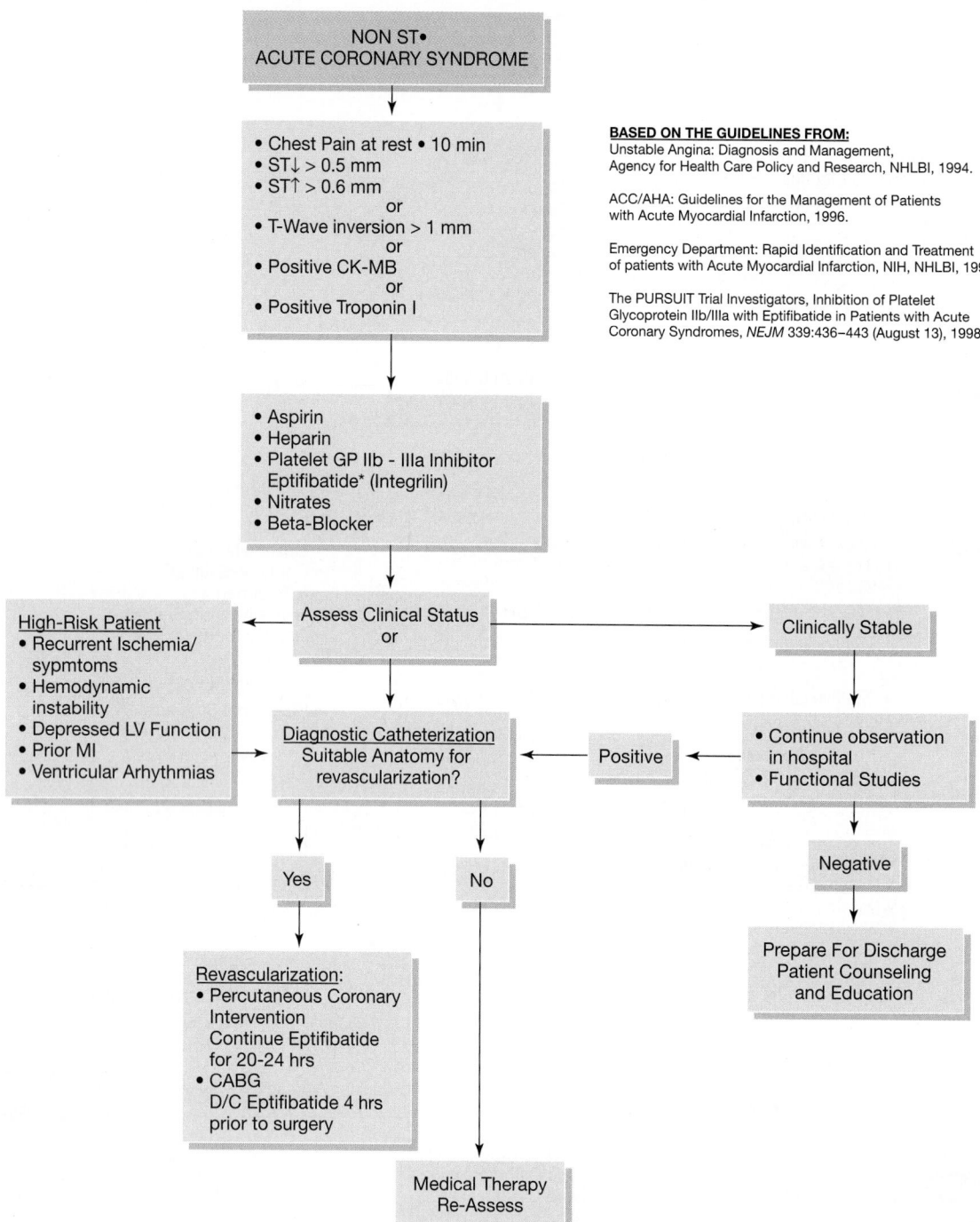

BASED ON THE GUIDELINES FROM:
Unstable Angina: Diagnosis and Management,
Agency for Health Care Policy and Research, NHLBI, 1994.

ACC/AHA: Guidelines for the Management of Patients
with Acute Myocardial Infarction, 1996.

Emergency Department: Rapid Identification and Treatment
of patients with Acute Myocardial Infarction, NIH, NHLBI, 1993.

The PURSUIT Trial Investigators, Inhibition of Platelet
Glycoprotein IIb/IIIa with Eptifibatide in Patients with Acute
Coronary Syndromes, *NEJM* 339:436–443 (August 13), 1998.

FIGURE 40–14 ■ Continued

therapy or revascularization with percutaneous coronary intervention (PCI) or coronary artery bypass graft (CABG) surgery. Chapter 39 🔗 discusses PCI.

Thrombolytic drug therapy is recommended for patients suspected of AMI who are younger than 75 years old, at low risk for bleeding, with symptoms lasting less than 12 hours. PCI is indicated when thrombolytic therapy is contraindicated or in patients with cardiogenic shock. PCI is recommended as an alternative first-choice therapy only if intervention can be performed within 60 to 90 minutes, by skilled clinicians (performed 75 procedures/

year), in high-volume centers (>200 PCI cases/year), and with demonstrated acceptable PCI success rates. Coronary artery bypass graft surgery (CABG) is recommended for patients with persistent pain or hemodynamic instability when treatment with PCI or if medical management including thrombolytic therapy fails (Antman et al., 2004).

Patients with unrelieved chest pain and ECG changes, pulmonary edema, hypotension, or new mitral regurgitation indicate a need for intensive care unit monitoring. However, patients without these features may be admitted to a noncritical care en-

CLINICAL PATHWAYS FOR MANAGEMENT
OF ACUTE MYOCARDIAL INFARCTION

CLINICAL PATHWAYS FOR MANAGEMENT
OF ACUTE CORONARY SYNDROMES

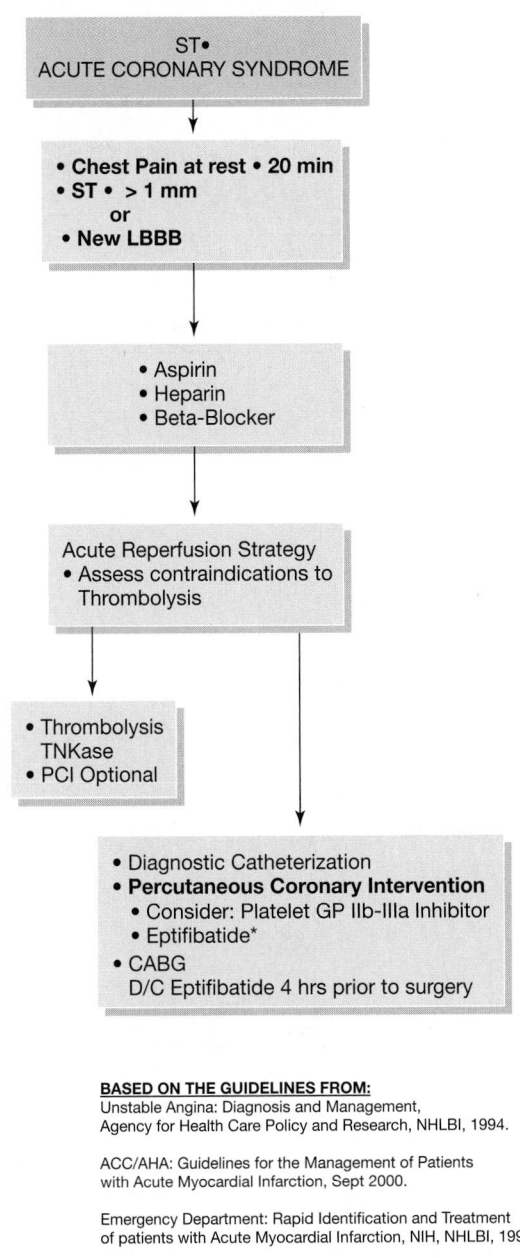

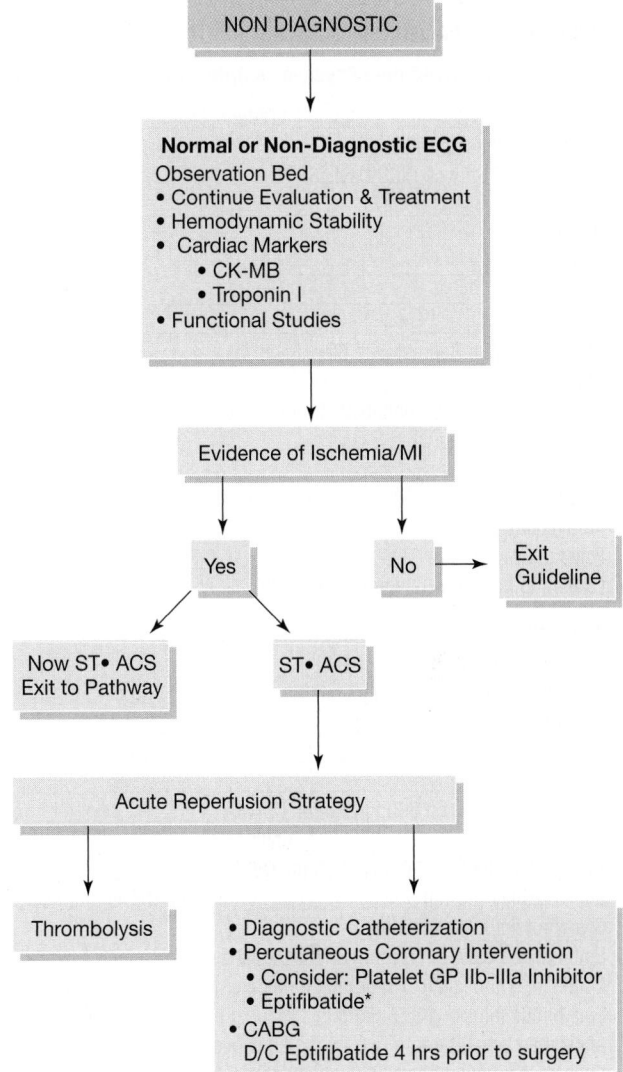

FIGURE 40–14 ■ Continued

vironment, depending on the health care provider's preference and hospital availability. Chart 40–13 (p. 1192) gives an example of a health care provider's orders used to treat ACS.

As part of the commitment to improving AMI outcomes, a number of studies have been conducted that bring teams of health care professionals together at the hospital and health system levels to evaluate treatment procedures, monitor resource utilization, identify patient-selection issues, and monitor outcomes. An example of this research is the National Registry of Myocardial Infarction (NRMI), sponsored by Genentech, Inc., which is one of the largest observational studies of acute myocardial infarction (AMI). As it is well known, AMI treatment

and intervention time is directly related to mortality. The faster the infarct-related artery is intervened on, the more myocardium is salvaged, thus, decreasing mortality. To track this, NRMI collects data on the four Ds: door, data, decision, and drug or dilation. From the time a patient presents to the emergency department door to the time the reperfusion drug is given should be 30 minutes or less, and the time from patient presentation to balloon dilation for reperfusion therapy should be 90 minutes or less. Since 1990, this study has collected data on more than 2.3 million AMI patients, helped more than 1,600 participating hospitals assess their approach to AMI treatment, and identified trends in patient outcome. Because of its size and

| CHART 40–13 | **Health Care Provider's Orders for Acute Coronary Syndrome** |

UNIVERSITY OF CALIFORNIA DAVIS MEDICAL CENTER, SACRAMENTO, CALIFORNIA PHYSICIAN'S ORDERS USE PATIENT PLATE

Acute Coronary Syndrome Physician's Orders AM2036 (4/04) MR#03/04896

DATE: _____ TIME: _____

Directions: Check or fill in _____ for orders to be completed.

Admit to HRT Service CICU Davis 6

Attending _____ Fellow _____

Resident _____ Pgr Pl# _____

Intern _____ Pgr Pl# _____

Diagnosis _____ Condition _____

Allergies _____ Diet: NPO _____

Activity: Bedrest Bedrest with BRP Up ad lib

Call HO for SBP > _____ ; DBP > _____ < _____ ; HR > _____ < _____ ; Temp > _____ ; O2 Sat < _____

Call For Old Records Continuous Cardiac Monitor

Daily Weight Strict I/O

Initiate Collaborative Pathway

Establish IV Access, 2 Sites if Possible, Prefer 18 g–20 g

Intravenous Fluids _____ at _____ mL/hr

Foley to Gravity

Oxygen to Maintain O2 Saturation > 92%

Medications

ASA 325 PO daily

Pantoprazole 40 mg PO daily

Beta Blocker _____

Ace Inhibitor _____

HMG-CoA Inhibitor _____

Nitroglycerin Infusion 50 mg/250 mL D5W @ _____ mcg/min, titrate for chest pain, keep SBP > _____

Heparin bolus _____ units

Heparin Infusion 25,000 units/250 mL D5W drip @ _____ units/hour

Enoxaparin (1 mg/kg) _____ mg sub Q every 12 hours

Glycoprotein IIb/IIIa Inhibitor:

Eptifibatide bolus (2 mg/mL) 180 mcg/kg IV over 1–2 minutes then start drip

Eptifibatide infusion (0.75 mg/mL) 2 mcg/kg/min (creat. < 2.0 mg/dL) @ _____ mL/hr X _____ hrs

Eptifibatide infusion (0.75 mg/mL) 1 mcg/kg/min (creat. > 2.0 mg/dL, CRCL < 50 ml/min) _____ mL/hr X _____ hrs

Abciximab bolus (2 mg/mL) 0.25 mg/kg IV over 1–2 minutes

Abciximab Infusion (9 mg/250 mL NS) 0.125 mcg/kg/min @ mL/hr x 12 hrs

Additional Medications:

_____

_____

_____

_____

PRN Medications

Morphine 0.3–5 mg IV Q 3–5 min max 15 mg Q 3 hr PRN chest pain

Meperidine 5–20 mg IV Q 3–5 min max 125 mg Q 3 hr PRN pain

Temazepam 15–30 mg PO H at bedtime prn insomnia

Droperidol 1.25–2.5 mg IV q 4 hrs PRN nausea

Alprazolam 0.25 mg PO q 8 hrs PRN anxiety

Atropine 0.5–1.0 mg IV for HR < 40 if SBP < 90

NTG 0.4 mg SL PRN chest pain X 3 **(Do not use nitrates within 24 hours of Viagra, Levitra, and Cilias use)**

Tests/Procedures CPK-MB q _____ hrs or until peak

Basic Chemistry Panel qam Troponin q _____ hrs or until peak

CBC qam APTT qam

CBC w/auto diff Comprehensive Chemistry Panel

Magnesium qam CXR PA & Lateral

Lipid Panel ECG qam and prn chest pain, arrhythmias, or ST changes

Ordering Physician Signature _____ Pl# _____ Pgr _____

Acute Coronary Syndrome

Source: University of California Davis Medical Center, Sacramento, CA.

scope, NRMI has had a profound impact on AMI treatment practices. Although this is not a controlled, randomized clinical trial, it does not test the effectiveness between therapeutic interventions, and so comparisons of outcomes across treatment groups must be interpreted with caution.

Pharmacologic and Nonpharmacologic Treatment of Acute Coronary Syndrome

Oxygen fuels the metabolic processes that support myocyte contractility and heart pumping. Adequate oxygen supply to working cells is threatened during reductions in coronary blood flow. Because ACS causes a reduction in blood flow to the myocardium, the goal for the treatment of ACS is focused on reducing the myocardial oxygen demand or increasing the supply of oxygenated blood delivered to the injured cardiac tissue. Specific medical and nursing interventions will decrease the heart's need for oxygen, whereas others will increase the supply of oxygen to the cardiac muscle. Myocardial oxygen demand or myocardial consumption is affected most by increases in heart rate, contractility, and heart wall tension. Myocardial demand is decreased by modifying activity level; ameliorating the effects of the autonomic stress response; promoting rest; and reducing heart rate, contractility, and vascular resistance through drug and interventional therapies.

Efforts aimed at increasing oxygen supply to ischemic myocardium revolve around five strategies: (1) Raise the amount of oxygenated blood delivered to the tissues with supplemental oxygen and blood transfusions; (2) relieve coronary smooth muscle vasoconstriction or spasm with vasodilators; (3) reperfuse ischemic tissue by dissolving thrombus with thrombolytic agents; (4) prevent thrombus formation with anticoagulant therapy; and (5) reestablish blood flow through invasive revascularization procedures such as coronary artery bypass graft surgery (CABG) and percutaneous coronary intervention (PCI). An in-depth discussion of PCI is found in Chapter 39 .

Activity Progression

Activity for patients with ACS is dictated by the emergence of anginal symptoms. Patients are advised to avoid certain activities, to refrain from sudden exertion, and to stop what they are doing if symptoms occur. Activity prescriptions, based on ischemic thresholds determined during exercise testing, are recommended to maintain or enhance exercise tolerance, strengthen ventricular wall motion, or reduce ischemic episodes.

Activity guidelines for patients following acute ischemic events have changed dramatically over the past 20 years. Historically patients were kept on bed rest for up to 8 weeks to allow for myocardial healing and reduce complications. Today AMI patients, without clinical signs of ischemia or depressed ventricular function, get out of bed after a 24-hour pain-free period. Certain self-care activities are allowed, such as toileting, feeding, bathing, weighing, transferring, and positioning, which require minimal energy expenditure and do not cause undue strain on the recovering heart. For elimination needs, during the first 24 hours, patients may use either a bedpan or a bedside commode, as both are equivalent in energy expenditure. Barring other limitations patients admitted with UA can advance their activity after symptoms are controlled and hemodynamic stability is achieved for 8 hours. After 24 hours AMI patients should be up in a chair, during which time an assessment for orthostatic changes should be done. A drop in systolic pressure of 20 mmHg or more, or a heart

rate increase of 20 beats per minute or more represents a positive orthostatic change indicating that the patient is deconditioned. Muscle deconditioning, as it relates to cardiac function, refers to the delayed or inadequate response of the leg muscles to contract reflexively to increase return of peripheral blood volume as the patient progresses from a lying to standing position. When a patient is deconditioned, blood pools in the legs, dropping systemic blood pressure and causing syncope or dizziness, risk of falls, and possible recurrence of ischemia. Orthostatic BP and heart rate changes can be ameliorated by timing activity apart from administration times of vasodilating and diuretic medications, and having the patient warm up with in-bed isotonic exercises, such as extending and flexing the feet, prior to rising. The National Guidelines for Cardiac Rehabilitation box (p. 1194) outlines activity guidelines from the American Association of Cardiopulmonary Rehabilitation.

Reducing Autonomic Stress Responses

Norepinephrine and epinephrine levels are elevated during the first few hours after an AMI. These catecholamines increase heart rate and systemic vascular resistance (SVR), both resulting in increases in myocardial oxygen demand. To lessen the cardiovascular impact of autonomic system overstimulation, interventions for patients with angina and myocardial infarction are aimed at identifying and eliminating triggers of autonomic nervous system stimulation. Following an acute event, patients are monitored for signs of excessive sympathetic nervous stimulation such as dysrhythmias, diaphoresis, cool/clammy skin, and elevations in hemodynamic parameters such as pulmonary artery wedge pressure (PAWP), afterload, heart rate, and BP. Conditions that may cause or potentiate excessive catecholamine release such as abnormal electrolyte levels, hypoxemia, acidosis, hyper/hypotension, tachy/bradycardia, fever, anemia, volume depletion, immobility, discomfort, pain, or psychoemotional stress are avoided or treated quickly. Pain is treated with intravenous (IV) morphine sulfate. Morphine sulfate has the added benefit of being a vasodilator, thereby reducing both preload and afterload. Anxiety is treated with oral or IV benzodiazepine such as lorazepam (Ativan) or midazolam (Versed), although morphine sulfate also will help decrease anxiety. Family interaction is either liberal or restricted depending on patient preference; tolerance, defined in terms of cardiac signs and symptoms, is scheduled around adequate rest periods for the patient. Sleep is promoted by maintaining a quiet environment, keeping the lights off or low during the night, minimizing interactions with the patient during sleep periods, and pharmacologic sleeping aids. Dietary modifications that reduce sympathetic stimulation include avoidance of caffeinated beverages and beverages of extreme hot or cold temperature.

Overstimulation of the parasympathetic nervous system can be equally deleterious to recovering an ischemic heart. Valsalva maneuvers such as bearing down, pain, or heightened emotional responses may stimulate the vagus nerve, causing a decrease in heart rate and electrical conduction through the heart. As opposed to healthy hearts, myocardium scarred from ischemia with a concomitant reduced blood supply cannot compensate for a drop in heart rate and cardiac output. Pain from procedures such as chest tube insertion or sheath pulling from angiography can cause local excitation of the vagus nerve, resulting in bradycardia

NATIONAL GUIDELINES for Cardiac Rehabilitation from the American Association of Cardiopulmonary Rehabilitation

Cardiac rehabilitation is a combination of exercise training, lifestyle modification, and nutrition. Each patient's training program is individualized based on her own physical abilities.

Beginning Level, Weeks 1–4

Aerobic Training

Activities

Walking, cycling, etc.

Intensity

60–70% maximum capacity

Duration

5–10 minutes initially, adding 1–2 minutes per session as tolerated by patient

Frequency

3–5 times per week

Strength Training

Activities

Dumbbell exercise, water therapy

Intensity

1 set, 8–10 repetitions

Duration

5–10 minutes

Frequency

4 times per week

Flexibility Training

Stretching should be done before each workout period

Improvement Level, Months 1–5

Aerobic Training

Activities

Walking, cycling, jogging, etc.

Intensity

60–70% maximum capacity up to 85%

Duration

20–45 minutes, adding 1–2 minutes per session as tolerated by patient

Frequency

5 times per week

Strength Training

Activities

Dumbbell exercise, water therapy, exercise bands

Intensity

1 set, 12–20 repetitions

Duration

10–15 minutes

Frequency

4 times per week

Flexibilty Training

Stretching should be done before each workout period

Maintenance Level, 6 Months and Beyond

Aerobic Training

Activities

Walking, cycling, jogging, etc.

Intensity

60–85% maximum capacity

Duration

20–60 minutes

Frequency

3 times per week to maintain fitness, although 5 times per week is encouraged

Strength Training

Activities

Dumbbell exercise, water therapy, exercise bands

Intensity

1 set, 8 repetitions

Duration

5–10 minutes

Frequency

3 times per week

Flexibilty Training

Stretching should be done before each workout period

Source: University of California, Davis Medical Center, Sacramento, California (2005).

---

and hypotension called a vasovagal reaction. Precautionary treatments to avoid overstimulation of the parasympathetic nervous system include small frequent feedings, stool softeners and laxatives, analgesics prior to painful procedures, and avoiding Valsalva maneuvers. The avoidance of taking rectal temperatures in patients following an AMI is based on the misconception that the rectal mucosa has vagal innervation, and that stimulation will result in hemodynamic or electrophysiological instability. No study

has demonstrated clinically significant cardiovascular changes resulting from rectal temperature taking. Chapter 24 describes all of the hemodynamic monitoring of cardiac patients.

Intra-Aortic Balloon Pump

Intra-aortic balloon pump (IABP) is used as an adjunct treatment for patients with ongoing ischemia, for those with complications related to AMI, and in high-risk patients who require prophylactic protection against ischemia prior to or during diagnostic, interventional, or surgical procedures. IABP employs a large catheter with a balloon, which is situated in the aorta between the left subclavian artery and the renal arteries takeoff branches. The balloon is inflated during the diastolic phase of the cardiac cycle and deflated right before systolic ejection. Inflating the balloon during diastole creates an elevated perfusion pressure back to the coronary artery located off the aortic route. This elevated perfusion pressure increases coronary blood flow, thereby enhancing oxygen delivery. The balloon is deflated during the contraction phase of the cardiac cycle so that ventricular pressure opens the aortic valve and blood is ejected out into the aorta. The deflation of the balloon just prior to systole creates a suction effect within the vessel that helps pull more blood from the left ventricle and decreases the resistance the blood encounters when leaving the heart (afterload). A lowered afterload resistance decreases workload on the heart and enhances forward ejection of blood. The goal when using an intra-aortic balloon pump is to increase the supply of oxygen to the myocardium and decrease the demand (Figure 40–15 ■).

Beta- (ß-) Adrenergic Blocking (ß-blockers) Agents

Inhibiting adrenergic stimulation by competitive binding sympathetic receptors with β-blocking agents has been shown to reduce myocardial ventilation oxygen consumption (MVO_2). β-blockers reduce heart rate at rest, attenuate heart rate with exercise, decrease myocardial fiber stretch and contractility, oppose platelet aggregation, and stabilize myocardial cellular membranes, thus,

reducing dysrhythmia occurrence. These actions slow the heart rate and decrease the oxygen demand. Patients with chronic stable angina, treated with β-blocker therapy, demonstrate reduced number, severity, and duration of ischemic episodes and increased exercise capacity (Adams, Josephsen, & Holland, 2005; Opie & Poole-Wilson, 2005). β-blockers are used to treat silent ischemia, angina associated with altered vasomotor tone, UA, and AMI. Whether administered IV or orally, early β-blocker therapy in the setting of AMI reduces infarct size, malignant ventricular dysrhythmia occurrence, chest pain, risk of cardiac arrest, and mortality without a greater incidence of heart failure or heart block. Because the risk of mortality is highest during the first year, therapy should begin soon after the first IV dose and continue for at least a year. When discontinuing β-blocker therapy, the drug should be weaned down with decreasing doses.

Therapeutic goals include reduction in frequency or suppression of anginal attacks, resting heart rate of 50 to 60 beats per minute, attenuated heart rate and BP response during exercise, and no adverse reactions. Contraindications and reasons for discontinuing therapy include hypotension, sinus bradycardia, bronchial asthma, AV nodal dysfunction, claudication or pain in legs from peripheral vascular disease, and hyperglycemia from diabetes. Patients should be advised against abruptly discontinuing β-blocking agents. Long-term therapy results in an increase in the number, affinity, and sensitivity of β-receptors. When no longer blocked, unopposed sympathetic stimulation is heightened, producing rebound tachycardia, hypertension, exacerbation of angina, ventricular ectopy, and greater risk of MI.

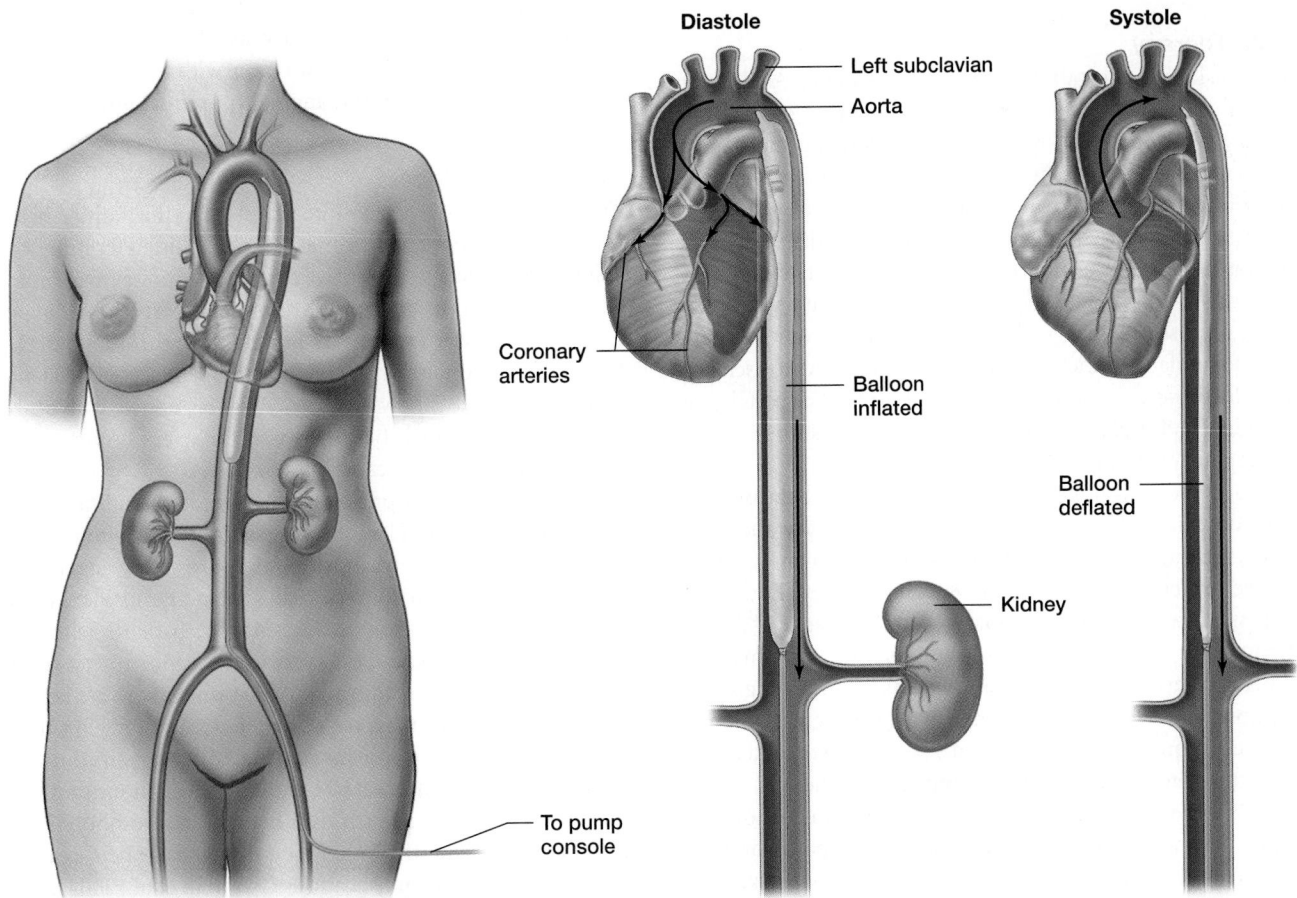

FIGURE 40–15 ■ Intra-aortic balloon pump catheter.

Angiotensin-Converting Enzyme Inhibitors

Low-dose angiotensin-converting enzyme inhibitors (ACEIs) started within 24 hours and continued indefinitely are part of the recommended therapy for patients suffering from an AMI because they reduce mortality and the incidence of left ventricular dysfunction and reinfarction (Antman et al., 2004). ACEIs are thought to be beneficial through a number of mechanisms: (1) increased production of superoxides by decreasing angiotensin II; (2) increasing endogenous nitric oxide, which increases vasodilation through ACEI inhibition of bradykinin degradation; and (3) positive influence on hemodynamic load, vascular function, myocardial remodeling, and neurohumoral regulation (Dendorfer, Dominiak, & Shunkert, 2005; Latini et al., 2003). Myocardial remodeling describes the process of replacing nonviable heart muscle tissue with nonelastic fibrinous collagen, which causes cardiac wall thinning, dilation, and subsequently an impaired ability for the ventricles to function normally. Side effects include hypotension, angioedema, persistent cough, and reduced creatinine clearance.

Angiotensin II Receptor Blockers in Myocardial Infarction

Angiotensin II receptor blockers (ARBs) have not been shown to be superior to ACEI alone, nor synergistic when added to ACEI, but are recommended for patients intolerant of ACEI therapy. The use of ACEI or ARBs is not advocated for patients with NSTEMI unless accompanied by persistent hypertension despite beta-blocker and nitrate therapy in patients with left ventricular dysfunction and in patients with diabetes (Libby, Bonow, Zipes, & Mann, 2008).

Nitrate Therapy

Once considered contraindicated in the setting of AMI, today nitrate therapy is a staple in drug management of occlusive coronary syndromes, regardless of the underlying mechanism triggering ischemia. Administration of nitrates causes the vascular smooth muscles to relax, resulting in dilation of venous, coronary, and, to a lesser degree, peripheral arterial vessels. Nitroglycerin dilates areas of arterial stenosis, especially in eccentric lesions, and can relieve spontaneous coronary vasospasm directly or possibly through the release of prostacyclin, another potent vasodilator, which improves collateral flow to ischemic areas. Nitroglycerin also has been shown to inhibit platelet aggregation, inhibit platelet adhesion, and cause disbursement of formed platelet clumps (Opie & White, 2005).

Nitrates are used alone or in combination with beta-blockers or calcium channel blockers to reduce the frequency and duration of angina symptoms, incidence of silent ischemia, and to improve exercise tolerance (Opie & White, 2005). Long-term benefits of nitrate therapy on mortality and incidence of AMI in patients with symptomatic and asymptomatic ischemia have not been determined. Short-term benefits of IV nitroglycerin with unstable angina and AMI are improved hemodynamics, decreased frequency and duration of symptoms, reduced infarct size, better patency rates following reperfusion therapy, greater residual left ventricular function, and decreased mortality. Long-acting nitrates such as oral, ointment, or patch preparations are used to treat patients with symptomatic CAD prophylactically. Faster acting nitrates such as sublingual tablets or spray-on nitroglycerin are used as needed to alleviate break-through angina. Patient are instructed to take up to 3 sublingual tablets or sprays spaced 5 minutes apart to relieve anginal attacks, which can be repeated in 30 minutes if symptoms return. If symptoms do not abate, or return despite rest and/or treatment, patients are instructed to activate the emergency medical system (EMS). Nitrates cannot be used within 24 hours after ingesting sildenafil citrate (Viagra) or like products because of the risk of severe vasodilation and death.

Other potential side effects of nitrate administration include reflex tachycardia, hypotension, headache, facial flushing, syncope, and cerebral ischemia. Over-the-counter analgesics usually relieve nitroglycerin-induced headaches. Patients should be cautioned about the potential for hypotension and reflex tachycardia when changing position from lying to standing. These same effects can be seem during IV nitroglycerin initiation and up-titration, especially in patients who present with hypovolemia, inferior wall MI, right ventricular infarction, or advanced age.

Vasodilator Therapy to Relieve Vasoconstriction or Vasospasm

Nitroglycerin is the drug of choice for relief of coronary vasoconstriction during chronic and acute myocardial ischemic syndromes. Sodium nitroprusside also produces coronary artery vasodilation. Unlike nitroglycerin, which is selective for venous and larger arterial beds, sodium nitroprusside affects only arterial vessels. Sodium nitroprusside is recommended as a second-line vasodilator if satisfactory blood pressure control is not obtained with nitroglycerin, and as the first-line therapy in the setting of AMI complicated with hypertension or acute heart failure.

Calcium channel blockers, such as diltiazem hydrochloride (Cardizem), are used in combination with nitrates in patients with Prinzmetal, or variant, angina to produce smooth muscle relaxation.

Thrombolytic Agents

Thrombus formation is an integral piece in the pathogenesis of myocardial ischemic syndromes. This has shifted treatment paradigms from simply supportive care and monitoring to rapid ischemia recognition, clot dissolution, and reperfusion of hypoxic tissue. Fibrinolytic therapy (treatment with thrombolytics) has been shown to establish reperfusion to the infarct-related artery successfully in a timely fashion. This has allowed myocardial muscle salvage, which has decreased the overall mortality rate for patients with a myocardial infarction.

Important general principles that guide the administration of thrombolytics are (1) contraindications, (2) timing of medication to time of event, and (3) monitoring for adverse reactions. Certain patient characteristics must be considered before administering thrombolytics. Essentially, patients who are at risk for bleeding because of a previous recent surgery, trauma, or history of recent bleeding complication, or who are hemodynamically unstable may be considered ineligible for thrombolytic therapy. An important aspect of administration is the delay from symptom onset to treatment. Every hour past symptom onset decreases the survival benefit of thrombolytic therapy. Past 12 hours, thrombolytic administration is associated with greater risk of complications (Antman et al., 2004).

Adverse reactions primarily focus on assessment of the patient for anaphylactic reactions, bleeding, and hemodynamic instability. Nurses need to watch for signs and symptoms of an allergic reaction, which include rash, wheezing, shortness of breath, flushing, and hypotension. Patients should be monitored for signs of bleeding from not only obvious sites such as IV catheter sites but also the mucous membranes of the oral pharynx, gums, nose, lungs, and rectum. Unnecessary catheter insertions and hypertensive states should be avoided. Neuro and vital sign checks should be performed according to institution protocol, monitoring for signs of intracranial hemorrhage and hemodynamic instability.

Anticoagulation Therapy

Procoagulant cells of the blood do not normally interact with the intact vascular endothelium. If vessel endothelium is injured or removed, blood contact with the elements of the subendothelial layer heralds the recruitment and activation of platelets and catalyzes the coagulation cascade. Anticoagulation therapies counteract thrombus formation in one or more of the following ways: deactivation of platelets, blocking of protein expression necessary for activation of the clotting cascade, and neutralization of thrombin generation or activity.

Plaque rupture causes the platelet surface glycoprotein (GP) Ib to adhere to subendothelial glycoproteins to form a monolayer of platelets over the plaque lesion. Additionally, activated platelets promote further platelet recruitment, aggregation, and activation by releasing stimulants from their granules and undergoing a change in shape, which allows expression of a binding protein. Activated platelets unleash other substances such as fibrinogen, thromboxane A_2, serotonin, and adenosine diphosphate (ADP) from granule stores, which in return attract and activate more platelets (Figure 40–16 ■). When a platelet is stimulated, it changes from a spherical contour to irregular shapes that result in the exposure of glycoprotein (GP) IIb/IIIa receptors and reactive phospholipids. The glycoprotein receptor sites bind with circulation fibrinogen to create a bridge between platelets, which then bind together to form a clot. Platelet surface phospholipids interact with plasma proteins of the clotting cascade, which also contributes to clot formation.

Antiplatelet agents deactivate platelets by either interfering with the production, release, or function of platelet-derived stimulants or the binding of GP IIb/IIIa receptors. Acetylsalicylic acid (ASA), clopidrogrel bisulfate (Plavix), and GP IIb/IIIa inhibitors form the constellation of antiplatelet agents currently used to treat ACS. Aspirin (ASA) has proven to be the most cost effective and least adverse antiplatelet agent used to date. ASA inactivates cyclo-oxygenase, an enzyme responsible for arachidonic acid oxidation into thromboxane A_2 and prostaglandins. ASA therapy has been effective in risk reduction with MIs and sudden death in patients with angina; reduced recurrence of ischemic symptoms in patients with UA; and reduced infarct size, rates of reinfarction, and mortality in patients with MI (Antman et al., 2004). Optimal dosing of ASA has not been determined. Following an initial dose of at least 160 milligrams, all patients with CAD should begin daily doses of 81 to 325 milligrams indefinitely, unless contraindications exist. Absorption is better with the chewable form of ASA, especially in patients who have received opiates. ASA suppositories can be safely used if nausea, vomiting, or known upper-gastrointestinal disorders are present. Patients with hypersensitivity to ASA can be started on Plavix as a substitute. Although commonly used alone as prophylaxis against thrombus formation in patients with stable CAD, in circumstances where plaque rupture is a definite risk, ASA is frequently used in combination with other antiplatelet agents.

Clopidrogrel bisulfate (Plavix), a thienopyridine, inhibits the platelet-stimulating effects of ADP. Plavix may be more effective than ASA in preventing thrombus formation following endothelial injury in that it inhibits both platelet adhesion and intimal proliferation, although Plavix has few side effects. It is given as a daily dose of 75 milligrams and is currently recommended as a first-line drug in addition to or in place of ASA for patients who present with NSTEMI.

Platelet adhesion to one another is dependent on fibrinogen contact with GP IIb/IIIa. Three GP IIb/IIIa antagonists are used in clinical practice: abciximab (ReoPro), eptifibatide (Integrelin), and tirofiban hydrochloride (Aggrastat). Abciximab is different from the others in that it is a monoclonal antibody that binds irreversibly to the GP IIb/IIIa receptor. Because it is an antigenic protein, there is a slight risk of anaphylaxis following administration. Once given, the antiplatelet effects of abciximab cannot be reversed despite administration of new platelets. Abciximab not only lasts the 10-day life cycle of the platelet but also affects newly formed platelets; eptifibatide and tirofiban are synthetic nonpeptide antagonists that compete with fibrinogen to bind with GP IIb/IIIa receptors. Unlike abciximab, the antiplatelet effects of eptifibatide and tirofiban can be reversed by withholding administration for 2 to 4 hours. All three GP IIb/IIIa inhibitors are administered intravenously by an initial bolus dose followed by a continuous infusion. Bleeding is the major complication and requires close monitoring and patient education for prevention. One major disadvantage of the GP IIb/IIIa blocking agents is that there is currently no simple, inexpensive method to monitor the extent of receptor blockade, which would allow dose titration and possibly reduce side effects. The lack of an oral preparation also limits the use of these agents to acute thrombotic events only.

Coagulation via the intrinsic and extrinsic clotting pathways is a dynamic process of a series of linked and interdependent reactions wherein one protein converts and activates another along a defined cascade of reactions that ultimately leads to thrombin generation. Activated thrombin detaches from the

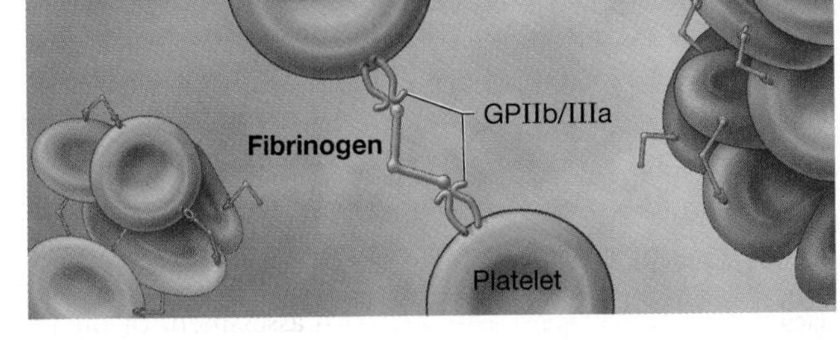

Platelet Aggregation

FIGURE 40–16 ■ Platelet aggregation.

phospholipids on the platelet surface and converts plasma fibrinogen to fibrin. Fibrin strands form a mesh that traps circulating blood elements to cause a clot. Inactivation of thrombin is achieved through the administration of (1) warfarin, which antagonizes the action of vitamin K–dependent clotting factors of the intrinsic clotting cascade; (2) unfractionated heparin, which when combined with the protein antithrombin III (AT III) adheres to and inactivates thrombin; (3) low molecular weight heparin (LMWH), which binds with factor X, effectively stopping the creation of thrombin through the clotting cascade; and (4) direct thrombin inhibitors such as hirudin, which bind directly to and inhibit thrombin activity.

Sodium warfarin (Coumadin) blocks an enzyme called vitamin K epoxide reductase necessary for the conversion of factors VII, IX, X, and II, and the proteins C and S into their activated forms. Wafarin's clinical use in the treatment of coronary syndromes is controversial and if used is limited to secondary prevention of thromboembolic complications following acute ischemic attacks and only in patients at low risk for serious bleeding complications. Because of this risk, warfarin therapy is not recommended in recent treatment guidelines for unstable angina or MI.

Intravenous heparin is an unfractionated combination of heparins with various densities and weights. The ability of heparin to bind with thrombin via the AT III protein depends on (1) the admixture of heparin molecules in the dose (high vs. low molecular weight), (2) circulating levels of AT III, (3) the presence of plasma proteins that inactivate heparin, and (4) the inability of heparin to reach thrombin sequestered within a fibrin clot. Plasma protein binding of unfractionated heparin contributes to a nonlinear, unpredictable, patient-specific anticoagulant response and heparin resistance. Using heparin doses adjusted according to patient weight and level of anticoagulation as measured by activated clotting time (ACT) or activated partial thromboplastin time (aPTT) produces better results with less bleeding complications. Most sources suggest a therapeutic aPTT range of 50 to 75 or 60 to 80 seconds with aPTT assessments drawn every 4 to 6 hours until a therapeutic range is achieved. Standardized nomograms, which prescribe how and when to adjust heparin dosage based on aPTT values, are extremely beneficial to nurses responsible for heparin titration (Figure 40–17 ■).

In summary, pharmacologic and nonpharmacologic measures to decrease oxygen demand and increase supply form the mainstay of initial management guidelines for patients with presenting signs of CAD, with resulting clinical manifestations of angina and ACS. Symptoms no longer controlled with pharmacologic agents are a clear indication of the need for more invasive procedures to revascularize the coronary arteries. These include either coronary artery angioplasty and/or surgical coronary revascularization. Decisions as to which treatment course is best, primarily depend on the severity of CAD and comorbid diseases, and their impact on the patient's lifestyle and risk for MI or death. Perhaps as important are patient preference and health care provider opinion in choosing treatment options. For emergent conditions, management may depend on the availability of cardiac catheterization and surgical services. See the Pharmacology Summary of Medications to Treat Coronary Disease box.

Medical Management of Complications of Acute Myocardial Infarction

Myocardial blood flow cut off for longer than 20 to 40 minutes initiates a dynamic process of cellular death, which extends over a period of several hours. Cell necrosis produces a loss of cell membrane integrity and degradation of connection tissue, which in turn causes cell swelling, protein leakage, and changes in cellular structure and function. In response, systemic catecholamine stimulation raises MVO_2 and taxes nonischemic tissue. With reestablishment of flow, initially cell necrosis continues and cell disruption and death ensue. Subsequent to cell death myocardial tissue undergoes remodeling characterized by the deposition of collagen in place of normal myocytes, muscle thinning, and dilation. These pathologic changes result in a myriad of complications that include recurrent angina, ventricular failure, dysrhythmias, and mechanical defects. Predictors of late major complications include the presence of early sustained ventricular tachycardia or fibrillation, presence of early sustained hypotension or cardiogenic shock, multivessel disease, and left ventricular dysfunction (Antman et al., 2004).

Recurrent Chest Pain from Ischemia

Chest pain that reemerges 12 hours to 6 days after an AMI, waxes and wanes, and is sometimes called stuttering or recurrent chest pain, may represent infarct extension. Recurrence of angina during recovery from AMI may depict coronary flow instability within the infarct-related artery. Pain, the most sensitive indicator

ACC/AHA Nomogram for Heparin Dosing

aPTT (s)	Bolus dose (u)	Stop infusion (min)	Rate change (mL/h)	Rate change (u/hr)	Repeat aPTT
<40	3,000	0	+1	100	6h
40–49	0	0	+0.5	50	6h
50–70	0	0	0	0	Next am
71–85	0	0	−0.5	50	Next am
86–100	0	30	−1	100	6h
101–150	0	60	−1.5	150	6h
>150	0	60	−3	300	6h

FIGURE 40–17 ■ Standardized nomograms for heparin dosage based on aPTT values.

PHARMACOLOGY Summary of Medications to Treat Coronary Artery Disease

Medication Category	Action	Application/Indication	Nursing Responsibility
Medical Management of Acute Coronary Syndrome (ACS)			

Calcium channel blockers:
  Diltiazem (Cardizem)
  Amlodipine (Norvasc)
	Inhibits calcium ion movement across the cell membrane in cardiac and vascular muscle, thereby relaxing the smooth muscle and dilating coronary and peripheral arteries.	Chronic stable angina.
		Vasospastic angina.
		Unstable angina.
		Hypertension.
		Postcoronary intervention.
		Dysrhythmias.
			Monitor blood pressure, heart rate, and rhythm.
			Monitor electrocardiogram (EKG) intervals.
			Monitor for response; i.e., decrease in angina, blood pressure, and dysrhythmias.
			Assess for increase in heart failure (HF), as edema may increase.

Nitrates:
  Nitroglycerin (NTG)
  Nitro-Bid
  Nitro-Dur
  Tridil
	Dilates coronary and systemic arteries, thereby decreasing preload and afterload.	Angina: chronic, unstable, or vasospastic.	Monitor blood pressure.
			Monitor for response; i.e., decrease in anginal pain, decrease in blood pressure.
			Assess patient for headache (known to cause headaches in some patients).
			Store drug in dark container, as it is sensitive to light.
			Do not administer within 24 hours of Viagra, Cialis, or Levitra.

Beta-adrenegic blockers:
  Metoprolol (Lopressor)
  Atenolol
	Selective: completely blocks beta-1 receptor stimulation in cardiac smooth muscle.
	Nonselective: causes a decrease in blood pressure through a mixture of beta-blocking effects but does not cause reflex tachycardia or decreased heart rate.
		Hypertension. Ventricular dysrhythmias.	Closely monitor blood pressure and heart rate.
			Monitor for response; i.e., decreased blood pressure, heart rate decreased, ventricular dysrhythmias.
			Monitor blood chemistries, especially those related to renal function.
			Use with caution in patients with chronic obstructive pulmonary disease (COPD), asthma, renal disease, or diabetes mellitus.

Angiotensin-converting enzyme inhibitors (ACE inhibitors):
  Benazepril (Lotensin)
  Captopril (Capoten)
  Enalapril (Vasotec)
	Inhibits the conversion of angiotensin I to angiotensin II; suppresses renin-angiotensin-aldosterone system.	Hypertension.
		Congestive heart failure.
			Monitor blood chemistries, specifically renal function and electrolytes.
			Monitor lower extremity edema.
			Monitor signs and symptoms of heart failure.
			Monitor response; i.e., decreased blood pressure, decreased shortness of breath (SOB), decreased rhonchi.
			Weigh patient every day.

Angiotensin II receptor blockers (ARBs):
  Candesartan (Atacand)
  Eprosartan (Teveten)
  Irbesartan (Avapro)
	Blocks the vasoconstrictor and aldosterone-secreting effects of angiotensin.	Hypertension.	Monitor for response; i.e., decrease in blood pressure (BP).
			Monitor blood chemistries.

Lipid Lowering Therapy			

HMG-CoA reductase inhibitors (statins):
  Atorvastin (Lipitor)
  Lovastatin (Mevacor)
  Simvastatin (Zocor)
  Pravastatin (Pravachol)
  Fluvastatin (Lescol)
  Rosuvastatin (Crestor)
	Inhibits HMG-CoA reductase enzyme, thereby preventing the formation of cholesterol in the liver. Statins lower total cholesterol, low density lipoproteins-cholesterol (LDL-C), and triglycerides while increasing high density lipoprotein-cholesterol (HDL-C). Statins have also been connected with stabilizing *rupture-prone* atherosclerotic plaque, improving vasomotor tone, decreasing levels of proinflammatory proteins, decreasing factors that contribute to thrombosis, and improving myocardial perfusion.	Hypercholesterolemia.	Monitor liver function studies.
			Monitor lipid panel.
			Monitor patient for myalgias.
			Administer medication in the evening to take advantage of the fact that the liver produces more cholesterol at nighttime than during the day.
			Patients may experience abdominal discomfort from gas or constipation, which usually subsides with continued therapy.
			Rarely causes elevated liver enzymes and muscle soreness, pain, and weakness, which may require changes in dose or discontinuance of statin therapy.
			Monitor liver function tests (LFT).

(continued)

PHARMACOLOGY Summary of Medications to Treat Coronary Artery Disease—*Continued*

Medication Category	Action	Application/Indication	Nursing Responsibility
Resins, or bile acid sequestrants: Cholestyramine (Questran) Colestipol (Colestid) Colesevelam (WelChol)	Binds with cholesterol-containing bile acids in the intestines and are then eliminated via stool.	Hypercholesterolemia.	Monitor lipid panel. Administered orally as powders or tablets and taken with water or fruit juice once, twice, or three times a day. May interfere with the absorption of other medications and, like statins, can cause constipation, bloating, nausea, and gas.
Fibrates: Gemfibrozil (Lopid) Fenofibrate (Tricor)	Fibrates lower triglycerides and can increase HDL-C levels.	Hypercholesterolemia.	Monitor serum LDL, very low density lipoprotein (VLDL), total cholesterol, and triglycerides. Monitor for gastrointestinal upset and bleeding. Assess for bloody stools, nosebleeds, cloudy or bloody urine, bleeding gums, and ecchyomoses.
Antihyperlipidemics: Ezetimibe (Zetia) Ezetimibe/Simvastatin (Zetia and Zocor) Combination drugs: Ezetimibe and Simvastatin (Vytorin) Work best when given with statin.	Ezetimibe: reduces blood cholesterol by inhibiting the absorption of cholesterol at the small intestine. This will decrease the level of cholesterol delivered to the liver. Simvastatin: inhibits HMG-CoA reductase enzyme, thereby decreasing cholesterol production; increases HDL-C and decreases VLDL and triglycerides.	Hypercholesterolemia.	Monitor liver function studies. Monitor lipid panel. Monitor patient for myalgias and headaches. Administer medication in the evening.
Niacin B vitamin	In high doses lowers triglycerides and LDL-C levels, and increases HDL-C.	Hypercholesterolemia. Increased triglycerides.	Patients should be advised not to start taking megadoses without being under the care of a clinician. Dose levels need to be gradually increased over time. Flushing or hot flashes (due to vasodilation) may occur, often requiring changes in antihypertensive medication dosage. Gastrointestinal symptoms of nausea, indigestion, gas, vomiting, diarrhea, and aggravation of peptic ulcers, liver problems, gout, and elevated blood sugar. Aspirin can be prescribed 30 minutes prior to the dose to decrease flushing.
Fibrinolytic (thrombolytic therapy)			
TNK	Modified human tissue plasminogen activator that binds to fibrin and converts plasminogen to plasmin. It is fibrin specific, thus decreasing the systemic activation of plasminogen.	Acute myocardial infarction.	Do not administer if the patient has active internal bleeding; history of cerebrovascular accident; intracranial or intraspinal surgery or trauma within 2 months; intracranial neoplasm, arteriovenous malformation, or aneurysm; known bleeding diathesis; or severe uncontrolled hypertension. Monitor for bleeding postdrug infusion. Administered as single bolus.
RPA	Nonglycoslated deletion mutein of tissue plasminogen activator, made by recombinant DNA technology.	Same as above.	Same as above. Administered as double bolus.

PHARMACOLOGY Summary of Medications to Treat Coronary Artery Disease—*Continued*

Medication Category	Action	Application/Indication	Nursing Responsibility
Antiplatelet Agents			
Acetylsalicylic acid aspirin (ASA)	Powerfully inhibits platelet aggregation by impairing hepatic synthesis of blood coagulation factors VII, IX, and X and possible inhibiting action of vitamin K.	Acute myocardial infarction and prevention of recurrence.	Monitor for gastrointestinal upset and bleeding. Assess for bloody stools, nosebleeds, cloudy or bloody urine, bleeding gums, and ecchyomoses. Administer with food. Do not administer if the patient has active internal bleeding. Discontinued use if ringing in ears. Maintain adequate fluid intake. Avoid medications with aspirin in them.
ADP receptor blockers: Clopidrogrel (Plavix) Ticlopidine (Ticlid)	Inhibits platelet aggregation by selectively preventing the binding of adenosine diphosphate to its platelet receptor.	Secondary prevention of myocardial infarction. Reduction in restenosis after stent placement.	Monitor for gastrointestinal upset and bleeding. Assess for bloody stools, nosebleeds, cloudy or bloody urine, bleeding gums, and ecchyomoses. Do not take other drugs that inhibit platelet aggregation.
Glycoprotein IIb/IIIa blockers: Eptifibatide (Integrilin) Abciximab (ReoPro) Tirofiban (Aggrastat)	Binds the IIb/IIIa receptor sites on platelets, preventing fibrinogen and von Willebrand factor from adhering to the platelet.	Treatment of acute coronary syndrome.	Monitor for bleeding. Stop infusion if bleeding occurs. Avoid invasive procedures including needle sticks.

Sources: Adams, M. P., Josephen, D. L., & Holland, L. N. (Eds.). (2005). *Pharmacology for nurses: A pathophysiologic approach.* Upper Saddle River, NJ: Prentice Hall Health; and Wilson, B. A., Shannon, M. T., & Stang, C. L. (2005). *Nurse's drug guide.* Upper Saddle River, NJ: Prentice Hall Health.

of infarct extension, may be accompanied by ECG changes, myocardial serum marker elevation (CK-MB, troponin I, and troponin T), hemodynamic instability, dysrhythmias, or worsening heart failure. Medical management for recurrent ischemic pain includes IV nitroglycerin (NTG), beta-adrenergic blockers, and calcium blockers. Refractory ischemic symptoms necessitate angiography to discern whether coronary occlusion is the cause and determine the appropriateness of repeat reperfusion therapy. Angiography is discussed in Chapter 39 ⊙ .

Pericarditis

Extension of myocardial wall necrosis through to the epicardium causes pericardial inflammation in some post-MI patients. Early or acute pericarditis occurs 48 to 72 hours after an AMI and is associated with larger infarcts and lower ejection fractions. Pericarditis often presents with pain accompanied by the following: pericardial friction rub, pericardial effusion, dyspnea, fever, elevated erythrocyte sedimentation rate (ESR), leukocytosis, and ECG changes of J point elevation with concave upward ST segment elevation in all leads except aVR and V_1, PR depression, persistently elevated T waves, or inverted T wave reversal. Absence of elevated CK-MB levels, symptom qualities, and ECG characteristics help differentiate pericarditis from ischemic pain. Pericarditis is discussed in detail in Chapter 41 ⊙ . The treatment of choice is the use of nonsteroidal anti-inflammatory drugs (NSAIDS) such as ibuprofen (Zipes et al., 2005). The use of indomethacin is discouraged because it can reduce coronary flow.

Dressler's syndrome (post-MI syndrome) connotes pericarditis that occurs 2 to 12 weeks after MI; it is thought to be an autoimmune or immunologic response to antimyocardial antibodies produced by myocardial necrosis (Zipes et al., 2005). Symptomology, diagnosis, and treatment are the same for early and late pericarditis except that symptoms developing later may reappear several times before resolving. The incidence of Dressler's syndrome has decreased with the era of thrombolytic therapy. Dressler's syndrome is discussed in detail in Chapter 41 ⊙ .

Heart Failure

Ischemia to myocardial tissue may cause transient or prolonged ventricular dysfunction requiring inotropic and vasodilation therapy to reduce myocardial oxygen demand and augment forward flow of blood. Reductions in blood flow to the myocardium trigger compensatory mechanisms whereby an ischemic muscle's ability to contract is lessened or down-regulated. Brief ischemic episodes, lasting less than 15 minutes, followed by reperfusion may not result in cellular necrosis but can produce a reversible transient depression of ventricular contraction that persists for hours or days called myocardial stunning (Zipes et al., 2005). Prolonged ischemia can produce compensatory down-regulation of contractile tissue, called myocardial hibernation, wherein oxygen debt requirements are matched to reduced oxygen supply (Zipes et al., 2005). (See the Pathophysiology of Myocardial Injury and Death section earlier in this chapter.) Partial or complete function is restored once reperfusion improves blood supply or therapy reduces myocardial oxygen demand. On cardiac imaging stunned and hibernating myocardium are reflected as areas of hypokinetic, akinetic or dyskinetic ventricular wall movement resulting in heart failure. This results in a temporary ventricular dysfunction without permanent myocyte damage, which may or may not present clinically as symptoms of ventricular failure. Prolonged ischemia without down-regulation of contractile ventricular function and reperfusion of ischemic tissue may cause cell membrane destruction, impaired cellular function and integrity, and eventually tissue necrosis. Heart failure is discussed in detail in Chapter 42.

Cardiogenic Shock

The incidence of cardiogenic shock in the setting of AMI is 7% and occurs when more than 40% of the left ventricle is infarcted, usually with severe three-vessel disease (Hochman et al., 2006). In patients presenting with AMI complicated by cardiogenic shock, survival has been reported between 20% and 50% when treated with thrombolytic agents, 40% and 70% with PCI, and 58% and 91% with emergency bypass surgery (Hochman et al., 2006). Emergency CABG is recommended for AMI patients with multivessel disease or cardiogenic shock who are not candidates for or have not undergone unsuccessful thrombolytic therapy and/or PCI, and who are within 4 to 6 hours from onset of AMI (Antman et al., 2004). Cardiogenic shock is discussed in Chapter 63.

Dysrhythmias

It is not uncommon for most patients with myocardial ischemia to experience some type of dysrhythmia. Dysrhythmia type depends on the location of arterial occlusion and the underlying electrical conduction tissue, which becomes ischemic. These dysrhythmias may be related to increased catecholamine activity, drug therapies, altered electrophysiological properties from hypokalemia, hypomagnesemia, intracellular hypercalcemia, and acidosis (Antman et al., 2004). Relative importance of each factor is unknown as is the efficacy of prophylactic treatments. Chapter 38 describes the cause and treatment of each of the dysrhythmias discussed next.

Supraventricular Tachycardia

The most common type of supraventricular tachycardia (SVT) that affects patients who have experienced an AMI is atrial fibrillation (AF); sinus tachycardia, premature atrial contractions, atrial flutter, atrial tachycardia, and accelerated junctional rhythms also occur. SVTs are managed by treating the underlying cause first. Additional treatments that may be necessary are synchronized cardioversion if the patient is severely compromised, slowing the rate with overdrive pacing or pharmacotherapy using primarily amiodarone, β-adrenergic blockers, calcium blockers, digoxin, or other antiarrhythmics.

Bradycardia

Bradycardia occurring from either an underperfused inferior wall myocardium or a heart block is treated using atropine, or cardiac pacing and withholding drugs that decrease the heart rate. Atropine is the drug of choice for treatment of symptomatic sinus bradycardia, ventricular asystole, and symptomatic heart block (Antman et al., 2004). Though cardiac pacing has not been shown to reduce mortality specifically, its use is recommended for patients with symptomatic bradycardia unresponsive to drug therapy (Antman et al., 2004).

Ventricular Dysrhythmias

Ventricular dysrhythmias, including premature ventricular contractions (PVCs), idioventricular and accelerated idioventricular rhythms, and nonsustained ventricular tachycardia (VT), can be expected in most patients early and within 48 hours during the course of recovery from AMI. Emergence of these dysrhythmias has not been shown to increase mortality nor warn of impending ventricular fibrillation (VF), unless the patient that is symptomatic is not treated.

Infarct Expansion, Ventricular Remodeling

Infarct expansion is the process of ventricular wall thinning and elongation of the infarct zone, which produces ventricular dyskinesia. Ischemia causes cellular inflammation, edema, and side-to-side cell slippage resulting in myocardial fibril changes. Ischemia causes myocardial cell fibers to become soft, distensible, and to rearrange in a wavy pattern, which results in a paradoxical fiber lengthening and wall bulging during systole and shortening during diastole. Eventually fibroblast proliferation causes collagen deposition and scar formation. Myofibrils are stretched and elongated and new fibrils are added, resulting in ventricular hypertrophy. The two processes of infarct expansion and ventricular hypertrophy cause ventricular remodeling, which can lead to development of heart failure and/or left ventricular rupture (Takemura & Fuiwara, 2004). Myocardial remodeling begins in the early stages of infarction and can continue for months and years. It is a predictor of increased mortality. Topographic changes from remodeling are identified using echocardiography and magnetic resonance imaging, described in Chapter 39. Limiting infarct size and maintaining patency of the infarct-related artery with reperfusion therapies are two primary strategies for preventing ventricular remodeling. Clinicians should avoid the administration of drugs that inhibit healing and scar formation, such as steroids, indomethacin, and ibuprofen. Reducing ventricular wall stress by decreasing preload with NTG and afterload with IABP and ACE inhibition is another means of limiting the extent of ventricular remodeling. Reduction in afterload and preload limits myocardial wall stress and subsequently infarct expansion and ventricular hypertrophy.

Left Ventricular Aneurysm and Thrombus Formation

Left ventricular aneurysm is a potential consequence of infarct expansion and remodeling. Aneurysm formation is associated with a greater risk of death, heart failure, angina, ventricular dysrhythmias, and embolization. Symptomatic patients may require temporary medical measures such as inotropic and afterload reducing agents, followed by surgical resection and/or endoventricular patching of the aneurysm, provided their remaining myocardial function is normal.

Mitral Valve Disruption

Papillary muscle ischemia can cause valve leaflet regurgitation or complete rupture, which accounts for 5% of deaths from MI (Massad & Geha, 2004). The posterior medial papillary muscle is affected more frequently because it receives blood supply only from the posterior descending artery (Figure 40–18 ■). Rupture can be complete, in which case rapid hemodynamic collapse ensues, or partial, with variable hemodynamic effects. Diagnosis of mitral valve disruption is made by two-dimensional echocardio-

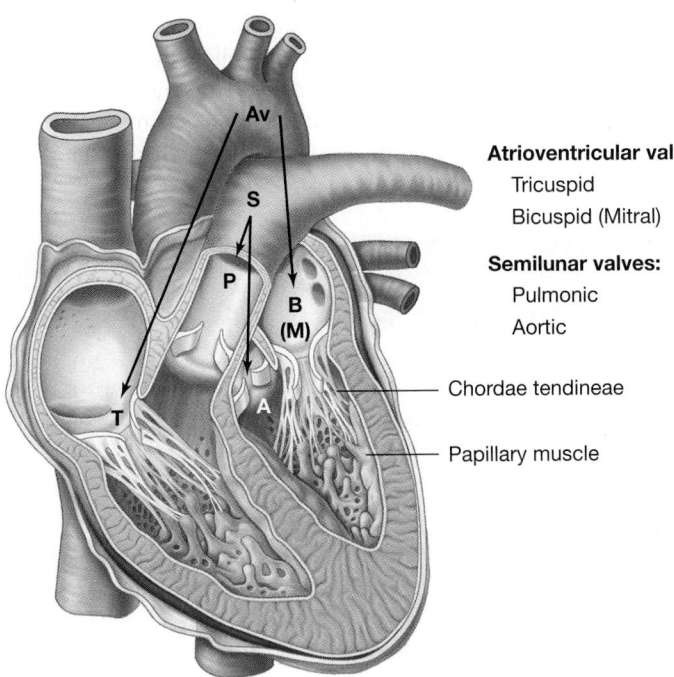

FIGURE 40–18 ■ Structures supporting the valves.

Atrioventricular valves:
Tricuspid
Bicuspid (Mitral)

Semilunar valves:
Pulmonic
Aortic

Chordae tendineae

Papillary muscle

graphy, cardiac catheterization, and ventriculography (Chapter 39 ☺). Afterload reduction with vasodilation therapy and IABP, preload reduction using nitrates and diuretics, and inotropic support may be necessary to stabilize the patient medically. Intermittent ischemic episodes may be treated with coronary artery bypass graft (CABG) surgery. Severe mitral valve disruption is treated with mitral valve repair or complete valve replacement. The diagnosis and treatment of valve disease is discussed in Chapter 41 ☺.

Ventricular Free Wall Rupture

Often fatal, rupture of the myocardial wall can be a result of an acute tear or a slow, incomplete rupture. It occurs in 1% to 3% of AMI patients and accounts for 10% of deaths from MI (Massad & Geha, 2004). Administration of thrombolytic therapy and intravenous β-adrenergic blockers has been linked to a decreased incidence of myocardial rupture following MI. Surgical repair is the only definitive treatment.

Ventricular Septal Defect (VSD)

Rupture of the ventricular septum results in a left-to-right shunting of the blood with symptoms of chest pain, syncope, and hypotension. Medical treatment includes the use of diuretics, vasodilators, inotropic agents, and IABP aimed at decreasing the amount of blood shunted from left to right and increasing forward flow. Emergency surgical repair involves debridement of infarcted tissue and suture of a septal patch to healthy septal tissue. This is indicated in the presence of pulmonary edema and cardiogenic shock.

■ Nursing Management

Nurses caring for AMI patients need to understand when and how to intervene to decrease the workload of the heart by increasing oxygen supply and decreasing oxygen demand. Nursing management of patients admitted to an intensive care unit depends on which method was used to reestablish coronary blood flow. Care of the patient following PCI is reviewed in Chapter 39 ☺. For patients treated medically, care is aimed at reducing myocardial oxygen demand, monitoring for signs indicative of adequate myocardial oxygen supply, administering and titrating medications to balance demand and supply, monitoring for and managing complications, and patient teaching. Hemodynamic monitoring with a balloon-tipped pulmonary artery (PA) catheter and intra-arterial pressure line is warranted for patients presenting with severe or progressive heart failure or pulmonary edema, cardiogenic shock or progressive hypotension, suspected mechanical/structural complications, or who are treated with vasoactive agents that affect blood pressure and therefore require titration. Pulmonary artery catheters and arterial lines are discussed in Chapter 24 ☺. Continuous cardiac monitoring in leads that will show ischemia or dysrhythmias is required. IABP therapy may be needed to reduce myocardial oxygen demand in the presence of heart failure, cardiogenic shock, or complications following an AMI. Serum tests such as complete blood count, chemistry panels, and coagulation profiles will be ordered to prevent complications and monitor response to treatments. Serial ECGs and serum cardiac markers are done to confirm the diagnosis of AMI and to determine the extent of infarction. Patients who have received thrombolytic therapy should be monitored for clinical signs of reperfusion including chest pain and ST segment elevation. Patients should be encouraged to inform the nurses of any new onset of chest pain or symptoms that were the same that occurred with the AMI. Anginal-type pain such as burning and pressure must be communicated between care providers. Commonly health care providers provide the nursing staff with "standing orders," which include contingency orders should certain complications such as a change in blood pressure or cardiac dysrhythmias occur. It is the nurse's responsibility to understand when to use these orders and how to assess the patient for effectiveness of the treatment.

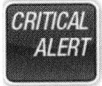 *It is not uncommon with cardiac patients for the health care provider to give a series of contingency orders that are implemented for a given clinical manifestation. An example is nitroglycerin (NTG) and 12-lead ECG orders for the occurrence of chest pain. It is important that the nurse obtain the ECG prior to administering the NTG because the medication will cause the ST segment to return to normal, thus, losing important diagnostic information.*

Patients are categorized as either high or low potential for complications, as well as either actual presence or absence of adverse sequelae. These categories determine the degree and duration of care and aggressiveness of the required treatment. For example, patients with no complications are low risk and can be fast-tracked within 24 to 48 hours to a lower level of care and discharged early. Patients with secondary complications and active comorbid diseases are at higher risk and will require longer hospital stays in areas with cardiac and hemodynamic monitoring capabilities.

No empiric data define the level of care the patient should receive once discharged from an area of intensive monitoring. Given that risk of sudden death is highest during the first 48 hours post-AMI and that intrahospital transfers can precipitate dysrhythmias, continuous cardiac monitoring for the first 48 hours of hospital stay and/or first 24 hours post–intensive care unit discharge is warranted. Other care needs required during convalescence on a step-down, telemetry, or intermediate unit for the AMI patient are the same as outlined for patients with unstable angina, with the exception of added attention to monitoring patient response to progressive activity.

The assessment data, which include sample questions specific to ACS, are found in the Nursing Process: Patient Care Plan for Acute Coronary Syndrome feature. Nursing diagnoses are developed from the assessment data and follow the assessment in the first column of the Nursing Process/Nursing Care Plan feature. This care plan applies the nursing process to the relevant nursing diagnoses and provides a comprehensive care plan for a patient with ACS in the acute period.

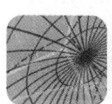

NURSING PROCESS: Patient Care Plan for Acute Coronary Syndrome

Assessment of Activity Tolerance

Subjective Data:
Are you able to complete your activities of daily living without fatigue?
Are you able to walk up a flight of stairs without getting short of breath?
Do you exercise on a regular basis?

Objective Data:
Monitor vital signs before and after walking in hall.
Assess heart sounds.
Monitor vital signs after completion of activities of daily living (ADLs).

Nursing Assessment and Diagnoses	Outcome and Evaluation Parameters	Planning and Interventions with *Rationales*
Nursing Diagnosis: *Activity Intolerance* related to insufficient oxygenation secondary to decreased cardiac output	**Outcomes:** Patient enrolls in cardiac rehabilitation program and attends post-MI lectures. ***Evaluation Parameters:*** Patient uses exercise log to record distances walked and symptoms experienced. Patient is able to monitor vital signs and adjust activity accordingly.	**Interventions and *Rationale:*** Encourage participation in cardiac rehabilitation program. Teach patient to use exercise log to monitor distances walked and symptoms. Teach patient how to monitor heart rate, blood pressure, and respirations as response to activity. *To increase endurance and strength and prevent weight gain.*

Assessment of Cardiac Output

Subjective Data:
Do you ever feel your heart beat fast, beat irregularly, or skip beats?
Do you ever feel light-headed?
Do you get short of breath when you walk distances?

Objective Data:
Assess heart rate and rhythm for abnormalities.
Monitor medications given and evaluate their response, especially those given for tachy/bradydysrhythmias.
Monitor blood pressure and respirations.

Nursing Assessment and Diagnoses	Outcome and Evaluation Parameters	Planning and Interventions with *Rationales*
Nursing Diagnosis: *Decreased Cardiac Output* related to dysrhythmias secondary to acute myocardial ischemia and infarction	**Outcomes:** Patient maintains normal and regular heart rate and rhythm. Patient verbalizes less fear and anxiety. ***Evaluation Parameters:*** Vital signs within normal limits. Exercise endurance increases. No anginal-type chest pain. Cardiac output within normal limits. No clinical manifestations of heart failure. Alert and oriented. Lungs clear.	**Interventions and *Rationales:*** Administer and teach antiarrhythmic medications, as ordered by health care provider *to ensure proper dosages and time intervals.* Provide comfort measures to patient and assurance *to decrease fear and anxiety.*

Assessment of Patient Ability to Cope

Subjective Data:
How are you feeling about your heart attack?
What are your thoughts about your future health?

Objective Data:
Evaluate patient response to written and verbal teaching materials about the patient's heart attack.
Evaluate patient response to discussion about current and future health concerns.

Nursing Assessment and Diagnoses	Outcome and Evaluation Parameters	Planning and Interventions with *Rationales*
Nursing Diagnosis: *Ineffective Coping* secondary to denial related to decreased physical status after myocardial infarction	**Outcome:** Patient verbalizes a decrease in problems and concerns. ***Evaluation Parameters:*** Vital signs within normal limits. Denies apprehension. Able to state an understanding of disease process.	**Interventions and *Rationale:*** Determine degree of denial; do not directly confront patient's denial; support patient's behavior. Provide active listening *to ensure patient you are working with her, not against her.*

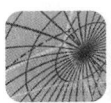

NURSING PROCESS: Patient Care Plan for Acute Coronary Syndrome—*Continued*

Assessment of Pain

Subjective Data:

Do you have chest pain?

Does your jaw hurt or throat hurt?

Does it radiate anywhere on your body?

Does it go away with a deep breath?

What makes the pain better or worse?

Objective Data:

Use pain scale (0–10) to quantify pain level.

Assess cultural or religious impact on the patient's response.

Assess location, duration, and onset of pain.

Nursing Assessment and Diagnoses	Outcome and Evaluation Parameters	Planning and Interventions with *Rationales*
Nursing Diagnosis: *Acute Pain* related to cardiac ischemia	**Outcome:** Pain free or controlled with medication. *Evaluation Parameters:* Patient notifies nurse immediately on experiencing pain. Patient's ECG is normal and pain is relieved with sublingual NTG. Patient is able to verbalize how to take sublingual NTG and its side effects.	**Interventions and *Rationale:*** Instruct patient to notify nurse immediately of chest pain. Implement health care provider's orders; i.e., ECG, sublingual NTG, morphine, oxygen. Teach patient about how to take sublingual nitroglycerin and its side effects. *This encourages the patient to participate in his own care and teaches one of the most important interventions for patients with CAD.*

Assessment of Fluid Status

Subjective Data:

Are you short of breath?

Do you monitor your weight?

Do you eat a lot of salt?

Objective Data:

Assess lung sounds for rales or crackles.

Monitor blood pressure, jugular venous distension (JVD), vital signs, urine output, daily weight, and peripheral edema.

Nursing Assessment and Diagnoses	Outcome and Evaluation Parameters	Planning and Interventions with *Rationales*
Nursing Diagnosis: *Excess Fluid Volume* related to fluid retention secondary to impaired myocardial contractility	**Outcomes:** Patient's body weight is within normal range; electrolytes will be maintained in normal range. *Evaluation Parameters:* Weight. Electrolyte values daily until stable. Lungs clear. No peripheral edema. Neck vein distention not present. Cardiac index and ejection fraction with normal limits.	**Interventions and *Rationales:*** Administer diuretics as ordered and teach patient rationale and side effects of medication. Weigh patient daily and stress to patient the importance of daily weights. Instruct patient to notify health care provider with greater than 2–3 pound gain. *This will allow the patient to identify weight gain from fluid.* Fluid restriction and low-sodium diet as ordered in order *to decrease excess fluid accumulation.*

Assess Patient/Family Knowledge of Disease and Treatment

Subjective Data:

Tell me what you know about your problems with your heart.

Tell me what you are doing about your risk factors.

Tell me about your dietary intake and your exercise program.

When do you develop chest pain and what makes it go away?

What medications are you on, when are you supposed to take them, and what are the side effects you should watch for?

When are you supposed to see your doctor?

Are you participating in a cardiac rehabilitation program?

Objective Data:

Patient/family may be anxious, confused, and need repeated information.

Mistakes being made with treatment plan.

Self-care deficit.

Nursing Assessment and Diagnoses	Outcome and Evaluation Parameters	Planning and Interventions with *Rationales*
Nursing Diagnosis: *Deficient Knowledge* related to disease and treatment plan	**Outcome:** Patient/family have an understanding of and comply with treatment plan. *Evaluation Parameters:* Patient and family understand treatment plan and safely become compliant. Patient and family understand the importance of risk factor control in preventing a progression of the disease. Patient and family participate in a cardiac rehabilitation program.	**Interventions and *Rationales:*** Describe the required diet, medications, activity, and limitations *to increase knowledge of disease and treatment.* Describe what clinical manifestations need to be reported to the health care provider and when to access the emergency medical system *to ensure immediate care when necessary.* Have patient/family repeat instructions *to assess understanding.* Provide information about the type, setting, and cost of a cardiac rehabilitation program, and assist with contacting the program *to decrease anxiety about the process.*

Sources: Wilkinson, J. M., & Ahearn, N. R. (2009). *Prentice Hall Nursing Diagnosis Handbook,* 9/E. Upper Saddle River, NJ: Prentice Hall.

Documentation of patient conditions is essential in order to assess normal progress following an AMI. Many institutions have developed a collaborative pathway as a mechanism for assessing this progress. The National Guidelines for an ACS Collaborative Pathway box includes an example of this pathway.

Collaborative Management

Patients who have experienced an acute myocardial infarction often recover best when a multidisciplinary approach is put into place. These patients benefit from several subspecialties such as physical therapy, respiratory therapy, dieticians, social workers, and of course the cardiologist and nurse. If a patient has suffered a large myocardial infarction he can spend several days to a few weeks in the hospital. When this happens the patient becomes weak from being in bed for such a long period of time as well as because his heart is not able to function at its previous level. Physical therapists can help bridge this gap and get the patient ambulating and performing activities of daily living before discharge so that he may function at home. Furthermore, they can help transition the patient into a cardiac rehabilitation program. Associated with prolonged bed rest comes the high risk of developing a respiratory infection. The respiratory therapist plays a key role in daily pulmonary toileting to prevent any nosocomial respiratory infections in these patients. The dietician focuses on proper in-hospital nutritional support as well as preparing the patient for dietary changes at home. The dietician emphasizes the need for a cardiac diet that is low in fat, cholesterol, and sodium intake. The social worker and discharge planner cannot go unnoticed in this collaborative approach. Oftentimes the myocardial infarction patient has a type A behavior pattern, is in denial, and is suffering from depression. Although the cardiologist can order some pharmacologic intervention, it is the social worker who can work best with these patients to help them understand their situation and learn effective coping mechanisms. They can assist these patients with behavior modification. The constant and consistent care provided by the nurse is the main link to these other disciplines. Only the nurse can provide an ongoing assessment of the patient

---

NATIONAL GUIDELINES for a portion of an ACS Collaborative Pathway

Acute Coronary Syndrome Collaborative Pathway

Collaborative Care Path Guidelines

Acute Coronary Syndrome

The **Collaborative Pathway** is part of the patient's medical record. For this reason, the physician, Registered Nurse, and other health-care professionals must collaborate together to insure that this Pathway is appropriately implemented. Utilizing the collaborative pathway supports the multi-disciplinary approach to patient care.

Upon admission, the RN will assess if the patient meets the criteria to be placed on this Pathway:

In general, any patient admitted with chest pain of unknown origin should be placed on the pathway.

Eligible Patients: *Chest pain of suspected cardiac origin, Angina Pectoris, Prinzmetal Angina, Unstable Angina/Rule-Out MI, MI.*

1. The RN is responsible to initiate the pathway and notify appropriate team members who will be involved in implementing patient care

2. The RN should collaborate with the admitting physician(s) regarding the patient's plan of care. This should be based on the pathway's standard of care while taking into consideration individualized patient care

3. It is the responsibility of the RN caring for the patient on each shift to:
   a. Review and document the progress of nursing and medical care as it occurs
   b. Review the pathway and evaluate whether the patient has met the expected outcomes
   c. Check off completion of care at the end of each day on the collaborative pathway
   d. Complete the "educational assessment" and "educational record" sections of the pathway
   e. Sign and date each page of the pathway
   f. Report to the upcoming shift the progress of the patient on the pathway, identify areas of concern, and outcomes that have not been met

4. It is the responsibility of the RN caring for the patient to document a Nursing Note on the Patient's progress on the pathway. A focus note is required if any pathway activity/outcomes are not met for any given day of the pathway.

Educational Record
Method of Teaching (MOT) Response (R)

AV – Audio-Visual V – Verbal 1 – Verbalizes/Indicates Understanding 2 – Further Instructions Needed

W – Written I – Interpreter 3 – Demonstrates Task 4 – Unable to Comprehend

D – Demonstration 5 – Refuses any information on Topic 6 – Other (see focus note for comments)

Teaching Topic Date Initials MOT Response Date Initials MOT Response

Explain Rationale For Admit to Hospital

Explain Reason for Tests and Procedures

Explain Chest Pain Scale of 1–10

Discuss Symptoms of Ischemia to Report to Nurse

Explain Collaborative Pathway

Provide Applicable Education Packet (Angina or MI)

Define ACS and Explain Causes
 View AHA educational videos for condition
 Discuss risk factors for CAD
 Discuss feelings pt./significant other experiencing
 Provide applicable printed information on discharge medications
 Review DC instructions: Activity level, clinic appt., prescriptions and symptoms to report
 Initials Signature Print Name Initials Signature Print Name
 Patient Addressograph

Source: University of California, Davis Medical Center.

COMPLEMENTARY & ALTERNATIVE THERAPIES Music Therapy

Description:

The prevention and psychosocial influences of cardiovascular diseases have been a focus for many in behavioral medicine, psychology, and nursing for the past 30 years. Music therapy is one method that provides a viable collaborative and complementary method to reduce risks for, and motivate rehabilitation from, cardiac events. During music therapy, the patient listens to music using headphones during hospitalization. Cardiac units should stock headphones, CD or other types of players, and a wide selection of musical CDs to fit patient preference, such as country-western, rock and roll, and classical. Prior to discharge, patients can be encouraged to continue listening to their music of choice at home during the recovery period.

Research Support:

Studies have shown that music modulates heart health measurements such as heart rate and blood pressure, enhances exercise programs, and relieves stress symptoms. In one study, a music therapy survey was administered to determine patients' current use and preference for music. The patients, who were in a cardiac rehabilitation program in a large city hospital, completed a survey on which they rated their level of use of music for exercise, relaxation, and enjoyment. The survey also gathered information on patients' musical preferences, musical experiences, and pertinent demographics. The patients, who were mostly white males over the age of 60, had positive, pleasurable responses to the aesthetic aspects of music. The researchers concluded that the use of music therapy in a cardiac rehabilitation program is warranted (Metzger, 2004).

A German study involved 15 patients in a coronary sport unit who listened to relaxation music while performing exercises adapted to their heart frequency. The patients' blood pressures were measured and their beta-endorphin blood levels were determined before the exercises and after listening to music. At the same time as having their blood samples collected, the participants had to perform two psychometric tests: Levenstein's perceived stress experience questionnaire (PSQ) to measure the graduation of subjective perceived stress and Spielberger's state-anxiety inquiry (STAI) as an indicator of coping. This protocol was performed 1 week prior to the mean trial, but the patients did not listen to music and had no blood collections or blood pressure measurements. There were no significant changes in PSQ-data in the test trial without music. However, in the mean trial (in which the participants listened to music), values in the section "worries" decreased. In addition, the STAI values were significantly lower, which indicates reduced anxiety after listening to music. Other results showed that beta-endorphin concentration and systolic blood pressure decreased significantly after participants listened to music. Researchers concluded that patients benefit from lower levels of worry and anxiety after music therapy (Vollert, Stork, Rose, & Mockel, 2003).

In patients having surgical procedures, music therapy has also been shown to reduce pain, anxiety, and physiological parameters. One study compared the effects of music therapy versus a quiet, uninterrupted rest period on pain intensity, anxiety, physiological parameters, and opioid consumption after cardiac surgery. Two randomized groups in a sample of 86 patients received either 20 minutes of music (intervention), or 20 minutes of rest in bed (control). The group that received music experienced a significant reduction in anxiety and pain as compared to the control group. However, there was no difference in systolic blood pressure, diastolic blood pressure, heart rate, nor a reduction in opioid usage in the two groups. (Sendelbach, Halm, Doran, Miller, & Gaillard, 2006).

References

Metzger, L. K. (2004). Assessment of use of music by patients participating in cardiac rehabilitation. *Journal of Music Therapy, 41*(1), 55–69.

Sendelbach, S. E., Halm, M. A., Doran, K. A., Miller, E. H., & Gaillard, P. (2006). Effects of music therapy on physiological and psychological outcomes for patients undergoing cardiac surgery. *Journal of Cardiovascular Nursing, 21*(3), 194–200.

Vollert, J. O., Stork, T., Rose, M., & Mockel, M. (2003). Music as adjuvant therapy for coronary heart disease. Therapeutic music lowers anxiety, stress and beta-endorphin concentrations in patients from a coronary sport group. *Deutsche Medizinische Wochenschrift, 128*(51–52), 2712–2716.

---

and the patient's response to these interventions. It is important that the nurses recognize they are the link and help collaborate all of these services, which will provide excellent patient care.

Health Promotion and Discharge Planning

The term *time is muscle* cannot be stressed enough in the care of the myocardial infarction patient. It is well known that the faster the infarct-related artery is opened, the more myocardium is salvaged. One reason early reperfusion is not established is because patients do not come into the hospital fast enough. The nurse is in a unique position to help with early treatment in a number of ways. First, nurses can collaborate with the community and establish educational programs that bring community awareness around the subject of timely treatment. Included in this is early recognition of symptoms and prompt initiation of emergency medical services. Nurses also can participate by teaching cardiopulmonary resuscitation so that, when an individual is suffering a heart attack, measures are being taken to ensure survival. A perfect place to offer these educational programs is in retirement communities because advanced age alone is a risk factor.

Once the patient enters the hospital system, the nurse again plays a key role in ensuring timely treatment. She can advocate on behalf of her patient to the health care provider. The nurse's physical assessment, as well as her interpretation of the ECG and laboratory tests, is vital in deciding the appropriate reperfusion strategy for these patients. Once the patient is discharged, again it is the nurse who plays a vital role in educating the patient and family in their recovery process. It is often the cardiac rehabilitation nurse who walks patients through lifestyle changes, behavior modification, and an exercise program to promote a full recovery. The nurse in this role teaches classes to small groups to educate them on topics such as nutrition, exercise, stress reduction, and even some new alternative therapies such as yoga, herbal medicines, and even acupuncture. It is important to include the family or another support system the patient has in this process so that others also can support optimal recovery. The Patient Teaching & Discharge Priorities box (p. 1208) presents the discharge needs for patients who have experienced a cardiac event.

■ Gerontological Considerations

The elderly population makes up the fastest growing portion of the American population. By the time a person reaches age 65, his heart has accomplished an amazing amount of work. To be specific the "adult heart beats more than 100,000 times a day,

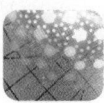

PATIENT TEACHING & DISCHARGE PRIORITIES for Coronary Artery Disease/Acute Coronary Syndrome

Need	Teaching
Knowledge of disease process and prognosis	Written and verbal instructions for: • Specific diagnosis/treatment; i.e., angioplasty, stent, heart attack, congestive heart failure, CAD • Follow-up labs, test, health care provider appointment • Medications • Diet • Activity. These instructions will reinforce the need to comply with therapy.
Understanding of medications	The patient and family are taught what the purposes of the medications are, their side effects, and their timing. These instructions will reinforce medication compliance and prevent over- or underdosing.
Safety	Stress the importance of wearing an identification bracelet to identify a heart problem to health care workers. Carry stent identification card in wallet to identify implant information to health care workers.
Disease prevention	Teach about dietary consumption. Stress the importance of a low-fat, low-cholesterol, low-salt diet. Teach about an exercise program. Stress the importance of exercise to prevent further CAD and keep current CAD from progressing. Offer cardiac rehabilitation program resources. Teach about behavior modification; decrease stress environment. Stress importance of smoking cessation and offer resources for community programs.
Reportable clinical manifestations	Teach to report chest pain or anginal equivalent. Stress how to take sublingual nitroglycerin should patient experience angina. Stress importance of using 911 emergency response system instead of driving self to emergency department (ED). Teach about fatigue and shortness of breath, as they too may be indicators of an unstable plaque or valve problem exacerbating. Teach about dental prophylaxis if patient was diagnosed with valve problem or had invasive coronary procedure.
Family/support system	Assess availability, knowledge, and compliance with treatment regimen. Assess discharge needs; i.e., home placement, medications, driving. Involve discharge planning if specific needs are not met to offer community resources.
Emotional adjustment of patient/family	Answer questions honestly. Encourage verbalization of frustrations and anger. Encourage positive reinforcement from the family. Provide active listening. Provide additional hospital and community resources, as necessary.

pumping roughly 2,000 gallons of blood through 60,000 miles of blood vessels every 24 hours" (Young, 1992). As one ages, one's heart undergoes physiological changes. These changes include stiffer ventricles due to the lack of the ability for the muscle to relax completely, decreased pumping function, decreased response to adrenaline, and decreased elasticity of the arteries. These changes can occur even in the absence of CAD but can be magnified in the presence of CAD.

CAD is the leading cause of death in the elderly. In fact, over half the people who suffer a heart attack are over age 65 (Young, 1992). Although men usually have a higher rate of CAD as compared to women during most of their lifetime, women have an equal, if not higher, rate after menopause. This may be due to the decrease in estrogen production. When one experiences a heart attack as an older individual, it may result in more complications and a longer hospital stay. Recovery is slower and presents many challenges. It may involve multiple systems in the body beyond just the cardiovascular system. This is often seen in patients with diabetes. The elderly also have a higher incidence of heart failure

and rhythm disturbances as a result of CAD alone or in conjunction with an AMI. For this reason it is imperative that the patient is monitored via a cardiac monitor and nursing management is directed appropriately to these changes.

Silent heart attacks are not uncommon in the elderly. This is attributed to the decreased sensation of pain. This is especially true again in the diabetic population, where it can occur at any age but increases in the elderly population. Instead of the typical "I feel like an elephant is sitting on my chest" symptoms, these patients may experience atypical symptoms such as heartburn or gastrointestinal discomfort and shortness of breath. Older individuals grow accustomed to illness and discomfort and thus frequently will overlook these otherwise overt symptoms. It is especially important to educate not only the elderly about these symptoms but also those who help with their daily care. Simple knowledge of this may prevent untoward outcomes among the elderly population.

Treatment options for the elderly often present challenges. Different considerations are given to the elderly when deciding on treatment options. For example, a patient who presents with a myocardial infarction who might otherwise meet the criteria for thrombolytics may in fact not meet the criteria simply based on age. For example, a patient who is 75 years or older is at a higher risk for an intracranial hemorrhage than is a 50-year-old patient. The health care provider critically assesses the risk benefit ratio in this instance, and the patient may or may not receive fibrinolytic therapy. The 50-year-old patient usually would receive fibrinolytic therapy because this is not as great a concern among the nonelderly population. Another example that demonstrates the differences in treating the elderly is a patient who presents with a ventricular dysrhythmia that might be treated with prophylactic lidocaine. Lidocaine can cause confusion and other side effects in elderly patients, thus negating its use in this patient population.

The management of these patients may also be different because they may be willing to accept a decrease in their quality of life. They may choose to refuse further invasive testing such as coronary angiography or bypass surgery. Instead they may accept some degree of limitation and just be managed through medications.

Should patients choose a more invasive treatment strategy, they must be willing to accept longer hospitalizations and complicated recovery patterns. Elderly patients often have other medical problems besides CAD disease. They may have multiple cardiac problems as well that include hypertension, atherosclerosis, calcified valves, and rhythm disturbances. These patients may have a more complicated recovery from procedures or surgery due to renal impairment, mobility limitations, mental status changes, and poor nutrition. All of this must be considered when deciding the pathway of care for these patients.

Lifestyle changes must not go unrecognized in the elderly. Risk factor modification such as smoking cessation, weight reduction, and proper diet may have a dramatic impact on their quality of life. Age-appropriate measures to help promote a healthy lifestyle have been suggested by the American Heart Association (AHA, 2008a). Physical inactivity is a modifiable risk factor for developing coronary artery disease. Lack of exercise also contributes to obesity, high blood pressure, a low level of HDL ("good") cholesterol, and diabetes. Even modest levels of physical activity are beneficial. The AHA states that a moderate amount of physical activity, preferably daily, is recommended for older adults. Healthly moderate activity for older persons includes:

- Longer sessions of moderately intense activities such as walking or swimming
- Shorter sessions of more vigorous activities such as fast walking or stair-climbing.

Coronary Artery Bypass Graft Surgery

For more than three decades, coronary artery bypass grafting (CABG) has been a mainstay for the treatment of coronary artery disease. During this time period, great advancements have occurred in both technique and technology. However, the basic concept of providing the heart with alternative methods of circulation has remained the same.

Prior to the advent of percutaneous coronary intervention (PCI), CABG was the only method of revascularization that showed success in alleviating symptoms, improving lifestyle, and improving mortality in select patient populations. PCI is discussed in detail in Chapter 39 ☉. Now that PCI is a widely accepted alternative, several research studies comparing the outcomes of CABG and PCI have helped develop an outline of which procedure is the most appropriate for different types of patients (Bypass Angioplasty Revascularization Investigation [BARI] 1996; Serruys et al., 2001). In short, the advantage of CABG is that it can provide more complete revascularization and show better long-term relief of symptoms. Less than 10% of patients who undergo CABG will need subsequent revascularization within 5 to 7 years (BARI, 1996). However, CABG patients also have more procedural-related pain, longer hospital stays, and more periprocedural myocardial infarctions (BARI, 1996). The final decision of CABG versus PCI is dependent on a number of factors and is important to review.

Indications

Patients who present with only mild symptoms of angina or who are even asymptomatic may benefit from CABG. However, there must be substantial evidence that CABG will prolong survival. In this scenario, a noninvasive test will show a very large area of myocardial ischemia. Despite the patient's being relatively asymptomatic, the test would suggest that the patient's anatomy is placing her at high risk. According to the American College of Cardiology (ACC) and the American Heart Association (AHA) guidelines for coronary artery bypass surgery, the following patients with mild or no symptoms are appropriate for CABG and are considered class 1 recommendations (Eagle et al., 2004):

- Significant left main coronary artery stenosis
- Left main equivalent: significant (greater than or equal to 70%) stenosis of the proximal left anterior descending artery (LAD) and proximal left circumflex artery
- Three-vessel disease. Survival benefit greater in patients with abnormal left ventricular function (less than 50%) or large areas of demonstrable myocardial ischemia.

Class 1 conditions are those for which there is evidence and/or general agreement that a given procedure or treatment is useful and effective. Patients with stable angina require a careful decision-making process as well. It is important that maximal medical therapy has been instituted and that risk factors have been addressed. The decision to proceed with surgery is driven by the likelihood that survival will be prolonged and symptoms will be relieved. It also is important to examine comorbidities. If a patient has diabetes or a reduced ejection fraction, a greater case can be made to proceed with surgery. According to the ACC/AHA guidelines, the following patients with stable angina are appropriate for CABG and are considered class 1 recommendations (Gibbons et al., 2002):

- Significant left main coronary artery stenosis
- Left main equivalent: significant (greater than or equal to 70%) stenosis of the proximal left anterior descending artery (LAD) and proximal left circumflex artery
- Three-vessel disease. Survival benefit greater in patients with abnormal left ventricular function (less than 50%)
- Two-vessel disease with significant proximal LAD stenosis and either left ventricular ejection fraction of less than 50% or demonstrable ischemia on noninvasive testing

- One- or two-vessel disease without significant proximal LAD stenosis but with a large area of viable myocardium and high-risk criteria on noninvasive testing
- Disabling angina despite maximal noninvasive therapy when surgery can be performed with acceptable risk.

The indications for CABG in a patient with unstable angina or non–ST segment elevation MI are similar to those in patients with stable angina. The critical factor that has to be considered with an unstable patient is the timing of the surgery. If a patient's symptoms are refractory and they are hemodynamically unstable, then revascularization should occur immediately. However, if a patient can be stabilized, there is some evidence that suggests a waiting period before performing surgery may improve outcomes. The following are class 1 recommendations for CABG by the ACC/AHA for unstable angina or non–ST segment elevation MI:

- Significant left main coronary artery stenosis
- Left main equivalent: significant (greater than or equal to 70%) stenosis of the proximal left anterior descending artery (LAD) and proximal left circumflex artery
- When percutaneous revascularization is not optimal or possible
- When ongoing ischemia not responsive to maximal nonsurgical therapy (Libby, Bonow, Zipes, & Mann, 2008).

The last group of patients would be those who are necessitating urgent intervention. Patients with ST elevation MI require immediate revascularization. These patients typically receive thrombolytics or undergo urgent PCI. In some cases PCI may fail or complications may occur. Performing surgery amid an acute MI greatly increases the risks of perioperative complications. Before the decision to undergo CABG is made, other acute therapies must be exhausted. The ACC considers the following to be class 1 recommendations for a patient with ST segment elevation MI to receive an urgent CABG:

- Failed angioplasty with persistent pain or hemodynamic instability in patients with coronary anatomy suitable for surgery
- Persistent or recurrent ischemia refractory to medical therapy in patients who have coronary anatomy suitable for surgery, who have a significant area of myocardium at risk, and who are not candidates for PCI
- If undertaking surgical repair of postinfarction ventricular septal rupture or mitral insufficiency
- Cardiogenic shock in patients less than 75 years old with ST segment elevation or left bundle branch block who develop shock within 36 hours of MI and are suitable for revascularization that can be performed within 18 hours of shock
- Life-threatening ventricular dysrhythmias in the presence of greater than or equal to 50% left main stenosis and/or triple vessel disease.

Standard Operative Techniques

Standard coronary artery bypass surgery is done via a median sternotomy using cardiopulmonary bypass (CPB), cold cardioplegia, and systemic hypothermia (28° to 32°C). CPB is a means to divert blood away from the heart and return it to the arterial system. The CPB machine temporarily performs the functions of the heart (circulation of blood) and lungs (gas exchange). This is accomplished by drainage of systemic venous blood directly to the CPB machine, usually via cannulation of the right atrium. The venous blood is then processed by the CPB machine. This entails a heat exchanger, which regulates the temperature of the blood; a filter, which does not permit air or atheroembolization to pass; and finally an oxygenator. Once the blood is oxygenated, it is then returned to the body via the arterial cannula, which usually is placed in the aorta. Further protection of the heart is achieved by cooling the heart with a cardioplegic solution. Infusions of cardioplegia allow surgeons to interrupt coronary flow safely for up to 20 minutes.

Once on CPB, anastomosis of the conduits will ensue (Figure 40–19 ■). The number of grafts usually varies from two to six. With the heart stopped, the surgeon can identify the obstructed artery and perform an arteriotomy to an area beyond the obstruction. An end-to-side anastomosis is then carried out with the chosen conduit. The proximal end of the graft is then anastomosed to the aorta using a similar technique.

Some surgeons perform coronary artery bypass without using CPB. This is generally referred to as beating heart bypass. Because CPB is not utilized, the heart remains beating. Mechanical stabilizers are placed on the area of the heart being bypassed to reduce motion. The advantage of this technique is the reduction of complications that can occur from CPB. The disadvantage is that the bypasses are more difficult to place accurately on a moving heart, which may lower the graft patency rate.

The left internal thoracic artery (ITA) is the preferred conduit as a graft to the LAD. The ITA (also commonly referred to as the IMA, or internal mammary artery) is the graft of choice due to its resistance to atherosclerosis and the ability to graft it as an *in situ* pedicle graft. This means that the artery remains connected proximally to the native subclavian artery. The 10-year patency rate for the ITA has been cited as 85% to 95% (Fitzgibbon et al., 1996; Goldman et al., 2004; Loop et al., 1986; Lytle et al., 1985). Because of the success of the ITA graft and its superiority over vein grafts, some surgeons are now performing bilaterally ITA grafting in nondiabetic patients. It is still too early to tell whether this will become common practice.

Vein grafts are typically the conduits used for the remaining bypasses. In most cases the greater saphenous vein is harvested from the leg. If the greater saphenous vein is not of good quality, the lesser saphenous vein and cephalic vein can be used. Up until just recently, a patient who required multiple bypasses would require an incision that extended over the entire length of the leg. A new technique wherein the vein is retrieved using an endoscope with one to three incisions is now being used in most large medical centers. The use of this technique has great advantages, including a decrease in incidence of leg wound infections and less pain.

Due to the success of ITA grafts, surgeons are exploring the use of other arteries as conduits. The most common arterial conduit other than the ITA is the radial artery. Before using the radial artery, Doppler studies must be done to assure adequate flow to the hand will resume with the radial artery gone. Unlike the ITA, the radial artery is used as a free graft. There is a greater incidence of spasm in radial artery grafts. The use of radial arteries has not replaced the use of vein grafts because most surgeons are waiting for more long-term data. Other arterial conduits that are being experimented with are the right gastroepiploic artery and the inferior epigastric artery. Use of these

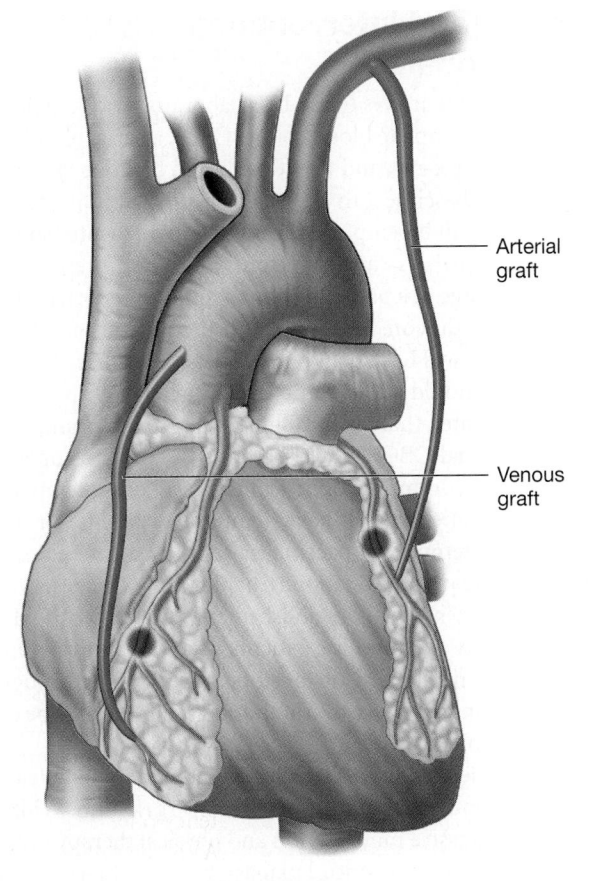

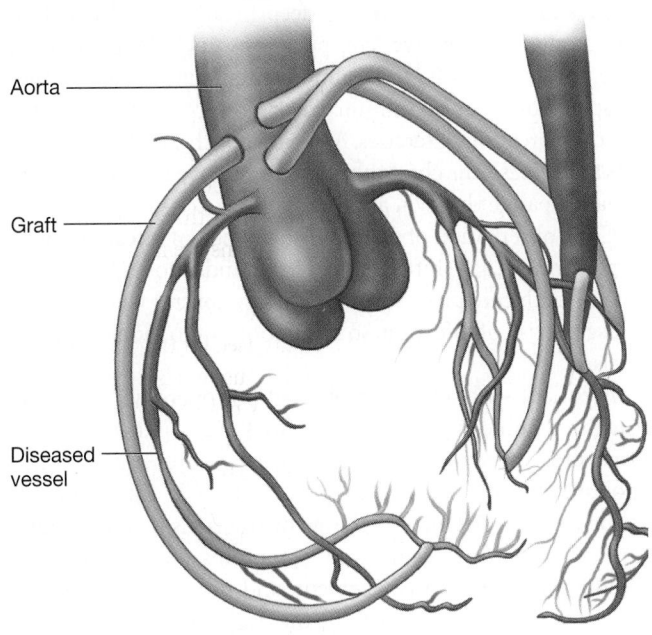

FIGURE 40–19 ■ Heart surgery grafts.

will require more research before determining whether they can be used as alternatives to vein grafts.

New Surgical Techniques

Advances in cardiac surgery have introduced new techniques. Although the use of these new techniques is not widespread, initial results seem to be encouraging. Minimally invasive direct coronary artery bypass surgery (MIDCAB) was first done in Europe but quickly spread to the United States. MIDCAB is done via only a small left anterior thoracotomy incision. Using a thoracoscope and mechanical stabilizers, the left internal thoracic artery can be directly harvested and anastomosed. Similar to beating heart bypass, this procedure is done off CPB so the heart remains beating. Medications are used to the slow the heart and the stabilizers to reduce motion. The advantage of this approach may be that it will reduce recovery time and potential postoperative complications such as CPB-related complications and wound infections. As with beating heart bypass, the disadvantage is that the bypasses are more difficult to place accurately on a moving heart, which may lower the graft patency rate. This technique is also usually limited to only one or two types of bypasses.

The latest development in cardiac surgery is called port-access technique. This procedure combines a minimally invasive approach with an endovascular cardiopulmonary bypass–cardioplegic arrest system. This technique uses peripheral CPB via femoral vessels with an endaortic occlusion device. The heart can then be bypassed and stopped without opening the chest. This allows for more accurate anastomosis as well as use of multiple grafts. This technique has also been used on patients with mitral valve disease for valve repair or replacement.

Postoperative Considerations

The overall rate of mortality for CABG is between 1% and 3%, with the risk increasing according to the number of risk factors a patient may have (Society of Thoracic Surgeons, 2006). As with any surgical procedure, complications can occur. Chapter 27 ∞ includes an in-depth discussion of common postoperative complications. Serious complications include stroke, myocardial infarction, and bleeding. Stroke can be a devastating complication that greatly affects recovery. Stroke is usually caused by an embolus from the ascending aorta or aortic arch. Surgeons are now employing the use of intraoperative echo to help detect irregularities within the aorta and avoid them while cannulating or clamping the aorta. Other postoperative complications to consider after CABG include tamponade, renal failure, respiratory failure, dysrhythmias, wound infection, and both pericardial and pleural effusions.

A patient with a completely uncomplicated postoperative period can be discharged as soon as 4 days. Most patients, however, will leave the hospital within 5 to 7 days. Once home, patients will gradually increase their activity levels and should be able to resume regular activity after 6 to 12 weeks. The amount of time is individualized and is dependent on a patient's age and other health problems. Risk factor modification is imperative, and all patients should be counseled on diet, exercise, weight control, and smoking cessation. Patients with hypertension, diabetes, and hyperlipidemia need aggressive management of these conditions.

■ Nursing Management

Skilled postoperative nursing management for the CABG patient is crucial for a successful recovery and prevention of complications. In the immediate postoperative period, patients are typically taken directly from the operating room to a specialized intensive care unit (ICU) with nurses who are trained in postcardiac surgery care. Depending on the institution and the patient's condition, some patients are extubated (removal of endotrachial tube) prior to leaving the operating room (OR). On arrival to the ICU, it is imperative for the nurse to receive a report from the OR on the patient, which should include the following: a summary of the surgery performed, amount of time the patient was "on pump," any intravenous drips that are running, recent laboratory values including arterial blood gases (ABG), any problems that occurred in surgery, and any coexisting illnesses that are pertinent. Knowing the type of surgery performed and the amount of time a patient was on cardiopulmonary bypass (CPB) are crucial to a patient's care. Prolonged bypass induces cytokine activation and an inflammatory response that results in red cell damage and hemoglobinuria, thrombocytopenia, clotting abnormalities, reduced pulmonary gas exchange, and cerebrovascular accidents.

Nursing Diagnoses

1. Pain related to surgery
2. Deficient knowledge related to disease and surgery
3. Potential for ineffective tissue perfusion related to fluid balance
4. Infection potential related to altered skin integrity

Assessment

Nursing assessment includes close monitoring of the patient's hemodynamic status. Continuous monitoring of cardiac output, cardiac index, pulmonary artery pressure, central venous pressure, and arterial pressure are assessed at regular intervals. Chapter 24 includes an in-depth discussion of these parameters. Close observation of the patient's heart rhythm, blood pressure, and oxygen saturation can detect new imbalances or hypoxia. Serum electrolytes and complete blood counts are assessed at regular intervals in order to intervene before complications occur. For example, an abnormal potassium or magnesium level can precipitate life-threatening cardiac dysrhythmias, and a low hemoglobin and hematocrit can decrease the oxygen-carrying capacity of the blood. Additionally, ventilator settings, chest tube drainage, and urine output are all assessed regularly.

Outcomes and Evaluation Parameters

Removal of the endotracheal tube (extubation) is an early outcome, and most hospitals will have protocols to wean the patient from ventilation as soon as possible. As a patient begins to wake up, it is important to prevent self-extubation and soft wrist restraints are usually required. Once a patient is extubated and hemodynamic parameters have remained stable, the next outcome is to get the patient weaned off all intravenous drips as tolerated and converted to oral medications. The patient's Swan-Ganz catheter is typically removed on postoperative day 1 if the patient is stable.

Neurological status is an essential evaluation parameter to establish, and once a patient begins to wake it is necessary to ask him to move each extremity and respond to simple questions. Early mobilization is important to reduce postoperative complications. It is standard for a patient to be out of bed and to a chair on post operative day 1 and transferred out of ICU if he is stable.

Planning and Interventions with Rationales

When the patient arrives to the ICU, laboratory work including chemistries, a complete blood count (CBC), arterial blood gases (ABGs), a chest x-ray, and an ECG should be done as soon as possible so a baseline can be established. Titration of intravenous drips will be employed to maintain adequate hemodynamic status such as cardiac output and blood pressure. Any abnormal change in a patient's status should be reported immediately to the surgeon. Depending on the institution and surgeon, a patient will have between 2 and 4 chest tubes. The chest tube output should be documented hourly. Any increase in output of greater than 100 milliliters per hour should be reported and serial CBCs should be done because postoperative bleeding most commonly occurs in the early postoperative period. Some patients will have temporary pacemaker wires placed, and a temporary pacemaker should be connected and tested to assure proper function (Chapter 36). These will be removed later when it is established that the patient will not need them. It is common for patients to develop dysrhythmias such as atrial fibrillation on postoperative days 2 through 5. Should a patient develop a dysrhythmia, an ECG should be done and the surgeon is notified.

Once a patient is out of ICU, he should remain on a telemetry floor to continue monitoring of his heart rhythm. While on telemetry, aggressive mobilization and physical therapy must be a focus. Adequate pain control management is important to encourage ambulation as well as deep breathing and coughing. Common postoperative complications include pneumonia, deep vein thrombosis, and pulmonary embolism. Each of these complications can be minimized or prevented by ambulation and deep breathing exercises. As a patient's chest tube output begins to decrease, the chest tubes will be removed and the amount of pain a patient has will also decrease.

Close observation of wounds for any sign of infection should be performed each shift. Changes in wounds should be reported to the health care provider. Poor glucose control will greatly increase the risk of infection, so it is important to monitor glucose levels.

A patient with an uncomplicated postoperative course will usually go home on postoperative day 4 or 5. Discharge medications most always include aspirin, beta-adrenergic blockers, cholesterol-lowering medications, and ACE inhibitors, described earlier. Detailed discharge instructions include medication management, signs and symptoms of infection and bleeding, risk factor management, and progression of activity levels. These instructions can be the deciding factor of whether a patient will succeed as an outpatient and should be reviewed thoroughly with the patient and his family.

Health Promotion

Discussing risk factors and employing secondary prevention measures will reduce the number of patients who have recurrent events after CABG. Patients will usually take medications such as cholesterol drugs, aspirin, beta-blockers, and ACE inhibitors long term. Daily exercise and adequate weight control will help reduce the risk of further coronary disease. If a patient smokes, it is imperative to use every measure possible to encourage cessation. Patients with diabetes are at a higher risk for recurrent cardiac events and should be monitored for this closely. A patient should be instructed on the signs and symptoms of angina and advised to report changes promptly.

Most patients will require repetitive counseling to change risk factors that have taken a lifetime to develop. Therefore, frequent follow-up with their primary health care provider and cardiologist is important to review risk factors and to monitor blood pressure, blood sugar, and cholesterol levels.

Research

Research is essential to improve the care, quality of life, and survival of patients with coronary artery disease. The goal of research is to identify areas where practice could improve and evaluate and test methods for these improvements. The research topics related to CAD are included in the Research Opportunities and Clinical Impact box. The list provides both medical and nursing research topics still under investigation. Electronic databases are a source for finding specific studies related to these topics.

RESEARCH OPPORTUNITIES AND CLINICAL IMPACT RELATED TO CORONARY ARTERY DISEASE

Research Area	Clinical Impact
Stem cell injection after acute myocardial infarction.	Stimulate new growth of myocardial cells and increase myocardial viability.
Gene therapy for chronic CAD patients who have no other alternatives.	Stimulate angiogenesis, thereby decreasing symptoms and increasing quality of life.
Facilitated percutaneous intervention for acute myocardial infarction.	Conjoined mechanical and pharmacologic interventions for AMI will decrease mortality and increase myocardial salvage.
Establish heart-healthy food supplements.	Decrease hyperlipidemia, thereby providing risk factor modification for some predisposed risk factors.
Identify predictors of vulnerable plaque and their impact.	Provide ability to manage plaque and prevent plaque rupture, thus future coronary events.
Establish standard of providing fibrinolytic therapy in the field.	Increase survival for acute myocardial infarction patient.
Effect of community awareness programs on patients with ACS emphasizing early symptom recognition and treatment.	Decrease adverse cardiovascular events and increase survival from out-of-hospital events.
Effect of immediately triaging women with ACS-like symptoms to chest pain unit.	Increase survival in the female population and bring awareness because their symptoms are often missed.
Behavior modification techniques and their effect on CAD and its events.	Lower all modifiable risk factors, thereby decreasing cardiovascular events in a high-risk population.
Effect on established grammar and high school education program teaching about CAD; i.e., signs and symptoms, treatments, outcomes.	Establish an aware and healthier population early on, thereby decreasing total cardiovascular events.

Clinical Preparation

CRITICAL THINKING

▶ Read
- History of Current Illness
- Past Medical History
- Physical Exam
- Admitting Medical Orders
- Laboratory Study Results

▶ Document
- Summary of Hospitalization
- Pathophysiology Form
- Laboratory Values
- Laboratory Results Explanation

▶ Apply
- List of Potential Nursing Diagnoses
- Concept Map
- Critical Thinking Questions

Log on to MyNursingKit.com to download forms you will need and to complete further steps in the Clinical Preparation assignment.

HISTORY OF PRESENT ILLNESS

You are a nurse in the coronary care unit (CCU) and have been notified that you will be receiving a patient from the cardiac catheterization lab with the diagnosis of ST segment elevation myocardial infarction (STEMI). You receive the following report from the nurse in the catheterization lab: Mr. Ray is a 43-year-old male with a history of hypertension, hypercholesterolemia, gastroesophageal reflux disease (GERD), and hepatitis C. He developed substernal chest pain while doing some yard work at approximately 1 p.m. today. His pain radiated to his left arm and was accompanied by shortness of breath, nausea, and vomiting. He rated his pain as a 10/10 in severity. He presented to the emergency department, and his first electrocardiogram (ECG) showed ST elevation in the anterolateral leads. He was initially treated with aspirin, nitro paste, morphine, and intravenous heparin. He was then emergently taken to the cardiac catheterization lab.

His cardiac catheterization showed a 100% thrombotic occlusion of his proximal left anterior descending artery. A drug eluting stent was placed, and the patient was placed on a ReoPro infusion.

On arrival to the CCU, the patient is awake and alert and denies any chest pain or shortness of breath. The patient denies any previous cardiac history. He is a pleasant man who appears in no acute distress.

Medical/Surgical History
No known allergies
Medications: none
Hypertension
GERD
Hepatitis C
Surgeries: knee and hip had "pins" placed

Social History
Family history: no premature heart disease; parents both alive and in good health
Last used tobacco 20 years ago and denies any ethanol use. He did use intravenous drugs approximately 15 years ago. He is employed as a landscaper.

Physical Exam
Temp: 97.6 BP 120/83 HR 80 RR: 14
Young Caucasian man with multiple tattoos, in no apparent distress
HEENT: scleras anicteric, oropharynx clear
Neck: supple, no lymphadenopathy
Lungs: clear to auscultation bilaterally
Cardiovascular: JVP not elevated; normal S_1 and S_2; regular rate and rhythm, no significant murmur, rub, or gallop; carotids 2+ without bruits
Abdomen: soft, nontender, nondistended, normoactive bowel sounds

Extremities: no edema
Neurological: normal, alert, and oriented $\times$ 3
CXR: normal
ECG: see history of present illness

Admitting Medical Orders
Admit to cardiology, coronary care unit
Condition guarded
Admitting diagnosis: acute coronary syndrome
Diagnosis: acute anterolateral STEMI
Vital signs and oxygen saturation q1h
Bed rest
Call house officer: pulse < 60 and > 100/minute; BP < 90 and > 160 systolic; temperature > 38.5; urine output < 30 mL/hr for 2 hours; respiratory rate > 30/minute; oxygen saturation < 92%
Sequential compression devices (SCD) to lower extremities
Diet: cardiac
Daily weight
Continuous cardiac monitor
Strict in/out
Foley to gravity
Oxygen per nasal cannula to maintain oxygen sat > 92%
IV: D5½NS @ 50 mL/hr

Scheduled Medications

ASA 325 mg po daily
Pantoprazole 40 mg po daily
Metoprolol 25 mg po bid
Lisinopril 20 mg po daily
Plavix 75 mg po daily
ReoPro gtt @ 0.125 mcg/kg/min for 12 hours
Lipitor 20 mg po daily

PRN Medications

Morphine 3–5 mg IV q3–5min, max 15 mg q3h prn pain
Temazepam 15–30 mg po qhs prn insomnia
Droperidol 1.25–2.5mg IV q6h prn nausea

Ordered Laboratory Studies

Troponin I q8h × 3
CPK–MB q8h × 3
Basic chemistry panel q a.m.
CBC q a.m.
Magnesium q a.m.
Lipid panel in a.m.

Ordered Diagnostic Studies

ECG q a.m.
Echocardiogram in a.m.

LABORATORY STUDY RESULTS

Test	Day 1	Day 2	Day 3
Sodium	135 mEq/L	136 mEq/L	137 mEq/L
Potassium	4.1 mEq/L	4.0 mEq/L	4.0 mEq/L
Chloride	103 mEq/L	104 mEq/L	103 mEq/L
Carbon dioxide (CO_2)	26 mEq/L	25 mEq/L	25 mEq/L
Blood urea nitrogen (BUN)	16 mg/dL	15 mg/dL	14 mg/dL
Creatinine	1.2 mg/dL	1.3 mg/dL	1.2 mg/dL
Glucose	85 mg/dL	96 mg/dL	89 mg/dL
Phosphorus	2.2 mg/dL	3.4 mg/dL	3.8 mg/dL
Calcium	9.1 mg/dL	8.7 mg/dL	9.1 mg/dL
Albumin	3.7 g/dL	3.7 g/dL	3.5 g/dL
Alkaline phosphorus	70 units/L	76 units/L	77 units/L
Aspartate aminotransferase	70 units/L	76 units/L	77 units/L
Bilirubin	1.8 mg/dL	1.4 mg/dL	1.2 mg/dL
Alanine phosphatase (ALT)	87 units/L	67 units/L	54 units/L
Magnesium	2.0 mEq/L	1.9 mEq/L	1.9 mEq/L
Creatine kinase	4368 units/L	2812 units/L	2000 units/L
Relative index	>6.9%	>10.7%	>9.4%
CK-MB	>300.00%	>300.00%	259.7%
Troponin I	>100 ng/mL	82.86 ng/mL	52.00 ng/mL
WBC	11.5/mm^3	10.9/mm^3	9.3/mm^3
RBC	4.89/mm^3	5.09/mm^3	4.92/mm^3
Hemoglobin	15.9 g/dL	16.5 g/dL	15.9 g/dL
Hematocrit	45.5%	47.8%	45.6%
Platelets	295/mm^3	256/mm^3	300/mm^3
Cholesterol	280 mg/dL		
High-density lipoproteins (HDL)	22 mg/dL		
Low-density lipoproteins (LDL)	198 mg/dL		
Very low-density lipoproteins (VLDL)	68%		
Apolipoproteins	162 mg/dL		
Triglycerides	210 mg/dL		

CRITICAL THINKING QUESTIONS

1. What is the purpose of Plavix for this patient?
2. Why were cardiac markers ordered?
3. What is the purpose of ReoPro in this patient?
4. When reviewing the ECG, what leads can you expect to be elevated with an acute anterolateral MI?
5. If the patient complains of chest pain that mimics the pain that he had before during the next couple of days, what steps would you take and anticipate?

Answers to Critical Thinking Questions appear in Appendix D.

NCLEX® REVIEW

1. Which of the following information reported by a patient indicates a non-modifiable risk to develop coronary heart disease?
   1. "I am trying to quit smoking, but it is difficult."
   2. "My blood sugars sometimes run a little high."
   3. "I walk at least one mile every day."
   4. "My father died of a heart attack at age 70."

2. A patient reports a history of having substernal chest pain. To help establish a diagnosis of stable angina, the nurse should ask which question.
   1. "Does your pain last for at least 15 minutes?"
   2. "Did your pain occur at rest?"
   3. "Was your pain precipitated by activity?"
   4. "Does your pain always radiate to the jaw?"

3. A patient seen in the clinic reports having episodes of left arm pain and chest tightness that started after having an argument. The nurse concludes the pain was most likely typical angina pain when the client also reports:
   1. The pain was relieved by taking nitroglycerin.
   2. Having just eaten a large meal prior to having the pain.
   3. Feeling very anxious when having the pain.
   4. Experiencing weakness and dizziness.

4. Because the electrocardiogram, ECG, of a patient admitted with acute coronary syndrome shows ST segment elevations, the nurse recognizes the patient has experienced:
   1. Mild cardiac ischemia.
   2. A myocardial infarction in the past.
   3. Subendocardial injury.
   4. Transmural ischemia.

5. A patient admitted with complaints of epigastric pain is evaluated for a myocardial infarction. Blood markers are negative but the electrocardiogram, ECG, shows deep Q wave changes without ST segment elevation. The nurse recognizes these changes indicate:
   1. Occurrence of an old myocardial infarction.
   2. Very recent myocardial ischemia.
   3. Pacemaker dysfunction.
   4. Ventricular hypertrophy.

6. The nurse concludes a patient has most likely experienced a myocardial infarction, MI, when blood work drawn four days following an episode of substernal pain with shortness of breath shows elevation of:
   1. Troponin I levels.
   2. Myoglobin levels.
   3. C-reactive protein.
   4. CK-MB.

7. A patient with severe three vessel disease experiences myocardial infarction, MI, causing occlusion to the left ventricle. The nurse places high priority on monitoring for sign of:
   1. Pericarditis.
   2. Cardiogenic shock.
   3. Dressler's Syndrome.
   4. Premature ventricular contractions.

8. The nurse recognizes a patient who is currently asymptomatic for cardiac ischemia may benefit from having coronary artery bypass graft, CABG, surgery since the patient has:
   1. A 50% occlusion of the circumflex artery.
   2. Been hospitalized with angina three times in the past year.
   3. Significant stenosis of the left anterior descending, LAD, and circumflex artery.
   4. A history of heart failure following a myocardial infarction a year ago.

9. Chest tube drainage output measures 200 mL in one hour in a patient recovering from a CABG. Which action should be taken by the nurse initially?
   1. Continue to monitor hourly outputs.
   2. Have the patient do cough and deep breathing exercises.
   3. Check the chest tube dressing for drainage.
   4. Report the findings to the primary care provider.

Answers for review questions appear in Appendix D

KEY TERMS

acute coronary syndrome (ACS) *p.1162*
akinesia *p.1187*
angina pectoris *p.1175*
arteriosclerosis *p.1159*
atherosclerosis *p.1159*
atheroma *p.1160*
cardiac risk factors *p.1164*
cholesterol *p.1165*
concentric *p.1162*
coronary artery disease (CAD) *p.1159*
creatine kinase (CK) *p.1184*
dyskinesia *p.1187*
eccentric *p.1162*
fibrous cap *p.1161*

high density lipoprotein *p.1167*
hypercholesterolemia *p.1165*
hyperlipidemia *p.1165*
hypokinesia *p.1187*
ischemia *p.1160*
low density lipoproteins *p.1166*
metabolic syndrome *p.1172*
MONA *p.1187*
myocardial hibernation *p.1164*
myocardial infarction (MI) *p.1181*
myocardial stunning *p.1164*
myoglobin *p.1184*
NSTEMI *p.1181*
oncosis *p.1164*

STEMI *p.1181*
sudden cardiac death (SCD) *p.1183*
thrombus *p.1162*
triglycerides *p.1167*
troponin *p.1184*
troponin I *p.1184*
troponin T *p.1184*
tunica adventitia *p.1159*
tunica intima *p.1158*
tunica media *p.1159*
unstable angina *p.1181*
variant, Prinzmetal, or vasospastic angina *p.1175*

PEARSON

EXPLORE **mynursingkit**™

MyNursingKit is your one stop for online chapter review materials and resources. Prepare for success with additional NCLEX®-style practice questions, interactive assignments and activities, web links, animations and videos, and more!

Register your access code from the front of your book at
www.mynursingkit.com

REFERENCES

Adams, M. P., Josephen, D. L., & Holland, L. N. (Eds.). (2005). *Pharmacology for nurses: A pathophysiologic approach.* Upper Saddle River, NJ: Prentice Hall Health.

Aggarwal, A., Schneider, D. J., Terrien, E. E., et al. (2004). Increased coronary arterial release of Interleukin-1 receptor antagonist and CD40 ligand indicative of inflammation associated with culprit coronary plaques. *American Journal of Cardiology, 93*(1), 6–9.

American Heart Association. (2008). *Inflammation markers signal rapidly advancing coronary disease.* Retrieved July 18, 2008, from http://www.americanheart.org/presenter.jhtml?identifier=3008009

American Heart Association. (2005a). Second International Conference on Women, Heart Disease, and Stroke. Orlando, FL, February 16–19.

American Heart Association. (2006a). *Facts about women and cardiovascular diseases.* Retrieved August 7, 2006, from http://www.americanheart. org/presenter.jhtml?identifier=2876

American Heart Association. (2006b). JAMA study: *Incidence and prognostic implications of stable angina pectoris among women and men: American Heart Association Media Advisory.* Retrieved July 18, 2008 from http://www. americanheart.org/presenter. jhtml?identifier=3038582

American Heart Association. (2006c). *Risk factors and coronary heart disease.* Retrieved August 16, 2006, from http://www. americanheart.org/presenter.jhtml?identifier=500

American Heart Association. (2006d). *Inflammation, heart disease and stroke: The role of C-reactive protein.* Retrieved August 16, 2006, from http://www.americanheart.org/presenter.jhtml?identifier=4648

American Heart Association. (2006e). *Triglycerides.* Retrieved August 16, 2006, from http://www. americanheart.org/presenter .jhtml?identifier=4778

American Heart Association. (2006f). *Heart disease and stroke statistics—2006 update.* Dallas, TX: Author. Retrieved August 8, 2006, from http://www.americanheart.org/presenter.jhtml? identifier=1928

American Heart Association. (2006g). *Physical activity and a healthy heart.* Retrieved September 17, 2006, from http://www.americanheart.org/ presenter.jhtml?identifier=1518

American Heart Association. (2008a). *Exercise (physical activity) for older people and those with disabilities.* Retrieved August 10, 2006, from http://www.americanheart.org/presenter.jhtml?identifier=4557

American Heart Association. (2008b). *Women, heart disease, and stroke.* Retrieved on July 18, 2008 from http://www.americanheart.org/presenter.jhtml?identifier=4786

American Heart Association. (2008c). *Women and Coronary Heart Disease.* Retrieved on July 18, 2008 from http://www.americanheart.org/ presenter.jhtml?identifier=2859

American Lung Association. (2006a). *Secondhand smoke fact sheet.* Retrieved August 16, 2006, from http://www.lungusa.org/ site/pp.asp?c= dvLUK900E&b=35422

American Lung Association. (2006b). *Statement on release of U.S. Surgeon General report on health consequences of secondhand smoke.* Retrieved August 16, 2006, from http://www.lungusa.org/ site/apps/nl/content3.asp?c=dvLUK900E&b=40407&ct=2689673

Antman, E., Anbe, D. T., Armstrong, P. W., Bates, E. R., Green, L. A., Hand, M., et al. (2004). ACC/AHA guidelines for the management of patients with ST-elevation myocardial infarction – Executive summary: A report of the American College of Cardiology/American Heart Association Task Force on Practice Guidelines (Committee to Revise the 1999 Guidelines for the Management of Patients with Acute Myocardial Infarction). *Circulation, 110*, 588.

Barandon, I., Couffinhal, I. T., Dufourcq, P., et al. (2004). Frizzled A, a novel angiogenic factor: Promises for cardiac repair. *European Journal of Cardiothoracic Surgery, 25*(1), 76–83.

Brown, T. A. (2001). Hibernating myocardium. *American Journal of Critical Care, 10*(2), 84–92.

Burke, A. P., Kolodgie, F. D., Farber, A., et al. (2002). Morphologic predictors of arterial remodeling in coronary atherosclerosis. *Circulation, 105*, 297.

Bypass Angioplasty Revascularization Investigation (BARI). (1996). Comparison of coronary bypass surgery with angioplasty in patients with multivessel disease. *New England Journal of Medicine, 335*, 217–225.

Castelli, W. P. (2001). Making practical sense of clinical trial data in decreasing cardiovascular risk. *American Journal of Cardiology, 88*(4), 16–20.

Clark, L.T., Ferdinand, K. C., Flack, J. M., et al. (2001). Coronary heart disease in African Americans. *Heart Disease, 3*, 97–108.

Coffey, M., Crowder, G. K., & Cheek, D. J. (2003). Reducing coronary artery disease by decreasing homocysteine levels. *Critical Care Nurse, 23*(1), 25–30.

Cohn, P. F., Fox, K. M., & Daly, C. (2003). Silent myocardial ischemia. *Circulation, 108*,1263–1277.

Dendorfer, A., Dominiak, P., & Schunkert, H. (2005). ACE inhibitors and angiotensin II receptor antagonists. *Handbook of Experimental Pharmacology, 170*, 407–442.

Diop, D., & Aghababian, R. V. (2001). Definition, classification, and pathophysiology of acute coronary ischemic syndromes. *Emergency Medicine Clinics of North America, 19*, 259–267.

Eagle, K. A., Guyton, R. A., et al. (2004). ACC/AHA guideline update for coronary artery bypass surgery. Retrieved July 15, 2008 from http://www.acc.org/qualityandscience/clinical/guidelines/news/bypass.htm

Fitzgibbon, G. M., Kafka, H. P., Leach, A. J., et al. (1996). Coronary bypass graft fate and patient outcome: Angiographic follow-up of 5,065 grafts related to survival and reoperation in 1,388 patients during 25 years. *Journal of the American College of Cardiology, 28*(3), 616–626.

Futterman, L. G., & Lemberg, L. (2000). The Framingham heart study: A pivotal legacy of the last millennium. *American Journal of Critical Care, 9*(2), 147–152.

Gene Analysis Service. (2005). Retrieved July 15, 2008 from http://www.gene-analysis-service.de/abcc6.htm

Gibbons, R., et al. (2002). *ACC/AHA guideline update for the management of patients with chronic stable angina.* Retrieved July 15, 2008 from http:// www.acc.org/qualityandscience/clinical/guidelines/stable/update%5Findex.htm

Goldfinger, T. M. (2003). Beyond the French paradox: The impact of moderate beverage alcohol and wine consumption in the prevention of cardiovascular disease. *Cardiology Clinics, 21*(3), 449–457.

Goldman, S., Zadina, K., Moritz, T., et al. (2004). Long-term patency of saphenous vein and left internal mammary artery grafts after coronary artery bypass surgery: Results from a Department of Veterans Affairs Cooperative Study. *Journal of the American College of Cardiology, 44*(11), 2149–2156.

Haskell, W. L. (2003). Cardiovascular disease prevention and lifestyle interventions: Effectiveness and efficacy. *Journal of Cardiovascular Nursing, 18*(4), 245–255.

Henning, R. J., & Olsson, R. A. (2001). Coronary blood flow and myocardial ischemia. In C. Rosendorff (Ed.), *Essential cardiology. Principles and practice.* Philadelphia: W. B. Saunders.

Higuchi, M. L., Reis, M. M., Sambiase, N. V., et al. (2003). Co-infection with *Mycoplasma pneumoniae* and *Chlamydia pneumoniae* in ruptured plaque with acute myocardial infarction. *Arquivos Brasileiros de Cardiologia, 81*(1), 12–22.

Hochman, J. S., Sleeper, L. A., Webb, J. G., et al. (2006). Early revascularization and long-term survival in cardiogenic shock complicating acute myocardial infarction. *Journal of the American Medical Association, 295*(21), 2511–2515.

Latini, R., Staszewsky, L., Maggioni, A., et al. (2003). Benefical effects of angiotensin-converting enzyme inhibitor and nitrate association on left ventricular remodeling in patients with large acute myocardial infarction: The delapril remodeling after acute myocardial infarction (DRAMI) trial. *American Heart Journal, 146*(1), 133–140.

Lewington, R., Clarke, N., Qizilbash, R., et al. (2002). Age-specific relevance of usual blood pressure to vascular mortality: A meta-analysis of individual data for one million adults in 61 prospective studies. *Lancet, 360*, 1903–1913.

Libby, Bonow, Zipes, & Mann. (2008). *Braunwald's Heart Disease, 8th Edition—A Textbook of Cardiovascular Medicine.* W. B. Saunders. Philadelphia.

Loop, F. D., Lytle, B. W., Cosgrove, D. M., et al. (1986). Free (aorta-coronary) internal mammary artery graft. Late results. *Journal of Thoracic and Cardiovascular Surgery, 92*(5), 827–831.

Lytle, B. W., Loop, F. D., Cosgrove, D. M., et al. (1985). Long-term (5 to 12 years) serial studies of internal mammary artery and saphenous vein coronary bypass grafts. *Journal of Thoracic and Cardiovascular Surgery, 89*(2), 248–258.

Massad, M. G., & Geha, A. S. (2004). Surgical repair of mechanical complications of myocardial infarction. *World Journal of Surgery, 28*(9), 847–856.

McSweeney, J., Cody, M., O'Sullivan, P., Elberson, K., Moser, D., & Garvin, B. (2003). Women's early warning symptoms of acute myocardial infarction. *Circulation, 108*(21), 2619–2623.

Morton, P. G., Fontaine, D. K., Hudak, C. M., & Gallo, B. M. (2005). *Critical care nursing: A holistic approach* (8th ed.). Philadelphia: Lippincott Williams & Wilkins.

Naghavi, M., Libby, P., Falk, E., et al. (2003a). From vulnerable plaque to vulnerable patient. A call for new definitions and risk assessment strategies: Part I. *Circulation, 108*, 1664–1672.

Naghavi, M., Libby, P., Falk, E., et al. (2003b). From vulnerable plaque to vulnerable patient. A call for new definitions and risk assessment strategies: Part II. *Circulation, 108*, 1772–1778.

Nash, D. (2004). Cardiovascular risk beyond LDL-C levels: Other lipids are performers in cholesterol story. *Post Graduate Medicine: online, 116*(3). Retrieved July 15, 2008 from http://www.postgradmed.com/issues/2004/09_04/nash.shtml

National Guidelines and Tools for Cardiovascular Risk Reduction. (2006). *Preventive cardiovascular nurses associations.* Philips Healthcare Communications.

Nomoto, K., Oguchi, S., Watanabe I., et al. (2003). Involvement of inflammation in acute coronary syndromes assessed by levels of high sensitivity C-reactive protein, matrix metalloproteinase-9 and soluble vascular-cell adhesion molecule-9. *Journal of Cardiology, 42*(5), 201–206.

Opie, L. H., & Poole-Wilson, P. A. (2005). β-*Blockers.* In L. H. Opie & B. J. Gersh (Eds.), *Drugs for the heart* (6th ed.). Philadelphia: W. B. Saunders.

Opie, L. H., & White, H. D. (2005). *Nitrates.* In L. H. Opie & B. J. Gersh, B. J. (Eds.), *Drugs for the heart* (6th ed.). Philadelphia: W. B. Saunders.

Pasterkamp, G., Fitzgerald, P. F., & de Kleijn, D. P. (2002). Atherosclerotic expansive remodeled plaques: A wolf in sheep's clothing. *Journal of Vascular Research, 39*, 514.

Pearson, T. A., Blair, S. N., Daniels, S. R., et al. (2002). *American Heart Association guidelines for primary prevention of cardiovascular disease and stroke: 2002 update.* Retrieved July 18, 2008 from http://circ.ahajournals.org/cgi/content/full/106/3/388

Pieniazek, P., Karczewska, E., Stepien, E., et al. (2001). Incidence of Chlamydia pneumoniae infection in patients with coronary artery disease subjected to angioplasty or bypass surgery. *Medicine Science Monitor, 7*(5), 995–1001.

Porth, C. M. (2005). *Pathophysiology: Concepts of altered health status* (7th ed.). Philadelphia: Lippincott Williams & Wilkins.

Rosenson, R. S., & Koenig, W. (2003). Utility of inflammatory markers in the management of coronary artery disease. *American Journal of Cardiology, 92*(1A), 10i–18i.

Sarwat, I., Krumholz, H., & Foody, J. A. (2004). Systolic hypertension in older persons. *Journal of the American Medical Association, 292,* 1074–1080.

Schoenhagen, P., Vince, D. G., Ziada, K. M., et al. (2002). Relation of matrix metalloproteinase 3 found in coronary lesion samples retrieved by directional coronary atherectomy to intravascular ultrasound observations on coronary remodeling. *American Journal of Cardiology, 89,* 1354–1359.

Serruys, P. W., Unger, F., Sousa, J. E., et al. (2001). Comparison of coronary-artery bypass surgery and stenting for the treatment of multivessel disease. *New England Journal of Medicine, 344*(15), 1117–1124.

Society of Thoracic Surgeons. (2006, Spring). *Adult cardiac database executive summary.* Retrieved July 15, 2008 from http://www.sts.org/documents/pdf/STS-ExecutiveSummarySpring2006.pdf

Takemura, G., & Fuiwara, H. (2004). Role of apoptosis in remodeling after myocardial infarction. *Pharmacology and Therapeutics, 104*(1), 1–16.

United States Department of Health and Human Services. (2006). *New Surgeon General's report focuses on the effects of secondhand smoke.* Retrieved August 16, 2006, from http://www.hhs.gov/news/press/2006pres/20060627.html

Venkat, A., Hekstra, J., & Lindsell, C. (2003). The impact of race on the acute management of chest pain. *Academic Emergency Medicine, 10*(11), 1199–1208.

Young, L. H. (1992). Yale University School of Medicine heart book. *Yale University School of Medicine, 21,* 263–271.

Zipes, D. P., Libby, P., Bonow, R. O., et al. (2005). *Heart disease: A textbook of cardiovascular medicine* (7th ed.). Philadelphia: W. B. Saunders.

41 CHAPTER

Caring for the Patient with Cardiac Inflammatory Disorders

Kathleen Osborn

Outcome-Based Learning Objectives

After studying this chapter, the learner will be able to:

1. Compare and contrast the etiology, pathophysiology, clinical manifestations, and medical and nursing management for the four inflammatory/infectious disorders.

2. Integrate the etiology, pathophysiology, clinical manifestations, and treatment for valve stenosis, regurgitation, and mitral valve prolapse.

3. Explain the rationale and type of preventive therapy necessary for patients with valve disease.

4. Differentiate valve repair and replacement procedures in terms of patient care and education needs.

5. Compare and contrast the four types of cardiomyopathy in terms of etiology, pathophysiology, clinical manifestations, and medical and nursing management.

6. Apply nursing diagnoses and the nursing process to the care of the patient with inflammatory and structural heart disease.

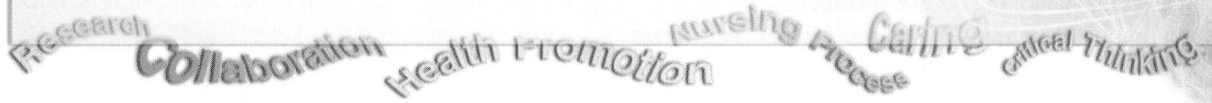

Research Collaboration Health Promotion Nursing Process Caring Critical Thinking

CARDIAC DISORDERS caused by inflammation or structural changes and abnormalities impact tissue perfusion due to altered myocardial pumping ability or abnormal blood flow through the heart. All three layers of the heart, the pericardium, myocardium, and endocardium, can be subject to inflammation and structural abnormalities. The manifestations differ depending on which layer is involved in the pathologic process. In recent years the incidence of cardiac structural disorders has increased due in part to advancements in the prevention and treatment of coronary artery disease. People are living long enough to develop the structural changes often associated with advanced age. An in-depth discussion of disorders affecting each layer of the heart is presented in this chapter.

INFLAMMATORY DISORDERS

The heart is susceptible to bacteria and microbes that may be infecting other organs of the body. The infection causes an inflammatory response that impacts the heart's ability to maintain a normal cardiac output. In the acute stages these infections are serious and potentially lethal. Additionally, damage to the heart during the infectious process can be long term and disabling. The inflammatory conditions affecting the heart—rheumatic heart disease, pericarditis, myocarditis, and endocarditis—are discussed next.

■ Rheumatic Heart Disease

Rheumatic heart disease is a complication of rheumatic fever. The pathologic process of **rheumatic fever** begins with a pharyngeal infection caused by Lancefield group A beta-hemolytic streptococcus (strep). If left untreated, approximately 3% of these pharyngeal infections result in rheumatic fever. The resulting rheumatic heart disease is thought to be caused by an abnormal autoimmune response to the original infection, but the exact pathogenesis remains unclear (Chin, 2006). The primary long-term damage is scarring and malfunction of the heart valves.

Epidemiology and Etiology

Until recently rheumatic fever was thought to be nearly eradicated from developed countries, although it continues to be a challenge because of its high prevalence in the developing world. It was the leading cause of death 100 years ago in the United States in people 5 to 20 years of age. Antibiotics and early treatment have made rheumatic fever rare in developed countries, although in recent years it has made a comeback in poor inner-city neighborhoods. Rheumatic fever occurs most frequently in children from 5 to 15 years of age and tends to affect connective tissues, especially those of the heart, brain, skin, and joints. The risk factors associated with the development and spread of streptococcal infections are outlined in the Risk Factors box. Rheumatic fever occurs equally among men and women, but the prognosis is worse for females because they are more likely to develop other conditions such as mitral valve prolapse (Chin, 2006).

Worldwide, chronic rheumatic heart disease is estimated to exist in 5 to 30 million children and young adults. Approximately 90,000 people die from this disease each year and the mortality rate remains 1% to 10% (Chin, 2006). Once rheumatic fever has occurred, a person is more susceptible to recurrent infections. With each infection more damage to the heart valve occurs.

Pathophysiology

As mentioned, rheumatic fever develops following pharyngitis from Lancefield group A beta-hemolytic streptococcus. The infecting organisms attach to the epithelial cells in the upper respiratory tract and produce enzymes that damage and invade other tissues of the body. These organisms elicit an acute inflammatory response after an incubation period of 2 to 4 days. Several weeks after the initial infection resolves, rheumatic fever results. Only infections of the pharynx initiate and reactivate rheumatic fever. Patients remain infected for weeks after the resolution of symptoms and may serve as a reservoir for infecting others.

In greater than half of the cases of rheumatic fever, an abnormal autoimmune response is thought to occur. It is theorized that the invading organism produces toxins that precipitate an antigen–antibody response. The antibodies appear to cross-react with connective tissues and bind to receptor sites on the heart, joints, skin, brain, and subcutaneous tissue, causing an acute inflammatory response. In the heart, all three layers, the endocardium, myocardium, and pericardium, become inflamed, giving rise to the term **pancarditis**. Microscopic lesions, referred to as Aschoff nodules are composed of a collection of lymphocytes and histocytes, are found in the fibrinous interstitial septa of the myocardium. Additionally, wartlike raised fibrinous lesions develop on the closure lines of the valve cusps. As Aschoff nodules age, they become more fibrinous scar tissue, contributing to the transient heart failure associated with rheumatic fever. As the inflammation subsides there is typically no long-term damage to the myocardium and pericardium. The long-term sequela of the inflammation is to the heart valves.

The inflammatory process causes swelling of the valves, and small bacterial vegetations form on the valve surface (Figure 41–1 ■), which leads to fibrous thickening and fusion of the valve leaflets, causing valve dysfunction. Damaged valves either do not completely open (stenosis) or close (regurgitation). The severity of the symptoms is dependent on the valve involved and the degree of dysfunction. Valve stenosis and regurgitation, described later in this chapter, cause an increase in the workload of the heart. The symptoms typically become worse over time with the most advanced condition leading to heart failure.

Clinical Manifestations

Clinical manifestations of rheumatic fever typically begin about 1 to 6 weeks after a bout of strep throat (pharyngitis), although in some cases the infection may have been too mild to be recognized. The diagnosis of rheumatic fever and rheumatic heart disease is based on a cluster of clinical manifestations and laboratory findings. Clinical manifestations of acute rheumatic fever and rheumatic heart disease are outlined in Chart 41–1.

The diagnosis of rheumatic fever and rheumatic heart disease is made by clustering signs and symptoms and analysis of laboratory and diagnostic tests. Carditis is the most significant manifestation of rheumatic fever. New or changing murmurs are one of the major signs of cardiac involvement. The murmur is caused by valve insufficiency or regurgitation. Murmurs typically found with acute rheumatic fever are (1) the apical pansystolic, high-pitched murmur, which has a blowing quality that radiates to the left axilla, indicating mitral regurgitation; (2) the apical diastolic murmur, which is low pitched and rumbling and is present with active carditis and accompanies severe mitral in-

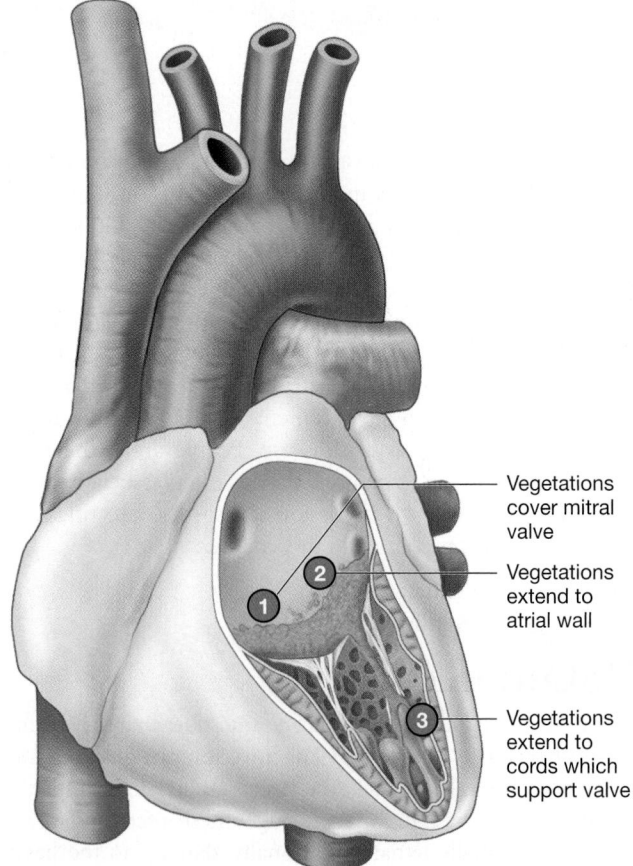

Vegetations cover mitral valve

Vegetations extend to atrial wall

Vegetations extend to cords which support valve

FIGURE 41–1 ■ Vegetative growth on a heart valve.

RISK FACTORS for Rheumatic Fever

Poor inner-city neighborhoods
Damp weather
Crowded living conditions
Malnutrition
Immunocompromised state
Poor access to health care

CHART 41–1	**Clinical Manifestations of Acute Rheumatic Fever and Rheumatic Heart Disease**

Clinical Manifestations of Acute Rheumatic Fever	**Clinical Manifestations of Rheumatic Heart Disease**
Fever	Chest pain
Malaise	Development of a new murmur or change in an existing murmur
Headache	Tachycardia and cardiac dysrhythmias
Erythema marginatum: red, raised, lattice-like rash, usually on the chest, back, and abdomen	Electrocardiogram (ECG) changes: prolonged PR interval
Swollen tender joints with small bony protuberances with or without the presence of subcutaneous nodules	Pericardial friction rub
	Symptoms of heart failure
May have weakness and shortness of breath	Cardiomegaly
Sydenham chorea: sudden, irregular, aimless involuntary movements that are self-limiting with no permanent damage	Mitral and aortic stenosis
Elevated white blood count (WBC)	

sufficiency; and (3) the basal diastolic murmur, a high-pitched, blowing, decrescendo murmur associated with aortic regurgitation (Chin, 2006). A complete description of murmurs is outlined in Chapter 37 .

> **CRITICAL ALERT**
> *If a new murmur is noted during the assessment of a patient with rheumatic fever, the nurse needs to report this to the health care provider. It may indicate the onset of rheumatic heart disease and requires further diagnostic testing. Where the murmur is heard depends on the valve that is involved.*

Heart failure may develop secondary to myocarditis or valve insufficiency. Another manifestation of cardiac involvement during rheumatic heart fever is pericarditis. A pericardial friction rub, distant muffled heart sounds, chest pain, and evidence of pericardial effusion are all consistent clinical manifestations of pericarditis.

Polyarthritis is the most common symptom and in 70% to 75% of the cases is the earliest manifestation of acute rheumatic fever (Chin, 2006). The arthritis typically begins in large joints of the lower extremities, such as the knees and ankles, and then migrates to other large joints of the lower and upper extremities. The affected joints are painful, swollen, erythematous, and have decreased range of motion. The arthritis reaches its most intense severity 12 to 24 hours after onset and persists for 2 to 6 days. Polyarthritis is not associated with any permanent disability.

Sydenham chorea is the major central nervous system (CNS) manifestation and may occur in patients with rheumatic fever (Chin, 2006). It is characterized by difficulty writing, involuntary grimacing, purposeless movements of the arms and legs (choreiform), speech impairment, generalized weakness, and emotional lability. Sydenham chorea is slightly more common in females under age 18 than males.

Laboratory and Diagnostic Procedures

When evaluating the patient with suspected rheumatic heart disease, a complete history and physical is necessary in order to evaluate the risk factors and the extent of the disease process. In addition to the clinical findings, a number of laboratory tests are useful when making the diagnosis. The Diagnostic Tests box (p. 1222) describes the laboratory and diagnostic tests and abnormalities associated with rheumatic fever and rheumatic heart disease.

Medical Management

Prevention is the primary goal in the management of rheumatic heart disease. Early treatment of the streptococcal infection with antibiotics will usually prevent the development of rheumatic fever. People with previous attacks are more susceptible to future episodes and each attack increases the amount of heart damage. Therefore, aggressive early treatment is essential in this population.

An antibiotic, typically penicillin, is used in the treatment of rheumatic fever. Oral penicillin V is the drug of choice, although erythromycin may be used when there is a penicillin allergy. Following the acute stage, prophylactic antibiotics are indicated to prevent further damage to the valves. The recommendation in the United States is that after the initial course of antibiotics, an intramuscular injection of penicillin G be given every 4 weeks. Although controversial, this schedule is continued indefinitely for high-risk patients or recurrent infections. Additional prophylactic antibiotics are indicated before and after any dental work or any surgical procedure.

Aspirin and nonsteroidal anti-inflammatory drugs (NSAIDs) are used to treat joint pain and fever. If symptoms of moderate to severe carditis are present as evidenced by cardiomegaly and heart failure, steroid administration is typically added to the therapy and continued for 2 to 4 weeks (Chin, 2006).

If heart failure with left ventricular dysfunction (ejection fraction less than 40%) occurs as a consequence of rheumatic fever, cardiac medications, such as angiotensin converting enzyme (ACE) inhibitors (or angiotensin receptor blockers), beta-adrenergic blockers, digoxin, or diuretics for congestion are indicated. See Chapter 42 for pharmacologic management of heart failure. See the Pharmacology Summary (p. 1236) for medications to treat inflammatory heart disease.

Bed rest is prescribed to reduce cardiac workload, especially during the acute phase. Once the carditis subsides the patient may begin a gradual schedule of increasing activity. Activity levels are dictated by the presence or absence of symptoms.

■ Nursing Management

Nursing management of the patient with rheumatic heart disease begins with an in-depth assessment of the clinical

DIAGNOSTIC TESTS for Cardiac Inflammatory Disorders

Test and *Normal Values*	Expected Abnormality	Rationale for Abnormality
White blood cells (WBC): *5000–10,000/mm³*	Elevated with rheumatic fever, pericarditis, and myocarditis. Mild elevation with infective endocarditis (IE).	Elevated levels are associated with inflammation and infection.
Red blood cells (RBC): *Male: 4.7–6.1 mm³* *Female: 4.2–5.4 mm³*	Mild to moderate decrease with rheumatic fever.	Occurs due to the inflammatory inhibition of erythropoiesis.
Erythrocyte sedimentation rate: *Male: up to 15 mm/hour* *Female: up to 20 mm/hour*	Elevated rheumatic fever, pericarditis, IE, and myocarditis.	The test measures inflammation. Chronic inflammation and infection cause an elevation.
C-reactive protein: *<10 mg/L*	Elevated rheumatic fever, pericarditis, IE, and myocarditis.	Acute-phase reactant protein used to indicate an inflammatory illness.
Antistreptolysin O titer (ASO): *<160 units/mL*	>250 unit/mL with rheumatic fever.	Streptococcal antibody test used to determine whether a previous streptococcal infection has caused a poststreptococcal infection such as rheumatic fever.
Cardiac marker: creatinine kinase MB (CK–MB), troponin T, and troponin I *CPK–MB: <3% or 0–7.5 ng/mL* *Troponin T: <0.2 ng/mL* *Troponin I: <0.35 ng/mL*	Elevated if carditis is present with all of the inflammatory disorders.	May be transiently elevated during the acute stages of myocardial cell damage.
BNP: *<100 pg/mL or <100 ng/L*	Elevated with ventricular hypertrophy, severe hypertension, and heart failure.	Marker of ventricular systolic and diastolic dysfunction. Useful to determine presence of heart failure.
Throat culture: *Negative or normal flora*	Positive for A beta-hemolytic streptococci with rheumatic fever.	Quantifies and differentiates bacterial from viral throat infections.
ECG: *Normal conduction time intervals (see Chapter 38)*	Prolonged PR interval with rheumatic fever. Diffuse ST segment abnormalities, T wave changes, dysrhythmias and heart block with myocarditis. ST segment changes associated with myocardial ischemia and the conduction delays typical of IE.	Conduction delays may be present with inflammation. ST segment changes may be present when myocardial ischemia is occurring.
Chest x-ray: *Clear lungs and normal heart size*	Enlarged heart and lung congestion with pancarditis and heart failure. May show cardiac enlargement if a pericardial effusion is present. Diagnoses of heart failure and in right-sided IE may show evidence of septic pulmonary emboli.	Cardiac enlargement occurs with inflammation, heart failure, and pericardial effusion. Congestion occurs with heart failure.
Echocardiogram (ultrasound): *Normal chamber size and normal cardiac structures*	Valve damage and dilated chamber size, abnormal pressure gradients, decreased ventricular function, and/or pericardial effusion with structurally abnormal valves. Depressed systolic function, dilated chambers, and mild to no pericardial effusion may occur with myocarditis. Determines the presence of pericardial fluid, motion of the heart walls, and the presence of restriction with pericarditis. Presence of thickening and calcification of the pericardium for IE.	The inflammation causes structural changes in cardiac chambers and function.
Cardiac catheterization: *Normal coronary arteries, chambers, and valve pressures*	Valve damage, enlarged chamber size, decreased ventricular and/or function with rheumatic fever. Valvular and ventricular function abnormalities, and assists in evaluating need for valve replacement surgery.	Inflammation causes changes in chamber size and valve function. Valve stenosis disrupts blood flow causing enlarged chamber size. Valve regurgitation causes a backflow of blood into the previous chamber.

DIAGNOSTIC TESTS for Cardiac Inflammatory Disorders—*Continued*

Test and *Normal Values*	Expected Abnormality	Rationale for Abnormality
Blood cultures: *Negative for organisms*	Positive and organism specific in 90–95% of cases with IE and therefore guide antibiotic therapy.	Organisms enter the bloodstream, adhere to the valve surface, and multiply.
Viral titers: *Negative*	Elevated.	Viral titers are present for 8 to 10 days after onset of illness.
Endomyocardial biopsy: *Normal tissue*	Presence of patchy cell necrosis and inflammatory changes confirm the diagnosis.	Often done within 6 weeks of acute illness while lymphocytic infiltration and myocyte damage is present.
Autoimmune serum markers: *Negative*	Presence of intracellular adhesion molecules on cardiac myocytes.	Intracellular adhesion molecules on cardiac myocytes is specific to autoimmune myocarditis.

Source: From *Laboratory Tests and Diagnostic Procedures with Nursing Diagnosis,* 6th edition, by J. V. Corbett, 2004, Upper Saddle River, NJ: Pearson Prentice Hall.

manifestations outlined in Chart 41–1, p. 1221. Further subjective and objective data related to clinical manifestations are outlined in the Nursing Process: Patient Care Plan for Inflammatory Heart Disease feature (p. 1224). The nurse must specifically note and report to the health care provider any progression of the clinical manifestations related to heart failure. In addition, any change in the loudness of the murmur must be documented and reported because this may indicate a progression of cardiac valve disorders.

The outcome for the patient with rheumatic fever is to make a full recovery with no residual cardiac pathology. As outlined in the nursing process patient care plan, nursing management focuses on resting the heart, pain relief, eradication of the infecting organism, and emotional support. Nursing interventions require critical thinking and sound clinical judgment because not all patients present with the same manifestations. It is essential to stress the importance of decreasing myocardial oxygen demand and cardiac workload. Strict bed rest is typically ordered, especially in the acute stages of these illnesses. The nurse must explain the importance of bed rest and activity restriction to the patient and family. Spacing care and activities to allow for periods of rest will decrease oxygen demand and, thus, cardiac workload.

Health Promotion

Prevention of a recurrence of the disease requires patient/family education about the need for prophylactic antibiotics, vigilant hygiene, good nutrition, and rest. The patient needs to be instructed to avoid individuals with upper respiratory infections to minimize exposure. The nurse should stress the risk for recurrence if a streptococcal infection occurs. A list of clinical manifestations that would indicate a need to seek medical help must be provided. It should be stressed that cardiac valve disease could develop and will require medical intervention. The Patient Teaching & Discharge Priorities box (p. 1227) outlines specific discharge priorities.

■ Pericarditis

Pericarditis, an inflammation of the pericardial sac, is the most common pathologic process affecting the pericardium. The pericardium or pericardial sac is a double-walled membranous sac that encloses the heart and the roots of the great vessels. The purpose of the pericardial sac is to prevent excessive dilation during diastole, to act as a barrier from infections in adjacent tissues, and to prevent displacement of the myocardium and great vessels. The inner serous layer of the pericardium is the visceral pericardium or epicardium and the outer layer is the parietal pericardium (Figure 41–2 ■, p. 1228). The space between these two layers is referred to as the pericardial space and normally it contains approximately 50 mL of fluid. The fluid serves to lubricate and decrease friction while the heart is moving during systole and diastole. Due to the inflammatory process, the two layers of the pericardium become inflamed and roughened, and the amount of fluid in the pericardial sac increases. Pericarditis can be acute and/or chronic constrictive (recurrent) and has several causes.

Epidemiology and Etiology

There are three general causes of pericarditis: infectious, noninfectious, and hypersensitive or autoimmune. These causes are listed in the Risk Factors box (p. 1228). If infectious, often the infection starts in some other organ in the body, usually the lungs and upper respiratory tract. The most common cause of pericarditis is caused by the coxsackie virus B and is referred to as Bornholm disease. People in their 20s and 30s who have had a recent upper respiratory infection and men ages 20 to 50 years are most likely to be affected. Frequently the cause of pericarditis is idiopathic. Noninfectious causes include uremia, which affects 6% to 10% of patients with advanced renal failure before initiation of dialysis. When patients with large effusions are studied, uremia may account for up to 20% of cases in some series. The widespread availability of dialysis has reduced the incidence of uremic pericarditis (Gowda, 2008). Noninfectious pericarditis also occurs after acute myocardial infarction (AMI) and following open heart surgery (postcardiotomy).

Hypersensitive or autoimmune responses are the third category of causes of pericarditis. This category includes connective tissue disorders, drug reactions, and rheumatoid diseases that affect the heart (Chart 41–5, p. 1250). **Dressler's syndrome,** also referred to as late pericarditis, occurs in 5% to 15% of the patients typically 1 to 4 weeks after an AMI. It is characterized by fever, pericarditis, chest pain, and pericardial friction rub and pleural

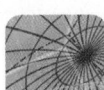

NURSING PROCESS: Patient Care Plan for Inflammatory Heart Disease

Assessment of Respiratory Status

Subjective Data:
Do you feel short of breath?
When does it occur?
How far can you walk before you have to rest due to shortness of breath?
Do you have a cough and, if so, do you cough anything up?
Do you become more short of breath when lying down?

Objective Data:
Acid–base balance.
Lung sounds.
Respiratory rate.
Assess for adventitious or diminished breath sounds.
Note presence of cough, and amount and color of sputum.
Monitor ABGs and oxygen saturation.
Monitor respiratory rate and depth.
Monitor restlessness and confusion.
Observe for cyanosis, especially in the mucous membranes.

Nursing Assessment and Diagnoses	Outcomes and Evaluation Parameters	Planning and Interventions with *Rationales*
Nursing Diagnosis: *Impaired Gas Exchange* related to heart failure	**Outcome:** Adequate gas exchange achieved. *Evaluation Parameters:* Normal arterial blood gases. No dyspnea: unlabored respirations < 24/minute. No ischemic ECG changes such as ST segment changes and dysrhythmias. Alert and oriented. Clear breath sounds. No restlessness, cyanosis, or fatigue. Oxygen saturation is within normal limits.	**Interventions and *Rationales:*** Monitor: ABG's, oxygen saturation, respiratory rate, lung sounds, and ECG Turn, cough, deep breathe, elevate head of bed. instruct on use of incentive spirometry. *Measures to promote gas exchange.* Administer humidified oxygen as prescribed *to increase oxygen levels.* Report respiratory distress to the health care provider. *Medical intervention may be indicated to prevent respiratory failure.* Assess need for suctioning and/or endotracheal intubation *to maintain adequate gas exchange.* Monitor fluid status *to assess heart failure.*

Assessment of Pain

Subjective Data:
Do you have problems with pain?
Where is the pain (joints, chest)?
What brings the pain on; what makes it go away?
What do you use to relieve it and is it effective?
Is the pain getting worse?

Objective Data:
Use pain scale (0–10) to quantify pain level.
Assess cultural and religious impact on patient's responses.
Assess the onset of increased pain to evaluate the presence of disease progression and/or an embolic event.

Nursing Assessment and Diagnoses	Outcomes and Evaluation Parameters	Planning and Interventions with *Rationales*
Nursing Diagnosis: *Pain, acute* related to fluid build up and inflammatory response	**Outcome:** Comfort level maintained. *Evaluation Parameters:* Patient able to communicate pain level and therapies that help alleviate it. Pain reduced and/or absent as evidenced by patient report and no pain behaviors: grimacing. Nonpharmacologic method of control is effective as evidenced by patient report and no pain behaviors. Patient reports satisfaction with pain management program. Patient is compliant with both antibiotics and pain medication schedule. Reports understanding of need to report a change in pain level to health care provider.	**Interventions and *Rationales:*** Instruct patient to inform nurse if pain is not relieved. *Indicates need to change pain management plan.* Obtain a clear description of source of discomfort. *This will assist in developing a pain management plan.* Correct misconceptions about risk of addiction and overdose *to decrease anxiety related to medication addiction.* Provide a supportive environment where patient is able to express pain level. *Opens communication and facilitates pain management.* Use pain control measures before pain becomes severe. *This increases comfort and decreases need for medication.* Teach nonpharmacologic method of control, i.e., guided imagery and massage, and breathing exercises. *These measures augment pain relief.* Teach the patient/family the correct dosage and time intervals for medication administration *to increase compliance and prevent complications.*

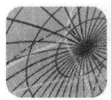

NURSING PROCESS: Patient Care Plan for Inflammatory Heart Disease—*Continued*

Assessment of Anxiety Related to Inflammatory Heart Disease

Subjective Data:
Has anyone explained your health problems to you?
Would you tell me what you know about your disease?
How does this disease affect your daily life?
Do you feel anxious about your health problems?
Do you have family members or close friends who provide emotional support?

Objective Data:
Observe for manifestations of anxiety: restlessness, apprehension, withdrawal.

Nursing Assessment and Diagnoses	Outcomes and Evaluation Parameters	Planning and Interventions with *Rationales*
Nursing Diagnosis: *Fear* and *Anxiety* related to inflammatory heart disease	**Outcomes:** Anxiety level minimized and manageable. **Evaluation Parameters:** Verbalizes anxious feelings. Verbalizes what relieves anxiety. Verbalizes absence of sensory perceptual disorders. Verbalizes absence of physical manifestations of anxiety. Behavioral manifestations of anxiety absent.	**Interventions and *Rationales:*** Provide factual information concerning diagnosis, treatment, disfigurement, disabilities, and prognosis. *Truthful explanations increase trust and potentially decrease anxiety.* Explain all procedures and allow time for mental preparation. *This decreases fear and anxiety of the unknown.* Allow time and encourage verbalization of fears related to illness *to assist in relieving anxiety.* Explore with the patient/family techniques to reduce anxiety. *This gives the patient a sense of control and opens communication about the subject.* Explore with patient effective ways to minimize anxiety. *This gives the patient a sense of control.* Instruct patient on use of relaxation techniques *to relieve anxiety.* Assess need for and administer antianxiety and pain medication. *If alternative measures are not effective, may need antianxiety agents.*

Assessment of Cardiac Output

Subjective Data:
Do you become short of breath at rest or with activity?
Has your shortness of breath become worse?
Do your legs become swollen at any time during the day?
Have you noticed a blue tinge in your nail beds?

Objective Data:
Determine heart rate and rhythm.
Assess:
Blood pressure   Capillary refill
Lung sounds   Right-sided heart failure (JVD,
Urine output   hepatomegaly, peripheral edema).

Nursing Assessment and Diagnoses	Outcomes and Evaluation Parameters	Planning and Interventions with *Rationales*
Nursing Diagnoses: *Decreased Cardiac Output* and *Ineffective Tissue Perfusion* related to infection, incompetent valves, and heart failure	**Outcome:** Sufficient cardiac output to perfuse organs. **Evaluation Parameter:** Minimal valve damage that decreases cardiac output.	**Interventions and *Rationales:*** Auscultate heart sounds for murmur and S_3, S_4 *to evaluate valve function and onset of heart failure.* Provide oxygen per order *to increase oxygen to the heart and peripheral tissues.* Administer diuretics, inotropics, and a low sodium diet *to treat heart failure.* Plan rest period *to reduce cardiac workload.*

Assessment of Tissue Perfusion

Subjective Data:
Do you have any pain in either leg?
Have you noticed any swelling or hard reddened areas?
Have you had any sudden chest pain that becomes worse when you take a deep breath?
Have you had any headaches, loss of consciousness, or dizzy spells?

Objective Data:
Assess:
Lung congestion   Skin and eyes
Urine output and color   Nail beds
Abdominal pain   Calf Deep Vein Thrombosis (DVT)
Neurological function   Glasgow Coma Scale.

(continued)

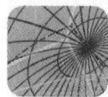

NURSING PROCESS: Patient Care Plan for Inflammatory Heart Disease—*Continued*

Nursing Assessment and Diagnoses	Outcomes and Evaluation Parameters	Planning and Interventions with *Rationales*
Nursing Diagnosis: *Ineffective Tissue Perfusion* related to dislodging of vegetative growths and immobility-related thrombophlebitis	**Outcome:** Occurrence of emboli diagnosed early and treatment instituted. ***Evaluation Parameter:*** Effective prevention of DVT.	**Interventions and *Rationales:*** Apply elastic compression stocking *to provide venous support.* Teach leg exercises *to promote venous return and decrease risk of DVT.* Report any new abnormal clinical manifestations to the health care provider. Monitor for therapeutic levels of anticoagulant therapy. Monitor for bleeding.

Assessment of Knowledge of Health Problems

Subjective Data:
What have you been told about your health problems?
Tell me what you know about your health problems.
What do you do when symptoms occur?
Do you see your health care provider on a regular basis?
Do you know what symptoms are important to report to your health care provider immediately?

Objective Data:
Assess knowledge of need to rest the heart and decrease the oxygen needs.
Explore patient's understanding of purpose of preventive antibiotic therapy.

Nursing Assessment and Diagnoses	Outcomes and Evaluation Parameters	Planning and Interventions with *Rationales*
Nursing Diagnosis: *Deficient Knowledge* related to disease process and prognosis	**Outcome:** Verbalizes understanding of prevention. ***Evaluation Parameter:*** Reports regular dental appointments and follow-up visits. Verbalizes adherence and compliance to therapy.	**Interventions and *Rationales:*** See Patient Teaching & Discharge Priorities feature for home care and remainder of teaching needs.

Assessment of Activity Tolerance

Subjective Data:
What type of activity fatigues you?
Has it been getting progressively worse?
Does activity increase joint tenderness and swelling?
Are you able to complete your ADLs without fatigue or shortness of breath?

Objective Data:
Assess for joint tenderness, swelling, and decreased range of motion.
Monitor vital signs during activity.

Nursing Assessment and Diagnoses	Outcomes and Evaluation Parameters	Planning and Interventions with *Rationales*
Nursing Diagnosis: *Activity Intolerance* related to decreased cardiac output, fatigue, and inflammation	**Outcome:** Able to complete ADLs without fatigue. ***Evaluation Parameter:*** Able to increase activity level with resolution of clinical manifestations.	**Interventions and *Rationales:*** Take 30- to 60-minute rest periods between all activities *to decrease cardiac workload.* Perform only essential activities until endurance improves *to decrease cardiac workload during the healing process.*

Assessment of Fever

Subjective Data:
Do you feel hotter than normal?
If so, how long have you been feeling that way?
Have you had the chills?

Objective Data:
Monitor temperature and WBC count.

Nursing Assessment and Diagnoses	Outcomes and Evaluation Parameters	Planning and Interventions with *Rationales*
Nursing Diagnosis: *Hyperthermia* related to the infection	**Outcomes:** Normal temperature. Absence of chills. ***Evaluation Parameters:*** Effective antibiotic treatment. Resolution of infection.	**Interventions and *Rationales:*** Administer antipyretics *to decrease temperature.* Administer antibiotics *to treat causative organism.* Cover patient *to prevent shivering and subsequent temperature elevation.*

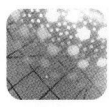

PATIENT TEACHING & DISCHARGE PRIORITIES for Inflammatory Heart Disease

Need	Teaching
Knowledge of disease process and prognosis	Home care needs include verbal and written instructions for: • Treatment plan • Follow-up care • Activity restriction These instructions will reinforce need to comply with therapy.
Understanding of medications	The patient/family are taught to administer the antibiotics and to care for the infusion site using aseptic technique. Teach the purpose, dose, and possible side effects of all medications to increase compliance and prevent over/underdosing.
Oral hygiene	Emphasize the importance of good dental hygiene and regular checkups to decrease the risk of pathogen entry via the mouth.
Disease prevention	Explain the need for antibiotic prophylaxis before invasive procedures to prevent reoccurrence. Encourage avoidance of people with upper respiratory infections to prevent an increased risk of infection. Avoid IV drug use.
Safety	Stress the importance of a medic alert bracelet to identify a heart problem to health care workers.
Reportable clinical manifestations	Instruct patient/family to report: • Change of exercise tolerance • New onset chest pain and fever • Clinical manifestations of heart failure
Family/Support system	Assess availability, knowledge, and compliance with treatment regimen. Assess respite needs and resources. Assess discharge placement needs: • Home • Rehabilitation facility • Extended care facility Assess home environment for need for assistive devices. Assess for need for professional home health needs. Assess need for follow-up appointments.
Emotional adjustment of patient/family due to the chronic nature of the disease.	Answer questions honestly. Encourage verbalization of frustrations and anger. Encourage positive reinforcement from the family. Stress that it is not uncommon to feel let down or depressed after discharge.

effusions. Dressler's syndrome may persist for weeks or even months after an AMI (Mayo Clinic, 2005a). Because it is thought to be an inflammatory process, treatment focuses on decreasing inflammation and treating the pain. NSAIDs such as aspirin treat the inflammation, and opioids are used to treat the pain.

Pathophysiology

With the infectious form of pericarditis, microbes causing the infection form an exudate of fibrin, white blood cells (WBCs), and endothelial cells. This exudate covers the pericardium, causing further inflammation of the surrounding tissues. Acute pericarditis can be either dry or exudative. If exudative, the pericardial sac fills with the serofibrinous exudate. Anywhere from 100 to 3,000 mL of fluid or exudate has been known to accumulate in the pericardial sac. This excess fluid accumulation restricts cardiac filling and emptying, therefore decreasing cardiac output and tissue perfusion. Without prompt treatment, shock and death will occur.

A number of causes of noninfectious pericarditis are listed in the accompanying Risk Factors box (p. 1228). Blunt trauma to the chest and heart surgery cause inflammation of the cardiac tissues. Small blood vessels may leak due to trauma, and the inflammation caused by tissue injury causes fluid to accumulate in the pericardial sac.

Chronic **constrictive pericarditis** occurs when the pericardial layers adhere to each other as a result of fibrosis of the pericardial sac. This usually occurs as a result of tuberculosis, typically found in the immigrant and prison populations, and people with acquired immunodeficiency syndrome (AIDS). Constrictive pericarditis also may develop secondary to surgery, uremia, or radiation. The fibrosis causes scarring and thickening of the pericardium, which decreases cardiac filling and contracting, leading to decreased cardiac output and heart failure.

Clinical Manifestations

Pain from pericarditis varies among patients with symptoms, ranging from mild to severe. The pain usually comes on suddenly,

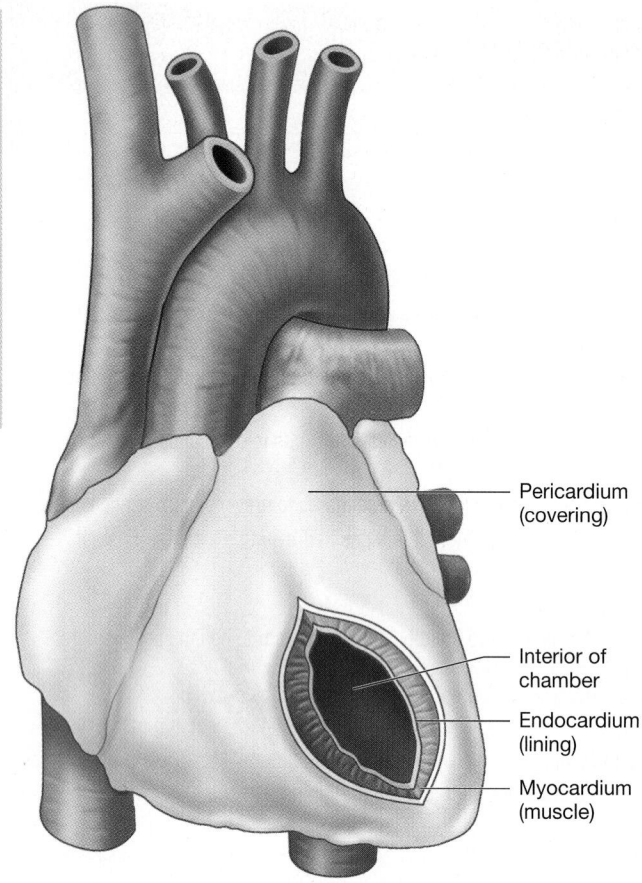

- Pericardium (covering)
- Interior of chamber
- Endocardium (lining)
- Myocardium (muscle)

FIGURE 41–2 ■ Layers of the heart wall.

RISK FACTORS for Pericarditis

Infectious	Bacterial: tuberculosis, streptococcus, staphylococcus, meningococcus, syphilis, pneumococcus, Lyme disease Viral: coxsackie virus B, echoviruses, endoviruses, adenoviruses, HIV, hepatitis Fungal Parasitic
Noninfectious	Chest trauma or injury Cardiac surgery Uremia Radiation therapy Cancer that has metastasized to the pericardium Acute myocardial infarction (AMI) (48–72 hr) Dissecting aortic aneurysm
Hypersensitive or autoimmune	Systemic lupus erythematosus Rheumatoid arthritis Scleroderma Polyarteritis nodosa Ankylosing spondylitis Myxedema MI (1–4 weeks, Dressler's syndrome) Drug reactions: procainamide, hydralazine, minoxidil

Source: American Heart Association. (2006c). *Sudden cardiac death.* Retrieved June 14, 2006, from http://www.americanheart.org/presenter.jhtml?identifier=4741.

often on the left side of the chest and radiates to the left shoulder, neck, and back. Some patients describe the pain in the same terms as anginal-type chest pain, while others describe it as a sharp pleuritic type pain. One way to differentiate the pain of pericarditis from angina is that it becomes worse with inspiration, coughing, movement of the trunk, and deep breathing. It also typically is worse when the patient is lying flat and tends to decrease when sitting up and leaning forward, when the heart is moved away from the diaphragmatic side of the lung pleura. This is often the key to the diagnosis. The chest pain often causes the patient to have dyspnea. Other causes of dyspnea also include compression of the bronchioles from the inflamed heart and fever.

The onset of bacterial pericarditis is associated with high fever (39.4°C [103°F]), chills, leukocytosis, malaise, joint pain, and a rise in the erythrocyte sedimentation rate (ESR). Anorexia, weight loss, and nausea also accompany the acute stages of the disease.

Electrocardiogram (ECG) changes also occur with pericarditis. ECG changes may include transient PR interval depression, tachycardia, bradycardia, and atrial fibrillation. Concurrent with the onset of chest pain, ST segment elevation in leads I, II, aVF, V_4, and V_6 occurs, followed by T wave inversion without Q wave changes. The T wave remains inverted for weeks to months later. ECG changes evolve over a period of weeks to months and are thought to be caused by superficial myocardial inflammation or epicardial injury. See Chapter 38 ✏ for a complete description of these ECG changes. Finally, the overall amplitude of the QRS complexes is typically decreased.

A **pericardial friction rub** is a key factor in the diagnostic assessment of a patient being evaluated for pericarditis. Friction rubs are described as a grating, scraping, squeaking, or crunching sound that is the result of friction between the roughened, inflamed layers of the pericardium. These sounds are best heard over the left sternal border in the 2nd, 3rd, or 4th intercostal space with the diaphragm of the stethoscope. The sounds become louder when the patient is sitting up and leaning forward. One way to distinguish it from a pleural friction rub is to ask the patient to momentarily hold her breath; if the rub persists, it is cardiac in nature. Pericardial friction rubs are often transient and may vary in intensity from hour to hour (Desai, 2002).

Pericardial effusion, an excess of pericardial fluid, is a threat to normal cardiac function. The fluid buildup in the pericardial sac is a result of an accumulation of infectious exudates or toxins, and/or blood. The clinical manifestations depend on the rate and amount of fluid collecting in the area. If the buildup is gradual, the pericardial sac will stretch and accommodate 1 to 2 liters without causing cardiac compression. Conversely, a rapid buildup of fluid does not allow the pericardial sac to stretch and, therefore, cardiac compression will occur with only 80 to 200 mL of fluid. If a pleural effusion is present, heart sounds are typically muffled and may be difficult to auscultate. Large effusions compress adjoining structures in the pleural cavity (e.g., pulmonary compression causes coughing, dyspnea, and tachypnea). Compression of the laryngeal nerve causes hoarseness, and compression of the phrenic nerve may induce hiccups (Desai, 2002).

Cardiac tamponade occurs when there is a rapid and large accumulation of fluid in the pericardial space. This is a medical emergency that is caused most frequently by bleeding, either from postoperative complications (thoracic surgery) or trauma. It also can be from an accumulation of pus or air and may be present with any type of pericarditis. This large collection of fluid raises the pressure in the pericardial sac, compressing the cardiac chambers, and prevents blood from entering the heart. Blood backs up into the venous system, raising venous pressure, while cardiac output and blood pressure fall because of a lack of blood filling the heart (decreased preload). See Chapter 24 🔗 for a complete explanation of preload. The drop in cardiac output and subsequent loss of tissue perfusion make this a life-threatening situation. The nurse must have knowledge of the clinical manifestations of cardiac tamponade and know how to intervene to prevent shock and death.

Clinical manifestations associated with tamponade are related to the decreased cardiac output and increased systemic venous congestion. A narrowing of the pulse pressure (systolic minus diastolic blood pressure to less than 30 mmHg) and tachycardia are hallmark signs of cardiac tamponade. The heart is attempting to compensate for the drop in cardiac output by increasing the rate. Without adequate preload, the increased rate cannot maintain a normal cardiac output, and the increased cardiac workload will lead to failure. Classic assessment findings for the patient with cardiac tamponade are referred to as **Beck's triad**, consisting of decreased blood pressure (BP), muffled heart sounds, and jugular venous distention. Additionally, weak peripheral pulses, and pulsus paradoxus are also present. A **pulsus paradoxus** is a greater than 10 mmHg drop in systolic BP during inspiration. The BP normally decreases during inspiration but does so by less than 10 mmHg. A paradox of greater than 10 mmHg is present when there is increased thoracic pressure as a result of pericardial swelling. This is an important diagnostic clue most frequently picked up by the nurse. The patient typically becomes restless and may have a decreased level of consciousness as the fluid accumulates and the cardiac output drops. Finally, the amplitude of the QRS complex of the ECG is low.

CRITICAL ALERT *The sudden onset of pulsus paradoxus is an indication that cardiac tamponade is occurring. The patient needs to be assessed for other signs of tamponade: tachycardia, diminished heart sounds, narrowed pulse pressure, and distended neck veins. The health care provider needs immediate notification to institute diagnosis and treatment. Cardiac tamponade is a life-threatening complication of pericardial effusion.*

Laboratory and Diagnostic Procedures

The patient's clinical manifestations and diagnostic and laboratory tests are used to confirm the diagnosis of pericarditis. There are no specific laboratory tests to diagnose pericarditis, but tests are performed to rule out other possible causes of the symptoms. The earlier box titled Diagnostic Tests for Cardiac Inflammatory Disorders (p. 1223) outlines the typical tests that are done to assist in confirming the diagnosis. In addition to the tests outlined in that box, antibody titers, blood urea nitrogen (BUN), and TB testing also are used to help determine the cause. An ECG and serial troponin and cardiac isoenzymes are done to rule out a myocardial infarction (Chapter 40 🔗). Computed tomography (CT) scans and

magnetic resonance imaging (MRI) also are used to identify pericardial effusions and/or the pericardial thickening characteristics of constrictive pericarditis (Chapter 39 🔗).

Hemodynamic monitoring is used with acute pericarditis to assess pulmonary artery pressures and cardiac output. Elevated central venous pressures and pulmonary artery pressures are seen due to inflammation. Cardiac output is decreased especially in the presence of cardiac tamponade.

A pericardiocentesis, the removal of fluid from the pericardial sac, is both diagnostic and therapeutic when effusion is present. The procedure is performed under sterile conditions with ECG, and hemodynamic monitoring capabilities. A health care provider inserts an 8-inch, 16- to 18-gauge needle into the pericardial sac and the fluid is aspirated (Figure 41–3 ■). The needle is attached to an ECG monitor to guide the depth of needle insertion. Once the needle touches the epicardial surface, ECG changes occur. The health care provider and the nurse observe the ECG monitor for ST segment and T wave changes that indicate the epicardial surface has been reached, and the needle is withdrawn slightly. When the needle is in the proper position, a catheter is placed, and the pericardial fluid is withdrawn. As the fluid drains, the pressures decrease and the clinical manifestations of tamponade begin to resolve. To assist in determining the cause of the pericardial effusion, the pericardial fluid is sent to the laboratory for culture and sensitivity analysis and cytology. If fluid buildup persists, the health care provider may choose to leave a catheter in the pericardium attached to a bag to allow for continuous draining of the fluid.

Medical Management

Medical management is directed toward finding the cause and instituting treatment to prevent complications. Because treatment is specific to the cause, it is essential that the cause of the pericarditis be determined. The diagnostic studies and clinical manifestations outlined above assist with determining the cause.

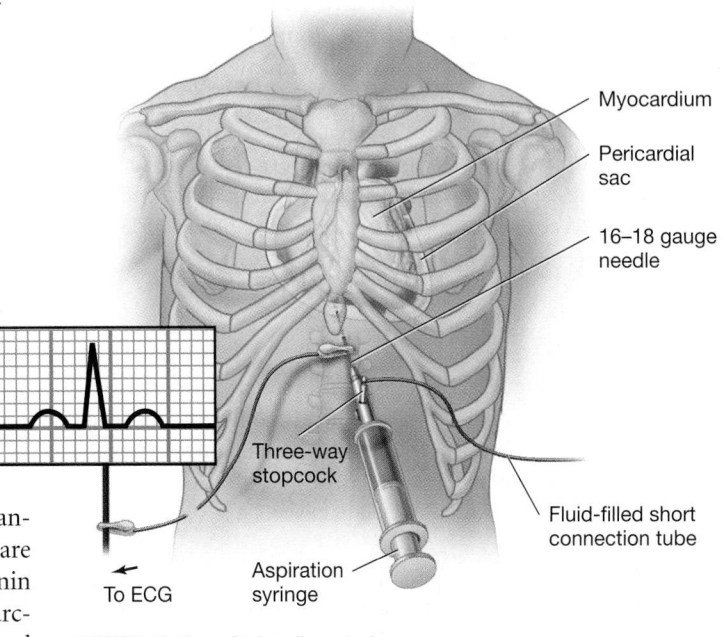

FIGURE 41–3 ■ Pericardiocentesis.

Myocardium

Pericardial sac

16–18 gauge needle

Three-way stopcock

Fluid-filled short connection tube

To ECG

Aspiration syringe

Antibiotic treatment is indicated if it is a bacterial infection and steroids are used when the pericarditis is secondary to systemic lupus erythematosus (SLE), a myocardial infarction (MI), or other immune system conditions. There is no specific curative treatment for viral pericarditis. It typically clears in 2 weeks to 3 months and symptom control treatments are indicated. Drugs known to treat tuberculosis are indicated if that is the cause of the pericarditis. If renal failure is the cause, more frequent and intense dialysis treatments are needed.

Pain must be assessed in order to differentiate pericarditis from a myocardial infarction, because treatment for myocardial infarction is time sensitive and would be contraindicated with pericarditis (Chapter 40). Pain control is managed with NSAIDs such as indomethacin (Indocin), ibuprofen, and aspirin in large doses. In addition to their analgesic properties, these medications reduce swelling. See the Pharmacology Summary (p. 1236) on medications to treat inflammatory heart disease.

Activity restriction is necessary until the swelling begins to subside and the pain is effectively managed. Bed rest is indicated with the head of the bed elevated to reduce cardiac workload. Symptoms and activity tolerance will dictate when increased activity is appropriate. Oxygen may be needed in the acute stages or in the presence of pericardial effusion. ECG monitoring is necessary to monitor for cardiac dysrhythmias and myocardial injury.

Because cardiac tamponade is a life-threatening complication of pericarditis, assessing for it is critical to patient survival. A pericardiocentesis is done to relieve the constricting effects of cardiac tamponade, and is indicated when the patient's blood pressure has decreased by 30 mmHg. Hemodynamic and ECG monitoring are necessary during and after the procedure to assess the patient's hemodynamic status. The amount of fluid removed is recorded on the output record in the patient's chart. Fluid replacement after pericardiocentesis is needed to increase cardiac output and tissue perfusion. Complications from a pericardiocentesis include dysrhythmias, pneumothorax, myocardial laceration, cardiac tamponade, and gastric fistula.

If recurrent effusions and tamponade occur or if there are adhesions from chronic constrictive pericarditis, the pericardium may have to be partially or completely surgically removed (**pericardiectomy**, **pericardial window**) to allow fluid to drain into the pleural space. This will relieve the compression on the heart and allow for adequate ventricular filling and cardiac output. Surgical resection of the pericardium is recommended in the early stages of constrictive pericarditis. Patients with advanced constrictive pericarditis have a 5% to 15% risk of mortality (Fauci et al., 1998).

■ Nursing Management

The goals of nursing management for the patient with pericarditis include pain and anxiety management; monitoring, treating, and reporting significant ECG changes; and evaluating the patient for the development of cardiac tamponade.

Assessment

The nurse must assess the patient's pain to distinguish it from angina-type chest pain as described earlier. It is important to assess the pain for the amount, quality, and location, to differenti-

ate it from the pain of an acute myocardial infarction. The ECG is monitored during pain because ST segment changes seen with an AMI are only seen in certain leads depending on the location of the infarction, whereas ST segment changes seen with pericarditis are present in all leads except aVR and V_1. Additionally, the patient is assessed for the clinical manifestations of cardiac tamponade including a decreased BP, muffled heart sounds, jugular venous distention, weak peripheral pulses, and pulsus paradoxus.

Nursing Diagnosis

Actual and potential nursing diagnoses related to pericarditis include:

- *Cardiac Output, Decreased*
- *Tissue Perfusion, Ineffective*
- *Anxiety*
- *Activity Intolerance*
- *Pain, Acute*

Outcomes and Evaluation Parameters

The desired outcomes for the patient with pericarditis include absence of pain and normal cardiac output. Finding and treating the cause will result in a relief of symptoms. Medical intervention with a pericardiocentesis, as described earlier, may be a lifesaving measure. Evaluation parameters include normal heart rate and blood pressure as well as a balanced intake and urine output. There should be an absence of any unusual fatigue and shortness of breath.

Planning, Interventions, and Rationales

Administration of the anti-inflammatory analgesics is essential, and helping the patient find a position of comfort also helps relieve the pain. Sitting up and leaning forward on a table in order to give the heart more room in the pleural cavity is typically the most comfortable position. A warm heating pad or hot water bottle also may help relieve the pain. Pain relief measures include elevating the head of the bed and administering anti-inflammatory agents as ordered.

> **CRITICAL ALERT**
>
> *When a patient complains of chest pain, it is essential that an assessment be done to determine if the pain is anginal-type pain associated with myocardial ischemia or if the pain is due to pericarditis. Anginal pain is typically described as a burning, pressure-type pain that is not associated with position change or deep breathing. It is relieved by nitroglycerin and rest.*
>
> *The chest pain associated with pericarditis is often described as sharp and gets worse with deep breathing. It is relieved by sitting up and taking anti-inflammatory drugs.*
>
> *The ECG needs to be assessed for ST segment changes associated with both types of pain. If the pain is unrelieved, the nurse needs to notify the health care provider for further orders.*

Nursing management of the patient during and following a pericardiocentesis includes monitoring the patient's response to the procedure. The nurse monitors the pulmonary artery, right atrial central venous pressure (CVP), pulmonary wedge pressures (Chapter 24), and the ECG during and after the procedure. As the effusion is relieved, the CVP and pulmonary artery wedge pressure will decrease and the blood pressure will increase. The amplitude of the QRS complex also increases as the pressure is relieved. Vital signs and urine output provide information about cardiac output and typically are monitored every 15 to 30 minutes for the first hour, then every 30 minutes for 1 hour, and then every hour for the first 24 hours. The amount of fluid removed is recorded on the output record and, if ordered, a specimen is sent to the laboratory for analysis. It is essential that the patient be monitored closely for a recurrence of tamponade. If the clinical manifestations prior to the pericardiocentesis return, a recurrence is suspected and the health care provider is immediately notified. The patient's anxiety is typically reduced when they are informed of what to expect in terms of clinical manifestations and treatment. The patient may require an antianxiety agent.

The remainder of the care is outlined in the Nursing Process: Patient Care Plan for Inflammatory Heart Disease feature (p. 1224).

Health Promotion

Health teaching for patients with pericarditis focuses on prevention. Teaching about the return clinical manifestations and when to seek medical help is essential. Identifying risk factors specifically related to the cause and outlining how to mitigate them will also help with disease prevention. The Patient Teaching & Discharge Priorities for Inflammatory Heart Disease box outlines specific patient teaching and discharge priorities (p. 1227).

Myocarditis

Myocarditis, a focal or diffuse inflammation of the myocardium or heart muscle, is an uncommon disorder that is frequently associated with pericarditis. The myocardium is the middle muscular layer of the heart. Its function is to provide the pumping action that propels the blood through the heart and into the peripheral circulation. Cardiac muscle contraction, referred to as systole, is when the blood is pumped out of the heart. Systole is followed by muscle relaxation or diastole, when blood flows into the cardiac chambers. Myocardial dysfunction can be systolic, diastolic, or both. Myocarditis affects the heart's ability to pump blood normally, thereby affecting cardiac output. Most cases of myocarditis originate from a viral infection, and often remain undiagnosed, due to the general lack of initial symptoms. In some cases the disease presents as an acute catastrophic illness requiring immediate attention. Myocarditis may be mistaken for ischemic, valvular, or hypertensive heart disease and can be both acute and chronic.

Epidemiology and Etiology

The incidence of myocarditis in the United States is estimated to be 1 to 10 per 100,000 people. It can occur at any age and is more common in men. Viral infections are the most common cause of myocarditis, followed by bacterial and fungal infections. Approximately 1% to 5% of patients with acute viral infections have myocardial involvement (Howes, 2008). A genetic predisposition for myocarditis is under investigation. Immunosuppressed patients are at a higher risk. Approximately 10% of patients with HIV develop myocarditis because the virus infiltrates the myocardium. The Risk Factors box outlines the infectious and noninfectious risk factors and causes of myocarditis. The occurrence of myopericarditis following a smallpox vaccination was investigated

RISK FACTORS and Causes of Myocarditis

Risk Factors	Autoimmune and connective tissue diseases
	Drug hypersensitivity or toxicity
	Sarcoidosis
	Hypersensitive immune reactions such as rheumatic fever
	Postcardiotomy syndrome
	Toxins
	Chemicals
	Alcohol use
	Nosocomial infections
	Large doses of radiation to the chest for treatment of malignancy
Causes	
Viral Infection	Coxsackie B virus accounts for 50% of the cases
	Coxsackie A virus
	Adenovirus
	Echovirus
	Mumps
	Rubella
	Influenza A and B
	Epstein-Barr
	Hepatitis
	HIV
	Hepatitis C
	Poliovirus
Bacterial infection	Diphtheria
	Typhoid fever
	Staphylococcus
	Pneumococcus
	Tuberculosis
	Tetanus
Fungal infection	Chagas' disease (South and Central America)
	Toxoplasmosis

using a sample of 230,734 first-time vaccinees. The results indicated that there were 18 cases of confirmed myopericarditis after a smallpox vaccination, an incidence of 7.8 cases per 100,000 per 30 days. No cases of myocarditis occurred in the group of 95,662 vaccinees who had previously been vaccinated. All cases were white males, ages 21 to 33 years, who presented with acute myocarditis 14 to 21 days after the vaccination (Halsell et al., 2003).

Pathophysiology

Myocarditis is an inflammatory disorder resulting from the causes outlined in the Risk Factors and Causes of Myocarditis box that typically occurs several weeks after the initial infection. The inflammatory process causes an infiltrate to build up in the cardiac myocytes, resulting in injury to the myocardial cells. Infectious agents infiltrate myocardial tissues, forming abscesses, and an autoimmune injury may occur when the immune system destroys both the invading organism and myocardial cells. The extent of damage determines the long-term effect on heart function. The majority of infections are self-limiting, and often subclinical, although severe or repeated infections may cause progressive deterioration in cardiac function. The most severe cases develop into cardiomyopathy, described later in this chapter.

Clinical Manifestations

The clinical manifestations of myocarditis vary, ranging from no overt clinical symptoms to severe heart involvement. Mild signs and symptoms include fatigue, malaise, shortness of breath, fever, gastrointestinal upset, and aching joints—very similar to flu symptoms. In contrast, myocarditis may appear suddenly with manifestations of heart failure or sudden cardiac death without prior symptoms. Symptoms of heart failure are discussed more thoroughly in Chapter 42 . When myocarditis and pericarditis occur simultaneously, manifestations may include a pericardial friction rub, chest pain, and a pericardial effusion. Blood clots on the heart wall (mural thrombi) may develop if blood stasis is present. Early cardiac symptoms typically appear 7 to 10 days after the initial infection.

Laboratory and Diagnostic Procedures

Several laboratory tests are done to diagnose both the cause and extent of the disease process with myocarditis. An evaluation of presenting symptoms followed by a thorough history and physical will determine the need for diagnostic and laboratory studies. The tests that assist in determining a definitive diagnosis are discussed in the Diagnostic Tests for Cardiac Inflammatory Disorders box (p. 1223). The WBCs must be monitored for elevations when diagnosing the disorder as well as periodically if symptoms reappear or worsen. Mild to moderate leukocytosis with atypical lymphocytes is common.

Medical Management

The primary aim of medical management for myocarditis is early diagnosis and treatment to mitigate the damage to the myocardial cells. Finding the cause and instituting timely and appropriate treatment is the cornerstone of the medical management for the patient with myocarditis. A complete history and physical including an assessment of the risk factors is indicated along with the diagnostic studies described above. Bed rest, a quiet environment, and a semi-Fowler's position are measures that decrease metabolic demand and reduce myocardial workload. Activity restrictions of varying levels depending on clinical manifestations may continue for up to 6 months. Oxygen may be needed when heart failure symptoms are present in the setting of hypoxemia. Medications for treating myocarditis include the following:

- Immunosuppressive therapy includes the use of steroids to prevent cardiac damage when the cause is autoimmune myocarditis.

- Antimicrobial medications are used when the myocarditis is caused by a bacterial infection.

- ACE inhibitors (or angiotensin receptor blockers), beta-adrenergic-blockers, digoxin, and diuretics are used if heart failure with left ventricular dysfunction occurs. See the Critical Alert regarding the use of digoxin with myocarditis.

- Antidysrhythmic medications are indicated to treat the dysrhythmias.

- Anticoagulants are used to prevent thromboembolism from mural wall blood clots.

- Antianxiety agents may be necessary for patients who are anxious due to the sudden onset heart disease and its impact on the quality of their life.

CRITICAL ALERT

- Digoxin: *Patients with myocarditis are sensitive to the effects of digoxin. Digoxin increases the force of cardiac contractions, thus, increasing the workload and oxygen demand of the heart muscle. These patients must be monitored closely for heart failure. Vital signs, lungs sounds, increasing shortness of breath, and peripheral edema need to be monitored on a frequent and ongoing basis.*
- NSAIDs: *The use of NSAIDs with myocarditis is contraindicated because they appear to increase cardiac damage.*

See the Pharmacology Summary of medications to treat inflammatory heart disease (p. 1236).

The prognosis for myocarditis caused by viral infections is excellent. Scarring and permanent myocardial damage from myocarditis vary from none to severe heart failure leading to death or requiring a heart transplant.

■ Nursing Management

The aim of nursing management is to rest the heart as much as possible. These patients are placed on strict bed rest and allowed minimal activities until the cause has been identified and treatment instituted. Increasing the level of activity can only progress when the symptoms subside with successful treatment.

Assessment and Nursing Diagnosis

Nursing assessment focuses on the clinical manifestations of heart failure. Alteration in cardiac output and altered tissue perfusion are the two sentinel nursing diagnoses for these patients.

The majority of patients experiencing myocarditis make a complete recovery without residual complications. Note, however, that cardiomyopathy can be a long-term complication of myocarditis. Nursing management and patient education are pivotal in preventing complications.

Outcomes and Evaluation Parameters

The desired outcomes for the patient with myocarditis include absence of pain and normal cardiac output. Finding and treating the cause will result in a relief of symptoms. Evaluation parameters include normal heart rate and blood pressure as well as a balanced intake and urine output. There should be an absence of any unusual fatigue and shortness of breath.

Planning, Interventions, and Rationales

As with other cardiac inflammatory diseases, resting the heart by spacing activities and by providing pain relief, emotional support, and a quiet environment will promote healing and assist in preventing compactions. As the patient's condition allows, active and passive range-of-motion exercises will help the patient regain strength and joint motion and should be performed regularly until activity levels increase. The nurse must teach the patient to avoid excessive fatigue and stop all activities immediately when light-headedness, dyspnea, or faintness occurs. Changes in activity restrictions are based on the patient's tolerance and the occurrence of clinical manifestations.

The remainder of the nursing management is outlined in the Nursing Process: Patient Care Plan for Inflammatory Heart Disease feature (p. 1224).

Health Promotion

Patient teaching goals focus on having the patient make a full recovery and preventing long-term complications. Gradually increasing activity levels promotes muscle tone and strength. The patient must be taught to stop activity and revise the plan if clinical manifestations recur. Additionally, it is essential for the nurse to outline the specific manifestations of heart failure and reinforce that the patient must seek medical care when they occur. Discharge medications need to be discussed and the nurse must assess the patient's understanding of the regimen. Specific discharge planning is outlined in the Patient Teaching & Discharge Priorities for Inflammatory Heart Disease box (p. 1227).

■ Endocarditis

Infective endocarditis (IE), previously known as bacterial endocarditis, is an infection of the cardiac endocardial layer of the heart, which may include one or more heart valves, the mural endocardium, and/or a septal defect. The endocardium is the inner lining of the heart and it is contiguous with the heart valves. Thus, an infection or inflammation of the endocardium affects the heart valve function. Figure 41–2 ■ (p. 1228) identifies the endocardium. IE is a life-threatening disease that occurs most often in persons with structural abnormalities of the heart or great vessels, but it also can occur with normal hearts.

There are two types of IE, acute and subacute. With acute IE the onset of symptoms is rapid, often in individuals with normal heart valves, and if untreated can lead to death within days to weeks. Acute IE is usually caused by a virulent organism and is more likely to follow infections of the respiratory, gastrointestinal, and genitourinary tracts, and following open heart surgery.

Subacute IE is the more common form and is usually caused by organisms of low virulence that have a limited ability to infect other organs. It is present in an inactive state for long periods of time in people with preexisting valve disease. It often becomes symptomatic after dental work or with an invasive procedure, but usually responds well to treatment.

Infective endocarditis is classified according to the causative organism, with hemolytic streptococci being the most common. Other causes and predisposing factors are outlined later in the Risk Factors box (p. 1234). The increasing use of contaminated needles by individuals using illegal intravenous (IV) drugs has increased the number of cases of IE in recent years. There is a high risk of bacteremia for these individuals due to the insertion of a contaminated needle into the venous blood. The tricuspid valve is the most frequently affected valve with IV drug use, especially cocaine use.

Epidemiology and Etiology

The incidence of IE continues to rise, with 15,000 to 20,000 new cases reported annually. Thus, IE is now the fourth leading cause of life-threatening infectious disease syndromes (after urosepsis, pneumonia, and intra-abdominal sepsis) (American Heart Association [AHA], 2006a). Internationally, the incidence of the disease is similar throughout developed countries. The greatest risk factor for the development of IE is preexisting heart damage. Infective endocarditis affects males twice as often as females and is distributed throughout all age groups. The mean age of patients has gradually risen during the last 50 years and cur-

rently more than 50% of the patients are greater than 50 years of age (Brusch, 2005). Infective endocarditis can develop in anyone and the most frequent bacteria are usually found in the mouth, intestinal tract, or urinary system. Nosocomial infections occur most often in patients who are debilitated and have long-term urinary and IV catheters. Patients who are immunosuppressed or who are receiving immunosuppressive therapy are at a higher risk for developing yeast or fungal IE. This population would include both cancer patients, people with human immunodeficiency virus, and IV drug users.

 CRITICAL ALERT Healthy People 2010 *(DHHS, 2004) established an important goal related to U.S. policy for the prevention of substance abuse among youth. The goal is to increase the percentage of young persons who reach adulthood without using tobacco, illicit drugs, or alcohol. Their focus is to strengthen the ability of children and teenagers to reject all such substances. To achieve overall prevention goals,* Healthy People 2010 *supports comprehensive community-based programs that include interventions that influence individual behavior and attitudes through education, and interventions that change environments through controls on the availability of substances. They recommend comprehensive programs that must be applied universally to the general population and in a more intensive fashion to selected and indicated groups and persons known to be at high risk for serious drug problems or to targeted groups of persons already exhibiting early signs of drug use. The prevention programs require coordination among schools, state and local governments, businesses, the faith community, civic groups, and other elements of the community.*

Prosthetic heart valve IE, which may develop in the early postoperative period (60 days or less) or later on (greater than 60 days), accounts for 10% to 20% of the cases. Common infecting organisms for early IE development are staphylococcus, gram-negative bacilli, and *Candida albicans. Staphylococcus epidermidis*, streptococci, and enterococci cause the later infections (Marill, 2006). Infective endocarditis affects males over 60 years old most frequently, and occurs most often with mitral valve replacements. Early prosthetic valve IE, usually due to a contaminated valve or preexisting bacteremia, has a rapid onset and high mortality. Late prosthetic valve IE follows the course of subacute IE. The Risk Factors box (p. 1234) outlines the risk factors and Chart 41–2 lists the organisms that cause IE.

Increased mortality is associated with increased age, infection of the aortic valve, development of heart failure, CNS

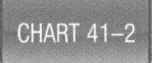

CHART 41–2 Etiologic Organisms that Cause Infective Endocarditis

Staphylococci (*Staphylococcus aureus, S. epidermidis*)

Streptococci (hemolytic streptococci, enterococci, *Streptococcus bovis, S. pneumoniae*)

Gram-negative bacteria (*Escherichia coli, Klebsiella*, pseudomonas)

Haemophilus

Actinobacillus

Cardiobacterium

Eikenella

Kingella

Aspergillus fumigatus

Candida albicans

complications, and other underlying diseases. Mortality rates also vary with infecting organism.

Pathophysiology

Several mechanisms are thought to contribute to the development of endocarditis. First a bacteremia (infection in the blood) occurs usually as a complication of an infection originating somewhere in the body (e.g., urinary tract infection, pneumonia, and cellulitis). Surgical procedures, dental work, and invasive diagnostics such as a colonoscopy also may allow bacteria to enter the bloodstream. Secondly, the narrowed orifice of a damaged valve reduces the movement of blood from the atria to the ventricle, allowing time for bacteria to grow and multiply. This increases the risk of bloodborne bacteria lodging on the endocardial valve surface, forming vegetative growths that adhere to the valve surface. These vegetative growths consist of fibrin, leukocytes, platelets, and the infecting microbe.

The infection spreads and becomes imbedded in the valve matrix, producing thinning and destruction of the valve and its supporting structures and ultimately causing valve dysfunction. Mechanical complications may occur, including rupture of chordae tendineae (Figure 41–4 ■; also see Figure 41–1 ■ (p. 1220) for vegetative growths on a valve surface), development of valve stenosis due to overgrowth of large vegetations, and perforation of a valve leaflet. The organisms then spread from the valve to the myocardium, culminating in myocardial dysfunction and heart failure.

The infection can be on either the right side or the left side of the heart or, in severe cases, both sides. Left-sided IE, which af-

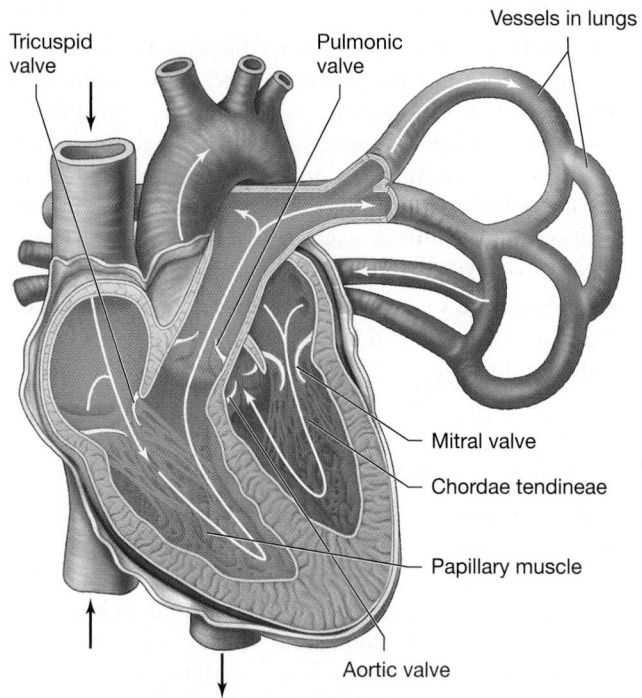

FIGURE 41–4 ■ Cardiac valves, chordae tendineae, and papillary muscle.

fects the mitral valve most often, is more common with bacterial infections and patients with underlying heart disease. Right-sided IE, which affects the tricuspid valve, is primarily a result of IV drug use, and most often is caused by *Staphylococcus aureus.*

The friable vegetative growths on the valves may break off into the circulation causing embolization. Left-sided emboli travel to the systemic circulation affecting the brain, kidneys, spleen, and causing limb infarction. Right-sided emboli travel to the lungs causing pulmonary complications. When the emboli become trapped in the organ, abscesses may form, further spreading the infection and impacting organ function.

Clinical Manifestations

Endocarditis may mimic almost any systemic disease depending on the infecting organism and the associated complications. The signs and symptoms of IE can be nonspecific but may involve many organs, often making it difficult to differentially diagnose. Fever occurs in about 90% of the patients and is typically accompanied by tachycardia, fatigue, malaise, anorexia, weight loss, headache, and chills (Candela, 2002). Bacterial IE is associated with high fevers, shaking chills, and night sweats. Arthralgias, myalgias, back pain, abdominal discomfort, headache, clubbing of fingers, anorexia and weight loss, and a low-grade fever often accompany subacute IE.

The cardiac assessment reveals a heart murmur, usually on the aortic or mitral valves. The mitral murmur is typically a midsystolic regurgitant type, whereas the aortic murmur may be early diastolic. Murmurs are uncommon with right-sided IE, because the pressures on the right side are too low to transmit the sound. (See Chapter 37 ☞ for a complete description of murmurs.) Dyspnea, cough, and chest pain are common complaints, especially if heart failure and decreased cardiac output have occurred. The accumulation of serous, purulent, and/or

---

RISK FACTORS for Infective Endocarditis

Recent dental surgery

Bleeding gums

Invasive procedures: oral surgery, gynecologic procedures, implantation of a cardioverter-defibrillator, hemodynamic catheters, insertion of an indwelling urinary catheter, or renal shunts

Illegal intravenous drug use

Long-term central line placement

Weakened cardiac valves

Prosthetic heart valve

Previous history of endocarditis

Complex cyanotic congenital heart disease

Urinary tract infection

Pneumonia

Cellulitis

Narrowed valve orifice

Rheumatic fever

Mitral valve prolapse with murmur

Marfan's syndrome

Degenerative valvular lesions

Aortic valve leaflet abnormalities

Asymmetric septal hypertrophy (hypertrophic cardiomyopathy)

Nosocomial infections

HIV

Chest trauma

hemorrhagic fluid in the pericardial sac causes a pericardial effusion and possibly tamponade. Tamponade causes a decrease in cardiac output, leading to shock, heart failure, and death. Heart failure occurs in approximately 50% of the patients with IE. ECG changes may include conduction delays (first-, second-, and third-degree heart blocks), diffuse ST segment changes, and PR interval depression. (Chapter 38 ☺ describes these and other ECG abnormalities.)

Vascular changes also may occur with IE including these:

- Splinter hemorrhages are black longitudinal streaks on the nail beds.
- Petechiae on the lips, buccal mucosa, palate, ankles, feet, antecubital space, and popliteal areas occur as a result of microembolization of vegetative lesions in these areas.
- Painful, red or purple, pea-size lesions, referred to as Osler's nodes, may be present on the fingertips or toes.
- Janeway's lesions, flat, painless, small, red spots, are found on the palms of the hand and soles of the feet.
- Roth's spots, round white spots surrounded by hemorrhage, may appear on the retina.

Finally, tiny emboli often break off of the heart valve and travel to distant organs, causing clinical manifestations associated with the specific organ: brain, heart, lungs, kidney, and/or spleen. Emboli also may travel to the limbs, interrupting peripheral perfusion. As many as 20% of the cases of IE have focal neurological complaints and stroke syndromes (Marill, 2006).

Laboratory and Diagnostic Procedures

The diagnosis of IE is typically based on a constellation of clinical findings. The history of clinical manifestations is variable, often with vague symptoms, making it difficult to diagnose. The Diagnostic Tests for Cardiac Inflammatory Disorders box (p. 1223) includes the tests used to diagnose IE. In addition to the standard tests described in that box, a positive rheumatoid factor and proteinuria are evaluated because they are present in some cases of IE. The echocardiogram evaluates the presence of thickening and calcification of the pericardium occurring most commonly with bacterial and fungal IE. Transesophageal echocardiography (TEE) is more sensitive than the traditional transthoracic echocardiogram particularly for detecting small vegetative growths and extension of the infection into the myocardial tissue and for assessing prosthetic valve function (Marill, 2006). A description of the TEE procedure and patient preparation is included in Chapter 39 ☺. If right-sided IE is suspected, a ventilation/perfusion (V/Q) scan may be useful to evaluate pulmonary function. A CT scan also is useful for localizing the area of the abscess.

Medical Management

Due to the complex nature of IE and its ability to mimic other diseases, diagnosing it is often difficult. Underdiagnosis can lead to clinical catastrophe and death, while overdiagnosis may result in weeks of unnecessary antimicrobial therapy with excessive costs and potentially avoidable drug-related side effects. It is imperative to make a definitive diagnosis and begin a treatment plan in a timely manner. Clinical management is both curative and supportive in nature. The priorities for management of IE are finding the cause and starting treatment to eradicate the infecting organism, minimize valve damage, and prevent heart failure. A thorough health history is required to evaluate risk factors including recent high-risk procedures (see earlier Risk Factors box) that may have precipitated an episode of IE. Most clinicians agree that patients who present with symptoms compatible with IE should be evaluated using the following criteria:

- When symptoms appear, blood cultures are obtained from separate sites that are repeated two to three times over a 24-hour period, and may be kept for up to 3 weeks to determine if the causative organism is slow growing. The cultures may be negative if the patient is currently on antibiotic therapy.
- TEE confirms a mass, abscess, or prosthetic valve damage.
- Clinical manifestations as outlined above include evidence of endocardial involvement.

Hospitalization is usually required for intravenous antibiotics and to administer supportive treatments for the clinical manifestations. Following the blood cultures, antibiotic therapy is initiated with drugs known to be specific to the organisms based on the laboratory sensitivity reports. Various classifications of antibiotics are used, including the penicillins, the cephalosporins, the aminoglycosides, and the antitubercular medications. If the cause is fungal, antifungal agents are used. Often a combination of these drugs is necessary to completely eradicate the organism.

Intravenous antibiotics are continued for 2 to 8 weeks depending on the organism, the blood culture, and the resolution of symptoms. The fibrin covering the vegetative growths protects the colonies from antibiotic therapy; therefore, an extended course of multiple antibiotics is typically required. Prosthetic heart valve IE usually requires combination antibiotic treatment for 6 to 8 weeks. Changes in antibiotic therapy may be necessary if allergic drug-related reactions occur and/or resistance to the medication develops. Resistance is measured by a repeated blood culture and sensitivity. The sensitivity portion of the test provides information about the medications' ability to kill the organism. Peak and trough drug levels also are measured to ensure that therapeutic levels of the drug are being given. Periodic blood cultures are done throughout the course of the illness. If the cultures remain positive, this indicates inappropriate therapy. Medications used to treat inflammatory heart disease are outlined in the Pharmacology Summary feature (p. 1236).

Surgical intervention is required for the following reasons: (1) to repair valvular regurgitation, which causes heart failure and is the most common reason for surgery; (2) to remove large vegetative growths that are at risk for embolization; (3) to treat fungal infections; (4) to replace a severely damaged valve; and (5) to remove a valve (native or prosthetic) that is a continuing source of infection and does not respond to antibiotic treatment. No response after 7 to 10 days of antibiotics is an indication that valve replacement is necessary.

Home care is appropriate once the symptoms are under control and the patient has adequate support systems at home. Intravenous antibiotic therapy can be continued at home once the patient/family has been taught the skills. Outpatient management is not advised for IV drug users due to issues with noncompliance. Patients with prosthetic valves typically stay in the hospital until the infection has resolved.

PHARMACOLOGY Summary of Medications to Treat Inflammatory Heart Disease

Medication Category	Action	Application/Indication	Nursing Responsibility
Inflammatory Heart Disease **Antibiotics** Erythromycin Penicillin Specific type depends on the organism	Inhibits protein synthesis of microorganisms by binding reversibly to a ribosome, thus interfering with transmission of genetic information.	*Rheumatic fever:* treats Lancefield group A beta-hemolytic streptococcus. *Pericarditis and myocarditis:* indicated if it is a bacterial infection. *Endocarditis:* indicated if infecting organism is bacterial and prophylactic for invasive procedures and dental work.	Assessment of history of drug allergies prior to administration. Assessment of clinical manifestations of allergic reaction. Assessment of relief of clinical manifestations to determine drug effectiveness. Patient education regarding need to complete the entire regimen and report any clinical manifestations of drug allergy.
Nonsteroidal Anti-Inflammatory Agents (NSAIDs) Indomethacin (Indocin) Ibuprofen Aspirin	Inhibits cyclooxygenase, an enzyme responsible for the formation of prostaglandins. When cyclooxygenase is inhibited, inflammation and pain are reduced.	*Rheumatic fever:* joint pain and fever. *Pericarditis:* chest pain and swelling. *Myocarditis:* pain. *Endocarditis:* fever.	Assess pain before and after administration to determine effectiveness. Medications should not be taken on an empty stomach. Monitor renal and liver function tests for abnormalities related to drug side effects. Assessment of bleeding and gastric ulcer development.
Steroids Solu-Cortef Cortisone Solu-Medrol	Stabilizes leukocyte lysosomal membrane; inhibits phagocytosis and release of allergic substances; reduces capillary dilation and permeability. Modifies immune response to various stimuli.	*Myocarditis:* to prevent cardiac damage when the cause is autoimmune.	Careful assessment of relief of clinical manifestations. Assessment of side effects: Infection due to depressed immune response. Blood glucose monitoring. Gastric bleeding. Emotional lability. Lack of wound healing. Patient education regarding need to eventually reduce dosage.
Cardiac Medications ACE inhibitors: Lisinopril Enalapril Ramipril Captopril	ACE inhibitor: Lowers peripheral resistance and reduces blood volume by enhancing the excretion of sodium by inhibition of angiotensin-converting enzyme.	*Myocarditis:* heart failure. *Rheumatic fever, pericarditis, and myocarditis:* to control atrial and ventricular dysrhythmias caused by inflammation and stretching of myocardium.	Monitor blood pressure carefully after first dose for hypotension. Educate patient that it takes 2 weeks for therapeutic effect. May experience dizziness.
Antiarrhythmic Agents Adenosine Amiodarone Atropine sulfate Sotalol	Alters the electrophysiological properties of the heart by either blocking flow through the channels or altering autonomic activity.	To control dysrhythmias.	There is a narrow margin between therapeutic effect and toxicity; therefore, careful and ongoing cardiac monitoring is essential. Patient teaching includes avoiding the use of alcohol, drugs, and tobacco.
Diuretics Furosemide Torsemide	Blocks reabsorption of sodium and chloride in the loop of Henle. Reduces edema associated with heart failure.	*Myocarditis:* heart failure.	Potassium levels also need monitoring because low levels are a side effect of certain diuretics, especially furosemide. May need potassium replacement. Measure urine output prior to administration to gauge the response to the medication.

PHARMACOLOGY Summary of Medications to Treat Inflammatory Heart Disease—*Continued*

Medication Category	Action	Application/Indication	Nursing Responsibility
Anticoagulant Therapy Coumadin Heparin Aspirin	Can either inhibit specific clotting factors in coagulation cascade or diminish the clotting action of platelets.	*Myocarditis:* to prevent thromboembolism from mural wall blood clots.	Ongoing assessment of therapeutic blood level per health care provider orders. Assess for bleeding including nosebleeds, bruising, "coffee-grounds" emesis, tarry stools, fatigue, and pale skin. Assess for decreases in hemoglobin, hematocrit, RBCs, and platelets.
Antianxiety Agents Valium Versed Xanax	Acts by binding with the gamma-aminobutyric acid (GABA) receptor-chloride channel molecule. This intensifies the effect of GABA, which is a natural inhibitory neurotransmitter.	*Rheumatic fever, pericarditis, myocarditis, and endocarditis:* may be necessary for anxiety-onset heart disease and its impact on the quality of life.	Assess patient's anxiety levels and ability to sleep. Assess for excessive sleepiness and respiratory depression as side effects.

Sources: Adams, M. P., Josephen, D. L., & Holland, L. N. (Eds.). (2005). Pharmacology for nurses: A pathophysiologic approach. Upper Saddle River, NJ: Pearson Prentice Hall; American Heart Association. (2005). Handbook of emergency cardiovascular care for health providers. Dallas, TX: Author; Wilson, B., Shannon, M., & Stang, C. (Eds.). (2005). Nurses drug guide. Upper Saddle River, NJ: Pearson Prentice Hall.

Prophylactic treatment for all persons who have the medical indications outlined on Chart 41–3 is critical to preventing an episode of IE. Moreover, other behaviors such as IV drug use need to be discussed with a patient who is at high risk for the development of IE. The use of an identification band would be helpful if an emergency situation occurred in which the patient was unable to speak for himself.

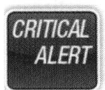 *Education of patients and families needs to stress the importance of informing health care providers of a valve disorder, history of infective endocarditis, or a prosthetic valve each time dental or invasive diagnostic procedures are performed. A medic alert bracelet would be useful.*

The emotional cost to the family and patient also cannot be overemphasized. This is a life-threatening illness, with the potential for permanent cardiac damage that has a significant impact on the quality of life.

Nursing Management

The goals of nursing management for a patient with IE include rest, pain management, and instituting the pharmacologic treatment and measures needed to reduce fever and other associated symptoms such as tachycardia, fatigue, malaise, anorexia, weight loss, headache, and chills. Patients with IE require a comprehensive plan of care. The nursing process serves as a template to develop the plan.

Assessment

Nursing care required for the patients with infective endocarditis includes an ongoing, in-depth physical assessment focusing on the patient's hemodynamic status, level of comfort, coping ability, and support from family or significant others. Nursing assessment is essential in order to prevent life-threatening complications. Frequent monitoring and assessment of trend changes in the vital signs and clinical manifestations will provide the most reliable information about the progress of these diseases. Careful monitoring of cardiac output and oxygenation also is necessary.

Nursing assessments specific to IE include murmurs, embolic events, and skin manifestations. Assessment for new and changing murmurs is essential because such changes indicate valve malfunction and are reportable to the health care provider. Heart sounds are assessed every 8 hours or more frequently if ordered by the health care provider. Assessing for embolic events also is

CHART 41–3   Indications for Prophylactic Antibiotic Therapy with Infective Endocarditis

Medical Indications	Procedural Indications
Prosthetic heart valve	A dental procedure in which bleeding is likely, including cleaning and extractions
Previous episodes of IE	Periodontal procedures/dental implants
Rheumatic heart disease	Bronchoscopy and/or pulmonary biopsy
Hypertrophic cardiomyopathy	Cystoscopy/colonoscopy
Mitral valve prolapse with regurgitation and murmur	Urinary catheterization when infection is present
Sclerotic aortic valve	Incision and drainage of infective tissue, especially soft tissue
Most congenital heart malformations	Vaginal delivery if infection is present
Surgically constructed systemic-pulmonary shunts or conduits	Most surgeries

Source: Eble, B. E., Reyeds, G., and Wiewall-Winkellmann, J. eMedicine—Endocarditis, Bacterial. http://intranet.santa.lt/thesaurus/REZIDENTUI/Valvular/endocarditis%20bacterial%20child.htm.

essential in that they may be life/organ threatening. Embolization of the spleen is manifested in localized abdominal tenderness and rigidity, sharp upper left quadrant pain, and splenomegaly. Emboli to the kidneys often cause flank pain, hematuria, and azotemia. Small peripheral blood vessels also may be affected by emboli, causing gangrene. Neurological deficits occur when emboli lodge in the brain, and finally, pulmonary emboli are common with right-sided IE. Skin assessment includes evaluating for splinter hemorrhages on the nail beds; petechiae on the lips, buccal mucosa, palate, ankles, feet, antecubital space, and popliteal areas; Osler's nodes, and Janeway's lesions (late finding).

Nursing Diagnosis

Nursing diagnoses that apply to patients with IE include:

1. Pain, acute
2. Fatigue
3. Altered cardiac output
4. Hyperthermia
5. Infection
6. Tissue perfusion ineffective

Outcomes and Evaluation Parameters

The desired outcomes for the patient with IE include absence of pain and normal cardiac output. Finding and treating the cause will result in relief of symptoms. Evaluation parameters include normal heart rate and blood pressure as well as a balanced fluid intake and urine output. There should be an absence of any unusual fatigue and fever. Education about prevention of a reoccurrence is critical. The patient/family needs to understand the importance of the preventive measures discussed next.

Planning, Interventions, and Rationales

The focus of nursing management is to provide an environment that supports decreasing myocardial oxygen demand and cardiac workload. The patient is encouraged to eat nutritious meals, drink lots of fluid, and rest both mentally and physically. Strict bed rest is only indicated with heart failure but restricted activity is necessary to decrease cardiac workload especially if there is valve incompetence. The nurse must explain the importance of bed rest and activity restriction to the patient and family. The nurse teaches the patient to avoid excessive fatigue and stop all activities immediately when chest pain, light-headedness, dyspnea, or faintness occurs. Changes in activity restrictions are based on the patient's tolerance and the occurrence of clinical manifestations. Fever, which typically persists for several days, is treated with antipyretics, forced fluids, cooling measures, and rest. Intravenous antibiotics and fluids are administered and as the antibiotics treat the infection, the discomfort level will decease.

Emotional support is essential for patients with IE. The patient needs to be given an opportunity to verbalize fears and concerns about a potentially life-threatening cardiac disorder that may cause permanent damage to the heart. Education about the clinical manifestations of heart failure and when it is necessary to seek medical attention also is essential. The Nursing Process: Patient Care Plan for Inflammatory Heart Disease feature (p. 1224) includes an in-depth care plan for patients with IE.

Health Promotion

Patient education includes information on how to avoid infection and making sure the patient knows that health care providers need to be informed that prophylactic antibiotics are necessary prior to the procedures outlined in Chart 41–3 (p. 1237). Patients are taught to use a soft toothbrush and to floss their teeth regularly to protect the gums from bleeding. Overall good hygiene will help prevent the reoccurrence of IE in high-risk patients. The patient must be taught the importance of seeking medical help if there is a return of clinical manifestations. In addition, it is important to stress seeking medical assistance if neurological or pulmonary symptoms occur, because these may indicate a serious complication. The specific education needed for management of the patient at home is outlined in the Patient Teaching & Discharge Priorities for Inflammatory Heart Disease box (p. 1227).

■ Collaborative Management

A collaborative care approach is optimal for management of patients with inflammatory heart disease. These conditions tend to be chronic with recurring remissions and exacerbations, thereby requiring lifelong management. Utilizing a multidisciplinary team approach, including health care providers, nurses, physical and occupational therapists, psychologists/psychiatrists, and pharmacists, will facilitate the best possible quality of life for the patient and the family.

In terms of medical care, in addition to the role of the cardiologist and surgeon, the patient may need psychiatric counseling to assist in lifestyle adjustments necessitated by a chronic disease process. The occupational therapist helps facilitate realistic occupational goals, while the physical therapist assists in the maintenance of optimum conditioning given the activity restrictions. Because much of the treatment for inflammatory cardiac disorders centers on medication, the role of the pharmacist is essential in educating the patient about how to manage the medications and their side effects. In addition to the nursing care described above, the nurse plays a pivotal role in coordinating the efforts of the health care team. In the inpatient setting the nurse facilitates communication between the members of the team and the patient/family. The nurse may also want to explore alternative therapies with the patient, such as music therapy, as discussed in the Complementary and Alternative Therapies box.

STRUCTURAL HEART DISEASE

Abnormalities in the physical structure of the heart impair blood flow and cardiac pumping ability. Therefore, these abnormalities result in decreased cardiac output and tissue perfusion. Structural abnormalities that affect the cardiac valves and heart muscle itself are discussed next.

CARDIAC VALVULAR DISORDERS

There are four valves in the heart: two semilunar valves, the aortic and the pulmonic; and two atrioventricular valves, the tricuspid and the mitral (Figure 41–5 ■). Each valve is located in a strategic position to provide unidirectional blood flow through

COMPLEMENTARY & ALTERNATIVE THERAPIES — Music Therapy

Description:

MUSIC THERAPY is a technique that involves multiple senses, including the hands, voice, emotions, mind, and spirit. There are two branches of music therapy: active and passive. An example of active music therapy is a patient with an inflammatory cardiac disorder who plays a musical instrument, or sings alone or with a choir. Active musical expression utilizes both motor and emotional responses. An example of passive music therapy is listening to specific music and/or sounds in order to relax, stimulate, motivate, or soothe the body and mind. Music therapy provides a simple, safe, and effective way to reduce potentially harmful physiological and psychological responses that arise from pain, fear, and anxiety.

Music therapy has been used successfully to decrease patient anxiety and provide better patient outcomes prior to diagnostic cardiac catheterization. Patient anxiety may have various causes, including feeling a lack of caring for them as individuals, excessive wait time before the procedure, and physical discomfort (McCaffrey & Taylor, 2005).

Research Support:

A Chinese study investigated the effect of music on the level of pain in patients undergoing C-clamp application after percutaneous coronary interventions. Surgical pain may create stress that affects physical and mental health. This randomized controlled study was conducted on 43 patients in the intensive care units of two acute care hospitals. Researchers collected both physiological and psychological variables at baseline and at 15, 30, and 45 minutes. At 45 minutes, the music group showed statistically significant reductions in heart rate, respiratory rate, and oxygen saturation than the control participants. The control group did not show these effects. The baseline comparison of the two groups showed no statistically significant differences; however, statistically significant differences in pain scores were found at 45 minutes for participants in the music group compared with the control group. The control group showed statistically significant increases in pain at 45 minutes compared with baseline (Chan et al., 2006).

Recovery time is prolonged due to the effects of anxiety experienced before, during, and after surgery, as this anxiety increases cardiovascular workload. Studies of music therapy as a nursing intervention have shown its ability to reduce anxiety. One randomized control trial evaluated the effect of music therapy on 60 postoperative adults older than 65 years of age. The experimental group listened to music during and after surgery, while the control group received standard postoperative care. Researchers administered the Spielberger State Trait Anxiety Inventory to both groups before surgery and 3 days postoperatively. In addition, mean intubation time was measured in both groups. The group that listened to music had lower anxiety scores and significantly fewer minutes of postoperative intubation after cardiovascular surgery. Researchers concluded that older adults undergoing cardiovascular surgery who listen to music have less anxiety and reduced intubation time than those who do not (Twiss, Seaver, & McCaffrey, 2006).

Children with cardiac disease can also benefit from music therapy. A Brazilian randomized clinical trial with placebo assessed 84 children during the first 24 hours of their postoperative period. The children's ages ranged from 1 day to 16 years. Each child received a 30-minute music therapy session with classical music. The child was then observed at the start and end of the session, and researchers recorded the child's heart rate, blood pressure, mean blood pressure, respiratory rate, temperature and oxygen saturation, plus a facial pain score. The two groups showed statistically significant differences in subjective facial pain scale and the objectives parameters of heart and respiratory rate after the intervention (Hatem, Lira, & Mattos, 2006).

References

Chan, M. F., Wong, O. C., Chan, H. L., Fong, M. C., Lai, S. Y., Lo, C. W., et al (2006). Effects of music on patients undergoing a C-clamp procedure after percutaneous coronary interventions. *Journal of Advanced Nursing, 53*(6), 669–679.

Hatem, T. P., Lira, P. I., & Mattos, S. S. (2006). The therapeutic effects of music in children following cardiac surgery. *Jornal de Pediatria, 82*(3), 186–192.

McCaffrey, R., & Taylor, N. (2005). Effective anxiety treatment prior to diagnostic cardiac catheterization. *Holistic Nurse Practitioner, 19*(2), 70–73.

Twiss, E., Seaver, J., & McCaffrey, R. (2006). The effect of music listening on older adults undergoing cardiovascular surgery. *Nursing in Critical Care, 11*(5), 224–231.

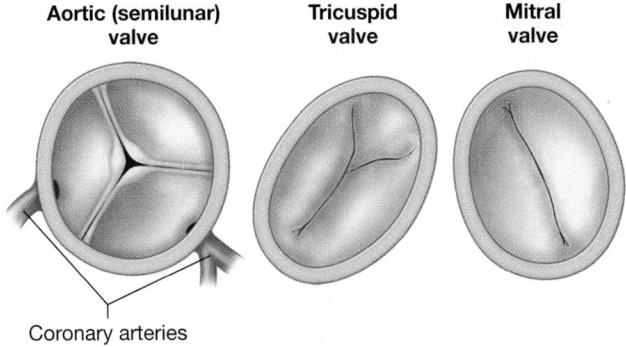

Aortic (semilunar) valve   **Tricuspid valve**   **Mitral valve**

Coronary arteries

FIGURE 41–5 ■ Normal cardiac valve shapes.

the heart (Figure 41–4, p. 1234). According to the AHA (2004), cardiac valve disease is the fifth most common cardiovascular disorder; the first four are coronary artery disease, heart failure, stroke, and hypertension. Although the incidence of rheumatic heart disease, a common causative factor in valve disease, has declined, no significant changes in the prevalence of valve disease have occurred (AHA, 2004). Three factors influence this lack of change:

(1) improvement in the assessment of valvular disorders, (2) an increased number of elderly, and (3) a greater number of recognized cases due to improvement in diagnostic testing technology.

Valvular heart disease is classified according to the valve involved and the functional alterations, which include stenosis and regurgitation. A regurgitant valve is one that is unable to close normally, causing a backward flow of blood, while a stenotic valve is unable to open normally, causing an impedance of blood flow. Valve regurgitation also is referred to as insufficiency or incompetence. When the valve is only mildly regurgitant or stenotic, the heart is initially able to adapt and maintain, but in time, chamber dilation and myocardial muscle hypertrophy occur, causing decreased contractility, reduced cardiac output, and finally heart failure. Valvular heart disease can be congenital or acquired, and it affects people of all ages (Wiegand, 2003). Most congenital valve repairs are performed immediately after birth or during early childhood. Significant advances have been made in the assessment and treatment of both congenital and acquired valve disease in the last several decades. Innovative diagnostic tools, pharmacologic developments, and improved invasive and surgical procedures have enhanced the quality of life for patients with valvular heart disease (Wiegand, 2003). The focus of medical and surgical intervention is to prevent heart failure and serious cardiac muscle damage.

Valvular Stenosis

Valvular stenosis is defined as a fibrotic thickening of the heart valve that causes fusion and calcification of the valve leaflet, resulting in a decrease in the size of the valve orifice (Figure 41–6 ■). The thickened leaflets interfere with the valve's ability to completely open, thus obstructing blood flow through the valve orifice and decreasing cardiac output. Valvular stenosis can occur in the mitral, aortic, and tricuspid valves. The degree of stenosis will determine the reduction in cardiac output and the presence and severity of clinical manifestations. Patients with mild to moderate stenosis are able to maintain cardiac output at rest but become symptomatic with exercise because the heart is unable to respond to the increased need for oxygen.

Valvular Regurgitation

Valvular regurgitation is defined as the inability of a valve to completely close during systole, resulting in a back flow of blood through the incompetent valve orifice into the previous chamber. In response to this, both of the chambers dilate and hypertrophy due to extra workload and the hypoxemia. This leads to progressive chamber failure and a decreased cardiac output. The development of failure is slow but it is the eventual outcome. Valve competence depends on normal leaflets, chordae tendineae, papillary muscles, and the valve annulus. A malfunction in any one of these structures will cause valvular regurgitation. Valvular regurgitation primarily affects the aortic, mitral, and on rare occasions the tricuspid valve and pulmonic valve.

MITRAL VALVE DISEASE

The mitral valve lies between the left atrium and the left ventricle, and controls blood flow between these two structures. Three diseases affect the mitral valve: stenosis, regurgitation, and prolapse. Each of these disorders is discussed next.

Mitral Valve Stenosis

Mitral valve stenosis (MVS), a common disorder of the mitral valve, is a progressive and chronic disease. The mitral valve assumes an abnormal funnel shape due to thickening and shortening of the valve structures as a result of calcification.

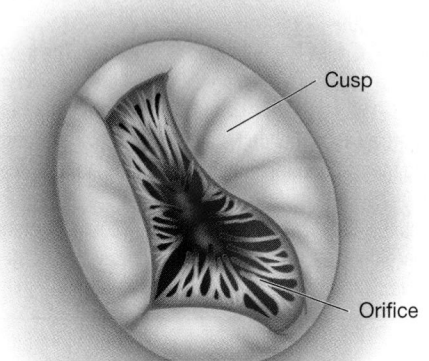

Normal Valve (open)
Normal valve opens widely and blood moves through freely.

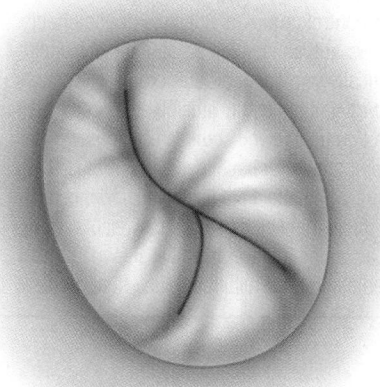

Normal Valve (closed)
Normal valve closes "water tight."

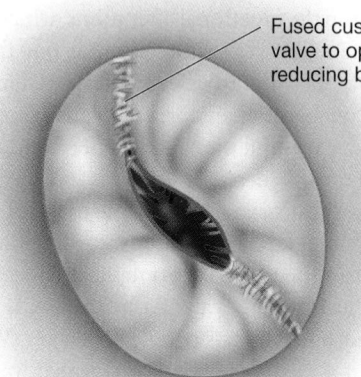

Fused cusps allow the valve to open only partly, reducing blood flow.

Stenosis (open valve)
Stenotic valve is thickened and bound down by scar tissue.

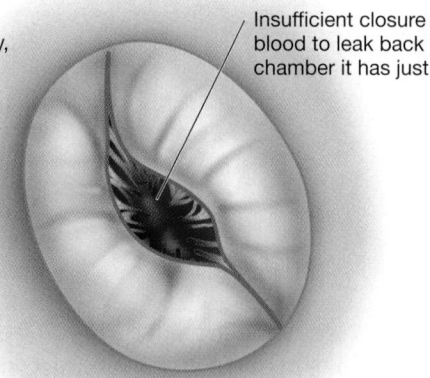

Insufficient closure allows blood to leak back into chamber it has just left.

Regurgitation (closed valve)
Valve leaflets are puckered and pulled apart by scar tissue—valve cannot close.

FIGURE 41–6 ■ Normal versus abnormal stenosed valve.

Contractures develop between the junctions or commissures (leaflets) of the valve (see Figure 41–6 ■). The stenosis narrows the opening of the valve, which obstructs blood flow from the left atrium to the left ventricle. The obstruction may be mild or severe. The normal orifice of a mitral valve is 4 to 6 cm and with stenosis it can become less than 1 cm.

Epidemiology/Etiology/Pathophysiology

Forty percent of persons with rheumatic heart disease develop mitral stenosis, making it the most common cause of this disease. Less common causes include infectious endocarditis, congenital mitral stenosis, rheumatoid arthritis, thrombus formation, calcification of the annulus, atrial myxoma (tumor), and SLE. Mitral stenosis is more common in women (66%) than men (Braunwald et al., 2005).

The inflammatory process caused by the infection results in fibrinous changes in the valve leaflet and chordae tendineae. The chordae tendineae shorten, causing narrowing of the outflow tract. The valve leaflets become fused, immobile, and are unable to completely open. The narrowed opening causes an obstruction to blood flow from the left atrium to the left ventricle during diastole, creating a pressure gradient. The obstruction causes the volume of blood and therefore the pressure to build up in the atrium, eventually backing up into the pulmonary system and causing increased pressure in the pulmonary vasculature. Consequently, it takes more pressure to pump blood and, thus, increases the workload of the heart. Eventually the prolonged rise in pressure and increased cardiac workload causes dilation and hypertrophy of the left atrium. Initially the heart is able to compensate, but eventually pulmonary capillary congestion occurs, causing pulmonary hypertension and subsequent backup into the right side of the heart. The increased pressure in the pulmonary vasculature causes fluid leakage across the alveolar membrane, leading to pulmonary edema. Finally, the increased pressure causes dilation and hypertrophy of the right ventricle and, if untreated, will lead to heart failure.

Clinical Manifestations

The size of the opening of the valve orifice determines the acuity of symptoms, and clinical manifestations depend on cardiac output and pulmonary vascular pressures. The most frequent complaint with mitral stenosis is dyspnea, which results from the pulmonary involvement.

Symptoms typically appear gradually over the course of a 20- to 30-year period and typically begin late in the fifth decade of life. In some cases, if rapid progression occurs, it usually takes 2 to 5 years for symptoms to appear. The early symptoms appear with exercise and in the later stages with rest. Specific clinical manifestations of mitral stenosis are outlined on Chart 41–4 (p. 1242).

■ Mitral Valve Regurgitation

Mitral valve regurgitation (MVR) or mitral insufficiency is defined as an inability of the mitral valve to close due to an abnormality in the structure and function of the valve. Fibrotic changes and calcification of the valve result in an inability to close completely during systole (see Figure 41–6 ■). There are two types of MVR, chronic and acute. In chronic MVR, the left atrium, left ventricle, and pulmonary vasculature dilate to accommodate the chronic volume overload. With acute MVR there is no chamber or vessel dilation so pressures rise in both the left atrium and ventricle, ultimately backing up into the pulmonary system, causing pulmonary edema.

Epidemiology/Etiology/Pathophysiology

Rheumatic heart disease is the primary cause of MVR and since it is on the decline with early and effective antibiotic treatment, the incidence of MVR also is declining. Mitral valve regurgitation from rheumatic heart disease is more common in women, although MVR from nonrheumatic causes is more common in men. Mitral valve regurgitation often is present with mitral valve stenosis. Other causes of MVR include connective tissue disorders (Marfan's syndrome), congenital valve malformation, coronary artery disease, endocarditis, dilated cardiomyopathy, mitral valve prolapse, amyloidosis, ankylosing spondylitis, and myocardial infarction.

With MVR there is an abnormality of one or more of the valve structures: leaflets, annulus (the valve ring that attaches to the leaflets), chordae tendineae, or papillary muscle. Valve leaflets and the chordae tendineae may shorten or tear, and the annulus may be stretched by heart enlargement to dilation and hypertrophy. Ventricular dilation and scarring from a myocardial infarction cause the papillary muscle to rupture, stretch, or be pulled out of position.

Due to the inability of the mitral valve to close, there is a backward flow of blood into the left atrium during systole. During diastole both the regurgitant blood and the normal blood flow into the ventricle, causing the left ventricle to be overfilled and dilated. This backward movement also increases the pressure in the left atrium and the pulmonary vasculature, resulting in varying degrees of chamber and vessel dilation and hypertrophy. The degree of involvement of these structures is determined by the etiology, severity, and duration of the MVR. For example, the acute MVR that occurs with myocardial infarction causes rupture of the papillary muscle and a sudden increase in left atrial distention and pressure. This increased pressure is transmitted to the pulmonary vasculature, resulting in rapid pulmonary edema and shock. In addition, cardiac output drops, thereby affecting organ and peripheral tissue perfusion. Conversely, in chronic MVR the volume overload on the left ventricle, left atrium, and the pulmonary vasculature allows for dilation and hypertrophy of these structures. Patients typically remain symptom free for several years until the development of left ventricular failure.

Clinical Manifestations

The clinical manifestations of mitral regurgitation depend on the cause and the degree of incompetence. In acute regurgitation, the left atrium has not had time to dilate and therefore the symptoms of pulmonary edema and shock appear quickly. The clinical manifestations of chronic MVR often take years to appear. Atrial fibrillation is a common and potentially deadly dysrhythmia associated with MVR (AHA, 2004). The remainder of the clinical manifestations for both acute and chronic MVR are outlined on Chart 41–4 (p. 1242).

■ Mitral Valve Prolapse

Mitral valve prolapse (MVP) is the most common form of heart valve disease in the United States (also referred to as Barlow's syndrome and floppy valve syndrome). Mitral valve prolapse occurs

CHART 41–4	**Clinical Manifestations of Cardiac Valve Disorders**

Valve/Disorder	Clinical Manifestation
Mitral valve stenosis	Atrial fibrillation (occurs 50% of the time), when present, causes an irregular, often weak pulse and a drop in cardiac output and blood pressure. Dyspnea, dyspnea on exertion, orthopnea, all due to pulmonary hypertension. Low-pitched rumbling crescendo–decrescendo diastolic murmur heard best with the bell of the stethoscope. Mural thrombi and stagnate blood found with atrial fibrillation causing embolization. Loud first heart sound heard (S_1). An opening snap reflecting high atrial pressures. Sound is best heard with the diaphragm of the stethoscope at the apex of the heart. Dry cough, dysphasia, and bronchitis occur due to bronchial irritation from the left atrial enlargement. Fatigue and weakness due to decreased cardiac output. Clinical manifestations of right-sided heart failure (Chapter 42). Palpitations and angina. Crackles in the lung bases. Hemoptysis.
Mitral valve regurgitation, acute	Sudden onset of dyspnea, thready peripheral pulses, and cool clammy skin. Pulmonary crackles. Decreased cardiac output. Atrial fibrillation with thrombus formation (occurs 75% of the time). Blowing high-pitched, systolic murmur. Left- and right-sided heart failure (Chapter 42).
Mitral valve regurgitation, chronic	Gradual onset of dyspnea, weakness, and fatigue gradually progressing to orthopnea, paroxysmal nocturnal dyspnea, and peripheral edema. S_3 and pansystolic (both systole and diastole) murmur at the apex radiating to the left axilla. Cough, pulmonary crackles. Atrial fibrillation with thrombus formation (occurs 75% of the time).
Mitral valve prolapse	Palpitations and irregular heartbeat. Sharp stabbing chest pain, especially during periods of stress. Paroxysmal atrial tachycardia, premature ventricular contractions, and ventricular tachycardia, precipitated by stress, caffeine, alcohol, and over-the-counter stimulants. Sharp stabbing chest pain usually occurs at rest but may occur with exercise. Panic attacks, anxiety, and impending doom. Fatigue, weakness, dyspnea. Chronically cold hands and feet and paresthesia (numbness and tingling) of arms and legs. Pansystolic murmur. Midsystolic to late-systolic click heard between S_1 and S_2. Light-headedness, dizziness, especially with position change; low blood pressure.
Aortic valve stenosis	Dyspnea, angina, fatigue, and syncope, which increase with exertion and are due to the fixed cardiac output. Harsh crescendo–decrescendo systolic murmur heard best in the second intercostal space on the right sternal border and the sound radiates to the carotid arteries. Palpable thrill is present. Increased pulmonary artery pressure and decreased cardiac output. Prominent S_4. Lung congestion. Left- and right-sided heart failure (Chapter 42). Palpitations.
Aortic valve regurgitation	High-pitched blowing, crescendo–decrescendo diastolic murmur. Decreased diastolic pressure and a widening of the pulse pressure. Pistol-shot pulse auscultated over the femoral arteries. Some patients have head bobbing with each heartbeat (Musset's sign). Palpitations and exaggerated carotid artery pulsations. Sudden sharp pulse, followed by a swift collapse of the diastolic pulse (waterhammer pulse). Exertional dyspnea, orthopnea, and paroxysmal nocturnal dyspnea. Nocturnal angina with diaphoresis. Bounding atrial pulse. Apical pulse is displaced to the left. Widened pulse pressure with an increased systolic pressure and a decreased diastolic pressure. Dizziness and exercise intolerance. Angina that occurs mostly at night and may not respond to conventional therapy. Left- and right-sided heart failure (Chapter 42).

CHART 41–4	Clinical Manifestations of Cardiac Valve Disorders—*Continued*
Valve/Disorder	**Clinical Manifestation**
Tricuspid valve stenosis (TVS) and regurgitation (TVR)	TVR: high-pitched blowing systolic murmur heard over the xiphoid area. TVS: low-pitched rumbling diastolic murmur heard best in the fourth intercostal space of the left sternal border. Right-sided heart failure (Chapter 42). Low cardiac output. Fatigue and weakness. Atrial fibrillation. Prominent waves in the neck veins due to vigorous atrial contraction. If in normal sinus rhythm, there are tall P waves.
Pulmonic valve stenosis (PVS) and pulmonic valve regurgitation (PVR)	Dyspnea and fatigue. PVR: high-pitched diastolic blowing murmur along the left sternal border. PVS: systolic crescendo–decrescendo murmur heard in the second left intercostal space (pulmonic area). Right-sided heart failure (Chapter 42). PVS: ECG has tall peaked T waves from atrial hypertrophy. Atrial fibrillation is common.

when one or more of the valve leaflets bulge or prolapse into the left atrium during systole (Figure 41–7 ■). This prolapse of the valve essentially results in valvular regurgitation. Varying degrees of valvular incompetence occur depending on the extent of the disorder. In many patients the disease is benign and they remain asymptomatic and undiagnosed; in others, serious complications result.

Epidemiology/Etiology/Pathophysiology

Mitral valve prolapse affects approximately 2% to 6% of the population, is eight times more common in women than men, and may be genetically inherited as a dominant gene (Grau, Pirelli, Yu, Galloway, & Ostrer, 2007). (Genetic predispositions to MVP are discussed in the Genetic Considerations box.) Other causes of MVP include endocarditis, coronary artery disease, myocarditis, connective tissue disorders, cardiomyopathy, hyperthyroidism, and cardiac trauma. The cause can also be idiopathic.

GENETIC CONSIDERATIONS for Mitral Valve Prolapse

There is a genetic predisposition with some forms of mitral valve prolapse. It is associated with Marfan's syndrome, a disorder present from birth, Graves' disease, and connective tissue disorders (University of Maryland, 2005).

MVP can result from abnormalities of the valve leaflets, chordae tendineae, papillary muscles, and left ventricular dysfunction. With MVP the leaflets of the valve are displaced upward into the left atrium during systole when the valve needs to be sealed shut to prevent a back flow of blood (see Figure 41–9 ■, p. 1248). The blood then regurgitates into the left atrium, as seen with mitral regurgitation. Severe mitral regurgitation is a complication of MVP. If progressive worsening of the regurgitation occurs, it can lead to heart failure.

Clinical Manifestations

Sixty percent of patients with MVP never have symptoms, 25% have mild clinical manifestations, 14% have moderate symptoms, and only 1% demonstrates severe symptoms (Orhon-Jech, 1999). Often the onset of symptoms is due to a major physiological stressor such as childbirth, or emotional situations such as divorce or death of a family member. The chest pain that accompanies MVP, which is described as sharp, is not due to inadequate blood flow to the heart muscle, but instead may be due to a stretching of the chordae tendineae and papillary muscle during prolapse. The chest pain may last for hours or days and is not brought on by exertion. Many patients experience panic attacks and a feeling of intense anxiety, and some feel an overwhelming sense of impending doom. The cause of these symptoms is unknown, but some clinicians believe that the anxiety felt during palpitations makes the body more sensitive to the stress hormones, which in turn increase palpitations and release of more stress hormone (Fung, 1999; Woods, Froelicher, & Motzer, 2000). These symptoms can last from a few seconds to a few minutes.

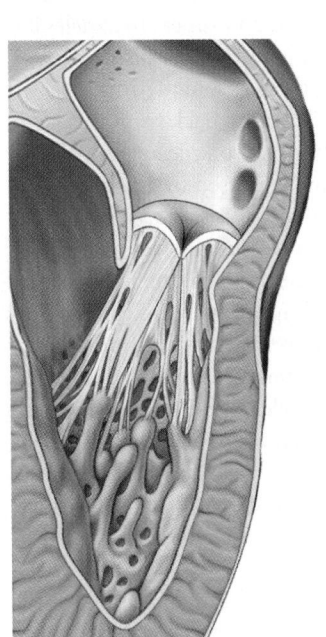
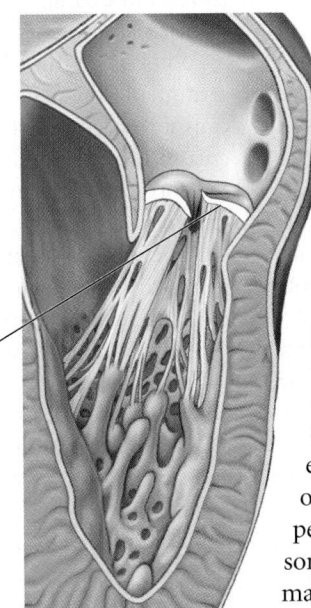

B: Valve prolapse

A: Normal

FIGURE 41–7 ■ Mitral valve prolapse.

If mitral regurgitation is present the patient will present with the associated symptoms. Patients with MVP have no activity restrictions except those mandated by the clinical manifestations. Patient teaching needs to include antibiotic prophylaxis for dental procedures and invasive testing (see Chart 41–3, p. 1237).

AORTIC VALVE DISEASE

The aortic valve lies at the root of the aorta in the left ventricle. It controls blood flow from the left ventricle through the aortic outflow tract into the systemic circulation. Diseases of the aortic valve include stenosis and regurgitation, both of which are discussed next.

◼ Aortic Valve Stenosis

Aortic valve stenosis (AVS) is similar to mitral stenosis in that there is a narrowing of the aortic valve orifice (see Figure 41–6 ◼, p. 1240). This stenosis results in an obstruction to blood flow from the left ventricle to the aorta during systole. AVS is a progressive, chronic disease, and if left untreated has a poor prognosis. Death is caused by sudden cardiac death (10% to 20% of cases) (Braunwald et al., 2005).

Epidemiology/Etiology/Pathophysiology

Causes of aortic stenosis include congenital leaflet malformation, rheumatic endocarditis, and degenerative changes associated with the aging process. It may also be idiopathic. Idiopathic aortic stenosis is typically mild and does not decrease cardiac output. Aortic stenosis is more common in males (80%) than females (Braunwald et al., 2005). In patients less than 30 years old, aortic stenosis is typically caused by a congenital malformation. When aortic stenosis is caused by rheumatic heart disease, typically the mitral valve also is involved and it occurs in persons between the ages of 30 and 70 years. Rheumatic heart disease destroys both valve leaflets with calcification and fibrosis, causing them to become scarred and rigid. In people older than 70 years of age, in the absence of rheumatic heart disease, atherosclerosis and degenerative calcification are the primary causes of aortic stenosis.

With aortic stenosis there is progressive narrowing of the valve orifice, typically over a period of several years or even decades (see Figure 41–6 ◼, p. 1240). The narrowed orifice makes it more difficult for the left ventricle to eject its load of blood. As the valve stenosis progresses, the left ventricle contracts more slowly and less forcibly in an attempt to maintain normal cardiac output. Even though the left ventricle attempts to increase blood flow, the stenotic valve blocks it, producing a fixed cardiac output. Prolonged increased pressure in the left ventricle causes hypertrophy, which is another cardiac muscle compensatory mechanism to maintain cardiac output. The increased cardiac workload results in increased cardiac oxygen consumption. Additionally, due to the decreased cardiac output, coronary artery blood flow is decreased. Thus, both the increased oxygen need and the decreased cardiac output result in myocardial ischemia. As ventricular end-diastolic pressure rises, the left atrial pressure increases and, over time, backs up into the pulmonary vasculature. Pulmonary vascular congestion and pulmonary edema eventually occur. If untreated, eventually pulmonary hypertension and right ventricular failure develop. With fixed cardiac output, the heart is unable to meet the oxygen demands during periods of increased activity and clinical manifestations begin to appear.

Clinical Manifestations

As aortic stenosis progresses, usually over several years, compensation fails, and symptoms begin to appear. Typically, the clinical manifestations begin to appear between the ages of 50 and 70 years and are a result of increased narrowing of the valve orifice and the onset of left ventricular failure. Symptoms generally develop when the valve orifice becomes one-third its normal size. Like mitral stenosis, dyspnea is the most frequent complaint and is usually accompanied by angina and exertional syncope. The clinical manifestations of aortic stenosis are outlined in Chart 41–4 (p. 1242).

◼ Aortic Valve Regurgitation

Aortic valve regurgitation (AVR) is similar to mitral valve regurgitation in that the blood regurgitates back into the left ventricle through a valve that is unable to completely close. This valve incompetence may be due to abnormal valve cusps or aortic root. The increased blood in the left ventricle causes dilation, hypertrophy, and eventually left ventricular dysfunction. Aortic valve regurgitation can be either chronic or acute.

Epidemiology/Etiology/Pathophysiology

The common causes of chronic AVR are rheumatic heart disease (67%), congenital valve malformation, and cardiomyopathy (Braunwald et al., 2005). Less common causes of chronic AVR include connective tissue disorders (Marfan's syndrome), rheumatoid arthritis, ankylosing spondylitis, chronic hypertension, and syphilitic aortitis. Abrupt dilation of the aortic root most commonly caused by a descending dissecting aortic aneurysm causes acute AVR. Other causes of acute AVR are blunt chest trauma and endocarditis. Except in cases caused by rheumatic heart disease, AVR is more common in men (75%) than women. In females it is commonly associated with coexisting mitral valve disease.

With AVR, the left ventricle receives blood from the left atrium and the regurgitant blood coming back from the aorta, causing the left ventricular end-diastolic volume to gradually increase. The regurgitant blood flow is caused by an inability of the aortic valve to close due to inflammation, scarring, and calcification of the valve leaflets from the causes listed earlier. With chronic AVR, as a compensatory mechanism, the left ventricle increases stroke volume in an attempt to increase cardiac output. The increased pressure causes ventricular dilation and hypertrophy (to increase muscle strength). As the condition progresses over time, the left ventricle loses its ability to compensate for the increased workload and cardiac output falls. The clinical manifestations of left ventricular heart failure begin to appear. Untreated, AVR will lead to increased left atrial pressures and dilation, pulmonary hypertension and congestion, and finally right-sided heart failure.

Much like acute mitral valve regurgitation, in acute AVR the left ventricle has not had time to develop the compensatory mechanisms. Therefore, with the extra blood volume the dramatic increase in cardiac workload results in a rapid decline in hemodynamic status, and patients develop fulminant pulmonary edema. If heart failure occurs rapidly, these patients often require emergent lifesaving measures.

Clinical Manifestations

Patients with chronic AVR may remain asymptomatic for as long as 20 years. The first complaints are typically an uncomfortable awareness of a heartbeat or palpitation. This bounding heartbeat is due to the large ventricular stroke volume and rapid diastolic runoff. The hallmark clinical manifestation of AVR is a diastolic murmur heard best at the second right intercostal space (aortic area) and radiating to the left sternal border. The remainder of the clinical manifestations for AVR are listed in Chart 41–4 (p. 1242).

Tricuspid Valve Disease

Tricuspid valve stenosis, which obstructs blood flow between the right atrium and the right ventricle, is an extremely rare and uncommon disorder (see Figure 41–6 ■, p. 1240). **Tricuspid valve regurgitation** is usually the result of pulmonary hypertension that increases right ventricular volume causing the ventricle to dilate and stretch. This stretching distorts the leaflets, chordae tendineae, and papillary muscle, preventing complete closure of the valve. The low pressure on the right side of the heart decreases the risk of inflammatory changes and calcification associated with high-pressure areas of the heart (left side).

Etiology/Epidemiology/Pathophysiology

Tricuspid stenosis occurs with rheumatic heart disease, IV drug use, and concurrently with mitral stenosis. Like aortic and mitral stenosis, the scarred and fibrosed valve leaflets are unable to completely open, creating the obstruction to blood flow. Right ventricular filling is decreased and right atrial pressure is increased due to the obstruction to blood flow. The right atrium enlarges and increased right atrial pressure is reflected backward into the systemic circulation causing congestion and clinical manifestations of right-sided heart failure. The decreased volume in the right ventricle reduces the blood flow to the lungs and left heart, resulting in a decreased cardiac output and tissue perfusion.

Like aortic and mitral regurgitation, with tricuspid regurgitation there is an inability of the valve to completely close during systole. The valve and its supporting structures become damaged by rheumatic heart disease, inferior myocardial infarction, blunt chest trauma, and infective endocarditis. Volume overload occurs in both the right atrium and right ventricle, causing a decreased cardiac output and right-sided heart failure.

Clinical Manifestations

Tricuspid stenosis increases the pressure in the right atrium, backing blood up into the venous circulation and resulting in right-sided heart failure. Atrial fibrillation is common due to the stretching of the atrium. If present, the patient is at a high risk for thrombus formation. The murmurs heard with both stenosis and regurgitation become more intense with inspiration.

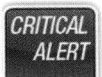

CRITICAL ALERT *Atrial fibrillation decreases cardiac output by 20% to 25%. If new-onset atrial fibrillation occurs, the nurse needs to assess tissue perfusion in the presence of a decreased cardiac output. Blood pressure, heart rate, respiratory rate, and presence of cyanosis need to be monitored frequently. Notification of the health care provider is necessary so measures can be instituted to terminate the abnormal rhythm (Josephson & McMullen, 2003).*

Pulmonic Valve Disease

Like aortic and mitral stenosis, **pulmonic valve stenosis** (PVS) restricts blood flow due to an inability of the valve to completely open (see Figure 41–6 ■, p. 1240). The blood from the right ventricle is obstructed from flowing into the pulmonary vasculature during systole. With **pulmonic valve regurgitation** (PVR) the valve is unable to completely close, causing blood to regurgitate back into the right ventricle (see Figure 41–6 ■, p. 1240). Like tricuspid disorders, the pulmonic valve is on the low-pressure right side of the heart; therefore, it is at a lower risk for developing the inflammatory changes and calcification associated with the high-pressure areas of the left side of the heart.

Epidemiology/Etiology/Pathophysiology

Disorders of the pulmonic valve are rare, and are usually caused by a congenital valvular malformation, although endocarditis, tumors, and rheumatic heart disease also have been implicated as causes. Pulmonic regurgitation is slightly more common than pulmonic stenosis and is typically caused by infective endocarditis, pulmonary artery aneurysm, syphilis, and pulmonary hypertension. The pulmonary hypertension dilates the pulmonary orifice, preventing complete valve closure.

With PVS the blood backs up into the right ventricle because of obstruction to blood flow through the narrowed valve orifice. Pulmonic valve regurgitation allows the blood in the pulmonary artery to regurgitate back into the right ventricle due to an inability to completely close. Therefore, both PVS and PVR prevent the blood from reaching the left side of the heart, thereby decreasing cardiac output. The increased blood volume in the right ventricle caused by both disorders increases ventricular volume and pressure, causing dilation and eventually hypertrophy. The final consequence of both disorders is right-sided heart failure (see Chapter 42 ☺).

Clinical Manifestations

Pulmonic valve disease is frequently associated with diseases of other valves. Therefore, the clinical manifestations may be complicated by multiple valve involvement. The clinical manifestations specifically associated with pulmonic valve disease are listed in Chart 41–4 (p. 1242).

CLINICAL MANAGEMENT FOR VALVE DISORDERS

Despite differences in pathophysiology the clinical management of patients with valve disease is similar. As always, the first priority is to find and treat the cause of the disorder and prevent complications and ultimately death. Treatment is based on the involved valve and the severity of the clinical manifestations and disease. Specifically, treatment focuses on preventing recurrent infective endocarditis, heart failure, and thromboembolism. Initially the patient is treated medically, but as the clinical manifestations become more disabling, surgical intervention is considered. Outlined next are the diagnostic studies and medical and surgical interventions for the treatment of valve disease.

Laboratory and Diagnostic Procedures for Cardiac Valve Disease

A heart murmur is usually the first indication of valve disease and once it has been identified by auscultation, diagnostic studies are done to determine the specific valve or valves involved and to confirm the progression of the disease. The most sensitive diagnostic test for valve disease is the echocardiogram because it provides information about the structure and function of the heart valves and enlargement of the chambers that is often a result of malfunctioning valves. It is able to identify thickened valve leaflets, vegetative growths, thrombus, myocardial function, and chamber size. In addition, the echocardiogram is able to measure pressure gradients across valves and pulmonary artery pressures can be estimated. Transesophageal echocardiography (Chapter 39 🔗) is particularly useful not only for diagnosing but also for tracking the progression of the disease (AHA, 2004). A discussion of additional diagnostic tests for cardiac valve disease is included in the Diagnostic Tests box.

Medical Management

Medical management begins with an in-depth history and physical. It is important to remember that a patient with valve disease may suddenly become ill or may slowly develop the symptoms over several years. The history needs to include information about the patient's health history, genetic factors, and social habits, such as IV drug use, that would increase the risk for developing valve disease. Specific questions need to be asked about a history of rheumatic fever and infective endocarditis. Each episode of these infections further increases valve dysfunction. The patient's fatigue level and ability to perform activities of daily living (ADLs), as well as the other clinical manifestations of valve disease need assessment during the physical exam.

After the cause has been identified and treatment begun, the medical management focuses on maintaining cardiac output, activity tolerance, and preventing complications. The treatment plan includes rest and medication. Pharmacologic management depends on the clinical manifestations and the progression of the disease. If heart failure is present with left ventricular dysfunction, ACE inhibitors (or angiotensin receptor blockers), digoxin, diuretics, and fluid and sodium restrictions are typically prescribed. See Chapter 42 🔗 for a complete description of the management of heart failure. For the remainder of the patient's life antibiotics are used prophylactically for dental work and invasive diagnostic studies as well as for the treatment of endocarditis. See the Pharmacology Summary of medications to treat cardiac valve disease (p. 1254).

Antidysrhythmic medications are used to manage the dysrhythmias that are common with valve disease. If atrial fibrillation occurs, every effort is made to terminate the dysrhythmia because it decreases cardiac output by as much as 25% in patients who may already have a compromised cardiac output due to their valve disease. Conversion to normal sinus rhythm is done with either drug

DIAGNOSTIC TESTS for Cardiac Valve Disease

Test and *Normal Values*	Expected Abnormality	Rationale for Abnormality
Echocardiogram and transesophageal echocardiography (TEE) Echocardiogram (ultrasound): *Normal chamber size and normal cardiac structures*	Abnormal structure and function of heart valves, able to identify thickened valve leaflets, vegetative growths, myocardial function, and chamber size. TEE is particularly useful not only for diagnosing but also for tracking the progression of the disease.	Vegetative growths and infection cause a thinning of valve leaflets leading to abnormal function.
Chest x-ray: *Clear lungs and normal heart size*	Pulmonary congestion, cardiac hypertrophy, chamber and great vessel enlargement, and calcification of the valves.	Abnormal valve function causes a change in blood flow leading to changes in chamber size and valve structure.
Cardiac catheterization: *Normal coronary artery blood flow, chamber size, and valve function*	The size of the valve opening and pressure gradients across valve surfaces is abnormal. Pressure in the heart chambers and pulmonary system is increased. Cardiac output typically is decreased.	Abnormal valve structure causes changes in openings leading to increased pressures in the cardiac chambers and decreased cardiac output.
Electrocardiogram (ECG): *Normal conduction time intervals*	Conduction delays, atrial and ventricular dysrhythmias, and the presence of cardiac ischemia. Is useful in detecting increased ischemia and the presence of life-threatening dysrhythmias.	Changes occur due to diminished blood flow to the myocardium due to decreased cardiac output caused by abnormal valvular function.
Cardiac MRI (CMR): *Normal heart valve function*	Valve size and competence.	Abnormal valve structure causes changes in openings, leading to increased pressures in the cardiac chambers and decreased cardiac output.

therapy (calcium channel blockers) or, if unsuccessful, synchronized cardioversion. After conversion, digoxin is typically prescribed to prevent further episodes of atrial fibrillation and control the heart rate. Chapter 38 describes atrial fibrillation. If atrial fibrillation persists, the blood stagnates in the quivering atrium and the patient is at a high risk for thrombus formation. Anticoagulant therapy is necessary to prevent strokes, pulmonary emboli, and deep venous thrombosis. Oral nitrates are prescribed for patients with aortic valve disease to increase peripheral dilation and decrease preload. This will decrease the pressure gradient in the left ventricle, thereby allowing it to pump more effectively and decreasing myocardial oxygen demand. Additionally, nitrates dilate the coronary arteries to increase perfusion to the myocardium.

The fixed and/or decreased cardiac output associated with valve disease limits physical activity. As the disease progresses the need for surgical intervention is in part determined by the patient's ability to perform the ADLs. Patients with asymptomatic aortic stenosis are placed on prophylactic antibiotics and instructed to get an echocardiogram every 6 months (Clarkston & Waldman, 2001). The echocardiogram serves as a guide for appropriate surgical intervention. Medical management of patients with aortic regurgitation includes prophylactic antibiotics, vasodilators to decrease ventricular afterload, and an echocardiogram every 6 months (Clarkston & Waldman, 2001).

In 1997, an association between diet medications (fenfluramine and phentermine) and valve regurgitation was identified in both left- and right-sided heart valves. The development of a new murmur in patients with no previous heart disease was noted, along with other symptoms of valve regurgitation. Based on these findings the federal Food and Drug Administration withdrew the drugs from the market.

Invasive Management of Valve Disease

When medical management is no longer effective and the hemodynamic status becomes unstable, invasive intervention is necessary to cure the problem or at least relieve symptoms. The need for intervention is determined in part by the impact of the clinical manifestations on the quality of life, the type and severity of valvular damage, and the patient's ability to tolerate the procedure. Options include either valve repair (annuloplasty, valvuloplasty, or commissurotomy) or valve replacement with a prosthesis. The reparative procedures do not result in a normal valve leaflet, but are associated with fewer side effects than valve replacement. The repaired valve functions more normally and cardiac output is improved, in essence buying the patient more time.

> **CRITICAL ALERT** *The patient is instructed to report to the health care provider when it is becoming too difficult to perform ADLs. This is one important indicator of the need for valve repair or replacement surgery.*

Annuloplasty

An **annuloplasty** corrects valve regurgitation by repairing the enlarged **annulus**, which is the fibrous ring at the junction of the valve leaflets and the muscular wall. This procedure is done when the valve leaflets are normal, but the valve fails to close due to this enlargement. The surgical procedure involves tightening the annulus with a prosthetic ring sutured in place, which reduces the size of the annulus (Figure 41–8 ■). Open heart surgery and cardiopulmonary bypass are required for an annuloplasty.

Valvuloplasty

The repair of the valve leaflet rather than replacement is referred to as a **valvuloplasty**. The torn or damaged leaflet, chordae tendineae, or papillary muscle is surgically repaired under general anesthesia and cardiopulmonary bypass. This procedure is primarily performed to treat mitral and aortic stenosis, although it has been used to treat tricuspid and pulmonic stenosis.

The most common valvuloplasty is a **commissurotomy**. The objective of this procedure is to separate fused valve leaflets. The site where leaflets meet each other is referred to as a **commissure**. With stenosis these commissures are abnormally fused either congenitally or due to calcification and scarring from inflammatory heart diseases. A closed commissurotomy requires general anesthesia but not cardiopulmonary bypass. After a midsternal incision is made a small hole is cut into the heart and the surgeon's finger or a dilator is used to break open the commissure. This procedure is useful for mitral, aortic, tricuspid, and pulmonic valve stenosis.

An open commissurotomy is performed with general anesthesia and cardiopulmonary bypass. This gives the surgeon direct

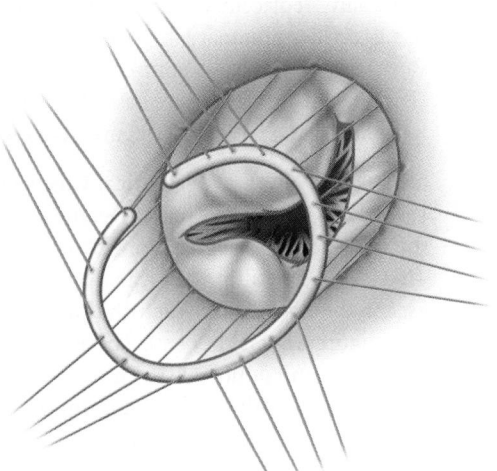
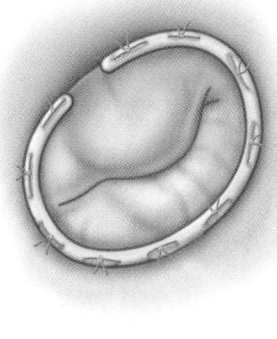

FIGURE 41–8 ■ Annuloplasty.

visualization of the valve and has the added advantages of allowing any thrombi to be removed and the degree of valve calcification to be identified. Additionally, if necessary, the chordae tendineae and papillary muscle can be repaired. The goals of this procedure are to improve leaflet mobility and to increase the size of the valve orifice. The procedure is most effective when the valve leaflets are thin and pliable (Wiegand, 2003).

Percutaneous Transluminal Balloon Valvuloplasty

Percutaneous transluminal balloon valvuloplasty (PTBV) is an invasive, nonsurgical commissurotomy used to dilate stenosed mitral and aortic valves (Figure 41–9 ■). In the heart catheterization

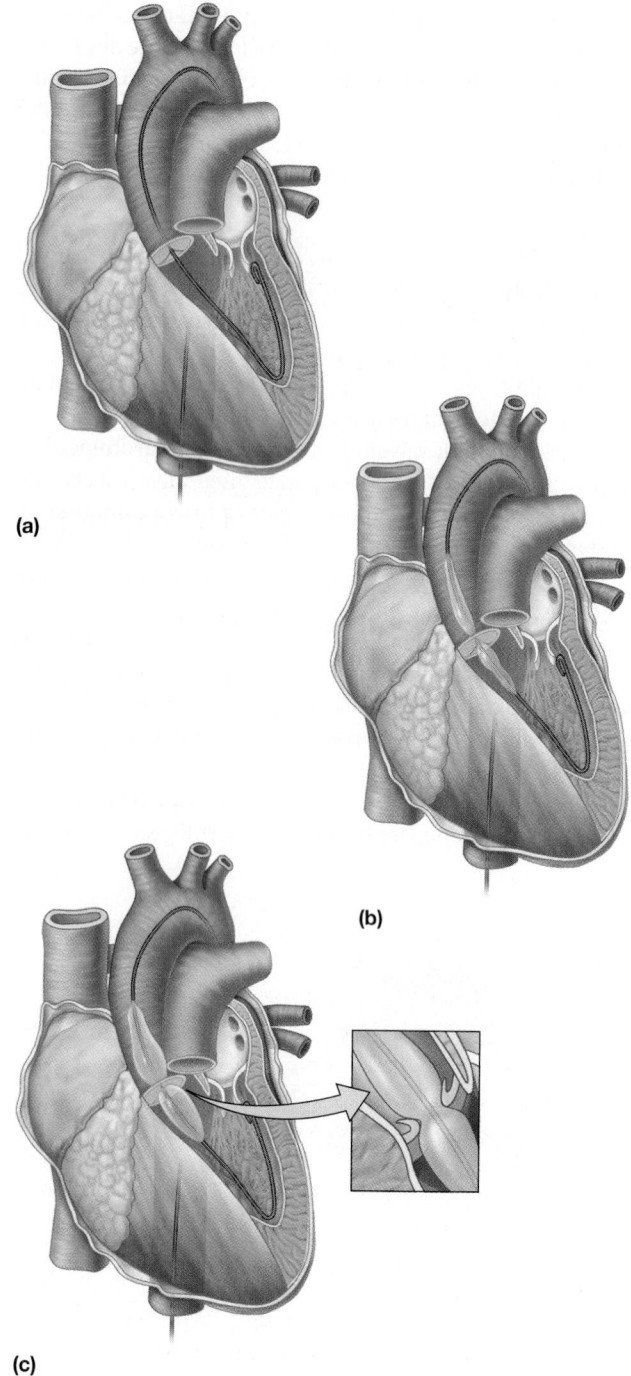

(a)

(b)

(c)

FIGURE 41–9 ■ Valvuloplasty.

laboratory with the patient under local anesthesia, a balloon-dilating catheter is inserted and positioned across the valve. To reach the mitral valve, the catheter is advanced through the femoral vein into the right atrium through the atrial septum and into the left atrium and across the mitral valve. The balloon is repeatedly inflated and deflated with dilute angiographic solution in order to dilate the stenosis. The valve is not completely occluded during inflation, thereby allowing some blood to flow to the left ventricle. The most common approach to treating aortic stenosis is to feed the catheter retrograde to blood flow in the femoral artery into the aorta until the valve is reached. To reach the tricuspid and pulmonic valves, a right-sided venous approach is used.

A balloon valvuloplasty will open the stenosis by 1 or 2 cm and reduce the pressure gradient across the valve. The aortic valve procedure is not as successful as that of the mitral valve. The rate of restenosis is approximately 50% in the first 12 to 15 months after the procedure (Braunwald et al., 2005). Some centers are reporting valve patency after 1 year and 60% to 70% required no intervention after 5 years. This procedure is useful to relieve symptoms in patients who are too high a surgical risk (Wiegand, 2003). Some degree of mitral regurgitation is present after the procedure. Other complications include emboli and rarely a left to right arterial shunt through the opening created by the catheter.

Prosthetic Heart Valves

Patients with cardiac valve disease must be monitored regularly by a cardiologist to determine the best time for valve replacement surgery. The general clinical state of the patient is usually appraised using the New York Heart Association classification system for functional disability (see Chapter 42). The goal is to replace the valve before permanent left ventricular damage occurs. Valve replacement is indicated when leaflets are calcified and immobile and when the clinical manifestations impact the patient's ability to perform ADLs.

Newer valves and improved surgical techniques have made valve replacement surgery safer. The goal for a valve is to be non-thrombogenic, durable, and create the least amount of stenosis. The type of valve used for a given patient is determined by the anatomic suitability, ease of insertion, the patient's age, contraindications to anticoagulant therapy (pregnancy), and patient preference. Valve replacement surgery is done under general anesthesia using cardiopulmonary bypass. After removal of the diseased valve, the new valve is sutured into the site of the native valve (Figure 41–10 ■). There are basically two different types of valves: mechanical and biological (Figure 41–11 ■).

Mechanical Valves **Mechanical valves** are commercially made valves. With the caged-ball valve, the ball floats up and occludes the valve opening when the pressure from the blood rises (Figure 41–11A ■). The tilting disk valve operates on the same principle except the disk closes when the pressure from the blood rises (see Figure 41–11B & D ■). There are two types of disk valves: single disk and double disk. The valve must have good hemodynamic design with the least amount of blood turbulence possible. The most frequently cited complications of mechanical valves are thromboembolism and anticoagulation-related problems (Aurigemma & Gaasch, 2002). Conversely, structural failure is relatively rare with mechanical valves as compared to

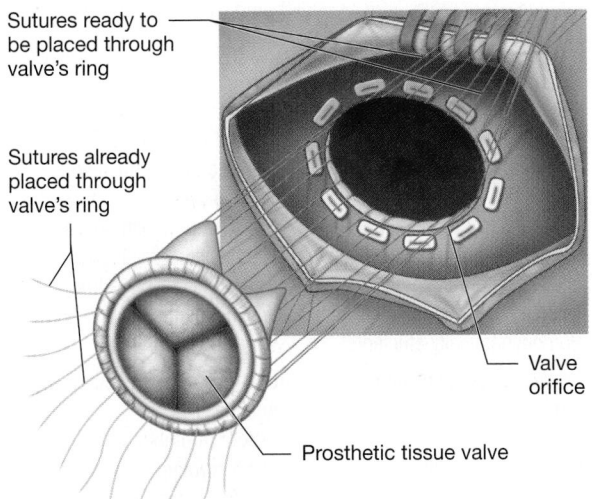

Sutures ready to be placed through valve's ring

Sutures already placed through valve's ring

Prosthetic tissue valve

Valve orifice

(a)

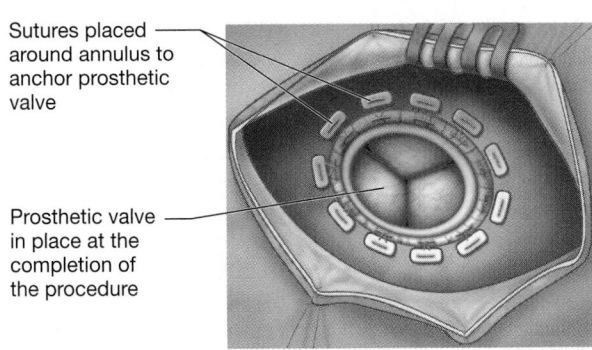

Sutures placed around annulus to anchor prosthetic valve

Prosthetic valve in place at the completion of the procedure

(b)

FIGURE 41–10 ■ Valve replacement surgery.

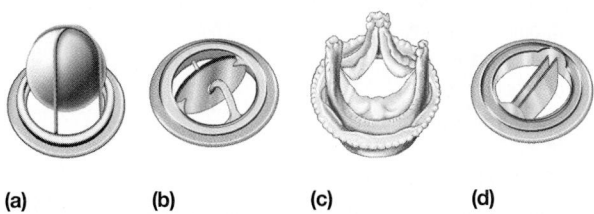

(a)   **(b)**   **(c)**   **(d)**

FIGURE 41–11 ■ Valve types: (A) caged-ball valve, (B) & (D) tilting-disc valve, and (C) porcine heterograph valve.

biological valves. Most mechanical valves are expected to last 20 to 30 years (Aurigemma & Gaasch, 2002). The specific valve description, advantages, and disadvantages are listed on Chart 41–5 (p. 1250).

Biological Valves **Biological valves**, most commonly come from pigs (porcine valves; see Figure 41–11C ■), although cow valves (bovine), and human valves also are used. Biological valves have a decreased incidence of clot formation compared to mechanical valves; therefore, long-term anticoagulation is not necessary. Biological valves do tend to wear out faster (7 to 10 years), especially in the younger populations who have increased amounts of calcium in the blood that break down the valve.

Note, however, that biological valves are useful for women of childbearing age because long-term anticoagulation is not feasible, preventing bleeding complications associated with menses, pregnancy, and childbirth. Biological valves also are used for the elderly population (greater than 70 years of age) and for patients with a history of peptic ulcer disease when anticoagulants are contraindicated.

There are two major types of biological valves: homograft valves and autograft valves. **Homograft** or **allograft valves** come from human cadaver donations and are used primarily to replace the aortic and pulmonic valves. The valves are harvested from a cadaver and stored cryogenically, although they are not readily available and are very expensive.

Autograft valves or autologous valves are obtained from the patient's own pulmonic valve and pulmonary artery. The pulmonic valve replaces the diseased aortic valve, and then the pulmonic valve is either replaced with a homograft or left without a valve. If the pulmonary pressures are normal, the surgeon may elect not to replace the valve.

■ Nursing Management

Nursing care of the patient with valve disease is aimed at assessing the clinical manifestations and progression of the disease, and conserving energy. The physical assessment begins with an in-depth history and an assessment of risk factors. Any episodes of rheumatic fever, endocarditis, or habits that increase the risk of valve disease are evaluated. The physical assessment includes vital signs, dysrhythmias, fluid status, anxiety, lung sounds, and the clinical manifestations of right- and left-sided heart failure, as described in Chapter 42 ☞ .

Nursing care focuses on conserving energy in order to maintain normal cardiac output and prevent the manifestations of heart failure and pulmonary congestion. Activity intolerance is a significant factor; therefore, the nurse spaces activities and visitors to allow for periods of rest. Because valve disease is a chronic debilitating disorder, it is important for the nurse to assess the patient's support systems. The Nursing Process: Patient Care Plan for Valve Disease (p. 1251) provides a comprehensive plan of care for a patient with valve disease. The Patient Teaching & Discharge box (p. 1253) outlines the patient teaching and discharge needs for a patient with valve disease.

The chronicity of valve disease and its atmosphere of uncertainty may produce anxiety, fear, and depression for the patient and family/significant others. A nursing assessment of the patient's ability to handle the situation and its impact on the quality of life is essential. The assessment findings are necessary in order to develop a comprehensive plan and help with the adjustment to the disease. The patient needs to be given an opportunity to express concerns and fears in a nonthreatening environment. Explanation of the medical regimen with rationales often decreases fear and frustration in patients.

The postoperative nursing care of the valve surgery patient includes monitoring for the usual complications such as hemorrhage, wound infection, and pulmonary complications. Additionally, the hemodynamic status and cardiac output must be closely monitored. For the first 24 to 48 hours after surgery, the patient is admitted to the critical care area where the ECG, cardiac

CHART 41–5	**Types of Prosthetic Heart Valves**			
Valve Type	**Types**	**Description**	**Advantage**	**Disadvantage**
Mechanical valve	Caged-ball: Starr-Edwards Smeloff-Cutter MaGovern-Cromie	Metal cage with struts mounted on ring, ball on inside of cage (Figure 41–11A ■, p. 1249).	Occupies less space in the ventricle. Requires less force to move the ball. Long-term durability up to 20 years. Hemodynamically efficient.	Lifetime anticoagulation. Audible click. Risk of thromboembolism. Infections harder to treat. Risk of hemorrhage from anticoagulants. Very large size.
	Tilting disc: Bjork-Shiley Lilehei-Kaster Medtronic Hall	Mobile disk attached to a circular ring by two struts (Figure 41–11B, D ■, p. 1249).	Produces central blood flow through orifice, like native valves. Long-term durability. Hemodynamically efficient.	Lifetime anticoagulation. Audible click. Risk of thromboembolism under pivoting points as a result of blood stasis. Infections harder to treat. Risk of hemorrhage from anticoagulants.
	Bileaflet valve: St. Jude Medical Duromedics	Two pivoting disks that open centrally attached to a ring.	Compact size, useful for children and patients with small aortic roots. Long-term durability. Hemodynamically efficient.	Lifetime anticoagulation. Audible click. Risk of thromboembolism. Infections harder to treat. Risk of hemorrhage from anticoagulants.
Biological tissue valve	Xenograft, porcine (pig): Hancock Carpenter-Edwards Medtronic	Harvested aortic valve from pig that is mounted on a sewing ring (Figure 41–11C ■, p. 1249).	Low incidence of thromboembolism. Need anticoagulation for only 3 months. Hemodynamically efficient. Quiet. Easier to treat infections.	Prone to deterioration. Frequent replacement required (5–7 years). Cumbersome structural design.
	Xenograft, bovine (cow): Ionescu-Shiley Carpenter-Edwards	Three leaflets composed of the pericardium of a 16- to 18-month-old calf that is mounted on a Dacron-covered frame.	Less resistant to blood flow. Useful for patients with small aortic roots. Low incidence of thromboembolism. Need short-term anticoagulation. Hemodynamically efficient. Quiet. Easier to treat infections.	Limited durability.
	Homograft/allograft: Cadaver	Harvested aortic valve from human cadaver that is sewn in place with special mounting material.	Low incidence of thromboembolism. Only rare need for anticoagulation. Excellent hemodynamics.	Limited durability. Not useful for mitral or tricuspid valve replacement. Not readily available. Very expensive.
Autograft valve	Autologous	Excised pulmonic valve and portion of pulmonary artery from patient.	Lasts 20 years. Nonthrombogenic, anticoagulation is unnecessary. Will grow with child. Useful for women in childbearing years, young adults, and for those who cannot tolerate anticoagulation.	Only possible if the aortic valve is normal. May require double valve replacement.

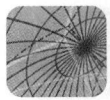

NURSING PROCESS: Patient Care Plan for Valve Disease

Assessment of Anxiety and Fear Related to Cardiac Valve Disease

Subjective Data:
What do you know about your disease process?
How do your health-related issues impact your daily life?
Do you feel anxious about your health?
Do you have family members or close friends who provide emotional support?

Objective Data:
Observe for manifestations of anxiety: restlessness, apprehension, withdrawal.

Nursing Assessment and Diagnoses	Outcomes and Evaluation Parameters	Planning and Interventions with *Rationales*
Nursing Diagnosis: *Anxiety* and *Fear* related to chronic disease process	**Outcome:** Anxiety level minimized and manageable. **Evaluation Parameters:** Verbalizes anxious feelings. Verbalizes what relieves anxiety. Demonstrates relief from anxiety by consistently controlling aggression, impulsiveness control, and self-mutilation restraint; and by improving coping and social interaction skills. Verbalizes absence of sensory perceptual disorders. Verbalizes absence of physical manifestations of anxiety. Behavioral manifestations of anxiety absent.	**Interventions and *Rationales:*** Provide factual information concerning diagnosis, treatment, disfigurement, disabilities, and prognosis. *Truthful explanations increase trust and potentially decrease anxiety.* Explain all procedures and allow time for mental preparation. *This decreases fear and anxiety of the unknown.* Allow time and encourage verbalization of fears related to illness *to assist in relieving anxiety.* Explore with the patient/family techniques to reduce anxiety. *This gives the patient a sense of control and opens communication about the subject.* Explore effective ways to minimize anxiety. *This gives the patient a sense of control.* Instruct the patient in the use of relaxation techniques *to relieve anxiety.* Assess need for and administer antianxiety and pain medication. *If alternative measures are not effective, may need antianxiety agents.*

Assessment of Activity Tolerance

Subjective Data:
What level of activity fatigues you?
Have you been becoming more fatigued with less activity recently?
Are you able to complete your ADLs without fatigue?

Objective Data:
Monitor tolerance to activities while on bed rest in order to obtain a baseline to plan activities.
Monitor for changes in symptoms and vital signs (VS) during activity.
Determine if pulse, respirations, and blood pressure (BP) return to normal within 3 minutes after stopping activity.

Nursing Assessment and Diagnoses	Outcomes and Evaluation Parameters	Planning and Interventions with *Rationales*
Nursing Diagnosis: *Fatigue* and *Activity Intolerance* related to decreased or fixed cardiac output	**Outcome:** Energy conservation. **Evaluation Parameters:** Endurance maintained. Balanced diet. Reports increased energy levels. Absence of clinical manifestations at rest.	**Interventions and *Rationales:*** Identify activities that increase fatigue *to avoid increasing cardiac workload.* Discontinue activity if chest pain, dyspnea, cyanosis, dizziness, hypotension, sustained tachycardia, or dysrhythmias develop *to aid in evaluating tolerance to activities.* Explore sedentary activities that the patient may enjoy *to provide a diversion that does not place a demand on the heart.* Maintain balanced nutrition to ensure adequate calories *to increase energy.*

(continued)

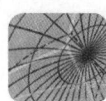

NURSING PROCESS: Patient Care Plan for Valve Disease—*Continued*

Assessment of Tissue Perfusion

Subjective Data:
Do you become short of breath? What causes it to occur?
How far can you walk before becoming short of breath?
Do you experience leg pain? If so, what brings it on and is it getting worse?
Do your hands and feet feel cold on a warm day?

Objective Data:
Assess:
Acid–base balance.
The presence of and/or change in a murmur.
Lung sounds.

Respiratory rate.
ECG.
Peripheral pulses.
Capillary refill.

Nursing Assessment and Diagnoses	Outcomes and Evaluation Parameters	Planning and Interventions with *Rationales*
Nursing Diagnosis: *Ineffective Tissue Perfusion* related to decreased cardiac output as a result of valve disease.	**Outcomes:** Maintenance of cardiac output. Adequate tissue perfusion. **Evaluation Parameters:** Absence of heart failure. Absence of atrial fibrillation and/or successful conversion to normal sinus rhythm.	**Interventions and *Rationales:*** Assess for adventitious or diminished breath sounds. *Indicates decreased gas exchange and heart failure.* Note presence of cough and amount and color of sputum. *Assessing for heart failure.* Monitor ABGs and oxygen saturation *to assess adequacy of gas exchange.* Monitor respiratory rate and depth *to assess for respiratory distress.* Monitor fluid status *to assess heart failure.* Monitor ECG for dysrhythmias, especially atrial fibrillation *to determine impact on cardiac output and risk for sudden death.* Monitor restlessness and confusion. *Indicators of inadequate gas exchange with resultant brain hypoxia.* Assess need for suctioning and/or endotracheal intubation. Suction when necessary *to maintain adequate gas exchange.* Observe for cyanosis, especially in the mucous membranes. *Indicators of inadequate gas exchange with resultant tissue hypoxia.* Turn, cough, deep breathe, elevate head of bed, instruct on use of incentive spirometry. *Measures to promote gas exchange.* Administer humidified oxygen as prescribed *to increase oxygen levels.* Report respiratory distress to the health care provider. *Medical intervention may be indicated to prevent respiratory failure.* Encourage low-sodium diet to *reduce fluid retention and heart failure.*

output, and pulmonary artery pressures can be monitored and ventilatory support can be provided if necessary.

Following repair or replacement of the valve, the heart requires time to adjust to the improved hemodynamic function. Vasoactive agents may be necessary in the immediate postoperative period to optimize cardiac output. Inotropic agents may be necessary to improve cardiac contractility, and vasodilators may be needed to decrease afterload (Wiegand, 2003). Continuous monitoring for cardiac dysrhythmias is essential because the mitral and aortic valves lie close to the conduction pathway. Transient or permanent heart blocks may occur due to edema, ischemia, or damage to the conduction pathway. A temporary or permanent pacemaker may be required. Additionally, atrial dysrhythmias are a common complication of cardiac surgery and are even more common after valve surgery (Wiegand, 2003). If indicated based on valve type, anticoagulant therapy is started within 48 hours of valve surgery.

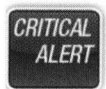 *Report to the health care provider an INR and/or PT that is either too low or too high. If the values are too low, there is increased risk of clot formation. If the values are too high there is an increased risk of excessive bleeding.*

Monitor and report decreases in hemoglobin and hematocrit, which may indicate bleeding. If the platelet count is less than 50,000/mm³, there also is an increased risk of bleeding.

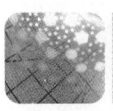

PATIENT TEACHING & DISCHARGE PRIORITIES for Cardiac Valve Disease

Need	Teaching
Knowledge of disease and progression of clinical manifestations	Detailed teaching materials about the disease process, medical regimen, and possible complications to increase knowledge and compliance.
Prevention	Antibiotics for dental work to prevent valve infection and repeated endocarditis.
Assess need for valve surgery	Seek medical help when unable to perform ADLs.
Safety	Medication dosages, frequency, side effects, and special considerations need to be explained to both the family and patient.
Postoperative learning needs to prevent complications	Anticoagulant therapy teaching needs to include: • Drug and dosage • Monthly International Normalized Ratio (INR) to determine correct dosage (ratio typically 2.0 to 3.0 depending on the diagnosis and health care provider preference). Prothrombin time (PT) also may be used to monitor anticoagulants (1.2 to 2 times greater than normal). Report bruising, bleeding, epistaxis, and hemoptysis. Avoid large amounts of yellow and dark green vegetables and fatty foods, which increase the absorption of vitamin K (clots blood). Avoid alcohol, aspirin, and anti-inflammatory drugs (NSAIDs). Inform health care providers of anticoagulant therapy. Test stools and vomitus for blood. Use soft-bristled toothbrush and an electric razor. To maintain an adequate level of anticoagulation without side effects.
Follow-up care	Medical follow-up continues for about a year to assess for complications, valve function, and compliance to therapy.

Source: From *Laboratory Tests and Diagnostic Procedures with Nursing Diagnosis,* 6th edition, by J. V. Corbett, 2004, Upper Saddle River, NJ: Prentice Hall.

A clinical pathway (Chapter 6) is frequently used during the early postoperative period as a guideline to achieve established outcomes within a prescribed length of stay for patients who are recovering from valve surgery. The protocols and guidelines outlined on the pathway provide useful tools for facilitating the coordination of care (Zevola, Raffa, & Brown, 2002).

Health Promotion

Due to the progressive nature of the disease, health promotion begins as soon as the patient is diagnosed with a valve abnormality. Patient/family education focuses on controlling the clinical manifestations, reducing physical activity, and preventing reoccurrences of an infection in the valve. Education includes information on medications, lifestyle choices, and preventive care. The patient needs to be given specific instructions about when to seek medical advice for surgical intervention. When the patient is no longer able to perform the ADLs, generally surgical intervention is discussed.

Once surgical intervention has occurred, formulating a teaching plan for the postoperative valve surgery also is an essential nursing function. The plan needs to include information about medications, activity, and the signs and symptoms that need to be reported to the health care provider.

 Following valve replacement surgery the patient is taught that if fever, increased heart rate, fatigue, malaise, anorexia, weight loss, headache, and chills, or night sweats occur, the patient needs to notify the health care provider. The clinical manifestations are a sign of postoperative infective endocarditis, which needs immediate medical attention.

Collaborative Management

Due to the chronic and progressive nature of cardiac valve disease, a collaborative care approach is optimal for management. Utilizing a multidisciplinary team approach, including health care providers, nurses, physical and occupational therapists, psychologists/psychiatrists, dieticians, and pharmacists, will facilitate the best possible quality of life for the patient and family. It is essential that the health care provider monitor the progress of the valve disease and determine when surgical intervention is necessary. Psychiatric counseling may be necessary to assist in lifestyle adjustments necessitated by a chronic disease process. The occupational therapist helps facilitate realistic occupational goals, while the physical therapist assists in the maintenance of optimum conditioning given the activity restrictions.

Because medication is an essential part of the management of valve disorders, the role of the pharmacist is crucial in educating the patient about how to manage the medications and their side effects. When cardiac valve disease is complicated by the presence of heart failure symptoms of congestion, diet and fluid restriction counseling are necessary. The dietitian can educate the patient/family about salt restrictions and help them learn about satisfying meals that do not increase the risk of fluid retention. In addition to the nursing care described earlier, the nurse plays a pivotal role in coordinating the efforts of the health care team. In the inpatient setting the nurse facilitates communication between the members of the team and the patient/family. The nurse also must include in the patient teaching the coordination of care after discharge (see Patient Teaching & Discharge Priorities box).

PHARMACOLOGY Summary of Medications to Treat Cardiac Valve Disease

Medication Category	Action	Application/Indication	Nursing Responsibility
Cardiac Medications			

Digoxin
Calcium channel blockers:
  Diltiazem (Cardizem)
  Verapamil (Calan)
ACE inhibitors
Antiarrhythmic agents
	Increases force and velocity of myocardial systolic contraction. Decreases conduction through AV node. Reduces automaticity in the SA node and slows impulse conduction through the AV node. Used for supraventricular dysrhythmias.
	ACE inhibitor:
	Lowers peripheral resistance and reduces blood volume by enhancing the excretion of sodium by inhibition of angiotensin-converting enzyme.
	Alters the electrophysiological properties of the heart by either blocking flow through the channels or altering autonomic activity.
		Convert and then control atrial fibrillation.
		Control atrial fibrillation.
		Manage heart failure if present.
		To manage the dysrhythmias that are common with valve disease.
			Digoxin requires periodic laboratory testing to ensure therapeutic drug level. Assess pulse prior to administration of digoxin. The pulse rate needs to be >60 beats/min.
			Never given if heart block, sick sinus syndrome, severe hypotension, and shock are present.
			Assess heart rate, blood pressure, lung sounds, and ECG monitor regularly.
			Monitor for hypotension especially when being given intravenously.
			Monitor blood pressure carefully after first dose for hypotension.
			Educate patient that it takes 2 weeks for therapeutic effect.
			May experience dizziness.
			There is a narrow margin between therapeutic effect and toxicity; therefore, careful and ongoing cardiac monitoring is essential.
			Patient teaching includes avoiding the use of alcohol, drugs, and tobacco.

Diuretics	Blocks reabsorption of sodium and chloride in the loop of Henle. Reduces edema associated with heart failure.	To manage heart failure if present.	Potassium levels also need monitoring because low levels are a side effect of certain diuretics, especially furosemide. May need potassium replacement. Measure urine output prior to administration to gauge the response to the medication.
Antibiotics	Inhibits protein synthesis of microorganisms by binding reversibly to a ribosome, thus interfering with transmission of genetic information.	Prophylactically for dental work and invasive diagnostic studies as well as for the treatment of acute endocarditis episodes.	Assessment of history of drug allergies prior to administration. Assessment of clinical manifestations of allergic reaction. Assessment of relief of clinical manifestations to determine drug effectiveness. Patient education regarding need to complete the entire regimen and report any clinical manifestations of drug allergy.
Anticoagulant Therapy			
Warfarin (Coumadin) Heparin	Can either inhibit specific clotting factors in coagulation cascade or diminish the clotting action of platelets.	Prevent strokes, pulmonary emboli, and deep venous thrombosis, especially if atrial fibrillation is occurring.	Ongoing assessment of therapeutic blood level per health care provider orders. Assess for bleeding including nosebleeds, bruising, "coffee-grounds" emesis, tarry stools, fatigue, and pale skin. Assess for decreases in hemoglobin, hematocrit, RBCs, and platelets.
Nitrates (nitroglycerin)	Relaxes both atrial and venous smooth muscle, causing decreased preload and afterload.	Used with aortic valve disease to increase peripheral dilation and decrease preload, thereby allowing the heart to pump more effectively, hence decreasing myocardial oxygen demand. Dilate the coronary arteries to increase perfusion to the myocardium.	Assess blood pressure before and during therapy. Hypotension could result. Should be given with other vasodilators. Patient education includes: No alcohol use. Rotate patches. Keep medication with you at all times and away from excessive heat and light. Report blurred vision, dry mouth, and severe headache.

Sources: Adams, M. P., Josephen, D. L., & Holland, L. N. (Eds.). (2005). *Pharmacology for nurses: A pathophysiologic approach.* Upper Saddle River, NJ: Pearson Prentice Hall; American Heart Association. (2005). *Handbook of emergency cardiovascular care for health providers.* Dallas, TX: Author; Wilson, B., Shannon, M., & Stang, C. (Eds.). (2005). *Nurses drug guide.* Upper Saddle River, NJ: Pearson Prentice Hall.

Cardiomyopathy

Cardiomyopathies (CMPs) are defined as diseases of the myocardial muscle fibers. The diseases result in progressive structural and functional abnormalities of the myocardium. The term *cardiomyopathy* was first introduced in 1957 and was defined simply as noncoronary artery heart disease of unknown etiology (Brigden, 1957). Currently, the World Health Organization defines cardiomyopathies as "diseases of the myocardium associated with cardiac dysfunction" (Richardson, 1996).

Cardiomyopathies are classified as primary and secondary. With primary CMPs, the etiology of the disease is unknown and the only abnormality is in the heart muscle itself. Secondary CMPs are caused by other disease processes such as ischemia, viral infections, alcohol intake and drug abuse, inherited disorders, and pregnancy. There are four types of CMPs: dilated, hypertrophic, restrictive, and arrhythmogenic. Each type is identified by differences in pathology, clinical manifestations, and treatment. All types of cardiomyopathy can lead to cardiomegaly and heart failure.

Dilated Cardiomyopathy

Dilated cardiomyopathy (DCM), the most common form of cardiomyopathy, is a disorder of the myocardium characterized by dilation and impaired contraction of one or more ventricles. When dilation becomes severe it may be accompanied by heart wall hypertrophy, which is an increase in myocardial wall thickness. Figure 41–12 ■ compares the ventricle size for each type of cardiomyopathy.

Epidemiology and Etiology

Dilated or congestive cardiomyopathy accounts for approximately 87% of all cardiomyopathies and is distributed throughout all age groups with the majority in the elderly population (Porth, 2005). The risk factors for the development of DCM are outlined in the Risk Factors box (p. 1256), although for 50% of cases no cause can be identified. Coronary artery disease is the most common cause of DCM in the United States, comprising 50% to 75% of patients with heart failure (Felker, Thompson, & Hare, 2000). This type of cardiomyopathy most frequently develops following a myocardial infarction and ventricular tissue remodeling. Prolonged ischemia causes a loss of myocytes that are replaced by noncontractile scar tissue, thereby leading to heart failure. These changes lead to irreversible myocardial dysfunction.

After initial diagnosis and onset of clinical manifestations, 50% of patients with DCM are alive in 5 years, and 25% are alive in 10 years. Mortality rates from DCM are highest in older persons, males, and the black race (Porth, 2004).

Pathophysiology

Some forms of DCM are idiopathic, but a genetic cause is present in as many as 30% of these patients (Hunt et al., 2005). Known risk factors for the development of DCM are outlined in the Risk Factors box (p. 1256). These factors cause the myocardial fibers to degenerate, become necrotic, and eventually be replaced by fibrotic tissue, referred to as tissue remodeling. Dilation of the cardiac chambers occurs due to the constant stress from overfilling. The stretching of the myocardial fibers increases the compliance of the ventricles but results in hypocontractility, reduced stroke volume, ejection fraction, and ultimately decreased cardiac output. Blood flows more slowly through the enlarged heart, causing mural thrombi (blood clots on the heart wall) to form, increasing the risk of atrial and ventricular emboli formation. Additionally, the extra blood that stays in the chambers after each contraction eventually backs up into the pulmonary system, causing heart failure symptoms and ultimately reducing blood flow to the tissues.

Cardiomyopathy during pregnancy or after pregnancy, referred to as peripartum cardiomyopathy (PPCM), is thought to be caused by an interaction of pericardium physiology with either infectious agents leading to myocarditis or by inflammatory, genetic, hormonal, or metabolic factors, and accounts for

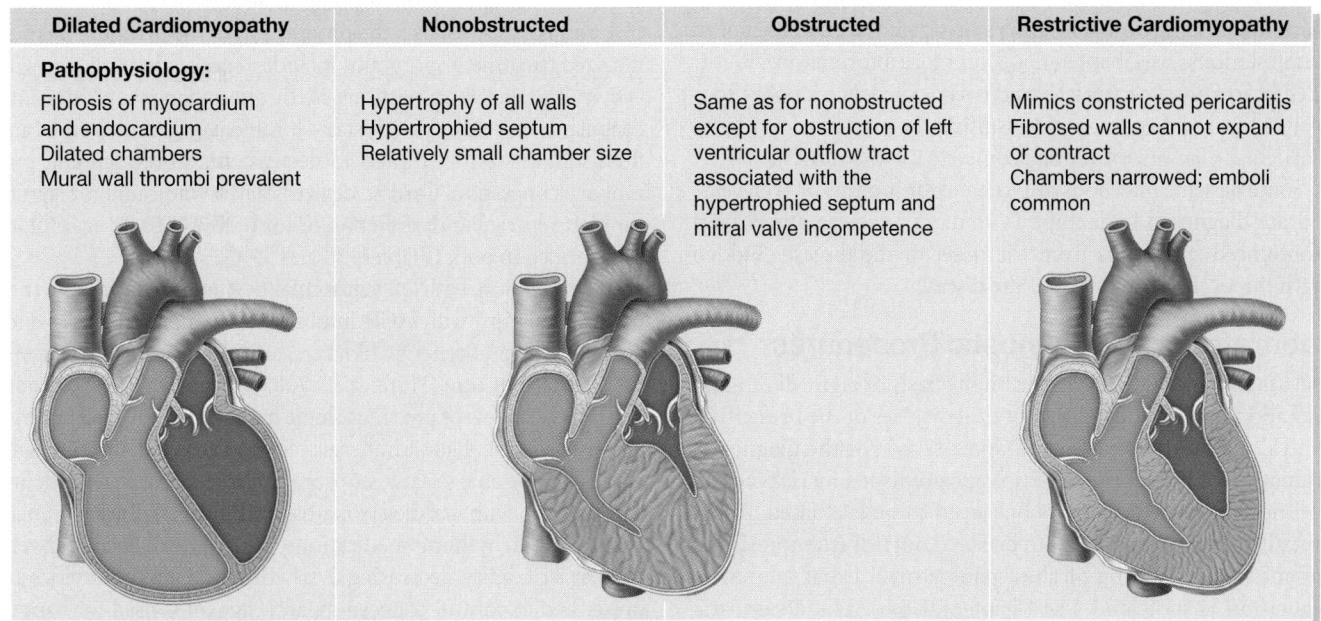

Dilated Cardiomyopathy	Nonobstructed	Obstructed	Restrictive Cardiomyopathy
Pathophysiology: Fibrosis of myocardium and endocardium Dilated chambers Mural wall thrombi prevalent	Hypertrophy of all walls Hypertrophied septum Relatively small chamber size	Same as for nonobstructed except for obstruction of left ventricular outflow tract associated with the hypertrophied septum and mitral valve incompetence	Mimics constricted pericarditis Fibrosed walls cannot expand or contract Chambers narrowed; emboli common

FIGURE 41–12 ■ Types of cardiomyopathy.

RISK FACTORS for Cardiomyopathy

Long-term uncontrolled hypertension
Cardiac valve disease
Coronary artery disease
Congenital heart disease
Viral myocarditis
Toxins (lead, mercury, carbon monoxide, arsenic)
Pregnancy and postpartum period
Connective tissue disorders (SLE, scleroderma, giant cell arthritis)
Alcohol abuse
Stress and sedentary lifestyle
Genetic predisposition
Nutritional deficiency (decreased thiamine, selenium, carnitine)
Sleep apnea
Cocaine
Chemotherapeutic agents
Bacterial/parasitic infections

Neuromuscular disorders (Duchenne's muscular dystrophy)
Endocrine disorders (diabetes, Cushing's disease)
Electrolyte abnormalities (hypocalcemia, hypophosphatemia, uremia)
Antiviral medications (zidovudine, didanosine)
Radiation therapy
Calcium overload
Amyloidosis and sarcoidosis
Hyperlipidemia
Sedentary lifestyle
Obesity
Smoking
Diabetes mellitus
Familial cardiomyopathies
Idiopathic
Cardiac surgery

Source: Afridi, H. R., & Hartnell, G. G. (2002). *Cardiomyopathy, dilated.* Retrieved August 3, 2006, from http://www.emedicine.com/radio/topic128.htm.

approximately 4% of the cases (Flutterman & Lemberg, 2000). The diagnosis of PPCM is based on (1) no other identifiable causes of heart failure, (2) heart failure within 5 months of delivery, (3) absence of heart disease prior to the last month of pregnancy, and (4) ECG revealing abnormal left ventricular systolic function. The majority of the cases of PPCM occur in the postpartum period, with up to 50% of the related deaths occurring within 3 months after delivery (Flutterman & Lemberg, 2000).

Clinical Manifestations

The clinical manifestations of DCM have an insidious onset. Findings depend on the area and the degree of structural dysfunction. Initial complaints typically include a complaint of increasing fatigue, dyspnea, and activity intolerance, classic symptoms of heart failure. The failing heart may include one or both sides of the heart, manifesting both left- and right-sided heart failure clinical manifestations (see Chapter 42 🔗 for more information). Right-sided heart failure occurs later and is associated with a poor prognosis. Mitral and/or tricuspid insufficiency may develop due to ventricular dilation, preventing complete valve closure.

Some patients may be asymptomatic for months or even years and are diagnosed by laboratory findings, whereas others have pronounced symptoms from the onset of the disease. Sudden death can occur at any stage of the disease.

Laboratory and Diagnostic Procedures

The diagnosis of DCM is made on the basis of an in-depth history and physical and ruling out other causes of the presenting clinical manifestations. (See Chapter 42 🔗 for the diagnostic evaluation of heart failure.) Etiologic predisposing risk factors outlined in the Risk Factors box need to be evaluated. Additionally other diseases need to be ruled out; for example, if the patient is complaining of chest pain, a myocardial infarction evaluation is indicated (see Chapter 40 🔗). The Diagnostic Tests box outlines the tests that are usually done to evaluate DCM. Because DCM is a progressive disease, frequent and ongoing monitoring is necessary. Clinical manifestations typically dictate the need for further testing and evaluation.

Medical Management

Because DCM is a chronic noncurable disease, management focuses on control of the disease, identifying precipitating factors, and control of clinical manifestations. Interventions are aimed at controlling progression of structural dysfunction that leads to heart failure, when possible. Treatment aims are more palliative than curative, and focus on decreasing cardiac workload.

The overall goals of medical management are to find the cause, improve contractile efficiency, and manage the symptoms and complications. If the cause can be identified and terminated, such as illicit drugs or alcohol, stopping these substances will help control, and possibly reverse, the progression of the disease. The multifaceted treatment program includes medications along with activity and dietary restrictions. Medication therapy includes anticoagulants for the blood stasis problems, and diuretics and fluid/sodium-restricted diets to decrease fluid overload and pulmonary congestion. Cardiac devices may be indicated for significant left ventricular dysfunction or for bradycardia or heart block as described in both Chapters 38 and 39 🔗 .

If heart failure with left ventricular dysfunction is present, then medical therapy with ACE inhibitors (or angiotensin receptor blockers), beta-adrenergic blockers, and aldosterone blockers are the standard of care (Hunt et al., 2005). Chapter 42 🔗 provides a complete review of pharmacologic management for left ventricular dysfunction. Beta-adrenergic blockers and ACE inhibitors together may be able to slow, stop, or even reverse tissue remodeling that occurs with cardiomyopathy and heart failure (Francis, 2004). Antiarrhythmic medications help control atrial and ventricular irritability, decreasing dysrhythmias. Finally, diuretics are prescribed to control congestion, and digoxin is used for continued symptoms of heart failure.

DIAGNOSTIC TESTS for Dilated Cardiomyopathy

Test with *Normal Values*	Expected Abnormality	Rationale for Abnormality
Chest x-ray: *Clear lungs and normal heart size*	DCM: Cardiomegaly and enlargement of the heart. Lung fields have pulmonary congestion and edema.	Cardiomyopathy causes an increase in heart size and predisposes heart failure.
Electrocardiogram (ECG): *Normal conduction time intervals* *(see Chapter 38)*	Dysrhythmias. Axis deviation. Left bundle branch block. ST segment changes. Sinus tachycardia.	Stretching of the myocardium may also cause conduction disturbances. Heart failure causes abnormal axis deviation. Ischemia associated with heart failure causes the dysrhythmias and ST segment changes.
Echocardiogram (ultrasound): *Normal chamber size and normal* *cardiac structures*	Enlarged chamber size, ventricular wall, and septum thickness. Sluggish wall motion. Decreased systolic and diastolic function.	The disease causes enlargement of the chamber, which results in sluggish wall motion and decreased systolic and diastolic function.
Cardiac catheterization to rule out coronary artery disease, assess hemodynamic status, and chamber size and function: *Normal coronary arteries, chambers,* *and valve pressures*	Enlarged chambers and decreased cardiac output.	The disease causes enlargement of the chamber, which results in a decreased force of muscle contraction leading to decreased cardiac output.
Endomyocardial biopsy occasionally done to rule out other causes of the clinical manifestations: *Normal myocardial tissue*	Myocardial cells positive for pathologic evidence of infiltration, fibrosis, or inflammation.	Changes due to disease process.
Radionuclide study: *Normal chamber volumes and blood* *perfusion to cardiac muscle*	Abnormally increased ventricular volume and deficits in myocardial muscle perfusion.	The disease causes enlargement of the chamber, which results in a decreased force of muscle contractions leading to an increase in blood being left in the chambers and thereby decreasing myocardial perfusion.

If left ventricular dysfunction is present with an ejection fraction of less than 35%, despite optimizing medications, an implantable cardioverter defibrillator (ICD) may be implanted (Chapter 39). A pacemaker with a lead in both ventricles, referred to as a biventricular pacemaker (or cardiac resynchronization therapy), is being used to treat heart failure when the ejection fraction is less than 35%, the QRS duration is greater than 120 milliseconds, and patients remain symptomatic despite optimal heart failure medicines. There are three leads, one in the right atrium and two in the ventricles. The pacemaker is able to synchronize cardiac contraction, beginning with atrial depolarization and ending with left ventricular depolarization. This produces significantly improved left ventricular performance, which results in an improved ejection fraction and cardiac output. Early studies have shown that because of improved blood flow and better emptying of the ventricles, the remodeling of tissue is reversing itself. The end result is an improved heart failure status. See Chapter 39 for complete descriptions of biventricular pacemakers. See the Pharmacology Summary of medications to treat cardiac valve diseases (p. 1254).

Activity restriction is essential during the acute illness, but over time, resuming activities that increase strength and endurance should be promoted. Early in the disease process patients may find the activity restrictions difficult to accept. Thus, patient/family education needs to stress that physical and emotional stress exacerbate the disease. As the disease progresses, most patients experience severe clinical manifestations that limit activity. Alcohol is discouraged for patients with DCM because it depresses myocardial contractility and further decreases cardiac output. End-stage therapies for patients who have progressive and refractory disease include heart transplantation or permanent mechanical assist devices. These therapies are fully described in Chapter 42 .

In 2003 the Centers for Disease Control and Prevention reported that two patients contracted dilated cardiomyopathy 3 months after receiving the smallpox vaccine. Smallpox vaccinations have not been previously associated with DCM. The AHA (2004) advises that these two adverse events should raise awareness that an inflammatory reaction from the vaccine could be a potential mediating factor in cardiomyopathy. Myocarditis, which involves an inflammatory reaction, has been seen in increased numbers in patients receiving smallpox vaccination.

Nursing Management

Nursing management begins with a detailed history and in-depth physical assessment. The nurse must inquire about possible risk factors and other diseases that may mimic DCM. Continuous monitoring of assessment parameters of the patient for changes in systemic perfusion include mental status, heart rate and rhythm, peripheral perfusion, oxygenation, fluid status, and vital signs. Since this is a progressive disease, an ongoing assessment is necessary to note significant trends.

The Impact of Repeated Episodes of Recurrent Tachycardia in Patients with Tachycardia-Induced Cardiomyopathy

Clinical Problem

Sudden death from cardiac arrest is a major health problem worldwide. Sudden cardiac death (also called sudden arrest) is death resulting from an abrupt loss of heart function (cardiac arrest). It occurs unexpectedly in individuals who may or may not have diagnosed heart disease. It occurs within minutes after symptoms appear. The most common underlying reason for patients to die suddenly from cardiac arrest is coronary heart disease although there is a significant incidence in both hypertrophic (HCM) and arrhythmogenic right ventricular cardiomyopathy (ARVC) (American Heart Association, 2006). For these patients, early detection, treatment, and prevention of sudden death are the focus of both patient and family education. Nurses must understand how to apply evidence-based findings when caring for patients with all types of cardiomyopathy, especially the younger population with HCM and ARVC because of the increased risk of sudden cardiac death.

Research Findings

Nerheim, Birger-Botkin, Piracha, and Olshansky (2004) conducted a study to assess the impact of repeated episodes of recurrent tachycardia in patients with tachycardia-induced cardiomyopathy. These authors hypothesized that although left ventricular ejection fraction measurements normalize after heart rate or rhythm control in patients with tachycardia-induced cardiomyopathy, recurrent tachycardia may have abrupt and deleterious consequences. The sample consisted of patients with tachycardia-induced cardiomyopathy that developed over years. Tachycardia episodes and outcomes were assessed. Twenty-four patients were identified, of which one-third were heart transplant candidates.

Within 6 months of rate control or correction of the rhythm, left ventricular ejection fraction improved or normalized and symptoms abated in all of the subjects. In the five patients who had tachycardia recur, the left ventricular ejection fraction dropped precipitously and heart failure ensued within 6 months, even though the initial impairment took years. Rate control eliminated heart failure and improved or normalized ejection fraction in 6 months. Three of 24 patients died suddenly and unexpectedly. The authors concluded that tachycardia-induced cardiomyopathy develops slowly and appears reversible by left ventricular ejection fraction improvement, but recurrent tachycardia causes rapid decline in left ventricular function and development of heart failure and the risk of sudden death increases.

Implications for Nursing Practice

This study clearly indicates a need for nurses to educate cardiomyopathy patients about the importance of maintaining a normal heart rate and rhythm. It appears from the study that controlling the heart rate and rhythm will slow the progression of the disease and reduce the risk for sudden cardiac death. Because both HCM and ARVC tend to occur in the younger population, which is more physically active, it is imperative that the importance of activity restriction be emphasized and reinforced. The family and significant others need to be included in the education process. Additionally, nurses need to understand that, when caring for this patient population, spacing of activities, allowing for rest periods, and careful monitoring of cardiac rhythms are essential. Ongoing nursing assessment of the heart rate and rhythm with activity will assist the patient and family in establishing parameters for a safe level of activity. The nurse needs to understand the importance of reporting the first signs of tachycardia so that treatment can be instituted.

Critical Thinking Questions

1. In order of priority, what are the most important points that would be included in an education plan for patients with cardiomyopathy and their families?

2. What method(s) would be effective in increasing compliance with activity limitations of young people with HCM and ARVC?

3. Identify nursing measures that would decrease the risk of tachycardia occurring.

Answers to Critical Thinking Questions appear in Appendix D.

References

American Heart Association. (2006e). *Sudden cardiac death*. Retrieved June 14, 2006, from http://www.americanheart.org/presenter.jhtml? identifier=4741.

Nerheim, P., Birger-Botkin, S., Piracha, L., & Olshansky, B. (2004). Heart failure and sudden death in patients with tachycardia-induced cardiomyopathy and recurrent tachycardia. *Circulation, 110* (3), 247–252.

The physical assessment focuses on an evaluation of the clinical manifestations and their impact on the patient's ability to perform ADLs. The basic assessment includes vital signs, fluid status, auscultation of a S_3, S_4, a murmur, pulmonary congestion, and an evaluation of peripheral perfusion. Typically the patient is on a cardiac monitor to detect dysrhythmias, conduction delays, and ST segment changes. The progressive nature of the disease requires that the patient have frequent ongoing nursing assessment in order to pick up ominous changes and worsening signs of heart failure.

Nursing care focuses on decreasing the workload of the heart. Pacing activities, restricting activity, positioning, and oxygen therapy will help conserve energy and diminish cardiac workload. Details of the nursing care for patients with cardiomyopathy are given in the Nursing Process: Patient Care Plan for Cardiomyopathy feature. The impact of repeated episodes of recurrent tachycardia in patients with tachycardia-induced cardiomyopathy is outlined in the Evidence-Based Practice feature.

Hypertrophic Obstructive Cardiomyopathy

Hypertrophic cardiomyopathy (HCM) is a disorder of the sarcomere, the contractile element of the cardiac muscle that is characterized by left ventricular and occasionally right ventricular hypertrophy, with greater hypertrophy occurring in the septum. This disorder is also referred to as idiopathic hypertrophic subaortic stenosis (IHSS) and hypertrophic obstructive cardiomyopathy (HOCM). The rationale for the variation in names is described below. Figure 41–13 ■ (p. 1262) demonstrates the difference between a normal ventricular wall and a hypertrophied wall.

Epidemiology and Etiology

Hypertrophic cardiomyopathy occurs in about 1 in 500 people in the general population, and it is the most common cause of sudden death in young people. In more than 50% of the cases, HCM is a genetic disorder, manifested by a defect in cardiac muscle development.

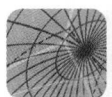

NURSING PROCESS: Patient Care Plan for Cardiomyopathy

Assessment of Knowledge of Disease

Subjective Data:

What have you been told about your health?

What is your understanding of the treatments you are on?

Do you drink alcohol or use any recreational drugs?

Do you take rest periods during the day?

What is your level of activity?

Do you feel any change in your ability to perform your activities of daily living (ADLs)?

How much activity can you do before you become short of breath?

What symptoms need to be reported to your health care provider?

Objective Data:

Assess:

Level of understanding of disease and treatment.

Compliance with therapy.

High-risk behaviors.

Lung sounds.

Vital signs.

Peripheral edema.

Shortness of breath.

Cough—type of sputum.

Nursing Assessment and Diagnoses	Outcomes and Evaluation Parameters	Planning and Interventions with *Rationales*
Nursing Diagnosis: *Deficient Knowledge* related to disease process, care needs, and complications	**Outcomes:** Understanding of disease process, care needs, and importance of compliance with treatment. **Evaluation Parameters:** Compliance with treatment plan. Activity level appropriate for cardiac workload.	**Interventions and *Rationales:*** Avoid high-risk behaviors (alcohol, cocaine). Report any increases in clinical manifestations to your health care provider. *To retard the progression of the disease.* Comply with therapy *to prevent progression of the disease.* Activity restriction *to decrease cardiac workload.*

Assessment of Heart Failure

Subjective Data:

How much activity are you able to do before becoming short of breath?

Do you have a cough? If so, is it productive?

Do your feet swell?

Objective Data:

Assess:

Vital signs.   Decreased urine output.

Lung sounds.   Orthopnea.

Jugular venous distention.   Pink frothy sputum.

Dyspnea.   Skin temperature.

Confusion.   Peripheral edema.

Nursing Assessment and Diagnoses	Outcomes and Evaluation Parameters	Planning and Interventions with *Rationales*
Nursing Diagnosis: *Tissue perfusion ineffective* related to hypercontractility and aortic outflow obstruction	**Outcome:** Prevention of heart failure. **Evaluation Parameters:** Lungs clear. Patient denies shortness of breath. Patient verbalizes understanding and willingness of treatment plan.	**Interventions and *Rationales:*** Monitor BUN, creatinine, liver enzymes, bilirubin *to assess blood supply to liver and kidneys.* Monitor fluid balance and record as prescribed *to assess fluid retention that would exacerbate the symptoms of heart failure.* Report significant imbalances to the health care provider *to obtain the necessary intervention(s) to correct the imbalance.*

Assessment of Anxiety

Subjective Data:

What do you know about your disease process?

How do your health-related issues impact your daily life?

Do you feel anxious about your health?

Do you have family members or close friends who provide emotional support?

Objective Data:

Observe for manifestations of anxiety: restlessness, apprehension, withdrawal.

(continued)

NURSING PROCESS: Patient Care Plan for Cardiomyopathy—*Continued*

Nursing Assessment and Diagnoses	Outcomes and Evaluation Parameters	Planning and Interventions with *Rationales*
Nursing Diagnosis: *Fear* and *Anxiety* related to disease process and sudden cardiac death	**Outcome:** Anxiety level minimized and manageable. *Evaluation Parameters:* Verbalizes anxious feelings. Verbalizes what relieves anxiety. Demonstrates anxiety-relief by consistently controlling aggression, impulsiveness, and self-mutilation, and by improving coping and social interaction skills. Verbalizes absence of sensory perceptual disorders. Verbalizes absence of physical manifestations of anxiety. Behavioral manifestations of anxiety absent.	**Interventions and *Rationales:*** Allow time and encourage verbalization of fears related to illness *to assist in relieving anxiety.* Explore with the patient/family techniques to reduce anxiety. *This gives the patient a sense of control and opens communication about the subject.* Provide factual information concerning diagnosis, treatment, disfigurement, disabilities, and prognosis. *Truthful explanations increase trust and potentially decrease anxiety.* Explain all procedures and allow time for mental preparation. *This decreases fear and anxiety of the unknown.* Explore effective ways to minimize anxiety. *This gives the patient a sense of control.* Instruct patient on use of relaxation techniques *to relieve anxiety.* Assess need for and administer antianxiety and pain medication. *If alternative measures are not effective, may need antianxiety agents.*

Assessment of Ability to Function in Usual Role

Subjective Data:
What is your role in your family?
Are you able to perform that role?
Who takes over your role function when you are not able to?
How do you feel about your inability to function in your role?

Objective Data:
Determine knowledge of health status (see *Deficient Knowledge* nursing diagnosis).
Assess level of functioning.
Assess alternatives or alterations in role function.

Nursing Assessment and Diagnoses	Outcomes and Evaluation Parameters	Planning and Interventions with *Rationales*
Nursing Diagnosis: *Powerlessness* over altered role function due to chronic progressive illness	**Outcomes:** Verbalizes a realistic perception of control. Verbalizes realistic perception of abilities to perform. *Evaluation Parameters:* Identifies health outcome priorities. Verbalizes powerlessness. Identifies actions that are within his/her control and demonstrates ability to perform those actions. Reports adequate support from staff and family.	**Interventions and *Rationales:*** Discuss realistic options for self-care. *Gives patient hope and realistic view of limitations.* Reinforce personal strengths. *Decreases sense of powerlessness.* Encourage verbalization of feeling of powerlessness. *Opens communication.* Assist patient to increase independence when realistic. *Decreases powerlessness.* Allow control over surroundings and schedule when possible. *Decreases powerlessness.* Keep items within reach. *Decreases powerlessness.* Set short-term realistic goals. *Decreases powerlessness.* Explore patient's support mechanisms: family, church, and friends. *Needed as a source of support.*

Assessment of Compliance with Treatment Regimen

Subjective Data:
What do you understand about your treatment plan?
Are you able to comply with the restrictions necessary to prevent further progression of your disease?
What can the health care team do to help you with treatment compliance?

Objective Data:
Assess motivation and willingness to comply with therapy.
Assess where health care team can assist with barriers to compliance.

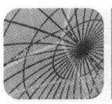

NURSING PROCESS: Patient Care Plan for Cardiomyopathy—*Continued*

Nursing Assessment and Diagnoses	Outcomes and Evaluation Parameters	Planning and Interventions with *Rationales*
Nursing Diagnosis: *Noncompliance* with medication and activity restrictions	**Outcomes:** Shows willingness to comply with therapy. ***Evaluation Parameters:*** Accepts imposed restrictions and complies with treatment plan.	**Interventions and *Rationales:*** Suggest alternative solutions to barriers *to determine interventions that will increase compliance.* Monitor and evaluate compliance with therapy *to determine patient's ability to sustain treatment.*

Assessment of Fatigue
Subjective Data:
What level of activity fatigues you?
Have you been becoming more fatigued with less activity recently?
Are you able to complete your ADLs without fatigue?

Objective Data:
Monitor tolerance to activities while on bed rest in order to obtain a baseline to plan activities.
Monitor for changes in symptoms and vital signs (VS) during activity.

Determine if pulse, respirations, and BP return to normal within 3 minutes after stopping activity.

Nursing Assessment and Diagnoses	Outcomes and Evaluation Parameters	Planning and Interventions with *Rationales*
Nursing Diagnosis: *Fatigue* and *Activity Intolerance* related to decreased cardiac output	**Outcomes:** No increase in fatigue or decrease in activity levels. ***Evaluation Parameters:*** Absence of or no progression of peripheral edema, congested lungs, decreased CO, dyspnea, pink frothy sputum, diaphoresis, and decreased renal and liver perfusion.	**Interventions and *Rationales:*** Identify activities that increase fatigue *to avoid increasing cardiac workload.* Discontinue activity if chest pain, dyspnea, cyanosis, dizziness, hypotension, sustained tachycardia, or dysrhythmias develop *to aid in evaluating tolerance of activities.* Explore sedentary activities the patient may enjoy *to provide diversion that does not place a demand on the heart.*

Assessment of Tissue Perfusion
Subjective Data:
Do you become short of breath? If so, what causes it to occur?
How far can you walk before becoming short of breath?
Do you experience leg pain? If so, what brings it on and is it getting worse?
Do your hands and feet feel cold on a warm day?

Objective Data:
Assess:
Acid–base balance.
Lung sounds.
Respiratory rate.

Nursing Assessment and Diagnoses	Outcomes and Evaluation Parameters	Planning and Interventions with *Rationales*
Nursing Diagnosis: *Ineffective Tissue Perfusion* related to decreased cardiac output	**Outcome:** Adequate gas exchange. ***Evaluation Parameters:*** Normal ABGs. No dyspnea: unlabored respirations < 24/minute. Alert and oriented. Clear breath sounds. No restlessness, cyanosis, or fatigue. Oxygen saturation is within normal limits.	**Interventions and *Rationales:*** Assess for adventitious or diminished breath sounds. *Indicates decreased gas exchange and heart failure.* Note presence of cough, and amount and color of sputum. *Assessing for heart failure.* Monitor ABGs and oxygen saturation *to assess adequacy of gas exchange.* Monitor respiratory rate and depth *to assess for respiratory distress.* Monitor fluid status *to assess heart failure.* Monitor restlessness and confusion. *Indicators of inadequate gas exchange with resultant brain hypoxia.* Assess need for suctioning and/or endotracheal intubation *to maintain adequate gas exchange.* Observe for cyanosis, especially in the mucous membranes. *Indicators of inadequate gas exchange with resultant tissue hypoxia.* Turn, cough, deep breathe, elevate head of bed, instruct on use of incentive spirometry. *Measures to promote gas exchange.* Administer humidified oxygen as prescribed *to increase oxygen levels.* Report respiratory distress to the health care provider. *Medical intervention may be indicated to prevent respiratory failure.*

(continued)

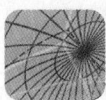

NURSING PROCESS: Patient Care Plan for Cardiomyopathy—*Continued*

Assessment of Cardiac Output

Subjective Data:
Do you feel weak or light-headed with activity?
Do you become short of breath? If so, what causes it to occur?
Is the shortness of breath getting worse?

Objective Data:
Assess:
Vital signs.
Lung sounds.
Weight.
Cardiac output.
Fluid intake and output.

Nursing Assessment and Diagnoses	Outcomes and Evaluation Parameters	Planning and Interventions with *Rationales*
Nursing Diagnosis: *Decreased Cardiac Output* related to hypercontractility and obstruction to outflow	**Outcomes:** Patient able to tolerate decreased cardiac output. Stabilization of cardiac output. *Evaluation Parameters:* Clear lung sounds. No dyspnea. Normal vital signs. Skin warm and dry. Normal heart rate and rhythm. No abnormal heart sounds (S_3 and S_4). No jugular venous distention, peripheral edema, and ascites. Normal urine output.	**Interventions and *Rationales:*** Monitor vital signs, lung sounds, skin, heart rate and rhythm, edema, JVD, and ascites *in order to monitor response and tolerance of altered cardiac output (CO).* Administer negative inotropic medications as ordered *to decrease the hypercontractility.* Avoid a Valsalva maneuver *because it impedes venous return (preload).*

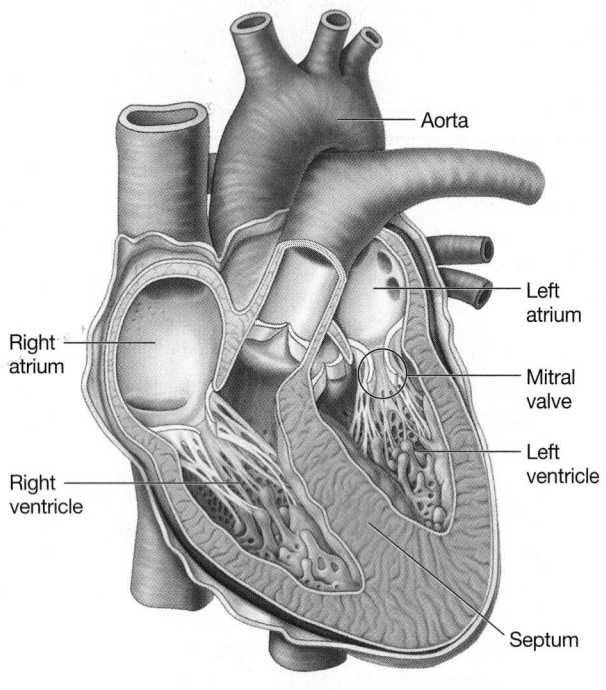

(a) Normal septum

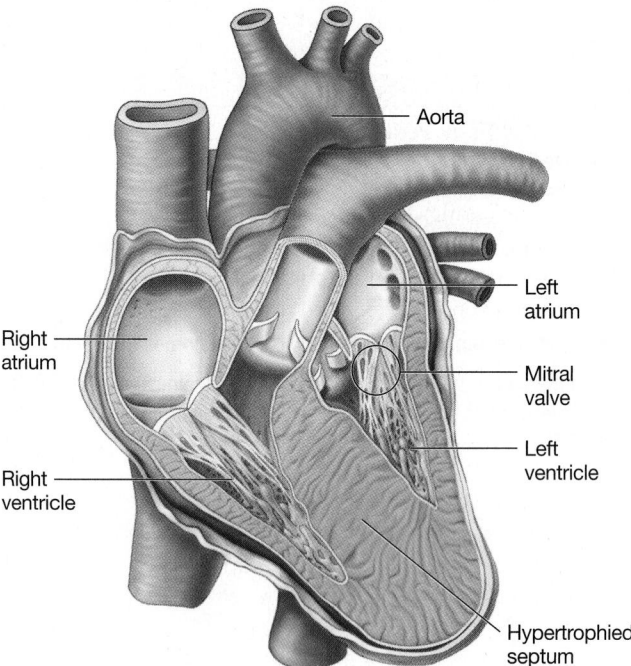

(b) Hypertrophied septum

FIGURE 41–13 ■ (a) Normal heart wall and (b) hypertrophied heart wall.

Close blood relatives (parents, children, or siblings) of someone with HCM often also have enlarged ventricular septums. In the majority of patients, hypertrophic cardiomyopathy is transmitted as an autosomal dominant trait.

Hypertrophic cardiomyopathy also can be caused by hypertension or hypoparathyroidism, and it frequently is idiopathic.

This condition is most commonly found in young adults, but it can also occur in the very young and in the aged population. Men and the black population are affected more by HCM. It is usually diagnosed in young adulthood in more active athletic individuals.

Hypertrophic obstructive cardiomyopathy has the same etiology as HCM, although these patients have the additional problem of having the left ventricular aortic outflow tract obstructed. This form of cardiomyopathy occurs in 1 in 500 persons with HCM in the United States (Lakkis, Nagueh, & Klieman, 1998). The pathophysiology of this type of cardiomyopathy is described next.

Pathophysiology

With HCM the walls of the ventricle hypertrophy or remodel, without an increase in the chamber size. Fibrotic infiltrates in the myocardium produce left ventricular stiffness and add to the hypertrophy of the wall and septum. One unique feature of HCM is that the cardiac muscle may not hypertrophy "equally." The interventricular septum, especially the upper portion, tends to have a greater increase in size than the free wall of the left ventricle. These changes result in a decreased ventricular chamber size and cause the ventricles to take a longer period of time to relax. The end result is diastolic dysfunction because the loss of ventricular compliance decreases the amount of blood that will flow into the ventricle during diastole. This has a direct negative effect on cardiac output and, thus, tissue perfusion. Another characteristic of HCM is hypercontractility of the muscle, rather than hypocontractility as seen in dilated cardiomyopathy. The hypercontractility occurs particularly in the intraventricular system.

A third characteristic of HCM is obstruction to the outflow tract of the left ventricle (LV) leading into the aorta. The site and extent of hypertrophy dictates the degree of obstruction. The hypertrophy distorts the septum, and in some patients, the anterior leaflet of the mitral valve is distorted, causing it to meet the septum, thus narrowing the left ventricular outflow tract during systole (Barkman & McCay, 2002). This occurs because of the inward movement of the septum during systole, which narrows the LV outflow and increases blood velocity. This increased velocity then pulls the mitral leaflet toward the septum (the venturi effect). Figure 41–14 ■ demonstrates how the septum and the anterior leaflet narrow the left ventricular outflow tract into the aorta.

Significant LV outflow obstruction is present in some patients at rest, while in others it is only evident during increased activity such as exercise. Reduced preload decreases chamber size and increased heart rate will increase LV outflow obstruction. Dehydration and suddenly sitting upright (orthostatic hypotension) are two examples of factors that will decrease preload, and fever and exercise are two factors that increase heart rate. The end result is a reduction in cardiac output that may range from minimal to severe and may lead to syncope, serious cardiac arrhythmias (ventricular tachycardia), and sudden death. Heart failure is the eventual outcome as the disease progresses. Not all individuals with HCM have obstruction to outflow, but if present, HCM is further classified as hypertrophic obstructive cardiomyopathy. If the obstructive process is present, the disorder is also referred to as idiopathic hypertrophic subaortic stenosis (see Figure 41–14 ■).

Clinical Manifestations

Clinical manifestations most commonly begin in late adolescence or early adulthood, but may appear at any age. Many of the clinical manifestations of HCM are similar to dilated cardiomyopathy. The most frequently reported manifestation is

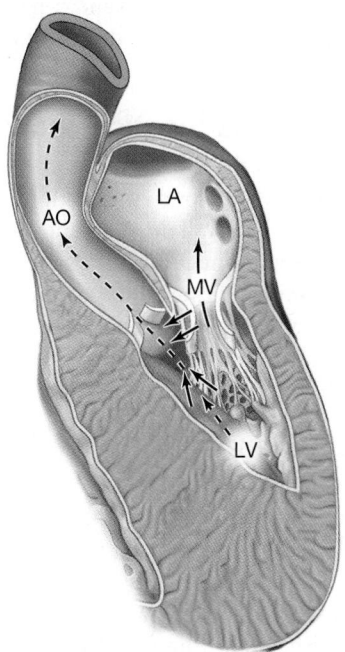

FIGURE 41–14 ■ Hypertrophic obstructive cardiomyopathy.

dyspnea, which is due to high pulmonary pressures created by the backup of blood from the restricted left ventricle. This type of cardiomyopathy also may occur without symptoms, although other frequently reported symptoms include chest pain, dizziness, presyncope or syncope, fatigue, orthopnea and paroxysmal nocturnal dyspnea, and palpitations. The symptoms appear gradually, will progress over time, and are associated with deterioration of LV function. Exercise tends to precipitate the symptoms and increases the risk of sudden death. But in some individual's sudden death or severe heart failure are the first clinical manifestations of the disease. Right- and left-sided heart failure may be present. The risk of sudden death, which appears most often in young adults, can be decreased by avoiding strenuous exercise. Sudden death is the most common cause of death for individuals with HCM.

Both supraventricular (primarily atrial fibrillation) and ventricular (tachycardia and fibrillation) dysrhythmias occur with HCM, along with sudden death. Additionally, it is common to have an abnormally forceful LV apical pulse, S_4, and a harsh crescendo–decrescendo systolic murmur of varying intensity that is heard best at the left lower sternal border and the apex. A systolic thrill may be palpated at the apex or lower left sternal border.

In severe cases of HOCM, pulmonary artery pressures are elevated because of increased backward pressure due to an inability of the left ventricle to empty. This eventually increases right ventricular pressure, causing the interventricular septum to shift to the left. The leftward shift causes further obstruction to the ventricular outflow tract (Barkman & McCay, 2002).

Adults with HCM were followed for 9 to 11 years by a group of researchers. The researchers found that patients who were asymptomatic had a lower cardiac mortality rate and a lower incidence of sudden cardiac death than those individuals with symptoms (Takagi, Yamakado, & Nakano, 1999). There is not a predictable correlation between the degree of obstruction and symptoms.

Laboratory and Diagnostic Procedures

The echocardiogram is the most useful tool when diagnosing both HCM and HOCM. It allows visualization of the LV hypertrophy and will also reveal wall motion abnormalities and diastolic dysfunction. Due to the progressive nature of the disease, bedside hemodynamic studies are done to monitor the pressures in cardiac chambers and the pulmonary system as well as providing ongoing cardiac output readings. The remainder of the tests are described in the Diagnostic Tests box.

Medical Management

Preventing heart failure and sudden cardiac death are the primary goals of treatment for patients with HCM. Improving the cardiac output is achieved by reducing ventricular contractility and relieving LV outflow obstruction. These measures improve ventricular filling and ultimately cardiac output and the quality of life. It is often difficult for young adults to adhere to a regimen of decreased activity. Emotional support and education are essential by both the nurses and the health care providers to help the individual understand and comply with the reduced activity levels.

If possible, finding and treating the underlying cause is the first priority of medical management. The remainder of medical care is directed toward controlling clinical manifestations, preventing progression of the disease, and improving the quality of life for the individual. The treatment plan, described below, consists of medications, activity restriction, fluid stabilization, surgical interventions, and possibly implanting electronic devices. Genetic testing for HCM is discussed in the Genetic Considerations box.

Negative inotropic medications, such as beta-adrenergic blocking agents and calcium antagonists, provide the mainstay of medical therapy and are used to decrease the hypercontractility and outflow obstruction. These medications also decrease the heart rate, which decreases cardiac workload and oxygen consumption. If the patient is in atrial fibrillation, anticoagulant medications are prescribed to assist in the prevention of clot formation. Antiarrhythmic medications are used to prevent life-threatening dysrhythmias and improve cardiac output and ICDs are used to prevent sudden cardiac death. Finally, HCM predisposes patients to endocarditis. Therefore, the health care

GENETIC CONSIDERATIONS for Hypertrophic Cardiomyopathy

Due to the genetic link of hypertrophic cardiomyopathy, the health care provider needs to test close family members for the disease. Family teaching needs to include CPR classes (National Institute on Alcohol Abuse and Alcoholism, 2002).

DIAGNOSTIC TESTS for Hypertrophic and Hypertrophic Obstructive Cardiomyopathy

Test with *Normal Values*	Expected Abnormality	Rationale for Abnormality
Chest x-ray: *Clear lungs and normal heart size*	Cardiac enlargement (cardiomegaly) specifically left atrial enlargement. If heart failure is present, pulmonary congestion and edema.	Due to progression of the disease process.
Resting and ambulatory ECG: *Normal conduction time intervals* (see Chapter 38)	*Resting:* Increased voltage and duration of the QRS complex. Both atrial and ventricular dysrhythmias. *Ambulatory:* ST segment changes that occur with increased activity. Increased hypercontractility that increases with activity.	Due to the ventricular hypertrophy and myocardial ischemia.
Echocardiogram (ultrasound): *Normal chamber size and normal cardiac structures*	Left ventricular hypertrophy. Hypercontractility. Asymmetrical wall size. Diastolic dysfunction.	The disease causes enlargement of the chamber and septum and hypercontractility, which results in abnormal valve function and cardiac output.
Cardiac catheterization to rule out coronary artery disease, assess hemodynamic status, and chamber size and function: *Normal coronary arteries, chambers, and valve pressures*	Increased chamber size and may see changes in valve function and cardiac output.	Tissue hypertrophy and hypercontractility cause abnormal valve motion, resulting in obstruction of the aortic outflow tract.
Radionuclide study: *Normal chamber volumes and blood perfusion to cardiac muscle*	Increased left ventricular and septal wall size. Asymmetrical hypertrophy. Hypercontractility.	Tissue hypertrophy and hypercontractility related to disease process.
Cardiac biopsy may be performed in order to analyze myocardial tissue: *Normal cellular size and function*	Tissue positive for infiltrations and fibrosis.	Changes due to disease process.

provider typically orders prophylactic antibiotics before dental work or invasive procedures (AHA, 2004).

Dehydration needs to be avoided because it will decrease preload and cardiac output. Patient and family education needs to stress the importance of consistent normal hydration. Activities, foods, and drinks (alcohol) that cause dehydration must be avoided. Surgical management is indicated for HCM if the patient has not responded positively to medical therapy and if marked obstruction to the aortic outflow tract is present due to the mitral valve meeting the enlarged septum. The surgical procedure is termed a ventriculomyotomy and involves excising some of the hypertrophied septal muscle. This widens the LV outflow tract, improves cardiac output, and relieves symptoms. Clinical manifestations and exercise tolerance are improved after this surgery in about 75% of cases (Braunwald, et al., 2005). A second surgical procedure sometimes used to decrease obstruction is the removal of the mitral valve, chordae tendineae, and the papillary muscle (see Figure 41–4 ■, p. 1234). The mitral valve is then replaced by an artificial valve. This procedure substantially reduces the space taken up by the mitral valve and supporting structures, allowing blood to move more easily around the enlarged septum. In addition to surgical complications, the primary problem of both of these procedures is dysrhythmias.

A nonsurgical treatment for HCM is alcohol ablation involving injection of alcohol down a small branch of the coronary artery feeding the area of muscle hypertrophy (septum). The alcohol destroys the extra cardiac muscle without having to surgically remove it, in effect causing an intentional myocardial infarction (Lewis, Boyd, Hubert, & Steele, 2001; Steinbis, 2003).

An implantable cardioverter defibrillator is useful for patients with HCM to treat ventricular tachycardia, ventricular fibrillation, and sudden death (American College of Cardiology [ACC], 2006; Saxton, Kumar, & DeMarco, 2006). If left ventricular dysfunction and ejection fraction less than 35% are present, a cardiac resynchronization therapy (CRT) (biventricular pacemaker) may help increase cardiac output (ACC, 2006; Saxton et al., 2006). Some experts believe with advanced heart failure a combination of an ICD and CRT is indicated (Saxton et al., 2006). Chapter 39 ⊚ provides complete descriptions of both the ICD and the pacemaker. Heart transplantation is the only long-term cure for the disease. Heart transplantation is described in Chapter 42 ⊚ .

■ Nursing Management

The primary goals of nursing care are to assess and monitor progress of the disease and to provide patient education and emotional support for individuals with this chronic progressive disease. The nursing process provides a framework for the care of these patients. A complete plan of care for HCM is outlined in this chapter in the Nursing Process: Patient Care Plan for Cardiomyopathy (p. 1259).

Assessment

Nurses must monitor and report changes in the assessment that indicate complications and progression of the disease. Specific nursing assessment data, interventions, rationales, and outcomes are outlined in the Nursing Process: Patient Care Plan for Cardiomyopathy (p. 1259) and are also reviewed in Chapter 42 ⊚ .

Monitoring the patient's hemodynamic status is essential as the disease progresses. Pulmonary artery pressure increases indicate the onset of heart failure, which increases the risk of further ventricular outflow obstruction. Moreover, the cardiac output needs ongoing monitoring to evaluate oxygenation and adequate tissue perfusion. The nurse needs to space activities for the hospitalized patient in order to allow for periods of rest.

The nursing diagnoses that apply to HCM include:

1. *Activity Intolerance, Risk for*
2. *Tissue Perfusion Ineffective, Cardiac and Peripheral*
3. *Coping*
4. *Fatigue*

Outcomes and Evaluation Parameters

Due to the risk of cardiac sudden death, both HCM and HOCM have a grave prognosis. End-stage therapies such as cardiac transplantation may be a viable option. The patient and family need to be given all options and the nurse must assess their understanding of the situation. Evaluation parameters would include a verbalization of the options including the lifestyle changes that would be necessary with organ transplantation.

Planning, Interventions, and Rationales

Providing emotional support for the patient with HCM is essential when planning the management of these patients, since this is a progressive chronic disease that could cause sudden death at anytime. Identifying perceived stressors for both the family and patient and assisting them in alleviating them will decrease the emotional stress. The patient and family need to feel free to verbalize fears and concerns and be reassured that these concerns are legitimate and that there are resources available to provide assistance. Providing realistic hope helps reduce anxiety and increase self-esteem; the patient needs to be encouraged to accomplish a goal no matter how small. If the patient is facing imminent death or waiting for a donor heart, an environment must be created in which the patient and family can openly express concerns and acknowledge fears. Encouragement, a caring touch, and a listening ear will improve the quality of life for patients and families dealing with HCM. See the Nursing Process: Patient Care Plan for Cardiomyopathy (p. 1259) for a complete nursing care plan to guide the care of patients with HCM and HOCM.

 *Families of patients with HCM and HOCM should be encouraged to learn CPR and how to access emergency care near their home.*

■ Restrictive Cardiomyopathy

Restrictive cardiomyopathy (RCM) is the least common type found in the United States. This disorder is characterized by endocardial scarring that usually affects one or both ventricles and restricts filling of blood, resulting in systolic dysfunction. The ventricle has normal wall thickness, but the walls are rigid, producing elevated filling pressures and dilated atria. Involvement of the valve is common, but the outflow tract is spared (see Figure 41–12 ■, p. 1255).

Epidemiology and Etiology

The cause of restrictive cardiomyopathy is divided into two classifications, primary and secondary. The cause of primary restrictive cardiomyopathy is idiopathic, whereas secondary cardiomyopathy is thought to be caused by a number of pathologic processes outlined below. Idiopathic restrictive cardiomyopathy can present at any age, but its incidence is increased in the elderly and is more common in women (Ammash, Seward, & Bailey, 2000).

The incidence of cocaine-related restrictive cardiomyopathy is on the rise. Cocaine causes both coronary artery and peripheral vasoconstriction and high levels of circulating catecholamines. The combined effect causes an increased workload for the myocardium and a decreased supply of oxygen, leading to myocardial ischemia and infarction. The cells of the myocardium become damaged, producing cardiomyopathy. These patients typically have a poor prognosis.

Pathophysiology

The development and progress of secondary RCM may be caused by amyloidosis, endomyocardial fibrosis, disorders in glycogen storage, hemochromatosis, and sarcoidosis or it may be idiopathic. With amyloidosis, a deposition of eosinophilic fibrinous protein buildup occurs in the heart, causing loss of an ability to stretch. Idiopathic restrictive cardiomyopathy is a poorly recognized entity of unknown cause characterized by nondilated, nonhypertrophied ventricles with diastolic dysfunction, resulting in dilated atria, with or without systolic dysfunction (Ammash et al., 2000). Contractility is unaffected by restrictive cardiomyopathy.

Microscopically, the endometrial changes that occur with restrictive cardiomyopathy include nonspecific patchy endocardial and interstitial fibrosis with increased collagen deposition and molecular hypertrophy. These changes result in the ventricle losing its ability to stretch, thereby decreasing compliance and an ability to fill, and causing a drop in cardiac output. As intraventricular pressures increase and cardiac output decreases,

manifestations of heart failure begin to appear. These manifestations typically progress rapidly, resulting in high mortality.

Clinical Manifestations

Patients with RCM have signs of pulmonary and systemic congestion. The most common symptom is dyspnea. In addition, patients complain of palpitations, fatigue, syncope, angina, generalized weakness, and exercise intolerance. In the advanced stages, clinical manifestations of either or both right- or left-sided heart failure are present. An S_3 is frequently present, and a systolic murmur from mitral and tricuspid regurgitation is common.

Laboratory and Diagnostic Procedures

As with all of the cardiomyopathies, the echocardiogram is the most useful diagnostic test for the diagnosis of restrictive cardiomyopathy. It reveals a thickened cardiac wall, a small ventricular chamber size, and dilated atria. This test also is able to evaluate diastolic filling changes as the disease progresses. The echocardiogram is also useful in distinguishing restrictive cardiomyopathy from constrictive pericarditis, the major disorder that mimics restrictive cardiomyopathy. Hemodynamic studies identify elevated left atrial and left ventricular pressures. The Diagnostic Tests box describes the remainder of the diagnostic tests for restrictive cardiomyopathy.

Medical Management

Currently there is no specific treatment or cure for RCM. Therefore, therapy is aimed at controlling symptoms to improve the quality of life. Like hypertrophic cardiomyopathy, restrictive cardiomyopathy patients are taught to avoid situations that impair venous filling, causing a further drop in cardiac output. The patient and family need to have a clear understanding that activity such as strenuous exercise, as well as any situation that causes dehydration, needs to be avoided.

Medical management is aimed at reducing pulmonary and systemic congestion and reducing the workload of the heart to di-

DIAGNOSTIC TESTS for Restrictive Cardiomyopathy

Test with *Normal Values*	Expected Abnormality	Rationale for Abnormality
Chest x-ray: *Clear lungs and normal heart size*	Cardiomegaly, specifically atrial enlargement. Pulmonary venous congestion. Pleural effusions may be present with heart failure.	Restriction of blood flow leading to pulmonary venous backup of blood and resulting in cardiac enlargement heart failure.
Electrocardiogram (ECG): *Normal conduction time intervals* (see Chapter 38)	Atrial fibrillation. Complex serious ventricular dysrhythmias. Tachycardia.	Distortion of the cardiac conduction system due to cardiomegaly. Cardiac ischemia causing dysrhythmias.
Echocardiogram: *Normal chamber size and normal cardiac structures*	Thickened cardiac wall. Small ventricular chamber size. Dilated atria. Decreased diastolic filling as disease progresses.	Restrictive nature of disease increases wall thickness and prevents myocardial fiber stretch to accommodate blood volumes. Blood backs up in atria causing it to dilate.
Radionuclide study: *Normal chamber volumes and blood perfusion to cardiac muscle*	Increased ventricular volume mass, decreasing chamber size. Areas of decreased perfusion.	Restrictive nature of disease prevents myocardial fiber stretch to accommodate blood volumes, causing decreased cardiac output and tissue perfusion.
Endomyocardial biopsy: *Normal myocardial tissue*	Presence of amyloidosis and/or sarcoidosis.	Causative agents for disease.

minish heart failure. There is not a medical cure for this disease, although treatment of the underlying cause of secondary restrictive cardiomyopathy may be beneficial.

The cornerstone of the medical treatment for RCM is drug therapy. Antiarrhythmic medications are prescribed, depending on the specific dysrhythmia. Diuretics are used to decrease pulmonary congestion, although the patient has to be monitored closely to prevent dehydration. Calcium channel blockers and beta-adrenergic blockers will decrease the heart rate, which then increases ventricular filling time. Anticoagulants are indicated for patients in atrial fibrillation to prevent thromboembolism (p. 1270). A low-sodium diet will decrease fluid retention and pulmonary congestion.

As with dilated cardiomyopathy, the heart failure from restrictive cardiomyopathy may be treated with a biventricular pacemaker. An implantable cardioverter defibrillator may be indicated to prevent sudden cardiac death (Chapter 39).

Both primary and secondary restrictive cardiomyopathies have a poor prognosis. Death is most frequently due to heart failure, sudden death, dysrhythmias, or stroke. End-stage heart failure strategies are more fully discussed in Chapter 42 .

PHARMACOLOGY   Summary of Medications to Treat Cardiomyopathy

Medication Category	Action	Application/Indication	Nursing Responsibility

Cardiomyopathy
 Cardiac Medications
 ACE inhibitors, angiotensin receptor blockers:
   Losartan
   Candesartan
   Irbesartan
   Valsartan
   Beta-adrenergic blockers
   Metoprolol tartrate
   (Carvedilol)
   Calcium channel blockers
   Antiarrhythmic agents
   Amiodarone
   Dofetilide
	ACE inhibitor:
	 Lowers peripheral resistance and reduces blood volume by enhancing the excretion of sodium by inhibition of angiotensin-converting enzyme.
	 Slows the heart rate. Decreases conduction through AV node. Increases force and velocity of myocardial systolic contraction. Reduces automaticity in the SA node and slows impulse conduction through the AV node. Used for supraventricular dysrhythmias.
		Dilated cardiomyopathy (DCM): slows or stops tissue remodeling and heart failure.
		 Decreases preload and afterload.
		 Arrhythmogenic right ventricular cardiomyopathy (ARVC): heart failure.
		 DCM: reduces heart failure symptoms; lower risk of mortality, sudden death; and delays need for transplant. Slow or stop tissue remodeling.
		 Hypertrophic cardiomyopathy/ hypertrophic obstructive cardiomyopathy (HCM/HOCM): decreases hypercontractility and outflow obstruction.
		 Also decreases the heart rate, which decreases cardiac workload and oxygen consumption.
		 Restrictive cardiomyopathy (RCM): decreases heart rate, which then increases ventricular filling time.
		 ARVC: tachyarrhythmias.
		 HCM/HOCM: decreases the hypercontractility and outflow obstruction.
		 Also decreases the heart rate, which decreases cardiac workload and oxygen consumption.
		 RCM: decreases heart rate, which then increases ventricular filling time.
		 DCM: helps control atrial and ventricular irritability, decreasing dysrhythmias.
		 HCM/HOCM/RCM: to prevent life-threatening dysrhythmias and improve cardiac output.
		 ARVC: tachyarrhythmias.
			Monitor blood pressure carefully after first dose for hypotension.
			 Educate patient that it takes 2 weeks for therapeutic effect.
			 May experience dizziness.
			 Monitor vital signs; observe for bradycardia, heart failure, or pulmonary edema.
			 Monitor orthostatic hypotension.
			 Assess fatigue and weakness.
			 Monitor intake and output.
			 Assess heart rate, blood pressure, lung sounds, and ECG monitor regularly.
			 Monitor for hypotension especially when being given intravenously.

Diuretics	Blocks reabsorption of sodium and chloride in the loop of Henle. Reduces edema associated with heart failure.	*DCM /HCM/HOCM/RCM:* to decrease pulmonary congestion. *ARVC:* right heart failure.	Potassium levels also need monitoring because low levels are a side effect of certain diuretics, especially furosemide. May need potassium replacement. Measure urine output prior to administration to gauge the response to the medication.

(continued)

PHARMACOLOGY Summary of Medications to Treat Cardiomyopathy—*Continued*

Anticoagulant Therapy Coumadin Heparin	Can either inhibit specific clotting factors in coagulation cascade or diminish the clotting action of platelets.	*HCM/HOCM/RCM:* if atrial fibrillation present, used to decrease clot formation.	Ongoing assessment of therapeutic blood level per health care provider orders. Assess for bleeding including nosebleeds, bruising, "coffee-grounds" emesis, tarry stools, fatigue, and pale skin. Assess for decreases in hemoglobin, hematocrit, RBCs, and platelets.
Nitrates (nitroglycerin)	Relaxes both atrial and venous smooth muscle, causing decreased preload and afterload.	*DCM:* decreases preload and afterload.	Assess blood pressure before and during therapy. Hypotension could result. Should be given with other vasodilators. Patient education includes: No alcohol use. Rotate patches. Keep medication with you at all times and away from excessive heat and light. Report blurred vision, dry mouth, and severe headache.
Antibiotics	Inhibits protein synthesis of microorganisms by binding reversibly to a ribosome, thus interfering with transmission of genetic information.	*HCM/HOCM:* predisposed to endocarditis so prophylactic antibiotics before dental work or invasive procedures are prescribed.	Assessment of history of drug allergies prior to administration. Assessment of clinical manifestations of allergic reaction. Assessment of relief of clinical manifestations to determine drug effectiveness. Patient education regarding need to complete the entire regimen and report any clinical manifestations of drug allergy.

Sources: Adams, M. P., Josephen, D. L., & Holland, L. N. (Eds.). (2005). *Pharmacology for nurses: A pathophysiologic approach.* Upper Saddle River, NJ: Pearson Prentice Hall; American Heart Association. (2005). *Handbook of emergency cardiovascular care for health providers.* Dallas, TX: Author; Wilson, B., Shannon, M., & Stang, C. (Eds.). (2005). *Nurses drug guide.* Upper Saddle River, NJ: Pearson Prentice Hall.

◼ Nursing Management

Nursing management focuses on decreasing the workload of the heart and conserving energy. Nursing care is similar to the care of the patient with the other types of cardiomyopathy. The Nursing Process: Patient Care Plan for Cardiomyopathy (p. 1259) outlines the care for all types of cardiomyopathy and the discharge priorities are presented in the Patient Teaching & Discharge Priorities box.

◼ Arrhythmogenic Right Ventricular Cardiomyopathy

Arrhythmogenic right ventricular cardiomyopathy (ARVC) is a newly recognized heart disease. It is defined as an electrical disturbance that develops when the muscle tissue in the right ventricle is replaced with fibrous scar and fatty tissues. In approximately 30% of patients, the left ventricle also is involved (Bruce, 2006).

ARVC has several different names, all of which refer to the same condition. These names include arrhythmogenic right ventricular dysplasia/cardiomyopathy (ARVD/C) and arrhythmogenic right ventricular dysplasia (ARVD). It is becoming usual practice for the disease to be known as ARVC (Cardiomyopathy Association, 2006).

Epidemiology and Etiology

The precise cause of ARVC is unknown, although it has a possible familial link in some patients. The onset of the disease typically is between the late teens to early 20s. It is rare for it to develop in early childhood or after age 40. It appears that men and women of any ethnic origin can be affected. When more than one member of the family is affected, the mode of inheritance appears to be an autosomal dominant gene (Bruce, 2006; Cardiomyopathy Association, 2006).

Because little is known about the disease, it is difficult to estimate how many people are affected. It is reasonable to estimate in the light of current knowledge that approximately 1 in 3,000 to 1 in 10,000 people are affected (Cardiomyopathy Association, 2006). Certain areas of the world have a higher incidence of the disease; these include Venice, Italy, and parts of Greece.

Pathophysiology

Patchy areas of fat develop primarily on the right ventricle, replacing functional cardiac muscle. The specific reason for this occurrence is under investigation. One theory suggests that an abnormal gene or genes leads to heart muscle cell damage and loss. The fibrous and fatty tissues are thought to replace these heart muscle cells as an attempt by the body to repair the dam-

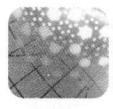

PATIENT TEACHING & DISCHARGE PRIORITIES for Cardiomyopathy

Need	Teaching
Prevention of disease progression	Teach the importance of following a treatment plan that includes medications (that slow disease progression) and lifestyle changes.
	Teaching includes:
	• Timed rest periods between activities.
	• Space activities to prevent dyspnea.
	• Avoid alcohol and drug use (cocaine).
	• Restrict sodium and fluid intake to prevent fluid overload.
Compliance with therapy	Teach the importance of complying with the treatment plan in order to slow the progress of the disease and prevent sudden death.
	Determine motivation factors for individual patients and create a plan that utilizes these factors.
	Comply with follow-up health care provider visits.
Prevent exacerbation of heart failure	Explain to patient/family what clinical manifestations to monitor and report to the health care worker:
	• Sudden increase in weight in a short period of time; i.e., greater than 2–3 lb in a few days
	• Shortness of breath at rest, possibly with chest pressure
	• Increased shortness of breath with activities
	• Persistent productive cough
	• Swelling ankles, feet, or abdomen
	• Waking breathless at night.
	Diet therapy: limit sodium to 2–3 g and 2 liters of fluid daily. Eat small, frequent meals.
	Plan rest periods between activities.
Reportable clinical manifestations	Clinical manifestations of heart failure (Chapter 42 ⊕).
	Clinical manifestations of infective endocarditis.
	New onset chest pain.

age. Once the muscle has been replaced, the areas become hypokinetic. Given the patchy nature of ARVC, abnormal areas may be surrounded by normal ones. Right ventricular thickening occurs early in the disease, and as the disease progresses it may involve the left ventricle. The patchy disorganized structure of the myocardium areas of the right ventricle may lead to one or more sites of abnormal electrical activity, accounting for abnormal ECG rhythm disturbances and abnormal contractile ability.

Clinical Manifestations

The degree and type of clinical manifestations and the risk of complications vary greatly among individuals with ARVC. Many patients report little to no difficulties or manifestations, whereas others have life-threatening problems. Typically, patients seek help for palpitations, light-headedness, and fatigue. More serious symptoms include syncope and symptoms of heart failure. The ECG exhibits complete or incomplete right bundle branch block. A signal-averaged ECG is abnormal. Patients may present with ventricular tachycardia that generally has a left bundle branch block contour, with T waves inverted over the right precordial leads. The ventricular tachycardia may be due to reentry. Supraventricular arrhythmias also can occur, and exercise can induce the ventricular tachycardia in some patients. Chapter 38 ⊕ provides an in-depth description of these dysrhythmias. Sudden cardiac death is the most serious complication of ARVC and at times the very first sign of the disease. It is generally believed that sporting activities do not cause ARVC, although the condition is reported more frequently among athletes compared to other groups of people (Cardiomyopathy Association, 2006).

Heart failure is a less common complication of ARVC and appears to occur later in the disease. Typically, right heart failure first is more common than left heart failure and is manifested by prominent visible veins in the neck; distention of the liver, which may lead to a sensation of fullness or discomfort in the upper abdomen; and swollen legs or ankles. Left heart failure occurs late when the disease is in the advanced stages and is manifested by fatigue and shortness of breath (see Chapter 42 ⊕).

Laboratory and Diagnostic Procedures

Research is showing that an MRI is a useful noninvasive test for diagnosis detection of right ventricular myocardial fibro-fatty changes in ARVD/C (Cardiomyopathy Association, 2006). The MRI has a strong correlation with histopathology and predicted inducible ventricular tachycardia (VT) on programmed electrical stimulation (Tandri et al., 2005). It has the unique ability to characterize tissue, specifically by differentiating fat from muscle. The echocardiogram also is a useful tool to assist in the diagnosis because it allows for visualization of the right ventricle and assessment of wall motion abnormalities. Due to the cardiac conduction changes that are associated with ARVC, serial ECGs are indicated to detect rhythm changes and serious life-threatening dysrhythmias. The remainder of the tests are described in the Diagnostic Tests box (p. 1270).

Medical Management

Other than heart transplant, there is no cure for ARVC, so medical management is aimed at controlling clinical manifestations and progression of the disease. Due to the familial nature of

DIAGNOSTIC TESTS for Arrhythmogenic Right Ventricular Cardiomyopathy

Test with *Normal Values*	Expected Abnormality	Rationale for Abnormality
Electrocardiogram (ECG): *Holter monitor:* ambulatory recording of the ECG over 24 to 48 hours. Exercise ECG: *Normal conduction time intervals* (see Chapter 38 ⊙)	Repolarization and depolarization abnormalities. Intraventricular conduction delay. Complete or incomplete right bundle branch block. Lethal ventricular dysrhythmias.	Dysrhythmias occur due to changes in the structure of the myocardial tissue causing abnormal conduction patterns. To detect exercise-induced ventricular dysrhythmias and assess functional capacity.
Cardiac catheterization and electrophysiological study (EPS)	Able to rule out coronary artery disease. Right ventricular dilation and dysfunction. *EPS:* able to induce the dysrhythmias. (Chapter 39 ⊙ discusses these tests.)	Determines the presence of other causes for the clinical manifestations. Fatty infiltration changes to myocardium cause ventricular dilation. Determines which drug will control the dysrhythmias.
Endomyocardial biopsy: *Normal cardiac tissue*	Fibrous scars and fatty infiltration changes to right ventricular myocardium.	Due to disease process.
Echocardiogram: *Normal chamber size and normal cardiac structures*	Dilated right and left ventricles with diminished contractility.	Due to fibrous scarring and fatty infiltrations to the myocardium.
Magnetic resonance imaging (MRI): *Normal cardiac tissue and chamber size*	Right ventricular myocardial fibro-fatty change.	Due to fibrous scarring and fatty infiltrations to the myocardium.
Exercise radionuclide study: *Normal chamber volumes and blood perfusion to cardiac muscle*	To detect exercise-induced ventricular dysrhythmias and assess functional capacity.	Detects changes that occur only with exercise.
Chest x-ray: *Clear lungs and normal heart size*	Cardiomegaly.	Due to fibrous scarring and fatty infiltrations to the myocardium.

Sources: Bruce, J. (2006). Getting to the heart of cardiomyopathy: Find out about the four types of cardiomyopathies. *Cardiac Insider,* pp. 16–20; Tandri, H., Saranathan, M., Rodriguez, E. R., Martinez, C., Bomma, C., Nasir, K., et al. (2005, January 4). Noninvasive detection of myocardial fibrosis in arrhythmogenic right ventricular cardiomyopathy using delayed-enhancement magnetic resonance imaging. *Journal of the America College of Cardiology, 45*(1), 98–103.

ARVC, medical management begins with an in-depth medical and family history. The heath care provider needs to assess any personal or family history of palpitations, light-headed sensation, or collapse.

Because the clinical manifestations and risk of sudden cardiac death vary with ARVC, there are no precise guidelines to determine which patients need to be treated and which is the best management approach. Established therapeutic options include beta-adrenergic blockers, antiarrhythmic drugs, catheter ablation, and an ICD. Pharmacologic therapy is the first choice of treatment for patients with well-tolerated and non–life-threatening ventricular arrhythmias. Treatment includes beta-adrenergic blockers and class I and III antiarrhythmic drugs (sotalol or amiodarone) alone or in combination with beta-adrenergic blockers. If heart failure is present, the patient is treated with diuretics and vasodilators. Typically, medication efficacy is based on symptom improvement, although a more reliable approach is the use of 24-hour Holter monitoring or stress testing to determine the effect of life activities and stress on arrhythmic events. Chapter 38 ⊙ discusses Holter monitoring.

Due to the risk for sudden cardiac death, in patients with sustained ventricular tachycardia (VT) and/or ventricular fibrillation (VF), antiarrhythmic drug treatment is indicated. Additionally, the need for electrophysiology (EPS) guided drug testing must be evaluated. The EPS is an invasive procedure that is done in the cardiac catheterization laboratory. It involves placing multiple multipolar catheter electrodes into the venous and sometimes the arterial side of the heart. These electrodes are positioned at various locations inside of the heart and they have two purposes: to record the electrical signal within the heart and to deliver an electrical stimulus at precisely timed intervals (programmed stimulation), which may or may not result in the initiation of VT/VF. This procedure identifies the location of the dysrhythmia. Antiarrhythmic drugs are administered followed by a second attempt to induce the dysrhythmia. If the dysrhythmia is not inducible, the drug is considered effective. Currently EPS is the standard test for reproducing dysrhythmias in a controlled environment in order to diagnose and treat the dysrhythmias.

Nonpharmacologic treatment is reserved for those patients with life-threatening ventricular dysrhythmias in whom drug treatment is either ineffective, is not applicable because of the inability to induce the clinical ventricular arrhythmias during EPS, or is associated with serious side effects. If the dysrhythmia remains inducible in patients with sustained VT and/or VF during EPS, other options are available. Pace mapping directed radio-frequency catheter ablation and ICD are the current options. Radio-frequency catheter ablation is a procedure done in the cardiac catheterization laboratory in which areas in the myocardium that initiate dysrhythmias are identified and destroyed with chemicals or electrical energy. The goal is to eliminate sites in the myocardium that initiate the dysrhythmia, thereby eliminating the dysrhythmia (AHA, 2006b). The implantable cardioverter defibrillator Radio-frequency ablation is a device that can automatically terminate potentially lethal dysrhythmias of VT and VF. It is considered safe and improves the long-term prognosis of ARVC patients at high risk of sudden death (Wichter et al., 2004). A complete description of ICDs is given in Chapter 39 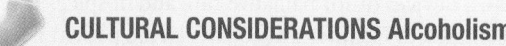. When all medical options have been exhausted, ARVC patients may be candidates for heart transplantation (Bruce, 2006).

Nursing Management

As with all types of cardiomyopathy, nursing management focuses on decreasing the workload of the heart and conserving energy. Additionally, these patients need to be monitored carefully for cardiac dysrhythmias. Nursing care is similar to the care of the patient with the other types of cardiomyopathy. The Nursing Process: Patient Care Plan for Cardiomyopathy feature (p. 1259) outlines the care of all four types of cardiomyopathy, and the discharge priorities are presented in the earlier Patient Teaching & Discharge Priorities box (p. 1269).

Health Promotion for the Cardiomyopathies

The chronicity of a cardiomyopathy has an impact on the quality of life for both the patient and the family/significant others. The nurse needs to evaluate the impact of the disease on the patient's role within the family and community. Additionally, the nurse needs to involve the family in the treatment plan and educational program. It is essential to identify stressors and attempt to work with the patient and family to relieve them.

Providing appropriate explanations of all treatments and interventions will increase compliance by both the patient and family. Home health nurses can provide the patient and family with an ongoing assessment of the effectiveness of the treatment plan and facilitate changes when necessary. The goal of therapy is to keep the patient functional and out of the hospital, and home health nurses are essential in the accomplishment of that goal.

When educating patients nurses must be knowledgeable about cultural factors that impact the development of cardiomyopathy. The dietary customs and social habits of certain cultures increase the risk for the development and progression of the disease. For example, excessive alcohol intake is a risk factor for the development and progression of dilated cardiomyopathy. Excessive alcohol intake is common in certain cultures. When developing a teaching plan, the nurse needs to evaluate the need for education related to alcohol intake and its impact on DCM. The Cultural Considerations box discusses cultural groups that have a higher rate of alcoholism.

For HCM and ARVC, patient education includes information on the importance of avoiding strenuous exercise in preventing symptoms, dehydration, and possibly lethal complications. Compliance with activity restriction is often difficult for the young adult with these disorders. Education also is necessary for increasing compliance with the medication regimen and dietary sodium restrictions. Patient compliance will help prevent the progression of the disease process and potentially improve the quality of life for the chronic disease. The Pa-

---

CULTURAL CONSIDERATIONS Alcoholism

Cultural Groups with the highest level of alcohol intake include:

American Indians

Alaska Natives

Native Hawaiians

Asian Americans

Note also that:

Alcohol use is increasing significantly among Hispanic adolescents.

Among all age and ethnic groups, men are more likely to drink than are women, and to consume large quantities in a single sitting.

---

tient Teaching & Discharge Priorities box (p. 1269) discussed the discharge priorities and learning needs for patients with cardiomyopathy. Due to the genetic predisposition of HCM and ARVC, family members need to be educated about being tested for the disease.

Collaborative Management

Due to the chronic and progressive nature of cardiomyopathy, a collaborative care approach is optimal for management. Utilizing a multidisciplinary team approach, including health care providers, nurses, physical and occupational therapists, psychologists/psychiatrists, dieticians, and pharmacists, will facilitate the best possible quality of life for the patient and the family. It is essential that the health care provider monitor the progression of the cardiomyopathy to determine the treatment plan. Psychiatric counseling may be necessary to assist in lifestyle adjustments necessitated by a chronic disease process. The occupational therapist helps facilitate realistic occupational goals, while the physical therapist assists in the maintenance of optimum conditioning given the activity restrictions.

Because medication is an essential part of the management of cardiomyopathy, the role of the pharmacist is crucial in educating the patient about how to manage the medications and their side effects. Given that heart failure is a common result of cardiomyopathy, the patient/family needs to consult with the dietician about dietary changes needed to control congestion that is exacerbated by excess salt and fluid intake. In addition to the nursing care described above and in the Patient Teaching & Discharge Priorities box (p. 1269) that discusses cardiomyopathy, the nurse plays a pivotal role in coordinating the efforts of the health care team. In the inpatient setting the nurse facilitates communication between the members of the team and the patient/family.

End-of-Life Issues with Cardiomyopathy

Due to the severity and progressive nature of the disease, the risk of sudden cardiac death increases as the disease progresses. Families and significant others need to be encouraged to learn cardiopulmonary resuscitation (CPR) and how to access emergency care near their home. When patients become end stage and are refractory to available therapies, they should be considered for advanced therapies such as cardiac transplantation or permanent mechanical assist devices or for palliative care and hospice. These options are discussed in Chapter 42 ⊕ . Finally, the patient needs to be asked about end-of-life wishes and an advance directive should be signed in advance of a sentinel life-threatening event.

National Guidelines for Cardiomyopathy

Controlling risk factors, healthy habits, and medication and device therapy will assist in the slowing and perhaps preventing the progress of all four types of cardiomyopathy. *Healthy People 2010* (U.S. Department of Health and Human Services [DHHS], 2004) serves as a prevention agenda for the nation with published guidelines for educating this patient population about risk factors such as substance abuse, blood pressure control, diet, and activity restrictions. Nurses need to be knowledgeable about these guidelines and use them for educating patients and families with cardiomyopathy. The National Guidelines box outlines the *Healthy People 2010* guidelines for two controllable causes of DCM.

◼ Gerontological Considerations

The effects of rheumatic fever and episodes of infective endocarditis are often not manifested until later in life. If valve stenosis or regurgitation occurs as a result of these infective processes, symptoms typically follow a slow stable course. In developed countries there is a latent period of 20 to 40 years from the occurrence of rheumatic fever to the onset of symptoms (AHA, 2006a,b). Then it is usually another decade before symptoms become disabling. Once significant limiting symptoms appear, however, survival rates drop to less than 3 years. This progression of the disease places the manifestations and need for treatment in the final decades of life. A decreased immune response and the existence of other debilitating diseases increase the risk for both medical and surgical complications in the elderly population. The stress of the illness and the normal physiological changes of aging put this group at risk for functional decline during hospitalization. Changes in cardiovascular, respiratory, and renal systems and the prevalence of comorbidities have been cited as possible causes (Cope & Hawley, 2001; Roche, Kramer, Hester, & Welsh, 1999).

Dilated cardiomyopathy is also a disease of the elderly. With the increasing geriatric population, more attention is being given to understanding diastolic failure induced by uncontrolled hypertension and cardiomyopathies. Researchers have demonstrated that the compensatory mechanisms associated with left ventricular diastolic dysfunction lead to elevated right heart pressures and eventually to right heart failure. When heart failure is present, the patient needs to be evaluated to differenti-

---

NATIONAL GUIDELINES for Two Controllable Causes of Dilated Cardiomyopathy

Risk Factor	Guideline
Alcohol intake	Moderate alcohol intake is defined as no more than 1 drink per day for women and no more than 2 drinks per day for men. However, some people should not drink any alcohol, including those who are:
	• Pregnant or trying to become pregnant
	• Taking prescription or over-the-counter medications that may cause harmful reactions when mixed with alcohol
	• Under the age of 21
	• Recovering from alcoholism or are unable to control the amount they drink
	• Suffering from a medical condition that may be worsened by alcohol
	• Driving, planning to drive, or participating in other activities requiring skill, coordination, and alertness.
	Over time, excessive alcohol use can lead to the development of chronic diseases, neurological impairments, and social problems. These include cardiomyopathy.
Substance abuse	Expand research to identify and locate any genetic components that would predispose individuals to the risk of alcoholism and drug addiction.
	Encourage middle/junior high and senior high schools to use science classes to instruct students about the deleterious effects of alcohol and drug abuse on the body.
	Adopt strategies to counter and prevent substance abuse in young people that recognize various risky behaviors on their part as making up a complex whole, to which integrated and congruent approaches are required.
	Ensure that parents are integrated into national strategies against substance abuse by young people as partners on an equal footing with schools, communities, and other concerned elements of society.
	Support studies to determine the long-term biologic consequences for children who are born to mothers addicted to drugs or alcohol.
	Urge all agencies and individuals involved in acting to control substance abuse to begin interventions as soon as possible after the first offense, when success in preventing recurrence is more likely.
	Direct studies toward establishing whether youth exposure to advertisements for alcoholic beverages is altering attitudes about underage drinking and whether this in turn increases underage alcohol use.
	Increase research to explicate the nature and persistence of biologic and electrophysiologic changes in the brains of adolescent and adult abusers of alcohol and drugs.

Source: U.S. Department of Health and Human Services. (2004). *Healthy People 2010 progress report: Substance abuse.* Retrieved June 3, 2006, from http://www.healthypeople.gov/data/2010prog/focus26/holisticonline.com/remedies/Heart/cm causes-of-cardiomyopathy.

ate between ventricular systolic and ventricular diastolic origins of the disease process. This is done to both understand the origins of the heart failure and to guide clinical management. Treatment goals must be directed toward controlling both systolic and diastolic pressures in order to achieve optimum outcomes (Bollinger & Sadar, 2003; Hunt et al., 2005). End-stage cardiomyopathy patients benefit from hospice support (see Chapter 42 ⊕). Chapter 17 ⊕ includes a complete description of services provided by hospice.

■ Research

Research is essential to improve the care, quality of life, and the survival of patients with both inflammatory and structural heart diseases. The goal of research is to identify areas where practice could improve and evaluate and test methods in these areas. The research topics related to inflammatory and the structural heart diseases are listed in the Research Opportunities and Clinical Impact box. The list includes both medical and nursing research topics under investigation. Electronic databases are a source for finding specific studies related to these topics.

RESEARCH OPPORTUNITIES AND CLINICAL IMPACT RELATED TO INFLAMMATORY AND STRUCTURAL HEART DISEASE

Research Area	Clinical Impact
Effect of immunosuppressive treatment on myocarditis.	Improvement in left ventricular ejection fraction and evidence of healed myocarditis.
Identify predictors of embolic risk among the clinical and laboratory data obtained on hospital admission in patients diagnosed as having definite infective endocarditis (IE).	To identify high-risk individuals for embolic events associated with IE.
Lyme carditis and the incidence of myocarditis and/or pericarditis.	Diagnostic and complication guidelines.
Identify link between teeth brushing and infective endocarditis.	Identification of safer methods of teeth cleaning for patients with IE.
Herbal and complementary medicine to treat heart disease.	Lowers cholesterol, saturated fats, low-density lipoproteins, triglycerides, and blood pressure.
Heart valves that are durable, nonthrombogenic, with a low incidence of endocarditis.	Decreases need for multiple valve replacement and decreases complications of valve replacement surgery.
Septal ablation for hypertrophic obstructive cardiomyopathy.	Decreases obstruction of blood flow from the left ventricle to the aorta.
Prevention of sudden cardiac death with hypertrophic cardiomyopathy.	Increases survival of patients with HCM.
Stem cell homing and tissue regeneration in ischemic cardiomyopathy.	Repair of damaged tissue from ischemia.
Alcohol consumption's impact on heart failure.	Determine amount that is cardioprotective.
Use of beta-blockers in the treatment of heart failure.	Slow the progression of heart failure and reduce mortality, including sudden cardiac death.
Thiamin status, diuretic medications, and the management of heart failure.	
Relationship of heart failure severity, left ventricular loading conditions, and repolarization length in advanced heart failure secondary to ischemic or idiopathic dilated cardiomyopathy.	
Nonsustained ventricular tachycardia in hypertrophic cardiomyopathy: an independent marker of sudden death risk in young patients.	Determine predictors of sudden death risk to institute preventive therapy, such as implantation of an ICD.
Improvement in hypertrophic cardiomyopathy after significant weight loss.	Associated with striking improvement in cardiac functional indices, which could have profound implications for long-term cardiovascular risk.

Clinical Preparation

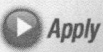

CRITICAL THINKING

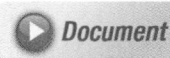

▶ Read

- History of Current Illness
- Past Medical History
- Physical Exam
- Admitting Medical Orders
- Laboratory Study Results

▶ Document

- Summary of Hospitalization
- Pathophysiology Form
- Laboratory Values
- Laboratory Results Explanation

▶ Apply

- List of Potential Nursing Diagnoses
- Concept Map
- Critical Thinking Questions

*Log on to MyNursingKit.com to download forms you will need and to complete further steps in the Clinical Preparation assignment.

HISTORY OF PRESENT ILLNESS

You are the nurse on the telemetry floor and you have been notified that you will be receiving a new patient from the emergency department (ED). The ED nurse calls the following report. Mr. H is a 26-year-old male brought in by ambulance, unconscious in the driveway of his home. He is initially seen by ED health care providers and the trauma team. Initial work-up included normal CT head, chest x-ray showing no pneumothorax, C-spine x-ray with no fractures, complete blood count (CBC), chemistry 7 panel, INR, UA; all were normal. ECG showed sinus tachycardia, low voltage, and nonspecific ST wave changes. Drug toxicology is still pending. A medicine consult was requested by the trauma service, for persistent shortness of breath (SOB) and an abnormal ECG.

At present, the patient is awake and alert. He feels weak and is short of breath. He denies assault. He denies a history of syncope and chest pain. He denies abdominal pain but has mild nausea. He denies fever, chills, and night sweats. He states he has a poor appetite but thinks he has gained weight due to swelling in his legs. He denies smoking cigarettes and denies crack/cocaine use. He states he drinks socially.

Of note, upon interviewing family, his mother states he is in good health and lives a very clean life. He is single, unemployed, and lives above her garage. She states he has no chronic health problems, but was told in his youth that he had a heart murmur. To her knowledge, the patient does not use any illegal drugs but does drink occasional alcohol. The patient's sister reports a very different story; she states the patient drinks at least six beers per day and frequently uses cocaine.

Medical–Surgical History

No known allergies
Medications: none
Illness: "heart murmur," no clinical problems
Surgeries: none

Social History

Family history: mom and dad healthy. The mother states that the patient does not use any illegal drugs but does drink occasional alcohol. The patient's sister reports a very different story; she states the patient drinks at least six beers per day and frequently uses cocaine.

Physical Exam

Young male overweight, mild discomfort due to SOB
Oxygen sat 90% on RA
BP 160/90 HR 115 RR 26
HEENT: normal but poor dentition
Neck: +JVD, no bruits
Heart: NL S_1, S_2, soft systolic murmur heard at PMI, S_3 present
Lungs: mild bibasilar rales
Abdomen: obese, soft, nontender
1+ lower extremity edema
Strong pulses throughout. Good cap refill
Normal neuro exam
No rash

Chest x-ray: cardiomegaly, mild interstitial edema
ECG: in history of present illness

Admitting Medical Orders

Admit to Cardiology–Telemetry Floor
Condition guarded
No known allergies
Admitting diagnosis: syncope unknown etiology: R/O dysrhythmia, ischemia, valvular disease; CHF probably due to cardiomyopathy via cocaine + alcohol abuse
Final diagnosis: cardiomyopathy and heart failure due to cocaine and alcohol abuse
Oxygen at 2–3 liters nasal cannula, keep oxygen saturation > 92%
Bed rest with bathroom privileges
Vital signs q2h with continuous ECG monitoring
Sequential compression device (SCD) to lower extremities
Incentive spirometry q hour while awake
Daily weight
Strict in/out
IV: saline lock; flush with NS q8h
Fluid restrict 1500 mL/day
Low Na diet
Call house officer: Pulse < 60 & > 110/minute; BP < 90 & > 160 systolic; temperature > 38.5; urine output < 30 mL/hr for 2 hours; respiratory rate > 30/minute; chest pain

Scheduled Medications

Lasix 40 mg IV every 12 hours for 2 days, then once a day

Nitropaste 1 inch q6h to chest wall topically

KCl 20 mEq po now and 20 mEq in 3 hours

Lisinopril 12.5 mg po daily

Lovenox 30 mg SQ bid

Magnesium sulfate 3 g IV dilute in 100 mL and give over 1 hour for a Mg level of less than 1.5 mEq/L $\times$ 1 now

PRN Medications

Phenergan 25 mg IV q6h prn nausea

Mylanta 30 mL q4–6h po prn dyspepsia

Triazolam 0.125–0.25 mg po q noc, prn sleep

Ativan 0.5–2 mg IV q6–8h prn anxiety (not to exceed 10 mg /24 hours)

Milk of Magnesia 30 mL daily, po prn constipation

Tylenol 650 mg po/pr q4h prn for pain

Ordered Laboratory Studies

Troponin I q3h $\times$ 3 days

Myoglobin q3h $\times$ 3 days

CPK–MB q8h $\times$ 3 days

Chemistry 20 and PO_4 on admission and Chemistry 7 q12h for first 2 days then daily

CBC q a.m.

Mg^{2+} q a.m.

Ordered Diagnostic Studies

Chest x-ray on admission and with adverse changes in O_2 saturation, increased shortness or breath, and/or increasing rales

Echocardiogram

Cardiac catheterization

12-lead ECG daily

LABORATORY STUDY RESULTS

Test	Day 1	Day 2	Day 3
Sodium	132 mEq/L	137 mEq/L	140 mEq/L
Potassium	3.0 mEq/L	4.0 mEq/L	3.8 mEq/L
Chloride	90 mEq/L	92 mEq/L	95 mEq/L
Calcium	8.6 mg/dL		
Venous carbon dioxide	25 mEq/L	24 mEq/L	26 mEq/L
Blood urea nitrogen (BUN)	28 mg/dL	25 mg/dL	22 mg/dL
Creatinine	2.0 mg/dL	1.7 mg/dL	1.2 mg/dL
Blood glucose	150 mg/dL	138 mg/dL	112 mg/dL
Total proteins	5.2		
Magnesium	1.0 mEq/L	2.0 mEq/L	2.0 mEq/L
Phosphorus	3.2 mg/dL		
Troponin I	0.26/0.23/0.28 ng/mL		
Myoglobin	110 µg/L		
Albumin	3.5 g/dL		
GGT	48 units/L		
T. Bilirubin	1.1 mg/dL		
CPK total	212 units/L		
CPK MB	1.8%		
LDH	166 units/L		
AST	38 units/L		
ALT	28 units/L		
WBC	14,000/mm³	12,000/mm³	11,000/mm³
Hemoglobin	10.2 g/dL	12.2 g/dL	13.8 g/dL
Hematocrit	32%	37%	40%
RBC	5/mm3		
Platelets	395/mm³	325/mm³	250/mm³
ABGs			
PO2	70 mmHg	78 mmHg	80 mmHg
O$_2$ saturation	90%	91%	93%
pH	7.30	7.34	7.38
PCO$_2$	50 mmHg	48 mmHg	43 mmHg
HCO$_3$	24 mEq/L	26 mEq/L	24 mEq/L

CRITICAL THINKING QUESTIONS

1. What is the purpose of the echocardiography for this patient?

2. Why did the doctor order cardiac marker laboratory tests?

3. Why was a cardiac catheterization done?

4. What is the importance of assessing the potassium level frequently?

5. The teaching plan for this patient needs to include specific information about lifestyle changes that will not cause a worsening of the heart disease. What information does this patient need to know and what referrals would be appropriate?

6. What is the goal of medical therapy for this patient? This answer drives much of the patient teaching and helps the nurse anticipate complications and potential problems with the patient as well as additional orders.

Answers to Critical Thinking Questions appear in Appendix D.

NCLEX® REVIEW

1. A patient's history indicates a past history of rheumatic fever. The nurse plans to assess the client for signs of:
    1. Pericarditis.
    2. Endocarditis.
    3. Mitral stenosis.
    4. Pulmonary fibrosis.

2. A patient presents to the emergency department with complaints of increasing dyspnea and chest pain. The nurse suspects the symptoms reflect aortic stenosis when the patient states:
    1. "I had a coronary artery bypass graft done five years ago."
    2. "I had rheumatic heart disease when I was a child."
    3. "I take a calcium channel blocker to treat an irregular heart rate."
    4. "I frequently experience palpitations."

3. The nurse should include the following teaching for a patient diagnosed with mitral valve prolapse.
    1. Avoid having any dental work until the valve is replaced.
    2. Plan for rest periods throughout the day.
    3. Take your oral temperature every morning.
    4. Keep a diary of all the high fat foods you eat.

4. A patient is scheduled for open surgical valvuloplasty of the mitral valve. When preparing the patient for surgery the nurse includes the following information.
    1. Cardiopulmonary bypass will not be required for this procedure.
    2. Anticoagulation therapy will not be necessary in the postoperative period.
    3. The valve will be repaired, but not replaced.
    4. This procedure will prevent the need for future valve surgeries.

5. A patient is diagnosed with restrictive cardiomyopathy secondary to cocaine abuse. The nurse plans nursing care recognizing treatment for this type of cardiomyopathy usually involves:
    1. Alcohol ablation.
    2. Insertion of an implantable automatic defibrillator, ICD.
    3. Aortic valve repair.
    4. Supportive therapy with medications.

6. The nurse suspects a patient having frequent episodes of chest pain has pericarditis. To help confirm the suspicion the nurse should ask which question.
    1. "Is the pain relieved by lying flat?"
    2. "Do you only experience the pain during the night?"
    3. "Does the pain become worse if you take a deep breath?"
    4. "Is the pain preceded by an episode of heart palpitations?"

Answers for review questions appear in Appendix D

KEY TERMS

allograft valve *p.1249*
annuloplasty *p.1247*
annulus *p.1247*
aortic valve regurgitation *p.1244*
aortic valve stenosis *p.1244*
arrhythmogenic right ventricular cardiomyopathy (ARVC) *p.1268*
autograft valve *p.1249*
Beck's triad *p.1229*
biological valve *p.1249*
cardiac tamponade *p.1228*
cardiomyopathies (CMPs) *p.1255*
commissure *p.1247*
commissurotomy *p.1247*

constrictive pericarditis *p.1227*
dilated cardiomyopathy *p.1255*
Dressler's syndrome *p.1223*
homograft valve *p.1249*
hypertrophic cardiomyopathy *p.1258*
infective endocarditis *p.1233*
mechanical valve *p.1248*
mitral valve prolapse *p.1241*
mitral valve regurgitation *p.1241*
mitral valve stenosis *p.1245*
myocarditis *p.1231*
pancarditis *p.1220*
pericardial effusion *p.1228*
pericardial friction rub *p.1228*

pericardial window *p.1230*
pericardiectomy *p.1230*
pericarditis *p.1223*
pulmonic valve regurgitation *p.1245*
pulmonic valve stenosis *p.1245*
pulsus paradoxus *p.1229*
restrictive cardiomyopathy *p.1265*
rheumatic fever *p.1219*
rheumatic heart disease *p.1219*
tricuspid valve regurgitation *p.1219*
tricuspid valve stenosis *p.1245*
valvular regurgitation *p.1240*
valvuloplasty *p.1247*

PEARSON
EXPLORE **mynursingkit**™

MyNursingKit is your one stop for online chapter review materials and resources. Prepare for success with additional NCLEX®-style practice questions, interactive assignments and activities, web links, animations and videos, and more!

Register your access code from the front of your book at
www.mynursingkit.com

REFERENCES

American College of Cardiology. (2006). *American College of Cardiology/European Society of Cardiology Clinical Expert consensus document on hypertrophic cardiomyopathy. A report of the American College of Cardiology Foundation Task Force on Clinical Expert Consensus Documents and the European Society of Cardiology Committee for Practice Guidelines.* Retrieved June 15, 2006, from http://www.acc.org/media/releases/highlights/2003/aug03/hcm.htm

American Heart Association. (2004). *2002 Heart disease and stroke statistics update.* Dallas TX: Author. Retrieved October 12, 2004, from http://www.americanheart.org/presenter.jhtml?identifier=4468

American Heart Association. (2006a). *Diagnosis and management of infective endocarditis and its complications—conclusions.* Retrieved June 15, 2006, from http://www.americanheart.org/presenter.jhtml?identifier=9350

American Heart Association. (2006b). *Endocarditis guidelines.* Retrieved August 7, 2006, from http://www.americanheart.org/presenter.jhtml?identifier=11078

American Heart Association. (2006c). *Pericardium and paricarditis.* Retrieved August 7, 2006, from http://www.americanheart.org/presenter.jhtml?identifier=4683

Ammash, N., Seward, J., & Bailey, K. (2000). Clinical profile and outcome of idiopathic restrictive cardiomyopathy. *Circulation, 101,* 2490–2494.

Aurigemma, G. P., & Gaasch, W. H. (2002). *Management of patients with prosthetic heart valves.* Retrieved June 6, 2006, from http://store.utdol.com/app/index.asp

Barkman, A., & McCay, J. (2002). Cardiogenic shock in a patient with hypertrophic obstructive cardiomyopathy after insertion of a pacemaker. *American Journal of Critical Care,* 11(6).

Bollinger, K., & Sadar, A. M. (2003). Care and management of the patient with right heart failure secondary to diastolic dysfunction: An advanced practice perspective and case review. *Critical Care Nursing Quarterly, 26*(1), 22–27.

Braunwald, E., Fauci, A. S., Kasper, D. L., Hause, S. L., Longo, D. L., & Jamison, J. L. (2005). *Harrison's principles of internal medicine* (16th ed.). New York: McGraw-Hill.

Brigden, W. (1957). Uncommon myocardial diseases. *Lancet, 2,* 1179.

Bruce, J. (2006). Getting to the heart of cardiomyopathy: Find out about the four types of cardiomyopathies. *Cardiac Insider,* pp. 16–20.

Brusch, J. L. (2005). *Infective endocarditis.* Retrieved August 2, 2006, from http://www.emedicine.com/med/topic671.htm

Candela, L. (2002). Caring for a patient with listeria endocarditis: Use of antibiotics desensitization. *Critical Care Nurse, 22*(5), 38–48.

Cardiomyopathy Association. (2006). *Arrhythmogenic right ventricular cardiomyopathy (ARVC).* Retrieved June 8, 2006, from http://www.cardiomyopathy.org/html/which_card_arvc_text.htm

Chin, T. K. (2006). Rheumatic heart disease, eMedicine. Retrieved on May 29, 2008 from http://www.emedicine.com/ped/topic2007.htm

Clarkston, N., & Waldman, A. R. (2001). Aortic valve replacement. *RN, 64*(1), 58–63.

Cope, S., & Hawley, R. (2001). Needs of the older patient in the intensive care unit following heart surgery. *Progressive Cardiovascular Nursing, 16*(2), 44–48.

Desai, K. (2002). *Pericardiocentesis.* Retrieved June 10, 2003, from http://www.emedicine.com/topic3560.htm

Fauci, A. S., Braunwald, E., Isselbacher, K. J., Wilson, J. D., Martin, J. B., Kasper, D. L., et al. (1998). *Harrison's principles of internal medicine* (14th ed.). New York: McGraw-Hill.

Felker, C. M., Thompson, R. E., & Hare, J. M. (2000). Underlying causes and long-term survival in patients with unexplained cardiomyopathy. *New England Journal of Medicine, 342,* 1077.

Flutterman, L. G., & Lemberg, L. (2000). Peripartum cardiomyopathy: An ominous complication of pregnancy. *American Journal of Critical Care, 9*(5).

Francis, G. (2004). *Halting remodeling in congestive heart failure.* The Cleveland Clinic Foundation, American College of Cardiology. Retrieved October 14, 2004, from http://www.chfpatients.com/heartbytes.htm#remodel

Fung, G. L., associate clinical professor of cardiology, University of California at San Francisco Medical School. (1999, June 7). Interview by Arlene Orhon-Jech.

Gowda, A. (2008). Pericarditis, uremic. *eMedicine Web MD.* Retrieved February 23, 2008, from http://www.emedicine.com/med/byname/pericarditis-uremic.htm

Grau, J.B., Pirelli, L., Yu, J.P., Galloway, A.C., & Ostrer, H. (2007). The genetics of mitral valve prolapse. *PubMed.* Retrieved on May 29, 2008 from http://www.ncbi.nlm.nih.gov/pubmed/17850623?ordinalpos=3&itool=EntrezSystem2.PEntrez.Pubmed.Pubmed_ResultsPanel.Pubmed_RVDocSum

Halsell, J. S., Riddle, J. R., Atwood, J. E. et al. (2003). Myopericarditis Following Smallpox Vaccination Among Vaccinia-Naive US Military Personnel. *JAMA: 289*(24):3283-3289.

Howes, D. S. (2008). Myocarditis. *eMedicine.* Retrieved on May 28, 2008 from http://www.emedicine.com/emerg/TOPIC326.HTM

Hunt, S. A., et al. (2005). ACC/AHA 2005 guideline update for the diagnosis and management of chronic heart failure in the adult: Summary article: A report of the American College of Cardiology/American Heart Association Task Force on Practice Guidelines (Writing Committee to Update the 2001 Guidelines for the Evaluation and Management of Heart Failure). *Journal of the American College of Cardiology, 46,* 1116–1143.

Jospehson, L., & McMullen, P. (2003). Atrial fibrillation: Beyond irregularly irregular. *Critical Care Choices: A Supplement to Nursing 2003 and Nursing Management,* pp. 6–10.

Lakkis, N. M., Nagueh, S. F., & Klieman, N. S. (1998). Echocardiography-guided ethanol septal reduction for hypertrophic obstructive cardiomyopathy. *Circulation, 98,* 1750–1755.

Lewis, P. S., Boyd, C. M., Hubert, N. E., & Steele, M. C. (2001). Ethanol-induced therapeutic myocardial infarction to treat hypertrophic obstructive cardiomyopathy. *Critical Care Nurse, 21*(2), 20–34.

Marill, K. (2006). *Endocarditis.* Retrieved August 3, 2006, from http://www.emedicine.com/emerg/topic164.htm

Mayo Clinic. (2005a). *Dressler's syndrome.* Retrieved August 2, 2006, from http://www.mayoclinic.com/health/dresslers-syndrome/DS00666

National Institute on Alcohol Abuse and Alcoholism. (2002, January). *Alcohol Alert,* No. 55. Retrieved August 3, 2006, from http://pubs.miaaa.nih.gov/publications/aa55.htm

Orhon-Jech, A. (1999). Mitral valve prolapse: What you need to know. *Nurse Week,* 16–17.

Porth, C. M. (2004). *Essential in pathophysiology: Concepts of altered health states.* Philadelphia: Lippincott Williams & Wilkins.

Porth, C. M. (2005). Pathophysiology: *Concepts of altered health states.* (7th ed.). Philadelphia: Lippincott Williams & Wilkins.

Richardson, P. (1996). Report of the World Health Organization/International Society and Federation of Cardiology Task Force on the Definition and Classification of the Cardiomyopathies. *Circulation, 93,* 841.

Roche, V. M. L., Kramer, A., Hester, E., & Welsh, C. H. (1999). Long-term functional outcome after intensive care. *Journal of the American Geriatrics Society, 47*(1), 18–24.

Saxton, L. D., Kumar, U. N., & DeMarco, T. (2006). *Cardiac resynchronization therapy (biventricular pacing) in heart failure.* Retrieved June 3, 2006, from Up to Date website: http://www.utdol.com/utd/store/index.do

Steinbis, S. (2003). Hypertrophic obstructive cardiomyopathy and septal ablation. *Critical Care Nurse, 23*(3), 47–58.

Takagi, E., Yamakado, T., & Nakano, T. (1999). Prognosis of completely asymptomatic adult patients with hypertrophic cardiomyopathy. *Journal of American College of Cardiology, 33,* 296.

Tandri, H., Saranathan, M., Rodriguez, E. R., Martinez, C., Bomma, C., Nasir, K., et al. (2005, January 4). Noninvasive detection of myocardial fibrosis in arrhythmogenic right ventricular cardiomyopathy using delayed-enhancement magnetic resonance imaging. *Journal of the America College of Cardiology, 45*(1), 98–103.

University of Maryland Medical Center (2005). *Mitral valve prolapse.* Retrieved May 28, 2006, from http://www.umm.edu/ency/article/000180.htm

U.S. Department of Health and Human Services. (2004). *Healthy People 2010 progress report: Substance abuse.* Retrieved June 3, 2006, from http://www.healthypeople.gov/data/2010prog/focus26/holisticonline.com/remedies/Heart/cm causes-of-cardiomyopathy

Wichter, T., Paul, M., Wollmann, C., Acil, T., Gerdes, P., Ashraf, O., et al. (2004). Implantable cardioverter/defibrillator therapy in arrhythmogenic right ventricular cardiomyopathy: Single-center experience of long-term follow-up and complications in 60 patients. *Circulation, 109*(12), 1445–1447.

Wiegand, D. L. (2003). Advance in cardiac surgery: Valve repair. *Critical Care Nurse, 23*(2): 72–91.

Woods, S. L., Froelicher, E. S. S., & Motzer, S. U. (2000). *Cardiac nursing.* (4th ed.). Philadelphia: Lippincott Williams & Wilkins.

Zevola, D. R., Raffa, M., & Brown, K. (2002). Using clinical pathways in patients undergoing cardiac valve surgery. *Critical Care Nurse, 22*(1), 31–50.

CHAPTER 42

Caring for the Patient with Heart Failure

Kismet Rasmusson
Jill Hall

Outcome-Based Learning Objectives

After studying this chapter, the learner will be able to:

1. Evaluate the etiology, incidence, and prevalence of heart failure.
2. Distinguish between systolic and diastolic dysfunction.
3. Describe the pathophysiology of heart failure and the compensatory neurohormonal responses that occur.
4. Compare and contrast right-sided versus left-sided symptoms of heart failure.
5. Evaluate the diagnostic workup used to determine the presence of heart failure.
6. Describe a comprehensive treatment plan including the medical, device, and surgical components to treatment, using the multidisciplinary team approach.
7. Describe the self-management concepts necessary for patients with heart failure.
8. Compare and contrast potential comorbidities associated with heart failure.
9. Describe components of end-of-life care for end-stage heart failure.

Research   Collaboration   Health Promotion   Nursing Process   Caring   Critical Thinking

HEART FAILURE is a common, chronic condition that has a significant impact, not only on patients living with the disease but also on care delivery systems. Current understanding of heart failure has matured from what was once thought to be a hemodynamic condition, to an understanding of complex neurohormonal changes resulting in an impairment of cardiac filling and/or ejection of blood. If left untreated, the disease will progress resulting in increased symptoms, hospitalizations, and possibly death. Leaders in heart failure care, such as the Heart Failure Society of America and the American Heart Association with the American College of Cardiology, have updated guidelines to help providers with delivering appropriate, evidence-based care.

Heart failure treatments have expanded significantly over the last 20 years and have been able to improve symptoms and reduce morbidity, mortality, and hospitalizations. Today, heart failure is treated with therapies of growing complexity: medications, cardiac devices, and surgical/interventional approaches. Special attention to controlling comorbid conditions and volume status is paramount. Medical therapy is aimed to reduce the detrimental neurohormonal cascade. Cardiac devices have an expanding role to prevent sudden cardiac death, to resynchronize dyssynchronous ventricles, and even to aid in the assessment of fluid status. End-stage therapies may offer the promise of extended life with modalities such as cardiac transplantation or mechanical assist devices for select patients. Palliative care and hospice will be essential for patients whose prognosis is poor.

Multidisciplinary teams providing care by using established disease management strategies improve outcomes. Nurses have been pivotal in patient care in providing self-management instruction, telephone management, and more (Rasmusson et al., 2006). The future of heart failure will come with understanding genetic implications and integrating clinical research into practice. Genetic implications are discussed in the Genetic Considerations box.

Epidemiology

Heart failure is a major public health problem affecting 5 million Americans (American Heart Association [AHA], 2006b). With over 550,000 new cases diagnosed each year in the United States, heart failure is reaching epidemic proportions. Contributing to the rising prevalence of heart failure are the aging U.S. population and increased survival rates among patients with hypertension and coronary artery disease (AHA, 2006b; Baker, 2002). Individuals who would have succumbed to an acute cardiac event in the past are now more likely to survive,

GENETIC CONSIDERATIONS for Heart Failure

Risk factors	Family history of early coronary artery disease (CAD), idiopathic or hypertrophic cardiomyopathy, sudden cardiac death. Virus exposure. African American race. Potential for thromboembolic events: atrial fibrillation, pulmonary embolism, intra-cardiac thrombi, or deep vein thrombosis.
Research	Familial Dilated Cardiomyopathy Research Project.[a] Viral genome; studying parvovirus B19. A-HeFT: African-American Heart Failure Trial: showed increased response to hydralazine and nitrates in addition to standard heart failure therapy. Genetic testing to assess warfarin dosing.
Counseling/screening	Counsel patients that their condition might pose a risk to their first-degree relatives. Appropriate screening would be recommended, then starting treatment if left ventricular dysfunction is found. To screen those with risk factors or a family history suggests simple screening of first-degree family members with a limited history, physical examination, 12-lead ECG, and echocardiogram. Genetic screening by blood testing is not yet well understood but may guide future treatment.

[a] Website: http://www.fdc.to.

Sources: Burkett, E. L., & Hershberger, R. E. (2005). State of the art: Clinical and genetic issues in familial dilated cardiomyopathy. *Journal of the American College of Cardiology, 45,* 969–981; Taylor, A. L., Ziesche, S., Yancy, C., et al. (2004). For the African-American heart failure trial investigators. Combination of isosorbide dinitrate and hydralazine in blacks with heart failure. *The New England Journal of Medicine, 351,* 2049–2057; and Wilson-Tang, W. H., & Francis, G. S. (2005). The year in heart failure. *Journal of the American College of Cardiology, 46,* 2125–2133.

albeit with impaired cardiac function (AHA, 2006b; Baker, 2002). With the rise of conditions such as diabetes, obesity, and the metabolic syndrome, increases in the risk of developing heart failure are significant (Hunt et al., 2005).

Mortality

Despite advances in heart failure treatments, mortality rates increased by 20.5% from 1993 to 2003. Nearly 290,000 people die annually of heart failure in the United States (AHA, 2006b). More than 75% of patients diagnosed with heart failure die within 8 years. Those with heart failure are six to nine times more likely than the general population to suffer from sudden death (AHA, 2006b).

Medical Impact

Heart failure is the most common diagnostic-related group (DRG) used for hospital admissions in the United States among the Medicare population (Hunt et al., 2005). Since 1979, the rate

of hospital discharges for patients with heart failure has increased by 174%, totaling more than 1 million annually (AHA, 2006b). Recurrences or exacerbations of symptoms are likely, particularly as the disease advances. An exacerbation often results in an acute crisis, leading to either emergency department visits or hospitalizations. Between 30% and 50% of patients discharged with acute heart failure are readmitted with an exacerbation to the hospital within 6 months. Although hospital readmissions may be preventable, such prevention is often accomplished at the expense of increasing resources, such as office visits and home monitoring by experienced nurses. Health delivery systems across the continuum of care are challenged to provide appropriate care to all patients, while limiting resource utilization. See the National Guidelines box (p. 1280) for the diagnosis and management of heart failure.

Economic Impact

Heart failure also is the most costly DRG in the United States with more dollars spent on it than on any other condition for the Medicare population (Hunt et al., 2005). Direct and indirect costs associated with heart failure amount to nearly $30 billion in the U.S. (AHA, 2007). Therapeutic pharmacologic advances in the treatment of heart failure, such as angiotensin-converting enzyme (ACE) inhibitors and beta-adrenergic blockers, have been shown to be cost-effective therapies. However, more complex and costly cardiac devices are adding to the expense of overall management. End-stage therapies, such as mechanical circulatory support and cardiac transplantation, in reality represent failures of early prevention and treatment, yet are used in selected, but few, patients. If the current trajectory of rising costs continues, heart failure expenditures could financially drain current health care resources.

Pathophysiology

Heart failure is best defined as a complex and debilitating clinical syndrome whereby there is "loss or dysfunction of the cardiac muscle" (Adams et al., 2006) or an "inability of the ventricle to fill or eject blood" (Hunt et al., 2005). The heart muscle is simply unable to pump adequately to supply enough blood to meet the body's metabolic needs, leading to significant impairment and often disability (Hunt et al., 2005). The syndrome of heart failure ultimately leads to common symptoms of poor activity tolerance, fluid retention, and fatigue, that limit quality of life.

Heart failure, the syndrome, should be distinguished from structural or functional causes, such as cardiomyopathy (any disease that affects the structure and function of the heart). The diagnosis, cause, and treatment of all cardiomyopathies are discussed in Chapter 41 .

Etiology

The leading etiologies of heart failure include hypertension, coronary artery disease, and dilated cardiomyopathies. Other factors that contribute to developing heart failure include well-established risk factors for cardiovascular disease or exposure to substances that are toxic to the cardiac muscle. Risk factors that may lead to heart failure are summarized in the Risk Factors box (p. 1280).

NATIONAL GUIDELINES for Heart Failure

Name of Guideline	Guideline Objectives
2005 American College of Cardiology and American Heart Association (ACC/AHA) Chronic Heart Failure Guidelines[a]	Characterizing the syndrome of heart failure.
	Initial and ongoing assessment.
	Therapies; stage based.
	Treating special populations.
	Treating concomitant disorders.
	End-of-life considerations.
	Implementation of practice guidelines.
Heart Failure Society of American (HFSA) 2006 Comprehensive Heart Failure Practice Guideline	Define heart failure.
	Discuss prevention strategies.
	Evaluating patients for heart failure.
	Managing asymptomatic patients.
	Nonpharmacologic treatments.
	Managing symptomatic patients.
	Disease management.
	Device therapies.
	Surgical therapies.
	Managing patients with preserved ventricular function.
	Managing acute decompensated heart failure.
	Managing patients with ischemic disease.
	Managing patients with hypertension.
	Managing special populations.
	Managing myocarditis.

[a] Website:http://www.hfsa.org/hf_guidelines.asp.

Sources: Adams, K. F., Lindenfeld, J., Arnold, J. M., et al. (2006). Executive summary: HFSA 2006 comprehensive heart failure practice guideline. *Journal of Cardiac Failure, 12*(1), 10–38; Hunt, S. A., Abraham, W. T., Chin, M. H., Feldman, A. M., Francis, G. S., Ganiats, T. G., et al. (2005). ACC/AHA 2005 guideline update for the diagnosis and management of chronic heart failure in the adult: Summary article: A report of the American College of Cardiology/American Heart Association Task Force on Practice Guidelines (Writing Committee to Update the 2001 Guidelines for the Evaluation and Management of Heart Failure). *Journal of the American College of Cardiology, 46,* 1116–1143.

RISK FACTORS for Heart Failure

Modifiable Risk Factors	Nonmodifiable Risk Factors
Atherosclerosis	Age
Cardiotoxic drug use (alcohol, illicit drugs, anthracyclines)	Positive family history of CAD
Diabetes	Gender
Hyperlipidemia	Genetics
Hypertension	
Metabolic syndrome	
Obesity	
Sedentary lifestyle	
Smoker	
Valvular abnormalities	

Sources: Adams, K. F., Lindenfeld, J., Arnold, J. M., et al. (2006). Executive summary: HFSA 2006 comprehensive heart failure practice guideline. *Journal of Cardiac Failure, 12*(1), 10–38; Hunt, S. A., Abraham, W. T., Chin, M. H., Feldman, A. M., Francis, G. S., Ganiats, T. G., et al. (2005). ACC/AHA 2005 guideline update for the diagnosis and management of chronic heart failure in the adult: Summary article: A report of the American College of Cardiology/American Heart Association Task Force on Practice Guidelines (Writing Committee to Update the 2001 Guidelines for the Evaluation and Management of Heart Failure). *Journal of the American College of Cardiology, 46,* 1116–1143.

Two very different pathologic processes may lead to heart failure as a result of a wide range of left ventricular functional abnormalities commonly referred to as systolic and diastolic dysfunction, discussed next. Both systolic and diastolic dysfunction may occur simultaneously and usually result in the same set of symptoms.

Systolic Dysfunction

Systolic dysfunction, also referred to as left ventricular systolic dysfunction (LVSD), is characterized by impaired ventricular function, which results in volume overload and decreased contractility. In the U.S., the most common cause of LVSD is coronary artery disease (CAD), followed by hypertension (Nohria, Lewis, & Stevenson, 2002). In an era of improved therapies to treat coronary artery disease and acute myocardial infarction, people now survive such events, but many remain with a dysfunctional ventricle. This may lead to the syndrome of heart failure. Other causes of systolic dysfunction include idiopathic, valvular, hypertrophic, and cardiotoxic substance use. LVSD is diagnosed when the **left ventricular ejection fraction (LVEF)** (the proportion of blood ejected during each ventricular contraction compared with the total ventricular filling volume) is below 40% to 45% (Cohn, 2000). A normal LVEF ranges from

55% to 70%. Chart 42–1 outlines the etiologies of heart failure. Once LVSD occurs, progressive adverse structural and neurohormonal changes occur within the heart, leading to deteriorating cardiac function and symptoms of low cardiac output and congestion (Jessup & Brozena, 2003). Neurohormones such as norepinephrine, endothelin, and cytokines are released, leading to an adverse condition called cardiac remodeling. This detrimental effect on the myocardium results from volume overload or cardiac injury and causes myocytes to revert to a fetal-type expression, ultimately changing the geometry from elliptical to spherical. These changes result in molecular, cellular, and interstitial changes of the cardiac muscle and are manifested clinically as changes in size, shape, and function of the heart, which leads to a reduction in ventricular function. Regardless of the etiology, once systolic dysfunction occurs, the heart is unable to pump enough blood to sustain the metabolic demands of the body. Right, left, and/or biventricular heart failure can occur, depending on the extent and anatomy of the damage (Figure 42–1 ■, p. 1282). Tissue remodeling is described in detail in Chapter 40 ☮ .

Left-sided heart failure, as the name suggests, is an abnormal cardiac condition characterized by the impaired pumping ability of the left side of the heart, which eventually backs the blood up into the pulmonary circulation. Elevated pressure and congestion in the pulmonary veins and capillaries result as the disease progresses. Symptoms that eventually follow impaired left ventricular function include fatigue, activity intolerance, shortness of breath, and cough. Often, orthopnea (an abnormal condition in which a person must sit or stand to breathe deeply or comfortably) and paroxysmal nocturnal dyspnea (a disorder characterized by sudden attacks of respiratory distress that awakens the person usually after several hours of sleep in a reclining position) will occur (Greenberg & Hermann, 2002; Nohria et al., 2002).

Right-sided heart failure is an abnormal cardiac condition characterized by the impairment of the pumping ability on the right side of the heart, leading to a backup of blood, followed by congestion and elevated pressure in the systemic veins and capillaries. The most common cause of right-sided dysfunction is left-sided dysfunction (Nohria et al., 2002). Other causes include a pathologic process in the lungs whereby blood cannot flow into the pulmonary vasculature, or result from an isolated right ventricular myocardial infarction. Symptoms of right heart failure result from volume overload leading to ascites and edema. Patients may complain of abdominal bloating and discomfort, often with a poor appetite and sometimes nausea and vomiting. Lower extremity edema occurs in many, but the absence of edema does not exclude volume overload in patients with heart failure.

Biventricular heart failure refers to a global inability of both ventricles of the heart to pump blood effectively. Forward blood flow is compromised, leading to right and left heart failure symptoms (Greenberg & Hermann, 2002). Symptoms are typically a combination of those from both right and left heart failure. Generalized malaise, activity intolerance, and even poor concentration are common as the disease progresses.

Diastolic Dysfunction

Diastolic dysfunction, also known as heart failure with preserved left ventricular ejection fraction (LVEF), is diagnosed when ventricular relaxation is slowed, with elevated filling pressures in the setting of normal ventricular volume and contraction (Hunt et al., 2005). Diastolic dysfunction is usually diagnosed when the clinical symptoms of heart failure are present with a normal LVEF (Jessup & Brozena, 2003). Diastolic dysfunction may account for 40% to 70% of all heart failure diagnosis (Jessup & Brozena, 2003). Patients with diastolic dysfunction are primarily elderly women, frequently with hypertension, diabetes, obesity, and atrial fibrillation (Adams at al., 2006). Although current understanding of diastolic dysfunction is limited due to a small body of research, it appears to have a burden similar to systolic dysfunction on health care resources

---

CHART 42–1   **Etiologies of Heart Failure**

Heart failure is a syndrome of symptoms that occurs from two pathologic processes: systolic dysfunction (when the heart is unable to contract normally) and diastolic dysfunction (when the heart is unable to relax normally). The etiologies leading to either process are noted here.

Systolic Dysfunction	Diastolic Dysfunction
Hypertension	Hypertrophic cardiomyopathy
Coronary artery disease (CAD)	Acute coronary insufficiency
Myocardial infarction	Systemic hypertension with hypertrophy
Ischemia (hibernating myocardium, stunned myocardium)	Acute and chronic CAD
Diabetes	Infiltrative cardiomyopathy
Alcoholic cardiomyopathy	Obstructive or nonobstructive disease
Peripartum cardiomyopathy	
Valvular cardiomyopathy	
Drug-induced cardiomyopathy	
Idiopathic cardiomyopathy	

Sources: Adams, K. F., Baughman, K. L., Dec, W. G., Elkayam, U., Forker, A. D., Gheorghiade, M., et al. (1999). Heart Failure Society of America (HFSA) practice guidelines. *Journal of Cardiac Failure, 5*(4), 357–382; Braunwald, E., Zipes, D. P., & Libby, P. (2001). *Heart disease: A textbook of cardiovascular medicine* (6th ed.). Philadelphia: W. B. Saunders; Greenberg, B. H., & Hermann, D. D. (2002). *Contemporary diagnosis and management of heart failure.* Newtown, PA: Handbooks in Health Care: Hunt, S. A., Abraham, W. T., Chin, M. H., Feldman, A. M., Francis, G. S., Ganiats, T. G., et al. (2005). ACC/AHA 2005 guideline update for the diagnosis and management of chronic heart failure in the adult: Summary article: A report of the American College of Cardiology/American Heart Association Task Force on Practice Guidelines (Writing Committee to Update the 2001 Guidelines for the Evaluation and Management of Heart Failure). *Journal of the American College of Cardiology, 46,* 1116–1143.

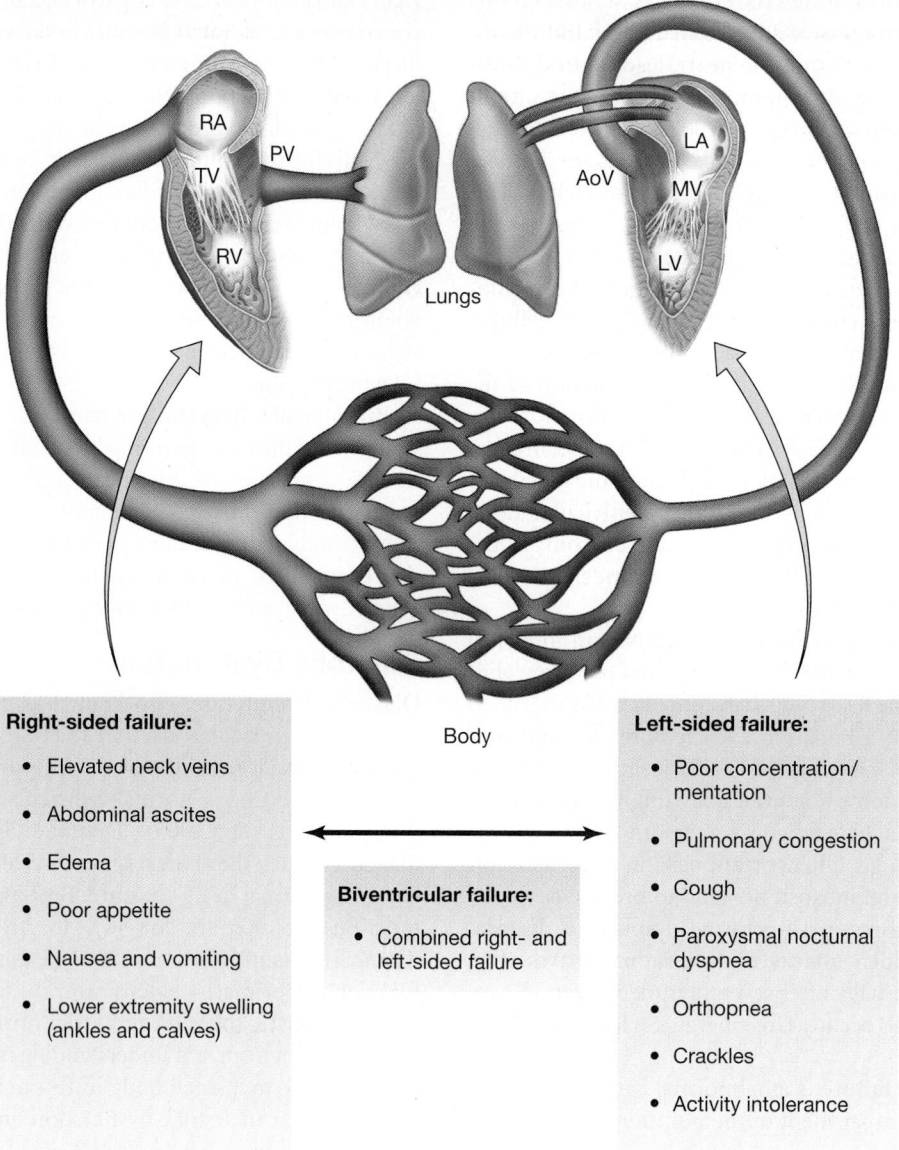

Right-sided failure:

- Elevated neck veins
- Abdominal ascites
- Edema
- Poor appetite
- Nausea and vomiting
- Lower extremity swelling (ankles and calves)

Biventricular failure:

- Combined right- and left-sided failure

Left-sided failure:

- Poor concentration/ mentation
- Pulmonary congestion
- Cough
- Paroxysmal nocturnal dyspnea
- Orthopnea
- Crackles
- Activity intolerance

FIGURE 42–1 ■ Right, left, and biventricular failure.

in terms of risk of admission, disability, and symptoms after hospitalization (Smith, Masoudi, Vaccarino, Radford, & Krumholz, 2003). Diastolic dysfunction seems to be related to a stiff, noncompliant heart with prolonged relaxation. The result is decreased filling, increased left ventricular end diastolic pressure, and reduced stroke volume at rest or during exercise (McKelvie, 2001). The increased susceptibility to changes in volume results in symptoms of "congestive" heart failure (Jessup & Brozena, 2003). Some causes of diastolic dysfunction include restrictive, obstructive, nonobstructive, hypertrophic, and infiltrative cardiomyopathies (see Chart 42–1, p. 1281). Principles of treatment focus on controlling hypertension, ischemia, and the ventricular rate when atrial fibrillation is present and on minimizing congestion (Adams et al., 2006). Given the robust data on systolic dysfunction and the lack of a standardized approach to treating diastolic dysfunction, this chapter focuses primarily on systolic dysfunction.

Neurohormonal Response

A series of compensatory mechanisms are triggered when the heart's pumping action is compromised. Regardless of the etiology of LVSD, the initial response to decreased cardiac output (the volume of blood expelled by the ventricles of the heart equal to the amount of blood ejected at each beat multiplied by the heart rate per minute) is the activation of the sympathetic nervous system (SNS) and the renin-angiotensin-aldosterone system (RAAS). Substances released with eventual detrimental cardiac effects include norepinephrine, angiotensin II, aldosterone, endothelin, vasopressin, and cytokines. Circulating levels play an important role in vasoconstriction, sodium retention, and toxic effects on the architecture of the heart described earlier (Hunt et al., 2005). In the early stages of heart failure, SNS and RAAS activation augments preload (the volume of blood being returned to the heart causing the stretch of myocardial fibers at end diastole), ventricular contractility, and heart rate, thereby maintaining cardiac output especially during exercise. But as cardiac function progressively worsens, these compensatory mechanisms are no longer able to maintain cardiac output and further compromise ventricular function (Greenberg & Hermann, 2002). Ventricular remodeling will result unless halted, which is a process by which detrimental effects are noted on the cardiac myocyte level.

Sympathetic Nervous System Activation

Increased SNS activity leads to elevated levels of norepinephrine. Norepinephrine causes vasoconstriction in the pulmonary and systemic vasculature and enhances venous tone, causing vasoconstriction. This initially maintains blood pressure and increases ventricular preload. Norepinephrine also causes renal vasoconstriction that allows for the glomerular filtration rate to remain stable despite decreased perfusion of renal blood flow. Circulating norepinephrine also increases sodium absorption leading to fluid retention that initially increases intravascular volume with subsequent temporary improvements in cardiac output and blood pressure. In addition, myocardial contractility and heart rate also are stimulated and therefore increase cardiac output. These neurohormonal effects provide short-term, necessary support to maintain cardiac output. In the long term, these deleterious effects cause increased cardiac wall stress, **hypertrophy** (an increase in the size of an organ caused by an increase in the size of the cells rather than in the number of cells), chamber dilation, increased myocardial oxygen consumption, worsening myocardial ischemia (a decreased supply of oxygenated blood to a body organ or part), and pulmonary and systemic congestion (Greenberg & Hermann, 2002).

Renin-Angiotensin-Aldosterone System Activation

Decreased renal perfusion triggers activation of the renin-angiotensin-aldosterone system (RAAS). Renin is released from the kidneys, causing a conversion of inactive angiotensin I into active angiotensin II. Angiotensin II is a potent vasoconstrictor that enhances venous tone and increases afterload (the load or resistance against which the left ventricle must eject its volume of blood during contraction). Angiotensin II also stimulates the secretion of aldosterone, causing sodium and fluid retention. In the short term, preload, cardiac output, and blood pressure are increased. However, long-term effects include increased cardiac workload, pulmonary and systemic congestion, and chamber dilation. Abnormal cell growth manifested by myocardial hypertrophy and adverse remodeling is also triggered by angiotensin II (Greenberg & Hermann, 2002).

Other Hormone Activation and Cytokine Release

Additional hormones that appear to be activated include the following: arginine vasopressin (from the pituitary hormone, which regulates free water clearance), endothelin (which is a potent vasoconstrictor released from endothelin cells), natriuretic peptides (released from cardiac tissue and vasculature, which cause vasodilation and natriuresis, which is the excretion of sodium), and cytokines, which have deleterious effects on cardiac remodeling (Greenberg & Hermann, 2002; Sha, Ali, Lamba, & Abraham, 2001).

▇ Course of Heart Failure

Once diagnosed, heart failure disease progression follows a predictable course (Figure 42–2 ■). Formal diagnosis usually occurs when symptoms develop and functional status is compromised. Treatment of patients with heart failure, regardless of their course, involves providing supportive care for presenting symptoms and addressing needs for patients with chronic disease. Once standard heart failure therapies including medications and/or devices are initiated, functional status is usually improved for a period of time. As the disease progresses, after a period of stability of unknown duration, many patients experience episodes of exacerbations followed by some periods of stabilization. Often, they are unable to regain their prior level of functional ability. Exacerbations become increasingly more frequent and stabilization more difficult, eventually leading to death unless the patient is a candidate for end-stage therapies.

Understanding the course of heart failure can help guide not only therapeutic decisions, but also discussions with patients and families for a comprehensive approach to care. Even those who respond to medical or device therapies with improvement of cardiac function may eventually decompensate, with a select few eligible for advanced therapies such as cardiac transplantation or mechanical circulatory support. End-of-life care is essential for those with a poor prognosis, who are otherwise not candidates for advanced therapies. Therefore, both patients and health care providers may better anticipate treatment options and the trajectory of the disease when they understand the course of heart failure.

Chronic Heart Failure

The onset of heart failure can either be insidious or acute. Clinical challenges relate to diagnosing and treating heart failure along the continuum from inpatient to outpatient settings. Chronic heart failure is recognized by patients as having a mixture of good and bad days, with ongoing dyspnea, fatigue, and activity intolerance. Patients typically complain of weight gain (despite a decreased appetite), nausea, vomiting, and slow changes in their ability to perform activities of daily living (ADLs). Patients may also complain of irritability, restlessness,

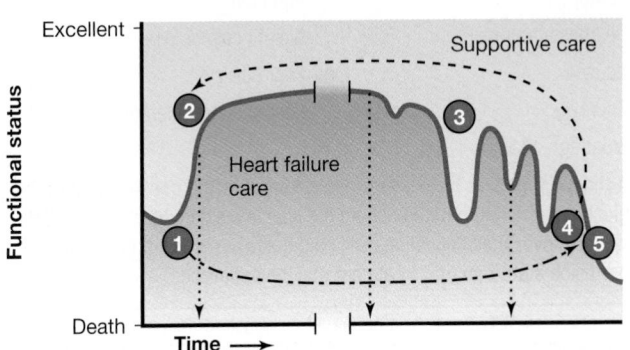

········ Sudden death event

- - - - Transplant or ventricular assist device

—·—· Non responders to medical management

FIGURE 42–2 ■ Course of heart failure.

or profound fatigue causing them to have poor energy. Increased urinary frequency and nighttime urination also are common (Greenberg & Hermann, 2002; Nohria et al., 2002). Symptoms will wax and wane in the majority of patients (Nohria et al., 2002). Heart failure is a chronic condition and, with suboptimal or lack of treatment, will lead to progressive cardiac dysfunction, progressive symptoms, and eventually death (Chart 42–2).

 **CRITICAL ALERT** *Subtle symptoms of heart failure include the following:*

1. *Crackles are absent in over 80% of those with elevated filling pressures.*
2. *Edema in the elderly is often unrelated to filling pressures.*
3. *The easiest vital sign used to assess perfusion is blood pressure.*
4. *Patients who fall asleep while interviewed may have poor perfusion.*
5. *Cool forearms and legs may be more specific of low cardiac output than are cold hands and feet.*

Stages of Heart Failure

The stages of heart failure, as defined and created by the American College of Cardiology (ACC) and the AHA (Figure 42–3 ■) (Hunt et al., 2005), have better defined the evolution and progression of heart failure, which in turn helps direct treatment strategies to assist in halting disease progression. Criteria were set forth for Stages A through D to (1) identify risk factors for developing heart failure, (2) detect the presence or absence of

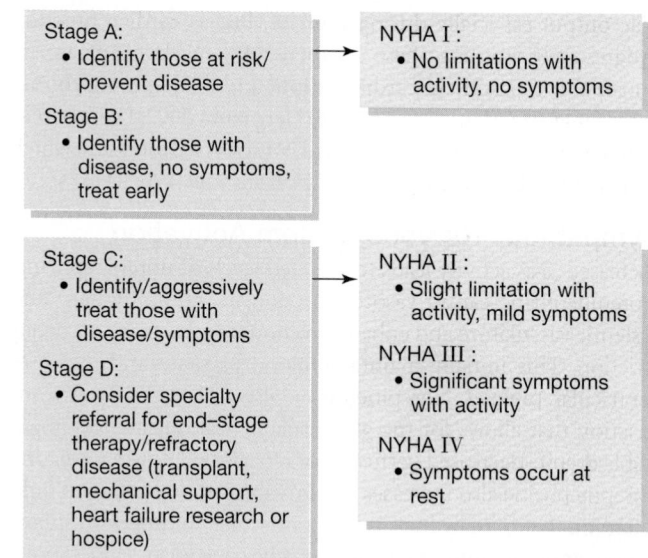

FIGURE 42–3 ■ The American College of Cardiology/American Heart Association (ACC/AHA) stages of heart failure vs. the New York Heart Association (NYHA) classes.

structural disease, and (3) treat based on well-proven strategies throughout the stages. The stages are described next.

Stage A

Stage A includes those at risk for developing the disease, but no structural abnormalities exist and no symptoms are present (Hunt et al., 2005). Risk factors for developing heart failure are similar to those for coronary artery disease: advancing age, diabetes, hypertension, hyperlipidemia, sedentary lifestyle, obesity, smoking, and excessive alcohol use (Greenberg & Hermann, 2002; Hunt et al., 2005). Risk factors for the development of coronary artery disease are described in detail in Chapter 40 ☕. Interventions for those in Stage A, aimed at reducing the risk of developing coronary artery disease, will likely prevent heart failure.

Stage B

Stage B includes asymptomatic patients who have structural heart disease. This is a difficult group to identify because symptoms are usually what will lead to the diagnosis of heart failure. Indiscriminately screening for heart failure is generally not recommended (Hunt et al., 2005) but could be selectively undertaken if risk factors were present. Persons with a prior myocardial infarction or significant coronary artery disease (CAD) or valvular disease are at particular risk in this stage. Evidence of structural disease can be detected on certain diagnostic tests including a 12-lead ECG (showing left ventricular hypertrophy); a chest x-ray showing **cardiomegaly** (enlargement of the heart); or an echocardiogram, chest CT, or MRI (showing ventricular hypertrophy or valvular dysfunction).

Evaluating a B-type natriuretic peptide (BNP) could be considered if there were clinical suspicions of heart failure, but an abnormally elevated value alone is not sufficient to diagnose heart failure. BNP is a 32-amino-acid polypeptide secreted by the ventricles of the heart in response to excessive stretching of myocytes in the ventricles. Levels of BNP are elevated in patients with left ventricular dysfunction, and levels correlate with both the severity of symptoms and the prognosis in congestive heart

---

CHART 42–2	**Heart Failure Symptoms**
Dyspnea	Abdominal distention
Exertional dyspnea	Right upper quadrant pain
Orthopnea	Swelling
Paroxysmal nocturnal dyspnea	Nocturia
Dyspnea at rest	Fatigue
Cough	Restlessness
Hemoptysis	Agitation
Decreased urine output	Weight gain or loss
Nausea	Poor energy
Anorexia	Poor exercise tolerance
Bloating	

A thorough patient history includes asking directed questions that may glean important information about the type and extent of symptoms individuals have. These questions will help guide assessment of volume and perfusion status, so that treatment may be optimized.

Sources: Adams, K. F., Baughman, K. L., Dec, W. G., Elkayam, U., Forker, A. D., Gheorghiade, M., et al. (1999). Heart Failure Society of America (HFSA) practice guidelines. *Journal of Cardiac Failure, 5*(4), 357–382; Braunwald, E., Zipes, D. P., & Libby, P. (2001). *Heart disease: A textbook of cardiovascular medicine* (6th ed.). Philadelphia: W. B. Saunders; Greenberg, B. H., & Hermann, D. D. (2002). *Contemporary diagnosis and management of heart failure.* Newtown, PA: Handbooks in Health Care; Hunt, S. A., Abraham, W. T., Chin, M. H., Feldman, A. M., Francis, G. S., Ganiats, T. G., et al. (2005). ACC/AHA 2005 guideline update for the diagnosis and management of chronic heart failure in the adult: Summary article: A report of the American College of Cardiology/American Heart Association Task Force on Practice Guidelines (Writing Committee to Update the 2001 Guidelines for the Evaluation and Management of Heart Failure). *Journal of the American College of Cardiology, 46,* 1116–1143.

failure. BNP may also be elevated with acute myocardial infarction, acute pulmonary embolus, and renal failure; it also elevates some with age alone. The BNP is most useful in its ability to exclude heart failure as a diagnosis, if the value is normal. Elevations in BNP values have correlated with significant heart failure symptoms and increased risk of mortality. Reducing BNP has been shown to improve clinical status, yet the role of serial BNP measurements to guide therapy remains unclear (Hunt et al., 2005). Treatments for Stage B patients include ACE inhibitors, angiotensin receptor blockers, and beta-blockers (and aspirin and a statin if CAD is present). Such treatments prevent further damage of the myocardium and delay progression to symptomatic disease. Treatments from Stage B should be coupled with the recommended preventive measures of Stage A (Hunt et al., 2005; Jessup & Brozena, 2003).

Stage C

Stage C refers to patients with symptomatic, structural heart disease. Recommended therapies include ACE inhibitors, angiotensin receptor blockers, beta-blockers, and digoxin. (See the Pharmacologic Management section (p. 1294) for more detail.) Diuretics are used to relieve congestive symptoms, and aldosterone blockade is added for persistent symptoms. Cardiac devices, such as internal cardioverter defibrillators and biventricular pacemakers, are used in appropriate candidates either to reduce the incidence of sudden cardiac death or to improve the synchronous contraction in the ventricles, or both. Chapter 39 🌐 discusses the pacemakers used for patients with heart failure.

Stage D

Stage D refers to patients with end-stage heart failure. When little hope of recovery exists, advanced interventions including heart transplantation, implantation of mechanical circulatory devices, enrollment in heart failure research studies, or hospice may be warranted (Hunt et al., 2005).

New York Heart Association Classification System

One measure used to quantify the degree of limitation and clinical symptoms of heart failure that are present in patients is the **New York Heart Association (NYHA) classification system**, a functional classification system that categorizes a patient's subjective degree of symptoms into NYHA classes I through IV (Cohn, 2000). It places patients in one of four classes dependent largely on the degree of dyspnea present when activities are performed (Hunt et al., 2005).

Class I: Patient has no symptoms.
Class II: Patient has symptoms with ordinary exertion.
Class III: Patient has symptoms with less than ordinary exertion.
Class IV: Patient has symptoms at rest.

Diagnosing Heart Failure

Heart failure is a complex clinical syndrome for which no stand-alone test has been able to establish the diagnosis (Adams et al., 2006; Hunt et al., 2005). Obtaining a full history, physical examination, and laboratory and diagnostic testing will help to understand the etiology, to assess the severity of symptoms, and to project the patient's prognosis.

History

A careful history of the onset, severity, and nature of symptoms will be critical in the initial evaluation when heart failure is suspected. Determine the patient's baseline ability to complete ADLs and his NYHA class. A patient with heart failure tends to present with symptoms of volume overload and low cardiac output (Chart 42–3, p. 1286).

Dyspnea continues to remain the most common presenting symptom, which patients largely identify as the key factor limiting their ADLs (Adams et al., 2006; Greenberg & Hermann, 2002; Hunt et al., 2005). Past medical history should include inquiring about potential comorbid conditions, such as coronary artery disease and the use of cardiotoxic substances. A thorough family history should also be reviewed to identify possible familial tendencies. Patients diagnosed with familial dilated cardiomyopathy may have up to a 30% chance of the same process in a first-degree relative (Burkett & Hershberger, 2005) (Charts 42–4 and 42–5, p. 1286).

■ Clinical Manifestations

The physical examination focuses largely on identifying signs of volume overload and decreased peripheral perfusion. As cardiac output deteriorates, specific physical manifestations become evident (Nohria et al., 2002) (Chart 42–6, p. 1287). General assessment may reveal a confused or disoriented patient due to low cardiac output and poor oxygen perfusion to the brain, but more commonly, patients complain of forgetfulness and loss of concentration. Patients with chronic heart failure may appear to have cardiac cachexia (general ill health and malnutrition marked by weakness and emaciation usually associated with severe disease). Evaluation of the neck may reveal **jugular venous distention** (blood pressure in the jugular vein, which reflects the volume and pressure of venous blood) if volume overload is present. Upon auscultation of the lungs, **crackles** (a common abnormal sound heard on auscultation of the lungs from the movement of fluid or exudate) may or may not be present for those in chronic heart failure. A cough may be present due to an elevation in pulmonary venous pressure. A cough may or may not be productive, but if pink frothy sputum is present, one should suspect pulmonary edema as a potential cause. Dull breath sounds may be heard in the presence of a pleural effusion.

Signs of abrupt decline in cardiac output include:

1. *Narrow pulse pressure*
2. *Cool extremities*
3. *Altered mentation*
4. *Hypotension*
5. *Cheyne–Stokes respiration*
6. *Resting tachycardia*
7. *Rise in BUN/creatinine*
8. *Oliguria.*

Patients may also have **tachypnea** (an abnormally rapid rate of breathing, more than 20 breaths per minute) while being examined. Palpation of the chest may reveal that the apical pulse is

CHART 42–3   Symptoms of Congestion Versus Symptoms of Low Cardiac Output

Heart failure symptoms typically are manifested in two categories: those of congestion, or excess fluid retention, and those of poor perfusion, resulting from diminished cardiac output. These symptoms can be categorized by body system or function, as noted here.

Organ System of Symptoms	Symptoms of Congestion	Symptoms of Low Cardiac Output
Pulmonary	Dyspnea, rest or exertional Paroxysmal nocturnal dyspnea Orthopnea Cough	
Cardiac	Chest pain/tightness/discomfort	Chest pain/tightness/discomfort Decreased urination
Abdominal	Epigastric distention General discomfort Discomfort with bending Abdominal distention Nausea or anorexia Early satiety	Nausea or anorexia
Extremities	Swelling; pedal, leg, sacral, scrotal/vulvar	Weakness, instability with ambulation
Cognitive	Fatigue	Impaired memory or concentration Confusion
Sleep	Sleep disturbance; air hunger, anxiety during sleep, need to sleep with head of bed elevated or in upright position	Sleep disturbance Daytime sleepiness
General	Fatigue Lack of energy Malaise	Lack of energy Easy fatigability Weight loss Malaise Decreased exercise tolerance Decreased urination

Sources: Braunwald, E., Zipes, D. P., & Libby, P. (2001). *Heart disease: A textbook of cardiovascular medicine* (6th ed.). Philadelphia: W. B. Saunders; Greenberg, B. H., & Hermann, D. D. (2002). *Contemporary diagnosis and management of heart failure.* Newtown, PA: Handbooks in Health Care; and Nohria, A., Lewis, E., & Stevenson, L. W. (2002). Medical management of advanced heart failure. *Journal of the American Medical Association, 287*(5), 628–640.

CHART 42–4   Past Medical History

Coronary artery disease	Alcohol consumption
Prior myocardial infarctions	Tobacco use
Hypertension	Obesity
Diabetes	Diabetes mellitus
Hyperlipidemia	Illicit drug use
Valvular disease	Collagen vascular disease
Peripheral vascular disease	Bacterial or parasitic infection
Rheumatic fever	Thyroid disease
Chest irradiation	Pheochromocytoma
Cardiotoxic agents	

Interviewing patients for a thorough past medical history will help the nurse understand what may be the leading etiology of heart failure. Once the etiology is known, treatment is based on treating or alleviating precipitating causes, instituting standard heart failure medications, and teaching self-management strategies.

Sources: Hunt, S. A., Abraham, W. T., Chin, M. H., Feldman, A. M., Francis, G. S., Ganiats, T. G., et al. (2005). ACC/AHA 2005 guideline update for the diagnosis and management of chronic heart failure in the adult: Summary article: A report of the American College of Cardiology/American Heart Association Task Force on Practice Guidelines (Writing Committee to Update the 2001 Guidelines for the Evaluation and Management of Heart Failure). *Journal of the American College of Cardiology, 46,* 1116–1143; Greenberg, B. H., & Hermann, D. D. (2002). *Contemporary diagnosis and management of heart failure.* Newtown, PA: Handbooks in Health Care.

CHART 42–5   Family History

Coronary artery disease	Valvular disease
Hypertension	Peripheral vascular disease
Diabetes	Conduction system disease
Hypercholesterolemia	Skeletal myopathies
Sudden cardiac death	Collagen vascular disease
Cardiomyopathies	

A thorough interview of a patient's history includes the medical history of the patient's family. This information will be important so the nurse can understand the risk factors posed to patients who may have a genetic or familial tendency for developing disease.

Sources: Adams, K. F., Baughman, K. L., Dec, W. G., Elkayam, U., Forker, A. D., Gheorghiade, M., et al. (1999). Heart Failure Society of America (HFSA) practice guidelines. *Journal of Cardiac Failure, 5*(4), 357–382; Greenberg, B. H., & Hermann, D. D. (2002). *Contemporary diagnosis and management of heart failure.* Newtown, PA: Handbooks in Health Care; and Hunt, S. A., Abraham, W. T., Chin, M. H., Feldman, A. M., Francis, G. S., Ganiats, T. G., et al. (2005). ACC/AHA 2005 guideline update for the diagnosis and management of chronic heart failure in the adult: Summary article: A report of the American College of Cardiology/American Heart Association Task Force on Practice Guidelines (Writing Committee to Update the 2001 Guidelines for the Evaluation and Management of Heart Failure). *Journal of the American College of Cardiology, 46,* 1116–1143.

Assessment of cyanotic patients includes the following:

1. *Obtain oxygen saturation.*
2. *Assess extremities for temperature and appearance of cyanosis.*
3. *Assess neurological status.*
4. *Place oxygen and notify provider.*
5. *If patient is currently on oxygen, assess connections, and, if correct, increase oxygen level and notify provider.*

CHART 42–6   Clinical Manifestations

Hypotension	Engorged liver
Jugular venous distention	Positive hepatojugular reflux
Rales	Splenomegaly
Pleural effusion	Cyanosis
Wheezing	Cool extremities
Tachypnea	Cachexia
Tachycardia	Confusion
Third heart sound	Disorientation
Ascites	

The physical examination of patients with heart failure should be focused on a thorough assessment of the entire body. Assessment of vital signs, lungs, heart, abdomen, extremities, and mental status will often provide physical evidence of the abnormalities noted here, although their absence does not mean heart failure is not present.

Sources: Braunwald, E., Zipes, D. P., & Libby, P. (2001). *Heart disease: A textbook of cardiovascular medicine* (6th ed.). Philadelphia: W. B. Saunders; Greenberg, B. H., & Hermann, D. D. (2002). *Contemporary diagnosis and management of heart failure.* Newtown, PA: Handbooks in Health Care; Hunt, S. A., Abraham, W. T., Chin, M. H., Feldman, A. M., Francis, G. S., Ganiats, T. G., et al. (2005). ACC/AHA 2005 guideline update for the diagnosis and management of chronic heart failure in the adult: Summary article: A report of the American College of Cardiology/American Heart Association Task Force on Practice Guidelines (Writing Committee to Update the 2001 Guidelines for the Evaluation and Management of Heart Failure). *Journal of the American College of Cardiology, 46,* 1116–1143.

displaced laterally due to left ventricular hypertrophy. On auscultation an **S₃** (abnormal third heart sound in the cardiac cycle) may be present with volume overload. An **S₄** (abnormal fourth heart sound in the cardiac cycle) may be heard when patients have significant hypertension. With increasing sympathetic stimulation, tachycardia (a condition in which the myocardium contracts at a rate greater than 100 beats per minute) may be present. Abdominal examination may reveal **ascites** (an abnormal intraperitoneal accumulation of fluid containing large amounts of protein and electrolytes) and also an engorged liver and spleen. A positive **hepatojugular reflux** (an increase in jugular venous pressure when pressure is applied over the abdomen suggestive of right-sided heart failure) may also be present if volume overload is found in the periphery. The extremities may exhibit edema measured by the degree of **pitting** (an indention that remains for a short time after pressing edematous skin with the finger). Cyanosis (bluish discoloration of the skin and mucous membranes caused by an excess of deoxygenated hemoglobin in the blood) and cooling of the extremities with a poor capillary refill can occur with shunting of blood to vital organs (Braunwald, Zipes, & Libby, 2001). Chapter 37 🔗 discusses cardiac assessment.

Assessment of tachypneic patients includes the following:

1. *Obtain oxygen saturation.*
2. *Assess extremities for temperature and appearance of cyanosis.*
3. *Assess neurological status.*
4. *Place oxygen and notify provider.*
5. *If patient is currently on oxygen, assess connections, and, if correct, increase oxygen level and notify provider.*

Laboratory and Diagnostic Procedures

Laboratory tests are obtained to evaluate for underlying disease or conditions that can cause or exacerbate heart failure. Other specific laboratory tests should be done to help the health care provider understand the etiology of heart failure, precipitating factors, and/or the degree of organ compromise when heart failure is present. Applicable tests are shown in the Diagnostic Tests box (p. 1288). Recommended blood work may give clues about the etiology and/or comorbidities of heart failure using a complete blood count, ferritin, troponin, lipid panel, and thyroid function tests. Other laboratory values may give an indication of the severity of the disease by assessing liver function tests, BNP, and renal function (Adams et al., 2006; Hunt et al., 2005).

Various cardiac imaging techniques are employed to identify structural abnormalities of the heart (see the Diagnostic Tests box, p. 1288). An echocardiogram, 12-lead electrocardiogram, and chest x-ray are indicated for all patients undergoing an evaluation for heart failure (Hunt et al., 2005). These are the least expensive and most accessible tests in many institutions. Further cardiac testing will provide information on the etiology of heart failure, extent of disease, measure of cardiac function, ejection fraction (EF), cardiac anatomy, and hemodynamics. Other means to assess ventricular function may be used, such as cardiac magnetic imaging (CMR). Both types of methods also examine cardiac wall motion, wall thickness, hypertrophy or enlargement of the ventricles, and valvular dysfunction, and may determine presence of infiltrative disease and estimate pulmonary pressures. Patients with angina should have an angiogram, but noninvasive imaging to detect myocardial ischemia may be used in patients for whom the diagnosis is less clear. An endomyocardial biopsy may be helpful in heart failure caused by infiltrative disease, collagen vascular disease, toxin exposure, or myocarditis, in which the diagnosis will guide specific treatment (Hunt et al., 2005). Other testing such as maximal oxygen consumption may be done to determine whether the symptoms are pulmonary in origin, as opposed to a cardiac etiology, or when assessing prognosis. Sleep disordered breathing should also be screened for, because this has increasingly become recognized as a common contributing factor of heart failure (Adams et al., 2006; Hunt et al., 2005).

Hemodynamic Monitoring

Hemodynamic monitoring has played an important role in assessing and guiding therapy in patients with acutely decompensated heart failure (Greenberg & Hermann, 2002). The ACC has recommended guidelines for the proper use of monitoring in the acute setting (Greenberg & Hermann, 2002). Hemodynamic monitoring has been found to be an adjunct to astute clinical assessment for the use of objective measures of cardiac

DIAGNOSTIC TESTS for Heart Failure

Test	Expected Abnormality	Rationale for Abnormality
LABORATORY TEST Complete blood count	Anemia Infection	Can determine whether anemia or infection is present, which can exacerbate heart failure symptoms. Anemia affects the oxygen carrying capacity, which could result in tissue hypoxia.
Serum electrolytes and creatinine	Renal insufficiency Electrolyte deficiencies	Can determine whether underlying renal disease or electrolyte deficiencies are present and also can obtain baseline measurements prior to the initiation of diuretic therapy.
Liver function tests	Hepatic congestion	Can determine the presence of hepatic congestion.
Urinalysis	Renal dysfunction Infection Diabetes	Can determine whether underlying renal disease, infection, or diabetes is present.
Thyroid function tests	Hypo-/hyperthyroidism	Can determine whether the etiology or the exacerbation of heart failure is related to hypo- or hyperthyroidism.
Serum ferritin	Hemochromatosis	Can determine whether the etiology of heart failure is related to iron overload.
B-type natriuretic peptide	Fluid volume overload	May be useful when the diagnosis is uncertain or to assess prognosis.
Lipid panel	Hypercholesterolemia Hyperlipidemia	May indicate the presence of coronary artery disease.
BNP	Elevated with left ventricular dysfunction	Levels correlate with both the severity of symptoms and the prognosis in congestive heart failure.
DIAGNOSTIC TEST Chest x-ray	Cardiomegaly Pleural effusion	Can determine presence of cardiac or great vessel enlargement, abnormal thoracic calcification, and pulmonary congestion.
Electrocardiogram	Left ventricular hypertrophy Left bundle branch block Pathologic Q waves	Can determine presence of dysrhythmias, left ventricular hypertrophy, and myocardial ischemia or insult.
Echocardiogram	Left ventricular dysfunction Myocardial infarction Diastolic dysfunction	Can determine size and function of atria and ventricles, segmental wall motion abnormalities, wall thickness, valvular structure and function.
Viability study	Coronary disease	Can determine extent of myocardial ischemia and viability.
Cardiac catheterization: right heart catheterization	Increased filling pressures, pulmonary artery pressures, cardiac output, and mixed venous blood gas	Can determine presence of volume overload or pulmonary hypertension.
Cardiac catheterization; left heart catheterization and selective coronary angiography	Evaluation of coronary arteries and assessment of ventricular function	Can determine whether coronary artery disease is present and whether intervention is possible.

Sources: Adams, K. F., Lindenfeld, J., Arnold, J. M., et al. (2006). Executive summary: HFSA 2006 comprehensive heart failure practice guideline. *Journal of Cardiac Failure, 12*(1), 10–38; Greenberg, B. H., & Hermann, D. D. (2002). *Contemporary diagnosis and management of heart failure.* Newtown, PA: Handbooks in Health Care; and Hunt, S. A., Abraham, W. T., Chin, M. H., Feldman, A. M., Francis, G. S., Ganiats, T. G., et al. (2005). ACC/AHA 2005 guideline update for the diagnosis and management of chronic heart failure in the adult: Summary article: A report of the American College of Cardiology/American Heart Association Task Force on Practice Guidelines (Writing Committee to Update the 2001 Guidelines for the Evaluation and Management of Heart Failure). *Journal of the American College of Cardiology, 46,* 1116–1143.

output, filling pressures, and systemic vascular resistance (Nohria et al., 2002).

Pulmonary artery occlusion pressure and cardiac output are both obtained with a pulmonary artery (Swan-Ganz) catheter. These readings give the heath care team information about the fluid volume and the patient's response to therapy such as diuretics. Specific values are discussed in the Nursing Process: Patient Care Plan for Heart Failure feature (p. 1302). Hemodynamic monitoring is discussed in detail in Chapter 24 .

Medical Management

Heart failure treatment options have evolved tremendously over time. Treating "dropsy," as it was referred to in the 1600s, with early forms of digitalis from the foxglove plant to advanced medications and device therapy to aid the failing heart (Figure 42–4). The rapid growth of heart failure treatment in the 21st century includes a combination of pharmacologic measures, cardiac devices, and surgical approaches. The most significant advances in heart failure management have occurred since 1985,

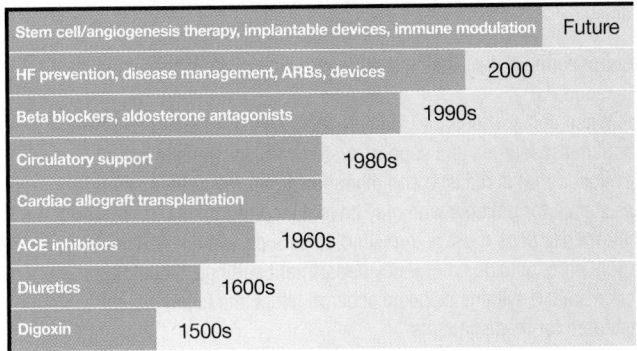

Evolution of Heart Failure Therapies

Stem cell/angiogenesis therapy, implantable devices, immune modulation	Future
HF prevention, disease management, ARBs, devices	2000
Beta blockers, aldosterone antagonists	1990s
Circulatory support	1980s
Cardiac allograft transplantation	
ACE inhibitors	1960s
Diuretics	1600s
Digoxin	1500s

FIGURE 42–4 ■ Evolution of heart failure therapies.

taking the role of medications as palliation for heart failure symptoms to those that improve that natural history of the disease (Konstam, 2004). Medications, such as ACE inhibitors and beta-adrenergic blockers, have become the current standard of care for their role in not only decreasing morbidity and mortality but also decreasing heart failure hospitalizations. Additionally, heart failure device therapies such as the biventricular pacemakers have a significant role, because they address the impact of sudden cardiac death and cardiac dyssynchrony. Chapter 39 discusses biventricular pacemakers in detail. Self-management and health promotion strategies will complete the heart failure treatment plan. Although a number of treatments have been shown to improve outcomes in patients with heart failure, the prognosis of these patients remains poor (Stewart, MacIntyre, Capewell, Mc-Murray (2003), resulting in frequent readmission to the hospital. Research is currently looking at the efficacy of using multidisciplinary strategies to improve outcomes for HF patients. This research is discssed in the Evidence-Based Practice Box (p. 1290).

Pharmacologic Management

Heart failure has no cure, but effective pharmacologic treatments have shown clear benefits of patient quality and length of life in both acute and chronic heart failure. Optimal pharmacologic management for patients with LVSD includes a combination of ACE inhibitors or angiotensin receptor blockers, beta-adrenergic blockers, diuretics, digoxin, and aldosterone antagonists. Despite advances in heart failure management, utilization of these proven therapies remains poor (Stafford & Radley, 2003). Strategies to keep patients on lifesaving medications are paramount, such as providing medication assistance programs to those in need, educating patients about the role of medical therapy, and addressing side effects that may limit quality of life.

The primary targets of pharmacologic therapies in chronic heart failure focus largely on inhibiting the neurohormonal response invoked by left ventricular dysfunction in addition to relieving the symptoms of congestion. Treatment goals for chronic heart failure include:

- Alleviate symptoms of congestion.
- Improve perfusion.
- Increase activity tolerance.
- Improve quality of life.

- Decrease hospitalizations.
- Reduce readmissions.
- Slow or reverse progression of cardiac dysfunction.
- Improve survival.
- Minimize risk factors.
- Provide palliative care.
- Decrease heart failure–related costs.
- Track outcomes (Greenberg & Hermann, 2002; Jessup & Brozena, 2003; McKelvie, 2001).

In acute heart failure, primary pharmacologic therapy is based on a rapid and thorough assessment of volume status, the extent of peripheral and organ perfusion, and the presence of precipitating and life-threatening conditions (Fonarow, 2001). Treatment goals are usually aggressive for acute heart failure and are aimed at:

- Relieving symptoms
- Stabilizing hemodynamic parameters
- Improving organ function
- Eliminating precipitating or exacerbating causes (Fonarow, 2001; Greenberg & Hermann, 2002; Nohria et al., 2002).

Angiotensin-Converting Enzyme (ACE) Inhibitors

All patients with left ventricular dysfunction, with evidence of an ejection fraction less than 40%, should be placed on an ACE inhibitor unless they have a known contraindication (Adams et al., 2006). This class of medication has shown improved survival, delayed progression of heart failure, and improved exercise tolerance (Hunt et al., 2005). ACE inhibitors work within the renin-angiotensin-aldosterone system (RAAS) to prevent the conversion of inactive angiotensin I into active angiotensin II, thus inhibiting the vasoconstricting action of angiotensin II and the angiotensin-mediated secretion of aldosterone (Teerlink & Massie, 2003). In preventing the vasoconstrictive properties of angiotensin II from occurring, blood vessels dilate and systemic vascular resistance is decreased. A decrease in systemic vascular resistance is generally referred to as *afterload reduction* (Teerlink & Massie, 2003). By blocking the effects of angiotensin II, ventricular hypertrophy and remodeling are inhibited and cardiac output is moderately improved (Teerlink & Massie, 2003). By lowering levels of aldosterone, which is responsible for sodium retention, intravascular volume is decreased, leading to a decreased preload.

Adverse effects from ACE inhibitors include cough, angioedema, renal insufficiency, and hyperkalemia. Hypotension may occur, and should be monitored for, as doses are increased. An ACE inhibitor–induced cough, due in large part to ACE inhibitor interference with the breakdown of bradykinin, is the most common cause for withdrawal. However, this occurs in only 5% to 10% of the population (Hardman & Limbird, 2001; Hunt et al., 2005). Switching from an ACE inhibitor to an angiotensin receptor blocker (ARB) is reasonable when a cough is thought to be related to the ACE inhibitor. Angioedema, a rare, potentially life-threatening condition, in which excessive mucous membrane edema occurs, will require withdrawal from the ACE inhibitor. Renal function and serum electrolytes must be

Heart Failure

Clinical Problem

Heart failure (HF) remains the most common discharge diagnosis in elderly patients, accounting for almost a quarter of all cardiovascular hospitalizations (Stewart et al., 2002). Heart failure patients commonly experience readmissions due to noncompliance, lack of understanding of self-management principles, inadequate treatment, and/or progressive disease. Although a number of pharmacologic treatments have been shown to improve outcomes in patients with HF (Jessup & Brozena, 2003), the prognosis of these patients remains poor (MacIntyre et al., 2000), resulting in frequent readmission to the hospital. Thus, there is a need for other approaches to management.

Research Findings

McAlister, Stewart, Ferrua, & McMurray (2004) conducted a study to determine whether multidisciplinary strategies improve outcomes for HF patients. The researchers searched electronic databases, bibliographies, and contacted experts to find multidisciplinary management programs in HF. Twenty-nine trials (5,039 patients) were identified. The researchers independently reviewed the results of the search strategy and selected all studies reporting the impact of outpatient-based multidisciplinary management strategies on mortality or hospitalization rates in patients with HF. Each type of intervention was then independently assigned to one of four groups: (1) multidisciplinary HF clinic; (2) multidisciplinary team providing specialized follow-up but not in a hospital or practice-based clinic; (3) telephone follow-up or telemonitoring and enhanced communication with primary health care provider (including advice to deteriorating patients to see their regular health care provider); or (4) educational programs designed to enhance patient self-care activities.

The study results reveal that these programs are associated with a 27% reduction in HF hospitalization rates and a 43% reduction in total number of HF hospitalizations. Those strategies that incorporate specialized follow-up by a multidisciplinary team or in a multidisciplinary HF clinic also reduce all-cause mortality by approximately one-quarter and all-cause hospitalizations by one-fifth.

Implications for Nursing Practice

In order to assist the patient in getting ready for discharge from the hospital, it is essential that the nurse have an understanding of the symptoms, diagnosis, and management (medical, device, and self-management). The nurse must stress the importance of compliance with every aspect of care. If the patient has been cared for using a multidisciplinary approach, the nurse typically coordinates each member of the team. The nurse must reinforce teaching and determine the patient/family's understanding of the disease and its management.

When doing discharge planning, the nurse must ask the patient about her resources and support system. A plan needs to be developed that is realistic and manageable for the patient and family. Assistance for patients who may have difficulties taking or obtaining their medications must be provided. Ensure patients have access to urgent care, outside emergency department settings. It could be beneficial if a system for postdischarge telephone follow-up were instituted for these patients.

Critical Thinking Questions

1. Your patient was discharged from the hospital 3 days ago after a heart failure hospitalization. You are the nurse calling him to see how he is feeling since discharge. He states that his daughter was supposed to pick up his medications, but had a family emergency and forgot. He still does not have his medications, and he was discharged 5 days ago. What do you do?

2. You are the nurse in a clinic, and a patient with heart failure says she is taking her medications appropriately and following a low-salt, fluid-restricted diet. Your patient's weight continues to rise, and symptoms are worsening. What do you do to help this patient?

3. Your patient is readmitted for heart failure 2 weeks after his last heart failure hospitalization. What can you do to understand what went wrong at home, and how you can prevent a third admission?

Answers to Critical Thinking Questions appear in Appendix D.

References

Jessup, M., & Brozena, S. (2003). Medical progress heart failure. *The New England Journal of Medicine, 348*, 2007–2018.

MacIntyre, K., Capewell, S., Stewart, S., et al. (2000). Evidence of improving prognosis in heart failure trends in case fatality in 66,547 patients hospitalized between 1986 and 1995. *Circulation, 102*, 1126–1131.

McAlister, F. A., Stewart, S., Ferrua, S., & McMurray, J. J. (2004). Multidisciplinary strategies for the management of heart failure patients at high risk for admission: A systematic review of randomized trials. *Journal of the American College of Cardiology, 44*(4), 810–819.

Stewart, S., Jenkins, A., Buchan, S., McGuire, A., Capewell, S., & McMurray, J. J. V. (2002). The current cost of heart failure to the National Health Service in the UK. *European Journal of Heart Failure, 4*, 361–371.

monitored within a week of initiating an ACE inhibitor and periodically thereafter, because hyperkalemia (serum levels greater than 5) and worsening renal insufficiency may occur (Hardman & Limbird, 2001; Hunt et al., 2005).

Blood pressure should be monitored frequently in patients started on ACE inhibitors. If a systolic blood pressure is found to be consistently less than 90 mmHg or if the patient complains of light-headedness, it generally warrants either a reduction in dose or stopping it completely. These symptoms may occur, especially in the setting of concomitant diuretic therapy. Initiation of ACE inhibitors is usually with short-acting agents, at low dose, with slow up-titration (Adams et al., 2006; Greenberg & Hermann, 2002).

Angiotensin II Receptor Blockers (ARB)

The RAAS system is only partially suppressed by the use of ACE inhibitors because angiotensin II is also produced by other pathways. ARBs cause inhibition by blocking RAAS activation at the angiotensin II receptor site. Angiotensin receptor blockers have been found to have clinical effects similar to those of ACE inhibitors with regard to the interference with the RAAS, yet they have not demonstrated superior results to ACE inhibitors in clinical trials. ARBs remain second-line therapy and may be considered when patients exhibit an ACE inhibitor–induced cough or angioedema (Hunt et al., 2005).

Beta-Adrenergic Blockers

Beta-adrenergic blockers, commonly referred to as beta-blockers, act primarily by blocking the sympathetic nervous system (SNS) in patients with heart failure and have been a major advance in heart failure treatment (Hunt et al., 2005). Patients placed on beta-adrenergic blockers who have had a myocardial infarction and/or left ventricular ejection fraction (LVEF) < 40% in addition to standard therapy of an ACE inhibitor, digitalis, and a diuretic, have been found to have an improved survival and reduced symptoms (Adams et al., 2006; Hunt et al., 2005). Other benefits include improved clinical status, decreased risk of sudden death, and improved overall exercise tolerance. Beta-adrenergic blockers have been found to be effective in all classes of heart failure, including patients with severe, but stable heart failure (Hunt et al., 2005).

Initially, sympathetic nervous system (SNS) activation assists the heart in maintaining a stable cardiac output. But eventually, these effects can cause increased vasoconstriction, decreased exercise capacity, decreased left ventricular efficiency, myocardial ischemia, increased potential for dysrhythmias, and worsening cardiac dysfunction. By blocking these effects, there is an improvement in coronary blood flow and less ischemia. There also is a decreased workload on the heart and less myocyte hypertrophy. Adverse cardiac remodeling is inhibited and the risk of sudden death by dysrhythmia is lessened (Sackner-Bernstein & Mancini, 1995).

Patients must be clinically stable prior to the initiation of a beta-adrenergic blocker because fluid retention may be precipitated (Hunt et al., 2005). Adjustments of diuretic management may be necessary if signs and symptoms of increasing congestion are noted. Beta-adrenergic blockers are generally initiated at low doses and increased slowly over time until target doses are achieved (Adams et al., 2006; Hunt et al., 2005). Beta-adrenergic blockers can also cause fatigue that may resolve spontaneously or be persistent enough to require the discontinuance or reduction of the medication (Hunt et al., 2005).

Nursing assessment includes observing for signs of hypotension, bradycardia, or congestion, because these conditions may require adjustment to the beta-adrenergic blocker dose or other background medications. Diabetic patients with recurrent hypoglycemia or those with resting leg ischemia should be educated to monitor for any increase of related symptoms. It is also imperative that nurses instruct patients on how to monitor their pulse, blood pressure, and symptoms of congestion, including helping them recognize when they should notify their health care provider for worrisome symptoms (Hardman & Limbird, 2001). Beta-adrenergic blockers can worsen bronchospasm in patients with reactive airway disease. If on nursing assessment wheezing is present, this may prompt the health care provider to discontinue beta-blocker therapy or then change to a beta-1 selective agent (type of beta-adrenergic blocker with less bronchospastic characteristics) at a low dose (Hardman & Limbird, 2001; Hunt et al., 2005). If patients experience hypotension while on both ACE inhibitors and beta-blockers, they might try

splitting the doses, or alternating the time of day one is taken in relation to the other. Smaller doses of the combination of ACE inhibitors and beta-blockers are preferred to higher doses of either medication alone.

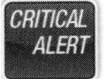 *Symptoms requiring adjustment of background medications or beta-blocker dose include:*

1. *Worsening shortness of breath*
2. *Weight gain*
3. *Fatigue*
4. *Hypotension*
5. *Light-headedness or syncope.*

Diuretics

The most effective method to relieve heart failure symptoms is to remove excess fluid with loop diuretics (Adams et al., 2006; Hunt et al., 2005). Patients with advanced heart failure needing enhanced diuresis may require the addition of chlorothiazides, such as metolazone, to loop diuretics. Hospitalized patients or those refractory to oral diuretics may require intravenous diuretics for rapid relief of congestive symptoms. The majority of diuretic agents work within the renal tubules to prevent sodium reabsorption and thereby cause natriuresis. Patients are started on a low diuretic dose, titrating subsequent doses to achieve the desired weight loss and symptom improvement. Primary management when using a diuretic will require the nurse to obtain laboratory work for close monitoring of serum electrolytes (because hypokalemia is common), to assess volume status (by evaluating symptomatology), to observe for excessive volume depletion (to ensure hypovolemia is prevented), and to monitor the response to diuretics (urine output and weight loss). Excessive volume depletion can also activate the RAAS system, negating the effect of the ACE inhibitor and ARB.

Patients placed on a diuretic will need nursing education regarding the mechanism of diuretic function and the importance of maintaining a euvolemic or "dry" weight (Greenberg & Hermann, 2002). If patient compliance with sodium and fluid restriction is poor, escalating diuretic doses may be needed to maintain **euvolemia** (when the body is in a state of equal fluid balance, without fluid retention). Often, by teaching patients the principles of diuretic self-adjustments, they are able to adjust their own dose, based on daily weights and symptoms, thus reducing the chance of volume overload. Patients who self-adjust diuretics must clearly understand how, when, and if their corresponding potassium supplementation is also increased. Patients who are unable to follow medication instructions, who are noncompliant, or who are challenged with more complicated multidrug regimens may not be candidates for adjusting their own diuretic dose due to the risk of dehydration or hypokalemia/hyperkalemia. A crucial point of education for congested patients is to emphasize the importance of sodium and fluid restriction (Greenberg & Hermann, 2002). Generally, a low-sodium diet of less than 2 to 3 grams combined with ingesting less than 2 liters of fluid per day is recommended.

Digitalis

Digitalis is a weak, positive inotrope that increases the contractility of the weakened heart muscle, thus, improving the volume of cardiac output (Teerlink & Massie, 2003). It has also been found to act as an antagonist to SNS activation (Greenberg & Hermann, 2002). It has been well studied and found to improve symptoms and exercise tolerance in patients with heart failure (Packer et al., 1993). Although there has been no mortality benefit identified with this medication, there is a decrease in hospitalizations with the greatest benefit in patients with NYHA class III and IV symptoms (Digitalis Investigation Group, 1997). Adverse effects of digitalis use are largely related to toxic serum concentrations, and therefore, patients should be placed on a low dose and be monitored to maintain a target therapeutic level < 1.0 ng/mL (Adams et al., 2006). Nursing assessment for patients on digitalis include monitoring for toxic drug levels that can cause cardiac dysrhythmias and conduction disturbances, bradycardia, gastrointestinal symptoms, and neurological complaints (Hardman & Limbird, 2001; Hunt et al., 2005). Certain medications can increase digitalis levels (Chart 42–7), and therefore, more frequent monitoring of serum concentrations is important in this subset of patients (Hardman & Limbird, 2001; Hunt et al., 2005).

Aldosterone Antagonists

Aldosterone antagonists are recommended for patients with heart failure and/or postmyocardial infarction with continued NYHA class III or IV symptoms treated with standard therapy of ACE inhibitors, beta-blockers, and diuretics. When the RAAS is activated, aldosterone release occurs. Aldosterone is a potent hormone secreted by the adrenal glands that, when activated in heart failure, causes sodium and fluid retention (Weber, 1999). Aldosterone also has neurohormonal effects including SNS activation and cardiac remodeling. Aldosterone antagonists provide a more complete blockade of the RAAS and reduce aldosterone release, resulting in a mortality benefit and a reduction in hospitalizations (Adams et al., 2006). Cautious use, with low doses of aldosterone antagonists, is encouraged. Strict monitoring of serum potassium and renal function is essential. It will

be necessary to reduce or discontinue potassium supplementation to maintain serum potassium at less than 5 mEq/L, and it should be discontinued if the serum creatinine is greater than 2.5 mg/dL (Adams et al., 2006). Gynecomastia (breast tenderness) is a troublesome adverse effect with spironolactone that is reversible when the medication is discontinued (Hunt et al., 2005). Eplerenone may be used as an alternative, due to its lower risk of causing gynecomastia. Because of the risk of hyperkalemia, aldosterone antagonists are not recommended in patients who are also on ACE inhibitors and ARBs.

Antiarrhythmic/Dysrhythmic Agents

Antiarrhythmic or dysrhythmic agents should not be used routinely to treat heart failure, but may be used for recurrent atrial fibrillation or symptomatic ventricular dysrhythmias (Hunt et al., 2005). Amiodarone, while effective in treating dysrhythmias, is associated with significant side effects such as thyroid and liver abnormalities, skin and visual abnormalities, pulmonary fibrosis, and nausea and vomiting. Careful monitoring during the course of therapy must be documented. Patients should be educated about increasing shortness of breath, bluish hue to nose or face, or other new symptoms.

Anticoagulant and Antiplatelet Agents

In patients with severe left ventricular dysfunction and an ejection fraction ≤ 35%, there is a potential for stasis within the ventricular chamber that could lead to the development of thrombi. It may be reasonable to anticoagulate such patients with warfarin therapy in the absence of a contraindication (Hunt et al., 2005). Patients with atrial fibrillation, mechanical heart valves, some mechanical assist devices, pulmonary embolism, transient ischemic attacks or cerebral vascular accidents, or other deep venous thrombosis also are candidates for anticoagulation therapy. Patients who have had a large anterior wall myocardial infarction or ventricular thrombus will often require anticoagulation therapy for 3 months (Hunt et al., 2005). Anticoagulation with warfarin requires frequent monitoring of the prothrombin time to keep patients in a therapeutic range measured by the international normalization ratio (INR) (Hardman & Limbird, 2001).

Nurses must assess a patient's "fall risk" because of potential bleeding in those taking oral anticoagulants and be sure the patient understands she may have an increased risk of bleeding. Patients must also receive instruction that frequent laboratory testing is required to maintain the INR in the desired target range. They should be instructed to call their health care provider with any signs of bleeding or with changes in their current medications, thus prompting additional assessment of changes that may occur to the INR. Antiplatelet agents, such as aspirin and clopidogrel, are indicated for patients with coronary artery, cerebral vascular, and peripheral vascular disease. Because patients may develop stomach upset and have increased bleeding risk with these agents, they should be alerted to associated warning signs.

CHART 42–7	**Medications That Increase Serum Digitalis Levels**
Quinidine	Captopril
Verapamil	Diltiazem
Spironolactone	Nifedipine
Flecainide	Nitrendipine
Propafenone	Cyclosporine
Amiodarone	

Any medication may have the potential of having an effect with other medications, leading to increased serum levels of one or both drugs. Even toxicity may result. This list includes those medicines known to increase serum digitalis levels. When digitalis levels become > 1.2, there is an associated increased risk of mortality. Those with levels > 2 are at risk of symptoms of digitalis toxicity, including nausea, vomiting, visual disturbance, or neurological changes.

Sources: Braunwald, E., Zipes, D. P., & Libby, P. (2001). *Heart disease: A textbook of cardiovascular medicine* (6th ed.). Philadelphia: W. B. Saunders; Hardman, J. G., & Limbird, L. E. (Eds.). (2001). *Goodman and Gilmans's The Pharmacological basis of therapeutics* (10th ed.). New York: McGraw-Hill; Hunt, S. A., Abraham, W. T., Chin, M. H., Feldman, A. M., Francis, G. S., Ganiats, T. G., et al. (2005). ACC/AHA 2005 guideline update for the diagnosis and management of chronic heart failure in the adult: Summary article: A report of the American College of Cardiology/American Heart Association Task Force on Practice Guidelines (Writing Committee to Update the 2001 Guidelines for the Evaluation and Management of Heart Failure). *Journal of the American College of Cardiology, 46,* 1116–1143.

 CRITICAL ALERT

1. Elderly patients with heart failure frequently void at night and therefore are at risk for falling if they arise suddenly.
2. Consider discussion with the health care provider about the different modalities to eliminate fall risks, including the use of indwelling catheter, bedside commode, or call light for assistance (for patients in the hospital) and home health and home needs–assessment for those at home.

Potential risks of anticoagulation therapy include the following:

1. *When international normalization ratio (INR) levels are supratherapeutic, bleeding may occur (hemoptysis, hematuria, bloody stool, epistaxis, or excessive bleeding from lacerations).*

2. *When INR levels are subtherapeutic, thrombi may form.*

3. *Discuss the risks and benefits of anticoagulant therapy, including what to watch for, dietary suggestions, and recommendations for monitoring.*

4. *Encourage compliance with medication dose changes and with the treatment plan.*

5. *Adverse effects may result if either of these is not followed closely.*

Inotropic, Vasopressor, and Vasodilator Therapeutic Agents

In patients with acute decompensated heart failure and critical hypoperfusion, intravenous diuretics, inotropes, vasopressor, or vasodilator agents have been found to be beneficial in improving hemodynamics, including stroke volume and cardiac output, and thereby improving blood pressure and perfusion to organs and tissues (Fonarow, 2001; Stevenson, 2003). When a patient presents with acute decompensated heart failure, the ideal drug would support blood pressure and improve cardiac hemodynamic pressures; that is, decrease pulmonary artery occlusion pressure and right atrial pressure, and increase cardiac output (Stevenson, 2003). Acute reduction in cardiac filling pressures is associated not only with symptomatic improvement but also with a reduction in mortality rates, whereas acute improvements in measured cardiac output or ejection fraction are not as closely associated with improved survival (Fonarow, 2001).

Intravenous inotropes, such as milrinone and dobutamine, have been found to improve hemodynamic pressures in the acute setting. However, when used chronically, they have been found to lead to increased mortality (Abraham et al., 2005). Inotropic agents may have use in a subset of patients with reduced blood pressure and severe symptoms with poor end-organ perfusion (Adams et al., 2006). Chronic inotropes may have a role in palliating symptoms for patients with end-stage disease, but are not recommended for intermittent use. Agents with vasodilating properties, such as intravenous nitroglycerine, sodium nitroprusside, and nesiritide, may be an alternative in select, diuretic-resistant patients to reduce ventricular filling pressures, decrease afterload, and improve symptoms of acute decompensation (Adams et al., 2006; Hunt et al., 2005).

Medications for Select Patients

Hydralazine/nitrates had been used in combination until ACE inhibitors showed superior results in patients with heart failure. Now, this combination is recognized as a reasonable alternative for patients who are unable to take an ACE inhibitor, ARBs, and/or beta-adrenergic blockers for whatever reason (Adams et al., 2006). African Americans patients with continued NYHA class III or IV symptoms, despite standard medical management with an ACE inhibitor or ARB and beta-adrenergic blockers, have improved outcomes with hydralazine/nitrates, which should be added if blood pressure allows. The Pharmacology Summary (p. 1294) reviews all of the medications used to treat heart failure.

Complementary and Alternative Therapies

Surveys have shown that at least 50% of patients with heart failure take some type of vitamins or herbal supplements to treat their disease or prevent other diseases (Greenberg & Hermann, 2002). The Complementary and Alternatives Therapies feature (p. 1296) presents a range of alternative therapies that are available. Although over 40 products are touted for cardiovascular benefits, little randomized-controlled clinical research supports claims, and safety and efficacy are not known. Despite the fact that supplemental therapies are widely used, there remains little understanding of how they interact with prescribed heart failure medications. Potentially harmful results may occur, especially in the elderly or those with impaired metabolism (Greenberg & Hermann, 2002). Chronically ill patients, especially those on diuretic therapy, should take a standard multivitamin daily (Hunt et al., 2005).

Patients may ask their health care providers questions such as the following about herbal medicine:

1. *Will this alternative or herbal therapy interfere with my heart failure medicines?*

2. *How much of this alternative or herbal therapy is safe for me to take?*

3. *Has this alternative or herbal therapy been tested for safety in people with heart failure?*

4. *Have research studies proven that this alternative or herbal therapy helps people with heart failure?*

A particularly dangerous supplement that patients with heart failure should avoid is *ma huang* (commonly known as ephedra), because it has been shown to be associated with deaths (Young, 2001). Garlic, ginseng, and *ginkgo biloba* may alter antiplatelet and anticoagulant effects, so those taking aspirin, other antiplatelet agents, or warfarin should be cautioned about bleeding (American Society of Consultant Pharmacists, 1999). Ongoing research is under way to learn whether hawthorn and coenzyme Q10 (CoQ10) have any role in heart failure, because they have been touted as effective treatments in improving symptoms. For a discussion of CoQ10 supplementation, see the Complementary and Alternative Therapies feature (p. 1296).

In summary, multiple medications are used in the management of heart failure with different indications, side effects, costs, and interaction profiles. The entire health care team must share the responsibility of emphasizing the importance of medical therapy to patients, their families, and their caregivers. The complexity of the heart failure medication regimen increases the risk of noncompliance and medication errors. Using creative methods to reinforce medication use with patients at every encounter, during the hospitalization, at discharge, and in outpatient venues will lead to the best possible outcomes.

Device Therapies for Heart Failure

Cardiac devices have a well-established role in the management of systolic dysfunction. These revolutionary devices have improved both length and quality of life when added to medical therapy for those with heart failure. Cardiac pacemakers and the expanded use of implantable cardioverter defibrillators (ICDs) have become the standard of care in select patients. Internal cardioverter defibrillators have shown superiority over medical

PHARMACOLOGY Summary of Medications to Treat Heart Failure

Medication Category	Action	Application/Indication	Nursing Responsibility
Angiotensin-converting enzyme (ACE) inhibitors: Benazepril Captopril Enalapril Lisinopril Quinapril Ramipril	Works within the renin-angiotensin-aldosterone system (RAAS) to inhibit the vasconstricting action of angiotensin II and the angiotensin-mediated secretion of aldosterone, thus causing blood vessels to dilate, and systemic vascular resistance is decreased. Results in decreased afterload, decreased sodium resorption, and increased contractility.	Use in all patients with reduced ventricular function; left ventricular ejection fraction (LVEF) < 40%. HF patients on ACE inhibitors have improved survival and delayed progression of heart failure due to the favorable blockade of the RAAS.	Monitor for ACE inhibitor-induced cough, dizziness, hypotension, hyperkalemia, and worsening renal insufficiency. Angioedema may also occur in rare settings.
Angiotensin II receptor blockers (ARBs): Candesartan cilexetil Eprosartan mesylate Irbesartan Losartan potassium Telmisartan Valsartan	Causes inhibition by blocking RAAS activation at the angiotensin II receptor site. Angiotensin receptor blockers have been found to have similar clinical effects as ACE inhibitors with regard to the interference with the RAAS. They decrease afterload, decrease sodium resorption, and increase contractility.	Use in heart failure (HF) patients who are intolerant to ACE inhibitors with an LVEF < 40%. HF patients on ARBs have improved survival and delayed progression of heart failure due to the favorable blockade of the RAAS.	Monitor for dizziness, hypotension, hyperkalemia, and worsening renal insufficiency.
Beta-adrenergic blockers: Carvedilol Metoprolol succinate	Acts primarily by blocking the sympathetic nervous system (SNS) in patients with heart failure. By blocking these effects, there is an improvement in coronary blood flow and less ischemia. There also is a decreased workload on the heart and less myocyte hypertrophy resulting in decreased myocardial ischemia and hypertrophy.	Use in HF patients with LVEF < 40% or postmyocardial infarction. HF patients on beta-blockers have been found to have improved survival, improvement in symptoms, a decrease in the risk of sudden death, and improved overall exercise tolerance.	Observe for signs of hypotension or bradycardia, as either condition may require adjustment to the beta-adrenergic-blocker dose or other background medications. Patient education is imperative about the initial response or up-titration of this drug, which can cause fatigue, dizziness, fluid retention, and worsening heart failure. It is also imperative that nurses instruct patients on how to monitor their pulse and blood pressure and to help them recognize when they should notify their provider if these parameters become too low. Beta-adrenergic blockers can worsen bronchospasm in patients with reactive airway disease and therefore should be monitored.
Diuretics: Bumetanide Furosemide Metolazone Torsemide	Interferes with the sodium retention of HF by inhibiting the reabsorption of sodium or chloride at specific sites in the renal tubules.	Use in HF patients exhibiting signs and symptoms of fluid overload. Diuretic drugs increase urinary sodium excretion and decrease physical signs of fluid retention in patients with HF.	Nursing assessment for patients on diuretics includes monitoring for signs of hypokalemia, hypotension, and dehydration. It is also imperative that nurses provide patient self-management instruction, including daily weights, sodium and fluid restrictions, and instruction on when to notify their health care provider about worsening symptoms.

PHARMACOLOGY Summary of Medications to Treat Heart Failure—*Continued*

Medication Category	Action	Application/Indication	Nursing Responsibility
Digitalis Digoxin	A weak, positive inotrope that increases the contractility of the weakened heart muscle thus, improving the volume of cardiac output. It has also been found to have an impact on enzyme inhibition in noncardiac tissues, thus, eventually leading to a suppression of renin secretion from the RAAS.	Use in HF patients with New York Heart Association (NYHA) class III or IV symptoms. This medication has been found to decrease hospitalizations and to improve symptoms, quality of life, and exercise tolerance.	Nursing assessment for patients on digitalis includes monitoring for toxic drug levels that can cause cardiac dysrhythmias and conduction disturbances, gastrointestinal symptoms, and neurological complaints.
Aldosterone antagonists: Spironolactone	Blocks the release of aldosterone hormone secreted by the adrenal glands that, when activated in heart failure, causes sodium and fluid retention.	Use in HF patients with continued symptoms, despite therapies listed above. Found to have a favorable mortality benefit and has shown to decrease hospitalizations. These benefits are greatest in those patients with NYHA class IV symptoms.	Monitor for signs of hyperkalemia and renal dysfunction. Should not be used in combination with ACE inhibitors and ARBs. Side effect of some aldosterone antagonists is gynecomastia, which may require a change in antagonist used. Nursing instruction should include a discussion with the health care provider regarding the reduction or discontinuation of potassium supplements and also the avoidance of high-potassium-containing foods. Nonsteroidal anti-inflammatory drugs and cyclooxygenase-2 inhibitors should be avoided, which can worsen hyperkalemia and renal dysfunction.
Hydralazine and isosorbide dinitrate	This combination of vasodilators acts on both arteries and veins. Theoretically, it may act as an antioxidant on nitric oxide.	African American HF patients on standard therapy (i.e., ACE inhibitors or ARBs) and beta-blockers may benefit when this combination is added. Patients unable to tolerate ACE inhibitor or ARB therapy may consider this alternative combination. This combination has shown improved survival, reduced hospitalizations, and improved quality of life.	Monitor for headache, hypotension, and gastrointestinal complaints. Should not be used in patients that have not had a trial of ACE inhibitor or ARBs. Compliance must be reinforced due to the multidose schedule required.
Antiarrhythmics: Amiodarone Bretylium Dofetilide Ibutilide Sotalol	This class III antiarrhythmic agent has sympatholytic (or antiadrenergic) effects on the heart and AV nodal blocking properties.	May be used for rate and rhythm control for patients in atrial fibrillation, and to suppress significant ventricular dysrhythmias, or may suppress implantable cardioverter defibrillator (ICD) shocks.	Possible side effects include pulmonary toxicities, skin discoloration, hepatic and/or thyroid derangements, corneal deposits, optic neuropathy, and interactions with warfarin and digoxin. May be proarrhythmic; monitor cardiac rhythm.

Sources: Adams, K. F., Lindenfeld, J., Arnold, J. M., et al. (2006). Executive summary: HFSA 2006 comprehensive heart failure practice guideline. *Journal of Cardiac Failure, 12*(1), 10–38; Crawford, P. A., & Lin, T. L. (2004). *The Washington manual cardiology subspecialty consult* (pp. 122–126). Philadelphia: Lippincott Williams & Wilkins; and Hunt, S. A., Abraham, W. T., Chin, M. H., Feldman, A. M., Francis, G. S., Ganiats, T. G., et al. (2005). ACC/AHA 2005 guideline update for the diagnosis and management of chronic heart failure in the adult: Summary article: A report of the American College of Cardiology/American Heart Association Task Force on Practice Guidelines (Writing Committee to Update the 2001 Guidelines for the Evaluation and Management of Heart Failure). *Journal of the American College of Cardiology, 46*, 1116–1143.

therapy alone in reducing sudden cardiac death. Cardiac pacemakers and ICDs are discussed in detail in Chapter 39.

Cardiac Resynchronization Therapy

Cardiac resynchronization therapy (CRT), also known as biventricular pacing, is useful in the treatment of heart failure in selected patients. The CRT device paces both ventricles simultaneously, thereby helping to restore a synchronized contraction that had been lost with the emergence of conduction abnormalities and dyssynchrony, which is present in approximately 25% to 30% of patients with heart failure (Abraham, 2003). CRT is most effective in patients with moderate to severe symptoms, despite optimal heart failure medication, with a LVEF < 35% and QRS duration > 120 milliseconds (Hunt et al., 2005). In a healthy heart, electrical impulses are generated from the sinus node in the right atrium, travel through the atrioventricular (AV) node, and then almost simultaneously down each bundle branch to cause a coordinated contraction of the left ventricle and efficient movement of blood through the heart. Heart failure patients with myocardial damage often have conduction abnormalities such as a bundle branch block, in which there is a delay in the transmission of the electrical impulse down one or the other bundle branch, causing a wide QRS complex on the ECG. This intraventricular conduction delay results in dyssynchronous movements between the ventricles, abnormal septal wall motion, suboptimal filling during diastole, poorly coordinated ventricular contraction, decreased left ventricular ejection fraction, and even impaired mitral valve function (Bakker et al., 2000;

Kerwin et al., 2000). Clinically, patients with a bundle branch block experience limited exercise tolerance, impaired quality of life, and poor functional capacity.

For CRT implantation, a pacemaker box is inserted surgically under the skin, usually in the left upper chest wall, and pacemaker leads are placed directly in the right ventricle and through a lateral vein into the left ventricle. These leads are programmed to coordinate contraction times between the ventricular leads while optimizing AV delay. Patients with atrial fibrillation may undergo AV junction ablation (rendering cells nonfunctional) and receive simple biventricular pacing (Abraham, 2003; Linde et al., 2002). The mechanical improvements seen with this kind of pacing in-

COMPLEMENTARY & ALTERNATIVE THERAPIES

Types of Therapies

Type of Therapy	Proposed Clinical Use	Evidence
Meditation	Inhibits sympathetic activation Improves quality of life (QOL)	In 17 elderly patients treated medically for heart failure, meditation led to a reduction in norepinephrine levels and improved QOL compared to control.
Relaxation	Improves some aspects of QOL	95 patients with moderately severe heart failure were randomized to 15 weeks of relaxation response therapy, to 15 weeks of cardiac education, or to usual care. Aspects of QOL that improved related to peace—spiritual and emotional scores, but not physical for the intervention group.
Inspiratory muscle training	Improves inspiratory muscle use, functional capacity, ventilatory response to exercise, and QOL	32 patients with heart failure with inspiratory muscle weakness were randomly assigned to either 12 weeks of inspiratory training or placebo training. Intervention group had improved inspiratory muscle strength, functional capacity, response to exercise, and QOL.
T'ai chi	Improves QOL Improves 6-minute walk test	30 patients with heart failure on standard therapy were randomized to 12 weeks of either t'ai chi or usual care. The intervention group had enhanced QOL and functional capacity.
Acupuncture	Inhibits sympathetic activation	15 advanced patients with heart failure underwent mental stress testing before and after (1) real acupuncture, (2) nonpoint acupuncture, and (3) no-needle acupuncture control. Acupuncture was found to attenuate sympathoexcitation during mental stress.
Nutraceuticals	Proposed to reduce risk of heart disease through antioxidant action	American College of Cardiology/American Heart Association (ACC/AHA) Chronic Heart Failure Guidelines 2005 ✓ **Not recommended to prevent or treat heart failure**
Hawthorn	Improved heart failure symptoms	A meta-analysis including 13 trials using hawthorn extract vs. placebo in chronic patients with heart failure showed significantly improved symptoms of dyspnea and fatigue.
Chelation therapy	Proposed to treat coronary artery disease	American Heart Association [a] ✓ **Not recommended for treating coronary artery disease**

[a] As per http://www.americanheart.org/presenter.jhtml?identifier=4493

Sources: Chang, B. H., et al. (2005). A relaxation response randomized trial on patients with chronic heart failure. *Journal of Cardiopulmonary Rehabilitation, 25*(3), 149–157; Curiati, J. A., et al. (2005). Meditation reduces sympathetic activation and improves the quality of life in elderly patients with optimally treated heart disease. *Journal of Alternative and Complementary Medicine, 11*(3), 465–472; Dall'Ago, P., Chiappa, G. R., Guths, H., Stein, R., & Ribeiro, J. P. (2006). Inspiratory muscle training in patients with heart failure and inspiratory muscle weakness: A randomized trial. *Journal of the American College of Cardiology, 47*(4), 757–763; Hunt, S. A., Abraham, W. T., Chin, M. H., Feldman, A. M., Francis, G. S., Ganiats, T. G., et al. (2005). ACC/AHA 2005 guideline update for the diagnosis and management of chronic heart failure in the adult: Summary article: A report of the American College of Cardiology/American Heart Association Task Force on Practice Guidelines (Writing Committee to Update the 2001 Guidelines for the Evaluation and Management of Heart Failure). *Journal of the American College of Cardiology, 46,* 1116–1143; Jeffrey, S. (2002). No evidence of benefit from chelation therapy. *HeartWire News.* Retrieved October 9, 2006, from http://www.theheart.org/article/277715.do; Middlekauff, H. F., Hui, K., Yu, J. L., Hamilton, M. A., Fonarow, G. C., Moriguchi, J., et al. (2002). Acupuncture inhibits sympathetic activation during mental stress in advanced heart failure patients. *Journal of Cardiac Failure, 8*(6), 399–406; Pittler, M. H., Schmidt, K., & Ernst, E. (2003). Hawthorne extract for treating chronic heart failure: Meta-analysis of randomized trials. *American Journal of Medicine, 114*(8), 665–674; and Yeh, G. Y., Wood, M. J., Lorell, B. H., Stevenson, L. W., Eisenberg, D. M., Wayne, P. M., et al. (2004). Effects of tai chi mind–body movement therapy on functional status and exercise capacity in patients with chronic heart failure: A randomized controlled trial. *American Journal of Medicine, 117*(8), 541–548.

COMPLEMENTARY & ALTERNATIVE THERAPIES

Coenzyme Q10 (CoQ10) Supplementation

Description:

Coenzyme Q10 (CoQ10) is an enzyme produced by the body that is a co-factor in mitochondrial energy production (Sander, Coleman, Patel, Kluger, & White, 2006). It is a solid, waxlike substance that is abundant in healthy heart tissue. Deficiencies of CoQ10—from 50% to 75% of normal levels—have been found in heart tissue biopsies of people with various heart diseases. The body produces less CoQ10 as a person ages and some cholesterol-lowering drugs also reduce levels of this vital enzyme. Supplement doses of CoQ10 range from 30 to 200 mg per day.

Heart failure (HF) is a condition that is greatly impacted by CoQ10 levels. HF impairs the heart's ability to maintain normal cardiac output. Following an initial cardiac insult, remodeling ensues, which results in left ventricular dilation and hypertrophy. Oxidative stress also increases after a cardiac insult, while CoQ10 levels decrease. This and other data led researchers to the hypothesis that CoQ10 may decrease oxidative stress, impair remodeling, and improve cardiac function (Weant & Smith, 2005)

Research Support:

A meta-analysis of trials by one team of researchers evaluated the impact of CoQ10 therapy on ejection fraction and cardiac output. The team conducted a systematic literature search to identify randomized, controlled trials of CoQ10 in heart failure between 1966 and June 2005. Researchers conducted a subgroup analysis to assess clinical heterogeneity between trials. The team identified 12 trials in which 10 evaluated ejection fraction and 2 evaluated cardiac output. Doses ranged from 60 to 200 mg/day, and treatment periods ranged from 1 to 6 months. Overall, ejection fraction showed a 3.7% net improvement. In addition, cardiac output increased an average of 0.28 L/minute. The researchers concluded that CoQ10 enhances systolic function in chronic heart failure; however, they noted that its effectiveness may be reduced with concurrent use of current standard treatments (Sander et al., 2006).

An Italian team conducted a double-blind, placebo-controlled crossover study of 23 patients with stable CHF secondary to ischemic heart disease. Researchers assigned patients to the following treatments, each of which lasted 4 weeks: oral CoQ10 (100 mg tid), CoQ10 plus supervised exercise training (ET) (60% of peak VO$_2$, five times a week), placebo, and placebo plus ET. There was significant improvement in both peak VO$_2$ and endothelium-dependent dilation of the brachial artery (EDDBA) after CoQ10 and after ET as compared with placebo. The researchers concluded that oral CoQ10 improves functional capacity, endothelial function, and LV contractility in CHF with no side effects. In addition, patients showed higher plasma CoQ10 levels and more pronounced effects on all the abovementioned parameters with a combination of CoQ10 and ET (Belardinelli et al., 2006).

The same research team, in a related study, found that CoQ10 supplementation resulted in a threefold increase in plasma CoQ10 level. Systolic wall thickening score index (SWTI) and left ventricular ejection fraction improved both at rest and peak dobutamine stress echo after CoQ10 supplementation (Belardinelli et al., 2005).

A New Zealand study examined 24 patients with stable, symptomatic heart failure and a left ventricular ejection fraction less than 40%. Each patient was randomized to 40 mg atorvastatin or placebo for 6 weeks, then the patient was crossed over to the other treatment arm for a further 6 weeks. Coenzyme Q10 was shown to be the significant variable that predicted improvement in endothelial function after adjusting for LDL-cholesterol levels (Strey et al., 2005).

References

Belardinelli, R., Mucaj, A., Lacalaprice, F., Solenghi, M., Principi, F., Tiano, L., et al. (2005). Coenzyme Q10 improves contractility of dysfunctional myocardium in chronic heart failure. *BioFactors, 25*(1–4), 137–145.

Belardinelli, R., Mucaj, A., Lacalaprice, F., Solenghi, M., Seddaiu, G., Principi, F., et al (2006). Coenzyme Q10 and exercise training in chronic heart failure. *European Heart Journal, 27*(22), 2675–2681.

Sander, S., Coleman, C. I., Patel, A. A., Kluger, J., & White, C. M. (2006). The impact of coenzyme Q10 on systolic function in patients with chronic heart failure. *Journal of Cardiac Failure, 12*(6), 464–472.

Strey, C. H., Young, J. M., Molyneux, S. L., George, P. M., Florkowski, C. M., Scott, R. S., et al. (2005). Endothelium-ameliorating effects of statin therapy and coenzyme Q10 reductions in chronic heart failure. *Atherosclerosis, 179*(1), 201–206.

Weant, K. A., & Smith, K. M. (2005). The role of coenzyme Q10 in heart failure. *Annals of Pharmacotherapy, 39*(9), 1522–1526.

---

clude less restrictive ventricular filling patterns, decreased mitral valve regurgitation, improved cardiac muscle contractile synchrony, increased LVEF, and improved cardiac index (Molhoek et al., 2002). Clinical improvements include improved NYHA class, peak oxygen uptake, quality-of-life scores, and 6-minute walk test scores (Abraham, 2003). The algorithm in Figure 42–5 ■ (p. 1298) illustrates how patients may be selected for CRT/automatic implanted cardioverter defibrillator (AICD) therapy. Cardiac resynchronization therapy is discussed in detail in Chapter 39 .

Implantable Cardioverter Defibrillators

Implantable cardioverter defibrillators (ICDs) are indicated for patients with heart failure at risk for sudden cardiac death due to significant reductions in ventricular function (LVEF < 35%). ICD implantation consists of a small generator box inserted surgically under the skin with leads extending into the heart. These programmable devices detect lethal ventricular dysrhythmias and respond by administering either overdrive pacing or an electric shock directly to the heart for sustained dysrhythmias. Mortality rates with the use of an ICD have decreased, even in the absence of a history of lethal ventricular dysrhythmias (Moss et al., 2002; Teerlink & Massie, 2003). Patients determined to be at risk of sudden death who also need a pacemaker can receive a combined pacemaker/ICD (Abraham, 2003; Bristow, Feldman, & Saxon, 2000; Teerlink & Massie, 2003). Selection criteria for identifying those appropriate for ICD implantation are summarized in Figure 42–5 ■ (p. 1298). Newer devices have advanced capabilities that couple diagnostic and treatment modes. Currently patients can be monitored from remote locations for their volume status, activity levels, and more. Chapter 39 discusses the indications for implantation of ICDs.

■ Nursing Management

Implantation of a pacemaker, ICD, or combined device is usually a less invasive procedure, requiring a simple incision to insert the control box and vascular insertion of the leads. Patients are usually admitted overnight for observation and then discharged after receiving a chest x-ray to ensure lead placement and to rule out a postprocedure pneumothorax. Recovery after placement of a pacemaker or ICD occurs over weeks, and patients should expect to experience some soreness of the chest wall and bruising. Appropriate pain management should be considered. Patients need instruction on wound care, to keep the site clean, and to

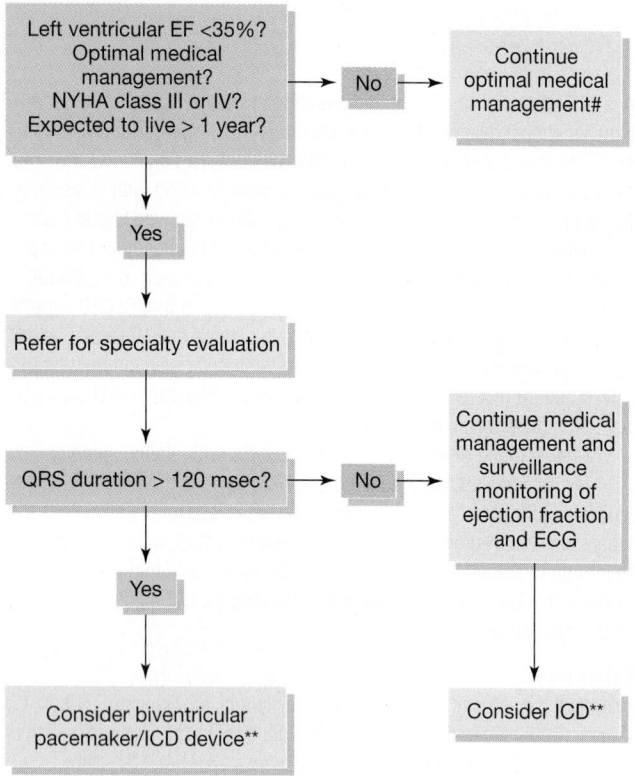

Notes:
** = Excluding risk of sudden cardiac death
# = ACE inhibitors or ARBs, beta blockers, diuretics, digoxin, spironolactone

FIGURE 42–5 ■ Algorithm for cardiac pacemaker and defibrillator.

monitor for signs and symptoms of infection or bleeding. An office visit to the health care provider to inspect the site usually occurs 1 week after implantation. To minimize the risk of dislodging the ventricular leads, patients are instructed not to raise the affected arm above the head and to avoid lifting of more than 10 to 15 pounds for approximately 3–4 weeks. Over time, they may resume usual activities.

Patients usually follow up with their electrocardiologist 1 month after their device implantation, and then every 6 to 12 months thereafter to ensure that the device is functioning properly and to have the battery life assessed. The device should be interrogated after any ICD discharges, to ensure that it is responding appropriately to a dysrhythmia, and then generally every 6 months. Patients are advised to carry their device identification card with them at all times and to avoid strong magnets, particularly those used in magnetic resonance imaging (MRI), and to alert airport security personnel. The Patient Teaching & Discharge Priorities box shows key points of the discharge plan after such procedures.

Percutaneous and Surgical Treatments for Coronary Artery Disease

Treating heart failure may include various catheter-based procedures. Procedures in the cardiac catheterization laboratory can provide diagnostic information (to assess the coronary tree, to assess for the presence of life-threatening dysrhythmias, and to assess hemodynamic measurements) and often provide opportunities

for treatment (revascularization for patients with coronary disease and treatments for dysrhythmia management). Balloon valvuloplasty (a percutaneous, catheter-based technique to relieve valvular stenosis) is sometimes considered for patients with a high mortality risk with surgical repair (Cohn, 2000; McKelvie, 2001). Balloon valvuloplasty is discussed in detail in Chapter 41 .

One of the leading causes of left ventricular dysfunction resulting in heart failure is from significant coronary artery disease. Percutaneous and surgical treatments will be employed based on the nature of the coronary lesions, the likelihood of achieving revascularization, and the patient's risk profile.

Percutaneous Coronary Interventions

Spanning from 1987 to 2003, cardiac catheterizations increased 326%, with 664,000 procedures performed on 652,000 patients (AHA, 2006b). Men accounted for 65% of these procedures, and 52% of the patients were over the age of 65. Percutaneous coronary interventions (PCIs) have become a modality of revascularization that is less invasive than coronary artery bypass graft (CABG) surgery, are associated with shorter recovery time, and have shown outcomes comparable to CABG (McKelvie, 2001). The elderly patient and those with significant left ventricular dysfunction may be better candidates for PCI over bypass surgery due to faster recovery rates and subsequent lower mortality rates.

PCIs include percutaneous transluminal coronary angioplasty (PTCA), atherectomy, laser angioplasty, implantation of intracoronary stents, and other catheter devices for treating CAD (Feldman et al., 2006). Patients with multivessel coronary disease treated with PTCA have 5-year survival rates, similar to those who undergo CABG, although patients with diabetes have a better survival rate when treated with CABG (McKelvie, 2001).

Adjunctive thrombolytic therapies (e.g., abciximab, tirofiban, and eptifibatide) with PTCA (and intracoronary stenting) have led to lower restenosis rates, fewer complications, and improved mortality (McKelvie, 2001). New directions in PCI will focus on the strategies to improve safety, reduce restenosis rates, and broaden eligibility criteria for patients with subsets of CAD that are currently excluded. Chapter 39 discusses in detail PCI procedures.

Coronary Artery Bypass Graft Surgery

Coronary artery bypass graft surgery competes with PCI to revascularize patients with significant coronary artery lesions. CABG surgery has been effective in treating significant CAD that is not amenable to catheter-based techniques in 50% to 70% of patients with heart failure (Nohria et al., 2002) (Figure 42–6 ■). As of 2003, 467,000 procedures were completed on 268,000 patients in the United States (AHA, 2006b). CABG may be considered in those with compensated heart failure with an ejection fraction greater than 20%. This procedure should be considered when there is a high likelihood that revascularization will decrease the amount of ischemic myocardium by improving blood flow and thereby improving cardiac muscle function (Kouchoukos, Blackstone, Doty, Hanley, & Karp, 2003). A complete description of CABG surgery is included in Chapter 40 .

 CRITICAL ALERT

Signs of stable heart failure include:

1. *On stable medications requiring little change*
2. *Normal hemodynamic parameters*
3. *Without recent acute decompensation*
4. *Acceptable blood pressure.*

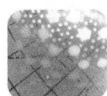

PATIENT TEACHING & DISCHARGE PRIORITIES for Pacemaker/Implantable Cardioverter Defibrillator Devices

A nursing care plan made for patients after implantation of cardiac devices includes monitoring patients postimplantation, teaching patients about the device, postoperative care, monitoring for adverse complications, and appropriate follow-up.

Need	Teaching
Patient/family • Provide patient education related to device and need for scheduled follow-up.	• Heart failure medical therapy will augment device therapy and will continue indefinitely. • Limit arm movement to affected side for 1 to 2 weeks (use of sling as needed). • No lifting with affected side for 3 to 4 weeks. • Assess site for signs and symptoms of infection/drainage/bleeding. • Call for abnormal sensation of chest wall muscle movement (indication of dislodged lead or diaphragmatic/pectoral pacing). • Follow-up will be in 1 week to assess site, at 1 month, and then every 6 months and as needed for device interrogation and battery life assessment.
Family/support system • Patients with an automatic implanted cardioverter defibrillator (AICD) may be shocked by the device.	• Family/supports need to understand this is the intended purpose, and that the patient will need follow-up with his cardiologist to assess appropriateness of device. • Patients may need support for anxiety due to the potential or real shocks from an implantable cardioverter defibrillator (ICD).
Setting • In hospital and at home: assess postoperative pain. • In hospital and at home: assess incision site.	• Have patient rate pain. • Provide pain medicines as ordered. • Continue to assess level of responsiveness and relief of pain. • Call cardiologist for unrelieved or new pain. • Assess for bleeding, other drainage. • Hematoma. • Call cardiologist for changes.

Sources: Bakker, P. F., Meijburg, H. W., de Vries, J. W., Mower, M. M., Thomas, A. C., Hull, M. L., et al. (2000). Biventricular pacing in end-stage heart failure improves functional capacity and left ventricular function. *Journal of Interventional Cardiac Electrophysiology, 4*(2), 395–404; and Vesty, J., Rasmusson, K. D., Hall, J., Schmitz, S., & Brush, S. (2004). Cardiac resynchronization therapy and automatic implantable cardiac defibrillators in the treatment of heart failure: A review article. *Journal of the American Academy of Nurse Practitioners, 16*(10).

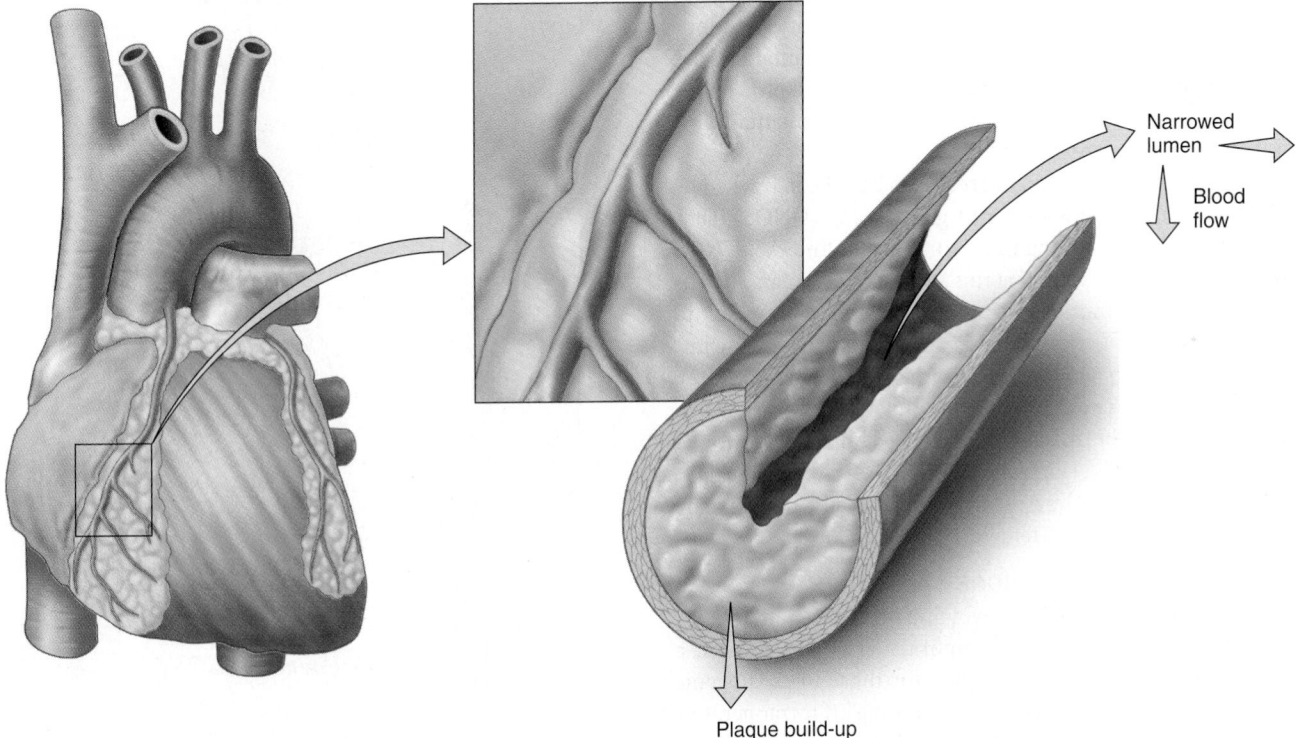

FIGURE 42–6 ■ Coronary artery disease.

Other Surgical Treatments for Systolic Heart Failure

Specific surgical procedures are utilized if they are likely to improve left ventricular function, clinical manifestations, and survival. The more chronically ill heart failure patient with significant comorbidities of renal, lung, and other vascular disease, however, will be placed at a higher surgical morbidity and mortality risk (Nohria et al., 2002). Surgical techniques to treat heart failure beyond CABG surgery include valve replacement or repair, cardiac transplantation, long-term mechanical assist devices, and investigational surgical therapies (Kouchoukos et al., 2003).

Valve Replacement or Repair

For those with significant cardiac valvular disorders, valve replacement or repair surgery may be performed to optimize hemodynamic parameters, limit symptoms, and improve survival (McKelvie, 2001). Timely consideration for valve replacement is the key to successful outcomes. When systolic dysfunction is severe, mitral regurgitant valve lesions are typically not replaced, because the advantage in this population has not been established (Nohria et al., 2002). Once the left ventricle becomes dilated with poor function, there is little hope for recovery by replacing the valve alone. Conversely, replacement or repair of stenotic valvular lesions is generally recommended. Chapter 41 ⊖ discusses the surgical management of valvular disorders.

Cardiac Transplantation

Heart transplant surgery was pioneered in 1967, leading to its widespread use for the treatment of end-stage cardiomyopathy in the early 1980s. Heart transplantation is a highly successful treatment for a select patient population whose 1- to 2-year prognosis is estimated to be less than 50% (Renlund & Taylor, 2002). Although heart transplantation remains the best long-term surgical treatment for heart failure in a small group of patients, it continues to be limited by the availability of donor hearts. An average of just over 2,000 heart transplantations are performed annually in the United States (AHA, 2006b). Thousands of patients would benefit from heart transplantation if more donor hearts were available.

Over 33,000 heart transplant recipients have been tracked by the national United Network for Organ Sharing (UNOS) database (2006). Average waiting times for those on the U.S. UNOS transplant list in a noncritical status are just over 1 year. The advent of modern immunosuppression (drug therapies used to prevent rejection of a transplanted organ) has dramatically improved survival rates over time (Greenberg & Hermann, 2002). First-year survival rates for patients undergoing heart transplantation are 86.4% (males) and 84.6% (females); and for 3-year survival, 78.9% (males) and 76.1% (females) (AHA, 2006b). Five-year survival rates for transplant patients are 72.2% (males) and 68.5% (females) (AHA, 2006b).

Mechanical Assist Devices

Circulatory support remains an evolving field with both temporary and permanent devices. Temporary assist devices are a means to provide circulatory support for those in cardiogenic shock or when difficulties occur when coming off intraoperative cardiopulmonary support (Greenberg & Hermann, 2002). Such support includes intra-aortic balloon pumps, centrifugal right and left ventricular assist devices (VADs), and percutaneous ventricular assist devices (PVADs). Longer term devices used to "bridge" patients who are declining as they await cardiac transplantation, or those for long-term or permanent use, include left ventricular assist devices (LVADs), total artificial hearts (TAHs), and right ventricular assist devices (RVADs).

Implantation of permanent or "destination" VADs has emerged as a promising surgical treatment option for those with end-stage heart failure (Figure 42–7 ■). Patients with such devices are able to return to their home settings, living with a significant improvement in length and quality of life. Implantable LVADs have been used since the mid-1980s in transplant candidates who continue to deteriorate in the setting of long waits for suitable donor hearts (Nohria et al., 2002). The devices were designed for short-term use for those needing a bridge to heart transplantation or as a bridge to myocardial recovery (Greenberg & Hermann, 2002). In 2001, results were published of the Randomized Evaluation of Mechanical Assist Treatment for Congestive Heart failure (REMATCH) trial, a landmark trial showing mortality and quality-of-life benefits for patients implanted with an LVAD versus those in the medical management arm (Rose et al., 2001). LVADs, as destination therapy, have been approved by the Food and Drug Administration for treating patients with end-stage heart failure who are not transplant candidates (Blue Cross Blue Shield Association, 2002). The future and success of this technology will be based on appropriate patient selection, improved devices durability, and coordinated teams who are able to provide long-term management to this specific population.

Investigational Surgical Therapies

Surgical techniques that reconfigure the heart's muscular geometry have had mixed results. Batista and other colleagues have

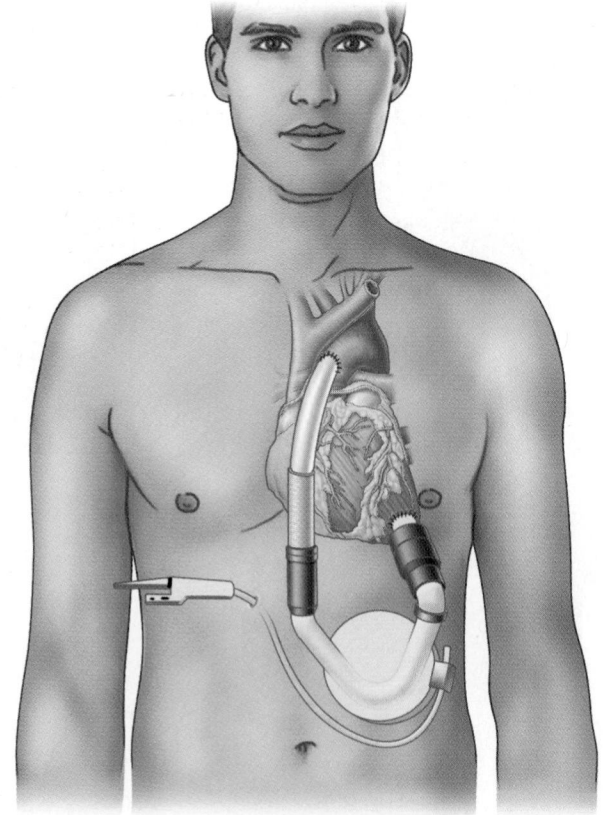

FIGURE 42–7 ■ Ventricular assist device.

performed a procedure of partial left ventriculectomy (Kouchoukos et al., 2003). This procedure involves resecting a segment of the left ventricle base on the premise that reduction in ventricular size will lead to improved function. Now known as the Batista procedure, it has grown out of favor as a treatment option for cardiomyopathy (Hunt et al., 2005; Nohria et al., 2002).

In contrast to the Batista procedure, in which weakened yet functional tissue is removed, ventricular aneurysm resection involves removal of nonfunctional myocardium (Kouchoukos et al., 2003). Ventricular restoration surgery is thought to reshape the misshapen geometry that occurs with systolic dysfunction. The future of this technique for patients with heart failure remains to be defined.

Research continues that examines the use of constraint devices that may change and support ventricular geometric configuration, thus leading to improved cardiac function. The Acorn cardiac support device is one such experimental device that is thought to cause improvements in function, symptoms, and degree of mitral valve regurgitation (Kouchoukos et al., 2003). Stem cell injection therapy during CABG is also under investigation.

Acute Decompensated Heart Failure

Acute heart failure contributes considerable expense to health care systems due to the need for frequent hospitalizations and has become a leading public health issue (Greenberg & Hermann, 2002; Jessup & Brozena, 2003; Nohria et al., 2002). Acute presentations of heart failure are manifestations of elevated ventricular filling pressures causing sudden congestion in the pulmonary vasculature and periphery, decreased cardiac output leading to poor perfusion of the periphery and kidneys, and increased systemic vascular resistance causing increased work for the heart (see Chart 42–1, p. 1281) (Adams et al., 2006; Fonarow, 2001; Greenberg & Hermann, 2002; Hunt et al., 2005; Nohria et al., 2002). Severe dyspnea (shortness of breath) is the leading symptom resulting in hospitalizations for heart failure, and its relief is usually a treatment priority (Greenberg & Hermann, 2002; Nohria et al., 2002). Paroxysmal nocturnal dyspnea, orthopnea, productive or nonproductive cough, bloating, right upper quadrant pain due to hepatic congestion, and palpitations due to excess volume in the atria may also present in the acute setting (Adams et al., 2006; Hunt et al., 2005; Nohria et al., 2002).

Nursing assessment of acute decompensated heart failure includes:

1. *Quick assessment of severity of symptoms*
2. *Vital signs*
3. *Hemodynamic status (peripheral pulses, temperature of skin, capillary refill time, and invasive hemodynamic parameters when available)*
4. *Oxygenation and work of breathing.*

Acute heart failure requiring intensive care monitoring:

1. *Evidence of myocardial infarction*
2. *Significant ventricular or supraventricular dysrhythmia*
3. *Compromised respiratory function*
4. *Evidence of low cardiac output*
5. *Anticipated need for hemodynamic monitoring*
6. *Severe comorbid disease.*

Acute decompensated heart failure can be precipitated by many conditions and situations (Chart 42–8). Cardiac decompensation generally may be attributed to issues with compliance, new or worsening comorbid conditions, and/or progressive disease (Greenberg & Hermann, 2002; McKelvie, 2001). Compliance issues that contribute to decompensated heart failure relate to failing to take medications at all or inappropriately, excess sodium and fluid intake, inadequate outpatient treatment, or inadequate follow-up, and they also may lead to acute decompensated symptoms (Greenberg & Hermann, 2002; Nohria et al., 2002). If acute decompensated heart failure is not treated, cardiogenic shock, multiorgan failure, and death may result. Patients with acute heart failure should be queried to understand better what circumstance(s) led to their decompensated state:

- Had they been self-monitoring at home?
- Did they know what actions to take if their clinical condition worsened?
- Did they have adequate access to outpatient care?
- Did they know who and when to call?
- Had they been taking medicines as prescribed?
- Did they understand how to follow a sodium and fluid restriction?
- Had they started any new medications recently?
- Had any other new medical problems been recently diagnosed?

Goals of acute decompensated heart failure include the following: to determine the reason for the decompensated state, relieve congestive symptoms, reverse hemodynamic compromise, treat dysrhythmias, assess for exacerbating comorbid conditions, use prognosis-altering medications, assess for their candidacy for cardiac devices or end-stage therapies, provide self-management education, and document that appropriate heart failure care was provided as mandated by regulatory entities. In preparing patients for life with heart failure outside the

CHART 42–8	**Precipitating or Exacerbating Factors for Developing Acute Heart Failure**
Noncompliance	Renal or hepatic insufficiency
Silent or overt ischemia	Pulmonary embolism
Dietary indiscretion	Substance abuse
Fluid indiscretion	Worsening valvular or cardiac function
Untreated hypertension	
Acute or chronic infection	Over-the-counter supplementation
Uncontrolled hyperglycemia	
Thyroid dysfunction	Iatrogenic factors
Inadequate follow-up	Pregnancy
Atrial fibrillation, new or rapid	Anemia
Other dysrhythmias	

Factors that may precipitate or exacerbate heart failure are numerous and may be related to new or poorly controlled comorbid conditions, noncompliance, iatrogenic causes, or lack of adequate follow-up.

Sources: Braunwald, E., Zipes, D. P., & Libby, P. (2001). *Heart disease: A textbook of cardiovascular medicine* (6th ed.). Philadelphia: W. B. Saunders; Greenberg, B. H., & Hermann, D. D. (2002). *Contemporary diagnosis and management of heart failure.* Newtown, PA: Handbooks in Health Care; and Nohria, A., Lewis, E., & Stevenson, L. W. (2002). Medical management of advanced heart failure. *Journal of the American Medical Association, 287*(5), 628–640.

hospital, one should consider which patients might benefit from the organized structure of a heart failure disease management program. On presentation, the patient can be classified based on degree of perfusion and volume status: well perfused and either hyper- or hypovolemic, or poorly perfused and either hyper- or hypovolemic (Figure 42–8 ■) (Nohria et al., 2002).

Nursing Management

The nursing care needs of a patient admitted with heart failure are directed at treating congestion and monitoring the patient's response to therapy. Fluid retention is the primary reason most patients with heart failure are admitted or readmitted to the hospital. Goals of treatment for acute decompensated heart failure include assessing response to diuresis, monitoring intake/output and daily weights, assessment of cardiac output, monitoring for dysrhythmias, encouraging increased levels of activity, performing ADLs, and enhancing patient knowledge of the disease process. Application of the nursing process will facilitate a comprehensive ap-

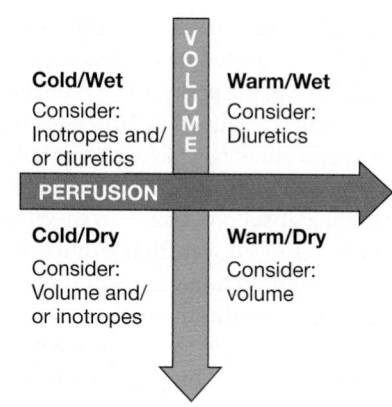

FIGURE 42–8 ■ Volume versus perfusion.

proach to patient assessment and care. The Nursing Process: Patient Care Plan feature applies the nursing process to the relevant nursing diagnosis of congestion and provides a comprehensive care plan for a patient with heart failure during hospitalization.

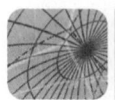

NURSING PROCESS: Patient Care Plan for Heart Failure

Assessment of Hypervolemia

Subjective Data:

Are you having difficulties breathing at rest or with activity?

How long have you had shortness of breath (SOB)?

Do you need to sleep with your head propped up, or do you awaken short of breath in the middle of the night?

Do you have a cough?

Do you have abdominal bloating or lower extremity swelling?

Have you had recent weight increase over a short period of time (2–3 days)?

Objective Data:

Vital signs: weight

blood pressure, heart rate (HR)

Oxygen saturation.

Dyspnea with exertion.

Lethargy.

Anxiety.

Lung sounds: crackles/wheezes.

Restlessness.

Elevated neck veins.

Ascites and/or lower extremity edema.

Daily weight.

Hemodynamic parameters:
1. Right atrial pressure (RAP) or central venous pressure (CVP)
2. Pulmonary artery pressure (PAP mean)
3. Pulmonary artery occlusion pressure (PAOP)
4. Cardiac output (CO) or cardiac index (CI).

Peripheral circulation:
1. Peripheral pulses
2. Presence of edema using the edema scale
3. Color and temperature
4. Capillary refill time.

Intake and output:
1. Assess volume of fluid intake by any route (e.g., oral, intravenous).
2. Assess volume of fluid expelled by any route (e.g., urinary, nasogastric (NG), drainage, blood).

Evaluate laboratory/diagnostic findings associated with hypervolemia:
1. Serum sodium (may be decreased, normal, or elevated based on cause of hypervolemia)
2. BUN (may be normal to decreased)
3. Urine specific gravity (may be decreased)
4. Hematocrit (may be decreased)
5. Chest x-ray (may show pulmonary congestion or cardiomegaly)
6. Right heart catheterization (may indicate elevated filling pressures).

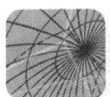

NURSING PROCESS: Patient Care Plan for Heart Failure—*Continued*

Nursing Assessment and Diagnosis	Outcomes and Evaluation Parameters	Planning and Interventions with *Rationales*
Nursing Diagnosis: Fluid volume excess related to ventricular dysfunction and sodium/water retention	**Outcomes:** Diuresis: improved volume status (i.e., euvolemia) and improved symptoms. ***Evaluation Parameters:*** Blood pressure target: 120/80 mmHg. Heart rate target: 60–100 beats/min. Improved New York Heart Association (NYHA) class. No signs of pulmonary congestion: airway patent; respiratory rate < 20 breaths/min; pattern regular and unlabored; lungs clear to auscultation all lobes bilaterally. Oxygen saturation > 90% in patients breathing room air. Hemodynamic parameters (normals): 1. RAP 1–7 mmHg or CVP 2–8 cm H_2O 2. PAP 10–20 mmHg 3. PCWP 6–12 mmHg 4. CO 3.5–5.5 L/min or CI 2.0–3.2 L/min/m². Peripheral circulation: 1. Pulse 2–3+ on pulse grading scale 2. No edema 3. Skin warm, natural color 4. Capillary refill time less than 3 seconds. Intake and output: 1. Intake/output difference greater than 1,000 mL/24 hours or as defined for diuresis per provider 2. Urinary output average of greater than or equal to 30mL/hr. Daily morning weight less than the day prior. Abdomen soft, nondistended; no ascites. Laboratory/diagnostic workup indicates: 1. Serum sodium 135–140 mEq/L 2. Blood urea nitrogen (BUN) 10–20 mg/dL 3. Urine specific gravity 1.005–1.030 4. Hematocrit, male: 42–52%, female: 37–47%.	**Interventions and *Rationales:*** Insert intravenous catheter. *To facilitate intravenous medication administration.* Administer and titrate intravenous (IV) medications. *To facilitate diuresis.* Record amount of Intravenous (IV) fluid infused. *To monitor intake.* Assess vital signs and urine output regularly (every hour or less). *To assess adequacy of diuresis.* Monitor central venous pressure and pulmonary artery occlusion pressure (PAOP), if possible. *To assess response to diuresis.* Obtain and track daily morning weight. *To monitor adequacy of diuresis.* Monitor serum electrolytes, hematocrit, serum creatinine, and report critical abnormalities to the provider. *To monitor hematological changes associated with hypervolemia, possibly hypovolemia, electrolyte changes, and diuresis.* Instruct patient on fluid and sodium restrictions. *To prevent excess oral intake, which negates the effect of diuresis.*

Assessment of Cardiac Output

Subjective Data:

How is your energy level?
Are symptoms limiting your level of activity?
Are you light-headed?
Are you having memory problems or trouble concentrating?
Are you making the same amount of urine as usual?

Objective Data:

Cardiovascular system:
1. Heart rate
2. Heart rhythm
3. Blood pressure
4. Peripheral pulses
5. Presence of edema using the edema scale
6. Color and temperature
7. Capillary refill time.
Heart sounds: murmurs, clicks, rubs, splitting.
Pulmonary status.
Oxygen saturation.
Hemodynamic parameters (as applicable):
1. Right atrial pressure (RAP) or central venous pressure (CVP)
2. Pulmonary artery pressure (PAP mean)
3. Pulmonary artery occlusion pressure (PAOP)
4. Cardiac output (CO) or cardiac index (CI).
Intake and output:
1. Assess volume of fluid intake by any route (e.g., oral, intravenous).
2. Assess volume of fluid expelled by any route (e.g., urinary, NG, drainage, blood).
ECG waveform (rhythm and intervals) as ordered (including cardiac rhythm, PR interval, QRS interval, QT/QTc interval, dysrhythmias).
Obtain weight.

(continued)

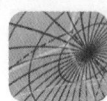

Evaluate laboratory/diagnostic findings associated with decreased cardiac output:

1. Serum BUN and creatinine (may be elevated)
2. Serum hematocrit, hemoglobin (may be decreased)
3. Echocardiogram (may show depressed ventricular function, pericardial effusion)
4. 12-lead ECG (may show dysrhythmias, myocardial infarction, heart block, tachycrdia, or bradycardia)
5. Blood gases (may show acidosis, hypoxemia)
6. Arterial–mixed venous blood gases may show an increased SaO_2/SvO_2 ratio.

Nursing Assessment and Diagnosis	Outcomes and Evaluation Parameters	Planning and Interventions with *Rationales*
Nursing Diagnosis: *Decreased Cardiac Output* related to ventricular dysfunction	**Outcome:** Adequate cardiac output as seen by improved organ, tissue, and cerebral perfusion related to ***Evaluation Parameters:*** Cardiovascular system: 1. Heart rate: 60–100 beats/min 2. Regular rhythm or patient's normal asymptomatic rhythm 3. BP: 120/80 mmHg 4. Pulses 2–3+ on pulse grading scale 5. No edema 6. Skin warm and natural color 7. Capillary refill time less than or equal to 3 seconds. Heart sounds: normal S_1 and S_2. Airway patent; respiratory rate < 20 per minute, pattern regular and unlabored; lungs clear to auscultation all lobes bilaterally. Oxygen saturation > 90% in patients breathing room air. Hemodynamic parameters: 1. RAP 1–7 mmHg or CVP 2–8 cm H_2O 2. PAP 10–20 mmHg 3. PCWP 6–12 mmHg 4. CO 3.5–5.5 L/min or CI 2.0–3.2 L/min/m². Intake and output: 1. Intake/output difference greater than 1,000 mL/24 hours or as defined for diuresis per provider 2. Urinary output average of greater than or equal to 30 mL/hr. ECG is stable, with regular rhythm or patient's normal asymptomatic rhythm, without evidence of ischemia, myocardial infarction, tachycardia/bradycardia, or heart block. Cardiac intervals are within normal limits: • PR interval: 0.12–0.20 second • QRS interval: < .10 second • QTc interval: 0.37–.047 second. Daily morning weight less than the day prior. Laboratory/diagnostic findings: 1. BUN 10–20 mg/dL 2. Creatinine 0.8–1.3 mg/dL 3. Hematocrit, male: 42–52%, female 37–47%; hemoglobin, male: 14–18 g/dL, female 12–16 g/dL 4. May show depressed ventricular function 5. Sinus rhythm, sinus dysrhythmia, or patient's normal asymptomatic rhythm 6. pH 7.35–7.45, PCO_2 35–45 mmHg, HCO_3 21–28 mEq/L, PO_2 80–100 mmHg, O_2 saturation 95–100%. 7. Normal SaO_2/SvO_2 ratio.	**Interventions and *Rationales:*** Insert intravenous catheter. *To facilitate intravenous medication administration.* Administer and titrate IV medications. *To facilitate diuresis and inotropic support.* Record amount of IV fluid infused. *To monitor intake.* Assess vital signs and urine output regularly (every hour or less). *To assess adequacy of diuresis and inotropic support.* Monitor hourly urine output. *To assess adequacy of diuresis.* Monitor central venous pressure and pulmonary artery occlusion pressures (PAOP, CO/CI), if possible. *To assess adequacy of diuresis and inotropic support of cardiac output.* Monitor integument and neurological status. *To assess for adequacy of tissue and cerebral perfusion.* Administer oxygen. *To ensure proper oxygenation and tissue perfusion.* Administration of medications. *To improve cardiac output, tissue perfusion, and diuresis.*

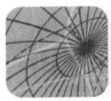

NURSING PROCESS: Patient Care Plan for Heart Failure—*Continued*

Assessment of Activity Tolerance

Subjective Data:

How much activity are you able to do (i.e., walk for 5, 10, 30+ minutes, or not at all)?

Are you more or less active now than 1, 3, and 6 months ago?

Are you able to walk up 1 or 2 flights of stairs without stopping?

Do you have symptoms during exercise (chest pain, shortness of breath, palpitations, and light-headedness)?

Objective Data:

Vital signs: blood pressure (BP) and heart rate (HR).

Oxygen saturation.

NYHA classification for heart failure assessment.

Pain scale.

6-minute walk.

Nursing Assessment and Diagnosis	Outcomes and Evaluation Parameters	Planning and Interventions with *Rationales*
Nursing Diagnosis: *Risk for Activity Intolerance* related to impaired cardiac function secondary to chronic heart failure	**Outcomes:** Activity tolerance stabilizes or improves as seen by improved NYHA classification for heart failure, and decreased symptoms. ***Evaluation Parameters:*** Normal vital signs. Oxygen levels are within normal range: oxygen saturation >= 90%. Patients have clear plan for activity, with reasonable goals. Patients have access to activity. Patients understand what symptoms to monitor during activity: increased shortness of breath, chest pain, palpitations, light-headedness. Symptoms during activity are minimal. Patients have action plan for symptoms that occur. NYHA classification for heart failure has improved. Indexes of quality of life are improved. Pain scale improves. Strength and balance improve. Nutrition improves. Weight reduction occurs (if needed). Stress is reduced. Smoking cessation is successful.	**Interventions and *Rationales:*** Monitor vital signs at rest and with activity and 3 minutes after activity (heart rate, BP, respiratory rate). *To obtain a baseline for comparison.* Monitor oxygenation before, during, and after activity. *To obtain a baseline for comparison.* Assess baseline activity level (including strength and balance) and tolerance to activity. *To use as basis for individualized plan.* Assess symptoms at rest and with activity. *To use as a baseline for comparison.* Monitor level of pain. Assess degree of symptoms (NYHA class). *To use as a baseline for comparison.* Assess quality of life (QOL). *To use as a baseline for comparison.* Promote activity: Start with reasonable daily plan, increasing slowly, set reachable goal, plan around periods of rest, and reassure that small improvements will lead to physical, emotional, and psychosocial benefits. *An individualized plan of care will promote change.* Promote exercise prescription: type, activity, duration, intensity. Monitor level of strength. *To individualize each patient's plan.* Teach appropriate diet to accompany activity plan. Assess body mass index (BMI). Monitor current level of nutrition and calorie content. *To enhance balance nutrition and promote weight loss as needed.* Teach strengthening exercises. *To promote muscular strength to improve balance.* Discuss level of stress and anxiety. Teach stress reduction techniques. *To facilitate well-being and foster activity plan.* Stress smoking cessation. *Smoking decreases oxygenation to muscles during activity.* Teach heart failure symptoms to monitor: shortness of breath, chest pain, light-headedness, and passing out, palpitation. *To obtain a baseline for comparison.*

(continued)

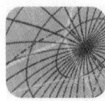

NURSING PROCESS: Patient Care Plan for Heart Failure—*Continued*

Assessment of Dysrhythmias

Subjective Data:

Do you experience palpitations or feel that your heart races?

Do you become light-headed or pass out?

Do palpitations or light-headedness occur at the same time?

Objective Data:

Vital signs: BP and HR.

Oxygen saturation.

Level of consciousness.

ECG.

Lab values: electrolytes and measures of acidosis.

Lung/cardiac.

Abdomen.

Integument.

Urine output.

Cardiac devices (if present).

Nursing Assessment and Diagnosis	Outcomes and Evaluation Parameters	Planning and Interventions with *Rationales*
Nursing Diagnosis: Cardiac output decreased due to dysrhythmias related to impaired cardiac function related to secondary to ischemia, acidosis, hypoxemia, electrolyte abnormalities, structural/conduction abnormalities, or device implantation.	**Outcome:** Absence of hemodynamically significant dysrhythmias. ***Evaluation Parameters:*** Heart rate is within normal range (60–80, or not > 100 beats per minute). Breath sounds are normal and clear, without respiratory distress. Oxygen levels are within normal range: Oxygen saturation >= 90%. Patient has no altered level of consciousness (LOC) or anxiety. ECG is stable, with regular rhythm or patient's normal asymptomatic rhythm, without evidence of ischemia, myocardial infarction, tachycardia/bradycardia, or heart block. Cardiac intervals are within normal limits: • PR interval: 0.12–0.20 second • QRS interval: < 0.10 second • QTc interval: 0.33–0.47 second. Lab values are within normal limits: 1. Potassium 3.5–5.1 mEq/L 2. Magnesium 1.3–2.1 mEq/L 3. Digoxin level, optimal = < 1.1 ng/mL, toxic: > 2.0 ng/mL 4. pH 7.35–7.45 5. $PaCO_2$ 35–45 mmHg 6. HCO_3 21–27 mEq/L 7. Base excess +/− 2 mEq/L Abdomen is soft, without pain, ascites, organomegaly. Urine output remains normal. Integument is dry, warm, well perfused. Cardiac device interrogation: shows properly functioning device with settings optimized and optimal battery life with leads intact.	**Interventions and *Rationales:*** Assess cardiovascular status: heart rate, regularity of rhythm (pattern), and blood pressure. *To assess baseline, monitor for changes and response to therapy.* Assess lung sounds. *To assess for presence of lung fluid from increased dysrhythmias.* Assess oxygenation saturation. *To monitor baseline, for changes with dysrhythmias and response to therapy.* Assess level of consciousness (LOC). *To assess for tissue perfusion.* Assess ECG and waveforms (rhythm, PR, QRS, and QTc intervals, dysrhythmias). *To establish a baseline, determine degree of abnormality and response to therapies.* Assess lab and blood gas values (potassium, magnesium, calcium, digoxin level, presence of acidosis). *To establish a baseline, determine degree of abnormality and response to therapies.* Assess abdomen. *To assess for ascites, abdominal pain, presence of bowel sounds, organomegaly.* Assess urine output. *To assess for decreases that may occur with dysrhythmias.* Assess integument. *To assess for cyanosis, pallor, or diaphoresis.* Assess cardiac device if present (i.e., pacemaker, cardiac defibrillator). *To assess proper position of leads and for appropriate device function.*

Assessment of Knowledge Deficit

Subjective Data:

Patient/family express concerns about the diagnosis of heart failure, in terms of prognosis, changes in lifestyle, and progression of disease.

Patient/family express lack of understanding of therapies to treat heart failure.

Patient/family express concerns about how to take medications and their potential side effects.

Patient/family express concerns what symptoms they might have and how to monitor them at home.

Patient/family express concerns about continuing a sexual relationship.

Patient/family express concerns about treatment options if medicines fail.

Patient/family express concerns about the mode of death.

Objective Data:

Patients may be anxious, confused, and may need repeated information.

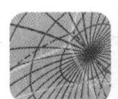

NURSING PROCESS: Patient Care Plan for Heart Failure—*Continued*

Nursing Assessment and Diagnosis	Outcomes and Evaluation Parameters	Planning and Interventions with *Rationales*
Nursing Diagnosis: *Deficient Knowledge* related to the diagnosis of heart failure.	**Outcomes:** Patient/family understand: The diagnosis of heart failure. Their prognosis. Treatments for heart failure. Lifestyle changes. Progression of the disease. Symptoms to monitor. Sexuality. End-stage treatment options. Mode of death. ***Evaluation Parameters:*** Patient/family will: • Ask appropriate questions about the course of heart failure. • Follow appropriate medication adjustments, and consider recommendations for surgical procedures and devices. • Come in with a completed self-care diary, following instructions between visits. • Call when their symptoms worsen for urgent evaluation when needed. • Express attempts at maintaining a sexual relationship. • Understand which end-stage therapies are available and for which they qualify. • Understand the usual mode of death of heart failure and have made appropriate plans with their health care team and family regarding their wishes. Advanced directives and power of attorney will have been filled out.	**Interventions and *Rationales*:** Discuss with patient/family the course of heart failure, using the diagram. *This will enhance their understanding of the chronic and progressive nature of the disease, which usually presents with periods of exacerbation and stabilization.* Discuss how heart failure is treated with the patient and family. *This will provide the fundamental treatment strategies for heart failure including medications, surgical strategies, and devices.* Discuss with patients/family the MAWDS-based curriculum of self-management support (see Figure 42–9 ■, p. 1311). *This will teach the basic concepts that will help them to understand their medications, about activity, the importance of daily weights, their diet, and what to do when their symptoms worsen.* Discuss the common symptoms of heart failure with the patient and family, describing shortness of breath, cough, fatigue, activity intolerance, weight gain/edema, palpitations, chest tightness, and poor concentration. *This will enable the patient to recognize her symptoms and reinforce calling early when her symptoms worsen, so she can be seen and have adjustments made in her medications, preempting an urgent hospitalization.* Discuss ways for the patient and significant other to maintain a sexual relationship. *Patients will understand that having sexual intercourse is about the amount of effort in climbing 2 flights of stairs. If they are able to complete this activity without significant symptoms, then sexual intercourse will likely be safe. Patients will understand other means of sexual intimacy and will understand what to do if symptoms worsen during sexual activities.* Describe end-stage treatment options to the patient and family. Those who fail standard therapy might be considered for cardiac transplantation, mechanical assist devices, and heart failure research studies or for hospice care. *The patient and family will understand which of the preceding end-stage therapies they might be considered for and why they might not be a candidate for others.* Describe the mode of death for patients with heart failure. *Most patients with heart failure die either by a sudden dysrhythmia (caused by ventricular tachycardia or fibrillation) or by progressive deterioration of the cardiac muscle and its function. Dying suddenly will be a fast, typically painless, way to die. Dying of progressive disease is typically associated with more symptoms that will require an individualized plan for symptom relief by medicines such as narcotics, anxiolytics, nitrates, diuretics, and oxygen.*

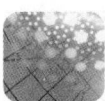

PATIENT TEACHING & DISCHARGE PRIORITIES for Heart Failure

Patients discharged from the hospital have multiple needs. Teaching strategies should be based on these needs, with the goal to prevent readmissions, decrease disease progression, and improve quality of life.

Need	Teaching
Patient/family • Prevent recurrent symptoms of congestion.	MAWDS self-management instruction (medications, activity, weights, diet, symptoms).
• Optimize medical therapy for heart failure and comorbid conditions.	Provide list of current medications to patients with dose and schedule, with clear instructions on changes from prehospitalization. Instruct purpose of medications; refill prescriptions before running out; do not double up for missed doses; call with adverse effects.
• Increase activity tolerance.	Increase activity as tolerated, monitoring for symptoms; become active most days; call with new or worsened symptoms.
• Minimize risk factors.	Review health maintenance strategies: smoking cessation, limited ethyl alcohol (ETOH), regular exercise, stress reduction, eating balanced diet, and optimally treating comorbid conditions.
• Provide palliative care.	Discuss chronic nature of disease; encourage multidisciplinary team meeting regarding overall plans for care.
Family/support system • Assess resources to assist with chronic illness in the home setting.	Provide resources based on individual's needs: home health, hospice, family/friends/neighbors to help with home care, meals, transportation.
Setting • Assess home needs.	Assess safety from falls for those who are weak and at risk for falling; use occupational therapy to assess home safety and for home aids for debilitated patients.

Once the patient is ready for discharge, it is essential that a teaching plan be implemented that will help prevent a recurrence of the heart failure. A practical approach, tailored to individual patients, will be needed to help patients integrate self-management strategies at home. The Patient Teaching & Discharge Priorities box outlines discharge care for patients with heart failure. It is also essential that cultural considerations be addressed because they potentially impact the patient's ability to prevent progression of the disease. The Cultural Considerations box presents necessary considerations related to various cultures.

Collaborative Management

Patients with heart failure need a multidisciplinary team approach to achieve optimal recovery and return to society. Nurses at all levels collaborate with health care providers, health care provider assistants, dietitians, pharmacists, social workers, and cardiac rehabilitation specialists across various care settings. Close scrutiny is required by the team to provide optimal, evidence-based care. Nursing assessment of subjective and objective measures of adequate diuresis will allow for a prompt notification to the health care provider if adjustments to the medical plan are needed. Nursing staff also can focus on the essential aspects of patient self-management, including instruction on medications, activity, daily weights, dietary guidance, and symptom management. A comprehensive nutritional plan should include helping patients follow a restricted salt and liquid diet. Dietitians help patients and families with a greater understanding of appropriate food and fluid guidelines. When hypervolemia is present, patients generally have a decline in physical activity, with dyspnea being their primary source of limitation in activity. Cardiac rehabilitation specialists help mobilize pa-

tients with monitored physical activity during their hospitalization and may provide a plan to follow after discharge. Social workers can evaluate and instruct on the psychosocial aspects of this diagnosis and also address any financial concerns.

Hospital Clinical Pathway

A focused clinical pathway, individualized to each patient, should be initiated at the beginning of a heart failure admission, guiding inpatient care in preparation for postdischarge management (Chart 42–9, p. 1310) (Greenberg & Hermann, 2002).

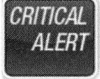 *Clinical discharge criteria include:*

1. *Achievement of euvolemia*
2. *Twenty-four-hour stability of fluid status, blood pressure, and renal function on oral medications*
3. *Walks without dyspnea*
4. *No complaints of light-headedness*
5. *Optimal blood pressure defined*
6. *Stable cardiac rhythm.*

Starting in 2002, the Joint Commission has mandated that patients admitted to the hospital with heart failure have documentation on their care related to the following: (1) a measure of ventricular function; (2) those with an LVEF less than 40% receive an ACE inhibitor (or ARB) unless contraindicated; (3) patients receive self-management instruction before discharge; and (4) smoking cessation counseling is provided to smokers. Adhering to these core measures has shown reductions in heart failure mortality (Kfoury, Hall, Rasmusson, Horne, & Renlund, 2006). Plans for optimal outpatient management should focus on ways to prevent readmissions for heart failure, to improve prognosis, to

CULTURAL CONSIDERATIONS for Risk Factors of Heart Failure

- At least 46% of African Americans and American Indians/Alaska Natives have at least two or more cardiovascular disease risk factors; and therefore, nursing care should include a thorough evaluation of their risk factors.

- The African-American Heart Failure Trial (A-HeFT) results suggest that African Americans have improved outcomes when isosorbide dinitrate and hydralazine are added to standard heart failure medications; and therefore, nursing care should entail a thorough review of their medications.

- Heart failure is more common in African Americans and appears to be of worse severity. The strongest risk factor for heart failure among African Americans is hypertension, which can also contribute to the pathology of their heart failure disease. African Americans experience a higher incidence of hospitalization. Nursing care for African American patients with heart failure may include hypertension education and also self-management strategies to prevent further rehospitalization.

- African Americans and Native Americans have higher incidences of renal disease than do Caucasians and Asians; and therefore, nursing care for these groups should include close monitoring of renal function because their heart failure management may need adjustment.

- Diabetes has been found to be the strongest risk factor for heart failure. The prevalence of diabetes in the American Indian or Alaska Native adult population was more than twice that of U.S. adults overall; and therefore, nursing care and management of patients with heart failure who are American Indians should entail an evaluation for diabetes.

- Cardiovascular disease is not a "man's" disease. It is the number-one killer of women and has killed more women than men, causing the death of over 500,000 women annually. Nursing care of both male and female patients should be consistent and thorough.

- Cardiovascular disease has been shown to cause an increased incidence of premature deaths greatest among American Indians or Alaska Natives (36%) and African Americans (31.5%), and the lowest among Caucasians (14.7%). Premature death was also higher among Hispanics (23.5%). Nursing care of these "at-risk" populations must be thorough, in particular with their discharge instructions, because cardiovascular mortality risk is greater among these populations.

Nursing care can be significantly enhanced when considering a patient's cultural background. This list describes pertinent cultural considerations that may need to be addressed.

Sources: American Heart Association. (2006a&b). *Heart and stroke statistics—2006 update.* Dallas, TX: Author; Smith, G. L., et al. (2005). Race and renal impairment in heart failure: Mortality in blacks versus whites. *Circulation, 111*(10), 1270–1277; Taylor, A. L. (2003). The African-American heart failure trial (A-HeFT): Rationale and methodology. *Journal of Cardiac Failure, 9,* S216–S219; Thomas, K. L., et al. (2005). Outcomes by race and etiology of patients with left ventricular systolic dysfunction. *American Journal of Cardiology, 96*(7), 1001–1013; Yancy, C. W. (2004). The prevention of heart failure in minority communities and discrepancies in health care delivery systems. *Medical Clinics of North America, 88*(5), 1347–1368; and Yancy, C. W., & Strong, M. (2004). The natural history, epidemiology, and prognosis of heart failure in African Americans. *Congestive Heart Failure, 10*(1), 15–18.

decrease mortality, to foster adherence, and to restore functional capacity (McKelvie, 2001). The power of educating patients with heart failure with standardized self-management techniques has led to reductions in mortality and should also be a focus prior to discharge (Hall et al., 2005).

Health Promotion

Heart failure management would be incomplete without the vital need for patients to receive self-management instruction and education from nurses and other members of the health care team. Research supports the importance self-management has on indexes such as quality-of-life, readmission rates, and functional status (Krumholz et al., 2002). Not only have heart failure medications altered patients' prognoses, but evidence exists showing the addition of self-management education can reduce mortality as well. Essential principles that focus on living with heart failure couple medications with nonpharmacologic therapies. Nonpharmacologic management strategies include appropriate diet and nutrition, health maintenance, and psychosocial/ lifestyle changes (Greenberg & Hermann, 2002).

The key concepts that patients must learn to incorporate into their daily lives can be summarized by an acronym called MAWDS: medications, activity, weights, diet, and symptoms, as depicted in Figure 42–9 ■ (p. 1311). If these concepts are followed, reductions in readmissions and costs associated with heart failure may occur (Krumholz et al., 2002). One community-based study has shown that patients who attended a MAWDS-based curriculum have improved knowledge of heart failure and an improved sense of quality of life (Rasmusson, Hall, Hofmann, Moore, & Renlund, 2002). This MAWDS-based self-management

education has even shown mortality benefits when documented during a heart failure admission (Hall et al., 2005).

 CRITICAL ALERT   *Self-management plan includes:*

1. *Patient and family education about MAWDS (medications, activity, daily weights, low-sodium diet, fluid restriction, and changes in symptoms)*
2. *Understands when to call provider with worsening symptoms*
3. *Follow-up appointment scheduled.*

Medications

Patients need instruction about their medications' action to improve symptoms, prevent hospitalizations, and prevent death. The typical patient with heart failure is on a complicated medical regimen for his heart condition along with therapy for his comorbid conditions. The more medications a person takes in a day, the more he is at risk for noncompliance or mistakes with his regimen. Patients need to understand the names of the medications, the time of the day they should be taken, their purpose, and what to do in case of missed doses and/or adverse reactions. Strategies aimed to increase long-term compliance and access to medications for those with limited resources must be planned.

Activity

Activity was long discouraged for those living with heart failure (Nohria et al., 2002). Exercise was thought to put an undue burden on the already weakened heart muscle. Now, it is increasingly evident that an optimal amount of activity can have significant benefits. Hemodynamic parameters, quality-of-life

CHART 42–9 **Heart Failure Clinical Pathway**

Once patients are hospitalized with heart failure, they need comprehensive care using a multidisciplinary approach such as the clinical pathway proposed here. Each day noted, progress should be made, looking forward to the anticipation of discharge. Planning should focus on medical and nursing therapies, education, physical therapy and dietary needs, consultations that may be needed, and discharge goals.

Aspect of Care	Day 1	Day 2	Day 3	Day 4
Inpatient Care	Admission weight vital signs (VS) q4h input and output (I & O) Physical assessment IV access Urinary catheterization optional Cardiac monitoring Oxygen Telemetry Begin admission medications to include IV diuretics Pain assessment	Daily weight by 0600 VS q4h I & O Physical assessment Continue meds: IV diuretics, change as indicated Increase ACEI if BP stable Adjust potassium supplementation Pain management	Daily weight by 0600 VS q4h I & O Physical assessment Continue meds/consider changing to oral diuretics if approaching euvolemia Increase ACEI, if tolerated Consider discharge urinary cath, cardiac monitor Pain management	VS q4h I & O Physical assessment Administer meds Increase ACEI Weigh on patient's home scale for discharge baseline Discharge IV access Pain management
Education	Self-management module I introduced Assess patients knowledge of heart failure (HF) (pre-test) Review: What is HF	Review HF pretest Teach self-management module I	Complete self-management module I Schedule patient/family conference	Post-test and review discharge instructions Smoking cessation
Nutrition/ Dietary	Notify dietary of: Na+ restriction Fluid restriction	Reinforce: Low Na+ foods Fluid restriction	Reinforce: Low Na+ foods Fluid restriction	Reinforce: Low Na+ foods Fluid restriction
Laboratory/ Diagnostics	Admit labs on admit orders Consider diagnostic tests: x-ray, ECG, MUGA, Echo, Pulse oximetry, etc.	Chem 7 PT/INR (if appropriate)	Chem 7 PT/INR	Chem 7 PT/INR
Activity	Bed rest/BP with assistance Initial Cardiac Rehab consult	OOB at least 30 minutes Cardiac Rehab	OOB for meals AMB qid Cardiac Rehab	OOB for meals AMB qid Cardiac Rehab
Consults	CONSULTS: Pharmacist Social Worker Dietitian Cardiac Rehab Other	CONSULT VISITS: Pharmacist Social Worker Dietitian Cardiac Rehab	CONSULT VISITS: Pharmacist Social Worker Dietitian Cardiac Rehab	F/U APPOINTMENTS WITH CONSULTS ARRANGED
Discharge Planning	Identify issues in the home setting	Assess self-care ability	Immunizations: pneumovax and influenza	Home scale Home health nursing Oxygen need Medications: ACEI, digoxin, spironolactone Follow up with CHF Clinic CHF support group referrals
Outcomes	Establish NYHA class Diagnostic evaluation of heart failure complete Estimate goal for baseline weight Establish extent of lung congestion Measurement of JVP HF pretest given Pain assessment complete	Improved NYHA class Relief of symptoms: improved breathing, lung sounds, decreased edema, weight Vital signs stable Improved JVP MAWDS understanding increased Pain management begun	Improved NYHA class Continued relief of symptoms Increase activity as tolerated Labs WNL for this patient Improved JVP MAWDS understanding increased Improved pain management	DISCHARGE CRITERIA: Symptoms improvement Without lung congestion Optimal JVP Decreased edema Decreased weight Stable labs Baseline weight achieved Cardiac rehab goal achieved Pain management has occurred Passed post-test Discharge instructions understood

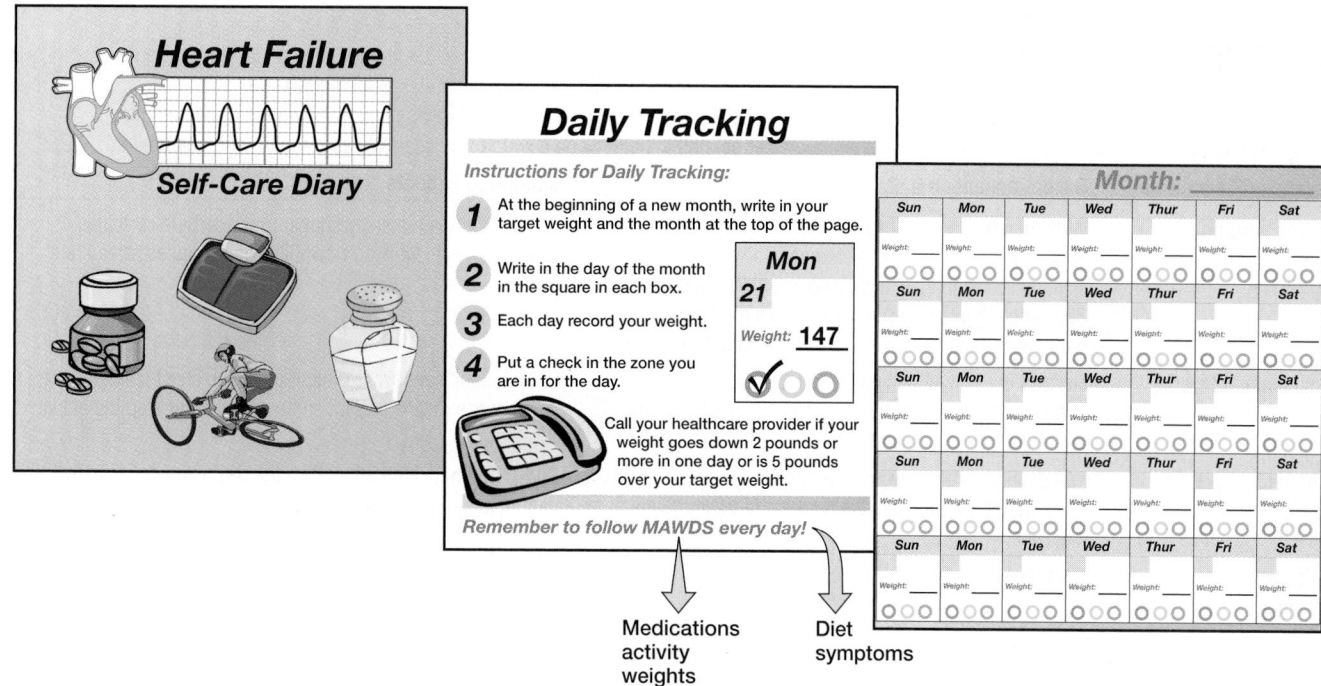

FIGURE 42–9 ■ Heart failure self-care diary.

indexes, functional status, and depression scores are all im-proved as persons with heart failure exercise on a consistent ba-sis (Adams et al., 2006). The reality of living with heart failure, however, is that the syndrome is fraught with a cycle of inactiv-ity that leads to further deconditioning. The challenge is, there-fore, to encourage a reasonable exercise program that will lead to clinical benefits. Cardiac rehabilitation may be started during a hospitalization in stable patients, but coverage by the Centers for Medicare & Medicaid Services (CMS) for outpatient cardiac rehab for heart failure remains limited. An exercise prescription given to patients must include the following components: type, frequency, duration, and intensity (Chart 42–10, p. 1312). Set-ting reasonable goals with patients is critical so that success with an exercise prescription may be achieved. Assessing behavioral and motivational issues is important for those patients who have struggled with maintaining an active lifestyle.

Weight

One of the most important aspects for patients to understand is to record their weight daily and know what to do when it devi-ates from a dry weight. The ultimate goal is to maintain a state of euvolemia, or when they are not retaining fluid, which means less congestion and fewer symptoms. As easy as this concept sounds, it is quite a challenge to health care providers to work out a plan with patients related to their weight. Some terms used to describe a "goal" weight when there is an absence of conges-tion are *optivolemic* and *euvolemic*. This weight needs to be de-termined in conjunction with the health care provider and may change over time with weight gain or loss from other causes than fluid. Patients not only feel better when they are not con-gested but also will likely stay out of the hospital (Greenberg & Hermann, 2002; Nohria et al., 2002).

Patients should be instructed to call their health care provider when their weight increases 2 or more pounds overnight, or more than 5 pounds from their "goal" weight.

Conversely, patients who lose too much weight are at risk of de-hydration and possibly syncope. A 5-pound or greater drop be-low their goal weight should prompt a call to their health care team. Patients should have an individualized plan for self-adjusted diuretic dosing regimens to achieve relief of congestion and limit the chance of readmission.

Diet

Activation of the RAAS leads to sodium and water retention. Pa-tients need instruction to help them understand that treating congestion with diuretics offers the best result when coupled with limiting dietary sodium (Greenberg & Hermann, 2002). Pa-tients with heart failure with congestive symptoms should be counseled to ingest less than 2 grams of sodium daily (Silver, 1998). Those with persistent evidence of volume overload should also ingest less than 2 quarts (or liters) of all fluids per day (Sil-ver, 1998). Following a low-sodium diet is challenging, because the American diet usually consists of 6 to 10 grams of sodium daily (Greenberg & Hermann, 2002). Most complain about food lacking in flavor when they change to the reduced sodium prepa-ration, yet herbs and spices should be encouraged to add flavor to foods to enhance their flavor. See Chart 42–11 (p. 1312) for a list of foods that are commonly know to be high in sodium con-tent with recommended alternatives. Patients often need help to understand how to read food labels, how to calculate their sodium intake, and how to make wise food selections when eat-ing out. Meeting with a dietitian and others to share shopping and food preparation tips will likely heighten success and com-pliance. Chapter 14 ⊙ includes a specific discussion of low-sodium diets.

Many patients with heart failure complain of "thirst." This mechanism is a neurohormonal response that tries to trick the body into seeking and retaining more fluids so that blood volume will increase, leading to increased flow to the renal system. Unfor-tunately, when heart failure is present, the heart is unable to keep

---

CHART 42–10 **Exercise Prescription**

Patients with heart failure usually fall into a cycle of inactivity, thus leading to further deconditioning. Exercise is usually limited by symptoms of congestion or poor perfusion. It is important to provide thorough instructions to patients on how to exercise safely as they live with heart failure.

Exercise Prescription	Recommendation to Patients	Caution to Patients
Type of exercise	Walk, run, bike, swim, hike. Factors such as personal preference, location, orthopedic challenges, and so on will help plan type. Choosing a type of exercise patient will enjoy should help her continue this activity over the long term.	Do not pursue an activity known to exacerbate certain conditions: e.g., walking downhill, which causes more knee pain.
Intensity of exercise	Discuss in terms of being able to maintain a conversation while exerting, yet having a high enough amount of energy expenditure.	Having significant symptoms of dyspnea, chest pain, or light-headedness means patient should back off or stop the activity.
Duration of exercise	Will depend on baseline level of fitness. Start slowly and increase the duration of their activity over time.	Reduce duration and intensity if the day following an activity, patient is too tired to perform activities of daily living (ADLs).
Frequency of exercise	Be active most days of the week.	Patient should not worry if he needs to skip a day occasionally. Just remember to try being active most days.

Sources: Adams, T. D., Fisher, A. G., Hansen, S. F., & Yanowitz, F. G. (2001). *Maintaining the miracle and owner's manual for the human body* (3rd ed.). Salt Lake City, UT: CAPP Publishing.

---

up with the body's demands and backward flow results in "volume-overloaded" patients and worsened symptoms. Low sodium intake, coupled with fluid restriction, will assist patients in maintaining their goal weight and may often lead to reductions in diuretic dosing (Greenberg & Hermann, 2002; Nohria et al., 2002).

Symptoms

Patients need to understand the typical symptoms of heart failure including exertional dyspnea, orthopnea, paroxysmal nocturnal dyspnea (PND), cough, edema, fatigue, and activity intolerance. Symptoms of heart failure lead to a poorer quality of life and re-

---

CHART 42–11 **Dietary Sodium Recommendations**

The sodium-restricted diet (2 g/day) is a well-known part of the heart failure patient's self-management, although the patient's ability to understand this diet and to comply with it remains a challenge in her care.

Food Group	High-Sodium Choice	Lower Sodium Alternative
Meats/fish/poultry	Cured meats (bacon, ham) Processed meats: jerky, salami, sausage Stews, casseroles, anchovies, pickled herring, King crab, canned meat/fish/poultry	Fresh lean meat seasoned with herbs/spices, roasted, baked, boiled, or poached
Fruits	Canned fruits, fresh fruit with salt added	Fresh fruit, no added salt, fruit juices
Vegetables	Canned soups or vegetables; canned vegetable juices; those in sauce or au gratin; canned beans: refried beans, pork and beans, kidney beans	Any vegetables; stewed, steamed, fresh, or boiled
Carbohydrates	Pretzels, potato chips, peanuts, popcorn, bagels, croissants, English muffins, oyster crackers, pita pockets, pancakes, stuffing, packaged puddings, pastries, cream pies, ice cream, creamed potatoes, noodles in cream sauce, fried rice	Fresh fruit, angel food cake, sherbert, frozen/nonfat yogurt, ice milk, gelatin, hard or soft rolls, plain bread or toast, unsalted crackers, breadsticks, mashed/baked/steamed/boiled potatoes, boiled or steamed rice, boiled noodles
Dairy/fats	Cottage cheese, Parmesan cheese, other hard and/or processed cheeses	Mozzarella
Condiments	Canned gravies, salad dressings, canned sauces, soy sauce, ketchup, mustard, olives, pickles, bouillon	Homemade gravy, other herbs/spices, oil and vinegar dressing, low-salt dressings
Fast foods	Hamburger, cheeseburger, fried chicken, pizza, onion rings, fish sandwich, burrito	Salad bars, baked potatoes, broiled chicken sandwich without sauce, fresh fruits/vegetables, sandwiches with low-salt meat and cheese options and limited spreads
Other	Frozen foods, milk shakes, chocolate or whole milk, cocoa, alcoholic drinks	Fruit juices, skim milk, soft drinks, tea, or coffee

Sources: Nephrogenic Diabetes Insipidus Foundation. (2006). *Low sodium diet basics.* Retrieved December 6, 2006, from http://www.ndif.org/pages/5-Low_Sodium_Diet_Basics; Silver, M. A. (1998). *Success with heart failure; Success and hope for those with congestive heart failure.* Reading, MA: Perseus Books.

sult in frequent hospitalizations (Nohria et al., 2002). Each patient should receive clear instruction on how to track her own symptoms and when to call if symptoms worsen. If a patient calls early enough, the issue may be managed on an outpatient basis, preventing an emergency room visit or hospitalization. Patients with heart failure need to understand that their symptoms will wax and wane, resulting in a combination of good and bad days. Listening to their bodies and keeping track of objective information (such as weight, blood pressure, and heart rate) that should be reported is critical. See Figure 42–9 ■ (p. 1311) for an example of a tool to help assist patients monitor and record weights, which may be used to communicate with their health care team about changes that occur outside predetermined parameters of weight and symptoms.

Family/Significant Other Support

Heart failure, like other chronic diseases, requires support from family, significant others, and also members of the community. Heart failure can pose both emotional and physical challenges to patients and those surrounding them. When patients are initially diagnosed, during times of exacerbations, and as they approach the end-of-life stage, patients with heart failure may need a significant amount of emotional and physical support. Patients and their loved ones need to understand the chronicity of the disease with which they live so they can make foreseeable adjustments to their daily activities to ensure an acceptable quality of life. This may include adjustments in all family-related activities such as family meal preparation and home maintenance. Meals should be planned that adhere to the sodium and fluid restrictions instructed for the patient. It also remains important for family members to encourage compliance with MAWDS recommendations (p. 1311). Available Internet resources, such as through the American Association of Heart Failure Nurses can help both patients and families better understand how to live with this common condition.

Lifestyles and Habits

Promoting healthy lifestyles is critical for all patients and is no different for patients with heart failure. General health promotion strategies that should be age and gender focused include:

- Smoking cessation
- Regular physical activity and weight control
- Limiting alcohol use and discouraging illicit drug use
- Stress management
- Dental care.

Health maintenance recommendations include:

1. *Vaccination for influenza and pneumonia*
2. *Regular exercise*
3. *Stress reduction techniques*
4. *Limitation of alcohol use*
5. *Discontinuance of nonsteroidal anti-inflammatory drugs (NSAIDs)*
6. *Regular health care follow-up.*

Patients with a chronic disease, such as heart failure, are recommended to follow additional disease prevention strategies for the following conditions: infection, CAD, hypertension, dia-

betes, hyperlipidemia, obesity, and malnutrition. Infection prevention includes recommendations for an annual influenza vaccination and a current pneumococcal vaccination. For those with valvular heart disease, endocarditis prophylaxis should be followed for dental and other invasive procedures. Primary prevention strategies for CAD include smoking cessation, regular exercise, and maintaining a healthy body weight. Additionally, CAD secondary prevention strategies focus on tight control of comorbid conditions that may influence the development or worsening of heart failure including diabetes, hypertension, hyperlipidemia, and obesity.

Hypertension and hyperlipidemia screening and treatment not only may prevent the development of CAD but also may prevent systolic dysfunction. Lifestyle changes including more exercise and better dietary choices will also help reduce hypertension and hyperlipidemia. Aggressively treating diabetes, targeting an optimal hemoglobin A_{1C} and prevention of target organ damage, will limit the risk of developing CAD and subsequent systolic dysfunction. Regular exercise and an improved diet will also prevent obesity and malnutrition.

Heart Failure Resources for Patients and Families

Many resources are available to help assist the nurse in educating the patient. It is also vital for nurses to instruct patients on how to access educational materials. In this multimedia era, patients with heart failure have numerous resource options available to them. The Internet alone has over 2 million sites to choose from on "congestive heart failure" for a search done through Google. Web-based sites for heart failure represent many different entities providing information: organizations specific to heart failure and cardiology, hospital systems providing heart failure care, governmental agencies with guidelines for treatment, drug and device companies with their product information and patient education, patients with their own websites, studies done on heart failure, and more. Help patients with tips about some of the more credible Internet sites, which are those ending in (dot) .edu, .gov, and .org. Well-established organizations providing valuable resources include the Heart Failure Society of America, the American Association of Heart Failure Nurses, and the American Heart Association.

Other resources on heart failure can be obtained through books from bookstores and hospital, university, or public libraries. Many companies have produced videos for patients to help them better understand heart failure. Drug and device companies and hospital systems often produce tools that focus on heart failure improvements. Community-based resources that are available include health care fairs, community lecture series, the local health department, the local chapter of the American Heart Association, and hospitals and care providers in the community. Patients with heart failure need resources sensitive to various cultures, in multiple languages, and at various levels of literacy.

■ Comorbidities of Heart Failure

Patients with heart failure commonly have comorbid conditions, requiring thoughtful and optimal treatment (Jessup & Brozena, 2003). The need for the evaluation of other comorbidities in the progression of heart failure has become increasingly more evident. Depression, anemia, renal insufficiency, diabetes, coronary artery disease, hypertension, and sleep apnea have all been found not only to worsen prognosis and increase morbidity and mortality rates, but also to confound heart failure treatment (Jessup & Brozena, 2003).

Depression

Depression is increasingly common among the elderly and especially in those with heart failure (Havranek, Ware, & Lowes, 1999). Patients with heart failure with untreated depression are at risk for increases in morbidity and mortality and also have reported poorer quality of life and functional capacity (Havranek et al., 1999; Nohria et al., 2002). A comprehensive treatment strategy, including counseling and the use of antidepressants, is important in managing patients with depression (Greenberg & Hermann, 2002). Counseling patients to enhance their understanding of the course of heart failure and helping the patient understand their treatment plan can significantly assist to decrease anxiety levels and to empower patients to be more proactive in their self-management. Drug therapy primarily involves antidepressants known as selective serotonin reuptake inhibitors (SSRIs) that are generally felt to be safe and therapeutic in patients with heart failure and do not alter hemodynamics (Greenberg & Hermann, 2002).

Anemia

Anemia is defined by the World Health Organization (WHO) as a hemoglobin of <12 g/dL in women or <13 g/dL in men (WHO, 1968). The prevalence of anemia is significant and increases with age, detected in up to 48% of the heart failure population (Kosiborod et al., 2003). Blood loss; iron, folate, or B_{12} deficiencies; infections; and medications have been common sources of anemia in patients with heart failure. Most commonly, chronic renal insufficiency leads to decreased erythropoietin production, resulting in anemia. The risk with anemia in patients with heart failure includes myocardial ischemia and increased need for higher cardiac output to maintain tissue metabolic oxygen requirements (which, in turn, can trigger the deleterious effects of the SNS system) (Greenberg & Hermann, 2002). Patients with heart failure and anemia have been found to have an increased risk of mortality (Horwich, 2002) and poorer prognosis (Dries, Exner, Domanski, Greenberg, & Stevenson, 2000). The treatment of choice is to correct the underlying disorder (Greenberg & Hermann, 2002). The use of blood transfusions or erythropoietin administration has not been supported in improving mortality but has been shown to improve clinical status (Greenberg & Hermann, 2002; Silverberg et al., 2001). Chapter 63 ☁ discusses anemia.

Renal Insufficiency

Renal insufficiency, as defined by a creatinine clearance of <60 mL/min, is prevalent in as many as 50% of patients with heart failure. It is present in at least 25% of patients hospitalized with heart failure (Krumholz et al., 2000). Poor renal perfusion, actual renal disease, or drug-induced disease have all been identified as sources of renal insufficiency in heart failure (Hunt et al., 2005). Renal insufficiency can cause increased activity by the RAAS system, triggering the vasoconstrictive properties of an-

giotensin II, causing blood vessels to constrict, and resulting in increased systemic vascular resistance and afterload (Braunwald et al., 2001). Renal insufficiency may prompt thoughtful reductions in heart failure medication therapies due to the greater risk of potential toxicities, such as with digitalis (Hunt et al., 2005). Worsening renal function can also be a prognostic indicator in heart failure and may require reductions in ACE inhibitors and beta-blocker therapies (Weinfeld, Chertow, & Stevenson, 1999). Treating renal insufficiency involves optimizing heart failure therapy (including ACE inhibitors, diuretics, and digitalis), optimizing renal hemodynamics, eliminating adverse medication use, and reversing identifiable causes if able (Braunwald et al., 2001). Chapter 47 ☁ discusses renal insufficiency.

Diabetes

There are 23.6 million children and adults in the United States, or 7.8% of the population, who have diabetes. While an estimated 17.9 million have been diagnosed with diabetes, unfortunately, 5.7 million people (or nearly one quarter) are unaware that they have the disease (American Diabetic Association, n.d.). Diabetes has a significant impact on cardiovascular function because of microvascular (endothelial proliferative changes of the arterioles) and macrovascular (atherosclerosis) changes in the vasculature promoted by the disease, leading to worsening ventricular dysfunction (Braunwald et al., 2001). Patients with diabetes are at greater risk of coronary artery disease, myocardial infarction, renal disease, hypertension, and heart failure (Braunwald et al., 2001). Patients who have strict glycemic control of their diabetes can significantly decrease their risk for coronary disease and subsequent risk of heart failure. Patients with diabetes and heart failure may halt the deleterious effects diabetes has on heart muscle function when optimal control is attained (Heart Outcomes Prevention Evaluation Study Investigators, 2000; Iribarren et al., 2001; Stratton et al., 2000). The cornerstone of diabetic therapy includes adjustments to diet and the use of insulin or oral hypoglycemic agents (Braunwald et al., 2001). Chapter 53 ☁ discusses diabetes.

Coronary Artery Disease

Coronary artery disease (CAD) is prevalent in over 13 million individuals in the United States (AHA, 2006b). It is the number-one killer of women and men alike. Coronary artery disease contributes to two-thirds of patients with heart failure (He et al., 2001). Approximately 22% of men and 46% of women will be disabled with heart failure postmyocardial infarction (AHA, 2006b). Coronary artery disease causes plaque buildup, which decreases perfusion to cardiac tissue (myocardial ischemia) and eventual inflammatory occlusion in the coronary arteries (myocardial infarction). Left ventricular pump function can be impaired, causing a depression in cardiac output and stroke volume that induces RAAS and SNS activation and their deleterious effects (Hunt et al., 2005). Therefore, primary prevention of coronary artery disease by preventing hypercholesterolemia becomes essential in preventing left ventricular dysfunction (Hunt et al., 2005). Secondary prevention of coronary disease with the use of hydroxy-methylglutaryl-coenzyme A (HMG-CoA, or "statins") medications and aspirin can significantly decrease the risk of heart failure by as much as

19% (Scandinavian Simvastatin Survival Study, 1994). Cardio-vascular disease is not a "man's" disease. It is the number-one killer of women and has killed more women than men since 1984, causing the death of over 500,000 women annually (AHA, 2006a). While all cancers combined kill only 260,000 females annually, 40,000 of these deaths are attributed to breast cancer (AHA, 2006a). The fear of developing breast cancer has led to a successful awareness campaign that has yet to be matched by a campaign to alert women of their even higher risk for heart disease. Chapter 40 💿 discusses CAD.

Hypertension

Hypertension is prevalent in over 50 million individuals in the United States (Chobanian et al., 2003). It is the primary diagnosis in 35 million office visits (Chobanian et al., 2003). It is a major risk factor for heart failure and is present in 10% of patients with diagnosed heart failure (Chobanian et al., 2003; He et al., 2001; Levy, Larson, Vasan, Kannel, & Ho, 1996). Hypertension causes increased workload on the heart due to increased systemic vascular resistance, leading to hypertrophy and dilation, and eventual worsening ventricular dysfunction (Braunwald et al., 2001). Patients who have their hypertension treated have demonstrated as high as a 51% risk reduction for developing heart failure (Dahlof et al., 1991; Kostis et al., 1997; Neal, MacMahon, & Chapman, 2000). Patients with hypertension are treated not only with pharmacologic agents but also with lifestyle modifications such as exercise, especially for weight reduction, a low-salt diet, and reducing alcohol consumption (Chobanian et al., 2003). Patients with heart failure along with persistent hypertension are placed on medications that not only control blood pressure but also treat heart failure (Adams et al., 2001; Baker, 2002). These medications include diuretics, ACE inhibitors, and also beta-adrenergic blockers (Baker, 2002). Chapter 21 💿 discusses hypertension.

Sleep Apnea

Sleep disordered breathing, including central or obstructive sleep apnea, has prevalence rates estimated as high as 50% in patients with heart failure (Javaheri, 2000; Javaheri et al., 1998; Sin et al., 1999). Sleep apnea can subsequently increase mortality rates in patients with heart failure (Hanly & Zuberi-Khokhar, 1996; Naughton 2006). Episodes of **apnea** (cessation of airflow for more than 10 seconds) and **hypopnea** (a reduction but not complete cessation of airflow to less than 50% of normal) while sleeping may result in oxygen desaturation, which causes transient increases in SNS activation leading to vasoconstriction, elevation of systemic blood pressure, and increased heart rate, all leading to ventricular hypertrophy, systolic dysfunction, and interstitial pulmonary edema (Bradley & Floras, 2003a, 2003b; Leung & Bradley, 2001). Patients may complain of irritability, excessive daytime fatigue, poor concentration, light or disrupted sleep, persistent PND, and orthopnea even when euvolemic on physical exam (Bradley & Floras, 2000; Naughton, 2006). Patients who present with these complaints should be screened for sleep apnea that is performed by overnight **polysomnography** (multichannel electrophysiological recording used to detect disturbances of breathing during sleep), evaluating for at least 10 to 15 episodes of apnea and hypopnea per hour of sleep (Bradley & Floras, 2003a & b). Treatment includes a continuous positive

airway pressure (CPAP) mask, which has been found to be beneficial in alleviating symptoms and improving abnormal respiratory patterns by reducing the degree of negative intrathoracic pressure required for respiration and decreasing left ventricular afterload, resulting in an improvement in left ventricular function (Kaneko et al., 2003; Naughton, 2006; Yan, Bradley, & Liu, 2001).

◼ Gerontological Considerations

Heart failure is generally a condition of the elderly, with the aging baby boomers contributing to the rise in heart failure incidence. There is little guidance in the literature on heart failure in the elderly, yet as the baby boomers continue to age and improvements are made in the treatment of CAD, those over age 65, living with heart failure will continue to grow. Although heart failure is the number-one discharge diagnosis in the elderly (Ahmed, 2003; Nohria et al., 2002), persons over age 65 are underrepresented in heart failure clinical trials (Heiat, Gross, & Krumholz, 2002; Jessup & Brozena, 2003). Although one epidemiologic study showed the average age at the time of first diagnosis to be 75 years of age, a review of randomized, controlled heart failure trials showed that only 3 of 59 studies included individuals in this age group (Heiat, Gross, & Krumholz, 2002). Some studies went so far as to exclude those over age 65 in the trial. Few studies have been done specific to the needs of this patient population; thus, the treatment approach comes from studies done in younger age groups (Heiat, Gross, & Krumholz, 2002; Nohria et al., 2002).

Due to the incidence of CAD and hypertension in the elderly, they are more likely to have heart failure with preserved systolic function. Logically, it follows that they will have more comorbid conditions and are thus victim to "polypharmacy," more so than those in younger age groups (Heiat, Gross, & Krumholz, 2002; McKelvie, 2001). Diastolic dysfunction is particularly common in obese, elderly women (Greenberg & Hermann, 2002; Jessup & Brozena, 2003). Whether the cause of heart failure is systolic dysfunction or diastolic dysfunction, the prognosis is poor once hospitalized, although mortality trends for systolic dysfunction have been found to be double those for diastolic dysfunction (McKelvie, 2001). The Gerontological Considerations box (p. 1316) summarizes prognostic predictors of increased mortality for those elderly patients with systolic dysfunction.

The common symptoms of heart failure are similar to those of any age: dyspnea (especially with exertion), cough, orthopnea, and dependent edema. The elderly, however, may present with less common or overt symptoms, such as fatigue, poor concentration, disorientation, and failure to thrive (McKelvie, 2001). Often, their symptoms may be confused with other disease processes or other concomitant comorbidities such as CAD, infection, or depression. A normal part of age-related changes of cardiac function may include modest decreases in systolic function and decreases in cardiovascular response with increased work load. As a result, stressors in the elderly may precipitate heart failure symptoms that might not present themselves in the younger population. These stressors include infection, hypothyroidism, hyperthyroidism, anemia, cardiac ischemia, hypoxia, hypothermia, hyperthermia, renal failure, nonadherence to drug or diet regimens, and potentially the use

GERONTOLOGICAL CONSIDERATIONS
for Poor Prognosis in the Elderly
with Systolic Dysfunction

High New York Heart Association (NYHA) class

Low exercise capacity

Very low ejection fraction (EF)

Severely dilated left ventricle

Ischemic etiology

Renal failure

Hyponatremia

Conduction system delays (left bundle branch block)

Ventricular dysrhythmias

Abnormal liver function tests

Shortened filling time of mitral filling pattern

Heart failure is a chronic disease that leads to death in 50% of patients within 5 years of diagnosis. Although difficulties remain with assessing prognosis, the indicators listed here, if present, provide objective evidence that suggests the patient's prognosis is poor.

Sources: Albert, N. M., Davis, M., & Young, J. (2002). Improving the care of patients dying of heart failure. *Cleveland Clinic Journal of Medicine, 69*(4), 321–327; and McKelvie, R. (2001). *Clinical evidence concise.* Kingsport, TN: BMJ Publishing Group.

of certain drugs (nonsteroidal anti-inflammatories, beta-blockers, and some calcium channel blockers) (McKelvie, 2001).

Given the limited available data in the literature related to treating diastolic dysfunction, most of the therapies should be aimed at treating CAD, hypertension, and volume overload (Ahmed, 2003; Jessup & Brozena, 2003). Therapeutic approaches for systolic dysfunction in the elderly should be based on general guidelines in the literature; start at low doses and titrate medications slowly to maximum tolerated doses (McKelvie, 2001). Because the elderly are at risk of hypotension in the setting of volume depletion, cautious use of antihypertensive agents that have vasodilatory properties is recommended in the setting of diuretic use (McKelvie, 2001) (see Chart 42–4, p. 1286). Toxicities to medications may occur in the elderly with renal insufficiency. Digoxin should be started at low doses (0.125 milligram daily) for those over the age of 70, monitoring levels because patients may be prone to toxicity because of reduced renal clearance (McKelvie, 2001; Nohria et al., 2002).

Coping with Heart Failure and End-of-Life Planning

Many challenges present themselves to those diagnosed with heart failure. There is the uncertainty related to prognosis, expectations related to response to medications, and possible loss of earning potential for those in the workforce. As with many chronic conditions, the impact of depression on heart failure is significant (Nohria et al., 2002). Persons diagnosed with heart failure need family or loved ones who participate actively in their life for the physical, psychological, and emotional support that is needed.

Despite medicine's best treatment options, those with heart failure will likely die from this disease process, as displayed in the course of heart failure (see Figure 42–2 ■, p. 1283). As usage

rates of medications that can alter the prognosis of heart failure improve, internal cardioverter defibrillators offer corresponding reductions in mortality. Using medications such as beta-adrenergic blockers can lead to a 5% to 15% increase in ejection fraction or even its normalization, which improves the patient's prognosis (Greenberg & Hermann, 2002). Many factors contribute to the unpredictability of a given patient's course, such as response to prognosis altering medications, compliance, and timing and level of care (Greenberg & Hermann, 2002).

When heart failure reaches a terminal stage and treatment options are limited, care should be geared toward comfort measures and reducing symptoms typically manifested as respiratory distress and pain (Albert, Davis, & Young, 2002). Palliative care is treatment done to reduce symptoms and suffering in end-of-life planning (Albert et al., 2002). Only recently has research focused on how best to treat patients in the final stages of heart failure (Albert et al., 2002; Brush, Zambroski, & Rasmusson, 2006). Optimally, palliative care should be included in the management of heart failure from the time of diagnosis, designed as part of comprehensive care across the continuum. Discussions about the level of care should be planned ahead of time, not during times of crisis. Advance directives, resuscitation wishes, living wills, formalizing estate planning, and discussing wishes with family and health care providers will lead to the best laid plans. Forward planning of this nature, however, is not often done.

Care providers have struggled with the ability to predict when death is near for patients with heart failure. It has become clear that patients with hypotension that require dose reductions of ACE inhibitors (or ARBs) and beta-adrenergic blockers, as well as increasing creatinine, and anemia, are all predictors of a poor prognosis. Albert and colleagues (2002) have proposed an algorithm with a scoring system based on identifiable criteria, as a means to assess readiness for palliative care. The criteria suggestive of a poor prognosis include NYHA class IV symptoms, tachycardia (heart rate > 100 beats per minute), serum sodium < 134 mmol/L, serum creatinine > 2.0 mg/dL, prior decompensation, use of inotropic infusion for hemodynamic stability, serious comorbid conditions, and dependence on others for assistance with ADLs. Others have used similar and additional prognostic indicators such as severe reductions in objective assessment of functional and exercise capacity. Those with 6-minute walk performance at 300 meters have higher mortality than those who can reach 450 meters (Greenberg & Hermann, 2002). Still, more evidence may be predictive of higher mortality (2 years; 60%) for those with left ventricular dimension > 85 millimeters (Nohria et al., 2002).

Patients and loved ones deserve an honest discussion related to caring for those who are near the end of life. Patients with heart failure will likely die of a sudden dysrhythmic event (if an ICD has not been implanted or has been deactivated) or the slower, progressive cardiac pump dysfunction (Nohria et al., 2002). Clear decisions should be made regarding symptom management (often done with narcotics, diuretics, nitrates, and anxiolytics) and can be planned ahead so medications are ready for use when needed (Albert et al., 2002; Nohria et al., 2002). Engaging home care, family and loved ones, community resources, and hospice can assist with facilitating the patient's individual preferences (Nohria et al., 2002). Discussing plans for turning off mechanical devices (pacemakers, defibrillators, ventricular assist devices) that may prolong life when little hope is present is often difficult, but will be necessary as their use becomes increasingly more common in treating heart failure (Albert et al., 2002). Planning for the end of life must account for the patient's spiritual, psychological, physical, social, and cultural needs. Ethical issues regarding heart failure care that must be considered thoughtfully are outlined in the Ethical Issues box.

Research

Cardiovascular research has led to tremendous advances in diagnosis and treatment. The Framingham Heart Study continues to be one of the research landmarks on which epidemiologic data on heart disease and treatment are based. In the past 30 years, studies that have been done on all the forms of heart failure treatment mentioned in this chapter have led to treatment guidelines for care. There has been an explosion of heart failure studies striving to find new treatments, hoping for methods to reduce mortality, to improve quality and length of life, and to reduce the cost. Understanding heart failure management will include a sensitivity and awareness of cultural aspects (see the Cultural Considerations box, p. 1309).

Comprehensive disease management strategies have been shown to improve outcomes associated with chronic heart failure. Such strategies include telephone follow-up with decision support software and protocol-driven pharmacologic management with close telephone nurse follow-up (Reigel et al., 2002; Whellen et al., 2001). Future directions for heart failure research studies can be found in the Research Opportunities and Clinical Impact feature (p. 1318).

ETHICAL ISSUES Related to Heart Failure

Specific ethical issues for heart failure (HF) patients and their families include:

- Quality of life after the initial onset of left ventricle (LV) dysfunction
- Employability after clinical stabilization
- When to withhold or withdraw care
- Dignified and comfortable death
- Psychological adjustment
- Considerations of futility
- Financial costs of end-stage therapies (i.e., transplant, mechanical circulatory support, intravenous medications)
- Turning off an implantable cardioverter defibrillator (ICD) device in chronic, severe, refractory HF patient
- Pregnancy in female HF patients
- Therapeutic potential of embryonic stem cells in HF
- Differences of care between male and female HF patients.

Sources: Adams, K. F., Lindenfeld, J., Arnold, J. M., et al. (2006). Executive summary: HFSA 2006 comprehensive heart failure practice guideline. *Journal of Cardiac Failure, 12*(1), 10–38; Kirkpatrick, J. N., & Kim, A. Y. (2006). Ethical issues in heart failure: Overview of an emerging need. *Perspectives in Biological Medicine, 49,* 1–9; and Lerou, P. H., & Daley, G. Q. (2005). Therapeutic potential of embryonic stem cells. *Blood Review, 19*(6), 321–331.

Genetic Considerations

Understanding genetic mechanisms of cardiomyopathy will broaden treatment approaches (Tang & Francis, 2005). Studies will evaluate genetic risk factors, therapies, legal implications, counseling, and screening issues. The Genetic Considerations box provides a more thorough review of genetic implications (p. 1279).

RESEARCH OPPORTUNITIES AND CLINICAL IMPACT RELATED TO HEART FAILURE CARE

Research Area	Clinical Impact
Depression and anxiety in patients with mechanical cardiac devices	Patients with heart failure are increasingly having cardiac devices implanted to prevent cardiac death or to improve contractility, or both. Understanding optimal treatment for anxiety or depression will be critical given the growing use of device therapy.
Caregiver support for end-stage heart failure	Heart failure is increasing in incidence and prevalence; thus, learning how to support the caregiver will be imperative.
Cost-effectiveness of heart failure therapies	Given the increasing evidence to support the use of cardiac devices, such as ICDs, pacemakers, and left ventricular assist device (LVADs), continual cost analysis of these therapies is essential.
Respiratory support for sleep disordered breathing	Patients with HF frequently experience abnormal respiratory patterns. Treatment or prevention of these abnormal respiratory patterns may lead to a reduction in the incidence of heart failure (HF).
External counterpulsation	This involves the use of a device that inflates and deflates around a patient's legs. This therapy has been shown to decrease the frequency of ischemic attacks in coronary artery disease (CAD) patients. Larger trials are underway to determine its routine use in HF care.
Implantable hemodynamic monitors	Implantable monitors are able to monitor ventricular filling pressures. This form of technology may be able to prevent HF exacerbations prior to their occurrence.
Cardiac support devices	Several surgical devices are currently in design stages to assist in the reduction of physical stresses on the left ventricle.
Myocardial regeneration by activation of stem cells	The possibility of reconstituting dead myocardium by activation of stem cells is a promising area of research.
Understanding the knowledge deficits of patients with heart failure	Patient understanding of his course of heart failure and self-management strategies is essential. Identifying the most significant barriers to patient understanding of his disease and self-management may likely improve outcomes.
Self-management strategies in heart failure	Identifying what improves patient compliance with self-management strategies may lead to improved outcomes.
The role of culture in patients with advanced heart failure	Identifying cultural barriers in providing patient care can help providers in formulating a comprehensive treatment plan.
Anthracycline-induced cardiomyopathy	Anthracyclines used to treat malignancies have been known to cause left ventricular dysfunction. More study is needed to learn how to prevent this, and to monitor and optimally treat this patient population.

Sources: Cohn, J. N., et al. (1997). Report of the National Heart, Lung, and Blood Institute special emphasis panel on heart failure research. *Circulation, 95,* 766–770; Garry, D. J., Masino, A. M., Naseem, R. H., & Martin, C. M. (2005). Ponce de Leon's fountain: Stem cells and the regenerating heart. *American Journal of Medical Science, 329*(4), 190–201; and Hunt, S. A., Abraham, W. T., Chin, M. H., Feldman, A. M., Francis, G. S., Ganiats, T. G., et al. (2005). ACC/AHA 2005 guideline update for the diagnosis and management of chronic heart failure in the adult: Summary article: A report of the American College of Cardiology/American Heart Association Task Force on Practice Guidelines (Writing Committee to Update the 2001 Guidelines for the Evaluation and Management of Heart Failure). *Journal of the American College of Cardiology, 46,* 1116–1143.

Clinical Preparation

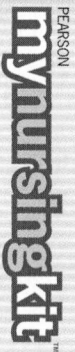

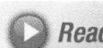 **Read**

- History of Current Illness
- Past Medical History
- Physical Exam
- Admitting Medical Orders
- Laboratory Study Results

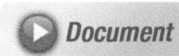 **Document**

- Summary of Hospitalization
- Pathophysiology Form
- Laboratory Values
- Laboratory Results Explanation

 **Apply**

- List of Potential Nursing Diagnoses
- Concept Map
- Critical Thinking Questions

Log on to MyNursingKit.com to download forms you will need and to complete further steps in the Clinical Preparation assignment.

HISTORY OF PRESENT ILLNESS

As the on-coming nurse on a telemetry cardiovascular care unit, you receive report about Mr. X, who was admitted with a diagnosis of heart failure 48 hours ago. He is a 56-year-old male who presented to his primary care provider with a 2-month history of worsening symptoms of dyspnea on exertion, a nonproductive cough, general fatigue, and decreased activity tolerance. Initially, the patient thought he had the flu, but when the symptoms persisted longer than expected, he sought medical attention. At the office Mr. X was found to have profound jugular ve-

nous distention, rhonchi in his lungs, and lower extremity swelling. After admission, he had an echocardiogram and a serum BNP that was 1,560 pg/mL. Coronary angiography was performed to provide a definitive diagnosis that revealed no evidence of coronary artery disease. Echocardiogram shows moderate concentric hypertrophy of the ventricles, moderate left ventricular dysfunction, ejection fraction 33%, mild to moderate mitral regurgitation. Angiogram: normal coronary arteries, ejection fraction 33%, confirmed reduction in ventricular function with a ventriculogram.

Medical Surgical History
Hyperlipidemia: diagnosed 3 years ago
Hypertension: diagnosed this past year
Type II diabetes: diagnosed this past year
Obesity: over 20 years
Hypothyroidism: diagnosed 12 years ago
Tonsillectomy: 40 years ago
Cholecystectomy: 4 years ago

Current Medications
Simvastatin 20 mg po qhs
Levothyroxine 0.125 mg po daily
Glipizide 500 mg po bid
Hydrochlorothiazide 25 mg po daily

Physical Exam
Vital signs: HR: 84 beats per minute; BP: 146/84 mmHg; temperature: 36.8°C; oxygen sat: 94% on 2 liters of oxygen.
He is a well-nourished male with appropriate affect and no apparent distress
All extremities have palpable pulses, are warm to touch, and have a capillary refill of less than 3 seconds.
3+ pitting edema is present in his lower ankles bilaterally, which extends to his midcalf; his lungs have bibasilar crackles without wheezing or retractions; he also has a nonproductive cough.
Normal S_1 and S_2 are present. S_3, and the point of maximal impulse is displaced laterally, into the anterior axillary line of his chest.
Positive hepatojugular reflux.
Bowel sounds present and palpation is nontender.

Admitting Medical Orders
Cardiology Service
Diagnosis: acute heart failure
Telemetry floor
Condition guarded
No known allergies
Full code
Bed rest with bathroom privileges
Call house officer: pulse < 60 and > 100/minute; BP < 90 and > 160 systolic; temperature > 38.5; urine output < 30 mL/hr for 2 hours; respiratory rate > 30/minute; oxygen saturation < 92%; Blood sugar < 60 or >120
Continuous cardiac monitor
Oxygen per nasal cannula to maintain oxygen sat > 92%
Vital signs and oxygen saturation q4hours
Daily a.m. weights
IV: saline lock-flush with NS q8h
Blood sugars ac and hs
Cardiac rehab evaluation and management
Low-sodium (< 2,000 mg/day), fluid-restricted (< 2 L/day) diet
Strict I&O
Sequential compression devices (SCD) to lower extremities when in bed
Incentive spirometry 2 hours while awake and q4 at night

Scheduled Medications
Simvastatin 20 mg PO qhs
Levothyroxine 0.125 mg PO daily
Glipizide 500 mg PO bid
Furosemide 80 mg PO bid
Potassium 40 mEq PO bid
Lisinopril 2.5 mg PO daily

PRN Medications

Morphine 3–5 mg IV q3–5min, max 15 mg q3h prn chest pain
Temazepam 15–30 mg PO qhs prn insomnia
Droperidol 1.25–2.5 mg IV q 6hours prn nausea

Ordered Laboratory Studies

Chemistry 7 panel daily
CBC now

BNP daily × 3
Lipid panel

Ordered Diagnostic Studies

Chest x-ray in a.m.
Echocardiogram
Angiogram

LABORATORY STUDY RESULTS

Test	Day 1 Admission	Day 1 Evening	Day 2 Morning
Potassium	4.8 mEq/L	3.5 mEq/L	3.8 mEq/L
Sodium	136 mEq/L	138 mEq/L	137 mEq/L
Chloride	103 mEq/L	104 mEq/L	103 mEq/L
Carbon dioxide (CO_2)	26 mEq/L	25 mEq/L	25 mEq/L
Calcium	8.8 mg/dL	8.7 mg/dL	9.1 mg/dL
Creatinine	1.8 mg/dL	1.4 mg/dL	1.2 mg/dL
(BUN)	30 mg/dL	24 mg/dL	18 mg/dL
Glucose	110 mg/dL	108 mg/dL	102 mg/dL
Hematocrit	40%	39%	44%
Hemoglobin	13.9 g/dL	13.5 g/dL	14.9 g/dL
Platelets	285/mm³	266/mm³	289/mm³
WBC	8.5/mm³	7.9/mm³	8.3/mm³
RBC	4.89/mm³	5.02/mm³	4.96/mm³
BNP	1,560 pg/mL	662 pg/mL	422 pg/mL
Cholesterol	260 mg/dL		
High-density lipoproteins (HDL)	36 mg/dL		
Low-density lipoproteins (LDL)	187 mg/dL		
Very-low-density lipoproteins (VLDL)	70%		
Apolipoproteins	160 mg/dL		
Triglycerides	196 mg/dL		

CRITICAL THINKING QUESTIONS

1. When reviewing Mr. X's orders when coming on shift, list them in order of priority.

2. Why would the patient receive daily a.m. weights?

3. Which laboratory values may require notification to the ordering provider?

4. What should you monitor for after giving lisinopril 2.5 mg PO daily?

5. Why is a beta-adrenergic blocker not listed on the ordered medications?

Answers to Critical Thinking Questions appear in Appendix D.

NCLEX® REVIEW

1. The nurse identifies the following risk factors in a patient admitted with symptoms of heart failure.
   1. A recent episode of acute pancreatitis
   2. Chronic fatigue syndrome
   3. Aortic stenosis
   4. Pleural effusion

2. When caring for a patient with systolic dysfunction the nurse anticipates the patient will exhibit symptoms related to which cardiac condition?
   1. Decreased cardiac output
   2. Aortic stenosis
   3. Mitral regurgitation
   4. Bradycardia

3. The nurse understands when a patient with heart failure experiences a decrease in cardiac output, the following neurohormonal responses will occur.
   1. Activation of the sympathetic nervous system, SNS
   2. Activation of the parasympathetic nervous system, PNS
   3. Inactivation of the renin angiotensin system, RAS
   4. Suppression of cytokine release

4. Which of the following symptoms should the nurse expect to see in a patient with left-sided heart failure?
   1. Weight gain
   2. Anorexia
   3. Dyspnea
   4. Peripheral edema

5. The nurse checks the brain naturietic peptide, (BNP) levels of a patient admitted with dyspnea and activity intolerance. Because the levels are normal, the nurse concludes:

   1. A diagnosis of heart failure can be excluded.

   2. The client has long standing heart failure.

   3. The client is most likely experiencing cardiac ischemia.

   4. The symptoms are related to pulmonary tissue damage.

6. The nurse should anticipate the treatment of a patient with stage B heart failure will include:

   1. ACE inhibitors and beta-blockers.

   2. Use of diuretics only.

   3. Insertion of an implantable cardiac defibrillator.

   4. Possible referral to hospice.

7. The nurse should incorporate the following key issues of a self-management program for a patient with heart failure:

   1. Medications, diet restrictions, weight reduction, and financial concerns.

   2. Medications, activity, weight, diet, and symptoms.

   3. Diet management, psychosocial concerns, and medications.

   4. Weight management, symptoms, social support, spirituality, and medications.

8. Because the following comorbidities can increase the mortality rate of patients with heart failure, the nurse assesses the patient for symptoms of:

   1. Diabetes and liver failure.

   2. Hypovolemic shock and anemia.

   3. Depression and anemia.

   4. Sleep apnea and deep vein thrombosis (DVT).

9. A patient is in end stage heart failure and the family asks what they should anticipate. The nurse recognizes the need to address the following:

   1. The lack of hearts available for heart transplants.

   2. Plans for treatment in the final stages of heart failure.

   3. Long-term home care management.

   4. Surgical interventions to correct structural abnormalities of the heart.

Answers for review questions appear in Appendix D

KEY TERMS

apnea *p.1315*
ascites *p.1287*
biventricular heart failure *p.1281*
cardiomegaly *p.1284*
crackles *p.1285*
diastolic dysfunction *p.1281*
euvolemia *p.1291*
heart failure *p.1279*

hepatojugular reflux *p.1287*
hypertrophy *p.1283*
hypopnea *p.1315*
jugular venous distention (JVD) *p.1285*
left-sided heart failure *p.1281*
left ventricular ejection fraction (LVEF) *p.1280*
New York Heart Association (NYHA) classification system *p.1285*

pitting *p.1287*
polysomnography *p.1315*
right-sided heart failure *p.1281*
S_3 (third heart sound) *p.1287*
S_4 (fourth heart sound) *p.1287*
systolic dysfunction *p.1280*
tachypnea *p.1285*

PEARSON
EXPLORE **mynursingkit™**

MyNursingKit is your one stop for online chapter review materials and resources. Prepare for success with additional NCLEX®-style practice questions, interactive assignments and activities, web links, animations and videos, and more!

Register your access code from the front of your book at
www.mynursingkit.com

REFERENCES

Abraham, W. T. (2003). Electrophysiological aids in congestive heart failure: Supporting and synchronizing systole. *Medical Clinics of North America, 87*(2), 509–521.

Abraham, W. T., Adams, K. F., Constanzo, M. R., Berkowitz, R. L., Cheng M. L., Fonarow, G. C., et al. (2005). In-hospital mortality in patients with acute decompensated heart failure requiring intravenous vasoactive medications. *Journal of the American College of Cardiology, 46*, 57–64.

Adams, K. F., Lindenfeld, J., Arnold, J. M., et al. (2006). Executive summary: HFSA 2006 comprehensive heart failure practice guideline. *Journal of Cardiac Failure, 12*(1), 10–38.

Adams, T. D., Fisher, A. G., Hansen, S. F., & Yanowitz, F. G. (2001). *Maintaining the miracle and owner's manual for the human body* (3rd ed.). Salt Lake City, UT: CAPP Publishing.

Ahmed, A. (2003). American College of Cardiology/American Heart Association chronic heart failure evaluation and management

guidelines: Relevance to the geriatric practice. *Journal of American Geriatric Society, 51*(1), 123–126.

Albert, N. M., Davis, M., & Young, J. (2002). Improving the care of patients dying of heart failure. *Cleveland Clinic Journal of Medicine, 69*(4), 321–327.

American Association of Heart Failure Nurses. (2007). *Patients are the heart of what we do.* Retrieved January 22, 2008, from http://www.aahfn.org/

American Diabetic Association. (N/D). *All about diabetes.* Retrieved July 23, 2008 from http://www.diabetes.org/about-diabetes.jsp.

American Heart Association. (2006a). *Facts about women and cardiovascular diseases.* Retrieved August 7, 2006, from http://www.americanheart. org/presenter.jhtml?identifier=2876

American Heart Association. (2006b). *Heart and stroke statistics—2006 update.* Dallas, TX: Author.

American Society of Consultant Pharmacists. (1999). *Consultant pharmacist forum; Herbal products and drug interactions.* Retrieved November 10, 2006, from http://www.ascp.com/public/pubs/tcp/1999/aug/forum.shtml

Baker, D. (2002). Prevention of heart failure. *Journal of Cardiac Failure, 8*(5), 333–346.

Bakker, P. F., Meijburg, H. W., de Vries, J. W., Mower, M. M., Thomas, A. C., Hull, M. L., et al. (2000). Biventricular pacing in end-stage heart failure improves functional capacity and left ventricular function. *Journal of Interventional Cardiac Electrophysiology, 4*(2), 395–404.

Blue Cross Blue Shield Association. (2002). *Left-ventricular assist devices as destination therapy for end-stage heart failure.* Assessment Program, 17(19). Retrieved November 10, 2006, from http://www.bcbs.com/tec/vol17/17_19.html

Bradley, T. D., & Floras, J. S. (2003a). Sleep apnea and heart failure: Part I. Obstructive sleep apnea. *Circulation, 107*, 1671–1678.

Bradley, T. D., & Floras, J. S. (2003b). Sleep apnea and heart failure: Part II. Central sleep apnea. *Circulation, 107*, 1822–1826.

Bradley, T. D. & Floras, J. S. (2000). Pathophysiologic interactions between sleep apnea and congestive heart failure. In T. D. Bradley & J. S. Floras (Eds.), *Sleep apnea: Implications in cardiovascular and cerebrovascular disease. Lung biology in health and disease* (Vol. 146, pp. 385–414). New York: Marcel Dekker.

Braunwald, E., Zipes, D. P., & Libby, P. (2001). *Heart disease: A textbook of cardiovascular medicine* (6th ed.). Philadelphia: W. B. Saunders.

Bristow, M. R., Feldman, A. M., & Saxon, L. A. (2000). Heart failure management using implantable devices for ventricular resynchronization: Comparison of medical therapy, pacing, and defibrillation in chronic heart failure (COMPANION) trial. *Journal of Cardiac Failure, 6*(3), 276–285.

Brush, S., Zambroski, C. H., & Rasmusson, K. (2006, Summer). Palliative care for the patient with end-stage heart failure. *Progress in Cardiovascular Nursing,* 166–170.

Burkett, E. L., & Hershberger, R. E. (2005). State of the art: Clinical and genetic issues in familial dilated cardiomyopathy. *Journal of the American College of Cardiology, 45*, 969–981.

Chobanian, A. V., Bakris, G. L., Black, H. R., Cushman, W. C., Green, L. A., Izzo, J. L., Jr., et al. (2003). The seventh report of the Joint National Committee on Prevention, Detection, Evaluation, and Treatment of High Blood Pressure. *Hypertension, 42*(6), 1206–1252.

Cohn, J. N. (2000). Pathophysiology and clinical recognition of heart failure. In J. T. Willerson & J. N. Cohn (Eds.), *Cardiovascular medicine* (2nd ed.). Philadelphia: Churchill Livingstone.

Dahlof, B., Lindholm, L. H., Hansson, L., Schersten, B., Ekborm, T., & Wester, P. O. (1991). Morbidity and mortality in the Swedish Trial in Old Patients with Hypertension (STOP-Hypertension). *Lancet, 338*, 1281–1285.

Digitalis Investigation Group. (1997). The effect of digoxin on mortality and morbidity in patients with heart failure. *The New England Journal of Medicine, 336*, 525–533.

Dries, D. L., Exner, D. V., Domanski, M. J., Greenberg, B., & Stevenson, L. W. (2000). The prognostic implications of renal insufficiency in asymptomatic and symptomatic patients with left ventricular systolic dysfunction. *Journal of the American College of Cardiology, 35*, 681–689.

Feldman, T. E., Hirshfeld, J. W., Jacobs, A. K., Kern, M. J., King, S. B., Morrison, D. A., et al. (2006). ACC/AHA/SCAI 2005 guideline update for percutaneous coronary intervention. *Journal of the American College of Cardiology, 47*, 216–235.

Fonarow, G. C. (2001). The treatment targets in acute decompensated heart failure. *Reviews in Cardiovascular Medicine, 2*(2), S7–S12.

Greenberg, B. H., & Hermann, D. D. (2002). *Contemporary diagnosis and management of heart failure.* Newtown, PA: Handbooks in Health Care.

Hall, J. A., Rasmusson, K. D., Kfoury, A. G., French, T. K., Rimmasch, H. L., Hofmann, L. C., et al. (2005). Successful implementation of heart failure self-management improves survival. *Journal of Heart and Lung Transplantation*, 24(Suppl. 2S), S68–S79.

Hanly, P. J., & Zuberi-Khokhar, N. S. (1996). Increased mortality associated with Cheyne–Stokes respiration in patients with congestive heart failure. *American Journal of Respiratory Critical Care Medicine, 153*, 272–276.

Hardman, J. G., & Limbird, L. E. (Eds.). (2001). *Goodman and Gilman's The Pharmacological basis of therapeutics* (10th ed.). New York: McGraw-Hill.

Havranek, E. P., Ware, M. G., & Lowes, B. D. (1999). Prevalence of depression in congestive heart failure. *American Journal of Cardiology, 84*, 348–350.

He, J., Ogden, L. G., Bazzano, L. A., Vupputuri, S., Loria, C., & Whelton, P. K. (2001). Risk factors for congestive heart failure in US men and women: NHANES I epidemiologic follow-up study. *Archives of Internal Medicine, 161*, 996–1002.

Heart Outcomes Prevention Evaluation Study Investigators. (2000). Effects of ramipril on cardiovascular and microvascular outcomes in people with diabetes mellitus: Results of the HOPE study and MICRO-HOPE sub study. *Lancet, 355*, 253–259.

Heiat, A., Gross, C. P., & Krumholz, H. M. (2002). Representation of the elderly, women, and minorities in heart failure clinical trials. *Archives of Internal Medicine, 162*, 1682–1688.

Horwich, T. B. (2002). Anemia is associated with worse symptoms, greater impairment in functional capacity and a significant increase in mortality in patients with advanced heart failure. *Journal of the American College of Cardiology, 39*(11), 1780–1786.

Hunt, S. A., Abraham, W. T., Chin, M. H., Feldman, A. M., Francis, G. S., Ganiats, T. G., et al. (2005). ACC/AHA 2005 guideline update for the diagnosis and management of chronic heart failure in the adult: Summary article: A report of the American College of Cardiology/American Heart Association Task Force on Practice Guidelines (Writing Committee to Update the 2001 Guidelines for the Evaluation and Management of Heart Failure). *Journal of the American College of Cardiology, 46*, 1116–1143.

Iribarren, C., Karter, A. J., Go, A. S., Ferrara, A., Liu, J. Y., Sidney, S., et al. (2001). Glycemic control and heart failure among adult patients with diabetes. *Circulation, 103*, 2668–2673.

Javaheri, S. (2000). Effects of continuous positive airway pressure on sleep apnea and ventricular irritability in patients with heart failure. *Circulation, 101*, 392–397.

Javaheri, S., Parker, T. J., Liming, J. D., Corbett, W. S., Nishiyama, H., Wexler, L., et al. (1998). Sleep apnea in 81 ambulatory male patients with stable heart failure: Types and their prevalences, consequences, and presentations. *Circulation, 97*, 2154–2159.

Jessup, M., & Brozena, S. (2003). Heart failure. *The New England Journal of Medicine, 348*, 2007–2018.

Kaneko, Y., Floras, J. S., Phil, D., Usui, K., Plante, J., Tkacova, R., et al. (2003). Cardiovascular effects of continuous positive airway pressure in patients with heart failure and obstructive sleep apnea. *The New England Journal of Medicine, 348*, 1233–1241.

Kerwin, W. F., Botvinick, E. H., O'Connell, J. W., Merrick, S. H., DeMarco, T., Chatterjee, K., et al. (2000). Ventricular contraction abnormalities in dilated cardiomyopathy: Effect of biventricular pacing to correct interventricular dyssynchrony. *Journal of the American College of Cardiology, 35*(5), 1221–1227.

Kfoury, A. G., Hall, J. C., Rasmusson, K. D., Horne, B., & Renlund, D. G. (2006). Incremental survival benefit with adherence to JCAHO heart failure measures. *Supplement to the Journal of Heart and Lung Transplant.*

Konstam, M. A. (2004). Heart failure training: A call for an integrative, patient-focused approach to an emerging cardiology subspecialty. *Journal of Cardiac Failure, 10*(5), 366–367.

Kosiborod, M., et al. (2003). The prognostic importance of anemia in patients with heart failure. *American Journal of Medicine, 114*, 112–119.

Kostis, J. B., Davis, B. R., Cutler, J., Grimm, R. H., Jr., Berge, K. G., & Cohen, J. D. (1997). Prevention of heart failure by antihypertensive drug treatment in older persons with isolated systolic hypertension. SHEP Cooperative Research Group. *Journal of the American Medical Association, 278*, 212–216.

Kouchoukos, N. T., Blackstone, E. H., Doty, D. B., Hanley, F. L., & Karp, R. B. (2003). *Kirklin/Barratt-Boyes cardiac surgery* (3rd ed., Vol. 2). Philadelphia: Churchill Livingston.

Krumholz, H. M., Amatruda, J., Smith, G. L., Mattera, J. A., Roumanis, S. A., Radford, M. J., et al. (2002). Randomized trial of an education and support intervention to prevent readmission of patients with heart failure. *Journal of the American College of Cardiology, 13*(1), 83–89.

Krumholz, H. M., Chen, Y. T., Vaccarino, V., et al (2000). Correlates and impact on outcomes of worsening renal function in patients > or = 65 years of age with heart failure. *American Journal of Cardiology, 85*, 1110–1113.

Leung, R. S. T., & Bradley, T. D. (2001). Sleep apnea and cardiovascular disease. *American Journal of Respiratory and Critical Care Medicine, 164*, 2147–2165.

Levy, D., Larson, M. G., Vasan, R. S., Kannel, W. B., & Ho, K. K. (1996). The progression from hypertension to congestive heart failure. *The Journal of the American Medical Association, 275*, 1557–1562.

Linde, C., Leclercq, C., Rex, S., Garrigue, S., Lavergne, T., Cazeau, S., et al. on behalf of the Multisite Stimulation in Cardiomyopathies study group (MUSTIC). (2002). Long-term benefits of biventricular pacing in congestive heart failure: Results from the Multisite Stimulation in Cardiomyopathy (MUSTIC) study. *Journal of the American College of Cardiology, 40*(1), 111–118.

McKelvie, R. (2001). *Clinical evidence concise.* Kingsport, TN: BMJ Publishing Group.

Molhoek, S. G., Bax, J. J., van Erven, L., Bootsma, M., Boersma, E., Steendijk, P., et al. (2002). Effectiveness of resynchronization therapy in patients with end-stage heart failure. *American Journal of Cardiology, 90*(4), 379–383.

Moss, A. J., Zareba, W., Hall, W. J., Klein, H., Wilber, D. J., Cannom, D. S., et al. for the Multicenter Automatic Defibrillator Implantation Trial II Investigators (MADIT-II). (2002). Prophylactic implantation of a defibrillator in patients with myocardial infarction and reduced ejection fraction. *The New England Journal of Medicine, 346*(12), 877–883.

Naughton, M. T. (2006). The link between obstructive sleep apnea and heart failure: Underappreciated opportunity for treatment. *Current Heart Failure Reports, 3*(4), 183–188.

Neal, B., MacMahon, S., & Chapman, N. (2000). Effects of ACE inhibitors, calcium antagonists, and other blood pressure-lowering drugs: Results of prospectively designed overviews of randomized trials. Blood Pressure Lowering Treatment Trialists' Collaboration. *Lancet, 356*, 1956–1964.

Nohria, A., Lewis, E., & Stevenson, L. W. (2002). Medical management of advanced heart failure. *Journal of the American Medical Association, 287*(5), 628–640.

Packer, M., Gheorghiade, M., & Young, J. B., et al., for the RADIANCE Study. (1993). Withdrawal of digoxin from patients with chronic heart failure treated with angiotensin-converting-enzyme inhibitors. *The New England Journal of Medicine, 397*, 1–7.

Rasmusson, K. D., Hall, J. A., Hofmann, L. C., Moore, S. V., & Renlund, D. G. (2002). Patient self-management knowledge and perceptions improve through community based heart failure teaching. *Journal of Cardiac Failure, 8*(4).

Rasmusson, K. D., Hall, J. A., & Renlund, D. G. (2006). Heart failure epidemic boiling to the surface. *Nurse Practitioner, 31*(11), 12–21.

Renlund, D. G., & Taylor, D. O. (2002). *Cardiac transplantation. Textbook of cardiovascular medicine* (2nd ed.). Philadelphia: Lippincott Williams & Wilkins.

Riegel, B., Carlson, B., Kopp, Z., LePetri, B., Glaser, D., & Unger, A. (2002). Effect of a standardized nurse case-management telephone intervention on resource use in patients with chronic heart failure. *Archives of Internal Medicine, 162*, 705–712.

Rose, E. A., Gelijns, A. C., Moskowitz, A. J., Heitjan, D. F., Stevenson, L. W., Dembitsky, W., et al. (2001). Long term use of a left ventricular assist device for end-stage heart failure. *The New England Journal of Medicine, 345*(20), 1435–1493.

Sackner-Bernstein, J. D., & Mancini, D. M. (1995). Rationale for treatment of patients with chronic heart failure with adrenergic blockage. *Journal of the American Medical Association, 274*, 1462–1467.

Scandinavian Simvastatin Survival Study. (1994). Randomised trial of cholesterol lowering in 4444 patients with coronary heart disease: The Scandinavian Simvastatin Survival Study (4S). *Lancet, 344*, 1383–1389.

Sha, M., Ali, V., Lamba, S., & Abraham, W. (2001). Pathophysiology and clinical spectrum of acute congestive heart failure. *Reviews in Cardiovascular Medicine, 2*(2), S2–S6.

Silver, M. A. (1998). *Success with heart failure; Success and hope for those with congestive heart failure.* Reading, MA: Perseus Books.

Silverberg, D. S., Wexler, D., Sheps, D., et al (2001). The effect of correction of mild anemia in severe, resistant congestive heart failure using subcutaneous erythropoietin and intravenous iron: A randomized controlled study. *Journal of the American College of Cardiology, 37*, 1775–1780.

Sin, D. D., Fitzgerald, F., Parker, J. D., Newton, G., Floras, J. S., & Bradley, T. D. (1999). Risk factors for central and obstructive sleep apnea in 450 men and women with congestive heart failure. *American Journal of Respiratory and Critical Care Medicine, 160*, 1101–1106.

Smith, G. L., Masoudi, F. A., Vaccarino, V., Radford, M. J., & Krumholz, H. M. (2003). Outcomes in heart failure patients with preserved ejection fraction. *Journal of the American College of Cardiology, 41*(9), 1510–1517.

Stafford, R. S., & Radley, D. C. (2003). The underutilization of cardiac medications of proven benefit, 1990–2002. *Journal of the American College of Cardiology, 41*(1), 56–61.

Stevenson, L. W. (2003). Clinical use of inotropic therapy for heart failure: Looking backward or forward. *Circulation, 108*, 367–372.

Stewart, S., MacIntyre, S., Capewell, S., McMurray, J. J. (2003). Heart failure and the aging population: an increasing burden in the 21st century? *Heart.* <javascript:AL_get (this,'jour,' 'Heart.');>. 2003 Jan; 89 (1): 49–53. <http://www.ncbi.nlm.nih.gov/entrez/utils/fref. fcgi?PrId=3051&itool=AbstractPlus-def&uid=12482791&db=pubmed&url=http://heart.bmj.com/cgi/pmidlookup?view-long&pmid=12482791> <http://www.ncbi.nlm.nih.gov/entrez/utils/fref.fcgi?PrId=3494&itol=AbstractPlus-nondef&uid=12482791&db=pubjed&url=http://www.pubmedcentral.nih.gov/articlerender.fcgi?tool=pubmed&pubmedid=12482791> Retrieved November 3, 2008 from http://www.ncbi.nlm.nih.gov/pubmed/1248279

Stratton, I. M., Adler, A. I., Neil, H. A., Matthews, D. R., Manley, S. E., & Cull, C. A. (2000). Association of glycaemia with macrovascular and microvascular complication of type 2 diabetes (UKPDS 35): Prospective observational study. *British Medical Journal, 321*, 405–412.

Tang, W. H., & Francis, G. S. (2005). The year in heart failure. *Journal of the American College of Cardiology, 46*(11), 2125–2133.

Teerlink, J. R., & Massie, B. M. (2003). Late breaking heart failure trials from the 2003 ACC meeting: EPHESUS and COMPANION. *Journal of Cardiac Failure, 9*(3), 158–163.

United Network for Organ Sharing. (2006). *It is all about life.* Retrieved December 1, 2006, from http://www.unos.org

Weber, K. T. (1999). Aldosterone and spironolactone in heart failure. *The New England Journal of Medicine, 341*, 753–755.

Weinfeld, M. S., Chertow, G. M., & Stevenson, L. W. (1999). Aggravated renal dysfunction during intensive therapy for advanced chronic heart failure. *American Heart Journal, 138*, 285–290.

Whellan, D. J., Gualden, L., Gattis, W. A., Granger, B., Russell, S. D., Blazing, M. A., et al. (2001). The benefit of implementing a heart failure disease management program. *Archives of Internal Medicine, 161*, 2223–2228.

World Health Organization. (1968). *Nutritional anaemias: Report of a WHO scientific group.* Geneva, Switzerland: Author.

Yan, A. T., Bradley, T. D., & Liu, P. P. (2001). The role of continuous positive pressure in the treatment of congestive heart failure. *Chest, 120*, 1675–1685.

Young, J. B. (2001). New therapeutic choices in the management of acute congestive heart failure. *Reviews in Cardiovascular Medicine, 2*(2), S19–S24.

Caring for the Patient with Peripheral Vascular Disorders

Brenda McCulloch

Outcome-Based Learning Objectives

After studying this chapter, the learner will be able to:

1. Describe the risk factors and clinical findings in peripheral arterial disease.
2. Develop a nursing care plan for the patient with peripheral arterial disease.
3. Compare and contrast the clinical findings and management of Raynaud's disease and Buerger's disease.
4. Discuss signs and symptoms of common potential complications of endovascular repair and surgery of the aorta, and appropriate nursing interventions for each.
5. Identify the risk factors, diagnosis, medical management, and nursing care for deep venous thrombosis.
6. Explain the actions of commonly used anticoagulants and antiplatelet agents used for patients with peripheral arterial disease and nursing management of the patient receiving them.
7. Identify the risk factors, diagnosis, medical management, and nursing care for varicose veins.
8. Identify the risk factors, diagnosis, medical management, and nursing care for aortic aneurysm and aortic dissection.

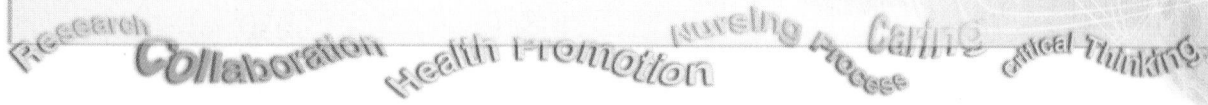

VASCULAR DISORDERS include disorders of the arterial, venous, and lymphatic systems of the body. Peripheral arterial disease includes occlusive, aneurysmal (dilated), and vasospastic disorders affecting the arterial system of the neck, abdomen, and extremities. Peripheral venous disease predominantly involves the legs and is usually due to thrombosis or insufficiency of the veins. Lymphatic disease leads to abnormal fluid collection, edema, and fibrosis. These peripheral vascular diseases may cause serious complications such as loss of limb or even loss of life.

Anatomy and Physiology Review

The peripheral vascular system is a network of branching blood vessels carrying oxygenated blood from the heart to the tissues of the body and returning deoxygenated blood to the lungs. The peripheral vascular system is made up of arteries, veins, and capillaries. The lymphatics, also considered part of the peripheral vascular system, help maintain adequate blood volume by returning tissue fluid to the bloodstream.

Arteries consist of three distinct layers: the tunica intima, the tunica media, and the tunica adventitia. The innermost lining of the tunica intima consists of the endothelium, which provides a smooth surface for flowing blood. The middle layer, or the tu-

nica media, is made up of smooth muscle cells, collagen, and elastin, providing elasticity and strength to the vessel. The tunica adventitia, or the outermost layer of the artery, consists of connective tissue and anchors the vessel in the surrounding tissue.

The largest artery in the body is the aorta. It ascends from the aortic root of the heart, passes through the chest, and descends into the abdomen, where it bifurcates about the level of the umbilicus. It branches off to various vital organs along the way. The major arteries are shown in Figure 43–1 ■ (p. 1324). Arteries branch sequentially from large to medium to the smallest arteries called arterioles, eventually reaching the capillary bed.

Capillaries are thin-walled structures consisting of a single layer of endothelial cells. Capillaries help facilitate rapid nutrient and waste product transport and removal. Venules are formed when several capillaries join together. Small venules form progressively larger veins and return blood from the periphery to the right atrium. The major veins are shown in Figure 43–2 ■ (p. 1325). Veins are thin-walled structures in contrast to arteries, and the venous system is comparably low pressure.

The lymphatic system is a network of vessels that transports lymph—a clear fluid that comes from the blood and bathes the tissues. Lymph contains water, protein, minerals, and white blood cells. Functions of the lymphatic system include the absorption of excess fluid and its return to the bloodstream, the

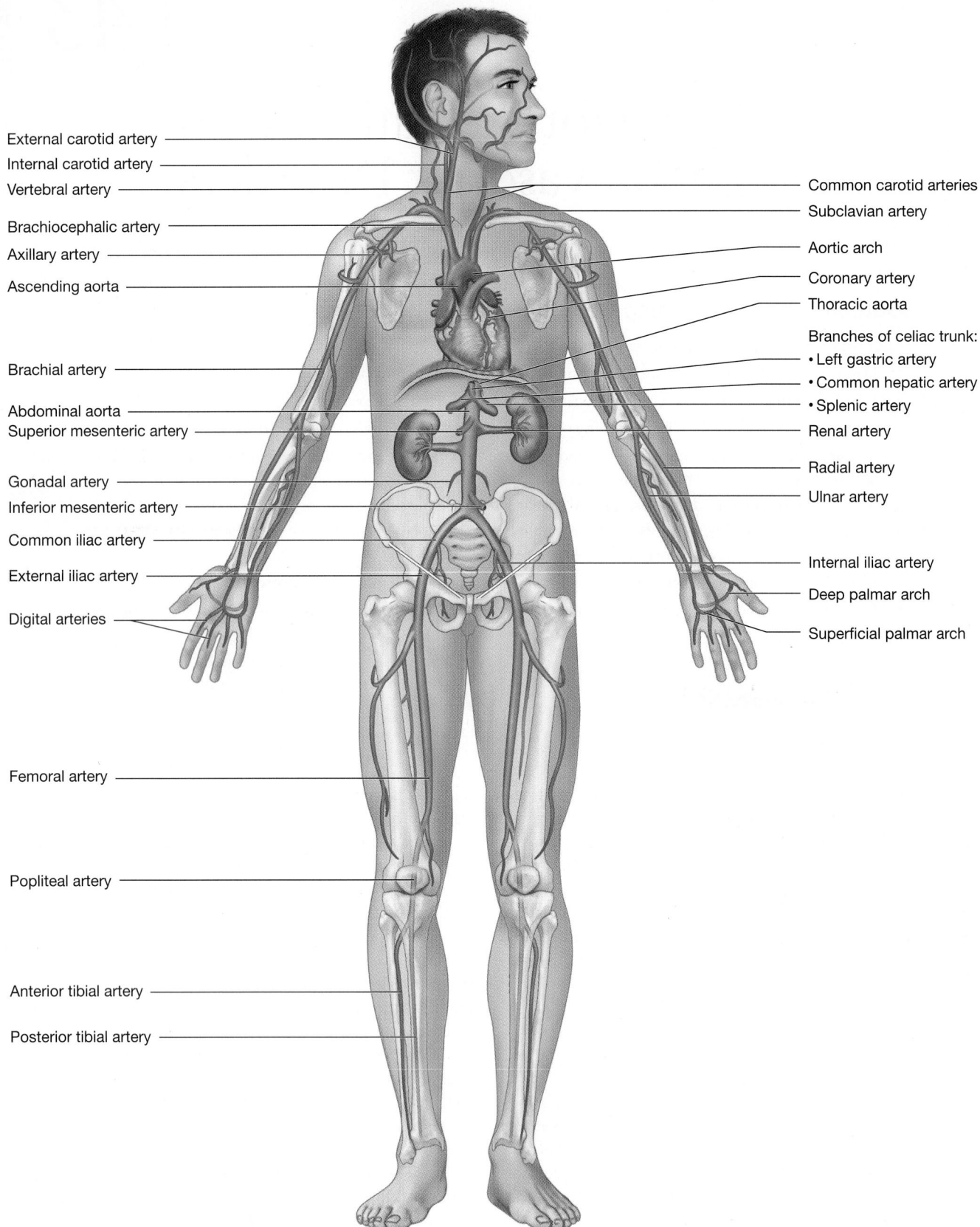

External carotid artery

Internal carotid artery

Vertebral artery

Brachiocephalic artery

Axillary artery

Ascending aorta

Brachial artery

Abdominal aorta

Superior mesenteric artery

Gonadal artery

Inferior mesenteric artery

Common iliac artery

External iliac artery

Digital arteries

Femoral artery

Popliteal artery

Anterior tibial artery

Posterior tibial artery

Common carotid arteries

Subclavian artery

Aortic arch

Coronary artery

Thoracic aorta

Branches of celiac trunk:
• Left gastric artery
• Common hepatic artery
• Splenic artery

Renal artery

Radial artery

Ulnar artery

Internal iliac artery

Deep palmar arch

Superficial palmar arch

FIGURE 43–1 ■ Major arteries of the body.

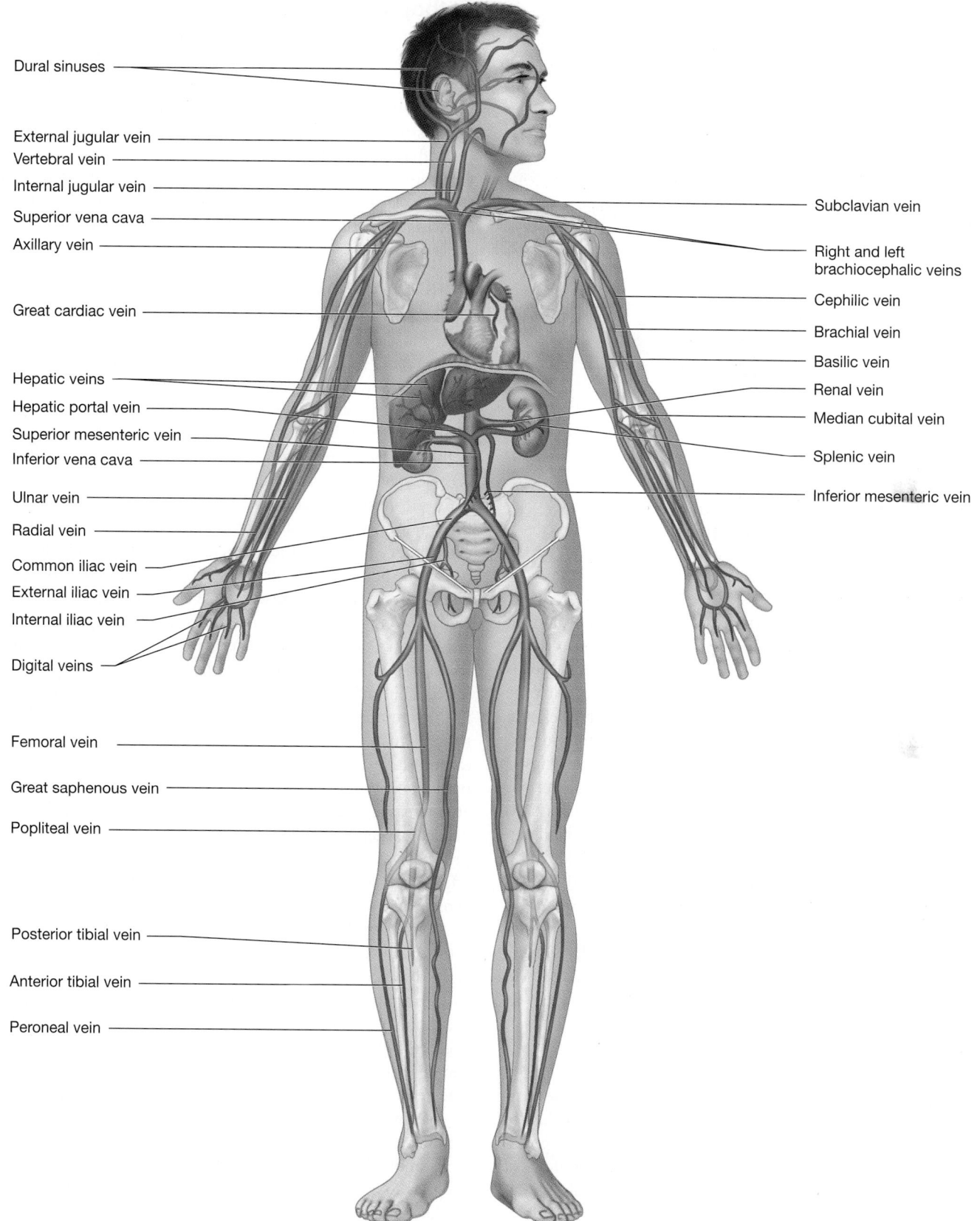

Dural sinuses

External jugular vein
Vertebral vein
Internal jugular vein
Superior vena cava
Axillary vein

Great cardiac vein

Hepatic veins
Hepatic portal vein
Superior mesenteric vein
Inferior vena cava

Ulnar vein

Radial vein

Common iliac vein
External iliac vein
Internal iliac vein

Digital veins

Femoral vein

Great saphenous vein

Popliteal vein

Posterior tibial vein

Anterior tibial vein

Peroneal vein

Subclavian vein

Right and left
brachiocephalic veins

Cephilic vein

Brachial vein

Basilic vein

Renal vein

Median cubital vein

Splenic vein

Inferior mesenteric vein

FIGURE 43–2 ■ Major veins of the body.

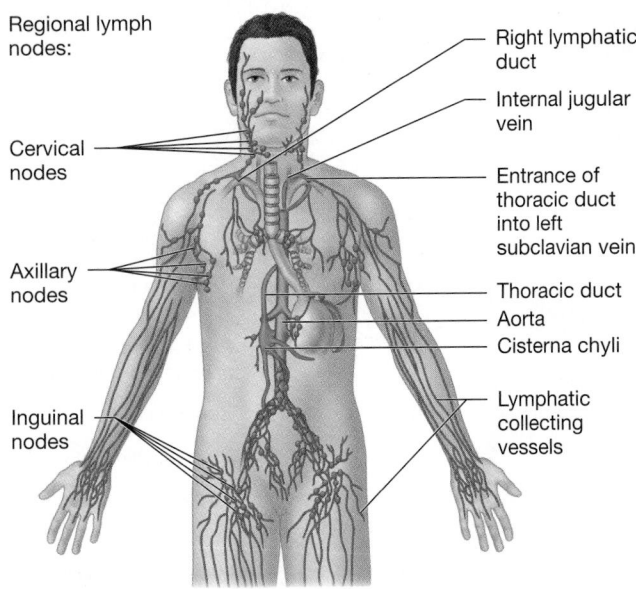

Regional lymph nodes:

Cervical nodes

Axillary nodes

Inguinal nodes

Right lymphatic duct

Internal jugular vein

Entrance of thoracic duct into left subclavian vein

Thoracic duct

Aorta

Cisterna chyli

Lymphatic collecting vessels

FIGURE 43–3 ■ The lymphatic system.

absorption of fat, and an immune system function. The lymphatic system is shown in Figure 43–3 ■.

Peripheral Arterial Disease

The American College of Cardiology (ACC) and the American Heart Association (AHA) define **peripheral arterial disease (PAD)** as "vascular disease caused primarily by atherosclerosis and thromboembolic pathophysiological processes that alter the normal structure of the aorta, its visceral arterial branches, and the arteries of the lower extremities." This chronic and progressive disorder is a largely underrecognized and underdiagnosed disease affecting 12 million Americans (AHA, 2007). Atherosclerosis has been defined as the process of fatty substances, cholesterol, cellular waste products, calcium, and fibrin building up in the inner lining of an artery, resulting in plaque buildup and a narrowing of the lumen of the artery (AHA, 2008b). PAD is defined as the development of this atherosclerotic process at various levels in the aortic bifurcation and the iliac arteries and the lower extremities, including the femoral, popliteal, peroneal, and tibial arteries. Atherosclerosis is further discussed in Chapter 40 ⊕.

Etiology and Epidemiology

The incidence of PAD increases with age, and approximately 5% of people 55 and older and 20% of those 70 and older have signs and symptoms. The incidence in men is slightly higher than in women, and it is more common in the African American population (Criqui et al., 2005). The risk factors, similar to those of heart disease and stroke, include cigarette smoking, diabetes, hyperlipidemia, hypertension, elevated C-reactive protein, and hyperhomocysteinemia (Hirsch et al, 2006; Sontheimer, 2006). Screening for PAD is recommended for patients with exertional leg pain, patients over age 50 who have associated risk factors such as smoking and diabetes, patients who have had diabetes for more than 20 years, and all patients over the age of 70 (Oka, 2006).

Pathophysiology

Atherosclerosis is a disease process that occurs over many years, usually beginning in childhood. Lipids (fats) collect under the inner lining of damaged artery walls, eventually narrowing or blocking the artery and obstructing blood flow. Over time, this fatty tissue can erode the wall of the artery, diminish its elasticity, and interfere with blood flow. Plaque deposits also can rupture, causing debris to migrate downstream within an artery. Clots can also form around the plaque deposits, further interfering with blood flow and posing added danger if they break off.

Clinical Manifestations

Signs and symptoms of PAD may include intermittent claudication, muscle/limb weakness with use, absent or diminished pulses, poor hair growth, cool skin, resting limb pain, **paresthesia** (an abnormal physical sensation such as prickling, tingling, or numbness), and poor healing of sores or ulcers.

Intermittent claudication (IC), or exercise-induced leg pain, is the most common symptom of peripheral arterial disease (Oka, 2006). The word *claudication* is derived from the Latin word for limp, or *claudico*. Descriptors patients may use about their pain include aching, cramping, tiredness, and/or fatigue. This pain can occur in the buttocks, hip, thigh, or calf, depending on the portion of the arterial tree affected by atherosclerotic disease. The muscle group distal to a stenotic (narrowed) or occluded (completely blocked) artery is affected by the decreased circulation. For example, more proximal lesions, such as aortoiliac lesions, will produce the pain of intermittent claudication in the hip, buttocks, or thigh, whereas the pain from lesions lower in the femoral or popliteal arteries produces calf pain. When a muscle is at rest, the metabolic needs are minimal, and even diseased arteries can provide adequate blood supply to maintain perfusion. With exercise, such as walking, metabolic demands are increased, and the diseased arteries are unable to deliver the needed oxygen to the muscles or to dispose of the metabolic byproduct lactic acid. The buildup of lactic acid causes pain in the affected muscle group of the leg. When the walking ceases, or shortly afterward, the pain resolves and exercise may resume.

Reproducibility of the ischemic pain is a hallmark finding of intermittent claudication. The pain occurs consistently at the same distance, and after resting, the pain subsides and exercise may continue. Time and distance to claudication, for example, the number of blocks a patient can walk before the pain starts, is useful information to obtain during the nursing assessment and can be used as a subjective measure of improved function after intervention.

Intermittent claudication can remain stable for years, and walking can improve muscle endurance, especially if the patient stops smoking tobacco. The atherosclerotic process can, however, progress to a point at which the patient experiences pain in the foot at rest. Rest pain is a sign of severe ischemia or lack of sufficient oxygen supply to the tissues. It is characterized by pain in the forefoot and toes, usually worse at night when lying flat in bed, and can either awaken a person from sleep or prevent sleep altogether. Patients will usually be more comfortable with the leg in a dependent position, such as dangling over the edge of the bed or chair, because gravity can enhance arterial circulation. Narcotic pain medicines, such as opiates, are indicated but may not control the pain well due to the severe nature of the ischemic rest pain.

Ulceration (skin breakdown) can occur as a result of poor blood supply, pressure, or trauma to an ischemic limb. A non-healing area of tissue injury is prone to necrosis or gangrene and infection. Arterial ulceration accounts for about 20% of all leg ulcers and is most likely to occur at the distal-most point of arterial flow. The toes are a common site for arterial ulceration (Sieggreen & Kline, 2004a). In arterial ulcerations, the base is pale, gray, or yellowish in color with little drainage and regular borders. Wounds are described in detail in Chapter 67 ⊚ . The foot pulses are diminished or absent, and the skin is pale and cool to touch. The patient typically complains of a burning, throbbing pain, unless he has peripheral neuropathy, most commonly seen in long-standing diabetes. Pain management can be challenging, requiring narcotics for relief (Sieggreen, 2005a).

 CRITICAL ALERT *Ongoing and regular nursing assessment of ulcerations and wounds in the patient with peripheral vascular disorders are essential, so that early signs and symptoms of infection can be detected and treated. Assessment finding in early localized infection can include low-grade temperature, warmth, tenderness, pain, edema, erythema, and new or increased drainage that may have a foul odor. If the patient develops mental status changes, hyperventilation, tachycardia, fever, chills, elevated white blood count, fatigue, or malaise, systemic infection (sepsis) may be occurring. These changes need to be reported to the health care practitioner.*

Laboratory and Diagnostic Procedures

The diagnosis of peripheral arterial disease is typically based on the patient's history; physical examination findings; and resting **ankle-brachial index (ABI)** results, which is a simple to perform, noninvasive test that detects peripheral arterial disease of the legs (Figure 43–4 ■). To determine the ABI, check the blood pressure of both arms with a Doppler and take the higher reading. Using a Doppler over the posterior tibial and dorsalis pedis pulses, determine the blood pressure in the foot, and take the higher of the two. It is the ratio of the highest ankle systolic pressure to the highest arm systolic pressure. An ABI ≥1.0 is considered normal, whereas a finding of ≤0.90 indicates peripheral arterial disease. A result less than 0.4 indicates severe arterial ischemia (Oka, 2006; Sieggreen, 2005a). The ABI may be falsely elevated in patients with diabetes (Olson & Treat-Jacobson, 2004). The Diagnostic Tests box (p. 1328) outlines the diagnostic tests performed for peripheral arterial disease.

Medical Management

According to the Seventh American College of Chest Physicians (ACCP) Conference on Antithrombotic and Thrombolytic Therapy (Hirsh, Guyatt, Alberts, & Schünemann, 2004), patients with PAD should receive lifelong antiplatelet therapy with aspirin. Aspirin has antithrombotic effects and inhibits platelet aggregation. Ticlopidine (Ticlid), clopidogrel (Plavix), and cilostazol (Pletal) or pentoxifylline (Trental) also may be indicated for some patients. Ticlopidine and clopidogrel are thienopyridine derivatives and inhibit adenosine diphosphate (ADP)-induced platelet aggregation. Cilostazol inhibits phosphodiesterase III, but its exact mechanism of action is not fully understood. It suppresses platelet aggregation and is a direct ar-

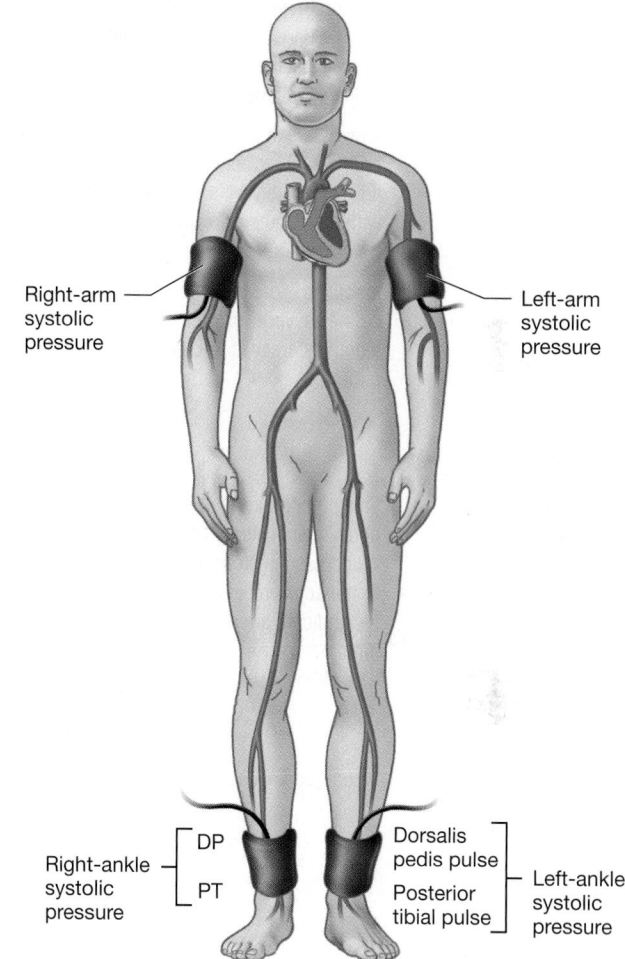

| Right ABI | $\dfrac{\text{Average right ankle pressure}}{\text{Average brachial artery pressure}}$ |
| Left ABI | $\dfrac{\text{Average left ankle pressure}}{\text{Average brachial artery pressure}}$ |

Interpretation of ABI	
>1.30	Noncompressible
0.91–1.30	Normal
0.41–0.90	Mild-to-moderate peripheral arterial disease
0.00–0.40	Severe peripheral arterial disease

FIGURE 43–4 ■ Ankle-brachial index chart.

terial vasodilator. Pentoxifylline has weak antithrombotic effects and lowers blood viscosity (Lipsitz & Kim, 2005). Additionally, cardiovascular risk reduction strategies are important for the patient with PAD and include the use of beta-adrenergic blockers, angiotensin receptor blockers, and lipid lowering agents. The Pharmacology Summary feature (p. 1335) provides a detailed list of pharmacologic therapies used to treat PAD.

Endovascular repair is the treatment of vascular disease from inside the blood vessel (endoluminal). It started as percutaneous balloon angioplasty for peripheral arterial disease in the 1960s and was further refined for coronary artery intervention 10 years later. Today, various endovascular options are available including angioplasty, stenting, and radiation therapy. Percutaneous transluminal angioplasty (PTA) is indicated for those patients who are limited by their pain, and there is a reasonable likelihood of

DIAGNOSTIC TESTS for Peripheral Arterial Disease (PAD)

Test	Expected Abnormality	Rationale for Abnormality
Ankle-brachial index (ABI)	0.95–1.1 normal. ≤0.9 indicative of PAD. ≤0.4 advanced ischemic disease with impending loss of tissue. Segmental arterial pressures and ankle-brachial indexes (ABIs) can be falsely elevated if the patient has calcified, noncompressible arteries. May be unreliable in patients with diabetes or patients with heavily calcified vessels. Suspect calcified arteries if the ABI is > 1.3 and/or if the ankle pressure is > 300 mmHg.	Noninvasive. Simple to perform. Cost effective. ABI compares ankle pressure with arm pressure. ABI is obtained by dividing the ankle pressure by the highest brachial blood pressure. Can also be assessed before and after exercise testing to evaluate arterial insufficiency.
Treadmill exercise arterial studies	A decrease in the ABI following exercise indicates arterial insufficiency. Patients with intermittent claudication (IC) will demonstrate 20 mmHg or more decrease in ABI within 1 minute following exercise.	Measures the lower extremity circulation's response to exercise. May be used to index severity of disease and assess a patient's response to an intervention, as well as for follow-up.
Duplex ultrasound	Identifies areas of stenosis in arterial vessels and defines severity of stenoses. Identifies areas of turbulent flow and abnormal flow patterns.	Noninvasive. Widely available. Portable. Uses sound waves reflected off of moving red blood cells and other tissues to evaluate the flow of blood. The different vascular beds have unique waveforms and variations from normal indicate disease.
Segmental arterial pressures	This procedure assesses the femoral, popliteal, dorsalis pedis, and posterior tibial arteries. A decrease in pressure of 20–30 mmHg from one segment to the adjacent, more distal segment implies a significant arterial obstruction in the vessels between the cuffs.	Noninvasive. More time-consuming than ABI to perform. Provides information about the anatomic location of vascular disease. Uses a sphygmomanometer and a Doppler at several areas, or segments, of the lower extremity. Pressures are recorded at the thigh, below the knee, and at the ankle and are compared to the brachial blood pressure. The blood pressure in the leg should equal the blood pressure in the arm.
Angiography	Visualizes anatomy, areas of stenosis, and/or occlusion.	Definitive method for anatomic evaluation. Invasive. Requires vascular access. Requires iodine-based contrast administration. Requires x-ray exposure. Accurate diagnosis. Requires skilled interpretation.
Computed tomography (CT)	Visualizes anatomy, areas of stenosis, and/or occlusion.	Noninvasive. Requires iodine-based contrast administration. Requires x-ray exposure. Expensive. Requires skilled interpretation. Less readily available. Useful for patients who cannot undergo magnetic resonance testing (pacemakers, defibrillators).
Magnetic resonance imaging (MRI) and magnetic resonance angiography (MRA)	Visualizes anatomy, areas of stenosis, and/or occlusion. Provides excellent anatomic detail. May be inaccurate in arteries treated with metal stents.	Noninvasive. Does not require vascular access. Does not require iodine-based contrast administration. Expensive. Requires skilled interpretation. Not widely available. May be difficult for claustrophobic patients. Cannot be used for some patients (pacemakers, defibrillators).

improvement with intervention. PTA is an invasive percutaneous procedure that can be done using local anesthesia with sedation. It is performed in the interventional radiology suite or in the cardiac catheterization laboratory by vascular surgeons, interventional radiologists, and/or cardiologists. A balloon-tipped catheter is inserted into the arterial vasculature, usually the femoral artery, and positioned at the area of obstruction. The balloon is then inflated, disrupting the plaque and stretching the media of the artery, thereby enlarging the opening. Stents—tubular metal devices made of stainless steel, nitinol, or titanium—are inserted to act as a mechanical scaffolding to hold a vessel open in the diseased area. Stents and other interventional devices are further discussed in Chapter 39 ∞ .

PTA is indicated for the treatment of arterial occlusive disease. It is most successful when performed for shorter lesions that are <5 cm (2 in.) in the iliac artery and <10 cm (4 in.) in the superficial femoral artery. PTA of lesions longer than these is more likely to restenose and also may be done in the smaller tibial vessels if the lesion is <2 cm (<1 in.)(Singh & Cousin, 2005). The long-term results of PTA for these lesions are less than optimal, but performing this procedure may allow enough improved blood flow to permit wound healing and/or limb salvage and to prevent or delay amputation.

Complications of percutaneous transluminal angioplasty are uncommon (2% to 5%) and include bleeding and hematoma at the access site, distal embolization, arterial dissection, or occlusion at the dilation site (Singh & Cousin, 2005). Other complications can include contrast allergy and contrast-induced renal failure. Following PTA, patients are discharged on aspirin and/or clopidogrel. Although the long-term results of this procedure are unknown at this time, PTA is rapidly becoming the initial intervention for revascularization of the lower extremities. The PTA technique is further discussed in Chapter 39 ∞ . Other adjunctive interventional techniques such as lasers, cutting balloons, atherectomy devices, and thermal devices can be useful in the iliac, femoral, popliteal, and tibial arteries.

Gene therapy may emerge as a treatment for peripheral arterial disease. Gene therapy, or therapeutic angiogenesis, augments collateral artery development by stimulating capillary growth and enhancing blood flow. Three growth factors are being studied in clinical trials: acidic fibroblast growth factor (aFGF), basic fibroblast growth factor (bFGF), and vascular endothelial growth factor (VEGF). The agents are delivered via intravascular catheter or intramuscular injection. Additional study is needed to determine the most effective agent and dosing (Hirsch et al., 2006).

Surgical Management

Arterial bypass is the surgical revascularization procedure performed for debilitating peripheral arterial disease. Surgery is done when a patient has disabling claudication and/or limb-threatening ischemia due to blocked arteries in the lower extremities. These reconstructive procedures are performed by a vascular surgeon and involve bypassing areas of occlusion with the patient's own vein (autogenous) or a synthetic graft. Numerous types of surgical procedures are available for the treatment of peripheral arterial disease, depending on the level of the disease within the aorta and distal leg arteries, and include aortoil-

iac bypass; aortobifemoral bypass; iliac endarterectomy, or iliofemoral bypass; femorofemoral bypass; and femoropopliteal bypass, the most commonly performed arterial bypass (Figures 43–5 through 43–9 ■, pp. 1330–1331). Following arterial bypass surgeries, frequent and careful assessment of circulation to the leg and foot is essential. Pulselessness distal to the graft site indicates decreased or no blood flow.

Amputation may be indicated for uncontrolled infection, uncontrolled pain, extensive tissue loss, and in cases in which adequate revascularization cannot be accomplished (Sieggreen & Kline, 2004a). Chapter 57 ∞ discusses amputation.

■ Nursing Management

Peripheral arterial disease (PAD) is a systemic process, and the majority of patients with PAD also have coronary artery disease (Oka, 2006). When assessing patients for PAD, the nurse needs to obtain subjective information from the patient about the

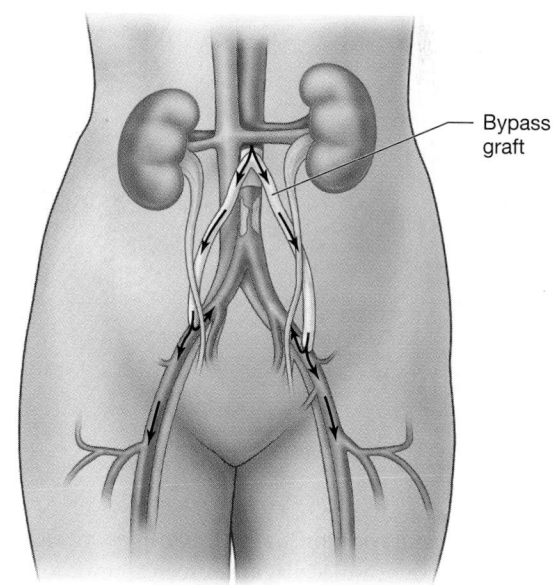

FIGURE 43–5 ■ Aortoiliac bypass.

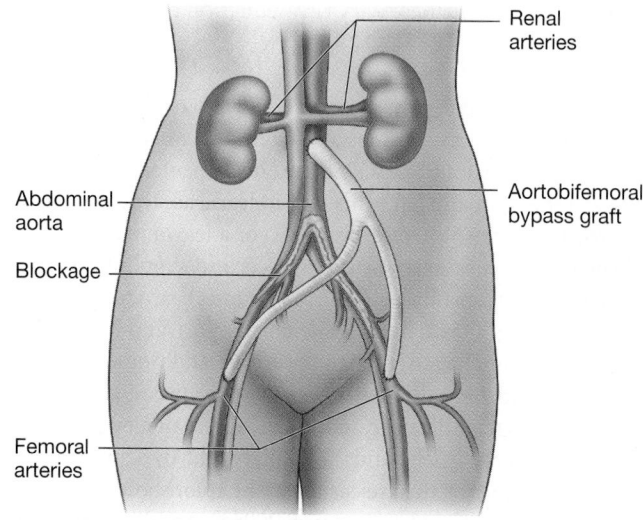

FIGURE 43–6 ■ Aortobifemoral bypass.

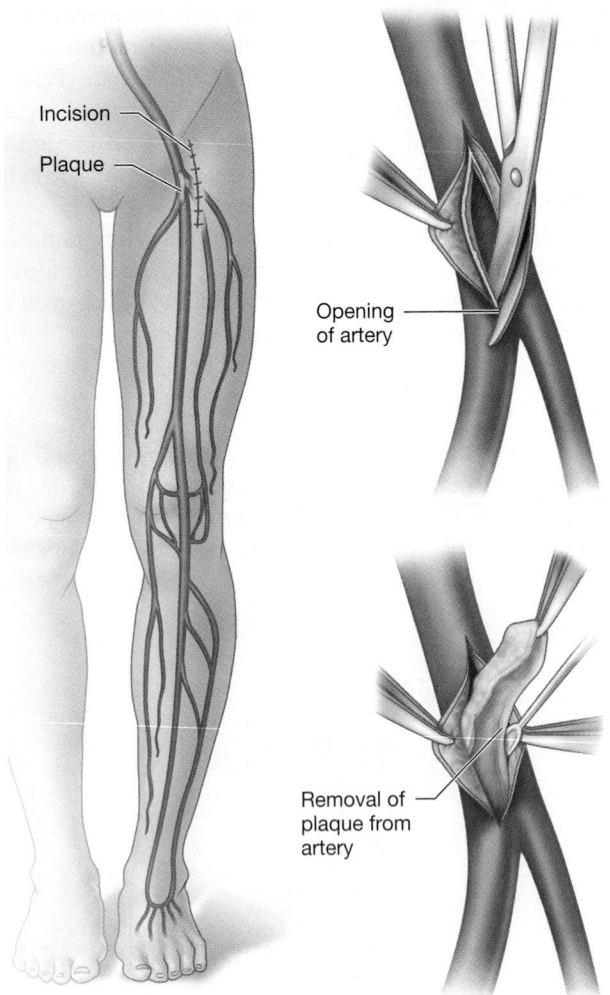

FIGURE 43–7 ■ Iliac endarterectomy.

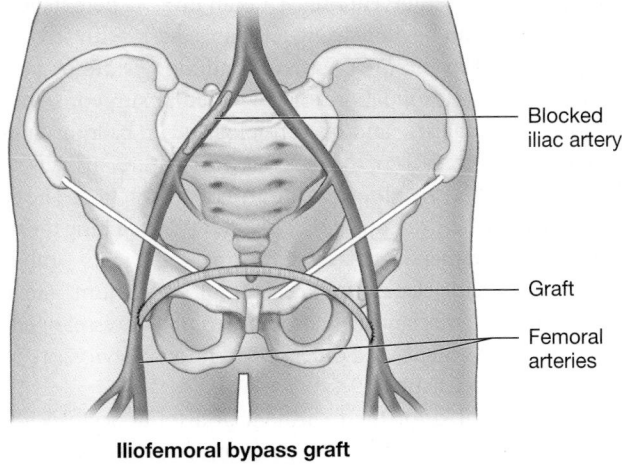

Iliofemoral bypass graft

(a)

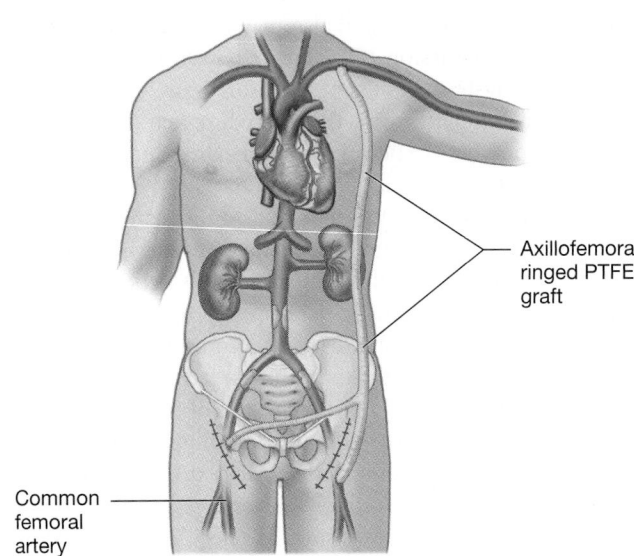

Axillofemoral bypass graft

(b)

FIGURE 43–8 ■ Femorofemoral bypass types: (A) iliofemoral bypass graft and (B) axillofemoral bypass graft.

present illness and symptoms, as well as the past medical history, especially previous cardiac diagnoses, such as myocardial infarction, hypertension, heart failure, and stroke. Obtaining information regarding the patient's history of smoking, hyperlipidemia, diabetes, family history, and activity level is important for planning necessary risk-reduction patient teaching.

Assessment

When assessing the patient for peripheral arterial disease, a thorough evaluation is essential. The measurement of bilateral blood pressure should be taken and documented. Differences between the right and left arms may indicate **aortic coarctation** (narrowing of the lumen of the aorta) or a lesion in a large vessel such as the subclavian artery. The carotid should be auscultated for vascular bruits, or abnormal sounds heard over areas of turbulent blood flow. The abdomen, flank area, and femoral arteries also should be auscultated for bruits. Additionally, the abdomen should be palpated to assess for signs of a pulsatile abdominal mass, indicating abdominal aortic aneurysm.

Assess fingers of each hand for capillary refill by depressing the nail until it blanches, then releasing it. The color should return to normal within 3 seconds (Sieggreen, 2005a). An Allen test (done to assess blood supply to the hand) should be performed to assess

for patency of the radial and ulnar arteries before the radial artery is cannulated for arterial blood gases or an arterial line insertion. To perform an Allen test, ask the patient to tightly clench her fist to produce blanching of the palm. While the fist is clenched, the nurse should occlude both the radial and the ulnar flow with his fingers or thumbs. While holding occlusive pressure, ask the patient to relax her fist and then release pressure over one of the arteries. Note the time it takes the palm to return to normal color. Repeat this while releasing pressure over the other artery. Failure of the color to return or a delay in return of color longer than 6 seconds is an abnormal finding that indicates narrowing or occlusion of the artery not being compressed. The Allen test also is discussed in Chapter 24 ☻.

Peripheral pulses are assessed in a systemic manner. Pulses—including the brachial, radial, femoral, popliteal, dorsalis pedis, and posterior tibial—are assessed for presence, rate, equality, regularity, and strength and are assessed and recorded as absent,

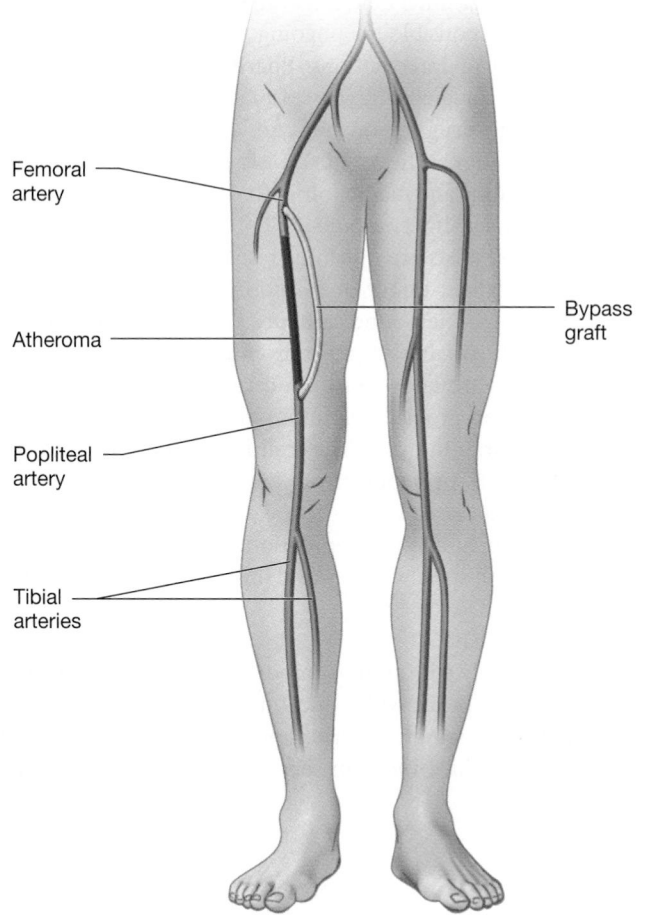

FIGURE 43–9 ■ Femoropopliteal bypass.

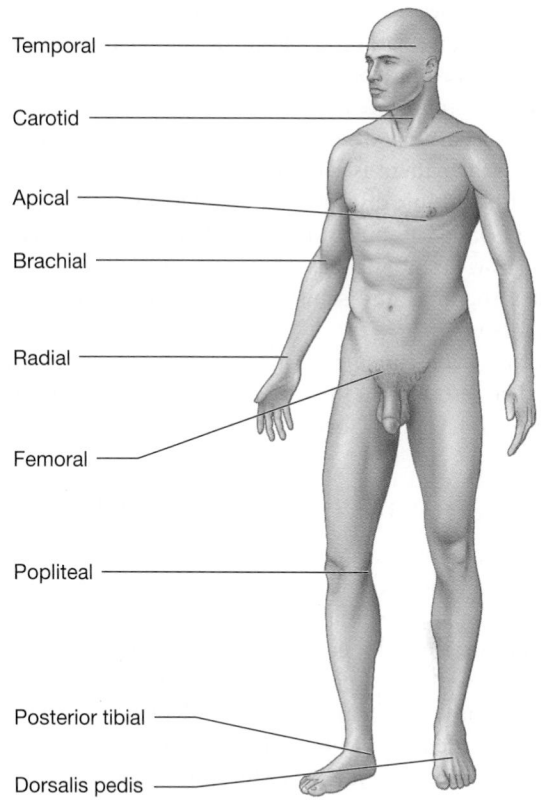

FIGURE 43–10 ■ Peripheral pulses.

diminished, normal, or bounding (Figure 43–10 ■). Occlusive arterial disease can impair blood flow and obliterate pulses in the affected extremity. Congenitally absent dorsalis pedis pulses occur in 10% of the population (Sieggreen, 2005a). Socks and shoes should be removed so that the feet can be inspected thoroughly. Note the color, temperature, and integrity of the skin, including any ulcerations. If ulcerations are present, ask the patient how long they have been there. Inspect the lower extremities for pallor, cyanosis, trophic changes—which include hair loss; thin, smooth, shiny skin; thick, brittle nails with or without fungal infection; tapering of toes or fingers—and any skin breakdown. Skin color should be examined carefully and with the patient in various positions. If arterial disease is present, pallor may be present when the legs are elevated. When patients hang their legs over the side of the exam table or bed, the legs become a deep red in color (dependent ruber) because blood is pooling in the arterioles. Hyperpigmentation of the skin is associated with venous, rather than arterial, disease. Additional physical findings may include decreased capillary refill, increased venous filling time, skin discoloration, decreased warmth, muscle or limb weakness with use, and poor healing. Pulse assessment is discussed in depth in Chapter 37 ⊙.

Nursing Diagnoses

Peripheral arterial disease results in decreased blood flow to the extremities causing tissue damage that can lead to ulceration, gangrene, infection, and amputation, causing disability and affecting quality of life. Many nursing diagnoses apply to these patients, including *Impaired Physical Mobility, Ineffective Tissue Perfusion, Impaired Skin Integrity, Readiness for Enhanced Comfort,* and *Deficient Knowledge.*

Interventions, Outcomes and Evaluation Parameters

Outcomes of nursing care of the patient with PAD include adequate vascular perfusion resulting in palpable pulses and warm extremities, sufficient tissue perfusion to promote healing of ulcers and reduce pain, and adequate knowledge of PAD so that the patient understands the disease process, how to manage her risk factors, and the current treatment plan.

It can be difficult to manage pain for some patients with PAD. The "six Ps" of arterial ischemia include the sudden onset of pain, pallor, pulselessness, poikilothermia (same as room temperature), paresthesia (sensation such as prickling, tingling, or numbness), and paralysis of the affected extremity. Patients with chronic pain may benefit from learning nonpharmacologic methods of pain control, such as intermittent rest periods while walking, guided imagery, and breathing exercises in addition to pharmacologic agents that may be prescribed.

Research has shown that regular structured exercise significantly improves the patient's functional capacity and is recommended as an initial treatment modality for patients with intermittent claudication. The most improvement was found when patients walked at least 30 minutes three times per week, walked until near maximal pain was reached, and continued this program for at least 6 months (Oka, 2006). Recruiting a walking partner or joining a group can facilitate compliance and increase consistency. For more on exercise as a way to help patients with PAD, see the Complementary and Alternative Therapies box.

Peripheral arterial disease is a lifelong disease. The more information the patient is provided, the better equipped he is to manage this chronic disorder. Be certain that the patient understands the basic pathophysiology of PAD, contributing risk factors and how best to manage them, prescribed medications and exercise programs, and signs and symptoms to report to his health care provider.

The applicable nursing diagnoses and nursing interventions are further described in the Nursing Process: Patient Care Plan for Peripheral Arterial Disease feature.

◼ Collaborative Management

A multidisciplinary team approach, including health care providers, advance practice nurses, such as nurse practitioners and/or clinical nurse specialists, staff nurses, pharmacists, physical therapists, wound specialists, and dietitians, is important in the management of the patient with peripheral arterial disease. Health care providers oversee the patient's plan of care by determining what medical or surgical therapies are needed, including diagnostic testing, surgical procedures, and pharmacologic and nonpharmacologic interventions. Nurses implement the plan of care and are responsible for ongoing monitoring, assessment, and evaluation of interventions. Pharmacists oversee the patient's pharmacologic profile, assessing for appropriateness of dosing, drug-to-drug interactions, and potential adverse reactions of medications. Physical therapists are essential in assisting patients in gaining and maintaining strength and mobility, especially after surgical interventions.

Wound specialists are a helpful resource for those patients who have sustained injury or infection and have wounds on their extremities. The wound care specialist assists with specialized treatments and dressings that promote healing. Whenever a patient has skin breakdown or wounds, a nutritional assessment by a dietitian can provide helpful insight into the patient's nutrition and hydration status. The dietitian can offer recommendations for foods or supplements that may promote healing. Patients with advanced PAD, who are dealing with pain, altered mobility, and/or potential amputation, may also benefit from interactions with social workers and hospital chaplains.

Health Promotion

Patient and family education is important in managing the patient with PAD. Begin with educating the patient and family about pathophysiology, intermittent claudication, and the mechanism by which the pain sensation occurs with walking,

COMPLEMENTARY & ALTERNATIVE THERAPIES — Exercise

Description:

An active exercise program can improve symptoms in patients with early peripheral vascular disease. A variety of exercises can improve peripheral vascular circulation, such as the use of treadmills, elliptical machines, plus walking and organized exercise classes.

Research Support:

While exercise rehabilitation has been effective, it is an underused therapy. Currently, however, exercise rehabilitation is the subject of several large research projects. Such projects are investigating mechanisms by which exercise therapy could benefit people with claudication and are also directly comparing exercise with other therapies (Regensteiner & Stewart, 2006).

One nonrandomized controlled study assessed the clinical and cost effectiveness of a supervised exercise program (SEP) in two groups of patients with intermittent claudication (IC). Thirty-seven patients (median age 69) received conservative medical therapy (CMT). Thirty-three patients (median age 67) received CMT plus a 3-month program of graduated physical exercise for 60 minutes, three times each week. Both groups of patients were assessed prior to and at 6 months following treatment. Patients were assessed using the SF36 questionnaire, which included walking distances (PRWD), treadmill claudication and maximal distances (ICD and MWD), ankle brachial pressure indices (ABPI) pre- and postexercise, and quality of life (QoL). Prior to intervention, the two groups reports on these areas were very similar. Following treatment, CMT patients demonstrated no significant change in PRWD or ICD; however, they did record a small but significant improvement in MWD. The exercise program patients demonstrated significant improvement in PRWD, ICD, and MWD. The researchers concluded that, compared to the conservative medical treatment group, the exercise program group increased walking distances, improved QoL, and was a highly cost-effective treatment for IC (Lee, Mehta, Ray, Heng, McCollum, & Chetter, 2006).

An effective treatment to improve walking capacity for individuals with peripheral arterial disease (PAD) is supervised treadmill-walking training. Another study examined the effect of a supervised treadmill-walking program on calf-muscle strength and endurance in individuals with PAD over the course of two stages. The first stage, a 12-week period, was a nonexercise, within-subject control stage. The second stage, a 12-week period, was an exercise training stage. Twenty-two subjects trained in the laboratory, 3 sessions per week for 12 weeks. Researchers measured walking capacity, calf-muscle strength and endurance, and peak oxygen uptake at the baseline and the end of each stage. The supervised treadmill-walking program significantly increased calf-muscle strength and endurance. There were also significant improvements in walking capacity and peak oxygen uptake following the training program. The results showed a significant correlation between the improved calf-muscle endurance and walking capacity (Wang, Zhou, Bronks, Graham, & Myers, 2006).

References

Lee, H. L., Mehta, T., Ray, B., Heng, M. S., McCollum, P. T., & Chetter, I. C. (2006, December 1). A non-randomised controlled trial of the clinical and cost effectiveness of a supervised exercise programme for claudication. *European Journal of Vascular and Endovascular Surgery,* Epub ahead of print.

Regensteiner, J. G., & Stewart, K. J. (2006). Established and evolving medical therapies for claudication in patients with peripheral arterial disease. *Nature Clinical Practice. Cardiovascular Medicine, 3*(11), 604–10.

Wang, J., Zhou, S., Bronks, R., Graham, J., & Myers, S. (2006). Effects of supervised treadmill-walking training on strength and endurance of the calf muscles of individuals with peripheral arterial disease. *Clinical Journal of Sport Medicine, 16*(5), 397–400.

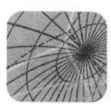

Assessment of Vascular Status

Subjective Data:

How far can you walk without stopping before you have pain?

Does leg discomfort or pain keep you from sleeping?

Does the pain wake you from your sleep?

Do you use an aid for walking such as a cane, walker, or wheelchair?

Do you need assistance to do your daily activities?

How many blocks (stairs) does it take to produce your pain?

Is the pain worse with elevation? Worse with cool temperatures?

Objective Data:

Peripheral pulses, temperature, and color of extremities.

Signs of ulceration, impaired healing, and trauma.

Walking distance.

Nursing Assessment and Diagnoses	Outcomes and Evaluation Parameters	Planning and Interventions with *Rationales*
Nursing Diagnosis: *Impaired Physical Mobility* related to disease and pain	**Outcome:** Adequate vascular perfusion. **Evaluation Parameters:** Palpable pulses. Warm extremities.	**Interventions and *Rationales:*** Teach patient importance of regular and structured ambulation *to enhance circulation and promote collateral development.* Teach patient importance of smoking cessation *to reduce the adverse vasospastic effects of nicotine.*

Assessment of Peripheral Vascular Perfusion and Skin Integrity

Subjective Data:

Do your extremities feel cold?

Do you have pain in your extremities?

Do you have any areas of sores or ulcerations?

Objective Data:

Assess extremities for perfusion: warmth, color, bilateral pulses, and edema.

Assess extent of wounds, if applicable.

Nursing Assessment and Diagnoses	Outcomes and Evaluation Parameters	Planning and Interventions with *Rationales*
Nursing Diagnoses: *Ineffective Peripheral Tissue Perfusion* and *Impaired Skin Integrity* related to diseased arteries	**Outcomes:** Sufficient tissue perfusion to perfuse extremities. Skin intact or ulcers healing. ***Evaluation Parameters:*** Warm extremities, palpable pulses, reduction in pain, and prevention of ulceration. No wounds or no signs of infection of the lower extremities. Demonstrates good foot care techniques. Eats well-balanced diet. Does not smoke or use smokeless tobacco.	**Interventions and *Rationales:*** Notify the heath care provider immediately if any of the six Ps of arterial ischemia occur abruptly: pain, pallor, pulselessness, poikilothermia (coldness), paresthesia, and paralysis of the affected extremity *to prevent tissue damage and loss.* Explain the importance of smoking cessation *to promote understanding and compliance.* Encourage patient to keep legs in dependent position *to enhance arterial perfusion.* Encourage patient to walk regularly and progressively *to promote conditioning and blood flow.* Teach patient risk factor modification *to prevent worsening of the atherosclerotic process.* Initiate wound care as directed *to promote healing and prevent infection and further tissue loss.* Teach patient to avoid trauma, heat, and sunburn to feet/legs *to prevent wounds and infection.* Teach patient about foot care: Keep feet and toes clean, mild soap only; dry well between toes; use lanolin emollient; inspect feet daily; clip toenails straight; wear proper fitting shoes; avoid walking barefoot. Avoid extremes in temperature to the extremities (hot baths, heating pads, cold water) *because sensation may be diminished.* Teach patient signs and symptoms of infection. Teach patient about good nutrition *to promote healing and prevent skin breakdown.* Smoking cessation counseling *to avoid detrimental effects of nicotine.*

Assessment of Discomfort

Subjective Data:

Do you have problems with pain when you are at rest?

Do you have problems with pain during activity, or when in a cold environment?

Where is the pain, what brings it on, and what makes it go away?

Is the pain getting worse?

Objective Data:

Use pain scale (0–10) to quantify pain.

Assess cultural and religious impact on patient's responses.

Assess the onset of increased pain to evaluate for disease progression or acute arterial obstruction.

(continued)

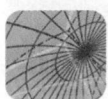

NURSING PROCESS: Patient Care Plan for Peripheral Arterial Disease—*Continued*

Nursing Assessment and Diagnoses	Outcomes and Evaluation Parameters	Planning and Interventions with *Rationales*
Nursing Diagnosis: *Readiness for Enhanced Comfort* related to tissue ischemia	**Outcome:** Comfort level maintained. **Evaluation Parameter:** Patient states adequate pain control has been obtained.	**Interventions and *Rationales:*** Assess pain so appropriate pain interventions can be initiated. Encourage periods of rest when walking *for pain relief.* Provide a supportive environment where patient is able to express pain level. Instruct patient to inform nurse if pain is not relieved. Use pain control measures before the pain becomes severe *to intervene early and with less medication.* Teach nonpharmacologic methods of pain control; that is, guided imagery and breathing exercises *to augment other treatments.*

Assessment of Knowledge of Self-Care Needs

Subjective Data:
How much do you smoke?
Are you willing to quit?
Has anyone explained your health problems to you?
How does this disease affect your daily life?
Are you able to care for yourself independently? If not, how much assistance do you need?

Objective Data:
Assess knowledge of disease process and progression, risk factors, and impact of smoking cessation.
Assess knowledge of patient's understanding of treatment plan, including medications and wound care, if indicated.
Assess needs for assistance.

Nursing Assessment and Diagnoses	Outcomes and Evaluation Parameters	Planning and Interventions with *Rationales*
Nursing Diagnosis: *Deficient Knowledge* of self-care needs and treatment plan related to tobacco use	**Outcome:** Adequate knowledge level. **Evaluation Parameters:** Patient/family are able to discuss disease process, risk factors, and current treatment plan. Verbalizes adherence to and compliance with treatment plan. Assistance is provided where deficiency exists. Patient/family verbalize understanding of disease, management, and prevention.	**Interventions and *Rationales:*** Provide factual information about diagnosis, treatment, risk factor modification, medications, and treatment plan *to ensure compliance.* Explain all procedures and allow patient to ask questions *to promote his understanding.* Provide information about care assistance *to ensure adequate help to provide a safe environment.*

and the important and ongoing need for risk factor modification. Compliance with the treatment plan is essential to help prevent the possible complications such as ulceration, gangrene, amputation, and myocardial infarction.

It is vital that the patient understand the risk factors that worsen PAD. Cigarette smoking is the single most important risk factor, and smoking cessation decreases the progression of PAD and improves the patient's functional status (Sieggreen, 2005a). Smoking cessation is fundamental because of the detrimental effects of tobacco on the arterial system. Endothelial function, lipoprotein metabolism, coagulation pathways, and platelet function are adversely affected by smoking tobacco. Smoking cessation decreases the risk of cardiovascular morbidity and mortality to levels that approach those who have never smoked. Abstinence from smoking as little as 8 weeks causes a gradual normalization of blood and plasma viscosity. Smoking cessation increases long-term survival in patients and decreases the amputation rate for patients with PAD (Cahall, 2004; Lu & Creager, 2004). The Agency for Healthcare Research and Quality (AHRQ, 2008) published "Treating Tobacco Use and Dependence," which is a set of evidence-based guidelines for treatment of nicotine dependence. The major steps of the AHCR guidelines to successful intervention are termed

the "five As": ask, advise, assess, assist, and arrange. Ask your patient if she smokes. If the patient is not a current smoker, ask about a past history of smoking or tobacco use. Advise her to quit in a clear, strong nonjudgmental manner. Assess her willingness to stop. Assist with counseling and pharmacotherapy. Arrange follow-up, preferably within the first week of quitting (Cahall, 2004).

Smokers trying to quit should receive pharmacotherapy and counseling. Approved medications for aiding smoking cessation include bupropion (Zyban), a nontricyclic antidepressant; nicotine replacement, available in gum, oral inhaler, nasal spray, and transdermal patch forms; and varenicline (Chantix), a drug that binds to nicotine receptors in the brain, blocking the full reinforcing effects of inhaled nicotine. Additionally, it slows the release of dopamine, which normally provides the feelings of pleasure from smoking. Nicotine replacement therapy is well tolerated and safe. The use of these agents doubles the rate of successful smoking cessation. Pharmacologic therapy alone is not enough; counseling also is needed. This can take the form of group meetings or individual behavioral therapy. Many hospitals and associations such as the American Lung Association and the American Heart Association offer ongoing group therapy for smoking cessation. For patients who are unwilling to quit, employ the five Rs: relevance of quitting, risks of smoking, rewards of quitting, roadblocks to quitting, and repetition. The Pharmacology Summary feature (p. 1337) outlines the pharmacologic agents that are used for smoking cessation.

For patients with diabetes, control of blood glucose is recommended. While there is no evidence that tight glycemic control (defined as a level of glycosylated hemoglobin < 7%) decreases intermittent claudication or critical limb ischemia, tight control of blood sugar levels has been demonstrated to decrease microvascular complications and the risk of myocardial infarction.

For PAD patients with hypertension, blood pressure control should be consistent with the evidence-based Seventh Report of the Joint National Committee on Prevention, Detection, Evaluation, and Treatment of High Blood Pressure (National Heart, Lung, and Blood Institute, 2004) recommendations of systolic blood pressure < 130 mmHg and diastolic blood pressure < 90 mmHg. Good blood pressure management has been found to decrease the risk of stroke, coronary artery disease, and mortality (Jacoby & Mohler, 2004). Chapter 21  discusses blood pressure guidelines and management.

Patients also need to be taught to avoid trauma, heat, and/or sunburn to their legs and feet to prevent the development of wounds and possible infection. Foot care information is essential for patients with PAD. The patient/caregivers need to be taught to keep feet and toes clean using mild soap. Thoroughly drying the feet and toes, and the use of a lanolin emollient regularly will help prevent skin breakdown. The feet need to be assessed daily for areas of potential pressure or breakdown. Toenails should be clipped straight across. Patients should not walk barefooted to avoid injury. Shoes should be properly fitted. Regular visits to a podiatrist may be beneficial for many patients with PAD.

Clinical trials have demonstrated the benefit of lipid lowering agents for patients who have PAD and coexisting cardiovascular and/or cerebrovascular disease (Gey, Lesho, & Manngold, 2004; Jacoby & Mohler, 2004; Rehring, Sandhoff, Stolepart, Merenich, & Whitton-Hollis, 2005). Normalizing lipid levels has been shown to reduce disease progression and the severity of intermittent claudication. According to the evidence-based National Cholesterol and Education Program III (2002 update), PAD patients should be managed the same as patients with coronary artery disease, whereby the primary goal is to lower the LDL-C levels to below 100 mg/dL. Coronary artery disease and dyslipidemia are discussed in Chapter 40 .

Complications

Acute arterial ischemia occurs when trauma, thrombosis, or embolism abruptly stops or greatly diminishes arterial flow. The most common cause is thromboembolism from the atrial appendage that occurs in patients with chronic atrial fibrillation, or from the left ventricle in the patient following acute myocardial infarction or chronic heart failure due to clot formation from stagnant blood.

> **CRITICAL ALERT** *Acute arterial ischemia is an emergency. Assessment findings in acute arterial ischemia include the "six Ps": pain, pallor, pulselessness, poikilothermia (coldness), paresthesia, and paralysis of the affected extremity.*

Immediate contrast angiography may be performed to determine the cause of the ischemia accurately. Management of the patient is dependent on the cause of the ischemia. If trauma, such as fractures or penetrating injuries, is the cause of the ischemia,

PHARMACOLOGY Summary of Medications to Treat Hypercholesterolemia

Medication Category	Action	Application/Indication	Nursing Responsibility
HMG-CoA reductase inhibitors (statins): Atorvastatin (Lipitor) Lovastatin (Mevacor) Simvastatin (Zocor) Pravastatin (Pravachol) Fluvastatin (Lescol) Rosuvastatin (Crestor)	Inhibits HMG-CoA reductase enzyme, thereby preventing the formation of cholesterol in the liver. Statins lower total cholesterol, LDL-C, and triglycerides while increasing HDL-C. Statins have also been connected with stabilizing *rupture-prone* atherosclerotic plaque (see the Etiology and Epidemiology of Carotid Artery Disease section later in this chapter), improving vasomotor tone, decreasing levels of proinflammatory proteins, decreasing factors that contribute to thrombosis, and improving myocardial perfusion.	Hypercholesterolemia.	Monitor liver function studies. Monitor lipid panel. Monitor patient for myalgias. Administer medication in the evening to take advantage of the fact that the liver produces more cholesterol at nighttime than during the day. Patients may experience abdominal discomfort from gas or constipation, which usually subsides with continued therapy. Rarely causes elevated liver enzymes and muscle soreness, pain, and weakness, which may require changes in dose or discontinuance of statin therapy. Monitor liver function tests (LFT).
Fibrates: Gemfibrozil (Lopid) Fenofibrate (TriCor)	Fibrates lower triglycerides and can increase HDL-C levels.	Hypercholesterolemia.	Monitor serum low density lipoprotein (LDL), very low density lipoprotein (VLDL), total cholesterol, and triglycerides. Monitor for gastrointestinal upset and bleeding. Assess for bloody stools, nosebleeds, cloudy or bloody urine, bleeding gums, and ecchymoses.

surgical repair is often required. Ischemia due to thrombosis or embolism is generally treated by immediate heparin therapy to stop the propagation of new clot and removal of the clot, either pharmacologically with catheter-based thrombolysis (streptokinase, urokinase, alteplase, reteplase) or mechanically with **embolectomy**, or mechanical removal of the clot.

Raynaud's Disease

Raynaud's disease (RD), first described in 1862, is an arterial vasospastic disorder caused by emotional distress or cold. The fingers and hands are most commonly affected, but the toes and feet also can be involved.

Etiology and Epidemiology

Individuals can have Raynaud's without any underlying disease associated with it, in which case it is called Raynaud's disease or primary Raynaud's. Or it can be part of another disease, in which case it may be referred to as Raynaud's phenomenon or secondary Raynaud's. Raynaud's disease is more prevalent in women and the typical onset is before age 30 (Mayo Clinic, 2006).

Pathophysiology

The precise pathophysiology of RD is unclear. It is caused by a transient spasm of the small cutaneous and subcutaneous arteries and arterioles, which results in a decreased blood flow to the affected extremity. Abnormalities of the endothelium may be responsible for initiating the vasospasm. RD is classified as primary or secondary. Primary or idiopathic RD has no known cause. Secondary RD is associated with many diseases, including connective tissue diseases, such as rheumatoid arthritis, scleroderma, and systemic lupus erythematosus (SLE), and myeloproliferative diseases, such as leukemia and polycythemia rubra vera. Occupational and environmental conditions are also associated with RD, particularly cold exposure, repetitive trauma, and vibration injury (chain saws, pneumatic drills).

Clinical Manifestations

The diagnosis of RD is made based on the patient's clinical manifestations. Usually during times of high stress/emotions or exposure to the cold, patients develop vasoconstriction of the arterial blood vessels causing cooling of the temperature of fingers, toes, and earlobes. As the temperature decreases, the skin color of the affected parts changes. There are three color changes that occur with RD (1) pallor (whiteness) in response to the vasospasms; (2) cyanosis (blue) due to the reduction of oxygenation of the blood; and (3) finally rubor (redness) when the vasospasms stop and the arterial blood returns (Reilly & Snyder, 2005). Other factors that may trigger ischemia include smoking, alcohol use, caffeine intake, cocaine, and amphetamines. The vascular changes also cause paresthesia to the affected parts. The episode ends when the arterial spasm relaxes and perfusion normalizes. Digits appear normal between attacks.

Diagnosis

A cold stimulation challenge may be administered to induce symptoms. The patient is exposed to cold temperatures by placing the hands in a basin of cold water. Patients with Raynaud's disease will quickly develop pallor and possibly cyanosis. When warmed, the patients experience redness and pain in their hands.

Nail-fold capillaroscopy can be performed to distinguish between primary and secondary Raynaud's disease (Reilly & Snyder, 2005). The nail bed is examined using a stereoscopic microscope or handheld ophthalmoscope to assess for the presence of enlarged, distorted, or deformed capillaries that may be associated with secondary RD.

Medical Management and Surgical Management

It is critical for the health care provider to obtain a complete history of the patient's past medical history to find out whether the patient has other connective tissue disorders, such as SLE and scleroderma. The signs and symptoms are vague: (1) malaise, (2) light sensitivity, (3) joint pain, and (4) skin lesions. Because the symptoms are vague, it is difficult to diagnosis. Treatment is based on signs and symptoms presented. Nonpharmacologic management of RD is directed toward avoiding known stressors (cold, emotional stress); controlling exposure to extremes in climate; dressing warmly in cold weather; and limiting tobacco, caffeine, and alcohol intake. Some patients may benefit from learning relaxation techniques. Regular physical exercise is important because it improves circulation and warms the body temperature. If pharmacologic treatment is needed to manage symptoms, the dihydropyridine calcium channel blocking agents, such as nifedipine, isradipine, amlodipine, and nicardipine, are used. Other agents that have been used to treat RD include prazosin (Minipress), fluoxetine, losartan, pentoxifylline, captopril, and topical nitroglycerin.

Surgical **sympathectomy**, removal of the sympathetic ganglia, has been performed for patients with severe symptoms of RD. It interrupts sympathetic nervous system stimulation to the affected vessels, decreasing vasoconstriction and spasm. Following this procedure, patients may experience relief of pain, decreased tissue loss, and improved wound healing. There is no cure for RD.

Complications

Complications of RD are not common. Digital ulcers may occur as a result of the disorder. Most digital ulcers will heal over several weeks to months with conservative therapy, provided the patient cares for his hands and/or feet carefully and seeks prompt treatment for signs and symptoms of infection. Surgery may be required when there is the threat of loss of a digit because of a nonhealing ulceration or gangrene.

Nursing Management

Careful history taking is important when assessing the patient with Raynaud's. Determine the patient's particular stressors and characteristics of attacks such as pain, numbness, color changes of the extremities, and frequency of attacks. The skin of the hands and toes should be assessed for the presence of ulcers and gangrene. Some medications, such as beta-adrenergic blockers, ergot alkaloids, and hormones, can precipitate episodes of vasospasm. It is important to obtain a detailed list of medications that the patient takes to assess for drug-induced vasospasm.

PHARMACOLOGY Summary of Medications for Smoking Cessation

Medication Category	Action	Application/Indication	Nursing Responsibility
Antidepressants Nontricyclic: Bupropion (Zyban, Wellbutrin)	Antidepressant neurochemical effect unknown.	Smoking cessation (off-label use for addiction to smokeless tobacco), depression.	Monitor for adverse effects: dry mouth, insomnia, sweating, blurred vision, weakness, vomiting, constipation, weight loss, or gain. Monitor for increased seizure potential if increasing dose, dose > 300 mg/day, or in presence of seizure disorder; head trauma history. Monitor for treatment-induced hypertension. Warn patient to avoid alcohol (increases seizure risk) and not to stop drug abruptly. Check hepatic and renal function for dose determination.
Tricyclic: Nortriptyline (Pamelor)	Antidepressant effect may be due to inhibition of norepinephrine reuptake.	Depression, smoking cessation (off-label use).	Monitor for adverse effects: orthostatic hypotension, urinary retention, constipation, confusion, or dry mouth. Monitor vital signs when initiating drug. Withhold and notify health care provider for systolic BP decrease is > 20mmHg or sudden increase in pulse. Be aware of drug interactions (alcohol, antihypertensives, hypnotics, and others). Monitor for adverse reactions. Contraindicated in patients during or within 14 days of treatment with monoamine oxidase inhibitor (MAOI).
Anxiolytic Alprazolam (Xanax)	Central nervous system (CNS) depressant effect may be due to limbic, thalamic, or hypothalamic action.	Anxiety disorders; short-term relief from anxiety symptoms.	Monitor for adverse effects: drowsiness, insomnia, and paradoxical excitement. Be aware of drug interactions (alcohol, CNS depressants, anticonvulsants, cimetidine, and others). Monitor for altered drug effect. Be aware drug should be reduced gradually when discontinued.
Smoking Deterrents Nicotine: Gum (Nicorette) Lozenge Transdermal patch (Habitrol, NicoDerm, Nicotrol) Nasal spray (Nicotrol NS) Vapor inhaler (Nicotrol inhaler)	Replaces nicotine.	Symptom reduction of nicotine-dependent smoker during cigarette withdrawal.	Monitor for adverse effects: headache, dizziness, and nausea. Monitor for route-specific adverse effects: gum: tongue, mouth, throat irritation; jaw pain; patch: skin irritation; nasal spray: nasal, throat irritation, or rhinorrhea. Be aware of drug interactions (theophylline, insulin, acetaminophen, and others). Monitor for decreased drug efficacy. Warn patient against smoking cigarettes or using smokeless tobacco while on replacement therapy.
Varenicline (Chantix)	Provides some nicotine effects through nicotine receptor agonist activity; blocks pleasurable effects of nicotine.	Nicotine withdrawal symptoms.	Monitor for adverse effects: nausea, diarrhea, anxiety, headache, sleep disturbance, arthralgia, and lethargy. Monitor for mood disturbances (depression, suicidal ideation).

Because the treatment of RD is supportive and there is no cure, patient and family teaching is very important to assist the patient in preventing and managing vasospastic episodes. It is important that patients clearly understand the disease process to avoid aggravating and alleviating events, such as cold environments and emotional stress. Smoking cessation counseling is essential. Patients may benefit from referrals for stress management class or relaxation techniques.

Health Promotion

Most patients have only mild to moderate symptoms and can manage sufficiently by avoiding exposure to cold and tobacco. Teach the patient to wear warm clothes and gloves, mittens, and/or hand warmers when required to be in cold environments. Exposure to cigarette smoke can cause symptoms. Patients with RD should avoid oral contraceptives, beta-adrenergic blockers, and ergot preparations because they have been known to exacerbate the symptoms of RD. Behavioral modification therapy may be helpful for some patients who have an emotional component to their RD.

Buerger's Disease (Thromboangiitis Obliterans)

Buerger's disease, or **thromboangiitis obliterans (TAO)**, is a nonatherosclerotic inflammatory vascular disease first described in 1879. It causes thrombus formation and occlusion bilaterally of the small vessels of the feet and hands. It is most common in young men who are heavy cigarette smokers.

Etiology and Epidemiology

The incidence of TAO has decreased overall in the last 50 years, but the incidence is increasing in women, most likely because of increased cigarette smoking among women (Arkkila, 2006). Although the cause of TAO is unknown, it is clearly associated with tobacco exposure.

Pathophysiology

In TAO, recurring inflammation of intermediate and small arteries and veins occurs predominantly in the lower extremities. This results in thrombus formation leading to occlusion of the vessels. Buerger's disease is thought to be an autoimmune disease. Immune assessment is discussed in Chapter 59 and immune disorders are discussed in Chapter 60.

Clinical Manifestations

Patients typically present with distal toe and/or finger ischemia and may have foot claudication. In advanced stages, ulcerations and gangrene of the fingers and toes may be present. Patients may also have superficial thrombophlebitis of the affected limb. Paresthesias of the feet and hands may also be present.

Diagnosis, Medical Management, and Surgical Management

There is no specific diagnostic testing for TAO, although an abnormal Allen test may be present. The diagnosis of TAO is based on clinical findings, and criteria for its diagnosis include smoking history, onset before age 50, ischemic ulcers, and pain. There is no cure for TAO. The primary treatment is directed toward smoking cessation and avoidance of secondhand smoke. Various medications are used, including steroids, antiplatelet agents, and anticoagulants, but there is no strong evidence of their effectiveness. Surgical revascularization is typically not feasible, although sympathectomy may be an option. Toe and finger ulceration, nonhealing wounds, and gangrene can occur, and amputation is required in up to 25% of patients (Arkkila, 2006). Chapter 67 discusses the incidence and care of ulcerations and non-healing wounds.

Complications

Complications of TAO include progressive ischemia and gangrene, leading to amputation. Infection of wounds can occur and patients can become septic. On rare occasion TAO also can affect other parts of the vasculature and cause occlusion of the cerebral, coronary, renal, splenic, or mesenteric arteries.

Nursing Management

Supportive nursing care of the patient with TAO is indicated. Smoking cessation counseling is essential for these patients, because continued smoking will keep the disease process progressing. Patients who continue smoking will likely require amputation. Nursing assessment of the patient with TAO is similar to that of the patient with peripheral arterial disease. The extremities should be closely assessed for abnormal findings such as pale or cyanotic skin, diminished or absent pulses, or skin ulcerations. Outcomes of care are directed toward improving circulation to the affected areas and to teach the patient to protect the limbs from injury and infection. Pain management and wound management may be indicated for patients with advanced stages of the disease. Pain management is discussed in detail in Chapter 15 and wound management in Chapter 67.

Health Promotion

Smoking cessation and the avoidance of all tobacco products, including chewing tobacco, are essential. Patient education is needed to teach the importance of avoiding injury to the feet and hands. Additionally, avoiding cold environments and medications that may cause vasoconstriction is required. If ulceration occurs, close monitoring for signs of infection is important to avoid subsequent gangrene and amputation. Skin assessment is discussed in Chapter 65 and wound management in Chapter 67.

Thoracic Outlet Syndrome

The thoracic outlet is a space between the thorax and the clavicle through which the main blood vessels and nerves pass from the neck and thorax into the arm. Thoracic outlet syndrome (TOS) is a rare disorder, more common in females, in which there is compression of the nerves and arteries of the arm in the thoracic outlet. It may be due to an extra first rib or an old fracture of the clavicle, which reduces the space of the outlet. Compression may occur with repetitive activities that require the arms to be held overhead.

Clinical manifestations include pain, paresthesias, muscular weakness and fatigue or swelling, and coldness in the arm and hand. The symptoms can be confused with those of other conditions, such as a herniated disk in the neck, carpal tunnel syndrome, and even bursitis of the shoulder.

The diagnosis of thoracic outlet syndrome is usually based on history and physical examination. Many patients will have history of an accident or trauma. To diagnose TOS, the elevated arm stress test (EAST) may be conducted. This is done by having the patient place both arms in 90 degrees of abduction and external rotation, then opening and closing her hands for 3 minutes. A positive EAST study is reproduction of symptoms (Chang, 2008). Other noninvasive testing that may be useful in diagnosing thoracic outlet syndrome includes cervical and chest x-ray to assess skeletal abnormality, color flow duplex scanning, MRI, and ulnar nerve conduction or electromyography. Invasive testing that may be performed includes an arteriogram and venography.

Treatment of TOS is initially directed toward nonsurgical interventions including physical therapy and pain management strategies. Physical therapy involves specific exercises aimed at strengthening the supporting muscles of the thoracic outlet structures. Muscle relaxants, nonsteroidal anti-inflammatory drugs such as aspirin or ibuprofen, moist heat, massage, analgesics, and short courses of steroids may be recommended. Surgical decompression of the thoracic outlet to remove the point of compression is indicated for patients with severe symptoms that limit their lifestyle.

Carotid Artery Disease

Stroke is a significant cause of death and disability in the United States and is the second leading cause of death worldwide. Stroke rates are higher for women and African Americans. Risk factors for stroke include hypertension, smoking, diabetes, atrial fibrillation, hyperlipidemia, physical inactivity, obesity, and illicit drugs, such as cocaine (American Stroke Association, 2006).

Etiology and Epidemiology

Stroke occurs when there is a sudden cessation of blood flow to an area of the brain resulting in cell death and loss of function to the involved area of the brain. The right and the left carotid and vertebral arteries supply blood to the brain.

Pathophysiology

The most common cause of stroke is atherosclerosis. The atherosclerotic process has previously been described in this chapter and in Chapter 40 ⊘. The bifurcation of the carotid artery and its branches is a common site for vascular turbulence and atherosclerotic plaque buildup, causing an obstruction to blood flow. When these plaques rupture, thrombosis can occur, causing altered blood flow to the area. This process can cause small thrombic clots to form, embolize, and occlude the carotid artery or branches of the carotid artery causing stroke.

Clinical Manifestations

A stroke may be preceded by a **transient ischemic attack (TIA)**. A TIA is a "warning stroke" or "mini-stroke" that produces stroke-like symptoms but no lasting damage. It occurs when the blood supply to part of the brain is briefly interrupted. Symptoms include numbness or weakness in the face, arm, or leg, especially on one side of the body; confusion or difficulty in talking or understanding speech; trouble seeing in one or both eyes; and difficulty with walking, dizziness, or loss of balance and coordination, which usually disappear within 1 to 5 minutes (American Stroke Association, 2006).

Neurological deficits associated with a stroke are dependent on where the damage to the brain has occurred. The clinical manifestations may include the abrupt onset of severe headache, confusion, transient monocular blindness, blindness, changes in speech such as slurring of words, and mono- or hemiparesis. Chapter 30 ⊘ provides a complete description of the pathophysiology, clinical manifestations, and treatment of stroke.

Diagnosis

Carotid artery disease may initially be found on physical exam when a bruit is auscultated over the artery. Patients who are experiencing clinical manifestations of carotid artery disease are typically referred for noninvasive testing with duplex ultrasound. Patients who are found on ultrasound to have significant lesions and are symptomatic may be further referred for invasive studies. Magnetic resonance imaging and/or computed tomography angiography (CTA) are replacing contrast angiography, once the gold standard for defining anatomy.

Medical Management

Medical therapy for patients with carotid disease includes antiplatelet therapy with aspirin. Endovascular therapy for carotid disease may be an option for patients who are not otherwise surgical candidates. It is a controversial procedure that requires skilled operators and careful patient selection. Carotid artery balloon angioplasty and stenting can be performed in the neurointerventional radiology laboratory or the cardiac catheterization laboratory. Using local anesthesia and minimal sedation, a balloon or stent is placed percutaneously across the lesion in the carotid artery to restore flow. Various cerebral protection devices have been developed and are being used to filter embolic particles that can break off during angioplasty or stent placement to decrease the risk of complications.

Surgical Management

Standard treatment for symptomatic carotid disease is **carotid endarterectomy (CEA)**, a surgical repair of carotid artery disease, which has been performed in this country since 1953. It is a commonly performed procedure done to prevent stroke in which atherosclerotic plaque and fatty deposits are removed from the carotid artery to restore blood flow to the brain. Operative stroke-death mortality has been reported to be 2.3% up to 7.4% for high-risk patients with severe coronary artery disease, chronic obstructive lung disease, and renal disease (Sullivan, 2005). Complications of CEA include perioperative stroke, blood pressure instability, cranial nerve injury, infection, restenosis, and death. Hyperperfusion syndrome, a rare complication of CEA, may occur in patients with bilateral carotid stenosis; it is the occurrence of ipsilateral temporal or frontal throbbing headache with or without nausea, vomiting, ipsilateral focal seizures, or focal neurological deficit without evidence of cerebral infarction (Abou-Chebl et al.,

2006). Contraindications to carotid endarterectomy surgery include acute hemorrhagic or major stroke, anatomy not accessible to the surgeon, and other technically challenging patients, such as those who have had prior radical neck dissection, radiation therapy, or severe cervical arthritis (LaMuraglia & Nigri, 2004).

■ Nursing Management

Following carotid endarterectomy, patients are monitored in various inpatient settings including neurological observation units, step-down units, or intensive care units.

Assessment

Beginning with assessment, the nursing process guides the care for the postoperative patient. In the immediate postoperative period, frequent cardiovascular and neurological assessments are done to monitor for complications such as carotid artery occlusion, cerebral embolization, or cranial nerve damage as well as incision site assessment and donor site assessment, if a venous graft was used. Frequent neurological assessment is aimed at assessing for cerebral ischemia, which may be evidenced by agitation, lethargy, visual disturbances, slurred speech, and paresthesias or paralysis. Nursing assessment includes facial symmetry, ability to swallow, tongue deviation, and shoulder strength to evaluate cranial nerve function.

Careful assessment of the patient's mental status, level of consciousness, pupillary responses, and motor/sensory function is needed to assess for perioperative stroke. In the event of stroke, motor and sensory changes would be noted on the contralateral side of the body. CEA may also interfere with cranial nerve function, which can be temporary or permanent. To assess for cranial nerve damage, observe for difficulty with speech, dysphagia, and upper airway obstruction, which may indicate hypoglossal nerve damage. Monitor facial muscles to assess the facial nerve. Ask the patient to shrug his shoulders and raise his arms to assess the accessory nerves. Loss of gag reflex and hoarseness may indicate damage to the vagus nerve or the recurrent laryngeal nerve. Nursing intervention includes notifying the health care provider promptly of changes in neurological status.

Nursing Diagnoses

The nursing diagnoses related to the postoperative carotid endarterectomy patient include:

- *Tissue Perfusion, Ineffective, Peripheral*
- *Risk for Infection*
- *Gas Exchange, Impaired.*

Interventions, Outcomes, and Evaluation Parameters

Careful monitoring for respiratory obstruction from edema or expanding hematoma at the surgical site is essential. If respiratory distress develops in the postoperative phase, nursing interventions include elevating the head of the bed, loosening the neck dressing if it appears to be constricting the neck, and administering oxygen as ordered. Stridor or deviation of the trachea from midline indicates an impending respiratory emergency and immediate intervention is required. Notification of the health care provider is done while suction supplies and equipment and a tracheostomy tray are being assembled. Outcomes of care include prevention of respiratory distress due to edema, and evaluation parameters include normal oxygen saturation levels, arterial blood gases, and no increased work of breathing.

Close monitoring of blood pressure is required in the early postoperative phase. Hypotension can occur because of stimulation of the carotid sinus during surgery. Hypertension can lead to bleeding or damage the arterial reconstruction.

Following CEA, patients are maintained on daily aspirin. The Patient Teaching & Discharge Priorities box provides discharge priorities for patients following carotid artery procedures. Nursing management of the stroke patient is discussed in detail in Chapter 30 ⚬.

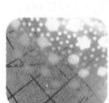

PATIENT TEACHING & DISCHARGE PRIORITIES for Carotid Artery Procedures

Need	Teaching

Knowledge of disease process	Home care needs include verbal and written instructions for:
	  Treatment plan, including wound care
	  Continued risk factor modification
	  Follow-up care
	  Activity instruction.

Understanding of medications	Teach the purpose, dose, and possible adverse effects of all medications to increase compliance and prevent over/underdosing.

Reportable clinical manifestations	Instruct patient/family to report:
	  Signs and symptoms of stroke, including sudden onset severe headache, visual disturbances or visual loss, weakness or paralysis of arms and/or legs
	  New onset fever, signs of wound infection.

Family/support system	Assess availability of, knowledge of, and compliance with treatment plan. Assess respite needs and resources. Assess discharge placement needs: home, skilled nursing care, rehabilitation facility, extended care facility. Assess for need for professional home health needs. Assess need for follow-up appointments.

Health Promotion

Patient teaching includes the importance of continuing daily aspirin, adequate blood pressure control, and risk factor modification. Patients and their families need to be instructed about reportable signs and symptoms, which include unilateral headache, neurological deficits, and seizure activity.

 ## Subclavian Steal Syndrome

Subclavian steal syndrome is a form of a transient ischemic attack (Chapter 30 ☿) that is caused by an obstruction of an extracranial artery that impairs blood flow to the vertebrobasilar arterial system. If the subclavian artery is occluded near its origin, the flow of blood in the vertebral artery is diverted or stolen from the basilar artery in the brain and shunted into the brachial circulation. Subclavian steal syndrome also can occur in the patient following coronary artery bypass grafting when a **stenosis**, or narrowing in the subclavian artery, is not corrected prior to use of the internal mammary artery as a bypass, causing the patient to have recurrent angina.

Clinical manifestations include complaints of dizziness, syncope, and vertigo due to the decreased circulation of the posterior cerebral circulation. Arm claudication also may occur. A difference in blood pressure between the right and left arm is found. It would be reduced on the same side as the subclavian stenosis. Blood pressure difference greater than 20 mmHg suggests subclavian stenosis. A carotid bruit may be audible as well.

Repair of the subclavian stenosis may be required for the symptomatic patient. Balloon angioplasty and stenting or carotid-subclavian bypass and axilloaxillary bypass may be done, depending on the patient's anatomy and surgical risk (Eisenhauer & Shaw, 2004).

Renovascular Disease

Renovascular diseases are disorders of the arteries of the kidneys, which result in systemic hypertension and kidney dysfunction.

Etiology and Epidemiology

Two disorders primarily affect the renal arteries: atherosclerotic renal artery stenosis (AS-RAS) and fibromuscular dysplasia (FMD). FMD is more common in girls and women between the ages of 15 and 50 and frequently involves the main renal artery and its branches (American Urological Association [AUA], 2002; Porth, 2007).

Atherosclerosis accounts for approximately 70% to 90% of renovascular disease (AUA, 2002). It is the cause of 1% to 2% of all cases of hypertension, making it the most common cause of secondary hypertension (Porth, 2007). The prevalence of AS-RAS increases with age, particularly in patients with diabetes, aortoiliac occlusive disease, coronary artery disease, or hypertension. However, many cases are never detected because hypertension or kidney failure does not develop (AUA, 2002). Hypertension is discussed in detail in Chapter 21 ☿ .

Pathophysiology

Patients with AS-RAS have progressive abnormal narrowing of the renal artery that occurs in 51% of the cases within 5 years after the initial diagnosis has been made. Anywhere from 3% to

16% of the arteries eventually become totally blocked, and shrinkage of the kidney occurs in approximately 20% of patients. The resulting hypertension is caused by reduced renal blood flow and activation of the renin-angiotensin-aldosterone mechanism. The diminished blood flow to the kidney causes a release of excessive amounts of renin, which increases the circulating levels of angiotensin II. Angiotensin II vasoconstricts the peripheral vessels and acts as a stimulus to increase aldosterone levels and sodium retention. The result of all of these changes is systemic hypertension. One or both kidneys may be affected (Porth, 2007). The renin-angiotensin-aldosterone system is discussed in detail in Chapter 21 ☿ .

Fibromuscular dysplasia is a noninflammatory, nonatherosclerotic disease that also can affect the renal arteries, which causes alterations in the intimal and/or medial layer leading to obstruction of blood flow and accounts for 10% to 25% of renovascular disease. This disorder is seen almost exclusively in women (Caulfield, Fernando, & Rosenfield, 2005; Porth, 2005). Unlike AS-RAS, FMD rarely leads to total renal artery blockage. The cause of FMD is unknown; a genetic predisposition, smoking, hormonal factors, and disorders of the blood supply to the renal artery itself are some of the causal theories associated with the disease.

Clinical Manifestations

Patients with renovascular disease present with significantly elevated blood pressure that is difficult to control, although it is not readily distinguishable from other forms of hypertension. Certain classic features such as lack of family history of hypertension, recent onset of hypertension, or onset of hypertension before age 50 are more suggestive of renovascular hypertension than of other forms of high blood pressure. It is frequently higher than 180/100 mmHg and may be resistant to two or more medications.

Diagnosis

The goal of diagnostic studies is to assess perfusion to the kidneys and the renin-angiotensin-aldosterone system. Duplex ultrasonography is recommended as the screening test to establish the presence of renal artery stenosis. CTA and magnetic resonance angiography (MRA) may also be used as screening tests. Contrast angiography may be performed to assess the renal-arterial vasculature. Angiographic findings of fibromuscular dysplasia demonstrate a very characteristic "string of beads" appearance in the lumen of the artery (Dickinson, Krishnan, Houlihan, & Walker, 2004).

Medical and Surgical Management

Medical therapy of atherosclerotic renal artery disease is directed toward careful blood pressure control, antiplatelet therapy, lipid management, smoking cessation, and weight reduction. Angiotensin-converting enzyme (ACE) inhibitors may be indicated in the presence of renal stenosis (Porth, 2007).

Endovascular therapy may be an option for select patients. Patients with fibromuscular dysplasia have good outcomes with renal angioplasty, obtaining improvements or cure in over 90% of patients. Percutaneous ballooning and stenting of renal artery atherosclerotic lesions have success rates of near 100% when performed by an experienced health care provider (Dickinson et al., 2004). Complications of renal artery angioplasty and stenting may include cholesterol embolization, vessel rupture, renal infarction, temporary deterioration in renal function, retroperitoneal hemorrhage, and access site vascular complications such as bleeding and hematoma (Dickinson et al., 2004).

Surgical management for renovascular disease is limited to those patients who present with severe hypertension in spite of maximal medical therapy and ischemic nephropathy. Procedures that may be performed include aortorenal bypass, the most common surgery performed for patients with renovascular disease, and renal artery thromboendarterectomy or renal artery reimplantation.

Health Promotion and Complications

Patients need to be instructed on the importance of regular and continuing medical follow-up. Close monitoring of blood pressure is required. Changes to the antihypertensive medication regime will likely be needed following stenting or surgical repair. Patients must be monitored for progression of renovascular disease and decline in renal function. Complications of untreated renovascular disease can include severely elevated blood pressure, stroke, renal insufficiency and failure, heart failure, retinopathy, and death.

■ Nursing Management

Caring for the patient who has undergone renal artery stenting is similar to the care of the patient who has undergone other types of peripheral angioplasty. Monitoring of blood pressure and urinary output is essential. Because renal stenting is performed by percutaneous arterial access, careful monitoring of the access site is needed, along with regular assessment of distal pulses. Follow-up laboratory testing of blood urea nitrogen (BUN) and creatinine levels is important to assess renal function.

Patients who have undergone surgical treatment of their renovascular disease, such as reconstruction of the renal arteries or aortorenal bypass, may require intensive care monitoring for several hours postoperatively. Postoperative monitoring includes frequent and ongoing assessment of the blood pressure. The remainder of postoperative nursing management is discussed in Chapter 27 ☺.

■ Aortic Aneurysm

An **aneurysm** is a diseased segment of an artery that becomes thin and dilated because of degenerative changes in the tunica media layer.

Etiology and Epidemiology

Arterial aneurysms can occur throughout the body. Aortic aneurysms can be saccular (extending over only part of the vessel circumference), projecting from one side of the aorta only, or fusiform (involving the entire circumference), which is symmetrical involvement of the aorta. The prevalence of aortic aneurysm in the United States varies with advancing age, family history, male gender, and tobacco use. The condition is more common in men, especially between ages 50 and 70. The incidence increases with age and develops more frequently in smokers. Additionally,

aortic aneurysms tend to have familial tendencies. The most common causes of aortic aneurysms are atherosclerosis and degeneration of the vessel media (Porth, 2005).

Pathophysiology

Aortic aneurysms can occur anywhere in the aorta, although the majority of them occur below the level of the renal arteries (infrarenal). These are referred to as abdominal aortic aneurysms (AAA). Thoracic aneurysms account for only 10% of the occurrences. The pathogenesis of an aortic aneurysm is not well understood. It is a localized area of the aorta that is weakened because of decreased elastin in the medial layer, loss of medial smooth muscle cells with thinning of the vessel wall. Inflammatory changes may also play a part. Causes include congenital weakness, trauma, and disease. Once the aneurysm is initiated, it will grow larger as the tension on the vessel wall increases. The pressure may increase to the point that it is putting pressure on the adjacent organs and interrupting blood flow. If a growing aneurysm is left untreated, it may rupture due to the increased tension (Porth, 2007).

Clinical Manifestations

The clinical manifestations of an aortic aneurysm depend on its size and location. Aneurysms of the thoracic area present with substernal, back, and neck pain. These patients also may have dyspnea, stridor, and brassy cough due to pressure on the trachea. If the laryngeal nerve is compressed, hoarseness may occur (Porth, 2007). Abdominal aortic aneurysms are typically asymptomatic. Frequently, an unknown aortic aneurysm is discovered during abdominal imaging performed for some other reason or during routine physical exam. Visual inspection may reveal a pulsatile abdominal mass near the umbilicus in the lean patient. Auscultation of this mass reveals a bruit (Chapter 37 ☺), caused by the turbulent flow in the widened area of the aorta.

Diagnosis

Diagnostic testing performed for aortic aneurysms includes abdominal ultrasound, CT scan, abdominal angiography, and MR angiography. The aortic aneurysm is followed by serial diagnostic tests to evaluate growth and impedance of surrounding organs. To be considered an AAA, the size must exceed 3 centimeters in diameter.

Medical Management

Medical management of the stable AAA includes ongoing surveillance with abdominal ultrasound performed every 6 months to assess the amount of aneurysmal growth, as well as smoking cessation, optimal blood pressure control, monitoring, and controlling fasting lipid values and discontinuance of steroids, if possible.

Endovascular stent graft covered with a thin layer of Dacron may be an option for some patients with an AAA. In endovascular repair of an AAA, the graft is placed into the aorta via access from the femoral artery. This procedure is performed in the operating room or in the cardiac catheterization laboratory using general, regional, or local anesthesia with sedation. Several endovascular stent graft systems are currently available (Figure 43–11 ■). Advantages for the patient include no long abdominal incisions, faster recovery time, and shorter length of stay. This ap-

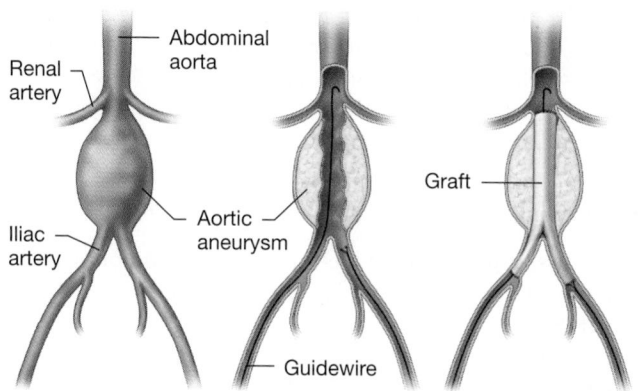

FIGURE 43–11 ■ Endovascular stent graft.

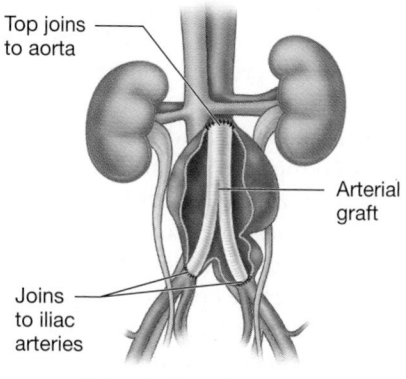

**Abdominal aortic aneurysm
surgical repair**

FIGURE 43–12 ■ Repair of abdominal aneurysm.

proach may be an option for the patient at very high risk for open-heart surgery because of extensive comorbidities, such as cardiac and or pulmonary disease. Complications of endovascular stent graft repair of an AAA include **endoleaks** (continued leaking of blood into the aneurysmal sac), arterial trauma, occlusion of the renal or hypogastric arteries, renal impairment due to contrast administration, device migration, structural failure, and/or infection. The long-term durability of these stent grafts is not known; lifelong follow-up is needed for these patients. The early mortality rate for endograft repair generally has been less than 3% (Hirsch, Haskal, Hertzer, Bakal, Creager, Halperin, et. al., 2006).

Surgical Management

Options for treating AAA are open surgical repair and endovascular repair. Surgical intervention for AAA has been performed for over 50 years. Patients with infrarenal AAAs measuring 5.5 centimeters or larger should undergo repair to eliminate the risk of rupture (Hirsch, Haskal, Hertzer, Bakal, Creager, Halperin, et. al., 2006). Elective AAA repair is a major surgical procedure with mortality rates reported between 2% and 6% and postoperative complication rates up to 32.4%. Cardiac complications are most common (Fleming, Whitlock, Beil, & Lederle, 2005). The perioperative administration of beta-adrenergic blockers, if not contraindicated, reduces the risk of adverse cardiac events and mortality in patients with coronary artery disease undergoing repair of atherosclerotic aortic aneurysms (Hirsch, Haskal, Hertzer, Bakal, Creager, Halperin, et. al., 2006).

The surgical approach is dependent on the location of the aneurysm, but the traditional approach is a midline or transverse incision with retroperitoneal dissection of the aneurysm. The aneurysm is resected, or removed, and replaced with Dacron graft material. The aneurysm wall is usually left in place to cover the Dacron graft. Aneurysms that extend above the renal arteries and into the thoracic aorta are more difficult to repair. If the ascending aorta is involved, cardiopulmonary bypass is required. Chapter 40 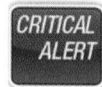 discusses cardiopulmonary bypass surgery. Figure 43–12 ■ shows the repair approach for AAA.

Immediate surgical repair is indicated for the patient who presents with expanding aneurysm or rupture. The mortality rate for emergency surgery for ruptured AAA is as high as 40% (Upchurch & Schaub, 2006).

Complications that can occur following open AAA repair include hemodynamic instability due to postoperative bleeding, hypothermia, myocardial ischemia and/or infarction, hypoxia due to atelectasis, fluid and electrolyte disturbances due to renal insufficiency, massive transfusions, inadequate hydration, ileus and abdominal distention due to ischemia or surgical manipulation of the bowel, and spinal cord ischemia due to interrupted blood flow during cross-clamping.

Complications

Complications that can occur from AAA include rupture, thrombosis, and embolization. The risk of rupture is related to the size of the aneurysm and is very high if the aneurysm is larger than 5.5 centimeters. Factors that can increase the risk of rupture include hypertension, smoking, and family history of ruptured AAAs. Embolization from the aneurysm can decrease perfusion to the lower extremities and is referred to as "blue toe syndrome." This syndrome, caused by emboli, is an indication for surgical repair of the AAA.

■ Nursing Management

Careful in-depth nursing assessment is essential for the patient undergoing surgical or endovascular repair of an abdominal aortic aneurysm. Prior to repair, the nurse needs to monitor the patient closely for signs and symptoms of impending rupture: restlessness, abdominal pain and tenderness, hypotension, and shock. Any of these symptoms should be reported immediately to the health care provider and the patient should be prepared for emergent surgery.

CRITICAL ALERT *The unstable patient who has experienced rupture of an abdominal aortic aneurysm (AAA) requires immediate fluid and blood resuscitation, blood pressure control with propranolol (Inderal) or nitroprusside (Nipride), and pain management while being prepared for emergency surgery.*

The nursing process guides the postoperative care of the patient immediately following the open AAA surgery. Nursing diagnoses that pertain to these patients include *Tissue Perfusion, Ineffective* related to the surgical procedure; *Decreased Cardiac Output,* and *Risk for Deficient Volume; Gas Exchange, Ineffective* related to anesthesia, possible fluid overload, and blood transfusions; *Readiness for Enhanced Comfort* related to surgical pain, immobility, and fear and anxiety; *Risk for Infection* related to the surgery; and *Deficient Knowledge* of postoperative care and discharge needs.

The postoperative patient is typically monitored in the intensive care setting for 6 to 24 hours. Priority nursing interventions include blood pressure and hemodynamic support, aggressive pulmonary toilet, and prevention and early detection of surgical complications. Hemodynamic instability can occur in the immediate postoperative phase, and patients are generally monitored invasively using an arterial line and central venous catheter and/or pulmonary artery catheter. Frequent and careful assessment of pulses and neurological function in the lower extremities is essential because normal blood flow may have been interrupted during surgery. Urine output also must be monitored closely if the aneurysm occurred above the renal arteries.

Postoperative complications can be caused by bleeding, hypovolemia, and third spacing of fluid, myocardial ischemia/infarction, hypertension, and hypothermia. Vasoactive drugs may be required in the immediate postoperative phase to support and control the blood pressure and other hemodynamic parameters. Patients are placed on bedside ECG monitors to assess cardiac dysfunction and the presence of dysrhythmias. The nurse should compare the postoperative cardiac rhythm to the preoperative ECG to assess for new changes that may indicate myocardial ischemia or infarction, such as ST segment depression or elevation. Hypothermia causes an increase in the systemic vascular resistance. Patients should be rewarmed 1 degree per hour until the core body temperature exceeds 36°C. Rewarming can be accomplished by using forced warm air blankets, administering warmed IV fluids/blood, warming the inspired ventilator air, and covering the patient's head with warm blankets.

Patients who have undergone open AAA repair require frequent assessment of their pulmonary status, including signs of poor oxygenation and ventilation as evidenced by abnormal arterial blood gases, cyanosis, sluggish capillary refill, use of accessory muscles to breathe, nasal flaring, and decreased level of consciousness. Regular assessment of the patient's airway is essential. Adequate pain management, frequent repositioning, and the regular use of incentive spirometry are essential to promote oxygenation and ventilation and prevent atelectasis.

Impaired renal function can occur due to decreased blood flow to the kidneys during surgery and with episodes of hypotension and hypovolemia. Monitor the urine output, BUN, and serum creatinine closely. Gastrointestinal disturbances can occur postoperatively because of ischemia and/or manipulation of the bowel during surgery. Assess for nausea, vomiting, abdominal pain/tenderness, distention, presence/absence of bowel sounds, blood in stools, and diarrhea. Spinal cord ischemia can occur because of an interruption of blood supply during cross-clamping of the aorta and cause sensory and motor deficits.

Health Promotion

Prior to surgery, patients should be taught the importance of blood pressure control and compliance with their medication regime. Risk factor reduction is important. Patients should be counseled to stop smoking. Following surgery, risk factor modification teaching is reinforced. Additionally, patients are taught wound care, activity restrictions, medication regime, and reportable symptoms, such as changes in sensation to the legs, which may indicate thrombosis of the graft, or gastrointestinal bleeding, which may indicate erosion of the graft into the duodenum.

 Spontaneous rupture of an aortic aneurysm causes sudden onset of abdominal and back pain accompanied by signs of hypotension, shock, and collapse. Once the aortic aneurysm ruptures, many patients die before arriving at a hospital for care.

■ Aortic Dissection

Aortic dissection (AD) is a life-threatening condition whereby the intimal layer of the aorta separates, creating a tear in the lumen of the aorta.

Etiology and Epidemiology

Blood flows into this space, referred to as a "false lumen," and diminishes the blood supply distal to the area of dissection. A dissection can occur anywhere in the aorta, although two-thirds of the dissections occur in the ascending aorta (Porth, 2005). As the dissection increases in size, pressure is placed on the surrounding organs, which may impact organ function. Risks for the development of AD include hypertension, degeneration of the medial layer of the vessel wall, trauma, Marfan's syndrome, and iatrogenic (treatment-induced) dissection caused by catheter-based interventions and aortic clamping during surgery. It occurs most frequently in those ages 40 to 60 and is more prevalent in males (Porth, 2007).

Pathophysiology

The exact cause of AD is unknown. Chronic stress from hypertension may play a significant role in the deterioration of the aortic wall. An aortic dissection begins with a tear in the intima, which allows blood to enter the aortic wall, stripping the intima from the adventitia of the aorta. Aortic dissection is classified according to its location. Dissection that involves the ascending aorta, which is the most common, is classified as Stanford type A or DeBakey type I. This type requires immediate surgical repair. Dissections that involve only the descending aorta are classified as Stanford type B or DeBakey type III. They do not generally require immediate surgery and are stabilized medically.

Clinical Manifestations

Most patients with AD present with sudden, sharp, shifting chest or back pain that can mimic acute myocardial infarction, pulmonary embolus, or ruptured AAA. The patient may describe it as "ripping" or "tearing." The pain is not affected by position changes and it may wax and wane. These patients also may have syncope or altered level of consciousness. About 25% of patients with AD present with signs of ischemia from blood flow obliterated by the dissection, such as stroke, anuria, and mesenteric and/or extremity ischemia that occurs because of the altered blood flow to the brain, kidneys, gut, and legs.

 *Rapid identification of aortic dissection is key in preventing death. Signs and symptoms of aortic dissection (AD) can mimic other disorders such as acute myocardial infarction and pulmonary embolus, making the diagnosis difficult. The most classic symptom of AD is the abrupt onset of severe, tearing chest pain that may radiate to the back. Patients may also present with sudden onset aortic insufficiency, neurological changes, and cardiac tamponade.*

Diagnosis

The diagnosis of aortic dissection begins with taking the patient's history and doing a physical examination. An assessment of risk factors is essential. Because aortic dissection is a life-threatening situation, prompt and careful assessment of the clinical manifestations also is essential. Diagnostic tests that will assist with the diagnosis include aortic angiography, transesophageal echocardiography, CT scan, and MRI studies. The Diagnostic Tests box outlines the diagnostic tests used to evaluate AD.

Medical Management

Medical therapy is recommended for type B dissections or those that are in the descending aorta, although surgery may be required when there is poor blood pressure control, inadequate pain relief, and/or progression of the dissection. Control of hypertension is essential for the patient with AD. Aggressive control of blood pressure is managed using beta-adrenergic blockers such as esmolol (Brevibloc), labetalol (Normodyne, Trandate), propranolol (Inderal), metoprolol (Lopressor), and nitroglycerine or nitroprusside (Nipride).

Endovascular repair of AD may also be an option for select patients. Because these procedures are less invasive, the patients have a shorter recovery period and a shorter length of stay. Complications, such as endoleaks, are similar to those seen in endovascular repair of AAA. Endovascular procedures are typically done with local anesthesia and procedural sedation.

Surgical Management

Surgical intervention is indicated for type A dissections, which are those that involve the ascending aorta when the patient develops ischemic complications and/or when medical management fails. If the proximal aorta is involved, the aortic valve may need to be replaced and the coronary arteries may need to be reimplanted. Surgical complications may include myocardial ischemia or infarction, arrhythmias, pulmonary atelectasis, renal failure, ischemic bowel, prolonged ileus, and leg ischemia.

Complications

The disruption of the aorta can cause life-threatening complications or death if not rapidly recognized and treated. Abnormal blood flow into the false lumen of the aorta results in occlusion of the branches of the aorta. If the dissection occurs proximally in the aorta, there is risk of shearing of the aortic valve and the coronary arteries, causing serious complications including myocardial infarction, acute aortic insufficiency, and pericardial tamponade. If the dissection moves distally in the aorta, there is risk of damage to the arteries that supply the kidneys, spine, abdomen, and legs.

■ Nursing Management

The nursing management of the patient following open AD repair is complex and very similar to the nursing management of

DIAGNOSTIC TESTS for Aortic Dissection

Test	Expected Abnormality	Rationale for Abnormality
ECG	May have ST segment changes if coronary arteries are affected in ascending aortic dissection.	Easily performed. Provides rapid information about coronary ischemia.
Chest x-ray	Widened mediastinum may be seen.	Easily performed. Not diagnostic.
TEE	Detects cardiac tamponade, involvement of coronary arteries, and damage to aortic valve.	Relatively easy to perform. Requires sedation.
CT scan	Quickly confirms location and extent of dissection.	Noninvasive. Requires contrast administration. Requires x-ray exposure. Expensive. Requires skilled interpretation. Less readily available. Provides no information about aortic valve involvement.
Angiography	Visualization of true and false lumen possible. Identification of coronary artery anatomy.	Invasive. Requires vascular access. Requires contrast administration. Requires x-ray exposure. Accurate diagnosis. Requires skilled interpretation.
MRI/MRA	Shows intimal tear, type and extent of dissection, and involvement of aortic valve.	Noninvasive. Does not require vascular access. Does not require contrast administration. Expensive. Requires skilled interpretation. Not widely available. May be difficult for claustrophobic patients.

the patient who has had open AAA repair. Patients spend the first 1 to 2 days in the intensive care unit for careful monitoring. Goals of therapy are directed toward airway and blood pressure management, and pain control. Care of the postoperative patient is discussed in detail in Chapter 27 ☺.

Health Promotion

Patients must be instructed to control their blood pressure carefully for the rest of their lives. Compliance with their medication regime is essential.

■ Venous Disorders

Venous disease is more likely to affect the lower extremities. The patient may experience intermittent swelling, tightness, and discomfort in one or both lower extremities due to a venous disorder. Unilateral extremity swelling may be associated with **deep venous thrombosis (DVT)**. Bilateral or diffuse edema may indicate that the patient has heart failure, valvular venous incompetence, or **lymphedema**, which is swelling due to obstruction of the lymphatic system.

The venous system of the lower extremities has two components: the superficial and the deep systems. Perforating of communicating veins transports blood from the skin and subcutaneous tissues from the superficial system to the deeper venous channels where it is then transported to the heart. The veins contain valves, which prevent retrograde flow, thereby maintaining normal flow of blood back to the heart. Muscle

function also assists in moving the blood back to the heart. There are more venous valves located in the lower legs than in the upper legs. Loss of valve function causes venous insufficiency, and venous hypertension can occur.

■ Varicose Veins

Varicose veins are dilated, tortuous veins that occur in the lower extremities as a result of the incompetence of valves of the deep and superficial venous system leading to valve reflux.

Etiology and Epidemiology

Risk factors for the development of varicose veins include older age, family history, female gender, occupations that requires standing, obesity, and history of phlebitis or clot. Other potential risk factors include constipation/low-fiber diet, smoking, hypertension, and injury. Pregnancy is likely a contributing factor for the increased incidence in females (Beebe-Dimmer, Pfeifer, Engle, & Schottenfeld, 2004). Varicose veins are subcutaneous veins that remain dilated when the patient is standing or sitting. Figure 43–13 ■ shows a normal venous structure and a varicose venous structure. In the general population, the incidence of varicose veins is between 5% and 30%, with a higher incidence in females (Eberhardt & Raffetto, 2005).

Clinical Manifestations

Some patients may have no symptoms whereas other patients experience sensations of heaviness, tiredness, itching, burning,

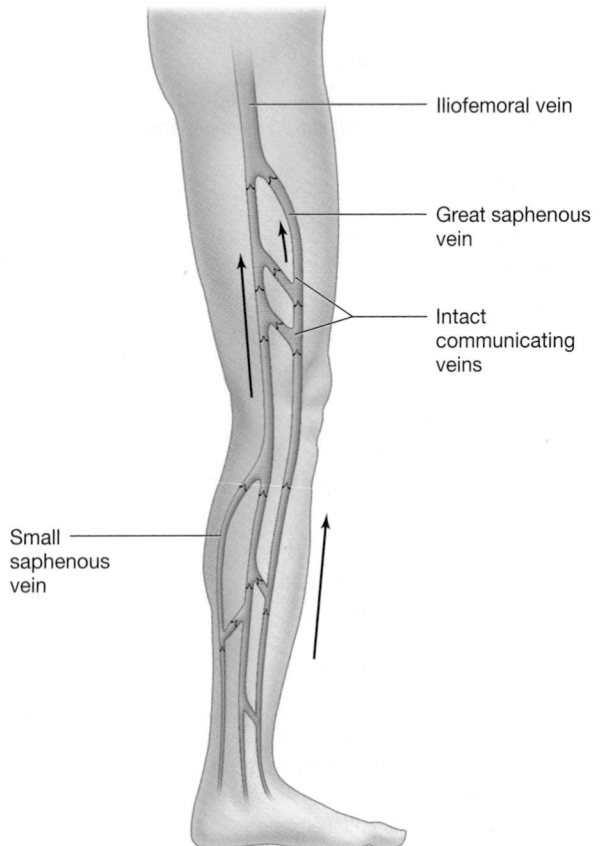

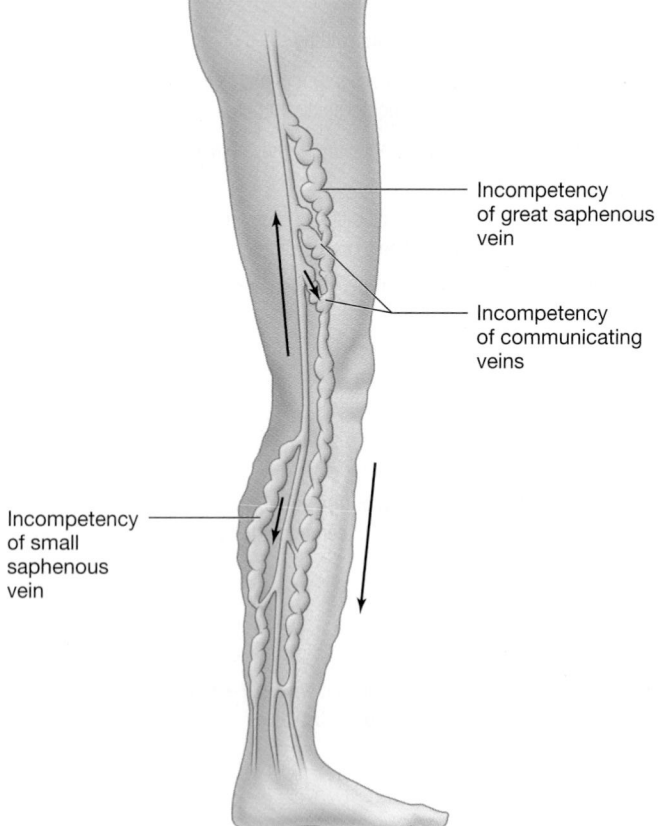

(a)   **(b)**

FIGURE 43–13 ■ (A) normal venous structure and (B) varicose veins.

or aching in their leg(s). Symptoms may intensify by the end of the day, especially after standing for long periods of time. Varicose veins may be prominent during pregnancy or menstruation.

Diagnosis, Medical Management, and Surgical Management

Diagnosis is made by physical examination and the patient's report of clinical manifestations. A frequent site of varicose veins is the greater saphenous vein. Doppler ultrasound may be used to assess blood flow in the large vessels, and angiography is used to assess valve function. Treatment may be required for patients with extensive varicose veins or those who are severely symptomatic. Interventional therapy, or nonsurgical alternatives to treatment for varicose veins, such as sclerotherapy, is performed less frequently because of the high incidence of reoccurrence. In sclerotherapy, generally reserved for small varicose veins and spider veins, the vein is injected with an irritating chemical, causing fibrosis and occluding the vessel lumen, which results in reduction of the varicose vein.

Surgical therapy for varicose veins may include ligation, stripping, laser therapy, or radiofrequency ablation of the vein, usually the saphenous vein (Teruya & Ballard, 2004). This is performed in the outpatient setting and the patient's recovery is generally a few days to 3 weeks at the most. Following venous sclerotherapy or surgery, patients must wear compression stockings to help prevent further varicosities. Complications of surgical repair of varicose veins may include hemorrhage, thrombophlebitis, edema, and infection.

Complications

Complications of untreated varicose veins can include increased risk of DVT and chronic venous insufficiency (CVI) leading to hyperpigmentation and ulceration of the feet and legs. This can increase the patient's susceptibility to injury and infection.

Nursing Management

Repair of varicose veins is generally scheduled as outpatient surgery, in either a hospital or a surgical clinic. Bed rest is suggested for the first 24 hours, with the foot of the bed elevated; then the patient is encouraged to walk short distances every 2 hours. Compression stockings are usually worn for several days following surgery. Surgical incisions should be inspected daily for signs of infection such as redness, tenderness, warmth, and drainage.

Patients should avoid showering or bathing the legs the first 24 hours and should avoid the use of lotions and creams on the legs until the incisions are fully healed.

Health Promotion

Prior to discharge, the patient should be taught to avoid activities that cause venous pooling, such as sitting for long periods of time and standing in one position for long periods of time. The nurse needs to explain the proper method for applying and wearing compression stockings. The patient should be encouraged to develop a walking program and to lose weight, if needed.

Venous Thromboembolism

Venous thromboembolism (VTE) consists of two conditions: deep venous thrombosis and pulmonary embolism (Tapson, 2005).

Etiology and Epidemiology

VTE is a common cardiovascular disorder affecting over 2 million in the United States each year, and an estimated 200,000 deaths in this country alone result from VTE (AHA, 2007). **Virchow's triad**—venous stasis, damage of the endothelium, and hypercoagulability—first described in 1846, remains the theory behind the thrombus formation of VTE. Multiple risk factors for the development of VTE are outlined in the Risk Factors box. **Pulmonary embolism (PE)** in this context is defined as the presence of a thrombus or blood clots in the pulmonary vessels, which obstructs blood flow and impedes gas exchange. The diagnosis and treatment of PE is discussed in detail in Chapter 36 .

Deep Venous Thrombosis

A deep venous thrombosis is defined as a clot that forms in the deep veins, usually those of the lower extremities and pelvis, although these clots can also occur in the upper extremities. Factors that contribute to the development of DVT include venous stasis, hypercoagulability, immobility, and thrombus formations. Figure 43–14 ■ (p. 1348) shows common locations for DVT occurrence. Risk factors for DVT are outlined in the Risk Factors for Venous Thromboembolism box.

Most hospitalized patients are at risk of developing DVT due to immobility, making risk assessment and prophylaxis extremely important. Medical and general surgery patients have a 10% to 40% risk of developing DVT during hospitalization, whereas orthopedic surgery patient have a 40% to 60% risk

---

RISK FACTORS for Venous Thromboembolism (VTE)

- Major abdominal, thoracic, gynecologic, and/or urologic surgeries
- Major orthopedic surgeries such as total hip or total knee procedures
- Spinal cord injuries; paresis
- Fracture of the pelvis, hip, or long bones
- Multiple trauma; burns
- Malignancy
- Myocardial infarction, heart failure, respiratory failure, sepsis, ulcerative colitis
- Intensive care unit admission

- Previous DVT/ Pulmonary embolism (PE)
- Age > 40 years
- Obesity
- Prolonged immobility of 3 days or more
- Varicose veins
- Pregnancy/postpartum
- Oral contraceptive use
- Acquired and inherited disorders of coagulation
- Presence of central venous catheters

Sources: Geerts, W. H., Pineo, G. F., Heit, J. A., Bergqvist, D., Lassen, M. R., Colwell, C. W., et al. (2004). Prevention of venous thromboembolism: The seventh ACCP conference on antithrombotic and thrombolytic therapy. *Chest, 126,* 338S–400S.

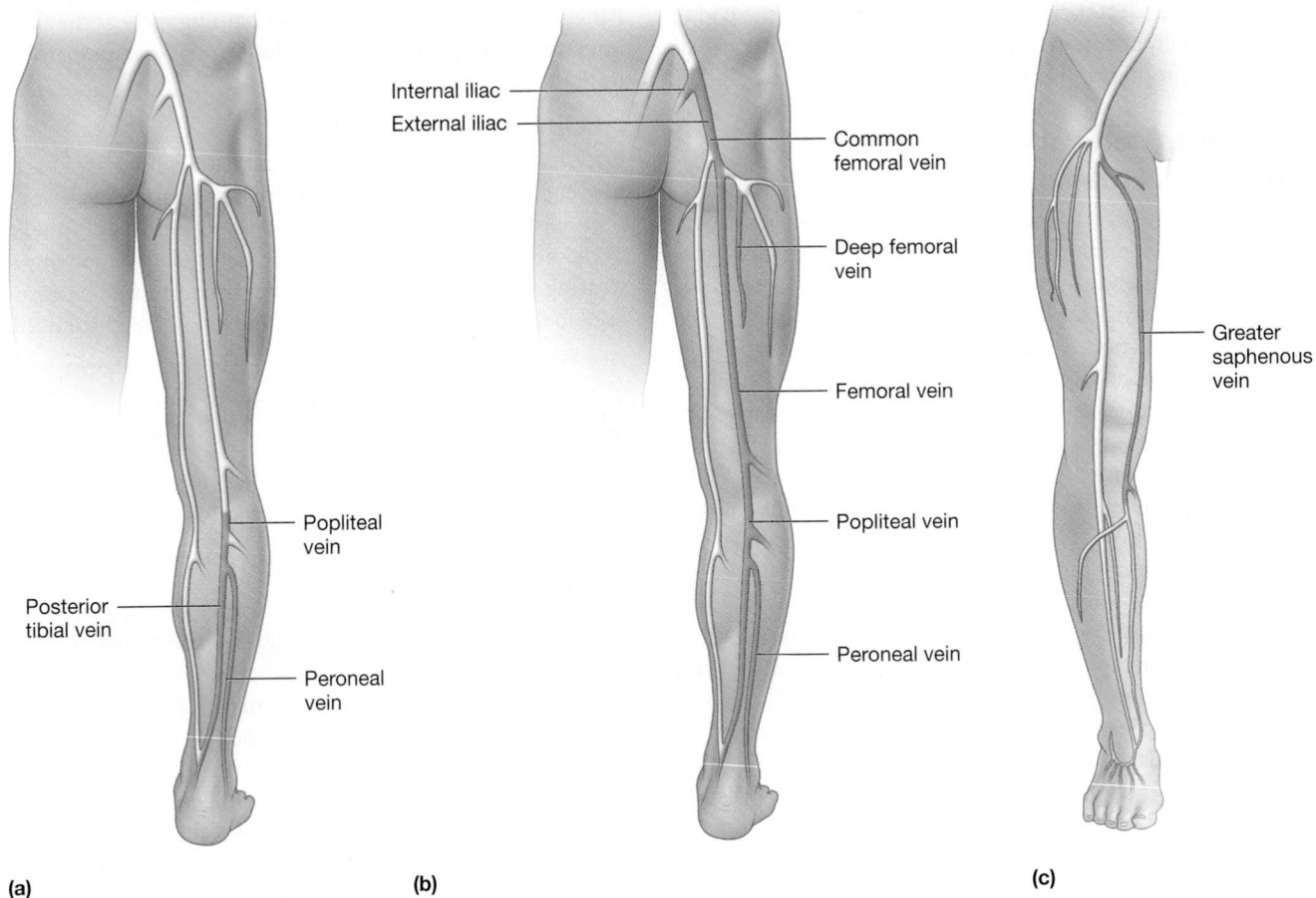

Internal iliac
External iliac
Common femoral vein
Deep femoral vein
Femoral vein
Popliteal vein
Peroneal vein
Popliteal vein
Posterior tibial vein
Peroneal vein
Greater saphenous vein

(a)   (b)   (c)

FIGURE 43–14 ■ Common locations of venous thrombosis.

MyNursingKit Animation: Drugs: Peripheral Vascular Drugs—Anticoagulant: Warfarin

(Kehl-Pruett, 2006). In 2004, the American College of Chest Physicians published its Seventh ACCP Conference on Antithrombotic and Thrombolytic Therapy guidelines (Hirsh et al., 2004) providing recommendations for DVT prophylaxis and treatment in medical and surgical patients. Despite these detailed guidelines, many hospitalized patients are not receiving adequate treatment to prevent DVT (Kehl-Pruett, 2006).

Clinical Manifestations

Signs and symptoms of DVT are variable, and the presence of a DVT may not be known until the patient develops a PE. Most DVTs begin in the deep veins of the calf. Some patients have no discomfort, whereas others may complain of unilateral extremity discomfort and pain, edema, warmth, tenderness, and redness. A palpable vein cord may be present. Homans' sign, or pain in the calf when the foot is dorsiflexed, is not a reliable indicator of DVT (Walsh & Rice, 2004).

Diagnosis, Medical Management, and Surgical Management

A number of diagnostic tests assist in identifying the presence and location of DVT. These tests are outlined in the Diagnostic Tests for Deep Venous Thrombosis box (p. 1350).

Pharmacological agents that can be added to the DVT prophylaxis regime include anticoagulants, such as intravenous or subcutaneous unfractionated heparin, subcutaneous low molecular weight heparin, intravenous or subcutaneous direct thrombin inhibitors, and oral warfarin. Aspirin has not been demonstrated to be effective in preventing DVT and is not recommended (Geerts

et al., 2004). According to the Seventh ACCP Conference on Antithrombotic and Thrombolytic Therapy guidelines (Hirsh et al., 2004), strict bed rest for confirmed DVT is not needed and patients may ambulate as tolerated. Additional interventions for confirmed DVT include extremity elevation 10 to 20 degrees above the level of the heart, local application of moist heat, avoidance of massaging affected extremity to prevent clot from breaking loose, and compression stockings. Anticoagulation with short-term intravenous or subcutaneous unfractionated heparin or subcutaneous low molecular weight heparin followed by long-term warfarin therapy for 3 to 6 months is initiated. The goal for the international normalized ratio (INR) is 2 to 3 (Rectenwald & Wakefield, 2005). Treatment regimes for DVT can be done in the outpatient setting as well as for the hospitalized patient. The Pharmacology Summary box outlines the pharmacologic treatment of VTE/DVT. The Evidence-Based Practice feature (p. 1356) discusses medications that prevent DVTs.

Some patients may require surgical intervention to prevent PE from occurring. Procedures include venous thrombectomy and interruption of the vena cava. Thrombectomy is not commonly performed. Vena cava interruption is done percutaneously by placement of an inferior vena cava filter device that captures thrombi, yet allows blood to flow through it. (Figure 43–15 ■, p. 1351). This is indicated for patients who have a contraindication to anticoagulation for DVT prophylaxis and treatment, such as the trauma patient or patients who have failed therapy by developing a clot while on anticoagulation (Marr, 2006). Complications of filter placement are rare. Trapped clots can eventually lead to venous

PHARMACOLOGY Summary of Medications to Treat Peripheral Vascular Disease

Medication Category	Action	Application/Indication	Nursing Responsibility
Anticoagulants			
Unfractionated heparin	Prevents clot formation by inhibiting thrombin, preventing the conversion of fibrinogen to fibrin.	Prevention of clot formation and extension in venous thrombosis and pulmonary embolism; prevention of postoperative DVT; treatment of DIC; maintenance of venous access device patency.	Monitor for adverse effects: bleeding, thrombocytopenia. Monitor aPTT, blood count, platelet count. Assess for presence of beef or pork allergy, history of heparin-induced thrombocytopenia (HIT), or active bleeding (contraindicated in these patients). Be aware of drug interactions (cephalosporins, penicillins, nitroglycerin (NTG), salicylate). Monitor for increased risk of bleeding. Preferred over low molecular weight heparin (LMWH) in presence of renal failure.
Low molecular weight heparin (LMWH): Enoxaparin (Lovenox) Dalteparin (Fragmin) Tinzaparin (Innohep)		Treatment of pulmonary embolism, DVT; prevention of venous thromboembolism.	Monitor for adverse effects: bleeding. Monitor for increased risk of bleeding in presence of reduced creatinine clearance. Contraindicated in patients who have or will receive epidural or spinal anesthesia or puncture.
Warfarin (Coumadin)	Inhibits hepatic synthesis of the vitamin K–dependent coagulation factors II, VII, IX, and X.	Long-term prophylaxis for thrombus formation; e.g., mitral valve replacement, atrial fibrillation, hypercoagulability disorders.	Monitor for adverse effects: bleeding, nausea, vomiting, and diarrhea. Monitor international normalized ratio (INR) and/or prothrombin time (PT). Be aware of multiple drug and food interactions (green leafy vegetables, alcohol, NSAIDs, acetaminophen, phenytoin, barbiturates, and many others). Assess current drug regime prior to initiating warfarin.
Antiplatelet Drugs			
Aspirin (acetylsalicylic acid, ASA)	Inhibits platelet aggregation.	Prevention of recurrent thromboembolism in MI, stroke; reduces progressive arterial obstruction in peripheral arterial disease (PAD).	Monitor for adverse effects: dyspepsia, nausea, heartburn, abdominal pain, gastrointestinal bleeding. Monitor for signs of toxicity (tinnitus, altered hearing). Increase blood sugar monitoring in presence of diabetes. Give with food. Warn patient to avoid alcohol and other drugs containing salicylates.
Clopidogrel (Plavix) Ticlopidine[a] (Ticlid) Cilostazol[b] (Pletal)	Inhibits adenosine diphosphate (ADP)-induced platelet aggregation. Promotes vasodilation.	Prevention of atherosclerotic event (e.g., myocardial infarction (MI), stroke, vascular death); intermittent claudication; may improve arterial ulcer healing.	Monitor for adverse effects: bleeding, abdominal pain, diarrhea, nausea, and headache. Monitor blood count, bleeding time, platelet function. Check neutrophil count if infection develops. Be aware of drug interactions (NSAIDs, diltiazem, vitamin A, anticoagulants, and others). Monitor for altered drug efficacy. Give with food.
Hemorheologic Drugs			
Pentoxifylline (Trental)	Prevents thrombus formation by decreasing blood viscosity; improves microcirculation by decreasing platelet aggregation.	Intermittent claudication.	Monitor for adverse effects: dyspepsia, nausea, vomiting, tremors, dizziness, and headache. Monitor for toxicity in presence of impaired renal function. Be aware of drug interactions (cimetidine, insulin, and theophylline). Monitor for drug toxicity or reduced efficacy. Give with food.

[a]Monitor for hematologic adverse reactions: agranulocytosis, aplastic anemia, thrombotic thrombocytopenic purpura.

[b]Warn patient to avoid grapefruit and grapefruit juice.

DIAGNOSTIC TESTS for Deep Venous Thrombosis

Test	Expected Abnormality	Rationale for Abnormality
Duplex ultrasound	Location and extent of clot or noncompressibility of the vein. Can identify floating, or unstable clot. May be difficult to perform in obese patient.	Most common diagnostic testing for deep venous thrombosis (DVT). 90% sensitive in the setting of symptomatic DVT. Noninvasive. Readily available; portable. Operator dependent.
Venography (also called phlebography)	Defines location and extent of the clot, which is seen as a filling defect. Identifies collateral circulation, if present.	Provides most accurate diagnosis of presence, location, and extent of clot. Invasive. Requires contrast administration. Costly. Risk of procedure induced thrombophlebitis. Invasive. Requires vascular access. Requires contrast administration. Requires x-ray exposure. Accurate diagnosis. Requires skilled interpretation.
CT scan	Useful to evaluate possible pelvic or abdominal thrombus. Useful for obese patients.	Noninvasive. Requires contrast administration. Requires x-ray exposure. Expensive. Requires skilled interpretation. Less readily available. May equal ultrasound in accuracy.
MRI	Useful for suspected iliac vein or inferior vena caval thrombosis.	Noninvasive. Sensitive for both acute and chronic DVT. Does not require vascular access. Does not require contrast administration. Expensive. Requires skilled interpretation. Not widely available. May be difficult for claustrophobic patients.
D-dimer	Elevated in DVT/PE due to release of degradation products released into the circulation when fibrin undergoes fibrinolysis.	Used to rule out the disorder, not confirm. A positive D-dimer test indicates that a DVT or pulmonary embolism (PE) is possible. Not diagnostic for DVT/PE, because the D-dimer is also elevated with recent surgery, trauma, and inflammation or any condition where clots may form.
Venous duplex imaging	Provides anatomic extent of venous disease. Detects DVT or venous obstruction. Provides information about valve function.	Noninvasive. Widely available. Portable. Uses sound waves reflected off of moving red blood cells and other tissues to evaluate the flow of blood. The different vascular beds have unique waveforms, and variations from normal indicate disease.
Photoplethysmography	A venous refill time < 20 seconds is indicative of venous disease.	Noninvasive testing. Provides overall assessment of venous physiology.
Venography	Determines venous patency.	Invasive testing. Requires contrast administration. Largely replaced by duplex scanning.
Ambulatory venous pressure	Pedal vein pressure measured before and after exercise to assess severity of venous disease.	Invasive testing. Seldom used in clinical practice.

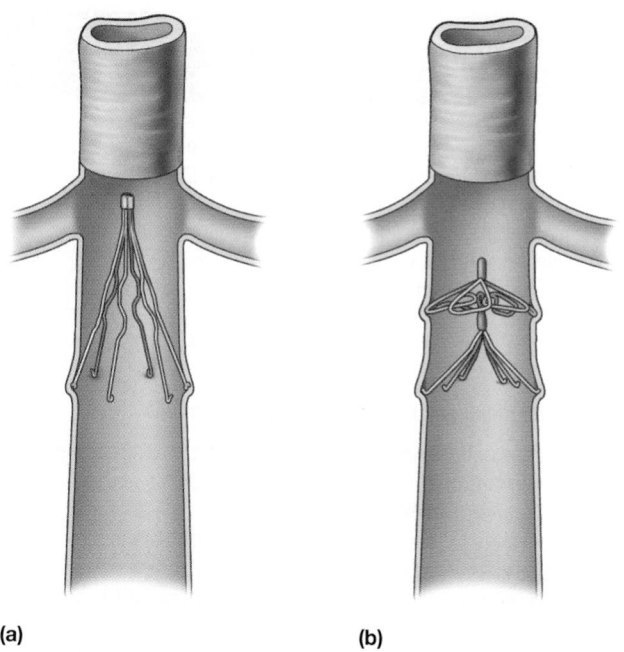

(a)   (b)

FIGURE 43–15 ■ Vena cava filters.

congestion and obstruction of the vena cava. Collateral vessels develop to maintain venous flow.

Nursing Management

Nurses play an active and important role in DVT prophylaxis and prevention. Nursing interventions include early ambulation whenever possible, active and passive range of motion exercises, extremity elevation, and mechanical methods of prophylaxis such as graduated compression stockings, intermittent pneumatic devices, and venous foot pumps. These mechanical devices increase venous outflow and/or reduce stasis in the leg veins (Geerts et al., 2004; Kehl-Pruett, 2006). Accurate leg length and calf circumference measurements are required to size graduated compression stockings correctly. Knee-high stockings are effective, less expensive, and easier to apply than are thigh-high stockings, which may enhance patient compliance with wearing stockings. Graduated compression stockings apply 18 mmHg at the ankle level and 8 mmHg at the thigh level. Intermittent and sequential compression devices decrease venous stasis and are often used in conjunction with graduated compression stockings (Figure 43–16 ■). Patients with underlying peripheral arterial disease should use compression stockings carefully. Complications of compression devices are rare and may include skin blisters. It is important that these devices are correctly sized and applied and that they are removed for only short periods of time.

The Nursing Process: Patient Care Plan (p. 1352) for Venous Thromboembolism feature outlines the nursing diagnoses and patient care needs that will provide a comprehensive plan of care for a patient experiencing a DVT.

Collaborative Management

A multidisciplinary team approach including health care providers, nurses, pharmacists, physical therapy, and dietitians is needed in providing care for the patient with VTE. Patients may benefit greatly from a nurse/pharmacist-directed antico-

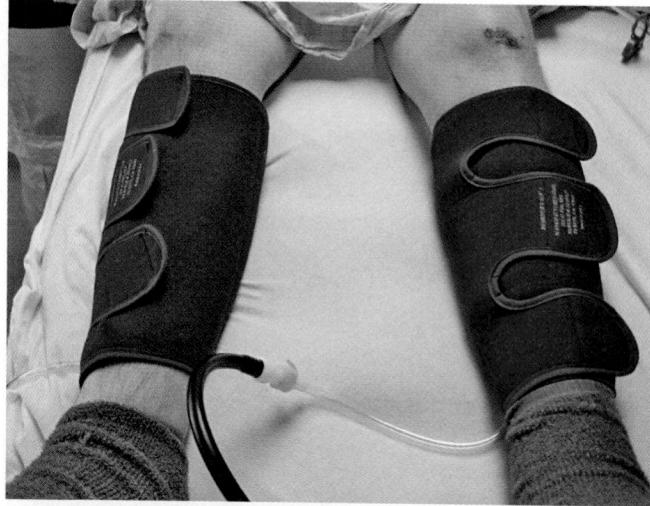

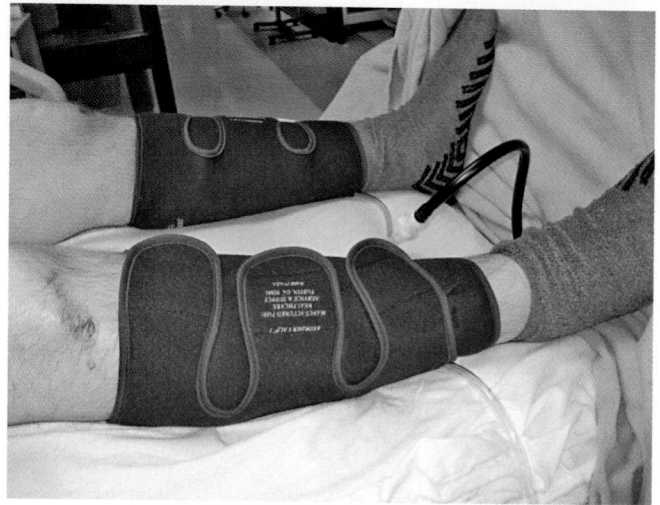

FIGURE 43–16 ■ Intermittent and sequential compression devices.
Source: Cheryl Wraa

agulation program to assist them in taking and monitoring their warfarin, if prescribed. Home health visits may be necessary for the patient undergoing outpatient treatment of DVT.

Health Promotion

To prevent DVT, patients should be taught the importance of regular walking, foot and ankle exercises, and foot elevation when hospitalized and during their recovery from hospitalization. If patients are discharged home on a pharmacologic prophylaxis plan such as unfractionated heparin, warfarin or enoxaparin, or direct thrombin inhibitors, they need to be taught their medication regime, which may include learning how to do injections, follow-up monitoring, and reportable adverse effects. The Patient Teaching & Discharge Priorities for Use of Anticoagulant Medications box (p. 1354) presents suggestions for teaching the patient who is on anticoagulating medications. The most common complications of these medications include bleeding and heparin-induced thrombocytopenia. Compression stockings should be worn to prevent venous pooling. The nurse needs to stress to patients to avoid prolonged sitting, standing, and to avoid crossing their legs. The Patient Teaching & Discharge Priorities for Deep Venous Thrombosis (p. 1355) outlines the discharge priorities that the nurse needs to include in the discharge teaching plan.

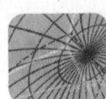

NURSING PROCESS: Patient Care Plan for Venous Thromboembolism

Assessment of Peripheral Vascular Status

Subjective Data:
Do you have pain, tenderness, or swelling in your legs or arms?
When did this occur and how long have you had it?
What is your activity level?
Have you traveled long distances recently?
Are you feeling short of breath?
Do you have pain in your chest?

Objective Data:
Assess for contributing factors for deep vein thrombosis (DVT)/pulmonary embolism (PE) development: immobility, major surgery, trauma, paralysis, history of previous DVT/PE episodes, and so on.
Assess extremities for pain, tenderness, erythema, and swelling.

Nursing Assessment and Diagnoses	Outcomes and Evaluation Parameters	Planning and Interventions with *Rationales*
Nursing Diagnosis: *Impaired Tissue Perfusion* related to DVT	**Outcomes:** Patient has adequate blood flow to extremities. Patient does not develop pulmonary clinical manifestations. Patient/family verbalize understanding of disease, management, and prevention. ***Evaluation Parameters:*** Warm skin, absence of edema, and absence of pain. Normal respiratory patterns, normal heart rate, and absence of chest pain.	**Interventions and *Rationales:*** Apply properly fitting compression stockings *to promote venous return and decrease venous stasis.* For confirmed DVT: Measure circumference of affected extremity daily *to monitor progression and/or resolution of DVT.* Maintain activity per order with affected limb elevated 10–20 degrees above the level of the heart *to reduce venous pooling and edema.* Maintain hydration *to prevent increased blood viscosity.* Explain the risk factors of venous thromboembolism (VTE), and the need for bed rest, limb elevation, compression stockings, and sequential compression; avoid rubbing/massaging calf *to prevent reoccurrences.* Monitor results of lab testing and noninvasive studies *to assess treatment effectiveness.*

Assessment of Pain Related to Impaired Circulation

Subjective Data:
On a scale of 0–10, how would you rate your pain at this time?
Where is your pain?
What brings it on?
What makes it go away?
How long have you had it, and is it getting worse or better?

Objective Data:
Use pain scale (0–10) to quantify pain.
Assess cultural and religious impact on patient's responses.
Assess the onset of increased pain to evaluate for disease progression or acute arterial obstruction.

Nursing Assessment and Diagnoses	Outcomes and Evaluation Parameters	Planning and Interventions with *Rationales*
Nursing Diagnosis: *Readiness for Enhanced Comfort* related to impaired circulation	**Outcome:** Relief of pain. ***Evaluation Parameters:*** Patient states adequate relief of pain. Patient understands measures necessary to prevent pain.	**Interventions and *Rationales:*** Obtain a clear description of source of discomfort. Provide moist heat *to help relieve pain and inflammation.* Keep affected extremity elevated above the level of the heart *to promote venous return and decrease venous stasis.* Provide a supportive environment where patient is able to express pain level. Instruct patient to inform nurse if pain is not relieved *in order to revise the care plan.* Use pain control measures before the pain becomes severe *to enhance comfort.* Teach nonpharmacological methods of pain control; that is, guided imagery and breathing exercises *to assist in relaxation and pain control.* Pain relief *to promote comfort.*

Assessment of Bleeding Related to Anticoagulant Therapy

Subjective Data:
Do your gums bleed when you brush your teeth?
Do you notice any blood in your urine or stool?
Do you notice any increased or unusual bruising?

Objective Data:
Assess aPTT or INR, and report subtherapeutic values and over therapeutic range.
Stool guaiac negative.
Assess for bleeding in mouth, nose, and urine.

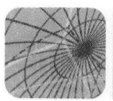

NURSING PROCESS: Patient Care Plan for Venous Thromboembolism—*Continued*

Nursing Assessment and Diagnoses	Outcomes and Evaluation Parameters	Planning and Interventions with *Rationales*
Nursing Diagnosis: *Fluid Volume Deficient, risk for*	**Outcomes:** Therapeutic aPTT or INR maintained in therapeutic range. No bleeding. **Evaluation Parameters:** No signs of bleeding in mouth, nose, urine, or stool.	**Interventions and *Rationales:*** Initiate and continue anticoagulant therapy *to prevent further clot development.* Monitor aPTT and/or INR prior to adjusting heparin or administering Coumadin *to optimize anticoagulation.* Assess for signs of bleeding *to ensure prompt identification and treatment.* Teach dietary restrictions of vitamin K *to avoid interactions with Coumadin.*

Assessment of Pulmonary Embolus Related to Embolization of Thrombus

Subjective Data:
Are you feeling short of breath?
Are you having chest pain? Are you coughing up blood-tinged sputum?
When did these symptoms begin?

Objective Data:
Rate, depth, and ease of respiration.
Assess lung sounds for adventitious or diminished sounds.
Assess sputum for blood.
Assess oxygen saturation levels.

Nursing Assessment and Diagnoses	Outcomes and Evaluation Parameters	Planning and Interventions with *Rationales*
Nursing Diagnosis: *Impaired Gas Exchange* related to VTE	**Outcomes:** No respiratory distress. Normal arterial blood gases. Normal oxygen saturation levels. **Evaluation Parameters:** No signs or symptoms of respiratory distress. No blood in sputum. No shortness of breath. No pain.	**Interventions and *Rationales:*** Instruct patient of reportable conditions: signs and symptoms of pulmonary embolus. Auscultate breath sounds for *assessment of crackles, rhonchi, or diminished sounds.* Provide oxygen per order *to increase oxygen to the heart, lungs, and periphery.* Administer anticoagulants or thrombolytic therapy *to treat VTE.*

Assessment of Self-Care Activities

Subjective Data:
Has anyone explained your health problems to you?
How does this disease affect your daily life?

Objective Data:
Assess knowledge of disease process and progression, risk factors, and need for compression stockings.
Assess knowledge of patient's understanding of treatment plan, including medications, if indicated.

Nursing Assessment and Diagnoses	Outcomes and Evaluation Parameters	Planning and Interventions with *Rationales*
Nursing Diagnosis: *Deficient Knowledge* of self-care needs related to disease	**Outcome:** Adequate knowledge level. **Evaluation Parameters:** Patient is able to discuss disease process, risk factors, and current treatment plan. Verbalizes adherence to and compliance with treatment plan.	**Interventions and *Rationales:*** Provide factual information about diagnosis, treatment, risk factor modification, medications, and treatment plan *to ensure compliance.* Explain all procedures and allow patient to ask questions *to promote his understanding.*

Complications

One of the complications of DVT is pulmonary embolism, which is described in Chapter 36 . Most thrombus come from the deep veins of the legs and can break loose spontaneously or be jarred loose by mechanical forces such as sudden standing and Valsalva. Pulmonary embolism may occur despite adequate anticoagulation. Clinical findings in PE may include dyspnea, tachypnea, pleuritic chest pain, cough, wheezing, syncope, hypotension, and cardiovascular collapse. The mortality associated with a large pulmonary embolism is 30% or more. A majority of patients with PE die within the first hour of symptom onset. Hypoxia occurs in these patients because of the imbalance or mismatch between blood flow and alveolar ventilation (Cardin & Marinelli, 2004).

CRITICAL ALERT *Signs and symptoms of pulmonary embolism (PE) include dyspnea, tachypnea, anxiety, apprehension, tachycardia, chest pain, hemoptysis, hypoxia, collapse, shock, and cardiac arrest. Right ventricular failure is the cause of death in patients who die of PE.*

A second complication following acute DVT is postphlebitic syndrome, which is chronic venous insufficiency (CVI). As many as 50% of patients develop this disorder following a DVT (Fahey, 2004; Rectenwald & Wakefield, 2005). To prevent postphlebitic syndrome from occurring, the use of elastic compression stockings with a pressure of 30 to 40 mmHg at the ankle is recommended for at least 2 years following the acute DVT episode (Büller et al., 2004). Chronic venous insufficiency occurs from

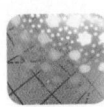

PATIENT TEACHING & DISCHARGE PRIORITIES for Use of Anticoagulant Medications

Medication Need	Teaching
All anticoagulant/antiplatelet agents	Take as directed by the health care provider.
	Do not skip doses.
	Consider an alert bracelet/necklace.
	Avoid activities that can cause injury or falling.
	Early warning signs of bleeding include bruising, nosebleeds, or bleeding gums. Serious bleeding can occur and includes:
	• Pink or brown urine
	• Red or black stool
	• Spitting up or coughing up bloody secretions or secretions that look like coffee grounds
	• Severe headache
	• Dizziness, fatigue, or weakness.
	Report any excessive bruising or bleeding to the health care provider.
Heparin	Patients need to be taught subcutaneous injection techniques.
Low molecular weight heparin	Patients need to be taught subcutaneous injection techniques.
	Frequent monitoring of lab work is generally not required for patients on low molecular weight heparin.
Warfarin/Coumadin	Patients need to take the exact dose as prescribed by their health care provider or pharmacist. They may need to take different doses of warfarin/Coumadin on different days of the week. Many patients taking warfarin are monitored by an interdisciplinary anticoagulation clinic rather than their health care provider. Instruct patients to know who is monitoring their warfarin/Coumadin.
	If patients miss two or more doses in a row, they should call whoever is managing their medication for further instructions.
	Regular blood testing of the INR level is required. Instruct patients to know their optimal INR range. For many cardiovascular patients, it is between 2 and 3.
	Drug interactions can occur. Patients should use care when taking many over-the-counter drug preparations. The most likely drugs to affect the INR include aspirin, ibuprofen, cold remedies, antacids, and vitamin supplements. Herbal supplements can impact the INR, especially dan shen, garlic, *Ginkgo biloba*, ginseng, green tea, or kava.
	Food interactions can occur. Because the drug reduces the liver's ability to use vitamin K, any foods that change the amount of vitamin K in the body can affect the INR. These foods include brussels sprouts, kale, green tea, asparagus, avocado, broccoli, cabbage, cauliflower, collard greens, liver, soybean oil, soybeans, certain beans, mustard greens, peas (black-eyed peas, split peas, chick peas), turnip greens, parsley, green onions, spinach, and lettuce.
	Patients may be advised to limit their alcohol intake.
	Warfarin/Coumadin can cause birth defects; it should NOT be taken by patients planning to become pregnant.

vein pathology, such as venous valvular incompetence, causing venous stasis and increased venous pressure in the lower extremities. Symptoms of CVI include dependent swelling, pain, and skin changes. Typical findings include hyperpigmentation, or brownish discoloration of the skin, edema, dermatitis, ulcerations, or scarring from healed ulcerations (Figure 43–17 ■). Patients may complain of cramping, heaviness, or aching of their legs.

Venous ulcerations are typically located near the medial malleolus or the lateral malleolus of the ankle, but can occur anywhere below the knee, including the foot (Brem, Kirsner, & Falanga, 2004). They are shallow, irregularly shaped, exudative wounds that are typically difficult. Pain may be worse when the legs are in a dependent position. Walking or elevating the legs may improve the pain of venous ulcers. Venous ulcers, which often recur, impact the patient's quality of life by causing pain and discomfort, decreased mobility, increased visits to the health care provider, or

hospitalizations, as well as the negative impact of managing a chronic condition: anxiety, fear, and depression.

Prior to treating venous ulcers, concomitant peripheral arterial disease must be ruled out. Compression therapy is the primary therapy used to treat venous ulcers. It is contraindicated in peripheral arterial disease; therefore, an ankle-brachial index (ABI) should be performed prior to compression therapy. A finding of ≤0.9 indicates peripheral arterial disease.

Compression therapy is provided using elastic or nonelastic dressings or wraps. An elastic dressing stretches with changes in leg size but will continue to compress, whereas a nonelastic dressing resists stretching. A rigid bandage, such as the **Unna's boot**, commonly used to treat venous ulcers, prevents edema while promoting healing and is worn for several days at a time.

The Unna's boot is being replaced in clinical practice by multilayer wrap compression, which is available in high and low compression pressures. An example of a multilayer wrap that

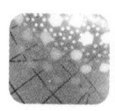

PATIENT TEACHING & DISCHARGE PRIORITIES for Deep Venous Thrombosis

Need	Teaching

Knowledge of disease process	Home care needs include verbal and written instructions for:
	  Treatment plan, including anticoagulation
	  Follow-up care
	  Activity restrictions, if any.

Understanding of medications	Teach the purpose, dose, and possible adverse effects of all medications to increase compliance and to prevent over/underdosing.
	Anticoagulant teaching: reason and importance, how to perform injections (if low molecular weight heparin prescribed), taking medications at the same time each day, not to skip a dose, frequent follow-up and lab testing, avoiding anything that might cause trauma/bleeding such as vigorous toothbrushing, contact sports.
Disease prevention	Explain the risk factors for DVT/PE development to prevent reoccurrences. The Risk Factors box (p. 1347) presents a detailed list of risk factors for venous thromboembolism.
	Avoid prolonged immobility, standing for long periods of time, car/airline flights > 6 hours; avoid constrictive clothing.
	Wear properly fitting and applied graduated compression stockings. If these stockings are recommended long term, teach patient to replace them every 3 months, because they lose their elasticity.

Reportable clinical manifestations	Instruct patient/family to report:
	  Increase in pain, tenderness, swelling of affected extremity
	  New onset pain, tenderness, swelling in another extremity
	  New onset shortness of breath, chest pain, anxiety, restlessness
	  New onset bleeding, headache, mental status changes.

Family/support system	Assess availability of, knowledge of, and compliance with treatment plan.
	Assess discharge placement needs.
	Assess for need for professional home health needs.
	Assess need for follow-up appointments.

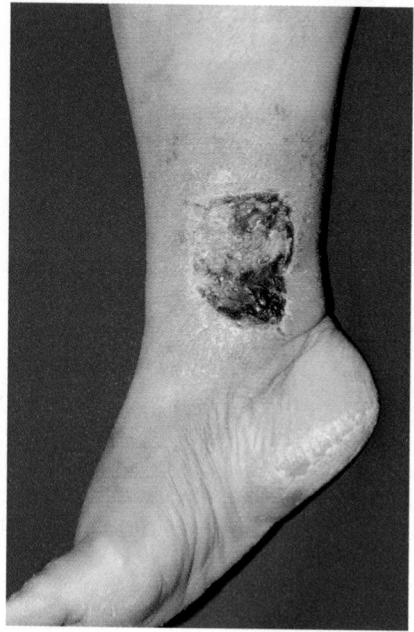

FIGURE 43–17 ■ Chronic venous insufficiency.
Source: Ribotsky/Custom Medical Stock Photo, Inc.

provides graded compression is Profore (Hunter, Langemo, Hanson, Anderson, & Thompson, 2005; Sieggreen, 2005a).

Venous ulcers require treatment using absorbent compresses, compression dressings, topical steroids, topical zinc oxide, or a broad-spectrum antifungal cream (rarely). The wound should be cleansed at each dressing change. The patient should be instructed to avoid known skin irritants and allergens. The application of eutectic mixture of local anesthetics (EMLA) cream may produce pain relief for sharp debridement, if needed. Adhesive hydrocolloid dressings have been found to be effective in healing venous ulcers. Topical antibiotics are generally not effective; a short course with a topical antimicrobial such as silver sulfadiazine may be beneficial. If signs of infection occur such as pain, fever, and drainage from the ulcer, a culture should be obtained and the appropriate systemic antibiotic started. Infections most commonly include gram-positive organisms such as *Staphylococcus* and *Streptococcus,* and gram-negative organisms such as *Pseudomonas* (Brem et al., 2004; Davis & Gray, 2005; Wound, Ostomy, and Continence Nurses Society, 2005).

An important component of wound assessment is ongoing photography of the wound and measurement of the wound size. This can readily be achieved by using a digital camera and single-use rulers that are available from various manufacturers. Having this objective history of the wound appearance and size makes it easier to follow trends in therapy and healing (Brem et al., 2004). An in-depth discussion of wound healing is presented in Chapter 67 ✪.

Patients with venous leg ulcers need to maintain adequate nutritional status to promote healing. A dietary consultation may be indicated. If indicated, the patient should be counseled about weight loss. Sufficient amounts of protein, vitamins A and C, and zinc are important. Decreased sodium intake is important to assist with managing edema. For patients with diabetes, tight

EVIDENCE-BASED PRACTICE

Medications for the Prevention of Deep Vein Thrombosis (DVT)

Clinical Problem

Homocysteine is a sulfur-containing amino acid found in the blood. Elevated levels of homocysteine have been linked to increased risk of premature coronary artery disease, stroke, and thromboembolism (venous blood clots), even among people who have normal cholesterol levels. Abnormal homocysteine levels appear to contribute to atherosclerosis in at least three ways: (1) direct toxic effect that damages the cells lining the inside of the arteries, (2) interference with clotting factors, and (3) oxidation of low density lipoproteins (LDL) (Barrett, 2003).

Elevated homocysteine levels also are associated with an increased risk of deep vein thrombosis and pulmonary embolism. According to den Heijer, Lewington, and Clarke (2005), up to now 24 case-control studies have been published with an overall relative risk for venous thrombosis of 1.60 (95% CI 1.10–2.34) for a 5 µmol/L higher homocysteine level. Moreover, three prospective studies showed an overall relative risk for venous thrombosis of 1.27 (95% CI 1.01–1.59), for a difference of 5 µmol/L. Recent meta-analyses on the effect of the MTHFR 677TT genotype on cardiovascular disease and venous thrombosis showed a modest increase in risk, supporting a hypothesis that homocysteine levels are causally related to thrombotic risk (den Heijer et al., 2005; Klerk et al., 2002; Wald, Law, & Morris, 2002).

Plasma homocysteine levels are strongly influenced by diet, as well as by genetic factors. The dietary components with the greatest effect in lowering the levels of homocysteine are folic acid and vitamins B_6 and B_{12}. Folic acid and other B vitamins help break down homocysteine in the body. Several studies have found that higher blood levels of B vitamins are related, at least partly, to lower concentrations of homocysteine (American Heart Association, 2008). Daily use of folic acid gives a 25% reduction in homocysteine levels, even at low doses of 0.5 milligram. The question is whether lowering of homocysteine by use of B vitamin supplementation also lowers the risk for venous thrombosis.

Research Findings

In 2006 den Heijer et al. (2007) conducted the VITRO (Vitamins and Thrombosis) study to investigate the effect of a combination preparation of 5 mg of folic acid, 50 mg of pyridoxine, and 0.4 mg of cyanocobalamin in the secondary prevention of deep venous thrombosis and pulmonary embolism in patients with a first event of venous thrombosis and hyperhomocysteinemia in a randomized, double-blind, and placebo-controlled setting. A secondary aim was to study the effect of vitamin supplementation in patients with a first event of venous thrombosis and a "normal" homocysteine concentration in an identical setting. The study concluded that B vitamin supplementation lowers homocysteine values, but it does not show a risk reduction in recurrent venous thrombosis. Elevated homocysteine blood levels remain a modest risk factor for recurrent thrombotic events.

Implications for Nursing Practice

The implication for nursing practice is that patients with elevated homocysteine levels are at a higher risk for DVT, a form of venous thromboembolism. Hospitalized patients are already at an increased risk of developing DVT due to immobility, advanced age, acute medical illness, and central venous catheters. Individuals who develop DVT are at further risk for serious complications such as pulmonary embolism and death. If a homocysteine level has been done, and the nurse is aware that the level is evaluated, it is imperative to institute timely nursing measures.

Treatment options, including high-dose anticoagulants and thrombolytics, may be contraindicated in certain inpatient populations; therefore, other methods of preventing DVT are imperative. Foot and ankle exercises encourage plantar and dorsiflexion, a very basic, natural technique. For those patients who are unable to perform foot and ankle exercises, passive range of motion is an appropriate substitute to reduce venous pooling by passively exercising muscles. Other measures for DVT prevention include active range of motion, early ambulation, graduated stockings, and pneumatic compression devices. Each improves venous return and reduces venous stasis in the leg veins. These measures are simple to use and do not increase the risk of bleeding, making them ideal for most hospital patients.

Nurses play key role in the prevention of DVT and its complications. Nursing management includes assessing every patient for risk factors for the development of the DVT. Admission assessments are an opportune time to evaluate risk factors such as mobility, age, previous history of DVT, and medical conditions that increase the risk of developing DVT in hospital patients. Patient risk assessment should be ongoing throughout hospitalization but especially with condition changes. Nurses must advocate for timely prevention and treatment measures. Following the intuition of these measures, the nurse must then evaluate their effectiveness (Kehl-Pruett, 2006).

Critical Thinking Questions

1. When a patient is admitted with an elevated homocysteine level, in order of priority, what nursing measures are essential?

2. Identify measures that would decrease the risk for the development of DVT.

3. What is the primary reason for instituting measures that prevent the development of DVT?

Answers to Critical Thinking Questions appear in Appendix D.

References

American Heart Association. (2008). *What is homocysteine?* Retrieved March 11, 2008, from http://www.americanheart.org/presenter.jhtml?identifier=535.

Barrett, S. (2003). *Homocysteine: A cardiovascular risk factor worth considering*. Retrieved March 11, 2008, from http://www.quackwatch.com/03HealthPromotion/homocysteine.html.

den Heijer, M., Lewington, S., & Clarke, R. (2005). Homocysteine, MTHFR and risk of venous thrombosis: A meta-analysis of published epidemiological studies. *Journal of Thrombosis Haemostasis, 3,* 292–299.

den Heijer, M., Williams, H. P. J., Blom, H. J., Gerrits, W. B. J., Cattaneo, M., Eichinger, S., et al. (2007). Homocysteine lowering by B vitamins and the secondary prevention of deep-vein thrombosis and pulmonary embolism. A randomized, placebo-controlled, double blind trial. *Blood, 109*(1), 139–144.

Kehl-Pruett, W. (2006). Deep vein thrombosis in hospitalized patients: A review of evidence-based guidelines for prevention. *Dimensions of Critical Care Nursing, 25*(2), 53–59.

Klerk, M., Verhoef, P., Clarke, R., Blom, H. J., Kok, F. J., & Schouten, E. G. (2002). MTHFR 677C->T polymorphism and risk of coronary heart disease: a meta-analysis. *JAMA, 288,* 2023–2031.

Wald, D. S., Law, M., & Morris, J. K. (2002). Homocysteine and cardiovascular disease: Evidence on causality from a meta-analysis. *British Medical Journal, 325,* 1202–1208.

glycemic control is essential to reduce infection and promote healing. An in-depth discussion of the nutritional aspects of wound healing is presented in Chapter 14 ☞ . Surgical intervention for venous ulcers is rarely required because no definitive procedure has been found for treatment.

Research into causes and treatment of DVT continues. See the Evidence-Based Practice box.

Lymphatic Disorders

The lymphatic system is composed of lymphatic vessels, lymph nodes, the spleen, and the thymus. This system filters bacteria and other particulate matter, thereby providing defense against disease. **Lymphangitis** is an acute inflammation of the lymphatic channels most commonly caused by an infection in one of the extremities. The associated lymph nodes become enlarged and tender. Recurrent episodes of lymphangitis can be associated with progressive lymphedema. The Diagnostic Tests box outlines the typical tests that are done to assist in confirming the diagnosis. Lymphedema can be primary or secondary. Primary lymphedema is inherited as an autosomal dominant trait. Secondary lymphedema occurs as a result of an acquired disorder, such as a malignancy, radiation, surgical removal of a component of the lymphatic system, trauma, or infection. Malignancy is the most common cause of secondary lymphedema in the United States (Sieggreen & Kline, 2004b). Figure 43–18 ■ shows lower extremity severe lymphedema.

Pathophysiology

Lymphedema occurs when there is an obstruction causing excess lymph buildup within the system, which ultimately overloads the transport capacity of the lymphatic system. This can progress to fibrosis and irreversible tissue damage. Lymphedema is classified into three stages. In Stage I, the edema is pitting and is reversible with elevation of the affected limb. In Stage II, fibrosis has occurred and the edema is nonpitting and nonreversible. In Stage III, the affected limb is greatly enlarged and the skin is thickened.

Clinical Manifestations

Lymphedema is the interstitial accumulation of lymph fluid that occurs when the lymphatic system is impaired. The affected

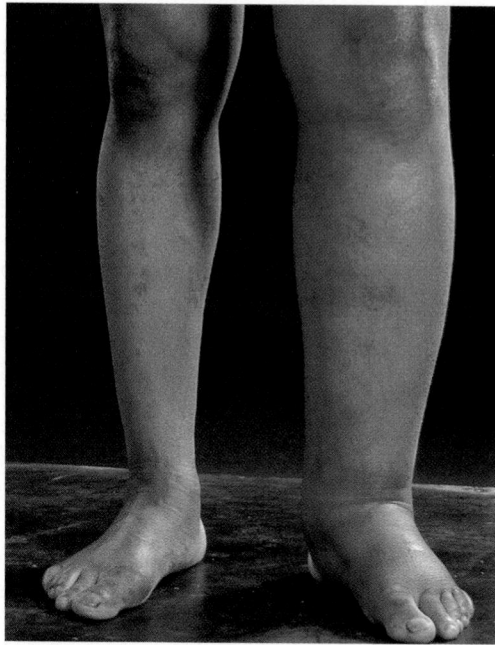

FIGURE 43–18 ■ Severe lymphedema.
Source: MSNB/Custom Medical Stock Photo, Inc.

limb(s) become edematous with thickened skin. Patients may complain of heaviness or fullness of the affected extremity.

Diagnosis and Medical Management

Diagnosis of lymphedema is based on the patient's history and clinical presentation. The patient should be asked about previous surgeries, radiation treatment, trauma, and infection. Medical therapy of lymphedema is directed toward controlling the fluid accumulation, maintaining skin integrity, and preventing infections. Bed rest, compression therapy, manual lymphatic drainage, short stretch compression wrapping, and limb elevation are the primary interventions for lymphedema.

Complications

Complications of lymphedema include recurrent cellulitis and/or lymphangitis, deep venous thrombosis, severe functional impairment, cosmetic embarrassment, and amputation (rare). Complications following surgery are common and include partial wound

DIAGNOSTIC TESTS for Lymphedema

Test	Expected Abnormality	Rationale for Abnormality
Lymphangiography	Obstructions in lymphatic communication visualized.	Requires contrast administration by injection into a small lymph channel in the dorsum of the foot. Complications of lymphangiography include acute lymphangitis. Rarely performed.
Lymphoscintigraphy	Obstructions in lymphatic communication visualized.	Most commonly performed diagnostic test for lymphedema. Requires injection of technetium 99m labeled colloid in the web spaces of the fingers or toes, and images are obtained at preset intervals. Complications are uncommon.

separation, seroma, hematoma, skin necrosis, and exacerbation of foot or hand edema. Patients with chronic lymphedema have a risk of developing lymphangiosarcoma. Although rare, this cancerous tumor is highly aggressive, requires radical amputation of the involved extremity, and has a very poor prognosis.

Nursing Management

Patients with lymphedema require limb elevation; compression garments (Figure 43–19 ■), which are custom fit garments that apply compression and prevent fluid from accumulating in the limb; and manual drainage, or the use of a lymph pump to reduce edema. The affected extremity is placed into the sleeve of the lymph pump, and it is then inflated to a preset pressure to help drain the extremity. The lymph pump may be used daily to reduce edema. Surgical options include resection of skin and subcutaneous tissue, skin grafting, drainage procedures, removal of tissue containing abnormal lymphatics, and less commonly, transplant of tissue from areas with normal lymphatic tissues to areas with abnormal lymphatic drainage. Rarely, bypass of abnormal lymphatic tissue is attempted, in some cases using vein grafts. Such procedures, which are frequently unsuccessful, are usually performed only under experimental protocols. Surgery has met with limited success and requires significant experience and technical expertise. Complications of surgery include poor healing, infection, prolonged hospitalization, poor cosmetic results, and failure to reduce the edema (Sieggreen & Kline, 2004b).

Health Promotion

Instruct patients on the importance of excellent skin hygiene and infection prevention. Good skin care with mild soaps and moisturizing creams is needed. Because patients with lymphedema are at risk of infection, particularly fungal infections, they need to be taught to inspect regularly for signs and symptoms of infection and to report them promptly.

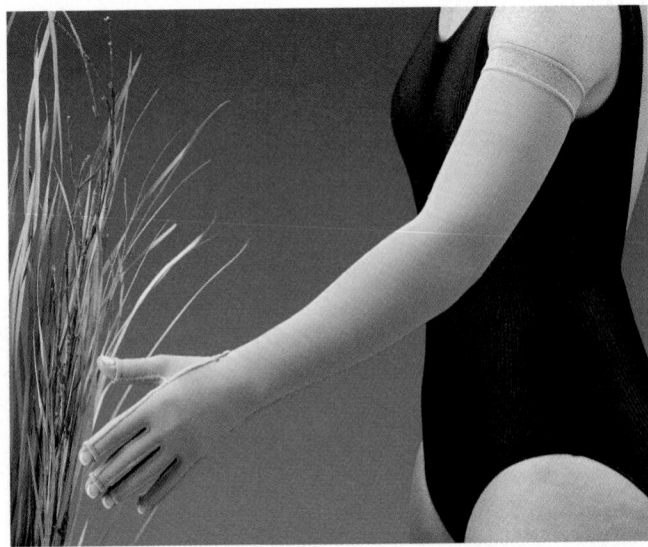

FIGURE 43–19 ■ Compression garment for lymphedema.
Source: © Gottfried Medical, Inc., used with permission

Gerontological Considerations

The prevalence of peripheral arterial disease, abdominal aortic aneurysm, deep venous thrombosis, and chronic venous insufficiency increases with age. Peripheral arterial disease, stroke, and myocardial infarction are the principal causes of death and disability in patients over age 50. Elderly patients with peripheral arterial disorders are at higher risk of coronary and cerebrovascular events, such as myocardial infarction and stroke. Elderly patients with acute and chronic venous disease are at higher risk of pulmonary embolus and death (AHA, 2006; Oka, 2006).

Peripheral vascular disease can cause functional limitations in the elderly, greatly affecting their quality of life. Physical training, strength training, and exercise programs can improve functional status. Low-intensity exercise programs, such as walking, golf, and shuffleboard, can be of great benefit for the elderly. Patients should be encouraged to continue to modify their risk factors for peripheral vascular disease by smoking cessation and controlling their blood pressure and blood sugar levels.

Special nursing care considerations for the elderly include a careful assessment of the cardiovascular and cerebrovascular systems. Myocardial ischemia and infarction can occur, leading to decompensation of the cardiovascular system. Stroke is a leading cause of death and disability in the elderly. The risk of having a stroke more than doubles for each decade of life after age 55. Following stroke, 25% of the elderly die and 25% will not be able to care for themselves. Teaching the patient and family members the signs and symptoms of TIA/impending stroke is essential (Federman, Bravata, & Kirsner, 2004).

Recovery from major vascular surgical procedures, such as abdominal aortic aneurysm repair or femoropopliteal bypass, can be prolonged in the elderly. Wound healing may be delayed and the elderly may be more likely to develop surgical complications, such as atelectasis, pneumonia, and wound infection. Elderly patients are more likely to develop complications of immobility, so turning, repositioning, and ambulating the patient as early as possible to maintain pulmonary function and promote independence also are important aspects of care. Careful assessment of the patient's nutritional intake is essential, in that it impacts wound healing and survival. Strict asepsis is critical because of the diminished immune response and increased susceptibility to infection.

Research

Peripheral vascular disorders affect millions of Americans, and the effects of these diseases can be limiting and potentially devastating. Research that further explores and defines nursing interventions and therapies for patients with peripheral vascular disease is needed. Nursing research in the area of peripheral vascular disorders and the application of evidence-based practice is essential for the continued refinement of care for the patients with peripheral vascular disorders. The research topics related to peripheral vascular disorders are outlined in the Research Opportunities and Clinical Impact box.

RESEARCH OPPORTUNITIES AND CLINICAL IMPACT RELATED TO PERIPHERAL VASCULAR DISORDERS

Research	Clinical Impact
Effects of gene therapy on peripheral arterial disease	Decrease in tissue loss and enhanced healing
Herbal and complementary medicine to treat peripheral arterial disease	Lowers blood lipids and blood pressure
Wound care in arterial and venous ulcers	Rapid and enhanced healing
Pressure reduction surfaces and devices	Rapid and enhanced healing; prevention of skin breakdown in patients with peripheral arterial disease (PAD) and other high-risk patients

Clinical Preparation

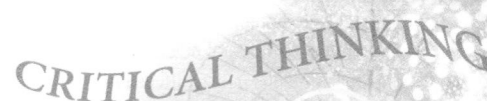

CRITICAL THINKING

 Read

- History of Current Illness
- Past Medical History
- Physical Exam
- Admitting Medical Orders
- Laboratory Study Results

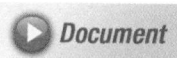 **Document**

- Summary of Hospitalization
- Pathophysiology Form
- Laboratory Values
- Laboratory Results Explanation

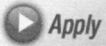 **Apply**

- List of Potential Nursing Diagnoses
- Concept Map
- Critical Thinking Questions

Log on to MyNursingKit.com to download forms you will need and to complete further steps in the Clinical Preparation assignment.

HISTORY OF PRESENT ILLNESS

As the on-coming nurse on the medical–surgical unit, you receive a report on Mr. Davis, a 68-year-old retired school-teacher admitted 2 days ago with peripheral arterial disease, rest pain in the right forefoot, and a nonhealing ulcer on the distal aspect of the right great toe. He was admitted from the ED and gave a 2-week history of persistent and severe pain, which has kept him from sleeping at night. He also noted redness and drainage from what had previously been a stable callus over the distal great toe.

You are told by the night nurse that Mr. Davis was stable throughout the night, was able to sleep at short intervals, although his pain level never decreased below 5/10 despite use of a morphine sulfate patient-controlled analgesia (PCA) pump and bolus doses of 5 mg twice.

Medical/Surgical History

His past medical history includes intermittent claudication after walking two blocks, type II diabetes, hypertension, hypercholesterolemia, and coronary artery disease. He is allergic to penicillin. Currently, he is a nonsmoker for 1 year after smoking 1 pack per day for 50 years. He has an alcohol intake of one glass of red wine with dinner. Past surgeries include three-vessel coronary artery bypass grafting 8 years prior and percutaneous transluminal angioplasty (PTA) and stenting of the right external iliac artery 1 year ago.

Social History

He is married with two grown children and a 2-year-old granddaughter. He is active in his church group and plays golf three times per week, although he is unable to walk the course because of leg pain and now uses a cart.

Current Medications

Atorvastatin (Lipitor) 40 mg po daily
Cilostazol (Pletal) 100 mg po bid
Aspirin 325 mg enteric-coated po daily
Metformin (Glucophage) 500 mg po bid
Benazepril (Lotensin) 20 mg po daily
Nitroglycerine 0.4 mg sublingual prn

Physical Exam

Physical exam findings reveal that Mr. Davis is alert and cooperative and oriented × 3. He currently rates his pain as 5/10 in the right foot. Vital signs: Blood pressure is 150/90 in the left arm, 160/100 in the right arm; heart rate 72; respiratory rate 18; temperature 37.5°C. His weight is 200 pounds. His height is 5'10". He has a left carotid bruit. His neurological exam is normal. He has a well-healed midline sternal incision. Heart tones are regular with no murmur heard. Lungs are clear with diminished breath sounds at the bases bilaterally. His abdomen is soft, nontender with active bowel sounds. He has bilateral femoral bruits. His femoral pulses are faintly palpable bilaterally and his popliteal, dorsalis pedis, and posterior pulses are absent bilaterally.

Dependent rubor is noted in the right foot, which blanches with elevation. Skin of the feet is dry and intact, except for the right great toe ulcer, which measures 1 cm. Capillary refill of the other toes is sluggish. Slight erythema is noted on the surrounding skin, and there is a small amount of serous drainage on the dressing. His toenails are thickened. 12-lead ECG: sinus rhythm with nonspecific ST segment changes.

Admitting Medical Orders

Vascular service
Admit to telemetry with continuous cardiac monitoring
Diagnosis: Peripheral arterial disease with ulceration, right toe
Allergy: penicillin
Vital signs q4h
Bilateral lower extremity pulse checks q4h
Bed rest with bathroom privileges
1,800-calorie ADA diet
Accuchecks ac and hs
Call house officer: pulse < 60 and > 130/minute; BP < 90 and
    > 160 systolic; temperature > 38.5; urine output < 30 mL/hr
    for 2 hours; respiratory rate > 40/minute; glucose > 150
IV saline lock: flush with NS q8h
NS wet-to-dry dressing changes to right great toe q8h

Scheduled Medications

Atorvastatin (Lipitor) 40 mg po daily
Cilostazol (Pletal) 100 mg po bid
Aspirin 325 mg enteric-coated po daily
Metformin (Glucophage) 500 mg po bid
Benazepril (Lotensin) 20 mg po daily
Nitroglycerine 0.4 mg sublingual prn chest discomfort/angina
Mylanta 30 mL q4h prn dyspepsia
Zolpidem (Ambien) 5 mg po qhs prn for sleep
Ativan 1 mg IV q6h prn anxiety
Milk of Magnesia 30 mL daily prn constipation
Tylenol 650 mg po/pr q4h prn for pain
Morphine sulfate PCA: 1 mg incremental dose q10min; if pain not
    well controlled, give morphine sulfate bolus 1–5 mg IV × 1

Ordered Laboratory Studies

CBC, basic metabolic panel, daily
Culture drainage right toe

Ordered Diagnostic Studies

12-lead ECG
PA and lateral chest x-ray
Carotid duplex today; also have vascular lab perform bilateral ABI
NPO at midnight for aortic angiography with runoff

LABORATORY STUDY RESULTS

Test	Admit	Day 2	Day 3
WBC	13.4/mm^3	14.0/mm^3	17.1/mm^3
RBC	3.66/mm^3	3.93/mm^3	3.67/mm^3
Hemoglobin	11.4 g/dL	12.1 g/dL	11.6 g/dL
Hematocrit	33.6%	35.8%	33.3%
Platelet count	172/mm^3	192/mm^3	221/mm^3
Sodium	137 mEq/L	134 mEq/L	135 mEq/L
Potassium	3.7 mEq/L	3.8 mEq/L	3.8 mEq/L
Chloride	101 mEq/L	96 mEq/L	97 mEq/L
Calcium	7.9 mg/dL	8.6 mg/dL	8.2 mg/dL
Blood sugar	306 mg/dL	255 mg/dL	203 mg/dL
BUN	34 mg/dL	36 mg/dL	34 mg/dL
Creatinine	1.7 mg/dL	1.8 mg/dL	1.7 mg/dL

CRITICAL THINKING QUESTIONS

1. What are the priorities of care for Mr. Davis?
2. What additional objective data would be helpful in assessing Mr. Davis?
3. What is the significance of the smoking history?
4. After morning rounds, Mr. Davis' health care provider orders an angiogram of the aorta and lower extremities. What is the rationale for these tests?
5. How will you prioritize Mr. Davis' nursing care following his angiogram?

Answers to Critical Thinking Questions appear in Appendix D.

NCLEX® REVIEW

1. A patient with a 30-year history of smoking tells the nurse that he can only walk a few blocks before the pain becomes severe in his lower legs. The nurse realizes this patient is describing:
   1. Intermittent claudication.
   2. Deep vein thrombosis.
   3. Peripheral neuropathy.
   4. Exercise intolerance.

2. A patient with peripheral arterial disease has intermittent claudication. Which of the following should the nurse include in this patient's plan of care?
   1. The use of moist heat.
   2. Keep legs elevated above the level of the heart.
   3. Teach importance of regular and structured ambulation.
   4. Remind that the legs will feel cool to the touch.

3. The nurse is instructing a patient with Raynaud's disease on self-management. Which of the following should be included in this instruction?
   1. Smoking cessation is the only treatment for this disease.
   2. Dress warmly in cold weather and limit alcohol intake.
   3. Avoid physical exercise.
   4. Prescribed medications have no effect on the disease.

4. A patient is having an endovascular stent graft to repair for an aortic abdominal aneurysm. Which of the following should the nurse include when assessing post-operative complications for this patient?
   1. Cerebrovascular embolus
   2. Abdominal surgical site infection
   3. Deep vein thrombosis associated with a longer hospital stay
   4. Renal impairment due to alterations in blood flow

5. A patient recovering from orthopedic surgery has developed a deep vein thrombosis in the left calf. Which of the following should the nurse include when instructing this patient?
   1. The need for early ambulation, use of compression stockings, and range of motion exercises.
   2. Avoid the use of compression stockings.
   3. Complete bed rest with the left leg elevated.
   4. Avoid unnecessary exercise.

6. A patient diagnosed with a deep vein thrombosis is started on low molecular weight heparin. Which of the following should the nurse instruct the patient about this medication?
   1. The need to avoid foods high in vitamin K
   2. The signs and symptoms of bleeding
   3. The need to have blood drawn to measure the INR
   4. Why this is the preferred medication for anyone with kidney failure

7. A patient with varicose veins is scheduled for radiofrequency ablation of the vein. Which of the following should the nurse include when providing pre-operative teaching to this patient?
   1. Complete bed rest will be required for 72 hours following this procedure to avoid stressing the suture line.
   2. Compression stockings will be worn to decrease venous stasis.
   3. Avoid showering until a week following the procedure to allow for maximum wound healing.
   4. Anticipate the use of anticoagulants to decrease the viscosity of the blood.

8. An elderly patient is assessed as having a pulsatile mass near the umbilicus. The nurse realizes that treatment will be according to which of the following?
   1. If an aortic aneurysm is diagnosed that is larger than 6 centimeters, surgery will be performed.
   2. If the abdominal ultrasound and CAT scan reveal a 4 centimeter abdominal aortic aneurysm, surgery will be performed.
   3. If diagnostic testing reveals the presence of an abdominal aortic aneurysm, steroids will be added to decrease the inflammatory response.
   4. If an abdominal aortic aneurysm is identified in the infrarenal area, the surgical approach is contraindicated.

Answers for review questions appear in Appendix D

KEY TERMS

aneurysm *p.1342*
ankle-brachial index (ABI) *p.1327*
aortic coarctation *p.1330*
aortic dissection (AD) *p.1344*
carotid endarterectomy (CEA) *p.1339*
deep venous thrombosis (DVT) *p.1346*
endoleaks *p.1343*

intermittent claudication (IC) *p.1326*
lymphangitis *p.1357*
lymphedema *p.1346*
paresthesia *p.1326*
peripheral arterial disease (PAD) *p.1326*
pulmonary embolism (PE) *p.1347*
stenosis *p.1341*

sympathectomy *p.1336*
thromboangiitis obliterans (TAO) *p.1338*
transient ischemic attack (TIA) *p.1339*
Unna's boot *p.1354*
varicose veins *p.1346*
venous thromboembolism (VTE) *p.1347*
Virchow's triad *p.1347*

PEARSON

EXPLORE **mynursingkit™**

MyNursingKit is your one stop for online chapter review materials and resources. Prepare for success with additional NCLEX®-style practice questions, interactive assignments and activities, web links, animations and videos, and more!

Register your access code from the front of your book at
www.mynursingkit.com

REFERENCES

Abou-Chebl, A., Yadiv, J. S., Reginelli, J. P., Bajzer, C., Bhatt, D., & Kreiger, D. W. (2006). Intracranial hemorrhage and hyperperfusion syndrome following carotid artery stenting. *Journal of the American College of Cardiology, 43*, 1596–1601.

Agency for Healthcare Research and Quality. (2008). *Treating tobacco use and dependence: 2008 update.* Rockville, MD: Author. Retrieved July 22, 2008, from http://www.ahrq.gov/path/tobacco.htm

American Heart Association. (2006). American Heart Association. Home Page Retrieved March, 28, 2006, from http://www.americanheart.org

American Heart Association. (2007). *Few Americans aware of dangerous peripheral arterial disease.* Retrieved on July 24, 2008 from http://www.americanheart.org/presenter.jhtml?identifier=3050383

American Heart Association. (2008b). *Atherosclerosis.* Retrieved July 24, 2008 from http://www.americanheart.org/presenter.jhtml?identifier=4440

American Stroke Association. (2006). *Learn to recognize a stroke.* Retrieved March 28, 2006, from http://www.strokeassociation.org/presenter.jhtml?identifier=1020

American Urological Association. (2002). *Renovascular disease.* Retrieved November 13, 2006, from http://www.urologyhealth.org/adult/index.cfm?cat=02&topic=126

Arkkila, P. E. (2006). Thromboangiitis obliterans (Buerger's disease). *Orphanet Journal of Rare Diseases, 1*, 14.

Beebe-Dimmer, J. L., Pfeifer, J. R., Engle, J. S., & Schottenfeld, D. (2004). The epidemiology of chronic venous insufficiency and varicose veins. *Annals of Epidemiology, 15*, 175–184.

Brem, H., Kirsner, R. S., & Falanga, V. (2004). Protocol for the successful treatment of venous ulcers. *The American Journal of Surgery, 188* (Suppl. 1A), 1S–8S.

Büller, H. R., Agnelli, G., Hull, R. D., Hyers, T. M., Prins, M. H. & Raskob, G. E. (2004). Antithrombotic therapy for venous thromboembolic disease: The seventh ACCP conference on antithrombotic and thrombolytic therapy. *Chest, 126*(3), 401S–428S.

Cahall, E. J. (2004). Assisting with tobacco cessation. *Journal of Vascular Nursing, 22*, 117–123.

Cardin, T., & Marinelli, A. (2004). Pulmonary embolism. *Critical Care Nursing Quarterly, 27*(4), 310–322.

Caulfield, M. T., Fernando, D., & Rosenfield, K. (2005). Renal and iliac intervention. In H. C. Herrmann (Ed.), *Interventional cardiology: Percutaneous noncoronary intervention* (pp. 295–320).Totowa, NJ: Humana Press.

Chang, A. K. (2008). *Thoracic outlet syndrome.* Retrieved July 25, 2008 from http://www.emedicine.com/emerg/TOPIC578.HTM

Criqui, M. H., Vargas, V., Depenberg, J., Ho, E., Allison, M., Langer, R. D., et al. (2005). Ethnicity and peripheral arterial disease: The San Diego population study. *Circulation, 112*, 2703–2707.

Davis, J., & Gray, M. (2005, May/June). Is the Unna's Boot bandage as effective as the four-layer wrap for managing venous leg ulcers? *Journal of Wound, Ostomy and Continence Nursing*, 152–156.

Dickinson, M. G., Krishnan, U., Houlihan, G., & Walker, C. M. (2004). Renal artery stenosis: Diagnosis and management. In G. S. Abela (Ed.), *Peripheral vascular disease: Basic diagnostic and therapeutic approaches* (pp. 270–282). Philadelphia: Lippincott Williams & Wilkins.

Eberhardt, R. T., & Raffetto, J. D. (2005). Chronic venous insufficiency. *Circulation, 111*, 2398–2409.

Eisenhauer, A. C., & Shaw, J. C. (2004). Atherosclerotic subclavian artery disease and revascularization. In G. S. Abela (Ed.), *Peripheral vascular disease: Basic diagnostic and therapeutic approaches* (pp. 283–294). Philadelphia: Lippincott Williams & Wilkins.

Fahey, V. A. (Ed.). (2004). *Vascular nursing* (4th ed.). Philadelphia: Elsevier.

Federman, D. G., Bravata, D. M., & Kirsner, R. S. (2004). Peripheral arterial disease: A systemic disease extending beyond the affected extremity. *Geriatrics 59*(4), 26–34.

Fleming, C., Whitlock, E. P., Beil, T. L., & Lederle, F. A. (2005). Screening for abdominal aortic aneurysm: A best-evidence systematic review for the U.S. Preventative Services Task Force. *Annals of Internal Medicine, 142*(3), 203–211.

Geerts, W. H., Pineo, G. F., Heit, J. A., Bergqvist, D., Lassen, M. R., Colwell, C. W., et al. (2004). Prevention of venous thromboembolism: The seventh ACCP conference on antithrombotic and thrombolytic therapy. *Chest, 126*, 338S–400S.

Gey, D. C., Lesho, E. P., & Manngold, J. (2004). Management of peripheral arterial disease. *American Family Physician, 69*, 525–533.

Hirsch, A. T., Haskal, Z. J., Hertzer, N. R., Bakal, C. W., Creager, M. A., Halperin, J, L., et al. (2006). ACC/AHA guidelines for the management of patients with peripheral arterial disease (lower extremity, renal, mesenteric, and abdominal aortic): A collaborative report from the American Association for Vascular Surgery/Society for Vascular Surgery, Society for Cardiovascular Angiography and Interventions, Society of Interventional Radiology, Society for Vascular Medicine and Biology, and the American College of Cardiology/American Heart Association Task Force on Practice Guidelines (Writing Committee to Develop Guidelines for the Management of Patients with Peripheral Arterial Disease). *Journal of the American College of Cardiology, 47*, 1–192.

Hirsh, J., Guyatt, G., Alberts, G. W., & Schünemann, H. J. (2004). The Seventh ACCP Conference on Antithrombotic and Thrombolytic Therapy: Evidence-based guidelines. *Chest, 126*, 172S–173S.

Hirsh, J., & Raschke, R. (2004). Heparin and low molecular weight heparin: the seventh ACCP conference on antithrombotic and thrombolytic therapy. *Chest, 126*(3), 188S–203S.

Hunter, S., Langemo, D., Hanson, D., Anderson, J., & Thompson, P. (2005). Compression therapy for venous ulcers. *Advances in Skin & Wound Care, 18*(8), 404–408.

Jacoby, D. S., & Mohler, E. R. (2004). Peripheral arterial disease: Risk factor identification and modification. In G. S. Abela (Ed.), *Peripheral vascular disease: Basic diagnostic and therapeutic approaches* (pp. 190–199). Philadelphia: Lippincott Williams & Wilkins.

Kehl-Pruett, W. (2006). Deep vein thrombosis in hospitalized patients: A review of evidence-based guidelines for prevention. *Dimensions of Critical Care Nursing, 25*(2), 53–59.

LaMuraglia, G. M., & Nigri, G. R. (2004). Surgery for peripheral vascular disease. In G. S. Abela (Ed.), *Peripheral vascular disease: Basic diagnostic and therapeutic approaches* (pp. 365–373). Philadelphia: Lippincott Williams & Wilkins.

Lipsitz, E. C., & Kim, S. (2005). Antithrombotic therapy in peripheral arterial disease. *Clinics in Geriatric Medicine, 22* 183–198.

Lu, J. T., & Creager, M. T. (2004). The relationship of cigarette smoking to peripheral arterial disease. *Reviews in Cardiovascular Medicine, 5*(4), 189–193.

Marr, J. (2006). Deep venous thrombosis recommendations. *Journal of Vascular Nursing, 24*(3), 91–93.

Mayo Clinic. (2006) *Raynaud's disease.* Retrieved October 15, 2007, from http://www.mayoclinic.com/health/raynauds-disease/DS00433

National Heart, Lung, and Blood Institute. (2004). *Seventh report of the Joint National Committee on Prevention, Detection, Evaluation, and Treatment of High Blood Pressure* (NIH Publication No. 04-5230, pp. 1–104). Bethesda, MD: Author.

Oka, R. K. (2006). Peripheral arterial disease in older adults: Management of cardiovascular risk factors. *Journal of Cardiovascular Nursing, 21*(55), S15–S20.

Olson, K. W., & Treat-Jacobson, D. (2004). Symptoms of peripheral arterial disease: A critical review. *Journal of Vascular Nursing, 22*(3), 72–77.

Porth, C. M. (2005). *Pathophysiology: Concepts of altered health status* (7th ed.). Philadelphia: Lippincott Williams & Wilkins.

Porth, C. (2007). *Essentials of pathophysiology* (2nd,ed.). St. Louis: Lippincott Williams & Wilkins.

Rectenwald, J. E., & Wakefield, T. W. (2005). The treatment of deep venous thrombosis, including the newer agents. *Disease of the Month, 51*, 104–111.

Rehring, T. F., Sandhoff, B. G., Stolepart, R. S., Merenich, J. A., & Whitton-Hollis, H. (2005). Atherosclerotic risk factor control in patients with peripheral arterial disease. *Journal of Vascular Surgery, 41*(5), 816–822.

Reilly, A., & Snyder, B. (2005). Raynaud's phenomenon. *American Journal of Nursing, 105*(8), 56–65.

Sieggreen, M. (2005a). Lower extremity arterial and venous ulcers. *Nursing Clinics of North America, 40*, 391–410.

Sieggreen, M. (2005b). Venous disorders: Overview of current practice. *Journal of Vascular Nursing, 23*(1), 33–35.

Sieggreen, M. Y., & Kline, R. A. (2004a). Arterial insufficiency and ulceration: Diagnosis and treatment options. *Nurse Practitioner, 29*(9), 46–52.

Sieggreen, M. Y., & Kline, R. A. (2004b). Current concepts in lymphedema management. *Advances in Skin & Wound Care, 17*(4), 174–180.

Singh, V. N., & Cousin, A. (2005). *Angioplasty, Peripheral.* eMedicince. Retrieved on July 24, 2008 from http://www.emedicine.com/radio/topic754.htm

Sontheimer, D. L. (2006). Peripheral vascular disease: Diagnosis and treatment. *American Family Physician, 73*(11), 1971–1976.

Sullivan, T. M. (2005). Surveillance and follow-up after carotid angioplasty and stenting. In M. A. Mansour & N. Labropoulos (Eds.), *Vascular diagnosis* (pp. 183–191). Philadelphia: Elsevier Saunders.

Tapson, V. F. (2005). The diagnosis of venous thromboembolism. *Disease of the Month, 51,* 86–93.

Teruya, T. H., & Ballard, J. L. (2004). New approaches for the treatment of varicose veins. *Surgical Clinics of North America, 84,* 1397–1417.

Upchurch, G. R., & Schaub, T. A. (2006). Abdominal aortic aneurysm. *American Family Physician, 73*(7), 1198–1204.

Walsh, M. E., & Rice, K. L. (2004). Venous thromboembolic disease. In V. A. Fahey (Ed.), *Vascular nursing* (4th ed.). Philadelphia: Elsevier.

Wound, Ostomy, and Continence Nurses Society. (2005). *Guideline for management of wounds in patients with lower-extremity venous disease.* Glenview, IL: Author.

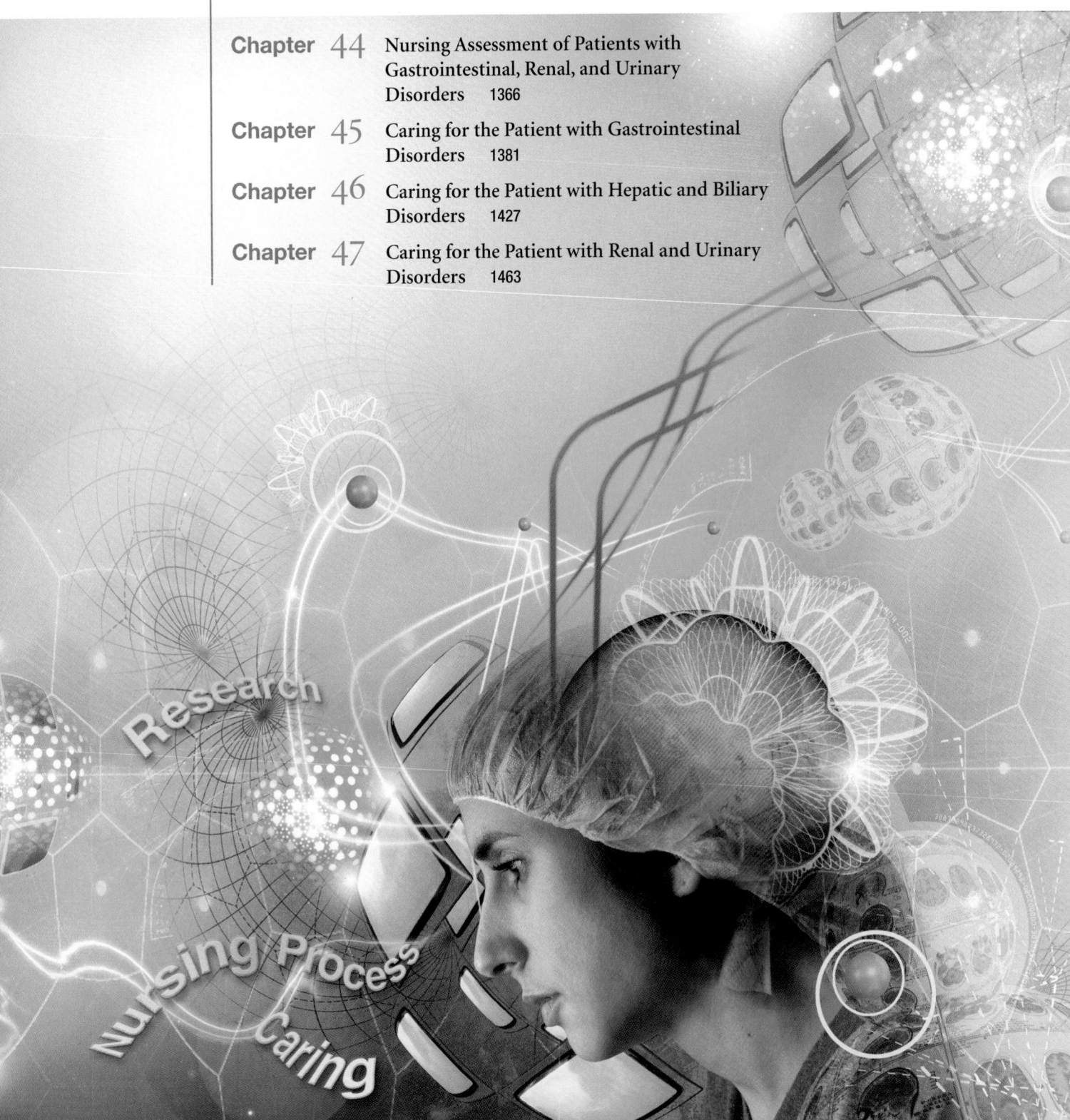

Profiles in Nursing

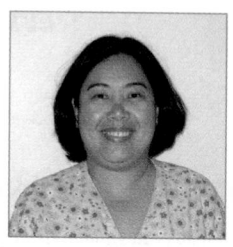

CELESTE I am Celeste May Padilla, clinical nurse III in the Renal Services Program at the University of California, Davis Medical Center. I am a member of the American Nephrology Nurses' Association and a certified nephrology nurse acknowledged by the Nephrology Nursing Certification Board. I have been working as a nephrology nurse since 1999, and give direct patient care to patients of different ages and varying diagnoses.

The nurses in the Renal Services Program are mobile—we go from different floors and units to provide dialysis. Most of our patients are adults with acute and chronic renal diseases, but we also care for pediatric and geriatric patients. Our average number of patients is 15 a day, but that number can rise to more than 20 patients on busy days. We also provide in-patient dialysis at Shriners Children's Hospital, which is adjacent to our facility.

We use the nursing process to direct the treatment of patients who are experiencing, or at risk for, renal disease. Our program provides different modalities such as *continuous renal replacement therapy* for patients in the intensive care unit (ICU) who are critically ill and diagnosed with acute renal failure. Patients who are at risk for renal impairment benefit from early dialytic management of fluid and solute imbalance. *Slow extended daily dialysis* (SLEDD) is another modality. SLEDD is used when ICU patients need gentle and slow dialysis so they can tolerate fluid removal and have electrolyte imbalances corrected. Intermittent hemodialysis, or regular dialysis, is a modality for patients in the medical–surgical units who can tolerate dialysis and maintain stable vital signs throughout the procedure. We provide interventions to improve patient outcomes based on the nurse's individual clinical judgment and knowledge.

As a nephrology nurse, it is part of my profession and daily life to follow the six components of caring. **Compassion** is being aware of my patient's needs, that is, willing to share and discover another person's meaning and purpose in life, sickness, and health. Providing care to patients who are in the denial stage of their diagnosis is one of my priorities. I show my **commitment** to my profession, department, and colleagues by my attendance on scheduled days to work and by my willingness to be called in to give prompt care to patients who need emergent dialysis.

On occasion, I have been called in the middle of the night to come to the emergency department (ED) to do emergent dialysis for a chronic patient who came in with hyperkalemia, severe chest pain, fluid overload, and very short of breath. The patient may be a noncompliant end-stage renal disease patient who didn't go to dialysis for several treatments and now is in the ED seeking emergent treatment. My **conscience** dictates that I suspend judgment; there is no choice based on whether the patient is compliant or not—we are always ready to render service.

I had one very young pediatric patient who required dialysis. The parents were always at the bedside 24/7, and they had never experienced dialysis before so they had many questions. I understood completely because they wanted to make sure that treatment was appropriate and the patient would be in good hands. As a **competent** nurse I answered them in a way they could easily understand. I showed them each step and demonstrated to them with **confidence** that I practice my profession without hesitation or doubt. My **comportment** helped them to accept the fact that their child needed dialysis.

Being a nephrology nurse involves giving direct care, educating, and coordinating. We complete a thorough assessment, and if a patient is stable enough to start dialysis, then we proceed. But if a certain modality is ordered for this particular patient and we know it's not safe, then we use our own judgment and inform our nephrologists of the patient's change in condition. Our nephrologists value our expertise and listen to our suggestions—after all, we are a team with one purpose: to deliver safe, excellent care.

> "As a nephrology nurse, it is part of my profession and daily life to follow the six components of caring. **Compassion** is being aware of my patient's needs, that is, willing to share and discover another person's meaning and purpose in life, sickness, and health."

Bonnie McCracken

Outcome-Based Learning Objectives

After studying this chapter, the learner will be able to:

1. Compare and contrast the significant subjective and objective data that pertain to the gastrointestinal and urinary systems obtained during history taking.
2. Identify the four components of the physical exam.
3. Describe techniques used during the physical assessment of the gastrointestinal and urinary systems.
4. Differentiate abnormal from normal findings of the physical assessment of the gastrointestinal and urinary systems.
5. Describe key aspects that should be included when documenting the physical examination.

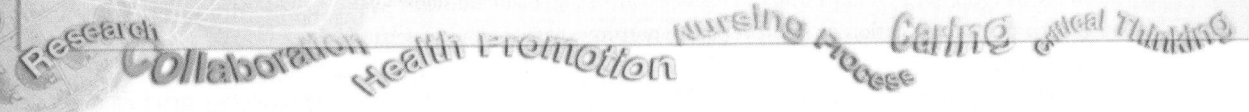

Research Collaboration Health Promotion Nursing Process Caring Critical Thinking

THE SYMPTOMS of abdominal pain are frequent presenting medical complaints. The symptoms may represent something very benign or something extremely serious and even life threatening. For example, the complaint of abdominal pain can be either gastroenteritis or an aortic aneurysm. The difference between the two diagnoses can be differentiated by a thorough history and physical examination. In order to perform a proper history and physical examination, the nurse must have a thorough understanding of the anatomy and physiology of the gastrointestinal system (Figure 44–1 ■). The nurse will then be able to determine what is occurring with the patient.

Anatomy and Physiology

For the nurse to complete a thorough assessment of the gastrointestinal and urinary systems, it is imperative to understand the anatomy and physiology of each system. This knowledge will assist the nurse in thinking critically and assimilating all data gathered during the assessment.

Gastrointestinal System

The primary purposes of the gastrointestinal (GI) system are to transport and deliver nutrition and water, and to support the function of cells throughout the body. The oral cavity or mouth is at the beginning of the GI tract. This is where food is taken in

and the process of digestion starts. The act of chewing and the mixture with saliva starts the breakdown of the food and makes it a size acceptable for passage through the esophagus. The salivary glands have several roles in this process. First, they add an aqueous component to the food bolus, making it easier to swallow, and second, they lubricate the mouth, facilitating the movement of the lips and tongue during swallowing. This aqueous environment assists in the distribution of the food across the taste buds dispersed across the tongue, making the food palatable and therefore more pleasing to eat. Without these taste buds, food would have no taste and be difficult to eat. An additional property of saliva is the reduction in bacteria in the oral cavity. Saliva contains large amounts of ions, such as chloride, bicarbonate, potassium, thiocyanate, hydrogen, and **immunoglobulin A**, a vital component for destroying oral bacteria (Urdan, Stacy, & Lough, 2006). There are three pairs of major salivary glands: the parotid, sublingual, and submandibular glands. The parotid gland secretes enzymes, which begins the chemical breakdown of large polysaccharides into dextrins and sugars.

The act of chewing is a complex process of using the teeth to masticate and the tongue to move the food bolus backward. Simultaneously, the soft palate lifts and covers the nasal passage while the epiglottis closes the opening, preventing aspiration of food. A change in any of these intricate movements can cause problems with the first step of digestion.

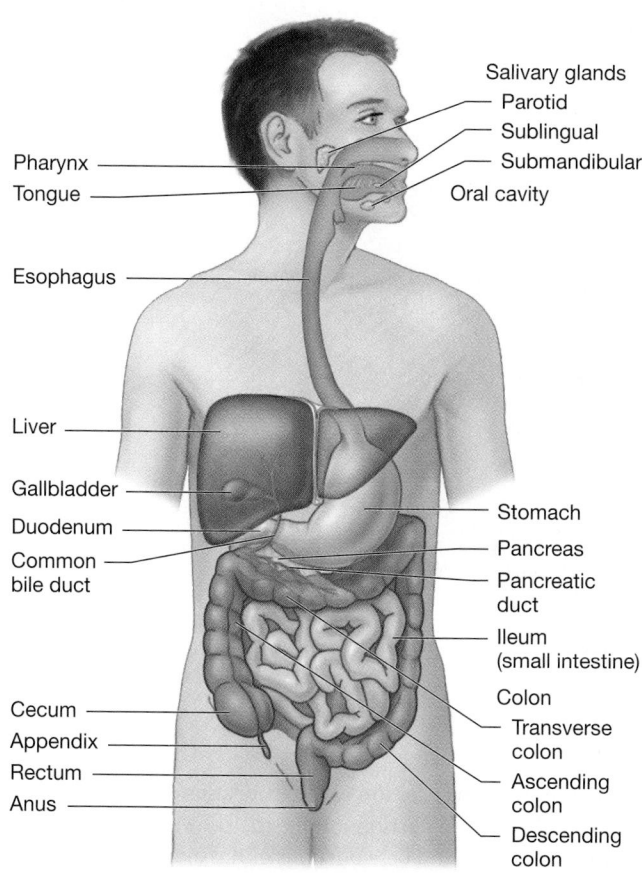

Salivary glands
— Parotid
— Sublingual
— Submandibular
Oral cavity

Pharynx ——
Tongue ——

Esophagus ——

Liver ——

Gallbladder ——
Duodenum ——
Common ——
bile duct

— Stomach
— Pancreas
— Pancreatic
duct
— Ileum
(small intestine)
— Colon
— Transverse
colon
— Ascending
colon
— Descending
colon

Cecum ——
Appendix ——
Rectum ——
Anus ——

FIGURE 44–1 ■ Organs of the gastrointestinal (GI) system.

The food bolus then passes through the **esophagus**. This tubular structure connects the oral cavity to the stomach. There is a segment of the esophagus in the cervical area, the thoracic area, and then it passes through the diaphragmatic hiatus into the abdominal cavity. There are two esophageal sphincters; the upper esophageal or **pharyngoesophageal**, which is created by the cricopharyngeus muscle, and the lower esophageal or **cardioesophageal**. The upper esophageal sphincter inhibits air from entering the esophagus during respiration, and the lower esophageal sphincter controls the food entering the stomach and prevents reflux of gastric contents. After swallowing, the esophageal sphincter in the upper portion closes, which increases the normal pressure within the esophagus. This phenomenon, along with peristalsis, moves the food bolus down to the stomach. **Peristalsis** is caused by the coordinated contraction of the circular and longitudinal muscle fibers making up the musculature of the esophagus. The pressure changes in the esophagus prevent reflux of the food bolus into the pharynx as well as gastric content from entering the lower portion of the esophagus. When reflux from the stomach into the esophagus occurs, it is known as **GERD, gastroesophageal reflux disease**. Commonly called "heartburn," it is a frequent patient complaint. Once the bolus has passed through the esophagus, the pressures return to normal.

The vagus nerve provides the parasympathetic innervation of the pharynx and the esophagus. Pharyngeal branches of the vagus nerve innervate the constrictor muscles of the pharynx with a small contribution by cranial nerves IX and XI. The upper esophageal sphincter and the upper portion of the esophagus are innervated by branches of the recurrent laryngeal nerves, which originate from the vagus nerve. Patients with injury to these nerves will have functional problems with their vocal cords as well as problems with the upper esophageal sphincter and motility of the esophagus, one of the causes of dysphasia, speech impairment resulting from a brain lesion or neurodevelopmental disorder. A problem with the upper esophageal sphincter also causes an increased risk of aspiration and further respiratory complications resulting from this condition.

The food bolus passes from the esophagus into the stomach. The stomach can be described as a muscular container where food is released into the intestine at a controlled rate. The stomach starts with the lower esophageal sphincter and ends with the pylorus. In between these two structures, the stomach can be divided into three portions: the cardia, the fundus, and the antrum (Figure 44–2 ■, 1368).

The **cardia** is where mucus and bicarbonate are secreted to protect the surface of the stomach from the acidic gastric juices. The lining of the stomach has multiple folds called rugae. Within this lining are deep gastric glands, which further differentiate the areas of the stomach. These glands are shallow in the cardia, medium depth in the antrum, and the deepest are found in the fundus. These deeper glands in the fundus contain secretory cells producing acid and pepsin, important components of the gastric juice. This capability establishes the primary purpose of the fundus as the secretory region of the stomach. The **antrum** is the place of the greatest motility with the purpose of mixing the gastric juices with the food particles and grinding them into smaller particles. The antrum then empties into the small intestine through the pylorus.

An understanding of the vasculature of the stomach is important in order to understand the significance of any bleeding in this area. This is the most vascularized portion of the gastrointestinal tract, which explains why a perforated ulcer can be life threatening due to rapid exsanguination. The largest artery supplying the stomach is the left gastric artery. This arises from the celiac trunk and is divided into the ascending and descending branches along the lesser curvature of the stomach. The second largest artery is the right gastroepiploic artery originating from the gastroduodenal artery. The left gastroepiploic artery arises from the splenic artery. These two arteries supply the greater curvature of the stomach. The fourth artery is the right gastric artery arising from the hepatic artery and runs along the distal stomach.

The venous system draining the stomach parallels the arteries. The left and right gastric veins drain into the portal vein, the right gastroepiploic veins drain into the superior mesenteric vein, while the left gastroepiploic vein drains into the splenic vein.

The nerve innervation of the stomach is with the anterior and posterior trunk of the vagal nerve. Approximately 90% of the nerve fibers are afferent, with the remaining 10% efferent.

The stomach empties through the pylorus into a portion of the small intestine called the duodenum. The duodenum has 12 sections and is responsible for the regulation of digestion and absorption. It is found almost entirely in the **retroperitoneal space**, the anatomic space behind the abdominal cavity. The

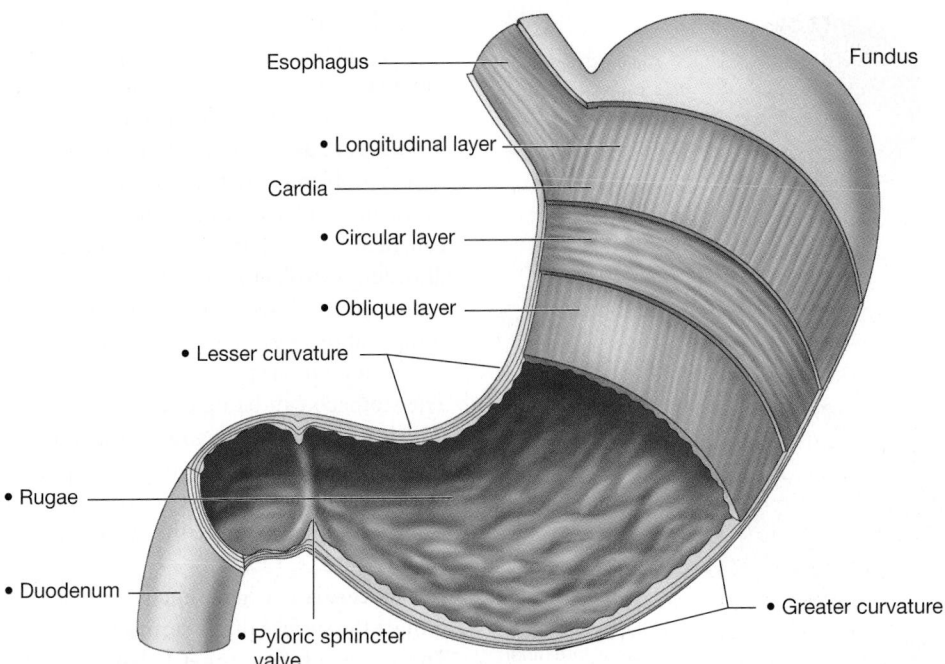

FIGURE 44–2 ■ The stomach.

primary purpose of this portion of the gastrointestinal tract is for the regulation of digestion and the absorption of the luminal contents. The duodenum is divided into four sections. The first, superior, part is approximately 5 centimeters from the pylorus to the second portion. It is in this area that a duodenal ulcer is found, usually along the anterior wall.

The second portion of the duodenum, known as the descending portion, is the area where the pancreatic and common bile ducts enter through the major duodenal papilla, or ampula of Vater. The pressure in the pancreatic duct is greater than in the bile duct to prevent reflux. To assist digestion, the pancreas secretes approximately 500 milliliters of fluid per day (Fisher, Andersen, Bell, Saluja, & Bruinicardi, 2005). The pancreatic juice is secreted from acinic and duct cells. The acinic cells secrete amylase, proteases, and lipases. These enzymes are responsible for the breakdown of carbohydrates, fats, and proteins. The duct cells secrete the water and electrolytes in the pancreatic juice. These cells keep a constant balance between the amount of bicarbonate/chloride and sodium/potassium that is secreted. The secretion of the pancreatic juice is the exocrine function of the pancreas. The endocrine function, although vital, is not discussed in this chapter.

The pancreatic duct carries the pancreatic juice, joins with the bile duct, and enters the duodenum where the contents assist the digestive process. The bile duct originates from the gallbladder, a muscular sac lying beneath and adjacent to the liver (Figure 44–3 ■). A simplistic way of thinking of it is as a conduit and storage receptacle for bile produced by the liver. The bile enters from the liver via the cystic duct and exits via the common bile duct, which then empties into the duodenum. Bile makes the fat molecules water soluble so the body may better utilize them.

The third and fourth portions of the duodenum are called the inferior/horizontal and are the ascending portions. This also describes the anatomic position of these portions of the duodenum. The second and third portions of the small bowel are called the jejunum and the ileum. These portions of the small bowel lie in the peritoneum but are tethered to the retroperitoneum. The surface of the small intestine is covered with small finger-like projections called villi. These in turn are covered with more projections called microvilli. This creates a larger surface area and a greater ability for absorption of nutrients before passing into the large intestine.

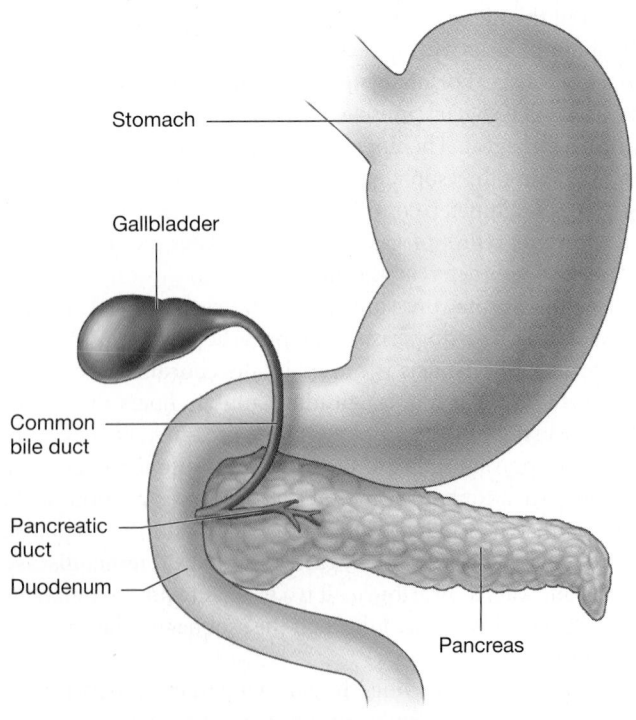

FIGURE 44–3 ■ The pancreas and gallbladder.

The large intestine starts at the ileocecal valve and ends at the anus. There are three anatomic and functional sections: the **colon** (the large intestine from the end of the ileum to the anal canal that surrounds the anus), the **rectum** (lower part of the large intestine between the sigmoid colon and the anal canal), and the **anal canal** (the last part of the large intestine situated between the rectum and the anus). The colon and rectum have five layers: the mucosa, submucosa, inner circular muscle, outer longitudinal muscle, and serosa. The serosa ends at the midrectum, and therefore there is no serosa in the mid and lower third of the rectum. The distal rectum also has inner smooth muscles, which join together to form the internal anal sphincter. The colon is also divided into sections. The cecum is the portion with the widest diameter and the thinnest muscle wall. It is the severe stretching of this thin wall that may lead to perforations. Paradoxically, the wide diameter makes it a rare location of obstruction.

The other terms commonly associated with the colon are *hepatic flexure, transverse colon, splenic flexure,* and *descending colon.* The ascending colon, on the right side of the abdomen, is fixed to the retroperitoneum. The transitional colon is more free and transverses the abdomen after the hepatic flexure. The greater omentum is attached to the superior and anterior portion of this part of the colon. The splenic flexure is the transition point to the descending colon, the portion on the left of the abdomen. The sigmoid colon is the narrowest and most mobile portion of the colon. It is because of this mobility that diseases of this portion of the colon may yield pain in the right lower abdomen, although the sigmoid is generally located in the left lower quadrant. Because of the lack of fixation, this part of the colon is subject to volvulus, when the colon turns into itself and the narrowness leads to common areas of obstruction.

The rectum is approximately 12 to 14 centimeters in length. It ends in the anal canal, which is 2 to 4 centimeters in length and is generally longer in men than in women. The differentiation between the anal canal and the rectum is at the dentate line. It is at this junction that the mucosa changes from the columnar rectal mucosa to the squamous anoderm. There are two sphincters: the internal sphincter and external sphincter at the distal rectum.

The function of the colon is primarily water absorption and electrolyte balance. This is why patients with diarrhea can have such imbalances in electrolytes. As the stool passes quickly through the colon when diarrhea is present, the normal function of absorption is gone. A large amount of water can be absorbed through the colon, up to 5,000 milliliters per day. Along with this is the transport of sodium, potassium, and chloride. Ammonia is produced when there is bacterial degradation of protein and urea. This ammonia is absorbed and transported to the liver, where it is metabolized. The absorption of ammonia is dependent on the intraluminal pH, which can be altered by a change in the bacteria levels leading to poor absorption of ammonia.

Stool is comprised of approximately 30% bacteria with the most prominent being *Escherichia coli,* known to cause grave illness when it contaminates food sources (Bullard & Rothenberger, 2005). Intestinal gas is primarily from swallowed air, but also is produced by intraluminal production and diffusion of blood. Nitrogen and oxygen are derived from the swallowing of air; carbon dioxide is from the breakdown of triglycerides and from the bicarbonate and hydrogen ions; and methane and hy-

drogen originate from the bacteria in the colon. The culmination of these gases is called flatus. The amount is dependent on the food intake, but 400 to 1,200 milliliters is released as flatus each day (Bullard & Rothenberger, 2005).

The motility of the bowel is what produces bowel sounds. Bowel sounds can be present without having a functioning bowel. For instance, with an ileus, there can be bowel sounds present, but as they are discoordinate; there is not resultant bowel movement or passing of gas. The movement of the intestine is called peristalsis. In the small intestine peristalsis occurs with the contraction of the longitudinal muscles causing the bowel to shorten and the contraction of the inner circular muscles resulting in luminal narrowing. This process moves the content along. In the colon the movement is slightly different. The movement of the colon is more in bursts with low and high amplitude contractions. The low amplitude movement moves the intraluminal content both antegrade and retrograde. It is thought this slows the process time through the colon, allowing for greater absorption. The high amplitude contraction is more coordinated, and the purpose is to move the stool mass along the colon to eventual elimination.

Defecation is the elimination of stool. This occurs with the stretching of the rectum, causing the relaxation of the internal sphincter with stool entering the rectal canal. Defecation can then occur as the rectum shortens and peristaltic waves force the stool out of the rectum. A problem with any of these steps can lead to constipation or incontinence.

Other organs involved in the process of digestion are the liver, pancreas, and gallbladder. Both the liver and the pancreas are multifunctional. The liver has functions that contribute to both metabolism and excretory functions. It is one of the largest organs and the largest gland. The pancreas has both endocrine and exocrine functions. The exocrine functions were discussed earlier. Although it is not within the scope of this chapter to discuss all the functions of the pancreas, an understanding of them is important and will be discussed in Chapter 46 🔗.

Related Structures

When examining the abdomen, it is important to have knowledge of all structures within the abdomen, even those that are not related to the gastrointestinal system. The abdomen is the only major cavity of the body not encased in bony structures. Although the lower ribs lend some support to the posterior cavity, the anterior cavity receives its structure from the muscle wall. The abdominal wall muscles consist of the rectus abdominus, the internal and external obliques, and the transverse abdominis (Figure 44–4 ■, p. 1370). These muscles support the abdomen, allow for movement, and when contracted increase the intra-abdominal pressure.

The vascular support of the gastrointestinal system was touched on earlier in this chapter. Another major artery to be aware of and examine when doing an abdominal assessment is the aorta. This is the major artery descending from the heart through the diaphragm, through the abdominal cavity, and bifurcating at the lower abdomen into the right and left iliac arteries. The aorta is discussed more thoroughly in Chapter 37 🔗.

The spleen can be found in the left upper quadrant and is protected by the lower left ribs. It is directly inferior to the diaphragm.

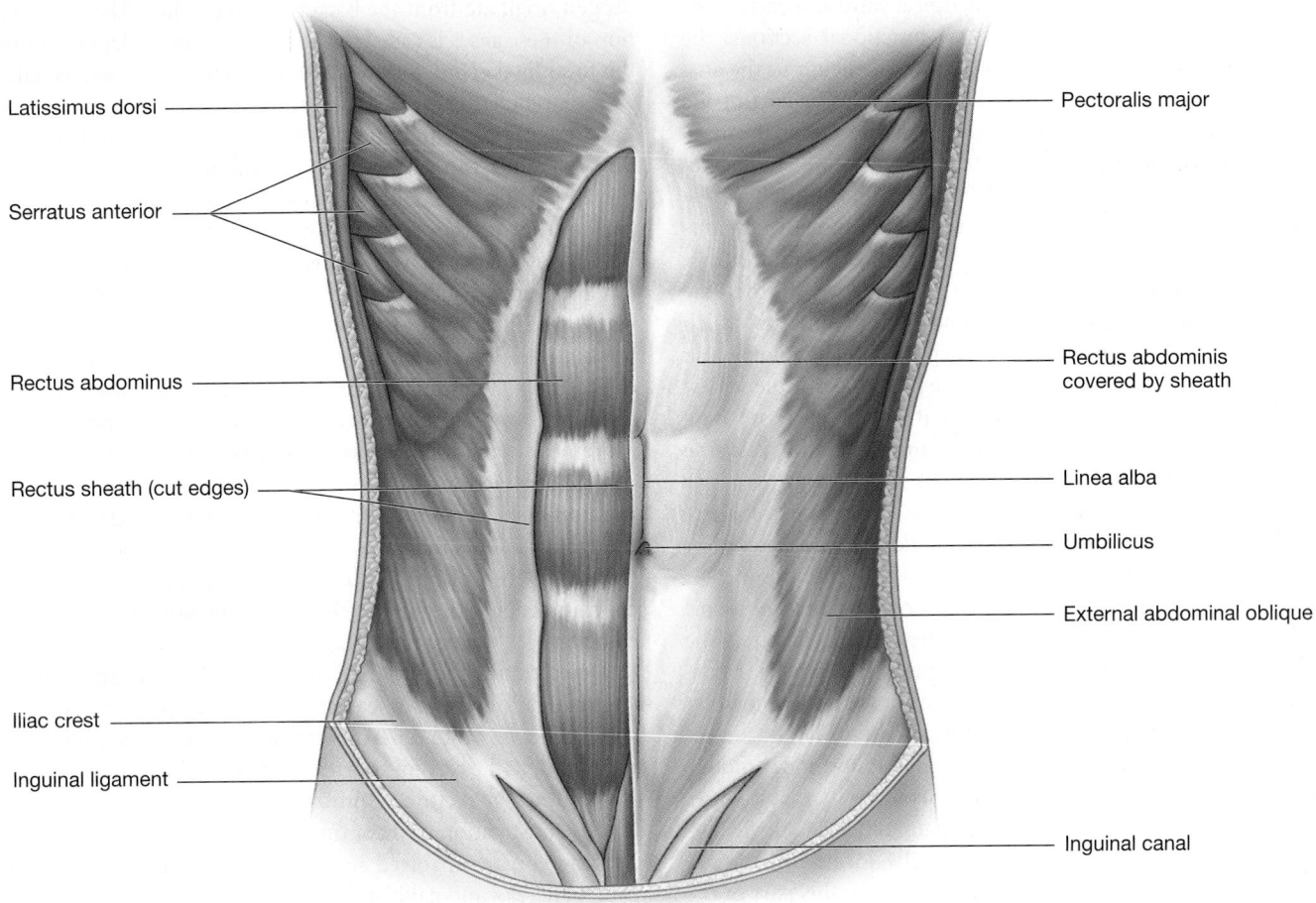

FIGURE 44–4 ■ Abdominal muscles.

The primary purpose of the spleen is to filter blood, destroy aged red blood cells, and return their by-products to the liver. Because of its vascular nature, this is an organ that when injured in a trauma to the abdomen, can be life threatening.

Urinary System

The organs of the urinary system lie within the abdomen. The kidneys and bladder lie within the space called the retroperitoneum. This is a space defined the by posterior peritoneum and the posterior body wall. Chart 44–1 lists the organs found in the peritoneal and retroperitoneal spaces.

The kidney is a complex organ and its function is discussed in detail in Chapter 47 ☻. The kidneys are a pair of organs located in the retroperitoneum on each side of the vertebral column. The right kidney is slightly lower than the left due to the presence of the liver. The kidneys are protected by the rib cage both anteriorly and posteriorly. They are also protected by a tough fibrous capsule, cushioned by perirenal fat and supported by the renal fascia. Put simply, the primary roles of the kidneys are to maintain fluid and electrolyte balance, help to achieve acid–base balance, and remove metabolic wastes. The renal system also has an important role in control of blood pressure, bone metabolism, and red blood cell synthesis (Figure 44–5 ■).

The urinary system also includes a drainage system: the ureters, bladder, and urethra. As urine is formed in the kidneys, it flows through the ureters, fibromuscular tubes, by peristalsis

CHART 44–1	Organs Found in the Peritoneal and Retroperitoneal Spaces		
Peritoneal Cavity	**Anterior Retroperitoneal Space**	**Posterior Retroperitoneal Space**
Omentum	Pancreas	Kidneys
Liver	Duodenum	Ureters
Stomach	Ascending colon	Adrenal glands
Gallbladder	Descending colon	
Spleen		
Jejunum		
Ileum		
Transverse and sigmoid colon		
Cecum		
Appendix		

into the bladder. The peristaltic action helps prevent reflux of the urine back into the kidneys. The bladder, which is also muscular, holds the urine and has a capacity of 280 to 500 milliliters. When the bladder is stretched the parasympathetic nervous system signals the smooth muscle of the bladder to contract and expel the urine through the urethra. When urine is expelled, the

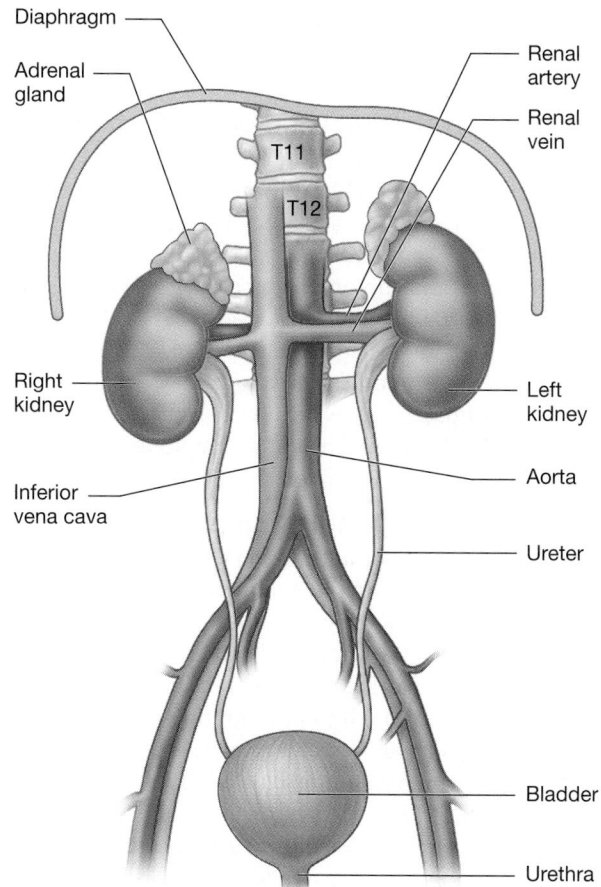

FIGURE 44–5 ■ The renal system.

voluntarily controlled external sphincter and the autonomically controlled internal sphincter must open. The length of the urethra is 3 to 5 centimeters in women and approximately 20 centimeters in men.

The reproductive organs are also found in the abdomen. These structures are found in the pelvic region in both males and females. Examination of this system will be addressed in Chapter 48 ⊙.

History

A thorough history will help the nurse identify gastrointestinal and urinary symptoms as well as current or potential problems that may affect system function. Information learned from a thorough history and physical exam could help prevent undesirable responses to current therapies and treatment plans. The essential assessment data included in the gastrointestinal and urinary history are outlined next.

Biographic and Demographic Data

Biographic and demographic data can lead to a myriad of information to assist the nurse in narrowing the questions, thinking of potential causes of the problem, and formulating how to pose questions and educational plans to meet the patient's needs.

Biographical data should include age, gender, culture, and educational background. Age and gender are important in narrowing the potential causes of the patient's initial complaint. For

instance, **intussusception** is a common cause of intestinal obstruction in children 2 years of age and younger, but is not seen in adults. It is also three times more commonly seen in male children than females (Hackman, Newman, & Ford, 2005). The same is true of **pyloric stenosis**, as this is a cause of regurgitation and poor feeding in infants, generally within the first month, but would not be the cause of similar complaints in adults. Pyloric stenosis is not more gender prominent. Alternately, if an infant were having left lower quadrant abdominal pain, the nurse would not be thinking about diverticulitis in children or adolescents, which would be a common cause in adults and more common in people older than age 40 (Bullard & Rothenberger, 2005).

Demographic data may also glean important information. If a patient lives in an agricultural area or has well water as a source of drinking water, *Giardia* and *Cryptosporidium* infections need to be considered in the case of ongoing diarrhea and abdominal cramping. This might not be the common differential diagnosis for a person who lives in a high-rise apartment in the city.

Cultural Considerations

Cultural background is important in understanding many aspects of communication and care, because it may greatly influence the patient's perception of the complaint, who to speak with in the family, and what interventions the patient may have sought on her own. Additionally, if the patient has recently traveled to her country of origin, it may provide a clue as to other causes not commonly seen. For example, certain types of parasites may be more prevalent in other countries than in the United States.

It is important to consider the patient's cultural background and be sensitive to other therapies the patient might have relied on to decrease his symptoms. In Japanese, Chinese, and East Indian cultures, ginger might have been used for complaints of abdominal pain or digestive issues (Erickson D'Avanzo & Geissler, 2003). If ginger has been used for a period of time, there is a concern regarding bleeding times, because this herb may inhibit platelet aggregation and decrease platelet thromboxane production. This could be catastrophic if the cause of the initial complaint were an ulcer and now the patient is at greater risk from internal bleeding.

Chief Complaint

It is important to allow the patient to express his concerns and explain his problem in his own words. Interruptions should be kept to a minimum, but clarifying questions should be asked. Keep an open mind, because sometimes information that is initially thought of as trivial can be the answer to the problem. A patient with chest pain has a thorough cardiac work-up without any indication of the source of the chest pain. The condition still remains troublesome and the patient mentions an intake of a half gallon of ice cream on a daily basis. Although the symptoms are not common to lactose intolerance, it turns out the chest pain symptoms are resolved after a trial of stopping the ice cream for 2 weeks. This would not have been recognized if the interviewer had not listened to what the patient was saying and kept an open mind.

Taking a history is a very important encounter with a patient. This is a time when a relationship with a patient is started. Therefore, it is vital to develop these skills early in nursing practice.

Because there are core questions when taking a history, it is best to develop a systematic approach that fits one's personal style and comfort level. As a beginner, the nurse should try different methods she has observed used by others. As the nurse becomes an expert, an individual style will emerge, allowing all important information to be gathered and a relationship with the patient established. Characteristics, duration, exacerbation or diminishment of symptoms, and what is wrong or feared by the patient define the chief complaint.

Present Symptoms

Asking the question, Tell me how your symptoms started, is an appropriate way to start an interview. This open-ended question allows the patient to tell the nurse the history of her complaint. Allow the patient the time to answer such questions while giving her nonverbal feedback such as nodding. This can be followed by more clarifying questions, such as, Are there any exacerbating events? Is it reproducible? What has changed since the onset of your symptoms? Does the pain get worse after you eat? Has the character or intensity of the pain changed over time? Can you do something that makes the diarrhea start or go away? These are a few examples of clarifying questions to assist in homing in on the problem. This further clarifies the complaint. If there is pain present, ask the patient to describe it. This is sometimes difficult, especially with children who do not have the verbal skills or the vocabulary to describe what they are feeling.

When interviewing adults, the nurse should have a number of adjectives in his repertoire in order to assist the patient. Typical terms are described in Chart 44–2. *Stabbing, crushing, dull, sharp, radiating, knifelike*, and *burning* are a few of the adjectives that will assist the patient in giving a better description of symptoms. Listen to the words the person uses in characterizing her symptoms, as this can lead to further clues. A complaint of burning or gnawing pain can be associated with ulcers emanating from the duodenum or the stomach. However, these ulcers can be differentiated by the timing and the cause of the symptoms. For example, duodenal ulcers are generally postprandial and awake the subject at night, whereas the pain of the gastric ulcer is precipitated by food. A complaint of burning with urination can be associated with a urinary tract infection.

Duration of Symptoms

How long the problem has been present is very revealing. Has the person waited 4 months to have something evaluated? Possibly there was a change in the characteristic that prompted the sudden attention. Are the symptoms short in duration, but continue to return? Is there something happening in common with the return of the symptoms? A female patient may have had mild symptoms of stress incontinence such as leaking when coughing or sneezing for some time but would just wear a panty liner. Now she is experiencing incontinence when she has the urge to void so the problem has worsened and she is now seeking care.

Exacerbation or Diminishment of Symptoms

Many times a patient will try "home remedies" before presenting for evaluation of a problem. Be open to asking about alternative therapies such as acupuncture, herbal remedies, or moxibustion (an Asian medicine therapy). Did anything the patient tried make the symptoms better or worse? Why did the patient think a certain action would work? The answer to this question can lead into what the patient thinks in wrong. For instance, if the patient thinks his obstructive symptoms were caused by constipation alone, the use of laxatives not only could be ineffective but also could make the symptoms worse by causing increased peristalsis.

What Is Wrong? What Is Feared?

This leads to a very important and sometimes missed area of exploration. What does the patient *think* is wrong with her? Many times, the patient will have a very good idea of what might be the cause of the problem, without really knowing it. Other times, the possibility of exploring the patient's fears of what might be the cause allows the nurse the opportunity to allay her anxieties. Does the patient's culture lead her to believe certain things? For example, in the Hmong culture, illness is believed to be caused by either evil spirits or the loss of a spirit; therefore, it might be difficult for a person of this culture to believe that the cause of diarrhea is from poorly prepared foods (Erickson D'Avanzo & Geissler, 2003).

Is the weight loss due to a fear of eating, or is the person eating frequently in order to make the symptoms subside? Weight loss can be associated with gastric ulcers because of the avoidance of the pain. On the other hand, patients suffering from duodenal ulcers might gain weight as they are eating more frequently to avoid the symptoms. Does the patient notice a change in his skin color or the color of his urine? This could be very important, as hepatitis A can lead to dark-colored urine.

By the end of this part of the interview, the nurse needs to have information regarding the following characteristics: location, quality of the discomfort or pain, severity of the symptoms, onset and duration of the complaint, any changes to the symptoms, and what makes it better or worse. If any of these questions are not answered, the nurse needs to use more focused questions. Examples of sample questions are listed in Chart 44–3.

Past Medical History

Past medical history should always include certain elements; childhood diseases, immunizations, major illnesses, hospitalizations, diagnostic procedures, surgeries, sexual history, medications, and allergies are all considered imperative when gathering data. If the patient is vague regarding the information or does not remember the name of a procedure, assist the patient by giving the best description. For instance, a childhood illness may have required hospitalization or surgery, but the patient might not know whether she had pyloric stenosis or a bowel obstruction. A surgery for a repair of pyloric stenosis is more common in the first 6 months of life, whereas a bowel obstruction from intussusception can be seen up to 2 years of age. Having knowledge regarding surgical procedures and age-

CHART 44–2	**Descriptive Terms**	
Gnawing	Burning	Ripping
Colicky	Stabbing	Dull
Sharp	Crushing	Aching
Localized	Diffuse	

CHART 44–3	**Examples of History Questions**
Location	Where does it hurt the most?
Severity	At the time it is the most painful, how would you rate the pain on a scale of 1–10, with 10 being the worst?
	Does the pain change as it becomes more severe?
Duration	How long does the pain last?
Quality	What does the pain feel like?
Onset	When did the pain start?
	What were the circumstances of the pain starting?
Aggravating factors	What makes the pain worse?
Alleviating factors	What do you do to make the pain better?
Changes	Have your symptoms changed over a period of time?
	Does your pain change from one episode to another?

related diseases can assist in helping the patient clarify possible childhood history.

It is important also to consider where the patient was raised. Practices and availability of medical care and hospitalization will differ between industrialized nations and third world countries. In some circumstances the availability of medical history might be difficult if not impossible to obtain.

Childhood Illnesses and Immunizations

Childhood illnesses should include a history of any significant illnesses. Patients with a history of celiac disease and cystic fibrosis commonly will have an association with stooling problems and obstruction due to the bulking of the stool. A history of streptococcal infection, hypoplastic kidneys, or obstructive uropathy can lead to urinary tract or renal dysfunction as an adult.

Specifically ask about immunizations commonly given for hepatitis, hepatitis B, and hepatitis A. There is also a hepatitis D vaccine, although it is less common. A history of a cholera vaccine may be less common, unless there has been recent travel or if the patient has been residing in another country.

Previous Illnesses and Hospitalizations

A history of major illnesses is important and may impact the chief complaint. For instance, a person whose diabetes is poorly controlled who presents with symptoms of a partial bowel obstruction may be having **gastroparesis,** a slowing in emptying of the stomach due to the diabetes. A patient with hypertension and diabetes may develop renal failure due to the vascular changes with decreased circulation to the kidneys. A history of

Crohn's disease not only can be related to multiple surgeries but also heightens the awareness of the potential for anal fissures and fistulas.

The nurse should ask the patient about medical problems for which the patient is currently being treated. Ask whether there is any diagnosis the patient has been given in the past. A patient may be treated for recurrent hemorrhoids due to intermittent bright-red blood from the rectum. However, if the patient has never had a colonoscopy, the atrioventricular (AV) malformation in the lower colon might be missed as the diagnosis. Chart 44–4 lists common major illnesses.

Diagnostic Procedures and Surgeries

A history of procedures is important in the history of gastrointestinal and urinary diseases. Frequent procedures may include endoscopic evaluations. Common endoscopic evaluations include the following: **endoscopic retrograde cholangiopancreatography (ERCP),** radiography following injection of a radiopaque material into the papilla of Vater; **flexible sigmoidoscopy,** a sigmoidoscope that uses fiber optics to inspect the sigmoid colon; and **colonoscopy,** visualization of the lower gastrointestinal tract through a flexible endoscope inserted through the anus. Patients might not remember what the name of the test is but would recall what symptoms led to the test. A person would not get an ERCP, which looks for gallbladder and pancreatic causes, if the chief complaint were blood in the stool.

As well as invasive testing, radiologic testing might be utilized in a work-up of GI symptomatology. Upper GI studies as well as a barium enema are common radiologic tests. An upper GI study might be the test of choice in a patient complaining of reflux. On the other hand, a **barium enema** is going to assist in evaluation of diverticular disease or possibly a tumor. For the renal system, a kidney-ureter-bladder (KUB) radiograph, intravenous pyelogram (IVP), renal ultrasound, computed tomography (CT), or magnetic resonance imaging, and renal angiography may help with a diagnosis.

When obtaining medical history from patients with gastrointestinal symptoms, past surgeries also play a major role. It is also important to correlate this information with the physical exam. At times patients will forget a surgery, especially if it was many years ago. Therefore, correlating the history with the scars on their abdomen is a helpful tool. When doing the abdominal examination, confirm what operation relates to which scar. This can also trigger more information from the patient. Pay particular attention to the area around the umbilicus, as laparoscopic scars are small and can be very faint. Chart 44–5 (p. 1374) lists common gastrointestinal surgeries.

Sexual History

A person's sexual practices can have an effect on certain gastrointestinal and urinary complaints. It is important to become comfortable with asking patients not only about their sexual

CHART 44–4	**Major Illnesses with GI-Related Complaints**			
Celiac sprue	Diabetes	Hirschsprung's disease	Crohn's disease	HIV
Alcoholism	Hyperlipidemia	Cystic fibrosis	Cancer	Hepatitis (A, B, C)
Inflammatory bowel disease	Thyroid problems	Hypertension	Hypercholesteremia	Depressive disorders

CHART 44–5	**Common Gastrointestinal Surgeries**

Appendectomy—removal of the appendix

Cholecystectomy—removal of the gallbladder

Choledochojejunostomy—opening between the common bile duct and the jejunum

Colostomy—opening of the colon through the abdominal wall

Gastrectomy—removal of part or all of the stomach

Ileostomy—opening of the ileum through the abdominal wall

Pyloroplasty—repair of the pylorus or to increase the opening

Vagotomy—resection of the branch of the vagus nerve

activity but also about their individual practices. The more self-conscious and uncomfortable the nurse is with asking these questions, the more the patient is going to be reluctant to self-disclose.

Anal intercourse can be related to disease of the anus and the rectum. Rectal cancer from human *papillomavirus* is important to catch and treat early. It is also possible to get other sexually transmitted diseases such as gonorrhea in the rectum. If the question is never asked, the problem will be overlooked with potential detrimental results for the patient. If a woman has frequent cystitis, it is important to ask and teach her that urinating shortly after intercourse is important to flush any bacteria that might have entered the urethra.

Medications

Medication history should include what is prescribed, what is taken over the counter, and also medications given to the patient by friends or family. Over-the-counter antacid is a commonly overused medication. What type and how often the medication is taken may also be important. Remember to include questions about laxatives and enemas. Inquire as to how frequently patients are using these agents. A frequent use of either can cause a decrease in bowel tone and thus increase the constipation and therefore the use of the laxative.

A history of frequent aspirin or nonsteroidal anti-inflammatory drug (NSAID) use is also significant. Make sure to ask about both. Are patients taking either of these frequently and then following it with an antacid in order to make the stomach pains subside so they can treat the discomfort from arthritis? NSAIDs, antihypertensive drugs that block angiotensin, and aminoglycoside antibiotics can cause an acute or chronic decline in kidney function.

Remember to ask about the use of herbal remedies or supplements. Some of the medications can be hepatotoxic or have other adverse effects not known to the patient. If the medication is a combination of medicines, it is sometimes difficult to verify exactly what the patient is taking, especially if the supplement is a combination of different types of herbs. At times further research is warranted to find all the different ingredients in a powder or tincture.

Allergies

A history of allergies should include not only the offending agent but also the allergic symptom it produces. Many patients mistake nausea as an allergic reaction when it is only a side effect. Also include any food or environmental allergies. Food allergies are especially important when examining a patient for gastrointestinal symptoms. Ask whether there is a certain food that is avoided due to undesirable effects.

Family History

A thorough family history is important and should include a relevant health history of the patient's siblings, parents, and grandparents. Some patients will include a medical history of a relative not related by blood. In other words, a patient may provide a medical history of an uncle, and the nurse may find out the uncle is married to the mother's sister. The nurse must make sure to clarify that she wants only direct relatives included in the history. Some diseases of the gastrointestinal system with hereditary components are Crohn's, familial polyposis, colon cancer, and malabsorption of nutrients such as fructose and folate. Adult onset diseases of the renal system with hereditary components include polycystic disease of the kidney, renal amyloidosis, and some renal cancers.

Social History

Social history includes any alcohol, tobacco, or recreational drug usage, including how often and how much of the substance is used or taken. For example, if a patient has a positive history of smoking, ask how many cigarettes he smokes per day. The same is true for alcohol use to determine whether he is at risk for hepatic disease due to the years of alcohol consumption. Some patients may be reluctant to discuss these habits. Ask these questions in a matter of fact way so the patient does not feel stigmatized or judged. Patients also need to know that this information is confidential and used only to assist in their care.

Habits

Changes in a patient's normal routine can provide clues to the nurse regarding the symptomology of the complaint. This information will also help to guide the nurse's line of questioning.

The nurse should ask the patient about her diet. Have there been any changes related to her current complaint? A recent change in diet can affect gastrointestinal illnesses. An example is the patient who completes a liquid fast and then starts eating again. This sudden stimulation may cause a first attack of cholecystitis, an inflammation of the gallbladder.

Stool patterns also should be included in this section. What is the patient's normal stool pattern? For some patients, stooling 1 to 2 times per week is very normal, whereas others need to have daily movement. Are there changes in consistency or color? Pencil-thin stools can be a concern for colon cancer but also can indicate large hemorrhoids. Is the act of defecation painful? Rectal fissures can be excruciating and lead to constipation due to the fear of defecation.

Patients who are developing renal failure may experience a metallic taste in their mouth from the uremia, which may cause a decrease in appetite. Also, rapid weight gain accompanied by orthopnea may be a sign of fluid overload from renal failure.

Recent Travel

Any recent history of travel is significant information to obtain. Certain gastrointestinal illnesses such as diarrhea are commonly linked to travel. Traveler's diarrhea is a common illness of many travelers both abroad and locally. This is a name commonly used when a person has diarrhea either while traveling or after; but it can be caused by many different agents including viral, bacterial, and parasitic organisms, and is generally contracted through contaminated food or water. It can be self-limiting or cause problems for an extended period of time. Certain organisms such as *Vibrio cholerae* may be common only in certain areas, but *Giardia* can be found in most countries, including the United States. Therefore, it is important to get a complete history of travel, both recent and as far back as several years, if necessary.

Physical Examination

When performing the physical examination of the patient with abdominal complaints, it is imperative that the nurse take a systematic approach to the examination. If it is done out of order, important findings may be obscured due to pain and the patient's subsequent inability to cooperate with the examination. The order is different than when assessing other systems. Inspection should come first, followed by auscultation, percussion, and finally palpation to avoid eliciting or increasing pain. It is important for the nurse to assess the patient's general state of health. Examining a patient experiencing pain from appendicitis is very different from examining a patient with complaints of mild diarrhea. Positioning the patient for the optimal examination does not always mean it is optimal for the examiner. For instance, a patient may not be able to lie flat in a supine position. A more comfortable position may be to have the knees bent. The nurse should work with the patient in establishing a comfortable position for the patient; this will make the examination more productive for both of them.

Inspection

The first element of the physical examination of the abdomen is inspection. This is done initially by just watching the patient. Is the patient able to walk with a normal posture, or is the person walking hunched over, protecting her abdomen? When the patient is sitting, is her posture normal? Is the patient able to sit or is she curled into a fetal position on the examination table or bed? Is the patient able to be still or must she move about due to the colicky pain of **renal calculi** (kidney stones)? These observations are the first part of the data collection and contribute to the ongoing collection of data.

Inspection should include the mouth. Inspect the mucosa for redness, any lesions, and moistness. The tongue should be inspected for any redness, inflammation, fissure, ulcerations, or lesions. The pharynx is evaluated by using a tongue blade to hold the tongue out of the way. Having the patient tilt his head back slightly assists in visualization of the soft palate, uvula, and movement of this structure. Inspect the uvula, tonsils, soft palate, and anterior and posterior pillars. Have the patient say "aah," and the soft palate and uvula should rise symmetrically. Inspection continues after the patient is lying flat and the abdomen is exposed. This might be difficult if the patient is unable to lie flat due to pain. However, inspection can be done with the patient in different positions, although this may not be as optimal.

Before the patient is touched, important data can be collected. Look at the contour of the patient's abdomen both obliquely and straight on. Sometimes masses, fluid waves, or change in contour can be seen. A **ventral hernia**, a hernia through the abdominal wall, is very distinct in an oblique view, particularly when the patient contracts the abdominal muscles. Look at the umbilicus, which is normally midline and inverted. The umbilicus will become everted with pregnancy, ascites, or an underlying mass. It can become enlarged and everted with an umbilical hernia. Observe the skin for any changes such as scars, color changes, hair patterns, or presence of striae. Note that hair patterns will vary between male and female patients. There can also be differences between different races. Female patients with hirsutism, excessive growth of hair in unusual places, may have increased hair growth along the pubic mons extending to the umbilicus. Asian women will demonstrate finer and scarcer patterns than Caucasian or African American women. The nurse should also be cognizant of coloration changes between skin tones. For example, what appears red on a light skin tone will have a different appearance on a darker skin tone. Observe the skin for redness with localized inflammation, jaundice with hepatitis, rashes, or cutaneous angiomas (spider nevi) that occur with portal hypertension or liver disease.

The inspection is the time to ask about the scars and the surgery related to them. Sometimes readdressing questions during this time will assist the patient in recalling further information. It also allows the nurse to ask a question in a slightly different manner, causing further recollection for the patient.

Auscultation

Auscultation is the second step in the physical examination process. This is an important step, and the nurse should become comfortable with auscultation and the sound of the abdomen. However, contrary to previous teaching, in the realm of an abdominal examination, bowel sounds may mean very little. A person can have acute peritonitis but still have bowel sounds. A patient with a postoperative ileus may have very loud bowel sounds, but the patient is distended and the bowels are not functioning in a coordinated pattern. Complete absence of bowel sounds would be significant, but keep in mind that the nurse would have to listen for a minimum of 5 minutes in all four quadrants. That being said, bowel sounds should be auscultated prior to palpation, as the deep palpation can affect the frequency of bowel sounds. The nurse should listen over all four quadrants for a period of 2 to 5 minutes. Note the frequency, pitch, and character of the bowel sounds. Ask the patient about passing flatus. Like all parts of the examination, it should be correlated with the history.

When placing a nasogastric tube, auscultation of the abdomen is imperative. The nurse should always listen over the epigastrium while pushing air in the tube after placement. A gurgling sound over this area should be heard if the nasogastric tube is in the correct position.

The epigastrium and bilateral upper quadrants should be auscultated with both the diaphragm and the bell of the stethoscope. This is the area to listen for the aorta and renal arteries. The nurse is listening for a bruit or schussing sound, which is an indication of an abnormality. Both groins should also be auscultated for bruits of the iliac arteries. Figure 44–6 ■ (p. 1376) indicates sites to listen for vascular sounds.

A ticklish patient may not tolerate the touch of the stethoscope. Having the patient place the stethoscope where the nurse

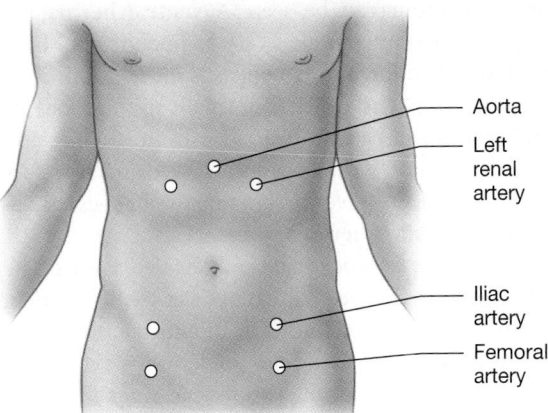

Aorta

Left renal artery

Iliac artery

Femoral artery

Sites to listen for vascular sounds

FIGURE 44–6 ■ Sites for vascular sounds.

directs will enhance the examination of this type of patient. This not only distracts the patient, but avoids tickling.

Percussion

Percussion, the third step in the physical examination process, is done by placing the nondominant hand flat on the surface of the abdomen. The first joint of the index or third finger is then struck gently with the index or third finger of the dominant hand (Figure 44–7 ■). The nurse should practice this on different types of surfaces and listen to the difference in the sound. A good example is on a melon or even a thigh. The nurse should be able to hear the difference. It is also important to have nails clipped short so as not to cause injury to self or the patient.

Percussing the abdomen will elicit different sounds. There should be the hollow sound, similar to that of tapping on a watermelon, over the epigastric area and sometimes over the bowels. If this hollow sound is throughout the entire abdomen, it is called **tympany** and is indicative of an obstruction or distention of the abdomen. This sound is produced by air in the intestine.

The liver and a full bladder give off a dull sound, similar to that when percussing a piece of meat. The liver edges can be determined by percussing from the lower right abdomen to the edge of the rib. At the transition of the hollow sound to the dull sound, the nurse will find the liver edge. Measure this area by determining how many finger breadths it is from the costal margin.

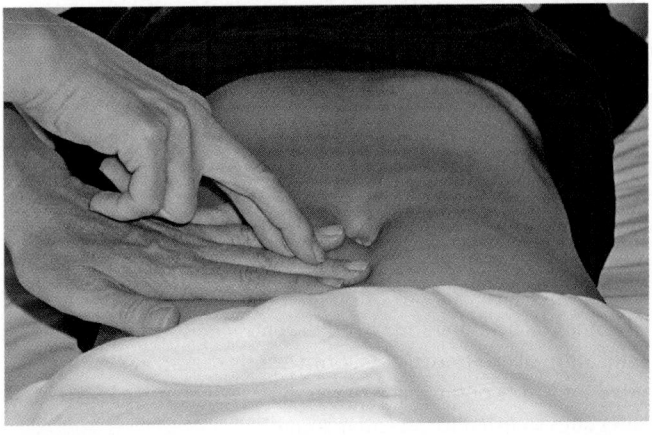

FIGURE 44–7 ■ Percussion of abdomen.
Source: Cheryl Wraa

Similarly, the spleen can be measured in the same fashion. However, the edge of the spleen should not be below the costal margin. It is more likely found near the 10th left rib. If it is below the rib, this is an indication of an abnormal enlargement. Palpation of the area should be done with great care. Percussion can also elicit pain particularly in patients with acute peritonitis, inflammation of the peritoneum.

The size of the bladder can be percussed especially if the patient has a full or distended bladder. In order to percuss the kidney, the patient must be lying on one side or be in a sitting position. The nurse should make a fist and gently strike the patient with the ulnar surface of the fist in the costal vertebral angle. This should be jarring to the patient, but should not elicit any pain. If this action causes pain, it is a sign of kidney infection or injury.

Case Study

A female patient presents with a history of nausea, vomiting, and abdominal pain. On further questioning she reveals she has been tired recently and thinks she has the flu because of generalized body aches. She usually smokes a pack a day but has had only 2 to 3 cigarettes in the past 2 days. She attributes this to not feeling well. She thinks she caught a flu virus because she recently spent over 10 hours on a plane while returning from a trip overseas.

On inspection the nurse notes that the patient has a yellowish tinge to her skin. She has diffused abdominal pain greater in the right upper quadrant. When the nurse percusses the right upper quadrant, there is a dull sound extending 3 finger breadths below the right costal margin. This indicates the patient has hepatomegaly. The most likely cause of this patient's complaints is hepatitis A.

The clinician reaches this conclusion by reviewing the information gathered from both the history and the physical examination.

Palpation

Palpation, the final step in the physical examination process, should start with the mouth and throat area. Any lesions or abnormalities of the oral pharynx should be palpated using a gloved finger. Lesions of the cheek are better felt by placing one finger inside the mouth and one on the cheek. By isolating the lesion between the fingers, the size and shape of the lesion is better defined.

Palpation of the abdomen should be done in a systematic pattern. Start with light palpation. This assists in the identification of muscle resistance and more superficial findings. In patients who are sensitive, even light palpation will cause muscle resistance. Maneuvers to relax the patient are having her bend her legs, using a stethoscope to palpate, or having the patient place her hand under the nurse's, using her hand to press down. After the patient becomes relaxed, the nurse can slide the nurse's hand under the patient's hand. When using the stethoscope to palpate, place the stethoscope on the abdomen, and while listening, the nurse can press harder on the abdomen, eliciting any pain the patient might sense.

The next step is deeper palpation. The nurse should use the palmar surface of the hand and palpate in all four quadrants. If the patient has a complaint of abdominal pain, palpate the area the patient identified as painful last.

The liver edge should be palpable. The nurse should recall where he first percussed the edges of the liver border and place his fingertips below this area. The hand should be placed lateral to the rectus muscle on the right hand side. Press gently down and up toward the ribs (Figure 44–8 ■). The nurse should have the patient take a deep breath. As the patient is inhaling, the liver edge will come down under the nurse's fingertips. A normal liver feels firm, sharp, and has a clear edge. A cirrhotic liver will feel stiffer and the edge will be irregular. The edge will also be palpable farther down on the abdomen.

To palpate the spleen, the nurse should be standing on the patient's right. Reach across with the left hand and place it on the lateral chest wall at the 10th rib. The hand should be placed below the costal margin. While supporting the rib with the left hand, gently palpate up toward and under the costal margin. As the patient takes a deep breath, the tip of the spleen might be palpated as it descends. The spleen is not always palpable, especially in adults. If it is easily palpated below the costal margin, the spleen is considered enlarged and medical staff should be notified.

Both the kidneys should be palpated, but the right kidney is easily palpated and the left kidney is rarely felt. When palpating the right kidney, place the left hand on the right flank area with gentle pressure toward the abdomen. Place the right hand on the abdomen parallel to the costal margin. Press the hands firmly together. The lower pole of the kidney should be felt as the patient takes a deep breath. At times the patient will have a sharp sensation as the kidney pole passes through the nurse's hands. This is not considered a painful sensation.

The left kidney is rarely palpable. However, this area should be examined for any abnormalities. The maneuver is the same. Place the left hand along the flank area. In some patients this can be accomplished from the right side of the table. However, if the patient is large or the left side cannot be reached in this fashion, perform this examination from the left side of the table (Figure 44–9 ■). The kidneys should feel firm and smooth. It is considered abnormal if an irregular surface is palpated, the kidney extends significantly lower than the rib cage, or obvious trauma is noted.

The aorta is palpated in the area above the umbilicus and slightly left. This may be difficult to palpate in the obese abdomen and can sometimes be seen as pulsating in the scaphoid

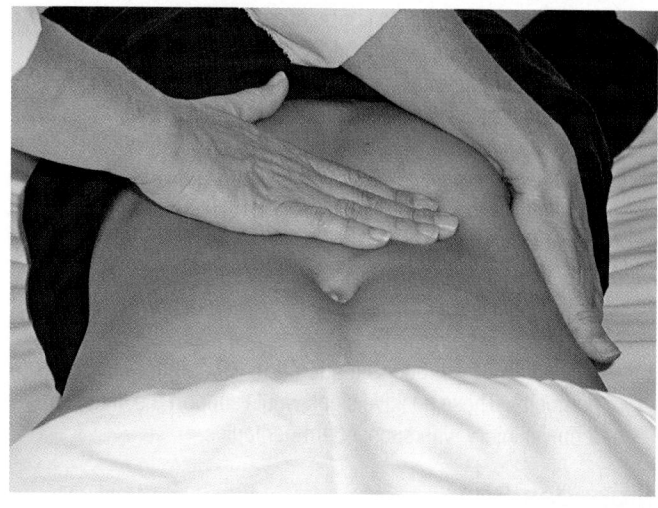

FIGURE 44–9 ■ Palpation of kidneys.
Source: Cheryl Wraa

abdomen. If the pulsation of the aorta is easily palpated, attempt to isolate it between the thumb and finger.

■ Adjunctive Physical Examinations

Certain physical examinations are specific to conditions of the abdomen in particular. These adjunctive exams will assist in narrowing or confirming the nurse's differential diagnosis.

Rebound Tenderness

Rebound tenderness describes tenderness greater when the pressure is released than when it is applied and is a reliable sign of peritoneal inflammation. To perform this test the nurse gently presses into the abdomen and then releases the pressure. Start light and then with greater firmness as the examination warrants. Start away from the area of pain and work toward the area identified by the patient as hurting the most. If a great deal of discomfort is found away from the identified source, stop. There is no further benefit of causing more pain to the patient.

Case Study

A 16-year-old male presents after a motor vehicle crash. On inspection an ecchymotic stripe is seen across the lower abdomen about 4 to 5 centimeters below the umbilicus. There are no other masses visualized. When palpating, the upper quadrants are palpated first, as the ecchymotic area will be the most tender. The initial examination reveals mild tenderness to palpation in the left lower quadrant. There is no rebound at the initial examination.

The continued work-up would include lab tests, primarily a complete blood count (CBC), to examine hemorrhagic anemia or leukocytosis to indicate an inflammatory process.

After several hours, this male patient complains of increased abdominal pain. The CT scan showed some free fluid in the pelvis, but no injury to the spleen or the liver. The concern would be a progressing injury. By reviewing all the information, the most likely cause for the increased pain is a possible bowel injury.

The method in which this patient is examined will be changed to meet his changing complaints. Palpation should always be farthest away from the point of identified pain. At this

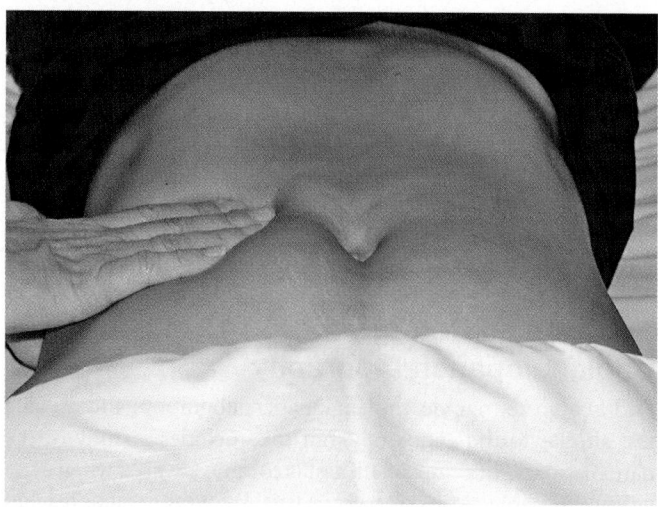

FIGURE 44–8 ■ Palpation of abdomen.
Source: Cheryl Wraa

juncture, palpation should not be done with the fingertips, but rather by placing the middle finger gently on the surface of the abdomen and tapping over the second joint with the finger of the other hand. Pain elicited with this maneuver is common in patients with peritonitis. If the patient has involuntary contraction of the abdominal muscles and pain with this examination, it may not be necessary to proceed further. However, if this does not indicate increased pain, examination for rebound tenderness may be required. This is done by pressing in gently with the fingertips of one hand and releasing rapidly. If the pain is worse at the time the fingertips are released, the examination is positive for rebound tenderness, yet another indication of peritonitis. These positive signs would support the diagnosis of a bowel injury with subsequent peritonitis.

Iliopsoas Sign

When this test is positive, it indicates an inflammation of the psoas muscle, which lies lateral to the lumbar vertebrae and passes deep into the inguinal ligament to the lesser trochanter of the femur. The lumbar plexus of nerves is embedded in the psoas. The iliacus muscle lies along the lateral side of the psoas muscle and extends across the sacroiliac joint to attach to the iliac fossa. Together these muscles form the iliopsoas, the chief flexor of the thigh. Clinically, the **iliopsoas** has relations to the kidneys, ureters, cecum, appendix, sigmoid colon, pancreas, lumbar lymph nodes, and nerves of the posterior abdominal wall. When there is intra-abdominal inflammation or disease of any of theses structures, movement of the iliopsoas causes pain. With the patient lying flat, have the patient flex the leg closest to the examiner. With the nurse's hand flat against the lateral surface of the thigh, have the patient push against the palm with some resistance applied. The test is positive if this causes the patient pain. Repeat on the other side.

Obturator Sign

This test is positive in patients with inflammation along the obturator internus muscle. Positive tests can be related to appendicitis, diverticulitis, and pelvic inflammatory disease, to name a few. The nurse should stand along the side of the bed while performing this test. Have the patient bend her knee and flex at the hip. While supporting the leg, flex the thigh to a right angle and externally and internally rotate the leg. Perform this on both sides.

Murphy's Sign

This test is positive when a person has inflammation of the gallbladder, as seen in cholecystitis. The nurse should stand on the right side of the bed. Place the hand flat on the abdomen with the fingertips just below the right costal margin. Have the patient gently inhale. As the liver and gallbladder descend into the fingertips, pain will be present when there is inflammation.

◼ Radiologic Testing

The use of radiologic testing is important in establishing the diagnosis of many abdominal complaints. Although it is not the goal of this chapter to provide education on all radiologic tests, a few will be listed.

Computed Tomography Scan of the Abdomen and Pelvis

The CT scan is very versatile in the information it provides to the clinician caring for the patient. Abscesses, fluid collections, vascular disorders, obstructions, and trauma can be seen. For trauma, however, this test is better for injury to solid organs such as the liver and spleen, rather than to hollow organs such of the bowel or bladder. This test can utilize intravenous, rectal, or oral contrast to enhance the images.

Ultrasound

Ultrasound is used for evaluation of the gallbladder, kidneys, and urinary tract, and at times the appendix. It can also be used for identification of free fluid in trauma patients with suspected intrabdominal injury.

Kidney-Ureter-Bladder (KUB) Versus Three-Way Abdominal Films

A **KUB** stands for kidney, ureters, and bladder and is also known as a "plain film of the abdomen." This is obtained with the patient lying flat and the x-ray plate placed beneath. It helps to determine position, size, and structure of the kidneys and urinary tract. It is useful in evaluating for the presence of calculi and masses. Also, this is an excellent test for obstruction, because it shows the air in the colon nicely. The three-way abdominal series not only incorporates the KUB view but also includes a picture of the abdomen with the patient on his side as well as one upright. This test helps differentiate air fluid levels in the intestinal tract.

Barium Enema

In this radiologic test, barium contrast is inserted in the rectum. The barium fills the colon and shows the contour of the intralumen. This test would enhance intraluminal processes such as colon cancer or diverticular disease.

◼ Invasive Procedures

Invasive procedures are uncomfortable and at times painful. For that reason, most of these procedures are done with conscious sedation.

Colonoscopy and Endoscopy

Colonoscopy and endoscopy allow the clinician to visualize the intraluminal space directly. The colonoscopy is a flexible tube with a small camera at the end that is inserted through the rectum and visualizes the intraluminal surface of the colon. This instrument also allows for biopsies to be taken. The same is true for the endoscopy; however, this similar flexible tube visualizes the upper GI tract and is inserted through the mouth.

Endoscopic Retrograde Cholangiopancreatography

Endoscopic retrograde cholangiopancreatography (ERCP) is a test similar to the endoscopy, but this includes a study of the pancreatic and bile ducts. This test is commonly used when evaluating for cholecystitis or pancreatitis. When the scope reaches the duodenum, the endoscopist locates the opening into the ducts or the ampulla. A small tube is placed in the ampulla, and contrast dye is injected that allows for visualization of the ducts. Removal of stones, biopsy, and sphincterotomy may be performed during this procedure.

Common Laboratory Studies

The significance of these laboratory tests (Chart 44–6) will be discussed in more detail in the disorder chapters. Chart 44–6 lists common studies used in the assessment of gastrointestinal, liver, pancreatic, renal, and urinary functions and their clinical significance.

Gerontological Considerations

The aging adult may have increased deposits of subcutaneous fat on the abdomen and hips as it redistributes away from the ex-

tremities. The musculature of the abdomen is thinner and has less tone. If the patient is thin, the nurse may be able to visualize peristalsis when the patient is lying supine. Also, the softer abdominal wall may make palpation of the organs easier. Because the lungs may be distended and the diaphragm depressed, the liver is palpated lower, appearing 1 to 2 centimeters below the costal margin with inhalation.

Summary

All nurses need to have the skills to understand and assess patients with abdominal and urinary complaints. Although these are common complaints of patients, the causes can be very complicated, with a large number of differential diagnoses. Therefore, it is important for the nurse to understand the underlying anatomy and physiology. With practice and further experience, the skills of the interview and examination will improve.

CHART 44–6   **Common Laboratory Studies**

Study	Clinical Significance
Studies of GI function	
• Stool culture	Detection of bacteria, ameba, or worms
	Large amounts of pus associated with ulcerative colitis, abscesses, and anorectal fistula
Studies of liver function	
• Alkaline phosphatase	↑ with biliary obstruction and hepatitis
• Aspartate aminotransferase (AST)	↑ with hepatocellular injury
• Alanine aminotransferase (ALT)	↑ with hepatocellular injury
• Lactate dehydrogenase (LDH)	↑ with hypoxic and primary liver injury
• Serum bilirubin	
• Indirect	↑ with hemolysis
• Direct	↑ with hepatocellular injury or obstruction
• Total	↑ with biliary obstruction
• Urine bilirubin	↓ with biliary obstruction
• Urine urobilinogen	↑ with hemolysis or shunting
• Albumin	↓ with hepatocellular injury
• Globulin	↑ with hepatitis
• Prothrombin time	↑ with chronic liver disease or vitamin K deficiency
• Partial thromboplastin time	↑ with severe liver disease or heparin therapy
Studies of pancreatic function	
• Serum amylase	↑ with pancreatic inflammation
• Serum lipase	↑ with pancreatic inflammation
• Urine amylase	↑ with pancreatic inflammation
• Stool fat	Decreased pancreatic lipase increases stool fat
Studies of renal function	
• Blood urea nitrogen (BUN)	↑ with poor renal function
• Serum creatinine	↑ with damage to nephrons
• Urine osmolality	↑ fluid volume deficit
	↓ fluid volume excess
• Serum osmolality	↑ fluid volume deficit
	↓ fluid volume excess

NCLEX® REVIEW

1. An adult patient is experiencing left lower quadrant pain. The nurse realizes this patient might be demonstrating:
   1. Acute appendicitis.
   2. Intussusception.
   3. Pyloric stenosis.
   4. Diverticulitis.

2. The nurse is preparing to conduct a physical examination on a patient. Which of the following should the nurse do first?
   1. Inspection
   2. Percussion
   3. Auscultation
   4. Palpation

3. When percussing a patient's bladder, the nurse hears a dull sound. Which of the following would this sound indicate?
   1. An empty bladder
   2. A bladder obstruction
   3. Kidney stones
   4. A full bladder

4. While assessing a patient, the nurse discovers rebound tenderness. This finding would be indicative of:
   1. Enlarged gallbladder.
   2. A negative obturator sign.
   3. Inflammatory process in the abdomen.
   4. A positive Murphy's sign.

5. A patient states she has had no abdominal surgeries but the nurse sees a large abdominal scar. Which should the nurse do?
   1. Document what the patient stated.
   2. Ask the patient what caused the abdominal scar.
   3. Assume the patient doesn't want to talk about the scar and change the subject.
   4. Palpate the scar.

Answers for review questions appear in Appendix D

KEY TERMS

anal canal *p.1369*
antrum *p.1367*
barium enema *p.1373*
cardia *p.1367*
cardioesophageal *p.1367*
colon *p.1369*
colonoscopy *p.1373*
endoscopic retrograde
   cholangiopancreatography
   (ERCP) *p.1373*

esophagus *p.1367*
flexible sigmoidoscopy *p.1373*
gastroparesis *p.1373*
GERD, gastroesophageal reflux
   disease *p.1367*
iliopsoas *p.1378*
immunoglobulin A *p.1366*
intussusception *p.1371*
KUB *p.1378*

peristalsis *p.1367*
pharyngoesophageal *p.1367*
pyloric stenosis *p.1371*
rectum *p.1369*
renal calculi *p.1375*
retroperitoneal space *p.1367*
tympany *p.1376*
ventral hernia *p.1375*

REFERENCES

Bullard, K.M., & Rothenberger, D. A. (2005). Colon, rectum and anus. *Schwartz's principles of surgery*. Retrieved February 26, 2006, from http://www. accessmedicine.com/content.aspx?aID=810060&searchStr=colon

Erickson D'Avanzo, C., & Geissler, E. (2003). *Mosby's pocket guide: Cultural health assessment*. St. Louis: Elsevier.

Fisher, W. E., Andersen, D. K., Bell, R. H., Saluja, A. K., & Bruinicardi, F. C. (2005). Pancreas. *Schwartz's principles of surgery*. Retrieved February 24, 2006, from http://www.accessmedicine.com/content.aspx?aID=812451&searchStr=pancreatic+juice#812451

Hackman, D. J., Newman, K., & Ford, H. R. (2005). Gastrointestinal tract. *Schwartz's principles of surgery*. Retrieved February 25, 2007,

from http://www.accessmedicine.com/content.aspx?aID=818606&searchStr=intussusception#818606

Urdan, L. D., Stacy, K. M., & Lough, M. E. (2006). *Thelan's critical care nursing* (5th ed.). St. Louis: Mosby.

Caring for the Patient with Gastrointestinal Disorders

Debera Thomas
Douglas Sutton

Outcome-Based Learning Objectives

After studying this chapter, the learner will be able to:

1. Describe the different causes of stomatitis and related nursing care.

2. Compare and contrast pathophysiology, clinical manifestations, and treatment with related nursing care of patients with peptic ulcer disease (PUD) and gastroesophageal reflux disease (GERD).

3. Develop a teaching plan for patients with celiac disease.

4. Analyze the similarities and differences between different types of inflammatory bowel disease.

5. List the risk factors for developing GERD.

6. Delineate nursing care for a patient with colon cancer.

7. Describe the different intestinal tubes and related nursing care for patients with intestinal obstruction.

8. Discuss the clinical manifestations of the complications of gastric surgery.

9. Outline the nursing care of a patient with an ileostomy, colostomy, and continent ileostomy.

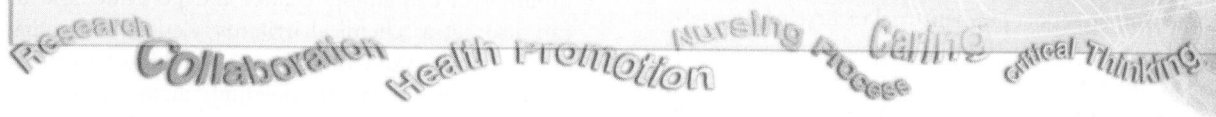

THE GASTROINTESTINAL (GI) tract consists of a hollow tube extending from the mouth to the anus and includes the esophagus, stomach, small intestine, large intestine, and rectum, as well as the accessory organs involved in digestion such as the pancreas, liver, and gallbladder. Anatomy of the gastrointestinal tract is presented in Chapter 44 ☺, and disorders of the liver, gallbladder, and pancreas are discussed in Chapter 46 ☺. Because the major functions of the GI tract are to prepare ingested food for absorption, absorb nutrients, and eliminate wastes, disorders of this system can have devastating effects on nutritional status, lifestyle, body image, and health in general. Most disorders of the GI tract can be classified as inflammatory, ulcerative, structural, or neural in nature.

DISORDERS OF THE MOUTH AND ESOPHAGUS

Disorders of the mouth and esophagus are the result of a variety of causes ranging from viral to nutritional. Likewise, diseases may be as common as a gastroesophageal reflux disease or as serious as esophageal cancer.

◼ Stomatitis

Stomatitis, the generalized inflammation of the oral mucosa, is classified according to the etiology. Similar to stomatitis is glos-

sitis, or inflammation of the tongue, which is caused by many of the same factors that cause stomatitis, so they may often coexist. These problems may be caused by a virus, bacteria, fungus, trauma, chemical agents, or nutritional deficiencies.

Pathophysiology

The oral mucosa consists of a thin, fragile layer of squamous epithelial cells with a rich blood supply. Cellular turnover is rapid, thus promoting quick healing but also providing an opportunity for cellular mutation and damage to these rapidly dividing cells. Because of the abundant blood supply and the fragility of the epithelial cells, the risks for infection, inflammation, and trauma are increased. Diagnosis is made by noting the history of current symptoms, including the presence of systemic illness or evidence of trauma (e.g., broken teeth, ill-fitting dentures), physical examination, culture, and/or biopsy.

Etiology

Etiology of disorders of the mouth and esophagus include the following: viral, bacterial, fungal, traumatic, chemical, and even nutritional deficiencies.

Viral Causes

Herpetic stomatitis is very common because herpes simplex viral (HSV) infection is widespread in the United States. It is estimated that between 30% and 100% of the U.S. population has HSV-specific antibodies, which indicate a past or dormant infection, and that up to 20% of the adult population is shedding the virus at any given time. Any previous infection of HSV (anywhere on the body) is the primary risk factor for all secondary manifestations of herpes simplex infection (McCaffrey, Thrush, Dunphy, & Porter, 2007).

Initial exposure to HSV results in consistently sized vesicles that are most commonly found on the tongue, on buccal and labial mucosae, and occasionally on the palate. The vesicles rupture and progress to painful ulcerations that are similar to aphthous ulcers and resolve in 10 to 14 days. Any condition that decreases the immune response, such as diabetes mellitus, HIV infection, cancer, chemotherapy, immunosuppressive medications, or aging, can increase the likelihood of viral reactivation causing recurrent stomatitis.

Bacterial Causes

Aphthous stomatitis (or **contact stomatitis**), commonly known as canker sores, is an ulcerative condition limited to the oral cavity. In fact, an estimated 20% of the population is affected at some time and 33% develops recurrent lesions that can continue for 40 years. Although the pathogenesis is unclear, an immunologic response to antigens in the buccal cavity is believed to be responsible for this type of stomatitis. Other possible causes and contributing factors are psychological stress, vitamin deficiencies, genetic predisposition, trauma, allergies, and viruses. The prevalence is higher in people with some autoimmune diseases, such as inflammatory bowel disease (Jackler & Kaplan, 2004), and some women report premenstrual recurrences.

There are four phases in the development of aphthous stomatitis. The premonitory phase is characterized by a tingling, burning, or hyperesthetic sensation that can last up to 24 hours. The preulcerative phase lasts from 18 hours to 3 days and is characterized by painful red macules or papules with erythematous halos. Next, the ulcerative phase, lasting from 1 to 16 days, is characterized by painful ulcers 2 to 10 millimeters in diameter and covered by a grayish yellow membrane. As this phase progresses, the pain ceases. The healing phase can last from 4 to 5 weeks, but the lesions are usually healed in 2 weeks.

Vincent's stomatitis, also known as acute necrotizing stomatitis or "trench mouth," is an acute bacterial infection of the gingiva oral mucous membranes caused most often by the bacteria *Borrelia vincentii*. It occurs in people with conditions that decrease the tissue's resistance, such as poor nutrition, extreme emotional stress, leukemia, severe systemic infections, and other conditions that decrease immunocompetence.

The clinical manifestations of Vincent's stomatitis include erythematous ulceration and necrosis of the gingival margins and oral mucosa. The interdental gingival papillae are red, reduced in size, and appear raw and painful. There is a characteristic purulent gray exudate, and the person complains of pain, increased salivation, gums that bleed easily, and bad breath. There may also be systemic manifestations such as malaise, anorexia, and enlarged lymph nodes in the neck (cervical).

Fungal Causes

Oral candidiasis is extremely common and occurs largely as a result of a compromised immune system or a disruption of the normal oral flora. This type of stomatitis results from an overgrowth of the yeast-like fungus *Candida albicans*. The overgrowth can result from antibiotic therapy, which destroys the normal flora in the oral cavity, as well as from the chronic use of inhaled steroids. When the immune system is compromised by such things as cancer chemotherapy treatments, radiation treatments to the head, immunosuppressive medications (glucocorticoids, antirejection drugs), aging, diabetes, emotional stress, malnourishment, or HIV/AIDS, *Candida* infection often occurs. The manifestations of oral candidiasis include white curd-like patches on the tongue, palate, and oral mucosa. Under the white patches, the surface of the tissue is red and sore, although the person usually complains that the lesions are dry or hot, rather than actually painful (Jackler & Kaplan, 2004).

Traumatic Causes

Traumatic oral ulcers are very common and occur most often at the tongue margins and buccal mucosa. It is often difficult to differentiate traumatic ulcers from aphthous stomatitis other than by history and the report of pain; traumatic ulcers are usually not as painful as aphthous ulcers. Common traumatic causes include thermal injury (hot beverage, hot pizza) and physical injury. Mechanical injury can result from ill-fitting dentures, malocclusion, broken teeth, and habitual cheek biting.

Chemical Causes

Chemical irritation can cause stomatitis. Common chemical irritants include spicy, acidic, or salty foods such as potato chips, pickles, and hot pepper sauce. Dental care products such as mouthwash containing alcohol and peroxide, and toothpaste can also act as chemical irritants. Cancer chemotherapy frequently causes stomatitis because, in addition to attacking cancer cells that are rapidly dividing, chemotherapy agents also attack other rapidly dividing cells, such as the mucous epithelial cells in the oral cavity. The chemical irritation from tobacco, whether smoking, dipping, or chewing, results in nicotinic stomatitis (McCaffrey et al., 2007). Bulimia can be a risk factor for stomatitis because of the repeated exposure of the oral mucosa to stomach acid from vomiting.

Nutritional Deficiencies

Several vitamin deficiencies can cause stomatitis, particularly angular stomatitis, glossitis, cheilosis, or, in other words, a sore mouth. The vitamin deficiencies, although rare in the United States, can be caused by malnutrition, malabsorption, alcoholism, restrictive dieting, and fad dieting. Stomatitis and glossitis are caused from deficiencies in many of the B vitamins. Both vitamin B_2 (riboflavin) and vitamin B_6 (pyridoxine) deficiency cause cheilosis and glossitis, whereas a deficiency in folate or B_{12} (cobalamin) can cause glossitis (Jackler & Kaplan, 2004).

No Known Cause

Benign migratory glossitis, also known as geographic tongue, erythema migrans, and stomatitis areata migrans, as the name implies, is a benign condition occurring in up to 3% of the population and is more frequently reported in people with psoriasis. It is characterized by the loss of papillae in some areas of the tongue. These areas are smooth and erythematous, giving the tongue a "maplike" appearance, hence the name *geographic tongue*. In addition, the areas can change in size, location, and appearance daily. Often the person with this condition complains of soreness or burning of the tongue exacerbated by hot, spicy, or acidic foods (Kelsch, 2007).

Medical Management

Medical management includes treatment of the causative factor if known and relief of symptoms.

Drug Therapy

The health care provider may order topical oral anesthetics such as 2% viscous lidocaine. The nurse should ensure that the patient rinse his mouth with the viscous lidocaine, then spit it out, because swallowing the solution may impair the ability to swallow. However, for patients who have lesions in the upper esophagus, the solution may be swallowed to relieve the pain of these lesions. The nurse should inform the patient that the lidocaine may be used every 3 hours as needed. Using lidocaine before meals may help improve oral intake. Agents that coat the oral mucosa may also be helpful in relieving the discomfort of stomatitis. Agents such as magnesium hydroxide (Milk of Magnesia) and kaolin (Kaopectate) may relieve the pain, particularly of aphthous ulcers, while providing protection of the lesions from further irritation. A mixed solution of 1 part diphenhydramine (Benadryl) for inflammation, 1 part aluminum-magnesium hydroxide (Maalox) for irritation and acidity, and 1 part viscous Xylocaine for pain is frequently ordered to relieve a combination of symptoms and improve appetite/nutritional status.

Anti-infectives will be ordered for the patient with stomatitis caused by viruses, bacteria, or fungus and are dispensed in topical, oral, or intravenous (IV) formulations. Antibiotics such as oral penicillin V potassium (Pen-Vee K) are usually effective for Vincent's stomatitis, but for severe gangrenous cases, IV antibiotics may be required. Antifungal agents such as nystatin suspension are prescribed for *Candida* infection. The nurse instructs the patient to swish the suspension around in the mouth for about 2 minutes and then swallow it. The antifungal agent may also be prescribed in a lozenge, which is held in the mouth until it is dissolved and swallowed. The nurse should instruct the patient to abstain from eating or drinking for 30 minutes after taking the medication.

Antiviral agents are prescribed for herpes simplex stomatitis. For patients with intact immune systems, oral acyclovir (Zovirax) is used. Continued use decreases the frequency and severity of the acute episodes. In patients with compromised immune systems, such as those with HIV/AIDS or those taking immunosuppressive medications, IV acyclovir may be needed. Nursing responsibilities include teaching the patient and the family that the medication does not cure the disease and that the virus remains latent in the body and may recur during times of physical or emotional stress. The Pharmacology Summary (p. 1384) feature outlines medications used to treat stomatitis.

Nursing Management

Assessment

Nursing care focuses on assessing the condition of the oral mucosa and determining how these inflammatory conditions are impacting the patient's well-being, specifically nutritional status.

Planning

The treatment of stomatitis and similar conditions is focused on treating the underlying cause, such as correcting vitamin deficiencies, removing the source of traumatic or chemical irritation, or medicating for the infecting organism.

Interventions and Rationales

For all causes of stomatitis, nursing care focuses on good oral hygiene. Frequent mouth care helps debride oral lesions and can decrease the chance of the patient's developing a superinfection. Mouth care using a soft toothbrush, toothette, or water pick should be done every 2 hours for stomatitis that is not controlled. It is essential to teach patients to avoid harsh mouthwashes, particularly those that contain alcohol, because these can irritate the ulcerated mucosa. The mouth can be rinsed with diluted hydrogen peroxide, warm saline, or sodium bicarbonate solution (1 teaspoon of baking soda per 8-ounce glass of water).

Another important nursing intervention for patients with stomatitis is nutritional assessment. It is often painful for patients to eat or drink when they have stomatitis, so the nurse should encourage a high-calorie, high-protein diet. Often, soft, bland foods are better tolerated and cool or cold foods may be soothing. Acidic foods such as citrus juices and tomatoes should be avoided, as well as spicy or hot foods. Weighing the patient daily can help establish the adequacy of the patient's caloric intake.

 *Contact stomatitis, or aphthous stomatitis, is an inflammatory reaction of the oral mucosa that occurs as a result of contact with irritants or allergens. Patients who report an allergy to latex may be susceptible to developing contact stomatitis if the nurse uses latex gloves when examining the oral mucosa. The incidence of latex allergy, in both patient and nurse populations, has been steadily increasing during recent years, thus requiring the nurse to determine the presence of latex allergy prior to implementing care (Lopes & Lopes, 2000).*

Oral Cancer

Oral cancer can occur on any surface of the mouth, including the lips, tongue, and pharynx. According to the Oral Cancer Foundation (2007), approximately 34,000 people in the United States would be newly diagnosed with oral cancer in 2007. Worldwide, the problem would be far greater, with more than 481,000 new cases expected. Of those diagnosed in 2007, only half will be alive in 5 years, and this number has not been improved in decades. The death rate for oral cancer is higher than that of the brain, liver, testes, kidney, or skin cancer (malignant melanoma). This is in part due to the fact that most oral cancers are found at a late stage. Only 5% of all cancers are oral cancer. The most prevalent risk factor for oral cancer is the use of tobacco, both smoking and smokeless (chewing tobacco). The use of tobacco is associated with 75% of all cases of oral cancer (Lynch, 2007). Other risk factors include drinking alcohol, Betel quid chewing, Areca nut use, human papillomavirus (HPV), abuse of narcotics, cannabis use, and human immunodeficiency virus (HIV) seropositivity. Predisposing risk factors include increasing age, male gender, and genetics (Lynch, 2007). Almost all oral cancers are attributed to lifestyle choices.

PHARMACOLOGY Summary of Medications Used to Treat Stomatitis

Medication Category	Action	Application/Indication	Nursing Responsibility
Anti-Infective Agents			
Antibiotics: Penicillin V potassium (Pen-Vee K)	Exerts bacteriocidal activity by destroying and inhibiting synthesis of bacterial cell wall.	Fusospirochetosis (Vincent's pharyngitis); pneumococcal, streptococcal, and nonpenicillinase-producing staphylococcal infections; endocarditis risk prophylaxis.	Monitor for adverse effects: nausea, vomiting, and diarrhea. Monitor for hypersensitivity reaction: pruititis, urticaria, fever, edema, arthralgia, and anaphylaxis. Give after a meal. Warn female patients that oral contraceptives may be rendered ineffective.
Metronidazole (Flagyl)	Exerts antibacterial and antiprotozoan activity by inhibiting DNA synthesis of infecting organism.	Intestinal amebiasis, colorectal surgery prophylaxis, *H. pylori* eradication, Crohn's disease, diverticulitis, pseudomembranous colitis, anaerobic bacterial infections.	Monitor for adverse effects: nausea, vomiting, anorexia, abdominal pain, dizziness, headache, peripheral neuropathy, seizures, and *Candida* overgrowth. Monitor liver function tests if hepatic dysfunction present. Be aware of multiple drug interactions; monitor for drug toxicities (theophylline, warfarin, disulfiram, and others). Instruct patient not to consume alcohol while taking drug and for at least 24 hours after last dose.
Ciprofloxacin (Cipro)	Exerts bacteriocidal activity on gram-negative and gram-positive bacteria by disrupting DNA replication.	Diverticulitis, infectious diarrhea, intra-abdominal infections.	Monitor for adverse effects: nausea, vomiting, diarrhea, rash, headache, peripheral neuropathy, seizures, and signs of *Candida* overgrowth. Monitor for acute onset of joint pain: notify health care provider. Monitor kidney and liver function if renal or hepatic impairment present. Be aware of multiple drug interactions; monitor for drug toxicities (theophylline, warfarin, procainamide, and others). Give medication 6 hours after or 2 hours before antacid or vitamin administration. Warn patient about possible photosensitivity and need for sunblock. Be aware of extensive IV drug incompatibilities.
Antifungal: Nystatin (Mycostatin, Nilstat)	Exerts fungistatic and fungicidal activity by disrupting permeability of fungal cell wall.	Local *Candida* infections, e.g., oropharyngeal, intestinal candidiasis.	Monitor for signs of contact dermatitis. Instruct patient not to eat or drink for 30 minutes after treatment for oral candidiasis.
Antiviral: Acyclovir (Zovirax)	Decreases viral shedding, formation of new lesions, and healing time by interfering with viral DNA synthesis.	Mucosal and cutaneous herpes simplex virus.	Monitor for adverse effects: headache, nausea, vomiting, and diarrhea. Monitor renal function, especially with IV administration.

Pathophysiology

Most oral cancers are squamous cell carcinoma, arising from the flat cells that line the oral cavity. This form of cancer is slow growing and may not produce symptoms until the tumor is well advanced, usually after invasion of the adjacent tissues and metastasis to other areas has occurred. The tumor ulcerates, produces pain, and may also present other symptoms such as irritation of the tongue, sore throat, and difficulty wearing dentures because of painful irritation. Oftentimes the patient with oral cancer will complain of otalgia (ear pain), which is referred from the oropharynx.

The second most common oral cancer is basal cell carcinoma, which occurs almost exclusively on the lips beyond the vermilion border. The characteristic lesion of this type of cancer is a nodule with an ulcerated center and raised pearly border. Although basal cell carcinoma does not metastasize, it can be locally invasive.

Etiology

The most widely recognized risk factor for the development of oral cancer is tobacco use. Tobacco contains chemicals that are known carcinogens, causing mutations in cellular DNA. Smokeless tobacco is particularly hazardous because the chemicals are absorbed directly through the oral mucosa. Heavy alcohol consumption is also a risk factor for oral cancer and has a synergistic effect with tobacco (Burgess, 2006). Other risk factors include marijuana use, infection with certain types of human papillomavirus, and repeated exposure to chemicals or irritation, such as poorly fitting dentures or broken teeth. Basal cell carcinoma is almost exclusively caused by prolonged sun exposure, placing people who work outdoors in sunny climates at greater risk for this type of cancer.

Medical Management

Elimination of causative factors or sources of irritation, such as all forms of tobacco or alcohol, is the initial treatment for oral cancer. Analgesics, coating agents, and oral anesthetic agents may be prescribed to relieve discomfort. (See the Stomatitis section earlier in this chapter (p. 1381) for a discussion of these agents.) Biopsy of the lesion is needed to diagnose the type of cancer. Tumor staging usually requires additional studies such as a magnetic resonance imaging (MRI) or computed tomography (CT) scan. Treatment is based on the extent of the cancer and presence of metastasis. Radiation may be prescribed before surgery in order to shrink the tumor. Radiation and chemotherapy may be appropriate postoperatively depending on the stage of the tumor and the patient's general health.

Excision of the tumor is usually the treatment of choice unless the tumor is very far advanced and considered unresectable. The goal of surgery is to remove the cancerous tissue, but the surrounding tissue and lymph nodes may also be removed to assure there is no local infiltration of cancerous cells. A radical neck dissection may be performed if the tumor is advanced. This procedure involves the removal of lymph nodes and muscles in the neck and is disfiguring. A tracheostomy will be performed during surgery to maintain adequate respiratory support and may become permanent depending on the extent of the neck dissection and subsequent respiratory function.

■ Nursing Management

Nursing management of the patient with oral cancer centers on elimination of causative factors, care of the oral mucosa, and the nutritional status of the patient before and after surgery. The Nursing Process: Patient Care Plan feature (p. 1386) outlines care for oral cancer.

Health Promotion

Eliminating tobacco use is the single most important factor in risk reduction of oral cancer. Because smokeless tobacco use is highest in males ages 15 to 22, the nurse should target this group for education. Smoking cessation, as well as limiting alcohol consumption, should be encouraged for everyone. Use of sunscreen on the face and lips can reduce the risk of basal cell carcinoma. Routine dental visits are also important in the early detection of oral cancers, as well as for keeping dentition in good repair.

Early detection is key to improving the prognosis of patients with oral cancer. In addition to identifying patients with risk factors, oral inspection may prove invaluable, as seen in the Evidence-Based Practice feature (p. 1387).

■ Hiatal Hernia

A **hiatal hernia** involves the herniation of the upper portion of the stomach into the thorax through the esophageal hiatus. There are two types of hiatal hernia. The most common, the **sliding (direct) hiatal hernia**, occurs 90% of the time (Huether, 2006). The second type is the **rolling (paraesophageal) hernia**. Hiatal hernia is believed to be a very common problem, but the majority of individuals have no symptoms. The incidence of hiatal hernia increases with age.

Gerontological Considerations

Hiatal hernias are more prevalent in Western countries, and the frequency increases with age. Up to 70% of patients who are 70 years of age will develop a hiatal hernia. It is thought that muscle weakening and a loss of elasticity are the primary factors that predispose the elderly patient to have an increased risk of developing a hiatal hernia. Physiologically, as the tissue elasticity is decreased due to aging, the gastric cardia may not return to its original position below the diaphragmatic hiatus. Hiatal hernias are more common in women, and it is thought that this may be due to the increased intra-abdominal pressures associated with pregnancy (Qureshi, 2006).

Pathophysiology/Etiology

The point at which the esophagus and vagus nerve pass through the diaphragm is an inherent area of weakness. In a sliding hiatal hernia, a portion of the fundus of the stomach moves upward through the esophageal hiatus into the thoracic cavity (Figure 45–1A ■, p. 1388). Several factors contribute to this condition, including a congenitally short esophagus, trauma, or weakening of the diaphragm at the gastroesophageal junction (Huether, 2006). The movement of the stomach upward occurs most often when the individual is lying down. Obesity and pregnancy exacerbate this type of hernia, as does anything that increases the intra-abdominal pressure, such as eating a large meal. When the individual assumes a standing position, the hernia slides back into the abdominal cavity. With this type of hernia, there is a **lower esophageal sphincter (LES)** pressure resulting in **gastroesophageal reflux** and esophagitis.

In a paraesophageal hernia (rolling hernia), there is herniation of the greater curvature of the stomach through the esophageal hiatus. The gastroesophageal junction remains in the normal position below the diaphragm (Figure 45–1B ■, p. 1388), and reflux is unusual. However, there can be congestion of the mucosal blood flow in the portion of the stomach in the thorax that can lead to gastritis and ulceration. In rare instances, there can be strangulation of the hernia, causing ischemia and hemorrhage, and this requires surgical intervention.

Both types of hiatal hernia produce similar symptoms, if symptoms are present at all. The primary symptom is reflux and heartburn. Patients often complain of feeling full, belching, and indigestion. Because the stomach herniates into the thoracic cavity near the midline, patients may complain of substernal chest pain and think they may be having a heart attack.

Medical Management

For patients with mild symptoms, the lifestyle changes mentioned earlier may provide symptom relief. The primary care provider may prescribe a **histamine₂ (H₂)-receptor blocker** (ranitidine, famotidine) or a **proton pump inhibitor (PPI)** (lansoprazole, omeprazole) to reduce gastroesophageal reflux.

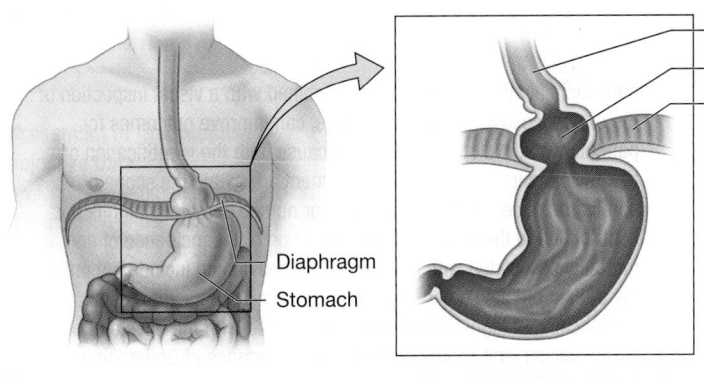

(a)

Herniation of the stomach through the hiatal opening

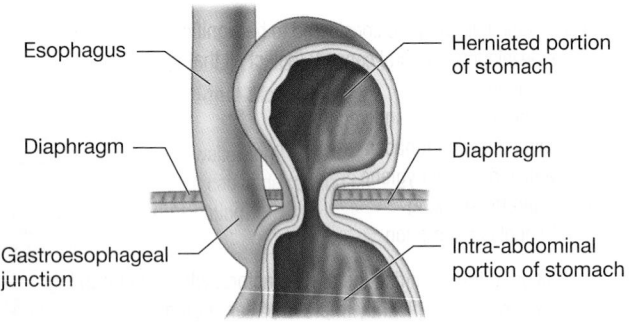

(b)

FIGURE 45–1 ■ (A) Hiatal hernia and (B) Paraesophageal hernia.

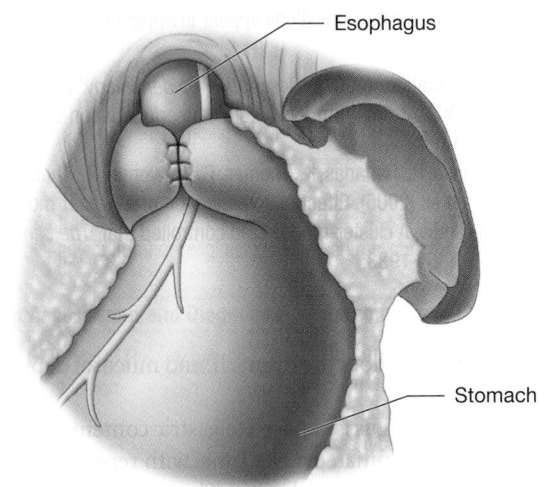

FIGURE 45–2 ■ Nissen fundoplication.

beta-adrenergic blockers (Inderal), calcium channel blockers (verapamil), estrogen, progesterone, diazepam (Valium), and theophylline. Nicotine also lowers LES, including the levels obtained via secondhand smoke (Thomas, 2007).

Clinical Manifestations

The most common symptom of GERD is heartburn, which can be mild to severe in nature. Additional symptoms that commonly occur are a sour taste in the morning on arising, regurgitation, dysphagia, coughing, belching, and chest pain. Atypical

symptoms include asthma or a sore throat. There are usually no outward physical signs that the patient has GERD, although the stool may test positive for occult blood due to possible microhemorrhages in the irritated esophageal mucosa.

Medical Management

The medical management of GERD is to educate patients regarding causative factors and assist them to make lifestyle changes. If the symptoms persist, then additional tests will be done to try to identify a cause.

Diagnostic Procedures

The diagnosis of GERD is most often made by symptomatology and predisposing risk factors. Unfortunately, the severity of the disease does not always correlate with the severity of the symptoms. In fact, severe disease may exist with few symptoms. If symptoms persist after 4 weeks of conservative treatment and lifestyle changes, an upper endoscopy may be done to visualize the esophagus directly and obtain tissue samples (Sherman, 2007). The tissue is examined for signs of Barrett's epithelium and malignancy. (Chart 45–1 details nursing care of the patient undergoing endoscopy.) Ambulatory esophageal pH monitoring is the most accurate way to diagnose GERD. In this test, a pH probe is placed 5 centimeters above the LES, and the pH is measured for 24 hours. If the pH is less than 4 above the LES, then GERD is diagnosed, especially if there are corresponding symptoms. Esophageal manometry measures the pressures of the LES and is used to determine its location before 24-hour ambulatory pH monitoring is done. Occasionally a barium swallow may be done to evaluate the esophagus and stomach and visualize a hiatal hernia.

Diet and Lifestyle Modifications

Lifestyle modifications including diet are key in the treatment of GERD. Many patients may have total symptom relief through these efforts alone. Foods that lower LES pressure (mentioned earlier) should be eliminated from the diet or ingested on an infrequent basis following use of medication to prevent symptoms. Because spicy foods may irritate the esophageal mucosa, they should be avoided as well. It is often helpful to eat small frequent meals with the largest meal at midday. The patient should avoid eating anything within 4 hours of bedtime, and the head of the bed should be elevated. Depending on the amount of caffeine an individual drinks, complete withdrawal may cause headaches so gradual elimination is preferred. Weight loss is important in patients who are overweight or obese. A regular exercise program such as daily walking can promote digestion as well as weight loss, thus diminishing symptoms. Tight garments or belts may increase symptoms by increasing intra-abdominal pressure and should be avoided. Smoking cessation should be considered a priority.

Medications

Medications for GERD can be purchased over the counter and prescribed. It is important to know whether the patient has been self-medicating, what the patient has used, and whether it has helped to relieve the symptoms.

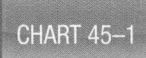

CHART 45–1   Nursing Care of a Patient Undergoing Endoscopy

PREPROCEDURE

- Explain the procedure again (should have been explained by the health care provider), and assure signed consent is in the chart.
- Assure NPO 8 to 12 hours prior to test.
- Record name of person driving the patient home after the test (patient CANNOT drive after the test).
- Place name band on wrist and have the patient change into a hospital gown.
- Have the patient remove any jewelry, dentures, or eyeglasses.
- Ensure the patient empties his bladder before the procedure.
- Take vital signs and start an IV for sedation.
- Answer any questions the patient has about the procedure, and explain that there may be a sensation of pressure as the endoscope is inserted and fullness in the stomach as air is injected to expand the stomach and allow for better visualization.

POSTPROCEDURE

- Frequent vital signs.
- Check gag reflex.
- NPO until gag reflex returns.
- Monitor for signs of complications: pain, dyspnea, tachycardia, or subcutaneous emphysema in the neck.
- Tell the patient to expect flatus or eructation resulting from the instillation of air during the procedure.
- Ensure that the patient does not drive himself home.

Antacids

Antacids are part of the initial treatment of GERD and often provide relief for mild to moderate symptoms. Antacids buffer (increase pH) the gastric contents and help to prevent further mucosal damage. Antacids are available without a prescription and are frequently used by individuals with heartburn even before they seek medical attention. Examples of antacids are Mylanta, Maalox, Tums, Rolaids, and Riopan. Gaviscon, an alginate-antacid, forms a floating barrier and prevents upright reflux.

Histamine$_2$-Receptor Blockers

Most H$_2$-receptor blockers, such as cimetidine (Tagamet), ranitidine (Zantac), nizatidine (Axid), and famotidine (Pepcid), are available without a prescription and are approved for the treatment of GERD. They are effective in reducing the secretion of gastric acid. They are usually taken twice a day for extended periods of time. The prescription strength of these drugs may be more beneficial if the patient has self-medicated with the lower doses before diagnosis.

Proton Pump Inhibitors

Gastric secretions can also be reduced by proton pump inhibitors such as omeprazole (Prilosec), lansoprazole (Previcid), rabeprazole (Aciphex), esomeprazole (Nexium), or pantoprazole (Protonix). These medications are very effective in treating GERD and have now been approved for long-term use. They may be needed for 6 months or longer. Proton pump inhibitors have been shown to heal the erosive lesions in addition to decreasing acid production.

Other Medications

Drugs such as metoclopramide (Reglan) promote gastric motility and speed gastric emptying, but do not affect acid secretion. By enhancing gastric motility, metoclopramide reduces the amount of time gastric contents have to potentially contact esophageal mucosa. Long-term use is not recommended, and use is associated with side effects such as fatigue, anxiety, ataxia, and even hallucinations. The Pharmacology summary feature (p. 1390) outlines medications used to treat gastroesophageal reflux.

Surgery

Most patients respond favorably to lifestyle modification and drug treatment, but there are some who require surgery to have resolution of GERD. Surgery involves increasing the pressure in the lower esophagus in order to prevent reflux of gastric contents. Several laparoscopic procedures are used either to tighten the LES with sutures or to cause scar tissue to form in the muscles surrounding the sphincter. The most common antireflux surgical procedure is the Nissen fundoplication (see Figure 45–2 ■).

■ Nursing Management

Nursing care for the patient with GERD focuses primarily on assessment, prevention of complications, and patient/family teaching. The Nursing Process: Patient Care Plan feature (p. 1391) shows a protocol for the patient with GERD.

Health Promotion

Teach patients and community members that frequent heartburn may be a sign of GERD and that they should seek treatment. The long-term consequences of untreated GERD can be serious and include esophageal strictures, Barrett's esophagus, and the possibility of esophageal cancer.

■ Achalasia

Achalasia is a motor disorder of the esophagus that is characterized by failure of the LES to relax properly and impaired peristalsis. This is caused by defective innervation of the smooth muscle of the esophagus and LES. Normally, the LES has tonic contractions with intermittent relaxation.

Pathophysiology

In the patient with achalasia, the LES fails to relax in response to swallowing as well as a loss of normal peristalsis. The etiology of this disorder is unknown, but it is believed to be a result of defective inhibitory pathways of the esophageal enteric nervous system. It results in a functional obstruction because the esophagus is unable to empty properly. The clinical manifestations include chronic and progressive dysphagia, regurgitation, and chest pain. Over time, the esophagus may be able to hold as much as 1 liter of material containing old, putrefying food, pus, and fluid. Aspiration pneumonia, esophageal ulceration, and rupture can result.

PHARMACOLOGY Summary of Medications Used to Treat Gastroesophageal Reflux

Medication Category	Action	Application/Indication	Nursing Responsibility
Histamine$_2$-Receptor Antagonists (H$_2$ Blockers)			
Ranitidine (Zantac) Famotidine (Pepcid) Cimetidine (Tagamet) Nizatidine (Axid)	Inhibits all phases of gastric acid secretion by blocking histamine receptors in gastric parietal cells; decreases volume and hydrogen ion concentration in gastric secretions.	GERD, duodenal ulcers, gastric ulcers, erosive esophagitis, symptomatic hiatal hernia, chronic hypersecretory conditions.	Monitor for adverse effects: rash, nausea, vomiting, constipation, diarrhea, abdominal pain, dizziness, and headache. Monitor blood count. Monitor elderly and patients with hepatic or renal disease for CNS effects. Administer 2 hours before or after administration of antacids. Consider need for B$_{12}$ replacement if given long term.
Proton Pump Inhibitors (PPIs)			
Lansoprazole (Prevacid), Omeprazole (Prilosec) Rabeprazole (Aciphex) Esomeprazole (Nexium) Pantoprazole (Protonix)	Decreases gastric acid by binding with H+/K+ ATPase in the gastric parietal cells, blocking final phase of acid production.	Short-term treatment of GERD (4–8 weeks), peptic ulcers, duodenal ulcers, erosive esophagitis, and symptomatic hiatal hernia; long-term treatment of chronic hypersecretory conditions.	Monitor for adverse effects: diarrhea, constipation, nausea, vomiting, stomach pain, headache, and dizziness. Monitor for altered absorption of medications, vitamins, and minerals requiring an acid environment. Be aware of multiple drug interactions (warfarin, diazepam, phenytoin, digoxin, theophylline, and others); monitor for signs of elevated serum levels. Evaluate need in elderly for calcium replacement, and evaluate for increased incidence of pneumonia. Instruct patient to take medication 30 minutes prior to meal.
Antacids			
Aluminum hydroxide (Amphojel) Calcium carbonate (Tums) Calcium Carbonate/magnesium hydroxide (Rolaids) Magnesium hydroxide (Milk of Magnesia) Magnesium Hydroxide/aluminum hydroxide (Maalox, Mylanta) Magaldrate (Riopan) Sodium bicarbonate (Alka-Seltzer)	Neutralizes gastric acid by increasing gastric pH.	GERD, esophagitis, gastritis, peptic ulcer disease, hyperacidity.	Monitor for constipation if taking calcium- or aluminum-based product, diarrhea if taking magnesium-based product. Monitor patients with renal or cardiac insufficiency for signs of accumulation of sodium, magnesium, or calcium from selected antacid. Monitor for hypophosphatemia if taking antacid containing aluminum. Be aware of multiple drug interactions; administer 2 hours before or after other oral medications if medication absorption may be affected.
Prokinetic Agent			
Metoclopramide (Reglan)	Increases gastric emptying and intestinal transit, apparently by sensitizing GI smooth muscle to acetylcholine; lowers esophageal sphincter tone; relaxes pyloric sphincter; blocks stimulation of medullary chemoreceptor trigger zone (CTZ) receptors for direct antiemetic effect.	Diabetic gastroparesis, GERD unresponsive to standard treatment, as an antiemetic postoperatively, and in chemotherapy and radiation therapy.	Monitor for adverse effects: restlessness, fatigue, drowsiness, insomnia, headache, dizziness, confusion, depression, hallucinations, involuntary movements, and diarrhea. Monitor for drug interaction (levodopa, digoxin, narcotics, tetracycline, and others). Monitor electrolytes for hypernatremia and hypokalemia, especially in patients with cardiac insufficiency or hepatic disease. Administer oral dose 30 minutes prior to meals. Warn patient to avoid alcohol, sedatives, and other CNS depressants. Be aware of multiple IV drug incompatibilities and light sensitivity.

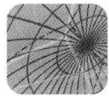

NURSING PROCESS: Patient Care Plan for GERD

Assessment of Discomfort/Pain
Subjective Data:
How often do you experience heartburn?
On a scale of 0–10, with 10 being severe, how would you rate your heartburn?
Do you have a sour taste in the morning when you get up?
Do you ever get a sour or burning sensation in your throat when you bend over or lie down after a meal?
Is your heartburn worse if you wear something tight around your waist?
Are there any foods that cause you discomfort? What are they?
Are you allergic to anything?
Does the pain improve when you eat?
Is your discomfort sharp, dull, gnawing, or burning?
What have you tried to relieve the pain?

Objective Data:
Epigastric tenderness.

Nursing Assessment and Diagnoses	Outcomes and Evaluation Parameters	Planning and Interventions with *Rationales*
Nursing Diagnosis: *Comfort, Readiness for Enhanced* related to esophageal mucosal injury from contact with gastric secretions	**Outcome:** No heartburn. **Evaluation Parameter:** Reports satisfactory control of discomfort.	**Intervention and *Rationale:*** Use pain scale (0–10) to quantify pain and discomfort. *To increase consistency in quantifying pain.*

Assessment of Knowledge of GERD and Treatment
Subjective Data:
What did you have for breakfast, lunch, and so forth?
Do you wear a tight belt or waistband?
Do you wear a girdle or panty hose with a tight waistband?
Do you eat within 2 hours of going to bed?
Do you lie down after eating?
Did you know that GERD is considered a chronic disease? And requires treatment?

Are you aware of the complications associated with GERD if left untreated?
Do you drink coffee, tea, alcohol, citrus juice, or cola?
What medications, OTC, prescription, or herbal, are you taking, and when do you take them?
How often do you eat foods containing mint or drink mint tea?
What are your plans for losing weight?

Nursing Assessment and Diagnoses	Outcomes and Evaluation Parameters	Planning and Interventions with *Rationales*
Nursing Diagnosis: *Knowledge, Readiness for Enhanced* related to treatment and long-term consequences of GERD	**Outcome:** Symptoms reduced. **Evaluation Parameters:** Able to verbalize lifestyle modifications to reduce reflux. Communicates a plan to lose weight. Understands the chronic nature of the disease and long-term consequences as evidenced by ability to articulate the nature of esophageal erosion and Barrett's epithelium.	**Interventions and *Rationales:*** Teach the importance of eating 4–6 small meals a day and to eliminate foods known to decrease lower esophageal sphincter (LES) pressure or cause irritation. *To decrease reflux.* Assess cultural and religious dietary practices. *To explore foods that are culturally based that may decrease LES pressure or cause irritation.* Explain the conversion of squamous epithelial cells to columnar epithelial cells and the possibility of developing cancer if reflux goes untreated over time. *To help the patient understand the consequences of GERD.* Instruct the patient to avoid lying down after eating. *To minimize reflux.* Educate the patient about medication regimen and possible side effects. *To improve adherence to medication regimen.*

Medical Management

The traditional treatment of achalasia has been the use of esophageal dilation or myotomy. Esophageal dilation is done using a balloon catheter (Figure 45–3 ■, p. 1392). The pneumatic dilator (balloon) is placed across the LES, usually under fluoroscopy with local anesthesia. The balloon is inflated to a predetermined level for about 30 to 60 seconds. This causes small tears in the esophageal sphincter muscle fibers, thereby reducing the pressure. The health care provider performs a myotomy using a laparoscope to incise the circular muscle

layer of the LES. A less invasive procedure is performed with the injection of botulinum toxin (**Botox**) into the LES through an endoscopic procedure. The disadvantage of this procedure is that it usually requires repeated treatment every 6 to 9 months.

■ Nursing Management

The nursing management for achalasia includes a detailed assessment of the patient's symptoms and nutrition. The focus

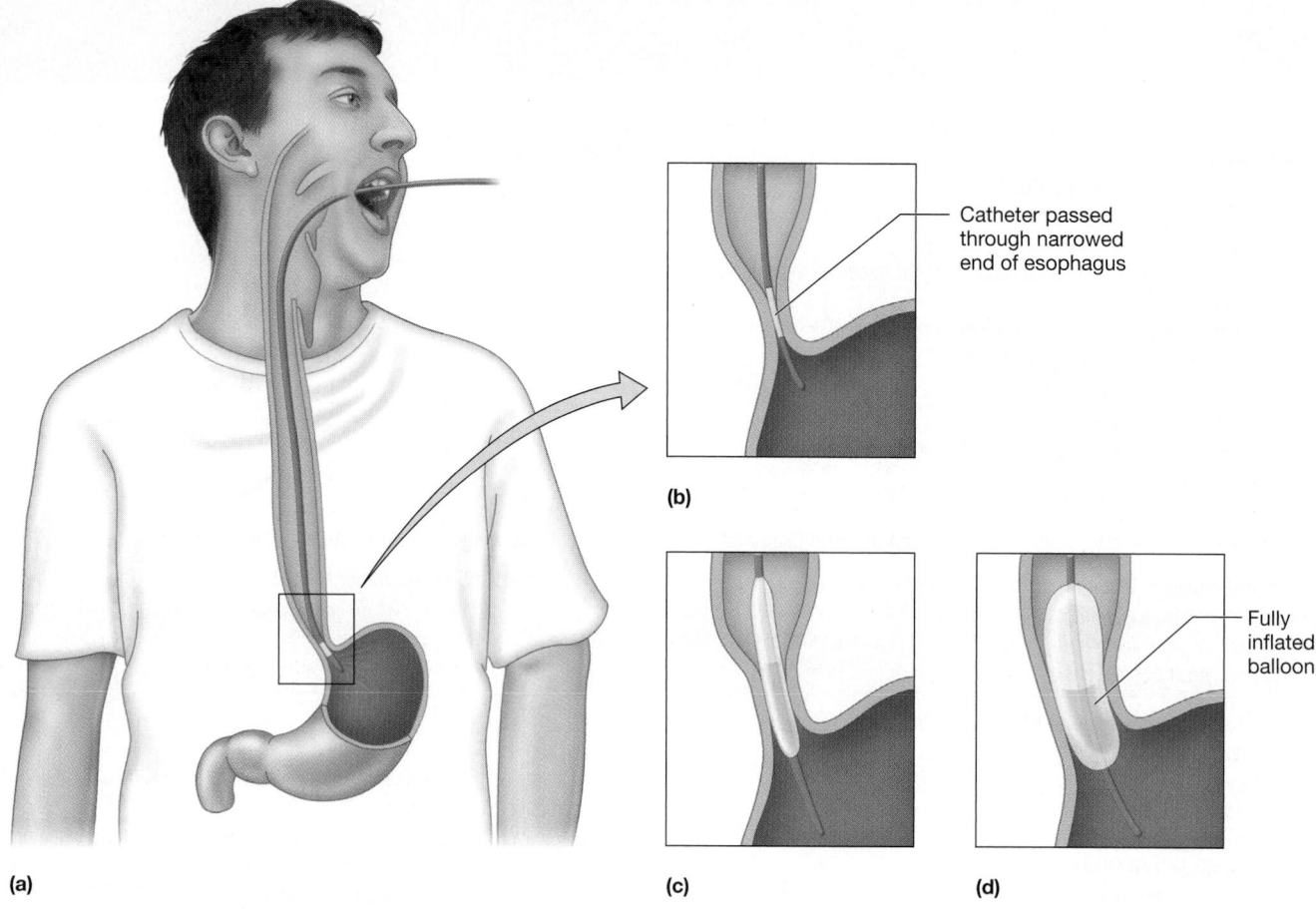

Catheter passed
through narrowed
end of esophagus

(b)

(c)

Fully
inflated
balloon

(d)

(a)

FIGURE 45–3 ■ Esophageal dilation.

then becomes teaching the patient regarding the disease process
and helpful dietary changes.

Assessment

Nursing assessment is the first step in caring for a patient with
achalasia. The nurse should determine the presence of primary
symptoms, their duration, the factors that increase their frequency or intensity, and what the patient has tried to relieve
them. A respiratory history is essential because of the potential
for aspiration pneumonia. A complete nutritional assessment,
including food tolerances and weight loss, will give the nurse an
idea of the impact of the esophageal symptoms. The patient
with achalasia may have halitosis (foul breath) because of the
putrefying food retained in the esophagus.

Interventions

Nursing interventions include advising the patient to try different foods because some foods may be better tolerated than others. Warm, soft foods or liquids are often better tolerated than a
standard diet, and small, frequent meals may aid in esophageal
emptying. Sleeping either with the head of the bed elevated or in
a semisitting position can help prevent nocturnal reflux.

The nurse may assist with endoscopic procedures that are
used to ease the pressure in the LES. The nurse should educate
the patient and family about what to expect regarding the procedure and symptoms that should be reported after the patient

has left the ambulatory center. The major nursing responsibility
is to monitor for respiratory distress and the return of swallowing after the procedure.

Esophageal Cancer

Although **esophageal cancer** is uncommon in the United States,
it is almost always fatal. The 5-year survival rate is less than 5%.
Survival increases if a diagnosis occurs in the early stages. Because the symptoms of esophageal cancer go unrecognized or are
associated with other more benign, conditions, it is usually not
diagnosed until late in the course of the disease.

Pathophysiology/Etiology

Cancer can occur anywhere along the esophagus, but it is more
common in the middle and distal portions. The most common
type of esophageal cancer is squamous cell and is more common
in African Americans than in whites, peaking at around age 60.
Adenocarcinoma is less common but is more common in whites
and is associated with the presence of Barrett's epithelium
(columnar rather than squamous epithelium) resulting from
chronic GERD.

The major risk factor for the development of esophageal cancer is long-term alcohol use. The risk increases as the amount of
alcohol consumed increases. Tobacco use increases the risk of
esophageal cancer, but pipe and cigar smokers have a higher risk

than cigarette smokers. Carcinogenesis is associated with deficiencies of trace elements and vitamins, particularly zinc and vitamin A, which may occur with malnutrition from poor economic conditions, special diets, or alcoholism.

The development of esophageal cancer is facilitated by any process that allows food and drink to remain in the esophagus for prolonged periods, by ulceration and metaplasia usually caused from esophageal reflux, and by long-term exposure of the esophagus to irritants. Malnutrition causes mucosal changes that promote neoplastic changes.

Clinical Manifestations

The clinical manifestations of esophageal cancer are similar to those of GERD, hiatal hernia, and achalasia, and include dysphagia, heartburn, chest pain, and regurgitation. Dysphagia, as the most common and most diagnostic symptom, is usually progressive, beginning with difficulty swallowing solid food, especially meat, and then progressing to difficulty swallowing soft foods and liquids. The dysphagia usually progresses rapidly over the course of weeks or months. Late in the disease, drooling may be noted because the patient can no longer swallow her saliva. Painful swallowing (odynophagia) is common and is described as a steady, dull, substernal pain.

Diagnostic Tests

Diagnosis of esophageal cancer is made with endoscopic visualization and biopsy. A barium swallow may be done initially to identify narrowing of the esophageal lumen or abnormal mucosa. After diagnosis is made, a CT scan or MRI is usually done to assess for metastasis to other organs. Other laboratory tests are done to assess for anemia (complete blood count, or CBC), nutritional status (serum albumin), liver function, and to detect liver metastasis (aspartate aminotransferase, or AST; alanine aminotransferase, or ALT; bilirubin; alkaline phosphatase).

Medical Management

The goal of therapy for the patient with esophageal cancer is to control dysphagia and maintain or improve nutritional status. Surgery is the only definitive treatment and is preferred in patients who are otherwise healthy. Radiation and chemotherapy, in addition to surgery, may enhance results.

Surgery for esophageal cancer involves removal of the affected area of the esophagus and reanastomosis of the remaining esophagus to the stomach. It is usually done in conjunction with radiation and chemotherapy. Radiation and chemotherapy done preoperatively can shrink the size of the tumor, making removal easier. If the cancer is extensive and has invaded the local tissue and metastasized to distant organs, surgery is done for palliation to relieve pain and dysphagia. Laser treatment and stents may be done to keep the esophagus patent in patients who have had surgery, or they may be used as palliation. Tumors in the upper esophagus usually require a tracheostomy and possibly a radical neck dissection with laryngectomy.

Complications following this radical surgery may include hemorrhage, shock, infection, and pneumonia. Additionally, there is the risk of leakage at the anastomosis sites or through the mediastinal space, and depending on the extent of the surgery, peritonitis may occur, leading to serious infection.

Nursing Management

Nursing care for the patient with esophageal cancer will focus on assessing the severity of the symptoms, providing support once diagnosis is made, and educating the patient and family on lifestyle changes needed to facilitate palliative care. Because the disease has a poor prognosis, produces symptoms that are frightening (feelings of choking), and requires a change in eating habits, the nurse assesses the patient's ability to cope, the patient's personal support systems, and acceptance of the diagnosis in order to make appropriate referrals. The nurse should encourage the patient to verbalize fears and feelings. Including the family members in the preoperative teaching and discussions can help the patient deal with the fear associated with the unknown.

Esophageal resection may be recommended, and if so, the nurse should prepare the patient for surgery. General preoperative care is discussed in Chapter 25 . Because the patient with esophageal cancer may be in a nutritionally poor state, nutritional support may be necessary before surgery is done. Patients usually require parenteral or tube feedings either before or after the procedure, and nursing responsibilities should include monitoring the patient's weight, intake and output, fluid and electrolyte balance, as well as assuring that the patient's questions are answered regarding the surgical procedure and postoperative changes. The Nursing Process: Patient Care Plan (p. 1394) presents the plan of care for postoperative patients with esophageal cancer.

DISORDERS OF THE STOMACH AND INTESTINES

The stomach is well suited for storing and mixing food with acid and enzymes. Alterations of the stomach lining or malignancies can cause painful and serious disease. The small intestine is the area of most of the digestion and absorption that occurs in the digestive tract, with the large intestine absorbing the remaining water and concentrating feces. Diseases of the intestines may manifest themselves as diarrhea, constipation, changes in the character of the stool, or in secondary diseases that arise as a result of poor nutrition.

Peptic Ulcer Disease

The word *peptic* comes from the Greek word meaning to digest. **Peptic ulcer** is a generic term used for any ulceration in the digestive surfaces of the upper GI tract. This includes gastric and duodenal ulcers. The word *ulcer* itself denotes disruption in the protective mucosal lining, thereby exposing the submucosal tissue to gastric secretions and digestion of the submucosa (autodigestion).

Gastric Ulcers

Gastric ulcers are more often seen in older patients between the ages of 55 and 70, occurring with equal frequency in men and women. Gastric ulcers occur less frequently than duodenal ulcers but tend to heal more slowly. A family history of ulcers is not usually associated with gastric ulcer disease.

NURSING PROCESS: Patient Care Plan for Postoperative Esophageal Cancer

Assessment of Airway and Gas Exchange

Subjective Data:
Assessing level of consciousness:
Do you know where you are?
What day is it?

What is your name?
Do you know what happened to you?

Objective Data:
Lung sounds.
Oxygen saturation.

Respiratory rate and character.
Color of skin and nail beds.

Nursing Assessment and Diagnoses	Outcomes and Evaluation Parameters	Planning and Interventions with *Rationales*
Nursing Diagnoses: *Airway Clearance, Ineffective* related to proximity of surgery to the trachea and thoracic incision *Gas Exchange, Impaired* related to possibility of aspiration and general anesthesia	**Outcome:** Adequate oxygenation. ***Evaluation Parameters:*** Alert and oriented. Normal pulse oximetry and arterial blood gases. Clear lung sounds. Ability to cough to clear secretions. Unlabored respiration.	**Interventions and *Rationales:*** Assess level of consciousness. *Indicates possible decrease in oxygenation and brain hypoxia.* Monitor ABGs and oxygen saturation. *To evaluate gas exchange.* Assess mucous membranes and nail beds for signs of cyanosis. *Indicators of inadequate gas exchange.* Assess for diminished or adventitious breath sounds. *Indicates possible aspiration or decreased inspiratory ability related to surgical pain.* Encourage deep breathing and coughing and use of incentive spirometer at least every hour. *To promote lung expansion, mobilize secretions, and prevent atelectasis.* Assess the need for suctioning. *To maintain a patent airway.* Monitor respiratory rate and character. *To assess for respiratory distress.* Report respiratory distress to the health care provider. *Early intervention can prevent respiratory failure.*

Assessment of Pain

Subjective Data:
What is your level of pain on a scale of 0–10, with 10 being the worst pain?
Are you allergic to anything?
Do you have any cultural or religious practices for dealing with pain?

Objective Data:
Restlessness.
Grimacing.

Moaning or groaning.
Shallow respirations.

Nursing Assessment and Diagnoses	Outcomes and Evaluation Parameters	Planning and Interventions with *Rationales*
Nursing Diagnosis: *Pain, Acute* related to surgery	**Outcome:** Comfort level maintained. ***Evaluation Parameters:*** Able to communicate level of pain and relief from medications. Able to take deep breaths without pain. Appears restful without restlessness or moaning.	**Interventions and *Rationales:*** Assess pain using pain scale (0–10) to quantify pain level. *To increase consistency in monitoring pain.* Assess level of pain 30 minutes and 1 hour after giving pain medication. *To assess effectiveness of medications.* Explore cultural and religious practices and beliefs about pain and illness. *Different cultures and religions have varying beliefs about pain, suffering, and disease.* Teach nonpharmacologic methods of pain control, such as guided imagery, meditation, and breathing exercises. *This may augment pain relief.*

Assessment of Nutrition

Subjective Data:
How much weight have you lost?
How long did you have difficulty swallowing?
What had you been able to eat?

Objective Data:
Body weight.
Body mass index.
Skin condition.

Wound healing.
Physical appearance.
Serum albumin.

Nursing Assessment and Diagnoses	Outcomes and Evaluation Parameters	Planning and Interventions with *Rationales*
Nursing Diagnosis: *Imbalanced Nutrition: Less than Body Requirements*	**Outcome:** Optimal nutrition. ***Evaluation Parameters:*** Maintains body weight or gains weight if underweight. Normal serum albumin. Skin is soft without evidence of dryness. Surgical incision healing. No evidence of skin breakdown.	**Interventions and *Rationales:*** Monitor body weight at same time every day. *Indicates a degree of adequate calorie intake and fluid balance.* Assess skin condition and healing. *Adequate dietary protein and calories are needed for wound healing and general skin condition.* Monitor laboratory values particularly serum albumin. Prepare and give parenteral or enteral nutrition as ordered. Assess for edema. *The presence of edema is one indicator of low serum proteins.* Check placement of feeding tube to prevent aspiration.

Pathophysiology/Etiology

Most gastric ulcers develop in the antrum, adjacent to the body of the stomach where acid is produced. Interestingly though, gastric ulcers are not associated with increased acid secretion, but rather with a defect in the mucosal barrier to hydrogen ions, allowing the ions to permeate the mucosa. Chronic gastritis may precipitate gastric ulcers by preventing the mucosa's ability to produce a protective layer of mucus. *Helicobacter pylori (H. pylori)*, a bacterium causing gastritis, is thought to be responsible for 60% of gastric ulcers (Wollner, 2004).

Another factor contributing to the formation of gastric ulcers is decreased prostaglandin secretion by the mucosa, therefore diminishing its protective ability. Medications such as aspirin and nonsteroidal anti-inflammatory drugs (NSAIDs) inhibit prostaglandin formation (O'Malley, 2003). Therefore, a strong association between the habitual use of these drugs and the development of gastric ulcers has been made.

Duodenal reflux of bile is another contributing factor in the development of gastric ulcers. Bile salts decrease the electrical potential across the gastric mucosal membrane, allowing hydrogen ions to diffuse into the mucosa where they disrupt permeability and cellular structure (Huether, 2006). An inflammatory response is established and histamine is released, stimulating an increase in acid, pepsinogen, blood flow, and capillary permeability leading to edema and minute hemorrhages.

Duodenal Ulcers

Duodenal ulcers are the most common type of peptic ulcer in the United States and are found more often in younger people. There is an association between people with type O blood and the development of duodenal ulcers, although the relationship is not yet clear. As with gastric ulcers, duodenal ulcers occur equally in men and women.

Pathophysiology/Etiology

Almost 80% of duodenal ulcers are caused by *H. pylori* gastritis (Wollner, 2004) and occur in the proximal duodenum. *H. pylori* thrives in the acid environment of the stomach once thought to be inhospitable to any bacteria. *H. pylori* produces urease, the enzyme that catalyzes the hydrolysis of urea to ammonia. Ammonia is toxic to the gastric epithelial cells and causes an inflammatory response that induces cytokine production leading to chronic gastritis.

Other factors contributing to duodenal ulcer formation include hypersecretion of acid and pepsin. The increased acid secretion may be in part related to a greater parietal cell mass, or to vagal activity stimulating the release of gastrin, which in turn stimulates the production of acid and pepsin. There may also be an inadequate secretion of bicarbonate by the duodenal mucosa, which in turn would result in increased secretion of acid (Huether, 2006). Cigarette smoke stimulates acid production, and NSAIDs inhibit prostaglandins, contributing to increased acid and decreased mucosal defenses.

Clinical Manifestations

The common characteristic of both gastric and duodenal ulcers is pain that is located in the upper abdomen. The pain is intermittent and described as gnawing, burning, aching, or hunger-like. Traditionally, the pain of gastric ulcers was considered to be related to food consumption and relieved by antacids and that of duodenal ulcers was relieved by food and commonly occurred before a meal or at night. However, there is wide variability in individual experiences of ulcer pain, and the pattern of pain is not diagnostic. Both duodenal and gastric ulcers produce pain when the stomach is empty that is most often relieved by food or antacids.

Other manifestations, particularly in the elderly, are not as easily associated with peptic ulcer disease (PUD). The patient may present with chest pain, dysphagia, or anemia. Anemia may be the presenting symptom in older adults, especially for those taking NSAIDs. Typically, gastric ulcers are more chronic in nature, whereas duodenal ulcers show periods of remission and exacerbation. Anorexia, weight loss, and vomiting are more common in patients with gastric ulcers, chiefly in older adults.

Complications

Complications of PUD include hemorrhage, perforation, and pyloric or gastric outlet obstruction. All of these complications can prove to be life threatening, but can be avoided with early diagnosis and treatment.

Bleeding is the most common complication of PUD, especially in the elderly, and may occur from an erosion of a small vessel producing a slow and insidious blood loss, or from an erosion of a larger vessel leading to severe hemorrhage and shock. Erosion occurs in smaller vessels; anemia and occult blood in the stool may be the only clinical manifestations. In the erosion of larger vessels, the patient may have bright-red emesis or emesis of partially digested blood, which has a "coffee-grounds" appearance. In addition, these patients usually have melena (dark, tarry stools).

Gastric outlet obstruction (or **pyloric obstruction**) is the result of edema, inflammation, scarring of the pylorus, or a combination of these conditions. As a slowly evolving process, it often begins with a feeling of epigastric fullness progressing to vomiting. If complete obstruction occurs, gastric acid, sodium, and potassium are lost in the vomitus, which can result in metabolic alkalosis and electrolyte imbalance.

The most serious complication of PUD is perforation. Perforation of the ulcer causes severe, sudden upper abdominal pain that radiates throughout the abdomen. Gastroduodenal contents containing acid, pepsin, bile, and pancreatic juice enter the abdominal cavity, causing peritoneal irritation and peritonitis, which triggers a massive inflammatory response. The classic manifestations of peritonitis, rigid boardlike abdomen and absence of bowel sounds, happen almost immediately following the perforation. However, the older adult may not exhibit these classic signs, but may have other nonspecific symptoms, thus delaying diagnosis and treatment.

Diagnostic Tests

The majority of peptic ulcers (80% to 90%) can be detected with a barium swallow (upper GI series), although small or superficial ulcers may be missed. Definitive diagnosis is made by direct visualization of the mucosa in the esophagus, stomach, and duodenum using an endoscope. See Chart 45–1 (p. 1389) for the nursing care of a patient undergoing endoscopy. Tissue specimens can be taken during the endoscopic procedure to detect *H. pylori* and malignancy. Because the majority of peptic ulcers are caused by *H. pylori* infection, testing for the organism is often done. The Diagnostic Tests box outlines the different tests that can be used to detect *H. pylori*.

Medical Management

Treatment for PUD is aimed primarily at relieving symptoms, eradicating *H. pylori* infection, and preventing complications such as hemorrhage, obstruction, or perforation. The health care provider makes the diagnosis of PUD by history and physical examination. With a high suspicion of the disorder, an initial course of drug therapy will be ordered and its effectiveness assessed in 1 month. In the event that there is no relief gained from treatment, or there is evidence of a complication, further diagnostic testing is done.

Medications

Most peptic ulcers can be successfully treated with medications. The goal of pharmacologic intervention is to eradicate *H. pylori* and has a success rate of 75% to 90% (Wollner, 2004). The standard therapeutic regimen at this time includes treatment with two antibiotics and a proton pump inhibitor for 10 to 14 days, but it may also include the use of a bismuth preparation. One regimen uses amoxicillin 1,000 milligrams bid with clarithromycin 500 milligrams bid; another uses metronidazole 500 milligrams bid and clarithromycin 500 milligrams bid; and the third option uses metronidazole 500 milligrams qid combined with tetracycline 500 milligrams qid. Usually after a course of treatment with antibiotics and proton pump inhibitors, the patient is maintained on a once daily dose of a proton pump inhibitor or H_2-receptor blocker (Wollner, 2004). Other medications that are used to treat PUD are antacids, prostaglandin analogs, and mucosal barrier fortifiers. See the Pharmacology Summary feature for drug therapy for *Helicobater pylori* eradication.

Lifestyle Modifications

There are no specific dietary modifications that individuals with PUD should follow because no food is considered ulcerogenic. It is generally believed that any food that does not cause the individual any discomfort can be consumed, and likewise, foods that cause discomfort should be avoided. The patient should be advised not to take NSAIDs or aspirin (or products containing aspirin; i.e., Excedrin, Alka-Seltzer). If the patient requires the anti-inflammatory action of NSAIDs, the health care provider may switch the patient to a COX-2 selective inhibitor, which is less likely to induce an ulcer. However, many of the newer studies show a significant portion of the normal population has similar symptoms when taking the COX-2 inhibitors, so monitoring the patient is paramount. Small amounts of alcohol do not cause harm, but large amounts should be avoided. The rate of healing is slowed and the recurrence rate increased in patients who smoke, so smoking should be discouraged. Because *H. pylori* is found in saliva and feces, increasing the possibility of person-to-person transmission through oral to oral and fecal to oral routes, good hand hygiene should be encouraged. Higher rates of *H. pylori* infection have been found in people living in close contact and where sanitation is not good.

Surgery

Fortunately, with the discovery of *H. pylori* infection as the major cause of peptic ulcers, and the development of medications to eradicate this organism, surgery is rarely necessary. Surgery may be required to treat the complications of PUD if medical treatment fails. (For the nursing care of the patient having gastric surgery, see the Nursing Process: Patient Care Plan for Gastric Cancer and Gastric Resection, p. 1401.)

■ Nursing Management

Most patients with PUD are treated with medications at home unless complications occur; then hospital admission is necessary. Nursing assessment should include a general health history with a focused assessment on complaints of epigastric pain and heart-

DIAGNOSTIC TESTS for *Helicobacter Pylori*

Test	Method	Results	Nursing Implications
Biopsy urease test	A tissue specimen is obtained during endoscopy and placed in a gel-containing urea.	*H. pylori* produces urease, which changes the color of the gel if the organism is present.	Endoscopy is an invasive procedure. See Chart 45–1 (p. 1389) for care of the patient undergoing endoscopy.
Biopsy examination	A tissue specimen is sent to the laboratory and examined under the microscope for evidence *of H. pylori*.	Presence of *H. pylori* indicates infection.	See Chart 45-1 (p. 1389) for care of the patient undergoing endoscopy
Enzyme-linked immunosorbent assay (ELISA)	A blood sample is tested for antibodies (IgG) against *H. pylori*.	Indicates current or past infection.	There are no food or fluid restrictions. Specimen is collected in a red-top tube.
Urea breath test	Radioactive carbon (C-13 or C-14) labeled urea is given in an oral preparation.	*H. pylori* metabolizes urea and produces carbon that then travels to the lungs and is exhaled. The amount of radioactive carbon in the breath is measured.	The nurse assures the patient that he will not be radioactive after this test and that the 13 C or 14 C is not harmful.
Fecal antigen immunoassay	Stool specimen is examined for *H. pylori*.	Determines active infection.	Confirms presence of *H. pylori*.

PHARMACOLOGY Summary of Drug Therapy for *Helicobacter Pylori* Eradication

Medication Category	Action	Application/Indication	Nursing Responsibility
Anti-Infective Agents Amoxicillin (Amoxil) Clarithromycin (Biaxin) Metronidazole (Flagyl)	Treatment protocols: Triple therapy (2 antibiotics + 1 PPI) Quadruple therapy (2 antibiotics + 1 PPI + bismuth) Sequential therapy (1 antibiotic + PPI followed by 2 antibiotics + 1 PPI) Causes bacterial cell death by inhibition of DNA or bacterial protein synthesis.	Active or inactive peptic ulcer with positive *H. pylori* test.	Monitor for adverse effects: rash, diarrhea, and nausea. Instruct patient to complete medications as ordered; contact health care provider if adverse reaction. Instruct patient not to crush extended-release forms of drug. Multiple drug interactions; monitor for signs of increased drug levels (theophylline, digoxin, warfarin, and others).

burn, including the nature of the pain and relationship to eating, the presence of any symptom associated with a complication (dysphagia, vomiting, and presence of blood in the vomitus), what relieves the pain, and what medications are in use, including NSAIDs or aspirin. The care plan for patients with peptic ulcer disease is presented in the Nursing Process: Patient Care Plan feature (p. 1398).

 CRITICAL ALERT *Peptic ulcer disease (PUD) is a common disorder that has a major impact on health care costs in the United States; it accounts for approximately 10% of all medical costs associated with digestive diseases. Currently it is thought that PUD is caused by Helicobacter pylori infection or the chronic use of nonsteroidal anti-inflammatory drugs (NSAIDs). The American Gastroenterological Association (2005) reported that approximately 30 million people take over-the-counter (OTC) and prescription NSAIDs daily for pain relief, headaches, and arthritis. Therefore, it is important for the nurse to determine whether the patient is taking an NSAID and to provide appropriate teaching related to dosage and side effects (Wilcox, Cryer, & Triadafilopoulos, 2005).*

Health Promotion

The thrust of health promotion to prevent PUD is to advise people to avoid known risk factors. As with chronic gastritis and GERD, these include cigarette smoking, excessive and prolonged alcohol ingestion, the use of oral corticosteroids, and the excessive use of NSAIDs and aspirin. Chronic gastritis and GERD do contribute to ulcer formation, and patients should be encouraged to seek treatment for these disorders. Nurses should use every opportunity to clarify misconceptions that ulcers are caused from eating spicy food; however, certain foods may precipitate symptoms in individuals with PUD.

Cancer of the Stomach

Gastric carcinoma is the second most common cancer in the world, but it is less common in the United States. It is twice as prevalent in men, with the highest incidences in Hispanics, African Americans, and Japanese Americans (who have retained the traditional diet). There seems to be a genetic predisposition to the development of gastric cancer. The majority of gastric cancer develops in the distal portions of the stomach and can be attributed to *H. pylori* infection. Chronic gastritis, gastric polyps, pernicious anemia, chronic gastric ulcer, and dietary factors, such as the use of nitrates (used to preserve meats) and smoked meats, may also contribute to the development of gastric cancer. Lack of hydrochloric acid (**achlorhydria**), atrophic gastritis, and history of gastric resection are also known to be risk factors for gastric cancer.

Pathophysiology

The most common type of cancer developing in the stomach is adenocarcinoma; and although it can develop on any mucosal surface, it is most common in the antrum and distal portions of the stomach. Early gastric cancer may involve the mucosa and submucosa and is usually asymptomatic. As the lesion progresses, it spreads to the gastric wall and regional lymph nodes. It may then advance to adjacent organs such as the liver, pancreas, and transverse colon. Because the stomach has a rich blood and lymphatic supply, the cancer spreads via the portal vein to the liver and through the systemic circulation to the lungs. Metastasis has also been found in bone, ovarian, and peritoneal tissue.

Clinical Manifestations

Regrettably, there are rarely any symptoms associated with gastric cancer. The patient may complain of anorexia, indigestion, heartburn, or early satiety, but these are vague and often the patient does not consider them serious. The patient may self-diagnose and self-treat with over-the-counter medications such as antacids, H_2-receptor antagonists, or proton pump inhibitors. Weight loss occurs as the disease progresses and the patient eventually becomes cachectic. When the patient's health fails, he usually seeks medical attention and diagnosis is made. By this time, the disease is far advanced and prognosis is poor.

Diagnostic Procedures

Definitive diagnosis is done through upper endoscopy and biopsy. See Chart 45–1 (p. 1389) for the nursing care of a patient undergoing endoscopy. Because the patient is usually ill at the time of diagnosis, other tests are done first. These include a CBC whereby a decreased hemoglobin and hematocrit may be the first indication of gastric cancer. Abdominal ultrasound may be done, particularly if a mass is felt on physical examination.

Medical Management

The medical management of gastric cancer involves identification of the cancer and in most cases is followed by surgical removal.

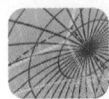

NURSING PROCESS: Patient Care Plan for Peptic Ulcer Disease

Assessment of Pain

Subjective Data:

On a scale of 0–10, with 10 being the worst pain, how would you rate your pain?

What does your pain feel like—burning, gnawing, aching, or stabbing?

When does your pain occur?

Does anything make it worse?

Does anything make it better?

Does eating make it better?

Does eating make it worse?

Does your pain occur before meals?

Does it wake you at night?

What have you used at home to relieve the pain?

Are you allergic to anything?

Do you take any medications such as aspirin, Excedrin, Motrin, or Advil?

If so, how much and for how long?

Do you smoke?

Have you felt nauseated?

Did you vomit?

Did the vomit contain blood or brown fluid?

Objective Data:

Vital signs.

Abdominal examination:
- Distention?
- Pain or tenderness on palpation?
- Bowel sounds?
- Soft or rigid?

Stool for occult blood.

Facial grimacing.

Restless, holding abdomen.

Nursing Assessment and Diagnoses	Outcomes and Evaluation Parameters	Planning and Interventions with *Rationales*
Nursing Diagnosis: *Pain, Acute* related to peptic ulceration and irritation of nerve endings	**Outcome:** Pain relieved. *Evaluation Parameters:* Able to communicate level of pain and therapies that relieve it. Able to verbalize need to quit smoking. No restlessness or facial grimacing.	**Interventions and *Rationales:*** Assess pain using scale (0–10) to quantify pain. *To increase consistency in pain measurement.* Assess pain, character and location, and its relationship to food intake, empty stomach, or other factors and what relieves the pain. *To establish a pattern to the pain and make a plan to control contributing factors.* Administer medications ordered *to reduce acid secretion and monitor effectiveness* (see the earlier Pharmacology Summary for details, p. 1390). Teach the importance of following through with medication regimen as ordered. *To increase the effectiveness of H. pylori eradication and decrease the risk of complications.* Provide information about the symptoms of complications of PUD and to have the patient call the health care provider immediately if any should occur. *To decrease the chances of a complication becoming life threatening.*

Surgery

Surgical resection of the stomach is considered the treatment of choice if gastric cancer is diagnosed early, or it may be performed for palliation if the cancer is more advanced. A partial gastrectomy, or removal of a portion of the stomach, can be done in several ways. The two most common partial gastrectomy procedures are the **gastroduodenostomy (Billroth I)**, whereby the lower portion of the stomach is removed and the remainder is anastomosed to the duodenum (Figure 45–4A ■); and the **gastrojejunostomy (Billroth II)**, which involves removal of a larger distal portion of the stomach with the remainder anastomosed to the jejunum (Figure 45–4B ■). In total gastrectomy, or the removal of the entire stomach, the esophagus is anastomosed to either the duodenum or the jejunum (Figure 45–4C ■).

Long-term complications of surgery are not uncommon. The most common problem is dumping syndrome, whereby the pylorus is bypassed and a food bolus enters the duodenum or jejunum rapidly. Because chyme (partially digested food in the stomach containing gastric acid and digestive enzymes) is hyperosmolar, water is pulled into the intestinal lumen to dilute it, causing a rapid decrease in blood volume. When the blood volume is decreased, there is a reflex sympathetic nervous system response manifested by tachycardia, orthostatic hypotension, dizziness, flushing, and di-

aphoresis. Additional symptoms such as nausea, epigastric pain, cramping, and loud, hyperactive bowel sounds (borborygmi) can occur within 5 to 30 minutes of eating. Diarrhea follows shortly.

In response to the hyperosmolar chyme being delivered to the jejunum, there is a rapid rise in blood sugar with a resultant release of excessive amounts of insulin. The insulin causes a secondary hypoglycemia to occur about 2 to 3 hours after eating. In most cases, dumping syndrome lasts from 6 to 12 months after surgery. The symptoms can be managed by eating small, more frequent meals. Carbohydrates should be reduced while increasing the amount of protein and fat in order to help slow the transit time. The patient should be instructed to lie down for 30 to 60 minutes after eating to slow transit time further.

Removal of any portion of the stomach can impact vitamin and mineral absorption. For example, iron is primarily absorbed from the duodenum and proximal jejunum. With the extensive surgery, coupled with the rapid gastric emptying, interference with iron absorption can manifest in anemia. Gastric resection may also decrease the amount of intrinsic factor produced by the parietal cells. Intrinsic factor is needed for the absorption of vitamin B_{12}. Only minute amounts of vitamin B_{12} are needed, and the liver stores enough for up to 2 years, so it may take that long for pernicious anemia to develop.

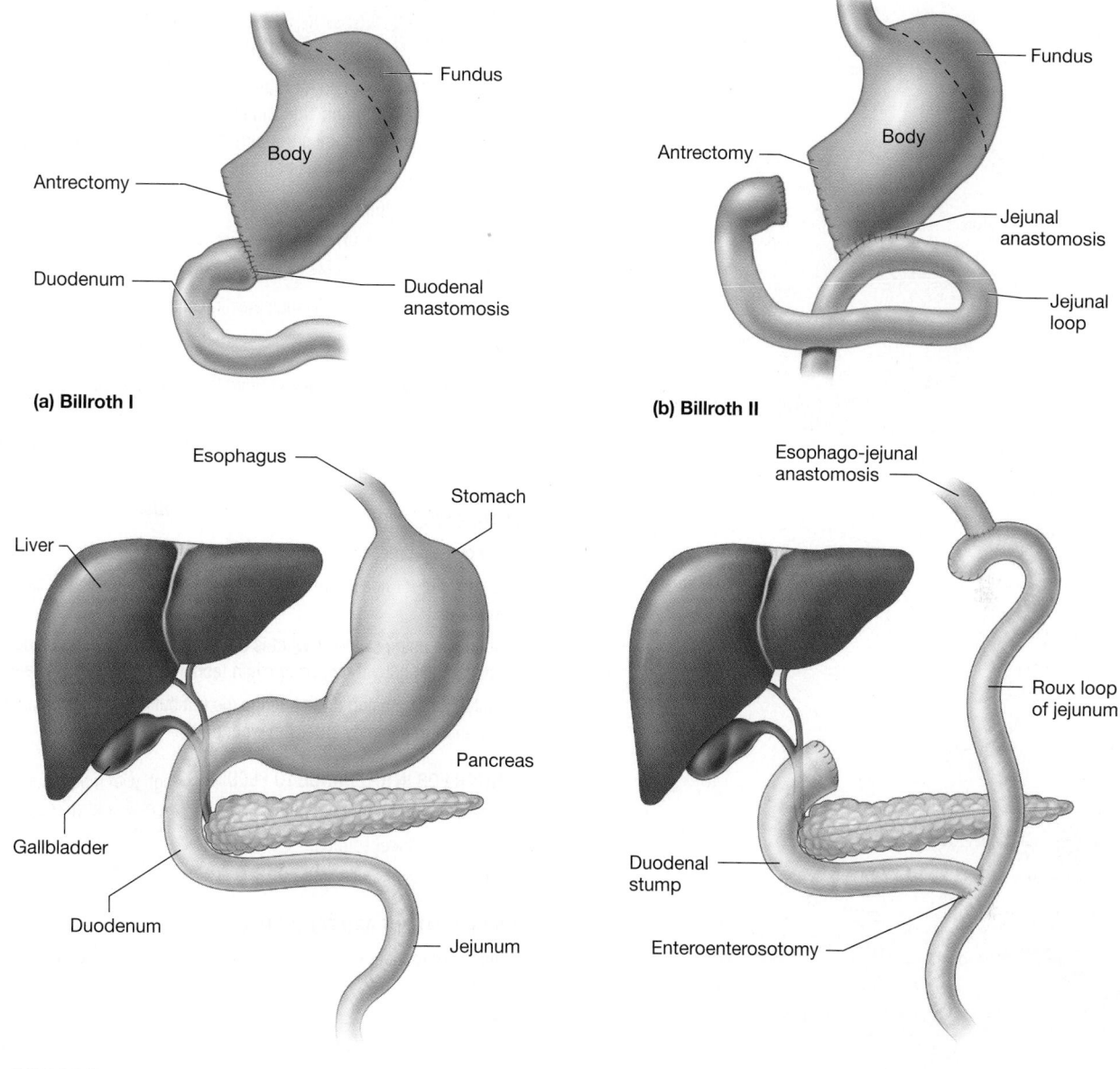

FIGURE 45–4 ■ (A) Billroth I, (B) Billroth II, and (C) total gastrectomy.

Radiation/Chemotherapy

Radiation or chemotherapy may be used to arrest metastatic or lymphatic spread of gastric carcinoma. It is considered palliative in patients with advanced disease to help shrink the tumor and provide some pain relief. However, because of the location of the cancer, these patients will require a feeding tube, in the form of either a gastrostomy tube, if the total stomach has been affected, or, if there is a sufficient portion of the stomach remaining, a jejunostomy tube (Figure 45–5 ■, p. 1400). Chart 45–2 (p. 1400) indicates nursing care of the patient with a feeding tube.

◼ Nursing Management

Nursing care of the patient with gastric cancer is mostly supportive. If there is no metastasis, surgical resection of the stomach is performed. For a detailed discussion on care of the patient with cancer, refer to Chapter 64 ☺. Application of the nursing process can facilitate a comprehensive approach to patient care. The Nursing Process: Patient Care Plan feature (p. 1401) covers the nursing management plan for patients with gastric cancer or having gastric resection.

Health Promotion

The nurse can educate the public about the contributing factors to the development of gastric cancer, such as avoiding or limiting foods containing nitrates, which include smoked meats, bacon, lunch meats, hot dogs, and any other meat product that does not require refrigeration. If a patient is known to have *H. pylori*, the nurse should encourage completion of the prescribed course of medications and return for follow-up to evaluate *H. pylori* eradication.

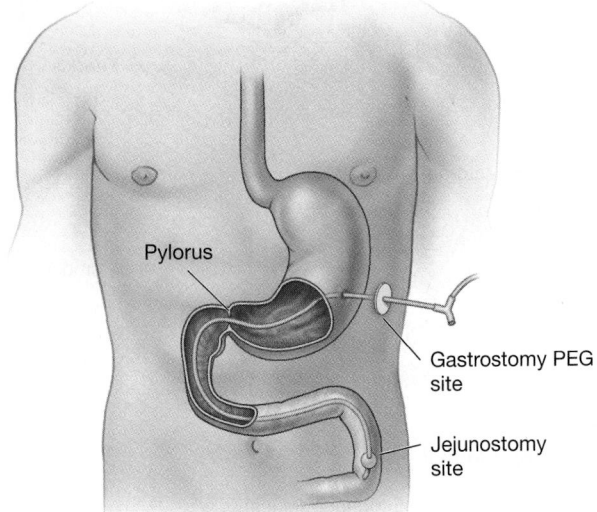

Pylorus

Gastrostomy PEG
site

Jejunostomy
site

(a) Gastrostomy

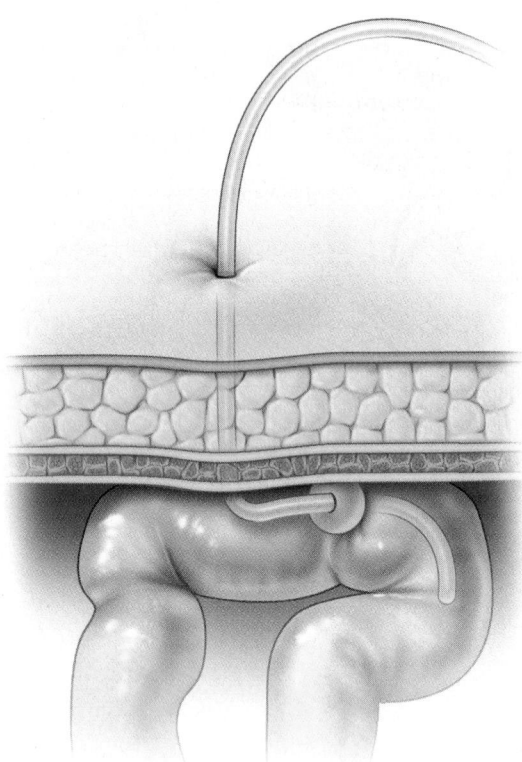

(b) Jejunostomy

FIGURE 45–5 ■ Gastrostomy and jejunostomy tube.

Malabsorption/Maldigestion Syndromes

Malabsorption is considered to be the failure of the small intestine to absorb nutrients from digested food, whereas **maldigestion** is the failure of chemical processes such as inadequate pancreatic enzymes or bile salts to break down food products. Maldigestive disorders result in the malabsorption of nutrients and thus are considered a form of malabsorption. In

---

| CHART 45–2 | **Nursing Care of the Patient with a Feeding Tube** |

The purpose of a gastrostomy tube or a jejunostomy tube is to provide complete nutrition through the alimentary system. It is safer and has fewer side effects than total parenteral nutrition (TPN), particularly when the patient is to have feedings at home.

CHECK TUBE PLACEMENT
- Aspirate and check pH or aspirate.
- A pH of 5 or less indicates gastric placement.
- A pH of 7 or higher usually indicates intestinal placement.

IRRIGATE TUBE
- *Gently* instill 30 to 50 milliliters of water before and after each feeding or as ordered.
- The lumen of some soft, small-diameter tubes may be cleaned with a special brush to maintain patency.

CLEANSE INSERTION SITE
- Remove old dressing (using clean gloves).
- Inspect site for healing or signs of infection (drainage, redness, or swelling).
- Clean site using saline or what is ordered, using sterile technique if the stoma is not yet healed or clean technique if the site is healed.
- Apply dressing using drain sponge (do not cut gauze dressing; it will fray and threads may enter the wound).

MONITOR FOR INTOLERANCE TO FEEDINGS
- Assess abdomen for distention.
- Auscultate bowel sounds.
- Palpate to assess for tenderness.

CONDUCT PATIENT AND FAMILY TEACHING
- Tube care (patient may clean site in the shower after stoma has healed).
- Feeding schedule.
- Monitoring for side effect of feeding.

---

addition to absorptive failure, malabsorption can be caused by surgical resection of the stomach and intestines, or by vascular disorders or intestinal diseases.

Celiac Disease (Sprue)

Celiac disease, also known as gluten-sensitive enteropathy and celiac sprue, is an autoimmune disorder in which there is a histologic change in the mucosal lining of the small intestine when food containing the gliadin component of gluten (wheat, rye, barley) is ingested (Landzberg, 2006; Young & Thomas, 2004). It was once considered to be a childhood illness and relatively rare. Health care providers now know that celiac disease occurs in individuals at any age and may affect as many as 1 in 200 people (Landzberg, 2006).

Pathophysiology

The development of celiac disease involves a genetic predisposition for the disease, gluten ingestion, and immune mediated

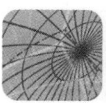

NURSING PROCESS: Patient Care Plan for Gastric Cancer and Gastric Resection

Nursing Assessment of Nutrition

Subjective Data:

What are your favorite foods?

How much did you weigh before you found out about your cancer?

Had you noticed any weight loss before that? How much?

Do you feel full after eating a small amount?

Are you nauseated?

Objective Data:

Daily weights.

Intake and output (I&O).

General appearance.

Laboratory studies:
- Serum albumin
- H & H

- Transferrin
- Ferritin
- TIBC
- Electrolytes.

Nursing Assessment and Diagnoses	Outcomes and Evaluation Parameters	Planning and Interventions with *Rationales*
Nursing Diagnosis: *Nutrition Imbalanced: Less than Body Requirements* related to removal of part of stomach	**Outcome:** Adequate nutrition. **Evaluation Parameters:** Body weight maintained or increased. Healing incision. Normal serum albumin. Normal serum electrolytes. Normal iron studies. Normal hemoglobin and hematocrit.	**Interventions and *Rationales:*** See Chart 45–2 for nursing interventions for patients with feeding tubes. Weigh daily at the same time and on the same scale. *To provide an accurate assessment of fluid balance and nutritional adequacy.* Measure and record accurate intake and output. *To estimate fluid balance.* Monitor laboratory indicators of nutritional status. *These are better indicators of nutritional status than body weight alone.* Assess skin for breakdown. *Can be an indicator of nutritional status, particularly protein.* Assess wound healing. *Decreased protein and vitamin C can hinder wound healing.* Medicate for nausea and pain as needed before meals. *Pain and nausea often produce anorexia and relief can increase the appetite.* Provide the patient with favorite foods or have family members bring home-prepared food when she is able to eat. *To increase the patient's nutritional intake.* Invite family or friends to visit at mealtime. Gathering for meals is a social function for many families and may improve the patient's intake.

Assessment of Emotional Status

Subjective Data:

What have the doctors told you about your cancer?

Who do you count on for support?

Do you have any religious, cultural, or spiritual beliefs that help you deal with your cancer?

Objective Data:

Family or friends visiting.

Clergy visiting.

Initiates conversations with the nursing staff.

Nursing Assessment and Diagnoses	Outcomes and Evaluation Parameters	Planning and Interventions with *Rationales*
Nursing Diagnosis: *Grieving, Complicated* related to diagnosis of cancer with poor prognosis	**Outcome:** Anxiety and fear controlled. **Evaluation Parameters:** Verbalizes fears about cancer and death. Communicates feelings with significant others.	**Interventions and *Rationales:*** Encourage family and significant others to spend as much time as possible with the patient, especially during difficult times such as visits from the health care provider, during chemo and radiation treatments. *To give purpose to the family and significant others and help them feel a part of the process.* Allow the patient to express any feelings without negating any of these feelings. *Allowing the patient to have hope may aid in coping behavior.* Inquire about the patient's cultural, religious, and spiritual beliefs about illness and death, and facilitate discussion with family and clergy where appropriate. *Spiritual and cultural beliefs can comfort the patient and family during this time.*

(continued)

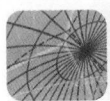

NURSING PROCESS: Patient Care Plan for Gastric Cancer and Gastric Resection—*Continued*

Assessment of Pain

Subjective Data:
On a scale of 0–10, with 10 being the worst pain, how would you rate your pain?
What does your pain feel like—burning, gnawing, aching, or stabbing?
Have you felt nauseated?
Did you vomit?
Did the vomit contain blood or brown fluid?

Objective Data:
Vital signs.
Abdominal examination:
• Distention?
• Pain or tenderness on palpation?

• Bowel sounds?
• Soft or rigid?
Stool for occult blood.
Facial grimacing.
Restless, holding abdomen.

Nursing Assessment and Diagnoses	Outcomes and Evaluation Parameters	Planning and Interventions with *Rationales*
Nursing Diagnosis: *Pain, Acute* related to surgical incision and metastatic cancer	**Outcome:** Pain relieved. **Evaluation Parameters:** Able to communicate level of pain and therapies that relieve it. Abdomen soft, nontender, and bowel sounds present. No restlessness or facial grimacing.	**Interventions and *Rationales:*** Assess pain using scale (0–10) to quantify pain. *To increase consistency in pain measurement.* Assess pain, character and location, and any related symptoms. *To give the nurse clues to the cause of the pain; i.e., incisional pain vs. infection, vs. peritonitis, vs. metastatic cancer.* Administer pain medications as ordered and assess pain level 30 minutes and 1 hour after administration. *To evaluate the effectiveness of the pain medication.*

responses. When a genetically susceptible individual ingests a gluten-containing product, there is a T-cell mediated immune response and chronic inflammation develops if ingestion is continued. Antibodies are produced in response to glutamic acid, which is a product of the digestion of gluten. The antibodies activate leukocytes and the cytokines that release interferon-γ, interlukin-4, and tumor necrosis factor (Young & Thomas, 2004). The microvilli and the brush border of the small intestine are destroyed by the release of cytokines. Continued ingestion of gluten will cause the eventual disappearance of the microvilli and the loss of brush border digestive enzymes, which results in malabsorption.

Clinical Manifestations

Although diarrhea is the most common symptom in children with celiac disease, up to 38% of adult patients are asymptomatic because the small intestine can compensate if the degree of involvement is limited (Presutti, Cangemi, Cassidy, & Hill, 2007). In fact, most adults have signs and symptoms that are unrelated to the GI tract, such as symptoms of rheumatoid arthritis, chronic hepatitis, dental enamel hypoplasia, iron deficiency anemia, neurological dysfunction, osteoporosis, short stature, and reproductive problems. It has been known since the 1970s that diarrhea may not be the primary symptom of celiac disease; however, the patient is usually diagnosed only if diarrhea is present.

Diagnostic Procedures

A biopsy of the small intestine is considered the gold standard for diagnosing celiac disease. When the tissue is examined, the mucosa appears flattened, with an absence of villi, indicating a degree of atrophy. Several new blood tests for celiac disease are proving to be sensitive and specific. They include antigliadin antibody (AGA), antiendomysium antibody (AEA), and tissue transglutaminase (tTG); however, tissue biopsy remains the definitive test (Young & Thomas, 2004).

Medical Management

At the present time, the only treatment for celiac disease is a total gluten-free diet. Gluten is found in wheat, barley, and rye grains (Chart 45–3). Some sources report that oats should also be avoided because they are contaminated by being processed in machines that also process wheat, rye, and barley without interim cleanings and decontamination. Additives, preservatives, and stabilizers may contain gluten, so many food and medicine sources may also cause symptoms.

■ Nursing Management

Support and education are the major nursing responsibilities in the care of individuals with celiac disease. Because the treatment is total elimination of gluten from the diet, the nurse needs to be well informed about foods that contain gluten in order to teach

CHART 45–3	Celiac Disease: Common Foods Containing Gluten That Should Be Avoided	
Barley malt	Gluten	Seitan
Beer	Kamut	Semolina
Bleached flour	Malt	Shoyu (soy sauce)
Bran	Malt extract	Soba noodles
Bread flour	Malt flavoring	Spelt
Brewer's yeast	Malt syrup	Sprouted wheat or
Bulgur wheat	Malt vinegar	barley
Coloring	Matzo	Udon (wheat noodles)
Couscous	Miso	Vegetable starch
Durum wheat	Pasta	Wheat
Edible starch	Pearl barley	Wheat germ
Farina	Rye	Wheat germ extract
Fillers	Seasoned French fries	Wheat germ oil
Food starch	(coated with flour)	Wheat grass

the patient diet modification. Potential hidden sources of gluten should be identified, such as canned or homemade cream soup, cream sauces, gravy, and some candies. Chart 45–3 lists the most common foods that contain gluten. Some items that contain gluten and are often overlooked include stamps, envelopes, and gummed labels; some toothpaste; vitamins; and laxatives. The nurse should be familiar with resources for support, such as the numerous organizations and websites that provide support, information, and gluten-free products.

Lactose Intolerance

Lactose intolerance is caused by a deficiency of lactase at the brush border of the small intestine, resulting in malabsorption. **Lactase** is an enzyme that aids in the breakdown of lactose, a disaccharide found in milk. The enzyme is needed to convert lactose into a monosaccharide, which can be absorbed in the small intestine. The deficiency is usually the result of a congenital defect, but intolerance does not usually develop until adulthood. Lactose intolerance can also be caused by several diseases of the intestine, including celiac disease and Crohn's disease.

Lactase deficiency is very common. In fact, it may affect as many as 90% of Asians and Native Americans and 70% of African Americans (McQuaid, 2004). Because of the lactase deficiency, there is undigested lactose in the intestines, which has two effects. First, intestinal bacteria cause fermentation of the undigested lactose, which produces gas. Second, because lactose is a large molecule, it increases the osmotic gradient in the intestines. These two processes produce the symptoms of lactose intolerance, which include bloating, abdominal distention, flatulence, crampy pain, and diarrhea. However, many individuals may remain symptom free unless large amounts of milk and milk-containing foods are ingested at one time.

Diagnostic Procedures

Lactase deficiency is diagnosed using the lactose breath test. This noninvasive test measures the amount of hydrogen gas exhaled after a 50-gram dose of lactose is given to a fasting patient. Hydrogen gas is a product of the fermentation of lactose in a lactase-deficient individual.

A lactose tolerance test can also be done to determine the degree of lactase deficiency. In this test, a dose of 100 grams of lactose is given orally, and the blood sugar is measured at 30, 60, and 120 minutes postadministration. In normal individuals, there should be an increase in the blood glucose, but in those with lactase deficiency, there is no increase.

Medical Management

Elimination of lactose from the diet will relieve the symptoms of this disorder. Some individuals may tolerate small amounts of lactose and may include in their diet foods that are lower in lactose, such as aged cheese and yogurt. They are cautioned to eliminate these foods if symptoms occur. There are lactase enzymes (Lactaid) available without a prescription to improve lactose tolerance, as well as milk containing lactase available commercially. Individuals, particularly women, may require calcium supplementation in order to get the minimum daily requirement of this mineral, if they must avoid all dairy products. The diet of most

Americans is more than adequate in protein, so eliminating dairy products should not cause protein deficiency.

■ Nursing Management

Nursing care for the patient with a lactase deficiency centers on educating the patient and family about sources of lactose and appropriate nutritional alternatives. Lactose is most concentrated in milk, ice cream, and cottage cheese, but is also found in other cheeses, milk chocolate, sherbet, custard, and cream soups. The nurse should teach the patient and family how to read labels in order to detect lactose in food.

Pancreatic Insufficiency

A deficiency of pancreatic enzymes can also cause malabsorption. Lipase, trypsin, chymotrypsin, and amylase are needed to digest fat, protein, and carbohydrates. If these pancreatic enzymes are insufficient, maldigestion occurs. A deficiency in pancreatic enzymes can be caused by pancreatitis, pancreatic cancer, cystic fibrosis, and pancreatic abscess. However, there must be significant pancreatic damage before insufficiency results.

Pancreatic insufficiency results in maldigestion of all nutrients, but because enzymes secreted by the intestinal brush border and salivary amylase help to digest carbohydrates and proteins, maldigestion of these nutrients is not profound. However, these enzymes do not aid in the digestion of fat, so there is a profound inability to digest fats. The consequence is **steatorrhea** (fat in the stools) and weight loss. There could also be problems with the absorption of fat soluble vitamins.

■ Nursing Management

Pancreatic insufficiency is treated with supplemental pancreatic enzymes. The nurse should administer the enzymes (Viokase) before meals. The Pharmacology Summary feature (p. 1404) outlines the use of supplemental enzymes. The nurse should teach the patient and family about the administration of the medication, to monitor for signs of vitamin deficiency, and to notify the health care provider if weight loss or steatorrhea occurs.

Short Bowel Syndrome

Short bowel syndrome results when there is a reduction in the surface of the small intestine from surgical resection of the small bowel, typically because of tumors, Crohn's disease, infarction, trauma, and radiation enteropathy. The degree of the resulting malabsorption depends on the location and extent of the resection. For example, if the duodenum, jejunum, or proximal ileum is removed, severe malabsorption usually occurs.

The absorption of water, nutrients, vitamins, and minerals is hindered in the early postoperative period after small bowel resection. If a large portion of the small intestine is removed, the transit time is significantly reduced. With time, the bowel adapts by enlarging and lengthening the villi that remain, thereby increasing the surface area available for absorption. Some patients may achieve digestion and absorption that is about the same as

PHARMACOLOGY Summary of Medications Used to Treat Pancreatic Insufficiency

Medication Category	Action	Application/Indication	Nursing Responsibility
Digestive Enzymes Pancrelipase (Viokase)	Breaks down fats, proteins, and starches in the final stage of digestion for easier absorption.	Steatorrhea from malabsorption syndrome, post pancreatectomy, gastrectomy, or GI surgery (e.g., Billroth II).	Monitor for adverse effects: nausea, abdominal cramps, and diarrhea. Assess for improved nutritional status and decreased steatorrhea. Be aware of religious considerations; drug is pork based.

it was before the resection. However, a significant number of patients have considerable malabsorption that leads to diarrhea, weight loss, dehydration, and nutrient deficiencies.

Medical Management

Treatment for short bowel syndrome focuses on relief of symptoms and methods to maintain nutrition. To maintain nutrition, small, frequent feedings of high-calorie, high-protein foods are usually prescribed if the patient can tolerate oral feedings. If oral feedings are not tolerated, then enteral tube feedings or total parenteral nutrition (TPN) will be ordered. Supplementation with vitamins and minerals is frequently necessary.

If diarrhea is a continued problem, antidiarrheal medications, such as Lomotil, which slows intestinal motility, will be ordered. Proton pump inhibitors such as omeprazole (Prilosec) may be ordered for patients who have gastric reflux or hypersecretion of gastric acid postoperatively. See the Pharmacology Summary feature (p. 1390) which outlines the use of proton pump inhibitors. See the Pharmacology Summary feature of medications used to treat diarrhea.

■ Nursing Management

Because the patient with short bowel syndrome is at risk for diarrhea, particularly in the early postoperative period, fluid and electrolyte imbalances are possible. Vital signs should be taken frequently and the nurse should monitor the condition of the patient's mucous membranes, daily weight, and record an accurate intake and output including measuring the volume of diarrhea.

The patient is also at risk for nutritional deficits. The health care provider may order total parenteral nutrition (TPN) to maintain the patient's nutritional status until the GI tract has recovered from surgical resection. The nurse monitors the patient's weight, laboratory values, central IV catheter, and insertion site. Once the patient's bowel sounds have returned, oral or enteral feedings may be started. It is important to monitor the patient's tolerance of the feeding once it is begun.

Educating the patient and family members is a major nursing responsibility. The patient will most likely have some problems with digestion and/or absorption for the rest of her life and will need guidance about the recommended diet and ways to maintain nutritional status. If the patient is able to tolerate oral feeding, small, frequent meals may be helpful. Resting in a reclining position after meals may help slow the GI transit time. The patient should be taught to monitor her body weight and to notify the health care provider if there is a consistent weight loss, which could signify either a fluid loss or inadequate calories.

Intestinal Obstruction

Intestinal obstruction can occur anywhere from the pylorus to the rectum and can be either partial or complete. There is impairment of forward movement of intestinal contents because of a mechanical cause (tumors [Figure 45–6C ■], adhesions [Figure 45–6A ■], Crohn's disease, diverticular disease, foreign bodies) or a functional cause (surgery, anesthesia, medications). Functional bowel obstructions are also called ileus, paralytic ileus, or adynamic ileus. Most bowel obstructions occur in the

PHARMACOLOGY Summary of Mediations Used to Treat Diarrhea

Medication Category	Action	Application/Indication	Nursing Responsibility
Antidiarrheal Agents **Opioids:** Codeine Camphorated opium tincture (Paregoric) Diphenoxylate/atropine (Lomotil) Loperamide (Imodium) **Other:** Bismuth subsalicylate (Pepto-Bismol)	Increases fluid and electrolyte absorption from the colon by slowing peristalsis. Reduces GI hypermotility by direct antibacterial effect and decreased prostoglandin synthesis.	Moderate to severe diarrhea. Traveler's diarrhea.	Monitor for signs and symptoms of dehydration and altered electrolyte levels. Observe for potential drowsiness. Instruct patient not to drive or perform other potentially hazardous activities until response to drug is known.

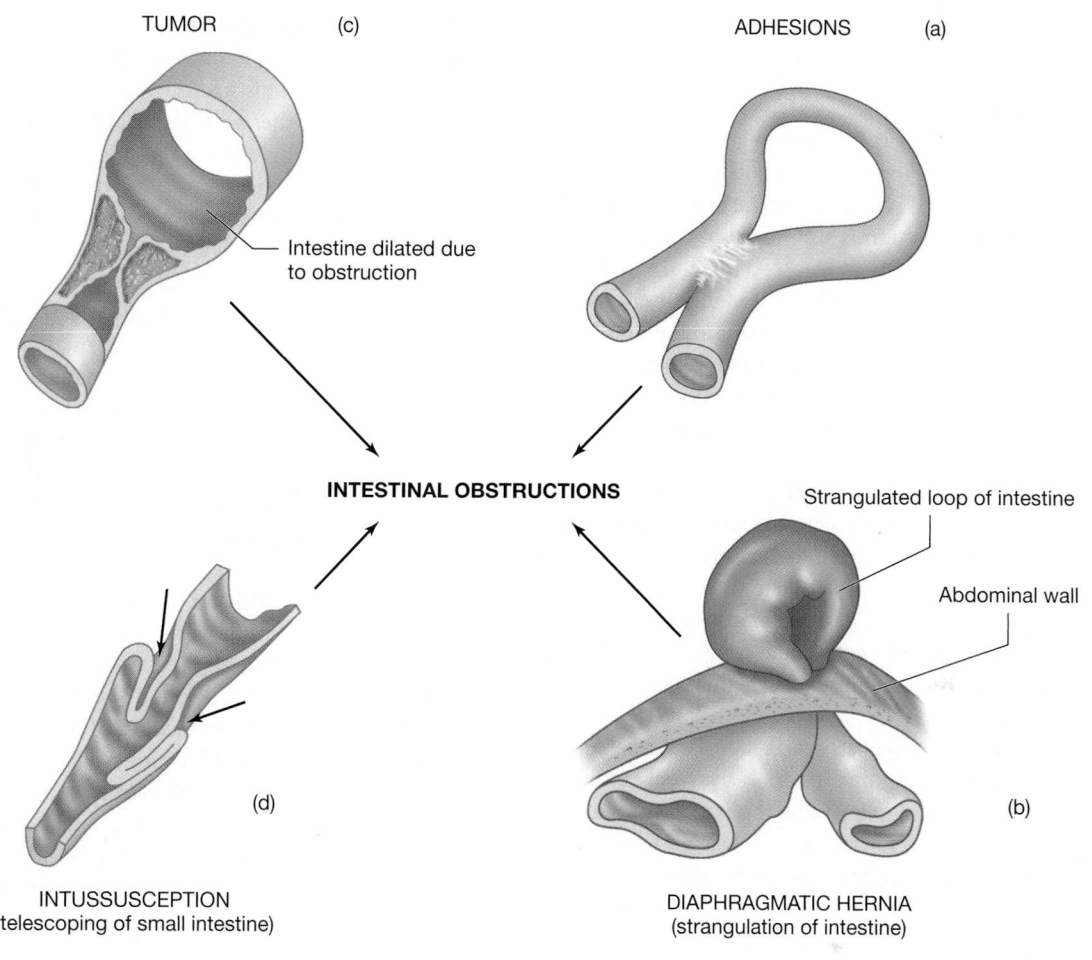

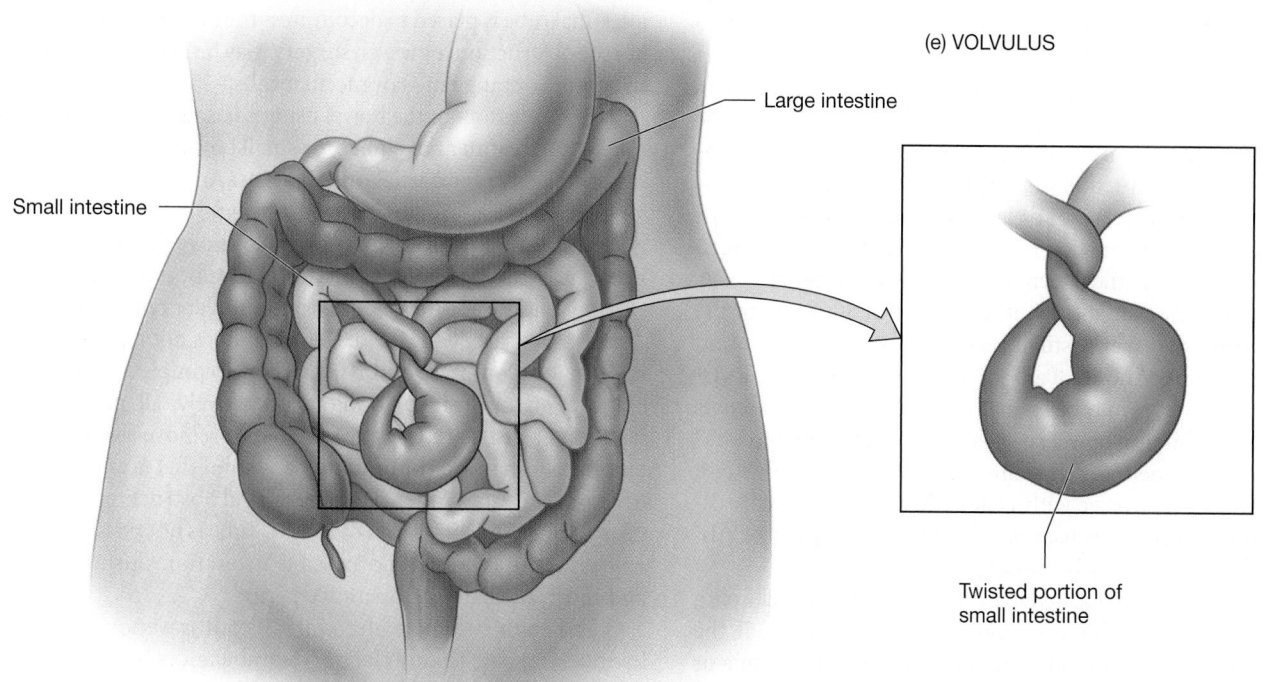

FIGURE 45–6 ■ Causes of intestinal obstruction (A) Adhesions, (B) Hernias, (C) Tumors, (D) Intussusception, (E) Volvulus.

small intestines, with only about 15% occurring in the large bowel.

Pathophysiology

The resultant physiology is the same regardless of the cause of the bowel obstruction. In mechanical obstructions, there is an increase in motility and secretions of the bowel, both proximal and distal to the obstruction. The amount of the secretions may exceed the intestine's ability to reabsorb this fluid, and it results in distention of the bowel. Both the distention and increased motility produce the characteristic cramping abdominal pain (Thomas, 2007). The bowel sounds become high pitched and tinkling, particularly distal to the obstruction. However, as the bowel obstruction progresses, there are diminished or absent bowel sounds.

Bowel obstructions can be classified as simple or strangulated. In a simple bowel obstruction there is no impairment of the vascular or neurological innervation to the intestine. Gas and intestinal secretions accumulate proximal to the obstruction and the distal bowel collapses. An inflammatory response is initiated and the bowel wall becomes edematous and congested. As the process continues there is the possibility of ischemia, necrosis, perforation, and death.

In a strangulated bowel obstruction there is an interruption of blood flow, both venous and arterial, by mechanical means (Thomas, 2007). A strangulated bowel obstruction is extremely serious. Impairment of arterial blood flow leads to ischemia, infarction progressing to gangrene, and perforation and death. This type of bowel obstruction is most often caused by hernias (Figure 45–6B ■), intussusception (telescoping of the bowel; Figure 45–6D ■), volvulus (twisting of the bowel; Figure 45–6E ■), or vascular occlusion, but can also result from surgical adhesions and tumor involvement.

Clinical Manifestations

The manifestations of a bowel obstruction vary depending on the location, type of obstruction, and rapidity of development. The most common symptom is pain. It is usually a cramping or colicky pain that increases as the obstruction progresses. Initially, it may be intermittent but becomes constant with the progression of the obstruction. If the obstruction is in the proximal small bowel, vomiting is common and metabolic alkalosis can result from the loss of gastric acid. If the obstruction is in the distal small bowel, the pain is usually intense and the patient may vomit fecal material.

Abdominal assessment reveals distention resulting from the accumulation of gas, intestinal secretions, and distended and edematous loops of bowel. Early in the obstructive process, visible peristaltic waves may be seen on inspection and hyperactive, high-pitched tinkling bowel sounds may be heard on auscultation of the abdomen. Bowel sounds cease later in the course of the obstruction. However, with a paralytic ileus, there may be diminished or absent bowel sounds throughout the process. Abdominal tenderness may be evident on palpation.

If the obstruction is located in the large intestine, colicky pain and constipation are the most common manifestations. If the pain is severe and continuous, it may indicate bowel ischemia or perforation. There can be massive dilation of the colon, causing pressure and impairing circulation leading to gangrene and perforation. If vomiting develops with a large bowel obstruction, it is usually late in the process.

Diagnostic Procedures

Bowel obstruction is determined with a careful history and physical exam. Confirmation of the diagnosis is made by x-rays and CT scan. Other laboratory tests, although not diagnostic, will be done to determine the presence of infection, fluid and electrolyte imbalances, and acid–base balance.

These laboratory studies usually include a CBC with a differential white blood cell (WBC) count. There will be varying degrees of leukocytosis, but a very elevated WBC count can indicate ischemia or impending strangulation. The serum amylase not only will be elevated in bowel obstruction but also will be elevated with pancreatitis, which has many of the same symptoms. Serum osmolality is elevated if dehydration is present from vomiting and sequestering of fluid in the bowel lumen. If vomiting is severe, hypokalemia and hypochloremia may also be present.

Abdominal x-rays will show distended loops of bowel. If it is a large-bowel obstruction, the entire intestine will be distended all the way to the level of the obstruction. In a small-bowel obstruction there is evidence of gas and fluid in the small bowel. In the upright abdominal x-ray, there are characteristic air–fluid levels within the bowel. Free air under the diaphragm on abdominal x-ray is indicative of bowel perforation.

CT scan with contrast media will be done to determine a mechanical obstruction. A barium swallow is contraindicated because of the possibility of intestinal perforation or a worsening of the obstruction. The contrast media used is diatrizoate meglumine (Gastrografin) and contains iodine. It cannot be used in patients who are allergic to iodine or seafood. A barium enema may be used to diagnose a large-bowel obstruction if there is no threat of perforation.

Medical Management

Treatment for bowel obstruction is centered on relieving the obstruction and resulting pressure in order to avoid perforation. An intestinal tube is placed to decompress the bowel, possibly relieving the obstruction; however, surgery may be necessary if the obstruction is strangulated or mechanical.

Decompression of the bowel using a nasogastric or intestinal tube is the treatment of choice for small bowel obstructions and is very effective for partial obstructions. An intestinal tube is a long tube that is usually inserted through the nose and has a weighted tip that works with gravity to move the tube into the intestine to the point of obstruction. The tube is attached to low suction and the accumulated gas and fluid are removed.

Surgery is needed if the obstruction does not respond to the intestinal decompression or if there is a complete mechanical obstruction or strangulation. Preoperatively, all patients will have a nasogastric (NG) tube inserted to remove stomach contents and to remove continuously any fluid that accumulates in the stomach (unless there is a mechanical obstruction involving the stomach; then insertion of the NG tube is not possible). This will prevent vomiting and possible aspiration during surgery and the immediate postoperative period.

The health care provider will order intravenous fluids to hydrate and correct any electrolyte imbalances before surgery. Isotonic IV fluids (NS, lactated Ringer's) will be given at a rate that will correct fluid balance rapidly but without risk of causing cardiac problems. Because potassium is lost in nasogastric suctioning, as well as through vomiting, potassium is usually added to the IV solution. Blood or blood products may be needed if the obstruction is strangulated or perforated because bleeding may occur. Intravenous antibiotics will be given preoperatively and during surgery to prevent the possibility of infection.

Surgery may involve several procedures including the lysing of adhesions, removal of infarcted or gangrenous bowel, removal of foreign bodies, or tumor resection. A bowel resection is done for most cases of obstruction, except when the cause of obstruction is adhesions. In that case, the adhesions are surgically released. A bowel resection involves removing the section of intestine that is involved and usually an end-to-end anastomosis is performed to reattach the sections of bowel. If a large section of small bowel is removed, the patient may have malabsorption postoperatively. Depending on the cause of the obstruction and the area of bowel affected, ileostomy or colostomy may be necessary.

Nursing Management

Nursing care for the patient with a bowel obstruction focuses on assessment of present condition, instituting fluid and electrolyte replacement, and bowel decompression, by placing either a nasogastric tube or an intestinal tube, and recording the forward progression of the latter. Chart 45–4 outlines care of the patient with a nasogastric tube or nasointestinal tube. If the bowel obstruction cannot be relieved, then surgery will be necessary. The nurse prepares the patient for possible surgery, both physically and emotionally. For complete nursing care for the patient with a bowel obstruction, see the Nursing Process: Patient Care Plan feature (p. 1408).

Diverticular Disease

Diverticular disease results from the occurrence of abnormal saclike outpouchings of the intestinal wall called diverticula. Diverticula can occur anywhere in the gastrointestinal tract except the rectum, but usually occur in the distal large intestine. Diverticular disease includes **diverticulosis**, which is the presence of one or more diverticula, and **diverticulitis**, which is inflammation of the diverticula with possible rupture into the colonic lumen.

Pathophysiology/Etiology

Where arteries penetrate the tunica muscularis are inherent weak points in the intestinal wall. It is at these points, particularly where pressures are normally high in order to push fecal material toward the rectum, that diverticula form. The mucosa herniates through the smooth muscle layers forming the diverticular sac. Diverticula themselves cause few problems; however, if undigested food or bacteria becomes trapped in the diverticula, they form a hard mass called a fecalith and intraluminal pressure increases, resulting in compromise of the blood supply. This results in ischemia of the diverticula and may lead to perforation.

Diverticular disease is common in developed countries, such as the United States, England, Australia, and France, where the diet consists mostly of refined foods. Diverticular disease was virtually unknown until about 1900 when modern grain milling practices began. This process removes two-thirds of the grain's fiber. Socially, only economically disadvantaged people ate brown (whole wheat) bread or brown rice. White, highly refined bread became a status symbol. The incidence of diverticular disease increases as people age and is quite common after age 60, but is rarely found in individuals younger than age 40.

CHART 45–4	**Care of the Patient with a Nasogastric (NG) or Nasointestinal (NI) Tube**

NG Tubes (Salem Sump)	**NI Tubes (Cantor, Miller-Abbott, Harris Tubes)**

• Maintain low intermittent suction.
• Check placement every 4 hours.
  1. Aspirate stomach contents and check pH.
  2. Insert 10 milliliters of air rapidly while listening with stethoscope over the stomach to hear the rush of air.
• Monitor skin integrity of nostril of insertion and provide skin care.
• Monitor bowel sounds (suction off).
• Irrigate tube with 30 milliliters NS every 4 hours or as needed to maintain patency.
• Measure NG drainage at least every 8 hours.
• Be sure that the "blue port" is patent, and never irrigate through the port. If the port leaks, do not let the tube hang down, but place it at the patient's shoulder. Do not plug the port unless ordered by the health care provider.
	• Before insertion of Cantor or Harris tube, fill the balloon reservoir with mercury. The balloon on the Miller-Abbott tube is filled with mercury once the distal end has reached the stomach.
	• Once inserted into the stomach, position the patient on his right side.
	• The health care provider may order the tube to be advanced 2–4 inches at a time or to let gravity move the tube into the small intestine.
	• Movement of the patient, either ambulation or changing positions in bed, will assist the forward movement of the tube.
	• The tube is not secured until it reaches the desired position.
	• The tube is not irrigated unless ordered by the health care provider.
	• Placement is checked by x-ray.
	• Low intermittent suction may be ordered once placement is confirmed.
	• Maintain NPO.
	• Mouth care at least every 2 hours.
	• Removal of the tube requires the mercury to be removed from the tube; then withdraw the tube 6 inches every hour until it is removed. The distal end of the tube may have a fecal taste and odor, so mouth care is essential.

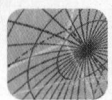

Assessment of Fluid, Electrolyte, and Acid–Base Balance

Subjective Data:
Have you been vomiting? How much? And for how long?
Has your belly become more distended?
Have you been urinating as much as usual?
Do you get dizzy when you stand up quickly?

Objective Data:
Vital signs.
Intake and Output (I&O):
- IV fluids
- Urine output
- NG or NI output
- Fecal output.

Skin color, temperature, turgor.
Abdominal assessment:
- Bowel sounds
- Distention
- Tenderness.

Nursing Assessment and Diagnoses	Outcomes and Evaluation Parameters	Planning and Interventions with *Rationales*
Nursing Diagnosis: *Fluid Volume, Deficient, Risk for* related to bowel obstruction and sequestration of fluid and nasogastric/intestinal suction	**Outcome:** Fluid balance maintained. **Evaluation Parameters:** Vital signs normal. Orthostatic blood pressure normal. Intake = output. Skin warm, moist, and pink. Abdomen soft; no increase in girth. Bowel sounds present.	**Interventions and *Rationales:*** Assess frequency and amount of vomiting. *To assess accurately fluid loss prior to hospitalization.* Assess urine frequency prior to hospitalization. *A decrease in urination is a sign of fluid sequestering in the gut.* Monitor orthostatic blood pressure and dizziness. *To assess hypotension and fluid volume deficit.* Monitor and record I&O from all sources every 2–4 hours. *Urine output less than 30 milliliters per hour indicates inadequate glomerular filtration rate, is an indicator of inadequate fluid volume, and is usually the first sign of fluid volume deficit. NG or NI tube drainage is figured into the fluid replacement needs.* Administer IV fluids as ordered to replace lost fluids. *Adequate fluid replacement is necessary to sustain tissue perfusion particularly to the heart and kidneys.* Assess skin color, temperature, and character at least every 4 hours. *When deficient fluid volume exists, cardiac output may decline, triggering a sympathetic nervous system response causing cool, clammy, and pale skin.* Measure abdominal girth at least every 8 hours. *To determine increasing distention and possible fluid sequestering in abdomen.* Assess abdomen for bowel sounds and tenderness. *Hyperactive, high-pitched bowel sounds are present early in a small bowel obstruction. In paralytic ileus there are diminished or absent bowel sounds.*

Assessment of Gastrointestinal Perfusion

Subjective Data:
On a scale of 0–10, with 10 being the worst pain, how would you rate your pain?
Has the character or intensity of your pain changed?
When was your last bowel movement? Was it normal for you?

Objective Data:
Vital signs.
I&O:
- NG or NI drainage
- Urine output
- Feces.

Abdominal assessment:
- Bowel sounds
- Distention
- Tenderness.

Nursing Assessment and Diagnoses	Outcomes and Evaluation Parameters	Planning and Interventions with *Rationales*
Nursing Diagnosis: *Tissue Perfusion, Ineffective Gastrointestinal* related to possible strangulation, volvulus, tumor, foreign body, or vascular congestion resulting from obstruction	**Outcomes:** Adequate GI tissue perfusion. Return of peristalsis. **Evaluation Parameters:** Normal bowel sounds. Normal bowel movements. Abdomen soft, nontender, and not distended. Pain free.	**Interventions and *Rationales:*** Assess level of pain every 1–2 hours using a scale of 0–10, with 10 being the worst pain. *A change in the intensity or character of the pain can indicate ischemia, infarction, gangrene, or perforation of the bowel.* Monitor vital signs every 1–2 hours. *Tachycardia can result from pain or a sympathetic response to tissue ischemia. Increased temperature may indicate impending sepsis from bowel perforation or gangrene. Falling blood pressure could signal shock and this. With a low blood pressure, it is difficult to perfuse the intestines, increasing the risk for infarction and possible perforation.* Monitor I&O with particular attention to urine output. *Urine output of less than 30 mL/hr indicates poor perfusion to the kidneys and inadequate glomerular filtration. Urine output declines before changes in the vital signs.* Monitor bowel sounds, abdominal distention, and tenderness. *Increasing abdominal girth and pain could signal perforation or sequestering of fluids in the intestines, causing congestion and impairing perfusion.*

Clinical Manifestations

Most people with diverticular disease are asymptomatic. When diverticulitis develops or the diverticulum hemorrhages, the clinical manifestations typically include left lower quadrant pain, fever with corresponding tachycardia, and possibly nausea, vomiting, and bowel changes, causing either diarrhea or constipation. The pain is usually located in the left lower quadrant because most diverticula form in this portion of the colon. It is initially intermittent, but becomes steady as the inflammatory process progresses and can be mild to severe in quality. The fever is low grade, usually less than 38.2°C (101°F), and can be accompanied by chills. Abdominal distention and flatulence may also occur. On palpation, the abdomen may be tender over the left lower quadrant. The complications of diverticular disease are relatively rare but can include hemorrhage, peritonitis, bowel obstruction, and fistula formation. Clinical manifestations in the elderly may be vague and nonspecific. They may have generalized abdominal pain as well as symptoms of a large bowel obstruction.

Diagnostic Procedures

Diverticular disease may be detected incidentally during diagnostic procedures for other problems or on routine colonoscopy. In the case of asymptomatic and uncomplicated diverticulosis, no other testing is usually indicated.

If symptoms develop, the health care provider will order a CBC with a differential to assess for bleeding and infection. The WBC count will increase and more immature cells will be evident (shift to the left) if the patient has diverticulitis because of inflammation and possible infection. The stool may also be tested for occult blood.

Neither a barium enema nor a sigmoidoscopy will usually be done during the acute phase of the process because of the risk of perforating an inflamed diverticulum. Ultrasonography is a noninvasive test that can detect an abscess or bowel thickening. CT scan not only can be used to detect an abscess but also can assess inflammation. If a perforation is suspected, abdominal x-rays can show free abdominal air, which is characteristic of perforation.

Medical Management

The treatment for diverticular disease can range from dietary modifications to surgical resection of the colon. Patients are usually managed as outpatients when symptoms are mild and fever is less than 38.2°C (101°F). Treatment includes rest, drug therapy, and dietary modifications. Hospital admission is required for higher fevers, persistent (more than 3 days) abdominal pain, dehydration, or the presence of lower GI bleeding. Treatment for more severe diverticulitis includes IV fluids, antibiotics, and possible nasogastric suction. Surgery may be necessary if the patient develops peritonitis from a ruptured diverticulum, abscess, bowel obstruction, fistula, or uncontrolled bleeding.

Dietary Modifications

While the patient is in the acute phase of diverticulitis, a clear liquid diet is recommended. If hospitalized, the patient is usually kept NPO initially and a nasogastric tube may be inserted. Once the acute phase has passed, dietary recommendations include eating a diet high in both soluble and insoluble fiber. The recommended fiber consumption for the general public of the United States is 25 to 30 grams and should be stressed for the person with diverticular disease. Chart 45–5 lists foods high in fiber. For patients with diverticular disease, foods containing small seeds, nuts, and foods with skins such as raisins, grapes, and corn are restricted, because they may become lodged in a diverticulum and cause inflammation and an exacerbation of diverticulitis. These foods are listed in Chart 45–6.

Drug Therapy

Acute diverticulitis is treated with broad-spectrum antibiotics. For mild attacks of diverticulitis, oral metronidazole (Flagyl) and ciprofloxacin (Cipro) may be used. When cost is an issue, trimethoprim-sulfamethoxazole (Bactrim) may be used in the place of the ciprofloxacin. If the diverticulitis is severe and the patient is hospitalized, IV antibiotics effective against gram-negative bacteria and anaerobes will be used. Refer to the Pharmacology Summary feature (p. 1397) for an outline of anti-infective agents.

CHART 45–5   **High-Fiber Foods Recommended for Patients with Diverticular Disease**

Grains and Cereals	Fruits and Vegetables*
Wheat bran	Cooked
Oat bran	
Rice bran	• Asparagus
Oatmeal	• Fresh beans (lima, green)
All-Bran Cereal	• Broccoli
Raisin bran	• Peas
Shredded wheat	
Whole wheat bread	• Squash
Multigrain bread	• Greens (kale, spinach)
Whole wheat crackers	• Potatoes
Bulgar (cracked wheat)	• Dried beans (pinto, kidney, navy, black-eyed peas)
Kasha (buckwheat groats)	
Brown rice	Raw
	• Carrots
	• Broccoli
	• Celery
	• Tomatoes
	Peaches
	Apples
	Nectarines
	Oranges
	Pears

* All fruits and vegetables should be eaten unpeeled when possible.

CHART 45–6   **Foods to Be Avoided by Persons with Diverticular Disease**

Popcorn	Berries
Corn	
Sesame seeds	• Strawberries
Poppy seeds	• Raspberries
Sunflower seeds	• Blueberries
Nuts	Figs
Cucumbers	Rye bread with caraway seeds
Okra	

For the patient with diverticulitis experiencing pain, analgesics will be ordered. If the pain is less severe, a mild analgesic is ordered. However, opioid analgesics may be necessary to relieve more severe pain. Meperidine hydrochloride (Demerol) or morphine is used. Pentazocine (Talwin) may cause less colonic pressure and is often used to relieve pain.

Bulk-forming agents, such as psyllium seed (Metamucil) or methylcellulose, are usually prescribed. Laxatives are avoided because they increase motility and intracolonic pressure, although stool softeners (Colace) may be used. See the Pharmacology Summary feature for stool softeners and bulk-forming agents. Enemas are also contraindicated because they increase the intraluminal pressure of the colon and risk diverticular perforation.

Rest

Rest is advocated during acute diverticulitis. The patient should avoid any activity that increases the intra-abdominal pressure, thereby risking perforation. Some of these activities include lifting, straining, coughing, sneezing, and bending.

Bowel rest may be necessary during the acute phase of the illness. Depending on the severity of the inflammation, the patient may be kept NPO. As feeding is resumed slowly, a low-roughage diet may be prescribed. This diet eliminates foods that are high in insoluble fiber, such as whole wheat foods, fruit, nuts, raw vegetables, and dried peas and beans. Fruit juices without pulp are usually permitted. On recovery, high-fiber foods are resumed.

Surgery

If the patient does not improve within 3 days of treatment, or there is deterioration in his condition, surgical intervention may be needed. About 20% to 30% of patients with diverticulitis require surgical treatment (Thomas, 2007). Surgery usually consists of a bowel resection with anastomosis. If surgery is required during the acute phase, a temporary colostomy may be necessary until the inflammation has subsided. The temporary colostomy is closed in 2 to 3 months.

Nursing Management

Because most patients with diverticular disease are symptom free, nursing care focuses on assessing for clinical symptoms of diverticulitis and secondary complications, as well as assessing the diet for fiber content. The Nursing Process: Patient Care Plan feature presents complete nursing care of the patient with acute diverticular disease.

Health Promotion

Health promotion is the number-one responsibility of the nurse. Primary prevention of diverticular disease can be accomplished the majority of the time through a high-fiber diet. Nurses can teach people in the community as well as patients in the hospital of the importance of a high-fiber diet. Nurses can work with local agencies to promote healthy eating, which includes a diet with 25 to 30 grams of fiber.

Inflammatory Bowel Disease

Inflammatory bowel disease (IBD) is an immunologic disease that results in idiopathic intestinal inflammation. It includes two distinct, yet similar conditions: **ulcerative colitis (UC)** and **Crohn's disease**. Both ulcerative colitis and Crohn's disease have common clinical manifestations as well as similar pathophysiology involving an inflammatory process. The cause of IBD remains under investigation, and it is now known that a constellation of factors contribute to the development of the disease. A combination of a genetic susceptibility, an abnormal immune response, an imbalance in beneficial and pathogenic bacteria in the intestines, and intestinal epithelial defects must be present for IBD to develop (Hampton, 2004).

Epidemiology

Approximately 2 million people in the United States are believed to have IBD (Biddle, 2003). The incidence of both ulcerative colitis (UC) and Crohn's disease is similar. The age of onset is usually between ages 15 and 25, although it can occur at any time. IBD is found worldwide, but is more prevalent in the United States, Canada, Europe, and Australia, yet rates are increasing in developing countries. Men and women are affected by IBD equally, although more men have UC and more women have Crohn's disease. The prevalence of IBD is reported for UC and Crohn's disease separately and is 229 per 100,000 for UC and 133 per 100,000 for Crohn's disease (Biddle, 2003).

PHARMACOLOGY Summary for Stool Softeners and Bulk-Forming Agents

Medication Category	Action	Application/Indication	Nursing Responsibility
Bulk-Forming Agents psyllium seed (Metamucil) methylcellulose	Improves bowel elimination by increasing stool bulk which promotes peristalsis	Constipation	Monitor for adverse effects: nausea, abdominal cramps, diarrhea. Be aware of drug interactions; monitor warfarin and digoxin levels. Instruct patient to follow each dose with an additional glass of water.
Stool Softeners docusate sodium (Colace)	Softens stool by allowing water and fat to penetrate	Constipation, prevention of straining	Monitor for adverse effects: abdominal cramps diarrhea. Instruct patient to increase fluid intake.

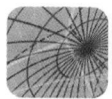

NURSING PROCESS: Patient Care Plan for Acute Diverticulitis

Assessment of Gastrointestinal Integrity

Subjective Data:
Are you having any bleeding?
Are you having any pain?
Have you noticed any abdominal bloating?

Objective Data:
Vital signs.
Abdominal assessment:
- Bowel sounds
- Abdominal girth
- Tenderness
- Guarding.

Stool assessment:
- Color
- Blood
- Consistency.

Nursing Assessment and Diagnoses	Outcomes and Evaluation Parameters	Planning and Interventions with *Rationales*
Nursing Diagnosis: *Tissue Integrity, Impaired* related to acute inflammatory process of diverticulitis	**Outcome:** Normal intestinal tissue. *Evaluation Parameters:* Normal vital signs. Normal bowel sounds in all quadrants. No abdominal distention. No abdominal tenderness. No abdominal guarding. Formed, soft stool. Stool negative for blood.	**Interventions and *Rationales:*** Assess vital signs every 4 hours for tachycardia and tachypnea, *which may indicate increased inflammation resulting in increased vascular leak syndrome and a fluid shift. Increasing fever may indicate perforation and peritonitis as well as increasing inflammation.* Assess abdomen every 4 hours for bowel sounds. *Decreasing bowel sounds may indicate peritonitis or bowel obstruction.* Measure abdominal girth and palpate abdomen for tenderness and guarding. *Increasing girth and/or tenderness and guarding can indicate a ruptured diverticulum, infection, peritonitis, or bleeding in the intra-abdominal cavity.* Examine stools for consistency and character as well as for evidence of blood, occult, or visual. *Diverticulitis can cause lower gastrointestinal bleeding.*

Assessment of Pain

Subjective Data:
On a scale of 0–10, with 10 being the worst pain, how would you rate your pain?
What does your pain feel like—dull, sharp, aching, or stabbing?
Have you felt nauseated?
Did you vomit?

Objective Data:
Vital signs.
Abdominal examination:
- Distention?
- Pain or tenderness on palpation?
- Bowel sounds?
- Soft or rigid?

Facial grimacing.
Restless, holding abdomen.

Nursing Assessment and Diagnoses	Outcomes and Evaluation Parameters	Planning and Interventions with *Rationales*
Nursing Diagnosis: *Pain, Acute* related to diverticulitis and possible ruptured diverticulum	**Outcome:** Comfort level maintained. *Evaluation Parameters:* Communicates reduced or absent pain. No pain behaviors evident: no facial grimacing, not holding abdomen. Abdomen soft with no distention, pain, or tenderness on palpation.	**Interventions and *Rationales:*** Assess pain using pain scale from 0–10, with 10 being the worst pain. *To increase consistency in quantifying pain.* Instruct the patient to inform the nurse if pain gets worse or is not relieved. *Can indicate complications or may need a change in pain medication.* Assess for associated symptoms that could indicate a complication. *Nausea and vomiting can indicate peritonitis.* Notify health care provider if pain increases or there are associated manifestations such as nausea, vomiting, or abdominal distention.

Pathophysiology

The causes of IBD may have a genetic link for some patients. For all, there develops an overly aggressive inflammatory response within the mucosa of the intestine.

Genetic Links

It is clear that some individuals are genetically predisposed to IBD even though only 10% to 15% of cases are familial (Hampton, 2004). The gene that encodes for a protein that possibly mediates epithelial cell-to-cell interactions is found on chromosome 10 and has been linked to Crohn's disease. Additionally, there is a gene on chromosome 7 that has been linked to Crohn's disease. Researchers are trying to identify other IBD-associated genes that mediate the immune response and epithelial integrity (Hampton, 2004).

Immune Response

In the normal intestine, the mucosal immune system works to protect against potentially harmful pathogens and distinguishes self-protein from non–self-protein structures. Antigens are presented to T lymphocytes and B lymphocytes by macrophages, or natural killer cells, and lymphokine-activated cells. The activated lymphocytes initiate the immune response, causing the release of cytokines, specific interleukins, and tissue necrosis factors. The antigen is transported through the lymphatics to the Peyer's patches, causing a release of lymphocytes into the lymph nodes and systemic circulation bound for the lamina propria of the intestines. Once in the intestines, there is an interaction between the lymphocytes and the endothelial cells resulting in the release of substances that support the inflammatory response. In people with IBD, there is a defect in this intestinal immune response (Smith & Bryant, 2002).

Immune Response to Bacteria

There is growing evidence to support that one aspect of IBD is the body's overly aggressive cell-mediated response to bacteria in the gut and/or a persistent infection. A few studies have identified *Mycobacterium paratuberculosis* as a possible pathogen associated with IBD, but further investigation is needed to confirm these studies (Hampton, 2004).

The Epithelium and Immune Response

The epithelial cells lining the intestines form a barrier for protection of the individual against a systemic bacterial infection. However, researchers now understand that the intestinal epithelium also has a role in the immune response. The epithelium communicates with the immune cells, and when the epithelial receptors recognize a bacterial product, they trigger the release of immunoregulatory proteins such as cytokines (Hampton, 2004).

Ulcerative Colitis

Ulcerative colitis (UC) is a disorder that involves chronic inflammation of the mucosal and submucosal layers of the colon and the rectum. It usually begins in the rectum and advances proximally, involving only the large intestine and usually only the sigmoid colon and rectum.

In UC, the inflammation begins at the base of the crypts of Lieberkühn and forms tiny mucosal hemorrhages with the development of abscesses that spread through the submucosa, causing necrosis. This, in turn, causes an increase in the release of inflammatory mediators, which results in congestion and edema leading to tissue friability and ulcer formation. The ulcers bleed easily causing bloody stools, a characteristic manifestation of UC. Atrophy and narrowing of the colon result from chronic inflammation.

Crohn's Disease

Crohn's disease differs from UC in that it can occur in any portion of the gastrointestinal tract from the mouth to the anus; however, it is usually limited to the ileum or ileocecal valve. Crohn's disease involves all layers (transmural) of the intestinal wall, but usually begins in the submucosa, spreading to the mucosa and serosa, while affecting some haustral segments and not others, producing what are called *skip lesions*. The lesions are granulomatous with areas of inflamed tissue circumscribed by scar tissue, giving the intestinal lumen a cobblestone appearance. As the disease progresses, the chronic inflammation causes fibrosis and loss of intestinal flexibility, resulting in obstruction, abscess, and fistula formation.

Malabsorption or malnutrition may develop in Crohn's disease for several reasons. First, Crohn's disease usually affects the jejunum and ileum where many nutrients are absorbed, and the presence of inflamed tissues and ulcers impairs absorption. Second, there may be a loss of exudate from the ulcerated area leading to not only protein loss but also occult or frank blood loss.

Clinical Manifestations

Ulcerative colitis and Crohn's disease have similar clinical manifestations that result from the inflammatory process in the intestines, and it can be difficult to distinguish between the two. Symptoms may be nonspecific and persist for years before diagnosis is made.

- Abdominal pain is usually present in both diseases and is characteristically a cramping type of sensation. The pain can be continuous or intermittent. The pain can be localized to either the right or left lower quadrant or be more diffuse, occurring over the entire lower abdomen.
- Diarrhea is usually present in both UC and Crohn's disease. There may be as many as 10 to 20 bowel movements per day. They can be loose and/or watery and may contain blood, although blood is more common in UC.
- Rectal urgency, incontinence, and tenesmus can be present in either UC or Crohn's disease.
- Systemic manifestations include fever, fatigue, joint pain, mouth sores, fatty liver, uveitis, autoimmune hepatitis, and primary sclerosing cholangitis. It is believed that these extraintestinal manifestations are of an immunologic nature similar to the IBD.

Diagnostic Procedures

Diagnosis of IBD can be difficult, especially when symptoms are nonspecific. The goal of treatment is to eliminate the intestinal inflammation and control the intestinal inflammatory response in the future.

Endoscopy

The gold standard for diagnosing IBD is colonoscopy. During colonoscopy, mucosal biopsy samples are taken at intervals and then examined microscopically for acute and chronic inflammation. UC and Crohn's disease can be differentiated on visualization. The inflammation in UC is continuous, whereas the pattern of inflammation in Crohn's disease is intermittent showing the characteristic skip lesions. An inflamed ileum can most always be attributed to Crohn's disease.

Radiography

A barium swallow with small-bowel follow-through and a barium enema are useful in detecting abnormalities such as ulcerations, strictures, colonic distention, obstruction, and fistulas. Radiography is used cautiously in patients with moderate to severe disease because there is a risk of colon perforation. Fistulas and abscesses, typical in patients with Crohn's disease, can be detected using MRI.

Blood Tests

No blood tests are available to diagnose IBD. A CBC is done to detect anemia resulting from blood loss, chronic inflammation, and malnutrition. An elevated WBC count results from the inflammatory process and abscess formation. The erythrocyte sedimentation rate (ESR) will be elevated but is not specific because it is elevated with any inflammation. Serum electrolytes, glucose, albumin, BUN, creatinine, and serum levels of vitamins are useful in monitoring the degree of malabsorption that may occur in Crohn's disease.

Genetic tests are now available but are not used widely. They are not diagnostic in themselves but are used in conjunction with other tests. Two genetic markers have been developed for clinical use. Anti–*Saccharomyces cerevisiae* antibodies (ASCA) are positive in about 60% of people with Crohn's disease. Perinuclear antineutrophil cytoplasmic antibodies (pANCA) are present in 60% to 80% of patients with UC or UC-like Crohn's disease (Biddle, 2003).

Medical Management

Medical management with medications and dietary changes is the first course of treatment. Only if medical management fails is surgery considered.

Drug Therapy

Medications are used in the treatment of IBD to halt acute exacerbations and minimize or eliminate recurrences. The most common medications act locally to control inflammation and systemically to suppress the immune response.

Sulfasalazine (Azulfidine) has been used to treat UC for more than 60 years. The active ingredient in this sulfonamide antibiotic is 5-aminosalicylic acid (5-ASA). It is safe and effective even when used long term. Patients with allergies to sulfa medications may be sensitive to sulfasalazine as well. This medication cannot be taken during pregnancy. There are now preparations that contain the 5-ASA without the sulfapyridine portion, which have fewer adverse effects, and include mesalamine (Asacol) and olsalazine (Dipentum). The 5-ASA inhibits prostaglandin production in the gut, thereby reducing the inflammatory process.

Corticosteroids, because of their potent anti-inflammatory effects, may be given to terminate an acute exacerbation of IBD. However, their use is avoided whenever possible because of the long-term side effects such as osteoporosis, diabetes mellitus, peptic ulcer disease, and cataracts. If the patient does not respond to 5-ASA treatment, prednisone is added at as low a dose as possible for the shortest time possible.

Immunomodulators such as azathioprine (AZA) and 6-mercaptopurine (6-MP) may be used for immunosuppression in place of corticosteroids. They are being used earlier in the course of IBD than in the past and may be used as a first line treatment. These medications need to be taken for at least 4 months before the full effect can be seen and can result in serious side effects such as bone marrow suppression, which may necessitate discontinuation of the drug if leucopenia or thrombocytopenia develops.

The most promising class of medications currently being developed is that of biologic modifiers. One drug, infliximab, a tumor necrosis factor-α (TNF-α) inhibitor, is approved for use in Crohn's disease. TNF-α is a cytokine that mediates components of the inflammatory process in Crohn's disease, thus, inhibiting TNF-α has proven beneficial in some patients (Rose, Armstrong, Klickstein, & Madsen, 2005). See the Pharmacology Summary feature (p. 1414) on the treatment of Inflammatory Bowel Disease.

Diet Therapy

There is no specific diet to follow for patients with IBD, other than one that is well balanced. Some patients with IBD report that certain foods exacerbate their condition. For example, milk and milk products may increase abdominal pain and diarrhea in some and should therefore be avoided if they cause problems. Conversely, a diet high in fiber may lessen diarrhea and improve tenesmus and rectal urgency. If the patient is known to have strictures or very severe acute symptoms, dietary fiber is contraindicated.

During an acute exacerbation of IBD, particularly Crohn's disease, the patient is allowed no food at all. This "bowel rest" helps relieve symptoms, which supports the theory that some foods and bacteria may be antigenic, causing inflammation in the gut. Total parenteral nutrition (TPN) is usually prescribed during the period of bowel rest. The Complementary and Alternative Therapies box (p. 1415) presents the use of hypnotherapy in treating irritable bowel syndrome.

Surgery

Patients who do not respond to the maximum doses of medication and/or who have complications such as malnutrition, anemia, bowel obstruction, and severe weight loss, are candidates for surgical intervention. The type of surgery will depend on the type of IBD and the location and extent of the lesions. As many as 66% of patients with Crohn's disease will undergo surgery for intractable disease with the average length of time from diagnosis to surgery of 3 years (Biddle, 2003). Only about 20% of people with UC require surgery, which is usually a total colectomy if the disease is extensive.

For patients with severe UC and for some patients with Crohn's disease, the surgical option is usually a total colectomy with an **ileal pouch anal anastomosis (IPAA)**. The entire colon, including the rectum, is removed, and a pouch is fashioned from the terminal ileum. The pouch is then anastomosed to the anus (Figure 45–7 ■, p. 1416). When healed, the pouch can hold enough fecal material to reduce bowel movements to 6 to 8 times a day. In order to allow time for the anastomosis to heal and the pouch to mature, a temporary loop **ileostomy** is done. A loop ileostomy involves bringing a loop of the ileum to the abdominal surface and creating a stoma to allow for the drainage of stool into a collection devise. After about 2 to 3 months, a second surgery is done to close the stoma and repair the bowel.

In patients with extensive Crohn's disease, an ileostomy, either permanent or continent, may be necessary. For these patients, an ileostomy is performed after removal of the entire colon, rectum, and anus. In a permanent ileostomy, fecal material is collected in an external collection bag. Fecal drainage is characteristically continuous and watery, because the large intestine is removed and this is where the majority of water is reabsorbed from feces. Another option is a **continent ileostomy**, also known as **Kock ileostomy or Kock pouch** (Figure 45–8 ■, p. 1417). During ileostomy surgery, the terminal ileum is folded back on itself and the inner wall removed, thereby forming a reservoir and a nipple valve. The end is then brought through the abdominal wall to form a stoma. The nipple valve prevents leaking of fecal contents through the stoma. The reservoir is emptied by a catheter inserted through the stoma. Nursing care of the patient with an ileostomy is outlined in the Nursing Process: Patient Care Plan feature (p. 1418) for patients with IBD.

PHARMACOLOGY Summary of Medications Used to Treat Inflammatory Bowel Disease (IBD)

Medication Category	Action	Application/Indication	Nursing Responsibility
5-Aminosalicylic Acid Agents Sulfasalazine (Azulfidine) Mesalamine (Asacol, Pentasa) Olsalazine (Dipentum)	Reduces inflammation by inhibiting prostaglandin production in the gut.	Mild to moderate inflammatory bowel disease (Crohn's disease, ulcerative colitis), proctosigmoiditis, remission maintenance in ulcerative colitis.	Monitor for adverse effects: headache, abdominal pain, cramps, and diarrhea. Evaluate for aspirin hypersensitivity, contraindicated in these patients. Sulfasalazine contraindicated in patients allergic to sulfa. Monitor BUN and creatinine, especially in presence of renal disease.
Corticosteroids Prednisone (Meticorten) Methylprednisolone (Medrol) Hydrocortisone (Cortef)	Decreases inflammation and immune response through inhibition of phagocytes, lymphocytes, histamine, and prostaglandin synthesis.	Moderate to severe IBD.	Monitor for adverse effects: mood swings, insomnia, nausea, hypertension, oral candidiasis, impaired wound healing, and symptoms of gastric ulcer. Monitor electrolytes and blood sugar. Warn patient not to stop drug abruptly.
Immunosuppressants Azathioprine (Imuran) Methotrexate (MTX)	Suppresses immune response by depressing T cell function.	Severe IBD.	Monitor for adverse effects: nausea, vomiting, and anorexia. Monitor CBC and platelet count. Observe for signs and symptoms of infection.
Biologic Response Modifier Infliximab (Remicade)	Monoclonal antibody that decreases inflammation by reducing production of proinflammatory cytokines.	Moderate to severe IBD.	Monitor for adverse reaction: fever, chills, pruritus, urticaria, chest pain, hypotension, hypertension, or dyspnea. Stop infusion and notify health care provider.
Coating Agents Sucralfate (Carafate) Bismuth subsalicylate (Pepto-Bismol)	Protects ulcer from gastric acid by forming a paste that adheres to ulcer; reduces pepsin.	Active duodenal ulcer, reflux esophagitis, acute erosive gastritis.	Monitor for adverse effects: constipation. Give sucralfate on an empty stomach, 1 hour before meals and at bedtime. Antacids should be given 30 minutes before or after administration. Warn patient about harmless darkening of stools when taking bismuth. Evaluate for aspirin hypersensitivity; bismuth subsalicylate contraindicated in these patients.
Bulk-Forming Agents Psyllium seed (Metamucil) Methylcellulose	Improves bowel elimination by increasing stool bulk, which promotes peristalsis.	Constipation	Monitor for adverse effects: nausea, abdominal cramps, and diarrhea. Be aware of drug interactions; monitor warfarin and digoxin levels. Instruct patient to follow each dose with an additional glass of water.
Stool Softeners Docusate sodium (Colace)	Softens stool by allowing water and fat to penetrate.	Constipation, prevention of straining.	Monitor for adverse effects: abdominal cramps and diarrhea. Instruct patient to increase fluid intake.

■ Nursing Management

Most patients with IBD are managed with medications, dietary changes, and stress reduction. Surgery is done usually as a last resort. Nursing care involves preparing the patient for diagnostic tests, managing the medication regimen, educating the patient about drug treatments and stress reduction, assessing the effectiveness of the interventions, and caring for the patient during the surgical experience, should surgery be necessary. Support networks are vitally important for this very life-disrupting disease. A number of resource groups are available, but the one recommended by most patients with IBD is the Crohn's & Col-

COMPLEMENTARY & ALTERNATIVE THERAPIES

Hypnotherapy

Description:

Irritable bowel syndrome (IBS) is a prevalent gastrointestinal disorder for which no clear cause has been found. Symptoms of IBS include abdominal pain, bloating, and altered bowel habits. Despite the great number of people afflicted with this disorder, there are few effective medical treatments (Tan, Hammond, & Joseph, 2005).

One theory as to the cause of IBS is stress. Hypnotherapy, which is also known as hypnosis, is a form of psychotherapy that uses the power of suggestion to help the patient achieve a deep state of relaxation. Hypnotherapy has been proven effective in many situations such as smoking cessation, headaches, pain, and insomnia.

Research Support:

In a clinical paper, a team of U.S. researchers reviewed 14 published studies to evaluate the effectiveness of hypnotherapy in treating IBS. Eight of the studies had no control group and six had a control group. The researchers found that hypnotherapy produced consistently significant results: Hypnotherapy improved IBS symptoms for the majority of patients. Researchers then evaluated the study results using the efficacy guidelines published by the Clinical Psychology Division of the American Psychological Association (APA). They found that the use of hypnotherapy for IBS qualifies for the APA's highest level of acceptance for both effectiveness and specificity. Researchers then sought to determine how hypnotherapy exerts its action on IBS. They found some evidence that supported both physiological and psychological mechanisms of action (Tan et al., 2005).

In another clinical paper, a team of researchers in Iran reviewed 15 studies on the use of hypnosis for IBS. The researchers based their criteria on the Rome Working Team recommendations for IBS trial design. The team's results showed that hypnosis improved IBS symptoms as well as quality of life, anxiety, and depression, and the improvements lasted from 2 to 5 years (Gholamrezaei, Ardestani, & Emami, 2006).

In a randomized controlled trial conducted in Britain, researchers studied the effect of gut-directed hypnotherapy on primary care IBS patients aged 18 to 65 years. Patients were diagnosed with IBS more than 6 weeks prior to the study and had no success with conventional management treatments. The intervention group received five sessions of hypnotherapy in addition to their usual IBS management. The control group received usual management only. Researchers collected symptom and quality of life data at baseline and again 3, 6, and 12 months posttest. At the 3-month mark, the intervention group showed significantly greater improvements in pain, diarrhea, and overall symptom scores. There were no significant differ-

ences in quality of life between the two groups. Patients in the intervention group, however, were significantly less likely to require medication. The majority of patients in the intervention group described an improvement in their condition. However, there was a lack of significant difference between groups beyond the 3-month mark. The researchers conclusions were that, although gut-directed hypnotherapy showed symptom reduction and reduced medication usage benefits, additional evidence is needed before clinicians can recommend the general introduction of hypnotherapy for IBS patients (Roberts, Wilson, Singh, Roalfe, & Greenfield, 2006).

The final study examined here involved 75 IBS patients in a nurse-led gut-directed hypnotherapy treatment program. Patients recorded their physical symptoms of IBS using 7-day diary cards. The patients' predominant symptoms included abdominal pain (61%), altered bowel habits (32.5%), and abdominal distension/bloating (6.5%). In addition, researchers administered an IBS-specific quality of life questionnaire as well as the Hospital Anxiety and Depression Scale. Statistics showed that patients' reported physical symptoms improved after hypnotherapy. Female patients who reported abdominal pain as their predominant physical symptom showed the most marked improvement. Six of the eight health-related quality of life domains that were measured (emotional, mental health, sleep, physical function, energy, and social role) also showed significant statistical improvement. Anxiety and depression also improved following treatment. Researchers concluded that hypnotherapy, when integrated into conventional care, provides a viable solution for the nursing management of irritable bowel syndrome (Smith, 2006).

References

Gholamrezaei, A., Ardestani, S. K., & Emami, M. H. (2006). Where does hypnotherapy stand in the management of irritable bowel syndrome? A systematic review. *Journal of Alternative and Complementary Medicine, 12*(6), 517–527.

Roberts, L., Wilson, S., Singh, S., Roalfe, A., & Greenfield, S. (2006). Gut-directed hypnotherapy for irritable bowel syndrome: Piloting a primary care-based randomised controlled trial. *British Journal of General Practice, 56*(523), 115–121.

Smith, G. D. (2006). Effect of nurse-led gut-directed hypnotherapy upon health-related quality of life in patients with irritable bowel syndrome. *Journal of Clinical Nursing, 15*(6), 678–684.

Tan, G., Hammond, D. C., & Joseph, G. (2005). Hypnosis and irritable bowel syndrome: A review of efficacy and mechanism of action. *American Journal of Clinical Hypnosis, 47*(3), 161–178.

---

itis Foundation of America. See the Nursing Process: Patient Care Plan feature (p. 1418) for the complete nursing care of the patient with inflammatory bowel disease.

■ Colon Cancer

Colon cancer is responsible for more than 56,000 deaths a year, second only to lung cancer with respect to cancer deaths. Men and women are affected equally, and the incidence increases after age 50. If the lesions are confined to the colon and rectum, the 5-year survival rate is as high as 90%. If there is spread to the adjacent tissues, the survival rate drops to 65%; and if there is involvement of distant sites, the survival rate is as low as 8% (Jemal et al., 2007). Early detection is therefore vital. Although the American Cancer Society (ACS) recommends sigmoidoscopy or colonoscopy after age 50, screening rates continue to be low, possibly because of the

personal and embarrassing nature of the test and the financial cost. The Cultural Considerations box (p. 1416) outlines the disparity in the rates of cancer, including colon cancer, among different racial and ethnic groups.

Pathophysiology/Etiology

There is a strong association between the development of colon cancer and genetic events. Researchers have linked an alteration in the p53 gene to 86% of colorectal cancers. Also, when there is an allelic deletion on chromosome 5, 17, or 18, the transformation from normal to malignant colon tissue is promoted (Huether, 2006).

Adenomatous polyps, which result from a mutation on chromosome 5, are considered premalignant tissue, and most colorectal cancers develop from this type of polyp (Huether, 2006). Three different types of polyps develop from mucosal epithelium: tubular, villous, and tubulovillous. Tubular polyps, the most common,

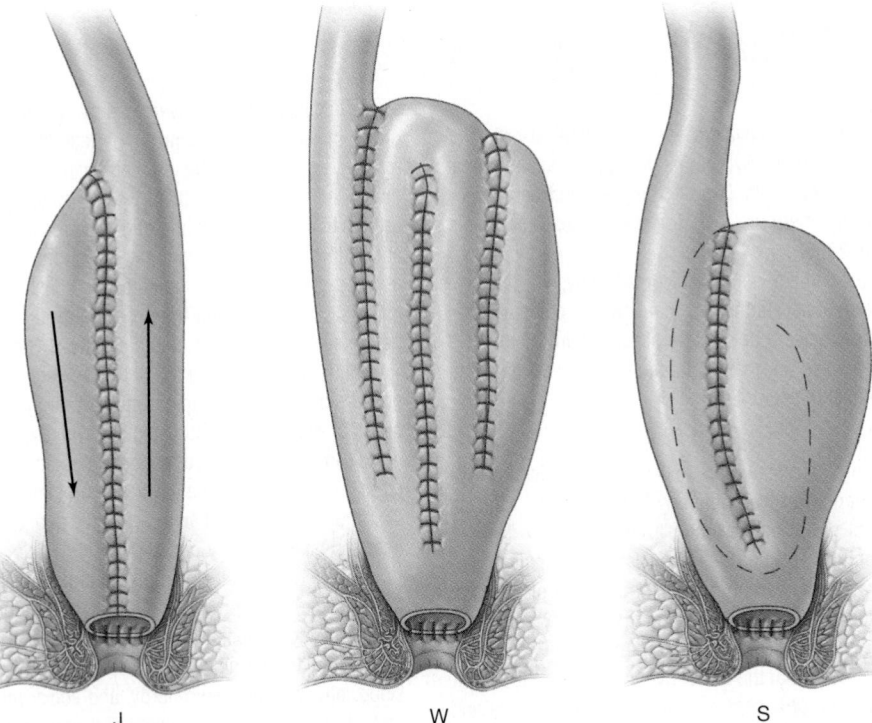

J   W   S

FIGURE 45–7 ■ Ileal pouch anal anastomosis.

CULTURAL CONSIDERATIONS Related to Colon Cancer

According to the American Cancer Society (2007), African Americans are more likely to develop and die from cancer than any other racial or ethnic population. Currently the death rate from cancer among African American males is 38% higher than among white males; for African American females, it is about 17% higher. Overall, racial and ethnic minorities face more obstacles in receiving health care services, including cancer prevention, early detection, and quality treatment. Statistics released from the American Cancer Society Surveillance Research reveal that African American males have the highest incidence and mortality associated with colorectal cancers (Jemal et al., 2007).

consist of a stalk and a spherical structure at the end. The stalk is attached to the intestinal wall. They are also called pedunculated polyps, and their numbers increase with aging. These polyps vary in size from less than 1 centimeter to as large as 5 centimeters. The larger the polyp, the more likely it will transform into malignant tissue. Villous adenomas are less common, are larger than 5 centimeters, and have a high malignant potential. In an autosomal dominant genetic disorder called familial polyposis, there are hundreds of adenomatous polyps present in the large intestine. The polyps in this disorder will transform to malignant tissue 100% of the time, usually by age 40.

There appears to be a link between dietary factors and the development of colorectal cancer. The disease is virtually unknown in poor countries where the diet consists mainly of unrefined grains, fruits, and vegetables. In countries like the United States, where the typical diet is high in animal protein, fat, and calories, the prevalence of colorectal cancer is higher. The largely animal source diet is believed to increase anaerobic bacteria in the colon, where they convert bile acids to carcinogens. The excess dietary animal fat also causes increased deposition of fatty acids within the cell membranes, and an increase in intestinal prostaglandins stimulates cell proliferation. Other nutrients that are associated with a lower risk for colon cancer are folic acid, selenium, vitamin D, and calcium. There is some research to indicate that the use of nonsteroidal anti-inflammatory drugs (NSAIDs), such as aspirin and ibuprofen, and hormone replacement therapy also decreases colon cancer risk. The role of physical inactivity remains controversial.

Recent research indicates that daily alcohol consumption increases the risk for colon cancer and is dose related. In fact, in one study the research found a 70% greater risk of colon cancer in people who drank alcohol daily when compared to their nondrinking counterparts (Su & Arab, 2004). There is also evidence to indicate a link between **C-reactive protein (CRP)** and colon cancer. CRP is a protein released from the liver in response to local inflammation or tissue injury. It has been known for a long time that CRP is a marker for inflammation but only recently discovered that there is a link between inflammation and colon cancer (Erlinger, Platz, Rifai, & Helzlsouer, 2004). This may help explain the association between anti-inflammatory agents and a reduced risk for colon cancer. The chronic inflammation of irritable bowel syndrome (IBS) is also known to increase the risk for developing colon cancer.

Adenocarcinoma is the most common type of colon cancer and accounts for 95% of colon tumors (Thomas, 2007). Adenocarcinomas grow irregularly and form hard, nodular areas. Colon cancer is classified by the tissue type, lymph node involvement, and stage of metastasis (TNM). The National Guidelines box (p. 1420) outlines two tumor classification systems. Colon cancer cells range from well differentiated to poorly differentiated. The cancer is spread first by local invasion and direct ex-

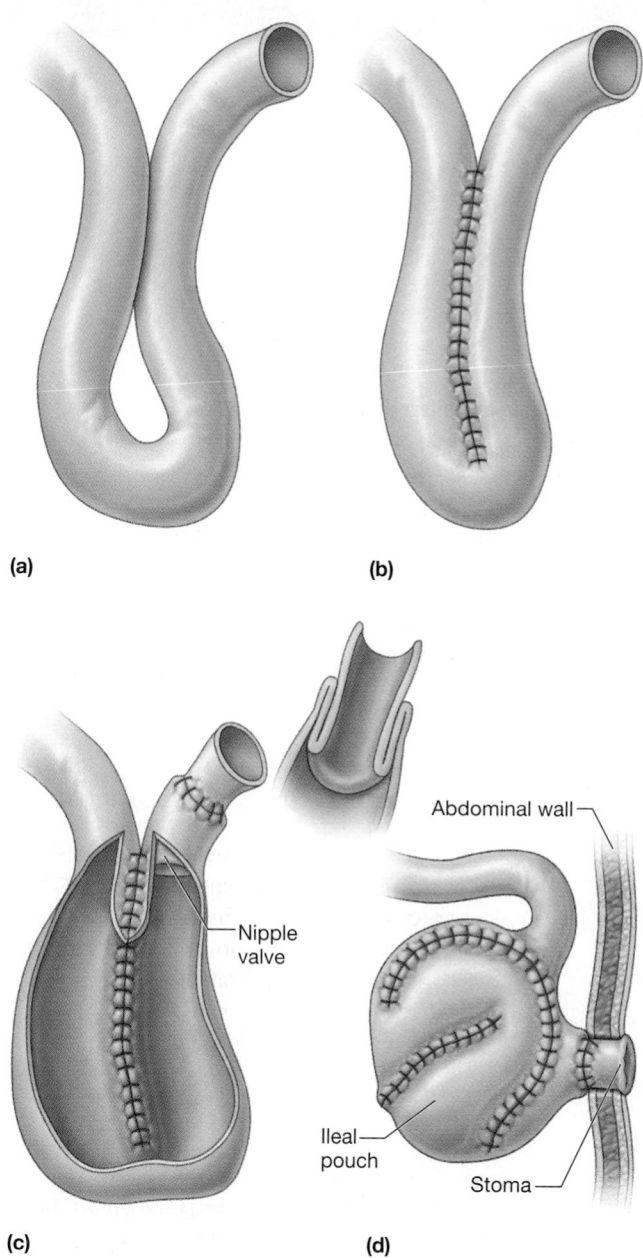

(a)

(b)

(c)

Nipple valve

(d)

Abdominal wall

Ileal pouch

Stoma

FIGURE 45–8 ■ Kock ileostomy.

tension. Any tissue or organ in the neighboring area can be affected, such as the liver, duodenum, small intestine, pancreas, and the abdominal wall. Because the lymph system is closely associated with the intestines, cancer is also easily spread to distant sites via this way. It can also reach distant sites by way of the circulation. The most common sites for metastasis of colon cancer are the liver, lungs, brain, and bones.

Clinical Manifestations

Colon cancer is usually asymptomatic until it is well advanced. Most types of colon cancer grow very slowly, taking 5 to 15 years of growth before symptoms are present, and even those symptoms are vague and often misdiagnosed. The symptoms will depend mostly on the location of the tumor and its stage of growth. The most common symptoms are a change in bowel habits, such as constipation or diarrhea, or a change in the caliber of the stools. The symptom that causes the most alarm, and usually prompts

the patient to see her health care provider, is bleeding in the stool. As the disease progresses, there may be weight loss, fatigue, abdominal pain, and anorexia. Anemia may also be a manifestation that presses the patient to seek attention. Some of the complications of colon cancer, such as bowel obstruction and bowel perforation, may be the first manifestations the patient notices.

Tumors in the ascending colon are usually polypoid and extend along one wall of the ascending colon. Because they are bulky tumors, a palpable mass can usually be felt. They tend to develop necrotic areas and ulcerate contributing to the slow blood loss and anemia. Pain is usually a late sign.

Descending colon tumors are usually small and button like. Rather than growing along one wall of the colon as tumors in the ascending colon do, these tumors grow around the circumference of the colon and spread along the entire bowel wall. Because of the circumferential nature of this type of colon cancer, obstruction is common. Constipation is the predominant symptom as the bowel lumen becomes smaller as the tumor grows.

Diagnostic Procedures

The American Cancer Society currently recommends that African American men be screened beginning at age 45 and that all others at age 50 have either an annual fecal occult blood test or a sigmoidoscopy every 5 years or a colonoscopy every 5 to 10 years (Irani & Krevsky, 2007). However, because sigmoidoscopy will detect cancer in only the sigmoid colon and the rectum, most health care providers recommend the colonoscopy, because it can establish the diagnosis of colon cancer with 100% accuracy (Thomas, 2007).

There are no laboratory tests that can establish the diagnosis of colon cancer; however, many tests are used to detect manifestations of colon cancer, such as chronic blood loss. A CBC will detect the anemia that results from blood loss and tumor growth, as well as the leukocyte response to inflammation. As mentioned previously, a C-reactive protein is also ordered to detect inflammation. **Carcinoembryonic antigen (CEA)** is found in 70% of people with cancer of the large intestine, but the test is too insensitive and nonspecific to be useful in screening or diagnosing colon cancer. CEA is useful in monitoring a patient's response to treatment.

The only definitive way to diagnose colon cancer is with a tissue biopsy. This is usually done using colonoscopy and is almost 100% accurate in diagnosing this type of cancer. As mentioned earlier, the TNM system for staging colon cancer is most often used to indicate the extent of the cancer and to judge prognosis. A CT scan is then done to detect possible metastasis in distant locations such as the liver or lungs.

Medical Management

Prevention of colon cancer is the primary goal of collaborative care, followed next by early detection and treatment. Prevention and early detection of colon cancer is done through educating the public about ways to decrease the risk, such as eliminating alcoholic beverages on a daily basis; increasing the amount of fruits, vegetables, and fiber; daily exercise and weight control; and possibly a daily low dose of aspirin.

Surgery

Surgery is the treatment of choice for individuals with colon cancer because it offers the only known cure. Even when metastasis

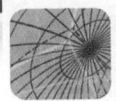

Assessment of Bowel Elimination

Subjective Data:

How many stools do you have a day?
What is the consistency and color?
Is there any blood?
Do you have any abdominal pain or cramping?
How long have you been having this problem?
When did it start?

Does stress in your life make it worse?
Does any food make the diarrhea worse?
Do you have any joint pain or fatigue?
Have you been treated before?
Do you take any home remedies, herbs, or over-the-counter medications?

Objective Data:

Vital signs.
Examination of abdomen:

- Bowel sounds
- Palpation
- Visual exam for contour, scars.

Visual inspection of stools.
Test stool for occult blood.

Nursing Assessment and Diagnoses	Outcomes and Evaluation Parameters	Planning and Interventions with *Rationales*

Nursing Diagnoses: *Diarrhea* related to irritable bowel syndrome (IBS). *Fluid Balance, Readiness for Enhanced* related to the diarrhea.	**Outcome:** Decreased diarrhea. ***Evaluation Parameters:*** Number of stools decreased by at least half. Consistency of stool: formed. Absence of blood in the stool. No abdominal cramping.	**Interventions and *Rationales:*** Take vital signs every 4 hours *to assess for signs of dehydration such as tachycardia, tachypnea, or fever.* Weigh daily *to assess for fluid losses.* Examine skin and mucous membranes *for evidence of dehydration, such as poor turgor, dry mucous membranes, or dry, cracked tongue.* Maintain NPO if ordered *to rest the bowel, which promotes healing and improves diarrhea.* Provide good perianal care with gentle cleansing agents, and apply protective cream or ointment to the area *to prevent skin breakdown.* Administer ordered medications, assess their effectiveness, and monitor adverse effects:
		
		• 5-ASA compounds (sufasalazine, mesalamine, olsalazine) are anti-inflammatory drugs that decrease inflammation of the intestinal mucosa.
		  1. Monitor for adverse effects, which include skin rashes, urticaria, pruritus, bleeding or easy bruising, fever, low WBC and platelet counts, low hemoglobin and hematocrit (bone marrow suppression), and decreased urine output (renal failure).
		  2. Give and teach patient to take these medications after eating to avoid gastric distress.
		  3. Encourage increased fluid intake (2 L/day) to prevent kidney damage.
		  4. Teach patient to notify the health care provider if any of the adverse effects occur.
		• Corticosteroids—adrenal hormones (prednisolone) that suppress the immune response and have anti-inflammatory properties:
		  1. Monitor for side effects such as elevated blood glucose, fluid retention (edema, weight gain, hypertension, heart failure), gastric ulcers, hypokalemia (muscle weakness, nausea, dysrhythmias), and mood swings.
		  2. Should be given only with meals to decrease the risk of ulcers and gastric distress.
		  3. Teach the patient to increase foods high in potassium (citrus fruit, bananas, potatoes) and reduce intake of sodium (canned soup, bottled salad dressing, processed meats, cheese).
		  4. Teach patient NOT TO STOP THE MEDICATION ABRUPTLY (the dose must be tapered).
		• Immunomodulators (azathioprine) suppress the immune system.
		  1. Be sure to tell the patient that these drugs must be taken for 4–5 months before the full effect is seen.
		  2. Monitor for adverse effects such as pancreatitis (usually within the first 2 months), and low WBC or platelet count.
		• Infliximab (tumor necrosis factor blocker) used for refractory Crohn's disease.
		  1. Given every 2–3 months and must be given intravenously.
		  2. Monitor for adverse effects such as infection serum sickness–like reaction and lupus-like syndrome (Biddle, 2003).

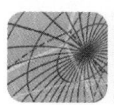

Assessment of Body Image

Subjective Data:
How has this disease/surgery affected your life?
Are you able to continue working? Socializing with friends? Shopping?
Has this affected how you feel about your personal relationships? Sexual activity?

Objective Data:
Facial expressions.
Body language.
Attitude toward stoma.

Nursing Assessment and Diagnoses	Outcomes and Evaluation Parameters	Planning and Interventions with *Rationales*
Nursing Diagnosis: *Disturbed Body Image* related to disease process and/or surgery	**Outcome:** Normal body image. ***Evaluation Parameter:*** Verbalizes acceptance of body image,	**Interventions and *Rationales:*** Assess the patient's current perception of self and demonstrate acceptance of where the patient is now. *Acceptance of the patient's feelings can help establish a caring and trusting nurse–patient relationship.* Provide an environment in which the patient feels comfortable talking about the disease and how it has impacted his life. To build caring nurse–patient relationship. Encourage the patient to talk about ways this disease has affected personal, work, social, and sexual relationships. *To provide understanding and demonstrate acceptance of the patient as a person.* Delineate possible treatment options, including graphic description of surgery and postop possibilities *to give the patient a sense of control.* Provide names and phone numbers of IBS support groups. If possible, arrange for the patient to meet with someone who has the disease. *This shows the patient that she is not the only person facing this problem.*

Assessment of Fecal Diversion (Ileostomy)

Subjective Data:
Are you having any cramping?
Are you passing any gas through the stoma?

Objective Data:
Vital signs.
Abdominal assessment:
- Stoma color
- Stoma drainage/bleeding
- Condition of skin surrounding stoma.
Condition of ostomy appliance.

Nursing Assessment and Diagnoses	Outcomes and Evaluation Parameters	Planning and Interventions with *Rationales*
Nursing Diagnoses: *Bowel Incontinence* related to fecal diversion. *Skin Integrity, Impaired, Risk for* related to ostomy drainage. *Knowledge, Deficient* related to fecal diversion.	**Outcome:** Normal functioning ileostomy. ***Evaluation Parameters:*** Stoma color pink and moist. No bloody effluent. Effluent dark green and viscous initially, gradually turning yellow-brown. Skin around stoma free of irritation and inflammation. Ileoanal skin without irritation or inflammation. Able to communicate necessary stoma care, dietary modification, and stress reduction techniques.	**Interventions and *Rationales:*** Monitor stoma color. *The stoma should be pink, beefy red, and moist with no obvious cyanosis or bleeding. It should extend about 2–3 centimeters from the abdominal wall. Impaired circulation will cause the stoma to be dark, blue, or very pale.* Assess stoma function. *Immediately postop there may be small amounts of blood.* Within 1 or 2 days the drainage will be dark green and viscous, gradually turning yellow-brown and developing an odor. Empty and measure ileostomy drainage when the pouch is one-third to one-half full and explain the procedure to the patient each time. *Emptying the pouch when it is not too full eliminates the possibility of the seal in the pouch breaking and causing leaking. Explaining the procedure to the patient each time gets the patient more comfortable with self-care.* Assess the skin surrounding the stoma and around the perianal area. The skin should be pink and remain free of irritation, excoriation, or inflammation. *Ileostomy drainage is irritating to the skin because it contains bile salts and digestive enzymes that normally get reabsorbed in the large intestine.* Apply a protecting skin barrier under the pouch *to prevent contact of drainage with skin.* Report abnormal assessment findings such as poor stoma color, bulging or retracted stoma, or rash around the stoma. Poor stoma color indicates poor circulation to the section of bowel that forms the stoma; bulging can indicate herniation or prolapse. Teach patient and family members to assess the stoma and to treat it gently. *Because there are no pain receptors in the stoma, it can become injured without feeling pain.* Teach patient to notify health care provider if there is a change in the stoma or if a rash develops in the skin surrounding the stoma. Assess the patient's ability to manage the ileostomy including knowledge of ostomy care, what medications to avoid (laxatives, enteric coated, or capsules), and signs and symptoms to report.

NATIONAL GUIDELINES for Tumor Classification

TNM Classification	American Joint Committee Classification
T (Tumor)	Stage 0:
	Carcinoma in situ.
Tx: tumor cannot be assessed.	Stage I:
T0: no tumor.	Invasion of submucosa (80–100% 5-year survival).
Tis: carcinoma in situ.	Invasion of muscularis propria.
T1: increasing tumor size.	Stage II (node negative disease) (50–75% 5-year survival):
T2: invades muscularis.	Invasion into the subserosa or into nonperitonealized pericolic or perirectal tissue.
T3: penetrates through bowel wall.	Tumor perforates the visceral peritoneum or invades other organs by direct extension.
T4: invades adjacent organs.	
N (Nodes)	Stage III (node positive disease) (30–50% 5-year survival):
Nx: cannot assess regional lymph nodes.	Bowel wall perforation with lymph node metastasis.
N0: no regional lymph nodes.	
N1: 1–3 pericolic or perirectal lymph nodes.	
N2: 4 or more pericolic or perirectal nodes.	
N3: lymph node metastasis along vascular trunk.	
M (Metastasis)	Stage IV (metastatic disease) (5% 5-year survival):
Mx: not assessed.	Presence of distant metastasis.
M0: no metastasis.	
M1: metastasis present at distant sites.	

Source: Adapted from Tierney, L. M., McPhee, S. J., & Papadakis, M. A. (2004). *Current medical diagnosis and treatment* (43rd ed.). New York: Lange Medical Books/McGraw-Hill.

has occurred, surgical resection can improve the chance of survival. There are several different surgical procedures for the patient with colon cancer depending on the stage, tumor size, and general health of the patient. Surgery can range from abdominoperineal resection with a colostomy to laser photocoagulation. With advances in surgical technique and equipment, thankfully, most patients do not require a colostomy, as was once the case. Tumors of the rectum, however, do usually require removal of the rectum, sigmoid colon, and anus, necessitating a sigmoid colostomy for fecal elimination.

Two procedures can be performed using an endoscope: laser photocoagulation and local excision and fulguration. During laser photocoagulation, an intense beam of laser light is aimed at the tumor where the heat generated destroys the cancerous tissue. This procedure is also helpful as palliative treatment for advanced tumors when the patient is not a good surgical candidate or to remove an obstruction. Local excision can be done by endoscopy or by laparoscopy. This surgical method is used if the tumor is small and well defined. Electrocoagulation or fulguration can reduce the size of a tumor in a patient who is not a good candidate for extensive colon resection.

Occasionally, an end-to-end anastomosis is not possible during colon resection, and the patient requires a colostomy for the diversion of fecal material. The type and permanence of the colostomy depends on the location of the tumor (Figure 45–9 ■). If there is a large bout of inflammation or tissue trauma, a temporary colostomy is created to give the bowel time to heal, and then the bowel is reanastomosed and the colostomy closed at a later date, usually in 3 to 6 months. A sigmoid colostomy, performed for cancer of the rectum, is most usually permanent.

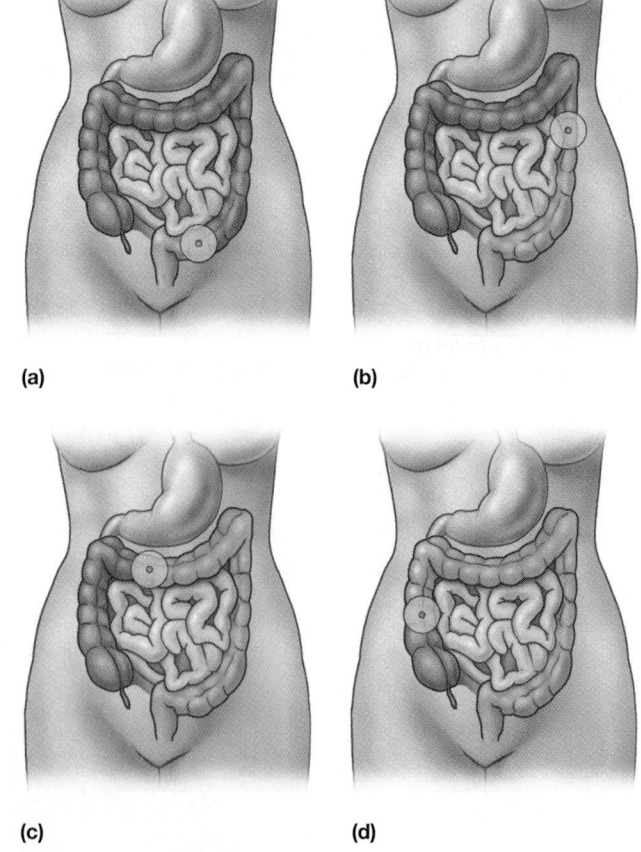

(a)

(b)

(c)

(d)

FIGURE 45–9 ■ Colostomy sites.

A double-barrel colostomy is created in the case of trauma to the colon or severe inflammation. The distal colon is bypassed but not removed, and may be reanastomosed. There are two stomas on the abdominal surface. The distal stoma, also called a mucous fistula because it drains mucus from the distal colon, usually requires only a gauze dressing. The proximal stoma will have fecal discharge and will require the application of an ostomy appliance (bag) to collect feces.

There are several other types of colostomies that are usually temporary in placement. In an emergency, a transverse loop colostomy may be performed. As the name implies, a loop of bowel is brought through the abdominal wall and suspended over a glass or plastic rod, preventing the bowel from slipping back into the abdomen. An ostomy is made in the loop of colon. The rod is removed usually in about 2 weeks. The Hartmann procedure is another technique for creating a temporary colostomy. In this procedure the distal colon is oversewn to close the lumen, and the proximal colon forms the colostomy. It is similar to the double-barrel colostomy, except that the lower portion does not have a stoma on the abdominal wall. Patients require the same care whether the colostomy is permanent or temporary. Nursing care of the patient with a colostomy is discussed in the Nursing Process: Patient Care Plan feature.

Chemotherapy and Radiation Therapy

Chemotherapeutic agents are used as an adjunctive therapy for colon cancer after colon resection. The patient is usually given a period of time to heal postoperatively before chemotherapy is started. Chemotherapy can be combined with radiation therapy to reduce the rate of recurrence. Radiation appears to prolong survival in patients with more advanced cancer, particularly rectal tumors. Radiation can also be used before surgery to shrink large tumors and make them easier to resect surgically.

Nursing Management

Because there is a link between lifestyle choices and the development of colon cancer, nursing can impact primary prevention of the disease by teaching and advising patients about lifestyle choices that may decrease the risk. Dietary modifications, including increasing the amount of dietary fiber and reducing the amount of fat, sugar, and meat, can help reduce colon cancer risk. However, it is not enough simply to tell a patient to increase fiber and decrease fat, sugar, and meat. The nurse must give specific information about what foods are high in fiber and those that are high in fat and sugar and should be eaten in limited quantities, and consider cultural, economic, and religious factors when making the suggestions.

Other important aspects of nursing care include teaching patients about the warning signs of colon cancer and when to seek treatment. A frank discussion with patients over age 40 about recommended screening and what each test involves can help dispel their fears and misconceptions.

Because the treatment of choice for patients with colon cancer is surgery, the focus of nursing care is on pre- and postoperative care, and support in dealing with a possible colostomy, chemotherapy, and radiation treatment, and possibly death. Emotional support throughout the course of the illness is paramount. See the Nursing Process: Patient Care Plan feature for complete nursing care of the patient with colon cancer.

Research

Research being done regarding gastrointestinal disorders is focused on less invasive approaches to surgical treatments; education regarding screening exams, particularly those with cultural barriers; and multiple alternative therapies. The Research Opportunities and Clinical Impact box (p. 1423) describes current research opportunities for gastrointestinal disorders.

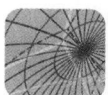

NURSING PROCESS: Patient Care Plan for the Patient with Colon Cancer Having Surgery

Assessment of Preoperative Readiness

Subjective Data:
What did the surgeon tell you about your surgery?
Do you have any questions that you would like to ask?

Objective Data:
Vital signs.
Signed consent.
Character of stool postbowel prep.
Has the enterostomal therapy nurse seen the patient?
Are all preop laboratory reports in the chart?

Nursing Assessment and Diagnoses	Outcomes and Evaluation Parameters	Planning and Interventions with *Rationales*
Nursing Diagnosis: *Fear* related to surgical procedure and diagnosis of cancer	**Outcome:** Ready for surgery. **Evaluation Parameters:** Signed consent. Lab reports in chart. Communicates fears and anxiety. Able to verbalize the nature and extent of the surgery.	**Interventions and *Rationales:*** Ask the patient to tell the nurse what will happen postoperatively. *This helps the nurse assess the patient's understanding of the procedure and what to expect in the postoperative period. It also assesses whether the patient understands what she signed for on the informed consent.* Administer the bowel prep as ordered and examine the stool to assess the effectiveness of the prep. Stool should be liquid and clear by the end of the prep. *The prep cleans the bowel and reduces the risk of infection postoperatively.* Contact the enterostomal therapist to arrange a preop visit with the patient *to help ease fear and anxiety about the possible colostomy.*

(continued)

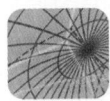

NURSING PROCESS: Patient Care Plan for the Patient with Colon Cancer Having Surgery—*Continued*

Assessment of Postoperative Pain

Subjective Data:
On a scale of 1–10, with 10 being the worst pain ever, how would you rate your pain?
Are you allergic to any pain medications?
Do you have any cultural or religious beliefs that might impact your pain control?

Objective Data:
Vital signs.
Restless and irritable.
Facial grimacing when moving.

Nursing Assessment and Diagnoses	Outcomes and Evaluation Parameters	Planning and Interventions with *Rationales*
Nursing Diagnosis: *Pain, Acute* related to surgical incision	**Outcome:** Comfort level maintained. *Evaluation Parameters:* Communicates pain level and effectiveness of analgesia. Reports adequate pain control. No facial grimacing.	**Interventions and *Rationales:*** Use pain scale (1–10) to quantify level of pain *in order to be consistent from nurse to nurse, and time to time, when assessing pain.* Teach the patient to inform the nurse if the pain is not relieved. *Indicates the need to change pain management plan.* Assess cultural and religious beliefs about pain and pain relief. *Different cultures and religions may view pain as punishment or may have nontraditional ways of treating pain.* Medicate the patient prior to ambulation. *Decreased pain increases exercise tolerance, and ambulation increases intestinal motility, preventing ileus, and enhances the respiratory effort, decreasing the chance of pneumonia.*

Assessment of Skin Integrity (Postoperative)

Subjective Data:
Ask the patient whether he has feeling around the stoma.

Objective Data:
Assess stoma and skin around stoma for:
- Redness
- Color of stoma
- Swelling
- Drainage.

Nursing Assessment and Diagnoses	Outcomes and Evaluation Parameters	Planning and Interventions with *Rationales*
Nursing Diagnosis: *Skin Integrity, Impaired* related to colostomy and surgical incision	**Outcome:** Good skin and stomal integrity. *Evaluation Parameters:* Stoma pink and moist. Skin surrounding stoma pink, no excoriation.	**Interventions and *Rationales:*** Inspect stoma and surrounding skin for color and edema. A healthy stoma is pink or beefy red and moist due to mucous production. The peristomal skin should be pink and show no signs of irritation, inflammation, excoriation, or rashes. *A bluish purple or dusky stoma indicates impaired blood flow to the stoma. Skin around the stoma can be irritated by the appliance, by a yeast infection, or from a leaking appliance.* Apply caulking agents (Stomahesive or Karaya paste) to maintain a leak-free secure ostomy appliance *to prevent leakage onto skin. Ostomy drainage is very irritating to the skin and can cause skin breakdown.* Assess surgical incision for bleeding, redness, and draining at least every 4 hours. Change dressing as ordered by surgeon to keep the incision clean and dry, *which helps prevent an infected incision.*

Assessment of Bowel Function

Subjective Data:
Are you passing any gas through the stoma?
Do you feel any rumbling in your abdomen?
Have you been nauseated?

Objective Data:
Examination of abdomen:
- Bowel sounds
- Palpation
- Visual exam for contour, condition of stoma, and any drainage.
Color, consistency, and frequency of colostomy drainage.
Test stool for occult blood.

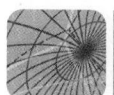

NURSING PROCESS: Patient Care Plan for the Patient with Colon Cancer Having Surgery—*Continued*

Nursing Assessment and Diagnoses	Outcomes and Evaluation Parameters	Planning and Interventions with *Rationales*
Nursing Diagnosis: *Bowel Incontinence* related to surgery and fecal diversion.	**Outcome:** Functioning colostomy. ***Evaluation Parameters:*** Stool from colostomy semiformed. Active bowel sounds.	**Interventions and *Rationales:*** Assess abdomen for bowel sounds, which indicate peristalsis has returned. *Manipulation and anesthesia have the potential for causing an ileus.* Assess for nausea and vomiting, which can also *indicate an ileus.* Assess the characteristics of the colostomy drainage. *Fecal-like drainage and flatulence from the stoma indicate the return of bowel function.*

RESEARCH OPPORTUNITIES AND CLINICAL IMPACT RELATED TO DISORDERS OF THE GASTROINTESTINAL TRACT

Area	Clinical Impact
Physiological Research	
Use of traditional Chinese medicine for gastrointestinal disorders.	Use of non-Western medicine for treatment of GI disorders may improve patient compliance due to fewer side effects and less cost.
Use of complementary and alternative medicine in patients with inflammatory bowel disease.	
Laparoscopic surgery for colon cancer.	Less invasive surgical techniques would decrease complications and patient length of stay.
Relationship between serum antibodies to bacterial antigens and clinical remission in Crohn's disease.	
Drugs for maintenance therapy in inflammatory bowel disease.	Medications or other treatments would decrease the long-term consequences of inflammatory bowel disease, thereby improving the quality of life and longevity.
More sensitive tests for assessing disease activity in inflammatory bowel disease.	
Surgical treatments for gastroesophageal reflux disease.	Because long-term GERD can lead to esophageal cancer, effective treatment can reduce mortality.
Emotional and Psychological Research	
Communicating about screening for colon cancer in culturally diverse groups.	Improved communication between health care providers and culturally diverse groups can increase screening in these groups and hopefully decrease mortality.
Patient satisfaction with photodynamic therapy for Barrett's esophagus.	
Quality of life after bariatric surgery.	
Quality of life after surgery for gastroesophageal cancer.	Understanding issues about quality of life can assist nurses to help patients cope better with life changes.
Music therapy to reduce anxiety before gastrointestinal procedures.	Improve psychological interventions to improve coping.

Clinical Preparation

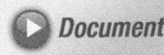 **Read**

- History of Current Illness
- Past Medical History
- Physical Exam
- Admitting Medical Orders
- Laboratory Study Results

 **Document**

- Summary of Hospitalization
- Pathophysiology Form
- Laboratory Values
- Laboratory Results Explanation

Apply

- List of Potential Nursing Diagnoses
- Concept Map
- Critical Thinking Questions

Log on to MyNursingKit.com to download forms you will need and to complete further steps in the Clinical Preparation assignment.

HISTORY OF PRESENT ILLNESS

As a nurse working on a GI floor in a large teaching hospital, you are receiving report about Ms. T, a 35-year-old woman who was admitted 2 days ago with hematemesis and abdominal pain. She reported symptoms of increasing epigastric pain for approximately 3 weeks, and the use of Tums, which had been working most of the time. She also reported taking aspirin daily for prevention of heart disease. The bleeding has stopped now, and she has just returned from an EGD (esophagogastroduodenoscopy), which confirmed a gastric ulcer.

Medical–Surgical History

Her past medical history includes gastroesophageal reflux disease for which she was prescribed Prilosec, but she could not afford to purchase the medication, so she has been taking Tums instead.

Social History

She has a 10 pack-year history of smoking, having quit 3 months prior to this admission. She reports being a "social" drinker. She reports an intentional weight loss of 50 pounds during the last year.

Physical Exam

Her vital signs are temperature 37°C; heart rate 90 and regular; respirations 16 and unlabored; and blood pressure 100/60 sitting. Her skin is pale and dry. Her lungs are clear to auscultation, and her heart is regular with no murmurs or extra heart sounds noted at this time. Her bowel sounds are present in all four quadrants, and her abdomen is soft with tenderness noted in the epigastrium. She has a nasogastric tube set to low intermittent suction that is draining green fluid.

Ms. T's current nursing care, medication schedule, and laboratory study results follow.

Admitting Medical Orders

Service: Medicine
Diagnosis: gastric ulcer
Allergies: none
Vital signs q15min × 4 then q1h × 2 then q4h with oxygen saturation
Activity: up to chair 4 times per day, may ambulate to bathroom
Diet: NPO, may have ice chips
Nasogastric tube to low wall suction; flush NG with 30 mL saline q8h
Call house officer: temp > 38.5°C, HR > 130 or < 60, RR > 30 or < 12, BP sys > 160 or < 90, O$_2$ sat < 92%, urine output < 120 mL in 4 hours, change in neurological or abdominal exam, any Hct result that is 5 less than the baseline ED Hct
IV: D5NS IV at 125 mL/hr
I&O: q8h
Test each stool for occult blood
Test NG drainage for occult blood q8h

Medications

Omeprazole 40 mg per NG daily (note: clamp NG tube for 2 hours)
Sucralfate 1 g susp daily (note: give through NG at least 3 hours after omeprazole and clamp for 1 hour)

PRN Medications

Hydromorphone 0.2 mg/mL concentration IV per PCA, incremental 0.2 mg, lock-out 6 minutes

Ordered Laboratory Studies

Type and cross match for 2 units packed RBCs (PRBCs)
CBC, electrolytes, retic count daily

LABORATORY STUDY RESULTS

Test	Admission	Day 1	Day 2
CBC	10.5 g/dL	9.5 g/dL	10 g/dL
• Hemoglobin (Hgb)	31%	27%	30%
• Hematocrit (Hct)	3.2 mm³	2.7 mm³	3 mm³
• RBC	2.0%	2.4%	2.4%
• Reticulocytes	72 µm³	68 µm³	70 µm³
• MCV	27 pg	25 pg	26 pg
• MCH	150 mm³	146 mm³	148 mm³
• Platelets	135 mEq/L	135 mEq/L	140 mEq/L
Electrolytes	3.6 mEq/L	3.5 mEq/L	3.9 mEq/L
• Sodium	9 mg/dL	9 mg/dL	9 mg/dL
• Potassium			
• Calcium			

CRITICAL THINKING QUESTIONS

1. What is the physiology mechanism behind the reason that aspirin causes peptic ulcers?

2. Why is omeprazole being given to Ms. T?

3. What is the impact of acute hemorrhage on the results of the CBC?

Answers to Critical Thinking Questions appear in Appendix D.

NCLEX® REVIEW

1. The nurse suspects a patient has Vincent's stomatitis when which clinical manifestation is assessed?

1. Increased salivation and bad breath
2. Painful red maculas with erythematous halos
3. White curd like patches on tongue
4. Oral ulcers covered with a grayish yellow membrane

2. A diagnosis of Barrett's esophagus is made following endoscopic examination of a patient experiencing symptoms of gastroesophageal reflux disease, GERD. The nurse understands this diagnosis is indicative of:

1. Premalignant tissue in the esophagus.
2. Presence of esophageal strictures.
3. Fine tears in the distal esophagus.
4. Ulcerated and inflamed esophageal tissue.

3. A patient is being evaluated for presence of celiac disease. The nurse explains the most definitive test will be a:

1. Gram staining of the stool.
2. Gastric pH analysis.
3. Antigliadin antibody.
4. Biopsy of the small intestine.

4. A patient with a history of irritable bowel disease, IBD, has been recently diagnosed with Crohn's disease. When planning care the nurse understands a manifestation of Crohn's that differs from ulcerative colitis includes:

1. Diarrhea can occur 10–20 times a day.
2. Abdominal pain is cramping in nature.
3. Malabsorption of nutrients often occurs.
4. Incontinence of stool may be a problem.

5. A patient complains of having frequent episodes of belching and heartburn secondary to GERD. The nurse determines the following could be contributing factors. The patient:

1. Has a BMI of 21.
2. Is lactose intolerant.
3. Drinks citrus juice with meals.
4. Eats a lot of high fiber foods.

6. The nurse is preparing education materials on colon cancer to present at a health fair. The following should be included as being risk factors. (Select all that apply.)

1. Daily alcohol intake
2. A low fat diet
3. A history of irritable bowel disease (IBD)
4. Use of daily calcium supplements
5. Daily use of NSAIDs

7. The blue port on a patient's Salem sump tube is leaking clear solution. The nurse should take which action?

1. Place the patient in a high Fowler's position.
2. Plug the port to prevent further leakage.
3. Irrigate the port with 30 mL of saline solution.
4. Place the tube at the shoulder level of patient.

8. A patient has been experiencing symptoms of dumping syndrome following a Bilroth II. The nurse should include which interventions in the plan of care?

1. Check for signs of hypoglycemia two hours after a meal.
2. Encourage ambulation in hall after meals.
3. Instruct patient to drink only cold liquids with meals.
4. Remove high fat food from the patient's tray.

9. The nurse is assessing the stoma on a patient with an ileostomy created three days ago. The nurse anticipates the stoma will appear:

1. Beefy red and moist.
2. Pale pink and extending 2–3 cm from abdominal wall.
3. Slightly purple and moist.
4. Pink and flat against the abdominal wall.

Answers for review questions appear in Appendix D

KEY TERMS

achalasia *p.1389*
achlorhydria *p.1397*
adenomatous polyps *p.1415*
anti-infectives *p.1383*
aphthous stomatitis (contact
    stomatitis) *p.1382*
Barrett's epithelium *p.1387*
Botox *p.1391*
carcinoembryonic antigen (CEA) *p.1417*
celiac disease *p.1400*
colon cancer *p.1415*
continent ileostomy (Kock ileostomy or
    Kock pouch) *p.1413*
C-reactive protein (CRP) *p.1416*
Crohn's disease *p.1410*
diverticular disease *p.1407*
diverticulitis *p.1407*
diverticulosis *p.1407*

duodenal ulcer *p.1395*
esophageal cancer *p.1392*
gastric carcinoma *p.1397*
gastric outlet obstruction (pyloric
    obstruction) *p.1395*
gastric ulcer *p.1393*
gastroduodenostomy (Billroth I) *p.1398*
gastroesophageal reflux *p.1385*
gastrojejunostomy (Billroth II) *p.1398*
Helicobacter pylori (*H. pylori*) *p.1395*
herpetic stomatitis *p.1381*
hiatal hernia *p.1385*
histamine$_2$ (H$_2$)-receptor blockers *p.1385*
ileal pouch anal anastomosis (IPAA) *p.1413*
ileostomy *p.1413*
inflammatory bowel disease (IBD) *p.1410*
intestinal obstruction *p.1404*

lactase *p.1403*
lactose intolerance *p.1403*
lower esophageal sphincter (LES) *p.1385*
malabsorption *p.1400*
maldigestion *p.1400*
oral cancer *p.1383*
oral candidiasis *p.1382*
pancreatic insufficiency *p.1403*
peptic ulcer *p.1393*
proton pump inhibitor (PPI) *p.1385*
rolling (paraesophageal) hernia *p.1385*
short bowel syndrome *p.1403*
sliding (direct) hiatal hernia *p.1385*
steatorrhea *p.1403*
stomatitis *p.1381*
ulcerative colitis (UC) *p.1410*
Vincent's stomatitis *p.1382*

REFERENCES

American Cancer Society. (2007). *Cancer facts & figures for African Americans 2007–2008.* Retrieved July 26, 2008, from http://www.cancer.org/docroot/STT/content/STT_1x_Cancer_Facts_Figures_for_African_Americans_2207-2008_08.asp

American Gastroenterological Association. (2005, January 16). Study shows long-term use of NSAIDs causes severe intestinal damage. *ScienceDaily.* Retrieved July 26, 2008, from http://www.sciencedaily.com/releases/2005/01/050111123706.htm.

Biddle, W. (2003). Gastroesophageal reflux disease: Current treatment approaches. *Gastroenterology Nursing, 26*(6), 228–236.

Burgess, J. A. (2006). Painful oral lesions: What to look for, how to treat: Part 1. *Consultant, 46*(13), 1497–1504.

Erlinger, T. P., Platz, E. A., Rifai, N., & Helzlsouer, K. J. (2004). C-reactive protein and the risk of incident colorectal cancer. *JAMA, 291*(5), 585–590.

Hampton, T. (2004). Scientists explore pathogenesis of IBD. *JAMA, 292*(22), 2708–2713.

Huether, S. E. (2006). Alterations of digestive function. In K. L. McCance & S. E. Huether, *Pathophysiology: The biologic basis for disease in adults and children* (5th ed., pp. 1385–1445). St. Louis: Mosby.

Irani, S., & Krevsky, B. (2007). Colorectal cancer screening: Which test, how often? *Consultant, 47*(2), 138–145.

Jackler, R. K., & Kaplan, M. J. (2004). Ear, nose, & throat. In L. M. Tierney, S. J. McPhee, & M. A. Papadakis (Eds.), *Current medical diagnosis and treatment* (pp. 175–211). New York: Lange Medical Books/McGraw-Hill.

Jemal, A., Siegel, R., Ward, E., Murray, T., Xu, J., & Thun, M. J. (2007). Cancer statistics, 2007. *CA: A Cancer Journal for Clinicians, 57*, 43–66.

Kelsch, R. (2007). *Geographic tongue.* Retrieved April 17, 2008, from http://www.emedicine.com/derm/topic664.htm

Landzberg, B. R. (2006). Celiac disease: Could you be missing the diagnosis? *Consultant, 46*(13), 1458–1465.

Lopes, M. H. B., & Lopes, R. A. M. (2000). Latex allergy in health care personnel. *AORN Journal, 72*(1), 42–3, 45–6, 55–6.

Lynch, D. P. (2007). Oral cancer risk and detection: The importance of screening technology. *RDH, 27*(9), 102–112.

McCaffrey, R., Thrush, S., Dunphy, L. M., & Porter, B. O. (2007). Eyes, ears, nose, and throat problems. In L. M. Dunphy, J. E. Winland-Brown, B. O. Porter, & D. J. Thomas, *Primary care: The art and science of advanced practice nursing* (2nd ed., pp. 229–303). Philadelphia: F. A. Davis.

McQuaid, K. R. (2004). Alimentary tract. In L. M. Tierney, S. J. McPhee, & M. A. Papadakis, *Current medical diagnosis and treatment* (pp. 515–622). New York: Lange Medical Books/McGraw-Hill.

O'Malley, P. (2003). Gastric ulcers and GERD: The new "plagues" of the 21st century update for the clinical nurse specialist. *Clinical Nurse Specialist, 17*(6), 286–289.

Oral Cancer Foundation. (2007). *Descriptive epidemiology.* Retrieved April 17, 2008, from http://www.oralcancerfoundation.org/cdc/cdc_chapter1.htm

Presutti, R. J., Cangemi, J. R., Cassidy, H. D., & Hill, D. A. (2007). Celiac disease. *American Family Physician, 76*(12), 1795–1802.

Qureshi, W. A. (2006). *Hiatal hernia.* Retrieved April 17, 2008, from http://www.emedicine.com/med/topic1012.htm

Rose, H. S., Armstrong, L. B., Klickstein, L. B., & Madsen, J. C. (2005). Pharmacology of immunosuppression. In D. E. Golan (Ed.), *Principles of pharmacology: The pathophysiologic basis of drug therapy* (pp. 667–681). Philadelphia: Lippincott Williams & Wilkins.

Sherman, C. (2007). Dyspepsia guidelines emphasize *H. pylori.* *The Clinical Advisor, 10*(2), 69–74.

Smith, M. M., & Bryant, J. L. (2002). Mind–body and mind–gut connection in inflammatory bowel disease. *Gastroenterology Nursing, 25*(5), 213–217.

Su, L. J., & Arab, L. (2004). Report: Alcohol consumption and risk of colon cancer: Evidence from the national health and nutrition examination survey I epidemiologic follow-up study. *Nutrition and Cancer, 50*(2), 111–119.

Thomas, D. J. (2007). Abdominal problems. In L. M. Dunphy, J. E. Winland-Brown, B. O. Porter, & D. J. Thomas, *Primary care: The art and science of advanced practice nursing* (2nd ed., pp. 473–561). Philadelphia: F. A. Davis.

Wilcox, C. M., Cryer, B., & Triadafilopoulos, G. (2005). Patterns of use and public perception of over-the-counter pain relievers: Focus on nonsteroidal antiinflammatory drugs. *Journal of Rheumatology, 32*, 2218–2224.

Wollner, T. (2004). Eradicate *H. pylori* with effective treatment regimens. *The Nurse Practitioner, 29*(6), 40–44.

Young, L. S., & Thomas, D. J. (2004). Celiac sprue treatment in primary care. *The Nurse Practitioner, 29*(7), 42–45.

Caring for the Patient with Hepatic and Biliary Disorders

Debera Jane Thomas
Douglas Sutton

Outcome-Based Learning Objectives

After studying this chapter, the learner will be able to:

1. Describe the different types of hepatitis virus and the mode of transmission for each one.
2. Discuss the clinical manifestations of hepatitis.
3. Compare and contrast pathophysiology, clinical manifestations, and treatment with related nursing care of patients with cirrhosis.
4. Outline the nursing care of a patient with hepatic encephalopathy.
5. Delineate nursing care for a patient with liver cancer.
6. List the risk factors for gallbladder disease.
7. Compare and contrast the nursing care for patients with an open cholecystectomy and laparoscopic cholecystectomy.
8. Analyze the similarities and differences between acute and chronic pancreatitis.
9. Discuss the causes, clinical manifestations, and treatment for pancreatic cancer.
10. Develop a teaching plan for patients with pancreatitis.

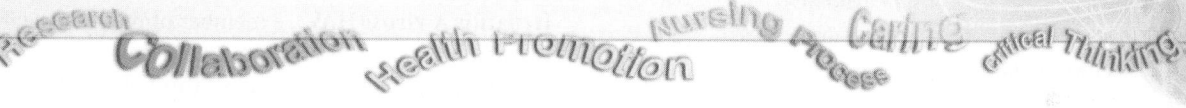

Research Collaboration Health Promotion Nursing Process Caring Critical Thinking

THE LIVER, gallbladder, and **exocrine pancreas** facilitate digestion by secreting hormones, enzymes, and other substances that are necessary for the breakdown of food (Figure 46–1 ■, p. 1428). For example, the liver secretes **bile** that contains salts needed for the breakdown and absorption of fats. Bile is stored and concentrated by the gallbladder for release in response to **cholecystokinin**, which is a hormone secreted from the mucosa of the small intestines. Cholecystokinin, in turn, stimulates the gallbladder to contract and eject bile, as well as stimulating the pancreas to secrete alkaline fluid. In addition to alkaline secretions that help neutralize the acidity of the chyme, the pancreas secretes enzymes that hydrolyze proteins, carbohydrates, and fats. **Trypsin**, **chymotrypsin**, and **carboxypeptidase** are enzymes secreted in inactive form from the pancreas that digest proteins. Pancreatic **alpha-amylase** and **lipase** digest carbohydrates and fats, respectively. This chapter discusses disorders of the liver, gallbladder, and pancreas.

DISORDERS OF THE LIVER

The liver is a complex organ with over 500 identified functions, including metabolic and regulatory functions. Because of its complexity, the clinical manifestations of liver problems can be varied and may include both physiological and psychological symptoms. One of the most amazing features of the liver is its ability to regenerate itself so some level of healing can occur. Liver disorders can result from infectious organisms, toxic substances, and/or tumors that produce either localized or diffuse **hepatocellular** inflammation or destruction.

Hepatitis

Hepatitis is simply defined as inflammation of the liver and is found to be a common problem throughout the world. It can be an acute or chronic infection that may be mild or life threatening, depending on the infectious agent. Inflammation of the liver may also be the result of lifestyle choices such as alcohol or drug abuse.

Etiology

Some of the many causes of liver inflammation include viruses, bacteria, metabolic and vascular disorders, drugs, alcohol, and other toxic substances such as cleaning fluids, industrial toxins, and plant poisons. Chart 46–1 (p. 1428) lists the many causes of hepatic inflammation.

Viral Causes

When most people hear the word *hepatitis*, they think of **viral hepatitis**. At least seven types of viruses are known to cause

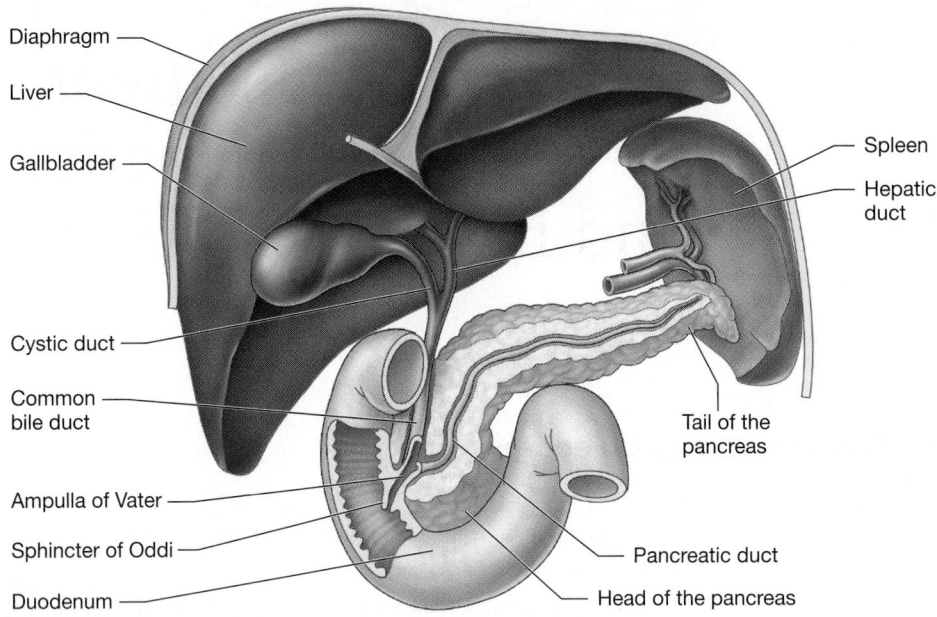

FIGURE 46-1 ■ Liver and biliary system.

CHART 46-1 Common Causes of Hepatic Inflammation

VIRAL

Hepatitis A, B, C, D, E
(HAV, HBV, HCV, HDV, HEV)

Cytomegalovirus

Epstein-Barr virus

Herpes and varicella-zoster viruses

Yellow fever virus

NONVIRAL

Amebic infiltration (amebic abscess)

Lyme disease

Syphilis

Bacteria

TOXINS

Ethanol (alcohol)

Carbon tetrachloride

Yellow phosphorus

Mushrooms (*Amanita phalloides*)

Herbs (comfrey)

METABOLIC DISORDERS

Alpha$_1$-antitrypsin deficiency

Wilson disease (copper metabolism)

VASCULAR DISORDERS

Budd-Chiari syndrome

Congestive heart failure

Severe hypotension

Shock

DRUGS

Acetaminophen

Allopurinol

Androgens and anabolic steroids

Aspirin (high doses)

Captopril

Carbamazepine

Chlorpromazine

Chlorpropamide

Cholecystographic dyes

Clindamycin

Erythromycin

Estrogen

Halothane

Imipramine

Isoniazid (INH)

Ketoconazole

L-asparaginase

Methotrexate

Methyldopa

Mithramycin

Monoamine oxidase inhibitors (MAOI)

Oral contraceptives

Para-aminosalicylic acid (PAS)

Phenytoin

Procainamide

Sulfonamides

Tetracycline

inflammation of the liver. Because of the diversity of liver function, the effects of hepatitis can be locally diffuse throughout the liver or can manifest as systemic disease. The Cultural Considerations box shows which groups are affected most by which viruses.

Hepatitis A

Hepatitis A virus (HAV), a member of the picornavirus family, is a small RNA virus (Thomas, 2007). It was once known as infectious hepatitis and is endemic throughout the world. Many cases go undiagnosed because symptoms are often nonspecific, mild, and flulike. In the United States, there were an estimated 3,579 cases in 2006, which indicates a steady decline since 2000, when there were 13,397 cases reported (CDC, 2008).

Transmission of HAV is usually through the fecal–oral route, meaning persons contract the virus by drinking water contaminated with sewage, eating uncooked food washed in this water, eating shellfish harvested from contaminated water, or eating food contaminated by a person who is infected and did not wash his hands after using the toilet. It is also considered a sexually transmitted disease, mainly through oral sex. Besides being found in the feces, the virus has been isolated from bile and sera of infected persons, meaning it is possible to transmit the disease through transfusion of infected blood (Huether, 2006). The incubation period (time between exposure and onset of symptoms) for HAV is anywhere from 2 to 6 weeks. The virus is found in the feces up to 2 weeks before symptoms occur and the week following the onset of symptoms, but may be as long as

CULTURAL CONSIDERATIONS Related to Hepatitis in the United States

Cultural groups with the highest reported infections of:

Hepatitis A: American Indians/Alaska Natives

Hepatitis B: non-Hispanic Blacks

Hepatitis C: similar across all racial/ethnic groups.

3 months and is most contagious during this time (Huether, 2006). It takes about 4 weeks for the body to develop antibodies to HAV (anti-HAV). **Serum immunoglobulin M (IgM)** is seen in the acute phase of the illness and begins to decline about 3 months after exposure. **Serum immunoglobulin G (IgG)** levels are slower to peak, but remain elevated years after exposure, conferring immunity against further infection by HAV. Hepatitis A usually causes no long-term damage and a chronic state is unknown for HAV.

Hepatitis B

Hepatitis B virus (HBV) is a DNA virus that replicates in the liver. It was once known as serum hepatitis. Hepatitis B occurs in most places in the world, but the rate of infection varies depending on location. HBV is a complex organism involving three basic components. The intact virus is sometimes called a Dane particle. It has a double-layered outer coat that carries the hepatitis B surface antigen (HBsAg), thereby allowing it to be detected by radioimmunoassay (Huether, 2006). Because of the protective coating, the core antigen (HBcAg) is not detectable in serum; however, a derivative of the core antigen, HBeAg, is detectable, and this serves as a marker of viral replication and infectivity.

HBV may be found in blood, semen, cervical secretions, saliva, and wound drainage with the highest concentration occurring in blood and blood products (Thomas, 2007). The virus is robust, living up to a week in an open environment (Thomas, 2007). Viral transmission is through direct contact with blood and blood products, sexual contact, and contact with contaminated inanimate objects. High-risk groups include health care workers, particularly those working in a laboratory, blood bank, or hemodialysis setting where there is frequent contact with blood and blood products. IV drug users, homosexual men, and people with multiple sex partners are also at risk. Transmission can also occur during pregnancy from mother to fetus, if the mother is infected in the 3rd trimester or at birth.

The incubation period for HBV is longer than that of other hepatic viruses, lasting anywhere from 2 to 6 months, during which time transmission is possible even when symptoms are absent. HBV can exist as a carrier state, and/or it can create a chronic active state of infection, which can progress to cirrhosis and liver failure, thus requiring liver transplantation. HBV infection can lead to an increased risk for developing liver cancer as well.

Hepatitis C

Hepatitis C virus (HCV), once known as non-A, non-B virus, is a large RNA virus with an incubation period of 60 to 150 days (Holloway & D'Acunto, 2006). It replicates at a very high rate, mutating readily, which causes the host immune system to have difficulty building a response. This in turn leads to a high rate of chronic infections.

There are six different genotypes of HCV with three of them occurring most often in the United States. The most common genotype found in the United States is genotype 1, with genotypes 2 and 3 occurring as well. The lack of viral replication is considered a sustained viral response (SVR), which is measured by HCV-RNA or viral load. Genotype 1 has the poorest response to treatment, about a 50% SVR, whereas genotypes 2 and 3 both respond to treatment with a 70% to 80% SVR (Deutsch, 2003).

Antibodies to HCV (anti-HCV) can be detected in acute, recovered, or chronic infection.

The rate of HCV infection has dropped drastically since 2000. The Centers for Disease Control reported that there were 3,197 new cases of HCV infection in 2000 but only 802 in 2006 (CDC, 2008). HCV is found predominantly in blood, blood products, and transplanted tissue. However, there is evidence that HCV can be transmitted sexually, particularly in those having multiple sex partners. In fact, for persons with hepatitis C, the risk appears to be similar for those that report drug use or multiple sex partners (Wasley et al., 2007). The most common cause of HCV transmission in the United States is attributed to injection drug use (CDC, 2008). It is also possible to transmit HCV through other percutaneous exposures, such as tattooing, body piercing, folk medicine practices, and barbering, although records of this transmission are not available.

 Of the reported cases of acute hepatitis C in 2005 (Wasley et al., 2007), the most common risk factor identified was injection drug use (50%). Other risk factors included multiple sexual partners (23%), surgical procedures (14%), and occupational exposure to blood (8%).

Hepatitis D

Hepatitis D virus (HDV), also known as delta virus, is an RNA virus that is defective and must have HBsAg present for its replication; therefore, simultaneous infection with HBV is necessary for HDV. The incubation period lasts from 1 to 6 months and transmission occurs in the same manner as for HBV. IV drug users have a high rate of HDV with a mortality rate of about 3% (Thomas, 2007).

Hepatitis E

Hepatitis E virus (HEV) is an RNA virus with an incubation period of 15 to 60 days (Huether, 2006). It is transmitted via the fecal–oral route and is similar to hepatitis A in clinical manifestations. Unlike HAV, however, the mortality rate for pregnant women who contract HEV is higher at 10% to 20% (Friedman, 2004). HEV is endemic in Southeast Asia, India, North Africa, and Mexico, but is uncommon in the United States.

Hepatitis G

Hepatitis G virus (HGV) is an RNA virus about which little is known. Transmission may occur percutaneously or through sexual contact. The virus has been detected in at least 50% of IV drug users, 30% of patients undergoing hemodialysis, and 15% of patients with chronic HBV or HCV. Infection of HGV is associated with a chronic viremia. Interestingly, it should be noted that if patients with HIV are also infected with HGV, their survival rate is improved (Friedman, 2004).

Pathophysiology

Once the liver is infected with any of these hepatitis viruses, an inflammatory response is initiated when the acini cells develop mononuclear inflammatory infiltrates. The inflammatory response causes edema within the liver and can obstruct the **bile canaliculi**, small channels adjacent to the hepatocytes that move bile toward the common bile duct. It is this intrahepatic obstruction of bile that causes obstructive jaundice. There may also be liver cell necrosis; **Kupffer cells**, cells that line the liver sinusoids and are phagocytic cells; hyperplasia; and scarring.

The cell-mediated immune response (cytokines, toxic T cells, natural killer cells) is responsible for the tissue injury that occurs. If the case of hepatitis is mild, there is little parenchymal damage, but hepatitis B and C usually cause the most severe liver inflammation and damage. Hepatitis C invades the liver cells, causing injury directly; therefore, the inflammation in the hepatocytes is directly related to the viral load. Although rare, acute fulminating hepatitis may be caused by hepatitis B (also coinfection with HDV), resulting in massive hepatocellular necrosis leading to liver failure. Even in severe cases of hepatitis, liver regeneration begins within 48 hours of the tissue injury.

For both HBV and HCV, asymptomatic carrier states may exist. Although these individuals may never develop an active disease process, they carry an increased risk for developing hepatocellular carcinoma (Thomas, 2007). Hepatitis B and C can produce chronic, active infections where the immune system is unable to clear the virus completely. About 10% of individuals infected with HBV will go on to develop chronic infection. In the case of HCV infection, 75% to 85% of those infected will go on to develop chronic HCV.

Additional agents can also cause liver inflammation (hepatitis). Bacteria and circulating bacterial endotoxins can invade the parenchyma during sepsis and cause liver injury. Some medications can also cause hepatitis. For example, toxic metabolites of acetaminophen can damage the cellular structure in the liver, leading to inflammation. Many chemotherapy drugs, such as methotrexate, vincristine, and the combination of 5-fluorouracil and levamisole, have a high potential for causing chemical hepatitis (Baldwin, 2003). But the most common toxic substance that causes chemical hepatitis is alcohol. Liver inflammation can occur after drinking large quantities in a relatively short time or from chronic consumption (alcohol abuse).

Clinical Manifestations

Regardless of the cause, the clinical manifestations of hepatitis are frequently very similar. The severity of the symptoms can range from almost none or asymptomatic, to fulminating hepatitis, progressing to liver failure and death. The patient is usually asymptomatic during the incubation period of viral hepatitis. With HBV infection, there is evidence of HBeAg in the blood, indicating a high degree of infectivity. Later in the incubation period, HBsAg (hepatitis B surface antigen) appears. Following the incubation period, there are three phases in the clinical course of viral hepatitis: the prodromal phase, the icteric phase, and (convalescent) recovery.

Prodromal Phase

It is often difficult to determine the beginning of the **prodromal phase**, the phase of acute hepatitis that occurs between exposure to the virus and the appearance of jaundice, because it starts about 2 weeks after exposure to the virus. Because the time of exposure is often unknown, the prodromal phase will vary depending on the incubation period. The prodromal phase can have either an insidious or a rapid onset. Symptoms may be vague, often flu-like, with anorexia, nausea, vomiting, and malaise, as well as frequent occurrences of myalgia, arthralgia, and easy fatigue (Thomas, 2007). Anorexia usually occurs early in this phase and is frequently accompanied by a distaste of smoking in those patients who are smokers. Additional manifes-

tations may include mild, but constant, abdominal pain in the right upper quadrant (RUQ) or epigastrium, as well as a fever less than 103°F (39.4°C).

Icteric Phase

The **icteric phase** begins with the onset of jaundice, which usually occurs 5 to 10 days after the initial symptoms, although some patients may never develop jaundice. The prodromal symptoms become worse with the onset of jaundice, but then a progressive clinical improvement follows. Due to the increased levels of conjugated **bilirubin**, a product in the breakdown of hemoglobin that is conjugated by the hepatocytes and is excreted in bile, the urine may be dark during this phase.

 In 2005, the CDC reported (Wasley et al., 2007) that overall 76% of persons infected with acute hepatitis A developed jaundice, 33% were hospitalized, and 0.6% died. Persons age 5 to 39 were more likely to report the development of jaundice (83%), whereas persons younger than 5 years and persons age 60 or older were less likely (58%).

Convalescent Phase

The **convalescent phase** is characterized by an increased sense of well-being, which usually begins after 2 to 3 weeks of acute illness. The phase is marked by additional signs of improvement such as increased appetite and energy level. The jaundice of the icteric phase and abdominal pain disappear. Complete clinical recovery varies depending on the type of hepatitis, but HAV is usually resolved in 9 to 10 weeks, while recovery may take up to 16 weeks.

Diagnostic Procedures

Tests that assess the degree of liver injury include:

- **Alanine aminotransferase (ALT)** is an enzyme released from hepatocytes when the liver is injured. The ALT is more specific for liver injury than the other enzymes mentioned next. In acute hepatitis, the serum ALT may exceed 1,000 IU/L.

- **Aspartate aminotransferase (AST)** is an enzyme found in hepatocytes and cardiac cells primarily, but it is also found in skeletal muscle cells, the kidneys, and the pancreas. It is released when there is cellular injury in these areas. When the liver is injured, the serum AST level can increase more than 10 times normal and will remain elevated for a longer period of time than in other injuries (Kee, 2002).

- **Alkaline phosphatase (ALP)** is an enzyme found mostly in liver cells and bone. Mild hepatocyte damage will cause a slight increase in the blood level of ALP. Acute hepatitis can cause marked elevations in the ALP, but the level rapidly returns to normal after the acute phase.

- **Gamma-glutamyltransferase (GGT),** an enzyme found mostly in the liver and the kidneys, is a good way to detect liver parenchymal disease. The GGT will increase 12 to 24 hours after heavy alcohol consumption and remain elevated for weeks after alcohol cessation; in fact, some alcohol rehabilitation programs are using this in planning care for these persons (Kee, 2002).

- **Lactic dehydrogenase (LDH),** an intracellular enzyme, is found in most cells, especially those in active metabolism such as the heart, skeletal muscle, liver, brain, and red blood cells. The subunit, LDH$_5$, is most specific for liver injury, with levels rising before jaundice develops.

- Serum bilirubin levels become elevated when there is hepatitis. Bilirubin is formed from the breakdown of hemoglobin and processed in the liver to form conjugated bilirubin. If there is intrahepatic edema or another obstruction (cirrhosis), conjugated bilirubin cannot enter the duodenum; therefore, levels of direct (conjugated) bilirubin will be elevated. If function is severely affected, the liver cannot conjugate bilirubin and the indirect (unconjugated) level will rise.

- Specific serological tests for viral antigens, antibodies, or the virus itself are available (Chart 46–2).

- Liver biopsy is done to evaluate chronic hepatitis due to HBV or HCV.

Medical Management

The goals of medical treatment for hepatitis are to identify the cause of the inflammation, either infectious or chemical, provide symptomatic treatment, monitor the damage to the liver, and support the liver's ability to regenerate and heal itself. Laboratory and diagnostic tests give clues to the cause of hepatitis, assess the degree of liver injury, and indicate the degree of healing.

Preventive Drug Treatment

Vaccines are available for HAV and HBV. The vaccine for HBV became available in 1982 and the vaccine for HAV in the early 1990s. In 2001 the Food and Drug Administration (FDA) approved a combination HAV and HBV vaccine that consists of a three-dose series (Wasley et al., 2007).

Anyone in a high-risk group should be vaccinated against HAV and HBV. High-risk groups include health care workers, day care workers, employees at correctional facilities, injection drug users, male homosexuals, and anyone traveling to an endemic area of HAV. Patients on hemodialysis and household and sexual contacts of persons with HBV should be vaccinated as well. Vaccine for HAV is given in 2 intramuscular (IM) doses 6 to 12 months apart. The most common side effect is pain at the injection site. HBV vaccine is given in a series of 3 IM doses, with the first dose followed in 1 month by the second one, and the third one given 5 months later. Side effects of HBV vaccine include pain at the injection site, fatigue, and headache.

Immune globulin (IG) is available for HAV and HBV postexposure prophylaxis. Postexposure prophylaxis is recommended for household and sexual contacts of people with HAV or HBV, health care workers after a needlestick injury, and others exposed to infected blood or body fluids. Postexposure prophylaxis for HAV is a single dose of IG, and it must be given within 2 weeks of exposure. For HBV, IG should be given as soon as possible, but may be given only up to 1 week after exposure, with a second dose given 1 month after exposure. It is recommended that the HBV vaccine be given at the same time as IG in the case of exposure.

Although there is no vaccine for hepatitis C, treatment is initiated to prevent chronic HCV once the diagnosis is made. The goal of treatment is to get a sustained viral response, which

| CHART 46–2 | Specific Tests for Viral Hepatitis |

Hepatitis A	Hepatitis B	Hepatitis C	Hepatitis D	Hepatitis E
HAV-RNA Is viral RNA and is found in stool; peaks 1–2 months after exposure and disappears before month 4.	**HBV-DNA** Is viral DNA and is found in serum just before the second month and disappears by month 5.	**HCV-RNA** Is viral RNA and indicates replicating virus.	**HDV-RNA** Is viral RNA and indicates acute infection.	**Anti-HEV** Is antibody and indicates infection.
Anti-HAV IgM Is found in serum during acute illness, peaking about 2–3 months after exposure and slowly decreasing. It is usually gone by 1 year after exposure.	**HBeAg** Is a marker for viral replication and appears about 2 months after exposure.	**Anti-HCV** Is antibody to the virus but does not indicate immunity.	**HDAg** Is hepatitis D antigen and indicates acute infection.	
Anti-HAV IgG Is found in serum during recovery and indicates immunity to the virus. It remains elevated for years.	**HBsAg** Is the surface antigen on the virus and is usually detected 1 week before HBeAg and disappears by month 5. Persistent levels indicate either a chronic or a carrier state.			
	Anti-HBc IgM Is antibody to HBcAg and is found during acute illness and convalescence but may persist for years.			
	Anti-HBs IgM Indicates acute illness and infectivity.			
	Anti-HBs IgG and **Anti-HBc IgG** Both indicate recovery from acute illness.			

means that HCV-RNA is undetectable 6 months after treatment is finished. Standard treatment is with PEG-Intron (pegylated interferon alfa-2b) subcutaneously and oral ribavirin 800 milligrams per day in divided doses for 6 to 11 months (Deutsch, 2003). The side effects of this treatment regimen may include fatigue, muscle aches, headache, fever, and chills. Drinking a lot of water and getting adequate rest can minimize these effects. Patients taking interferon preparations have also reported depression.

Supportive Treatment

Treatment for hepatitis is primarily supportive, regardless of the cause. The keystone of therapy is rest, adequate nutrition, proper diet, and avoidance of alcohol. Few patients require hospitalization, which may be necessary for patients with fulminant liver failure.

The diet recommended for patients with hepatitis is a low-fat, high-calorie diet, with a large portion of the calories coming from complex carbohydrates, such as whole grains, fruits, and vegetables. Depending on the level of functional liver impairment, increased protein intake may also be recommended. Good sources of protein with lower fat concentrations are foods such as egg whites, tofu, beans, and fat-free dairy products. Alcohol and other agents toxic to the liver must be avoided.

Because fatigue can be a common complaint for patients with hepatitis, planned rest periods throughout the day are essential. Although activity is usually restricted during the acute phase of hepatitis, bed rest is rarely indicated. Strenuous activity is discouraged, but may be gradually resumed as the healing process progresses.

Complementary Therapies

Several herbal preparations that have been used for centuries have been shown to be beneficial to the liver. Milk thistle (Silybum marianum) is one of the oldest therapies for liver disease. Its active ingredient, silymarin, has demonstrated its ability to promote hepatocyte growth and reduce liver inflammation, as well as protecting the liver cells from toxic damage (Pelc, 2003). Another herbal preparation for hepatitis uses licorice root, which has both anti-inflammatory and antiviral properties. However, long-term use may cause hypertension and edema because of its chemical resemblance to aldosterone. For patients with HCV receiving the standard treatment, ginger root may help relieve the nausea associated with interferon.

■ Nursing Management

Nursing care for the patients with hepatitis involves supportive measures and education. Most patients with hepatitis are not hospitalized, but are managed in their own homes. Those requiring hospitalization would be those with fulminant hepatitis, or chronic hepatitis that has progressed to cirrhosis, liver cancer, or liver failure.

Health Promotion

One of the primary responsibilities of nursing with regard to viral hepatitis focuses on prevention and reducing the spread of infection through education. For all types of viral hepatitis, but especially for HAV and HEV, good hand hygiene practices after using the bathroom and before handling food are crucial to pre-

vent transmission. Because many types of hepatitis can be spread through sexual activity, education should include encouraging patients to use safer sexual practices, including barrier protection (condoms), abstinence, and monogamy. There is a high risk of transmitting viral hepatitis through shared needles and other equipment. Some communities therefore participate in a needle exchange program, in which used needles can be traded for sterile ones, thereby reducing the risk of viral hepatitis and HIV.

Nurses are influential in educating the public about vaccinations for HAV and HBV. All people in moderate- and high-risk groups should be encouraged to be vaccinated. Many public health departments offer these vaccines at a reduced cost or no cost for individuals at risk. Postexposure prophylaxis is available for people who have known or probable exposure to HAV or HBV.

Assessment

The focus of the nursing assessment is to identify the patient's responses to hepatitis, both physically and emotionally, and to try to determine the sources of transmission that are controllable if the patient has viral hepatitis. Assessment should include a history of manifestations related to hepatitis, such as complaints of anorexia, nausea, vomiting, abdominal pain, and fatigue. Complaints may also include muscle or joint pain, and patients with hepatitis may notice that their stools become pale or almost white. This results from intrahepatic obstruction of the flow of bile into the duodenum. Conversely, their urine may be dark for the same reason. It is important to assess the onset and duration of symptoms in order to attempt to help patients identify their exposure to hepatitis. The history should include asking questions about sexual practices, injection drug use, chemical exposure, travel history, alcohol use, and dietary practices. Because many drugs and herbal preparations can have adverse effects on the liver, it is important to inquire about these substances, including over-the-counter (OTC) medications and other nonprescription preparations.

Physical assessment should include vital signs, color of the skin, sclera and mucous membranes, color of the stool and urine, and examination of the abdomen for tenderness and contour. Because an elevated bilirubin causes pruritus, there may be evidence of lesions from scratching or a report of generalized urticaria. If liver function is compromised, there may be problems affecting blood clotting factors, and the patient should be observed for signs of bleeding, such as bruising or petechiae.

Interventions

As mentioned earlier, the nursing interventions for patients with hepatitis are mainly supportive. Patients with hepatitis need education about the importance of rest and scheduling rest periods into their daily routines. Diet teaching should include information about specific foods high in complex carbohydrates and protein, low in fat, and abstinence from alcohol, often referred to as a "liver friendly" diet. These diet instructions should consider individual dietary preferences as well as cultural traditions. Specific information about disease transmission should also be included. Because pruritus may be a problem for some patients with hepatitis, specific ways they can relieve the itching and preserve their skin integrity is essential. The Nursing Process: Patient Care Plan

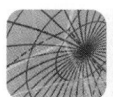

NURSING PROCESS: Patient Care Plan for Hepatitis

Assessment of Fatigue

Subjective Data:
How long have you felt tired or fatigued?
Are you able to maintain your activities of daily living?
How much activity can you tolerate before you feel fatigued?
What makes you feel better?

Objective Data:
Musculoskeletal examination:
- Muscle strength
- Activity tolerance
- Vital signs

Nursing Assessment and Diagnoses	Outcomes and Evaluation Parameters	Planning and Interventions with *Rationales*
Nursing Diagnoses: *Fatigue. Activity Intolerance* related to inadequate liver function	**Outcome:** Reduced fatigue. ***Evaluation Parameters:*** Ability to perform activities of daily living. Increased activity tolerance.	**Interventions and *Rationales:*** Encourage frequent rest periods during the day. *Energy conservation is necessary for tissue rebuilding and regaining well-being.* Facilitate the identification of essential activities and delegate tasks to others. *Energy conservation is necessary for tissue rebuilding and regaining well-being.* Encourage increased activity as fatigue improves. *A feeling of improvement can enhance well-being, self-concept, and a sense of control.*

Assessment of Nutritional Status

Subjective Data:
Are you having trouble eating?
Have you lost any weight?
How is your appetite?
Have you lost a taste for any foods?
Are there foods that you have a taste for?
Has your food consumption changed?
Do you drink alcohol?

Objective Data:
Body weight and appearance
Skin turgor
Skin and hair condition

Nursing Assessment and Diagnoses	Outcomes and Evaluation Parameters	Planning and Interventions with *Rationales*
Nursing Diagnosis: *Nutrition, Readiness for Enhanced* related to anorexia and reduced liver function	**Outcome:** Adequate nutrition. ***Evaluation Parameter:*** No weight loss.	**Interventions and *Rationales:*** Instruct the patient to eat foods that appeal to her, but stress the importance of high-calorie carbohydrates and proteins. *Carbohydrates are necessary for sufficient energy, and proteins are needed for healing.* Explain the importance of avoiding substances that can be toxic to the liver, such as alcohol and acetaminophen *in order to prevent further liver damage or inflammation.* Teach the patient to read food labels and choose foods that are low in fat and have adequate levels of vitamins and minerals, such as Instant Breakfast drink mix, *to improve nutritional status and promote healing.*

Assessment of Skin

Subjective Data:
Does your skin itch?
Have you been scratching your skin?
Have you noticed a change in the color of your skin?

Objective Data:
Examine skin for:
- Jaundice
- Lesions from scratching
- Dryness
- Bruises
- Petechiae

Nursing Assessment and Diagnoses	Outcomes and Evaluation Parameters	Planning and Interventions with *Rationales*
Nursing Diagnosis: *Skin Integrity, Risk for Impaired* related to jaundice and resultant pruritus	**Outcome:** Skin integrity maintained. ***Evaluation Parameters:*** Reports diminished itching. No bruising or petechiae. No lesions from scratching.	**Interventions and *Rationales:*** Instruct the patient to use cool, lightweight, nonrestrictive clothing and avoid woolens. *Clothing made from lightweight fabrics causes less itching.* Explain that a cool environmental temperature and cool water for bathing may increase comfort related to pruritus. Instruct the patient to keep her fingernails trimmed and well cared for *to decrease the likelihood of excoriating when scratching.* Instruct the patient to take antihistamine medication as ordered *to reduce pruritus.*

(continued)

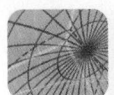

NURSING PROCESS: Patient Care Plan for Hepatitis—*Continued*

Assessment of Infection Transmission

Subjective Data:
Have you ever had a blood transfusion?
Do you have any tattoos or body piercings?
Do you use injectable drugs?
Where have you traveled recently?
Have you eaten any raw fish or seafood?
Where do you work? Child care facility? Correctional facility? Hemodialysis unit?
Do you handle blood or body fluids for your job?
Has anyone you know been sick or had yellow skin?
Do you have multiple sex partners?
When did your symptoms begin?

Objective Data:
Enlarged lymph nodes
Tender liver

Nursing Assessment and Diagnoses	Outcomes and Evaluation Parameters	Planning and Interventions with *Rationales*
Nursing Diagnosis: *Infection, Risk for* related to the transmission of viral hepatitis.	**Outcome:** No spread of the infection. **Evaluation Parameter:** Verbalizes modes of transmission and ways to prevent spread.	**Interventions and *Rationales:*** Use standard or universal precautions when handling blood or body fluids. *Viral hepatitis is transmitted by direct contact with infected feces, body fluids, and blood.* Explain that the time of highest infectivity is before symptoms appear, and that *good hand hygiene can prevent the spread of the disease.* Teach about safe and safer sex practices *to prevent the spread of the virus.* Encourage prophylactic treatment for close contacts and/or vaccination against HAV and HBV. *These measures decrease the risk of contracting the disease or decrease the severity of the illness.*

feature includes specific interventions and application of the nursing process to a patient with hepatitis.

Cirrhosis

Cirrhosis, the 12th leading cause of death in the United States (Askey, 2006), is an irreversible, progressive deterioration of the liver that results from chronic liver disease. Cirrhosis is the result of hepatocellular injury and inflammation usually occurring over time. If the injury or inflammation is short lived, the liver is usually able to regenerate itself. However, severe acute injury, as that seen in hepatitis, can result in cirrhosis. Cirrhosis may be brought about by a variety of causes including chronic hepatitis; alcoholism; prolonged, severe right heart failure; and long-term obstruction to biliary flow. Chart 46–3 lists the causes of cirrhosis. The most common cause of cirrhosis in the United States is alcoholic cirrhosis.

Pathophysiology

Prolonged liver injury from toxins, inflammation, and metabolic derangements causes liver cell damage and cell death. The damaged or dead liver cells are repaired or replaced with tissue that is more fibrous than the original tissue. Fibrotic scarring is the result. Liver cells continue to regenerate but do so in an abnormal pattern. This abnormal liver regeneration creates regenerative nodules. The fibrotic scarring and nodular development

alter the normal lobular architecture. Diffuse, disorganized fibrous bands result, and then as the surviving hepatocytes regenerate, more nodules are formed. The development of cirrhosis depends on several factors, including the length of time the liver is subjected to the injury, the severity of the injury, and the liver's reaction to the assault (Thomas, 2007). As the liver repairs itself, there is distortion in the microcirculation. Collateral vessels develop in the newly regenerated nodule connecting the portal vein to the hepatic artery (Figure 46–2 ■). This results in increased resistance to the flow of blood throughout the liver, causing portal venous hypertension because these vessels are inefficient.

As mentioned earlier, cirrhosis can result from a variety of causes, one of which is alcohol abuse. The ingestion of alcohol causes metabolic changes in the liver in which there is a decrease in the utilization of fatty acids by the liver, increased fatty acid synthesis, increased esterification of fatty acids into triglycerides, and a decreased secretion of fat from the liver (Friedman, 2004). This condition, called fatty liver, can possibly be reversed if no further alcohol is consumed. Continued alcohol use causes liver inflammation leading to necrosis, fibrosis, regenerative nodules, and structural changes.

Prolonged obstruction to the flow of bile within the liver or biliary system can also cause cirrhosis. When the bile ducts within the liver are obstructed, the proximal hepatocytes are injured. There is an inflammatory response to the injury with inflammatory cells infiltrating the liver, leading to fibrosis and

CHART 46–3 Causes of Cirrhosis

INFECTIOUS AND DISEASE-RELATED CAUSES

Autoimmune chronic active hepatitis

Biliary cirrhosis

Chronic pancreatitis

Cholelithiasis

Cystic fibrosis

Diabetes mellitus

Hepatitis B and C

Hypertriglyceridemia

Obesity

Sclerosing cholangitis

Syndrome "X" (insulin resistance syndrome)

HEPATOTOXINS

Direct:
- Alcohol
- Carbon tetrachloride
- Phosphorus

Indirect:
- Acetaminophen
- Alkylated anabolic steroids
- Mushroom toxin (*Amanita phalloides*)
- Methotrexate
- Tetracycline

Genetic diseases:
- Galactosemia
- Hemochromatosis
- Wilson disease

Vascular disorders of the liver:
- Budd-Chiari syndrome
- Ischemic hepatitis
- Right heart failure (chronic)

---

regenerative nodules. This is essentially the same pathway that chronic hepatitis B and C cause cirrhosis; that is, chronic inflammation leading to fibrosis and regenerative nodules.

Clinical Manifestations

Cirrhosis can be asymptomatic until liver function is severely affected and, even then, the onset of symptoms is gradual. Cirrhosis may be found incidentally on the annual physical exam. The manifestations of cirrhosis can be nonspecific and are the result of the hepatocellular damage and portal hypertension. Initially the patient might complain of fatigue, weakness, anorexia, and weight loss, which is caused from the decreased metabolic functions of the liver. Because the liver produces bile, which is needed for the digestion of fat and the formation of fat soluble vitamins, impaired liver function may result in fat soluble vitamin deficiency, particularly of vitamin K. Deficiency of vitamin K

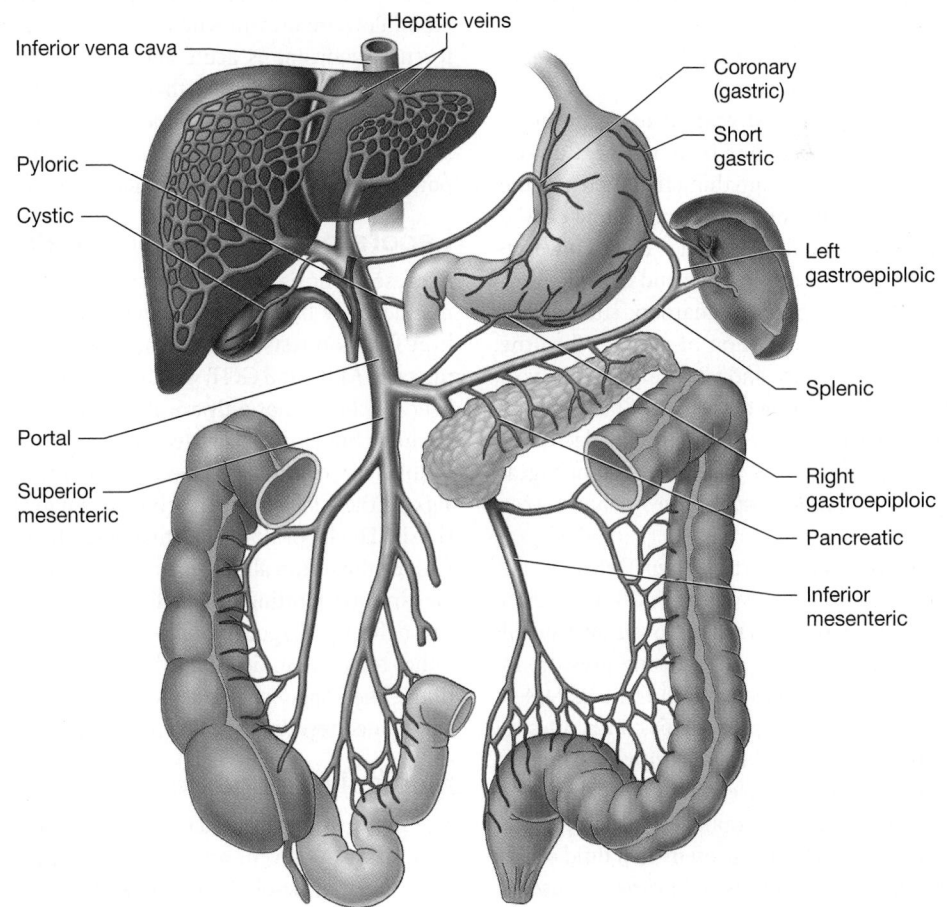

FIGURE 46–2 ■ Portal circulation.

causes problems with blood clotting and fat malabsorption. Other metabolic functions of the liver include **gluconeogenesis** (the making of glucose from noncarbohydrate sources), glycogen storage, synthesis of albumin, clotting factors, and other blood proteins. When liver function is severely compromised and the liver is unable to make albumin, **hypoalbuminemia** leads to edema. Both ascites and peripheral edema develop in part because of the decrease in colloidal osmotic pressure. Because of the architectural changes in the cirrhotic liver structure, there is obstruction to the flow of bile out of the liver, causing jaundice of the skin and sclera. Chart 46–4 contains a list of clinical manifestations of cirrhosis and the physiological basis for each.

Complications

As cirrhosis progresses, severe systemic complications occur, the most significant of which are **portal hypertension**, **hepatic encephalopathy**, and **hepatorenal syndrome**. Each of these conditions has further clinical manifestations and complications.

Portal Hypertension

As the internal architecture of the liver is distorted as a result of scarring, venous blood flow through the portal venous system is impeded. This increases the portal venous blood pressure, from a normal of about 3 mmHg to at least 10 mmHg. Because the portal veins carry blood from the GI tract, spleen, and pancreas to the liver, the obstruction of this blood flow from cirrhosis causes increased pressure in the vessels in the aforementioned organs. The increased pressure causes increased blood flow in collateral vessels, which normally have lower pressure. This causes varices (distended, tortuous, collateral veins) to develop particularly in the esophagus and rectum.

Esophageal varices are thin-walled veins that are prone to rupture, causing massive, life-threatening hemorrhage. Rupture of esophageal varices can result from anything that increases the pressure in the vessel, such as coughing, or from trauma caused by something as simple as eating high-roughage food. However, bleeding from esophageal varices can be slow and chronic leading to anemia and **melena**, the black or maroon, sticky, foul-smelling feces resulting from the digestion of blood. When the varices rupture, there is hemorrhage and vomiting of large volumes of dark-red blood. Contributing to the risk of hemorrhage is erosion by gastric acid, elevated venous pressure, and decreased clotting factors. Individuals who have recurrent esophageal bleeding from portal hypertension usually die within a year (Huether, 2006).

Another consequence of portal hypertension is splenomegaly, or enlargement of the spleen. The splenic vein branches from the portal vein, so when blood flow is obstructed through the portal vein, the subsequent increasing pressure in the splenic vein causes an enlarged spleen as well as the increased rate of blood cell destruction by the spleen. This contributes to the occurrence of anemia. More platelets are removed from circulation and sequestered in the spleen, leading to impaired clot formation, all of which contribute to esophageal bleeding.

Ascites is simply the accumulation of protein-rich fluid in the abdominal cavity. Portal hypertension is the primary cause of ascites, but hypoalbuminemia and accumulation of aldosterone aid in the fluid accumulation. The low serum albumin decreases the colloidal osmotic pressure in the blood vessels causing fluid to escape into the interstitial space, which decreases the circulating blood volume. This, in turn, causes the kidneys to retain sodium and water to increase the blood volume, leading to an increase in hydrostatic pressure and accelerating portal hypertension and ascites formation.

Hepatic Encephalopathy

Hepatic encephalophathy, also known as portosystemic encephalopathy, is the result of an increased level of circulating neurotoxins. The most abundant neurotoxin is ammonia, which forms as the end product of protein digestion. Normally, the hepatocytes convert ammonia to urea, which is then excreted by the kidneys. However, when liver function is impaired, ammonia builds up in the blood causing altered cerebral energy metabolism, interfering with neurotransmitters, and causing cerebral edema. The accumulation of other substances, such as short-chain amino acids, serotonin, and tryptophan, is thought to cause additional symptoms of encephalophathy including **asterixis**, a flapping tremor of the hands when the arms are outstretched, believed to be caused by the accumulation of substances normally detoxified by the liver, agitation, restlessness, and changes in mentation (Huether, 2006).

Hepatorenal Syndrome

Hepatorenal syndrome is characterized by the occurrence of azotemia in a patient with liver failure when other causes of renal failure have been excluded. The cause of this syndrome is unknown, but intense renal vasoconstriction and decreased renal blood flow are present while renal tissue is normal. Type I hepatorenal syndrome is acute and occurs when there is increased serum creatinine to more than 2.5 mg/dL in less than 2 weeks. Type II hepatorenal syndrome is chronic and progresses more slowly. The presence of oliguria, sodium and water retention, hypotension, and peripheral vasodilation indicates a poor prognosis.

Laboratory and Diagnostic Procedures

Because cirrhosis has systemic consequences, nonspecific abnormalities may be found in many laboratory tests. For example, liver function tests (LFTs)—including ALT, AST, alkaline phosphatase (ALP), and GGT, which are indications of liver injury not liver function—not only are all usually elevated in patients with cirrhosis but also are elevated in hepatitis, sclerosing cholangitis, gallbladder disease, and because of some medications. Conversely, these lab results may be normal in the early stages of cirrhosis. The laboratory tests that actually measure liver function include the serum albumin, prothrombin time, partial thromboplastin time, clotting time, bilirubin, and serum ammonia level. The definitive diagnosis of cirrhosis is made through liver biopsy. Other tests give indications of severity and associated complications. The Diagnostic Tests box (p. 1438) outlines the tests and anticipated results for patients with cirrhosis.

Medical Management

The first priority in medical management for the patient with cirrhosis is to prevent or minimize complications such as portal hypertension, esophageal varices, hepatic encephalopathy, and hepatorenal syndrome. This is accomplished through holistic care that addresses physical, spiritual, and psychosocial aspects

CHART 46–4 **Clinical Manifestations of Cirrhosis and Physiological Causes**

Clinical Manifestation	Physiological Cause
Integumentary	
• Jaundice	Blocked outflow of bile from liver due to structural change.
• Palmar erythema	Altered sex hormone metabolism (high estrogen).
• Spider angioma	High capillary pressure.
• Decreased body hair	Altered sex hormone metabolism.
• Pruritus	High levels of bilirubin cause itching.
• Ecchymosis	↓ clotting factors, ↑ platelet destruction by spleen, ↓ vitamin K.
• Caput medusae	Intrahepatic obstruction to portal blood flow.
• Edema	Low serum albumin, high hydrostatic pressure, sodium and water retention.
Gastrointestinal	Intrahepatic obstruction to portal blood flow.
• Esophageal varices	Stretching of Glisson's capsule or ascites.
• Abdominal pain	Increased venous pressure in GI tract.
• Anorexia	Hypoalbuminemia, ↑ lymph production, ↑ capillary filtration pressure, ↑ renal absorption of sodium and water.
• Ascites	Intrahepatic obstruction of bile flowing into duodenum.
• Light-colored stools	Esophageal varices bleed.
• GI bleeding	Portal hypertension causes venous congestion.
• Hemorrhoids	
Neurological	Hepatocytes unable to convert ammonia (by-product of protein metabolism) to urea to be excreted by the kidney
• Hepatic encephalopathy	(↑ ammonia).
• Sensory disturbances	High serum ammonia levels are neurotoxic.
• Asterixis (liver flap)	Caused by high serum ammonia levels.
Cardiovascular	Intrahepatic obstruction to portal blood flow.
• Portal hypertension	Increased fluid volume from sodium and water retention and ↑ aldosterone.
• Bounding pulse	Fluid and electrolyte imbalance.
• Dysrhythmias	
Hematologic	Liver unable to synthesize clotting factors and vitamin K.
• Decreased clotting factors	Enlarged spleen causes ↑ destruction of platelets.
• Thrombocytopenia	↑ RBC destruction in spleen, bleeding.
• Anemia	
Hepatic	Scarring.
• Atrophic, nodular liver	Intrahepatic obstruction to portal blood flow causes engorgement of spleen.
• Splenomegaly	
Respiratory	Ascites cause pressure on diaphragm.
• Dyspnea	
Reproductive	Altered sex hormone metabolism.
• Oligomenorrhea (female)	Altered sex hormone metabolism (high estrogen).
• Testicular atrophy	Altered sex hormone metabolism (high estrogen).
• Gynecomastia (male)	Altered sex hormone metabolism.
• Loss of libido	
Metabolic	Liver unable to synthesize albumin.
• Hypoalbuminemia	Altered renal excretion.
• Hypokalemia	Related to low serum protein levels.
• Hypocalcemia	Impaired metabolism of nutrients.
• Malnutrition	Muscles are used as protein source.
• Muscle wasting	

DIAGNOSTIC TESTS for Cirrhosis

Test	Description	Anticipated Results in Cirrhosis
LIVER FUNCTION TESTS		
ALT (alanine aminotransferase)	Enzymes released during liver injury. Primarily found in liver cells.	May be 200–4,000 units/L. The higher elevations result from drug- or chemical-induced liver damage.
AST (aspartate aminotransferase)	Mainly found in liver and heart muscle.	10 times or more above the normal (8–38 units/L) and stays elevated for longer period.
ALT/AST	Normally the ALT is more elevated than the AST in liver disease.	In alcoholic cirrhosis, the AST is more elevated.
ALP (alkaline phosphatase)	Primarily found in liver and bone. ALP[1] isoenzyme found in liver. ALP[2] isoenzyme found in bone.	Markedly elevated in severe liver disease—normal is 42–136 units/L; ALP[1] 20–130 units/L.
TESTS THAT INDICATE LIVER FUNCTION		
Bilirubin	Bilirubin is formed from the breakdown of red blood cells (RBCs) and is not water soluble (unconjugated). It is transported to the liver where it is conjugated by the hepatocytes and is then water soluble.	Normal values: 0.1–1.2 mg/dL (total bilirubin); 0.1–0.3 mg/dL direct bilirubin (conjugated). Obstruction to bile flow either within the liver or extrahepatic (gallbladder disease) will cause an increase in direct bilirubin. Indirect bilirubin may be elevated from hemolysis or hepatocyte damage where the liver is unable to conjugate the bilirubin.
Serum ammonia	Ammonia is nitrogenous waste from the breakdown of protein. Liver cells convert ammonia to urea for excretion by the kidneys. Compromised liver function causes ammonia levels to increase.	Normal values: 15–45 mcg/dL; elevated in hepatic failure, hepatic encephalopathy, portacaval shunt, and high-protein diet with liver failure.
Prothrombin time (PT)	PT measures clotting ability that is influenced by factors I (fibrinogen), V, VII, and X.	Prothrombin time: normal is 10–13 seconds or 70–100%. Because the liver makes clotting factors, including prothrombin, compromised liver function will decrease clotting.
Serum albumin	Albumin is synthesized by the liver and makes up more than half of the plasma proteins.	Normal values: 3.5–5.0 g/dL; 52–68% to total protein. Diminished liver function will decrease albumin levels.
Serum glucose	Stored in the liver as glycogen. Decreased liver function may impair glycogen storage.	Normal values: 70–110 mg/dL. Serum glucose may be low due to inadequate glycogen storage.
Serum cholesterol	The liver synthesizes cholesterol.	Normal values: <200 mg/dL. May be decreased in liver failure. May be increased in biliary cirrhosis and cholangitis.
TESTS FOR OTHER SYSTEMIC EFFECTS		
CBC and platelets	Nutritional status may be compromised in patients with liver disease. Folic acid and B$_{12}$ deficiencies are common in alcoholic cirrhosis. Esophageal varices cause bleeding. Splenomegaly, caused by portal hypertension, causes increased destruction of platelets.	Normal values: Hb—male = 13.5–18 g/dL, female = 12–16 mg/dL. Hct—male = 40–54%, female = 36–46%. RBCs—male = 4.5–6 mcg/L, female = 4–5 mcg/L. Platelets—150,000–400,000 mcg/L. These values may all be decreased due to bleeding, folate and B$_{12}$ deficiency, and increased platelet and RBC destruction.
Serum electrolytes	Serum electrolytes include sodium, potassium, magnesium, and phosphate; are affected by malnutrition, fluid retention, and altered renal excretion all due to cirrhosis.	Normal values: Sodium—135–145 mEq/L Potassium—3.5–5.3 mEq/L Magnesium—1.5–2.5 mEq/L Phosphate—1.7–2.6 mEq/L Chloride—95–105 mEq/L Decreased values indicate malnutrition, hemodilution, and altered renal excretion caused from cirrhosis.
OTHER TESTS TO ASSESS THE LIVER		
Abdominal ultrasound	Sound waves are reflected back from tissues and converted to electrical signs by a computer. It is used to determine the size of organs.	The liver may be enlarged earlier in cirrhosis, but is usually small and nodular in advanced disease.
Esophagastroscopy	Endoscopic examination of the esophagus.	This test is used to visualize esophageal varices and may be used to sclerose bleeding varices.
Liver biopsy	A tissue sample is taken via a needle puncture of the liver. It is used to determine the type of liver disease.	In early cirrhosis the histologic changes seen are micronodular. Histologically, there are hepatocellular necrosis and mallory bodies (hyaline endoplasmic reticulum), which indicate the onset of fibrosis. Fatty infiltration and fibrosis are also seen.

of the patient. The Complementary and Alternative Therapies box presents the importance of spiritual care of the patient.

Because alcoholism is a major cause of cirrhosis in the United States, efforts at alcohol abstinence are encouraged. This requires the involvement of the family as well as other forms of support. Comprehensive treatment of cirrhosis includes medications, surgical intervention, diet, and counseling.

Treatment for Ascites

Most medications given to a patient with cirrhosis target the complications of cirrhosis. For example, most patients with cirrhosis have portal hypertension with or without ascites, low serum albumin, and increased renin-angiotensin-aldosterone secretion, complicated by the liver's inability to inactivate aldosterone; and therefore they require diuretic therapy. Spironalactone (Aldactone) is usually given because this diuretic inhibits aldosterone action and increases reabsorption of potassium,

making it a potassium-sparing diuretic. The dose is usually 100 milligrams per day. Furosemide (Lasix), 40 to 60 milligrams per day, may also be given to augment diuresis (Friedman, 2004). Some patients with massive ascites, who also have respiratory compromise, may be given intravenous albumin to increase their oncotic pressure (pressure generated by plasma proteins to maintain vascular fluid volume), but this treatment is very expensive, and the benefits may be minimal. The Pharmacology Summary feature later in the chapter (p. 1446) outlines the medications used to treat hepatic disorders.

Medical Treatment

Many medical therapies for patients with ascites involve a reduction in dietary sodium, which is usually accomplished by restrictions on the patient's fluid and sodium intake. Initially, the sodium restriction is quite severe, with sodium limits of no more than 400 to 800 milligrams per day. Once diuresis occurs,

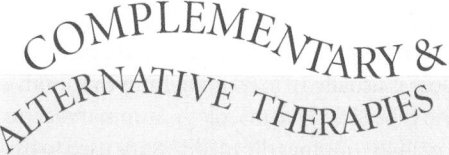

COMPLEMENTARY & ALTERNATIVE THERAPIES **Spiritual Care**

Description:

Although the concept of "sense of belonging as connectedness" is abstract, there is great potential to positively impact the mental health of many populations when the nurse can gain an understanding of this concept within a cultural worldview. A sense of belonging as connectedness is part of the dynamic nature of human life. Most cultures emphasize the social significance of a sense of belonging to interpersonal relationships and the well-being of individuals, family, and community (Hill, 2006). Some conditions have few allopathic or alternative therapies that are effective. In these cases, the best approach is through spiritual guidance and support, and in some cases, prayer.

Research Support:

An exploratory study identified four nursing competencies for spiritual care: (1) the nurse's role as both a professional and an individual person; (2) delivery of spiritual care using the nursing process; (3) communication with patients, interdisciplinary team members, and clinical/educational organizations; and (4) ensuring ethics in nursing care. Results of this study showed that spiritual care is complex, and requires that nurses be aware of patients' individual uniqueness, including each patient's unique connection between mind, body, and spirit. The study also concluded that nurses must assess each patient's spiritual status during illness and implement holistic care as recommended by the Nursing Code of Ethics (Baldacchino, 2006).

The treatment of Hepatitis C presents many physical and emotional challenges for patients. One study explored patients' experiences during hepatitis C treatment. In order for the nurse to ensure the patient's well-being, it is important for the nurse to understand the patient's experience from a holistic nursing perspective. In this study, patients undergoing treatments for hepatitis C engaged in a dialogue with investigators. The investigators then analyzed the dialogue content, reflection, and pre-understanding. Investigators found that patients' treatment experiences shared four common emotions: sadness, anger, fear, and frustration. This analysis uncovered two themes: (1) "That is not who I am," from patients who rejected the notion of being a "typical" patient, saw treatment as tolerable, felt "different" during treatment, and felt abandoned due to treatment; and (2) "looking beyond the experience" from patients who sought faith and understanding beyond conventional health care (Sheppard & Hubbert, 2006).

The HeartTouch technique is an internal method of changing thoughts and feelings. One study tested the effects of nurses who practice this technique on patients' perceived stress, hardiness, and spiritual well-being. The study used experimental and control groups. The control group participated in an educational session that discussed the effects of thoughts and feelings on stress and health. The experimental group also learned the Heart-Touch technique and practiced it for 1 month. Study results showed that nurses who practiced HeartTouch experienced a greater improvement in outcome variables than those who did not practice HeartTouch. Researchers concluded that patients can reduce stress, increase hardiness, and increase spiritual well-being by learning about the power of thoughts and feelings, then using HeartTouch to change them (Walker, 2006).

Eastern spiritual practices emphasize the interconnectedness of body, mind, and spirit. A review paper by Chan and colleagues (2006) proposed that this spirituality does not need to be restricted to any specific religious practice, nor does it need to be pursued in a highly abstract way. Researchers found that nurses can use the body-mind-spirit framework in a flexible way to engage more clients and facilitate the important process of individual exploration and change. Researchers identified key components that include exploring the inner self, utilizing all senses, connecting the body with the mind, and rebalancing one's relationship with the natural and social environment. Researchers concluded that the ultimate goal is to help patients create meaning in their lives and "reach a state of mature spirituality of tranquility and transcendence" (Chan, Ng, Ho, & Chow, 2006).

References

Baldacchino, D. R. (2006). Nursing competencies for spiritual care. *Journal of Clinical Nursing, 15*(7), 885–896.

Chan, C. L., Ng, S. M., Ho, R. T., & Chow, A. Y. (2006). East meets West: Applying Eastern spirituality in clinical practice. *Journal of Clinical Nursing, 15*(7), 822–832.

Hill, D. L. (2006). Sense of belonging as connectedness, American Indian worldview, and mental health. *Archives of Psychiatric Nursing, 20*(5), 210–216.

Sheppard, K., & Hubbert, A. (2006). The patient experience of treatment for hepatitis C. *Gastroenterology Nursing, 29*(4):309–315.

Walker, M. J. (2006). The effects of nurses' practicing of the HeartTouch technique on perceived stress, spiritual well-being, and hardiness. *Journal of Holistic Nursing, 24*(3), 164–175.

sodium intake may be increased slightly. Fluid restrictions are usually set to between 800 and 1,000 milliliters per day.

Some patients with extensive ascites may have difficulty breathing because diuretic therapy was ineffective and the amount of fluid remaining limits movement of the diaphragm. In these patients, a paracentesis may be performed. **Paracentesis** involves removing fluid from the abdominal cavity. After cleansing the lower abdomen, the health care provider will apply local anesthesia and insert a small bore trocar into the peritoneal cavity. Vacuum tubing is connected to the trocar and fluid is drained into a collection bottle. Daily removal of 500 to 1,000 milliliters through paracentesis may be effective without increasing the risk of fluid and electrolyte imbalance. However, large-volume paracentesis, or the removal of 4 to 6 liters of fluid, may be needed and is usually effective in relieving the respiratory symptoms. This can be performed daily as well but increases the risk of fluid and electrolyte imbalance. Intravenous albumin is usually given with a large-volume paracentesis to replace the proteins contained in ascitic fluid. If these are not replaced, a reduction in blood volume because of a shift in oncotic pressure could occur. Chart 46–5 covers nursing care of the patient undergoing paracentesis.

Although it is not a true surgical procedure, a transjugular intrahepatic portosystemic shunt (TIPS) may be used to relieve refractory ascites. This procedure relieves portal hypertension and involves insertion of a catheter into the jugular vein, through which an expandable stent is placed between the hepatic vein and the portal vein. The stent allows blood to flow from the portal vein into the hepatic vein, therefore bypassing the liver and effectively reducing portal pressure. The TIPS procedure has replaced the previous procedure that used peritoneovenous shunts (Friedman, 2004).

Treatment for Hepatic Encephalopathy

Hepatic encephalopathy is a complication of cirrhosis that results from increased levels of ammonia causing a disturbance in mental status. Lactulose, a nonabsorbable synthetic disaccharide that causes the contents of the colon to become more acid, is the most commonly used medication to reduce ammonia levels in the blood. When the colon contents are more acidic, a nonabsorbable form of ammonia (NH_4^+) is created and it is excreted in feces. Lactulose also decreases the presence of those bacteria in the colon that form ammonia when they digest protein in the stool. The standard dose of this medication is 30 milliliters of liquid 3 to 4 times a day. The dose is titrated to a level that results in the patient having two or three loose stools per day. If the patient cannot take oral medication, then 300 milliliters of lactulose is mixed with about 700 milliliters of saline and given as a retention enema, with repetition every 4 to 6 hours (Friedman, 2004). Some patients may also receive neomycin sulfate, which destroys the ammonia-forming bacteria in the intestines, but this practice is used less now than it once was.

Patients with hepatic encephalopathy are often agitated and combative because of the increased level of ammonia and other toxic substances. Oxazepam (Serax), a benzodiazepine that is not metabolized by the liver, is used cautiously to treat marked agitation. The standard dose is usually 10 to 30 milligrams by mouth or through a nasogastric tube. The Pharmacology Summary feature later in the chapter (p. 1446) outlines the medications used to treat hepatic disorders.

Helicobacter pylori generates ammonia in the stomach. There is some evidence that eradicating the *H. pylori* may improve hepatic encephalopathy. The medication regimen for *H. pylori* eradication is discussed in Chapter 45 .

Patients with hepatic encephalopathy will have dietary protein withheld during acute episodes. Once oral intake is resumed, protein is reintroduced slowly into the diet. Vegetable protein is tolerated better than animal protein. Initially, about 20 grams per day is introduced, increasing the amount 10 grams a day to a maximum of 60 to 80 grams per day (Friedman, 2004).

Treatment for Esophageal Varices

Because many cirrhotic patients with esophageal varices are prone to developing bacterial infections, prophylactic antibiotic medication is often given. Quinolone antibiotics, such as norfloxacin, are preferred. The drug is given orally, via nasogastric tube, or intravenously, twice a day for 7 days.

Medications to reduce portal pressure may be given. The only medication approved in the United States is octreotide, and it is given intravenously as a bolus and then followed by an infusion. It is unclear how the drug works, but it seems to reduce blood flow to the spleen and liver, therefore reducing portal pressure in patients with cirrhosis. Use of this drug in combination with endoscopic therapy has been shown to improve survival (Friedman, 2004).

Vitamin K is often given to patients with cirrhosis and esophageal varices because intrahepatic obstruction to bile flow (from the change in hepatic architecture) causes a vitamin K deficiency (because bile is needed to emulsify fats and vitamin K is fat soluble). Because the healthy liver produces clotting factors, many of which are vitamin K dependent, the person with a cirrhotic liver demonstrates an abnormal prothrombin. The recommended dose of vitamin K is 10 milligrams given subcutaneously. Folic acid and ferrous sulfate are given to treat any underlying anemia.

CHART 46–5 | **Nursing Care of the Patient Undergoing Paracentesis**

PREPROCEDURE
- Weigh patient.
- Take vital signs and measure abdominal girth.
- Have the patient empty his bladder.
- Place sitting in an upright position, seated in a chair if possible.
- Assemble needed equipment.

DURING PROCEDURE
- Monitor blood pressure, pulse, and respiratory rate and effort.
- Reassure the patient and family.

POSTPROCEDURE
- Monitor vital signs, especially blood pressure and respiratory effort.
- Monitor for bleeding or excessive drainage from the puncture site.
- Administer albumin if ordered.
- Send specimens to the laboratory for analysis if ordered.
- Change dressing as needed.
- Monitor for infection.

In the case of severe bleeding from esophageal varices, a transfusion of red blood cells, fresh frozen plasma, or platelets may be given. The Pharmacology Summary feature later in the chapter (p. 1446) outlines the medications used to treat hepatic disorders.

The bleeding from esophageal varices must be stopped as quickly as possible. The preferred method is banding. Banding, or variceal ligation, is done during endoscopy and involves the placement of tiny rubber bands on the varices to occlude blood flow. Another treatment done during endoscopy is **sclerotherapy**. This is done by injecting the varices with an agent that causes the vessel to become sclerotic, most commonly ethanolamine or tetradecyl sulfate (Friedman, 2004). Banding has fewer complications than sclerotherapy, but the latter is preferred during active bleeding because of the inability to visualize the varices for banding.

Balloon tamponade of bleeding varices may be used only as a short-term measure in cases in which endoscopy is not immediately available or when bleeding cannot be controlled with pharmacologic or endoscopic techniques. A special three-lumen nasogastric tube (Sengstaken-Blakemore and Minnesota tubes) that has an esophageal balloon, a gastric balloon, and a lumen that opens into the stomach is inserted through the nose. Once in the stomach, the gastric balloon is inflated, applying pressure to the cardiac sphincter at the distal esophagus. Then the esophageal balloon is inflated and tension is applied to the tube. This effectively applies direct pressure to any bleeding vessels. Complications of this treatment, such as aspiration, ulceration and perforation of the esophagus, and airway obstruction, are not uncommon, so this method is rarely used.

Treatment for Hepatorenal Syndrome

Drug therapy for hepatorenal syndrome is generally ineffective. An intravenous infusion of a long-acting vasoconstrictor (ornipressin) and albumin may improve the condition temporarily, but there are numerous ischemic side effects of this therapy. Other combinations of albumin and vasopressors may be used, but they do not improve survival. The Pharmacology Summary feature later in the chapter (p. 1446) outlines the medications used to treat hepatic disorders.

Very few interventions are effective in treating hepatorenal syndrome. A type of modified dialysis, the molecular absorbent recirculating system (MARS), selectively removes substances that are bound to albumin and may prolong survival. Patients with hepatorenal syndrome may also benefit from the TIPS procedure.

Surgical Treatment for End-Stage Liver Disease

Liver transplantation is indicated for patients with end-stage liver disease resulting from cirrhosis; chronic hepatitis B and C; **sclerosing cholangitis**, an inflammatory disorder of the biliary tract that leads to fibrosis and strictures in the biliary system; **primary biliary cirrhosis**, an autoimmune disease where there is inflammation and destruction of the intrahepatic biliary system that results in fibrosis; small hepatocellular carcinoma; and some metabolic diseases where the defect is in the liver. Absolute contraindications for liver transplant include active alcoholism or drug abuse, malignancy, and advanced cardiopulmonary disease. In some cases, transplant is considered for patients over age 70, those with alcohol abstinence of less than 6 months, and patients who are HIV positive. Transplant is not usually considered until the patient demonstrates a deteriorating functional status,

increasing bilirubin, decreasing serum albumin, refractory ascites, recurrent variceal bleeding, or worsening encephalopathy.

Survival rates for liver transplantation have steadily improved in the past 2 decades and currently the 5-year survival is about 80%. The increased survival is due to advances in surgical technique and improved immunosuppression. Immunosuppression is accomplished with a combination of cyclosporine or tacrolimus, prednisone, azathioprine, and mycophenolate mofetil (Friedman, 2004). Side effects of the medications are numerous and include infection, hypertension, hyperlipidemia, neuropsychiatric effects, and weight gain.

■ Nursing Management

Nursing management of the patient with cirrhosis involves a thorough assessment of risk factors, education regarding lifestyle changes, and developing a plan of care to minimize complications.

Assessment

The focus of the nursing assessment is to evaluate the patient's risk factors and underlying cause of cirrhosis as well as to assess the clinical manifestations of cirrhosis in order to plan care. A thorough health history should consist of an accurate social history (alcohol and substance abuse), sexual history (risk behaviors, lack of libido, impotence), previous exposure to blood products during surgery, and employment history. A review of symptoms by system will help the nurse establish nursing diagnoses. The physical assessment should include vital signs, level of consciousness, skin color and condition, as well as generalized urticaria. The nurse should pay close attention to areas of bruising or **caput medusae**, a term used to describe the engorged, tortuous, and visible blood vessels radiating from the umbilicus in patients with severe liver disorders, which indicate severe liver disease. A methodical abdominal assessment will include general appearance, shape, contour, and girth as well as percussion for the liver margins, noting the size of the liver and palpating for tenderness and a fluid wave.

Interventions

Nursing interventions for the patient with cirrhosis may be directed at many body systems because most body systems are affected when liver function is compromised. The Nursing Process: Patient Care Plan feature (p. 1442) applies the nursing process to a patient with cirrhosis. The Discharge Priorities box (p. 1444) describes the discharge priorities for patients with cirrhosis.

Health Promotion

Because most cases of cirrhosis are preventable, educating the patient and community, especially children and young adults, about high-risk behaviors is essential. The most common cause of cirrhosis in the United States is alcohol abuse, so limiting alcohol intake, especially for women, is the number-one topic for health education. Hepatitis B and especially hepatitis C are risk factors for the development of cirrhosis. Prevention of bloodborne hepatitis is accomplished by sexual abstinence or safe sex practices, and avoidance of injection drug use, as well as unnecessary exposure to blood and bodily fluids.

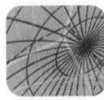

NURSING PROCESS: Patient Care Plan for Cirrhosis

Assessment of Fluid Volume

Subjective Data:

Have you noticed your ankles or feet swelling? For how long?

Have you noticed that your belly has gotten bigger? When did you notice this?

Have you vomited any blood?

Do you have hemorrhoids?

Objective Data:

Vital signs

Abdominal assessment:
- Bowel sounds
- Contour
- Girth
- Liver size
- Tenderness
- Fluid wave

Stool assessment.

Laboratory values:
- Serum albumin
- Serum electrolytes
- Hematocrit
- Creatinine
- BUN

Peripheral edema

Body weight

Jugular venous distention

Intake and output (I&O)

Urine specific gravity

Nursing Assessment and Diagnoses	Outcomes and Evaluation Parameters	Planning and Interventions with *Rationales*
Nursing Diagnosis: *Fluid Volume, Excess* related to portal hypertension and possible hepatorenal syndrome	**Outcome:** Fluid status normal. **Evaluation Parameters:** Decreasing abdominal girth. No peripheral edema. Normal laboratory results. No evidence of active bleeding. No jugular venous distention. Urine specific gravity normal. Urine output at least 30 mL/hr.	**Interventions and *Rationales:*** Weigh daily at the same time of day on the same scale, and monitor I&O. *This gives an accurate assessment of fluid status because a daily change in body weight can be attributed to water retention (or loss).* Measure abdominal girth at the same location on the abdomen at least once a day, but preferably every 8 hours *to monitor progression of ascites.* Restrict dietary sodium to less than 2 grams per day and fluid as ordered. *Sodium promotes water retention, aggravating ascites and portal hypertension.* Monitor lab values and report abnormalities. *Low serum albumin can contribute to ascites and edema. Hyponatremia and hematocrit may indicate hemodilution. Rising BUN and creatinine can indicate impending hepatorenal syndrome.* Examine neck veins for distention and extremities for edema. *Distended jugular veins indicate fluid overload, and edema can result from excess fluid and low serum albumin.* Give prescribed diuretics *to reduce body water.*

Assessment of Nutrition

Subjective Data:

Are you having trouble eating?

Have you lost any weight?

How is your appetite?

Do you drink alcohol? How much?

Objective Data:

Body weight and appearance

Skin and hair condition

Nursing Assessment and Diagnoses	Outcomes and Evaluation Parameters	Planning and Interventions with *Rationales*
Nursing Diagnosis: *Nutrition, Imbalanced: Less than Body Requirements* related to anorexia, impaired protein metabolism, and reduced absorption of fat soluble vitamins because of reduced liver function	**Outcome:** Adequate nutrition. **Evaluation Parameter:** No weight loss.	**Interventions and *Rationales:*** Provide a high-calorie, low-protein, low-sodium diet with 6 small meals per day as ordered. *Protein may be restricted if there is evidence of GI bleeding or encephalopathy in an effort to reduce nitrogenous waste products from protein metabolism.* Weekly weights after discharge. *Short-term fluctuations are usually associated with fluid balance, whereas long-term changes are a better indicator of nutritional status.* Explain the importance of avoiding substances that can be toxic to the liver, such as alcohol and acetaminophen, *in order to prevent further liver damage.* If there is no protein restriction, teach the patient to read food labels and choose foods that are high in protein and have adequate levels of vitamins and minerals, such as Instant Breakfast drink mix, *to improve nutritional status and prevent breakdown of skeletal muscle.*

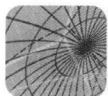

NURSING PROCESS: Patient Care Plan for Cirrhosis—*Continued*

Assessment of Skin

Subjective Data:

Does your skin itch?

Have you been scratching your skin?

Have you noticed a change in the color of your skin?

Objective Data:

Examine skin for:

- Jaundice
- Lesions from scratching
- Dryness
- Bruises
- Petechiae

Nursing Assessment and Diagnoses	Outcomes and Evaluation Parameters	Planning and Interventions with *Rationales*
Nursing Diagnosis: *Skin Integrity, Risk for Impaired* related to jaundice and resultant pruritus	**Outcome:** Skin integrity maintained. **Evaluation Parameters:** Reports diminished itching. No bruising or petechiae. No lesions from scratching.	**Interventions and *Rationales:*** Instruct the patient to use cool, lightweight, nonrestrictive clothing and avoid woolens. *Clothing made from lightweight fabrics causes less itching.* Explain that a cool environmental temperature and cool water for bathing may increase comfort related to pruritus. *Hot water causes more pruritus.* Instruct the patient to keep his fingernails trimmed and well cared for *to decrease the likelihood of excoriating when scratching.* Instruct the patient to take antihistamine medication as ordered *to reduce pruritus.*

Assessment of Bleeding Potential

Subjective Data:

Have you vomited blood?

Have your stools been dark and tarry looking?

Have you noticed that you bruise easily?

Objective Data:

Vital signs

Test stool for occult blood.

Laboratory values:

- Coagulation studies
- Platelet count
- Hemoglobin and hematocrit

Nursing Assessment and Diagnoses	Outcomes and Evaluation Parameters	Planning and Interventions with *Rationales*
Nursing Diagnosis: Fluid Volume, Deficit: Risk for related to the liver's ability to synthesize clotting factors, portal hypertension with resultant esophageal varices, and hemorrhoids	**Outcome:** No hemorrhage. **Evaluation Parameters:** Stool negative for occult blood. No vomiting blood. Coagulation studies normal. Hemoglobin and hematocrit normal. Vital signs normal.	**Interventions and *Rationales:*** Give vitamin K as ordered. *Vitamin K is synthesized in the liver and may be decreased in cirrhosis.* Teach patient to use a soft toothbrush and avoid using dental floss *because decreased clotting factors make the patient more prone to bleeding.* Monitor for bleeding (stool, skin, urine, and mucous membranes) *because decreased clotting factors make the patient more prone to bleeding.* Instruct patient to refrain from eating rough foods that can cause *trauma to the esophagus and cause varices to bleed.*

Assessment of Mental Status

Subjective Data:

Can you tell me your name, what day it is, and where you are?

Objective Data:

Assess cognitive function

Reflexes

Nursing Assessment and Diagnoses	Outcomes and Evaluation Parameters	Planning and Interventions with *Rationales*
Nursing Diagnosis: Confusion: Risk for related to hepatic encephalopathy	**Outcome:** No disruption in mental status. **Evaluation Parameters:** Alert and oriented to person, place, and time. Able to perform simple computations. Behavior appropriate. Normal reflexes. MMSE score of 25 or better.	**Interventions and *Rationales:*** Administer Mini-Mental Status Exam (MMSE). *Hepatic encephalopathy can cause changes in mentation even in the prodromal phase.* Provide a low-protein diet as ordered *to reduce the nitrogen metabolites of protein digestion.* Administer medications to reduce ammonia level as ordered. *Lactulose, oral or enema, promotes diarrhea and the elimination of ammonia in the feces.* Monitor deep tendon reflexes. *As hepatic encephalopathy progresses, reflexes become exaggerated.*

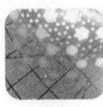

PATIENT TEACHING & DISCHARGE PRIORITIES for Cirrhosis of the Liver

Need	Teaching
Knowledge of disease process and prognosis	Home care needs include verbal and written instructions for: The treatment plan Follow-up care Nutritional and fluid needs.
Diet therapy	Many patients with cirrhosis have special dietary needs and restrictions, particularly related to protein, sodium, and fluid intake. Teaching should focus on each patient's specific dietary plan developed by the health care provider or dietician (Lutz & Przytulski, 2006).
	Frequently, these patients develop abdominal ascites and fluid retention; the nurse should reinforce the importance of adhering to a sodium-restricted diet (Afdhal, 2007).
	For the most part, patients with chronic liver disease are protein depleted, which tends to worsen as the disease progresses. The nurse should reinforce the importance of consuming small, frequent meals that are well balanced in order for the body to have sufficient kilocalories and nutrients to prevent catabolism of tissue protein for energy (Afdhal, 2007).
Drug therapy	The nurse should recognize that drug therapy is focused on the alleviation of symptoms and the prevention of complications, but it cannot reverse cirrhosis (Chisholm-Burns et al., 2008).
	Current drug therapy is available to treat the complications of ascites, varices, spontaneous bacterial peritonitis, hepatic encephalopathy, and coagulation abnormalities (Chisholm-Burns et al., 2008).
	Patients with liver disease may have several types of medications prescribed; however, commonly prescribed medications include beta-blockers, diuretics and lactulose syrup. It is important for the nurse to provide teaching related to expected effects, prescribed dosage, as well as any side effects in order to improve compliance and promote optimal patient outcomes. Emphasis should be placed on the importance of reporting side effects to the health care provider immediately for further evaluation.
Alcohol abstinence	Abstinence from alcohol is critical and should be reinforced during discharge teaching.
	The nurse should provide information regarding local support groups and counseling services to facilitate adherence to this critical component of the treatment plan.

Sources: Afdhal, N. H. (2007). *Epidemiology of and risk factors for gallstones.* Retrieved April 24, 2008, from http://www.uptodate.com/patients/content/topic.do?topicKey=~5rphinkcGz/zys; Chisholm-Burns, M. A., Wells, B. G., Schwinghammer, T. L., Malone, P. M., Kolesar, J. M., Rotschafer, J. C., et al. (2008). *Pharmacotherapy principles & practice.* New York: McGraw-Hill; and Lutz, C., & Przytulski, K. (2006). *Nutrition and diet therapy: Evidence-based applications.* Philadelphia: F. A. Davis.

Liver Cancer

Cancer of the liver accounts for less than 2% of all deaths from cancer in the United States. Primary liver cancer is rare in the United States but is common in densely populated areas in southern Africa, Asia, and Greece (Huether, 2006). However, the liver is a common site of metastatic spread from cancer in other parts of the body. People with chronic hepatitis B or C are at a high risk for developing primary liver cancer.

Pathophysiology

Cancer of the liver develops from the liver's parenchymal cells (hepatocellular carcinoma) or from the cells in the bile ducts (**cholangiocarcinoma**). Up to 90% of all primary liver tumors are hepatocellular carcinoma. This type of cancer can be nodular, massive, or diffuse, and is most closely related to cirrhosis or hepatitis B and C. Hepatocellular carcinoma metastasizes to the heart, lungs, brain, kidneys, and spleen. Cholangiocarcinoma is more common in southeast China, where liver fluke infestation is common, and has a similar metastatic profile to hepatocellular carcinoma.

Primary liver cancer arises when there is damage to the hepatocellular DNA. Both hepatitis B and C viruses can act as carcinogens especially in the presence of cirrhosis. Exposure to mycotoxins, such as those produced by *Aspergillus flavus* (mold on corn, peanuts, and grain), causes the mutation of the p53 suppressor gene (Huether, 2006). Other risk factors for the development of liver cancer include heavy smoking and drinking, prolonged use of anabolic steroids, and arsenic-contaminated water.

Clinical Manifestations

The clinical manifestations of liver cancer are often general and nonspecific. Symptoms may include weakness, anorexia with weight loss, fatigue, and malaise. These usually occur early, but as the tumor enlarges or more of the liver becomes involved, manifestations include abdominal pain, ascites, jaundice, and a palpable mass in the right upper quadrant. There may also be signs of liver failure such as portal hypertension.

Laboratory and Diagnostic Procedures

There are no specific tests for liver cancer, although most tumors can be identified by magnetic resonance imaging (MRI) and computed tomography (CT) scans. Once a suspicious area is found, a liver biopsy is done to determine the tumor type. Liver enzymes, AST and ALT, are measured and are usually elevated in people with liver cancer. Patients with advanced hepatocellular cancer will have an elevated alpha-fetoprotein (AFP). An elevated AFP is strongly correlated with chronic hepatitis B infection, rapid tumor growth, and poorly differentiated tumors (Huether, 2006).

Medical Management

Surgical resection of the liver is possible only if the tumor is localized and in a lobe of the liver that can be removed. For example, if the tumor is in the posterior section of the right lobe, it

Medications Used in Palliative Care

Clinical Problem

When a patient develops acute or chronic liver failure, the metabolism of medications commonly used for palliation becomes abnormal, requiring a careful and frequently changing dosing regimen. Decreased hepatic blood flow and the shunting of blood cause the medications to be metabolized more slowly and to have an increased bioavailability. For instance, benzodiazepines such as midazolam that are used for sedation may have an increased effect due to the presence of unmetabolized toxins, increased sensitivity to the drug, stimulation of the gamma-aminobutyric acid (GABA) receptors, and reduced cerebral blood flow (Rhee & Broadbent, 2007).

Research Findings

To facilitate care of the patient with liver failure, Rhee and Broadbent (2007) conducted an extensive literature search, as well as a review of major textbooks in pharmacology, palliative care, hepatology, and gastroenterology. From these data they developed a table of functional groups of medications commonly used in palliative care: the pharmacologic half-life with normal liver function and with cirrhosis. When data were available, the medications affected by cirrhosis were further broken down following the Child-Pugh criteria of liver disease. This information may assist in the decision-making process of which medications to use, reduce potential complications, and improve palliation of symptoms for patients with liver failure. As an example, here are the findings for opioid analgesics and nonopioid analgesics. Within the article, the complete table includes comments and

recommendations for changes in dose and frequency with the references used for each drug.

Implications for Nursing Practice

It is important for the nurse to understand the degree of decreased function of the liver and to understand the affect on the metabolism of medications. Patients with end-stage liver disease require palliation. Knowing the expected increase in the half-life of analgesics will allow the nurse to administer medications safely.

Critical Thinking Questions

1. Discuss the effect of liver failure on the metabolism of palliative medication.

2. The health care team prescribes morphine IV for a patient with acute liver failure. Before initiating the prescription, what is most important for the nurse to do?

Answers to Critical Thinking Questions appear in Appendix D.

Reference

Rhee, C., & Broadbent, A. M. (2007). Palliation and liver failure: Palliative medications dosages guidelines. *Journal of Palliative Medicine, 10*(3), 677–687.

Source: Adapted from Rhee, C. & Broadbent, A. M. (2007). Palliation and liver failure: Palliative medications dosages guidelines. *Journal of Palliative Medicine, 10(3),* 677–687.

Medication	Half-Life Normal Liver	Half-Life Cirrhosis	Half-Life Child-Pugh A	Half-Life Child-Pugh B	Half-Life Child-Pugh C
Opioid Analgesics					
Fentanyl	4.4 minutes	5.1 minutes			
Hydromorphone	2.5 hours	No data			
Methadone	18.8 hours	No data	11.3 hours	13 hours	35.5 hours
Morphine (IV)	1.7 hours	4.2 hours	3.4 hours	4.35 hours	4.47 hours
Morphine (oral)	3.3 hours	5.5 hours	6.4 hours	6.85 hours	4.4 hours
Morphine (SR)	4.01 hours	No data	7.36 hours		
Oxycodone	3.4 hours	13.9 hours			
Nonopioid Analgesics					
Aspirin	7.9 hours	7.3 hours			
Ibuprofen	2.2 hours	No data	1.9 hours		2.6 hours
Naproxen	14.14 hours	20.36 hours			

EVIDENCE-BASED PRACTICE

cannot be removed because the right hepatic vein is located in this area. Chemotherapy agents may be given directly into the liver or systemically. Liver transplant is an option for small tumors without evidence of spread. Overall, the survival prospects for patients with liver cancer are less than 6 months.

■ Nursing Management

A goal of nursing care for patients with liver cancer is prevention whenever possible. Nurses can encourage alcohol abstinence

and prevention of HBV and HCV. In those patients who have a risk factor for liver cancer, such as chronic infection with HBV or HCV, the risk for developing liver cancer can be reduced if they abstain from alcohol. Most of the nursing interventions for a patient with liver cancer are similar to those for patients with cirrhosis and liver failure. Nursing care includes helping patients with liver cancer prepare for death, supporting the family, and providing comfort. Refer to Chapter 17 ☺ for nursing management at end of life. See Evidence-Based Practice box for specific medications for palliative care.

PHARMACOLOGY Summary of Medications Used to Treat Hepatic Disorders

Medication Category	Action	Application/Indication	Nursing Responsibility
Antiviral Agents			
Interferons: Peginterferon alfa-2b (PEG-Intron) Interferon alpha-2a (Pegasys)	Inhibits viral replication in infected cells, activates cellular immunity.	Management of chronic hepatitis C.	Monitor for adverse effects: fatigue, muscle aches, headache, fever, and chills. Monitor complete blood count (CBC) with differential, platelets, and renal function. Monitor for severe reactions: depression, psychoses, suicidal ideation, and pancreatitis. Be aware theophylline level may increase. Monitor drug level.
Noninterferons: Adefovir (Hespera)	Exerts antiviral effects by interfering with viral DNA.	Treatment of chronic hepatitis B.	Monitor for adverse effects: muscle weakness, abdominal pain, diarrhea, dyspepsia, nausea, hematuria, headache, and rash. Monitor electrolytes, renal and hepatic function, especially in presence of liver or kidney dysfunction.
Lamivudine (Epivir)	Exerts antiviral effects by interfering with viral DNA replication.	Treatment of chronic hepatitis B.	Monitor for adverse effects: neuropathy, insomnia, dizziness, fever, nausea, and diarrhea. Monitor liver and renal function, CBC with differential. Observe for lactic acidosis.
Oral ribavirin (Rebetol)	Antiviral effect thought to be due to interference with viral RNA synthesis.	Management of hepatitis C in combination with interferon alpha-2b.	Monitor for adverse effects: fatigue, myalgia, nausea, insomnia, headache, irritability, and depression. Monitor hemoglobin, neutrophil count. Observe for development or worsening of cardiac or pulmonary dysfunction.
Diuretics			
Potassium sparing: Spironolactone (Aldactone)	Promotes diuresis through sodium and chloride excretion in distal tubule without loss of potassium.	Hepatic cirrhosis, ascites.	Monitor for adverse effects: hyperkalemia, menstrual irregularities, gynecomastia, and impotence. Monitor electrolytes and I&O. Be aware of multiple drug interactions (digoxin, ACE inhibitors, corticosteroids, NSAIDs, and others). Monitor for altered drug efficacy or toxicity. Monitor digoxin level if given concurrently.
Loop diuretic: Furosemide (Lasix)	Diuretic effect due to reduced reabsorption of sodium and chloride in loop of Henle, proximal tube, and distal tubule.	Edema associated with hepatic cirrhosis.	Monitor for adverse effects: hypotension, hypokalemia, hyponatremia, hypochloremia, hypocalcemia, and metabolic alkalosis. Be aware of multiple drug interactions (digoxin, insulin, NSAIDs, and others). Monitor for altered drug efficacy or toxicity. Be aware of ototoxicity potential with patients on aminoglycoside or if rapid IV administration, especially in presence of decreased renal function or high drug dose. Monitor electrolytes and I&O. Be aware of multiple drug incompatibilities when given IV.
Hyperosmotic Laxative Lactulose	Increases ammonia excretion by acidifying colon contents, reducing diffusion of ammonia from colon to blood.	Prevention and treatment of hepatic encephalopathy.	Monitor for adverse effects: nausea, vomiting, and hypernatremia. Monitor electrolytes. Monitor fluid status.
Aminoglycoside Antibiotic Neomycin sulfate	Reduces blood ammonia by destroying ammonia-forming bacteria.	Cirrhosis, hepatic coma.	Monitor for adverse effects: diarrhea, nausea, and vomiting. Observe for severe adverse reactions: respiratory paralysis, ototoxicity, and nephrotoxicity. Monitor renal function and serum drug levels.

PHARMACOLOGY Summary of Medications Used to Treat Hepatic Disorders—*Continued*

Medication Category	Action	Application/Indication	Nursing Responsibility
Synthetic Hormone			
Octreotide (Sandostatin)	Reduces portal blood flow by inhibiting release of vasodilatory hormone.	Variceal bleeding.	Monitor for adverse effects: nausea and diarrhea. Monitor electrolytes, blood glucose.
Sedative-Hypnotic			
Oxazepam (Serax)	Causes sedative effect by potentiating inhibitory neurotransmitter GABA.	Anxiety, acute withdrawal symptoms in chronic alcoholism, agitation.	Monitor for adverse effects: drowsiness, ataxia, paradoxical stimulant response, and sleep disturbances, especially in elderly. Monitor for drug interactions (other CNS depressants, cimetidine, phenytoin, smoking, and others). Monitor for altered drug efficacy or toxicity. Be aware prolonged use requires slow withdrawal of medication. Caution patient sedative effect is increased with alcohol.
Immunosuppressants			
Cyclosporine[a] (Sandimmune, Neoral) Tacrolimus[a] (Prograf, Protopic) Mycophenolate[a] (CellCept) Azathioprine (Azasan, Imuran)	Suppresses immune response by inhibiting lymphocyte replication or disrupting helper T cells or inhibiting antibody formation.	Adjunct therapy with corticosteroids for transplant rejection, oral form—biliary cirrhosis, Crohn's disease, ulcerative colitis.	Monitor for adverse effects: hypertension, nausea, vomiting, and infection. Observe for signs of toxicity: tremors, seizures, altered mental status, visual disturbances, nephrotoxicity, and neurotoxicity. Monitor CBC, liver, and renal function tests, electrolytes, and blood sugar. Be aware of multiple drug specific interactions (digoxin, NSAIDs, erythromycin, verapamil, cimetidine, allopurinal, ACE inhibitors, warfarin, and others). Monitor for altered drug levels, nephrotoxicity, or leukopenia.

[a]*Monitor blood sugar.*

DISORDERS OF THE GALLBLADDER

The gallbladder is a saclike structure that concentrates and stores bile. Bile is produced by the liver and is necessary for the absorption of dietary fat and fat soluble vitamins. Most gallbladder disorders result in obstructed bile flow from the liver to the gallbladder or from the gallbladder to the duodenum. The most common cause of obstructed flow is gallstones, or **cholelithiasis**. When a gallstone either forms in or migrates to the common bile duct, the resultant condition is called **choledocholithiasis**. Cirrhosis can obstruct the flow of bile from the liver to the gallbladder (Figure 46–3 ■, p. 1448). Other causes of obstructed flow include tumors (rare) and abscesses.

■ Cholelithiasis

Gallstones may form from a combination of factors. If the stone is large, it may obstruct flow from the gallbladder to the duodenum, causing pain.

Etiology and Epidemiology

Gallstones result from a combination of factors including biliary stasis, inflammation of the gallbladder, and abnormal bile com-

position and reabsorption. There are two types of gallstones: those predominantly composed of cholesterol and those composed of calcium bilirubinate. Cholesterol gallstones are the more commonly occurring, with 80% of gallstones in the United States and Europe being this type. In Japan, however, 30% to 40% of gallstones are the calcium bilirubinate type (Friedman, 2004).

Cholelithiasis is more common in women, but the incidence in both men and women increases as people age. In fact, 20% of women and 10% of men have gallstones by the age of 65. Certain ethnic groups are at a higher risk for gallstones. For example, 75% of Native American Indian women over the age of 25 have gallstones (Chart 46–6, p. 1448). Other risk factors for the development of cholelithiasis are obesity, especially in women; high estrogen states; diabetes; hyperlipidemia; cirrhosis; and Crohn's disease. Rapid weight loss is also associated with gallstone formation, and there is an increased incidence after bariatric surgery. Many drugs can increase the risk for gallstone formation, such as clofibrate, ceftriaxone, oral contraceptives, and hormone replacement therapy.

Pathophysiology

Cholesterol is a normal component of bile, but when the bile is supersaturated with cholesterol, the chances increase for cholesterol crystal formation. The cholesterol crystals aggregate to

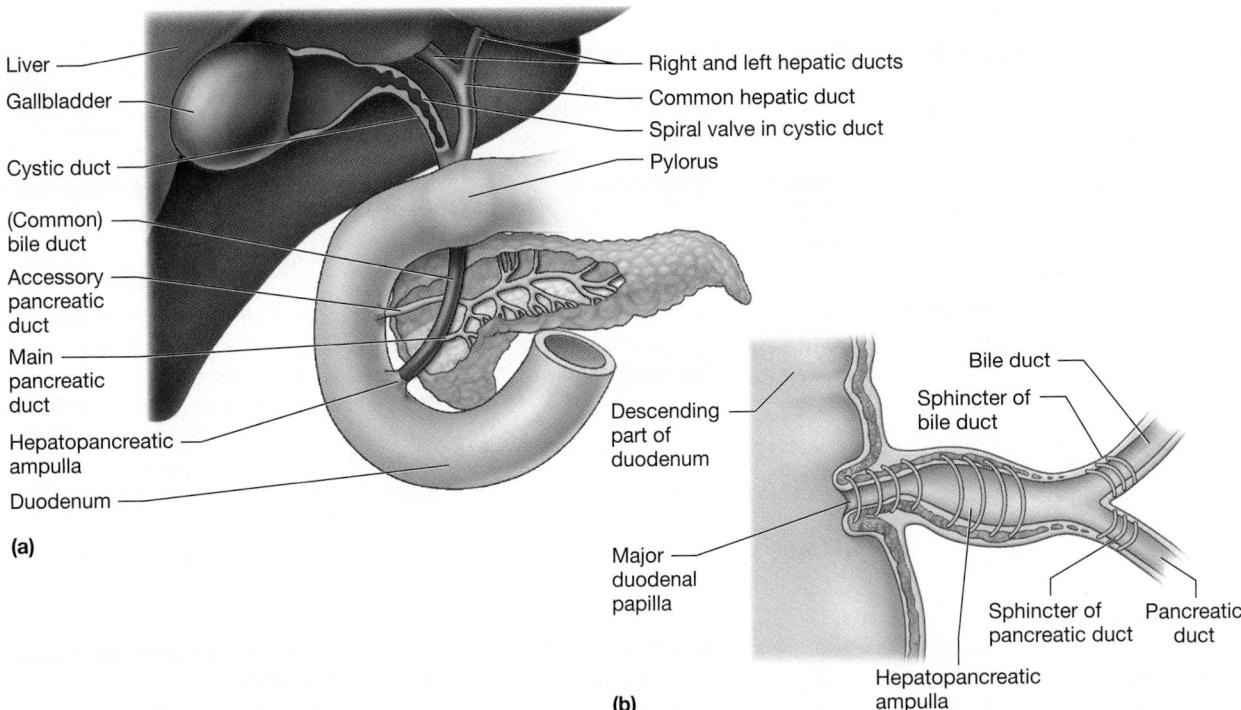

(a)

(b)

FIGURE 46–3 ■ (A) Extrahepatic bile passages, gallbladder, and pancreatic ducts. (B) Entry of the pancreatic and bile ducts into the hepatopancreatic ampula, then into the duodenum.

form larger stones. When these "macrostones" obstruct the cystic or common bile duct, the gallbladder becomes inflamed and **cholecystitis** results. It is unclear why the hepatocytes form bile with a high concentration of cholesterol, but it is most likely a combination of factors, including the presence of a defective enzyme that influences the liver cells' synthesis of cholesterol, a decreased secretion of bile acids, and a decreased reabsorption of bile salts from the ileum.

Clinical Manifestations

The most common manifestation of cholelithiasis is epigastric and/or right upper quadrant pain. Most patients also complain of intolerance to fatty foods and nausea. Other symptoms include flatulence, bloating, abdominal distention, diarrhea, and chest pain. Often the pain associated with gallstones is steady and severe with radiation to the mid-upper back, right scapula, and shoulder. Pain usually occurs within 1 hour after eating, may be accompanied by nausea and vomiting, and may last for 4 to 5 hours. If a stone becomes lodged in the common bile duct, the patient may also develop jaundice as a result of hepatocyte damage from bile refluxing into the liver.

■ Cholecystitis

Cholecystitis is simply inflammation of the gallbladder and can be an acute or chronic problem. The most common cause of both acute and chronic cholecystitis is a gallstone lodged in the cystic duct. When the flow of bile out of the gallbladder is obstructed, the gallbladder becomes distended and an inflammatory response is initiated.

Pathophysiology

In at least 90% of the patients with cholecystitis, cholelithiasis is the cause. If the gallstones are in the cystic duct, pressure in the gallbladder increases, causing ischemia of the mucosal wall and inflammation. Prolonged ischemia leads to necrosis and in severe cases gangrene can result. In a severely inflamed gallbladder, or in the case of gangrene, perforation with resultant peritonitis is possible. In patients who are immunosuppressed, infectious organisms such as cytomegalovirus and cryptosporidiosis can cause acute cholecystitis. Chronic cholecystitis can result from persistent irritation of the gallbladder by either repeated bouts of acute cholecystitis or constant presence of many small gallstones in the gallbladder.

Clinical Manifestations

The clinical manifestations of cholecystitis are similar to those of cholelithiasis. Pain is the predominant symptom and is usually severe and steady, lasting up to 12 to 18 hours. As with gallstones, the pain is usually in the right upper quadrant and may radiate to the mid-upper back, right scapula, and shoulder. Unlike cholelithiasis, the patient with cholecystitis can have a fever and chills. The gallbladder may be palpable on abdominal exam if it is extremely inflamed, and there may be tenderness with possible guarding on palpation of the RUQ. Jaundice may be present as well.

■ Biliary Dyskinesia

Biliary dyskinesia is a term applied to motility disorders of the gallbladder. Although they are uncommon disorders, the clinical manifestations are almost indistinguishable from other problems of the gallbladder. The most common clinical manifestation is episodic abdominal pain. The pain is usually epigastric or in the right upper quadrant and may radiate to the back and right scapula. As with the pain in cholelithiasis, the pain from biliary dyskinesia occurs following a fatty meal and may be accompanied by nausea and vomiting.

Laboratory and Diagnostic Procedures

The diagnostic test of choice for cholelithiasis is an *ultrasound of the gallbladder*. This test is noninvasive and can detect gallstones, dilated ducts, wall inflammation, and abnormal fluid presence. It can also be used to assess the emptying of the gallbladder for patients that may have biliary dyskinesia. Other tests may be performed to identify possible complications or to rule out other possible causes of the symptoms.

- *Serum bilirubin,* both direct (conjugated) and indirect (unconjugated), is measured. If the direct bilirubin is elevated (normal = 0.3 to 1.2 mg/dL), this is most indicative of an obstructive process within the liver or biliary system. Gallstones, cirrhosis, or hepatitis can cause this type of obstruction. On the other hand, indirect bilirubin is elevated when there is RBC hemolysis or when the hepatocytes are unable to conjugate bilirubin, usually due to cellular damage.
- *Serum amylase and lipase* are measured to determine whether the pancreas is involved, possibly due to common bile duct obstruction, or whether pancreatitis is present.
- *AST and ALT* will usually be measured to determine whether any liver injury has occurred as a result of a stone in the common bile duct.
- A *CBC* may indicate an infectious process in the gallbladder if the WBC count is elevated.
- An oral cholecystogram is rarely done any longer. For this test, the patient is given an oral dye that concentrates in the gallbladder, making any stones visible.

Medical Management

Patients with asymptomatic cholelithiasis are usually treated conservatively with dietary modifications and lifestyle changes. However, if the patient has frequent symptoms, very severe symptoms, or cholecystitis, surgery to remove the gallstone and the gallbladder is indicated.

Dietary and Lifestyle Management

For mild cases of cholelithiasis, diet (low fat) and lifestyle changes may be effective in managing the condition. For more severe cases, diet and lifestyle changes are only a part of treatment that will include surgery. For either case, dietary fat intake is limited. Chart 46–7 lists foods with a high fat content. Patients with obstructed bile flow may require supplementation with the fat soluble vitamins A, D, E, and K. For patients who are obese, a weight loss program that includes exercise is recommended. Other contributing factors such as hyperlipidemia and diabetes are treated to minimize recurrence of gallstones.

Surgery

Surgery is the treatment of choice for most patients with cholelithiasis, cholecystitis, and biliary dyskinesia. Removal of the gallbladder, or **cholecystectomy**, is done most often using the laparoscopic surgical method, which is minimally invasive, has fewer complications, and requires a much shorter length of hospital stay than the traditional open cholecystectomy. Patients with a very large or infected gallbladder may not be candidates for laparoscopic cholecystectomy and may require an open cholecystectomy. During the laparoscopic procedure, the surgeon may find it necessary to convert the procedure to an open cholecystectomy. If stones are located in the common bile duct, an exploration of this duct is done, and a T-tube is placed in the common bile duct to maintain patency, allowing bile to pass from the liver into the duodenum until the edema from surgery diminishes. Chart 46–8 (p. 1450) outlines the nursing care of a patient with a T-tube.

Medications

Some patients may not be good surgical candidates or they may refuse surgery. Drugs are available to dissolve the gallstones by reducing the cholesterol content of the stone. Ursodiol (Actigall) or chenodiol (Chenix) may be used but are effective only if the gallstones contain a high concentration of cholesterol and are less than 1.5 to 2 centimeters in diameter. Treatment with these agents is expensive and usually lasts for 1 to 3 years, with recurrent stone formation occurring in 50% of patients after

CHART 46–7 Foods High in Fat Content

Full fat dairy products:
- Whole milk
- Cheese
- Cream
- Ice cream
- Cottage cheese
- Sour cream

Cooking and salad oil:
- Olive oil
- Canola oil
- Corn oil
- Sunflower oil

Salad dressing (regular, not lite)

Snack foods:
- Potato chips
- Corn chips
- Pork rinds

Fried food:
- Doughnuts
- French fries
- Hamburgers
- Bacon
- Fried fish, chicken

Nuts

Peanut butter

Chocolate

Gravy

Some cuts of meat:
- Ham
- Pork shoulder
- Lunch meat
- Ground meat

CHART 46–8   Care of the Patient with a T-Tube

- Attach tube to sterile gravity drainage.
  - Place patient in Fowler's position to maximize gravity drainage.
- Monitor drainage and record the amount every 8 hours.
  - The amount may be between 500 and 1,000 milliliters on the first day, decreasing to about 200 milliliters by the 3rd day.
  - Drainage may be blood tinged at first but becomes green-brown.
  - Drainage in excess of 500 milliliters by the 3rd day is excessive, and the surgeon must be notified.
- Monitor color of the stools.
  - Pale stools indicate obstruction of flow of bile to duodenum.
- Clamp the T-tube as ordered, and monitor the patient's response to clamping.
- Keep skin clean and free from bile drainage.
  - Bile is irritating to the skin. Skin can be protected with zinc oxide, karaya, or other barrier.
- Teach the patient how to care for the tube during activities of daily living.
  - The patient may be discharged with the tube in place and should be informed of the signs of infection, such as fever, redness, swelling, or drainage from the site, as well as care for the tube, avoiding any direct pulling or traction on the tube.
  - A daily shower is usually permitted, but a tub bath is not.

treatment is stopped. The Pharmacology Summary feature later in the chapter (p. 1457) outlines medications used to treat biliary disorders.

Other drug treatment for cholelithiasis and cholecystitis includes antibiotics if an infection is suspected. Bile salts accumulate on the skin when the patient is jaundiced and this causes pruritus. Cholestyramine (Questran) binds these bile salts, which are then excreted in the stool. For acute cholecystitis a narcotic analgesic may be needed to relieve the pain.

Ultrasound Therapy
Extracorporeal shock wave lithotripsy (ESWL) is a method to break up large gallstones by using ultrasound waves. After the procedure, the patient may have biliary colic pain when the gallbladder attempts to expel the stone fragments. Patients undergoing ESWL also require oral dissolution therapy to help dissolve the stone fragments. This method of treating cholelithiasis is more than 5 times more expensive than surgery.

Complementary Therapy
The use of the herb goldenseal to treat cholecystitis has had limited research. The active ingredient berberine has been shown to decrease the symptoms of cholecystitis. It appears to stimulate the secretion of bile. Use in pregnancy is contraindicated because of the stimulatory effects on the uterus and should not be used during breast-feeding.

Nursing Management

Nursing care for patients with cholelithiasis or cholecystitis includes assessment, assuring pain relief, preparing the patient for possible surgery, preventing infection, and education regarding future prevention, postoperative care, and dietary modifications.

Assessment
Nursing assessment includes a complete history and physical examination. The history should focus on risk factors for cholelithiasis and cholecystitis; previous history of symptoms; character, duration, and relationship of pain with meals; presence of associated symptoms such as nausea and vomiting; and current medications, activity, and diet. If the patient reports dark-colored urine and light-colored stools, there is a strong suspicion of a gallstone obstructing the common bile duct, the cystic duct, or the hepatic duct.

The physical exam should include a head-to-toe assessment, including body weight and BMI (body mass index). Scleral color, skin color and condition, abdominal palpation for tenderness or guarding, and a visual examination of stool and urine should also be included. The physical exam should include a thorough heart and lung assessment as well, because the patient will most likely be scheduled for surgery.

Interventions
Most patients who have acute cholelithiasis will eventually require surgery, either laparoscopic cholecystectomy or open cholecystectomy. Nursing care centers on comfort measures and preventing complications such as pneumonia, infection, and nausea. The Nursing Process: Patient Care Plan feature presents the complete care for the patient with cholelithiasis and surgery.

Health Promotion
Several risk factors for cholelithiasis can be controlled, such as obesity, hyperlipidemia, and diabetes. Increasing exercise and maintaining a well-balanced low-fat, low-calorie diet can modify obesity. However, rapid weight loss should be discouraged because it could contribute to gallstone formation. Hyperlipidemia can be controlled through medication, by a low-fat, low-cholesterol diet, and with at least 30 minutes per day of regular exercise. Good control of blood sugar in patients with diabetes may also decrease the recurrence of gallstones.

DISORDERS OF THE EXOCRINE PANCREAS

Disorders of the pancreas that will be discussed are pancreatitis, acute and chronic, and cancer of the pancreas.

▪ Pancreatitis

Pancreatitis, or inflammation of the pancreas, can be acute or chronic and is a potentially serious disease. Most cases of pancreatitis occur between age 50 and 60 with incidence the same for men and women. Risk factors for the development of pancreatitis include alcoholism, biliary obstruction, peptic ulcers, trauma, extreme hyperlipidemia, hypertriglyceridemia, and the use of some medications (Huether, 2006). Mortality is high if the patient develops cardiac, pulmonary, or renal complications.

Acute Pancreatitis
Many cases of acute pancreatitis are mild, are self-limiting, and do not require hospitalization. However, about 20% of patients

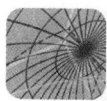

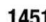

NURSING PROCESS: Patient Care Plan for Cholelithiasis and Surgery

Assessment of Pain:
Acute Cholelithiasis/Cholecystitis; Preoperatively

Subjective Data:
What is your level of pain on a scale of 0–10, with 10 being the worst pain?
Are you allergic to anything?
Do you have any special cultural or religious practices for dealing with pain?
Do you have pain when you eat certain foods, particularly high-fat foods?
Have you ever had this type of pain before? If yes, how long did it last? What relieved the pain in the past?
Do you take oral contraceptives? Or hormone replacement therapy?
Could you possibly be pregnant?

Objective Data:
Vital signs q4h:
- Temperature
- BP
- Pulse
- Respirations

Abdominal examination:
- Bowel sounds
- Tenderness
- Guarding
Restlessness
Grimacing
Moaning or groaning
Shallow respirations

Nursing Assessment and Diagnoses	Outcomes and Evaluation Parameters	Planning and Interventions with *Rationales*
Nursing Diagnosis: *Pain, Acute* related to cholelithiasis/cholecystitis	**Outcome:** Comfort level maintained. **Evaluation Parameters:** Able to communicate level of pain and relief from medications. Able to take deep breaths without pain. Appears restful without restlessness or moaning.	**Interventions and *Rationales:*** Assess pain using pain scale (0–10) to quantify pain level. *To increase consistency in monitoring pain.* Administer pain medication, usually meperidine or morphine (research indicates that morphine does not cause sphincter of Oddi spasms), and assess level of pain 30 minutes and 1 hour after giving medication. *To assess effectiveness of medications.* Explore cultural and religious practices and beliefs about pain and illness. *Different religions have varying beliefs about pain, suffering, and disease.* Teach nonpharmacologic methods of pain control, such as guided imagery, meditation, and breathing exercises. *This may augment pain relief.* Discuss foods that are high in fat and may cause nausea and GI distress even after surgery. *Foods high in fat stimulate contractions of the gallbladder and may cause pain if stones are present.* (See Chart 46–7 (p. 1449) for a list of high-fat foods.)

Assessment of Nutrition

Subjective Data:
How is your appetite?
Are you nauseated?
Are there any foods that make you nauseated?
Have you lost a lot of weight lately?

Objective Data:
Height and weight measurements
BMI

Laboratory results:
- Bilirubin
- Serum albumin
- Glucose
- Cholesterol
- Urinalysis

Nursing Assessment and Diagnoses	Outcomes and Evaluation Parameters	Planning and Interventions with *Rationales*
Nursing Diagnosis: *Nutrition: Readiness for Enhanced* related to anorexia, pain, and nausea from impaired bile flow	**Outcome:** Adequate nutrition. **Evaluation Parameters:** No weight loss. Serum albumin normal. Fasting glucose normal. No reported nausea. No evidence of bleeding.	**Interventions and *Rationales:*** Obtain diet history, history of large rapid weight loss, and height and weight measurements *to help establish current status and possible imbalanced diet with fat soluble vitamin deficiency.* Assess laboratory results and report any abnormal values to the patient's health care provider. *Bilirubin in the urine indicates an obstruction to bile flow and will be reflected in an elevated serum bilirubin. Patients with diabetes mellitus and high serum cholesterol are at risk for gallstones. Protein malnutrition is reflected in a low serum albumin.* Give supplemental vitamins as ordered. *Bile is necessary for the absorption of fat soluble vitamins, so supplements may be necessary.* Educate the patient about avoiding foods that contain a large amount of fat. *Even after removal of the gallbladder, high-fat foods may cause nausea.* Refer to a dietitian for a low-fat diet plan that promotes slow weight loss. *Many patients with gallbladder disease are overweight or obese and will benefit from a sensible weight loss plan.*

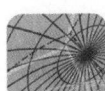

NURSING PROCESS: Patient Care Plan for Cholelithiasis and Surgery—*Continued*

Assessment of Postoperative Status

Subjective Data:

What is your level of pain on a scale of 0–10, with 10 being the worst pain?

Are you nauseated?

How active were you before surgery?

Objective Data:

Vital signs:
- Temperature
- BP
- Pulse
- Respirations

Abdominal examination:
- Bowel sounds
- Tenderness

- Guarding
- Wound inspection

Laboratory values:
- CBC
- Coagulation studies
- Bilirubin

Nursing Assessment and Diagnoses	Outcomes and Evaluation Parameters	Planning and Interventions with *Rationales*
Nursing Diagnoses: *Comfort: Readiness for Enhanced* related to surgical incision. *Nutrition: Readiness for Enhanced* related to postoperative nausea. *Airway Clearance, Ineffective* related to decreased lung expansion, immobility, and anesthesia. *Infection: Risk for* related to surgical incision and ineffective airway clearance.	**Outcome:** Discharge 1–2 days postoperatively. ***Evaluation Parameters:*** Hemoglobin and hematocrit normal. Vital signs normal. No complaints of nausea. Bowel sounds and bowel movement. Eating soft food without nausea.	**Interventions and *Rationales:*** Assess pain using pain scale (0–10) to quantify pain level, and administer pain medication as ordered or monitor the PCA (patient controlled analgesia) if the patient has an IV pump. *To increase consistency in monitoring pain.* Give antiemetic as ordered *to prevent vomiting that may result from anesthesia.* Discuss previous activity level, and instruct to resume normal activity slowly over 2–3 days after discharge. *An otherwise sedentary patient cannot be expected to be more active after surgery than before.* Give vitamin K as ordered. *Vitamin K is a fat soluble vitamin and may be ordered postoperatively to prevent bleeding.* Position in semi-Fowler's and ambulate as ordered when the patient is alert. *Early ambulation promotes lung expansion and helps prevent postoperative pneumonia, as well as promoting intestinal motility. The upright position allows for fuller lung expansion.* Monitor vital signs every 2–4 hours × 4, then every 4–8 hours as ordered *to detect any complications. Tachycardia, increased respiratory rate, or elevated temperature can indicate pain, bleeding, or infection.* Examine abdomen for return of bowel sounds, signs of peritonitis, and assess wound for drainage and infection. *Increasing abdominal tenderness, guarding, and rigid abdomen may be signs of an intra-abdominal leak of bile or blood.* Assess laboratory results for signs of over-/underhydration, bleeding, biliary obstruction, and infection, and notify the health care provider. *Early detection of complications of surgery, such as hemorrhage, infection, edema of the common bile duct, and fluid overload/dehydration, makes treatment more efficient.*

develop severe pancreatitis, which can lead to necrosis of the pancreas, and must be hospitalized.

Pathophysiology

The precise cause of pancreatitis is unknown, but most cases are associated with either biliary tract obstruction or heavy alcohol use. It is believed that activated pancreatic enzymes, particularly trypsin, leak into the pancreatic tissue and begin the process of autodigestion; the pancreas begins to digest itself. If bile refluxes into the pancreas as a result of biliary obstruction, this activates the pancreatic enzymes and the process of autodigestion. Activated trypsin and lipase begin to break down the cell membranes, which results in edema, vascular leakage, hemorrhage, and necro-

sis. In response to this autodigestion, tissue necrosis factor-alpha (TNF-α), substance P, and many interleukins and kinins enter the systemic circulation causing damage to tissue in the lungs, blood vessels, and kidneys, which results in increased mortality.

Clinical Manifestations

The most prominent manifestation of acute pancreatitis is sudden, severe, steady epigastric pain. The pain is worse when the patient is lying supine or when walking. It may radiate to the right or left side of the back and is made better by sitting, leaning forward with the knees bent. The patient usually complains of nausea and vomits. During a severe attack the patient may appear anxious and sweaty. The patient may also have abdominal distention, decreased bowel sounds, and rigidity. In 3 to 6 days Turner's sign (ecchymosis in the flanks) and Cullen's sign (bruising around the umbilicus) may appear as a result of retroperitoneal bleeding.

Circulating pancreatic enzymes can cause pleural effusions, atelectasis, or pulmonary edema in a small number of patients. Manifestations of these complications include tachypnea, tachycardia, and hypoxia. In addition, transient hyperglycemia may result from glucagon secretion from damaged cells in the pancreatic islets.

Chronic Pancreatitis

Chronic pancreatitis is an irreversible process of gradual destruction of pancreatic tissue with 50% to 80% of the cases attributed to chronic alcohol use (Fox, 2006). However, less than 10% of alcoholics develop chronic pancreatitis. Additional causes of chronic pancreatitis include cystic fibrosis, a genetic mutation in the cystic fibrosis transmembrane conductance regulator gene, and an autosomal dominant trait with high penetrance (Fox, 2006). Obesity, type II diabetes mellitus, and insulin resistance are also associated with chronic pancreatitis (Fox, 2006). Approximately 10% of cases of chronic pancreatitis have no identifiable cause.

Pathophysiology

The pathogenesis of chronic pancreatitis from alcohol ingestion is believed to cause the secretion of insoluble pancreatic proteins that go on to calcify and obstruct the pancreatic duct. As the pancreatic ducts become blocked, inflammation and fibrosis occur, destroying the function of the pancreatic tissue. The resulting pancreatic insufficiency leads to malabsorption and diabetes mellitus may also develop. Other theories as to the pathogenesis of chronic pancreatitis include embryonic defects, resulting in a relative obstruction of pancreatic flow, or trauma causing inflammation in the ductal epithelium, triggering the characteristic inflammatory changes (Fox, 2006).

Clinical Manifestations

The predominant manifestation of chronic pancreatitis is recurrent epigastric and left upper quadrant pain that may be referred to the left lumbar region. Other common symptoms may include anorexia, nausea, vomiting, weight loss, flatulence, and constipation. The pain in chronic pancreatitis is less severe than in the acute disease. The abdomen is usually tender with mild muscle guarding over the pancreas. The attacks initially last from several hours to 2 weeks, but generally become almost continuous as the disease progresses. A late manifestation is **steatorrhea**, which is bulky, fatty, and foul stools from the lack of pancreatic lipase.

Diagnostic Tests for Acute Pancreatitis

The diagnosis of acute pancreatitis is based on a complete history and physical exam, and elevated levels of serum amylase and lipase, and urine amylase. Other tests, such as serum bilirubin and serum alkaline phosphatase, indicate obstruction of the common bile duct, which can result from stones or edema, resulting in acute pancreatitis. An elevated ALT (>80 units/L) in patients with symptoms of acute pancreatitis indicates a biliary pancreatitis.

- Serum amylase increases just hours after the onset of the disease to levels two to three times normal. It will return to normal (25 to 125 units/L) within 3 to 4 days, or sooner in mild cases.
- Serum lipase levels rise rapidly, remain elevated up to 14 days, and then return to normal (<200 units/L).
- Serum alkaline phosphatase will be elevated if there is compression or obstruction of the common bile duct causing the acute pancreatitis. Normal values are 30 to 90 units/L.
- Serum bilirubin will also be elevated in cases of compression or obstruction of the common duct.
- Serum calcium levels may be decreased because of saponification, and this correlates with the severity of the disease. Levels below 7 mg/dL are associated with a poor prognosis (Friedman, 2004).
- C-reactive protein (CRP) elevations after 48 hours indicate the possibility of pancreatic necrosis (Friedman, 2004).
- White blood cell elevation (leukocytosis) is usually present in acute pancreatitis and indicates inflammation.

Imaging tests are ordered for the patient with acute pancreatitis. An abdominal x-ray may show signs of acute pancreatitis such as gallstones, a segment of small intestine in the left upper quadrant that is filled with air, or a gas-filled segment of transverse colon that ends at the area of pancreatic inflammation (Friedman, 2004). A CT scan is ordered after 3 days in order to identify necrotizing pancreatitis. A fluid collection in the pancreas seen on CT scan is an ominous sign and is associated with an increased mortality rate.

Laboratory and Diagnostic Procedures for Chronic Pancreatitis

Laboratory values for patients with chronic pancreatitis are usually similar to those of acute pancreatitis; however, the amylase and lipase may be normal. Most patients with chronic pancreatitis (80%) will develop diabetes after having the disease for 25 years and have elevated blood sugar levels and glycosuria. Stool samples usually show an elevation in fecal fat content as a result of pancreatic insufficiency.

The most sensitive test for chronic pancreatitis is the endoscopic retrograde cholangiopancreatography (ERCP), an imaging test to locate the cause of a biliary obstruction. Contrast media is injected into the duodenal papilla, and the biliary and pancreatic ducts are viewed. It will show dilated ducts, intraductal stones, strictures, or pseudocysts. Newer tests such as **magnetic resonance cholangiopancreatography (MRCP)**, a noninvasive imaging test, and endoscopic ultrasonography with tissue sampling are becoming more common and may replace the ERCP (Swaroop, Chari, & Clain, 2004).

Medical Management of Acute Pancreatitis

Treatment of acute pancreatitis involves resting the pancreas. This includes keeping the patient NPO (nothing by mouth), so a nasogastric tube frequently is inserted and connected to low intermittent suction. This keeps normal secretions from stimulating the pancreas to release digestive enzymes, therefore causing pain. Bed rest may be ordered until the acute phase has subsided. When the patient is free from pain and bowel sounds have returned, a diet of clear liquids is usually ordered. The diet is then advanced slowly to low fat. In severe cases, particularly necrotizing pancreatitis, large amounts of intravenous fluids may be required to maintain the patient's fluid volume. This may require the patient to be transferred to the intensive care unit.

Medications

Pain relief is of primary importance and is usually achieved with narcotic analgesics. Meperidine or morphine sulfate may be ordered every 3 to 4 hours. Antibiotics such as Imipenem or cefuroxime may be prescribed if there is evidence of infection, or in the case of pancreatic necrosis, to prevent infection. In the patient with severe pancreatitis who has been NPO for 7 to 10 days, total parenteral nutrition may be needed to maintain adequate nutritional status. Patients that are hypocalcemic will be given calcium gluconate intravenously to prevent tetany. The Pharmacology Summary feature later in the chapter (p. 1457) outlines medications used to treat biliary disorders.

Surgery

Surgery to debride the pancreas and surrounding tissue is indicated for patients that have infected necrotizing pancreatitis. This process may improve survival for those with multiorgan failure if the pancreatitis does not respond to other treatment within 4 to 6 weeks. If pancreatic abscesses develop, then the patient may require a percutaneous or open surgical drainage. Occasionally, patients with acute pancreatitis develop pseudocysts, which require drainage if persistent pain develops or if there is ductal obstruction.

Medical Management of Chronic Pancreatitis

Patients with chronic pancreatitis require lifelong changes in their lifestyle. Abstinence from alcohol is mandatory because it often will precipitate an acute attack. A low-fat diet should be maintained because of the lack of the pancreatic enzyme lipase, which is responsible for fat synthesis. During an acute exacerbation of chronic pancreatitis, the patient will be treated in much the same way as a patient with acute pancreatitis.

Medications

Although pain is a major manifestation of chronic pancreatitis, narcotic analgesia is avoided when possible because opioid addiction is common in these patients. These patients will require nutritional supplementation with pancreatic enzymes (Chart 46–9). If steatorrhea becomes a major problem, a dietary supplement with a high concentration of lipase will be prescribed. The supplements should be taken with meals. If the medication is not enteric coated, then an H$_2$-receptor antagonist such as ranitidine or a proton pump inhibitor such as omeprazole is given once or twice a day.

Surgery

Surgical intervention may be needed in patients with chronic pancreatitis to eradicate biliary tract disease, make sure that bile can freely flow into the duodenum, or eliminate obstruction of the pancreatic duct (Friedman, 2004). Pancreatic pseudocysts may need to be drained if they are over 6 centimeters in diameter. Surgery may also be attempted to try and relieve pain.

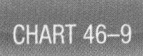

CHART 46–9 **Pancreatic Enzyme Supplement Preparations**

Pancreatic enzymes are purified from pig pancreases.

- Actions:
  - Contains protease, lipase, and amylase
  - Digests proteins, fats, and carbohydrates
- Contraindications:
  - Allergy to pork protein
  - Jews keeping kosher
  - Vegetarians

CONVENTIONAL PREPARATIONS

Viokase

Ilozyme

Cotazym

ENTERIC-COATED PREPARATIONS

Creon

Pancrease

Cotazym-S

Ultrase

■ Nursing Management

The major focus of nursing care for the patient with pancreatitis is pain control, nutrition, and health teaching about alcohol abstinence.

Assessment

Subjective data for both acute and chronic pancreatitis should include a history of the present condition including a comprehensive assessment of the pain and associated symptoms. A social history can give clues to alcohol intake, amount, and duration. For a complete assessment, see the Nursing Process: Patient Care Plan feature for pancreatitis.

Nursing Diagnoses and Interventions

The Nursing Process: Patient Care Plan feature also outlines the nursing diagnoses and interventions for the patient with pancreatitis. The National Guidelines box (p. 1457) presents the practice guidelines for acute pancreatitis.

Health Promotion

Because most cases of pancreatitis are related to alcohol abuse, the focus of prevention is on abstinence from alcohol. After diagnosis, it is essential that patients with pancreatitis abstain from alcohol to prevent future painful episodes. Referral to Alcoholics Anonymous or other treatment programs is recommended.

■ Cancer of the Pancreas

Cancer of the pancreas is the fourth leading cause of cancer death overall. It is estimated that in 2008, 37,680 patients in the United States will be diagnosed with pancreatic cancer and

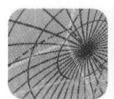

NURSING PROCESS: Patient Care Plan for Pancreatitis

Assessment of Pain

Subjective Data:

What is your level of pain on a scale of 0–10, with 10 being the worst pain?
Are you allergic to anything?
Do you have any special cultural or religious practices for dealing with pain?
Describe the character of your pain? Burning? Steady? Radiate?
Is your pain worse when you are lying down?
Do you have pain when you eat?
Does vomiting relieve the pain?
Have you ever had this type of pain before? If yes, how long did it last? What relieved the pain in the past?
Do you have a history of gallbladder disease?
Do you drink alcohol? How much? How often?

Objective Data:

General appearance:
- Looks distressed
- Sits with knees pulled toward chest
- Restlessness
- Grimacing
- Moaning or groaning
- Clenched fists

Pulse—tachycardia
Shallow rapid respirations
Abdominal tenderness or guarding
Flank or periumbilical ecchymosis
Diaphoresis

Nursing Assessment and Diagnoses	Outcomes and Evaluation Parameters	Planning and Interventions with *Rationales*
Nursing Diagnosis: *Pain: Acute* related to pancreatitis	**Outcome:** Comfort level maintained. **Evaluation Parameters:** Able to communicate level of pain and relief from medications. Appears restful without restlessness or moaning.	**Interventions and *Rationales:*** Assess pain using pain scale (0–10) to quantify pain level. *To increase consistency in monitoring pain.* Administer pain medication, usually meperidine or morphine, and assess level of pain 30 minutes and 1 hour after giving medication. Notify health care provider if pain is unrelieved. *To assess effectiveness of medications.* Explore cultural and religious practices and beliefs about pain and illness. *Different religions have varying beliefs about pain, suffering, and disease.* Teach nonpharmacologic methods of pain control, such as guided imagery, meditation, and breathing exercises. *This may augment pain relief.* Maintain a quiet, darkened, comfortable environment. *This can help decrease physical and mental stimulation, which can lead to decreased pancreatic secretions and less pain.* Maintain bed rest and position the patient in a sitting position *to decrease the pain caused by stretched abdominal muscles that are irritated by inflammation.* Close the patient's door during mealtime *because the smell of food can stimulate pancreatic secretions.* Place a nasogastric tube if ordered, and/or monitor drainage and relief of pain. *This helps to "rest" the pancreas and removes secretions that can stimulate the pancreas to produce enzymes.*

Assessment of Nutrition

Subjective Data:

Are you nauseated?
Have you vomited?
Have you noticed any weight loss?

Objective Data:

Height and weight measurements
BMI
Abdominal examination:
- Diminished or absent bowel sounds

Laboratory results:
- Serum albumin
- Glucose
- Transferrin
- Hemoglobin and hematocrit (H & H)

(continued)

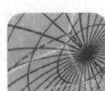

NURSING PROCESS: Patient Care Plan for Pancreatitis—*Continued*

Nursing Assessment and Diagnoses	Outcomes and Evaluation Parameters	Planning and Interventions with *Rationales*
Nursing Diagnosis: *Nutrition, Imbalanced: Less than Body Requirements* related to nausea, vomiting, pain, and possible lack of pancreatic enzymes for digestion	**Outcome:** Adequate nutrition. ***Evaluation Parameters:*** No weight loss. Serum albumin normal. Fasting glucose normal. Hemoglobin and hematocrit normal. No reported nausea.	**Interventions and *Rationales:*** Weigh daily on same scale at the same time. *Fluctuations in weight from day to day are an indicator of fluid balance, but changes over a week reflect nutritional status.* Assess laboratory results and report any abnormal values to the patient's health care provider. *The pancreas produces enzymes that aid in the digestion of protein, fat, and carbohydrates. Protein malnutrition is reflected in a low serum albumin. Transferrin is a protein that transports iron, so this level may be low. The H & H may be decreased in cases of malnutrition. Serum glucose may be elevated if the pancreatitis affects the endocrine function of the gland.* Monitor the frequency, color, consistency, and odor of stools. *Lack of lipase from the pancreas results in poor fat digestion and steatorrhea results. The presence of steatorrhea indicates severe pancreatitis with impaired pancreatic function.* Provide oral hygiene at least every 2 hours while the nasogastric tube is in place *to decrease discomfort and maintain the integrity of the oral and nasal mucosa.* Offer small, frequent meals, beginning with clear liquids once bowel sounds return and pain is relieved. *Smaller meals reduce the secretion of pancreatic enzymes.*

Assessment of Fluid and Electrolyte Status

Subjective Data:
Do you feel dizzy or light-headed?

Objective Data:

Cardiac status:
- Rhythm
- Pulmonary artery pressure
- Peripheral pulses
- Capillary refill

Vital signs:
- BP
- Pulse
- Respirations

Renal function:
- Hourly urine output
- Daily body weight

Neurological function:
- Mental status
- Level of consciousness
- Behavior

Laboratory values:
- Electrolytes
- Hematocrit
- BUN and creatinine

Nursing Assessment and Diagnoses	Outcomes and Evaluation Parameters	Planning and Interventions with *Rationales*
Nursing Diagnoses: *Fluid Volume Deficit* related to vascular leak syndrome resulting from inflammation, and fluid accumulation in the abdominal cavity. Potential for electrolyte imbalance related to nasogastric suction	**Outcomes:** Adequate fluid volume and electrolyte balance. ***Evaluation Parameters:*** Normal blood pressure with no orthostatic changes. Normal sinus rhythm. Stable daily weight with moist mucous membranes. Pulmonary artery pressure 8–12 mmHg. Cardiac output at least 5 L/min. Brisk capillary refill. Good peripheral pulses. Urine output 30 mL/hr. Alert and oriented.	**Interventions and *Rationales:*** Evaluate cardiac status: heart rate and rhythm at least every 4 hours; orthostatic blood pressure, pulmonary artery pressure usually every 4 hours as indicated; peripheral pulses; capillary refill; skin color. *These assessments help establish fluid volume. The body compensates for diminished volume by increasing the heart rate to maintain cardiac output. Capillaries constrict to force more fluid into the general circulation and the signs are weak peripheral pulses and pale skin color. A decreased cardiac output means a decrease in the renal perfusion and decreased urine output and possibly early prerenal renal failure.* Monitor renal function by measuring urine output every hour and notifying the health care provider if the level is less than 30 mL/hr. Daily body weight *is an indicator of fluid status.* Monitor neurological function by assessing level of consciousness and behavior. *Cerebral perfusion may be diminished if there is a fluid volume deficit and the cardiac output is low. Electrolytes, particularly sodium, can cause confusion when the levels are low.* Monitor laboratory values for electrolyte status and renal function. *Electrolytes are lost in nasogastric suction or vomiting. The BUN and creatinine will rise if renal function is compromised.*

NATIONAL GUIDELINES for Acute Pancreatitis

Priorities of Care	Guideline
Supportive care	The nurse should anticipate the need for supportive care with particular attention to the assessment and prevention of hypoxemia and the need to ensure adequate fluid balance. Nursing interventions would include: • Frequent assessment of vital signs. • Frequent assessment of bedside oxygen saturation. • Accurate assessment of fluid status (strict I&O). • Administration of supplemental oxygen therapy, particularly when narcotic agents are being used for pain control. • Aggressive IV fluid therapy is critical to counteract hypovolemia caused by third space losses, vomiting, diaphoresis, and an increased vascular permeability secondary to the presence of inflammatory mediators. • The nurse should also monitor serum laboratory values for signs of inadequate fluid balance and hemoconcentration.
Level of nursing care	A patient with acute pancreatitis who develops organ failure or severe pancreatitis should be transferred to an intensive care or step-down unit to accommodate the evolving high acuity needs. Common indicators of organ failure or increased severity include: • Sustained hypoxemia • Hypotension refractory to IV therapy • Signs of renal insufficiency (such as a serum creatinine > 2 mg/dL) • Hemoconcentration in an elderly client with a history of cardiovascular disease who requires aggressive fluid resuscitation. Additional danger signals that warrant increased evaluation, but may not necessitate transfer to a high acuity bed, include: • Obesity (BMI > 30) • Oliguria (urine output < 50 mL/hr) • Tachycardia with pulse ≥ 120 beats/min • Encephalopathy • Increased need for narcotic analgesics.
Nutritional support	When pancreatitis is mild, oral intake is typically restored in 3 to 7 days, thus negating the need for nutritional support. However, during more prolonged periods of inadequate nutritional intake, enteral feedings are preferred over total parenteral nutrition (TPN). Enteral nutrition, administered into the distal jejunum, avoids the stimulation of pancreatic secretions and does not exacerbate the disease. In general, enteral feedings have been found to be safer and less expensive than TPN.

Source: Banks, P. A., & Freeman, M. L. (2006). Practice guidelines in acute pancreatitis. *American Journal of Gastroenterology, 101*(10), 2379–2400.

PHARMACOLOGY Summary of Medications Used to Treat Biliary Disorders

Medication Category	Action	Application/Indication	Nursing Responsiblity
Gallstone-Solubilizing Agents			
Ursodiol (Actigall) Chenodiol (Chenix)	Dissolves gallstones by reducing the cholesterol content of the stone or blocking cholesterol production.	Prevention, dissolution of noncalcified cholesterol gallstones, primary biliary cirrhosis.	Monitor for adverse effects: nausea, vomiting, and dyspepsia. Be aware of drugs that reduce efficacy: bile acid sequestrants, aluminum antacids, estrogens, some lipid lowering agents.
Bile Acid Sequestrants			
Cholestyramine (Questran, LoCholest) Colestipol (Colestid)	Decreases pruritus by decreasing circulation bile acids and decreasing bile acid deposits in skin tissue.	Relief of pruritus secondary to partial biliary stasis.	Monitor for adverse effects: constipation, abdominal pain, nausea, vomiting, indigestion, and headache. Be aware long-term use may require supplementation of fat soluble vitamins. Give 1 hour after or 4–6 hours before other drugs.

34,290 will die from the disease (American Cancer Society, 2008). Risk factors include obesity, chronic pancreatitis, family history of pancreatic cancer, history of abdominal radiation, and cigarette smoking. In fact, smokers have twice the incidence of pancreatic cancer as nonsmokers. There is some evidence that a high-fat diet and diabetes mellitus increase the risk as well, particularly in women. The risk of developing pancreatic cancer increases with age.

Pathophysiology

Most pancreatic cancer is ductal adenocarcinoma that develops from the exocrine cells in the ducts. Rarely, cancer develops in the endocrine cells, and these types of tumors, which are always fatal, are called **apudomas**. Ductal adenocarcinoma begins in the ducts, slowly invades the glandular tissue, and then extends into the surrounding tissue. Roughly 75% of these cancers arise in the head of the pancreas, although they can occur anywhere in the pancreas. When the tumor arises in the head of the pancreas, it usually causes obstruction of the common bile duct early in the course of the disease with resultant jaundice. Survival is longer in these patients, probably because they seek treatment earlier than those with cancer in the body or tail of the pancreas. Because of the vascular structure of the area, cancer cells infiltrate the portal vein, mesenteric artery, vena cava, and aorta, with metastasis to the liver (Huether, 2006).

Clinical Manifestations

Most cases of pancreatic cancer are asymptomatic until the tumor invades surrounding tissue or obstructs the common bile duct. Jaundice may be the first sign. In about 70% of cases, patients recall vague, diffuse epigastric pain that did not cause them alarm. Once jaundice occurs, stools become light in color and the urine becomes dark. Pruritus results from the bilirubin in the skin. The blockage of pancreatic enzymes into the duodenum results in problems of fat and protein digestion and absorption, so the patient may exhibit weight loss, steatorrhea, and malnutrition.

Laboratory and Diagnostic Procedures

Diagnosis of pancreatic cancer is done by history and physical examination. When there is a suspicion of pancreatic cancer, a dual-phase spiral CT or an MRI is done to detect the tumor. The dual-phase method detects 80% of tumors. The next step is to perform a percutaneous needle aspiration to get samples of the tissue for cytologic study (Friedman, 2004). If the CT or MRI is inconclusive, an ERCP may be done to identify any neoplasm. In

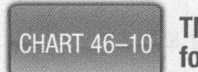

CHART 46–10 **TNM Classification for Pancreatic Cancer**

Tis: Carcinoma in situ.

T1: Tumor is limited to the pancreas and is less than 2 centimeters in size.

T2: Tumor is larger than 2 centimeters but limited to the pancreas.

T3: Tumor spread beyond the pancreas but no involvement of the celiac axis or superior mesenteric artery.

T4: Tumor invasion of the celiac axis or superior mesenteric artery.

about 30% of patients, a laparotomy is performed to establish a definitive diagnosis and determine the extent of the disease. Tumor staging is done based on the TNM system of classification. Chart 46–10 outlines the TNM staging for pancreatic cancer.

Medical Management

Treatment of pancreatic cancer is varied, ranging from surgical intervention to palliation. If the tumor is limited to the head of the pancreas and there is no lymph node involvement or metastasis, then radical **pancreaticoduodenal (Whipple) resection** is done. This procedure has a 5-year survival rate of 20% to 25%. The Whipple procedure involves removal of the head of the pancreas, the duodenum, a distal portion of the stomach, a part of the jejunum, and the lower half of the common bile duct. Unfortunately, most pancreatic cancer is too advanced when first diagnosed for the Whipple procedure to be effective. Radiation and chemotherapy may be used after surgery to enhance recovery efforts or for palliation in patients with unresectable cancer.

Patients with pancreatic cancer require nursing care that focuses on palliation, comfort, and support. Chapter 64 presents the care of patients with cancer, and Chapter 45 discusses the care of patients with gastrointestinal surgery.

Research

Research is necessary for improvement in the care of patients with liver, gallbladder, and pancreatic disorders. The goal of research is to identify areas in practice where innovations can impact the patient's health and well-being, and then to develop and test interventions that address the identified problems. The Research Topics Related to Patients with Liver, Gallbladder, or Pancreatic Disorders feature presents a list of research opportunities related to these disorders.

RESEARCH TOPICS RELATED TO PATIENTS WITH LIVER, GALLBLADDER, OR PANCREATIC DISORDERS

Research	Clinical Impact
Physiological Research	
Vaccine for hepatitis C.	Development of a vaccine would decrease the number of people with chronic hepatitis C and possible liver failure.
Drugs to treat hepatitis C genotype most common in the United States.	Effective drug treatment can help decrease the spread of hepatitis C and improve morbidity and mortality.
Drugs to reverse hepatic encephalopathy.	
Effective treatments for hepatorenal syndrome.	Medications or other treatments would decrease the complications of cirrhosis, thereby improving the quality of life and longevity of patients with cirrhosis.
Drugs to prevent esophageal varices.	
Herbal preparations to boost liver function in patients with a compromised liver.	Patient comfort is enhanced with less dependence on narcotics.
The management of pain in patients with pancreatitis.	
Use of acupuncture as an adjunct to pain management in pancreatitis.	

Emotional and Psychological Research	Clinical Impact
Living With the Uncertainty of Chronic Hepatitis C	
Music therapy to reduce anxiety before, during, and after painful procedures such as paracentesis, ERCP, and surgical intervention.	Nurses can help patients cope with an uncertain future and increase patient well-being.
Quality of life after liver transplant.	The goal is to improve psychological interventions to improve coping.
	Understanding the issues after liver transplant can help nurses plan interventions for patients to maximize their recovery.

Clinical Preparation

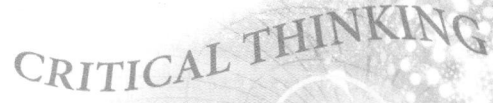
CRITICAL THINKING

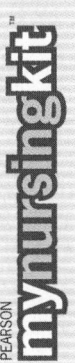
PEARSON mynursingkit™

Read

- History of Current Illness
- Past Medical History
- Physical Exam
- Admitting Medical Orders
- Laboratory Study Results

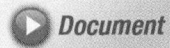
Document

- Summary of Hospitalization
- Pathophysiology Form
- Laboratory Values
- Laboratory Results Explanation

Apply

- List of Potential Nursing Diagnoses
- Concept Map
- Critical Thinking Questions

Log on to MyNursingKit.com to download forms you will need and to complete further steps in the Clinical Preparation assignment.

HISTORY OF PRESENT ILLNESS

As the nurse on a medical–surgical floor in a community hospital, you receive report about Mr. M., a 60-year-old construction worker who was admitted 2 days ago with a diagnosis of cirrhosis of the liver.

Medical–Surgical History

According to his wife, Mr. M.'s past medical history includes hepatitis A infection as a young man. He has no history of any other diseases. He has had a "beer belly" for at least 20 years, but his wife notices that it has been getting larger during the last week.

Social History

Mr. M. drinks 6 to 10 beers each night after work and greater amounts on the weekends. He has smoked three packs of cigarettes a day for the last 30 years. He does not take any prescription medications, but uses Tylenol occasionally for headache.

Physical Exam

In report the nurse leaving states that Mr. M. is confused and restless in bed. His vital signs are temperature of 37°C; pulse of 120 beats per minute; respirations 26 and labored; blood pressure of

140/76. She states that he is slightly jaundiced and diaphoretic. His lungs are clear to auscultation, and gynecomastia is noted on the chest exam. His heart sounds indicate a regular rhythm, tachycardia, with no murmurs or gallops.

Mr. M.'s abdomen is large and distended with hypoactive bowel sounds. It is tender to palpation with a positive fluid wave. His spleen is enlarged. His abdominal girth is 56 inches and his stool tests positive for blood. He is confused and oriented to person only. The nurse reports that he has asterixis and hyperactive reflexes.

Admitting Medical Orders

Service: medicine
Diagnosis: cirrhosis of the liver
Allergies: none known
Vital signs q4h including oxygen saturation
Neurological checks q4h
Abdominal girth q shift
I&O q shift
Daily weight
Activity: bed rest
DVT prophylaxis: sequential compression device to lower extremities

Incentive spirometer: q1h while awake
Diet: sodium restriction: 2 g/day; fluid restriction: 1,500 mL/day; high-calorie, low-protein, 20 g/day diet
Call house officer: temp > 38.5°C, HR > 110 or < 60, RR > 30 or < 12, BP sys > 160 or < 90, O_2 sat < 92%, urine output < 120 mL in 4 hours, change in neurological or abdominal exam, any Hct result that is 5 less than the baseline ED Hct
IV: D5NS IV at 10 mL/hr

Scheduled Medications

Multivitamin 1 po daily
Lactulose 30 mL po qid × 3 days then bid
Spironolactone (Aldactone) 100 mg po daily
Lasix 40 mg po daily
Oxazepam (Serax) 10 mg po tid

Ordered Laboratory Studies

Hgb and Hct
Electrolyte panel
Liver function tests
Serum ammonia qam
Chart and test stool for occult blood

LABORATORY STUDY RESULTS

Test	Admission	Day 1	Day 2
Hemoglobin (Hgb)	12.5 g/dL	12.0 g/dL	11.8 g/dL
Hematocrit (Hct)	38%	36%	34%
Bilirubin—total	1.5 mg/dL	1.5 mg/dL	1.5 mg/dL
• Direct	0.6 mg/dL	0.6 mg/dL	0.6 mg/dL
• Indirect	0.9 mg/dL	0.9 mg/dL	0.9 mg/dL
AST	400 unit/L	386 unit/L	352 unit/L
ALT	150 unit/L	149 unit/L	147 unit/L
Alkaline phosphatase	150 unit/L	144 unit/L	144 unit/L
Electrolytes:			
• Sodium	138 mEq/L	140 mEq/L	141 mEq/L
• Potassium	3.5 mEq/L	3.4 mEq/L	3.5 mEq/L
• Calcium	8.6 mg/dL	8.8 mg/dL	8.8 mg/dL
Serum ammonia	50 µ/dL	58 µ/dL	46 µ/dL
Serum albumin	3.0 g/dL	3.2 g/dL	3.0 g/dL

CRITICAL THINKING QUESTIONS

1. What signs and symptoms of hepatic encephalopathy is Mr. M. manifesting?

2. Describe the pathophysiology of cirrhosis and how it relates to each of his clinical manifestations.

3. Why is Mr. M. on a low-protein diet?

4. Why is lactulose given to Mr. M.?

Answers to Critical Thinking Questions appear in Appendix D.

NCLEX® REVIEW

1. A patient is being evaluated for hepatitis C infection. Which question will best assist the nurse in identifying if exposure has occurred?
   1. "Have you traveled outside the country recently?"
   2. "Do you eat a lot of uncooked shellfish?"
   3. "Have you ever had a tattoo?"
   4. "Do you share eating utensils with anyone infected with hepatitis A?"

2. During the prodromal phase of hepatitis the nurse expects to assess which of the following symptoms in the patient:
   1. Hypothermia.
   2. Increased appetite.
   3. Dark colored urine.
   4. Constant epigastric pain.

3. The nurse identifies a patient with cirrhosis of the liver with an albumin level of 2.5 gm/dL is at risk for the development of:
   1. Peripheral edema.
   2. Prolonged blood coagulation.
   3. Jaundice of the skin.
   4. Vitamin A malabsorption.

4. A patient with cirrhosis develops hepatic encephalopathy and is extremely confused and agitated. The nurse places priorty on administering which ordered medication?
   1. Lactulose, Chronulac
   2. Oxazepam, Serax
   3. Propanolzole, Protonix
   4. Phytonadione, Vitamin K

5. A patient diagnosed with liver cancer three months ago has elevated alpha-fetoprotein levels, AFP. The nurse should incorporate which of the following interventions into the plan of care.
   1. Provide supportive and comfort measures to the patient and family.
   2. Explain how the transhepatic portosystemic shunt, TIPS will relieve symptoms.
   3. Prepare the patient and family for the likelihood of a liver transplant.
   4. Restrict dietary proteins and foods high in sodium.

6. The nurse identifies the following factor would have increased the risk to develop stones in a patient diagnosed with cholelithiasis.
   1. The patient consumes a high fiber diet.
   2. The patient recently was treated with aminoglycosides for a urinary tract infection.
   3. The patient has had rapid weight loss secondary to crash dieting.
   4. The patient is of northern European descent.

7. A patient who had a cholecystectomy 2 days ago complains of abdominal pain which is unrelieved by the opioid analgesic given one hour ago. Which action should be taken initially by the nurse?
   1. Administer a second dose of analgesia.
   2. Encourage the patient to ambulate in order to expel flatus.
   3. Examine abdomen for rigidity and tenderness.
   4. Position patient in a side lying fetal position.

8. A patient admitted with complaints of mid epigastric and abdominal pain is being evaluated for pancreatitis. The nurse recognizes which finding would support a diagnosis of chronic pancreatitis rather than acute pancreatitis?
   1. Stools are clay colored.
   2. Amylase level is normal.
   3. Blood sugar is within normal limits.
   4. Abdomen is tender to palpation.

9. A patient who is experiencing jaundice has just been diagnosed with pancreatic cancer. The nurse anticipates the patient will display which other symptoms?
   1. Pale dilute urine
   2. Clay colored stools
   3. Weight gain
   4. Easy bruising

10. When providing discharge instructions for a patient recovering from chronic pancreatitis, the nurse should plan to include which instructions?
    1. Avoid using all over-the-counter analgesics.
    2. Eat a diet low in fat.
    3. Limit alcohol drinks to one a day.
    4. Avoid sharing any eating utensils.

Answers for review questions appear in Appendix D.

KEY TERMS

alanine aminotransferase (ALT) *p.1430*
alkaline phosphatase (ALP) *p.1430*
alpha-amylase *p.1427*
apudomas *p.1458*
aspartate aminotransferase (AST) *p.1430*
asterixis *p.1436*
bile *p.1427*
bile canaliculi *p.1429*
biliary dyskinesia *p.1449*
bilirubin *p.1430*
caput medusae *p.1441*
carboxypeptidase *p.1427*
cholangiocarcinoma *p.1444*
cholecystectomy *p.1449*
cholecystitis *p.1448*
cholecystokinin *p.1427*
choledocholithiasis *p.1447*
cholelithiasis *p.1447*
chymotrypsin *p.1427*

cirrhosis *p.1434*
convalescent phase *p.1430*
esophageal varices *p.1436*
exocrine pancreas *p.1427*
gamma-glutamyltransferase (GGT) *p.1430*
gluconeogenesis *p.1436*
hepatic encephalopathy *p.1436*
hepatitis A virus (HAV) *p.1428*
hepatitis B virus (HBV) *p.1429*
hepatitis C virus (HCV) *p.1429*
hepatitis D virus (HDV) *p.1429*
hepatitis E virus (HEV) *p.1429*
hepatocellular *p.1427*
hepatorenal syndrome *p.1436*
hypoalbuminemia *p.1436*
icteric phase *p.1430*
Kupffer cells *p.1429*
lactic dehydrogenase (LDH) *p.1430*
lipase *p.1427*

magnetic resonance
   cholangiopancreatography
   (MRCP) *p.1453*
melena *p.1436*
pancreaticoduodenal (Whipple)
   resection *p.1458*
pancreatitis *p.1450*
paracentesis *p.1440*
portal hypertension *p.1436*
primary biliary cirrhosis *p.1441*
prodromal phase *p.1430*
sclerosing cholangitis *p.1441*
sclerotherapy *p.1441*
serum immunoglobulin G (IgG) *p.1429*
serum immunoglobulin M (IgM) *p.1429*
steatorrhea *p.1453*
trypsin *p.1427*
viral hepatitis *p.1427*

PEARSON
EXPLORE mynursingkit™

MyNursingKit is your one stop for online chapter review materials and resources. Prepare for success with additional NCLEX®-style practice questions, interactive assignments and activities, web links, animations and videos, and more!

Register your access code from the front of your book at
www.mynursingkit.com

REFERENCES

Afdhal, N. H. (2007). *Epidemiology of and risk factors for gallstones.* Retrieved April 24, 2008, from http://www.uptodate.com/patients/content/topic.do?topicKey=~5rphinkcGz/zys

American Cancer Society. (2008). *Pancreatic cancer.* Retrieved August 9, 2008, from http://www.cancer.org/docroot/CRI/content/CRI_2_4_1X_What_are_the_key_statistics_for_pancreatic_cancer_34.asp?rnav=cri

Askey, B. D. (2006). Managing cirrhosis in a primary-care setting. *The Clinical Advisor, 9*(12), 22–28.

Baldwin, P. D. (2003). Chemical hepatitis. *Clinical Journal of Oncology Nursing, 7*(1), 99–103.

Centers for Disease Control and Prevention (CDC). (2008). *Viral hepatitis.* Retrieved August 9, 2008, from http://www.cdc.gov/hepatitis/

Chisholm-Burns, M. A., Wells, B. G., Schwinghammer, T. L., Malone, P. M., Kolesar, J. M., Rotschafer, J. C., et al. (2008). *Pharmacotherapy principles & practice.* New York: McGraw-Hill.

Deutsch, K. F. (2003, May). Hepatitis C: The silent epidemic. *The Clinical Advisor,* 10–18.

Fox, K. M. (2006). Chronic pancreatitis. *Clinician Reviews, 16*(6), 46–52.

Friedman, L. S. (2004). Liver, biliary tract, and pancreas. In L. M. Tierney, S. J. McPhee, & M. A. Papadakis, *Current medical diagnosis & treatment* (pp. 623–668). New York: Lange Medical Books/McGraw-Hill.

Holloway, M., & D'Acunto, K. (2006). An update on the ABCs of viral hepatitis. *The Clinical Advisor, 9*(6), 26–37.

Huether, S. E. (2006). Alterations of digestive function. In K. L. McCance & S. E. Huether, *Pathophysiology: The biologic basis for disease in adults and children* (5th ed., pp. 1385–1445). Philadelphia: Mosby.

Kee, J. L. (2002). *Laboratory and diagnostic tests with nursing implications* (6th ed.). Upper Saddle River, NJ: Prentice Hall.

Lutz, C., & Przytulski, K. (2006). *Nutrition and diet therapy: Evidence-based applications.* Philadelphia: F. A. Davis.

Pelc, C. E. (2003). Milking it! *Hepatitis, 5*(3), 15–17.

Rhee, C., & Broadbent, A. M. (2007). Palliation and liver failure: Palliative medications dosages guidelines. *Journal of Palliative Medicine, 10*(3), 677–687.

Swaroop, V. S., Chari, S. T., & Clain, J. E. (2004). Severe acute pancreatitis. *JAMA, 291*(23), 2865–2868.

Thomas, D. J. (2007). Abdominal problems. In L. M. Dunphy, J. E. Winland-Brown, B. O. Porter, & D. J. Thomas, *Primary care: The Art and Science of Advanced Practice Nursing* (2nd ed., pp. 473–561). Philadelphia: F. A. Davis.

Wasley, A., Miller, J. T., & Finelli, L. (2007). Surveillance for acute viral hepatitis—United States, 2005. *Morbidity and Mortality Weekly Report, 56*(SS-3), 1–24. Retrieved April 24, 2008, from http://www.cdc.gov/mmwr/preview/mmwrhtml/ss5603a1.htm

Caring for the Patient with Renal and Urinary Disorders

Cheryl Wraa

Outcome-Based Learning Objectives

After studying this chapter, the learner will be able to:

1. Discuss the function of the kidney in relation to regulating fluid, electrolyte, and acid–base balance.
2. List common diagnostic tests used to determine kidney function and related diseases.
3. Identify the major diseases of the kidney.
4. Discuss complications of kidney-related diseases.
5. Recognize the signs and symptoms associated with urinary tract disorders.
6. Compare and contrast the underlying principles of hemodialysis and peritoneal dialysis.

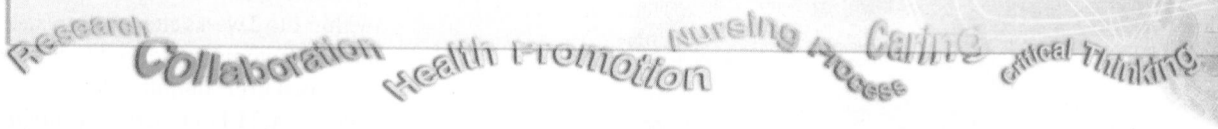

Research Collaboration Health Promotion Nursing Process Caring Critical Thinking

THE KIDNEYS play an important role in maintaining constancy of the internal environment of the body through multiple functions, including:

- Maintaining electrolyte balance, which is a major factor for normal nerve and muscle physiology.
- Helping to regulate acid–base balance through the reabsorption and elimination or conservation of sodium, potassium, hydrogen, chloride, and bicarbonate ions.
- Production of **erythropoietin**, a hormone that stimulates the production of red blood cells in the bone marrow.
- Secretion of **renin** that converts angiotensinogen to angiotensin, which stimulates the release of aldosterone by the adrenal cortex. Aldosterone plays a part in the regulation of sodium and water reabsorption to help elevate blood pressure.
- Activating vitamin D, and regulating calcium and phosphate conservation and elimination, which contribute to the metabolic functions of the skeletal system.
- Regulating the osmolality of the extracellular fluid through action of the antidiuretic hormone (ADH).
- Elimination of metabolic wastes: urea, uric acid, creatinine, and drugs and their metabolites.

Throughout the day the two kidneys process approximately 1,700 liters of blood and combine the waste products to produce approximately 1.5 liters of urine. To put it another way, the kid-

neys filter a person's entire blood volume 60 to 70 times a day (Porth, 2005; Urden, Stacy, & Lough, 2006).

Physiology

To better understand the disease processes, it is important to be familiar with the physiology of the renal system. The **nephron** is the functional unit of the kidney, and each kidney encompasses approximately 1 million nephrons (Urden et al., 2006). Each nephron consists of a **glomerulus**, a compact tuft of capillaries where blood is filtered (Figure 47–1 ■, p. 1464). The glomerulus is encased in a thin double-walled capsule called **Bowman's capsule**. The capillary walls of the glomerulus are very thin, and the blood pressure within them is higher than the pressure in Bowman's capsule; therefore, fluid from the plasma is filtered into the capsule. This fluid is initial urine, and in the healthy nephron, neither red blood cells nor protein should pass through the filter. Nutrients and water are then reabsorbed by the proximal convoluted tubule and taken back into the capillaries that surround the tubules. Two important electrolytes, sodium and chloride, are reabsorbed during this time according to the body's needs. The waste products of protein metabolism, urea, and creatinine, along with substances that are in excess in body fluids, such as hydrogen ions, are secreted into the distal tubules to be excreted. Finally, urine empties into the renal pelvis, moves down the ureters, is stored in the bladder, and then leaves the body through the urethra.

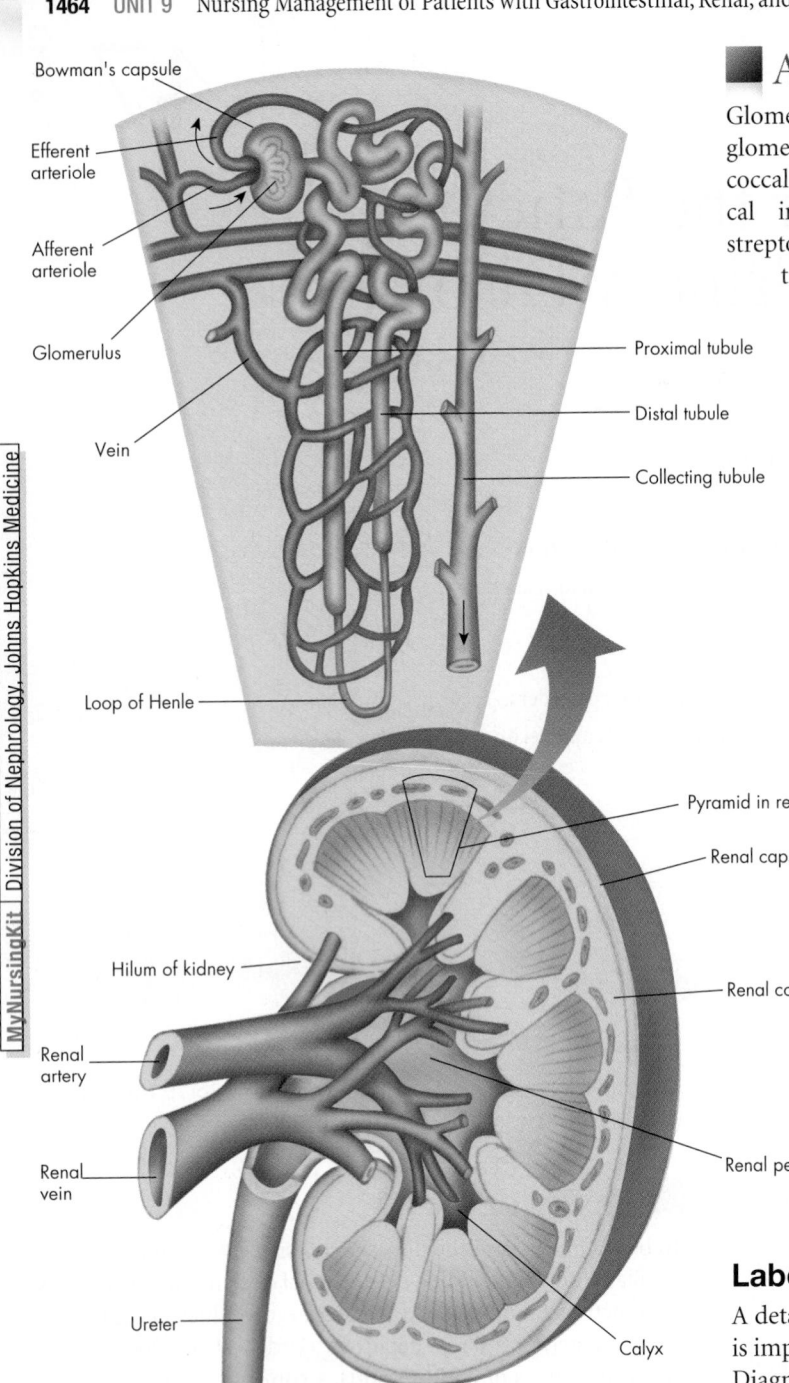

Bowman's capsule
Efferent arteriole
Afferent arteriole
Glomerulus
Vein
Loop of Henle
Proximal tubule
Distal tubule
Collecting tubule

Hilum of kidney
Renal artery
Renal vein
Ureter

Pyramid in renal medulla
Renal capsule
Renal cortex
Renal pelvis
Calyx

FIGURE 47–1 ■ The kidney and nephron.

DISORDERS OF THE KIDNEY

There are multiple diseases of the kidney, all of which cause loss of filtration capacity. Some are rapidly reversible and others cause permanent damage to the kidneys. When approximately two-thirds of filtration capacity is lost, symptoms of renal failure appear, with end-stage renal disease being the loss of approximately seven-eighths of filtration capacity. The goal of care for all the disease processes is to stop the source of damage to the kidneys and preserve what filtration capacity remains (Walser, 2004).

Acute Glomerulonephritis

Glomerulonephritis is a degenerative inflammation of the glomeruli and most commonly results from a previous streptococcal infection, usually of the respiratory tract. The streptococcal infection triggers antibody production against the streptococcal antigen. The antigen–antibody complexes become trapped in the glomeruli, causing an inflammatory response. Other causes can be immunoglobulin A (IgA) nephropathy, thin basement membrane disease, hereditary nephritis (Alport syndrome), lupus, and mesangial proliferative glomerulonephritis (Follin & Lenker, 2004; Post & Rose, 2008c). There is no pus formation associated with glomerulonephritis, nor are any bacteria found. As neutrophils collect in the inflamed loops of the glomeruli, the blood flow to the nephrons is reduced, and less filtration into Bowman's capsule occurs with less urine being formed. The glomeruli begin to degenerate along with the nephron, and the kidney tissue shrinks. The remaining functioning glomeruli become permeable, allowing red blood cells and albumin to appear in the urine. The disease is most common in young males, but can occur at any age (Follin & Lenker, 2004).

Acute glomerulonephritis usually occurs within 1 to 3 weeks after an untreated pharyngitis. Symptoms include mild edema; **oliguria**, decreased urine output of less than 400 milliliters in a 24-hour period; **proteinuria**, the presence of protein in the urine; **azotemia**, an increase in the blood urea nitrogen (BUN) caused when the kidneys are unable to excrete normally; **hematuria**, blood present in the urine; and fatigue.

Laboratory and Diagnostic Procedures

A detailed patient history and assessment of clinical symptoms is important for the diagnosis of acute glomerulonephritis. The Diagnostic Tests box presents tests that are helpful in supporting the diagnosis of acute glomerulonephritis.

Goodpasture's Syndrome

Another cause for acute or rapidly progressive glomerulonephritis is Goodpasture's (anti-GBM antibody) syndrome. In this disorder, circulating antibodies are directed against an antigen intrinsic to the glomerular basement membrane (GBM), resulting in acute glomerulonephritis. It is unknown what stimulus triggers the production of the circulating autoantibodies, and the disease is rare, with an estimated less than one case per million population (Pusey & Kalluri, 2008).

The syndrome presents similarly to other forms of rapidly progressive glomerulonephritis with relatively acute renal failure, urinalysis showing proteinuria, and a nephritic sediment characterized by white cells, dysmorphic red cells, and granular casts. What is different is that 60% to 70% of patients will also pre-

DIAGNOSTIC TESTS for Acute Glomerulonephritis

Test	Expected Abnormality	Rationale for Abnormality
Urinalysis	Presence of protein, red blood cells, white blood cells, and mixed cell casts	Increased permeability of the functioning glomeruli
Serum creatinine	Elevated serum creatinine	Impaired glomerular filtration
Urine creatinine clearance	Decreased	Impaired glomerular filtration
Serum antistreptolysin-O titer	Elevated	Recent streptococcal infection
Throat culture	May show group A beta-hemolytic streptococci	Recent streptococcal infection

sent with pulmonary involvement, usually consisting of alveolar hemorrhage (Pusey & Kalluri, 2008). The patients will complain of shortness of breath, cough, and some will have hemoptysis. Chest radiograph will exhibit pulmonary infiltrates. Goodpasture's syndrome is usually idiopathic, but it can occasionally follow pulmonary infections or be associated with pulmonary injury.

Goodpasture's syndrome should be suspected in any patient with acute glomerulonephritis, especially if the patient also exhibits rapid progression and pulmonary hemorrhage. To diagnose the syndrome, there must be demonstration of anti-GBM antibodies in either the serum or the kidney. Normally a renal biopsy is performed, as it provides information regarding the activity and chronicity of renal involvement.

The medical management of Goodpasture's syndrome is plasmapheresis combined with prednisone and cyclophosphamide (Kaplan, Appel, & Pusey, 2007). The plasmapheresis removes the circulating anti-GBM antibodies and other mediators of inflammation. The immunosuppressive medications minimize new antibody formation. This disorder is typically associated with severe renal injury and, if untreated, progresses quickly to end-stage renal failure.

Alport Syndrome

Alport syndrome, or hereditary nephritis, is a progressive glomerular disease that is genetically heterogeneous with X-linked, autosomal recessive and autosomal dominant variants (see Chapter 11 🔗). The prevalence of the disease is approximately 1 in 50,000 live births (Kashtan, 2007). The disorder occurs from mutations in genes encoding several members of the type IV collagen protein family, the predominant collagenous constituent of basement membranes. The secondary changes in glomerular basement membrane composition that occur due to the mutations predispose to the development of glomerulosclerosis. The histologic changes increase in severity with age.

Patients with Alport syndrome will initially present with asymptomatic microhematuria and episodes of gross hematuria. The plasma creatinine level and blood pressure are normal early in the disease, but hypertension, increasing proteinuria, and renal insufficiency occur with time. End-stage renal disease usually appears in males between age 16 and 35. In females, renal failure may be delayed until age 45 to 60. Patients may also exhibit several extrarenal manifestations including sensorineural hearing loss beginning in the high tones and progressing over time to frequencies in the range of conversational speech; and eye changes such as white or yellow flecking of the perimacular region of the

retina, corneal lesions such as posterior polymorphous dystrophy, and recurrent corneal erosions (Kashtan, 2007).

Diagnosis is usually suspected with a family history of renal failure and deafness. Up to 15% of cases have no family history of renal disease, and the diagnosis is made by renal biopsy with analysis of type IV collagen expression (Kashtan, 2007). There is no specific treatment for Alport syndrome. For patients who develop end-stage renal failure, dialysis or transplantation can be performed, although 3% to 4% of patients develop de novo anti-GBM antibody disease after transplantation (Kashtan, 2007).

Medical Management

The goals of treatment for acute glomerulonephritis are relief of symptoms and prevention of complications. Supportive care includes fluid restrictions, bed rest, dietary sodium restrictions, and correction of electrolyte imbalances. Medical treatment includes diuretics to reduce extracellular fluid and antihypertensives if needed. The Pharmacology Summary feature on page 1490 presents medications used to treat renal disorders.

▮ Nursing Management

Although patient care is primarily supportive, it is important to monitor the patient and watch for signs of acute renal failure. Critical assessments include strict monitoring of intake and output, daily weight, assessment of renal function through serum creatinine, blood urea nitrogen (BUN) levels, and urine creatinine clearance. Consult the dietary department to provide a high-caloric, low-protein, low-sodium, and low-potassium diet. Instruct the patient that follow-up examinations are necessary to detect renal failure. The patient should have his blood pressure, urine protein, and renal function assessed for at least 1 year following to detect recurrence. More detail will be given in the Nursing Management section for the patient with chronic glomerulonephritis later in this chapter.

Although the prognosis for acute glomerulonephritis is generally good, with normal kidney function returning after a period of time, repeated occurrences can lead to chronic glomerulonephritis.

▮ Chronic Glomerulonephritis

Chronic glomerulonephritis is a slow, progressive disease caused by inflammation of the glomeruli that results in sclerosis and scarring. This leaves the remaining glomeruli to do all of the filtration. An elevation of blood pressure is necessary for this to be accomplished; therefore, hypertension often accompanies this disease (Follin & Lenker, 2004).

Common causes of chronic glomerulonephritis include membranoproliferative glomerulonephritis, membranous glomerulopathy, focal segmental glomerulosclerosis, and rapidly progressive glomerulonephritis. Systemic disorders include lupus erythematosus, Goodpasture's syndrome, and diabetes mellitus.

Laboratory and Diagnostic Procedures

Chronic glomerulonephritis usually remains subclinical until the progressive phase begins, which may take years. At any time the disease may become progressive, and the patient will exhibit hypertension, proteinuria, and hematuria. As the disease continues to progress, the patient may exhibit azotemia, nausea, vomiting, pruritus, dyspnea, and fatigue. During the late stages of the disease, mild to severe edema and anemia may develop. The ensuing severe hypertension may cause the heart to hypertrophy and will lead to heart failure, which will accelerate the development of renal failure necessitating dialysis or potential for kidney transplantation. Tests that are helpful in the diagnosis of chronic glomerulonephritis are outlined in the Diagnostic Tests box.

Medical Management

The goals of treatment are control of hypertension with antihypertensives and a sodium restrictive diet; correction of electrolyte imbalances through dietary restrictions and supplements; and reduction of edema and the prevention of heart failure with diuretics. For end-stage glomerulonephritis, treatment may include antibiotics for urinary tract infections, dialysis for renal failure, and potential for transplantation. The Pharmacology Summary feature on page 1490 presents medications used to treat renal disorders.

◼ Nursing Management

Because treatment is primarily supportive, close observation and monitoring of the patient's blood pressure, strict intake and output, and daily weight are necessary to evaluate fluid retention and possible fluid overload. Monitor blood work for signs of electrolyte and acid–base imbalances. Consult the dietary department to plan a low-sodium, high-caloric diet with adequate protein.

Assessment

The nurse should inquire as to the following during the nursing history:

- Amount and frequency of urination
- Headaches, swelling of the lower extremities
- Recent high-risk episodes such as an infection; cardiac, vascular, or biliary surgery; significant trauma; ingestion of aspirin, antibiotics, or other drugs; and allergic response to food, drugs, or a blood transfusion
- Pain in the flank area
- Fatigue or longer than usual sleep periods
- Muscle cramps or difficulty breathing during exercise.

The nurse should assess the patient for the following physical findings:

- Oliguria (less than 400 mL/day)
- Abnormal urine color, clarity, or smell
- Lethargy
- Normal or high blood pressure
- Dyspnea
- Fine crackles with auscultation of the lung fields.

Nursing Diagnoses

Nursing diagnoses for the patient with glomerulonephritis include:

- *Fluid Volume, Excess* related to sodium and water retention
- *Infection, Risk for*
- *Nutrition, Imbalanced: Less than Body Requirements* related to anorexia, nausea, and restricted dietary intake.

Planning

The overall goals for the patient with glomerulonephritis are to prevent further damage to the kidney and prevent renal failure.

Outcomes and Evaluation Parameters

Outcomes and evaluation parameters for the patient with glomerulonephritis include:

- The patient will maintain serum electrolyte levels within acceptable limits.
- The patient will be normovolemic, as exhibited by vital signs and hemodynamic readings within acceptable parameters,

DIAGNOSTIC TESTS for Chronic Glomerulonephritis

Test	Expected Abnormality	Rationale for Abnormality
Urinalysis	Presence of protein, red blood cells, and red blood cell casts	Impaired filtration
Serum creatinine	Rising serum creatinine	Indicates advanced renal insufficiency
Blood urea nitrogen (BUN)	Rising serum BUN	Indicates advanced renal insufficiency
X-ray or ultrasonography	Shows smaller kidneys	Atrophy of the kidney
Biopsy of the kidney	Identifies the underlying disease	Needed to guide therapy

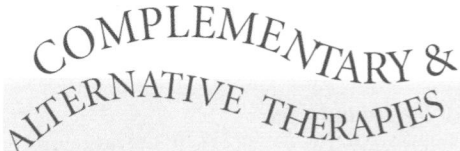

COMPLEMENTARY & ALTERNATIVE THERAPIES   Cranberries

Description:

Urinary-tract infections (UTIs) are very common, and recurrent UTIs have significant implications. Antibiotics are the most prevalent conventional treatment, but antimicrobial resistance and side effects result from frequent use. UTIs result from the colonization and adherence of uropathogens in the urinary tract. It has been shown that cranberries (*Vaccinium macrocarpon*) interfere with uropathogen adherence. Therefore, cranberries provide a promising alternative in the treatment and prevention of UTIs (Beerepoot et al., 2006).

Research Support:

Two randomized controlled trials involved 300 young women with recurrent UTIs who consumed cranberry juice or tablets daily. Results showed that daily use of cranberry reduced the relapse rate for UTI. Of 100 women who consumed cranberry juice or tablets daily for 1 year, 15 to 33 women prevented at least one urinary tract infection. Daily doses of cranberry ranged from 7.5 g of concentrate in 50 mL of water, to 750 mL of juice, to two tablets of concentrate. This same research paper examined two trials that involved elderly patients in hospitals or nursing homes who used cranberry-based products. Results from these studies showed a small reduction in UTI relapse frequency. However, it is important to note that cranberry juice or tablets may interact with warfarin, and may cause bleeding problems for patients taking warfarin concurrently ("Cranberry and Urinary Tract Infections," 2006).

Anthocyanins are components in cranberry that are believed to exert a therapeutic effect on UTIs. In order to determine the amount of absorption and excretion of anthocyanins, another study conducted by a Japanese research team analyzed urine samples from 11 healthy volunteers after they ingested cranberry juice. Volunteers consumed 200 mL of cranberry juice that contained 650.8 mcg of anthocyanins. Researchers collected urine samples within 24 h before and after consumption. Results showed

that cranberry anthocyanins are well absorbed and excreted in human urine (Ohnishi et al., 2006).

Sweetened dried cranberries are popular food items available in most grocery stores. Another study determined whether consumption of this type of cranberry product elicited the same urinary antiadherence effect against uropathogens as previously demonstrated with cranberry juice. *Escherichia coli* is one of the most common uropathogens that causes UTI. Levels of *E. coli* were analyzed from urine samples of five women with culture-confirmed UTIs. Of the urine samples collected after the women consumed approximately 42.5 g of dried cranberries, one demonstrated 50% antiadherence activity, two demonstrated 25% activity, and two showed no increased activity. Although this was a very small study, results suggest that sweetened dried cranberries may offer similar therapeutic effects as cranberry juice (Greenberg, Newmann, & Howell, 2005).

References

Beerepoot, M. A., ter Riet, G., Verbon, A., Nys, S., de Reijke, T. M., Geerlings, S. E. (2006). Non-antibiotic prophylaxis for recurrent urinary-tract infections. *Nederlands Tijdschrift voor Geneeskunde, 150*(10), 541–544.

Cranberry and urinary tract infections: Slightly fewer episodes in young women, but watch out for interactions. (2006). *Prescrire International, 15*(84), 145–146.

Greenberg, J. A, Newmann, S. J., & Howell, A. B. (2005). Consumption of sweetened dried cranberries versus unsweetened raisins for inhibition of uropathogenic Escherichia coli adhesion in human urine: A pilot study. *Journal of Alternative and Complementary Medicine, 11*(5), 875–878.

Ohnishi, R., Ito, H., Kasajima, N., Kaneda, M., Kariyama, R., Kumon, H., et al. (2006). Urinary excretion of anthocyanins in humans after cranberry juice ingestion. *Bioscience, Biotechnology, and Biochemistry, 70*(7), 1681–1687.

---

clear lung sounds, minimal peripheral edema, normal skin turgor, and maintenance of weight gain and loss.

- The patient will not show signs of infection, as exhibited by a normal temperature, clean, dry access sites for lines and catheters, negative cultures, and completion of the antibiotic regime.

- The patient will be able to understand and agree to comply with dietary modifications and activity restrictions.

Interventions and Rationales

Nursing interventions and rationales for the patient with glomerulonephritis include:

- Continually assess for signs of infection. Document and report any signs to the health care team. *Uremic syndrome (which may occur) suppresses normal cell metabolism and immune response, placing the patient at greater risk for infection.*

- Provide skin care and use preventive measures to protect against shearing or decubitus formation. Turn the patient every 2 hours, maintain wrinkle-free linens, and use protective pads to bony areas. Provide site care and dressing changes for intravenous lines according to hospital policy. *Skin integrity is compromised due to the edema and accumulation of waste products in the tissues because of the altered metabolism.*

Site care will assist to prevent accumulation of moisture, which serves as growth media for infective organisms.

- Collaborate with the health care team to implement a high-carbohydrate diet that provides small amounts of high-quality proteins; limits fluids, sodium, and potassium; and includes vitamin supplements. *A high-carbohydrate diet supplies calories for energy needs; limiting proteins prevents protein catabolism, as the kidneys are unable to excrete the waste products at this time; fluids and sodium are limited to prevent volume overload, while potassium is limited because the kidneys are unable to excrete it.*

- Administer diuretics as needed and ordered. Document administration and results. *Diuretics may be given to reduce fluid overload and increase fluid volume through the kidneys in an attempt to prevent acute renal failure.*

Evaluation

The patient will remain free of infection, maintain fluid and electrolyte balance, and maintain her weight while following the diet regimen. Topics that should be addressed with patients who have glomerulonephritis and/or their families before discharge are described in the Patient Teaching & Discharge Priorities box (p. 1468).

Pyelonephritis

Pyelonephritis, one of the most common renal diseases, is a sudden inflammation of the kidney and renal pelvis caused by bacteria (Follin & Lenker, 2004). The inflammation is **suppurative** (associated with the formation of pus). The bacteria that usually cause pyelonephritis are normal intestinal and fecal floras that grow readily in urine. Pyelonephritis is more common in women because they have a shorter urethra, and the proximity of the meatus to the vagina and rectum allows the bacteria to reach the urethra and bladder more easily. The most common causative bacteria are *Escherichia coli*, followed by *Proteus, Pseudomonas, Staphylococcus aureus*, and *Streptococcus faecalis* (Hager & Mills, 2008).

The infection usually starts in the bladder and then spreads to the kidney through the ureters. The bacteria can also be introduced by instrumentation such as catheterization, cystoscopy, or urologic surgery; by bacteria translocated by the blood, as in septicemia or endocarditis; and from lymphatic infections. Risk factors for increased incidence of pyelonephritis are included in the Risk Factors box.

Laboratory and Diagnostic Procedures

The signs and symptoms of pyelonephritis include urinary urgency, frequency, and burning; dysuria; nocturia; and hematuria. The urine may appear cloudy and have the odor of ammonia or fish. Due to the inflammatory response to the bacteria, the patient usually experiences high fever, chills, flank pain, and fatigue. If the bacterial infection is not severe, the symptoms may subside within a few days, but a residual bacterial infection is common and may cause recurrence of symptoms if untreated. Tests that are helpful in the diagnosis of pyelonephritis are listed in the Diagnostic Tests box.

Medical Management

Treatment consists of identification of the infecting organism and treatment with the appropriate antibiotics. Intravenous antibiotics are often used initially to control the growth of bacteria. Commonly used antibiotics include sulfa drugs, cephalosporins, amoxicillin, levofloxacin, and ciprofloxacin. If the patient is experiencing urinary urgency and frequency, urinary analgesics such as phenazopyridine are appropriate. The Pharmacology Summary feature on page 1490 presents medications used to treat renal disorders. See

---

RISK FACTORS for Pyelonephritis

- Inability to empty the bladder. Examples include neurogenic bladder, urinary obstruction due to tumor, kidney stone, prostatic hyperplasia, or urinary stasis.
- Being female due to the proximity of the urinary meatus to the vagina and rectum. Females also lack the antibacterial prostatic secretions produced in males.
- Sexually active women due to the increased risk of bacterial contamination from intercourse.
- Pregnant women. Approximately 5% develop asymptomatic bacteriuria and, if untreated, approximately 40% develop pyelonephritis (Follin & Lenker, 2004).
- Diabetes due to the development of neurogenic bladder, which causes incomplete emptying and urinary stasis. Also, glucose in the urine may support bacterial growth.
- Compromised renal function from other renal diseases increases the susceptibility.

The bacteria that reach the kidney create colonies of infection within 24 to 48 hours. Abscesses frequently form and when they rupture, pus enters the renal pelvis and appears in the urine. Untreated, the abscesses can continue to form and fuse until the entire kidney is filled with pus. If this continues, renal failure occurs and uremia develops. If the infection is less severe, the kidney can heal but will form scar tissue that tends to contract and cause the kidney to shrink and become granular, making it less efficient.

Complementary & Alternative Therapies feature (p. 1467) for nonpharmaceutical adjuncts for prevention of infection.

 **CRITICAL ALERT** *If the patient is pregnant, be sure that the prescribed antibiotic is safe to use during pregnancy.*

If the infection was caused by an obstruction, surgery may be necessary to relieve the obstruction.

Nursing Management

If the patient has a high fever, administer antipyretics. Encourage the patient to drink enough fluids to maintain a urine output of more than 2,000 mL/day to empty the bladder of contaminated

---

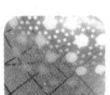

PATIENT TEACHING & DISCHARGE PRIORITIES for Glomerulonephritis

Need	Teaching
Nutrition	Have patient/family work with dietitian to plan a low-sodium, high-caloric diet with adequate protein.
Medications	Stress to the patient the importance of taking prescribed antihypertensives as scheduled, even if patient is feeling better.
	Suggest that diuretics be taken in the morning to decrease disruption of sleep due to need to void.
Skin care	Stress to the patient the importance of good skin care, as the pruritus and edema may cause skin breakdown.
	Teach the patient how to assess ankle edema.
Avoidance of continued infections and scarring	Stress to patient/family the importance of reporting signs of infection, particularly urinary tract infection, and to avoid contact with people who have infections.
	Stress importance of follow-up appointments to assess renal function.

DIAGNOSTIC TESTS for Pyelonephritis

Test	Expected Abnormality	Rationale for Abnormality
Urinalysis	Pyuria: pus in urine; leukocytes appear singly, in clumps, and in casts.	Rupture of abscesses, allowing pus to empty into the urine.
	Low specific gravity and osmolality.	Decreased ability to concentrate urine.
Urine culture	Bacteriuria: more than 100,000 organisms/mcL of urine.	Bacterial growth in urine.
X-ray films of the kidneys, ureters, and bladder (KUB)	May reveal cause of obstruction: renal calculi, tumor, or cysts.	Obstruction causes urinary retention and stasis, increasing risk for infection.

urine but not to drink more than 3 liters of fluid, as that may decrease the effectiveness of the antibiotics. When collecting urine for urinalysis and culture, teach the proper technique for a clean-catch urine specimen, and send the culture within 30 minutes of collection to prevent overgrowth of the bacteria.

Assessment

When taking a patient history, the nurse should consider the following: age; sex; whether a female patient is sexually active; whether the patient has had a recent procedure such as catheterization, cystoscopy, or urologic surgery; and whether the patient has a history of neurogenic bladder. Physical assessment findings may include fever (usually 38.9°C or higher), burning with urination, general fatigue, hematuria, flank pain, and urinary frequency and urgency.

Nursing Diagnoses

Nursing diagnoses that apply to pyelonephritis include:

- *Infection, Risk for* related to insufficient knowledge to avoid exposure to pathogens, neurogenic bladder, or urinary obstruction
- *Urinary Incontinence, Urge* due to infection
- *Fatigue* due to inflammation.

Planning

The goals for the patient with pyelonephritis are to treat the infection and prevent further infections.

Outcomes and Evaluation Parameters

Outcomes and evaluation parameters include:

- The patient is free from infection, as exhibited by follow-up urine culture that is free of growth.
- The patient does not experience urgency or urinary urge incontinence.

- The patient does not suffer fatigue, as exhibited by the ability to do normal activities without tiring.

Interventions and Rationales

Nursing interventions and rationales for the patient with pyelonephritis include:

- The nurse should teach the patient the importance of completing the patient's prescribed antibiotic therapy and the need to drink enough fluids to produce more than 2,000 milliliters of urine per day. *Stopping antibiotics early, even when symptoms subside, may allow the infectious agent to remain. Drinking plenty of fluid helps to empty the bladder of contaminated urine.*
- The nurse should teach the patient to plan activities in short increments to allow for rest time. *Planning activities to allow for rest periods in between will prevent further fatigue.*
- If the patient is having urinary urgency and burning with urination, administer urinary analgesics. *Urinary analgesics relieve the pain of burning, frequency, and urgency arising from irritation of urinary tract mucosa.*

Evaluation

The patient should have a normal temperature, have no burning or frequency with urination, and have no growth on culture of the urine.

Topics that should be addressed with patients who have pyelonephritis and/or their families before discharge are outlined in the Patient Teaching & Discharge Priorities box.

Hydronephrosis

If an obstruction occurs in the ureter, bladder, or urethra, the kidney can become extremely dilated with urine. The most common

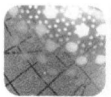

PATIENT TEACHING & DISCHARGE PRIORITIES for Pyelonephritis

Need	Teaching
Prevention	Instruct female patients to wipe the perineum from front to back after defecation.
	Instruct female patients to void after sexual intercourse to flush the bladder and urethra.
Antibiotic therapy	Instruct the patient to complete the prescribed antibiotics even after symptoms subside.
Follow-up treatment	Encourage follow-up care for high-risk patients.
	Teach patients the signs and symptoms of infection: cloudy urine, burning with urination, urgency, frequency, and fever.

causes of obstruction are an enlarged prostate gland, urethral strictures, and renal calculi. Other causes may include stricture or stenosis of the bladder outlet or ureter, abdominal tumors, tumors of the ureter and bladder, blood clots, neurogenic bladder, and congenital abnormalities. If the site of the obstruction is the urethra or bladder, then both kidneys are usually affected. If the obstruction occurs in one ureter, then the hydronephrosis will be unilateral. When the obstruction is in the urethra, distal to the bladder, first the bladder dilates with urine acting as a buffer, which delays the hydronephrosis.

Hydronephrosis is most commonly a chronic condition with slow changes in the kidney that occur with pain or other symptoms. If the obstruction is severe and prolonged, fibrotic changes occur in the kidney, and there is a loss of function of the nephrons that are involved. The finding of hydronephrosis is often accidental, occurring when a radiograph or ultrasound of the abdomen is ordered for another reason.

Laboratory and Diagnostic Procedures

Signs and symptoms of hydronephrosis vary depending on the cause of the obstruction and the extent of the blockage. Symptoms may be as mild as slight discomfort and slightly decreased urine flow. Other patients may experience severe, colicky renal pain or flank pain that radiates to the groin. If the hydronephrosis is unilateral, the pain is only on the affected side. If infection occurs due to stagnation of urine, then the patient will develop fever, nausea, and pain on urination. Tests that are helpful in the diagnosis of hydronephrosis are presented in the Diagnostic Tests box.

Medical Management

Treatment consists of identifying and treating the cause of the obstruction in order to preserve renal function and prevent infection. Removal of the obstruction may include dilation for stricture of the urethra, prostatectomy for prostatic hypertrophy, or surgical removal of calculi or tumor. Inoperable obstructions may require drainage of the kidney using a nephrostomy tube.

Nephrostomy Tube

Nephrostomy tubes are placed percutaneously under fluoroscopy or surgically. The tube is placed through the flank area into the renal pelvis and secured to a closed drainage system to allow drainage via gravity flow. Preprocedure, several precautions are taken: A broad-spectrum antibiotic is given to prevent infection; coagulopathy should be corrected; and uncontrolled hypertension should be corrected. It is important to assess the tube for kinks or clots that may impede drainage. If the tube becomes dislodged, the fistula that was created closes quickly, and it may be impossible to insert another catheter in as little as 30 minutes. Nursing management of the patient that has had a nephrostomy tube placed includes:

- Assess for complications such as bleeding at the site, hematuria, fistula formation, and infection.
- Assess skin at nephrostomy site for signs of inflammation, infection, bleeding, leakage of urine, and skin irritation.
- Assess tube patency. If obstructed, the patient will complain of pain and pressure.
- Use aseptic technique when replacing dressings.
- Encourage oral intake of fluids to promote flushing of the kidney and nephrostomy tube.
- Never clamp a nephrostomy tube.
- Never irrigate a nephrostomy tube without specific orders.

■ Nursing Management

If the hydronephrosis has already affected renal function, a diet low in protein, sodium, and potassium is indicated to prevent progression of renal failure prior to surgery. Refer to the earlier Nursing Management section for the patient with glomerulonephritis. Prior to the patient's diagnostic tests, inquire regarding allergies to dye or foods that contain iodine such as shellfish. Hydronephrosis can be very painful; administer pain medication as needed. Topics that should be addressed with patients who have hydronephrosis and/or their families before discharge are presented in the Patient Teaching & Discharge Priorities box.

■ Polycystic Kidney Disease

Polycystic kidney disease is a congenital anomaly that is characterized by multiple clusters of fluid-filled cysts that grossly enlarge the kidneys. The cysts are dilated kidney tubules that do not open into the renal pelvis. As the cysts enlarge and fuse, they usually be-

DIAGNOSTIC TESTS for Hydronephrosis

Test	Expected Abnormality	Rationale for Abnormality
Intravenous pyelogram (IVP)	Identification of stricture or obstruction.	Decrease in or cessation of flow.
	Dilation of the renal pelvis.	Inability to drain renal pelvis.
Renal ultrasonography	Identification of fluid accumulation.	Inability of urine to drain from renal pelvis.
	Identification of area of obstruction.	Stricture, tumor, or calculi will be visible.
Renal function studies:		
Blood urea nitrogen (BUN)	Increased.	Decreased filtration.
Serum creatinine	May rise slightly.	Nephron function loss.
Creatinine clearance	Decreased.	Decreased glomerular function.

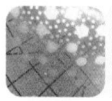

PATIENT TEACHING & DISCHARGE PRIORITIES for Hydronephrosis

Need	Teaching
Prevention	Teach older men, especially those with prostatic hypertrophy, to have routine checkups to monitor progression. Also instruct them to recognize and report symptoms of hydronephrosis, such as colicky pain, blood in the urine, or urinary tract infections.
Nephrostomy tube care	Instruct patient/family in the care of the nephrostomy tube. Teach the importance of checking for bleeding and patency. Stress importance of immediate notification of the health care provider if the tube becomes dislodged.
Signs and symptoms of postoperative complications	Instruct patient/family during hospitalization and at home after discharge.
	Instruct patient/family to report any sign of impending hemorrhage and shock: tachycardia; cold, clammy skin; and a feeling of anxiousness or decreased level of consciousness.
Antibiotic therapy	If there was concurrent infection, instruct the patient to complete the prescribed antibiotics even after symptoms subside.

come infected. The cysts compress and gradually replace the functioning renal tissue, leading to fatal uremia. The disease appears in two forms, infantile or adult, with both types affecting males and females equally (Follin & Lenker, 2004; Hager & Mills, 2008).

Infantile polycystic kidney disease is inherited as an autosomal recessive trait and may cause stillbirth or early neonatal death. If the infant survives, he usually develops fatal renal, respiratory, or heart failure by the age of 2.

Adult polycystic kidney disease is inherited as an autosomal dominant trait and affects 1 of 500 to 1,000 individuals (see Chapter 11). The disease usually becomes symptomatic between ages 30 and 50 (Hager & Mills, 2008). This is because, in the adult form, renal deterioration not only is more gradual but also progresses to fatal uremia. Unless the patient receives treatment with dialysis, a kidney transplant, or both, once uremic symptoms develop the disease is usually fatal within 4 years.

Laboratory and Diagnostic Procedures

Adult polycystic kidney disease may go undiagnosed for some time because the symptoms are nonspecific, such as hypertension, polyuria, and urinary tract infections. As the disease progresses, the patient will develop signs and symptoms related to the enlarging kidneys. These include lumbar pain, swollen or tender abdomen, and abdominal pain that is exacerbated by exertion and relieved by lying down. Signs and symptoms that

manifest in the advanced stages are recurrent hematuria, retroperitoneal bleeding from a ruptured cyst, proteinuria, and abdominal pain caused by ureteral passage of clots or calculi.

The diagnosis of polycystic kidney disease is made from both family history and examination revealing grossly enlarged and palpable kidneys. Tests that are helpful in the diagnosis of polycystic kidney disease are outlined in the Diagnostic Tests box.

Medical Management

The goal of treatment is to preserve renal function and prevent infectious complications. Adequate control of hypertension is necessary to help prevent rapid deterioration in function. As the disease progresses, the patient will require dialysis. The Pharmacology Summary feature on page 1490 presents medications used to treat renal disorders.

■ Nursing Management

Young adult patients should be encouraged to seek genetic counseling. Approximately half of the children born to a patient with polycystic kidney disease will have the disease (Walser, 2004). Because the disease is progressive, comprehensive patient teaching and emotional support are extremely important. For more detail, refer to the Nursing Management section for the patient with acute renal failure later in this chapter. Topics that

DIAGNOSTIC TESTS for Polycystic Kidney Disease

Test	Expected Abnormality	Rationale for Abnormality
Ultrasonography, tomography, and radioisotope scans	Enlargement of the kidneys and cysts.	Enlargement is caused by the fluid-filled cysts that displace the renal tissue.
Retrograde ureteropyelography	Enlarged kidneys with elongation of the renal pelvis, flattening of the calyces, and indentations.	Enlargement is caused by the fluid-filled cysts that displace the renal tissue.
Urinalysis	Presence of protein, red blood cells, and red blood cell casts.	Impaired filtration.
Serum creatinine	Rising serum creatinine.	Indicates advanced renal insufficiency.
Blood urea nitrogen (BUN)	Rising serum BUN.	Indicates advanced renal insufficiency.

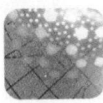

PATIENT TEACHING & DISCHARGE PRIORITIES for Polycystic Kidney Disease	
Need	**Teaching**
Asymptomatic stage	Monitor kidney function carefully: • Obtain a creatinine clearance test every 6 months. • Obtain a urine culture every 6 months.
Follow-up care	Patient/family at home: • Monitor filtration capacity and progression of the disease. • If infection detected, patient should receive antibiotic treatment even if she is asymptomatic.

should be addressed with patients who have polycystic kidney disease and/or their families before discharge are presented in the Patient Teaching & Discharge Priorities box.

Renal Infarction

An occlusion of a renal blood vessel results in renal infarction and an area of necrosis in one or both kidneys. The location of the infarction depends on the site of the occlusion. In approximately 75% of infarctions, the vessel that becomes occluded is the renal artery. The embolic event is secondary to a predisposing cardiovascular disease such as mitral stenosis, atrial fibrillation, microthrombi in the left ventricle, rheumatic valvular disease, endocarditis, or a recent myocardial infarction. Less common causes include atherosclerosis of the renal vasculature, thrombus from flank trauma, sickle cell anemia, and scleroderma (Follin & Lenker, 2004).

The degree of occlusion and rate of decreased blood flow to the kidney determine whether the event will be acute or become chronic as the narrowing progresses. Signs and symptoms include severe upper abdominal pain or constant flank pain with tenderness, fever, nausea, and vomiting. Renovascular hypertension may occur several days after infarction due to the reduced blood flow, which stimulates the renin-angiotensin mechanism.

Renal infarction may also arise from renal vein thrombosis (RVT). A spontaneous renal vein thrombosis is rare in patients who are ambulatory but has been reported in patients with trauma, women taking oral contraceptives, patients with hypovolemia or dehydration, and those with inherited procoagulant defects (Radhakrishnan, 2008). RVT can be unilateral or bilateral, is usually chronic, and may extend into the inferior vena cava. Pulmonary embolus may be the first clue that the patient

has chronic RVT. Acute RVT typically presents with flank pain, microscopic or gross hematuria, a marked elevation in serum lactate dehydrogenase, and an increase in the size of the affected kidney on radiographic study. If the acute RVT is bilateral, the patient may present with acute renal failure.

Laboratory and Diagnostic Procedures

Any patient with predisposing cardiovascular disease, flank trauma, sickle cell anemia, or scleroderma who develops typical signs and symptoms should be further evaluated for renal infarction. Renal vascular angiography or venogram will show the exact location and extent of obstruction, but it is a high-risk procedure due to the adverse effects of the dye load on renal function. Tests that are helpful in the diagnosis of renal infarction are listed in the Diagnostic Tests box.

Medical Management

Therapies to remove the occlusion include administration of intra-arterial streptokinase, lysis of blood clots, catheter embolectomy, and heparin therapy. If the infarcted area becomes infected or is very large, causing hypertension, surgical repair of the occlusion or removal of the kidney may be necessary.

Nursing Management

It is important to monitor the patient's intake and output, daily weight, and electrolyte levels to assess renal function. Encourage the patient to schedule follow-up appointments to monitor return of renal function. Refer to the Nursing Management section for the patient with acute renal failure later in this chapter.

DIAGNOSTIC TESTS for Renal Infarction

Test	Expected Abnormality	Rationale for Abnormality
Urinalysis	Presence of protein, red blood cells, and red blood cell casts	Impaired filtration
Serum enzyme levels	Elevated lactate dehydrogenase (LD), alkaline phosphatase, and aspartate aminotransferase	Result of tissue destruction
Excretory urography	Reveals diminished or absent excretion of contrast	Indicates diminished or nonfunctioning kidney
Isotopic renal scan	Reveals absent or reduced blood flow to kidneys	Indicates the area and extent of occlusion

Renal Carcinoma

Carcinoma of the kidney causes enlargement of the organ and eventually destroys it. Approximately 80% to 85% of all primary renal cell carcinomas originate within the renal cortex. Transitional cell carcinomas of the renal pelvis account for 8%, with other parenchymal epithelial tumors, collecting duct tumors, and renal sarcomas occurring infrequently (Atkins, 2006b). Renal carcinoma represents approximately 2% of total cancer incidence and mortality (Atkins, 2006b). The Risk Factors box presents the risk factors that have been associated with renal carcinoma. The influence of genetic disorders on the risk of developing renal carcinoma is outlined in the Genetic Considerations box.

Laboratory and Diagnostic Procedures

Many patients are asymptomatic until the disease is advanced, and when diagnosed, 25% have either metastases or advanced disease (Atkins, 2006a). The most common presenting symptoms are hematuria, pain, abdominal mass, and weight loss. There is an increasing amount of patients who are diagnosed as an incidental finding of a radiologic procedure performed for another indication. Metastasis to other organs often occurs, with common metastatic sites being the lungs, lymph nodes, liver, bones, and the brain.

Medical Management

Treatment consists of surgical removal. Renal carcinoma is radiation resistant, so this form of treatment is used only if the cancer has spread to the perinephric region or lymph nodes. Chemotherapy has not been shown to be effective against renal cancer. Biotherapy using lymphokine-activated killer cells with recombinant interleukin-2 has shown promise but also causes adverse reactions (Hager & Mills, 2008). Refer to Chapter 64 ⊕ for the care of the patient with cancer.

Nursing Management

This nursing management section pertains to the immediate preoperative and postoperative care for the patient undergoing a nephrectomy.

Assessment

During the health history, the nurse should focus on:

- Any history of comorbidities such as diabetes, hypertension, or vascular disease
- Any concerns or fears the patient may have regarding normal kidney function after the surgery
- Concerns regarding activity and diet restrictions after the surgery
- Patient's level of weight loss, nausea or vomiting, and fatigue.

During the physical assessment, the nurse should focus on:

- Signs of fluid overload: peripheral edema and distended neck veins
- Hypertension
- Signs of hypovolemia: decreased blood pressure; pale, cool skin; agitation
- Adventitious breath sounds
- Dysuria, hematuria, oliguria, or polyuria
- Skin color, temperature, and turgor.

Nursing Diagnoses

The primary nursing diagnoses for the patient undergoing nephrectomy are:

- *Knowledge, Deficient* related to the procedure
- *Pain, Acute*
- *Fluid Volume, Imbalanced, Risk for*
- *Gas Exchange, Impaired*

Planning

The overall goals for the patient undergoing nephrectomy include understanding of the procedure and postoperative plan

---

RISK FACTORS for Renal Carcinoma

- Cigarette smoking. Smoking increases the risk of renal carcinoma by twofold.
- Occupational exposure to toxic compounds. Exposure to compounds such as cadmium, asbestos, and petroleum by-products has been suggested to increase the risk of renal carcinoma. The exposure may be associated with mutations in genes associated with the pathogenesis of renal carcinoma.
- Obesity. There appears to be a direct correlation between obesity and an increased risk of developing renal carcinoma.
- Acquired cystic disease of the kidney. Patients on dialysis who develop polycystic kidney disease have been estimated to have a risk of developing renal carcinoma that is 30 times greater than that of the general population. The cancer typically develops after 8 to 10 years of dialysis.

Source: Atkins, M. (2006b). *Epidemiology, pathology, and pathogenesis of renal cell carcinoma.* Retrieved April 16, 2007, from http://www.uptodate.com

---

GENETIC CONSIDERATIONS for Renal Carcinoma

Patients with certain inherited disorders show an increased risk of developing renal carcinoma (see Chapter 11 ⊕). Included are hereditary papillary renal cancer, characterized by a predisposition to development of multiple, bilateral, papillary renal tumors. The inherited papillary cancers usually occur late in life with most patients being in their 70s. Hereditary leiomyoma, or Reed syndrome, is characterized by cutaneous leiomyomas (benign soft tissue neoplasms that arise from smooth muscle), uterine fibroids, and renal carcinomas that may be single, multiple, and bilateral. The renal tumors are aggressive and may metastasize. Von Hippel-Lindau syndrome is an autosomal dominant disorder that has a predisposition to neoplasm. Approximately one-third of patients with this disease develop renal cell carcinoma. Birt-Hogg-Dube syndrome is characterized by skin lesions that develop on the skin of the head and neck, lung cysts with spontaneous pneumothoraces, and a predisposition to kidney neoplasms.

Source: Atkins, M. (2006b). *Epidemiology, pathology, and pathogenesis of renal cell carcinoma.* Retrieved April 16, 2007, from http://www.uptodate.com

(cough and deep breathe, use of incentive spirometer, etc.), control of postoperative pain, and prevention of postoperative complications.

Outcomes and Evaluation Parameters

The major outcomes and evaluation parameters for the patient undergoing nephrectomy are:

- Patient is able to verbalize understanding of operative procedure.
- Patient is able to demonstrate ability to cough and deep breathe, splint the incision site, use the incentive spirometer, and perform leg exercises.
- Postoperative pain is controlled as evidenced by patient rating pain low on a 0–10 scale. Patient maintains vital signs within normal limits.
- The patient's fluid and electrolytes will be balanced as exhibited by a urine output greater than 30 mL/hr initially and 60 mL/hr or greater by time of discharge. Electrolytes will be within normal limits.
- The patient will maintain adequate oxygenation as evidenced by unlabored respirations, clear breath sounds in all lobes, and arterial blood gases within normal limits.
- The patient will have normal bowel function as evidenced by normal, active bowel sounds, ability to eat a regular diet, and ability to have a regular bowel movement.

Interventions and Rationales

Nursing interventions and rationales for the patient undergoing nephrectomy include:

- Discuss with the patient where the incision will be made, if the patient will have a chest tube or any drains, and the effects of positioning after surgery. *Knowledge of what to expect postoperatively will decrease the patient's fear and anxiety, and increase her ability to participate in her postoperative care.*
- Teach the patient regarding postoperative pain management. Let the patient know whether he will have patient-controlled analgesia or epidural infusion. Discuss potential adverse effects and the importance of requesting pain medication before the pain becomes severe. *The patient will be able to better control his pain with an understanding of the plan.*
- Protect the remaining kidney by maintaining adequate hydration. Monitor urine output and specific gravity. Minimize the use of nephrotoxic medications. *Preservation of the remaining kidney is paramount. Appropriate hydration preserves renal function and the removal of waste products. Use of nephrotoxic drugs may damage the remaining kidney.*
- Assist the patient to perform incentive spirometry, encourage the patient to cough and deep breathe, splint the incision site, promote early ambulation, and check pulmonary status frequently. *Atelectasis is an inherent risk of general anesthesia. Also, the patient with a flank incision is at risk because the intercostal muscles were spread and the 12th rib may be removed. Pain involved with this incision limits deep breathing. If atelectasis develops and is not treated, it can lead to pneumonia.*
- Encourage early and frequent ambulation. Encourage fluids and progression of diet as tolerated. Assess the abdomen for

distention and bowel sounds. Monitor nasogastric tube drainage. *Manipulation of the bowel during surgery increases the risk of paralytic ileus.*

Evaluation

The patient's pain will be controlled postoperatively, respiratory effort will be unlabored, and breath sounds will be clear in all lobes. The patient will be able to advance her diet and have return of normal bowel function. The patient will be able to take adequate food and fluid orally and will maintain normal fluid and electrolyte imbalance.

■ Acute Tubular Necrosis

Acute tubular necrosis (ATN) results from damage to the renal tubular epithelium from a nephrotoxic or ischemic injury. ATN is the most common form of intrinsic renal failure and accounts for the majority of acute renal failure admissions to the hospital (Urden et al., 2006). The damage to the epithelium prevents normal concentration of urine, filtration of waste products, regulation of acid–base balance, electrolyte hemostatsis, and fluid balance.

The common causes of ATN can be divided into two categories:

1. Toxic injury is the result of damage from nephrotoxins that cause uniform, widespread damage. Nephrotoxins are usually drugs, chemical agents, or bacterial endotoxins. Sources of nephrotoxins include:
   - Rhabdomyolysis
   - Nephrotoxic medications: cephalosporins, analgesics containing phenacetin, antineoplastic agents, aminoglycosides
   - Contrast media
   - Insecticides, fungicides
   - Methanol
   - Heavy metals: arsenic, mercury, lead, uranium
   - Phencyclidine (PCP).
2. Ischemic injury occurs when perfusion to the kidneys is severely reduced. The damage to the tubular membrane is irregular and causes cast formation. Causes of ischemic injury include:
   - Hemorrhage
   - Severe dehydration
   - Shock: hypovolemic, septic, cardiogenic
   - Crush injuries
   - Transfusion reaction
   - Obstetric complications: severe toxemia, placenta previa, abruptio placentae, uterine rupture.

Laboratory and Diagnostic Procedures

ATN commonly occurs in patients that are debilitated or critically ill. Therefore, it can be difficult to diagnose in the early stages because effects of the primary disease or injury may mask the symptoms. The first sign may be decreased urine output, although only 50% of patients become oliguric (Urden et al., 2006). Oliguria is more common in ischemic damage and carries a higher mortality rate when present.

Accurate diagnosis tends to occur in the advanced stage, as the glomerular filtration is greatly reduced leading to increased uremia, electrolyte abnormalities, and metabolic acidosis. Tests that are helpful in the diagnosis of acute tubular necrosis are outlined in the Diagnostic Tests box.

Medical Management

The acute phase of ATN often requires total support of renal function with hemodialysis. Initially treatment may be the infusion of large volumes of fluid in conjunction with administration of a diuretic to flush the tubules of cellular casts and debris, but the patient must be carefully monitored for fluid overload. Infection is the leading cause of death in patients with ATN (Follin & Lenker, 2004), so the patient must be assessed frequently for any signs of fever and the infection treated with the appropriate antibiotics. The Pharmacology Summary feature on page 1490 presents medications used to treat renal disorders.

With appropriate treatment, renal function will slowly return with the glomerular filtration rate at 70% to 80% of normal within 1 to 2 years. Although most patients recover normal renal function, 33% will have residual renal insufficiency, and approximately 5% will require ongoing hemodialysis (Urden et al., 2006).

◼ Nursing Management

Maintenance of fluid balance is important in the patient with ATN, with fluid overload a common complication of therapy. Therefore it is important to accurately document daily weight, intake and output, including loss from wound drainage, and dialysis balances. Maintain electrolyte balance by monitoring laboratory results, enforcing dietary restriction of foods containing sodium and potassium, and assessing for potassium content in prescribed medications such as penicillin.

The debilitated patient is vulnerable to infection, and because infection is the leading cause of death in patients with ATN, use of aseptic technique is paramount. Monitor for fever, chills, delayed wound healing, and flank pain. Encourage the patient to cough and deep breathe to prevent pulmonary complications. For a more detailed review of additional interventions, refer to the Nursing Management section for the patient with acute renal failure later in this chapter.

◼ Renal Failure

Renal failure is the inability of the kidneys to clear the blood of the waste products of protein metabolism: urea and creatinine. Urea, an end product of protein catabolism resulting from the breakdown of ammonia in the liver, is the primary method of nitrogen excretion from the body. If the body is unable to excrete the urea, it accumulates and toxicity develops.

Acute Renal Failure

Acute renal failure (ARF) develops suddenly and can usually be reversed with treatment, but if the condition causing the failure is not treated, the patient will progress to end-stage renal disease, uremic syndrome, and death. The causes of acute renal failure can be classified into three categories: (1) prerenal, (2) intrinsic, and (3) postrenal. Chart 47–1 (p. 1476) lists causes within the three categories. The mortality rate remains high for acute renal failure, with rates ranging from 25% to 90%. Influencing factors include the increasing age of patients and the comorbid conditions that accompany aging, such as vascular disease and diabetes (Dirkes & Hodge, 2007).

Laboratory and Diagnostic Procedures

Acute renal failure is a sudden and critical event with early signs being oliguria, azotemia, or **anuria**, a total loss of urine production. As the patient becomes more uremic, he will develop systemic signs and symptoms including headache, irritability, confusion, nausea, vomiting, diarrhea, pruritus, pallor, purpura; hypotension early in the process and then hypertension; **anasarca** (total body edema); altered clotting mechanisms; and bleeding. Reduced tubular hydrogen excretion produces hyperchloremia of low anion gap acidosis. If the glomerular filtration rate becomes severely impaired, the retention of acidic wastes may produce a high anion gap acidosis (see Chapter 19 ⌾). As a result of the acidosis, the patient's breath will have the odor of ammonia, and the patient may exhibit **Kussmaul's respirations**,

DIAGNOSTIC TESTS for Acute Tubular Necrosis

Test	Expected Abnormality	Rationale for Abnormality
Urinalysis	Presence of red blood cells and red blood cell casts	Impaired filtration
	Low specific gravity (1.010)	Decreased ability to concentrate urine
	Low osmolality (less than 400 mOsm/kg)	
Serum creatinine	Rising serum creatinine	Indicates advanced renal insufficiency
Blood urea nitrogen (BUN)	Rising serum BUN	Indicates advanced renal insufficiency
Arterial blood gases (ABG)	Metabolic acidosis	Impaired filtration
	pH < 7.35	
	HCO_3 < 24 mEq/L	
Electrolytes	Hyperkalemia	Impaired filtration
	Hyperphosphatemia	
	Hypocalcemia	

CHART 47–1 Types of Acute Renal Failure

Category	Causes
Prerenal failure	Diminished blood flow to the kidneys causes prerenal failure. The decreased flow may result from: <ul><li>Hypovolemia</li><li>Sepsis</li><li>Embolism</li><li>Heart failure</li><li>Idiopathic thrombocytopenic purpura</li><li>Transfusion reactions</li><li>Malignant hypertension</li><li>Scleroderma.</li></ul>
Intrinsic failure	Intrinsic (parenchymatous) failure results from damage to the kidney. The damage may be a result of: <ul><li>Acute tubular necrosis</li><li>Acute poststreptococcal glomerulonephritis</li><li>Systemic lupus erythematosus</li><li>Polyarteritis nodosa</li><li>Vasculitis</li><li>Sickle cell disease</li><li>Bilateral renal vein thrombosis</li><li>Nephrotoxins</li><li>Ischemia</li><li>Renal myeloma</li><li>Acute pyelonephritis.</li></ul>
Postrenal failure	Postrenal failure is the result of bilateral obstruction of urine outflow. Obstruction may be caused by: <ul><li>Renal calculi</li><li>Clots</li><li>Papillae from necrosis</li><li>Tumors</li><li>Benign prostatic hyperplasia</li><li>Strictures</li><li>Urethral edema from catheterization.</li></ul>

which are deep, sighing respirations. The most immediately life-threatening electrolyte imbalance that occurs with acute renal failure is severe **hyperkalemia**, an excess of potassium in the blood. The accompanying muscle weakness will cause heart failure and possible cardiac arrest. Sources of potassium should be identified and regulated if possible. Endogenous sources include cell lysis, hematoma reabsorption, and tissue breakdown. Exogenous sources include medications that interfere with potassium regulation, intravenous fluid, and diet. Water and sodium imbalances are common, because the patient can neither conserve nor excrete sodium or water optimally. Hyponatremia and fluid overload are common. The ability of the kidney to excrete phosphorus is impaired when the glomerular filtration rate

drops below one-third of normal. The resulting phosphorus retention leads to the formation of insoluble calcium phosphorus salts that can precipitate in soft tissue.

The progress and severity of the failure can be assessed by measurement of the glomerular filtration rate (GFR). The GFR is evaluated through clearance tests of the waste product creatinine. When the GFR is impaired, the serum creatinine level rises, and the creatinine clearance rate falls.

$$Creatinine\ clearance\ =$$
$$\frac{Urine\ creatinine\ concentration\ (mg\,\%) \times Urine\ volume\ (mL/min)}{Plasma\ creatinine\ concentration\ (mg\,\%)}$$

The test consists of a 12- or 24-hour urine collection and a blood sample. Normal levels are 88 to 128 mL/min in women and 97 to 137 mL/min in men. Values are slightly decreased in the elderly due to reduced renal plasma flow with aging. A creatinine clearance less than 40 mL/min is suggestive of moderate to severe renal impairment (Kee, 2005). Tests that are helpful in the diagnosis of acute renal failure are outlined in the Diagnostic Tests box.

Medical Management

The goal of treatment is to identify and treat reversible causes. Supportive measures include:

- Restrict protein intake to 0.25 to 0.5 g/kg per day to prevent increased urea synthesis.
- Provide nutrition to ensure a caloric intake of > 400 kilocalories per day to reduce tissue catabolism.
- Monitor potassium. If hyperkalemia occurs, therapy can include hypertonic glucose and insulin infusions, administration of intravenous calcium, and oral or rectal administration of potassium exchange resin. If the patient continues to be hyperkalemic, dialysis may be necessary.
- Restrict free water intake to avoid water overload and hyponatremia.
- Avoid exposure to or administration of nephrotoxic agents (Chart 47–2).
- Adjust doses of all medications that are excreted by the kidneys.
- Avoid nonsteroidal anti-inflammatory drugs (NSAIDs), and angiotensin-converting enzyme inhibitors (ACE inhibitors), as they interfere with potassium regulation.
- Avoid magnesium-containing drugs (antacids).
- Reduce the risk of hospital-acquired infection by using strict aseptic technique and removing indwelling urinary and vascular catheters when feasible.
- Use intermittent hemodialysis or continuous renal replacement therapy.

Continuous Renal Replacement Therapy

Continuous renal replacement therapy (CRRT) is a mode of dialysis that may be used in the hospital to treat acute renal failure. CRRT is a way to remove solute and fluids slowly and continuously in a patient that may be hemodynamically unstable. Described simply, CRRT includes blood flowing from a vascular access point; the blood is then purified in some manner outside the body by use of filters, creating an effluent and returning the purified blood to the body through another vascular access.

DIAGNOSTIC TESTS for Acute Renal Failure

Test	Expected Abnormality	Rationale for Abnormality
Blood urea nitrogen (BUN)	Increased	Impaired glomerular filtration
	Not as reliable an indicator of renal damage as serum creatinine levels, because the BUN is easily changed by protein intake, blood in the gastrointestinal tract, and cell catabolism	
Serum creatinine	Increased	Impaired glomerular filtration
Serum electrolyte levels:		
Potassium	Increased	Impaired filtration
Sodium	Decreased	Dilutional
Phosphorus	Increased	Impaired filtration
Calcium	Decreased	Response to increased phosphorus
Urinalysis	Presence of red blood cell casts, proteinuria	Impaired filtration
	Low specific gravity (1.010)	Decreased ability to concentrate urine
	Low osmolality (less than 400 mOsm/kg)	
Radiography:		
Renal ultrasound	Identification of size of the kidneys	Changes may signify damage to the kidney
Computed tomography *should be done without contrast*	Characterization of the parenchyma and collecting systems	May identify cause of kidney dysfunction
Retrograde pyelography	Identifies urinary tract obstruction	Will identify damage to kidney
Isotopic renal scan	Assesses renal perfusion and function	

CHART 47–2 Nephrotoxic Agents

Antibiotics
- Amphotericin B
- Colistin
- Gentamicin
- Kanamycin
- Neomycin
- Phenazopyridine
- Polymyxin B

Antineoplastic agents

Heavy metals
- Arsenic
- Lead
- Mercury

Iodinated radiographic contrast

Miscellaneous
- Acetaminophen
- Amphetamines
- Cyclosporine
- Heroin
- Silicon

Nonsteroidal anti-inflammatory drugs

Pesticides

Poisonous mushrooms

Solvents
- Carbon tetrachloride
- Ethylene glycol
- Methanol

High-efficiency membranes are used for maximum water and waste removal. The membranes are synthetic and biocompatible. In all forms of CRRT, as blood flows through the hemofilter, water is filtered through the pores in the membrane and produces the ultrafiltrate. The ultrafiltrate is composed primarily of water, electrolytes, wastes, and some dialyzable medications. Indications for use include hypervolemic or edematous patients unresponsive to diuretic therapy, multiple organ dysfunction syndrome (MODS), and large fluid volume removal in hemodynamically unstable patients. Terms that are commonly used with CRRT are:

- **Ultrafiltration**— Process of removing excess water by creating a pressure differential between the blood and fluid compartments. Positive pressure in the blood path and negative pressure in the dialysate path cause the excess water to move from the patient to the dialysate. The negative pressure is a suctioning force applied to the membrane.
- **Diffusion**—Spontaneous movement of solute from an area of higher concentration to an area of lower concentration.
- **Convection**—Movement of solutes through a membrane via an action called a solvent drag.
- **Osmosis**—Spontaneous movement of water from an area of lower concentration to an area of higher concentration.
- **Hemofiltration**—Movement of large amounts of fluid via ultrafiltration, and some movement of solutes via convection.
- **Replacement fluid**—Approximates normal plasma to meet the patient's needs. Fluids given may include lactated Ringer's solution, normal saline, albumin, bicarbonate, and electrolytes.

- **Dialysate**—Solution that surrounds the patient's blood, separated by a filter, and allows solute to cross from one side to the other.

There are several forms of CRRT. The four most frequently used are:

- **Continuous arteriovenous hemofiltration (CAVH)**—The blood is circulated by the patient's own arterial pressure, so a pump is not necessary. There is no concentration gradient, so only filtration of fluid occurs. Electrolytes are eliminated only as they are pulled along with the fluid. Replacement fluid is infused into the venous port to approximate fluid removal or to maintain weight balance.

- **Continuous arteriovenous hemodialysis (CAVHD)**—As with CAVH, the blood is circulated by the patient's own arterial pressure, so a pump is not necessary. CAVHD uses dialysate, which adds the advantages of the filtering properties of dialysis, providing a better clearance of urea. The dialysate solution is infused along with the hemofiltered blood.

- **Continuous venovenous hemodialysis (CVVHD)**—Diffusion and ultrafiltration are used to remove waste products. Dialysate is infused countercurrent to the blood flow in the outside compartment of the hemofilter to provide diffusion of wastes from the blood. CVVHD requires the use of a blood pump to control the flow at specific rates to optimize diffusion.

- **Slow continuous ultrafiltration (SCUF)**—This form of CRRT is used primarily for fluid removal. No dialysate or replacement fluids are used as wastes; electrolyte balance and acid–base balance are not as critical an issue. SCUF is the hemofiltration therapy of choice when the only goal is fluid removal and the patient is not azotemic, as in patients who are refractory to diuretics.

Nursing implications for CRRT include monitoring of fluid and electrolyte balance. Vital signs, hemodynamic status, and intake and output should be monitored hourly. The amount of hourly ultrafiltrate removed depends on an hourly fluid-balance calculation and assessment of the patient's volume status. Excess fluid volume to be removed is ordered by the health care provider and is usually termed as net loss. It may be ordered as 50 to 200 mL/hr more than hourly intake. This would be calculated as the patient's non-CRRT intake, such an intravenous infusions, medications, and feedings, plus fluid loss ordered by the health care provider minus non-CRRT system output, such as chest tube drainage, blood loss, and urine. The CRRT system infuses and removes fluid after the fluid balance is calculated and the desired volumes are input into the system. The system then monitors the amount of replacement fluids and/or dialysate to be infused and the volume of fluid removed. The patient's weight should be checked daily. Assessment and care of the vascular access sites is very important, because patency of the catheter can affect the effectiveness of the therapy.

◼ Nursing Management

Fluid balance is critical for the patient with acute renal failure. Intake, output, and daily weight should be closely monitored and documented. Intake of fluids should match the amount of urine output plus 500 to 750 milliliters a day for insensible losses and 400 milliliters a day for metabolic processes (Hogan, 2007). Strict measurement of output should include all body fluids, such as wound drainage. The patient should be instructed to follow the National Renal Diet that contains food exchanges for protein, sodium, potassium, and phosphorus. Monitoring of intake includes the patient's nutritional status. A high-calorie, low-protein, low-sodium, low-potassium diet is key in preventing further progression of the disease. Restrictions should be as follows:

- Sodium intake should only be what is needed to replenish losses, which is approximately 20 to 40 mEq/day (2 to 3 g/day).

- Limit protein to 0.25 to 0.5 g/kg body weight per day to minimize azotemia or nitrogen retention if not being dialyzed. If on dialysis, may increase protein to 1.2 g/kg daily.

- Limit diet potassium to 25 to 40 mEq/day to prevent hyperkalemia until urine volume increases during recovery.

- Parenteral iron may be needed to enhance erythropoiesis.

- Dietary phosphate may need to be restricted, although low-phosphate diets may be poorly accepted. Phosphate-binding antacids may be used to decrease the amount.

- If the patient is anorexic, give her small, frequent meals. (Hogan, 2007)

The patient with acute renal failure is susceptible to infectious complications. The use of aseptic technique is of significant importance in preventing hospital-acquired infections. Prevent complications of immobility with frequent position changes, coughing and deep breathing, and passive range-of-motion exercises. Provide frequent mouth care to prevent stomatitis.

If the patient is uremic, he may be confused and unsteady. Provide safety measures, such as having the bed in low position, three side rails up and one down to prevent falls, and soft restraints, if necessary.

Assessment

Focused nursing assessment during history taking should include:

- Amount and frequency of urination
- Change in urine color and smell
- History of headaches, dependent edema, or palpitations
- Pain around the flank or costal margin areas
- Nausea, loss of appetite, odd taste in mouth
- Weight gain or loss
- Weakness and fatigue
- Inability to concentrate or confusion
- Any job-related exposure to nephrotoxic agents
- Cessation of menstruation or impotence
- Increased irritability.

Focused nursing assessment during physical exam should include:

- Abnormal urine color, clarity, or smell
- Oliguria (<400 mL/day) or anuria (<50 mL/day) or nonoliguric ARF (1 to 2 L/day)
- Lethargy, apathy
- Tremors
- Bounding, rapid pulse with normal or high blood pressure, distended neck veins

- Orthostatic hypotension
- Tachypnea, dyspnea, or adventitious breath sounds
- Kussmaul's respirations (found when patient is acidotic)
- Dependent edema (with hypervolemia), poor skin turgor (with hypovolemia)
- Thin, brittle hair and nails.

Nursing Diagnoses

Key nursing diagnoses for the patient with acute renal failure include:

- *Fluid Volume, Excess*
- *Infection, Risk for*
- *Nutrition, Imbalanced: Less than Body Requirements*
- *Injury, Risk for*
- *Knowledge, Deficient* related to ARF and possible dialysis.

Planning

The overall goals for the patient with ARF are to identify and treat reversible causes, prevent further damage to the kidneys, and maintain fluid and electrolyte balance.

Outcomes and Evaluation Parameters

Patient outcomes and evaluation parameters for the patient with acute renal failure include:

- Maintenance of serum electrolyte levels as evidenced by results of lab work being within normal limits.
- Maintenance of fluid volume as evidenced by vital signs and hemodynamic readings being within acceptable limits.
- The patient will maintain balanced nutrition as exhibited by limited weight loss, muscle wasting, or edema.
- The patient will remain free of infection as exhibited by white blood count (WBC) being within normal range, no increase in temperature, and clean, dry access sites for lines and catheters.
- The patient will not be at risk for injury as exhibited by no signs or symptoms of uremia, such as confusion and tremors.
- The patient will have a clear understanding of the disease process and the plan of care by expressing knowledge of and commitment to comply with treatments.

Interventions and Rationales

Nursing interventions and rationales for the patient with ARF include:

- Monitor and document electrolyte levels as ordered. *The kidneys have lost the ability to regulate electrolyte excretion and reabsorption. This is expecially true of potassium, phosphate, calcium, and magnesium. The levels can change quickly and result in complications.*
- Monitor the ECG continuously. Notify the health care team and document any changes. *Electrolyte imbalances can cause dysrhythmias and cardiac arrest.*
- If hyperkalemia is present, notify the health care team and be prepared to administer the following, as ordered: *The kidneys' inability to excrete potassium released by normal cellular metabolism can cause very high potassium levels.*

1. 50% Glucose intravenously and insulin solution. *In an emergent situation, glucose and insulin may transport potassium into the cells, temporarily lowering the serum potassium level.*
2. Calcium chloride or calcium gluconate intravenously. *To protect the heart from the effect of hyperkalemia on the cardiac rhythm, calcium competes with potassium for entry into cardiac cells.*
3. Administration of cation-exchange resins such as sodium polystyrene sulfonate (Kayexalate with sorbitol) orally or rectally as ordered. *Sodium polystyrene sulfonate removes potassium at a rate of 1 mEq/g of medication by exchanging it for sodium in the bowel. The sorbitol helps to remove the bound potassium from the bowel by acting as an osmotic diarrhetic.*

- Limit dietary and drug intake of potassium (penicillin VK or potassium-containing antacids). Limit intake of magnesium-containing antacids. *The kidneys are unable to excrete the potassium or magnesium.*
- Assess for signs of fluid overload, such as weight gain, hypertension, tachypnea, adventitious breath sounds, peripheral edema, and low hematocrit. Maintain a strict record of intake and output. *During ARF the kidneys are unable to maintain normal fluid balance resulting in fluid overload during the oliguric stage and a potential for dehydration during the diuretic stage.*
- Restrict fluid intake to measure output plus 400 mL/day. Compare intake and output records with daily weights. If fluid losses have increased or the patient is losing weight, consult the health care team. *The kidneys are unable to eliminate excess fluids; therefore, intake must be restricted to replacement of lost fluids plus 400 mL/day to cover insensible losses (through lungs and skin).*
- Provide hard candies and frequent mouth care. *Restricting fluids may cause dry mouth and thirst. Hard candy will stimulate salivation, and mouth care will remove debris and add comfort.*
- Administer diuretics as ordered. Document administration and results. Administer vasodilators as ordered, such as low-dose dopamine. *During prerenal conditions, diuretics may be administered in an attempt to prevent ARF by increasing fluid volume through the kidneys. If the kidneys are marginally functioning, diuretics may cause ARF. Vasodilators expand the vascular bed, lessening the congestion and the risk of pulmonary edema. Low-dose dopamine increases renal perfusion by dopaminergic stimulation of the renal blood vessels.*
- Assess for signs of infection (increased temperature, increased WBC, signs of infection at IV and catheter sites). Practice strict asepsis and provide site care and dressing changes according to policy. *The uremic syndrome that develops with ARF suppresses normal cell metabolism and immune response, placing the patient at increased risk for infection. Careful hand hygiene and the use of aseptic technique during procedures help to prevent infection. Site care prevents the accumulation of secretions that serve as growth media for infective organisms. Regular assessment of all site areas and general assessment of the skin will allow for early identification and treatment of infection.*
- Provide skin care and use preventive measures to protect against shearing or decubitus formation. Turn the patient every 2 hours, maintain wrinkle-free linens, and use protective pads to bony areas. Provide site care and dressing changes

for intravenous lines according to hospital policy. *Skin integrity is compromised due to the edema and accumulation of waste products in the tissues due to the altered metabolism. Site care will assist to prevent accumulation of moisture, which serves as a growth medium for infective organisms.*

- Collaborate with the health care team to implement a high-carbohydrate diet that provides small amounts of high-quality proteins; limits fluids, sodium, and potassium; and includes vitamin supplements. *A high-carbohydrate diet supplies calories for energy needs; limiting proteins prevents protein catabolism, as the kidneys are unable to excrete the waste products at this time; fluids and sodium are limited to prevent volume overload, while potassium is limited because the kidneys are unable to excrete it.*

- Monitor BUN, creatinine, uric acid, and pH levels as ordered. Assess for signs and symptoms or uremia (headache, confusion, change in mentation, pruritus, nausea and vomiting, weight loss with muscle wasting, Kussmaul's respirations, seizures). *The accumulation of metabolic waste products and increasing acidosis reflect worsening kidney function. Uremia affects all systems in the body, but the changes may initially be subtle.*

- Assess for signs and symptoms of hemorrhage. *Uremic syndrome places the patient at high risk for stress ulcers and coagulopathy.*

- Monitor the patient for anemia (hematocrit and hemoglobin levels). Administer folic acid and iron supplements, or administer blood as ordered. *In ARF the kidneys' ability to produce erythropoietin, a hormone that stimulates the production of red blood cells (RBCs), diminishes, resulting in anemia. Folic acid and iron supplements stimulate RBC production. Administration of packed red blood cells provides RBCs without causing fluid overload.*

- Provide information and teaching for the patient and significant others as needed regarding the process and stages of ARF, signs and symptoms that should be reported immediately, dietary modifications, activity restriction, and an explanation of any procedures, including dialysis. *Knowledge and understanding of the disease process and the treatment plan help to decrease anxiety and may enhance recovery. If the patient is acutely ill, teaching may need to be done in small time frames.*

Evaluation

The patient should be able to verbalize her understanding of the disease process and the plan of care. The patient will maintain serum electrolyte levels and vital signs within acceptable limits. The patient will not display signs of uremia. The patient will remain free of infection with clean, dry access sites for lines and catheters. The patient will have only limited weight loss with no signs of muscle wasting or edema.

Chronic Renal Failure

Chronic renal failure is generally not reversible and often gets progressively worse. The symptoms of renal failure usually appear when approximately two-thirds of filtration capacity is lost. When the loss of filtration ability reaches approximately seven-eighths, the survival of the patient depends on maintenance dialysis or kidney transplantation. When a patient reaches this stage of failure, the patient is said to have **end-stage renal disease (ESRD)** (Follin & Lenker, 2004; Walser, 2004). If the patient continues

without treatment, uremic toxins accumulate and cause potentially fatal physiological changes in all of the major organ systems.

In the United States, over 300,000 patients have ESRD and are currently on dialysis. Outside of the United States there are another 300,000 to 400,000 patients on dialysis, with many hundreds of thousands of patients in third world countries who suffer from ESRD but do not have dialysis available for economic reasons. In the United States, the number of patients on dialysis increases each year, and it is estimated that by 2010 there will be approximately 650,000 patients with ESRD (Walser, 2004).

Many patients who are developing kidney disease and early renal failure are unaware due to the lack of symptoms in the early stages. There are those who are at risk for renal failure due to inherited susceptibilities or dangerous behaviors. At-risk groups include:

- **Being African American**—This population has almost twice the frequency of ESRD than the population at large and comprises 30% of patients with ERSD (Walser, 2004).

- **Genetics**—Many first-degree relatives, such as siblings or children, of patients with ESRD have signs of renal disease. The explanation is not yet clear, but statistics reveal a strong familial factor (Walser, 2004).

- **Polycystic kidney disease**—As stated earlier in this chapter, polycystic kidney disease is an inherited condition, with half of the children of patients with the disease developing the disorder.

Diseases that lead to an increased risk of renal failure include:

- **Diabetes**—In the United States today, patients with diabetes comprise the largest group of patients starting dialysis (Walser, 2004). The cardiovascular changes that develop with diabetes gradually decrease the circulation to the kidneys and eventually cause irreversible damage. Recent studies have revealed that close control of blood glucose levels in those patients with insulin-dependent diabetes reduces the incidence of renal failure (Follin & Lenker, 2004; Walser, 2004).

- **Hypertension**—Hypertension is one of the most common disorders in the United States (Walser, 2004). Vascular changes with this disease cause a decrease in circulation to the kidneys, gradually damaging the nephrons.

- **Potassium deficiency**—Chronic diarrhea or an overuse of laxatives can cause chronic potassium deficiency. The kidney's ability to produce concentrated urine, and to decrease output in response to dehydration, is impaired by potassium deficiency. Patients with potassium deficiency tend to excrete large amounts of urine even though they have reduced kidney function. If the potassium deficiency is severe, the kidney may never recover and renal failure will occur (Walser, 2004).

- **Urinary tract obstruction**—Diseases that obstruct outflow of urine, such as enlarged prostate in men, will cause back pressure and hydronephrosis. If not treated, the hydronephrosis will distort the shape of the kidney and diminish the function.

- **Chronic glomerular disease**—Chronic glomerulonephritis scars and eventually destroys the ability of the glomeruli to function.

- **Chronic infection**—Chronic infections such as pyelonephritis or tuberculosis will also cause scarring and eventually destroy the ability of the kidney to function.

Laboratory and Diagnostic Procedures

The presence of any type of chronic kidney disease should be established as early as possible and be based on the presence of kidney damage and level of renal function through measurement of the glomerular filtration rate (GFR). Chronic kidney disease in adults is defined as evidence of structural or functional kidney abnormalities as revealed by abnormal urinalysis, imaging studies, or histology; or GFR < 60 mL · min⁻¹ · (1.73 m²)⁻¹ that persists for at least 3 months (Post & Rose, 2008c; Michigan Quality Improvement Consortium, 2006). The extent of the disease is classified based on the level of renal function. The National Kidney Foundation defines the stages as:

Stage 1: Kidney damage with normal or increased GFR, GFR ≥ 90 mL · min⁻¹ · (1.73 m²)⁻¹

Stage 2: Kidney damage with mild decrease in GFR, GFR = 60 to 89 mL · min⁻¹ · (1.73 m²)⁻¹

Stage 3: Moderate decrease in GFR, GFR = 30 to 59 mL · min⁻¹ · (1.73 m²)⁻¹

Stage 4: Severe decrease in GFR, GFR = 15 to 29 mL · min⁻¹ · (1.73 m²)⁻¹

Stage 5: Kidney failure, GFR < 15 mL · min⁻¹ · (1.73 m²)⁻¹ or dialysis.

(Michigan Quality Improvement Consortium, 2006)

Diagnosis of chronic renal failure is made through clinical assessment and a history of progressive debilitation with gradual deterioration of renal function. One of the earliest symptoms of chronic renal failure, and also the most common, is fatigue. The patient may describe feeling tired all of the time or tiring quickly with mild activity. The patient may also describe a loss of the sense of well-being. The cause of fatigue is unclear and is disproportionate to the anemia that develops with chronic renal disease. Fatigue is one of the most prevalent causes of disability in patients with chronic renal failure (Walser, 2004).

Muscle cramps, typically involving the calf muscles, are the second most common complaint of patients with chronic renal failure (Walser, 2004). The cramps can be very painful and are often experienced at night. The exact cause is unknown, but a decreased potassium or sodium level can make the cramps worse.

As the blood urea concentration increases, the patient may have a loss of appetite with accompanying nausea and vomiting. Intensive nutritional counseling and calculation of dietary needs to prevent weight loss are very important for the well-being of the patient with chronic renal failure and will be discussed later in this chapter.

Chronic renal failure eventually produces changes throughout all body systems.

- Cardiovascular changes
  - Hypertension
  - Cardiomyopathy
  - Uremic pericarditis
  - Pericardial effusion
  - Heart failure
  - Peripheral edema
  - Arrhythmias
- Respiratory changes
  - Increased susceptibility to infection due to pulmonary macrophage activity
  - Pulmonary edema
  - Pleural effusions
  - Uremic pleuritis
  - Uremic pneumonitis
  - Dyspnea due to heart failure
  - Kussmaul's respirations due to acidosis
- Gastrointestinal changes
  - Inflammation and ulceration of gastrointestinal mucosa
  - Ulceration and bleeding gums
  - Esophagitis
  - Gastritis
  - Duodenal ulcers
  - Uremic colitis
  - Pancreatitis
  - Proctitis
  - Uremic fetor: ammonia smell to breath
  - Anorexia
  - Nausea and vomiting
- Neurological changes
  - Peripheral neuropathy causing pain, burning, and itching in the legs and feet; eventually progresses to paresthesia and footdrop from motor nerve dysfunction
  - Shortened memory and attention span
  - Drowsiness
  - Irritability
  - Confusion
  - Coma
  - Seizures
- Endocrine changes
  - Stunted growth in children
  - Infertility and decreased libido in both sexes
  - Amenorrhea
  - Impotence and decreased sperm production in men
  - Increased aldosterone secretion due to increased renin production
  - Increased blood glucose levels due to impaired carbohydrate metabolism
- Hematopoietic changes
  - Anemia
  - Decreased red blood cell survival time
  - Blood loss from dialysis and gastrointestinal bleeding
  - Mild thrombocytopenia
  - Platelet defects
  - Increase in bleeding and clotting disorders
- Skeletal changes
  - Calcium–phosphorus imbalance and parathyroid imbalance cause:
    - Skeletal pain
    - Skeletal demineralization
    - Pathologic fractures
    - Calcifications in the brain, eyes, gums, joints, myocardium, and blood vessels

- Cutaneous changes
  - Skin appears yellowish bronze, dry, and scaly
  - Itching
  - Purpura
  - Ecchymosis
  - Petechiae
  - Thin, brittle fingernails with lines
  - Dry, brittle hair that may fall out easily

Tests that are helpful in the diagnosis of chronic renal failure are presented in the Diagnostic Tests box.

Medical Management

Treatment is aimed at slowing the progression of the disease by treating any underlying condition that may be contributing to or causing the failure; treating specific symptoms; and minimizing complications. As the disease progresses, identification of potential patients for dialysis is necessary to prepare them adequately.

Reversible causes of decreased renal function in the patient with chronic renal failure include hypovolemia from vomiting, diarrhea, diuretic use, or bleeding, and hypotension due to myocardial dysfunction, sepsis, or pericardial disease. In the case of hypovolemia, fluid replacement may result in the return of renal function to the previous baseline.

For patients with chronic renal failure, the administration of drugs or diagnostic contrast will adversely affect renal function. The use of drugs that lower the glomerular filtration rate (such as NSAIDs and ACE inhibitors), aminoglycoside antibiotics, and radiographic contrast should be avoided.

Medical Management to Slow Progression

To slow the progression of the failure, protective mechanisms are employed. Studies have suggested that progression may be due in part to secondary factors such as intraglomerular hypertension and hypertrophy; glomerular scarring; hyperlipidemia;

metabolic acidosis; and tubulointerstitial disease (Post & Rose, 2008c). Therefore, antihypertensive therapy is given for both renal protection and cardiovascular protection, because there is a marked increase in cardiovascular risk with chronic renal failure. Patients are usually administered angiotensin-converting enzyme (ACE) inhibitors or angiotensin II receptor blockers (ARBs). The goal is a reduction in blood pressure to less than 130/80 mmHg (Post & Rose, 2008c). If the goal is not reached with an ACE inhibitor or an ARB, then a diuretic is added and, if necessary, diltiazem, verapamil, or a beta-blocker.

 *ACE inhibitors and angiotension II receptor blockers (ARBs) can cause a decrease in renal function and an increase in plasma potassium soon after the onset of therapy. Repeat plasma creatinine and potassium within 3 to 5 days.*

Patients with chronic renal failure without dialysis should have dietary interviews every 3 months with measurement of serum albumin and body weight. The deterioration of the patient's nutritional status often begins early in the course of the disease. Malnutrition in patients that are about to begin maintenance dialysis is a strong predictor of poor clinical outcome (Hogan, 2007). For patients who are not undergoing dialysis, a low-protein diet consisting of 0.60 g/kg per day should be considered. When well monitored, a low-protein, high-energy diet maintains nutritional support while limiting the potentially toxic nitrogenous metabolites, development of uremic symptoms, and occurrence of other metabolic complications. Low-protein diets can decrease the effects of hyperphosphatemia, metabolic acidosis, hyperkalemia, and other electrolyte disorders.

The energy expenditure and requirements of a nondialyzed patient with chronic renal failure is similar to that of healthy adults. A diet providing approximately 35 kcal/kg per day has been shown to maintain neutral nitrogen balance, to promote higher serum albumin concentrations, and to reduce the urea nitrogen appearance (Hogan, 2007). Patients who are age 60 or older tend to be

DIAGNOSTIC TESTS for Chronic Renal Failure

Test	Expected Abnormality	Rationale for Abnormality
Serum electrolytes:		
Urea nitrogen	Increased	Impaired glomerular filtration
Creatinine	Increased	
Potassium	Increased	
Sodium	Increased	
Hemoglobin and hematocrit	Decreased	Insufficient production of erythropoietin
Arterial pH and bicarbonate levels	Decreased	Impaired glomerular filtration
Urinalysis	Presence of red blood cell casts, proteinuria	Impaired filtration
	Low specific gravity (1.010)	Decreased ability to concentrate urine
	Low osmolality (less than 400 mOsm/kg)	
Radiography:		
Renal ultrasound	Reduced kidney size	Permanent damage to the kidney
Computed tomography *should be done without contrast*	Characterization of the parenchyma and collecting systems	
	Reveals decreased function	
Isotopic renal scan	May show decreased perfusion	
Kidney biopsy	Histologic identification of underlying pathology	Identifies pathology

less physically active, so an intake of 30 to 35 kcal/kg per day may be sufficient. It may be difficult for patients to achieve this level of energy intake, and nutritional supplements with high energy density may be necessary.

The patient who is on maintenance dialysis, either hemodialysis or peritoneal dialysis, is recommended to have a dietary protein intake of 1.2 g/kg per day with at least 50% of the protein being of high biologic value. Protein that is considered of high biologic value has an amino acid composition similar to human protein, is usually an animal protein, and tends to be utilized more efficiently by humans to conserve body proteins. Daily energy intake for the patient requiring dialysis is the same as for the patient without dialysis.

Medical Management of Complications of Renal Failure

As stated, renal failure affects many body systems. Multiple complications may arise due to the loss of renal function. The patient should be monitored closely and have any complication treated.

The kidneys are able to maintain sodium and intravascular volume balance until the GFR falls below 10 to 15 mL/min. Even though the patient with mild to moderate failure is able to maintain fluid balance, he is less able to respond to a rapid infusion of sodium and is prone to fluid overload. Most patients with renal failure who experience fluid overload respond to a combination of dietary sodium restriction and diuretic therapy with a loop diuretic given daily.

Hyperkalemia usually develops in the patient who is oliguric and has a high intake of potassium in her diet, increased tissue breakdown, or hypoaldosteronism due in part to the administration of an ACE inhibitor. Hyperkalemia in conjunction with administration of an ACE inhibitor usually occurs when the serum potassium is elevated prior to therapy. If this is the case, institution of a low-potassium diet or use of a loop diuretic in conjunction often decreases the degree of hyperkalemia. For some patients, a low dose of Kayexalate (5 grams with each meal), can lower the serum potassium concentration.

Patients with chronic renal failure tend to retain hydrogen ions and progressively develop metabolic acidosis with serum bicarbonate concentrations between 12 and 20 mEq/L. Treatment of even mild acidemia is desirable, because bone buffering of some of the excess hydrogen ions is linked with the release of calcium and phosphate from the bone, worsening the bone disease. Also, uremic acidosis can increase skeletal muscle breakdown and diminish albumin synthesis, eventually causing loss of lean body mass and weakness. Treatment consists of administration of sodium bicarbonate 0.5 to 1 mEq/kg per day. Sodium citrate may also be used but is avoided in a patient taking aluminum-containing antacids, as it enhances intestinal aluminum absorption.

Phosphate retention starts early in renal disease due to decreased filtration. The condition remains mild with hyperphosphatemia occurring late, but the retention is related to the development of secondary hyperparathyroidism. The parathyroid gland hypersecretes parathyroid hormone (PTH) to correct both hyperphosphatemia and hypocalcemia, and in the early stages of renal disease maintains a phosphate balance in the patient with a GFR greater than 30 mL/min. Dietary phosphate restriction may delay the development of secondary hyperparathyroidism, but this can be accomplished only by limiting protein intake, which is

not acceptable to many. Once the GFR falls below 25 to 30 mL/min, oral phosphate binders are usually required. Guidelines recommend keeping serum phosphorus levels between 2.7 and 4.6 mg/dL in patients with chronic renal failure and between 3.5 and 5.5 mg/dL in patients with end-stage renal disease. The most widely used phosphate binder is calcium carbonate. The dose ranges from 2.5 to 20 g/day and is increased gradually until the serum phosphate falls or hypercalcemia ensues. Close monitoring of the serum calcium concentration is needed, as hypercalcemia is a common complication of this therapy.

 *Phosphate binders are most effective when taken with meals to bind dietary phosphate.*

There is also a nonabsorbable agent, sevelamer, that does not contain calcium or aluminum. Sevelamer is a cationic polymer that binds with phosphate through ion exchange. It is used in patients who cannot tolerate calcium carbonate or who exhibit a persistent hyperphosphatemia. Other phosphate binders such as aluminum hydroxide, magnesium hydroxide, and calcium citrate should be avoided due to their side effects of aluminum toxicity and hypermagnesemia with the magnesium hydroxide. All phosphate binders have limited binding capacity and should be used in conjunction with a carefully planned diet that restricts phosphorus when possible.

Hypertension is present in 80% to 85% of chronic renal failure patients (Post & Rose, 2008c). Fluid retention contributes to the elevation of blood pressure; therefore, control is usually achieved with a combined therapy of ACE inhibitor or ARB and a diuretic. As stated previously, the recommended blood pressure goal is less than 130/80 mmHg.

The anemia associated with chronic renal failure is due primarily to reduced production of erythropoietin and shortened red cell survival. Although anemia is present in most patients with chronic renal failure, the patient should be evaluated for all other causes prior to instituting a therapy. In patients with end-stage renal disease, epoetin alfa (EPO) or darbepoetin alfa therapy helps to correct the anemia. Erythropoietic agents are given to patients who are predialysis with a hemoglobin concentration less than 11 g/dL. Guidelines suggest that the initial erythropoietin dose should be approximately 80 to 120 units/kg per week (Post & Rose, 2008c). The hemoglobin level should be tested weekly, and the dose or frequency adjusted. Darbepoetin alfa, another erythropoietic agent, has a longer half-life and greater biologic activity than recombinant erythropoietin and can be scheduled weekly, every 2 weeks, or monthly. The recommended starting dose for patients with chronic renal failure is 0.45 mcg/kg per week. The drug can be given intravenously or subcutaneously.

For an adequate response to erythropoietin or darbepoetin, the patient must have sufficient iron stores. This usually requires the administration of oral or intravenous iron to maintain a serum ferritin level of greater than 100 ng/mL. Patients are most commonly given 325 milligrams of ferrous sulfate three times daily. Severe anemia may require the infusion of fresh frozen packed cells or washed packed cells.

A tendency to bleed is present in both acute and chronic renal failure due to platelet dysfunction. If the patient is asymptomatic, no therapy is indicated. If the patient is actively bleeding or is scheduled for an invasive procedure, then therapy may consist of the administration of desmopressin acetate (DDAVP), which improves platelet function by increasing levels of factor VIII; cryoprecipitate; and the initiation of dialysis.

Patients with advanced renal failure may present with uremic pericarditis. They will complain of fever, pleuritic chest pain, and have a pericardial friction rub. Because it is a metabolic pericarditis and epicardial injury is uncommon, the electrocardiogram will usually not show the typical diffuse ST and T wave elevation seen with other forms of pericarditis. This development is an indication to institute dialysis. With dialysis, most patients will have a resolution of chest pain and a decrease in the size of the effusion.

If end-stage renal disease goes untreated, the patient will develop uremic neuropathy with dysfunction of the central and peripheral nervous systems, including encephalopathy leading to seizures and coma. Signs of sensory dysfunction, such as restless leg or burning feet syndrome, are frequent presentations of uremic neuropathy. These signs and symptoms are usually absolute indications for the initiation of dialysis.

Nursing Management

With chronic renal failure, management is aimed at slowing the progression of the disease to end-stage renal disease and avoiding complications. Patient education regarding control of underlying causes such as diabetes and hypertension is key. Infection, volume depletion, and the taking of nephrotoxic medications must be avoided to prevent further deterioration of renal function. As the patient reaches end-stage renal disease, management moves to dialysis or renal transplantation. The Nursing Process: Patient Care Plan outlines nursing care for chronic renal failure.

 *Medications that are excreted primarily by the kidneys require modification of dosage and/or frequency. Elderly patients with chronic renal failure that are taking digitalis must have careful dosage titration, as 85% of the drug is excreted by the kidneys.*

Collaborative Management

Working with a renal dietician is very beneficial. To slow progression of the disease, protein and phosphorus are restricted. Carbohydrates are increased to ensure that the patient has adequate caloric intake to prevent tissue catabolism. As the disease progresses, sodium intake is limited and fluids may be restricted. The kidneys' ability to excrete potassium is decreased; therefore, potassium intake is also limited. Providing a fact sheet listing foods that are restricted or limited is helpful. Provide sample menus to help the patient plan daily menus that incorporate these restrictions.

Patients may also benefit from psychological counseling to help them cope with a chronic illness and the uncertain future it entails.

Initiation of Maintenance Dialysis

For patients with chronic renal failure, the decision to initiate maintenance dialysis or renal transplantation involves discussion between the patient and the health care provider with consideration of subjective and objective data. It is important to explore with the patient his perception of his quality of life and the changes that will occur, in the case of dialysis, with a therapy that is technologically complex. With hemodialysis, the treatment regimen is based on two factors: the restriction of certain nutrients and the removal of waste metabolites from the blood by regular dialysis. The management is effective only if the patient adheres closely with the therapeutic regimen. Although hemodialysis can effectively contribute to long-term survival of patients with ESRD, morbidity and mortality of patients on dialysis remain high, especially due to cardiovascular disease. Approximately 33% of patients on hemodialysis survive past 5 years of treatment, whereas 70% of recipients of kidney transplant are alive after 5 years (Denhaerynck et al., 2007).

The absolute clinical indications to initiate renal replacement therapy include:

- Pericarditis
- Volume overload or pulmonary edema that is refractory to diuretics
- Increasing hypertension that is minimally responsive to antihypertensive medications
- Progressive uremic encephalopathy or neuropathy
- Persistent nausea and vomiting
- Plasma creatinine concentration above 12 mg/dL or blood urea nitrogen greater than 100 mg/dL (Ismail, 2008).

Early recognition of chronic renal failure allows for renoprotective therapy such as rigorous blood pressure control and protective dietary changes, as discussed earlier. Early recognition enables dialysis to be initiated at an optimal time and may also permit the recruitment and evaluation of family members for the placement of a renal allograft before the need for dialysis arises (Post & Rose, 2008c).

Relative indications to initiate renal replacement therapy include:

- Anorexia progressing to nausea and vomiting
- Decreased attentiveness
- Decreased cognitive tasking
- Depression
- Severe anemia that is unresponsive to erythropoietin
- Persistent pruritus or restless leg syndrome (Ismail, 2008).

The advantage of starting dialysis when relative indications are present is to enhance the quality of life and to prolong survival. Dialysis has also been shown to improve multiple nutritional indexes including serum albumin, iron, transferrin saturation, creatinine, and the nPNA (protein nitrogen appearance) over the first 6 months of therapy (Ismail, 2008).

When the decision has been made to begin renal replacement therapy, discussion should commence with the patient regarding the advantages and disadvantages of hemodialysis, peritoneal dialysis (continuous or intermittent), and renal transplantation (living or deceased donor).

Hemodialysis

To perform hemodialysis, the patient must have vascular access. For acute access a dual-lumen venous catheter may be used. The outflow openings are proximal to the inflow openings on the opposite side to avoid dialyzing the same blood that was just returned to the vessel. The subclavian, internal jugular, and femoral veins are usually used for this short-term access, and the catheters can be inserted at the bedside. Percutaneous catheters

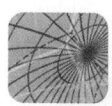

Assessment of Fluid Status

Subjective Data:
How much fluid have you been taking in?
Have you felt short of breath?
Have you gained weight?

Objective Data:
Assess:
Patient weight
Skin turgor

Presence of edema
Blood pressure
Respiratory effort and lung sounds

Nursing Assessment and Diagnoses	Outcomes and Evaluation Parameters	Planning and Interventions with *Rationales*
Nursing Diagnosis: *Fluid Volume, Excess* related to compromised regulatory mechanisms secondary to renal failure	**Outcome:** Neither fluid volume excess nor deficient volume will occur. **Evaluation Parameters:** Demonstrates no rapid weight changes. Absence of edema. Normal skin turgor. Reports no difficulty breathing.	**Interventions and *Rationales:*** Assess dietary intake and habits that may contribute to excess fluid volume. *To identify potential sources of fluid such as foods high in sodium, medications that contain fluid, or amount of fluid taken with medications.* Teach patient/family rationale for restrictions. *Understanding promotes cooperation.* Teach and encourage need for frequent oral hygiene. *To minimize dry mouth associated with fluid restriction.*

Assessment of Nutritional Intake

Subjective Data:
Describe your usual intake pattern.
Is this intake sufficient?
Do you have religious dietary restrictions or practices?
How often do you exercise?
Who prepares your meals?
Do you feel you have enough energy?

Objective Data:
Assess:
General appearance
Weight

Hair, nails, and skin
Muscle mass
Edema

Nursing Assessment and Diagnoses	Outcomes and Evaluation Parameters	Planning and Interventions with *Rationales*
Nursing Diagnosis: *Nutrition, Imbalanced: Less than Body Requirements*	**Outcome:** The patient will maintain adequate nutrition. **Evaluation Parameter:** Maintenance of weight without loss of muscle mass.	**Interventions and *Rationales:*** Facilitate education with a renal dietary consultant. *Consultation can ensure a diet that provides optimal caloric and nutrient intake.* Encourage frequent oral hygiene. *Poor oral hygiene leads to bad breath and taste in the mouth, which decreases the appetite.* Provide the patient with printed material outlining the dietary needs and restrictions. *To aid the patient in selecting the proper foods.* Promote the intake of protein foods with high biologic value: eggs, meats, and dairy products. *Complete proteins provide positive nitrogen balance needed for growth and healing.*

Assessment of Activity Tolerance

Subjective Data:
Are you able to perform activities of daily living?
Do you experience pain that interferes with activity?
Are there activities you feel you are unable to do?

Objective Data:
Assess strength and balance.
Assess response to activity by taking vital signs at rest and then after performing an activity.
Assess coping strategies.

Nursing Assessment and Diagnoses	Outcomes and Evaluation Parameters	Planning and Interventions with *Rationales*
Nursing Diagnosis: *Activity Intolerance* related to fatigue, anemia, and altered metabolic state	**Outcome:** Patient will have a balance of rest and activity to aid participation without fatigue. **Evaluation Parameters:** Alternates rest and activity. Reports a decrease in fatigue and an increased sense of well-being. Participates in self-care activities.	**Interventions and *Rationales:*** Promote independence in self-care as tolerated. *To promote self-esteem.* Encourage naps between activities. *To promote activity within patient's limits.* Assess factors that may be contributing to fatigue: Fluid and electrolyte imbalances Anemia Depression. *To identify factors contributing to fatigue.*

(continued)

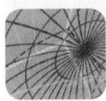

NURSING PROCESS: Patient Care Plan for Chronic Renal Failure—*Continued*

Assessment of Knowledge of Disease Process

Subjective Data:
What causes renal failure?
What is the relationship of fluid and dietary restrictions to renal disease?
What is your understanding of renal failure?

Objective Data:
Patient follows treatment regimen and is able to articulate understanding of disease process.

Nursing Assessment and Diagnoses	Outcomes and Evaluation Parameters	Planning and Interventions with *Rationales*
Nursing Diagnosis: *Therapeutic Regimen Management, Ineffective* related to lack of knowledge of disease process and treatment	**Outcome:** Understands cause of renal failure and need for treatment. *Evaluation Parameters:* Patient can explain fluid and dietary restrictions and their relationship to kidney failure. Uses written information to clarify questions.	**Interventions and *Rationales:*** Assess understanding of disease process. *To provide baseline for teaching needs.* Assist patient to identify ways to incorporate treatment into his lifestyle. *To help build self-esteem.* Assist patient to obtain written information about renal disease. *To give the patient information that can be reviewed at home.*

in the subclavian or jugular vein may be left in place for 1 to 3 weeks. Catheters placed in the femoral vein can remain for up to 1 week.

For patients who require long-term or maintenance dialysis, vascular access is imperative and often a major problem. There are various forms of access, including arteriovenous fistula, arteriovenous graft, and arteriovenous shunt (Figure 47–2 ■). All of these allow access to the arterial circulation and return to the venous circulation.

Arteriovenous (AV) graft is the most common form of access for treating chronic renal failure. The graft consists of a Gortex tube that is surgically implanted into the forearm. A surgical in-

cision is made; an artery and vein are identified; then a tunnel, either straight or U-shaped, is created; and the graft is anastomosed to the artery and vein. After the surgical site is closed, the graft creates a raised area that looks like a large peripheral vein. During dialysis two large-bore needles are placed for outflow from and inflow to the graft. When the needles are removed, firm pressure is required until bleeding subsides.

An AV fistula is formed by creating a surgical incision, identifying a peripheral artery and vein, then creating an opening in both the artery and vein, and anastomosing the two openings. The anastomosis may be side to side, end to end, or end to side. The high pressure from the arterial flow creates a pseudo-

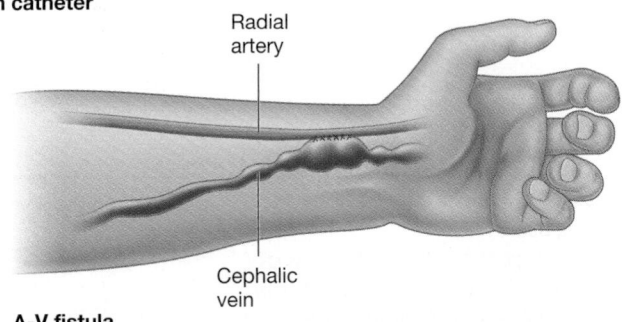

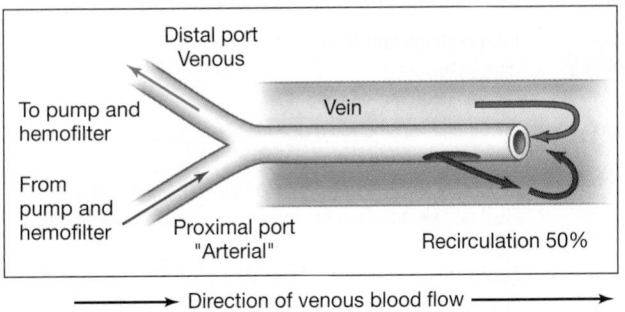

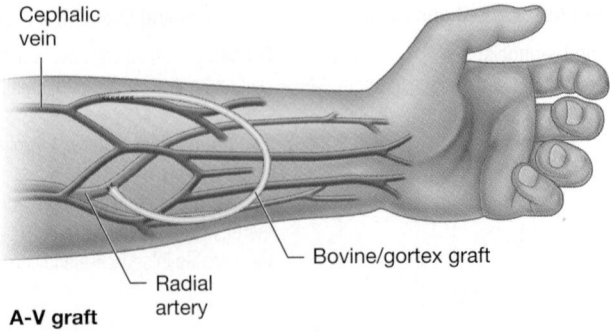

FIGURE 47–2 ■ Types of vascular access.

aneurysm of the vein that, when healed, a large-bore needle can be inserted into for dialysis. The fistula must mature and may require weeks to months before developing sufficient flow. If the fistula is accessed before it is developed, painful vascular spasm may occur. AV fistulas also have the potential of creating arterial insufficiency due to the high arterial blood flow diverted for dialysis. The symptoms that occur are known as vascular steal syndrome. The extremity becomes pale, cool, and painful. The nurse may assess patency of the fistula by palpation or auscultation. A patent fistula has a thrill when palpated and a bruit when auscultated with a stethoscope. The extremity should also be assessed and should be warm to the touch with good color.

AV external shunts are created by performing a cutdown over a peripheral artery and then a vein; a Teflon silicone cannula is implanted in both the artery and vein and is connected to silicone rubber tubing that exits from the skin. The two ends are then connected by an external U-shaped shunt that has a connector at the midpoint. The connection can be opened after both sides of the shunt are clamped, and then both sides are attached to the dialysis machine. External shunts are associated with complications such as infection and bleeding. Because of these, external shunts are rarely used for chronic maintenance dialysis.

The nursing implications for access devices are to protect the patency of the device and prevent infection. Complications involving access devices are one of the leading causes for hospitalization of patients on renal dialysis. Nursing management of complications of AV fistulas and grafts is described in Chart 47–3.

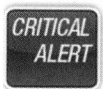 *Blood pressure measurements, blood draws, and intravenous lines should never be performed on the arm that has the access device.*

To initiate dialysis, two large-bore needles are placed in the fistula or graft. Arterial blood is sent from the patient to the dialyzer with the assistance of a pump. Prior to dialysis, the machine is primed with saline so no air is in the system. At the beginning of dialysis, the saline is discarded as the blood fills the dialyzer circuit. Heparin is added to the blood as it enters the dialyzer, because blood has a tendency to clot when it encounters a foreign substance. The blood then enters the extracorporeal circuit, a long plastic cartridge that contains thousands of parallel hollow fibers, which are a semipermeable membrane made of a synthetic material. Dialysis fluid, called dialysate, is pumped into the cartridge, bathing the fibers; and through osmosis and diffusion, exchanges of fluid, electrolytes, and toxins from the blood enter the dialysate. The dialysate and blood are pumped in opposite directions through the dialyzer to maintain a high osmotic and chemical gradient. After the blood leaves the dialyzer, it is returned to the patient via the venous line through the second needle. At the end of the procedure, the dialysis machine is filled with saline to return all of the patient's blood to her. Each dialysis treatment takes between 3 and 4 hours, and most patients require treatment three times a week. Although dialysis is very efficient, it does not remove all metabolites. In between each dialysis treatment, electrolytes, toxins, and fluids increase. Contraindications to hemodialysis include hemodynamic instability, lack of access, and inability to anticoagulate. Chart 47–4 lists the complications of hemodialysis. The research topics related to dialysis are outlined in the Research Opportunities and Clinical Impact box (p. 1488). The Evidence-Based Practice box (p. 1488) discusses the success of hemodialysis.

Peritoneal Dialysis

Peritoneal dialysis is the infusion of sterile dialyzing fluid through an implanted catheter in the abdominal cavity. The dialysate fluid bathes the peritoneal membrane that covers the abdominal organs and overlies the capillary beds. As occurs with hemodialysis, excess fluid and solutes travel via osmosis, diffusion, and active transport from the peritoneal capillary fluid through the capillary walls, through the peritoneal membrane, into the dialyzing fluid. After a prescribed amount of time, the fluid is drained from the abdomen by gravity.

Peritoneal dialysis may be performed as continuous or intermittent. Continuous ambulatory peritoneal dialysis, or CAPD, requires multiple exchanges during the day and a continuous

CHART 47–3	Nursing Management of Complications of AV Fistulas and Grafts
Complication	**Nursing Management**
Grafts and Fistulas	
Infection	Use aseptic technique when cannulating access.
Bleeding	Do not cannulate new access too early.
Thrombosis	Teach patients not to wear anything constrictive on the accessed arm.
Pseudoaneurysm	Avoid multiple cannulations in the same area.
Pain from vascular steal syndrome	Apply warm compresses and administer analgesia.
Fistulas	
Inadequate blood flow	Teach patients to develop blood flow through daily exercises such as squeezing a ball while applying slight impedance to the flow distal to the access point.

CHART 47–4	Complications of Hemodialysis
Complication	**Cause**
Hypotension	Rapid removal of vascular volume Decreased systemic vascular resistance Decreased cardiac output
Loss of blood	Residual blood not rinsed from the dialyzer Accidental separation of vascular tubing Dialysis membrane rupture Bleeding from access site after removal of needles
Muscle cramps	Rapid removal of sodium and water
Hepatitis	Blood transfusions IV drug abuse
Sepsis	Infection of the vascular access site Introduction of bacteria during dialysis due to poor technique or interruption of tubing
Disequilibrium syndrome (development of cerebral edema)	Rapid changes in the composition of the extracellular fluid due to removal of solutes from the blood more rapidly than from the cerebrospinal fluid and the brain

EVIDENCE-BASED PRACTICE

Hemodialysis

Clinical Problem

Registries within the United States and Europe show an increase in the prevalence and incidence of end-stage renal disease. Only 32% to 33% of patients on hemodialysis survive beyond their fifth year of treatment. In comparison, 70% of patients who have kidney transplants survive beyond their fifth-year post transplant (Denhaerynck et al., 2007). The success of hemodialysis depends on following a regimen of fluid restriction, dietary guidelines, medication prescriptions, and attendance at hemodialysis sessions.

Research Findings

Denhaerynck et al. (2007) reviewed the literature looking at the four aspects of success with hemodialysis. Results of nonadherence regarding fluid restriction, dietary guidelines, medication prescriptions, and attendance at hemodialysis sessions varied greatly depending on how the study was conducted and which country the subjects were from. Most of the studies concentrated on adherence to fluid restriction, but adherence to the entire prescribed medical regimen is crucial for achieving good therapeutic results and reducing morbidity and mortality. Fluid nonadherence can result in fluid overload and provoke shortness of breath, dizziness, anxiety, panic, lung edema, and hypertension. Nonadherence to medication and dietary regimens can result in elevated serum levels of phosphate, which plays a role in the development of secondary hyperparathyroidism and renal osteodystrophy. Elevated levels of phosphate also contribute to coronary artery disease, which significantly increases the risk for mortality. Skipping or shortening dialysis is associated with increased mortality. Denhaerynck and colleagues found in their review of the literature that "In studies in which the delivered dialysis dose was determined by assessing appointment nonadherence, the relationship between the dose and higher mortality or higher blood pressure was significant. Skipping at least one dialysis session per month has been associated with a 25% to 30% higher risk of death."

Implications for Nursing Practice

After reviewing the literature, Denhaerynck et al. (2007) believed that "The prevalence of nonadherence with the different aspects of the dialysis regimen seems considerable. However, assessment of nonadherence has two major obstacles: inconsistencies in definitions and invalid measurement methods." Despite these issues, the evidence suggests that the behavioral dimension of hemodialysis should be considered to guarantee adherence to the treatment regimen and adequate treatment results. Nurses are in an excellent position to affect the behavioral dimension by assessing adherence and by implementing adherence-enhancing interventions and patient teaching that have the ultimate goal of improving clinical outcomes.

Critical Thinking Questions

1. Discuss the consequences of nonadherence to fluid, dietary, and medication regimens.

2. How can the nurse help the patient to be adherent with his hemodialysis regimen?

Answers to Critical Thinking Questions appear in Appendix D.

Reference

Denhaerynck, K., Manhaeve, D., Dobbels, F., Garzoni, D., Nolte, C., & De Geest, S. (2007). Prevalence and consequences of nonadherence to hemodialysis regimens. *American Journal of Critical Care, 16*(3), 222–235.

Source: Adapted from: Denhaerynck, K., Manhaeve, D., Dobbels, F., Garzoni, D., Nolte, C., & De Geest, S. (2007). Prevalence and consequences of nonadherence to hemodialysis regimens. American Journal of Critical Care, 16(3), 222–235.

RESEARCH OPPORTUNITIES AND CLINICAL IMPACT RELATED TO DIALYSIS

Research Area	Clinical Impact
What are the optimum serum bicarbonate and blood pH levels for patients on maintenance dialysis?	Data available for patients without renal insufficiency indicate that a mid-normal or high-normal blood pH range maintains better nutritional status than the low-normal range.
What are the long-term effects of correcting acidemia on clinical and nutrition-related outcomes?	Tight control of acidemia may improve nutritional status, but in the long term how will it affect morbidity and mortality?
Development of a simple and inexpensive method for determining the energy expenditure in individual acutely ill patients.	A simple method would enhance the monitoring of patients with renal failure. It would assist in defining how energy needs may vary with different protein and amino acid intakes.
The effects of different levels of protein intake on outcome and nutritional markers of patients on dialysis.	Increasing protein intake can alter dialysis requirements. It would be valuable to define the effect of higher levels of protein intake on the optimal dose of dialysis.
Which energy sources (protein, amino acids, carbohydrates, and fat) are associated with optimal clinical outcomes for patients with renal failure?	Maintaining optimal nutritional status and energy is crucial to the patient's progression and quality of life.

dwell overnight. The nighttime dwell can be accomplished with an exchange device, which would then perform two exchanges overnight. Continuous cyclic peritoneal dialysis, or CCPD, has a continuous daytime dwell with an exchange device exchanging several cycles overnight.

Intermittent peritoneal dialysis, or IPD, has periods in which dialysate is in the abdomen (wet abdomen) and periods in which the peritoneal cavity has been drained (dry abdomen). Patients who are unable to tolerate the full volume of dialysate or who leak at the catheter site may use a technique called tidal peritoneal dialysis, or TPD. TPD uses exchanges whereby the peritoneal cavity always contains some dialysate, usually up to half the regular amount. TPD is used infrequently, because it requires larger amounts of dialysate, which becomes very expensive.

Nursing Management

The amount of, concentration of, and dwell time for the dialysate are determined by the health care provider. When performing IPD, it is important to obtain baseline vital signs and weight for comparison at the end of the drainage. Measurement of abdominal girth and respiratory status is helpful as an indication of fluid retention. Assess for the presence of edema and obtain lab work for status of electrolytes, hematology, and blood glucose levels. When connecting or disconnecting the solution to the catheter, it is imperative to use good aseptic technique to prevent entry of bacteria into the peritoneal cavity. Dialysate fluid should be at least body temperature to provide comfort and enhance exchange. When the fluid is removed, it is important to assess its appearance. The outflow fluid should be straw colored and not be cloudy or blood tinged, which might indicate peritonitis. Compare the amount of dialysate infused to the outflow amount to determine whether less fluid drained out, and the patient is fluid balance positive; or whether there was more outflow volume than was infused, and the patient is fluid balance negative.

If it is anticipated that the patient will be doing CAPD or CCPD, the nursing focus is on teaching the patient/family how to perform the dialysis. Use of aseptic technique and signs and symptoms of infection are particularly important aspects to be taught.

Kidney Transplantation

Kidney transplantation is the treatment of choice for end-stage renal disease because it improves the quality of life and reduces the mortality risk for most patients (Post & Rose, 2008a). Restoring kidney function reverses many of the pathophysiological changes that occur with renal failure. Transplantation eliminates the dependence on and restrictions associated with dialysis. Maintenance of a successful kidney transplant costs much less than the continued need for dialysis.

A kidney for transplantation may be from a living donor, such as a relative with compatible tissue type, or a human cadaver. The success of the transplant is increased if it is received before dialysis is initiated. The success of the transplant is dependent on careful tissue typing before the transplant and immunosuppression after the transplant. Rejection is the major complication related to transplant surgery. These rejections are potentially reversible and are treated with increased immunosuppression. Signs of rejection are oliguria, sudden weight gain, fever, a rise in BUN and serum creatinine, hypertension, and pain over the graft site. The long-term complications, which occur secondary to the use of immunosuppressive drugs, include infection, hypertension, chronic liver disease, bone demineralization, cardiovascular disease, cancer, cataracts, and gastrointestinal hemorrhage.

Nursing Management

The greatest risk to patients who have undergone transplantation is infection. Risk for infection occurs from invasive procedures, immunosuppression, and exposure to infected individuals. When caring for transplant patients, use of aseptic technique is paramount. It is important to teach the patient/family that due to the immunosuppressive medications the patient's response to infection will be muted. Teach them the importance of being sensitive to low-grade temperature elevation, any fever, and unexplained tachycardia. Also stress the importance of avoiding exposure to individuals known to have infections. See Chapter 27 ☺ for care of the postoperative patient. A listing of resources about renal failure is included in the National Guidelines box.

NATIONAL GUIDELINES for Renal Failure Resources

- **KDOQI clinical practice guidelines and clinical practice recommendations for anemia in chronic kidney disease. (2) 2007 update of hemoglobin target.**—National Kidney Foundation—Disease Specific Society. 1997 (updated 2006 May; addendum released 2007 Sep). Original guideline: 145 pages; addendum: 60 pages. (NGC:006019)

- **Diagnosis and management of adults with chronic kidney disease.**—Michigan Quality Improvement Consortium - Professional Association. 2006 Nov. 1 page. (NGC:005685)

- **NKF-K/DOQI clinical practice guidelines for peritoneal dialysis adequacy: Update 2006.**—National Kidney Foundation—Disease Specific Society. 1997 (updated 2006). 32 pages. (NGC:005330)

- **NKF-K/DOQI clinical practice guidelines for vascular access: Update 2006.**—National Kidney Foundation—Disease Specific Society. 1997 (updated 2006). 26 pages. (NGC:005331)

- **NKF-K/DOQI clinical practice guidelines and clinical practice recommendations for anemia in chronic kidney disease: 2007 update of hemoglobin target.**—National Kidney Foundation—Disease Specific Society. 1997 (updated 2007). 145 pages; addendum 60 pages. (NGC:006019)

- **NKF-K/DOQI clinical practice guidelines for hemodialysis adequacy: Update 2006.**—National Kidney Foundation—Disease Specific Society. 1997 (updated 2006). 85 pages. (NGC:005329)

Source: National Guideline Clearinghouse. Retrieved August 10, 2008, from http://www.guideline.gov

PHARMACOLOGY Summary of Drugs Used in Renal Disorders

Medication Category	Action	Application/Indication	Nursing Responsibility
Anti-infectives Quinolone Ciprofloxacin (Cipro) Norfloxacin (Noroxcin)	Inhibits DNA gyrase, an enzyme necessary for bacterial replication.	Urinary tract infections, acute pyelonephritis.	Obtain culture and sensitivity prior to administration. Assess for skin rash or other signs of hypersensitivity reaction. Patient teaching: Increase fluid intake while taking mediation. Do not take the following within 2 hours of taking the medication: aluminum or magnesium antacids, iron supplements, multivitamins with zinc, or sucralfate. Avoid exposure to excess sunlight or artificial UV light. Avoid NSAIDs. Do not breast-feed.
Antineoplastic alkylating agent Chemotherapy	Thought to be the result of cross-linkage of DNA strands blocking synthesis of DNA, RNA, and protein.	Cancer.	Monitor leucopenia. Assess for signs of infection. Monitor and report hematuria or dysuria. Protect patient from potential sources of infection. Patient teaching: Adhere to dosage regimen; and do not omit, increase, decrease, or delay doses. Hair loss occurs in some patients and will be noted 3 weeks after therapy begins. Amenorrhea may last up to 1 year after medication is stopped. Do not breast-feed.
Loop diuretic Furosemide (Lasix) Bumetanide Torsamide	Decreases renal vascular resistance. May increase renal blood flow.	Treatment of edema associated with kidney disease, including nephrotic syndrome.	Monitor for signs of hypokalemia: malaise, depressed reflexes, muscle weakness, rapid irregular pulse, hypotension, vomiting, and mental confusion. Monitor blood pressure. Monitor serum and urine electrolytes. Monitor input and output (I&O) ratio and pattern. Patient teaching: Consult health care team regarding allowable salt and fluid intake. Eat potassium-rich foods daily; bananas, oranges, peaches, and dried dates. Signs and symptoms of hypokalemia. Make position changes slowly to prevent dizziness or imbalance. Avoid prolonged exposure to direct sun. Do not breast-feed.
Corticosteroid: Dexamethasone Decadron Prednisolone (Prelone) Delta-Cortef	Immediate-acting synthetic analog of hydrocortisone. Effect depends on biotransformation to prednisolone.	May be used in cancer therapy, in inflammatory conditions, and as an immunosuppressant.	Monitor blood pressure; Report an ascending pattern. Monitor serum electrolytes. Monitor for signs of infection: Use of steroids may mask infection and delay healing. Assess for oral Candida infection. Long-term use: Monitor bone density. Patient teaching: Do not alter dosing regimen or stop medication suddenly. Appetite will improve and a slight weight gain is expected. Avoid alcohol and caffeine, as they may contribute to steroid ulcer development. Report any symptoms of GI distress to the health care team. Do not breast-feed.
Antihypertensives	Refer to Chapter 21 ☄.	Refer to Chapter 21 ☄.	Refer to Chapter 21 ☄.

DISORDERS OF THE BLADDER AND URINARY TRACT

The bladder stores urine and controls the elimination. Disorders affecting storage and elimination can result in incontinence or obstruction of urinary flow, which ultimately will affect renal function.

◼ Nephrolithiasis

Renal and ureteral calculi are formed when substances in the urine come out of solution and form a precipitate that accumulates and grows in size. The calculi may form anywhere in the urinary tract but most commonly develop in the renal pelvis or calyces of the kidneys and are generally referred to as *kidney stones*. In the United States, 1 in 1,000 people require hospitalization for renal calculi, with its being more prevalent in males than in females (Hager & Mills, 2008).

The calculi vary in size and may be single or multiple. They can remain in the renal pelvis or pass through the ureter to the bladder. Small calculi are often passed spontaneously in the urine, whereas larger calculi, when entering the ureter, may damage the renal parenchyma or become lodged and cause pressure necrosis. If the calculi cannot pass through the ureter, they will cause obstruction leading to hydronephrosis, as the kidney is unable excrete urine. A **staghorn calculus** is a calculus or stone that remains in the renal pelvis and becomes so large that it fills the pelvis completely, blocking the flow of urine.

As stated earlier, the calculi are formed from precipitation of substances normally dissolved in the urine. Eighty percent of patients form calcium stones, the most common being calcium oxalate and less commonly calcium phosphate (Curhan, Aronson, & Preminger, 2008). Other types include magnesium ammonium phosphate or, occasionally, urate or cystine. The exact cause is unknown, but predisposing factors include:

- **Infection**—The pH changes provide a favorable medium for formation of calculi, especially magnesium ammonium phosphate or calcium phosphate. Infected tissue also provides a site for the development. Bacteria may serve as the nucleus in calculus formation, which is common in magnesium ammonium phosphate or staghorn calculi.

- **Dehydration**—The decrease in urine production leads calculus-forming substances to become concentrated and to form calculi more easily.

- **Metabolic factors**—Predispositions to the formation of calculi from metabolic abnormalities are hyperparathyroidism; renal tubular acidosis; gout, due to the elevated uric acid levels; defective metabolism of oxalate; genetic defect in the metabolism of cystine; and excessive intake of vitamin D or dietary calcium.

- **Obstruction**—Any condition that results in urinary stasis, such as spinal cord injury, allows the calculus-forming substances to remain and adhere. Stasis also promotes infection, which compounds the problem.

There are also several hereditary diseases by which the patient may develop renal calculi. In patients who have a rare disease called renal tubular acidosis, 70% develop renal calculi. Cystinuria and hyperoxaluria are two other rare, inherited metabolic disorders that also tend to develop calculi. Hypercalciuria is an inherited disease that causes calcium from food to be absorbed in excess and lost into the urine. This high level of calcium in the urine causes calcium oxalate or calcium phosphate crystals and the formation of calculi.

Laboratory and Diagnostic Procedures

Pain is the primary symptom and is usually the result of obstruction. As the calculi attempt to pass, they may occlude the opening to the ureter, increasing the number and force of peristaltic contractions. Typically the pain is severe and colicky, and it travels from the costovertebral angle to the flank, and then to the suprapubic area and external genitalia. If the calculi remain in the renal pelvis and calyces, the pain will be more constant and dull in nature. Because the pain is severe, nausea and vomiting usually occur. The patient may also have hematuria from damage by the calculi. Tests that are helpful in the diagnosis of calculi are outlined in the Diagnostic Tests box (p. 1492).

Medical Management

The majority of renal calculi are smaller than 5 millimeters in diameter and are able to pass without invasive intervention. Treatment focuses on promoting the passage with vigorous hydration and pain control. Diuretics may be given to prevent urinary stasis and continuing calculus formation. The Pharmacology Summary feature on page 1496 presents medications used to treat bladder and urinary tract disorders.

If calculi are too large to pass, surgical intervention or lithotripsy may be required. A cystoscope may be inserted through the urethra to retrieve calculi from the ureter. A ureteroscope may be inserted through the ureter to remove calculi from the kidney. If the attempt to capture the stone is unsuccessful, electrohydraulic lithotripsy or laser lithotripsy may be used to break the stone apart into smaller particles that can pass naturally. Extracorporeal shock-wave lithotripsy is the use of acoustic shock waves that travel through soft tissues to shatter the calculi into fragments, which can then pass normally. The procedure may be performed with the patient immersed in a tank of water and is then called hydrolithotripsy.

◼ Nursing Management

It is important to try to determine the composition of the calculi to prevent further formation. Have the patient strain all urine through a urine strainer and send all solid material obtained to the lab for analysis. Encourage intake of fluids to facilitate passage and encourage the patient to walk. Renal calculi are very painful and frequent monitoring of pain level and administration of analgesics will assist with passage. In the past, patients who form calcium calculi were told to avoid dairy products and foods with high calcium content. Recent studies have shown that foods high in calcium may help prevent calcium calculi, but taking calcium in pill form may increase the risk of developing calculi (National Institute of Diabetes and Digestive and Kidney Diseases [NIDDK], 2007). Also, antacids that have a calcium

DIAGNOSTIC TESTS for Calculi

Test	Expected Abnormality	Rationale for Abnormality
Kidneys/ureters/bladder (KUB) radiograph	Most will show renal calculi.	Calculi are the precipitation of substances and will appear on x-ray.
Excretory urography, Abdominal CAT scan Renal MRI scan	Any of these imaging tests will reveal the obstruction and help determine the size and location of the calculi.	Calculi are the precipitation of substances and will appear on imaging.
Renal ultrasonography	May detect obstructive changes such as hydronephrosis.	If the obstruction is total, urine will be unable to drain, causing hydronephrosis.
Calculus analysis	Reveals mineral content.	Assists in diagnosing cause of calculi.
Urinalysis	Increased specific gravity and acid or alkaline pH. Hematuria. Crystals: calcium, urate, or cystine.	Suitable environment for different types of calculi formation. Damage from the calculi. Precipitate from the calculi.
Blood uric acid levels	May be increased.	Indicates gout as the cause of the calculi formation.

base may need to be avoided. Patients prone to calcium oxalate calculi should limit their intake of the following foods:

- Beets
- Chocolate
- Coffee
- Cola
- Nuts
- Rhubarb
- Spinach
- Strawberries
- Tea
- Wheat bran.

Assessment

Assessment for the patient with renal or ureteral calculi includes:

- Any past history or family history of calculi, gout, or other renal problems
- Blood in the urine
- Painful, urgent, and frequent urination
- Decreasing urine output
- Severe pain in the pelvis; can be dull, constant pain or intermittent, excruciating pain radiating anteriorly down to the vulva in women or testes in men.

Nursing Diagnoses

Major nursing diagnoses for the patient with calculi include:

- *Pain, Acute*
- *Urinary Elimination, Impaired*
- *Knowledge, Deficient* related to disease process

Planning

Overall goals include pain control, passage and identification of the calculi, and understanding of potential causes of calculus formation and the possible need for dietary restrictions and increased fluid intake.

Outcomes and Evaluation Parameters

Outcomes and evaluation parameters for the patient with calculi include:

- Pain is decreased to a tolerable level as evidenced by the patient rating the pain as less than 3 on a 0–10 scale.
- The patient will not exhibit impaired urinary elimination as evidenced by voiding more than 200 milliliters of clear amber urine each void.
- The patient will understand the disease process and plan of care as evidenced by his ability to articulate how calculi are formed and the need for dietary restrictions.

Interventions and Rationales

Nursing interventions and rationales for the patient with calculi include:

- Administer analgesics and antispasmodics as ordered. *Narcotic analgesia is warranted due to the severity of the pain. Antispasmodics relax tense muscles and reduce reflex spasms.*
- Monitor the volume and character of each void. Strain all urine for calculi. Encourage intake of fluid (12–17 eight-ounce glasses of fluid daily). *Adequate urine output indicates proper kidney function. Increased fluid intake is necessary to flush the calculi through the kidney and ureters. The characteristics of the urine can indicate the presence of infection (odorous, cloudy) and hemorrhage.*
- Provide information to the patient and significant others regarding dietary limitations for specific calculi, the need for regular activity, adequate fluid intake, and signs and symptoms of recurrence, such as pain and hematuria. *The patient needs an understanding of preventative strategies in order to comply with the regimen.*

Evaluation

The patient will have a tolerable level of pain as evidenced by a low pain rating on a 0–10 scale. The patient will void more than 200 milliliters of urine each void. The urine will be clear and without foul odor. The patient will be able to articulate an understanding of preventative measures and will agree to comply.

Topics that should be addressed with patients who have renal calculi and/or their families before discharge are presented in the Patient Teaching & Discharge Priorities box.

 Cystitis and Urethritis

Cystitis is an inflammation of the urinary bladder and is more common in women than in men due to their urethra being shorter. The most common cause is the introduction of *Escherichia coli* from fecal material into the urethra. The bacteria then travel up to the bladder. Cystitis may also develop following sexual intercourse when organisms around the vaginal opening enter the urethra.

Urethritis is an inflammation of the urethra. As with cyctitis, the most common causative microorganism is *Escherichia coli*, followed by *Klebsiella*, *Enterobacter*, *Proteus*, and *Pseudomonas*. Sexually transmitted infections, such as gonorrhea, can also cause cystitis and urethritis (Frazier & Drzymkowski, 2007).

Acute nongonococcal urethritis (NGU) is one of the most common sexually transmitted infections affecting men (Bradshaw et al., 2005). In a study conducted by Bradshaw and colleagues (2005), they found that the cause of the urethritis differed with different clinical and behavioral association. Adenoviruses and herpes simplex virus were associated with sex with men and insertive oral sex. *Chlamydia trachomatis* and *Mycoplasma genitalium* infections were associated with sex with women and unprotected vaginal sex. Insertive oral sex was highly associated with NGU, in which no pathogen was detected.

Laboratory and Diagnostic Procedures

The signs and symptoms of cystitis include increased urinary frequency with a sense of urgency, burning with urination, and at times hematuria. Urinalysis reveals bacteria, pus, and casts in the urine.

 Nursing Management

Nursing management for the patient experiencing bladder infections includes treatment of the source and education regarding ways to prevent recurrent infections.

Interventions and Rationales

The nursing interventions and rationales for cystitis include the following. The nurse should encourage the patient to increase fluids. *Fluids assist in flushing bacteria out of the urethra.* Treatment usually consists of an appropriate antibiotic and, if urination is very painful, phenazopyridine, which is taken orally and when excreted by the kidney produces a topical analgesia. Inform the patient that the phenazopyridine will turn urine a bright-orange color that will stain clothing. If the patient is female, discuss the importance of cleansing the genital area from front to back to avoid contamination by fecal material. Also, encourage the female patient to void as soon as possible after having sexual intercourse. *This will flush contaminates that may have entered the urethra.* Encourage male patients to have protected sex. The Pharmacology Summary feature on page 1496 presents medications used to treat bladder and urinary tract disorders.

 Neurogenic Bladder

As the renal system creates urine, it is stored in the bladder to be released. For the system to function properly, muscles and nerves work together to hold urine in the bladder and then release it when desired. When the bladder becomes full, nerves carry messages to the brain to let it know. The nerves then carry messages from the brain to tell the muscles either to tighten to block the release of urine or to release to allow the urine to flow out. Problems that affect the ability of the nerves to relay these messages may cause difficulty with bladder control. The most common causes of damage to nerves and nerve pathways are:

- Diabetes: autonomic neuropathies
- Cerebral disorders: stroke, brain tumor, dementia
- Vaginal childbirth
- Infections of the brain or spinal cord
- Traumatic injury to the brain or spinal cord
- Multiple sclerosis, Parkinson's disease
- Heavy metal poisoning
- Collagen diseases: systemic lupus erythematosus
- Herpes zoster. (Follin & Lenker, 2004; NIDDK, 2008)

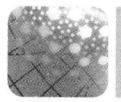

PATIENT TEACHING & DISCHARGE PRIORITIES for Renal Calculi

Need	Teaching
Prevention of further stones	Encourage patient intake of fluids to maintain a urine output of 3 to 4 liters a day. Patient's urine should be diluted and appear colorless.
Acidify urine	If the patient's urine is consistently alkaline (7.2 to 7.7), calcium phosphate or magnesium ammonium phosphate calculi may develop.
	Encourage the patient to drink fruit juices, especially cranberry juice.
Dietary restrictions with gout	Uric acid calculi may develop.
	Instruct patient/family to avoid alcohol and purine-rich foods, such as anchovies, liver, sardine, kidneys, sweetbreads, and lentils.

Bladder Control Problems

Three different kinds of bladder control problems arise from nerve damage:

1. **Urinary retention**—The nerves and pathways are damaged, and the bladder muscles do not receive the message that the bladder is full and it is time to release urine. The bladder then becomes too full, and urine may back up resulting in hydronephrosis, stagnant urine leading to infection, and overflow incontinence.

2. **Poor control of sphincter muscles**—There are sphincter muscles that surround the urethra keeping it closed to hold urine in the bladder. If the nerves or pathways to the sphincter muscles are damaged, the muscles will either become loose, allowing leakage, or remain tight, preventing the release of urine.

3. **Overactive bladder**—The damaged nerves and pathways may send signals to the bladder at inappropriate times causing the muscles to contract without warning. Symptoms of an overactive bladder include urinary frequency, urinating eight or more times a day or two or more times a night; urinary urgency, a strong and sudden need to urinate immediately; and urge incontinence, the leaking of urine that follows a strong, sudden urge.

Laboratory and Diagnostic Procedures

If the history and physical examination lead health care providers to suspect nerve damage, the tests outlined for neurogenic bladder in the Diagnostic Tests box are helpful in supporting the diagnosis.

Treatment for Overactive Bladder

The goal of treatment is to protect the kidney and upper urinary tract, prevent infection, and prevent urinary incontinence by evacuating the bladder. If the patient has an overactive bladder, bladder training may be the first course of treatment.

For bladder training, the patient keeps a diary to include fluid intake, times the patient voids, and any episodes of urine leakage. The diary helps to identify any patterns and helps in planning to avoid incontinence. The patient plans to void at certain times of the day and, as he gains more control, may increase the interval of time between voiding. For women, Kegel exercises are also part of bladder training and are used to strengthen the muscles that hold urine in. The following explains how to do Kegel exercises:

- Have the patient identify the correct muscles by imagining that she is sitting on a marble and wants to pick it up with her vagina. Have her picture sucking the marble into the vagina. Instruct the patient not to tighten her stomach, buttocks, or thigh muscles. Tightening the wrong muscles can put increased pressure on the muscles that control the bladder. Instruct the patient to squeeze the pelvic muscles and not to hold her breath.

- Instruct the patient to tighten the pelvic muscles and hold for a count of 3. Then relax the muscles for a count of 3. Initially tell the patient to do a few sets and gradually work up to 3 sets of 10 repeats. If it is difficult to do in a sitting position, have the patient try the exercise lying down.

- Inform the patient that bladder control may not improve for 3 to 6 weeks. Some patients have noticed an improvement after the first few weeks.

Bladder control treatment may include electrical stimulation of the nerves that control the bladder and sphincter muscles. Depending on which nerves are being treated, the electrical stimulus can be given through the vagina or through patches placed on the skin. Also, a wire can be surgically placed near the coccyx and connected to a stimulator that can be placed under the skin. This device, marketed as the InterStim system, has been approved by the Food and Drug Administration (FDA) to treat urge incontinence, urgency-frequency syndrome, and urinary retention in patients for whom other treatments have failed (NIDDK, 2008).

Medications that help to relax the bladder muscles and prevent bladder spasms include anticholinergics such as oxybutynin chloride (Ditropan), hyoscyamine (Levsin), propantheline bromide (Pro-Banthine), and tolterodine (Detrol). The most common side effect is dry mouth, but larger doses can cause blurred vision, tachycardia, flushing, and constipation. Administering time-release formulations helps to decrease the side effects. The Pharmacology Summary feature on page 1496 presents medications used to treat bladder and urinary tract disorders.

If urinary incontinence is severe and other treatments have failed, a surgery known as augmentation cystoplasty may be considered. The surgery enlarges the bladder by replacing diseased bladder with a section taken from the bowel. This improves the ability to store urine but may make it more difficult to empty, requiring regular catheterization.

Treatment for Urinary Retention

Urinary retention can occur due to the inability of the bladder wall muscle to contract or the inability of the sphincter muscle to relax. Patients can be taught techniques of bladder evacuation including Credé's method, Valsalva's maneuver, and intermittent catheterization.

DIAGNOSTIC TESTS for Neurogenic Bladder

Test	Expected Abnormality	Rationale for Abnormality
Voiding cystourethrography	Vesicoureteral reflux and continence	Poor nerve innervation to the muscles of the neck of the bladder
Uroflow	Diminished urine flow	Lack of muscle contraction
Cystometry	Poor bladder muscle tone with decreased pressures during filling and contraction	Poor nerve innervation with diminished tone
Sphincter electromyography	Decreased sphincter and bladder tone	Poor nerve innervation causing decreased bladder tone or involuntary spasms

Credé's method is the application of manual pressure over the lower abdomen; Valsalva's maneuver is performing a forced exhalation against a closed glottis. Both are used to promote complete emptying of the bladder. Although most patients can learn these methods, they are not always successful, and the patient may still need to perform catheterization.

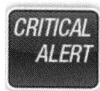 *Patients with spinal cord injuries who perform Credé's method may develop autonomic dysreflexia, a rise in blood pressure to potentially fatal levels due to the stimulation of the sympathetic nervous system.*

Patients and/or their family members can be taught to perform intermittent catheterization at regular intervals to empty the bladder. If patients are unable to catheterize themselves and there is no other family member or caregiver to assist them, then they may need to have an indwelling catheter that can be changed less often. There are several risks associated with indwelling catheters, including infection, bladder stones, and bladder tumors.

When nerve signals to the sphincter muscles that squeeze the urethra shut and the bladder are not coordinated, the bladder and urethral sphincter may contract at the same time, making it difficult to pass urine easily. Medications may be used to reduce muscle spasms and help relax the sphincter. Baclofen (Lioresal) is used to prevent muscle spasms or cramping in patients with multiple sclerosis and spinal injuries. Diazepam (Valium) can also be used as a muscle relaxant. Alpha-adrenergic blockers such as terazosin (Hytrin) and doxazosin (Cardura) can be used to relax the sphincter. Side effects can include low blood pressure, dizziness, and nasal congestion.

Urethral stents, which are small tubelike devices, can be inserted into the urethra and expanded, like a spring, widening the opening for urine to flow out. Risks associated with stents include movement of the stent and infection.

Male patients may consider surgery to prevent urinary retention. The surgeon passes a thin instrument through the urethra to deliver electrical or laser energy to burn away sphincter tissue. The patient may have a sphincter resection, or removal of a section of the sphincter, or a sphincterotomy, which is complete removal of the external sphincter. The surgery causes loss of urine control, and the patient will need to wear an external catheter that fits over the penis like a condom and drains the urine to a leg bag for collection. Complications of the surgery can include bleeding, infection, and problems obtaining an erection.

If conservative treatment has failed and the patient is experiencing frequent urinary retention with damage to the kidney, urinary diversion may be needed. Urinary diversion via an ileal conduit is described in the next section, Cancer of the Bladder. Another form of urinary diversion is the replacement of the bladder with a urinary reservoir, an internal pouch made from sections of bowel or other tissue. The urine is stored inside the body, and a catheter is passed through a stoma to empty the pouch. A third option is an orthotopic neobladder, which consists of a detubularized segment of intestine used to construct a reservoir for urine storage. The ureters are implanted into the reservoir, and the reservoir is anatomosed to the native urethra. The patient is able to control continence via the external sphincter of the urethra.

Nursing Management

Nursing care for patients with neurogenic bladder varies depending on the underlying cause and the method of treatment. It is very important to explain and review the treatment plan frequently. Topics that should be addressed with patients who have neurogenic bladder and/or their families before discharge are outlined in the Patient Teaching & Discharge Priorities box.

Cancer of the Bladder

Bladder cancer is the fourth most common cancer in men and the ninth leading cancer in women in the United States (McGrath, Michaud, & DeVivo, 2006). Tumors may develop on the surface of the bladder wall or grow within the bladder wall. Those that grow within the wall are invasive and usually infiltrate the bladder wall, invading the underlying muscles. Approximately 90% of bladder tumors are transitional cell carcinomas that arise from the transitional epithelium of mucous membranes (Davis, 2006; Follin & Lenker, 2004). Bladder tumors are most common in males over the age of 50 and are more common in populated industrial areas.

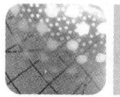

PATIENT TEACHING & DISCHARGE PRIORITIES for Neurogenic Bladder

Need	Teaching
Prevention of calculi formation and infection from urinary stasis	Encourage the patient to increase fluid intake to prevent formation of calculi and infection.
Bladder evacuation	Teach and have patient/family perform evacuation techniques, such as Credé's method, Valsalva's maneuver, and intermittent catheterization. To assist the female patient in learning self-catheterization, use a mirror.
Prevent infection	Teach patient/family the importance of strict aseptic technique during catheterization.
	If the patient has an indwelling catheter, teach the need for cleaning the catheter insertion site with soap and water at least twice a day.
	Teach patient/family to watch for signs of infection including: • Fever • Cloudy or foul-smelling urine.
Enterostomal care	If a urinary diversion procedure has been done, arrange for consultation with an enterostomal therapist.

PHARMACOLOGY Summary of Drugs Used in Bladder and Urinary Tract Disorders

Medication Category	Action	Application/Indication	Nursing Responsibility
Opioid Analgesics			
Morphine sulfate	Binds with and activates opioid receptors in brain and spinal cord to produce analgesia and euphoria.	Treatment of pain.	Regular, frequent assessment of pain and nonpain symptoms: i.e., shortness of breath, anxiety, etc. Safe and timely reduction of pain and symptom levels. Barriers to effective pain management should be addressed, including inappropriate fears of risk of side effects, addiction, and respiratory depression.
Urinary Analgesic			
Phenazopyridine (Pyridium)	Azo dye: exact mechanism of action not known. Therapeutic effect: local anesthetic action on urinary tract mucosa.	Symptomatic relief of pain, burning, frequency, and urgency caused by irritation of the urinary tract mucosa.	Instruct patient: The drug will turn urine a bright-orange color and will stain clothing. Stop use immediately, and contact health care team if skin or sclerae appear to have a yellowish color. Do not breast-feed while taking medication.
Anti-infectives			
Cephalosporins Cefazolin Ancef Kefzol Cefuroxime Kefurox Zinacef Ceftriaxone Rocephin	Binds to one or more of the penicillin-binding proteins located on cell walls of susceptible organisms. This inhibits the final stage of bacterial wall synthesis, killing the bacteria.	Infections of genitourinary tracts.	Determine prior hypersensitivity to cephalosporins and penicillins. Perform culture and sensitivity tests prior to therapy. Monitor input and output (I&O) pattern, especially with patients with impaired renal function and patients older than age 50. Monitor patients for antibiotic-associated pseudo-membranous enterocolitis caused by *Clostridia difficile*. Avoid use of alcohol during and for 48 to 72 hours after taking drug. Yogurt or buttermilk may help protect against intestinal superinfection by maintaining normal intestinal flora. Do not breast-feed while taking medication. For third-generation cephalosporins: Do not give within 2 hours of aluminum- or magnesium-containing antacids or iron supplements.
Sulfonamide Sulfamethoxazole Bactrim Sulfasoxazole Gantrisin	Believed to interfere with folic acid biosynthesis (required for bacterial growth) by competitive inhibition of aminobenzoic acid.	Acute, recurrent, and chronic urinary tract infections.	Obtain culture and sensitivity prior to administration. Monitor I&O. Fluid intake should be enough to create urinary output of at least 1,500 milliliters a day to prevent crystalluria and stone formation. Monitor urine pH daily. Acidic urine increases risk of crystalluria. Monitor temperature. Increased temperature may signify sensitization or hemolytic anemia. Assess for skin lesions, popular or vesicular, especially on sun-exposed areas. Observe patients with diabetes taking oral hypoglycemic medication for hypoglycemic reactions. Patient teaching: may make hormonal contraceptives unreliable. Avoid exposure to ultraviolet light and excessive sunlight. Do not breast-feed while taking medication.
Quinolone Ciprofloxacin (Cipro) Norfloxacin (Noroxcin)	Inhibits DNA gyrase, an enzyme necessary for bacterial replication.	Urinary tract infections, acute pyelonephritis.	Obtain culture and sensitivity prior to administration. Assess for skin rash or other signs of hypersensitivity reaction. Patient teaching: Increase fluid intake while taking mediation. Do not take the following within 2 hours of taking the medication: aluminum or magnesium antacids, iron supplements, multivitamins with zinc, or sucralfate. Avoid exposure to excess sunlight or artificial UV light. Avoid NSAIDs. Do not breast-feed.

PHARMACOLOGY Summary of Drugs Used in Bladder and Urinary Tract Disorders—*Continued*

Medication Category	Action	Application/Indication	Nursing Responsibility
Aminopenicillin Ampicillin Amoxicillin	Inhibits mucoprotein synthesis in cell wall of rapidly multiplying bacteria.	Urinary tract infections.	Obtain culture and sensitivity prior to administration. Determine previous hypersensitivity to penicillins and cephalosporins. Assess for urticarial rash: sign of hypersensitivity. Assess for diarrhea to rule out pseudomembranous colitis. Patient teaching: Take medication as prescribed; do not miss a dose and continue until all medication is taken. Do not breast-feed.
Anticholinergic (parasympatholytic) Oxybutynin (Ditropan)	Exerts direct antispasmodic action, and inhibits muscarinic effects of acetylcholine on smooth muscle.	Relieve symptoms associated with voiding in patients with neurogenic bladder.	Monitor patients for expected responses to therapy. Assess patients with colostomy or ileostomy for abdominal distention and onset of diarrhea—may be early signs of obstruction or toxic megacolon. Patient teaching: Do not drive or engage in potentially hazardous activities until the patient is aware of how the medication affects her. Do not overexert in hot environments; medication suppresses sweating and may cause heatstroke. Do not breast-feed.

Environmental carcinogens such as 2-naphthylamine, benzidine, tobacco, and nitrates have been found to predispose a person to transitional cell tumors. Therefore, those who work in industries where they are exposed to these carcinogens are at high risk for development of this type of tumor. These industries include rubber workers, weavers, leather finishers, hairdressers, aniline dye workers, petroleum workers, and spray painters. The time period between exposure and development of symptoms is approximately 18 years (Follin & Lenker, 2004).

Women also develop bladder cancer but tend to be diagnosed at more advanced stages. Bladder cancers that occur in women include a higher portion of rare cell types such as adenocarcinoma, small cell carcinoma, and squamous cell carcinoma (see Chapter 64 🖱). Also, older women have a thin bladder wall, which may permit a more rapid spread of the tumor. Risk factors for women are for those who smoke, use hair dye, and ingest tap water containing nitrates (Follin & Lenker, 2004).

Laboratory and Diagnostic Procedures

The first sign is most commonly gross, painless, intermittent hematuria. Patients with invasive tumors may have suprapubic pain after voiding.

Diagnostic tests include cystoscopy with anesthesia, so a bimanual examination can be done to determine whether the bladder is fixed to the pelvic wall. Biopsy of the tumor will confirm the type of cancer. Tests that are helpful in the diagnosis of bladder cancer are listed in the Diagnostic Tests box (p. 1498).

Staging and Grading the Tumor

Bladder cancer is categorized according to stage, the tumor's anatomic progression or depth, and to grade, the cell differentiation and aggressiveness. The American Joint Committee on Cancer (AJCC) developed the tumor, nodes, metastasis system, which includes the following stages:

- Stage 0: Cancer cells are found only on the inner surface of the bladder wall.
- Stage I: Cancer cells have invaded the layer of connective tissue under the bladder wall but have not penetrated muscle or spread to lymph nodes or distant sites.
- Stage II: Cancer cells have invaded the muscle layer but have not passed through the muscle to reach the tissue layer surrounding the bladder, nor have cancer cells spread to lymph nodes or distant sites.
- Stage III: Cancer cells have spread into the outer layer of tissue surrounding the bladder and may also invade surrounding structures, but lymph nodes and distant sites are not involved.
- Stage IV: Cancer cells have spread to the pelvic or abdominal wall or metastasized to a distant location such as the lungs, liver, or bones.

Grading compares how abnormal the cancer cells appear in relation to normal tissue of the same type and how aggressive the cells seem to be. Well-differentiated cells resemble normal cells more closely, tend to be less aggressive, grow slowly, and are termed low-grade tumors. Poorly differentiated cells are termed higher grade and are more aggressive (Davis, 2006).

Medical Management

If the tumor has not invaded the muscle, the tumor can be removed by transurethral resection and electrical destruction. If there are superficial tumors in multiple sites, intravesicular chemotherapy is used. The bladder is directly washed with an antineoplastic drug. Tumors may reoccur, and as long as they do

DIAGNOSTIC TESTS for Bladder Cancer

Test	Expected Abnormality	Rationale for Abnormality
Urinalysis	Red blood cells	Invasion of the bladder wall
	Malignant cells	
Excretory urography	Identifies tumor infiltration	Damage by the tumor to the bladder and surrounding structures
	Delineates problems in the upper urinary tract	
	Displays hydronephrosis	
	Detects deformity of the bladder wall	
CAT scan	Displays the thickness of the involved bladder wall	Progression of the cancer
	Detects enlarged retroperitoneal lymph nodes	
Ultrasonography	May detect metastasis outside of the bladder	Progression of the cancer

not invade the muscle layer, treatments may be repeated as needed. Intravesical immunotherapy is a treatment similar to intravesicular chemotherapy except the agent that is instilled to treat the cancer is bacillus Calmette-Guérin (BCG), a form of inactivated tuberculosis bacterium. BCG immunotherapy works by triggering the body's own immune system to destroy the cancer cells. This treatment is indicated for lower stage tumors that have not invaded the muscle wall.

Tumors that are too large to remove transurethrally and are away from the bladder neck and ureteral orifice, require a segmental bladder resection. Tumors that have infiltrated the muscle require a radical cystectomy, removal of the entire bladder. Due to the incidence of metastasis, the surgery involves removal of the bladder, lymph nodes, urethra, the prostate and seminal vesicles in males, and the uterus, ovaries, and adnexa in females. A urinary diversion is created using the intestinal tract and is usually an ileal conduit (Figure 47–3 ■). A segment of ileum is separated from the small intestine and formed into a tubular pouch with the open end being brought to the skin surface, forming a stoma. The ureters are then connected to the pouch and the patient will need to wear an external pouch to collect the urine.

Following a radical cystectomy, another option is the creation of a neobladder, or internal urine collection reservoir formed from the small intestine and connected to the urethra. The patient learns to void normally through the urethra by tightening the abdominal muscles in a Valsalva-type maneuver. The advantage of the neobladder is that the patient can maintain a relatively normal lifestyle. Because the neobladder does not fully empty, the patient will need to learn to perform self-catheterization twice a day to remove residual urine and prevent infection. The patient may also need to irrigate the bladder through the catheter to remove mucus that can accumulate from the neobladder wall.

Following the cystectomy, bladder cancers that are advanced will also require radiation therapy and chemotherapy. Refer to Chapter 64 ⊙ for nursing care of the patient undergoing radiation therapy and chemotherapy.

Nursing Management

For general nursing management of the postoperative patient, refer to Chapter 27 ⊙. Following radical cystectomy, one of the most important postoperative nursing responsibilities is to monitor urine output. Urine output that drops below 30 mL/hr may indicate shock, hemorrhage, obstructed ureters, or renal dysfunction. Encourage the patient to look at the stoma, and involve the patient in the care of the stoma as soon as possible. Advise the patient that as soon as she can she may participate in most activities except heavy lifting and contact sports. Prior to discharge, referral for home health care or an enterostomal therapist should be made to help coordinate the patient's care. Males will be impotent because the surgery damages the sympathetic and parasympathetic nerves that control erection and ejaculation. The patient may, at a later date, have a penile implant placed that will allow for sexual intercourse without ejaculation. Refer patients with an ostomy to resources such as the United Ostomy Association and the American Cancer Society.

Summary

The key to most renal and urinary disorders is the recognition and treatment of the cause and the preservation of renal function. The nurse is a critical member of the health care team in monitoring changes in the patient's condition and reporting and acting on these changes. Many renal and urinary disorders require lifestyle changes by the patient. The nurse's role in teaching, discussing, and evaluating the patient's understanding is critical to the success of long-term treatment and preservation of renal function.

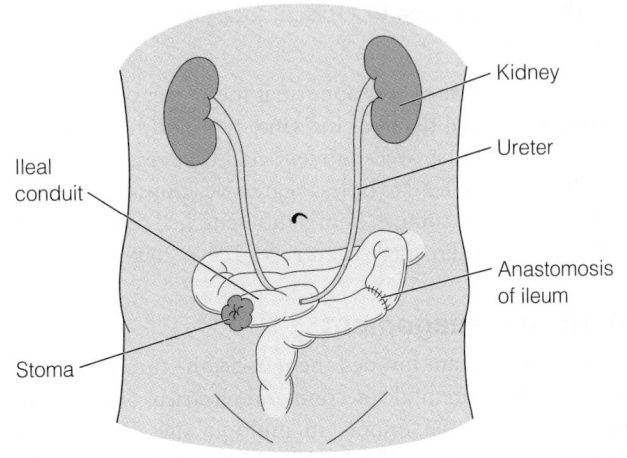

Kidney

Ureter

Ileal conduit

Anastomosis of ileum

Stoma

FIGURE 47–3 ■ Ileal conduit.

Clinical Preparation

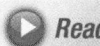 **Read**

- History of Current Illness
- Past Medical History
- Physical Exam
- Admitting Medical Orders
- Laboratory Study Results

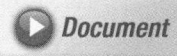 **Document**

- Summary of Hospitalization
- Pathophysiology Form
- Laboratory Values
- Laboratory Results Explanation

 **Apply**

- List of Potential Nursing Diagnoses
- Concept Map
- Critical Thinking Questions

Log on to MyNursingKit.com to download forms you will need and to complete further steps in the Clinical Preparation assignment.

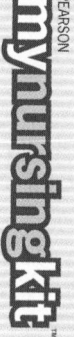

HISTORY OF PRESENT ILLNESS

A 72-year-old male came to the emergency department (ED) complaining of right lower abdominal/groin pain. He stated that the pain was 8/10 and started suddenly after returning from the airport where he had lifted heavy luggage. He was found to have an incarcerated right inguinal hernia with bowel necrosis. He was taken to the operating room for bowel resection and repair of his hernia. Of note, in the ED he received 100 mL of normal saline IV and 300 mL of blood product. His output was 110 mL of urine via Foley catheter and 200 mL gastric content via nasogastric tube.

After the surgery he was admitted to the medical–surgical ward. On postoperative day 1, the patient's total urine output for the day was 230 mL. Despite receiving multiple fluid boluses, his urine output remained low and he had a rise in his serum creatinine and BUN. On the morning of postoperative day 2 he was transferred to the ICU for fluid management and strict monitoring of his intake and output.

Medical–Surgical History

He has no significant medical history and takes aspirin, multivitamins, fish oil, folic acid, and calcium daily. Family history is significant for adult-onset diabetes.

Social History

The patient has never smoked and occasionally drinks alcohol. He is married and lives with his wife.

Physical Exam

You receive the patient in bed with the head of the bed up 30 degrees. He opens his eyes to voice and follows commands. He complains of lethargy and a mild headache. Breath sounds are clear bilaterally. His abdomen is soft and slightly tender at the surgical site. The surgical site is clean, dry, and intact. His bowel sounds are decreased. The extremities are warm with 3+ pulses to all. You note 2+ dependent edema to the lower extremities.

Admitting Medical Orders

Service: surgical ICU service
Diagnosis: incarcerated right inguinal hernia, acute renal failure
Allergies: penicillin
Diet: renal diet; restrict protein intake to 0.25 to 0.5 g/kg per day; caloric intake of > 400 kcal/day; low sodium and potassium; restrict free water intake
Vital signs every 1–2 hours and prn with O_2 saturations
Accu-Cheks: before meals and at bedtime
Activity: bed rest; up to chair bid

Call house officer; temp > 38.5°C; SBP > 180 or < 90; pulse > 110 or < 50; resp rate > 30 or < 8; O_2 sat < 92%, urinary output < 30 mL/hr × 2 hours; blood sugar < 70 or > 150
IVs: D5.45NS; titrate fluids to equal output plus 400 mL/day
Foley to gravity drainage
Strict I&O
Weight daily
Respiratory care: incentive spirometer every hour when awake
DVT prophylaxis: sequential compression device to lower extremities

Scheduled Medications

Metoprolol 5 mg IV q6h
Famotidine 20 mg IV bid
Regular insulin SC sliding scale
Hydromorphone 0.2 mg/mL concentration IV per PCA, incremental 0.2 mg, lock-out 6 min

PRN Medications

Diphenhydramine 12.5 mg IV q6h prn itching

Ordered Laboratory Studies

Electrolyte panel qam
Complete blood count qam

LABORATORY STUDY RESULTS

Test	Day 1	Day 2	Day 3
WBC	$17.8/mm^3$	$21.7/mm^3$	$12.3/mm^3$
RBC	$5.97/mm^3$	$5.80/mm^3$	$5.25/mm^3$
Hgb	17.1 g/dL	16.8 g/dL	15.4 g/dL
Hct	51.1%	49.6%	46.2%
Platelets	$867/mm^3$	$815/mm^3$	$658/mm^3$
Na	138 mEq/L	139 mEq/L	140 mEq/L
K	4.0 mEq/L	4.2 mEq/L	4.9 mEq/L
Cl	104 mEq/L	106 mEq/L	109 mEq/L
Total CO_2	26 mEq/L	25 mEq/L	26 mEq/L
BUN	14 mg/dL	25 mg/dL	33 mg/dL
Creatinine	1.0 mg/dL	1.9 mg/dL	2.1 mg/dL
Glucose	175 mg/dL	151 mg/dL	173 mg/dL

CRITICAL THINKING QUESTIONS

1. What contributed to the patient's acute renal failure?

2. What serum electrolyte changes would you expect to see?

Answers to Critical Thinking Questions appear in Appendix D.

NCLEX® REVIEW

1. The urine output of a patient in cardiogenic shock has been 200 mL for the last 24 hours and serum creatinine level is 1.5 mg/dL. The nurse suspects the patient is in acute renal failure when laboratory values indicate:

1. BUN is 16 mg/dL.
2. Calcium is 8.7 mg/dL.
3. Sodium level is 152 mg/dL.
4. Potassium is 4.8 mEq/L.

2. A patient with suspected pyelonephritis has urine sent for analysis and culture. The nurse checks for which result to substantiate the diagnosis?

1. High specific gravity
2. Low leukocyte count
3. Casts in the urine
4. Presence of protein

3. A patient has been diagnosed with the onset of acute renal failure. The nurse recognizes a prerenal precipitating cause in the patient is:

1. Urinary calculi.
2. Recent intravenous pylogram with contrast dye.
3. Congestive heart failure.
4. Crushing injury.

4. In order to prevent the cardiovascular complications associated with chronic renal failure, the nurse should include which interventions in the plan of care?

1. Apply a non-drying lotion to the skin.
2. Maintain a low fat, low carbohydrate diet.
3. Evaluate ankles for edema daily.
4. Restrict fluid and salt intake.

5. A patient has a neobladder created following a radical cystectomy. The nurse plans to teach the patient which technique?

1. Manual Credé
2. Kegel exercises
3. Self-catheterization
4. Stoma wafer change

6. A patient receiving hemodialysis tells the nurse that the worst part of the treatment is the severe leg cramps that he gets a few hours after the procedure. Which of the following should the nurse instruct this patient?

1. The leg cramps are because of the blood transfusions that you receive.
2. The leg cramps are because of an infection that will need to be treated.
3. The leg cramps are because of the extra water and salt that is being removed.
4. The leg cramps are because you aren't eating enough protein.

Answers for review questions appear in Appendix D

KEY TERMS

anasarca *p.1475*
anuria *p.1475*
azotemia *p.1464*
Bowman's capsule *p.1463*
end-stage renal disease (ESRD) *p.1480*
erythropoietin *p.1463*

glomerulus *p.1463*
hematuria *p.1464*
hyperkalemia *p.1476*
Kussmaul's respirations *p.1475*
nephron *p.1463*

oliguria *p.1464*
proteinuria *p.1464*
renin *p.1463*
staghorn calculus *p.1491*
suppurative *p.1468*

PEARSON
EXPLORE **mynursingkit**™

MyNursingKit is your one stop for online chapter review materials and resources. Prepare for success with additional NCLEX®-style practice questions, interactive assignments and activities, web links, animations and videos, and more!

Register your access code from the front of your book at
www.mynursingkit.com

REFERENCES

Atkins, M. (2006a). *Clinical manifestations, evaluation, and staging of renal cell carcinoma.* Retrieved April 16, 2007, from http://www.uptodate.com

Atkins, M. (2006b). *Epidemiology, pathology, and pathogenesis of renal cell carcinoma.* Retrieved April 16, 2007, from http://www.uptodate.com

Bradshaw, C. S., Tabrizi, S. N., Read, T. R., Garland, S. M., Hopkins, C. A., Moss, L. M., et al. (2005). Etiologies of nongonococcal urethritis: Bacteria, viruses, and the association with orogenital exposure. *The Journal of Infectious Diseases, 193,* 336–345.

Curhan, G., Aronson, M., & Preminger, G. (2008). *Diagnosis and acute management of suspected nephrolithiasis in adults.* Retrieved August 4, 2008, from http://www.uptodate.com/patients/content/topic.do?topicKey=~PEEs8wkDGf.awB&selectedTitle=1~150&source=search_result

Davis, C. B. (2006). Bladder cancer: Revealing news about a hidden threat. *Nursing 2006 36*(4), 54–57.

Denhaerynck, K., Manhaeve, D., Dobbels, F., Garzoni, D., Nolte, C., & De Geest, S. (2007). Prevalence and consequences of nonadherence to hemodialysis regimens. *American Journal of Critical Care, 16*(3), 222–235.

Dirkes, S., & Hodge, K. (2007). Continuous renal replacement therapy in the adult intensive care unit. *Critical Care Nurse, 27*(2), 61–81.

Follin, S., & Lenker, D. (Eds.). (2004). *Handbook of diseases* (3rd ed.). Philadelphia: Lippincott Williams & Wilkins.

Frazier, M. S., & Drzymkowski, J. W. (2007). *Essentials of human diseases and conditions* (4th ed.). St. Louis: Elsevier.

Hager, L., & Mills, E. J. (Eds.). (2008). *Nursing: Understanding diseases.* Philadelphia: Lippincott Williams & Wilkins.

Hogan, M. A. (2007). *Nutrition & diet therapy* (2nd ed.). Upper Saddle River, NJ: Prentice Hall Health.

Ismail, N. (2008). *Indications for initiation of dialysis in chronic renal failure.* Retrieved August 9, 2008, from http://www.utdol.com/online/content/topic.do?topicKey=dialysis/18787&selectedTitle=23~150&source=search_result

Kaplan, A., Appel, G., & Pusey, C. (2007). *Treatment of anti-GBM antibody (Goodpasture's) disease.* Retrieved August 3, 2008, from http://www.uptodate.com/patients/content/topic.do?topicKey=~OaJEblyepxfF.0&selectedTitle=1~150&source=search_result

Kashtan, C. E. (2007). The wages of thin. *Journal of the American Society of Nephrology, 18,* 2800–2802.

Kee, J. L. (2005). *Handbook of laboratory and diagnostic tests with nursing implications.* Upper Saddle River, NJ: Prentice Hall Health.

McGrath, M., Michaud, D. S., & DeVivo, I. (2006). Hormonal and reproductive factors and the risk of bladder cancer in women. *American Journal of Epidemiology, 163*(3), 236–244.

Michigan Quality Improvement Consortium (2006). *Diagnosis and management of adults with chronic kidney disease.* Retrieved August 10, 2008, from http://www.guideline.gov

National Institute of Diabetes and Digestive and Kidney Diseases (NIDDK). (2007). *Kidney stones in adults.* Retrieved January 26, 2007, from http://kidney.niddk.nih.gov/kudiseases/pubs/stonesadults/

National Institute of Diabetes and Digestive and Kidney Diseases (NIDDK). (2008). *Nerve disease and bladder control.* Retrieved August 2, 2008, from http://kidney.niddk.nih.gov/kudiseases/pubs/nervedisease/

Porth, C. (2005). *Pathophysiology: Concepts of altered health states* (7th ed.). Philadelphia: Lippincott Williams & Wilkins.

Post, T. W., & Rose, B. D. (2008a). *Diagnostic approach to the patient with acute or chronic kidney disease or renal failure.* Retrieved August 10, 2008, from http://www.uptodate.com

Post, T. W., & Rose, B. D. (2008b). *Diagnostic approach to the patient with acute or chronic kidney disease.* Retrieved August 10, 2008, from http://www.uptodate.com

Post, T. W., & Rose, B. D. (2008c). *Overview of the management of chronic kidney disease in adults.* Retrieved August 10, 2008, from http://www.uptodate.com

Pusey, D. C., & Kalluri, R. (2008). *Pathogenesis and diagnosis of anti-GBM antibody (Goodpasture's) disease.* Retrieved August 3, 2008, from http://www.uptodate.com/patients/content/topic.do?topicKey=~3F_i7b5xj4DwvF&selectedTitle=2~52&source=search_result

Radhakrishnan, J. (2008). *Diagnosis and treatment of renal infarction.* Retrieved August 10, 2008, from http://www.utdol.com/online/content/topic.do?topicKey=renldis/17093&selectedTitle=1~32&source=search_result

Stevens, L., & Perrone, R. (2008) *Assessment of kidney function: Serum creatinine; BUN; and GFR.* Retrieved August 10, 2008, from http://www.uptodate.com

Urden, L. D., Stacy, K. M., & Lough, M. E. (Eds.). (2006). *Critical care nursing* (5th ed.). St. Louis: Mosby.

Walser, M. (2004). *Coping with kidney disease.* Hoboken, NJ: John Wiley.

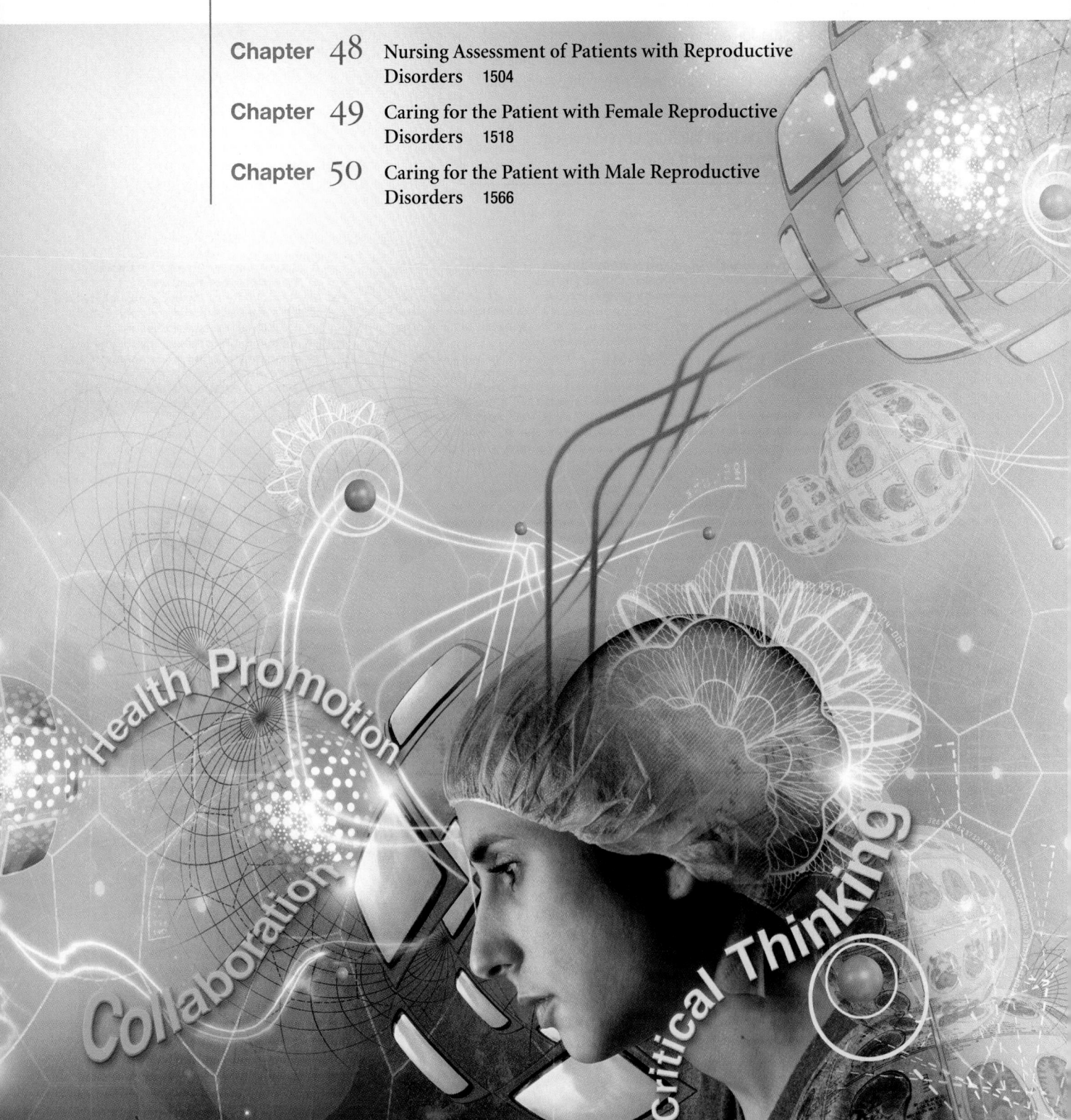

UNIT 10

Nursing Management of Patients with Reproductive Disorders

Health Promotion

Collaboration

Critical Thinking

LESLIE My name is Leslie Theilen and I work on the High Risk Maternity Antepartum unit of a large medical center in a metropolitan area. The unit's population spans the spectrum of pregnancy disorders including preterm labor, gestational diabetes, preeclampsia, and premature rupture of membranes. Women stay on the unit from hours to months before they deliver, often experiencing a sense of loss and independence due to separation from their homes and families.

I have worked in this hospital for 17 years. I am a member of the American Association of Women's Health, Obstetrics, and Neonatal Nurses, and hold several national certifications. My practice roles include providing direct patient care, precepting new nurses and nursing students, conducting unit-based audits for performance improvement, participating on the Joint Commission preparation team and staff nurse council, teaching classes as a service excellence adviser, and serving as a mentor coordinator for my unit.

I have wanted to be a nurse since the first time I saw a baby born. I made a **commitment,** to myself and my patients, to be the best nurse I could be. As a nurse caring for pregnant women, I am not only responsible for the well-being of the patient but also that of her unborn child(ren). I have cared for women of childbearing ages from 12 to 50, the poor and wealthy, married and single, addicted and sober, and treated each one as I would want to be cared for. I regularly attend classes and seminars in order to stay up to date with research findings and changes in clinical practice. Recently, I completed my bachelor's degree in nursing from California State University, Sacramento.

A typical day is anything but. I may be the charge nurse for the day, assigned to precept a nursing student or orient a new hire. Or I may be assigned to care for three patients with different needs and acuities. Recently, I cared for a patient who was 22 weeks pregnant with bulging membranes. She arrived on the unit via wheelchair, coming from the doctor's office after a routine ultrasound found her cervix dilated 5 centimeters with the bag of water bulging through into her vagina. She was crying and obviously upset. Offering reassurance, I placed her in the Trendelenburg position in the hopes that gravity would assist with the recession of the bag of water. I explained to her that the first goal was to stop the continued dilation of the cervix, then to get the pregnancy to the 24-week mark that constitutes viability. The patient was alone and had no one to call. I spent most of my time talking with her and listening to her fears. Although I tried for several hours to stop her contractions, her bag of water ruptured. Worried that she had advanced in dilation and the baby would easily pass through the cervix, I notified the doctor and then explained what was happening to the patient, emphasizing that our goal was to keep her pregnant as long as possible. Upon examination, the doctor explained to the patient there was nothing we could do to prevent the birth from happening. The patient began sobbing. I held her hand and promised not to leave her.

The doctor wanted to transfer the patient to labor and delivery to give birth since delivery was not normally done on our unit. I could not in all good **conscience** let this women be moved from her surroundings where she felt safe. This was a time for **compassion** not routine. There was no question; she would stay and I would help her give birth. I knew I had the **competence** to assist the doctor in her delivery and the **confidence** to provide her with the best care I could give. Her labor was short and after a few pushes, she gave birth to a son. He was given a name, pictures of the two of them were taken, and his mother held him until he died. I stayed with her as she counted his fingers and toes, kissing him while she told him how perfect he was. I found myself crying with my patient over the loss of her son. Later, I thanked her for letting me care for her and sharing that very sacred moment in her life. She thanked me for letting her stay on the unit and deliver with the only nurse she had come to know and trust. I was proud that my **comportment** had made an impression and that in thinking outside the box I had made a good decision for my patient.

At the end of each of my workdays, I look back at the people who invited me into their lives. It is with great gratitude that I am allowed to be the hand that calms the anxious, the comforting voice that soothes the ache, the attentive ear that listens to the worries. I am a counselor, care provider, safe haven, and friend. I am a nurse.

> "I made a **commitment,** to myself and my patients, to be the best nurse I could be. As a nurse caring for pregnant women, I am not only responsible for the well-being of the patient but also that of her unborn child(ren)."

Nursing Assessment of Patients with Reproductive Disorders

Patricia Caudle
With contribution by:
Laurie Kaudewitz

Outcome-Based Learning Objectives

After studying this chapter, the learner will be able to:

1. Describe the structures and function of the male and female reproductive systems.
2. Identify pertinent subjective and objective data related to the reproductive systems and information about the sexual function that should be obtained.
3. Identify risk factors for reproductive system disorders.
4. Differentiate normal from abnormal findings obtained from the physical assessment for males and females.
5. Describe age-related changes in the male and female reproductive systems.
6. Discuss the implications for health promotion related to the reproductive systems of females and males.

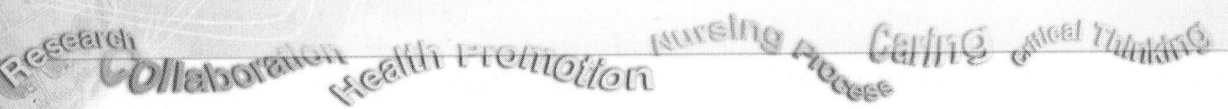

ASSESSMENT OF the female and male reproductive systems requires an understanding of the anatomy, open communications, a nonjudgmental attitude, gentleness, and a high degree of empathy and compassion. Most women and men consider the genital area very private, and many may be reluctant to talk about concerns or to allow examination by the nurse. The nurse should not be offended if the patient asks for an examiner of the same gender. Privacy and confidentiality are very important and should be maintained at all times.

The reproductive systems of the female and male include sexual organs, the lower urinary system, and the anorectal area. This means that assessment of the reproductive system is complex and must include history and physical examination that is inclusive of the three systems. This chapter outlines the important components of the female and male reproductive system assessment. Concepts discussed here introduce the learner to assessment skills needed to care for patients with disorders of the female and male reproductive systems discussed in Chapters 49 and 50 ✑.

Female Reproductive System

The female breast tissue extends from the second to the sixth rib on either side of the sternum and covers the pectoralis major

muscle (Figure 48–1 ■). The skin over the breasts is the same color as other skin and may have striae (stretch marks). The nipples are on the anterior surface of each breast, surrounded by the areola (pigmented skin around the nipple). The areola has sebaceous glands that may be raised and more active during pregnancy (Montgomery's tubercles). Sebaceous glands help to moisturize the nipple to make it more pliable (Stables & Rankin, 2005). Occasionally, supernumerary nipples are seen along a line (the "milk line") from the axilla to the upper thigh on either side (Figure 48–2 ■). These small nipples may be mistaken for moles. They are considered normal variants and are benign (Bickley & Szilagyi, 2007).

Each breast is made up of glandular, connective, and adipose (fatty) tissue. The glandular tissue includes 15 to 20 lobes suspended from ducts that drain into sinuses. The sinuses are near the nipple and are drained by smaller ducts on the nipple surface. The lobes are further divided into lobules where the milk is produced during lactation. The connective tissue provides support via ligaments within the breast (also called Cooper's ligaments). Adipose tissue completes the structure of the breasts and determines the size of the breast (see Figure 48–1 ■) (Bickley & Szilagyi, 2007).

Physiologically, breast tissue responds to estrogen (steroid female hormone produced by the ovary and placenta),

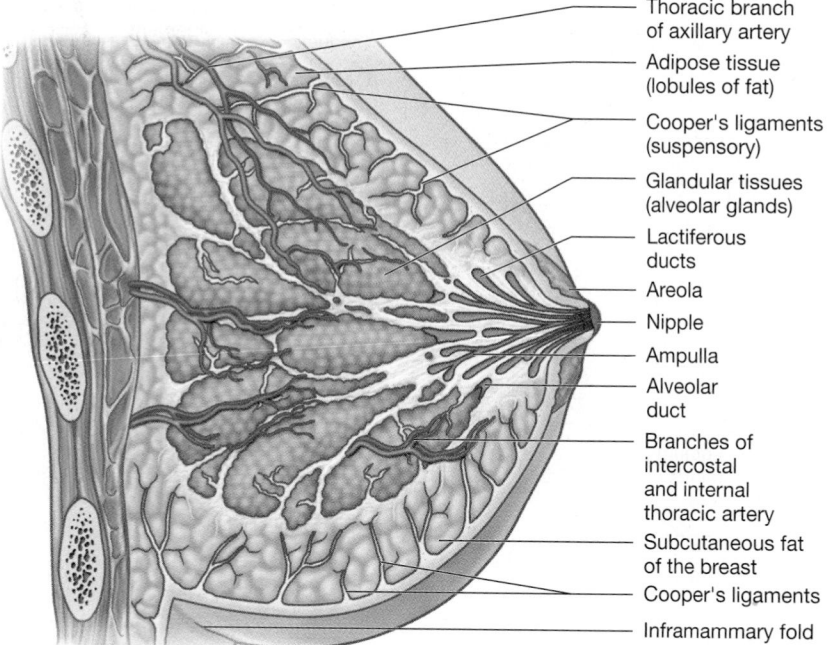

Thoracic branch of axillary artery

Adipose tissue (lobules of fat)

Cooper's ligaments (suspensory)

Glandular tissues (alveolar glands)

Lactiferous ducts

Areola

Nipple

Ampulla

Alveolar duct

Branches of intercostal and internal thoracic artery

Subcutaneous fat of the breast

Cooper's ligaments

Inframammary fold

FIGURE 48–1 ■ The female breast.

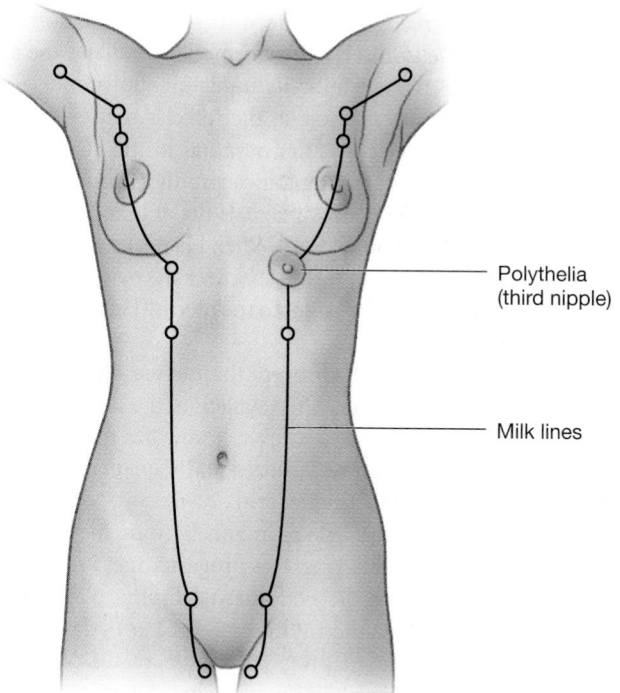

Polythelia (third nipple)

Milk lines

FIGURE 48–2 ■ Supernumerary nipples.

progesterone (steroid female hormone produced by the ovary and placenta), **prolactin** (hormone produced in the anterior pituitary), and **oxytocin** (hormone produced in the hypothalamus and released by the posterior pituitary) in the processes of **galactogenesis** (the manufacture of milk from available nutrients) and **lactation** (breast-feeding). The cyclic changes in estrogen and progesterone levels each month cause changes in the breasts as they prepare for lactation, even though a pregnancy does not always occur. This cyclic exposure to hormonal change is thought to be a factor in the development of breast cancer (American Cancer Society, 2006b).

Lymph nodes drain the breasts to the axilla, clavicular area, mediastinum, the opposite breast, and into glands in the liver (Stables & Rankin, 2005). The lymph nodes of the axilla and clavicular area are accessible to physical examination.

The female external genitalia depicted in Figure 48–3 ■ (p. 1506) have several components that are important to recognize during examination. These include the mons, the vulva (labia majora and labia minora), the clitoris (erectile tissue at apex of labia minora), the urinary meatus (urinary opening above the vaginal opening), and the introitus (opening to the vagina). The introitus is surrounded by an elastic line of connective tissue called the hymenal ring (Stables & Rankin, 2005).

Internally, the female reproductive organs include the uterus (muscular, hollow organ where the embryo matures before birth), the fallopian tubes (hollow tube from the uterus to the ovaries, where fertilization occurs), and the ovaries (female gonad). The uterus sits between the rectum and the bladder. The opening to the uterus is the cervix, found at the internal end of the vagina (Stables & Rankin, 2005) (Figure 48–4 ■, p. 1506).

The lymph nodes of the female external and internal reproductive organs that are accessible to examination are the superficial inguinal nodes, including the horizontal grouping and the vertical grouping. These nodes are found in the groin on each side. The horizontal group is below the inguinal ligament, and the vertical group lines up along the great saphenous vein. The horizontal group drains the lower abdomen, the superficial external genitalia, the anal canal, the perineum, and the lower vagina. The vertical group drains the upper leg (Bickley & Szilagyi, 2007).

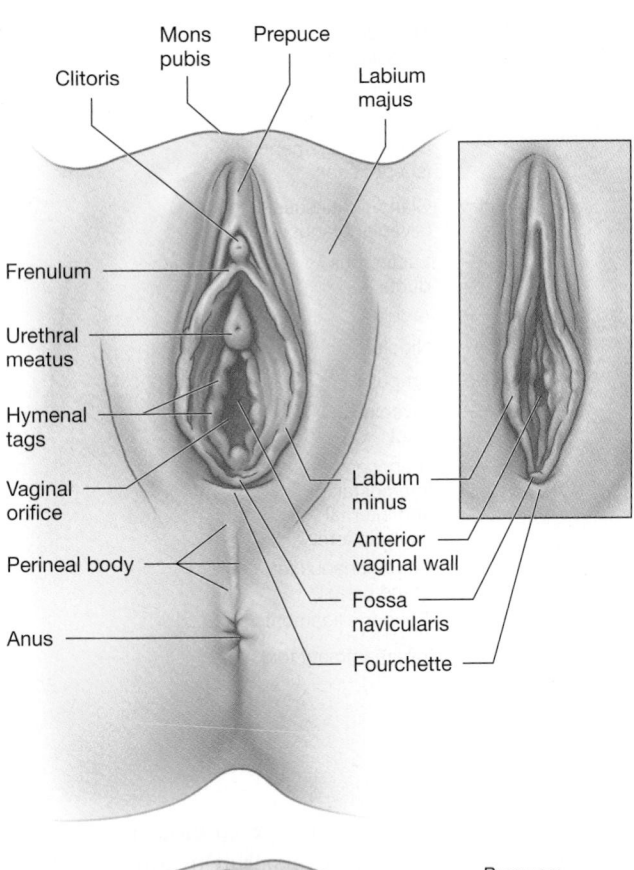

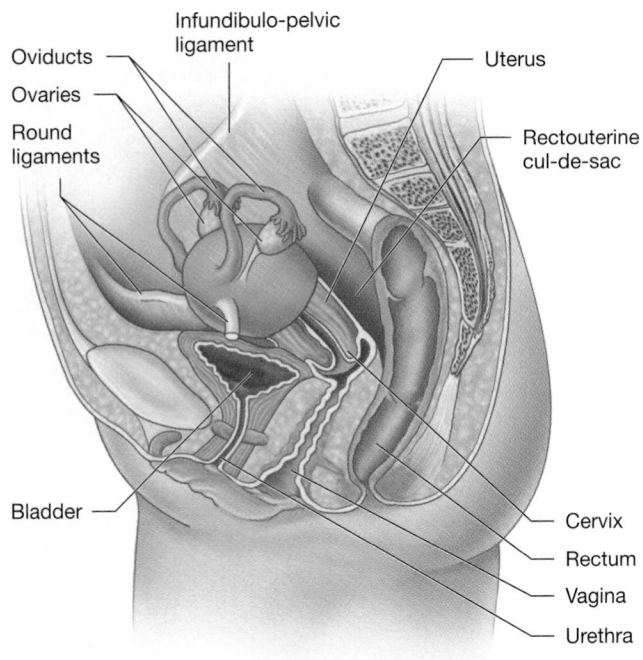

FIGURE 48–4 ■ Female internal genitalia.

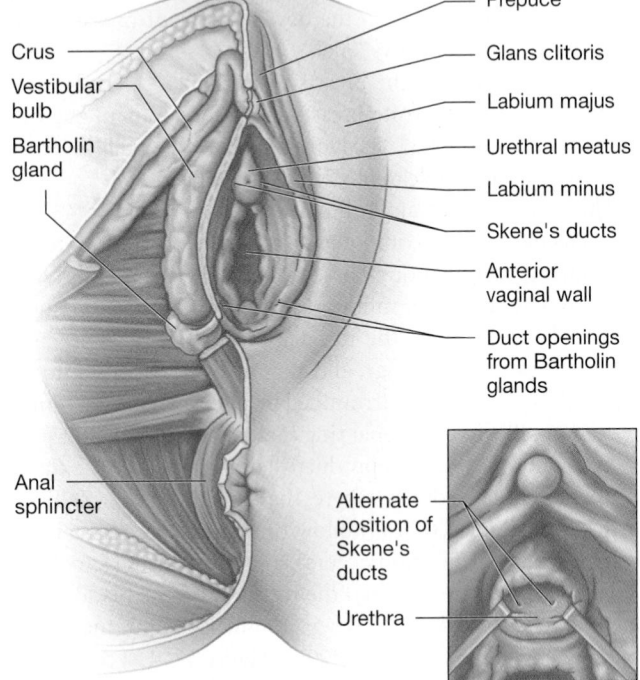

FIGURE 48–3 ■ Female vulva including anus.

Physiology of the Menstrual Cycle

The menstrual cycle is a complex physiological process that involves the hypothalamus, pituitary gland, ovaries, and endometrium. The cycle begins with the first day of menses. Menses, or vaginal bleeding, is the result of the thickened endometrial lining that was constructed during the previous cycle that is being sloughed or shed. As this occurs, the hypothalamus (through

complex signals) recognizes a need to secrete gonadotropin-releasing hormone (GnRH). This hormone stimulates the anterior pituitary to release follicle-stimulating hormone (FSH), which in turn stimulates a few of the follicles that exist on the ovary. From the follicles that first respond to the FSH, one becomes dominant. This growing follicle produces and secretes estrogen. When estrogen peaks, it signals the anterior pituitary to release luteinizing hormone (LH). When LH peaks, ovulation occurs. That is, the dominant follicle extrudes the ovum. The ovum travels to the fallopian tube and into the uterus (Hughes, Steele, & Leclaire, 2006).

Under the influence of estrogen, the uterine lining has been thickening before ovulation. After ovulation, the lining begins to proliferate; that is, it gets even thicker. It now has more nutrients available should the ovum be fertilized and implantation into the endometrial lining occur (Hughes et al., 2006).

After ovulation, the follicle remnants become the corpus luteum (yellow body), which secretes progesterone. Progesterone causes the "fluffing" of the endometrial lining. If a fertilized ovum does not implant, then at the end of 12 to 14 days the corpus luteum regresses and progesterone decreases. When this happens, the endometrial lining sloughs and menses begins (Hughes et al., 2006). Figure 48–5 ■ is a graph that shows when in the cycle each event occurs.

■ Male Reproductive System

The male breast is a small nipple and areola. There is a small amount of undeveloped breast tissue that may enlarge (gynecomastia) in response to certain drugs or illicit drug use. Breast cancer rarely occurs in male breast tissue (Slovik, 2006).

The male external genitalia are pictured in Figure 48–6 ■. External genitalia include the penis and scrotum (skin pouch that contain the testes). The penis is made up of erectile tissue

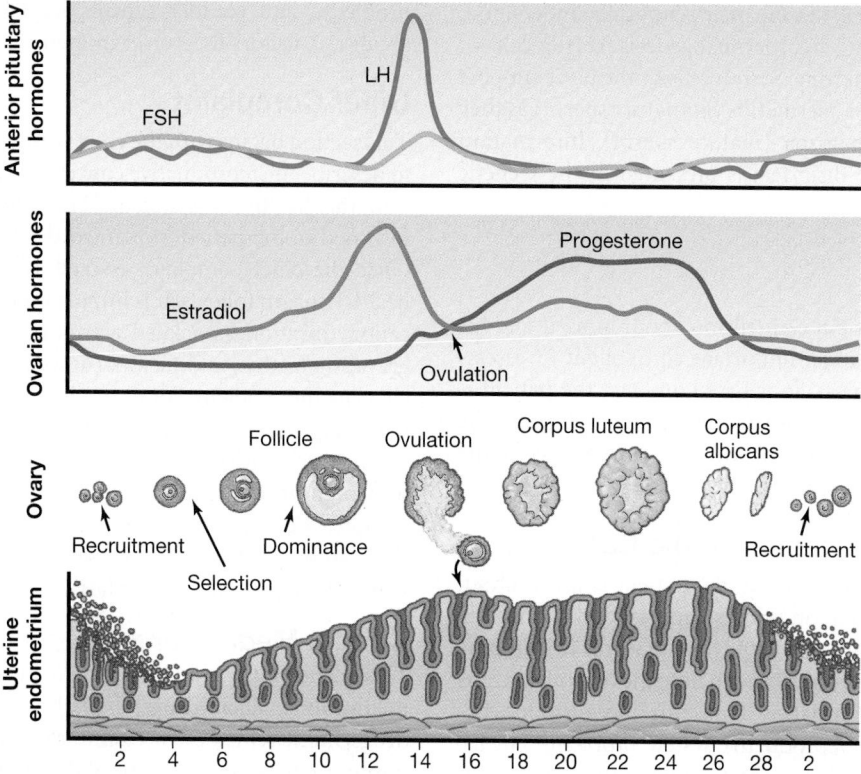

FIGURE 48–5 ■ The menstrual cycle.

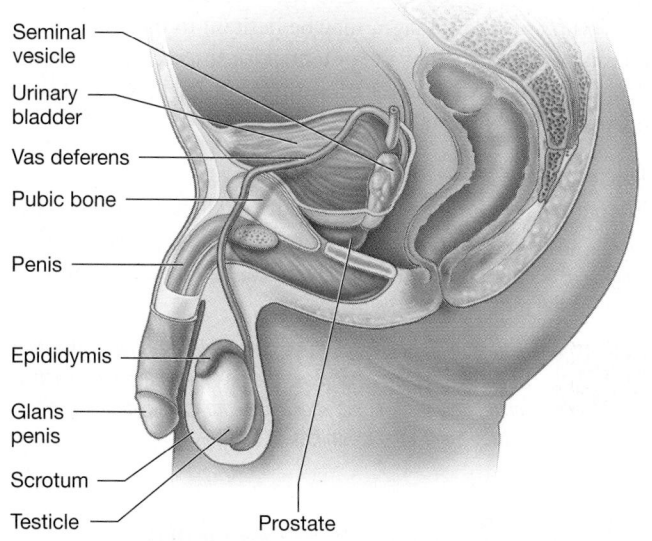

FIGURE 48–6 ■ Male genitalia.

and contains the urethra. At the tip of the penis is the urinary meatus (opening of the urethra to the outside). Within the scrotum are the testis, the epididymis (anatomic structure on the posterior of the testicle), and the spermatic duct. The spermatic duct is surrounded by blood vessels and together they form the spermatic cord (Bickley & Szilagyi, 2007). As the spermatic cord ascends into the abdomen via the inguinal canal, it becomes the vas deferens (duct that carries sperm and semen to the seminal vesicles and prostate). Sperm pass through the vas deferens to the seminal vesicles (finger-like structures behind the prostate), which produce 60% of semen

(Stables & Rankin, 2005), and into the prostate (a gland at the bladder neck; the urethra passes through it) to be mixed with prostate fluid before ejaculation during intercourse. The prostate is about 2.5 centimeters long with a median sulcus (groove) between two lateral lobes. A third, anterior, lobe is not palpable. The prostate is fibrous and firm to touch (Bickley & Szilagyi, 2007).

The inguinal canal (tunnel for vas deferens) is medial to the inguinal ligament and has two openings: the external and internal inguinal rings. The external inguinal ring is accessible to examination. The inguinal canal is the site for direct and indirect inguinal hernias, which are common in men (Bickley & Szilagyi, 2007). Chapter 50 ◉ includes an in-depth discussion of hernias.

Inguinal lymph nodes are located below the inguinal ligament in a horizontal configuration at the groin and along the femoral and great saphenous veins vertically on the upper thigh. The horizontal group drains the lower abdomen, buttock, external genitalia, anal canal, and perianal area. The vertical group drains the upper thigh. The testicles drain into lymph nodes in the abdomen. The abdominal lymph nodes are not accessible to palpation (Bickley & Szilagyi, 2007).

Physiology of Male Reproduction

Male reproductive physiology begins with an interaction between the hypothalamus, the pituitary gland, and the testis. The hypothalamus secretes gonadotropin-releasing hormone (GnRH) based on signals from the central nervous system and blood levels of testosterone. The GnRH travels to the anterior pituitary gland and causes the release of luteinizing hormone (LH) and follicle-stimulating hormone (FSH). LH stimulates testosterone and other hormone synthesis in the Leydig cells of the testicle. The role of FSH in the male is not fully understood. It appears to be necessary for spermatogenesis. Leydig cells of the testis produce testosterone. Sertoli cells of the testis support and provide nutrients for spermatids (immature sperm) as they grow to become spermatozoa (mature sperm). Information about sex chromosome disorders is presented in the Genetic Considerations box.

History

History, or what the patient can tell you about himself and his health concerns, is the most important component of assessment. Much of what nurses do is based on what the patient is able to convey about how he or she feels and the symptoms he or she is having. In this section, the health history related to the reproductive system is discussed.

Biographical and Demographic Data

After introductions are completed, the patient is asked about age, marital status, occupation, address, and other data that will identify this history as specifically for this patient. It is important to date and time the history and to note the reliability of the person providing the information. From this interview clues begin to emerge related to reproductive system problems. For instance, the older the female patient, the higher the risks are for breast, endometrial, and uterine cancer. See Chapter 49 for more about risks for cancer in women. The older the male patient, the higher the risks are for sexual dysfunction, prostate

problems, and bladder cancer. See Chapter 50 for more about risk factors for cancer in men.

Chief Complaint

This section begins with the chief complaint. The patient is asked to describe the reproductive concern that has brought her or him into the health care system. The chief complaint is usually recorded in the patient's own words (Bickley & Szilagyi, 2007). Once the chief complaint is established, a description of the health concern follows. It is important to ask about the onset, location, duration, associated symptoms, any treatments tried, aggravating factors, and factors (other than treatments) that may alleviate the problem. For example, a male may complain of urinary frequency, urgency, difficulty beginning the urinary stream, and nocturia with gradual onset when he is describing symptoms of benign prostatic hyperplasia (BPH). See Chapter 50 for a complete description of BPH. Chart 48–1 lists specific questions that can be used to elicit history of present illness from a man with benign prostatic hyperplasia.

Current Medications

This section of the history should include a list of prescribed medications, illicit drugs, herbal remedies, over-the-counter drugs, home remedies, or vitamins that the patient is taking. It is important to record the name of the drug or herb, the dosage, and how often it is being taken. Some women who are taking birth control pills may forget to mention this, so it is a good habit to ask women of childbearing age about birth control pills. Ask men with prostate problems whether they are taking saw palmetto. Men who are taking Viagra may be hesitant to discuss this with the nurse. This drug has the potential for interacting with other drugs, such as cardiac medications, and causing harm, so it is important to ask about it.

Allergies

All patients should be asked about allergies to drugs, latex, foods, and environmental substances. For those patients with allergies, the chart should be clearly marked so that the health care team is alerted.

> **CRITICAL ALERT** *Examination of a patient using latex gloves when that patient has a latex allergy increases the risk for an adverse reaction, including anaphylactic shock. Be sure to ask about possible allergy before the examination begins.*

GENETIC CONSIDERATIONS for Sex Chromosome Disorders

Normal sperm occur in two types. One type has 22 autosomes and an X chromosome, and the other has 22 autosomes and a Y chromosome. Only one type of ovum is ready for fertilization, and it has 22 autosomes and an X chromosome. Therefore, it is the sperm contribution to the coupling that will determine the sex of the child. In the assessment of the female and the male, the examiner may examine individuals who have a sex chromosome disorder. The two most common examples are Klinefelter's syndrome and Turner's syndrome.

Klinefelter's syndrome occurs in about 1 in 1,000 births and is usually an extra one or two X chromosomes (XXY or XXXY). This is generally not identified until puberty when the secondary sexual characteristics do not occur. These individuals will have decreased testosterone, testicular atrophy, long legs and arms, feminine hair distribution, gynecomastia, a feminine voice, infertility, and mental retardation (Banasik, 2005).

Turner's syndrome is a monosomy disorder in which the sex chromosome has only one X chromosome and no corresponding X or Y. The phenotype (how the person will look or will display the abnormality) is female, but the ovaries do not develop and secondary sex characteristics such as breast development and pubic hair do not appear. This abnormality is rare, occurring in about 1 in 3,000 live births (Banasik, 2005). Other physical characteristics include short stature, webbing of the neck, amenorrhea (no menses), a wide chest, and heart defects.

Sources: Banasik, J. (2005). Genetic and developmental disorders. In L. Copstead & J. Banasik, *Pathophysiology* (3rd ed., pp. 123–148). Philadelphia: W. B. Saunders; and Moore, K., & Persaud, T. (2003). *Before we are born: Essentials of embryology and birth defects* (6th ed.). Philadelphia: W. B. Saunders.

CHART 48–1 Interview Questions for History of Present Illness

After introductions, Mr. Davis tells you he has come to the hospital for surgery on his prostate. Here are some questions that would be asked to find out about his symptoms:

Have you been troubled with frequency of urination?

How often do you have to urinate?

Is this keeping you up at night?

Do you have difficulty starting the urinary stream?

Have you had to be catheterized because you could not void?

Does dribbling of urine occur after you void?

Are you ever incontinent?

Past Medical History

This section of the history includes childhood and adult illnesses; comorbid conditions; immunizations; hospitalizations; surgeries; and menstrual, obstetric, sexual, and social histories. Here the discussion is about some parts of the patient's past history that may affect reproductive health.

Childhood Illnesses and Immunizations

For women, childhood diseases that would have affected her health, fertility, or the health of her children would need to be considered. For instance, any communicable disease that affected her health severely would affect her ability to have children. This could mean that she would need to prevent pregnancy or to have special care if she were to become pregnant. Another example is the woman of childbearing age who has not had rubella or immunization for rubella. If she develops rubella while she is pregnant, this could cause birth defects in her child.

The childhood disease of concern for men is mumps. This viral illness has the potential for affecting the testicles, causing sterility. See Chapter 50 🔗 for further discussion of mumps orchitis.

Previous Illnesses and Hospitalizations

Medical comorbidities that may impact the reproductive system would include diabetes, hypertension, hepatitis, and HIV. The male with diabetes or hypertension treated with certain antihypertensive drugs may experience impotence. Hepatitis and human immunodeficiency virus (HIV) are sexually transmitted infections (STIs) that may be life threatening. Patients (female or male) who have hepatitis or HIV may pass these diseases to their sexual partners. The nurse should determine whether the patient has been diagnosed and treated for a sexually transmitted infection such as chlamydia, gonorrhea, syphilis, or herpes. For women, it is also important to ask whether they have ever had pelvic inflammatory disease (Narrigan, 2006). Ask about hospitalizations for any reproductive health concerns or chronic health problems. Find out when the hospitalization occurred, what the problem was, and how it was treated.

Diagnostic Procedures and Surgeries

Past surgeries that may affect the woman with a reproductive system problem may include breast surgeries, hysterectomy, bilateral tubal ligation, cervical laser or cryosurgery, or any surgery for **endometriosis** (presence of uterine lining in sites other than within the uterus). See Chapter 49 🔗 for further discussion of surgeries of the reproductive system.

Procedures of particular interest in this section of the history for women include screenings or tests for breast cancer and cervical cancer. Mammograms, lump biopsies, or any other procedures for breasts would need to be dated and recorded in the history. It is also important to note the date of the last cervical cancer screening and the results of the Papanicolaou (Pap) smear. If the patient has ever been diagnosed with cervical dysplasia or treated for an abnormal Pap smear, it should be documented.

Men who have had prostate surgery may have increased incontinence or impotence. Other surgeries that may impact the reproductive system or lower urinary system include orchidectomy, vasectomy, or penile reconstruction due to epispadias (the urinary meatus is at the top or dorsal surface of the penis, between the penis and bladder) or **hypospadias** (the urinary opening is on the ventral or bottom of the penis, between the scrotum and the distal end of the penis). See Chapter 50 🔗 for further discussion of surgeries of the reproductive system.

Menstrual History

For women, the menstrual and obstetric history should be included in the health history. The menstrual history should include age at **menarche** (first menstruation), length of time from first day of menstrual flow to first day of next menstrual flow (one cycle), number of days and characteristics of menses, regularity of cycles, **molimenal** symptoms (symptoms accompanying menstruation), and the first day of her last menstrual period. For older women, ask about menopause including age at onset and symptoms such as hot flashes, vaginal dryness, night sweats, and insomnia (Narrigan, 2006).

Obstetric History

Obstetric history includes the number of pregnancies, premature and term births, and spontaneous and therapeutic abortions. It is also important to determine whether the deliveries were spontaneous vaginal births or cesarean sections and whether there were any complications (Narrigan, 2006).

Sexual History and Risks for Sexually Transmitted Infection

Healthy People 2010 set 10 high-priority public health issues for this decade. Responsible sexual behavior is number 5 on this list of the most important changes people can make to help everyone in the United States be healthier (U.S. Department of Health and Human Services [DHHS], 2007). The steps toward achieving this goal include identifying people who are engaging in risky sexual behavior and helping them to choose safer practices. In working toward this goal, the examiner can ask the patient about the last time the patient had intimate physical contact or sex with someone; whether the patient is happy with her or his sex life; whether the patient has sex with men, women, or both; and any concerns the patient may have about sexual health. If the patient is in a mutually monogamous relationship, then the risks are decreased for sexually transmitted infection (Narrigan, 2006).

In settings where the patients may be at risk for sexually transmitted infection or HIV, more in-depth exploration of sexual practices may be indicated. The Centers for Disease Control and Prevention (CDC) has published a list of five areas to be explored along with counseling about the prevention of sexually transmitted infection and HIV. Chart 48–2 (p. 1510) lists specific questions that the CDC suggests be used to elicit this history.

Family History

Explore the family history of women for mother, sister, maternal grandmother, or aunts with breast cancer. The occurrence of breast cancer in any of these relatives increases the risks for the patient (Lashley, 2005). This is also true of about 10% of cases of ovarian cancer.

There is the possibility that there may be women who are daughters of women who took diethylstilbestrol (DES) to prevent a miscarriage during that pregnancy. These daughters are at 40 times the risk of developing cancer of the vagina and cervix (Wallace & Sanford, 2006). Therefore, it is important to ask women born between 1940 and 1971 whether they were exposed to DES while *in utero*.

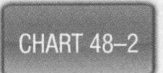

CHART 48–2

Exploring the Five Areas of Concern in the Prevention of Sexually Transmitted Infection (STI)

PARTNERS

"Do you have sex with men, women, or both?"

"In the past 12 months, how many partners have you had sex with?"

PREVENTION OF PREGNANCY

"Are you or your partner trying to get pregnant?" If "no":

"What are you doing to prevent pregnancy?"

PROTECTION FROM STIS

"What do you do to protect yourself from STIs?"

PRACTICES

"To understand your risks for STIs, I need to understand the kind of sex you have had recently."

"Have you had vaginal sex, meaning 'penis in vagina sex'"? If "yes":

"Do you use condoms: never, sometimes, or always?"

"Have you had anal sex, meaning 'penis in anus sex'"? If "yes":

"Do you use condoms: never, sometimes, or always?"

"Have you had oral sex, meaning 'mouth on penis/vagina sex'"?

For Condom Answers

If "never": "Why do you not use condoms?"

If "sometimes": "In what situations or with whom, do you not use condoms?"

PAST HISTORY OF STIS

"Have you ever had an STI?"

"Have any of your partners had an STI?"

Additional Questions to Identify Human Immunodeficiency Virus (HIV) and Hepatitis Risk

"Have you or any of your partners ever injected drugs?"

"Have any of your partners exchanged money or drugs for sex?"

"Is there anything else about your sexual practices that I need to know about?"

Source: Workowski, K., & Berman, S. (2006). Sexually transmitted disease treatment guidelines. *Morbidity and Mortality Weekly Report, 55*(RR-11), 2–3.

Men should be asked whether their father or brother has prostate cancer. Early onset prostate cancer seems to occur in some families. African American men are particularly susceptible. See further discussion of inheritance of susceptibility to prostate cancer in Chapter 50 ☺.

Social History

Occupations or hobbies by which patients have been exposed to hazardous materials increase their risks for infertility (female and male) and prostate cancer. Ask the patient whether he works around hazardous materials such as excessive heat, radiation, heavy metals, or organic solvents and how he protects himself (Quallich, 2006).

Cigarette Smoking and Substance Abuse

Habits such as cigarette smoking, alcohol use, or illicit drug use should be explored. There is evidence from cohort and case-control research that cigarette smoking and secondhand smoke

increase the risks for cervical cancer (National Cancer Institute, 2007). Alcohol and illicit drug use have been shown to increase the incidence of sexually transmitted infection and HIV (Fogel, 2006b).

It is best to ask directly, "Tell me about your use of alcohol," or "When was your last drink of alcohol?" If the patient answers in such a way that the examiner is suspicious of problem drinking, then screening questions such as the CAGE questionnaire (Chart 48–3) can be used to help identify alcohol abuse. CAGE stands for "cutting down, annoyance if criticized, guilty feelings, eye-openers" (Bickley & Szilagyi, 2007).

The same direct approach should be used in questioning about illicit drug use. Direct questions, such as "Have you ever used any drugs other than those required for medical reasons?" and "Have you ever injected a drug?" work best to elicit this information from the patient (Bickley & Szilagyi, 2007).

Domestic Violence

Violence affects people of all ages, both genders, and of all religions, races, and socioeconomic groups. Domestic violence, whereby intimate partners inflict physical, sexual, or emotional injury, is very prevalent (Harley, 2006; Mick, 2006). In fact, *Healthy People 2010* lists injury and violence as number 7 of the top 10 high-priority health issues in the United States (DHHS, 2007). People who suffer intimate partner violence are more likely to abuse alcohol and drugs, and to have HIV or a sexually transmitted infection (Fogel, 2006b; Wingood, 2006).

Domestic violence is difficult to discuss, but questions about abuse should be asked of all patients, both women and men. The only way to begin to change behavior is to uncover the abuse. Make it a habit to ask patients questions, such as "Are there times in your relationship that you feel unsafe or afraid?" or "Within the last year, have you been hit, kicked, punched, or otherwise hurt by someone you know?" (Bickley & Szilagyi, 2007). Try to conduct the interview in private, away from family or the abusive partner (Harley, 2006).

■ Physical Examination

After the history is completed, the examiner should ask the patient to disrobe and put on a gown for the physical examination. The gown should open in front for better access to the breasts and genitals of both the female and male patient. Assemble the equipment needed for the pelvic examination. The examiner should step out of the room while the patient changes. Hand hygiene and donning of gloves by the examiner needs to occur in the room, in front of the patient.

CHART 48–3   The CAGE Questionnaire

1. Have you ever felt the need to **C**ut down on drinking?
2. Have you ever felt **A**nnoyed by criticism of your drinking?
3. Have you ever felt **G**uilty about drinking?
4. Have you ever taken a drink first thing in the morning (**E**ye-opener) to steady your nerves or get rid of a hangover?

Source: From Mayfield, D., McLeod, G., Hall, P.: The CAGE questionnaire: Validation of a new alcoholism screening instrument. *American Journal of Psychiatry, 131,* 1121–1123, 1974.

Female Examination

Chart 48–4 lists the equipment needed for the female examination. The nurse examiner should be accompanied by an assistant because of the sexual nature of this examination. This is true regardless of the gender of the nurse. During the physical assessment, the nurse should teach the patient about healthy lifestyles and choices.

Breasts

The breast examination is best done with the woman sitting at the end of the examination table. For inspection of the breast, she should be asked to open the gown so that her breasts are fully visible to the examiner. The examiner should inspect the breasts for size, shape, contour, dimpling, and inverted nipples; areas of increased vascularity; and erosion or inflammation of the nipple or areola. The inspection should be carried out while the patient's arms are at her side, then again when she raises her arms above her head or presses her hands to her hips to contract the pectoralis muscle. These maneuvers will move the breast and pull the suspensory ligaments in such a way that a tumor would cause dimpling or a bulge. If the woman has large, pendulous breasts, a bimanual (palpating breast tissue between the two hands of the examiner) examination of the breasts as she leans forward will help to palpate any masses (Narrigan, 2006).

The next portion of the breast examination is palpation. Ask the patient to lie down and raise one arm over her head. Place a small pillow or folded towel beneath the shoulder on the side of the breast to be examined, and palpate all the breast tissue. Palpate in a circular pattern, in smaller circles as you near the center of the breast. Be sure to include all four quadrants of the breast, including the upper outer quadrant and the tail of Spence (a section of breast tissue that extends toward the axilla). End the palpation with a gentle pressure on the nipple between the thumb and forefinger to determine whether there is discharge from the nipple. Repeat the procedure for the other breast. Palpate for masses or tenderness. If there is nipple drainage, collect a specimen on a slide and send it to the laboratory for evaluation (Narrigan, 2006).

Inspect the axilla for lesions, masses, or inflammation. Hold the patient's arm in a relaxed position and palpate for the axillary nodes by grasping the axillary fold and feeling for pectoral nodes along the pectoral muscle. Reach high in the axilla and feel along the humerus for the lateral lymph nodes. Then, change hands so that the arm is supported and the opposite hand can examine for subscapular nodes by feeling inside the posterior axillary fold. Examine along the top and below the clavicle for supra- and infraclavicular nodes. Repeat the entire procedure for the opposite adnexa (Bickley & Szilagyi, 2007).

External Genitalia

While the patient is still lying down, examine the groin for swollen inguinal lymph nodes. When this is completed on both sides, help her move down on the table and to put her feet into the stirrups for the external genitalia and internal genitalia examinations. Her buttocks should be right at the edge of the end of the examination table with her knees flexed and legs spread so that the external genitalia are accessible to examination. This is the **lithotomy** position (Figure 48–7 ). Raise the head of the examination table to help her be more comfortable and drape her lower body and legs.

The nurse examiner should sit on a stool for the examination and lower the drape so that the nurse can see the patient's face during the examination. Inspect the external genitalia. The nurse tells the patient the nurse is going to touch her before the nurse moves a gloved hand to the vulva to spread the tissues for inspection of the entire vulva and perineum. Look for lesions, warts, vesicles, changes in pigmentation, signs of abuse such as bruises or lacerations, swollen Bartholin glands, or vaginal discharge or blood at the introitus. Figure 48–8 ■ (p. 1512) illustrates the technique for examining the Bartholin glands. Ask the patient to bear down as if to move her bowels, and observe for any bulges of cystocele (relaxation of the anterior vagina wall under the urinary bladder) or rectocele (relaxation of the posterior vaginal wall over the rectum) or prolapsed uterus at the introitus. Cystocele and rectocele are discussed in Chapter 49 ✍. Palpate bulges to differentiate the cystocele from the rectocele. Palpate the Bartholin glands at 7 and 5 o'clock to the introitus. Palpate with one finger for the location of the cervix within the vagina (Bickley & Szilagyi, 2007).

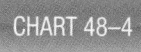 *Discovery of very painful swelling of the Bartholin gland should be referred immediately to a gynecologist for treatment (Birnbaum, 2006).*

Vagina and Cervix

The nurse places a small amount of water soluble lubricant on the speculum and tells the patient that the nurse is about to insert the speculum to visualize the cervix. Grasp the speculum in the dominant hand, spread the labia with the opposite hand, and

CHART 48–4	**Equipment Needed for the Female Genitalia Examination**

1. Examination gloves (latex or nonlatex, depending on patient allergy)
2. A good light source (gooseneck lamp or light that attaches to the speculum)
3. Speculum (choose size most appropriate for the patient)
4. Water soluble lubricant
5. Pap smear equipment
6. Culture tubes for STIs or other bacterial infection

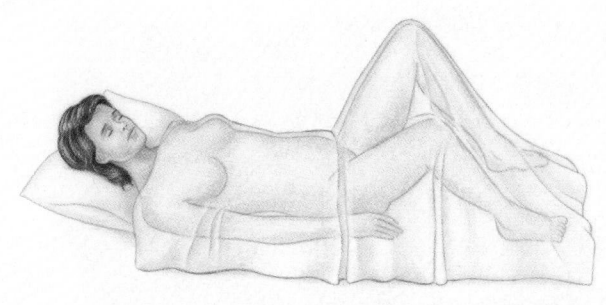

FIGURE 48–7 ■ Female lithotomy position.

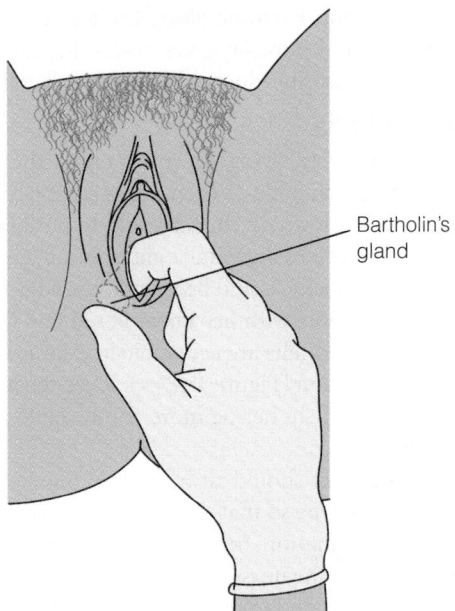

FIGURE 48–8 ■ Palpation of the Bartholin glands.

insert the speculum, pointing it down and back toward the cervix (Figure 48–9 ■). Open the speculum to visualize the cervix. Look for any lesions, warts, or increased vascularization on the cervix or the vaginal walls. Look at the cervical os (opening) for drainage. Obtain specimens for Pap smear or STI cultures as appropriate (Figure 48–10 ■). Note whether the cervix bleeds slightly on contact with the specimen collector. If blood is present, this means that the cervix is **friable** (easily damaged). Rotate the speculum to visualize the remainder of the vagina before removing it. Discard the speculum appropriately (Bickley & Szilagyi, 2007).

Uterus and Adnexa

Lubricate the forefinger and long finger of the dominant hand for the bimanual examination. Explain to the patient that the examination of the uterus and ovaries is next. Insert the lubricated fingers into the vagina and palpate the cervix for motion tenderness by moving it side to side. Perform a bimanual examination with one hand on the lower abdomen just above the symphysis

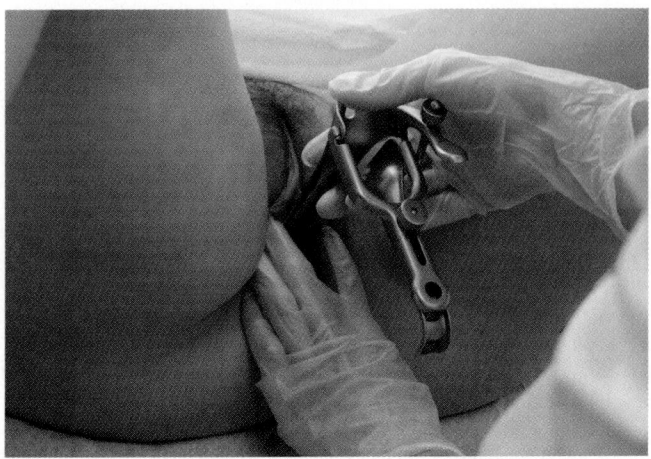

FIGURE 48–9 ■ Speculum insertion.

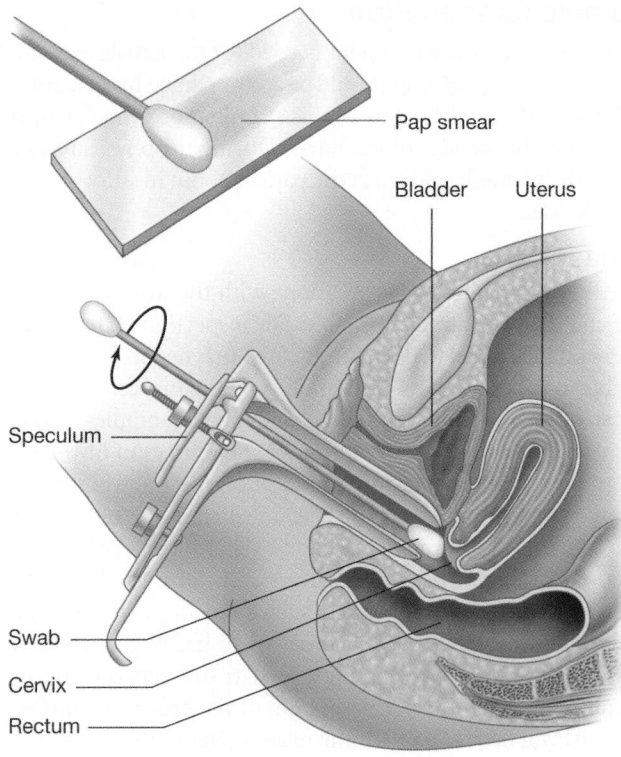

FIGURE 48–10 ■ Obtaining Pap smear.

(pubic bone) and the fingers in the vagina pressing the cervix and uterus upward toward the abdominal hand to determine uterine tenderness, position, size, and shape. Figure 48–11 ■ shows the bimanual exam of the female. Move the hands to the right adnexa and examine bimanually for masses or tenderness. Move the hands to the left adnexa and repeat the examination for masses or tenderness. Figure 48–12 ■ depicts the palpation of the adnexa (Bickley & Szilagyi, 2007).

Rectum

If the woman's history or examination indicates a reason, then a rectal examination should be done. Put on clean examination gloves. Inspect the anal area for hemorrhoids, fissures, lesions, or warts. Lubricate the index and long fingers of the dominant hand, and then place the long finger over the anus and ask the patient to bear down as if for a bowel movement. Insert the finger as the anus opens. Place the forefinger into the vagina. Palpate for lesions, a retroverted uterus, or a fistula between the vagina and rectum. Remove the forefinger from the vagina and palpate the entire rectal wall with the long finger for rectal lesions. After removal of the long finger, place any stool obtained on a hemoculture card and test for occult blood (Bickley & Szilagyi, 2007).

Help the patient to move back on the table before sitting up, so that she is supported by the examination table. Help her down from the examination table, give her some tissue to remove the excess lubricant from the genitalia, and leave the room to give her privacy to dress.

Male Examination

The male breast should be inspected for lesions, piercing, or gynecomastia. If the history or inspection has revealed a problem with the male breast, palpation for masses and tenderness is indicated.

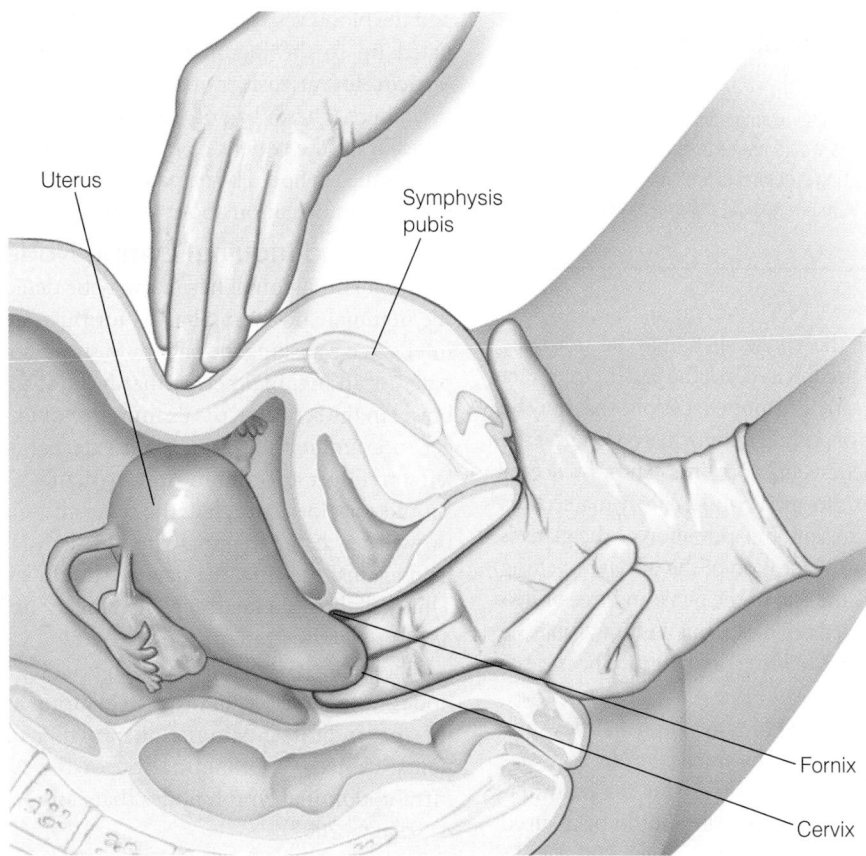

FIGURE 48–11 ■ Bimanual exam female.

The male external genital examination should occur in a warm, private room after the examiner has washed and warmed the examining hands. The patient should be asked whether the room is warm enough. A cold room or cold examining hands will activate the **cremasteric reflex** (testicles rise in the scrotum to the abdominal cavity when the thigh is stroked or the room is cold). The nurse should introduce herself or himself and ask permission before proceeding. This will give the patient an opportunity to ask for a same-sex examiner, if he wishes. During the examination, the patient may be standing or lying down. Drape and gown the patient so that the genitalia can be visualized by having the patient hold up the gown if he is standing or

to have a cover over his chest and legs if he is lying down. The examiner should be accompanied by an assistant or the patient's wife because of the sexual nature of the examination (Ceo, 2006). The Cultural Considerations box (p. 1514) notes the importance of respecting cultural attitudes about privacy.

External Genitalia

The examination of the male external genitalia is completed by inspection followed by palpation. Chart 48–5 (p. 1514) lists the equipment that may be needed. With the male standing, the examiner can sit on a stool in front of him and inspect the genitalia for lesions in the pubic hair, on the penis, or on the front or back of the

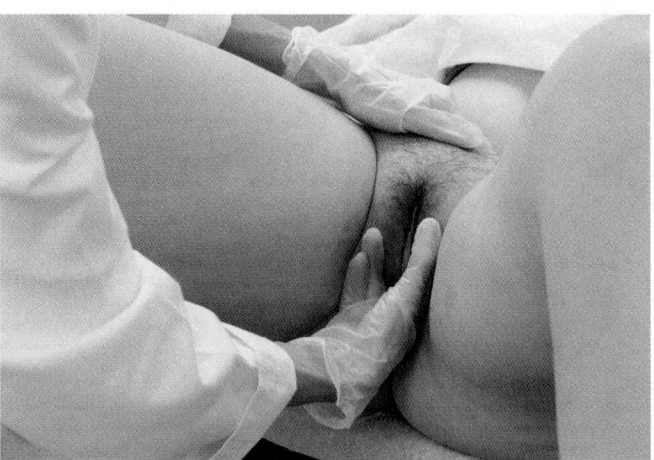
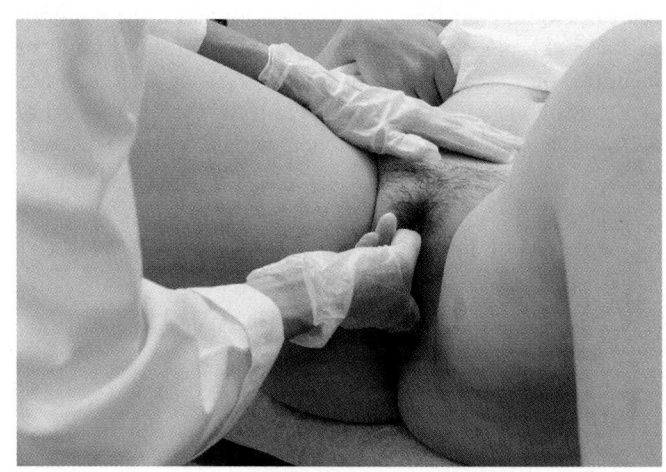

FIGURE 48–12 ■ Palpation of adnexa.

CULTURAL CONSIDERATIONS for Genital Examinations

Before proceeding with a male genital examination with the wife present, ask the wife whether she would prefer to leave. In certain cultures, the wife's presence during a genital examination of her husband would be considered taboo or against cultural mores (Ceo, 2006).

scrotum. The dorsal vein of the penile shaft may be normally prominent. If the male is not circumcised, ask the patient to retract the foreskin so that the glans can be inspected. Lesions that may be seen include **chancres** (ulcers of syphilis), abnormal contour of the scrotum, cancer, warts, herpetic vesicles, or infestation by lice or other insects in the pubic hair. Smegma (white, cheesy material) is a normal finding under the foreskin. Inflammation of the glans is called balanitis. Inspection for the location of the urinary opening follows. Normally, it will be at the end of the penis and free of discharge. If the patient has reported discharge, but it is not visible, he should be asked to strip the penis to bring discharge to the meatus for culture (Bickley & Szilagyi, 2007).

Palpation of the penis is reserved for any abnormalities such as tenderness or plaque formation. The nurse should be aware that the male patient may have an erection during the examination. This is often beyond his control, and he should be assured that this is a normal occurrence (Bickley & Szilagyi, 2007).

If the contour of the scrotum is suspicious, palpation for **cryptorchidism** (an undescended testicle), scrotal **hydrocele** (swelling due to fluid accumulation in the scrotum), or hernia should be done. A hernia with a loop of bowel in the scrotum can be differentiated from hydrocele by translumination (with a light source behind the swelling, look for a glow of clear fluid or no light penetrance). One can also auscultate the scrotal mass with the aid of the stethoscope for bowel sounds (Ceo, 2006).

> **CRITICAL ALERT** *Discovery of an undescended testicle in a teenager would warrant immediate referral to an urologist. The incidence of testicular cancer is increased when the testicle is undescended (Goroll & Mulley, 2006).*

Palpation of the testis is accomplished by grasping it between the thumb and forefinger and feeling for nodules or masses. The examiner should be aware that too much pressure on the testis can cause deep pain. The epididymis is found on the posterior surface and is palpated in the same way. Cysts or tumors may be identified on the testicle or epididymis. Cysts or tumors in this area may be malignant or benign. From the epididymis, a cord will ascend upward toward the abdomen. This is the vas deferens

CHART 48–5 Equipment Needed for the Male Genitalia Examination

1. Examination gloves (latex or nonlatex, depending on patient allergy)
2. Water soluble lubricant
3. Flashlight or other light source for translumination
4. Stethoscope

and the blood vessels of the spermatic cord. This structure is palpated up to the inguinal ring where it enters the abdomen. **Varicocele** (varicosities of the veins of the scrotum) may be identified here. These "bag of worms" abnormalities are more likely to occur on the patient's left side. Both sides of the scrotum and both testicles should be palpated (Ceo, 2006). See Chapter 50 for more information about varicoceles.

Hernia and Inguinal Lymph Nodes

Femoral and inguinal hernias may be detected by inspection of the inguinal and femoral areas for bulges. These bulges can be intensified by asking the patient to strain down or cough. To palpate for an inguinal hernia that has not presented as a loop of bowel in the scrotum, the examiner should use the right forefinger to examine the patient's left external inguinal ring and the left forefinger to examine the patient's right. This maneuver should start low enough in the scrotum to assure that the fingertip will reach the inguinal ring. While the examining finger is held against the ring, the patient should cough or strain down. This will bring a mass against the examining finger. Figure 48–13 ■ demonstrates this maneuver.

The superficial inguinal lymph nodes are palpated, and if the nodes in the horizontal or vertical group are swollen or tender, this may indicate inflammation or malignancy of the scrotum or penis. Cancer or inflammation of the testicles would affect intra-abdominal lymph nodes that cannot be palpated (Bickley & Szilagyi, 2007).

Prostate

To palpate the prostate, a rectal examination is required. The patient will need to lean over the examining table or lie on his left side with his right knee drawn up (Figure 48–14 ■). The anal area is inspected by spreading the buttocks. The examiner should look for lesions, external hemorrhoids, or warts in this area. The examiner should lubricate the forefinger of the dominant hand generously. To decrease discomfort, the nurse should tell the patient what is about to be done, have the patient bear down as if moving his bowels, and move the examining finger into the anal canal as it opens. The posterior surface of two lobes of the prostate is palpated through the anterior rectal wall. The examiner should identify the median sulcus and note the size and firmness of the prostate, and the presence of any masses or tenderness. When the examination is complete, the examiner removes the

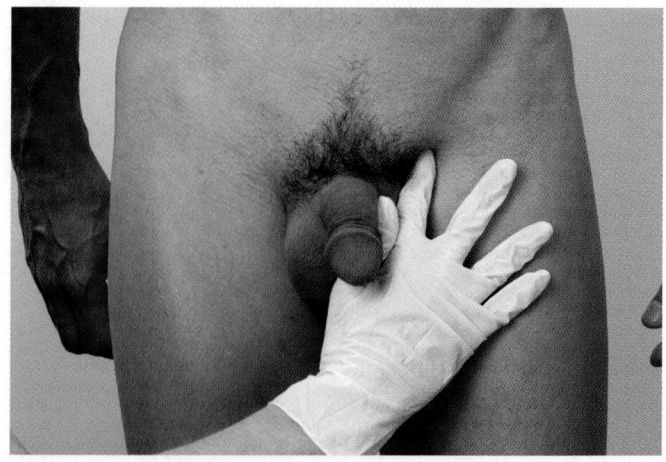

FIGURE 48–13 ■ Palpation for inguinal hernia.

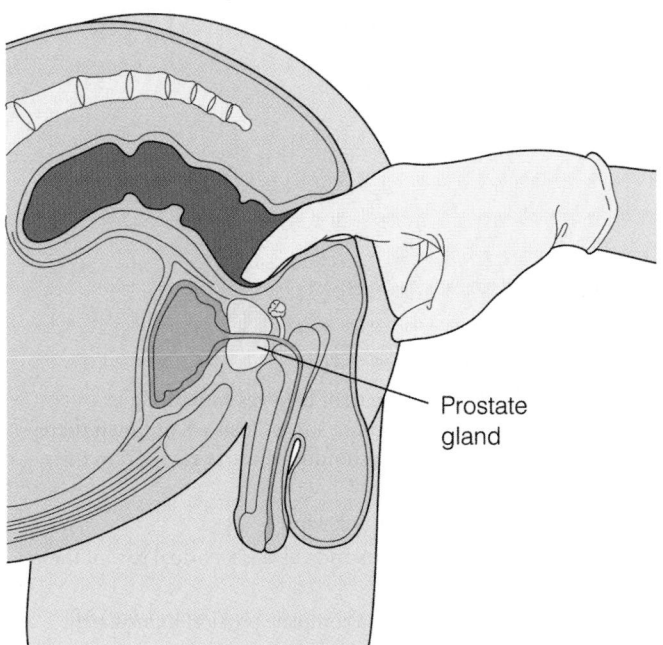

FIGURE 48–14 ■ Digital rectal exam prostate.

finger and wipes the excess lubricant from the anus (Bickley & Szilagyi, 2007; Ceo, 2006).

Gerontological Considerations

As with all systems of the body, the reproductive system undergoes changes with aging. Psychologically, there is reduced libido and decreased sexual satisfaction. This does not mean that men and women over age 65 are not sexual or that they do not enjoy sexual activity. It just means that sex is not as intense or frequent (Fogel, 2006a). On the other hand, libido and sexual feelings may decrease due to loss of a significant other, social isolation related to loss of mobility, or other factors. Some elders experience incontinence of urine, which decreases their willingness to exercise or to socialize with others (Stanley, Blair, & Beare, 2005).

Women experience menopause and the loss of estrogen usually in the early part of the fifth decade. The decrease in estrogen may cause symptoms such as hot flashes (which usually come and go during the first 5 years of menopause) and drying of the vaginal mucosa. Drying of the vaginal mucosa will make sexual intercourse and vaginal examinations uncomfortable. Less frequently, the woman may experience sleep disturbances, decreased ability to concentrate, and depression. Over time, decreased estrogen will contribute to loss of muscle mass and bone, and increased fat of the abdomen. The breast will atrophy as the glandular tissue is replaced by fat. The vulva will lose fat and the mons and vulva will lose hair. There may also be graying of the pubic hair (Ebersole, Hess, Touhy, & Jett, 2005).

Changes in mobility brought on by aging may necessitate a change in the positioning for vaginal examinations. For those women who cannot open their legs at the hips for the lithotomy position, alternate positioning may be needed. A side-lying position with the top leg drawn up will allow for small speculum examination of the vagina and cervix. Another option is to have two assistants support the patient's legs during the examination (Bickley & Szilagyi, 2007).

Men experience **andropause** (decrease in testosterone) beginning gradually in about the third decade. This causes decreased spermatogenesis and a shortening of the penis; the penis is slower to erection, and the scrotum hangs lower. Chronic disease may affect the testicles, causing them to shrink. Depression and a decrease in cognition may occur, just as with women in menopause. Men may have loss of muscle mass and bone mass, but not as much as seen in women (Stanley et al., 2005).

Loss of mobility or inability to stand for long periods may necessitate that the patient lie down for the prostate examination. Lying on the left side, bending at the hips, and drawing the right leg up so that the anal area is accessible to the examiner, is the recommended position (Bickley & Szilagyi, 2007).

Health Promotion

Health promotion means following a lifestyle that is conducive to health. Sexual health requires a healthy mind and body, open communications with the partner, and capacity to enjoy and control sexual impulses according to social norms (Fogel, 2006a). To be sexually healthy is to have a good body image and sexual identity. Sexual health is promoted by mutually monogamous relationships with uninfected partners. It also entails the avoidance of substances such as alcohol or illicit drugs that would decrease inhibitions and cause the female or male to engage in risky sexual behaviors.

National Guidelines for Disease Screening and Self-Examination

Early detection of disease through screening examinations is a tactic for health promotion. For women, cervical and breast cancer screening are recommended. The United States Preventive Services Task Force (USPSTF) recommends that sexually active women have annual Pap smears until age 65. At this point, the benefit of screening seems to diminish (USPSTF, 2003a). For breast screening, the USPSTF recommends screening mammography every 1 to 2 years for women age 40 and older (USPSTF, 2003b). According to the USPSTF, the research to date (worldwide) has not demonstrated that breast self-examination reduces mortality from breast cancer. The USPSTF does not recommend routine screening for ovarian cancer with serum CA-125 levels or transvaginal ultrasound, because research has not established that the benefits outweigh the potential harm (USPSTF, 2003d). The American Cancer Society, however, recommends that women with a strong family history of ovarian cancer be screened with both transvaginal ultrasound and serum CA-125 levels (American Cancer Society, 2006b).

For adolescents and young men, the USPSTF recommends against testicular self-examination and routine screening by clinicians (USPSTF, 2003c). Studies demonstrate that routine examination of the testicles has caused more harm than benefit.

For older men, the USPSTF has found that there is insufficient evidence to recommend for or against routine screening for prostate cancer with serum levels of prostate-specific antigen (PSA) and digital rectal examination (DRE) of the prostate (USPSTF, 2003e). Routine screening has been shown to cause unnecessary anxiety, biopsies, and treatments with severe side effects for a cancer that may never have affected the patient. In addition, there continue to be many false-positive PSAs.

Summary

Assessment of the reproductive systems of women and men has been described. Readers are encouraged to use what has been presented in this chapter in management plans for women and men with reproductive health care concerns, as presented in Chapters 49 and 50 ⊚ .

NCLEX® REVIEW

1. The nurse is instructing a teenage patient about menstruation and hormone regulation. Which of the following should the nurse include in this instruction?
   1. The next menstrual cycle begins on the last day of the current menses.
   2. The uterine lining becomes thicker because of estrogen.
   3. Estrogen causes ovulation.
   4. After ovulation, the lining of the uterus becomes thinner.

2. A male patient seeks medical care for a new onset of impotence. Which of the following should the nurse assess in this patient?
   1. Any other chronic illnesses such as diabetes
   2. Past medical history including mumps
   3. History of sexually transmitted infections
   4. Date of first sexual experience

3. A 35-year-old female is having difficulty conceiving. Which of the following can the nurse assess in this patient to aid in determining the cause of the infertility?
   1. Smoking history
   2. Occupations and hobbies
   3. Amount of daily exercise
   4. Amount of daily sleep and rest

4. While assessing the penis of an uncircumcised male, the nurse notes a white cheesy substance under the foreskin. The nurse realizes this finding indicates:
   1. Smegma, a normal finding.
   2. Syphilis.
   3. Inflammation.
   4. Discharge.

5. A 50-year-old female patient believes something is "drastically wrong" because she is "losing hair down there." Which of the following should the nurse respond to this patient?
   1. There could be something wrong.
   2. Hair loss over the mons and vulva is a normal part of the aging process.
   3. I suggest you schedule a complete physical immediately.
   4. Hair doesn't really serve a purpose there anyway.

6. A 70-year-old male patient tells the nurse that he "hates his annual physical" because every year he worries what his PSA level is going to be. Which of the following does this anxiety suggest?
   1. The patient does not like his primary physician.
   2. Routine screening for prostate cancer can lead to unnecessary anxiety.
   3. The patient thinks he has prostate cancer.
   4. The patient is hiding a health concern.

Answers for review questions appear in Appendix D

KEY TERMS

andropause *p.1515*
chancres *p.1514*
cremasteric reflex *p.1513*
cryptorchidism *p.1514*
endometriosis *p.1509*
friable *p.1512*

galactogenesis *p.1505*
hydrocele *p.1514*
hypospadias *p.1509*
lactation *p.1505*
lithotomy *p.1511*
menarche *p.1509*

molimenal *p.1509*
oxytocin *p.1505*
progesterone *p.1505*
prolactin *p.1505*
varicocele *p.1514*

EXPLORE **mynursingkit**
PEARSON

MyNursingKit is your one stop for online chapter review materials and resources. Prepare for success with additional NCLEX®-style practice questions, interactive assignments and activities, web links, animations and videos, and more!

Register your access code from the front of your book at
www.mynursingkit.com

REFERENCES

American Cancer Society. (2006a). *Can ovarian cancer be found early?* Retrieved February 27, 2008, from http://www.cancer.org/docroot/CRI/content/CRI_2_4_3X_Can_ovarian_cancer_be_found_early_33.asp?sitearea=CRI

American Cancer Society. (2006b). *What are the risk factors for breast cancer?* Retrieved April 27, 2007, from http://www.cancer.org/docroot/CRI/content/CRI_2_4_2X_What_are_the_risk_factors_for_breast_cancer_5.asp?sitearea

Bickley, L., & Szilagyi, P. (2007). *Bates' guide to physical examination and history taking* (9th ed.). Philadelphia: Lippincott Williams & Wilkins.

Birnbaum, S. (2006). Medical evaluation of female sexual dysfunction. In A. Goroll & A. Mulley. (2006), *Primary care medicine: Office evaluation and management of the adult patient* (5th ed., pp. 792–795). Philadelphia: Lippincott Williams & Wilkins.

Ceo, P. (2006). Assessment of the male reproductive system. *Urologic Nursing, 26*(4), 290–296.

Ebersole, P., Hess, P., Touhy, T., & Jett, K. (2005). *Gerontological nursing and healthy aging* (2nd ed.). St. Louis: Mosby.

Fogel, C. (2006a). Sexuality. In K. Schuiling & F. Likis (Eds.). *Women's gynecologic health* (pp. 149–167). Boston: Jones & Bartlett.

Fogel, C. (2006b). Sexually transmitted infections. In K. Schuiling & F. Likis (Eds.), *Women's gynecologic health* (pp. 421–468). Boston: Jones & Bartlett.

Goroll, A., & Mulley, A. (2006). *Primary care medicine: Office evaluation and management of the adult patient* (5th ed.). Philadelphia: Lippincott Williams & Wilkins.

Harley, A. (2006). Domestic violence screening: Implications for surgical nurses. *Plastic Surgical Nursing, 26*(1), 24–28.

Hughes, N., Steele, N., & Leclaire, S. (2006). Gynecologic anatomy and physiology. In K. Schuiling & F. Likis (Eds.), *Women's gynecologic health.* Boston: Jones & Bartlett.

Lashley, F. (2005). *Clinical genetics in nursing practice* (3rd ed.). New York: Springer.

Mick, J. (2006). Identifying signs and symptoms of intimate partner violence in an oncology setting. *Clinical Journal of Oncology Nursing, 10*(4), 509–513.

Narrigan, D. (2006). Gynecologic history and physical examination. In K. Schuiling & F. Likis (Eds.), *Women's gynecologic health* (pp. 101–126). Boston: Jones & Bartlett.

National Cancer Institute (NCI). (2007). *Cervical cancer (PDQ): Prevention, health professional version.* Retrieved February 27, 2008, from http://www.cancer.gov/cancertopics/pdq/prevention/cervical/HealthProfessional

Quallich, S. (2006). Examining male infertility. *Urologic Nursing, 26*(4), 277–288.

Slovik, D. (2006). Evaluation of gynecomastia. In A. Goroll & A. Mulley, *Primary care medicine: Office evaluation and management of the adult patient* (5th ed., pp. 707–710). Philadelphia: Lippincott Williams & Wilkins.

Stables, D., & Rankin, J. (Eds.). (2005). *Physiology in childbearing* (2nd ed.). Edinburgh, UK: Elsevier.

Stanley, M., Blair, K., & Beare, P. (2005). *Gerontological nursing: Promoting successful aging with older adults* (3rd ed.). Philadelphia: F. A. Davis.

U.S. Department of Health and Human Services. (2007). *Healthy People 2010 leading health indicators: Priorities for action.* Retrieved February 27, 2008, from http://www.healthypeople.gov/LHI/Priorities.htm

U.S. Preventive Services Task Force (USPSTF). (2003a). Recommendations and rationale: Screening for cervical cancer. In *Guide to Preventive Services* (2nd ed.). (Publication No. 00-P046). Rockville, MD: Agency for Healthcare Research and Quality. Retrieved February 27, 2008, from http://www.ahcpr.gov/clinic/3rduspstf/cervcan/cervcan.htm#clinical

U.S. Preventive Services Task Force (USPSTF). (2003b). Recommendations and rationale: Screening for breast cancer. In *Guide to Preventive Services* (2nd ed.). (Publication No. 00-P046). Rockville, MD: Agency for Healthcare Research and Quality. Retrieved February 27, 2008, from http://www.ahcpr.gov/clinic/3rduspstf/breastcancer/brcanrr.htm

U.S. Preventive Services Task Force (USPSTF). (2003c). Recommendations and rationale: Screening for testicular cancer. In *Guide to Preventive Services* (2nd ed.). (Publication No. 00-P046). Rockville, MD: Agency for Healthcare Research and Quality. Retrieved February 27, 2008, from http://www.ahcpr.gov/clinic/3rduspstf/testicular/testiculrs.htm

U.S. Preventive Services Task Force (USPSTF). (2003d). Recommendations and rationale: Screening for ovarian cancer. In *Guide to Preventive Services* (2nd ed.). (Publication No. 00-P046). Rockville, MD: Agency for Healthcare Research and Quality. Retrieved February 27, 2008, from http://www.ahcpr.gov/clinic/3rduspstf/ovariancan/ovcanrs.htm

U.S. Preventive Services Task Force (USPSTF). (2003e). Recommendations and rationale: Screening for prostate cancer. In *Guide to Preventive Services* (2nd ed.). (Publication No. 00-P046). Rockville, MD: Agency for Healthcare Research and Quality. Retrieved February 27, 2008, from http://www.ahcpr.gov/clinic/3rduspstf/prostatescr/prostaterr.htm

Wallace, M., & Sanford, A. (2006). Gynecologic cancers. In K. Schuiling & F. Likis (Eds.), *Women's gynecologic health.* Boston: Jones & Bartlett.

Wingood, G. (2006). Efficacy of an HIV prevention program among female adolescents experiencing gender-based violence. *American Journal of Public Health, 96*(6), 1085–1090.

CHAPTER 49

Caring for the Patient with Female Reproductive Disorders

Katherine Kelly
Kathleen Osborn

With Contributions by:
John M. Osborn
Laurie Kaudewitz

Outcome-Based Learning Objectives

After studying this chapter, the learner will be able to:

1. Differentiate the cause, mode of transmission, prevention, and treatment of sexually transmitted infections.
2. Discuss risk factors, diagnosis, and treatment of breast cancer.
3. Describe the procedure for a breast self-examination.
4. Differentiate the pathophysiology of the most common female reproductive disorders.
5. Discuss the medical treatment and nursing care for the most common female reproductive disorders.
6. Discuss the common causes and treatment of infertility and the related nursing care.
7. Discuss common diagnostic surgical procedures related to female reproductive disorders.
8. Describe key components of the interview of a patient who has been victimized by intimate partner violence.

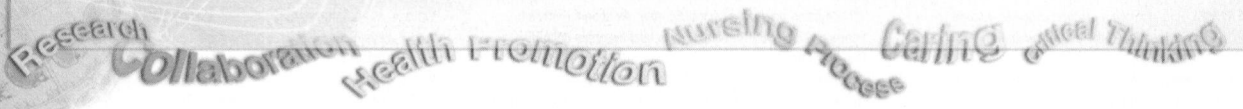

MANY HEALTH concerns of women relate to normal changes that occur in the reproductive cycle, but others involve alterations in normal reproductive functioning. Still others are cancer-related or sexually transmitted problems. This chapter will address specific diseases and disorders that affect the reproductive system and its functioning. It includes the expected signs, symptoms, and treatments as well as the psychosocial impact of each disease or disorder. *Healthy People 2010* guidelines are incorporated throughout the chapter with an emphasis on improving the health of women.

Sexually Transmitted Infections

Sexually transmitted infections (STIs) are also referred to as sexually transmitted diseases (STDs). They are more accurately identified as infections rather than diseases. STIs include more than 25 infections that are passed from person to person during sexual contact (CDC, 2008f).

One of the 28 focus areas in *Healthy People 2010* includes reducing or preventing sexually transmitted infections. Specifically, the goal of this focus area is promoting responsible sexual behavior, strengthening community capacity, and increasing access to quality services in an attempt to prevent sexually transmitted in-

fections (STIs) and their complications. The government recognizes that social, cultural, and behavioral factors play a role in the spread of these infections, and that access to health care is critical to preventing the spread of disease. The Centers for Disease Control and Prevention estimates that 19 million new sexually transmitted infections occur each year, almost half of them among young people ages 15 to 24 (CDC, 2005b). Women comprise two-thirds of these diagnoses (Johnson-Mallard, 2007).

Sexually Transmitted Infections Characterized by Cervicitis

Infectious disease of the cervix is primarily a result of sexual transmission. These infections, although easily transmitted through sexual contact, are often asymptomatic; therefore, women of childbearing age are routinely screened for them. Women are diagnosed with about two-thirds of these diseases, and it is women who suffer the morbidity of these infections in the form of loss of fertility (Johnson-Mallard, 2007).

Chlamydia Infections

The Centers for Disease Control and Prevention (CDC) reports that **chlamydia** is the most frequently reported infectious disease

1518

in the United States with 2.8 million new cases each year (CDC, 2008c). Chlamydia is known as a "silent™" disease because about three-quarters of infected women have no symptoms (CDC, 2008c). It is caused by *Chlamydia trachomatis* and transmitted during sexual intercourse. The bacteria initially infect the cervix and the urethra. Women who do notice symptoms often complain of burning urination, vaginal discharge, and mild lower abdominal cramps. Like gonorrhea, it is important to perform routine screening to prevent chlamydia from spreading. Also like gonorrhea, chlamydia that is left untreated can develop into pelvic inflammatory disease up to 40% of the time. Chlamydial infections cannot be distinguished from other urogenital infections by symptoms alone. Laboratory testing is needed to differentiate chlamydial infection from other lower genital tract infections such as urinary tract infection, bacterial vaginosis, and trichomoniasis. Figure 49–1 ■ shows typical objective signs of a chlamydia infection. To test for chlamydia, a small amount of vaginal fluid is needed to culture for the presence of the causative organism. A new urine test also is available that provides a noninvasive, quick mechanism for diagnosis (Quest Diagnostics, 2005). Chlamydia is treatable with antibiotics, typically azithromycin orally in a single dose or doxycycline orally for 7 days. In all diagnosed cases, partner treatment is necessary, and use of condoms is recommended until the infection is gone. Due to the prevalence of the disease, the CDC recommends routine screening for the following groups:

- Women with multiple sexual partners
- Sexually active women under 20 years of age
- Women over 24 years of age who are inconsistent with the use of barrier contraception, or have had new or more than one sex partner during the last 3 months.

The Pharmacology Summary of Medications to Treat Female Reproductive Disorders feature (p. 1552) includes the medications used to treat chlamydia infections.

Lymphogranuloma Venereum

Lymphogranuloma venereum (LGV) is an invasive, systemic infection that is caused by *Chlamydia trachomatis*. The most common clinical manifestation of LGV among heterosexuals is tender inguinal and/or femoral lymphadenopathy that is typi-

cally unilateral. Rectal exposure in women can result in proctocolitis, which causes anal pain, constipation, fever, and/or tenesmus. If not treated, LGV proctocolitis might lead to chronic colorectal fistulas and strictures. Treatment with doxycycline or erythromycin cures the infection and prevents further tissue damage. Sexual partners with whom the patient has had sexual contact in the preceding 60 days should also be treated.

Gonorrhea

Gonorrhea is the second most commonly reported sexually transmitted infection in the United States, with 339,593 cases reported in 2005 (CDC, 2005b). It is estimated that only one-half of the actual number of infections are reported. There has been a steady decline in the rate of reported cases of gonorrhea over the past 30 years (since 1975); however, the decline has leveled off in the past 5 to 6 years. Women ages 15 to 19 have the highest rate of infection. Increased prevalence is also noted in those living in the southern United States and African Americans. The incidence of gonorrhea is most prevalent in high-density urban areas among persons who have multiple sex partners and engage in unprotected sexual intercourse.

Gonorrhea is caused by the bacterium *Neisseria gonorrhoeae*, which infects the warm moist environment of the reproductive tract, along with any other mucous membranes in the body, such as the oral mucosa and the mucosa of the eye in a newborn. It is spread by sexual contact with another infected individual. Ejaculation does not have to occur for the infection to be transmitted. Gonorrhea can also be spread from mother to baby during delivery. Gonorrhea in women is often an incidental diagnosis, as it can very often be asymptomatic. For that reason, routine screening is important for all women of childbearing age. Symptoms in women include burning with urination, a vaginal discharge, or vaginal bleeding between periods. Occasionally, patients will have some pelvic pain and fever indicating a more serious pelvic inflammatory disease that has resulted from gonorrhea. Untreated gonorrhea can develop into pelvic inflammatory disease causing damage to the fallopian tubes in the form of scar tissue, which in turn causes infertility or increased risk of ectopic pregnancy.

Gonorrhea is easy to diagnose if the patient presents for care. Cervical discharge can be cultured to confirm the presence of infectious bacteria, when present; then antibiotic therapy is initiated. Some resistance has been detected to the commonly used antibiotics, so the Centers for Disease Control and Prevention (CDC) has updated the recommended regimens. Currently CDC recommendations include ceftriaxone or cefixime. These medications can be given as a single dose. This one-treatment dose is so successful that a follow-up culture is not necessary, but if desired, the most cost-effective approach is to culture 1 to 2 months after treatment. Gonorrhea is highly communicable, and partner treatment is essential. The CDC recommends concomitant treatment for chlamydia, because it frequently coexists most with gonorrhea. Condoms are recommended to prevent reinfection during sexual relations.

Etiology, Epidemiology, and Pathophysiology of Pelvic Inflammatory Disease

Pelvic inflammatory disease (PID) is an infection of the uterus, fallopian tubes, and ovaries. It is a common and a serious complication of many sexually transmitted infections, with up to 80% of cases being related to chlamydia and gonorrhea infections. The

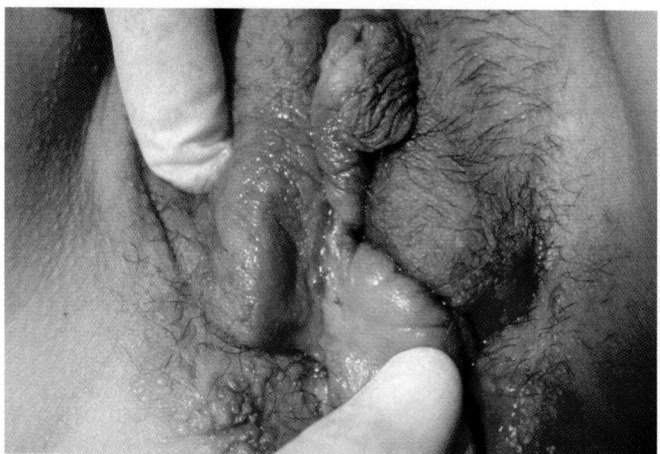

FIGURE 49–1 ■ Chlamydia.
Source: Courtesy, Director-General and Programme Manager Prevention of Blindness, World Health Organization

highest risk for the development of PID is seen in women of child-bearing age who are sexually active. This population tends to have a higher incidence of STIs and bacterial infections that cause PID (CDC, 2008e). It is estimated that more than 1 million women experience an episode of acute PID each year, with more than 100,000 becoming infertile and 300,000 requiring hospitalization as a result. Annually, more than 150 women die from PID or its complications (CDC, 2008e). The Risk Factors box outlines the risk factors for the development of pelvic inflammatory disease. PID is more likely to occur during the first days of the menstrual cycle, so sexual intercourse during menstrual bleeding is also a risk.

Clinical Manifestations of Pelvic Inflammatory Disease

Symptoms vary from none to severe, including lower abdominal pain, fever, foul-smelling vaginal discharge, painful intercourse, painful urination, and irregular menstrual bleeding. Objective findings include fever (38.3°C), abnormal cervical or vaginal discharge, elevated white blood count (WBC) and erythrocyte sedimentation rate (ESR), and pain with palpation of the adenexal areas and/or the cervix. Patients with suspected PID need to have cultures of vaginal secretions to confirm diagnosis and a pelvic ultrasound to rule out a tubo-ovarian abscess and ectopic pregnancy.

Medical Management of Pelvic Inflammatory Disease

PID is curable with antibiotics. Because the causative organism is often unclear, it is important to treat with at least two different broad-spectrum antibiotics that cover a wide range of organisms. Bed rest helps with pain control, but the patient needs to placed in a high Fowler's position to help control spread of infection to the upper abdominal area. Universal precautions need strict adherence if the patient has purulent vaginal drainage and shares a bathroom. Patient teaching should include restriction of sexual relations if vaginal drainage is present. Use of a condom to prevent reinfection is important if an individual is not in a long-term, monogamous relationship with an uninfected partner. A patient's partner should be referred for evaluation and treatment of any sexually transmitted infection. Nurses should provide emotional support and stress the importance of follow-up care and evaluation. Patients should return for a follow-up evaluation 48 to 72 hours after the medication is started and again in 7 to 10 days.

Health Promotion for Diseases Characterized by Cervicitis

Patient and partner education is essential to the prevention and spread of the diseases characterized by cervicitis. The following facts are necessary components of the teaching plan:

- Cervicitis is most often transmitted during vaginal, anal, or oral sex.

> **RISK FACTORS for the Development of Pelvic Inflammatory Disease**
>
> Age (adolescent and young women)
> Nonwhite women
> Multiple sex partners
> History of sexually transmitted infection
> Intercourse with a partner who has untreated urethritis
> Recent intrauterine device insertion
> Nulliparity

- Ejaculation does not have to occur in order for infection to occur.
- These infections can be passed from infected mother to baby during vaginal birth.
- The greater number of sex partners, the greater risk of infection.
- Teenagers and young women are most at risk for cervicitis infections if sexually active.
- Sex partners must be treated in order to prevent recurrence and spread.
- Complications from cervicitis infections include pelvic inflammatory disease, ectopic pregnancy, and infertility.
- Routine screening for cervicitis should occur during yearly exams.
- A single dose of the appropriate antibiotic can cure cervicitis infections.
- Prevention of cervicitis infections is accomplished by being in long-term, mutually monogamous relationship with a partner who has been tested and is known to be uninfected.
- Latex condoms when used consistently and correctly can reduce the risk of transmission of cervicitis.

Sexually Transmitted Infections Characterized by Ulcers

Ulcers found in the genital area can be suspicious for three conditions primarily. Multiple painful vesicles are often herpes simplex virus (HSV). HSV is the most frequently occurring ulcerative disease of the genitals. However, a group of flesh-colored cauliflower-like lesions can be human papillomavirus (HPV), and a single chancroid-type lesion may be indicative of primary syphilis.

Etiology and Epidemiology of Syphilis

Syphilis is a complex sexually transmitted infection that can lead to serious systemic illness and even death if untreated. **Syphilis,** caused by the *Treponema pallidum* bacterium, is a systemic infection and is referred to as the "great imitator" because its symptoms often mimic those of other STIs (CDC, 2008f). Between 2003 and 2004, the cases of syphilis increased in the United States by 8% (CDC, 2004). In 2005 there were 8,724 cases, representing an increase of 9.3% (CDC, 2005b). Most cases occurred in persons 20 to 39 years of age; the incidence of infectious syphilis was highest in women 20 to 24 years of age, with the rate of 3 cases per 100,000 (CDC, 2005b). Rates are very high among young adult African Americans in urban areas and in the southern United States. Experts have attributed current syphilis infections to crack cocaine use, which is accompanied by the practice of exchanging sex for money and drugs (Nakashima, Rolfs, Flock, Kilmarx, & Greenspan, 1996). The CDC also reports that in 2005, 50% of the total number of primary and secondary syphilis cases was reported from 19 counties and 2 cities.

Pathophysiology and Clinical Manifestations of Syphilis

There are three primary stages of syphilis. In the first stage, a painless chancre (Figure 49–2 ■) develops soon after being infected, but will disappear on its own. If identified at this stage, a single dose of penicillin G can cure the infection (CDC, 2008f). If the in-

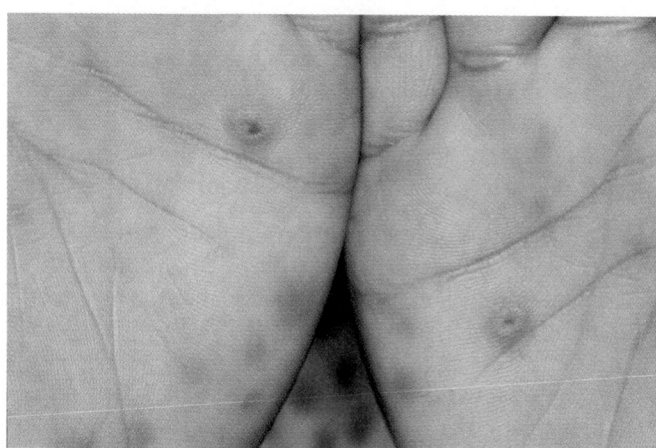

FIGURE 49–2 ■ Syphilis chancre.
Source: Zeva Oelbaum/Peter Arnold, Inc.

fection progresses to the secondary stage, a rough rash will appear on various parts of the body, but in particular on the soles of the feet and the palms of the hands. Other symptoms of the second stage may include fever, weight loss, swollen lymph glands, and muscle aches. A cure is still possible at this stage, but will require larger doses of antibiotics. Without treatment, the infection progresses to the latent and final state of the disease. Latent syphilis is defined as syphilis characterized by seroreactivity without other evidence of disease. The final stage begins after secondary symptoms disappear. The infection remains in the body for years and slowly damages the brain, nerves, eyes, heart, blood vessels, liver, bones, and joints. Symptoms, which typically progress to what is termed *neurosyphilis*, include muscle weakness, difficulty coordinating muscle movements, paralysis, numbness, blindness, dementia, and eventual death. Genital sores (chancres) caused by syphilis make it easier to transmit and acquire HIV infection. There is an estimated two- to fivefold increased risk of acquiring HIV infection when syphilis is present (CDC, 2008f).

Transplacental transmission of an infected mother to her fetus is very possible. If pregnancy occurs while a woman has syphilis, the fetus could develop deformities or could be stillborn. Routine screening of pregnant women is widely performed in the United States (CDC, 2008g). Providers can diagnose syphilis by examining material from a chancre (infectious sore) or using a blood test. Shortly after being infected, the body produces syphilis antibodies that can be detected. Every pregnant woman should have a blood test for syphilis.

Medical Management of Syphilis
A single intramuscular injection of penicillin will cure a person who has had syphilis for less than 1 year. Treatment with penicillin during pregnancy is necessary. If the woman is allergic to penicillin, she may require skin testing with desensitization treatment in order to receive penicillin, because alternate drug choices, such as doxycycline, tetracycline, and erythromycin, are contraindicated in pregnancy (CDC, 2008f). See the Pharmacology Summary feature (p. 1552).

Etiology, Epidemiology, and Pathophysiology of Genital Herpes
Genital herpes is caused primarily by the herpes simplex virus (HSV). It presents as painful multiple vesicular or ulcerative lesions found on the labia, perineum, and vaginal areas. Once one

is infected, HSV becomes a chronic, lifelong viral infection. There are two types of herpes simplex virus. Type 1 has historically been the source of cold sores or fever blisters on the mouth and lips. Type 2 HSV usually refers to herpes infection of the genitals. This distinction, however, has become blurred in recent years. It is no longer uncommon to find HSV types 1 and 2 in both areas of the body.

Genital herpes is considered a sexually transmitted infection; most infections are caused by HSV-2. At least 50 million persons in the United States have genital HSV infection. Many persons have mild or unrecognized infections but shed virus intermittently in the genital tract (CDC, 2008d). Generally, a person can get HSV type 2 only by sexual contact with someone who has a genital HSV type 2 infection. Unfortunately, the infected person does not have to have open lesions to transmit the virus to a partner. This makes it very difficult to prevent transmission between partners. Many people infected with HSV-2 are not aware of their infection.

Clinical Manifestations of Genital Herpes
The signs and symptoms may be transient and very mild. The first outbreak usually occurs within 2 weeks after the virus has been transmitted, and the sores heal within 2 to 4 weeks. During a first outbreak, the patient may have some mild flu-like symptoms including low-grade fever, inguinal lymphadenopathy, and fatigue in addition to the ulcerative lesions in the genital area (Figure 49–3 ■). More women than men are infected with HSV-2, probably because transmission is more likely from man to woman than it is from woman to man (CDC, 2008d). Most people diagnosed with a first episode of genital herpes can expect to have several outbreaks within a year. Over time these recurrences usually decrease in frequency.

Medical Management of Genital Herpes
Diagnosis of HSV-2 can often be made by visual exam; however, cultures from an open lesion can provide confirmation. If there

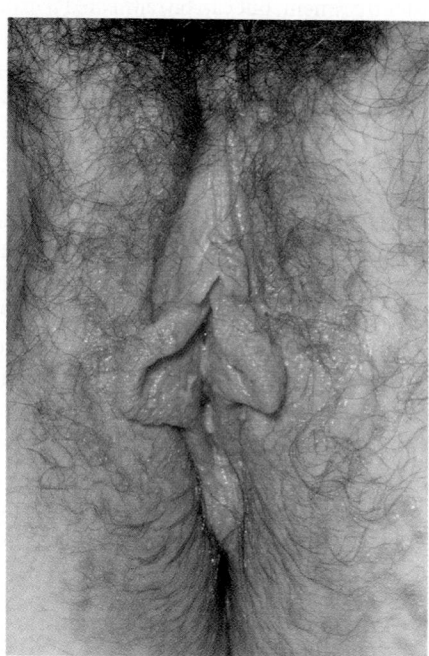

FIGURE 49–3 ■ Herpes simplex virus type 2.
Source: Mediscan/Visuals Unlimited

are no open sores at the time of exam, certain blood tests detect HSV-1 or HSV-2 infection. Although genital herpes causes recurrent outbreaks that are painful and worrisome, the condition is not life threatening unless the patient is immunosuppressed. Potentially lethal infections can occur in patients with HIV. HSV infections can make people more susceptible to HIV. Additionally, HSV-2 can also make HIV-infected individuals more infectious. Pregnant women with HSV-2 risk transmission of HSV to the infant during delivery; therefore, women with HSV-2 frequently deliver by cesarean.

Treatment of HSV-2 can be accomplished with antiviral medications (acyclovir or valcyclovir). These medications cannot cure HSV-2, but they can shorten and prevent outbreaks. Daily suppressive therapy is used for some patients who continue to have repeated outbreaks and to reduce transmission to uninfected partners. Treatment recommendations also include cleaning of lesions daily to prevent secondary infections, sitz baths to increase comfort, loose cotton underwear, and analgesics for discomfort. Abstinence from the first sign of recurrence through complete healing of the lesions is the recommendation, along with condoms between episodes.

Etiology, Epidemiology, Pathophysiology, and Medical Management of Chancroid

A **chancroid** is a bacterial sexually transmitted infection that occurs rarely outside of tropical climates. Although this infection may occur with any sexually active person, it is more common in men, especially those that are uncircumcised. The first symptom is typically a sore or raised bump on the genital organs. Within 5 to 10 days of the initial lesion, the glands on one or both sides of the groin become enlarged, hard, and painful. This infection is transmitted through intercourse as long as there is an open sore. There is no evidence of any natural resistance, and reinfection can occur immediately after treatment with antibiotics, with the lesions healing within about 2 weeks of treatment. Because there is no natural immunity to a chancroid, the individual is considered cured after treatment, but can be reinfected if exposed to the bacterium. Prevention techniques that include limiting the number of sex partners, using a condom, and thorough hygiene after sexual contact will help decrease the spread of this infection.

Etiology and Epidemiology of Human Papillomavirus

Human papillomavirus (HPV), also referred to as genital warts, infection is the most common sexually transmitted viral infection in the United States. The best estimate is that there are over 20 million people infected with HPV in the United States. It is anticipated that there will be 6.2 million new infections yearly. The highest rate of infection occurs in sexually active adolescents, but by age 50, at least 80% of women will have acquired a genital HPV infection (Allred, Cox, & Mahoney, 2006). Approximately 100 types of HPV have been identified. About 30 high-risk forms of HPV are known to cause genital tract cancers including cervical cancer. Many other types are known to cause genital warts, but not cancer.

Pathophysiology and Clinical Manifestations of Human Papillomavirus

Most people who have HPV do not know they are infected. The virus causes **genital warts** that appear as cauliflower-like growths in the genital, anal, and vaginal areas. They can be raised or flat, single or multiple; some are small and some are large. Genital warts are transmitted via sexual contact with an infected person. The warts may appear within weeks or months, or not at all (Figure 49–4 ■). Itching, increased vaginal discharge, and abnormal vaginal bleeding after intercourse are typical symptoms.

Medical Management of Human Papillomavirus

Most women are diagnosed with HPV based on abnormal Papanicolaou smear (Pap smear). A Pap smear, the primary method of screening for cervical cancer, detects precancerous changes in the cervix that may occur as a result of HPV infection. The warts can be treated with topical medications, such as Podofilox solution or Imiquimod cream. Genital warts can also be removed with minor surgery, known as cryotherapy, with liquid nitrogen, or with a shave excision.

On June 8, 2006, the Food and Drug Administration approved the use of a vaccine developed to prevent cervical cancer caused by HPV. The vaccine, known as Gardasil, protects against the four HPV types that are responsible for 70% of cervical cancers and 90% of genital warts. The vaccine is recommended for females aged 9 to 26. Ideally, the vaccine should be administered before the onset of sexual activity. However, females who are sexually active also may benefit from vaccination. The vaccine is recommended at a younger age because research studies demonstrated that titers were higher for young girls than for older females participating in the efficacy trials. The duration of vaccine protection is unclear. Current studies indicate that the vaccine is effective for at least five years (CDC, 2008f). The advent of the HPV vaccine does not change any of the recommendations for cancer screening outlined in the National Guidelines box. The American Cancer Society recommends beginning of screening for cervical cancer within 3 years of initiation of sexual activity or by age 21. Repeat exams should be done every 2 years for women until age 70. Women that have 3 consecutive normal exams and are in a monogamous relationship may extend testing to every 3 years. Likewise, women who are over 70 years of age and have had 3 or more normal cervical screenings in the previous 10 years may opt to discontinue the screenings. Women who have had a total abdominal hysterectomy may be able to discontinue testing if their surgeon agrees. For women who have had a subtotal hysterectomy, cervical cancer screenings should continue (American Cancer Society, 2008).

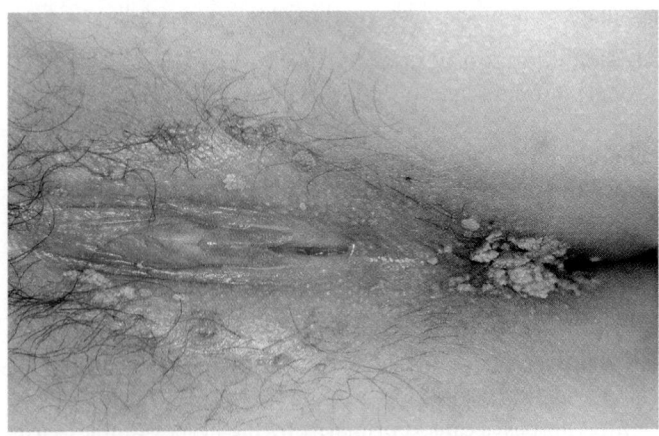

FIGURE 49–4 ■ Human papillomavirus (HPV) genital warts.
Source: ISM/Phototake NYC

NATIONAL GUIDELINES for Cervical Cancer Screening from the American Cancer Society

Criteria	ACS Guidelines
Age to initiate screening	3 years after the onset of sexual activity, no later than age 21
Screening frequency	Screening should be done every year with the regular Pap test or every 2 years using the newer liquid-based Pap test. After age 30, women with 3 consecutive normal tests and in a monogamous relationship may be screened every 2 to 3 years.
	Another option for women over 30 is to get screened every 3 years (but not more frequently) with either the conventional or liquid-based Pap test, plus the HPV DNA test.
	Women who have certain risk factors such as diethylstilbestrol (DES) exposure before birth, HIV infection, or a weakened immune system due to organ transplant, chemotherapy, or chronic steroid use should continue to be screened annually.
Screening after hysterectomy	Women who have had a total hysterectomy (removal of the uterus and cervix) may also choose to stop having cervical cancer screening, unless the surgery was done as a treatment for cervical cancer or pre-cancer.
	Women who have had a hysterectomy without removal of the cervix should continue to follow the guidelines.
Discontinuation of screening	After age 70 and 3 normal cytology exams in previous 10 years, screening can be discontinued.
	Women with a history of cervical cancer, DES exposure before birth, HIV infection, or a weakened immune system should continue to have screening as long as they are in good health.
Routine screening HPV infection	Test for HPV DNA is FDA approved as an adjunct to cervical screening among women age 30 and over.

Source: "American Cancer Society Guidelines for the Early Detection of Cancer: Cervical Cancer" adapted and reprinted by the permission of the American Cancer Society, Inc. from www.cancer.org. All rights reserved.

Health Promotion for Diseases Characterized by Ulcers

Patient and partner education is essential to the prevention and spread of the diseases characterized by genital ulcers. The following facts are necessary components of the teaching plan:

- Any unusual discharge, sore, or rash, particularly in the groin area, should be a signal to refrain from having sex and to seek the care of a health care provider.

- Prevention of sexually transmitted infections is best accomplished by abstaining from sexual contact or being in a long-term, mutually monogamous relationship with a partner who has been tested and is known to be uninfected.

- Condoms are not fully effective in preventing the spread of genital ulcer diseases. Persons with HSV and HPV should abstain from sexual activity with uninfected partners when lesions or other symptoms are present.

- An HSV-infected person who does not have any symptoms can still infect sex partners by shedding virus between outbreaks.

- HPV infection can lead to cervical cancer.

- Avoidance of alcohol and drug use may also help prevent transmission of STIs, as these activities may lead to risky sexual behavior.

- It is important that sex partners talk to each other about their HIV status and history of other STIs so that preventive action can be taken.

- Transmission of an STI cannot be prevented by washing the genitals, urinating, and/or douching after sex.

- Ulcerative STIs that cause sores, ulcers, or breaks in the skin or mucous membranes, disrupt barriers that provide protection against infections such as HIV.

Sexually Transmitted Infections Characterized by Vaginitis

Vaginitis is usually characterized by a vaginal discharge and/vulvar itching and irritation. A vaginal odor might be present. Three infections are associated with vaginitis conditions: trichomoniasis, bacterial vaginosis, and candidiasis.

Etiology, Epidemiology, Pathophysiology, Clinical Manifestations, Diagnosis, and Medical Management of Trichomoniasis

Trichomoniasis is a very common protozoan infection caused by *Trichomonas vaginalis*. Trichomoniasis affects both men and women, but symptoms are more common in women. Symptoms often include burning and itching in the vaginal area. Objective findings include a malodorous, yellow-green vaginal discharge with vulvar irritation, although some women experience minimal symptoms.

Microscopic examination of vaginal secretions can reveal flagellated protozoa, but this method has a sensitivity of only 60% to 70% (Figure 49–5 ■, p. 1524). A nucleic acid probe test is also available and has a higher sensitivity. Vaginal culture is the most sensitive and specific method of diagnosis. This infection is considered the most common curable STI in young people (CDC, 2008f). It is treated with a single dose of metronidazole and abstinence until both partners are asymptomatic. See the Pharmacology Summary feature (p. 1552).

Etiology, Epidemiology, Pathophysiology, Clinical Manifestations, Diagnosis, and Medical Management of Bacterial Vaginosis

Bacterial vaginosis (BV) is the most common bacterial infection in women of childbearing age, and it is seen in 16% of pregnant

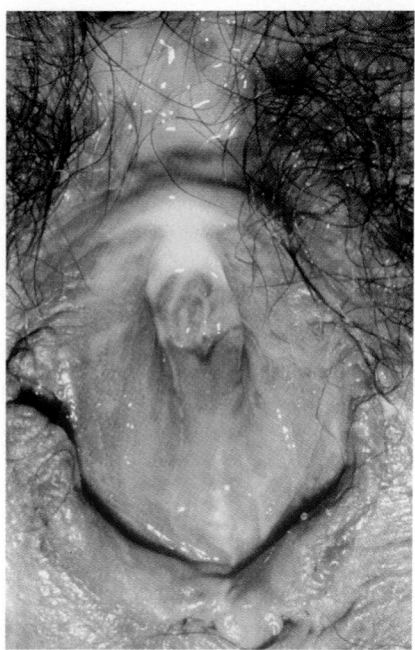

FIGURE 49–5 ■ Trichomoniasis.
Source: NMSB/Custom Medical Stock Photo, Inc.

women (CDC, 2008f). It is not the typical STI, that is, transmitted from one person to the other, although the CDC does list it under the sexually transmitted infection area. The cause of BV is not clearly understood, but it is known that an imbalance in the normal bacteria growth found in the vagina can cause an overgrowth of anaerobic bacteria known as *Gardnerella vaginalis.*

BV is associated with having multiple sex partners, a new sex partner, douching, use of an intrauterine device to prevent contraception, and a lack of vaginal lactobacilli. Women who have never been sexually active are rarely affected. Women with BV have an increased white/gray, typically thin vaginal discharge, with an unpleasant odor. These women may also experience burning on urination or vaginal itching. Objective findings include a thin, white discharge, the presence of clue cells on microscopy, and a fishy odor of vaginal discharge.

There are no complications associated with BV except in pregnancy. Babies are often born prematurely or are of low birth weight. BV can migrate upward and infect the uterus and fallopian tubes, increasing the risk of ectopic pregnancy or infertility and pelvic inflammatory disease (PID). The reason is unclear, but BV increases the woman's susceptibility to HIV, chlamydia, and gonorrhea.

Treatment is necessary to avoid PID because it can lead to infertility and damage to the fallopian tubes, which increases the risk of ectopic pregnancy. Two different medications are prescribed, metronidazole and clindamycin, both being safe if needed during pregnancy. The medications can be either oral or a topical vaginal route. See the Pharmacology Summary feature (p. 1552). BV can recur after treatment. Treatment of male sex partners has not been beneficial in preventing the recurrence of BV.

Etiology, Epidemiology, Pathophysiology, Clinical Manifestations, Diagnosis, and Medical Management of Candidiasis

Candidiasis is a fungal infection, more commonly referred to as a yeast infection. *Candida* organisms are typically found in the

genital tract, the gastrointestinal tract, and the mouth. Symptoms develop when there is an overgrowth of *Candida* caused by multiple factors such as pregnancy, diabetes mellitus, and the use of antibiotics and/or corticosteroids that disturbs the pH or hormone balance in these areas (CDC, 2008b). Other causes can include tight-fitting undergarments that maintain a moist environment for fungal growth and frequent douching that may alter the pH balance that is needed to prevent it.

The normal *Candida* flora is rarely passed from person to person (CDC, 2008b), but can be transmitted through oral or genital sexual contact, when a disturbance in pH or hormone balance occurs. Symptoms include a white, cheesy discharge, often with intense itching, a burning sensation, and painful urination. A culture of the genital area is usually sent for testing to confirm the presence of candidiasis.

The treatment of choice is a 3- or 7-day course of antifungal drugs taken orally, topically, or vaginally (CDC, 2008b). Self-treatment is becoming common as more over-the-counter drugs become available. The CDC (2008b) indicates that as many as two-thirds of women who self-treat do not have the disease, leading to an increasing number of resistant infections. Women who have recurrences of what they believe to be candidiasis should seek medical diagnosis to rule out another cause of their symptoms. Recurrent or unresponsive episodes of candidiasis may be due to diabetes mellitus or HIV. Untreated infections may lead to persistent symptoms and an increased chance of passing the infection between partners. Wearing cotton undergarments that allow for better absorption of moisture and limiting douching may decrease the incidence of *Candida* growth in prone individuals.

Health Promotion for Diseases Characterized by Vaginitis

Patient and partner education is essential to the prevention and spread of the diseases characterized by vaginitis. The following facts are necessary components of the teaching plan:

- Observe for changes in color, odor, and amount of vaginal discharge.
- Wear light cotton underwear.
- If a presumed yeast infection does not improve with over-the-counter (OTC) treatment, seek medical care.
- Changes in the environment of the vagina may occur with changes in diet, medications, and new sex partner.
- Recurrent vaginitis or vaginitis that is nonresponsive to treatment requires further consultation with a health care provider.
- Avoid douching.

Acquired Immunodeficiency Syndrome

Acquired immunodeficiency syndrome (AIDS) is a result of an infection with the human immunodeficiency virus (HIV). HIV/AIDS is primarily transmitted by sexual contact, but it also can be acquired through a transfusion with infected blood, by an infant through the childbirth process, via contaminated needles, or through breast-feeding from an infected mother. The HIV virus attacks the immune system, which then places the individual at high risk for opportunistic infections. Due to altered immunity, these individuals are often unable to fight infections and eventually succumb to this disease. Certain medications have been successful at slowing the disease process, but, as of yet, there is no cure (CDC, 2008f).

The CDC (2008f) estimates there are 40,000 new cases in the United States each year and the fastest growing population are heterosexuals under the age of 25. HIV/AIDS is a deadly combination, and to decrease the incidence, a concerted effort must be made on the part of all people. The CDC has initiated an HIV prevention program that details the implemented activities for 2008, evaluation, communication, and plans for 2009. Chapter 60 ⊘ includes an in-depth discussion of HIV/AIDS.

◼ Nursing Management

Care of patients with sexually transmitted infections is primarily aimed at health education that prevents infections. Patients should receive results of testing as soon as possible and be encouraged to follow up for treatment. Nurses, who are responsible for revealing results of testing for STIs to patients, should be extremely careful to protect the confidentiality of their patients. Leaving messages on phones or with domestic partners or other family members is strictly prohibited. The Nursing Process: Patient Care Plan feature outlines nursing care specific to sexually transmitted infections (p. 1526).

◼ Collaborative Management

Sexually transmitted infections are a sensitive topic for many patients. Patients are reluctant to seek treatment for these issues and instead hope they will resolve on their own. Nurses and health care providers must work together to help patients feel comfortable discussing possible STIs and the source of infections. Patients should be encouraged to disclose their infection to sexual partners, and for some infections, the disease may be reportable to the public health department (i.e., syphilis, gonorrhea, and chlamydia). On occasion, patients will realize that an STI is the result of an unfaithful partner. At that time it may be reasonable to offer psychological counseling to the patient.

Health Promotion for Sexually Transmitted Infections

The specific information for patient/partner teaching is included under each STI section when described earlier. In general, health promotion for sexually transmitted infections should be directed at prevention. Once the disorder occurs, the care is directed toward symptom management, decreasing progression when possible, prevention of recurrence, and prevention of infection of others. The care and education need to be individualized to both the type of STI and the patient's needs.

The CDC (2008f) maintains that the primary preventative measure of sexually transmitted infections is to abstain from sexual intercourse and contact (including vaginal, anal, and oral sex) or in being in a long-term, monogamous relationship with an uninfected partner. Because neither of these measures is always followed, safer sex practices are the most common preventative measure. Once the infection is present, early treatment can assist in decreasing its progression. Some STIs are curable,

such as gonorrhea, syphilis, and trichomoniasis, and others are only treatable. To assist with prevention of both transfer to another partner and recurrence, safer sex practices are encouraged.

◼ Breast Disorders

Breast disorders are most often manifested by pain, lumps, or nipple discharge. Sixteen percent of women between the ages of 40 and 69 will have one of these breast complaints (Klein, 2005). Most lumps are benign and are a result of fibrocystic changes, mastitis, or intraductal disorders. Breast malignancies are the most commonly occurring cancer in women and the second leading cause of death in women in the United States (Klein, 2005). The following section will discuss specific common breast disorders.

Pathophysiology of Fibrocystic Breast Abnormalities

Most breast masses are benign and are caused by fibrocystic changes. Fibrocystic breast changes most often occur as a result of hormone shifts around the time of the menses. However, the condition can also be exacerbated by stress or anxiety, nutritional factors, and physical or environmental stimuli.

Fibrocystic breast changes are characterized by an increase in glandular and fibrous tissues in the breast. This increase in fibrous tissue is palpable on examination and also may be seen on mammography. Fibrocystic changes are thought to be caused by estrogen dominance, which is why the changes wax and wane with menses and usually disappear after menopause, but the exact cause is unknown. When the fibrous tissue blocks milk ducts, fluid-filled cysts form. Typically, this condition affects women between the ages of 30 and 50.

Clinical Manifestations of Fibrocystic Breast Abnormalities

The manifestations of fibrocystic breast changes include a smooth, mobile, well-defined, tender lump usually found in the upper outer quadrant of the breast. The mass exhibits no redness, warmth, or overlying skin changes. Patients may sometimes note that coffee, tea, cola soft drinks, and chocolate aggravate the masses and cause increased tenderness. Breast pain (**mastalgia**) may be experienced in women with fibrocystic disease premenstrually but usually disappears after the menses when the influence of hormones diminishes.

Medical Management of Fibrocystic Breast Abnormalities

Fibrocystic changes are not precancerous and do not increase the woman's risk of developing breast cancer, but they can cause pain and anxiety (ACOG, 2000). Medical treatment for pain and tenderness associated with fibrocystic breasts may involve decreasing the estrogen level. Danazol (Danocrine), an antiestrogenic, can be given in severe cases. See the Pharmacology Summary feature (p. 1552).

◼ Nursing Management

Nursing care should include obtaining a focused history of the patient with a breast mass to determine the risk of breast cancer. The Risk Factors box (p. 1527) outlines hormonal and nonhormonal

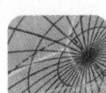

NURSING PROCESS: Patient Care Plan for Sexually Transmitted Infections

Assessment of Impaired Tissue Integrity

Subjective Data:
When did your symptoms begin?
Have you ever had this before?
Describe your symptoms.
Tell about the habits of your sex partner or partners.

Objective Data:
Skin appearance (color, texture, temperature, discharge, etc.)
Describe lesions (type, location, distribution, size, etc.)
Assess for edema and pain

Nursing Assessment and Diagnoses	Outcomes and Evaluation Parameters	Planning and Interventions with *Rationales*
Nursing Diagnosis: *Impaired Tissue Integrity* related to effects of disease process of STIs	**Outcome:** Tissue integrity will be restored. *Evaluation Parameters:* Skin tissue will be without breaks or lesions. Skin tissue will be pink without redness, excoriation, pain, or damage.	**Interventions and *Rationales:*** Assess damaged skin. *Gives baseline data to determine healing process.* Instruct patient on healthy hygiene. *Keeping clean and dry will decrease organism growth.* Instruct patient on use of sitz bath or warm soaks. *To cleanse area, increase circulation, and increase healing.* Administer and do home teaching on prescribed medications. *To decrease organism growth and increase healing.*

Assessment of Anxiety

Subjective Data:
Describe for me how you feel about this diagnosis.
What is your greatest concern?

Objective Data:
Verbal statements that indicate concern and anxiety
Nonverbal clues such as facial expressions showing concern or worry, wringing of hands, nervousness, etc.
Is the patient withdrawn/quiet/apathetic?

Nursing Assessment and Diagnoses	Outcomes and Evaluation Parameters	Planning and Interventions with *Rationales*
Nursing Diagnosis: *Anxiety* related to diagnosis of sexually transmitted infection (STI)	**Outcome:** Patient's anxiety level will be reduced. *Evaluation Parameters:* Patient will verbalize feeling less anxious. Patient affect will appear less stressed.	**Interventions and *Rationales:*** Assess patient concerns. *Gives baseline for intervention needs.* Provide open atmosphere and nonjudgmental attitude for communication/discussion. *To maintain relaxed atmosphere and nonjudgmental attitude to encourage patient verbalization.* Identify support systems for patient. *To identify whom patient can rely on for encouragement.* Answer questions honestly and openly. *To provide therapeutic environment.*

Assessment of Knowledge

Subjective Data:
What do you know about the prevention/transmission of STIs?
Are you sexually active?
If so, do you have more than one partner?
Do you want to get pregnant?
Do you use birth control?
Do you use any protection from diseases such as condoms?

Objective Data:
Patient's level of knowledge related to STIs
Patient's willingness to learn more about the importance of and the types of protection

Nursing Assessment and Diagnoses	Outcomes and Evaluation Parameters	Planning and Interventions with *Rationales*
Nursing Diagnosis: *Deficient Knowledge* related to disease prevention/transmission	**Outcome:** Disease transmission will be reduced or prevented. *Evaluation Parameters:* Patient will verbalize understanding of ways to prevent/reduce transmission. Patient will verbalize understanding of need for partner treatment to reduce reinfection. Patient verbalizes commitment to safer sex practices.	**Interventions and *Rationales:*** Assess knowledge level. *Must have baseline for teaching.* Teach ways to prevent/reduce disease transmission such as abstinence or condoms. *Both ways will decrease direct contact.* Encourage questions. *Giving information increases chance of compliance.* Provide information regarding treatment of partners to reduce reinfection. *Important to reduce transmission.*

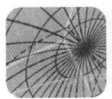

NURSING PROCESS: Patient Care Plan for Sexually Transmitted Infections—*Continued*

Assessment of High-Risk Behaviors

Subjective Data:
Are you aware of the dangers of unprotected sexual contact?
Are you concerned about either contracting or transmitting an STI?

Objective Data:
Evidence of STI based on culture results and/or clinical examination.

Nursing Assessment and Diagnoses	Outcomes and Evaluation Parameters	Planning and Interventions with *Rationales*
Nursing Diagnoses: Self Neglect Related to Ineffective Health Maintenance due to sexual behaviors	**Outcome:** Patient will verbalize understanding of safer sex practices. **Evaluation Parameters:** Patient will verbalize understanding of use of condoms. Patient will advise partner of need for treatment. Patient will avoid further exposure to sexually transmitted infection.	**Interventions and *Rationales:*** Assess understanding of how STIs are transmitted. *Must have baseline for teaching.* Assess understanding of use of condoms. *Must have baseline for teaching.* Supply condoms as needed. *To supply condoms for use with subsequent sexual contacts.* Encourage questions and frank discussion of risks of unprotected sexual contact. *Information provided in a nonjudgmental manner will increase potential for compliance.* Provide resources for pregnancy planning. *To encourage patient to prevent unplanned pregnancy.* Provide resources for treatment of sexual partners. *To emphasize the importance of partner treatment to prevent reinfection.*

risk factors for breast cancer. Relevant history includes family history, age of menarche and menopause, history of breast-feeding, and number of pregnancies and live births. Documentation of oral or transcutaneous contraceptives or hormone replacement therapy is also pertinent.

During the physical assessment, lump characteristics should be documented, including changes in size over time, changes relative to the menstrual cycle, duration, pain, swelling, redness, fever, or discharge from the nipples. A clinical breast exam should be performed to evaluate the mass. Clinical breast exam is described in Chapter 48 ☞. Often masses can be preliminarily determined to be benign or malignant based on clinical exam, but mammogram and/or ultrasound, followed by fine needle aspiration, is used to gain definitive diagnosis. Chart 49–1 outlines the differences between benign versus malignant breast masses.

Nursing management includes suggesting a well-fitting support bra, decreasing salt and caffeine, which can increase the size of the cysts, taking ibuprofen (Motrin) (see Pharmacology Summary feature on p. 1552) as an anti-inflammatory agent for the pain, and applying local heat to the area of the mass. More importantly, the nurse needs to allow the patient to express concerns and ask questions regarding the source and implications

RISK FACTORS for Breast Cancer

Hormonal Risks	Nonhormonal Risks
Long menstrual histories	Women with a family history of breast cancer
Use of birth control pills	Lack of regular exercise
Hormone replacement therapy	Post menopausal obesity
Early menarche (<12 years)	Increased use of alcohol
Late menopause (> 55 years)	Night shift workers
Age at first full term pregnancy (after 30 years)	Age (65 years +)
	Caucasian women after age 40
	High breast tissue density
	No full term pregnancies
	Never breast-fed
	Higher socioeconomic status
	Tall
	Jewish heritage
	Two or more first-degree relatives with breast cancer at an early age

Source: "American Cancer Society. Breast Cancer Facts and Figures 2007–2008. Atlanta: American Cancer Society, Inc." "Breast Cancer: What are the Risk Factors for Breast Cancer" adapted and reprinted by the permission of the American Cancer Society, Inc. from www.cancer.org. All rights reserved.

CHART 49–1   Differentiation of Breast Masses by Clinical Exam

Benign Mass	Malignant Mass
No skin changes are noted. Breasts are symmetrical.	The mass is fixed to surrounding skin and soft tissue, causing skin dimpling and asymmetry of the breasts.
When palpated, the lump is smooth.	The mass is irregularly shaped.
The consistency of the lump is soft to firm.	The consistency is hard.
The lump is mobile beneath the skin.	The mass is immobile beneath the skin.
The margins are well defined and easily delineated.	The margins are poorly defined and irregular.
The mass is tender to palpation.	The mass is usually nontender.

of the mass. Ensure that the patient understands the terms *benign* and *malignant* and the types of diagnostic evaluations that will be used to make a definitive diagnosis. Impress on the patient the importance of reporting any change in the mass immediately to the treating health care provider.

Etiology, Pathophysiology, Clinical Manifestations, and Treatment of Mastitis

Mastitis, which is an inflammation of the breast tissue, occurs most frequently in women who are breast-feeding. Microorganisms invade the tissue through a portal of entry such as a crack or a fissure in the nipple, or through a duct. Symptoms include breast tenderness, redness typically at the site of inflammation, and edema. The woman may also experience fatigue, malaise, fever, or chills.

Treatment includes rest, fluids, alternating warm and cold compresses, and continued breast-feeding. Alternating warm and cold compresses aids in pain relief and increases circulation to the area.

Continuation of breast-feeding was controversial many years ago because it was thought the infection could cause harm to the nursing infant. Mastitis is inflamed breast tissue, not the milk ducts, and it is often caused from clogged milk ducts in breast-feeding women. Therefore, emptying the breasts frequently and completely is a successful intervention. Antibiotics are prescribed when the infection does not clear with nonpharmacologic methods, or when the health care provider feels the infection may cause additional problems. The woman is instructed to wear a support bra. Nursing care is aimed at prevention of breast tissue damage from engorgement by encouraging breast-feeding, relieving discomfort, treating the infection causing the inflammation, and prevention of recurrence. Women who are nursing infants should use lanolin creams to the nipples regularly to avoid cracking of the nipples and thus preventing invasion of bacteria into the breast tissue. Mastitis occurs primarily in breast-feeding mothers, so instruction on feeding technique and symptoms may prevent progression of this problem.

Etiology and Epidemiology of Breast Cancer

Breast cancer is defined as the formation of a malignant glandular tumor as a result of an uncontrolled growth of abnormal cells in the breast tissue. The malignant cells over time destroy normal breast tissue. Other than skin cancer, breast cancer is the most common cancer in women, with more than 212,000 new cases occurring in 2006 and 41,000 deaths (American Cancer Society [ACS], 2007). Breast cancer accounts for nearly 1 in 3 cancers diagnosed in U.S. women (ACS, 2005). The overall incidence of breast cancer appears to have increased since 1975 when there was both a shift in delaying childbearing and the advent of breast mammography, which detected cancers earlier (ACS, 2005; CDC, 2008a). Therefore, a goal of *Healthy People 2010* is to "reduce the numbers of new cancers as well as the illness, disability, and death caused by cancer" (DHHS, 2000).

Risk Factors for Breast Cancer

The etiology of breast cancer is based on a number of risk factors (Chart 49–2). Several factors are associated with increased risk of breast cancer including age, family history, age at first pregnancy, age of menarche, and age of menopause. These are nonmodifiable risk factors. Modifiable risk factors include obesity, hormone replacement therapy, alcohol consumption, and sedentary lifestyle.

Besides being female, age is the most important risk factor for breast cancer (Osteen, 2001). The risk increases with age from 1 in 1,984 at age 20 to 1 in 24 at age 70. Currently, a woman living in the United States has a 1 in 8 lifetime risk of developing breast cancer. This has gradually increased over the past three decades in part due to longer life expectancy and more complete diagnosis through the use of mammography screening (ACS, 2005).

Family history is also a significant etiologic factor. Women with a family history of breast cancer, especially in a first-degree relative (mother, sister, or daughter), have an increased risk of developing breast cancer (Loman et al., 2001). Families with extensive history of breast and ovarian cancers are often screened for mutation of the BRCA1 gene. The BRCA1 is a tumor suppression gene when it functions normally. However, the BRCA1 gene can undergo mutation or alteration that causes increased susceptibility of the patient to not only breast cancer but ovarian cancer as well. The BRCA1 gene is located on chromosome 17; a similar gene, the BRCA2 gene, is located on chromosome 11. Five percent to ten percent of breast cancers are related to BRCA1 and BRCA2 gene mutations. Women with BRCA1 and BRCA2 gene mutations have a 40% to 80% lifetime risk of developing breast cancer. BRCA1 and BRCA2 gene mutations are also associated with early onset of breast cancer (Ford et al., 1998).

Reproductive hormones, specifically estrogen and progestin, are thought to influence breast cancer risk through effects on cell proliferation and DNA damage. Early menarche (<12 years of age) and menopause at > 55 years of age increase the exposure to estrogen. Being over age 30 at the time of a first full-term pregnancy and a low number of pregnancies may increase a woman's risk of breast cancer by affecting the endogenous reproductive hormones her body produces (Hulka & Moorman, 2001). The prolonged use of combination hormone replacement (estrogen and progestin) has also been shown to increase the risk of breast cancer (Rossow et al., 2002). The use of oral contraceptives may increase the risk of breast cancer slightly; however, once the woman stops using oral contraceptives for 10 years or more, she has the same risk as the woman who never used oral contraceptives. (Li et al., 2003).

Other modifiable risk factors can be considered in the prevention of breast cancer. There is, of course, no guaranteed way to prevent breast cancer, but decreasing risk factors is an effective strategy in reducing the risk of breast cancer. Obesity increases the risk of postmenopausal, but not premenopausal, breast cancer (Boyles, 2006). In postmenopausal women, circulating estrogen is primarily produced in fat tissue; therefore, having more adipose tissue increases estrogen levels and supports potential tumor formation. A recent American Cancer Society (2005) study showed that women with a body mass index (BMI) of > 25 are 1.3 to 2.1 times more likely to die from breast cancer compared to women with normal weight (BMI of 18.5 to 24.9). Recent studies also indicate that physical activity appears to have a protective effect on women with regard to breast cancer. The protective effect is most apparent in lean women, women who have carried children to term, and premenopausal women (Bianchini, Kaaks, & Vaino, 2002; McTiernan et al.,

| CHART 49–2 | Overview of Risk Factors for Developing Breast Cancer |

Nonmodifiable Risk Factors	Modifiable Risk Factors	Uncertain, Controversial, or Unproven Risk Factors
Gender: • 100 times more common in women.	**Childbirth:** • Having children later than age 30. • Not having any children.	**High-fat diets:** • Most studies found that breast cancer is less common in countries where the typical diet is low in total fat, low in polyunsaturated fat, and low in saturated fat. • Many studies of women in the United States have not found breast cancer risk to be related to dietary fat intake.
Age: • About 1 out of 8 invasive breast cancer diagnoses are younger than 45. • Two out of 3 women are age 55 or older.	**Oral contraceptive use:** • Women now using oral contraceptives have a slightly greater risk. • Risk seems to decline once their use is stopped.	**Antiperspirants:** • One small study recently found trace levels of parabens (used as preservatives in antiperspirants and other products), which have weak estrogen-like properties, in a small sample of breast cancer tumors. The study did not look at whether parabens had caused the tumors. • A large study of breast cancer causes found no increase in breast cancer in women who used underarm antiperspirants or who shaved their underarms.
Genetics: • Women with mutated breast cancer genes BRCA1 and BRCA2 have an 80% chance of developing breast cancer during their lifetime. **Ethnicity:** • Caucasian women are slightly more likely to develop breast cancer than are African American women. • African American women are more likely to die from this cancer. • Asian, Hispanic, and Native American women have a lower risk of developing and dying from breast cancer. BRCA mutations are found most often in: • Jewish women of Ashkenazi (Eastern European) population • African American women • Hispanic women	**Postmenopausal hormone therapy (PHT):** • Combined postmenopausal hormone therapy increases the risk of developing and may also increase the chances of dying from breast cancer. **Breast-feeding:** • Some studies suggest that breast-feeding may slightly lower risk, especially if continued for 1.5 to 2 years.	
Family history of breast cancer: • Having one first-degree relative (mother, sister, or daughter) with breast cancer approximately doubles a woman's risk. • Having two first-degree relatives increases her risk about fivefold. • A family history of breast cancer in a father or brother increases a woman's risk. • 20–30% of women with breast cancer have a family member with this disease. • 70–80% of women who get breast cancer do not have a family history.	**Alcohol:** • One alcoholic drink a day has a very small increase in risk. • Two to 5 drinks daily have about 1½ times the risk. • Also known to increase the risk of developing cancers of the mouth, throat, esophagus, and liver.	**Night work:** • Several studies have suggested that women who work at night may have an increased risk. This is a fairly recent finding, and more studies are in progress to look at this issue. According to some researchers, the effect may be due to disruption in melatonin, a hormone that is affected by light, but other hormones are also being studied.

(continued)

CHART 49–2	Overview of Risk Factors for Developing Breast Cancer—*Continued*

Nonmodifiable Risk Factors	Modifiable Risk Factors	Uncertain, Controversial, or Unproven Risk Factors

History of breast cancer:
• Cancer in one breast has a three- to fourfold increased risk of developing a new primary cancer in the other breast or in another part of the same breast. This is different from a *recurrence* of the first cancer.
 	
Abnormal breast biopsy results:
• The *proliferative lesions with atypia* (those with excessive growth of cells in the ducts or lobules of the breast tissue, and in which the cells no longer appear normal) increase risk 4 to 5 times. They include:
  • Atypical ductal hyperplasia (ADH)
  • Atypical lobular hyperplasia (ALH).
 	
Menstrual periods:
• Menstruating at an early age (before age 12).
• Menopause after age 55 has a slightly higher risk.
 	
Previous chest radiation:
• Radiation therapy to the chest area as treatment for another cancer (such as Hodgkin's disease or non-Hodgkin's lymphoma) significantly increases risk.
 	
Diethylstilbestrol (DES) exposure:
• Slightly increased risk.
	Overweight or obese:
	• Increased breast cancer risk, especially for women after menopause due to once the ovaries stop making estrogen, most of a woman's estrogen comes from fat tissue. Having more fat tissue after menopause can increase estrogen levels and thereby increase the risk.
	
	Physical activity:
	• Evidence is growing that physical activity in the form of exercise reduces breast cancer risk. The only question is how much exercise is needed. The Women's Health Initiative (WHI) found that as little as 1.25 to 2.5 hours per week of brisk walking reduced a woman's risk by 18%.
	• Walking 10 hours a week reduced the risk a little more.	

Source: "American Cancer Society. Breast Cancer Facts and Figures 2007–2008. Atlanta: American Cancer Society, Inc."

2003). The underlying mechanism is not well understood at this time. Alcohol consumption is consistently associated with increased breast cancer risk (Li et al., 2003). Alcohol appears to increase estrogen and androgen levels; therefore, the equivalent of two drinks a day may increase breast cancer risk by 21% (Singletary & Gapstur, 2001).

Pathophysiology of Breast Cancer

Breast tissue is made up of glands for milk production, called lobules, and ducts that connect the lobules to the nipple. Cancer arises from the epithelial cells that line the ducts and the lobules. Breast cancers can be *in situ*, which is the term that describes a cancer confined to the ducts or lobules. In 2005, there were 58,490 cases of *in situ* breast cancer (American Cancer Society, 2005). This type of breast cancer is not usually palpable on exam, so it is most often discovered by mammogram. The rates of *in situ* breast cancer have increased markedly since 1980, largely due to the increased diagnostic ability of mammography. Most cases of ductal carcinoma *in situ* (DCIS) are detectable only through mammography (National Cancer Institute, 2000). Approximately 22% of breast cancers are *in situ* (ACS, 2005). Lobular cancer *in situ* (LCIS) is not considered a true cancer by many

oncologists, but more of an indicator of increased risk of invasive cancer. Nearly all cancers at the *in situ* stage can be cured (ACS, 2005).

Invasive or infiltrative cancer starts in the lobules or ducts, but breaks through the walls to invade the surrounding fatty tissue of the breast. The most common type of breast cancer is invasive ductal carcinoma. In 2005 there were 211,240 cases of invasive ductal cancer (ACS, 2005). Once cancer is identified as invasive, it is staged according to the American Joint Committee on Cancer. The National Guidelines box outlines the staging of breast cancer.

Paget's disease is a rare form of breast cancer that is characterized by infiltration of the nipple epithelium. The patient may have itching, burning, and bloody nipple discharge. Some ulceration may be present as well. Treatment delays can be caused by misdiagnosis as infection or dermatitis. Prognosis is good for Paget's disease when the cancer is localized in the nipple.

Another form of breast cancer that is very rare is inflammatory breast cancer. This is a very malignant form of cancer because of its aggressive nature and fast growing character. This type of cancer is described by a finding of *peau d'orange* on the skin of the breast. The skin of the breast, which looks red, feels warm and has a thickened appearance resembling an orange peel.

NATIONAL GUIDELINES for the Staging of Breast Cancer

Stage	Tumor Size	Lymph Node	Metastasis
I	<2 centimeters	No involvement	None
IIA	No evidence of primary tumor	0–3 Axillary or internal mammary nodes	None
IIB	2–5 centimeters	0–3 Axillary or internal mammary nodes	None
IIIA	No evidence of tumor ranging to > 5 centimeters	Yes; 4–9 axillary or internal mammary nodes	None
IIIB	Any size with extension to chest wall or skin	Yes; 4–9 axillary or internal mammary nodes	None
IIIC	Any size	Yes; 10 or more axillary, internal mammary, or infraclavicular nodes	None
IV	Any size	Any type of nodal involvement	Yes

Source: American Joint Committee on Cancers. (2005). *AJCC cancer staging manual.* Retrieved February 27, 2008, from http://www.cancerstaging.org/products/ajccproducts.html

Clinical Manifestations of Breast Cancer

Early stage breast cancer or *in situ* cancer typically produces no symptoms when the tumor is small and most treatable. The most significant finding in breast cancer is a painless mass. The lump is most often in the upper outer quadrant of the breast where the majority of glandular tissue is found. The mass may be noted as a thickening in the breast tissue found during self-breast exam or showering. Other symptoms are an unusual lump in the axilla or above the clavicle. A persistent skin rash near the nipple area can signal Paget's disease, along with flaking or eruption near the nipple. Some tumors can cause dimpling, pulling, or retraction in one breast, creating an asymmetrical appearance. Some patients will complain of a burning, stinging, or prickling sensation in the breast. Nipple abnormalities such as spontaneous discharge, erosion, inversion, or tenderness can occur less commonly (American Cancer Society, 2005).

Diagnosis of Breast Cancer

The key to survival from breast cancer is early detection and intervention, with a 5-year survival rate of 97% for women diagnosed in Stage I (ACS, 2005). Mammography and breast self-exam are the two primary keys to early diagnosis. Breast self-exams, described in Chart 49–3, should be performed monthly beginning in the early 20s. Breast self-examination, along with mammography, can detect breast cancer early, with the cure rate being nearly 100% with early detection (CDC, 2008a). Once an abnormality has been detected, more invasive diagnostic techniques such as breast biopsy are used to make a definitive diagnosis. Diagnostic techniques are discussed next.

Mammography

The CDC (2008a) maintains that mammography is the most effective way to detect breast cancer when it is at a treatable stage. **Mammography** is a low-dose x-ray procedure that allows visualization of the internal structure of the breast. Mammography can identify cancer several years before physical symptoms develop. Modern screen-film units used today result in higher quality images with a considerably lower x-ray dose than the general-purpose x-ray equipment used in the past. The National Cancer Institute (NCI) (2007) and the CDC (2008a) recommend that all women over age 40 have a mammogram every 1 to 2 years. This alone could reduce breast cancer mortality by 20% to 25% over 10 years (CDC, 2008a). Mammography can

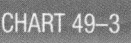 **CHART 49–3**   **Breast Self-Exam (Self-Breast Exam)**

Beginning in their 20s, women should be told about the benefits and limitations of breast self-exam (BSE). Women with breast implants can do BSE. It may be helpful to have the surgeon help identify the edges of the implant so that you know what you are feeling. Women who are pregnant or breast-feeding can also choose to examine their breasts regularly.

ESTABLISH A REGULAR SCHEDULE

- Perform on day 4–7 of menstrual cycle.
- If no periods, choose a regular day (i.e., the first of each month).
- Know how breasts normally look and feel and report any new breast changes to a health professional as soon as they are found.
- Best time to examine breasts is when the breasts are not tender or swollen.

INSPECT BREASTS

- Lie down and place your right arm behind your head. The exam is done while lying down, not standing up. This is because when lying down the breast tissue spreads evenly over the chest wall and is as thin as possible, making it much easier to feel all the breast tissue.
- Use the finger pads of the 3 middle fingers on left hand to feel for lumps in the right breast.
- Use overlapping dime-sized circular motions of the finger pads to feel the breast tissue.
- Use 3 different levels of pressure to feel all the breast tissue. Use each pressure level to feel the breast tissue before moving on to the next spot.
  - Light pressure is needed to feel the tissue closest to the skin.
  - Medium pressure to feel a little deeper.
  - Firm pressure to feel the tissue closest to the chest and ribs. A firm ridge in the lower curve of each breast is normal.

IMPORTANT POINTS TO REMEMBER

- Many lumps are benign.
- Early detection through breast self-exam and mammography increases the survival rate.

Source: "How to Perform a Breast Self-Exam adapted and reprinted by the permission of the American Cancer Society, Inc. from www.cancer.org. All rights reserved."

detect about 80% to 90% of breast cancers in women without symptoms; testing is somewhat more accurate in postmenopausal than in premenopausal women (Kerlikowski & Barclay, 1997). Approximately 60% of women over the age of

40 have had a mammogram within the previous year; however, a woman who has no health insurance, who has not graduated from high school, or who has recently immigrated to the United States is much less likely to have access to mammogram or clinical breast exam.

Terms associated with mammography include *screening* versus *diagnostic* and *film* versus *digital*. A screening mammogram simply indicates that the breast is being evaluated for any lumps or signs of potential cancer. A diagnostic mammogram is utilized when the screening mammogram or a clinical breast exam finds a suspicious area of the breast requiring closer evaluation. The diagnostic mammogram is often specific to the area in question and may utilize an enhancement mechanism to better view this area. Film mammography uses a film to both capture and display the breast tissue being evaluated. Film mammography is limited with dense breast tissue, seen in a population at higher risk for breast cancer (NCI, 2007). Digital mammography stores the electronic image in a way that allows for it to be enhanced, magnified, or manipulated to evaluate areas in question more fully.

Breast Ultrasound

Breast ultrasound is not as effective a screening tool as is mammography. It is used more often in the office setting for further characterization and guided biopsy of breast masses and suspicious axillary nodes. Ultrasound is very useful in differentiating solid masses and cystic lesions. Sound waves bounced off of the cystic lesion reveal lobulated and nonechogenic lesions with well-defined borders. The surgeon can use ultrasound to aid in locating and excising nonpalpable breast lesions and achieving clean lumpectomy margins. The future may find ultrasound being used to ablate tumors.

Breast Biopsy

A breast biopsy is performed to evaluate a lump or cyst that is found to be of a suspicious nature on mammography. There are four primary types of biopsies: fine needle aspiration biopsy, incisional biopsy, excisional biopsy, and stereotactic needle biopsy. Each is unique in its own way and used for specific reasons.

A fine needle aspiration (FNA) biopsy uses a fine gauge (typically 22 or 25 gauge) needle to pierce the skin and remove fluid from a cyst or remove cells from a solid mass. The tissue is removed by inserting the needle in the mass and aspirating fluid or cells, which are then sent to a pathology lab for analysis. The procedure is done under mammography or ultrasound guidance to pinpoint the exact location of the mass. This is usually an outpatient procedure, not requiring any stitches, and many patients resume normal activities that same day. Prior to discharge from the outpatient facility, assessment of the puncture site, vital signs, and pain evaluation are done. Discharge instructions include signs and symptoms of infection, pain-relief measures, and health care provider follow-up appointment. An FNA is considered the easiest form of breast biopsy, with rapid results (Imaginis, 2006). It is limited in that it samples only a small portion of tissue or cells.

Impalpable lesions are often evaluated using an image guided core needle biopsy. The patient needs to understand that the lesion will only be sampled, not excised. The core needle biopsy is less expensive than open biopsy, takes less time, and leaves only a tiny scar. Limitations of the procedure include the possibility of a sampling error that will cause the examiner to miss the lesion, causing equivocal findings that will require follow-up.

An open surgical incisional biopsy is considered the gold standard against which other methods are compared (Imaginis, 2006). Surgical incisional biopsies involve a less than 2-inch incision in the breast done under local anesthetic or intravenous (IV) sedation, and, like FNA, are usually considered an outpatient procedure. Prior to the procedure the surgeon will use mammography to locate and mark the specific area. Marking is done by several methods. If the abnormality can be felt by examination, the surgeon will mark the area using a marker or skin dye. If it cannot be felt by examination, the surgeon will use ultrasound to insert a small hollow needle into the mass, followed by insertion of a thin wire into the hollow bore of the needle. The needle is removed once the wire is placed. The patient is taken to the operating room for removal of all or part of the abnormality.

An excisional biopsy is done when complete removal of the abnormality and some surrounding tissue is planned. In this case, the pathologist will evaluate whether the margins of the lesion are free of abnormal cells, indicating that the entire lesion was removed. An incisional biopsy is performed when the lesion is large enough that removal through the small incision is not possible. A part of the lesion is removed in this case and sent for pathology evaluation, with follow-up surgery or treatment based on the pathology report. Pain control, vital signs, incisional assessment, and emotional needs are evaluated by the nurse. A follow-up appointment is made with the health care provider.

A stereotactic needle biopsy refers to the method in which the needle is guided into the abnormality. Stereotactic mammography is a three-dimensional mammography whereby the woman lies on her stomach on a mammography table with her breast protruding through a hole in the table. The breast is compressed as with a mammogram and an image taken. A biopsy is taken under a local anesthetic using a fine gauge needle. This procedure does not require surgery and is only mildly uncomfortable, but will produce a biopsy sample similar to the surgical route. The disadvantage is that the size of the abnormality is not clearly understood with this method. There are no special discharge instructions for the patient, and follow-up is scheduled with the health care provider.

Treatment of Breast Cancer

Breast cancer treatment is usually multileveled. Most women will require some form of surgery, and this may be followed by radiation, chemotherapy, hormone therapy, or monoclonal antibody therapy. A **lumpectomy**, removal of the cancerous growth and a small amount of surrounding normal tissue, is the least invasive form of surgery and is usually followed by 6 to 7 weeks of radiation. This is coupled with axillary node dissection and radiation therapy to improve long-term survival. A woman who chooses lumpectomy and radiation therapy will have the same expected long-term survival as if she had chosen a more invasive surgery such as mastectomy (American Cancer Society, 2005; Fisher et al., 2002).

Other surgical techniques include a simple (also called a total) **mastectomy**, which is removal of the entire breast, or a modified radical mastectomy, which is removal of the entire breast along with the surrounding lymph nodes. This surgery does not include removal of the chest wall muscles, as is done in radical mastectomy. Radical mastectomy is very rarely used today because of the disfiguring nature of the surgery. Radical mastectomy is not any more effective than other procedures. A complication of axillary node dissection is the problem of lymphedema, a serious swelling of the arm caused by retention of lymph fluid (Bumpers, Best, Norman, & Weaver, 2002).

Radiation is used to destroy cancer cells remaining in the breast tissue, chest wall, or underarm lymph nodes. Currently technology increases the ability to target radiation therapy accurately and decrease the side effects from radiation therapy. Radiation therapy can be used in conjunction with surgery and chemotherapy to improve long-term survival in women with lymph node positive disease.

Chemotherapy is a systemic method of destroying cancer cells that may have migrated to other parts of the body. Chemotherapy also is used to reduce the size of a tumor to allow a more conservative, rather than radical, approach to surgery. Hormone therapy is used to block the effects of estrogen on the growth of breast cancer cells. Tamoxifen, the most common medication used in breast cancer, blocks the tumor's ability to utilize estrogen in both pre- and postmenopausal women. Tamoxifen has been shown to reduce the rate of recurrence by 26%, and has reduced the death rate by 14% (American Cancer Society, 2005). Another group of antiestrogen agents known as aromatase inhibitors (anastrozole, letrozole) has been successfully used to block estrogen production by tissues other than the ovaries in postmenopausal women (ACS, 2005). Trastuzumab, a monoclonal antibody, targets a protein of breast tumors called HER2. Trastuzumab has been shown to improve survival for women with metastatic disease as well as late stage and recurrent disease (ACS, 2005; National Cancer Institute, 2000). See the Pharmacology Summary feature (p. 1552). A complete discussion of monoclonal antibodies is found in Chapter 59. Additional information on aspects of diagnosis and treatment of breast cancer may be found in Chapter 64 .

Breast Reconstruction

Reconstructive breast surgery occurs after mastectomy for breast cancer. Advances in techniques have made breast reconstruction a more desirable procedure for women requiring mastectomy. Reconstructive surgery can be done at the time of the mastectomy or it can be delayed, based on the woman's preference. Immediate breast reconstructive surgery does not delay administration of chemotherapy or radiation, nor does it prevent detection of recurrent disease. It is now thought to be beneficial to perform the breast reconstruction immediately after the mastectomy. An immediate breast reconstruction is more cost-effective, allows for a quicker recovery, and makes for reduced inconvenience, as well as greater satisfaction, for the patient (Harcourt & Rumsey, 2001). (Breast reconstruction is discussed in detail in the Diagnostic and Surgical Procedures section later in the chapter.)

Predicting Breast Cancer Survival

Breast cancer survival is dependent on multiple factors. The time since diagnosis is a factor; eighty-eight percent of women survive 5 years after diagnosis, 80% survive 10 years after diagnosis, 71% survive 15 years after diagnosis, and 63% survive 20 years after diagnosis (Smigal, et al, 2006). The 5-year survival

rate is slightly lower among women diagnosed with breast cancer before age 40. This may be due to tumors in this age group being more aggressive and less responsive to hormonal therapy (Kroman et al., 2000).

The stage of cancer at diagnosis also determines survival rate. Naturally, the survival rate is lower among women with more advanced state of disease; the 5-year survival rate is 98% for localized disease and 81% for regional disease with only a 26% survival rate for women diagnosed with distant-stage disease (Smigal, et al., 2006). In addition, larger tumor size at diagnosis is associated with decreased survival. A tumor is considered to be large when it is greater than 5.0 centimeters. Survivability can also depend on race or ethnicity and socioeconomic factors. African American women with breast cancer are less likely than Caucasian women to survive 5 years (Smigal, et al., 2006). Aggressive tumor characteristics associated with poorer prognosis appear to be more common in African American women (Chlebowski, Prentice, & Adams-Campbell, 2005). The presence of additional illnesses, lower socioeconomic status, unequal access to medical care, and disparities in treatment may contribute to the observed differences in survival between lower and higher income breast cancer patients. Chapter 64 provides an in-depth discussion of cancer staging and treatment.

◼ Nursing Management

The patient with breast cancer requires a comprehensive interdisciplinary care plan to address the complex nature of the disease. The Nursing Process: Patient Care Plan feature (p. 1534) provides a complete care plan for the patient with breast cancer. The Patient Teaching & Discharge Priorities box (p. 1536) outlines the discharge teaching for the patient with breast cancer.

Health Promotion for Breast Cancer

Patient and family education is essential for the prevention of breast cancer. The following facts are necessary components of the teaching plan:

- Self-breast exam
- Weight management
- Avoidance of excessive alcohol use
- Mammograms every 2 years after age 40
- Caution with use of hormone replacement therapy during menopause.

The United States (U.S.) Preventive Services Task Force recommends screening mammography, with or without clinical breast examination, every 1 to 2 years for women aged 40 or older. This task force found evidence that mammography screening every 12 to 33 months significantly reduces mortality from breast cancer. Evidence is strongest for women aged 50 to 69, the age group generally included in screening trials. For women aged 40 to 49, the evidence is weaker that screening mammography reduces mortality from breast cancer, and the absolute benefit of mammography is smaller, than it is for older women (U.S. Preventive Services Task Force, 2002).

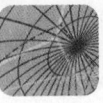

NURSING PROCESS: Patient Care Plan for Breast Cancer

Assessment of Patient History

Past medical history, relative risk factors, menstrual history, pregnancy history, reproductive cancers, such as ovarian or endometrial, benign breast disease, previous breast cancer.

Subjective Data:
Do you have pain in your back or other bone?
How is your appetite?
Have you had any change in breast size or symmetry, or skin changes over the breast?

Objective Data:
Signs of anxiety or stress, axillary or supraclavicular lymphadenopathy, changes in lung sounds (indicative of lung metastasis); hepatomegaly, jaundice, or ascites; obesity; or cachexia.

Nursing Assessment and Diagnoses	Outcomes and Evaluation Parameters	Planning and Interventions with *Rationales*
Nursing Diagnosis: *Deficient Knowledge* related to disease process, medications, treatment options, and complications	**Outcome:** Increased understanding of diagnosis, disease process, and treatment. *Evaluation Parameter:* Patient asks pertinent questions related to disease process, treatment, and symptoms.	**Interventions and *Rationale:*** Provide information to patient regarding disease process, medications, and treatment options. Encourage patient to ask questions regarding disease process, medications, and treatment options. Explain assessment findings to patient and encourage her to relate changes in signs and symptoms. *To increase knowledge about the disease.*

Assessment of Signs and Symptoms of Pain

Subjective Data:
Tell me your level of pain on a scale of 0–10, with 10 being the worst pain you have ever had.
Describe the location, intensity, and quality of your pain.

Objective Data:
Assess vital signs
Signs of stress and tension due to pain

Nursing Assessment and Diagnoses	Outcomes and Evaluation Parameters	Planning and Interventions with *Rationales*
Nursing Diagnosis: *Acute Pain* related to breast cancer and surgical intervention	**Outcomes:** Comprehensive pain management. Patient reports tolerable pain. Patient uses analgesic and nonanalgesic measures appropriately. *Evaluation Parameters:* Reduction in pain to patient acceptance. Patient reports pain is under control.	**Interventions and *Rationales:*** Perform a comprehensive pain assessment. Provide for quiet and restful environment. Reposition for comfort as needed. Provide for diversion with music, television, or relaxation techniques. Provide patient teaching regarding use of analgesics or PCA as appropriate. Advocate for patient when needed to change or increase pain medications. Encourage patient to use pain control measures before pain becomes severe and out of control. *To ensure the patient is as comfortable as possible.*

Assessment of Coping Abilities

Subjective Data:
Do you have a history of reproductive cancers?
Do you have any questions about your treatment plan?
Do you feel less anxious with more or less information?
Tell me what you are feeling regarding your illness?
Who are your support systems?

Objective Data:
Signs of anxiety and stress
Reduced communicative efforts
Withdrawal from social support
Insomnia
Crying

Nursing Assessment and Diagnoses	Outcomes and Evaluation Parameters	Planning and Interventions with *Rationales*
Nursing Diagnosis: *Disturbed Body Image* related to anticipated physical effects of treatment modalities	**Outcomes:** Development of effective coping behaviors. Development of attitude of realistic hope. *Evaluation Parameters:* Patient verbalizes feelings and fears about illness. Patient accepts social support. Patient reports decrease in symptoms of stress and anxiety. Patient reports increase in psychological well-being.	**Interventions and *Rationales:*** Encourage verbalization of feelings, perceptions, and fears *to reduce stress and anxiety.* Encourage patient to seek social support in the form of outreach groups *to feel less alone.* Encourage interaction with other women with breast cancer *to feel less alone.* Encourage patient to verbalize feelings of helplessness, and provide information regarding progress with treatments *to decrease stress level.* Encourage family members to verbalize concerns regarding the diagnosis, treatment, and potential complications *to decrease stress level.*

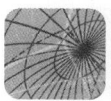

NURSING PROCESS: Patient Care Plan for Breast Cancer—*Continued*

Assessment of Signs and Symptoms of Infection

Subjective Data:
Do you have any increased pain, redness, or drainage from surgical site?

Objective Data:
Fever and chills
Changes in white blood count (WBC)
Drainage from the wound
Positive wound cultures
Decreased healing

Nursing Assessment and Diagnoses	Outcomes and Evaluation Parameters	Planning and Interventions with *Rationales*
Nursing Diagnosis: *Risk for Infection* related to neutropenia	**Outcome:** Avoidance of infection. **Evaluation Parameters:** Healed wound. No fever. Diminishing or absent pain.	**Interventions and *Rationales:*** Instruct patient and family members in hand hygiene *to prevent wound contamination.* Monitor surgical site for signs of infection for redness, odor, drainage, and lack of healing *that would indicate an infection.* Provide patient education about infection signs and symptoms and what to report to the surgeon. *To institute medical intervention as soon as possible.*

Assessment of Acceptance of Body Image

Subjective Data:
How do you feel about the changes in your body since surgery?
Do you plan to have reconstruction done?
Do you have any questions?

Objective Data:
Ability to participate in care
Willingness to interact with social support persons
Willingness to touch affected breast

Nursing Assessment and Diagnoses	Outcomes and Evaluation Parameters	Planning and Interventions with *Rationales*
Nursing Diagnosis: *Disturbed Body Image* related to anticipated physical effects of treatment modalities	**Outcome:** Acceptance of body image. **Evaluation Parameters:** Patient exhibits willingness to touch affected breast. Patient shows acceptance of social support. There is an interaction with individuals with similar change in body image. Patient discusses changes in body image. Patient demonstrates willingness to use strategies to enhance appearance.	**Interventions and *Rationales:*** Encourage patient to interact with Reach to Recovery volunteer *to develop hope for the future.* Encourage patient to attend breast cancer support group where she can draw on experiences of other women with breast cancer. Provide information on support groups available to patient. Facilitate contact with individuals with similar change in body image.

Female Reproductive System Disorders

Reproductive system disorders are varied and do not have age barriers. This section will discuss the more common disorders, their clinical manifestations, and treatment modalities, along with some prevention methods where applicable. Further information on general reproductive assessment can be found in Chapter 48 .

Etiology, Epidemiology, Pathophysiology, and Clinical Manifestations of Uterine Fibroid Tumors

Fibroid tumors of the uterus, also known as leiomyomas and myomas, occur in more than 30% of women 40 to 60 years of age but are almost always benign (Evans & Brunsell, 2007). They occur with higher prevalence in African American women, and some studies indicate that African American women are more likely than Caucasian women to have more symptomatic tumors (Kjerulff, Langenberg, Seidman, Stolley, & Guzinski, 1996). Leiomyomas are the most common female reproductive tract tumors (Evans & Brunsell, 2007). The lesions are growths aris-

ing from the tissue of the uterine muscle for unknown reasons (Figure 49–6 ■, p. 1536). They develop slowly in women ages 25 through 40, and tend to enlarge during pregnancy and after menopause; fibroids often decrease on their own, due to decreased estrogen production. Fibroids often cause no symptoms, so many are undiscovered unless the patient has dysfunctional uterine bleeding, pelvic pain, and infertility or pregnancy loss. Uterine tumors can add pressure to surrounding organs, causing pain, constipation, urinary problems, menorrhagia (heavy bleeding), and metrorrhagia (irregular bleeding). Risk factors for uterine fibroid tumors include 40 years of age or older, nulliparity, obesity, family history, African American, and hypertension.

Diagnosis and Medical Management of Uterine Fibroid Tumors

Diagnosis is accomplished based on an internal examination using transvaginal ultrasonography and hysteroscopy to help visualize the tumor and determine its exact location and size. The surgeon can then determine the best approach for treatment. The options for treatment of uterine fibroid tumors have increased substantially in the last 20 years. There are currently multiple treatment options that depend on the size of the tumor,

PATIENT TEACHING & DISCHARGE PRIORITIES for Breast Cancer

Need	Teaching
Analgesics	Take analgesics as prescribed.
Patient	Encourage patient to take analgesics as prescribed.
Family/support system	Advise patient to report to health care provider if analgesics are inadequate.
Activity	Range of motion exercises to maintain muscle tone and improve lymph and blood circulation.
Patient	Assist patient with items that are heavy and discourage strenuous activity.
Family/support system	
Diet	Regular, well-balanced diet as soon as desired.
Patient	Adequate amount of protein to ensure healing and immunity.
Family/support system	Encourage a healthy diet.
Postoperative	The value of a well-fitting prosthesis.
Patient	Provide resources for prosthetic bra.
Family/support system	Assist patient as needed with resources and provide emotional support.
Coping needs	Explain implications of a loss of a breast as it relates to self-image. Provide resources for counseling.
Patient	Spouse may need assistance in dealing with emotional needs of patient. Provide resources for counseling.
Family/support system	
Complications	Signs and symptoms of complications to include surgical site changes that indicate infection.
Patient	New or worsening pain, especially back pain (bone metastasis), shortness of breath, or change in sensorium.
Family/support system	Advise family members of important findings for which they should notify the patient's health care provider or seek emergency care.

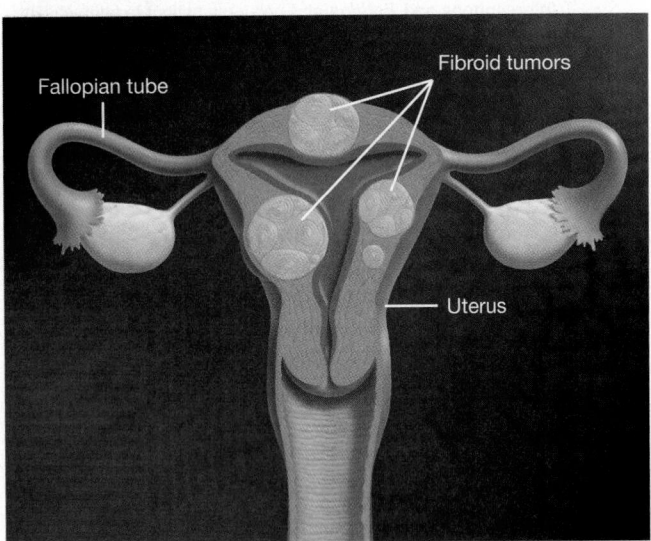

FIGURE 49–6 ■ Uterine fibroid tumor.
Source: Jane Hurd/Phototake NYC

the age of the patient, and the severity of symptoms. Choice of options also depends on whether fertility needs to be preserved. Observational management is increasingly recognized as a reasonable course for women with asymptomatic tumors. Conservative treatment involves drug therapy such as nonsteroidal anti-inflammatory drugs (NSAIDs) to control pain, birth control pills, and hormone therapy to decrease the size of the fibroids and the associated discomfort.

Uterine fibroid embolization, a nonsurgical treatment done under intravenous sedation that shrinks the fibroid, may also be used. This procedure is minimally invasive and avoids surgery. It is an interventional radiologic procedure that occludes the uter-

ine arteries that feed the fibroid. Intravenous (IV) conscious sedation is needed to assure patient comfort during the embolization procedure and is usually adequate, although some operators may prefer epidural or spinal analgesia. Patients usually experience pelvic pain immediately after the procedure. Nursing personnel are responsible for monitoring sedated patients and should be prepared to manage sedation and the analgesia required immediately after the procedure. This procedure will not preserve fertility.

In women whose symptoms are severe, or if the fibroid is very large, treatment can range from simple fibroid removal (myomectomy) to hysterectomy. Laser surgery is often used for myomectomy. A new technique that may prevent the need for a hysterectomy consists of destroying the uterine lining with heated water that is circulated into the uterus (MedlinePlus Medical Encyclopedia, 2007). This procedure is advantageous in that it can preserve fertility. Hysterectomy is the procedure that is used the most often for fibroid tumors. Justification for this recommendation includes the risk that tumors that are large could potentially mask other adnexal pathology and increase operative complication rates.

Etiology and Epidemiology of Endometriosis

Endometriosis affects approximately 10% of women in the United States (Mounsey, Wilgus, & Slawson, 2006). That makes it one of the most common health problems for women. Generally, women who have endometriosis are in the age range of 20 to 30 with the average age being 27. Women have symptoms for an average of 2 years before a definitive diagnosis is made.

Pathophysiology of Endometriosis

Endometriosis is a condition in which endometrial-like cells that are normally found only in the uterus are found outside of the uterus. These cells attach to ovaries, fallopian tubes, the bowels, or abdominal organs. During the menstrual cycle, these cells respond to hormone production and may swell and bleed. In response, the body will surround these lesions with scar tissue, which can form adhesions on the area of attachment. These adhesions respond to the hormones that stimulate the monthly period with the proliferation of blood and tissue. Tissue and blood that are shed into the body cause inflammation, scar tissue, and subsequently pain. As the misplaced tissue grows, it can cover and grow into the ovaries and block the fallopian tubes, causing problems of infertility (U.S. Department of Health and Human Services, Office on Women's Health, 2006).

Clinical Manifestations of Endometriosis

Endometriosis can produce mild symptoms of discomfort, to severe symptoms of pain, and infertility. The symptoms include pain in the lower abdomen and pelvis radiating down the thighs and to the lower back. There is often a feeling of rectal pressure and discomfort when defecating. Patients with endometriosis have dysmenorrhea and pain with sexual intercourse (dyspareunia) along with abnormal uterine bleeding. These women also have difficulty conceiving a child. Endometriosis is associated with infertility because of adhesions that distort the pelvic anatomy and cause impaired ovum release and implantation. A meta-analysis of 22 studies evaluating *in vitro* fertilization (IVF) outcomes found that patients with endometriosis had a pregnancy rate of nearly one-half that of patients without endometriosis (Barnhart, Dunsmoor-Su, & Coutifaris, 2002).

Risk Factors for Endometriosis

Risk factors for endometriosis include a family history, menstrual flow of greater than 6 days, and menstrual cycle of less than 28 days. Women at risk for endometriosis experienced menarche at an early age and have very heavy menses; they also have periods that last more than 7 days. Some studies suggest that women may lower their chances of developing endometriosis if they exercise regularly and avoid alcohol and caffeine.

Diagnosis and Medical Management of Endometriosis

Endometriosis is diagnosed using pelvic ultrasound and laparoscopy. Treatment ranges from palliative over-the-counter pain medications to prescription medications and surgery. The most commonly prescribed medication is oral contraceptives. Other medications prescribed include high-dose progesterone, gonadotropin-releasing hormone (Gn-RH), and danazol, all of which alter the production of hormones causing the symptoms associated with endometriosis, or shrink the sites of adhesions that will reduce symptoms. See the Pharmacology Summary feature (p. 1552). Laparoscopic surgery to examine reproductive organs and remove or obliterate endometrial tissue is an alternative treatment. A hysterectomy may be indicated in extreme cases.

▪ Nursing Management and Health Promotion

Nursing management for the patient with endometriosis is primarily about patient education. The patient needs to understand the disease process and the accompanying signs and symptoms. Patients need to understand the treatment options and the use of medications that are used to treat endometriosis. NSAIDs and heat are often helpful. Hormone medications may stop periods but can cause side effects similar to menopause (hot flashes and vaginal dryness). Sometimes these side effects will subside if patients take an estrogen pill every day. Patients should not get pregnant while taking medications for endometriosis. Women who want to get pregnant may need surgery to treat their endometriosis. Even with surgery, women with endometriosis may still need fertility treatments. Endometriosis will probably go away with the onset of menopause.

Nursing Diagnoses

Nursing diagnoses associated with endometriosis include:

1. Potential for *Tissue Perfusion, ineffective* from prolonged and heavy periods
2. *Fatigue* related to anemia
3. *Chronic Pain* and *Acute Pain* related to pelvic lesions
4. *Deficient Knowledge* related to management of symptoms and treatment options
5. *Ineffective Sexuality Pattern* related to dyspareunia
6. *Anxiety* and *Grieving* related to decreased fertility.

Outcomes

Expected outcomes associated with endometriosis include:

- A normal menstrual pattern with periods lasting up to 5 days and menstrual cycles extending to 28 days.
- Menstrual bleeding that does not require more than 1 pad in 2 hours.
- Menstrual discomfort that is controlled and does not interfere with patient's normal activities.
- Patient verbalizes understanding of management of the symptoms and treatment options.
- Patient reports less discomfort with sexual intercourse.
- Patient seeks specialized care for infertility as indicated.

Interventions

Nursing interventions associated with endometriosis include:

- Monitoring of complete blood count (CBC) to determine changes in hemoglobin and hematocrit. Report a drop of 1 gram or more in the hemoglobin or a drop of 3% or more in the hematocrit.
- Encourage the patient to pace activities to avoid fatigue.
- Instruct patient in pain management techniques, including use of NSAIDs and heat, along with relaxation techniques and diversion.
- Provide a nonjudgmental environment in which to discuss problems with dyspareunia and sexual dysfunction. Provide resources for further counseling.
- Provide resources for infertility counseling as indicated.

Etiology, Epidemiology, Pathophysiology, Clinical Manifestations, and Medical Management of Cystocele and Rectocele

A **cystocele** occurs when the wall between the bladder and the anterior vagina weakens and the bladder protrudes into the vaginal vault (Figure 49–7 ■). This frequently occurs following multiple vaginal deliveries. Symptoms include urine leakage when the woman sneezes, coughs, or laughs, or incomplete emptying of the bladder. The woman will often describe a feeling of pelvic pressure. When cystoceles are large, the bladder may not empty completely, and the patient will be susceptible to urinary tract infections.

A **rectocele** occurs when the posterior vaginal wall is weakened and the rectum bulges into the vagina (Figure 49–8 ■). The most frequent symptom is difficulty initiating a bowel movement, with resultant constipation, and rectal pressure. This can occur in women who have had conditions that involve repetitive bearing down, such as chronic constipation, chronic coughing,

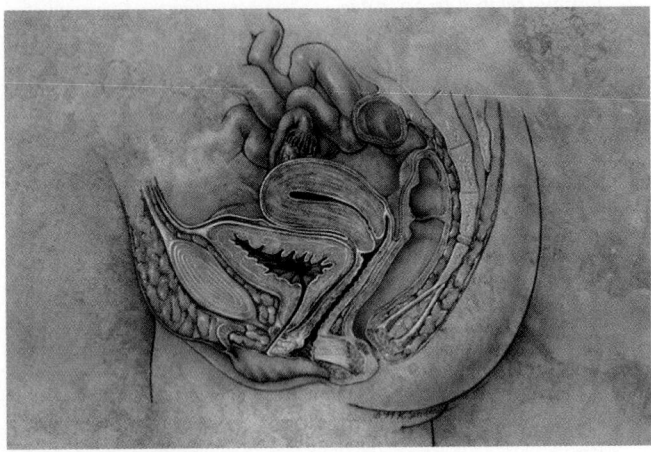

FIGURE 49–7 ■ Cystocele with uterine prolapse.
Source: Kevin A. Somerville/Phototake NYC

Cystocele   Rectocele

Urethrocele   Enterocele

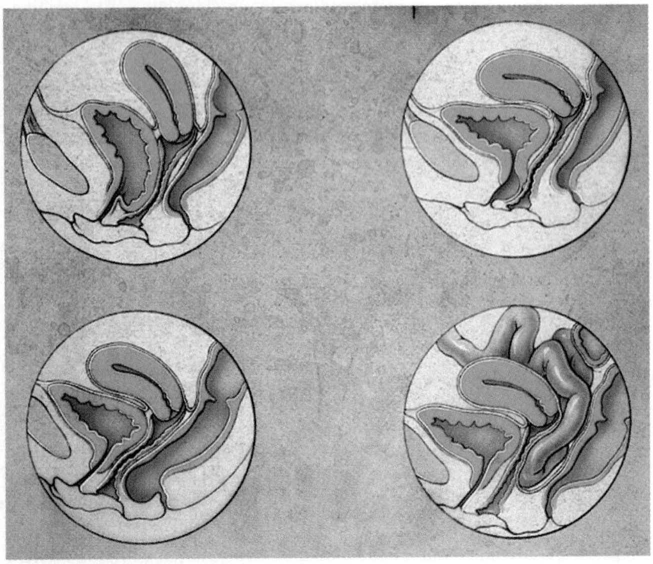

FIGURE 49–8 ■ Rectocele.
Source: Kevin A. Somerville/Phototake NYC

or repetitive heavy lifting. Simple Kegel exercises (intermittent tightening of the perineal and vaginal muscles) will help to prevent the development of these problems.

For women with mild to moderate symptoms, a pessary may be an option. A **pessary** is a device that, when inserted into the vagina, will help support the vaginal walls, reducing the bulging into the vagina; therefore, it is used for management of pelvic support defects such as cystocele, rectocele, and uterine prolapse. The pessary is also used before and after pelvic surgery such as hysterectomy to support the pelvic floor muscles. For those patients who are not good candidates for extensive surgery to repair defects of the pelvic floor, the pessary is an important management option. The pessary is one of the oldest medical devices available. Currently, there are a number of different types of pessaries and health care providers are becoming reacquainted with their use. Pessaries should not be used if there is evidence of active pelvic infection such as vaginitis or pelvic inflammatory disease. Patients should be compliant with follow-up visits.

Complications of pessaries include vaginal irritation, infection, discharge, pressure sores, or allergy to the components of the pessary. Patients should know that although the pessary can be worn during sexual intercourse, it does not provide any method of birth control or protection against sexually transmitted infections. Last, the patient must be taught effective placement and removal of the pessary and how to care for and clean it.

Surgery can correct the issues of cystocele and rectocele when the symptoms are moderate to severe. Cystoceles and rectoceles are repaired using a procedure called a colporrhaphy, also referred to as an anterior/posterior (A&P) repair, depending on whether one or both procedures are done. The anterior wall repair, done for a cystocele, involves repair and resultant strengthening of the weakened area by either shortening the pelvic muscles providing greater support for the bladder or suspending the urinary bladder in the proper position. The posterior repair is used for the rectocele and tightens the pelvic floor muscles to provide greater support for the rectum. Risks are minimal but can include bleeding and infection. Postoperative assessment includes monitoring vital signs, observing vaginal bleeding greater than simple spotting, signs of infection, and adequate hydration. The woman will have a Foley catheter for 1 or 2 days, and intake and output should be monitored accordingly. Stool softeners may be needed to avoid straining with bowel movements, and encouraging a well-balanced, high-fiber diet will assist in maintaining normal bowel function. Discharge instruction should include avoiding activities that might stress the incision, including intercourse or placing anything in the vagina until released by the health care provider. Avoiding long periods of standing, coughing, and sneezing will also decrease strain on the surgical site. Adequate fluids and continuing a well-balanced, high-fiber, high-protein diet will aid in healing and regaining normal bowel function.

Etiology, Epidemiology, Pathophysiology, Clinical Manifestations, and Treatment of Uterine Prolapse

Uterine **prolapse** is another common structural disorder that occurs as a result of weakening of the pelvic floor musculature. The structures supporting the uterus are sometimes weakened during pregnancy and childbirth. There is an increased risk for uterine prolapse with obesity, chronic coughing, and straining during bowel movements. In addition, multiple pregnancies, congenital weakness, and loss of elasticity and muscle tone due to the aging process can contribute to the problem. The result is the uterus is displaced downwardly into the vaginal canal. The uterus can prolapse enough to be seen outside the vagina. The prolapse pulls on surrounding structures and puts pressure on the bladder and rectum. This pressure can cause symptoms of incontinence or retention, and may be aggravated by coughing or lifting heavy objects. Generally, the treatment of choice is surgery to suture the uterus into place and tighten the musculature supporting it. Occasionally, a hysterectomy is done, although a pessary to support the uterus can be inserted into the vagina to support the uterus.

Etiology, Epidemiology, Pathophysiology, Clinical Manifestations, and Medical Management of Ectopic Pregnancy

An **ectopic** pregnancy is implantation of the products of conception outside the uterine endometrium (Figure 49–9 ■). Approximately 2% of all pregnancies are ectopic (Sepilian, 2007). The most common location for an ectopic pregnancy is the fallopian tube (95%). The other 5% may occur in such places as the cervix, ovary, or abdomen. Causes of ectopic pregnancy are varied but often include problems that may leave scar tissue or prevent movement of the fertilized ovum appropriately down the fallopian tube and into the uterine cavity. These problems include pelvic inflammatory disease (PID), previous ectopic pregnancy, endometriosis, tubal surgery, and use of an intrauterine device (IUD) for birth control. Also contributing to the risk of ectopic pregnancy are procedures used in infertility treatments, including *in vitro* fertilization and embryo transfer.

Any condition that leaves residual scar tissue can cause partial or complete blockage of the fallopian tubes. The scar tissue impedes the passing of the fertilized egg into the uterus. As the cells divide, the gestational sac expands against the tubal wall. If allowed to continue, the tube expands until it ruptures, causing acute lower abdominal pain and internal bleeding.

Often the patient will present with typical symptoms of pregnancy, including an elevated quantitative human chorionic gonadotropin (HCG), amenorrhea, and nausea, but with pelvic pain and in some cases light vaginal bleeding. The prime time for the manifestations of ectopic pregnancy is at approximately 7 weeks after a missed period. These findings are very nonspecific and are certainly common to patients who may be having a spontaneous abortion, acute appendicitis, ovarian torsion, pelvic inflammatory disease, and renal calculi. Therefore, the positive HCG is very important to making the diagnosis of ectopic pregnancy. Because the implantation is not inside the uterus where space for the growth of the embryo is adequate, the growth puts pressure on the surrounding tissues and structures causing discomfort and pain. If the fallopian tube ruptures, the patient experiences intense, sharp, unilateral pain with pain referred to the shoulder as a result of irritation of the diaphragm by blood in the abdominal cavity. When this happens, there is risk of hemorrhage and hypovolemic shock. This is treated as a medical emergency.

Due to the life-threatening potential of ectopic pregnancy, all women of childbearing age who present with lower abdominal or pelvic pain should be tested for pregnancy. If the test is positive, then the patient will need a transvaginal ultrasound to examine the ovaries, uterus, and fallopian tubes. Quantitative HCG is a serum test used to determine the duration of the pregnancy. Under normal circumstances, this value doubles every 48 hours in early pregnancy. If the HCG level fails to double, the pregnancy is not viable, and an ectopic pregnancy is assumed until proven otherwise. The transvaginal ultrasound will be accurate in determining the presence of an intrauterine pregnancy when the quantitative HCG has reached 1,500 to 2,000 mLU/m. (Lozeau & Potter, 2005).

Medical treatment of ectopic pregnancy is preferred over surgical treatment. Methotrexate, a drug often used in cancer treatment, is the current drug of choice and will act on the ectopic cells as it does in cancer treatment: to destroy the cells. It is given if the ectopic is unruptured and the patient is in stable condition. It is given intramuscularly and often as an outpatient procedure. Successful treatment may require more than one dose of methotrexate.

Failure of beta HCG levels to decrease by at least 15% from day 4 to day 7 after methotrexate administration indicates the need for an additional dose of methotrexate or surgery (ACOG, 1998).

If surgery is indicated with a ruptured ectopic pregnancy, it consists of repair of the tube if future pregnancies are desired. Removal of the tube may be necessary if repair is not possible or may be desired if future pregnancies are not planned. Approximately 30% of women treated for ectopic pregnancy later have difficulty conceiving. Rates of recurrent ectopic pregnancy are between 5% and 20% (Lozeau & Potter, 2005).

Reproductive System Cancers

Reproductive system cancers include cervical, vulvar, endometrial, ovarian, and vaginal cancers. See Chart 49–4 (p. 1540) for a comparison of these cancers. Chapter 64 ⏎ has an in-depth discussion of the pathophysiology of cancer development and progress.

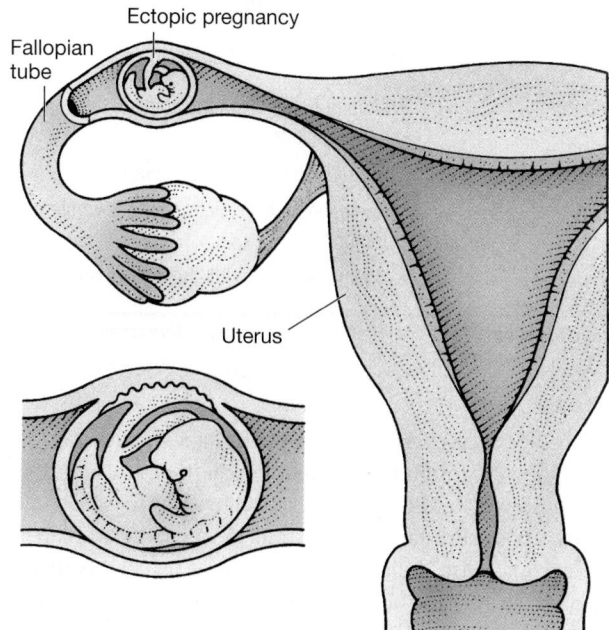

FIGURE 49–9 ■ Ectopic pregnancy.
Source: © Dorling Kindersley

CHART 49–4	**Comparison of Female Reproductive Cancers**	
Etiology	**Assessment**	**Interventions**
Cervical Cancer		
Third most common reproductive cancer. 90% Squamous cell. 10% Adenocarcinoma. Average age 40–50. Increased risk with human papillomavirus (HPV) and herpes 2, multiple partners, and decreased socioeconomic status. Increased in African American and Hispanic women.	Preinvasion is often asymptomatic. Invasive shows postcoital bleeding and abnormal bleeding. Late symptoms include rectal bleeding, hematuria, back and leg pain, and anemia. Pap smear is the single most reliable diagnostic test (it will show 90% of early cervical cancers). Other diagnostic tests include colposcopy, biopsy, and conization.	Preinvasive lesions often entail cryosurgery, laser surgery, or loop electrosurgical excision procedure (LEEP: an electrically charged thin wire is used to remove a thin layer of cells from the cervix). Typically done as an outpatient procedure. Invasive treatment is hysterectomy with internal or external radiation.
Vulvar Cancer		
Fourth most common gynecologic cancer. Average age 60–70. Those under 35 are linked to condolymata. 90% Squamous cell. Slow growing. 90% Survival even with late diagnosis if nodes are negative. Less than 50% survival with node involvement.	Lesion usually asymptomatic until 1–2 centimeters. Symptoms include vulvar pruritus and burning pain. Diagnosed by biopsy with histologic evaluation using toluidine blue.	Local, wide excision, or vulvectomy. External radiation.
Endometrial Cancer		
Most common gynecologic malignancy. Average age 50–65. Risk factors include obesity, nullipara, infertility, diabetes mellitus, hypertension, family history, Caucasian, and hormone imbalance, which is the most significant risk factor.	Symptoms include abnormal uterine bleeding, lower back pain, lower pelvic pain, uterine enlargement, and positive Pap smear. Diagnosis by fractional curettage or endometrial biopsy.	Total abdominal hysterectomy with bilateral salpingectomy and oophorectomy. Radiation (internal or external) before or after surgery. Chemotherapy with advanced stage or recurrent.
Ovarian Cancer		
Second most frequent gynecologic cancer. Causes more deaths than any other reproductive cancer. Risks include nullipara, infertility, and family history. Affects all ages but increased in the 50s.	No definitive tests. Often diagnosed in late stage. Symptoms include lower abdominal discomfort and digestive complaints. Increased pain, weakness, and malnutrition are late signs.	Treatment varies from removal of the ovary to total hysterectomy. Chemotherapy. Antineoplastic drugs. Radiation is controversial.
Vaginal Cancer		
Rare. Two types: squamous cell (increased in ages 60–80) and adenocarcinoma (increased in ages 12–30). Risks include young women of mothers who received diethylstilbestrol (DES) in 1945–1970 as a treatment for miscarriage.	Bleeding or discharge not related to menstruation. Pain during intercourse (dyspareunia). Pelvic pain.	Treatment depends on the stage of the cancer and may include: • Surgery (to remove the cancer) • Radiation (to kill cancer cells and/or shrink tumors) • Chemotherapy (to kill the cancer cells).

Source: "Detailed Guides for Cervical, Vulva, Endometrial, Ovarian and Vaginal Cancer" adapted and reprinted by the permission of the American Cancer Society, Inc. from www.cancer.org. All rights reserved.

Etiology, Epidemiology, Pathophysiology, Clinical Manifestations, and Treatment of Orgasmic Dysfunction

One phase of the sexual response cycle is the orgasmic phase. When there is difficulty reaching orgasm, it is called orgasmic dysfunction, or **anorgasmia**. Anorgasmia is considered to be one of the most common sexual problems among women; however, less than 20% of cases are related to physiological issues. Anorgasmia is frequently found to be psychological in nature and results from unresolved conflicts about sexual activity or marital conflict (Phillips, 2000). Primary dysfunction is when the woman has never had an orgasm following any means of sexual stimulation. Secondary dysfunction occurs when the woman has had orgasms in the past, but is unable to achieve them now. Causes of anorgasmia can be disease that results in general debility such as multiple sclerosis, diabetes, spinal cord injuries, and hormonal conditions that affect sexual response. Drugs such as antidepressants, alcohol, and other central nervous system (CNS) depressants can also inhibit sexual response. Chart 49–5 outlines medications that interfere with sexual function.

Menopause and oophorectomy (surgical removal of the ovaries) create a hypoestrogenic state, which may increase the likelihood of orgasmic dysfunction. Testosterone decreases with menopause and oophorectomy, and is considered an essential female hormone for sexual desire as well as in males. Testosterone appears to have a direct role in sexual desire. However, studies are limited at this point, so there are no guidelines for testosterone replacement therapy for women with disorders of desire (Phillips, 2000). Use of testosterone supplementation in conjunction with estrogen replacement therapy has shown success in increasing sexual desire and orgasm (Phillips, 2000). Orgasmic disorders can be treated with Kegel exercises and masturbation. The purpose is to maximize stimulation and minimize inhibition.

Treatment of both physical and psychological circumstances may benefit from counseling therapy. When medical conditions prevent the ability to reach orgasm, therapy may be directed at alternative ways of satisfaction, such as simple holding each other close, touching, or exploring individual ways that make each other feel satisfied. When secondary dysfunction is the cause, counseling is directed at the couple and the root of their discord.

CHART 49–5	**Medications That Interfere with Sexual Function**

PSYCHOACTIVE MEDICATIONS

Antipsychotics

Barbiturates

Benzodiazepines

Selective serotonin reuptake inhibitors

Lithium

Tricyclic antidepressants

CARDIOVASCULAR AND ANTIHYPERTENSIVE MEDICATIONS

Antilipid medications

Beta-blockers

Clonidine

Digoxin

Spironolactone

CENTRAL NERVOUS SYSTEM AGENTS

Anticholinergics

Antihistamines

H_2 blockers

Methyldopa

Amphetamines

Anorexic drugs

Narcotics

Phenytoin

Etiology, Epidemiology, Pathophysiology, Clinical Manifestations, and Treatment of Dyspareunia

Dyspareunia, painful intercourse, can be a result of several factors including both physiological and psychological ones. Endometriosis is an example of a physiological cause, which is due to displaced endometrial tissue in the peritoneal cavity. Menopause is another physiological cause, resulting from a decrease in hormone production, which in turn decreases the normal lubricating mechanism of the vagina. In addition, the vagina may become somewhat smaller during menopause, causing a more difficult penetration. Other physiological causes may include an imperforate hymen or vaginal scarring.

Psychological causes may be related to early traumatic events such as sexual abuse or rape, triggering an involuntary reflex known as vaginismus. **Vaginismus** is a condition in which the vaginal muscles at the introitus contract very tightly, making vaginal penetration painful.

Hormonal treatment of endometriosis, often with danazol (Danocrine), an androgenic steroid, has been successful in regression of the displaced endometrial tissue. Hormone replacement therapy and lubricating gel can assist in the treatment of dyspareunia related to menopause. Psychological causes require counseling.

■ Nursing Management

Use of the nursing process provides an effective framework to guide the nursing management for patients experiencing the various disorders of the reproductive system. During the nursing assessment it is important to obtain a history from the woman about the type of reproductive disorder that is occurring. The nurse should be careful not to ask questions in a manner so as to allude to bias toward heterosexuality or homosexuality. Establishment of the patient's sexual orientation is necessary for appropriate evaluation and management. Nonjudgmental, direct questions best achieve this goal (Phillips, 2000). The interviewer must be careful to ensure privacy and confidentiality. During the interview the nurse gains a complete history of the patient symptoms include timing, situation, and duration. Questioning the patient about her insight into the cause may be very helpful. It is important to collect history regarding chronic illness, injuries, and a psychiatric history. Prescription and over-the-counter medications as well as the use of recreational drugs and alcohol must be listed accurately. Surgical interventions and malignancies such as breast cancer can alter self-image and cause decreased sexuality. Questions regarding relationships should be asked to determine level of partner support and previous problematic or violent relationships.

A complete physical needs to be done with a pelvic exam to determine the existence of vaginismus, vulvar dystrophy, dermatitis, vaginal atrophy, infectious disease, scar tissue, postoperative changes, fibroids, masses, endometriosis, tenderness, or structural defects. The goal of the examination is detection of disease; however, the examination also provides an opportunity to educate the patient about normal anatomy and sexual function, and to reproduce and localize pain encountered during sexual activity (Phillips, 2000).

Nursing Diagnoses

Nursing diagnoses associated with female reproductive dysfunction include:

- *Disturbed Body Image*
- *Ineffective Sexuality Pattern*
- *Risk for Situational Low Self-Esteem* related to sexual difficulties
- *Chronic Pain*
- *Compromised Family Coping*
- *Decisional Conflict* related to treatment options
- *Deficient Knowledge* related to disease process
- *Disturbed Thought Process* related to sense of inadequacy
- *Fear*

Outcomes

Expected outcomes of care for patients experiencing reproductive dysfunction include:

- Enhanced knowledge related to sexual functioning
- Decreased anxiety and fear
- Acceptance of body image
- Adequate decision making regarding treatment options
- Improved family coping
- Adequate health seeking behaviors
- Adequate sexual functioning and identity
- Enhanced self-esteem related to sexual difficulties
- Adequate pain relief and ability to cope with pain.

Planning and Intervention

Care of the patient with sexual dysfunction requires education, support, and therapeutic interventions. Information regarding normal anatomy, sexual function, and the normal changes of aging, pregnancy, and menopause are important. Encourage discussion of sexual issues in the context of a medical condition or a new medication agent prescribed. Depression is frequently associated with reproductive disorders; therefore, psychological counseling may be necessary. Women with long-standing dysfunction, multiple dysfunctions, or history of sexual abuse need to be referred to a gynecologist and/or psychological counseling.

Health Promotion
for Female Reproductive Disorders

Patients frequently have difficulty discussing sexual problems with their health care provider. But up to 70% of couples have a problem with sex at some time during their relationship. Promoting good sexual health is dependent on providing an accepting environment in which patients can discuss problems with sexual response. Encouraging patients to explain their problems openly and honestly with their health care provider can result in possible treatments. It is also important for couples to communicate regarding concerns. A mutually satisfying relationship that includes respectful and caring behaviors on the part of both partners provides the best hope for a gratifying sex life.

■ Menstrual Disorders

Menstrual disorders involve not only physical symptoms but emotional symptoms as well. Because the menstrual cycle is related to the reproductive ability of a woman, any problems may be a cause of great concern. Almost all women will experience some form of menstrual disorder in their lifetime, such as missing a period, heavy periods, or painful periods. The most common ones are discussed next.

Etiology, Epidemiology, Pathophysiology, Clinical Manifestations, and Medical Management of Amenorrhea

Amenorrhea is defined as the absence of menstruation. It is considered primary when the girl/woman has not started her menstrual cycles by the age of 16. It is secondary when menstruation has been present but ceases for more than 3 months and is not related to pregnancy. Secondary amenorrhea is more common than primary amenorrhea. Causes of amenorrhea are varied and may be related to stress, athleticism, weight changes, and disease/hormonal processes. Chart 49–6 outlines the various causes of amenorrhea.

Primary amenorrhea can be caused by a congenital absence of a part of the reproductive tract such as ovaries, uterus, or vagina. Another cause could be the presence of the imperforate hymen. Imperforate hymen is a congenital defect in which the opening to the vagina does not form, and as a result there is no exit from the vagina. Imperforate hymen occurs in 1 in 1,000 women. A procedure using local anesthetic can correct the defect.

In adolescence, stress, eating disorders, exercise, and ovulation abnormalities can cause irregular periods. This is especially pertinent in the patient in which fat comprises less than 10% of the body. Bulimia, anorexia, obesity, and malnutrition may alter the hormone balance in the body, as some are produced by fat cells. This change in hormone production or utilization may cause amenorrhea. Excessive exercise, usually more than 20 hours a week for a prolonged number of weeks, triggers a reduction in reproductive hormones, in particular, leptin. Decreased leptin can interfere with the production of luteinizing hormone, which is necessary for ovulation.

There is a triad of symptoms that has been identified in the female athlete that reflects the health issues of females who exercise more than 20 hours week. The components include amenorrhea or oligomenorrhea, eating disorder (anorexia or bulimia), and decreased bone mineral density (Sherman & Thompson, 2004). Alternatively, women who are obese also have a higher incidence of amenorrhea.

Elevated prolactin levels may inhibit ovulation and consequently cause amenorrhea. The elevated levels may be related to pituitary tumors and can cause breast milk production not related to pregnancy (galactorrhea). Elevated prolactin levels need to be evaluated by an endocrinologist. Treatment of amenorrhea depends on the cause. Frequently, correcting pituitary disorders, thyroid disorders, or inducing appropriate nutrition and exercise levels can result in normal menstruation.

CHART 49–6 Causes of Amenorrhea

Hormone Alteration

Thyroid disease: hypothyroidism
Pituitary dysfunction
Menopause
Pregnancy
Cushing's syndrome
Polycystic ovary syndrome

Chronic Disease

Liver failure
Renal failure
Cancer (bronchogenic, renal cell CA)
Autoimmune diseases
Chemotherapy
Pelvic radiation
Central nervous system tumor
Diabetes
Immunodeficiency
Inflammatory bowel disease
Thyroid disease
Severe chronic depression

Structural Defects

Imperforate hymen
Congenital defect causing absence of ovaries, fallopian tubes, or uterus
Cervical stenosis
Transverse vaginal septum

Medications

Oral contraceptives
Antipsychotics
Antidepressants
Antihypertensives
Histamine H_2-receptor blockers
Opiates, cocaine

Exercise and Nutrition

Anorexia or bulimia nervosa
Excessive exercise
Excessive weight loss
Malnutrition

Alterations in Growth and Development

Constitutional delay of growth and puberty
Acromegaly
Congenital adrenal hyperplasia
Mumps
Genetic defects

Etiology, Epidemiology, Pathophysiology, Clinical Manifestations, and Treatment of Polycystic Ovary Syndrome

Polycystic ovary syndrome (PCO or PCOS) is an endocrine disorder that results from high levels of androgens (male hormones), especially testosterone. The incidence of PCOS is relatively common at 5% to 10% (U.S. Department of Health and Human Services, Office on Women's Health, 2007). It is the most commonly occurring endocrine disorder in women of childbearing age and the most common cause of infertility (U.S. Department of Health and Human Services, Office on Women's Health, 2007). The causes of PCOS are unknown at this time, but scientists are studying genetic mutations that may be at the root. It is known that there is a familial tendency for PCOS. It is also known that poor utilization of insulin increases production of the male hormones (androgens) that cause many of the manifestations of PCOS.

The high level of male hormones often causes an associated low follicle-stimulating hormone (FSH) production, which prevents mature egg production. Egg production is required for the stimulation of progesterone. Without progesterone a woman's menstrual cycle is irregular or absent. When there is no mature egg produced, the follicles fill with fluid and form cysts. The cysts that form make male hormones, which also prevent ovulation. As cysts continue to form, some may become the size of grapefruit.

The associated low or absent progesterone production, increased estrogen levels, and increased androgen production may produce the following manifestations: increased facial hair and acne, oligomenorrhea (few periods), infertility due to anovulation, pelvic pain due to ovarian cyst formation, anxiety or depression due to appearance and infertility, obesity, and elevated lipids and blood glucose. On rare occasions PCOS may produce the male characteristics of deepening voice and clitoral enlargement.

It is important that the woman maintain a regular schedule of medical visits so the growth of the cysts can be monitored. Treatment is directed at the symptoms causing the most concern and may involve pharmacologic interventions or surgery. Oral contraceptives are used to suppress ovulation by inhibiting the release of luteinizing hormone (LH) and decreasing testosterone levels. In addition, this often improves hirsuitism. Gonadotropin-releasing hormone (Gn-RH) may be used if the oral contraceptives do not reduce the size of the cysts. If a pregnancy is desired, the use of oral contraceptives is replaced by ovulation-inducing medications.

Cysts that are greater than 8 centimeters are typically surgically removed. Analgesics may be used for pain management associated with pressure from the enlarging cysts. Additionally, the patient should be treated with oral hypoglycemics such as metformin to control blood glucose and lower testosterone production. This will aid in slowing abnormal hair growth and ovulation may return after a few months. Metformin will also decrease body mass and improve cholesterol levels. See the Pharmacology Summary feature (p. 1552).

Nursing interventions are directed toward pain management and education in the areas of treatment options. Women who adopt a healthy lifestyle by maintaining normal weight and getting regular exercise can help manage PCOS. Even 10% loss in body weight can restore a normal period and make a woman's cycle more regular (Master-Hunter & Heiman, 2006).

Women with PCOS have a 4 to 7 times' higher risk of coronary artery disease and myocardial infarction than do women of the same age without PCOS. Additionally, PCOS patients are at greater risk of having high blood pressure. The increased risk for the development of endometrial cancer is another concern for women with PCOS. Irregular menstrual periods and the absence of ovulation cause women to produce the hormone estrogen, but not the hormone progesterone. Progesterone causes the endometrium to shed its lining each month as a menstrual period. Without progesterone, the endometrium becomes thick, which can cause heavy bleeding or irregular bleeding. Over time, this can lead to endometrial hyperplasia and the potential for cancer cells to develop (U.S. Department of Health and Human Services, Office of Women's Health, 2007). Resources for women looking for more information about PCOS include the Polycystic Ovarian Syndrome Association, Inc. and the American Association of Clinical Endocrinologists.

Etiology, Epidemiology, Pathophysiology, Clinical Manifestations, and Treatment of Dysmenorrhea

Dysmenorrhea is defined as painful menstruation. It is generally described as cramping-type pelvic pain that begins shortly before or at the onset of the monthly menses. Most women experience the discomfort for approximately 3 days. Adolescents report the highest incidence of dysmenorrhea. A recent study in Sweden found a prevalence of dysmenorrhea of 90% in women 19 years of age and 67% in women 24 years of age (French, 2005). Dysmenorrhea is classified as primary, which is associated with increased uterine contractility, or secondary, which is caused by some form of pelvic pathology, such as endometriosis or fibroid tumors.

With primary dysmenorrhea, there is an increase in uterine muscle contractions due to an increase in the prostaglandin level in the second half of the menstrual cycle. Systemic response to increased prostaglandin levels is manifested in pain in the lower back and lower abdomen, nausea, diarrhea, headache, and weakness. It is seen only with ovulatory cycles because both estrogen and progesterone are necessary for it to occur. It is also seen primarily in adolescents and women in their early 20s, with the incidence and severity often declining with age. Risk factors for dysmenorrhea include adolescent age, nulliparity, heavy menstrual flow, attempts to lose weight, depression and anxiety, and smoking.

Evaluation of the patient with dysmenorrhea should include a history of symptoms and menstrual cycles, including age of menarche and level of flow. An abdominal exam alone is performed on the adolescent who is not yet sexually active. A pelvic examination should be performed in females who have been sexually active to screen for sexually transmitted infections. A transvaginal ultrasound can be used to rule out anatomic abnormalities such as masses, ovarian cysts, and endometriosis. Laparoscopic surgery may be needed to further identify and define causes of dysmenorrhea.

Management varies depending on the severity of symptoms. Chart 49–7 shows the nonpharmacologic therapies most often prescribed. The pharmacologic therapies are listed in the Pharmacology Summary feature (p. 1552). Being cognizant of the increased incidence of bleeding that occurs with certain pain relievers is essential.

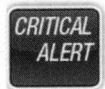

CRITICAL ALERT *Do not use nonsteroidal anti-inflammatory drugs (NSAIDs) for patients with hemophilia, those with bleeding ulcers, those allergic to aspirin or other NSAIDs, or those taking anticoagulant medications. Be sure to take NSAIDs with milk or food to help prevent gastric irritation and possible bleeding.*

Secondary dysmenorrhea is pain associated with a specific condition, such as endometriosis, pelvic inflammatory disease, or

CHART 49–7 Nonpharmacologic Therapies for Dysmenorrhea

Therapy	Rationale
Heating pad/hot bath and fetal position	Increases vasodilation Relaxes uterine muscle Decreases uterine ischemia
Lower back massage	Relaxes paravertebral muscles Increases pelvic blood supply
Effluerage (rhythmic rubbing)	Distraction and focal point
Exercise	Increases vasodilation Decreases ischemia Releases natural endorphins Decreases prostaglandins Decreases stress
Dietary changes: Decreased salt Increased water intake	Reduces fluid retention Natural diuretic

Source: Lowdermilk, D. L., & Perry, S. E. (2004). *Maternity & women's health care* (8th ed.). St. Louis: Mosby.

uterine fibroids. In contrast to primary dysmenorrhea, this discomfort is often characterized by dull, lower abdominal aching that radiates to the back and thighs, bloating, and pelvic fullness.

Management is directed at removing the underlying cause, often necessitating surgery to excise the displaced tissue or remove the fibroids. Pharmacologic pain-relief measures are the same as with primary dysmenorrhea. Nursing care is directed at education of the woman regarding the cause or treatment modalities. Patients should be advised to maintain a healthy diet and exercise level, take in plenty of fluids, and use heat and NSAIDs in moderation to help with symptoms. Patients who do not respond to simple measures should seek care to determine the possibility of secondary causes. Also patients should seek care for dysmenorrhea that occurs later in life, pain that occurs at other times besides the first couple of days of a period, any vaginal discharge, or abnormal bleeding between periods.

Etiology, Epidemiology, Pathophysiology, Clinical Manifestations, and Treatment of Menorrhagia

Menorrhagia is defined as excessive or prolonged menstruation. The menses of young women may vary from month to month, and a single heavy period is not necessarily cause for concern. However, high-volume periods that last more than 7 days are cause for concern. A woman who requires pad or tampon changes every 1 to 2 hours is considered to have menorrhagia. Menorrhagia can be caused by endometriosis, pelvic inflammatory disease, intrauterine devices for birth control, uterine fibroids, or functional ovarian cysts. Also women with hypothyroid conditions can have very heavy periods. Health care providers will also check for clotting disorders.

Treatment is dependent on the cause. Alternative contraceptive methods may be utilized if that is the cause. Fibroids may be surgically removed or shrunk through use of medications. Infections may indicate the need for antibiotic drug therapy. Assessment of the amount of bleeding is done through saturated pads or tampon counts. Hemoglobin analysis can be used to determine the extent of blood loss. Other pertinent laboratory values include a thyroid-stimulating hormone to determine the presence of a hypothyroid condition, and serum or urine HCG to test for pregnancy.

Etiology, Epidemiology, Pathophysiology, Clinical Manifestations, and Treatment of Metrorrhagia

Bleeding between menstrual periods is called **metrorrhagia**. A small amount of spotting may be seen around the time of ovulation and is considered normal. Use of low-dose oral contraceptives reduces the amount of hormones available in the body and is also associated with breakthrough bleeding. Pathologic causes of metrorrhagia include endometritis, STIs, pregnancy-related problems, ovarian cysts, or uterine fibroid tumors. Postmenopausal bleeding may be caused by uterine polyps, inappropriately prescribed hormone therapy, or uterine cancer. Early evaluation of this concern is extremely important. The hormone frequently in deficient status and causing metrorrhagia is progesterone, which is accompanied by a relative excess of estrogen. This results in hyperplasia of the endometrial lining of the uterus. Without adequate progesterone, sloughing of the lining occurs, resulting in vaginal bleeding that is not in accordance with the woman's monthly cycle. Hormone imbalances can be caused by anovulation, stress, and emotional upheavals. However, of utmost concern is that abnormal bleeding from the vagina, whether menorrhagia or metrorrhagia, can be an indicator of neoplasm and should be evaluated urgently.

Treatment is directed at the cause, such as drug therapy for endometritis and STIs; removal or shrinkage of cysts and fibroids; and surgery, drug, or chemotherapy/radiation for cancers. Pregnancy-related problems must be dealt with on an individual basis. Nursing care involves education regarding the causes of and treatments for metrorrhagia and addressing the fatigue associated with anemia and the relative dehydration.

Etiology, Epidemiology, Pathophysiology, Clinical Manifestations, and Treatment of Premenstrual Syndrome

Premenstrual syndrome (PMS) is a common, but complex, often misunderstood condition, involving physical, psychological, and behavioral symptoms. The Committee on Gynecologic Practice of the American College of Obstetricians and Gynecologists (ACOG) indicates that up to 80% of women of childbearing age have physical symptoms during menstruation: Twenty percent to forty percent have symptoms consistent with PMS; 2% to 4% indicate that their symptoms cause severe disruption of their daily activities (ACOG, 2005). These symptoms vary widely among women, so much so that it is difficult to define PMS. When present, the symptoms occur in the luteal phase, the time from ovulation until the start of the menstrual period of the cycle. Chart 49–8 shows the more common symptoms related to PMS, but symptoms can number 100 (Cronje & Studd, 2002). The diagnosis of PMS should meet specific criteria: symptoms occur in the luteal phase and resolve with menses; no symptoms occur during the follicular phase; and symptoms recur with repeated cycles (Lowdermilk & Perry, 2004).

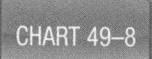

CHART 49–8 Symptoms Commonly Associated with Premenstrual Syndrome

Abdominal bloating

Lower extremity edema

Breast tenderness

Weight gain

Depression

Irritability

Loss of concentration

Food cravings/binges

Headache

Fatigue

Backache

Mood swings

Source: Cronje, W., & Studd, J. (2002). Premenstrual syndrome and premenstrual dysphoric disorder. *Primary Care, 29*(1), 1–12.

The etiology and pathophysiology of PMS is poorly understood. There is a biologic trigger that is exacerbated by psychosocial factors. Serotonin neurotransmitter is also considered to be a factor. It does appear there is a genetic or familial tendency associated with PMS. Additionally, estrogen and progesterone imbalances may play a role as well as nutritional deficiencies such as of vitamin B_6 and magnesium.

Management of PMS symptoms is difficult because of the diversity of symptoms in different women. Diet and exercise provide some relief for some women, along with the reduction of salt, sugar, and caffeinated beverages. The diet needs to be high in carbohydrates, limited in simple sugar, and limited in alcohol use to minimize hypoglycemia. Caffeine intake should be limited to decrease irritability. Women who exercise regularly appear to have fewer symptoms of anxiety and depression due to the increase in endorphin levels. Education is by far the most important part of management. The nurse can assist the woman in symptom evaluation, in cyclic relationships, and in counseling and support. Alternative and complimentary therapies have been found to help manage symptoms for some women. For example, the use of black cohosh root helps relieve anxiety and depression by suppressing estrogen, as presented in the Complementary and Alternative Therapies box (p. 1546). Bugleweed decreases prolactin levels and decreases breast discomfort (Lowdermilk & Perry, 2004). Medications may be used when other treatments fail to improve the PMS symptoms. Diuretics, prostaglandin inhibitors, which are the nonsteroidal anti-inflammatory drugs (NSAIDs), progesterone, and oral contraceptives have been shown to relieve symptoms. Fluoxetine (Prozac), 20 milligrams a day, is the only FDA-approved drug for PMS (Jones, 2001). See the Pharmacology Summary feature on p. 1552.

Etiology, Epidemiology, Pathophysiology, Clinical Manifestations, and Treatment of Premenstrual Dysphoric Disorder

Premenstrual dysphoric disorder (PMDD) is recognized as a separate syndrome, with similar, but more severe symptoms, often overwhelming the woman (Elliot, 2002). PMDD is a severe form of PMS that includes five or more symptoms of depression for most of the time during the last week of the luteal phase that begin to remit within a few days after onset of the follicular phase of the menstrual cycle (Bhatia & Bhatia, 2002). Symptoms include those of atypical severe depressive disorders (depressed mood, interpersonal rejection, hypersensitivity, carbohydrate craving, and hypersomnia). Women have depressed mood with feelings of hopelessness, anxiety, tension, and feelings of being "on edge." Many women describe marked anger or irritability and increased interpersonal conflicts. Friends and family notice decreased interest in usual activities and hypersomnia. Patients also complain of lethargy, easy fatigability, and marked lack of energy with changes in appetite and food cravings. Women with PMDD state they feel overwhelmed and out of control. Physical symptoms include breast tenderness and swelling, headaches, joint and muscle pain, and bloating.

There is a significant correlation between depression and PMDD; however, not all patients have depressive symptoms, so PMDD is not considered just a variant of depression. The etiology of PMDD is a combination of biologic, psychological, environmental, genetic, and social factors. Seventy percent of women whose mothers have been affected by PMS and PMDD have the disorders as well. Additionally, there is a 93% correlation rate in monozygotic twins compared with a rate of 44% in dizygotic twins (Bhatia & Bhatia, 2002). It is also reasonable to believe that PMDD has a hormonal basis because PMDD affects only women of childbearing age.

Treatment of PMDD must incorporate lifestyle changes, nutritional supplements, stress management, and pharmacologic interventions. Lifestyle changes include aerobic exercise and dietary changes that include small frequent balanced meals rich in complex carbohydrates, decreasing caffeine and sodium, restricting alcohol, and smoking. Nutritional supplements that are recommended include vitamin B_6, calcium carbonate, magnesium, and tryptophan. Nonpharmacologic treatments are also pertinent recommendations and include stress management, anger management, individual and couple's therapy, and patient education regarding the cause of, diagnosis of, and treatment for PMS and PMDD. Psychologists also recommend light therapy with 10,000 lux cool-white fluorescent light. Pharmacologic treatments include antidepressant and anxiolytic medications. Selective serotonin reuptake inhibitor (SSRI) antidepressants are considered first line. Fluoxetine 20 milligrams per day may be used during the luteal phase or throughout the full menstrual cycle (Bhatia & Bhatia, 2002). Alprazolam or another anxiolytic has also been shown to be effective in patients with PMS and PMDD. There is an issue with dependency on benzodiazepine-type medications, so this should be used for a short term only and only as a second line therapy if SSRIs fail. Hormonal therapies that are used are the gonadotropin-releasing hormone agonists; these suppress ovulation and cause amenorrhea, thereby providing significant relief of symptoms in those who do not also have significant depressive symptoms. These medications can cause symptoms of menopause such as hot flashes, vaginal dryness, and fatigue and irritability, so use is limited. Danazol is a weak androgen that is sometimes prescribed for women with endometriosis and fibrocystic breast disease. It is sometimes used to treat PMDD. Danazol can reduce symptoms, but has side effects of anovulation and masculinization. Gonadotropin-releasing hormone agonists and danazol have limited use due to the side effects and cost. See the Pharmacology Summary feature (p. 1552).

COMPLEMENTARY & ALTERNATIVE THERAPIES

Black Cohosh for Menopausal Symptoms

Description:

Many women seek complementary and alternative treatments as well as lifestyle modifications for their menopausal symptoms instead of using prescription HRT (Nachtigall et al., 2006). Black cohosh, in particular, is very commonly used as an herbal medicine for menopausal symptoms in both America and Europe over the past several decades. However, its bioactive components are still unknown (Jiang, Kronenberg, Balick, & Kennelly, 2006).

Research Support:

A review of randomized controlled trial evidence showed that black cohosh had a high level of support for treatment of menopausal symptoms (Dennehy, 2006). Another review of clinical trials showed that black cohosh significantly reduced menopause-related depression and anxiety in all studies reviewed (Geller & Studee, 2006).

A research team in the Czech Republic investigated a black cohosh extract to assess its effect on endometrial tissue of 400 postmenopausal women. Over the course of 52 weeks, participants received a daily dose of 40 mg of black cohosh extract. Results showed a lack of endometrial proliferation as well as improvement of menopausal complaints after the 1-year treatment period (Raus, Brucker, Gorkow, & Wuttke, 2006).

References

Dennehy, C.E. (2006, November–December). The use of herbs and dietary supplements in gynecology: An evidence-based review. *Journal of Midwifery and Womens Health,* 51(6), 402–409.

Geller, S. E., & Studee, L. (2006, December 28). Botanical and dietary supplements for mood and anxiety in menopausal women. *Menopause.* [Epub ahead of print]

Jiang, B., Kronenberg, F., Balick, M. J., & Kennelly, E. J. (2006). Analysis of formononetin from black cohosh (Actaea racemosa). *Phytomedicine,* 13(7), 477–486.

Nachtigall L., E., Baber, R. J., Barentsen, R., Durand, N., Panay, N., Pitkin, J., et al. (2006). Complementary and hormonal therapy for vasomotor symptom relief: A conservative clinical approach. *Journal of Obstetrics and Gynaecology Canada,* 28(4), 279–289.

Raus, K., Brucker, C., Gorkow, C., & Wuttke, W. (2006, July-August). First-time proof of endometrial safety of the special black cohosh extract (Actaea or Cimicifuga racemosa extract) CR BNO 1055. *Menopause,* 13(4), 678–691.

Nursing Management

Ideally all women should be screened for PMS and PMDD on a routine basis. Incorporate screening questions into a self-assessment that is routinely collected during intake. Much of the basic subjective data can be collected via a structured questionnaire. The following screening questions are effective:

- Do you ever have pelvic pain or cramps during or around the time of your period?
- Are you able to treat this pain so it does not bother you?
- Do you ever have other physical or mood discomforts during or around the time of your period?
- Are you able to treat these discomforts so they do not bother you?

Assessment of PMS and PMDD

Conduct a focused nursing assessment for women with PMS and PMDD for whom current treatments or self-care therapies are ineffective. An interview by a nurse can confirm self-report data as well as collect additional data. Start with a focused health history whenever possible to identify the individual woman's pattern of PMS or PMDD. The menstrual cycle may be divided into three phases: premenstrual, early menstrual (days 1 to 3 or days of heavy flow), and late menstrual (day 4 and onward or days of lighter flow).

The following areas should be assessed:

- Pattern of severity of PMS or PMDD across premenstrual and early menstrual phases
- Rating of overall distress caused by PMS or PMDD
- Pattern of severity of other cyclic discomforts across premenstrual and early menstrual phases
- Rating of overall distress caused by cyclic discomforts
- Influences on the cyclic pain symptoms; for example, work stress, diet, or exercise.

Identify the individual woman's pattern of symptom management by gathering the following information:

- Interventions, including self-care strategies
- Pattern of use across premenstrual and early menstrual phases
- Rating of relief obtained from intervention
- Rating of satisfaction with pain and symptom control
- Rating of adherence (i.e., consistent use of treatment).

Conduct a focused history and physical assessment using data from the history as a basis. The assessment data need to be organized into symptom patterns. Chart 49–9 provides a template for this organization.

Planning Expected Outcomes and Care for PMS and PMDD

Review assessment data together with the woman, and identify the outcomes important to the woman and amenable to nursing intervention. Expected outcomes for PMS and PMDD management may include the following:

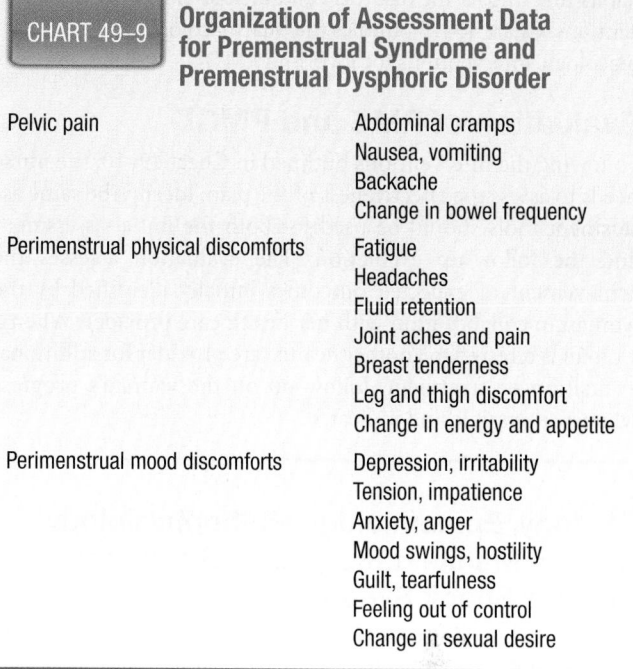

CHART 49–9   Organization of Assessment Data for Premenstrual Syndrome and Premenstrual Dysphoric Disorder

Pelvic pain	Abdominal cramps Nausea, vomiting Backache Change in bowel frequency
Perimenstrual physical discomforts	Fatigue Headaches Fluid retention Joint aches and pain Breast tenderness Leg and thigh discomfort Change in energy and appetite
Perimenstrual mood discomforts	Depression, irritability Tension, impatience Anxiety, anger Mood swings, hostility Guilt, tearfulness Feeling out of control Change in sexual desire

- Improvements in PMS and PMDD symptoms' frequency, severity, distress, and pattern
- Improvements in discomfort symptoms' frequency, severity, distress, and pattern
- Increased comfort level (physical and psychosocial well-being)
- Successful use of treatments to manage symptoms
- Relief of pain and discomfort
- Enhanced role performance (work, family, friends, school, leisure)
- Patient understanding of the cost of various forms of treatment.

Review symptom patterns and establish expected outcomes through mutual goal setting with the woman. Use the assessment as an opportunity to educate women about managing pain and discomfort. Develop an individualized treatment plan, incorporating the multimodal treatment strategies and participant involvement through personal choice whenever possible.

Interventions for PMS and PMDD

Because PMS and PMDD are a complex mixture of physiological and psychological clinical manifestations, is it essential to implement a comprehensive plan that focuses on symptom management interventions. This plan will provide the patient with the knowledge and interventions to manage the disorder. The nurse along with the patient must identify goals of care and explore ways to best achieve the goals. To enhance coping, the nurse must provide an atmosphere of acceptance and give factual information concerning diagnosis, treatment, and prognosis. Mutual goal setting is essential for the plan to be successful.

Keeping a log of when and what stressors increase the clinical manifestations will assist in identifying appropriate interventions. The patient needs to be instructed to self-monitor stressors and habits that impact the disorders and then identify effective interventions. Chart 49–10 outlines the pharmacologic and nonpharmacologic interventions for PMS and PMDD.

Evaluation of PMS and PMDD

Following the interventions outlined in Chart 49–10, the nurse needs to assess the effectiveness of the plan. Ideally, the same assessment tools should be used for both the initial assessment and the follow-up evaluation. The evaluation assesses the achievement of expected outcomes initially identified by the woman in collaboration with her health care provider. When a woman is referred to another health care provider for additional evaluation or treatment, follow up on the woman's progress whenever possible and indicated.

Etiology, Epidemiology, Pathophysiology, Clinical Manifestations, and Treatment of Toxic Shock Syndrome

Toxic shock syndrome (TSS) affects 1 to 2 women in every 100,000 in the United States, from 15 to 44 years of age (CDC,

2005a). It is caused by the *Staphylococcus aureus* (*S. aureus*) bacterium, which is thought to be found in tampons and intravaginal contraceptive devices. Although *S. aureus* is colonized commonly on skin surfaces, it can cause multisystem problems when it invades the body through a break in the skin. Symptoms of TSS include sudden onset of fever, chills, vomiting, diarrhea, intense muscle pain, and a diffuse red rash. Chart 49–11 outlines the signs and symptoms associated with TSS.

Toxic shock is an urgent condition that can rapidly progress to severe and intractable hypotension and multisystem dysfunction. Desquamation of the palms of the hands and the soles of the feet are later signs. This infection can lead to shock and kidney and liver failure (McKinley Health Center, 2002). Hospitalization is often recommended if there is a rapid progression of severe symptoms requiring intravenous fluids and antibiotics. Mortality rate will vary, depending on the organism involved. Although *S. aureus* is the primary organism involved, TSS has been associated with *Streptococcus pyogenes exotoxin*. The mortality rate with *S. aureus* is less than 3%, but with *S. pyogenes exotoxin* it is as high as 70% (Salandy & Brenner, 2002). Primary prevention techniques include avoiding the super plus tampons and/or changing them every 2 to 4 hours, and using the smallest size tampon that will ab-

---

CHART 49–10 **Interventions for Premenstrual Syndrome and Premenstrual Dysphoric Disorder**

Self-Monitoring Interventions

Tracking symptoms.
Tracking stressors, function, and health status.

Pharmacologic Symptom Management

Over-the-counter (OTC) pain medication:
- Nonsteroidal anti-inflammatory drugs (NSAIDs).
- Timing and strength of the medication are critical to pain relief.
- Take an adequate dose of medication at the first sign of pain or before bleeding occurs.
- Manufacturers' recommendations for OTC medications should not be exceeded.
- Read labels of other OTC medications taken concomitantly, particularly cold and sleep remedies.
- Be advised regarding appropriate duration of use because of the potential for gastrointestinal distress or other side effects.

Hormones:
- Combination estrogen–progestin oral contraceptives.
- Progesterone intrauterine device.

Nutritional supplements:
- Calcium: 1,200 mg/day (do not exceed 2,500 mg/day).
- Magnesium: 250 mg/day (do not exceed 500 mg/day).
- Essential fatty acids.
- Vitamin B complex: B_6 50–200 mg/day, B_1 100 mg/day.

Antidepressant medication:
- Refer to a mental health professional as indicated for symptoms of depression.

Topical/cutaneous symptom management:
- Heat application: heating pad, hot baths, disposable heat wraps.
- Therapeutic massage.
- Acupressure and acupuncture.
- Transcutaneous electrical nerve stimulation (TENS).

Behavioral/Cognitive Symptom Management

Behavioral relaxation:
- Breathing exercises.
- Stretching exercises.
- Progressive muscle relaxation.
- Autogenic training.

Cognitive relaxation:
- Thought-stopping strategies.
- Thought substitution.
- Decreased negative self-talk.
- Meditation.
- Mindfulness meditation.
- Guided imagery.
- Prayer.
- Affirmations.
- Biofeedback.
- Distraction.

Lifestyle Modifications as Indicated

General dietary modification:
- Decreasing intake of caffeine, simple sugars, and salt.
- Eating frequent, small meals.
- Increasing water and fluid intake to 6–8 glasses per day.
- Reducing alcohol intake.
- Increasing intake of foods that can decrease symptoms such as:
  Those that are rich in essential fatty acids
  Those that are rich in B complex vitamins
  Those that are rich in calcium and magnesium.
- Use a daily multivitamin and mineral supplement.
- Use a premenstrual syndrome formula vitamin and mineral supplement during premenses.
- Smoking cessation.
- Exercise. Encourage one or more of the following types of exercise as indicated and as can be tolerated:
  Regular aerobic exercise
  Nonaerobic exercise (e.g., yoga, t'ai chi, stretching/relaxation
  Exercise modification across the menstrual cycle.

Environmental modification interventions:
- Environmental stress management.
- Time management.
- Social support.

CHART 49–11   Signs and Symptoms of Toxic Shock Syndrome

Sudden high fever
Low blood pressure
Vomiting and/or diarrhea
A rash similar to a sunburn, found mostly on the palms of hands and soles of feet; may also see peeling of the skin on hands and feet
Confusion/delirium
Muscle aches
Redness of eyes, mouth, and throat
Seizures
Headache

sorb the menstrual flow without leakage for 2 to 4 hours. Once toxic shock has been diagnosed or suspected, the woman should avoid tampons altogether and use sanitary pads exclusively.

Diagnosis of TSS is based on fever, low blood pressure, rash that peels after 1 to 2 weeks, and at least 3 organs with signs of dysfunction. In some cases, blood cultures may be positive for growth of *S. aureus* (MedlinePlus Medical Encyclopedia, 2006b). Treatment includes intravenous fluids, vasopressors to control hypotension, antibiotics, and dialysis as needed for acute renal failure.

Patient education regarding toxic shock syndrome should include information regarding signs and symptoms and when the patient should seek care. Women should be advised that superabsorbent tampons that are left in place for too long become a breeding ground for bacteria and put young women at risk for toxic shock syndrome. Women should also be advised that using a diaphragm or contraceptive sponge can cause toxic shock syndrome. One can reduce chances of developing toxic shock syndrome by changing a tampon every 4 to 8 hours and using the lower absorbency tampon. It can also help to alternate using tampons and sanitary napkins whenever possible.

Etiology, Epidemiology, Pathophysiology, and Medical Management of Menopause

Menopause is the process by which the ovaries cease to function. The process can take 10 to 15 years as the regression of follicles within each ovary starts to accelerate after age 35. Symptoms begin as early as age 42 and end usually by age 58. More than 90% of women have ceased having periods by their early 50s. This process is accelerated by smoking. Once a woman has experienced 1 year of amenorrhea, she is considered postmenopausal. The average age of natural menopause is 51. A hysterectomy is referred to as surgical menopause. **Perimenopause** is the time during which periods may increase, decrease, and become irregular as the function of the ovaries waxes and wanes. As the ovaries become nonfunctional, the follicles cease to respond by producing estrogen. As the estrogen levels are depleted, a number of signs and symptoms appear. Irregular vaginal bleeding is common, and vasomotor symptoms manifest as hot flashes. Patients may experience vaginal drying and thinning of the mucosa, which causes atrophic vaginitis causing dyspareunia. The same mucosal changes occur in the bladder as well, causing a de-

crease in bladder capacity and loss of tone. These changes can cause dysuria and frequency even when no infection is present. This is often a somewhat difficult time for many women psychologically, as they experience emotional lability and changes in sleep patterns.

Health problems can become an issue at this time of life because the cardiovascular, musculoskeletal, and endocrine systems are affected. Cholesterol levels may begin to change, increasing the cardiovascular risks. The high density lipoproteins (good cholesterol) decrease and the low density lipoproteins (bad cholesterol) increase. The loss of estrogen, which begins a steady decline in bone density, puts the woman at risk for osteopenia, osteoporosis, and the potential for fractures.

The symptoms that the perimenopausal or menopausal woman may present should be considered carefully before determination of menopause. The possibility of thyroid dysfunction, anemia, and depression can present with many of the same symptoms. Laboratory tests that are valuable include an estrogen level and FSH level. The FSH (>35 international units per liter) is elevated and the estrogen level is decreased with menopause.

The most significant concern for the woman presenting with menopausal symptoms is how to manage her symptoms. Women have received volumes of conflicting information regarding hormone therapy during menopause. Most women know that hormone therapy provides relief from symptoms, but they also know that there are increased risks of breast cancer, stroke, heart disease, deep venous thrombosis, and pulmonary emboli. Thus, women are very conflicted about using hormone therapy to help with symptoms. If women want to consider taking hormone therapy for short-term treatment of menopausal symptoms, the risks and benefits should be explained fully. All options should be considered. Estrogen alone may be prescribed for the woman that has had her uterus removed. Estrogen and progesterone must be prescribed for the woman who still has a uterus. Unopposed estrogen causes hyperplasia of the endometrial lining and places the patient at risk for endometrial cancer. Progesterone has side effects that are problematic including increased appetite, weight gain, irritability, depression, headache, and breast tenderness. There are numerous preparations of hormone therapy, combination preparations with estrogen and progesterone, separate preparations and topical creams, gels, rings, and dermal patches. Vaginal creams are usually specific for atrophic vaginitis, but do not provide relief from vasomotor symptoms. One very important aspect of patient teaching for the woman considering hormone therapy is the high risk of fatal pulmonary emboli in the women who smoke and take hormone therapy.

Other therapies are available; for example, antidepressants can be used to help with situational depression that can accompany menopause. Fluoxetine, paroxetine, and venlafaxine are sometimes effective alternatives to hormone therapy in managing symptoms. Vasomotor symptoms can be relieved even if the patient is not depressed. Selective estrogen receptor modulators (SERMs) such as raloxifene can be used to prevent bone loss in patients at risk for osteoporosis. See the Pharmacology Summary feature (p. 1552).

Nonpharmacologic therapies can often be a better alternative for the woman with family history of endometrial, ovarian, or breast cancer. Managing the environment and reducing caffeine and alcohol can reduce the effects of vasomotor symptoms. Vitamin E (800 international units) may also help reduce vasomotor symptoms. Kegel exercises and lubricants can aid in vaginal dryness and associated dyspareunia. Well-balanced nutrition, exercise, and good sleep habits can decrease anxiety and depression and maintain a sense of well-being. Weight-bearing exercise also reduces the loss of bone density and prevents weight gain. Aerobic exercise helps the patient manage her weight and improves cardiovascular health. The patient who takes calcium supplements and maintains a diet high in complex carbohydrates and vitamin B complex will maintain optimal weight and minimize symptoms. The American Cancer Society recommends yearly exams after 40 to detect cancers. Health teaching should address alcohol and tobacco abuse, diet, and exercise.

Etiology, Epidemiology, Pathophysiology, and Medical Management of Infertility

Infertility is generally considered a viable diagnosis when a couple has been unable to achieve a pregnancy after 12 months of unprotected intercourse, and it affects about 10% of the reproductive population (American Society for Reproductive Medicine [ASRM], 2002). Primary infertility refers to a couple who has never been pregnant, whereas secondary infertility refers to a couple who has been pregnant in the past but has been unable to achieve another pregnancy. There are many religious and cultural considerations necessary when discussing infertility with couples. For instance, the Roman Catholic Church deems technical procedures such as *in vitro* fertilization, donor insemination, and the freezing of embryos as unacceptable. Protestant and Muslim groups support *in vitro* fertilization with the husband's sperm, and Christian Scientists support both husband and donor insemination (Lowdermilk & Perry, 2004). Many cultures blame the woman for fertility difficulties and sometimes believe her infertility is caused by her sins or due to evil spirits (D'Avanzo & Geissler, 2003).

Both male and female factors are involved with infertility. The American Society for Reproductive Medicine (2002) simplifies the statistics and states that one-third is male related, one-third is female related, and one-third is a combination or unexplained. In male infertility, the cause is most commonly related to a decreased sperm count, but could be related to retrograde ejaculation, impotence, hormone deficiency, a varicocele (distended testicular veins), or scarring from a sexually transmitted infection. Female-related causes are most commonly related to ovulatory dysfunction. Other causes may include hormone imbalance, ovarian cysts, or pelvic infections. Age has also been associated with fertility difficulties. The woman reaches peak fertility in her early 20s, and the likelihood of conceiving after age 35 or 40 is less than 10% per month (MedlinePlus Medical Encyclopedia, 2008). In addition to age-related factors, couples at risk for infertility involve those with multiple sexual partners, those with a sexually transmitted infection, endometriosis, men with a history of orchitis or a history of undescended testicles, past history of diethylstilbestrol (DES) exposure for both men and women, and those with chronic diseases such as diabetes or thyroid disorders.

Diagnosis is determined through a complete history and physical examination of both partners, and the reported inability of a couple to conceive after 1 year of unprotected intercourse. The year time frame is often decreased in older couples due to the premium time frame for conception. The Diagnostic Tests box presents the typical diagnostic tests for reproductive disorders.

Treatment for infertility must be directed at the cause. Sometimes all that is necessary is counseling regarding timing of intercourse. As much as 85% to 90% of couples can be treated with conventional methods that involve medications or surgical repair of reproductive organs (ASRM, 2002). Assisted reproductive therapies (ARTs), for example, *in vitro* fertilization, have brought hope and success to many infertile couples. These procedures are used less than 5% in the treatment of infertility (ASRM, 2002), in part because of the cost, which can run into the thousands of dollars. Chart 49–12 (p. 1553) outlines the assisted reproductive therapies available to infertile couples.

Etiology, Epidemiology, Pathophysiology, and Medical Management of Abortion

Abortion is defined as the ending of a pregnancy before what is thought to be the age of fetal viability. This age of viability is decreasing due to an increase in medical technology; it ranges from 22 to 24 weeks' gestation (Lowdermilk & Perry, 2004). Some literature even supports the age of viability as low as 20 weeks' gestation (MedlinePlus Medical Encyclopedia, 2006a). There are two types of abortions: spontaneous, the naturally occurring loss of the pregnancy, and elective or induced, the intentional termination of the pregnancy. A miscarriage is considered a "lay term" for spontaneous abortion.

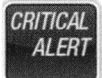 *Because of the negative connotation associated with the term abortion, when asking the patient about her pregnancy history, it might be beneficial to ask whether she has ever had a spontaneous loss or an elective loss of a pregnancy, rather than use the single term abortion or miscarriage. A patient may say yes to a miscarriage, but may not include the fact that she has also had an elective abortion, because the lay public often confuses the terms.*

Spontaneous abortion has four classifications: incomplete, complete, threatened, and inevitable (Chart 49–13, p. 1553). Not all symptoms will end in a spontaneous loss of the pregnancy. For example, only 30% of women with vaginal bleeding during the first trimester, with or without abdominal cramping, will have their pregnancy end in abortion (MedlinePlus Medical Encyclopedia, 2006a). When spontaneous abortion does occur, it is usually because the fetus has died, often due to chromosomal or developmental abnormalities (MedlinePlus Medical Encyclopedia, 2006a). Other causes of spontaneous abortion include maternal endocrine disease, such as thyroid or diabetes, or infection. It is thought that up to 50% of pregnancies may be spontaneously lost, most before the woman even realizes she is pregnant, and a 10% loss for known pregnancies (MedlinePlus Medical Encyclopedia, 2006a).

Symptoms of all types of spontaneous abortion include cramping and vaginal bleeding associated with a pregnancy, and they occur between what would be considered normal menstrual periods. Low back or abdominal pain, described as dull,

DIAGNOSTIC TESTS for Reproductive Disorders

Test	Expected Abnormality	Rationale for Abnormality
Herpes simplex virus (HSV)	Positive viral culture. Positive serologic test.	Indicates presence of HSV-1 or HSV-2.
Chlamydia	Positive culture.	Indicates presence of bacteria.
Syphilis	Venereal Disease Research Laboratories (VDRL): positive. Rapid plasma reagin (RPR): positive.	Indicates presence of serologic markers indicative of *Treponema*.
Gonorrhea	Positive culture.	Growth of *N. gonorrhoeae* bacteria from specimen.
Bacterial vaginosis	Positive vaginal culture.	Presence of *G. vaginalsis* from specimen.
Trichomoniasis	Microscopy positive for flagellates.	Indicative of presence of *Trichomonas* in specimen.
Vulvovaginal candidiasis	Microscopy positive for pseudohyphae. Positive culture of vaginal discharge.	Presence of *Candida* in specimen.
Human papillomavirus (HPV)	Nucleic acid probe positive for specific type of HPV. Liquid-based cytology with positive HPV finding. Carcinoma *in situ* noted from Pap smear.	Presence of genital warts, also known as HPV.
Mammogram	Positive for breast mass.	Suspicious for breast cancer. Mammography can detect 80–90% of breast cancers in women without symptoms. Requires biopsy for confirmation.
Breast cancer genes BRCA1 BRCA2	Positive for gene mutation.	Increases lifetime risk of developing breast cancer by 40–80%.
Transvaginal ultrasound Pelvic ultrasound	Positive for uterine mass, ectopic pregnancy, or ovarian cyst. Positive for fetal demise.	Determines size and location of masses and helps with the decision for or against surgery. Determines presence of ectopic pregnancy.
Urine human chorionic gonadotropin (HCG) Serum HCG Quantitative HCG	Positive: indicative of pregnancy. A quantitative HCG that doubles in 48 hours is indicative of pregnancy that is continuing. A quantitative HCG that fails to double in 48 hours is indicative of fetal demise.	Serum HCG is most accurate. Quantitative HCG is helpful in determining the length of pregnancy, and serial quantitative HCG tests are performed to determine the possibility of spontaneous abortion.
Blood culture	Positive for *S. aureus*.	Possible toxic shock syndrome.
Follicle-stimulating hormone	Greater than 35 international units per liter.	Indicative for menopause.
Semen analysis	2–3 days after complete abstinence.	Determines adequacy of volume, viscosity, sperm count, and motility.
Basal body temperature	Daily temperature of the woman before rising.	Determines ovulation if temperature rise of 0.5–1 degree is noted during the cycle.
Cervical mucus	Daily or every other day.	Notes cyclic changes in mucus to determine whether sperm can pass. Ideally needs thin, stretchy mucus for optimal sperm movement.
Serum progesterone	Late cycle (day 20–25).	Determines corpus luteum production of progesterone necessary for maintenance of a pregnancy.
Postcoital test	1–2 days before ovulation and 2–8 hours after intercourse.	Evaluates sperm motility in cervical mucus.
Commercial urine test for ovulation	Around the time of ovulation.	Determines luteinizing hormone, which is necessary for ovulation.
Hysterosalpingogram	Day 7–10 of cycle.	Assesses patency of uterine cavity and fallopian tubes.
Laparoscopy	Anytime.	Direct visualization of the pelvic cavity.

Sources: Adapted from Lowdermilk, D. L., & Perry, S. E. (2004). *Maternity & women's health care* (8th ed.). St. Louis: Mosby; MedlinePlus Medical Encyclopedia. (2008). *Infertility*. Retrieved February 28, 2008, from http://www.nlm.nih.gov/medlineplus/ency/article/001191.htm; and Mount Sinai Medical Center. (2008). *Reproductive endocrinology*. Accessed August 8, 2008, from http://www.mountsinai.org/Patient%20Care/Service%20Areas/Women/Procedures%20and%20Health%20Care%20Services/Reproductive%20Endocrinology

PHARMACOLOGY Summary of Medications to Treat Female Reproductive Disorders

Medication Category	Action	Application/Indication	Nursing Responsibility
Antibiotics: Azithromycin or erythromycin (Zithromax or ERY-C)	Disrupts cell wall synthesis of susceptible bacteria.	Chlamydia infection.	Large single dose given. Consider prevention for nausea. Take with food.
Doxycycline (Doryx)	Disrupts cell wall synthesis of susceptible bacteria.	Chlamydia infection.	Take with large glass of water. Not for patients under 18 years of age.
Penicillin G	Disrupts cell wall synthesis of susceptible bacteria.	Syphilis.	Intramuscular (IM) injection.
Metronidazole (Flagyl)	Disrupts cell wall synthesis of susceptible bacteria.	Trichomoniasis.	Caution patient not to drink alcohol while taking.
Clindamycin (Cleocin)	Disrupts cell wall synthesis of susceptible bacteria.	Bacterial vaginosis.	Can be given po or as vaginal ovules.
Nonsteroidal anti-inflammatory drug (NSAID): Ibuprofen (Motrin)	Cyclooxygenase-1 (COX-1) inhibitor with anti-inflammatory, analgesic, and antipyretic effects.	Premenstrual syndrome (PMS), premenstrual dysphoric disorder (PMDD), fibrocystic breast disease.	Caution patient to take with food to avoid stomach irritation.
Antineoplastic hormone antagonist: Tamoxifen (Nolvadex)	Nonsteroidal gonad-stimulating drug with potent antiestrogenic activity.	Palliative or adjunctive treatment for advanced breast cancer. Can reduce the recurrence or incidence of breast cancer in women at high risk.	Monitor white blood count for neutropenia.
Antiestrogen agents: Aromatase inhibitors Anastrozole (Arimidex) Letrozole (Femara)	Nonsteroidal competitive inhibitor of the enzyme system that converts androgens to estrogens.	Blocks estrogen production by other tissues in women who are postmenopausal.	Menopausal symptoms may increase.
Monoclonal antibody antineoplastic agent: Trastuzumab (Herceptin)	Recombinant DNA monoclonal antibody that selectively binds to the human epidermal growth factor to inhibit tumor growth.	Treatment of patients with metastatic breast cancer whose tumors express a protein known as HER2/neu.	Monitor for congestive heart failure. Not for use in patients with preexisting cardiac disease or dysfunction.
Antineoplastic antimetabolite: Methotrexate (Rheumatrex)	Antimetabolic and folic acid antagonist, thereby interfering with mitotic processes.	Nonsurgical treatment of ectopic pregnancy.	Generally one or two doses given. Most adverse effects are seen in long-term use such as with rheumatoid arthritis. Methotrexate will be excreted in breast milk.
Androgen: Danazol (Danocrine)	Mild androgenic effects that suppress follicle-stimulating hormone (FSH) and luteinizing hormone (LH).	Treatment of endometriosis and fibrocystic breast disease.	Monitor for masculinity effects, virilization, menstrual irregularities, and gastrointestinal (GI) distress.
Female hormones: Estrogen	Natural or synthetic steroid hormone secreted by the ovaries.	Treatment of menopausal symptoms from natural occurrence or surgical occurrence. Low doses can be used to control metrorrhagia.	Monitor for irregular vaginal bleeding and breast tenderness. Increased potential for deep venous thrombosis, especially if patient is a smoker.
Progesterone	Steroid hormone that opposes estrogen.	Prevents endometrial hyperplasia. Treatment for anovulation.	Monitor for dysfunctional or irregular vaginal bleeding.
Oral hypoglycemic: Metformin (Fortamet)	Increases binding to insulin receptor sites.	Lowers testosterone production in the patient with polycystic ovary syndrome.	Monitor for hypoglycemia and GI distress.
Antidepressants: Fluoxetine (Prozac) Paroxetine (Paxil) Venlafaxine (Effexor)	Selective serotonin reuptake inhibitor.	Approved for PMS and PMDD.	Avoid abrupt withdrawal of the medication. Avoid alcohol. Take in the morning to avoid insomnia.

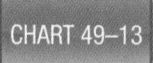 **Assisted Reproductive Therapies**

Reproductive Therapy	Indications	Procedure
In vitro fertilization (IVF) *In vitro* fertilization and embryo transfer (IVF-ET)	Blocked fallopian tubes; severe male infertility/sterility; cervix has an unfavorable environment due to acidic secretions. Shortens life span of sperm.	Ova retrieved from female and sperm from male; fertilization takes place in laboratory; fertilized eggs transferred a few days later to uterus in hopes of implantation (50% success rate for women under age 40).
Intrauterine insemination (IUI)	Severe male infertility/sterility; cervical hostile environment.	Husband or donor sperm are passed through a catheter into the uterus at the time of ovulation.
Intracytoplasmic sperm injection (ICSI)	Severe male infertility or failure to inseminate via IVF.	Harvest a single sperm and inject into ova and then inseminated via IVF.
Gamete intrafallopian transfer (GIFT)	Same as IVF but must have at least one tube patent.	Ova retrieved from ovary and fertilized in catheter with washed motile sperm; immediate transfer to fimbriated ends of fallopian tube.
Zygote intrafallopian transfer (ZIFT)	Same as GIFT.	Same as IVF but fertilized ova transferred to fallopian tube during zygote stage.

Sources: Adapted from Lowdermilk, D. L., & Perry, S. E. (2004). *Maternity & women's health care* (8th ed.). St. Louis: Mosby; and Mount Sinai Medical Center. (2008). *Reproductive endocrinology.* Accessed August 8, 2008, from http://www.mountsinai.org/Patient%20Care/Service%20Areas/Women/Procedures%20and%20Health%20Care%20Services/Reproductive%20Endocrinology

---

CHART 49–13   Classification of Spontaneous Abortions

Incomplete. Not all products of conception are expelled.

Complete. All productions of conception are expelled.

Threatened. Signs/symptoms of abortion are present and indicate the loss could happen.

Inevitable. Signs/symptoms of abortion cannot be stopped and the loss will eventually happen.

Symptoms of all types of abortion include vaginal bleeding with or without abdominal cramping.

Source: Lowdermilk, D. L., & Perry, S. E. (2004). *Maternity & women's health care* (8th ed.). St. Louis: Mosby.

---

sharp, or cramping, may be constant or intermittent. If tissue is passed, the abortion is usually considered inevitable. It is worth noting that up to 20% of all women experience some vaginal bleeding in the first trimester, but less than half of them experience an abortion (MedlinePlus Medical Encyclopedia, 2006a).

On examination, the cervix is often thin and dilated, and there may be evidence of rupture of the amniotic membranes. Human chorionic gonadotropin (HCG) levels will drop after a fetal death. Other laboratory tests that may be beneficial with a pregnancy loss include a complete blood count (CBC) to determine blood loss and a white blood count (WBC) to identify any infection. An ultrasound, transvaginal or abdominal, will assist with the diagnosis of fetal death and/or the presence of placental fragments that may have been retained in the uterus after a pregnancy loss.

Nothing can be done to treat an abortion that is inevitable, although there are palliative interventions that may help maintain the integrity of a pregnancy by providing a quiet uterine environment. These interventions include bed rest and abstaining from intercourse.

When an abortion occurs, it must be determined that all placental fragments and products of conception were fully expelled.

If not, a procedure called a dilation and curettage (D&C) may be performed to scrape the uterine lining clean of fragments. The amount of postprocedure uterine bleeding must be monitored. It is expected after a complete abortion or a D&C that the amount of bleeding is about the same as a normal menstrual period. Bleeding that continues longer, is heavier, or contains tissue fragments or any signs of infection, such as fever or foul-smelling vaginal discharge, should be reported to the health care provider. It is recommended to prevent another pregnancy for approximately the length of gestation of the current loss (i.e., if 8 weeks' gestation, then wait 8 weeks before attempting another pregnancy).

The second type of abortion is elective or induced. This may be done because of the desire of the woman to terminate the pregnancy due to not desiring a child or because of the results of fetal medical tests; for example, the potential for Down syndrome or a congenital illness such as hemophilia. The woman herself may have an illness that would put the fetus or herself at risk for harm, such as a serious heart condition, cancer, or advanced diabetes. When done for medical necessity, the term *therapeutic abortion* is often used. *Roe v. Wade* is the hallmark case in 1973 that legalized abortion in the United States for any reason before the 24th week of gestation. Third-trimester abortions may be performed only when the life or health of the mother is endangered by the pregnancy.

Induced abortions may be completed through the use of drugs or surgery. Surgical abortion methods include uterine evacuation, vacuum aspiration, dilation and curettage (D&C), and induced procedures. With uterine evacuation, a small cannula is inserted through the cervix. The products of conception are suctioned out of the uterus using a syringe during the 4th through 8th weeks of gestation. A vacuum aspiration is normally used from the 6th through the 14th week of gestation. The cervix is dilated and a cannula is inserted into the uterus. This canula is attached to a vacuum device that will remove the products of conception. Uterine evacuation and vacuum aspiration are procedures often done in an office setting. A D&C can be performed between the 6th and 16th weeks of gestation. The procedure involves dilating the cervix and scraping the lining of the uterus with a curette to remove the contents. A variation of this procedure is a D&E, dilation and evacuation, which is more difficult but can be done up to the 24th week of gestation. An induced abortion is the usual procedure between the 16th and 24th weeks of gestation. To perform an induced abortion, a small amount of amniotic fluid is replaced with a prostaglandin or pitocin solution. Approximately 24 to 48 hours later, the uterus will begin to contract and expel the fetus. The D&C, D&E, and induced abortion are done under general anesthesia.

Complications of any abortion procedure include bleeding, infection, cervical or uterine tear, retained products of conception, or even missed abortion whereby the pregnancy continues. Along with these physical complications, the woman may experience emotional upset surrounding the circumstances, which may require counseling to come to terms with the decision or necessity of the abortion. Nursing care involves education on complications, referral as needed, and emotional support.

◼ Diagnostic and Surgical Procedures

There are several surgical procedures specific to women's health. These include exploratory laparoscopy, colposcopy, bladder suspension, and hysterectomy. An exploratory laparoscopy is a minimally invasive procedure that involves a small incision through which a laparoscope is inserted that allows visualization of the internal organs and structures to assess for disease processes. Carbon dioxide is instilled into the abdomen to elevate the abdominal wall and create a larger work area. After the procedure, the incision is sutured to secure the edges for healing. The patient may experience shoulder pain as the carbon dioxide dissipates from the abdomen. Instruct the patient to sit up and walk to promote gas diffusion and reduce pain. The nurse should be careful to assess the following:

- Incisions and any drainage
- Vital signs, bowel sounds
- Nutrition.

A **colposcopy** is a test to evaluate the cells of the cervix. The cervix is visualized with the use of a bright light and magnification, in order to see abnormal cells. Biopsies of unusual cells can be taken at precise spots. The procedure can be done in an office setting. The patient is encouraged to take ibuprofen or extra strength Tylenol shortly before the procedure to help control the pain of the procedure. It is important to remind the patient not to insert anything into the vagina, including not having intercourse, for 24 to 48 hours before the procedure. Spermicides, tampons, and semen can interfere with test results. Risks and complications are rare but can include slight spotting to heavy bleeding after the procedure. The patient should be taught signs and symptoms of infection and that she should report any pelvic or abdominal pain.

A **bladder suspension**, or Burch procedure, is done to suspend the bladder and correct urinary incontinence. During childbirth, the bladder ligaments are sometimes weakened and cause the bladder to sink in the pelvic cavity, causing leakage of urine, or incontinence. This is a common complaint of women typically over 40 years of age that have given birth to one or more children. The bladder suspension can be done using an abdominal incision, or it can be done utilizing a laparoscope, which lessens the length of hospitalization. As with any surgery, bleeding is a complication that needs assessing, and the patient is instructed that normal bladder function often does not return for up to 2 months. Specific discharge instructions for a bladder suspension that the nurse should carefully review with the patient are outlined in the Patient Teaching & Discharge Priorities box.

Hysterectomy

Hysterectomy is a surgical procedure to remove the uterus. Approximately 600,000 hysterectomies are performed each year in the United States (CDC, 2008h). The surgery can be done as a total abdominal hysterectomy removing the uterus, ovaries, and fallopian tubes, or as a vaginal hysterectomy in which the uterus is removed through the vagina. Hysterectomies are performed for four conditions primarily: uterine fibroids (leiomyoma, myoma), endometriosis, cancer, and uterine prolapse. Other reasons necessitating a hysterectomy include severe, chronic pelvic pain; long-term, chronic vaginal bleeding; or cancers involving the cervix, ovaries, or uterus.

A hysterectomy involves removal of the uterus, which can be done in one of three ways: through an abdominal incision, through the vagina, or through laparoscopic incisions in the abdomen. The reason for the removal will determine which procedure to use and whether other organs besides the uterus are to be removed. A partial hysterectomy is the removal of the upper portion of the uterus, leaving the cervix intact. A total hysterectomy involves removal of the entire uterus and the cervix. A radical hysterectomy is the removal of the uterus, the cervix, and the upper part of the vagina. The procedure chosen will depend on the extent of the pathology necessitating the surgery. For example, uterine fibroids may require only a partial hysterectomy, whereas extensive cancer could require a total or radical hysterectomy.

Nursing care for the woman having a hysterectomy includes addressing the following nursing diagnoses:

Anxiety related to fear of surgery and related diagnosis

Risk for Infection related to surgical procedure

Readiness for Enhanced Fluid Balance from electrolyte imbalance related to urinary retention

Potential for *Altered Tissue Perfusion* related to hemorrhage

Potential for *Altered Tissue Perfusion* related to deep venous thrombosis

Deficient Knowledge related to surgical procedure and risks and benefits

Acute Pain related to incision

Fatigue related to blood loss

Disturbed Body Image related to perceived loss of femininity.

Risks associated with hysterectomy are the same as those related to any major abdominal surgical procedure including reactions to medications, bleeding, infection, and bladder and bowel injury. Recovery is fastest with the vaginal or laparoscopic procedure, and the patient may experience less pain. The patient usually has a urinary catheter for 1 to 2 days while hospitalized,

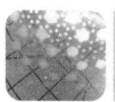

PATIENT TEACHING & DISCHARGE PRIORITIES for a Bladder Suspension

Need	Teaching
Analgesics	Take analgesics as prescribed.
Patient	Encourage patient to take analgesics as prescribed.
Family/support system	Advise patient to report to health care provider if analgesics are inadequate.
Activity	Avoid lifting, straining, driving, or other strenuous activity for 2–4 weeks.
Patient	Assist patient as needed to allow adequate rest and avoidance of strenuous activity.
Family/support system	
Diet	Regular, well-balanced diet as soon as desired.
Patient	Avoid spicy foods, caffeine, and alcohol, as they may irritate the bladder during healing.
Family/support system	Encourage a healthy diet.
Bladder/catheter care	Urinate regularly and use self-catheterization as taught (as often as after each void until residual amount is less than 100 milliliters).
Patient	
Family/support system	Assist patient as needed.

Sources: University of Maryland Medical Center. (2004). *Anterior vaginal wall repair.* Retrieved February 27, 2008, from http://www.umm.edu/ency/article/003982.htm

and some health care providers order injectable heparin for those at higher risk for blood clots. Ambulation is essential as soon as feasible, and a regular diet is encouraged after bowel function returns. Discharge instructions should include no heavy lifting, regular diet, rest, and nothing in the vagina, including intercourse, until released by the health care provider in 6 to 8 weeks. Menopause is immediate for women who also have their ovaries removed during the hysterectomy, and estrogen replacement therapy should be discussed with the patient.

The Maryland Women's Health Study and the Maine Women's Health Study were large, prospective studies designed to measure outcomes of hysterectomy for benign conditions. These studies demonstrated that hysterectomy substantially improves symptoms and quality of life in women with multiple and severe symptoms associated with gynecologic disorders. Medical therapy for abnormal bleeding and chronic pelvic pain produced significant improvements, but one-quarter of the nonsurgical group subsequently underwent hysterectomy (Kjerulff et al., 2000).

Salpingo-oophorectomy is the procedure whereby the fallopian tubes and ovaries are removed. Removal of just the fallopian tube is a salpingectomy. Oophorectomy is the removal of just the ovary. These can be unilateral or bilateral depending on the pathology that requires the procedure. These surgeries are done for ectopic pregnancy, ovarian cysts, or cancers of the ovary. In the case of cancer of the endometrium or ovaries that is spreading, the salpingo-oophorectomy may be done in conjunction with a total abdominal hysterectomy and the procedure may be abbreviated as TAH-BSO (total abdominal hysterectomy and bilateral salpingo-oophorectomy). A procedure such as this creates surgical menopause. The symptoms can be more intense than the gradual menopause that occurs naturally. The patient may be treated for these symptoms with a variety of estrogen replacements if the surgery is not done for cancer. Remember that estrogen is generally not given to women with reproductive cancer because many of these types of cancer are estrogen dependent. The care of these patients is very similar to that of the patient with a hysterectomy.

Mammoplasty

Cosmetic and reconstructive surgery on the breast is performed to increase or decrease its size, to lift the breast tissue, or for replacement after mastectomy. Augmentation or enlargement of the breast is generally done for cosmetic purposes. Breast reduction is often done for functional reasons because large breasts can cause back and shoulder pain and contribute to poor posture, possibly allowing this surgery to be covered financially by insurance. A mastopexy is a surgical procedure performed to improve drooping (ptotic) breasts. Breast reconstruction following mastectomy also is possible and is usually covered by insurance.

Breast Augmentation

Augmentation of the breast involves the implantation of a manufactured silicone shell implant filled with either silicone gel or saline, or, in some cases, a double lumen implant consisting of each of these substances. The implants are placed in a surgically created pocket either subglandular (beneath the breast tissue but in front of the muscle fascia) or submuscular (under the pectoralis muscle and sometimes the serratus anterior and upper part of the rectus abdominus muscles). The surgery is typically done on an outpatient basis either under local anesthesia and conscious sedation or under general anesthesia. Surgical incisions are made in one of four areas: around the periareolar margin; in or just above the inframammary fold; in the axilla; or in and around the umbilicus. Figure 49–10 ■ (p. 1556) shows a patient both before and after an augmentation mammoplasty.

Complications are rare and include hypertrophic scars, hematoma formation, infection, deflation or rupture of the implant, asymmetry of the breasts, temporary or permanent loss of sensation, and contracture of scar tissue. Formation of scar tissue around the implant is normal to "wall it off" as a foreign body. However, the scar tissue can sometimes thicken and contract, making a smaller pocket, which can then lead to breast firmness referred to as capsule contracture. The cause of this condition is usually unknown, but the incidence is thought to be increased by hematoma and seroma formation,

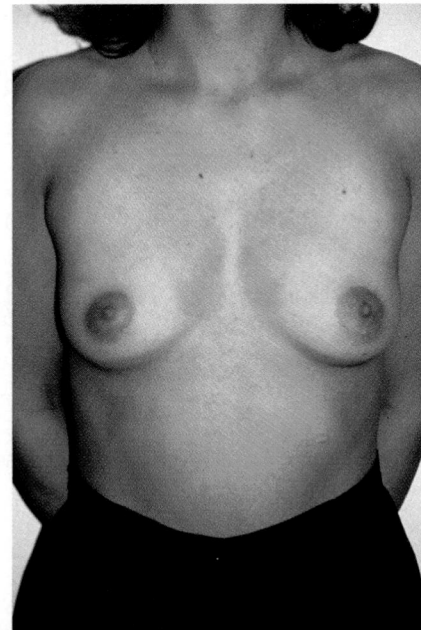

(a)

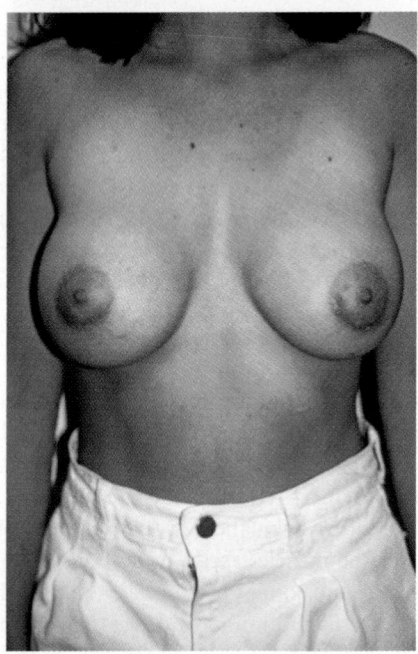

(b)

FIGURE 49–10 ■ Breast augment (A) before and (B) after.
Source: Custom Medical Stock Photo, Inc.

or subclinical infections. Treatment is usually surgical, incising the scar to allow the surrounding tissues to expand and create a larger pocket, thus, allowing the implants to feel softer and drape more naturally. Recently the Erchonia laser is being used to soften the capsules, resulting in a more natural feel and appearance of the breasts. The long-term effects of laser use are yet to be determined, and the results are variable among patients. Women with breast augmentation have the same incidence of developing a malignancy as those without implants and therefore should continue to do regular breast self-examination and mammograms (American Cancer Society, 2007).

Silicone is used to make breast implants because it is the least reactive substance placed in the body and is not rejected, as most

foreign bodies are. For this reason, it is also used for facial, testicular, penile, and joint implants. It is used for shunts, pacemakers, and as a coating to lubricate needles and syringes. However, in 1990, concerns were raised about the safety of the breast implants and the possibility that they might be contributing to many of the immunologic diseases that usually occur in women, such as chronic fatigue syndrome, fibromyalgia, lupus, scleroderma, and so forth. In 1992, the FDA restricted the use of the gel-filled implants only to women undergoing breast reconstruction following mastectomy for cancer, to those having replacement of previously placed gel implants, or to those undergoing augmentation with a mastopexy at the same time. Women undergoing augmentation only were restricted to using saline-filled implants. This restriction was lifted in 2006, 14 years later, after the FDA became reassured that there did not seem to be confirmation of these concerns either scientifically or statistically.

Breast Reduction

Breast reduction is usually done for complaints of pain and discomfort related to large breasts but can be done for cosmetic reasons as well. Breast reduction relieves pain in the back, neck, and shoulder; increases the patient's feelings of self-worth; and potentially decreases anxiety and depression (Iwuagwu et al., 2006). Breast reduction is a surgical procedure in which breast tissue and skin are removed from the center and lower parts of the breast. Usually the nipple and areolar complex are relocated superiorly, keeping the complex attached to the subcuticular breast tissues to retain circulation and sensation. In women with very large breasts, it may be necessary to remove the nipple and areolar complex completely during the procedure and relocate the complex as a full thickness skin graft after the breast tissue and skin have been removed and the remaining breast tissue and skin sculpted to give a natural-looking breast appearance.

Breast reduction also can be performed using liposuction if much of the breast is made up of fat cells. Liposuction may or may not use ultrasonic energy to emulsify fat cells. This technique removes a significant volume of breast fat, and in younger patients with good elasticity, it lifts the breast while leaving minimal scarring. Liposuction for breast reduction is not indicated for older women or for women with very large breasts.

Breast reduction is usually done under general anesthesia and, depending on the patient's age and condition, can be done as either an outpatient or an inpatient. Complications include blood loss, infection, hematoma, asymmetry of breasts, loss of sensation, and hypertrophic scarring. In childbearing women, this surgical procedure may result in the inability to breast-feed. The scar from this procedure extends around the areola and straight down from the center of the inferior portion of the areola to the inframammary fold. Sometimes there is also a scar across the inframammary fold. Women tend to be extremely satisfied with the results because of the increased comfort and appearance.

Mastopexy

Mastoplexy is a surgical procedure performed in women who have nursed, have lost weight, or have breasts that have settled due to the aging process. This procedure lifts the nipple and areolar complex superiorly, excises excess skin, and reshapes the remaining skin without removing breast tissue. An implant may be inserted during a mastopexy to improve breast fullness and give a more natural shape. This procedure does have some degree of visible scarring.

Breast Reconstruction

There are several approaches for reconstructing the breast following a mastectomy. The goal of breast reconstruction is to create a mound that creates a normal appearance in a bra or a bathing suit and improves the woman's self-image. It also is possible to re-create a pigmented circle with a mound in the center that looks like a normal nipple and areola in thin clothing. It is not possible to restore the normal breast function of lactation or nipple sensation or erectility. The process of reconstructing the breast can begin immediately when the mastectomy is being performed, or it can be delayed and begun in a separate surgery later. The timing is based on patient and surgeon preference, along with the possible need for chemotherapy and/or radiation.

Symmetry of the breasts is usually easier to achieve when doing bilateral reconstruction. No matter which technique is used, it is sometimes difficult to match a normal side that is too large, ptotic, or has had other changes associated with the aging process. Sometimes a mastopexy, augmentation, or reduction is

done on the normal side for symmetry. In some states the law mandates that both breasts' procedures be covered by the patient's insurance carrier.

Tissue Expanders and Implant Reconstruction

Breast reconstruction using an implant is usually a multistep process. It begins after the mastectomy with the placement of a tissue expander under the skin and pectoral, serratus anterior, and rectus abdominus muscles in order to stretch the muscle and skin and create a pocket for subsequent placement of an implant. The tissue expander is minimally inflated on insertion and gradually filled with weekly injections of saline inserted into a self-sealing valve in the expander. This facilitates a gradual expansion of skin and muscle tissue until the desired breast size is reached (Figure 49–11 ■). Once the size is reached, the expander is surgically removed and a permanent implant is inserted. Although not commonly used, some expanders are designed also to be the permanent implant, thereby eliminating the need for a second surgery.

Tissue Transfer Reconstruction

It is possible to use the patient's own tissue to reconstruct the breast by using tissue transferred from other areas of the body. The three types of tissue transfers include the latissimus dorsi muscle of the back, the transverse rectus abdommis muscle (TRAM) of the lower abdomen, and the microvascular free flaps from the lower abdomen or buttocks. The placement of this tissue will replace skin and breast tissue removed during the mastectomy.

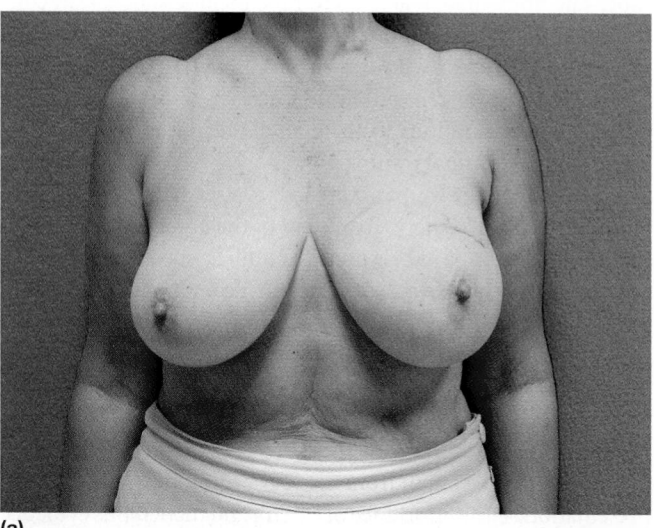
(a)

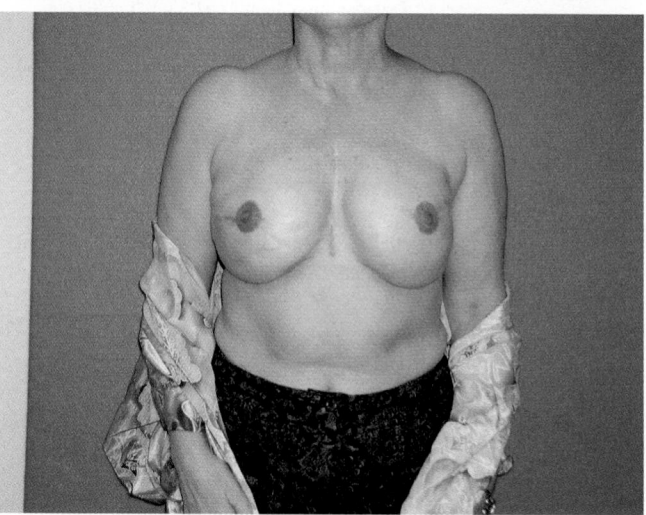
(b)

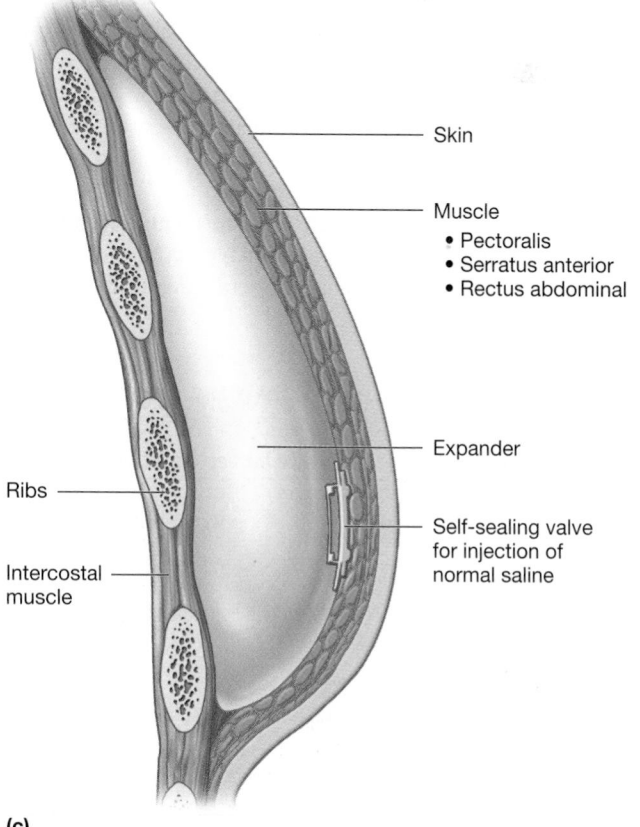
(c)

FIGURE 49–11 ■   Tissue expander (C) and breast reconstruction photos (A) before, (B) after.
Source: (a) and (b): Kathleen Osborn

A latissimus dorsi flap consists of a skin island attached to the latissimus dorsi muscle, which gets its blood supply from axillary vessels to which it is attached. Usually an implant is inserted beneath muscle to augment the volume when a latissimus dorsi flap is used.

A TRAM flap consists of skin from the lower abdomen left attached to the rectus abdominus muscle for its blood supply that is then tunneled up under the remaining abdominal skin and carefully inserted and sculpted into the deficient breast area to create a mound that resembles a breast. If there is sufficient abdominal tissue, this technique can be used to reconstruct both breasts at the same time, splitting the skin in the center and leaving each half attached to its respective rectus muscle. The main trade-off for this procedure is that it does weaken the abdominal musculature. Implants may or may not be used with a TRAM flap, depending on the amount of fatty tissue available, the patient's preference for size, and the amount of volume required for symmetry.

Some patients may be better candidates for a microvascular free flap reconstruction in which skin and fat are taken from either the abdomen or the buttock, along with their vascular supply, which are then sutured using microvascular techniques to the surrounding recipient vessels for circulation. Patients who smoke, patients with diabetes, and patients with some previous abdominal scars may not be good candidates for this procedure, because of the already compromised vascular supply to the skin and muscle.

Nipple-Areolar Reconstruction

Once the mound is reconstructed, there are several methods for reconstructing the nipple and areolar complex. The techniques used involve various combinations of local flaps, skin grafts, and sometimes tissue from the nipple on the normal side, if it is of adequate size. After the nipple and areola have been reconstructed, the final step is to use micropigmentation (tattooing) to darken the area to match the contralateral breast for unilateral reconstruction. This completes the reconstruction and helps to make women feel "whole" again.

Complications of breast reconstruction include wound infection, hematoma, dehiscence, asymmetry, rupture of the expander or implant, and capsule contracture. Wound infection

may occur especially if the woman is immunosuppressed due the cancer itself and/or is under treatment with chemotherapy. Capsule contracture was discussed earlier in this chapter. Previous radiation may result in various degrees of fibrosis of the skin and muscle and may make expansion more difficult.

Papanicolaou (Pap) Smears

Annual Papanicolaou (Pap) smears are highly successful in diagnosing early cancer of the cervix (NCI, 2007). The National Cervical Cancer Coalition (2005) recommends women begin Pap smears 3 years after becoming sexually active or by age 21. There are two primary classification systems in use, the cervical intraepithelial neoplasia (CIN) and the Bethesda systems. A comparison of these systems will help with understanding of Pap smear results (Chart 49–14).

■ Interpersonal Violence

Sexual assault is an act of violence. It is defined as the forcible perpetration of a sexual act on a person without his or her consent. According to the National Violence Against Women Survey (2005), 1 in 6 women will be the victim of rape or attempted rape. The immediate reactions to rape include shock, fear, confusion, and disbelief. Some who have been raped may deny the incident occurred or withdraw from rescuers. Those who have been raped may sustain physical injuries as well, which include bruising and lacerations to the genital area, head and neck injuries, and abdominal trauma.

Initial care of the woman who has been sexually assaulted centers on the person's safety. Treatment of the urgent and emergent injuries and emotional responses requires specifically trained professionals who have experience in dealing with those who have been sexually assaulted and can provide not only the crisis intervention that makes a difference at the time of the incident but also the continuing care over the course of her recovery. Readily available rape advocates, specially trained law enforcement personnel, and sexual assault nurse examiners (SANEs) should be involved with the patient from the very beginning of the patient's presentation. The importance of careful and meticulous evidence collection is the second priority after assuring the patient's safety

---

CHART 49–14	Classification of PAP SMEARS (CIN Versus Bethesda System)

Description	Cervical Intraepithelial Neoplasia (CIN Grading)	Bethesda System (2001)
Normal	Normal	Normal
Atypia	Atypia	Atypical squamous cells of undetermined significance (ASCUS)
Human papillomavirus (HPV)	HPV	Low-grade squamous intraepithelial lesion (SIL)
Atypia with HPV	Atypia (condylomatous atypia)	Low-grade SIL
Mild dysplasia	CIN I	Low-grade SIL
Moderate dysplasia	CIN II	High-grade SIL
Severe dysplasia	CIN III	High-grade SIL
Carcinoma *in situ*	CIS	High-grade SIL
Invasive cancer	Invasive cancer	Invasive cancer

Source: National Cervical Cancer Coalition. (2005). *Cervical cancer.* Retrieved February 28, 2008, from http://www.nccc-online.org/patient_info/cervical_cancer.html

and treatment of injuries. Sexual assault nurse examiners are specially trained to collect this evidence according to the protocol of the local jurisdiction. Sexual assault exams are for the express purpose of collecting evidence and have no bearing on the patient's medical care. The victim of a sexual assault must consent to the collection of evidence in total or in part. The process is laborious and time consuming, and many who have been victimized become exhausted and frustrated with the process without the appropriate support from the rape advocate and the sexual assault examiner. The evidence that should be collected and usually included in local protocols includes a history of the assault, collection of seminal fluid and possible sperm, combing pubic hair for foreign hair and matter, fingernail scrapings, collecting the patient's blood for typing and DNA screening, collecting torn or stained clothing, taking photographs of the injuries, and creating an accurate body map of the injuries. The handling of evidence is critical, and therefore, the sexual assault nurse examiner carefully labels all evidence and seals it for transfer to law enforcement. This is referred to as "creating a chain of evidence," which is critical to maintaining the integrity of the evidence. No unnecessary personnel should be involved in handling evidence.

Assessment findings of the victim of rape may be unpredictable. Emotionally, some victims of rape may be extraordinarily calm and controlled. Others may be hysterical and difficult to calm. Many cry uncontrollably and express anger and fear; others may be silent and withdrawn. Physical findings include oral, vaginal, and rectal injuries, bruises to the neck and arms, head injuries, and multiple scrapes and cuts. One of the most important findings in a woman who has been raped is a slight tear to the posterior fourchette of the vaginal opening. This small physical indication is frequently an indication of forced penetration. Many victims of rape show very few or no injuries because they cooperate with their attacker out of fear for their life. All these women should be monitored carefully during evidence collection for delayed response to the assault. Decreasing level of consciousness or changes in vital signs will require that evidence collection be halted and the patient be assessed for occult injuries. Most evidence collection protocols include toxicology and blood alcohol levels to determine whether the person who was raped was under the influence of drugs or alcohol, which may have impacted her ability to fight off her attacker. Screening for sexually transmitted infections is also part of the exam, and prophylactic treatment with antibiotics is offered to the patient. Additionally, the patient is offered emergency contraception. Victims of sexual assault should never be allowed to leave the hospital alone after treatment. Rape advocates should be available to ensure the patient's safety once released from the hospital. A safe house, family member's home, or women's shelter may be possible options for the patient.

Nurses can help prevent sexual assaults by educating young women about self-defense and avoiding risky situations. Encouragement of patients to participate in self-defense classes can improve situational awareness and confidence. Female patients should also be encouraged to practice safe habits in lighting entrances to home, locking doors, and avoiding opening doors to strangers. Women patients should protect their identification as a single occupant in phone books, in mailbox listings, and on answering machines. Remind patients of the dangers of walking in deserted areas especially after dark. Encourage patients to pay attention to suspicious behaviors and avoid being alone in offices or elevators with unknown persons. In social situations, patients should avoid becoming intoxicated or accepting mixed drinks from casual acquaintances. All women should proceed very cautiously with online correspondence. Providing resources to female patients for obtaining whistles or pepper spray and encouraging them to keep it accessible will add to the general safety of women.

Many communities have rape crisis centers or phone lines that are staffed 24 hours a day. The programs provide counseling and advocacy and ensure appropriate treatment during medical and legal procedures. Victim financial assistance can be arranged to offset lost time from work and added expenses for medical care, psychological counseling, transportation, and housing. In 2002 the Association for Genitourinary Medicine established national guidelines for the treatment of adult victims of sexual assault, which are outlined in the National Guidelines box (p. 1560). Recent research that improves practice is discussed in the Evidence-Based Practice feature (p. 1561).

Gerontological Considerations

As women age, they are more prone to some conditions and less prone to others. In general, the geriatric population is rapidly growing, and health issues need to be addressed by the health care providers. Information on the effects of aging on the female population is widely available. For example, much information exists on menopause and the effects it has on sexual desire and sexual response. There is a plethora of information on breast cancer and the need for screening mammography, even in the aging population. The National Institute on Aging provides information on many topics, including women's health issues.

Research

Research on women's health issues has been in the forefront for many years. Both the Office of Research on Women's Health and the National Institute on Aging are involved in research on menopause, fibroids, and cancer, to name only a few topics. The Research Opportunities and Clinical Impact box (p. 1561) outlines potential research topics related to female reproductive disorders and trends in the care of women.

NATIONAL GUIDELINES for the Management of Adult Victims of Sexual Assault

Ensure local law enforcement is aware of patient.

Forensic exam is useful up to 7 days postassault.

The orifices used in the assault, the timing of the assault, prior and subsequent consenting sexual intercourse, use of condoms by the assailant, and whether or not ejaculation had occurred should be documented.

Signed consent is essential if any information is subsequently disclosed to the police. This should be with the understanding that the court may order disclosure of all information divulged during the legal proceedings.

Injuries requiring immediate attention will take precedence over any other examination.

If the assault is recent, accurately document injuries found on the genital inspection. Petechial hemorrhages on the palate should be sought with a history of forced oral penetration. Anal examination including proctoscopy should be performed if there is a recent history of forced anal penetration, noting any trauma.

A full screening for sexually transmitted infections at presentation is recommended.

Exam should include cultures for *Neisseria gonorrhoeae* and tests for *Chlamydia trachomatis* from any sites of penetration or attempted penetration.

Vaginal slides for microscopy and yeasts, bacterial vaginosis, and *Trichomonas vaginalis*.

Blood should be drawn for syphilis serology.

Hepatitis B, HIV, and hepatitis C testing should be offered.

Sexually transmitted infection (STI) prophylaxis:
    Ciprofloxacin 500 milligrams immediately, doxycycline 100 milligrams twice daily bid for 7 days, or
    ciprofloxacin 500 milligrams immediately and azithromycin 1 gram immediately.
    Hepatitis B vaccination should be offered if the patient has not received it previously.
    A discussion about HIV infection should be part of the interview with the patient and follow-up testing and counseling. The patient can be offered
        postexposure prophylaxis in line with the postexposure prophylaxis guidelines for occupational exposure. This should be started within 72 hours
        after a high-risk exposure.

Pregnancy prevention:
    Postcoital oral contraception can be issued if within 72 hours of the assault and no risk of preexisting pregnancy.
    Levonorgestrel 0.75 milligram for 2 doses 12 hours apart.

Counseling:
    Post-traumatic stress disorder is common following sexual assault; however, there is no evidence that brief psychological debriefing reduces this.
    Links with local victim support organization, rape crisis groups, and local psychologist should be present to facilitate referral if needed.
    As psychological sequelae may develop months or years later, communication with the general health care provider to ensure continuity of care
        should be encouraged.

Source: Andrews, R. T., Spies, J. B., Sacks, D., Worthington-Kirsch, R. L., Niedzwiecki, G. A., Marx, M. V., et al. (2002). *National guidelines on the management of adult victims of sexual assault.* London: Association for Genitourinary Medicine (AGUM), Medical Society for the Study of Venereal Disease.

Sexual Assault Nurse Examiners (SANE)

Clinical Problem

Care of individuals who have been a victim of sexual assault is complex and multifaceted. There are obvious emotional needs along with physical as well as legal issues. Research is need to evaluate the most effective approach to ensure a comprehensive plan is in place. These researchers evaluated the use of sexual assault nurse examiners (SANEs) as opposed to staff nurses and health care providers.

Research Findings

Plichta, Clements, and Houseman (2007) conducted a study to assess the impact of SANE programs in the care of victims of sexual assault. The findings of this study include evidence that emergency departments with forensic nurse examiners for victims of sexual assault generally provide better and timelier care to these patients and are also better at conducting the forensic exam. Those emergency departments with full coverage models of SANE programs were significantly more likely to offer a full forensic exam, to have a relationship with a rape crisis center, and to participate in a community-wide sexual assault response team (SART). They are also more likely to offer victims emergency contraception and shower facilities as well as fresh clothing. Additionally, emergency departments with SANE programs were more likely to offer staff training and annual in-services on the care of victims of sexual assault.

Implications for Nursing Practice

Sexual assault nurse examiners and emergency department nurses have been proactive in the development of standards of care for victims of sexual violence. The potential for improving care and determining referrals for those who have been sexually assaulted will create the opportunity for the victim to recover more fully from the event with fewer complications. The SANE model allows for comprehensive services to victims and a coordinated response from law enforcement, district attorney, health care, and advocacy services. The follow-up care includes crisis intervention and witness protection. The forensic exam that is conducted using the guidelines for forensic exams is more effective in aiding in the subsequent prosecution of the sexual offender. Each emergency department needs a written policy regarding the care of survivors of sexual assault and written protocols on the care of the victim and the training of the staff. There should be well-defined working relationships with other agencies and cooperation between agencies to achieve the best outcome for the victim of sexual assault.

Critical Thinking Questions

1. The following priorities should be addressed for the patient entering the emergency department with a chief complaint of sexual assault:
   a. A phone to contact a friend for a ride home
   b. Assessment of injuries
   c. Reassurance of her safety
   d. Report to law enforcement for possible investigation
   e. B, C, D
   f. A and C

2. The chain of evidence in a sexual assault exam:
   a. Must be kept as clear as possible with as few people as possible handling the evidence
   b. Dictates that rape kits must not be opened until the forensic exam begins
   c. Requires the nurse performing the forensic exam to sign the rape kit over to the investigating officer when complete
   d. Allows the rape kit to be left alone in the nurses' station while awaiting collection by the investigating officer
   e. A and D
   f. A, B, C

3. The role of the rape advocate in a sexual assault includes:
   a. Providing emotional support to the patient during and after the forensic exam
   b. Explaining findings from the forensic exam to family members
   c. Ensuring safe shelter for the patient immediately after the forensic exam
   d. Explaining investigative procedures to the victim
   e. A and B
   f. A, C, D

Answers to Critical Thinking Questions appear in Appendix D.

Reference

Plichta, S. B., Clements, P. T., & Houseman, C. (2007). Why SANES matter: Models of care for sexual violence victims in the emergency department. *Journal of Forensic Nursing, 3*(1), 15–23.

RESEARCH OPPORTUNITIES AND CLINICAL IMPACT RELATED TO FEMALE REPRODUCTIVE DISORDERS

Research Area	Clinical Impact
Clinical Trials	
Hormone replacement therapy	Will assist with information on the impact of short- versus long-term therapy on heart disease, breast cancer, Alzheimer's disease, stroke, and dementia
Physiologic Research	
Research on why some fibroids grow to become problems and others do not	May help develop strategies to prevent fibroids and to develop new strategies to decrease the need for hysterectomy
Breast cancer	Cause, treatment, prevention, and survival
Menopause	Treatment options for prevention of symptoms
Pregnancy	Prenatal care and prevention of complications and fetal abnormalities and death
Infertility	Ability to have children

Source: Office of Research on Women's Health. (2008). *Annual NIH research priorities for women's health.* Retrieved August 10, 2008, from http://orwh.od.nih.gov/research/priorities.html

Clinical Preparation

Read

- History of Current Illness
- Past Medical History
- Physical Exam
- Admitting Medical Orders
- Laboratory Study Results

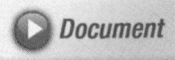

Document

- Summary of Hospitalization
- Pathophysiology Form
- Laboratory Values
- Laboratory Results Explanation

Apply

- List of Potential Nursing Diagnoses
- Concept Map
- Critical Thinking Questions

Log on to MyNursingKit.com to download forms you will need and to complete further steps in the Clinical Preparation assignment.

HISTORY OF PRESENT ILLNESS

Mrs. G is a 54-year-old admitted early yesterday morning for a scheduled total abdominal hysterectomy and bilateral salpingo-oophorectomy. The patient has had heavy menstrual periods all her life, but for the last 2 years she has felt confined to the house due to the amount of bleeding she experienced. Her health care provider has put her on various medications in an attempt to control the heavy bleeding without success. Mrs. G also has several uterine fibroid tumors that cause severe discomfort. She and her health care provider decided a total abdominal hysterectomy with bilateral salpingo-oophorectomy was warranted.

During morning report, it was reported that the occlusive dressing on the abdominal incision has been marked for a moderate amount of bleeding, but that it appears to have stopped as the drainage marks have gotten no bigger in the last 6 hours. The patient was scheduled for a hemoglobin and hematocrit this morning. She is currently receiving patient-controlled analgesia with morphine. The day nurse enters the patient's room at 0745 and begins the initial assessment. Temp: 99.4°F P: 96 RR: 22 BP: 108/62. IV D5½ NS with 20 KCL infusing at 125 mL/hr, without signs of redness or swelling at the IV site. Lung sounds: clear to auscultation.

Patient is lying quietly in bed, eyes closing as if she is very tired. Patient reports pain is increasing, is 7 on a 1–10 scale. When the covers are pulled back to examine the dressing, the nurse notes bright-red blood oozing from the edges of the dressing. Further assessment reveals approximately 20 milliliters of bright-red blood staining the top sheet that was covering the patient. The nurse pushes the patient call light and asks the secretary to please page the attending surgeon. The surgeon arrives and requests a suture kit and local anesthetic to put in retention sutures in an attempt to control the bleeding. The equipment arrives, and the surgeon removes the occlusive dressing to reveal an oozing incision, without redness, edema, slight ecchymosis, and edges remain approximated with staples. The surgeon asks for the most recent laboratory work that was drawn earlier in the morning. After placing 6 retention sutures and observing that the oozing has stopped, the surgeon leaves the floor after writing orders for antibiotics every 6 hours.

Medical/Surgical History

Mrs. G had 3 vaginal deliveries of live children. She had an appendectomy at age 15.

Social History

Mrs. G lives with her husband and has 3 grown children who all live in the local area. She has never smoked or used illicit drugs. She has a glass of wine in the evening with her dinner. Mrs. G runs an average of 20 miles per week.

Physical Exam

Temp: 97.4°F P: 82 RR: 16 BP: 108/62

Oxygen sat 98% on RA

HEENT: normal

Heart: regular rate and rhythm, normal S_1, S_2

Lungs: clear to auscultation in all fields

Abdomen: soft, nontender, bowel sounds present

Normal neuro exam

No rash

Chest x-ray: clear

ECG: WNL

Weight: 130 lb

Height: 5.4 ft

Admitting Medical Orders

Surgical service

Admit to surgical floor

Admitting diagnosis was menorrhagia and uterine fibroid tumors. Status post total abdominal hysterectomy with salpingo-oophorectomy.

No known allergies

Call house officer: pulse < 60 and > 130/minute; BP < 90 and > 160 systolic; temperature > 38.5; urine output < 30 mL/hr for 2 hours; respiratory rate > 30/minute

Ambulate qid beginning postoperative day 1

IV D5½ NS with 20 KCL at 125 mL/hr

Vital signs q4hours

Sequential compression device (SCD) to lower extremities until ambulating without assistance
Incentive spirometer q2h while awake
I&O q8hours
Progressive postoperative diet as tolerated post-nausea

Scheduled Medications
PCA: morphine sulfate 1mg/mL, incremental dose 1mg, lock out 6 minutes
Unasyn 2 grams IV q6h.

PRN Medications
Phenergan 25 mg q6h prn nausea
Ativan 0.5–2 mg IV q6–8h prn anxiety (not to exceed 10 mg/24 hours)
Tylenol 650 mg PO/PR q4h for pain
Benadryl 25-50 mg IV q6hours PRN insomnia or itching

Ordered Laboratory Studies
CBC morning after surgery

LABORATORY STUDY RESULTS

Test	1 Day Prior to Surgery	4 Hours After Surgery	0500 Today
HGB	14.3 g/dL	11.9 g/dL	9.5 g/dL
HCT	43%	38%	32%
Platelets	230,000/mm³	165,000/mm³	90,000/mm³
WBC	8,000/mm³	12,000/mm³	14,000/mm³
RBC	4.9/mm³	4.1/mm³	3.92/mm³

CRITICAL THINKING QUESTIONS

1. What action by the nurse would be top priority?

2. What should the nurse do next?

3. Based on this situation and the 3 days of lab values, which of the interventions outlined below should receive the highest nursing priority?

- Assess incision q30min × 2, then q1h × 2, then q2h × 2, then prn for signs of bleeding or infection.
- IV at 200 milliliters q1h for 4 hours, then decrease to 150 milliliters per hour.
- Administer analgesic as prescribed.
- Unasyn 2 grams IV q6h.
- Vital signs and oxygen saturation q4h.
- CBC stat.
- Call laboratory results to the health care provider.
- Educate patient on safety measures for low hemoglobin and platelets.
- Change patient linens to provide comfortable environment.
- Encourage oral fluids and increased protein and iron in diet.

Answers to Critical Thinking Questions appear in Appendix D.

NCLEX® REVIEW

1. A female patient is diagnosed with a chlamydia infection. The nurse realizes that this patient will most likely be treated with:
1. Penicillin G.
2. Flagyl.
3. Doryx.
4. Cleocin.

2. A female patient wants to reduce her risk of developing breast cancer. Which of the following should the nurse instruct this patient?
1. Do not have any children.
2. Do not use underarm antiperspirants.
3. Limit dietary fat intake.
4. Have children before the age of 30.

3. The nurse is reviewing the technique for self-breast examination with a post-menopausal female. Which of the following should be included in this instruction?
1. Do the exam at least one time each month.
2. Use a mirror to examine the shape and size of each breast.
3. Always examine in a lying down position.
4. If you feel a lump, prepare yourself emotionally for the diagnosis of breast cancer.

4. A patient with uterine fibroids was told that the size of the fibroids has decreased. The nurse realizes that the decrease in size could be due to:
1. Constant uterine bleeding.
2. Decreased estrogen production.
3. Pregnancy.
4. Menopause.

5. A patient is diagnosed with an unruptured ectopic pregnancy. The nurse realizes this patient will most likely be treated with:

1. Surgical removal of the fallopian tube.

2. Methotrexate.

3. A pessary.

4. Colporrhaphy.

6. The nurse is assessing a 24-year-old female's reproductive status. Which of the following assessment findings would increase this patient's risk of infertility?

1. Type I diabetes mellitus.

2. Diagnosis of scoliosis.

3. Menses began at the age of 13.

4. Parents had 4 children, all live births.

7. A patient is recovering from an exploratory laparoscopy. Which of the following should the nurse instruct this patient to reduce the pain caused by carbon dioxide?

1. Splint the incision before moving.

2. Ambulate.

3. Lay flat in bed for at least 16 hours.

4. Ingest clear liquids only for at least one day.

8. A female victim of personal violence is brought into the emergency department by the local police. Which of the following should the nurse do first?

1. Have the patient sign a consent form to collect evidence.

2. Obtain the patient's name and address.

3. Find three additional staff members to be with the patient during the assessment.

4. Locate a SANE immediately.

Answers for review questions appear in Appendix D

KEY TERMS

abortion *p.1550*
anorgasmia *p.1540*
bacterial vaginosis (BV) *p.1523*
bladder suspension *p.1554*
breast cancer *p.1528*
candidiasis *p.1524*
chancroid *p.1522*
chlamydia *p.1518*
colposcopy *p.1554*
cystocele *p.1538*
dysmenorrhea *p.1544*
dyspareunia *p.1541*
ectopic *p.1539*
endometriosis *p.1536*

fibrocystic breast *p.1525*
fibroid tumor *p.1535*
genital herpes *p.1521*
genital warts *p.1522*
gonorrhea *p.1519*
human papillomavirus (HPV) *p.1522*
hysterectomy *p.1554*
lumpectomy *p.1532*
lymphogranuloma venereum (LGV) *p.1519*
mammography *p.1531*
mastalgia *p.1525*
mastectomy *p.1532*
mastitis *p.1528*

menorrhagia *p.1544*
metrorrhagia *p.1545*
pelvic inflammatory disease (PID) *p.1519*
perimenopause *p.1549*
pessary *p.1538*
premenstrual dysphoric disorder (PMDD) *p.1545*
premenstrual syndrome (PMS) *p.1545*
prolapse *p.1538*
rectocele *p.1538*
syphilis *p.1520*
trichomoniasis *p.1523*
vaginismus *p.1541*

EXPLORE PEARSON mynursingkit™

MyNursingKit is your one stop for online chapter review materials and resources. Prepare for success with additional NCLEX®-style practice questions, interactive assignments and activities, web links, animations and videos, and more!

Register your access code from the front of your book at
www.mynursingkit.com

REFERENCES

Allred, S., Cox, J. T., & Mahoney, M. (2006). HPV prevention and the promise of the new vaccines. *Journal of the American Academy of Nurse Practitioners, 18*(Suppl. 2), 1–11.

American Cancer Society (ACS). (2003). *Updated breast cancer screening guidelines released.* Retrieved February 27, 2008, from http://www.cancer.org/docroot/NWS/content/ NWS_1_1x_Updated_Breast_Cancer_Screening_Guidelines_ Released.asp

American Cancer Society (ACS). (2005). *Breast cancer facts and figures 2005–2006.* Retrieved February 27, 2008, from http://www.cancer. org/downloads/STT/CAFF2005BrF.pdf

American Cancer Society (ACS). (2007). *What are the risk factors for breast cancer?* Retrieved February 27, 2008, from

http://www.cancer.org/docroot/CRI/content/CRI_2_4_2X_What_are _the_risk_factors_for_breast_cancer_5.asp?rnav=cri

American Cancer Society (ACS). (2008). *Cervical cancer: Prevention and early detection.* Retrieved August 12, 2008, from http://www. cancer.org/docroot/CRI/content/CRI_2_6x_cervical_cancer_ prevention_and_early_detection_8.asp?sitearea=PED

American College of Obstetricians and Gynecologists (ACOG). (1998). Medical management of tubal pregnancy (Number 3, December 1998). Clinical management guidelines for obstetricians- gynecologists. *International Journal of Gynecology & Obstetrics, 165,* 97–103.

American College of Obstetricians and Gynecologists (ACOG). (2000). *Fibrocystic breast changes.* Retrieved February 27, 2008, from

http://www.rgoa.yourmd.com/ypol/user/userMain.asp?siteid=1744 043&content=userViewContentInFramework&bcx=My+Doctor ^TAB~Web+Site^MNU~ROCHESTER+GYNECOLOGIC+%26+ OBSTETRIC+ASSOCIATES%2C+P.C.^PST^1744043~Our+Practice ^CAT^1~Article^MAP^ZZZLF2SXODC&cid=ZZZLF2SXODC&secure =2&rndm=0.4799626

American College of Obstetricians and Gynecologists (ACOG). (2005). *Premenstrual syndrome* (ACOG Practice Bulletin No. 15). Washington, DC: Author.

American Joint Committee on Cancers. (2005). *AJCC cancer staging manual.* Retrieved February 27, 2008, from http://www. cancerstaging.org/products/ajccproducts.html

American Society for Reproductive Medicine (ASRM). (2002). *Frequently asked questions about infertility*. Retrieved February 27, 2008, from http://www.asrm.org/Patients/faqs.html

Andrews, R. T., Spies, J. B., Sacks, D., Worthington-Kirsch, R. L., Niedzwiecki, G. A., Marx, M. V., et al. (2002). *National guidelines on the management of adult victims of sexual assault*. London: Association for Genitourinary Medicine (AGUM), Medical Society for the Study of Venereal Disease.

Barnhart, K., Dunsmoor-Su, R., & Coutifaris, C. (2002). Effect of endometriosis on *in vitro* fertilization. *Fertility and Sterility, 77*, 1148–1155.

Bhatia, S. C., & Bhatia, S. K. (2002). Diagnosis and treatment of premenstrual dysphoric disorder. *American Family Physician, 66*(7), 1235–1251.

Bianchini, F., Kaaks, R., & Vainio, H. (2002). Weight control and physical activity in cancer prevention. *Obesity Reviews, 3*(1), 5–8.

Boyles, S. (2006). Age, Obesity, and Breast Cancer Risk: Extra Weight May Lower Risk for Younger Women. *WebMD*. Retrieved August 16, 2008 from http://www.webmd.com/breast-cancer/news/20061127/breast-cancer-risk-age-and-obesity

Bumpers, H. L., Best, I. M., Norman, D., & Weaver, W. L. (2002). Debilitating lymphedema of the upper extremity after treatment of breast cancer. *American Journal of Clinical Oncology, 25*(4), 365–367.

Centers for Disease Control and Prevention (CDC). (2004). *Trends in reportable sexually transmitted diseases in the United States, 2004*. Retrieved February 27, 2008, from http://www.cdc.gov/std/stats04/04pdf/trends2004.pdf

Centers for Disease Control and Prevention (CDC). (2005a). *Toxic shock syndrome*. Retrieved February 28, 2008, from http://www.cdc.gov/ncidod/dbmd/diseaseinfo/toxicshock_t.htm

Centers for Disease Control and Prevention (CDC). (2005b). *Trends in reportable sexually transmitted diseases in the United States, 2005*. Retrieved August 12, 2008, from http://www.cdc.gov/std/stats05/trends2005.htm

Centers for Disease Control and Prevention (CDC). (2008a). *Breast cancer*. Retrieved August 12, 2008, from http://www.cdc.gov/cancer/breast/

Centers for Disease Control and Prevention (CDC). (2008b). *Candidiasis*. Retrieved February 28, 2008, from http://www.cdc.gov/nczved/dfbmd/disease_listing/candidiasis_gi.html#21

Centers for Disease Control and Prevention (CDC). (2008c). *Chlamydia*. Retrieved February 27, 2008, from http://www.cdc.gov/std/chlamydia/the-facts/default.htm

Centers for Disease Control and Prevention (CDC). (2008d). *Genital herpes*. Retrieved February 28, 2008, from http://www.cdc.gov/std/Herpes/default.htm

Centers for Disease Control and Prevention (CDC). (2008e). *Pelvic inflammatory disease—CDC fact sheet*. Retrieved February 28, 2008, from http://www.cdc.gov/std/PID/STDFact-PID.htm#What

Centers for Disease Control and Prevention (CDC). (2008f). *Sexually transmitted diseases*. Retrieved February 27, 2008, from http://www.cdc.gov/nchstp/dstd/disease_info.htm

Centers for Disease Control and Prevention (CDC). (2008g). *STDs and pregnancy—CDC fact sheet*. Retrieved February 28, 2008, from http://www.cdc.gov/std/STDFact-STDs&Pregnancy.htm#test

Centers for Disease Control and Prevention (CDC). (2008h). *Women's reproductive health: Hysterectomy*. Retrieved August 13, 2008, from http://www.cdc.gov/reproductivehealth/WomensRH/Hysterectomy.htm

Chlebowski, R. T., Prentice, R., & Adams-Campbell, A. (2005). Re: Ethnicity and breast cancer: Factors influencing differences in incidence and outcome. *Journal of the National Cancer Institute, 97*(21), 1619–1620.

Cronje, W., & Studd, J. (2002). Premenstrual syndrome and premenstrual dysphoric disorder. *Primary Care, 29*(1), 1–12.

D'Avanzo, D., & Geissler, E. (2003). *Mosby's pocket guide to cultural health assessment* (3rd ed.). St. Louis: Mosby.

Elliot, H. (2002). Premenstrual dysphoric disorder. *North Carolina Medical Journal, 63*(2), 72–75.

Evans, P., & Brunsell, S. (2007). Uterine fibroid tumors: Diagnosis and treatment. *American Family Physician, 75*(10), 1503–1507.

Fisher, B., Anderson, S., Bryant, J., Margolese, R. G., Deutsch, M., Fisher, E. R., et al. (2002). Twenty-year follow-up of a randomized trial comparing total mastectomy, lumpectomy, and lumpectomy plus irradiation for the treatment of invasive breast cancer. *The New England Journal of Medicine, 347*, 1233–1241.

Ford, D., Easton, D. F., Stratton, M., Narod, S., Goldgar, D., Devilee, P., et al. (1998). Genetic heterogeneity and penetrance analysis of the BRCA1 and BRCA2 genes in breast cancer families. *American Journal of Human Genetics, 62*, 676–689.

French, L. (2005). Dysmenorrhea. *American Family Physician, 71*(2), 285–290.

Harcourt, D., & Rumsey, N. (2001). Psychological aspects of breast reconstruction: A review of the literature. *Journal of Advanced Nursing, 35*(4), 477–487.

Hulka, B. S., & Moorman, P. G. (2001). Breast cancer: Hormones and other risk factors. *Maturitas, 28*, 103–113.

Imaginis. (2006). *Breast cancer diagnosis*. Retrieved February 28, 2008, from http://www.imaginis.com/breasthealth/biopsy/core.asp

Institute for Clinical Systems Improvement (ICSI). (2006). *Initial management of abnormal cervical cytology (Pap smear) and HPV testing*. Bloomington, MN: Author.

Iwuagwu, O. C., Walker, L. G., Stanley, P. W., Hart, N. B., Platt, A. J., & Drew, P. J. (2006). Randomized clinical trial examining psychosocial and quality of life benefits of bilateral breast reduction surgery. *British Journal of Surgery, 93*(3), 291–294.

Johnson-Mallard, V. (2007). Increasing knowledge of sexually transmitted infection risk. *Nurse Practitioner, 32*(2), 26–32.

Jones, C. (2001, March). Premenstrual dysphoric disorder. *Advances for Nurse Practitioners*, 87–90.

Kerlikowski, K., & Barclay, J. (1997). Outcomes of modern screening mammography. *Journal of the National Cancer Institute, Monographs, 22*, 105–111.

Kjerulff, K. H., Langenberg, P., Rhodes, J. C., Harvey, L. A., Guzinski, G. M., & Stolley, P. D. (2000). Effectiveness of hysterectomy. *Obstetrics & Gynecology, 95*, 319–325.

Kjerulff, K. H., Langenberg, P., Seidman, J. D., Stolley, P. D., & Guzinski, G. M. (1996). Uterine leiomyomas. Racial differences in severity, symptoms and age of diagnosis. *Journal of Reproductive Medicine, 41*, 483–490.

Klein, S. (2005). Evaluation of Palpable Breast Masses. *American Family Physician: A peer reviewed journal of the American academy of family physicians*. Retrieved August 15, 2008 from http://www.aafp.org/afp/20050501/1731.html.

Kroman, N., Jensen, M. B., Wohlfahrt, J., Mouridsen, H. T., Andersen, P. K., & Melbye, M. (2000). Factors influencing the effect of age on prognosis in breast cancer: Population based study. *British Medical Journal, 320*, 474–478.

Li, C. et al. (2003). The Relationship between Alcohol Use and Risk of Breast Cancer by Histology and Hormone Receptor Status among Women 65–79 Years of Age. *Cancer Epidemiology Biomarkers & Prevention* Vol. 12, 1061-1066, American Association for Cancer Research. Retrieved on August 14, 2008 from http://cebp.aacrjournals.org/cgi/content/abstract/12/10/1061

Loman, N., Johannsson, O., Kristoffersson, U., et al. (2001). Family history of breast and ovarian cancers and BRCA1 and BRCA2 mutations in a population-based series of early-onset breast cancer. *Journal of the National Cancer Institute, 93*, 1215–1223.

Lowdermilk, D. L., & Perry, S. E. (2004). *Maternity & women's health care* (8th ed.). St. Louis: Mosby.

Lozeau, A. M., & Potter, B. (2005). Diagnosis and management of ectopic pregnancy. *American Family Physician, 72*(9), 1707–1714.

Master-Hunter, T., & Heiman, D. L. (2006). Amenorrhea: Evaluation and treatment. *American Family Physician, 73*(8), 1374–1382.

McKinley Health Center. (2002). *Toxic shock syndrome and tampons*. Retrieved February 28, 2008 from http://www.mckinley.uiuc.edu/Handouts/toxic_shock_syndrome.html

McTiernan, A., Kooperberg, C., White, E., Wilcox, S., Coates, R., Adams-Campbell, L., et al. (2003). Recreational physical activity and the risk of breast cancer in postmenopausal women. *JAMA, 290*(10), 1331–1336.

MedlinePlus Medical Encyclopedia. (2006a). *Abortion—spontaneous*. Retrieved February 28, 2008, from http://www.nlm.nih.gov/medlineplus/ency/article/001488.htm

MedlinePlus Medical Encyclopedia. (2006b). *Toxic shock syndrome*. Retrieved February 28, 2008, from http://www.nlm.nih.gov/medlineplus/ency/article/000653.htm

MedlinePlus Medical Encyclopedia. (2007). *Hysterectomy*. Retrieved February 28, 2008, from http://www.nlm.nih.gov/medlineplus/ency/article/002915.htm

MedlinePlus Medical Encyclopedia. (2008). *Infertility*. Retrieved February 28, 2008, from http://www.nlm.nih.gov/medlineplus/ency/article/001191.htm

Mounsey, A. L., Wilgus, A., & Slawson, D. C. (2006). Diagnosis and management of endometriosis. *American Family Physician, 74*(4), 594–600.

Mount Sinai Medical Center. (2008). *Reproductive endocrinology*. Accessed August 8, 2008, from http://www.mountsinai.org/Patient%20Care/Service%20Areas/Women/Procedures%20and%20Health%20Care%20Services/Reproductive%20Endocrinology

Nakashima, A. K., Rolfs, R. T., Flock, M. L., Kilmarx, P., & Greenspan, J. R. (1996). Epidemiology of syphilis in the United States, 1941–1993. *Sexually Transmitted Diseases, 23*(1):16–23.

National Cancer Institute (NCI). (2000). *SEER summary staging manual—2000*. Retrieved February 28, 2008, from http://seer.cancer.gov/tools/ssm/

National Cancer Institute (NCI). (2007). Screening Mammograms: Questions and Answers. Retrieved on January 1, 2009 from http://www.cancer.gov/cancertopics/factsheet/detection/screening-mammograms

National Cervical Cancer Coalition. (2005). *Cervical cancer*. Retrieved February 28, 2008, from http://www.nccc-online.org/patient_info/cervical_cancer.html

Osteen, R. (2001). Breast cancer. In R. E. Lenhard, R. T. Osteen, & R. Gansler (Eds.), *Clinical oncology* (pp. 251–268). Atlanta, GA: American Cancer Society.

Phillips, N. (2000). Female sexual dysfunction: Evaluation and treatment. *American Family Physician, 62*(1), 127–136, 141–142. Retrieved February 28, 2008, from http://www.aafp.org/afp/20000701/127.html

Plichta, S. B., Clements, P. T., & Houseman, C. (2007). Why SANES matter: Models of care for sexual violence victims in the emergency department. *Journal of Forensic Nursing, 3*(1), 15–23.

Quest Diagnostics. (2005). *Chlamydia tests*. Retrieved February 28, 2008, from http://www.questdiagnostics.com/kbase/topic/medtest/hw4046/howdone.htm

Roussow, J. E., Anderson, G. L., Prentice, R. L., LaCroix, A. Z., Kooperberg, C., Stefanick, M. L., et al. (2002). Risks and benefits of estrogen plus progestin in healthy postmenopausal women: Principal results from the Women's Health Initiative randomized controlled trial. *JAMA, 288*(3), 321–333.

Salandy, D., & Brenner, B. (2002). *Toxic shock syndrome*. Retrieved February 28, 2008, from http://www.emedicine.com/emerg/topic600.htm

Sepilian, V. P. (2007). Ectopic Pregnancy. *eMedicine*. Retrieved August 16, 2008 from http://www.emedicine.com/med/topic3212.htm.

Sherman, R. T., & Thompson, R. A. (2004). The female athlete triad. *The Journal of School Nursing, 20*(4), 197–202.

Singletary, K. W., & Gapstur, S. M. (2001). Review of epidemiologic and experimental evidence and potential mechanisms. *JAMA, 286*(17), 2143–2151.

Smigal, C. et al. (2006). Trends in Breast Cancer by Race and Ethnicity: Update 2006. *Cancer Journal*; 56:168-183 doi: 10.3322/canjclin.56.3.168

University of Maryland Medical Center. (2004). *Anterior vaginal wall repair*. Retrieved February 27, 2008 from http://www.umm.edu/ency/article/003982.htm

U.S. Department of Health and Human Services (DHHS). (2000). *Healthy People 2010 understanding and improving health*. Washington, DC: Author.

U.S. Department of Health and Human Services (DHHS), womenshealth.gov. (2006). *Endometriosis*. Retrieved February 28, 2008, from http://www.4woman.gov/faq/endomet.htm

U.S. Department of Health and Human Services (DHHS), womenshealth.gov. (2007). *Polycystic ovarian syndrome (PCOS)*. Retrieved February 28, 2008, from http://www.4woman.gov/faq/pcos.htm

U.S. Preventive Services Task Force. (2002). Screening for breast cancer: Recommendations and rationale. *Annals of Internal Medicine, 137*(5, Pt. 1), 344–346.

Caring for the Patient with Male Reproductive Disorders

Patricia Caudle

With contributions by:
Laurie Kaudewitz

Outcome-Based Learning Objectives

After studying this chapter, the learner will be able to:

1. Identify the most common male reproductive disorders.
2. Discuss the etiology, pathophysiology, clinical manifestations, and treatments of testicular, penile, and prostatic disorders.
3. Interpret diagnostic test results for male reproductive disorders.
4. Identify nursing management goals when caring for males with reproductive disorders.
5. Apply nursing diagnoses and nursing process to the care of the male patient with testicular and prostatic cancer.
6. Discuss health education, health promotion, and disease prevention specific for male health.

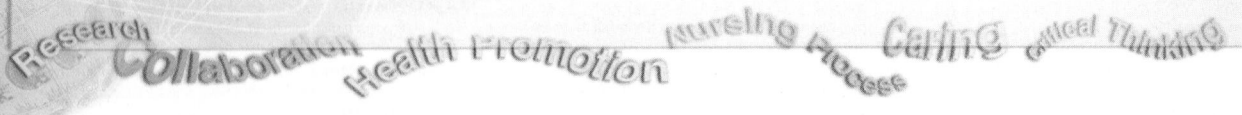

MALE REPRODUCTIVE disorders are often complex as they involve both sexual functioning and the urinary system. Disorders of the male reproductive system may also be a source of embarrassment for the male. Nursing care should include both the physical and emotional aspects associated with these disorders. This chapter will differentiate some of the major male reproductive disorders and will discuss both medical and nursing management. Figure 50–1 ■ portrays the normal anatomy of the male genitourinary system.

Testicular Disorders

Testicular disorders may arise from inflammation, infection, trauma, or cancer. The most common disorders are discussed here, along with appropriate treatment modalities and nursing care. Health education and prevention are important aspects of nursing care in this section.

Epididymitis: Etiology

Epididymitis is an infection or inflammation of the ductus epididymidis, a crescent-shaped structure found on the posterior aspect of each testicle (Cole & Vogler, 2004). The epididymis functions in the transport of sperm from the testicle to the vas deferens.

An infection of the epididymis may originate at the prostate, the urethra, or the urinary bladder and migrate via the urinary system to the vas deferens and the epididymis (see Figure 50–1 ■).

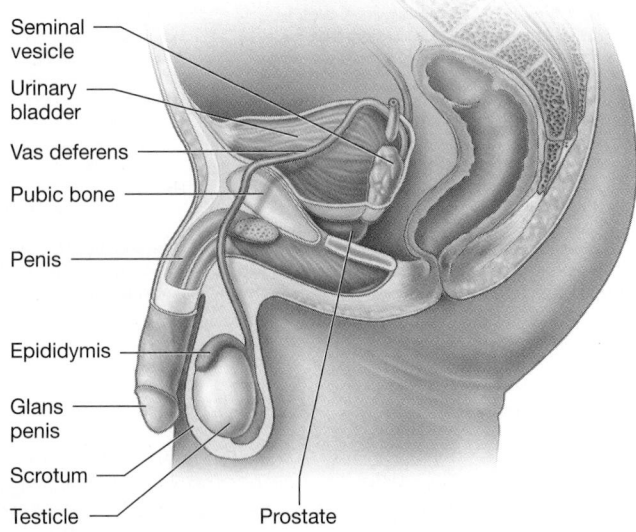

Seminal vesicle
Urinary bladder
Vas deferens
Pubic bone
Penis
Epididymis
Glans penis
Scrotum
Testicle
Prostate

FIGURE 50–1 ■ Normal anatomy of the male genitourinary system.

Infection of the epididymis in men younger than age 35 is more likely to be the result of gonococcal, chlamydial, or ureaplasma organisms. In older men, infection is more likely to be the result of prostatitis, instrumentation of the urinary system, or a structural lesion such as carcinoma of the testis (Goroll & Mulley, 2006). In these cases, the coliform bacteria, especially *Escherichia coli*, are most frequently identified as causative (Cole & Vogler, 2004).

Clinical Manifestations

Symptoms include tenderness and swelling of the epididymis that may spread to the testicle causing a large, tender scrotal mass (Goroll & Mulley, 2006). When a sexually transmitted organism is the cause, dysuria, penile discharge, fever, and pus in the urine or semen may be seen. Inguinal lymph nodes may be enlarged, especially on the side where the location may be situated. The tests outlined in the Diagnostic Tests box can be used to determine a diagnosis of epididymitis.

Medical Management

Medical management of epididymitis includes antibiotics specific to the causative organism identified, analgesics, and nonsteroidal anti-inflammatory agents (NSAIDs). See Chapter 15 🔗 for a discussion of pain assessment and management. The Pharmacology Summary feature (p. 1585) presents medications used to treat male reproductive disorders.

■ Nursing Management

Nursing management includes encouraging the patient to maintain bed rest and elevating the scrotum with a towel sling. Elevation and the application of cold to the scrotum will help decrease swelling and pain. Figure 50–2 ■ (p. 1568) depicts one form of towel sling. Ambulation requires a soft scrotal support that keeps the scrotum close to the body (Karlowicz, 1995). Patients need education about epididymitis, the medications used, and how to avoid a recurrence of the ailment.

Orchitis: Etiology

Orchitis is an inflammation or infection of one or both testes. Infection may be caused by viral or bacterial agents. One viral cause is mumps orchitis which may be seen 7 to 10 days after mumps parotitis or, rarely, it may occur spontaneously (Goroll & Mulley, 2006). Mumps orchitis usually is unilateral and may cause infertility. Men who have never had the mumps and are exposed to the mumps virus require treatment. Like epididymitis, the causative bacterial agents include gonorrhea, chlamydia, and *Escherichia coli*.

 CRITICAL ALERT   *Men exposed to the mumps virus who have never had mumps should receive gamma globulin immediately to aid in decreasing the severity of the disease and preserving fertility.*

Clinical Manifestations

Symptoms and diagnostic testing are the same as for epididymitis. It is important to be aware that the symptoms of orchitis closely resemble testicular torsion, a surgical emergency described in the next section of this chapter.

Medical Management

Medical treatment includes the use of antibiotics when appropriate, analgesics, and NSAIDs (see the Pharmacology Summary feature, p. 1585). Viral causes are treated with rest, fluids, and NSAIDs.

■ Nursing Management

Nursing management includes minimizing activity, elevation of the scrotum using a towel sling or soft support (see Figure 50–2 ■, p. 1568), and cold compresses to decrease edema and pain. The goal of treatment is to prevent testicular atrophy, infertility, abscess, and impotence. Emotional support is important because of the reproductive concerns. In cases in which antibiotics are needed, teaching should stress the importance of completing the full course of medication prescribed.

Testicular Torsion: Epidemiology and Etiology

Testicular torsion occurs when a mobile testicle causes a twisting of the spermatic cord, essentially closing off the blood supply to the testicle. Loss of blood supply to the testicle will cause ischemia, necrosis, and loss of the testicle if it is not relieved within 6 to 12 hours (Cole & Vogler, 2004).

DIAGNOSTIC TESTS for Epididymitis

Test and Normal Values	Expected Abnormality	Rationale for Abnormality
Urinalysis: *Normally will not have any white blood cells or bacteria*	Elevated white count.	Due to inflammatory/infectious process.
Cultures of any discharge: *Normally will be negative for bacteria*	May be positive for chlamydia, gonorrhea, *Escherichia coli*, etc.	Sexually transmitted infections and coliforms may cause epididymitis.
White blood cells (WBC): *Normal = 5,000–10,000/mm³*	Elevated white count. Shifts indicating acute infection.	Due to inflammatory/infectious process.

Sources: Adapted from Cole, F., & Vogler, R. (2004). The acute, nontraumatic scrotum: Assessment, diagnosis and management. *Journal of the American Academy of Nurse Practitioners, 16*(2), 50–56; and Fischbach, F. (2003). *A manual of laboratory and diagnostic tests* (7th ed.). Philadelphia: Lippincott Williams & Wilkins.

Towel sling scrotal support

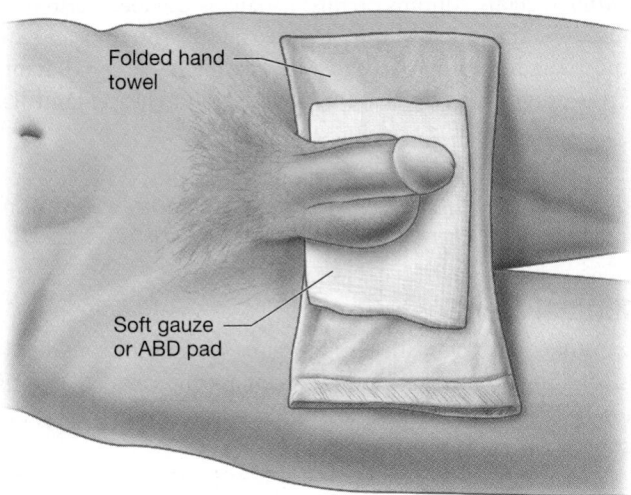

Folded hand
towel

Soft gauze
or ABD pad

FIGURE 50–2 ■ Scrotal supports.

 **CRITICAL ALERT** *Sudden onset of scrotal/testicular pain without injury in an adolescent should be considered testicular torsion until proven otherwise. Surgical intervention to preserve the testicle should occur within 6 to 12 hours of occurrence.*

Annually, 1 in 4,000 males under the age of 25 experience testicular torsion (Ringdahl & Teague, 2006). The process for the development of this problem begins with the congenital absence of attachment of the testicle to the tunica vaginalis. Without this attachment, the testicle hangs freely and can easily twist on the cord (Cole & Vogler, 2004). The left testicle is more at risk because of the longer spermatic cord.

Clinical Manifestations

Clinical manifestations include sudden, severe pain in one testicle, nausea, vomiting, and light-headedness. On examination, the testicle will be high in the scrotum due to the shortening of the spermatic cord. Figure 50–3 ■ depicts the twisting and shortening of the spermatic cord. The affected testicle may also feel larger than normal, and the cremasteric reflex (the testicle will rise in the scrotum when the thigh near the scrotum is stroked) will be absent (Ringdahl & Teague, 2006). Diagnosis is confirmed with Doppler ultrasound.

Medical Management

Medical treatment for testicular torsion is immediate surgery. The testicle and cord are untwisted, and if the testicle is viable, it is anchored to the scrotum (**orchiopexy**) to prevent recurrence. If the testicle is nonviable, then it is removed (**orchiectomy**). Before and after surgery, the patient will require analgesia (Ringdahl & Teague, 2006). See Chapter 15 🔗 for a discussion of pain assessment and management.

■ Nursing Management

Nursing care of boys and men experiencing testicular torsion usually begins in the postoperative period and includes bed rest, observation for bleeding or drainage on the dressing, monitor-

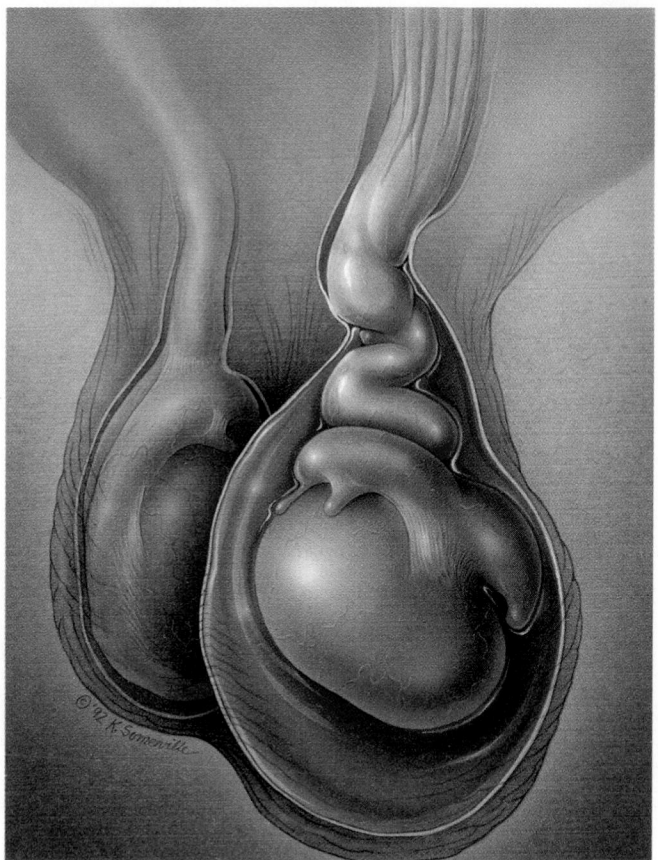

FIGURE 50–3 ■ Testicular torsion.
Source: Kevin A. Somerville/Phototake NYC

ing vital signs, administering analgesics, and providing scrotal support. The towel sling (see Figure 50–2 ■) can be used while the patient is in bed. Ambulation will require a soft scrotal support that keeps the scrotum close to the body (Karlowicz, 1995). Education of the patient and his parents would include information about the analgesic action and side effects and the importance of follow-up visits with the urologist or surgeon. When the adolescent reaches ages 14 to 16, a testicular prosthesis can be implanted if desired (Ringdahl & Teague, 2006).

Hydrocele: Epidemiology and Etiology

The space between the tunica vaginalis and the testicle may fill with fluid causing a hydrocele (Goroll & Mulley, 2006). This is the most common cause of scrotal swelling. In the newborn male, hydrocele develops when fluid that surrounds the testicles does not absorb after the closure of the tunica vaginalis *in utero*. In older males, hydrocele may develop after infection in the scrotum, injury, radiation, or testicular cancer. There are also incidences of idiopathic hydrocele among elderly males (Every, Mikkelsen, & Bailey, 2005).

Clinical Manifestations

Clinical manifestations include scrotal swelling that transluminates (light source behind the swollen scrotum will cause a glow as the light penetrates the fluid). The swelling is not painful unless there is so much fluid that it causes increased pressure on the testes (Goroll & Mulley, 2006).

Medical Management

Medical management is usually conservative, as the fluid will be reabsorbed in time. Should the swelling increase to painful levels, the fluid can be aspirated or surgically drained to prevent damage to the testes (Every, Mikkelsen, & Bailey, 2005).

■ Nursing Management

Nursing care depends on the extent of the hydrocele. For newborns with hydrocele, the care is the same as for all newborns. For adults, elevation of the scrotum may help. If surgery is required, postoperative care is similar to the postoperative care for testicular torsion.

Spermatocele: Etiology, Epidemiology, and Clinical Manifestations

Spermatoceles are painless, sperm-containing cysts that occur on the upper portion of the testis near the epididymis. These cysts are thought to be caused by an occlusion of the efferent (outflow) spermatic ducts of the testis. Usually only one testis is affected and the cyst is 1 centimeter or less in size (Scrotal Masses, 2005).

While most spermatoceles go unnoticed, some become large enough to annoy the male or the cyst may be found coincidentally in males who seek help for infertility (Bazar et al., 2003). On physical examination, the cyst is palpable and transluminates. Translumination helps differentiate this fluid-filled cyst from a solid nodule that is more likely to be testicular cancer. Diagnosis is verified by ultrasound (Goroll & Mulley, 2006).

Medical Management

Medical management for those rare spermatoceles that grow large enough to disfigure or cause pain is inguinoscrotal surgery to remove the mass (Bazar et al., 2003). Patients who require surgery can be reassured that the procedure does not affect fertility or virility (Goroll & Mulley, 2006).

Varicocele: Epidemiology and Etiology

A varicocele is an enlargement of the veins of the pampiniform plexus within the scrotum. It develops because of incompetent venous valves just like varicose veins in the legs. Varicoceles are most likely to occur on the left because the left spermatic vein empties directly into the renal vein causing increased hydrostatic back pressure within the vein when the patient stands (Goroll & Mulley, 2006). About 15% of all males and 40% of males who have infertility have varicocele (Quallich, 2006). The cause is unknown and there are no specific risk factors.

Clinical Manifestations

Signs and symptoms of varicocele include a "bag of worms" appearance to the scrotum that decreases in size when the patient is recumbent. The varicocele is usually not painful, but some men will notice a dull ache and fullness or pulling to the affected side of the scrotum after prolonged standing (Quallich, 2006).

Medical Management

Medical management is not necessary unless there are symptoms or infertility. Surgical treatment may be used to seal the affected vein and redirect blood flow to a normal vein if the varicocele is painful. Surgery has not improved fertility (Quallich, 2006).

Undescended or Mispositioned Testicles: Epidemiology, Etiology, and Clinical Manifestations

When one or both testes are not in the scrotum at birth, it is called cryptorchidism. During gestation, the testes form inside the abdomen and, normally, move down into the scrotum at term. Occasionally, the testicle may be misdirected as it emerges from the inguinal canal into areas other than the scrotum (Every, Mikkelsen, & Bailey, 2005). Figure 50–4 ■ depicts some of the extrascrotal sites.

Cryptorchidism occurs in 0.7% to 1% of male infants at birth (Every, Mikkelsen, & Bailey, 2005). The cause may be a testicular or hormonal defect. Undescended testicles become fibrotic and spermatogenesis does not occur. In addition, there is an increased risk for testicular cancer in the cryptorchid testes.

Medical Management

Medical treatment is usually postponed until the child is 1 year of age. If the testis is still undescended at this time, the testis is brought down into the scrotum and orchiopexy is performed. This is an outpatient procedure with few side effects and the baby recovers quickly.

Testicular Cancer: Etiology and Epidemiology

Cancer that forms in the tissue of the testis usually occurs in men between the ages of 20 and 39. It is the most common form of cancer in Caucasian men between the ages of 15 and 34 (National Cancer Institute [NCI], 2007c). It is estimated that testicular cancer will occur in 7,920 men in the United States in 2007. Of these, approximately 380 will die of the disease (NCI, 2007c). Men of Scandinavian descent are at greatest

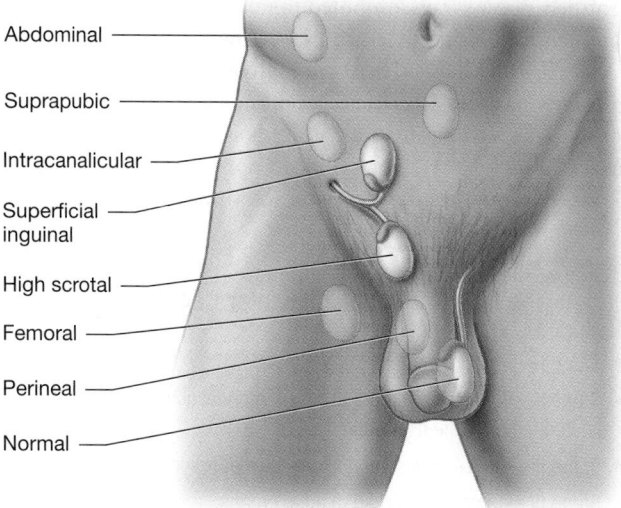

Ectopic testes Cryptorchism

Abdominal
Suprapubic
Intracanalicular
Superficial inguinal
High scrotal
Femoral
Perineal
Normal

FIGURE 50–4 ■ Extrascrotal testicular sites.

risk, but overall the rate of occurrence has increased by 200% in the last 40 years. Other risk factors include familial history (especially siblings), prior personal history, cryptorchidism, Klinefelter's syndrome, natural exposure to gestational estrogen, and exposure to insecticides (Brown, 2004; Goroll & Mulley, 2006).

Pathophysiology

Testicular cancer may arise from a germ cell, stromal cell, or nongerm cell of the testes. Nongerminal neoplasms originate from Leydig cells or stromal cells and occur less frequently. Germinal tumors account for 95% of testicular tumors and are generally divided into two groups: seminomas that are slow growing and nonseminomas that are more aggressive. Nonseminomas have four subtypes: embryonal, yolk sac, choriocarcinoma, and teratoma (Every, Mikklesen, & Bailey, 2005; Stevenson & McNeill, 2004). Teratoma subtypes are the least likely to metastasize, whereas choriocarcinomas are the most likely to metastasize (NCI, 2007c).

Clinical Manifestations

Usually, a solid, painless, nontransluminating lump is found on the testicle of a young man. Some men will have a dull discomfort or heaviness in the scrotum and lower abdomen. Occasionally, the scrotum will swell. Many testicular cancers are first diagnosed as epididymitis or orchitis and treated with antibiotics. When the lump does not resolve, further studies reveal the malignancy. Testicular tumors have also been found coincident to sports injuries to the groin or genitals. A small number of men may first seek medical advice because of **gynecomastia** (enlargement of the male breast) caused by testicular tumors that secrete beta human chorionic gonadotropin (HCG) (Brown, 2004). Men with metastatic disease may complain of cough, hemoptysis, and weight loss. Chapter 64 ☞ has an in-depth discussion of the diagnosis and treatment of cancer.

Diagnostic Testing and Staging

The first line of diagnostic testing after a lump is found is ultrasonography of the scrotum. Ultrasound is excellent for differentiating cancer from epididymitis or hydrocele. Once the tumor is identified, chest x-ray, computed tomographic (CT) scan of the abdomen, and serum markers are obtained in order to stage the cancer (Brown, 2004). The commonly used staging system appears in Chart 50–1. Testicular cancer produces a predictable spread to the retroperitoneum, lungs, and mediastinum (Stevenson & McNeill, 2004). Fine needle or open biopsy is never done because of the danger of seeding the scrotum with the cancer cells

---

> **CHART 50–1** **Staging of Testicular Cancer**
>
> - **Stage I**—Cancer is confined to the testicle.
> - **Stage II**—Cancer has spread to retroperitoneal nodes, but disease is limited to below the diaphragm.
> - **Stage III**—Cancer has spread above the diaphragm.
> - **Stage IV**—Tumor has spread to other organs.
>
> *Source:* Adapted from Goroll, A., & Mulley, A. (2006). *Primary care medicine: Office evaluation and management of the adult patient* (5th ed.). Philadelphia: Lippincott Williams & Wilkins.

---

and causing a more rapid dissemination of the cancer to the abdomen and lungs (Goroll & Mulley, 2006; NCI, 2007c).

Serum tumor markers include beta human chorionic gonadotropin (secreted by most choriocarcinomas and about 50% of other nonseminomas), alpha-fetoprotein, and lactate dehydrogenase. These serum markers are used to detect disease, to monitor response to treatment, and as a surveillance tool following treatment (NCI, 2007c). A rise in the serum markers during chemotherapy indicates relapse or failure to respond to treatment. An elevation in serum markers a year after treatment indicates recurrence and the need for chemotherapy. The Diagnostic Tests box offers further explanation of tumor markers.

Medical Management

Medical management decisions depend on the type of tumor, the stage of the disease, and tumor markers. Seminomatous testicular tumors, Stages I and II, are treated by orchiectomy via an inguinal route and retroperitoneal node irradiation (NCI, 2007c). This combination will result in 100% cure rates. Side effects of radiation therapy include fatigue, skin changes, loss of appetite, nausea, diarrhea, and reduced sperm production. Sperm production from the remaining testicle does recover, but it will take 1 to 2 years after radiation. Seminomatous tumors at Stage III or above may be treated pre- and postorchiectomy with cisplatin-based chemotherapy that results in cure rates of about 90% (Goroll & Mulley, 2006). See the Pharmacology Summary feature (p. 1585).

Nonseminomatous testicular tumors in Stages I and II require only the surgical removal of the affected testicle. The cure rate for surgery is about 95% (Goroll & Mulley, 2006). Higher stages of the nonseminomatous tumors require chemotherapy. Cisplatin-based multiple-agent chemotherapy is highly effective, even in patients with metastatic disease. This newest chemotherapy for testicular cancers has decreased the need for wide lymphadenectomy.

Follow-up medical surveillance is very important. For the first year, the patient is seen monthly. For years 2 and 3, he is evaluated every other month; every 3 months in the third year; and every 6 months in the fourth and fifth years. The majority of recurrences will occur within the first 2 years, but relapse can occur even beyond that time. Examinations should include physical examination, tumor markers, chest x-ray, and CT scans of the abdomen and pelvis should be done every 3 to 6 months (NCI, 2007c; Segal et al., 2001).

◾ Nursing Management

Nursing care for men newly diagnosed with testicular cancer requires a high degree of emotional support. The men experiencing this cancer face altered sexuality, body image, role function, and fertility. They often fear loss of masculinity and must come face to face with their own mortality. Reassurance that orchiectomy does not cause **impotence** (problems associated with ejaculation or orgasm, in addition to erectile dysfunction) or infertility and that masculinity will remain intact is important. Open discussion of sexuality and the genitalia will allow the patient to express his worries without embarrassment. Review of the surgical procedure, the treatment planned, and the cure rates of these treatments will also help alleviate fear. Keep communications with the patient clear, concrete, and open.

DIAGNOSTIC TESTS for Testicular Cancer Using Tumor Markers

Test and *Normal Values*	Expected Abnormality	Rationale for Abnormality
Human chorionic gonadotropin (HCG): *Produced in the syncytiotrophoblasts* *Normal range < 2 ng/mL or no measurable amount*	Increased in seminoma, embryonal, and choriocarcinoma tumors.	Used to detect tumors too small to be detected by x-ray or computed tomography (CT) scan.
Alpha-fetoprotein (AFP): *Produced in the liver, GI tract, fetal yolk sac* *Normal range < 15 ng/mL*	Elevated in yolk sac tumors.	Used to detect tumors too small to be detected by x-ray or CT scan. Also elevated when there is liver damage.
Lactate dehydrogenase (LDH): *Normal range 70–250 units/L*	Nonspecific.	Useful in staging of seminomas and nonseminomatous germ cell tumors. Also elevated in hemolysis, liver and muscle disease, and myocardial infarction.

Source: Adapted from National Academy of Clinical Biochemistry (NACB). (2006). *Tumor markers PDF. Practice guidelines and recommendations for use of tumor markers in the clinic: Testicular Cancer (section 3A).* Retrieved March 30, 2007, from http://www.aacc.org/Pages/default.aspx

Nursing Interventions and Health Promotion

Preoperatively, the patient will need information about postoperative incision care, analgesia, and pulmonary toileting. Presurgical laboratory tests will need to be obtained. See Chapter 25 ☞ for review of preoperative teaching. The possibility for testicle prosthesis may be discussed, should the patient feel that this would improve his body image (Brown, 2004).

There is usually bowel preparation because an abdominal inguinal incision is used, even for simple orchiectomy. This may be done at home before admission for surgery or after admission. The patient needs to know that he should avoid aspirin and other NSAIDs about a week prior to surgery to decrease bleeding risks (Stevenson & McNeill, 2004). This is a very stressful time and education will need to be repeated and reinforced.

Some patients with testicular cancer may be receiving chemotherapy before surgery. If one of the agents used is bleomycin, lung toxicity may have occurred and pulmonary risks are increased. Close monitoring of respiratory function will be needed.

Postoperatively, emotional support is needed as staging the cancer proceeds. Anxiety and fear may require that the nurse continue to repeat information. If the surgery includes extensive retroperitoneal lymph node removal, the patient may be in the hospital for about a week. During the recovery time, pain control, fluids, monitoring the incision for bleeding or infection, pulmonary toileting, and monitoring vital signs for elevated temperature or shortness of breath are all part of routine care. (See Chapter 27 ☞ for postoperative care and Chapter 15 ☞ for pain assessment and management.) All postoperative patients are at increased risk for deep venous thrombosis and should begin to ambulate on the first day. Pain management before ambulation will ease the discomfort and help them to be more willing to move.

Patients who have seminomas will begin radiation therapy before discharge. Radiation therapy will involve the retroperitoneal area and will require education for the patient about what to expect. Side effects of irradiation include nausea, vomiting, diarrhea, fatigue, skin changes, and loss of appetite (Brown, 2004; NCI, 2007d). An antidiarrheal and an antiemetic will be needed. Cisplatin-based multiagent chemotherapy will begin for patients with nonseminomas or cancers that have spread outside the testicle. Chemotherapy offers systemic therapy, reaching cancer cells anywhere in the body. Common side effects are nausea, hair loss, fatigue, diarrhea, vomiting, fever, chills, cough, mouth sores, and skin rash. Other, less common side effects include numbness, loss of reflexes, impaired hearing, and decreased to absent sperm production (NCI, 2007c). Nursing care will include emotional support, assistance with oral hygiene, antidiarrheal and antiemetic medications such as Zofran (ondansetron), and skin care. See the Pharmacology Summary feature (p. 1585).

Discharge priorities for the patient with testicular cancer are delineated in the Patient Teaching & Discharge Priorities box (p. 1572).

Health Promotion

Young men at risk for testicular cancer are not likely to receive education about self-testicular examination. In addition, they are not likely to have a testicular examination on routine physical or during a visit to the health care provider for another reason (Brown, 2004). Nurses are in a key position to encourage and to teach self-testicular examination in their community. The Testicular Cancer Resource Center has patient instruction programs to help nurses reach young men with this important information (Testicular Cancer Resource Center, 2007).

It has been recommended that men over age 50 receive Digital rectal exam (DRE) and PSA tests every year. If the screening tests indicate a need, then transrectal ultrasound guided biopsy should be done and repeated every 3 years (Gray & Sims, 2006).

Health fairs or community programs designed to include the African American man can be especially beneficial. African American men have the highest incidence of prostate cancer in the world (NCI, 2007b). In addition, they are less likely to seek care. A culturally sensitive program within the community is more apt to attract these men and to save lives (Ward-Smith, 2006).

■ Prostate Disorders

The prostate gland is located under the urinary bladder at the bladder neck and in front of the rectum in men (see Figure 50–1 ■, p. 1566). It is primarily made up of smooth muscle and

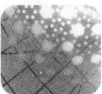

PATIENT TEACHING & DISCHARGE PRIORITIES for Testicular Cancer

Need	Teaching
Knowledge of disease process and prognosis	Home care needs include verbal and written instructions for: 1. The treatment plan, including continued radiation therapy or chemotherapy appointments 2. Follow-up care and appointments with the health care provider 3. Activity restriction.
Understanding of medications	If chemotherapy is to continue, patient/family is taught how to care for the infusion site using aseptic technique. Teach the purpose, dose, timing, and possible side effects of all medications.
Reportable clinical manifestations	Instruct patient/family to report: 1. Bleeding or drainage at the incision site 2. Fever 101°F 3. Signs of deep venous thrombosis 4. Signs of pulmonary embolism or other lung problems.
Patient/family support system	Assess availability of, knowledge of, and compliance with treatment regimen. Assess home environment for need for assistive devices. Assess for need for professional home health services. Offer cancer support resources.
Emotional adjustment of patient/family due to diagnosis of cancer	Answer questions honestly. Encourage verbalization of frustration and anger. Discuss adjustments that will need to be made at home.

collagen enclosed in a fibrous capsule. The urethra passes through the prostate. When semen moves through the prostatic portion of the urethra, the prostate secretes prostatic fluid that increases the pH of semen to help sperm survive in the more acidic female reproductive system (Every, Mikkelsen, & Cagle, 2005). Disorders of the prostate include inflammation, infection, hyperplasia, and cancer. This section discusses each of these disorders.

Prostatitis: Etiology

Inflammation of the prostate gland (**prostatitis**) may be acute, chronic, infectious, or noninfectious. Chronic prostatitis is more common and may persist long after the bacteria are eradicated. In fact, 90% of patients with chronic prostatitis have sterile ejaculate and urine (Goodson, 2006). The National Institutes of Health has developed a consensus classification system for prostatitis, which is outlined in the National Guidelines box.

Acute prostatitis may arise from ascending urinary infection, rectal infection, or bloodborne pathogens. Gram-negative coliforms are the usual causative bacteria, especially *Escherichia coli*,

Proteus, Klebsiella, and enterococci. Less frequently, sexually transmitted *Chlamydia*, ureaplasma (virus), or *Trichomonas* may be the causative agent (Goodson, 2006). Causes of chronic or abacterial prostatitis are not always identifiable. It has been theorized that increased levels of purine, uric acid, or pyrimidine may have gotten into the prostatic ducts causing inflammation. Some health care provider researchers believe it may be an autoimmune disorder (McNaughton Collins, MacDonald, & Wilt, 1999/2008).

Clinical Manifestations

The clinical presentation differs depending on the type of prostatitis the patient has contracted. Chart 50–2 summarizes the symptoms according to prostatitis type.

Laboratory and Diagnostic Procedures

Diagnostic testing for prostatitis would include urinalysis, pre- and postprostatic massage urine, and a digital rectal examination (DRE). For older men, a urine cytology should also be done.

NATIONAL GUIDELINES for the Classification of Prostatitis

   I. Acute bacterial prostatitis

  II. Chronic bacterial prostatitis

 III. Chronic prostatitis/chronic pelvic pain syndrome

 IIIa Inflammatory

 IIIb Noninflammatory

 IV. Asymptomatic inflammatory prostatitis (discovered incidentally)

Source: Adapted from NIH Consensus Classification System for Prostatitis in Prostatitis: Prostate disease (2005). *Merck manual professional*. Retrieved March 30, 2007, from http://www.merck.com/mmpe/sec17/ch240/ch240c.html

---

CHART 50–2 **Clinical Manifestations of Acute and Chronic Prostatitis**

Acute Prostatitis	Chronic Prostatitis
Flu-like symptoms: fever, chills, myalgia, malaise	Recurrent episodes of infection
	Symptoms same but milder
Pain in genitalia, pelvis, or low back	Abacterial prostatodynia
Dysuria, nocturia, urgency, frequency	Pain in pelvis
	Painful ejaculation
Hematuria	
Painful ejaculation	

Sources: Adapted from Porche, D. (2006). Prostatitis. *Journal of Nurse Practitioners, 2*(10), 662–663; and Prostatitis: Prostate disease (2005). *Merck manual professional*. Retrieved March 30, 2007, from http://www.merck.com/mmpe/sec17/ch240/ch240c.html

Prostate Cancer

Clinical Problem

Early diagnosis and treatment of prostate cancer has increased the time the patient and his spouse must cope with treatment regimens for the cancer. These treatments cause severe side effects including fatigue, incontinence, sexual dysfunction, threatened body image, and loss of masculinity. These insults to quality of life have a profound effect on the patient and his wife. Sometimes the health care team does not include the spouse in the patient's care. This can also have a pervasive effect on the wife and the patient. Nurses, especially, should be attuned to the needs of the spouse and assist her whenever possible.

Research Findings

Hawes et al. (2006) conducted a descriptive, cross-sectional study of 66 couples in their homes as part of an experimental intervention program in problem-solving therapy. The spouses of patients were asked to report two problems they believed were important to solve during the study. From this descriptive arm of the study, it was learned that the spouse issue of maintaining a balanced life and emotional wellness was most often listed as a concern. Second most listed was the patient's issue of lack of communication, fear, and depression. The third most frequently listed issue was treatment and side-effect issues.

Implications for Nursing Practice

Wives of men with prostate cancer need support and guidance. Nurses should recognize that the problems wives face when their husbands are ill are not solely from the husband's diagnosis and treatment regimen. Wives should be given the opportunity to discuss problems with balancing their lives and maintaining emotional wellness. If there are problems within the relationship, such as lack of

communication, these could undermine the couple's ability to cope with treatment-related issues. Nurses can begin a discussion with the wife, explore what she finds stressful, and offer problem-solving guidelines.

Anticipating problems when a new treatment regimen is planned and initiating discussions with the patient and his wife will help them both to cope and problem solve.

Critical Thinking Questions

1. Why should spouses of men with prostate cancer be offered support and be included in care planning for the patient?

2. In this descriptive study, the investigators discovered three leading problems identified by the participants. Using these identified problems as a guide, describe the most important points about guiding and nurturing spouses and patients with prostate cancer.
   a. Help the wife balance multiple demands and maintain emotional balance.
   b. Help the wife by anticipating problems and preparing her for challenges.
   c. Initiate discussions with spouses and patients to help them problem solve.
   d. Involve the spouse in medical decision making along with her husband, the patient.

Answers to Critical Thinking Questions appear in Appendix D.

Reference

Hawes, S., Malcarne, V., Ko, C., Sadler, G., Banthia, R., Sherman, S., et al. (2006). Identifying problems faced by spouses and partners of patients with prostate cancer. *Oncology Nursing Forum, 33*(4), 807–814.

EVIDENCE-BASED PRACTICE

The urinalysis is collected in four different sterile containers. The first 10 milliliters of urine is from the urethra, the midstream urine is from the bladder, and the last few drops are premassage prostatic urine. After massage of the prostate, another urinalysis is obtained. All of the urine samples are cultured, with the infective agent to the prostate recovered from the postmassage specimen (Goodson, 2006; Porche, 2006). A prostate-specific antigen (PSA) test may be done. It is expected to be higher and it is nonspecific, but it does give supporting evidence for a diagnosis of prostatitis.

Medical Management

Medical management decisions depend on the type of prostatitis the patient has and the infective agent identified. Bacterial prostatitis is treated with appropriate antibiotics. The Pharmacology Summary feature (p. 1585) gives more details about antibiotic treatment. Antibiotics are given orally for a period of 30 days in an attempt to prevent chronic prostatitis. If the patient becomes septic, he may be admitted for care and be given IV antibiotic therapy until he is afebrile for 24 to 48 hours (Prostatitis: Prostate Disease, 2005). When the patient is discharged, oral therapy will continue for 4 to 6 weeks.

Some health care providers will use other drugs such as alpha blockers, NSAIDs, muscle relaxants, stool softeners, and in the

case of chronic pelvic pain, anxiolytics (Porche, 2006; Prostatitis: Prostate Disease, 2005). Symptomatic treatments may include sitz baths, prostate massage, pelvic floor exercises, and microwave therapy. Microwave therapy is a transurethral heat treatment used more often in benign prostatic hyperplasia, which is discussed later in this chapter.

■ Nursing Management

Nursing care for patients with prostatitis includes education about the disease, the medications used, and the treatments to help decrease pain and swelling of the prostate. If the patient is admitted for sepsis related to prostatitis, IV antibiotic therapy will be given. This will require education of the patient about the medication and its side effects and close monitoring of the patient for signs of worsening condition. The nurse will also help with sitz baths and other comfort measures. When the patient is discharged, he and his family will need education about the disease; the medications; the need to continue the antibiotic for 4 to 6 weeks as prescribed and why; and the importance of follow-up visits with the health care provider. The Patient Teaching & Discharge Priorities box (p. 1574) lists some teaching points important for the patient with prostatitis.

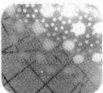

PATIENT TEACHING & DISCHARGE PRIORITIES for Prostatitis

Need	Teaching
Patient/Family/support system	Continue antibiotics as prescribed.
Patient/Family/support system	Report continuation or worsening of symptoms to health care provider.
Patient	Regular voiding and complete emptying of bladder.
Patient	Increase fluids, such as water, to 64 to 128 ounces per day to flush the bladder.
Patient	Avoid beverages and food that are irritating to the bladder: • Alcohol • Caffeine • Citrus juices • Hot/spicy foods.

Benign Prostatic Hyperplasia

Benign prostatic hyperplasia (BPH) is nonmalignant, nodular growth of prostatic tissue that eventually compresses the urethra, causing lower urinary tract symptoms (LUTS) (Beckman & Mynderse, 2005; McVary, 2006). BPH is a common disorder of aging men, occurring in as many as 90% of men ages 85 and older (Kuritzky, Rosenberg, & Sadovsky, 2006; McVary, 2006).

Etiology and Epidemiology

The exact cause of BPH is not known; however, one theory is that BPH may result from a "restart" of the same induction process of the prostate that occurs in the embryo (McVary, 2006). Another theory is that testosterone and estrogens levels change with age (Alper & Crawford, 2005).

Pathophysiology

Nodules form at the transition zone, or innermost aspect of the prostate gland, along the urethra in response to the change in hormones (McVary, 2006). Because the prostate is expandable and elastic, urethral constriction may not occur until the prostate is significantly enlarged. Also, neuronal control over prostatic smooth muscle differs among men, making lower urinary tract symptoms unpredictable.

As the urinary urethra constricts, it causes increased pressure to urinate, thereby causing bladder distention, eventual hypertrophy of the detrusor muscle, bladder diverticula, urinary stasis, infection, and bladder stone formation. If the obstruction is prolonged, **hydronephrosis** (backflow of urine into the renal pelvis) will occur and cause damage to the kidneys (Benign Prostatic Hyperplasia, 2005).

Clinical Manifestations

Clinical manifestations of BPH are varied. Some men who have BPH do not develop lower urinary tract symptoms (LUTS) or acute urinary retention (AUR) (O'Leary, 2006). Others will present with obstructive or irritative symptoms that significantly affect their quality of life. Chart 50–3 lists the signs and symptoms of BPH. The American Urological Association (AUA) has developed a symptom index tool that can be used to quantify the symptoms of BPH for each patient. The AUA Symptom Score is used both in diagnosing and for monitoring therapeutic response. It is a seven-question exploration of symptoms that

---

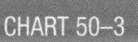

CHART 50–3 **Clinical Manifestations of Benign Prostatic Hyperplasia**

Urinary hesitancy and intermittency

Weak urine stream

Nocturia, frequency, and urgency

Sensation of incomplete bladder emptying

Terminal dribbling of urine

Overflow incontinence

Complete urinary retention

Hematuria if straining at urination is severe

Enlarged, rubbery prostate that has lost the median furrow

Full urinary bladder palpable on abdominal examination

Urinary tract infection

Bladder stones and diverticuli

Renal damage, insufficiency, and failure after prolonged urinary retention

---

Sources: Adapted from Benign prostatic hyperplasia (BPH). (2005). *Merck manual professional.* Retrieved April 4, 2007, from http://www.merck.com/mmpe/sec17/ch240/ch240b.html; O'Leary, M. (2006). Treatment and pharmacologic management of BPH in the context of common comorbidities. *American Journal of Managed Care, 12*(Suppl. 5), S129–S140; and McVary, K. (2006). BPH: Epidemiology and comorbidities. *American Journal of Managed Care, 12*(Suppl. 5), S122–S128.

---

the patient can answer while waiting to be seen. The score allows the health care provider to match treatment options with the severity of the symptoms for each patient (Beckman & Mynderse, 2005; Benign Prostatic Hyperplasia, 2005).

Laboratory and Diagnostic Procedures

Diagnostic testing for BPH begins with the AUA Symptom Index. The next step is history and physical examination, including evaluation for neurological deficits and a digital rectal examination (DRE) of the prostate gland. Chapter 48 🔗 describes the DRE more fully. Other tests that may be used include urinalysis, serum blood urea nitrogen and creatinine, postvoid residual urine measurement, and uroflow rate studies that assess voiding patterns. If hematuria, urinary tract infection, or signs of renal failure are discovered, then renal imaging, urine cytology studies, and cystoscopy may be done (Alper & Crawford, 2005). The prostate-specific antigen (PSA) is sometimes used to differentiate BPH from prostate cancer. The PSA is described more fully in the Cancer of the Prostate section later in this chapter.

Medical Management

Patients who have developed LUTS seek medical advice because of the discomfort. Treatment will depend on the impact on the patient's quality of life, the presence of comorbidities such as diabetes or heart disease, and the severity of the urinary problem (O'Leary, 2006). Treatment modalities vary from watchful waiting to radical surgery.

Medication and Treatments

Patients with mild symptoms who are willing to make some lifestyle changes can usually postpone medical or surgical intervention for a time. Lifestyle changes would include such things as decreasing fluid intake at bedtime to decrease nocturia, decreasing caffeine and alcohol intake because of the irritation to the urinary system, and limiting prescription and over-the-counter drugs that may affect urination (Beckman & Mynderse, 2005; O'Leary, 2006). Chart 50–4 lists medications that may affect urination. Patients who choose watchful waiting are evaluated annually or when worsening symptoms occur.

Medication therapy has replaced surgery as the most common treatment of BPH (Beckman & Mynderse, 2005). Two primary drug types are used to reduce LUTS: alpha-adrenergic antagonists and 5-alpha reductase inhibitors. Alpha-adrenergic antagonists work by relaxing the bladder neck and prostatic muscle tone, thereby relieving obstruction. Newer alpha-adrenergic antagonists selectively reduce the prostatic smooth muscle tone and do not affect the blood pressure (Barry, 2006).

The second class of medication for BPH is the 5-alpha reductase inhibitors that work by reducing the conversion of testosterone. This slows prostate growth; however, it takes 6 to 12

CHART 50–4	**Medications That May Affect Urination**

Diuretics cause urinary frequency.

Sympathomimetic agents such as ephedrine cause increased urethral sphincter contractility.

Anticholinergic drugs such as atropine, Spiriva, and Vesicare cause decreased detrusor contractility.

Antihistamines and antidepressants have caused lower urinary tract symptoms (LUTS) in older men.

Over-the-counter drugs, especially cold remedies, cause LUTS by various mechanisms.

Opiates (Oxymorphone, meperidine) may cause urinary retention and urinary tract spasms.

Skeletal muscle relaxants (methocarbamol) may cause renal impairment.

Sources: Adapted from Alper, B., & Crawford, E. (2005). Benign prostatic hyperplasia. *The Clinical Advisor, 8*(10), 119–121; and Beckman, T., & Mynderse, L. (2005). Evaluation and medical management of benign prostatic hyperplasia. *Mayo Clinic Proceedings, 80*(10), 1356–1362.

months of drug therapy to see the full effect (Beckman & Mynderse, 2005). More about the different drugs used for BPH can be found in the Pharmacology Summary feature (p. 1585).

Many men wanting to prevent or decrease symptoms of BPH choose herbal remedies such as *Pygeum africanum* (African star grass), African plum tree bark, rye grass pollens, stinging nettle, and cactus flower (Buck, 2004). The most popular of the herbal remedies is saw palmetto (*Serenoa repens*). The Complementary and Alternative Therapies box presents some types of alternative therapies that are available. Saw palmetto has been studied in

COMPLEMENTARY & ALTERNATIVE THERAPIES

Types of Therapies

Type of Therapy	Proposed Clinical Use	Nursing Responsibility
Nutriceuticals Vitamin E Vitamin K (para-aminobenzoate) Lycopene, selenium, Vitamin E, calcium, green tea, phytoestrogens	Varied success in treatment of Peyronie's disease. Decrease risk for prostate cancer, under study.	Fat soluble vitamins in excess are harmful. Investigate the amount the patient is taking. Not associated with adverse affects and good for overall health.
Saw palmetto (*Serenoa repens*)	Antiandrogenic, anti-inflammatory, and antiproliferative actions have been claimed. A recent study seems to show there is no difference in lower urinary tract symptoms (LUTS) among men who take this herbal versus placebo.	Ask the patient with prostate problems whether he has been taking saw palmetto. This will cause changes in the prostate-specific antigen (PSA).
Pygeum Africanum	Antiandrogenic action slows growth of prostate; relieves nocturia.	Ask the patient whether he is using this alternative. No adverse effects but questionable efficacy.

Sources: Adapted from Argyriou, A., Chroni, E., Koutras, A., Iconomou, G., et al. (2006). A randomized controlled trial evaluating the efficacy and safety of vitamin E supplementation for protection against cisplatin-induced peripheral neuropathy: Final results. *Supportive Care in Cancer: Official Journal of the Multinational Association of Supportive Care in Cancer, 14*(11), 1134–1140; Bent, S., et al. (2006). Saw palmetto for benign prostatic hyperplasia. *New England Journal of Medicine, 354*(6), 557–566; Buck, A. (2004). Is there a scientific basis for the therapeutic effects of *Serenoa repens* in benign prostatic hyperplasia? Mechanisms of action. *The Journal of Urology, 172*(5, Pt. 1), 1792–1799; Gray, M., & Sims, T. (2006). Prostate cancer: Prevention and management of localized disease. *The Nurse Practitioner, 31*(9), 15–28; Ishani, A., MacDonald, R., Nelson, D., Rutks, J., & Wilt, T. (2000). *Pygeum africanum* for the treatment of patients with benign prostatic hyperplasia: A systematic review and quantitative meta-analysis. *American Journal of Medicine, 109*(8), 654–664; and Peyronie's disease: Penile and scrotal disorders. (2005). *Merck manual professional.* Retrieved March 31, 2007, from http://www.merck.com/mmpe/print/sec17/ch239/ch239f.html

Europe and the United States and has been proven safe. However, a double-blind, randomized trial that included 225 men over age 49 studied the effects of saw palmetto versus placebo and found that the two groups had similar LUTS at the end of 1 year (Bent et al., 2006).

Surgery

Although many men with BPH respond to medication therapy, there are those who do not want to take the medication for life, who are unable to tolerate the medications, or whose prostate continues to enlarge. These men are candidates for more invasive therapy. The mainstay of surgeries for BPH is transurethral resection of the prostate (TURP), wherein a resectoscope is passed through the urethra, a cystoscope is passed through the resectoscope to visualize the bladder and urethra, and a removable loop of resectoscope cuts prostate tissue and coagulates bleeding vessels. Continuous irrigation is needed to prevent blood clotting. Postoperative side effects may include erectile dysfunction, **retrograde ejaculation** (backflow of semen into the bladder at ejaculation), and, in about 1% of cases, incontinence (Benign Prostatic Hyperplasia, 2005; Nickel, 2006).

Transurethral microwave heat treatment (TUMT) and transurethral needle ablation (TUNA) are forms of thermoablation of the prostate. These are alternative operative therapies wherein microwave heat is used to coagulate prostate tissue. A microwave antenna is placed in the urethra and radiofrequency is passed into the prostate via needles. The device is surrounded by a cooling jacket to protect the urethra. These outpatient procedures are cheaper than TURP and there is less bleeding, but heat ablation usually has to be repeated in 1 to 2 years (Goroll & Mulley, 2006; Nickel, 2006).

Other treatments include transurethral vaporization of the prostate (TUVP) and transurethral incision of the prostate (TUIP). In TUVP, the urologist uses laser or electrical vaporization to destroy or remove prostate tissue. TUIP involves making surgical incisions in the prostate to enlarge the urethral opening. TUIP is less destructive than TURP and TUVP, making it a better choice for younger men. It is less likely to cause retrograde ejaculation or erectile dysfunction (Goroll & Mulley, 2006).

Acute urinary retention of BPH can rapidly become an emergent condition, requiring catheterization. If a standard catheter cannot be passed through the urethra, a stiffer catheter may be used. It the blockage still cannot be penetrated, the patient must undergo cystoscopy and the use of dilators to open the urethra and drain the bladder. Eventually, an overfull bladder will cause hydroureter, hydronephrosis, and renal failure (Benign Prostatic Hyperplasia, 2005).

■ Nursing Management

When a patient with BPH comes to the hospital because of LUTS, bladder infection, urinary retention, or hydronephrosis, he is seeking relief and is anxious about any procedures that may have been planned with his health care provider. The nurse will need to do a careful assessment of the patient's condition, elimination patterns, medications, and the patient's knowledge of his condition and any planned procedure. He and his wife or family will need to receive education about the procedure, medications that will be used, and what to expect from the proce-

dure. Preoperative preparation is similar to that of other surgeries and is discussed more fully in Chapter 25 ⊘.

If the patient is admitted with acute urinary retention, catheterization is needed. It is very important to maintain a closed, sterile system while the catheter is in place. As for any patient with a renal or urinary problem, intake and output records should be maintained. Review Chapter 44 ⊘ for care of the patient with urinary impairment.

Postsurgical care following a TURP will include maintenance of continuous bladder irrigation to decrease clot formation and bleeding. A three-way catheter is placed after surgery and a steady flow of saline is used to flush the bladder. The nurse should be sure that the catheter is secured to the patient's thigh with a Velcro strap to prevent injury to the urethra and bladder neck. The irrigation and drainage tubing should be checked often for kinks that would block flow. Clot formation will cause obstruction and fluid retention. If a clot should occlude the catheter, the system can be opened and direct irrigation with saline can be done, but this should be a sterile procedure and avoided unless absolutely necessary.

Monitoring for bleeding is very important. If the output becomes redder, the irrigation should be increased. Bright-red heavy bleeding would indicate an arterial bleed requiring that the health care provider be called.

TURP is painful surgery and bladder spasms occur because the catheter irritates the bladder mucosa (Karlowicz, 1995). The patient should be encouraged not to strain against the catheter or try to urinate around the catheter, as this will increase the spasm. Also, straining at stool will be very uncomfortable for the patient. Analgesia and stool softeners are indicated. Review Chapter 15 ⊘ on pain assessment and treatment for more information about care of patients with postoperative pain.

Prevent infection by keeping the irrigation system closed and cleaning the urinary meatus with soap and water at least twice a day. Monitor the vital signs and the patient for any indication of infection. Encourage increased fluid intake to keep urine output at about 50 milliliters above the irrigation fluid being used. Encourage ambulation and pulmonary toilet as with all patients who have had surgery.

In 24 to 48 hours, the irrigation will stop if the bleeding has stopped. The catheter may be removed in 1 to 5 days (Benign Prostatic Hyperplasia, 2005). The patient should be monitored for urinary retention and assisted as needed when he attempts to void. Some men prefer to stand to void. Some may be able to void if sitting in a warm bath.

Discharge planning and education should begin early so that the patient and his family have time to ask questions. The Patient Teaching & Discharge Priorities box lists the discharge teaching needed for the patient with BPH who has experienced TURP.

Cancer of the Prostate: Etiology and Epidemiology

A man's lifetime risk for prostate cancer is 1 in 6, making this disease the most common cancer in men in the United States and the second leading cause of death. It is estimated that there will be 218,890 new cases and 27,050 deaths due to prostate cancer in 2007 (NCI, 2007a, 2007b). The incidence is increasing as

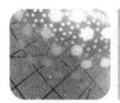

PATIENT TEACHING & DISCHARGE PRIORITIES for Transurethral Resection of the Prostate (TURP) Used to Treat Benign Prostatic Hyperplasia

Need	Teaching

Knowledge of disease process and prognosis	Home care needs including verbal and written instructions for:
	    Urinary incontinence, lower urinary tract symptoms (LUTS), and sexual function will improve.
	    Rest; avoid lifting heavy objects or sitting for long periods.
	    Practice pelvic exercises, stopping urinary stream, and contracting and relaxing pelvic muscles.
	    Follow-up with the health care provider in 1 week.

Understanding of medication	Use of analgesic for bladder pain; how much and how often.
	Purpose, dose, and possible side effects of alpha-adrenergic blocker if ordered for improvement of voiding.
Safety	Pain medication and alpha-adrenergic blocker may cause hypotension.
	Rise slowly and move carefully to avoid falls.
Danger signs	Inability to void, shortness of breath, and bleeding from the urinary tract are signs of emergent conditions; and patient needs to come to the emergency department.
Family/support system	Assess availability of, knowledge of, and compliance with the treatment plan.
	Assess home environment for need of assistive devices.
	Assess for need for professional home health care.
Emotional adjustment	Answer questions honestly.
	Encourage verbalization of frustrations with LUTS.
	Encourage positive reinforcement from the family.

the population ages. In fact, aging is the most powerful risk factor for prostate cancer. African American men have a 60% higher incidence rate of it than do Caucasian men. The Genetic Considerations box outlines the influence of mutated genes on developing prostate cancer. Other risk factors for this cancer are presented in the Risk Factors box.

Pathophysiology

The prostate has three zones: central zone, peripheral zone, and transitional zone. These zones are surrounded by a fibromuscular casing. The peripheral zone, where prostate cancer usually originates, occupies about 70% of the gland. The cause of prostate cancer is unknown (Gray & Sims, 2006).

Prostate cancer occurs in two forms: latent or slow growing and aggressive or fast growing. The aggressive form is more likely to occur in African American and younger men (Gray & Sims, 2006).

Clinical Manifestations

Prostate cancer may be asymptomatic if it is of the slow-growing type. Some men have prostate cancer for many years and die of other causes. Often signs and symptoms are not noticed until

GENETIC CONSIDERATIONS for BRCA2 Mutation

About 10% to 15% of cases of prostate cancer may result from mutated breast cancer genes. BRCA2 mutations are linked with an increased risk for early onset prostate cancer.

Although this association is not as strong as the association between BRCA1 and breast cancer, it is advisable for men with a potential for BRCA2 mutation to begin screening prostate-specific antigen (PSA) and digital rectal examination (DRE) as early as age 40. Men with a brother or father who had prostate cancer are more likely to have the BRCA2 mutation.

Source: Adapted from Lashley, R. (2005). *Clinical genetics in nursing practice* (3rd ed.). New York: Springer.

RISK FACTORS for Prostate Cancer

Age: usually occurs in men over age 65.

Ethnicity: African American men.

Family history: especially father or brother with the disease; 5% to 10% may be due to high-risk inherited gene factors.

Diet: high fat and meat consumption.

Body weight.

Smoking increases risk of fatal prostate cancer.

Sources: Adapted from Gray, M., & Sims, T. (2006). Prostate cancer: Prevention and management of localized disease. *The Nurse Practitioner, 31*(9), 15–28; and National Cancer Institute. (2007d). *Prostate cancer.* Retrieved April 7, 2007, from http://www.cancer.gov/cancertopics/types/prostate

after metastasis has occurred. Chart 50–5 (p. 1578) lists the more common signs and symptoms of prostate cancer.

Diagnostic Testing and Staging

With the advent of prostate-specific antigen (PSA) as a screening tool, many men with asymptomatic, early prostate cancer have been identified. PSA is a serum kinase that originates from the prostate epithelial cells. It is not specific enough to diagnose prostate cancer as a single test and must be used with digital rectal examination (DRE) to increase the likelihood of identifying a cancer. PSA levels less than 4 ng/mL are normal and levels higher than 10 ng/mL have a 67% predictive value for prostate cancer (Mahon, 2005).

An abnormal DRE and an elevated PSA level indicate a need for further testing. A transrectal ultrasound guided biopsy is used to identify and help stage and grade the disease. There is one system for staging and one system for grading: the tumor, node, metastasis (TNM) staging system and the Gleason histologic grading system (Gray & Sims, 2006). Chart 50–6 (p. 1578) outlines the TNM system.

CHART 50–5	**Common Signs and Symptoms of Prostate Cancer**

Frequent urination

Urinary retention

Trouble starting or holding back urine

Weak or interrupted urine stream

Dysuria

Hematuria

Painful ejaculation

Nocturia

Pain in the lower back, hips, or upper thigh if cancer has metastasized

Source: Adapted from National Cancer Institute. (2007d). *Prostate cancer.* Retrieved April 7, 2007, from http://www.cancer.gov/cancertopics/types/prostate

CHART 50–6	**Tumor, Node, Metastasis (TNM) Staging System for Prostate Cancer**

T1 = microscopic, not visible by transrectal ultrasound

T2 = palpable, appears confined to the prostate

T3 = protruding beyond the capsule or into the seminal vesicles

T4 = fixed and extends well beyond the prostate

Source: Adapted from Walsh, P., Retik, A., Vaughan, E., & Wein, A. (Eds.). (2007). *Campbell's urology* (9th ed.). Philadelphia: W. B. Saunders. Cited in Gray, M., & Sims, T. (2006). Prostate cancer: Prevention and management of localized disease. *The Nurse Practitioner, 31*(9), 15–28.

The Gleason grading system is based on histologic patterns in the cellular structure of the prostate. The pathologist looks at the two most common patterns within the sample and gives a grade to the first and second most frequently occurring patterns. This gives a score such as 4 + 3 or 3 + 4 with the 4 + 3 being the sample with the poorest prognosis. Gleason scores of less than 7 indicate a lower risk of metastasis, and scores higher than 7 indicate a higher risk (Gray & Sims, 2006).

The PSA and the Gleason score are used in planning further medical diagnostic testing and intervention (Goroll & Mulley, 2006). If the PSA is greater than 20 ng/mL, then bone metastasis is probable and a bone scan is recommended. CT scans are used only for men whose Gleason scores are over 6.

Medical Management

Once the diagnosis is established and the tests for staging and grading are completed, then the next step is medical intervention. Compounding factors include the patient's age and any comorbidities. If the tumor is slow growing and the patient's life expectancy is affected by other health problems, the decision may be to do nothing or to begin a program of watchful waiting. In this case, a DRE and serum PSA would be done every 3 to 12 months, and the patient would be monitored for LUTS and signs that the cancer may have metastasized. Transrectal ultrasound guided biopsy may be done every 3 years, but these examinations are painful and the patient may choose not to have them done (Gray & Sims, 2006). During this time, lifestyle interventions to improve diet, exercise, and stress management can be instituted. Group support may be helpful, also. The Complementary and Alternative Therapies box discusses the benefits of a healthy lifestyle.

Radiation therapy is used for localized tumors and can be delivered by external beam radiation or implant therapy (brachytherapy). Brachytherapy has fewer side effects than radical surgery or external beam radiation, including less frequent occurrence of erectile dysfunction and urinary incontinence. This therapy will cause swelling of the prostate that will alter urination patterns and can last up to 12 months (Goroll & Mulley, 2006; Zeroski, Abel, Butler, Wallner, & Merrick, 2005). External beam radiation occurs over about 6 weeks, and there are several side effects including cystitis, proctitis, and dermatitis that occur near the end of the treatment period and may last for as much as 6 weeks after the treatments have stopped (Gray & Sims, 2006). External beam radiation is discussed in Chapter 64 👁. Patients who choose either of the radiation treatments have the potential for needing medication to help them to void and reduce the risk of urinary retention. Conversely, these patients may need medication to alleviate frequency and urgency.

If the tumor is the more aggressive type and the patient is younger, he may choose radical **prostatectomy** or removal of the prostate, seminal vesicles, and adjacent tissues. This can be done as open surgery or by laparoscopic or robot-assisted open surgery. Robot-assisted laparoscopic radical prostatectomy offers smaller incisions, less blood loss, and shorter hospital stays but requires a high degree of skill for the surgeon and it is more expensive (Gray & Sims, 2006; Rigdon, 2006).

Hormone therapy (androgen suppression) or orchiectomy is used to decrease the level of testosterone, thereby slowing disease progression (Goroll & Mulley, 2006). This therapy is being used in localized disease and for advanced, symptomatic metastatic disease. Often, it helps to relieve the pain and other symptoms of advanced disease. Medications used to decrease testosterone include estrogen and the Gn-RH agonist. Chemotherapy is a last resort in prostatic cancer. Its use does not seem to alter survival rates significantly (Goroll & Mulley, 2006).

A new development has just been announced by the American Cancer Society. A vaccine called Provenge is being studied and may soon be approved by the United States Food and Drug Administration (FDA) for use in treating advanced prostate cancer. This vaccine is the first to be designed to treat existing cancer. It is made of the patient's own cells and a protein that stimulates the immune system and causes it to attack the cancer. If approved, this vaccine will offer a treatment option for men who have metastatic disease (ACS, 2007).

Treatment guidelines for prostate cancer and support of the senior oncology patient may be accessed via links in the National Guidelines box (p. 1580).

■ Nursing Management

The nurse's role in the diagnostic stage of prostate cancer may include assisting with the diagnostic examinations, education of the patient and his partner about the diagnostic tests and what to expect, physical care postbiopsy, and emotional support. If the patient and his partner should choose watchful waiting, the nurse may educate them concerning the timing of follow-up vis-

COMPLEMENTARY & ALTERNATIVE THERAPIES

Healthy Lifestyle

Description:

Many herbal products claim to enhance male virility and overall health, such as saw palmetto seed. However, these claims have little validation in the scientific research. Considering this absence of evidence-based data on herbal products, the best approach to ensuring optimal male reproductive health includes the well-validated behaviors of regular exercise, weight management, and a healthy diet.

Research Support:

The lifestyle habits of smoking and obesity cause a large burden of disease, including a negative impact on male reproductive health. However, one study showed that, although eliminating smoking and obesity does increase good health, it may not absolutely reduce morbidity (van Baal, Hoogenveen, de Wit, & Boshuizen, 2006).

Another study evaluated the effects of changes in health behaviors including reduction in dietary fat intake, increase in exercise, and stress management on coronary risks and psychosocial factors. Over the course of 3 months, 869 nonsmoking CHD patients enrolled in the health insurance-based Multisite Cardiac Lifestyle Intervention Program. Results showed that patients experienced a significant overall improvement in coronary risk as well as perceived stress and hostility. These results suggest that multicomponent programs that focus on diet, exercise, and stress management may benefit patients (Daubenmier et al., 2007).

The Health Professionals Follow-up Study monitored 42,847 men for a period of 16 years. Participants, who were from 40 to 75 years of age and free of disease, completed questionnaires that assessed five lifestyle factors that were identified as low risk. The five lifestyle factors were (1) the absence of smoking, (2) body mass index less than 25 kg/m², (3) moderate-to-vigorous activity of at least 30 minutes per day, (4) moderate alcohol consumption of 5 to 30 grams per day, and (5) the top 40% of the distribu-

tion for a healthy diet score. Over the course of the study, researchers found that men who were at low risk for these five lifestyle factors had a lower risk of coronary heart disease (CHD) as compared to men who were at low risk for no lifestyle factors. Sixty-two percent of coronary events in this cohort may have been prevented with better adherence to these 5 healthy lifestyle practices. Among men taking medication for hypertension or high cholesterol, 57% of all coronary events may have been prevented with a low-risk lifestyle. Compared to men who did not make lifestyle changes, those who adopted at least two additional low-risk lifestyle factors had a 27% lower risk of CHD. Results showed that adherence to lifestyle practices including exercise, weight management, not smoking, moderate alcohol consumption, and a healthy diet may prevent a majority of CHD events among U.S. men. In addition, men that are healthier as a result of these lifestyle behaviors will likely have better reproductive health (Chiuve, McCullough, Sacks, & Rimm, 2006).

References

Chiuve, S. E., McCullough, M. L., Sacks, F. M., & Rimm, E. B. (2006). Healthy lifestyle factors in the primary prevention of coronary heart disease among men: Benefits among users and nonusers of lipid-lowering and antihypertensive medications. *Circulation, 114*(2), 160–167.

Daubenmier, J. J., Weidner, G., Sumner, M. D., Mendell, N., Merritt-Worden, T., Studley, J., et al. (2007). The contribution of changes in diet, exercise, and stress management to changes in coronary risk in women and men in the multisite cardiac lifestyle intervention program. *Annals of Behavioral Medicine, 33*(1), 57–68.

van Baal, P. H., Hoogenveen, R. T., de Wit, G. A., & Boshuizen, H. C. (2006). Estimating health-adjusted life expectancy conditional on risk factors: Results for smoking and obesity. *Population Health Metrics, 4*, 14l.

---

its with the health care provider for DRE, PSA, and transrectal ultrasound (TRUS) guided biopsy. The nurse may also guide the patient in improving his diet, exercise regimen, and stress management. Referrals to groups in the local community for support of patients with newly diagnosed prostate cancer would also be appropriate. See Evidenced-Based Practice box on page 1573.

Patients with prostate cancer may be seen in the emergency department for urinary retention. The nurse's role here is to offer emotional support, to educate about the catheter's being used to relieve the retention, and the need for slowed release of urine from a distended bladder. The patient and his partner will need emotional support and education about the catheter and the use of any incontinence pads or devices.

When the medical plan is for radiation therapy in the form of external beam radiation or brachytherapy, the nurse's role will be teaching about the procedure and the side effects. Chapter 64 discusses the various types of radiation therapy. The patient and his partner should be alert to signs of urinary retention secondary to prostate swelling and should seek care immediately if it occurs. The patient will need education about proctitis, cystitis, and dermatitis and demonstrations on how to use the skin protectant and the medications ordered (see the Pharmacology Summary feature, p. 1585).

Radical prostatectomy may be chosen. In this event, the preoperative preparation is much the same as for other surgeries.

Refer to Chapter 25 for preoperative preparation. The patient will need to know about the use of the suprapubic catheter and the pain management plan for him. He will need emotional support as he faces some of the complications such as urinary incontinence, erectile dysfunction (depending on the operative approach), possible rectal injury, and anal damage. Urinary incontinence is most likely right after surgery and will improve over the next 6 months to 2 years by about 50% (Gray & Sims, 2006).

Reinforcement of education and repeated information is needed for the anxious patient and his partner. The diagnosis is a difficult one and will change their lives substantially. His body image is changing and the patient will have many life adjustments to make.

Hormone therapy or orchiectomy may be done if the cancer has spread beyond the prostate. If orchiectomy is chosen, the surgery is quick and usually recovery goes well. The loss of the testicles, however, may have a profound effect on the patient. The loss of masculinity can mean depression due to altered body image and function. Hormone therapy in the form of diethylstilbestrol or luteinizing hormone-releasing hormone agonists will lower the testosterone level, but the side effects may be further debilitating to the patient. The nurse can help find ways of decreasing the side effects and offer support to the couple as they cope with the changes.

NATIONAL GUIDELINES for Treatment and Support of Patients with Prostate Cancer

Principles of Expectant Management

Expectant management means that active monitoring of the course of the disease with the expectation to intervene if the cancer progresses.
Localize cancer monitoring includes:

- Digital rectal exam (DRE) and prostate-specific antigen (PSA) every 6 months, or at least every 12 months.
- Needle biopsy of prostate may be repeated within 6 months of diagnosis if initial biopsy was < 10 cores or palpable tumor contralateral to the side of the positive biopsy.
- Needle biopsy of the prostate may be repeated within 18 months of diagnosis if initial biopsy was > 10 cores.

Cancer progression may have occurred if:

- Primary Gleason grade 4 or 5 is found with repeat prostate biopsy.
- Prostate cancer is found in a greater number of prostate biopsies or occupies a greater extent of prostate biopsies.
- PSA doubling time < 3 or PSA velocity is > 0.75.

A repeat prostate biopsy is indicated for signs of disease progression by exam or PSA.
Advantages of expectant management:

- Avoid unnecessary therapy and its side effects
- Quality of life maintained
- Risk of unnecessary treatment of small, indolent cancers is reduced

Disadvantages of expectant management:

- Chance of missed-opportunity for cure
- Risk of progression and/or metastases
- Subsequent treatment may be more intense with increased side effects
- Nerve sparing may be more difficult, which may reduce chance of potency preservation after surgery
- Increased anxiety
- Requires frequent medical exam and periodic biopsies
- Uncertain long-term history of prostate cancer

Source: National Comprehensive Cancer Network. (2008). *Clinical practice guidelines in oncology: Prostate cancer* [V.1.2008]. Retrieved August 11, 2008, from http://www.nccn.org/professionals/physician_gls/PDF/prostate.pdf

---

Chemotherapy may be needed if the patient's disease has spread to other organs. Nursing care for cancer patients is discussed in Chapter 64 ∞.

The Nursing Process: Patient Care Plan feature provides further information about treating a patient who has undergone radical prostatectomy. Refer to the Patient Teaching & Discharge Priorities box for information on discharge planning after radical prostatectomy (p. 1584).

Collaborative Management

Prostate cancer is a complex disease and requires a team approach for optimal care. The urologist is assisted by nurses, the oncologist, anesthesiologists, nutritionists, counselors, and community resources. Open communication between specialties will facilitate the best care possible for the patient. The health care team should include the spouse or partner and the patient's family in all aspects of the plan of care.

The urologist is a specialist in the care of patients with renal and urinary disorders. The urologist is the team leader and responsible for surgery. Nurses assist in the many roles discussed earlier. The oncologist, a specialist in chemotherapy and radia-

tion treatment for cancer, will be called if the tumor has grown outside the prostate and metastasized to other organs. Anesthesiologists direct the general anesthesia or epidurals needed during surgery or as a palliative measure for severe pain. Nutritionists help the patient and his spouse to choose nutritious foods that help in healing and restoration of the body. Counselors help the couple to cope with this stressful life event. The counselor may help with problem-solving methods, stress relief, or biofeedback and relaxation techniques. Community resources include the different institutions that offer information and support groups, such as the American Cancer Society and the National Cancer Institute. Other community resources may be home health care, physical therapy, massage therapists, and local support groups for the spouse or the couple.

Penile Disorders

There are a number of penile disorders, many of which may cause an alteration in sexual functioning. Treatment for the various disorders may range from simple medication to radical surgery. Psychological counseling is an integral part of the treatment and follow-up phases of care for patients with these conditions. The most common penile disorders are discussed in this section.

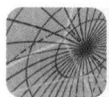

NURSING PROCESS: Patient Care Plan for Prostate Cancer After Radical Prostatectomy

Assessment of Anxiety and Fear

Subjective Data:
Tell me about your concerns.
Are you concerned that treatments may affect your quality of life?
Do you understand your diagnosis?
Do you understand your health care provider's plan for you?
Who are your support people?
Have you ever had cancer before?
How have you coped with stress in the past?
Are you aware that there will be a loss of sexual function that may or may not be permanent?

Objective Data:
Body language: look of concern or anguish

Nursing Assessment and Diagnoses	Outcomes and Evaluation Parameters	Planning and Interventions with *Rationales*
Nursing Diagnoses: *Anxiety* related to diagnosis, treatment plan, and prognosis *Ineffective Sexuality Pattern* related to prostate cancer and treatments *Disturbed Body Image* related to diagnosis, orchiectomy, and side effects of other treatments	**Outcome:** Reduced stress and improved ability to cope. *Evaluation Parameters:* Appears more relaxed. States that he feels less anxious. Reiterates information about diagnosis, treatment, and prognosis in calm manner.	**Interventions and *Rationales:*** Clarify information and help patient to cope by helping him to understand. *Often anxious patients are not able to understand as well.* Be there for him. *Quiet presence helps alleviate fear.* Offer support and open communication with him and his partner. *An atmosphere of acceptance and openness will help him to be more willing to talk.* Answer questions honestly and reiterate information often and in concrete terms. *Anxiety reduces cognition.* Encourage him to verbalize his concerns about sex and changes in his physical appearance. *Verbalizing fear is the first step in alleviating fear.*

Assessment of Pain

Subjective Data:
Do you have pain?
Where is the pain?
Is it getting worse?
On a pain scale of 1–10, with 10 being the worst, how would you rate your pain?
Assess gender, cultural, and religious impact on patient response to pain.

Objective Data:
Body language, facial grimace, confusion, and anxiety may be signs of pain

Nursing Assessment and Diagnoses	Outcomes and Evaluation Parameters	Planning and Interventions with *Rationales*
Nursing Diagnosis: *Readiness for Enhanced Comfort* related to postoperative prostatectomy pain	**Outcome:** Comfort level maintained. *Evaluation Parameters:* Patient will be able to communicate pain level and therapies that help alleviate it. Pain reduced and/or absent as evidenced by patient report and no pain behaviors. Nonpharmacologic method of pain control is effective, as evidenced by patient report and no pain behaviors. Patient reports satisfaction with pain management.	**Interventions and *Rationales:*** Instruct patient not to strain against the catheter in an attempt to void. *Straining will cause bladder spasms and increased pain.* Instruct patient to inform the nurse if the pain is not relieved. *Indicates need to change pain management plan.* Obtain clear description of location of pain. *To assist in developing a pain management plan.* Provide supportive atmosphere so that patient is comfortable asking for assistance with pain. *Open communications facilitate pain management.* Ask the patient about pain and encourage him to use the pain medication prescribed. *Men are more stoic and less likely to request medication for pain.* Use pain control measures before pain becomes severe. *To increase comfort, decrease anxiety, and decrease need for pain medication.* Record patient response to pain medication. *Record of relief or lack of relief helps health care team plan for better pain relief.*

(continued)

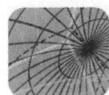

Assessment of Knowledge

Subjective Data:

Tell me what you understand about the surgery planned for you.

Have you had surgery before?

Do you know what to expect after surgery?

What is your understanding about the catheter used after surgery?

Do you know how to use an incentive spirometer?

Do you know how to use support hose?

Objective Data:

Patient unable to answer questions correctly

Patient asks questions that indicate lack of knowledge

Nursing Assessment and Diagnoses	Outcomes and Evaluation Parameters	Planning and Interventions with *Rationales*
Nursing Diagnosis: *Deficient Knowledge* related to the treatment plan and care needs	**Outcome:** Patient will be more cooperative and willing to participate in his care. **Evaluation Parameters:** Patient verbalizes understanding of surgical procedure planned. Patient verbalizes understanding of need for pulmonary toilet, support hose, early ambulation, and need for catheter, and the pain management plan. Patient demonstrates use of incentive spirometer. Patient verbalizes understanding of how to use and why to use support hose.	**Interventions and *Rationales:*** Provide education in simple terms. *Simplicity enhances the anxious patient's ability to learn.* Explain what to expect with surgery and the recovery period. *Knowledge assists the patient to be less fearful.* Explain that the urinary catheter is also a splint to help maintain the surgical reconnection of the urethra. *Knowing the reason for the catheter increases tolerance of the discomfort.* Explain what will be experienced. *Knowing a little about how it will feel will reduce fear.* Allow to ask questions. *Open communication enhances learning.* Allow patient to become familiar with spirometer. *Handling equipment makes it familiar and easier to use after surgery.* Demonstrate how support hose are used. *Support hose are used to help prevent thrombosis and pulmonary embolism.*

Assessment of Urinary Elimination

Subjective Data:

Preoperative:

    What is your usual pattern of urination?

    When was the last time you voided?

    Does your bladder feel full?

    Are you dribbling urine?

Postoperative:

    Is the catheter uncomfortable?

Objective Data:

Preoperative:

    Bladder distention, dribbling urine, or incontinence

Postoperative:

    Yellow, pink-tinged urine

    Catheter and tubing intact and free of kinks

    Catheter secured to inner thigh

Nursing Assessment and Diagnoses	Outcomes and Evaluation Parameters	Planning and Interventions with *Rationales*
Nursing Diagnosis: *Urinary Retention* due to urethral obstruction secondary to prostate enlargement	**Outcome:** Normal urinary output. **Evaluation Parameters:** Preoperative: Urinary retention relieved. Patient is dry and comfortable. Postoperative: Output at 50 milliliters or more per hour. Balance to intake and output. No retention related to kinks in catheter tubing. Patient does not strain against catheter. Catheter is secured to inner thigh at all times.	**Interventions and *Rationales:*** Preoperative: Usual pattern gives baseline. *Return to usual pattern is goal to work toward.* Relieve urinary retention. *Urinary retention will cause damage to the bladder, and, if severe and prolonged, hydroureter, hydronephrosis, and renal failure.* Postoperative: Maintain strict intake and output records. *High output is needed to clear blood from bladder to prevent clots and obstruction. Output less than intake indicates retention.* Monitor color and amount of output. *Increased bleeding must be identified early and corrected.* Keep catheter secured to thigh and prevent dislodging. *Dislodging the catheter can cause damage to the urethra anatomosis or bladder neck.* Keep tubing coiled on the bed and free of kinks. *To facilitate urine flow and prevent obstruction.* Use incontinence pads and other equipment to keep patient dry. *Urine is irritating and can cause skin breakdown.*

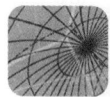

NURSING PROCESS: Patient Care Plan for Prostate Cancer After Radical Prostatectomy—*Continued*

Assessment of Bowel Elimination

Subjective Data:
When was your last BM?
Are you using a stool
softener or laxatives?

Objective Data:
Frequency and consistency of bowel movements
Type and amount of stool softeners and/or laxatives

Nursing Assessment and Diagnoses	Outcomes and Evaluation Parameters	Planning and Interventions with *Rationales*
Nursing Diagnosis: Potential for Pain, Acute, related to Constipation and straining at stool	**Outcome:** Regular bowel movement (BM) without straining. *Evaluation Parameter:* Patient reports regular BM that is soft and passed without straining.	**Intervention and *Rationale:*** Administer stool softener and encourage increased fluids. *Straining at stool can cause bleeding and increased pain.*

Assessment of Skin and Fluid Volume

Subjective Data:
Have you had problems with urine leaking from your catheter?
Are you able to keep you skin dry?
Are you thirsty?
Does your urine appear concentrated?
Have you had a fever or chills?
Does your urine appear cloudy or clear?

Objective Data:
Inspect skin exposed to urine or tape
Inspect incision and catheter site
Vital signs

Nursing Assessment and Diagnoses	Outcomes and Evaluation Parameters	Planning and Interventions with *Rationales*
Nursing Diagnoses: *Risk for Impaired Skin Integrity* related to urinary incontinence *Risk for Infection* related to surgery and urinary retention *Risk for Deficient Fluid Volume* related to blood loss	**Outcomes:** No skin breakdown. No infection at the incision. *Evaluation Parameters:* Skin is intact. Patient has no complaints of skin itching or burning. Vital signs are normal for the patient.	**Interventions and *Rationales:*** Inspect skin. Keep skin clean and dry. *Clean, dry skin does not break down.* Monitor surgical wound and drain sites for infection or signs of healing. *Early identification of infection decreases morbidity.* Monitor vital signs for elevated temperature. *Indication of infection.* Monitor pulse and blood pressure for signs of blood loss. *High pulse and lower blood pressure indicate blood loss.* Assist in early ambulation. *Ambulation improves circulation and enhances healing.*

Phimosis and Paraphimosis

Phimosis occurs when a tight foreskin cannot be retracted over the penile glans (Figure 50–5 ■, p. 1586). Phimosis is usually the result of inflammation or infection secondary to poor hygiene. Treatment includes antibiotics for infection and circumcision if the phimosis interferes with urination (Every, Mikkelsen, & Bailey, 2005).

Paraphimosis occurs when a retracted foreskin becomes trapped over the glans (see Figure 50–5 ■, p. 1586). The retracted foreskin causes a tourniquet effect, decreasing the circulation to the glans. Swelling develops swiftly, further tightening the foreskin band. Compressing the glans and moving the foreskin forward should be attempted as soon as possible. If the foreskin cannot be manually reduced, circumcision is needed and may have to be done as an emergency procedure to prevent ischemia and necrosis of the glans (Every, Mikkelsen, & Bailey, 2005).

Nursing care includes education about hygiene, emotional support, monitoring vital signs for evidence of a worsening condition, and administration of analgesics. Circumcision is usually an outpatient surgery and does not require hospitalization.

Peyronie's Disease

Peyronie's disease is a penile condition where palpable, fibrous plaque forms on the corpora cavernosa. The plaque will cause abnormal curvature of the penis and painful, incomplete erections. Peyronie's disease affects middle-aged and older men (Figure 50–6 ■, p. 1586). The cause is unknown.

There are no completely effective treatments for this condition. Limited success has occurred with vitamin E and aminobenzoate potassium (Potaba). Alternative therapies may be helpful. Surgery is a last resort, but removing the plaque and repairing the corpora cavernosa with a graft has offered relief of pain (Every, Mikkelsen, & Bailey, 2005).

Nursing management would include emotional support, education about the condition and medications used, preoperative care, and postoperative care for those who have surgery. If the surgery is extensive, a suprapubic catheter may be placed so that the penis can heal more quickly.

Urethral Stricture

The urethra is the most distal portion of the urinary tract (see Figure 50–1 ■, p. 1566). It allows urine and semen to pass out of the body. Stricture within the urethra may occur as the result of trauma, an enlarged or nodular prostate, instrumentation, or infection that causes scarring. Strictures will block the flow of urine and ejaculate. Urinary retention may result, and if the stricture is severe enough, hydronephrosis may result. Signs and

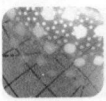

PATIENT TEACHING & DISCHARGE PRIORITIES for Prostate Cancer After Radical Prostatectomy

Need	Teaching
Knowledge of self-care and need for follow-up visit with health care provider	Home care needs including verbal and written instructions for: May go home with catheter in place. Needs education about home including maintaining patency of the tubing and cleansing the urinary meatus. Urinary incontinence may follow removal of catheter but will improve. Rest; avoid lifting heavy objects, sitting for long periods, or straining at stool. Maintain increased oral intake at about 2–3 quarts a day, unless medically contraindicated. Practice pelvic exercises, stopping urinary stream, and contracting and relaxing pelvic muscles. Follow-up with the health care provider in 1 to 3 weeks.
Understanding of medication	Use of analgesic and antimuscarinic for bladder pain; how much and how often and what the side effects may be. Purpose, dose, and possible side effects of alpha-adrenergic blocker if ordered for improvement of voiding.
Safety	Pain medication and alpha-adrenergic blocker may cause hypotension. Rise slowly and move carefully to avoid falls.
Danger signs	If the catheter comes out before it is supposed to, if unable to void after the catheter is removed, if patient experiences any shortness of breath, bleeding from the urinary tract, or high fever, he should be sent to his health care provider.
Family/support system	Assess availability of, knowledge of, and compliance with the treatment plan. Assess home environment for need of assistive devices. Assess for need for professional home health care. Seek support groups for spouse or partner to help her cope. Respite care may be needed.
Emotional adjustment	Answer questions honestly. Encourage verbalization of frustrations and fears. Encourage positive reinforcement from the family.
Institutional and community resources and support groups	Suggest National Cancer Institute, American Cancer Society as resources. Offer community-based programs and support group addresses and phone numbers.

symptoms include decreased urinary stream, spraying of urine, urethral discharge, bladder infection secondary to retrograde urination, and urinary retention. Diagnosis is made by cystoscopy or urethrography (Every, Mikkelsen, & Bailey, 2005).

Medical management includes surgical procedures to dilate or reconstruct the urethra. These procedures may be done under general or epidural anesthesia on an outpatient basis. Chapter 47 includes a discussion of the treatment for urinary disorders.

Nursing care depends on the extent of the stricture and surgical procedures to correct the stricture. Most of the patients will need pre- and postoperative teaching, analgesia, careful monitoring of vital signs, and observation for bleeding or drainage. See Chapter 15 for information about pain assessment and management. Many of these patients need emotional support if the stricture has become severe enough to warrant surgery.

Epispadias

An epispadias is an abnormal urethral opening on the dorsal or top of the penile shaft just under the urinary bladder. It is a congenital condition that usually occurs with exstrophy of the bladder where the abdominal wall fails to form below the umbilicus (Every, Mikkelsen, & Bailey, 2005).

Medical management involves staged surgical procedures to reconstruct the bladder and urethra. Usually these repairs are completed by school age, but if the congenital disorder was severe, particularly with exstrophy of the bladder, there may be problems with incontinence, impotence, and fertility.

Nursing management includes emotional support of the child and his parents, education, and preoperative and postoperative care. Chapter 47 includes a discussion of the treatment for urinary disorders.

Hypospadias: Etiology

Hypospadias is a congenital disorder wherein the urinary opening occurs on the ventral or lower portion of the penis. Embryonic development of the male urethra begins as a cleft in the genital area during gestation at about 8 to 14 weeks of life. Incomplete closure of the cleft will cause the meatus to occur anywhere along the lower penis, including the scrotum and the perineum (Carmichael et al., 2005).

Medical management includes staged reconstruction of the penis. For those infants in which the meatus occurs on the scrotum or perineum, studies are conducted to determine whether there is insufficient masculinization (Every, Mikklesen, & Bailey, 2005).

Nursing care includes emotional support of the baby and his parents, education about the defect, and preoperative and postoperative care. Chapter 47 includes a discussion of the treatment for urinary disorders.

PHARMACOLOGY Summary of Medications to Treat Male Reproductive Disorders

Medication Category	Action	Application/Indication	Nursing Responsibility
Antibiotics: Macrolides (Biaxin) Penicillin (Pen-Vee K) Fluoroquinolones (Cipro) Trimethoprim-sulfamethoxazole (Bactrim) Doxycycline (Doryx) Specific type depends on causative agent.	Varies with antibiotic; may be bactericidal or bacteristatic.	Used for infections of susceptible organisms including sexually transmitted infection, epididymitis, orchitis, prostatitis, coliforms, and any postoperative infections.	Assess for drug allergies before beginning any antibiotic. Assess for any manifestation of allergic reaction. Assess for improvement of symptoms, especially decreased fever and pain. Educate patient concerning importance of completing full course of antibiotics.
Nonsteroidal anti-inflammatory agents (NSAIDs): Ibuprofen (Advil) Naproxen sodium (Aleve)	Prostaglandin synthetase inhibition.	Used for fever reduction, for pain relief, and for decreasing inflammation.	Assess for drug allergies before beginning any drug. Give with food. Assess for gastrointestinal side effects, including ulcer and gastrointestinal (GI) bleeding. Assess for relief of symptoms.
Chemotherapy: Cisplatin (Platinol-AQ) Bleomycin (Blenoxane), Etoposide (Toposar)	Alkylates DNA, RNA; inhibits enzymes that allow synthesis of amino acids in proteins; activity is not cell cycle phase specific.	Used for testicular cancer.	Assess for drug allergies. Prepare for anaphylactic reaction with first dose. Monitor renal and liver function tests for abnormalities related to chemotherapy side effects. Side effects of cisplatin include nausea, vomiting, alopecia, fatigue, neutropenia, azoospermia, peripheral neuropathy, and ototoxicity. Bleomycin may cause fibrosis, pneumonitis, and lung toxicity. Etoposide may cause hepatotoxicity and nephrotoxicity.
Antiemetics and antidiarrheals (especially for side effects of chemotherapy): Ondansetron (Zofran)	Ondansetron blocks serotonic 5-HT3 receptor, decreasing nausea. Antidiarrheals work directly at intestinal muscle to decrease peristalsis or increase bulk.	Side effects of chemotherapy include vomiting and diarrhea. Ondansetron (Zofran) has been especially efficacious for this type of nausea.	Assess for drug allergies. Assess for untoward effects such as headache and dizziness. Assess for relief of symptoms.
Benign Prostatic Hyperplasia			
Alpha blockers: Doxazosin (Cardura) Terazosin (Hytrin) Tamsulosin (Flomax) Alfuzosin (Uroxatral) 5-Alpha reductase inhibitors: Finasteride (Proscar) Dutasteride (Avodart)	Alpha blockers work by relaxing the bladder neck and prostatic smooth muscle tone. Blocks conversion of testosterone to androgen, thereby decreasing size of the prostate.	Improves urinary flow; relieves hesitancy, urgency, and frequency. Blocks conversion of testosterone to potent androgen, thereby reducing size and growth of prostate. More efficacious for men with larger prostates.	Assess for drug allergies. Monitor blood pressure and heart rate. Assess for side effects such as dizziness, headache, and nausea. Observe for improvement of symptoms. Warn patients to limit Viagra to 25 milligrams at least 4 hours before or after using alpha blockers. Assess for allergies before administering. Monitor for side effects such as decreased libido, ejaculatory problems, and lower prostate-specific antigen (PSA) levels.
Medications for Side Effects of Radiation Therapy			
Antimuscarinics: Tolterodine (Detrol LA) Oxybutynin (Ditropan) Phenazopyridine (Baridium) Trypsin, castor oil, and balsam of Peru (Xenaderm)	Relaxes smooth muscle in urinary tract: Exerts analgesic, anesthetic action on the urinary mucosa. Antispasmodic. Skin protectant.	Radiation cystitis: helps relieve frequency and urgency. Relieves discomfort of bladder irritation. For relief of proctitis symptoms. Skin irritation due to radiation. Soothes and promotes healing.	Assess for allergies to any drugs. Monitor for side effects. Assess for relief of symptoms. Encourage diet low in irritants such as coffee, spicy foods, and alcohol. Encourage diet high in fluid intake and roughage to keep stool soft and movements regular.

(continued)

PHARMACOLOGY Summary of Medications to Treat Male Reproductive Disorders—*Continued*

Medication Category	Action	Application/Indication	Nursing Responsibility
Hormone Therapy for Prostate Cancer			
Diethylstilbesterol (DES) Leuprolide Eligard® Lupron® Lupron Depot®	Antiandrogen. Luteinizing hormone-releasing hormone agonist.	Slows or stops prostate cancer growth by lowering androgen levels to those of castration. Lowers androgen levels to those similar to castration.	Monitor for side effects: feminization and loss of libido. Erectile dysfunction. Explain side effects. Help patient find ways to cope. Monitor for side effects such as hot flashes, impotence, and loss of libido.

Sources: Adapted from Barry, M. (2006). Approach to benign prostatic hyperplasia. In A. Goroll & A. Mulley, *Primary care medicine: Office evaluation and management of the adult patient* (5th ed., pp. 909–914). Philadelphia: Lippincott Williams & Wilkins; Gray, M., & Sims, T. (2006). Prostate cancer: Prevention and management of localized disease. *The Nurse Practitioner, 31*(9), 15–28; Kuritzky, L., Rosenberg, M., & Sadovsky, R. (2006). Efficacy and safety of alfuzosin 10 mg once daily in the treatment of symptomatic benign prostatic hyperplasia. *International Journal of Clinical Practice, 60*(3), 351–358; National Cancer Institute (NCI). (2007d). *Treatment choices for men with early-stage prostate cancer.* Retrieved April 9, 2007, from http://www.cancer.gov/cancertopics/prostatecancer-treatment-choices.; RxList the Internet Drug Index. (2007a). *Cisplatin.* Retrieved March 31, 2007, from http://www.rxlist.com/cgi/generic/cisplatin_ids.htm; RxList the Internet Drug Index. (2007b). *Motrin.* Retrieved March 31, 2007, from http://www.rxlist.com/cgi/generic/ibup.htm; RxList the Internet Drug Index. (2007c). *Zofran injection.* Retrieved March 31, 2007, from http://www.rxlist.com/cgi/generic/ondansetron.htm; and Wilt, T., Howe, R., & Rutks, I. (2000). Terazosin for benign prostatic hyperplasia. *Cochrane Database Systematic Reviews 2000.* In *The Cochrane Library,* 2007, Issue 1. Retrieved March 31, 2007, from www.thecochranelibrary.com

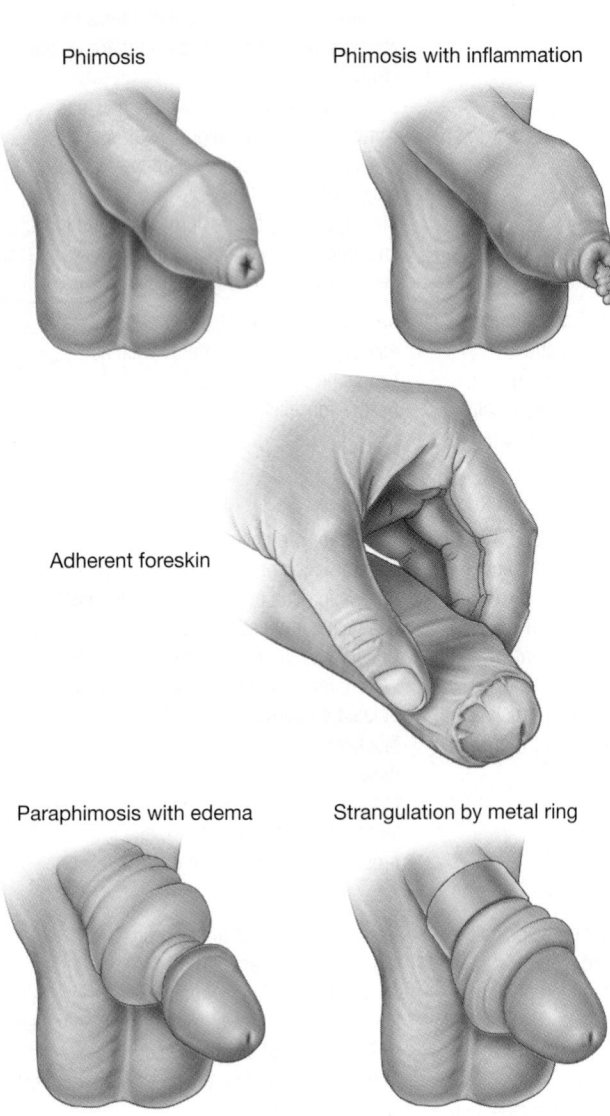

Phimosis

Phimosis with inflammation

Adherent foreskin

Paraphimosis with edema

Strangulation by metal ring

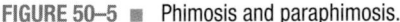

FIGURE 50–5 ■ Phimosis and paraphimosis.

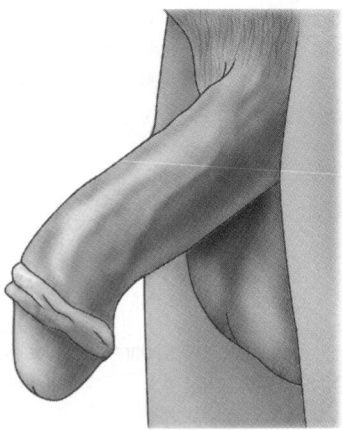

FIGURE 50–6 ■ Peyronie's disease.

Penile and Scrotal Injuries

Men are more likely than women to experience genital trauma. Scrotal injuries may be the result of infections, burns, or gunshot wounds. Testicular injuries are more likely to be blunt trauma that may cause hematoma or even rupture of the testicle. Penile injuries may occur from pant zippers, amputations, animal bites, gunshot wounds, battlefield injuries, or ruptures of the corpus cavernosum caused by severe bending of the penis during an erection (Genital Trauma: Genitourinary Tract Traumas, 2005/2007).

Medical care includes identification of the extent of the injury and surgical repair as needed. Antibiotic therapy and analgesia will be needed. Nursing care depends on the extent of the injury. Preoperative and postoperative education and emotional support are imperative.

Cancer of the Penis

Penile cancer is very rare in North America and Europe, accounting for approximately 0.2% of cancers in men and 0.1% of cancer deaths in men in the United States. Penile cancer is more common in some parts of Africa and South America, where it accounts for up to 10% of cancers in men (American Cancer Society, 2008). More than 95% of penile carcinomas are squamous cell carcinomas (Goodman, Hernandez, & Shvetsov, 2007).

Causes of the various types of penile cancer are not known. Research has shown that two proteins produced by high-risk human papillomavirus can interfere with tumor suppressor genes, thereby allowing cancer to grow (ACS, 2007). Risk factors for penile cancer are listed in the Risk Factors box.

Medical care for penile cancer is usually surgery. This may be circumcision or laser ablation for smaller lesions or partial or total **penectomy** (removal of part of or the entire penis) for larger lesions. Radiation therapy is used if the cancer has not spread beyond the local lymph nodes. Chemotherapy is used when the cancer is widely spread, with little success (Penile Cancer: Genitourinary Cancer, 2005).

Nursing care depends on the extent of the cancer. Preoperative and postoperative education and emotional support are imperative. Care of the patient undergoing cancer treatment is discussed in detail in Chapter 64 .

Sexual Functioning

In order to impregnate a female, a male must have normal **spermatogenesis** (the manufacture of normal sperm in high numbers), and he must have the ability to transmit the sperm into a woman's vagina. This means that he needs to be able to have and sustain an erection and to have a normal ejaculation (Hatcher et al., 2004). If a male does not want to produce children but wishes to continue sexual relations, he can use condoms or undergo sterilizing surgery called vasectomy. This section will explore selected topics related to male sexual function, including erectile dysfunction, male infertility, andropause, and vasectomy.

Erectile Dysfunction

Erectile dysfunction (ED) is the inability to achieve or sustain an erection firm enough for intercourse. In the United States, it is estimated based on imprecise data that 10 to 20 million men over age 18 have had at least a few instances of ED. The prevalence increases to 50% of men aged 40 to 70 (Male Sexual Dysfunction, 2005).

Epidemiology and Etiology

ED may be primary (a man has never achieved erection) or secondary (a man has had erections but is no longer able). It is estimated that about 80% of ED events are physiological and the remaining events have a psychological cause, including but not

limited to guilt, depression, performance anxiety, and fear of intimacy (Male Sexual Dysfunction, 2005).

The major organic causes include diabetes, stroke, atherosclerosis, spinal cord injuries, and complications of prostate surgery. Hormones, significant smoking, drugs, and structural problems may also contribute to ED. Chart 50–7 lists some drugs that may cause ED.

Laboratory and Diagnostic Procedures

Diagnostic tests will include a complete history to reveal disease, congenital defects, medication use, and any associated psychological concerns. The physical examination would focus on secondary sexual characteristics, any evidence of circulatory problems, anatomical abnormalities of the penis, and neurological deficits. Laboratory tests may include testosterone serum levels, prolactin levels, tests for diabetes, a lipid profile, and thyroid function tests, depending on the findings of the history and physical examination (Male Sexual Dysfunction, 2005). Chapter 48 on reproductive assessment details male reproductive history and physical examination.

Medical Management

Medical management of ED depends on the underlying cause. Contributory drugs can be changed or discontinued, depression can be treated, and patients and their partners can be educated about ED and sexual intimacy alternatives to intercourse (Krebs, 2006).

Devices are available to help achieve and sustain an erection. If mechanical devices are not acceptable to the patient and his partner, drug therapy may be used. The most popular of these drugs is sildenafil (Viagra), which enhances nitric oxide release needed for an erection. Sildenafil will cause coronary vasodilation and hypotension and should not be used with other nitrates such as nitroglycerine. Also, it should be used in lower dosage and with extreme caution if the patient is taking an alpha blocker for BPH (Male Sexual Dysfunction, 2005).

Other drugs may be injected into the urethra or into the penis to produce an erection. These medications have a higher incidence of injury to the penis and are more likely to cause **priapism** (an erection that lasts more than 4 hours). There are also penile prostheses that may be surgically implanted.

Collaborative Management

Collaborative management is indicated for men with ED. First on the team is his sexual partner. Education, counseling, emotional support, acceptance, and open communication are essential.

Health care providers, nurses, counselors, and community support groups may have a role in providing holistic care for this couple on a long-term basis.

Male Infertility

General information about infertility may be found in Chapter 49 🌐. Achieving a pregnancy requires both male and female contributions. When a couple cannot achieve a pregnancy after 1 year of unprotected intercourse, the male factor alone is the cause in about 20% of cases and will contribute in 30% to 40% of all couples who seek medical help for infertility (Quallich, 2006). There are reversible and irreversible causes of male infertility, many of which are listed in Chart 50–8.

The most common test for evaluating male infertility is semen analysis. This test gives information about male hormone cycle integrity, spermatogenesis, and the patency of the genital tract. Refer to Chart 50–9 for the parameters for semen analysis.

Medical care for infertility depends on the underlying cause and is highly specialized. Most of the medical interventions are completed on an outpatient basis from infertility clinics.

Andropause

Unlike women, men begin to decrease the production of sex hormones at about age 30. The decrease is gradual and the rate of decline varies greatly among individual men. Both cross-sectional and longitudinal studies have demonstrated that about 25% of men over age 70 have a significant testosterone deficiency (Seidman, 2006). Whether or not this age-dependent reduction in testosterone levels requires hormone replacement is under debate.

Physiologically, men aged 40 to 70 experience a decrease in total, free, and bioavailable testosterone and an increase in sex hormone-binding globulin (SHBG). The decrease in testosterone is associated with an increase in follicle-stimulating hormone (FSH) and a modest increase in luteinizing hormone (LH). These changes suggest an age-related impairment in the secretion of hypothalamic gonadotropin-releasing hormone (Tan & Pu, 2004). Unlike women in menopause who stop ovulating, men with lower levels of testosterone remain fertile.

Androgen decline in aging males (ADAM), or andropause, may cause mood changes, decreased libido, decreased muscle mass, increased abdominal fat, thinning of bones, decreased en-

ergy, slowed mathematical thinking, and lower blood counts (Organon, 2002a). Often, the symptom severity does not correlate with the level of testosterone in serum (Tan & Pu, 2004).

Diagnostic and Laboratory Procedures

After a thorough history and physical, laboratory measurement of **bioavailable testosterone** (both free testosterone and testosterone that is loosely bound to albumin) is the most appropriate test to diagnose andropause in men over age 65. Testing methods include radioimmunoassay and saliva testing. The Endocrine Society Andropause Consensus Statement has recommended treatment with androgen replacement if the older man has both significant symptoms and a low bioavailable testosterone level. Serum levels of testosterone are highest soon after awakening, so test results should be evaluated based on the timing of the sample (Tan & Pu, 2004).

Medical Management

Testosterone replacement therapy has not proven effective in reversing most andropause symptoms (Seidman, 2006). Haren et al. (2005) assessed the effect of 12 months of oral testosterone on self-reported andropause symptoms in older men with low plasma testosterone levels and found that testosterone undecanoate (Andriol) 80 milligrams twice a day did not improve symptoms. There was some evidence that Andriol may preserve mood and some erectile function, but only in men with the lowest testosterone levels before treatment (Haren et al., 2005).

Andriol should not be used if the older male has ever had breast or prostate cancer, allergies to androgens, or use of anticoagulant medications. It is used with caution if there is preexisting liver disease, heart or blood vessel disease, edema, prostatic hyperplasia, kidney disease, or diabetes mellitus (Organon, 2002b).

Men experiencing andropause seem to benefit from counseling, decreasing stress, losing excess weight, increasing zinc intake, adequate nutrition, and weight training to build muscle mass. Weight training and increased muscle mass have increased endogenous testosterone levels (Tan & Pu, 2004).

◼ Nursing Management

Nursing care of older men with andropause symptoms includes education about what andropause is and the lifestyle changes that can improve symptoms. An excellent website for information about andropause and the use of androgen replacement therapy is produced by Organon, the pharmaceutical company that manufactures Andriol.

CHART 50–8 Causes of Male Infertility

Reversible Causes	Irreversible Causes
Varicocele	Klinefelter's syndrome
Heavy smoking	Congenital bilateral absence of vas deferens
Hypercholesterolemia	
Some forms of erectile dysfunction	Spinal cord injuries
	Antisperm antibodies
Hypogonadism	Some forms of erectile dysfunction
Obesity	Impaired spermatogenesis
Recreational drug use	
Alcohol intake	

Source: Adapted from Quallich, S. (2006). Examining male fertility. *Urologic Nursing, 26*(4), 277–288.

CHART 50–9 Semen Analysis Parameters

Volume	2–5 milliliters
pH	7–8
Sperm count	>20 million/mL
Motility	>50%
Morphology	>14% with normal morphology (World Health Organization [WHO] criteria)
White blood count (WBC)	1–3 per high-power field

Source: Adapted from Sperm disorders. (2005). *Merck manual professional.* Retrieved April 4, 2007, from http://www.merck.com/mmpe/sec18/ch256/ch256b.html

Vasectomy

Vasectomy is male sterilization surgery whereby the vas deferens on each side is identified, cut, and the cut ends are ligated or cauterized closed (Sterilization, 2007). Vasectomy is highly effective in preventing pregnancy if at least two semen-free ejaculates have been analyzed and documented. This is needed to assure that the vas deferens was cut and closed and that all sperm have been cleared from the system. The procedure can be done in the health care provider's office under local anesthesia in about 20 minutes.

Inguinal Hernia

Abdominal **hernias**, protrusions of abdominal contents through a weakness in the abdominal wall, are very common. About 700,000 surgeries for abdominal hernia occur in the United States each year (Hernias of the Abdominal Wall, 2005). About half of all abdominal hernias are **indirect inguinal hernias** (present via the inguinal canal and exit at the external inguinal ring) and another 25% are **direct inguinal hernias** (occur above the inguinal ligament, close to the pubic tubercle and the external inguinal ring). See Figure 50–7 ■ for a depiction of direct and indirect inguinal hernias.

Inguinal hernias are usually congenital but may become symptomatic due to trauma or chronic cough (Goroll & Mulley, 2006). Signs and symptoms depend on the severity of the hernia and include a visible bulge, discomfort or pain, tenderness, bowel obstruction, and infarction. Chart 50–10 lists clinical manifestations specific to inguinal hernias.

Medical Management

Medical management includes diagnosis and surgery to repair the hernia with placement of mesh to reinforce the repair. Surgery for hernia repair may be conventional or laparoscopic depending on the skill of the surgeon. Occasionally, when the hernia is small and asymptomatic, a watchful waiting approach will be taken. Hernia repair surgery is considered elective unless incarceration occurs (Goroll & Mulley, 2006; Hernias of the Abdominal Wall, 2005).

Nursing Management

Nursing care depends on the severity of the hernia. Education is of particular importance because the patient who is scheduled for surgery will need to know the signs and symptoms of incarceration and strangulation so that he can seek help immediately. Patients

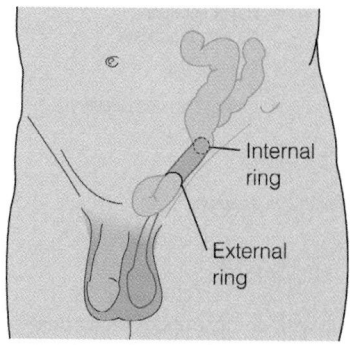 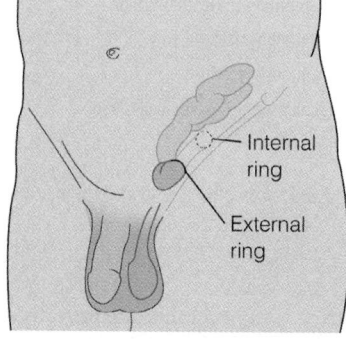

Internal ring
External ring
Internal ring
External ring

FIGURE 50–7 ■ Direct and indirect inguinal hernia.

| CHART 50–10 | **Clinical Manifestations of Inguinal Hernias** |

Reducible; Mass appears on standing, reduces when supine.

Incarcerated: Contents cannot be replaced into the abdomen, even when supine.

Strangulated: Irreducible hernia where blood supply to trapped bowel has been cut off and bowel obstruction has occurred.

Source: Adapted from Goroll, A., & Mulley, A. (2006). *Primary care medicine: Office evaluation and management of the adult patient* (5th ed.). Philadelphia: Lippincott Williams & Wilkins.

| CHART 50–11 | **Sexually Transmitted Infections by Presenting Sign** |

Presenting Sign	Sexually Transmitted Infection
Urethritis	Gonococcal Nongonococcal: chlamydia, trichomoniasis
Genital ulcers	Herpes, primary syphilis, chancroid, granuloma inguinale, lymphogranuloma venereum
Genital warts	Human papillomavirus (HPV)
Immune deficiency	Human immunodeficiency virus (HIV); acquired immunodeficiency syndrome (AIDS)

Source: Adapted from Centers for Disease Control and Prevention. (2006). Sexually transmitted disease treatment guidelines, 2006. *Morbidity and Mortality Weekly Report,* 55(RR-11), 1–94. Retrieved April 7, 2007, from http://www.cdc.gov/mmwr/preview/mmwrhtml/rr5511a1.htm

usually want to know that they will be up the same day of surgery, return to light work in 2 to 3 weeks, and return to full activity in 3 to 6 weeks. There should be no effect on sexual function (Goroll & Mulley, 2006). Many hernia surgeries are done in outpatient surgery. See Chapter 25 for a review of preoperative nursing.

If the hernia is strangulated, it may require bowel resection as well as hernia repair. Postoperatively, analgesia, pulmonary toilet, and monitoring of vital signs and for bleeding or drainage on the dressing will be needed. Patients who have bowel surgery usually have a nasogastric tube and require IV therapy. See Chapter 45 for a description of care of the patient after bowel surgery.

Sexually Transmitted Infections

Surveillance data from the Centers for Disease Control and Prevention (CDC) indicate that the incidence of sexually transmitted infections (STIs) continues to increase each year. The CDC has categorized STIs by their primary presentation. Chart 50–11 refers to each abnormality and the STIs it may involve.

Treatment of STIs should include both the patient and his partner. Both should receive an examination for any coexisting STI; medication as appropriate; and education and counseling to prevent reinfection, complications, and spreading the infection to others. Male condom use does protect the male from infection, and it prevents the transmission of sperm and infection to his partner. A more complete discussion of STIs can be found in Chapter 49 on female reproductive disorders and Chapter 60 on immune response disorders.

Gerontological Considerations

As discussed earlier, diseases of the prostate are most likely to occur in older men. This is also a time that other diseases tend to occur, complicating the prostate condition and treatment. Because of the changes in the body caused by aging, special consideration for skin care and bowel elimination become more important to nursing care for older men presenting with reproductive disorders. Nursing assessment of the older male should also include hearing and vision. If the older male is hard of hearing or unable to see as well as he used to, then education must be modified to fit his needs. Communication must be clear, simple, and direct.

Research

To improve care of males experiencing abnormalities with their reproductive system, it is imperative that nurses be knowledgeable and that research continue to refine this knowledge. The Research Opportunities and Clinical Impact box outlines potential research topics related to male reproductive disorders.

RESEARCH OPPORTUNITIES AND CLINICAL IMPACT RELATED TO MALE REPRODUCTIVE DISORDERS

Research Area	Clinical Impact
Examination of why prostate cancer risks are higher for African American men.	African American men are much more likely to develop and die from prostate cancer.
Determination of whether selenium and vitamin E may help prevent prostate cancer.	Research currently underway. Prevention of prostate cancer is much preferred to treating it.
Use of complementary and alternative therapies among patients with cancer.	Nurses should know more about complementary and alternative therapies so that they can give information about safety and efficacy to their patients.
Prostate cancer outcomes study (PCOS) is examining the impact of treatments for prostate cancer on quality of life.	Important for the patient to know all about his options and potential outcomes before choosing a treatment.
Identifying problems faced by partners of men with prostate cancer.	Nurses are recognized support persons, and wives or partners will turn to them when they need help dealing with decreased affection from or depression in their partner. Support of the partner helps in support of the patient.
Predicting the use of complementary and alternative therapies among patients with cancer.	Nurses need to be asking patients about the complementary and alternative therapies they may be using such as herbs, vitamins, and homeopathic medications that may impact their medical care.

Clinical Preparation

CRITICAL THINKING

PEARSON mynursingkit™

 Read

- History of Current Illness
- Past Medical History
- Physical Exam
- Admitting Medical Orders
- Laboratory Study Results

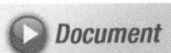 **Document**

- Summary of Hospitalization
- Pathophysiology Form
- Laboratory Values
- Laboratory Results Explanation

 **Apply**

- List of Potential Nursing Diagnoses
- Concept Map
- Critical Thinking Questions

Log on to MyNursingKit.com to download forms you will need and to complete further steps in the Clinical Preparation assignment.

HISTORY OF PRESENT ILLNESS

You are the nurse receiving report on Mr. Hyatt, a 60-year-old male patient who is 3 days postoperative from a suprapubic prostatectomy. The patient was first seen 2 weeks ago in his health care provider's office with complaints of increasing difficulty voiding during the past 4 months. The physical exam and elevated PSA strongly suggested prostate cancer, and a transrectal ultrasound guided biopsy was done. The results showed a T2, Gleason 2 + 2 tumor. The patient was given the option of radiation therapy or surgery. The patient opted for an immediate prostatectomy. The patient was admitted early yesterday morning for surgery.

You begin your shift rounds and greet the patient as you enter the room. You note an IV in the right forearm, without redness or edema, infusing at 100 mL/hr. A suprapubic catheter is in place and draining well. The outflow bag contains red-tinged fluid. The patient is in a semi-Fowler's position with the overbed table in front of him. The tray on the table contains unopened apple juice, chicken broth, and coffee. When questioned about his untouched food, he states he is just not hungry. You continue the assessment and examine the occlusive suprapubic dressing, which appears moist under the tape. Patient states that his pain on a 1–10 point scale, with 10 being the worst, is 6 mostly around the suprapubic catheter. You give the patient an analgesic and help him to a more comfortable position.

You change the suprapubic dressing around the catheter and note a thick yellow odorous discharge on the dressing with a streak of red on the gauze. A sterile dressing is reapplied to the site, which appears inflamed, with slight edema, minimal bruising, with pale yellow drainage at the catheter insertion site. A suture is visible that is holding the catheter in place. When you return to the nurses' station, the laboratory results for the patient have returned. The health care provider is notified of the CBC values.

Medical–Surgical History

Past medical history was on the chart and is remarkable for hypertension and insulin-dependent diabetes. The patient had all the "usual" childhood illnesses including measles, mumps, and rubella. He had a broken arm requiring casting at age 15 as a result of a baseball injury. There were no major illnesses or medical events until the patient was in his 40s. At age 42, the patient was diagnosed with hypertension requiring 150 milligrams of irbesartan (Avapro) once daily. At age 48, the patient was diagnosed with diabetes, which was controlled with diet therapy until 3 years ago when he started taking a sliding-scale insulin lispro (Humalog) with meals. His blood sugars average in the 120s most days.

Social History

Lives with wife independently. Has three adult children all of whom live out of state. He smoked for 30 years and quit about 10 years ago. He drinks alcohol socially.

Physical Exam

Vital signs: temp 100°F, P 88, R 18, and BP 134/90
Cardiovascular: JVP not elevated; normal S_1 and S_2; regular rate and rhythm, no significant murmur, rub, or gallop; carotids 2+ without bruits
Lung sounds: clear
Bowel sounds: hypoactive in all four quadrants; abdomen is tense
HEENT: scleras anicteric, oropharynx clear
Neck: supple, no lymphadenopathy
Lungs: clear to auscultation bilaterally
Extremities: no edema
Neurological: normal, alert, and oriented × 3
CXR: normal
ECG: normal sinus rhythm with bundle branch block
   Admitting Medical Orders
   Diagnosis: cancer of the prostate; prostatectomy
   Surgery/urology
   Admit to surgical floor
   No known allergies
   Vital signs and oxygen saturation q4h
   Call house officer: pulse < 60 and > 130/minute; BP < 90 and > 160 systolic; temperature > 38.5; urine output < 30 mL/hr for 2 hours; respiratory rate > 30/minute; oxygen saturation < 92%: blood sugar > 120

IV: D51/2NS at 100 mL/hr
Clear liquids postnausea; advance to regular diet as tolerated
Ambulate qid beginning postoperative day 1
Sterile dressing change daily and prn beginning postoperative day 1
Continuous sterile NS bladder irrigation
Fingerstick glucose ac and at bedtime beginning on postoperative day 1
I&O q8h
Incentive spirometer q2h during the day and q4h at night
Sequential compression devices (SCDs) to lower extremities
Scheduled Medications
Humalog S_0 sliding scale per patient home routine
Unasyn (ampicillin sodium) 1.5 g IV daily
Avapro 150 mg po daily beginning postoperative day 1
PRN Medications
Demerol 100 mg IM q4h prn pain
Lortab 7.5 mg po q4h prn pain
Phenergan 25 mg IV or IM q4h prn nausea
Ordered Laboratory Studies
CBC and glucose daily

LABORATORY STUDY RESULTS

Test	Postoperative Day 1	Postoperative Day 2	Postoperative Day 3
White blood cell count (WBC)	12,000/mm³	15,000/mm³	18,000/mm³
Platelets	410,000/mm³	380,000/mm³	378,000/mm³
Hemoglobin (HGB)	14 g/dL	12 g/dL	10 g/dL
Hematocrit (HCT)	48%	42%	39%
Red blood cells (RBC)	4.92/mm³	4.2/mm³	3.5/mm³
Platelets	298,000 mm³	308,000 mm³	310,000 mm³
Hemoglobin A1c	7.2 %	—	—
Serum glucose	114 mg/dL	105 mg/dL	114 mg/dL

CRITICAL THINKING QUESTIONS

1. Which nursing assessment should take priority for this patient?

2. Why should the nurse assess the suprapubic catheter when assessing the patient's pain?

3. What significance is there to the thick yellow drainage at the suprapubic insertion site?

4. What impact do the hemoglobin and diabetes have on the patient's recovery?

5. What significance does the temperature have at this point in the patient's postoperative course?

Answers to Critical Thinking Questions appear in Appendix D.

NCLEX® REVIEW

1. The nurse is caring for a young male patient with an infection of the epididymis. The nurse realizes this infection is most likely the result of:
   1. Inflammation from a sports-related injury.
   2. Exposure to the mumps.
   3. Sexually transmitted infections.
   4. *Escherichia coli* spread from the urinary tract.

2. A 30-year-old male patient is admitted with symptoms of cancer. The nurse realizes that the most common type of reproductive cancer in males under 35 years of age is:
   1. Prostate.
   2. Testicular.
   3. Penile.
   4. Urethral.

3. The nurse working in a urology clinic asks a male client to complete an AUA Symptom Index Tool for the purpose of:
   1. Assisting to diagnose sexual dysfunction disorders.
   2. Determining risk factors for urinary tract malignancy.
   3. Assessing the symptoms associated with incontinence.
   4. Quantifying the symptoms of benign prostatic hypertrophy.

4. The nurse is providing care to a male patient with continuous bladder irrigation after a TURP. The care priority for this patient would be:
   1. Running in one liter per hour of irrigation fluid.
   2. Securing the catheter to the bedrail to promote drainage.
   3. Manually irrigating the catheter several times per shift.
   4. Checking the drainage tubing for kinks on a regular basis.

5. The nurse is providing care to a patient recovering from an orchiectomy for testicular cancer. Which of the following nursing diagnoses should the nurse include when planning this patient's care?
   1. Risk for Infection
   2. Altered Mobility
   3. Disturbed Body Image
   4. Impaired Urinary Elimination

6. The nurse is instructing a 52-year-old male on reproductive health. Which of the following should this instruction include?
   1. Encourage to receive a DRE and PSA test annually.
   2. Teach testicular self-examination.
   3. See a health care provider only if experiencing changes in urinary elimination patterns.
   4. Educate that a lifetime risk for prostate cancer is 1 in 10.

Answers for review questions appear in Appendix D

KEY TERMS

benign prostatic hyperplasia (BPH) *p.1574*
bioavailable testosterone *p.1588*
direct inguinal hernia *p.1589*
epididymitis *p.1566*
erectile dysfunction (ED) *p.1587*
gynecomastia *p.1570*
hernia *p.1589*
hydronephrosis *p.1574*
impotence *p.1570*

indirect inguinal hernia *p.1589*
orchiectomy *p.1568*
orchiopexy *p.1568*
orchitis *p.1567*
paraphimosis *p.1583*
penectomy *p.1587*
Peyronie's disease *p.1583*
phimosis *p.1583*

priapism *p.1587*
prostatectomy *p.1578*
prostatitis *p.1572*
retrograde ejaculation *p.1576*
spermatocele *p.1569*
spermatogenesis *p.1587*
testicular torsion *p.1567*
vasectomy *p.1589*

PEARSON

EXPLORE mynursingkit™

MyNursingKit is your one stop for online chapter review materials and resources. Prepare for success with additional NCLEX®-style practice questions, interactive assignments and activities, web links, animations and videos, and more!

Register your access code from the front of your book at
www.mynursingkit.com

REFERENCES

Alper, B., & Crawford, E. (2005). Benign prostatic hyperplasia. *The Clinical Advisor, 8*(10), 119–121.

American Cancer Society (ACS). (2007). *ACS News Center. Prostate cancer vaccine one step closer to approval.* Retrieved April 7, 2007, from http://www.cancer.org/docroot/NWS/content/NWS_1_1x_Prostate_Cancer_Vaccine_One_Step_Closer_to_Approval.asp

American Cancer Society (ACS). (2008). *Detailed guide: Penile cancer.* Retrieved April 4, 2007, from http://www.cancer.org/docroot/CRI/CRI_2_3x.asp?dt=35

Argyriou, A., Chroni, E., Koutras, A., Iconomou, G., et al. (2006). A randomized controlled trial evaluating the efficacy and safety of vitamin E supplementation for protection against cisplatin-induced peripheral neuropathy: Final results. *Supportive Care in Cancer: Official Journal of the Multinational Association of Supportive Care in Cancer, 14*(11), 1134–1140.

Barry, M. (2006). Approach to benign prostatic hyperplasia. In A. Goroll & A. Mulley, *Primary care medicine: Office evaluation and management of the adult patient* (5th ed., pp. 909–914). Philadelphia: Lippincott Williams & Wilkins.

Bazar, H., Baydar, S., Boyunaga, H., Batislam, E., Basar, M., & Yilmaz, E. (2003). Primary bilateral spermatocele. *International Journal of Urology, 10,* 59–61.

Beckman, T., & Mynderse, L. (2005). Evaluation and medical management of benign prostatic hyperplasia. *Mayo Clinic Proceedings, 80*(10), 1356–1362.

Benign prostatic hyperplasia (BPH). (2005). *Merck manual professional.* Retrieved April 4, 2007, from http://www.merck.com/mmpe/sec17/ch240/ch240b.html

Bent, S., et al. (2006). Saw palmetto for benign prostatic hyperplasia. *New England Journal of Medicine, 354*(6), 557–566.

Brown, C. (2004). Testicular cancer: an overview. *Urologic Nursing, 24*(2): 83–93.

Buck, A. (2004). Is there a scientific basis for the therapeutic effects of *Serenoa repens* in benign prostatic hyperplasia? Mechanisms of action. *The Journal of Urology, 172*(5, Pt. 1), 1792–1799.

Carmichael, S., Shaw, G., Laurent, C., Lammer, E., Olney, R., & the National Birth Defects Prevention Study. (2005). Hypospadias and maternal exposure to cigarette smoke. *Paediatric and Perinatal Epidemiology, 19,* 406–412.

Cole, F., & Vogler, R. (2004). The acute, nontraumatic scrotum: Assessment, diagnosis and management. *Journal of the American Academy of Nurse Practitioners, 16*(2), 50–56.

Every, M., Mikkelsen, D., & Bailey, D. (2005). Alterations in male genital and reproductive function. In L. Copstead & J. Banasik, *Pathophysiology* (3rd ed., pp. 790–805). St. Louis: Elsevier Saunders.

Every, M., Mikkelsen, D., & Cagle, C. (2005). Male genital and reproductive function. In L. Copstead & J. Banasik, *Pathophysiology* (3rd ed., pp. 772–789). St. Louis: Elsevier Saunders.

Fischbach, F. (2003). *A manual of laboratory and diagnostic tests* (7th ed.). Philadelphia: Lippincott Williams & Wilkins.

Genital trauma: Genitourinary tract traumas. (2005/2007). *Merck manual professional.* Retrieved April 4, 2007, from http://www.merck.com/mmpe/print/sec21/ch314/ch314c.html

Goodman, M.T., Hernandez, B. Y. & Shvetsov, Y. B. (2007). Demographic and Pathologic Differences in the Incidence of Invasive Penile Cancer in the United States, 1995–2003. *Cancer Epidemiology Biomarkers & Prevention* 16, 1833-1839. doi: 10.1158/1055-9965.EPI-07-0221. *American Association for Cancer Research.* Retrieved August 17, 2008 from http://cebp.aacrjournals.org/cgi/content/abstract/16/9/1833?ck=nck

Goodson, J. (2006). Management of acute and chronic prostatitis. In A. Goroll & A. Mulley, *Primary care medicine: Office evaluation and management of the adult patient* (5th ed., pp. 914–919). Philadelphia: Lippincott Williams & Wilkins.

Goroll, A., & Mulley, A. (2006). *Primary care medicine: Office evaluation and management of the adult patient* (5th ed.). Philadelphia: Lippincott Williams & Wilkins.

Gray, M., & Sims, T. (2006). Prostate cancer: Prevention and management of localized disease. *The Nurse Practitioner, 31*(9), 15–28.

Haren, M., Chapman, I., Coates, P., Morley, J., & Wittert, G. (2005). Effect of 12 month oral testosterone on testosterone deficiency symptoms in symptomatic elderly males with low-normal gonadal status. *Age and Aging, 34*(2), 125–130. Retrieved November 5, 2007, from *Cochrane Central Register of Controlled Trials* (*CENTRAL*), 2007, Issue 4.

Hatcher, R., et al. (2004). *Contraceptive technology.* New York: Ardent Media.

Hawes, S., Malcarne, V., Ko, C., Sadler, G., Banthia, R., Sherman, S., et al. (2006). Identifying problems faced by spouses and partners of patients with prostate cancer. *Oncology Nursing Forum, 33*(4), 807–814.

Hernias of the abdominal wall. (2005). *Merck manual professional.* Retrieved April 4, 2007, from http://www.merck.com/mmpe/print/sec02/ch011/ch011f.html

Ishani, A., MacDonald, R., Nelson, D., Rutks, J., & Wilt, T. (2000). *Pygeum africanum* for the treatment of patients with benign prostatic hyperplasia: A systematic review and quantitative meta-analysis. *American Journal of Medicine, 109*(8), 654–664.

Karlowicz, K. (Ed.). (1995). *Urologic nursing: Principles and practice.* Philadelphia: W. B. Saunders.

Krebs, L. (2006). What should I say? Talking with patients about sexuality issues. *Clinical Journal of Oncology Nursing, 10*(3), 313–315.

Kuritzky, L., Rosenberg, M., & Sadovsky, R. (2006). Efficacy and safety of alfuzosin 10 mg once daily in the treatment of symptomatic benign prostatic hyperplasia. *International Journal of Clinical Practice, 60*(3), 351–358.

Lashley, R. (2005). *Clinical genetics in nursing practice* (3rd ed.). New York: Springer.

Mahon, S. (2005). Screening for prostate cancer: Informing men about their options. *Clinical Journal of Oncology Nursing, 9*(5), 625–627.

Male sexual dysfunction. (2005). *Merck manual professional.* Retrieved April 4, 2007, from http://www.merck.com/mmpe/sec17/ch227/ch227c.html

McNaughton Collins, M., MacDonald, R., & Wilt, T. (1999). Interventions for chronic abacterial prostatitis (review). *Cochrane Database of Systemic Reviews.* In *The Cochrane Library,* 2007, Issue 1. Retrieved August 11, 2008, from http://www.mrw.interscience.wiley.com/cochrane/clsysrev/articles/CD002080/frame.html

McVary, K. (2006). BPH: Epidemiology and comorbidities. *American Journal of Managed Care, 12*(Suppl. 5):, S122–S128.

National Academy of Clinical Biochemistry (NACB). (2006). *Tumor markers PDF. Practice guidelines and recommendations for use of tumor markers in the clinic: Testicular Cancer (section 3A).* Retrieved March 30, 2007, from http://www.aacc.org/members/nacb/lmpg/onlineguide/draftguidelines/tumormarkers/pages/tumormarkerspdf.aspx

National Cancer Institute (NCI). (2007a). *Genetics of prostate cancer (PDQ).* Retrieved April 7, 2007, from http://www.cancer.gov/cancertopics/pdq/genetics/prostate/HealthProfessional/

National Cancer Institute (NCI). (2007b). *Prostate cancer.* Retrieved April 7, 2007, from http://www.cancer.gov/cancertopics/types/prostate

National Cancer Institute (NCI). (2007c). *Prostate cancer treatment (PDQ): Stage information.* Retrieved August 11, 2008, from http://www.cancer.gov/cancertopics/pdq/treatment/prostate/HealthProfessional/page4#Section_88

National Cancer Institute (NCI). (2007d). *Testicular cancer: Questions and answers.* Retrieved March 22, 2007, from http://www.cancer.gov/cancertopics/factsheet/sites-types/testicular#5

National Cancer Institute (NCI). (2007e). *Treatment choices for men with early-stage prostate cancer.* Retrieved April 9, 2007, from http:/ /www.cancer.gov/cancertopics/prostate-cancer-treatment-choices

National Comprehensive Cancer Network. (2008). *Clinical practice guidelines in oncology: Prostate cancer* [V.1.2008]. Retrieved August 11, 2008, from http://www.nccn.org/professionals/physician_gls/PDF/prostate.pdf

Nickel, J. C. (2006). BPH: Costs and treatment outcomes. *The American Journal of Managed Care, 12*(Suppl. 5), S141–S148.

O'Leary, M. (2006). Treatment and pharmacologic management of BPH in the context of common comorbidities. *American Journal of Managed Care, 12*(Suppl. 5), S129–S140.

Organon. (2002a). *Impact of low testosterone.* Retrieved November 5, 2007, from http://www.andropause.com/about_andropause/impact.asp

Organon. (2002b). *Understanding risks.* Retrieved November 5, 2007, from http://www.andropause.com/treatment_options/understanding.asp

Penile cancer: Genitourinary cancer. (2005). *Merck manual professional.* Retrieved April 4, 2007, from http://www.merck.com/mmpe/print/sec17/ch241/ch241d.html

Peyronie's disease: Penile and scrotal disorders. (2005). *Merck manual professional.* Retrieved March 31, 2007, from http://www.merck.com/mmpe/print/sec17/ch239/ch239f.html

Porche, D. (2006). Prostatitis. *Journal of Nurse Practitioners, 2*(10), 662–663.

Prostatitis: Prostate disease. (2005). *Merck manual professional.* Retrieved March 30, 2007, from http://www.merck.com/mmpe/sec17/ch240/ch240c.html

Quallich, S. (2006). Examining male fertility. *Urologic Nursing, 26*(4), 277–288.

Rigdon, J. (2006). Home study program: Robotic-assisted laparoscopic radical prostatectomy. *AORN Journal, 84*(5), 759–762, 764, 766–774.

Ringdahl, E., & Teague, L. (2006). Testicular torsion. *American Family Physician, 74,* 1739–1743.

RxList the Internet Drug Index. (2007a). *Cisplatin.* Retrieved March 31, 2007, from http://www.rxlist.com/cgi/generic/cisplatin_ids.htm

RxList the Internet Drug Index. (2007b). *Motrin.* Retrieved March 31, 2007, from http://www.rxlist.com/cgi/generic/ibup.htm

RxList the Internet Drug Index. (2007c). *Zofran injection.* Retrieved March 31, 2007, from http://www.rxlist.com/cgi/generic/ondansetron.htm

Scrotal masses. (2005). *Merck manual professional.* Retrieved November 3, 2007, from http://www.merck.com/mmpe/print/sec17/ch239/ch239i.html

Segal, R., Lukka, H., Klotz, L., Eady, A., Bestic, N., & Johnston, M. (2001). Cancer Care Ontario Practice Guidelines Initiative Genitourinary Cancer Disease Site Group. Surveillance programs for early stage nonseminomatous testicular cancer: A practice guideline. *Canadian Journal of Urology, 8*(1), 1184–1192. In *Database of Abstracts of Reviews of Effects,* 2007, Issue 1. Retrieved March 29, 2007, from http://www.mrw.interscience.wiley.com/cochrane/

Seidman, S. (2006). Normative hypogonadism and depression: Does "andropause" exist? *International Journal of Impotence Research, 18,* 415–422.

Sperm disorders. (2005). *Merck manual professional.* Retrieved April 4, 2007, from http://www.merck.com/mmpe/sec18/ch256/ch256b.html

Sterilization. (2007). *Merck manual professional.* Retrieved August 14, 2008, from http://www.merck.com/mmpe/sec18/ch255/ch255c.html

Stevenson, T. D., & McNeill, J. A. (2004). Surgical management of testicular cancer. *Clinical Journal of Oncology Nursing, 8*(4), 355–360.

Tan, R., & Pu, S. (2004). Is it andropause? Recognizing androgen deficiency in aging men. *Postgraduate Medicine, 115*(1), 62–66.

Testicular Cancer Resource Center. (2007). *How to do a testicular self examination.* Retrieved April 1, 2007, from http://tcrc.acor.org/tcexam.html

Walsh, P., Retik, A., Vaughan, E., & Wein, A. (Eds.). (2007). *Campbell's urology* (9th ed.). Philadelphia: W. B. Saunders.

Ward-Smith, P. (2006). Cultural disparities in the diagnosis and treatment of prostate cancer. *Urologic Nursing, 26*(5), 397–405.

Wilt, T., Howe, R., & Rutks, I. (2000). Terazosin for benign prostatic hyperplasia. *Cochrane Database Systematic Reviews 2000.* In *The Cochrane Library,* 2007, Issue 1. Retrieved March 31, 2007, from www.thecochranelibrary.com

Zeroski, D., Abel, L., Butler, W. M., Wallner, K., & Merrick, G. S. (2005). Factors affecting patient selection for prostate brachytherapy: What nurses should know. *Clinical Journal of Oncology Nursing, 9*(5), 553–560.

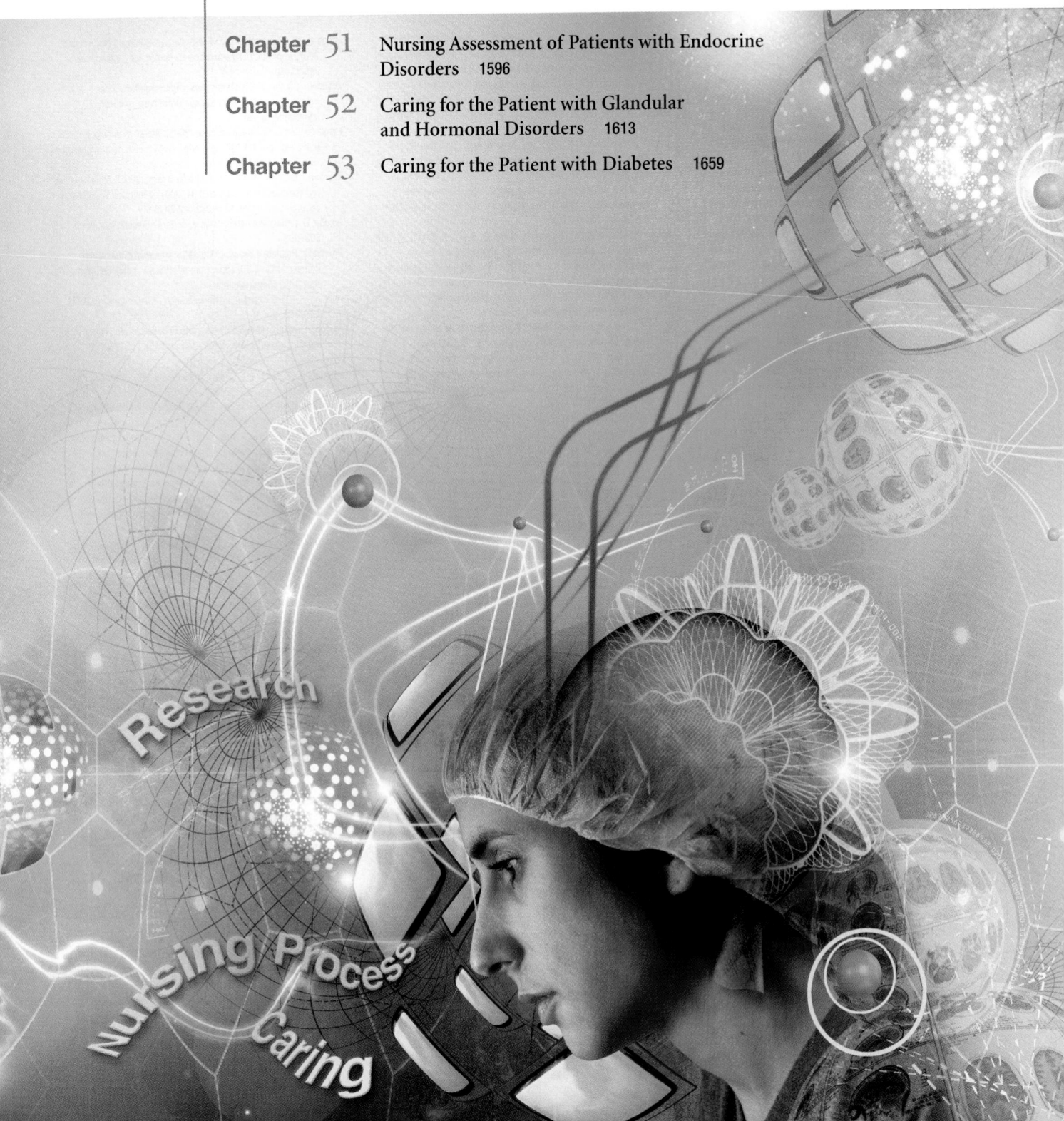

Research

Nursing Process

Caring

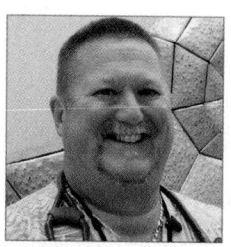

RICH My name is Rich and I am a clinical resource nurse (CN III) on a medical–surgical unit at a 540-bed teaching hospital. As a tertiary facility, we receive patients from all of Northern California as well as a large population of underserved patients who seek health care when they are at their sickest. As a resource nurse, I do patient care and precept new nurses. I care for patients with diabetes, pancreatitis, acute liver failure, chronic renal failure, antibiotic-resistant serious infections, and for those who require long-term ventilator support.

I chose to work at this hospital because it is a teaching facility where state-of-the-art practices are implemented, and it has a nursing body that encourages personal growth and career movement and doctors who value the input of the nursing staff and truly work as a team to provide the utmost in quality patient care. This hospital uses the primary nursing model, in which the nurse is at center stage when orchestrating the care required by each patient. As their primary nurse, I am able to help patients understand what the plan of treatment is for them.

I also teach in a local nursing program as a clinical instructor. Both as a clinical nurse and as part-time faculty, I have the opportunity to teach new nurses and students the six components of caring. I also value the importance of these six components in the care that I give to my patients. On a typical day, I can be caring for three to four patients with complex problems. My **commitment** to each of the patients is that I will do my utmost to provide them the nursing care that will enable them to heal and ultimately be discharged from the hospital. We care for long-term ventilator patients and our commitment to them as a unit is to provide the highest level of care to afford them the ability to have quality time with their families as we attempt to wean them from the ventilator or, in some cases, as we prepare both the patient and families for a life of being ventilator dependent.

Compassion is an integral part of my daily interactions with my patients. Patients come to our unit with a variety of unhealthy habits, such as alcohol and drug abuse, that over time have put them into various states of organ failure. It can be very easy to become jaded when dealing with this type of patient. My compassion for these individuals allows me to provide them with the nonjudgmental care that is required to bring them back to their prior state of wellness. Often these patients have become so debilitated that they are no longer able to do the simplest of activities of daily living and my **conscience** dictates that I assist them with these tasks in a dignified manner.

Because I have 26 years of experience as a nurse, I am able to perform my nursing care in a **confident** manner. In doing so, I put patients at ease by letting them know that I have performed my nursing skills many times. My confidence in performing procedures serves to decrease patients' anxiety levels. I pride myself in being a very **competent** nurse. I have had physicians tell me that they have been glad that I was caring for their patients because they know my level of competence. This also allows me to feel comfortable precepting a novice nurse. As a preceptor, I am able to guide new nurses in applying what they have learned and can help make their transition to this busy and often demanding unit less stressful. My **comportment**, or how I interact with my patients and their families, is a professional nurse–patient relationship. I let them know that I will be their advocate while they are under my care.

Being able to think critically is essential, because it is the nursing assessments that indicate when a patient is not doing well and what information needs to be communicated to physicians. Critical thinking is essential when caring for the complex ventilator patient because they can decompensate at any given moment during the weaning stages. Clinical reasoning also is paramount in dealing with the patients who have illnesses or comorbidities that may hamper their efforts at a full recovery. It is the task of nurses to use their broad nursing knowledge to prioritize the care required of the particular patient. Nurses must be able to communicate with the health care team in a concise and focused manner about these priorities. I have had the opportunity on many occasions to analyze patients' vital signs and physical appearance and demeanor and been able to summon the medical team to evaluate any patient who in my estimation has taken a turn for the worst. This ability is something that has evolved over time as I have evolved into the professional nurse that I am today.

> "My **commitment** to each of the patients is that I will do my utmost to provide them the nursing care that will enable them to heal and ultimately be discharged from the hospital."

Nursing Assessment of Patients with Endocrine Disorders

Corinne Harmon

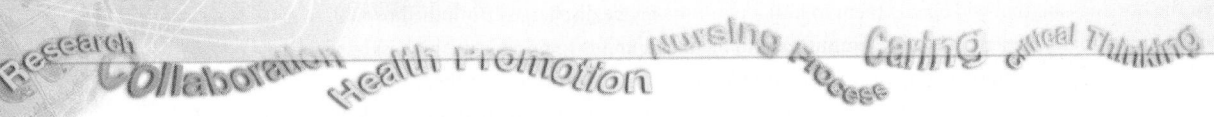

THE ENDOCRINE SYSTEM is truly a marvel. This system of glands and specialized tissue located throughout the body is involved in maintaining the body's overall function and homeostasis. This is accomplished through the release of hormones. Hormones exert their effect only on specific target tissues. This specificity of action and the fact that glands are ductless makes the endocrine system unique.

■ Anatomy and Physiology Review

The endocrine system is composed of glands, glandular tissue, and target tissue or receptors. The organs of the endocrine system are known as glands. Glands arise from glandular epithelial tissue during embryonic development. These glands include

- Hypothalamus
- Pituitary gland
- Adrenal glands
- Thyroid gland
- Parathyroid glands
- Islet cells of the pancreas
- Gonads.

The term **endocrine** refers to the process of an active biological agent being secreted into the bloodstream. These biological agents are known as hormones. The functions of the glands and their production of hormones may be age contingent as is discussed sequentially under each gland and hormone produced.

General Structure and Function of Hormones

Hormones are chemical substances that have a regulatory action on target tissues. They act as chemical messengers to stimulate certain functions while retarding others. Because glands are ductless, hormones are released directly into the circulation. The hormone then travels thorough the bloodstream where it will exert its action on target cells or receptors. Target tissues (cells) or **receptors** represent those tissues or organs upon which the specific hormone acts. The receptors within the endocrine system are able to distinguish a specific hormone from all other chemicals in circulation and bind to it in a lock-and-key type manner. This binding process then triggers the target tissues or organs to produce the desired response. The organs and target tissue of the endocrine system are located throughout the body.

The endocrine system's functioning is intimately connected to that of the nervous system. Together, these systems provide a mechanism for communication between cells and organs. This connection is referred to as *neuroendocrine regulation*. The systems work synergistically to regulate overall physiological functioning by regulating responses to the internal and external environment. Through the combined efforts of the two systems, growth and development, maintenance of homeostasis, the adaptability to changes in the external environment, and reproduction can occur.

Hormone Classification and Function

Hormones travel through the bloodstream to reach target tissues or receptors. They exist as proteins, peptides, lipids, or amino acid analogues. As they circulate in the bloodstream, they may be free or bound. The majority of hormones are secreted in their active form. Others must undergo metabolic conversion to their active form in peripheral tissue. Hormones also function in other ways. If hormones affect cells within the vicinity of their release, it is known as **paracrine functioning**. Hormones are said to have **autocrine functioning** when the hormones produced act on the cells that created them.

General Hormone Regulation

All hormones are interrelated to some degree, and a number of complex interactions control their secretion. Overall, hormone regulation involves the interplay of individual hormone responses, while counterbalancing the influence of other hormones by integrating mechanisms for terminating or attenuating their response. These mechanisms operate to maintain an intricate balance of the internal environment, ensuring precise control in order to maintain homeostasis. Hormone release may be regulated by one or more mechanisms. Common regulatory mechanisms at work within the endocrine system include basal hormone release, circadian or infradian rhythms, brain-mediated neural stimulation or inhibition of hormone release, and feedback systems.

In basal hormone release, small amounts of hormones are released continuously. **Circadian rhythms** refer to cyclical biological activities. The phenomenon denotes that there is an orderly change or variation in hormonal activity during a 24-hour period. An example of this is the release of cortisol, whose peaks and troughs have been demonstrated by serum analyses. **Infradian rhythms** are those that last for more than 24 hours. This is seen in females in the menstrual cycle. Neural regulation of hormone secretion, suppression, or release also occurs.

A feedback system is a regulatory system that keeps certain body functions within a prescribed range to sustain homeostasis (Figure 51–1 ■). Feedback systems can be positive or negative. In **negative feedback**, an alteration in a hormone level stimulates a series of changes to return the level to normal. **Positive feedback** occurs when the increased secretion of a hormone causes another gland to release a hormone. The best example of this is the release of leuteinizing hormone in response to higher estrogen levels.

Feedback loops can be simple or complex. A simple loop is seen with insulin and glucagon; with hyperglycemia, insulin is released, whereas with hypoglycemia, glucagon is released. In more complex loops, control is accomplished by releasing factors made in the hypothalamus as well as by stimulating factors made in the pituitary.

Hypothalamus Gland

The hypothalamus gland is located in the third ventricle of the brain and is composed of nervous tissue. It shares its circulatory system with the anterior pituitary, and it plays a role in the func-

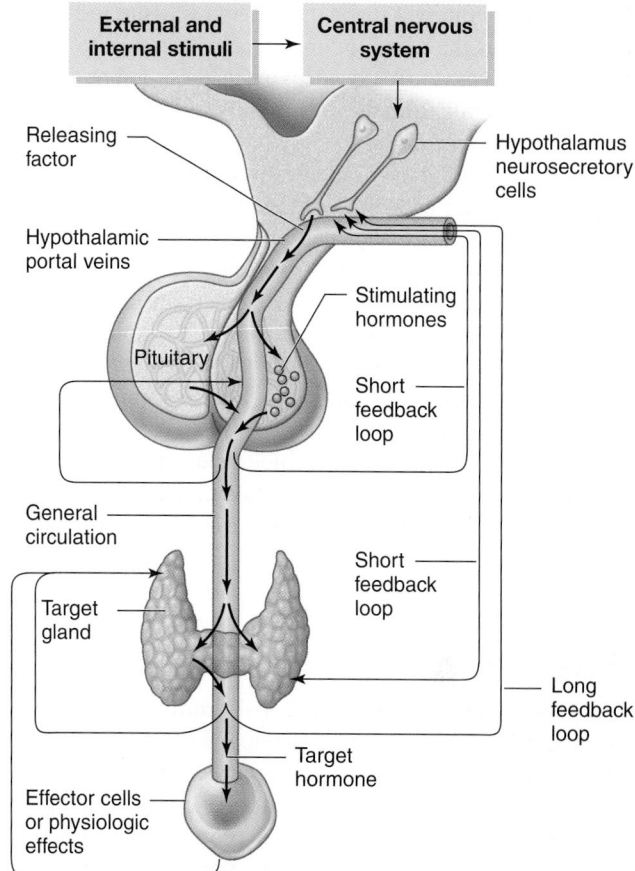

FIGURE 51–1 ■ General feedback loop.

tion of both the anterior and posterior pituitary. The hormones produced in the hypothalamus are secreted directly into the anterior pituitary gland via the hypothalamic-hypophyseal portal system. These hormones, called neurohormones, may be stimulatory or inhibitory. They act directly on the tissues of the pituitary gland to control the secretion of the anterior pituitary hormones. Inhibiting hormones are released by the hypothalamus to stop the formation and secretion of target hormones; the most important of these is prolactin inhibitory factor. Tropic or stimulating hormones, which are made by the pituitary, act on target tissue or glands to release hormones needed for homeostasis, growth maturation, and reproduction of the individual.

The hypothalamus receives signals from almost all possible sources, including the cerebral cortex. These sources send pain and psychological messages, causing release of tropic hormones. Therefore, prolonged stress can alter cortisol, thyroid, and growth hormone levels and cause menstruation to cease. Because of this interrelation and the wide range of functions that these hormones exert in maintaining the body's function, the hypothalamus is considered by some to be the true "master gland."

Pituitary Gland

The pea-sized pituitary gland is located at the base of the brain above the sphenoid bone. It is divided into two parts, the anterior pituitary (adenohypophysis) and the posterior pituitary (neurohypophysis). The anterior pituitary is glandular tissue and the posterior pituitary is actually an extension of the hypothalamus.

The posterior pituitary is made up of nervous tissue and its primary function is the release of antidiuretic hormone, to be discussed later, and oxytocin. Oxytocin in females is responsible for the secretion of milk from the breasts and causes the contraction of the uterus during labor.

The anterior pituitary originates from epithelial tissue and comprises approximately 80% of the gland's mass. Its cells secrete hormones that are regulated by the releasing and inhibiting hormones produced by the hypothalamus. Five specialized cell types within the anterior pituitary are responsible for the secretion of the six major hormones: growth hormone, thyroid-stimulating hormone or thyrotropin, adrenocorticotropin hormone or corticotropin, prolactin, follicle-stimulating hormone, and luteinizing hormone. Most of these hormones are tropic hormones. Releasing and inhibiting hormones produced by the hypothalamus control the secretion of the hormones produced by the anterior pituitary (Chart 51–1). Each of these is discussed under a separate section.

Assessment

Hormones are involved in the use and production of energy, growth and development, sexual development and maturation, and maintaining homeostasis. These vast, encompassing functions make it clear that the assessment of endocrine function is an involved task. Disorders may not produce any associated symptoms or may be so vague as to be attributed to any number of problems other than endocrine dysfunction. Abnormalities are produced by five indistinct mechanisms: difficulty with the appropriate transport of a hormone, production of hormones by hypersecretion (excessive production) or hyposecretion (decreased production), inability of target tissues to respond to a secreted hormone, and inappropriate stimulation of target tissue.

Health History

Assessing for normal and abnormal hormonal variations entails a thorough assessment of the patient's history along with a systematic, complete physical examination. Assessment should include examination of past medical history, family history, current complaints, general and functional health evaluation, and diagnostic testing. General health screening and focused screening of chief complaints will assist in the identification of the origin of suspected endocrine disorders.

Exploration of the patient's history is essential. Questioning should seek to assess the onset, characteristics, and severity of symptoms. The nurse also should seek to identify any alleviating or aggravating factors, associated symptomatology, and timing of symptoms. The patient is asked about previous head injuries, hospitalizations, illnesses, surgeries and treatments, changes in appearance, sleep and rest patterns, elimination problems, sexual dysfunction, changes in diet or appetite, and medication usage. Cognitive function, including sensory and perception, along with affect, also may be altered with endocrine dysfunction.

Along with a review of the entire medical history, family, occupational, and social histories are evaluated. Disorders of the endocrine system tend to occur in a familial pattern. There is a high correlation of diabetes, thyroid disorders, and obesity among families. Knowing this information should assist the interviewer in conducting a more focused assessment. Dietary patterns and involuntary weight losses and gains should be explored. Exposure to chemicals, use of drugs and alcohol, smoking, coping with stress, and behavioral patterns are all areas to be investigated.

Health Assessment Across the Adult Life Span

Generally endocrine disorders should be assessed for all patients across the adult life span. However, certain hormonal disorders are prone to develop in certain age groups. For example, disorders of the pituitary and related hormones tend to affect chil-

---

CHART 51–1 **Anterior Pituitary Hormone Production and Function**

Cell Type	Hormone Produced	Hormone Function
Somatotropic	Growth hormone (GH) or somatotropin	• Stimulates growth and development of skeletal muscle and long bones. • Metabolizes carbohydrates, fats, and protein.
Lactotrophic	Prolactin	• Stimulates the production of breast milk following childbirth. • Increases response of the follicles to luteinizing hormone (LH) and follicle-stimulating hormone (FSH).
Thymotrophic	Thyroid-stimulating hormone (TSH)	• Stimulates the production and synthesis and release of thyroid hormone from the thyroid.
Corticotrophic	Adrenocorticotrophic hormone (ACTH)	• Stimulates the release of hormones from the adrenal cortex.
Gonadotrophic	Follicle-stimulating hormone (FSH) Luteinizing hormone (LH)	• In women, stimulates the development of ovarian follicles and estrogenic female sex hormones. • In men, functions in the development and maturation of sperm. • In women, stimulates ovulation and formation of corpus luteum from an ovarian follicle. • In men, stimulates production of male sex hormones.
Melanocytic	Melanocyte-stimulating hormone (MSH)	• Stimulates the production and release of melanin (melanogenesis) by melanocytes in skin and hair.

dren and young adults. Hyperpituitarism, or oversecretion of the growth hormone is evident in adulthood after puberty. Gigantism begins before the epiphyseal closure of the bones; the disease is progressive. It affects children as evidenced by an increasing growth rate. Acromegaly develops between the ages of 30 and 50; and dwarfism occurs as a result of failure of the pituitary gland and is evident in young adults. Deficiency in hormones produced by the pituitary gland also may affect sexual development of males and females and cause consequences in postpartum lactation.

Age differences also are noted in diabetes mellitus (DM), type 1 and type 2, generated by decreased production of insulin by the pancreas or by decreased ability to use insulin. Type 1 DM typically occurs in people before the age of 30, peaking at ages 5 to 11. Type 2 usually develops after the age of 30, often in middle age. Gestational diabetes starts or is first recognized during pregnancy, usually becoming apparent during the 24th to 28th weeks of pregnancy. It is important to recognize these age variations in assessing patients because they can help guide the assessment process and recognition of presenting symptoms.

Relative to the aging population the most frequent sign of hormonal imbalance is hypothyroidism (Bharaktiya, Orlander, Woodhouse, & Davis, 2007). This is discussed in detail under the discussion of the thyroid gland. Disorders related to each of the hormonal imbalances referenced above are discussed in Chapters 52 and 53 ☺.

Current Health Problems

Because the endocrine system functions in the storage and production of energy, the patient should be asked about energy levels and the ability to carry out activities of daily living (ADLs) independently. The patient may report not being able to "do what I used to" or may complain of generalized weakness and fatigue." Patients are more likely to report a gradual decline than an abrupt change in activity tolerance. Assessment of a patient's energy level also will be important in developing the ongoing plan of care. Thyroid and adrenal dysfunction are common reasons for altered energy levels (see these sections later in this chapter).

Physical Examination

The only endocrine glands that can be palpated are the thyroid, ovaries, and testes. All others are located within the body and examination of function relies on the examination of the end result of hormone function on target tissue and diagnostic testing. The physical exam should be thorough and systematic. This section provides a general overview. More findings are included in the specific endocrine disorder section.

General appearance, skin, hair, nails, facial contours, and body symmetry can provide clues to the endocrine gland experiencing dysfunction. Normal growth and development patterns are compared to physical findings in the client. Alterations of temperature, heart rate, and blood pressure all may be attributed to endocrine dysfunction. Comparisons to normal stature and usual body weight may yield clues to pituitary or thyroid dysfunction.

The physical exam should begin with vital sign measurement, height and weight, and mental status exam. The skin and its appendages also are examined. The skin is assessed for temperature, color, homogeneous pigmentation pattern, turgor,

texture, edema, and presence of masses. The skin also is assessed for the presence of lesions or striae. Nail angle, thickness, and pigmentation are reviewed for abnormalities. Hair distribution pattern and texture are noted. The presence of acne, hirsutism, ecchymosis, striae, thinning skin, and alopecia may be associated with steroid-excess states. Excessive sweating and coarse dry skin also can be associated with endocrine dysfunction.

Assessment of the head and neck involves both internal and external examination. Visually, the examination begins with the inspection of the face and neck for contours, symmetry, and masses. The oral cavity is examined for color, size, intactness, lesions, and condition of teeth, tongue, and gums. The neck also is examined for bulging and masses along with the position of the trachea. The eyes are assessed for bulging. Visual acuity, field of gaze, and lid movement should be evaluated.

The chest is visualized for its overall appearance. Symmetry of chest movement is noted. Heart sounds are auscultated and the patient is examined for the presence of bruits (turbulent blood flow through a vessel or artery). Heart rhythm is assessed for regularity and the presence of abnormality and is compared to peripheral pulses. Lung sounds are assessed. Measurement of oxygen saturation will provide information that may be important in evaluating mental status and cognitive function. The size of the heart can be affected by endocrine disease. The presence of adventitious (abnormal) breath sounds may indicate increased fluid retention that may be seen in patients with endocrine dysfunction.

Peripheral pulses are palpated and pulse volume is noted. The abdomen usually is assessed for skin color, pigmentation pattern, and presence of striae. It also is inspected for distention, masses, pulsations, and dilated veins. Bowel sounds are auscultated, noting frequency and character. Palpation is done to assess for the presence of masses, tenderness, or pain. Unintentional weight loss due to loss of appetite, weight gain, constipation, and bouts of diarrhea can all be seen in patients experiencing endocrine dysfunction. Liver impairment also may be seen in the endocrine disorders of diabetes and myxedema. Abdominal obesity has been associated with metabolic syndrome.

The upper and lower extremities are examined visually for general appearance, pigmentation pattern, skin texture, and hair distribution. Symmetry of muscle mass along with appropriateness of size as dictated by normal parameters of growth and development are assessed. Deep tendon reflexes, motor movement, sensation, and strength are assessed. Proprioception, coordination, and the presence of tremors are noted.

Nervous system complaints are common in endocrine dysfunction because nearly all hormones have a demonstrated influence on the central nervous system. Headache is a common complaint. Patients also may display tremors, lethargy, and convulsions. Electrolyte imbalances produced by endocrine disorders can produce considerable muscle weakness or spastic muscle activity. Neuropathies, myopathy, osteoporosis, osteomalacia, gouty arthritis, and distortion of bone growth all can be seen in endocrine dysfunction.

A number of endocrine disorders are associated with urinary dysfunction. Patients may complain of frequency, urgency, and nocturia with diabetes mellitus or insipidus. Nephrolithiasis (kidney stones) can occur with hyperparathyroidism, Cushing's disease, and acromegaly. Patients with diabetes mellitus are prone to urinary tract infections. Congenital urinary abnormalities are seen in Turner's syndrome. The next section focuses on specific subjective and objective findings for different endocrine disorders.

Specific Hormonal Functions and Assessment of Hormonal Imbalances

Each hormone has a specific function. Hormones act on the target tissue by different mechanisms. They can alter the function of the target tissue by interacting with chemical receptors located either on the cell membrane or in the interior of the cell. Imbalances, either hypersecretion or hyposecretion of the hormone, can lead to specific hormonal disorders.

Growth Hormone

Like the other hormones controlled by the pituitary in a complex feedback loop, growth hormone (GH) is secreted by the pituitary directly into the blood throughout the life cycle in a double feedback loop. GH synthesis and release is controlled by the hypothalamus through growth hormone releasing factor (GHRF) and growth hormone release-inhibiting hormone (GHRIH), which stimulate the pituitary to release GH. Once released into circulation, GH stimulates the production of insulin-like growth factor-1 (IGF-1), also known as somatomedin C (SM-C). Growth hormone stimulates growth of all tissues. When the epiphyses of the bones close at approximately age 21, bone growth will cease.

Assessment

A tumor of the pituitary with GH hypersecretion can cause excess growth or gigantism in children. The nurse should take a careful history of size of other family members to rule out genetic causes for very tall children. The nurse assessing extremes in size should consider a tumor of the pituitary as the source.

In adults, the name for hypersecretion of GH is acromegaly. More than 95% of acromegaly cases are caused by a pituitary adenoma that secretes excess amounts of GH. Ectopic production of GH and GHRH by malignant tumors accounts for other causes (Khandwala, 2005). Hypersecretion causes growth of the carti-lage, resulting in enlargement of the ears and jaw, protrusion of the tongue, and disproportionately large hands and feet with thick fingers and toes. There is skeletal thickening, hypertrophy of the skin, and enlargement of the heart and liver. Other findings include weakness, delayed onset of puberty, and irregular menstruation. Because GH is an insulin antagonist, the nurse should assess for hyperglycemia. Because tumors of the pituitary may erode into the oral mucosa, the mouth needs careful inspection.

Insufficient GH causes a child to be a perfectly proportioned midget, in contrast to dwarfism, a genetic defect in which there is failure of the long bones to grow. Children who are not on the growth chart need referral to an endocrinologist.

Laboratory and Diagnostic Procedures

Growth hormone (somatotropin) is increased in gigantism and acromegaly, and decreased in dwarfism. However, random GH measurements are often not diagnostic because of the episodic secretion of GH, its short half-life, and the overlap between GH concentration in patients with acromegaly and healthy subjects. Because IGF-1 has a long half-life, its measurement is useful to gauge integrated GH secretion, to screen for acromegaly, and to monitor the efficacy of therapy (Khandwala, 2005). A computerized tomography (CT) or magnetic resonance imaging (MRI) scan will show pituitary tumor in gigantism. X-rays may show spotting or stippling near the epiphyses of the bones in dwarfism. Chart 51–2 summarizes growth hormone testing.

Antidiuretic Hormone

Antidiuretic hormone (ADH) or vasopressin is synthesized in the cell bodies of neurons located in the hypothalamus and transmitted to the posterior pituitary along axons in response to neural stimulation. ADH is responsible for the reabsorption of water in the renal tubules resulting in an increase in circulatory volume, and is released in response to increased osmolality of the blood. Excessive ADH, secreted by tumors or ectopic sources, causes fluid retention and is known as syndrome of inappropriate ADH (SIADH). Lack of ADH causes fluid loss and is known as diabetes insipidus.

Assessment

The nurse should take a careful history of the cardiac and renal systems when assessing fluid balance to eliminate these as causes for fluid retention. Excessive weight gain without overt edema is

CHART 51–2	Growth Hormone Testing		
Laboratory Test and Normal Values	**Gland Tested Diagnostic Significance**	**Disorders Associated with Abnormal Levels *(symptoms are italicized)***	
		Increased	**Decreased**
Growth hormone (somatotropin) Adult (fasting and at rest) 2–5 ng/mL	Anterior pituitary (origin) Muscle and bone (target)	*Gigantism in children, acromegaly in adults,* benign pituitary gland tumor, severe malnutrition states, hyperpituitarism, multiple endocrine neoplasia, neurofibromatosis	*Dwarfism in children,* hypopituitarism, Seckel's syndrome, congenital GH deficiency, pituitary fibrosis, or calcification
IGF-1 Concentrations vary with age. An assay in which reference ranges have been stratified in such a manner is required.	Anterior pituitary (origin) Muscle and bone (target)	*Gigantism in children, acromegaly in adults,* benign pituitary gland tumor, severe malnutrition states, hyperpituitarism, multiple endocrine neoplasia, neurofibromatosis	*Dwarfism in children,* hypopituitarism, Seckel's syndrome, congenital GH deficiency, pituitary fibrosis, or calcification

characteristic of SIADH, as are hyponatremia, nausea, vomiting, muscle cramps, confusion, convulsions, inappropriately elevated urine osmolality (>200 mOsm/kg), excessive urine sodium excretion (UNa >30 mEq/L), and decreased serum osmolality. These findings occur in the absence of diuretic therapy; in the presence of normal volume without edema; and in the setting of otherwise normal cardiac, renal, adrenal, hepatic, and thyroid function (Rafailov, 2007). This syndrome may occur as a result of ectopic secretion in association with oat-cell lung cancer, pancreatic cancer, prostate cancer, and Hodgkin's disease as well as a number of other disorders.

 Hyponatremia with serum sodium < 115 mEq/L causes osmotic shifts of fluid from the blood into the brain. This increases the pressure and can cause lethargy, headaches, decreased responsiveness, seizures, and coma.

Excessive urination, decreased urine specific gravity, thirst, and dehydration are found with lack of ADH, known as diabetes insipidus (DI). The term *insipidus* means lacking character, referring to the clear colorless urine. Trauma or autoimmune response can cause a lack of ADH. The most common form is central DI. Central DI results from damage to the pituitary gland, which disrupts the normal storage and release of ADH. Nephrogenic DI results when the kidneys are unable to respond to ADH. Rarer forms occur because of a defect in the thirst mechanism (dipsogenic DI) or during pregnancy (gestational DI) (National Kidney and Urologic Diseases Information Clearinghouse, 2006).

 Trauma to the head may damage the pituitary and result in decreased production of ADH, resulting in extreme diuresis or diabetes insipidus. Trauma patients who produce excessively large amounts of urine are at risk of hypovolemic shock.

Laboratory and Diagnostic Procedures

Serum osmolarity testing is done to determine ADH balance. Increased serum osmolality indicates lack of ADH and dehydration; decrease in serum osmolality indicates SIADH and fluid overload. Serum sodium is also decreased when fluid is retained; it is increased with diabetes insipidus and dehydration. Urine osmolality testing will be decreased in diabetes insipidus due to large volumes of very dilute urine. Chart 51–3 summarizes antidiuretics hormone tests of the posterior pituitary used to determine disorders of associated abnormal levels.

Gonads

The gonads are the body's primary source of sexual hormones. They are controlled in a triple feedback loop. The hypothalamus makes follicle-stimulating hormone releasing factor (FRF) and luteinizing hormone releasing factor (LRF). FRF from the hypothalamus causes release of follicle-stimulating hormone (FSH) and luteinizing hormone (LH) from the anterior pituitary gland. FSH in women promotes maturation of the ovarian follicle, which produces estrogen. As levels of estrogen rise, there is an increase in LH. Together FSH and LH induce ovulation. In men, FSH produces spermatogenesis, and the LH stimulates secretion of androgens.

Gonads are important for the progression into puberty and they control other physical traits that differentiate men from women. The principal hormone produced by the testes is testosterone. The primary hormones produced by the ovaries are estrogen and progesterone. For males, testosterone maintains reproductive functioning and secondary sexual characteristics. Sexual hormones also promote the production and maturation of sperm and stimulate most cells into protein synthesis.

In women, the ovaries secrete estrogen and progesterone to maintain reproductive functioning and secondary sexual characteristics. Progesterone in females also promotes the growth of the lining of the uterus for the implantation of a fertilized ovum and prepares the mammary glands for lactation. Some sexual hormones, called androgens, also are produced by the adrenal gland.

Assessment

Assessment of reproductive and sexual functioning entails the visualization of age-appropriate sexual development along with questioning concerning changes in libido, fertility, impotence, and menstrual irregularities. Hair distribution and character also are noted, particularly pubic hair, which decreases with decreased sex hormones. The breasts are observed for contours, masses, tenderness, and the presence of inappropriate lactation. Males are assessed for gynecomastia (enlarged breasts), which occurs when the liver does not destroy female hormones made by the adrenal gland. The testes are palpated in males and a pelvic examination conducted in females. Clitoral enlargement in women may indicate an endocrine disorder. Precocious puberty in the young may be caused by premature release of gonadotropin-releasing hormone (GnRH) by the hypothalamus. Lack of secondary sexual characteristics in adults may be seen in pituitary hypofunction.

The patient should be assessed for sexual maturation using Tanner's stages (Estes, 2002); (Chart 51–4, p. 1602). Failure to develop secondary sexual characteristics of pubic hair and genital growth by the age of 16 should be investigated and referred by the nurse.

CHART 51–3	Antidiuretic Hormone Testing		
Laboratory Test and Normal Values	**Gland Tested Diagnostic Significance**	**Disorders Associated with Abnormal Levels** *(symptoms are italicized)*	
		Increased	**Decreased**
Antidiuretic hormone If serum osmolarity is >290 mOsm/kg: 2–12 pg/mL or SI: 1.85–11.1 pmol/L If serum osmolarity is <290 mOsm/kg: <2 pg/mL or SI: <1.85 pmol/L	Posterior pituitary (origin) Kidneys (target) Used to diagnose diabetes insipidus and syndrome of inappropriate antidiuretic hormone release (SIADH)	Pituitary hyperplasia, drugs, severe pain, stress, hyperthermia, *SIADH, weight gain, hyponatremia,* ectopic production from cancer, pneumonia, tuberculosis, cerebrovascular disease	Pituitary failure, *diabetes insipidus, psychogenic polydipsia, enuresis, nephrotic syndrome*

CHART 51–4	Tanner's Stages		
Tanner Stage	**Pubic Hair (Both Male and Female)**	**Genitals (Male)**	**Breasts (Female)**
I	No pubic hair at all (prepubertal state) (ages 10 and under)	Prepubertal (testicular volume is less than 1.5 mL; small penis of 3 cm or less).	No glandular tissue; areola follows the skin contours of the chest (prepubertal).
II	Small amount of long, downy hair with slight pigmentation at the base of the penis and scrotum (males) or on the labia majora (females) (ages 10–11)	Testicular volume between 1.6 and 6 mL; skin on scrotum thins, reddens, and enlarges; penis length unchanged.	Breast bud forms, with small area of surrounding glandular tissue; areola begins to widen.
III	Hair becomes more coarse and curly, and begins to extend laterally (ages 12–14)	Testicular volume between 6 and 12 mL; scrotum enlarges further; penis begins to lengthen to about 6 cm.	Breast begins to become more elevated, and extends beyond the borders of the areola, which continues to widen but remains in contour with surrounding breast.
IV	Adult-like hair quality, extending across pubis but sparing medial thighs (ages 13–15)	Testicular volume between 12 and 20 mL; scrotum enlarges further and darkens; penis increases in length to 10 cm and circumference.	Increased breast size and elevation; areola and papilla form a secondary mound projecting from the contour of the surrounding breast.
V	Hair extends to medial surface of the thighs (ages 16+)	Testicular volume greater than 20 mL; adult scrotum and penis of 15 cm in length.	Breast reaches final adult size; areola returns to contour of the surrounding breast, with a projecting central papilla.

Laboratory and Diagnostic Procedures

Testing involves FSH and LH levels. Pituitary malfunction causes a lack of these hormones, which will result in lack of menses in women and lack of secondary sexual characteristics in boys and girls. Testosterone levels are done when there is precocious puberty or delayed male sexual development. Refer to Chart 51–5.

Adrenal Glands

The triangular-shaped adrenal glands sit on the upper poles of the kidneys. Within the adrenal glands there are two distinct layers that have specialized functions. The outer layer is known as the adrenal medulla. The inner layer is the adrenal cortex. These glands are responsible for secretion of catecholamines and steroids, which are released to assist the body in maintaining homeostasis when exposed to stressors.

The adrenal medulla produces the catecholamines epinephrine and norepinephrine, substances that play an important role in the body's physiological response to stress. Epinephrine is a potent vasoconstrictor that, when released, increases heart rate, force of cardiac contraction, and blood pressure. Epinephrine also stimulates release of glucocorticoids in order to increase the serum glucose. Norepinephrine is an even more potent vasoconstrictor, mostly released at the neuromuscular junction, which also increases the heart rate and force of cardiac contractions. It constricts blood vessels throughout the body. Essential hypertension is sometimes caused by benign adrenal medulla tumors, called pheochromocytoma (see Chapter 21 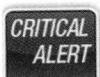).

The adrenal cortex secretes corticosteroids of which there are two types, mineralocorticoids and glucocorticoids; both are essential to life. Mineralocorticoids, such as aldosterone, exert control over the retention of sodium and water in maintaining blood pressure and body fluid volume. The glucocorticoids function in carbohydrate metabolism, assist in immune func-

tion, are released in response to stress, and are controlled by a complex feedback loop. A drop in the cortisol level to the hypothalamus stimulates the release of cortisol releasing factor (CRF), a neurohormone that subsequently causes the pituitary to release adrenocorticotropic hormone (ACTH). ACTH then directly stimulates an increase in cortisol by the adrenal cortex. If the cortex is not responsive (primary failure or Addison's disease), the pituitary increases production of ACTH in an effort to raise cortisol levels. Increased ACTH stimulates melanocytes, causing darkening of the skin with Addison's disease. The perception of stress impacts the hypothalamus, and increased stress from illness, surgery, or psychological trauma can increase cortisol levels up to 30 times normal levels. Figure 51–2 ■ illustrates the adrenal gland feedback loop.

> **CRITICAL ALERT** *When patients take cortisone, the increased levels in the blood inhibit production of CRF and ACTH, and the patient's adrenal gland stops functioning. Because ACTH stimulates the release of the mineralocorticoid aldosterone, a sudden cessation of the medication may result in cardiovascular collapse.*

Assessment

The nurse must complete a careful history about the onset of symptoms and medications taken to eliminate other possible etiologies. Two major disorders may be caused by adrenal cortex malfunction. The first adrenal cortex disorder is Cushing's disease, caused by an excess of cortisol. Cortisol causes breakdown of fat and muscle from the extremities for conversion to glucose (gluconeogenesis), which is subsequently deposited as fat in the abdomen and face and back. Symptoms of Cushing's disease include truncal obesity, thin arms and legs, moon face, buffalo hump, severe fatigue and muscle weakness, hyperglycemia, easy bruising, gastrointestinal bleeding, depression, and osteoporosis. Because hyperfunction of the adrenal cortex also can include increased aldosterone and androgens, hypertension may be present.

CHART 51–5	Gonadal Gland Testing		
Laboratory Test and Normal Values	**Gland Tested Diagnostic Significance**	**Disorders Associated with Abnormal Levels (symptoms are italicized)**	
		Increased	**Decreased**
Follicle-stimulating hormone (FSH) *Males:* 4–15 mU/mL *Females:* 4.6–22.4 mU/mL pre- and postovulation 13–41 mU/mL midcycle peaks	Anterior pituitary (origin) Ovaries and testes (target) Controls the growth and maturation of ovarian follicles in women and the production of sperm in men	Ovarian failure of menopause, hysterectomy, castration, anorchism, hyperthyroidism, hyperpituitarism, hypothalamic tumor, acromegaly, *primary amenorrhea*	*Infertility*, adrenal hyperplasia, *secondary amenorrhea*, anorexia nervosa, neoplasm, hypogonadotropism, hypophysectomy
Luteinizing hormone (LH) *Males:* 3–18 mU/mL *Females:* 2.4–34.5 mU/mL pre- and postovulation 43–187 mU/mL midcycle peaks	Anterior pituitary (origin) Ovaries and testes (target) In women, responsible for the ovulation and stimulation of the ruptured follicle to produce progesterone. In men, stimulates the production of androgens, which support development of secondary sexual characteristics	Menopause, anorchism, hyperpituitarism, Klinefelter, liver disease, pituitary tumors	*Hypogonadism (primary or secondary)*, pituitary insufficiency, adrenal hyperplasia or tumor, *amenorrhea* (pituitary failure, *secondary gonadal insufficiency*), malnutrition, hypophysectomy
Testosterone *Males:* 270–1,070 ng/dL *Females:* 8–86 ng/dL	Gonads (origin) Assesses precocious sexual development in young males; assesses the activity of ovaries and testes in adults	*Precocious puberty (in boys)*, *masculinization in women and girls*, *adrenogenital syndrome*, adrenal hyperplasia, adrenal tumor, testicular tumor	*Failure of the testes to develop*, pituitary insufficiency, *male impotence*, cirrhosis, *hypogonadism*, orchiectomy, *gynecomastia*, *obesity*

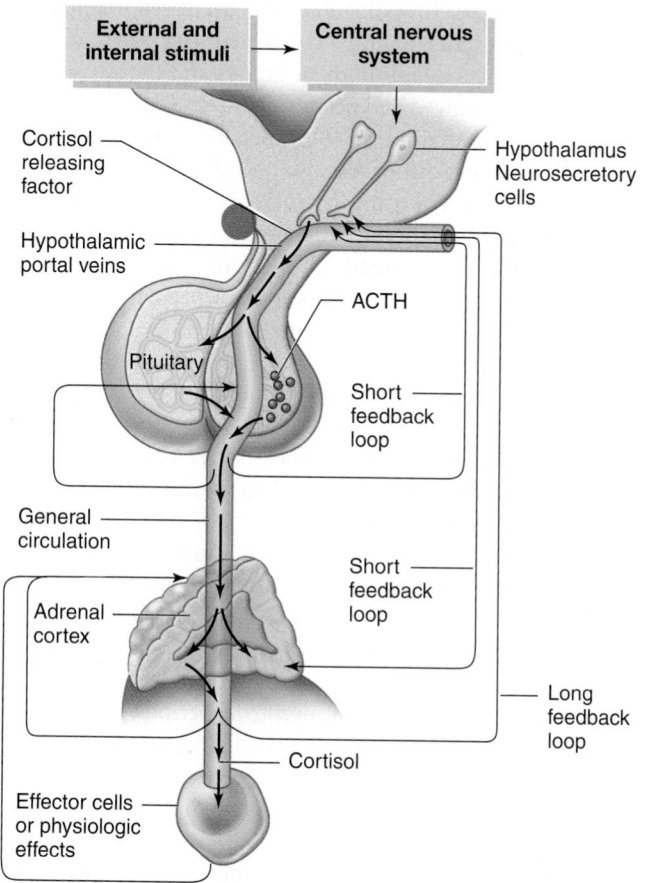

FIGURE 51–2 ■ Adrenal gland feedback loop.

Distribution and location of facial hair should be noted. The presence of hirsutism and deepening of the voice in women can occur with androgen excesses. Cushing's disease is caused by tumor or trauma and is to be differentiated from Cushing's syndrome, an iatrogenic condition caused by exogenous administration of cortisone.

The second cortex disorder is Addison's disease, caused by an autoimmune response that destroys the adrenal cortex. It is characterized by lack of aldosterone, a mineralocorticoid responsible for sodium and water reabsorption from the kidney tubules. Aldosterone, a mineralocorticoid, acts at the level of the distal tubular sodium/potassium exchange system to increase potassium excretion while facilitating sodium reabsorption. Mineralocorticoid deficiency causes increased urinary losses of sodium, chloride, and water, along with decreased excretion of potassium. The results of hyponatremia are loss of extracellular fluid, decreased cardiac output, and hyperkalemia. Hyperkalemia results as the kidney tubules reabsorb other cations because they cannot absorb sodium ions. The nurse should assess for hypotension, muscle weakness, dysrhythmias, and fatigue. The heart may be smaller in Addison's disease due to a reduction in volume of circulating fluid (Odeske & Nagelberg, 2006).

If the disorder is caused by primary adrenal cortex failure, the resulting increase in ACTH causes a dark skin color or tanned appearance that is most prevalent on the areas exposed to sun. Increased pigmentation of the oral mucosa also may indicate Addison's disease. Hypoglycemia and weight loss are symptoms caused by decreased levels of cortisol from primary failure of the entire adrenal gland. Lack of androgen causes decreases in body, axillary, and pubic hair, especially in women who have no other source of androgen hormones. Other symptoms include nausea, vomiting, anorexia, a craving for salty foods, and the inability to tolerate stress.

 **CRITICAL ALERT** *Acute adrenal insufficiency is called Addisonian crisis and is a life-threatening event triggered by a stressful situation such as surgery, trauma, or severe infection. The patient may die from hypotension from volume depletion.*

Hyperaldosteronism (Conn's syndrome) is most commonly caused by adrenal adenoma and is characterized by increased secretion of aldosterone. This mineralocorticoid causes increased sodium retention with potassium and hydrogen ion excretion. The nurse should assess for increased blood pressure, hypernatremia, hypokalemia, and metabolic alkalosis.

If assessment includes severe hypertension and other symptoms including shakiness, anxiety, cold diaphoresis, and headache, the nurse should consider an adrenal medulla disorder. Pheochromocytoma is a benign tumor of the adrenal medulla that produces excess adrenaline and accounts for less than 1% of all hypertensive cases. It can occur at any age, but is most common in people between the ages of 40 and 60. Ninety percent of cases are sporadic. However, 10 percent can be linked to hereditary causes (American Urological Association, 2007).

Laboratory and Diagnostic Procedures

Laboratory tests ordered for adrenal cortex disorders first include checking cortisol levels, which follow a diurnal pattern in the body. If there is an abnormal level, ACTH stimulation tests determine if the disorder is caused by adrenal (primary failure) or pituitary (secondary failure) malfunction. Normally, the ACTH stimulation test will cause an increase in cortisol levels. If the pituitary is not functional (secondary failure), the hypothalamus increases production of CRF, but the ACTH and cortisol levels will still be low. In tertiary failure of the hypothalamus, all three hormone levels will be low. Another test is 17 ketosteroids; it measures the urinary excretion of metabolites from cortisol and is elevated with hypersecretion or Cushing's and low with Addison's. Aldosterone levels will also be depressed with Addison's. X-rays and CT scans may show an adrenal tumor. Tuberculosis testing can eliminate TB of the kidney as a cause of failure.

Testing for adrenal medulla disorders includes urinary catecholamines and metanephrines, measured in a 24-hour urine collection. If these are more than two times the normal level, imaging studies are usually done to look at the adrenal glands. Levels are elevated with pheochromocytoma and decreased with adrenal gland hypofunctioning. Chart 51–6 summarizes adrenal gland tests. See Chapter 59 for additional information 🔗.

Thyroid Gland

The thyroid gland is located in the neck anterior to the upper part of the trachea and just inferior to the larynx. It has two lobes, which are in the shape of a butterfly connected by a structure known as the isthmus. The thyroid has both glandular and follicular tissue, which produces the hormones secreted by the thyroid, triiodothyronine (T_3) and thyroxine (T_4), as well as calcitonin hormones, which are responsible for cellular metabolism, for growth and development in children, and for the regulation of calcium levels.

The thyroid is controlled by a complex feedback loop. A drop in thyroid levels to the hypothalamus stimulates production of thyroid releasing factor (TRF), a neurohormone that subsequently causes the pituitary to release thyroid-stimulating hormone (TSH), which then causes release of thyroid hormone (TH). In primary failure of the thyroid gland, there is low TH with increased TSH, the pituitary's attempt to increase TH levels. In secondary failure of the pituitary, there is low TH and low TSH with increased TRF, the hypothalamus's attempt to increase TH levels. In tertiary failure of the hypothalamus, all three hormones are low: low TRF results in low TSH, which results in low TH. Figure 51–3 ■ (p. 1606) shows the thyroid feedback loop.

Assessment

Thyroid malfunction is one of the most common endocrine disorders. Congenital hypothyroidism, formerly known as cretinism, can be endemic, genetic, or sporadic. If untreated, it results in mild to severe impairment of both physical and mental growth and development. Infants are screened at birth for this condition. Short stature may indicate insufficient thyroid hormone in a child. Lack of secondary sexual characteristics in adults may be caused by lack of thyroid hormone.

Because thyroid hormone controls the metabolic rate, the nurse should assess the patient for fatigue and weight gain. Elevated cholesterol levels are common with hypothyroidism. There may be heavy menstrual periods and constipation from decreased peristalsis. There are decreased deep tendon reflexes. The hair is thinned and dry and loses its shine, and the skin is dry. Patients with hypothyroidism may complain of cold intolerance and have bradycardia. Because hypothyroidism causes slow mentation, cognitive disorders, and decreased orientation, a mental status exam should be completed. Hypothyroidism is sometimes associated with nodular goiters and the swallowing process may be involved and needs to be assessed.

Profound hypothyroidism is associated with myxedema, which refers to a deposit of mucopolysaccharides that causes a nonpitting edema. The cardinal manifestation of myxedema coma is a deterioration of the patient's mental status, which may be subtle, manifesting as apathy, neglect, or a decrease in intellectual function (Wall, 2000). Typically, patients with myxedema have primary hypothyroidism manifested by low T_4 levels and elevated TSH levels.

Graves' disease is the most common cause of hyperthyroidism, accounting for 60% to 80% of all cases. It is an autoimmune disease caused by an antibody, active against the TSH receptor, which stimulates the gland to synthesize and secrete excess thyroid hormone (Reid & Wheeler, 2005). Hyperthyroidism increases the metabolic rate and causes vasodilation in attempts to decrease body temperature. Patients complain of heat intolerance and may have lower blood pressure and compensatory tachycardia, palpitations, and functional heart murmurs. The increased metabolism causes weight loss and fatigue. Diarrhea and shorter or lighter menstrual periods may be seen in clients with hyperthyroidism. The patient may have difficulty sleeping. There may be exaggerated deep tendon reflexes. Hyperthyroid disorders may impair coping ability and are known to cause psychosis (Fenton & Gold, 2006).

Hyperthyroidism is associated with "fullness" in the neck. The swallowing process is observed along with the character and

CHART 51–6 Adrenal Gland Testing

Laboratory Test and Normal Values	Gland Tested Diagnostic Significance	Disorders Associated with Abnormal Levels *(symptoms are italicized)*	
		Increased	**Decreased**
ACTH stimulation *Rapid test:* cortisol levels increase > 7 mg/dL above baseline *24-hour test:* cortisol level > 40 µg/dL *3-day test:* cortisol level > 40 µg/dL	Adrenals (target) Pituitary (origin) Evaluates the ability of the adrenal gland to respond to ACTH administration	Exaggerated response: Cushing's syndrome Bilateral adrenal hyperplasia: more cortisol is released in response to ACTH dose	Normal or below response: adrenal insufficiency (Addison's) results in less cortisol release in response to stimulation because the gland is not functioning
Serum ACTH *a.m.:* <80 pg/mL or <18 pmol/L (SI units) *p.m.:* <50 pg/mL or <11 pmol/L (SI units)	Anterior pituitary (origin) Adrenals (target) To assess etiology of either overproduction (Cushing's disease) or underproduction of cortisol (Addison's disease)	Ectopic ACTH producing tumors, stress, Addison's disease (primary adrenal insufficiency), surgical removal of the adrenals, adrenal suppression with long-term exogenous steroid therapy. If the adrenal glands are less functional, ACTH production increases via the feedback loop	Pituitary insufficiency; Cushing's syndrome, (exogenous steroid administration) or Cushing's disease caused by bilateral adrenal hyperplasia will cause decreased levels via feedback loop
Serum cortisol *8 a.m.:* 5–23 µg/dL or 138–635 nmol/L (SI units) *4 p.m.:* 3–13 µg/dL or 83–359 nmol/L (SI units)	Adrenals (origin) Measures serum cortisol levels Diurnal functioning with peak levels of 6–8 morning and lowest levels around midnight	*Cushing's disease*, stress including burns, ectopic ACTH producing tumors, *obesity*, hyperpituitarism, hyperthyroidism, pregnancy	*Addison's disease*, hypopituitarism, hypothyroidism; low cortisol levels cause hypoglycemia
Urinary cortisol 20–70 µg/ 24 hr or 25–95 ng/mg of creatinine	Adrenals (origin) Assess for adrenal hyperfunction	Cushing's syndrome, stress, ectopic ACTH-secreting tumors, pregnancy, hyperthyroidism, obesity	Addison's disease, hypopituitarism, hypothyroidism
17-Hydroxycorticosteroids (Porter–Sibler test, 17-OCHS) *Males:* 4–10 mg/24 hr or 8.3–27.6 µmol/day (SI units) urine specimen *Females:* 2–8 mg/24 hr or 5.2–22.1 µmol/day (SI units) urine specimen	Adrenals (origin) Assess for adrenal hyperfunction	Cushing's syndrome, cortisone administration, ACTH-secreting ectopic tumors, obesity, hyperthyroidism, Cushing's disease	Addison's disease, congenital adrenal hyperplasia or lack of cortisol, hepatic disorders, renal disorders, hypopituitarism, hypothyroidism
17-Ketosteroids (17KS) *Males:* 6–20 mg/24 hr or 20–70 µmol/day (SI units) *Females:* 6–17 mg/24 hr or 20–60 µmol/day (SI units)	Adrenals (origin) Measures the metabolites of steroids from both the adrenal cortex and the testes except for the androgen testosterone	Adrenogenital syndrome, tumors of the adrenal cortex and testes, ACTH administration, hyperpituitarism, *Cushing's syndrome*	*Addison's disease*, severe debilitating disease, severe stress and infection, chronic disease, hypogonadism, castration, certain adrenal adenomas, hypopituitarism
Aldosterone *Serum* *Supine:* 3–10 ng/dL or 0.08–0.30 nmol/L (SI units) *Sitting upright for at least 2 hours:* *Males:* 6–22 ng/dL or 0.17–0.61 nmol/L (SI units) *Females:* 5–30 ng/dL or 0.14–0.80 nmol/L (SI units) Urine 2–26 units/24 hr or 6–72 nmol/24 hr (SI units)	Adrenals (origin) Kidney tubules (target) To diagnose hyperaldosteronism Hyponatremia and hyperkalemia stimulate increased aldosterone release Decreased aldosterone results in less reabsorption of sodium from the renal tubules causing hyponatremia	Primary or secondary hyperaldosteronism (Conn's), adrenal tumor or hyperplasia, laxative abuse, poor perfusion states, pregnancy, oral contraceptives, *hypertension*	Addison's disease, primary hypoaldosteronism salt-wasting syndrome, antihypertensive therapy; steroid therapy may interfere with feedback loop, *hypotension*

(continued)

| CHART 51–6 | **Adrenal Gland Testing—*Continued*** |

Laboratory Test and Normal Values	Gland Tested Diagnostic Significance	Disorders Associated with Abnormal Levels *(symptoms are italicized)* Increased	Decreased
Plasma renin assay *Supine:* 0.3–3.0 ng/mL per hour *Upright:* 1.0–9.0 ng/mL per hour	Adrenals (target) Glomerulus (origin) Evaluation of hypertension To make differential diagnosis of primary versus secondary hyperaldosteronism. In primary, both renin and aldosterone are increased; in secondary, renin is decreased and aldosterone is increased	*Hypertension*, Addison's, secondary hyperaldosteronism, hypokalemia, cirrhosis, salt-losing GI disease, renal disease	Primary hyperaldosteronism, congenital adrenal hyperplasia, steroid therapy
Urinary Catecholamines *Dopamine:* 65–400 mcg/24 hr *Epinephrine:* 1.7–22.4 mcg/24hr *Norepinephrine:* 12.1–85.5 mcg/24 hr *Metanephrines:* 24–96/mcg/24hr *Vanillylmandelic acid (VMA):* 1.4–6.5 mg/24hr *Homovanillic acid (HVA):* 0.0–15.0 mg/d	Adrenal medulla (origin) To assess adrenal medullary function	Pheochromocytoma, neuroblastomas, adrenocortical adenoma, *seizures, stress (severe anger or anxiety)*	Profound hypofunctioning, Addison's disease, chronic disease

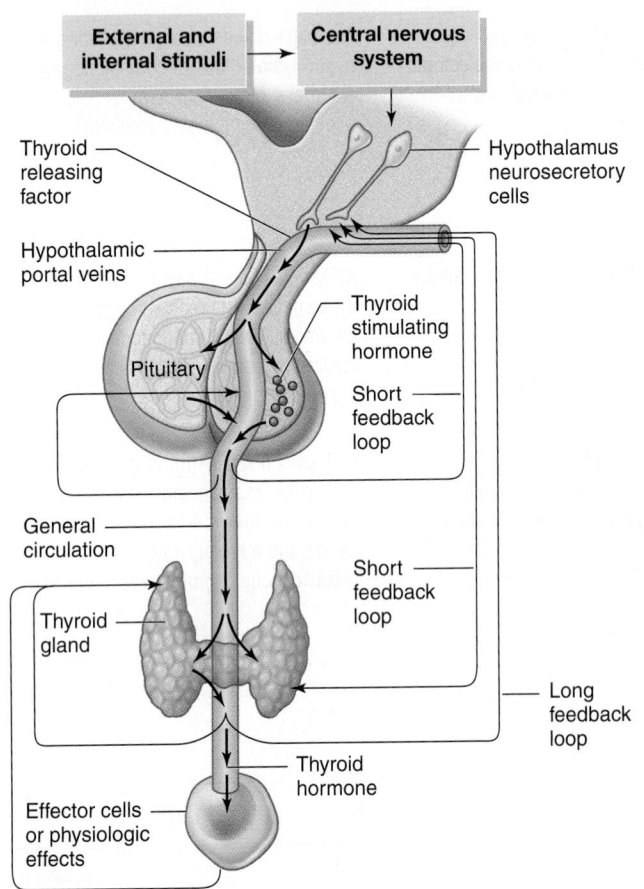

FIGURE 51–3 ■ Thyroid gland feedback loop.

quality of voice. When patients experience thyroid enlargement, they will have palpable or visible enlargement of the thyroid, which can displace the trachea and thus affect breathing and swallowing.

Because of the close association to catecholamines, the patient may experience nervousness and anxiety, shaking, irritability, tremors, and diaphoresis. Prolonged hyperthyroidism causes deposits of fat in the pads behind the eyes, causing bulging of the eyes (exophthalmos) and, occasionally, double vision or loss of vision. Any of these symptoms should motivate the nurse to investigate further.

Laboratory and Diagnostic Procedures

There is no consensus on screening for thyroid disease (see the Health Promotion section on the next page). T_3 and T_4 levels are lower in hypothyroidism and elevated in hyperthyroidism. TSH levels are commonly checked to determine thyroid homeostasis; they are elevated with primary failure of the thyroid gland. TRF (made by the hypothalamus) is elevated with secondary failure (of the pituitary). Because of the connection to the hypothalamus, increased perception of stress can alter TH production. Chart 51–7 summarizes types of glandular failure and related

| CHART 51–7 | **Differentiation of Thyroid Gland Hormone Testing and Glandular Failure** |

	T_3 and T_4	TSH	TRH
Primary failure (thyroid gland)	Low	High	High
Secondary failure (pituitary gland)	Low	Low	High
Tertiary failure (hypothalamus gland)	Low	Low	Low

diagnostic test results of thyroid stimulating hormone (TSH) and thyrotropin-releasing hormone (TRH). Chart 51–8 summarizes different thyroid function tests. The Gerontological Considerations box (p. 1608) discusses the effects of hypothyroidism and hyperthyroidism on elderly patients.

 CRITICAL ALERT *Severe hyperthyroidism (thyrotoxicosis or Graves' disease) can cause tachycardia in excess of 150 beats per minute and is considered a medical emergency; beta-blockers are given to decrease the heart rate until ablation of the thyroid gland is accomplished.*

Health Promotion Related to Thyroid Imbalances

Hypothyroidism can be associated with obesity. According to new guidelines issued by the American Thyroid Association (ATA), everyone should be screened at 5-year intervals at a minimum, for thyroid problems beginning at age 35 (Ladenson et al., 2000). Those

with symptoms should be checked even more frequently. The American College of Physicians has been recommending thyroid screening for women ages 50 and older for the past few years because it is estimated that thyroid dysfunction affects 5% to 15% of women (Helfand & Redfern, 1998). Although men are less affected by this problem, the ATA is suggesting screening of both sexes, because the blood test used to detect levels of TSH is inexpensive. They state that screening is important because thyroid problems can easily go undetected and can lead to other serious conditions.

Parathyroid Glands

There are four to six parathyroid glands embedded on the posterior surface of the lobes of the thyroid gland. The chief cells secrete parathyroid hormone (PTH) in response to a drop in calcium levels. PTH is responsible for the regulation of the serum calcium level through a simple feedback loop. This balance is maintained by the excretion of phosphorus and reabsorption

CHART 51–8 Thyroid Gland Testing

Laboratory Test and Normal Values	Gland Tested Diagnostic Significance	Disorders Associated with Abnormal Levels (symptoms are italicized)	
		Increased	**Decreased**
Antithyroglobin antibodies (thyroid autoantibody) Titer < 1:100	Thyroid (origin) Presence of antibodies to several components, which may cause inflammation and destruction of thyroid gland	Thyroiditis, rheumatoid arthritis, pernicious anemia, *hypothyroidism* or hyperthyroidism, thyroid cancer, Graves' disease, Hashimoto's thyroiditis, systemic lupus erythematosus	Normal is a negative titer or titer of less than 1:100
Thyroxine index, Free (FT$_4$) 0.8–2.4 ng/dL or 10–31 pmol/L (SI units)	Thyroid (origin) Evaluates thyroid function	*Hyperthyroidism, acute psychiatric illness*	*Hypothyroidism, anorexia nervosa,* severe illness
Triiodothyronine uptake (T$_3$ resin uptake) 24–34% or 24–34 AU (arbitrary units, SI units)	Thyroid (origin) Measures amount of T$_3$ bound to protein and the evaluation of thyroid function	Hyperthyroidism, hypoproteinemia	Hypothyroid, hypothyroid states, hepatitis, cirrhosis
Thyrotropin releasing hormone (TRH) Euthyroid < 10	Thyroid function Hypothalamus (origin) Pituitary (target) Evaluation of thyroid function	Primary hypothyroidism (thyroid disease), secondary hypothyroidism (pituitary disease) or TRH secreting tumor in hypothalamus	Hyperthyroid, secondary hyperthyroidism (pituitary disease) or nonfunctional hypothalamus
Thyroid stimulating hormone (TSH) assay 2–10 mU/L (SI units)	Anterior pituitary (origin) Thyroid (target) Differentiate primary and secondary hypothyroidism	Primary hypothyroidism (thyroid dysfunction), Addison's, anti-TSH antibodies, goiter, hyperpituitarism or pituitary adenoma, postop thyroidectomy	Secondary hypothyroidism (pituitary disorder with decreased secretion); high doses of dopamine or corticosteroids, Hashimoto's, primary hyperthyroidism
Thyroxine (T$_4$) *Males:* 51–154 nmol/L (SI units) *Females:* 64–154 nmol/L (SI units) *>60 yr:* 64–124 nmol/L (SI units)	Thyroid (origin) Assess thyroid function, monitor replacement and suppression therapy	Hyperthyroidism, acute thyroiditis, porphyria, cirrhosis, excess dietary intake of iodine, goiter, Graves', thyrotoxicosis	Hypothyroidism, pituitary insufficiency, hypothalamic failure, protein malnutrition, iodine insufficiency, Hashimoto's thyroiditis, nephrotic syndrome, thyroidectomy
Thyroid scan Homogeneous uptake of radioactive tracer and normal size, shape, and position of gland	Thyroid gland (origin) Differentiates between causes of nodules	Increased uptake in hyperfunctioning nodule or "hot nodules"; not usually malignant	Normal uptake; decreased uptake in "cold nodules"; are more likely to be malignant

GERONTOLOGICAL CONSIDERATIONS Related to Thyroid Disorders

In the elderly, symptoms of thyroid disorders are difficult to diagnose. Hypothyroidism is not unusual but may go unrecognized for a variety of reasons including mistaking the nonspecific signs and symptoms as a part of the "normal aging" process or other medical conditions that may exist in the elderly (Singh, 1999). Symptoms common to both the aging process *and* to hypothyroidism include anorexia, cognitive decline, cold intolerance, constipation, dry skin, fatigue, hearing loss, hoarseness, paresthesias, slowed reflexes, and weakness. In a large study, the following symptoms of hyperthyroidism were present in less than half of the elderly: tremor, nervousness, hyperactive reflexes, increased sweating, polydipsia, heat intolerance, and increased appetite (Trivalle et al., 1996). In this same study, tachycardia, fatigue, and weight loss were present in more than half of elderly thyrotoxic patients.

and excretion of calcium in the urine, gastrointestinal tract, and from bone. Increases in phosphorus, which bind to and lower calcium ions, stimulate PTH release.

A sudden decreased PTH level can result in tetany (carpopedal spasm), a life-threatening condition. This most commonly occurs due to accidental removal of the glands during thyroid surgery, or from autoimmune destruction. A reduced total serum calcium can also result from a decrease in albumin secondary to liver disease, nephrotic syndrome, or malnutrition.

Increased PTH levels can be primary from tumor, resulting in hypercalcemia, or secondary, resulting from hypersecretion. Renal failure causes hyperphosphatemia, leading to hypocalcemia, and subsequent secondary hyperparathyroidism. Calcitonin is released from the thyroid gland in response to hypercalcemia; it shifts calcium from the blood into the bones. Homeostasis of calcium balance is dependent on normal levels of vitamin D.

Assessment

Hypocalcemia causes neuromuscular irritability and tetany. Patients usually complain of numbness and tingling sensations in the perioral area or in the fingers and toes. Muscle cramps are common in the back and lower extremities and may progress to tetany. Neurological symptoms, including irritability, impaired intellectual capacity, depression, and personality changes, may be present. Respiratory disturbances may develop from laryngospasm and bronchospasm.

Hypocalcemia seen in parathyroid disorders can produce spastic contraction of the arm when a blood pressure cuff is applied (Trousseau's sign) or facial muscle contraction when the facial nerve is tapped (Chvostek's sign). Alkalosis induces tetany due to a decrease in ionized calcium. In severe cases, hypocalcemia may lead to arrhythmias, hypotension, and heart failure. Seizures of all types can occur in patients with hypocalcemia.

CRITICAL ALERT *Hyperventilation causes respiratory alkalosis, which drops the ionized calcium in the blood and can result in tetany and respiratory arrest. Carpopedal spasm (Trousseau's sign) and spasm of the facial nerve when tapped (Chvostek's sign) are earlier signs of impending tetany.*

Hypercalcemia is caused by overactive parathyroid glands and also by metabolic cancers to the bone and from some medications. The nurse should assess for symptoms of dehydration,

dry skin, confusion, thirst, nausea and vomiting, constipation, fatigue, and decreased deep tendon reflexes.

Laboratory and Diagnostic Procedures

Calcium levels help evaluate calcium metabolism, ionized and nonionized calcium in serum, and parathyroid functioning. PTH levels can also be measured; they will be elevated if calcium levels are decreased, and decreased with hypercalcemia. Because a gradual drop does not create symptoms, a low serum calcium does not always correlate with tetany. The nurse must correlate the clinical picture with the blood levels. Calcitonin and serum phosphorous levels also help evaluate parathyroid functioning. Chart 51–9 outlines the laboratory tests used to evaluate the parathyroid gland (Porth, 2007).

Pancreas

The pancreas lies beneath the peritoneum and behind the stomach, with its head and neck in the curve of the duodenum. Its body extends horizontally across the horizontal posterior abdominal wall and its tail touches the spleen. The pancreas is unique in that it has both endocrine and exocrine functions. The islet cells within the pancreas provide endocrine functioning. These cells are responsible for carbohydrate metabolism and regulation of glucose levels through secretion and inhibition of insulin and glucagons. There are four types of islet cells: alpha, beta, delta, and PP cells.

Alpha cells are responsible for the production of glucagon. This hormone decreases the oxidation of glucose and promotes an increase in the serum glucose level by signaling the liver to release glucose from the glycogen stores. Beta cells are responsible for the production of insulin. Insulin facilitates the uptake and use of glucose by the cells and prevents excessive breakdown of glycogen in the liver and muscle. Together, insulin and glucagon control blood sugar levels by a simple feedback loop. Delta cells produce somatostatin, which inhibits GH, TSH, and gastrointestinal hormones, such as glucagon and insulin, by the alpha and beta cells of the pancreas. PP cells produce pancreatic polypeptide, or digestive enzymes, which are responsible for the exocrine activity of the pancreas.

Assessment

Diabetes mellitus is a disorder characterized by either lack of insulin (type 1) or impaired use of insulin (type 2). Either results in hyperglycemia, which in turn creates an osmotic pull of fluid off the tissues, causing polyuria, polydipsia, dehydration, and confusion leading to stupor or coma. The patient may have severe dehydration with volume depletion and hypotension. Hyperglycemia also causes osmotic fluid shifts in the vitreous fluid resulting in blurred vision. Because insulin normally suppresses breakdown of fat, and there is no insulin in type 1 diabetes, this disorder is also characterized by acidosis from conversion of stored fat to fatty acids. Acidosis causes nausea, vomiting, hunger, low pH, and compensatory Kussmaul's respirations. The nurse should assess for rapid, shallow respirations, as well as a fruity odor to the breath and urine.

The risk factors for type 1 DM include genetic factors plus a viral infection causing autoimmune destruction. Type 2 DM has been linked genetically with, and is strongly correlated to, obesity, age, ethnic minorities, physical inactivity, and gestational diabetes (National Diabetes Information Clearinghouse

CHART 51–9	Parathyroid Gland Testing		
Laboratory Test and Normal Values	**Gland Tested Diagnostic Significance**	**Disorders Associated with Abnormal Levels** *(symptoms are italicized)*	
		Increased	**Decreased**
Parathyroid hormone (PTH) 10–65 pg/mL or 10–65 ng/L (SI units)	Parathyroid (origin) Bone and gut (target) Evaluation of hypocalcemia and hypercalcemia; also monitored in patients with chronic renal failure	Increased as a response to low serum calcium levels: *hypocalcemia, rickets,* malabsorption syndrome, vitamin D deficiency, parathyroid adenoma, ectopic PTH producing tumors, *renal hypercalciuria,* chronic renal failure (secondary hyperparathyroidism)	Decreased as a response to high serum calcium levels: hypercalcemia of malignancy, metastatic bone tumor, sarcoidosis, vitamin D intoxication; hypoparathyroidism due to surgical ablation or immunoablation
Osteocalcin Adults > 22 *Males:* 5.8–14 ng/mL *Females:* 3.1–13.4 ng/mL	Parathyroid function Bone (origin) Evaluation of bone turnover in diseases that affect bone density	Hyperparathyroidism, osteoporosis, Paget's disease, acromegaly, hyperthyroidism, low calcium intake, low estrogen production	Hypoparathyroidism, steroid therapy, multiple myeloma, hypercalcemia from malignancy
Total serum calcium 9–10.5 mg/dL or 2.25–2.75 mmol/L	Parathyroid function Bone (origin) Evaluation of calcium metabolism, ionized and nonionized calcium in serum and parathyroid functioning	Hyperparathyroidism, bone metastasis, hypercalcemia, Addison's, acidosis, hypervitaminosis, immobility, renal calculi	Hypoparathyroidism, renal failure, rickets, vitamin D deficiency, osteomalacia, alkalosis, burns, chronic renal disease, parathyroidectomy, hypoproteinemia
Calcitonin *Males:* 3–26 pg/mL or 3–26 ng/L (SI units) *Females:* 2–17 pg/mL or 2–17 ng/L (SI units)	Thyroid (origin) Parathyroid (target) Responsible for lowering the calcium ion levels	Anemia, cancer, chronic renal failure, parathyroid adenoma or hyperplasia; *increased levels result in hypocalcemia*	autoimmune thyroiditis; *decreased levels result in hypercalcemia*
Serum phosphorus 3–4.5 mg/dL or 0.97–1.45 mmol/L (SI units)	Parathyroid function Diet (origin) Evaluation of parathyroid and calcium abnormalities	Hypoparathyroidism, renal failure, bone tumors, hyperthyroidism, diabetic acidosis, increased dietary intake of phosphorus; *increased levels result in hypocalcemia*	Hyperparathyroidism, chronic antacid ingestion, chronic alcoholism, burns, malnutrition, vitamin D deficiency and myxedema, Crohn's, dialysis, sprue
Serum alkaline phosphatase (ALP) 30–120 unit/L	Parathyroid function Multiple origins Evaluation of bone and liver diseases	Hyperparathyroidism, primary cirrhosis, biliary obstruction, *healing fractures,* Paget's disease, rheumatoid arthritis, hyperthyroidism	Hypophosphatemia, malnutrition, pernicious anemia, scurvy, celiac disease, malnutrition, hypothyroidism

[NDIC], 2006. Long-term changes associated with DM include retinopathy, nephropathy, vascular and cardiac disease, and hypertension. The nurse needs to take a careful history about the onset of symptoms and complete a thorough examination of the heart, extremities, kidneys, and eyes.

Because of regulatory mechanisms, it is unusual for a nondiabetic patient to have episodes of severe hypoglycemia. When this occurs, the nurse should suspect an islet-secreting tumor of the pancreas. Low blood sugar causes release of epinephrine, which stimulates hunger, tachycardia, diaphoresis, and feelings of nervousness. Hypoglycemia can cause confusion, sudden unconsciousness, seizures, and brain injury.

Laboratory and Diagnostic Procedures

DM is diagnosed in the presence of any random blood sugar higher than 200 mg/dL and/or a fasting blood sugar of >125 mg/dL (NDIC, 2006). Prediabetes is diagnosed with a fasting blood sugar of between 110 and 125 mg/dL. One test done to diagnose borderline diabetes is a glucose tolerance test (GTT). A carbohydrate load is given and then blood sugars are checked prior to and at intervals afterward. Fasting and before meals blood test-

ing is done in the home and hospital setting. The most accurate test of long-term control of blood sugar is the hemoglobin A1c test, which measures the glucose attached to hemoglobin and gives information about the average blood sugar level in the previous 6-week period. A microalbuminuria test is the best indicator of early renal involvement. Chart 51–10 (p. 1610) summarizes pancreatic gland testing.

In type 2 diabetes, there may be insulin resistance at the cellular level, resulting in high blood sugar despite increased insulin levels. Insulin resistance has been linked to metabolic syndrome. In 1999, the World Health Organization criteria for metabolic syndrome required the presence of diabetes mellitus, impaired glucose tolerance, impaired fasting glucose, or insulin resistance, *and* two of the following:

- Blood pressure $\geq$ 140/90 mmHg

- Dyslipidemia: triglycerides $\geq$ 1.695 mmol/L and/or high-density lipoprotein cholesterol $\leq$ 0.9 mmol/L (male), $\leq$ 1.0 mmol/L (female)

- Central obesity: waist-to-hip ratio > 0.90 (male), > 0.85 (female), and/or body mass index > 30 kg/m^2

| CHART 51–10 | **Pancreatic Gland Testing** | | |

Laboratory Test and Normal Values	Gland Tested Diagnostic Significance	Disorders Associated with Abnormal Levels *(symptoms are italicized)*	
		Increased	Decreased
Fasting glucose <100 mg/dL normal fasting glucose 100–126 mg/dL impaired fasting glucose >126 mg/dL diagnostic for diabetes	Pancreas (target) Diet (origin) Glucose homeostasis	*Impaired fasting glucose*, *hyperglycemia*, diabetes mellitus, IV fluids, physiological stress	*Hypoglycemia*, insulinomas
Oral glucose tolerance test <140 mg/dL normal glucose tolerance 140–200 mg/dL impaired glucose tolerance >200 mg/dL diagnostic for diabetes	Pancreas (target) Diet (origin) Glucose metabolism	Diabetes mellitus, *impaired glucose tolerance*, Cushing's syndrome, hepatic tumors, pregnancy, pheochromocytoma, hyperthyroidism	Insulinomas, Addison's, celiac disease, hepatic disease, hypothyroidism
Hemoglobin A1c or glycosylated hemoglobin 4–6%; <7% for diabetics	Pancreas (target) Diet (origin) Glucose metabolism	Diabetes mellitus, gestational diabetes	Insulinomas, Addison's, celiac disease, hepatic disease, hypothyroidism

- Microalbuminuria: urinary albumin excretion ratio ≥20 mg/min or albumin-to-creatinine ratio ≥30 mg/g (Harmel & Mathur, 2003).

Critical Thinking Related to Assessment Data

As previously noted, when conducting a focused endocrine assessment, it is critical to begin with a thorough history of the patient's chief complaints. The nurse needs to elicit any experience with signs or symptoms of endocrine disease or disorders. Symptoms usually are manifested according to which endocrine hormone is being overproduced and secreted or underproduced and secreted. Thus, it is incumbent on the nurse to understand the functions on the endocrine system.

When assessing the endocrine system, the nurse likely will perform a problem-focused assessment, following a comprehensive assessment. The focused assessment may need to be repeated periodically when an interval or abbreviated assessment shows a change in status from the last assessment or report received. When a new symptom emerges or the patient experiences some distress, a focused endocrine assessment also should be considered.

Physical exam techniques consist of the same techniques used in a general exam: inspection, auscultation, palpation, and percussion. With inspection, the nurse is looking forward for anything that can be observed with eyes, ears, or nose, for example, skin color, locations of lesions, bruises or rashes, symmetry, size of body parts, and abnormal sounds or odors.

Auscultation is used in the focused endocrine assessment before palpation or percussion. Findings that may be auscultated include murmurs, cardiac irregularities, adventitious breath sounds, and alterations in bowel sounds.

Palpation is another physical exam technique that is used in the focused endocrine assessment. Palpation allows the nurse to assess for texture, tenderness, temperature, moisture, pulsations, masses, and internal organs (Porth, 2007).

Percussion is used to allow the nurse to elicit tenderness or sounds that point to underlying problems. When percussing directly over suspected areas of tenderness, the patient should be monitored for signs of discomfort.

Examples of Data Collection

Data is acquired through the history and physical exam and is enhanced with laboratory testing. With endocrine disorders, the history is the most essential piece of data collection. Many times, patients will have a constellation of symptoms that do not clearly fit into one hormone imbalance. The nurse is in a unique position to analyze the data to determine the relevance of each symptom to the underlying disorder. Abnormal findings need to be reported to the primary care provider and patient education initiated. With proper education, patients can be empowered to manage and improve their personal health.

Diagnostic Evaluation

Providing patient education, allaying patient's fears regarding the testing process, and ensuring that testing is done appropriately are parts of the nurse's role in diagnostic assessment and evaluation of the endocrine system. Proper preparation for diagnostic testing is essential for ensuring accurate evaluation of endocrine system function. Testing may require special diets, fasting, or use of drugs in order to assess proper functioning. It is the nurse's role to assist the patient in preparing for these tests.

Laboratory and Diagnostic Procedures

Laboratory tests for endocrine function involve serum hormone levels, suppression and stimulation, and urine hormone levels. In most cases, elevated hormone levels are associated with increased function of the gland. Suppression and stimulation testing is used to determine glandular function in feedback loops.

Urine hormone levels give information about increased and decreased function of specific glands. Radiological examinations also are used to made diagnostic decisions.

Serum Hormone Levels

Diagnostic testing of the endocrine system begins with examination of serum hormone levels. Some tests may involve a single specimen, whereas others require multiple blood samples. Laboratory testing of a specific endocrine organ involves the measurement of the specific hormone or tropic hormones. If the serum concentration of hormone is deficient, further testing is needed to assess whether the deficiency is related to dysfunction of the associated gland; this is known as primary dysfunction. If the deficiency is due to the dysfunction of another gland or a stimulating hormone, it is known as secondary dysfunction. If the deficiency is due to dysfunction of the neurohormone, as in TRF or CRF, it is known as tertiary dysfunction.

Suppression and Stimulation Testing

Suppression and stimulation testing also may be used to assess endocrine function. This type of testing is accomplished by the administration of a drug that stimulates or suppresses the release of hormones. This type of testing is especially useful in differentiation of primary or secondary dysfunction. Numerous tests may be necessary to definitively confirm an endocrine system disorder.

A record of the medications that the patient is receiving as well as those that should be withheld, foods that should be avoided during testing, and instructions regarding the purpose and procedure for the test are provided by the nurse. Special materials may need to be obtained from the laboratory for the specimen collection. Special handling of the specimens also may be necessary (e.g., adding acid to the specimen or keeping the specimen on ice).

Urine Hormone Levels

Measurements of urinary hormone or hormone metabolite excretion often are done on a 24-hour urine sample which provides a better measure of hormone levels during that period than hormones measured in an isolated blood sample. The advantages of a urine test include the relative ease of obtaining the urine sample and the fact that blood sampling is not required, though it is recognized that reliability timed urine collections often are difficult to obtain. Because many urine tests involve the measure of a hormone metabolite, rather than the hormone itself, drugs or disease states that alter hormone metabolism may interfere with the test results. Some urinary hormone metabolite measurements include hormones from more than one source and are of little value in measuring hormone secretion from a specific source. "For example, urinary 17-ketosteroids are a measure of both adrenal and gonadal androgens" (Porth, 2007, page 671).

Radiologic Examination

Radiologic examination with simple x-rays, CT scanning, or MRI scanning can be used to visualize endocrine glands to assess for size, atrophy, hypertrophy, or neoplasm. The nurse provides explanations of the purpose and procedures for radiologic exams. Allergies to iodine, shellfish, or contrast media also must be determined prior to examination by CT scans requiring contrast. Pregnancy should be ruled out for female patients prior to any type of x-ray examination. If the patient is to have an MRI, nurses should inquire about claustrophobia, previous surgeries, implantable devices, and any previous injuries involving metals such as gunshot wounds or pellet injuries.

In summary, conducting the health history, physical examination, and preparation for and interpretation of laboratory tests and procedures takes experience and practice. It is not enough to simply ask the right questions and perform the physical exam. The nurse must critically analyze all of the data obtained, synthesize the data into a relevant problem focus, and then identify a plan of care for the patient based on this synthesis. Examples of plans of care based on assessment data are found in Chapters 52 and 53 📖.

Health Promotion

Health promotion in general is based on knowing and identifying the risk factors and overt symptoms of hormonal imbalances. These vary with the type of hormonal imbalance experienced, but the public should be made aware of common symptoms, such as headache, sudden weight gain or loss, thinning of hair, lethargy, localized pain, nausea, irritability, nocturia, heat intolerance, insomnia, and others. The public should be made aware of the Internet sources or health promotion pamphlets available through health care providers' offices or localized outlets that provide information related to specific hormonal imbalances. An annual physical examination may alert patients to potential problems. Patients also should be counseled as to when to report aberrant symptoms to the physician or health care provider.

■ Summary

In conclusion, endocrine disorders cause changes in almost every system in the human body. The nurse must carefully assess each system for alterations in function and appearance to discern the system involved. Some physical changes can be caused by more than one endocrine imbalance. Careful examination and laboratory testing are essential to accurate diagnosis and treatment.

NCLEX® REVIEW

1. A patient with diabetes does not understand how an injection of insulin can take the place of insulin secreted from the pancreas. Which of the following should the nurse respond to this patient?

   1. It does not; insulin is for another purpose.
   2. Insulin helps the pancreas work well.
   3. It works by a negative feedback mechanism.
   4. Insulin is a hormone and works through the bloodstream.

2. The nurse is explaining to a patient how the hormones secreted by the ovaries work on the ovaries to cause an egg follicle to mature. This nurse is instructing the patient on which of the following?

   1. Neuroendocrine regulation
   2. Paracine functioning
   3. Autocrine functioning
   4. Basal hormone release

3. A patient has been diagnosed with cancer that has metastasized to the outer layer of his adrenal glands. Which of the following hormones will be affected by this disease?

   1. Mineralcorticoids
   2. Glucocorticoids
   3. Epinephrine
   4. Calcitonin

4. During an assessment a patient says "I eat but am losing weight! And I'm so thirsty and seem to always have to pass water." Which of the following should the nurse say in response to this patient?

   1. Does frequent urination keep you up at night?
   2. Do you use tobacco?
   3. Everyone thinks that they weigh less than they really do.
   4. Does anyone in your family have diabetes?

5. A 50-year-old female patient asks the nurse why a follicle-stimulating hormone test was done. Which of the following should the nurse respond to this patient?

   1. It measures the amount of hormones your adrenal glands are making.
   2. It measures the hormones being made by your thyroid.
   3. It checks for ovarian function and might indicate if you are approaching menopause.
   4. It predicts how well you metabolize carbohydrates, proteins, and fats.

Answers for review questions appear in Appendix D

KEY TERMS

autocrine functioning *p.1597*
circadian rhythm *p.1597*
endocrine *p.1596*

infradian rhythm *p.1597*
negative feedback *p.1597*
paracrine functioning *p.1597*

positive feedback *p.1597*
receptors *p.1596*

EXPLORE PEARSON **mynursingkit**™

MyNursingKit is your one stop for online chapter review materials and resources. Prepare for success with additional NCLEX®-style practice questions, interactive assignments and activities, web links, animations and videos, and more!

Register your access code from the front of your book at
www.mynursingkit.com

REFERENCES

American Thyroid Association. (2008). *NACB thyroid guidelines.* Retrieved June 9, 2008, from http://www.thyroid.org

American Urological Association. (2007). *Pheochromocytoma.* Retrieved September 12, 2007, from http://urologyhealth.org/adult/index.cfm?cat=02&topic=114

Bharaktiya, S., Orlander, P. R., Woodhouse, W. T., & Davis, A. B. (2007). *Hypothyroidism.* Retrieved June 9, 2008, from http://www.emedicine.com/med/topic1145.htm

Estes, M. E. (2002). *Health assessment and physical exam* (2nd ed.). New York: Delmar Publishing.

Fenton, C. L., & Gold, J. G. (2006). *Hyperthyroidism.* Retrieved June 8, 2008, from http://www.emedicine.com/ped/TOPIC1099.HTM

Harmel, A., & Mathur, R. (2003). *Davidson's diabetes mellitus.* St. Louis: Elsevier.

Helfand, M., & Redfern, C. C. (1998). Screening for thyroid disease: An update. *Annals of Internal Medicine, 129*(2), 144–158.

Khandwala, H. M. (2005). *Acromegaly.* Retrieved September 2007 from http://www.emedicine.com/med/topic27.htm

Ladenson, P. W., Singer, P. A., Ain, K. B., et al. (2000). American Thyroid Association guidelines for detection of thyroid dysfunction. *Archives of Internal Medicine, 160*(11), 1573–1575.

National Diabetes Information Clearinghouse. (2006). *Am I at risk for diabetes?* Retrieved September 12, 2007, from http://diabetes.niddk.nih.gov/dm/pubs/riskfortype2/index.htm#6

National Kidney and Urologic Diseases Information Clearinghouse. (2006). *Diabetes insipidus.* Retrieved September 2007 from http://kidney.niddk.nih.gov/kudiseases/pubs/insipidus/index.htm

Odeske, S. & Nagelberg, S. B. (2006). Addison disease. *eMedicine.* Retrieved June 8, 2008, from http://www.emedicine.com/med/TOPIC42.HTM

Porth, C. M. (2007). *Essentials of pathophysiology: Concepts of altered health states.* Philadelphia: Lippincott Williams & Wilkins.

Rafailov, A. (2007). *Syndrome of inappropriate antidiuretic hormone secretion.* Retrieved September 2007 from http://www.emedicine.com/emerg/topic784.htm

Reid, J. R. & Wheeler, S. F. (2005). Hyperthyroidism: Diagnosis and treatment. *American Family Physician, 72*(4). Retrieved June 9, 2008, from http://www.aafp.org/afp/20050815/623.html

Singh, S. (1999). Low levels of thyroid hormone blamed on age. *Geriatrics and Aging, 2*(6). Retrieved June 9, 2008, from http://www.geriatricsandaging.ca/fmi/xsl/article.xsl?-lay=Article&-recid=220&-find=-find

Trivalle, C., Doucet, J., Chassagne, P., et al. (1996). Differences in the signs and symptoms of hyperthyroidism in older and younger patients. *Journal of the American Geriatrics Society, 44*(1), 50–53.

Wall, C. R. (2000). Myxedema coma: Diagnosis and treatment. *American Family Physician, 62*(11). Retrieved September 2007 from http://www.aafp.org/afp/20001201/2485.html

Caring for the Patient with Glandular and Hormonal Disorders

Abby Heydman

With contributions by:
Annita Watson
Kathleen Osborn

Outcome-Based Learning Objectives

After studying this chapter, the learner will be able to:

1. Describe the anatomic location and function of the endocrine glands, including the physiological effects of the hormones that each gland produces.
2. Compare the common pathophysiological syndromes caused by under- and overproduction of hormones for each of the endocrine glands, including the thyroid, parathyroid, hypothalamus and pituitary, and adrenal glands.
3. Identify clinical manifestations, treatment, and nursing interventions for hypo- and hypermetabolic conditions.
4. Describe the complex neurological and immunologic effects of common glandular disorders.
5. Develop a plan of care for patients with each of the common endocrine gland disorders, including the patient teaching and discharge needs.
6. Describe the potential gerontological implications for each glandular disorder.
7. Identify implications for nursing research when caring for persons with glandular disorders.

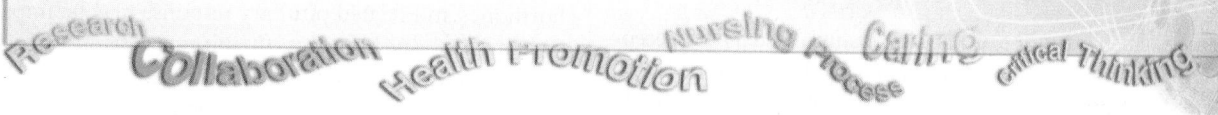

THE HUMAN BODY is a complex organism that functions as a result of exquisite control by the glandular system in constant interaction with the neurological and immune systems. All major organ systems and physiological processes such as cell metabolism, bone metabolism, growth, homeostasis, regulation of energy, and reproduction are regulated by the glandular system and its feedback control systems. This chapter focuses on disorders of the major endocrine glands: the thyroid, parathyroid, hypothalamus and pituitary, and the adrenal glands. Disorders of the thyroid gland are emphasized because these are the most common problems seen by nurses in clinical practice.

Endocrinology

Endocrinology is a broad field of science and medicine that involves the study of the glands and tissues that produce hormones that serve as chemical messengers orchestrating a multitude of physiological processes. The endocrine glands specifically include the thyroid, parathyroid, adrenals, pituitary, hypothalamus, thymus, pancreas, pineal, ovaries, and testes. The ovaries and testes are discussed in Chapters 48, 49, and 50 . The thymus gland is involved in regulation of the immune system and is discussed in Chapters 59, 60, and 61 . The pan-

creas produces insulin and it is discussed in Chapter 53 . The pineal gland is a tiny structure located in the middle of the brain and it secretes melatonin, which is involved with biological rhythms and reproductive functions. Researchers are still learning about the role of the pineal gland and it has not been cited as a major factor in human disease. For this reason, the pineal gland is not discussed in this chapter. The anatomic location of each of the endocrine glands is illustrated in Figure 52–1 ■, (p. 1614).

Hormones

Hormones are substances that circulate like chemical messengers to produce cellular actions and to regulate physiological processes throughout the body. Hormones include amino acid derivatives, small neuropeptides, large proteins, steroid hormones, and vitamin derivatives, which act primarily by stimulating target cells that are uniquely responsive to them. The target tissue for a hormone includes all of the cells that have receptor sites for that hormone. Sometimes target tissue is localized in a single gland and, in some cases, the target tissue is located throughout the body.

Hormone Production

Hormone production is stimulated by the body in three ways. First, several hormones are controlled by a **negative feedback**

The endocrine glands secrete hormones which regulate various functions throughout the body

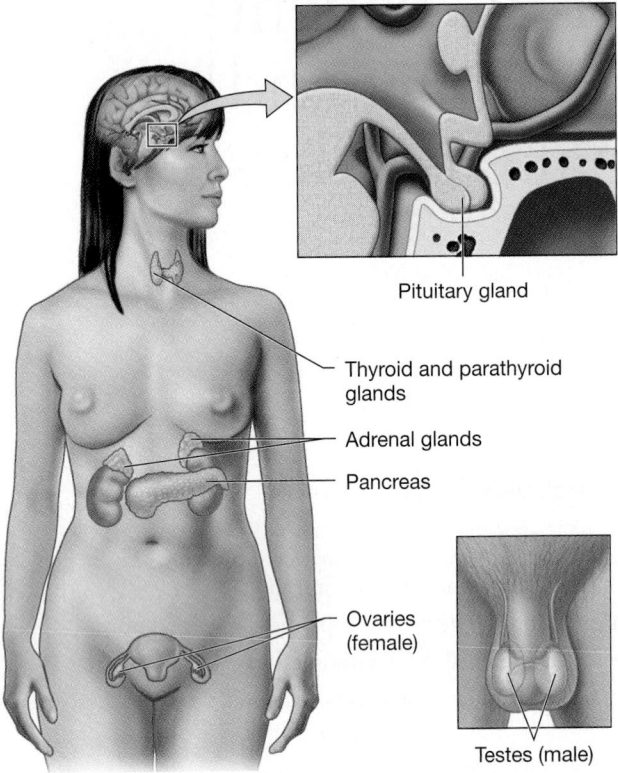

Pituitary gland

Thyroid and parathyroid glands

Adrenal glands

Pancreas

Ovaries (female)

Testes (male)

FIGURE 52–1 ■ Location of the endocrine glands in the male and female bodies.

system in which hormone production is stimulated if body receptors indicate that the concentration of a needed hormone is low. Second, hormone production can be stimulated by a hormone produced by another organ. Hormone-stimulating hormones are called tropic hormones. For example, the pituitary gland produces thyroid-stimulating hormone (TSH), which acts on the thyroid gland to stimulate production of thyroid hormone. Third, hormones can be produced by direct nervous system stimulation.

Hormones are produced by both the endocrine glands and the exocrine glands, which include specialized tissues in the gut and other parts of the body (Braunwald et al., 2001). Hormones produced by the endocrine glands, also known as ductless glands, are secreted internally into the blood, whereas hormones secreted by the exocrine system are secreted through ducts or tubes (Chart 52–1). An example of an endocrine hormone is thyroxine, a hormone that is produced by the thyroid gland. An example of an exocrine hormone is gastrin, which is produced by the gastric mucosa for the purpose of stimulating the production of hydrochloric acid and the enzyme pepsin to aid in the digestion of food. Other exocrine glands include the small intestine, which secretes the hormones secretin and cholecystokinin; the heart, which produces atriopeptin; and the placenta of a pregnant woman, which produces chorionic gonadotropin. In recent years, research has demonstrated that peptide hormones also are produced by brain tissue, leading to a new field of neuroendocrinology. This chapter focuses on common disorders of the major endocrine glands and the clinical situations nurses are most likely to see in practice.

Endocrine Disorders

Endocrine disorders are linked to several factors including aging, illness, stress, environmental substances, congenital birth defects, and genetics. In addition, surgery, trauma, cancerous and benign tumors, infection, and autoimmune disorders may all trigger endocrine dysfunction. The major clinical problems seen in the endocrine glands are those related to underproduction or overproduction of hormone, and those cases in which there is resistance to the action of the hormone. Generally, hormone underproduction can be treated by hormone replacement therapy and overproduction can be treated by reducing hormone levels through surgical intervention or the use of medications to lower hormone levels.

The endocrine system is studied by measuring hormone levels in the blood. Endocrine disorders are classified as primary, secondary, or tertiary based on the particular physiological system involved in causing the disease. Primary endocrine disease occurs when the organ itself is diseased. Secondary disease occurs when the pituitary and its stimulating hormones are affected by some pathology. Tertiary disease occurs when dysfunction occurs within the hypothalamus. Chart 52–2 (p. 1617) shows disorders of the endocrine system.

The Effect of Aging on the Endocrine System

The aging process takes a toll on normal cells and gradually leads to altered hormone production and secretion, changes in hormone metabolism and hormone levels, slowed response of target cells to hormones, and changes in physiological body rhythms such as menstruation. Secretion of some hypothalamic hormones and related pituitary response may be impaired due to aging. As a person ages, the pituitary gland often becomes smaller and may fail to work as effectively, leading to decreased muscle mass, decreased heart function, and osteoporosis. Infections or trauma may quickly destabilize older patients because the aging body is less capable of responding to either internal or external stressors due to a decline in endocrine functioning.

■ Disorders of the Thyroid Gland

The thyroid gland is a small butterfly-shaped and highly vascular organ located in the front of the neck with lobes connected by an isthmus resting on the anterior side of the trachea (Figure 52–2 ■, p. 1618). The primary function of the thyroid gland is to produce thyroid hormone, which regulates body metabolism.

Disorders of the thyroid gland are the most common of the diseases of the endocrine system, and include hypothyroidism, hyperthyroidism, and thyroid nodules. **Hypothyroidism** is a condition in which the thyroid gland produces an inadequate amount of thyroid hormone. **Hyperthyroidism** occurs when an excess of thyroid hormone is secreted. Thyroid nodules are lumps in or on the thyroid gland and they may be small or large. Thyroid nodules are of four general types: overgrowth of normal thyroid tissue, a fluid-filled cyst, or a benign or malignant tumor (American Association of Clinical Endocrinologists [AACE], 2005d). Because the thyroid gland affects the functioning of most of the body processes, signs and symptoms may be diffuse and difficult to diagnose. For this reason, the health care provider will need to rely on discriminating laboratory tests of

| CHART 52–1 | **Glands and Their Hormones** |

Endocrine Gland and Hormone Source	Hormone(s)	Action Site	Physiological Effects
Hypothalamus	Thyrotropin-releasing hormone (TRH)	Anterior pituitary	Stimulates release of TSH and prolactin.
	Gonadotropin-releasing hormone (GnRH)	Anterior pituitary	Responsible for release of FSH and LH.
	Growth hormone-releasing hormone (GHRH)	Anterior pituitary	Promotes growth hormone secretion.
	Corticotropin-releasing hormone (CRH)	Anterior pituitary	Promotes release of ACTH.
	Somatostatin	Pituitary Pancreas GI tract	Inhibits secretion of GH, TSH, gastric hormones. Prolongs gastric emptying. Suppresses pancreatic hormones.
	Dopamine	Anterior pituitary	Inhibits release of prolactin.
Pituitary gland			
Anterior lobe (adenohypophysis)	Human growth hormone (GH)	Systemic	Stimulates growth and cell reproduction.
Posterior lobe (neurohypophysis)	Thyroid-stimulating hormone (thyrotropin) (TSH)	Thyroid	Stimulates release of thyroid hormone.
	Adrenocorticotropin (ACTH)	Adrenal cortex	Stimulates the cortex of the adrenal gland and boosts the synthesis of corticosteroids, mainly glucocorticoids, and also mineralocorticoids and sex steroids (androgens).
	Follicle-stimulating hormone (FSH)	Ovaries	Stimulates growth of immature graafian follicles to maturation.
		Testes	Essential in spermatogenesis.
	Luteinizing hormone (LH)	Ovaries	Stimulates production of the sex hormones. Triggers ovulation and development of the corpus luteum during the menstrual cycle.
	Prolactin	Mammary glands	Stimulates mammary glands to produce milk.
	Melanocyte-stimulating hormone	Skin and hair	Stimulates production and release of melanin by melanocytes in skin and hair.
	Antidiuretic hormone (ADH) (vasopressin)	Kidneys	Causes kidneys to concentrate urine. Stimulates thirst.
	Oxytocin	Breasts Uterus Testes	Causes milk to "let down" into mammary ducts. Aids uterine contraction and cervical dilation during labor and delivery. Facilitates sperm transport in ejaculation.
Thyroid gland	Thyroxine (T_4) Triiodothyronine (T_3)	Systemic	Controls metabolic rate, metabolism, growth, and development.
	Thyrocalcitonin (calcitonin)	Bone	Reduces the level of calcium in the blood. Lowers bone reabsorption.
Parathyroid gland	Parathyroid hormone (parathormone) (PTH)	Bone, kidney, and intestine	Increases calcium absorption, raises calcium levels in blood, promotes bone reabsorption.
Adrenal glands Cortex Medulla	Mineralocorticoids (aldosterone and similar hormones)	Kidneys	Stimulates active reabsorption of sodium, passive reabsorption of water, and the active secretion of potassium in the distal convoluted tubule, thus increasing blood pressure and blood volume.
	Glucocorticoid (cortisol)	Receptors in most tissues and cells	Regulates or supports cardiovascular, metabolic, immunologic, and homeostatic functions.
	Androgens (including testosterone)	Gonads	Stimulates or controls the development and maintenance of masculine characteristics. Is the precursor for estrogen.
	Epinephrine (adrenalin)	Cardiac muscle, smooth muscle, glands	Increases heart rate and stroke volume, dilates the pupils, constricts arterioles in the skin and gut while dilating arterioles in leg muscles. Elevates the blood sugar level by increasing hydrolysis of glycogen to glucose in the liver, and begins the breakdown of lipids in fat cells.
	Norepinephrine (noradrenalin)	Sympathetic nervous system	Activates the sympathetic nervous system to directly increase heart rate, release energy from fat, and increase muscle readiness.

(continued)

| CHART 52–1 | **Glands and Their Hormones—*Continued*** |

Endocrine Gland and Hormone Source	Hormone(s)	Action Site	Physiological Effects
Thymus	Thymosin	Immune system	Aids in development of the body's immune system.
Pineal gland	Melatonin	Gonads	Can suppress sexual desire. Influences the circadian rhythm.
Pancreas Islets of Langerhans	Insulin	Muscles and tissues	Lowers blood sugar, controls utilization and storage of carbohydrates. Increases glycogen synthesis.
	Glucagons	Liver	Raises blood glucose, glycogenolysis.
	Somatostatin		Lowers blood glucose by interfering with release of growth hormone and glucagon.
Gonads Testes (males)	Androgens (testosterone)	Gonads Muscle tissues	Stimulates male sex characteristics. Promotes enlargement of muscle mass.
Ovarian follicle (females)	Inhibin	Ovaries, pituitary, placenta	Inhibits FSH synthesis and secretion and participates in the regulation of the menstrual cycle.
	Oestrogens (estrogen)	Breasts Uterus	Promote the development of female secondary sex characteristics, such as breasts, and are also involved in the thickening of the endometrium and other aspects of regulating the menstrual cycle.
Corpus luteum	Testosterone	Endometrium	Responsible for the thickening of the endometrium and its development in pregnancy.
	Progesterone	Endometrium	Converts the endometrium to its secretory stage to prepare the uterus for implantation.
Placenta	Human chorionic gonadotropin (HCG)	Endometrium	Prevents disintegration of the corpus luteum of the ovary and thereby maintains progesterone production that is critical for a pregnancy.
	Human placental lactogen (hPL)	Placenta	Ensures nutrient supply to the fetus.
	Progesterone	Placenta	Supports gestation and embryogenesis.
	Corticotropin-releasing hormone (CRH)	Placenta	Helps determine duration of the pregnancy.
Gastrointestinal tract (stomach and intestines)	Gastrin	Stomach	Produces gastric juices.
	Enterogastrone	Stomach	
	Secretin	Liver and pancreas	Inhibits secretion and motility.
	Pancreozymin	Pancreas	Produces pancreatic juices rich in enzymes.
	Ghrelin	Pituitary	Is associated with growth hormone release and appetite stimulation.
	Cholecystokinin (CCK)	Gallbladder	Provides for contraction and emptying of the gallbladder.
Liver	Insulin-like growth factor	Nerve, muscle, and other cells	Has insulin-like effects. Regulates cell growth and development.
	Angiotensinogen	Vascular	Constricts blood vessels and raises blood pressure.
		Brain	Increases thirst.
		Kidneys	Increases glomerular filtration rate.
		Adrenals	Increases production of aldosterone.
	Thrombopoietin	Bone marrow, platelets	Regulates the production of platelets.
Kidney	Calcitriol (1,25-dihydroxyvitamin D)	Intestine	Stimulates calcium absorption from the gut.
	Renin	Kidneys	Stimulates the renin-angiotensin-aldosterone system.
	Erythropoietin (EPO)	Bone marrow	Increases red blood cell production.
Brain	Peptide hormones	Brain and nervous system	May be used as neurotransmitters in the nervous system.
Heart	Atrial-natriuretic peptide (atriopeptin) (ANP)	Heart	Is involved in the homeostatic control of body water and sodium.

Glands and Their Hormones—*Continued*

Endocrine Gland and Hormone Source	Hormone(s)	Action Site	Physiological Effects
Adipose tissue	Leptin	Brain and nervous system	Decreases appetite and food intake, reduces insulin secretion and fat storage, increases sympathetic activity and metabolic rate.
	Resistin	Adipose cells	Suppresses insulin's ability to stimulate glucose uptake by adipose cells.
Skin	Calciferol (vitamin D)	Kidneys Intestines Bones	Contributes to the maintenance of normal levels of calcium and phosphorus in the bloodstream. Aids in the absorption of calcium for the formation of bones and teeth.
Bones	Osteocalcin	Pancreas and fat cells	Aids in sugar metabolism.

Sources: Braunwald, E., Hauser, S. L., Fauci, A. S., Longo, D. L., Kasper, D. L., & Jameson, J. L. (2001). *Harrison's principles of internal medicine* (15th ed.). New York: McGraw-Hill; Colorado State University, (2000). *Pathophysiology of the endocrine system.* http://www.colostate.edu; EndocrineWeb. (2002a). *Hyperthyroidism, overactivity of the thyroid gland. Part 2: Causes of hyperthyroidism.* Retrieved September 19, 2005, from http://endocrineweb.com/hyper2.html; EndocrineWeb. (2002b). *Pheochromocytoma.* Retrieved March 10, 2006, from http://endocrineweb.com/pheo.html; Hormone Foundation. (2006). *Endocrine glands.* Retrieved January 24, 2006, from http://www.hormone.org/endo101/index.html.

Disorders of the Endocrine System

Gland	Disorders of Hypometabolism	Hormone Involved	Disorders of Hypermetabolism
Thyroid	Hypothyroidism Cretinism Hashimoto's thyroiditis Postpartum thyroiditis	Thyroid hormone	Hyperthyroidism Graves' disease Postpartum thyroiditis Toxic goiter Hot nodules
Parathyroids	Hypoparathyroidism	Parathyroid hormone	**Hyperparathyroidism**
Anterior Pituitary	Hypopituitarism Sheehan's syndrome* Infertility	Growth hormone Prolactin ACTH	**Hyperpituitarism** Gigantism (children and youths) **Acromegaly (adults)** **Prolactin adenoma** Cushing's syndrome
Posterior Pituitary	Diabetes insipidus*	ADH	**SIADH***
Adrenal Cortex	Adrenal insufficiency* Addison's disease Congenital adrenal hyperplasia	Cortisol Aldosterone	**Cushing's syndrome** **Primary aldosteronism/Conn's disease***
Adrenal Medulla		Adrenalin (epinephrine)	**Pheochromocytoma***

*Described in an abbreviated form in the chapter.

thyroid function. Chart 52–3 (p. 1618) shows hypo- and hypermetabolic disorders of the thyroid.

■ Hypothyroidism

Hypothyroidism is a common endocrine disorder resulting from deficiency of thyroid hormone. It usually is a primary process, but also may be a secondary process. Primary hypothyroidism, caused by thyroid gland malfunction, is a common condition in which the thyroid gland fails to produce sufficient thyroid hormone to sustain normal metabolic function. This type of hypothyroidism may be caused by Hashimoto's disease, an autoimmune disease, surgical removal of the organ, therapeutic radiation as a result of treatment for hyperthyroidism, congenital hypothyroidism (**cretinism**, a condition caused by congenital absence that affects 1 in 4,000 newborns), or atrophy of the thyroid gland (Bharaktiya, Orlander, Woodhouse, & Davis, 2007).

Other causes include aging, iodine deficiency, tumors of the thyroid gland, or discontinuation of thyroid hormone replacement therapy or supplementation in cases where this therapy is being used (Greco, 2001). Secondary hypothyroidism occurs when the cause is related to pituitary tumors and other pituitary disorders and results from alterations in the hypothalamic–pituitary axis (Elliott, 2000; Greco, 2001). Tertiary thyroid disease originates at the level of the hypothalamus (Holcomb, 2002c).

Epidemiology and Etiology

Primary hypothyroidism is much more common than secondary and tertiary hypothyroidism (Porth, 2007). Hypothyroidism is defined as a deficiency in the production of TSH and is found in approximately 4.6% of the population (Kajantie et al., 2006). It is more common in women with small body size at birth and low body mass index during childhood. Generally, thyroid disease is much more common in females than in males,

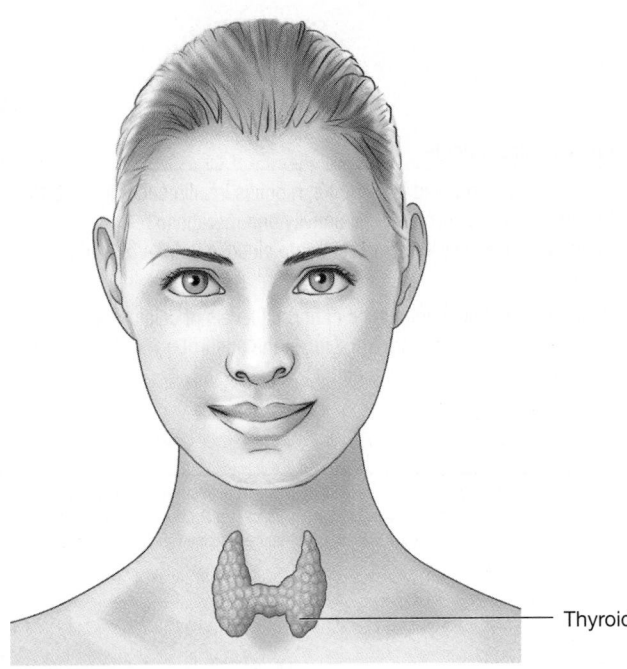

FIGURE 52–2 ■ The thyroid gland.

with reports of prevalence being two to eight times higher in females (Bharaktiya et al., 2007). Note also that the frequency of hypothyroidism, goiters, and thyroid nodules increases with age. Hypothyroidism is most prevalent in elderly populations, with as much as 2% to 20% of older age groups having some form of hypothyroidism (Bharaktiya et al., 2007). From a racial perspective the prevalence of hypothyroidism has been reported to be higher in Caucasians than in people of Hispanic descent or African Americans (Hollowell et al., 2002).

Primary hypothyroidism may result from **thyroidectomy** (removal of the thyroid) or ablation of the gland with radiation. Certain goitrogenic agents such as lithium carbonate and the antithyroid drugs propylthiouracil and methimazole in continuous dosage can produce hypothyroidism and goiter, as can iodine deficiency (which is very uncommon in the United States) (Porth, 2007).

The most common cause of hypothyroidism is a condition known as **Hashimoto's thyroiditis**, also known as **chronic lymphocytic thyroiditis**, a disorder in which the body's own immune system attacks the thyroid gland. The inflammatory response damages thyroid tissue and reduces the thyroid gland's ability to produce thyroid hormone. Studies in China indicate

CHART 52–3	**Hypothyroid and Hyperthyroid Metabolic Disorders**	
	Hypothyroidism	**Hyperthyroidism**
Types of Thyroid Disorders and Therapy	A hypometabolic condition in which the thyroid gland fails to produce adequate thyroid hormone, resulting in a slowdown of metabolism and cellular function.	A hypermetabolic condition in which the thyroid gland produces an excess of thyroid hormone and the body increases cellular function in response.
Primary Disease (causative source is the thyroid gland itself)	*Hashimoto's thyroiditis:* an autoimmune disease leading to underproduction of thyroid hormone. May result from surgical removal of the thyroid, therapeutic radiation of the thyroid gland, endemic cretinism, and postpartum thyroiditis.	*Graves' disease:* an autoimmune disease causing overproduction of thyroid hormone. May result from postpartum thyroiditis and a "hot" thyroid nodule. Stress also may be a contributing factor.
Secondary Disease (causative source is largely due to pituitary dysfunction)	The pituitary gland becomes unable to produce adequate TSH, thus thyroxine levels drop, causing hypothyroidism. Causes include adenoma, infarction, infiltrative disease, surgery, and trauma.	The pituitary continues to produce TSH, stimulating the thyroid gland to produce more T_3 and T_4, leading to hyperthyroidism.
Tertiary Disease	Caused by impaired production of TRH from the hypothalamus, which fails to stimulate the pituitary to produce TSH.	
Pharmacologic Intervention	Administer synthetic thyroid hormone. Patient should take drug (usually levothyroxine) daily in the early morning on an empty stomach.	Administer antithyroid drugs: propylthiouracil, methimazole, or potassium iodide to inhibit thyroid hormone secretion. Hydrocortisone may be given to block TSH and for adrenal insufficiency. Calcium channel blockers and beta-blockers may be given to slow the heart rate and reduce atrial fibrillation.
Medical Intervention	*Primary disease:* administer synthetic thyroid hormone. Monitor thyroid levels regularly. *Secondary disease:* assess and treat pituitary disease. *Tertiary disease:* treat problem arising from the hypothalamus.	*Primary disease:* administer antithyroid drugs or radioactive iodine to partially or completely eliminate thyroid hormone production. *Secondary disease:* administer antithyroid drugs and treat pituitary disease.
Surgical Intervention	*Primary disease:* surgical removal of the thyroid if large goiter or nodules present.	*Primary disease:* surgical removal of part or all of the thyroid gland to reduce or eliminate hormone production.

Sources: Adapted from Holcomb, S. (2002). Thyroid diseases: A primer for the critical care nurse. *Dimensions of Critical Care Nursing, 21*(4), 127–133; Porth, C. M., 2007.

that excessive intake of iodine may increase the incidence and prevalence of autoimmune thyroiditis (Teng et al., 2006).

Pathophysiology

The thyroid gland functions with a negative feedback system through the involvement of three organs, the hypothalamus, the anterior pituitary, and the thyroid glands. The hypothalamus secretes thyrotropin-releasing hormone (TRH), the initiating hormone, which stimulates the anterior pituitary to release TSH, causing the thyroid to secrete thyroid hormone (T_3, T_4) (Larson, Anderson, & Koslawy, 2000; Porth, 2007). The dynamic feedback regulatory and compensatory responses of the pituitary and the thyroid gland are known as the hypothalamus–pituitary–thyroid axis (Holcomb, 2002c).

Follicles within the thyroid gland produce thyroxine (T_4), which constitutes approximately 95% of the thyroid hormone initially produced by this gland, as well as triiodothyronine (T_3) and calcitonin. Much of the T_4 is eventually converted into T_3, thus these are referred to collectively as thyroid hormone (Larson et al., 2000; Porth, 2007). Both thyroxine and triiodothyronine require iodine for their synthesis. With iodine deficiency, the thyroid is unable to secrete sufficient thyroid hormone. Calcitonin, also known as thyrocalcitonin, is secreted in response to high levels of calcium, reducing plasma calcium by depositing calcium in the bones. The pathophysiology of thyroid disease can involve autoimmune response disorders, inflammation, infection, atrophy of the gland, hyperplasia of tissues, tumor growth, or genetic mutations or abnormalities. See the Risk Factors for Hypothyroidism box.

Clinical Manifestations

Vague complaints of fatigue, weight gain, cold intolerance, constipation, and mental lethargy may make diagnosis of hypothyroidism difficult until the disease has progressed significantly. Dry skin, hair thinning or loss, and enlargement of the thyroid gland may be observed on physical examination. In cases of primary thyroid disease, laboratory tests will reveal a high level of TSH, because the pituitary will respond to an underproduction of thyroid hormone. In such cases, free T_4 (FT_4) (thyroxine) will be lower than normal. A major problem is that symptoms are very insidious and patients may have chronic **thyroiditis**, an inflammation of the thyroid gland, for years before a diagnosis is made and intervention initiated.

Long-standing or severe hypothyroidism may lead to a serious condition known as **myxedema**, a term used to describe the accumulation of mucopolysaccharides in tissues. This condition is characterized by signs of serious physiological compromise, including profound lethargy, muscle weakness, facial edema, thick tongue, mental decline, and personality change. Infection or trauma may precipitate myxedema as the body becomes increasingly compromised and unable to respond due to inadequate thyroid hormone.

Laboratory and Diagnostic Procedures

Thyroid function is evaluated using laboratory tests, thyroid scanning, fine-needle biopsy, and ultrasonography. Measurement of TSH in the blood and also the thyroxine level is a key diagnostic tool in suspected cases of hypothyroidism. Measurement of the FT_4 serum level reflects the amount of unbound

RISK FACTORS for Hypothyroidism

Risk factors for hypothyroidism include familial history of thyroid disease, a history of autoimmune disease, pernicious anemia, aging, an inadequate supply of dietary iodine, and previous treatment for hyperthyroidism. Hypothyroidism can occur at any age but is particularly common in older adults, affecting 17% of women and 9% of men over age 60 (Thyroid Federation International, 2003). An iodine-deficient diet also is a risk factor in the development of hypothyroidism. Iodine is needed as a raw material for the production of thyroid hormone and an inadequate supply leads to a decrease in thyroid hormone production. This condition results in overstimulation of the thyroid gland through the production of TSH by the pituitary gland, resulting in an enlarged gland or a goiter. A **goiter** is a significant enlargement of the thyroid gland.

Fortunately, goiters caused by iodine deficiency are rarely seen in developed countries due to the addition of iodine to salt and other foods, but may be seen in underdeveloped countries where natural sources of iodine are low and nutrition is poor. Patients who have had previous treatment for hyperthyroidism also are at risk following treatment, because radiation therapy or surgery may significantly reduce the production of thyroid hormone over time. Some drugs and foods inhibit thyroid production and are known as **goitrogens**. For example, lithium, a drug commonly used for the treatment of bipolar disorders, may cause hypothyroidism. Similarly, the drug rifampin, which is used to treat tuberculosis, is known to impair thyroid secretion (Takasu, Takara, & Komiya, 2005). Another drug implicated in thyroid dysfunction is amiodarone. Used for cardiac arrhythmias, amiodarone may cause abnormal results on thyroid tests and either thyrotoxicosis or hypothyroidism (Porsche & Brenner, 2006).

thyroxine in the blood and is considered the best clinical measure of thyroxine levels. Total T_3 and total T_4 are considered to be less reliable indicators of thyroid level because they are affected by drugs and other protein-binding factors.

The pituitary–thyroid negative feedback loop quickly responds when a low level of thyroid hormone is perceived. Small decreases in thyroid hormone level will result in a rapid increase in output of TSH, and increases in thyroid hormone will lead to a decrease in TSH production. Low levels of T_3 and T_4 (or FT_4) in the presence of high levels of TSH indicate that the problem is due to disease of the thyroid gland. Low levels of TSH in combination with low levels of T_3 and T_4 (or FT_4) indicate potential problems with the pituitary gland. Treatment for primary hypothyroidism, in which the thyroid gland itself is functioning poorly, is directed at hormone replacement therapy. When the problem is caused by failure of the pituitary to release TSH, further diagnostic work will be required to determine a course of therapy. Symptoms and physical findings in thyroid disease are shown in Chart 52–4 (p. 1620).

Monitoring of TSH and FT_4 will continue to be important during hormone replacement therapy as a means to evaluate the effectiveness of treatment over time. A test for thyroid antibodies also may reveal Hashimoto's thyroiditis (hypothyroidism) or Graves' disease (hyperthyroidism). In addition, thyroid scanning can be used by the health care provider when evaluating thyroid nodules, which are fairly common, occurring in 1% to 4% of the population over age 50 (AACE, 2005a). A scan involves administration of a small dose of radioactive isotope, which becomes concentrated in the thyroid tissue. Following the

CHART 52–4	**Symptoms and Physical Findings for Thyroid Disease**	
Physiological System	**Symptoms of Hypothyroidism**	**Symptoms of Hyperthyroidism**
Cardiopulmonary	Slowed heartbeat/pulse, high blood pressure, high cholesterol levels, cardiac enlargement, congestive heart failure, ascites	Rapid heartbeat/pulse, palpitations, angina, irregular heart rhythm, heat intolerance, and hot flashes
Neuromuscular	Drowsiness, fatigue, mental lethargy, forgetfulness, depression, muscular weakness, emotional lability, and paranoia	Insomnia, jitteriness, shaking, nervousness, irritability, hand tremors, muscle weakness, myalgia, and muscle cramps
Gastrointestinal	Enlarged tongue, constipation, reduced bowel sounds	Difficulty swallowing, more frequent bowel movements, diarrhea
Skin/hair	Dry patchy skin, coarse and thinning hair (alopecia), fluid retention in skin, cold intolerance, decreased perspiration, edema of face and eyelids	Thinning hair or alopecia, warm, moist skin (sweating), heat intolerance
Other	Weight gain, fatigue, heavy and irregular menstrual periods, lowered body temperature	Unexplained weight loss, change in or lighter menstrual cycles, bulging eyes (exophthalmos), goiter (thyroid enlargement), accelerated loss of calcium from bones
Diagnostic lab values	Elevated cholesterol levels Serum TSH (will be low if the pituitary is involved and high if the thyroid gland is the affected tissue) Decreased or absent T_4 and T_3 levels Low basal metabolic rate (BMR) Presence of thyroid antibodies	Low level of TSH Elevated serum free T_4 and free T_3 Elevated BMR

Source: Adapted from American Association of Clinical Endocrinologists. (2005b). *Hyperthyroidism: Information for patients.* Retrieved September 19, 2005, from http://www.aace.com/members/ brochures.php; American Association of Clinical Endocrinologists. (2005c). *Hypothyroidism: Information for patients.* Retrieved September 19, 2005, from http://www.aace.com/members/brochures. php; Hadley, M. E. (2000). *Endocrinology* (5th ed.). San Francisco: Benjamin Cummings.

ingestion or injection of the isotope, a picture is taken of the gland to determine the nature of the nodule, a majority of which are benign. The thyroid scan shows whether a nodule is hot or cold (nonfunctioning). Ultrasound also can be useful in evaluating the size and shape of nodules, whether a nodule is a cyst (cysts are normally benign) or solid, but it is less useful in differentiating benign from malignant growths. A fine-needle biopsy is the most accurate method used to determine whether a nodule is malignant or benign. Ultrasonography of the thyroid may be most useful in guiding the placement of a needle for biopsy to obtain a good specimen (AACE, 2005b; Larson et al., 2000). See the Diagnostic Tests for Thyroid Disorders box.

Medical Management

The treatment for hypothyroidism involves the replacement of thyroid hormone as indicated by the physiological functioning of the gland. In hypothyroidism, therapeutic actions are directed at stimulating the production of or replacing thyroid hormone. Hypothyroidism is easily treated with the administration of the synthetic thyroid hormone levothyroxine. The dosage is determined by the amount needed to bring TSH levels into the normal range and to provide abatement of symptoms. Approximately 70 to 100 mcg of levothyroxine is given daily based on age, weight, hormone levels, and symptoms. Initial adult doses vary from 25 to 100 mcg, with smaller doses given to the elderly and patients with diabetes or cardiac disease.

To ensure maximum absorption of the hormone, it is advised that levothyroxine be taken in the early morning on an empty stomach. Synthetic thyroid hormone can be taken safely concurrently with some medications, but patients taking medications such as anticoagulants, beta-blockers, cholesterol-lowering

drugs, or seizure control drugs should check with the pharmacist for potential drug interactions. Although administration of levothyroxine will bring thyroid hormone levels within normal limits, it may suppress TSH, which increases the risk of osteoporosis, a side effect that can be avoided by the ingestion of calcium carbonate. However, if the two preparations are taken together, the calcium can interfere with absorption of thyroid hormone. Thus patients should be advised to take any over-the-counter (OTC) vitamins, minerals (including iron), and antacids at least 4 hours earlier or later than thyroid hormone (Neafsey, 2004). Patients also need to be advised that they will be taking thyroid replacement hormone for life.

- *Because the absorption of the synthetic thyroid hormone levothyroxine is altered by food and selected drugs, herbs, vitamins, and minerals, the nurse should advise the patient to take this drug on an empty stomach, usually as a single dose before breakfast and to hold food intake for at least 1 hour. Patients should ingest this medication at least 4 hours before taking antacids, iron, or vitamin/mineral supplements.*

- *Because the bioavailability of the drug varies with different manufacturers, patients should continue taking the same brand continuously or should have thyroid function studies done 6 to 8 weeks after a change in prescription.*

- *Patients should be advised they will be taking thyroid replacement therapy for the remainder of their lives and not to discontinue this medication without consulting with their health care provider.*

Symptoms of hypothyroidism gradually fade over a period of 3 to 6 weeks as therapy is initiated. Blood levels of TSH and FT_4 should be tested 6 to 8 weeks after therapy is initiated and regularly thereafter until hormone levels stabilize and symptoms disappear.

DIAGNOSTIC TESTS for Thyroid Disorders

Test	Nature of the Test	Normal Ranges*	Use in Diagnosis	Nursing Implications
Thyroid-stimulating hormone (TSH) test	Laboratory test of blood.	*Adults:* 2–12 microinternational unit/mL	Differentiating primary from secondary hypothyroidism. Elevation of TSH occurs in primary hypothyroidism. In secondary hypothyroid states where pituitary pathology exists, TSH may be absent or very low, even with low levels of T_3 and T_4.	Prepare patient for blood test. Does not require fasting. Recent administration of radioisotopes for other diagnostic tests may affect test results.
TSH stimulation test	A laboratory examination of the blood.	Evidence of increased thyroid function with administration of TSH.	Helps differentiate primary and secondary hypothyroidism. Patients with primary disease are unable to increase the production of thyroid hormone when stimulated with TSH.	Prepare patient for blood test. Fasting is not required.
Thyrotropin-releasing hormone (TRH) test	An IV bolus of TRH is given.	A quick rise in TSH levels within 30 minutes after receiving TRH.	Reveals the responsiveness of the anterior pituitary to TRH. Confirms the presence of primary hyperthyroidism because little or no increase in TSH is seen due to the suppression effect of excess circulation of thyroid hormone. A TSH level that rises too high may indicate early hypothyroidism.	Prepare patient for blood test. Does not require fasting. Explain procedure to patient. Check site of drug administration.
Thyroxine (T_4) screen	A laboratory test with blood.	*Adults:* 4–11 mcg/dL	Provides a direct (but not always reliable) measure of T_4 in the blood. Increased levels indicate hyperthyroidism and low levels indicate hypothyroidism.	Results may be affected by iodine contrast scans. Level also may be affected by medications such as estrogen, oral contraceptives, seizure medications, and opiates such as heroin, lithium, steroids, and antithyroid drugs.
Thyroxine index, free (FT$_4$ index)	A laboratory test of blood.		Measures the amount of free T_4, which is not affected by thyroid-binding globulin abnormalities. Reflects the real hormonal status more effectively than does a total T_4 or T_3 blood test. Increased levels indicate hyperthyroidism and decreased levels indicate hypothyroidism.	Explain the procedure to the patient.
Triiodothyronine (T_3) radioimmunoassay	A laboratory test of blood.		Accurately measures thyroid function. When levels are below normal, hypothyroidism generally exists.	May be affected by pregnancy, recently administered radioisotope administration, and selected drugs. Does not require fasting.

(continued)

DIAGNOSTIC TESTS for Thyroid Disorders—*Continued*

Test	Nature of the Test	Normal Ranges*	Use in Diagnosis	Nursing Implications
Triiodothyronine (T$_3$) uptake test	A laboratory test of blood.	25–35%	Indirectly quantifies thyroid-binding globulin and thyroid-binding prealbumin, which may be elevated due to pregnancy, oral contraceptive use, or genetic factors. Adds information in the diagnosis of hypothyroidism and hyperthyroidism.	May be affected by recent radioisotope scans and selected drugs. Does not require fasting.
Iodine uptake scan	Patient takes an oral dose of radioactive iodine on an empty stomach. The amount of iodine that is taken up by the thyroid gland is measured during the next several hours.	Measures how much iodine is taken up by the thyroid gland.	Hypothyroid patients take up little iodine and hyperthyroid patients take up a lot of iodine.	Patient should be NPO before exam. Usually done in conjunction with thyroid lab studies.
Thyroid scan	A radioactive substance is given to enhance visualization of the gland. An image of the gland is recorded as the scan passes over the gland.	Reveals normal size, shape, position, and function. No areas of decreased or increased uptake are apparent.	Particularly useful in differentiating thyroid nodules, Graves' disease from Plummer's disease, and metastatic tumors.	Contraindicated in pregnancy and with allergies to iodine.
Thyroid ultrasound	Ultrasound.	Reveals normal size, shape, and position of gland.	Useful in differentiating cystic from solid thyroid nodules. Can be used to aid in placement of needle for biopsy. A safe procedure when thyroid scan cannot be done due to pregnancy.	Prepare patient for procedure.

*Normal ranges are best determined by the laboratory administering the tests.

Sources: Adapted from EndocrineWeb.com. (2008). Retrieved August 29, 2008 from http://www.endocrineweb.com/; Larson, J., Anderson, E., & Koslawy, M. (2000). Thyroid disease: A review for primary care. *Journal of the American Academy of Nurse Practitioners, 12*(6), 226–232.

Following stabilization, thyroid hormone levels then should be checked annually to ensure that the appropriate medication level has been reached and to avoid drug-induced hyperthyroidism.

Nursing Management

Nursing care for patients with hypothyroidism is guided by the severity of the disease process and related symptoms. Typically, the nurse is an objective observer and recorder of patient signs and symptoms, both during diagnosis and following treatment, a role that is particularly important given the frequency with which the diagnosis of hormonal disorders is delayed or missed. Patients with hypothyroidism will report weight gain, dry skin and hair, constipation, fatigue, and mental lethargy. In cases of long-standing disease or seriously decreased hormone levels, cardiac problems may be apparent as evidenced by bradycardia, high blood pressure, high cholesterol levels, cardiac enlargement, and congestive heart failure.

Nursing care should be directed at symptom management and improvement of the patient's physiological status with hormone replacement therapy. Patients should be instructed on the nature of the hormone replacement and the importance of taking thyroid hormone on an empty stomach. The primary goal of treatment is to return patients to a **euthyroid**, or normal thyroid, status. Patients are started on small to moderate doses of levothyroxine to begin their hormone replacement therapy. Patients with diabetes should be monitored carefully during this period because their blood sugars may be more labile due to hypothyroidism. See the Nursing Process: Patient Care Plan for Hypothyroidism, which details the nursing process used in caring for patients with hypothyroidism.

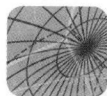

NURSING PROCESS: Patient Care Plan For Hypothyroidism

Assessment of Current Body Characteristics

Subjective Data:

Is your pulse slower than normal?

Has your weight changed, either increased or decreased in recent months?

Do you feel energetic or fatigued much of the time? Are you sleeping a great deal but still feeling tired?

Has there been any change in your activity tolerance?

How would you describe your mental alertness and memory?

Describe your menstrual pattern. Has there been any change in the frequency or flow during your menstrual periods?

Objective Data:

Weight gain

Edema around eyes and facial puffiness

Thick tongue

Bradycardia and dyspnea

Low body temperature

Enlargement of the thyroid gland (goiter)

TSH level high

FT_4 low

Unable to process thoughts rapidly

Nursing Assessment and Diagnoses	Outcomes and Evaluation Parameters	Planning and Interventions with *Rationales*
Nursing Diagnosis: *Fatigue*, and *Activity Intolerance* secondary to hypometabolic state with decreased cardiac output	**Outcome:** Patient is able to manage self-care and explain rationale for therapeutic plan, including medication regime and instructions. **Evaluation Parameters:** Patient is able to repeat instructions for taking medications and can describe symptoms of both hypo- and hyperthyroidism. TSH and FT_4 levels return to normal range. **Outcome:** Patient does not use sedatives or opiates during acute phase of illness. **Evaluation Parameter:** Patient and health care team express awareness of risks associated with use of sedatives, opiates, or alcohol.	**Interventions and *Rationales:*** Instruct patient on administration of hormone replacement medication, signs and symptoms of hypo- and hyperthyroidism, and self-care practices. *To ensure patient takes hormone replacement medication on an empty stomach for optimal absorption. To inform patient to be alert for signs of hypo- or hyperthyroidism.* Patient and health care providers are warned to avoid use of sedatives, opioids, analgesic medications, or alcohol products, which would further depress metabolic functions and increase risk of myxedema crisis. *To prevent further suppression of the patient's metabolic state and possible serious complications such as coma, particularly in the elderly.*

Assessment of Skin and Nail Characteristics and Wound Healing

Subjective Data:

Have you noticed any change in your skin, hair, or nails lately?

Are your nails brittle, thick, and often breaking or splitting?

Is your skin cold, dry, or itchy? Do you bruise easily? Do wounds heal slowly?

Objective Data:

Skin cool and dry

Evidence of itching skin

Brittle nails

Hair dry, sparse, coarse, and brittle

Generalized interstitial edema

Nursing Assessment and Diagnoses	Outcomes and Evaluation Parameters	Planning and Intervention with *Rationales*
Nursing Diagnosis: *Risk for Impaired Skin Integrity* secondary to thyroid hormone deficiency	**Outcome:** Verbalizes satisfaction with improved condition of skin, hair, and nails, with less itching and breaking. **Evaluation Parameters:** Skin intact, soft, and moist with no evidence of patient itching or scratching. Patient's hair is soft and thick.	**Interventions and *Rationales:*** Avoid use of soaps, astringents, or other agents such as alcohol. Liberally apply emollient skin lotion. Consider using an alternating air mattress if needed. *To counteract drying of skin, hair, and nails due to hormone loss and to protect skin from injury.*

Assessment of Gastrointestinal Function and Disturbances

Subjective Data:

Have you observed any changes in your bowel habits?

Have you experienced frequent constipation or abdominal pain?

Is your cholesterol high?

Objective Data:

Abdomen distended

Bowel sounds decreased

Weight gain

Increased TSH level

Decreased T_4

Presence of thyroid antibodies

Nursing Assessment and Diagnoses	Outcomes and Evaluation Parameters	Planning and Interventions with *Rationales*
Nursing Diagnosis: *Constipation* secondary to lethargy, activity intolerance, and hypometabolic state	**Outcome:** Observed bowel function is normal with no reports of constipation or abdominal pain. **Evaluation Parameters:** Abdomen soft, not distended. Active bowel sounds. Patient's normal bowel pattern is resumed.	**Interventions and *Rationales:*** Administer stool softeners as prescribed. Gradually increase fluid intake and fiber in diet. Increase activity level with short, frequent walks and mild exercise. *To maintain or regain normal bowel function and to prevent bowel obstruction or megacolon.*

(continued)

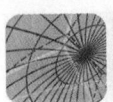

NURSING PROCESS: Patient Care Plan For Hypothyroidism—*Continued*

Assessment for Hypothermia

Subjective Data:
Are you feeling too cold or too hot?
Do you feel anxious or restless?

Objective Data:
Wearing multiple layers of clothing
Skin is cool and dry
Hypothermia (in severe myxedema) with low body temperature

Nursing Assessment and Diagnoses	Outcomes and Evaluation Parameters	Planning and Interventions with *Rationales*
Nursing Diagnosis: *Hypothermia* secondary to metabolic dysfunction	**Outcome:** Patient is able to tolerate typical ambient temperatures without distress. **Evaluation Parameters:** Body temperature within normal range. Patient appears comfortable with no reports of distress related to ambient temperature.	**Interventions and *Rationales:*** Monitor the environment to provide a warm room for patient comfort. *To minimize patient discomfort while patient's body is adapting to stabilization of hormone levels.*

Assessment of Cognition Level and Memory Impairment

Subjective Data:
Do you feel mentally alert?
Are your thought processes slowed?
Is your short- or long-term memory impaired?
Are you irritable or confused?

Objective Data:
Responds appropriately to questions
Able to follow directions
Recalls objects when asked to
Recognizes individuals by name and/or position

Nursing Assessment and Diagnoses	Outcomes and Evaluation Parameters	Planning and Interventions with *Rationales*
Nursing Diagnosis: *Confusion, Acute* secondary to hypothyroidism	**Outcomes:** Patient oriented to time, place, and circumstances. Able to recall instructions regarding medications and activity prescriptions. Mood stable. **Evaluation Parameters:** Alert and oriented. Evidence of effective short- and long-term memory. Family reports stable affect and mood.	**Interventions and *Rationales:*** Reduce stimuli and mental demands while hormone deficiency is replaced. Instruct family about potential mood swings, depression, and irritability. Provide instructions to patient and family in writing as well as orally. *To minimize distress and disorientation while patient's body is adapting to stabilization of hormone levels.*

Discharge Priorities

Discharge priorities include ensuring patient's understanding of the need for lifelong hormone replacement therapy and annual monitoring of hormone levels once a stable, therapeutic level of hormone has been reached. Some authorities advise patients to be wary of changing brands or suppliers of hormone replacement drugs because of the variability in bioavailability of the drug in different products (American Thyroid Association, 2005; Holcomb, 2002c; Thyroid Foundation of America, 2004b). If the brand name drug or generic drug is changed, the patient should be retested about 6 weeks after starting on the new medication. Consultation with an endocrine specialist is advised, particularly if the patient is diabetic or pregnant.

Gerontological Considerations

Hypothyroidism is seen clinically at an increasing rate in women over age 50. Clinical manifestations, unless severe, may be too subtle to easily recognize, thus making diagnosis and intervention more difficult. In rare cases, **myxedema coma**, a rare life-threatening complication in which there is overwhelming cardiopulmonary failure, may be seen in elderly patients, usually precipitated by some untoward event such as infection, trauma, surgery, or neurological disorder (Figure 52–3 ■). Patients

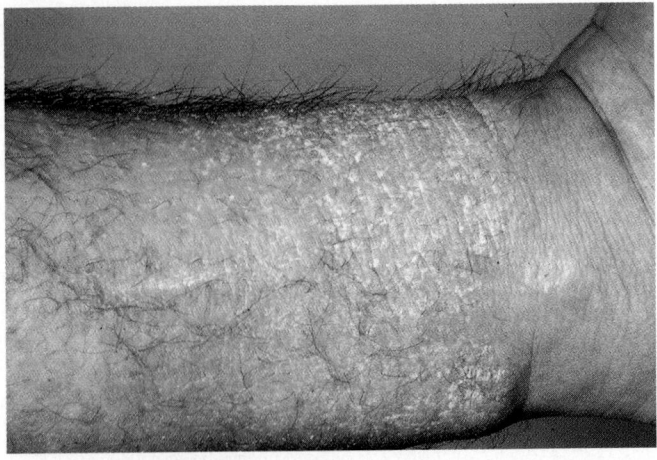

FIGURE 52–3 ■ Patient with myxedema.

present with all the usual, but exacerbated and serious symptoms of hypothyroidism, and they typically have body temperatures below normal as well. Hypothermia, with body temperature lower than 35°C (95°F), is a key sign that myxedema coma may be impending. In addition, patients with myxedema coma may demonstrate serious cardiac symptoms, impaired ventilation, and neuromuscular weakness. Timely diagnosis and intervention is essential in such cases because mortality rates are high.

In addition, it is essential that the underlying problem be identified and treated since patients may have other problems such as myxedema megacolon, an abnormal dilation of the colon that is not caused by mechanical obstruction, due to reduced intestinal motility caused by hypothyroidism. This condition may lead health care providers to consider surgery when the primary need is for hormone replacement therapy.

Fortunately, abdominal symptoms usually subside when synthetic thyroid hormone is administered to the patient (Greco, 2001). In emergency situations, levothyroxine sodium, a more powerful injectable form of triiodothyronine, may be administered intravenously for treatment of myxedema coma. Nurses must be particularly vigilant in assessment and reporting of cardiac symptoms, impaired ventilation, and neuromuscular weakness in these cases. Patients may require ventilator assistance and other support measures to ensure survival.

- *Immediately report signs of myxedema, a severe, life-threatening illness with symptoms including facial edema, thick tongue (macroglossia), mental confusion, irritability, severe mood swings, significant hypothermia (91°F to 95°F), severely slowed pulse and respirations, decreased blood pressure, profound neuromuscular weakness, anemia, and signs of psychosis, because the mortality rate is high.*
- *Avoid use of sedatives, opiates, or alcohol to prevent congestive heart failure and circulatory collapse.*
- *Provide respiratory support with administration of oxygen and ventilation if needed.*
- *Administer intravenous fluids with care, observing for plural effusion and congestive heart failure.*
- *Be prepared to administer fast-acting intravenous thyroid hormone to restore the body's thyroxine level.*
- *Slowly rewarm the patient to avoid causing refractory hypotension and increased oxygen demand.*
- *Observe for signs of infection and treat infections immediately to avoid further compromise of the patient.*

Health Promotion

The thyroid gland requires iodine to manufacture thyroid hormone. Until iodine was added to salt sometime in the 1920s, hypothyroidism was not uncommon in some parts of the United States. Patients should be encouraged to eat a healthy diet, to purchase salt enhanced with iodine, and ensure that iodine is ingested regularly. Another food source high in iodine is seafood. Health promotion for patients with thyroid disease most often revolves around instruction regarding medications for hormone replacement therapy since therapy will be required for the remainder of the patient's lifetime. Some patients will find it difficult to accept the notion that lifetime drug therapy is advised

for treatment of this disorder. For this reason, it is important for the nurse to assess the patient's understanding of the disorder and the need for hormone replacement therapy.

The Genetic Considerations for Hypothyroidism box discusses the nurse's role if a familial predisposition to hypothyroidism is suspected.

Collaborative Management

Patients with thyroid disease will need the support of several members of the health care team. Following diagnosis, the patient with hypothyroidism will benefit from instruction by the pharmacist regarding medication for replacement of thyroid hormone and medications to treat other symptoms such as anemia. The nutritionist or dietitian can provide helpful consultation on diet to address the hypometabolic needs of the patient's body while therapy corrects and stabilizes thyroid hormones.

Hyperthyroidism

Hyperthyroidism, a condition in which there is excess production of thyroid hormone, is caused by an increase in thyroid function for any reason. This condition may lead to **thyrotoxicosis**, a clinical syndrome that results when tissues are exposed to high levels of circulating thyroid hormone (Greenspan, 2004).

Epidemiology and Etiology

Hyperthyroidism may be due to Graves' disease, toxic multinodular goiter, painful subacute thyroiditis caused by a viral infection, other types of thyroiditis, adenomas of the thyroid gland, and excessive iodine or thyroid hormone intake. **Graves' disease**, a disorder named for an Irish physician who described the syndrome, is an autoimmune disorder that is the most common cause of hyperthyroidism, with it being more prevalent in women (Porth, 2007; Yeung & Habra, 2007). In Graves' disease, thyroid stimulating immunoglobulins (TSIs) activate TSH receptors on the thyroid follicular cells, resulting in increased production of thyroid hormones and symptoms of hyperthyroidism such as increased appetite, unexplained weight loss, heat intolerance, exertional dyspnea, increased heart rate, fatigue, nervousness, goiter, and palpitations (Waltman, Brewer, & Lobert, 2004). Generally, thyroiditis involves the entire thyroid gland and is eight times more common in women than men between the ages of 30 and 50 years (Figure 52–4 ■, p. 1626).

Other causes of thyroiditis with resulting temporary hyperthyroidism include subacute thyroiditis (also known as De Quervain's thyroiditis), and silent thyroiditis (lymphocytic and postpartum thyroiditis). These may be caused by a viral infection, and there are indications that trauma and stress, such as

GENETIC CONSIDERATIONS for Hypothyroidism

Patients should be advised of any familial predisposition to thyroid disease based on a family history of thyroid and autoimmune disorders in order to advise other family members of this particular health risk.

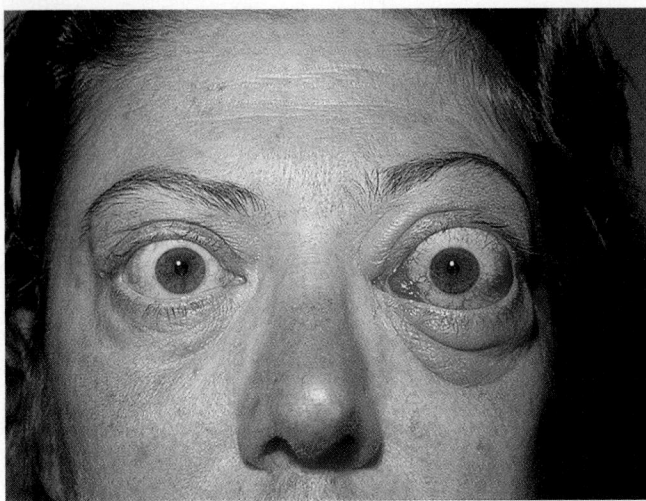

FIGURE 52–4 ■ Patient with Graves' disease.

pregnancy, also may influence the development of the disease. In subacute thyroiditis, patients often experience pain as well as enlargement of the thyroid gland. Many patients with these conditions will resume normal thyroid function over time, but sometimes treatment is required for subsequent hypothyroidism (AACE, 2005d).

Multiple or single "hot" nodules in the thyroid gland may excrete excess thyroid hormone. These conditions are called toxic multinodular goiter or toxic nodule. Thyroid nodules are fairly common and only a small percentage are malignant. Nodules may occur simply due to excess growth of normal thyroid tissue, fluid-filled cysts, inflammation (thyroiditis), or benign or cancerous tumors. A single enlarged nodule may cause hyperthyroidism because it can produce a very large amount of thyroid hormone. For more information, see the Risk Factors for Hyperthyroidism box.

Pathophysiology

Hyperthyroidism is a condition in which excessive levels of thyroid hormone stimulate the body's metabolic processes, resulting in symptoms indicative of the hypermetabolic state, including loss of weight, nervousness, rapid pulse, and warm, moist skin. Thyrotoxicosis is an inclusive term that describes severe hypermetabolic conditions caused by the thyroid hormones. Hyperthyroidism may be due to primary disease

RISK FACTORS for Hyperthyroidism

There appears to be a genetic predisposition to autoimmune disorders that cause hyperthyroidism, or Graves' disease. Situational physiological changes such as the stress of pregnancy or viral illness can stimulate the onset of the disease. Excessive iodine intake and excessive thyroid hormone replacement therapy can also be predisposing factors (Holcomb, 2002c). A history of amiodarone therapy for cardiac arrhythmias is also a risk factor for hyperthyroidism because amiodarone is 37% iodine by weight (Porsche & Brenner, 2006). Hyperthyroidism occurs most often in women in their middle years but can occur in older adults and children as well.

involving the thyroid itself or it may be caused by unchecked pituitary secretion of TSH. In primary hyperthyroidism, inflammation of thyroid cells occurs due to thyroiditis with accumulation of white blood cells and fluid causing thyroid enlargement. In secondary hyperthyroidism, increased growth and proliferation of thyroid cells may also occur due to stimulation by TSH produced by the pituitary. Long-standing or very acute illness states can lead to cardiac complications and **exophthalmus**, bulging of the eyes.

Clinical Manifestations

The clinical signs of hyperthyroidism will vary depending on the severity of thyrotoxicosis, patient age, and individual response to high levels of thyroid hormone. Key indications of hyperthyroidism are unexplained weight loss, fine tremors of the hand and tongue, hyperactivity, heat intolerance, palpitations, tachycardia (with heart rate greater than 100 beats/min), fatigue, and weakness. See Chart 52–3 (p. 1618) for a comparison of signs and symptoms in hypothyroidism and hyperthyroidism. The symptoms of hyperthyroidism may be very subtle initially in elderly patients, presenting with complaints of fatigue and/or weight loss. Elderly patients are easily misdiagnosed and may be thought to have depression, given that they report insomnia, fatigue, and impaired concentration and memory.

Graves' Disease During Pregnancy

Pregnant women normally have some increase in thyroid stimulation during pregnancy and the thyroid gland will enlarge somewhat. However, significant **thyromegaly**, abnormal growth in thyroid tissue, and goiter are unusual physical findings and should cause the clinician to evaluate a pregnant woman for possible hyperthyroidism. Graves' disease is the most common endocrine disorder other than diabetes in pregnancy and may put mother and fetus at risk for preterm delivery, perinatal morbidity, heart failure, and thyroid storm. During pregnancy, Graves' disease is managed best with antithyroid drugs (medications that inhibit the production of thyroxine), because radioactive iodine will affect the fetus's thyroid gland and surgery will increase the risk of miscarriage or preterm delivery (Waltman et al., 2004).

Laboratory and Diagnostic Procedures

The same diagnostic tests described earlier in the section on hypothyroidism are used in the assessment of patients with suspected hypermetabolic thyroid states. Measurements of TSH and FT_4 are commonly used to assess patients with suspected hyperthyroidism. A decrease in TSH in combination with a high level of FT_4 indicates hyperthyroidism. Refer to the earlier Diagnostic Tests for Thyroid Disorders box (p. 1621) for an overview of the thyroid tests used to assess thyroid functioning during diagnosis and treatment of thyroid disorders.

Medical Management

Hypermetabolic thyroid states, including Graves' disease, can be difficult to treat, depending on the responsiveness of thyroid tissue to treatment modalities (Fenton, Gold, & Sadeghi-Nejad, 2006). There are three common ways to treat Graves' disease:

- Antithyroid drugs, which inhibit production or conversion of active thyroid hormone

- Radioactive iodine, which destroys all or part of the thyroid gland and makes it unable to produce excessive thyroid hormone
- Subtotal thyroidectomy, in which most of the thyroid gland is removed, making it unable to produce excessive thyroid hormone.

Medical options usually are tried first since complications, including hemorrhage, damage to the parathyroid glands, and impairment of the vocal cords, can occur with surgical intervention. Antithyroid drug therapy has the benefit of lower cost and is safer for patients such as pregnant women, adolescents, and children. Moreover, antithyroid drugs can be of great value in autoimmune diseases such as Graves' disease because antithyroid drugs improve the autoimmune process (Cooper, 2005). However, selection of treatment for hyperthyroidism will depend on age, physical condition, pregnancy, degree of illness, and personal preferences.

Antithyroid drugs, such as propylthiouracil (PTU) and methimazole (Tapazole, Carbimazole), may be used in both the initial and long-term treatment of hyperthyroidism. Methimazole, taken in just one daily dose, has an advantage over PTU, which must be given in three divided doses. Thus, methimazole, which yields more rapid improvement in serum concentrations of thyroxine and triiodothyronine, also enhances better patient compliance.

Short-term use of antithyroid drugs may be prescribed to reduce thyroid hormone levels over a period of a few weeks since radioactive iodine can initiate acute thyroiditis, causing the release of more stored thyroid hormone. Iodine solutions may also be given orally for up to 2 weeks to reduce thyroxine production prior to surgery but this approach is of short-term benefit. Antithyroid drug therapy is also used in vulnerable, elderly patients at risk for cardiac complications and for pregnant patients for whom other therapies present a special risk (Holcomb, 2002c; Waltman et al., 2004). It is essential that when such patients are hospitalized, careful attention be given to ensuring that they are receiving their antithyroid medications (Harris, 2007).

Antithyroid drugs are associated with a variety of side effects. Skin rashes may be managed with the administration of an antihistamine. Other minor side effects include arthralgias, nausea, and abnormal taste or smell. PTU and methimazole can cause more serious side effects such as liver inflammation, a severe deficiency of white blood cells, and polyarthritis, thus patients should be advised to stop the drug and notify their health care provider if they experience jaundice of the skin, fever, or sore throat. Propylthiouracil is the preferred antithyroid drug in pregnancy because methimazole is known to cause rare congenital anomalies (Cooper, 2005).

Antithyroid drugs may be effective over a period of several months to a few years and the hyperthyroidism may subside. However, patients with severe hyperthyroidism often require more aggressive therapy because antithyroid drugs may not manage symptoms adequately. Patients whose antithyroid drugs have been discontinued should have their thyroid function evaluated regularly since reoccurrence of hyperthyroidism may occur (Cooper, 2005). Medications used to treat hyperthyroidism are shown in the Pharmacology Summary (p. 1628).

Graves' disease also is routinely treated with radioactive iodine therapy (except in pregnancy as noted) and offers the advantage of rapid oblation of the thyroid gland. Radioactive iodine concentrates in thyroid tissues, thus it does not present a risk to the rest of the body. It has the additional advantage that it can be taken on an outpatient basis, thus the patient may avoid hospitalization. Outcomes, including partial or complete elimination of thyroid hormone production, depend on the dosage of the radioactive iodine and sensitivity of tissues. Because of the potential for permanent elimination of all thyroid hormone production over time, patients should be given both oral and written instructions on symptoms of hypothyroidism, and thyroid hormone levels should be taken at regular intervals until the patient has stabilized over a period of several months. In rare cases, treatment may need to be repeated.

Surgical intervention may be selected if antithyroid drugs are ineffective or if the patient is not a candidate for either drug therapy or radioactive iodine therapy for some reason. Surgery is warranted when there is suspicion of malignancy, compression of the trachea or esophagus due to thyroid enlargement, difficult-to-manage hyperthyroidism during pregnancy, or substernal thyroid. Lifetime replacement of thyroid hormone is needed when a major portion or all of the thyroid gland has been removed or oblated through surgery or radioactive iodine. Other drugs such as beta-blockers or calcium channel blockers also will be prescribed during episodes of hyperthyroidism in order to control cardiac arrhythmias such as tachycardia and/or atrial fibrillation.

A rare, but serious complication of hyperthyroidism is **thyroid storm**, a life-threatening condition in which the body decompensates in overwhelming thyrotoxicosis. The most vulnerable patients for thyrotoxicosis are the elderly and those patients who are prone to infection or postsurgical complications, are pregnant or postnatal, and those subject to antithyroid medication withdrawal (Harris, 2007). Thyrotoxicosis is characterized by sinus or supraventricular tachycardia, hyperpyrexia (with temperature above 40°C [104°F]), confusion, delirium, and coma. Immediate treatment is essential to prevent fatalities, which occur in 20% to 30% of cases (Waltman et al., 2004).

◼ Nursing Management

The goal in nursing management of the patient with hyperthyroidism is to support the treatment plan, which is directed at reducing or eliminating the output of thyroid hormone and addressing the symptoms attendant to the hypermetabolic state. Instruction on the action, benefits, and side effects of antithyroid drugs is a key role for the nurse. It is essential that patients understand that therapy should not be abruptly halted unless there are signs of serious side effects. Immediate consultation with the health care provider should occur if antithyroid drugs are discontinued. This is a vulnerable time when thyroid storm could occur, thus patients must be advised to observe for worsening signs of hyperthyroidism and report such signs to their health care provider. Should the patient be hospitalized, the nurse must note signs of significant change in a patient's condition and alert the health care provider so that immediate action can be taken to counteract the cascade of thyroid hormone to prevent fatalities, which occur in a significant percentage of those patients who develop thyroid storm.

PHARMACOLOGY Summary of Medications to Treat Thyroid Disorders

Medication	Action	Side Effects	Nursing Care
Propylthiouracil (PTU)	Controls hyperthyroidism by slowing thyroid hormone production. May be given over several months and may cause temporary or long-term remission of hyperthyroidism.	Allergic reaction with rash, hives, fever, joint pain. Decrease in white blood cells, sore throat, fever, joint aches, infection. Impaired liver function, jaundice, fever, loss of appetite, and abdominal pain.	Instruct patient to have regular follow-up of thyroid function since hyperthyroid activity may reoccur. Monitor white blood cell count. Monitor liver function. Report fever or sore throat to health care provider immediately.
Methimazole (Tapazole, Carbimazole)	Inhibits synthesis of thyroid hormone.	Caution in patients with liver disease, bone marrow disorders, and previous allergies to other antithyroid drugs. Congenital anomalies.	Instruct patient to take at same time daily at regular intervals. Monitor liver function. Avoid giving when the following drugs are being taken: anticancer drugs, iodine-containing drugs, lithium, sulfonamides, interferon.
Iodide or iodide products (Lugol's solution, sodium iodide, potassium iodide)	Inhibits synthesis and release of thyroid hormone and decreases size and vascularity of the thyroid. Effective for relatively short-term therapy (7–14 days).	Diarrhea, vomiting, nausea, abdominal pain. Skin rash, GI bleeding may signal adverse reaction.	Advise patient to drink all of solution, to use a straw to avoid discoloration of teeth, and not to withdraw drug abruptly. Discourage use of OTC drugs without health care provider consultation. Have patient report symptoms of iodism: abdominal symptoms.
Propranolol (Inderal)	Beta-adrenergic blocking agents. Decreases the effects and some symptoms of excess thyroid hormone.	Decreases heart rate and myocardial oxygen consumption. Lowers blood pressure.	Contraindicated in patients with asthma, sinus bradycardia, and heart block. Instruct patient not to discontinue abruptly. Discourage use of OTC drugs without health care provider consultation.
Radioactive iodine (sodium iodide [I-131], Iodotope)	Radioactive iodine destroys thyroid tissue with maximum benefit apparent in 3–6 months. Radioactive iodine concentrates in thyroid tissues and is excreted in a few days.	No serious complications reported so this has become the treatment of choice.	Instruct patient to: Have thyroid hormone levels monitored regularly. Take thyroid replacement hormone on an empty stomach. Take hormone replacement for life. Do not change brands of hormones without follow-up monitoring. Follow radiation precautions as directed.

Sources: Adapted from EndocrineWeb.com. (2007). Endocrine disorders & endocrine surgery. Retrieved August 29, 2008 from http://www.endocrineweb.com/; Jordan, S. (2005). Prescription drugs: Uses and effects. Thyroid disorders: Symptom control. Nursing Standard, 19(23), 56–58; Medline Plus. (2001). Cabergoline (systemic). Retrieved March 7, 2006, from http://www.nlm.nih.gov/medlineplus/druginfo/uspdi/203584.html; Physician's drug handbook (11th ed.). (2005). Philadelphia: Lippincott Williams & Wilkins; Sachse, D. (2001). Acromegaly. American Journal of Nursing, 101(11), 69, 71, 73–75.

CRITICAL ALERT

- *Thyroid storm occurs in severe hyperthyroidism and may be triggered by surgery, trauma, infection, postpartum status, or withdrawal of antithyroid drugs, resulting in severe tachycardia, heart failure, hyperthermia, and shock.*
- *Ensure adequate oxygen and ventilation.*
- *Control dysrhythmias if they occur.*
- *Administer IV fluids, monitoring glucose and electrolyte levels.*
- *Administer antithyroid drugs to inhibit the biosynthesis and block the release of thyroid hormone. (Iodide preparations should not be given for at least 1 hour after other antithyroid medications because they may be used to synthesize more T₄.)*

Patients choosing radioactive iodine therapy as their treatment option need both instruction and reassurance regarding the benefits of this therapy, as well as any information about radiation pre-cautions that must be taken during the first few days after therapy is initiated. Specific instructions will be provided to patients by the health care provider or the radiology staff but generally patients will be instructed to avoid close contact with other persons for a period of days. Patients with small children will need to arrange alternative care during this period. Patients should use a private toilet and be instructed to flush two times after each use. They should not be involved in handling food preparation for others and should launder towels and linens they use separately from others. Use of disposable eating utensils and plates is suggested (AACE, 2005c).

Patients will need to know the signs and symptoms of hypothyroidism because radioactive iodine treatment is likely to result in hypothyroidism over a period of several weeks to months. Written instructions regarding signs of hypothyroidism and the need for regular evaluation of thyroid function should be given to the patient at discharge. In addition, it is essential to stress the importance of continuous hormone replacement in the event of hypothyroidism since inadequate thyroid hormone replacement increases the risk of hyperlipidemia and increased heart disease (Franklin, Sheppard, & Maisonneuve, 2005).

If surgical intervention is planned in the case of hyperthyroidism, the nurse prepares the patient for surgery and provides immediate postoperative care. Surgical intervention may include a subtotal thyroidectomy, a partial resection, or removal of the thyroid gland. Postoperatively the nurse should pay particular atten-

tion to the patient's airway, because hemorrhage and swelling may compromise respiratory status. It is advisable to have emergency supplies such as a tracheostomy tray available at the bedside or close by on an emergency response cart. Accidental removal of the parathyroids is also a potential risk, thus intravenous calcium also should be available if needed. The critical response team should be alerted as early as possible should there be indications that the patient will need rapid intervention. The patient care plan for patients with hyperthyroidism is shown in the Nursing Process: Patient Care Plan for Hyperthyroidism. Chart 52–5 (p. 1631) shows life-threatening conditions related to thyroid disease.

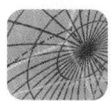

NURSING PROCESS: Patient Care Plan for Hyperthyroidism

Assessment of Cognition Level

Subjective Data:
What medications have you been taking?
Does your family have a history of any particular disease(s)?
Has your weight changed during the past year?
Is there unexplained change in body weight?
Do you feel anxious, nervous, or restless?
Have you noticed any insensitivity to changes in room temperature?
Are you "wound up" or "feeling like you are in overdrive"?
How much exercise are you getting?
Are you experiencing any muscle weakness?
Is there anything affecting your ability to be active?

Objective Data:
Skin warm and diaphoretic
Hair loss
Agitation, hand tremors
Enlarged thyroid, exophthalmos of the eyes
Hyperthermia Tachypnea, Tachycardia (heart rate >100 beats/min)
Hyperreflexia
Elevated serum T_3, T_4

Nursing Assessment and Diagnoses	Outcomes and Evaluation Parameters	Planning and Interventions with *Rationales*
Nursing Diagnosis: *Anxiety* and restlessness, fine hand tremors, and insomnia secondary to hypermetabolism	**Outcome:** Patient expresses relief from symptoms of excess thyroid hormone. **Evaluation Parameters:** Patient reports less anxiety and restful sleep through the night. Patient's tremors and blood levels of free T_3 and free T_4 decrease and stabilize. Patient is comfortable in an environment with a normal range in ambient temperature. Patient's vital signs are within normal range.	**Interventions and *Rationales:*** Decrease environmental stimuli and promote a restful environment. Eliminate chemical stimulants such as caffeine from diet. Administer antithyroid drugs as prescribed. *To eliminate stimulants that will exacerbate sleep deprivation and anxiety.*

Assessment of Understanding of Disorder

Subjective Data:
Have you lost or gained weight during the past year?
Did you take any specific steps to cause this change in your weight?
Describe your appetite for me.
How do you feel most of the time: anxious? calm?

Objective Data:
Patient underweight for height
Clothing too large for size/frame

Nursing Assessment and Diagnoses	Outcomes and Evaluation Parameters	Planning and Interventions with *Rationales*
Nursing Diagnosis: *Imbalanced Nutrition* secondary to anxiety, restlessness, and hypermetabolic state	**Outcomes:** Patient regains normal weight and reports resumption of appetite. Patient can describe symptoms of hypo- and hyperthyroidism. **Evaluation Parameters:** Patient's weight is maintained or returned to normal. Nutritional deficiencies eliminated. Patient reports appetite and intake are satisfactory. Patient able to describe symptoms of hypo- and hyperthyroidism.	**Interventions and *Rationales:*** Monitor weight daily. Offer patient a well-balanced diet with nutritional supplements and nutritional consultation as needed. Teach patient about effects of hypo- and hyperthyroidism on weight. *To ensure patient regains health and lost weight if desirable and to enable patient to report early signs of change in metabolic state that might indicate a need for further medical intervention.*

(continued)

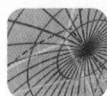

NURSING PROCESS: Patient Care Plan for Hyperthyroidism—*Continued*

Assessment of Ocular Characteristics and Function

Subjective Data:
Have you noticed any facial changes, swelling, redness, or protrusion of the eyes?

Objective Data:
Eyes appear dry and reddened
Eyes protrude (exophthalmos)
Patient unable to close eyelids completely
Visible sclera

Nursing Assessment and Diagnoses	Outcomes and Evaluation Parameters	Planning and Interventions with *Rationales*
Nursing Diagnosis: *Risk for Injury* to eyes secondary to exophthalmos and inability to close eyelids completely	**Outcome:** Eyes are moist and patient reports no eye pain or discomfort. ***Evaluation Parameter:*** No evidence of eye damage or corneal ulceration or abrasion.	**Interventions and *Rationales:*** Encourage patient to flush eyes with warm water at intervals while awake, to use artificial tears to keep eyes moist, and to cover eyes while sleeping and as needed if patient is unable to close eyes completely. *To keep eyes moist and to prevent corneal ulceration or abrasion.*

Assessment of Cardiac Function

Subjective Data:
Have you noticed any change in your pulse or heart rate?
Have you experienced any chest pain recently?
Have you observed any swelling in your feet?
What is your energy level?

Objective Data:
Tachycardia with heart rate >100 beats/min
Atrial fibrillation
Edema
Cardiac enlargement
Chest pain

Nursing Assessment and Diagnoses	Outcomes and Evaluation Parameters	Planning and Interventions with *Rationales*
Nursing Diagnosis: *Decreased Cardiac Output* related to hypermetabolic state	**Outcomes:** Cardiac function within normal limits. Patient free from symptoms of pulmonary edema and heart failure. ***Evaluation Parameters:*** Assessment reveals that heart rate has decreased and stroke volume has increased. No dyspnea present. No coughing and wheezing present. Tissues free from edema. Patient verbalizes feeling less tired and free of anxiety. Patient expresses having an appetite. Patient oriented to time, place, and person. No evidence of pink frothy sputum.	**Interventions and *Rationales:*** Evaluate vital signs frequently. Administer antithyroid and cardiac medications as prescribed. Maintain a restful, calm supportive environment. Assess toleration of physical activity and work with patient to gradually increase activity as tolerated. *To reduce risk of congestive heart failure in patients with a hypermetabolic state.*

CRITICAL ALERT

- *Following a thyroidectomy, it is essential that during the immediate postoperative period, the patient be observed closely for signs of hemorrhage or swelling in the operative site, as well as damage to the vocal cords or parathyroid glands. Check behind the neck for signs of pooling blood.*

- *The postop patient should be readily observable by the nurse and have a call bell in order to get immediate attention should symptoms of respiratory distress be noted. The location of the thyroid gland in proximity to the trachea and vocal cords also presents a threat to the airway, should swelling or hemorrhage cause obstruction. A tracheostomy set should be readily available in case of this emergency.*

- *In the event of accidental removal of part or all of the parathyroid glands, intravenous calcium should also be readily available.*

Discharge Priorities

Discharge priorities with thyroid disease include patient education about thyroid functioning, particularly symptoms of both hypothyroid disease and hyperthyroid disease since treatments for either condition may result in the opposite condition. Patients need to understand that they should receive regular follow-up laboratory work to assess thyroid function since treatments for hyperthyroidism, including antithyroid drugs, radioactive iodine, and surgery, may result in a significant decrease or cessation in thyroid hormone production over time. On the other hand, administration of levothyroxine in dosages that are too high may lead to symptoms of hyperthyroidism. Patients need careful instruction about the need for follow-up after treatment for thyroid disorders until there is evidence that hormone levels are normal and have stabilized. Certain vulnerable patients with hyperthyroidism or hypothyroidism should be instructed to avoid additional stress or infections until their disease is under control. Postsurgical patients should receive instruction about wound care and signs and symptoms of infection that should be reported immediately to the health care provider. Hyperthy-

CHART 52–5	Life-Threatening Complications of Thyroid Disorders	
	Hypothyroidism Myxedema Coma	**Hyperthyroidism Thyroid Crisis/Storm**
Life-Threatening Conditions	Myxedema coma occurs when a precipitating event such as trauma, infection, or sedation compromises the *hypothyroid* patient (usually older adults with long-standing primary thyroid disease).	Acute thyrotoxicosis/thyroid crisis/thyroid storm occurs when there is failure of the compensatory metabolic, thermoregulatory, and cardiovascular systems in the *hyperthyroid* patient.
Early Symptoms	Weight gain, extreme fatigue or lack of energy, bradycardia, lethargy, mental dullness, memory impairment, cold intolerance.	Significant unexplained weight loss, warm, moist skin, heat intolerance, cardiac palpitations and tachycardia. Tachypnea and dyspnea on exertion.
Signs or Symptoms of Serious Complications	Very low body temperature (32.8°–35°C [91°–95°F]) Skin very cool and dry Seizures, severe bradycardia, delayed deep tendon reflexes Nonpitting edema (particularly around face and eyes), enlarged tongue, decreased awareness and loss of consciousness Profound mood disturbance and psychosis may occur	Tachycardia (greater than 140 beats/min), atrial fibrillation, arrhythmias, increased stroke volume, symptoms of high output heart failure with pulmonary edema. Very high body temperature (up to 40°C [105°F]) restlessness, agitation, abdominal pain, nausea, vomiting, coma, emotional lability, exophthalmos, goiter, and coma.
Laboratory Values	Low TSH (if the pituitary is involved) and very high TSH (if the thyroid gland is the affected tissue) Low serum FT_4 Hyponatremia, hypoglycemia, hyperlipidemia Respiratory acidosis ECG: prolonged QT intervals Pleural and pericardial effusions Presence of antithyroid antibodies	Low level of TSH High serum FT_4 Elevated liver function tests Elevated alkaline phosphatase
Assessment	Vital signs, level of consciousness, lab work	Body temperature, blood glucose levels
Treatment	Hormone replacement therapy	Antithyroid drugs Surgery

Sources: Adapted from Greco, L. K. (2001). Hypothyroid emergencies. *Topics in Emergency Medicine, 23*(4), 44–50; Dahlen, R. (2002). Managing patients with acute thyrotoxicosis. *Critical Care Nurse, 22*(1), 62–69; Holcomb, S. (2003). Detecting thyroid disease, Part 1. *Nursing, 33*(8), 32cc1–32cc4; Waltman, P. A., Brewer, J. M., & Lobert, S. (2004). Thyroid storm during pregnancy: A medical emergency. *Critical Care Nursing, 24*(2), 74–79.

roidism in the elderly population is addressed in the Gerontological Considerations box.

Health Promotion

Optimal health in terms of endocrine function requires a healthy diet, including a reliable source of iodine for the production of thyroid hormone. Patients should be encouraged to plan a healthy diet that includes fish and foods supplemented with iodine such as iodized salt. Health promotion for patients with thyroid disorders requires careful attention to prescribed medications such as

hormone replacement therapy or antithyroid drugs. Symptoms of the hypo- or hypermetabolic state will reoccur if appropriate hormonal levels are not maintained. Patients may be advised to avoid additional stress when experiencing acute thyroid disease until such time as their condition stabilizes. For more on hyperthyroidism in certain populations, see the Cultural Considerations and Genetic Considerations boxes.

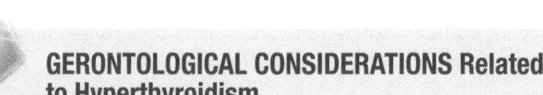

GERONTOLOGICAL CONSIDERATIONS Related to Hyperthyroidism

Hyperthyroidism is more common among the 30- to 50-year-old age group, whereas hypothyroidism is a more common problem in patients over age 50. Elderly patients are most vulnerable to serious complications from either hypothyroidism or hyperthyroidism. Diagnosis may be difficult until metabolic function is significantly altered due to the insidious nature of the disease. Infection, trauma, surgery, and stress may precipitate a serious crisis in elderly patients with hypo- or hypermetabolic diseases of the thyroid. Use of medications such as sedatives or opiates also may put these patients at great risk. The nurse must consider the potential for myxedema coma or thyroid crisis in elderly patients and those made more vulnerable due to coexisting illness or stress.

CULTURAL CONSIDERATIONS for Hyperthyroidism

Patients with thyroid disorders may have to take long-term drug therapy or lifelong hormone replacement therapy. Chronic illness is not well accepted in some cultures and poor understanding of the outcomes of rejecting medical therapy may lead to life-threatening consequences. The nurse will need to assess patient and family acceptance and understanding of the disease in order to tailor patient instruction and support appropriately.

GENETIC CONSIDERATIONS for Hyperthyroidism

Researchers know that there is a genetic predisposition to thyroid disease, although the exact genetic problem has not yet been identified. Parents affected by thyroid disease should be advised to share that information with their children so that they are alerted to potential health problems in the future.

Complementary and Alternative Approaches

Patients with thyroid disease may find complementary care such as meditation, massage therapy, and acupuncture to be beneficial in balancing the immune system and in improving one's sense of well-being. However, herbal therapies should be used with extreme caution at this time and only with consultation with the patient's primary care physician, given the potential for drug interactions. Overall, complementary and alternative therapy should not be seen as a replacement for traditional medical therapy in thyroid disease. For more about one type of complementary therapy, aromatherapy, see the Complementary and Alternative Therapies box.

◼ Collaborative Management

As noted when discussing collaborative management of patients with hypothyroidism, patients with hyperthyroidism also will need the support of several members of the health care team. The pharmacist has a role in instruction of hyperthyroid patients who may have to take antithyroid drugs and beta-blockers or calcium channel blockers if they have cardiac symptoms. A radiologist specializing in radiation therapy may administer radioactive io-

dine, which is the preferred treatment for hyperthyroidism. In some cases, the patient with hyperthyroidism may be referred to a surgeon for surgical removal of the thyroid gland if the patient is not a candidate for radioactive iodine therapy or if surgery is needed to remove a large goiter or malignant nodule. The nutritionist also can provide helpful consultation on diet to address the hypermetabolic needs of the patient's body while therapy corrects and stabilizes thyroid hormones.

◼ Disorders of the Parathyroid Gland

The parathyroid glands are four small, highly vascular glands located behind the thyroid gland (Figure 52–5 ◼). Anatomic variation in the number and location of parathyroid glands occurs with some frequency. Approximately the size of a grain of rice, the parathyroid glands regulate the blood calcium level within a very narrow range (8.5 to 10.5 mg/dL) to maintain the effective functioning of the body's muscles and nerves. Calcium-sensing receptors in the parathyroid glands are stimulated to release parathyroid hormone into the blood when serum calcium levels

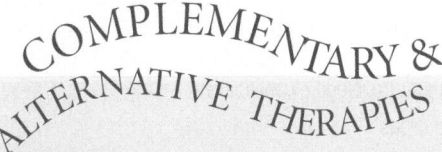

COMPLEMENTARY & ALTERNATIVE THERAPIES   Aromatherapy

Description:

Aromatherapy literally means using a scent (aroma) as healing therapy. The products used in aromatherapy are made from herbs and flowers that have been reduced to their aromatic essence. These aromatic essences are then combined with a "carrier oil" such as almond oil, and either applied to small areas of the skin or inhaled. These products are then used as an inhalant. Aromatherapy may be either self-administered, or administered by aromatherapy practitioners (aromatherapists) who are trained in the use of the inhalant, including its indication, quality and dose, and the length of time the patient should use the inhalant. Aromatherapy is often used to treat conditions such as dysmenorrhea, stress, and insomnia—all of which can be related to glandular and hormonal problems.

Research Support:

One randomized placebo-controlled trial explored the effect of aromatherapy with lavender, clary sage, and rose on dysmenorrhea symptoms. The trial involved 67 female college students whose primary dysmenorrhea symptoms were menstrual cramps. Participants rated their menstrual cramps as greater than 6 on a 10-point visual analogue scale. Participants had no systemic or reproductive diseases and were not taking contraceptive drugs. Three groups of participants were randomized: an experimental group who received aromatherapy, a placebo group, and a control group. The aromatherapy procedure involved applying two drops of lavender (*Lavandula officinalis*), one drop of clary sage (*Salvia sclarea*), and one drop of rose (*Rosa centifolia*) in 5 mL of almond oil to the abdomen. In the placebo group, the same treatment was used but only with almond oil. The control group received no treatment. Participants rated their menstrual cramp levels with a visual analogue scale. The aromatherapy group showed significantly improved menstrual cramps than the placebo and control groups at both post-test time points (first and second day of menstruation after treatment). Researchers concluded that the topical application of aromatherapy with lavender, clary sage, and rose is an effective

part of nursing care to women experiencing dysmenorrhea (Han, Hur, Buckle, Choi, & Lee, 2006).

Another study examined the use of aromatherapy with lavender to improve mild insomnia. This small, single-blind, randomized pilot study involved 10 participants (5 males and 5 females). Participants inhaled lavender using an Aromastream® electric diffuser over the course of the 4-week trial. Researchers measured outcomes using the Pittsburgh Sleep Quality Index. Results showed that aromatherapy with lavender created an improvement of insomnia. Women and younger volunteers with a milder insomnia experienced the largest improvement. Researchers concluded that, although a larger trial is needed to draw definitive conclusions, outcomes favor aromatherapy with lavender for mild insomnia (Lewith, Godfrey, & Prescott, 2005).

Cortisol is known as the "stress hormone." A third study examined the use of aromatherapy with lavender and rosemary on cortisol levels. Participants included 22 healthy volunteers who inhaled the lavender and rosemary aromas for 5 minutes. Then, saliva samples were collected from each participant and cortisol levels were tested. Results showed that lavender and rosemary decrease cortisol (Atsumi & Tonosaki, 2007).

References

Atsumi, T., & Tonosaki, K. (2007, February 28). Smelling lavender and rosemary increases free radical scavenging activity and decreases cortisol level in saliva. *Psychiatry Research, 150*(1), 89–96.

Han, S. H., Hur, M. H., Buckle, J., Choi, J., & Lee, M. S. (2006, July-August). Effect of aromatherapy on symptoms of dysmenorrhea in college students: A randomized placebo-controlled clinical trial. *Journal of Alternative and Complementary Medicine, 12*(6), 535–541.

Lewith, G. T., Godfrey, A. D., & Prescott, P. (2005, August). A single-blinded, randomized pilot study evaluating the aroma of Lavandula augustifolia as a treatment for mild insomnia. *Journal of Alternative and Complementary Medicine, 11*(4), 631–637.

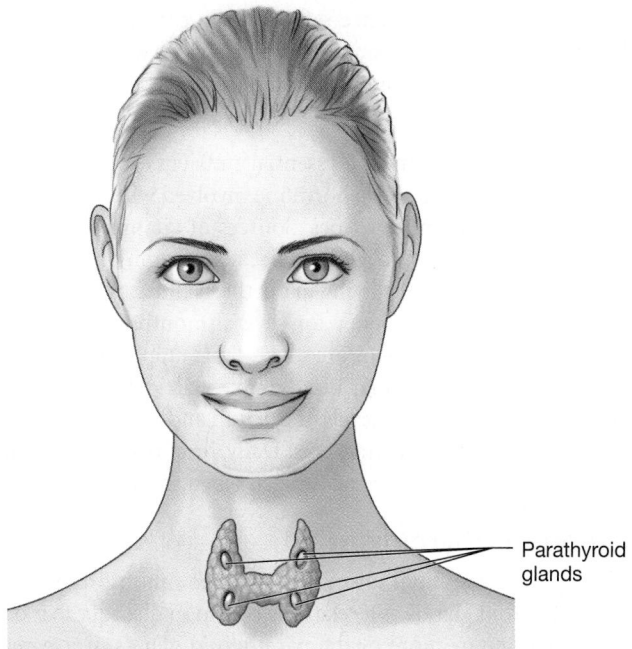

FIGURE 52–5 ■ The parathyroid glands.

drop below a normative level. Parathyroid hormone (PTH) is a small protein that acts directly on both the bone and kidneys where it stimulates release and reabsorption of calcium. It also acts indirectly on the intestines, causing them to reabsorb calcium. Thus PTH contributes to the finely tuned homeostasis of calcium in the body (Braunwald et al., 2001).

As is true with the other endocrine glands, disorders of the parathyroid gland include **hypoparathyroidism**, in which there is inadequate secretion of parathyroid hormone, and **hyperparathyroidism**, in which there is excessive secretion of PTH. Both conditions are rare, frequently missed for long periods because of vague symptoms, and may be identified through routine laboratory testing for other conditions. Genetics may play a role in parathyroid disorders, as discussed in the Genetic Considerations for Parathyroid Disorders box.

◼ Hypoparathyroidism

Hypoparathyroidism is a rare condition that occurs when the parathyroid glands do not make enough parathyroid hormone.

Parathyroid hormone helps regulate the levels of calcium and phosphorus in the blood.

Epidemiology and Etiology

When a deficient amount of PTH is produced, hypocalcemia (lower than normal levels of calcium in the blood) results, and there is too little phosphorus in the blood. This syndrome typically results from iatrogenic causes or is one of many rare diseases (Gonzalez-Campoy, 2007). Hypoparathyroidism may be either inherited or acquired (from injury to the glands or, more rarely, from surgery on the thyroid gland).

Pathophysiology

Patients with primary hypoparathyroidism have a low level of serum calcium with a high level of phosphorus in the absence of renal failure or tissue trauma. Pseudohypoparathyroidism (PHP), a hereditary syndrome that becomes apparent in adolescence, involves target tissues that are unresponsive to PTH, causing symptoms like those of hypoparathyroidism (Braunwald et al., 2001). Acquired hypoparathyroidism may occur due to complications from thyroid or neck surgery, but this is seen infrequently because surgical techniques have improved.

When other factors are at play in the cause of hypoparathyroidism, PTH may simply be ineffective (as with renal failure) or overwhelmed (due to severe hyperphosphatemia). Medications, severe trauma, sepsis, and acute pancreatitis are all factors that can cause acute, transient hypocalcemia but may be short term and not require treatment. Chronic hypocalcemia on the other hand, caused by hereditary hypoparathyroid disease, typically becomes symptomatic and does require intervention. See the Risk Factors for Hypoparathyroidism box.

Clinical Manifestations

Typically, hypoparathyroid patients complain about weakness; muscle cramps, particularly of wrists and feet; abnormal paresthesias with tingling, numbness, and burning of hands; excessive nervousness; loss of memory; and headaches. Nerve excitability, triggered by low blood calcium, causes continuous nerve impulses, which stimulate nerve contraction.

Other symptoms may include malformations of the teeth and fingernails, spasms of facial muscles (**Chvostek's sign**), and contraction of carpal muscles with mild compression of the nerves (**Trousseau's sign**)(Urbano, 2000). Chvostek's sign can be induced by tapping on the inferior margin of the zygoma, which

GENETIC CONSIDERATIONS for Parathyroid Disorders

Research is shedding new light on the genetic variations associated with parathyroid disease. At present, this information is useful primarily in diagnosis of new cases of the disease. Genetic counseling is advisable for families with hereditary parathyroid disease but patients may be reluctant to initiate this step if hereditary conditions are considered to be shameful or something to be hidden due to poor cultural acceptance. Families may become more open to genetic counseling with appropriate information about the benefits of this service.

RISK FACTORS for Hypoparathyroidism

Risk factors for hypoparathyroidism include family history and heredity, neck surgery, or the presence of other disease. The precise cause is unknown except in those cases where the parathyroid glands have been removed. The disease may occur singularly or concomitantly with other endocrine disorders. Hypoparathyroidism affects both genders equally, and generally is seen in children under age 16 and adults over age 40. Symptoms of hypocalcemia in older persons should be explored fully because these are more likely due to nutritional deficiencies, renal failure, intestinal disorders, or neck surgery than to primary hypoparathyroidism (Braunwald et al., 2001).

will cause facial spasms, and Trousseau's sign can be elicited by inflating the blood pressure cuff and maintaining the cuff pressure above systolic, which will produce carpal spasms if the serum calcium level is low. Transient cases of hypocalcemia occur due to trauma, burns, medications, and a variety of serious illnesses, and these must be differentiated from true hypoparathyroidism because transient symptoms require little intervention, whereas chronic hypoparathyroidism requires lifetime treatment.

Laboratory and Diagnostic Procedures

Diagnosis begins with a careful history including attention to nutritional history and calcium intake, a history of hereditary disease, the presence of other endocrine disorders, duration of illness, clinical signs and symptoms, renal failure, and an analysis of medications the patient is taking. Diagnostic tests, in addition to serum calcium and phosphatase, include PTH immunoassay and tests for vitamin D metabolites. In primary hypoparathyroidism, the level of PTH is low in spite of low levels of serum calcium.

Medical Management

Treatment of hypoparathyroidism is managed with supplementation of calcium, calcitriol (an active form of an artificial vitamin D), and high doses of oral vitamin D daily. Two or 3 grams of calcium are given daily to patients with primary hypoparathyroidism.

 Nursing Management

Nursing care for patients with hypoparathyroidism is directed at hormone replacement, symptom management, and support of patient self-care. Because primary disease lasts a lifetime, patients require thorough explanations about their condition and long-term treatment. Instruction on calcium and vitamin D supplements and their role in disease management should begin early after diagnosis. Patients also may find support from patient networks established by others who have the same disease, such as the Hypoparathyroid Association; thus a nursing referral to community groups is suggested. The Gerontological Considerations box gives more information about the effects of hypoparathyroidism on elderly patients.

Discharge Priorities

Discharge priorities for patients with parathyroid disease are focused on compliance with the prescribed medication regime and safety related to falls and fracture prevention. Follow-up home visits are warranted to assess how the patient has modified

> ### GERONTOLOGICAL CONSIDERATIONS Related to Hypoparathyroidism
>
> Older patients are particularly vulnerable to bone fractures, so the condition of hypoparathyroidism must be carefully managed as adults age. Careful attention to nutrition, with a high intake of calcium and vitamin D is important. Compliance with the medical regime, which includes high doses of oral calcium, calcitriol, and vitamin D, may be difficult but is essential in the elderly. The nurse will want to initiate a fall prevention program to decrease the risk of fractures. Patients should be encouraged to do a careful analysis of their home environment to remove throw rugs or other items that might put them at risk for a fall.

the environment to enhance safety and to determine whether the patient needs further support in compliance with prescribed calcium and vitamin D supplementation.

Health Promotion

Vitamin D and calcium are essential nutrients in the human diet. Vitamin D is actually a hormone involved with the metabolism of bone and other tissues. Sources of vitamin D include both diet and exposure to sunlight because vitamin D is synthesized by the skin. Patients living in northern climates are susceptible to vitamin D deficiency for several months out the year during which daylight hours are short. Thus supplementation of the diet with vitamin D may be advisable, particularly for those with lower than desirable levels of calcium and those considered to be vulnerable to bone fractures. Daily, brief periods of exposure to sunlight should be encouraged when this is feasible.

Hyperparathyroidism

Primary hyperparathyroidism, the most common problem of the parathyroid glands, is a relatively common disorder that occurs when one or more of the parathyroid glands oversecrete parathyroid hormone.

Epidemiology and Etiology

The incidence of hyperparathyroidism is 1 in 500 to 1,000, and it tends to occur in those over age 50 and in women more than men (Tangiera, 2004). Secondary hyperparathyroidism occurs when another medical condition causes the parathyroid glands to produce too much PTH in response to chronically low levels of circulating calcium. Kidney failure, malabsorption problems, and rickets, a disease caused by severe vitamin D deficiency, are the main causes of this type of hyperparathyroidism.

Physiology and Risk Factors

Hyperparathyroidism results in excessive PTH, leading to hypercalcemia, an excessive level of calcium, and hypophosphatemia, a low level of phosphatase, in the blood. Primary hyperparathyroidism is most commonly caused by a benign tumor, an adenoma, or hyperplasia in one or more of the parathyroid glands. Cancer is the cause of hyperparathyroidism in less than 1% of cases. When one parathyroid gland oversecretes PTH, the other glands will become dormant, responding to the high levels of calcium in the blood (Porth, 2007). Symptoms may be mild or severe depending on the size and impact of the tumor. Hyperparathyroidism may cause **osteitis fibrosa cystica**, a complication in which bone softens and becomes deformed or forms cysts. Secondary hyperparathyroidism may be due to rickets, vitamin D deficiency, or chronic renal failure (Gonzales-Campoy, 2007). Hypercalcemia also may develop secondary to malignancies in the body, in which parathyroid hormone-related peptide is released by tumor cells. This results in a syndrome that mimics hyperparathyroidism (Braunwald et al., 2001).

Primary hyperparathyroidism is rare but more common in middle-aged and older women. Evidence suggests that there is a genetic factor in its development. Neck radiation increases the incidence of the disease.

Clinical Manifestations

Patients with hyperparathyroidism may present with symptoms of bone tenderness, bone cysts, or polyuria due to excretion of high levels of calcium. In severe cases of the disease, the bones may lose significant calcium, seriously affecting bone density, and become brittle, with overt signs of osteopenia (mild loss of bone density) and osteoporosis (moderate to severe loss of bone density resulting in "brittle bones"). This may lead to susceptibility to bone fractures, a particular problem for older patients. High levels of calcium in the blood also may cause inflammation of the gastric lining and the pancreas, leading to a higher risk for ulcers and acute pancreatitis. Kidney stones, caused by high blood levels of calcium and the constant effort of the kidneys to excrete excess calcium, are another potential problem for patients with hyperparathyroidism. Parathyroid pathology often produces vague symptoms over a long period and may simply be discovered in laboratory blood work associated with routine physical examinations.

Laboratory and Diagnostic Procedures

A diagnosis of hyperparathyroidism is most accurately determined with tests of the parathyroid hormone, serum calcium, and alkaline phosphatase levels. In hyperparathyroidism, the blood parathyroid hormone level and the serum calcium level will be elevated and the alkaline phosphatase level will be abnormally low.

Medical Management

At one time invasive surgery under general anesthesia was required to remove a diseased parathyroid tumor. Locating the diseased parathyroid gland could be a problem because of its small size as well as the fact that the gland may have migrated to another location during fetal development. Such surgeries always carried the risk of hemorrhage, as well as damage to the vocal cords. Today, expert surgeons can remove the diseased parathyroid gland under local anesthesia by doing a minimally invasive, radioguided parathyroidectomy. Radioactive tracers facilitate faster and safer surgical intervention. Function of the hyperparathyroid glands can be assessed during surgery using radioactive ratios or PTH assays.

In cases of secondary hyperparathyroidism, the objective is to treat the underlying cause, although chronic kidney failure is the most common etiologic factor (Gonzalez-Campoy, 2007). Damaged kidneys cannot convert vitamin D to the active form, so an active form of vitamin D is used to reduce the production of PTH. After many years, vitamin D treatment can lose its effectiveness in some people, and excessively high levels of both calcium and phosphorus may occur. The drug cinacalcet (Sensipar) can reduce PTH levels, which lowers the chance of this occurring.

A new drug, paricalcitol (Zemplar), has recently been approved for administration orally as well as by injection during hemodialysis therapy. Dosage is determined by serum plasma parathyroid hormone levels, which are tested, along with serum calcium and serum phosphorus, at 2-week intervals for the first 3 months, then monthly for 3 months. Once it has been determined that the patient is stable, testing can be reduced to a quarterly schedule. Patients taking this drug should avoid medications that include large amounts of aluminum such as Maalox, Mylanta, Gaviscon, and Amphojel (Pavlovich-Danis, 2006).

■ Nursing Management

Nursing management for the patient with hyperparathyroidism is focused on patient teaching about the disease, preparation and follow-up for surgical intervention, and instruction about medications and the need for laboratory studies for regular

follow-up. Because minimally invasive surgery is the intervention of choice, the patient will be discharged quickly. Thus discharge planning and postoperative instructions should include instruction on dressing changes and follow-up medical visits with regular evaluation of serum calcium levels. If the glands have been completely removed, patient instruction prior to discharge should include information about foods that are good sources of calcium such as milk and other dairy products, tofu, broccoli, kale, mustard greens, oysters, salmon, and sardines.

If the patient and health care provider choose long-term follow-up for milder cases of the disease, the patient should drink lots of water, get plenty of exercise, and avoid diuretics, such as those in the thiazide classification. Immobilization and gastrointestinal illness with vomiting or diarrhea can cause calcium levels to rise. If these conditions develop, patients with hyperparathyroidism should seek medical attention.

Discharge Priorities

Discharge priorities include patient instruction on postsurgical care including observation of the operative site and dressing changes as indicated by the health care provider. The importance of follow-up with laboratory studies to monitor serum calcium levels should be stressed in concert with follow-up visits with the surgeon and endocrinologist.

Surgical removal of the affected gland provides relief of major symptoms and problems related to hypercalcemia. Close follow-up of patients is warranted to ensure that serum levels of calcium are maintained within recommended ranges.

Health Promotion

Following surgery, patients should feel a significant improvement in their health status. With return to normal or near-normal parathyroid functioning, patients should maintain a healthy diet with good sources of calcium and vitamin D essential for a healthy musculoskeletal system. As noted earlier, optimal synthesis of vitamin D in the body warrants at least brief exposure to sunlight daily. Outdoor activity, such as walking, would be beneficial to patients and accomplish both their need for vitamin D synthesis and cardiovascular benefits.

■ Collaborative Management of Parathyroid Disorders

Patients with parathyroid disorders can benefit from care provided by a wide array of health care providers, including the pharmacist, the nutritionist, the endocrinologist, and the genetic counselor, as well as the nurse. Parathyroid problems are rare and typically should be dealt with by an endocrinologist and highly trained surgeons who have experience working with the parathyroid glands. The pharmacist will provide essential information on drug therapies and vitamin and mineral supplementation, not only to the patient but to members of the health care team.

Complementary Care Related to Parathyroid Disorders

Complementary therapies may aid the patient's overall sense of well-being and should be encouraged for this reason. However, such therapies do not substitute for traditional Western medical therapies such as surgery for hyperparathyroidism or calcium and vitamin supplementation for hypoparathyroidism.

Symptom management is very important for patient comfort and well-being. Complementary therapies may be particularly useful in the management of parathyroid disease symptoms, such as fatigue, myalgia, and paresthesias. Acupuncture has been found to ease the symptoms of hyperthyroidism, and may be useful if used alongside traditional medical techniques. Aromatherapy also is considered helpful. Substances such as clove or myrtle are recommended for problems of the thyroid, and they can be made up into oils that are burned. The vapors can then be inhaled or used as bath oils or lotions. In addition, reducing stress and improving the body's immune response are desired outcomes because it may take several months for the body to respond to traditional therapy and for hormone levels to return to normal.

Disorders of the Hypothalamus and Pituitary Glands

Although the pituitary gland is often referred to as the "master" gland because it is responsible for cellular homeostasis and growth, the pituitary gland is so anatomically and physiologically connected with the hypothalamus that it is really the integrated functioning of these glands that affects most of the body's physiological processes. For this reason, this section provides a brief overview of the integrated functioning of these two glands, followed by common disorders that nurses may see in clinical practice.

Diseases of the hypothalamus and pituitary glands may become apparent early or late in life and include conditions caused by insufficient production and overproduction of hormones. As is true for many endocrine disorders, signs and symptoms of hypothalamic or pituitary disease may be subtle and insidious, leading to delayed or missed diagnosis.

Physiological Integration of the Hypothalamus and Pituitary Glands

Located in the middle of the base of the brain, the hypothalamus encapsulates the ventral portion of the third ventricle. The pituitary gland lies immediately beneath the hypothalamus, lying in a depression of the sphenoid bone of the skull called the sella turcica (Figure 52–6 ■). The pituitary is composed of two structures, the anterior pituitary, or adenohypophysis, and the posterior pituitary, called the neurohypophysis. Hormones produced by the hypothalamus control secretions of the anterior pituitary through a rich and direct vascular network that enables the pituitary to respond to miniscule amounts of concentrated hypothalamic hormone. The posterior pituitary, which is more of an extension of the hypothalamus, is composed of neurological cells and tissues (Dorton, 2000; Porth, 2007).

The hypothalamus produces a variety of releasing hormones that stimulate the production of other hormones by the pituitary gland. Secretion of the releasing hormones in the hypothalamus is affected by the perceived level of circulating pituitary hormones. When the level of a circulating pituitary hormone falls, the hypothalamus increases production of a releasing hormone, stimulating hormone production by the pituitary in what is called a

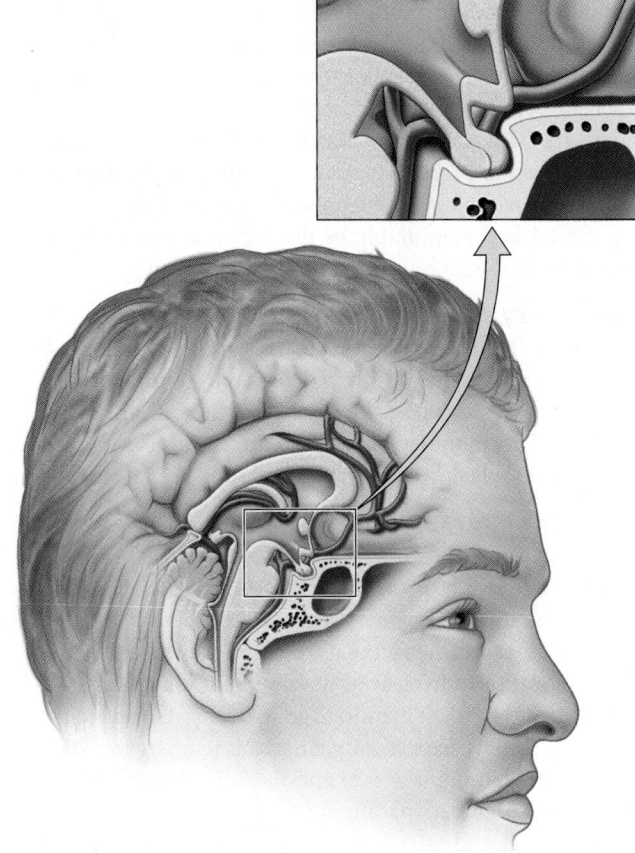

The pituitary secretes hormones that are essential to growth and reproduction

FIGURE 52–6 ■ The pituitary gland.

negative feedback system. Releasing hormones secreted by the hypothalamus include thyrotropin-releasing hormone (TRH), gonadotropin-releasing hormone (GnRH), growth hormone-releasing hormone (GHRH), corticotropin-releasing hormone (CRH), and somatostatin and dopamine. Should the hypothalamus be unable to produce one or more of the releasing hormones or should disease cause overproduction of a releasing hormone, pituitary gland functioning would be altered, leading to symptoms of pituitary dysfunction.

Hypothalamic Disorders

Disorders of the hypothalamus, as well as the pituitary, result from birth defects, genetic abnormalities, trauma (including hemorrhage), neoplasms, vascular disruptions, inflammatory disorders, infiltrative disease (such as tuberculosis), or radiation exposure.

Symptoms usually occur because of failure of the pituitary gland to secrete tropic hormones due to suppression of hypothalamic-releasing hormones. Thus, treatment is generally sought by patients because of metabolic problems related to an underproduction or overproduction of pituitary hormones. A key role for the health care provider is to determine whether the etiology of the endocrine problem is one related to the hypothalamus or the pituitary gland. In some cases, both glands may be affected by the disease process. Although there are a few, very rare genetic disorders and birth defects of the hypothalamus, most nurses will not see these in the clinical setting, thus the focus of this section is on common pituitary disorders that result from an excess or a deficit of the pituitary tropic hormones.

Hypometabolic Disorders of the Anterior Pituitary Gland: Hypopituitarism

Pituitary disorders result in inadequate secretion of one or more pituitary hormones. **Hypopituitarism** is a term used to describe the inadequate secretion of some of the hormones produced by the anterior pituitary gland, whereas **panhypopituitarism** is a term used to describe a disorder in which there is inadequate secretion of all of the anterior pituitary hormones. The pituitary hormones are shown in Chart 52–6.

Epidemiology and Etiology

The most common cause of pituitary disorders is pituitary tumors, which are described as secretory and nonsecretory. Secretory tumors cause problems with excessive secretion of one or more hormones. Nonsecretory, endocrine-inactive, or null tumors, as they are sometimes described, do not produce hormones but may create problems of hyposecretion of hormones if size and mass of the tumor impairs normal pituitary functioning (Pituitary Network Association [PNA], 2006b). A high percentage of hypopituitary disorders are due to pituitary adenomas. Acute pituitary insufficiency may also occur after severe postpartum hemorrhage in a syndrome called Sheehan's syndrome or infarction of a pituitary tumor (Kattah, 2006; Mayo Clinic, 2006). Congenital malformation, exposure to radiation or chemicals, and other unknown factors may also cause pituitary dysfunction.

In the United States, the prevalence of pituitary adenomas is high (10% to 20%); however, the actual presence of clinical disease is quite uncommon. Approximately 2 to 6 in 100,000 persons per year present with symptoms attributed to pituitary tumors (PNA, 2006a). There do not appear to be significant differences between genders in developing adenomas, with the exception of postpartum pituitary necrosis.

Risk Factors

Congenital malformations of the pituitary may develop during fetal growth and are the cause of some hypopituitary problems in infants and children. DNA mutations leading to tumors may also occur due to exposure to radiation or carcinogens, but idiopathic factors also cause pituitary tumors. Some purport that a few types of pituitary tumors appear to run in families, but the precise mechanism is not clear (Ferry & Shim, 2006).

Pathophysiology of the Anterior Pituitary

Each of the two pituitary structures has very distinct functions. The anterior pituitary, or adenohypophysis, produces growth hormone (GH), also known as somatotropin, TSH, adrenocorticotropic hormone (ACTH), prolactin, luteinizing hormone (LH), follicle-stimulating hormone (FSH), and melanocyte-stimulating hormone.

Normally growth hormone is produced episodically in short bursts, followed by periods of inactivity. Growth hormone production is more frequent and of higher volume in youth and gradually declines with age (Sachse, 2001). Protein, lipids, and carbohydrate metabolism are all influenced by growth hormone. TSH acts on target tissue in the thyroid gland, causing the release of thyroid hormones that influence metabolism. Similarly, ACTH acts on target tissue in the adrenal cortex, stimulating steroid biosynthesis and secretion. Prolactin stimulates milk production in the mammary gland and is thought to have some action on testicular function. FSH and LH act on tissue in the ovaries and testes, stimulating production of ovarian follicles in females, and the first steps of sperm production in males.

CHART 52–6	**Pituitary Hormones**			

Pituitary Source	Hormone	Location of Target Tissue	Role/Function
Posterior pituitary/ neurohypophysis	Oxytocin	Mammary glands Uterus Ovaries Testes	Milk ejection Uterine contractions
	Antidiuretic hormone (arginine, vasopressin)	Kidney	Water conservation
Anterior pituitary/ adenohypophysis	Adrenocorticotropic hormone (ACTH)	Adrenal cortex	Steroid biosynthesis and secretion
	Growth hormone (somatotropin)	Liver Adipose tissue	Growth promotion
	Thyroid-stimulating hormone (TSH)	Thyroid gland	Triggers thyroid hormone release
	Melanocyte-stimulating hormone	Melanocytes	Production of melanin in the fetus and infant
	Follicle-stimulating hormone (FSH)	Ovaries Testes	Development of ovarian follicles Spermatogenesis
	Prolactin	Mammary glands	Milk production
	Luteinizing hormone (LH)	Ovaries Testes	Reproduction Spermatogenesis

Melanocyte-stimulating hormone acts on melanocytes, enhancing melanin production (Dorton, 2000).

Clinical Manifestations

The clinical picture of hypopituitarism is dependent on disease causation and which hormone(s) is (are) being undersecreted and the degree to which secretion has been affected. For example, deficiency in growth hormone may occur because this seems to be one of the first hormones to be decreased in patients with pituitary tumors. GH continues to be important after childhood and is essential to an individual's optimal sense of physical and emotional well-being. Patients with depressed GH levels will complain of fatigue and lack of energy and vitality and will report the need to sleep during the day. Deficiency in growth hormone is evident in symptoms of central obesity, reduced muscle mass, and increased body fat. Other patient complaints may include reduced capacity for exercise, impaired psychological well-being, poor body image, and social isolation. Deficiency in GH is the most common of the selective hypopituitary problems with gonadotropin deficiency occurring less frequently (Porth, 2007).

When pituitary tumors are present, clinical signs are likely to include headache and visual disturbances, as well as symptoms indicative of hyposecretion of specific pituitary hormones. Nonsecretory tumors, which suppress pituitary function because of their size or mass, may lead to symptoms such as vomiting, decreased mental alertness, loss of libido, infertility, and amenorrhea (PNA, 2006b).

Panhypopituitarism, a complete hypopituitarism that causes metabolic dysfunction, sexual immaturity, and growth retardation, can be caused by failure of either the pituitary or the hypothalamus. In this syndrome, there is inadequate secretion of all of the anterior pituitary hormones. It can occur early in life or in adulthood and may become apparent only during extreme stress when the body is unable to respond effectively to maintain homeostasis (Anderson, 2002; Kattah, 2006).

Laboratory and Diagnostic Procedures

Magnetic resonance imaging (MRI) or computerized tomography (CT) scans are indicated to identify the size and location of a pituitary tumor. Laboratory blood tests also are used to evaluate levels of the pituitary hormones affected by the tumor such as GH, ACTH, FSH, LH, TSH, and antidiuretic hormone (ADH). Because blood levels of GH vary throughout the day, blood testing for GH must be done after a stimulus to GH production is initiated. Stimulation tests include the insulin tolerance test or an arginine stimulation test. Hypoglycemia normally increases GH secretion. Blood levels of GH are tested in 30-minute intervals following administration of insulin. Failure to secrete growth hormone in response to hypoglycemia is an indicator of impaired GH secretion. Arginine stimulation may be used as a diagnostic tool for patients for whom hypoglycemia might be a risk. Failure to produce growth hormone following administration of arginine is indicative of pituitary disease. The effects of some of these tests on the elderly is discussed in the Gerontological Considerations box.

Medical Management

Hormone replacement may be needed for any of the pituitary hormones that are being undersecreted due to tumor growth, trauma, or congenital deformity. Cortisol replacement is partic-

GERONTOLOGICAL CONSIDERATIONS Related to Tests for Hypopituitarism

Older patients and patients with a history of cardiac disease may not endure the insulin tolerance test well, so other diagnostic measures such as the arginine stimulation test should be considered. Given the complexity of endocrine clinical problems, consultation with an endocrine specialist is advised.

ularly important in those cases where this hormone is suppressed because it regulates blood glucose and blood pressure. Treatment of hypopituitary function involving growth hormone insufficiency is by administration of synthetic GH by injection. Patients are taught how to self-administer growth hormone. Initial dosage is based on body weight and size, with long-term dosage determined by laboratory studies and patient response. Surgery for removal of a pituitary tumor may be warranted and this treatment is discussed under the treatment section for hyperpituitarism later in this chapter.

◾ Nursing Management

Instruction in self-care, particularly administration of hormone replacement medications, may require that the nurse teach the patient how to give injections safely because some hormones are available only in injectable form. Low hormone production may make the patient more vulnerable to stress, both physical and psychological, so patients should be advised to report signs and symptoms of impending illness promptly to their health care provider.

Discharge Priorities

Understanding of the disease process and related symptoms is important for the patient. Change in symptoms may occur only over a period of several months after treatment is initiated, so patients must continue to update their health care provider on current symptoms and state of well-being. Synthetic growth hormone has been available for treatment of adult growth hormone deficiency for approximately two decades but it is expensive. Patients on limited incomes may need assistance in applying to pharmaceutical firms for free or low-cost supplies of the drug.

Health Promotion

Head trauma is a potential cause of pituitary gland dysfunction. Helmets should be worn by individuals who participate in sports that have the risk of head injury, including bicycling, motorcycling, or skateboarding. Nurses are important role models and teachers with regard to public safety including the use of helmets during high-risk activities.

Hypermetabolic Disorders of the Anterior Pituitary Gland: Prolactinomas and Acromegaly

Prolactinoma is a condition in which a noncancerous tumor (adenoma) of the pituitary gland in the brain overproduces the hormone prolactin. The major effect of increased prolactin is a decrease in normal levels of sex hormones—estrogen in women and testosterone in men. Although prolactinoma isn't life-threatening, it can cause visual impairment, infertility and other effects. Prolactinoma is one of several types of tumors that can develop in the pituitary gland.

Acromegaly is a hormonal disorder that results from too much growth hormone (GH) in the body. In acromegaly, the pituitary produces excessive amounts of GH. Usually the excess GH comes from benign, or noncancerous, tumors on the pituitary. These benign tumors are called adenomas.

Epidemiology and Etiology

Pituitary tumors are the most common cause of hyperpituitary disorders. According to some authorities, the most common type of pituitary adenoma is a prolactin-secreting prolactinoma, leading to problems with fertility and lactation (Braunwald et al., 2001). A second type of hyperpituitary disorder is one that involves the overproduction of growth hormone, resulting in one of two syndromes depending on the age at which the disorder occurs.

Prolactinomas account for 30% to 50% of pituitary tumors. In women, symptoms include absence of menstrual periods, infertility, and **galactorrhea**, the spontaneous flow of milk in a breast unassociated with childbirth or nursing. In men, symptoms include loss of libido, infertility, or signs of central nervous system compression. Goals of treatment are reduction in hyperprolactinemia, reduction in tumor size, resumption of menses and fertility, and improvement of galactorrhea (Braunwald et al., 2001).

Diagnosis of this specific type of pituitary tumor is done by measuring the prolactin level, and in men, measuring the testosterone level (Medline Plus, 2004). Prolactinomas are treated like other types of pituitary tumors as described later in this chapter.

Pituitary tumors also may produce an excess of growth hormone. The overproduction of GH results in two conditions that present with different physical manifestations depending on the timing of the disorder in one's physical development. **Gigantism** occurs in children when overproduction of pituitary hormone occurs before the closure of epiphysial plates in the long bones. Such children may grow as tall as 8 feet in height. On the other hand, **acromegaly** is a disorder that occurs when there is overproduction of pituitary hormone in adults whose epiphysial plates have closed.

Pathophysiology of Hyperpituitary Disorders

Tumors that produce growth hormone account for up to 15% of pituitary adenomas (Ferry & Shim, 2006). Normally, the hypothalamus produces GHRH, which stimulates the anterior pituitary to produce GH. GH stimulates the liver to produce insulin-like growth factor-1 (IGF-1), a hormone that causes bones and other tissues to grow and signals the pituitary to reduce production of GH. Continued production of GH by the pituitary gland leads to unwanted growth of bones and organs, as well as elevation of blood glucose levels, resulting in glucose intolerance (Sachse, 2001).

Hyperpituitarism evolves as two different syndromes depending on the age at which gland dysfunction occurs. As mentioned above, gigantism is the syndrome in which oversecretion of growth hormone begins early in life before there is closure of

the epiphysial plates. Without treatment, growth in height and weight continue throughout adulthood, leading to extremely abnormal height. Over time the physiological demands on the body exceed its capacity to maintain cardiovascular and musculoskeletal homeostasis and the individual typically dies a premature death of cardiovascular failure. Acromegaly, which occurs when there is an excess of growth hormone in adulthood, results in gradual but marked changes in facial characteristics, hands, feet, and ears (Figure 52–7■, p. 1640) (Chan, Ziebert, Maas, & Chan, 2005). The most common cause of gigantism and acromegaly is a pituitary adenoma; only in rare instances are these disorders caused by a nonpituitary tumor.

Risk Factors

About 3% of pituitary adenomas run in families and are due to inherited DNA mutations. Acquired mutations can occur due to exposure to radiation or cancer causing chemical agents. Other genetic mutations occur for unknown reasons (American Cancer Society, 2006).

Clinical Manifestations

As is true in pituitary disorders leading to hypopituitarism, the clinical picture in hyperpituitarism depends on the size of the adenoma and the type of hormone secretion, if any, that it produces. As noted previously, the most common pituitary adenoma, accounting for about 30% to 50% of tumors, is a prolactin-secreting prolactinoma. The primary symptom of this tumor is lactation. Growth hormone-secreting tumors, which cause acromegaly, also are seen with some frequency (Braunwald et al., 2001; Pituitary Disorders Education and Support, 2006a). Acromegaly causes excessive bone and soft tissue growth, leading to subtle and gradual coarsening of facial features over a period of years. The periorbital ridge, lips, and nose enlarge, and skin becomes coarse and oily (see Figure 52–7 ■, p. 1640). Patients may experience weakness and fatigue, headaches, loss of peripheral vision, and intermittent sweating as well as separation of teeth and a change in facial appearance (Ferry & Shim, 2006; Song & Weil, 2005). Complaints of osteoarthritis and myalgia are common. The physical changes caused by acromegaly are insidious because they occur gradually and may be attributed to a number of physical findings. Patients may have hyperpituitarism for years before a diagnosis is made.

Laboratory and Diagnostic Procedures

Diagnosis of hyperpituitary disease is based on the clinical picture, patient history, and laboratory results. Tests may be done to evaluate each of the target hormones produced by the pituitary gland in order to determine the extent of pituitary impairment. If a prolactin adenoma is suspected, prolactin hormone levels are tested, and in men, testosterone levels are evaluated because production of testosterone is inhibited in the presence of high levels of prolactin. With suspected growth hormone-secreting tumors, the plasma GH level is measured by radioimmunoassay.

Stimulation tests, such as an insulin tolerance test (ITT), arginine stimulation test, and GHRH test, may be given to assess the pituitary response and the ability to produce hormones. Elevation in GH level following a glucose suppression test will lead to concerns about the possibility of acromegaly. In addition, the IGF-1 level, which is a more stable measure, also is evaluated. Elevated IGF-1 levels are almost always indicative of acromegaly

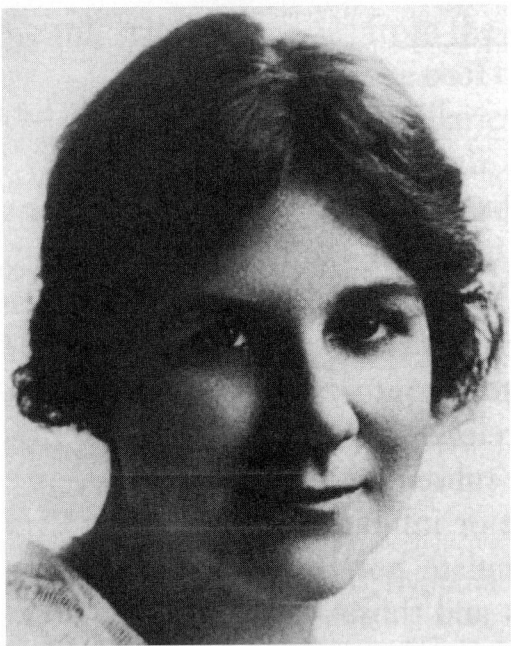

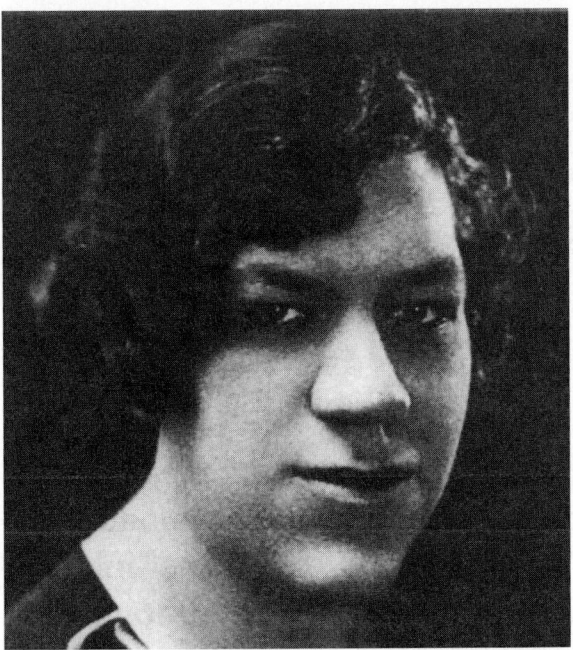

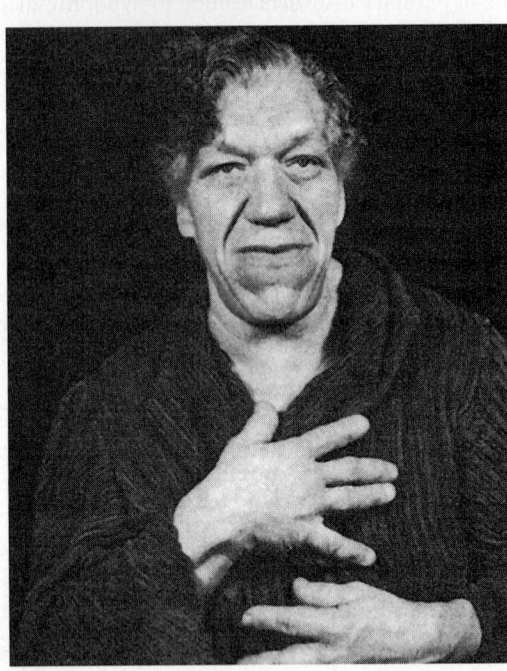

FIGURE 52–7 ■ Patient with development stages of acromegaly.
Source: (a) and (b) © Dr. William H. Daughaday, University of California/Irvine. American Journal of Medicine (20) 1956. With permission of Excerpta Medica Inc.; (c): Reproduced by permission from American Journal of Medicine 20:133, 1956 Copyright © 1956 by Elsevier Science Ltd.

(Sachse, 2001). Examination of the field of vision is another examination that can be done because patients with pituitary tumors sometimes experience a loss of peripheral vision due to the tumor pressing on nerves leading into the eye (Pituitary Disorders Education & Support, 2006a).

Medical Management

Primary treatment of acromegaly and many other hyperpituitary disorders is surgical intervention to remove the adenoma. This surgery is most successful with patients who have a small, localized tumor. Radiation therapy and pharmacologic intervention following surgery will depend on patient response to the initial surgery. Tumor resection frequently reduces growth hormone production significantly and patients subsequently will experience a reduction in serum GH and alleviation of symptoms. Unfortunately, facial characteristics will remain largely unchanged.

Transsphenoidal microsurgery, with the surgical approach through the nose, along the front of the nasal septum, or under the lip and through the upper gum, into the sphenoid sinus cavity, is the most common treatment for removal of pituitary tumors. This surgical procedure usually eliminates the need for a craniotomy and permits much shorter hospital stays.

Radiation may be selected as a treatment modality if the patient is not a good candidate for surgery. A number of targeted radiosurgery approaches are available, including gamma knife and proton beam therapies. In these approaches, an MRI scan is used to create an image of the brain and the exact location of the tumor. The MRI is used to map locations for application of high-dose radiation beams, which are used to destroy tumor tissue while avoiding surrounding healthy tissue. This approach may take several months for resolution of symptoms and for this reason, radiation therapy is typically used as an adjunct to other treatments.

Radiation therapy may be the primary method of treatment for patients who are poor surgical risks. With this method, however, reduction in growth hormone levels takes much longer, often a period of years. Radiation therapy also is used when the hormone level remains high if surgical intervention is unable to remove all of the adenoma. Medications, including somatostatin analogues or dopamine agonists, which lower serum growth hormone, may also be used in treatment. Medications used to treat hyperpituitary disorders are shown in the Pharmacology Summary.

Octreotide is a somatostatin analogue medication that has proven effective in the treatment of acromegaly. The drug usually causes a marked reduction in symptoms of headache, sweating, and joint pains. Administered by intramuscular or subcutaneous injection, this medication is typically used as adjunctive therapy for patients who have residual tumor following surgery (Katznelson, 2006).

PHARMACOLOGY Summary of Medications to Treat Pituitary Disorders

Medication	Action	Side Effects	Nursing Care
Hyperpituitary Disorders			
Bromocriptine (oral tablet or capsules) Initiate therapy with small doses moving to 20 mg daily.	A dopamine agonist. Decreases sweating and soft tissue edema. Reduces high prolactin levels and restores ovulation and ovarian function in women with amenorrhea.	GI upset: nausea and vomiting, postural hypotension, depression, and nightmares. May cause intolerance to alcohol. Contraindicated in patients with uncontrolled hypertension or toxemia of pregnancy and those with hypersensitivity to ergot derivatives.	Explain that it may take several weeks for menses to resume. Take with meals to avoid GI distress. Rise slowly from supine position to avoid fainting, dizziness. Avoid use of alcohol. Avoid pregnancy (use mechanical barrier methods, not birth control pills).
Pergolide (oral tablet) 0.05 mg given orally daily for 2 days increasing gradually as directed to maximum dose of 5 mg/day. Doses should be divided into 3 doses daily.	Dopamine agonist. Inhibits prolactin secretion and decreases growth hormone levels.	GI distress/pain, constipation, light-headedness, sedation, hypotension, dry mouth.	Increases risk of atrial premature contraction and sinus tachycardia in patients with history of arrhythmia. Administer first dose at night with patient lying down to decrease dizziness. Reduced oral salivation requires good oral hygiene.
Cabergoline (oral tablet) 0.25 mg two times per week. May be increased every 4 weeks up to 1 mg two times per week.	Dopamine agonist. Antihyperprolactinemic. Stops pituitary secretions of prolactin hormone. Will resolve menstrual problems. Reduces lactation.	Abdominal pain, vertigo, changes in vision, difficulty concentrating, dizziness, swelling of hands or feet.	Do not drive until you know how this drug affects you. Get up slowly from supine position to avoid fainting. Avoid pregnancy (see above).
Octreotide 50–500 mg tid (available in forms that can be administered subcutaneously or by IM injection)	Somatostatin analogue. Relieves symptoms such as headache, sweating, and joint pain.	Gallstones, nausea, abdominal pain, diarrhea.	Tell patients to report GI symptoms because drug may cause gallstones.

Sources: Adapted from EndocrineWeb.com. (2007). Endocrine disorders & endocrine surgery. Retrieved August 29, 2008 from http://www.endocrineweb.com/; Jordan, S. (2005). Prescription drugs: Uses and effects. Thyroid disorders: Symptom control. *Nursing Standard, 19*(23), 56–58; Medline Plus. (2001). *Cabergoline (systemic).* Retrieved March 7, 2006, from http://www.nlm.nih.gov/medlineplus/druginfo/uspdi/203584.html; *Physician's drug handbook* (11th ed.). (2005). Philadelphia: Lippincott Williams & Wilkins; Sachse, D. (2001). Acromegaly. *American Journal of Nursing, 101*(11), 69, 71, 73–75.

Dopamine agonists are a second class of drugs used to treat hyperpituitary disorders. They inhibit prolactin secretion and also cause a decrease in growth hormone. Dopamine agonists such as bromocriptine, pergolide, and cabergoline have varying mechanisms of action but can be useful in the management of symptoms caused by an excess of prolactin and GH in hyperpituitarism. Common side effects include drowsiness, headache, nausea, vertigo, and hypotension, particularly when therapy is initiated and if the client is supine. Gradual dosage titration is necessary with dopamine agonists to minimize side effects. Taking the medication with meals or milk helps patients avoid nausea. Patients should be advised to use care in driving until they know how the drug will affect them. These medications should not be given with estrogen preparations or birth control pills, and women of childbearing age should be advised to use mechanical barrier forms of birth control while taking the drug to avoid pregnancy. Patients taking dopamine agonists should be advised to consult with a pharmacist to ensure that other drugs they are taking do not counteract their action or cause untoward drug interactions (Medline Plus, 2005).

■ Nursing Management

Nursing assessment of patients with hyperpituitarism is critical to providing effective patient care. This condition often is associated with visual field defects and bony erosion. Thus, the nurse is assessing for mass effects of hormone excess including: headache, double vision, excessive sweating, hoarseness, milk secretion from the breast, sleep apnea, carpal tunnel syndrome, joint pain, limitation of motion, muscle weakness, and numbness or tingling of the skin (Porth, 2007).

Nursing Diagnosis

A diagnosis of hyperpituitarism may be made when evidence of hormonal imbalance surfaces during a time of stress such as hospitalization for other problems. The diagnosis of hyperpituitarism may be missed for years unless patients have severe headaches or marked physical changes in a short period of time. Nurses can offer strong support during the diagnostic period with explanation of and preparation for diagnostic tests. A primary nursing goal is to prepare patients for surgery and postoperative recovery for adenoma tumor resection. The fact that minimally invasive surgery is available may not lessen the patient's and family's fears about surgery.

Interventions and Rationales

Preoperative nursing care includes installation of antibiotic nose drops, discussion about mouth breathing, oral hygiene, early ambulation and activity, pain management, and hormone replacement therapy. A skilled neurosurgeon can remove the tumor with transsphenoidal microsurgery if the tumor is small and localized. Padding may be required for a brief period after surgery but sometimes this is not necessary. Postoperative complications include increased intracranial pressure due to cerebrospinal fluid (CSF) leak, meningitis, transient diabetes insipidus, and hypopituitarism with hormone replacement for life (Pituitary Network Association, 2006c).

Postoperative nursing care includes neurological assessment due to the risk of increased intracranial pressure, observations of temperature, pupils, vital signs, and fluid balance. The head of the patient's bed should always be elevated at a 30-degree angle to reduce headaches and pressure on the entry point in the sella turcica. The patient should be cautioned to avoid coughing, sneezing, straining at stool, or other activities that would initiate the Valsalva maneuver to prevent leakage of cerebrospinal fluid. Leaking of CSF, which is signaled by complaints of persistent generalized or supraorbital headache, increases the risk of meningitis and warrants prophylactic antibiotics, bed rest, and continued elevation of the head of the patient's bed. Nasal drainage, if present, should be tested by the lab for glucose, which indicates leakage of CSF.

Caution should be taken with provision of oral hygiene to avoid trauma to the surgical site. Use of a toothbrush should be discontinued for up to 10 days, and oral hygiene should be provided by the nurse at 4-hour intervals. Seizure precautions should be taken and mild analgesia provided for pain. Because transient diabetes insipidus may occur following surgery due to loss of ADH stored in the pituitary, urine output and serum and urine osmolality should be monitored (Laws, Vance, & Thapar, 2000). Patients generally will have a short hospital stay and should be advised to avoid exercise and unusual activities at home until cleared to do otherwise by the health care provider.

Somatostatin analogues and dopamine agonists are used in pharmacologic therapy to inhibit secretion of pituitary hormones. Patients who are prescribed medications to counteract hormone overload may need repeated explanations of the pharmacologic benefit of these preparations and instructions on potential side effects. Consultation with the pharmacist on dosage, timing, and route of administration, as well as common side effects and contraindications, is advised given that nurses typically are not administering these medications with great frequency in their practice.

Discharge Priorities

Changes in physical appearance and energy levels may have a long-term effect on patient relationships. Patients often report that quality of life is significantly altered by this disorder, even after treatment (Baird, Sullivan, Zafar, & Rock, 2003). Contin-

ued follow-up of patients is required after initial treatment to ensure that hormone levels return to normal and that efforts are made to address patient symptoms and complaints. Nurses may be able to offer vital emotional support for patients during diagnosis, treatment, and follow-up.

Gerontological Considerations

Older patients may be overwhelmed when trying to understand the nature of this rare disease. If the pituitary adenoma is large and cannot be entirely removed, or if the patient is not a candidate for surgery, medications may have to be used to inhibit hormone production. Older patients may need simple but clear instructions on medications and potential side effects. Resolution of symptoms may take some time leading to discouragement, and lack of change in physical appearance may be particularly disheartening and lead to depression. Patients may experience improvement in their field of vision with tumor excision, but failure to remove the tumor, even if other symptoms are controlled, may lead to diminished quality of life for patients who are unable to drive.

Health Promotion

Case studies indicate that patients with pituitary adenoma can have an improved quality of life with appropriate follow-up and case management (Carr, 2001). Patients should be instructed on signs of hypopituitarism, including severe chronic fatigue, central obesity, and reduced muscle mass, because they may experience this syndrome following treatment of the pituitary adenoma. Management of related endocrine disorders also is important. Referrals to support groups and organizations devoted to the needs of patients with pituitary problems may be another health promotion strategy for nursing consideration.

Disorders of the Posterior Pituitary Gland

The posterior pituitary, composed largely of axons of hypothalamic neurons, produces both antidiuretic hormone and oxytocin. Oxytocin stimulates uterine smooth muscle contraction at birth and also stimulates milk ejection and let-down in lactating mothers. Research also has indicated that oxytocin plays some role in the birth process and maternal behavior, but further research is needed on this action. The clinical disorders that the nurse is most likely to see in practice are those that involve an insufficient production of or insensitivity to ADH or an excess of ADH.

Hypometabolic Disorders of the Posterior Pituitary

Diabetes insipidus (DI) is a hypometabolic condition characterized by excretion of large amounts of severely diluted urine, which cannot be reduced when fluid intake is reduced. It signifies inability of the kidney to concentrate urine. There are four types of DI and treatment of the syndrome depends on the particular cause of the disease.

Epidemiology and Etiology

Diabetes insipidus is caused by a deficiency of antidiuretic hormone, also known as vasopressin, due to the destruction of the back or "posterior" part of the pituitary gland where vasopressin is normally released from, or by an insensitivity of the kidneys to that hormone. It can also be induced iatrogenically by various drugs.

This hypometabolic syndrome is not common, with a prevalence of 1 case per 25,000 people (Cooperman, 2008). The etiology of disorders related to the secretion of ADH may be linked to the pituitary gland itself or they may be caused by several other physiological disorders. There are no significant sex differences in DI. Male and female prevalences are equal. Mortality is rare in adults as long as water is available. Severe dehydration, hypernatremia, fever, cardiovascular collapse, and death can ensue in children, elderly people, or in those with complicating illnesses.

Pathophysiology and Risk Factors

Antidiuretic hormone is essential in maintaining fluid and electrolyte balance in the human body. ADH controls the concentration of urine through action on the collection tubules within the kidneys. Diabetes insipidus involves a permanent or transient deficiency in the synthesis or release of ADH or a decreased renal responsiveness to ADH. The four types of diabetes insipidus are discussed next.

Neurogenic Diabetes Insipidus

Neurogenic diabetes insipidus (also known as central, primary, or pituitary DI) is caused by a deficiency of ADH. Risk factors can include damage to the posterior pituitary by tumors, infection, head trauma, infiltrations, and genetic abnormalities. About half of the cases appear to be genetic in origin and half are idiopathic, that is, they occur for unknown reasons. Symptoms of this disorder may be apparent in early childhood or may suddenly appear later in life. Patients typically report constant thirst, along with polyuria, and the patient's urine is almost clear in color. Symptoms can be managed with synthetic hormone replacement using desmopressin (DDAVP), usually administered intranasally or orally. Once treatment is initiated, patients should be monitored for fluid overload and hypernatremia (Holcomb, 2002a).

Nephrogenic Diabetes Insipidus

Nephrogenic diabetes insipidus (NDI) is caused by resistance of the kidneys to ADH, rendering the ADH ineffective. This syndrome may be chronic if caused by a genetic defect or it may be acquired and transient if it occurs as a side effect of drugs such as lithium, colchicine, methoxyflurane, amphotericin B, gentamicin, and more. Eliminating selected medications may resolve acquired NDI. Inherited NDI usually appears early with symptoms of polyuria and polydipsia, but there are genetic patterns that differ, leading to mild or more serious symptoms. Diagnosis may be more difficult in such cases.

Genetically induced NDI is treated by prevention of dehydration through the provision of adequate fluid intake, dietary sodium restriction, and the use of a thiazide diuretic alone or in combination with a prostaglandin inhibitor to reduce urine output. Paradoxically, the thiazides tend to have an antidiuretic effect in DI (Loffing, 2004). Patients may require potassium supplementation to avoid depletion of potassium (Nephrogenic Diabetes Insipidus Foundation, 2005a).

Gestational Diabetes Insipidus

Gestational diabetes insipidus is caused by a deficiency of ADH that occurs only during pregnancy if the pituitary is damaged or if the placenta destroys the hormone too quickly. Treatment involves short-term hormone replacement therapy because the disease disappears 4 to 6 weeks after delivery. It may reoccur with future pregnancies.

Dipsogenic Diabetes Insipidus

Dipsogenic diabetes insipidus is a syndrome that causes primary polydipsia, abnormal thirst, and extreme intake of water and other fluids. It is caused by disease or damage to the part of the brain that regulates thirst. This is the one form of DI in which patients are not dehydrated. Patients ingest a large volume of water leading to water intoxication, decreased plasma osmolality, and a decrease in sodium concentration.

Symptoms include headache, loss of appetite, and nausea. Rarely, this disorder may be caused by **psychogenic polydipsia** in which excessive thirst occurs for psychogenic reasons. Hormone replacement may help manage symptoms but does not address the underlying cause of the disease (Nephrogenic Diabetes Insipidus Foundation, 2005a).

Tumors, trauma, surgery, infection, pregnancy, congenital defects, and genetic disorders are all factors that contribute to the development of diabetes insipidus but there is a significant percentage of cases with idiopathic etiology.

Clinical Manifestations

Each of the different forms of diabetes insipidus is characterized by polyuria (excretion of large amounts of dilute urine) and polydipsia (excessive thirst). Patients with DI present with dry mucous membranes, poor skin turgor, and other signs of dehydration. In untreated cases, symptoms of tachycardia and hypotension signal impending hypovolemic shock, which can be life threatening (Innis, 2002b).

Laboratory and Diagnostic Procedures

Diagnostic tests will help to determine the origin of diabetes insipidus and direct the appropriate therapy since treatment varies depending on the etiology. Blood and urine levels of ADH will be taken before and during a water deprivation or dehydration test, which will determine whether DI is neurogenic or nephrogenic in nature. Serum electrolytes and the osmolality of serum and urine will be determined. Serum will reveal an elevated osmolality and high sodium level (hypernatremia). Urine will be poorly concentrated, with low osmolality and decreased specific gravity (Holcomb, 2002b). An MRI will be used to rule out the presence of a pituitary tumor. A family history and genetic testing will be done to determine whether the disease has been inherited or whether there has been recent stress or trauma to the pituitary (Holcomb, 2002a).

A stimulus test such as fluid deprivation or administration of DDAVP, a synthetic replacement for antidiuretic hormone, to assess the impact of secretion of vasopressin may be done to differentiate neurogenic DI from dipsogenic DI. Unlike pituitary DI, DDAVP eliminates both excessive urination but not the symptoms of increased thirst and fluid intake in dipsogenic DI. In fact, water intoxication is a serious concern with this disorder. Patients will complain of headache, lethargy, and nausea and will have low levels of plasma sodium concentration (hyponatremia).

Medical Management

Treatment is dependent on the type of DI the patient is experiencing. Neurogenic DI may be treated by resolving the pituitary problem causing the disorder. For example, surgery for a pituitary tumor may be indicated. If irreparable damage has been done to pituitary tissues by tumor, infection, head injury, a congenital defect, or some other unexplained factor, then DI is likely to be permanent and must be managed with drugs including desmopressin or DDAVP. These will control the symptoms of constant thirst, drinking, and urination. On the other hand, gestational DI will generally resolve within 4 to 6 weeks following the conclusion of pregnancy but is likely to reoccur with subsequent pregnancies.

Nephrogenic DI, caused by genetic defects, drugs, or kidney disease, can be managed through a combination of hydration strategies, a low-sodium and sometimes low-protein diet, and the use of diuretics to reduce the volume of urine output. A thiazide diuretic, alone or in combination with a prostaglandin inhibitor, or a potassium-sparing diuretic may be ordered as part of the treatment regimen. If diuretics are used, potassium levels should be monitored. Potassium supplements may be needed to prevent hypokalemia. If DI is a side effect of lithium or other drugs, it is important to ensure that the therapeutic drugs selected for treatment do not impair their excretion (Nephrogenic Diabetes Insipidus Foundation, 2005b). It may be necessary to modify drug therapy for patients unable to tolerate lithium due to diabetes insipidus (Innis, 2002a).

■ Nursing Management

The primary goal in nursing care for patients with neurogenic, gestational, and nephrogenic DI is to prevent serious dehydration by ensuring that patients have an adequate fluid intake. Intravenous fluid replacement and an abundance of oral fluids should be readily available and administered. Vital signs and intake and output should be monitored very closely. Hormone replacement therapy is provided when appropriate, and electrolytes may be supplemented as needed. Diuretics may be used in nephrogenic DI to help kidneys eliminate sodium and decrease the glomerular filtration rate, resulting in conservation of urine. Patients will have a lifetime commitment in the management of hyperpituitarism unless the treatment resolves the underlying problem by pituitary tumor resection, or termination of pregnancy.

Discharge Priorities

Discharge priorities focus on patient instruction regarding the nature of the disease and the importance of hydration and strategies to ensure the availability of fluid at all times. Medic alert jewelry and a medical identification card should always be carried by the patient so that the patient's condition is known and in emergency situations the treatment is efficient. Patients should be made aware of community resources, including organizations that promote education and research on DI.

Hypermetabolic Disorder of the Posterior Pituitary: SIADH

The posterior pituitary secretes the hormones ADH and oxytocin. An excess of oxytocin has not been reported to be problematic, but oversecretion of ADH does occur and is considered potentially life threatening if untreated. This disorder is called **syndrome of inappropriate antidiuretic hormone (SIADH)**.

Epidemiology and Etiology

SIADH results from a failure of the negative feedback system that regulates the release and inhibition of ADH. In persons with this syndrome, ADH secretion continues even when serum osmolality is decreased, causing marked water retention and dilutional hyponatremia (Bayless, 2003; Porth, 2007). It occurs in adults and premature infants, and is caused by a variety of pathophysiological conditions.

Although SIADH is not unusual in adults, it is rare in the pediatric population, and other causes of hyponatremia are more common. It is the most common cause of hypotonic normovolemic hyponatremia in children. Exact incidence figures are not available.

The presence of hyponatremia, its severity, and delay in initiating adequate treatment appear to be the main indicators for both morbidity and mortality. The mortality rate in hyponatremic patients is 50-fold higher than in patients who do not develop hyponatremia. Moreover, the mortality rate in patients with serum sodium concentrations of less than 120 mmol/L is 25%, or twice that, of patients with mild hyponatremia. Acute decreases in serum sodium in adults are associated with a cited mortality rate of 5% to 50%, depending on the severity and rate of development, whereas in children it is only about 8%. Infants probably tolerate cerebral edema with fewer untoward effects because of their expandable cranium. Symptomatic postoperative hyponatremia can result in high morbidity and mortality rates in children of both sexes, which is due, in large part, to inadequate brain adaptation and lack of timely treatment (Ferry & Pascual-y-Baralt, 2007). Controlled studies in adults have shown that women and men are equally likely to develop hyponatremia and hyponatremic encephalopathy after surgery. Menstruating women who develop hyponatremic encephalopathy are 25 times more likely to die or have permanent brain damage than either men or postmenopausal women. The Risk Factors box addresses the risk factors for SIADH.

Although genetic factors may be involved in the etiology of pituitary disorders, not enough is known at present to offer dis-

---

RISK FACTORS for SIADH

SIADH occurs in patients who have central nervous system disorders, patients who have experienced shock, trauma, stress, or surgery, and patients with malignancies or pulmonary infections such as TB, bacterial pneumonia, or a lung abscess. Selected drugs including narcotics, tranquilizers, barbiturates, general anesthetics, thiazide diuretics, hypoglycemic agents, antidepressants, and some chemotherapeutic agents also are associated with rare cases of SIADH. A high percentage of patients with SIADH have a malignancy, often a small cell or oat cell carcinoma lung cancer, but other forms of cancer also have been found to cause this disorder. Malignant cells can secrete ADH or ADH-like chemicals, which serve as an ectopic source of ADH. Seriously ill ventilated patients and the elderly may experience an increase in the release of ADH (Langfeldt & Cooley, 2003; Terpstra & Terpstra, 2000).

ease prevention strategies. Consultation with the health care provider on the potential benefit of genetic screening should be considered but may offer limited benefit at this time.

Pathophysiology

Several mechanisms regulate sodium and water balance in the human body. The hypothalamus contains strategically located osmoreceptors that maintain a feedback control system for ADH secretion. Changes in the extracellular fluid resulting from a decrease or increase in the sodium ion concentration stimulate the osmoreceptors to increase or decrease the firing rate of the osmoreceptor cells, which stimulates or reduces production of ADH accordingly. Circulating ADH increases the permeability of distal tubules and the collecting duct by attaching to receptor sites in these tissues. Thus when stimulated by increasing plasma osmolality, the osmoreceptors of the hypothalamus secrete ADH and the kidneys respond by reabsorbing more water into the capillary network. As a consequence, a smaller volume of concentrated urine is excreted. When plasma osmolality is low, ADH secretion decreases and little water reabsorption occurs, resulting in the excretion of a large volume of dilute urine.

Decreases in blood pressure and volume, which are communicated by stretch receptors in the heart and large arteries, also stimulate the secretion of ADH. Thus if a patient has experienced extreme blood loss, the body will respond by increasing the output of ADH significantly (Colorado State University, 2003). SIADH occurs when ADH hormone continues to be secreted in spite of hyponatremia (low serum sodium levels).

Clinical Manifestations

Symptoms develop due to gradual water intoxication as evidenced by low serum sodium levels, and patients will exhibit headache, nausea, anorexia, thirst, increase in weight, oliguria, muscle cramps, weakness, and fatigue. As hyponatremia increases, mental confusion, irritability, and disorientation will occur. Seizures and coma can occur along with cerebral edema. When serum sodium drops below 110 to 115 mEq/L, the risk of death is high (Langfelt & Cooley, 2003). Critical care nurses should be alert to symptoms in patients who are known to be at risk for development of SIADH. Culture may play a part in a patient's response to the symptoms of pituitary disorders, as discussed in the Cultural Considerations for Pituitary Disorders box.

Laboratory and Diagnostic Procedures

Laboratory tests of electrolytes, serum and urine osmolality, urine specific gravity, and blood urea nitrogen (BUN) can be useful in the diagnosis of SIADH. Serum sodium is usually moderately or severely low depending on patient condition. Clinical diagnostic measures will be focused on eliminating other potential causes for hyponatremia and fluid retention such as congestive heart failure and cirrhosis. Once the syndrome is identified, the underlying cause should be explored with further diagnostic studies as needed.

Medical Management

Treatment is first directed at the problem of hyponatremia and water intoxication through fluid restriction and gradual correction of the serum sodium level with intravenous electrolytes,

CULTURAL CONSIDERATIONS for Pituitary Disorders

Both hypopituitarism and hyperpituitarism can cause symptoms that will be problematic for patients in terms of cultural acceptance. In patients with long-standing hypersecretion of growth hormone, changes in facial characteristics present a special problem. Body image may be distorted due to coarsening of facial features and may cause the patient particular problems in those cultures where appearance is highly valued. Unexplained lactation is another untoward symptom that may create cultural complications for patients since this typically occurs independent of pregnancy and normal lactation. In addition, the fact that it may take several months for hormone levels, let alone symptoms, to return to normal is often very disturbing for patients.

food, and fluids. The degree of fluid restriction is dependent on the severity of hyponatremia. Lower levels of serum sodium require more aggressive fluid restriction. Too rapid a correction of hyponatremia is ill advised because a complication can occur that will result in cerebral edema, seizures, permanent brain damage, and death a few days after treatment. If a patient is ambulatory, the health care provider may prescribe the use of medications that will block the action of ADH, such as demeclocycline or lithium, in order to avoid strict fluid restriction.

Along with efforts to correct fluid and electrolyte balance, efforts must be made to address the underlying cause of SIADH. Surgical excision of the tumor mass, radiation therapy, or chemotherapy to decrease tumor size may be attempted. Antibiotics should be initiated if the cause is believed to be an infection. Drugs suspected in the etiology of SIADH should be discontinued (Carr, 2001).

Nursing Management

Nurses in critical care and oncology settings should be particularly alert in their physical assessment of patients at high risk for SIADH. Assessment of hydration including skin turgor, mucous membranes, intake and output, daily weight, and monitoring for fluid overload is important. Nursing care for patients with suspected SIADH includes meticulous recording of intake and output, urine specific gravity, weight, and vital signs.

During the acute phase of SIADH, the nurse should monitor the patient's neurological status and take seizure precautions. The nurse also should work with the patient and family on a plan for monitored fluid intake and restriction throughout the day. Fluids that are relatively high in sodium such as tomato juice, milk, or broth should be encouraged. Dry mouth may be addressed with sugarless gum or candies, mouth moisturizers, or artificial saliva products (Langfelt & Cooley, 2003).

Patient and family education should include strategies to deal with SIADH as well as the underlying disease and related nursing care. Patients or their caregivers should be instructed on how to record the patient's daily weight and intake and output measurements for ongoing evaluation. Increased weight and decreased output should be reported because further treatment may be required.

Discharge Priorities

Discharge priorities include attention to postoperative instructions and routine follow-up with the health care provider. If patients are taking antipituitary drugs to counteract excess hormone production, instructions should include signs and symptoms of drug side effects. It is not uncommon for further treatment to be required if the tumor is not completely removed and continues to grow over time. Patients should be advised to continue follow-up evaluations with the endocrinologist so that additional treatment such as radiation therapy or medications can be used to reduce symptoms and to improve quality of life (Carr, 2001).

Collaborative Management

Care of patients with pituitary disorders typically will require close teamwork between and among the endocrinologist, neurosurgeon, primary care provider, nurses, and diagnostic imaging staff at the very least. Pharmacists and dietitians also may be involved in planning the care of the patient. The goal of treatment should be to eliminate the pituitary tumor, stabilize hormone production, and improve quality of life for the patient, which often has been severely compromised over time. Research and surgical advances in the field of treatment of neurological and endocrine disorders will require that health professionals work together and update their knowledge of contemporary standards of care when patients present with these rare clinical diagnoses.

Complementary and Alternative Approaches

Complementary approaches to care may offer considerable enhancement of the well-being of patients following treatment for diseases of the pituitary gland. Elimination of symptoms may take several months following initiation of treatment and complementary measures may offer particular benefit during this period. Again, complementary measures do not substitute for medical treatment aimed at eliminating causative factors such as benign tumors, but they can be important in improving quality of life. Some studies have shown that patients with pituitary tumors report quality of life to be diminished even after hormone levels return to normal following traditional treatment (Baird et al., 2003). This suggests that additional study is needed to determine how these patients can be restored to optimal health, potentially with the use of complementary approaches.

Disorders of the Adrenal Gland

The adrenal glands, like the other endocrine glands, can be affected by a variety of conditions including congenital malformations, genetic disorders, autoimmune disease, infection, hemorrhage, and tumors, all of which can cause either hypofunction or hyperfunction of the glands. The adrenal glands produce hormones that are essential to the body's "fight-or-flight" response and general adaptation to stress (see Chapter 12). Thus hypo- or hypersecretion of hormones of the adrenal glands can have significant and pervasive effects on health.

Although each adrenal gland is described as one unit, in reality, the gland is composed of two very distinct parts, the cortex and the medulla, with cells and tissues that secrete different hormones and have different functions. Chart 52–7 lists hypo- and hyper-metabolic disorders of the adrenal gland. Note that hypometabolic disorders have been identified involving the adrenal cortex but not the adrenal medulla, but hypermetabolic disorders occur in both the adrenal cortex and adrenal medulla.

Hypometabolic Adrenal Disorders: The Adrenal Cortex

Hypofunction of the adrenal glands can occur for many reasons and the degree of dysfunction determines whether the symptoms are mild, moderate, or life threatening. However, any level of impairment puts the individual at risk during times of stress or disease because the body's ability to produce essential hormones to maintain homeostasis has been compromised. Although this condition is fairly rare, adrenal insufficiency may be acute or chronic. The two major hypometabolic disorders of the

CHART 52–7	Hypometabolic and Hypermetabolic Disorders of the Adrenal Glands		
Adrenals	**Disorder**	**Hormones**	**Clinical Picture**
Adrenal cortex, hypometabolic disorders	Congenital adrenal hyperplasia	Cortisol and aldosterone deficiency with an excess in androgen hormone	Adrenal crisis with dehydration and shock Masculinization of females and early puberty; short stature
	Adrenal insufficiency	Cortisol deficiency	Adrenal crisis
	Addison's disease	Cortisol deficiency	Adrenal crisis
Adrenal cortex, hypermetabolic disorders	Cushing's syndrome Primary aldosteronism/Conn's disease	Cortisol excess Aldosterone excess	Hypertension Abdominal obesity Muscle wasting Hypertension with hypokalemia
Adrenal medulla, hypometabolic disorders	None identified	None identified	None identified
Adrenal medulla, hypermetabolic disorders	Pheochromocytoma	Adrenalin excess	Hypertension

adrenals are primary adrenal hyperplasia and Addison's disease. Congenital adrenal hyperplasia is hereditary and becomes apparent at birth or childhood, whereas Addison's disease usually occurs later in life. Adrenal insufficiency caused by long-term administration of corticosteroid drugs is not a disease per se, but is a disorder with symptoms like those of Addison's disease.

Addison's disease is adrenocortical insufficiency due to the destruction or dysfunction of the entire adrenal cortex. It affects both glucocorticoids and mineralocorticoid function. The onset of disease usually occurs when 90% or more of both adrenal cortices are dysfunctional or destroyed (Odeke & Nagelbereg, 2006).

Epidemiology and Etiology

In the mid-19th century, primary adrenal insufficiency was first described by a physician, Thomas Addison, for whom the condition was later named. At that time, the most common cause of the disease was tuberculosis (TB) infection and this remains the second most common cause today. However, the incidence of Addison's disease secondary to an increase in opportunistic infections related to human immunodeficiency virus (HIV) is rising (Holcomb, 2006). Addison's disease is a rare condition caused by a severe or total deficiency of hormones produced by the adrenal cortex, and results from partial or complete destruction of the adrenal glands. In a normal state, when the body perceives the need for greater energy, the pituitary gland secretes ACTH, which stimulates the release of cortisol by the adrenal glands. In adrenal gland insufficiency, secretion of cortisol is impaired leading to a serious imbalance in homeostasis. The body becomes unable to respond to new and differing demands for adrenal hormones. In most cases of adrenal insufficiency, the adrenal cortex is primarily affected but when the medulla is involved, catecholamine deficiency also may occur. A patient with Addison's disease is shown in Figure 52–8 ■.

The leading cause of Addison's disease is autoimmune disease in which the body's immune system makes antibodies that gradually destroy the cells of the adrenal cortex (Odeke & Nagelbereg, 2006). Autoimmune destruction of the cortex involves a long process, typically occurring over months and years. Chronic infections such as TB, histoplasmosis, or cytomegalovirus may cause Addison's disease, but infection is much less commonly involved today. Cancer (usually caused by metastasis from other tissues such as the breast), hemorrhage into the adrenal gland, tumors, bilateral adrenalectomy, and sudden withdrawal of long-term corticosteroid therapy are other, less frequently noted causes of Addison's disease (Anderson, 2002; National Adrenal Diseases Foundation, 2006a).

Currently the prevalence of Addison's disease in the United States is 40 to 60 cases per 1 million population. Internationally, the condition is rare, and is not associated with a racial predilection. Idiopathic autoimmune Addison's disease tends to be more common in females and children. The most common age at presentation in adults is 30 to 50 years, but the disease could present earlier in patients with any of the polyglandular autoimmune syndromes, congenital adrenal hyperplasia (CAH), or if onset is due to a disorder of long-chain fatty acid metabolism (Odeke & Nagelbereg, 2006).

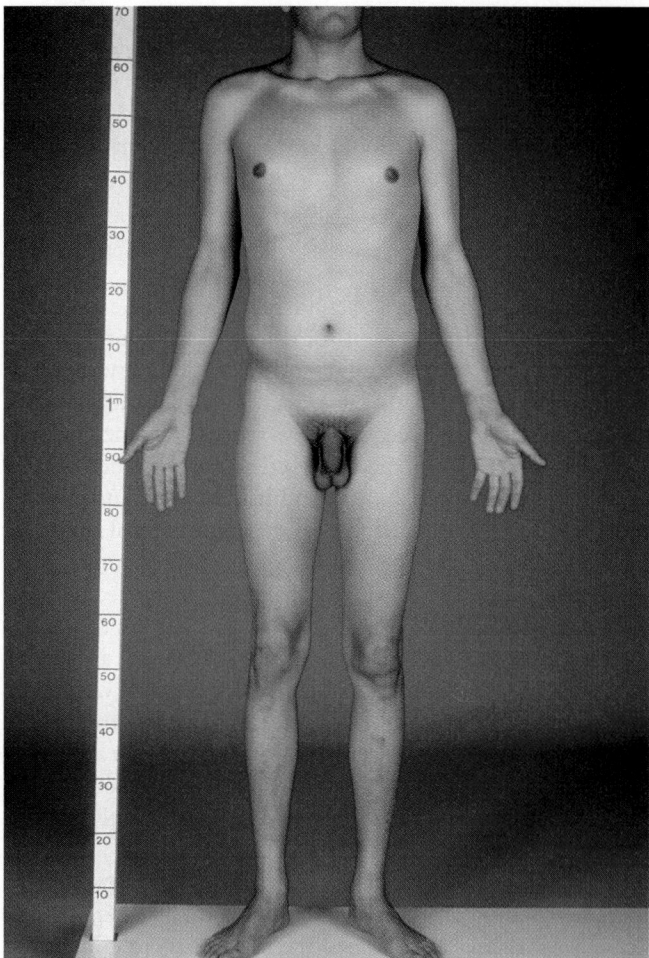

FIGURE 52–8 ■ Patient with Addison's disease.
Source: Bart's Medical Library/Phototake NYC

Pathophysiology

There are two adrenal glands, one located above each kidney in the human body, and they have two distinct parts: the cortex, which is the outer portion, and the medulla, the inner portion. The adrenal cortex produces two essential hormones: cortisol and aldosterone. These hormones are key to the body's general adaptation to stress and illness. The adrenal cortex also produces androgens, which are important in the development of the gonads and male sexual characteristics. Cellular receptors for cortisol exist in cell cytoplasm throughout the entire body. Thus the presence of a normal level of the adrenal hormone cortisol is essential for maintaining cell homeostasis and viability (Coursin & Wood, 2002).

The medulla produces the hormones epinephrine (also known as adrenalin) and norepinephrine. Adrenalin increases heart rate and stroke volume, dilates the pupils, and constricts arterioles in the skin and gut while dilating arterioles in leg muscles. Adrenalin also elevates the blood sugar level by increasing hydrolysis of glycogen to glucose in the liver, and begins the breakdown of lipids in fat cells. Norepinephrine activates the sympathetic nervous system to directly increase heart rate, release energy from fat, and increase muscle readiness.

The hormones of the adrenal glands are produced through the interaction of the negative feedback control of both the hypothalamus and the pituitary glands (Figure 52–9 ■). The hypothalamus produces CRH, which stimulates the pituitary to produce ACTH, to signal the need for production of glucocorticoids in the adrenals. Glucocorticoid levels vary naturally throughout the day, with lower levels typically being produced in the evening hours and production peaking in the early morning hours. Under conditions of stress such as illness, surgery, or trauma, the normal body can dramatically increase the synthesis of cortisol (Coursin & Wood, 2002).

Adrenal insufficiency is a condition in which the body fails to produce adequate amounts of adrenal hormones. **Primary adrenal insufficiency** occurs in conditions when most (up to 90%) of the adrenal gland has been destroyed, resulting in an absence of sufficient glucocorticoids (cortisol), mineralocorticoids (aldosterone), and androgens. The disease process originates within the adrenal gland and may involve autoimmune disease, infection, or hemorrhage. Congenital adrenal hyperplasia is an inherited form of adrenal insufficiency. **Secondary adrenal insufficiency**, caused by impaired pituitary secretion of ACTH, occurs when there is an inadequate secretion of cortisol but an adequate amount of aldosterone. The diseases are similar in that in both conditions there is a loss of cortisol (Coursin & Wood, 2002). Primary adrenal hyperplasia differs from these forms of adrenal insufficiency in that the adrenals are able to respond to signals from the pituitary and attempt to compensate for a decline in cortisol and aldosterone by significantly increasing production of androgen.

Although Addison's disease is rare, a more common problem that may occur in critically ill adults is secondary adrenal insufficiency, which can occur when the patient has received long-term administration of therapeutic glucocorticoids, such as prednisone. These drugs commonly are given for inflammatory conditions and autoimmune disorders such as rheumatoid arthritis, asthma, and ulcerative colitis. Administration of cortisone drugs suppresses the normal stimulation response of the hypothalamus to release CRH and the pituitary to release ACTH, which would trigger the production of increased cortisol in the adrenals. Disruption in the hypothalamic–pituitary–adrenal

(HPA) axis function may last for a long period and is a major reason why abrupt withdrawal of cortisone therapy is ill advised and may put the patient at serious risk (Pfadt & Carlson, 2006). Resumption of normal HPA activity after a long period of hormone therapy may take up to a year (Coursin & Wood, 2002). Thus cortisone drugs should always be discontinued with gradually diminishing doses over an extended period of time. The risk factors for adrenal disorders are discussed in the Risk Factors box.

Clinical Manifestations

Patients with Addison's disease experience severe and chronic fatigue and loss of appetite and weight. Nausea, vomiting, and diarrhea occur in many cases. Patients feel light-headed because their blood pressure is low, and they may experience orthostatic hypotension, that is, low blood pressure upon standing (Løvås & Husebye, 2005). Hyperpigmentation of skin is common, with scars, skinfolds, and pressure points such as elbows, knees, and knuckles becoming characteristically dark. In women, menstruation cycles and patterns may change. Patients may crave salt and may experience low blood sugars. **Addisonian crisis** (or **adrenal crisis**) occurs when symptoms of the disease become exacerbated due to stress, causing severe pain in the lower back, abdomen, or legs; vomiting, or diarrhea with severe dehydration; and low blood pressure and loss of consciousness (Pituitary Network Association, 2006a). Patients with adrenal insufficiency for any reason may experience adrenal crisis if hormone replacement is not initiated, is inadequate, or if other factors increase the physiological demand for adrenal hormones.

Laboratory and Diagnostic Procedures

The physical examination and patient history give the first indications of adrenal insufficiency. The most specific laboratory test is the short ACTH stimulation test, an exam in which a baseline blood sample is drawn and then a synthetic form of ACTH is given by injection, followed by the measurement of blood and, in some cases, urine cortisone levels at 30, 60, and 90 minutes. Patients with adrenal insufficiency are unable to respond to stimulation by producing more cortisol, and do not produce more cortisol (Whiteman, 2006). A prolonged ACTH stimulation test may be given to clarify whether the disease is primary or secondary. A CT scan may be ordered to enhance diagnosis in terms of cause of the disease (Luken, 1999).

Medical Management

Patients with Addison's disease or adrenal insufficiency are treated with hormones designed to replace cortisol (Cortef, prednisone, or cortisone) and aldosterone (fludrocortisone [Florinef]). In addition, the doctor may recommend treating

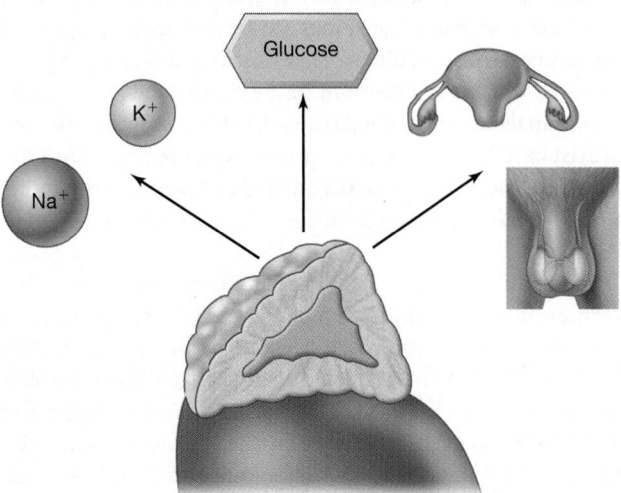

Adrenal glands secrete hormones which help regulate chemical balance, regulate metabolism, and supplement other glands

FIGURE 52–9 ■ Adrenal gland hormone secretion.

androgen deficiency with an androgen replacement called dehydroepiandrosterone. Some studies indicate that, for women with Addison's disease, androgen replacement therapy may improve their overall sense of well-being, libido, and sexual satisfaction.

Oral doses of hydrocortisone or cortisone acetate, 20 to 30 mg/day, are given in divided doses morning and evening. Typically, two-thirds of the medication is given in the morning and one-third in the evening to mimic the normal output of cortisol throughout the day. Hydrocortisone should be taken with meals, milk, or antacids to avoid increasing gastric acidity and distress. Aldosterone is replaced with a synthetic aldosterone steroid, fludrocortisone tablets (Florinef), taken once daily to prevent loss of sodium, hyperkalemia, and intravascular depletion. If the patient is unable to take replacement therapy by mouth, medications are administered intravenously.

Patients in adrenal crisis are seriously ill and require fluid replacement with intravenous saline and dextrose in saline solution immediately, along with intravenous hydrocortisone for 48 to 72 hours. Patients should be monitored for their electrolyte balance, blood count, and plasma as a means to determine appropriate adjustments to drug dosages. In children with primary adrenal hyperplasia, androgen blocking drugs and growth hormone may be used to block the effects of excess androgen production and to enhance growth in height (National Adrenal Diseases Foundation, 2006b).

Nursing Management

Nurses play a key role during adrenal crisis in managing fluid replacement, administering hormone replacements, and measuring vital signs, weight, and fluid intake and output. Once the crisis is resolved, a plan for patient and family education must be developed in cooperation with the medical staff. Patients will require instruction on lifetime drug therapy and risks during periods of stress and illness. Patients should be encouraged to keep a small amount of medications with them at all times in the event of a disaster because interruption of drug therapy can be catastrophic. It is advisable that patients learn how to administer intramuscular injections so that they can self-administer hydrocortisone if unable to take medications by mouth due to nausea or vomiting. Patients should consult with their physician about the advisability of carrying a syringe and a dose of injectable cortisol with them in case of emergency. Cortisol hormone replacements will need to be increased during stress and illness to avoid complications and the mineralocorticoid fludrocortisone acetate should be increased during summer months or periods of intense exercise when sweating increases. The Nursing Process: Patient Care Plan for Acute Adrenal Insufficiency explains the nursing process to be used in caring for patients with this disorder, and the Gerontological Considerations box (p. 1650) addresses additional teaching for the elderly with this disorder.

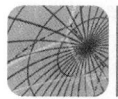

NURSING PROCESS: Patient Care Plan for Acute Adrenal Insufficiency

Assessment of Cognitive Level, Muscle Strength, and Ability to Perform ADLS Independently

Subjective Data:
Have you been taking any steroid medications, such as prednisone, cortisone, or any other steroid drugs?
What other medications, herbs, or dietary supplements have you been taking?
Have you been able to maintain your usual activities of daily living?
What has your appetite been like?
Have you noticed any food cravings lately?
How much salt or sodium do you get in your diet?
Have you experienced any nausea or vomiting?
Do you feel mentally alert?
Are you sleeping well?
Have you experienced any stress, trauma, or illness recently?

Objective Data:
Low blood pressure
Orthostatic hypotension
Poor skin turgor
Tender abdomen
Face appears round, edematous
Muscle weakness noted
Low serum sodium, high potassium noted

Nursing Assessment and Diagnoses	Outcomes and Evaluation Parameters	Planning and Interventions with *Rationales*
Nursing Diagnosis: *Deficient Fluid Volume* and *Hyponatremia* secondary to adrenal insufficiency	**Outcomes:** Free of symptoms of adrenal insufficiency. ***Evaluation Parameters:*** Vital signs within normal limits. Patient able to stand at bedside without vertigo. Abdomen soft, bowel sounds normal. Patient reports appetite has returned with no food cravings. Patient verbalizes feeling less fatigued. Skin turgor appears elastic. Serum sodium and sodium serum levels within normal range. No evidence of nausea, vomiting, or diarrhea.	**Interventions and *Rationales:*** Administer IV therapy, which may include 0.09% saline solution or 5% dextrose in saline to improve fluid and electrolyte balance *to raise blood pressure and improve perfusion of oxygen to tissues.* Administer IV hydrocortisone for first 48–72 hours, followed by oral administration for essential hormone replacement to be taken with meals *to provide hormone needed due to suppression of HPA axis due to long-term corticosteroid therapy and to prevent GI distress.*

(continued)

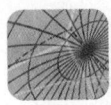

Nursing Process: Patient Care Plan for Acute Adrenal Insufficiency—*Continued*

Assessment of Emergency Preparedness in the Event of Adrenal Insufficiency Crisis

Subjective Data:

Do you carry a medical identification card with a list of your medications on it?

Do you wear a medical ID bracelet or other jewelry?

Have you informed family members or caregivers of your history with corticosteroid drugs?

Tell me what your understanding is about how corticosteroid drugs affect your body.

Are you experiencing any pain?

Please describe the location and intensity.

Objective Data:

Blood pressure: 84/40

Temperature: 101°F

Heart rate: 124

Diaphoretic

Appears confused, disoriented as to time and place

Vomited during interview

No medic alert noted on patient on admission to ICU

Family members report patient has been taking corticosteroids for rheumatoid arthritis

Medications found in patient's purse

Nursing Assessment and Diagnoses	Outcomes and Evaluation Parameters	Planning and Interventions with *Rationales*
Nursing Diagnosis: *Risk of Ineffective Therapeutic Regimen Management*	**Outcomes:** Prepared to care for self and to prevent insufficiency crisis. ***Evaluation Parameters:*** Patient wears a medical alert bracelet on next clinic visit and shows nurse her medical ID in purse. Patient reports notifying other health care providers (podiatrist, ophthalmologist, and dentist) of medication regimen. Patient able to describe rationale for safety precautions related to long-term use of corticosteroid drugs and the need for gradual tapering off of drugs when they are discontinued.	**Interventions and *Rationales:*** Develop teaching plan with patient and family to ensure adequate understanding of benefits and risks of corticosteroid therapy and measures to be taken for patient safety, including use of medical alert jewelry and ID card, notification of other health care providers, and need for gradual tapering off of corticosteroid medications when these are discontinued. *To enable patient to manage self-care with better understanding of medications and side effects, to enhance safety of patient when undergoing medical procedures with other health care providers, and to alert health care providers to patient's history of corticosteroid use in the event of emergency.*

GERONTOLOGICAL CONSIDERATIONS Related to Adrenal Insufficiency

Older patients are more vulnerable to serious problems with adrenal insufficiency and may require more frequent monitoring and observation. The nurse will want to instruct not only the patient, but a spouse or other caregiver about signs and symptoms of impending crisis so that assistance can be obtained if the patient is unable to seek medical assistance in a timely way, for example, when there is infection or nausea and vomiting.

Discharge Priorities

Preparation of patients for discharge must include instruction regarding the need to take hormone replacement therapy for life. Of particular importance is for patients to understand that stress or illness is likely to increase their need for hydrocortisone. In such situations, they should increase the dosage of hormone as advised by their health care provider.

Persistence of vomiting or diarrhea indicates a need for urgent care, which may include intravenous saline and intramuscular hydrocortisone. Flu-like symptoms should never be ignored because they may be the initial indicators of adrenal crisis. The nurse should coordinate care with a home care or community health agency because effective patient and caregiver education may require the patient to be in more optimal health and because sufficient time must be provided to cover key aspects of care.

Health Promotion

Patients with a history of adrenal insufficiency should wear a medical identification bracelet or necklace and keep an identification card with medical instructions in their wallet or purse. A medical alert in the form of medical identification may enable health care personnel to respond to a patient's need for immediate hormone and fluid replacement and could be life saving. Knowledge about the disease is essential for self-management, particularly during illness or added stress. Thus the patient and a reliable family member should have appropriate follow-up with home care to ensure that they have adequate information and skill to manage the demands of the chronic form of the disease. Patient referral to the appropriate support group is suggested.

Collaborative Management

It is important for the pharmacist, rehabilitation professional, and home health nurse to be involved in providing follow-up care with the patient diagnosed with an adrenal crisis. The patient must be advised about permanent hormone injections and the method of self-administration of intramuscular injections. The pharmacist also should be involved in providing instructions on how to take medications, which is particularly important during periods of stress and illness. It is advisable to have a physical therapist or rehabilitation professional collaborate with the patient in establishing an exercise regimen that can be adapted throughout the year to accommodate seasonal changes.

Hypermetabolic Disorders of the Adrenal Cortex: Cushing's Syndrome

Hypermetabolic disorders of the adrenal cortex include **Cushing's syndrome**, which involves an excess of cortisol, and primary aldosteronism, which involves an excess of aldosterone, which is discussed later in the chapter.

Epidemiology and Etiology

Cushing's syndrome occurs with long-term secretion or exposure to excessive adrenocortical hormones, particularly cortisol and related corticosteroids, and to a lesser extent androgens and aldosterone. Factors known to trigger Cushing's syndrome include problems in the HPA axis that cause excess cortisol release from the adrenal glands, iatrogenic sources such as prednisone therapy, and ectopic courses such as tumors outside of the pituitary that produce ACTH (Holcomb, 2005).

The female-to-male incidence ratio is approximately 6:1 for Cushing's syndrome due to an adrenal or pituitary tumor. Ectopic ACTH production is more frequent in men than in woman because of the increased incidence of lung tumors in the population. The peak incidence of Cushing's syndrome due to either an adrenal or pituitary adenoma occurs in persons ages 25 to 49 years. Ectopic ACTH production due to lung cancer occurs later in life (Holcomb, 2005).

Pathophysiology

An excess of cortisol stimulates anti-inflammatory effects and rapid catabolism of protein and peripheral fat to support hepatic glucose production. One of two mechanisms may be at play. Excess cortisol may be produced because of elevated ACTH levels from the pituitary, which stimulate the adrenal cortex to produce more hormones. Or an excess of cortisol may be produced independent of ACTH production, due to the presence of hormone-producing tumor cells or the administration of cortisone and steroid drugs. The presence of excess cortisone causes systemic physiological manifestations including lipidosis, hypertension due to retention of water and sodium, increased gastric secretions and decreased gastric mucus, increased hepatic gluconeogenesis and insulin resistance, increased antibody formation and lymphocyte production, suppressed inflammatory response, and osteoporosis. These physiological alterations in turn lead to heart disease and/or heart failure, peptic ulcer, impaired glucose tolerance, frequent infections and poor wound healing, and pathologic fractures (Kirk, Hash, Katner, & Jones, 2000).

A majority (approximately 70%) of Cushing's syndrome cases are caused by overproduction of ACTH by the pituitary. Other cases are due to the presence of a tumor outside of the pituitary. Such tumors are usually malignant and often involve a small cell carcinoma of the lung or a pancreatic tumor. Another common cause of Cushing's syndrome is administration of synthetic glucocorticoids or steroids, which are commonly used for chronic inflammatory or immune diseases such as rheumatoid arthritis, ulcerative colitis, systemic lupus, and asthma.

Clinical Manifestations

Patients with Cushing's syndrome will present with a particular pattern of fat deposition on their face and bodies. The face will be round and typically referred to as "moon face" and the trunk will appear large and the patient will be obese with slender arms and legs (Figure 52–10 ■). Acne and purple striae will appear on the face. Fat will be concentrated in fat pads above the clavicle and over the upper back in what is sometimes described as a "buffalo hump." Patients may report a history of poor health, frequent infections with poor wound healing, and sudden weight gain (Holcomb, 2005). Vital signs will indicate hypertension and further evaluation may reveal left ventricular hypertrophy.

Androgen production will cause emphasis of secondary sex characteristics in women with hirsutism, virilism, hypertrophy of the clitoris, and amenorrhea or oligomenorrhea. Muscle wasting and pathologic fractures complete the picture in males and females affected with Cushing's disease (National Adrenal Diseases Foundation, 2006b). Family members also may report that the patient has been irritable and emotionally labile, and cases of steroid-induced psychosis may be seen (Shirk, 2003).

Laboratory and Diagnostic Procedures

Specific laboratory tests of blood and urine will be done to test for excess levels of cortisol. Cortisol production is usually low in the evenings, thus high levels will support a diagnosis of Cushing's syndrome. Specialized suppression tests, such as the dexamethasone suppression test, will be used to help differentiate ACTH-dependent Cushing's syndrome (pituitary dependent or ectopic) from non–ACTH-dependent (adrenal tumor) forms. Blood chemistry for sodium, potassium, and glucose will reveal abnormalities such as high serum sodium and glucose levels. A 24-hour urine sample will be collected for determining free cortisol. A CT scan and MRI will help localize tumors if these are

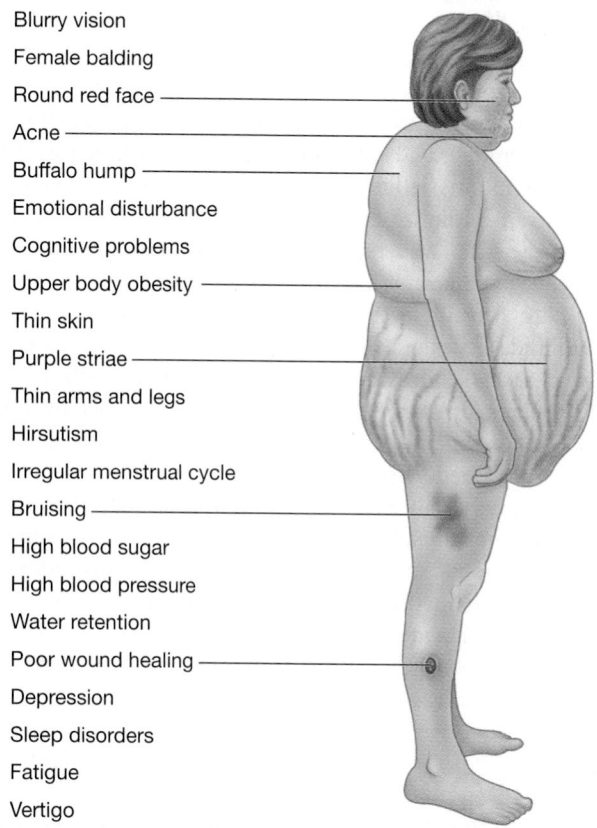

Blurry vision
Female balding
Round red face
Acne
Buffalo hump
Emotional disturbance
Cognitive problems
Upper body obesity
Thin skin
Purple striae
Thin arms and legs
Hirsutism
Irregular menstrual cycle
Bruising
High blood sugar
High blood pressure
Water retention
Poor wound healing
Depression
Sleep disorders
Fatigue
Vertigo

FIGURE 52–10 ■ Patient with Cushing's syndrome.

DIAGNOSTIC TESTS for Cushing's Syndrome

Test	Clinical Value
Urinary free cortisol excretion	Shows excess cortisol excreted in urine, indicating Cushing's syndrome.
Low-dose dexamethasone suppression tests	Helps distinguish pituitary from ectopic corticotrophin-dependent Cushing's syndrome.
Late night serum and salivary cortisol	Demonstrates presence of Cushing's syndrome if late night levels of cortisol are high.
CRH stimulation test	Aids in diagnosing ectopic corticotrophin production.
Inferior petrosal sinus sampling	Localizes the site of ACTH production.
CT scan	Provides evidence of pituitary or other tumor/malignancy.
MRI	Provides evidence of pituitary or other tumor/malignancy.

Sources: Adapted from Boscaro, M., Barzon, L., Fallo, F., & Sonino, N. (2001). Cushing's syndrome. *Lancet, 357,* 783–791; Kirk, L. F., Hash, R. B., Katner, H. P., & Jones, T. (2000). Cushing's disease: Clinical manifestations and diagnostic evaluation. *American Family Physician, 62*(5), 1119– 1127, 1133–1134; Porth, 2007.

causing the disease. Refer to the Diagnostic Tests for Cushing's Syndrome box for a list of the tests that can be used for differential diagnosis in hypermetabolic adrenal states.

Medical Management

Management of Cushing's syndrome is directed at the etiology of the disease. Surgery is the primary intervention for tumors of the adrenal or pituitary glands or other tissue such as the lung. Transsphenoidal microsurgery, as described earlier in this chapter, is used to remove pituitary tumors that are stimulating excessive ACTH production. Radiation therapy also may be used for tumors in the pituitary or other locations. In some cases, surgery may not be indicated and drugs may be used to counter the effect of excess production of adrenal hormones. One such drug is Mitotane (Lysodren), an adrenal cytotoxic preparation, which suppresses adrenal gland function and helps to reduce blood glucose and blood pressure. Mitotane decreases the size of adrenal tumors and reduces symptoms caused by excess hormone secretion. Aminoglutethimide (Cytadren) is another adrenal steroid inhibitor, which can be used to decrease production of adrenal hormones. Side effects of both drugs include gastrointestinal symptoms, lethargy, dizziness, depression, and vertigo. Patients can minimize effects by taking the medication with meals or a snack (Anderson, 2002). Caution should be used in the event a patient experiences trauma, infection, or other physiologically stressful event while taking mitotane or aminoglutethimide since these drugs may seriously impair the patient's ability to increase hormone production in response to the stress.

In patients for whom Cushing's syndrome is caused by longterm administration of corticosteroid drugs, a plan for gradual withdrawal or reduction of medication is indicated. Corticosteroids cannot be abruptly withdrawn because the patient may experience an adrenal crisis with symptoms of hypoadrenal function. Gradual reduction in dosage and administration of medications on alternate days will help minimize the suppression of normal hormone production.

The Gerontological Considerations box discusses elderly patients with Cushing's syndrome.

Nursing Management

Nursing care for patients with transsphenoidal surgery, indicated for patients whose Cushing's syndrome is caused by

GERONTOLOGICAL CONSIDERATIONS Related to Cushing's Syndrome

Quality of life for patients with Cushing's syndrome is often compromised by changes associated with the disorder, including distorted body image and the physical and psychological symptoms of excess hormone production. Elderly patients are most vulnerable to stress and other factors that may precipitate a crisis to which their bodies cannot readily respond because of a disorder of the adrenal glands. Observation and careful assessment of elderly patients with Cushing's syndrome will reduce the incidence of complications and death in this population. Elderly patients may be poor surgical risks, thus medical management of Cushing's syndrome is the preferred treatment option.

ACTH stimulation from the pituitary gland, was described earlier in this chapter. Routine nursing care will focus on regular assessment of vital signs, symptoms of hormone or drug toxicity, signs of fever or infection, and complications such as cardiovascular events, diabetes mellitus, depression, and suicide.

Assessment

Specific nursing assessments for suspected Cushing's syndrome will relate to the presence of excess cortisol and ACTH. When taking a patient history for Cushing's syndrome the nurse must be alert for potential precipitating factors such as hypothalamus or pituitary dysfunction or corticosteroid therapy. Face and body distribution of fat must be noted. Acne and purple striae on the face may be present, as well as the development of secondary sex characteristics in women such as hirsutism, virilism, and menstrual dysfunction. Vital sign assessments may indicate the presence of hypertension. Musculoskeletal strength should also be noted. Subjective complaints of weight gain are important, as are family reports of irritability and emotional changes.

Nursing Diagnosis

Primary nursing diagnoses for the patient with Cushing's syndrome will focus on improvement of self-esteem and body image, as well as complications of the disease process. Interpersonal relationships may also have been affected by body changes in patients. Problems related to cardiovascular and musculoskeletal complications may also be present.

Planning

Planning care of the patient with Cushing's syndrome will relate to nursing diagnoses that focus on body image, self-esteem, and relationships. The nurse must prepare the client for multiple diagnostic testing, which will include both serum and urine samples. Some treatment protocols involve surgery, as well as radiation and other pharmacologic interventions. Planning for the management of side effects from treatment must be a priority for the nurse.

Outcomes and Evaluation Parameters

As mentioned in the medical management section, the goals of treatment for Cushing's syndrome focus on the etiology of the disease. Because surgery is often the primary intervention, the nurse should establish goals related to pre- and postoperative patient care and the prevention of complications following surgery. Radiation and or pharmacologic therapy may also be indicated.

The nurse should then establish patient care goals related to adherence to a medical regimen, as well as goals that foster an improvement in the patient's body image, self-esteem, and interpersonal relationships.

Interventions and Rationales

The nurse should monitor the patient for baseline and ongoing measurements related to body characteristics and vital signs. Cardiovascular and musculoskeletal assessments should be monitored. Educational sessions for teaching must be a priority to assist the patient and family members to understand the changes that have occurred in the patients' bodies. Interventions to enhance self-esteem and interpersonal relationships will also be a priority. In the case of surgery, nursing interventions related to both pre- and postoperative care must be implemented.

Evaluation

While undergoing medical care for Cushing's syndrome, the patient should verbalize the rationale for adhering to the treatment regimen. Patients and family members should be able to verbalize what is causing the changes to their bodies, and how these changes have an impact on their physical and emotional well-being. When surgery is indicated, the patient should verbalize an understanding of the procedure, as well as the pre- and postoperative care required.

Discharge Priorities

The goal of care is to return adrenal function to normal and to stabilize hormone levels within a normal range. Prevention and early identification of infection is another goal in light of the body's compromised ability to respond to such stress. Patients who have had a long-standing surplus of corticosteroid hormone are likely to be emotionally labile and subject to serious depression and psychosis. Suicide precautions may be necessary and family members should be alerted to the need to report signs of worsening emotional stability to health care providers.

Hypermetabolic Disorders of the Adrenal Cortex: Hyperaldosteronism

Hyperaldosteronism is a disorder in which the adrenal cortex overproduces the hormone aldosterone, leading to hypertension in affected individuals. Primary hyperaldosteronism occurs when the adrenal gland itself is diseased and secondary hyperaldosteronism occurs when the etiology is outside of the adrenal glands. At one time it was believed that this disorder was responsible for a very small percentage of patients with hypertension, but improvements in screening techniques indicate the incidence is more prevalent (Mayo Clinic, 2005; Mulatero et al., 2004).

Pathophysiology, Risk Factors, and Clinical Picture

Primary aldosteronism, which is responsible for up to 70% of cases, usually is caused by a benign adenoma that produces excess aldosterone or stimulates adjacent cells to secrete excess hormone. Conn's disease, a condition in which the kidneys retain sodium and excrete potassium, is the name given to the disorder when it involves an adrenal adenoma. Other, less common causes of the disease are adrenal cancers and genetic mutations (which are rare) and adrenal hyperplasia (overactivity of both glands).

Patients present with hypertension, which does not respond well to medication or other treatment, as well as headache, orthostatic hypotension, muscle weakness and cramps, fatigue, temporary paralysis, constipation, numbness, pricking, tingling sensations, excessive thirst, and urination (HealthAtoZ, 2002). Hypokalemia and low plasma renin also are noted. Hypertension in combination with hypokalemia should receive further investigation for aldosteronism because the presence of hypokalemia is often indicative of high levels of aldosterone (Shah, 2006). A condition that causes high blood pressure in children and young adults is a rare type of this disease that runs in families and is called glucocorticoid-remediable aldosteronism (GRA) (Mayo Clinic, 2005).

Laboratory and Diagnostic Procedures

Laboratory measurements of aldosterone and renin levels are taken to measure hormone levels. An adrenal vein sample of blood may be drawn by the radiologist from the right and left adrenal veins to determine if aldosterone levels are high in one or both adrenal glands. This will help determine which gland has an adenoma or whether both glands are affected by hyperplasia. An oral salt or saline loading test or fludrocortisone suppression test (FST) may be administered to determine whether the aldosterone level remains high when it would normally decline. A CT scan will help to confirm the presence and location of an adenoma. Screening and detection of aldosteronism is important because studies indicate a high incidence of cardiovascular events such as stroke in patients with the disease.

Medical Management

Surgical removal of the aldosteronoma can bring significant symptom relief and is the treatment of choice. Hypertension may continue to be a problem, but it can often be controlled more effectively with medications. Management of hypertension will reduce the risk of kidney disease, as well as strokes and other cardiovascular problems (HealthAtoZ, 2002). Antihypertensive drugs such as calcium channel blockers may be prescribed for treatment. Potassium-sparing diuretics are another treatment option to reduce blood volume through diuresis. Potassium levels should be monitored for patients on diuretics.

A widely used drug for this condition is spironolactone, however, it is not advised in patients with kidney disease. Long-term spironolactone drug therapy causes impotence and gynecomastia in men, so this medication is generally used only for women. Another drug, amiloride, is the drug of choice for control of symptoms in men (Shah, 2006).

Nursing Management

Patients' vital signs should be monitored frequently and they should be advised to check their blood pressure at home in order to provide regular reports to their health care provider. In addition to monitoring vital signs and dressings postoperatively, the nurse should work with the patient and family to develop an instructional plan to cover monitoring medications, diet, and activity at home. If hypertension continues to be a problem, the nurse will recommend stress reduction strategies, including meditation, biofeedback, yoga, massage therapy, and diet and exercise to assist in reduction of blood pressure.

Hypermetabolic Disorder of the Adrenal Medulla: Pheochromocytoma

Pheochromocytoma is a rare, usually nonmalignant tumor of the adrenal medulla that causes a hypermetabolic condition characterized by excess production of the hormones of the adrenal medulla.

Pathophysiology, Risk Factors, and Clinical Manifestations

The adrenal medulla produces hormones known as catecholamines, including the hormones epinephrine and norepinephrine. Epinephrine stimulates the heart rate and stroke volume and raises blood sugar levels. Norepinephrine stimulates the sympathetic nervous system. Pheochromocytoma, a rare tumor of the adrenal medulla, causes hypertension by producing an excess of epinephrine (adrenalin) and norepinephrine. The disease typically strikes men and women equally between 40 and 60 years of age. About 5% to 10% of cases appear to have a hereditary component, particularly those cases in which there is involvement of both glands (American Urological Association, 2006; Braunwald et al., 2001). Hypertension may be episodic or long standing, and it can become life threatening. Hypertensive paroxysms in which the patient experiences dangerously high blood pressure, profuse sweating, nausea, and other symptoms may be triggered by specific events such as emotional stress, trigger foods, abdominal pressure, tobacco, and selected drugs, including histamine and glucagon. In addition to hypertension, patients with pheochromocytoma may experience headache, tachycardia, and palpitations (American Urological Association [AUA], 2006).

Laboratory and Diagnostic Procedures

Diagnostic tests include 24-hour blood and urine measurements of catecholamine metabolites. Upper limits for catecholamines are 590 to 885 nmol per 24 hours. In patients with pheochromocytoma, values of 1480 nmol and higher are seen. Assays of free or unconjugated catecholamines are also helpful in diagnosis. CT scans and MRI can be used to determine location and size of the tumor (Braunwald et al., 2001).

Medical Management

Treatment involves laparoscopic surgical removal of the tumor, which may involve one or both adrenal glands. A laparoscopic approach minimizes scarring, lowers the risk of hernias at the surgical site, reduces postoperative pain, and provides for shorter hospital stays and recovery time. Surgery is more successful in reducing blood pressure if symptoms have been of short duration. Long-standing hypertension is more difficult to reverse, even with surgery (AUA, 2006). Medical management of hypertension may be required following surgery, and drugs such as alpha-adrenergic blockers may be given to block excess hormone and lower blood pressure.

Nursing Management

Most surgical procedures for adrenal tumor removal today are non-invasive in nature; therefore, making the patient's recovery course and period easier than open surgery. Postoperatively, the nurse will be concerned with observation of the operative site, management of the patient's pain, and management of the patient's blood pressure and vital signs. Postoperative teaching includes informing the patient that she may engage in light activity while at home after surgery and can remove any dressings and shower the day after the operation. Normal routine activities, such as driving, may be resumed within a week. Typical postoperative care is discussed at length in Chapter 27 ✆ .

Health Promotion in Hypermetabolic Adrenal Disorders

Adrenal hormone levels will decline and begin to return to normal with treatment whether it is through elimination of a tumor or gradual withdrawal of corticosteroid therapy. Physiological and psychological changes may occur in the patient over several weeks. Patients should be encouraged to maintain a low-sodium, moderate-carbohydrate, low-fat diet to counteract the effects of excess hormone.

An exercise plan should be initiated with gradual resumption of activities. Such a program enhances cardiovascular health and builds muscle and bone tissues that become weakened in cases of Cushing's syndrome. Hypertension should be monitored on a long-term basis because treatment may be required for persistent hypertension in spite of removal of tumor tissue.

Collaborative Management in Adrenal Disorders

Collaborative care will involve the primary care provider, endocrinologist, surgeon, pharmacist, and nutritionist. Management of these rare disorders will require specialized expertise for optimal results. Communication and coordination among members of the health care team will be essential as the patient moves from clinic to hospital to home settings. Patient support and instruction on these complex medical problems will help to allay anxiety and decrease stress. Instruction and involvement of family members is essential given that patients may have to rely on family members for assistance in the event of a medical crisis.

Cultural and Genetic Considerations for Adrenal Disorders

Individuals with congenital or long-term adrenal insufficiency and patients with successful surgical treatment of pituitary tumors may require a lifetime of replacement hormone therapy. In some cultures, a need for continued therapy will stigmatize the individual as "sick" or illness prone, making it more difficult for the individual to maintain a normal life. Patient's and families may not be aware that one of the most famous U.S. presidents, John F. Kennedy, had Addison's disease and in spite of a heavy regimen of medications he was able to stand for election and serve in one of the most demanding jobs in the world. Patients should be encouraged to become as well informed about their disease as possible to enhance effective self-care of adrenal insufficiency.

Autoimmune disorders and congenital adrenal hyperplasia, genetics, and pituitary tumor development cause adrenal insufficiency through either hypo- or hypermetabolic function of the adrenal glands. Early screening of newborns will help to prevent avoidable deaths due to adrenal crisis that may go unrecognized. Parents also may benefit from genetic counseling, which will explain how a disease such as congenital adrenal hyperplasia or other disorders are inherited and options for future pregnancies. Research on genetic causes of adrenal disorders and potential gene therapies offer much potential for the future.

Research

Significant advances have been made in the diagnoses and treatment of endocrine disorders in recent years due to the development of new diagnostic imaging technologies, an immunoassay test of hormones, improved laboratory techniques for genetic studies, and new synthetic hormones and hormone agonists. The development of minimally invasive surgeries for pituitary, parathyroid, and adrenal tumors has been beneficial in the treatment of endocrine disorders. There have also been significant advances in the understanding of genetic factors underlying many endocrine disorders. The role of infection, stress, autoimmune disease, and genetics continues to impact the exploration of endocrine disease etiology and pathology. The field of genetics, genetic counseling, and gene therapy all hold significant promise in endocrinology in the future.

Improvement in clinical management of endocrine diseases is another important frontier in research. Although medical and surgical interventions, as well as hormone replacement therapy, have reaped big rewards in patient management and outcomes, some patients report decreased quality of life despite treatment. This suggests that although hormone levels may appear to be normal after therapy is initiated in endocrine disease, other complex physiological and psychological factors are at play in restoring patients to optimal health. Nurses in ambulatory clinics could play a role in investigating quality-of-life issues for patients with endocrine disease.

Many of the endocrine problems described in this chapter are rare, but they are very debilitating and even life threatening when they occur. Prevention of these diseases offers the most hope for optimal clinical impact because usually when endocrine disorders are established, the treatment is for a lifetime. Increasing the genetic screening of infants at birth for potentially treatable endocrine diseases such as congenital adrenal hyperplasia would certainly save lives. Studies on the genetic etiology of endocrine disease and potential gene therapy also offer significant potential benefits in terms of disease prevention. However, ethical questions abound and funding for this kind of research may not be seen as a top priority.

Other avenues of research that could have a significant clinical impact are those that focus on early identification and treatment of hormonal disorders such as severe hypo- or hyperthyroidism, Cushing's syndrome, gigantism, and acromegaly. Early diagnosis would prevent some of the irreversible physiological changes that occur with such diseases. Studies to determine the etiology of autoimmune disorders of the endocrine glands also hold promise for prevention and treatment. The endocrine system is exquisitely designed to maintain homeostasis in the body in spite of rapidly changing environmental conditions. Disease disrupts and interferes with the exquisite balance and adaptability that exists in an optimally functioning endocrine system. In this situation, regaining optimal health is a bit like putting Humpty Dumpty back together again. Advances in biochemistry, technology, genetics, and pharmacology all offer hope in the search for cures and care of the patient with endocrine problems.

Clinical Preparation

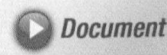

Read

- History of Current Illness
- Past Medical History
- Physical Exam
- Admitting Medical Orders
- Laboratory Study Results

Document

- Summary of Hospitalization
- Pathophysiology Form
- Laboratory Values
- Laboratory Results Explanation

Apply

- List of Potential Nursing Diagnoses
- Concept Map
- Critical Thinking Questions

Log on to MyNursingKit.com to download forms you will need and to complete further steps in the Clinical Preparation assignment.

HISTORY OF PRESENT ILLNESS

Mrs. B is a 49-year-old female who has been seen in your clinic for her primary health care needs for several years. On a recent visit, you note that she has gained approximately 20 pounds during the past year. She complains of constant fatigue, cold intolerance, and difficulty concentrating. She indicates that her performance at work has declined, that she does not feel as mentally alert as usual, and that she is slower to complete tasks than previously.

Medical–Surgical History

Mrs. B has had an unremarkable medical history with the exception of a short episode of rheumatoid arthritis in her early 30s. The disease responded well to treatment and she has been in remission since that time. Until now she has maintained good physical health. She takes no medications except a daily multivitamin and an occasional aspirin. She has had no surgeries. Regular Pap smears and mammograms have been negative for disease.

Social History

Mrs. B does not smoke, and drinks alcohol only rarely. She works as an administrative assistant in a local engineering firm. She is divorced and a single parent with two healthy adult children.

Physical Examination

Physical examination reveals dry skin and hair that is dry and thinning in spots. The thyroid gland appears enlarged upon palpation. Lungs are clear. The abdomen is slightly distended. Abdominal sounds are diminished and, upon questioning, the patient reports recent bouts of constipation. Vital signs are within normal limits.

Laboratory Studies

Laboratory studies to assess the level of free T_4 and TSH are completed. The TSH level is high and the free T_4 level is low, indicating an underfunctioning thyroid.

Nursing Care

The patient is given a prescription for thyroid hormone replacement therapy and instructed about its use. She is to take levothyroxine each day early in the morning on an empty stomach. Follow-up appointments are scheduled for 8-week intervals during the next 6 months for continued evaluation of hormone levels to determine whether the dosage is adequate, symptoms abate, and the thyroid gland changes in size. The patient is encouraged to increase fluid and dietary fiber intake and exercise to reduce constipation and to aid in weight loss.

CRITICAL THINKING QUESTIONS

1. Identify prevailing symptoms of Mrs. B, with underlying rationale, that led to assessing her for hypothyroidism.

2. Explain the relevance of a low T_4 level and high TSH level in arriving at a diagnosis of hypothyroidism.

3. In developing an outpatient plan of care for the home setting, what key elements with rationale would you consider discussing with Mrs. B?

Answers to Critical Thinking Questions appear in Appendix D.

NCLEX® REVIEW

1. A patient is diagnosed with gastric and duodenal ulcers. The nurse realizes that this patient might experience alterations in which of the following hormones?
   1. Progesterone
   2. Enterogastrone
   3. Angiotensinogen
   4. Calcitriol

2. A 13-year-old patient is diagnosed with an overproduction of a hormone produced by the anterior pituitary gland. The nurse realizes this patient is experiencing:
   1. Gigantism.
   2. Acromegaly.
   3. Sheehan's syndrome.
   4. Infertility.

3. A patient with hypothyroidism is prescribed levothyroxine. Which of the following should the nurse instruct this patient?
   1. Take with an antacid.
   2. Take the medication first thing in the morning on an empty stomach.
   3. Expect the symptoms to subside immediately.
   4. This medication is taken temporarily until the symptoms subside.

4. A patient is admitted with palpitations, hand tremors, muscle weakness, and muscle cramps. Which of the following endocrine disorders should be considered as the cause of this patient's symptoms?
   1. Pheochromocytoma
   2. Hyperthyroidism
   3. Hypothyroidism
   4. Diabetes insipidus

5. The nurse is planning discharge instructions for a patient with diabetes insipidus. Which of the following should be included in these instructions?
   1. The need for frequent rest periods
   2. Strategies to have access to fluids at all times
   3. Availability of high sodium foods
   4. Progressive ambulation activities

6. An elderly patient recovering from back surgery is demonstrating signs of hypothermia. Which of the following should the nurse do to assist this patient?
   1. Increase fluids.
   2. Provide oxygen.
   3. Consider the onset of myxedema coma and contact the health care provider.
   4. Provide warm blankets.

7. A patient recovering from an endocrine disorder tells the nurse that even though the hormone levels are considered "normal," she still feels "terrible." Which of the following should the nurse respond to this patient?
   1. What part of your life is terrible?
   2. That is to be expected.
   3. Everyone goes through this.
   4. I'm sure that you will feel better in time.

Answers for review questions appear in Appendix D

KEY TERMS

acromegaly *p.1639*
Addisonian crisis (adrenal crisis) *p.1648*
Addison's disease *p.1647*
adrenal insufficiency *p.1648*
chronic lymphocytic thyroiditis *p.1618*
Chvostek's sign *p.1633*
cretinism *p.1617*
Cushing's syndrome *p.1651*
diabetes insipidus (DI) *p.1642*
euthyroid *p.1622*
exophthalmus *p.1626*
galactorrhea *p.1639*
gigantism *p.1639*

goiter *p.1619*
goitrogen *p.1619*
Graves' disease *p.1625*
Hashimoto's thyroiditis *p.1618*
hyperparathyroidism *p.1633*
hyperthyroidism *p.1614*
hypoparathyroidism *p.1633*
hypopituitarism *p.1637*
hypothyroidism *p.1614*
myxedema *p.1619*
myxedema coma *p.1624*
negative feedback *p.1613*
osteitis fibrosa cystica *p.1634*

panhypopituitarism *p.1637*
pheochromocytoma *p.1654*
primary adrenal insufficiency *p.1648*
psychogenic polydipsia *p.1643*
secondary adrenal insufficiency *p.1648*
syndrome of inappropriate antidiuretic hormone (SIADH) *p.1644*
thyroid storm *p.1627*
thyroidectomy *p.1618*
thyroiditis *p.1619*
thyromegaly *p.1626*
thyrotoxicosis *p.1625*
Trousseau's sign *p.1633*

REFERENCES

American Association of Clinical Endocrinologists. (2005a). *Hashimoto's thyroiditis: Information for patients.* Retrieved September 19, 2005, from http://www.aace.com/members/brochures.php

American Association of Clinical Endocrinologists. (2005b). *Hyperthyroidism: Information for patients.* Retrieved September 19, 2005, from http://www.aace.com/members/brochures.php

American Association of Clinical Endocrinologists. (2005c). *Hypothyroidism: Information for patients.* Retrieved September 19, 2005, from http://www.aace.com/members/brochures.php

American Association of Clinical Endocrinologists. (2005d). *The thyroid nodule: Information for patients.* Retrieved September 19, 2005, from http://www.aace.com/members/brochures.php

American Cancer Society. (2006). *Do we know what causes pituitary tumors?* Retrieved June 12, 2008, from http://www.cancer.org/docroot/CRI/content/CRI_2_4_2X_Do_we_know_what_causes_pituitary_tumors_61.asp?rnav=cri

American Thyroid Association. (2005). *ATA Alliance for Thyroid Patient Education.* Retrieved September 19, 2005, from http://www.thyroid.org/patients/links.html

American Urological Association. (2006). *Pheochromocytoma.* Accessed March 7, 2006, from http://www.UrologyHealth.org.adult/index

Anderson, T. (2002). *Atlas of pathophysiology.* Springhouse, PA: Springhouse Corporation.

Baird, A., Sullivan, T., Zafar, S., & Rock, J. (2003). Quality of life in patients with pituitary tumors: A preliminary study. *Quality Management in Health Care, 12*(2), 97–105.

Bayless, P. (2003). The syndrome of inappropriate antidiuretic hormone secretion. *International Journal of Biochemistry and Cellular Biology, 35,* 1495–1499.

Bharaktiya, S., Orlander, P. R., Woodhouse, W. R., & Davis, A. B. (2007). Hypothyroidism. *eMedicine.* Retrieved June 19, 2008, from http://www.emedicine.com/med/topic1145.htm

Boscaro, M., Barzon, L., Fallo, F., & Sonino, N. (2001). Cushing's syndrome. *Lancet, 357,* 783–791.

Braunwald, E., Hauser, S. L., Fauci, A. S., Longo, D. L., Kasper, D. L., & Jameson, J. L. (2001). *Harrison's principles of internal medicine* (15th ed.). New York: McGraw-Hill.

Carr, S. (2001). Acromegaly management in the community. *Journal of the American Geriatric Society, 50*(5), 970–972.

Chan, M., Ziebert, M., Maas, D., & Chan, P. (2005). Photo quiz: "My rings won't fit anymore." *American Family Physician, 71*(9), 1766–1767.

Colorado State University. (2000). *Pathophysiology of the endocrine system.* Retrieved on March 6, 2003, from http://www.colostate.edu

Colorado State University. (2003). *Congenital adrenal hyperplasia.* Retrieved March 8, 2006, from http://www.colostate.edu

Cooper, D. S. (2005). Antithyroid drugs. *New England Journal of Medicine, 352*(9), 905–917.

Cooperman, M. (2008). Diabetes insipidus. *eMedicine.* Retrieved June 12, 2008, from http://www.emedicine.com/med/topic543.htm

Coursin, D. B., & Wood, K. E. (2002). Corticosteroid supplementation for adrenal insufficiency. *Journal of the American Medical Association, 287*(2), 236–240.

Dahlen, R. (2002). Managing patients with acute thyrotoxicosis. *Critical Care Nurse, 22*(1), 62–69.

Dorton, A. M. (2000). The pituitary gland: Embryology, physiology, and pathophysiology. *Neonatal Network, 19*(2), 9–17.

Elliott, B. (2000). Diagnosing and treating hypothyroidism. *The Nurse Practitioner, 25*(3), 92–103.

EndocrineWeb. (2002a). *Hyperthyroidism, overactivity of the thyroid gland. Part 2: Causes of hyperthyroidism.* Retrieved September 19, 2005, from http://endocrineweb.com/hyper2.html

EndocrineWeb. (2002b). *Pheochromocytoma.* Retrieved March 10, 2006, from http://endocrineweb.com/pheo.html

Ezell, J. (2006). What is secondary adrenal insufficiency? *Nursing, 36*(5).

Fenton, C. L., Gold, J. G., & Sadeghi-Nejad, A. (2006). Hyperthyroidism. *eMedicine.* Retrieved June 8, 2008, from http://www.emedicine.com/ped/TOPIC1088.HTM

Ferry, R. J., & Pascual-y-Baralt, J. F. (2007). Syndrome of inappropriate antidiuretics hormone secretion. *eMedicine.* Retrieved June 12, 2008, from http://www.emedicine.com/ped/topic2190.htm

Ferry, R. J., & Shim, M. (2006). Hyperpituitarism. *eMedicine.* Retrieved June 12, 2008, from http://www.emedicine.com/PED/topic1092.htm

Franklin, J. A., Sheppard, M. C., & Maisonneuve, P. (2005). Thyroid function and mortality in patients treated for hyperthyroidism. *Journal of the American Medical Association, 294*(1), 71–80.

Gonzalez-Campoy, J. M. (2007). Hypoparathyroidism. *eMedicine.* Retrieved June 12, 2008, from http://www.emedicine.com/MEDS/Topic1131.htm

Greco, L. K. (2001). Hypothyroid emergencies. *Topics in Emergency Medicine, 23*(4), 44–50.

Greenspan, F. S. (2004). The thyroid gland. In F. S. Greenspan & D. G. Gardner (Eds.), *Basic and clinical endocrinology* (7th ed., pp. 215–294). New York: Lang Medical Books/McGraw-Hill.

Harris, C. (2007). Recognizing thyroid storm in the neurologically impaired patient. *Journal of Neuroscience Nursing, 39*(1), 40–42, 57.

HealthAtoZ. (2002). *Hyperaldosteronism.* Retrieved March 8, 2006, from http://www.healthatoz.com

Holcomb, S. (2002a). Diabetes insipidus. *Dimensions of Critical Care Nursing, 21*(3), 94–97.

Holcomb, S. (2002b). Stopping the cascade of diabetes insipidus. *Nursing, 32*(3), 32cc1–32cc2, 32cc4, 32cc6.

Holcomb, S. (2002c). Thyroid diseases: A primer for the critical care nurse. *Dimensions of Critical Care Nursing, 21*(4), 127–133.

Holcomb, S. (2003). Detecting thyroid disease, Part 1. *Nursing, 33*(8), 32cc1–32cc4.

Holcomb, S. (2005). Confronting Cushing's syndrome. *Nursing, 35*(9), 32hn1–32hn6.

Holcomb, S. (2006). Do the clues add up to Addison's disease? *Nursing 2006, 36*(3), 64hn1–64hn4.

Hollowell, J. G., Staehling, N. W., Flanders, W. D., Hannon, H., Gunter, E. W., Spencer C. A., et al. (2002). Serum TSH, T_4, and thyroid antibodies in the United States population (1988 to 1994): National Health and Nutrition Examination Survey (NHANES III). *Journal of Clinical Endocrinology & Metabolism, 87*(2), 489–499.

Hormone Foundation. (2006). *Endocrine glands.* Retrieved January 24, 2006, from http://www.hormone.org/endo101/index.html

Innis, J. (2002a). Recognizing lithium induced diabetes insipidus. *Nursing, 32*(6), 32cc12, 32cc15.

Innis, J. (2002b). Treating nephrogenic diabetes insipidus. *Dimensions of Critical Care Nursing, 21*(3), 98–99.

Jordan, S. (2005). Prescription drugs: Uses and effects. Thyroid disorders: Symptom control. *Nursing Standard, 19*(23), 56–58.

Kattah, J. (2006). Pituitary tumors. *EMedicine.* Retrieved August 28, 2008 from http://www.emedicine.com/NEURO/topic312.htm

Kajantie, E., Phillips, D. I., Osmond, C., Barker, D. J., Forsen, T., & Eriksson, J. G. (2006). Spontaneous hypothyroidism in adult women is predicated by small body size at birth and during childhood. *Journal of Endocrinology Metabolism, 91*(12), 4953–4958.

Katznelson, L. (2006). *Medical management of acromegaly with octreotide.* Retrieved March 7, 2006, from Massachusetts General Hospital website: http://pituitary.mgh.edu/e-f-943.htm

Kirk, L. F., Hash, R. B., Katner, H. P., & Jones, T. (2000). Cushing's disease: Clinical manifestations and diagnostic evaluation. *American Family Physician, 62*(5), 1119–1127, 1133–1134.

Langfeldt, L. A., & Cooley, M. E. (2003). Syndrome of inappropriate antidiuretic hormone secretion in malignancy: Review and implications for nursing management. *Clinical Journal of Oncology Nursing, 7*(4), 425–430.

Larson, J., Anderson, E., & Koslawy, M. (2000). Thyroid disease: A review for primary care. *Journal of the American Academy of Nurse Practitioners, 12*(6), 226–232.

Laws, E. R., Vance, M. L., & Thapar, K. (2000). Pituitary surgery for the management of acromegaly. *Hormone Research, 53*(Suppl. 3), 71–75.

Loffing, J. (2004). Paradoxical antidiuretics effect of thiazides in diabetes insipidus: Another piece in the puzzle. *Journal of the American Society of Nephrology, 15,* 2948–2950.

Løvås, K., & Husebye, E. S. (2005). Addison's disease. *Lancet 365*(9476), 2058–2061.

Luken, K. K. (1999). Pearls for practice: Clinical manifestations and management of Addison's disease. *Journal of the American Academy of Nurse Practitioners, 11*(4), 151–154.

Mayo Clinic. (2005). *Primary aldosteronism.* Retrieved from http://www.mayclinic.com/health/primary-aldosteronism

Mayo Clinic. (2006). *Sheehan's syndrome.* Retrieved February 10, 2006, from http://www.mayoclinic.com/health/sheehans-syndrome/AN01084

Medline Plus. (2001). *Cabergoline (systemic).* Retrieved March 7, 2006, from http://www.nlm.nih.gov/medlineplus/druginfo/uspdi/203584.html

Medline Plus. (2004). *Prolactinoma.* Retrieved March 7, 2006, from http://www.nlm.nih.gov/medlineplus/ency/article/000336.htm

Medline Plus. (2005). *Octreotide (systemic).* Retrieved March 7, 2006, from http://www.nlm.nih.gov/medlineplus/druginfo/uspdi/202421.html

Mulatero, P., Stowasser, M., Loh, K., Fardella, C., Gordon, R., Mosso, L., et al. (2004). Increased diagnosis of primary aldosteronism, including surgically correctable forms, in centers from five continents. *The Journal of Clinical Endocrinology & Metabolism, 80*(3), 1045–1050. Retrieved March 8, 2006, from http://jcen.endojournals.org

National Adrenal Diseases Foundation. (2006a). *Adrenal diseases—Addison's disease.* Retrieved January 24, 2006, from http://www.medhelp.org/nadf/diseases/addisons.htm

National Adrenal Diseases Foundation. (2006b). *Adrenal diseases—Cushing's syndrome.* Retrieved January 24, 2006, from http://www.medhelp.org/nadf/diseases/cushings.htm

Neafsey, P. J. (2004). Levothyroxine and calcium interaction: Timing is everything. *Home Health Nurse, 22*(5), 338–339.

Nephrogenic Diabetes Insipidus Foundation. (2005a). *Facts and statistics: Definition.* Retrieved February 12, 2006, from http://www.ndif.org/facts/html

Nephrogenic Diabetes Insipidus Foundation. (2005b). *Facts and statistics: Description.* Retrieved February 12, 2006, from http://www.ndif.org/facts/html

Odeke, S., & Nagelbereg, S. B. (2006). Addison disease. *eMedicine.* Retrieved June 8, 2008, from http://www.emedicine.com/med/TOPIC42.HTM

Pavlovich-Danis, S. (2006). Zemplar: New treatment option for secondary hyperparathyroidism. *Nursing Spectrum, 16*(6), 23.

Pfadt, E., & Carlson, D. (2006). Action stat: Acute adrenal crisis. *Nursing 2006, 36*(8), 80.

Physician's drug handbook (11th ed.). (2005). Philadelphia: Lippincott Williams & Wilkins.

Pituitary Disorders Education & Support. (2006a). *Pituitary conditions and treatment.* Retrieved February 10, 2006, from www.pituitarydisorder.net/pituitary_conditions_treatments.html

Pituitary Network Association. (2006a). *Adrenal insufficiency: Secondary Addison's or Addison's disease.* Retrieved February 10, 2006, from http://www.pituitary.org/disorders/addisons_disease.aspx

Pituitary Network Association. (2006b). Adult growth hormone (GH). Deficiency. Retrieved February 10, 2006, from http://www.pituitary.org/disorders/gh_deficiency.aspx

Pituitary Network Association. (2006c). *Endocrine—inactive (i.e., non-functional tumors).* Retrieved February 10, 2006, from http://www.pituitary.org/disorders/non-functioning_tumors.aspx

Pituitary Network Association. (2006e). *Hypopituitarism.* Retrieved February 10, 2006, from http://www.pituitary.org/disorders/hypopituitarism.aspx

Porsche, R., & Brenner, Z. (2006). Amiodarone-induced thyroid dysfunction. *Critical Care Nurse, 26*(3), 34–42.

Porth, C. M. (2007). *Essentials of pathophysiology: Concepts of altered health states* (2nd ed.). Philadelphia: Lippincott Williams & Wilkins.

Sachse, D. (2001). Acromegaly. *American Journal of Nursing, 101*(11), 69, 71, 73–75.

Shah, N. (2006).Unexplained weakness in a newly diagnosed hypertensive. *Clinical Advisor for Nurse Practitioners, 9*(10), 106.

Shirk, M. (2003). Hallelujah! A case of steroid psychosis and unorthodox intervention. *American Journal of Nursing, 103*(9), 31.

Song, J. K., & Weil, R. J. (2005). Pathologic quiz case: An unusual cause of acromegaly. *Archives of Pathology and Laboratory Medicine, 129*(3), 415–416.

Takasu, N., Takara, M., & Komiya, I. (2005). Rifampin-induced hypothyroidism in patients with Hashimoto's thyroiditis. *New England Journal of Medicine, 352*(5), 518–519.

Tangiera, E. C. (2004). Hyperparathyroidism. *American Family Physician, 69,* 333–340.

Teng, W., et al. (2006). Effect of iodine intake on thyroid diseases in China. *New England Journal of Medicine, 354*(26), 2783–2793.

Terpstra, T. L., & Terpstra, T. L. (2000). CESieries: Syndrome of inappropriate antidiuretic hormone secretion: Recognition and management. *MEDSURG Nursing, 9*(2), 61–68.

Thyroid Federation International. (2003). *Thyroid videos online.* Retrieved September 19, 2005, from http://www.thyroid-fed.org./intro/thyroidvideos.html

Thyroid Foundation of America (2004a). Thyroid disorders and treatments: Overview. Retrieved August 21, 2005, and September 19, 2005, from http://www.allthyroid.org/disorders/ondex.html

Thyroid Foundation of America (2004b). Thyroid patient organizations. Retrieved September 19, 2005, from http://www.allthyroid.org/resources/patient.html

Urbano, F. L. (2000). Signs of hypocalcemia: Chvostek's and Trousseau's signs. *Hospital Physician,* March 2000, 43–45.

Waltman, P. A., Brewer, J. M., & Lobert, S. (2004). Thyroid storm during pregnancy: A medical emergency. *Critical Care Nursing, 24*(2), 74–79.

Whiteman, K. (2006). ACTH stimulation: Testing the Adrenals. *Nursing, 36*(7), 24–25.

Yeung, S. C. J., & Habra, M. A. (2007). Graves' disease. *eMedicine.* Retrieved June 12, 2008, from http://www.emedicine.com/med/TOPIC929.HTM

Caring for the Patient with Diabetes

Laurie Quinn

With contributions by:
Cynthia Fritschi

Outcome-Based Learning Objectives

After studying this chapter, the learner will be able to:

1. Discuss the epidemiology of diabetes and pre-diabetes (impaired glucose tolerance and impaired fasting glucose).
2. Differentiate between the classifications of pre-diabetes and diabetes as they relate to clinical manifestations and health care management.
3. Compare and contrast the pathophysiology of pre-diabetes and diabetes.
4. Identify the major acute and chronic complications associated with diabetes.
5. Identify risk factors for adults associated with the development of pre-diabetes and diabetes.
6. Discuss the pharmacologic and nutritional management of diabetes as contrasted between diabetes type 1 and type 2.
7. Discuss the role of physical activity and exercise in the prevention and treatment of diabetes.
8. Describe the clinical signs and symptoms, diagnosis, medical therapy, nursing assessment, and management of diabetes.
9. Compare and contrast the clinical signs and symptoms, diagnosis, treatment, nursing assessment, and management of diabetic ketoacidosis, hyperglycemic hyperosmolar syndrome, and hypoglycemia.
10. Describe the prevention, progression, clinical signs and symptoms, nursing assessment, and management of lower extremity disease as it relates to diabetes.

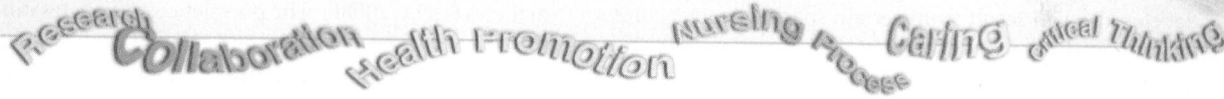

Research Collaboration Health Promotion Nursing Process Caring Critical Thinking

DIABETES MELLITUS (DM) is a disorder of carbohydrate, protein, and fat metabolism resulting from an imbalance between insulin availability and insulin need. It is not actually a single disease but a group of metabolic disorders characterized by **hyperglycemia** (high blood glucose) resulting from defects in insulin secretion, insulin action, or both (DeFronzo, 2004). The hormone **insulin,** which is secreted by the beta cells of the islets of Langerhans, is used by the body to break down blood sugars and starches into energy. Diabetes can represent an absolute insulin deficiency, impaired release of insulin by the **pancreatic beta cells,** inadequate or defective insulin receptors, or the production of defective insulin that is destroyed before it can carry out its action (Porth, 2007). The intent of this chapter is to discuss diabetes mellitus and abnormal glucose tolerance generally, and then specifically as the concepts apply to the hospitalized patient with diabetes.

The most recent criteria for the diagnosis and classification of diabetes and abnormal glucose tolerance were published by the American Diabetes Association (ADA) in 1997 with minor updates since that time (American Diabetes Association, 2007). These newer criteria are based on the etiology of diabetes rather than the phenotypical presentation of the disease. In the past when an understanding of the mechanisms underlying the cause of diabetes was less mature, its classification was either related to age or conventional treatment regimens (e.g., diet, insulin, oral medications). These newer classification criteria allow for the diagnosis and classification of five types of diabetes and pre-diabetes: type 1 diabetes, type 2 diabetes, gestational diabetes mellitus, other types of diabetes, and pre-diabetes. Type 1 and type 2 diabetes are the most common forms of diabetes. The development of both type 1 and type 2 diabetes is initiated by interplay between genetics and the environment.

Type 1 diabetes mellitus (DM) is a catabolic, autoimmune disorder in which circulating insulin is very low or absent and plasma glucagon is elevated. The pancreas shows lymphocytic infiltration and destruction of insulin-secreting cells of the islets of Langerhans, causing insulin deficiency. Patients need exogenous insulin to reverse this catabolic condition, prevent ketosis, decrease hyperglucagonemia, and normalize lipid and protein metabolism (Hussain & Vincent, 2007). Type 1 diabetes, previously referred to as juvenile diabetes mellitus, insulin-dependent diabetes mellitus, and type I diabetes mellitus, affects 5% to 10%

of the diabetes population (Centers for Disease Control and Prevention [CDC], 2005). This type of diabetes is associated with destruction of the pancreatic beta cells, the cells that secrete insulin. In the majority of people with type 1 diabetes, the destruction is mediated by an autoimmune process. Because individuals with type 1 diabetes produce no insulin, they require pharmacologic insulin therapy for survival.

Type 1 diabetes can occur at any age, but is frequently diagnosed before 30 years of age; however, there is an adult form of autoimmune type 1 diabetes termed **latent autoimmune diabetes in adults (LADA)** (Pozzilli & Di Mario, 2001). In addition, there are uncommon forms of non–immune-mediated forms of type 1 diabetes. Individuals with type 1 diabetes are usually thin or normal weight at diagnosis and have an abrupt onset of symptoms. In addition, those with type 1 diabetes are more prone to the development of diabetic ketoacidosis, an acute life-threatening complication.

Type 2 diabetes mellitus, previously referred to as adult-onset diabetes or non–insulin-dependent diabetes mellitus (NIDDM) or simply type 2 diabetes, describes a condition of hyperglycemia that occurs despite the availability of insulin (referred to as relative insulin deficiency). Unlike type 1 diabetes mellitus, patients are not absolutely dependent on insulin for life, even though many of these patients are ultimately treated with insulin (Ligaray & Isley, 2007). Type 2 diabetes usually is diagnosed after the age of 30 years, but is beginning to occur more frequently at younger ages. Individuals with type 2 diabetes are not dependent on exogenous insulin to sustain life; however, insulin therapy and/or oral medications may be needed to control hyperglycemia. These individuals are often obese and have a strong family history of type 2 diabetes.

Diabetes also can result from certain specific genetic conditions (e.g., maturity onset-diabetes of the young), surgery (e.g., pancreatectomy), drugs (e.g., corticosteroids), infections (e.g., congenital rubella), and other illness. The initial diagnosis and clinical presentation of the diabetes in this group varies with the underlying disorder. **Maturity onset diabetes of the young (MODY)** is an autosomal dominant subtype of type 2 diabetes that is often diagnosed at younger ages (Tattersall, 1998). An important point is that MODY is not early-onset type 2 diabetes; it is instead a group of monogenetic (single-gene) defects resulting in impaired insulin secretion (Malecki & Klupa, 2005). The clinical presentation of MODY usually is associated with mild hyperglycemia. MODY typically presents in children or during young adulthood and is inherited as an autosomal dominant pattern (Velho & Robert, 2002).

Gestational diabetes mellitus (GDM) refers to a condition in which the onset of diabetes is first diagnosed during pregnancy. This form of abnormal glucose tolerance affects about 4% of pregnancies or 135,000 women in the United States annually (CDC, 2005). Though a specific cause has not been identified, it most commonly affects women with a family history of diabetes, those with glycosuria, and those with a history of stillbirth or spontaneous abortion. Other possible considerations include advanced maternal age and five or more previous pregnancies (Porth, 2007). It also is believed that the hormones produced during pregnancy reduce a woman's sensitivity to insulin, resulting in high blood sugar levels.

Those diagnosed with GDM require dietary treatment and possibly insulin therapy to control hyperglycemia. Uncontrolled hyperglycemia during pregnancy can result in fetal and maternal complications. Gestational diabetes mellitus poses an increased risk for the development of type 2 diabetes with as many as 50% of women with GDM developing type 2 diabetes later in life (CDC, 2005).

Pre-diabetes is a term used to identify people who are at increased risk for developing diabetes. Pre-diabetes can be determined in two different ways. Patients may have fasting plasma glucose levels above normal or they may have abnormal results on an oral glucose tolerance test. In either case the results are abnormal but do not meet the diagnostic criteria for diabetes. The two types of glucose intolerance included in this category include **impaired fasting glucose (IFG)** (a condition that exists when blood sugar levels are higher than normal but not high enough to say that one has diabetes) and **impaired glucose tolerance (IGT)**. IGT is a pre-diabetic state of dysglycemia that is associated with insulin resistance and increased risk of cardiovascular pathology. Individuals with pre-diabetes are at increased risk for developing type 2 diabetes. Approximately 41 million individuals in the United States have pre-diabetes (CDC, 2005).

Epidemiology and Etiology of Diabetes and Other Forms of Glucose Intolerance

The prevalence of diabetes for all age groups worldwide has been estimated to be 6.0% or 246 million in the year 2007 (International Diabetes Federation, 2006). Approximately 23.5 million or 10.7% of the U.S. population over 20 years of age has diabetes (ADA, 2008f). The prevalence of diabetes differs by factors such as race, ethnicity, and geographic location. Some of these factors are explored in the following paragraphs.

Its increasing prevalence has deemed diabetes mellitus a major public health problem in the United States that is affecting millions of individuals, of which an estimated 6.6 million are undiagnosed. From 2002 to 2007, the number of individuals diagnosed with diabetes increased from 12.1 to 17.5 million. In addition, an estimated 54 million individuals have abnormalities in glucose tolerance that place them at high risk for developing diabetes (ADA, 2008f). The global prevalence of diabetes is expected to increase from 171 million in the year 2000 to 366 million in the year 2030 (Wild, Roglic, Green, Sicree, & King, 2004). Among those born in the United States during the year 2000, the lifetime probability of developing diabetes is 32.8% for males and 38.5% for females (Narayan, Boyle, Thompson, Sorensen, & Williamson, 2003). Obesity, population growth, aging, urbanization, and physical inactivity are primary factors accounting for this epidemic.

A variety of serious acute and chronic complications are associated with diabetes. The acute complications are medical emergencies and include diabetic ketoacidosis, hyperosmolar hyperglycemic syndrome, and hypoglycemia. The chronic complications include disorders associated with **microvascular** (small vessel) changes in the eyes, nerves, and kidneys, along with **macrovascular** (large vessel) changes in the heart, veins and arteries. These changes result in retinopathy (eye disease), neuropathy (nerve disease), nephropathy (kidney disease), and accelerated development of coronary heart disease (CHD), cerebrovascular disease, and peripheral vascular disease (PVD). These complications are associated with excessive morbidity and mortality from heart disease, blindness, kidney failure, extremity amputations, and other chronic conditions.

Diabetes and its related complications are associated with significant personal, social, and economic costs. The economic impact of diabetes and diabetic complications on the U.S. economy is substantial. Medical expenditures attributed to diabetes in 2007 were estimated at $174 billion including $116 billion dollars in medical costs and $58 billion dollars in indirect costs (ADA, 2008f). *Direct* medical costs include expenditures related to hospital inpatient care, diabetes medications and supplies, retail prescriptions for diabetes complications, and health care provider office visits. *Indirect* medical costs include costs resulting from increased absenteeism from work, reduced productivity at work and home, unemployment, disability, and loss of productivity due to premature death (ADA, 2008f). Successful treatment of diabetes is essential for reducing the personal, social, and economic costs associated with this disorder. As the prevalence of diabetes increases, the complications of diabetes also will increase, unless aggressive treatment strategies are employed. Because patients with diabetes are so frequently seen in clinical practice, it is essential for nurses to be knowledgeable about the care and treatment of patients with diabetes. The hospitalized patient with diabetes presents a series of unique challenges. The purpose of this chapter is to explore the clinical management of the medical–surgical patient with diabetes.

Type 1 DM accounts for approximately 5% to 15% of all diagnosed diabetes (CDC, 2005; Hussain & Vincent, 2007). Approximately 1 in every 400 to 600 children and adolescents has type 1 diabetes (CDC, 2005) making it one of the most common severe chronic disorders of childhood. Type 1 diabetes affects 0.22% or 176,500 thousand people under the age of 20 years (CDC, 2005). In addition, type 1 diabetes affects approximately 1.4 million in the United States and perhaps 10 million to 20 million individuals globally (Wild et al., 2004).

Type 2 diabetes accounts for approximately 90% to 95% of all diabetes, both nationally and globally (CDC, 2005). There has been a dramatic increase in the prevalence of type 2 diabetes, especially among newly Westernized countries. Only India and China exceed the United States in the number of individuals diagnosed with diabetes (International Diabetes Federation, 2006).

Cultural and Ethnic Considerations of Diabetes Development

The prevalence of diabetes increases with age and varies among different ethnic groups. Approximately 10.6 million, or 20.9%, of the U.S. population ages 60 years or older have diabetes. Age-adjusted rates for diabetes among Mexican Americans and non-Hispanic blacks are 1.7 and 1.8 times, respectively, greater than the rate for non-Hispanic whites (CDC, 2005). In general, the U.S. prevalence of diabetes is highest in Native Americans. The total age-adjusted prevalence of diabetes among Alaska Natives and American Indians in the southern United States is 8.1% and 27%, respectively. Total prevalence data are not available for Asian Americans or Pacific Islanders. In Hawaii, however, Native Hawaiians, Asians, and other Pacific Islanders over 20 years of age have age-adjusted rates of diagnosed diabetes that are more than two times those of non-Hispanic whites (CDC, 2005).

Type 2 diabetes, a disease traditionally associated with adults, has been increasing among children and adolescents. There are no large-scale epidemiologic studies on the prevalence of type 2 diabetes in children and adolescents. A variety of clinic-based reports and small population studies, however, indicate that this increased prevalence of type 2 diabetes among youth is highest among Native American, African American, and Hispanic youth (Bobo et al., 2004; Fagot-Campagna et al., 2000; Rosenbloom, House, & Winter, 1998; Rosenbloom, Joe, Young, & Winter, 1999; Young & Rosenbloom, 1998). In these reports, the percentage of type 2 diabetes among children and adolescents with pediatric diabetes has increased from <5% before 1994 to 30% to 50% in subsequent years (Fagot-Campagna et al., 2000; Kaufman, 2002; Ligaray & Isley, 2007).

■ Normal Physiology of Fuel Metabolism

The pancreas is located in the posterior portion of the upper abdomen and is divided into the exocrine and endocrine pancreas. Chapters 51 and 52 ⊙ provide more information on endocrine assessment and glandular and hormonal disorders. The exocrine pancreas produces hormones primarily involved in digestion, whereas the endocrine pancreas produces hormones associated with endocrine function.

The exocrine pancreas primarily is composed of small glands called acini, whereas the endocrine pancreas is made up of small cells called islets of Langerhans. These islet cells are distributed throughout the exocrine pancreas and are divided into the alpha cells, beta cells, delta cells, and F cells. Alpha cells secrete the hormone **glucagon**, beta cells secrete the hormone insulin, delta cells secrete the hormone somatostatin, and F cells (or pancreatic polypeptide cells) secrete the hormone **pancreatic polypeptide**. Somatostatin is a hormone that is produced in the delta cells of the pancreas and other locations, including the gastrointestinal tract and the hypothalamus. Somatostatin inhibits the release of insulin from the beta cells and glucagon from the alpha cells of the pancreas. Pancreatic polypeptide is a complex peptide hormone whose role is not entirely understood. In relation to diabetes, the most important of these hormones are insulin and glucagon. These hormones are discussed in greater detail throughout the chapter.

Interrelationships among insulin, glucagon, cortisol, growth hormone, and the catecholamines epinephrine and norepinephrine control fuel metabolism. The effects of insulin are most prominent in liver, adipose tissue, and muscle. The primary functions of insulin in these tissues include the synthesis of **glycogen** (the storage form of glucose) in liver and muscle, the synthesis of protein (a large complex molecule made up of one or more chains of amino acids) in liver and muscle, and the synthesis of triglycerides (molecules consisting of a glycerol backbone with three fatty acids) in adipose tissue and to a smaller extent in muscle.

Insulin is necessary for **glycolysis**, the biochemical pathway that results in the generation of high-energy compounds such as adenosine triphosphate (ATP) and nicotinamide adenine dinucleotide NAD and for glucose transport, the movement of glucose into insulin-sensitive tissues, such as muscle. Most importantly, insulin suppresses **gluconeogenesis** (formation of glucose from noncarbohydrate substrates), **glycogenolysis** (breakdown of glycogen to glucose), and **lipolysis** (breakdown of triglycerides to free fatty acids [FFAs] and glycerol). Insulin promotes glucose uptake and utilization in tissues. Skeletal muscle is the major site of insulin-mediated glucose disposal during the fed state (period following meals) and is critical for preventing hyperglycemia and maintaining glucose homeostasis.

Collectively, glucagon, cortisol, growth hormone, epinephrine, and norepinephrine are referred to as **counterregulatory hormones** because their actions oppose the effects of insulin. The functions of each of these hormones in intermediary metabolism are presented in Chart 53–1. Glucagon is secreted from the alpha cells of the pancreas. The primary functions of glucagon include hepatic gluconeogenesis, glycogenolysis, lipolysis, and **ketogenesis** (formation of ketones [energy substrates] from FFAs). Cortisol, a hormone secreted by the adrenal cortex, causes protein catabolism and lipolysis, therefore, providing precursors for gluconeogenesis and ketogenesis. Growth hormone, secreted by the anterior pituitary, causes lipolysis and provides precursors (glycerol and FFAs) for gluconeogenesis and ketogenesis. Of the catecholamines, epinephrine has the greatest role in fuel metabolism. This hormone is secreted by the adrenal medulla and is associated with glycogenolysis, gluconeogenesis, and lipolysis.

The primary goal following a meal is maintenance of normal blood glucose levels. Following the ingestion of carbohydrates (CHO), mainly sugars and starches, insulin levels rise and stimulate glucose uptake into insulin-sensitive tissues, primarily muscle. Glucagon levels decrease, so there is a higher ratio of insulin to glucagon. Glucose is the primary oxidative fuel for all tissues during the absorptive state. Glucose that is in excess of the oxidative needs of the major tissues is stored as glycogen or lipids.

The primary goal of fuel metabolism during the fasted state is to provide glucose for the brain and nervous tissue. The fasted state is generally considered to be 10 to 12 hours following an overnight fast. The ratio of glucagon to insulin is higher during this time. Hepatic glycogenolysis and gluconeogenesis increase plasma glucose levels. Free fatty acids, released from adipose tissue lipolysis, are oxidized by muscle for energy. As fasting continues, insulin remains suppressed, glucagon levels remain elevated, and the principal source of hepatic glucose production is gluconeogenesis. In addition, ketones can be oxidized by the brain for energy.

In summary, normal fuel metabolism is regulated by a series of complex relationships among insulin, glucagon, and other counterregulatory hormones. Normal plasma glucose levels are tightly regulated by the following three processes: hepatic glucose production, glucose uptake and utilization by peripheral tissues (primarily skeletal muscle), and the actions of insulin and counterregulatory hormones, primarily glucagon. Insulin and glucagon have opposing effects on glucose metabolism. Higher glucagon levels and lower insulin levels facilitate hepatic gluconeogenesis and glycogenolysis during fasted states, thereby preventing hypoglycemia. Fasting plasma glucose levels are determined primarily by hepatic glucose production. Plasma insulin levels increase and glucagon levels decrease as blood glucose levels rise during the fed state.

Pathophysiology and Fuel Metabolism in Diabetes

The hormonal-fuel relationships described above are abnormal in all types of diabetes. In type 1 diabetes, there is a nearly complete loss of insulin production, whereas in type 2 diabetes, there is decreased insulin production and insulin resistance. **Insulin resistance** is generally described as the inability of either endogenous or exogenous insulin to achieve its normal biologic response in its target tissues. The abnormalities of fuel metabolism associated with diabetes result from a deficiency in insulin and an increase in glucagon and other counterregulatory hormones. These hormonal abnormalities most profoundly affect the muscle, liver, and adipose tissue. Hyperglycemia results from decreased glucose transport into insulin-sensitive tissues (e.g., skeletal muscle), hepatic gluconeogenesis, and hepatic and muscle glycogenolysis. In type 1 diabetes, the increased mobilization of free fatty acids from adipose tissue leads to increased hepatic synthesis of ketone bodies and results in the acute complication of diabetic ketoacidosis. In type 2 diabetes, the amount of free fatty acids that are converted to ketone bodies is usually not sufficient for the development of diabetic ketoacidosis.

Physiological Manifestations of Systemic Complications of Diabetes Mellitus

Diabetes complications affect major body systems and organs. These major complications are discussed next.

Insulin Resistance	Insulin	Glucagon ↑	Cortisol ↑	Growth ↑ Hormone	Epinephrine/ ↑ Norepinephrine
Glycogen Synthesis	↑	↓			↓
Glycogenolysis	↓				↑
Gluconeogenesis	↓	↑	↑	↑	↑
Lipolysis	↓		↑	↑	↑
Ketogenesis	↓	↑			
Protein Synthesis	↑	—	↓	↑	
Proteolysis	↓		↑		

CHART 53–1 **Effects of Insulin and Counterregulatory Hormones on Intermediary Metabolism**

Note: ↓ = inhibits or decreases; ↑ = stimulates or increases.

Diseases of Heart and Vessels

CHD, PVD, and cerebrovascular disease are more common, occur earlier, and are more severe in people with diabetes. Heart disease death rates in adults with diabetes are about 2 to 4 times higher than in adults without diabetes (CDC, 2005). The risk for stroke is 2 to 4 times higher among people with diabetes, and about 65% of deaths among people with diabetes are due to heart disease and stroke (CDC, 2005). CHD is the leading cause of diabetes-related deaths. In the United States, more than 60% of nontraumatic amputations are in patients with diabetes and usually result from the combination of PVD and neuropathy (CDC, 2005). In 2002 about 82,000 nontraumatic lower limb amputations were performed on people with diabetes (CDC, 2005). About 75% of adults with diabetes have blood pressure readings ≥130/80 mmHg or use prescription medications for hypertension (CDC, 2005).

Kidney Disease

Diabetes is the leading cause of chronic kidney disease (CKD) in the United States, accounting for 44% of new cases annually (CDC, 2005). In 2002, in the United States and Puerto Rico, 44,400 people with diabetes began treatment for end-stage renal disease (ESRD) (CDC, 2005). In the same year, a total of 153,730 people in the United States and Puerto Rico with diabetes-related ESRD were living on chronic dialysis or with a transplanted kidney. The Third National Health and Nutrition Examination Survey (NHANES III), conducted from 1988 to 1994, obtained information on the health and nutritional status of the U.S. population through interviews and direct physical examinations. Data from NHANES III demonstrated that approximately 25% to 30% of adults with type 2 diabetes have evidence of early renal disease, as evidenced by **microalbuminuria,** small amounts of protein (30 to 299 mg/24 hours) in the urine, whereas another 5% to 13% have evidence of overt nephropathy, as evidenced by albuminuria ≥300 mg/24 hours (Harris, 2001).

Blindness and Other Visual Disorders

Diabetes remains the leading cause of new cases of blindness among adults 20 to 74 years old (CDC, 2005). Visual impairment among persons older than 50 years of age with and without diabetes has been estimated at 23.5% and 12.4%, respectively (CDC, 2004). The primary causes of visual impairment and blindness among patients with diabetes include diabetic retinopathy, cataracts, macular degeneration, and glaucoma (CDC, 2004). The prevalence of diabetic retinopathy among persons older than 50 years of age is approximately 10.2%. People with diabetes have substantially greater age-adjusted prevalence of cataracts (31.8% vs. 21.2%) and glaucoma (8.0% vs. 4.3%) than the general population (CDC, 2004). Visual disorders are discussed more in Chapter 71 🔗.

Neuropathy

About 60% to 70% of people with diabetes have mild to severe forms of nervous system damage (CDC, 2005). The results of such damage include, but are not limited to, peripheral neuropathy (e.g., impaired sensation or pain in the hands, legs, and feet) and autonomic neuropathy (e.g., delayed gastric emptying, bladder dysfunction, impotence, orthostatic hypotension, and cardiac abnormalities). Approximately 6% of U.S. hospitalizations for diabetes result from some form of neuropathy (CDC, 2005).

Complications of Pregnancy

Elevated glucose levels prior to conception and during the first trimester of pregnancy can cause major birth defects in 5% to 10% of pregnancies and spontaneous abortions in 15% to 20% of pregnancies (CDC, 2005). In addition, chronic hyperglycemia diabetes during the second and third trimesters of pregnancy can result in macrosomia (excessively large babies), resulting in neonatal and obstetrical risks (CDC, 2005).

Diabetic Ketoacidosis

Diabetic ketoacidosis (DKA) is a state of absolute or relative insulin deficiency aggravated by ensuing hyperglycemia, dehydration, and acidosis-producing derangements in intermediary metabolism. The most common causes are underlying infection, disruption of insulin treatment, and new onset of diabetes. DKA is typically characterized by hyperglycemia greater than 300 mg/dL, low bicarbonate level (<15 mEq/L), and acidosis (pH <7.30) with ketonemia and ketonuria (Porth, 2007; Rucker, 2008).

It is one of the most serious complications of diabetes and is most commonly associated with type 1 diabetes. This complication is listed on approximately 3% to 4% of all hospital discharges among people with diabetes (National Center for Chronic Disease Prevention and Health Promotion, 2004). The highest mortality rates from DKA are noted among African American males (36.8%) and elderly men and women older than 75 years of age (ADA, 2001). From 1980 to 2001, the number of deaths with DKA as the underlying cause has remained relatively stable. In 1980 there were 1,772 deaths due to DKA, and in 2001 that number was 1,871 (National Center for Chronic Disease Prevention and Health Promotion, 2004).

Hyperosmolar Hyperglycemic Syndrome

Hyperosmolar hyperglycemic syndrome (HHS) is a hyperglycemic crisis characteristically found in the elderly infirm who are unable to meet their fluid needs; however, this syndrome is beginning to occur at younger ages (ADA, 2001; Nugent, 2005). An estimated 11,000 hospital discharges mention HHS and 70% occur in those older than 64 years of age. Mortality rates for HHS range from 10% to 50% and are largely attributed to underlying illnesses (ADA, 2001).

Hypoglycemia

Hypoglycemia (low blood glucose) in patients with diabetes results from pharmacologic treatment with insulin or oral hypoglycemic medications. Prevalence rates for mild hypoglycemia are difficult to estimate because some degree of hypoglycemia is characteristically associated with intensive diabetes management. In the **Diabetes Control and Complications Trial (DCCT),** approximately 6% of the intensively treated patients had episodes of moderate to severe hypoglycemia (DCCT Trial Research Group, 1993).

▪ Risk Factors and Pathophysiology of Type 1 Diabetes

Type 1 diabetes appears to result from an interaction between genetics, environment, and autoimmunity. There is a great deal of research involving the etiology of this disorder, but the prevailing theories are detailed next.

Genetics

A familial predisposition to the development of type 1 diabetes does exist; however, the exact mode of genetic inheritance remains unclear. Among U.S. Caucasian populations, the overall risk of developing type 1 diabetes is approximately 0.2% to 0.4% (Hussain & Vincent, 2007; Porth, 2007; Muir, Schatz, & Maclaren, 1992). A sibling of a person with type 1 diabetes has a 6% risk of developing the disorder (Muir et al., 1992). The offspring of a father with type 1 diabetes has a greater chance of developing the disorder (6%) than the offspring of a mother (3%) (Muir et al., 1992). Most significantly, however, is that there is a higher concordance for type 1 diabetes among monozygotic twins (25% to 50%) than dizygotic twins (6%) (Muir et al., 1992). If the development of type 1 diabetes were determined completely by genetic inheritance, the concordance rate would be 100%. This fact that the concordance rate among identical twins is 25% to 50% supports the fact that there is an environmental trigger that initiates the transition from genetic predisposition to type 1 diabetes. The Genetic Considerations box discusses the genes involved in the development of type 1 diabetes.

Environmental

A triggering event in those at risk for developing type 1 diabetes initiates a series of autoimmune events ending in pancreatic beta-cell destruction. A variety of environmental triggers have been proposed as initiating events, but no single factor has been consistently associated with the risk of type 1 diabetes. Among the many possible initiating events, viral infections, dietary factors, and toxins have been identified as possible environmental triggers in the development of type 1 diabetes.

Congenital rubella syndrome is strongly associated with the development of type 1 diabetes, but this syndrome represents a small number of cases (Lammi, Karvonen, & Tuomilehto, 2005). The observation that children frequently develop type 1 diabetes following a viral illness has provided anecdotal evidence that a virus may be the initiating event in type 1 diabetes. In particular, it has been postulated that enteroviruses may initiate the development of type 1 diabetes in those genetically at risk for the disorder (Akerblom, Vaarala, Hyoty, Ilonen, & Knip, 2002).

Of the possible dietary etiologic factors, cow's milk proteins have received the main attention. Studies indicate an association between early exposure to dietary cow's milk proteins and an increased risk of type 1 diabetes, but the data remain controversial (Akerblom et al., 2002; Dahlquist, 1997; Gerstein, 1994; Knip, 2003). Toxins that have gained attention as possible environmental triggers for type 1 diabetes are the N-nitroso compounds. Nitrate is found in vegetables, and nitrate and nitrite are found in meat products. In the gut, nitrate is reduced to nitrite. Nitrite is transformed in the gut by reaction with amines and amides to nitrosamines and nitrosamines. Evidence such as this suggests that there is a relationship between nitrates and nitrites in type 1 diabetes, but this relationship is under investigation.

Autoimmunity

A number of circulating autoantibodies to pancreatic beta-cell components have been identified in those with type 1 diabetes. These autoantibodies include cytoplasmic islet cell antibodies (ICAs), insulin autoantibodies (IAAs), antibodies directed against the enzyme glutamic acid decarboxylase (GAD), and antibodies against islet tyrosine phosphatase (i.e., IA2 and IA2beta) (Kaufman & ADA, 2008). Unaffected relatives are at risk for the development of type 1 diabetes. The presence of two or more antibodies, together with alterations in insulin secretion, is highly predictive of the development of type 1 diabetes within 5 years (Kaufman & ADA, 2008). These autoantibodies serve as markers of an ongoing autoimmune process.

Sequence in the Development of Type 1 Diabetes

The proposed scheme for the development of type 1 diabetes is detailed in Figure 53–1 ■.

Environmental factors trigger an immune response with the development of ICAs, IAAs, and other islet cell antigens, such as GAD (Kaufman & ADA, 2008). These antibodies are markers of a progressive loss of pancreatic beta-cell mass. These can be helpful in the diagnosis of type 1 diabetes. As noted in Figure 53–1 ■, when the beta-cell mass is reduced by 80% to 90%, marked *impairments in insulin release* and *overt* type 1 diabetes develop. This is followed by a period of endogenous insulin production

GENETIC CONSIDERATIONS for Type 1 Diabetes

Approximately 40% to 50% of the genetic predisposition to the development of type 1 diabetes is conferred by genes on the short arm of chromosome 6, either within or in proximity to the Class II human leukocyte antigen (HLA) region of the major histocompatibility complex (MHC) (Kaufman & ADA, 2008). The inheritance of particular HLA alleles can account for more than half of the genetic risk of developing type 1 diabetes. HLA-DR and HLA-DQ are most strongly linked with type 1 diabetes. In type 1 diabetes at least one allele of DR3 or DR4 is found in 95% of Caucasians, and individuals with both DR3 and DR4 are particularly susceptible to type 1 diabetes. Conversely, the DR2 allele is protective against type 1 diabetes. (Kaufman & ADA, 2008).

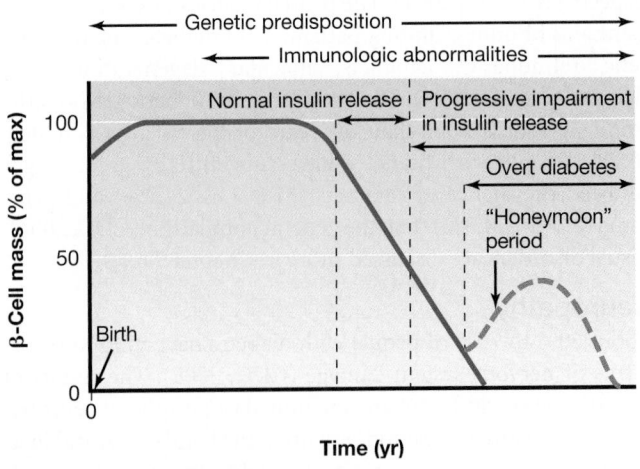

FIGURE 53–1 ■ Proposed scheme of natural history of the beta-cell defect.

called the **honeymoon period**. This "honeymoon period" represents the period of time during which exogenous insulin requirements are reduced. The clinical presentation of the honeymoon period varies from moderate reductions in insulin requirements to normalization of glucose tolerance (Harmel, Mathur, & Davidson, 2004). This period is relatively short lived, usually a few weeks to several months (Harmel et al., 2004) and is followed by loss of insulin production and dependence on exogenous insulin secretion.

Relationship Between Environmental Triggers and Beta-Cell Destruction

The question remains as to how the environmental trigger actually initiates the cascade of events leading to pancreatic beta-cell dysfunction. Currently two theories have been proposed to explain how an environmental trigger can initiate the autoimmune process.

The first theory is that an environmental trigger, such as a virus, directly induces tissue damage and inflammation. This subsequently leads to the release of beta-cell antigens and the recruitment and activation of lymphocytes and additional inflammatory leukocytes to the tissue.

The second theory, known as **molecular mimicry**, postulates that an environmental trigger, such as a virus, produces an immune response against autoantigens. This theory suggests that a susceptible host encounters an environmental trigger, such as a virus, that has antigens that are immunologically similar to the host antigens; however these antigens differ sufficiently enough to induce an immune response when presented to T cells. As a result, the tolerance to autoantigens breaks down, and the immune response cross reacts with host structures to cause tissue damage and disease (Albert & Inman, 1999).

◼ Risk Factors and Pathophysiology of Type 2 Diabetes

A number of risk factors are associated with the development of type 2 diabetes, as discussed next.

Genetics

Though there are genetic determinants of both type 1 and type 2 diabetes, the genetic linkage is stronger in those with type 2 diabetes. A small number of cases of type 2 diabetes are caused by a single-gene defect, such as MODY. The genetic component of the more common form of type 2 diabetes appears to be complex, involving the interactions of several genes and environmental factors (So et al., 2000).

Ethnicity

There is wide variability in the risk of type 2 diabetes among different racial and ethnic groups. Ethnic differences were described earlier in this chapter in the Epidemiology and Etiology of Diabetes and Other Forms of Glucose Intolerance section.

Racial Admixture

Data from populations whose origins are a mixture of different ethnic groups with varying risks for type 2 diabetes have provided *indirect* evidence that there is a genetic predisposition to this disease. Many Hispanics living in the southwestern United States share genes with Native Americans, such as the Pima Indians, and with non-Hispanic Caucasians, who are at much lower risk for developing diabetes. A study of Mexican Americans indicated that the prevalence of type 2 diabetes in this group is associated with the proportion of Native American genes in this population (Gardner et al., 1984). Though dated, the results of this study still are relevant to understanding the etiology of diabetes. The prevalence of type 2 diabetes in the group with the lowest amount of Native American admixture had a prevalence of diabetes at 5%, whereas the group with the highest Native American admixture had a prevalence of 14.5%. The Strong Heart Study, which examined the prevalence of cardiovascular disease (CVD) among three groups of Native Americans, noted that the prevalence of type 2 diabetes in adults ages 45 to 74 years increased with increasing levels of Native American ancestry (Lee et al., 1995).

Family History

Family history is an established risk factor for the development of type 2 diabetes. Twin studies have demonstrated that type 2 diabetes is highly concordant in monozygotic twins, but to a lesser degree in dizygous twins (Newman et al., 1987). The high concordance rate for type 2 diabetes among monozygotic twins supports the evidence that genetic factors play a significant role in the development of type 2 diabetes.

Diet

During times of reduced caloric intake, such as in food shortages during wars, there is a decline in morbidity and mortality from type 2 diabetes (ADA, 2001). Therefore, there appears to be an association between the amount of caloric intake and development of type 2 diabetes. However, the independent effects of caloric restriction on prevention of type 2 diabetes are difficult to discern from the effects of reducing or maintaining normal body weight. The exact dietary composition of diet in the prevention of type 2 diabetes also is not clear. High-CHO and low-fat diets appear to deteriorate insulin sensitivity, but high-fat and low-CHO diets may decrease satiety and lead to higher energy intake.

Obesity

Obesity is strongly associated with the development of type 2 diabetes (Gregg et al., 2004). There has been an increased emphasis on the role of central or visceral obesity (weight centered around the abdomen) in the development of type 2 diabetes. Central body obesity appears as a prognostic marker for glucose intolerance, hyperinsulinemia, and hypertriglyceridemia. Type 2 diabetes and pre-diabetes are manifestations of an underlying disorder termed *metabolic syndrome* (Burant & ADA, 2008).

Metabolic syndrome refers to a group of metabolic abnormalities that predisposes individuals to CVD and type 2 diabetes. The primary abnormalities included in this syndrome include insulin resistance, glucose intolerance, hyperinsulinemia, increased triglycerides and decreased HDL cholesterol, central obesity, and hypertension. The most common criteria used to define metabolic syndrome were developed by the Adult Treatment Panel III (ATP III) National Cholesterol Education Program Expert Panel on Detection, Evaluation, and Treatment of High Blood Cholesterol in Adults (Ford & Giles, 2003). Three or more of the following abnormalities must be present:

- High blood pressure ≥130/85 mmHg
- Hypertriglyceridemia ≥150 mg/dL
- Low high density lipoprotein cholesterol: ≤40 mg/dL in men; ≤50 mg/dL in women
- Abdominal obesity: waist circumference ≥102 cm in men; ≥88 cm in women
- Elevated fasting glucose ≥100 mg/dL.

Physical Inactivity

A number of epidemiologic studies during the last two decades have demonstrated that high levels of physical activity protect against the development of type 2 diabetes (Haffner, 1997; Helmrich, Ragland, Leung, & Paffenbarger, 1991; Hu et al., 2001; Manson et al., 1991, 1992). Two intervention studies have confirmed the value of lifestyle changes in the prevention of type 2 diabetes (Knowler et al., 2002; Tuomilehto et al., 2001). The Finnish Diabetes Prevention Study examined whether type 2 diabetes could be prevented through lifestyle modification in subjects with impaired glucose tolerance (IGT) (Tuomilehto et al., 2001). In this study, subjects were assigned to either an intervention or a control group. Subjects in the intervention group received individualized counseling aimed at weight reduction, dietary fat reduction, saturated fat reduction, increased dietary fiber, and increased physical activity. The risk of diabetes was reduced by 58% in the intervention group.

In the U.S. **Diabetes Prevention Program (DPP),** approximately 3,234 adults with elevated fasting and postload plasma glucose concentrations (i.e., those with pre-diabetes) were randomized into three groups: placebo, medication metformin (an oral hypoglycemic medication), or a lifestyle modification program (Knowler et al., 2002). The lifestyle intervention program reduced the incidence of diabetes by 58% and metformin reduced the incidence by 31% when compared with placebo. The study concluded that to prevent one case of diabetes during a 3-year period, 6.9 persons would have to participate in the lifestyle intervention program, and 13.9 would have to receive metformin. Therefore, the lifestyle intervention was more effective than the metformin.

Urbanization

When certain populations migrate from rural to urban settings, they have an increased prevalence of type 2 diabetes when compared to those whose relatives remain in the original setting. Because urbanization is associated with changes in diet, physical activity, socioeconomic activity, and obesity, the risk of type 2 diabetes increases. This is best exemplified by the Pima Indians of the Southwestern United States, who have a greater than 50% chance of developing type 2 diabetes in their lifetime, but whose relatives in Mexico (who have a traditional lifestyle) have a very low risk of diabetes (Valencia et al., 1999).

Socioeconomic Status and Education

Socioeconomic status (SES) also is associated with the development of type 2 diabetes. Individuals in the lowest SES brackets have the highest risk of type 2 diabetes (ADA, 2001). In addition, lower levels of education also are inversely related to diabetes risk in the United States (ADA, 2001).

Intrauterine Environment

Intrauterine factors may increase the risk of type 2 diabetes. For example, low birth weight has been associated with an increased risk for developing diabetes. It has been hypothesized that this relationship is the result of undernutrition *in utero*, which causes a limited development of pancreatic beta cells, whose number is fixed at birth (Rich-Edwards et al., 1999).

Sequence in the Development of Type 2 Diabetes

Type 2 diabetes is a heterogeneous group of disorders characterized by decreased liver, muscle, and adipose tissue sensitivity to insulin, and a defect in insulin secretion from the pancreatic beta cell. Because both insulin resistance and a reduction in insulin secretion are present at diagnosis of type 2 diabetes, it is difficult to determine which of these metabolic abnormalities the initial defect is. Nonetheless, the development of type 2 diabetes follows a typically evolving course, which can be divided into three distinct stages.

In the first stage, genetic factors probably influence both insulin sensitivity and insulin secretion. As noted previously, environmental factors, such as obesity and physical inactivity, are usually associated with the development of insulin resistance. There is an initial period of hyperinsulinemia in which the pancreatic beta cell is able to overcome insulin resistance and maintain normal glucose tolerance. At this stage, although there is an underlying defect in insulin secretion, the pancreatic cell is able to produce a high level of insulin, and normal glucose homeostasis is maintained by a compensatory hyperinsulinemia (Figure 53–2 ■).

In the second stage, insulin resistance increases and this compensatory hyperinsulinemia becomes insufficient to maintain normal glucose homeostasis. Under conditions of insulin resistance, visceral adipose tissue is very sensitive to the effects of catecholamines and is associated with enhanced lipolysis. This leads to increased free fatty acids (FFA) production and mobilization, exacerbating insulin resistance in liver and muscle. In addition, impairments in insulin-mediated glucose uptake, particularly at the muscle, become evident. Insulin-mediated glucose transport into skeletal muscle, the major target for glucose disposal, becomes impaired. Fasting plasma glucose levels remain normal but postprandial (after a meal) plasma glucose levels rise (Figure 53–3 ■).

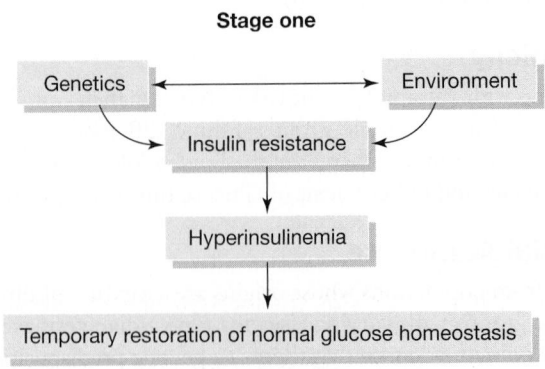

FIGURE 53–2 ■ Stage 1 development of type 2 DM.

Stage two

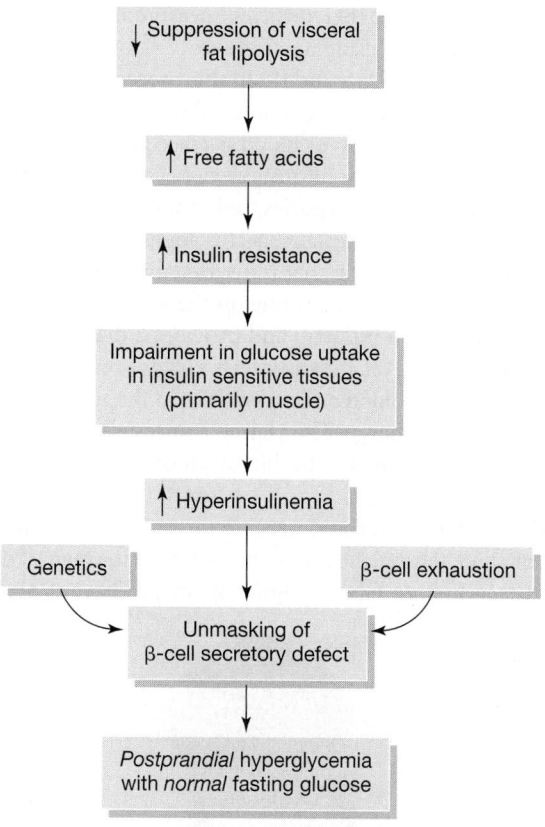

FIGURE 53–3 ■ Stage 2 development of type 2 DM.

Stage three

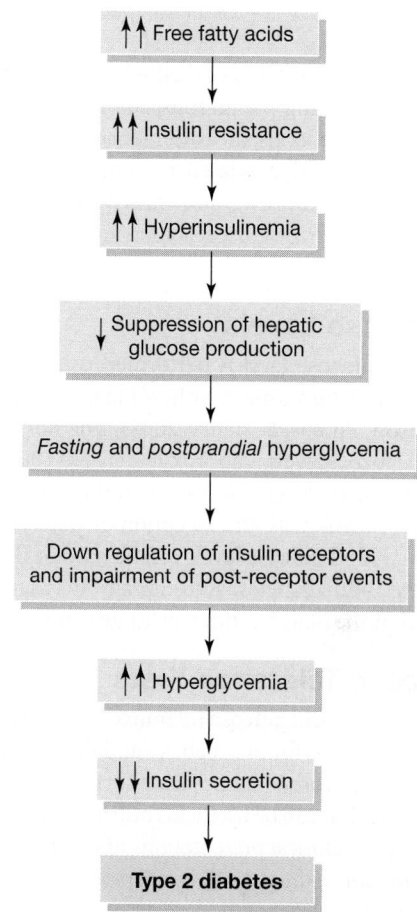

FIGURE 53–4 ■ Stage 3 development of type 2 DM.

In the third stage, there is a further increase in insulin resistance. The restraining effects of insulin on hepatic glucose production become impaired and plasma glucose levels increase. In addition, the worsening hyperglycemia has toxic effects on the pancreatic beta cell, and insulin secretion subsequently declines. With increasing insulin resistance, there is an even greater increase in FFA production and mobilization. The increase in FFAs causes a further increase in insulin resistance. Fasting and postprandial hyperglycemia result from increased insulin resistance, unrestrained hepatic glucose production, and glucose toxicity (Figure 53–4 ■).

Clinical Manifestations

In general, the clinical signs and symptoms of type 1 diabetes originate from hyperglycemia and ketosis, whereas the clinical signs and symptoms of type 2 diabetes originate from hyperglycemia. HHS is a medical emergency primarily associated with type 2 diabetes. The following are signs and symptoms of diabetes *uncomplicated* by DKA or HHS:

- *Glucosuria* (glucose in urine) is associated with an **osmotic diuresis,** an increase in urine volume caused by an osmotic substance (glucose) in the renal tubules.
- *Polyuria* (increased urination) is the primary clinical manifestation of the osmotic diuresis.
- *Nocturia* is frequent urination at night associated with *polyuria.*

- *Osmotic diuresis* is associated with dehydration and volume depletion.
- *Hypotension* (low blood pressure) occurs as a result of dehydration and volume depletion.
- *Tachycardia* (increased heart rate) also occurs as a result of dehydration and volume depletion.
- *Polydipsia* (increased thirst) is a compensatory response to the dehydration and volume depletion.
- *Polyphagia* (increased appetite) results from the significant loss of calories that occurs through the loss of calories in the urine. For example, the amount of glucose in the urine can exceed over 300 kcal/day (Funk, 2003).
- Weight loss occurs through dehydration, volume depletion, and the loss of calories in the urine.
- Fatigue is most likely related to alterations in CHO, protein, and lipid metabolism, especially protein catabolism.

Laboratory and Diagnostic Procedures

Diabetes is a chronic disease requiring frequent monitoring of blood glucose levels so that appropriate diagnoses are made and therapeutic goals can be accomplished through adjustments in diet, physical activity, and pharmacologic therapy. These determinations are performed in a clinical laboratory setting. Following the initial diagnosis of diabetes, patients are taught to measure blood glucose levels several times each day using portable glucose meters. This is called self-monitoring of blood glucose. In the following paragraphs, the laboratory measurement of blood glucose levels, measurement of longer term blood glucose control (e.g., glycosylated proteins), measurement of short-term glucose control, and miscellaneous indices of glycemic status (e.g., urine glucose, blood and urine ketones) are discussed.

Blood Glucose Levels

A fasting blood glucose level is performed using whole blood, plasma, and serum glucokinase, or hexokinase enzymatic methods (McPherson, Pincus, & Henry, 2007). The normal range of fasting blood glucose levels is approximately 60–100 mg/dL. The fasting blood glucose level is measured following an overnight fast (no food or drink with the exception of water) for 10 to 12 hours. Fasting blood glucose levels can be used in the diagnosis of pre-diabetes and diabetes. Additionally it is an important measurement in the daily monitoring of glycemic control.

Oral Glucose Tolerance Tests

As noted previously, **oral glucose tolerance tests (OGTTs)** can be used as diagnostic tools for pre-diabetes and diabetes in nonpregnant adults. Oral glucose tolerance tests normally are not used to diagnose diabetes, but can be useful in confirming the diagnosis of diabetes in atypical clinical presentations of diabetes. Patients are asked to fast for approximately 10 hours prior to the OGTT; they are asked to make certain that their intake of CHO is 150 g/day for the 3 days prior to the test (Joslin & Kahn, 2005). In addition, they are asked to refrain from smoking during the test and participate in their usual activity on the day prior to the test. In the standard OGTT, blood glucose levels are drawn prior to and 1/2, 1, 2, and 3 hours following ingestion of 75 grams of glucose (as in a commercial glucose preparation of glucose dissolved in water). As noted earlier, the diagnosis of pre-diabetes or diabetes is made on the 2-hour value ($\geq$140 to <200 mg/dL; and $\geq$200 mg/dL, respectively). The intermediate glucose levels (1/2, 1, and 3 or more hours) are used primarily for research purposes. Note that different criteria are used for the diagnosis of diabetes in pregnant women (Joslin & Kahn, 2005).

Self-Monitoring of Blood Glucose

One of the most important developments in the management of diabetes is self-monitoring of blood glucose (SMBG). The process of SMBG allows patients to measure blood glucose levels at any time and make changes in diet, physical activity, and pharmacologic therapy. The information can be used to make immediate decisions (e.g., insulin dose prior to meals) or this information can be used to make decisions on therapeutic changes based on blood glucose trends over time. Patients routinely are instructed to perform preprandial blood glucose measurements (i.e., immediately prior to meals and snacks), postprandial blood glucose measurements (i.e., approximately 2 hours after a meal or snack), or in the assessment of clinical symptoms (e.g., hypoglycemia). Patients and health care

providers can review the results of SMBG measurements together and discuss overall changes in management.

The process of SMBG involves measurement of capillary blood glucose levels using a variety of portable blood glucose meters (Figures 53–5A ■ and B). In this process, patients puncture their fingers with a small lancet device, obtaining a small drop of blood. This drop of blood is placed on a strip that has been placed in a small monitoring device. The meter technology falls into two general categories, reflectance and sensor methods. In meters using reflectance technology, the blood is placed directly on a reagent strip that is inserted over a glucose sensor. The blood reacts with an enzyme on the reagent strip; the meter shines a light on the strip and provides a digital readout of the blood glucose level. In sensor technology, a reaction between the glucose in the blood and an enzyme in the test strip generates an electrical charge. The charge is measured by the meter and a digital readout of the blood glucose level is provided (Harmel et al., 2004).

Whether blood glucose levels are measured in a home, hospital, or clinic setting, the meters need to have the highest degree of accuracy. In hospitals and clinics, strict quality control proce-

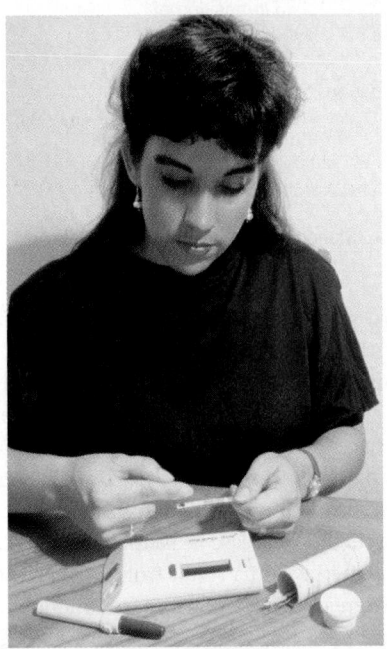

(a)

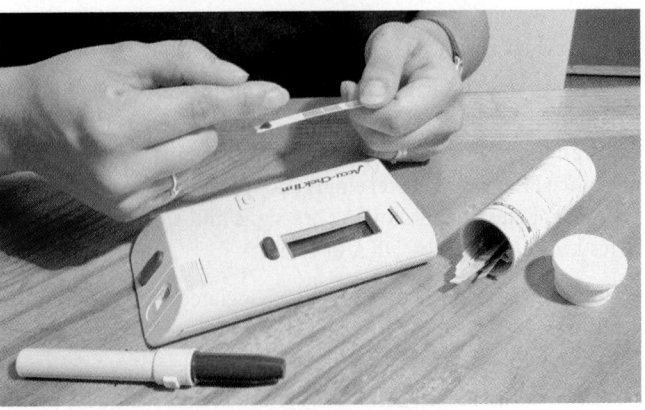

(b)

FIGURE 53–5 ■ Blood glucose monitor.
Source: Tony Freeman/PhotoEdit Inc.

dures are needed to maintain the accuracy of these devices, which are used by multiple operators on several patients. Each hospital or clinic has detailed quality control procedures to ensure that the meters are measuring blood glucose levels accurately and the operators are performing the test correctly. At minimum the procedures will include checking the meters against high, normal, and low standard solutions and periodically assessing operator technique. The standard solutions have specific glucose concentrations in the high, normal, and low ranges. When these solutions are placed on glucose test strips, they should yield a specific concentration. The nursing staff often is responsible for maintaining quality control checks and assessing their own performance. In addition to strict quality control procedures, the following steps are important in obtaining accurate blood glucose levels (Harmel et al., 2004):

- Strips must be current and properly stored at appropriate temperatures.
- The meter must be calibrated to the correct lot number of strips.
- The meter must be clean. This is particularly true of reflectance meters.
- An adequate amount of blood must be placed on the strip.
- The finger must be clean and dry prior to the puncture.

The timing of blood glucose measurements should correlate with the patient's meal status, clinical condition, and insulin regimen.

 A hospitalized patient eating four times (three meals and a bedtime snack) per day should have a blood glucose measurement performed prior to each meal or snack. There should not be major gaps between glucose determinations and administration of food. For example, when calculating the prebreakfast dose of rapid-acting insulin, the calculation should be based on a glucose determination made shortly before breakfast, not several hours prior. Patients who are not eating also should have their glucose levels checked four times per day, but it may be more appropriate to check blood glucose levels every 6 hours, depending on their insulin regimen. In addition, patients who are more unstable may need determinations more frequently (e.g., every 2 hours).

Continuous Blood Glucose Monitoring

During the past few years, blood glucose sensing devices have been developed that provide continuous intermittent measurement of the glucose level in interstitial fluid. The continuous blood glucose monitoring system (Medtronics, Inc.) measures glucose levels in interstitial fluid every 10 seconds and provides an average blood glucose level every 5 minutes (Figure 53–6 ■). The sensor is a small device with tubing and a small cannula; the cannula is inserted into the subcutaneous tissue, usually in the abdomen. The sensor is connected to a small monitor, roughly the size of a pager. At least three times each day the patient takes a fingerstick blood glucose level and programs it into the monitor for calibration purposes. The patient also programs events, such as meals and exercise, into the monitor.

In older versions of the sensor, the patient removes the device after 3 days and returns it to the health care provider who

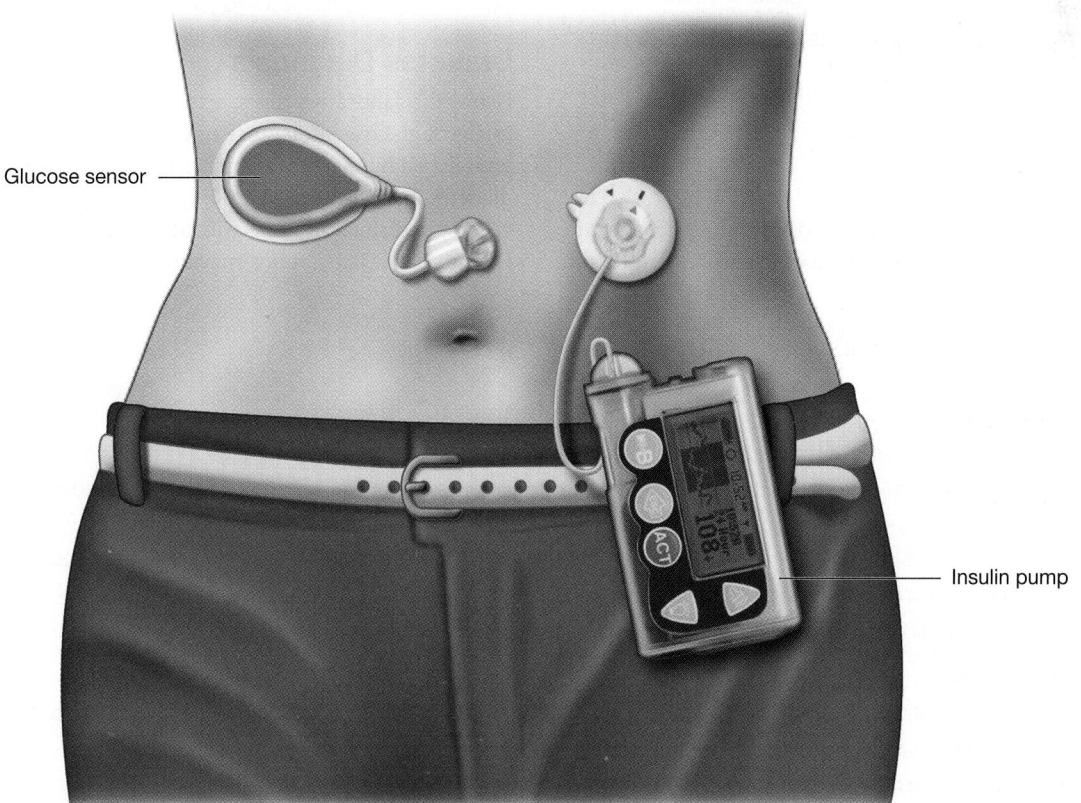

FIGURE 53–6 ■ Continuous blood glucose monitoring system.

downloads the blood glucose data. Together the patient and the health care provider discuss trends in the blood glucose patterns. Mutual decisions between the health care provider and the patient can be made regarding treatment decisions. Newer versions of the sensing device will allow the data to be accessed by the patients.

Hemoglobin A$_{1c}$ Test

The primary laboratory test used for monitoring longer term glucose control is the **hemoglobin A$_{1c}$ (HbA$_{1c}$) test**. A normal HbA$_{1c}$ is <6%. This test also is known as glycated hemoglobin or glycosylated hemoglobin, although it is most often referred to as "A1C." Hemoglobin A$_{1c}$ is formed when glucose in the blood binds irreversibly to hemoglobin to form a stable glycated hemoglobin complex. Protein glycation is the nonenzymatic reaction of sugars with proteins. Because the normal life span of red blood cells is 90 to 120 days, the HbA$_{1c}$ reflects the average blood glucose values of the previous 2 to 3 months and is directly proportional to the ambient concentration of plasma glucose in the blood over the life span of the red blood cells. This test is the most widely used measure for assessment of glucose control (Goldstein et al., 2004).

Glycated Serum Proteins

In addition to hemoglobin, there are a number of additional **glycated serum proteins** (GSPs) in diabetes. In particular, glycated albumin constitutes approximately 80% of the major proteins that undergo glycosylation (Barr, Nathan, Meigs, & Singer, 2002; McFarland, Catalano, Day, Thorpe, & Baynes, 1979). Because the half-life of albumin is 17 to 20 days, measurement of glycated albumin reflects short-term glycemic control (Harmel et al., 2004). Measurements of total GSPs and glycated serum albumin correlate can be useful, particularly in situations where the HbA$_{1c}$ cannot be measured or may not be of use (e.g., in the presence of hemolytic anemias). The fructosamine assay is the most widely used method of quantifying total GSPs or total glycated hemoglobin (Barr et al., 2002), reflecting short-term glycemic control.

Urinary Glucose

SMBG has replaced the measurement of urinary glucose as the measure of glycemic control. The urinary measurement of glucose involves the semiquantitative measurement of glucose, usually in a single urine specimen. Prior to the introduction of blood glucose monitoring devices, patients would make several assessments throughout the day of urinary blood glucose using chemical reagents to assess glycemic control. Urinary glucose is no longer used to routinely monitor glucose control; however, it is part of a routine urinalysis. Ordinarily, glucose should not be detectable in the urine. If glucose is present in a urine specimen, further evaluation is warranted.

Urinary and Blood Ketones

Urinary ketone testing is an essential part of diabetes self-management for patients with type 1 diabetes, pregnancy with preexisting diabetes, and gestational diabetes (Goldstein et al., 2004). Patients use chemical reagents to provide an estimate of urinary ketones, usually ranging from "trace" to "large" amounts. Normally ketones are not detectable in the urine. Urinary ketones may be present in nondiabetic individuals following fasting. In addition, urinary ketones may be present in the first morning urine of pregnant women.

The presence of detectable amounts of urinary ketones in the urine of patients with diabetes is reflective of impending large amounts of serum ketones, which are associated with the development of DKA. It is recommended that patients with type 1 diabetes test their urine for ketones, during times of stress or infection, when blood glucose levels are consistently elevated (>300 mg/dL) and when classic symptoms of DKA (e.g., abdominal pain, nausea, and vomiting) are present (Goldstein et al., 2004). In addition to urinary ketone assessment, bedside and self-testing kits can be used to quantify blood ketone (e.g., beta hydroxybutyrate) levels in a manner similar to those used to test capillary blood glucose levels (Bektas, Eray, Sari, & Akbas, 2004).

Diabetes Diagnosis

Using the laboratory tests just described, diabetes and other forms of glucose intolerance can be diagnosed using the criteria established by the ADA, which serve as a national guideline for diabetes diagnoses (ADA, 2007). Typically, any one of the three criteria described in the National Guidelines for Establishing a Diagnosis of Diabetes box may be used.

NATIONAL GUIDELINES for Establishing a Diagnosis of Diabetes

Diabetes Diagnosis

Any one of the following three criteria may be used to establish a diagnosis of diabetes:

- A random plasma glucose (PG) concentration of ≥200 mg/dL with symptoms of hyperglycemia, for example, polydipsia (excessive thirst), polyuria (excessive urination)
- A fasting plasma glucose (FPG) concentration of ≥126 mg/dL on more than one occasion with or without symptoms of hyperglycemia
- An elevated PG concentration (≥200 mg/dL) at 2 hours following consumption of 75 grams of glucose during an OGTT.

   Important: In the absence of unequivocal hyperglycemia, these criteria should be confirmed by repeat testing on a different day.

Pre-Diabetes Diagnosis

Pre-diabetes includes two categories: impaired fasting glucose (IFG) and impaired glucose tolerance (IGT). The criteria for each are as follows:

- Impaired fasting glucose is a condition in which the FPG is ≥100 and <126 mg/dL on two occasions.
- Impaired glucose tolerance is a 2-hour plasma blood glucose level ≥140 and <200 mg/dL following 75 grams of oral glucose.

Source: American Diabetes Association. (2007). Nutrition recommendations and interventions for diabetes: A position statement of the American Diabetes Association. *Diabetes Care, 30*(Suppl. 1), S48–S65.

Medical Management

The current philosophy of diabetes management is based primarily on the results of two major studies, the Diabetes Control and Complications Trial (DCCT) (DCCT Trial Research Group, 1993) and the **United Kingdom Prospective Diabetes Study (UKPDS)** (U.K. Prospective Diabetes Study Group [UKPDSG], 1998b). The DCCT and the UKPDS demonstrated in type 1 and type 2 diabetes, respectively, that any level of hyperglycemia is associated with the development of diabetes-related complications. In both of these studies, improvements in glycemic control were associated with reductions in microvascular complications (i.e., neuropathy, nephropathy, and retinopathy). The Evidence-Based Practice box (p. 1672) discusses glycemic control and its relationship to diabetes-related complications in more detail.

In the UKPDS, hypertension was associated positively with the development of microvascular complications, and improved blood pressure control was associated with reductions in microvascular disease (UKPDSG, 1998b). Thus the overall goal of diabetes management is the prevention of chronic long-term complications (such as those previously described), with distinctions between short-term and long-term goals. The short-term goals of diabetes management include prevention of severe hypoglycemia, hyperglycemia, and acute complications such as DKA and HHS. Long-term glycemic goals include normalizing blood glucose levels and preventing systemic complications. Laboratory tests for the monitoring short- and long-term glycemic control are detailed in Chart 53–2 (p. 1673).

Although the DCCT (DCCT Trial Research Group, 1993) and the UKPDS (UKPDSG, 1998b) demonstrated that improved glycemic control resulted in reductions in CVD, these reductions did not reach statistical significance. This suggests that the development of diabetes-related CVD is caused by a variety of factors, including glycemic control, dyslipidemias, hypertension, and prothrombotic factors. The target glycemic and metabolic goals for patients with diabetes are as follows (McCarren & ADA, 2007):

- Glycemic goals:
  - HbA_{1c}: <7.0% (These goals are individualized; some patients may establish more stringent glycemic goals, e.g., a normal A1C of <6%.)
  - Preprandial blood glucose: 90 to 130 mg/dL
  - Postprandial blood glucose: <180 mg/dL (The postprandial measurements are generally made 1 to 2 hours following the meal.)
- Blood pressure goals: <130/80 mmHg
- Lipid goals:
  - Low density lipoprotein (LDL) cholesterol: <100 mg/dL
  - Triglycerides: <150 mg/dL
  - High density lipoprotein (HDL) cholesterol: > 40 mg/dL

Current management strategies for the treatment of diabetes include a combination of exercise, nutrition, miscellaneous lifestyle changes (e.g., smoking cessation), and pharmacologic therapy directed toward normalization of blood glucose, blood pressure, and blood lipid levels. An extensive review of antihypertensive and lipid-lowering drugs is beyond the scope of this chapter, however, the role of glucose-lowering drugs is discussed next.

Pharmaceutical Management of Hyperglycemia

The pharmacologic treatment of both types 1 and 2 diabetes has undergone a revolution during the past two decades. The exact relationship between blood glucose levels and the development of chronic diabetes-related complications was debated for several years. Some researchers thought that these complications were the result of poor glycemic control, whereas others believed that there was no relationship. The DCCT (DCCT Trial Research Group, 1993) and the UKPDS (UKPDSG, 1998a) clarified that diabetes-related chronic complications could be prevented or reduced by maintaining **normoglycemia** (normal blood glucose levels). Patients with diabetes now use intricate pharmacologic regimens (along with medical nutrition therapy and exercise) to normalize blood glucose levels. Newer insulin preparations, insulin delivery systems, and oral medications have been developed to assist patients in maintaining normal blood glucose levels.

Because the basic pathophysiological defect in type 1 diabetes is a deficiency of insulin production, the pharmacologic treatment of type 1 diabetes involves the use of exogenous insulin to replace the insulin deficiency. Type 2 diabetes is characterized by insulin resistance and reduced insulin secretion, so the pharmacologic therapy of type 2 diabetes involves oral medications, insulin, or a combination of both. The general mechanisms of insulin and oral diabetes medication are discussed next, followed by discussion as to more specific pharmacologic treatment regimens for both type 1 and type 2 diabetes. This information is presented not to replace a pharmacologic text, but to highlight the important aspects of pharmacologic management.

Insulin Preparations

Until the mid-1980s insulin was produced from beef (bovine) and pork (porcine) sources. Beef and pork insulin preparations are no longer manufactured or marketed in the United States and current insulin products are produced synthetically.

Human insulin is produced by recombinant DNA technology; the structure of recombinant human insulin matches the amino acid sequence of human insulin. Insulin analogs have been developed through amino acid rearrangement, substitution, addition, and deletion in the structure of this synthetically produced human insulin. Insulin **analogs** are altered forms of insulin, different from the insulin secreted by the human pancreas, but still available to the human body for performing the same action as human insulin in terms of glycemic control. These insulin analogs have absorption and biologic activity that mimic the normal physiological pattern of endogenous insulin secretion more precisely than traditional insulin preparations.

Time Profile of Insulin Preparations

Insulin preparations are characterized by *onset, peaks, and duration* of action. Normal physiological insulin secretion involves both basal and meal-stimulated insulin release. Under normal physiological conditions, serum glucose and insulin responses are closely matched; when glucose levels rise, there is a corresponding rise in insulin levels. Under basal conditions (i.e., overnight, between meals, and during fasting) plasma glucose is maintained within a narrow range with a comparable response in insulin secretion. Following a meal, plasma glucose levels rise

Glycemic Control

Clinical Problem

Patients with diabetes often develop severe diabetes-related complications (neuropathy, nephropathy, retinopathy, and an accelerated development of all forms of cardiovascular disease). Nurses and other health care providers must apply evidence-based findings to reduce the development of these complications.

Research Findings

Two major studies have examined the relationship between glycemic control and the development of diabetes complications: the Diabetes Control and Complications Trial (DCCT Trial Research Group, 1993) and the United Kingdom Prospective Diabetes Study (UKPDSG, 1998a, 1998b). The results of these studies changed diabetes management and are the primary foundation for our current recommendations for glycemic control in diabetes.

The DCCT and UKPDS were prospective, randomized, controlled trials of intensive versus standard glycemic control of patients with type 1 and 2 diabetes, respectively. The DCCT demonstrated definitively that improved glycemic control is associated with sustained, decreased rates of microvascular complications (retinopathy, nephropathy, and neuropathy) in type 1 diabetes. The UKPDS demonstrated that, in patients with newly diagnosed type 2 diabetes, intensive use of medications (metformin, sulfonylureas, insulin) and lifestyle interventions reduced the development of microvascular disease. In the UKPDS there was a trend toward reduction in CVD, as noted by a statistically nonsignificant reduction ($p = 0.052$) in the risk for combined fatal and nonfatal myocardial infarction and sudden death.

In both of these studies, the mean HbA_{1c} of the intensive group was approximately 7%. Thus, the American Diabetes Association recommends that the target HbA_{1c} in patients with diabetes is 7%. Epidemiologic data have demonstrated an incremental benefit (although small in absolute terms) to lowering HbA_{1c} into the normal range (Stratton et al., 2000); however, this reduction must be balanced against the risk of hypoglycemia and other comorbidities.

The recommendations of the ADA (2008e) regarding glycemic control are as follows:

- Lowering HbA_{1c} to an average of ~7% has clearly been shown to reduce microvascular complications of diabetes and, possibly, macrovascular disease. Therefore, the HbA_{1c} goal for nonpregnant adults in general is <7%.

- Epidemiologic studies have suggested an incremental benefit to lowering HbA_{1c} from 7% into the normal range. Therefore, the HbA_{1c} goal for selected individual patients is as close to normal (<6%) as possible without significant hypoglycemia.

- Less stringent HbA_{1c} goals may be appropriate for patients with a history of severe hypoglycemia, patients with limited life expectancies, children, individuals with comorbid conditions, and those with long-standing diabetes with minimal or stable microvascular complications.

Implications for Nursing Practice

Attaining tight glycemic control in patients with diabetes requires a balance of diet, physical activity, and medications. This is not an easy task! Nurses are in a unique position to help patients self-manage their diabetes. Nurses need to develop strong assessment skills that examine the patient from clinical, cultural, behavioral, and psychosocial perspectives. Appropriate plans of care can be structured from this assessment.

Critical Thinking Questions

1. Joe S. is a 16-year-old patient with newly diagnosed type 1 diabetes. He refuses to check his blood glucose levels on a regular basis. When he asks "What is the big deal about checking my blood sugar?" which of the following would be your response?
   a. Keeping your blood glucose levels in the normal range is necessary to prevent diabetes complications!
   b. We know that keeping your blood sugar in the normal range is important in preventing complications and overall making you feel better, but let's talk about how things are going with your diabetes, in general.

2. Mary B. is a 44-year-old patient with type 2 diabetes. When she states "I have the adult form of diabetes; it is not a problem. I don't really need to check my blood sugar," how do you respond?
   a. There is a relationship between blood glucose levels and the development of complications that can occur regardless of the age at which you develop diabetes. Do you have the strips and a meter to check your sugar?
   b. You are correct! Diabetes that is diagnosed as an adult is far less serious than diabetes that is diagnosed as a child.

3. Sally J. is a 90-year-old women who was recently hospitalized for a hip fracture that occurred following a fall. During a home visit, the nurse finds that the patient (with the help of the family) is checking her blood glucose level two times per day and administering multiple daily injections of insulin. When you ask the family about this treatment regimen, they reply that they have a grandson with type 1 diabetes and understand the importance of "tight" glucose control. The patient has a HbA_{1c} of 6.0%. On discussions with her primary health care provider, you find that he has tried to have the patient and family target Sally's insulin therapy to a more reasonable goal of 7% to 7.5% but has had no success. How would you approach this?
   a. Tell the family that the risk of hypoglycemia (and falling again) is greater than the risk of developing complications.
   b. Organize a meeting with the social worker, physician, and other health care providers to discuss the best way to approach the patient and family, knowing (as above) that the risk of falling is greater than that of developing complications. If the patient and family still want "tight" glycemic control, then a monitoring plan should be developed to prevent hypoglycemia (accessible snacks, more frequent monitoring).

Answers to Critical Thinking Questions appear in Appendix D.

References

American Diabetes Association. (2008e). Standards of medical care in diabetes—2008. *Diabetes Care, 31*(Suppl. 1), S12–S54.

DCCT Trial Research Group. (1993). The effect of intensive treatment of diabetes on the development and progression of long-term complications in insulin-dependent diabetes mellitus. *New England Journal of Medicine, 329*(14), 977–986.

Stratton, I. M., Adler, A. I., Neil, H. A., Matthews, D. R., Manley, S. E., Cull, C. A., et al. (2000). Association of glycaemia with macrovascular and microvascular complications of type 2 diabetes (UKPDS 35): Prospective observational study. *British Medical Journal, 321,* 405–412.

U.K. Prospective Diabetes Study Group. (1998a). Effect of intensive blood-glucose control with metformin on complications in overweight patients with type 2 diabetes (UKPDS 34). *Lancet, 352*(9131), 854–865.

U.K. Prospective Diabetes Study Group. (1998b). Tight blood pressure control and risk of macrovascular and microvascular complications in type 2 diabetes (UKPDS 38). *British Medical Journal, 317*(7160), 703–713.

EVIDENCE-BASED PRACTICE

CHART 53–2   **Tests Used to Monitor Glycemia and Ketosis in Diabetes**

Test	Results	Comments
Blood glucose levels	70–110 mg/dL prior to meals <120 mg/dL 2 hours after a meal	
Hemoglobin A$_{1c}$ (HbA$_{1c}$ or A1c)	≤5%	Normal ranges may vary slightly depending on the laboratory used; reflects glucose control over the previous 3 months.
Glycosylated serum proteins (GSPs) Fructosamine Glycated albumin	0–285 µmol/L* 0.6–3%*	Reflects glucose control over the previous 2–3 weeks; higher levels reflect worsening glucose control.
Urine glucose	Negative	
Urine ketones	Negative	Often reported as "trace," "small," "moderate," or "high" with higher levels reflecting a greater degree of ketosis.
Serum ketones	Negative	Often reported in dilutions (e.g., 1:8, 1:16) with higher dilutions reflecting a greater degree of ketosis.

*Values from Associated Regional and University Pathologists, Inc. (ARUP) Laboratories, http://www.aruplab.com/guides.

---

and there is a rapid increase in insulin secretion. Therefore, insulin secretion often is referred to as basal or meal stimulated. The goal of insulin therapy is to mimic this normal pattern of insulin secretion. Therefore, pharmacologic insulin preparations are often characterized by their ability to mimic basal or meal-stimulated properties. In clinical practice the amount of insulin that is given to match the meal-stimulated insulin response is provided as an insulin "bolus."

Commercial insulin preparations are divided into rapid-, short-, intermediate-, and long-acting preparations based on

onset, peak (highest concentration of insulin), and duration of action. The comparative actions of each preparation are detailed in Chart 53–3.

Five insulin analogs are currently available: lispro, aspart, glulisine, detemir, and glargine. Insulins lispro, aspart, and glulisine have rapid absorption profiles, whereas insulins detemir and glargine have delayed insulin absorption. The actions of insulins lispro, aspart, and glulisine most closely resemble meal-stimulated insulin responses, whereas insulins glargine and detemir most closely resembles basal insulin secretion.

CHART 53–3   **Comparative Effects of Common Insulin Preparations**

Type/Generic Name	Brand Name(s)	Onset (hours)	Peak (hours)	Duration (hours)
Rapid Acting				
Insulin lispro (analog) Insulin aspart Insulin glulisine	Humalog NovoLog Apidra	<0.25	1–2	3–4
Short Acting				
Regular	Humulin R Novolin R Humulin R (U-500)*	0.5–1.0	2–3	3–6
Intermediate Acting				
NPH (isophane)	Humulin N Novolin N	2–4	4–10	12–18
Long Acting	Lantus	2–4	Peakless	20–24
Insulin glargine Insulin detemir	Levemir	0.8–2	Relatively flat	~ 24
Combinations				
50% lispro protamine/50% insulin lispro	Humalog Mix 50/50	0.5–1	Dual	~18–24
70% NPH/30% regular	Humulin 70/30 Novolin 70/30	0.5–1	Dual	~18–24
50% NPH/50% regular	Humulin 50/50	0.5–1	Dual	~18–24
75% aspart protamine/25% aspart	NovoLog Mix 75/25	<0.25	Dual	~18–24
75% lispro protamine/25% lispro	Humalog Mix 75/25	<0.25	Dual	~18–24

*The concentration of commercial insulin in the United States is 100 units/mL (U-100); however, regular insulin is also available as 500 units/mL (U-500). This concentration is usually used only in patients who are extremely insulin resistant.

Rapid-Acting Insulin The time-action profiles of the rapid-acting insulin analogs are detailed in Chart 53–3 (p. 1673). These preparations have an onset of action of approximately 15 minutes after injection, and reach peak biologic action within approximately 1 to 2 hours. They are most effective in reducing postprandial glycemia.

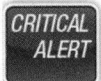 **CRITICAL ALERT** *Because the onset of action of rapid-acting insulin preparations is so quick, they should be injected as close to the meal or snack as possible to avoid hypoglycemia. A critical role of the nurse is to be alert for signs and symptoms of hypoglycemia and educate patients and family about how to prevent and treat hypoglycemic reactions.*

Rapid-acting insulin preparations are routinely administered before a meal or snack; however, in certain situations these agents may be administered following a meal. For example, often it is difficult to predict the caloric intake of patients who are acutely or chronically ill because they may have changes in taste or appetite. In these situations, the actual amount of food consumed (particularly the CHO content) can be determined and a postmeal dose of rapid-acting insulin administered. This method helps to reduce the potential for hypoglycemia since the food intake and amount of insulin are more accurately matched.

Short-Acting Insulin The only available short-acting insulin preparation is Regular insulin, which is injected prior to meals. To match the peak action of insulin with the postprandial rise in glucose, Regular insulin should be injected approximately 30 to 45 minutes prior to a meal. The use of Regular insulin has been largely replaced by rapid-acting insulin analogs. Because the rapid-acting preparations have a more rapid onset of action and a greater peak effect, they resemble meal-stimulated endogenous insulin secretion more closely than Regular insulin.

Intermediate-Acting Insulin The only intermediate-acting insulin preparation currently available is Neutral Protamine Hagedorn (NPH) insulin. With a slow onset of action, prolonged peak effect, and lengthened duration of action, NPH insulin traditionally has been used to provide basal insulin coverage (usually with two injections per day). However, the use of NPH as basal insulin is somewhat limited due the high plasma insulin concentrations during peak action, thus increasing the risk of hypoglycemia.

Long-Acting Insulin Long-acting insulin was produced to provide basal insulin coverage with relatively small peak biologic action. Glargine is a long-acting acting insulin analog that has no "peak" action, mirroring basal insulin secretion more precisely. Detemir, a newer long-acting insulin analog that has a relatively flat peak, also is used as basal insulin. Slight differences are seen in the onset, peaks, and duration of these preparations. These differences are detailed in Chart 53–3 (p. 1673).

Premixed Insulins
Premixed insulins are combinations of rapid- or short-acting insulin preparations mixed with intermediate-acting insulin in specific proportions. The most common premixed insulin contains 70% NPH and 30% Regular insulin (70/30). Other forms of premixed combinations are listed in Chart 53–3 (p. 1673). These premixed insulins are helpful in patients who have difficulty mixing insulin doses, however, they do not permit easy adjustment of premeal and basal insulin. For example, if a patient using 70/30 insulin needed an increase in pre-meal Regular insulin, it would be impossible to make this adjustment without also increasing the dose of NPH.

Incretin Mimetics
Exenatide injection (Byetta) (Amylin Pharmaceuticals, 2007) is an injectable medication used as adjunctive mealtime therapy to improve glycemic control in patients with type 2 diabetes mellitus who are taking metformin, sulfonylureas, or a combination of metformin and sulfonylureas. This medication belongs to a class of medications called **incretin mimetics**. An incretin mimetic enhances glucose-dependent insulin secretion from the pancreatic beta cell. Therefore, the greatest effect of exenatide is a reduction in postprandial glucose levels. In addition, the incretins suppress elevated glucagon levels, promoting satiety, decreasing food intake, and slowing gastric emptying.

The primary side effect of exenatide is nausea. The nausea may be minimized by increasing the medication dosage slowly. Exenatide should be administered subcutaneously 60 minutes prior to meals. Exenatide may decrease the rate at which orally administered drugs are absorbed. Therefore, oral medications that require rapid absorption that are dependent on threshold concentrations for effective action (e.g., antibiotics and oral contraceptives) should be administered 1 hour prior to administration of the exenatide.

Amylin Analog
Pramlintide acetate injection (Symlin) (Amylin Pharmaceuticals, 2007) is a synthetic analog of human amylin, a hormone secreted by the pancreatic beta cell. Pramlintide can reduce postprandial blood glucose control by slowing gastric emptying, suppressing glucagon secretion, and promoting satiety. Pramlintide is injected subcutaneously immediately before meals (Gutierrez, 2008) and is indicated for improving glycemic control in type 2 diabetes. It also can be used as adjuvant mealtime therapy for the treatment of type 1 diabetes. Pramlintide may decrease the rate at which drugs affecting gastrointestinal motility and alpha-glucosidase inhibitors are absorbed. Such medications should be administered 1 hour before or 2 hours after administration of pramlintide.

Insulin Delivery Devices
A number of insulin delivery devices are available for the administration of insulin. These vary from syringes to pens to cartridges. The ADA publishes a product directory every January in its *Diabetes Forecast* magazine. This is an excellent resource for exploring the ever-changing spectrum of diabetes products (e.g., insulin pumps, sensors, pens, cartridges, and meters).

The traditional method of delivering insulin is a disposable insulin syringe and needle. Recently, however, a variety of pens and insulin cartridges have been developed to add flexibility in insulin dosing and administration. The spectrum of pens and cartridges include disposable and reusable devices and a variety of insulin preparations.

Insulin Pumps
Continuous subcutaneous insulin infusion (CSII) is a method of intensive insulin therapy that is used in the management of diabetes. An insulin pump is made up of a pump reservoir (syringe) filled with insulin, a small battery-operated pump, and a

computer chip that allows the patient to program and deliver a specific amount of insulin on a regular basis (Figure 53–7 ■). The reservoir is connected to tubing with a needle or flexible cannula at the end, through which the insulin is delivered. The cannula is inserted subcutaneously, usually on the abdomen. The entire infusion set is changed routinely every 2 days.

The pump delivers insulin 24 hours a day in programmed rates specific to each patient. Insulin pumps are designed to help mimic the basal and meal-stimulated patterns of endogenous insulin secretion. During insulin pump therapy, a small amount of short- or rapid-acting insulin is infused continuously. This rate helps to maintain blood glucose levels within a normal range between meals and during the night.

The pump can be programmed to infuse differing basal rates throughout the 24-hour period. For example, a patient who exercises every day at a particular time may elect to decrease the basal rate during the exercise period. Prior to meals and snacks, the patient injects a specific calculated dose or "bolus" of insulin through the pump. This dose of insulin is calculated based on the premeal/snack blood glucose levels and the CHO content of the meal/snack and reflects meal-stimulated insulin secretion.

Oral Diabetes Medications

Currently six classes of oral medications are approved for the treatment of type 2 diabetes in the United States: *sulfonylureas, meglitinides, α-glucosidase inhibitors, biguanides, thiazolidinediones,* and *dipeptidyl peptidase-4 (DPP-4) inhibitors.* Broadly these medications are grouped into those that enhance insulin secretion (sulfonylureas and rapid-acting secretagogues), reduce hepatic glucose production (biguanides), delay digestion and absorption of intestinal CHO (alpha-glucosidase inhibitors), improve insulin sensitivity (thiazolidinediones and biguanides), and increase postprandial insulin secretion (DPP-4 inhibitors).

The general characteristics of medications within these classes are detailed in the Pharmacology Summary (p. 1678). General information regarding the major classes of drugs used to treat type 2 diabetes is also provided in the Pharmacology Summary (p. 1678). More detailed information regarding drugs within each of these classes is included in the following paragraphs. This information is not meant to replace a pharmacology text, but to highlight important information.

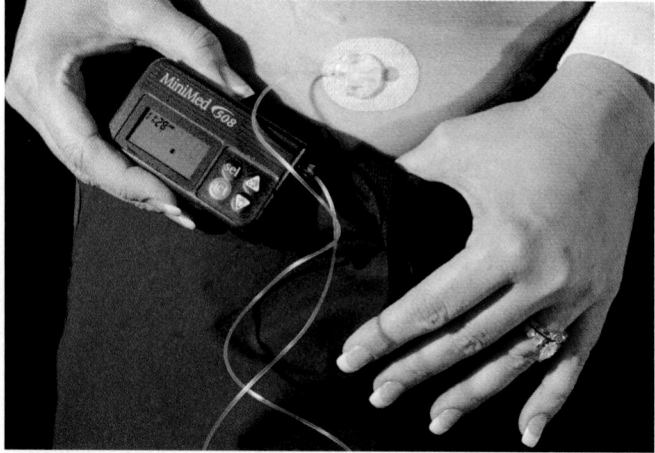

FIGURE 53–7 ■ Insulin pump.
Source: Spencer Grant/Photo Researchers, Inc.

Sulfonylureas

Sulfonylureas are indicated for the treatment of type 2 diabetes and have been an important part of diabetes therapy for several decades. These medications are grouped into first-generation and second-generation compounds. The first-generation products are associated with greater adverse events and interactions. These compounds have been replaced largely by the second-generation compounds.

The primary mechanism through which sulfonylureas exert their effects is by stimulating insulin secretion from the pancreatic beta cell. The secretion of insulin is regulated by ATP-dependent potassium channels, located in the plasma membrane of the pancreatic beta-cell. Sulfonylureas bind to the sulfonylurea receptor and close ATP-dependent potassium channels. As potassium accumulates within the beta cell membrane, the beta cell depolarizes, leading to an influx of calcium. The increased concentration of calcium causes insulin granules to migrate to the cell surface, where the granules rupture and release the insulin by exocytosis (Campbell & White, 2000).

The most common side effect of oral sulfonylureas is hypoglycemia. In addition, there are two specific issues that are important to note. First, there is some cross-sensitivity with sulfa medications, suggesting that some patients who are allergic to sulfa will also be allergic to sulfonylureas. Second, the combination of chlorpropamide and alcohol can result in a disulfiram (medication used in the treatment of alcoholism) reaction characterized by warmth, flushing, headache, nausea, vomiting, sweating, and thirst (Harmel et al., 2004). Although chlorpropamide is seldom used, patients are still advised to avoid alcohol when prescribed second-generation sulfonylureas are used (e.g., glipizide, glyburide, glimepiride).

Meglitinides

Meglitinides are indicated as an adjunct to nutrition and exercise in patients with type 2 diabetes to reduce hyperglycemia. Meglitinides comprise a new class of insulin secretagogues that are structurally and pharmacologically distinct from sulfonylureas (Krentz & Bailey, 2005). This class of medications causes rapid secretion of insulin from the pancreatic beta cells. They are given prior to meals in order to reduce postprandial hyperglycemia.

Meglitinides bind to the sulfonylurea receptor on the plasma membrane of the pancreatic beta cell at a site distinct from the sulfonylurea binding site. This results in the closure of ATP-dependent potassium channels. The closure of these channels inhibits potassium efflux from the cell, and causes membrane depolarization and calcium influx (Campbell & White, 2000). This influx of calcium stimulates the secretion of insulin from the beta cell as described previously with respect to sulfonylureas. There are distinct differences, however, between the onset and duration of action of sulfonylureas and meglitinides. Whereas, sulfonylureas cause insulin to be released in a sustained fashion and are associated with a longer duration of action, meglitinides cause insulin to be released rapidly and are associated with a shorter duration of action (Campbell & White, 2000). The rapid absorption pattern of meglitinides makes them ideal agents to be administered prior to each meal to reduce postprandial hyperglycemia.

Because the meglitinides induce a rapid insulin response, hypoglycemia is a potential risk. Patients need to be counseled to eat within 20 minutes after oral administration to prevent hypoglycemia.

Alpha-Glucosidase Inhibitors

There is increasing emphasis on the contribution of postprandial hyperglycemia to the development of diabetes-related complications. Alpha-glucosidase inhibitors have the ability to reduce the postprandial rise in blood glucose levels and improve glucose control.

Alpha-glucosidase inhibitors are named for their ability to reversibly bind to alpha-glucosidase enzymes (i.e., sucrase, maltase, isomaltase, and glucoamylase) in the brush border of the small intestine. The alpha-glucosidase enzymes break down disaccharides and oligosaccharides into glucose and other monosaccharides that can be absorbed in the small intestine. The competitive reversible binding by the alpha-glucosidase inhibitors to these enzymes delays the absorption of CHOs from the gastrointestinal tract, which leads to a more even absorption of sugars throughout the gut. As a result, there is a blunting of the normally sharp rise in postprandial blood glucose levels that follow a meal.

The gastrointestinal side effects, such as softer stools, diarrhea, flatulence, and bloating, are self-limiting and can be reduced with a lower initial starting dose and a slower dose titration. However, alpha-glucosidase inhibitors are contraindicated in a number of gastrointestinal problems including inflammatory bowel disease, colonic ulceration, and partial intestinal obstruction (Campbell & White, 2000). In addition, alpha-glucosidase inhibitors are contraindicated in the presence of any chronic intestinal disease associated with marked alterations in digestion and absorption and any gastrointestinal conditions that may deteriorate as a result of increased intestinal gas formation (Campbell & White, 2000). Hypoglycemia can occur with alpha-glucosidase inhibitors; hence, patients need to be counseled to use pure glucose, such as fruit juices, glucose tablets, and glucose gels to treat their reactions because the absorption of other CHO may be delayed.

Biguanides

Biguanides are a class of medications that has been used extensively in Europe since the 1950s. One of the earlier compounds, phenformin, was approved for use in the United States in 1959. Federal approval for this medication was withdrawn in 1976 after several cases of fatal lactic acidosis (Krentz & Bailey, 2005). Metformin is another biguanide that has been used extensively in Europe for several decades and has a well-established safety profile. In 1995, this compound was approved for use in the United States.

Metformin has a number of effects on CHO and lipid metabolism. Metformin enhances the sensitivity of peripheral and hepatic tissues to insulin. This compound has multiple effects on the liver, reducing both hepatic glycogenolysis and gluconeogenesis and increasing glycogen synthesis. This reduction in hepatic glycogenolysis and gluconeogenesis results in decreased hepatic glucose production and lowers blood glucose concentrations.

The primary side effects of metformin are gastrointestinal disturbances such as nausea, vomiting, and diarrhea. These side effects can largely be prevented through slow titration of the dosage. A rare but important adverse reaction associated with metformin is lactic acidosis. As noted previously, metformin is excreted primarily by the kidney. Therefore, in the presence of renal insufficiency, the medication accumulates and the risk of lactic acidosis increases. Although lactic acidosis is not a frequent complication of metformin therapy, when it does occur, it can be life threatening. Therefore, careful screening of patients at greatest risk for developing lactic acidosis is the best prevention.

 *Metformin is contraindicated in patients with acute or chronic metabolic acidosis, who have known hypersensitivity to metformin, heart failure requiring pharmacologic management, renal disease or dysfunction as evidenced by serum creatinine levels ≥1.5 mg/dL (males) and ≥1.4 mg/dL (females) or abnormal creatinine clearance, and age >80 years with an abnormal creatinine clearance.*

 Radiological studies often are associated with nephrotoxic contrast dyes. The diabetic kidney is particularly vulnerable to these dyes. In patients treated with metformin, deterioration in renal function can result in accumulation of lactic acid and development of lactic acidosis. Metformin should be withheld for at least 48 hours after procedures in which iodinated radio contrast dyes are used and restarted when serum creatinine levels are normal. In addition, metformin should be discontinued temporarily for any surgical procedure and should be reinstituted only after it has been established that postprocedure renal function is normal.

A number of medical conditions, such as heart failure, acute myocardial infarction, and septic shock, are associated with hypoxia, decreased tissue perfusion, and lactic acidosis. As such, metformin is contraindicated during these situations. Because patients who consume excess alcohol have a greater propensity for lactic acidosis, metformin should be used cautiously in chronic alcohol abusers. Impaired hepatic function also is associated with lactic acidosis and thus metformin should be used cautiously in such patients.

Thiazolidinediones

The thiazolidinediones are a unique class of antihyperglycemic medications that improve insulin sensitivity through multiple actions on gene regulation. These drugs, which are often termed *insulin sensitizers*, require that circulating levels of insulin be present for these drugs to be effective.

The action mechanisms of thiazolidinediones are not completely understood. The effects of thiazolidinediones are mediated through a family of nuclear receptors, called the peroxisome-proliferator-activated (PPAR) receptors. The PPAR family of receptors is responsible for the modulation of lipid homeostasis, adipocyte differentiation, and insulin action. In particular, thiazolidinediones bind and activate the PPAR isoform, improving blood glucose control through enhancement of hepatic and peripheral insulin sensitivity. The thiazolidinediones also show some cross reactivity with other isoforms in the PPAR family, which accounts for their potential roles in a variety of cellular processes, such as regulation of lipid metabolism.

The first thiazolidinedione, troglitazone, was associated with fatal liver toxicity and was withdrawn from the U.S. market in 2000. Because pioglitazone and rosiglitazone are biochemically related to troglitazone, strict guidelines were developed by the U.S. Food and Drug Administration (FDA) regarding how frequently liver function should be monitored. Active liver disease does remain a contraindication to the use of thiazolidinediones, even though pioglitazone and rosiglitazone have not been associated with hepatotoxicity (Krentz & Bailey, 2005). In 2004, the FDA recommendation for monitoring of liver enzymes was relaxed. Liver enzymes must be drawn prior to the initiation of thiazolidinediones and periodically thereafter, based on the clinical judgment of the health care provider.

Fluid retention and weight gain are the main adverse effects in human trials of thiazolidinediones. The fluid retention can result in edema and cases of heart failure have been precipitated. Patients who had significant heart failure, categorized as New York Heart Association (NYHA) class III and IV, were excluded from phase III trials of rosiglitazone and pioglitazone because troglitazone was associated with volume expansion, increased preload, and adverse cardiac effects in animal models of hypoglycemia (Campbell & White, 2000). Therefore, the thiazolidinediones are contraindicated in patients with NYHA class III and IV heart failure.

Dipeptidyl Peptidase-4 Inhibitors

The newest class of oral diabetes medications is the DPP-4 inhibitors. These medications are a part of incretin-related therapies that exert their effects by increasing meal-related insulin secretion and reducing postprandial blood glucose levels.

Incretin hormones, including glucagon-like peptide 1 (GLP-1) and glucose-dependent insulinotropic polypeptide (GIP), are released by the intestine throughout the day, and levels are increased in response to a meal. These hormones are rapidly inactivated by the enzyme dipeptidyl peptidase 4. When blood glucose concentrations are normal or elevated, GLP-1 and GIP increase insulin synthesis and release from pancreatic beta cells. GLP-1 also lowers glucagon secretion from pancreatic cells, leading to reduced hepatic glucose production.

Sitagliptin currently is the only DDP inhibitor approved in the United States; however, a number of newer DDP inhibitors are in clinical trials. One rare complication of sitagliptin is Stevens-Johnson syndrome, a life-threatening hypersensitivity reaction affecting the skin (Burant & ADA, 2008). In general, no dosage adjustment is needed for patients with mild to moderate liver or kidney disease; however, lower dosages are recommended for patients with moderate and severe kidney disease or ESRD requiring hemodialysis.

Approach to Insulin Therapy in Type 1 Diabetes

As previously noted, patients with type 1 diabetes rely on exogenous insulin to sustain life. The goal of insulin therapy in type 1 diabetes is the normalization of blood glucose levels. This is best achieved using combinations of insulin in a manner that most closely resembles basal and meal-stimulated insulin release. See the Pharmacology Summary of Medications to Treat Type 2 Diabetes (p. 1678).

Some of the options for insulin regimens are presented next.

Twice-Daily Injection Regimen

The insulin regimens discussed in this section are examples of a two-injection regimen, combining Regular or rapid-acting insulin (lispro) with an intermediate-acting insulin (NPH) prior to breakfast and prior to supper (Figure 53–8 ■).

The lispro peaks when the blood glucose level rises after breakfast and dinner and the NPH insulin provides basal insulin coverage. The Regular insulin peaks later and the peaks are not

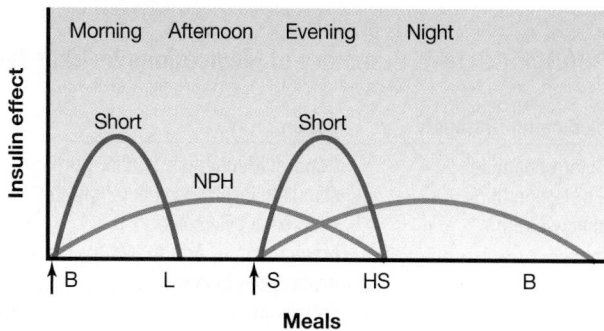

(a)

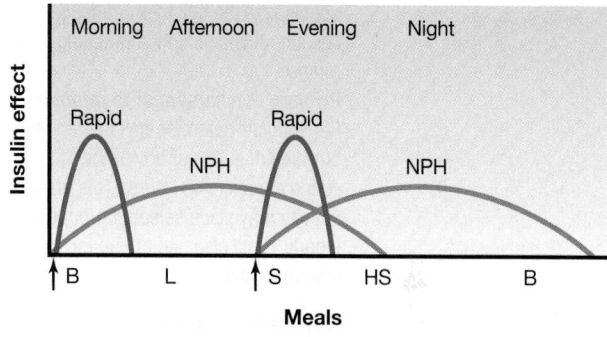

(b)

FIGURE 53–8 ■ Twice-daily split and mixed insulin regimen.

as high. Because no rapid-acting insulin is provided at lunch, the peak of the NPH insulin helps to reduce blood glucose levels following lunch. Using this regimen, patients with type 1 diabetes can attain *adequate* glucose control. The peak effect of NPH predisposes patients to hypoglycemia if meals are skipped. This regimen provides the patient little flexibility in changing mealtimes.

Three-Times-Daily Injection Regimen

The regimen discussed here is an example of a three-times-daily injection regimen (Figure 53–9 ■, p. 1682), combining Regular or rapid-acting insulin with NPH prior to breakfast, Regular or rapid-acting insulin prior to dinner, and NPH prior to bedtime. The major difference in this method with the method described in the previous paragraph is that the NPH is injected prior to bedtime. The movement of the NPH to bedtime means that the NPH will peak in the middle of the night, when the glucose is rising in response to the normal increase in endogenous growth hormone secretion. This method has value in individuals who have high fasting glucose levels on awakening.

There are two major causes of fasting hyperglycemia, the **dawn phenomenon** and the **Somogyi effect**. The dawn phenomenon is defined as fasting hyperglycemia without prior nocturnal hypoglycemia, and the Somogyi effect is defined as fasting hyperglycemia with prior hypoglycemia (Sheehan, 2004). The dawn phenomenon occurs when growth hormone, a counterregulatory hormone, is secreted during the night. Patients awake with elevated fasting blood glucose levels, precipitated, in part, by growth hormone. Moving the timing of the NPH insulin to bedtime means that the NPH insulin will peak as growth hormone rises.

PHARMACOLOGY Summary of Medications to Treat Type 2 Diabetes

Medication/Category	Action	Application/Indication	Nursing Responsibility
Chlorpropamide (First-generation sulfonylurea)	**General Mechanism:** Sulfonylureas stimulate insulin secretion from the pancreatic beta cells. **Mechanism of Action (MOA):** These medications bind with a cell surface protein on the pancreatic beta cell. The binding of the sulfonylurea with the sulfonylurea receptor (SUR) results in the closure of potassium channels and depolarizes the cell membrane, opening calcium channels and stimulating insulin release. **Primary Mechanism of Clearance:** Renal chlorpropamide has the longest duration of action of any of the sulfonylureas (>48 hours). This enhanced activity may place selected groups (e.g., elderly, renal disease) at risk for hypoglycemia.	Used to lower blood glucose in patients with type 2 diabetes.	Assess patient for allergy to other sulfonylureas or sulfa medications. Assess patient for renal or liver disease. Assess patients who are at high risk for injury from hypoglycemia (e.g., elderly). Assess patient for signs and symptoms of hyponatremia (chlorpropamide specific effect). Assess patient for weight gain. Instruct patient on the signs and symptoms of hypoglycemia. Instruct patient on the treatment of hypoglycemia. Instruct patient to avoid ingesting alcohol with medication to prevent a disulfiram reaction.
Tolbutamide (First-generation oral sulfonylurea)	**General Mechanism:** Sulfonylureas stimulate insulin secretion from the pancreatic beta cells. **MOA:** See above **Primary Mechanism of Clearance:** Hepatic	Lowers blood glucose in patients with type 2 diabetes.	As above
Tolazamide (First-generation sulfonylurea)	**General Mechanism:** Sulfonylureas stimulate insulin secretion from the pancreatic beta cells. **MOA:** See above **Primary Mechanism of Clearance:** Hepatic and renal	Lowers blood glucose in patients with type 2 diabetes.	As above
Glyburide (Second-generation sulfonylurea)	**General Mechanism:** Sulfonylureas stimulate insulin secretion from the pancreatic beta cells. **MOA:** See above **Primary Mechanism of Clearance:** Hepatic and renal	Lowers blood glucose in patients with type 2 diabetes.	As above
Glipizide (Second-generation sulfonylurea; available in extended-release formulations)	**General Mechanism:** Sulfonylureas stimulate insulin secretion from the pancreatic beta cells. **MOA:** See above **Primary Mechanism of Clearance:** Hepatic	Lowers blood glucose in patients with type 2 diabetes.	As above *In addition:* Instruct patient to take glipizide with meals.
Glimepiride (Second-generation sulfonylurea)	**General Mechanism:** Sulfonylureas stimulate insulin secretion from the pancreatic beta cells. **MOA:** See above **Primary Mechanism of Clearance:** Hepatic and renal	Lowers blood glucose in patients with type 2 diabetes.	As above

PHARMACOLOGY Summary of Medications to Treat Type 2 Diabetes—*Continued*

Medication/Category	Action	Application/Indication	Nursing Responsibility
Metformin (Biguanide) (available in extended-release formulations)	**General Mechanism:** Metformin reduces hepatic glucose production and improves insulin sensitivity. **MOA:** Metformin reduces hepatic glucose production through decreased hepatic glycogenolysis and decreased hepatic gluconeogenesis. It also improves insulin sensitivity through mechanisms that are not entirely clear. **Primary Method of Clearance:** Metformin is not metabolized but is cleared rapidly from the kidney. Metformin is contraindicated in patients with renal, cardiorespiratory, hepatic dysfunction, and alcohol abuse. These conditions may precipitate lactic acidosis, which is a rare, but life-threatening, complication. Renal dysfunction is defined as: Serum creatinine: $\geq$1.5 mg/dL in males; $\geq$1.4 mg/dL in females; or abnormal creatinine clearance. Elderly patients need a 24-hour urine for creatinine clearance prior to starting on metformin.	Lowers blood glucose in patients with type 2 diabetes.	Assess patient for allergy to metformin. Assess patient for contraindications to metformin (renal, cardiorespiratory, hepatic dysfunction, and alcohol abuse). Assess patient for the development of gastrointestinal symptoms, such as diarrhea, nausea, vomiting, flatulence, abdominal discomfort, and indigestion. Encourage patients to report continued gastrointestinal symptoms to their health care provider, because the symptoms may resolve with slower titration of the metformin dose. Discuss with patient the risk of lactic acidosis. Instruct patient on the signs and symptoms of hypoglycemia. In general, metformin does not cause hypoglycemia as monotherapy. However, hypoglycemia may occur when metformin is combined with other medications. Discuss with patients the need to discontinue metformin prior to any procedure using a radiocontrast dye, and to resume the medication only when normal renal function has been assessed.
Acarbose (Alpha-glucosidase inhibitor)	**General Mechanism:** Alpha-glucosidase inhibitors reduce postprandial hyperglycemia. **MOA:** The actions of the alpha-glucosidase inhibitors occur in the intestinal lumen where they competitively inhibit enzymes that convert polysaccharides into simple sugars. The alpha-glucosidase inhibitors delay the absorption of dietary carbohydrates until they reach the distal bowel. As a result, these inhibitors reduce postprandial hyperglycemia. **Primary Method of Clearance:** Renal and feces	Lowers postprandial hyperglycemia in patients with type 2 diabetes.	Assess patient for allergy to alpha-glucosidase inhibitors. Assess patient for any gastrointestinal conditions (e.g., inflammatory bowel disease, colonic ulceration, partial intestinal obstruction) that may deteriorate as a result of increased intestinal gas formation. Instruct patient to contact her health care provider for continued bloating and flatulence, because the symptoms may resolve with slower titration of the alpha-glucosidase dose. Instruct patient to take the medication with the first bite of each meal. Instruct patient to recognize the signs and symptoms of hypoglycemia. In general, alpha-glucosidase inhibitors do not cause hypoglycemia when used as monotherapy. Hypoglycemia can occur when used in combination with other hypoglycemic medications. Instruct patient on the treatment of hypoglycemia. Patients using alpha-glucosidase inhibitors need to treat their reactions with pure glucose, such as glucose gels, glucose tablets, or fruit juice, because the absorption of other carbohydrates may be delayed.

(continued)

PHARMACOLOGY Summary of Medications to Treat Type 2 Diabetes—*Continued*

Medication/Category	Action	Application/Indication	Nursing Responsibility
Miglitol (Alpha-glucosidase inhibitor)	**General Mechanism:** Alpha-glucosidase inhibitors reduce postprandial hyperglycemia. **MOA:** See above **Primary Method of Clearance:** Renal	Lowers postprandial hyperglycemia in patients with type 2 diabetes.	As above
Repaglinide (Meglitinide)	**General Mechanism:** Meglitinides cause a rapid increase in insulin secretion. **MOA:** Meglitinides are nonsulfonylureas medications that act through the SUR on the pancreatic beta cells. The meglitinides bind with the SUR at a site distinct for the traditional sulfonylureas (see above). The binding of the sulfonylurea with the SUR results in the closure of potassium channels and depolarizes the cell membrane, opening calcium channels and stimulating insulin release. The meglitinides differ from the sulfonylureas in that the insulin response is rapid and exerts it major effect on postprandial hyperglycemia. **Primary Method of Clearance:** Hepatic	Lowers postprandial hyperglycemia in patients with type 2 diabetes.	Assess patient for any allergies to meglitinide. Instruct patient to take the medication at the start of the meal and to withhold the dose if no meal is eaten. Instruct patient on the signs and symptoms of hypoglycemia. Instruct patient on the treatment of hypoglycemia.
Nateglinide (Meglitinide)	**General Mechanism:** Meglitinides cause a rapid increase in insulin secretion. **MOA:** See above **Primary Method of Clearance:** Hepatic and renal	Lowers postprandial hyperglycemia in patients with type 2 diabetes.	As above
Sitagliptin (Dipeptidyl peptidase-4 [DPP-4] inhibitor)	**General Mechanism:** DPP-4 inhibitors lower postprandial hyperglycemia. **MOA:** Glucagon-like peptide 1 (GLP-1) is a hormone that is secreted by the intestinal L-cell, which suppresses elevated glucagon levels, promotes satiety, decreases food intake, and slows gastric emptying. DPP-4 is an enzyme that inactivates the GLP-1 peptide. DPP-4 inhibitors slow the breakdown of GLP-1 and thereby extend the effects of the hormone. **Primary Method of Clearance:** Hepatic and renal	Lowers postprandial hyperglycemia in patients with type 2 diabetes.	Assess patient for allergies to DPP-4 inhibitors. Instruct patient to notify health care provider if a skin rash develops.
Pioglitazone (Thiazolidinedione)	**General Mechanism:** Thiazolidinediones improve insulin sensitivity. **MOA:** The actions of thiazolidinediones occur through the actions of a group of nuclear regulatory proteins, peroxisome-proliferator-activated (PPAR) receptors, which are important in fat and carbohydrate metabolism. Thiazolidinediones bind and activate the PPARγ isoform and improve insulin sensitivity. **Primary Method of Clearance:** Hepatic	Lowers postprandial hyperglycemia in patients with type 2 diabetes.	Assess patient for the presence of liver disease. Monitor patient for weight gain and fluid retention. Instruct patient to contact his health care provider if shortness of breath, edema, and fatigue develop. Instruct patient to contact her health care provider if signs and symptoms develop of liver disease: nausea, vomiting, fatigue, jaundice, and dark urine. Instruct anovulatory premenopausal women (e.g., polycystic ovarian syndrome) that these medications may cause ovulation to resume and pregnancy to occur.

PHARMACOLOGY Summary of Medications to Treat Type 2 Diabetes—*Continued*

Medication/Category	Action	Application/Indication	Nursing Responsibility
Rosiglitazone (Thiazolidinedione)	**General Mechanism:** Thiazolidinediones improve insulin sensitivity. **MOA:** See above **Primary Method of Clearance:** Hepatic	As above	As above
Exenatide (Incretin mimetics)	**General Mechanism:** Exenatide reduces postprandial hyperglycemia. **MOA:** Exenatide is an analog of GLP-1 (see DPP-4 inhibitors) that suppresses elevated glucagon levels, promotes satiety, decreases food intake, and slows gastric emptying. The medication is injected prior to meals to reduce postprandial hyperglycemia. **Primary Method of Clearance:** Renal	Lowers postprandial hyperglycemia in patients with type 2 diabetes.	Assess patient for any allergies to incretin mimetics. Instruct patient on proper injection techniques. Instruct patient to check the injection site for swelling and irritation. Instruct patient to inject medication prior to meals. Instruct patient on the signs and symptoms of hypoglycemia. Instruct patient on the treatment of hypoglycemia. Instruct patient to call his health care provider with continued gastrointestinal symptoms, because slower titration of the dose may alleviate this problem.
Pramlintide (Amylin analog)	**General Mechanism:** Pramlintide reduces postprandial hyperglycemia. **MOA:** Amylin is a neuroendocrine hormone that is secreted with insulin from the pancreatic beta cells. This hormone can reduce postprandial blood glucose control through slowing gastric emptying, suppressing glucagon secretion, and promoting satiety. Pramlintide is an amylin analog that is injected prior to meals to reduce postprandial hyperglycemia. **Primary Method of Clearance:** Renal	Pramlintide is used in patients with type 1 diabetes and insulin-treated type 2 diabetes. Patients with type 1 diabetes are amylin deficient. Patients with type 2 diabetes have a poor amylin response to meal. Treatment with pramlintide can address each of these problems,	Assess patient for any allergies to pramlintide. Assess patient for gastroparesis and hypoglycemic unawareness because these conditions may predispose the patient to severe hypoglycemia. Instruct patient on proper injection techniques. Instruct patient to check the injection site for swelling and irritation. Instruct patient to inject medication prior to meals. Instruct patient on the signs and symptoms of hypoglycemia. Instruct patient on the treatment of hypoglycemia.

Sources: American Diabetes Association. (2008a). *Diabetes forecast resource guide 2008.* Alexandria, VA: Author; Burant, C. F., & American Diabetes Association. (2008). *Medical management of type 2 diabetes* (6th ed.). Alexandria, VA: American Diabetes Association; Campbell, R. K., & White, J. R., Jr. (2000). *Medications for the treatment of diabetes.* Alexandria, VA: American Diabetes Association; Gutierrez, K. (2008). *Pharmacotherapeutics: Clinical reasoning in primary care* (2nd ed.). St. Louis: W. B. Saunders; Kaufman, F., & American Diabetes Association. (2008). *Medical management of type 1 diabetes* (5th ed.). Alexandria, VA: American Diabetes Association; Youngkin, E. Q., Sawin, K. J., Kissinger, J. F., & Isreal, D. S. (Eds.). (2005). *Pharmacotherapeutics* (2nd ed.). Upper Saddle, NJ: Pearson Prentice Hall.

Prior to initiating this regimen, it probably is best to assess whether the patient has dawn phenomenon or the Somogyi effect. In the Somogyi effect, hypoglycemia occurs during the middle of the night. When the hypoglycemia occurs there is a release of glucose from the liver. This release of glucose from the liver is associated with a rise in glucose and an elevated fasting blood glucose level. As a result, patients awake with an elevated fasting blood glucose level. The best way to assess for whether this is the Somogyi effect or the dawn phenomenon is to test the blood glucose levels in the middle of the night. If hypoglycemia is present in the middle of the night, it is likely that the elevated morning blood glucose level is rebound hyperglycemia or the

Somogyi effect. If hypoglycemia is not present during this time, it is more likely that the elevated morning blood glucose level is a result of the dawn phenomenon.

Four-Times-Daily Injection Regimen

The regimen described here requires four injections of insulin per day (Figure 53–10 ■, p. 1682): NPH is given at breakfast and bedtime, while the rapid- or short-acting insulin is give prior to each meal. The premeal insulin helps reduce the postprandial hypoglycemia. The NPH provides "basal" insulin. As noted previously, NPH has a characteristic peak action that predisposes the patient to hypoglycemia.

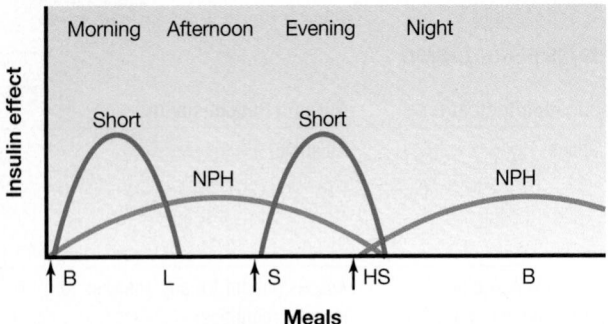

(a)

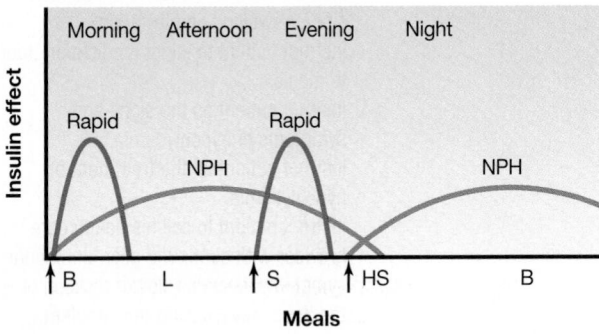

(b)

FIGURE 53–9 ■ Three-times-daily insulin injection regimen.

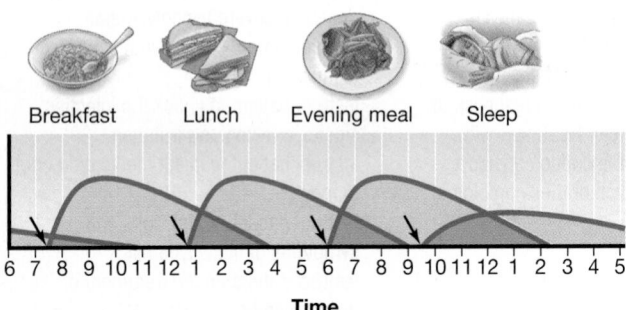

FIGURE 53–10 ■ Four-times-daily insulin injection regimen.

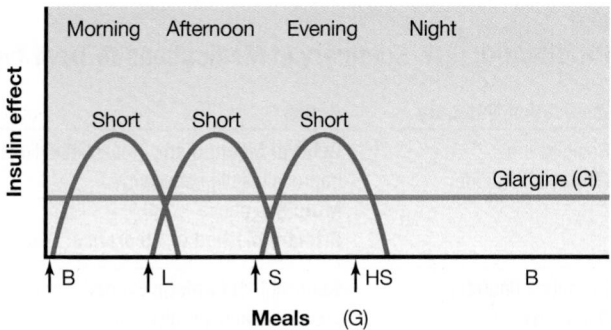

(a)

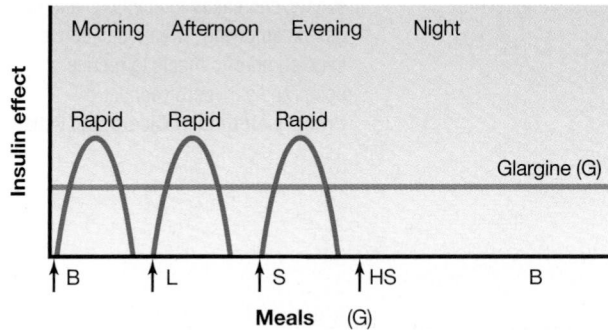

(b)

FIGURE 53–11 ■ Multiple daily dose regimen.

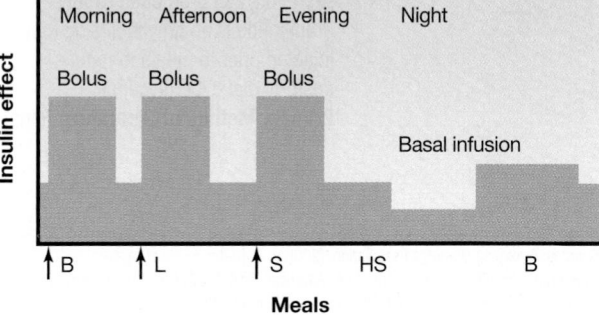

(a)

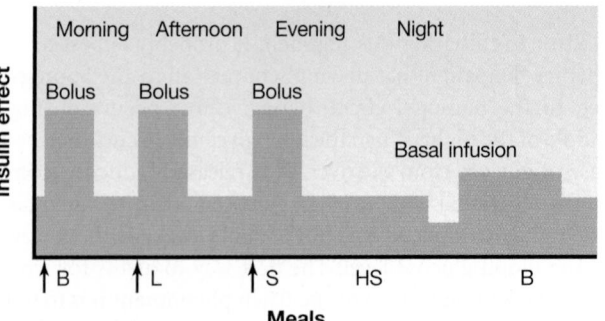

(b)

FIGURE 53–12 ■ Continuous subcutaneous insulin infusion.

"Peakless" insulins, such as glargine, provide better basal insulin coverage. The multiple-dose regimen using glargine is widely used by patients with diabetes and is illustrated in Figure 53–11 ■. In this regimen, long-acting insulin (i.e., glargine) is used in combination with a rapid-acting insulin (lispro) prior to each meal. The glargine insulin has no peak; therefore, it resembles endogenous insulin more precisely.

One of the most effective ways to mimic normal insulin secretion is through the use of an insulin pump, which can provide continuous subcutaneous insulin infusion. The insulin pump, described earlier, is programmed to infuse rapid doses of short-acting insulin continuously at a basal rate, with patients determining bolus insulin injections prior to meals and snacks. The actions of the insulin pump are shown (Figure 53–12 ■). One of the important features of this insulin delivery system is that the basal rate can be changed to match the needs of individual patients. For example, higher rates of insulin can be delivered throughout for those patients who have high fasting glucose levels, presumably due to counterregulatory hormone secretion (e.g., growth hormone) during the night.

Pharmacologic Treatment of Type 2 Diabetes

The traditional approach to the treatment of type 2 diabetes has employed diet and exercise as a "first-line" therapy, introducing pharmacologic therapy when patients cannot meet their glycemic goals with diet and exercise alone. During the past decade, there have been some fundamental differences in the understanding of diabetes that have caused reevaluation of this approach.

Health care providers often are faced with the question as to when to initiate sequential (i.e., diet and exercise, followed by pharmacologic therapy, if indicated) or complementary therapy (i.e., introduction of simultaneous pharmacologic, diet, and exercise therapy) in the treatment of hyperglycemia. The majority of patients with type 2 diabetes are obese, having attempted to lose weight over several years. Increasingly, health care providers are introducing medications at the diagnosis of diabetes to be used in combination with diet and exercise. Some of the newer medications (biguanides and thiazolidinediones) used in the treatment of type 2 diabetes are unlikely to produce hypoglycemia when used as monotherapy; these medications can be safely used at diagnosis in patients with mild to moderate hyperglycemia. Metformin may be used in combination with diet and exercise in patients who have been diagnosed with pre-diabetes.

Although many patients with type 2 diabetes initially are treated successfully with monotherapy, eventually one type of medication is not sufficient to maintain normal blood glucose levels. Because medications have specific mechanisms of action that revolve around several major processes (e.g., augmenting insulin supply, decreasing insulin resistance, decreasing glucose absorption), these medications can be used in combination to maintain normoglycemia. Some of these combinations include sulfonylureas and metformin, sulfonylureas and alpha-glucosidase inhibitors, sulfonylureas and thiazolidinediones, and metformin and meglitinides. Additionally, there are a number of newer medications that combine different medications in one pill. These include metformin and Glyburide (Glucovance), metformin and rosiglitazone (Avandamet), metformin and Glipizide (Metaglip), metformin and pioglitazone (ACTOplus Met), metformin and sitagliptin (Janumet), pioglitazone and glimepiride (Duetact), and rosiglitazone and glimepiride (Avandaryl). The specific properties of each of the classes (e.g., thiazolidinediones, sulfonylureas) are detailed in the Pharmacology Summary (p. 1678) earlier in this chapter.

Oral Medications

Some general principles apply when combining oral medications (Riddle, 1999). First, when a patient fails oral monotherapy, combining drugs of different classes is usually more effective than stopping one and substituting another. Second, when a patient requires near-maximum doses of one medication, adding another drug usually is better than increasing the dosage of the original medication. Third, secondary failure of the two-drug combination in patients with type 2 diabetes is expected eventually. In these patients, a three-drug combination is potentially useful, but one should consider the addition of insulin to the existing regimen or insulin alone should be considered.

Insulin Therapy in Type 2 Diabetes Mellitus

The purpose of insulin therapy in patients with type 2 diabetes is to provide adequate insulin to supplement the reduction in insulin secretion and to overcome insulin resistance. Type 2 diabetes is a progressive disease with patients responding to oral medications early in their disease, but requiring insulin treatment for adequate glucose control over time (UKPDSG, 1998a). Insulin therapy remains a viable and often necessary option for achieving optimal glucose control. When introducing insulin therapy for patients with type 2 diabetes, any of the previously described regimens are useful.

Insulin also may be provided in combination with selected oral medications. For example, sulfonylureas may be provided throughout the day with a dose of NPH or glargine given at bedtime. The goal of this regimen is to suppress hepatic glucose production during the night. Theoretically, the patient awakes with a lower fasting blood glucose level and the sulfonylureas are more effective during the day. In addition, insulin can be added to regimens consisting of metformin and thiazolidinediones. However, edema is a side effect of thiazolidinediones, particularly when combined with insulin. Both patients and health care providers should be cognizant of the risk of heart failure when thiazolidinediones are used in patients with type 2 diabetes.

Nutrition and Diabetes

Nutrition and physical activity also fall within the realm of medical management, as well as nursing management and self-management. Historically, the American Diabetes Association attempted to identify the "ideal diabetes diet" based on estimated caloric needs and percentages of **micronutrients** (nutritional components such as vitamin or minerals that are needed in small quantities for living organisms) and **macronutrients** (nutritional components such as protein, CHO, and fat that are needed in larger quantities for living organisms). Currently, **medical nutrition therapy** (**MNT**) in diabetes consists of meal planning approaches that are determined by clinical evidence, cultural, social, and ethnic preferences, and patient motivation. There is greater liberalization of macronutrient content, particularly in the amount of CHOs, as long as both glycemic and lipid goals are met. See Chapter 14 🔵 for more information on nutrition.

The American Diabetes Association has extensively reviewed and revised their dietary guidelines (ADA, 2007). These national guidelines now include recommendations for the role of nutrition in the prevention of diabetes (primary prevention), the prevention of complications (secondary prevention), and the treatment of complications (tertiary prevention). These goals are outlined in the National Guidelines for MNT in Individuals at Risk for Diabetes or Pre-Diabetes box (p. 1684).

Target Micronutrients and Macronutrients in the Diet

The ADA recommendations for treatment of pre-diabetes, diabetes, and diabetes complications are fairly extensive and beyond the scope of this chapter. However, the recommended micronutrients and macronutrients are summarized in Chart 53–4 (p. 1684). It is extremely important to note that the macronutrient (i.e., CHO, fats, and protein) content is highly individualized, and may need to be modified in response to lipid and blood pressure goals.

NATIONAL GUIDELINES for MNT in Individuals at Risk for Diabetes or Pre-Diabetes

The goals for MNT for individuals at risk for diabetes or pre-diabetes are as follows:

- To decrease the risk of diabetes and CVD by promoting healthy food choices and physical activity leading to moderate weight loss.
- To decrease the risk of diabetes and CVD through maintenance of this weight loss.

The goals of MNT for individuals with diabetes are as follows:

- Achieve and maintain blood glucose levels in the normal range or as close to normal as is safely possible.
- Achieve and maintain a lipid and lipoprotein profile that decreases the risk for the development of CVD.
- Achieve and maintain normal blood pressure levels in the normal range or as close to normal as is safely possible.
- Prevent or decrease the rate of the development of chronic diabetes complications by modifying nutrient intake and adapting healthy lifestyle changes.
- Address nutritional needs, taking into account each individual's personal and cultural references and willingness to change.
- Maintain the pleasure of eating by only limiting food choices where there is scientific evidence in support of excluding these choices from the diet.

The goals of MNT that apply to specific situations are as follows:

- Provide adequate calories to ensure normal growth and development in youth with type 1 diabetes, youth with type 2 diabetes, and in pregnant and lactating women.
- Provide self-management training for safe conduct of exercise, including the prevention and treatment of hypoglycemia in individuals treated with medications that cause hypoglycemia.
- Provide self-management training for diabetes treatment during acute illness.

Source: American Diabetes Association. (2007). Nutrition recommendations and interventions for diabetes: A position statement of the American Diabetes Association. *Diabetes Care, 30* (Suppl. 1), S48–S65.

CHART 53–4 **General Macronutrient and Micronutrient Recommendations in Individuals with Diabetes**

CARBOHYDRATES (CHO)

- Dietary patterns including CHO from fruits, vegetables, whole grains, legumes, and low-fat milk are encouraged.
- Low-CHO diets, restricting total carbohydrate to <130 g/day, are not recommended in the management of diabetes.
- Monitoring CHO (e.g., CHO counting, exchanges, experience) is an important strategy in the nutritional treatment of diabetes.
- The use of the glycemic index (i.e., a ranking system that evaluates the effect of CHO on blood glucose levels; higher glycemic index foods are associated with a higher postprandial rise in blood glucose) and load (i.e., a ranking system that takes into consideration the glycemic index and portion size) may provide a modest additional benefit over that observed when total carbohydrate is considered alone.
- Sucrose-containing foods can be substituted for other CHO in the meal plan. If these foods are an addition to the meal plan, they can be covered with insulin or other glucose-lowering medications.
- Many more choices are available today than in the past for including the CHO intake into the diet of individuals with diabetes; however, care should be taken to avoid increased caloric intake.
- Sugar alcohols and nonnutritive sweeteners are considered safe as long as they are consumed within the daily intake levels established by the FDA.

FAT AND CHOLESTEROL

- Limit saturated fat to <7% of total calories.
- Intake of *trans* fat should be minimized.
- Dietary cholesterol should be limited to <200 mg/day.

PROTEIN

- In diabetic patients with normal renal function, there is little evidence to suggest that usual protein intake (15–20% of caloric intake) should be modified.
- Ingested protein can increase the plasma insulin response without increasing blood glucose levels; therefore, protein should not be used to treat acute or prevent nocturnal hypoglycemia in patients with type 2 diabetes.
- High-protein diets are not recommended as a method for weight loss at this time.

ALCOHOL

- If adult patients with diabetes consume alcohol, their daily intake should be limited to a moderate amount (women: ≤1 drink per day; men: ≤2 drinks per day).
- Alcohol should be consumed with food to reduce the risk of nocturnal hypoglycemia in individuals using insulin or oral medications that enhance insulin secretion.
- Moderate alcohol consumption (ingested alone) has no acute effect on blood glucose and insulin concentrations; when CHO is combined with alcohol (i.e., in a mixed drink), the blood glucose level may rise.

MICRONUTRIENTS

- Vitamin or mineral supplementation in patients with diabetes (compared with the general population) does not provide any additional medical benefits.
- Supplementation with antioxidants, such as vitamins E and C and carotene, is not advised; the benefits have not been established and there are concerns about safety.
- Chromium supplementation is not recommended because the benefits have not been established.

Source: American Diabetes Association. (2007). Nutrition recommendations and interventions for diabetes: A position statement of the American Diabetes Association. *Diabetes Care, 30* (Suppl. 1), S48–S65.

Medical Nutrition Therapy

There is no longer a single "diabetes diet"; patients work as partners with their diabetes care team to attain and maintain healthy eating habits that foster the goals of MNT. Meal plans are individualized for each patient, taking into account the patient's lifestyle, culture, food preferences, and ability to make changes. Different educational resources and approaches may be needed during different phases of the educational process. Ideally, every patient with diabetes should be referred to a dietician with training in diabetes MNT. Nurses, physicians, and other members of the health care team are important players in reinforcing healthy eating habits.

Specific considerations need to be addressed when developing meal plans. These primary considerations include glycemic and lipid goals, the type of diabetes, and the pharmacologic treatment regimen being used. In patients with type 1 diabetes using intensive insulin therapy, such as CSII and multiple daily injections (MDIs), meals and physical activity can be coordinated with their insulin doses. Meal planning in the patient using CSII or MDI can be relatively flexible, whereas meal planning in patients with more traditional insulin regimens (e.g., split-mixed insulin) needs to be consistent. For example, patients using CSII or MDI may elect to delay meals for a period of time by maintaining a basal insulin rate and administering the short-acting insulin dose immediately before the meal. In contrast, patients using split-mixed insulin dosing (NPH and short-acting insulin prior to breakfast and prior to dinner) cannot easily change the time of the insulin dose to accommodate meals.

Meal planning for patients with type 2 diabetes also is dependent on the pharmacologic treatment regimen. As noted previously, the patient with type 2 diabetes may use a variety of pharmacologic treatment regimens including oral medications and insulin therapy. In addition, some patients with type 2 diabetes may control their blood glucose levels with a combination of diet and exercise without medications. Many patients with type 2 diabetes are obese and require caloric restriction and weight loss. Diet, weight loss, and pharmacologic therapy need to be finely coordinated. For example, dosages of medications often need to be decreased with caloric restriction or weight loss to prevent hypoglycemia. Otherwise the amount of caloric intake needed to prevent and treat hypoglycemia may interfere with weight loss. With both type 1 and type 2 diabetes, frequent blood glucose testing is necessary to determine the effectiveness of pharmacologic treatment combined with MNT.

Many patients who have been diagnosed with diabetes for a long period of time were taught a system of meal planning using "ADA Exchange Lists." In the ADA Exchange List method all foods were categorized into groups (e.g., bread/starches, meats, fruits, vegetables, fats) and assigned portion sizes representing "1 exchange" or "1 serving" of a particular food. Each exchange had a specific amount of carbohydrates, proteins, and fats. Patients were prescribed a daily meal plan based on a total amount of daily calories (e.g., 1,200 calories per day) equaling a predetermined number of servings from each exchange group.

The ADA Exchange List is not used extensively anymore; however, the principles of the exchange system still may be used for easily determining CHO servings. Because one serving of CHO is 15 grams, patients may be given a meal plan with a specified number of CHO servings at each meal or snack. The pa-

tients are free to choose among all CHO foods of equal CHO value. This method is simple, requiring little calculation. Books are available that list portion sizes of commonly eaten CHO-containing foods. (Evert, Hess-Fischl, & ADA, 2006; Fairview Health Services, 2003; McCarren & ADA, 2007).

Individuals using insulin therapy may learn how to adjust their premeal rapid-acting insulin based on the amount of CHO in the meal. Carbohydrate counting is a method of tracking nutritional intake of CHO and relating the CHO quantity to an insulin dosage. Patients use this ratio to calculate the dose of insulin they must take with meals or snacks. Most adults with type 1 diabetes require 1 unit of rapid-acting insulin (such as insulin lispro or aspart) for every 10 to 15 grams of CHO. The ratio may be different with each meal and change with varying levels of physical activity. The following example shows how a patient with type 1 diabetes can calculate her insulin dose:

> Prelunch blood glucose level: 104 mg/dL
>
> Insulin-to-CHO ratio: 1:12
>
> Prelunch insulin dose: 4 units

Food	CHO Amount (grams)
1 cup black bean chili	32
1 1/2 cups green salad with tomatoes	10
2 tbsp vinaigrette dressing	6
Total CHO grams:	48

As can be seen from the calculations, the total amount of CHO from a variety of food sources is 48 grams. Because the ratio of insulin to CHO (grams) in the preceding example is 1:12, the premeal dose of rapid-acting insulin is 4 units.

Patients are instructed to read food labels (Figure 53–13 ■, p. 1686) to determine the total amount of CHO in a food item. Serving size must also be monitored because food choices may contain several servings in one item (e.g., 2 servings of CHO in a 12-ounce can of soda pop). This method requires calculations prior to each meal and is an essential skill for those using insulin pump therapy or intensive MDI therapy. As noted in the previous example, the amount of insulin required to cover a specified number of CHO grams is called the insulin-to-CHO, or insulin:CHO, ratio. The ratio is determined through careful monitoring of blood glucose levels before and after meals, frequent communication between all members of the health care team, and trial and error (Bode, 2004).

Nutritional Needs of Hospitalized Patients

As in any catabolic illness, nutritional needs in diabetic patients are compromised. In patients with diabetes, there is an added dilemma of providing adequate calories to maintain nutritional status and promote healing while maintaining glycemic control. The caloric needs of most hospitalized patients can be met through provision of 25 to 35 kcal/kg body weight (McMahon & Rizza, 1996). Protein requirements are variable based on the degree of physiological stress. For example, mildly stressed patients with normal hepatic and renal function require 1.0 g/kg body weight, whereas moderately to severely stressed patients with normal hepatic and renal function may need 1.5 g/kg body weight (McMahon & Rizza, 1996).

Nutrition Facts

Serving Size 1 container (170 grams)

Amount Per Serving	
Calories 170	
	% Daily Values*
Total Fat 1.5g	**2%**
Saturated Fat 1g	**5%**
Cholesterol 10mg	**3%**
Sodium 130mg	**5%**
Potassium 300mg	**9%**
Total Carbohydrate 33g	**11%**
Fiber 0g	**0%**
Sugars 30g	
Protein 6g	**12%**
Calcium	**20%**
Vitamin B$_{12}$	**10%**
Riboflavin	**15%**
Phosphorus	**15%**

FIGURE 53–13 ■ Example of food nutrition label.

The preferred route of feeding is the oral route, however, if adequate intake is not possible, then enteral or parenteral feedings will be needed. CHO counting is integrated into the diet of the hospital patient in various ways. For example, in some hospital protocols, a specific amount of CHO is provided with each meal and an estimated insulin:CHO ratio is determined. Therefore the nursing staff can administer the insulin dose immediately prior to the meal. In other hospital protocols, the estimated insulin:CHO ratio is determined and administered based on the variable amount of CHO in the meal. In general, such protocols provide provisions for patients who have poor appetites, nausea, vomiting, and other gastrointestinal disorders. In these cases, the nurse may administer the rapid-acting insulin dose at the end of the meal, when he can observe the amount of CHO eaten. For information about how the diet of patients with diabetes is affected by cultural and aging considerations, see the Cultural Considerations and Gerontological Considerations boxes.

Exercise and Physical Activity

Regular exercise and a physically active lifestyle provide numerous benefits for people with type 1 and type 2 diabetes, as well as those at risk for developing diabetes. Results of a recent multicen-

CULTURAL CONSIDERATIONS Related to Diet for Patients with Diabetes

An important factor in adherence to a dietary plan is to develop diets that best reflect the ethnic practices of each individual. The ADA website provides a number of useful materials about dietary instruction. The materials, which can be downloaded and printed, are available in a variety of languages and provide information on various ethnic and regional dietary habits. These are very important because a patient's adherence to dietary recommendations may increase when traditional foods, practices, and cultural, and dietary customs are included in educational instruction.

GERONTOLOGICAL CONSIDERATIONS Related to Diet for Patients with Diabetes

Many elderly patients are undernourished due to a variety of physiological, psychological, social, and economic considerations. These may include, but are not limited to, changes in smell, taste, and thirst; side effects of medications; inability to shop for food or prepare meals; cognitive impairment, depression, isolation, and loneliness; and inadequate resources to purchase food (Gilden, 1999). For elderly patients it may be necessary to modify their nutritional diet by changing the nutrient composition or density, modifying the food consistency, or using supplements.

ter research trial clearly demonstrated that lifestyle intervention including regular exercise is superior to metformin at preventing the onset of diabetes in high-risk individuals (Knowler et al., 2002). Benefits for those already diagnosed with type 1 or type 2 diabetes include lower blood glucose levels, improved insulin sensitivity, improvements in cardiovascular risks such as blood lipids and blood pressure levels, improved cardiac conditioning, increased strength and flexibility, and improved personal well-being. Exercise also may help in weight loss when used in conjunction with a calorie-restricted diet (Lebovitz & ADA, 2004).

Although the benefits of exercise outweigh the risks of exercise in most instances, many factors must be taken into account prior to initiating an exercise program. In nondiabetic individuals substrate metabolism is tightly balanced by neuroendocrine mechanisms to maintain normoglycemia. Fuel mobilization from muscle and liver stores during exercise may be 20-fold higher than during sedentary activity to maintain normal blood glucose levels. During exercise, glucose transport into working muscles is enhanced, while cellular resistance to insulin is decreased. Plasma insulin levels decrease, while levels of circulating counterregulatory hormones such as glucagon, cortisol, epinephrine, and norepinephrine increase to maintain glucose homeostasis and avoid hypo- or hyperglycemia. However, individuals with diabetes may have impaired neuroendocrine responses to exercise.

In general, patients with diabetes using pharmacologic therapy are at greater risk for hypoglycemia during and following exercise. In fact, the hypoglycemic effect of exercise can persist for several hours; therefore, patient education about preventing and treating exercise-related hypoglycemia is essential.

Individuals with type 1 diabetes can participate in all levels of physical activity, including leisure time activities and professional sports, if they are in good metabolic control and do not have complications (Zinman, Ruderman, Campaigne, Devlin, & Schneider, 2004). For these individuals, the metabolic response to exercise may vary dramatically in relation to plasma glucose levels at the time of exercise, timing of the last food eaten, type of exercise, and level of insulin usage. The use of exogenous insulin plays a key role, potentiating hypoglycemia in those who are overinsulinized and hyperglycemia with possible ketosis in those who are underinsulinized. Exercise-induced hypoglycemia is common, and may occur for many hours after the exercise is completed. Individuals in poor metabolic control are at risk for worsening of hyperglycemia and ketosis. Guidelines for exercise in this population include the following (Zinman et al., 2004):

- Avoid exercise if blood glucose is >250 mg/dL and ketones are present; use caution if blood glucose levels are >300 mg/dL without ketosis.

- Ingest CHO-containing foods if blood glucose levels are <100 mg/dL prior to exercise.

- Monitor blood glucose levels before, after, and more frequently during the postexercise period because the blood glucose-lowering effects of exercise may last many hours after exercise.

- Self-monitor blood glucose responses to different activity levels to determine appropriate changes to diet and insulin.

- Maintain a supply of readily available CHO-containing foods during and after exercise.

The use of intensive insulin therapies, such as MDI therapy or CSII, allows for greater flexibility in making appropriate adjustments to insulin and food, thus decreasing the risk of exercise-induced hypo- or hyperglycemia. The importance of blood glucose monitoring and record keeping cannot be overemphasized because these are the primary means of monitoring glycemic responses to exercise and determining the necessary insulin and dietary changes required to avoid hypo- or hyperglycemia.

For individuals with type 2 diabetes, regular exercise plays a key role in improving long-term metabolic control due to its positive impact on insulin resistance. Exercise, like insulin, decreases blood glucose levels by enhancing glucose uptake into skeletal muscles. Enhanced glucose utilization and insulin sensitivity may last for up to 24 hours after the exercise bout (Devlin, Hirshman, Horton, & Horton, 1987). Although exercise-induced hypoglycemia is less problematic in individuals with type 2 diabetes, those treated with insulin or insulin secretagogues need the same precautions for prevention of hypoglycemia as those with type 1 diabetes.

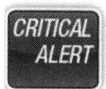 ***CRITICAL ALERT*** *Patients with diabetes can learn to decrease their insulin dose prior to intense exercise to prevent hypoglycemia; however, most exercise is unplanned and patients are often unable to make such adjustments. Because the glucose-lowering effects of exercise can persist for several hours after an exercise bout, patients (especially those using exogenous insulin) are at particular risk for postexercise hypoglycemia. Therefore, nurses should counsel patients to monitor blood glucose levels closely following exercise to prevent hypoglycemia. In particular, patients should monitor their blood glucose prior to sleep to prevent nocturnal hypoglycemia.*

Exercise and Diabetes Complications

The long-term complications associated with diabetes pose special concerns and require extra consideration when planning an exercise program. The ADA recommends that all individuals with diabetes undergo a detailed medical evaluation with appropriate diagnostic studies prior to beginning an exercise program (Zinman et al., 2004). Recommendations include use of a graded exercise test in high-risk individuals. A preexercise assessment for all individuals with diabetes should include an evaluation of PVD, retinal examination, evaluation of renal function, and assessment of autonomic and peripheral neuropathy. The presence of complications does not preclude participation in exercise, but does require attention by members of the health care team.

Exercise Prescriptions

Exercise prescriptions should be individualized to each person, with an emphasis on enjoyment of the activity. Generally, an exercise bout should include 5 to 10 minutes of warm-up, such as low-intensity walking or cycling, 5 to 10 minutes of gentle stretching, a period of aerobic activity, such as swimming, walking, or dancing, and 5 to 10 minutes of cooldown. Moderate to vigorous aerobic activity should be prescribed based on individual preferences, current level of fitness, and risk factors. For example, an individual with decreased or absent lower extremity sensation should be instructed to participate in non–weight-bearing activities such as swimming or bicycling (Zinman et al., 2004). The exercise bouts should be done three to five times per week to achieve cardiovascular conditioning and glycemic control. If weight loss is a goal, the frequency should be increased (Lebovitz & ADA, 2004).

Health Promotion

Exercise offers many benefits for individuals with diabetes and should be encouraged as part of a healthy lifestyle. Although exercise does pose special risks for patients with diabetes, individualized exercise plans can be developed for the majority of patients with diabetes. Through careful clinical assessment and planning, most risks can be minimized or prevented so that most people with diabetes can enjoy the benefits of regular physical activity. Exercise education should include a review of the signs, symptoms, and treatment for hypoglycemia, ketone testing for individuals with type 1 diabetes, proper hydration during exercise, and foot protection measures including proper footwear and self-assessment prior to and immediately after exercise. Positive reinforcement and inclusion of friends and family members in the exercise plan may help to improve motivation.

■ Complementary and Alternative Medicine and Glycemic Control

An extensive systematic review of published literature on the efficacy and safety of herbal therapies and vitamin/mineral supplements for glycemic control in patients with diabetes was published in 2003 (Yeh, Eisenberg, Kaptchuk, & Phillips, 2003). Results of the review concluded that there is insufficient evidence to actively recommend or discourage the use of any particular supplement; however, most appeared to be generally safe. In addition, the review concluded that the seven most promising supplements included *Coccinia indica*, American ginseng, *Momordica charantia*, nopal, L-carnitine, *Gymnema sylvestre*, aloe vera, and *vanadium*. The Complementary and Alternative Therapies box (p. 1688) discusses the antidiabetic potential of certain spices.

Randomized clinical trials are needed to assess the efficacy of these types of supplements. Most importantly, sound clinical judgment is needed when patients report the use of these plant foods for treatment for diabetes treatment. In particular, nurses and other health care professionals must understand that these medications are supplemental therapy; such supplements claim to enhance insulin secretion, but do not take the place of exogenous insulin. Because patients with type 1 diabetes lack the ability to produce insulin, claims that a supplement will increase insulin secretion in type 1 diabetes are misleading and can be dangerous. In the future, however, as we refine our knowledge of these supplements, there may be a place for them in diabetes treatment.

Management of Hospitalized Patients with Diabetes

For several decades the management of diabetes in the hospitalized patient has focused on the treatment of the acute complications of diabetes, DKA and HHS. The stress of critical illness, however, worsens glycemic control in patients with diabetes and often precipitates hyperglycemia in individuals with no history of diabetes or glucose intolerance. During the last decade, the deleterious effects of hyperglycemia on the clinical outcomes of acutely ill patients with and without diabetes have been estab-

lished. The following paragraphs focus on the treatment of hyperglycemia in patients who are acutely ill along with general treatment strategies for DKA, HHS, and hypoglycemia.

Hyperglycemia in Acute Illness

Physiological stress, such as acute illness, causes an increase in counterregulatory hormones, glucagon, cortisol, growth hormone, and catecholamines. These hormones increase insulin resistance and hepatic glucose production and decrease glucose transport, resulting in hyperglycemia. Investigations into the relationship between hyperglycemia and poor recovery from acute illness have gained momentum during the past few years; however, hyperglycemia has been known to interfere with recovery from infections and wound healing for several decades.

In clinical practice alterations in immune response contribute to the severity of common infections, such as lower extremity ulcers (Lioupis, 2005) along with the development of more severe infections. Recent studies have shown that hyperglycemia also has deleterious effects on recovery from critical illness (Van den Berghe & Bouillon, 2004), myocardial infarction (Malmberg, 2004), stroke (Capes, Hunt, Malmberg, Pathak, &

COMPLEMENTARY & ALTERNATIVE THERAPIES   Garlic and Other Spices

Description:

It is well established that diet plays a large role in the management of diabetes mellitus. Although garlic and spices are well known as a vital part of flavoring foods for increased taste enjoyment, some spices also have therapeutic effects including antidiabetic effects.

In addition to providing flavor and therapeutic physiological properties, spices can partially or wholly replace less health-promoting ingredients such as salt, sugar, and added saturated fat. Current nutritional guidelines for patients with diabetes include increasing intake of vegetables, yet many people do not enjoy eating vegetables. Spices can improve the flavor of vegetables and help patients to adhere to dietary guidelines (Tapsell et al., 2006).

Research Support:

Diabetes mellitus is characterized by increased protein glycation and advanced glycation end product (AGEP) formation. Glycation and AGEP formation have been implicated in diabetic complications, as well as the formation of damaging free radicals through glucose and protein autoxidation. Compounds that have both antiglycation and antioxidant properties may have therapeutic potential in the treatment of diabetes mellitus. Several studies have shown that aged garlic extract (AGE) is a potent antioxidant and can inhibit the formation of AGEPs *in vitro*. AGE may also inhibit the formation of glycation-derived free radicals (Ahmad & Ahmed, 2006).

Another study identified the following spices as having antidiabetic and hypoglycemic properties:

- Fenugreek seeds (*Trigonella foenumgraecum*)
- Garlic (*Allium sativum*)
- Onion (*Allium cepa*)
- Turmeric (*Curcuma longa*)
- Cumin seeds (*Cuminum cyminum*)
- Ginger (*Zingiber officinale*)
- Mustard (*Brassica nigra*)

- Curry leaves (*Murraya koenigii*)
- Coriander (*Coriandrum sativum*) (*Srinivasan, 2005*).

Onion (*Allium cepa L.*) and garlic (*Allium sativum L.*) have a long history as both spices and medicine. One study found that the therapeutic properties of garlic and onion can be attributed to volatile sulfur compounds called thiosulfinates, which also create the strong odor and flavor of these spices (Lanzotti, 2006).

Another study investigated the effects of garlic oil on glycemic control in rats with streptozotocin-induced diabetes. Diabetic rats were fed garlic oil by gavage (100 mg/kg body weight) every other day for 16 weeks after the induction of diabetes. Although garlic oil did not affect oral glucose tolerance, it significantly improved oral glucose tolerance at 4, 8, 12, and 16 weeks. The researchers concluded that garlic oil can be used in the long-term treatment of diabetes to improve oral glucose tolerance (Wong, Lii, Hse, & Sheen, 2006).

References

Ahmad, M. S., & Ahmed, N. (2006, March). Antiglycation properties of aged garlic extract: Possible role in prevention of diabetic complications. *Journal of Nutrition 136* (3 Suppl), 796S–799S.

Lanzotti, V. (2006). The analysis of onion and garlic. *Journal of Chormatograpy A, 1112* (1–2), 3–22.

Srinivasan, K. (2005). Plant foods in the management of diabetes mellitus: Spices as beneficial antidiabetic food adjuncts. *International Journal of Food Science and Nutrition, 56* (6), 399–414.

Tapsell, L. C., Hemphill, I., Cobiac, L., Patch, C. S., Sullivan, D. R., Fenech, M., et al. (2006, August 21). Health benefits of herbs and spices: The past, the present, the future. *Medical Journal of Australia, 185* (4 Suppl), S4–S24.

Wong, P. L., Lii, C. K., Hse, H., & Sheen, L. Y. (2006). Antidiabetic effect of garlic oil but not diallyl disulfide in rats with streptozotocin-induced diabetes. *Food Chemistry and Toxicology, 44* (8), 1377–1384.

Gerstein, 2001), and cardiac surgery (Furnary, Wu, & Bookin, 2004). Evidence supports the fact that normoglycemia in hospitalized patients results in decreased morbidity and mortality in patients (Umpierrez et al., 2002).

Target Glycemic Goals for Hospitalized Patients

During a consensus conference on inpatient diabetes and metabolic control (Garber, Seidel, & Ambruster, 2004), target glycemic goals for hospitalized patients were established. The upper limits for these goals are as follows:

- Intensive care unit (ICU): 110 mg/dL
- Non–critical care units: preprandial, 110 mg/dL
- Maximum blood glucose: 180 mg/dL.

Insulin Protocols Designed to Meet Treatment Goals in Hospitalized Patients

Evidence supports the use of intravenous insulin infusions in the ICU among hyperglycemic critically ill patients (e.g., during myocardial infarction, following surgeries) regardless of whether or not there is a history of diabetes. In addition, evidence also supports the use of intravenous (IV) insulin in patients who have fluctuating blood glucose levels regardless of whether the patients are treated in the ICU or another unit. However, it is not always practical or standard hospital policy to have IV insulin infusions on non–critical care units.

Various protocols are used to maintain target glucose levels during hospitalization. There is no one standard protocol because each individual's response to insulin depends on a variety of factors. In general, the protocols include infusion of glucose to help prevent hypoglycemia and wide fluctuations in blood glucose levels. Insulin infusion protocols have been found to be of importance in use with patients who are NPO (nothing by mouth), receiving parenteral nutrition, and receiving enteral tube feedings. The use of an IV insulin infusion allows for greater flexibility in changing the insulin dosage and preventing hypoglycemia. An example of an insulin infusion algorithm is described in Chart 53–5.

As can be noted in Chart 53–5, there are three *hypothetical* insulin dosing schemes or algorithms. Patients are started on algorithms based on individual characteristics. For example, "algorithm 1" may be most appropriate for the majority of hospitalized patients. "Algorithm 2" may be most appropriate for patients who have had coronary artery bypass grafting (CABG) or a solid organ transplant or have been treated with glucocorticoids. Ordinarily patients may not be initially treated on "algorithm 3," but this algorithm may be used if blood glucose control is suboptimal on algorithm 2. Each set of algorithms is accompanied by a set of strict criteria as to when to move up or down *within* algorithms or *between* algorithms.

In addition, protocols are currently available for the use of subcutaneous insulin to meet target glucose levels, to transition from IV insulin infusions to subcutaneous insulin (especially when transferring from the ICU to non–critical care units), or to use subcutaneous insulin as a starting point to meet target glycemic control. Standardized insulin protocols have three major components: a premeal insulin dose (e.g., 3 units lispro), a basal insulin dose (e.g., 20 units Glargine qhs), and a "correction factor" (e.g., 5 units lispro). The *correction factor* is an additional amount of insulin that is provided with each meal based on the premeal blood glucose. For example, if a patient routinely uses 3 units of lispro prior to lunch, but her prelunch blood glucose is 250 mg/dL, an additional 5 units of lispro may be administered. In the outpatient setting, patients work with their health care provider to determine their premeal correction factor. In the hospital setting, the determination of the correction factor is based largely on predetermined protocols (Moghissi & Hirsch, 2005).

Diabetic Ketoacidosis

As mentioned earlier, diabetic ketoacidosis is a life-threatening complication precipitated by an acute or relative deficiency in insulin secretion and characterized by profound disturbances in CHO, fat, and protein metabolism. Typically, DKA is treated in the ICU. DKA and HHS have been considered complications of

---

CHART 53–5 **Hypothetical Algorithmic Approach to Diabetes Treatment in the Hospitalized Patient**

Algorithm 1		Algorithm 2		Algorithm 3	
Blood Glucose (mg/dL)	Insulin Infusion Rate (units/hr)	Blood Glucose (mg/dL)	Insulin Infusion Rate (units/hr)	Blood Glucose (mg/dL)	Insulin Infusion Rate (units/hr)
<70	No infusion	<70	No infusion	<70	No infusion
70–110	0.2	70–110	0.4	70–110	0.8
111–120	0.5	111–120	1.0	111–120	2.0
121–150	1.0	121–150	2.0	121–150	4.0
151–180	1.5	151–180	3.0	151–180	6.0
180–210	2.0	180–210	4.0	180–210	8.0
211–240	2.5	211–240	5.0	211–240	9.0
241–270	3.0	241–270	6.0	241–270	10.0
271–300	3.5	271–300	7.0	271–300	11.0
301–330	4.0	301–330	8.0	301–330	12.0
331–360	4.5	331–360	9.0	331–360	14.0
< 360	6.0	< 360	12.0	< 360	16.0

Sources: John, R., & Fogelfeld, L. (2004). Inpatient management of diabetes and hyperglycemia. *Disease-a-Month, 50*(8), 438–479; Moghissi, E. S., & Hirsch, I. B. (2005). Hospital management of diabetes. *Endocrinology Metabolism Clinics of North America, 34*(1), 99–116.

type 1 and 2 diabetes, respectively. Although generally this is true, DKA and HHS can occur in both types of diabetes (Umpierrez & Kitabchi, 2003). The overlap is becoming more apparent as type 2 diabetes occurs with increasing frequency at younger ages (Harmel et al., 2004).

Hyperosmolar Hyperglycemic Syndrome

Hyperosmolar hyperglycemic syndrome is a life-threatening complication characterized by serum hyperosmolarity, dehydration, and hyperglycemia; it is usually restricted to patients who cannot recognize their thirst or express their need for water. Such patients may include the infirm; people who are neglected, very young, very old, or institutionalized; and those who have mental deficiencies. In addition, this syndrome also is seen in patients with excessive unreplaced fluid losses, secondary to massive glycosuric diuresis, and following gastrointestinal fluid losses and limited fluid intake.

Hypoglycemia

Hypoglycemia results from an imbalance between glucose production and glucose utilization that occurs when glucose use exceeds glucose production. Hypoglycemia results in a low blood glucose level (<60 mg/dL) and is associated with a variety of adrenergic and neuroglycopenic symptoms.

Hypoglycemia Unawareness

Hypoglycemia unawareness is defined as the loss of autonomic nervous system responses to hypoglycemia. Symptoms, such as tachycardia, sweating, or palpitations, normally prompt patients to eat in order to prevent progression to severe hypoglycemia. Hypoglycemia unawareness results from altered counterregulation, particularly deficient glucagon and epinephrine responses to hypoglycemia. Subjects with hypoglycemic unawareness are clearly at risk for severe hypoglycemia and injury. The probability of hypoglycemic unawareness and its associated risks should be considered in patients with an increased emphasis on normalization of blood glucose control using intensive insulin regimens and oral hypoglycemic combination therapy.

Etiology and Precipitating Factors of DKA, HHS, and Hypoglycemia

A number of precipitating factors are associated with the development of DKA, HHS, and hypoglycemia, as detailed in Chart 53–6.

Pathophysiology

Short synopses of the pathophysiology of each of the three major complications are given next, starting with DKA.

Diabetic Ketoacidosis

The development of DKA is related to the effects of insulin deficiency on CHO, fat, and lipid metabolism. Although these derangements occur simultaneously, it is helpful to consider them individually in order to correlate the pathophysiology, clinical symptoms, and treatments. The separate effects of insulin lack on CHO, fat, and protein metabolism are described in the following subsections.

Insulin Deficiency and CHO Metabolism

A relative or absolute insulin deficiency results in decreased glucose use by the peripheral tissues, particularly adipose tissue and muscle. Blood glucose levels increase as a result of decreased glucose transport, hepatic and muscle glycogenolysis, and hepatic gluconeogenesis. Glycosuria and osmotic diuresis occur when blood glucose levels exceed the renal threshold. The osmotic diuresis occurs because there is increased urine flow due to an abnormally high concentration of glucose that is reabsorbed incompletely by the proximal tubule. As water reabsorption occurs in the proximal tubule, secondary to Na^+ reabsorption, the concentration of glucose builds up and its osmotic presence impedes the reabsorption of water. In addition, the failure of water to follow Na^+ causes the Na^+ concentration in the proximal tubular lumen to fall below that of the interstitial fluid. The concentration difference between the proximal tubular lumen and the interstitial fluid impedes some Na^+ reabsorption. Thus both Na^+ and water reabsorption are impeded in an osmotic diuresis. This osmotic diuresis results in volume depletion and a reduced glomerular filtration rate (GFR). Reductions in GFR cause decreased renal excretion of glucose, further increasing the hyperglycemia.

CHART 53–6	Common Precipitating Factors of Diabetic Ketoacidosis, Hyperosmolar Hyperglycemic Nonketotic Syndrome, and Hypoglycemia[a]	
Diabetic Ketoacidosis	**Hyperosmolar Hyperglycemic Syndrome**	**Hypoglycemia**
• Infection	• Undiagnosed diabetes	• Excessive insulin
• Cessation of insulin	• Acute infection	• Wrong type of insulin (e.g., administering rapid-acting instead of long-acting insulin)
• Undiagnosed diabetes	• Cerebrovascular accident	• Missing meals or snacks
• Myocardial infarction	• Myocardial infarction	
• Pancreatitis	• Acute pancreatitis	
• Trauma/shock	• Acute pulmonary embolus	
• Stroke	• Hemodialysis	
	• Peritoneal dialysis	
	• Renal failure	
	• Total parenteral nutrition	
	• Medications (e.g., cimetidine, phenytoin thiazide diuretics)	

[a]Patients treated with insulin or oral diabetes medications.

Adults with an intact thirst mechanism and normal renal function initially may become only mildly hyperglycemic during DKA since the kidneys are able to excrete some of the filtered glucose load. Adults *without* intact thirst mechanisms (e.g., following a stroke) may not be able to compensate for their fluid loss and become severely hyperglycemic. This loss of water and electrolytes leads to dehydration and hemoconcentration. There is a marked reduction in circulating blood volume leading to peripheral circulatory failure progressing to shock, hypotension, and anuria. In addition, there is generalized tissue anoxia, with a shift to anaerobic metabolism, resulting in increasing concentrations of lactic acid in the blood. Coma and death subsequently result after the development of peripheral circulatory failure. See Chapter 42 ☺.

Insulin Deficiency and Fat Metabolism

Insulin deficiency results in mobilization of depot fat in the blood. The liver is flooded with FFAs, which are converted to ketone bodies (acetoacetate and beta-hydroxybutyrate). These ketone bodies are weak acids that are buffered after release from the liver, decreasing the body's buffering capacity. The developing ketonemia leads to progressive metabolic acidosis, which in turn initiates the characteristic deep and rapid respirations accompanied by an acetone odor to the breath (Kussmaul breathing). These Kussmaul respirations are a compensatory response to metabolic acidosis, designed to reduce CO_2. As ketonemia exceeds the renal threshold for ketone body reabsorption, ketones appear in the urine. The ketones are excreted with sodium, which contributes to the net sodium loss. A severe metabolic acidosis results in depression of the respiratory vasomotor center, compromised cardiovascular output, and reduced vascular tone. This may result in cardiovascular collapse with the generation of lactic acid, which adds to the existing acidosis.

Insulin Deficiency and Protein Metabolism

Insulin deficiency results in decreased protein synthesis and promotes net protein catabolism, particularly in muscle. This results in a net loss of nitrogen from the body and increased blood urea nitrogen (BUN) levels. This is accompanied by net loss of K^+, particularly from muscle protein breakdown. Progressive dehydration results in protein catabolism and additional K^+ is subsequently lost in the urine. The final result is that there is a net body loss of K^+.

Counterregulatory Hormones

DKA causes increased plasma glucagon levels, resulting in accelerated rates of hepatic glucose production and ketogenesis. *Catecholamines* stimulate both hepatic and muscle glycogenolysis and adipose tissue lipolysis. The FFAs and glycerol resulting from the lipolysis are converted subsequently to ketones and contribute to glucose production in the liver through ketogenesis and gluconeogenesis, respectively. *Cortisol* increases proteolysis, providing amino acid precursors for gluconeogenesis. *Growth hormone* causes an increase in lipolysis, contributing to ketogenesis and glucose production. *Catecholamines, cortisol,* and *growth hormone* all cause insulin resistance and decreased peripheral glucose uptake.

Hyperosmolar Hyperglycemic Syndrome

The pathogenesis of HHS is similar to that of DKA, but there are specific differences. The pathogenesis of HHS includes hyper-

glycemia and severe dehydration, but does not include metabolic acidosis. Individuals with HHS have a significant reduction in GFR related to dehydration and volume depletion. The reduction in GFR results in an inability to dispose of some of the excess glucose through the kidneys and potentiates hyperglycemia.

The metabolic acidosis does not develop, presumably because the underlying plasma insulin levels are sufficient to inhibit unrestrained lipolysis, but not sufficient to normalize plasma glucose levels. Theoretically, the amount of FFAs that reach the liver is less than in DKA and the production of ketones is restrained. The emergent symptoms associated with metabolic acidosis, are not present to prompt early medical intervention. HHS may evolve over a period of days to weeks, leading to more profound hyperglycemia, dehydration, and hyperosmolality than is seen in DKA.

Hypoglycemia

Glucose is the obligate fuel for the brain and central nervous system. The brain is not able to synthesize or store glucose and must rely on circulating blood glucose levels for survival. Normal blood glucose levels are maintained through the complex interplay between insulin, glucagon, and other counterregulatory hormones. In patients who do not have diabetes, plasma insulin levels decline as blood glucose levels decline; and serum insulin levels increase as plasma glucose increase. However, in patients using exogenous insulin and insulin secretagogues, plasma insulin levels and blood glucose are not appropriately suppressed. Therefore, blood glucose levels may decrease, but the insulin levels remain elevated.

Clinical Manifestations of DKA, HHS, and Hypoglycemia

There are a variety of clinical signs and symptoms of DKA, HHS, and hypoglycemia. In general, these signs and symptoms result predominantly from hyperglycemia, dehydration, hyperosmolality, metabolic acidosis, and electrolyte disturbances. There is overlap between the signs and symptoms of DKA and HHS, with some exceptions. As noted previously, HHS is not associated with a metabolic acidosis. In addition, the degree of hyperglycemia, dehydration, and hyperosmolality is much more severe in HHS than DKA. The general causes of these clinical signs and symptoms are listed in Chart 53–7 (p. 1692).

Laboratory and Diagnostic Procedures

Hyperglycemia is present in both DKA and HHS due to a relative or absolute deficiency of circulating insulin. The hyperglycemia associated with HHS generally is greater than in DKA (Chart 53–8, p. 1692). Because HHS is not associated with emergent symptoms of metabolic acidosis and many of the affected patients are unable to articulate their needs, the course of the disease may evolve over a longer period of time. Additionally, the reduction in GFR during the severe dehydration of HHS decreases urinary loss of glucose, further increasing the blood glucose level.

- **Metabolic acidosis**—Metabolic acidosis is present in DKA as reflected in a *reduced arterial pH, reduced plasma bicarbonate,* and *increased anion gap* and is due primarily to the accumulation of ketone bodies. In addition, some degree of lactic acidosis exists from hypoperfusion, which also contributes to the acidosis.

- **Ketoacids**—The ketoacids beta-hydroxybutyrate and acetoacetate accumulate in the serum causing metabolic acidosis. The

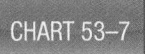

Signs and Symptoms of Diabetic Ketoacidosis, Hyperosmolar Hyperglycemic Syndrome, and Hypoglycemia

CHART 53–7

Diabetes Ketoacidosis

- *Polyuria* is caused by an osmotic diuresis induced by hyperglycemia.

- *Polyphagia* is caused by inability to use energy substrates (CHO, protein, and fats) appropriately.

- As the metabolic acidosis progresses, *polyphagia* is generally replaced by *anorexia*, due to the effects of ketones.

- *Polydipsia* is a compensatory response to dehydration and volume depletion.

- *Weight loss* results from *dehydration* and altered utilization of CHO, protein, and fats.

- *Fatigue* occurs in response to altered CHO, protein, and lipid metabolism, especially protein catabolism, but likely other factors (e.g., dehydration) also contribute to fatigue.

- *Blurred vision* occurs in response to hyperglycemia. Fluid accumulates in the lens of the eye, causing refractory changes.

- *Hypotension, tachycardia,* and *poor skin turgor* result from dehydration and volume depletion.

- As the *metabolic acidosis, dehydration*, and *volume depletion* progress, orthostatic hypotension develops.

- *Cardiac arrhythmias* result primarily from electrolyte disturbances, such as abnormal K^+.

- *Nausea and vomiting* are thought to result from the accumulation of serum ketones. The cause of abdominal pain is not certain but may be related to potassium depletion. Nausea and vomiting also may be related to the precipitating cause of DKA or HHS.

- *Kussmaul's respirations* (deep rapid respirations) are a compensatory mechanism to decrease $PaCO_2$.

- The *red, flushed face*, seen along with Kussmaul's respirations, is due to the increased levels of $PaCO_2$, which have a vasodilating effect.

- *Decreased mental status* and *coma* are primarily due to dehydration and serum hyperosmolality.

- *Hypothermia* results from a variety of causes, the most common being peripheral vasodilation, severe dehydration, and in DKA, metabolic acidosis. In addition, *hypothermia* may be a manifestation of the precipitating event (e.g., sepsis).

Hyperosmolar Hyperglycemic Syndrome

- *Polyuria* (as above).

- *Polyphagia* (as above).

- *Polydipsia* (as above).

- *Weight loss* and *dehydration* (as above).

- *Fatigue* (as above).

- *Blurred vision* (as above).

- *Hypotension, tachycardia,* and *poor skin turgor* (as above).

- *Cardiac arrhythmias* (as above).

- *Decreased mental status* and *coma* are primarily due to dehydration and serum hyperosmolality.

- *Hyperglycemia, dehydration,* and *serum hyperosmolality* are usually much more severe than in DKA. This results in *cerebral dehydration,* which is associated with neurological symptoms such as hemiparesis, seizures, and coma.

- *Hypothermia* results from a variety of causes, the most common being peripheral vasodilation and severe dehydration. In addition, hypothermia may be a manifestation of the precipitating event (e.g., sepsis).

- *Vascular thrombosis* results from severe dehydration. Patients with HHS are at greater risk because of the severity of dehydration and hyperosmolality.

Hypoglycemia

- The clinical symptoms of hypoglycemia are generally divided into autonomic and neuroglycopenic categories.

- The autonomic symptoms are subdivided into adrenergic (e.g., tremors, palpitations, nervousness, anxiety) and cholinergic (e.g., sweating and hunger) categories.

- The neuroglycopenic symptoms (irritability, confusion, drowsiness, weakness, difficulty speaking, unresponsiveness, unconsciousness, seizures, and coma) result from glucose deprivation to the central nervous system.

Laboratory Values in Diabetic Ketoacidosis, Hyperosmolar Hyperglycemic Nonketotic Syndrome, and Hypoglycemia

CHART 53–8

Diabetic Ketoacidosis	Hyperosmolar Hyperglycemic Syndrome	Hypoglycemia
Random plasma glucose (>250 mg/dL)	Random plasma glucose (usually >600 mg/dL)	Random plasma glucose (usually <60 mg/dL)
Arterial pH <7.3	Arterial pH: >7.3	
7.25–7.30: associated with mild DKA	Serum bicarbonate: >15 mEq/L	
7.00–7.24: associated with moderate DKA	Anion gap: <12	
<7.00: associated with severe DKA	Serum ketones: negative or small	
Serum bicarbonate <15 mEq/L (decreases with moderate to severe DKA)	Urine ketones: negative or small	
Anion gap: >10 (increases with moderate to severe DKA)	Serum osmolality: (>340 mOsm/kg)	
Serum ketones: positive		
Urinary ketones: positive		
Serum osmolality: variable		

hydrogen ions of the ketoacids are buffered by bicarbonate, which causes reduced serum bicarbonate.

- **Serum Na⁺**—The serum Na⁺ in DKA or HHS may be low, normal, or high. The presence of increased levels of glucose in the extracellular space causes the movement of water from the intracellular to the extracellular space; this dilutes and lowers the serum Na⁺ concentration. As the fluid volume deficit increases, water in the extracellular space is lost in excess of Na⁺ and the serum Na⁺ concentration increases.

 The serum K⁺ level may be low, normal, or elevated at the initial clinical presentation of both DKA and HHS. In both DKA and HHS, there is a loss in total body stores of K⁺ from cellular destruction and urinary losses. In an attempt to buffer the metabolic acidosis, however, K⁺ shifts from the intracellular to extracellular space in exchange for hydrogen ions, which move from the extracellular to the intracellular space. With initiation of insulin therapy, K⁺ moves back into the cell and the serum K⁺ drops from the initial serum level. Therefore, insulin infusion and K⁺ are usually begun simultaneously.

- **Serum PO₄⁻**—The serum PO₄⁻ level may also be normal on clinical presentation of DKA or HHS. However, as in DKA, these levels do not reflect actual body deficits that exist when phosphate shifts from intracellular to extracellular during DKA or HHS.
- **Serum creatinine**—The serum creatinine levels are elevated in both DKA and HHS due to severe dehydration and hyperosmolality. The serum creatinine levels in HHS usually are elevated above those in DKA, reflecting possible renal impairment.
- **BUN**—The serum BUN levels are elevated in both DKA and HHS due to dehydration, serum hyperosmolality, and protein catabolism. As with serum creatinine, the BUN levels in HHS usually are elevated above those in DKA, reflecting possible renal impairment.
- **Serum osmolality**—The serum osmolality may be elevated in both DKA and HHS, and is typically higher in HHS than DKA. The rising plasma glucose level increases serum osmolality.
- **White blood count (WBC)**—The WBC may be elevated in DKA. This may reflect a normal leukocytosis that frequently accompanies DKA or the presence of actual infection.

Medical Management of DKA, HHS, and Hypoglycemia

The overall treatment of DKA and HHS revolves around general measures, insulin treatment, fluids, and electrolytes. Overall general measures in the treatment of DKA and HHS include the following:

- Identification of those patients who require hemodynamic monitoring
- Protection of airway in stuporous or comatose patients
- Insertion of a nasogastric tube in patients with a vulnerable airway
- Hourly measurement of serum glucose
- Frequent (every 1 to 4 hours) measurement of arterial blood gases (ABGs), serum ketones, and electrolytes
- ECG monitoring for dysrhythmias (e.g., hypokalemia and hyperkalemia)

- Hourly assessment of urinary output, vital signs, and neurological status
- Chest x-ray and imaging studies as indicated
- Use of a flow sheet to monitor vital signs, urine output, glucose, ABGs, serum ketones, blood chemistries, electrolytes, and IV fluids
- Hourly assessment and documentation of clinical status as treatment progresses.

Insulin Treatment

The preferred method of insulin delivery in DKA and HHS involves Regular insulin as a low-dose IV infusion. The continuous insulin infusion helps to prevent both rapid changes in serum glucose along with hypokalemia and hypoglycemia. In addition, the insulin infusion allows for flexible adjustment of the infusion rate in response to changes in plasma glucose. An IV bolus injection of Regular insulin (0.1 unit/kg body weight) is usually administered prior to beginning the insulin infusion. This bolus should be followed by a continuous infusion of $0.1 \text{ unit} \cdot \text{kg}^{-1} \cdot \text{hr}^{-1}$ (approximately 5 to 10 units/hr) until the plasma glucose concentration is 250 to 300 mg/dL and the arterial pH is ≥7.3 or HCO₃⁻ is ≥18 mEq/L. Important points of this insulin therapy are as follows:

- Blood glucose levels should be monitored hourly during the insulin infusion with a goal of reducing the plasma glucose gradually at a rate of $80 \text{ to } 100 \text{ mg} \cdot \text{dL}^{-1} \cdot \text{hr}^{-1}$.
- The insulin infusion should be decreased to 2 to 3 units/hr until the blood glucose is 250 to 300 mg/dL and the bicarbonate is HCO₃⁻ is ≥18 mEq/L. The plasma glucose is likely to be corrected prior to the correction of acidosis.
- The insulin infusion should be continued in the presence of acidosis even if the glucose level is continuing to decline toward normal levels. Glucose should be administered at 5 to 10 g/hr intravenously to prevent hypoglycemia.
- Subcutaneous insulin should be given approximately 30 minutes prior to stopping the infusion to make certain that there is no delay that could cause relapse of DKA.

Fluid Therapy

Increased plasma glucose, as seen in DKA and HHS, results in a shift of water from the intracellular to the extracellular space. There is an initial deficit in intracellular fluid, followed by extracellular (intravascular compartment) fluid loss, precipitated by osmotic diuresis. In addition, there may be ongoing losses of fluid (e.g., nausea and vomiting), which further dehydration and volume contraction.

The first goal of fluid therapy in DKA or HHS is the restoration of intravascular fluid volume, thereby, maintaining adequate blood pressure, treating or preventing shock, and reestablishing renal perfusion. The use of isotonic normal saline (0.9 NS) is necessary as a first-line treatment in DKA and HHS. As hyperglycemia is corrected, water is shifted back into the intracellular space. This could potentially lead to circulatory collapse, if 0.9 NS, which remains in the intravascular space, is not administered concurrently with insulin.

After correcting the intravascular fluid losses, the second goal of fluid therapy is to restore the free water deficit by infusing hypotonic solutions such as 0.45 NS. As dehydration is corrected in HHS, normal renal perfusion is established and glucose is lost through urinary glucose disposal. Therefore, patients with HHS may have significant reductions in serum glucose during the process of rehydration alone, requiring less insulin to correct hyperglycemia.

In adult patients (with no underlying comorbidities such as cardiac, renal, and liver disease), 1 to 2 liters of 0.9 NS should be infused for prompt correction of hypotension and hypoperfusion over the first hour. During hours 1 through 4, 750 to 1,000 mL/hr of 0.9 NS or 0.45 NS should be infused for severe volume depletion; or 250 to 500 mL/hr of 0.9 NS or 0.45 NS should be infused for moderate volume depletion. During hours 4 through 24, the infusion rate should be adjusted depending on the patient's intake, urinary output, and hydration status. The composition of the fluid is dependent on serum sodium and plasma osmolality measurements. In addition, the rate of fluid replacement does depend on each patient's overall cardiopulmonary status and the presence of comorbidities.

Electrolyte Management

Phosphate replacement is not recommended routinely in either DKA or HHS, although other electrolytes such as magnesium and calcium may be supplemented as needed. With insulin treatment during DKA and HHS, however, potassium is shifted from the intracellular to the extracellular space, thus placing patients at particular risk for hypokalemia. Some important points regarding potassium replacement are discussed next.

The results of the admission serum K^+ level should be obtained prior to initiating K^+ replacement therapy. If the patient is anuric, the K^+ supplementation should be held. If the patient is anuric and hypokalemic, adults may be given 10 to 30 mEq KCl over 1 to 2 hours, provided close ECG monitoring can be established and serum potassium levels can be assessed frequently. During hours 2 through 8, K^+ supplementation usually is added as 20 to 40 mEq KCl/L is infused depending on the serum K^+ level and estimated K^+ deficit during hours 8 through 48. Bicarbonate therapy is recommended only in the following situations: life-threatening hyperkalemia, severe lactic acidosis, and severe acidosis (pH < 6.9).

Hypoglycemia Management

As noted previously, the blood glucose level in DKA may normalize faster than resolution of the metabolic acidosis. This necessitates the infusion of IV glucose (D10%W or D5%W) for prevention of hypoglycemia. In HHS the glucose level may decline fairly quickly; as renal function improves urinary glucose disposal increases. Patients in this situation need close monitoring to avoid rapid shifts in blood glucose, serum osmolality, and hypoglycemia. This involves slowing the insulin infusion rate as the blood glucose levels decline and providing IV glucose as indicated. When patients with DKA and HHS treated with IV insulin infusions develop hypoglycemia, the lower blood glucose level can be treated with intravenous glucose (D50%W), unless the patient is able to eat and drink appropriately.

 In hospital settings, insulin drips have been used for DKA and HHS for many years. Currently, insulin drips are being used to maintain normal blood glucose levels in non-DKA or non-HHS patients to maintain normal blood glucose levels. As a result, nurses must assess patients on insulin drips frequently for signs and symptoms of hypoglycemia and assess blood glucose levels on a planned basis (more intense insulin regimens require more frequent monitoring) and anytime hypoglycemia is suspected.

As just mentioned, in the hospital setting, D50%W is available to treat severe hypoglycemia (or hypoglycemia in patients who cannot eat); at home, however, patients are taught to inject intramuscular or subcutaneous glucagon for severe insulin reactions. Occasionally, glucagon may be administered in the hospital setting. The usual adult dose is 1 mg S_Q or IM; since the major adverse effect of glucagon is nausea and vomiting, patients should rest on their side following administration to prevent aspiration. Adult patients with mild or documented asymptomatic hypoglycemia can be treated with 10 to 20 grams of glucose in the form of juice, soda, liquid glucose, or glucose tablets. If these patients are using alpha-glucosidase inhibitors, they need to be treated with 10 to 20 grams of pure glucose, such as glucose gels and glucose tablets; this is because there will be delayed absorption of other forms of CHO. Following treatment, the patient's blood glucose level should be checked and treatment repeated every 10 to 20 minutes until the blood glucose level returns to normal (Harmel et al., 2004).

Management of Acute Diabetes Complications

A number of complications can occur in patients with DKA and HHS. The most common complications include electrolyte imbalances such as hypokalemia, hypoglycemia, and hypercalcemia. The most emergent and dreaded complication of DKA is cerebral edema (Brown, 2004). The development of cerebral edema typically occurs approximately 6 to 12 hours after therapy has begun when the severe acidosis has been partially corrected, the blood glucose has been reduced, blood pressure restored, and the patient appears to be recovering. This complication most commonly occurs in children (Harmel et al., 2004).

 *The development of cerebral edema is marked by abrupt changes in mental status, abnormal neurological signs, progression to coma, and brain herniation and death.*

There have been a number of proposed causes of cerebral edema. Such causes include a rapid fall in glucose with movement of water from the extracellular to intracellular space, causing brain swelling; a rapid decrease in plasma oncotic pressure resulting from the use of protein-free solutions; and altered cerebral pH with paradoxical cerebrospinal cord acidosis resulting from bicarbonate administration. The failure of serum sodium to rise despite correction of hyperglycemia appears to signify excessive administration of free water and such patients are at risk for cerebral brain swelling (Dunger et al., 2004; Hale et al., 1997).

Despite the fact that no one particular cause of cerebral edema in DKA has been identified, it appears prudent to avoid a rapid fall in plasma osmolality by using 0.9 NS as the initial hydrating solution as in the protocol described previously. In addition, it appears prudent to allow the plasma glucose levels to fall slowly as described previously. If cerebral edema occurs, therapeutic measures include the use of mannitol and dexamethasone.

Medical Management of Chronic Complications of Diabetes

As noted previously, various chronic complications are associated with diabetes. These complications are broadly divided into macrovascular and microvascular complications.

Macrovascular Complications

The leading cause of death among patients with type 2 diabetes mellitus is CVD, with the majority of these deaths attributed to

CHD. The process through which the metabolic derangements of diabetes accelerate the development of CVD in diabetes has yet to be determined and remains an area of intense investigation, focusing on hyperglycemia and insulin resistance (particularly in type 2 diabetes) as major underlying contributors. The topic of CVD is discussed in Chapter 40 ⊙, so it is not discussed extensively in this chapter. As in all complications of diabetes, early detection of CVD is likely to yield better outcomes. Lifestyle interventions including increasing physical activity, weight loss, eating a healthy diet, smoking cessation, and management of prothrombotic factors (through the use of daily aspirin if not contraindicated) are most likely to decrease the risk of macrovascular disease; however, the management of dyslipidemias and hypertension are of the utmost importance.

Microvascular Complications

The microvascular complications of diabetes include retinopathy, neuropathy, and nephropathy. These complications were discussed earlier in the chapter, and also are discussed in other chapters in the text (see Chapters 43, 47, and 71 ⊙).

Retinopathy   The national guidelines proposed by the ADA recommend that health care providers work closely with patients and families (Burant & ADA, 2008). For more details, see National Guidelines for Diabetic Retinopathy box.

Nephropathy   The development of diabetic nephropathy is often asymptomatic, such that it usually is detected on routine laboratory screening tests. The natural history of diabetic nephropathy is a progression from a period of hyperfiltration, which is characterized by an increased GFR, to ESRD, which is characterized by nephrotic range proteinuria, decreasing GFR, and increasing creatinine. The development of diabetic nephropathy is largely dependent on duration of disease and level of glycemic control. The DCCT clearly demonstrated that there is a relationship between level of glycemia and the development and progression of nephropathy. The first sign of developing nephropathy is the presence of microalbuminuria (>30 mg albumin/24 hours) (Burant & ADA, 2008). Microalbuminuria should prompt the health care provider to aggressively treat even minor elevations in blood pressure in order to preserve renal function. In particular, angiotensin-converting enzyme (ACE) inhibitors and angiotensin receptor blockers (ARBs) are most beneficial in delaying the progression of nephropathy in patients with diabetes and microalbuminuria. In addition to hypertension, other factors such as neurogenic bladder, infections, and nephrotoxic drugs, including selected radiocontrast dyes, are associated with a decline in renal function among those patients with diabetes (see Chapter 45 ⊙).

The ADA guidelines, as listed in the National Guidelines for Diabetic Nephropathy box, highlight the information considered to be the most important in the treatment of nephropathy (Burant & ADA, 2008).

Neuropathy   Diabetic neuropathy can affect any area of the body and exists primarily as diabetic polyneuropathy, autonomic neuropathy, or combinations of both. It is beyond the scope of this text to explore this topic in detail; however, attention will focus on some major issues associated with autonomic and peripheral neuropathy.

Autonomic Neuropathy   Diminished autonomic nerve function can cause a variety of symptoms. In particular, autonomic polyneuropathy is associated with the development of gastroparesis, neurogenic bladder, diabetic diarrhea, and impaired cardiovascular reflexes (e.g., orthostatic hypotension and tachycardia) and sexual dysfunction (e.g., impotence).

Cardiovascular autonomic neuropathy is associated with a variety of clinical manifestations, most particularly resting tachycardia (>100 beats per minute), orthostasis (a decrease in systolic blood pressure of >20–30 mmHg on standing) (ADA, 2008c). Patients may complain of dizziness or weakness, nausea, vomiting, and syncope when standing up quickly (Harmel et al., 2004). Patients with severe orthostasis may need fludrocortisone and/or compression stockings.

Gastrointestinal disturbances are common in diabetes and may include esophageal disturbances, gastroparesis, diarrhea, and fecal incontinence (ADA, 2008c). *Gastroparesis* is a syndrome

---

NATIONAL GUIDELINES for Diabetic Retinopathy

- Instruct patients to report visual symptoms promptly.
- Instruct patients about the relationship between hyperglycemia, hypertension, and diabetic retinopathy, focusing on risk factor control to preserve eyesight.
- Inform patients about the importance of an annual dilated examination.
- Inform patients that isometric exercise can raise intraocular pressure; as such, these exercises can worsen proliferative retinopathy.
- Inform patients about support programs and community services for patients with visual impairments and visual loss.

Source: Burant, C. F., & American Diabetes Association. (2008). *Medical management of type 2 diabetes* (6th ed.). Alexandria, VA: American Diabetes Association.

NATIONAL GUIDELINES for Diabetic Nephropathy

- Optimizing glycemic control can prevent or delay the progression of diabetic nephropathy.
- Annual tests for microalbuminuria can detect early diabetic nephropathy.
- Regular blood pressure checks can identify hypertension; hypertension can damage the kidney, precipitate the onset of nephropathy, and accelerate the progression.
- Treatment of hypertension with medication, weight loss, and sodium restriction can prevent the development and decrease the progression of diabetic nephropathy.
- The increased risk of infections in patients with chronic hyperglycemia can result in infections, such as pyelonephritis, with decline in renal function. Patients need to report signs and symptoms of infection to their health care provider.
- Patients who have progressive diabetic nephropathy need to explore options such as dialysis and transplantation with their health care provider.

Source: Burant, C. F., & American Diabetes Association. (2008). *Medical management of type 2 diabetes* (6th ed.). Alexandria, VA: American Diabetes Association.

characterized by the impaired transit of food from the stomach to the duodenum in the absence of a mechanical obstruction. This condition is characterized by early satiety, nausea, vomiting, and abdominal discomfort. These symptoms are often accompanied by fluctuations in blood glucose levels due to delayed gastric emptying or retention of food products. These fluctuations are most pronounced in individuals on insulin therapy. Insulin may peak during periods of delayed gastric emptying causing hypoglycemia; the absorption of food while the actions of insulin are waning may cause hyperglycemia. Treatment of gastroparesis largely relies on diet and medications, and nutritional support may be needed in the most severe cases. Improved glycemic control may actually improve gastric emptying. Frequent (six to eight per day) low-fat, low-fiber meals, especially liquids, may be indicated in gastroparesis (Harmel et al., 2004). Metoclopramide, a dopamine agonist, improves gastric emptying time and has a central antiemetic action (Harmel et al., 2004). Erythromycin is a motilin agonist that stimulates gastric motor activity and can provide some symptomatic relief in the treatment of gastroparesis (Harmel et al., 2004).

Diabetic diarrhea is characterized by the frequent passage of loose stools occurring primarily after meals and during the night. Some patients have alternating periods of diarrhea and constipation. The cause of the diarrhea is unknown and diagnosis is made after other causes of diarrhea (e.g., infection) are excluded. The treatment is largely empirical involving the use of antidiarrheal agents, such as loperamide.

Diabetic autonomic neuropathy also is associated with genitourinary track disturbances. These may include bladder and and/or sexual dysfunction. Neurogenic bladder is characterized by a pattern of frequent, small voiding, and incontinence leading to urinary retention. An evaluation of bladder dysfunction should be performed in patients with diabetes who have recurrent urinary tract infections, pyelonephritis, urinary incontinence, or a palpable bladder (ADA, 2008c). In males, diabetic neuropathy may result in the loss of penile erection and/or retrograde ejaculation (ADA, 2008c). Therapy with selective phosphodiesterase-5 inhibitors (e.g., sildenafil, vardenafil) is now the first line of therapy for male erectile dysfunction (Joslin & Kahn, 2005). However, vacuum devices, intrapenile injections of vasodilating substances (e.g., papaverine), and the implantation of an inflatable or semirigid prosthesis may allow the patient to resume sexual activity.

Polyneuropathy Polyneuropathy is most commonly seen in the legs, feet, and hands. This is called **diabetic peripheral neuropathy (DPN)** and is clearly a significant factor in the pathway leading to lower extremity ulceration (Burant & ADA, 2008). Although DPN is predominantly associated with sensory loss, motor and autonomic nerve fibers also can be affected. Distal symmetric sensorimotor polyneuropathy is the most common form of DPN. As the name implies, it usually appears first in the distal portions of the extremities, moving proximally in a "stocking-glove" distribution. It encompasses both sensory and motor nerve damage and affects both limbs.

Clinical symptoms associated with sensory nerve damage may include numbness, pain, burning, tingling, and eventual partial or total loss of sensation. The pain associated with DPN is first felt distally, in the lower legs, and usually worsens at night. The pain can be persistent or intermittent, occurring over periods of weeks or months. This pain is usually described as aching or burning in nature. Improvement of pain without medication is usually accompanied by the loss of protective sensation and an increase in the risk of foot and lower limb injuries, including ulceration.

Vascular and Neuropathic Complications Leading to Lower Extremity Amputations

Lower extremity amputations in patients with diabetes result from a combination of pathologic events working in tandem. Most diabetic lower extremity amputations originate from diabetic foot ulcers, peripheral arterial disease (PAD), PVD, peripheral neuropathy, minor trauma, deformity, increased plantar pressures, and infection contributing to the development and progression of these ulcers.

Assessment of Sensory Loss Testing for large fiber sensory changes in the diabetic foot can be cost effective and easily performed in any setting with a Semmes-Weinstein monofilament (Mayfield, Reiber, Sanders, Janisse, & Pogach, 2004). The monofilament is a single nylon fiber attached to a handle that buckles under a specified amount of force. A range of monofilaments are available, but the preferred is the 5.07, or 10 grams. The patient is asked to close his eyes and the monofilament then is applied bilaterally to various points on the plantar surface of the toes and metatarsal heads where discriminatory ability is best appreciated. The patient is then asked to give a verbal cue when the monofilament is felt. The inability to perceive the monofilament in any area is considered loss of protective sensation (LOPS). A screening form can be used to document and track where there is loss of protective sensation (Chart 53–9).

Loss of protective sensation also can be established by testing the vibratory perception threshold (VPT), a technique used to measure sensory neuropathy. The simplest and least expensive method uses a 128-Hz tuning fork that is rapped against the clinician's hand and then held to a bony prominence on the foot or the hallux. The patient is asked to indicate when she stops feeling the vibration. If she is unable to feel vibration, she is considered at risk for ulceration.

Treatment for Neuropathic Pain Neuropathic pain is often refractory to traditional analgesic therapy and provides a challenge in pain management. The primary classes of medications used to treat DPN include tricyclic drugs (e.g., amitriptyline, nortriptyline, imipramine), anticonvulsants (e.g., gabapentin, carbamazepine, pregabalin), 5-hydroxytryptamine and norepinephrine uptake inhibitor (e.g., duloxetine), and substance P inhibitor (e.g., capsaicin cream) (ADA, 2008c).

Charcot Deformity Together, distal symmetric polyneuropathy and peripheral autonomic neuropathy can lead to neuropathic osteoarthropathy, or *Charcot deformity*. The underlying assumption is that autonomic neuropathy damages the sympathetic nerves innervating the small blood vessels of the lower extremities. This causes a loss of constrictive tone resulting in vasodilation, increased peripheral perfusion, and expedited

CHART 53–9 Diabetic Foot Screening Using the Semmes-Weinstein Monofilament

PLANTAR SENSORY TESTING

Fill in the following blanks with an "R", "L", or "B" to indicate positive findings on the right, left, or both feet, respectively:

Has there been a change in the foot since the last evaluation?	Yes___	No___
Is there a foot ulcer now, or history of foot ulcer?	Yes___	No___
Does the foot have an abnormal shape?	Yes___	No___
Are the nails thick, too long, or ingrown?	Yes___	No___
Does the patient currently perform daily foot care?	Yes___	No___

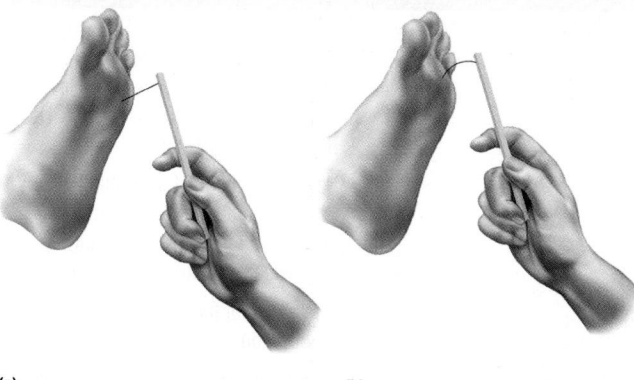

(a) (b)

Picture of Semmes-Weinstein Monofilament being used

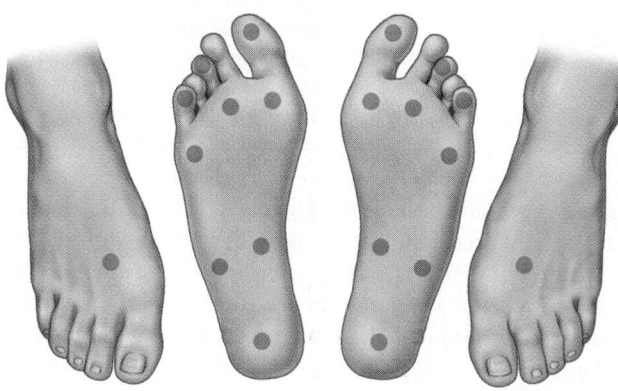

Marked areas indicative of loss of protective sensation as determined by use of monofilament

Risk Category		Action
0	No loss of protective sensation	0 and 1: Teach foot care guidelines.
1	Loss of protection sensation (no deformity, callus, preulcer, or hx of ulceration)	
2	Loss of protective sensation with deformity, preulcer, callus, or corn	2 and 3: Refer immediately to primary care provider/ foot care specialist.
3	History of plantar ulceration	

bone resorption and osteopenia. The salient features and therapy for Charcot deformity are detailed in Chart 53–10 (p. 1698).

Peripheral Vascular Disease Inadequate perfusion to the lower extremities deprives the tissues of oxygen, nutrients, and antibiotics, and impairs waste removal, thus placing the limb at risk for impaired wound healing and gangrene. Clinical findings in PVD include diminished or absent peripheral pulses and intermittent claudication (pain with walking that is relieved by rest). If patients complain of deep, aching pain at night or with rest, severe vascular disease may be present and ulceration or gangrene may follow soon. Additionally, pain may not be present in patients with concurrent neuropathic sensory loss. Unfortunately, gangrene may be the first sign of severe PVD.

Additional signs and symptoms of PVD are shown in Chart 53–11 (p. 1698). Peripheral vascular disease also is discussed in Chapter 43 .

Assessment of vascular status is important to adequately determine risk in a healthy foot, to define the underlying problem in the presence of an ulcer, and to determine the location of a blockage prior to bypass surgery. After gathering data about the patient's medical history and current self-described pain, the health care provider should proceed with a general inspection of the extremities. The dorsalis pedis and posterior tibial pulses should be assessed and graded as palpable or nonpalpable. In the event the pulse is diminished or absent, a second evaluation should be made by another health care provider. The continued absence of a pulse warrants further work-up. The last step in the assessment is to auscultate for femoral bruits. If bruits are present, an arterial brachial index (ABI) should be performed. The ABI is a test that measures the blood pressures in the arm and ankle both at rest and during treadmill walking; a numerical calculation is performed that is used to predict the severity of PVD.

Literature on the diabetic foot has indicated that, by instituting a regular, organized plan of foot care, most diabetic foot problems can be prevented, but the first step is assessment of risk. Following is a list of the factors that have been associated with increased risk for lower extremity ulcers and amputations (Burant & ADA, 2008):

- Patients who have been diagnosed with DM > 10 years
- Male gender
- Patients with poor glucose control
- Patients with cardiovascular, retinal, or renal complications.

Conditions related to the feet that are associated with higher risk for amputations include:

- Peripheral neuropathy with loss of protective sensation
- Altered biomechanics (in the presence of neuropathy)
- Evidence of increased pressures (erythema, hemorrhage under a callous)
- Bony deformity
- Peripheral vascular disease
- A history of ulcers or amputation
- Severe nail pathology.

The ADA recommends that all patients with diabetes should receive a thorough foot examination annually. The foot examination

CHART 53–10	Stages, Clinical Findings, and Therapy for Charcot Deformity		
Charcot Stage	**Features**	**Clinical Findings**	**Therapy**
1. Acute	• Weakened ligaments are allowed to stretch beyond their normal range of motion, causing spontaneous dislocation of the foot • Joint effusions and bone resorption also occur • Easily confused with osteomyelitis	**Physical Exam** • Visible reddening of foot • Warmth • Edema • Easily palpable pulses • May require advanced imaging technologies because microfractures and joint effusions may be missed by x-ray	• Immediate elimination of weight-bearing on affected limb • If compliance is questioned, hospitalization may be necessary • Continue until redness, edema, and foot temperatures return to normal
2. Progressive	• Dislocation and fragmentation of bone • Further fracture • Osseous tissue and muscle have been weakened from nonuse and will need progressive return to full weight-bearing rather than an abrupt return	Radiography usually shows fractures at the metatarsal joints	• Total non–weight-bearing • Crutches and walkers are not recommended, because they may overstress the contralateral limb. Use of a wheelchair is a better option • Use of total contact or walking casts assure immobilization of joint, but can be walked in, thus undermining non–weight-bearing
3. Advanced	• Collapse of the plantar arch from multiple fractures and joint collapse	"Rocker-bottom" foot	• Prevention of foot ulcer and amputation • Referral for custom orthotic footwear • Surgical intervention may be warranted to reduce or excise bony prominences and/or ulcers if present • Fusion of unstable joints or severely deformed feet may provide a safer base for accepting weight-bearing stress and reducing the risk for further ulceration and collapse

CHART 53–11	Signs and Symptoms of Peripheral Vascular Disease

• Feet cold to touch
• Blanching on elevation
• Dependent rubor
• Loss of hair on foot or toes
• Atrophy of subcutaneous fatty tissue
• Absent or diminished pulses
• Delayed venous filling time after elevation (>25 sec)
• Shiny skin
• Thickened nails, often with fungal infection
• Blue toe syndrome

does not need to be time consuming or require expensive or specialized equipment. All health care providers who treat patients with diabetes should be proficient in conducting simple screening examinations. The findings from this risk assessment should guide the plan for prevention and care of foot problems.

During the initial encounter, and throughout the process, the health care provider should assist the patient to change any modifiable risk factors such as smoking, home foot care practices, activity levels, and glycemic control. A variety of home foot care practices have been devised that help decrease the development of foot ulcers and amputation in patients with diabetes and neuropathy. These practices are detailed in the next section.

It is important to note practices that place the patient at higher risk for injury. These include walking without shoes, walking with ill-fitting shoes, decreased attention to daily inspections, and cutting toenails when vision is too poor to visualize the extremity. Activities such as jogging on concrete sidewalks may be contraindicated in patients with diabetes and neuropathy because they may result in trauma to the extremities. Poor glycemic control is associated with poor wound healing and infection. Care for the high-risk foot should not be delayed while waiting on lifestyle changes or glycemic improvement.

Patient Education for Prevention of Lower Extremity Disease As the foundation for all intervention, patient diabetes self-management education should be a priority in every clinical setting. Patients should be taught the following principles of foot care (Ahroni, 2003):

1. **Inspection**—The feet and interdigital areas should be checked daily for blisters, sores, cuts, and calluses. A magnifying glass or handheld mirror may be helpful in viewing the tops, sides, and bottoms of the feet. If patients have cognitive

or visual impairments, a family member should be instructed in assisting or performing the foot examination. The shoes and socks also should be inspected for foreign objects, holes, or raised seams that could cause skin breakdown.

2. **Daily care**—Feet should be washed with warm, soapy water and dried thoroughly; soaking of the feet in water is not advisable. Water temperature should be checked by forearm or elbow to avoid burns. Minor calluses may be *gently* removed with a pumice stone. Thick calluses should be inspected and reduced by a foot care specialist. Nails should be trimmed straight across and the edges filed. If a patient has any visual difficulty, he should not attempt to trim nails. Lotion should be applied daily or more often if skin is dry, avoiding the area between the toes.

3. **Footwear**—Patients should be taught never to go barefoot to prevent injury to their feet. The decreased sensation associated with neuropathy may cause an injury to go unnoticed. Shoes and slippers should be inspected prior to use to make certain that no objects (e.g., coins) have accidentally dropped into them. In addition, when purchasing shoes, patients should ensure that the size is correct. Patients should be advised to break their shoes in slowly, always wear socks or hose, and replace socks rather than attempt to darn them. Because garters restrict blood flow, they should be avoided.

4. **Special care**—Patients should be taught not to use over-the-counter chemical agents to remove corns and warts.

The irritation caused by such chemicals may result in irritation and subsequent ulceration. In addition, sharp instruments or razor blades should never be used to self-treat foot problems such as ingrown toenails. The health care provider should be notified if any problem arises (cuts, blisters, nonhealing wounds, signs of infection, redness, or swelling).

■ Nursing Management

The nursing care needs of hospitalized patients with type 1 or type 2 diabetes, regardless of their admitting diagnosis, require ongoing attention to subjective and objective changes in diabetes status. The nurse often will be the first to notice improvement or deterioration in blood glucose control, which ultimately can hasten or delay recovery. The assessment data, which include sample questions specific to diabetes, are found in the Nursing Process: Care Plan for the Hospitalized Patient with Diabetes (p. 1700). The care plan applies the nursing process to the relevant nursing diagnoses and provides a comprehensive nursing approach for any hospitalized patient with type 1 or type 2 diabetes. This care plan should be used in conjunction with the care plans for concomitant diagnoses.

The nurse should also be aware of the discharge priorities associated with patients who have diabetes. Some examples are listed in the Patient Teaching & Discharge Priorities box.

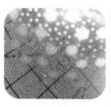

PATIENT TEACHING & DISCHARGE PRIORITIES for Diabetes

Need	Teaching
Physiological teaching needs	Discharge education needs should be evaluated as soon as possible when patients are admitted to the hospital.
	The education needs should be individualized to each patient, but should minimally address those "survival skills" necessary for the patient to be able to self-manage his or her diabetes in the outpatient setting.
	Education should be an ongoing process throughout the hospitalization and nurses should take advantage of every possible "teachable moment" to reinforce learning.
	Survival skill assessment and education should result in the patient or the patient's caregiver being able to: • Describe medication name, dosage, timing, side effects, and refill information. • Demonstrate appropriate technique for preparation and administration of insulin injection (if patient requires insulin). • Demonstrate appropriate technique for monitoring capillary blood glucose levels at home, and verbalize when testing should be done. • Verbalize target blood glucose goals and when to call the health care provider. • Describe the signs, symptoms, and treatment for hypoglycemia. • Describe the signs and symptoms and action to take for hyperglycemia. • Describe how to manage diabetes during illnesses such as the flu. • Verbalize basic understanding of healthy-eating concepts and timing of meals if insulin-requiring. • Verbalize when to call a health care provider.
	If patients are newly diagnosed with diabetes or pre-diabetes during this admission, or they have never received formal diabetes self-management education, or if they have had changes in their health or therapy, they should be referred for further outpatient diabetes education and follow-up.
Psychosocial teaching needs	Patients with diabetes must learn to cope with the daily stress of caring for a chronic disease. The incidence of depression and other psychological disturbances is much higher in people with diabetes than the general population. It is important for the nurse to assess psychosocial needs, family support, and coping skills to foster the patient's ability to self-manage his diabetes, while maintaining optimal quality of life.
	Discharge planning for patients who need further psychosocial support may include: • Referral for social work services • Information about local diabetes support groups • Referral for psychological evaluation.

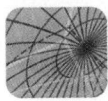

NURSING PROCESS: Patient Care Plan for Hospitalized Patient with Diabetes

Assessment of Blood Glucose Level

Subjective Data:

"I feel shaky."

"I am so thirsty and I am urinating every few hours."

"I can't get any sleep because I am urinating all night long."

Objective Data:

Elevated blood glucose	Palpitations
Polyuria	Mood changes
Polyphagia	Irritability
Weight loss	Unresponsiveness
Fatigue	Unconsciousness
Diaphoresis	Convulsions
Tremors	Coma

Nursing Assessment and Diagnoses	Outcomes and Evaluation Parameters	Planning and Interventions with *Rationales*
Nursing Diagnosis: *Risk for Unstable Blood Glucose*	**Outcome:** Patient will have an acute reduction in hyperglycemia. ***Evaluation Parameters:*** Evidence of a decrease in blood glucose levels. Common target blood glucose levels are: *Critically ill patients:* 110–180 mg/dL *Non–critically ill patients:* 90–130 mg/dL premeal; <180 mg/dL at 2 hours postmeal. **Outcome:** Patient will have resolution of hypoglycemia. ***Evaluation Parameter:*** Evidence of normalization of blood glucose levels.	**Interventions and *Rationales:*** In the event of hyperglycemia, administer medications to reduce blood glucose as ordered. These may include insulin, incretin mimetics or oral diabetes medications alone or in combination. In critically ill settings insulin may be administered intravenously (see text). *All of the medications listed above have a glucose-lowering effect.* **Interventions and *Rationales:*** In the event of hypoglycemia, administer medications or food to raise the blood glucose levels. Examples of foods that raise blood glucose levels include: 3–4 glucose tablets 1/2 cup of fruit juice 5–6 pieces of hard candy. Medications to raise blood glucose levels include: Dextrose 50% H$_2$O Glucagon *All of the medications listed above will increase blood glucose levels.* **Interventions and *Rationales:*** Check the blood glucose level prior to administering glucose-lowering medications. Consult with the medical team if a change in dose may be indicated due to abnormally low (hypoglycemic) or high (hyperglycemic) values. *Because blood glucose levels are affected by factors such as medications (in general), diabetes medications, diet, exercise and physiological stress, fluctuations in blood glucose levels are common in hospitalized patients.* Sustained hyperglycemia in response to treatment may reflect a poor response to therapy, necessitating a change in treatment plan. As the illness resolves, blood glucose levels decline; this may result in hypoglycemia, necessitating a change in the treatment plan. Check blood glucose as ordered. *The frequency and the timing of the blood glucose monitoring will differ depending on the therapy (see text).* Monitor for signs and symptoms of hypoglycemia or worsening hyperglycemia; if either is suspected, test blood glucose levels immediately. *Bedside blood glucose monitoring allows the nurse to verify if the patient has hypoglycemia or hyperglycemia and treat accordingly.*

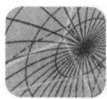

NURSING PROCESS: Patient Care Plan for Hospitalized Patient with Diabetes—*Continued*

Assessment of Fluid Volume Alterations

Subjective Data:
"I feel weak and light-headed."
"My mouth is very dry and I am always thirsty."

Objective Data:
Hypotension
Orthostatic hypotension
Tachycardia

Poor skin turgor
Decreased urine output

Nursing Assessment and Diagnoses	Outcomes and Evaluation Parameters	Planning and Interventions with *Rationales*
Nursing Diagnosis: *Deficient Fluid Volume* with potential for hypoglycemic shock	**Outcome:** The patient will have restoration of fluid volume. *Evaluation Parameters:* Resolution of hypotension. Resolution of orthostatic hypotension. Resolution of tachycardia. Improved skin turgor.	**Interventions and** *Rationales:* General measures include: Encourage fluid intake (in awake and alert patients). Rehydrate with 0.9 NS for intravascular fluid loss. Rehydrate with 0.45 NS for intracellular fluid loss (if indicated). *0.9 NS will reestablish extracellular fluid volume losses; 0.45 NS will restore intracellular volume losses.* Monitor oral fluid intake. Monitor vital signs. Monitor urine output. *To assess hydration status or adequacy of fluid replacement.*

Assessment of Acid–Base Imbalances

Subjective Data:
"I'm breathing fast."
Complaints of headache, altered sleeping pattern, and occasional chest pain

Objective Data:
Decreased arterial pH
Increased anion gap
Decreased serum bicarbonate
Positive serum ketones
Positive urinary ketones

Kussmaul's respirations
Acetone odor to breath
Red, flushed face
Decreased mental status

Nursing Assessment and Diagnoses	Outcomes and Evaluation Parameters	Planning and Interventions with *Rationales*
Nursing Diagnosis: *Risk for acute confusion related to alteration in Acid–Base Balance*	**Outcome:** Patient will have resolution of acid–base imbalance by: *Evaluation Parameters:* Normal arterial pH. Normal anion gap. Normal serum bicarbonate. Negative urinary ketones. Negative serum ketones. Improvements in mental status. Resolution of Kussmaul's breathing, facial flushing, and acid odor to breath.	**Interventions and** *Rationales:* Administer intravenous insulin as ordered. *Insulin will correct the metabolic acidosis.* Obtain the following laboratory tests as ordered and monitor the results closely: ABGs, anion gap, serum ketones, urinary ketones, and serum bicarbonate. The timing of the laboratory tests will change based the acuity of the patient and response to treatment. *The monitoring of these values will help monitor the patient's response to treatment.* Monitor for resolution of the following signs and symptoms: Kussmaul's respirations; fruity odor to breath; red, flushed face; and mental status changes. *Monitoring for resolution in signs and symptoms will help to assess the response to therapy.*

Assessment of Electrolyte Imbalances

Subjective Data:
Experience of muscle spasms.
Describes feelings of weakness, twitching, or confusion.

Objective Data:
Decreased serum potassium level (hypokalemia)

(continued)

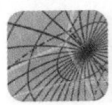

NURSING PROCESS: Patient Care Plan for Hospitalized Patient with Diabetes—*Continued*

Nursing Assessment and Diagnoses	Outcomes and Evaluation Parameters	Planning and Interventions with *Rationales*
Nursing Diagnoses: Decreased cardiac output related to alteration in serum potassium levels (lower than normal) Increased serum potassium level, higher than normal (hyperkalemia) Decreased serum sodium level (hypokalemia)	**Outcome:** Normalization of serum potassium level. ***Evaluation Parameter:*** Serum potassium level is within normal limits.	**Interventions and *Rationales:*** Administer IV potassium (as ordered), usually in the form potassium chloride or potassium phosphate. *Total body potassium stores are often decreased in DKA or HHS. Patients often present with normal or increased potassium levels. Regardless, when exogenous insulin is administered, the serum potassium levels will decrease (see text). Administration of IV potassium is usually indicated to maintain normal potassium levels.* Monitor patients for signs and symptoms of hypokalemia such as: Muscle weakness Anxiety Lethargy Depression Confusion Fatigue Muscle cramps Constipation Abnormal cardiac rhythms such as T-wave flattening, inverted T waves, prominent U wave, ST segment depression, ventricular arrhythmias (e.g., premature ventricular contractions), and atrial arrhythmias. Monitor patients for signs and symptoms of hyperkalemia such as: Muscle twitching Paralysis Gastrointestinal hypermotility Abdominal cramping Diarrhea Muscle cramps Irritability Anxiety Abnormal cardiac rhythms such as tall peaked T waves, widened QRS, and ventricular fibrillation. *Monitoring for signs and symptoms of hypokalemia and hyperkalemia will help assess patient response to treatment.*

Note: This list is not meant to be all inclusive but reflects common issues in the hospitalized patient with diabetes.

Health Promotion, Diabetes Education, and Cultural Implications

Much of the previous portion of this chapter has focused on the clinical presentation and the acute management of patients with diabetes. Diabetes care is a complex balance between the patient and health care providers. The majority of diabetes management decisions are made by the patient, far from the supervision of health care providers. The patients must be provided with the tools necessary to manage their disease.

Diabetes self-management education is an interactive and collaborative process between the patient and the health care team than leads to better diabetes control and health outcomes. Strategies of diabetes self-management education include providing the patient and significant other with the knowledge necessary to the successful management of diabetes. This information may include, but is not limited to (ADA, 2008d):

- Describing the pathophysiology of diabetes and treatment options

- Incorporating nutritional management and physical activity into lifestyle

- Using diabetes medication(s) safely to achieve maximum therapeutic effectiveness

- Monitoring blood glucose and other parameters and interpreting and using the results to make self-management decisions

- Preventing, detecting, and treating acute and chronic complications

- Developing personal strategies to address psychosocial issues and concerns to promote health and behavior changes.

The behavioral context on which the patient learns diabetes self-management skills is based on the complex interplay between culture and perceptions of health and illness. According to

Fleury-Milfort (2004), "the culture and the religious background of a patient and (of the diabetes educator) provide the context in which the patient develops certain values, beliefs, behaviors, attitude, self-care habits and relationships with health-care providers." When a nurse is engaged in diabetes self-management teaching, she should assess the patient's beliefs about the causes of diabetes and diabetes complications, perceptions of the effect of diabetes and diabetes treatment on one's life, the role of family members on health care decisions and responsibilities, and the importance of customs and observances influencing the treatment plan (Fleury-Milfort, 2004). An understanding of such issues can form the basis of culturally sensitive self-management educational experiences.

Collaborative Management

Optimal care of patients with diabetes requires a multidisciplinary team approach to their care. Physicians, nurses, and dieticians work as a team to monitor blood glucose results, make changes in medication or nutrition therapies, and assess the response to those changes. As the health status of the patient improves or deteriorates, diabetes status also may change rapidly. Healing of infections or increases in mobility (and, thus, ambulation) may cause rapid lowering of blood glucose levels. Addition of some medications, such as corticosteroids may cause elevations in blood glucose levels, requiring alterations in medication dosage by the health care provider. Hyperglycemia, if left untreated, will delay healing and may lead to longer hospitalizations. Careful assessment and monitoring by the nurse is crucial in alerting other members of the health care team to changes in diabetes status that can change the course of patient recovery. The dietitian plays a key role in adjusting diets and nutrients. The physical therapist and occupational therapist also may be involved in the case of mobility and self-care issues.

Summary

Diabetes is a chronic disease and the occurrence and progression of diabetes-related complications can be decreased through intensive glucose, hypertension, and lipid control. In addition, there is mounting evidence that the actual development of diabetes can be decreased through lifestyle modification including increased physical activity and weight maintenance or weight loss (if indicated). Acute complications of diabetes can be avoided through careful monitoring and attention to precipitating factors; yet when these acute complications occur, intensive medical management can decrease mortality and morbidity from these complications. Because the incidence of diabetes is increasing worldwide, health care professionals need to stay current with new treatment measures to address the personal, social, and economic problems associated with diabetes.

Clinical Preparation

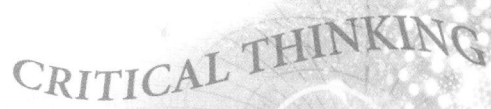

 Read

- History of Current Illness
- Past Medical History
- Physical Exam
- Admitting Medical Orders
- Laboratory Study Results

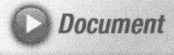 **Document**

- Summary of Hospitalization
- Pathophysiology Form
- Laboratory Values
- Laboratory Results Explanation

 **Apply**

- List of Potential Nursing Diagnoses
- Concept Map
- Critical Thinking Questions

Log on to MyNursingKit.com to download forms you will need and to complete further steps in the Clinical Preparation assignment.

HISTORY OF PRESENT ILLNESS

The patient is a 20-year-old college student who presented to the local emergency department (ED). He reported that he and several other students had a gastrointestinal virus over the past few weeks. The primary symptoms were nausea, vomiting, and diarrhea, which usually resolved within 24 to 48 hours. John reported that he never completely recovered from his illness, feeling tired and listless during the previous week. During the past 2 to 3 days he noted increased thirst and increased urination, along with fatigue during this time period. John has been nauseated and vomiting during the last 2 hours, and has vomited twice in the ED.

The following medications were administered in the ED: an initial bolus of regular intravenous insulin (10 units) followed by an intravenous regular insulin drip of 6 units/hour. In addition, a potassium chloride (KCl) rider (20 mEq/hr) was initiated after it was established that the patient had adequate urinary output (>30 mL/hr).

Nursing care while in the ED revolved around assessing and providing interventions for any emergency needs (i.e., vascular fluid replacement); obtaining the diagnostic laboratory values: arterial blood gases (ABGs), serum ketones, complete blood count

(CBC), serum blood chemistries, serum electrolytes, and urinalysis (UA). In this particular patient, the current nursing care plan calls for initiating fluid replacement therapy (0.9 normal saline at 1 L/hr); obtaining a capillary glucose reading; performing an electrocardiogram (ECG); and sending a stool specimen to the laboratory for culture and sensitivity.

The patient was transferred to the medical intensive care unit (MICU) where you are assigned to care for him.

Medical–Surgical History

The patient's general medical history is noncontributory. There is no history of major medical illnesses, surgeries, or traumas. He does not use any medications, but does report using an "over-the-counter" drug to stop diarrhea during the previous episode of the "flu."

Mother (age 45) has rheumatoid arthritis; father (age 50) has hypertension. Siblings: brother (age 16) has no major illnesses; sister (age 14) has no major illnesses; and brother (age 10) has type 1 diabetes.

Social History

Patient reports social drinking (4 to 6 beers on weekends); has never smoked cigarettes, but smokes approximately 1 to 2 cigars every 2 to 3 months; he indicates that he has never used recreational drugs.

Physical Exam

Patient is a thin acutely ill male; 6'0" and 155 lbs. The following clinical signs are noted: poor skin turgor, dry mucous membranes, facial flushing, and deep rapid breathing with fruity odor to breath. His chest is clear to auscultation; his heart examination reveals tachycardia and is otherwise normal; the abdominal examination reveals a diffusely tender abdomen; the neurological examination reveals increasing lethargy, otherwise his neurological status is normal.

Vital signs: temperature is 99°F. In a supine position, his blood pressure is 100/70, pulse 100 beats per minute, and respirations 32. In a standing position, his blood pressure is 90/60; pulse, 115 beats per minute, and respirations are 32.

Admitting Medical Orders

Admit to Medical ICU

Admitting diagnosis: newly diagnosed type 1 diabetes; diabetic ketoacidosis (mild to moderate)

Allergies: none noted

Vital signs q1h

Neuro checks q1h

Activity: bed rest with bathroom privileges

I&O q8h

Sequential compression stockings (SCDs) to lower extremities

Diet: 1,800-calorie diabetic diet

Call house officer: HR < 60 or > 120, systolic BP < 90 or > 160, temperature > 38.5°C, RR < 10 or > 30, urinary output < 240 mL in 8 hours, O_2 saturation < 92%, glucose level < 70 or > 130, serum sodium level < 135 or > 145, serum potassium level < 3.8 or > 4.5, increased lethargy per neuro checks

IVs: normal saline 0.45 at 100 mL/hr

Scheduled Medications

Insulin drip at 6 units/hour

Potassium chloride (KCl) IV at 20 mEq/hr

PRN Medications

Phenergan for nausea 25 mg IV q4–6h prn

D50%W 25 g IV prn if Accu-Chek less than 70 mg/dL

Ordered Laboratory Studies

Serum K, Na, Cl, HCO_3 q2h

Serum K every hour if unstable

ABGs, CBC, Chem panel, serum acetone, and urine ketones q4h

Accu-Cheks q1h

Stool culture q24h × 3 days

Ordered Diagnostic Studies

ECG on admission and q4h

The patient has a relatively uneventful course during hospitalization with one exception. After approximately 8 hours of treatment, the patient was noted to be increasingly lethargic and confused. The two primary differential diagnoses for this condition include hypoglycemia and cerebral edema. A capillary blood glucose level taken at that time revealed a blood glucose level of 60 mg/dL, which confirms the hypoglycemia. The patient is given 25 g of dextrose 50% in water (D50%W). After administration of the D50%W, the patient is alert and oriented and the subsequent blood glucose reading is 100 mg/dL. The results of other pertinent tests at this time are shown below in the Laboratory Study Results table.

Because the patient's diabetic ketoacidosis has resolved and the patient is able to take fluids and food, the insulin drip is discontinued. Prior to discontinuing the drip, the patient is started on an insulin protocol with an initial starting dose of Glargine 20 units subcutaneously. The premeal lispro dose will be titrated depending on the meal and overall appetite of the patient. In general an insulin:carbohydrate (CHO) ratio of 1:20 (1 unit of lispro insulin to 20 mg of CHO) will be used.

The nursing care at this time is centered on (1) monitoring response to therapy and (2) patient education. In particular, patient education revolves around teaching survival skills (insulin injection, basic nutrition teaching, blood glucose monitoring) and helping to transition to an outpatient education program.

LABORATORY STUDY RESULTS

Test	Result on Admission	4 Hours Post-Admission	8 Hours Post-Admission
Serum glucose	450 mg/dL	250 mg/dL	60 mg/dL
Arterial pH/PO_2/PCO_2	7.1/105/22	7.2/100/35	7.4/100/38
Serum bicarbonate (HCO_3)	9 mEq/L	13 mEq/L	20 mEq/L
Serum Na^+	135 mEq/L	138 mEq/L	142 mEq/L
Serum K^+	5.3 mEq/L	5.0 mEq/L	4.8 mEq/L
Serum Cl^-	98 mEq/L	100 mEq/L	100 mEq/L
Serum acetone	1.16 dilutions	1.8 dilutions	Negative
Serum creatinine	1.4 mg/dL	1.2 mg/dL	—
Serum blood urea nitrogen (BUN)	25 mg/dL	20 mg/dL	—
Hemoglobin	17 g/dL	15 g/dL	14 g/dL
Hematocrit	47%	44%	42%
White blood count	15,000 cells/mm^3	10,000 cells/mm^3	5,000 cells/mm^3
Urine ketones	Large	Moderate	Negative
ECG	Normal sinus tachycardia	Normal sinus rhythm	Normal sinus rhythm
Stool (culture)	Negative		

CRITICAL THINKING QUESTIONS

1. What are the four major biochemical derangements in diabetic ketoacidosis?

2. What are the clinical signs and symptoms (as noted in this scenario) that are derived from these biochemical derangements?

3. How do nursing interventions for diabetic ketoacidosis (DKA) develop from identification of each of these derangements?

4. The patient in this scenario has mild to moderate DKA. How might clinical signs, symptoms, laboratory tests, and treatments differ if the patient had severe DKA?

5. What discharge plans would you anticipate for this patient?

Answers to Critical Thinking Questions appear in Appendix D.

NCLEX® REVIEW

1. The nurse recognizes the following is true regarding the prevalence of diabetes.
   1. The most common form is type 1.
   2. Approximately 20% of Americans over age 60 have diabetes.
   3. The lowest prevalence occurs among Native Americans.
   4. The highest incidence worldwide is in the United States population.

2. The nurse determines a patient has the criteria for pre-diabetes when the following are identified on assessment:
   1. The patient is 20 years old and requires therapy with oral hypoglycemic agents.
   2. The patient was diagnosed with gestational diabetes with her last pregnancy.
   3. Fasting blood sugar (FBS) level is 130 mg/dL.
   4. Glucose tolerance test shows normal blood sugar levels.

3. The nurse identifies the following patient to be most at risk to develop type 1 diabetes:
   1. The adolescent who had chronic bacterial ear infections as a child
   2. A school age child whose mother has type 1 diabetes
   3. A toddler with a monozygotic twin who has type 1 diabetes
   4. A pre-school age child with a dizygotic twin who has type 1 diabetes

4. The nurse recognizes the following assessment findings in a patient with type 2 diabetes are associated with the metabolic syndrome.
   1. Elevated triglycerides and HDL levels
   2. Abdominal obesity and decreased HDL level
   3. Elevated LDL level and hypertension
   4. Elevated blood sugar and decreased triglyceride level

5. A patient with type 1 diabetes is experiencing early signs of proliferative retinopathy. The nurse includes the following instructions for management and prevention of further complications.
   1. "Be sure to have a dilated eye examination every two years."
   2. "Avoid doing any isometric exercises."
   3. "Restrict protein in the diet to 10 grams a day."
   4. "Keep your blood sugar level less than 150 mg/dL."

6. The nurse incorporates the following interventions in the plan of care for a patient receiving a meglitinide oral hypoglycemic agent.
   1. Administer the medication with meals.
   2. Check for signs and symptoms of hyperglycemia one hour after the meal.
   3. Check for allergies to sulfa.
   4. Instruct patient to eat within 20 minutes of taking the medication.

7. The nurse should give the following instructions to a patient with Type 2 diabetes who takes oral hypoglycemic agents and is planning to begin an exercise program.

   1. "You will be at increased risk for hyperglycemia up to two hours after exercising."
   2. "Avoid eating anything before you start exercising."
   3. "Exercise may lower your blood sugar for several hours after completing the activity."
   4. "Eat only simple carbohydrates if you become hypoglycemic after exercising."

8. The nurse determines a patient is experiencing side effects of an alpha-glucosidase inhibitor when these symptoms are manifested sixty minutes after taking the medication.

   1. Abdominal bloating and diarrhea
   2. Elevated temperature
   3. Tremors and palpitations
   4. Fatigue

9. An elderly patient is seen in the emergency department. The family reports the patient has "diabetes" and has not eaten well for the past few days; the patient's blood sugar is 475 mg/dL. Which assessment finding would indicate the patient is experiencing diabetic ketoacidosis (DKA) rather than hyperosmolar hyperglycemic syndrome (HHS)?

   1. Face is flushed and red.
   2. Skin turgor is inelastic.
   3. Patient is lethargic and difficult to arouse.
   4. Blood pressure is 80/40.

10. The nurse recognizes which of the following patients with diabetes is most at risk to develop lower extremity ulcers and/or amputation.

    1. A male who was diagnosed with diabetes two years ago
    2. An elderly female who maintains her blood glucose between 100–140 mg/dL
    3. A male patient with chronic renal failure (CRF)
    4. A female patient who recently had a myocardial infarction (MI)

Answers for review questions appear in Appendix D

KEY TERMS

analog *p.1671*
continuous subcutaneous insulin infusion (CSII) *p.1674*
counterregulatory hormones *p.1662*
dawn phenomenon *p.1677*
Diabetes Control and Complications Trial (DCCT) *p.1663*
Diabetes Prevention Program (DPP) *p.1666*
diabetic ketoacidosis (DKA) *p.1663*
diabetic peripheral neuropathy (DPN) *p.1696*
gestational diabetes mellitus (GDM) *p.1660*
glucagon *p.1661*
gluconeogenesis *p.1662*
glycated serum proteins (GSPs) *p.1670*
glycogen *p.1661*
glycogenolysis *p.1662*
glycolysis *p.1661*

hemoglobin A$_{1C}$ (Hb A$_{1C}$) test *p.1670*
honeymoon period *p.1665*
hyperglycemia *p.1659*
hyperosmolar hyperglycemic syndrome (HHS) *p.1663*
hypoglycemia *p.1663*
hypoglycemic unawareness *p.1690*
impaired fasting glucose (IFG) *p.1660*
impaired glucose tolerance (IGT) *p.1660*
incretin mimetics *p.1674*
insulin *p.1659*
insulin resistance *p.1662*
ketogenesis *p.1662*
latent autoimmune diabetes in adults (LADA) *p.1660*
lipolysis *p.1662*
macronutrients *p.1683*
macrovascular *p.1660*

maturity onset diabetes of the young (MODY) *p.1660*
medical nutrition therapy (MNT) *p.1683*
microalbuminuria *p.1663*
micronutrients *p.1683*
microvascular *p.1660*
molecular mimicry *p.1665*
normoglycemia *p.1671*
oral glucose tolerance test (OGTT) *p.1668*
osmotic diuresis *p.1667*
pancreatic beta cells *p.1659*
pancreatic polypeptide *p.1661*
pre-diabetes *p.1660*
Somogyi effect *p.1677*
type 1 diabetes mellitus *p.1659*
type 2 diabetes mellitus *p.1660*
United Kingdom Prospective Diabetes Study (UKPDS) *p.1671*

REFERENCES

Ahroni, J. H. (2003). Diabetic foot care and education. In M. J. Franz (Ed.), *Diabetes and complications* (5th ed., pp. 67–83). Chicago: American Association of Diabetes Educators.

Akerblom, H. K., Vaarala, O., Hyoty, H., Ilonen, J., & Knip, M. (2002). Environmental factors in the etiology of type 1 diabetes. *American Journal of Medical Genetics, 115*(1), 18–29.

Albert, L. J., & Inman, R. D. (1999). Molecular mimicry and autoimmunity. *New England Journal of Medicine, 341*(27), 2068–2074.

American Diabetes Association. (2001). *Diabetes: Vital statistics* (p. v). Alexandria, VA: Author.

American Diabetes Association. (2007). Nutrition recommendations and interventions for diabetes: A position statement of the American Diabetes Association. *Diabetes Care, 30*(Suppl. 1), S48–S65.

American Diabetes Association. (2008a). *Diabetes forecast resource guide* Alexandria, VA: Author.

American Diabetes Association. (2008b). National standards for diabetes self-management education. *Diabetes Care, 31*(Suppl. 1), S97–S104.

American Diabetes Association. (2008c). Standards of medical care in diabetes—2008. *Diabetes Care, 31*(Suppl. 1), S12–S54.

American Diabetes Association. (2008d). *Total prevalence of diabetes and pre-diabetes.* Retrieved June 27, 2008, from http://www.diabetes.org/diabetes-statistics/prevalence.jsp

American Diabetes Association. (2008e). Standards of medical care in diabetes—2008. *Diabetes Care, 31*(Suppl. 1), S12–S54.

American Diabetes Association. (2008f). Total prevalence of diabetes and pre-diabetes. Retrieved June 27, 2008, from http://www.diabetes.org/diabetes-statistics/prevalence.jsp

Amylin Pharmaceuticals. (2007). *Product information.* Retrieved June 9, 2007, from http://www.amylin.com

Barr, R. G., Nathan, D. M., Meigs, J. B., & Singer, D. E. (2002). Tests of glycemia for the diagnosis of type 2 diabetes mellitus. *Annals of Internal Medicine, 137*(4), 263–272.

Bektas, F., Eray, O., Sari, R., & Akbas, H. (2004). Point of care blood ketone testing of diabetic patients in the emergency department. *Endocrine Research, 30*(3), 395–402.

Bobo, N., Evert, A., Gallivan, J., Imperatore, G., Kelly, J., Linder, B., et al. (2004). An update on type 2 diabetes in youth from the national diabetes education program. *Pediatrics, 114*(1), 259–263.

Bode, B. W. (Ed.). (2004). *Medical management of type 1 diabetes.* Alexandria, VA: American Diabetes Association.

Brown, A. F. (2004). Aetiology of cerebral oedema in diabetic ketoacidosis. *Emergency Medicine Journal, 21*(6), 754–755.

Burant, C. F., & American Diabetes Association. (2008). *Medical management of type 2 diabetes* (6th ed.). Alexandria, VA: American Diabetes Association.

Campbell, R. K., & White, J. R., Jr. (2000). *Medications for the treatment of diabetes.* Alexandria, VA: American Diabetes Association.

Capes, S. E., Hunt, D., Malmberg, K., Pathak, P., & Gerstein, H. C. (2001). Stress hyperglycemia and prognosis of stroke in nondiabetic and diabetic patients: A systematic overview. *Stroke, 32*(10), 2426–2432.

Centers for Disease Control and Prevention. (2004). Prevalence of visual impairment and selected eye diseases among persons aged >/=50 years with and without diabetes—United States, 2002 *Morbidity and Mortality Weekly Report, 53*(45), 1069–1071.

Centers for Disease Control and Prevention. (2005). *National diabetes fact sheet: General information and national estimates on diabetes in the United States, 2005.* Retrieved from http://www.cdc.gov/diabetes/pubs/factsheet05.htm

Dahlquist, G. G. (1997). Viruses and other perinatal exposures as initiating events for beta-cell destruction. *Annals of Medicine, 29*(5), 413–417.

DCCT Trial Research Group. (1993). The effect of intensive treatment of diabetes on the development and progression of long-term complications in insulin-dependent diabetes mellitus. *New England Journal of Medicine, 329*(14), 977–986.

DeFronzo, R. A. (2004). Pathogenesis of type 2 diabetes mellitus. *Medical Clinics of North America, 88*(4), 787–835, ix.

Devlin, J. T., Hirshman, M., Horton, E. D., & Horton, E. S. (1987). Enhanced peripheral and splanchnic insulin sensitivity in NIDDM men after single bout of exercise. *Diabetes, 36*(4), 434–439.

Dunger, D. B., Sperling, M. A., Acerini, C. L., Bohn, D. J., Daneman, D., Danne, T. P., et al. (2004). ESPE/LWPES consensus statement on diabetic ketoacidosis in children and adolescents. *Archives of Disease in Childhood, 89*(2), 188–194.

Evert, A. B., Hess-Fischl, A., & American Dietetic Association. (2006). *Pediatric diabetes: Health care reference and client education handouts.* Chicago, IL: American Dietetic Association.

Fagot-Campagna, A., Pettitt, D. J., Engelgau, M. M., Burrows, N. R., Geiss, L. S., Valdez, R., et al. (2000). Type 2 diabetes among North American children and adolescents: An epidemiologic review and a public health perspective. *Journal of Pediatrics, 136*(5), 664–672.

Fairview Health Services. (2003). *Guide to carbohydrate counting: A simple meal-planning method for people with diabetes* (3rd ed.). Minneapolis: Fairview Publications.

Fleury-Milfort, E. (2004). Diabetes self-management education. In A. P. Harmel & R. Matchur (Eds.), *Davidson's diabetes mellitus: Diagnosis and treatment.* Philadelphia: W. B. Saunders.

Ford, E. S., & Giles, W. H. (2003). A comparison of the prevalence of the metabolic syndrome using two proposed definitions. *Diabetes Care, 26*(3), 575–581.

Funk, J. (2003). Pathophysiology of disease: An introduction to clinical medicine. In S. McPhee, V. Lingappa, & W. Ganong (Eds.), *Disorders of the endocrine pancreas.* New York: McGraw-Hill.

Furnary, A. P., Wu, Y., & Bookin, S. O. (2004). Effect of hyperglycemia and continuous intravenous insulin infusions on outcomes of cardiac surgical procedures: The Portland diabetic project. *Endocrinology Practice, 10*(Suppl. 2), 21–33.

Garber, A. J., Seidel, J., & Armbruster, M. (2004). Current standards of care for inpatient glycemic management and metabolic control: Is it time for definite standards and targets? *Endocrinology Practice, 10*(Suppl. 2), 10–12.

Gardner, L. I., Jr., Stern, M. P., Haffner, S. M., Gaskill, S. P., Hazuda, H. P., Relethford, J. H., et al. (1984). Prevalence of diabetes in Mexican Americans. Relationship to percent of gene pool derived from Native American sources. *Diabetes, 33*(1), 86–92.

Gerstein, H. C. (1994). Cow's milk exposure and type I diabetes mellitus. A critical overview of the clinical literature. *Diabetes Care, 17*(1), 13–19.

Gilden, J. L. (1999). Nutrition and the older diabetic. *Clinics in Geriatric Medicine, 15*(2), 371–390.

Goldstein, D. E., Little, R. R., Lorenz, R. A., Malone, J. I., Nathan, D., Peterson, C. M., et al. (2004). Tests of glycemia in diabetes. *Diabetes Care, 27*(7), 1761–1773.

Gregg, E. W., Cadwell, B. L., Cheng, Y. J., Cowie, C. C., Williams, D. E., Geiss, L., et al. (2004). Trends in the prevalence and ratio of diagnosed to undiagnosed diabetes according to obesity levels in the U.S. *Diabetes Care, 27*(12), 2806–2812.

Gutierrez, K. (2008). *Pharmacotherapeutics: Clinical reasoning in primary care* (2nd ed.). St. Louis: W. B. Saunders.

Haffner, S. M. (1997). Impaired glucose tolerance, insulin resistance and cardiovascular disease. *Diabetic Medicine, 14*(Suppl. 3), S12–S18.

Hale, P. M., Rezvani, I., Braunstein, A. W., Lipman, T. H., Martinez, N., & Garibaldi, L. (1997). Factors predicting cerebral edema in young children with diabetic ketoacidosis and new onset type I diabetes. *Acta Paediatrica, 86*(6), 626–631.

Harmel, A. P., Mathur, R., & Davidson, M. B. (2004). *Davidson's diabetes mellitus: Diagnosis and treatment* (5th ed.). Philadelphia: W. B. Saunders.

Harris, M. I. (2001). Racial and ethnic differences in health care access and health outcomes for adults with type 2 diabetes. *Diabetes Care, 24*(3), 454–459.

Helmrich, S. P., Ragland, D. R., Leung, R. W., & Paffenbarger, R. S., Jr. (1991). Physical activity and reduced occurrence of non-insulin-dependent diabetes mellitus. *New England Journal of Medicine, 325*(3), 147–152.

Hu, F. B., Manson, J. E., Stampfer, M. J., Colditz, G., Liu, S., Solomon, C. G., et al. (2001). Diet, lifestyle, and the risk of type 2 diabetes mellitus in women. *New England Journal of Medicine, 345*(11), 790–797.

Hussain, A. N., & Vincent, M. T. (2007). *Diabetes mellitus, type* Retrieved July 1, 2008, from http://www.emedicine.com/MED/topic546.htm

International Diabetes Federation. (2006). *Diabetes atlas* (3rd ed.). Brussels, Belgium: International Diabetes Federation.

Joslin, E. P., & Kahn, C. R. (2005). In C. Ronald Kahn et al. (Eds.), *Joslin's diabetes mellitus* (14th ed.). Philadelphia: Lippincott Williams & Wilkins.

Kaufman, F., & American Diabetes Association. (2008). *Medical management of type 1 diabetes* (5th ed.). Alexandria, VA: American Diabetes Association.

Kaufman, F. R. (2002). Type 2 diabetes mellitus in children and youth: A new epidemic. *Journal of Pediatric Endocrinology and Metabolism 15*(Suppl 2), 737–744.

Knip, M. (2003). Cow's milk and the new trials for prevention of type 1 diabetes. *Journal of Endocrinological Investigation, 26*(3), 265–267.

Knowler, W. C., Barrett-Connor, E., Fowler, S. E., Hamman, R. F., Lachin, J. M., Walker, E. A., et al. (2002). Reduction in the incidence of type 2 diabetes with lifestyle intervention or metformin. *New England Journal of Medicine, 346*(6), 393–403.

Krentz, A. J., & Bailey, C. J. (2005). Oral antidiabetic agents: Current role in type 2 diabetes mellitus. *Drugs, 65*(3), 385–411.

Lammi, N., Karvonen, M., & Tuomilehto, J. (2005). Do microbes have a causal role in type 1 diabetes? *Medical Science Monitor, 11*(3), RA63–69.

Lebovitz, H. E., & American Diabetes Association. (2004). *Therapy for diabetes mellitus and related disorders* (4th ed.). Alexandria, VA: American Diabetes Association.

Lee, E. T., Howard, B. V., Savage, P. J., Cowan, L. D., Fabsitz, R. R., Oopik, A. J., et al. (1995). Diabetes and impaired glucose tolerance in three American Indian populations aged 45–74 years. The strong heart study. *Diabetes Care, 18*(5), 599–610.

Ligaray, K. P. L., & Isley, W. O. (2007). *Diabetes mellitus, type 2.* Retrieved July 1, 2008, from http://www.emedicine.com/med/topic547.htm

Lioupis, C. (2005). Effects of diabetes mellitus on wound healing: An update. *Journal of Wound Care, 14*(2), 84–86.

Malecki, M. T., & Klupa, T. (2005). Type 2 diabetes mellitus: From genes to disease. *Pharmacologic Reports, 57*(Suppl.), 20–32.

Malmberg, K. (2004). Role of insulin-glucose infusion in outcomes after acute myocardial infarction: The diabetes and insulin-glucose infusion in acute myocardial infarction (DIGAMI) study. *Endocrinology Practice, 10*(Suppl. 2), 13–16.

Manson, J. E., Nathan, D. M., Krolewski, A. S., Stampfer, M. J., Willett, W. C., & Hennekens, C. H. (1992). A prospective study of exercise and incidence of diabetes among U.S. male physicians. *Journal of the American Medical Association, 268*(1), 63–67.

Manson, J. E., Rimm, E. B., Stampfer, M. J., Colditz, G. A., Willett, W. C., Krolewski, A. S., et al. (1991). Physical activity and incidence of non-insulin-dependent diabetes mellitus in women. *Lancet, 338*(8770), 774–778.

Mayfield, J. A., Reiber, G. E., Sanders, L. J., Janisse, D., & Pogach, L. M. (2004). Preventive foot care in diabetes. *Diabetes Care, 27*(Suppl. 1), S63–S64.

McCarren, M., & American Diabetes Association. (2007). *American Diabetes Association guide to insulin and type 2 diabetes.* Alexandria, VA: American Diabetes Association.

McFarland, K. F., Catalano, E. W., Day, J. F., Thorpe, S. R., & Baynes, J. W. (1979). Nonenzymatic glucosylation of serum proteins in diabetes mellitus. *Diabetes, 28*(11), 1011–1014.

McMahon, M. M., & Rizza, R. A. (1996). Nutrition support in hospitalized patients with diabetes mellitus. *Mayo Clinic Proceedings, 71*(6), 587–594.

McPherson, R. A., Pincus, M. R., & Henry, J. B. (2007). *Henry's clinical diagnosis and management by laboratory methods* (21st ed.). Philadelphia: W. B. Saunders.

Moghissi, E. S., & Hirsch, I. B. (2005). Hospital management of diabetes. *Endocrinology Metabolism Clinics of North America, 34*(1), 99–116.

Muir, A., Schatz, D. A., & Maclaren, N. K. (1992). The pathogenesis, prediction, and prevention of insulin-dependent diabetes mellitus. *Endocrinology Metabolism Clinics of North America, 21*(2), 199–219.

Narayan, K. M., Boyle, J. P., Thompson, T. J., Sorensen, S. W., & Williamson, D. F. (2003). Lifetime risk for diabetes mellitus in the United States. *Journal of the American Medical Association, 290*(14), 1884–1890.

National Center for Chronic Disease Prevention and Health Promotion. (2004). *Data and trends: National diabetes surveillance system: Mortality due to diabetic ketoacidosis.* Retrieved June 9, 2007, from http://www.cdc.gov/diabetes/statistics/mortalitydka/source.htm

Newman, B., Selby, J. V., King, M. C., Slemenda, C., Fabsitz, R., & Friedman, G. D. (1987). Concordance for type 2 (non-insulin-dependent) diabetes mellitus in male twins. *Diabetologia, 30*(10), 763–768.

Nugent, B. W. (2005). Hyperosmolar hyperglycemic state. *Emergency Medical Clinics of North America, 23,* 629–648.

Porth, C. M. (2007). *Essentials of pathophysiology: Concepts of altered health states.* Philadelphia: Lippincott Williams & Wilkins.

Pozzilli, P., & Di Mario, U. (2001). Autoimmune diabetes not requiring insulin at diagnosis (latent autoimmune diabetes of the adult): Definition, characterization, and potential prevention. *Diabetes Care, 24*(8), 1460–1467.

Rich-Edwards, J. W., Colditz, G. A., Stampfer, M. J., Willett, W. C., Gillman, M. W., Hennekens, C. H., et al. (1999). Birth weight and the risk for type 2 diabetes mellitus in adult women. *Annals of Internal Medicine, 130*(4, Part 1), 278–284.

Riddle, M. C. (1999). Oral pharmacologic management of type 2 diabetes. *American Family Physician, 60*(9), 2613–2620.

Rosenbloom, A. L., House, D. V., & Winter, W. E. (1998). Non-insulin dependent diabetes mellitus (NIDDM) in minority youth: Research priorities and needs. *Clinical Pediatrics (Philadelphia), 37*(2), 143–152.

Rosenbloom, A. L., Joe, J. R., Young, R. S., & Winter, W. E. (1999). Emerging epidemic of type 2 diabetes in youth. *Diabetes Care, 22*(2), 345–354.

Rucker, D. W. (2008). *Diabetic ketoacidosis.* Retrieved July 1, 2008, from http://www.emedicine.com/emerg/topic135.htm

Sheehan, J. P. (2004). Fasting hyperglycemia: Etiology, diagnosis, and treatment. *Diabetes Technology and Therapeutics, 6*(4), 525–533.

So, W. Y., Ng, M. C., Lee, S. C., Sanke, T., Lee, H. K., & Chan, J. C. (2000). Genetics of type 2 diabetes mellitus. *Hong Kong Medical Journal, 6*(1), 69–76.

Tattersall, R. (1998). Maturity-onset diabetes of the young: A clinical history. *Diabetic Medicine, 15*(1), 11–14.

Tuomilehto, J., Lindstrom, J., Eriksson, J. G., Valle, T. T., Hamalainen, H., Ilanne-Parikka, P., et al. (2001). Prevention of type 2 diabetes mellitus by changes in lifestyle among subjects with impaired glucose tolerance. *New England Journal of Medicine, 344*(18), 1343–1350.

U.K. Prospective Diabetes Study Group. (1998a). Effect of intensive blood-glucose control with metformin on complications in overweight patients with type 2 diabetes (UKPDS 34). *Lancet, 352*(9131), 854–865.

U.K. Prospective Diabetes Study Group. (1998b). Tight blood pressure control and risk of macrovascular and microvascular complications in type 2 diabetes (UKPDS 38). *British Medical Journal, 317*(7160), 703–713.

Umpierrez, G. E., Isaacs, S. D., Bazargan, N., You, X., Thaler, L. M., & Kitabchi, A. E. (2002). Hyperglycemia: An independent marker of in-hospital mortality in patients with undiagnosed diabetes. *Journal of Clinical Endocrinology and Metabolism, 87*(3), 978–982.

Umpierrez, G. E., & Kitabchi, A. E. (2003). Diabetic ketoacidosis: Risk factors and management strategies. *Treatments in Endocrinology, 2*(2), 95–108.

Valencia, M. E., Bennett, P. H., Ravussin, E., Esparza, J., Fox, C., & Schulz, L. O. (1999). The Pima Indians in Sonora, Mexico. *Nutrition Reviews, 57*(5, Part 2), S55–S57; discussion S57–S58.

Van den Berghe, G., & Bouillon, R. (2004). Optimal control of glycemia among critically ill patients. *Journal of the American Medical Association, 291*(10), 1198–1199.

Velho, G., & Robert, J. J. (2002). Maturity-onset diabetes of the young (MODY): Genetic and clinical characteristics. *Hormone Research, 57*(Suppl. 1), 29–33.

Wild, S., Roglic, G., Green, A., Sicree, R., & King, H. (2004). Global prevalence of diabetes: Estimates for the year 2000 and projections for 2030. *Diabetes Care, 27*(5), 1047–1053.

Yeh, G. Y., Eisenberg, D. M., Kaptchuk, T. J., & Phillips, R. S. (2003). Systematic review of herbs and dietary supplements for glycemic control in diabetes. *Diabetes Care, 26*(4), 1277–1294.

Young, R. S., & Rosenbloom, A. L. (1998). type 2 (non-insulin dependent) diabetes in minority youth: Conference report. *Clinical Pediatrics (Philadelphia), 37*(2), 63–65.

Zinman, B., Ruderman, N., Campaigne, B. N., Devlin, J. T., & Schneider, S. H. (2004). Physical activity/exercise and diabetes. *Diabetes Care, 27*(Suppl. 1), S58–S62.

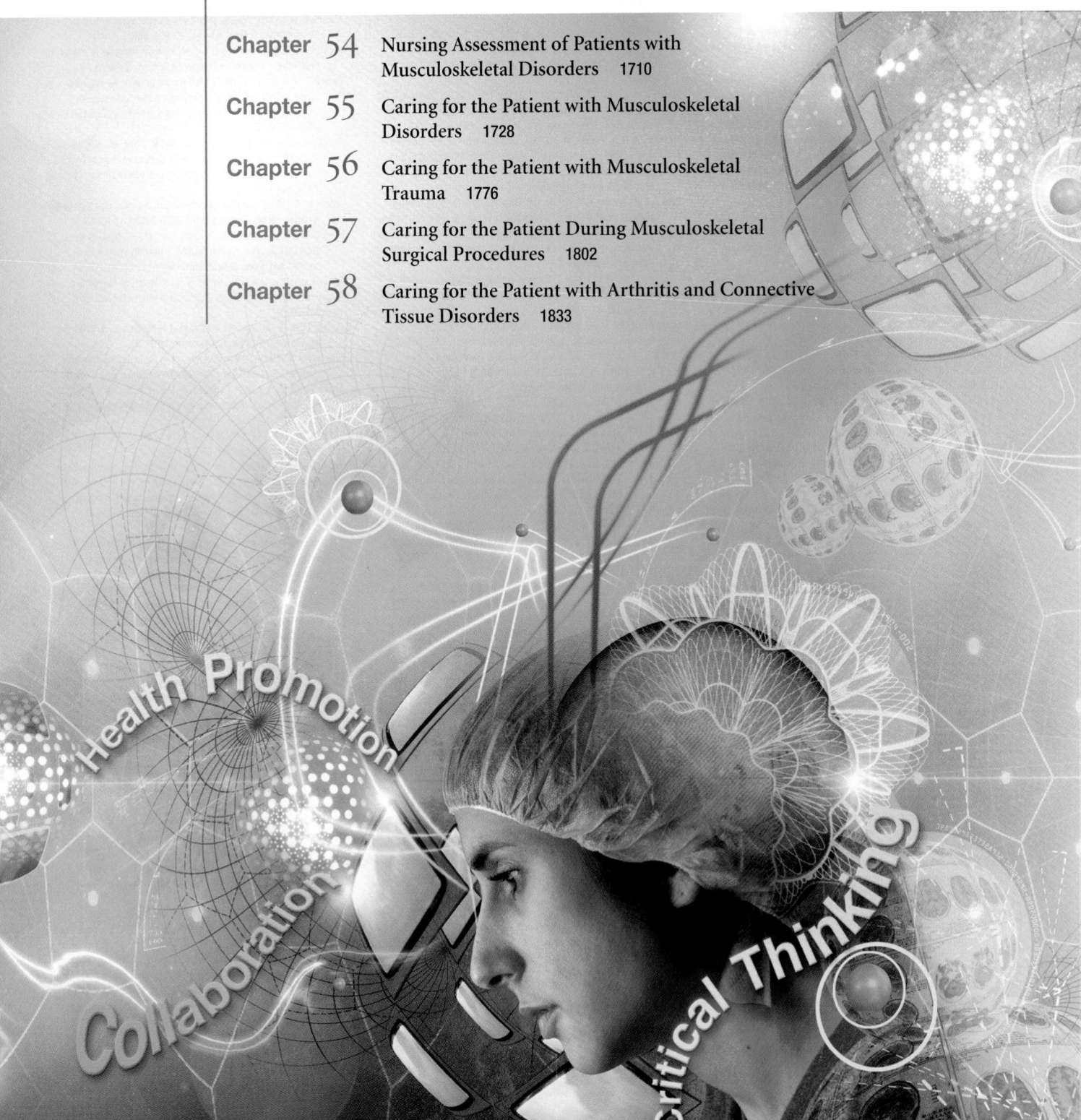

UNIT 12

Nursing Management of Patients with Musculoskeletal Disorders

Health Promotion

Collaboration

Critical Thinking

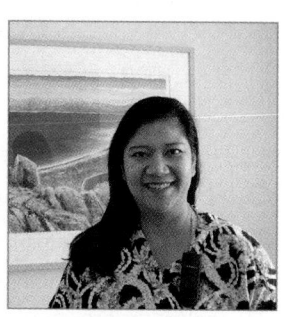

MELISA My name is Melisa Agustin Jager and I am a clinical resource nurse for a 36-bed orthopedic unit at a Level 1 trauma center that facilitates care to patients in the quickly growing area of Northern California. The orthopedic unit population encompasses the range of orthopedic/trauma practice. The orthopedic nursing staff provides wide-ranging types of care to patients having routine and scheduled orthopedic knee, hip, and spine surgeries to the traumatic injuries, including multiple fractures, sustained from motor vehicle crashes.

As a clinical resource nurse on the unit, I engage in a multitude of key practices including these: assisting with the implementation of quality assurance and problem-solving techniques to help employees meet their professional goals; providing methodology for the technological advances and equipment we use during our daily orthopedic practices, including devices to improve range of motion and the intricacy of fixators and tractions; arranging routine in-service programs for staff that will impart shared knowledge so staff can keep up with the ever-changing dynamics of medicine; and encouraging collaborative care by achieving interpersonal communication with ancillary staff such as the physical/occupational therapist in order to receive guidance regarding safe mobility transfers and developing a plan with the pain pharmacist for the orthopedic patient to achieve comfort during his hospital stay.

A day in the life of an orthopedic nurse has the instrumental characteristics of caring. **Compassion** should be common practice in your nursing care. One example is to speak to patients with soft and empathetic tones—as you would speak to a loved one. Compassionate nursing goes beyond the mere implementation of medical techniques/practices; it involves providing a positive, interactive environment in which rapport and trust develop between nurse and patient. Particularly in orthopedic nursing, the patient who is immobile and not able to care for herself often looks to the nurses for strength and hope.

Resource nurses are leaders who have had significant experience and **competence** in the implementation of orthopedic procedures. Being competent when providing direct care for a patient with posterior hip precautions is distinctly different than anterior precautions to prevent dislodging the hip. Often as a resource nurse, I act as a mentor for less experienced nurses by demonstrating the appropriate techniques involved in caring for patients with specialized needs.

As a resource nurse it is important for me to show **confidence** when speaking with patients and their families. Patients and their families trust a confident/assertive nurse rather than a nurse who cannot articulate a clear plan of care or is not able to explain a procedure effectively.

When caring for a patient, if something is not ethically right, I act with **conscience** and provide tactful advocacy. I facilitate calling a care conference with the health care team, ancillary staff, and family. With long-term patients on the orthopedic unit in particular, a conference facilitates updating the plan of care and provides optimal health services. Our population is culturally diverse so it is important to be culturally sensitive and acknowledge the patient's beliefs.

It is important for me to show pride and **commitment** to my profession. I demonstrate my commitment with a positive attitude when stress is high on the unit. It is important to boost morale and commitment to team building when another person exhibits toxic behavior. On the orthopedic unit critical thinking skills are life-saving attributes. If a nurse on our unit does not recognize the signs and symptoms of compartment syndrome, the patient is at great risk of loss of circulation to that limb, leading to amputation.

At this hospital, the hallmark is its teaching environment. Clinical resource nurses are motivated to instill proactiveness and commitment and to develop a sense of autonomy in order to achieve a higher standard of proficiencies among the employees and most importantly to incorporate excellence in patient care.

> "Compassionate nursing goes beyond the mere implementation of medical techniques/practices; it involves providing a positive, interactive environment in which rapport and trust develop between nurse and patient."

Nursing Assessment of Patients with Musculoskeletal Disorders

Helene Harris

Outcome-Based Learning Objectives

After studying this chapter, the learner will be able to:

1. Identify basic anatomy and physiology of the musculoskeletal system.

2. Analyze the process of obtaining a history on the musculoskeletal system.

3. Identify the general guidelines required for a musculoskeletal examination.

4. Identify the process of assessment of the following structures: temporomandibular joint, shoulders, elbows, wrists, hands, fingers, neck, spine, hips, knees, ankles, and feet, as well as assessment of gait.

5. Compare and contrast normal and abnormal findings associated with the temporomandibular joint, shoulders, elbows, wrists, hands, fingers, neck, spine, hips, knees, ankles, feet, and gait.

6. Compare and contrast the normal and abnormal range of motion for the temporomandibular joint, shoulders, elbows, wrists, hands, fingers, neck, spine, hips, knees, ankles, feet, and gait.

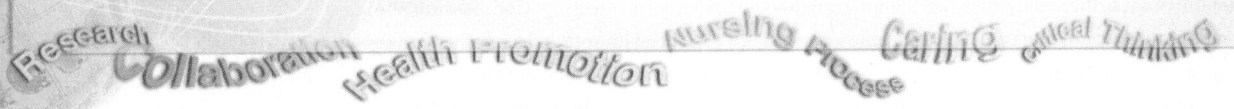

THE MUSCULOSKELETAL system is composed of bones, joints, ligaments, tendons, and cartilage. Each one of these parts plays a key role in the maintenance of a healthy, functioning system. The musculoskeletal system plays a definitive role in determining a person's quality of life because it not only allows movement but also protects inner organs, produces red blood cells, and supports the body.

People in every age group at some time in their lives may be afflicted with either temporary or permanent disabilities related to musculoskeletal problems. Injuries can occur in all stages of life, but children are particularly prone to accidents, and the elderly are inclined to succumb to falls and subsequent fractures. In a study by Lillicrap, Byrne, and Speed (2003), it was noted that out of 100 patients hospitalized for reasons other than orthopedic problems, 63% of them had some degree of musculoskeletal dysfunction.

▓ Anatomy and Physiology of the Musculoskeletal System

Because of the importance of the musculoskeletal system, and the number of patients with primary or secondary orthopedic problems, it is imperative for the nurse to understand how to conduct a musculoskeletal assessment. Each component of the musculoskeletal system must undergo a thorough and systematic evalua-

tion to identify abnormalities so that they can be treated or so further problems can be prevented.

Bones

Bones are composed of collagen fibers, which, in turn, are made up of calcium and phosphate. The human skeleton is constructed of 206 separate bones that have the ability to change structure according to their current function. The skeletal system develops from the middle layer of embryonic tissue. Development begins at approximately the fourth week in the embryo and continues to grow during the first two decades of life. Bones also have the ability to repair themselves after injury through a process of resorption and regeneration. The process involves formation of a hematoma that provides the basis for blood vessel and fibroblast infiltration, proliferation of osteoblasts, callus formation, ossification of the callus, and remodeling of the fracture site. The bone is made up of osteoblasts, which are cells that form the bone itself, and osteoclasts, which are cells that reabsorb bone during repair, for instance, of a fracture (Porth, 2007).

Bones in the human body can be classified into three types: (1) long bones, which have a tubular shaft and articular surfaces, or surfaces that form a joint, at each end; (2) flat bones, which are thin with broad surfaces; and (3) short or irregular bones that vary in size and shape (Bickley, 2003). Chart 54–1 provides examples of the three types of bones.

The functions of bone are many: They provide support for the body; protect internal organs from injury; store calcium, phosphorus, and other minerals; provide for movement in conjunction with muscles; and, in long bones, produce red and white blood cells (Porth, 2007).

Muscles

Muscles are contractile tissues that are attached by tendons to bone and other body parts. They are found in three types throughout the body.

Smooth muscle is stimulated by the autonomic nervous system, meaning it is not under voluntary, or conscious, control. Smooth muscle is found in the skin, internal organs, reproductive system, major blood vessels, and the excretory system. These muscles contract when needed to perform the function of the particular organ system, such as peristalsis. Skeletal, or striated, muscles are called voluntary muscles because they are under conscious control and are supplied with nerves from the central nervous system.

Skeletal muscles are connected to bones via tendons. The skeletal muscles, together with the bones they attach to, allow the body to move, such as in walking or picking objects up with the fingers.

Cardiac muscle, comprising most of the heart, is under autonomic system control and not voluntary control. Like the skeletal muscle, cardiac muscle is striated and contains actin and myosin filaments. The filaments are smaller and more compact than skeletal muscle cells and contain many large mitochondria due to the continuous energy needs. The contractions of the cardiac muscle provide the heartbeat and the pumping of blood through the heart (Porth, 2007).

Cartilage

Cartilage is an elastic, flexible connective tissue. The main function of cartilage is as a "cushioner." It covers the surfaces of joints, protecting them when sliding or moving over one another and thus preventing damage and friction to the joints. For instance, costal cartilages join the ribs to the sternum and vertebrae. The articular cartilages, such as those in the shoulder or hip joint, protect the bone ends and allow easy movement of the joint. Once damaged, cartilage cannot be repaired (Weber & Kelley, 2007).

Ligaments

Ligaments play a crucial role in the function of the skeletal joints in that they bind the ends of different bones together, preventing **dislocations** (displacement of a bone from its normal position). An example is the knee joint connecting the femur with the patella, tibia, and fibula (Bickley, 2003) (Figure 54–1 ■).

Tendons

Tendons connect muscle to bone. The dense tissue is composed largely of intercellular bundles of collagen fibers arranged in the same direction. This provides great tensile strength and can withstand tremendous pull in the direction of fiber alignment. If the musculotendinous unit is stretched to injury, it is called a strain. The most common sites for strains are the lower back and the cervical area of the spine (Porth, 2007).

Joints

A joint is where two or more bones meet or come together. Joints are responsible for a person's **range of motion (ROM)**, or extent and type of movement. In assessing joints it is important to understand and differentiate between three different mechanical configurations of joints: spheroidal joints, hinge joints, and condylar joints. *Spheroidal joints* are located in the shoulders and hip. They have a ball-and-socket contour, which allows for a broad range of motion—not just in a back-and-forth direction, but also swiveling actions. *Hinge* joints are flat and slightly curved. The hinge joint allows movement in only one axis, namely, flexion and extension, as in the elbow. Examples of *condylar joints* include the knee, where the articulating ends of the bones are not connected directly but are linked by a strong fibrous capsule that surrounds the joint and is continuous with the periosteum. There is also additional support from ligaments that extend between the bones of the joint (Bickley, 2003; Weber & Kelley, 2007). Figure 54–2 ■ (p. 1712) illustrates the three

CHART 54–1	**Types of Bones**	
Long Bones	**Flat Bones**	**Short/Irregular Bones**
Femur	Ribs	Vertebral column
Tibia	Scapula	Carpal
Fibula	Sternum	Tarsal
Humerus	Ilium	
Radius		
Ulna		
Clavicle		
Metacarpals		
Metatarsals		
Phalanges		

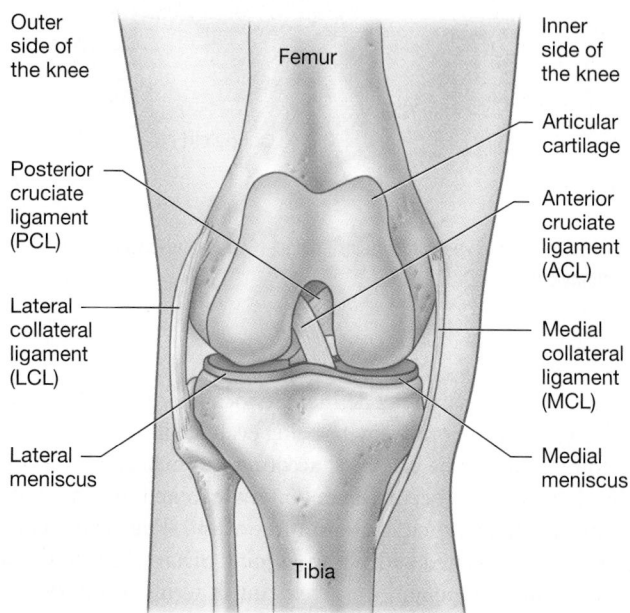

FIGURE 54–1 ■ Ligaments of the knee joint.

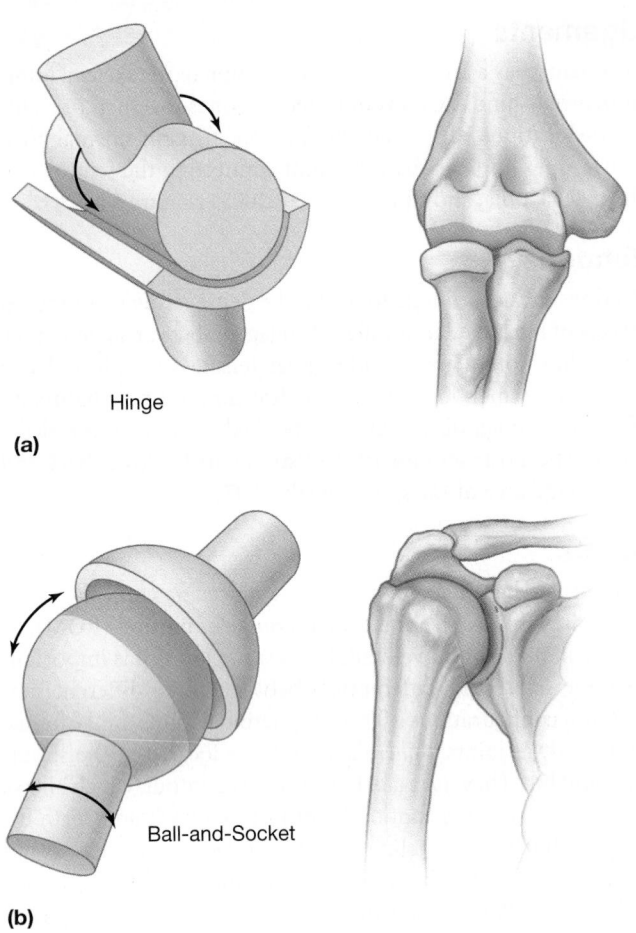

(a) Hinge

(b) Ball-and-Socket

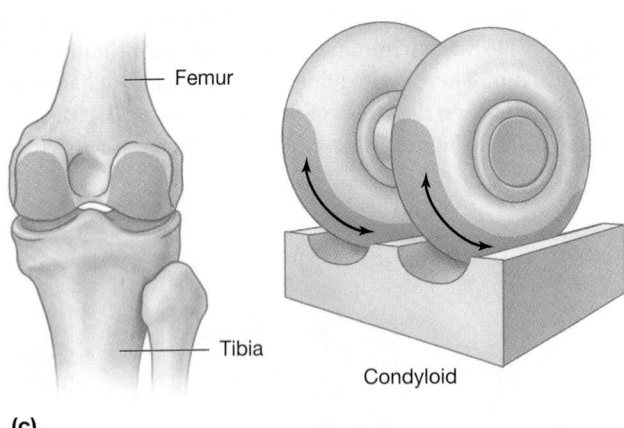

Femur

Tibia

Condyloid

(c)

FIGURE 54–2 ■ Types of joints: (A) hinge; (B) ball-and-socket; (C) condyloid.

CHART 54–2	**Vocabulary of Range of Motion**
Abduction	Moving an extremity away from the midline of the body
Adduction	Moving an extremity toward the midline of the body
Circumduction	Moving an extremity in a circular motion
Extension	Straightening the extremity of a joint; increasing the angle of the joint
Hyperextension	Moving a joint beyond its normal range
Flexion	Bending an extremity at a joint; decreases the angle of the joint
Eversion	Moving the foot outward
Inversion	Moving the foot inward
Pronation	Facing downward
Supination	Facing upward
Plantar flexion	Placing the foot downward
Dorsal flexion	Placing the foot upward
External rotation	Turning away from the midline of the body
Internal rotation	Turning toward the midline of the body

Sources: Adapted from Kozier, B., Erb, C., Berman, A., & Snyder, S. (2008). *Fundamentals of nursing. Concepts, process and practice* (8th ed.). Upper Saddle River, NJ: Pearson Prentice Hall; Magee, D. (2008). *Orthopedic physical assessment* (5th ed.). Elsevier; Weber, J., & Kelley, J. (2007). *Health assessment in nursing* (3rd ed.). Philadelphia: Lippincott Williams & Wilkins.

slide over one another, such as the knee. The bone surfaces of these joints are covered with cartilage, which allows the two bones to slide over one another and be freely movable. The bones of the joint are separated by a synovial capsule, which surrounds the joint and secretes synovial fluid, a lubricant that also promotes the sliding movement of the bones.

A further aid to movement in the synovial joints is the **bursae** (sacs containing viscous lubricating fluid; singular, *bursa*), which lie between the skin and surface of the bone or joint, contain synovial fluid, and are located in areas where tendons, muscles, and bones have the tendency to rub against one another, such as the acromion process in the shoulder, wrists, knees, hips, and ankles. *Cartilaginous joints* are only slightly movable and are located between the vertebrae and the symphysis pubis. They are separated by a fibrous disk and joined by interosseous ligaments (Bickley, 2003; Weber & Kelley, 2007).

■ History

The nursing assessment of a patient presenting with a musculoskeletal complaint should start with a thorough history and physical assessment of the musculoskeletal system. A detailed history of the system is vital in determining a patient's ability to function and perform activities of daily living (ADLs). In turn, this determination plays an important role in developing an effective plan of care, because disabilities related to musculoskeletal disorders can affect every aspect of a patient's life.

In gathering subjective data, the nurse should ask the patient a series of open-ended questions regarding past and present mus-

types of joints. Chart 54–2 defines the vocabulary used when describing the type of movement being evaluated.

Joints can also be classified according to material composition. *Fibrous joints* occur where bones are joined together with connective tissue, such as the sutures of the skull. There is no movement associated with a fibrous joint. *Synovial joints* are the most common type and most relevant in terms of injury and loss of range of motion. The synovial joints are the joints between bones that do not come in contact with one another but

culoskeletal illnesses, injuries, related diagnostic procedures, surgeries, and treatments. The questioning should start with the chief complaint, or the symptom or condition that has compelled the patient to seek medical care. These questions should be formulated to allow the patient to describe her own impressions of the condition. Next, the past medical history of the patient is important because previous musculoskeletal injuries or disorders can have lingering effects on the neurological system, leading to new conditions. Chronic health conditions can also have a profound effect on the musculoskeletal system, and questions that reveal these disorders will help in the diagnosis of the presenting symptom. Social history and psychosocial history add to the fullness of the patient's medical history by revealing lifestyle habits, such as smoking or level of exercise, and coping mechanisms that can be important both in diagnosis and in treatment of the condition.

History taking is an important part of assessment. During this time the nurse establishes a caring relationship with the patient. It is important to let the patient describe his issues in his own words. Keep an open mind and listen carefully as this information will direct your clarifying questions.

Biographical and Demographic History

Biographical data should include age, gender, culture, and educational background. This information will assist the nurse in narrowing the questions, thinking of potential causes of the problem, and formulating how to pose questions and educational plans to meet the patient's needs. Demographic data may be helpful in determining causes of injury. For instance, if the patient has a job where she is sitting and typing on a computer all day, she may complain of back and neck pain from sitting in a chair that does not support her back, or pain in the joints of the hand, wrist, or arm from the repetitive motion during typing or improper height of the desk placing strain on the joints.

Cultural Considerations

It is important to take into consideration the patient's cultural background and conversational norms. Refer to Chapter 9 ∞ for a more detailed discussion on cultural norms. Ask the patient if he has used any healing herbs or other alternative treatments such as acupuncture.

Chief Complaint

Characteristics, length of duration, exacerbation or diminishment of symptoms, and what is wrong or feared by the patient helps to define the chief complaint. Ask the patient open-ended questions. Allow her time to answer fully, giving encouragement with nonverbal cues such as nodding your head. Clarifying questions that may be useful include the following:

- What brings you to the facility/office/hospital today?
- How long have you had this symptom?
- When did it start?
- What have you done to alleviate it?
- What makes it better? What makes it worse?
- How has it affected your lifestyle?
- Has the symptom gotten worse since it first started? In what way has it gotten worse? When did it get worse? Did anything precipitate it getting worse? If so, what?

- Is pain associated with the symptom? If the patient answers "yes," ask this follow-up question: Are you experiencing any pain associated with the symptom?
- Where is the pain?
- Does it radiate anywhere?
- How long does it last?
- Have you taken any medication for the pain? What have you taken? How much? How often? Does the medication alleviate the pain? Does it reduce the intensity of the pain?
- How does the pain affect your daily lifestyle?
- What other treatments besides pain medication have you used?
- Do you have any other symptoms? Swelling? Can you describe the type of weakness?

Past Medical History

When obtaining a past medical history, the patient may be asked the following questions:

- Have you had any past surgeries? Where? When? For what reason?
- Do you have any permanent problems associated with past injuries or surgeries?
- Do you know if you have any other health problems that may affect medication therapy, or, due to respiratory problems or fatigue, inhibit ambulation or performance of ADLs ?
- Do you have diabetes? Sickle cell anemia? Systemic lupus erythematosus (SLE)? These are important questions because diabetes can cause neuropathies that can affect ambulation, and sickle cell anemia and SLE can lead to osteoporosis and osteomyelitis (Weber & Kelley, 2007).
- Does anyone in your family have rheumatoid arthritis or osteoporosis? These diseases tend to be hereditary and may predispose a patient to these conditions (Weber & Kelley, 2007).
- Have you had a tetanus or polio vaccine recently? Recent tetanus and polio vaccines may cause joint stiffness. If the patient has never had a polio vaccination, ask if he has traveled to a third world country recently; if so, the patient may have contracted the disease at that time.
- What medications do you take regularly? Include all over-the-counter (OTC) medications.
- Do you have any allergies? If so, to what? (Be specific: medications, environmental.)
- *If the patient is female:* Have you started menopause? Are you on hormone replacement therapy? The lack of estrogen in a menopausal woman can lead to osteoporosis.

A social history provides additional information about the patient's lifestyle that may affect the potential disorder or complaint. The nurse should consider the following questions:

- Do you smoke? If so, how much and how often? Smoking raises the risk of osteoporosis.
- Do you drink alcohol? If so, how much? Excessive alcohol intake raises the risk of osteoporosis.

- Do you have a regular exercise regime? Can you describe it? Do you engage in exercise outside of a routine? How often? What type of exercise?

- Please describe your occupation. Does it involve heavy lifting, pushing, or pulling, or do you sit at a desk all day? Heavy strenuous activities may precipitate back problems, while sitting may lead to posture anomalies, which can lead to other problems such as respiratory disorders.

- Do you use an **assistive device** such as a cane, walker, or brace? If so, which do you use? Why?

- Does your musculoskeletal problem affect your lifestyle or activities of daily living? How?

The nurse should ask the patient how she copes with the injury or illness and whether the illness/injury affects family and personal relationships. Observe the patient's nonverbal cues, note whether the patient appears depressed, angry, or anxious when the history is taken.

■ Physical Examination

In the physical examination, the nurse uses inspection and palpation to collect objective data. These data are then recorded and made available to the health care team. A full musculoskeletal exam will take time; document findings during the exam for accuracy.

General Guidelines for Musculoskeletal Assessment

General guidelines for conducting a musculoskeletal assessment are as follows:

- Inspect for deformities.
- Inspect and palpate any swelling.
- Feel the area for increased temperature and observe for redness.
- Palpate for tenderness around a joint.
- Assess for range of motion.

 **CRITICAL ALERT** *Do not force a body part past its normal range. Discontinue ROM when the patient complains of pain or discomfort.*

Inspection

Abnormal appearance of a joint may be due to a musculoskeletal or neuromuscular disease, dislocation, tumor, mass, degenerative change, contracture, or atrophy of the muscle. When inspecting compare corresponding paired joints for symmetry. The nurse observes for skin color, scars, shape of the site, deformities, **muscle atrophy** (shortening of a muscle), masses, or swelling. Also inspect for **fasciculations** (an abnormal contraction or shortening of a bundle of muscle fibers) and **tremors** (an involuntary movement of a body part), which can be related to neuromuscular disorders.

Swelling may be due to an inflammation of the joint (reaction of tissue to irritation, injury, or infection), intra-articular swelling or effusion (escape of fluid into the tissue), a swollen bursa, synovial membrane thickening, or a bony overgrowth. A "boggy" feeling over an edematous area may indicate an edematous synovial membrane, which can be indicative of a soft tissue injury (Magee, 2008). If there is swelling, the nurse should note the size and shape of the edematous area, the site, and signs of inflammation such as redness. When inspecting a joint, observe for alignment.

Palpation

The nurse will feel the skin at the site with the back of his fingers to assess the skin's temperature. Note whether the skin is hot, warm, cool, or cold to the touch. Heat and redness over a joint may be indicative of inflammation or a septic joint (infection of a joint). Cold or cool temperatures may indicate a circulation problem (Weber & Kelley, 2007). The nurse will feel for skin texture, dryness, or moisture. Excessive dryness may indicate an acute, **gouty joint** (inflammation of a big toe, heels, elbows, ankles, dorsum), whereas moisture is often associated with a septic joint (Magee, 2008).

Palpate the muscles surrounding the joint and bony articulations. Note any tenderness, swelling, or masses. A normal joint is not tender to palpation. The patient should be asked if the palpation causes any tenderness or pain. Tenderness around a joint may be due to arthritis, a septic joint, inflammation, bursitis, or osteomyelitis (Weber & Kelley, 2007).

Palpate for **nodules** (small raised areas) that may not be visible. While palpating inquire about any numbness, tingling, or weakness in the area.

Range of Motion

Range of motion may be decreased due to pain, muscle spasms, weakness, and atrophy. Decreased ROM occurs in joints where there is inflammation, arthritis, lack of use, dislocation, masses, or pain.

The nurse can test the ROM of all joints by asking the patient to actively move the joints one at a time. Compare each joint for flexibility and mobility, and assess the patient's ability to move the joint through its normal full range of motion. Familiarize yourself with the normal ROM for each type of joint so you will recognize a limitation.

 **CRITICAL ALERT** *When assessing joints, muscles, and movements, always assess on both sides of the body for purposes of comparison.*

A **goniometer** measures the angle of the joint in degrees, and can assist in the assessment of ROM of a joint (Figure 54–3 ■).

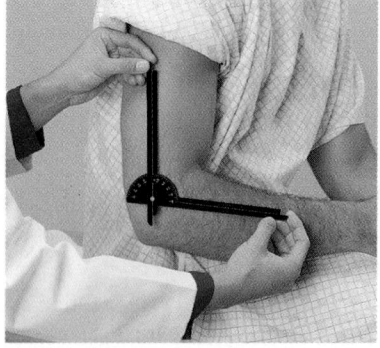

FIGURE 54–3 ■ Goniometer.

To measure the joint angle, place the goniometer exactly at the angle of the joint. The nurse will document, for example, "the right knee flexes from 20–60 degrees." This is important in describing the degree of decreased ROM from normal and also provides a baseline for future measurement (Magee, 2008).

Testing Muscle Strength

Muscle strength is measured by placing your hand firmly against the body part in question and asking the patient to push hard against your hand. Perform the test on both sides and compare your findings, knowing that the dominant side of the body will be stronger. For example, if the nurse is testing the trapezius muscle in the shoulders, she will place her hand against the patient's shoulder and push to allow resistance for the patient and then ask the patient to push against her hand. The nurse will then document the strength of the patient's ability to push by describing the strength as *normal, slightly weak, weak,* or *severely weak* or by recording that the patient was unable to push at all. Chart 54–3 describes a grading system for the documentation of muscle strength.

■ Head-to-Toe Musculoskeletal Assessment

It is important to be methodical when assessing the musculoskeletal system so as not to miss any abnormalities.

Temporomandibular Joint

The temporomandibular joint (TMJ) is the hinge of the jaw. It is located anterior to the external ear and is constantly opening and closing when a patient talks, eats, chews, and yawns (Bickley, 2003). To examine the TMJ, have the patient in a sitting position. Examination includes inspection and palpation. To assess the TMJ, the nurse should place his index and middle fingers anterior to the external ear, just in front of the tragus. The patient is asked to open her mouth as wide as possible. At this time the nurse's fingers should slide into the "groove" or joint space. The nurse moves the patient's jaw back and forth, palpating for masses or nodules. The nurse also inspects the area for redness and swelling indicating inflammation.

CHART 54–3	Muscle Strength Grading	
Functional Level		**Grade**
No evidence of contractibility (inability to contract muscles)—paralysis		0
Slight contractibility—severe weakness		1
ROM without gravity—passive ROM performed by examiner		2
Active ROM with gravity—moderate weakness		3
Complete active ROM against gravity with some resistance—minimal weakness		4
Complete ROM against gravity with resistance—normal		5

Source: Adapted from Bickley, L. (2003). *Bates' guide to physical assessment and history taking* (8th ed.). Philadelphia: Lippincott; Kozier, B., Erb, C., Berman, A., & Snyder, S. (2008). *Fundamentals of nursing. Concepts, process and practice* (7th ed.). Upper Saddle River, NJ: Pearson Prentice Hall; Weber, J., & Kelley, J. (2007). *Health assessment in nursing* (3rd ed.). Philadelphia: Lippincott Williams & Wilkins.

The patient is then asked to open and close the mouth. While the patient does this, the nurse notes the range of motion and questions the patient as to any tenderness. The nurse also listens for any "clicking" sounds. Soft clicking sounds without any complaints of discomfort or ROM difficulty may not be indicative of any problems; however, if the clicking sounds are hard or grating, accompanied by pain or discomfort, and are affecting range of motion, this can be indicative of arthritic changes or a possible dislocation (Magee, 2008).

Normal Findings

- Patient is able to open and close the mouth without difficulty about 2.5 to 5 cm (1 to 2 in.).
- Jaw moves laterally without pain or tenderness.
- Some clicking may be heard and felt during movement.

(Weber & Kelley, 2007).

Abnormal Findings

- Unable to open mouth 2.5 to 5 cm (1 to 2 in.).
- A grating, clicking, or popping sound is noted with a TMJ problem, possibly a dislocation.
- Patient complains of pain, tenderness with opening and closing of the mouth, which may indicate arthritis.
- Masses, nodules felt during palpation.
- Inability to hold mouth open.
- Decreased muscle strength.

Shoulders

The shoulder is composed of the clavicle, acromion process, and the humerus and is able to move in many directions due to various joints, bones, and muscle groups called the shoulder girdle. The clavicle and acromion process are responsible for the stability of the shoulder girdle.

The nurse will need to inspect the shoulders **anteriorly** (the front plane of the body) and **posteriorly** (the back plane of the body). Observe for any swelling, change in skin color, deformity, atrophy, fasciculations, and **asymmetry** (unequal in size and proportion). Patients with scoliosis may have one shoulder higher than the other, causing asymmetry. Inspect for swelling or redness over the joint capsule anteriorly or a bulge under the deltoid, which may be indicative of a problem in the bursa (Bickley, 2003).

Assess range of motion to include **abduction** (away from the midline of the body—in this case, raising the arm away from the body), **adduction** (moving toward the midline of the body—in this case, moving the arm across the front of the body), flexion, extension, hyperextension, internal rotation, and external rotation. Explain to the patient that you will be testing the range of motion of the shoulders and will ask them to perform seven movements (Figure 54–4 ■, p. 1716).

1. Begin by having the patient stand straight with arms at the sides. Observe the area for symmetry.

2. To test for abduction, ask the patient to raise the arms to shoulder level.

3. To test for adduction, ask the patient to raise the arms above the head with the palms facing each other.

4. To test for flexion and extension, ask the patient to bend and straighten out the elbows.

5. To test for external rotation, ask the patient to place both hands behind the neck with elbows out to the side.

6. To test for internal rotation, ask the patient to place the hands behind the lower back.

7. Ask the patient to clasp his hands and bring them around the lower back as far as he can.

Normal Findings

The patient should be able to:

- Raise the arms 90 degrees to the shoulder level.

- Flex arms to 180 degrees and fully extend the arms.

- Hyperextend arms behind the back 50 degrees.

- Place hands behind the neck and lower back at 90 degrees without crepitus, pain, or decreased ROM.

- Shrug shoulders against resistance.

(Weber & Kelley, 2007)

Abnormal Findings

- Pain and decreased ROM are associated with rotator cuff tears, tendonitis, sprains, and bursitis.

- Decreased ability to shrug shoulders or inability to shrug shoulders against resistance may indicate a lesion of cranial nerve XI.

- Weakness in performance of ROM exercises indicates joint disease or muscle disuse.

- Shoulders that are flat or asymmetrical may be dislocated.

- Any redness, heat, or swelling may be associated with sprains, strains, degenerative joint disease, and arthritis.

- Atrophy is associated with nerve damage or disuse.

(Bickley, 2003; Magee, 2008; Weber & Kelley, 2007)

While the patient is performing these tasks, palpate the joints for **crepitus** (grating produced by bone rubbing against bone), and question the patient regarding any associated pain (Jarvis, 2008; Magee, 2008; Weber & Kelley, 2007).

To test the muscle strength of the shoulders, the nurse asks the patient to perform a number of movements and exercises. To assess the deltoid muscle, the patient should hold her arms upward while you try to push them down. To assess the biceps, the patient should flex the arm while you try to extend it. To assess the triceps, the patient should extend the arm while you try to flex it. Finally, to assess the trapezius muscle, the patient should shrug her shoulders while you try to hold the shoulders down (Bickley, 2003; Weber & Kelley, 2007).

Normal Findings with Muscle Grading

- Muscle strength of 3 or greater.

- Muscle strength greater in dominant side.

- Coordinated and painless movements.

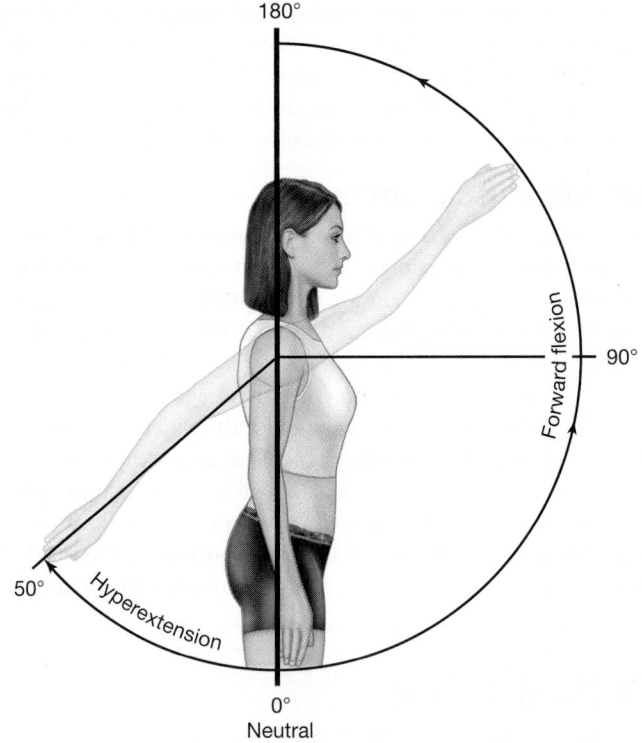

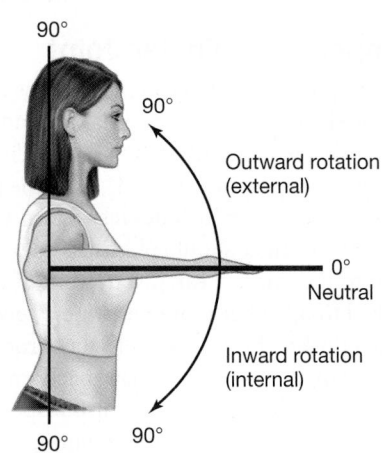

FIGURE 54–4 ■ Shoulder ROM.

Abnormal Findings

- Muscle strength is less than 3.

- Patient is unable to push against resistance.

- Assistance is required to perform exam.

 CRITICAL ALERT *Some patients who complain of shoulder pain can be experiencing or possibly already have had a cardiac event. Further assessment is required.*

Elbows

The elbow is a complex joint where the humerus, radius, and ulna come together and are enclosed in a synovial capsule. The elbow can move in extension and flexion, using the joint of the humerus and ulna (humeroulnar joint), and in pronation (palm downward) and supination (palm upward), using the radius. The ulnar nerve passes through the elbow, around the medial epicondyle of the humerus (Bickley, 2003).

During inspection it is best to support the patient's arm with your nonexamining hand. Flex the patient's elbow to approximately 70 degrees. This prevents the patient's muscles from tightening during the examination. Inspect the elbow for shape, deformities, size, redness, swelling, nodules, and bulging. With the tips of your middle fingers and thumb, palpate the olecranon process, epicondyles, and the grooves on either side of the olecranon process. Assess for heat, swelling, tenderness, and nodules (Bickley, 2003; Weber & Kelley, 2007).

To test for range of motion, ask the patient to flex the elbow and bring the hand to the forehead, then extend or straighten the elbow (Figure 54–5 ■). Note any deviations in the angle or deformities. Ask the patient to hold the arm out and supinate (turn the palms up) and pronate (turn the palms down). Have the patient then flex and extend the arm with your resistance. Repeat flexion and extension with the patient supinating and pronating the palms. Assess for deformities, tenderness, swelling, and nodules (Bickley, 2003; Magee, 2008).

 *Never force a patient to perform ROM tests if the patient is unable or unwilling.*

Normal Findings

- The elbows are symmetrical without nodules, deformities, swelling, or redness.
- Patient is able to perform flexion, extension, supination, and pronation without evidence of swelling, tenderness, or any visible nodules.

Abnormal Findings

- Redness, swelling, deformity over the olecranon process may indicate injury, arthritis, or bursitis.
- Inability to perform range of motion without pain, swelling, deformity, or nodules needs further investigation. Nodules noted during ROM exercises may indicate rheumatoid arthritis (an autoimmune disease that causes inflammation to the joints) or rheumatic fever. Pain and tenderness on movement may indicate tennis elbow, which is due to overuse of the elbow.
- Deformity or displacement of the joint during palpation or range of motion may indicate a fracture (broken bone) or dislocation of the elbow.

Wrists

The wrist joint contains the articulation of the distal radius and double row of carpal bones intertwined to form a malleable hinge. The wrist is a condyloid articulation that allows 3 degrees of freedom. Its movements include flexion, extension, abduction, adduction, and circumduction (Figure 54–6 ■). The joint is surrounded by a capsule and strengthened by multiple ligaments.

The examination should start with the nurse inspecting and palpating the wrist. Inspect the wrist for symmetry, size, shape, deformities, nodules, and swelling. Palpate the wrist for nodules, movement, and tenderness by holding the patient's wrist between your two hands and palpating the lateral and medial surfaces, as well as the groove of each wrist joint with your thumbs.

Normal Findings

- The wrist is symmetrical, without any deformities, swelling, or nodules.

Abnormal Findings

- Swelling, tenderness, and nodules may indicate rheumatoid arthritis.
- Pain, tenderness, and a deformity may indicate an injury or trauma to the wrist.
- A round, painless, swollen, fluid-filled area may indicate a ganglion cyst.

(Jarvis, 2008; Weber & Kelley, 2007)

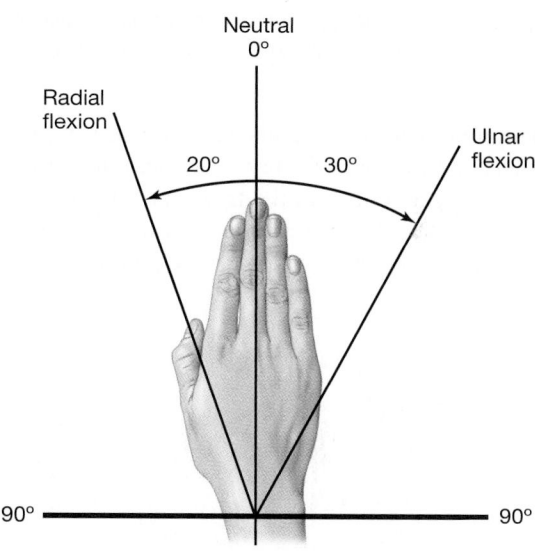

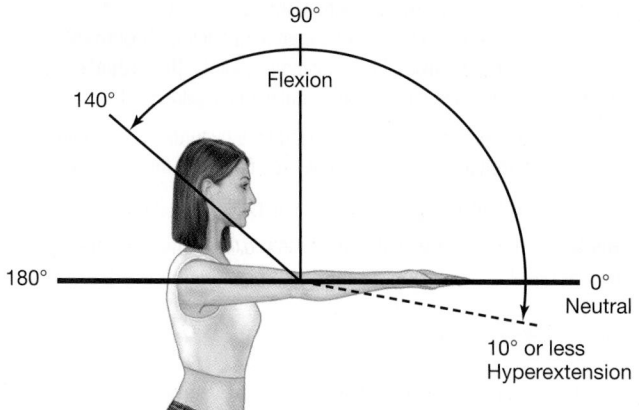

FIGURE 54–5 ■ Elbow ROM.

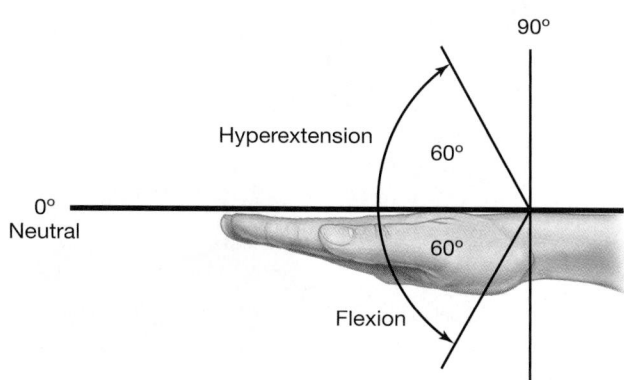

FIGURE 54–6 ■ Wrist ROM.

Next, the nurse should test the patient's range of motion in the wrist. To test for flexion and extension, ask the patient to bend the wrist back and forth. To test for ulnar or radial deviations, ask the patient to hold the wrist straight out in front of his body, with the palm downward, and move the hand inward toward and outward from the body. Finally, the nurse should palpate the anatomic snuffbox, just lateral to the thumb toward the middle of the hand.

Now repeat the exercises, but with resistance. The nurse should stabilize the patient's forearm on a table or hard surface, place the patient's wrist in extension, and then place her fingertips in the patient's palm. Ask the patient to flex the wrist against gravity. Stabilize the patient's forearm and ask the patient to flex the wrist. The nurse places her hand on the patient's dorsal metacarpals, just below the wrist, and asks the patient to extend the wrist against gravity.

Normal Findings

- Patient should have 90 degrees of flexion and the ability to hyperextend to 70 degrees without pain or swelling.
- Patient should be able to move the wrists laterally and medially.
- Patient should be able to have full range of motion against resistance (Magee, 2008).

Abnormal Findings

- Inability to perform full ROM needs further investigation. An example of a common abnormal condition of the wrist is carpal tunnel syndrome.

Carpal tunnel syndrome occurs when the median nerve is compressed as it travels with the flexor tendons through a canal made by the carpal bones and the transverse carpal ligament (Figure 54–7 ■). Carpal tunnel syndrome is caused by repetitive motion with the wrist flexed, such as with typing. Patients with carpal tunnel syndrome complain of numbness, tingling, and pain in the wrists and fingers.

To assess for carpal tunnel syndrome, the patient is asked to perform three tests:

1. **Thumb abduction**—Ask the patient to raise the thumb perpendicular to the palm. The nurse applies pressure to the distal phalanx. If the patient has difficulty performing this maneuver, the median nerve may be compressed.
2. **Tinel's sign**—With your finger, percuss lightly over the course of the medial nerve, located in the medial, inner aspect of the wrist.
3. **Phalen's test**—Ask the patient to place the back of each hand against one another while flexing the wrists 90 degrees for 60 seconds (Bickley, 2003; Magee, 2008; Weber & Kelley, 2007).

Abnormal findings include numbness, tingling, or pain at the wrist or fingers.

Hands and Fingers

The joints of the hands include the **metacarpophalangeal joint** (the joint between the metacarpal bones of the hand and the phalangeal bones of the fingers), the proximal interphalangeal joint and the distal **interphalangeal joint** (the joints between the phalanx bones of the fingers). Because there is very little protection to the bones in the fingers and hands, they are susceptible to trauma and disability. Inspection and palpation are the techniques used in examination of the hands and fingers (Bickley, 2003).

Inspect the palmar and dorsal surfaces of the hands and fingers for size, shape, deformity, color, swelling, nodules, and tenderness. Assess the fingers at rest and while in motion. Palpate the metacarpophalangeal joints at the distal fingers. Then palpate the proximal, middle, and distal interphalangeal joints using your thumb and index finger.

Normal Findings

- The fingers are in a straight line and symmetrical, without deformity, swelling, or nodules.
- Swelling, nodules, and complaints of tenderness are not noted on palpation.

Abnormal Findings

- Swelling of the phalanges, in addition to stiff tender fingers, may indicate acute rheumatoid arthritis.
- Hard, painless nodules at the joints of the fingers may indicate osteoarthritis (progressive loss of cartilage at a joint). **Bouchard's nodes** are found over the proximal interphalangeal joints. **Heberden's nodes** are seen over the distal interphalangeal joints (Figure 54–8 ■).
- "Swan neck" deformity is characterized by a hyperextension of the proximal interphalangeal joint with a fixed flexion of the distal joint.
- Swelling and thickening of the metacarpophalangeal joint.
- **Boutonniére deformity** is flexion of the proximal interphalangeal joint (Figure 54–9 ■).

(Bickley, 2003; Weber & Kelley, 2007)

Test range of motion of the fingers and hands. To test for abduction, ask the patient to extend and spread the fingers apart. To test for adduction, ask the patient to make a fist. To text for

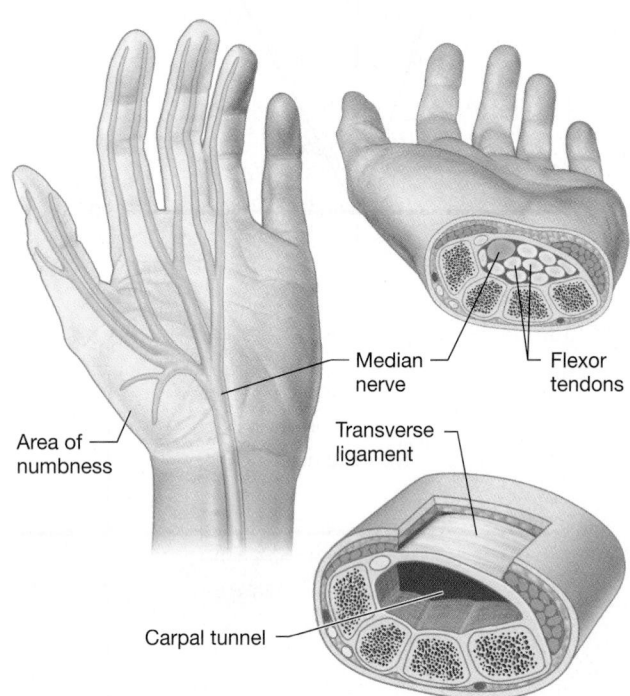

Median nerve

Flexor tendons

Area of numbness

Transverse ligament

Carpal tunnel

FIGURE 54–7 ■ Carpal tunnel.

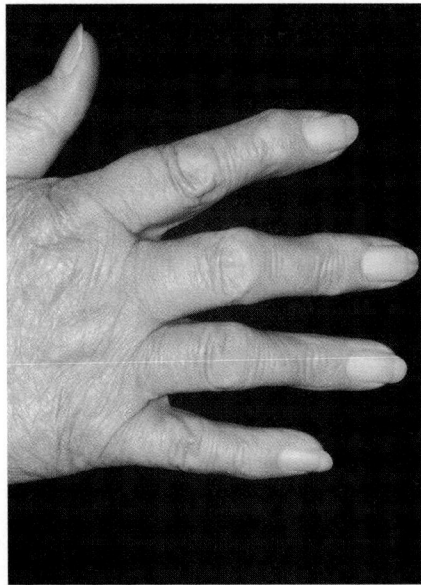

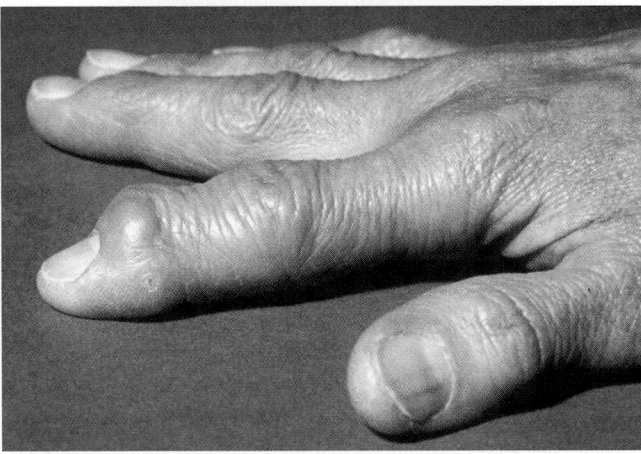

FIGURE 54–8 ■ Bouchard's nodes and Heberden's nodes.
Source: (top): © Pulse Picture Library/CMP Images/Phototake All rights reserved; (bottom): Bart's Medical Library/Phototake All rights reserved.

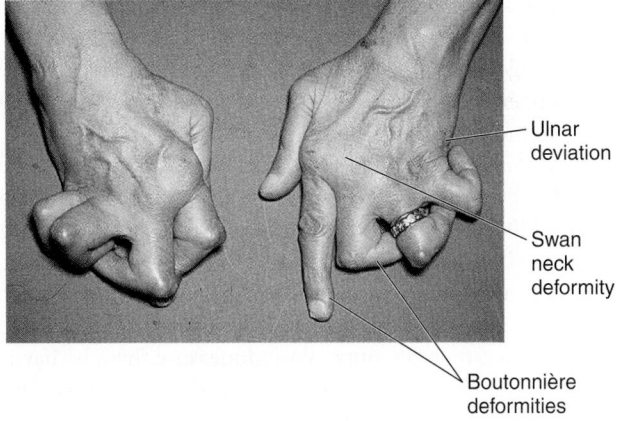

Ulnar deviation

Swan neck deformity

Boutonnière deformities

FIGURE 54–9 ■ Deformities of the hand.

flexion and hyperextension, ask the patient to bend the fingers down and then hold them up.

To test for flexion of the thumb, ask the patient to move the thumb across the palm and touch the fifth finger. To test for extension of the thumb, ask the patient to move the thumb across the palm away from the rest of the fingers. To test for abduction

and adduction of the thumb, ask the patient to move the thumb anteriorly away from the palm, then back. To test for opposition, or movement of the thumb across the palm, ask the patient to touch each of the fingertips with the thumb.

Normal Findings

- Patient is able to perform all ROM exercises without pain or swelling.
- The thumb should move to and away from the other fingers without difficulty.
- All fingers should abduct and adduct without pain and swelling.
- Hyperextension should occur without any difficulty at about 30 degrees.

Abnormal Findings

- Inability to perform any of the ROM tests without discomfort, swelling, and deformity needs further investigation.
- Difficulty or an inability to extend the ring or fifth finger is a sign of **Dupuytren's contracture**.
- Slight flexion of a finger, pain on extension, swelling, and tenderness may be indicative of acute **tenosynovitis**, an infection of the flexor tendon sheaths.

(Bickley, 2003; Weber & Kelley, 2007)

Neck and Spine

The spine or vertebral column is composed of alternating vertebrae and fibrocartilaginous disks that are connected by ligaments and supported by muscles that extend from the skull to the pelvis. This provides axial support to the body. The bony vertebra is composed of an anterior body and a posterior arch made up of two pedicles and two laminae that are united to form the spinous process. On either side of the arch is a transverse process and superior and inferior articular processes. The articular processes articulate with the adjacent vertebrae to form synovial joints. The articular processes account for the degree of flexion, extension, or rotation possible in each segment of the vertebral column. The transverse and spinous processes act as levers for the muscles attached to them.

As the spinal column progresses from the head, the vertebral body size increases. The intervertebral disks connecting the vertebral bodies act like shock absorbers for stresses applied to the vertebral column. There are four distinct curvatures to the vertebral column: (1) the cervical curve, which is concave; (2) the thoracic curve, which is convex; (3) the lumbar curve, which is concave; and (4) the sacral curve, which is convex (Bickley, 2003).

Examination of the spine includes inspection and palpation. Have the patient stand straight with arms at the sides and begin by examining the curvature of the cervical, thoracic, and lumbar areas from the right and left sides of the patient as well as behind the patient. Observe for differences in the height of the shoulders and iliac crests.

Palpate the spinous processes of each vertebra with the thumb, the paravertebral muscles on both sides of the spine and over the sacroiliac joint on the posterior superior iliac spines. If the patient complains of pain moving from the lower back down one or both legs, perform Lasègue's test: Have the patient in a relaxed, supine position. Ask the patient to raise the affected leg until pain is felt, then lower the leg until the pain is relieved; at this point the foot is dorsiflexed to reproduce the pain. Pain that shoots down one or both legs during dorsiflexion may indicate sciatic nerve involvement, a condition that may be caused by a herniated disk or pressure on the spinal cord (Magee, 2008; Weber & Kelley, 2007).

Normal Findings

- The cervical and lumbar curves should be concave; the thoracic and sacral curves should be convex when observed on either side of the patient.

- The spine is straight when observed from behind the patient.

- The shoulders, iliac crests, and gluteal folds should be aligned.

(Weber & Kelley, 2007)

Abnormal Findings

- *Scoliosis:* Lateral deviation or curvature of the thoracic spine, with a downward slant of the thoracic cage on the affected side. The pelvis tilts upward on the opposite side, usually at the chest level. Noticed first in adolescents (Figure 54–10B ■).

- *Kyphosis:* An extreme thoracic curve (hunchback or humpback) often occurs with aging (Figure 54–10D ■).

- *Lordosis:* Excessive inward curve of the spine. Patient appears to be swaybacked.

- Flattening of the lumbar spine may be indicative of a herniated disk at the lumbar area or **ankylosing spondylitis** (inflammation of the spine and the sacroiliac joints).

- Pain between the spinous processes may indicate arthritis, fracture or other trauma, infection, or herniated disks.

- Tenderness on palpation of the posterior superior iliac spine (the dimple just above the buttocks) may indicate ankylosing spondylitis.

- Pain on palpation of the paravertebral muscles may indicate degenerative changes or inflammation to the muscles.

- Pain radiating down one or both legs may indicate sciatic nerve involvement.

(Bickley, 2003; Magee, 2008; Weber & Kelley, 2007)

Range of Motion of the Neck

To test the range of motion of the cervical spine, have the patient touch the chin to the chest (flexion) and then look up at the ceiling (extension). To test rotation of the neck, have the patient turn the head from side to side, looking over the shoulder. To test lateral bending of the neck, have the patient tilt the head and touch the ear to the corresponding shoulder.

Normal Finding

- Full range of motion without pain.

Abnormal Findings

- Decreased range of motion can result from arthritis, muscle spasms, or cervical strain.

- Pain in the neck, shoulders, and arms can be due to spinal cord compression.

- Numbness may indicate spinal cord compression.

- Neck pain with decreased ROM accompanied by fever and chills may be due to an infection, such as strep throat or meningitis.

(Bickley, 2003; Magee, 2008)

Range of Motion of the Spine

To test for flexion, ask the patient to bend forward and touch the toes. To test for hyperextension, stabilize the patient's hips from behind the patient, and ask the patient to bend backward. To test for lateral bending of the spine, ask the patient to bend sideways, and to test for rotation, ask the patient to twist the shoulders to the right and then to the left and vice versa.

Normal Findings

- Patient is able to perform full ROM exercises without pain/deformity.

- When bending down to touch toes, the back flattens.

- No exaggerated curvatures of the spine are noted.

- Muscles display symmetry.

Abnormal Findings

- Pain on movement in the thoracic and lumbar areas can be due to muscle or soft tissue injury, osteoarthritis, ankylosing spondylitis, and any **congenital** (describes a condition that was present at birth) conditions.

- Deformity of the thorax on bending indicates scoliosis.

- Lumbar lordosis indicates ankylosing spondylitis.

- Asymmetrical muscle movements, fasciculations, and decreased or exaggerated angles need further investigation.

- Pain radiating from the lower back to one or both legs may indicate nerve involvement.

(Bickley, 2003; Magee, 2008; Weber & Kelley, 2007)

Hip

The hip is located inside the pelvis. The bones that make up the pelvis include the sacrum, pubis, ileum, and ischium. The hip joint is a ball-and-socket joint formed by the articulation of the rounded head of the femur and the cuplike acetabulum of the pelvis. It forms the primary connection between the bones of the trunk and pelvis with the lower extremity. Both joint surfaces are covered with a strong but lubricated articular hyaline cartilage. The hip is important because it bears the weight of the upper body and it contains the hip joint, which allows the leg to move freely.

To examine the hip, inspect the patient's anterior and posterior pelvis for bruising, asymmetry in height, and muscle atrophy. In addition, inspect the buttocks for symmetry. Observe the patient's **gait**, or way of walking. Ask the patient to remove all clothing except underwear and examine the patient walking to and from you barefooted. If one of the patient's legs is longer than the other, then the nurse should measure them by having the patient lie down with the legs extended. The nurse then measures from the anterior superior iliac spine across the leg medially to the medial malleolus (Weber & Kelley, 2007).

Observe for the hip motion, knee flexion, and a heel-to-heel distance of 5 to 10 cm (2 to 4 in.). Inspect the spine for any abnormal curvatures. Question the patient regarding pain; specifically, where in the gait phase the pain occurs. With the patient standing, palpate the hips and pelvis for tenderness, crepitus (grating sound), and nodules (Bickley, 2003; Weber & Kelley, 2007).

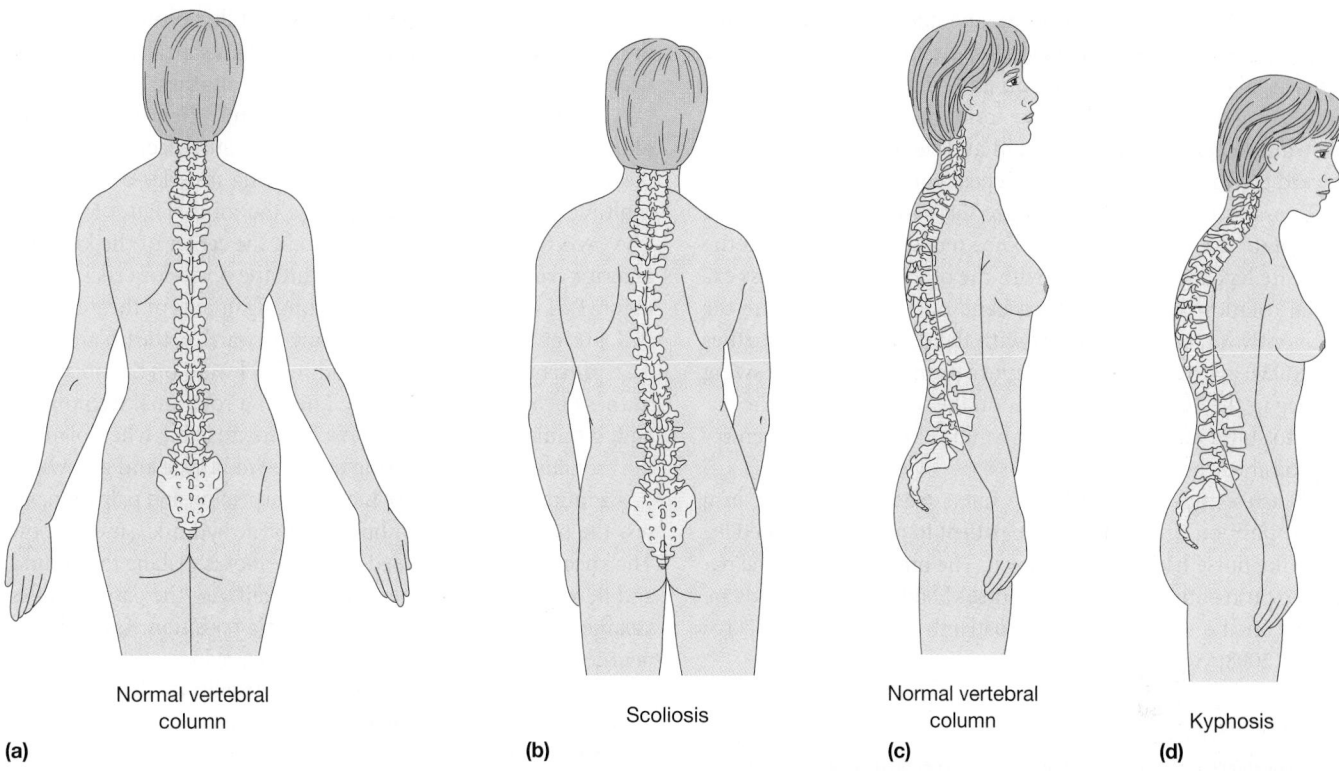

Normal vertebral column	Scoliosis	Normal vertebral column	Kyphosis
(a)	**(b)**	**(c)**	**(d)**

FIGURE 54–10 ■ Normal spine and its deformities: (A) normal vertebral column, posterior view; (B) scoliosis; (C) normal vertebral column, lateral view; (D) kyphosis.

Normal Findings

- The pelvis, on anterior and posterior inspection, is symmetrical in height and shape.
- The buttocks are equal in size.
- Patient is able to bear weight on both legs without pain.
- The gait is rhythmic, nonstaggering, and without a limp.
- The feet are lifted off the ground and are then replanted firmly on the ground.
- Crepitus is not noted by the patient during walking.
- The arm swing is in conjunction with the walking gait.
- During walking the patient's hips are equal and move rhythmically with the gait.
- Patient is able to walk on his toes and on his heels without difficulty or pain.
- Both legs are the same length.
- The knee is flexed while walking, except when the heel touches the ground.
- With the feet forward in a normal standing position, the heel-to-heel distance is 5 to 10 cm (2 to 4 in.).

Abnormal Findings

- An asymmetric pelvis is indicative of hip dislocation, fractured hip, arthritis, **degenerative joint disease** (osteoarthritis), muscle weakness, or atrophy.
- Difficulty in ambulation with an irregular gait may indicate a dislocation or fracture of the hip, degenerative joint disease, or muscle weakness.
- Abnormal curvature of the spine during ambulation may indicate scoliosis or lordosis.
- Leg shortening could mean muscle deformities or hip fracture.
- Unequal leg length may indicate scoliosis.
- Wide heel-to-heel base may indicate a foot or cerebellar problem.

(Weber & Kelley, 2007)

Range of Motion of the Hip

To test ROM of the hip, have the patient lie in the supine position (Figure 54–11 ■). Raise one leg above the body while keeping

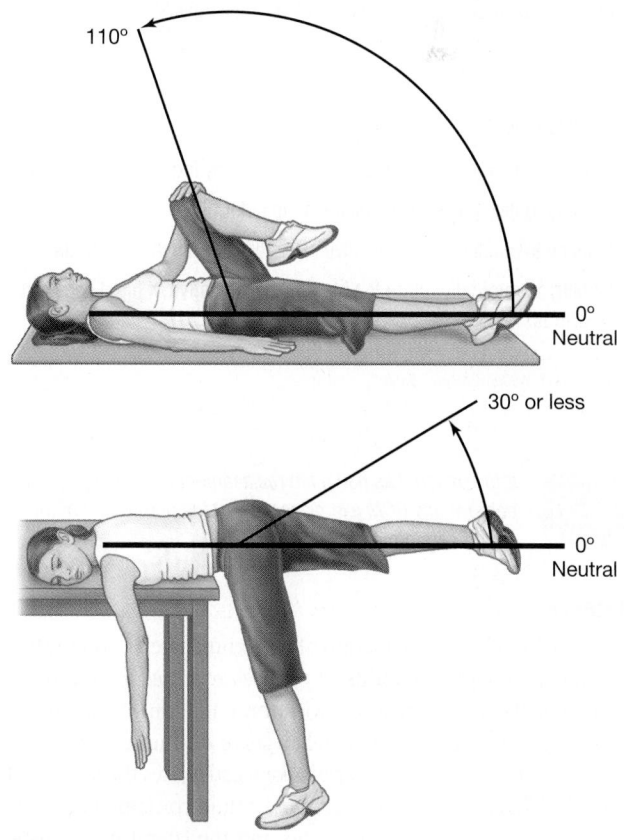

FIGURE 54–11 ■ Hip ROM.

the knee extended and then bring one knee to the chest while keeping the other leg extended. Repeat the exercise with the other leg. To assess for abduction and adduction, have the patient swing one leg laterally away from the body as far as possible while keeping the knee straight and then bring the leg back toward the midline of the body. Repeat with the other leg.

To assess internal rotation, have the patient bend one knee and rotate the knee so that the knee moves inward toward the opposite leg, and then repeat with the other knee. To assess external rotation, have the patient bend one knee and rotate the knee outward, and then repeat with the other knee. To further test ROM, ask the patient to assume a prone position and swing one leg in the air, and then repeat on the other side. Ask the patient to stand and swing one leg behind the body, and then repeat on the other side.

To assess muscle strength, the nurse places the patient in a supine position, and then asks the patient to raise an extended leg while the nurse tries to hold it down. The nurse then asks the patient to push both legs against the nurse's hands while the hands are placed on the outer side of the patient's knees (Bickley, 2003; Magee, 2008; Weber & Kelley, 2007).

Normal Findings

- Patient should be able to raise the legs to at least 90 degrees of flexion with the knee straight and to 120 degrees of flexion with the knee flexed.

- Patient should be able adduct leg to 20 to 30 degrees and abduct it 45 to 50 degrees.

- Patient should be able to internally rotate to 40 degrees and externally rotate to 45 degrees.

- Patient should be able to hyperextend the leg at least 15 degrees.

- Patient should be able to move the extremities against resistance.

(Magee, 2008; Weber & Kelley, 2007).

Abnormal Findings

- Deformity of one or both hips during flexion may indicate a hip deformity.

- Inability to flex knees may indicate a hip deformity.

- Inability to abduct hip is indicative of hip disease, such as arthritis.

- Inability to internally rotate the hip may be indicative of hip disease, such as arthritis.

(Bickley, 2003; Weber & Kelley, 2007)

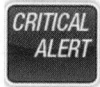 **CRITICAL ALERT** *If the patient has had a hip replacement or hip surgery, do not perform any ROM exercises without the permission of the health care provider.*

Knees

The knee joint is the articulation of the femur, patella, and the tibia. The knee is actually two joints: (1) The *femoropatellar joint* consists of the patella, a bone that sits within the tendon of the anterior quadriceps muscle, and the patellar grove on the femur through which it slides. (2) The *femorotibial joint* articulates the femur with the tibia. The joint is bathed in synovial fluid contained inside the joint capsule. The medial meniscus and the lateral meniscus are

two cartilaginous menisci within the joint that protect the ends of the bones from rubbing on each other, act as shock absorbers, and deepen the tibial sockets where the femur attaches.

The knee allows flexion, extension, and slight rotation. The muscles that help move the joint are the quadriceps muscles on the front of the knee and the hamstring muscles on the back. Multiple ligaments help to stabilize the joint (Figure 54–12 ■). The two cruciate ligaments located in the center of the knee, the anterior cruciate ligament (ACL) and the posterior cruciate ligament (PCL), are the major stabilizing ligaments of the joint. The PCL prevents the femur from sliding forward on the tibia, and the ACL prevents the femur from sliding backward on the tibia. Both of these ligaments stabilize the knee in a rotational fashion also and, if damaged, the knee may become unstable when planting the foot and pivoting, causing the knee to buckle and give way.

Examination of the knee includes inspection and palpation. Assess the patient during ambulation for a rhythmic, smooth flow. The knee should be extended when the foot is striking the ground, and flexed during the other phases of gait. Ask the patient to first assume a supine position and then a sitting position. Assess the patient for symmetry of the knees, swelling, redness, size, shape, deformities, and alignment. Assess for atrophy of the quadriceps muscles and the hollows on either side of the knee (Bickley, 2003; Weber & Kelley, 2007).

Palpate the knee while the patient is sitting on the edge of the table with the legs dangling. Palpate for tenderness, heat, swelling, crepitus, and nodules. Begin by palpating 10 cm (about 4 in.) above the patella. Using fingers and thumb, move

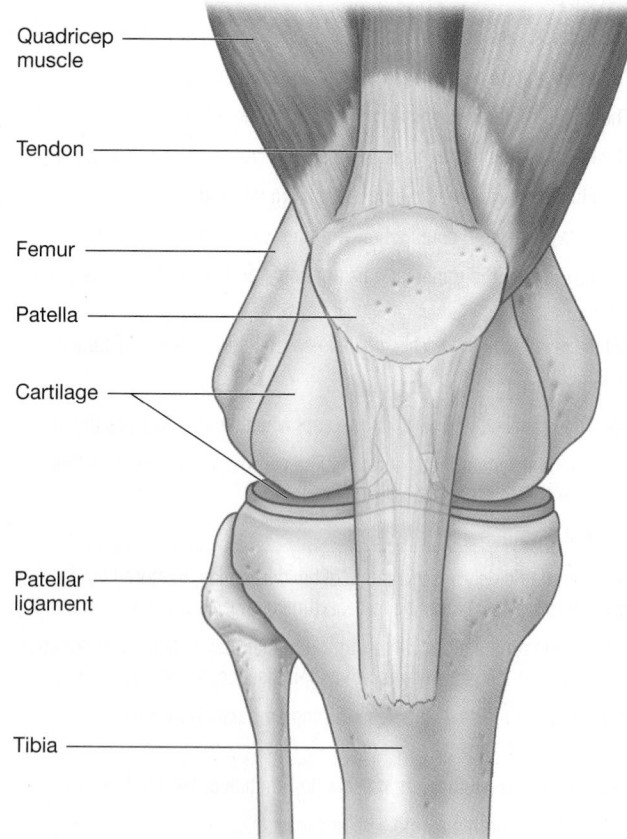

FIGURE 54–12 ■ Knee joint.

Quadricep muscle

Tendon

Femur

Patella

Cartilage

Patellar ligament

Tibia

downward toward the knee (Bickley, 2003). If swelling is encountered, the following further tests are performed with the patient in the supine position:

1. The *bulge sign* is used to detect fluid in the knee. Place the hand on the medial aspect of the patient's knee and push upward two to four times to displace the fluid. Then place the hand on the lateral side of the knee and look for a bulge of fluid in the hollow area medial to the patella.

2. The *balloon sign* is performed by placing the thumb and index finger of one hand on each side of the patella while the other hand compresses the suprapatellar pouch against the femur. This allows the nurse to feel the fluid entering the spaces next to the patella.

3. The *ballottement test* is used to assess large amounts of fluid, particularly in the suprapatellar pouch. Press against the sides of the patella with the thumb and index finger of one hand, while pushing the patella against the femur with the opposite hand. While pressing on the sides of the patella, fluid is displaced in the suprapatellar pouch. While pushing the patella against the femur, the fluid returns to the pouch and the nurse is able to feel a "wave" as the fluid returns to the pouch (Bickley, 2003; Weber & Kelley, 2007).

Normal Findings

- Both knees are symmetrical.
- Both legs are the same length.
- The hollows are present on both sides of the patella.
- There is no redness, swelling, or tenderness.
- No deformities are noted.
- No nodules are noted.
- The muscles are firm and taut.
- No crepitus is felt or heard.

Abnormal Findings

- Knees turn outward, called bowlegs or genu varum.
- Knees turn inward, called knock-knees or genu valgum.
- Irregular bony ridges may be indicative of osteoarthritis.
- Pain and tenderness may be indicative of bursitis.
- Heat may be indicative of osteoarthritis.
- Pain and crepitus may indicate a rough surface between the femur and the back of the patella.
- Pain on movement by means of quadriceps contraction may indicate a degenerative patella.
- Pain over a tendon or an inability to extend the leg may indicate a tear of a tendon or ligament.
- Thickness, warmth, and bogginess on the sides of the patella may indicate synovitis or osteoarthritis.
- Swelling or bulges of the lateral or medial aspects of the knee or above the knee may indicate an effusion (leaking of fluid into the knee) of the knee or synovial thickening.
- Inability to walk without stumbling or pushing the knee into extension may indicate a weakening of the quadriceps.

Range of Motion of the Knee

To test for ROM of the knee, have the patient in a sitting position and do the following tests. To test for flexion, ask the patient to bend the knee. To test for extension and hyperextension, ask the patient to straighten the knee. To test for internal and external rotation, ask the patient to rotate the foot medially and laterally (Figure 54–13 ■).

To test muscle strength, the nurse asks the patient to extend the leg as the nurse tries to bend it. This tests quadriceps muscle strength. Then the nurse asks the patient to flex the knee while the nurse tries to straighten it. This tests hamstring muscle strength.

Normal Findings

- Patient should be able to flex the knee to 120 to 130 degrees (Weber & Kelley, 2007).
- Patient should be able to extend the knee without difficulty and hyperextend the knee to 15 degrees.
- Patient should have full ROM against resistance.

Abnormal Findings

- Difficulty with ROM may indicate osteoarthritis or a muscle or joint problem.
- Crepitus is noted in osteoarthritis.

Be aware that pain and abnormal or decreased ROM may also indicate a ligament injury or meniscus tear to the anterior or posterior cruciate ligaments and the medial and lateral collateral ligaments. Pain on the lateral sides of the knee, "popping" or "clicking" sounds with movement, patient complaints of the knee "locking," or difficulty in fully extending the knee may indicate damage to the meniscus. To assess for a torn meniscus, perform the McMurray test. With the patient in a supine position, the nurse asks the patient to flex one knee and hip. The nurse then cups one hand over the knee and places her index finger and thumb on opposite sides of the knee. With the other hand, the nurse grasp the patient's heel and rotates the lower leg and foot laterally and medially. Gently and slowly extend the knee, and note any abnormal sounds (Weber & Kelley, 2007).

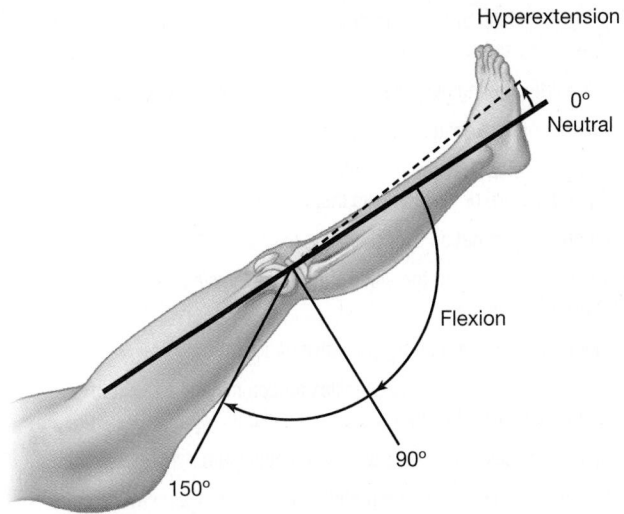

FIGURE 54–13 ■ Knee ROM.

CRITICAL ALERT *If the patient is complaining of severe pain, it is best to let a physician, nurse practitioner, or physician's assistant assess the patient and perform the McMurray test.*

Ankles and Feet

The ankle is the joint between the lower tibia, the fibula, and the talus. The feet are made up of many small bones. Both the ankle and foot have many ligaments and thick padding to cushion the foot against the weight of the body during ambulation (Bickley, 2003).

Ask the patient to stand, walk, and sit. Observe the ankles and feet for shape, deformities, nodules, corns, calluses, bunions, and swelling. Note the position of the toes. Ask the patient to walk barefoot and note the ability to walk normally on the heels and on the toes. Ask the patient to walk placing one foot in front of the other and to walk backwards. Ask the patient to sit with the feet dangling at the sides of the table. Observe the position of the feet and toes. Inspect for roundness and smoothness of the medial malleolus.

Assess ROM by asking the patient to point his toes toward the floor (plantar flexion), point toes toward his nose (dorsiflexion),

Normal Findings

- The toes should point straight ahead and be in alignment with the feet, though some may point slightly inward or slightly outward.
- No nodules, calluses, corns, or bunions are noted.
- The medial malleolus should be round and smooth.
- No pain elicited on palpation.
- The Achilles tendon is without nodules or tenderness.

Abnormal Findings

- A great toe that is deviated medially and abducted to the first metatarsal with an inflamed bursa or bunion on the medial side is indicative of hallux valgus.
- A hot, tender, red, swollen metatarsophalangeal joint is indicative of gouty arthritis.
- A flattened longitudinal arch, so that the sole is very close to the ground or touches the ground may be indicative of flat foot (evident only when patient is ambulating).
- An abnormally high arch may be indicative of cavus foot.
- Hyperextension of the metatarsophalangeal joint of the second toe is referred to as hammer toe.
- Painful thickening over the skin over a bony prominence is a corn.
- An area of thickened skin over a region of pressure points is a callus.
- A wart located over the thick skin of the sole of the foot is referred to as a plantar wart, or verruca vulgaris.
- Painful, inflammation over the great toe may be indicative of gout.
- Tenderness between the ankle joints is indicative of arthritis, infection, or injury to the ankle.
- Painful movement may be indicative of arthritis.
- Pain or nodules around the Achilles tendon may be a result of rheumatoid arthritis, bursitis, or tendonitis.
- Pain at the calcaneus may be due to bone spurs.
- Pain and tenderness of the metatarsals and grooves may indicate arthritis or circulatory compromise.

(Bickley, 2003; Magee, 2008; Weber & Kelley, 2007)

turn the soles of the feet out, then in (eversion, inversion), and then flex and straighten the toes (Figure 54–14 ■).

Palpate with your thumbs at the anterior aspect of each ankle joint, the heel, and the posterior and anterior calcaneus. Palpate the metatarsophalangeal joints, as well as in between them for tenderness, and the Achilles tendon for tenderness, swelling, heat, and nodules (Bickley, 2003; Magee, 2008; Weber & Kelley, 2007).

Gait (Ambulation)

To assess gait, or ambulation, ask the patient to walk away from you using the heel-to-toe gait, swinging her arms. Next have the patient walk toward you. Then ask the patient to walk on tiptoes toward you, and away from you on her heels. Observe the patient during the two phases of walking: The first is the stance phase of gait. This occurs when the foot is on the ground and the patient is weight bearing or walking on the foot. The second phase is the swing phase. This occurs when the patient moves the foot forward and is not bearing weight. Observe for difficulty in weight bearing, gait anomalies, symmetry of legs, rate, rhythm, and arm motion.

Inspect the patient during ambulation for ability to walk heel to toe; arm swing in conjunction with walking; base of support; and posture; limping, or leaning to one side; inability to bear weight on one or both legs.

Normal Findings

- Patient is able to ambulate with smooth, rhythmic movement; arms swing in conjunction with walking.
- No leaning or limping noted; patient is able to keep balance.
- Toes point straight ahead.
- Patients is able to walk heel to toe.
- Back is straight with a wide base of support.

Abnormal Findings

- Leaning or limping may indicate a neurological problem.
- Toes pointing inward or outward may be indicative of bunions or arthritis.
- Arms extended to sides to maintain balance may indicate a neurological problem.
- Shuffling or the inability to take coordinated steps may indicate Parkinson's disease.

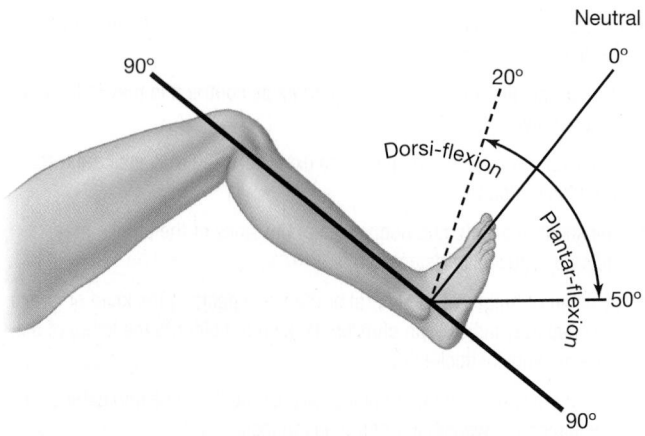

FIGURE 54–14 ■ Ankle ROM.

Gerontological Considerations

As "baby boomers" age, persons 50 years and older will make up the largest population group in the United States, so it is important to understand the numerous changes in the musculoskeletal system that occur with age. When assessing older patients with musculoskeletal ailments, the nurse needs to recognize several important aspects:

1. Flexibility and strength tend to decrease as people age.

2. Because of changes to bone and muscle, older people may find it hard to maintain the various positions required for a proper assessment. Lying supine for a long period of time is difficult for patients with cardiopulmonary problems.

3. Bones become weaker as calcium reabsorption lessens with age.

4. As the bones become weaker, fractures can become more prevalent.

5. Women who are menopausal or postmenopausal are subject to osteoporosis.

6. Articular hyaline cartilage becomes thinner at the joints, restricting ROM.

7. Osteoarthritic changes occur with age, particularly in postmenopausal women. Osteoarthritis causes smooth articular surfaces to become rough and painful.

8. Rheumatoid arthritis causes inflammation and decreased or limited movement of the fingers. The condition is painful and affects a person's ability to perform ADLs.

9. The elderly are prone to **pathologic fractures** (fractures that occur without trauma) due to thinning of the bones.

10. Skeletal muscle mass decreases with age, leading to cramping and severe pain.

Assessing the Elderly Patient

Obtain a current history to include all medications, including OTC drugs. Inquire about pain, discomfort, limitation in movement, and any difficulty performing ADLs. Assess the patient as he ambulates, walks, grasps your hand, and bends over. Note any weakness. Inspect the hands and fingers for rheumatoid nodules or swelling and note any circulatory impairment by blanching the finger/toe nails. Chart 54–4 provides more details for assessing elderly patients.

 *Note any signs of depression (crying, monotone voice, lethargy). A limitation in mobility may cause a person to become depressed and possibly suicidal.*

Documentation

Documentation of the examination of the musculoskeletal system entails noting subjective data as well as objective data. Include the patient's response to various parts of the examination, including the patient's inability to perform a particular task of an examination or the performance of only part of the task. Note complaints of pain and tenderness, swelling, redness, nodule formation, noticeable deformity, or dizziness.

CHART 54–4	Assessing the Elderly Patient
System	**Difference with the Elderly**
Shoulders	Inability to perform ROM without discomfort
Elbows	Inflammation, swelling, and decreased ROM due to arthritis
Wrist	Decreased ROM, swelling
Hands/fingers	Swelling and thickening of the metacarpophalangeal joint and the proximal interphalangeal joint, decreased ROM, due to rheumatoid arthritis Heberden's nodules over the distal interphalangeal joint and Bouchard's nodes over the proximal interphalangeal joints due to osteoarthritis
Neck	May have difficulty performing ROM
Spine	Kyphosis
Hip	Decreased ROM, crepitus due to arthritis and degenerative joint disease
Knee	Bowleggedness due to loss of muscle control
Ankles	Decreased strength and ROM due to bone thinning and decreased muscle mass
Gait	Wider base of support; slower paced, nonrhythmic walking; use of assistive devices

Sources: Adapted from Magee, D. (2008). *Orthopedic physical assessment* (5th ed.). Elsevier; Weber, J., & Kelley, J. (2007). *Health assessment in nursing* (3rd ed.). Philadelphia: Lippincott Williams & Wilkins.

Nursing Diagnoses

Nursing diagnoses for the musculoskeletal system are based on the subjective and objective data obtained. Nursing diagnoses applicable for the musculoskeletal examination include the following:

- *Activity Intolerance* related to difficulty with ambulation, decreased ROM, pain, swelling, muscle weakness, pain, joint deformity

- *Mobility, Impaired* related to difficulty with ambulation, decreased ROM, pain, swelling, muscle weakness, pain, joint deformity

- *Pain, Acute* related to a specific condition

- *Pain, Chronic* related to a specific condition

- *Disuse Syndrome, Risk for* related to difficulty with mobility, decreased ROM

- *Injury, Risk for* related to difficulty with mobility, decreased ROM, pain

- *Trauma, Risk for* related to difficulty with mobility, decreased ROM

- *Activity Intolerance, Risk for* related to difficulty with ambulation, decreased ROM, pain, swelling, muscle weakness, pain, joint deformity

- *Falls, Risk for* related to decreased mobility, decreased ROM

- *Powerlessness* related to loss of independence.

Health Promotion

Many musculoskeletal disorders are due to individual behaviors as well as social and environmental factors. Many individuals do not participate in regular physical activities, such as jogging, bicycling, or walking. Physical activity is important for many reasons, but as far as the musculoskeletal system is concerned, regularly scheduled physical activity increases muscle and bone mass. Physical activity can prevent thinning of bones as well as muscle atrophy. The increase in muscle mass coincides with a decrease in falling in the elderly, which allows for independence and an ability to perform ADLs.

Obesity also affects the musculoskeletal system in that people who are overweight and obese have a difficult time engaging in physical activity as they become short of breath and fatigued more easily. Cigarette smoking causes lung problems, which again can affect an individual's ability to participate in physical activity.

To maintain one's quality of life, it is important for everyone to engage in some degree of regular physical activity to help maintain a strong musculoskeletal system.

Summary

The musculoskeletal system plays a major role in a patient's mobility and quality of life. As a nurse it is imperative to understand all of the components and how to conduct a thorough assessment of the system. Performing a systematic evaluation to identify abnormalities will assist with timely treatment and the prevention of future complications.

NCLEX® REVIEW

1. A patient sustains a fracture to the ribs. The nurse realizes that the type of bone injured is considered:
   1. Long.
   2. Short.
   3. Flat
   4. Irregular.

2. While assessing a patient with a musculoskeletal injury the nurse asks if the patient uses any assistive devices. This question would be considered as being a part of which of the following areas of the patient's history?
   1. Chief complaint
   2. Social
   3. Demographic data
   4. Biographical data

3. During the musculoskeletal assessment, the nurse notes atrophy of the patient's left thigh muscles. The assessment technique the nurse used to determine this finding would be:
   1. Palpation.
   2. Percussion.
   3. Inspection.
   4. Range of motion.

4. The nurse asks a patient to raise the arms above the head with the palms facing each other. The body area that the nurse is currently assessing would be the:
   1. Elbow.
   2. Shoulders.
   3. Wrist.
   4. Hand.

5. The nurse is assessing a patient's feet. Which of the following would be considered a normal finding during this assessment?
   1. Hallux valgus
   2. Cavus foot
   3. Verruca vulgaris
   4. Toes pointing inward

6. The nurse is assessing a patient's hip range of motion. Which of the following is considered a normal finding?
   1. Leg adduction 10 degrees
   2. Leg abduction 25 degrees
   3. External rotation 45 degrees
   4. Internal rotation 20 degrees

Answers for review questions appear in Appendix D

KEY TERMS

abduction *p.1715*
adduction *p.1715*
ankylosing spondylitis *p.1720*
anteriorly *p.1715*
asymmetry *p.1715*
assistive device *p.1714*
asymmetry *p.1715*
Bouchard's nodes *p.1718*
boutonniére deformity *p.1718*
bursae *p.1712*
carpal tunnel syndrome *p.1718*

congenital *p.1720*
crepitus *p.1716*
degenerative joint disease *p.1721*
dislocation *p.1711*
Dupuytren's contracture *p.1719*
fasciculations *p.1714*
gait *p.1720*
goniometer *p.1714*
gouty joint *p.1714*
Heberden's nodes *p.1718*

interphalangeal joint *p.1718*
metacarpophalangeal joints *p.1718*
muscle atrophy *p.1714*
nodules *p.1714*
pathologic fractures *p.1725*
posteriorly *p.1715*
range of motion (ROM) *p.1711*
tenosynovitis *p.1719*
tremors *p.1714*

REFERENCES

Bickley, L. (2003). *Bates' guide to physical assessment and history taking* (7th ed.). Philadelphia: Lippincott.

Jarvis, C. (2008). *Pocket companion for physical examination and health assessment* (5th ed.). St. Louis: W. B. Saunders.

Lillicrap, M. S., Byrne, E., & Speed, C. A. (2003). Musculoskeletal assessment of general medical in-patients—joints crying out for attention. *Rheumatology, 42,* 951–954.

Magee, D. (2008). *Orthopedic physical assessment* (5th ed.). St. Louis, MO: Elsevier, Inc.

Porth, C. M. (Ed.). (2007). *Pathophysiology: Concepts of altered health states* (7th ed.). Philadelphia: Lippincott Williams & Wilkins.

Weber, J., & Kelley, J. (2007). *Health assessment in nursing* (3rd ed.). Philadelphia: Lippincott Williams & Wilkins.

Caring for the Patient with Musculoskeletal Disorders

Helene Harris
Karen Bawel-Brinkley
Cheryl Wraa

Outcome-Based Learning Objectives

After studying this chapter, the learner will be able to:

1. Compare and contrast the etiology, pathophysiology, clinical manifestations, and medical and nursing management for bone diseases.

2. Explain the rationale and type of preventive therapy necessary for patients with bone disease.

3. Describe the unique treatment and prevention needs of the gerontological population.

4. Compare and contrast the etiology, pathophysiology, clinical manifestations, and medical and nursing management for muscular diseases.

5. Differentiate between the five types of myopathies, various treatment modalities, and nursing care of a patient diagnosed with a myopathy.

6. Discuss the causative factors, treatment modalities, and nursing care related to a patient diagnosed with fibromyalgia.

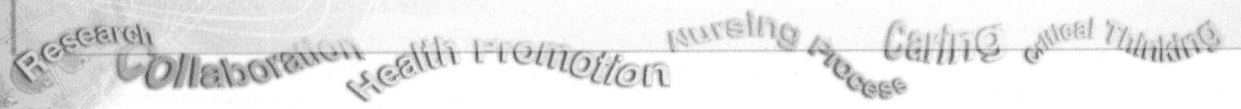

THE MUSCULOSKELETAL system consists of bones, muscles, ligaments, tendons, and other connective tissue. Organic (collagen fibers), inorganic materials (mineral salts), and water combine to form bone tissue that provides protection for crucial internal organs, storage for calcium and other minerals, and sites for formation and development of the cells of the blood (Copstead & Banaski, 2005; Seeman, 2002).

Bone disorders can result from disuse, nutritional deficiencies, chemotherapy, genetic or environmental influences, and traumatic injuries or accidents. Because individuals with bone disease may experience loss of function and independence, the nurse must have a clear understanding of the effects of bone disease and how the disorder or disease will impact the patient's life.

■ Bone Physiology

This section presents a brief overview of bone physiology and bone formation. Because anatomy and physiology provide the foundation for medical and nursing goals and care, the reader is encouraged to review bone physiology and formation.

Characteristics

The study of bones and bone structure of the human body is referred to as **osteology**. The human body consists of the axial and appendicular skeleton comprising 206 bones. These bones have some degree of elasticity and toughness that provide an anchor against which muscles, connected by means of ligaments and tendons, can exert force.

The bone/bone marrow system includes bone cells, fat cells, blood vessels, and nonliving materials including water and minerals. Bones are classified as osseous tissue that is formed from calcium phosphate. This tissue is considered to be a hard **endoskeletal** connective tissue. The body has 80 axial bones (head, facial, hyoid, auditory, trunk, ribs, and sternum) and 126 appendicular bones (arms, shoulders, wrists, hands, legs, hips, ankles, and feet) (Porth, 2005). Bones provide structural support, protect vital organs, act as attachment sites for muscles that permit the mechanics of human motion, and serve as a mineral reservoir and a way to catch unsafe minerals (e.g., lead). Chart 55–1 presents a summary of the classification of bones and their characteristics.

Bone Tissue

Bone tissue has the ability to be strong, lightweight, and adaptable to meet the functional needs of the body (Beers & Porter, 2006; Chan & Duque, 2002). Bone is covered with a fibrous membrane known as the **periosteum**. The blood supply to bone is achieved through blood vessels running through two layers of

CHART 55–1	**Classification of Human Bones and Characteristics**	
Classification of Bone	**Example Bone in Human Body**	**Characteristic of Bone**
Long bones	Femur Tibia	• Tubular • Regions of the bone: diaphysis, epiphysis, and metaphysis • Hollow with bone marrow • Shaft made of compact hard bone and thickest in the middle • Trabecular bone toward the end of the bone • Increases in size in one dimension during growth
Short bones	Wrist Ankle Carpal Tarsal	• Cuboidal in shape • Cancellous bone in the center and compact bone outer shell
Flat bones	Cranium Scapula	• Spongy bone between two layers of compact bone • Generally curved in structure (inner and outer diploe)
Irregular bones	Bones of the face Vertebrae	• Irregular shape • Does not fit into any other category
Sesamoid	Patella	• Occur in tendon leading to exposure to friction

the periosteum: the thick outer layer, which is composed of connective tissue, and the inner layer, which is composed of elastic fibers. In addition, fine nerves and lymphatic vessels run through the thick fibrous tissue covering the bone. The periosteum tightly covers the bone and is connected to both ends of the bone with the epiphyseal cartilage except where tendons and ligaments attach to the bone, and then the periosteum is integrated with them. Two results of the aging process are that the periosteum becomes thinner and vascularity declines (Porth, 2005).

The human body has three types of bone tissue: compact, cancellous, and subchondral tissue (Figure 55–1 ■) **Compact**

(or **cortical**) **bone** is resistant to compression, is dense, and is laid down in concentric layers. **Cancellous** (having a hard outer casing with the interior being porous, spongy, and meshwork-like in structure) or **trabecular** (cancellous bone found at the ends of the long bones [e.g., femur], in vertebrae, and in the flat bones of the pelvis) **bone** is laid down in response to stress and shape to accommodate loads placed on the bone (Figure 55–2 ■). The arrangement of plates, rods, arches, and braces in the interior of trabecular bone provides the strength needed for weight bearing. **Subchondral bone** is the smooth tissue at the ends of bones that is covered with cartilage. Cartilage is the specialized, tough connective tissue that is present in adults, and the tissue from which most bones develop in children. Both compact and trabecular bone are **lamellar bone** or mature bone. In the human body, lamellar bone is a slow-forming bone with cellular distribution being orderly and the direction of the collagen fibers standardized (Gupta et al., 2005).

Cortical (outer layer) or compact bone provides about 80% of the skeletal mass and is the major component of tubular bones. Cortical bone has a densely packed, calcified intercellular matrix that makes it more rigid than cancellous bone. **Haversian canals**, which contain one or two capillaries and nerve fibers that serve as the transport systems for nutrients, are located in the cortical bone.

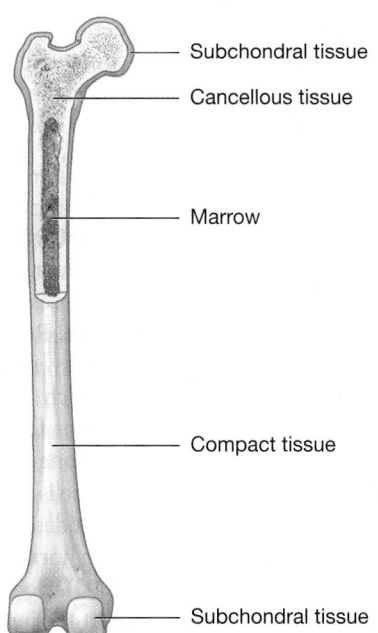

Subchondral tissue

Cancellous tissue

Marrow

Compact tissue

Subchondral tissue

FIGURE 55–1 ■ Bone tissues.

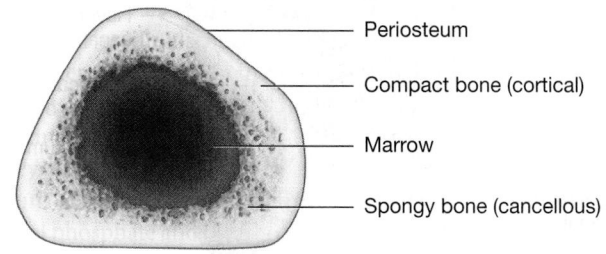

Periosteum

Compact bone (cortical)

Marrow

Spongy bone (cancellous)

FIGURE 55–2 ■ Cortical and cancellous bone.

CHART 55–2	**Hormonal Effects on the Bone**	
Gland	**Hormones**	**Actions on Bone Tissue**
Anterior pituitary gland	Growth hormone and somatotropin	• Stimulate the production of IGFs by the osteoblasts by stimulating longitudinal bone growth. • Increases the rate of mitosis of chondrocytes and osteoblasts. • Increases the rate of protein synthesis (collagen, cartilage matrix, and enzymes for cartilage and bone formation).
	Thyroid-stimulating hormone (TSH)	• Controls the rate of thyroxine production from the thyroid gland.
	Gonadotropins: luteinizing and follicle-stimulating hormones	• Controls growth and reproductive activities of the gonads.
Thyroid gland	Thyroxine (T_4) and triiodothyronine (T_3)	• Regulates the body's metabolic rate. • Increases the rate of protein synthesis. • Increases energy production from all food types.
	Calcitonin	• Peptide hormone. • Acts on the kidneys and bones to lower serum calcium levels. • Antagonist to PTH, which leads to lowering of the number of osteoclasts absorbed. • Delays calcium absorption from the intestine and increases calcium in the urine.
Parathyroid gland	Parathyroid hormone (PTH)	• Maintains normal serum calcium levels by secreting PTH, which increases bone resorption of calcium from bones to the blood, thereby raising blood calcium levels. • Increases the absorption of calcium by the small intestine and kidneys.
Adrenal glands	Glucocorticoids: cortisol	• Assist in the body's response to stress; suppressing inflammation, increasing serum glucose, and regulating metabolism of carbohydrates, fat, and protein. • Enhances protein synthesis. • Increases the breakdown of protein and fatty acids.
	Mineralocorticoids: aldosterone	• Regulates electrolyte concentrations (Na^+, K^+) in the extracellular fluid.
	Androgens: dehydroepiandrosterone sulfate and androstenedione	• Produce and maintain secondary sexual characteristics.

CHART 55–3	**Other Organ Systems and Hormones That Influence Bone Growth**	
Organ	**Hormone**	**Actions on Bone Tissue**
Kidney	Vitamin D	Produced in the kidneys and affected by PTH, dietary intake of vitamin D (fat-soluble vitamin), and skin exposure to sunlight.
Ovaries or testes	Estrogen or testosterone	• Promotes closure of epiphyses of long bones, thereby stopping growth. • Assists with the retention of calcium in the bones, thereby maintaining a strong bone matrix.

glucocorticoid levels exceed normal concentration they have deleterious effects on the skeletal system. Either by direct or indirect means, high levels of glucocorticoids can reduce bone mass by (1) decreasing calcium absorption from the intestines, (2) reducing bone formation, (3) increasing bone resorption, (4) excreting calcium from the kidneys, and (5) decreasing the production of sex steroid (Copstead & Banaski, 2005; Fajardo & Di Cesare, 2005; Takeda et al., 2004). For example, high-dose glucocorticoids for infection can cause osteoporosis through the combination of decreasing bone formation and increasing bone resorption.

Vitamin D (1,25-dihydroxyvitamin) is produced by the kidneys and is a hormone. This hormone is under the influence of three factors: (1) PTH, (2) dietary intake of vitamin D (fat-soluble vita-

min), and (3) skin exposure to sunlight, or ultraviolet-B (UVB) radiation. Receptors to vitamin D are located in the bone, kidneys, intestines, and other cells. Vitamin D hormone is necessary for bone mineralization by promoting gastrointestinal absorption of calcium and phosphorus. When given in high doses, vitamin D can increase bone resorption (Fajardo & Di Cesare, 2005).

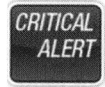 **CRITICAL ALERT** *Women in northern latitudes have been shown to have a decline in their vitamin D levels during the winter months.*

Gonadal steroids are produced in the ovaries and testes. These include estrogen in females and androgens in males. Both contribute to maintaining bone metabolism by regulating rates of bone formation and bone resorption. These hormones are necessary for bone strength and decrease with aging (see the Gerontological Considerations box). Chart 55–4 summarizes hormone function and action on bone tissue.

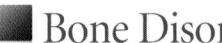 Bone Disorders

Bone disorders can result from disuse, genetic or environmental influences, and traumatic injuries or accidents. Loss of function and independence may be experienced by an individual with bone disease. As a result the nurse must have a clear understanding of the effects of bone disease and how the disorder or disease will influence the individual. The focus of this section of the chapter is on the care of individuals with bone disease.

Osteoporosis

Bone is a matrix-mineral–like substance with varying degrees of density at various points within the structure. **Osteoporosis** is a skeletal disease that is characterized by low bone mass and deterioration of the bone tissue. This continued deterioration results

GERONTOLOGICAL CONSIDERATIONS Related to Changes in Bone Tissue

Changes in bone tissue that occur with aging include:

- Decline in muscle mass and connective tissue
- Reduction in cancellous bone (volume, number of cells, and width)
- Decline in bone density
- Reduction in gonadal status
- Reduction in estrogen levels
- Increase in osteoclast numbers and life expectancy
- Increased adiposity of bone marrow
- Decrease in blood vessels
- Reduction in cortical bone tissue related to bone absorption on the endosteal surface
- Increased porosity and decline in ability to deposit new bone on the endosteal surface
- Decline in hormonal response.

CHART 55–4	Hormone Function and Action on Bone Tissue	
Hormone	**Function**	**Clinical Manifestations**
Anterior pituitary gland: growth hormone (somatropins)	Hypofunction	• *Children:* Delayed growth, fine features, and short stature proportionate • *Adult:* May be associated with hyposecretion of other pituitary hormones
	Hyperfunction	• *Children:* Increase linear growth and tall stature • *Adult:* acromegaly or giantism
Pituitary hyperstimulation of the adrenal cortex	Hypercortisolism or Cushing's syndrome	• Muscle weakness • Muscle wasting • Osteoporosis • Fractures
Thyroid-stimulating hormone (TSH)	Hyposecretion	• Retarded development • Dwarfism
Thyroxine (T$_4$) and triiodothyronine (T$_3$)	Hyposecretion	• Poor muscle tone • Growth retardation • Delayed bone development • Dwarfism • Loss of cortical and trabecular bone
	Hypersecretion	• Muscle weakness
Parathyroid	Hyposecretion	• Low serum calcium levels • Paresthesias, cramps, and spasms • Tetany • Chvostek's sign • Trousseau's sign
	Hypersecretion	• High serum calcium levels • Bone demineralization
Glucocorticoids		• Decline in bone formation and increased bone resorption • Osteoporosis • Fractures

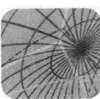

NURSING PROCESS: Patient Care Plan for a Fractured Hip—*Continued*

Nursing Assessment and Diagnoses	Outcomes and Evaluation Parameters	Planning and Interventions with *Rationales*
Nursing Diagnosis: *Nutrition, Imbalanced: Less Than Body Requirements*	**Outcome:** The patient will maintain adequate nutrition to assist with healing. ***Evaluation Parameter:*** Maintenance of weight without loss of muscle mass.	**Interventions and *Rationales:*** Facilitate education with a dietary consultant. *Consultation can ensure a diet that provides optimal caloric and nutrient intake.* Encourage frequent oral hygiene. *Poor oral hygiene leads to bad breath and a bad taste in the mouth, which decreases the appetite.* Provide the patient with printed material outlining dietary needs and restrictions. *Aids the patient in selecting the proper foods.* Promote the intake of protein foods with high biologic value: eggs, meats, and dairy products. *Complete proteins provide the positive nitrogen balance needed for growth and healing.* If the patient has osteoporosis, encourage intake of foods rich in calcium: Low-fat dairy products Spinach Kale Beans and other legumes Broccoli Tofu Salmon Sardines. Also encourage foods rich in vitamin D: Cod liver oil Fatty fish Eggs Fortified foods such as milk and cereals. *Calcium adds strength and stiffness to bones. Vitamin D is essential for calcium absorption and normal bone mineralization.*

Assessment of Skin Integrity

Subjective Data:
Is the discomfort in the area of your surgical incision decreasing?
Have you noticed any drainage from the surgical site?
Inquire if the patient is experiencing pain, itching, or discomfort to any area on the skin.

Objective Data:
Assess the patient's skin and surgical site for redness, swelling, or drainage.

Nursing Assessment and Diagnoses	Outcomes and Evaluation Parameters	Planning and Interventions with *Rationales*
Nursing Diagnosis: *Skin Integrity, Impaired: Risk for* related to immobility and surgical incision	**Outcome:** Patient will achieve wound healing and not develop a pressure ulcer. ***Evaluation Parameters:*** The patient will relate minimal discomfort at the surgical site, and the incision will remain without signs of infection. The patient will show no signs of redness over bony prominences.	**Interventions and *Rationales:*** Monitor vital signs and lab results. *Temperature, pulse, and white blood cell count may increase in response to infection.* Maintain use of aseptic technique. *Use of aseptic technique avoids the introduction of infectious organisms.* Assess surgical site for appearance and character of drainage. *Redness, edema, and drainage at the surgical site indicate infection.* Reposition the patient every 2 hours and assess skin for redness or change in sensation. Add padding to bony prominences. *Repositioning and adding padding relieves pressure on the bony prominences. Redness or a change in sensation on the skin may indicate the development of a pressure ulcer.*

falling, especially for the elderly population. It is recommended that pathways in the house be cleared of furniture, throw rugs, and clutter. For the older adult adequate lighting and proper footwear are essential in preventing unnecessary falls causing fractures.

Evidence-Based Practice

As stated earlier, screening for risk factors and falls assessment will identify those who are at risk for osteoporosis and/or falls and fractures. The New Zealand Guidelines Group developed a best practice, evidence-based guideline that provides recommendations for appropriate and effective processes for assessment of personal, social, functional, and clinical needs in older people. The Evidence-Based Practice box includes the evidence-based guideline for the prevention of hip fractures in people ages 65 years and older.

Prevention of Hip Fracture in People Ages 65 Years and Older

Clinical Problem

Older people are at a high risk for falls and hip fracture. Guidelines for evaluation of risk factors and preventive strategies will decrease the prevalence of the problem.

The following guideline from the New Zealand Guideline Group provides an evidence-based summary of the clinical aspects of hip fracture prevention and preventive strategies for those older people at high risk of hip fracture.

Research Findings

The consequences of hip fractures in older people create a significant and increasing burden of illness in the community, and can precipitate a dramatic decline in physical function. Twenty percent of older people who sustain a hip fracture die within a year. Two years after the fracture, survivors are more than four times likely to have limited mobility than people of similar age without a fracture and are more than twice as likely to be functionally dependent. Evidence shows that women are at greater risk of hip fracture than men, and this risk increases steadily and substantially with age. In addition to gender, other factors that increase the risk of hip fracture are:

- Living in institutional care
- Significant cognitive impairment
- Certain medications (e.g., anticonvulsants, corticosteroids)
- Personal history and lifestyle factors
- Certain medical conditions (e.g., type II diabetes in women)
- Low bone mineral density.

The guideline makes recommendations on risk assessment and effective preventive strategies for reducing hip fractures. A second guideline has been developed for acute management and immediate rehabilitation after hip fracture in people ages 65 years and over and is available from the New Zealand Guideline Group.

Recommendations for Risk Assessment of Individuals at High Risk of Hip Fracture

Individuals at high risk of sustaining a hip fracture include the following:

- Women ages 80 years and older and men ages 85 years and older
- Women ages 70 years and older and men ages 75 years and older:
  - Living in institutional care OR
  - With significant cognitive impairment.
- Women ages 70 years and older and men ages 75 years and older with one or more of the following conditions:
  - Visual acuity 0.2 (6/30)
  - History of a fall with fracture in the previous year
  - History of frequent falling

- Type II diabetes (evidence available for women only)
- If currently using any of the following medications:
  - Anticonvulsant therapy
  - Opioids (including propoxyphene containing pain medication)
  - Corticosteroids (doses greater than prednisone 5 mg/day or equivalent)
  - Any psychotropic drug
  - Type Ia antiarrhythmics.
- Women ages 70 years and over with three or all of the following four personal history/lifestyle factors:
  - Smoking history
  - Personal history of any previous fracture
  - History of maternal hip fracture
  - Low body mass index.
- Women ages 65 years and older are at high risk if their bone mineral density (BMD) is 2 standard deviations (SDs) below normal for age (Z-score > −2.0), and 75 years and older if BMD is 1 SD below normal for age (Z-score > −1.0). The decision on prevention/treatment should take into account Z-score *AND* other risk factors.
- Men ages 75 years and older with any of the following personal history/lifestyle factors:
  - Low body mass index
  - Smoking history
  - History of spine, hip, or wrist fracture
  - History of stroke.
- Men ages 70 years and older are at high risk if their BMD is 2 SDs below normal for age (Z-score > −2.0), and 80 years and older if BMD is 1 SD below normal for age (Z-score > −1.0). The decision on prevention/treatment should take into account Z-score *AND* other risk factors.

Screening

- The available evidence does not support the use of BMD measurement for population screening of asymptomatic individuals.
- At present, there is only limited evidence that the use of BMD measurement in selected individuals is effective in reducing the risk of future fractures.

Recommendations for Preventive Strategies

Preventing Falls

- A program of muscle strengthening and balance training, individually prescribed by a trained health professional in a New Zealand primary health care setting, reduces the frequency of falls in high risk community-dwelling older people.

(continued)

Prevention of Hip Fracture in People Ages 65 Years and Older—*Continued*

RISK ASSESSMENT & PREVENTIVE STRATEGIES
FOR HIP FRACTURE IN OLDER PEOPLE

SUMMARY ALGORITHM

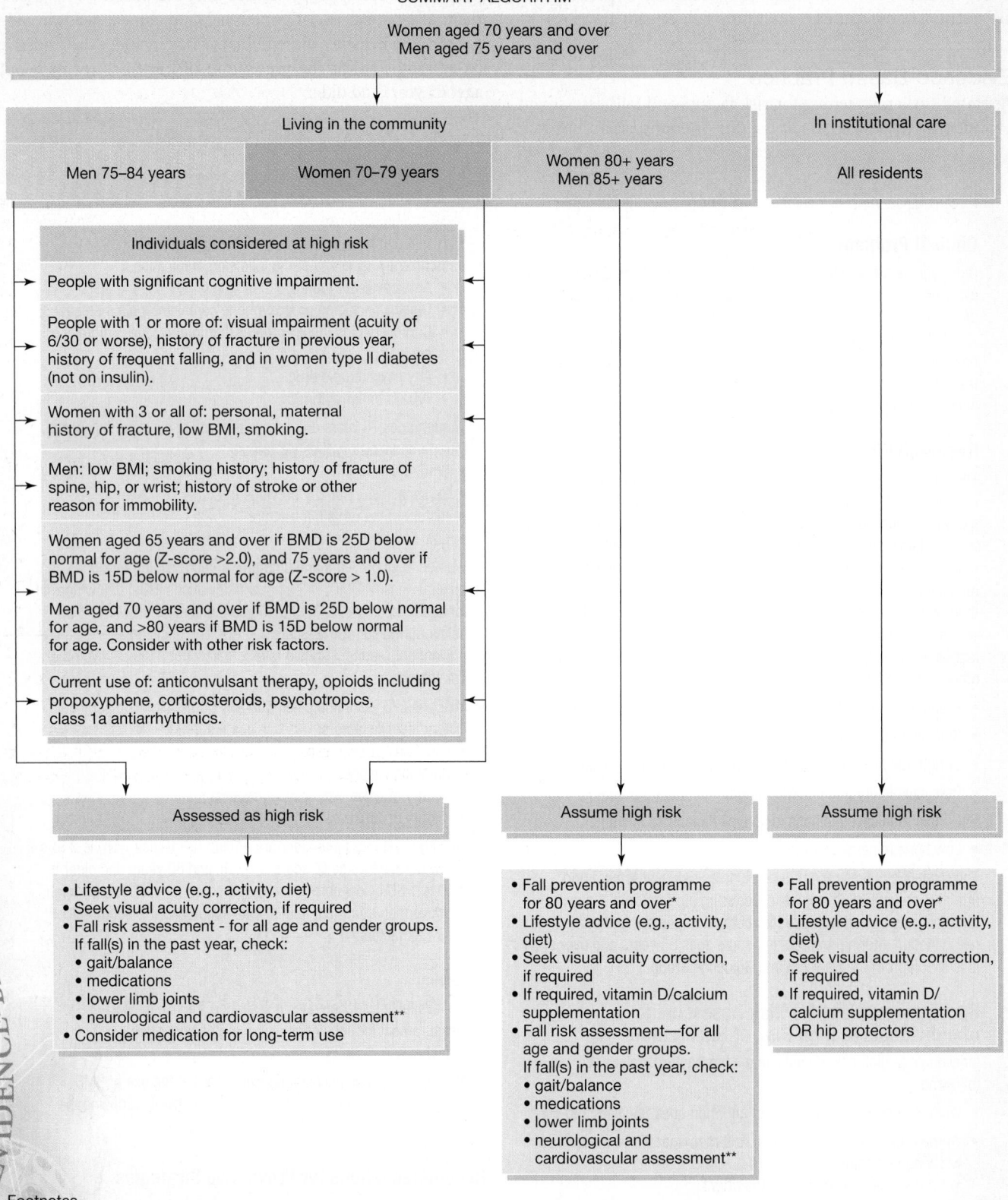

Women aged 70 years and over
Men aged 75 years and over

Living in the community | **In institutional care**

| Men 75–84 years | Women 70–79 years | Women 80+ years / Men 85+ years | All residents |

Individuals considered at high risk

People with significant cognitive impairment.

People with 1 or more of: visual impairment (acuity of 6/30 or worse), history of fracture in previous year, history of frequent falling, and in women type II diabetes (not on insulin).

Women with 3 or all of: personal, maternal history of fracture, low BMI, smoking.

Men: low BMI; smoking history; history of fracture of spine, hip, or wrist; history of stroke or other reason for immobility.

Women aged 65 years and over if BMD is 25D below normal for age (Z-score >2.0), and 75 years and over if BMD is 15D below normal for age (Z-score > 1.0).

Men aged 70 years and over if BMD is 25D below normal for age, and >80 years if BMD is 15D below normal for age. Consider with other risk factors.

Current use of: anticonvulsant therapy, opioids including propoxyphene, corticosteroids, psychotropics, class 1a antiarrhythmics.

Assessed as high risk

- Lifestyle advice (e.g., activity, diet)
- Seek visual acuity correction, if required
- Fall risk assessment - for all age and gender groups. If fall(s) in the past year, check:
  - gait/balance
  - medications
  - lower limb joints
  - neurological and cardiovascular assessment**
- Consider medication for long-term use

Assume high risk

- Fall prevention programme for 80 years and over*
- Lifestyle advice (e.g., activity, diet)
- Seek visual acuity correction, if required
- If required, vitamin D/calcium supplementation
- Fall risk assessment—for all age and gender groups. If fall(s) in the past year, check:
  - gait/balance
  - medications
  - lower limb joints
  - neurological and cardiovascular assessment**

Assume high risk

- Fall prevention programme for 80 years and over*
- Lifestyle advice (e.g., activity, diet)
- Seek visual acuity correction, if required
- If required, vitamin D/ calcium supplementation OR hip protectors

EVIDENCE-BASED PRACTICE

Footnotes
*From Figure 1, p666: American Geriatrics Society, British Geriatrics Society, and American Academy of Orthopaedic Surgeons Panel on Falls Prevention Guideline for the prevention of falls in older persons *Journal of the American Geriatrics Society 2001; 49:* 664-672.
**Refer.[24]

Source: This guideline was developed by William Gillespie (Convenor), John Campbell, Melinda Gardner, Lesley Gillespie, Jan Jackson, Clare Robertson, Jean-Claude Theis, and Raymond Jones. The consultation group included Marion Robinson, Heather Thomson, and Jim Reid. Published by New Zealand Guidelines Group Inc. Reproduced with permission from New Zealand Guidelines Group. Prevention of Hip Fracture amongst People aged 65 years and over. Guideline summary. Wellington: 2003.

- Multidisciplinary, multifactorial health/environmental screening/intervention programs reduce the frequency of falls in high-risk community-dwelling older people.

- Assessment, advice, and facilitation of home environment modification, when conducted in an experimental situation by a trained occupational therapist, reduces the frequency of falls in high-risk community-dwelling older people.

Medication for Bone Protection

- Daily supplementation with vitamin D and calcium reduces the hip fracture rates among high-risk older people in institutional care, or who have already sustained a hip fracture.

- Bisphosphonates (alendronate, risedronate) reduce hip and other fracture rates in community-dwelling older women under 80 years of age.

- Evidence for the effectiveness of hormone replacement therapy (HRT) in reducing hip fracture rates in women ages 65 years and older is conflicting. In view of more recent evidence on the risks of HRT, it is not recommended for first-line prevention of hip fracture. (Refer to Appendix C in full guideline or HRT Update Summary from the New Zealand Guidelines Group.)

Hip Protectors

- Hip protectors appear to reduce the incidence of hip fractures in older people in institutional care provided that compliance/adherence is achieved.

Choosing a Prevention Strategy— Current Estimates of Cost Effectiveness

- In frail older people in residential or nursing home care, calcium and vitamin D supplementation appears more cost effective than the use of hip pads, although both approaches have similar efficacy.

- The cost effectiveness of bisphosphonates compared with HRT is sensitive to compliance and the incidence of adverse events, and is unclear. (Refer to Appendix C in full guideline for current advice on HRT from the New Zealand Guidelines Group.)

- The overall cost effectiveness of fall prevention programs, compared with other strategies used for hip fracture prevention, is not known.

Implications for Nursing Practice

Nurses should screen older patients for risk factors for falling and increased potential for fractures. Using the findings, the nurse will educate the patient and family regarding ways to decrease their risks and to increase mobility and safety within their environment.

Critical Thinking Questions

1. How does screening for risk factors help to prevent hip fractures?

2. Why is exercise important in preventing fractures of the hip?

Answers to Critical Thinking Questions appear in Appendix D.

Osteomyelitis

Osteomyelitis is an infection of the bone that requires aggressive early treatment to decrease the amount of bone or joint damage.

Epidemiology

Unlike the "silent" onset of osteoporosis, osteomyelitis can have an acute, subacute, or chronic onset. The acute and chronic forms can present the same clinical picture. The bones that are most commonly involved include the upper ends of the humerus and tibia and the lower end of the femur. Occasionally the spinal vertebrae may be affected (Frazier & Drzymkowski, 2009).

The first line of defense for the bone is the skin; however, bones can become infected through the bloodstream, direct invasion, and infections in adjacent bone or soft tissues. One in 5,000 children may experience acute osteomyelitis (King et al., 2006). In general, children tend to have a higher incident of acute osteomyelitis and adults tend to present with subacute and chronic osteomyelitis (King et al., 2006; Mayo Clinic, 2007). Individuals with diabetes have a 16% risk factor for acquiring osteomyelitis. The problem with osteomyelitis is that symptoms develop over time and may go unnoticed for several days to a week. Individuals who experience vertebral osteomyelitis have a 10% to 15% risk of developing neurological problems due to spinal cord compression from the inflammatory process (King et al., 2006).

Etiology and Pathophysiology

The cause of the inflammatory process results from pyogenic organisms such as *Staphylococcus aureus, Staphylococcus epidermidis, Escherichia coli, Mycobacterium tuberculosis, Neisseria gonorrhoeae,* Pseudomonas, Salmonella, fungi, and mycobacteria. These organisms are not age discriminate and can affect anyone at any age. *Staphylococcus aureus* is responsible for 90% of

the infections followed by streptococcal bacteria (Frazier & Drzymkowski, 2009). Individuals who are at risk for developing osteomyelitis include individuals having a compromised immune system, diabetes, peripheral vascular disease, malignancies, and the presence of prosthetic hardware within the bone (Frazier & Drzymkowski, 2009).

Acute osteomyelitis falls into two categories: hematogenous and direct contact. Hematogenous osteomyelitis is an infection caused by bacterial infection from a distant site migrating by way of the bloodstream to the bone. It is commonly seen in children. Two common bone sites provide a rich environment for organism growth: the vascular metaphysic of growing bones and the distal metaphysic. The pyrogenic organism finds the rich blood supply of the metaphysic of the growing bone an ideal environment for receiving needed nutrients for growth and proliferation. A sharp angle at the distal metaphysic structure slows the blood, causing stagnation and thrombosis formation. The thrombosis formation can result in ischemia, leading to necrosis and bacterial growth (King, et al., 2006).

The other category of acute osteomyelitis, direct contact, results from direct trauma or surgery. It is the direct contact of bacteria or the implanting of bacteria from the outside environment that can cause infection. For example, osteomyelitis can be diagnosed following a surgical procedure. In this case, the disease process is localized to a specific bone but can potentially spread to surrounding tissues. Osteomyelitis resulting from direct trauma, injury, or surgery involves many organisms and the clinical manifestations tend to be more localized than those of hematogenous osteomyelitis (King et al., 2006).

Chronic osteomyelitis is typically associated with other disease processes. It is the primary disease process that predisposes the individual to bone infections. For example, individuals with diabetes have a higher incidence of osteomyelitis because of the poor circulation in the lower extremities and high level of blood sugar. Peripheral vascular disease, sickle cell anemia, and immune deficiency syndrome are just a few examples of other primary disease processes that predispose an individual to osteomyelitis (King et al., 2006).

In summary, osteomyelitis is a complex bone disorder with the potential for chronic and long-term effects. Therefore, medical diagnosis must be on the accurate classification of the cause (direct or indirect) and the organism involved. In some cases, young, rapidly growing, normal cells and cells subjected to inflammation and change in their blood supply can exhibit characteristics that may indicate bone tumor.

Clinical Manifestations

Clinical manifestations of osteomyelitis include the following symptoms: fever, edema at involved site, warmth to touch, tenderness at site, and movement or joint limitations at the involved site (i.e., contractures). The patient may have generalized complaints of fatigue and malaise. As the infection progresses a subperiosteal abscess may develop. The purulent material causes pressure and eventual fracturing of small pieces of bone.

Laboratory and Diagnostic Procedures

Lab tests that will help in the diagnosis of osteomyelitis include CBC and blood cultures. For the CBC, the white blood cells and leukocytes (leftward shift with increased polymorphonuclear leukocyte) will be elevated and the hemoglobin will be decreased. The erythrocyte sedimentation rate is also elevated. Needle aspiration of bone with culture of material taken is essential to identifying the causative organism.

Radiographic images in the initial stages may not be helpful. Eventually, the x-rays will demonstrate a swelling of overlying tissues and about 40% to 50% focal bone loss. An MRI may be helpful in making the diagnosis. MRI will differentiate soft tissue from bone marrow involvement and is useful for surgical localization of the osteomyelitis. Other tests include a bone scan and ultrasonography. The ultrasonograph can demonstrate soft tissue abscess or fluid collection and periosteal elevation.

Medical Management

Medical management in the acute phase focuses on treating the underlying cause for full recovery with minimal loss of function. Pharmacologic and surgical interventions are possible strategies. Management is geared toward preventing nonhealing of the wound, sepsis, immobility, and amputation.

Medical intervention may include immobilization of the affected bone and prescribing medications such as pain medicines and antibiotics. Pharmacologic interventions include the use of broad-spectrum antibiotics until organism sensitivity is obtained. Generally, antibiotics will be administered intravenously and may extend over a course of 4 to 6 weeks. Oral antibiotics may be prescribed following the completion of the intravenous (IV) antibiotics.

Surgery may be considered to incise the site and drain the abscess. If it is chronic osteomyelitis, surgery is recommended to remove the dead bone. The wound may require repeated debridement followed by frequent sterile dressing changes. It is suggested that patients be placed on drainage and secretion precautions.

Physical therapy may be ordered to maintain the patient's activity level and teach the patient how to use assistive devices during the no-weight-bearing stage. Healing requires adequate nutrition. A nutritionist may be consulted to assess caloric and protein intake. Dietary planning is based on the patient's need for calories, protein, and vitamins to promote healing.

A social worker or case manager may be another key member of the multidisciplinary team providing coordination of appropriate inpatient and outpatient care. When the patient is discharged, the home health nurse becomes important for following medical treatment in the home environment. In this disease process, strict adherence to the medical regimen is imperative to prevent the chronicity of the disease. Therefore, it is essential for the home health nurse to reinforce education on medication and appropriate lifestyle changes.

◼ Nursing Management

Nursing care focuses on rest, immobilization of the affected part, and administration of analgesics, antipyretics, and antibiotics. The affected extremity should be supported to facilitate adequate circulation and proper alignment to prevent contractures (Christensen & Kockrow, 2003). Preventive care will include monitoring the wound, performing prescribed wound care, preventing dehydration, reinforcing adherence to the antibiotic regimen, and regular follow-up. See the Nursing Process: Patient Care Plan for Osteomyelitis feature for more details.

Education focuses on information about the disease process, medications, signs of inflammation, and changes that might indicate worsening of the condition. If osteomyelitis is not treated properly, it can become chronic. In such cases the individual may go home with an indwelling catheter or PICC line for antibiotics. The patient and family members will need education on how to care for the intravenous types of lines. The Patient Teaching & Discharge Priorities for Osteomyelitis box (p. 1748) lists other aspects of patient education.

Osteitis Deformans (Paget's Disease)

Osteitis deformans is a chronic disorder that causes irregular bone breakdown and formation, which in turn causes the bones to weaken. This results in pain, bone deformities, fractures, and arthritis.

Epidemiology and Etiology

The cause of osteitis deformans is unknown. It can occur in only a portion of one bone, the entire bone, or many bones throughout the skeletal system. The most common sites are the pelvis and tibia. Other less affected areas include the femur, clavicle, skull, and spine. The disease usually presents in patients older than 40 years of age and becomes increasingly more common with age (Frazier & Drzymkowski, 2009).

Pathophysiology

With this disease, the affected areas of bone produce new bone faster than old bone can be broken down. The disease usually occurs in two stages: the vascular stage, in which bone tissue is broken down but the spaces are filled with blood vessels and fibrous tissue rather than new bone; and the sclerotic stage, in

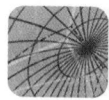

NURSING PROCESS: Patient Care Plan for Osteomyelitis

Assessment of Pain
Subjective Data:
On a scale of 1–10 with one being a little pain and 10 being the worst pain you have ever felt, at what level is your pain?
Do you routinely take pain medication at home? If yes, what is the name of the medication and why do you take it?
Are you allergic to any medications?

Objective Data:
Monitor patient for:
Facial grimacing
Change in breathing pattern
Change in blood pressure and/or pulse rate
Diaphoresis
Agitation

Nursing Assessment and Diagnoses	Outcomes and Evaluation Parameters	Planning and Interventions with *Rationales*
Nursing Diagnosis: *Pain, Acute* related to inflammation	**Outcome:** Pain level will be tolerable. *Evaluation Parameter:* Patient will not exhibit symptoms of pain and will verbalize pain control.	**Interventions and *Rationales:* Nonpharmacologic:** Reduce lighting and noise, and provide room for the patient's significant others. Cultural and spiritual factors such as prayer, ritual, and music can also increase the patient's comfort. *Promotes relaxation and comfort.* **Pharmacologic:** Medicate the patient with narcotics and nonsteroidal anti-inflammatory drugs as ordered. Assess for effectiveness. *Bone pain is usually severe.* Elevate and support the affected extremity. *Elevating the extremity reduces edema by enhancing venous return. Supportive positioning protects against muscle strain.* Teach the patient to report increasing or uncontrolled pain. *Increasing pain may indicate ineffective therapy or worsening infection.*

Assessment of Knowledge of Treatment Regimen
Subjective Data:
Do you understand which medications you are taking and when to take them?
Can you tell me what osteomyelitis is?
What is your weight-bearing status?

Objective Data:
Patient takes medications as prescribed.
Patient demonstrates proper wound care.
Patient reports no elevation of temperature or recurrence of pain or other symptoms at the site.

Nursing Assessment and Diagnoses	Outcomes and Evaluation Parameters	Planning and Interventions with *Rationales*
Nursing Diagnosis: *Knowledge, Deficient* related to treatment regimen	**Outcome:** The patient will comply with therapeutic plan. *Evaluation Parameters:* The patient will take medications on time, demonstrate proper wound care, and report signs or symptoms of complications quickly.	**Interventions and *Rationales:*** Teach the patient and family the importance of adhering to the therapeutic regimen. *Knowledge regarding the reasons for the therapeutic plan and the consequences that may occur if not followed will motivate the patient to adhere.*

Assessment of Nutritional Intake
Subjective Data:
Describe your usual intake pattern.
Is this intake sufficient?
Do you have religious dietary restrictions or practices?
How often do you exercise?
Who prepares your meals?
Do you feel you have enough energy?

Objective Data:
General appearance
Weight
Hair, nails, and skin
Muscle mass
Edema

(continued)

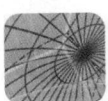

NURSING PROCESS: Patient Care Plan for Osteomyelitis—*Continued*

Nursing Assessment and Diagnoses	Outcomes and Evaluation Parameters	Planning and Interventions with *Rationales*
Nursing Diagnosis: *Nutrition, Imbalanced: Less Than Body Requirements*	**Outcome:** The patient will maintain adequate nutrition to assist with healing. ***Evaluation Parameter:*** Maintenance of weight without loss of muscle mass.	**Interventions and *Rationales:*** Facilitate education with a dietary consultant. *Consultation can ensure a diet that provides optimal caloric and nutrient intake.* Encourage frequent oral hygiene. *Poor oral hygiene leads to bad breath and a bad taste in the mouth, which decreases the appetite.* Provide the patient with printed material outlining the dietary needs and restrictions. *Aids the patient in selecting the proper foods.* Promote the intake of protein foods with high biologic value: eggs, meats, diary products. *Complete proteins provide the positive nitrogen balance needed for growth and healing.* Promote the intake of foods high in protein and vitamins A, B, and C. Common food sources include meat, fish, poultry, fortified cereals, dairy products, dark green and yellow vegetables, citrus fruits/juices, potatoes, cauliflower, and tomatoes. *Promotes cell regeneration.*

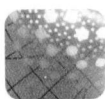

PATIENT TEACHING & DISCHARGE PRIORITIES for Osteomyelitis

Need	Teaching
Nutrition: • Patient and family	Work with dietitian to plan a high-protein diet rich in vitamins A, B, and C to promote cell regeneration.
Medications: • Patient	Stress importance of taking prescribed antibiotics as scheduled even if patient is feeling better. Teach the patient the signs and symptoms of any side effects that may occur.
Safety: • Patient and family	Stress importance of a safe environment to prevent falls and possible fractures. Teach the proper use of any assistive devices that may be required.
Avoidance of continued infections: • Patient and family	Stress the importance of reporting signs of infection. If patients require long-term antibiotics they will require a special intravenous line such as a PICC. Education for maintenance of the catheter and the importance of aseptic technique should be emphasized. Stress importance of follow-up appointments to assess therapeutic effectiveness.

which the vascular fibrous tissue hardens and is similar to bone but is fragile, leading to pathologic fractures (Frazier & Drzymkowski, 2009).

Clinical Manifestations

Osteitis deformans rarely causes symptoms. When symptoms do occur they usually include bone pain at the site. The pain can become disabling because it is constant and worse at night. Patients may experience edema or deformity at the affected site. If the ossicles of the ear are involved, hearing loss or deafness will occur. Complications of the disease include pathologic fractures, hypercalcemia, renal calculi, spinal cord injury, and occasionally development of bone sarcoma (Frazier & Drzymkowski, 2009).

Laboratory and Diagnostic Procedures

Radiographic imaging, bone scanning, and a bone marrow biopsy assist with diagnosis. Serum lab results will show an elevated alkaline phosphatase, and urinalysis will reveal an elevated hydroxyproline concentration. Both results indicate a high rate of bone production.

Medical Management

Treatment of osteitis deformans is symptom based. Treatment goals are the relief of pain and prevention of bone loss. Injections of the hormone calcitonin may be given to regulate the level of calcium in the blood and help prevent bone loss. A diet high in protein, calcium, and vitamin D also helps to prevent bone loss, especially if the use of bisphosphonate medications has been added to the treatment plan (Frazier & Drzymkowski, 2009).

◼ Nursing Management

The goals of nursing management include education regarding the disease process and palliative treatment of symptoms. It is important to teach the patient that exercise is an important part of the treatment plan to stimulate bone growth and maintain flexibility and strength. Maintaining a healthy weight is also important to avoid undue stress on affected bones.

Benign Bone Tumors

Bone tumor is an abnormal growth of the bone cells and can be benign or cancerous. The tumors can be from cartilage (chondrogenic), from bone (osteogenic), or from fibrous tissue (fibrogenic). Benign bone tumors do not spread to other tissues or organs.

Epidemiology

Generally, adults over the age of 40 years and children ages 10 years or younger are at a higher risk for developing bone tumors. Examples of benign bone tumors include aneurysmal bone cyst, osteochondroma, fibrous dysplasia, chondroblastoma, and osteoid osteoma.

Etiology and Pathophysiology

Bone tumors can be classified according to their origins or as benign or malignant. Benign bone tumors generally are not life threatening, present few symptoms, and do not result in death. A tumor in the bone causes the normal bone tissue to react by osteolytic response (bone destruction) or osteoblastic response (bone formation). Bone tissue cells are very active and new bone is constantly forming and old bone is dissolving. Bone tumors result from an abnormal growth of cells that can originate from bone cells, cartilage, fibrous tissue, marrow, or vascular tissue.

Generally benign tumors illustrate the geographical pattern by having a slow symmetrical growth pattern. Slow erosion can cause bone destruction and may cause the adjacent normal bone to respond to the tumor by altering its normal pattern of remodeling. The bone's surface changes and the contours enlarge in the tumor areas. Because adjacent tendons and muscles provide structural support for the bone, as the adjacent tissues are displaced, the bone becomes weakened and fracture can result. A few examples of benign bone tumors include nonossifying fibroma, osteochondroma, osteoma, osteoblastoma, enchondroma (Ollier's disease), bone cyst, chondroblastoma, and giant cell tumor (McCance & Huether, 2006). Osteochondroma accounts for 35% to 50% of all benign tumors (Copstead & Banaski, 2005). Pathologic characteristics of bone tumors include bone destruction, attrition, or expansion of the cortex and also periosteal response to changes in underlying bone (McCance & Huether, 2006).

Clinical Manifestations

There are two predominant clinical manifestations for benign tumors: Pressure around surrounding tissues may cause pain, and range of motion may be affected if the tumor becomes too large. Pain is usually the presenting symptom and is often worse at night or after exercise. At times bone tumors produce no symptoms and are detected when the weakened bone fractures.

Diagnostic Procedures

Radiographs, CT scan, radionuclide bone scan, and/or MRI can be used to diagnose the tumor.

Medical Management

The treatment for bone tumors, whether benign or malignant, is surgical excision. Surrounding muscle and other tissue are of-

ten removed and bone grafting may be needed. Amputation may be required depending on the tumor site and extent. Surgical removal alone is enough to treat benign bone tumors.

◼ Nursing Management

The care of patients with bone tumors is preventive in nature. Health promotion revolves around monitoring the size of the bone tumor. If the tumor is removed surgically, nursing and collaborative care will focus on preparing the patient for surgery followed by monitoring and prevention of postop complications. For the care of the patient undergoing orthopedic surgery, refer to Chapter 57 ⊕ .

Bone Cancer and Bone Metastases

The most common types of primary bone cancer include osteosarcoma, chondrosarcoma, and Ewing's sarcoma (Frazier & Drzymkowski, 2009).

Epidemiology

In the year 2008 it was estimated that 2,380 new cases of bone and joint cancer would be diagnosed. Approximately 1,470 deaths are expected from these cancers. Osteosarcoma is the most common bone cancer (35% of the reported cases), followed by chondrosarcoma (26% of the reported cases) and Ewing's sarcoma (16% of the reported cases) (American Cancer Society [ACS], 2008).

Osteosarcoma usually presents in young people between the ages of 10 and 30. A small percentage of cases (10%) develop in people who are greater than 60 years of age (ACS, 2008). Osteosarcoma has a greater incidence in males than females and the tumor most often develops in the arm, leg, or pelvis.

Chondrosarcoma is a cancer of cartilage cells and is uncommon in people younger than 20 years of age. After the age of 20, the risk of developing the cancer continues to rise until the person reaches the age of 75. The incidence is equal for men and women (ACS, 2008). Chondrosarcoma may present anywhere in the body where there is cartilage, but the most common sites are the pelvis, leg, and arm bone. It will occasionally present in the trachea, larynx, and chest wall.

Ewing's sarcoma is a primary malignant bone tumor in the pediatric and adolescent population. It usually occurs in the second decade of life and approximately 80% of cases are in people younger than 20 years of age (Lahl, Fisher, & Laschinger, 2007). Although there is no significant difference between the races in the incidence of osteosarcoma, there is a significantly higher incident of Ewing's sarcoma in Caucasian children when compared to children of the same age from the African American population (Lahl et al., 2007). Ewing tumors form in the cavity of the bone and most often present in the long bones of the leg and arm.

Etiology and Pathophysiology

Bone metastasis and primary bone cancer are two separate disease processes and are treated differently. Secondary tumors arise from cells that have broken off from the original tumor site and enter the lymph system or bloodstream and travel to that specific area. Bone metastases are generally observed in patients who have had a relapse in their cancer. Approximately 75% of the bone metastases originate from carcinomas of the prostate, breast, kidney, and lung. To a lesser extent, other cancers that spread to the bone can come from the following cancers: thyroid, colon, and melanoma. The bones most commonly affected are the pelvis, vertebrae, ribs, femur, and humerus (Frazier & Drzymkowski, 2009).

Malignant bone tumors that are primary tumors are rare and typically emerge from connective and supportive tissue cells. Primary malignant bone tumors account for greater than 85% of bone tumors in the pediatric population, but are rarely seen after the age of 30 (Frazier & Drzymkowski, 2009). The exact cause of bone cancer is unknown.

Recent findings suggest that an individual's DNA can become defective or mutated. Oncogenes promote cell division and tumor suppressor genes cause cells to die or slow down cell division. DNA mutations can activate oncogenes or inactivate tumor suppressor genes. Also, it has been determined that individuals with bone cancer can inherit mutations from their parents. As a result, cancerous cells form a tumor and invade and destroy adjacent bone tissue. The rate of growth of the tumor and the response to treatment depends on the type of cancer involved. Most bone cancers are not inherited, but a result of mutations acquired. For instance, radiation is used as a treatment for some cancers, but can also cause cancer by damaging DNA. Bones that are exposed to radiation as a treatment are more likely to develop bone cancer later (ACS, 2008; see Chapter 11).

Bone destruction from the tumor can result in one of three different types of patterns: (1) geographic pattern, (2) moth-eaten pattern, or (3) permeative pattern. With the geographic pattern, the tumor edges have well-defined margins. In the moth-eaten pattern, the margins are less defined and are easily separated from the bone. When the margins are not clear and abnormal lytic bone merges with normal bone, this is suggestive of the permeative pattern (McCance & Huether, 2006). Bone tumors that are considered malignant include osteosarcoma, chondrosarcoma, chordoma, and Ewing tumor. Lymphoma and multiple myeloma also start in the bones, but are not considered bone cancer because they develop in the lymph nodes and in the plasma cells, respectively.

Osteosarcoma is the most common primary bone cancer and usually presents between the ages of 10 and 15 years old. It usually develops in the distal femur, followed by the proximal tibia and humerus. Most patients die within 2 years due to metastasis to the lung. Risk factors include Paget's disease, PTH injections for osteoporosis, and radiation therapy for other forms of cancer (Frazier & Drzymkowski, 2009).

Ewing's sarcoma involves the pelvis and lower extremity. The tumor usually presents between the ages of 4 and 25 years of age. The tumor is invasive and extends into the soft tissue. Metastasis occurs early and is usually to the lungs and other bones (Frazier & Drzymkowski, 2009). Chondrosarcoma also involves the pelvis and lower extremity, but usually presents between the ages of 30 and 60 years old. The tumor grows slowly and is locally invasive (Frazier & Drzymkowski, 2009).

Clinical Manifestations

Due to the destruction, erosion, and expansion of the tumor, pain is the primary symptom. The intensity of the pain can be mild to severe. If a fracture is sustained, the patient will have acute pain. As a result of swelling, the patient may experience range-of-motion (ROM) limitation and joint effusion. The area may be tender to palpation and warm to touch with superficial blood vessels noticeable. Osteosarcoma begins with pain and swelling and a "sunburst" appearance on radiograph. Ewing's sarcoma presents with pain and swelling, fever, fatigue, anemia, and leukocytosis. On radiograph the tumor has an "onion skin" appearance. Chondrosarcomas are slow growing so the pain is intermittent and dull. The tumor presents a lobular pattern on radiograph.

Laboratory and Diagnostic Procedures

Radiographs are useful in demonstrating tumor activity and will show increases and decreases in bone density. A bone scan can detect the extent of the malignancy and help follow the planned therapy. CT and MRI will demonstrate soft tissue involvement and the exact location of the tumor.

Lab tests will include chemistry and CBC. Serum alkaline phosphatase is generally elevated. In some situations, the hematologic lab values will be altered. Other tests include bone biopsy, arteriography, chest x-ray, and lung scan to detect metastasis.

Medical Management

The treatment of bone cancer is best achieved by a multidisciplinary team. The objective or the goal is to slow the growth of the tumor by destroying and removing the lesion. Depending on the specific type of bone tumor, chemotherapy, surgery, radiation, or a combination of these treatments may be used.

■ Nursing Management

The care of the patient with bone cancer is challenging. Therapeutic management might include chemotherapy, radiologic therapy, surgery, and pharmacologic interventions. Chemotherapy may be administered prior to having surgery done and then to prevent metastases. A combination of therapies may be used to achieve optimal response and minimize potential drug resistance. Immunotherapy and hormone therapy may also be used. Supportive care may need to be given during the course of the disease and involves case workers, social workers, and hospice.

The primary focus of nursing care is relief of pain, prevention of pathologic fractures, and provision of a supportive environment. The nursing care will involve the patient's response to pain control measures, side effects of the pain medications, chemotherapy, and radiation therapy. Nursing care that focuses on preoperative and postoperative care may be implemented if a surgical procedure is indicated (see Chapter 57). If the stage of cancer is advanced, pathologic bone fractures may occur; therefore, inactivity would be encouraged. For a detailed discussion of care for the patient with cancer, refer to Chapter 64 .

■ Muscular Disorders

This section of the chapter details various types of muscle diseases. Although several of these diseases are not very common, it is important for nurses to understand both the pathophysiology of the conditions and the associated nursing care considerations that are required to fully care for these patients. After completion of this section, the nurse will be able to formulate critical thinking skills associated with these uncommon but debilitating and sometimes chronic disorders.

Muscular Dystrophies

Muscular dystrophies are a group of genetic myopathies caused by a protein deficiency in muscle membranes. In other words, a person's DNA is not producing a particular protein named dystrophin that is required by muscles and muscle membranes to function properly. Therefore, a person with a muscular dystrophy has progressive muscle weakness leading to an inability to control any voluntary movement (Figure 55–5 ■). The muscles eventually atrophy from nonuse. Skeletal muscles are not the only muscles affected by muscular dystrophy. The cardiac muscle and diaphragm may be affected as well (Muscular Dystrophy Association [MDA], 2008).

Genetics

Genetics play the key role in whether a child develops muscular dystrophy (MD). Muscular dystrophy occurs when a gene on the X chromosome fails to make the protein dystrophin. Without dystrophin, muscle cells are unable to function properly, leading to skeletal muscle weakness or failure. Most children afflicted with muscular dystrophy are males, because male children have only one X chromosome (from the mother). If that X chromosome is not producing dystrophin, then the child will develop MD. Female children receive X chromosomes from both parents, so even if one X chromosome is flawed, it is likely that the other X chromosome can provide the dystrophin, and she will have few or no symptoms, but will be a carrier (Figure 55–6 ■). Even though the incidence of MD is mostly in males, MD weakness develops in 2.5% to 20% of females. The incidence in male children is about 1 in 3,500 live male births (Centers for Disease Control and Prevention [CDC], 2008a; MDA, 2008).

Duchenne Muscular Dystrophy

In children, especially male children, the most prevalent muscular dystrophy is Duchenne muscular dystrophy (DMD). In

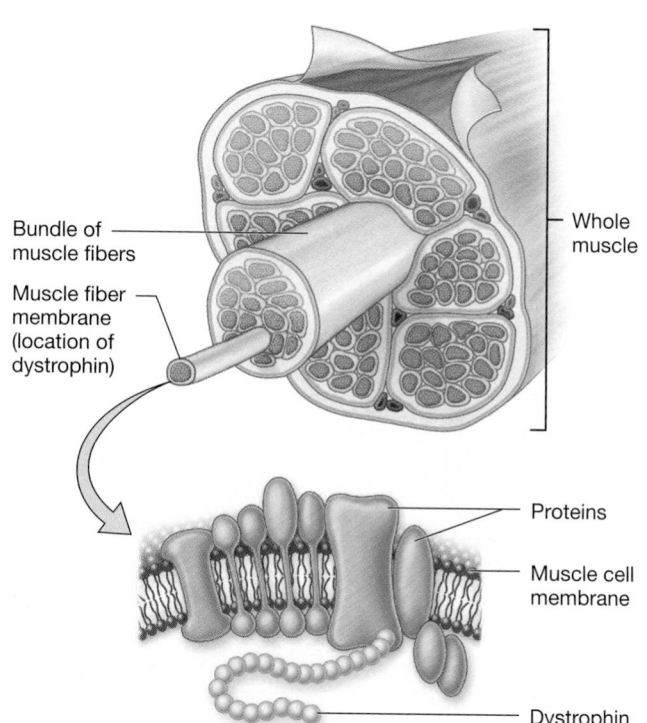

FIGURE 55–5 ■ Muscle fiber membrane.

Bundle of muscle fibers
Muscle fiber membrane (location of dystrophin)
Whole muscle
Proteins
Muscle cell membrane
Dystrophin

Example of X-linked recessive inheritance

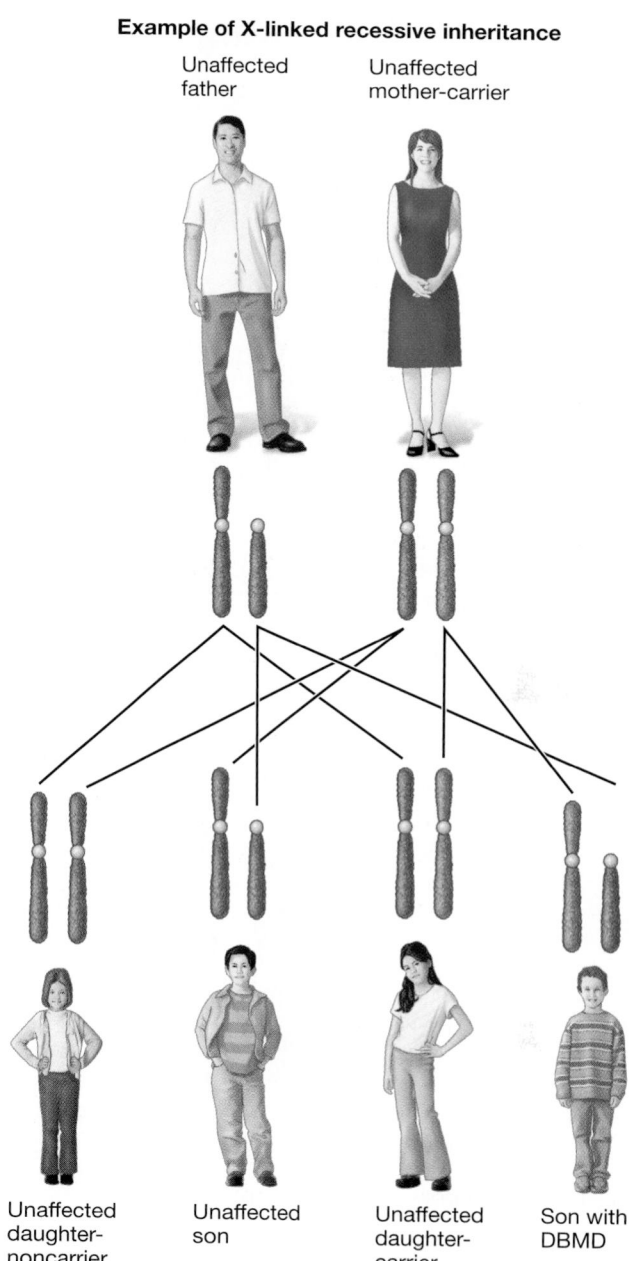

Unaffected father
Unaffected mother-carrier

Unaffected daughter-noncarrier
Unaffected son
Unaffected daughter-carrier
Son with DBMD

FIGURE 55–6 ■ Muscular dystrophy inheritance pattern.

Duchenne muscular dystrophy, there is a complete absence of dystrophin. Muscle weakness and loss of muscle develop gradually, with signs usually first appearing when the child is 2 through 6 years old, but symptoms generally are exhibited about age 3 (CDC, 2008a). Weakness starts near the trunk then progresses to the extremities about 3 to 5 years after the initial weakness is experienced. Most commonly, the lower extremities are affected before the upper extremities (Figure 55–7 ■, p. 1752).

The weakness begins with the child having difficulty with simple tasks, such as maintaining his or her balance, and it leads to an inability to perform activities such as climbing stairs or getting up from a bed or chair. Children afflicted with DMD are late starters in learning to walk and as toddlers have enlarged calf muscles. By school age, the child has an unsteady gait and falls quite often, almost appearing clumsy. The child uses the Gowers' maneuver to rise up from the floor (Figure 55–8 ■, p. 1752). The

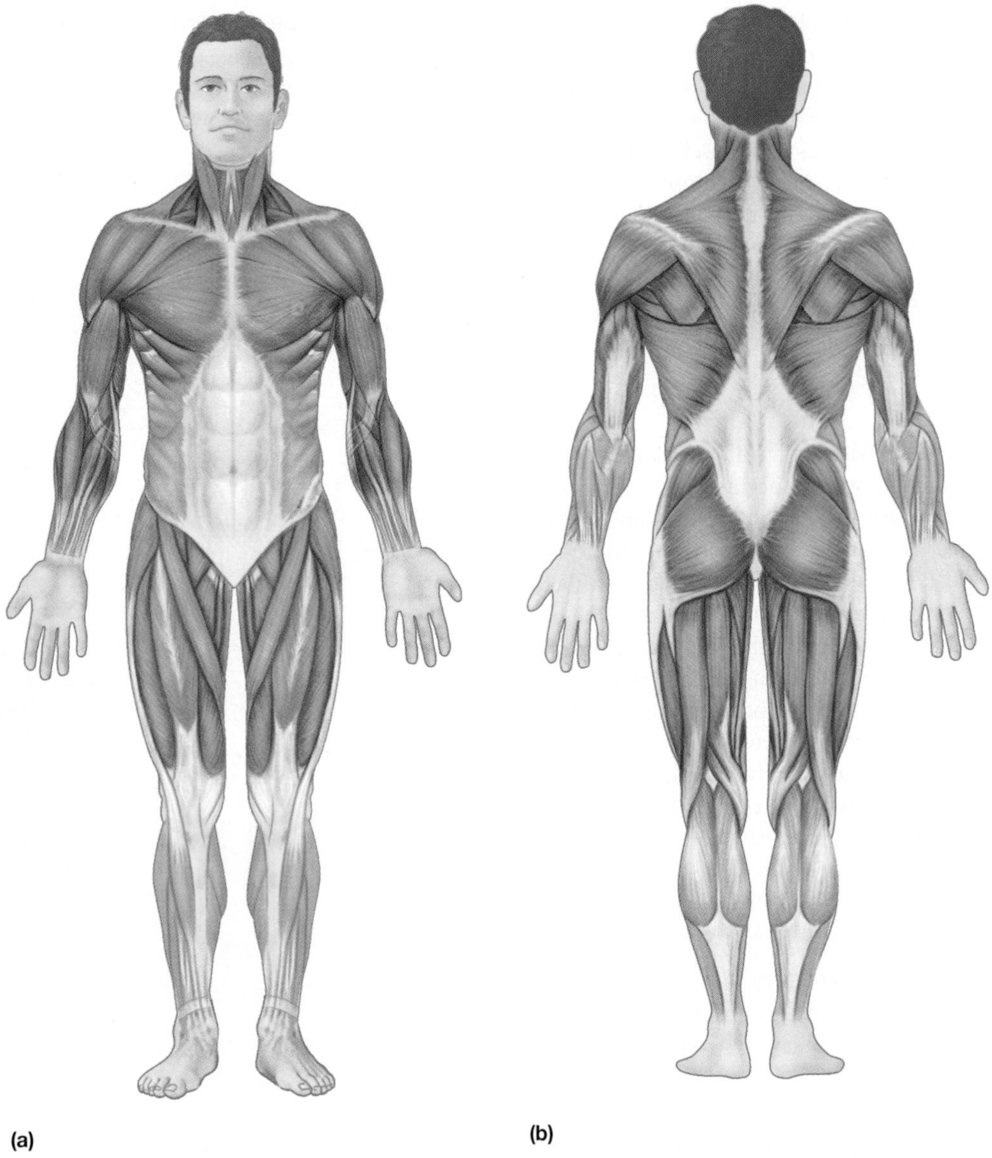

(a) (b)

FIGURE 55–7 ■ Muscles affected by muscular dystrophy.

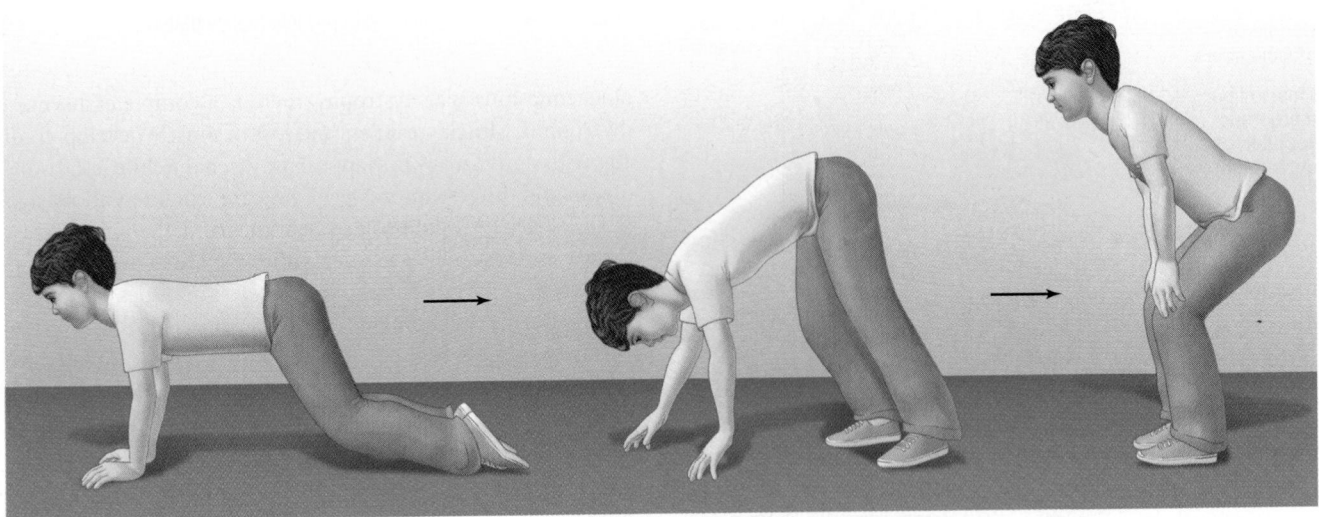

FIGURE 55–8 ■ Gowers' maneuver.

Gowers' maneuver involves the child getting on his hands and knees, then raising his rear end, which allows the child to walk on his hands and knees, and then achieving a standing position. The child often walks on the toes or balls of his feet with a waddling gait. To compensate for a lack of balance, the child sticks his abdomen out and puts his shoulders back (MDA, 2008). The child also has difficulty running, and generally is unable to jump or hop. Between the ages of 7 and 12, the child will no longer be able to walk and will use a wheelchair. Adolescents are usually unable to perform daily tasks, such as eating, with their arms, hands, or fingers. The course of the disease is progressive and usually fatal in the teens or early 20s. Death is usually due to respiratory or heart problems (CDC, 2008a).

Becker Muscular Dystrophy

Becker muscular dystrophy (BMD) is a less common type of MD, and the disease is generally milder than DMD. In BMD, some dystrophin is produced and it does not manifest itself until a person is in his teens or young adulthood when the person notices himself becoming weaker than usual when engaging in physical exercise or activities. This weakness is usually first noticed in the pelvic and hip area, the thighs, and the shoulders. The severity and progression of the disease vary depending on the amount of dystrophin that is being released. The child/adolescent generally has a normal IQ for age.

Complications Associated with Duchenne or Becker Muscular Dystrophy

Several serious and sometimes life-threatening complications may result from DMD or BMD.

Cardiomyopathy
The most serious complications involve the cardiac and respiratory systems. As discussed in Chapter 41 ⊙, cardiomyopathy is due to cardiac muscle weakening, a direct result of the absence or lack of dystrophin. Cardiomyopathy leads to heart failure, which is a major cause of death in patients with muscular dystrophy. Primary dilated cardiomyopathy and conduction abnormalities develop with DMD. Most MD patients usually do not become symptomatic until they are in their teens, probably due to their lack of ability to exercise. Approximately 70% of those with BMD develop cardiomyopathy. As discussed in Chapter 41 ⊙, patients with cardiomyopathy have shortness of breath, fluid in the lungs characterized by crackles or rhonchi, and lower extremity edema due to the heart muscle's inability to pump. Boys afflicted with muscular dystrophy often die from heart failure by the time they are in their 20s (CDC, 2008a).

Respiratory Distress
Children with muscular dystrophy have an increased risk for weakness of the diaphragm and other ancillary muscles that assist in ventilation (MDA, 2008). If the diaphragm and other muscles are weak, then the child will have trouble expanding the chest to allow for effective inspiration and expiration. These children also have trouble coughing. Difficulty coughing coupled with weak, poor inspiratory/expiratory effort places MD patients at high risk for respiratory infections. Simply being in a room with someone who has a mild rhinitis or cold can predispose these children to pneumonia. With progression of the disease, many of the children will require long-term assisted mechanical ventilation or a tracheostomy. In addition, because patients with muscular dystrophy are prone to respiratory infections, it is extremely important for them to be current with their pneumococcal and flu vaccinations.

Muscle Atrophy and Contractures
When a muscle is weak and unused, it deteriorates and shortens, leaving the associated joint prone to a permanent flexed position called a *contracture*, the shortening of a muscle attached to a joint. Contractures can affect the knee, elbow, wrist, hip, and finger joints. If preventive measures are not taken, contractures can become permanent, causing total loss of mobility to the affected joint, as well as discomfort. To prevent such contractures, it is important for all joints to be passively exercised.

Cognitive Effects
Around one-third of the boys affected with Duchenne muscular dystrophy have some form of a progressive learning disability (MDA, 2008). In addition, some children with DMD have some level of mental retardation. Researchers believe that the lack of dystrophin in the brain affects the child's cognitive, behavioral, and intellectual abilities. Specific cognitive and intellectual skills affected are verbal skills, memory, attention, and focusing skills. In addition, some boys have difficulty with emotional interaction (MDA, 2008). School counselors, psychologists, and neuropsychologists can educate the family in techniques that may assist with learning and interaction skills.

Spinal Abnormalities
Exaggerated curvature of the spine is prevalent in young adults with Duchenne muscular dystrophy. The three types of curvatures are **lordosis**, or swayback, noticed mostly in those young men who are still able to ambulate; **scoliosis**, or a lateral curvature of the spine; and **kyphosis**, or hunchback. Scoliosis that is severe can lead to respiratory problems, sleeping problems, and the inability to sit straight or remain seated for prolonged periods of time.

Treatment for spinal curvatures consists of attaching metal rods to the spine to help keep the spine in straight alignment.

Osteoporosis
Normally, muscles exert pressure on the bones they are attached to, which helps to maintain the strength of the bones. The weakening of muscles from muscular dystrophy can lead to weakening of bones, or osteoporosis. The bones become very thin and brittle, which can lead to pathologic fractures. In patients with muscular dystrophy, simple daily activities, such as lifting a heavy object or twisting, may cause a bone to break. Many patients in wheelchairs experience pathologic fractures due to their inability to bear weight.

Laboratory and Diagnostic Procedures

Diagnosis of muscular dystrophy is based on signs and symptoms noted specifically in toddlers in the prewalking or walking phase. Observance of the Gowers' maneuver is a telltale sign of muscular dystrophy. Other affirmation of the disease includes an elevated level of serum creatinine kinase (CK), an enzyme that is found in skeletal muscles. Normally there are high levels of CK in the muscle and low levels in the blood. With MD, there is a breakdown of the muscle membrane and CK leaks out into the blood. The patient with MD will have a CK level that is 20 to 200 times higher than normal and is increased from the time of birth (CDC, 2008a).

Genetic testing may be done to look for a mutation in the dystrophin gene. The test first looks for large pieces of the gene that are missing or duplicated. If a deletion or duplication is found in the dystrophin gene, the diagnosis is confirmed. Sixty-five to 70% of patients with DMD or BMD will have a deletion or duplication (CDC, 2008a).

Other diagnostic tests include a muscle biopsy of the involved muscle to document the absence of dystrophin. An **electromyelogram (EMG)** will differentiate between a myopathy and neuropathy. An electromyelogram is important in the diagnosis of muscular dystrophy because it measures electrical activity in muscles and can demonstrate the muscle damage that is associated with muscular dystrophy.

Pulmonary function tests and an electrocardiogram (ECG) may be done to evaluate degree of respiratory or cardiac involvement.

Medical Management

At this time there is no specific treatment for muscular dystrophy; however, modalities such as medications, exercise, and diet may enhance the mobility of the patient and ability to move and function independently as long as possible.

Medications A glucocorticoid such as prednisone, which has an anti-inflammatory effect, has been shown to delay the progression of the disease and to improve muscle mass (Frazier & Drzymkowski, 2009). Prednisone must be prescribed cautiously, however, due to its numerous side effects.

Exercise Exercise is important in people afflicted with muscular dystrophy. The function of ambulating should be encouraged because it maintains the motion of a joint and prevents the joint from contracting. Passive range-of-motion (PROM) exercises are helpful in preventing contractures of the joints if the patient cannot actively exercise. PROM exercises must be performed on each joint at least every 4 hours while the patient is awake to prevent the muscles and tendons associated with the joints from shortening or atrophying. A child who can walk should continue to walk, even if only short distances, for as many months or years as he is able. Walking is an exercise that helps to maintain muscle strength and mobility. If the child cannot or does not walk, the muscles will lose strength and atrophy more quickly.

An alternative exercise therapy method called Watsu is being utilized by people with physical disabilities. Watsu involves the person doing limb and muscle stretching while floating in warm water, either actively or passively. The stated benefits of Watsu include total relaxation and a calming effect, not only to the limbs and muscles but to the patient as well (Osborn, 2005). General aquatic therapy in warm water also maintains the muscle tone.

Diet The nurse should assess dietary considerations for patients with muscular dystrophy. Patients with muscular dystrophy have certain specific nutritional requirements for health maintenance. A well-balanced diet is imperative for several reasons. Because the muscles are in the process of breaking down, and because maintenance of muscle mass is necessary to keep MD patients in good health, the muscles have high energy requirements. Moreover, they require high protein intake. MD patients typically require 68% more protein in their diets than average healthy adults (Leighton, 2003).

It is also important for MD patients to maintain a reasonable body weight. Obesity can cause exacerbation or worsening of respiratory and cardiac dysfunction, whereas weight loss can signify muscle wasting and decreasing energy stores and can further complicate an already weakened cardiac and respiratory system. Constipation due to immobility is also a potential complication of muscular dystrophy. Therefore, it is important that people diagnosed with muscular dystrophy consume at least eight glasses of water a day (unless contraindicated by other health conditions) and eat a diet high in fiber, which may avoid constipation.

Nursing Implications Regarding Diet It is important for weight measurement and monitoring to be a part of the patient's care plan. When assisting a patient with meal planning, the nurse should encourage a diet high in protein, fiber, minerals, and vitamins. A referral to a dietitian may be warranted if weight loss or significant weight gain is noted. It is also important for the nurse to be cognizant of upper extremity involvement in a patient with MD, because the patient will need to be fed.

Physical Therapy Physical therapy is aimed at prolonging muscle strength and thus preventing contractures. Both active and passive ROM exercises are indicated, and walking is encouraged if possible to enhance strength and stamina. Physical therapy should also focus on gait training and transfer training. When ambulation is lost, the patient needs to see a physical therapist for customization of a wheelchair, for recommendations about devices that assist with ADLs, and for help accomplishing tasks.

Occupational Therapy Occupational therapy focuses on exercises that allow the patient with MD to perform ADLs such as eating, dressing, or brushing teeth. Whereas physical therapy focuses on gross motor movements, occupational therapy focuses more on the maintenance of fine motor movements.

Braces and Standing Walkers Braces may be used to support the ankles and feet of an ambulatory child with MD. Braces are also utilized to prevent plantar flexion, a type of contracture. A standing walker can assist the patient to stand, thus promoting circulation and allowing the patient to bear weight on her joints.

Research

Current medical research into muscular dystrophy is focusing on several areas:

- **Protein repair**—Boosting the functions of proteins may help repair damage to muscle cells.
- **"Gene-silencing"**—This research is aimed at attempting to "turn off" the cells that harbor an elongated stretch of DNA thought to cause a type of MD.
- **Miniaturized genes for dystrophin**—These types of genes have been shown to improve the muscles of mice with Duchenne muscular dystrophy.
- **DNA testing**—Better DNA testing might reveal mutations in the dystrophin gene (MDA, 2008).

Myotonic Muscular Dystrophy

Myotonic dystrophy or Steinert's disease is the most common adult form of muscular dystrophy. It, like Duchenne muscular dystrophy, is caused by a defective gene that is transferred from one generation to another. The manifestations of myotonic dystrophy involve muscle wasting of the distal extremities, including hands, forearms, and feet and also the face and neck. The *myotonic* part of the term myotonic dystrophy refers to a delay in the relaxation phase after muscle contraction. An example would be a person who is unable to release his hand after gripping something. Fifty percent of the cases of myotonic dystrophy are diagnosed by age 20; however, many cases are not diagnosed until 50 years of age (MDA, 2008).

Clinical Manifestations

Myotonic dystrophy is a multisystem disease because it affects organs and tissues other than muscles. Myotonic dystrophy can affect the eyes, specifically in the manifestation of cataracts; the muscles involved in swallowing, resulting in dysphagia; the respiratory system, involving weakness of the diaphragm and an adverse reaction to anesthesia; the gastrointestinal system, including decreased peristalsis; and the endocrine system, resulting in alteration or inappropriate insulin secretion, increased carbohydrate metabolism, and excessive sleeping (MDA, 2008). Unlike with other dystrophies that can usually be diagnosed based on muscle wasting symptoms alone, myotonic dystrophy is often diagnosed based on presentation of other symptoms. In some cases, the patient's initial complaint to her health care provider may be a change in vision or difficulty swallowing.

Laboratory and Diagnostic Procedures

Myotonic muscular dystrophy is diagnosed by a complaint of distal weakness and myotonia. A muscle biopsy will determine the diagnosis. DNA testing will also delineate a diagnosis of myotonic dystrophy by finding an abnormality on chromosome 19. Some patients in the early stages of the disease have the "classic" look of myotonic dystrophy: muscle wasting of the face, jaw, neck, hands, feet, and forearms.

Medical Management

Treatment is based on support of the wasting muscles. In addition, avoiding complications such as constipation from decreased gastric peristalsis, aspiration from difficulty swallowing, and decreased visual acuity from resulting cataracts should be addressed.

Medications used for myotonic dystrophy include phenytoin (Dilantin), mexiletine (Mexil), carbamazepine (Tegretol), quinine, and procainamide (Pronestyl). All of these medications may be useful in treating the delayed muscle relaxation that generally occurs in patients with myotonic dystrophy (Mayo Clinic, 2007).

Research

Medical research is focused on isolating and mapping the genetic defect. The defect for myotonic dystrophy is in the arm of chromosome 19. Knowledge of the exact chromosome may allow for better genetic testing and reveal avenues for further research for treatment modalities.

Limb Girdle Muscular Dystrophy

This type of muscular dystrophy primarily affects the pelvis and shoulder areas. Limb girdle muscular dystrophy generally has a slow progression rate, but it is not uncommon in some patients for it to progress rapidly. Muscle weakness and wasting may begin at the upper extremities and progress to the lower extremities or have just the opposite pattern of progression. The signs and symptoms are usually noted during childhood, but they can also begin during the teen years and into adulthood. The incidence of male-to-female cases is about equal.

Facioscapulohumeral Disease

Facioscapulohumeral disease (FSHD) is a rare type of muscular dystrophy that affects the face, shoulder girdle, and upper arms and is more common in females than males. Diagnosis is made based on specific symptoms, which include weakness in the muscles that open and close the eyes; the muscles that allow a person to purse the lips, to smile, and to whistle; and the muscles that stabilize the scapula. Other affected muscles include the muscles of the hip girdle, foot, and abdomen. The diagnosis of FSHD is usually made by the time a person is in her 20s. The progression of this type of muscular dystrophy is insidious, with extended periods where the disease seems to be arrested.

Oculopharyngeal Muscular Dystrophy

This type of muscular dystrophy generally strikes people who are in their 50s and 60s. The most prominent feature is bilateral ptosis, in which the eyelids droop to the level of the pupil or below the level of the pupil. The patient has a contraction of the occipitofrontal muscle (muscle at the forehead) that is evident on observation and he tends to tip the forehead back in order to compensate for the ptosis, which can impair vision. The patient also has ocular muscle weakness, which prevents lateral eye movement, and weakness of the pharyngeal muscles (ineffective gag reflex), leading to dysphagia for solid foods.

Patients with oculopharyngeal muscular dystrophy also have weakness in their leg muscles and proximal hip girdle. The long-term problems associated with oculopharyngeal muscular dystrophy have less to do with the muscle weakness than with the dysphagia and the resulting possibility of aspiration pneumonia. With supplemental nutrition, modification to food consistency, and proper positioning, patients with this type of muscular dystrophy can have a good quality of life. Chart 55–10 (p. 1756) summarizes the differences in the types of muscular dystrophies.

■ Nursing Management for the Patient with Muscular Dystrophy

Nursing care for patients with muscular dystrophy is aimed at supporting the patient's independence level, preventing complications, and preventing injury, as discussed in the Nursing Process: Patient Care Plan for Muscular Dystrophy feature (p. 1756).

■ Collaborative Management

Many aspects of care are required for patients with muscular dystrophies. For the patient, the care of a nurse, nutritionist, physical therapist, occupational therapist, and orthotics technician will assist the patient to maintain mobility for as long as possible. For the caregiver, assistance from a financial counselor, psychologist, home health nurse, and access to respite care will decrease the chance of severe caregiver role strain.

Gerontological Considerations

Some patients diagnosed with myotonic muscular dystrophy are over the age of 50 and patients diagnosed with oculopharyngeal muscular dystrophy are usually in their 50s or 60s. Nursing considerations for these patients include safety issues, because as a person ages, muscle mass and muscle tone decrease. In addition to the weakness caused by the muscular dystrophy, the nurse must be aware of the normal aging process. Referrals to physical therapy or the use of assistive devices, such as canes or walkers, may be necessary.

CHART 55–10 **Differences in the Types of Muscular Dystrophies**

Type of Dystrophy	Signs/Symptoms	Onset and Progression
Duchenne	Mostly males Late walkers Unsteady gait Gowers' maneuver	Noticeable at 2–6 years of age Wheelchair bound by 7–12 years of age Many develop respiratory and cardiac problems and die by the mid-20s
Becker	Weakness after engaging in physical exercise or activities Begins in pelvic area, thighs, hips, and shoulders	Teens or young adults Generally will require assistive devices
Myotonic	Muscle wasting in upper extremities, face, neck, hands, forearms, feet	Adults Multisystem effects with chronic problems
Limb-girdle	Muscle wasting in hips and shoulders	Childhood, teen, or adult Cardiopulmonary complications
Facioscapulohumeral	Muscle wasting in face, shoulder girdle, and upper arms	Young adulthood
Oculopharyngeal	Bilateral ptosis Patient tips the head back Dysphagia for solid food	50s–60s

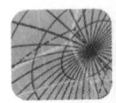

NURSING PROCESS: Patient Care Plan for Muscular Dystrophy

Assessment of Muscle Strength

Subjective Data:
Are you experiencing weakness in any muscle groups?
Are you having difficulty walking or feel off balance?

Objective Data:
Assess strength in upper and lower extremities.
Observe patient as she ambulates.

Nursing Assessment and Diagnoses	Outcomes and Evaluation Parameters	Planning and Interventions with *Rationales*
Nursing Diagnosis: *Activity Intolerance Impaired Physical Mobility*	**Outcome:** Ability to maintain enough muscle strength to ambulate as long as possible. *Evaluation Parameter:* Ability to stand with assistive devices.	**Interventions and *Rationales:*** Teach family to perform PROM exercises. Have them do the exercises three times a day. *Maintains joint mobility and prevents contractures.* Administer prednisone if prescribed. *May improve muscle mass and prolong ambulation.* Teach patient and family the need to maintain appropriate weight. *Obesity makes it difficult for the patient to move and support herself.* Teach patient/family the importance of maintaining safety in the home by keeping it uncluttered *to prevent injury.*

Assessment of Nutritional Status

Subjective Data:
Do you have difficulty swallowing?
What types of food do you eat?
Who prepares your meals?

Objective Data:
Assess patient's skin turgor and fragility.
Assess for excessive loss of hair.

Nursing Assessment and Diagnoses	Outcomes and Evaluation Parameters	Planning and Interventions with *Rationales*
Nursing Diagnosis: *Nutrition, Imbalanced: Less Than Body Requirements*	**Outcome:** The patient/family will be able to understand the rationale for and provide well-balanced meals three times a day. *Evaluation Parameters:* The patient will not experience weight loss of 2.5 kg in a 24-hour period. The patient will drink at least one supplement per day.	**Interventions and *Rationales:*** Ensure a well-balanced meal high in protein, carbohydrate, fiber, vitamins, and minerals *to promote healthy bones, muscles, and tissues and to provide energy.* Weigh daily, using the same scale and the same type of clothing. *Weight loss may indicate muscle-mass wasting, as well as possible malnutrition.* Provide carbohydrate and/or protein supplements as needed. *Supplements assist in maintaining adequate nutrition, which is required to maintain a healthy musculoskeletal system.*

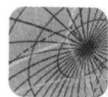

NURSING PROCESS: Patient Care Plan for Muscular Dystrophy—*Continued*

Assessment of Elimination

Subjective Data:
How often do you have a bowel movement?
Is it difficult for you to have a bowel movement?

Objective Data:
Document frequency and quality of bowel movements.

Nursing Assessment and Diagnoses	Outcomes and Evaluation Parameters	Planning and Interventions with *Rationales*
Nursing Diagnosis: *Constipation, Risk for*	**Outcome:** The patient will not be constipated. **Evaluation Parameter:** The patient will not have difficulty having a bowel movement.	**Interventions and *Rationales:*** Provide a high-fiber diet. *Fiber adds bulk to the stool.* Encourage the patient to drink 2,500 mL fluid per day (unless contraindicated by a medical condition). *Fluids help to maintain a soft stool.* Administer stool softener as ordered *to maintain a soft stool.* Reposition the patient every 2–4 hours *to facilitate peristalsis.*

Assessment of Self-Care

Subjective Data:
Are you able to bathe yourself?

Objective Data:
Observe ability to get in and out of the bath and wash body or body parts.

Nursing Assessment and Diagnoses	Outcomes and Evaluation Parameters	Planning and Interventions with *Rationales*
Nursing Diagnosis: *Self-Care Deficit: Bathing/Hygiene*	**Outcome:** The patient will participate in all aspects of care and ADLs. **Evaluation Parameters:** The patient will be able to wash body with minimal assistance.	**Interventions and *Rationales:*** Allow as much independence as possible, allowing the patient to assist in tasks that maintain or build self-esteem. *Maintenance of a positive attitude will allow for a better quality of life.*

Assessment of Swallowing Ability

Subjective Data:
Do you have difficulty swallowing?
Do you ever choke on your food?

Objective Data:
Depressed cough and gag reflexes
Impaired swallowing

Nursing Assessment and Diagnoses	Outcomes and Evaluation Parameters	Planning and Interventions with *Rationales*
Nursing Diagnosis: *Aspiration, Risk for*	**Outcome:** The patient will not aspirate. **Evaluation Parameters:** The patient will have an intact gag reflex. The patient will have clear lung sounds before and after eating and drinking.	**Interventions and *Rationales:*** Assess the patient's gag reflex prior to administering food or fluids. *A gag reflex that is not intact is a precursor to aspiration.* Assess lung sounds before and after meals/drinking. *A new onset of adventitious lung sounds may indicate aspiration.* Assess respiratory status before and after meals/drinking. *Shortness of breath, difficulty breathing, and increased respiratory rate may be indicative of aspiration.* Provide thickened liquids. *Thickened liquids are easier to swallow through esophagus and into stomach.* Teach the patient and family to eat small bites of food. *Patient is less likely to choke.*

Assessment of Cardiac Function

Subjective Data:
Do you experience shortness of breath with physical activity?

Objective Data:
Assess patient's activity tolerance by noting onset of shortness of breath or pain.

(continued)

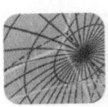

NURSING PROCESS: Patient Care Plan for Muscular Dystrophy—*Continued*

Nursing Assessment and Diagnoses	Outcomes and Evaluation Parameters	Planning and Interventions with *Rationales*
Nursing Diagnosis: *Cardiac Output, Decreased*	**Outcome:** Patient will demonstrate increasing tolerance for physical activity. **Evaluation Parameters:** The patient will have audible S_1 and S_2 heart sounds. The patient will not have any cyanosis or pallor. The patient's capillary refill will be 3 seconds or less.	**Interventions and *Rationales:*** Monitor heart sounds. *Muffled heart sounds may be indicative of cardiomyopathy.* Assess color. *Pallor, cyanosis may be indicative of decreased cardiac output.* Assess capillary refill. *Capillary refill greater than 3 seconds may indicate decreased cardiac output.* Schedule rest periods between activities *to decrease the workload of the heart.* Restrict fluids *to decrease the workload of the heart.*

Assessment of Breathing

Subjective Data:	Objective Data:
Do you have difficulty breathing? Do you feel short of breath?	Ineffective chest excursion Nasal flaring Orthopnea Use of accessory muscles to breathe

Nursing Assessment and Diagnoses	Outcomes and Evaluation Parameters	Planning and Interventions with *Rationales*
Nursing Diagnosis: *Breathing, Ineffective*	**Outcome:** The patient will demonstrate effective breathing patterns. **Evaluation Parameters:** The patient will have eupneic respirations and normal color and will breathe without the use of accessory muscles. The patient will have an oxygen saturation level of between 90% and 100%.	**Interventions and *Rationales:*** Observe for dyspnea (difficulty breathing), pallor or cyanosis, rate and depth of respirations, use of accessory muscles. *Tachypnea (rapid respiratory rate, usually greater than 24 per minute), bradypnea (slow respiratory rate, usually less than 10 per minute), and shallow respirations will indicate respiratory dysfunction.* Monitor oxygen saturation levels via pulse oximeter. *Levels below 90% may indicate hypoxia.* Encourage rest periods as needed *to allow for easier respirations.* Teach purse-lipped and deep breathing exercises *to expand lungs for maximum oxygen intake and expel carbon dioxide.*

Assessment of Caregiver Role

Subjective Data:	Objective Data:	
Are you having any difficulty with any of the caregiver tasks? How is your health? Are you having trouble sleeping? Do you have any concerns regarding your loved one's care?	The caregiver is: Experiencing headaches Has lost or gained weight	Is angry Is feeling depressed

Nursing Assessment and Diagnoses	Outcomes and Evaluation Parameters	Planning and Interventions with *Rationales*
Nursing Diagnosis: *Caregiver Role Strain, Risk for*	**Outcome:** The caregiver will demonstrate emotional health. **Evaluation Parameters:** Free of anger. Free of depression. Less frustrated. Verbalizes a sense of control and self-esteem.	**Interventions and *Rationales:*** Refer patient/family to the Muscular Dystrophy Association and other local support groups. *Discussing concerns with others in the same situation provides a support network.* Allow the patient/family to verbalize fears/concerns. *Provides support.*

As people with muscular dystrophy age, they experience many associated symptoms that adults without muscular dystrophy also experience. Eyesight often decreases. Cataracts are more prevalent in older people, as is arcus senilis, a thin gray-white ring that surrounds the eye margin and may affect the vision. Peristalsis slows down and appetite and nutritional caloric needs decrease with age. Because protein is so important for maintenance of healthy muscles, especially in a patient with MD,

the nurse should take care to assist patients in meal planning or refer them to a dietitian. See the Patient Teaching & Discharge Priorities for Muscular Dystrophy box for more information.

Myopathies

Myopathy refers to any disease of the muscle (National Institute of Neurological Disorders and Stroke [NINDS], 2008). There are various forms of myopathies, which can be inherited or can

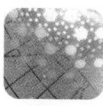

PATIENT TEACHING & DISCHARGE PRIORITIES for Muscular Dystrophy

Need	Teaching
Safety: • Setting (home)	Maintain a safe environment by not having clutter on the floor. Remove throw rugs, electrical wires, clutter toys, etc.
Proper nutrition: • Patient	Eat a well-balanced diet to include protein, carbohydrates, minerals, vitamins.
Self-care activities: • Patient and family	Provide as much of own care as possible to maintain independence, but rest when needed.
Maintain mobility: • Patient and family	Move joints as much as possible.
Prevent constipation: • Patient and family	Eat a diet high in fiber and drink at least 2500 mL fluid/day.

occur in later years (Chart 55–11). Myopathies can also be secondary complications due to endocrine disorders, metabolic disorders, muscle inflammation or infection, certain drugs, or gene mutations (NINDS, 2008).

Clinical Manifestations

The main sign of generalized myopathy is weakness of limbs. In some cases, exercise increases the weakness; in other cases, exercise improves the weakness or even causes it to disappear (NINDS, 2008). Affected muscle groups vary by patient.

Medical Management

Treatment varies according to the type of myopathy. Some patients may require symptomatic treatment only, whereas others may require supportive care, such as braces or other orthotic devices, medications, or physical therapy National Institute of Neurological Disorders & Stroke (2008). The prognosis for myopathies again varies depending on the type. Some patients do not have a disrupted quality of life, whereas to others the myopathy may be disabling.

Types of Myopathies

Following are descriptions of the types of myopathies, clinical presentation, and medical management. Nursing management for the patient with myopathies is presented at the end of the section.

Congenital Myopathy

This type of myopathy is due to a chromosomal defect leading to **hypotonia**, an absence of muscle tone resulting in flaccid, weak muscles in infancy and weakness and delayed motor activity in later childhood years. Diagnosis of a congenital myopathy is made by muscle tissue sampling, which indicates changes in the structure and morphology of the muscle. Treatment is supportive.

Hypokalemic Myopathy

Hypokalemic myopathy is common in the elderly and is due to a low serum potassium level caused by long-term diuretic use (Merck, 2003). Other causes of hypokalemic myopathy include potassium deficiency in the diet, excessive alcohol consumption, aldosteronism, intestinal wasting of potassium (malabsorption), and licorice intoxication (Merck, 2003). Hypokalemic paralysis can occur with diabetic ketoacidosis, after an amphotericin B treatment, chronic diarrhea, renal tubular acidosis, or other chronic conditions that cause hypokalemia.

Clinical Manifestations   Muscle weakness due to hypokalemic myopathy develops gradually and usually affects the proximal muscles of the legs, arms, trunk, and neck. In some cases the thoracic muscles and diaphragm are also affected (Merck, 2003). In patients with hypokalemic myopathy, the potassium level is less

CHART 55–11   Types of Myopathies

Type	Signs/Symptoms
Congenital	Chromosomal defect leading to hypotonia in infancy and weakness and delayed motor activity in later childhood years.
Hypokalemic	Common in the elderly and due to an electrolyte imbalance caused by long-term diuretic use. Affects proximal muscles of the legs, arms, trunk, and neck; may affect thoracic muscles and diaphragm.
Mitochondrial	Affects the ocular muscles; may cause encephalomyopathies.
Steroidal	Chronic use of prednisone can lead to muscle weakness, increased risk for pathologic fractures.
Inflammatory:	
• Polymyositis	Acquired diseases of the skeletal muscle.
• Dermatomyositis	Generalized muscle weakness.
• Inclusion body myositis	Identified by a heliotrope (bluish-purplish in color) rash and muscle weakness. Progressive inflammation of the muscles, usually in men over 50 years of age.

than 3 mEq/L (normal is 3.5 to 5.0 mEq/L). Deep tendon reflexes are less active than normal or may be inactive. The only complaint the patient has is of lethargy; there are no complaints of pain or discomfort (Merck, 2003).

Medical Management   Potassium replacement therapy reverses hypokalemic myopathy within 1 month. Chronic hypokalemic myopathy may need to be treated with oral potassium supplements and the patient should be encouraged to eat foods rich in potassium such as avocado, banana, cantaloupe, dates, figs, orange juice, potato, prunes, and some salt substitutes.

Mitochondrial Myopathy

Mitochondrial myopathy is named for the part of the cell it affects, the mitochondria that are responsible for producing most of the energy that is needed for cells to function. A mitochondrial disease can shut down some or all the mitochondria, depleting the essential energy supply. Because muscle cells and nerve cells have especially high energy needs, muscular and neurological problems are common features of mitochondrial disease. Symptoms can include muscle weakness, exercise intolerance, hearing loss, trouble with balance and coordination, seizures and learning deficits (MDA, 2003).

Medical Management   Treatments aim at fixing or bypassing the defective mitochondria. These treatments are dietary supplements based on three natural substances involved in the production of the energy molecule ATP. One supplement is creatine, which normally acts as a reserve for ATP by forming a compound called *creatine phosphate*. When a cell's demand for ATP exceeds the amount its mitochondria can produce, creatine can release phosphate to rapidly enhance the ATP supply. Another substance is carnitine, which improves the efficiency of ATP production by helping import certain fuel molecules into mitochondria, and cleaning up some of the toxic by-products of ATP production. Carnitine is available as an over-the-counter supplement called L-carnitine. The last supplement is coenzyme Q10 (coQ10), which is a component of the electron transport chain that uses oxygen to manufacture ATP. Some mitochondrial diseases are caused by coQ10 deficiency, and there is evidence that coQ10 supplementation is beneficial in these cases (MDA, 2003).

Steroid-Induced Myopathy

Long-term corticosteroid usage can lead to muscle weakness and increased risk for pathologic fractures. Patients on corticosteroids for more than 1 year are at risk for steroid myopathy. The manifestations of the muscle weakness are insidious, particularly with a daily dose for more than 6 months (Younger, 2003).

Medical Management   Unless contraindicated, the patient should be changed to alternate-day usage of corticosteroids as soon as possible. If the weakness is primarily due to steroid usage, then the symptoms should subside in about 2 to 3 months after the steroid dosage is decreased, and complete recovery is expected (Merck, 2003). A daily exercise regimen is recommended to promote muscle tone.

Inflammatory Myopathies

The inflammatory myopathies are a group of acquired diseases of the skeletal muscle (Dalakas & Hohfield, 2003). These types of myopathies have in common moderate to severe muscle weakness, but all are treatable. The three types of inflammatory my-

opathies are polymyositis, dermatomyositis, and inclusion body myositis. See the Pharmacology Summary on Muscular Disorders.

Polymyositis

Polymyositis (PM) is a type of myopathy that occurs slowly over weeks and months. It is an autoimmune connective tissue disorder that causes damage to muscle fibers. Polymyositis usually affects proximal muscles and causes weakness to those muscles. Complaints include decreasing ability to perform simple tasks, such as combing hair or rising from a chair, or tasks involving fine motor movement (Dalakas & Hohfield, 2003).

Polymyositis affects predominantly women, and African Americans, ages 45 to 65 years old (Merck, 2003). The cause of PM is unknown, but may be triggered by viral, bacterial, or parasitic agents, drugs, vaccinations, or even stress.

Clinical Manifestations   Symptoms that accompany polymyositis may be systemic, as well as muscular. Generalized muscle weakness is the main complaint from patients. The weakness is more prevalent in the hips and thighs and the weakness begins as an "ache." For most patients the initial complaint that brings them to see the health care provider is weakness in the upper and lower extremities. Patients with PM also may experience fatigue, weight loss, and changes in nails or skin, including a rash or redness. Systemic involvement includes dysphagia, cardiac involvement, and respiratory involvement. Polymyositis may also occur with another connective tissue disorder known as an overlap syndrome.

Laboratory and Diagnostic Procedures   Diagnosis of polymyositis is based on symptomology, the exclusion of other neuromuscular diseases, muscle biopsy findings, elevated serum CK levels (muscle enzymes), and an abnormal electromyography. The confirmatory diagnosis is made with five criteria: proximal muscle weakness, elevated CK, EMG changes, positive muscle biopsy, and a typical skin rash.

Medical Management   The treatment for polymyositis depends on the severity of the symptoms and involvement of other systems. The goal of treatment is to improve the patients' quality of life, thus allowing them to carry out their normal ADLs. Various medications are used to treat polymyositis, including prednisone and immunosuppressive drugs, such as methotrexate and azathioprine (Imuran).

The prognosis is poor if the muscle weakness is progressive and severe. This may lead to aspiration pneumonia, dysphagia, malnutrition, and respiratory failure. The patients benefit from physical therapy and a scheduled exercise routine. Frequent monitoring for progression of muscle weakness is warranted.

Dermatomyositis

Dermatomyositis is an autoimmune disease that affects the small blood vessels and capillaries in muscles. It is identified by a heliotrope (bluish-purplish in color) rash and muscle weakness. Degeneration of the skin and muscle ultimately occur, leading to bilateral muscle weakness and some muscle atrophy, mostly of the proximal limb muscles. The heliotrope rash is noted on the eyelids, while an erythematous rash is noted on the chest, face, and neck. Gottron's rash, a reddish raised rash or papules, is noted on the metacarpophalangeal joints and the interphalangeal joints. The nail beds are thick and cracked. Dermatomyositis affects women more than men, and approximately

PHARMACOLOGY Summary for Muscular Disorders

Medication Category	Action	Application/Indication	Nursing Responsibilities
Anticonvulsant			
Phenytoin: (Dilantin)	Helps stabilize the neurons by regulating voltage-dependent sodium and calcium channels, inhibiting calcium movement across neuronal membranes, and enhancing sodium-potassium ATP activity in neurons and glial cells.	To treat delayed muscle relaxation	• Preferred administration routes are oral and intravenous injection. • If patient has difficulty swallowing, open the rapid-release capsules and mix with food or fluid. • To minimize gastric distress, give medication with or just after meals. • If administering through a nasogastric tube, minimize drug absorption in tubing by diluting suspension threefold with sodium chloride or sterile water. After administration, flush tube with at least 20 mL of diluent. • Long-term therapy may increase the patient's requirements for folic acid or vitamin D supplements.
Class IB Antiarrhythmic			
Mexiletine: (Mexil)	Inhibits fast sodium channels in myocardial cell membranes.	To treat delayed muscle relaxation	• Assess for signs of thrombocytopenia, which can occur within a few days of starting mexiletine therapy. • Teach patient to take drug at evenly spaced intervals, to avoid missing doses. • To minimize gastric distress, give medication with food.
Analgesic, Anticonvulsant			
Carbamazepine: (Tegretol)	Slows nerve impulse transmission by blocking sodium channels thus preventing sodium from entering the cell.	To treat delayed muscle relaxation	• Drug is metabolized by the liver—use with caution in patients with impaired hepatic function. • Monitor white blood cell and platelet counts. Decreased counts may indicate bone marrow depression. • To minimize gastric distress, give medication with food. • Teach patient to wear sunscreen to prevent photosensitivity reactions. • Teach patient and family to notify health care provider if they experience unusual bleeding or bruising, fever, rash, or mouth ulcers.
Antiarrhythmic			
Procainamide: (Pronestyl)	Inhibits sodium influx through cell membranes.	To treat delayed muscle relaxation	• Teach patient to swallow extended release tablets whole, without crushing or chewing them. • If patient has difficulty swallowing, have patient crush regular-release tablets or open capsules and mix with food or fluid. • Teach patient to take medication 1 to 2 hours after meals with a full glass of water. • Teach patient and family to notify health care provider if patient experiences unusual bleeding or bruising, fever, rash, or diarrhea.
Antipsoriatic, Antirheumatic			
Methotrexate	Inhibits dihydrofolate reductase, the enzyme that reduces folic acid to tetrahydrofolic acid. Inhibition of the acid interferes with DNA synthesis and cell reproduction.	Immunosuppressant	• Follow policy for preparing and handling drug. Avoid skin contact. • Increase patient's fluid intake to reduce risk of gastric distress. • Assess patient for signs of bleeding and infection.

(continued)

PHARMACOLOGY Summary for Muscular Disorders—*Continued*

Medication Category	Action	Application/Indication	Nursing Responsibilities
Antimetabolite, Immunosuppressant Azathioprine: (Imuran)	May prevent proliferation and differentiation of activated B and T cells. Intefees with DNA and RNA synthesis.	Immunosuppressant	• Teach patient to take oral drug with food or meals to minimize gastric distress. • Therapy increases risk of viral, fungal, bacterial, and protozoal infections. Monitor for signs of infection especially in patients with cardiac insufficiency or hepatic disease. • Administer oral dose 30 minutes prior to meals. • Warn patient to avoid alcohol, sedatives, and other CNS depressants. • Be aware of multiple IV drug incompatibilities and light sensitivity.

10% of the patients have some type of malignancy, with breast and lung tumors being the most common (Merck, 2003).

Clinical Manifestations The patient presents with one or more of the following signs: the heliotrope rash; Gottron's papules, which are violet-colored plaques at the finger joints; or **Gottron's sign**, a reddened smooth, scaly rash at the finger joints; thickened fingernails; and muscle weakness. The rash, however, may be noted without muscle weakness. The weakness is a gradual process, usually developing over several months. The proximal limb muscles are affected and are weaker than the distal muscles. In addition, neck muscles are weak. Other muscles involved are those involved with swallowing, leading to possible dysphagia. Other complaints include myalgia and muscle tenderness. Other organs may also be involved, including the respiratory system, which may lead to interstitial lung disease; the cardiac system, which may lead to cardiomyopathy and conduction anomalies; and the gastrointestinal tract, leading to delayed emptying. Microvasculopathy (very small capillaries, veins, and arteries that do not allow for adequate perfusion) of the gastrointestinal tract occurs, leading to ulcerations and perforations of the intestine.

Laboratory and Diagnostic Procedures Diagnosis of dermatomyositis is determined by signs and symptoms, elevated CK levels, an elevated eosinophil sedimentation rate, and an elevated antinuclear antibody titer. Muscle biopsy shows atrophy of muscle fibers, a decreased number of capillaries and **perivascular** (around blood vessels) infiltrates. An EMG shows muscle inflammation (Merck, 2003).

Medical Management Treatment is the same as for polymyositis. The patient should be monitored for tumors, and additional tests to rule out breast and lung cancer should be anticipated.

Inclusion Body Myositis

Inclusion body myositis (IBM), like the other myopathies, is an autoimmune disorder that is characterized by a progressive inflammation of the muscles. It occurs mostly in men over age 50 and is a common inflammatory myopathy in the elderly.

Clinical Manifestations The patient complains of asymmetric muscle weakness, usually beginning in the wrists, finger flexors, and knee extensors. Muscle atrophy usually develops early compared to the other myopathies. In some cases facial muscles are involved, as is dysphagia. Patients with IBM may remain ambulatory for many years, even after the symptoms begin (Merck, 2003).

Medical Management Elevated CK levels and muscle biopsies that show eosinophilic and cytoplasmic inclusion bodies are the main two diagnostic tools for IBM. As of this writing, there is no known treatment for IBM, however, prednisone and immune globulin have been shown to be effective. Prevention of footdrop and wrist drop is an important aspect in the maintenance of quality of life. This is achieved by bracing and physical therapy.

◼ Nursing Management

The object of nursing care is to encourage as much independence as the patient can tolerate, teaching safety measures and the importance of adhering to the prescribed medication regime.

Assessment

It is essential that the nurse listen and document the patient's complaints. Question the patient on:

- When the symptoms began
- Whether there are any accompanying symptoms
- Whether the symptoms have affected the patient's ability to maintain ADLs
- What type of medications the patient is taking, both prescription and OTC
- Whether the patient has noticed any change in his nutritional status
- Whether the patient has noticed any changes in the skin (i.e., rash, redness, etc.).

The nurse must assess the patient's condition by physical examination. Test muscle strength resistance of the affected limb, the unaffected limb, and compare both sides. Auscultate heart and lung sounds. Test deep tendon reflexes (biceps, triceps, patellar). Inspect the extremities for footdrop or wrist drop. Assess the skin for color and the presence of any rashes. Observe gait, balance, and the patient's ability to participate in the exam. For further nursing management, refer to the Nursing Process: Patient Care Plan for Muscular Myopathies.

Gerontological Considerations for Patients with a Myopathy

It is common for myopathies to develop in people in their 50s and 60s. As with all patients with muscle diseases, safety concerns are a priority. The older a person becomes, the more brittle the bones become. Muscle mass and tone decrease and combined with the effects of aging, the added muscle weakness associated with myopathy puts the patient at risk for falls and other injuries. In creating a plan of care for a patient diagnosed with a myopathy, safety must be a priority. For more information, see the Research Opportunities and Clinical Impact Related to Muscular Myopathies (p. 1765).

Many of these patients are diagnosed at an age when they might be contemplating retirement and future plans with their spouse. A medical diagnosis of a myopathy will alter their lifestyle and many may become depressed. Nurses should anticipate patients reacting negatively to this new diagnosis and need to be aware of mood swings that are typical for a patient with a myopathy. For more information, see the Patient Teaching & Discharge Priorities for Muscular Myopathies box (p. 1765).

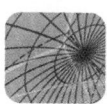

NURSING PROCESS: Patient Care Plan for Muscular Myopathies

Assessment of Muscle Strength

Subjective Data:
Have you experienced weakness in any extremity?
Have you had difficulty swallowing?

Objective Data:
Assess patient's ability to perform ROM on all limbs.
Assess patient's ability to perform resistance tests on all four limbs, flexion of the biceps and extension of the triceps:

- Hand grip
- Flexion of the hip
- Adduction at the hip
- Abduction at the hip
- Extension at the hips
- Extension at the knee
- Flexion at the knee
- Dorsiflexion and plantar flexion

Nursing Assessment and Diagnoses	Outcomes and Evaluation Parameters	Planning and Interventions with *Rationales*
Nursing Diagnosis: *Disuse Syndrome, Risk for*	**Outcome:** The patient is able to perform ROM on all extremities. **Evaluation Parameter:** The patient is able to perform resistance on all four limbs.	**Interventions and *Rationales:*** Provide a physical or occupational therapy referral as needed. *Physical therapists and occupational therapists are able to provide the patient with additional exercises for isotonic muscle movement.* Encourage the patient to eat a well-balanced diet (protein, carbohydrates, vitamins, and minerals) *to maintain a healthy musculoskeletal system.* Teach patient and family the need to maintain appropriate weight. *Obesity makes it difficult for the patient to move and support himself.* Teach patient/family the importance of maintaining safety in the home by keeping it uncluttered *to prevent injury.*

Assessment of Activity Tolerance

Subjective Data:
Do you become fatigued after performing simple tasks?

Objective Data:
Test patient's muscle strength before and after performing physical tasks.

Nursing Assessment and Diagnoses	Outcomes and Evaluation Parameters	Planning and Interventions with *Rationales*
Nursing Diagnosis: *Activity Intolerance*	**Outcome:** The patient is able to perform ADLs without extreme fatigue. **Evaluation Parameter:** The patient and family have implemented an activity/rest period schedule.	**Interventions and *Rationales:*** Instruct the patient and family to pace activities per patient tolerance by assisting in devising an exercise plan that is tolerable and does not cause fatigue. *To decrease muscle fatigue and patient exhaustion.* Encourage the patient to eat a well-balanced diet (protein, carbohydrates, vitamins, and minerals) *to maintain a healthy musculoskeletal system.*

Assessment of Ability to Perform Self-Care

Subjective Data:
What activities are difficult for you to perform?
Do you require assistance with activities?

Objective Data:
Observe patient and evaluate ability to perform ADLs.

(continued)

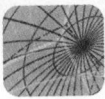
Nursing Assessment and Diagnoses	Outcomes and Evaluation Parameters	Planning and Interventions with *Rationales*
Nursing Diagnosis: If progressive, *Self-Care Deficit: Bathing/Hygiene* and *Dressing/Grooming*	**Outcome:** The patient is able to perform ADLs without extreme fatigue. ***Evaluation Parameters:*** The patient has developed a schedule for performing ADLs. The patient will perform active ROM exercises on all joints three times a day.	**Interventions and *Rationales:*** Teach patient/family to pace daily hygiene practices *to allow the patient to maintain independence.* Encourage active ROM exercises to all joints as prescribed *to maintain joint mobility.* Set up exercise plan with the patient, keeping in mind the patient's limitations. *Exercise helps maintain a healthy musculoskeletal system.*

Assessment of Fall Risk

Subjective Data:
Do you have difficulty with balance?
Have you fallen recently?

Objective Data:
Have the patient walk and observe for balance and muscle weakness.

Nursing Assessment and Diagnoses	Outcomes and Evaluation Parameters	Planning and Interventions with *Rationales*
Nursing Diagnosis: *Falls, Risk for*	**Outcome:** The patient will not fall. ***Evaluation Parameters:*** Patient/family understand the importance of safety and will ensure safety measures are taken in the home. Patient demonstrates slower ambulation and verbalizes understanding about taking designated rest periods in between ambulation, if required.	**Interventions and *Rationales:*** Discuss with the patient/family safety issues in the home, such as throw rugs or other obstacles that may precipitate falls. *Such obstacles can lead to more serious injury.* Discuss with the patient/family the importance of taking time when ambulating. *May prevent serious injury and maintain level of independence.*

Assessment of Swallowing

Subjective Data:
Do you ever choke on your food?
Do you have difficulty swallowing?

Objective Data:
Have speech pathology do a swallow study.
Observe patient swallowing liquid and watch for coughing.

Nursing Assessment and Diagnoses	Outcomes and Evaluation Parameters	Planning and Interventions with *Rationales*
Nursing Diagnoses: *Swallowing, Impaired* and/or *Aspiration, Risk for*	**Outcome:** The patient will not aspirate. ***Evaluation Parameters:*** If required, the patient will see a speech pathologist. The patient and family demonstrate cutting foods into smaller pieces.	**Interventions and *Rationales:*** Refer to speech pathology. *Speech pathologists are able to detect various types of swallowing abnormalities.* Teach the patient and family to eat small bites of food. *Patient will be less likely to choke.* Provide thickened liquids to prevent aspiration. *Thickened liquids are easier to swallow directly into esophagus and stomach.*

Assessment of Coping

Subjective Data:
Do you feel unusually fatigued?
Have you been able to communicate your concerns?

Objective Data:
Observe for:
Decreased use of social support
Destructive behavior toward self and others
Inability to meet basic needs
Inadequate problem solving
Lack of goal-directed behavior
Poor concentration

Nursing Assessment and Diagnoses	Outcomes and Evaluation Parameters	Planning and Interventions with *Rationales*
Nursing Diagnosis: *Coping, Ineffective*	**Outcome:** The patient demonstrates effective coping. ***Evaluation Parameters:*** The patient: Takes actions to manage stressors. Shows self-restraint regarding compulsive or impulsive behaviors. Seeks information concerning illness and treatment. Reports decrease in negative feelings.	**Interventions and *Rationales:*** Allow the patient/family to verbalize fears and concerns. *Provides a support network.* Refer to local and national support system. *Provide support of other people in similar situations.*

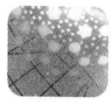

PATIENT TEACHING & DISCHARGE PRIORITIES for Muscular Myopathies

Need	Teaching
Safety considerations	Pace exercise and performance of ADLs with rest periods.
Importance of maintaining joint flexibility	Perform active ROM exercises on all joints three times a day.
Eat a well-balanced diet	Eat foods high in protein, vitamins, minerals, and carbohydrates.
Regular checkups	If symptoms worsen, see primary care provider immediately. Maintain follow-up appointments.

Rhabdomyolysis

Rhabdomyolysis is defined as a syndrome involving muscle necrosis or breakdown. The injured muscle fibers release myoglobin into the bloodstream. The myoglobin then alters the filtration in the kidneys, causing damage and failure. The degree of illness ranges in severity from elevations in muscle enzymes without any symptoms noted by the patient to severe life-threatening symptoms such as electrolyte imbalances and acute renal failure. Some of the causes of rhabdomyolysis include trauma with muscle compression, surgical procedures in which there is a long period of muscle compression, immobilization due to a comatose or postictal state (usually occurring after seizure activity when the patient has been unconscious and unresponsive to stimuli) in which the patient is lying in one position for long periods of time, extreme physical exertion, snakebite, toxins, and viral, bacterial, or fungal infection (Bartelmo & Lockhart, 2008).

Clinical Manifestations and Diagnosis

The patient typically presents to the hospital with muscle pain (myalgia), fatigue, fever, nausea and vomiting, and dark-colored urine. The diagnosis of rhabdomyolysis is based on elevated serum CK levels, which typically are 100 times normal or higher. The high levels of CK come primarily from the necrosis of skeletal muscle. Myoglobinuria (the presence of myoglobin in the urine) results from muscle tissue breakdown and the muscle substances entering the urine and represents an extremely abnormal condition. Myoglobin may be detected in the urine when the serum level is 1,500 to 3,000 ng/mL.

Complications

Numerous complications are associated with rhabdomyolysis:

- Acute renal failure due to tubular obstruction secondary to the myoglobulin pigments
- Electrolyte imbalance:
  - Hyperkalemia (elevated potassium levels in the blood) and hyperphosphatemia (elevated phosphate levels in the blood) can result due to the release of potassium and phosphate from the damaged muscles.
  - Hypocalcemia (low serum calcium level) due to deposited calcium salts in the muscle tissue. This electrolyte imbalance can be severe and patients often show other symptoms associated with hypocalcemia, such as disturbances in cardiac conduction or blood coagulation.
  - Hyperuricemia (elevated uric acid level in the bloodstream) is a result of purine metabolism, resulting in an elevated serum uric acid concentration. Purines are present in nucleic acids, which are both obtained from endogenous and dietary sources.
  - Metabolic acidosis (electrolyte imbalance involving shift of the acid–base balance toward the acid side) can also occur.
  - Compartment syndrome (increased pressure in muscle compartment, may lead to permanent disability of the associated joint) due to edema of a limb and muscle.

Medical Management

The treatment of rhabdomyolysis involves identifying and addressing the underlying cause. Prompt management and prevention of acute renal failure related to the muscle breakdown that causes the myoglobinuria is essential. Increased fluids are administered to hydrate the patient, thereby avoiding or preventing obstruction of the renal filtration process by the myoglobin, which could result in acute renal failure.

◼ Nursing Management

Patients with acute or severe rhabdomyolysis are hospitalized and, due to the severity of the kidney involvement, may be closely monitored in an intensive care unit (ICU). Nursing care will focus on hydration, strict fluid management, and close attention to the impact of possible abnormal electrolyte levels. Bicarbonate is given intravenously to prevent myoglobin from breaking down into toxic compounds in the kidney. Refer to Chapter 47 😊 for

RESEARCH OPPORTUNITIES AND CLINICAL IMPACT RELATED TO MUSCULAR MYOPATHIES

Research Area	Clinical Impact
If the patient maintains his regular regime (at a slower pace), could the disease progression be delayed?	Maintenance of the patient's "normal" routine may promote a better quality of life.
How does a patient's support system affect the progression of the disease?	A positive family support system may prevent depression or a lack of self-esteem related to the disease.

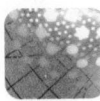

PATIENT TEACHING & DISCHARGE PRIORITIES for Rhabdomyolysis

Need	Teaching
Safety	Ensure home is free of obstacles.
	Take time with ADLs.
Monitor urine output	Inform primary care provider if urine output is low.
	If on a fluid restriction, explain to the patient the importance of maintaining the restriction, so as not to overload heart and lungs.
Follow-up care for kidney and electrolyte monitoring	Stress importance of notifying primary care provider if developing difficulty breathing, swelling, very dry skin, low urinary output, and discolored urine.

nursing management of the patient in acute renal failure. See the box titled Patient Teaching & Discharge Priorities for Rhabdomyolysis for more information.

Eaton-Lambert Syndrome

Eaton-Lambert syndrome is an autoimmune disease that affects muscular activity and function. It is usually associated with small cell carcinoma of the lung and affects men more often than women. Eaton-Lambert syndrome is caused by a decrease in acetylcholine release. In addition, serum from patients with this syndrome contains circulating immunoglobulin antibodies that block calcium channels. Calcium is required by motor nerve fibers to function (Merck, 2003).

Clinical Manifestations

Patients with Eaton-Lambert syndrome complain of muscle fatigue primarily in the leg and trunk muscles. Other symptoms include occasional hyporeflexia, or weak tendon reflex, but muscle contraction restores the tendon reflex. Autonomic symptoms are also present, such as dry mouth, impotence, decreased lacrimation and sweating, orthostatic hypotension, and decreased pupillary reaction to light accommodation (Merck, 2003).

Laboratory and Diagnostic Procedures

Diagnosis of Eaton-Lambert syndrome is made by electrophysiological responses to nerve stimulation. Affirmation of Eaton-Lambert syndrome is also determined by an elevated level of antibodies to the voltage-gated P/Q-type calcium channel. Elevations of these types occur in practically all cases due to lung cancer.

Medical Management

Patients with a diagnosis of lung carcinoma should be monitored frequently for muscle weakness. In some cases, the neuro-

muscular transmission improves after the tumor is removed. Drugs that increase acetylcholine release are also used as well as drugs that control immune-mediated diseases. These drugs include prednisone, azathioprine, and immune globulin.

Nursing Management

The object of nursing management is to teach patients safety measures and adherence to their medication regime. If the cause of Eaton-Lambert syndrome is lung cancer, then the nurse should provide symptomatic care and education. For more information, see the Patient Teaching & Discharge Priorities for Eaton-Lambert Syndrome box.

Muscle Cramps

Muscle cramps are sudden involuntary contractions in one or more muscle that last for a few seconds to minutes. Muscle cramps can be caused by a nerve that malfunctions, as in spinal cord injury, or from dehydration, lack of minerals in the body, overuse or straining of the muscle, and a decreased blood supply to the muscle (MedLine Plus, 2008).

The bundles of fibers that make up the muscle contract and expand to produce movement. It is important to keep the fibers stretched out so that they may respond vigorously during exercise. If the muscle is poorly conditioned, then it is more likely to become fatigued, which can change the spinal neural reflexes causing cramping. Overexertion of the muscle depletes the oxygen supply to the muscle cells, leading to waste products that cause muscle spasm (AAOS, 2008).

Exercise-induced muscle cramps are manifested by pain and involuntary muscle contractions that occur either during exercise or immediately after exercise (Dumke, 2003). The pain is often spasmodic and episodic. Exercise-induced muscle cramps

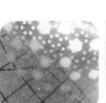

PATIENT TEACHING & DISCHARGE CONSIDERATIONS for Eaton-Lambert Syndrome

Need	Teaching
Safety	Ensure home is free of obstacles.
	Take time with ADLs.
Mobility	Maintain joint mobility by performing active ROM exercises on all joints three times a day.

CHART 55–12	**Muscle Cramps**	
Type	**Cause**	**Treatment**
Fatigue	Inadequate stretching prior to exercise Dehydration	Stretching of the affected muscle Adequate hydration with electrolyte-based beverage
Exercise	Inadequate training	Training with warm-up exercise, hydration, well-balanced diet
Hypocalcemia	Low calcium level	A diet that includes foods high in calcium or calcium supplements Monitor electrolytes
Idiopathic	Unknown; occurs during bedtime	Stretching exercise after cramps begin or before bedtime

occur more frequently during hot weather as sweat drains the body of fluid, sodium, and other minerals such as potassium and calcium. The lack of these nutrients may cause the muscle to spasm. It is also thought that muscle cramps primarily occur over muscles that span two joints (AAOS, 2008; Dumke, 2003).

Calcium plays an important role in the musculoskeletal system. One of its primary roles is in regulating muscle contraction and relaxation. A person who has hypocalcemia is at risk for muscle spasms of the face and extremities. Hypocalcemia also results in hyperactive deep tendon reflexes. Hypercalcemia, in turn, can cause generalized muscle weakness and flaccidity of the muscles.

Idiopathic muscle cramps are muscle cramps that occur with no particular etiology. The cramps are usually without accompanying weakness. Idiopathic muscle cramps generally affect healthy, middle-aged or elderly adults and generally occur during the nighttime or when the person is sleeping. The most common muscles affected are of the calf or foot muscles, causing plantar flexion to the afflicted foot. The various types of muscle cramps are summarized in Chart 55–12.

Medical Management

Diagnosis is made on the patient's subjective complaints and lack of any weakness or disability. The treatment is prophylactic, in that the patient is instructed to stretch prior to exercise and to maintain balanced nutrition and fluid intake. Patients who have night cramps should be encouraged to perform stretching exercises on the legs prior to falling asleep. When muscle cramps occur, the patient is instructed to stretch directly after the pain begins.

◼ Nursing Management

The nursing plan of care involves education regarding safety issues and measures to prevent the occurrence of muscle cramps. Research into the efficacy of electrolyte-based drinks is addressed in the Research Opportunities and Clinical Impact Related to Muscle Cramps box.

Assessment

The nurse should assess the patient's condition through a physical examination. Observe the patient during ambulation. Test resistance on all four extremities. Monitor electrolyte levels. Obtain a daily "diary" of the patient's intake and output. Obtain a history regarding the cramps by asking do they only occur with exercise, are they relieved by stretching, is there a family history of muscle cramps? Although most muscle cramps are benign, they can be signs of underlying disease such as spinal nerve irritation or compression, thyroid disease, or liver disease (AAOS, 2008). Note that the elderly are prone to muscle cramps for reasons discussed in the Gerontological Considerations box.

Fibromyalgia

Fibromyalgia is a syndrome of chronic musculoskeletal pain. It is common in the elderly population and a major cause of disability. The exact cause is unknown, but one theory suggests that

GERONTOLOGICAL CONSIDERATIONS Related to Muscle Cramps

In addition to the decreased muscle mass and tone that are inherent to the aging process, many elderly people do not drink enough fluids due to the fear and embarrassment of incontinence. Therefore, it is imperative that the nurse teach the older patient the importance of hydrating, exercising in moderate temperatures to prevent the onset of muscle cramps, and performing some mild stretching exercises. Before suggesting electrolyte-based drinks, the nurse should know the patient's laboratory values of sodium and potassium. If a patient has a history of hypernatremia or hyperkalemia, then recommending these drinks on a daily basis may be detrimental to his health. The older patient needs to eat a well-balanced diet with vitamins and minerals to maintain bone and muscle integrity. Encourage the patient to have regular checkups in which electrolyte levels are monitored.

RESEARCH OPPORTUNITIES AND CLINICAL IMPACT RELATED TO MUSCLE CRAMPS

Research Need	**Clinical Impact**
In exercise-induced muscle cramps, will drinking one to two glasses of an electrolyte-based drink prior to exercising prevent muscle cramps?	A decreased incidence of muscle cramps due to dehydration, as well as longer endurance levels.

stress is responsible for fibromyalgia. Other theories suggest that the patient has an abnormal amount of pain-related chemicals in the nervous system; the patient has a conscious or subconscious tension, resulting in sleep disturbances; or the patient has a lowered pain threshold.

Recent studies have shown that patients with fibromyalgia have a "skewed" central pain processing function in their body (Peeke, 2003). Research has also shown that patients with fibromyalgia have elevated levels of a nerve growth factor and a chemical signal called *substance P* in the spinal fluid. Also, the amount of serotonin, the chemical produced in the brain that has an effect on nerves, is low (Frazier & Drzymkowski, 2009). These patients become extremely sensitive to even minor pain. Fibromyalgia is not associated with any type of musculoskeletal disorder, nor does it predispose a patient to a musculoskeletal disorder, but it may coexist with certain rheumatologic diseases such as lupus or arthritis.

Clinical Manifestations

The main signs and symptoms of fibromyalgia are pain in the back, neck, forearms, and knees. Besides joint and muscle pain, other symptoms are headaches, inability to sleep which leads to daytime fatigue, dizziness, alternating constipation and diarrhea, generalized weakness, depression, numbness and tingling of hands and feet, and memory loss. The onset of symptoms may be associated with psychological distress, trauma, or infection. The symptoms are aggravated by poor posture, strenuous exercise, and smoking (Frazier & Drzymkowski, 2009).

Laboratory and Diagnostic Procedures

The diagnosis of fibromyalgia is based on the patient's subjective symptoms, as well as a medical and surgical history. Patients with fibromyalgia do not have any other associated musculoskeletal disorder; therefore, arthritis, inflammations, and bursitis should be ruled out. Patients with this condition complain not only of muscle and joint aches but are extremely tender in these specific areas: at the antecubital area, below the clavicles, at the posterior neck, at the posterior top of the buttocks, and at the lateral pelvis. The American College of Rheumatology (2008) uses criteria for classification of fibromyalgia. This criteria includes widespread pain for a minimum of 3 months, and pain at 11/18 tender points on palpation. These points include the occipital, low cervical trapezius, supraspinatus, rib, epicondyle, and gluteal and knee areas.

Medical Management

The treatment of fibromyalgia is based on the severity of pain, stress level, and overall health of the patient. There is no cure for fibromyalgia but treatment will help to alleviate symptoms and restore function. The plan of care will involve patient education, stress reduction, physical exercise, and medications to reduce pain and improve the quality of sleep.

The federal Food and Drug Administration has approved the use of pregabalin (Lyrica) for patients with fibromyalgia. Two double-blinded studies indicated that people using the medication showed rapid and sustained pain reduction and improved sleep patterns for 6 months (Arthritis Foundation, 2008).

A scheduled exercise plan is important for increasing the blood supply, oxygen, and nutrients to joints and muscles. Recommended exercises include walking, bike riding, swim-ming, or aerobic exercise. Watsu, an exercise regimen performed in warm water, has been shown to be effective in patients with fibromyalgia (Osborn, 2005). The patient with fibromyalgia may require assistance in eliminating or controlling the stress that is causing symptoms. Anxiety and depression must be controlled in order to control fibromyalgia. Sometimes an antidepressant may be ordered to assist the patient through the "rough spots" and can promote the balance of pain-producing chemicals. A continuing medication regimen and an exercise plan are helpful in maintaining healthy muscles and joints.

■ Nursing Management

Nursing care should focus on assisting the patient to participate in a regimen that alleviates or minimizes the discomfort, as well as methods to deal with the patient's current stressors. Education about the illness, the importance of sleep, use of pain management strategies, adaptation to their illness, and promotion of regular exercise should be the nurse's role in assisting patients with this illness. See the Nursing Process: Patient Care Plan for Fibromyalgia feature and the Gerontological Considerations for Fibromyalgia box.

Alternative Treatments for Patients with Fibromyalgia

Massage therapy and relaxation techniques have been shown to help relieve the pain, stiffness, and sleep disturbances associated with fibromyalgia, as discussed in more detail in the Complementary and Alternative Therapies box (p. 1770).

Other alternative treatments used for patients with fibromyalgia include acupuncture, herbal products, reflexology, biofeedback, meditation and prayer, and **transcutaneous electrical nerve stimulation** (TENS) (pain relief via low-voltage electrical stimulation over a painful area).

Poliomyelitis

The onset of polio occurred in the 1950s with devastating outcomes for patients, such as flaccid paralysis of the legs. People contracted polio through a virus that is spread from infected

---

GERONTOLOGICAL CONSIDERATIONS
for Fibromyalgia

As people get older, sleep patterns change and many people do not sleep soundly throughout the night. Inadequate sleep is exacerbated in patients diagnosed with fibromyalgia, and so, besides the usual safety issues related to pain in the joints, they are particularly at risk for falls because of fatigue.

Older patients need to be aware that as the liver function decreases with age, medications are not filtered as quickly, leading to a faster rate of toxicity. This is particularly important when taking nonsteroidal anti-inflammatory agents, which can lead to ulcerations of the stomach and intestinal wall. Tylenol can cause altered liver function, which is especially dangerous to a patient who already has decreased liver function.

Lastly, chronic or acute pain, coupled with stress, may cause an older patient to feel hopeless, helpless, and alone, which may lead to depression.

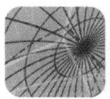

NURSING PROCESS: Patient Care Plan for Fibromyalgia

Assessment of Pain

Subjective Data:
On a scale of 1–10 with 1 being a little pain and 10 being the worst pain you have ever felt, at what level is your pain?
Do you routinely take pain medication at home? If yes, what is the name of the medication and why do you take it?
Are you allergic to any medications?

Objective Data:
Pain assessed during ROM to all joints. Pain greater when bending and turning the neck.
Monitor patient for:
Facial grimacing
Change in breathing pattern
Change in blood pressure and/or pulse rate
Diaphoresis
Agitation

Nursing Assessment and Diagnoses	Outcomes and Evaluation Parameters	Planning and Interventions with *Rationales*
Nursing Diagnosis: *Pain, Acute* or *Chronic*	**Outcome:** Pain level will be tolerable. *Evaluation Parameters:* Diminished or absent level of pain through patient's self-report. Absence of physiological indicators of pain.	**Interventions and *Rationales:*** Assess the patient's pain level on a scale of 1–10. Assess the pain level with bending the back, ROM of all joints. *Determining a specific pain level in relation to certain movements is helpful in devising an exercise plan, and prescribing a medication regime.* Assist the patient in developing an exercise plan that is not too strenuous. Teach medication regime and the importance of adherence to the medication plan, as well as reporting of side effects related to NSAIDs: gastric upset, rectal, or oral bleeding, bruising, abdominal discomfort. If on Tylenol, monitor liver enzymes. *Long-term Tylenol use or high-doses of Tylenol may cause liver damage.*

Assessment of Coping

Subjective Data:
Do you feel unusually fatigued?
Have you experienced altered sleep patterns?
Have you been able to communicate your concerns?

Objective Data:
Observe for:
Decreased use of social support
Destructive behavior toward self and others
Inability to meet basic needs
Inadequate problem solving
Lack of goal-directed behavior
Poor concentration

Nursing Assessment and Diagnoses	Outcomes and Evaluation Parameters	Planning and Interventions with *Rationales*
Nursing Diagnosis: *Coping, Ineffective*	**Outcome:** The patient will demonstrate effective coping. *Evaluation Parameters:* The patient: Takes actions to manage stressors. Shows self-restraint regarding compulsive or impulsive behaviors. Seeks information concerning illness and treatment. Reports decrease in negative feelings.	**Interventions and *Rationales:*** Allow the patient/family to verbalize fears and concerns. *Provides a support network.* Assist the patient in finding ways to cope with stress: Refer to social services or a therapist to assist the patient in managing stressful situations. *Social services and/or therapy can assist the patient in dealing with stress via several techniques.* Refer to local and national support system. *Provides support of other people in similar situations.* If the patient is placed on antidepressants, teach the patient the importance of maintaining the dose schedule and not to change or discontinue the medication without talking to her primary care provider. *Abruptly discontinuing antidepressants can exacerbate the symptoms of clinical depression.*

oropharyngeal secretions or fecal matter. Although polio has been fairly well eradicated in the United States, many Third World countries are struggling to control the onset and outbreak of polio (CDC, 2008b).

Epidemiology and Etiology

The polio virus infects the anterior horn cells of the gray matter of the spinal cord, which causes selective destruction of the motor neurons. The virus enters the body through the nasal and oral passages, crosses into the gastrointestinal tract, and enters the bloodstream traveling to the central nervous system. The incubation period is 7 to 21 days. It is highly infectious but up to 95% of patients who have the virus have no symptoms. Approximately 6% will have flu-like symptoms and fewer than 1% result in permanent paralysis. Of the patients who progress to paralysis, 5% to 10% die as a result of the virus affecting the respiratory muscles (CDC, 2008b; Frazier & Drzymkowski, 2009).

Clinical Manifestations

The poliovirus damages the nerves that control muscles. Because of the nerve damage, patients with polio have extreme muscle weakness and at times paralysis of an extremity. The patient will present with a low-grade fever, discharge from the sinuses, and malaise. As the disease progresses, the patient will complain of muscle weakness, stiff neck, nausea and vomiting, and flaccid paralysis of the muscles involved. The muscles affected atrophy and decreased tendon reflexes and joint deterioration evolve. Many patients with polio require assistive devices, such as canes, walkers, and crutches. In some cases, the paralysis affects the respiratory muscles, causing death.

Medical Management

The treatment for polio is immunization. Two forms of immunization are currently used against the polio virus: an injected polio vaccine (IPV) or a live, oral polio vaccine (OPV). Both vaccines are effective in preventing transmission of the disease from person to person, but in some cases the OPV can cause polio. For this reason, many health professionals recommend the IPV vaccine instead.

The vaccine schedule against polio varies for children and adults:

- **Children**—Children receive four doses of IPV at 2 months of age, 4 months of age, 6 to18 months of age, and a booster at 4 to 6 years of age.
- **Adults**—For adults who have not previously received the vaccine, it is important to administer it if they (1) plan to travel to countries where polio is active, (2) work with the polio virus, or (3) care for patients with polio.

For the patient who actually has active polio, the treatment is supportive. Analgesics and moist heat application are administered for pain. In the acute phase bed rest is indicated followed by physical therapy and evaluation for the use of assistive devices such as braces.

Post-Polio Syndrome

Post-polio syndrome (PPS) is acquired by patients who previously had polio. In some patients who have had polio, some of the undamaged nerves grow branches that connect to muscles that have lost their nerve connection, allowing some movement to the muscle. However, it is now being noted that the nerve connections are

COMPLEMENTARY & ALTERNATIVE THERAPIES   Massage

Description:

The general definition of massage therapy is the use of one's hands, fingers, elbows, forearm, or feet on another's body to elicit relaxation, reduce stress, promote health, or to treat a specific condition of the musculoskeletal system. Most U.S. states require a massage therapist to be licensed in order to practice. Massage therapy has evolved during the twentieth century to become a well known, respected therapy.

Research Support:

One study examined the impact of massage applied after exercise on muscle soreness. The study involved 10 healthy participants who performed 10 sets of 6 arm exercises. Three hours later, each participant then received 10 minutes of massage on only one arm; the other arm received no treatment. Although researchers found that massage had no effect on muscle function, they did find a significant decrease in muscle soreness in the arm that received massage (Zainuddin, Newton, Sacco, & Nosaka, 2005).

Massage that is performed on the patient's hand (or hand massage) is a simple, nonintrusive nursing intervention that the nurse can incorporate into routine nursing care activities. The nurse who utilizes hand massage can convey caring, promote comfort, and facilitate nurse–patient communication. One study evaluated the effect of hand massage on older adults residing in a nursing home. Outcomes were measured in terms of comfort and satisfaction. Over specific time periods, researchers found significant group differences in comfort and satisfaction between control and intervention groups. However, researchers found no significant differences in comfort levels or satisfaction with care over time (Kolcaba, Schirm, & Steiner, 2006). This may, in part, be due to the prevalence of memory impairment in older adults.

A review of 13 published randomized and quasi-randomized studies aimed to examine the effect of massage therapy on low-back pain, which is one of the most common musculoskeletal problems. Many people seek relief of their low-back pain through massage therapy. These studies showed that massage may be beneficial for patients with low-back pain, particularly when combined with exercise and education. However, researchers felt that more studies are needed to confirm these conclusions (Furlan, Imamura, Dryden, & Irvin, 2008).

References

Furlan, A. D., Imamura, M., Dryden, T., & Irvin, E. (2008, October). Massage for low-back pain. *Cochrane Database Systematic Reviews, 8*(4), CD001929.

Kolcaba, K., Schirm, V., & Steiner, R. (2006). Effects of hand massage on comfort of nursing home residents. *Geriatric Nursing, 27*(2), 85–91.

Zainuddin, Z., Newton, M., Sacco, P., & Nosaka, K. (2005). Effects of massage on delayed-onset muscle soreness, swelling, and recovery of muscle function. *Journal of Athletic Training, 40*(3), 174–180.

not as strong as once thought and therefore start to break down again after a time. This breakdown causes renewed weakness of the muscle they control. The progressive weakness is not noted until 15 years or more after the initial disease and involves already affected muscles (Frazier & Drzymkowski, 2009; WebMD, 2007).

Clinical Manifestations

Manifestations include new muscle weakness, fatigue, and muscle and joint pain. Some patients may develop dysphagia, respiratory difficulty, and decreased ability to tolerate cold. Those at risk for developing PPS are patients who had polio as a teenager or adult, still have muscle weakness, are female, and have had respiratory difficulty related to damage to the nerves that control breathing (WebMD, 2007).

Medical Management

Continuation of an active lifestyle is important for patients with PPS. The goals of treatment are to learn ways to stay active despite muscle weakness and to control muscle and joint pain with analgesics, heat and cold, and a balanced diet. The patient may require the use of assistive devices in order to maintain their ADLs and normal routine.

Nursing Management

Nursing care is directed to supportive care, safety measures, and adherence to an exercise regimen.

Assessment

The nurse should listen to the patient's subjective complaints and ask about the following:

- The patient's medical–surgical history
- When the symptoms began
- Whether there are any accompanying symptoms
- Whether the symptoms have affected the patient's ability to maintain ADLs
- What type of exercise the patient engages in and how often the patient exercises
- Whether the patient has traveled to any Third World countries
- What type of medications the patient is taking, both prescription and OTC
- Whether the patient has had any respiratory difficulty, back pain, or dysphagia.

The nurse should objectively assess the patient by performing a physical examination. Observe the patient during ambulation. Test resistance of all four limbs. Auscultate lung sounds. Have the patient bend forward and backward (if able) to test the strength of the back muscles.

Nursing Diagnosis

The primary diagnoses for the patient with poliomyelitis or PPS include:

- *Physical Mobility, Impaired*
- *Fatigue*

- *Falls, Risk for*
- *Airway Clearance, Ineffective*
- *Disuse Syndrome, Risk for*

Outcomes and Evaluation

Outcomes include maintenance of a clear airway as exhibited by the patient's ability to swallow and cough, maintenance of current muscle use as exhibited by the patient's ability to perform scheduled exercises, and maintenance of functional alignment of all joints. Due to muscle weakness, the patient is at risk for falls. Outcome criteria would include no falls. Fatigue will be evaluated by the patient's ability to plan rest periods throughout the day to maintain strength.

Planning, Interventions, and Rationales

Patient education is key to the prevention of polio. Parents should be encouraged to have their children vaccinated and any adult who has not been vaccinated and is traveling to a Third World country is advised to receive the vaccine.

The patient with polio or PPS will be evaluated for factors that increase the risk of muscle and joint complications, such as preexisting conditions such as arthritis or surgery, that would reduce mobility. Muscle function depends on activity to maintain and increase muscle strength and maintain balance and muscle tone. Disuse will cause atrophy and lead to shortening of muscle fibers and reduce joint motion.

An active exercise program should be developed, as the patient's condition permits, including complete ROM to all joints at least four times daily. Active exercise promotes maximum muscle contraction and helps to maintain muscle strength and endurance. Full ROM exercises to all joints stretches the surrounding muscle fibers and maintains the coordinated function of the joint structures.

It is important to plan rest periods between activities to prevent fatigue. Rest periods assist with endurance and the ability to participate in the plan of care.

Administer analgesics and warm and cold compresses to areas of discomfort. Promoting comfort permits physical activity.

Instruct the patient on the use of mobility aids (canes, braces, walkers). Educating the patient regarding the importance of mobility aids helps her adjust to using them. Mobility aids help to prevent injury and can offer the patient a sense of security.

Evaluation

Prognosis for the patient with poliomyelitis is fair depending on the muscles that are involved. The prognosis for PPS is good. Evaluation of the plan of care will include the patient's statement that pain is controlled and an assessment of muscle strength along with the patient's ability to participate in the exercise regimen. If the patient requires mobility aids, evaluation will include proper use of the device as exhibited by the patient and a lack of falls or injury as reported by the patient. For more information, see Patient Teaching & Discharge Priorities for Post-Polio Syndrome (p. 1772).

Health Promotion for Patients with Musculoskeletal Disorders

All of the ailments discussed in this section have some type of permanent disability and/or an acute or chronic discomfort or

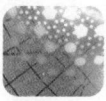

PATIENT TEACHING & DISCHARGE CONSIDERATIONS for Post-Polio Syndrome

Need	Teaching
Need for exercise regime	Maintain and plan a daily exercise regime that promotes bone and muscle activity, but is not physically exhausting, such as walking or bike riding.
Eat a well-balanced diet	Set up a dietary menu that includes, vitamins, minerals, protein, calcium, and carbohydrates.
Maintain body mass index for height (ideal body weight)	Weigh weekly. If gaining weight, modify diet to decrease carbohydrates.
Rest periods	Rest if tired or in between activities and exercise programs.

weakness associated with them. Healthy living, to include not being overweight, eating a healthy diet, and practicing some type of exercise plan, is mandatory for preventing further complications in patients with these conditions. A scheduled exercise program is prescribed in order to maintain joint mobility, to increase circulation and oxygenation to the muscles and tissues, and to strengthen bone. Patients should maintain a weight that is appropriate for their height, because added weight causes stress to an already impaired musculoskeletal system. Maintenance of weight is predicated on a good exercise plan, plus a diet low in fats.

The concept of the federal government's *Healthy People 2010* campaign is not just for healthy individuals but can benefit everyone, even those with chronic or disabling conditions. It is a framework of national health objectives designed to identify preventable threats to health and establish goals to reduce these threats. The leading health indicators that correlate with this chapter are as follows: Engage in an exercise program, abstain from tobacco use and substance abuse, maintain weight per body mass index (ideal weight), receive immunizations for polio if traveling to a Third World country, and maintain regular visits with a health care provider. Therefore, nursing responsibilities should include health teaching to include dietary management, weight control, abstinence from smoking, and a viable exercise program.

Clinical Preparation

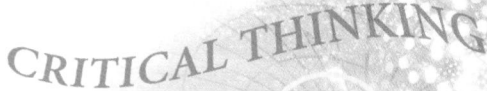

CRITICAL THINKING

PEARSON mynursingkit

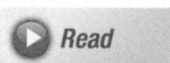 **Read**

- History of Current Illness
- Past Medical History
- Physical Exam
- Admitting Medical Orders
- Laboratory Study Results

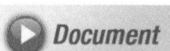 **Document**

- Summary of Hospitalization
- Pathophysiology Form
- Laboratory Values
- Laboratory Results Explanation

 **Apply**

- List of Potential Nursing Diagnoses
- Concept Map
- Critical Thinking Questions

Log on to MyNursingKit.com to download forms you will need and to complete further steps in the Clinical Preparation assignment.

HISTORY OF PRESENT ILLNESS

You are the nurse on a medical–surgical unit. You have been notified that you will be receiving a patient from the emergency department (ED). The ED nurse calls the unit and gives report on the 72-year-old female being admitted. She was found by her daughter in her home on the floor of her bedroom approximately 12 hours after a fall. The patient states she does not clearly remember what led to the fall and is complaining of sharp, constant right hip discomfort.

Medical–Surgical History
The patient has a history of hypertension. She states she has never had an operation.

Social History
The patient states she has never smoked. She drinks alcohol occasionally. She walks for 20 minutes daily and takes a t'ai chi class on Tuesday afternoons.

Physical Exam
The patient is orientated to person, place, and time. Pupils are equal and react to light. Bilateral grasps are equal and strong. She rates her right hip pain at an 8 on a scale of 0 (no pain) to 10 (most pain ever). Vital signs: temp: 99°F; BP: 180/90 mmHg; heart rate: 104 bpm; 22 respirations per minute, even and relaxed. Bilateral breath sounds are present and clear in all lobes; however, bilateral

breath sounds are slightly diminished in the lower lobes. Right leg is adducted and internally rotated, but patient denies numbness or tingling of her right foot. Right pedal pulses palpated less than left, but right pedal pulse strong by Doppler. She states that she takes high blood pressure medication and on occasion an aspirin for joint discomfort.

Admitting Medical Orders

Service: orthopedic surgery
Diagnosis: fracture right hip
Allergies: no known allergies
Vital signs: every 4 hours including oxygen saturation
Call house officer: temp > 38.5°C, HR > 110 or < 60, RR > 30 or < 12, BP sys > 160 or < 90, O₂ sat < 92%, urine output < 120 mL in 4 hours, change in neurological exam, any Hct result that is 5 less than the baseline ED Hct
Activity: bed rest
Diet: nothing by mouth
IVs: D5.45NS with 20 mEq of KCl at 100 mL/hr
I&O: every shift
Respiratory care: incentive spirometer every hour when awake
DVT prophylaxis: sequential compression device to lower extremities bilaterally
Treatments: skin traction to right lower extremity
Consent to be signed for open reduction and internal fixation of right trochanter

To the operating room tomorrow on call
Insert Foley catheter
Daily weight

Scheduled Medications

Atenolol 50 mg po every day
Preop medication per anesthesiologist

PRN Medications

Phenergan 25 mg IV every 6 hours prn nausea
Morphine 2–4 mg IV every 4 hours prn pain
Ativan 0.5 mg IV every 6 hours prn anxiety
Tylenol 650 mg PO every 4 hours for pain

Ordered Laboratory Studies

Complete blood count and Chem panel every morning

Ordered Diagnostic Studies

Chest x-ray every morning

LABORATORY STUDY RESULTS

Test	ED Initial	ED 2nd (4 hours)	On Admission to Floor
CBC			
Hemoglobin (Hgb)	10.5 g/dL	9.5 g/dL	9.5 g/dL
Hematocrit (Hct)	34%	33%	32%
RBC	3.2/mm³	3/mm³	3/mm³
Reticulocytes	2.0%	2.4%	2.4%
MCV	72 µm³	68 µm³	68 µm³
MCH	27 pg	25 pg	25 pg
Platelets	150/mm	146/mm³	146/mm³
Electrolytes			
Sodium	135 mEq/L	135 mEq/L	140 mEq/L
Potassium	3.6 mEq/L	3.6 mEq/L	3.9 mEq/L
Calcium	9 mg/dL	9 mg/dL	9 mg/dL
BUN	14 mg/dL	14 mg/dL	16 mg/dL
Creatinine	0.8 mg/dL	1 mg/dL	1.2 mg/dL
Glucose	150 mg/dL	148 mg/dL	140 mg/dL

CRITICAL THINKING QUESTIONS

1. What pertinent information can be assessed by the medical–surgical nurse?

2. What are the patient's risk factors for sustaining a fracture?

3. What other lab tests might the nurse anticipate?

4. What are the goals of medical management for this client?

5. What are two priority nursing diagnoses?

6. What are some postoperative instructions for this client?

Answers to Critical Thinking Questions appear in Appendix D.

NCLEX® REVIEW

1. The mechanical properties of bone are based on which of the following?
   1. Age and flexibility
   2. Nutritional status and body weight
   3. Stress and strain
   4. Gravity and circumference

2. A nurse is providing a preventive health care seminar related to ways to decrease the effects of osteoporosis. Which of the following risk factors does the nurse discuss which apply to both men and women?
   1. Anorexia
   2. Diet low in calcium and Vitamin D
   3. History of maternal hip fracture
   4. Low body weight and low body mass index

3. A nurse has provided an overview of evidence-based care for prevention of hip fracture in older people. Which statement made by a participant warrants further education?
   1. "Living at my own home increases my chance of a fracture."
   2. "Taking anticonvulsants may increase my possibility of falling."
   3. "Insulin-dependent diabetic patients are more at risk."
   4. "Women experience more hip fractures than men."

4. All forms of muscular dystrophies have what element in common?
   1. The cause of death is due to systemic infection.
   2. The average life expectancy is into the fourth decade.
   3. Muscle membranes have a protein deficiency or absence of dystrophin.
   4. Cognitive development and functioning are not at a full level.

5. A 75-year old male with long-term alcohol abuse would likely experience which of the following myopathies?
   1. Hypokalemic
   2. Polymyositis
   3. Steroid-induced
   4. Inclusion body myositis

6. The diagnosis of fibromyalgia is based on the patient's report of:
   1. long-term arthritis history.
   2. treatment for depression.
   3. familial tendency of the condition.
   4. subjective symptoms.

Answers for review questions appear in Appendix D

KEY TERMS

cancellous (trabecular) bone *p.1729*
compact (cortical) bone *p.1729*
dermatomyositis *p.1760*
electromyelogram (EMG) *p.1754*
endoskeletal *p.1728*
Gottron's sign *p.1762*
Haversian canals *p.1729*
hypotonia *p.1759*

kyphosis *p.1753*
lamellar bone *p.1729*
lordosis *p.1753*
modeling *p.1730*
osteoblasts *p.1730*
osteoclasts *p.1730*
osteocytes *p.1730*
osteoid *p.1730*

osteology *p.1728*
osteoporosis *p.1733*
periosteum *p.1728*
perivascular *p.1762*
scoliosis *p.1753*
subchondral bone *p.1729*
transcutaneous electrical nerve stimulation (TENS) *p.1768*

EXPLORE PEARSON mynursingkit™

MyNursingKit is your one stop for online chapter review materials and resources. Prepare for success with additional NCLEX®-style practice questions, interactive assignments and activities, web links, animations and videos, and more!

Register your access code from the front of your book at
www.mynursingkit.com

REFERENCES

American Academy of Orthopaedic Surgeons. (2008). *Muscle cramps.* Retrieved May 24, 2008, from http://orthoinfo.aaos.org/topic.cfm?topic=A00200#Cause

American Cancer Society. (2008). *Detailed guide: Bone cancer.* Retrieved May 17, 2008, from http://www.cancer.org/docroot/CRI/content/CRI_2_4_1X_What_Is_bone_cancer

American College of Rheumatology. (2008). *Fibromyalgia.* Retrieved May 24, 2008, from http://www.rheumatology.org/publications/classification/fibromyalgia/fibro.asp

Arthritis Foundation. (2008). *Fibromyalgia.* Retrieved May 24, 2008, from http://www.arthritis.org/new-fibro-treatment.php

Bartelmo, J. M., & Lockhart, A. (Eds.). (2008). *Nursing: Understanding diseases.* Philadelphia: Lippincott Williams & Wilkins.

Beers, M. H., & Porter, R. S. (Eds.). (2006). *The Merck manual of diagnosis and therapy* (18th ed.). Whitehouse Station, NJ: Merck Research Laboratories.

Canalis, E. (2004). Mechanisms of glucocorticoid induced osteoporosis. *Arthritis Research Therapy, 6*(Suppl. 3), 37.

Centers for Disease Control and Prevention. (2008a). *Duchenne and Becker muscular dystrophy.* Retrieved May 24, 2008, from http://www.cdc.gov/ncbddd/duchenne/

Centers for Disease Control and Prevention. (2008b). *Polio.* Retrieved May 25, 2008, from http://www.cdc.gov/vaccines/vpd-vac/polio/in-short-both.htm

Chan, G. K., & Duque, G. (2002). Age-related bone loss: Old bone, new facts. *Gerontology, 48*(2), 62–71.

Christensen, B., & Kockrow, E. (2003). *Adult health nursing* (4th ed.). St. Louis: Mosby.

Copstead, L. E., & Banaski, J. L. (2005). *Pathophysiology* (2nd ed.). St. Louis: Elsevier.

Cosman, F., Nieves, J. W., Zion, M., Woelfert, L., Luckey, M., & Lindsay, R. (2005). Daily and cyclic parathyroid hormone in women receiving alendronate. *New England Journal of Medicine 353*, 566–575.

Dalakas, M. C., & Hohfield, R. (2003). Polymyositis and dermatomyositis. *Lancet, 363*.

Dumke, C. L. (2003). Muscle cramps are not all created equal. *Athletic Therapy Today*, pp. 42–43.

Fajardo, M., & Di Cesare, P. E. (2005). Disease-modifying therapies for osteoarthritis: Current status. *Drugs and Aging, 22*(2), 141–161.

Forsblad D'Elia, H., Larsen, A., Waltbrand, E., Kvist, G., Mellström, D., Saxne, T., et al. (2003). Radiographic joint destruction in postmenopausal rheumatoid arthritis is strongly associated with generalized osteoporosis. *Annals of Rheumatic Disease, 62*(7), 617–623.

Frazier, M. S., & Drzymkowski, J. W. (Eds.). (2009). *Essentials of human diseases and conditions* (4th ed.). St. Louis: Saunders.

Gupta, R., Caiozzo, V., Cook, S. D., Barrack, R. L., & Skinner, H. B. (2005). *Current diagnosis and treatment in orthopedics* (4th ed.). New York: McGraw-Hill Medical.

Hogan, M. A., DeLeon, E., Gingrich, M. M., & Willcutts, K. (2007). *Nutrition and diet therapy* (2nd ed.). Upper Saddle River, NJ: Pearson Prentice Hall.

Hunter, D. J., & Sambrook, P. N. (2000). Bone loss: Epidemiology of bone loss. *Arthritis Research, 2*, 441–445.

Jochems, C., Islander, U., Erlandsson, M., Verdrengh, M., Ohlosson, C., & Carlsten, H. (2005). Osteoporosis in experimental postmenopausal polyarthritis: The relative contributions of estrogen deficiency and inflammation. *Arthritis Research and Therapy, 7*, R837–R843.

King, R. W., Johnson, D., Stearns, D. A., Talavera, F., Weiss, E. L., Halamka, J., et al. (2006). *Osteomyelitis.* Retrieved January 22, 2007, from http://www.emedicine.com/emerg/topic349/htm

Lahl, M., Fisher, V. L., & Laschinger, K. (2007). Ewing's sarcoma family of tumors: An overview from diagnosis to survivorship. *Clinical Journal of Oncology Nursing, 12*(1), 89–97.

Leighton, S. (2003). Nutrition for boys with Duchenne muscular dystrophy. *Nutrition & Dietetics, 60*, 1.

Lim, S., Joung, H., Sin, C. S., Lee, H. K., Kim, K. S., Shin, E. K., et al. (2004). Body composition changes with age have gender-specific impacts on bone mineral density. *Bone, 35*, 792–798.

MacLean, C., Newberry, S., Maglione, M., McMahon, M., Ranganath, V., Suttorp, M., et al. (2008). Systematic review: Comparative effectiveness of treatments to prevent fractures in men and women with low bone density or osteoporosis. *Annals of Internal Medicine, 148*, 197–213.

Majumdar, S. R., Johnson, J. A., McAlister, F. A., Bellerose, D., Russell, A. S., Hanley, D. A., et al. (2008). Multifaceted intervention to improve diagnosis and treatment of osteoporosis in patients with recent wrist fracture: A randomized controlled trial. *Canadian Medical Association Journal, 178*(5), 569–575.

Marcus, R., & Gopalakrishnan, G. (2005). Secondary forms of osteoporosis. In F. L. Coe & M. J. Favus (Eds.), *Disorders of bone and mineral metabolism.* Philadelphia: Lippincott Raven Publishers.

Mayo Clinic. (2007). *Muscular dystrophy.* Retrieved May 25, 2008, from http://www.mayoclinic.com/health/muscular-dystrophy/DS00200

McCance, K., & Huether, S. (2006). *Pathophysiology: The biologic basis for disease in adults and children* (5th ed.). St. Louis: Mosby.

MedlinePlus. (2008). *Muscle cramps.* Retrieved May 24, 2008, from http://www.nlm.nih.gov/medlineplus/musclecramps.html

Merck. (2003). *Merck manual of geriatrics.* (2003). Whitehouse Station, NJ: Author.

Muscular Dystrophy Association. (2008). *Facts about Duchenne and Becker muscular dystrophies.* Retrieved August 17, 2008, from http://www.mda.org/publications/fa-dmdbmd-what.html

Muscular Dystrophy Association (MDA). (2003). *Facts about mitochondrial myopathies.* Retrieved August 27, 2008, from http://www.mda.org/Publications/mitochondrial_myopathies.html#whatare

National Institutes of Health. (2007). *Osteoporosis.* Retrieved May 25, 2008, from http://www.niams.nih.gov/Health_Info/Bone/Osteoporosis/default.asp

National Institute of Neurological Disorders and Stroke. (2008). *Myopathy.* Retrieved May 24, 2008, from http://www.ninds.nih.gov/disorders/myopathy/myopathy.htm

Osborn, K. (2005). *Water, watsu, and wellness.* Retrieved May 25, 2008, from http://www.massageandbodywork.com/Articles/OctNov2005/Water.html

Peeke, P. M. (2003). 90 days to fibromyalgia relief. *Prevention.* Retrieved August 17, 2008, from http://www.prevention.com/cda/article/90-days-to-fibromyalgia-relief/dff472e50d803110VgnVCM10000013281eac____/health/conditions.treatments/fibromyalgia

Porth, C. (2005). *Pathophysiology: Concepts of altered health states* (7th ed.). Philadelphia: Lippincott Williams & Wilkins.

Raisz, L. G. (2005). Pathogenesis of osteoporosis: Concepts, conflicts, and prospects. *Journal of Clinical Investigation, 115*(12), 3318–3325.

Seeman, E. (2002). Pathogenesis of bone fragility in women and men. *Lancet, 359*, 1841–1850.

Takeda, E., Taketani, Y., Sawada, N., Sato, T., & Yamamoto, H. (2004). The regulation and function of phosphate in the human body. *Biofactors, 21*(1–4), 345–355.

U. S. Department of Health and Human Services. (2004). *Bone health and osteoporosis: A report of the surgeon general.* Retrieved June 20, 2008, from http://www.surgeongeneral.gov/library/bonehealth

WebMD. (2007). *Post-polio syndrome.* Retrieved May 25, 2008, from http://www.webmd.com/brain/tc/post-polio-syndrome-topic-overview

Younger, D. S. (2003). The myopathies. *Medical Clinics of North America, 87*, 899–907.

Caring for the Patient with Musculoskeletal Trauma

Miki Patterson
Cheryl Wraa

Outcome-Based Learning Objectives

After studying this chapter, the learner will be able to:

1. Describe the incidence, prevalence, and prevention strategies for musculoskeletal trauma.
2. Explain the pathophysiological stages of bone healing.
3. Compare and contrast the various types of fractures and methods for fracture treatment.
4. Apply nursing diagnoses and the nursing process to the care of the patient with musculoskeletal trauma.
5. Discuss potential complications related to musculoskeletal trauma.
6. Identify research implications for nursing practice in caring for the musculoskeletally injured patient.

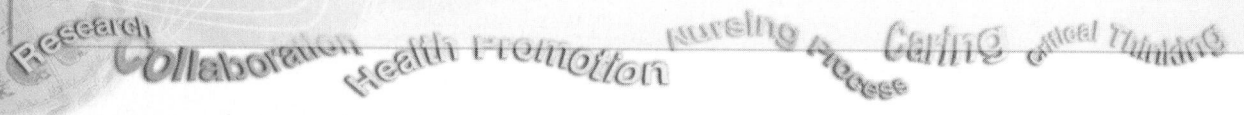

MUSCULOSKELETAL TRAUMA affects most people at some point in their lifetime. Musculoskeletal injuries are a frequent occurrence in blunt trauma, such as motor vehicle crashes, falls, crush injuries, sports injuries, and auto versus pedestrian collisions. Musculoskeletal injuries can also be a result of penetrating trauma such as gunshot or stab wounds (Bongiovanni, Bradley, & Kelley, 2005). Injuries to the musculoskeletal system occur in 85% of patients who sustain blunt trauma (American College of Surgeons (ACS), 2004). Prevention is the only method to decrease the effects of injuries to the muscles, tendons, ligaments, and bones. Whether at home, in the workplace, at play, or on the road, many strategies have been designed to reduce or prevent injuries. Helmets and seat belts; bike, gun, and water safety; and reduced alcohol consumption are major strategies addressed by the Centers for Disease Control and Prevention (CDC) and Emergency Nurses Association (ENA) to prevent injuries. Every 30 minutes someone in the United States dies in an alcohol-related crash (ENA, 2006). Public awareness and education can affect social change and help to decrease the incidence of alcohol-related injuries.

Half of all sports-related injuries are also preventable. Education and awareness surrounding protective equipment, safer playing environments, and rules designed to prevent injury are important in reducing the frequency and severity of sports in-

juries (National Safe Kids Campaign, 2003). Stretching, warm-up exercises, and strengthening and balance training regimens are key in preventing sports injuries.

Etiology

Musculoskeletal trauma results from injuries that are accidental and nonaccidental to a person's bones, joints, and soft tissues. "Accidental" trauma is caused by overuse, impact, sports injuries, and vehicle crashes. Motor vehicle crashes, bicycle and pedestrian injuries, and falls are the most common etiology for musculoskeletal trauma. Nonaccidental or inflicted trauma is seen as a result of domestic violence, child abuse, and altercations and may take the form of blunt trauma, whereby impact is made between the body and an object or force, or penetrating trauma, when an object such as a knife or bullet enters the body. The most common musculoskeletal injuries are strains, sprains, contusions, and fractures.

Health Promotion

The best cure for musculoskeletal trauma is prevention. For athletes, a proper warm-up, stretching, training, supervision, equipment, and surfaces help to prevent common sports injuries. Environmental factors may also play a role in sports safety. For instance, playing on wet or uneven turf may cause athletes to lose their footing and fall, injuring or twisting a joint or extremity. Properly trained coaches and trainers are important in preventing musculoskeletal trauma. They should understand the nutrition and hydration needs of athletes as well as developmental differences and norms. For example, children with open **physes** (growth plates) should perform very limited fastball pitching, because the movement involved with this type of pitching can permanently deform their elbows due to stress on the physis or growth plates.

It is also important not to allow athletes to compete with pain or injuries unless a clinician has evaluated them. Nurses united in the mission "to advance the quality of musculoskeletal health care by promoting excellence in research, education and nursing practice" have formed the National Association of Orthopedic Nurses (NAON) and provide information and educational materials on a wide variety of topics and issues.

Prevention of trauma related to motor vehicle crashes is a major health care issue. Health education that stresses prevention of the problems associated with alcohol consumption and driving is a common goal of public health and other groups such as MADD (Mothers Against Drunk Driving) and SADD (Students Against Destructive Decisions, founded as Students Against Driving Drunk). To fight the high incidence of teen crashes nationwide, the Recording Artists, Actors and Athletes Against Drunk Driving (RADD) Coalition and the National Highway Traffic Safety Administration (NHTSA), both members of the National Organizations for Youth Safety (NOYS), have joined forces with others to develop programs to educate teens regarding this issue.

■ Pathophysiology

Understanding the mechanism and physiological affect of an injury will assist the nurse in prioritizing the assessment and care of the patient with a musculoskeletal injury. Following are descriptions of common injuries found in musculoskeletal trauma.

Contusions

A **contusion** is an injury to soft tissue caused by trauma in which the skin is not broken. A contusion is characterized by pain, discoloration (bruising), and swelling. The initial treatment is ice for 48 hours to constrict the capillaries and impede blood and edema in tissue, later followed by warm moist applications to assist increasing circulation to resorb the edematous fluid.

Sprains and Strains

A **strain** is an injury to the muscle belly or its tendon attachment to bone, typically caused by excessive force or load on a joint or muscle. The associated pain may be described as dull or sharp pain that increases with movement of the muscle. With intramuscular bleeding, it can take up to 24 hours for any bruising to become visible because the blood remains primarily within the muscle sheath, causing pain and local swelling (Anscomb, 2007).

Sprains are similar in nature to strains, but they occur at the **ligaments** (strong fibrous bands of connective tissue) that attach bone to bone. Sprained ankles are one of the most common musculoskeletal injuries in people of all ages, athlete and sedentary alike (Harvard Women's Health Watch, 2007). The

most common type of ankle sprain occurs when the foot rolls inward, damaging the ligaments of the outer ankle (Figure 56–1 ■). Medial ankle sprains, which affect the ligaments of the inner ankle, occur most often in contact sports and are more likely to cause chronic ankle instability with subsequent sprains. The severity of the sprain depends on the degree of damage to the ligaments and how unstable the joint becomes. Chart 56–1 (p. 1778) describes the three grades for this type of injury. Oftentimes a Grade 3 sprain is accompanied by an **avulsion fracture** whereby the ligament breaks off a small piece of the bone at its attachment. The area may have an effusion, ecchymosis, and be very tender to palpation.

Both strains and sprains are diagnosed by a physical exam and history. A radiograph of the affected extremity may be used to rule out an associated fracture.

Medical Management

The initial treatment follows the acronym **PRICE**:

- **Protection**—Immobilize and prevent weight bearing. Grade 2 and 3 sprains are protected from further injury by splints, braces, or casts.
- **Rest**—This is important during the first 24 to 48 hours after the injury to prevent further damage.
- **Ice**—The use of ice has many benefits. Cold helps to relieve pain by reducing nerve conductivity, slowing metabolism of oxygen at the injury site, and reducing cell death and inflammation. An ice pack should be applied to the affected area with the limb elevated and remain in place for 10 to 15 minutes, three to four times a day for the first 3 to 4 days postinjury. Contraindications to ice therapy are cold sensitivity (Raynaud's disease), skin lesions, and peripheral vascular disease.
- **Compression**—Compression aids in the control of edema at the injury site by applying direct pressure and increasing venous return. The pressure should be graduated. When patients begin to bear weight on the extremity, they should wear a compression bandage only when the foot is on the floor and not when elevated. Patients should only need to use a compression bandage for the first 4 to 5 days because the acute inflammatory phase should be over.
- **Elevation**—Elevation is only effective if the affected limb is raised above the heart.

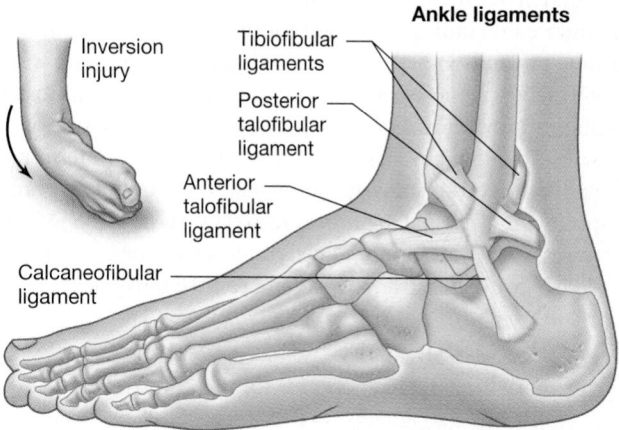

FIGURE 56–1 ■ Ankle ligaments and inversion injury.

CHART 56-1	**Grades of Sprain Severity**			
Severity	**Degree of Ligament Damage**	**Symptoms**	**Recovery Time**	**Treatment**
Grade 1	Ligament stretched	Mild pain, swelling, and tenderness. Bruising uncommon. Joint stable with no difficulty bearing weight.	1–3 weeks	Mild injury PRICE
Grade 2	Partial tear 20–75%	Moderate pain, swelling, and tenderness. Some bruising. Joint may have mild to moderate joint instability. Patient will have some decreased ROM and function. Patient will experience pain with weight bearing and walking.	3–6 weeks	PRICE Restrict weight bearing Splint Cast Brace
Grade 3	Complete tear or rupture	Severe pain, swelling, tenderness, and bruising. Unstable joint with loss of function and ROM. Patient will be unable to bear weight or walk.	Several months	PRICE Restrict weight bearing Splint Cast Brace May require surgical intervention

Source: Adapted from Harvard Women's Health Watch. (2007). *Recovering from an ankle sprain.* Retrieved April 5, 2008, from http://www.health.harvard.edu.

The most commonly used analgesic for sprains and strains is a nonsteroidal anti-inflammatory drug (NSAID). Medical attention should be sought immediately for any loss of function, sensation, pallor, or pain that is disproportionate to the injury.

Nursing Management

The nursing management of strains and sprains initially focuses on protection of the limb and pain control. Patient teaching regarding exercises to help restore function and prevent injury are essential to the patient's recovery.

Assessment

The nurse should obtain a thorough history to help differentiate a soft tissue injury from a possible fracture. The circumstances leading up to and the mechanism of the injury should be explored. Strains and muscle ruptures usually occur from a sudden stretch on a muscle that is actively contracting, such as during a sport or when lifting a heavy object. A sprain is usually the result of a sudden trauma such as tripping. A pop or snap felt at the time of injury could indicate ligament rupture or fracture. Inquire regarding previous injury to determine if the joint may have weakness. During physical examination, compare both extremities to distinguish any deformity or asymmetry. Complete rupture of the muscle is identified by a break in the normal muscle outline, particularly with resisted movement. Evaluate the extremity for range of motion. It is normal to have decreased function as the swelling increases, so it is important to determine a baseline assessing the difference between active, passive, and resisted movement.

Nursing Diagnoses

The primary nursing diagnoses for sprains and strains include:

- *Pain, Acute*
- *Physical Mobility, Impaired*
- *Knowledge, Deficient* related to plan of care.

Outcomes and Evaluation Parameters

The desired outcomes for the patient with a strain or sprain are relief of pain, protection of the joint, and return of strength and mobility. Following the PRICE regimen described above will help to control pain and swelling. Rehabilitative range-of-motion (ROM), stretching, and strengthening exercises, as described in Figures 56–2 ■ and 56–3 ■, will help to strengthen and protect the joint. Evaluation parameters include pain control as described by the patient, resolution of edema, and return of strength and range of motion.

Planning, Interventions, and Rationales

Administration of anti-inflammatory medication, elevation, application of an elastic bandage for compression, and application of an ice pack for 15- to 20-minute intervals four to five times a day will assist in decreasing the swelling and pain. Teaching the patient ROM, stretching, and strengthening exercises like those shown in Figures 56–2 ■ and 56–3 ■ will help the patient regain strength and mobility to the joint, hence restoring function and preventing further injury.

Health Promotion

Health teaching for patients with contusions, strains, and sprains centers on restoration of function and prevention of further injury. Balance training is found to reduce injury to the ankle and the knee. Balance training in the form of t'ai chi improves balancing ability and muscular cocontraction around the ankle joint, which is helpful in reducing injury in older adults who are balance impaired. Balance training in conjunction with strength and agility training has been used to enhance the neuromuscular responses to stabilize the knee joint in female athletes, thus reducing injury (Hrysomallis, 2007). The Complementary and Alternative Therapies feature (p. 1780) discusses the use of chiropractic care for extremities.

Range of motion, stretching, and strengthening: First 1–2 weeks

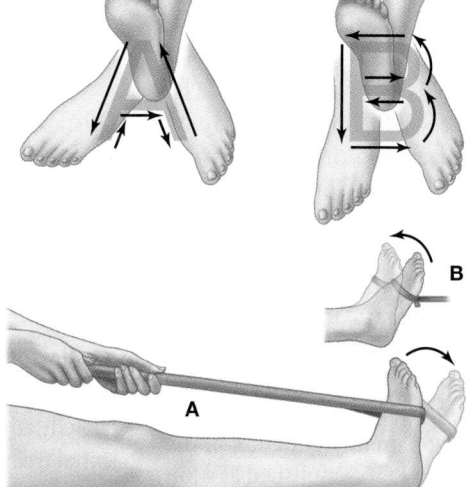
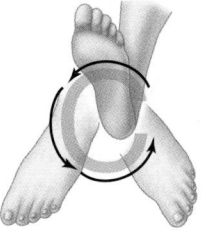

Ankle alphabet. With the heel on the floor, write all the capital letters of the alphabet with your big toe, making the letters as large as you can.

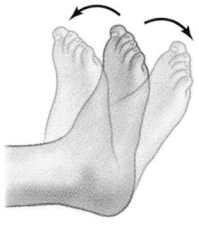

Flexes. Rest the heel of the injured foot on the floor. Pull your toes and foot toward your body as far as possible. Release. Then point them away from the body as far as possible. Release. Repeat as often as possible in the first week.

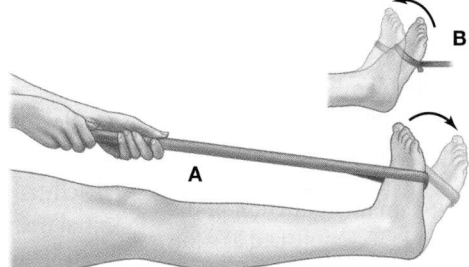

Press down, pull back. Loop an elasticized band or tubing around the foot, holding it gently taut (A). Press your toes away and down. Hold for a few seconds. Repeat 30 times. Tie one end of the band to a table or chair leg (B). Loop the other end around your foot. Slowly pull the foot toward you. Hold for a few seconds. Repeat 30 times.

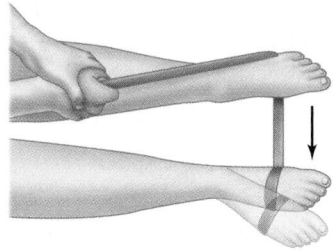

Ankle eversion. Seated on the floor, with an elasticized band or tubing tied around the injured foot and anchored around your uninjured foot, slowly turn the injured foot outward. Repeat 30 times.

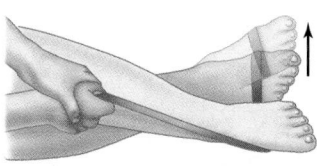

Ankle inversion. Seated on the floor, cross your legs with your injured foot underneath. With an elasticized band or tubing around the injured foot and anchored around your uninjured foot, slowly turn the injured foot inward. Repeat 30 times.

FIGURE 56–2 ■ Range of motion, stretching, and strengthening of the ankle. Perform the first 1 to 2 weeks after injury.
Source: Harvard Women's Health Watch. (2007). *Recovering from an ankle sprain.* Retrieved April 5, 2008, from http://www.health.harvard.edu

Stretching and strengthening: Weeks 3–4

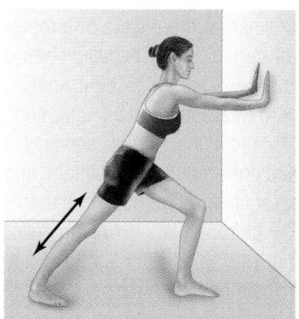

Standing stretch. Stand one arm's length from the wall. Place the injured foot behind the other foot, toes facing forward. Keep your heels down and the back knee straight. Slowly bend the front knee until you feel the calf stretch in the back leg. Hold for 15–20 seconds. Repeat 3–5 times.

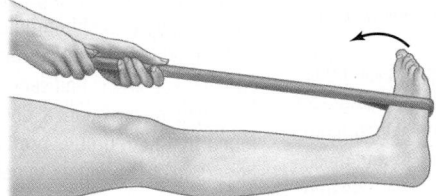

Seated stretch. Loop an elasticized band or tubing around the ball of the foot. Keeping the knee straight, slowly pull back on the band until you feel the upper calf stretch. Hold for 15 seconds. Repeat 15–20 times.

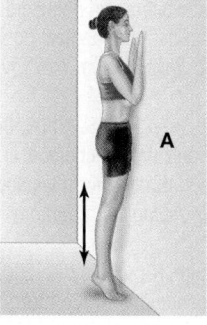

Rises. Stand facing a wall with your hands on the wall for balance (A). Rise up on your toes. Hold for 1 second, then lower yourself slowly to the starting position. Repeat 20–30 times. As you become stronger, do this exercise keeping your weight on just the injured side as you lower yourself down.

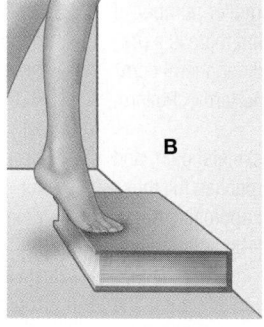

Stretches. Stand with your toes and the ball of the affected foot on a book or the edge of a stair (B). Your heel should be off the ground. Use a wall, chair, or rail for balance. Hold your other foot off the ground behind you, with knee slightly bent. Slowly lower the heel. Hold the position for 1 second. Return to the starting position. Repeat up to 15 times, several times a day. This exercise can place a lot of stress on the ankle, so get your clinician's go-ahead before trying it.

FIGURE 56–3 ■ Stretching and strengthening exercises for the ankle. Perform 3 to 4 weeks after injury.
Source: Harvard Women's Health Watch. (2007). *Recovering from an ankle sprain.* Retrieved April 5, 2008, from http://www.health.harvard.edu

Dislocations

A **dislocation** is a displacement of a bone from its normal position in a joint. With a dislocation, injuries to the ligaments and capsule of the joint are present. A compound dislocation occurs when soft tissue is torn and the joint is exposed to air, which can result in contamination and requires surgical intervention. The dislocation is very painful and requires reduction as soon as possible to reduce pain and avoid vascular and/or nerve damage. For example, a dislocated hip pulls against the soft tissue capsule that contains the vessels that feed the femoral head. This force can occlude the blood supply to the femoral head, which leads to severe complications such as **avascular necrosis (AVN)**, in which the bone tissue dies due to a temporary or permanent loss of blood supply to the bone. Dislocation may also cause significant neurological injury due to the proximity of the nerve to the joint. For example, an anterior shoulder dislocation may cause axillary nerve injury. As with vascular damage, reduction of the bone to its normal position in the joint is accomplished as soon as possible.

 *A dislocation is considered an orthopedic emergency.*

Etiology

The cause of a dislocation is usually an injury that exerts force great enough to tear the joint ligaments such as a fall, motor vehicle crash, or sports-related impact. A fracture may also be associated with the dislocation.

Clinical Manifestations

The patient will usually present with a deformity of the extremity. He will have severe pain and may have decreased sensation and or circulation distal to the injury.

Diagnostic Procedure

A radiograph of the joint and surrounding bones may be done to rule out an accompanying fracture.

Medical Management

Initial treatment consists of protection and reduction of the dislocation by a trained individual as soon as possible. Ideally, repositioning of the joint should occur within 15 to 30 minutes (Frazier & Drzymkowski, 2007). After that time frame, the joint may be so edematous and painful that the reduction may be impossible without general anesthesia.

COMPLEMENTARY & ALTERNATIVE THERAPIES — Chiropractic

Description:

Chiropractic is a health care profession that involves manual manipulation of the musculoskeletal system to correct vertebral subluxation (a misalignment) or joint dysfunction. Conventional chiropractic uses corrective thrusts of the hands that are called adjustments. Other forms of chiropractic may use an "activator," which is a small instrument that aligns bone positions with less force.

Research Support:

There is a scarcity of higher-level research designs in chiropractic studies, such as randomized controlled trials. The studies discussed below represent the best studies of chiropractic care to date.

One review of literature by a group of Australian researchers sought to document both the quantity and type of research on the use of chiropractic care for lower extremity conditions. All articles that the research team chose for inclusion were those with a lower extremity diagnosis, and those in which doctors of chiropractic performed the treatment. The research team conducted an analysis on the 1,652 articles identified to assess those that included peripheral and/or spinal treatment. The research team found that there were a large number of case studies and a smaller number of higher-level publications. The research team also found that there is a predominance of multimodal management of both spinal and peripheral components in the peer-reviewed literature (Hoskins, McHardy, Pollard, Windsham, & Onley, 2006).

One study focused on patients with chronic musculoskeletal pain, and compared the clinical outcomes of two chiropractic approaches for these patients. The two approaches included the most common approach, diversified spinal manipulation, and a nonmanipulative mind–body approach, the Bioenergetic Synchronization Technique. The study involved 81 patients, of which 74 were females, and the median age was 66 years. The patients were treated for 4 weeks, followed by a 3-week nontreatment interval. Results showed similar mean improvements in the Pain Disability Index for both the Bioenergetic Synchronization Technique group and the diversified technique group (Hawk, Rupert, Colonvega, Boyd, & Hall, 2006).

The goal of another study focused on attitudes regarding chiropractors and chiropractic care. The study involved two groups: persons who had used chiropractic services and those who had not. The first objective of the study was to determine whether there were differences in attitudes and other determinants of care-seeking behavior between the two groups of persons. This study also aimed to determine whether members of these two groups were interested in choosing nonmedical doctors (such as chiropractors) for providing routine services. The results showed different attitudes and preferences about health and health care in people who had seen a doctor of chiropractic before than in those who had never seen a doctor of chiropractic. However, researchers found that both groups preferred physician assistants and nurse practitioners to chiropractors to perform routine health care services (Gaumer & Gemmen, 2006).

References

Gaumer, G., & Gemmen, E. (2006). Chiropractic users and nonusers: Differences in use, attitudes, and willingness to use nonmedical doctors for primary care. *Journal of Manipulative and Physiological Therapy, 29*(7), 529–539.

Hawk, C., Rupert, R. L., Colonvega, M., Boyd, J., & Hall, S. (2006, September). Comparison of bioenergetic synchronization technique and customary chiropractic care for older adults with chronic musculoskeletal pain. *Journal of Manipulative and Ohysioliogical Theraphy, 29*(7), 540–549.

Hoskins, W., McHardy, A., Pollard, H., Windsham, R., & Onley, R. (2006). Chiropractic treatment of lower extremity conditions: A literature review. *Journal of Manipulative and Physiological Theraphy, 29*(8), 658–671.

Nursing Management

Nursing management consists of assessment and protection of the extremity, pain control, and education to regain strength and mobility of the affected joint.

Assessment

Complete a thorough examination of the extremity involved including a peripheral nerve assessment to determine neurological impairment and continual reassessment for any progression. Chart 56–2 describes common nerve involvement for specific dislocations. Assess capillary refill and pulses distal to the injury to determine vascular impairment.

Nursing Diagnoses

Primary nursing diagnoses for the patient with a dislocation include:

- *Acute Pain*
- *Risk for Injury*
- *Impaired Physical Mobility.*

Outcomes and Evaluation Parameters

The desired outcomes for the patient with a dislocation are relief of pain, prevention of damage to the nerves and vasculature, and restoration of strength and mobility of the affected joint. Evaluation parameters include control of pain as described by the patient, restoration of nerve and vascular function, and return of strength and mobility to the joint as exhibited by range of motion and strength assessment.

Planning, Interventions, and Rationales

As stated earlier, a dislocation is an orthopedic emergency. The nurse should quickly assess and immobilize the affected joint and extremity to prevent further damage and to recognize any vascular or nerve involvement. The patient will require intravenous pain medication because the pain is severe. The nurse should anticipate and prepare the patient for conscious sedation because this will most likely be needed for reduction. Postreduction, the patient will require a stabilization splint to prevent the joint from reinjury until the tissues have healed.

Health Promotion

Teaching the patient ROM exercises to maintain mobility and strengthening exercises for the muscles that surround the joint is essential for optimal outcome. Repeated dislocation is potentially damaging to the joint. Review with the patient the proper use of splinting devices and the plan of care for timing or resumption of activities.

Fractures

A quick review of bone basic anatomy is helpful to understand terminology use in the description of fractures and injuries. Long bones are found in the upper and lower extremities and are classified as such because they have certain anatomic features in common as shown in Figure 56–4 ■ (p. 1782). The shaft of the long bone is mainly compact bone hollowed out to form a marrow-filled medullary canal. All long bones have an **epiphysis**, the bone end beyond the physis; physis, growth plate; **metaphysis**, an area of widening between the diaphysis and physis; and **diaphysis**, the shaft between both metaphysis on each end. Bone ends typically form a joint with another bone end and are differentiated as the proximal (closest to a person's head or core) and distal.

Short bones are found in the wrist and ankle. They are irregularly shaped and, except for the compact bone on the surface, they are spongy throughout. Flat bones are found where protection of underlying structures is needed, such as the skull and ribs, or a large area for muscle attachment, such as the scapula. They consist of a layer of spongy bone between two layers of compact bone.

Healing of Fractures

Fractures are a discontinuity of the bone that may be complete or incomplete (Porth, 2005). A fracture or break in the bone causes a healing cascade beginning with the blood that leaks out at the fracture site. This hematoma is rich in osteoclasts, which make bone. Clotting factors that remain due to the hematoma initiate the formation of a fibrin meshwork that serves as a framework for the fibroblasts and new capillary buds. Granulation tissue is formed and gradually replaces the clot.

During cellular proliferation and callus formation, the osteoblasts, or bone-forming cells, multiply and differentiate into the fibrocartilaginous callus. This process begins distal to the

CHART 56–2	**Peripheral Nerve Assessment**			
Injury	**Nerve**	**Motor**	**Sensation**
Wrist dislocation	Median distal	Thenar contraction with opposition	Index finger
Anterior shoulder dislocation	Musculocutaneous	Elbow flexion	Lateral forearm
Distal humeral shaft, anterior shoulder dislocation	Radial	Thumb, finger MCP extension	First dorsal web space
Anterior shoulder dislocation, proximal humerus fracture	Axillary	Deltoid	Lateral shoulder
Knee dislocation	Posterior tibial	Toe flexion	Sole of foot
Fibular neck fracture, knee dislocation	Superficial peroneal	Ankle eversion	Lateral dorsum of foot
Posterior hip dislocation	Superior gluteal	Hip abduction	

Source: Adapted from American College of Surgeons. (2004). *Advanced Trauma Life Support Student Course Manual.* Chicago: American College of Surgeons.

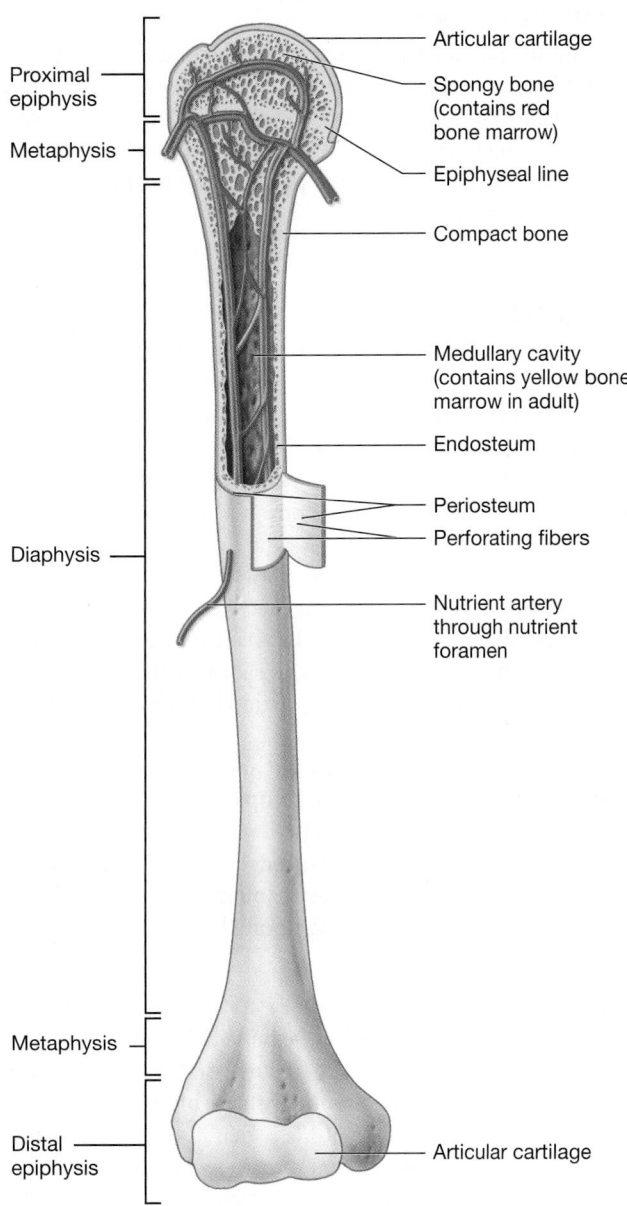

FIGURE 56–4 ■ Long bone.

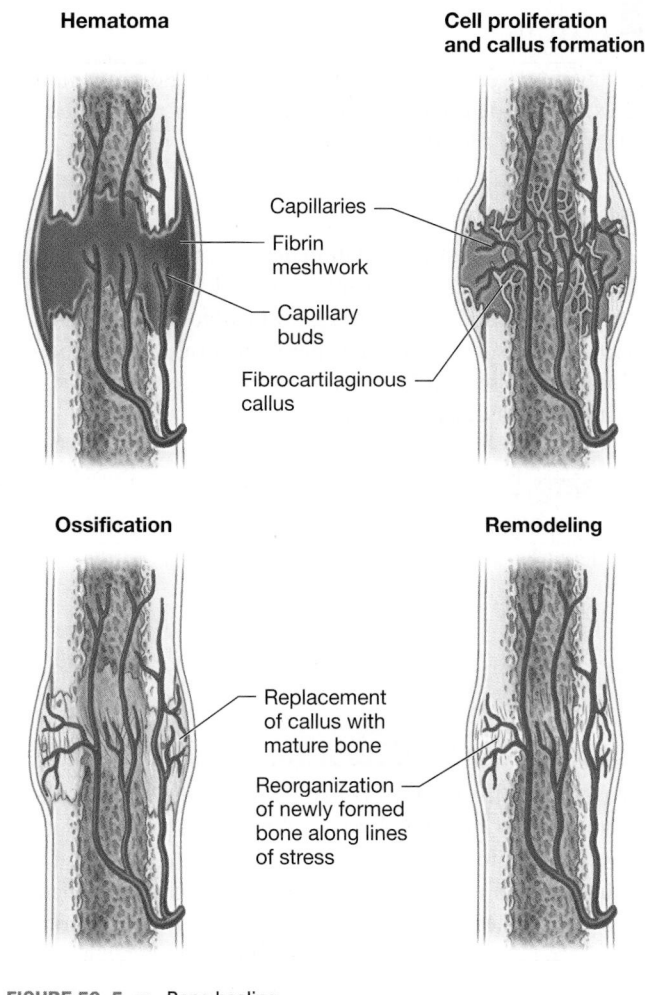

FIGURE 56–5 ■ Bone healing.

fracture where there is greater blood supply. Within a few days a cartilage "collar" is evident around the fracture site. The edges of the collar that are on either side of the fracture unite to form a bridge that connects the bone fragments. Initially the callus is soft but within the third to fourth week of fracture healing, the bone calcifies as mineral salts are deposited.

Ossification is the final lying down of bone after the fracture has been bridged and the fragments are united. Mature bone replaces the callus, and the fracture site feels firm and appears united on radiograph. It is at this point that a cast may be removed. The remodeling process involves resorption of the excess callus in the marrow space and the external aspect of the fracture. The process is directed by mechanical stress and weight bearing becoming stronger in relation to its function (Figure 56–5 ■). Healing time is dependent on the site and type of the fracture and on the underlying health of the patient. With long bones, displaced fractures, and fractures with less surface area, strength and

function usually return within 6 months after bone union is complete. Small nondisplaced fractures require less time to heal and the patient will usually have full function within 2 to 4 weeks.

Classification of Fractures

Fractures are classified in various ways; the simplest is whether a fracture is open or closed. A closed fracture is when the soft tissue envelope, which may be damaged, does not communicate with the outside; in effect, there is no skin opening. An open fracture means there is a tear in the soft tissue, exposing the bone to the outside environment. The important concept is that all open fractures have the potential to be contaminated, and this increases the morbidity (or frequency of complications or poor outcome) and mortality (fatal outcome) of the injury. The time frames vary by institution but many consider 6 to 8 hours the maximum time that a contaminated fracture can wait to be taken to the operating room and "washed out," a process that is often referred to as an *inspection and debridement* (I&D) (Feliciano, Mattox, & Moore, 2008). During the I&D the fracture and soft tissue are washed out with a pulsed lavage, typically with antibiotic solution. The soft tissue is inspected, debris is removed, and any damaged or necrotic tissue is debrided to try to reduce the possibility of infection. Chart 56–3 shows a grading classification for open fractures.

Grade I is typically an "inside-out" fracture, that is, one in which the end of the fractured bone pokes through the skin and

CHART 56–3	**Grading of Open Fractures**
Grade	**Description**
Grade I	Wound less than 1 cm with minimal soft tissue injury. Wound bed is clean. Bone injury is simple with minimal comminution.
Grade II	Wound is greater than 1 cm with moderate soft tissue injury. Wound bed is moderately contaminated. Fracture contains moderate comminution.
Grade III	Following fractures automatically results in classification as type III: • Segmental fracture with displacement • Fracture with diaphyseal segmental loss • Fracture with associated vascular injury requiring repair • Farmyard injuries or highly contaminated wounds • High-velocity gun shot wound (GSW) • Fracture caused by crushing force from fast moving vehicle.
Grade IIIA	Wound less than 10 cm with crushed tissue and contamination. Soft tissue coverage of bone is usually possible.
Grade IIIB	Wound greater than 10 cm with crushed tissue and contamination. Soft tissue is inadequate and requires regional or free flap.
Grade IIIC	Fracture in which there is a major vascular injury requiring repair for limb salvage.

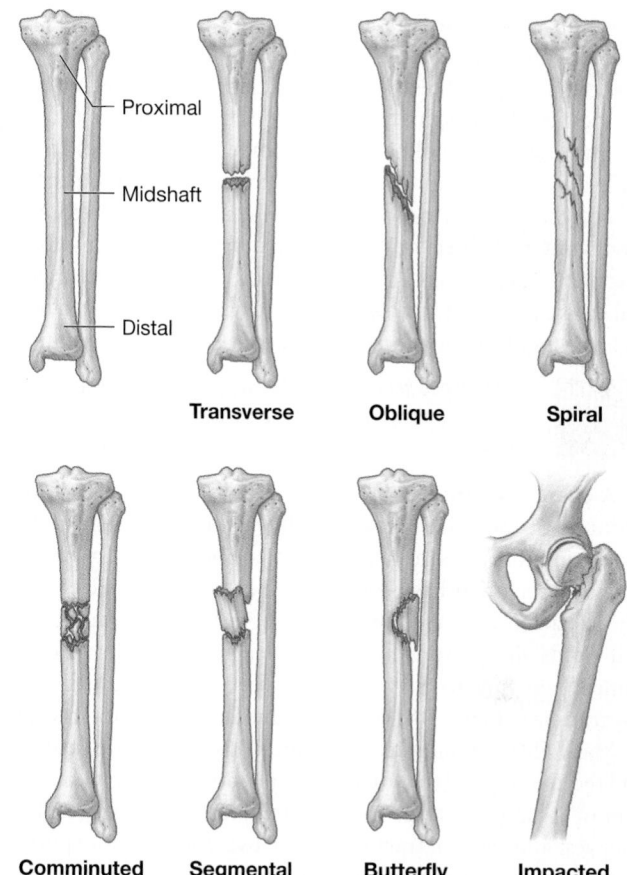

FIGURE 56–6 ■ Classification of fractures by direction of fracture.

returns. This is considered the cleanest fracture with limited risk for deep infection. A Grade II fracture occurs when a soft tissue wound is greater than 1 cm with moderate contamination and soft tissue injury. A Grade III fracture has a greater than 10-cm wound opening, is severely contaminated, and involves comminution of the bone, soft tissue loss, and vascular injury (*Gustillo classification of fracture*, 2004).

There are other ways to classify fractures such as by appearance, apposition angulation, and mechanism of injury. Long bone fractures may be described by their appearance, which also gives some indication of the mechanism of injury. Descriptors such as *transverse, oblique, spiral, comminuted, segmental, butterfly,* and *impacted* are commonly used (Figure 56–6 ■).

Transverse fractures are horizontal to the bone shaft and usually result from a direct blow. Healing of nondisplaced transverse fractures is usually uneventful because the muscle pulls and compresses the bone ends together, which is key in bone healing. Oblique fractures are diagonal in nature and may allow shortening of the bone due to the muscle pulls. The diagonal configuration may allow the bone ends to slide down on each other. A spiral fracture is as described: spiral, typically caused by rotatory torsion. These fractures are suspicious of inflicted injury in nonambulating children, because they typically occur as a result of limb twisting. Segmental fractures describe bone that is broken in more than one place. These fractures are difficult to

manage without surgical intervention to stabilize the bone fragments. In butterfly fractures, large pieces of the bone are shaped like a butterfly with one side longer than the other. Impacted fractures occur when broken ends of bone are forced together. These fractures have a high rate of healing and limited pain because most pain of fractures comes from the innervated periosteum portion of the bone ends rubbing against each other. Impacted fractures do not readily move but need to be protected from displacing until healing occurs.

Fracture apposition speaks to the relation of the bone ends to each other; for example, if half of each bone end is touching the other, it is considered 50% opposed. If the bones ends are not in contact at all, it may be referred to as 100% displaced or 0% apposition. Nondisplaced fractures keep anatomic alignment. Fracture angulation describes the angle at the apex of the fracture in relation to the proximal fragment of bone. Some fracture descriptions are specific to the particular bone such as spine and pelvis fractures.

Spinal fractures can occur in the 7 cervical vertebrae, frequently referred to as the C-spine, 12 thoracic vertebrae or T-spine, and 5 lumbar vertebrae or L-spine, and are classified as stable or unstable using a three column theory. This theory divides the vertebrae into three columns, the anterior, middle, and posterior columns. If any two of these columns are disrupted, the spine is considered to be unstable.

 **CRITICAL ALERT** *When two vertebral columns are disrupted, the spinal cord and nerve roots are no longer protected from serious neurological injury.*

An unstable spine is typically treated with complete bed rest with log rolling, a Roto Rest bed or Stryker frame bed, or surgical fixation. The special beds allow the patient to be turned without flexing the patient's spine. Changes in position are needed to avoid pressure areas and pooling of fluids. Some spine fractures are described by the mechanism of injury, such as a **burst fracture** that occurs when an axial load is placed on the spine and a vertebra explodes out in all directions. This form of fracture may push bone fragments into the spinal canal and has the potential for neurological damage. Burst fractures are unstable, and patients need to be watched for any neurovascular changes in the lower extremities.

 *Any changes in exam should be reported to attending surgeons immediately, because deficits can become permanent.*

A **chance fracture** is one through bony and or ligamentous portions of the spine caused by distraction of vertebrae. The most common scenario is a person in the back seat of a car with only a lap belt that has been involved in a motor vehicle crash. The impact forces the person's upper body forward, while the lap belt holds the person down, producing tearing through the spine. These injuries may not be visible on plain spine films so any trauma patient with back pain should be suspect for injuries.

Many C-spine fractures or ligamentous injuries are unstable and require surgical treatment and or treatment in cervical traction or a halo vest to prevent neurological compromise. Both halo vest and cervical traction rely on two, four, or more pins to be placed in a ring around the patient's head and torqued to 6 to 8 pounds of pressure, which enable the pins to penetrate the outer table of the skull, securing them in place. Care of the pin site includes watching for any drainage, erythema, or movement. For a detailed discussion of spine and spinal cord injuries, refer to Chapter 32 .

 *Clear drainage from a pin site or ear could represent cerebrospinal fluid and must be reported to the attending surgeon immediately.*

Medical Management

Initial management of an extremity fracture consists of immobilization that includes the joint above and the joint below the fracture. After the extremity is splinted, neurological and vascular status is reassessed and a plan for definitive care is accomplished:

- Femoral fractures are temporarily immobilized with a traction splint that applies force distally at the ankle as the splint is pushed proximally into the perineum. Excessive traction for long periods of time may cause skin damage to the foot, ankle, or perineum.
- Tibia fractures are immobilized with padded cardboard long-leg splints or a splint made with plaster immobilizing the lower leg, knee, and ankle.
- Ankle fractures may be immobilized with a pillow splint or padded cardboard. It is important to avoid pressure over bony prominences.
- The hand is temporarily splinted in an anatomic functional position with the wrist slightly dorsiflexed and the fingers gently flexed. This can be done by placing the hand over a roll of gauze or rolled towel and then securing a short arm splint.

- Forearm and wrist fractures are immobilized flat on padded cardboard splints or a pillow.
- The elbow, upper arm, and shoulder are usually immobilized to the body in a flexed position using a sling.

Narcotics are generally needed for effective pain relief and should be given in small frequent doses. The patient will be further evaluated to determine the extent of the injury and if she will require simple casting or surgical intervention for open reduction and internal fixation.

There are typically five treatment options for fractures: closed treatment with casting, traction, surgical treatment with external fixation, open reduction with internal fixation, or intramedullary rod. A combination of these options may also be used. There are risk, benefits, and indications for each, which are discussed next.

Casting, Bracing, and Splinting

The easiest and sometimes most cost-effective treatment for fractures is the cast. A **cast** is a rigid circumferential encasement device made of plaster or fiberglass. Casting material (plaster or fiberglass and Webril/cotton padding) is relatively inexpensive and readily available. Casting does not completely keep bones from moving and it may allow shortening or displacement of fractures. Patients may complain of hearing or feeling crepitus, crunching or grinding of their bone ends moving in the cast.

A cast must include the joint above and the joint below a fractured long bone. This restricts joint motion for the length of time needed for fracture healing but renders those joints stiff when treatment is complete and frequently requires rehabilitation of atrophied muscles. However, this form of treatment is not optimal in the immediate postinjury period because it is rigid and does not allow for the swelling of tissues, which typically occurs for the first 3 days after a fracture. Fractures can be painful until the bone ends begin to granulate and get "sticky" around 10 to 14 days in the average, well-nourished, nonsmoking patient. Another problem with casting is there is no access to soft tissues to observe for pressure points or skin breakdown. Most cast material must stay dry so it is difficult for the patient to take a bath or shower. Fiberglass casting tape used with a waterproof Gortex liner is now used for certain applications allowing casts in showers or chlorinated swimming pools.

A splint or brace is manufactured or made by the caregiver with casting material. It allows the fractured bone to rest within a firm surface to decrease motion, but is not circumferential. The splint or brace is secured by straps or wrapped circumferentially with a bandage. This allows for adjustment if there is increased swelling and removal for visualization of the soft tissues.

Traction

Traction is a treatment option that is used in most underdeveloped countries but is not the treatment of choice in the United States due to the cost of long hospital stays and the complications associated with the immobilization involved with traction. The purpose of traction is to maintain alignment of the bone with an axial pull along the axis of the bone to counteract the pulls of the muscles. **Skin traction** or **Buck's boots traction** consists of straps or foam boots secured to lower extremities with a cord pulling no more than 6 pounds and is frequently used for comfort in patients with hip fracture. No more than 6 pounds should be placed on this kind of traction because pressure areas will develop. The nurse should examine the skin under the boot or bandage wrap every 4 to 6 hours looking for any reddened areas.

Skeletal traction entails placement of a skeletal pin that is drilled through the bone such as a distal femur or proximal tibia. The portions of the skeletal pin exiting the skin on either side of the limb are attached to a bail. A cord is secured to the bail and runs through pulleys to a weighted bag suspended at the end of the bed. The purpose of the weight is to pull along the axis of the bone to counteract the muscle forces (spasm) in an attempt to bring bones "out to length" and/or maintain anatomic alignment. A trapeze on the bed may help the patient move in the bed; however, it should not be used if the patient has a spine fracture.

Pin site care is an important nursing function. Skeletal traction pins are exposed to the environment where they protrude through the skin and can allow bacteria to travel down to the bone. Skeletal pins are generally not painful except when placed or removed or if the pin sites become infected. It is expected that the pin site will be red, tender, and have bloody or serosanguineous drainage for the first 24 to 72 hours. After that time any tenderness or drainage should be suspect for infection. Pin sites should also remain flat and not be allowed to tent on the pin. Pin releases are performed to keep the skin off the pin. The tent provides a warm moist dark area for bacteria (always present at the pin skin interface) to accumulate and grow. For more on pin site care, see the box titled Evidence-Based Practice.

Traction has high morbidity and mortality risks, especially in elderly patients. The problems with traction stem from the immobilization involved, which can produce complications such as skin breakdown, urinary tract infection, pneumonia, deep venous thrombosis (DVT), and pulmonary embolism (PE). The cost of hospitalization for traction in the United States far exceeds that of surgical treatment. Traction is labor intensive, from setting up traction beds, repeating x-rays frequently, and changing the axis of the pull to change the angulation of the fracture.

External Fixation

External fixation refers to a form of treatment in which the bones or bone ends of a fracture are held in place by skeletal pins, which are screwed into the bone and attached to a frame worn on

---

Pin Site Care

Clinical Problem

Infection of pin sites is one of the most common complications associated with the use of skeletal pins, wires, and external fixation (Walker, 2007). An infection at the pin site is painful and will delay mobilization of the patient. The infection may also lead to other severe complications including osteomyelitis, nonunion of the bone at the fracture site, delayed fracture healing, loss of fracture alignment, or systemic infection. All of these complications can result in long-term pain and possible disability. Due to the significance of pin site care, it is important to base the care and technique on evidence.

Research Findings

Hydrogen peroxide was commonly used in the past to cleanse pin sites, especially to remove crusts from around the pin site. Currently, the use of hydrogen peroxide is discouraged because it may cause damage to the healthy tissue surrounding the pin. It has also been associated with increased infection rates and the disruption of the skin's normal flora (Walker, 2007).

In 2005, the National Association of Orthopaedic Nurses completed a systematic analysis of the research literature on skeletal pin site care and sought opinions of an expert panel to develop guidelines for skeletal pin site care (Holmes & Brown, 2005). They found that there were two experimental studies regarding pin site care, but they explored different aspects: one study explored cleansing solutions and the other addressed frequency of site care. The panel also reviewed five case series studies in which one that reported comparison of two methods of site care was judged to be of high quality. Using the methodology of expert consensus, the panel developed the following major recommendations:

- Pins located in areas with considerable soft tissue should be considered at greater risk for infection.
- After the first 48 to 72 hours when drainage may be heavy, pin site care should be done daily or weekly for sites with mechanically stable bone–pin interfaces.

- Chlorhexidine 2 mg/mL solution may be the most effective cleansing solution for pin site care.
- Patients and their families should be taught pin site care before discharge from the hospital. They should be required to demonstrate whatever care needs to be done and should be provided with written instructions that include signs and symptoms of infection.

Implications for Nursing Practice

Guidelines reflect the state of current knowledge within the health care literature regarding the effectiveness of current practice. Clinical practice guidelines are developed by reviewing these findings and seeking the opinions of known experts in that field of practice. The expert consensus is vital in practice that has little or no research to review.

Although there was little research regarding care of the skin immediately surrounding the skeletal pin site, some of what had been done was judged to be of good quality and therefore useful. It is clear that (1) the solution used to cleanse pin sites should be chlorhexidine and (2) nurses should not use peroxide.

Critical Thinking Questions

1. What risks are involved if pin sites are not kept clean and dry?

2. Which assessment findings would the nurse expect a patient with an infected pin site to exhibit?

Answers to Critical Thinking Questions appear in Appendix D.

References

Holmes, S. B., & Brown, S. J. (2005). Skeletal pin site care: National Association of Orthopaedic Nurses guidelines for orthopaedic nursing. *Orthopaedic Nursing, 24*(2), 99–107. Retrieved August 5, 2008, from http://www.guidelines.gov/summary/summary.aspx?doc_id=7420&nbr=004379&string=pin+AND+site+AND+care.

Walker, J. A. (2007). Evidence for skeletal pin site care. *Nursing Standard, 21*(45), 70–76.

EVIDENCE-BASED PRACTICE

the outside of the body. External fixation devices (EFDs) have become the treatment of choice for many fractures, especially when soft tissues are damaged and access is needed for wound care.

Unlike casting, external fixation allows for greater mobility and joint motion above or below the fracture. External fixation may be used for emergent stabilization of fractures or as definitive treatment. Scars are minimal compared to open reduction internal fixation or intramedullary rodding. For some the pins may be removed in a clinic.

The most common complication of external fixation is pin site infection. Skeletal pins protrude though an opening in the skin, which creates a foreign body reaction. The body reacts by forming a bursal lining between the pin and skin. This protective membrane produces fluid to reduce the friction at the pin/skin interface. This fluid is easily contaminated by the bacteria skin flora and needs to be allowed to drain out at the pin site to reduce the concentration of microorganisms. (See the Evidence-Based Practice box, p. 1785.)

Another complication of external fixation or skeletal traction is a plantar flexion contracture of the foot. Without support the foot will rest in plantar flexion and this can result in Achilles tendon shortening or tightness. This deformity can be avoided with frequent stretching and the use of a foot plate.

Open Reduction Internal Fixation

A very common method of fracture fixation is **open reduction internal fixation (ORIF)**, in which a fracture is exposed by an incision in the skin directly over the fracture. Implants such as plates (strips of metal), screws, and wires are placed directly on or in the bone to anatomically stabilize a fracture (Figure 56–7 ■). This method of fracture fixation allows direct visualization of the fracture but can disrupt the circulation to the bone and leave large surgical scars.

Complications associated with this method are wound infection and hardware failure or breakage. It is not optimal for use with comminuted or osteoporotic bone or damaged or suboptimal soft tissues. Patients with conditions such as peripheral vascular disease, diabetes, and obesity frequently encounter healing problems. Screw heads may be prominent and irritate tissue, and hardware may need to be removed following healing.

Intramedullary Rod

Intramedullary (I-M) rodding refers to a method of fracture fixation that entails sliding a metal rod down the medullary canal of a long bone (Figure 56–8 ■). This form of fixation allows for anatomic alignment and is helpful for segmental fractures. I-M rods allow for early weight bearing because they share the load and leave joints free to move. They may need to be removed after healing is complete. The holes left by the screws are stress risers and fractures may occur through them when an I-M rod is removed.

The benefits of this fixation method include small surgical scars in less obvious places than with other methods. For example, the rod in Figure 56–8 ■ was placed through a 4-cm incision above the hip, and small stab incisions were made to place the screws. There is a slight increased risk of fat embolism with this method because of the pressure exerted in the canal by the reamer or from hammering the I-M rod down, which may force fat into the bloodstream.

■ Nursing Management

Nursing management of the patient with an extremity fracture involves relief of pain and frequent reassessment of neurovascular status. Patients with femur fractures require frequent monitoring of their vascular status because femoral shaft fractures are associated with significant blood loss of up to 1,500 to 2,000 mL and the patient can develop hypovolemic shock (Feliciano et al., 2008).

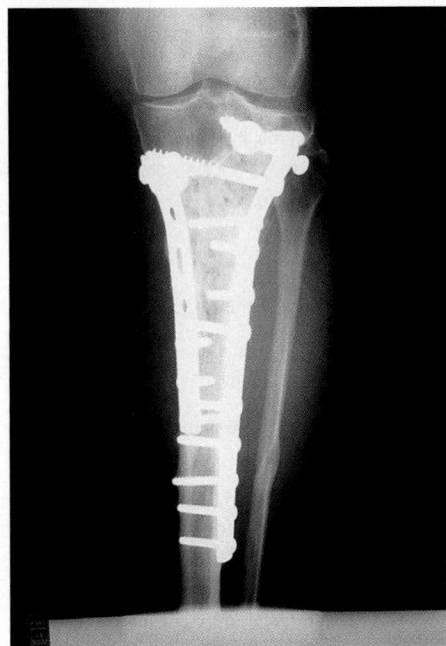

FIGURE 56–7 ■ Open reduction internal fixation.
Source: Cheryl Wraa

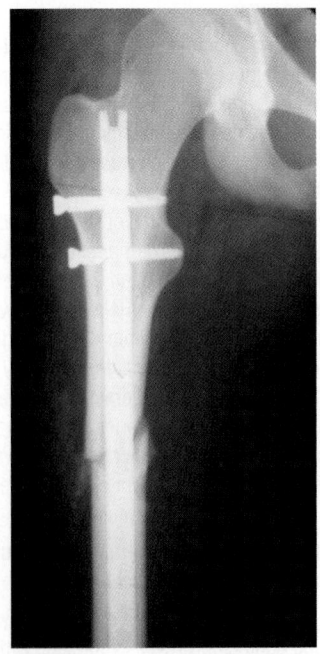

FIGURE 56–8 ■ Intramedullary rodding.
Source: Cheryl Wraa

Assessment

Initial assessment of an extremity fracture includes observation for deformities, breaks in the skin, and a thorough assessment of vascular and sensory status distal to the extremity. Frequent reassessment of neurovascular status is necessary to prevent complications.

Nursing Diagnoses

The primary nursing diagnoses for the patient with an extremity fracture include:

- *Pain, Acute*
- *Physical Mobility, Impaired*
- *Injury, Risk for*
- *Fluid Volume, Risk for Deficient*
- *Infection, Risk for.*

Outcomes, planning, intervention, and evaluation are discussed under pelvic fractures.

Pelvic Fractures

A large amount of force is required to fracture the pelvis. Therefore, the nurse should be anticipatory and assess for other serious injuries. The pelvis consists of two innominate bones and the sacrum, which form a ring of bone. The bones are held in a structural unit primarily by the ligaments of the pelvis (Figure 56–9 ■). The strongest ligamentous structures are in the posterior aspect of the pelvis at the sacroiliac (SI) joints. These ligaments have to hold up the weight-bearing forces from the lower extremities to the spine that are transferred to the SI joints. Major blood vessels are located on the inner wall of the pelvis (Figure 56–10 ■). Whenever the pelvis is fractured, these arteries and associated veins can be damaged and extensive bleeding will occur. The lumbar and sacral plexus of nerves run through the posterior pelvis and can be affected with pelvic trauma

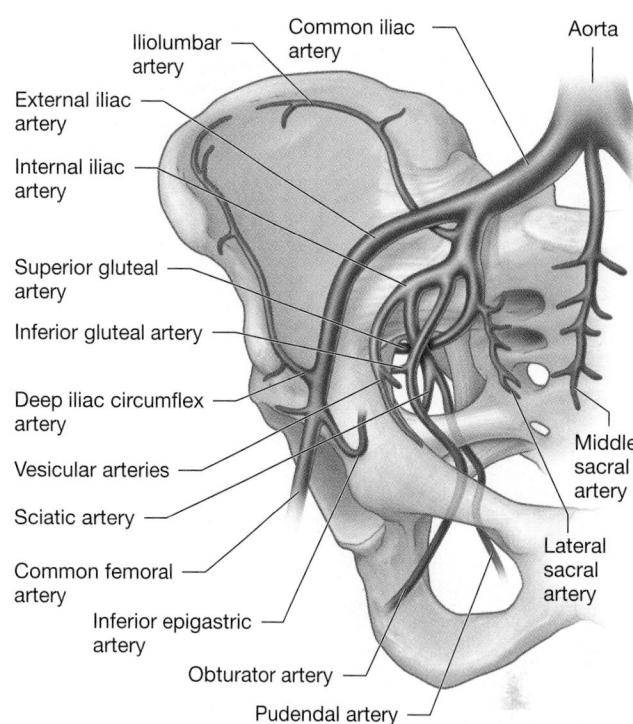

FIGURE 56–10 ■ Vascular anatomy of the pelvis.

(Figure 56–11 ■). Organs that can be injured during a trauma with pelvic fracture are the bladder and urethra, vagina, prostate, and gastrointestinal system.

Three types of forces cause damage to the pelvis. The first and most common is lateral compression (Figure 56–12 ■, p. 1788). Examples include a pedestrian hit on his side by a motor vehicle, a fall from a height where the patient lands on her side, and a motor vehicle crash where intrusion of the vehicle compresses the pelvis.

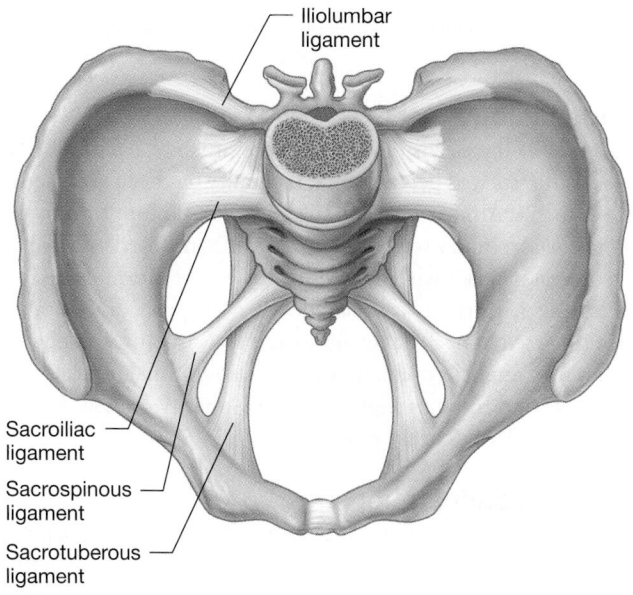

FIGURE 56–9 ■ Ligaments of the pelvis.

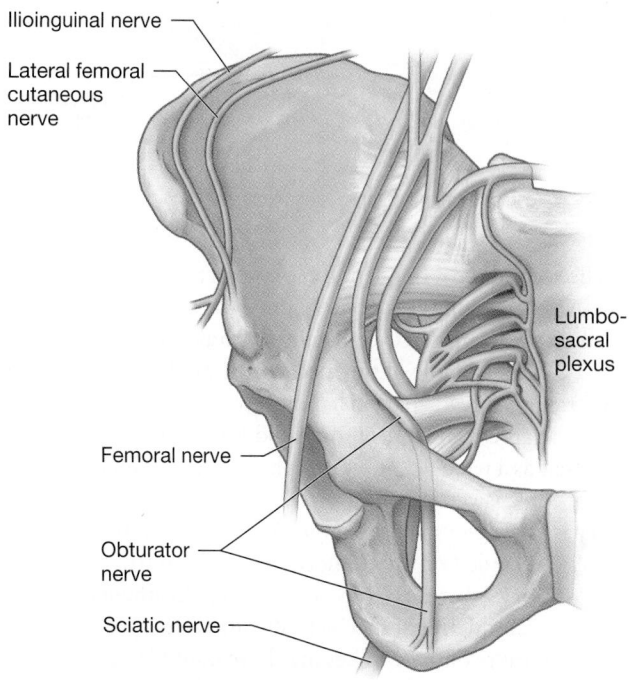

FIGURE 56–11 ■ Neuroanatomy of the pelvis.

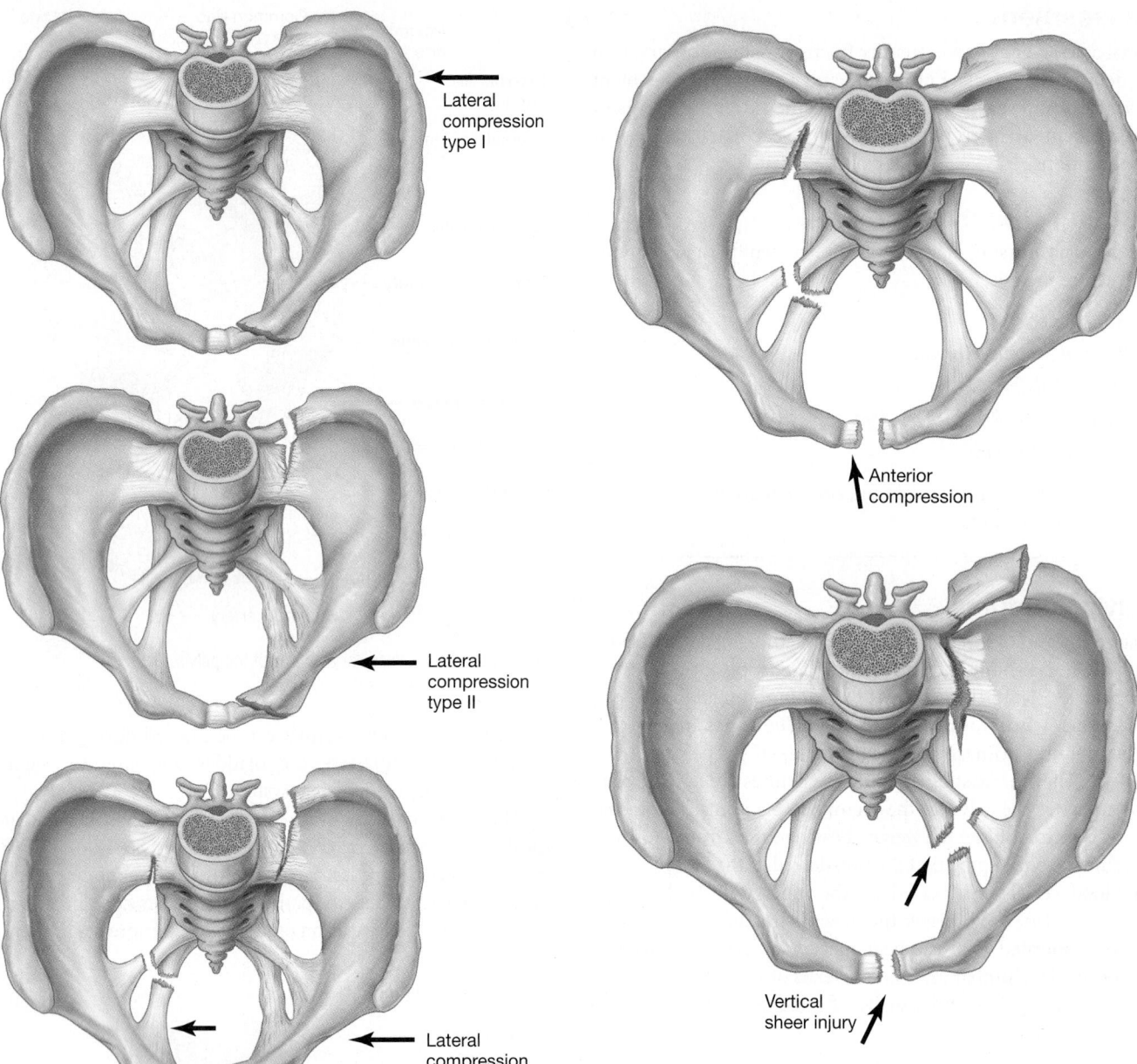

FIGURE 56–12 ■ Lateral compression fractures.

FIGURE 56–13 ■ Anterior compression and vertical shear injuries.

The second most frequent force is from an anterior or posterior (AP) direction. This occurs from either direct contact with the iliac spine or force transmitted from the femur (Figure 56–13 ■). An example of the mechanism would be when a person's legs are spread apart in a motorcycle crash. The injury can involve ligament disruption only and the injury usually manifests itself as a widened pubic symphysis and SI joints. The third type of force is vertical shear (see Figure 56–13 ■). This type of injury is most commonly seen in patients who jumped from a height and landed on an extended lower extremity. The vertical shear injury disrupts the restraining ligaments of the hemipelvis, rendering it mechanically unstable.

One or more of these forces may have injured patients at one time. It is important for the nurse to inquire as to the mechanism of injury to be anticipatory of the type of injury the patient may have sustained.

Epidemiology

Fractures of the pelvis comprise approximately 2% of all fractures. With isolated pelvic injury, mortality has been reported to be 1% to 2%. Almost 20% of multiple injured blunt trauma patients have an injury to the pelvic ring. When closed pelvic fractures are associated with multiple injuries, the mortality rises to 10% to 15%. Mortality associated with open pelvic fractures has been reported to be 30% to 50%, and pelvic fractures associated with intracranial hemorrhage or severe abdominal injuries have been reported to be as high as 50% (Mohanty, Musso, Powell, Kortbeek, & Kirkpatrick, 2005).

Clinical Manifestations

During physical examination, the nurse should inspect the pelvis to see if there is a rotation of the iliac crest and/or any difference in leg length. When palpating, exert gentle lateral compression and distraction of the iliac crests and inward compression of the symphysis pubis to determine pelvic stability.

It is critically important to be careful when maneuvering the pelvis so as not to cause damage to the vasculature or neural bundles.

If the pelvis feels unstable, alert the health care team so others will not attempt to manipulate the pelvis and cause further damage or increased bleeding. Inspect the skin and skin folds to identify any open fractures. Observe the meatus to check for blood signifying a possible urethral injury.

 If there is blood at the meatus, do not attempt to insert a Foley catheter.

The health care team will perform a digital rectal exam to evaluate for sensation, sphincter tone, presence of blood, and position of the prostate. Female patients will undergo a vaginal exam to look for tears in the vagina signifying an open fracture. The lower extremities should be evaluated for pulses, motor, and sensation.

Diagnostic Tests

Initially, an AP radiograph of the pelvis will show most fractures and associated dislocations. This view, however, does not allow the health care team to determine the degree of bone displacement and small factures may be missed. Additional views called inlet and outlet views may be obtained. The inlet view is taken at a 60-degree angle from the head toward the feet. This will show the posterior and cephalic displacement of fractures of the posterior arch, widening of the SI joint, and displacement of the anterior arch. The outlet view is a 45-degree angle taken from the foot of the bed directed toward the head. This helps in identifying a displacement or leg-length discrepancy, disruptions of the SI joints, and sacral factures.

Computed tomography (CT) of the pelvis assists with the diagnosis of crushing, shearing injuries, SI joint displacement, acetabular injuries, and posterior osseous ligamentous structure of the pelvis. The scan will also assist in diagnosing associated visceral injuries and bleeding.

Medical Management

The most important factors that direct management of pelvic injury are the patient's hemodynamic status and stability of the pelvic ring. In the patient who is both hemodynamically and mechanically unstable and the bleeding is thought to be from the pelvic fracture, external stabilization of the pelvis is a priority. The main sources of bleeding are the presacral venous plexus and fractured bony surfaces. External stabilization with a pelvic binder decreases the hemorrhage by reducing the volume of the pelvic basin and approximating the fracture ends. Pelvic binders are cloth and go around the pelvis circumferentially (Figure 56–14 ■). They are simple to apply, inexpensive, and can be placed in the prehospital setting. Potential complications of the binder include skin necrosis if left in place for a long period or applied too tightly. If a binder is applied too tightly with lateral compression injuries with sacral fractures, it may cause visceral or neural injury.

The source of bleeding from pelvic fractures is usually venous but arterial injury can occur and account for hemodynamic instability in 10% to 20% of patients (Mohanty et al., 2005). For the patients who remain hemodynamically labile after external stabilization, pelvic angiography may be performed for identification and embolization of the source of bleeding. Patients who are hemodynamically stable but exhibit an arterial

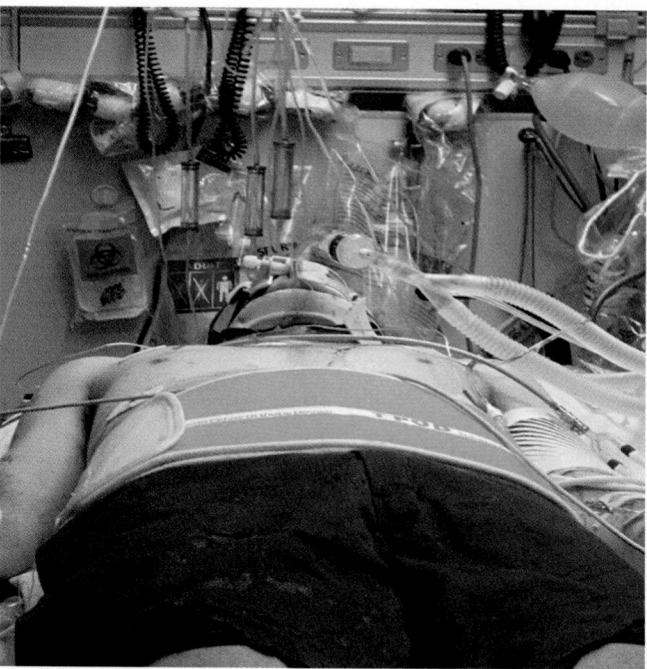

FIGURE 56–14 ■ Pelvic binder.
Source: Cheryl Wraa

blush on CT scan, signifying bleeding at the site, may also undergo angiography for embolization.

Minimally displaced pelvic fractures that have ligamentous stability of the pelvic ring are treated with protected weight bearing on the affected side and pain medication. If displacement at the fracture site occurs when the patient begins to bear weight, further surgical treatment may be necessary. Fractures that have marked displacement of the anterior ring without complete posterior ring disruption are usually treated with reduction and surgical anterior ring stabilization. Patients who have complete disruption of the posterior ring will require surgical stabilization of both the anterior and posterior pelvic ring.

■ Nursing Management

Initial nursing management of the patient with a pelvic fracture includes continued reassessment for potential complications, pain control, and keeping the patient still after a binder is applied. If the patient requires surgical stabilization, postfixation nursing management includes pain control, continued assessment for complications such as bleeding, infection at the incised site, DVT, PE, and pneumonia. For care of the orthopedic surgical patient, refer to Chapter 57 ☺.

Assessment

Initial nursing management of the patient with a pelvic fracture includes continued assessment of the patient for concomitant injuries, and signs and symptoms of potential complications.

Nursing Diagnoses

The primary nursing diagnoses for the patient with pelvic fracture include:

- *Pain, Acute*
- *Physical Mobility, Impaired*

- *Injury, Risk for*
- *Fluid Volume, Deficient, Risk for*
- *Infection, Risk for.*

Outcomes and Evaluation Parameters

The desired outcomes for the patient with a fracture of any type are relief of pain, prevention of damage to the nerves and vasculature, and restoration of strength and mobility. Evaluation parameters include control of pain as described by the patient, restoration of nerve and vascular function as demonstrated by exam, and return of strength and mobility as noted by assessment.

Planning, Interventions, and Rationales

With all fractures, the nurse should quickly assess and immobilize the affected extremity or pelvis to prevent further damage and to recognize any vascular or nerve involvement. Figure 56–15 ■ illustrates how to quickly assess for sensory and motor function.

The patient will require intravenous pain medication because fracture pain is severe. In the postresuscitative phase, pain control is critical to assist with rehabilitation to normal activities of daily living. Studies have shown that patients who receive adequate pain relief recover more quickly (Bongiovanni et al., 2005). Patients are better able to participate with physical therapy if their pain is appropriately managed.

If the patient presents with an open fracture, apply a sterile dressing immediately to help protect the open wound from further contamination. Postoperatively any wounds, dressings, or splints should be monitored for signs of infection such as warmth and redness, drainage with a foul odor, purulent drainage, increased pain, and fever. If signs of infection are noted, notify the health care team immediately.

For the patient who has an unstable pelvic fracture, the nurse should anticipate the need for a blood transfusion and ensure the patient has been typed and crossmatched for blood products. If the patient is placed in a pelvic binder, the nurse should assess position of the binder and ensure smooth, direct contact between the patient and binder to avoid skin breakdown. Chart 56–4 shows an example of a patient care standard for pelvic binder management.

The nurse is critical in monitoring the patient for signs that would indicate the onset of hypovolemic shock and the need for resuscitative measures. An orthopedic trauma patient who has experienced fractures of the pelvis or long bones is at risk for significant bleeding. The nurse should monitor the patient's hemodynamic status including vital signs and laboratory values. A patient may lose as much as 20% of his blood volume before exhibiting signs and symptoms of shock. The nurse should monitor the vital signs for an increase in heart rate, decrease in blood pressure, increase in respiratory rate, and a decrease in urine output. Laboratory results will show a decrease in the hemoglobin and hematocrit. Refer to Chapter 61 🌐 for a detailed discussion of shock.

Nerve	Sensory function		Motor function	
Peroneal	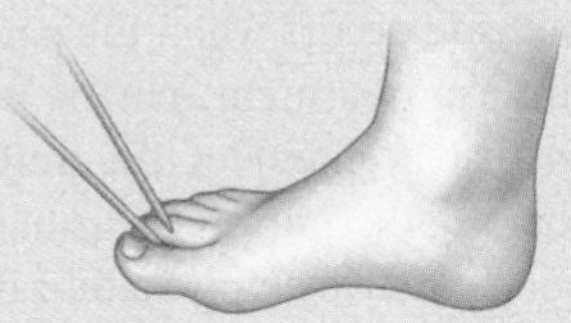	Prick the lateral surface of the big toe and the medial surface of the second toe.	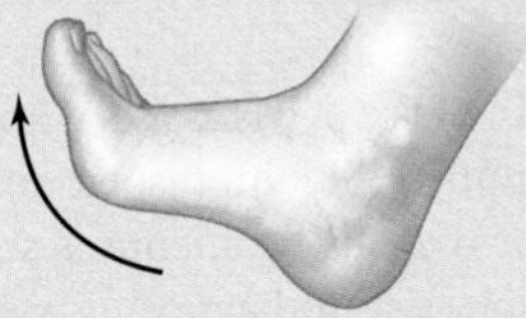	Ask the patient to dorsiflex his ankle and extend his toes.
Tibial	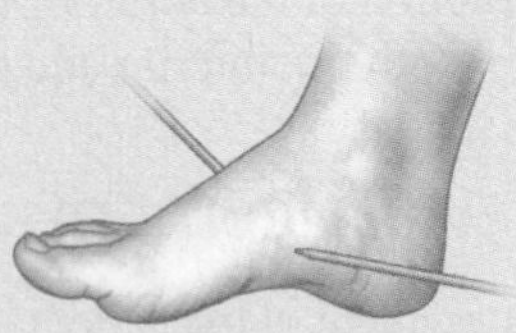	Prick the medial and lateral surfaces of the foot.	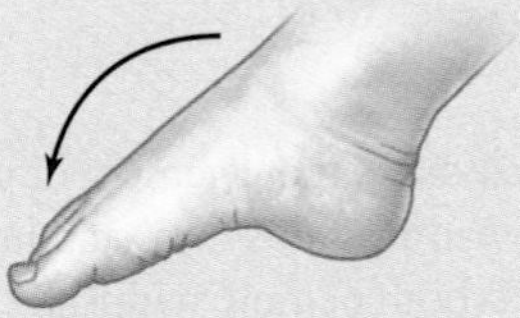	Ask the patient to plantarflex his ankle. Note whether the patient can flex his toes.
Radial	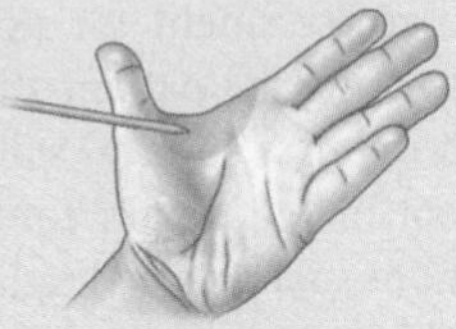	Prick the web space between the thumb and index finger.	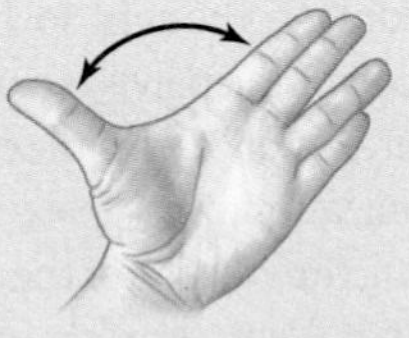	Ask the patient to hyperextend his wrist or thumb.
Ulnar	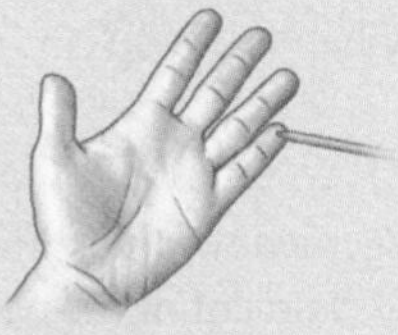	Prick the distal fat pad of the fifth (small) finger.	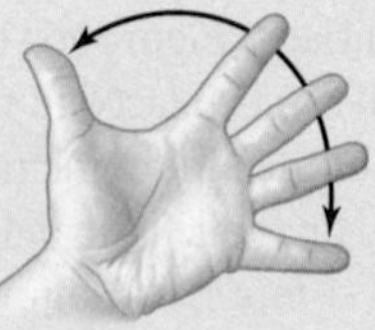	Ask the patient to abduct all his fingers.
Median	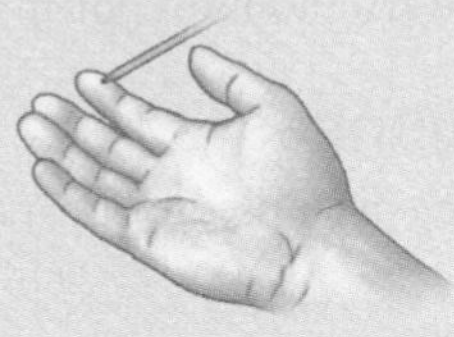	Prick the distal surface of the index finger.	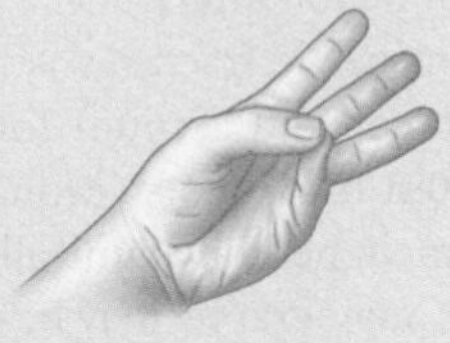	Ask the patient to oppose his thumb and fifth finger. Note whether patient can flex his wrist.

FIGURE 56–15 ■ Motor and sensory assessment.

CHART 56–4   Pelvic Binder Management

UC Davis Health System
Pelvic Binder Management
Patient Care Standards VI-10
Revised 2/11/07

I. SETTING
Emergency Department and Intensive Care Units
Performed by: Independent function by RN after binder has been placed by health care provider.

II. OUTCOME STANDARDS
  A. Provide a quick, safe and effective method in initial treatment of pelvic fractures.
  B. Lower mortality rate.
  C. Aid in pain management due to disruption of pelvis.
  D. The patient will not develop skin breakdown due to compressive nature of binder.
  E. Patient will maintain alignment and hemodynamic stability as exhibited by: systolic blood pressure >90, will maintain integrity of distal pulses, warmth of distal extremitites.

III. SUPPORTIVE DATA
Unstable pelvic fractures in the poly-traumatized patient are a significant source of blood loss and mortality. Evidence supports the use of a stabilization device (pelvic binder), which applies anterior/posterior pelvic compression, for use in initial treatment to stabilize a suspected pelvic fracture to help prevent blood loss and aid in pain control. The pelvic binder is a temporary device until definitive treatment can be accomplished.

IV. PROCEDURE
  A. Initial Placement
    1. Initial Placement will typically occur in the Emergency Department and is placed by the MD.

  2. Upon arrival to admitting unit and throughout the patient stay, assess position of the binder, ensure smooth, direct contact between patient and binder. Assure that there are no creases or wrinkles in binder, which could quicken skin breakdown.
  B. Ongoing care:
    1. Once the pelvic binder has been placed, it should not be removed or adjusted for 72 hours, unless the patient requires operative intervention for the region covered by the binder, or other contraindications are noted.
    2. If, after 72 hours, the patient is hemodynamically stable, (SBP shall remain >90 mmHg, x 4 hours and hemoglobin remains stable) the health care provider should be at the bedside for the first release of compression, then the nurse shall:
       a. Routinely release the pulley-tab by detaching the Velcro tab from the belt and allow the draw strings to relax 1cm, without losing compression of pelvis every 2 hours.
       b. If visible, assess as much skin integrity as possible with each 1cm release as listed above. If the health care provider wishes to assess full circumference skin integrity of the pelvis/torso, the binder may be log-rolled, otherwise, the binder shall remain in place and the maximum release by the nurse will be as stated in #1 above.
    3. Report any changes to the health care provider team.
    4. Document on the appropriate department tool the following:
       a. Time of pelvic binder application.
       b. Initial status of skin integrity in pelvic region.
       c. Every 2 hour release of pulley system.
       d. Skin assessment with each release.
       e. Notification of health care provider if patient condition changes or skin breakdown noted.

Source: UC Davis Health System, University of California, Davis (2007).

Health Promotion

Rehabilitation is an important aspect of the care of the patient with a fracture. The patient should be mobilized as soon as possible to prevent further complications. Physical therapy should begin early to prevent contractures and increase mobility and strength to the extremity.

Traumatic Amputations

Traumatic amputations are when part or all of a digit or limb is severed from the body. These are upsetting to patients as well as staff. Many emergency service members bring the amputated part to the hospital in hopes of possible reattachment.

Surgical reattachment of a severed limb is done only under certain circumstances because the surgery is difficult. It is not attempted with a digit of the hand unless it is a thumb or index finger needed for function and the wound has clean borders. Crush-type amputations are not attempted due to the poor outcome. Only cleanly separated traumatic amputations in patients without significant risk factors for impaired healing such as smoking are considered for reimplantation. For adults, it is nearly impossible for nerves to regenerate in the lower extremity, and the reattached limb may be painful and dysfunctional (Feliciano

et al., 2008). Complete amputation and a prosthesis could allow a patient to return to normal activities in days to weeks, whereas reconstruction of mangled limbs can span over years with a huge psychological strain and impact on function and occupation. For a complete discussion of amputation refer to Chapter 57 .

There are as many physical/mobility issues to deal with as there are emotional issues for the patient with an amputation. The patient may need to have wound care to the stump and have trouble just looking at it. The patient may have bizarre sensations such as feeling like her foot is cold or itchy when it is not there. These are called phantom limb sensations. Patients may need to retrain their brains to distinguish where their body ends. Most will also need to grieve the loss of their limb and counseling should be initiated prior to discharge. Prostheses will be made and a great deal of physical and occupational therapy may be needed to adapt to a missing limb or digit.

Complications of Musculoskeletal Trauma

Most all complications of musculoskeletal trauma are detected early by an accurate complete nursing assessment. Assessment of the injured patient begins with the ABC's of airway, breathing, and circulation. Orthopedic assessment consists of vital signs, pain assessment, inspection, palpation, and the extremely important neurovascular exam. Inspection is head to toe, appraising skin integrity and discoloration such as bruising.

Palpate for areas of tenderness, crepitus, or swelling. The neurovascular exam consists of assessing the color, temperature, capillary refill, pulses, edema, sensory and motor function, and pain level of an extremity such as a hand or foot. The neurovascular exam of the extremities should be performed and documented with each vital sign assessment (or as ordered), and changes need to be reported to the health care team. Many acute care centers have a neurovascular check sheet for patient assessment. Figure 56–16 ■, A–F, shows examples of the neurovascular documentation section of an electronic medical record. When assessing an extremity, comparison of the affected extremity to the nonaffected extremity is important.

Pulses are assessed at typical points such as the radial pulse at the wrist and the dorsalis pedis pulse on the mid-dorsum of the foot. Posterior tibial pulses can be felt just posterior to the medial malleolus.

Sensory and motor function of each nerve branch should be assessed. The upper extremity nerves are the radial, ulnar, and median nerves. Lower extremity nerves are the peroneal and tibial. Muscle strength (graded 5–0) and joint range of motion, both passive (the nurse moves the joint for the patient) and active (the patient moves the joint), are assessed and documented and expressed as a ratio such as 4/5 (4 out of 5).

Pain should be assessed frequently, and there are many methods to do this including observation of facial grimace, guarding postures, limp, and vital sign changes such as elevated blood pressure and pulse. Refer to Chapter 15 ☜ for a complete discussion of pain assessment.

Orthopedic injuries are very painful. Broken bones hurt until they stop moving, which may be 14 days or longer. Pain management is paramount for injured patients for many reasons including comfort level, adequate ventilation, rehabilitation, and aiding with sleep. Most patients, including children, will require narcotics. Children have historically been undermedicated, which can have long-term implications. Physiological predictors of post-traumatic stress disorder (PTSD) in children have shown that the strongest of the physiological correlations appears to be patients' perception of their pain. The worse the degree of early pain, the more likely that they will exhibit PTSD after the injury (Norman, Stein, Dimsdale, & Hoyt, 2007). Orthopedic patients frequently have physical therapy ordered and will need to get out of bed as soon as possible to prevent the complications of bed rest and immobilization. It is helpful to have patients premedicated 30 to 60 minutes prior to physical therapy.

Mobility

Patients with musculoskeletal trauma may have mobility issues. Even a sports injury may require crutches and a change in weight-bearing status. Many assistive devices, such as wheelchairs, walkers, crutches, canes, or reachers, are available. Wheelchairs need to

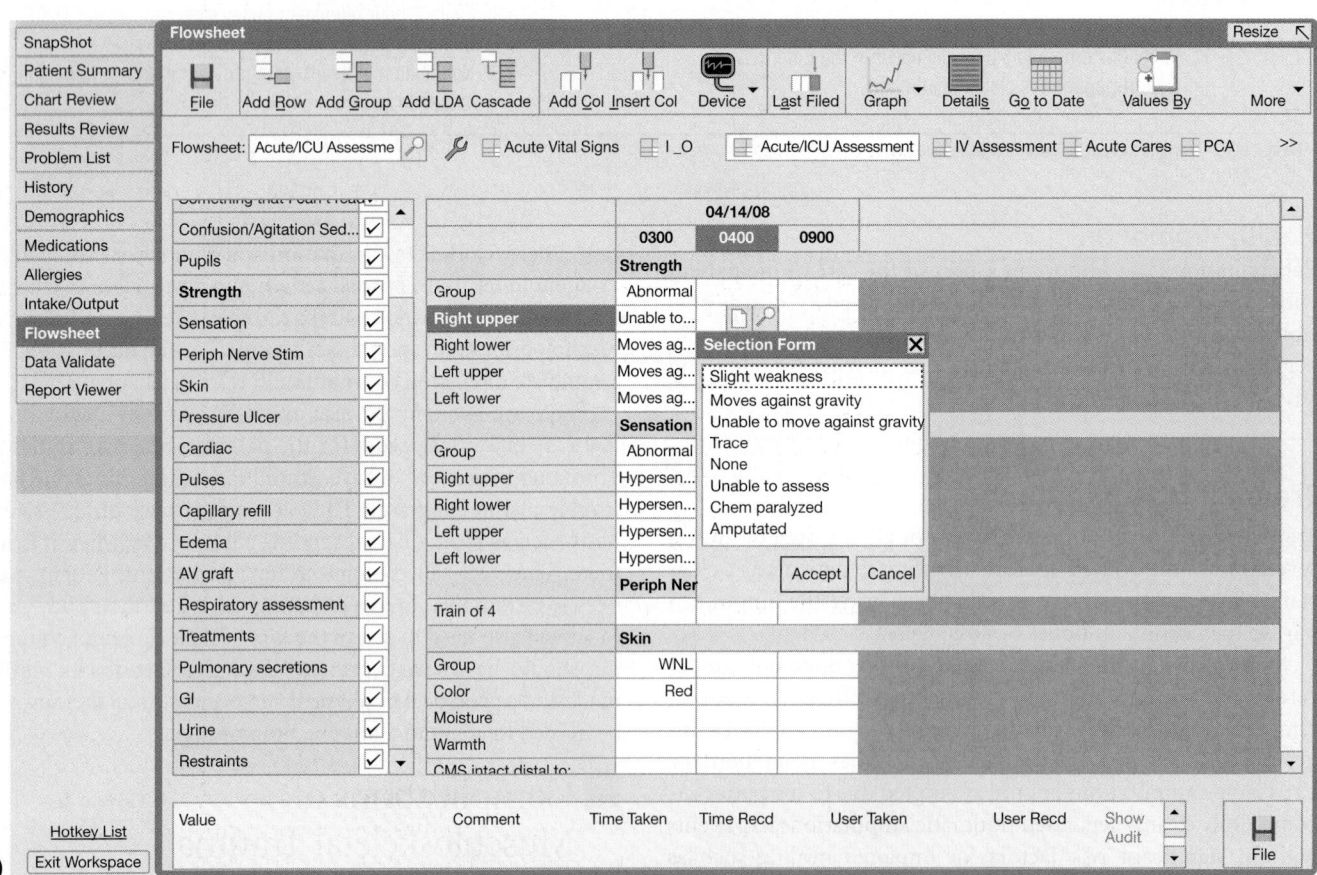

FIGURE 56–16 ■ Neurovascular assessment: (A) strength; (B) sensation; (C) skin; (D) pulses; (E) capillary refill; (F) edema.

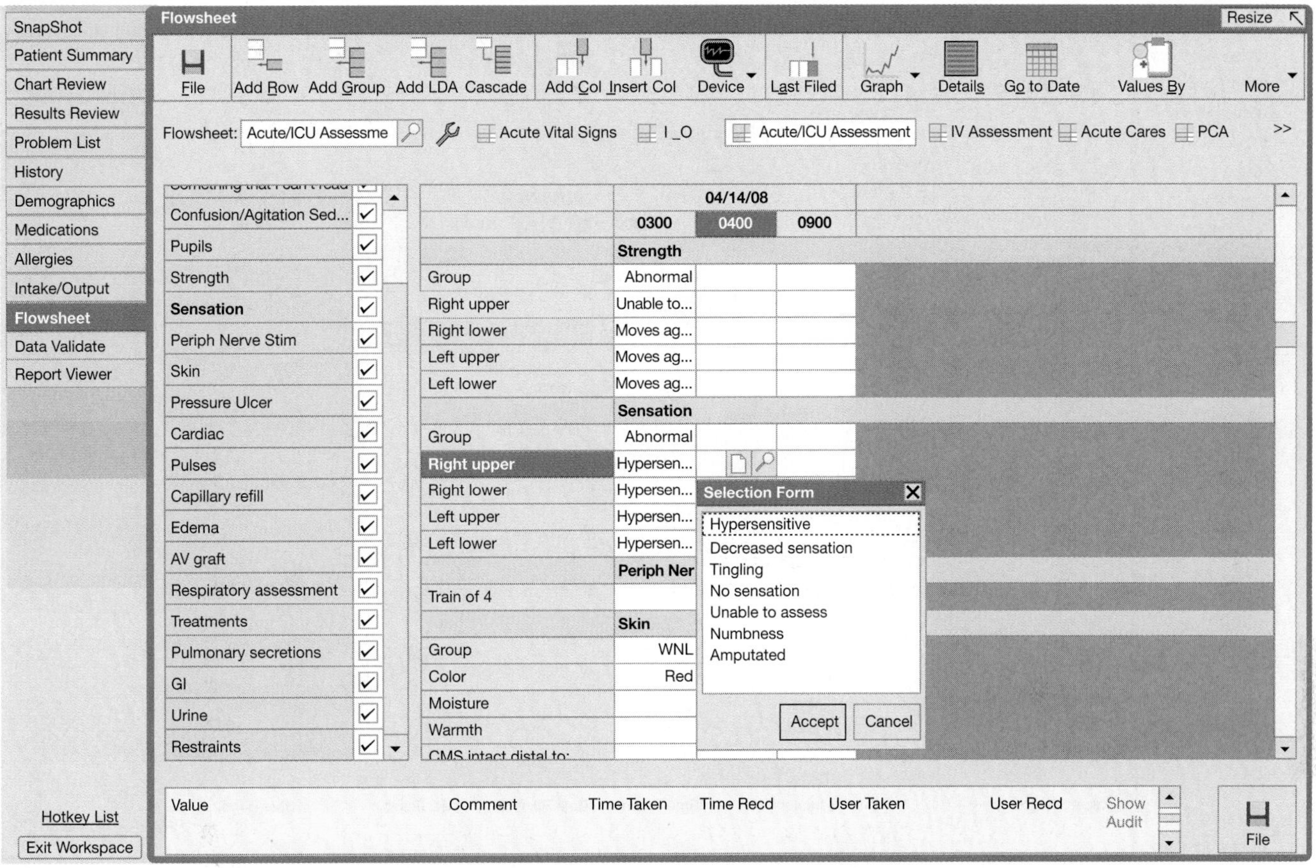

(b)

FIGURE 56–16 ■ Neurovascular assessment: (A) strength; (B) sensation; (C) skin; (D) pulses; (E) capillary refill; (F) edema.—*Continued*

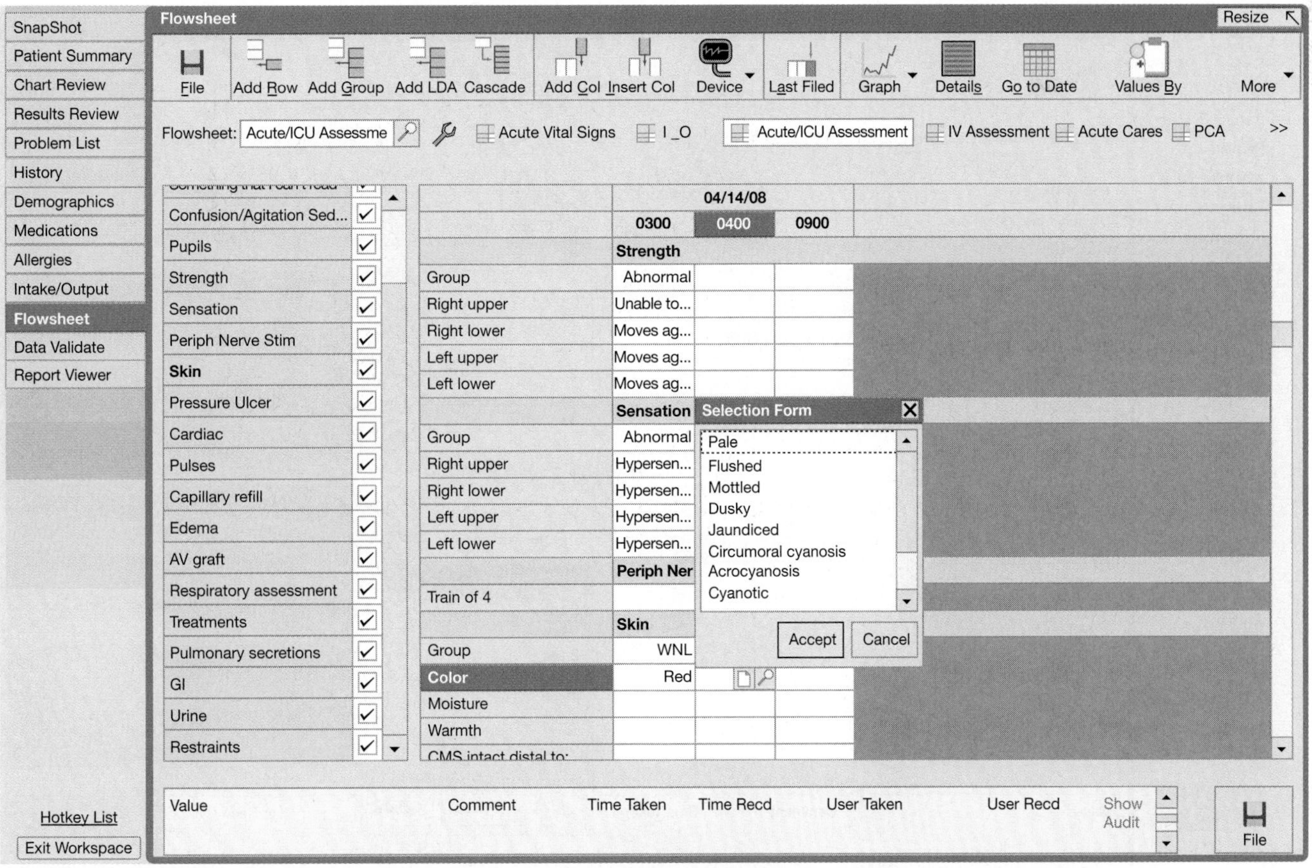

(c)

FIGURE 56–16 ■ Neurovascular assessment: (A) strength; (B) sensation; (C) skin; (D) pulses; (E) capillary refill; (F) edema.—*Continued*

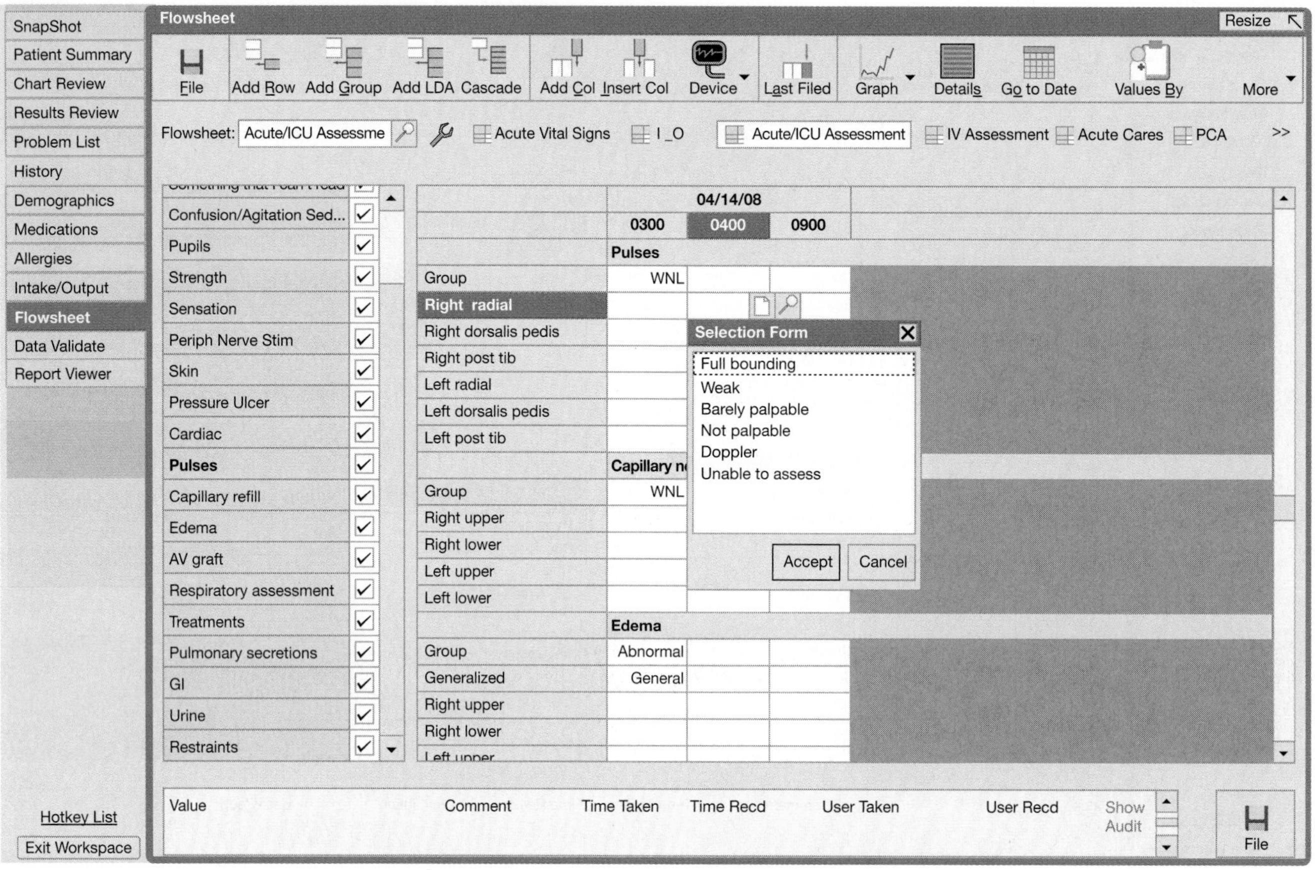

(d)

FIGURE 56–16 ■ Neurovascular assessment: (A) strength; (B) sensation; (C) skin; (D) pulses; (E) capillary refill; (F) edema.—*Continued*

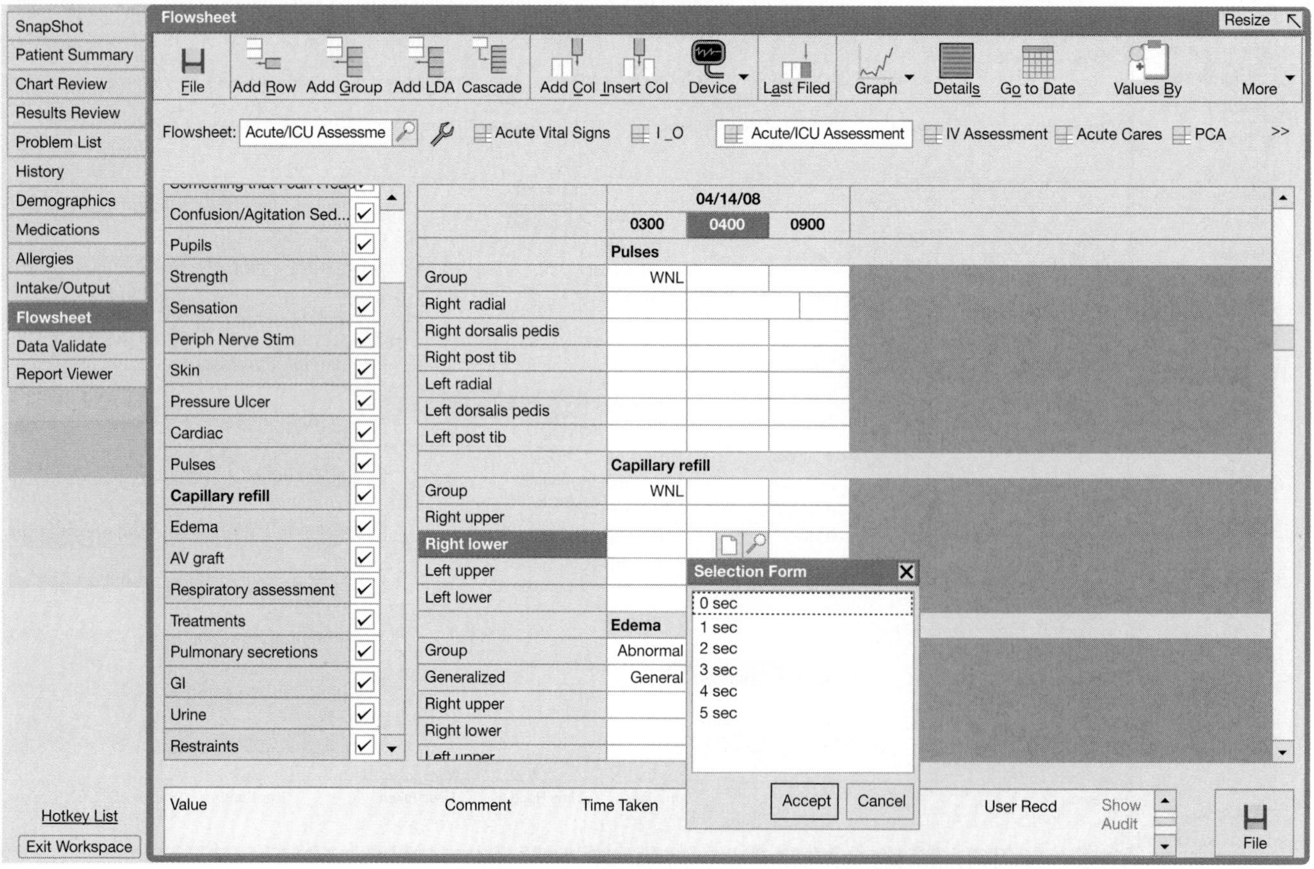

(e)

FIGURE 56–16 ■ Neurovascular assessment: (A) strength; (B) sensation; (C) skin; (D) pulses; (E) capillary refill; (F) edema.—*Continued*

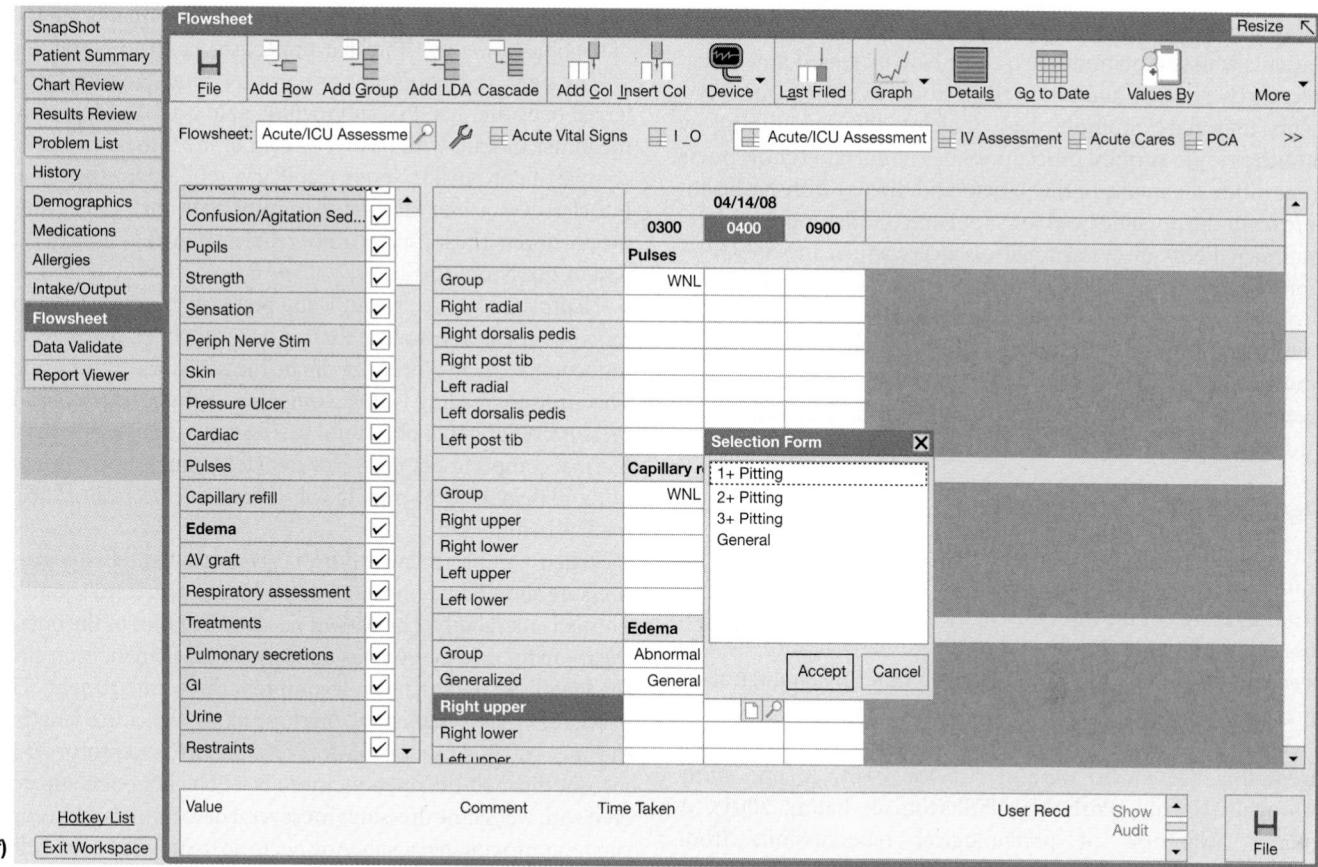

FIGURE 56–16 ■ Neurovascular assessment: (A) strength; (B) sensation; (C) skin; (D) pulses; (E) capillary refill; (F) edema.—*Continued*

be fit to the patient and can come with elevating leg rests and reclining backs. Manual, one-side drive, and electric wheelchairs are available depending on patients' abilities and the time they will be expected to use one.

Walkers are frames with four posts and handgrips usually made of aluminum. They may be required by elderly patients or those who are large or have difficulty with balance and need to have restricted weight bearing. Walkers may have wheels on the front legs for patients who cannot lift them.

Crutches are devices used in pairs to aid ambulation by transferring weight to upper extremities. Crutches come in two types—axillary crutches and forearm (also referred to as loftstrand or Canadian) crutches. The axillary crutches can be made of wood or aluminum. When patients are fitted for axillary crutches (allowing for four fingerwidths between axilla and crutch top) they should be encouraged not to rest their armpits on the crutch. Most of the weight can be carried on the palms of the hand if there is no injury to hand or arm. If such an injury exists, a platform crutch may be more appropriate. The weight of a patient for these crutches is limited to 113 kg (250 pounds) for most manufacturers of wooden crutches. It is very important to teach the patient the proper use and to observe them using the crutches.

A cane is a wooden or metal stick with a curved graspable handle at the top. A cane should be used on the opposite side of the injury to "unload" an extremity or aid with balance. In addition, it should be measured to fit to the palm of a nearly fully extended arm when laterally placed 8 to 12 inches from the foot.

Many musculoskeletal conditions will require a specific weight-bearing status. This is a directive on how much weight the clinician would—or would not—like the patient to put on an extremity (Chart 56–5).

CHART 56–5	**Weight-Bearing Status**	
NWB	Nonweight bearing	Should not put any weight on extremity (not even to push up in bed).
TDWB, TTWB	Touch down or toe touch	Allowed to let toe touch the ground for balance and allows leg to be rested on the ground but no weight should be placed on it.
PWB	Partial weight bearing	Usually a percentage of the person's weight, for example, 25–50%.
WBAT	Weight bearing as tolerated	The patient may begin to put weight on the extremity as pain recedes.
FWB	Full weight bearing	Allowed to walk normally on the extremity; does not require crutches.

Nutrition

Patients who sustain multiple trauma have increased nutritional needs to heal tissue injuries. In the resuscitative phase, many patients may have multiple days of being allowed nothing by mouth prior to surgical procedures. It is important for the nurse to monitor the intake of the patient and discuss with the health care team the possible need for supplement nutrition. Multiple-trauma patients are at risk for stress ulcers, which are sores or lesion on the lining of the stomach or duodenum and may be prophylactically treated with H_2-receptor antagonists, proton pump inhibitors, and sucralfate. Frequently patients involved in trauma have social issues such as drug or alcohol abuse and poor dietary habits. These will need to be taken into consideration and addressed individually.

Psychological Recovery

The psychological impact and sequelae of musculoskeletal trauma are not well known. There are more factors involved than just the trauma of the injury itself; there are medical treatments, loss of mobility or school or work time, financial burdens, and even changes in self-concept. PTSD and other psychological sequelae can be seen months after physical recovery.

Wishful thinking as a coping mechanism was distinctive in predicting those who were at risk for PTSD in one study (Dougall, Ursano, Posluszny, Fullerton, & Baum, 2001). A greater awareness of psychological repercussions from trauma, especially inflicted or disfiguring injuries, is needed. There are early identifiable risk factors for post-traumatic maladjustment: panic during or immediately after the trauma, reexperiencing symptoms, avoidance, sleep disturbance, injury from an assault, previous trauma and psychiatric history, and blaming someone else for the injury. Rusch, Gould, Dzwierzynski, and Larson (2002) discussed that any reexperiencing of symptoms, avoidance, trauma-related phobias, depression, irritability, and increased substance use suggests psychological impairment. Younger children may regress or exhibit changes in play or sleep including night terrors, aggression, irritability, avoidance, and emergence of new fears (Rusch et al., 2002).

Compartment Syndrome

Compartment syndrome is a common complication and the cause of poor outcomes and much litigation. **Compartment syndrome** is a condition whereby increasing pressure within the muscle compartments compromises circulation and the function of soft tissues, nerves, and vessels in that compartment, which leads to anoxia of the tissue and necrosis, which in turn leads to more edema in the compartment and a subsequent increase in pressure.

Compartment syndrome is cyclical and builds until a surgical release of the fascial envelope is performed. If pressure is not reduced, irreversible muscle damage and nerve damage can occur within hours and can also lead to life-threatening complications such a rhabdomyolysis and renal failure. Compartment syndrome can occur due to increasing internal pressure, for example, from bleeding into the compartment by fractured bone and torn muscle tissue or overhydration or from the external pressure applied by the trauma itself, casts, dressing, burns (tight eschar), or even clothing. The most commonly affected compartments are those of the tibia (lower leg), forearm, upper arm, hand, foot, and thigh.

The signs and symptoms of compartment syndrome are referred to as the "five Ps," and include pain out of proportion to the injury or pain with passive stretch of the muscle within that compartment, pallor, poor capillary refill, paresthesia, and pulselessness in the affected extremity. Pain that seems out of proportion to the injury or is not relieved by analgesia is the earliest of the symptoms.

Neurovascular assessment is the best way to note early symptoms because it is typically a clinical diagnosis, but if there is doubt intracompartmental pressure can be measured with a transducer. This pressure reading is then compared to the patient's diastolic pressure. A difference of 30 mmHg is essential for tissue perfusion. Normal compartment pressures are 0 to 8 mmHg and a pressure of more than 30 to 45 mmHg will cause tissue necrosis if the patient's diastolic reading is low.

When compartment syndrome is suspected, all sources of pressure should be removed and the health care team should be notified emergently. The patient needs to be taken to the operating room for an emergent **fasciotomy**, which is an incision along the length of the fascia to decompress the compartment. This procedure opens the fascial envelope along the entire length of the muscle. The muscle is allowed to expand, frequently protruding out through the open incision. It will be left open and covered with wet saline dressings for several days until the skin edges can be approximated again. Any necrotic tissue will be debrided. Skin grafts or amputations may be required for severe cases.

Rhabdomyolysis

Rhabdomyolysis occurs when the injured skeletal muscle fibers break down and leak inflammatory mediators, such as myoglobin and creatinine kinase, into the circulation. It is most commonly seen with crush injuries but can occur with any massive soft tissue injury.

Complications associated with rhabdomyolysis include acute renal failure. This occurs due to renal tubular obstruction from the filtration of the released myoglobin. The patient may also exhibit respiratory distress due to muscle weakness and fluid and electrolyte imbalances.

Signs and symptoms of rhabdomyolysis include pain, tenderness, swelling, bruising, and weakness within the affected muscles. Upon assessment the muscles involved may feel soft and flabby. The patient's urine will also become dark in color (referred to as myoglobinuria) as the renal system attempts to filter the myoglobin. Patients may also develop systemic symptoms including general malaise, fever, nausea and vomiting, confusion, agitation, and anuria as the acute renal failure progresses. Diagnosis is confirmed by a creatinine kinase level. The level will be increased to five times or more of the normal value.

Treatment consists of administration of IV fluids to maintain circulating blood volume and perfuse the kidneys while flushing the myoglobin from the kidneys. Creatinine kinase levels should be obtained and high rates of fluid continued until the levels decrease to 1,000 units/L. The patient's associated acidosis is treated with a sodium bicarbonate infusion to alkalinize the urine. Fifty percent to 70% of patients who develop acute renal failure will require dialysis to treat the electrolyte imbalances and fluid overload (Bongiovanni et al., 2005). Most patients have a complete recovery of renal function after treatment.

Deep Venous Thrombosis and Pulmonary Embolism

Deep venous thrombosis is a blood clot in the venous circulatory system typically in the lower extremity. Virchow's triad—venous stasis, intimal damage, and hypercoagulability—combines to a state of thrombogenesis. A recent analysis of 1,602 patients who developed DVT and PE identified in the American College of Surgeons National Trauma Data Bank revealed the following significant risk factors: age greater than 40; lower extremity fracture with an abbreviated injury scale (AIS) > 3 (scale is from 1 to 6, with 1 being lowest severity and 6 being highest severity); head injury with an AIS > 3; exceeding 3 ventilator days; venous injury; and a major operative procedure (Knudson, Ikossi, Khaw, Morabito, & Speetzen, 2004). Other risk factors have been identified that reflect the hypercoagulable state. Higher levels of homocysteine and plasminogen activator-1 levels correlate with DVT in a study of patients with spinal cord injury (Aito, Abbate, Marcucci, & Cominelli, 2007). Prophylaxis for DVT consists of early ambulation, use of serial compression devices (SCDs) of the lower extremities, and administration of low-molecular-weight heparin or unfractionated heparin for anticoagulation. If the clot extends proximally, a portion may break loose and cause a pulmonary embolism.

Pulmonary embolism is a blood clot that has broken free from a site that travels through venous circulation, through the right side of the heart to the lungs where it lodges in one or both branches of the pulmonary artery to obstruct or partially obstruct circulation. The most common signs and symptoms are anxiety or a feeling of impending doom coupled with dyspnea. For a detailed discussion of PE, see Chapter 35 ⊘.

Fat Embolism Syndrome

Fat embolism syndrome (FES) occurs when fat globules released from long-bone fractures enter the circulatory system. Up to 90% of long-bone fractures have some release of fat emboli associated with the fracture, only 3% to 4% progress to FES (Feliciano et al., 2008). In the most severe cases, the emboli can produce multiple-organ failure from both a direct embolic effect and from activation of the inflammatory cascade. The most commonly noted triad of symptoms is acute respiratory failure, neurological dysfunction, and a petechial rash (Chart 56–6). Acute respiratory failure may be the only symptom in a large number of patients.

Cast Syndrome

Cast syndrome or superior mesenteric artery syndrome (SMAS) can be fatal. SMAS occurs when there is compression of the superior mesenteric artery at the duodenum, from anterior pressure such as a body cast or brace and posteriorly resisted by the descending aorta and spine (Shetty, 2004). This compression impedes the blood flow to the bowel, causing ischemia and eventually necrosis of the gastrointestinal tract and vessel walls that can result in hemorrhage and death. This is most often seen in children in body casts or hip spica casts; however, it also is seen in adults with casts or back braces especially if they have

CHART 56–6	Classic Triad for Signs and Symptoms of Fat Embolus	
Early Findings	**Later Findings**	**Last Component**
Hypoxemia Dyspnea Tachypnea	Neurologic abnormalities: Confusion Altered LOC Focal deficits Possible seizures	Petechial rash found most often on the head, neck, anterior thorax, subconjunctiva, and axillae.

Source: Weinhouse, G. (2008). Fat embolism syndrome. Retrieved August 10, 2008, from http://www.utdol.com/online/content/topic.do?topicKey=cc_medi/13397&selectedTitle=1~27&source=search_result.

had spine injury or surgery where there is any hyperextension of the lumbar spine or distraction injuries of the spine.

The first symptoms are vague abdominal pain, pressure, distention, and irritability; this is followed by nausea, projectile vomiting, and bowel obstruction. SMAS may occur postoperatively or days or weeks later especially with very young children growing larger in hip spica casts. Early treatment is essential, begun by bivalve (cutting both sides of the cast to relieve pressure), window (cutting a section of the cast away from a pressure point), or removal of the cast (or brace). Decompression of the stomach is achieved with a nasogastric (NG) tube to continuous intermittent suction.

Pressure Ulcers

Skin integrity and prevention of pressure areas is key to orthopedic nursing. Keeping heels off the bed is crucial, as is padding of bony prominences. Providing adequate nutrition and hydration and keeping the skin clean and dry are measures aimed at promoting good skin turgor.

Complex Regional Pain Syndrome

Complex regional pain syndrome (CRPS), formerly known as reflex sympathetic dystrophy (RSD), is a diffuse persistent pain usually associated with vasomotor, trophic, and bony changes and limited mobility of an extremity following a local injury. Early referral to physical therapy for movement and pain clinic personnel who specialize in this disorder is crucial.

■ Gerontological Considerations

The nurse should be aware of specific gerontological considerations for musculoskeletal trauma. Hip and wrist fractures are the most common types of fractures in elderly patients. Conditions such as osteoporosis or tumor may predispose the elderly to a pathologic or insufficiency fracture. In such a fracture the bone is not strong enough for its function and it breaks through the weakened framework with little trauma. Fractures in the elderly may occur prior to, or as a result of, a fall. A high mortality rate is associated with hip fracture in the elderly; more than 4% die during hospitalization and 10% to 35% die within a year of the injury (Meehan, 2002; Morris & Zuckerman, 2002). Delay in surgical repair of hip fracture is associated with complications of bed rest including atelectasis, thromboembolism, urinary tract infection, and pressure ulcers (Orosz et al., 2004). Early weight bearing and return to preferred living situation with adequate services has been associated with better medical, psychosocial, financial, and cultural outcomes (Meehan, 2002).

Prevention of fractures is a key nursing initiative. Fall prevention, nutrition evaluation, and encouraging screening and osteoporosis treatment for elderly patients are essential for good quality-of-life outcomes.

Elderly patients have other considerations such as sensory and metabolic deficits and delays in medication absorption and healing. Constipation is a major concern for the elderly who sustain musculoskeletal fracture and are immobilized or who require narcotics or undergo surgery. There are psychosocial issues for the elderly such as fear of becoming infirm, being in pain, running out of money, having to be dependent on family, asking for help, appearance concerns such as assistive devices making them look old, sexuality, being alone, and that the road back to recovery may be too much. They may grieve over loss of function, friends, or lifestyle. Most will lose a functional level after a hip fracture; for example, if they were ambulatory within their community, they may only be ambulatory at home after the injury.

Research Opportunities

Both physiological and psychosocial opportunities exist for research in orthopedic nursing. The Research Opportunities chart includes a sample of topics for further nursing research.

Summary

Orthopedic injuries are a frequent occurrence because of blunt trauma and increasingly of penetrating trauma. The nurse plays a crucial role within the health care team in providing timely care for this population. The nurse will be the one to frequently assess and monitor the patient's orthopedic injury and is in the position to recognize and intervene when potential life- and limb-threatening conditions occur.

RESEARCH OPPORTUNITIES AND CLINICAL IMPACT RELATED TO ORTHOPEDIC NURSING

Research Area	Clinical Impact
Physiological Research	
The management of pin sites placed for skeletal traction and external fixation.	Nurses do not have sufficient evidence on which to base best care of pin sites to prevent infection.
Use of alternative methods to manage pain on the orthopedic unit.	Alternative methods of pain management such as acupuncture, acupressure, and massage could be used by nurses to help manage pain.
Development of guidelines to manage pain treatment when patients are transferred to rehab/extended care facilities or home.	There are no guidelines and reported poor pain control of patients after discharge from acute care.
Psychosocial, Ethical, and Legal Research	
Effectiveness of discharge teaching and plans of care and reality of resource availability in the home or community for postoperative patients or those with musculoskeletal injuries.	Many patients are discharged quickly without sufficient resources in place or without understanding plans of care. For example, what is ordered for home and what actually occurs may not be the same. Identify areas for improvement in teaching information and methods, as well as community resources for the postoperative or injured orthopedic patient, especially the elderly, uninsured, and underinsured.
	Prevent the return of underinsured patients who use the emergency department for their health care.
	Decrease return visits and get patients into the appropriate health care systems, decreasing costs.

Clinical Preparation

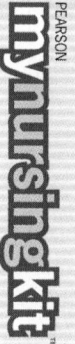

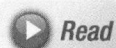 **Read**

- History of Current Illness
- Past Medical History
- Physical Exam
- Admitting Medical Orders
- Laboratory Study Results

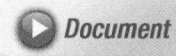 **Document**

- Summary of Hospitalization
- Pathophysiology Form
- Laboratory Values
- Laboratory Results Explanation

 **Apply**

- List of Potential Nursing Diagnoses
- Concept Map
- Critical Thinking Questions

Log on to MyNursingKit.com to download forms you will need and to complete further steps in the Clinical Preparation assignment.

HISTORY OF PRESENT ILLNESS

The patient is a 17-year-old female who was involved in a high-speed, single-vehicle frontal crash and had a negative toxicology/drug screen. Multiple injuries include a concussion and a forehead laceration that has been sutured. She has had her right open tibia fracture washed out with application of an external fixator. She has had an IM rod placed in her right femur fracture. Head CT was negative. Her admitting diagnoses include multiple trauma, right femur fracture, right open tibia/fibular fracture with soft tissue loss, chest contusion, loss of consciousness at the scene, and a forehead laceration.

Medical–Surgical History

The patient takes no medications. Previous surgeries include an appendectomy at age 10.

Social History

The patient is a junior in high school and lives with her parents. The patient denies smoking, drinking, or use of illicit drugs.

Physical Exam

The patient opens her eyes to voice and is oriented. Pupils are equal, round, and reactive to light and accommodation. Suture line on forehead is clean, dry, and intact. Breath sounds are equal bilaterally with equal chest rise. The patient complains of pain to right chest wall with deep breath, no crepitus noted. Heart sounds are normal. Abdomen is soft and nontender with diminished bowel sounds in all quadrants. Right thigh is edematous; suture line is dry and intact. External fixator to right lower leg is intact; pin sites exhibit slight redness and small amount of serous drainage. Motor and sensory to extremities are intact. Peripheral pulses are slightly decreased in the right lower extremity. The patient complains of pain in the right leg at a 6 on a 0–10 scale.

Admitting Medical Orders

Service: trauma service with orthopedic consultation
Diagnosis: concussion, right femur fracture, right open tibia/fibular fracture with soft tissue loss, chest contusion, forehead laceration
Allergies: amoxicillin
Vital signs with oxygen saturations q4h × 24 hours
Call house officer: temp > 38.5°C, HR > 130 or < 60, RR > 30 or < 12, BP sys > 160 or < 90, O_2 sat < 92%, urine output < 120 mL in 4 hours, change in neurological or abdominal exam, any Hct result that is 5 less than the baseline ED Hct, any change in neurovascular exam of the right lower extremity
Activity: patient's weight-bearing status is touch down to right leg; up to chair with assistance
Diet: advance diet as tolerated
Intravenous fluids: D5/0.45 NS with 20 mEq of KCl at 100 mL/hr
Foley catheter to gravity drainage
I&O: every shift
Respiratory care: incentive spirometer every hour when awake
DVT prophylaxis: sequential compression device to left lower extremity

Wound care: pin site care tid, clean forehead laceration with half-strength H_2O_2 and apply bacitracin, elevate right lower extremity

Scheduled Medications

Hydromorphone PCA 0.2 mg/mL, incremental dose 0.4 mg, lock-out 10 minutes
Vancomycin 1 g IV q8h
Docusate capsule 100 mg by mouth twice daily
Enoxaparin 30 mg subcutaneously q12h

PRN Medications

Phenergan 25 mg IV q6h prn nausea
Morphine 2–4mg IV q4h prn pain
Ativan 0.5 mg IV q6h prn anxiety
Ondansetron 4 mg IV q12h if needed for nausea

Ordered Laboratory Studies

CBC every morning
Chem 7 panel every other day

LABORATORY STUDY RESULTS

Test	Preop	Postop, Immediate	Postop, 4 Hours
WBC	28.5/mm³	19.3/mm³	22.4/mm³
RBC	4.40/mm³	4.33/mm³	4.65/mm³
Hemoglobin	13.9 g/dL	12 g/dL	14.5 g/dL
Hematocrit	41%	40%	43%
Platelet count	412/mm³	357/mm³	399/mm³
APTT	20.3 seconds		
INR	0.98		
Sodium	140 mEq/L		
Potassium	3.6 mEq/L		
Chloride	109 mEq/L		
Carbon dioxide	23 mEq/L		
Urea nitrogen	11 mg/dL		
Creatinine blood	0.8 mg/dL		
Glucose	179 mg/dL		
Calcium	8.1 mg/dL		
Lipase	17 unit/dL		

CRITICAL THINKING QUESTIONS

1. On initial admission to the floor postoperatively, which complications should you assess for?
2. In what position should the right leg be placed?

Answers to Critical Thinking Questions appear in Appendix D.

NCLEX® REVIEW

1. The nurse is planning a health promotion program for sports injuries. Which of the following would be the most important for the nurse to emphasize in this program?
   1. How to use new equipment
   2. Prevention of injuries
   3. Why sports need to be supervised
   4. How injuries are related to the time of day
2. A patient with a fracture is able to have his cast removed. The nurse realizes this patient is in which phase of the fractured bone healing process?
   1. Fibroblast framework
   2. Callus formation
   3. Bone calcification
   4. Ossification
3. A victim of a motor vehicle crash has an open fracture of the left femur. Which of the following is a priority of care for this patient?
   1. Provide pain relief.
   2. Prevent damage to surrounding tissue.
   3. Decrease the potential for contamination.
   4. Cast the affected bone immediately.
4. The nurse is planning care for a patient with a fractured pelvis and femur. Which of the following would be a priority for this patient's care?
   1. Monitoring hemodynamic status.
   2. Arranging for a traction set-up.
   3. Providing explanation of nursing care to follow.
   4. Administering oral narcotic analgesics.
5. A patient sustained a crushing injury to both legs. Which of the following would indicate to the nurse that rhabdomyolysis has occurred?
   1. Muscle spasms of the affected extremities
   2. Dark colored urine
   3. Excessive thirst
   4. Double or blurred vision
6. The patient who had a right above-the-knee amputation tells the nurse "I keep wanting to scratch my right foot." Which of the following should the nurse respond to this patient?
   1. It's a side effect of your pain medication.
   2. You are experiencing something called phantom sensations.
   3. Your leg was amputated and it isn't there anymore.
   4. I can get a psychiatrist for you to talk with.

Answers for review questions appear in Appendix D

KEY TERMS

avascular necrosis (AVN) *p.1780*
avulsion fracture *p.1777*
Buck's boots traction *p.1784*
burst fracture *p.1784*
cast *p.1784*
chance fracture *p.1784*
compartment syndrome *p.1796*
contusion *p.1777*
diaphysis *p.1781*

dislocation *p.1780*
epiphysis *p.1781*
external fixation *p.1785*
fasciotomy *p.1796*
fractures *p.1781*
intramedullary (I-M) rodding *p.1786*
ligament *p.1777*
metaphysis *p.1781*

open reduction internal fixation
    (ORIF) *p.1786*
physes *p.1777*
PRICE *p.1777*
skeletal traction *p.1785*
skin traction *p.1784*
sprain *p.1777*
strain *p.1777*

PEARSON
EXPLORE **mynursingkit**™

MyNursingKit is your one stop for online chapter review materials and resources. Prepare for success with additional NCLEX®-style practice questions, interactive assignments and activities, web links, animations and videos, and more!

Register your access code from the front of your book at
www.mynursingkit.com

REFERENCES

Aito, S., Abbate, R., Marcucci, R. & Cominelli, E. (2007). Endogenous risk factors for deep-vein thrombosis in patients with acute spinal cord injuries. *Spinal Cord, 45*(9), 627–631.

American College of Surgeons. (2004). *Advanced Trauma Life Support Course Manual.* Chicago: American College of Surgeons.

Anscomb, S. (2007). Managing sprains and strains. *Practice Nurse, 33*(5), 44–49.

Bongiovanni, M. S., Bradley, S. L., & Kelley, D. M. (2005). Orthopedic trauma critical care nursing issues. *Critical Care Nursing Quarterly, 28*(1), 60–71.

Dougall, A. L., Ursano, R. J., Posluszny, D. M., Fullerton, C. S., & Baum, A. (2001). Predictors of posttraumatic stress among victims of motor vehicle accidents. *Psychosomatic Medicine, 63*(3), 402–411.

Emergency Nurses Association. (2006). *Alcohol and injury facts.* Retrieved September 11, 2007, from http://www.ena.org/ ipinstitute/fact/ENAIPFactSheet-Alcohol.pdf

Feliciano, D. V., Mattox, K. L., & Moore, E. E. (Eds.). (2008). *Trauma* (6th ed.). New York: McGraw-Hill.

Frazier, M. S., & Drzymkowski, J. W. (Eds.). (2007). *Essentials of human diseases and conditions* (4th ed.). St. Louis: W. B. Saunders.

Gustillo classification of fracture. (2004). Retrieved January 1, 2004, from http://www.wheelessonline.com/oa2/60.htm

Harvard Women's Health Watch. (2007). *Recovering from an ankle sprain.* Retrieved April 5, 2008, from http://www.health.harvard.edu

Holmes, S. B., & Brown, S. J. (2005). Skeletal pin site care: National Association of Orthopaedic Nurses guidelines for orthopaedic nursing. *Orthopaedic Nursing, 24*(2), 99–107.

Hrysomallis, C. (2007). Relationship between balance ability, training and sports injury risk. *Sports Medicine, 37*(6), 547–555.

Knudson, M. M., Ikossi, D. G., Khaw, L., Morabito, D., & Speetzen, L. (2004). Thromboembolism after trauma: An analysis of 1602 episodes from the American College of Surgeons National Trauma Data Bank. *Annals of Surgery, 240*(3), 490–498.

Meehan, A. J. (2002). National Consensus Conference on improving the continuum of care for patients with hip fracture. *Orthopaedic Nursing, 21*(1), 16–22.

Mohanty, K., Musso, D., Powell, J. N., Kortbeek, J. B., & Kirkpatrick, A. W. (2005). Emergent management of pelvic ring injuries: An update. *Canadian Journal of Surgery, 48*(1), 49–56.

Morris, A. H., & Zuckerman, J. D. (2002). National Consensus Conference on improving the continuum of care for patients with hip fracture. *Journal of Bone & Joint Surgery—American Volume, 84-A*(4), 670–674.

National Safe Kids Campaign. (2003, 7/2003). *Sports and recreation.* Retrieved September 1, 2003, from http://www.safekids.org/tier2_rl.cfm?folder_id=178

Norman, S. B., Stein, M. B., Dimsdale, J. E., & Hoyt, D. B. (2007). Pain in the aftermath of trauma is a risk factor for post-traumatic stress disorder. *Psychology Medicine, 10,* 1–10.

Orosz, G. M., Magaziner, J., Hannan, E. L., Morrison, R. S., Koval, K., Gilbert, M., et al. (2004). Association of timing of surgery for hip fracture and patient outcomes. *Journal of the American Medical Association, 291*(14), 1738–1743.

Porth, C. M. (Ed.). (2005). *Essentials of pathophysiology.* Philadelphia: Lippincott Williams & Wilkins.

Rusch, M. D., Gould, L. J., Dzwierzynski, W. W., & Larson, D. L. (2002). Psychological impact of traumatic injuries: What the surgeon can do. *Plastic and Reconstructive Surgery, 109*(1), 18–24.

Shetty, A. (2004). *Superior mesenteric artery syndrome.* Retrieved January 2, 2005, from http://www.emedicine.com/ped/topic2175.htm

Walker, J. A. (2007). Evidence for skeletal pin site care. *Nursing Standard, 21*(45), 70–76.

57

Caring for the Patient During Musculoskeletal Surgical Procedures

Karen Cooper
Kathleen Osborn

With contributions by:
Cheryl Wraa

Outcome-Based Learning Objectives

After studying this chapter, the learner will be able to:

1. List components of the neurovascular assessment appropriate for a patient who has had orthopedic surgery.
2. Discuss the types of precautions required to prevent hip dislocation in the postoperative hip replacement patient.
3. Describe the nursing actions appropriate for a patient with symptoms of complications, including compartment syndrome.
4. Describe the appropriate use of assistive devices utilized for orthopedic patients.
5. Discuss the importance of optimal pain control in the postoperative orthopedic patient.

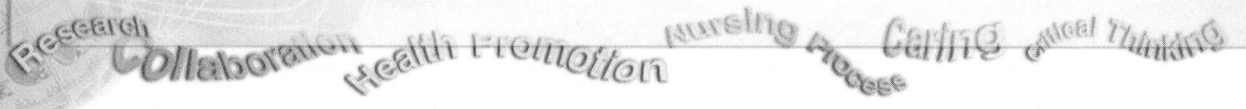

PATIENTS UNDERGOING musculoskeletal surgery generally fall into two categories: (1) those that have experienced increasing pain or disability over time causing them to seek a surgical resolution to their complaints, or (2) patients who have had a traumatic event. The patient who enters the hospital for an elective orthopedic procedure often has the benefit of preoperative teaching and preparation for the procedure. The patient who has experienced a traumatic event may present unique challenges for the nurse, both preoperatively and postoperatively. The nurse is in a unique position to recognize potential problems and prevent complications that have a direct impact on the ability of the patient to improve or maintain functional status and return to a productive lifestyle. Orthopedic surgical patients face recovery from both the sequelae of surgery and anesthesia as well as potential complications specific to the orthopedic problem encountered. The nursing process provides a systematic approach to the identification of actual or potential problems that impact the patient's recovery. These actual and potential problems are identified from assessment data and are utilized to develop a plan of care specific to the patient's needs.

The orthopedic surgeon performs a physical assessment and diagnostic testing to determine whether the diseased/traumatized bone or joint requires surgical replacement of the joint or simple repair. Repair may include removal of bone and ligament particles, smoothing of joint surfaces, reconnection of torn ligaments, or replacement of ligaments with allograft (cadaver) or autograft (tissue from another area to replace damaged ligaments or bone). Replacement of the joint may include repair as well as the implantation of a new joint.

Traumatic injuries play a large part in the need for orthopedic surgery in patients of all ages. Congenital deformities are generally repaired in the pediatric population. Spinal surgery for scoliosis is usually performed in the early adolescent period, whereas spinal surgery for disk repair or laminectomy is performed in young and middle adulthood. Hip fractures are a common traumatic injury for the elderly, as is joint replacement surgery. The life of an artificial joint and the surrounding bone tissue is shorter than that of a natural joint, with current artificial hips and knees lasting approximately 20 years. Knowledge of biographic and demographic data is important in planning appropriate care for the patient. Elder patients are at risk for postoperative delirium. Knowledge of the patient's prior experiences, abilities, and accomplishments can assist the nurse in providing patient-specific interventions to maintain orientation and prevent cognitive function alterations.

Preoperative Assessment of the Orthopedic Surgical Patient

The assessment of the preoperative orthopedic surgical patient must take into account both the health history as well as the history surrounding the surgical event. Knowledge of patient demographics, related to the injury, general health, and medical and social history, is often obtained from the preoperative history and physical exam. The nurse must be diligent in obtaining information regarding the presurgical status of the patient. The mechanism of injury is important for the nurse to know to be able to formulate a plan of care for the patient with appropriate attention to patient safety and necessary interventions and precautions for the patient. For example, did the patient fall because he had a stroke and now has residual weakness on one side of his body? Was the patient in a skilled nursing facility and fell from bed because she was confused? Did the patient trip and fall as an unpreventable accident? The time of injury to surgery also impacts the focus of nursing assessment and care planning. If the patient fell and fractured a hip, was taken to the emergency department, and was not allowed to eat or drink for many hours prior to surgery, closer attention to intake and output and potential hypovolemia is a greater concern. If the patient was injured in a motor vehicle crash, there may be other associated injuries that will complicate care. The type of surgery performed has inherent risks and complications that the nurse must anticipate and utilize in focusing the patient assessment specific to the patient and his needs.

Clinical Manifestations

Pain, loss of function, and deformity are the three major complaints associated with musculoskeletal conditions that cause the patient to seek surgical care. It is important to utilize a consistent pain scale when assessing the patient's pain level. Chapter 15 🔗 includes an in-depth discussion of pain. Loss of function may be directly related to the injury or indirectly related to nerve damage or pain.

The mechanism of injury is also an important factor because treatment may be necessary as an emergency procedure for a traumatic injury. Patients having elective surgical procedures, such as a total knee replacement for osteoarthritis or below knee amputation for peripheral vascular disease, may have very different expectations regarding the proposed surgery. The patient electing to have a knee replacement may see the surgery as desired to relieve chronic pain and deformity and to restore function. The patient facing an amputation may have unresolved issues regarding the decision to have surgery and fears loss of function. The psychological preparation, physical abilities, and function of the patient preoperatively are important to consider in providing care in the postoperative period.

Past Medical History

The past medical history gives important information regarding potential complications that may occur during the postoperative period. For example, patients with a history of cardiovascular disease may suffer perioperative myocardial infarction, dysrhythmias, or delay in surgical healing. Patients with diabetes may be more prone to postoperative infection and need for altered glucose control. Patients with a prior history of deep venous thrombosis (DVT) are at greater risk for developing postoperative DVT. If the patient has asthma or chronic obstructive pulmonary disease (COPD), she may be at greater risk for pulmonary complications.

Medications

All medications should be reviewed with the patient prior to surgery. Cardiac, pulmonary, and renal medications should alert the nurse to potential complications and the need for anticipatory planning in the care of the patient. In addition, medications that increase bleeding tendencies should be discontinued prior to surgery. Aspirin, heparin, and nonsteroidal anti-inflammatory drugs (NSAIDs), which are platelet inhibitors, need to be discontinued prior to surgery.

Oral bisphosphonates such as alendronate (Fosamax) are used to prevent bone loss from osteoporosis and may be discontinued during hospitalization. Hormone replacement therapy for postmenopausal females may increase the risk of postoperative deep venous thrombosis, so it is also frequently discontinued during hospitalization. Calcium supplements of 1,000 to 3,000 milligrams daily and calcitonin nasal spray may also be prescribed to prevent bone loss.

The nurse should ask the patient specifically about over-the-counter medications and dietary supplements. Ginseng, garlic, and *Ginkgo biloba* dietary supplements interact with platelets and may increase bleeding during surgery. Chart 57–1 (p. 1804) discusses herbal supplements that may impact surgery.

Allergies

The nurse must be knowledgeable of the patient's allergies to prevent potential anaphylactic reactions to medications administered pre- and postoperatively. Patients may also report prior negative reactions to medications as allergies. For example, if morphine causes gastric upset the patient may report this as an allergy. If a morphine patient-controlled analgesia (PCA) is ordered for the patient, the nurse must teach the patient that adverse reactions are not always present with decreased dosages of the medication. The nurse must also be aware of potential allergic reactions to medications that may have cross sensitivity, such as penicillin allergies possibly related to cephalosporin allergy. Patient allergies should be recorded on the health care provider order forms and medication administration record to prevent medication errors.

Prior Surgeries and Hospitalizations

The patient's prior hospital and surgical experiences should be explored with the patient. If the patient has had negative experiences in the past, the nurse should utilize knowledge of these problems in the care planning process to communicate patient needs and attempt a positive current hospital experience. Expectations of the current hospitalization should be elicited and clarified if necessary. The plan of care for the current hospitalization and surgery should be reviewed with the patient and specific daily goals should be negotiated.

Cardiovascular Disease

Knowledge of preexisting cardiovascular disease is an important consideration in planning the care of the orthopedic surgical patient. Many anesthetic agents cause myocardial suppression and increase the risk of surgical cardiac events. Preoperative

CHART 57–1	**Herbal Supplements and the Orthopedic Surgical Patient**	
Herbal Supplement	**Reported Use**	**Nursing Considerations**
Garlic	Treat high blood pressure. Treat atherosclerosis.	Increases risk of bleeding especially if other anticoagulants, antiplatelet, or anti-inflammatory medications are administered. May affect glycemic control. Discontinue 1–2 weeks prior to surgery.
Ginkgo biloba	May decrease plaque formation in atherosclerosis to reduce peripheral vascular disease.	May increase effects of anticoagulants and antiplatelet medications to increase bleeding postoperatively. Discontinue 2 days–2 weeks prior to surgery.
Ginseng	Improve concentration and stamina.	Inhibits platelet aggregation and may potentiate bleeding especially if additional anticoagulants or antiplatelet medications are administered. Discontinue 1–2 weeks prior to surgery.
Glucosamine	Decrease joint discomfort, increase joint flexibility, and "rebuild" cartilage.	May affect serum glucose levels and interact with insulin effect. Monitor serum glucose. May increase blood pressure and heart rate, thereby masking signs of hypovolemia in the postoperative patient.

evaluation of chest pain should be carried out, and a 12-lead ECG is performed to determine whether the patient has signs of myocardial ischemia. Patients with a history of dysrhythmias may require telemetry monitoring before and after surgery. Antidysrhythmic medications should be continued during the postoperative period. If the patient has a pacemaker or implantable cardioverter defibrillator (ICD), magnetic resonance imaging (MRI) is contraindicated.

Pulmonary Disease

Patients with preexisting pulmonary disease are at greater risk of developing pulmonary complications in the postoperative period. Patients with chronic obstructive pulmonary disease (COPD) may have lower baseline arterial oxygen levels that may delay wound healing. This population may also be at greater risk for carbon dioxide retention and decreased respiratory drive. Frequent assessments of respiratory status including respiratory rate, depth, and oxygen saturation should be performed. Supplemental oxygen may be necessary to promote adequate oxygenation; however, low flow rates are generally prescribed to prevent suppression of the respiratory drive. Unit 7 ⊕ includes in-depth discussion of pulmonary disorders.

Diabetes

Surgical stress and alterations in a patient's normal eating patterns can affect blood glucose levels. Surgical stress may increase insulin needs in the postoperative period. Nothing by mouth (NPO) status increases the risk of hypoglycemia. The patient's capillary blood glucose levels should be assessed at regular intervals to monitor glucose levels. Patients may be placed on sliding scale coverage for blood glucose in addition to their regular insulin or oral hypoglycemic regimen, as elevated blood glucose levels increase wound healing time. Patients with diabetes may also be at greater risk for infection. Surgical wounds should be carefully inspected for signs and symptoms of infection.

Functional Status

The patient's previous functional status should be evaluated preoperatively and goals set for the postoperative period that are equal to or better than the preoperative functional status. Elders who undergo surgery are at risk for functional decline because they may be dependent on the nurse for all activities. Patients should be encouraged to engage in activities to their full potential. More time should be allotted for elder activities, as they frequently require more time to complete activities of daily living. Patients with a prior history of stroke may have residual weakness that impedes the patients' ability to perform postoperative rehabilitation exercises and activities of daily living. The stroke may have been the original cause of injury for the patient.

Genetic Factors

Osteogenesis imperfecta (OI), commonly called "brittle bone" syndrome, is an extremely rare genetic disorder affecting type I collagen formation. There are several types. Type I is the mildest form of the disease. Patients are prone to fractures, have collagen deficiency, and females have an increased risk of postmenopausal osteoporosis. Type II OI is nearly always fatal during the neonatal period due to birth injuries. Type III (severe) OI patients have severe bone deformities, have sufficient but abnormal collagen, and are prone to bone fractures. Respiratory insufficiency related to rib fractures and thoracic cage deformity is a major complication in this group. They may fracture a rib simply by coughing. Type IV, or "moderate OI with short stature" patients, is similar to type III, but has less skeletal deformity. With this disease the treatment of fractures is often complicated by delayed union.

Occupational History

Occupation is an important factor in musculoskeletal injuries in terms of both causation and recovery. Depending on the injury, the patient may be unable to return to work for weeks or months after injury or surgery. If injured at work and now unable to return to work on a permanent basis, the patient may need vocational rehabilitation. If the injury is unrelated to work, but the patient must now be off from work to recover, this may cause financial hardship.

Culture

Patients' cultural history should be included in the plan of care for the patients. If they have specific requirements for the gender of the nurses and caretakers assigned to them, these should be accommodated whenever possible. Knowledge of a patient's pain expression should be included in the plan of care. Cultural accommodations for activities of daily living (ADL) and cultural dietary accommodations may be necessary and should be communicated. The patient should be offered spiritual affiliation if desired.

Anesthetic

The anesthetic agents utilized for orthopedic surgery depend on the type of surgery planned and the duration of the surgery. General anesthesia usually involves a combination of inhaled anesthetic agents, paralytics, and narcotics. Epidural anesthesia may be utilized in the patient undergoing lower extremity or low back surgery. When epidural anesthesia is utilized, the administration of narcotics, sedatives, and hypnotics is generally restricted to prevent respiratory compromise. The type of epidural anesthetic should be reported and the time of the last dose clearly recorded so that patients do not receive opioid narcotics during the period specified for the epidural agent used.

Subcutaneous pain pumps may be used in some orthopedic procedures. These devices deliver a slow, continuous infusion of local anesthetic into the operative or suture site to prevent or relieve postoperative pain. The nurse and patient should anticipate that the area surrounding the insertion site will be numb. The goal of such pumps is to decrease the need for oral or intravenous postoperative pain medication, which may contribute to respiratory depression or drowsiness. Adverse reactions are related to sensitivity or allergy to the local anesthetic. A complete discussion of the various types of anesthesia, along with the medical and nursing management of the patient, is in Chapter 26 ☺.

Surgical Procedures

Prior to surgery the surgical site, level, or digit should be marked by initialing the correct operative site with indelible pen or other means such as an adhesive strip according to hospital protocol. This is a Joint Commission requirement for patient safety (called the universal protocol) to prevent surgery at the wrong site. The marking may be part of a preoperative patient check at the time of admission or at the time that the surgical consent is signed. The nurse verifies the patient's understanding of the operative procedure as well as confirming the correct site or side, limb, or digit of the surgery. Chapter 26 ☺ outlines the Association of periOperative Registered Nurses (AORN) and the American College of Surgeons national standards for prevention of wrong-site surgery.

Preprocedure education should include the surgery itself, its inherent risks and benefits, and options for blood donation. Elective patients frequently are scheduled for same-day surgery, so that the responsibility for preoperative preparation falls on the outpatient or office nurse.

There are commercially available preoperative and surgery-specific films and pamphlets for patients to view prior to surgery that can be helpful in providing portions of preoperative education to the patient. Chapter 24 ☺ includes a complete discussion of blood administration. It is not within the scope of this chapter to review all types of orthopedic surgery. Selected orthopedic surgical approaches that require hospitalization will be covered.

Upper Extremity Surgery

Upper extremity surgeries include total shoulder or elbow joint replacement, rotator cuff repair, and open reduction or stabilization of fractures of the humerus, radius, or ulna. Most elective upper extremity surgeries below the elbow are performed on an outpatient basis. Shoulder and elbow surgery may require one or more inpatient hospital days to ensure that nerve entrapment does not occur from postoperative edema. Reduction and stabilization of fractures are discussed in detail in Chapter 56 ☺.

The shoulder is a ball-and-socket joint that is made up of three bones: the upper arm bone (humerus), shoulder blade (scapula), and collarbone (clavicle). The top of the humerus fits into the small socket (glenoid) of the shoulder blade to form the shoulder joint (glenohumeral joint). The socket of the glenoid is surrounded by a soft-tissue rim (labrum). The articular cartilage and a thin inner lining (synovium) of the joint allow the smooth motion of the shoulder joint. The upper part of the shoulder blade (acromion) projects over the shoulder joint. One end of the collarbone is joined with the shoulder blade by the acromioclavicular (AC) joint, and the other end of the collarbone is joined with the breastbone (sternum) by the sternoclavicular joint. The joint capsule, which is a thin sheet of fibers that surrounds the shoulder joint, allows a wide range of motion, yet provides stability. The rotator cuff is a group of four muscles—the supraspinatus, infraspinatus, teres minor, and subscapularis—that along with the tendons attaches the upper arm to the shoulder blade. A saclike membrane (bursa) between the rotator cuff and the shoulder blade cushions and helps lubricate the motion between these two structures. The rotator cuff stabilizes the humeral head in the glenoid fossa. The muscles attached to the rotator cuff enable arm motion that allows an individual to take part in activities such as throwing or swimming.

Rotator Cuff Repair

Rotator cuff tears can occur from a single traumatic injury (Figure 57–1 ■, p. 1806). These patients often report recurrent shoulder pain for several months and can recall the specific injury that triggered the onset of the pain. A cuff tear may also happen at the same time as another injury to the shoulder, such as a fracture or dislocation. Of note, most tears are the result of overuse of the muscles and tendons over a period of years. People who are especially at risk for overuse are those who engage in repetitive overhead motions such as baseball, tennis, weight lifting, and rowing. Rotator cuff tears are most common in people over the age of 40 (American Academy of Orthopaedic Surgeons [AAOS], 2007a). Partial thickness or full-thickness tears may occur (Figure 57–2 ■, p. 1806). Partial thickness rotator cuff tears are associated with chronic inflammation and the development of spurs on the underside of the acromion or the acromioclavicular joint. Full-thickness tears are most often the result of impingement, partial thickness rotator cuff tears from heavy lifting or falls. Clinical manifestations include:

- Atrophy or thinning of the muscles about the shoulder
- Pain in the front of the shoulder that radiates down the arm when lifting the arm or when lowering the arm from a fully raised position
- Weakness when lifting or rotating the arm
- Crepitus or crackling sensation when moving the shoulder in certain positions

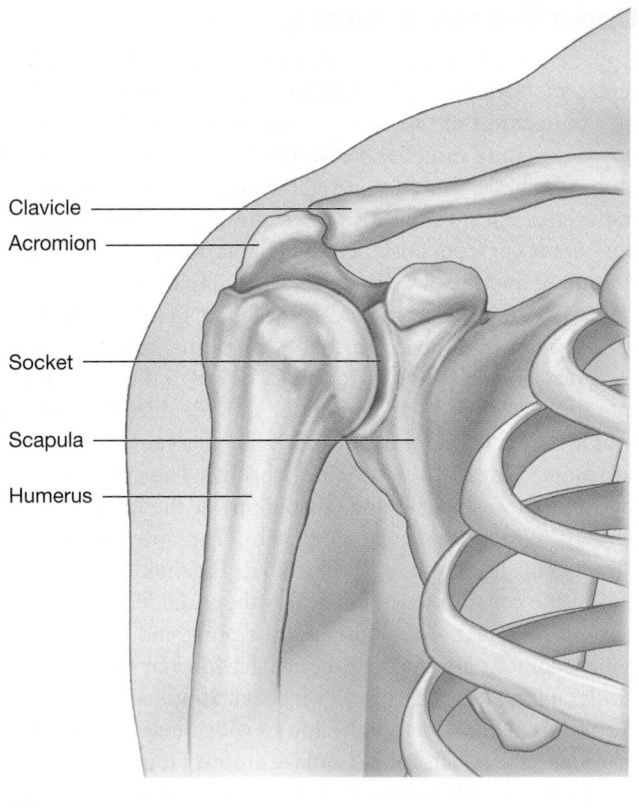

Clavicle
Acromion

Socket

Scapula

Humerus

(a)

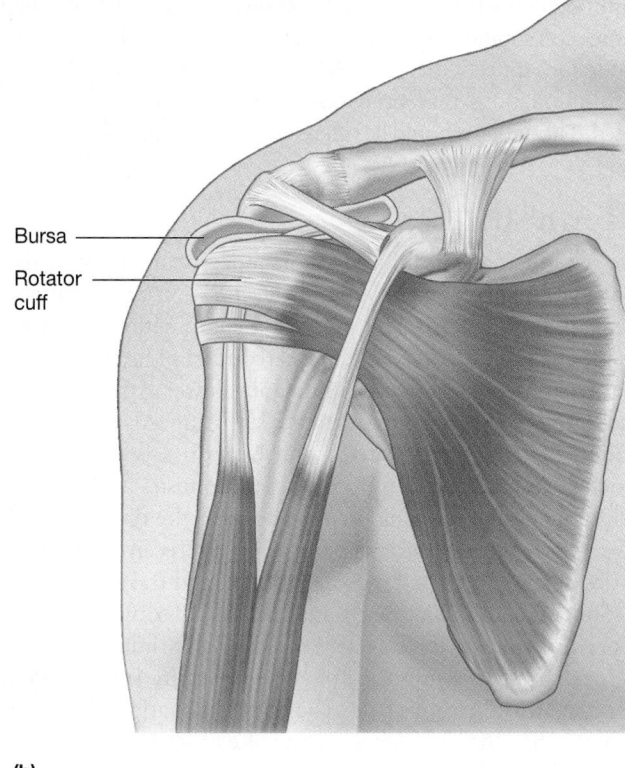

Bursa
Rotator cuff

(b)

FIGURE 57–1 ■ Shoulder anatomy.

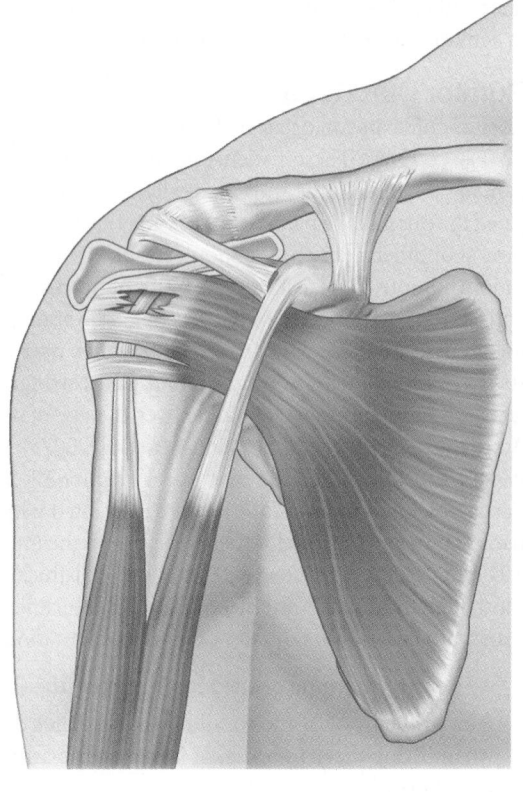

(a)

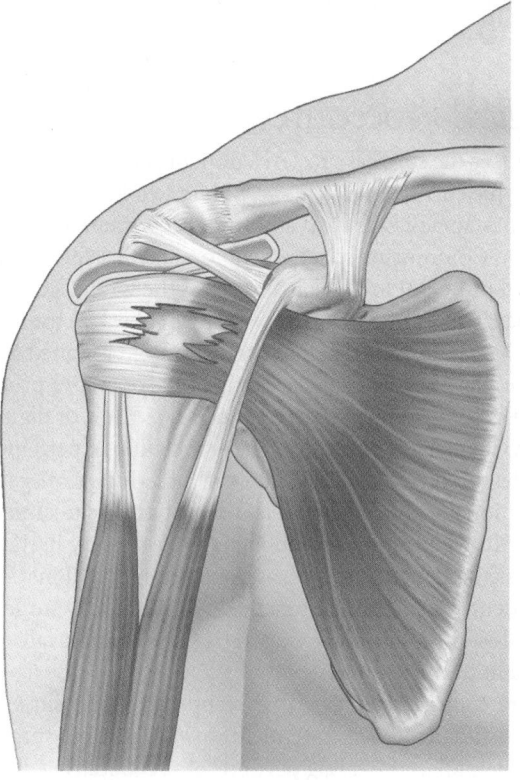

(b)

FIGURE 57–2 ■ (A) Impingement with partial tear. (B) Full-thickness tear.

- When the tear occurs with an injury, there may be sudden acute pain, a snapping sensation, and an immediate weakness of the arm.

Symptoms may develop right away after a trauma, such as a lifting injury or a fall on the affected arm, or they may develop gradually with repetitive overhead activity or following long-term wear.

The type of surgical repair depends on the size, shape, and location of the tear. A partial tear (see Figure 57–2A ■) may require only a trimming or smoothing procedure, called a *débridement*. A complete tear (see Figure 57–2B ■) within the thickest part of the tendon is repaired by suturing the two sides of the tendon back together. If the tendon is torn away from where it inserts into the bone of the humerus, it is repaired directly to bone (AAOS, 2007a). There are two approaches to the surgical procedure: open or arthroscopic. The open surgical approach is described in Chart 57–2. With an arthroscopy the orthopedic surgeon inserts a pencil-thin device with a small lens and lighting system into tiny incisions to look inside the joint. The images inside the joint are relayed to a TV monitor, allowing the surgeon to make a diagnosis. Other surgical instruments can be inserted to make repairs, based on findings. Many of these surgical repairs can be done on an outpatient basis.

Shoulder Arthroplasty

Arthroplasty refers to restoration of a joint either by **total joint replacement**, replacement of a joint with a prosthesis, or by resurfacing bone and removing damaged bone and cartilage. Total replacement of the shoulder and elbow is not as common as of the hip and knee. An indication for the surgery is severe pain resulting from rheumatoid arthritis, osteoarthritis, avascular necrosis, or post-traumatic arthritis. Osteoarthritis and rheumatoid arthritis can destroy the shoulder joint and surrounding tissue. Arthritis is discussed in detail in Chapter 58 ⚭.

Clinical manifestations include pain that progressively worsens and is aggravated by activity. When the glenohumeral shoulder joint is affected, the pain is centered in the back of the shoulder and frequently intensifies with changes in the weather. If the acromioclavicular joint is involved, the pain is focused in the front of the shoulder. A person with rheumatoid arthritis of both shoulders may have pain in all these areas. Limited motion is another problem. It may become more difficult to lift the arm to comb hair or reach up to a shelf. A clicking or snapping sound (crepitus) may be heard with movement. As the disease progresses, any movement of the shoulder causes pain. Night pain is common and sleeping may be difficult. The involved arm is typically weak due to muscle atrophy, is tender to touch, and has limited range of motion. Crepitus (a grating sensation inside the joint) may be felt with movement. X-rays of an arthritic shoulder will show a narrowing of the joint space, changes in the bone, and the formation of bone spurs (osteophytes) (American Academy of Orthopaedic Surgeons, 2007b).

The surgical approach used to treat the arthritis of the glenohumeral joint is by replacing the entire shoulder joint with a prosthesis (total shoulder arthroplasty) or by replacing the head of the upper arm bone (hemiarthroplasty) (see Chart 57–2). The goal of surgery is to restore the best possible function to the joint by removing scar tissue, balancing muscles, and replacing the joint surfaces. Figure 57–3 ■ shows the artificial joint components including the humeral ball (which is made of metal) and the glenoid component (which is made of plastic). The humeral ball is fixed to the humerus with the humeral stem, and the glenoid component is attached to the shoulder blade using a small amount of bone cement. Shoulder range of motion is

---

CHART 57–2   **Shoulder Arthroscopy**

- Incision is made approximately 6–10 inches in length to expose the shoulder joint.
- The humeral head is dislocated from the socket.
- The head of the humerus is shaved/removed to shape the bone to fit the implant, and the bone canal is drilled to prepare for the prosthesis implant.
- The implant is inserted into the humerus.
- The glenoid socket is shaved to create a smooth articular surface or is shaved and a concave disk implanted to replace the glenoid socket surface. Holes may be drilled into the glenoid surface to secure the implanted glenoid socket.
- Debris (torn ligaments, bone fragments, and clots) are removed, and ligaments are adjusted.
- The surgical site is sutured closed after the joint is tested for smooth motion.

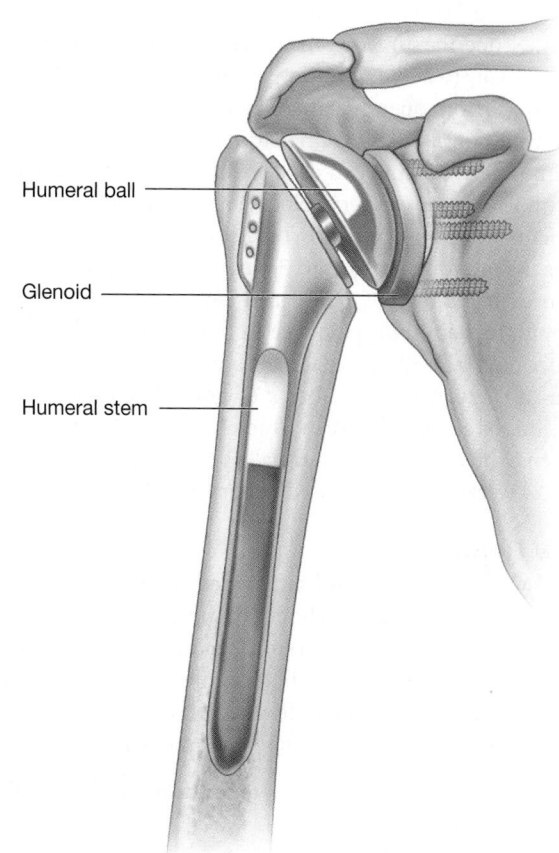

Humeral ball

Glenoid

Humeral stem

FIGURE 57–3 ■ Shoulder arthroplasty.

started immediately after the procedure, and patients are usually discharged from hospital 3 days after surgery if they are comfortable and have a good range of passive motion. The recovery of strength and function may continue for up to 1 year after surgery (Matson & Warme, 2008). Hemiarthroplasty is a shoulder replacement wherein only the humeral head is replaced with an artificial joint.

The most common surgical procedure used to treat arthritis of the acromioclavicular joint is a resection arthroplasty. A small piece of bone from the end of the collarbone is removed, leaving a space that later fills with scar tissue. Surgical treatment of arthritis of the shoulder is generally very effective in reducing pain and restoring motion (American Academy of Orthopaedic Surgeons, 2007b).

Shoulder Subluxation and Dislocation Repair

Shoulder instability or subluxation and shoulder dislocation are potentially painful and disabling conditions. Subluxation and dislocation both represent problems that occur when the humeral head does not stay centered correctly in the socket (or *glenoid*). These problems may manifest themselves with pain from doing the normal activities of daily living, to the inability to lift the arm without dislocating the joint.

The treatments for these conditions vary widely depending on the severity of symptoms and signs. Many patients will improve with the appropriate bracing and physical therapy. However, for those patients who require surgery, arthroscopic surgery is used to diagnose the exact nature of the joint instability. The goal of surgery is to reestablish the stability of the humeral head in the shallow glenoid socket without compromising the shoulder motion. Using the scope, the surgeon can evaluate the entire shoulder joint and can usually treat the conditions leading to the instability with this approach. Infrequently, patients may require an open surgery, using an incision about 8–13 cm (3 to 5 inches) long to correct the problem. The procedure can usually be performed within a few hours under general (or nerve block) anesthesia.

Patients undergoing arthroscopic shoulder stabilization will require a sling for usually 2 to 3 weeks, and simple range-of-motion exercises may be performed daily. Outpatient physical therapy for reestablishing pain-free motion and strengthening the shoulder muscles will be needed for a few months. Normally, a person can return to most forms of normal activity within 6 weeks, limited athletics between 10 and 14 weeks, and all activities and even contact athletics can usually be accomplished between 14 and 24 weeks, depending on the sport (Wahl & Slaney, 2005).

Elbow Repair

The elbow is a hinge and ball-and-socket joint made up of the humerus, ulna, and radius. The positioning and interaction of the bones in the joint allow for a small amount of rotation as well as hinge action. The primary stability of the elbow is provided by the ulnar collateral ligament on the medial (inner) side of the elbow. As muscles contract and relax, two unique motions occur:

- The hinge joint allows the elbow to bend and straighten (flexion and extension, respectively).
- Rotation through the ball-and-socket joint allows the hand to be rotated palm down and palm up (pronation and supination, respectively).

Osteoarthritis of the elbow occurs when the cartilage surface is damaged or becomes worn. This can happen because of a previous injury such as elbow dislocation or fracture, or it may also be the result of degeneration of the joint cartilage. Osteoarthritis usually affects the weight-bearing joints, such as the hip and knees; therefore, the elbow is one of the least affected joints because of its well-matched joint surfaces and strong stabilizing ligaments. As a result, the elbow joint can tolerate large forces across it without becoming unstable. The most common cause of osteoarthritis is a previous injury, such as a fracture that involved the surface of the joint or an elbow dislocation. Injury to the ligaments resulting in an unstable elbow can also lead to osteoarthritis, even if the elbow surface is not damaged, because the normal forces across the elbow are altered, causing the joint to wear out more rapidly. Of note, one of the most common injuries to the elbow occurs on the lateral, or outer, side of the elbow, referred to as lateral epicondylitis (tennis elbow) (American Academy of Orthopaedic Surgeons, 2007c).

The most common clinical manifestations of elbow arthritis are pain and loss of range of motion. Patients also report a "grating" or "locking" sensation in the elbow. The grating is due to loss of the normal smooth joint surface caused by cartilage damage or wear. The locking is caused by loose pieces of cartilage or bone that dislodge from the joint and become trapped between the moving joint surfaces, blocking motion. As the disease progresses, joint swelling may also occur. The swelling may also cause numbness in the ring finger and small finger due to ulnar nerve pressure. Finally, if the elbow cannot be moved through its normal range of motion, it may stiffen into a position in which it is bent (flexion) (American Academy of Orthopaedic Surgeons, 2007c).

Arthroscopy, which removes loose bodies or inflammatory/degenerative tissue in the joint, provides symptom improvement at least in the short term. It also attempts to smooth out irregular surfaces. Multiple small incisions are used to perform the surgery. It can be done as an outpatient procedure, and recovery is reasonably rapid. If the joint surface has worn away completely, the most definitive treatment is joint replacement. For patients who are too young or too active to have prosthetic joint replacement, there are other surgical options. If loss of motion is the primary symptom, the surgeon can release the contracture and smooth out the joint surface. At times, a new surface made from the patient's own body tissues can be made. These procedures can provide years of symptom improvement (American Academy of Orthopaedic Surgeons, 2007c).

Elbow Dislocation

Elbow dislocations are a common injury that typically occurs when a person falls onto an outstretched hand. On impact the force is sent to the elbow, and usually there is a turning motion in this force that can rotate the elbow out of its socket. Because the elbow is stabilized with the combined effects of bone surfaces, ligaments, and muscles, when it dislocates, any or all of these structures can be injured to different degrees. There are three basic types of elbow dislocation: a simple, a complex, and a severe dislocation. A simple dislocation does not have any major bone injury. A complex dislocation can have severe bone and ligament injuries. With a severe dislocation, the blood vessels and nerves that travel across the elbow may be injured. If this happens, there is a risk of losing the arm.

A complete elbow dislocation is extremely painful, and the arm will look deformed and may have an odd twist at the elbow. A partial elbow dislocation can be harder to detect; because the elbow is only partially dislocated, the bones can spontaneously relocate and the joint may appear fairly normal. The elbow usually will move fairly normally, but it is painful. There may be bruising on the inside and outside of the elbow where ligaments may have been stretched or torn. Partial dislocations can continue to recur over time if the ligaments never heal. The pulses on the injured side must be checked. If the artery is injured, the hand will be cool to touch and may have a white or purple hue due to the diminished blood supply. If nerves were injured during the dislocation or from subsequent swelling, some or all of the hand may be numb and not able to move. Over time, following a dislocation, there is an increased risk for arthritis in the elbow joint if the alignment of the bones is not good; the elbow does not move and rotate normally; or the elbow continues to dislocate.

An elbow dislocation should be considered an emergency injury. The goal of immediate treatment is to return the elbow to its normal alignment, and the long-term goal is to restore function to the arm. With a complex elbow dislocation, surgery may be necessary to restore bone alignment and repair ligaments. Blood vessel or nerve injuries will also need surgical repair.

After surgery, the elbow may be protected with an external hinge. This device protects the elbow from dislocating again. Late reconstructive surgery can successfully restore motion to some stiff elbows. This surgery removes scar tissue and extra bone growth. It also removes obstacles to movement.

Carpal Tunnel Repair

The wrist is an extremely complex joint that provides the mobility to give the hand a full range of motion, while at the same time providing the strength for heavy gripping. There are 15 bones from the end of the forearm to the hand. The wrist has 8 small bones, called carpal bones. These bones are grouped in 2 rows across the wrist. The proximal row begins with the thumb side of the wrist and is made up of the scaphoid, lunate, triquetrum, and pisiform bones. The distal row of carpal tunnel bones is made up of the trapezium, trapezoid, capitate, and hamate bones.

The proximal row connects the radius and the ulna (forearm) to the bones of the hand. The bones of the hand are called the metacarpal bones. These are the long bones that lie within the palm of the hand. The metacarpals attach to the phalanges, which are the bones in the fingers and thumb (eOrthopod, 2003).

The carpal tunnel is a narrow, tunnel-like structure in the wrist (Figure 57–4 ■). The bottom and sides of this tunnel are formed by wrist (carpal) bones and the top of the tunnel is covered by the transverse carpal ligament. The median nerve and tendons travel from the forearm into the hand through this tunnel. With carpal tunnel syndrome, tendons in the wrist swell and put pressure on the median nerve, causing hand numbness and pain. Carpal tunnel syndrome is more common in women than in men and affects up to 10% of the entire population (American Academy of Orthopaedic Surgeons, 2007d). The causes of carpal tunnel syndrome include:

- Heredity
- Repetitive motions of the hands or wrist over a very long period of time

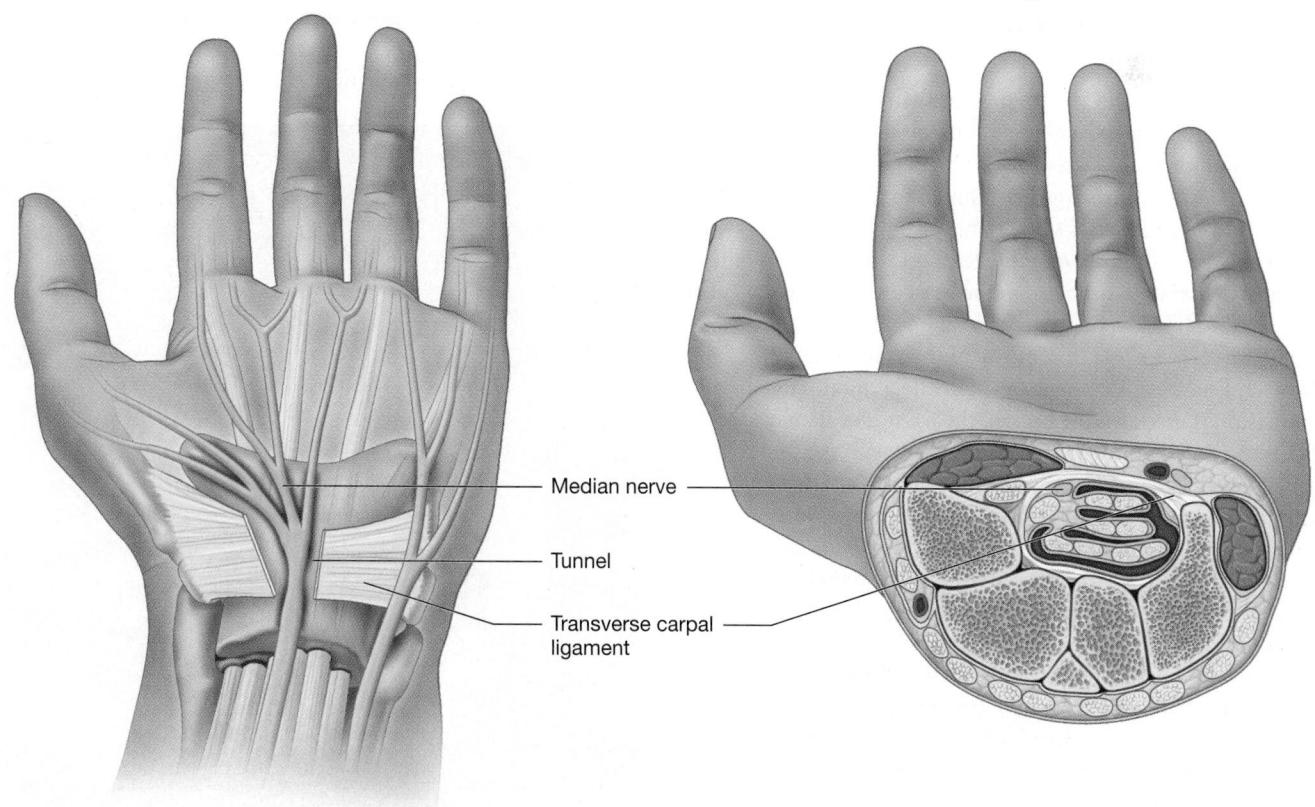

(a)   (b)

FIGURE 57–4 ■ Carpal tunnel syndrome.

Median nerve

Tunnel

Transverse carpal ligament

- Hormonal changes related to pregnancy and menopause
- Diabetes, rheumatoid arthritis, and thyroid gland imbalance
- In some cases idiopathic

The clinical manifestations are pain, numbness, and tingling in the hand. Patients describe an electric-shock-type pain in the fingers or hand. The thumb side of the hand is usually most involved. Movement of the hand and wrist such as when holding an object like a phone, or when reading or driving makes the pain occur. Shaking the hand often helps decrease symptoms. Clinical manifestations initially are intermittent, but over time they may become constant. Fine motor coordination such as is needed to button a button can be difficult. When the condition is very severe, muscles in the palm may become visibly wasted.

Treatment begins with a brace or splint worn at night to keep the wrist in a natural position. Splints can also be worn during activities that aggravate symptoms. Anti-inflammatory medications such as ibuprofen help with pain relief. As the disease progresses and the individual becomes more disabled, surgery may become necessary. The decision whether to have surgery is primarily based on the severity of the symptoms. In more severe cases, surgery is considered sooner because other treatment options are less helpful. In very severe cases, surgery may be recommended to prevent irreversible damage. The surgeon uses an endoscope to access and open the top of the carpal tunnel, which increases the size of the tunnel and decreases pressure on the nerve. Typically the surgery is done on an outpatient basis under local anesthesia. Recovery is gradual; on average, grip and pinch strength generally return by about 2 months after surgery. Complete recovery may take up to 1 year, although it may be longer if the nerve is severely affected before treatment is attempted (American Academy of Orthopaedic Surgeons, 2007d).

Wrist Arthroplasty

Both osteoarthritis and rheumatoid arthritis affect the strength of the fingers and hand, making it difficult to grip or pinch. The typical candidate for wrist replacement surgery has severe arthritis. However, the surgery is limited to individuals who do not need to use the wrist to meet heavy demands in daily use. The primary reasons for wrist replacement surgery are to relieve pain and to maintain function in the wrist and hand. It may also improve the ability to perform daily living activities.

The surgery consists of removal of the worn-out ends of the bones and their replacement by an artificial joint (prosthesis). An incision is made on the back of the wrist. The damaged ends of the lower arm bones are removed, along with the first row of carpal bones. The radial component of the prosthesis is inserted into the center of the radius bone on the outside of the lower arm. The carpal component is then inserted into the center hand bone (third metacarpal) or screwed into the remaining row of carpal bones. Bone cement may be used to hold the components in place. Wrist arthroscopy surgery is often combined with other procedures to correct deformities or disorders in the tendons, nerves, and small joints of the fingers, and the thumb.

After surgery a cast is worn for the first several weeks, followed by a protective splint that will need to be worn for the next 6 to 8 weeks. Gradual exercises will need to be done for several weeks to restore movement and, eventually, to increase power and endurance. Wrist arthroplasty can improve motion to about 50% of normal. The physical demands that are placed on the wrist pros-

thesis will have an effect on how long the implant lasts. Use of a hammer or pneumatic tools may need to be avoided, and the amount of weight lifted must be limited. A fall on the outstretched hand may break the prosthesis, so activities such as roller sports, which could result in a fall, should be avoided. The average wrist replacement can be expected to last 10 to 15 years with careful use (American Academy of Orthopaedic Surgeons, 2007e).

Postoperative Assessment

Initial assessment during the initial postoperative period should focus on the potential problems of hypovolemia, bleeding complications, hypoxemia, and neurovascular compromise. After upper extremity surgery, the nurse must perform a neurovascular assessment that includes all digits of the hand, specifically the thumb and fourth and fifth fingers in order to test for ulnar nerve function (Figure 57–5 ■). Ask the patient to make an "OK" sign with his thumb and index finger to check motor integrity related to the ulnar nerve. The assessment of function of the operative extremity should be compared to that of a nonoperative/noninvolved site.

Upper extremity surgeries frequently utilize slings, immobilizing dressings, splints, and binders postoperatively. Slings may be used to elevate the extremity above the level of the heart to decrease edema formation. An elastic and Velcro shoulder immobilizer is generally used with rotator cuff repair surgery. The patient may remove the immobilizer for hygiene purposes or for performing the prescribed exercises with the affected arm until the formal physical therapy program is begun. The patient with a shoulder arthroplasty will have a shoulder immobilizer or sling after surgery. External fixator devices and splints may be utilized to immobilize and retain alignment of the arm. The length of immobilization depends on the severity of the type of surgery and the surgeon's preference. An exercise program will help regain motion and strength in the involved extremity. This program be-

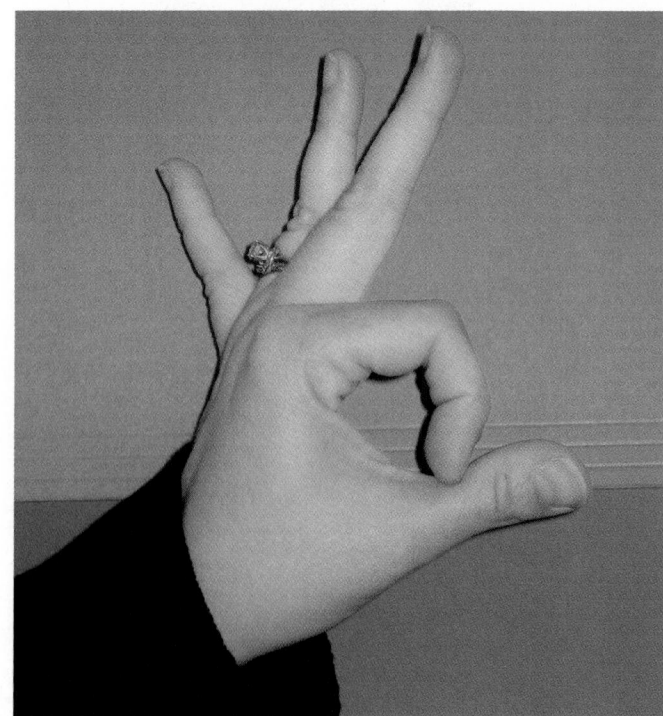

FIGURE 57–5 ■ OK sign for ulnar integrity.
Source: Cheryl Wraa

MyNursingKit | Journal of Bone and Joint Surgery

gins with passive motion, advances to active and resistive exercises, and is typically coordinated by the surgeon and the physical therapist. Complete recovery may take several months. A strong commitment to rehabilitation is important to achieve a good surgical outcome. The surgeon will examine the outcome to advise when it is safe to return to overhead work and sports activity.

Total Hip Arthroplasty

The most common cause of severe hip pain is arthritis. It is estimated that 40 million people in the United States have some form of arthritis (Arthritis Foundation, 2008). The three most common types of arthritis that cause joint pain are osteoarthritis, rheumatoid arthritis, and trauma-related arthritis, which is a result of joint injury causing inflammation and joint damage (Arthritis Foundation, 2008). Hip replacement is also used for patients with bone tumor or bone loss from insufficient blood supply to the bone (avascular necrosis).

The hip joint is formed where the top of the femur meets the acetabulum, or socket of the pelvic bone (Figure 57–6 ■). The top of the femur is ball shaped and fits into the socket formed by the acetabulum. The bones are covered by a layer of smooth cartilage that cushions and protects the bones and allows easy motion. Also surrounding the joint is the synovial lining, which produces a moisturizing lubricant. Ligaments connect the bones of the joint and hold them in place. The ligaments also add strength and elasticity for movement. Large muscles attached by tendons keep the joint stable.

Arthritis or inflammation causes the surfaces of the joint to become rough, causing the severe pain. When conservative treatment fails to provide adequate relief from pain, radiographs show destruction of the joint, and mobility is impaired, total hip replacement is considered. If the patient is active, the artificial hip joint may need to be replaced in 15 or 20 years. Revision total hip surgery, or redo, is a more complex procedure, and in general the surgery takes longer and there is greater blood loss.

Osteolysis is the term used to describe previously repaired joints whose components have worn out or become damaged.

Hip replacement surgery involves removal of the femoral head, creation of a "posthole" in the femur for the implant or femoral stem, acetabular repair with implant of cup and liner, and finally, placement of the femoral head on the stem (Figure 57–7 ■ and Chart 57–3). Hip replacement surgery may involve the use of cement, particularly if there is poor bone quality. Bone cement ingredients may include antibiotics, but are primarily polymers that improve adhesion. This is particularly useful for patients who have high potential for delayed healing or infection. The use of cement may decrease the healing time for surgery, as bone growth and regeneration to secure the joint are not necessary. If the patient has the potential for repeated surgery, however, the use of cement will require that a greater area of revision and removal of bone occur, and this must be considered in the decision of whether cement should be used. Elderly patients who will not require further surgery for repair or replacement are therefore more likely to receive surgery that includes the use of cement.

> **CHART 57–3**   **Hip Replacement Surgical Procedure**
>
> - Open surgical incision is 10–14 inches.
> - Minimally invasive hip replacement incisions are made—one or two 1–2-inch incisions.
> - The femoral head is dislocated from the acetabular socket.
> - The acetabular socket is shaved to resurface and shape the bone to receive the shell implant (a dome-like surface, which may include a liner).
> - The femoral head is removed and shaved to shape the bone. The femoral canal is drilled to receive the implant stem.
> - The stem of the implant is inserted into the femur.
> - A surgical drain is implanted and the surgical site closed with sutures.

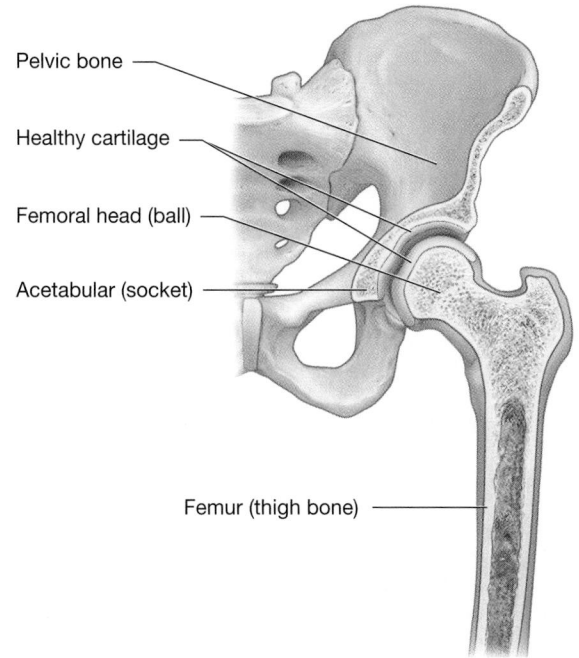

FIGURE 57–6 ■ Hip joint.

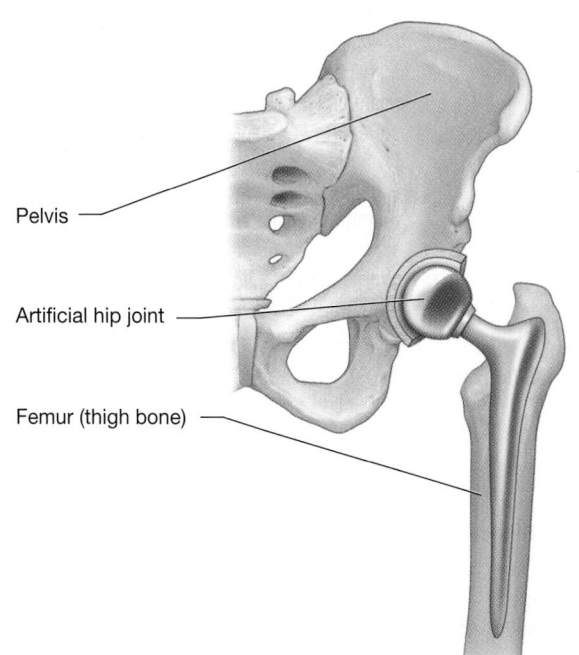

FIGURE 57–7 ■ Artificial hip joint.

Postoperative Assessment

Initial assessment during the postoperative period should focus on the potential problems of hypovolemia, bleeding complications, hypoxemia, and neurovascular compromise. After hip arthroplasty or closed reduction, the patient will be placed on hip precautions (Chart 57–4). The type of precautions required depends on the approach that was utilized. For instance, if a posterior approach was used, the patient will be placed on posterior hip precautions. The goal of the precautions is to prevent the hip from dislocating posteriorly. Anterior hip precautions involve avoiding activities that would allow the hip to dislocate anteriorly. Chart 57–4 outlines the specific precautions for both posterior and anterior approaches. The immediate postoperative nursing management of hip surgery patients is outlined in Chart 57–5, which

---

CHART 57–4 **Hip Precautions**

Posterior Hip Precautions	Anterior Hip Precautions
Hip abductor pillow while in bed.	Hip abductor pillow while in bed.
Do not bend hip greater than 90 degrees.	Take mini steps when walking.
Use an elevated toilet seat.	Do not assume a straddle position—like mounting a horse.
Do not sit in low chairs.	Do not twist or turn the body away from the operative side.
Do not twist or turn the body toward the operative side.	Do not turn leg and foot outward.
Do not turn leg and foot inward.	Do not lift operative leg up and out.
Keep operative leg straight when getting up and use one's arms to push up.	

CHART 57–5 **Total Hip Arthroplasty Clinical Pathway**

Activity	Operative Day	Postoperative Day 1	Postoperative Day 2	Postoperative Days 3–5
General	Admit to postoperative unit. Intake and output (I&O). Urinary catheter to gravity, surgical drain, empty prn; notify health care provider of drainage >200 mL/shift. Posterior hip precautions. Sequential compression device. Abduction pillow while in bed. Diet: clear liquids; progress to regular diet. Medications: patient-controlled analgesia (PCA); antinausea; stool softener; IV antibiotic every 8 hours for 6 doses. Nursing: neurovascular checks; monitor dressing drainage; monitor surgical drain output; vital signs every hour × 2 hours, then every 4 hours. Turn and position every 2 hours; pressure ulcer prevention.	Low-molecular-weight heparin (LMWH) 40 milligrams subcutaneous daily. Surgical drain discontinued by health care provider.	Discontinue urinary catheter. Oral pain medication. Discontinue PCA. Confirm surgical drain has been discontinued. Saline lock IV when taking 2,000 milliliters of fluids in 24 hours.	Laxative if no bowel movement (BM). Discontinue IV prior to discharge.
Physical Activity	Bed rest 8 hours. Out of bed (OOB) to chair in 8 hours. Incentive spirometry every 2 hours while awake.	OOB to chair. Meals tid. Ambulate bid.	OOB to chair tid. OOB to bathroom. Ambulate tid.	Independent ambulation with walker.
Diagnostic Tests	Hemoglobin and hematocrit.	Hemoglobin and hematocrit.		
Discharge Planning/Patient Education	Abduction pillow. Walker. Instruct patient on hip precautions and transfer technique.	Raised toilet seat. Reinforce patient education on hip precautions.	Discuss discharge plan with patient: skilled nursing facility (SNF) versus home.	Instruct patient/family on LMWH injection and wound care if home discharge.

describes a clinical pathway for hip arthroplasty. Discharge planning is complex for hip surgery patients. The general considerations for discharge planning and home modifications specific for hip surgery are discussed in Chart 57–6.

Refer to Chapter 55 for a complete discussion of the repair and management of fractured hips.

Pelvic Surgery

The pelvis is comprised of the iliac crest, ilium, sacrum, coccyx, ischial tuberosities, and acetabulum. The symphysis pubis is the anterior joint of the pelvis, and the sacroiliac joint is the posterior joint. Pelvic fractures are frequently associated with other traumatic injuries from motor vehicle crashes. It is essential to know the mechanism of injury because it assists the health care team in anticipating additional injuries, especially with motor vehicle crashes. Common additional injuries that are associated with pelvic fractures are femur fracture, bladder rupture, and risk for retroperitoneal bleed.

Simple fractures that are not displaced are considered to be stable fractures. Unstable fractures are fractures in which ligaments are torn, there are multiple fractures, or there is movement of the pelvic girdle with downward pressure with the patient in a supine position. If the pelvic fracture is unstable, it may be treated with external fixation or internal fixation. Pelvic fracture surgery, along with the nursing and medical management, is described in detail in Chapter 56 .

Knee Surgery

The knee is the largest joint in the body and one of the most easily injured. It is made up of four bones: the femur, the tibia, the fibula, and the patella (Figure 57–8 ■). The knee contains four main ligaments: the inner medial collateral ligament (MCL); the outer lateral collateral ligament (LCL); the anterior cruciate ligament (ACL); and the posterior cruciate ligament (PCL). The function of the ligaments is to help control motion by connecting bones and by bracing the joint against abnormal types of motion. The knee muscles that go across the knee joint are the quadriceps (front of knee) and the hamstrings (back of knee). Another important structure, the meniscus, is a wedge of soft cartilage between the femur and the tibia that serves to cushion the knee and helps it absorb shock during motion.

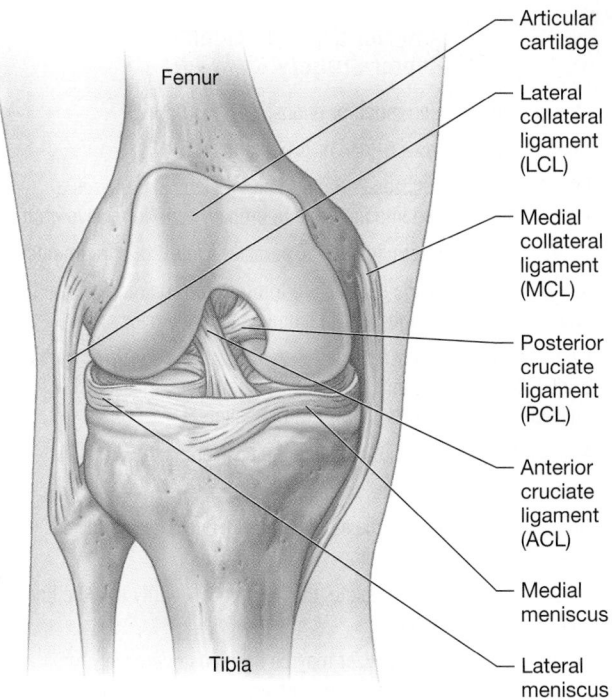

FIGURE 57–8 ■ Knee anatomy.

Common sports injuries occur with the ligaments. Ligaments may be stretched predisposing the joint to dislocation. Ligaments may also be torn if overextension or trauma occurs. Ligaments do not regenerate. If they are torn and disability or frequent dislocations occur, they must be repaired or replaced. The anterior cruciate ligament (ACL) and the medial collateral ligament (MCL) are frequently injured in sports. The posterior cruciate ligament (PCL) may also be injured.

Anterior Cruciate Ligament (ACL) Repair

Changing direction rapidly, slowing down when running, and landing from a jump may cause tears in the ACL. Athletes who participate in skiing, basketball, and those who wear cleats, such as football players, are susceptible to ACL injuries. The goal of the ACL reconstruction surgery is to prevent instability and restore the function of the torn ligament, creating a stable knee. Patients treated with surgical reconstruction of the ACL have long-term success rates of 82% to 95%. Recurrent instability and graft failure are seen in approximately 8% of patients (American Academy of Orthopaedic Surgeons, 2007f). The ACL is not usually repaired because of failure over time with this approach. The ACL is generally replaced by a substitute graft made of tendon. The sources of tendon include patellar, hamstring, or quadriceps tendon autograft (from patient); or patellar tendon, Achilles tendon, semitendinosus, gracilis, or posterior tibialis tendon allograft (taken from a cadaver). There also are synthetic grafts available. The surgery procedure is described in Chart 57–7 (p. 1814).

Knee Arthroplasty

If osteoarthritis wears away a knee joint's articular cartilage, arthroplasty (replacement) is a common and successful procedure that improves knee motion and allows a patient to resume relatively normal activities without pain. The surgeon resurfaces

---

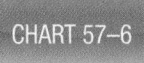 **CHART 57–6** **Home Modifications for Hip Surgery Patients**

- Securely fastened safety bars or handrails for the bath and shower
- A stable armchair with a firm seat cushion allowing the knees to remain lower than the hips
- A raised toilet seat
- A shower bench or chair
- A sock aid and a long-handled shoe horn for putting on and taking off shoes and socks without excessively bending at the hip
- A "reacher" to access items without bending at the hip
- Removal of all loose carpets and electrical cords from walkways
- Food and household items up to waist level to prevent bending

CHART 57–7   Anterior Cruciate Ligament Repair Surgery

- May be done as open repair or endoscopic procedure.
- Open repair requires a 6-inch or greater incision.
- Endoscopic repair utilizes 2–3 one-inch incisions and utilizes a surgical drill inserted into incisions to prepare bone to receive graft.
- Debris is removed (torn ligaments, particles, clots, bone fragments).
- Meniscus and cartilage injuries are trimmed or repaired, and the torn anterior cruciate ligament (ACL) stump is then removed.
- Ligaments are typically replaced with allograft, autograft, or synthetic graft. If bone attachments are necessary, surgical drills may be utilized to prepare the bone for graft attachment.
- ACL graft is placed in almost the same position as the torn ACL.
- Graft may be secured with sutures or screws.
- Open repair entrance site is sutured closed, and a drain may be inserted for blood collection.
- Before the surgery is complete, the surgeon will verify that the knee has full range of motion.
- Elastic support or immobilizer may be used postoperatively for simple repairs, to contain movement, and to prevent surgical site stress.
- Continuous passive motion (CPM) devices may be used postoperatively for extensive repairs or anterior cruciate ligament surgeries to prevent shortening of the ligament and prevent joint stiffening and loss of range of motion.
- ACL repairs are usually done on an outpatient basis.

CHART 57–8   Knee Arthroplasty

- Thigh tourniquet is applied to decrease bleeding during surgery.
- Incision is made in anterior knee approximately 10 inches in length.
- Femoral head and tibia are surgically shaved to prepare for prosthetic implant.
- The patella is shaved or replaced to allow free movement after joint prosthesis is implanted.
- Debris in surgical site is removed.
- A drain may be inserted to remove blood from surgical area.
- Prosthesis is implanted.
- Surgical site is sutured closed.
- Continuous passive motion (CPM) may be utilized postoperatively utilizing progressive angles of flexion and extension as prescribed by the health care provider.

the knee joint, replacing damaged and worn weight-bearing surfaces with a prosthesis (implant) made of metal alloys, ceramic material, or high-density plastic parts that may be joined to bone by acrylic cement (Figure 57–9 ■). Up to three bone surfaces may be replaced during the total replacement of the knee: the lower condyles of the femur, the top surface of the tibia, and the back surface of the kneecap. Chart 57–8 presents the surgical procedure.

Postoperatively early mobilization is important. Initially, there is a bulky dressing around the knee and a drain to remove any fluid buildup. The drain will be removed in a day or two. A continuous passive motion exercise machine that will slowly and smoothly straighten and bend the knee is typically applied after surgery. Although pain after surgery is quite variable and not entirely predictable, it can be controlled with medication. The hospital stay may last from 3 to 7 days. The goal for discharge is to have the patient get in and out of bed independently, bend the knee up to approximately 90 degrees, extend the knee fully, walk with crutches or a walker, and demonstrate knowledge of the prescribed home exercises.

Nursing management of the patient with a total knee replacement is multifaceted and requires a comprehensive plan to ensure a return to pain-free function. General aspects of care for patients requiring orthopedic surgery are discussed in the Nursing Management of the Postoperative Patient section and outlined in the Nursing Process: Patient Care Plan feature later in this chapter (p. 1822). Use of a clinical pathway for the specific management

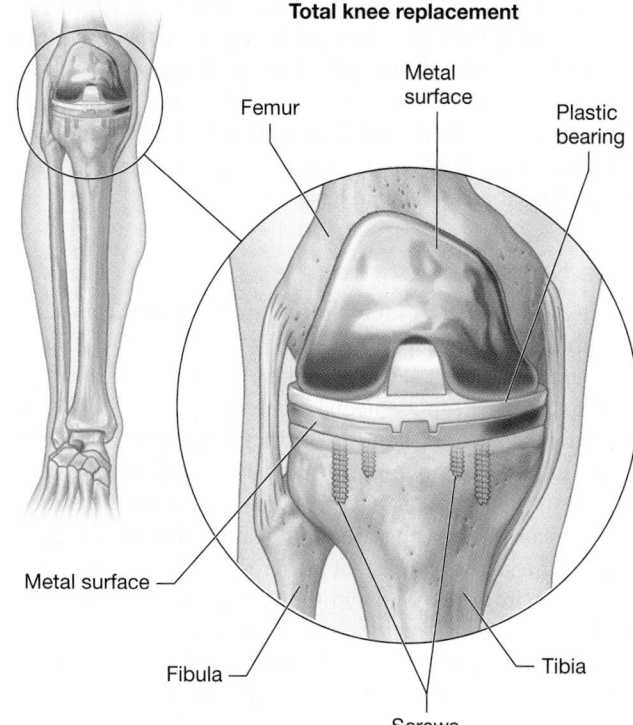

Total knee replacement

Femur · Metal surface · Plastic bearing · Metal surface · Fibula · Screws · Tibia

FIGURE 57–9 ■ Knee arthroplasty.

provides the health care team with an organized, comprehensive approach to nursing management (Chart 57–9).

Meniscus Repair

The meniscus is a wedge-like rubbery cushion located where the femur and tibia meet at the knee joint (see Figure 57–8 ■, p. 1813). The meniscus helps the knee joint carry weight, glide, and turn in many directions. It also keeps the femur and tibia from grinding against each other. Meniscal tears can occur with twisting, pivoting, and decelerating motions of the knee. These injuries often occur in combination with other injuries such as a torn anterior cruciate ligament. As the cartilage weakens and wears

| CHART 57-9 | **Total Knee Arthroplasty Clinical Pathway** | | | |

Activity	Operative Day	Postoperative Day 1	Postoperative Day 2	Postoperative Day 3 Discharge
General	Admit to postoperative unit. Intake and output (I&O). Urinary catheter to gravity, surgical drain, empty prn; notify health care provider of drainage > 100 mL/shift. Continuous passive motion (CPM) machine while in bed; antiembolism stocking; sequential compression device to nonoperative leg. Diet: clear liquids; progress to regular diet. Medications: patient-controlled analgesic (PCA); antinausea; stool softener; IV antibiotic every 8 hours for 6 doses. Nursing assessment: neurovascular checks; monitor dressing drainage; monitor surgical drain output; vital signs every hour × 2 hours, then every 4 hours. No pillow under knees.	Discontinue urinary catheter. Saline lock IV. Low-molecular-weight heparin (LMWH) 40 milligrams subcutaneous daily. Health care provider to discontinue surgical drain.	Confirm surgical drain has been discontinued.	Laxative if no bowel movement (BM). Discontinue IV.
Physical Activity	Bed rest. Dangle at bedside.	Out of bed (OOB) to chair tid for meals. Ambulate with crutches bid.	OOB to chair tid for meals. Ambulate with crutches tid.	Independent ambulation with crutches.
Diagnostic Tests		Hemoglobin and hematocrit.		
Discharge Planning/Patient Education	Obtain crutches. Instruct patient on performance of foot pump exercises. Inform about CPM machine.	Crutch walking instruction. No weight bearing. Instruct in transfer technique.	Discuss discharge plan with patient: skilled nursing facility (SNF) versus home. Order home CPM machine for patient.	Instruct patient/family on LMWH injection and wound care if home discharge. Instruct on CPM application.

thin over time, a degenerative tear can occur without any significant trauma.

Clinical manifestations typically include a "popping" sensation when the tear occurs followed by inflammation, stiffness and swelling, pain, buckling, and fluid collection. Without treatment, a fragment of the meniscus may loosen and drift into the joint, causing it to slip, pop, or lock; and the knee may lock at a 45-degree angle, until it is manually moved or otherwise manipulated. Initially the treatment includes rest and pain medication. If the tear does not heal on its own and the knee becomes painful, stiff, or locked, a surgical repair may be necessary. The surgeon can examine the area arthroscopically and trim off damaged pieces of cartilage. A cast or brace is typically used to immobilize the knee after surgery. A course of rehabilitation exercises is necessary before resuming previous activities.

Postoperative Assessment
Initial assessment during the initial postoperative period should focus on the potential problems of hypovolemia, bleeding com-

plications, hypoxemia, and neurovascular compromise. After lower extremity surgery, the nurse must perform a neurovascular assessment that includes all toes on the affected side.

Lower extremity surgeries frequently utilize splints, slings, immobilizing dressings, and binders postoperatively. The extremity needs to be elevated above the level of the heart to decrease edema formation. The patient may remove the immobilizer for hygiene purposes or for performing the prescribed exercises with the affected joint until the formal physical therapy program is begun. The length of immobilization depends on the severity of the type of surgery and the surgeon's preference. An exercise program will help regain motion and strength in the involved extremity. This program begins with passive motion, advances to active and resistive exercises, and is typically coordinated by the surgeon and the physical therapist. Complete recovery may take several months. A strong commitment to rehabilitation is important to achieve a good surgical outcome. The surgeon will examine the outcome to advise when it is safe to return to overhead work and sports activity.

Amputation

Amputation is the surgical removal or traumatic loss of a part. In the upper extremities amputation is rare and often associated with trauma, meningococcemia, and osteosarcoma. Osteosarcoma necessitates the removal of the bone in which the cancer is present. Chapter 55 discusses osteosarcoma and other types of bone cancer. In the lower extremities, peripheral vascular disease, diabetes, and gangrene are the frequent causes for elective amputation. Below knee amputation (BKA) is preferred to above knee amputation because balance and coordination are more stable, gait is more natural, and there is a better potential for revisions, if needed. Above knee amputation (AKA) requires more energy to ambulate. The AKA patient must raise the hip and swing the prosthesis/leg forward for clearance because the leg plus prosthesis must remain straight. In the elderly this may be a safety risk, and wheelchair mobility is a safer practice.

Traumatic amputation is a sudden loss of the part and may require more extensive removal of tissue, bone, and muscle than amputation due to vascular insufficiency. Traumatic amputation is discussed in Chapter 56 . Traumatic amputation may be associated with increased potential for phantom limb pain, body image disturbance, and grief/loss disturbance than amputation resulting from chronic disease processes.

Chart 57–10 describes the surgical procedure for amputation. The Evidence-Based Practice feature provides information regarding stump and phantom limb pain.

Postoperative Assessment

Because many amputations are the result of peripheral vascular insufficiency, the patient must be monitored closely for skin integrity and with particular care given to prevent pressure ulcer development. The remaining heel should be floated off of the mattress with pillows or a heel protection device. In the immediate postoperative period, stump care usually involves elevation of the stump and compression wrapping of the extremity to prevent edema. A figure-of-eight method beginning at the distal stump is utilized to wrap the stump.

Phantom limb pain is a common complication of amputation. Current research is attempting to define characteristics and causative factors of phantom limb pain and to determine whether specific treatments may be performed prior to and during surgery to prevent phantom limb phenomena. Current treatments for phantom limb pain include pain medication, antiseizure medication, antidepressants, nerve block, spinal stimulation, use of transcutaneous electrical nerve stimulation (TENS) units, and biofeedback or other cognitive pain-relief modalities. Pain management is discussed in Chapter 15 .

CHART 57–10   Surgical Amputation

- A tourniquet (pneumatic or other restrictive device) is applied above the area to be amputated.
- A skin flap is prepared by excising the skin from the muscle and folding it back (away from the area to be amputated).
- A guillotine device or saw is used to perform the amputation.
- The skin flap is utilized to close the surgical wound.

CRITICAL ALERT   *The stump should be elevated for the first 24 hours to prevent postoperative edema. After 24 hours, keep the stump flat while in bed or extended while out of bed in a chair to prevent contracture of the nearest joint.*

Spinal Surgery

Back pain is the cause of more lost work hours than any other medical condition and is the second leading cause of work absences. Most back pain occurs between the ages of 45 and 64, and it is more common among men than women (eMedicineHealth, 2008). The spine can be divided into three categories: the vertebral bony column, intervertebral disks, ligaments, and muscles; spinal cord and nerves; and the spinal cord vasculature. The bony vertebral column consists of 33 vertebrae separated and cushioned by the intervertebral disks. The bony vertebrae and disks are joined together by ligaments. The disks allow a degree of flexibility to the spine. They temporarily flatten out and bulge when compressed, acting as shock absorbers. If the disk is under an extreme load, the central nucleus can rupture through the surrounding cartilaginous fibers resulting in a herniated disk, which places pressure on the nerve root. Approximately 25% of people who have back pain have a herniated disk (eMedicineHealth, 2008). The most common site of back pain is in the lower back with more than 95% of operations being performed on the fourth and fifth lumbar vertebrae.

Discectomy refers to surgery in which the diseased disk is removed. **Laminectomy** refers to surgery in which only part of the disk, usually only the herniated portion, is removed. It is called a laminectomy because the surgeon must cut through the lamina to access the herniated disk. During the procedure, the surgeon will make an incision over the vertebrae and down to the bony arches of the vertebrae. The ligament joining the vertebrae along with all or part of the lamina is removed to see the involved nerve root. The surgeon will then pull the nerve root back toward the center of the spinal column and remove part of or the entire disk. The incision will be closed, and the large back muscles will protect the spine and nerve roots. Traditional discectomy or laminectomy surgical procedures usually involve 3- to 4-day hospital admissions. Patients are generally placed on a patient-controlled analgesia (PCA) machine to control their pain postoperatively. Initially patients are kept flat in bed for 24 hours and logrolled, ensuring that spinal alignment is maintained, every 2 hours to prevent pressure ulcers.

Minimally invasive surgery can be done through arthroscopic procedures and with the use of lasers. Procedures done arthroscopically include:

- **Foraminotomy**—This procedure is used to relieve pressure on nerves being compressed by the intervertebral foramen, the space where a nerve root exists in the spinal canal. The compression can be caused by bone, bulging disk, or scar tissue. A small incision is made and the scope is placed. With the use of small surgical instruments and or a laser, the bone or tissue that is compressing the nerve is removed. The patient is ambulated within 2 hours of the procedure.

- **Laminotomy**—This procedure is used to relieve the pressure on the spinal canal for the exiting nerve roots and spinal cord by increasing the amount of space available. The pressure

Stump and Phantom Limb Pain

Clinical Problem

A significant problem following amputation is acute stump pain and phantom limb pain. Phantom limb pain during the first year following surgery is reported by up to 70% of amputees (Lambert et al., 2001). Pain in the affected limb prior to surgery is correlated to the degree of stump and phantom limb pain postoperatively.

Research Findings

Lambert et al. (2001) completed a randomized prospective study comparing preoperative epidural and intraoperative perineural analgesia. Preoperative epidural patients received epidural bupivacaine and diamorphine 24 hours before surgery, during surgery, and 3 days postoperatively. The intraoperative perineural patients received an intraoperatively placed perineural catheter for intra- and postoperative administration of bupivacaine. During the surgery all of the patients received general anesthesia. Their results showed that, during the first 3 days postoperatively, pain scores were significantly higher in the perineural group. After 3 days, 29% of the patients in the epidural group and 44% of patients in the perineural group reported phantom pain. In 6 months phantom pain was reported in 63% of the epidural group and 88% of the perineural group. In 1 year phantom pain was reported in 38% of the epidural group and 50% of the perineural group. When comparing the two groups, the study did not show a significant difference in limb pain but did show that the epidural group had significantly better pain control immediately postoperatively.

Another study (Jahangiri, Jayatunga, Bradley, & Dark, 1994) looked at the combination of drugs that were used in the epidural infusion. Because the infusion of morphine and bupivacaine can cause hypotension, it can make the patient difficult to manage on a ward and may require a higher level of care for monitoring. The study compared the effectiveness in reducing stump and phantom limb pain with epidural infusion containing bupivacaine, clonidine, and a lower dose of diamorphine. The control group received opioid analgesia on demand. There were 13 patients in the study group and 11 patients in the control group. Pain was assessed postoperatively at 7 days, 6 months, and 1 year. At 1 year, 1 patient in the study group and 8 patients in the control group had phantom limb sensation. The researchers concluded that perioperative epidural infusion of bupivacaine, clonidine, and diamorphine is safe and effective in reducing phantom pain after amputation.

In 2003, Gehling & Tryba conducted an analysis of factors contributing to the results of phantom limb pain prophylaxis. They analyzed all published articles on phantom limb pain prophylaxis from 1966 to 1999. Their results found an association between regional analgesia via epidural infusion pre-, intra-, and postoperatively and a significant reduction of phantom limb pain 12 months after amputation.

Implications for Nursing Practice

Studies show a significant reduction in acute postoperative stump pain and the development of phantom limb pain with pre-, intra-, and postoperative analgesia via epidural infusion. Patient education regarding epidural infusion and knowledge regarding the effects and side effects of the medication used is of great importance. Advocating having the infusion started preoperatively appears to benefit the patient especially with regard to phantom limb pain 12 months following surgery.

Critical Thinking Questions

1. What is the reasoning for beginning the epidural infusion prior to surgery and continuing 3 days after surgery?

2. Why is it important to prevent or decrease the incidence of phantom limb pain?

Answers to Critical Thinking Questions appear in Appendix D.

References

Gehling, M., & Tryba, M. (2003). Prophylaxis of phantom pain: Is regional analgesia ineffective? *Der Schmerz, 17*(1), 11–19.

Jahangiri, M., Jayatunga, A. P., Bradley, J. W., & Dark, C. H. (1994). Prevention of phantom pain after major lower limb amputation by epidural infusion of diamorphine, clonidine, and bupivacaine. *Annals of the Royal College of Surgery in England, 76*(5), 324–326.

Lambert, A. W., Dashfield, A. K., Cosgrove, C., Wilkins, D. C., Walker, A. J., & Ashley, S. (2001). Randomized prospective study comparing preoperative epidural and intraoperative perineural analgesia for the prevention of postoperative stump and phantom limb pain following major amputation. *Regional Anesthesia Pain Medicine, 26*(4), 316–321.

EVIDENCE-BASED PRACTICE

may be caused by bone spurs, spinal stenosis, arthritis, a bulging or herniated disk, or scar tissue. The procedure is done in the same manner as the foraminotomy. The patient is able to ambulate within 2 hours of the procedure.

- **Percutaneous arthroscopic discectomy**—This procedure is the removal of a bulging or herniated disk that is pressing on a nerve root or the spinal cord. The procedure is done in the same manner as the foraminotomy. The patient is able to ambulate within 2 hours of the procedure.

Spinal fusion (fusing vertebrae together with bone graft or plates and screws so that an area of the spine cannot move) surgery may be performed after traumatic, unstable injuries to stabilize the spine and prevent further injury and loss of function

(Figure 57–10 ■, p. 1818). In some cases it may also be performed to treat vertebral fractures, kyphosis, or scoliosis. Bone grafts are used like cement to weld the vertebrae together, or the bones are held together by plates and screws so that they can no longer move. If an autologous bone graft is used, the piece of bone is generally taken from the iliac crest during the back surgery. Allograft bone donations are obtained from donor banks or stored in the operating room in a refrigerator or freezer. Allograft bones are obtained from cadavers and are sterilized and frozen, or stored in sterile packaging. There are several types of spinal fusion surgery options, including:

- **Posterolateral gutter fusion**—The procedure is done through the back.

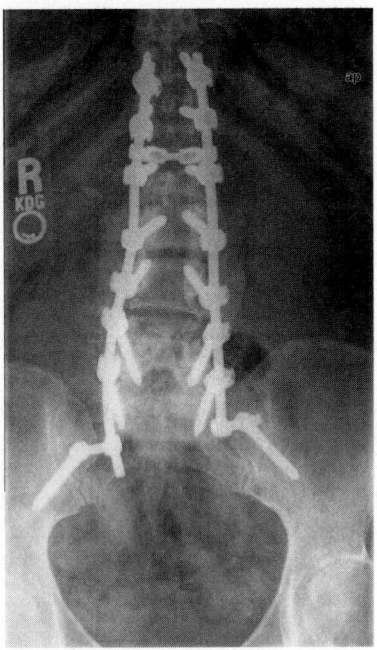

FIGURE 57–10 ■ Spinal fusion with plates and screws x-ray.
Source: Karen Cooper RN, MSN, CCRN, CNS

- **Posterior lumbar interbody fusion (PLIF)**—The procedure is done from the back and includes removing the disk between two vertebrae and inserting bone into the space created between the two vertebral bodies.
- **Anterior lumbar interbody fusion (ALIF)**—The procedure is done from the front and includes removing the disk between two vertebrae and inserting bone into the space created between the two vertebral bodies.
- **Anterior/posterior spinal fusion**—The procedure is done from the front and the back.

Postoperative Assessment

After surgery, until the bones fuse, the patient may need to wear a brace to maintain alignment of the spine. The operative site must remain in strict anatomic alignment. For example, if the patient with back surgery is to be turned, the back must remain in a straight line during turning so there is no torque or twisting of the operative site. The surgeon may order the patient to be flat in bed after surgery for a specified amount of time. Prior to getting the patient out of bed, a back brace must be placed on the patient while lying flat. This is done by logrolling the patient, applying the pieces of the brace, and securing the Velcro straps. A thoracolumbosacral orthosis (TLSO) is the type of brace generally utilized (Figure 57–11 ■). It is specially created from a mold of the patient and made of durable plastic, using Velcro straps to hold the two sides together. The TLSO is also used as the postoperative brace for other types of back surgery. In order to ensure that the patient can achieve a standing position without bending, the patient should be assisted from the flat-in-bed position in the raised bed to the erect position with two-person support.

Postoperative complications after spinal surgery may include transient bowel and bladder dysfunction due to edema of the spine causing compression of the sympathetic and parasympathetic nerve tracts. The nurse will monitor the pa-

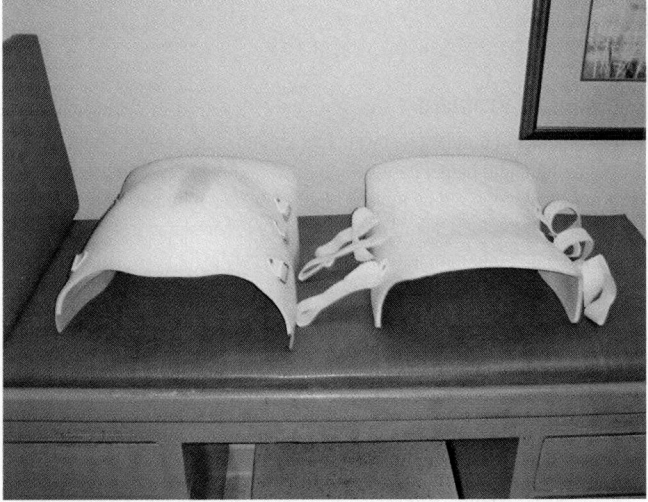

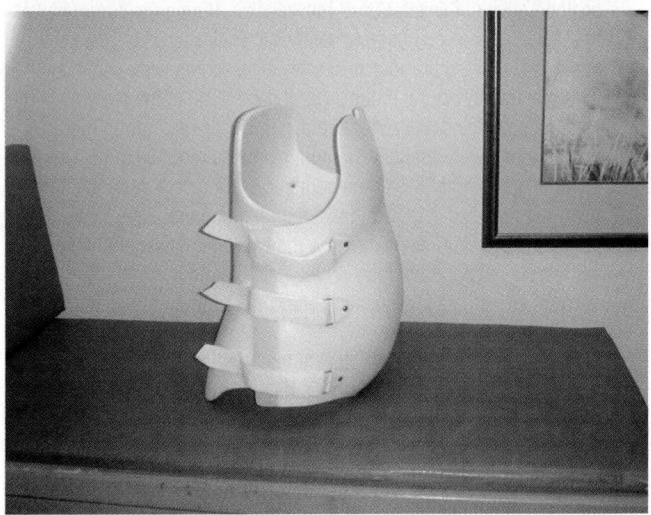

FIGURE 57–11 ■ Thoracolumbosacral orthosis brace (TLSO).
Source: Karen Cooper RN, MSN, CCRN, CNS

tient for return of bowel sounds, and the patient should not receive a diet until bowel sounds return. If the patient has difficulty emptying her bladder after surgery, she may require intermittent urinary catheterization. The spinal dressing must be monitored for both bleeding and possible cerebrospinal fluid (CSF) leak.

A CSF leak may occur if the dura is opened during the surgical procedure. During spinal surgery, the dura of the spinal cord is invaded and there is a potential for the surgical site to leak CSF. CSF leaks appear as a clear fluid that forms a halo around any serous drainage on the dressing. CSF leaks increase the potential for development of meningitis and often cause a postoperative headache that is worse when the patient is upright. The surgeon should be notified if a CSF leak is present or suspected. A blood patch may be used to treat the CSF leak from the surgical site. An anesthesiologist injects 5 to 20 milliliters of unclotted blood into the surgical site (into the epidural space). After the blood patch is performed, the patient should remain flat in bed for 2 hours to ensure that the blood does not migrate and is allowed to clot and prevent further CSF leakage.

 CRITICAL ALERT *Cerebrospinal fluid leak in the spinal surgery patient should be reported immediately and precautions to prevent meningitis instituted.*

COMPLEMENTARY & ALTERNATIVE THERAPIES   Healing Touch

Description:

Healing touch is an energy healing technique in which practitioners use their hands to therapeutically affect the patient's energy field. Despite the name, healing touch practitioners never actually touch the patient; instead, they keep their hands about 3 inches above the patient's skin, tapping into—and aligning and balancing—the energy field that surrounds the body. Although the body is never physically touched, patients report an improvement in musculoskeletal conditions. Therapeutic effects can include relieving pain, accelerating wound healing, preventing illness, promoting relaxation, and easing the dying process. Healing touch, which emerged in the 1970s from other energy healing techniques such as therapeutic touch, is now performed by practitioners all over the world, including nurses.

Research Support:

One article cited a patient's improvements after trauma, including improvements in physiological and psychological complaints, health perception, and well-being (Burr, 2005). A clinical study involved 56 patients who received healing touch and completed the Healing Touch Comfort Questionnaire. Of the 56 patients, 51 were women, and 5 were men, with an average age of 51. Study results showed that participants who received more than four healing touch treatments had higher comfort levels than those with fewer than four treatments (Dowd, Kolcaba, & Steiner, 2006).

A pilot study assessed the effect of healing touch on chronic neuropathic pain in patients with spinal cord injury. The study involved the administration of both healing touch as well as guided progressive relaxation on 12 veterans over the course of six weekly home visits. The instruments used to assess outcomes showed sensitivity, such as the Diener Satisfaction with Life Scale, which showed increased well-being in the healing touch group and no change in the control group. However, there was a large variation among the groups. Researchers concluded that healing touch may benefit chronic pain (Wardell, Rintala, Duan, & Tan, 2006).

References

Burr, J. P. (2005, September-October). Jayne's story: Healing touch as a complementary treatment for trauma recovery. *Holistic Nurse Practitioner, 19*(5), 211–216.

Dowd, T., Kolcaba, K., & Steiner, R. (2006, May-June). Development of the healing touch comfort questionnaire. *Holistic Nurse Practitioner, 20*(3), 122–129.

Wardell, D. W., Rintala, D. H., Duan, Z., & Tan, G. (2006). A pilot study of healing touch and progressive relaxation for chronic neuropathic pain in persons with spinal cord injury. *Journal of Holistic Nursing, 24*(4), 231–240.

If the patient has had back pain for many years, it may be difficult to manage his pain postoperatively. Chronic pain follows different neural pathways. Refer to Chapter 15 😊 for an in-depth discussion of pain assessment and treatment. Control of the environment to encourage relaxation and alternative therapies such as healing touch, described in the Complementary and Alternative Therapies box, are interventions the nurse can use to help relieve the patient's pain.

Ankle and Foot Surgeries

The act of walking can put up to 1.5 times one's body weight on one's foot. During 1 hour of strenuous exercise, the feet will cushion up to 1 million pounds of pressure (American Academy of Orthopaedic Surgeons, 2005). The foot has 26 bones. The ankle joint is comprised of the talus and the ends of the tibia and fibula. It is supported by three groups of ligaments. The movement of the foot and ankle is supported by the muscles and tendons. Most injuries of the foot and ankle are caused by overuse, poor conditioning, and improperly fitting shoes.

Ankle pain is most commonly due to a sprain but also can be caused by arthritis, gout, bone fracture, tendonitis, infection, poor structural alignment of the leg or foot, or chronic ankle joint instability from a severe injury or multiple injuries. The most common injury of the ankle is a sprain. During a fall or jump, the foot is likely to turn inward (inversion) and stretch or tear ligaments. Every day approximately 25,000 people sprain their ankle (American Academy of Orthopaedic Surgeons, 2005). The ankle joint is held together and protected from abnormal movement by the ligaments. Normally, a ligament will stretch within its limits and then return to normal position. When a ligament is forced to stretch beyond its limits, a sprain occurs. A severe sprain will actually cause tearing of the elastic fibers of the ligament. The ligament that is most commonly injured is the lateral ligament on the lateral aspect

of the ankle. For a detailed discussion of sprains, refer to Chapter 56 😊.

Tendon Injuries

Tendons connect muscle to bone. Two tendons run along the outer aspect of the ankle and foot to help stabilize the ankle joint. These tendons are called the peroneal tendons (Figure 57–12 ■). Peroneal tendon injuries can be acute or chronic and occur most often in patients who participate in sports that involve repetitive ankle motion. The tendon may have an acute tear or fray from overuse. The tendons can also sublux out of their normal position.

The largest and strongest tendon of the lower leg is the Achilles tendon. The tendon connects muscles in the lower leg with the calcaneus bone. A complete or partial tear of the Achilles tendon is called a rupture (Figure 57–13 ■, p. 1820). Jumping, pivoting, or sudden acceleration to a run can stretch the tendon beyond its capacity and cause a tear.

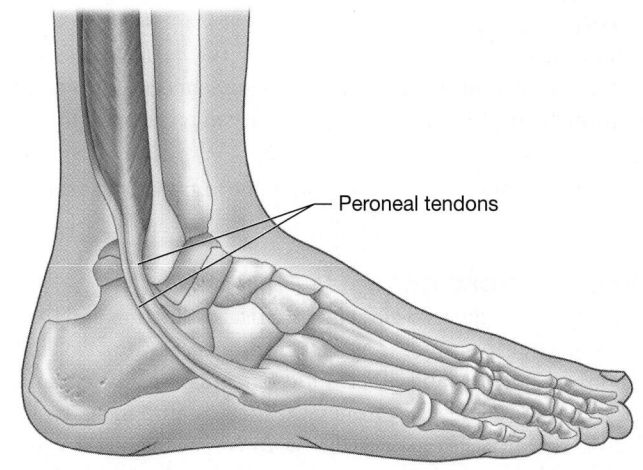

FIGURE 57–12 ■ Peroneal tendons.

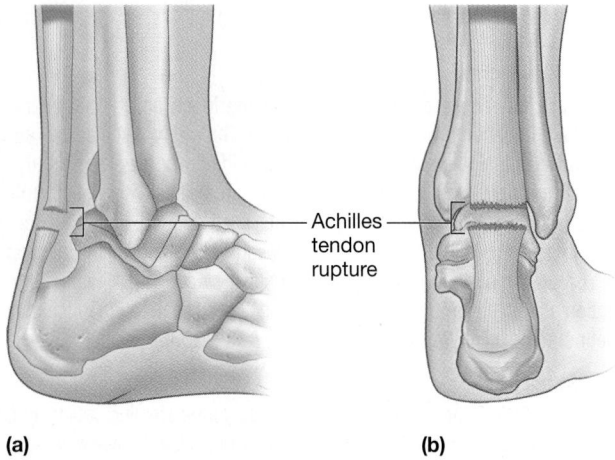

(a)   (b)

FIGURE 57–13 ■ Achilles tendon rupture.

Injury to the tendons or ligaments of the ankle will cause severe pain, swelling, and difficulty with mobilization, because weight bearing will increase the pain. Without proper healing, the joint will become unstable, injury will reoccur, and the patient will develop chronic ankle pain. Other causes of chronic ankle pain include arthritis of the joint, synovitis (inflammation of the joint lining), an injury to the nerves that pass through the ankle, and development of scar tissue after a sprain, which takes up space in the joint and places pressure on the ligaments.

Symptoms of chronic ankle pain include pain on the lateral side of the ankle, swelling, stiffness, difficulty walking on uneven ground or high heels, tenderness, and repeated ankle sprains.

Nonsurgical management for minor sprains and strains is covered in Chapter 56 👁. If conservative treatment does not bring relief, then surgery may be required. Surgical treatment for ankle injuries is rare, but it is used for injuries that fail to respond to nonsurgical treatment and for persistent instability after months of rehabilitation and nonsurgical treatment. Surgical options include:

- **Arthroscopy**—A surgeon examines the joint to see whether there are any loose fragments of bone or cartilage, or part of the ligament caught in the joint, and cleans debris and makes repairs.
- **Reconstruction**—A surgeon repairs the torn ligament or tendon with suture, or uses other ligaments and/or tendons found in the foot and around the ankle to repair the damaged ligaments.
- **Arthroplasty**—A surgeon replaces the joint with an artificial joint.

Ankle Arthroscopy

Arthroscopy of the ankle includes surgical evaluation and treatment for multiple conditions. During the arthroscopy, small incisions are made and fiber-optic cameras with very small surgical tools are placed through the incision into the joint and used to perform the repair. Arthroscopy is used to remove debris in the ankle joint from torn cartilage or from a bone chip. It can

also be used to repair or reattach tendons and ligaments damaged during a severe sprain.

Ankle Reconstruction

Ankle reconstruction is the repair of the torn ligament or tendon with sutures, or the use of other ligaments and/or tendons found in the foot and around the ankle to repair the damaged ligaments. The procedure may be done through arthroscopic surgery or as an open procedure.

Ankle Arthroplasty

Ankle arthroplasty is the replacement of the joint with an artificial joint (Figure 57–14 ■). Although ankle arthroplasty is done much less frequently than knee or hip replacement, it can reduce the pain from arthritis. To fit the metal socket in place, the ends of the tibia and the fibula are shaped first. Following that, the top of the talus is shaped so the metal talus component can be inserted. After the bones are prepared, all the different pieces of the artificial ankle joint are put into place. To make sure that the ankle socket or the tibial component fits tightly, two screws are placed through the fibula and the tibia just above the artificial ankle joint. To prevent any motion that could loosen the artificial joint, bone is grafted between the fibula and the tibia to fuse them. The bone graft is taken from the bone that was removed earlier during the shaping procedure.

Postoperative Assessment

Weight-bearing status will be determined by the surgeon and will depend on the extent of the repair. Some patients will be allowed to bear weight with crutches; others will be placed in an immobilizer for as long as 6 weeks. If the surgery was extensive, such as remodeling of the ankle, a cast may be applied to prevent the patient from moving the joint too early and to promote healing. The nurse should instruct the patient to keep the incisions clean and dry and to observe for any signs of infection such as redness, increased pain, and drainage. The ankle should be elevated and iced to minimize swelling and prevent increased pain.

Surgical Management for the Foot

The most common foot surgeries are for the treatment of bunions and hammer toes. A bunion, also called hallux valgus, is a turning outward of the big toe (Figure 57–15 ■). The first metatarsal be-

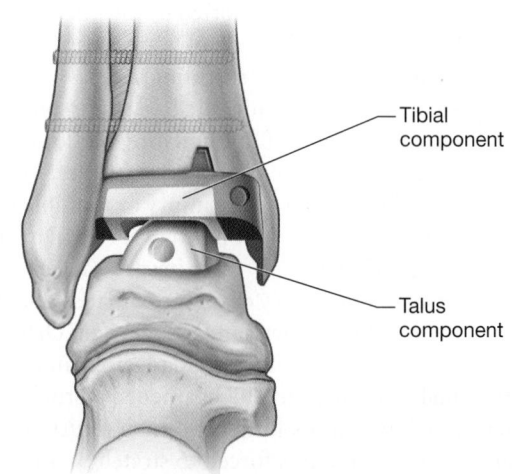

FIGURE 57–14 ■ Ankle arthroplasty.

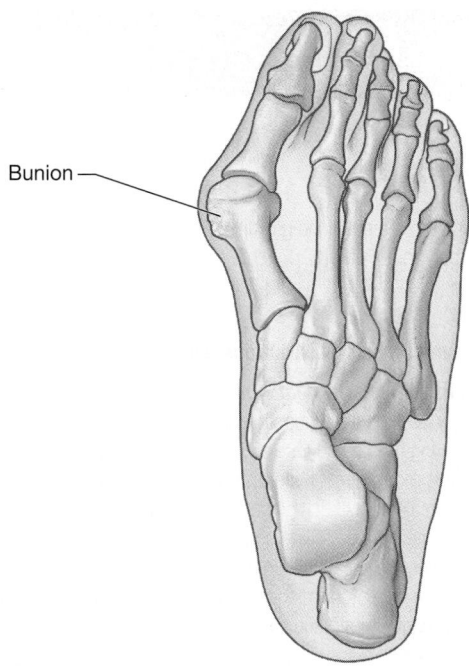

FIGURE 57–15 ■ Bunion.

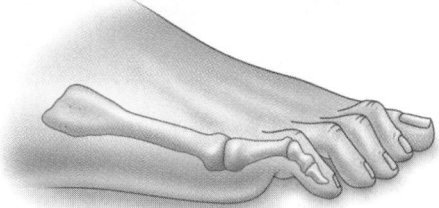

Hammer toes

FIGURE 57–16 ■ Hammer toe.

comes prominent on the inner border of the foot. This bump is the bunion and is made up of bone and soft tissue. The larger the bunion becomes, the more pressure is exerted on the joint while walking and the more pain develops. The big toe may angle toward and even move under the second toe. The deformity may even progress to force the second toe out of alignment, at times overlapping the third toe, and the foot will appear deformed. As the bunion progresses, arthritis may develop in the joint.

The bunion is painful and can make it difficult to wear shoes and affect mobility. Bunions can be caused by polio or arthritis, but most commonly are caused by ill-fitting shoes and heels that squeeze the toes into an unnatural position. A study by the American Orthopaedic Foot & Ankle Society found that 88% of women in the United States wear shoes that are too small, and 55% have bunions. Bunions are nine times more common in women than in men (American Academy of Orthopaedic Surgeons, 2001).

A hammer toe is a deformity of the second, third, fourth, or fifth toe. The toe is bent at the middle joint and resembles a hammer (Figure 57–16 ■). Initially, hammer toes are flexible and can be corrected with simple measures but, if untreated, they become fixed and require surgery. Hammer toe results from shoes that do not fit properly or a muscle imbalance. Muscles work in pairs to straighten and bend the toes. If the toe is bent and held in one position for a long period of time, muscles tighten and cannot stretch out.

Multiple surgical procedures may be done alone or in combination depending on the degree of deformity. The goal of surgery is to realign the joint, relieve pain, and correct the deformity. The procedures include:

- **Repair of the tendons and ligaments around the toe**—With a bunion, the tissues may be too tight on one side and too loose on the other, creating an imbalance that causes the big toe to drift toward the others. This procedure shortens the loose tissues, lengthens the tight ones, and is usually combined with an osteotomy.
- **Osteotomy**—The surgical cutting of bone and realignment of the joint.
- **Exostectomy**—Removal of the excess bone on the toe joint; used only for an enlargement of the bone with no drifting of the big toe.
- **Arthrodesis**—Removal of the damaged joint surfaces, followed by the insertion of screws, wires, or plates to hold the surfaces together until it heals.
- **Resection arthroplasty**—Removal of the damaged portion of the joint to create a flexible "scar" joint.

■ Nursing Management

The plan of care for the orthopedic patient is formulated by the registered nurse in conjunction with the patient. The nursing process provides the framework to ensure that all aspects of patient management are being addressed. The nurse caring for the patient after surgery must consider the time since surgery (postoperative days since surgery) in setting priorities and determining patient progress toward discharge. Pain control in the postoperative period is a major focus, because it can indicate potential problems or prevent the patient from completing necessary exercises and reaching goals that are necessary to recover and rehabilitate. (See the Pain Management section later in this chapter.) General postoperative assessment is discussed in Chapter 27 ⊘.

The nursing assessment of the patient is both holistic and focused. The nurse must rely on the patient's self-report to provide the necessary information to determine the patient's current status accurately. The Nursing Process: Patient Care Plan feature (p. 1822) provides examples of subjective and objective assessment and evaluation data for the patient with a musculoskeletal disorder as a foundation for providing care to this population. The nurse collects this assessment data to evaluate factors such as pain, neurovascular status, wound appearance, and drains and dressings, specific therapeutic modalities, and exercising.

Neurovascular Assessment

The neurovascular assessment is a requirement in the assessment of patients with musculoskeletal injury and surgery. The neurovascular assessment should be performed bilaterally so

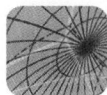

NURSING PROCESS: Patient Care Plan for the Orthopedic Surgical Patient

Assessment of Airway and Gas Exchange

Subjective Data:
Are you having difficulty breathing?
Can you take a deep breath and cough for me?
Do you feel like you are getting enough air?
Do you use an inhaler or have a history of lung problems?

Objective Data:
Lung sounds
Oxygen saturation, arterial blood gas analysis
Respiratory rate, depth, effort
Mental status

Nursing Assessment and Diagnoses	Outcomes and Evaluation Parameters	Planning and Interventions with *Rationales*
Nursing Diagnosis: *Gas Exchange, Impaired* related to anesthetic or narcotic effect, fluid overload, pulmonary or fat emboli, pneumonia, or preexisting pulmonary or cardiovascular disease exacerbation	**Outcomes:** Airway open. Adequate gas exchange. ***Evaluation Parameters:*** Breath sounds clear, without evidence of snoring or stridor. Oxygen saturation > 94% or as ordered by health care provider. Arterial blood gas demonstrates PaO$_2$ > 80 mmHg and PaCO$_2$ 35–45 mmHg. Respiratory rate 12–20 per minute, unlabored with good chest expansion. Alert and oriented to person, place, time, and situation.	**Interventions and *Rationales:*** Initially a jaw thrust maneuver may be necessary to maintain an open airway if the patient has snoring breath sounds indicating airway obstruction from tongue. If this maneuver is necessary, the patient may require additional reversal agents such as naloxone or flumazenil. The anesthesiologist or surgeon may need to be contacted for orders for these medications. *To maintain open airway.* Assess patient for adequacy of respiratory rate and depth, auscultate breath sounds, and monitor oxygen saturation. Analyze arterial blood gas when results are available. *Indicates gas exchange is adequate.* Assess patient's level of consciousness and orientation to person, place, time, and situation. *Confusion, agitation, restlessness, or difficult arousal may indicate hypoxia.* Encourage patient to perform incentive spirometry (ICS) every 1–2 hours for 10 breaths while awake. Have patient cough and deep breathe after utilizing ICS. Assist patient out of bed (OOB) to chair and ambulating at least three times a day. *To promote adequate gas exchange, promote airway clearance, and prevent atelectasis.*

Assessment of Neurovascular Status

Subjective Data:
Can you move your (name part distal to surgery)?
Where do you feel me touching you? Is this sharp or dull?
Are you in pain? Can you describe your pain using a scale of 0 to 10?
Do you have any numbness or tingling?

Objective Data:
Strength of movement   Color of skin
Sensation   Skin temperature
Pulses   Capillary refill time

Nursing Assessment and Diagnoses	Outcomes and Evaluation Parameters	Planning and Interventions with *Rationales*
Nursing Diagnosis: *Neurovascular Dysfunction, Peripheral: Risk for* related to edema, vascular insufficiency, nerve damage, or surgical complication	**Outcomes:** Absence of neurovascular deficits. Skeletal structures in alignment. ***Evaluation Parameters:*** Full strength. Sensation intact. No numbness, tingling, or pain. Pulses 2–3+ palpated. Skin warm, pink, and dry. Capillary refill time < 3 seconds.	**Interventions and *Rationales:*** Perform neurovascular assessment every 2–4 hours. Assess bilateral extremities. *To give indication of normal findings for patient.* Elevate limb above level of heart in position of function. *To decrease edema formation and prevent contracture.* Evaluate sensation using a dermatome chart for patients with epidural anesthesia/catheters and patients with spinal surgery. *Dermatome chart describes level of anesthesia or deficit.* Evaluate strength and range of motion during planned postoperative activities. *Postoperative exercise improves circulation, improves healing, and prevents contractures and deconditioning.*

Assessment of Volume Status

Subjective Data:
Are you thirsty?
Do you need to urinate?
Do you feel cold?
How is your breathing?
Do you feel anxious? Or that your heart is beating faster than normal?

Objective Data:
Urine output, color, specific gravity
Blood loss from surgical drains/dressing
Intake and output balance
Heart rate, blood pressure, respiratory rate (RR)
Blood urea nitrogen (BUN)/creatinine
Hemoglobin (Hgb) and hematocrit (HCT)
Skin turgor, capillary refill

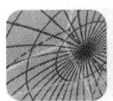

NURSING PROCESS: Patient Care Plan for the Orthopedic Surgical Patient—*Continued*

Nursing Assessment and Diagnoses	Outcomes and Evaluation Parameters	Planning and Interventions with *Rationales*
Nursing Diagnoses: *Fluid volume, Deficient* related to blood loss and inadequate fluid intake *Fluid volume, Imbalanced: Risk for* due to impaired renal function and fluid intake in excess of output	**Outcome:** Adequate and balanced intake and output. **Evaluation Parameters:** Vital signs within normal limits. Intake and output balance. Lungs clear. Urine output adequate. BUN and creatinine normal. Hgb and HCT stable. Drainage from wound < 50 milliliters in 24 hours.	**Interventions and *Rationales:*** Strict intake and output (I&O) to include all po liquids, IV fluid intake and urine, gastric, and wound drainage output. Maintain shift and ongoing totals. Assess wound drainage. Frankly bloody drainage may be present on the first postoperative day, but should change to serosanguinous after that. Notify health care provider of excessive blood loss. *To give an accurate reflection of fluid balance.* Obtain vital signs as ordered. *Tachycardia and low blood pressure may indicate hypovolemia. Increased respiratory rate or adventitious breath sounds may indicate volume overload.* Monitor laboratory studies for signs of hypo-/hypervolemia. *The hemoglobin and hematocrit, BUN, and creatinine levels provide information on volume status.*

Assessment of Pain

Subjective Data:
Can you describe your pain for me using a 0–10 scale with 0 being no pain and 10 being the worst pain you have ever had?
Using that 1–10 scale, what is your comfort level?

Objective Data:
Patient pain score
Type of pain-relief modality

Nursing Assessment and Diagnoses	Outcomes and Evaluation Parameters	Planning and Interventions with *Rationales*
Nursing Diagnosis: *Pain, Acute* related to surgical procedure, compartment syndrome, osteoarthritis, or cerebrospinal fluid (CSF) leak (in spinal surgery patient)	**Outcomes:** Patient will have pain controlled and will be able to participate in all aspects of rehabilitation program. **Evaluation Parameter:** Pain scale score at or below predetermined comfort level score.	**Interventions and *Rationales:*** Medicate patient for pain score greater than comfort level. Notify health care provider if symptoms unrelieved by ordered medication. *Patients have a right to pain control within their described comfort level. Pain that is not relieved may indicate development of complications such as compartment syndrome.* Place spinal patient in supine position if he complains of headache. *CSF leak headache increases with drainage, upright position.*

Assessment of Wound Status and Potential for Infection

Subjective Data:
Are you having more or less pain in your (name surgical site) today?
Do you feel as though you have fever or chills?
Are you having urinary frequency or urgency?

Objective Data:
Temperature and vital signs
Wound drainage appearance, odor
Suture site redness, edema, warmth
Urine appearance, odor
Wound/urine culture results
White blood count (WBC) results

Nursing Assessment and Diagnoses	Outcomes and Evaluation Parameters	Planning and Interventions with *Rationales*
Nursing Diagnosis: *Infection, Risk for* and delayed wound healing related to age, open surgery, compound fracture, and comorbid condition	**Outcomes:** Wound/bone healing within expected time frame. No evidence of infection. **Evaluation Parameters:** Surgical incision is clean, dry, and approximated, without redness. Urine clear, no odor. Vital signs within normal limits (WNL). WBC count < 11,000/mcL.	**Interventions and *Rationales:*** Obtain vital signs as ordered or every 4 hours, including temperature. *To provide early indication of changes indicating infection.* Assess surgical site and drainage each shift. *To provide early indication of changes indicating infection.* Monitor lab values, especially WBC count. *Elevations in WBC indicate infection.*

Assessment of Functional Status

Subjective Data:
How do you feel today?
Are you able to bathe and perform your postoperative exercises unassisted, or do you need some help?
How far did you walk yesterday?

Objective Data:
Amount in feet that patient is able to ambulate
Time in hours that patient is out of bed
Amount of persons needed to get patient out of bed or to assist with ambulation
Assistive devices needed for mobility

(continued)

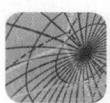

NURSING PROCESS: Patient Care Plan for the Orthopedic Surgical Patient—*Continued*

Nursing Assessment and Diagnoses	Outcomes and Evaluation Parameters	Planning and Interventions with *Rationales*
Nursing Diagnosis: *Self-Care, Readiness for Enhanced* related to surgery, pain, immobility, or decreased mental status	**Outcome:** Patient able to care for self. *Evaluation Parameters:* Able to perform postoperative exercises including transfers, ambulation, and pulmonary toilet at prescribed intervals. Able to ambulate with walker 50 feet with steady gait; able to ambulate unassisted for 50 feet with steady gait. Able to complete toilet and hygiene functions unassisted.	**Interventions and *Rationale:*** Patient should be assisted out of bed as soon as feasible. Follow health care provider orders/clinical pathway instructions for mobility and activities. If health care provider does not order progressive mobilization of the patient, notify health care provider to obtain activity orders. *To prevent deconditioning and maintain or improve functional status.*

Assessment of Skin Integrity

Subjective Data:
Are you able to turn and position yourself?
Do you have any painful areas while you are in bed?
Do you have any reddened areas that you are aware of?

Objective Data:
Skin appearance
Patient position
Presence of pressure relief device

Nursing Assessment and Diagnoses	Outcomes and Evaluation Parameters	Planning and Interventions with *Rationales*
Nursing Diagnoses: *Skin Integrity, Risk for Impaired* related to decreased sensorium and immobility.	**Outcome:** Patient will have no evidence of skin breakdown. *Evaluation Parameters:* Skin surface clean, dry, pink, and intact. Patient position change is performed or observed at least every 2 hours while in bed or every 15 minutes while seated.	**Interventions and *Rationales:*** Turn and position patient every 2 hours while in bed (logroll, maintaining spinal alignment if patient with spinal surgery). Float heels off of bed with pillows or heel lift device. Follow hospital protocol for use of pressure relief mattresses and overlays. *To prevent pressure ulcer development.* Assess skin integrity and document each shift and with each change in position. Assess areas over bony prominences, where prostheses, casts, traction, or splints contact. *To provide early detection of potential for skin breakdown.*

Assessment of Patient's Understanding of Treatment Plan and Continuing Care Needs

Subjective Data:
Do you have any questions about your plan of care?
What are your goals for today?
Do you have anyone at home to assist you?
Tell me about your home so that I have a good picture of it.

Objective Data:
Observation of activities
Verbalization of continuing care plan

Nursing Assessment and Diagnoses	Outcomes and Evaluation Parameters	Planning and Interventions with *Rationales*
Nursing Diagnoses: *Knowledge, Deficient* of self-care needs and treatment plan related to postoperative delirium *Therapeutic Regimen Management, Ineffective related to* postoperative exercises, administration of deep venous thrombosis (DVT) prophylaxis, and self-care activities without assistance related to age, obesity, decreased functional capacity, and lack of home support	**Outcome:** Patient is able to discuss a realistic plan for self-care after hospital discharge. *Evaluation Parameters:* Patient verbalizes knowledge of plan of care and goals. Patient demonstrates ability to perform postoperative exercises correctly in the appropriate frequency. Patient verbalizes a plan for assistance with activities of daily living (ADL) and ongoing therapeutic requirements if needed. Demonstration of ability to ambulate at least 100 feet and perform self-care activities.	**Interventions and *Rationales:*** Assess patient's readiness to learn and provide patient education regarding patient procedures, activities, medications, and care needs. *Assessment of patient readiness enables the nurse to provide education at appropriate times.* Begin discharge planning on admission. Encourage significant other/family participation in plan. Evaluate care needs compared with patient abilities. Patient/significant other should be able to verbalize/demonstrate essential activities prior to discharge. *To ensure that sufficient time is allotted to provide education and training so that patient/family are able to perform activities after discharge.* Prior to discharge, ensure that patient understands plan of care and is able to verbalize important aspects in her own words and to verbalize a plan for obtaining medications, equipment, and assistance in the home environment. *To help ensure compliance with treatment plan.*

that the affected extremity can be compared to the unaffected extremity. If the patient undergoes spinal surgery, the neurovascular assessment is performed on the parts of the body distal to the surgical site. The neurovascular assessment includes assessment of the five Ps: pain, pulse, paresthesia, paralysis, and pallor. A complete assessment of circulation, motor, and sensory functions must be performed. Neurovascular compromise or deterioration should be reported to the surgeon immediately. The nurse should anticipate performing the neurovascular assessment in conjunction with vital signs.

The neurovascular assessment should proceed systematically. Activities that may cause pain should be performed last. The nurse should first inspect the extremities for general appearance including color and presence of edema. Skin color should be described as pink or normal, pale, or cyanotic. Red or ruddy skin may indicate venous engorgement. Skin temperature and presence of moisture should be assessed. Normally the skin is warm and dry. Coolness of the skin may indicate decreased circulation. Excessive warmth or heat may indicate an early sign of infection or cellulitis. Moist skin is frequently found in the skin folds of obese persons and may require interventions to prevent fungal infection or skin maceration. Moist skin may also indicate venous insufficiency, excessive effort, or fever.

The pulse strength provides information regarding blood supply to the affected extremity and surgical site. Pulses most distal to the surgical site should be palpated. If no pulse is present, the nurse should obtain Doppler pulses and systematically attempt to palpate the presence of a pulse in a proximal direction. For example, if no dorsalis pedis or posterior tibial pulse is present, the nurse should next palpate for a popliteal pulse. Pulses in the lower extremities include the dorsalis pedis, posterior tibial, and popliteal. Pulse points in the upper extremities include the radial and brachial. The pulse should be described as grade 0–4 or as a Doppler pulse (Chart 57–11).

Skin turgor indicates hydration status and also helps describe the fullness of tissue in the operative extremity. After surgery, the inflammatory process causes vasodilation of vessels supplying the site, which results in tissue swelling. Because the part may be immobilized after surgery, venous return is decreased because of decreased muscle pump action. Skin turgor may be described as normal/brisk, slow, or tense. The skin of the distal extremity should be compressed between the nurse's thumb and index finger to a tent-like projection and released to test turgor. The skin should return to its normal state briskly. Slowed skin turgor indicates low volume status or dehydration. Tense skin cannot be tested. Edema in the surgical area is assessed regularly. Right after surgery, edema is a normal occurrence due to tissue manip-

ulation during surgery, and it gradually diminishes over time. If skin is tense or the extremity edematous, the patient should be instructed to elevate the part above heart level and perform appropriate exercises to increase muscle pump action and venous return. Patients with shoulder or arm surgery should perform finger exercises or hand squeezes with a rubber ball. Patients with lower extremity surgery should perform dorsiflexion and plantar flexion (foot pumps). The reoccurrence of edema may indicate infection.

Capillary refill testing is used to evaluate arterial filling in the small vessels supplying the skin. It can be assumed that if the capillary refill is normal, the circulation in the larger vessels is also intact. Capillary refill is described in seconds. Either a nail bed or distal skin may be tested. The nail bed or skin is depressed with one finger until the skin blanches and then is released. The test site is then observed for the time it takes for skin color to return to normal. Normal capillary refill time is less than 3 seconds. Delayed capillary refill (greater than 3 seconds) indicates decreased tissue perfusion.

The sensory and motor assessments evaluate nerve function. Prior to testing sensation, the nurse should have the patient close her eyes, or the area to be tested should be obstructed from view with the bedsheets. This will prevent the patient from giving information based on what she sees instead of what she actually feels. If the patient underwent extremity surgery, testing of sensation distal to the surgical site is required. If the patient underwent spinal surgery or epidural anesthesia, a more comprehensive evaluation utilizing dermatomes should be performed. Nerve impulses may be delayed due to surgical complications or from compression of nerves by postoperative edema. When assessing sensation, the nurse should apply light touch and ask the patient "where" she feels the touch. If the patient is repeatedly asked, "Do you feel this?" the patient may reply yes because she feels that is the expectation and therefore gives inaccurate responses.

Motor strength is assessed by asking the patient to perform specific activities. These activities involve testing the patient's ability to move the part, the strength of the part in moving against gravity, and the strength of the part against resistance. Motor strength should be graded on a scale of 0 to 5. If the patient is unable to move the part, he receives a score of zero. If full strength is demonstrated and is equal to the unaffected part, the patient should receive a score of 5.

Pain Management

Patients are entitled to be in their "comfort zone" at all times. The nurse must assess the patient for the specific cause of pain and provide appropriate interventions. Knowledge of the medications administered during surgery and the timing of the last dose of pain medications is important for the nurse accepting the patient in the postanesthesia care unit (PACU) and the orthopedic unit. Pain medication may be administered via the epidural, oral, intramuscular, cutaneous, or intravenous route. Patient-controlled analgesia (PCA) or around-the-clock pain medication is often utilized in the early postoperative period. The PCA can be set to deliver a constant or basal rate in addition to the patient's being able to self-administer a preset dose at prescribed intervals to achieve pain control.

CHART 57–11	Pulse Strength Chart
0	No palpable pulse
1+	Weak, barely palpable, or easily obliterated
2+	Palpable
3+	Strong, easily palpable
4+	Bounding

Surgical pain is concentrated at the surgical site and is generally described as sharp and nonradiating. Pain assessment should be based on a consistent scale. Many scales are available for use using a numeric scale or pictures to help the patient describe her pain level. Each patient has a particular comfort level or pain tolerance level. Pharmacologic and nonpharmacologic interventions should be utilized to ensure that the patient's pain score is maintained within the comfort range. Pain may be anticipated prior to physical therapy or other activities and the patient offered pain medication prior to these activities. Pain is assessed with each set of vital signs and after administering pain medications.

Atypical pain requires a comprehensive assessment. The nurse should have the patient describe the location and quality of pain with each assessment. It should not be assumed that all pain is related to the surgical site. Chest pain, pain at sites other than the operative site, and increased pain should be evaluated to determine the cause. The underlying cause should be corrected to relieve the pain. For example, if the pain is cardiac in origin, interventions to relieve myocardial ischemia should be performed. Chapter 15 includes an in-depth discussion of pain management.

Appearance of Surgical Site and Dressing

The surgical dressing should be inspected for the presence of blood and drainage. In the immediate postoperative period, oozing of blood may be expected. The area of drainage should be marked using a pen or indelible marker so that the rate of bleeding can be objectively assessed. Excessive bleeding may indicate that a blood vessel has not been sufficiently contained during surgery. The surgeon should be notified if there is excessive bleeding. The surgeon may order additional reinforcement of the dressing, or it may require pharmacologic therapy such as vitamin K, cryoprecipitate, or discontinuation of anticoagulant therapy. In some cases, the patient may need to be returned to the operating room. Surgical wound drainage should be described as sanguineous if it is frankly bloody or serosanguineous if it is pinkish or blood mixed with plasma. Wound drainage may increase with patient movement, and the nurse should assess the patient's activity to determine whether the activity is causing strain on the suture line. Activities and positions that place stress or strain on the suture line should be avoided. The dressing of a spinal surgery patient should be assessed for the presence of cerebrospinal fluid (CSF). If CSF is present, the surgeon should be notified.

The surgeon is frequently the first person to change the primary surgical dressing. Symptoms of wound infection generally appear within 3 days of surgery and should be assessed within this time period. The suture line should be assessed to determine whether the skin is approximated and the sutures and staples are intact. Purulent or malodorous drainage should be reported to the surgeon. Infection is discussed later in this chapter in the Complications section.

Surgical Tubes and Drains

Postoperative orthopedic patients will frequently have surgical drains and urinary catheters. The urinary catheter should be discontinued as soon as the patient is able to get out of bed and ambulate, to reduce the risk of a urinary tract infection. The patient should be able to urinate within 8 hours after the urinary catheter is discontinued. Surgical drains may be discontinued 24 hours after surgery if output is less than about 50 milliliters in 24 hours. Many surgical drains use suction to withdraw blood and fluid. The nurse should ensure that the suction device used is activated. For example, a Hemovac or Jackson Pratt drain must be compressed to create suction. Chapter 67 includes an in-depth description of the various surgical drains.

Therapeutic Modalities

Many therapeutic modalities are commonly ordered for patients undergoing orthopedic surgery. **Continuous passive motion devices** (machines into which the affected extremity or joint is placed to perform slow, continuous passive range of motion to avoid stiffness and prevent a decrease in range of motion) may be utilized for patients who have knee surgery to prevent loss of range of motion of the joint. Sequential compression devices or compression stockings may be utilized in patients at risk for DVT. Cryotherapy units or ice bags may be utilized to decrease pain and swelling in the joint after surgery. Physical therapy as well as active and passive range of motion may be required to prevent loss of function and to maintain strength and range of motion in the orthopedic patient.

Exercise

Planned exercise is an important part of the recovery plan for the orthopedic surgical patient. Specific exercises, often called therapeutic exercises, will be prescribed to promote and maintain range of motion and function. The plan of care for the patient should include specific measurable goals for the patient. Because orthopedic surgery is generally performed to improve function or repair a defect, typical goals include range of motion, the strength of the limb, or ability to participate in the rehabilitation exercise program. Specificity and measurability of the goal are important so that it is clear whether the patient has attained it or not. For example, if the goal for a patient is that he will be able to ambulate independently 50 feet by day 2 after surgery is not met and the patient ambulates with assistance for only 20 feet, there is an objective starting point for the analysis of why the goal was not accomplished. The patient should be encouraged to continue the exercises prescribed in the hospital after discharge. An overall general health exercise program should be encouraged as well to ensure cardiovascular and bone health.

Discharge Planning

Knowledge of where the patient resides, the physical aspects of the residence such as number of stairs or size of bathrooms (is the bathroom large enough for the patient to turn around in with a walker?), is information necessary to plan for the patient's safe discharge. Presence of children or significant others who are willing to assist the patient after hospitalization will influence the discharge plan. Elder patients who have had joint replacement surgery frequently require skilled nursing care beyond hospitalization. If the hospitalized elder is a primary caregiver for a spouse now left at home without assistance, the patient will need to make arrangements to provide care for the spouse during the current hospitalization. Anxiety related to home and financial concerns can impede the patient's recovery and rehabilitation.

Postoperative precautions and exercises may also be taught prior to surgery. Precautions and exercises to be performed depend on the surgical site (back, lower extremity, upper extremity, and pelvis). In some cases the patient may be asked to perform exercises such as walking to build endurance, specific exercises to improve circulation, or exercises to increase strength and range of motion.

Environment

The physical environment of the home should be discussed with the patient. Specific accommodations may be necessary, and the patient should plan for these prior to discharge. For example, the patient may require a hospital bed after surgery, and friend or family assistance should be elicited to configure the environment for this. Throw rugs should be removed, if necessary, to prevent falls. Postoperative equipment such as cryotherapy, hospital bed, elevated toilet seat, or continuous passive motion (CPM) devices should be ordered and their presence in the home assured prior to discharge. If the patient will have activity restrictions or precautions after surgery, the physical environment in the home may need simple alterations such as the movement of articles for activities of daily living to an accessible area. If the patient resides in a physical environment that prevents activity prescribed for recovery or ability to obtain access to health care appointments or supplies, the nurse must assist the patient to develop an alternate plan for home care. If friends or family are unable to assist with an alternate living situation for the recovery period, assistance from discharge planning or social work may be needed to assist patient placement in a rehabilitation, assisted living, or skilled nursing facility.

■ Complications

The nurse should be knowledgeable regarding not only potential complications related to general surgery but also complications specific to orthopedic surgery. The nurse must be alert to subtle, early signs and symptoms of complications and respond quickly to prevent permanent disability, decompensation, or delays in recovery.

Respiratory Insufficiency

Pulmonary complications in the orthopedic surgical patient may be related to a variety of causative factors. **Fat embolus** is a complication specific to orthopedic injuries involving long bone fracture. Fat globules from the bone marrow travel into the venous system and to the pulmonary vessels. Fat blocks the pulmonary vessels and inactivates surfactant, which promotes the development of acute respiratory distress syndrome (ARDS). The patient will develop respiratory distress: tachypnea, air hunger, and hypoxia. Other signs and symptoms associated with fat embolus are fever, tachycardia, restlessness, decreased mental status, and petechiae. Arterial blood gas findings demonstrate an initial decrease in $PaCO_2$ followed by increased $PaCO_2$ and low PaO_2. Other diagnostic tests such as chest x-ray and ventilation/perfusion scan are nonspecific for fat embolus. Patients with suspected fat embolus should be intubated and placed on mechanical ventilation with positive end-expiratory pressure (PEEP). Treatment is largely supportive until the condition resolves. A detailed discussion of the diagnosis and management of ARDS is in Chapter 36 😊 .

Pulmonary embolus may also cause respiratory insufficiency and is usually associated with deep venous thrombosis. Signs and symptoms are similar to fat embolus, but pulmonary embolus is not generally associated with the development of ARDS.

After arrival to the medical–surgical floor, the patient should be monitored closely for the first 4 to 12 hours to ensure that the vital signs remain stable and the respiratory rate and effort appropriate. Routine vital signs and respiratory status are then observed for the remainder of hospitalization. Incentive spirometry is typically ordered for the postoperative period to promote lung expansion and prevent respiratory complications such as atelectasis and pneumonia. Typically, the patient is encouraged to perform incentive spirometry every 1 to 2 hours while awake. Coughing and deep breathing should follow use of the incentive spirometer to assist in the removal of secretions from smaller airways. Patients are now assisted out of bed as soon as they are able, depending of the type of surgery. Sitting in a chair enables the patient to expand the thorax to a greater degree than while in bed and also acts to promote respiratory function. Pneumonia is a serious complication, particularly for the gerontological postoperative patient. The patient may be at risk for aspiration pneumonia related to decreased mental status, use of nasogastric (NG) tubes, or preexisting medical conditions such as stroke or dysphagia. Elevations in temperature should alert the nurse to the potential that the patient has atelectasis or pneumonia. Aggressive pulmonary toilet is needed to remove secretions and improve airway exchange.

Venous Thromboembolism

Venous thromboembolism (VTE) includes both deep venous thrombosis (DVT) and pulmonary embolism. Risk factors in the orthopedic surgical population include immobility of a limb, long surgical times in a single position, hypercoagulablity of blood due to activation of the clotting cascade from surgical stimulation and from being NPO, as well as endothelial disruption from the surgery or trauma itself. The three factors of venous stasis, hypercoagulability, and vessel injury make up Virchow's triad for VTE risk. Virchow's triad is discussed in Chapter 43 😊 .

Patients undergoing total hip and total knee repair/replacement surgery are at high risk for DVT, and current standards of practice include providing DVT prophylaxis in these patient populations. Prevention strategies to decrease the incidence of DVT include the administration of heparin (unfractionated or low molecular weight), the use of antiembolism stockings, and the use of sequential compression devices. Most pulmonary emboli occur as the result of DVT. Additional risk factors for VTE include obesity, use of oral contraceptives, old age, varicose veins, prior VTE, and Factor V Leiden (FVL) gene mutation. Factor V Leiden disorder is the most common blood coagulation disorder. Approximately 4% to 7% of the population is heterozygous for Factor V Leiden disorder. The risk of VTE in a heterozygous patient is increased in the presence of other risk factors such as obesity or use of oral contraceptives. Homozygous Factor V Leiden disorder severely increases the risk of thromboembolic event, and these patients are placed on anticoagulants (Edmonds, Crichton, Runciman, & Pradhan, 2004; Folsom et al., 2002; Ornstein & Cushman, 2003).

In spite of appropriate therapy, the incidence of DVT in orthopedic patients is still prevalent, and nurses must be diligent in assessing patients for signs and symptoms of DVT. DVT symptoms may be nonspecific. The patient may complain of pain in an extremity. The extremity may become swollen, edematous, and tender at or distal to the clot. Although the legs are the most common site for DVT, immobile arms are also at risk to develop clots. Pain associated with DVT may increase with exercise of the part. A positive Homans' sign is associated with lower leg DVT. Homans' sign is considered positive when plantar and dorsiflexion on the affected side cause calf pain. DVT is discussed in detail in Chapter 43 .

Symptoms of VTE may range from dramatic to nonspecific. The patient with pulmonary embolism may have acute onset of chest pain, shortness of breath, decreased sensorium, and pink, frothy sputum. Typically, the patient with pulmonary embolism will demonstrate tachycardia and tachypnea. Arterial blood gases may be normal or demonstrate hypoxia. Oxygen saturation may be normal or decreased in pulmonary embolism. Pulmonary embolism is discussed in detail in Chapter 36 .

Compartment Syndrome

Compartment syndrome is a rare condition occurring when swelling within an anatomical compartment restricts blood flow. An anatomical compartment is one in which the fascia or an external device such as a cast prohibits expansion of the compartment as edema and engorgement increase. This causes compression of vascular and nervous system structures. As edema and engorgement increase, pain increases and is unrelieved by narcotic pain medication administration. The area affected will be swollen and tense. Pain significantly increases with extension or flexion of the affected part. There may be changes in the neurovascular assessment of the patient indicating that compartment syndrome is present. The patient may have pain, paresthesia, pulselessness, paralysis, and/or pallor of the part. If compartment syndrome in an extremity is suspected, the extremity should not be elevated, but should be maintained at the level of the heart to improve perfusion. Normal tissue pressure is less than 15 mmHg. Numerous devices may be utilized to determine tissue or compartment pressure. If the tissue or compartment pressure is greater than 30 mmHg, compartment syndrome should be suspected. Treatment of compartment syndrome requires release of the constriction to accommodate swelling. If a cast is causing the restriction, it should be bivalved (cut down both sides). If the constriction is at the fascial level, the patient will require surgery. There are devices available that can be inserted through the skin to measure the actual compartment pressure. If the nurse suspects compartment syndrome is present, the surgeon should be notified immediately to prevent permanent disability or loss of limb.

Pressure Ulcers

Patients with orthopedic injuries are also at particular risk for the development of preventable pressure ulcers. For example, patients with hip surgery are at particular risk for heel pressure ulcers. The heels should be floated off of the mattress utilizing pillows. If the pillows are insufficient to maintain the heels off of the bed, assistive devices such as heel lift boots or specialty pressure relief beds or mattresses may be utilized. The best tool to prevent pressure ulcer development is repositioning the patient

at least every 2 hours. Frequent assessment of the skin allows early detection of potential impairments in skin integrity requiring more aggressive interventions. The orthopedic patient may also develop pressure ulcers in areas where prosthetic devices, casts, splints, or traction causes friction. If there is evidence of friction, extra padding may be needed, or adjustment of the splint, prosthesis, or cast may be necessary.

Infection

Patients with traumatic injuries such as open fractures, preexisting infection, cardiovascular disease or diabetes, and extremes of age are at risk of developing postoperative infections. Postoperative infection will increase the duration of hospitalization and may precipitate sepsis. Prior to surgery the skin over the surgical site is prepped with an antibacterial solution such as povidone-iodine; or if there is an existing wound, it is irrigated copiously with normal saline. Although prophylactic antibiotic therapy, typically a cephalosporin, is given preoperatively and postoperatively, infection may occur. The nurse should be alert to the signs and symptoms of postoperative surgical site infection. Signs of surgical infection include redness, erythema, warmth, edema, purulent drainage, dehiscence of the suture site, and fever. A wound culture may be obtained to determine the organism responsible for the infection and appropriate antibiotic coverage. The sutures or staples may be removed to promote local therapy with wound dressings.

Osteomyelitis is infection of the bone itself. The incidence of osteomyelitis is highest in patients who have had compound fractures, external fixator devices, and open orthopedic procedures. This infection may be related to invasion by bacteria, fungus, or virus. Tuberculosis infection may occur in the bone tissue as a result of exposure to tuberculosis. The patient may complain of deep bone pain. Failure of the surgical site or pressure ulcer to heal may be the first indication that osteomyelitis is present. Confirmation that osteomyelitis is present may be obtained from MRI, CT, x-ray, bone biopsy, or bone scan. Treatment for osteomyelitis requires long-term, generally 6 weeks of, antibiotic therapy.

Late complications of orthopedic surgery include infection of the surgical hardware. The decision to remove the hardware is dependent on the impact on patient mobility, pain level, age, and potential complications such as neurovascular injury, deformity, and inability to replace the implant, which may have significant impact on the patient's mobility and ability to continue working in her current occupation. In cases of external fixator devices or screw implants, removal of hardware is less complicated and does not necessarily impact the patient's activities of daily living. If bone has healed and the screws or plates are no longer necessary for joint or bone stability, the surgery has far less impact on patient mobility and ability to carry out activities of daily living or occupational activities.

Joint Dislocation

Dislocation may occur due to overextension of the joint. Complications of dislocation include pain, decreased range of motion, and neurovascular compromise. Strict adherence to joint precautions can prevent complications of dislocation. Signs and symptoms of joint dislocation include swelling, pain, immobility, and shortening (the extremity appears shorter than the unaffected extremity).

Heterotrophic Ossification

Heterotrophic ossification (HO) is the development of bone tissue in areas where bone tissue is not normally present. Myositis ossificans progressiva develops in childhood and is the progressive development of bone tissue (ossification) in soft tissues throughout the body. The life span of patients with myositis ossificans progressiva is severely shortened, and patients frequently die from complications of compression of vital organs from lesions in the second or third decade. Heterotrophic ossification is a late complication that may be seen in musculoskeletal and spinal cord injury. The exact mechanism of bone formation is not known, but it is thought to be an inflammatory reaction of intramuscular and connective tissue after injury or surgery. Sepsis or infection may predispose the patient to the development of HO. Symptoms associated with heterotrophic ossification depend on the site and size of the lesion. In spinal cord injury, the site of the anomalous bone lesion is always lower than the level of injury. Frequent sites of post-traumatic heterotrophic ossification are the soft tissues surrounding the hips, knees, shoulders, or elbows. Patients may be asymptomatic if the lesion is small; or they may experience pain, decreased range of motion, and signs of inflammation or infection if the lesion is large or interferes with joint motion. Signs and symptoms in an extremity with a heterotrophic lesion may include pain, swelling, rubor, pain, and fever. Because these signs and symptoms are similar to those of venous thrombosis, the patient will have radiologic studies such as a bone scan and x-rays to determine whether the patient has heterotrophic ossification, as well as testing for VTE such as D-dimer and ultrasound flow studies of the extremity.

Treatment of heterotrophic ossification includes administration of nonsteroidal anti-inflammatory medications and indomethacin for pain, in addition to focused radiation to the joint. These medications may decrease the development of heterotrophic ossification as well. Etidronate disodium may be administered to patients prone to the development of heterotrophic ossification to prevent lesion formation, and is administered preoperatively and postoperatively when the HO lesions are surgically excised.

Osteonecrosis or Avascular Necrosis

Osteonecrosis (avascular necrosis) is the death of bone tissue and may occur at any time after injury to bone due to impairment of circulation. Patients at high risk of osteonecrosis include patients taking steroids, receiving radiation therapy, or with alcohol dependence. Many medical conditions such as sickle cell anemia, HIV, gout, and osteoporosis may be predisposed to osteonecrosis.

Collaborative Management

A multidisciplinary team approach is necessary to optimize care for the orthopedic surgical patient. The surgeon determines the activity prescription for the patient, and the nurse works collaboratively with the physical therapists to enable the patient to perform activities to the level of his capabilities. It is important that any required restrictions to activity and precautions to prevent hip dislocation or spinal torque be taken. Because many patients will have comorbid conditions, this collaboration ensures patient safety. Adequate nutrition is necessary for wound healing and to maintain patient strength. The clinical dietician is a valuable team member to provide input regarding adequate caloric intake that adheres to dietary restrictions that may be present for patients with cardiovascular, endocrine, or renal disease. Because many hip replacement and amputation patients may require home care assistance and assistive devices, or skilled care after discharge, discharge planners and/or social work assistance is helpful. Individual patients may also require psychiatric consultation depending on their response to their surgery or the event that caused the surgery to be necessary. Spiritual support for patients during hospitalization may also assist the patients in adapting successfully to their current situation and maintaining a positive outlook necessary to participate fully in rehabilitation efforts.

Health Promotion

The greatest impact that nurses can have regarding musculoskeletal injuries and surgery is that of prevention. Patients who have musculoskeletal surgery generally receive explicit instructions on how to prevent the recurrence of their injury. It would be a great service to elders to provide information on home safety before they become injured and have surgery. Safety devices to prevent injury such as bathroom safety bars should be made available to elders by their health plans or should be a requirement for installation by landlords.

Another method in which health care providers can improve eldercare is by reviewing medications at each visit and in pharmacies. Over-the-counter medications should be included in the pharmacy medication lists so that better prevention of polypharmacy reactions is achieved.

Health promotion includes regular exercise. Walking not only is an excellent cardiovascular exercise but also maintains bone mass. Obesity is increasing in the United States, and education on the effects of obesity on knee and hip joints may assist in promoting the maintenance of appropriate weight maintenance.

Hormone replacement therapy to prevent osteoporosis remains controversial. Women who are postmenopausal should be encouraged to perform exercises and maintain calcium levels with supplements, or oral bisphosphonates may assist in preventing bone loss. Women should receive education by their health care providers on the options available.

The nurses in the presurgical clinic, the postanesthesia care unit, and the surgical unit, the home care nurse, and the skilled nursing facility all play a pivotal role in the care of the patient undergoing musculoskeletal surgery. The nurse who is knowledgeable about the patient's history, needs, preferences, and available resources is in a unique position to promote a positive surgical experience for the patient. Holistic and focused assessments and early intervention act to prevent postoperative complications and ensure that the patient receives prompt treatment to prevent permanent disability or prolonged rehabilitation times. A comprehensive knowledge of the potential complications associated with particular injuries and surgeries enables the nurse to focus on prevention and early detection of potential problems. The nurse who understands the importance of postoperative activities such as turning and positioning, exercise, and assessment of neurovascular status will provide vigilant care that assists the patient in achieving care goals. Through interaction with the patient in obtaining the history and assisting the patient with activities, the nurse can obtain data and utilize information to create and implement a plan of care specific to the patient as an individual.

Research

There are multiple opportunities for research available in the realm of musculoskeletal surgical complications and therapies.

It is an exciting time in nursing research, and important practice changes are beginning to rely on new evidence. Any of the questions listed in the Research Opportunities and Clinical Impact box lend themselves to study that may impact the future of orthopedic nursing care.

RESEARCH OPPORTUNITIES AND CLINICAL IMPACT RELATED TO MUSCULOSKELETAL SURGICAL PROCEDURES

Research Opportunities	Clinical Impact
Prophylactic antibiotic therapy is commonplace for orthopedic surgical procedures. Studies could be performed comparing the infection rates in low-risk patients, comparing the use of prophylactic antibiotics versus placebo.	Is the use of prophylactic antibiotic therapy necessary, or should it be reserved for patients who are at high risk of infection?
Which therapy is more effective in preventing deep venous thrombosis (DVT): sequential compression devices or elastic compression stockings? Many institutions utilize both. Is this overkill or an added expense? Research studies could compare the use of sequential compression devices alone versus the use of elastic compression stockings alone versus the use of both.	Possible cost savings for the institution and the patient.
Is there a difference in discharge date or ability to participate in postoperative activities in patients who receive regional/epidural anesthesia versus those who receive general anesthesia? Are there differences in the perceived ability to participate in postoperative activities between the two groups? Are there differences in the postoperative pain scores between the two groups? Is there a difference in the pain scores reported between patients receiving pain-controlled analgesia (PCA) versus those who received epidural anesthesia?	Possibility of decreased hospital stay for the patient.
Is there a difference in the range of motion, distance ambulated between patients who receive preoperative exercise counseling prior to elective joint replacement and those who do not?	Possibility of decreased hospital stay for the patient. Decreased rehabilitation time.

Clinical Preparation

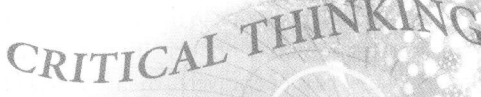

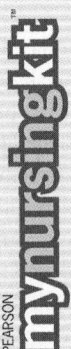

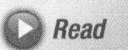 **Read**

- History of Current Illness
- Past Medical History
- Physical Exam
- Admitting Medical Orders
- Laboratory Study Results

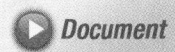 **Document**

- Summary of Hospitalization
- Pathophysiology Form
- Laboratory Values
- Laboratory Results Explanation

 **Apply**

- List of Potential Nursing Diagnoses
- Concept Map
- Critical Thinking Questions

Log on to MyNursingKit.com to download forms you will need and to complete further steps in the Clinical Preparation assignment.

HISTORY OF PRESENT ILLNESS

Mrs. T. is a 72-year-old patient who was admitted to the hospital for right total hip replacement. She has right hip osteoarthritis as the result of osteonecrosis secondary to prednisone use for polymyalgia rheumatica. She has painful right knee arthritis and end-stage right hip osteoarthritis not responding to conservative management and was scheduled for right total hip replacement. A posterior approach total hip replacement was performed under general anesthesia. Estimated blood loss during the procedure was 1,000 mL. Cell Saver was utilized during the procedure and shed blood returned to the patient as was planned preoperatively. The patient was sent to the recovery room in stable condition.

Medical–Surgical History

The patient has a history of hypertension, mild cardiovascular disease, obesity, polymyalgia rheumatica, and right knee arthritis. Her surgical history includes a hysterectomy at age 50 due to fibroid tumors, and removal of her gallbladder at age 35 due to gallstones.

Social History

Mrs. T. is a retired teacher who lives alone in a retirement community. She has two daughters and one son who all live in the area. She has never smoked and has a glass of wine each evening.

Physical Exam

You receive the patient on day 1 postoperatively from her right total hip replacement. She is awake, alert, and oriented. Her vital signs are within normal limits. Breath sounds are equal bilaterally, diminished at the bases with rales. Her abdomen is slightly distended, soft, nontender with minimal bowel sounds. The patient states that she has not passed flatus or had a bowel movement since the surgery. The patient has a Foley catheter that is draining clear, yellow urine. Motor and sensory of all extremities are intact. Her surgical site is clean, dry, and intact. She complains of pain to the right hip at a 6 on the scale of 1–10.

Admitting Medical Orders

Service: orthopedic surgery

Diagnosis: right hip replacement

Allergies: none

Vital signs: every 4 hours including oxygen saturation, and neurovascular checks to right lower extremity

Call house officer: temp > 38.5°C, HR > 110 or < 60, RR > 30 or < 12, BP sys > 160 or < 90, O_2 sat < 92%, urine output < 120 mL in 4 hours, change in neurovascular exam to right lower extremity, any Hct result that is 5 less than the baseline postoperative Hct

Activity: up to chair 4 times per day with assistance; ambulate with physical therapy twice daily

Posterior hip precautions:
- Hip abductor pillow while in bed
- Do not bend hip greater than 90 degrees
- Use an elevated toilet seat
- Do not sit in low chairs
- Do not twist or turn the body toward the operative side
- Do not turn leg and foot inward
- Keep operative leg straight when getting up and use your arms to push up

Diet: low-sodium, low-fat diet

IV: D5/.45NS with 20 mEq KCl IV at 100 mL/hr

Foley to gravity drainage

I&O: every shift

Respiratory care: use incentive spirometer hourly when awake

DVT prophylaxis: low-molecular-weight heparin, sequential compression devices to lower extremities

Scheduled Medications

Atenolol 50 mg po daily

Nifedipine 30 mg po daily

Lisinopril 10 mg po daily

Cefazolin sodium 1 g IV q8h for 6 doses

Enoxaparin 30 mg subcutaneously q12h

Oxycodone HCl 10 mg po q12h around the clock (hold for delirium)

Docusate sodium 100 mg po bid

PRN Medications

Magnesium hydroxide (laxative) oral 2,400 mg po prn

Morphine sulfate 1–3 mg IV q2h prn for severe pain

Metoclopramide hydrochloride (Reglan) 10 mg IV q6h prn for nausea and vomiting

Ordered Laboratory Studies

CBC and electrolyte panel every morning

LABORATORY STUDY RESULTS

Test	Preop	Postop, Immediate	Postop Day 1
WBC	8/mm³	12/mm³	9 K/mm³
RBC	4.55/mm³	4.27/mm³	4.30/mm³
Hemoglobin	11 g/dL	9.8 g/dL	9.5 g/dL
Hematocrit	32%	29%	28%
Platelet count	221/mm³	196/mm³	196/mm³
APTT	30 seconds	31 seconds	
INR	1.2	1.0	1.0
Sodium	135 mEq/L	140 mEq/L	138 mEq/L
Potassium	3.4 mEq/L	3.1 mEq/L	3.5 mEq/L
Chloride	102 mEq/L	105 mEq/L	103 mEq/L
Carbon dioxide	23 mEq/L	25 mEq/L	24 mEq/L
Urea nitrogen	11 mg/dL	12 mg/dL	12 mg/dL
Creatinine blood	0.8 mg/dL	1.0 mg/dL	1.0 mg/dL
Glucose	130 mg/dL	140 mg/dL	120 mg/dL
Calcium	8.1 mg/dL	8.1 mg/dL	8.3 mg/dL
Lipase	17 unit/dL	20 unit/dL	19 unit/dL

CRITICAL THINKING QUESTIONS

1. How can you distinguish the difference between expected postoperative pain and the pain caused by compartment syndrome?

2. What areas of assessment must be performed immediately upon a patient's admission to the nursing unit after orthopedic surgery?

3. What types of precautions are necessary for a patient who has had a total hip replacement?

4. How are pulmonary complications prevented during the postoperative period?
   What assessments and actions do you perform for a confused elderly postoperative patient?

Answers to Critical Thinking Questions appear in Appendix D.

NCLEX® REVIEW

1. A patient has undergone surgery for a fractured tibia. The nurse plans to complete a neurovascular assessment. Which of the following aspects will be included? Select all that apply.
   1. Pain level
   2. Pulse quality
   3. Sensation and movement
   4. Color of extremity
   5. Level of consciousness
   6. Use of muscles

2. A nurse is reviewing home care with a patient following a hip replacement procedure. Which of the following instructions would be included?
   1. Slightly bend the operative leg when getting up from the chair or bed.
   2. Exercise the affected extremity by turning the leg inward 5–10 times.
   3. Progressively increase the amount of bending at the waist daily.
   4. Use an elevated toilet seat in the main bathroom at home.

3. The nurse strongly suspects the occurrence of compartment syndrome in a patient wearing a long-leg cast. In preparation for the health care provider to come and perform the necessary treatment; the nurse would gather what supplies or equipment?
   1. Ace bandages to wrap around the bivalved cast
   2. Extra pillows to elevate the casted leg above the heart

3. Syringe, needle and topical anesthetic to aspirate the hematoma
4. A percussion hammer to physically assess reflexes for damage

4. Of the following assistive devices, which would be the most appropriate for home use for a patient who has undergone a total hip replacement procedure?
   1. Heel lift boot
   2. A "reacher" tool
   3. Continuous passive motion (CPM) machine
   4. Wheelchair

5. A nurse is serving as a preceptor for a new graduate on an orthopedic unit. As they enter a patient's room using patient's-controlled analgesia (PCA), the nurse states, "This pump is delivering a 2 mg basal rate of morphine sulfate, along with prn doses." The new graduate reflects understanding of the order through which statement?
   1. "The patient receives 2 mg of the drug when he pushes the delivery button."
   2. "Every hour 2 mg of morphine is delivered continuously."
   3. "The maximum amount of morphine to be received is 2 mg per hour."
   4. "The pump administers a beginning dose of 2 mg and increases the amount hourly."

Answers for review questions appear in Appendix D

KEY TERMS

amputation *p.1816*
arthrodesis *p.1821*
arthroplasty *p.1807*
compartment syndrome *p.1828*

continuous passive motion device *p.1826*
discectomy *p.1816*
fat embolus *p.1827*
heterotrophic ossification (HO) *p.1829*

laminectomy *p.1816*
osteolysis *p.1811*
osteonecrosis *p.1829*
total joint replacement *p.1807*

REFERENCES

American Academy of Orthopaedic Surgeons (AAOS). (2001). *Bunion surgery*. Retrieved May 28, 2008, from http://orthoinfo.aaos.org/topic.cfm?topic=A00140

American Academy of Orthopaedic Surgeons (AAOS). (2005). *Sprained ankle*. Retrieved May 27, 2008, from http://orthoinfo.aaos.org/topic.cfm?topic=A00150

American Academy of Orthopaedic Surgeons (AAOS). (2007a). *Rotator cuff tears*. Retrieved May 29, 2008, from http://orthoinfo.aaos.org/topic.cfm?topic=A00064

American Academy of Orthopaedic Surgeons (AAOS). (2007b). *Arthritis of the shoulder*. Retrieved May 30, 2008, from http://orthoinfo.aaos.org/topic.cfm?topic=A00222

American Academy of Orthopaedic Surgeons (AAOS). (2007c). *Osteoarthritis of the elbow*. Retrieved May 31, 2008, from http://orthoinfo.aaos.org/topic.cfm?topic=A00421

American Academy of Orthopaedic Surgeons (AAOS). (2007d). *Carpal tunnel syndrome*. Retrieved June 2, 2008, from http://orthoinfo.aaos.org/topic.cfm?topic=A00005#Anatomy

American Academy of Orthopaedic Surgeons (AAOS). (2007e). *Wrist joint replacement (wrist arthroplasty)*. Retrieved June 2, 2008, from http://orthoinfo.aaos.org/topic.cfm?topic=A00019

American Academy of Orthopaedic Surgeons (AAOS). (2007f). *ACL injury: Does it require surgery?* Retrieved June 2, 2008, from http://orthoinfo.aaos.org/topic.cfm?topic=A00297

Arthritis Foundation. (2008). *Arthritis and related diseases*. Retrieved August 29, 2008, from http://www.arthritis.org/faq.php

Edmonds, M. J., Crichton, T. J., Runciman, W. B., & Pradhan, M. (2004). Evidenced-based risk factors for postoperative deep vein thrombosis. *ANZ Journal of Surgery, 74*, 1082–1097.

eMedicineHealth. (2008). *Lumbar laminectomy*. Retrieved June 10, 2008, from http://www.emedicinehealth.com/lumbar_laminectomy/article_em.htm

eOrthopod. (2003). *Wrist anatomy*. Retrieved June 2, 2008, from http://www.eorthopod.com/public/patient_education/6607/wrist_anatomy.html

Folsom, A. R., Cushman, M., Tsai, M. Y., Aleksic, N., Heckbert, S. R., Boland, L. L., et al. (2002). A prospective study of venous thromboembolism in relation to Factor V Leiden and related factors. *Blood, 99*(8), 2720–2725.

Matson, F. A., III, & Warme, W. J. (2008). *Total shoulder joint replacement for shoulder arthritis: Surgery with a dependable, time-tested conservative prosthesis and accelerated rehabilitation can lessen pain and improve function in shoulders with arthritis*. Retrieved May 30, 2008, from http://www.orthop.washington.edu/uw/shoulderreplacement/tabID__3376/ItemID__62/Articles/Default.aspx

Ornstein, D. L., & Cushman, M. (2003). Factor V Leiden. *Circulation, 107*, e94–e97.

Wahl, C. J., & Slaney, S. L. (2005). *Arthroscopic shoulder surgery for shoulder dislocation, subluxation, and instability: Why, when and how it is done*. Retrieved May 30, 2008, from http://www.orthop.washington.edu/uw/arthroscopic/tabID__3376/ItemID__162/Articles/Default.aspx

Caring for the Patient with Arthritis and Connective Tissue Disorders

Kathy Riccosa

With contributions by:
Cheryl Wraa
Kathleen Osborn

Outcome-Based Learning Objectives

After studying this chapter, the learner will be able to:

1. Differentiate autoimmune disease from connective tissue disease.
2. Utilize the nursing process when planning care for each autoimmune disease.
3. Compare and contrast the etiology, pathophysiology, clinical manifestations, nursing management, and prevention of the various types of arthritis.
4. Identify the four highest priority nursing diagnoses for rheumatoid arthritis and osteoarthritis.
5. Describe nursing management for patients experiencing gout.
6. Compare and contrast the clinical manifestations and nursing management of each of the following connective tissue diseases: (a) myositis, (b) polymyositis, and (c) dermatomyositis.

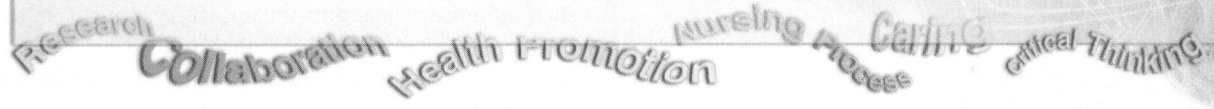

CONNECTIVE TISSUE consists of cells surrounded in an extracellular matrix of fibers, which serves to add strength and support, bind, and protect the various organs of the body. Three types of fibers make up the various connective tissues found in the body: collagen fibers, reticular fibers, and elastic fibers. Any inflammation of these tissues in joints can cause connective tissue disorders. Common connective tissue disorders include lupus erythematosus, gout, and Lyme disease. It is frequently very difficult to make a definitive diagnosis because signs and symptoms are often vague. It is projected that 37% of the population in the United States, or 1 million people, have a heritable connective tissue disorder (WrongDiagnosis.com, 2008). Connective tissue disorders are not just one disease, but a collection of more than 100 unique conditions that can destroy the connective tissue of the joints and have results ranging from daily pain to complete immobility.

Arthritis

Arthritis is a common descriptive term that applies to the collection of rheumatic diseases that can be localized, self-limiting conditions or systemic, autoimmune processes (Porth, 2005). It is estimated that by the year 2030, 67 million Americans 18 years of age and older will be diagnosed by a health care provider as having arthritis (Centers for Disease Control and Prevention [CDC], 2007).

Osteoarthritis: Epidemiology and Etiology

Osteoarthritis (OA), the most common form of arthritis, is a chronic condition that accompanies aging, most commonly affecting weight-bearing joints. OA is a leading cause of pain and disability in the elderly. Seventy percent of people age 40 and older and 80% of those age 65 and older are afflicted with this chronic condition (FamilyPracticeNotebook.com, 2008; Porth, 2005). Osteoarthritis (OA) was previously thought to be a normal consequence of aging; however, it is now realized that osteoarthritis results from a complex interplay of multiple factors, including joint integrity, genetic predisposition, local inflammation, mechanical forces, and cellular and biochemical processes. The disease can occur as a primary idiopathic disorder that is localized or generalized (involves more than three joints). Secondary OA is due to an underlying cause such as congenital defects of joint structure, single severe trauma or multiple traumas, inflammatory diseases, or metabolic disorders. The disease is usually diagnosed by an overall clinical impression based on the patient's age, history, findings on physical examination, and radiographic findings (Kalunian, 2007; Porth, 2005).

Pathophysiology

Joint degeneration with OA occurs on the articular surfaces of the cartilage with bony formations at the edges of weight-bearing joints, such as the knees and hips. OA also involves the joints of the fingers at the proximal interphalangeal joints (Figure 58–1 ■), and can affect the wrists, elbows, ankles, spinal vertebrae and joints of the pelvis. OA results in significant changes in both the composition and the mechanical properties of cartilage. Early in the disease the cartilage contains more water and fewer concentrations of proteoglycans, the large molecules that afford elasticity and stiffness and allow cartilage to

resist compression. There is also a decrease in local synthesis of new collagen and an increase in the breakdown of existing collagen. It is thought that the changes are a result of the release of cytokines that stimulate production and the release of enzymes that are destructive to joint structures. This damage predisposes the cartilage tissue to more injury and impairs the cells' ability to repair the damage by producing new collagen and proteoglycans (Porth, 2005).

Clinical Manifestations

Patients will complain of a brief interval of morning stiffness, pain on motion with overuse of affected joint, and over time the possibility of joint bone deformity (FamilyPracticeNotebook.com, 2008). Joints most frequently affected are the knees, hips, cervical and lumbar vertebrae, proximal and distal joints of the hand, and the first metatarsophalangeal joints of the feet (Porth, 2005).

Laboratory and Diagnostic Procedures

According to the Hospital for Special Surgery (2005) three different radiologic techniques are used to determine the diagnosis of arthritis: plain radiographs of the affected joint, computed tomography (CT), and magnetic resonance imaging (MRI). See the Diagnostic Tests box for these diagnostic tests as well as the radiologic tests used to identify OA and the expected abnormalities that would be found.

Medical Management

Initially, the best treatment for weight-bearing joints is rest. As the condition becomes more progressive, then nonsteroidal anti-inflammatory agents may be taken to alleviate discomfort of the affected joints. Medications used would include classifications such as nonsteroidal anti-inflammatory drugs (NSAIDs), cyclooxygenase-2 (COX-2) inhibitors, and antimalarials to relieve symptoms. The Pharmacology Summary feature on page 1839 outlines medications used to treat arthritis and connective tissue disorders. A multidisciplinary approach may include a nutritionist to help with weight reduction and a physical therapist to develop an exercise program to include range-of-motion exercises.

Once the patient exhausts previous options and the patient's quality of life is further compromised, surgical intervention

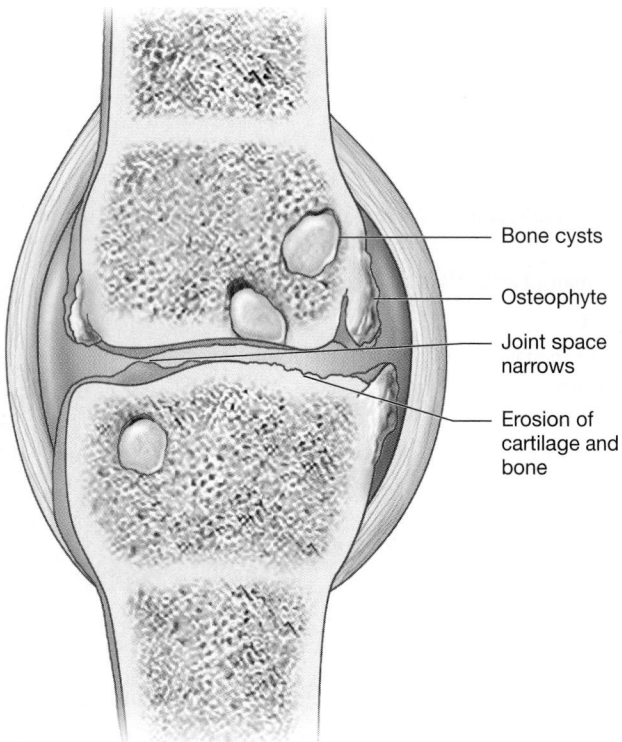

Bone cysts

Osteophyte

Joint space narrows

Erosion of cartilage and bone

FIGURE 58–1 ■ Joint degeneration with OA.

DIAGNOSTIC TESTS for Osteoarthritis

Test	Expected Abnormality	Rationale for Abnormality
DIAGNOSTIC TEST		
Bone density	Increased. Asymmetrical joint cartilage loss.	Subchondral sclerosis. Confirmation of bone on bone contact.
Erythrocyte sedimentation rate (ESR)	Increased.	Presence of inflammatory disease.
Rheumatoid factor	Negative.	No rheumatoid arthritis.
RADIOLOGIC TEST		
X-ray	Degenerative changes. Narrowing of bone space.	Articular surfaces are worn where bone rubs against bone.
Computed tomography (CT)	Bone spurs.	Bone cyst and sclerosis are common with disease progression.
Magnetic resonance imaging (MRI)	Reactive bone edema. Soft tissue swelling. Bone fragments within the joint.	Very sensitive test to bony and soft tissue changes. Able to identify early degenerative changes.

should be considered. There are three kinds of surgical procedures that can improve the health of patients suffering from osteoarthritis: synovectomy, arthrodesis, and reconstructive surgery. A synovectomy is the removal of the swollen synovial casing prior to damage to the bone and cartilage taking place. Fusion of the joint is called arthrodesis. An arthrodesis is done when there is severe destruction of the surfaces of the joint. Joint replacements, usually total knee or total hips, are done when these weight-bearing joints have been completely damaged. It is important that the patient be aware of options in order to make an informed decision about the care received. For a detailed discussion regarding orthopedic surgery, refer to Chapter 57 .

■ Nursing Management

The nursing process provides a framework to create a comprehensive plan of care for the patient with OA. The nursing process will lead the nurse in utilizing the problem-solving approach in caring for patients with OA. The nurse begins with the general assessment and then concentrates on the clinical manifestations specifically related to OA.

Assessment

When assessing the patient with osteoarthritis, subjective symptoms include pain, tenderness in joints, fatigue, generalized weakness, anorexia, cold intolerance, and parasthesia. Objective symptoms include joint changes such as being enlarged, limited movement, stiffness, swelling, redness, localized heat around the joint, shiny stretched skin over and around the joint, and **subcutaneous nodules**. Other objective assessments are weight loss, elevated temperature, crepitus of joints, deformities or contractures, and cold and clammy extremities. Decreased hemoglobin and elevated white blood count (WBC) could support the diagnosis of osteoarthritis.

Nursing Diagnoses

For the patient with OA, the following are the highest priority nursing diagnoses. Based on these nursing diagnoses, plans and expected outcomes can be generated.

1. *Pain, Chronic* related to bone rubbing against bone, inflammation, or deformity
2. *Mobility: Physical, Impaired* related to stiffness
3. *Falls, Risk for* related to malaise and weakness
4. *Body Image, Disturbed* related to arthritic changes in joints
5. *Readiness for Enhanced Self-Care* related to inability to perform activities of daily living independently
6. *Imbalanced Nutrition: More than Body Requirements* related to obesity
7. *Powerlessness* related to changes in disease process, financial status, and role of the family.

Planning

The interdisciplinary team is critical to the success of treating the patient with OA because the collaborative method will provide assistance to the patient in a holistic approach. Based on the degree and severity of symptoms, the nurse should assist the patient with comfort, exercise, and pharmacologic therapies to reduce pain with a variety of medication choices, such as nonsteroidal anti-inflammatory drugs (NSAIDs). Discussing other options will be helpful in regard to surgical intervention to ease discomfort and improve mobility. See the Gerontological Considerations box on page 1836 for additional information.

Outcomes and Evaluation Parameters

The desired outcomes for the patient with OA include control of pain and stiffness, maintenance of quality of life, and ability to perform self-care activities. Evaluation parameters include the patient's expression that the pain is controlled, the patient reports no falls, and the patient is able to perform daily self-care activities.

Interventions and Rationales

With OA, pain relief from spasms, inflammation, or swelling is of the highest priority. Medications are instituted to help with the relief of the symptoms. The nurse needs to teach the patient to read the adverse effects of the medication and take precautions to prevent gastrointestinal upset, such as having food in one's stomach before taking the drug. See the Pharmacology Summary feature on page 1839 for specific drugs for treating OA.

Nonpharmacologic interventions include the use of heat to reduce muscle spasms and cold to reduce inflammation and pain. In addition, there are multiple alternative therapies, as described in the Complementary and Alternative Therapies box (p. 1836). For the prevention of contractures, the patient should be active in exercise, sleep on a firm mattress, and use splints to maintain alignment. Elevation of the extremity and rest will reduce swelling, and splints will maintain alignment to prevent contractures. A physical activity program should range from passive and active range of motion to swimming, which is critical in minimizing the complications of immobility. Also, the use of splints and/or supportive devices may be useful in maintaining alignment and promoting function.

If a patient is at risk for falls, it is critical that that be identified on admission. A fall protocol should be implemented with frequent observation of the patient, toileting often, offering nourishments, and responding quickly to the patient call light. Review the hospital's policy and procedure to ensure patient safety. This practice will assist in keeping the patient safe while hospitalized. The family should also be made aware of the risk and taught how to keep the patient safe while at home, such as by removing scatter rugs, removing clutter, and providing assistance when the patient is ambulatory.

If the patient is unable to perform activities of daily living, there might be issues related to care. Encourage the patient to be as independent as possible, and offer assistance when needed. Provide support and positive feedback each time the patient makes an effort to perform activities.

Managing weight loss can be challenging. Consulting a nutritionist will help provide a low-calorie, balanced, appealing diet plan to reduce weight. It is important to realize that weight reduction is a slow process, and weight loss may take a long period of time depending on the amount the patient needs to lose. Incorporate ethnic foods when possible.

As a person loses function, powerlessness may follow. Empowerment is critical to the patient's well-being. Encourage the patient to verbalize any concerns, and listen actively. Utilize reflective communication, as it will assist the patient to discover how best to function. In fact, it is important to encourage the patient to be as independent as possible and be proud of accomplishments made. Because OA is a chronic disease, discharge instructions are important to ensure compliance with the health care plan. For more details, see the Patient Teaching & Discharge Priorities box for the patient with osteoarthritis.

Evaluation

Explore the implications of having this debilitating disease and its effects on the patient's life, such as living with pain and creating an environment where the patient is safe. Encourage weight reduction in patients who are obese as well as promoting exercise. Promote independence and offer assistance when needed. Allow the patient to become empowered to take control by keeping informed about the latest therapeutic, pharmacologic, and surgical interventions.

Rheumatoid Arthritis: Epidemiology and Etiology

Rheumatoid arthritis (RA) is a chronic inflammatory process that affects the peripheral joints and surrounding muscles, liga-

GERONTOLOGICAL CONSIDERATIONS

Because a large number of baby boomers are reaching an average age of 55 and older, and obesity continues to increase, it seems likely that more patients will be experiencing osteoarthritis and become inactive because it is difficult to move. Teaching health promotion is critical to maintaining well-being: Diet and exercise should be the priorities of education.

ments, tendons, and blood vessels. It is thought to be an autoimmune disorder that not only involves tissue hypersensitivity but also has a genetic component. Antiglobulin antibodies combine with immunoglobulin in the synovial fluid and form complexes. Neutrophils are then attracted to the joint space and cause destruction.

RA most commonly affects women between ages 20 and 40, and is present in 2% to 3% of the population. One out of every 6 people, or 2.1 million Americans, have RA (InnerVibrance, 2006). As the baby boomers age, it is estimated that 60 million people will be affected with RA by the year 2020 (InnerVibrance, 2006). RA is noted worldwide as affecting three times more women than men, although it can occur at any age, with the peak incidence being between ages 25 and 55 (Frazier & Drzymkowski, 2009).

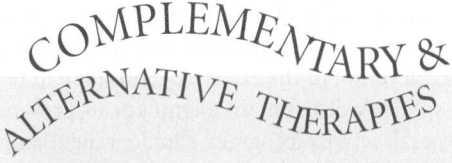

COMPLEMENTARY & ALTERNATIVE THERAPIES for Osteoarthritis and Rheumatoid Arthritis

Description:
Some conditions have shown improvement from many different CAM therapies. Therefore, nurses would be remiss to recommend only one CAM therapy to their patients. Osteoarthritis (OA) and rheumatoid arthritis (RA) are conditions for which multiple approaches have benefit.

Research Support:
A study by an English research team aimed to better understand CAM use among patients with RA. The researchers identified three goals of the study: to assess the impact of a patient's use of CAM therapy on the patient's perspective of health and well-being, to understand why a patient chooses a CAM therapy, and to learn which forms of CAM therapies were most commonly used by patients. Researchers found that the most commonly used CAM therapies were herbal remedies and supplements, and aromatherapy massage. Results showed that, compared to conventional treatments, CAM therapies had advantages due to a lower incidence of adverse reactions, greater patient choice, psychological comfort, and an increased quality in the patient–therapist relationship. Researchers concluded that the high incidence of CAM use by patients with RA indicates a need for more evidence-based information about its use and safety (Rose, 2006).

Guided imagery with relaxation (GIR) is a commonly used CAM therapy by patients with OA. A randomized pilot study tested the effect of GIR on health-related quality of life in women with OA. Study participants used GIR for 12 weeks. Results showed that GIR significantly increased participants' health-related quality of life in comparison to the control group (Baird & Sands, 2006). Results of other studies suggest that acupuncture, several herbal medicines, and capsaicin cream have an encouraging risk-benefit profile (Ernst, 2006).

Another study assessed the Benson Relaxation Technique (BRT) used concurrently with medication to determine its effect on disease activity in patients with RA. The experimental group received BRT combined with medication and the control group received medication only. The two groups showed a significant difference in anxiety, depression, and feeling of well-being. Although the two groups' clinical symptoms and laboratory findings were not statistically significant, they did indicate a decline in disease progress. Researchers concluded that BRT can be an effective technique in improving symptoms in patients with RA (Bagheri-Nesami, Mohseni-Bandpei, & Shayesteh-Azar, 2006). Another study examined the impact of a nurse-led rheumatology clinic on patients with RA. Researchers concluded that such clinics can be not only a source for empowering patients with RA to adopt new stances to alternative actions, but they can also help patients achieve a higher level of faith in their own abilities (Arvidsson et al., 2006).

References
Arvidsson, S. B., Petersson, A., Nilsson, I., Andersson, B., Arvidsson, B. I., Petersson, I. F., et al. (2006). A nurse-led rheumatology clinic's impact on empowering patients with rheumatoid arthritis: A qualitative study. *Nursing and Health Sciences, 8*(3), 133–139.

Bagheri-Nesami, M., Mohseni-Bandpei, M. A., & Shayesteh-Azar, M. (2006). The effect of Benson Relaxation Technique on rheumatoid arthritis patients: Extended report. *International Journal of Nurse Practitioners, 12*(4), 214–219.

Baird, C. L., & Sands, L. P. (2006). Effect of guided imagery with relaxation on health-related quality of life in older women with osteoarthritis. *Research in Nursing and Health, 29*(5), 442–451.

Ernst, E. (2006). Complementary or alternative therapies for osteoarthritis. *Nature Clinical Practice Rheumatology, 2*(2), 74–80.

Rose, G. (2006). Why do patients with rheumatoid arthritis use complementary therapies? *Musculoskeletal Care, 4*(2), 101–115.

PATIENT TEACHING & DISCHARGE PRIORITIES for Osteoarthritis

Need	Teaching
Because the joints affected are weight bearing, it is important not to contribute to stress of those joints by additional weight.	Encourage patients who are obese to reduce weight.
Increase mobility.	Promote the patient to participate in an exercise program (stretching, passive and active range of motion, swimming, t'ai chi)
Maintain range of motion.	
Do not exacerbate symptoms.	
Joint protection.	Modify work or home environment to accommodate limited weight bearing.
Reduce pain and avoid complications of drug therapy.	Pharmacologic therapy: Teach about each drug classification, how to take the medication, drug interactions, adverse effects, and reporting any complications to health care provider.

Pathophysiology

RA begins with an inflammatory process in the synovial membrane and joint capsule with swelling causing the infiltration of lymphocytes, macrophages, and neutrophils that perpetuate the inflammatory response. These cells produce enzymes that cause the destruction of cartilage, which then becomes fibrous, causing calcification of the fibrous tissue (InnerVibrance, 2006). The inflammatory response has four signs: redness, heat, swelling, and pain. In some RA patients, pannus (development of an extensive network of new blood vessels in the synovial membrane that is destructive) is experienced (Figure 58–2 ■). Pannus is a feature that differentiates RA from other forms of inflammatory arthritis (Porth, 2005).

Clinical Manifestations

An assessment is critical in making a diagnosis of RA. Assessment of the joints is to observe inflammation and deformity in affected joints. With RA, patients experience remissions and ex-acerbations of the disease. Remissions are periods of time that the disease process is inactive, and exacerbations are flare-ups or when the disease becomes active. During exacerbations, patients may experience the following: fatigue, low-grade fever, anorexia, joint pain and swelling due to inflammation, and symmetrical joint deformity. Most often the joints of the hands are affected (MedicineNet.com, 2008a).

RA not only affects the joints but also may affect organs of the entire body. Glands may become swollen, and the patient's mouth may become dry. Other organs affected may include the lungs, blood, and spleen. RA can cause rheumatoid nodules in the lungs, causing pleuritis. There is a decrease of red blood cells, causing anemia, and a decrease of white blood cells due to spleen enlargement (MedicineNet.com, 2008a). Frequently, vasculitis may occur, which results in an impairment of blood supply and potentially causes necrosis of tissues of the nail beds and dermal ulcers (MedicineNet.com, 2008a).

Laboratory and Diagnostic Procedures

Diagnostic imaging is important for patients to undergo to determine the presence and severity of rheumatoid arthritis (MedicineNet.com, 2008a). The Diagnostic Tests box (p. 1838) outlines the laboratory and diagnostic tests commonly used to diagnose rheumatoid arthritis.

Medical Management

RA is a chronic condition without a cure. However, certain measures are used to control this disease and treat symptoms, such as pain control, maintaining joint function, reducing damage to joints and reducing deformity (MedicineNet.com, 2008a). Early intervention will improve outcomes, so patients should be seen as soon as possible to reduce complications. Treatment includes the following: pharmacologic interventions, rest, exercises, safeguarding joints, and patient teaching. Sometimes it is more effective to use a blend of medications to treat the discomfort associated with RA such as NSAIDs and corticosteroids. Other drugs may be considered based on the patient's severity of disease and the response to the disease. Common medications given would include antineoplastics (methotrexate) or antimalarials (Plaquenil). Patient education regarding medication should include information about its actions, adverse effects, and interactions with food or other medications in order to ensure proper medication administration. Some of these medications are long acting, and the patient

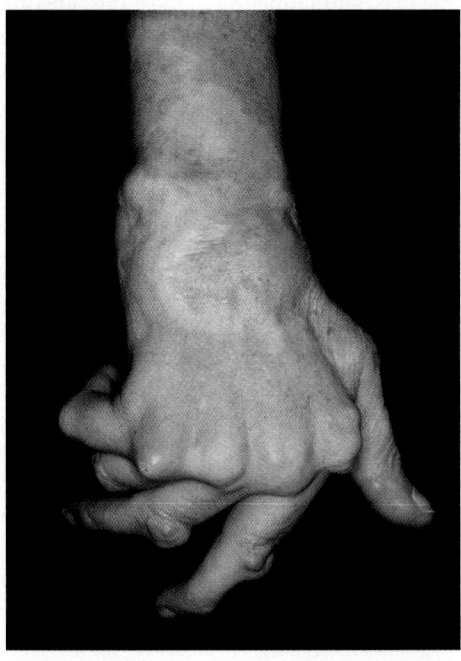

FIGURE 58–2 ■ In some RA patients, pannus (development of an extensive network of new blood vessels in the synovial membrane that is destructive) is experienced.
Source: Princess Margaret Rose Orthopaedic Hospital/Photo Researchers, Inc.

DIAGNOSTIC TESTS for Rheumatoid Arthritis

Test	Expected Abnormality	Rationale for Abnormality
LABORATORY TEST		
Rheumatoid factor	Positive or can be negative	Indicates presence or absence of rheumatoid arthritis (RA)
Anticitrulline antibody	Positive	Indicates presence of RA in the absence of rheumatoid factor
Antinuclear antibodies	Positive	Indicates presence of RA
Sedimentation rate	Increased	Presence of inflammation in joints
DIAGNOSTIC TEST X-ray	Abnormal joint space with erosion of articular surface	Presence of RA in affected joints

needs to be compliant and take the medications as directed to maximize their effect. See the Pharmacology Summary of Medications used to treat arthritis and connective tissue disorders feature.

Nursing Management

The nursing process provides a framework to create a comprehensive plan of care for the patient with RA. The nursing process will lead the nurse in utilizing the problem-solving approach in caring for patients with RA. The nurse begins with the general assessment and then concentrates on the clinical manifestations specifically related to RA. Nursing management for the patient with RA also includes education to assist the patient with progression of the disease and maintenance of quality of life.

Assessment

During a subjective assessment, the patient may complain of joint stiffness, pain, and swelling. Also, there may be complaints of being tired and fatigued. Some patients experience weight loss due to anorexia. An objective assessment includes subcutaneous nodules over bony prominences and symmetrical, bilateral involvement of joints, which can cause creaking or crackling in the affected joints called crepitus. Over time, some patients experience contractures and muscle atrophy.

Nursing Diagnoses

The highest priority nursing diagnoses for the patient with RA are:

1. *Pain, Chronic* related to bone rubbing against bone, inflammation, or deformity
2. *Mobility: Impaired Physical* related to stiffness
3. *Falls, Risk for* related to malaise and weakness
4. *Body Image, Disturbed* related to arthritic changes in joints
5. *Activity Intolerance* related to fatigue
6. *Self-Care, Readiness for Enhanced* related to inability to perform activities of daily living independently
7. *Nutrition: Imbalanced, Less than Body Requirement* related to anorexia
8. *Powerlessness* related to changes in disease process, financial status, or role of the family

Planning

During the planning stage, goals are to prevent contractures/deformities and provide health teaching. A multidisciplinary team is critical for the success of treating a patient with RA. Health care team members would include health care providers, nursing staff, occupational therapists, physical therapists, and dietitians. Collaborative and coordinated care is essential for the patient to meet both short- and long-term goals.

Outcomes and Evaluation Parameters

The desired outcomes for the patient with RA include control of pain and stiffness, maintenance of patient's quality of life, and ability to perform self-care activities. Evaluation parameters include the patient's expression that the pain is controlled, the patient reports no falls, and the patient is able to perform daily self-care activities.

Interventions and Rationales

Maintaining joint mobility is critical. Active range of motion may promote maximum function in the joints. Encouraging patients to participate in passive range of motion also encourages independence and active patient participation to promote independence. Water exercise works well with this disease as it allows the body to move easily and does not put stress on the joints. Therefore, the patient will be able to optimize joint function.

For RA it is necessary to provide rest during times when the disease process flares up. Encourage the patient to perform active range of motion, as well as providing passive range of motion to prevent contractures. Provide scheduled activities with planned rest periods to prevent fatigue. Offer heat to reduce the inflammatory process and encourage motion. Offer medications to control pain, such as nonsteroidal anti-inflammatory drugs, corticosteroids, high dosages of acetylsalicylic acid, or narcotics.

This debilitating disease causes visible deformities most often in the hands. Patients may experience issues with the appearance evident with body changes and limited movement. The nurse needs to provide an atmosphere in which a rapport can be built with the patient. Time must be made for the patient to feel comfortable to verbalize feelings or concerns by listening actively. Assist the patient in making realistic short- and long-term goals; support the patient by providing referrals to local chapters of the American Arthritis Association and other organizations.

PHARMACOLOGY Summary of Medications Used to Treat Arthritis and Connective Tissue Disorders

Medication Category	Action	Application/Indication	Nursing Responsibility
Nonsteroidal Anti-Inflammatory Drugs Ibuprofen (Motrin, Advil) Diclofenac (Voltaren) Naproxen (Naprosyn)	Exerts anti-inflammatory, analgesic action by inhibition of prostaglandin synthesis; antipyretic effects by action on hypothalamus.	Rheumatoid arthritis, osteoarthritis, mild to moderate pain. Off-label use: psoriatic arthritis, systemic lupus.	• Monitor for adverse effects: nausea, vomiting, diarrhea, constipation, blurred vision, and tinnitus. • Monitor for exacerbation in patients with asthma or existing renal, liver, or hematopoietic dysfunction. • Be aware of multiple drug interactions (aminoglycosides, anticoagulants, beta-blockers, and others). • Warn patient that alcohol and smoking increase incidence of gastrointestinal (GI) bleeding. • Be aware of increased risk of myocardial infarction, stroke, and cardiovascular thrombosis, especially in the presence of existing cardiovascular disease.
Cyclooxygenase-2 (COX-2) Inhibitor Celecoxib (Celebrex)	Exerts anti-inflammatory, analgesic, and antipyretic effects by inhibiting prostaglandin synthesis.	Rheumatoid arthritis, osteoarthritis, ankylosing spondylitis, postoperative pain.	• Monitor for adverse effects: dyspepsia, abdominal pain, nausea, and headache. • Monitor for signs of hepatotoxicity (nausea, vomiting, itching, abdominal pain), and GI bleeding (tarry stools, upper GI distress). • Be aware of drug interactions (diuretics, aminoglycosides, warfarin, angiotensin-converting enzyme [ACE] inhibitors, and others). • Monitor for altered drug efficacy or toxicity. • Monitor hematocrit (HCT), hemoglobin (Hgb), electrolytes, and liver and renal function. • Be aware of increased risk of myocardial infarction, stroke, and cardiovascular thrombosis, especially in the presence of existing cardiovascular disease. • Give 2 hours before or after antacids.
Disease-Modifying Antirheumatic Drugs (DMARDs): **Antineoplastic** Methotrexate (MTX, Rheumatrex)	Exerts immunosuppressive effect by inhibiting T lymphocytes and depleting folate needed for DNA, RNA, and protein synthesis.	Severe, disabling rheumatoid arthritis. Off-label use: psoriatic arthritis, systemic lupus.	• Monitor for adverse effects: headache, rash, nausea, vomiting, diarrhea, stomatitis, and alopecia. • Observe for signs of severe adverse effects: bone marrow suppression; liver, lung, kidney, or GI toxicities. Monitor complete blood count (CBC), renal and hepatic function, metabolic profile, and chest x-ray at regularly scheduled intervals. • Be aware of multiple drug interactions (acetylsalicylic acid [ASA], NSAIDs, digoxin, phenytoin, and others). Observe for altered drug efficacy or toxicity. • Advise patient of increased toxicity with alcohol and caffeine consumption. Contact health care provider before using over-the-counter (OTC) drugs. • Warn patient of photosensitivity and to use sun block.

(continued)

PHARMACOLOGY Summary of Medications Used to Treat Arthritis and Connective Tissue Disorders—*Continued*

Medication Category	Action	Application/Indication	Nursing Responsibility
Immunosuppressants Cyclosporine (Sandimmune, Neoral) Mycophenolate (CellCept) Azathioprine (Imuran)	Suppresses immune response by inhibiting lymphocyte replication or disrupting helper T cells.	Treatment of rheumatoid arthritis unresponsive to conventional therapy, systemic lupus.	• Monitor for adverse effects: hirsutism, hypertension, nausea, vomiting, and infection. • Observe for signs of toxicity: tremors, seizures, altered mental status, visual disturbances, nephrotoxicity, and neurotoxicity. • Monitor CBC, magnesium, potassium, blood sugar, liver, and renal function tests. • Be aware of multiple drug interactions (digoxin, NSAIDs, erythromycin, verapamil, cimetidine, allopurinol, and others). Monitor for altered drug levels, nephrotoxicity, or leukopenia.
Cyclophosphamide (Cytoxan)	Blocks DNA, RNA, and protein synthesis.	Off-label use: treatment of severe rheumatoid arthritis.	• Monitor for adverse effects: dizziness, nausea, vomiting, alopecia, hyperkalemia, and hyponatremia. • Monitor for severe adverse effects: leukopenia, pulmonary emboli, interstitial pulmonary fibrosis, nephrotoxicity, and hemorrhagic cystitis. • Monitor leukocyte and platelet counts, HCT, electrolytes, and renal function including urinalysis.
Sulfonamide Antibiotic Sulfasalazine (Azulfidine)	Reduces inflammation by decreasing production of arachidonic acid metabolites.	First line treatment for rheumatoid arthritis.	• Monitor for adverse effects: rash, headache, nausea, vomiting, and bloody diarrhea. • Observe for serious adverse effects (bone marrow suppression, hepatitis). Monitor CBC, and renal and liver function tests.
Tumor Necrosis Factor (TNF) Inhibitors Etanercept (Enbrel) Infliximab (Remicade)	Reduces inflammation by preventing TNF mediated cellular response.	Rheumatoid arthritis management, psoriatic arthritis, ankylosing spondylitis.	• Monitor for adverse effects: infection, nausea, headache, and injection/infusion site reactions. • Monitor for signs of severe adverse effects: blood dyscrasia, demyelinating diseases, sepsis, especially in poorly controlled diabetes and other predisposing diseases. • Monitor CBC, chest x-ray, urinalysis, and C-reactive protein. • Be aware of drug interactions (methotrexate, azathiopine, leflunomide, and others). Monitor for increased risk of blood dyscrasia.
Antimalarials Hydroxychloroquine (Plaquenil) Chloroquine (Aralen) Quinacrine	Exerts anti-inflammatory effect by inhibiting prostaglandin synthesis.	Treatment of rheumatoid arthritis.	• Monitor for adverse effects: hypotension, nausea, diarrhea, pruritus, irritability, headaches, weakness, hair loss, or bleaching. • Monitor electrocardiogram (ECG), CBC, and liver and kidney function. • Observe for potential exacerbation of disease when given in presence of blood, liver, GI, or neurological disorders. • Monitor for irreversible retinal damage. Warn patient of importance of regular eye exams. • Be aware of multiple drug interactions (antacids, cimetidine, methotrexate, and others). • Give with food to decrease adverse GI effects.

PHARMACOLOGY Summary of Medications Used to Treat Arthritis and Connective Tissue Disorders—*Continued*

Medication Category	Action	Application/Indication	Nursing Responsibility
Glucocorticoids			
Prednisone (Meticortin) Prednisolone (Delta-Cortef)	Anti-inflammatory, immunosuppressant activities due to inhibition of prostaglandin synthesis, histamine release, and phagocyte and lymphocyte function.	Acute exacerbation of rheumatoid arthritis, pulse therapy.	• Monitor for adverse effects: mood swings, anxiety, insomnia, nausea, vomiting, weight gain, acne, and delayed wound healing. • Observe for increased risk of GI bleeding and, in rheumatoid arthritis patients, pneumonia. • Monitor blood count, glucose, and electrolytes. • Be aware of drug interactions (theophylline, warfarin, and others). Monitor for toxicity or decreased efficacy. • Warn patient of potential need for dose adjustment if ill or if stress increases. Do not abruptly stop drug.
Chelating Agent			
D-penicillamine	Antirheumatic effect likely due to inhibition of collagen formation and depression of immunoglobin M (IgM), rheumatoid factor, and immune complexes.	Rheumatoid arthritis. Off-label use: scleroderma.	• Monitor for adverse effects: rash, pruritus, fever, arthralgia, nausea, vomiting, abdominal pain, and diarrhea. • Monitor for severe adverse effects: ptosis, diplopia (myasthenia gravis syndrome), exertional dyspnea, cough, wheezing (bronchiolitis obliterans), hematuria, proteinuria (nephritic syndrome), or decreased platelets or leukocytes (bone marrow depression). • Observe for reactivation of previous peptic ulcer, hepatic dysfunction, or pancreatitis. • Monitor CBC and urine tests monthly. • Give 1 hour before or 2 hours after eating. Avoid antacids or iron preparations. • Advise patient to increase fluid intake.

Because many of the patients with RA are young, surgical intervention may be appropriate when dialoguing about different treatment options for maintaining or improving the quality of life. Surgical treatment options for those with RA such as the following may be discussed: synovectomy, arthrodesis, and/or reconstructive surgery. Information is critical when considering all of the alternatives for treatment. Because this is a chronic disease, discussing discharge priorities is essential. For more information, see the Patient Teaching & Discharge Priorities box (p. 1842) about rheumatoid arthritis.

Evaluation

When evaluating the patient's status, the goal is to have the patient become as independent as possible by having minimal loss of mobility and increased ability to perform the activities of daily living. The installation of safety devices in the home, such as guardrails in the bathrooms and shower areas will assist the patient in living independently, as well as in gaining confidence in his abilities. The patient is to remain adverse-effect free from the use of medications to treat this disease. Finally, if there is no sign of recovery, provide the patient with information on ways to have the best quality of life possible using adaptive equipment or information regarding joint surgery. Examine the ability to

continue working or the ideas of retirement, financial status, and changes in the role of the family.

Health Promotion

Health teaching should include education regarding the adverse effects of NSAIDs because gastrointestinal upset, as well as gastric bleeding, is common. Signs of gastric bleeding are black tarry stools.

 Ringing in the ears (tinnitus) is a toxic side effect of aspirin use. Be sure to monitor these adverse effects with patients taking a high dosage of aspirin.

Encourage patients to remain as independent as possible. This is achieved by using assistive devices such as splints, walkers, or canes for performing activities of daily living and ambulation. Encourage patients to pace activities with rest in order to prevent fatigue. Teach patients to use body mechanics for body posture. Allow patients to verbalize frustrations and encourage them to adapt to their disabilities. Self-determination should also be encouraged to achieve the highest level of function with the patient with rheumatoid arthritis. Knowledge is power when making critical decisions about all types of treatment choices. See the Gerontological Considerations box on page 1842 for more information.

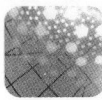

PATIENT TEACHING & DISCHARGE PRIORITIES for Rheumatoid Arthritis

Need	Teaching
Pain control	Teach the patient about medications that assist the patient's pain.
Maintaining joint function	Active range of motion.
	Passive range of motion.
	Gentle exercise, such as swimming or moving joints in a Jacuzzi.
Rest	Alternate activities with period of rest.
	Elevate affected joint to optimize circulation.

GERONTOLOGICAL CONSIDERATIONS for Rheumatoid Arthritis

Rheumatoid arthritis is a debilitating condition that affects the whole person. The goal of treatment is to treat the patient holistically and attempt to control the signs and symptoms of the disorder. The patient's safety is critical and assisting her with activities of daily living is important while maintaining her dignity. Families may need to be involved in caregiving as a patient becomes incapacitated.

Psoriatic Arthritis: Epidemiology and Etiology

Psoriatic arthritis is an inflammatory process associated with psoriasis. For a detailed explanation of psoriasis, refer to Chapter 66 ⊙. Initially psoriatic arthritis was considered a variant of rheumatoid arthritis, but it is now recognized as a distinct clinical entity (Gladman, 2007).

Psoriatic arthritis does not favor either gender. Among patients with psoriasis, estimates of prevalence vary from 4% to 6% up to 30% (Gladman, 2007). Psoriatic arthritis carries an incidence of approximately 6 per 100,000 per year, and a prevalence of approximately 1 to 2 per 1,000 (Gladman, 2007). The exact cause of psoriatic arthritis and of psoriasis itself is not known. It is thought that certain genetic, immunologic, and environmental factors contribute to the disease. It is known that psoriasis occurs in families, with approximately 40% of patients having a family history of the disease in first-degree relatives (Gladman, 2007).

Psoriatic arthritis had not been considered an autoimmune disease, but a number of immune abnormalities have been identified in patients with psoriasis and psoriatic arthritis. Included are:

- Elevated serum levels of immunoglobulins and antinuclear antibodies.
- T cell expression of HLA-DR molecules and receptors for interleukin-2 with a variety of adhesion molecules and the secretion of proinflammatory cytokines.
- Fibroblasts from the synovium show enhanced proliferative activity and platelet-derived growth factors (Gladman, 2007).

Environmental factors that have been associated with the development of psoriasis and psoriatic arthritis include both bacterial and viral infections, and trauma (Gladman, 2007). Patients that develop psoriatic arthritis have given a history of trauma to that joint prior to the onset of the disease. It is not clear how the trauma is related to psoriatic arthritis.

Pathophysiology

Psoriatic arthritis is an autoimmune disease with a known human leukocyte antigen (HLA)–associated risk factor. Psoriatic arthritis affects the ligaments, tendons, fascia, and joints. This disease occasionally develops even in the absence of detectable psoriasis. Psoriatic arthritis may occur at higher frequencies when skin involvement is more severe, especially when pustular psoriasis is present; however, recent studies suggest that this may not be valid (Hammadi, 2008).

Clinical Manifestations

Patients present with pain and stiffness in the affected joints. The stiffness worsens with prolonged immobility and is alleviated with physical activity. The affected joints will be tender, painful when the joint is stressed, and present with effusions. Most frequently the patients present with polyarthritis, followed by oligoarthritis. Distal arthritis and arthritis mutilans are considered most specific for psoriatic arthritis (Gladman, 2008). Other common features include soft tissue inflammation at the site of tendon insertion into the bone of the Achilles tendon, the plantar fascia, and the pelvic bones; tenosynovitis of the flexor tendons of the hands, the extensor carpi ulnaris tendon, or other sites; and **dactylitis**, a uniform swelling of the soft tissues between the metacarpophalangeal and interphalangeal joints. With dactylitis, there is diffuse swelling of the entire digit, which is often referred to as "sausage digit." Dactylitis occurs in approximately one-half of patients with psoriatic arthritis and is associated with an increased risk of progressive joint damage (Gladman, 2008). The patient may also have nail involvement characterized by pits in the nail plate and onycholysis (separation of the lateral edges of the nail plate from the nail bed).

Laboratory and Diagnostic Procedures

There is no specific diagnostic laboratory test for psoriatic arthritis. In approximately one-third of patients there is an elevated sedimentation rate and leukocytosis showing an inflammatory response. Rheumatoid factor (RF) is found in only 2% to 10% of cases of psoriatic arthritis. The presence of joint damage radiologically is seen in two-thirds of patients on diagnosis. Radiologic findings show both erosive changes and new bone formation in the distal joints. Magnetic resonance imaging (MRI) reveals inflammation in the adjacent bone marrow and soft tissues with the appearance of inflammation of entheses in joints that may not be clinically inflamed. These findings suggest that **enthesitis** (inflammation at the site of tendon insertion into bone) is the primary lesion in psoriatic arthritis. Psoriatic arthritis is also associated with decreased bone mineral density, which may lead to osteoporosis and increased risk of fractures.

Medical Management

The first line of treatment for psoriatic arthritis is usually the administration of nonsteroidal anti-inflammatory medications (NSAIDs). The use of both selective cyclooxygenase-2 (COX-2) inhibitors and nonselective NSAIDs is noted, and the choice is usually a health care provider or patient preference. This class of drug controls the mild inflammatory features of psoriatic arthritis. The combination of nonselective NSAIDs with an antiulcer drug may reduce the risk of gastroduodenal damage from the drug. Antiulcer drugs are discussed in Chapter 45 .

If the arthritis does not respond to NSAIDs and the patient exhibits polyarticular involvement, the patient may benefit from early use of disease-modifying antirheumatic drugs (DMARDs). Also, patients whose psoriasis and arthritis are of equal severity may benefit from medications used for control of psoriasis. Although there is a lack of evidence in regards to its efficacy, methotrexate has been the drug of choice for psoriatic arthritis (Gladman, 2008). The most serious potential side effects of methotrexate include liver toxicity, bone marrow suppression, and interstitial lung disease. Because of the liver toxicity, patients must not consume alcohol when taking methotrexate. If the patient refuses to give up alcohol, sulfasalazine may be used as long as there is no known allergy to sulfa drugs. If the disease does not improve after 3 months of treatment with a DMARD, then an anti–tumor necrosis factor (anti-TNF) agent may be introduced. Etanercept and infliximab have received regulatory approval for the treatment of psoriatic arthritis. See the earlier Pharmacology Summary for Arthritis and Connective Tissue Disorder on p. 1839.

Any patient with psoriasis with the complaint of joint discomfort should be evaluated for psoriatic arthritis. The patient's goals include relief of pain, treatment of the infection, rehabilitation of the joint after the infection subsides, and knowledge of treatment regimen. Evaluation parameters include control of pain as expressed by the patient, decrease in the signs and symptoms of infection, and the ability of the patient to articulate the plan of care. Patients may obtain complete relief of joint tenderness and swelling and, with continued use of medication, avoid a relapse. Patients who present with mild disease, less disability, and male gender are associated with a greater likelihood of achieving remission (Gladman, 2008). Assessment and protection of the affected joint are important to the success of treatment.

◼ Nursing Management

Nursing management focuses on the same issues as with all types of arthritis: early recognition, pain relief, and protection of the joint from further damage. The nurse may support and immobilize the affected joint in a splint. Because the inflammatory process can cause scar tissue within the joint, it is important to splint the joint in a functional position. Analgesics are prescribed to control pain and anti-inflammatory medication such as NSAIDs may be used to control joint inflammation.

The nurse instructs the patient on the process of psoriatic arthritis so he may understand the therapeutic regimen. Of importance is the adherence to the therapeutic regimen, support of the affected joint, and adherence to weight-bearing and activity restrictions during the inflammatory process to prevent permanent damage to the joint. If assistive devices are to be used, the nurse will help the patient in learning safe use of the devices. Evaluation includes decreased pain and swelling. The patient will report adequate pain relief and an increase in physical mobility with demonstrated safe use of assistive devices.

Gouty Arthritis: Epidemiology and Etiology

Gouty arthritis is a condition in which there is an imbalance in purine metabolism, which increases uric acid in the joints with the formation of uric acid crystals (MedlinePlus Medical Encyclopedia, 2007). Gout can affect any joint but most commonly affects those of the feet, especially the great toe. According to the National Institutes of Health, approximately 275 people out of 100,000 are affected (MedlinePlus Medical Encyclopedia, 2007). Based on all of the different types of arthritis, gouty arthritis accounts for 5% (National Institute of Arthritis and Musculoskeletal and Skin Diseases, 2008). Primary gout most commonly occurs in men over age 30 and postmenopausal women. Secondary gout occurs in the elderly (Frazier & Drzymkowski, 2009).

The cause of primary gout is unknown but is thought to have a hereditary component with a defect in purine metabolism. This disease is more common in men than in women and those who are overweight. Onset of an acute attack of gout sometimes follows excessive eating or drinking (MedlinePlus Medical Encyclopedia, 2007). Risk factors include heredity, an enzyme defect, and exposure to lead (MedlinePlus Medical Encyclopedia, 2007).

Pathophysiology

With gouty arthritis, there is an imbalance with purine metabolism. Instead of the uric acid crystals being excreted through the kidneys, they accumulate in the joints. These crystals are needle-like causing excruciating pain, usually in the joints of the elbows, wrist, fingers, knees, ankles, and toes, with 75% of patients affected in the great toe (Figure 58–3 ◼) (National Institute of Arthritis and Musculoskeletal and Skin Diseases, 2008). Gout

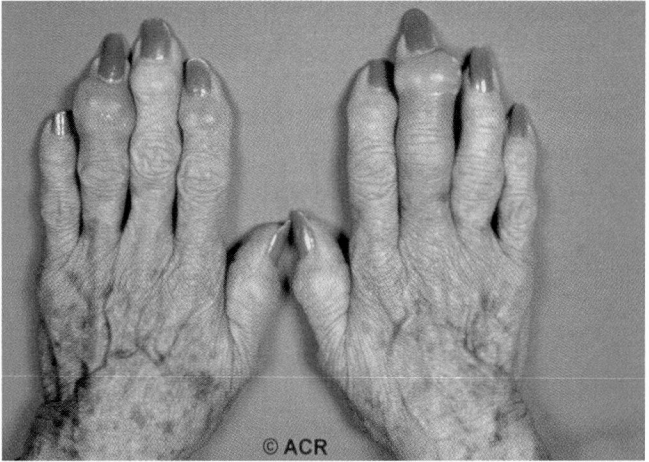

FIGURE 58–3 ◼ Instead of the uric acid crystals being excreted through the kidneys, they accumulate in the joints. These crystals are needle-like causing excruciating pain, usually in the joints of the elbows, wrists, fingers, knees, ankles, and toes, with 75% of patients affected in the great toe.
Source: © 1972–2004 American College of Rheumatology Clinical Slide Collection. Used with permission.

follows an intermittent course and a patient can be free from symptoms for years between attacks.

Clinical Manifestations

According to Meiner (2001), gout has a four-stage progression: asymptomatic, acute gout episode, interval gout, and chronic tophaceous gout. During the asymptomatic phase, there is an elevation of uric acid in the blood, but no symptoms (MedlinePlus Medical Encyclopedia, 2007). In the second stage, called acute gout episode, there is an increase of uric acid crystals accumulating in the space of the joints. These uric acid crystals can also settle in cartilage in the earlobes. This is called **tophi**. During this stage, the patient experiences a sudden onset of severe pain, usually in the night. Other manifestations include increased swelling and inflammation, which cause the affected part to feel hot. Some will experience knife-like pain in the earlobe, elbow, or feet. This sudden attack can be triggered by stress, illness, or the consumption of alcohol or drugs. Without treatment, this phase can last from 3 to 10 days. Interval gout is the period of time this condition is in remission. Finally, the fourth stage, called chronic tophaceous gout, occurs when the illness is not treated, which results in disabling effects such as permanent damage to the joints and kidneys (Meiner, 2001).

Laboratory and Diagnostic Procedures

Elevated blood levels of uric acid occur in some individuals, but are normal in approximately 10% of people during an acute attack of gouty arthritis. Moreover, uric acid levels are elevated in 5% to 8% of the general population, so the presence of an elevated level does not necessarily mean that gout is the cause of an inflamed joint. X-ray examination of the joint is primarily used to assess underlying joint damage, especially in patients who have had multiple episodes of gouty arthritis. The most useful and accurate test is joint aspiration. A needle is inserted into the joint to withdraw a sample of fluid, which is examined to see whether there are gout crystals or bacterial infection present. Sometimes other crystals can be found in the joint fluid, such as calcium pyrophosphate, which is caused by an entirely different condition called pseudogout ("like gout"). Joint aspiration is the ultimate method of being certain of a diagnosis of gouty arthritis, as opposed to other causes such as an infection in the joint (eMedicineHealth, 2008).

Medical Management

Medical management focuses on mitigating the clinical manifestations of gouty arthritis. Medications used specifically for gout include colchicine and allopurinol. These drugs reduce uric acid production, thus reducing the inflammatory process. It is important to monitor uric acid levels while on medication (Frazier & Drzymkowski, 2009).

Patients with gout must adhere to a dietary regimen to reduce the consumption of purines. Foods that should be avoided are dried beans and peas, organ meats, wheat germ, anchovies, and seafood. Patients should consume a moderate amount of protein. The recommendation is to eat only 200 grams of meat, poultry, or fish twice weekly and to eliminate organ meats. Alcohol consumption should be limited to 1 drink 3 times a week, whereas beer ingestion should be completely discontinued, as it has a high purine count and increases gout risks regardless of amount (Hogan, 2007). It is not recommended for individuals to follow a high-protein, low-carbohydrate diet because this can worsen the symptoms. Because fat intake should also be limited, patients should select low-fat meats and use nonsaturated oils. Increasing fluid intake is critical to dilute urinary uric acid crystals. Patients should consume between 2 and 3 liters of fluid daily (Hogan, 2007). See the Pharmacology Summary of medications used to treat gouty arthritis.

PHARMACOLOGY Summary of Medications Used to Treat Gouty Arthritis

Medication Category	Action	Application/Indication	Nursing Responsibility
Antigout Agents			
Colchicine Allopurinol (Aloprim, Zyloprim) Probenecid (Benemid)	Exerts anti-inflammatory effect; decreases pain and swelling by interrupting the inflammatory response. Reduces uric acid; has no direct anti-inflammatory or analgesic action.	Treatment of acute gout, prophylaxis, and recurrent gouty arthritis. Off-label use: scleroderma. Treatment of chronic gout.	• Observe for early signs of toxicity (colchicine): weakness, anorexia, nausea, vomiting, diarrhea, especially in presence of cardiac, renal, or hepatic disease. • Observe for severe adverse effects: nausea, sore throat or mouth, fever, fatigue, unusual bleeding, or bruising (bone marrow depression). • Monitor serum uric acid, CBC, electrolytes, urinalysis, and renal and hepatic function. • Monitor IV site to prevent extravasation when colchicine given IV. • Monitor for drug interactions (vitamin B_{12}, erythromycin, NSAIDs, and others with colchicine; theophylline, ampicillin, thiazide diuretics, and others with allopurinol; some antibiotics, vitamin C, and cranberry juice with probenecid). • Advise patient to increase fluid intake. • Give after a meal to reduce gastric distress.

Nursing Management

Utilization of the nursing process will guide the nurse in understanding the method for organizing critical thinking skills when providing patient care in the presence of specific illness. When planning care, the short-term goals should be directed at pain reduction or comfort based on the causative factors. Because gouty arthritis is a chronic disease and there are interventions that help control the clinical manifestations, developing a health plan is essential. See the Evidence-Based Practice for the Treatment of Gouty Arthritis feature for a discussion of the literature regarding the treatment of gouty arthritis. Long-term goals should be focused on patients becoming compliant to medication and dietary regimens. The Nursing Process: Patient Care Plan feature (p. 1846) outlines the nursing management of the patient with gouty arthritis.

Health Promotion

Because gouty arthritis is caused by indulging in foods high in purines, it can be controlled by eating a well-balanced, low-calorie, low-purine diet and by reducing alcohol consumption. Foods to be avoided are alcohol, organ meats, and rich foods such as gravies, dried legumes, and anchovies. These foods will increase uric acid in the blood and can lead to uric acid crystal buildup most often resulting in uric acid crystals located in the joint of the great toe. Pain medications are not the treatment of choice, rather antigout medications and dietary therapy to reduce the uric acid level.

Compared to other connective disorders, gouty arthritis has been noticeably understudied in the literature (Mikuls & Saag, 2005). On reviewing the literature, it is determined that there are no formal national guidelines for the *risks* of gouty arthritis. It is important to determine that the main vulnerability factor for acquiring gouty arthritis is an increased uric acid level in the blood. However, based on a review of many articles and websites, the National Guidelines box (p. 1847) offers guidelines for *reducing* the incidence of gouty arthritis.

Collaborative Management

To achieve optimal functioning, patients with gouty arthritis need a multidisciplinary team approach, including health care providers, nurses, social workers, physical therapists, pharmacists,

---

Treatment of Gouty Arthritis

Clinical Problem

An acute attack of gouty arthritis is very painful. The drug colchicine has been used to decrease the symptoms related to gout but has gastrointestinal side effects that may increase the patient's distress.

Research Findings

A comparison was done to determine whether the effectiveness of colchicine was preferred over that of the placebo with a sample size of 43 patients (Schlesinger, Schumacher, Catton, & Maxwell, 2006). For those patients who had taken colchicine, there was a reduction of the following symptoms: pain (34%) and tenderness on palpation, swelling, redness (30%). However, all patients on colchicine (100%) developed gastrointestinal (GI) symptoms: vomiting and/or diarrhea.

Implications for Nursing

The actual medication improved acute gout attacks, but caused GI adverse effects with all who took this medication due to the frequency necessary to reduce pain, swelling, and other symptoms causing the gout attack. Encouraging patients to maintain a low purine diet and avoid excessive use of alcohol in order to prevent an acute attack may be a better alternative for the patient.

Critical Thinking Questions

1. How can you maximize the effect of antihyperuremic medications and reduce the gastrointestinal side effects?

2. Are there other classifications of medications other than antihyperuremics that could work in the treatment of gout?

Reference

Schlesinger, N., Schumacher, M. C., Catton, M., & Maxwell, L. (2006). Colchicine for acute gout. *Cochrane Database of Systematic Reviews*, 2006, Issue 4. Retrieved June 20, 2007, from http://mrw.interscience.wiley.com/cochrane/clsysrev/articles/CD006190/frame.html.

Clinical Problem

There is no consensus among rheumatologists about the standardized treatment of patients who have gouty arthritis.

Research Findings

On a literature search, 310 potential articles for review were identified. Many articles were eliminated due to their not being relevant or being written in a language other than English. Thus, 120 articles were included in the database. Finally, twenty-three (19%) articles that were randomized controlled trials were used in this study (Mikuls et al., 2004). In a breakdown of these pharmaceutical studies, 48% discussed nonsteroidal anti-inflammatory drugs (NSAIDs) in treatment of gouty arthritis, 8% studied colchicines, and 43% discussed urate-lowering medications for long-term therapy. The expert panel in this study examined both articles on medication (urate-lowering medications and NSAIDs) as well as on other process indicators (lifestyle modifications). The literature suggested that the topic of gouty arthritis was understudied as a connective tissue disorder, compared to other connective tissue disorders that have been studied and reported in the literature.

Implications for Nursing Practice

The topic of gouty arthritis is understudied and presents as an opportunity to nurses to explore ways to improve patient plans of care in regards to gouty arthritis.

Critical Thinking Question

1. What type of research can be conducted by nursing in the area of gout?

Answers to Critical Thinking Questions appear in Appendix D.

Reference

Mikuls, T. R., MacLean, C. H., Olivieri, J., Patino, F., Allison, J., Farrar, J.T., et al. (2004). Quality of care indicators for gout management. *Arthritis & Rheumatism, 50*(3), 937–943.

EVIDENCE-BASED PRACTICE

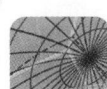

NURSING PROCESS: Patient Care Plan for Gouty Arthritis

Assessment of Pain

Subjective Data:
Do you have pain?
Is it constant or intermittent?
What brings it on and what makes it go away?
What intensity is it (numeric, colors, or faces), including location, character?

Objective Data:
Monitor:
Uric acid levels
Onset of pain
Relieving factors

Nursing Assessment and Diagnoses	Outcomes and Evaluation Parameters	Planning and Interventions with *Rationales*
Nursing Diagnoses: *Comfort, Readiness for Enhanced Pain, Acute* related to uric acid crystal deposits in affected joints	**Outcome:** Comfort level maintained. ***Evaluation Parameters:*** Uric acid levels are within normal limits. Pain controlled with or without nonpharmacologic therapies or with or without medication. Joint swelling decreased.	**Interventions and *Rationale:*** Assess pain on a scale. Monitor uric acid levels. Alternative pain interventions: position, elevation, ice, distraction. Medicate as ordered by the health care provider. *As there is an increase in blood uric acid levels, uric acid crystals form in joints causing discomfort, usually affecting one affected joint: warm and swollen.*

Assessment of Nutrition

Subjective Data:
What kinds of foods do you eat on a daily basis?
Have you gained or lost weight in the last year?
Do you eat at home or in restaurants?
Who prepares the meals?
What is your knowledge of foods containing purines?

Objective Data:
Monitor:
Weights at specified interval
Meal selections
Verbalizing foods consumed high in purines

Nursing Assessment and Diagnoses	Outcomes and Evaluation Parameters	Planning and Interventions with *Rationales*
Nursing Diagnosis: *Nutrition: Imbalanced, More than Body Requirements* related to increased intake of foods high in purine and increased calories	**Outcome:** Patient adherence to a low-purine diet. ***Evaluation Parameters:*** Patient will be able to verbalize appropriate meal planning with foods low in purine. Weight loss at reasonable amount weekly based on baseline weight (about 1–2 pounds per week).	**Interventions and *Rationales:*** Obtain a sample of patient's meal choice selections in a week to determine baseline purine intake. Create low-purine weight loss meal plan to include cultural foods in order to decrease uric acid, such as grains, fruits, vegetables, and beans. Teach the patient to avoid the following foods high in purines: cheese, wine, organ meats, and shellfish. Encourage the patient to drink plenty of liquids, about 2,000–3,000 milliliters daily, *to reduce potential creation of kidney stones.* Encourage the patient to have alkaline-ash diet *to increase the urine pH and decrease the precipitation of uric acid, and to improve the action of gouty medications, such as probenicid.*

Assessment of Therapeutic Regimen

Subjective Data:
Explain your dietary needs.
Explain why and when you take your medications.

Objective Data:
Patient is able to verbalize low-purine foods and the incorporation of these foods into low-calorie diet plan
Weight loss
No joint discomfort

Nursing Assessment and Diagnoses	Outcomes and Evaluation Parameters	Planning and Interventions with *Rationales*
Nursing Diagnosis: *Therapeutic Regimen Management, Effective*	**Outcome:** Patient will adhere to therapeutic regimen to control exacerbations. ***Evaluation Parameter:*** Verbalizing compliance to the prescribed therapeutic regimen.	**Interventions and *Rationale:*** Patient will verbalize compliance with the following: Foods low in purine and calories Compliance to medication Comfort Management of weight loss Exercise: passive and active range of motion. *Compliance to the above therapeutic regimen will empower the patient to take control of this disease by providing knowledge about therapeutic treatment.*

NATIONAL GUIDELINES for Health Promotion for Gouty Arthritis

Healthy People 2010 is a set of government objectives that encourages a healthy lifestyle in order to promote health. Its two main goals are (1) increasing the quality of years of a healthy life and (2) eliminating health disparities (DHHS, 2000). It is important when caring for a patient with gouty arthritis to provide the proper education that will enhance his health promotion. With gout, there is an increase of uric acids from purine metabolism. It has been discussed that diets high in purine can cause gout. Two of the health indicators identified by *Healthy People 2010* are overweight/obesity and substance abuse. Most often, people who are overweight are typically consuming foods high in purines, thus making this population of people more at risk for gouty arthritis. It is imperative for the patient to understand that behavioral changes will reduce, if not eliminate, this disease process and thus promote a healthy lifestyle. By consuming

an increased amount of alcohol, uric acid will be metabolized from the liver and passed in the bloodstream to be excreted in the kidneys. However, excretion can be inhibited with gouty arthritis, causing the uric acid crystals to remain in the tissues (Chemocare.com, 2005).

Thus, it is important to remember two factors when caring for a patient with gout. One is that the increased consumption of foods high in purines results in high uric acid in the blood. Second, the decreased ability to excrete uric acids from the kidneys causes a buildup of uric acid crystals in the tissues. Healthy lifestyle choices can make the difference between one acute attack of gouty arthritis and a lifetime of gout attacks. Educating the patient is powerful, but having the patient incorporate behavioral changes can be life altering by promoting healthy choices.

Sources: Chemocare.com. (2005). *Hyperuricemia.* Retrieved July 30, 2007, from http://www.chemocare.com/managing/hyperuricemia-high-uric-acid.asp; and U.S. Department of Health and Human Services (DHHS). (2000). *Healthy People 2010.* Retrieved July 30, 2007, from http://www.healthypeople.gov.

---

occupational therapists, psychologists/psychiatrists, and dieticians. Ongoing physical therapy will help increase range of motion in the joints. The occupational therapist assists the patient with exercises that will enhance fine motor movements, whereas the social worker and a psychologist/psychiatrist are used to help the patient adjust to a chronic illness. Finally, a comprehensive plan for nutrition is important for teaching the patient and family about dietary restrictions. The pharmacist helps the team coordinate the medication regimen.

Reactive Arthritis

Reactive arthritis is caused by a reaction to an infection somewhere else in the body (National Institute of Arthritis and Musculoskeletal and Skin Diseases, 2002). This disease has several other names, such as Reiter's syndrome or undifferentiated spondylarthropathy. Many conditions refer to a spectrum of diseases that share certain clinical manifestations; among the most common is the spondyloarthropathy family, called undifferentiated spondylarthropathy, whereas reactive arthritis and Reiter's syndrome encompass a small amount of cases (Yu, 2008). Reactive arthritis characteristically causes inflammatory response in the genitourinary tract, the joints, and the eyes (National Institute of Arthritis and Musculoskeletal and Skin Diseases, 2002).

Epidemiology

This disease is more common in men than in women. Men between ages 20 and 40 more frequently develop reactive arthritis. When the trigger is a sexually transmitted infection, men still outnumber women by 9%. Food-borne infections do not discriminate between genders in transmitting reactive arthritis. However, women experience a milder case with remissions and exacerbations (National Institute of Arthritis and Musculoskeletal and Skin Diseases, 2002).

Etiology

This is a noncontagious disease. On the other hand, for this disease to be communicable, one must pass the bacterium that triggers the disease from person to person (National Institute of Arthritis and Musculoskeletal and Skin Diseases, 2002). Reactive arthritis usually begins between 1 and 3 weeks after becoming

infected. One organism, called *Chlamydia trachomatis*, is spread through sexual contact and without treatment can cause reactive arthritis and respiratory infection, called *Chlamydia pneumoniae* (National Institute of Arthritis and Musculoskeletal and Skin Diseases, 2002).

Gastrointestinal infections, such as *Salmonella*, *Shigella*, *Yersinia*, and *Campylobacter*, also are responsible for causing reactive arthritis (National Institute of Arthritis and Musculoskeletal and Skin Diseases, 2002).

Pathophysiology

A patient develops a bacterial infection as identified earlier. Spondyloarthropies cause inflammation and bone destruction at the site of insertion (Yu, 2008). Reactive arthritis most commonly causes secondary conditions, such as arthritis, uveitis, and urethritis (Yu, 2008). However, a variety of symptoms can occur affecting the following: musculoskeletal system, enthesopathy, inflammatory spine pain, genital lesions, skin lesions, inflammatory eye disease, inflammation of the bowel mucosa, cardiac disease, amyloidosis, and evidence of preceding infection (Yu, 2008).

Clinical Manifestations

Asymmetrical joint swelling often occurs, especially in the lower extremities (knees and ankles). Enthesopathy is the inflammation around the insertion of ligaments, tendons, joint capsule, or fascia near the bone (Yu, 2008). Other symptoms that may occur are dactylitis, inflammation of the neck and low back, painless skin lesions called **circinate balanitis**, unilateral uveitis, Crohn's-like bowel inflammation, aortic regurgitation, amyloidosis, and rheumatic infections.

Laboratory and Diagnostic Procedures

Confirmation of this disease examines both laboratory data and diagnostic imaging. Laboratory tests that can confirm reactive arthritis are as follows: (1) HLA-B27, (2) alpha E beta 7 in T lymphocytes (for patients with spondylarthropathy and Crohn's), (3) epithelial E-cadherin, (4) CD163-positive macrophages, (5) lymphocytes with T helper-2 phenotype, (6) immunoglobin A (IgA) antibodies, (7) proteinuria, (8) erythrocyte sedimentation rates, (9) ligase chain reaction, (10) polymerase chain reaction, and (11) stool cultures for the presence of diarrhea (Yu, 2008). Diagnostic tests that also can confirm reactive arthritis include MRI for bone confirmation, slit lamp examination for eye involvement, x-ray, and computed tomography (Yu, 2008).

Accurate diagnosis tends to occur in the advanced stage, because the glomerular filtration is greatly reduced, leading to increased uremia, electrolyte abnormalities, and metabolic acidosis. More information is provided in the Diagnostic Tests box for undifferentiated spondylarthropathy.

Medical Management

Treatment is symptomatic control and prevention. The medications most commonly used are as follows: (1) nonsteroidal anti-inflammatory drugs to reduce joint inflammation, (2) glucocorticoids to reduce severe joint inflammation, (3) topical glucocorticoids to reduce skin lesions and promote healing, (4) anti-infectives to rid infections, (5) immunosuppressants to suppress the immune system when previous medications have not been effective, and (6) tumor necrosis factor inhibitor drugs to reduce a protein involved with inflammation when other medication therapies are again ineffective (National Institute of Arthritis and Musculoskeletal and Skin Diseases, 2002). See the earlier Pharmacology Summary for Arthritis and Connective Tissue Disorders featured on p. 1839.

Physical activity is needed to promote range of motion in the affected joints. Range-of-motion exercises reduce stiffness and promote flexibility. Using hydrotherapies also assists the patient in maximizing movement of the joints of the body, especially the limbs and spine.

Nursing Management

The nursing process provides the framework for a nurse to offer knowledgeable and sound patient care. The *assessment* includes evaluating the clinical manifestations associated with reactive arthritis, as described earlier. It is also important to complete a head-to-toe assessment when evaluating the patient's current condition. The nurse needs to question the patient and family about their knowledge of the disease, the associated risk factors, and necessary treatments. Identifying the *nursing diagnoses* pro-

vides a method to analyze the priorities in providing patient care. These include:

1. *Pain, Acute* related to joint and spine inflammation
2. *Knowledge, Deficient* related to lack of information about pathophysiology, difficulty to confirm diagnosis, and treatment options
3. *Activity Intolerance* related to polyarthritis
4. *Skin Integrity, Impaired* related to skin lesions
5. *Diarrhea* related to bowel inflammation
6. *Sensory Perception: Disturbed Visual* related to uveitis.

The *outcome* goals of treatment are to have the patient symptom free and compliant with therapy. *Evaluation parameters* include to treat infection, keep the condition in remission by complying with the therapeutic regimen and avoiding risk factors, and to avoid exacerbations.

Nursing planning and interventions include teaching the patient about the risk factors, medications, and supportive treatments; for example, the importance of exercise because it is essential to maintain or promote joint function of the lower extremities and the spine. Finally, reactive arthritis is difficult to diagnose, so the nurse needs to encourage the patient to have patience during the diagnosis phase of the illness and utilize the multidisciplinary team. The *outcome* is to improve the quality of life by mitigating and preventing symptoms with the treatment plan. The goals for *evaluation* include no infection, the patient complies with the therapeutic regimen to remain in a state of remission, and absence of exacerbation.

Collaborative Management

Specialists must be incorporated in caring for a patient with reactive arthritis based on symptoms, Those participating, for example, would be an ophthalmologist for eye disease, gynecologist for female genital disease, urologist to treat genitourinary disease in both males and females, dermatologist for skin lesions, orthopedist for surgical intervention with joint

DIAGNOSTIC TESTS for Undifferentiated Spondylarthropathy

Test	Expected Abnormality	Rationale for Abnormality
Urinalysis	Presence of red blood cells, red blood cell casts Low specific gravity (1.010) Low osmolality (less than 400 mOsm/kg)	Impaired filtration Decreased ability to concentrate urine
Serum creatinine	Rising serum creatinine	Indicates advanced renal insufficiency
Blood urea nitrogen (BUN)	Rising serum BUN	Indicates advanced renal insufficiency
Arterial blood gases (ABGs)	Metabolic acidosis pH < 7.35 $HCO_3 < 24$ mEq/L	Impaired filtration
Electrolytes	Hyperkalemia Hyperphosphatemia Hypocalcemia	Impaired filtration

disease, rheumatologist for arthritis, and physical therapist for promoting joint function.

Ankylosing Spondylitis

Ankylosing spondylitis (AS) is a type of arthritis that affects the spine and the sacroiliac joints. This systemic inflammatory disease is usually progressive and affects primarily the spinal column (Figure 58–4 ■). The patient may also experience fatigue, weight loss, fever, diarrhea, and eye pain and photophobia due to uveitis (Frazier & Drzymkowski, 2009).

Epidemiology and Etiology

In the United States, AS affects 129 out of 100,000 people, mainly adolescents and young adults. It is most common among Native Americans but also affects other ethnicities (American College of Rheumatology, 2008). It is more common in men and typically begins in the sacroiliac area and adjacent soft tissues (Frazier & Drzymkowski, 2009).

It is not certain how a patient gets AS. There is a common genetic marker, called HLA-B27, in affected individuals. Some individuals become predisposed after exposure to bowel or urinary tract infections (American College of Rheumatology, 2008).

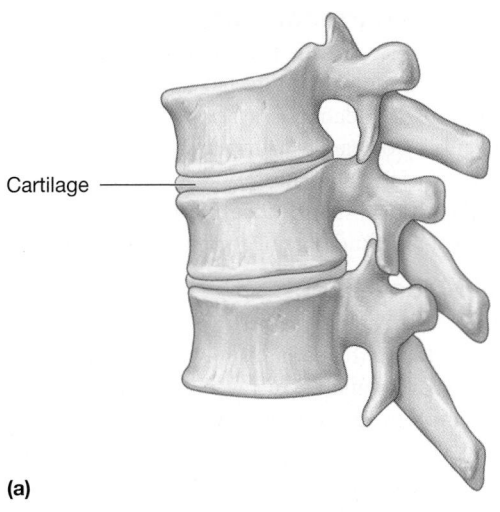

(a)

Cartilage

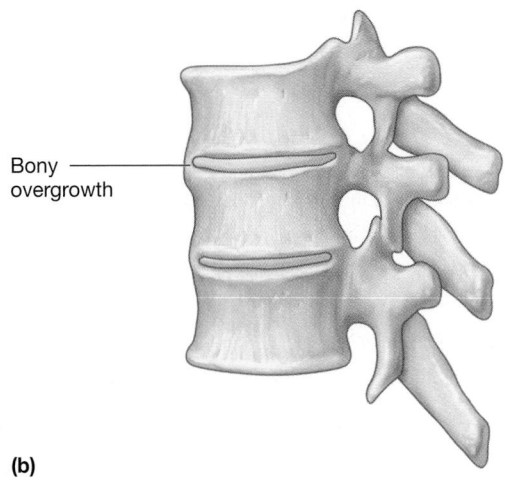

Bony overgrowth

(b)

FIGURE 58–4 ■ Bony overgrowth of ankylosing spondylitis. (A) Normal vertebrae (B) Vertebrae with bony overgrowth typical of ankylosing spondylitis.

Clinical Manifestations

Ankylosing spondylitis usually occurs first in the sacroiliac area. The patient may experience low back pain and stiffness in the morning that improves with activity. An early sign is that a patient will have a loss of flexibility in the lumbar spine. Arthritis can occur in attaching joints, tendons, and ligaments as in the shoulder, hips, and feet. As the inflammation increases and healing occurs, new bone growth fuses the bones together such as in the ribs and vertebrae (American College of Rheumatology, 2008). With restriction of the ribs, lung capacity may be impaired as well as normal functioning with activities of daily living. As the condition advances, there can be involvement of the eye inflammation and the valves of the heart can be affected (American College of Rheumatology, 2008). The patient may also have a history of inflammatory bowel disease or a family history of arthritis (Frazier & Drzymkowski, 2009).

Laboratory and Diagnostic Procedures

Laboratory data include the following tests: sedimentation rate indicating inflammation, hemoglobin and hematocrit to determine anemia, and HLA-B27 assay, indicating an increase to confirm the diagnosis of AS. Diagnostic tests that are helpful to confirm the diagnosis are x-rays and bone scans (American College of Rheumatology, 2008).

Medical Management

Early detection, diagnosis, and treatment are the best plan in controlling AS (American College of Rheumatology, 2008). Medications that are helpful in treating AS include nonsteroidal anti-inflammatory medications and methotrexate (an oncology chemotherapeutic agent). See the earlier Pharmacology Summary for Medications Used to Treat Arthritis and Connective Tissue Disorders on p. 1839.

Rest is just as important as having physical activity. The patient needs to plan rest periods. The patient needs to sleep an ample amount of time during the night as well (American College of Rheumatology, 2008).

■ Nursing Management

The use of the nursing process will assist the nurse in being able to understand the disease and provide appropriate patient care. The specific disease process will be featured under each stage of the nursing process.

Assessment

Nursing assessment includes evaluating the specific joint and back manifestations described earlier. The assessment also needs to include an in-depth assessment of the other organs such as the heart valves. Chapter 9 ⊙ includes a description of an in-depth nursing assessment.

Nursing Diagnoses

The priority nursing diagnoses for the patient with AS include:

1. *Pain, Chronic* related to arthritic joint discomfort
2. *Activity Intolerance* related to musculoskeletal changes
3. *Breathing Pattern, Ineffective* related to changes in rib cage affecting lungs
4. *Fatigue* related to anemia.

Outcomes, Planning, and Evaluation

Outcomes for the patient with AS include relief of pain as expressed by the patient; relief of edema as noted on assessment; and maintenance of posture and mobility through physical therapy and moderate exercise. When planning care, it is important to treat joint symptoms as they present themselves. Utilizing the multidisciplinary team to assist the patient in maintaining function is essential. Physical therapy and occupational therapy can assist the patient in remaining functional. Encourage the patient to remain as independent as possible with therapeutic and nontherapeutic measures, such as understanding of and compliance with the medication regimen and balancing the therapeutic regimen of physical activity. Exercise programs can maintain posture and joint flexibility (American College of Rheumatology, 2008). Respiratory therapy will assist the patient in maintaining lung function. The patient can enhance lung capacity by swimming or aerobic activities. Because ankylosing spondylitis is a progressive condition, it is critical that the patient maintain a program of continuing care (American College of Rheumatology, 2008). The goals for the evaluation are to have the pain managed effectively and the patient able to continue to perform activities of daily living, breathe effectively, and have decreased fatigue.

Septic Arthritis: Epidemiology and Etiology

Nongonococcal bacterial arthritis (**septic arthritis**) is the most destructive form of acute arthritis and can result from trauma, from direct inoculation of bacteria during joint surgery, from spread of infection from another part of the body (hematogenous), or when an infection from an adjacent bone extends through the cortex into the joint space (Goldenberg & Sexton, 2007).

The incidence of septic arthritis is estimated to be 2 to 5 per 100,000 persons (Kherani & Shojania, 2007). Predisposing factors include being over age 80, rheumatoid arthritis, diabetes, skin infection, recent joint surgery or a prosthetic joint, and oral carriage of *Staphylococcus aureus* (Goldenberg & Sexton, 2007; Kherani & Shojania, 2007). Each of the predisposing factors has a modest impact on the risk, but combinations of the factors lead to a substantially increased risk.

Pathophysiology

In the majority of cases, septic arthritis arises from hematogenous spread of bacteria to the joint. Common sources of the infection include intravenous drug use, indwelling catheters, and an underlying immunocompromised state such as HIV infection. Bacteria are more likely to localize in a joint with preexisting arthritis, with patients with rheumatoid arthritis being especially susceptible (Goldenberg & Sexton, 2007). Any microbial pathogen can cause septic arthritis, but organisms such as *Staphylococcus aureus* and *Streptococcus* more commonly cause joint infections than do gram-negative bacilli. Most joint infections are monomicrobial with rare polymicrobial infections occurring in patients with penetrating trauma that involves the joint space. Initially the bacteria deposit in the synovial membrane and produce an acute inflammatory response. The bacteria quickly enter the synovial fluid, creating purulent joint inflammation. Within 1 week the synovial membrane develops hyperplasia, and the cytokines and proteases that were released cause cartilage degradation and inhibit cartilage synthesis. With large effusions, pressure necrosis can result in further cartilage and bone loss. Chart 58–1 outlines causes of infectious arthritis with clinical clues.

Clinical Manifestations and Laboratory and Diagnostic Procedures

Patients with septic arthritis present with a single swollen and painful joint. Common joints affected are the knee (>50%), wrist, ankles, and hips (Goldenberg & Sexton, 2007). Systemic chills, fever, and leukocytosis are usually present. There may also be evidence of an associated skin, urinary, or respiratory infection. The definitive diagnostic test is the identification of bacteria via a culture of the synovial fluid obtained from joint aspiration.

Medical Management

The infection is treated with broad-spectrum intravenous antibiotics initially and then organism-specific antibiotics after the culture results are available. Intravenous antibiotics are continued until symptoms disappear. A typical duration of therapy is 3 to 4 weeks with approximately 2 weeks of intravenous antibiotics and the remainder with oral antibiotics. Progressive range-of-motion exercises will be needed once the infection has subsided. The patient also is treated with antipyretics and pain medication as necessary.

CHART 58–1 **Causes of Septic Arthritis**

Organism	Clinical Clues
Staphylococcus aureus	Healthy adult with skin breakdown, previously damaged joint, or prosthetic joint
Streptococcus	Healthy adult, splenic dysfunction
Neisseria gonorrhoeae	Healthy sexually active adult, associated tenosynovitis, vesicular pustules, and negative synovial fluid culture and gram stain
Aerobic or anaerobic gram-negative bacteria	Immune-compromised patients, gastrointestinal infection
Mycobacterium species	Immune-compromised patient with recent travel to or residence in an endemic area
Fungal	Immune-compromised patients
Spirochete	Exposure to ticks

Source: Adapted from Goldenberg, D., & Sexton, D. (2007). Bacterial (nongonococcal) arthritis in adults. *UpToDate.* Retrieved October 23, 2007, from http://www.uptodate.com/patients/content/topic.do?topicKey=~hcmhzYL2SL2ACJ&selectedTitle=7~147&source=search_result.

Nursing Management

Nursing management focuses on early recognition, pain relief, and protection of the joint from further damage. The nursing process provides a framework for organizing and managing the care of patients with septic arthritis.

Assessment

Patients with septic arthritis present with a warm, painful, and swollen joint with decreased range of motion. Patients at risk are those who are elder, are diabetic, have RA, or have preexisting joint disease or joint replacement. Elderly patients and those taking immunosuppressive or steroid medications may not exhibit as dramatic a reaction to the infection. If there is a risk of infection, the patient must have ongoing assessment to detect it as early as possible.

Nursing Diagnoses

The highest priority nursing diagnoses for the patient with septic arthritis are:

1. *Pain, Acute* related to inflammation and swelling
2. *Mobility: Physical, Impaired* related to pain and swelling of joint
3. *Falls, Risk for* related to pain and swelling of joint
4. *Infection, Risk for*
5. *Knowledge, Deficient* related to treatment regimen.

Outcomes and Evaluation Parameters

The patient's goals include relief of pain, treatment of the infection, rehabilitation of the joint after the infection subsides, and knowledge of treatment regimen. Evaluation parameters include control of pain as expressed by the patient, decrease in the signs and symptoms of infection, and the ability of the patient to articulate the plan of care.

Planning, Interventions, and Rationales

The nurse must support and immobilize the affected joint in a splint. Because the inflammatory process can cause scar tissue within the joint, it is important to splint the joint in a functional position. Analgesics are prescribed to control pain; and after the infection has responded to antibiotic therapy, anti-inflammatory medication such as NSAIDs may be used to limit joint damage.

Evaluation

Evaluation includes absence of infection exhibited by decreased pain and swelling, normal temperature, normal white blood cell count, and negative wound cultures. The patient will report adequate pain relief and an increase in physical mobility with demonstrated safe use of assistive devices. The patient will also be able to articulate an understanding of the continued therapeutic regimen and demonstrate compliance by taking medications as prescribed, demonstrating proper wound care, and reporting signs and symptoms of complications promptly.

Septic joints that are diagnosed and treated early usually recover normal function. Assessment and protection of the affected joint are important to the success of treatment. If the articular cartilage is damaged during the inflammatory response to the infection, joint fibrosis and decreased function may result.

Health Promotion

The nurse instructs the patient on the process of septic arthritis so the patient may understand the therapeutic regimen. Of importance is the adherence to the antibiotic regimen, support of the affected joint, and adherence to weight-bearing and activity restrictions during the inflammatory process to prevent permanent damage to the joint. If assistive devices are to be used, the nurse will help the patient in learning safe use of the devices.

If joint fluid was surgically drained, the nurse teaches the patient aseptic techniques for dressing changes and wound care. The patient should be given instruction for range-of-motion exercises and encouraged to perform them after the infection subsides to maintain optimal joint function.

Systemic Lupus Erythematosus: Epidemiology and Etiology

Systemic lupus erythematosus (SLE) is a chronic inflammatory autoimmune disease that attacks connective tissue or organs. SLE is characterized by remissions and exacerbations, which are common during the spring and summer months. SLE affects mostly women from 30 to 40 years old (Frazier & Drzymkowski, 2009). The etiology is unknown, but it is thought that there is a defect in the body's immunologic mechanism, a predisposition genetically, or an environmental stimulus. Chapter 60 ⊘ includes a complete discussion of the immune mechanisms related to SLE.

Pathophysiology

Certain immune complexes deposit in blood vessels, among collagen fibers, and on organs that cause necrosis and inflammation in the major organs, such as the kidneys, brain, eyes, lymphatic system, gastrointestinal (GI) tract, lungs, and skin. A significant feature with SLE is the body's ability to form antibodies against many different tissue components. For a patient who is genetically susceptible, there are multiple predisposing factors associated with SLE. These include physical or mental stress, exposure to sunlight or ultraviolet light, viral or streptococcal infections, pregnancy, and abnormal estrogen metabolism. SLE can also be aggravated or triggered by specific medications such as procainamide, anticonvulsants, hydralazine, and, less commonly, sulfa drugs, penicillins, and hormonal contraceptives.

Clinical Manifestations

Subjective assessment includes weakness, sensitivity to light, and pain in the joints. Objective assessment may reveal elevated temperatures; butterfly rash on the face and the palms of the hands, a type of Raynaud's disease; loss of weight; and dysfunction in one or any of the organs of the renal, gastrointestinal, cardiac, respiratory, or neurological system. Raynaud's disease is discussed in Chapter 43 ⊘. With gastrointestinal involvement, patients often experience ulcers in the mouth and nasopharyngeal areas, with 90% of patients experiencing joint pain similar to that of RA. In addition, renal complications are common such as glomerulonephritis. Central nervous system changes occur, such as headaches, irritability, and depression.

Laboratory and Diagnostic Procedures

Two specific tests are used to confirm the diagnosis of SLE: lupus erythematosus preparation (LE prep) and antinuclear antibodies (ANAs). Other laboratory tests would include the following: anti-DNA, anti-Sm antibody, serum complement test, and complement proteins C3 and C4. For more details, see the Diagnostic Tests box for SLE.

Medical Management

There is no permanent cure for SLE; therefore, the goal of treatment is to relieve symptoms and protect organs by decreasing inflammation and/or the level of autoimmune activity in the body. Many patients with mild symptoms may need no treatment or only intermittent courses of anti-inflammatory medications. Those individuals with more serious illness involving damage to internal organs may require high doses of corticosteroids in combination with other medications that suppress the body's immune system (MedicineNet.com, 2008d). See the earlier Pharmacology Summary feature of Medications Used to Treat Arthritis and Connective Tissue Disorders on p. 1839.

Patients with SLE need more rest during periods of active disease. Lack of sleep has been found to be a significant factor in developing fatigue in these patients. The health care provider needs to work with the patient and family to develop a plan that addresses sleep quality and the effects of underlying depression, lack of exercise, and self-care coping strategies on overall health. During these periods, carefully prescribed exercise is still important to maintain muscle tone and range of motion in the joints.

Nonsteroidal anti-inflammatory drugs (NSAIDs), such as aspirin, ibuprofen (Motrin), naproxen (Naprosyn), and sulindac (Clinoril), are effective in reducing inflammation and pain in muscles, joints, and other tissues. Corticosteroids are more potent than NSAIDs; therefore, they are used to restore function when the disease is active and are particularly helpful when internal organs are involved. Corticosteroids can be given by mouth, injected directly into the joints and other tissues, or administered intravenously. Unfortunately, corticosteroids have serious side effects

when given in high doses over prolonged periods, and the health care provider must monitor the activity of the disease in order to use the lowest doses that are safe (MedicineNet.com, 2008d).

Hydroxychloroquine (Plaquenil) is an antimalarial medication found to be particularly effective for SLE patients with fatigue, skin, and joint disease. It has been found to be significantly effective in reducing the frequency of abnormal blood clots in SLE patients. For resistant skin disease, other antimalarial drugs, such as chloroquine (Aralen) or quinacrine, are considered and can be used in combination with hydroxychloroquine (MedicineNet.com, 2008d).

Immunosuppressive medications are used for treating patients with more severe manifestations of SLE with damage to internal organs. Examples of immunosuppressive medications include methotrexate (Rheumatrex, Trexall), azathioprine (Imuran), cyclophosphamide (Cytoxan), chlorambucil (Leukeran), and cyclosporine (Sandimmune). All immunosuppressive medications can seriously depress blood cell counts and increase risks of infection and bleeding. Most recent research is indicating benefits of rituximab (Rituxan) in treating lupus. Rituximab is an intravenously infused antibody that suppresses a particular white blood cell, the B cell, by decreasing their number in the circulation. B cells have been found to play a central role in lupus activity, and when they are suppressed, the disease tends toward remission (MedicineNet.com, 2008d).

Recently, mycophenolate mofetil (CellCept) has been used as an effective medication for lupus when it is associated with kidney disease. It helps reverse active lupus kidney disease (lupus renal disease) and helps maintain remission after it is established. Additionally, it has fewer side effects than the traditional immunosuppressive medications (MedicineNet.com, 2008d).

In SLE patients with serious brain or kidney disease, plasmapheresis is sometimes used to remove antibodies and other immune substances in order to suppress immunity. Some SLE patients develop seriously low platelet levels, thereby increasing the risk for spontaneous bleeding. Because the spleen is believed to be the major site of platelet destruction, surgical removal of the spleen is sometimes performed to improve platelet levels. Plasmapheresis has also been used to remove proteins (cryoglobulins) that can lead to vasculitis. End-stage kidney damage from SLE requires dialysis and/or a kidney transplant (MedicineNet.com, 2008d).

DIAGNOSTIC TESTS for Systemic Lupus Erythematosus

Test	Expected Abnormality	Rationale for Abnormality
Lupus erythematosus (LE) prep	Elevated	Presence of systemic lupus erythematosus (SLE).
Antinuclear antibody (ANA)	Elevated	Presence of autoantibodies in blood.
Anti-DNA	Present	Conclude whether there are antibodies in the genetic materials in the cell.
Anti-Sm antibody	Present	Antibodies present on the ribonucleoprotein on the cell nucleus.
Serum complement test	Present	Presence of total group proteins, which can be consumed in immune reactions.
Complement proteins C3 and C4	Present	Examine specific levels of proteins present.
Urinalysis (UA)	Hematuria Proteinuria	Evidence of kidney involvement.

Nursing Management

The goals of nursing management are to limit complications from the disease which vary with each patient. The nursing process provides the framework for the development of the plan of care.

Assessment

Nursing management of the patient with SLE includes ongoing assessments for signs of infection and any dysfunction of the renal, gastrointestinal, cardiac, respiratory, and neurological systems. It is essential to observe patients for signs or symptoms of organ complications. Watch for signs of cardiac involvement such as tachycardia. With respiratory involvement, a patient may experience increased respirations, dyspnea, tachypnea, or orthopnea. Diarrhea, abdominal pain, or distention may indicate gastrointestinal disturbances. Renal involvement may manifest itself as weight gain, scanty urine, and decreased specific gravity; ataxia or ptosis may also indicate neurological involvement. Notify the health care provider immediately about any hematologic signs such as malaise, weakness, chills, and/or epistaxis.

Nursing Diagnoses

Nursing diagnoses related to the patient with SLE are listed in priority order:

1. *Injury, Risk for* related to weakness
2. *Comfort, Readiness for Enhanced* related to joint and/or nerve pain
3. *Activity Intolerance* related to weakness and anemia
4. *Skin Integrity, Impaired* related to photosensitivity
5. *Oral Mucous Membrane, Impaired* related to mouth and nasopharyngeal ulcers
6. *Nutrition: Imbalanced, Less than Body Requirements* related to anorexia and weight loss
7. *Fluid Volume, Excess* related to kidney dysfunction and/or corticosteroid use
8. *Anxiety* related to fear of the disease process
9. *Therapeutic Regimen Management, Readiness for Enhanced* related to exacerbation of disease process.

Outcomes and Evaluation Parameters

Outcomes for the patient with SLE include adaptation to the physical and psychological changes brought about by the disease. The goal is to reduce or limit complications of SLE. The evaluation parameters include the patient's verbalizing an understanding of the changes that are occurring and identifying strategies to cope. The patient should also be able to explain the current therapeutic regimen and identify strategies to prevent complications and reduce side effects of medications.

Planning, Interventions, and Rationales

Planning includes developing a comprehensive health maintenance plan. Interventions include teaching the patient about ways to reduce injuries, controlling discomfort, balancing rest with activity, maintaining skin integrity, reducing oronasopha-ryngeal ulcers, improving diet, restoring fluid volume, reducing anxiety, and complying with the medication regimen.

When implementing care, one of the most important measures to promote is rest. Patients should try to sleep between 8 and 10 hours a night. Encourage the patient to pace activities and plan rest. Stress should be avoided and an unhurried environment is preferred. Teaching the patient and family the importance of rest and decreased stress is paramount.

It is important to provide passive or active range of motion to promote joint movement. Ensure that the patient has not sustained any injuries or falls. Determine whether the patient experiences pain normally or while on medications, and if he remains physically active within his ability to do so. Additionally, the nurse needs to promote proper skin care, which includes hygiene, use of mild soap, use of sunscreen when outdoors, and avoidance of exposure to the sunlight. Observe the skin and oropharyngeal cavities to determine whether they are intact and without lesions. Encourage mouth care a couple times a day if the patient has mouth ulcers, and encourage the patient to change the consistency of his diet to reduce irritation and promote nutritious meals while he has stomatitis.

The diet should be balanced with all of the food groups, which will promote nutritional status, as well as counteract nutritional interactions with corticosteroids. A diet low in sodium is encouraged for patients who have edema, which could indicate renal involvement. Patients should have daily weights, intake, and output to determine fluid volume balance. Encourage the intake of vitamin C, as it is essential in the biosynthesis of collagen and increases total collagen synthesis. Ascertain whether the patient maintains her weight, maintains fluid balance, and can tolerate her diet of choice. Keep the patient calm and allow her to verbalize concerns about the disease process. With the proper diet and precautions, the patient should remain in a state of remission, while simultaneously keeping the organs intact and healthy. The Patient Teaching & Discharge Priorities box (p. 1854) outlines discharge planning for the patient with SLE.

Health Promotion

Providing adequate health teaching is also a goal in the plan of care. It is critical that the patient understand about medications, such as the different classifications, actions, adverse effects, and any interactions with food or other medications. Common medications used for SLE are analgesics, nonnarcotic analgesics, corticosteroids, oncologic drugs, and antimalarials. In addition to understanding about medications, it is important that the patient understand the disease process, diagnosis, prognosis, and treatments available. Teach the patient ways to avoid sun, changing doses of medications, fatigue, infections, and pregnancy without approval from her health care provider. Promote regular exercise and prevent fatigue. Medic alert bracelets should be worn.

Scleroderma: Epidemiology and Etiology

Progressive systemic sclerosis or scleroderma is a progressive autoimmune disease that affects women four times more than men, with peak incidence between ages 35 and 50 (Frazier &

PATIENT TEACHING & DISCHARGE PRIORITIES for Systemic Lupus Erythematosus

Need	Teaching
Safety	Stress the need to reduce injuries. Teach the patient and family ways to reduce risks in their environment to prevent falls.
Integrity of oral mucosa	Explain the importance of reducing irritation of the nose, mouth, and throat to reduce oronasopharyngeal ulcers.
Rest	Encourage the patient to balance rest with activity.
Skin integrity	The patient should maintain skin integrity to prevent integumentary involvement.
Diet	Provide the patient with plan for a balanced diet to maintain health.
Adequate fluid volume	Stress the importance of restoring fluid volume to prevent dehydration.
Low stress	Encourage the patient to reduce stress to prevent a flare-up of systemic lupus erythematosus (SLE). Encourage support groups.
Medications	Teach the patient and family the importance of the patient's medications and the need to comply with medication regimen to prevent further organ damage.

Drzymkowski, 2009; Porth, 2005). Scleroderma crosses all ethnic backgrounds. However, those of European descent are afflicted more than African Americans (National Institute of Arthritis and Musculoskeletal and Skin Diseases, 2006; Porth, 2005). Again, as with other diseases covered in this chapter, the cause is unknown and believed to be autoimmune. With scleroderma, the immune system stimulates the production of an excess of fibroblasts, the cells that produce collagen. In limited scleroderma the hardening of the skin is limited to the hands and face. Diffuse scleroderma also involves the trunk and proximal extremities. The diffuse scleroderma is a severe and progressive disease with early onset of organ involvement including the gastrointestinal tract, heart, lungs, and kidneys (Frazier & Drzymkowski, 2009; Porth, 2005).

Pathophysiology

Scleroderma causes fibrotic changes in connective tissue throughout the body. It can involve any of the following systems: integumentary, circulatory, joints, alimentary canal, cardiac, respiratory, renal, and/or gastrointestinal tract. As the disease becomes more involved, the acronym CREST syndrome identifies a group of symptoms affiliated with the disease's getting advanced with a poor recovery or chance of remission. C stands for calcium deposits in organs; R stands for Raynaud's type symptoms; E stands for esophageal dysfunction; S stands for sclerodactyly, meaning scleroderma of the fingers and toes; and T stands for telangiectasia, which is a vascular lesion formed by dilation.

Clinical Manifestations

The disease is characterized by inflammatory and then degenerative and fibrotic changes in the skin, blood vessels, synovial membranes, skeletal muscles, and internal organs.

Subjective clinical findings are verbalized by the patient who complains of joint pain and muscle weakness. Objective clinical findings note hard skin that fixes to underlying structures. The affect becomes flat and general body movements are rigid. Telangiectases are noted on the lips, fingers, face, and tongue. Some patients develop dysphagia and Raynaud's-type symptoms.

Laboratory and Diagnostic Procedures

Initially, the diagnosis of the scleroderma syndrome is based on the clinical manifestations of the illnesses. Laboratory data would consist of positive LE prep with elevated gamma globulin levels, and the presence of antinuclear antibodies. A particular antibody, the anticentromere antibody, is found almost exclusively in the CREST form of scleroderma. Anti-Scl-70 antibody (antitopoisomerase I antibody) is most often seen in patients with the diffuse form of scleroderma. Other tests that help evaluate the presence or extent of any internal disease include upper and lower gastrointestinal examinations; chest x-rays, lung function testing, and CAT scanning to examine the lungs; and ECG, echocardiograms, and sometimes heart catheterization to evaluate the pressure in the arteries of the heart and lungs.

Medical Management

Because this is a chronic disease, medical management focuses on symptom control and improving the patient's quality of life. Medications are utilized to assist the patient with symptoms of the disease. Corticosteroids help with the inflammation, and salicylates or narcotics are used for joint discomfort. For Raynaud's-type symptoms, vasodilators are used to increase circulation. Most commonly, immunosuppressants and D-penicillamine are also administered. Hand warming and protection from cold temperatures may be all that is necessary for mild Raynaud's disease. Low-dose aspirin is frequently prescribed to prevent tiny blood clots in the fingers, especially in patients with a history of fingertip ulcerations. Medications that dilate the arteries, such as nifedipine (Procardia, Adalat) and nicardipine (Cardene), or topical nitroglycerin applied to the side of the affected digit is frequently used to treat moderate Raynaud's disease. Gently applied finger splints can protect tender tissues. A class of medications that is typically used for depression, the selective serotonin reuptake inhibitors, such as fluoxetine (Prozac), can sometimes improve the circulation of the affected digit. In cases of severe Raynaud's disease, surgical procedures, such as those used to interrupt the nerves of the finger that stimulate constriction of the blood vessels (digital sympathectomy), may be necessary. Ulcerations of the fingers can require topical or oral antibiotics (MedicineNet.com, 2008b).

Medications used to treat esophagus irritation and heartburn are omeprazole (Prilosec), esomeprazole (Nexium), and lansoprazole (Prevacid). Antacids can also be helpful. Elevating the head of the bed can reduce the backflow of acid into the esophagus that causes inflammation and heartburn. Avoiding caffeine and cigarette smoking also helps. Constipation, cramping, and diarrhea are sometimes caused by bacteria that can be treated with tetracycline or erythromycin. Increased fluid intake and fiber intake are good general measures to help with constipation (MedicineNet.com, 2008b).

Medications that are used to suppress the overly active immune system include penicillamine, azathioprine, and methotrexate. Serious inflammation of the lungs (alveolitis) can require immune suppression with cyclophosphamide (Cytoxan) along with prednisone. Approximately 10% of patients with the CREST variant that develop scleroderma have pulmonary hypertension (Chapter 36 ⊘), which is often treated with calcium antagonist medications, such as nifedipine, and anticoagulation (MedicineNet.com, 2008b).

Irritated, itchy dry skin can be helped by emollients such as Lubriderm, Eucerin, or Bag Balm. Colchicine may be helpful in decreasing the inflammation and tenderness that periodically accompany the calcinosis nodules in the skin. Telangiectasias, such as those on the face, can be treated with local laser therapy. Sun exposure should be minimized as it can worsen telangiectasias (MedicineNet.com, 2008b). Medications used to treat scleroderma are addressed in the earlier Pharmacology Summaries on p. 1839.

◼ Nursing Management

The nursing process provides the framework necessary to develop a comprehensive health care plan. The goals of nursing care involve control of pain and support of the patient and family.

Assessment

As with all of the joint diseases, nursing assessment focuses on the extent of joint range of motion and pain. With scleroderma, the nurse must also assess for organ involvement. The lungs, heart, skin, and gastrointestinal system must be assessed for involvement. Chapter 9 ⊘ outlines the essential components of the nursing assessment for each of these organs.

Nursing Diagnoses

The highest priority nursing diagnoses for the patient with scleroderma are as follows:

1. *Pain, Chronic* related to joint pain
2. *Skin Integrity, Impaired* related to skin lesions
3. *Body Image, Disturbed* related to flat affect, skin lesions, and telangiectases
4. *Falls, Risk for* related to limited motion and rigidity
5. *Therapeutic Regimen Management, Ineffective* related to noncompliance with medications
6. *Mobility: Physical, Impaired* related to rigidity and limited movement
7. *Anxiety* related to poor prognosis.

Planning, Interventions, Rationales, and Evaluation

When planning the treatment for the patient with scleroderma, the goal is to support the patient and family and improve the quality of life, because there is no cure. When implementing the care, the nurse must be knowledgeable about which organs are involved and the associated clinical manifestations. The nurse must continually monitor function of all vital organs, such as the heart, lungs, and kidneys, to determine the perfusion. Explain the purpose of each medication and the importance of compliance. Advise the patient about the adverse effects of all of the medications.

Engage in regular inspection of skin and oropharyngeal areas to maintain skin integrity. Because skin manifestations are common, it is essential that the patient be taught to use mild soap and lotion on the skin. The use of emollient lotions is helpful as is strict adherence to sunscreens. The nurse should stress to avoid exposure to the cold due to vasoconstriction of vessels, thereby decreasing peripheral circulation. If there is lung involvement, provide education on the importance of not smoking, and deep breathing exercises should be encouraged to improve oxygenation.

Include the multidisciplinary team in assisting the patient to be independent for as long as possible. Physical therapy can usually provide assistance to keep the patient moving and aid with mobility. Ensure joint pain is managed with or without medication, and combine with physical therapy in order to improve physical mobility. Occupational therapy can provide assistance with activities of daily living. Evaluate the patient for signs of increased muscle weakness and rigidity. Make certain the patient is compliant with medications and understands the importance of the treatment regimen. The patient needs to be reminded to keep himself away from situations that may lead to falls or high levels of anxiety.

Finally, have discussions with the patient about the physical changes that are occurring to help her be better able to cope with changes in her body image as the disease progresses. Explain which symptoms need to be reported to the health care provider, and stress the importance of regular medical examinations. Evaluation of the health plan includes an assessment of the patient's knowledge of the disease, the importance of compliance with the treatment plan, and limitations.

◼ Lyme Disease

Lyme disease is a bacterial infection that affects the organs and joints that is transmitted from black-legged ticks. In the city of Lyme, Connecticut, a group of children spontaneously developed a debilitating arthritis. The Centers for Disease Control and Prevention (CDC) was alerted to this phenomenon, and research into the progression of illness and disease vectors was underway. In 1977, at the conclusion of the investigation, it was found that deer ticks were transmitting a degenerative disease to humans, which was subsequently named Lyme disease, after the city that had brought medical attention to it (Centers for Disease Control and Prevention, 2008).

Epidemiology

In 2006, 19,931 cases of Lyme disease were reported, showing a national average of 8.2 cases per 100,000 persons (Centers for Disease Control and Prevention, 2008). The deer tick bites the host (human) and transmits the disease. In the United States, Lyme disease is heavily concentrated in the areas of the Northeast, Southeast, and West Coast (Centers for Disease Control and Prevention, 2008).

Etiology

Lyme disease is caused by bacteria, called *Borrelia burgdorferi*, which are found in infected black-legged ticks. There are two species of black-legged ticks: *ixodes scapularis* located in the Northeast and north central United States and *ixodes pacificus* in the western parts of the United States. These ticks are much smaller than the ticks that animals such as dogs and cattle carry. Ticks feed by placing their mouth on the human and sucking the blood. The bacteria are transferred slowly by transmitting the infection over a couple of days of feeding (Centers for Disease Control and Prevention, 2008).

Those individuals who live in rural areas near trees and overgrown shrubs may be at risk for Lyme disease. Outdoor activities, such as hiking, camping, gardening, working in forestry, and wildlife/parks management in specified areas, expose participants to a higher risk of being infected (Centers for Disease Control and Prevention, 2008).

Pathophysiology and Clinical Manifestations

An infected tick attaches to a human, sucks the person's blood, and transfers the disease. There are three stages of the disease, which can affect many systems of the body.

1. Early localized disease, occurring a few days to 1 month after the tick bite.
   - Erythema chronicum migrans (reddened area where the tick bite occurred) occurs in 70% to 80% of patients.
   - Associated symptoms and signs may include fatigue, malaise, lethargy, headache, stiff neck, myalgias, arthralgias, and regional or generalized lymphadenopathy.
2. Early disseminated disease occurring days to 10 months after the tick bite.
   - Carditis. Occurs in approximately 5% of untreated patients. Manifestations include conduction defects, mild cardiomyopathy, or myopericarditis.
   - Neurological disease. Occurs in approximately 15% of untreated patients. Manifestations include lymphocytic meningitis; encephalitis; cranial neuropathy (most often facial, can be bilateral), peripheral neuropathy, or radiculoneuropathy; or myelitis.
   - Musculoskeletal involvement. Occurs in approximately 60% of untreated patients. Manifestations include migratory polyarthritis and/or polyarthralgias.
   - Skin involvement. Multiple erythema chronicum migrans lesions, erythema nodosum.
   - Lymphadenopathy. Regional and/or generalized.
   - Eye involvement. Conjunctivitis, iritis, choroiditis, vitritis, retinitis.
   - Liver disease. Liver function test abnormalities, hepatitis.
   - Kidney disease. Microhematuria, asymptomatic proteinuria.
3. Late or chronic disease, occurring months to years after the tick bite.
   - Musculoskeletal symptoms. Approximately 60% of untreated patients develop intermittent monoarticular or oligoarticular arthritis; approximately 10% of untreated patients develop persistent monoarthritis, usually affecting the knee.
   - Neurological disease. Incidence is rare but may be exhibited by chronic, often subtle, encephalopathy, encephalomyelitis, and/or peripheral neuropathy (Sexton, 2008).

Laboratory and Diagnostic Procedures

It is important to obtain the correct diagnosis before treating this condition. Be sure that the patient obtains a blood test that can be used to detect the presence of antibodies from the bacterium to corroborate the diagnosis. Antibiotics can be given to cure the disease if caught early. The most common classifications of anti-infectives are tetracyclines and penicillins. Another goal is to prevent this disease for further progression. It is important to talk to patients about prevention and health promotion.

Medical Management

For early-stage Lyme disease, oral antibiotics are the standard treatment. These usually include doxycycline for adults and children older than 8, or amoxicillin or cefuroxime axetil for elder adults, younger children, and pregnant or breast-feeding women. These drugs often clear the infection and prevent complications. A 14- to 21-day course of antibiotics is usually recommended. If the disease has progressed, intravenous antibiotic for 14 to 28 days is an effective treatment plan for eliminating infection, although it may take some time to recover symptomatically (MayoClinic.com, 2008).

The flu-like symptoms are treated with supportive measures, depending on the presenting symptoms. For example, fever is treated with antipyretics and rest, and the joint pain is treated with NSAIDs and rest.

◼ Nursing Management

The nursing process provides the framework for the management of patients with Lyme disease. Nursing management focuses on treatment of the infection and education of the patient and family on ways to avoid exposure to ticks and possible reinfection.

Assessment

Assessment of the early localized disease, the first stage, which occurs between days 7 and 10, includes evaluating for a growing rash called erythema chronicum migrans (ECM). ECM looks like a bull's eye on the affected part. Assess for flu-like symptoms: headache, confusion, forgetfulness, stiff neck, irregular heartbeat, achy and swollen joints, and swollen lymph glands

(Frazier & Drzymkowski, 2009). During the second stage, which occurs a couple of weeks to months after being infected, the nurse needs to focus the assessment on the neurological system. Assessment findings could include severe headaches, poor motor balance, and temporary facial paralysis. During the late stage of the disease, which can occur from months to years after being infected, the musculoskeletal system is attacked. Arthritis is a complication of this disease. Approximately 5% of the people infected will develop chronic arthritis (Centers for Disease Control and Prevention, 2008).

Nursing Diagnoses

The following are the high-priority nursing diagnoses for the patient with Lyme disease:

1. *Infection, Risk for* related to tick contamination
2. *Pain, Acute* related to neurological symptoms of the disease
3. *Knowledge, Deficient* related to unfamiliarity of Lyme disease.

Interventions, Outcomes, and Evaluation Parameters

Nursing interventions are dependent on the stage of the disease and the patient's clinical manifestations. For example, early in the disease process, the management would focus on treating the flu-like symptoms. The later stages of the disease are more complex, and the nursing care is dependent on what systems are involved. For example, if there is neurological involvement and muscle weakness, the nurse must focus on protection of the airway and prevention of patients falling or injuring themselves. The outcome of care is to have the patient free of infection as exhibited by a decrease in symptoms. It is imperative that the patient and family understand ways to protect themselves from exposure and reinfection. During this phase of the nursing process, the evaluation parameters would include educating the patient about the disease and its cause, signs, symptoms, treatment, and prevention by examining discharge priorities. For more information, see the Patient Teaching & Discharge Priorities box about Lyme disease.

Health Promotion

It is important to teach individuals about ways to prevent disease. Many things can be done to promote protection from Lyme disease. During the summer months, avoid areas where ticks are contaminated. Be sure to wear long sleeve shirts, long pants, and socks. Tuck socks into pants and tuck shirts into pants to minimize exposure of the skin. By wearing light color clothing, ticks

are easily seen and can be removed before getting bit. It is important to use tick repellents, such as DEET. Be careful not to overuse these products. Avoid high grassy trails when walking. Once individuals are finished being outdoors, they should remove their clothing and wash it. Also, they should examine their body thoroughly and remove any attached ticks. Use tweezers to carefully remove them. Once the tick is removed, be sure that antiseptic is used to clean the area. Check pets to be certain that they do not have ticks. Tick collars can be put around the neck of the pets.

■ Sjögren's Syndrome: Epidemiology and Etiology

Sjögren's syndrome (SS) is an autoimmune disease. SS immune cells attack and destroy the glands that produce tears and saliva (Frazier & Drzymkowski, 2009). In the United States, SS affects 1 million to 4 million people. Usually the ratio of women to men is 9 to 1 (Borenstein, 2007). Sjögren's syndrome is found more commonly in patients with a family history of other autoimmune illnesses.

Pathophysiology

SS is an inflammatory disease that can affect different parts of the body. SS features inflammation in the glands of the body resulting in dryness in the affected areas. SS is characterized by the increased production of more antibodies in the blood that are directed against various tissues of the body. This particular autoimmune illness is caused by inflammation of the glands that produce tears (lacrimal glands), leading to decreased water production for tears and eye dryness. Inflammation of the glands that produce the saliva in the mouth (salivary glands, including the parotid glands) leads to mouth dryness (MedicineNet.com, 2008c). SS is not considered a connective tissue disease when it involves the glands affecting the eyes and mouth only. However, when SS is associated with RA, then it is considered a connective tissue disease (MedicineNet.com, 2008c).

Clinical Manifestations

The two symptoms that are the hallmark of Sjögren's syndrome are dry eyes and dry mouth (Sjögren's Syndrome Foundation, 2008). The disease can also cause dryness in other body organs including the kidneys, gastrointestinal tract, lung, and blood vessels. Many patients have debilitating joint pain and fatigue. The symptoms can wax and wane and go into remission. Some

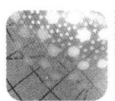

PATIENT TEACHING & DISCHARGE PRIORITIES for Lyme Disease

Need	Teaching
Knowledge of disease process	Encourage understanding of the infectious process of Lyme disease. Early detection is critical for early treatment and prevention of complications.
Prevention	Those who live in highly infected areas should be taking precautions to reduce the risk of getting infected. Teach patient the importance of using insect repellant when out of doors in high risk areas.
Medications	Encourage compliance with medication regimen. If infected, it is imperative to continue to take entire prescription as ordered by health care provider.

patients may have only mild symptoms where others are severely affected and experience a poor quality of life.

Laboratory and Diagnostic Procedures

According to Sjögren's Syndrome Foundation (2008), 70% of individuals with SS will have an elevated antibody (ANA), which measures antibodies that react against normal components of the cell nucleus. Sjögren's syndrome antigens (SSA and SSB) are also elevated; with 70% of the population having SS, the rheumatoid factor is elevated, measuring positive. The erythrocyte sedimentation rate is also elevated, indicating an active inflammatory process. Immunoglobulins measure normal blood proteins and are also elevated with SS (Sjögren's Syndrome Foundation, 2008).

Other tests that may be used are the following: the Schirmer's test, measuring tear production; Rose Bengal and Lissamine green, using dyes to observe abnormal cells on the surface of the eye; slit lamp exam, magnifying the volume of tears of the eye by viewing it in its resting state; parotid gland flow, measuring the amount of saliva produced over a certain period of time; salivary scintigraphy, measuring salivary gland function; sialography, an x-ray of the salivary duct system; and lip biopsy, used to confirm lymphocytic infiltration of the minor salivary glands (Sjögren's Syndrome Foundation, 2008).

Medical Management

There is no cure for SS at this time. However, symptoms can be treated. Patients can use moist replacement therapies for symptoms of dryness. Increasing fluid intake, using oral sprays, and chewing sugarless gum may help oral dryness. Wearing sunglasses to protect the eyes and using artificial tears are recommended (Frazier & Drzymkowski, 2009). Many classifications of medications are helpful, such as nonsteroidal anti-inflammatory drugs for musculoskeletal symptoms, and corticosteroids and immunosuppressive therapies for severe complications (National Institute of Neurological Disorders and Stroke, 2008d).

Nursing Management

When utilizing a nursing problem-solving approach, the nursing process will lead the nurse to understand the disease process while prioritizing care for those with SS.

Assessment

For subjective assessments, patients will complain of feeling dryness in the following locations: mouth, mucous membranes, and skin. Objective assessments include irritation, a gritty feeling, or painful burning in the eyes; dry mouth; dysphagia; swelling of saliva glands; and dryness of nasal passage or throat, or vagina or skin (National Institute of Neurological Disorders and Stroke, 2008d). There are periods of remissions and exacerbations. Exacerbations usually occur after an illness.

Patients also may experience blurred vision, recurrent mouth infections, swollen parotid glands, hoarseness, dysphagia, debilitating fatigue, and joint pain (National Institute of Neurological Disorders and Stroke, 2008d).

Nursing Diagnoses

The following is a list of high-priority nursing diagnoses for the patient with Sjögren's syndrome:

1. *Nutrition: Imbalanced, Less than Body Requirements* as related by dysphasia
2. *Pain, Chronic* related to dried secretions in mucous membranes and joint pain
3. *Knowledge, Deficient* related to unfamiliarity of educational resources
4. *Communication: Verbal, Impaired* related to hoarseness
5. *Self-Care, Readiness for Enhanced* related to debilitating fatigue.

Interventions, Outcomes, and Evaluation Parameters

Interventions include protecting the affected tissues, assisting in preventing complications, avoiding irritation to the tissues, monitoring for signs and symptoms of infection, and assessing for the development of complications. Outcomes for the patient with SS include relief of symptoms of dryness in the oral cavity and eyes. Evaluation parameters include adequate nutritional status, pain abatement, awareness of educational resources, ability to communicate effectively, and care for self.

■ Myositis: Epidemiology and Etiology

Myositis is an uncommon disease wherein the immune system inflames the body's own healthy muscle tissue. There are four kinds of myositis: polymyositis (PM), dermatomyositis (DM), inclusion body myositis (IBM), and juvenile myositis (JM) (National Institute of Neurological Disorders and Stroke, 2008a, 2008b, 2008c). PM can occur at any age, but affects those between ages 40 and 50. DM, like PM, can arise at any age, but is more prevalent between ages 40 and 60 and between ages 5 and 15. Both are more common in African Americans than in Caucasians and affect more women than men (Frazier & Drzymkowski, 2009; National Institute of Neurological Disorders and Stroke, 2008a, 2008c). Myositis occurs more readily with patients who have lupus. IBM typically begins after age 50 and is more common in women than in men. Globally, DM and PM together affect 5 to 10 people out of 100,000 (MayoClinic.com, 2007). Theses conditions are usually caused by an injury, infection, or autoimmune condition (Ariel & Teitel, 2007).

Pathophysiology

Myositis is a disease where the immune system causes chronic inflammation of the voluntary muscles of the body. Voluntary muscles are consciously controlled to help move the body. Myositis may be triggered by an injury, infection, or an autoimmune disease. PM consists of muscle weakness. DM has the same symptoms as PM; but DM differs because of the skin involvement with a distinctive rash over the face, shoulders, arms, and bony prominences (MayoClinic.com, 2007).

Clinical Manifestations

Symptoms for PM include muscle weakness especially proximal to the trunk, such as in the hips and shoulders. Patients have difficulty getting up out of chairs, climbing stairs, lifting objects, and reaching overhead (National Institute of Neurological Disorders and Stroke, 2008c). As the condition advances, some patients have dysphasia.

With DM, patients have the same symptoms as PM, but a rash exists. This rash is purplish blue discolorations on the face, eyelids, bridge of nose, neck, shoulders, elbows, knees, knuckles, upper chest, and back (American Association of Orthopedic Surgeons, 2008; National Institute of Neurological Disorders and Stroke, 2008a). Some patients develop calcium deposits under the skin that manifest as bumps under the skin. IBM has a gradual onset of muscle weakness all over the body. Atrophy of the muscles can occur in wrists or fingers, forearms, and thighs. Some people may develop dysphagia. JM is a combination of the three other kinds of myositis: PM, DM, and IBM.

Laboratory and Diagnostic Procedures

A laboratory test that can assist with the diagnosis of myositis is the creatine kinase. This test measures autoantibodies and the muscle enzymes. Two diagnostic tests that also can confirm the diagnosis are the electromyogram and magnetic resonance imaging to identify the inflamed muscles (MayoClinic.com, 2007).

Medical Management

The health care provider needs to reassure the patient that there are treatments available, but no cure. Prompt treatment consists of reducing inflammation and restoring strength. Some methodologies can curb muscle atrophy. First, medications may improve myositis. Corticosteroids act to suppress the immune system and slow the attack on healthy muscles (MayoClinic.com, 2007). Nonsteroidal anti-inflammatory medications are given to reduce pain. Physical therapy will help the patients strengthen muscles. An exercise program may be beneficial to prevent muscle atrophy and promote range of motion. Utilizing a whirlpool bath, heat, and gentle massage may be beneficial (MayoClinic.com, 2007). Rest can assist this condition. Pacing activities and planning rest are valuable in reducing inflammation of muscles (MayoClinic.com, 2007).

◼ Nursing Management

Utilization of the nursing process will provide the nurse with the tools necessary to provide safe and sound patient care. The nurse must assess for muscle weakness, as this is the most common symptom. Varying degrees of loss of muscle strength may cause difficulty in getting up from a sitting position, climbing stairs, or lifting an object above the shoulders. Some patients may complain of muscle aches and tenderness to touch.

Nursing Diagnoses

Nursing diagnoses that are a priority for a patient with myositis include:

1. *Self-Care, Readiness for Enhanced* related to muscle weakness
2. *Activity Intolerance* related to muscle atrophy
3. *Body Image, Disturbed* related to rash
4. *Falls, Risk for* related to inability to support body's weight
5. *Pain, Chronic* related to muscle atrophy.

Interventions, Outcomes, and Evaluation Parameters

Nursing interventions include assisting the patient with activities of daily living and spacing care to allow for periods of rest. Outcomes for the patient with myositis include restoring strength and reducing muscle weakness in order to prevent atrophy of muscles. Promote independence by encouraging the patient to perform activities of daily living to the fullest extent while balancing rest and physical activity. Evaluation parameters are that the patient is able to provide own self-care, report activity tolerance, accept body image changes, have no falls, and have no pain with or without medications.

◼ Research

Many clinical trials are taking place on a variety of connective tissue diseases, such as arthritis and lupus. Several connective tissue diseases are also inherited. These trials examine the effects of medication on the disease itself, whereas others examine the issue of stem cells to correct the condition. Many of these disorders can be controlled by changes in behavior or lifestyle changes in which diet and exercise play a critical role. For specific information about research that is being conducted, go to the National Institutes of Health's website to search for the most up-to-date information and research on specific diseases.

MyNursingKit | National Institute of Health

Clinical Preparation

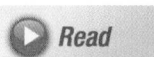 **Read**

- History of Current Illness
- Past Medical History
- Physical Exam
- Admitting Medical Orders
- Laboratory Study Results

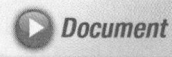 **Document**

- Summary of Hospitalization
- Pathophysiology Form
- Laboratory Values
- Laboratory Results Explanation

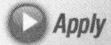 **Apply**

- List of Potential Nursing Diagnoses
- Concept Map
- Critical Thinking Questions

Log on to MyNursingKit.com to download forms you will need and to complete further steps in the Clinical Preparation assignment.

HISTORY OF PRESENT ILLNESS

EA is a 48-year-old Caucasian male who works as a pastry chef at one of the most prestigious hotels in San Francisco. He is married and has 13 children. He weighs 378 pounds and has a history of kidney stones on the left side. He came into the emergency department when he had completed work after the dinner crowd. He presented symptoms of an elevated temperature of 101°F, chills, malaise, and excruciating pain in his right great toe.

Medical–Surgical History

Upon interview: The patient revealed that his father and grandfather had gout.

Physical Exam

Patient verbalized, "I feel real tired and have had a temperature of 100 degrees for two days." His toe was swollen, red, and hot. On a pain scale, the patient indicated his pain was an "11." Laboratory tests were collected and the only elevations were a serum uric acid level and a low pH in the urine. Tophi are located in the following places: (1) his ear lobes bilaterally, (2) right elbow, and (3) bilateral knees. The physician ordered the patient to have the following medications: allopurinol and colchicine and a diet low in purines.

CRITICAL THINKING QUESTIONS

1. What risk factors presented in this scenario indicate gout?
2. What types of food may cause an acute attack of gouty arthritis?
3. What are three objective assessments that lead you to believe the patient may have gout?
4. What is a complication of having too much serum uric acid and low pH? Which organ is most commonly involved?

Answers to Critical Thinking Questions appear in Appendix D.

NCLEX® REVIEW

1. A patient was told she has lupus erythematosus. Which of the following should the nurse instruct this patient?
   1. It's a term to describe rheumatic disease.
   2. It's a chronic inflammatory process that affects joints.
   3. It's a common connective tissue disorder.
   4. It's an inflammation associated with psoriasis.

2. Which of the following should the nurse include when planning the care of a patient with rheumatoid arthritis?
   1. Increase activity
   2. Maximize activities of daily living
   3. Restrict calories
   4. Prevent deformities

3. A patient is admitted with circinate balanitis and uveitis. The nurse realizes this patient is most likely experiencing:
   1. Reactive arthritis.
   2. Rheumatoid arthritis.
   3. Osteoarthritis.
   4. Septic arthritis.

4. The nurse has completed the assessment of a patient with osteoarthritis. Which of the following nursing diagnoses would be applicable to this patient?
   1. *Knowledge Deficit*
   2. *Ineffective Coping*
   3. *Imbalanced Nutrition: More than Body Requirements*
   4. *Fluid Volume Deficit*

5. A patient is diagnosed with gout. The nurse should instruct this patient to avoid which of the following foods?

1. Lettuce
2. Gravies
3. Broccoli
4. Chicken

6. A patient is admitted with muscle weakness and a blue-tinted rash on his face, neck, and back. The nurse realizes this patient is most likely experiencing:

1. Myositis.
2. Polymyositis.
3. Dermatomyositis.
4. Inclusion body myositis.

Answers for review questions appear in Appendix D

KEY TERMS

ankylosing spondylitis *p.1849*
circinate balanitis *p.1847*
dactylitis *p.1842*
enthesitis *p.1842*
gouty arthritis *p.1843*
Lyme disease *p.1855*

myositis *p.1858*
osteoarthritis (OA) *p.1833*
psoriatic arthritis *p.1842*
reactive arthritis *p.1847*
rheumatoid arthritis (RA) *p.1836*

septic arthritis *p.1850*
Sjögren's syndrome *p.1857*
subcutaneous nodules *p.1835*
systemic lupus erythematosus *p.1851*
tophi *p.1844*

EXPLORE PEARSON **mynursingkit™**

MyNursingKit is your one stop for online chapter review materials and resources. Prepare for success with additional NCLEX®-style practice questions, interactive assignments and activities, web links, animations and videos, and more!

Register your access code from the front of your book at
www.mynursingkit.com

REFERENCES

American Association of Orthopedic Surgeons (AAOS). (2008). *Myositis.* Retrieved September 1, 2008 from http://orthoinfo.aaos.org/topic.cfm?topic=A00198

American College of Rheumatology. (2008). *Ankylosing spondylitis.* Retrieved May 24, 2008, from http://www.rheumatology.org/public/factsheets/as.asp

Ariel, D., & Teitel, M. D. (2007). Myositis. *Healthline.* Retrieved July 23, 2007, from http://www.healthline.com/adamcontent/myositis

Arthritis-FAQ.com. (2007). *Gout overview.* Retrieved July 18, 2007, from http://www.arthritis-faq.org/gout.html

Borenstein, D. (2007). Epidemiology, diagnostics and management. *Medscape Today.* Retrieved July 23, 2007, from http://www.medscape.com/viewarticle/423760

Centers for Disease Control and Prevention (CDC). (2007). *Prevalence of arthritis.* Retrieved May 24, 2008, from http://www.cdc.gov/arthritis/data_statistics/arthritis_related_statistics.htm#1

Centers for Disease Control and Prevention (CDC). (2008). *Lyme disease.* Retrieved May 24, 2008, from http://www.cdc.gov/ncidod/dvbid/lyme/ld_statistics.htm

Chemocare.com. (2005). *Hyperuricemia.* Retrieved July 30, 2007, from http://www.chemocare.com/managing/hyperuricemia-high-uric-acid.asp

eMedicineHealth. (2008). *Gout.* Retrieved May 23, 2008, from http://www.emedicinehealth.com/gout/article_em.htm

FamilyPracticeNotebook.com. (2008). *Osteoarthritis.* Retrieved August 25, 2008, from http://www.fpnotebook.com/Rheum/Osteoarthritis/Ostrthrts.htm

Frazier, M. S., & Drzymkowski, J. W. (Eds.). (2009). *Essentials of human diseases and conditions* (4th ed.). St. Louis: Saunders Elsevier.

Gladman, D. (2007). Pathogenesis of psoriatic arthritis. *UpToDate.* Retrieved October 23, 2007, from http://www.uptodate.com/patients/content/topic.do?topicKey=~nKkKMlvosxI56.&selectedTitle=1~78&source=search_result

Gladman, D. (2008). Clinical manifestations and diagnosis of psoriatic arthritis. *UpToDate.* Retrieved August 21, 2008, from http://www.uptodate.com/patients/content/topic.do?topicKey=~FFX.7DwCxZDGbF&selectedTitle=2~150&source=search_result

Goldenberg, D., & Sexton, D. (2007). Bacterial (nongonococcal) arthritis in adults. *UpToDate.* Retrieved October 23, 2007, from http://www.uptodate.com/patients/content/topic.do?topicKey=~mchmzYL2SL2ACJ&selectedTitle=7~147&source=search_result

Hammadi, A. A. (2008). Psoriatic arthritis. *eMedicine.com.* Retrieved May 23, 2008, from http://www.emedicine.com/MED/topic1954.htm

Hogan, M. A. (2007). *Nutrition & diet therapy* (2nd ed.). Upper Saddle River, NJ: Pearson Prentice Hall.

Hospital for Special Surgery. (2005). *Osteoarthritis.* Retrieved May 1, 2006, from http://www.imaginghss.org/imaging-of-orthopaedic-conditions/osteoarthritis.htm

InnerVibrance. (2006). *Rheumatoid arthritis.* Retrieved February 28, 2006, from http://www.innervibrance.com/rheumatoid_arthritis.html

Kalunian, K. C. (2007). *Pathogenesis of OA: Diagnosis and classification of OA.* Retrieved August 28, 2008, from http://www.utdol.com/online/content/topic.do?topicKey=osteoart/3785&selectedTitle=1~150&source=search_result

Kherani, R., & Shojania, K. (2007). Septic arthritis in patients with preexisting inflammatory arthritis. *Canadian Medical Association Journal, 176*(11), 1605–1608.

MayoClinic.com. (2007). *Polymyositis.* Retrieved May 24, 2008, from http://www.mayoclinic.com/health/polymyositis/DS00334

MayoClinic.com. (2008). *Lyme disease: Symptoms.* Retrieved May 23, 2008, from http://www.mayoclinic.com/health/lyme-disease/DS00116/DSECTION-2

MedicineNet.com. (2008a). *Rheumatoid arthritis.* Retrieved May 23, 2008, from http://www.medicinenet.com/rheumatoid_arthritis/article.htm

MedicineNet.com. (2008b). *Scleroderma.* Retrieved May 21, 2008, from http://www.medicinenet.com/scleroderma/article.htm

MedicineNet.com. (2008c). *Sjogren's syndrome.* Retrieved May 23, 2008, from http://www.medicinenet.com/sjogrens_syndrome/article.htm

MedicineNet.com. (2008d). *Systemic lupus erythematosus (SLE or lupus).* Retrieved May 23, 2008, from http://www.medicinenet.com/systemic_lupus/article.htm

MedlinePlus Medical Encyclopedia. (2007). *Acute gouty arthritis.* Retrieved May 23, 2008, from http://www.nlm.nih.gov/medlineplus/ency/article/000422.htm

Meiner, S. (2001). Gouty arthritis: Not just a big toe problem. *Geriatric Nursing, 22*(3), 132–134.

Mikuls, T. R., MacLean, C. H., Olivieri, J., Patino, F., Allison, J., Farrar, J. T., et al. (2004). Quality of care indicators for gout management. *Arthritis & Rheumatism, 50*(3), 937–943.

Mikuls, T. R., & Saag, K. G. (2005). Gout treatment: What is evidence-based and how do we determine and promote optimized clinical care? *Current Rheumatology Reports, 7*(3), 242–249.

National Institute of Arthritis and Musculoskeletal and Skin Diseases (NIAMS). (2002). *Reactive arthritis.* Retrieved December 18, 2004, from http://www.niams.nih.gov/hi/topics/reactive/reactive.htm

National Institute of Arthritis and Musculoskeletal and Skin Diseases (NIAMS). (2006). *Scleroderma.* Retrieved August 21, 2008, from http://www.niams.nih.gov/hi/topics/scleroderma/scleroderma.htm

National Institute of Arthritis and Musculoskeletal and Skin Diseases (NIAMS). (2008). *Arthritis: Causes and risk factors—Gout.* Retrieved August 21, 2008, from http://nihseniorhealth.gov/arthritis/causesandriskfactors/01.html

National Institute of Neurological Disorders and Stroke. (2008a). *Dermatomyositis information page.* Retrieved August 21, 2008, from www.ninds.nih.gov/disorders/dermatomyositis/dermatomyositis.htm

National Institute of Neurological Disorders and Stroke. (2008b). *Inclusion body myositis information page.* Retrieved August 21, 2008, from http://www.ninds.nih.gov/disorders/inclusion_body_myositis/inclusion_body_myositis.htm

National Institute of Neurological Disorders and Stroke. (2008c). *Polymyositis information page.* Retrieved August 21, 2008, from http://www.ninds.nih.gov/disorders/polymyositis/polymyositis.htm

National Institute of Neurological Disorders and Stroke. (2008d). *Sjögren's syndrome information page.* Retrieved August 28, 2008, from http://www.ninds.nih.gov/disorders/sjogrens/sjogrens.htm

Porth, C. (2005). *Pathophysiology: Concepts of altered health states* (7th ed.). Philadelphia: Lippincott Williams & Wilkins.

Schlesinger, N., Schumacher, M. C., Catton, M., & Maxwell, L. (2006). Colchicine for acute gout. *Cochrane Database of Systematic Reviews,* 2006, Issue 4. Retrieved June 20, 2007, from http://mrw.interscience.wiley.com/cochrane/clsysrev/articles/CD006190/frame.html

Sexton, D. H. (2008). Clinical manifestations of Lyme disease. *UpToDate.* Retrieved April 30, 2008, from http://www.uptodate.com/patients/content/topic.do?topicKey=~9197/aelfkcit3&selectedTitle=2~133&source=search_result

Sjögren's Syndrome Foundation. (2008). *Sjögren's syndrome.* Retrieved September 1, 2008, from http://www.sjogrens.org/syndrome/diagnosis.html

U.S. Department of Health and Human Services (DHHS). (2000). *Healthy People 2010.* Retrieved July 30, 2007, from http://www.healthypeople.gov

WrongDiagnosis.com (WD.com). (2008). *Prevalence and incidence of connective tissue disorders.* Retrieved June 30, 2008, from http://www.wrongdiagnosis.com/c/connective_tissue_disorders/prevalence.htm

Yu, D. (2008). *Reactive arthritis.* Retrieved September 1, 2008, from http://www.utdol.com/online/content/topic.do?topicKey=spondylo/7349&selectedTitle=1~86&source=search_result

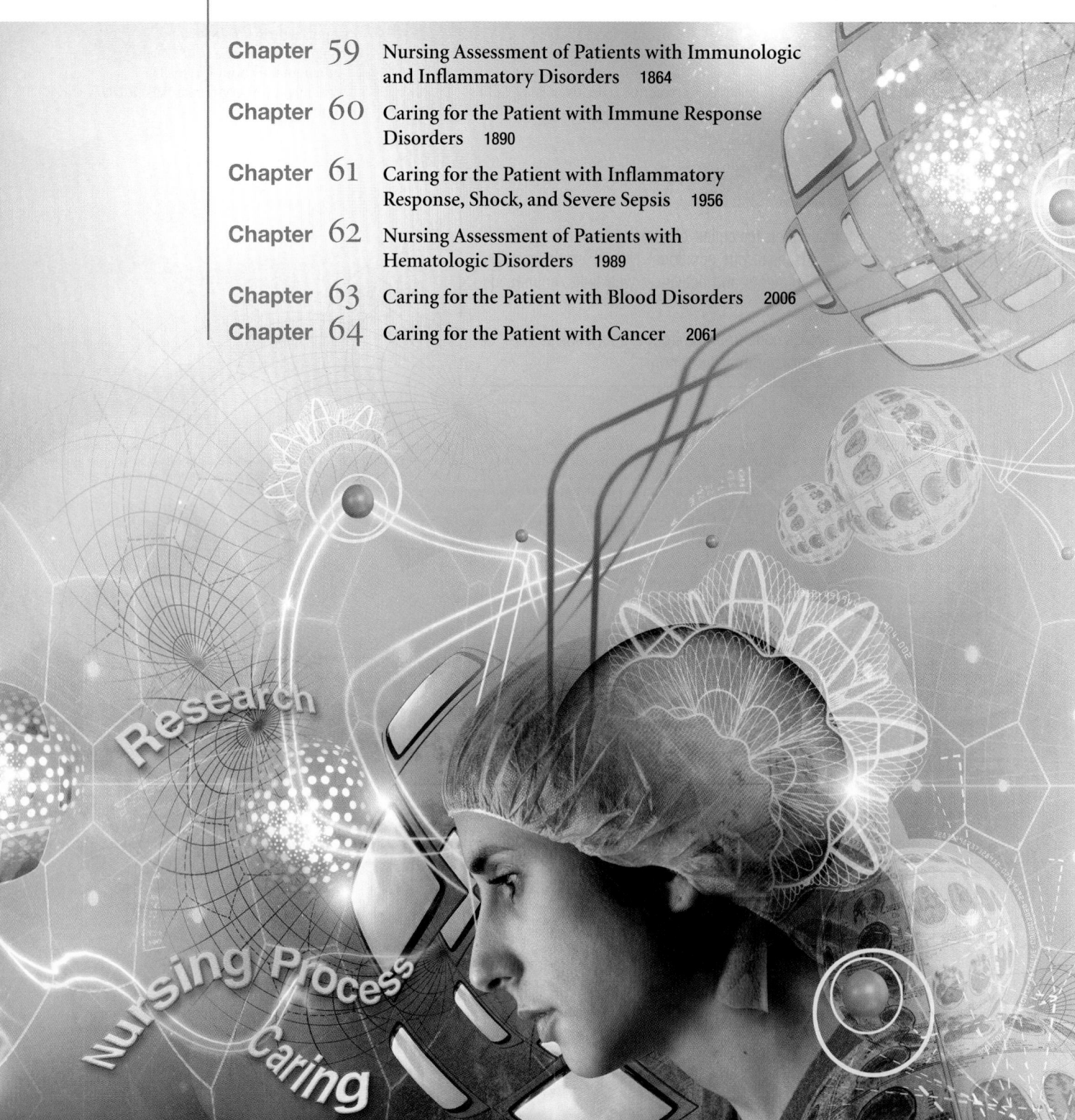

UNIT 13

Nursing Management of Patients with Immunologic, Inflammatory, and Hematologic Disorders

Research

Nursing Process

Caring

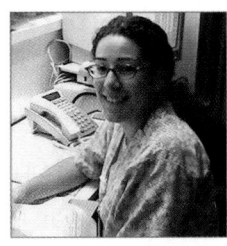

SOLEDAD SANCHEZ   My name is Soledad Sanchez and I always knew I wanted to be a nurse. This feeling came from my mother who left an indelible mark on my career choice. She cared for her children and others with a calming, warm sense that easily transmitted to other people. Trained as a nurse by religious sisters in her native country, she continued to use those skills in the United States as she helped others in need. Before attending nursing school, I did not really understand what it meant to be a nurse. Through my education, I soon developed a love for physiology and pathophysiology and gained a deeper understanding of the full scope of the healing process from a biological and humanitarian perspective. In 2001 I received my associate degree in nursing from Cerritos College. Later I attended Cal State Long Beach for a BS degree. I have been a registered nurse for 7 years, the last two of which I have been employed at a large medical center in Northern California. My experience has challenged me and nurtured a deeper understanding and compassion for people's most vulnerable moments in life.

I work on a 27-bed unit caring for patients from a number of specialties including oncology and neuroscience. I care for a wide diversity of oncology patients. For example, there are the young adults with new diagnoses of cancer whose emotional state is very fragile. Virtually every aspect of their lives as well as that of their families is affected. It is essential to establish a rapport with them and to assess their coping mechanisms. Only then will they open themselves up to you, making the patient–nurse relationship more comfortable, which allows for better communication and the implementation of optimal care delivery options. It becomes easier to discuss their fears and show compassion—just the mere action of sitting by their bedside and talking to them at eye level shows that we care. **Compassion** is a powerful healing tool.

As a registered nurse, I am part of a collaborative team of health care providers that includes physicians, social workers, dieticians, and pharmacists who strive to deliver quality patient care with the patient's desired goals in mind. As a certified chemotherapy and biotherapy provider, I am able to provide curative and palliative care to our patients who have cancer. Patient education is vital to this role, as is evaluating and understanding the orders. The integrity of the therapy is maintained by two independent checks of the dosages and assessment factors. This **confidence** is one facet of the six components of caring; having confidence not just in oneself, but in one's fellow colleagues helps create an environment of teamwork, trust, and dependability.

My approach to nursing is framed by the six components of caring: **compassion**, **competence**, **confidence**, **conscience**, **commitment**, and **comportmen**t. While the daily routine of oncology nursing centers on assessing and administering chemotherapy to patients, one key aspect is examining and assessing the side effects of chemotherapy and patients' tolerance. For example, a male patient in his early thirties with sarcoma in his second cycle of chemotherapy reported that with his last cycle he developed severe nausea, vomiting, and constipation. After discussing his previous medication regimen and past history, I developed a clear image of a possible regimen. After consulting with the chemotherapy pharmacist, a treatment plan was established that was very effective in treating his side effects. **Competence** was demonstrated by obtaining a detailed history of the patient, knowledge of the medication, and collaboration with the interdisciplinary team.

Another example of incorporating the components of caring is that of an elderly patient admitted for generalized weakness and subsequently diagnosed with non-Hodgkin's lymphoma. Knowing the prognosis was poor and the patient was in a frail state, I was concerned and uncomfortable with the oncologist's orders for chemotherapy. I proceeded to call the patient's partner and physician. After explaining the chemotherapy agents and possible side effects, a social worker was called to conduct a family conference. The patient was later discharged home with hospice care. I could not in good **conscience** blindly follow the initial orders. Ultimately, my professional **commitment** to the patient was demonstrated by advocating for the best possible quality of life.

Clinical reasoning is achieved after collecting and evaluating all pertinent patient assessment data. During initial report of the day, you begin using critical thinking and clinical reasoning to establish a plan of care for the patient and with your assessment you refine your plan on an ongoing basis.

Oftentimes, nursing is bittersweet because you enter people's lives when they are most vulnerable. Through that vulnerability you can encounter immense strength, which is the sweetest part for me. I see my role as using my abilities to access and foster that strength, and being humbled by it. Strength is found in the most extraordinary places. Helping someone during their time of suffering is an art in itself.

> "My experience has challenged me and nurtured a deeper understanding and compassion for people's most vulnerable moments in life."

CHAPTER 59

Nursing Assessment of Patients with Immunologic and Inflammatory Disorders

Debra Brady
Kathy Yeates

With contributions by:
Kathleen Osborn

Outcome-Based Learning Objectives

After studying this chapter, the learner will be able to:

1. Describe the function of the organs, tissues, and cellular components of the immune system.
2. Compare and contrast the significance of self antigens versus non-self antigens and immune tolerance.
3. Compare and contrast cell-mediated and humoral immunity in relationship to the type of lymphocytes involved, response to antigens, and role in immune protection.
4. Compare and contrast the actions of cytokines, lymphokines, interleukins, interferons, complement, and tumor necrosis factor on immune function.
5. Explain the action and significance of acquired immune response through immunizations.
6. Explain the action and significance of antigen presentation in B-cell activation, stimulation of immunoglobulin production, and secondary immune response.
7. Discuss the effects of aging on the immune system.
8. Apply the assessment skills of inspection, palpation, percussion, and auscultation in evaluating body systems and determining the status of immune function.
9. Interpret and relate immune-related laboratory tests when assessing immune function.

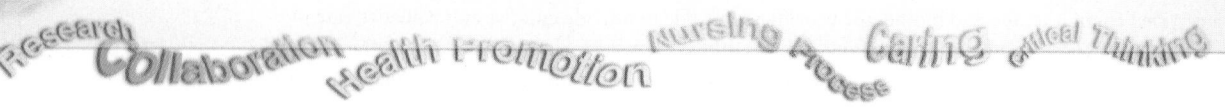

Research   Collaboration   Health Promotion   Nursing Process   Caring   Critical Thinking

AN INTACT and functioning immune system is critical for survival. The immune system functions to protect the body from invasion of microorganisms and foreign substances, in addition to eliminating damaged or mutant cells such as cancer cells. The protective process of response to a foreign substance is referred to as **immunity**. To function appropriately, it is essential that the immune system be able to differentiate between "self" cells and an infinite number of "non-self" substances and foreign cells such as bacteria, viruses, or tumor proteins. Any substance that the immune system recognizes as foreign is referred to as an **antigen**. The ability to differentiate self from non-self is referred to as **immune tolerance**. Loss of immune tolerance is the basis for numerous immune abnormalities, which are discussed in Chapter 60 ☞.

The immune system includes central and peripheral lymphoid tissues and immune cells that function to defend the body against disease through natural and acquired immunity as well as the inflammation process. Chart 59–1 provides an overview of the immune response.

Natural immunity is accomplished through specific organs, cells, and chemicals that are present at birth or shortly after, as discussed below. Acquired immunity includes antibodies, immunocompetent T cells and B cells, and cytokines that act to remove antigens that are considered non-self (Rote, 2006). Immune cells also include a variety of white blood cells such as macrophages, neutrophils, and eosinophils. This chapter focuses on the anatomy and physiology of normal immune function and assessment of the immune system. A complete description of inflammation is available in Chapter 61 ☞.

Genetic factors play a key role in immune function. Abnormalities in gene development that affect the immune system will be discussed in Chapter 60 ☞ as they relate to the development of specific disease processes.

▮ Anatomy of the Immune System

The major components of the immune system include the bone marrow, the lymphatic system including lymph nodes and lymphatic circulation, and the spleen. These organs and tissues are located throughout the body in order to provide systemic immune response.

CHART 59–1	**Overview of Inflammation and Natural and Acquired Immunity**
	Key Features
INFLAMMATION	Initial response to injury of any kind. Includes cells, such as neutrophils and macrophages, and chemical mediators, such as histamine, complement, and clotting cascade. Inflammation produces the symptoms of redness, swelling, heat or fever, pain, and loss of function.
NATURAL IMMUNITY	Organs such as skin, lymphatic system as well as immune tolerance to self antigens. Mechanical processes such as cough can help remove debris from the body. Gastric pH helps protect the stomach from bacteria. Mucous membranes wash debris away and may have lysozyme secretions that can eliminate debris and bacteria.
ACQUIRED IMMUNITY	System of cells such as B and T cells that protect through immunoglobulins and cell-mediated immune response. Antibodies produced by B cells can attach to antigens and stimulate phagocytosis. T cells regulate the production of antibodies and release other lymphokines that direct immune cells to eliminate antigens or destroy mutant cells.

Sources: DeFranco, A. L., Locksley, R., & Robertson, M. (2007). *Immunity: The immune response in infectious and inflammatory disease.* Sunderland, MA: Sinauer Associates; McCance, K., & Heuther, S. (2006). *Pathophysiology: The biological basis for disease in adults and children* (5th ed.). St. Louis: Mosby; Porth, C. (2007). *Essentials of pathophysiology* (7th ed.). Philadelphia: Lippincott Williams & Wilkins.

Bone Marrow

Knowledge of the functions of bone marrow is important in understanding the development of the immune system. As demonstrated in Figure 59–1 ■ (p. 1866), bone marrow is rich in *stem cells*, cells that can differentiate into a variety of cell lines that are critical for immune function. Stem cells have the capacity to produce any type of cell that they are chemically directed to make. For example, stem cells differentiate into white blood cells such as granulocytes, lymphocytes, and monocytes. Granulocytes become neutrophils, eosinophils, and basophils. Lymphocyte precursors in bone marrow become B- and T-cells lines. Monocytes differentiate from white blood cell precursors. Monocytes circulate in the blood and mature into macrophages. Bone marrow stem cells also differentiate into red blood cells (erythrocytes) and platelets (thrombocytes) (Twite & Gaspard, 2007).

Granulocytes

Granulocytes are the line of white blood cells that differentiate into neutrophils, basophils, and eosinophils. They are named granulocytes because their cell cytoplasm contains granules of chemicals such as histamine. These granules can be seen on Gram stain, and are used to identify and count the cells microscopically.

Neutrophils

Neutrophils are important phagocytic cells. Their function is to consume cellular debris, immune complexes, and bacterial and viral particles. Neutrophils are the first group of white blood cells to arrive at the site of injury or cell death. They have a short life span, approximately 72 hours or less.

Basophils

Basophils migrate from the bloodstream into tissue and mature into mast cells. Mast cells are filled with granules of histamine and are important in initiating the inflammatory response following injury. When a body cell is injured, mast cells in the immediate vicinity release large quantities of histamine, stimulating the inflammatory response (DeFranco, Locksley, & Robertson, 2007).

Eosinophils

Eosinophils comprise a very small portion of the total number of white blood cells. They are stimulated to increase their numbers in the presence of parasites. The number of eosinophils also increases in the presence of allergies. Eosinophils are responsible for increasing the immune and inflammatory response.

Nongranulocytes

The **nongranulocyte** cell lines include lymphocytes and monocytes. These cells are identified microscopically by their large nucleus and the lack of granules in their cytoplasm. Nongranulocytes are highly effective phagocytic white blood cells that can engulf large numbers of foreign antigen, such as bacteria.

Monocytes

Monocytes circulate in the blood and migrate into tissue to mature as macrophages. The primary function of monocytes and macrophages is phagocytosis. They arrive at the site of cell injury hours to days after neutrophils. Macrophages have a longer life span, have a higher tolerance for an acidic environment, and are capable of consuming larger amount of debris for an extended period of time than other monocytes (Rote, 2006).

Lymphocytes

Lymphocytes differentiate into T lymphocytes and B lymphocytes. Microscopically T and B lymphocytes appear similar, with a large nucleus and no granules in the cytoplasm. T lymphocytes, also known as CD4 cells, are responsible for regulating and initiating the immune response. The primary function of B cells is the production of antibodies such as immunoglobulins (Ig): IgE, IgG, IgA, IgM, and IgD (DeFranco et al., 2007).

Deficiencies in functional bone marrow and stem cells can lead to immune deficiency disorders. Primary immune dysfunction such as an IgG deficiency is an example of the incorrect maturation of B cells that cannot produce immunoglobulin G (Twite & Gaspard, 2007).

Lymphatic System

The **lymphatic system** is comprised of the vessels, lymph nodes, and lymph tissue. This system of vessels drains lymph fluid, referred to as chyle, through the entire body and returns it to venous circulation in the chest. The vessels drain **chyle** (a milky fluid comprised of serous fluid, white cells, and fatty acids) into the thoracic and lymphatic ducts in the mediastinum. The

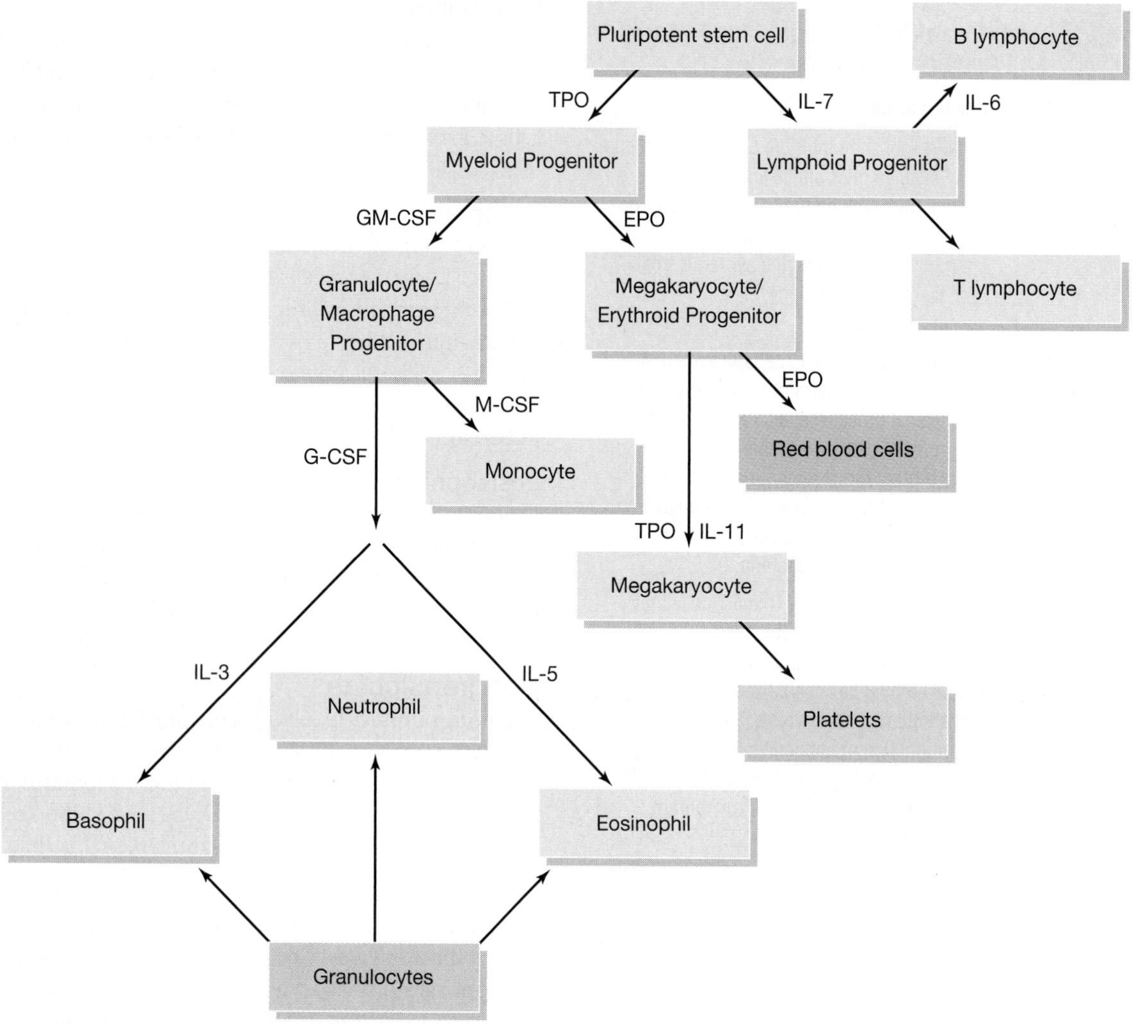

```
                                    Pluripotent stem cell              B lymphocyte

                          TPO                          IL-7        IL-6

                    Myeloid Progenitor              Lymphoid Progenitor

              GM-CSF                     EPO

          Granulocyte/               Megakaryocyte/                 T lymphocyte
          Macrophage                 Erythroid Progenitor
          Progenitor
                                                        EPO
                        M-CSF
          G-CSF                                    Red blood cells
                        Monocyte

                                             TPO   IL-11

                                          Megakaryocyte

              IL-3                 IL-5

                    Neutrophil                      Platelets

    Basophil                      Eosinophil

                    Granulocytes
```

FIGURE 59–1 ■ Cell line differentiation in bone marrow.

lymph vessels follow the same route as veins and arteries and run parallel to veins. Chyle then drains from the mediastinum into the heart through the superior vena cava.

Lymph nodes and lymph tissue filter debris from the breakdown of cells, bacteria, virus, and fungal antigens. Lymphocytes such as T and B cells are found in lymph nodes. Lymph nodes and tissue contain or house macrophages that ingest cells, bacteria, and debris. Two-thirds of fixed lymph tissue is located in the abdomen surrounding the intestinal tissue, and is referred to as Peyer's patches. This is important because the vessels that deliver blood to the intestines facilitate the entry of large molecules of digested materials into the circulatory system. Vessels able to absorb large food particles may also allow the entry of viral and bacterial particles. Hence, immune protection by Peyer's patches is vital (Twite & Gaspard, 2007). A high concentration of lymph tissue also is located in the lungs. Alveolar macrophages function with lymph tissue to protect the lungs from bacteria, virus, and debris from the outside environment (DeFranco et al., 2007).

Lymph nodes are consolidated groups of lymph tissue and are found throughout the body. Lymph nodes located in the neck, axilla, and groin may be palpated. Like lymph tissue, they contain macrophages and lymphocytes, and are able to filter and remove dead cells, bacteria, and other debris from the system as well as assist in mounting the immune response (Figure 59–2 ■).

During infection, inflammation, or injury, lymph nodes in the area of injury will become swollen. An example of this is the swelling of lymph nodes in the axilla and neck during pneumonia (Rote, 2006).

 Patients with compromised immune function such as HIV/AIDS or cancer patients on chemotherapy need to have lymph nodes examined even if no other complaint is present. Nodes swollen by cell debris of any kind warrant further investigation.

Tonsils and Adenoids

Tonsils and adenoids are consolidated lymph tissue located in the throat. They function to remove and filter debris, bacteria, and viruses from the upper airways and mouth. Like all consolidated lymph tissue, they contain B and T cells as well as macrophages (DeFranco et al., 2007).

Spleen

The spleen plays a significant role in immune function as part of the lymphatic system. It is comprised of white and red pulp and is involved in hematologic filtration, sequestering of red and white cells, and immune response. The white pulp of the spleen is rich in lymphocytes that can be activated in an immune response. The red pulp is responsible for filtering out

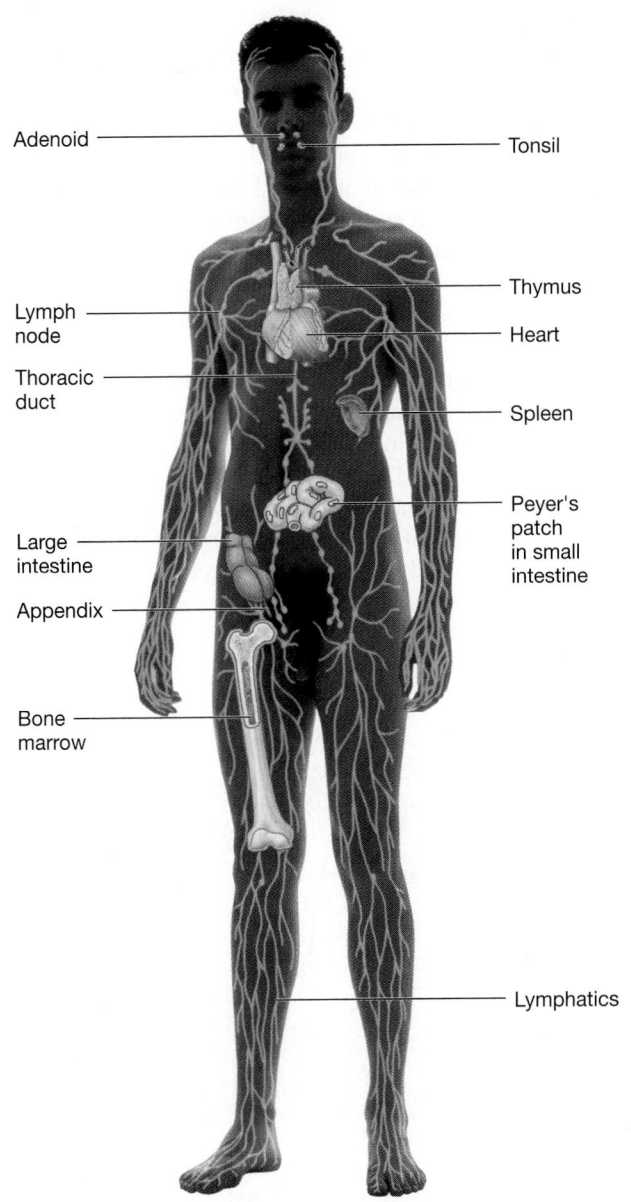

Adenoid

Tonsil

Lymph node

Thymus

Heart

Thoracic duct

Spleen

Large intestine

Peyer's patch in small intestine

Appendix

Bone marrow

Lymphatics

FIGURE 59–2 ■ Lymphatic system with lymph nodes.

old or damaged red blood cells. The spleen may also sequester red and white blood cells and platelets, and thereby decrease these levels in the circulating blood volume. The spleen may become enlarged in acute inflammatory or infectious disease processes because of the stimulation of the immune response. An enlarged spleen (splenomegaly) can be involved in a plethora of disease processes such as trauma, cancer, infection, portal hypertension, thrombosis, cysts, and mononucleosis, and this assessment finding warrants further investigation (Twite & Gaspard, 2007).

To assess the spleen, place the patient on the right side, and percuss down the midaxillary line from an area of resonance over the lung to dullness over the spleen. The spleen is normally not detected on palpation. If detected, the spleen should not be percussed more than 6 to 8 cm (about 2 to 3 in.) above the left costal margin. An enlarged spleen is diagnosed if there is a greater than 8-cm finding above the costal margin (Dillon, 2007).

Physiology of the Immune System

The physiology of the immune system includes the function of the lymphatic tissues, cells, and chemicals that provide protection from infectious agents, antigens, and mutated cells and enable the body to differentiate self from non-self. The immune response includes both natural and acquired immunity.

Natural Immunity

Natural immunity is the responsibility of a group of body organs, cells, and chemicals that are present at birth or shortly after. These include the cells and chemicals of the inflammatory response, barriers such as skin, and chemicals such as complement. **Natural immunity** is defined as the organs, cells, and secretions of the body that provide protection from foreign proteins, chemicals, and other non-self particles. Natural immunity includes the integumentary system, the lymphatic system, and secretions such as lysozymes, immunoglobulins, and subcellular receptors such as toll-like receptors. The white blood cells and chemicals of the inflammatory response are an important part of natural immunity. All of these components of natural immune function are present at birth (Figure 59–3 ■, p. 1868).

Physical and Chemical Barriers

Anatomic and chemical barriers provide the first line of defense in immune protection. Physical barriers include the skin and the mucous membranes. Natural immune system chemical barriers include lysozymes, acidic pH of the stomach, and toll receptors, all of which are discussed below.

Skin

Natural immunity starts with the skin. Skin is physically the largest organ of the human body. It acts as a barrier to debris, bacteria, and other organisms. It protects soft organs and tissue from changes in the environment. Skin is capable of inhibiting bacterial growth. Bacteria are always present on the surface of the skin in varying quantities. The small amount of moisture and pH of the skin protect it from bacterial growth. Therefore, intact skin is critical to the survival of the organism. Even small breaks in the integrity of skin can lead to large wounds or infections locally or systemically because organisms are able to enter the body (Rote, 2006).

Careful examination of the skin is an essential part of every physical assessment of patients. Patients may require education about maintaining skin integrity. When a rash or skin breakdown occurs, patients need to be educated to report to their health care provider the onset of the symptoms, where on the body it is occurring, and any attempted home treatment.

Mucous Membranes

Mucous membranes also form part of the first line of defense in natural immunity. Mucous membranes assist in protecting the body from attack by washing dirt and debris from the body. Ciliated cells in the trachea move bacteria and dirt from the trachea through a wavelike motion. In addition, mucous membranes in the mouth secrete lysozymes and immunoglobulins that are mildly antibiotic and assist in protecting the

The immune system

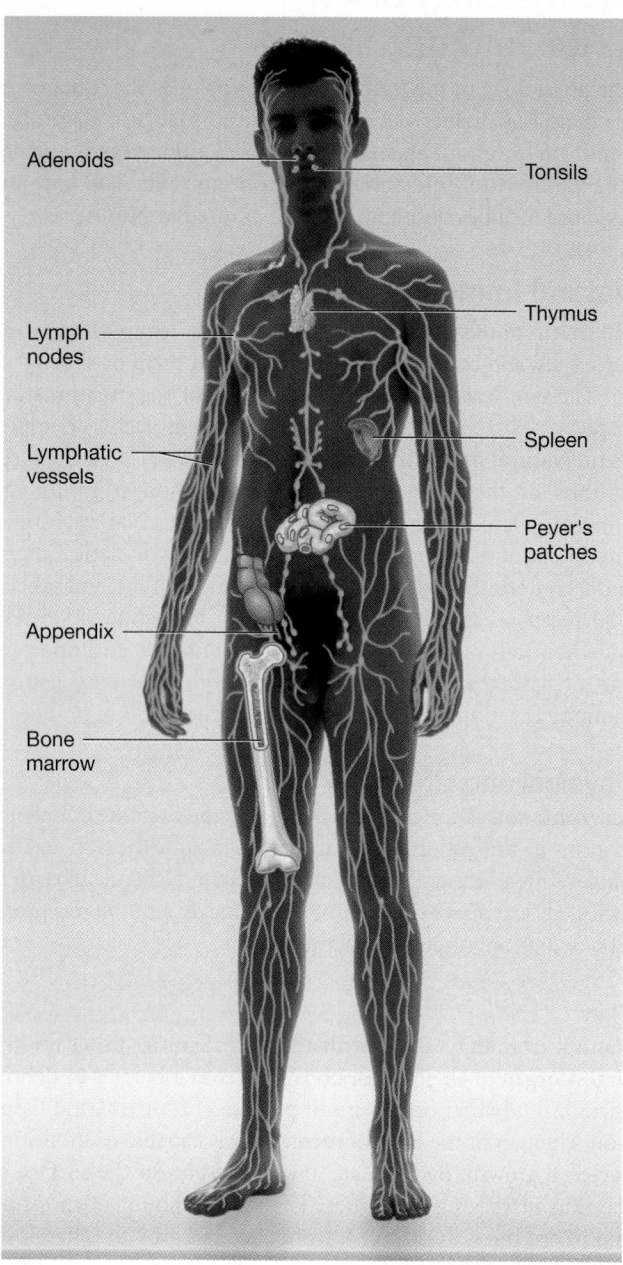

FIGURE 59–3 ■ Immune system with organs.
Source: Michael Freeman/Phototake NYC

mouth from bacterial infection (Sommer, 2007). Oral care is essential in preventing infections in the oral cavity.

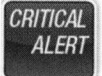 **CRITICAL ALERT** *Patients who are receiving supplemental oxygen by mask or ventilator need frequent oral care. Although oxygen by mask and ventilator can be humidified, patients may not be able to keep oral mucosa moist and clean. Gentle swabbing with soft swabs and water or mouthwash can help keep the mouth moist. Patients receiving oxygen by mask may require assistance with brushing their teeth. Patients on a ventilator are dependent on the nurse for oral care. There is growing evidence that oral bacteria can lead to nosocomial pneumonia (Tablan et al., 2004).*

Gastric pH

Immune protection is also provided in the stomach. The pH of the stomach ranges from approximately 1.0 to 3.0. This pH is so acidic most bacteria, fungi, and viral particles are unable to survive.

Toll Receptors

Finally, **toll receptors** present at the cellular level are small receptors on the surface of many types of immune and tissue cells that are able to initiate immune responses when pieces of bacterial cell walls attach to them. Humans are born with these toll receptors and they comprise an important innate protection for the body because they act as a gate or point of initiation of certain cell functions (Figure 59–4 ■). Toll receptors are shaped to accept the lipopolysaccharide portion of the cell wall of bacteria, while others are shaped to accept the wall of a fungal cell (DeFranco et al., 2007).

Toll receptors not only stimulate the immune system, they also can signal a cell to start **apoptosis**, or programmed cell death. Infected cells can often be induced to undergo apoptosis and destroy themselves (Rote, 2006). Additionally, cells stimulated by the attachment of a lipopolysaccharide piece of bacterial wall are able to stimulate the release of tumor necrosis factor, a key chemical in initiating immune and inflammatory responses. This response is critical in alerting the system to the presence of non-self antigens such as bacteria (DeFranco et al., 2007).

Toll-like receptors

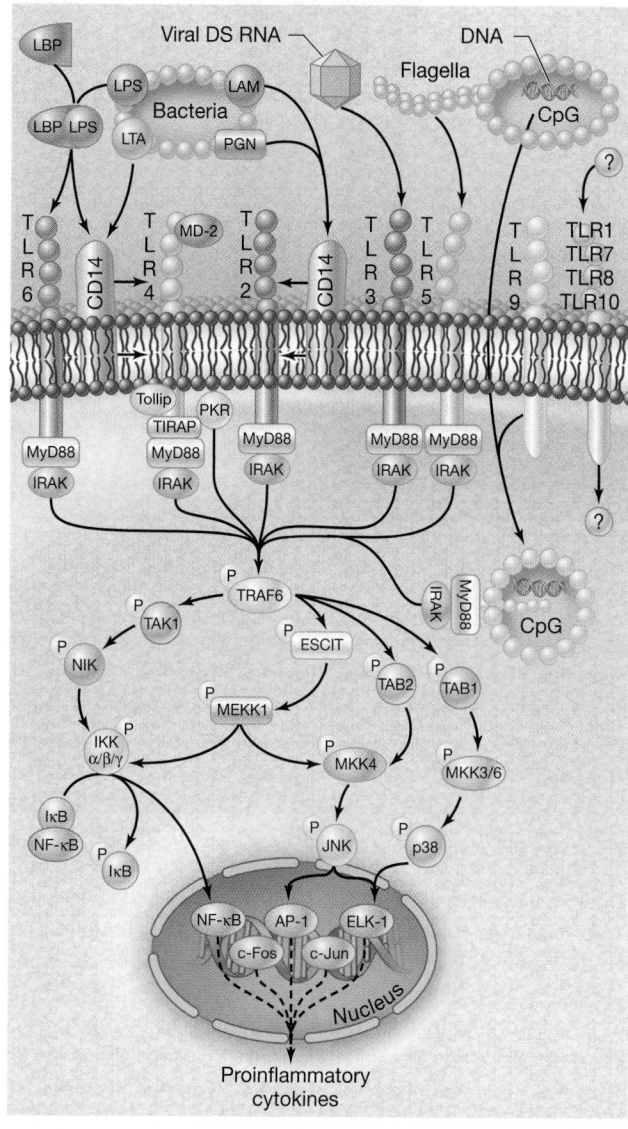

FIGURE 59–4 ■ Toll receptors.

Self Versus Non-Self

Self is defined as all cells of the body and the receptors on those cells that are recognized as unique to that individual. Major histocompatibility complex (MHC) receptors on cells are an example of a marker used by the immune system to determine if a cell belongs to the organism or not. Additionally, **human leukocyte antigens (HLAs)** are protein markers on the cell wall of white blood cells that alert the immune system to the appropriateness of a cell belonging to the system. These are the markers that are tested for matching in organ transplant because an exact HLA match will minimize the immune response and the risk of transplant rejection (Rote, 2006).

Non-self is any protein, antigen, or the stimulatory part of any foreign cell that the immune system does not recognize as self. Antigens are small proteins that can signal the immune system to mount a response and eliminate the foreign cell, bacteria, virus, or fungus (DeFranco et al., 2007).

Bacteria, virus, fungi, and amoebic parasites are major threats to the survival of the human body. The immune system is constantly looking for cells and proteins that are not self. Cancer cells frequently lack specific markers, thus, the immune system may or may not recognize the mutant cell as non-self (Figure 59–5 ■). If the immune system does not identify the mutated malignant cells, a tumor may develop. Chapter 64 ⊙ discusses the development of a cancerous tumor in detail.

Immune Tolerance

Immune tolerance is defined as the ability of the immune system to tolerate all **self antigens** while retaining the ability to mount an immune response to **non-self antigens**. Immune tolerance begins during embryonic development of the immune system. Lymphocytes that react with self antigens are selectively eliminated as the immune system develops. This leaves the newborn with B-cell and T-cell lines that do not attack self antigens. Self antigens include HLAs and MHC, as well as several other antigenic particles that are often cell receptors. When the body reacts to self receptors or other cell parts as an antigen, autoimmune disease may result (DeFranco et al., 2007). Chapter 60 ⊙ discusses autoimmune diseases.

Inflammatory Response

The inflammatory response is an important part of the body's response to any injury and an integral part of the immune response. White blood cells such as neutrophils and macrophages travel to the site of injury in response to the chemicals of inflammation such as histamine, complement, and bradykinin. Inflammation presents with symptoms of redness, edema, pain, and heat from increased blood flow to the area of injury (Sommer, 2007).

The inflammatory response is seen in cell injury, allergy reactions, anaphylaxis, and many disease processes. Cells and chemicals of the inflammatory response also stimulate the activity of T cells and B cells to mount an immune response. For a complete discussion of inflammation see Chapter 61 ⊙.

Acquired Immunity

Acquired immunity occurs after birth and includes antibodies, immunocompetent T cells and B cells, and cytokines that act to remove antigens that are considered non-self. Acquired immunity also includes immunizations received as a child or an adult. Acquired immunity can be described as the ability of the immune cells to correctly produce antibodies, regulate the immune response, and respond only to non-self antigens (DeFranco et al., 2007). **Active acquired immunity** involves the production of antibodies by the immune system in response to specific foreign antigens, such as bacteria. This immunity is considered acquired because the body develops the ability to regulate the immune system and produce antibodies after birth and after exposure to antigens in the environment. Active immunity is acquired by either contracting the disease or through a vaccination. Acquired immunity involves lymphocyte cells and chemicals that can confer long-term permanent protection against the disease for which the antibodies have been produced. Figure 59–6 ■ (p. 1870) describes immune cell differentiation from precursor cells.

Lymphocytes include **T cell** and **B cells**. **T lymphocytes** are involved in the cellular immune response and are responsible for stimulating and regulating the immune response. The **B lymphocytes** are involved in the humoral immune response and are responsible for the creation and release of antibodies and development of long-term immune protection.

Cellular Immune Response

The cellular immune response is initiated by white blood cells called T cells. T cells are vital in regulating immune function (Figure 59–7 ■, p. 1870). T-cell lymphocytes are responsible for stimulating or decreasing the immune response through the production of chemicals called cytokines that can directly destroy cells, help macrophages find the antigen and consume it, and protect cells from viral attachment (Twite & Gaspard, 2007).

T Lymphocytes

T-cell precursors in the bone marrow differentiate into types of T lymphocytes. Immature T cells travel from the bone marrow via the bloodstream to the thymus gland and other lymphatic tissues. T cells mature and differentiate primarily in the thymus during childhood. Following puberty the thymus gland shrinks, and T-cell differentiation and maturation predominantly occurs in other lymphatic tissue such as the white pulp of the spleen and the lymph nodes.

T lymphocytes are the regulatory cells of the immune system whose function is to start and stop the immune processes. These processes include phagocytosis, cytokine secretion, and activation of B cells (Sommer, 2007). As a consequence, the functions

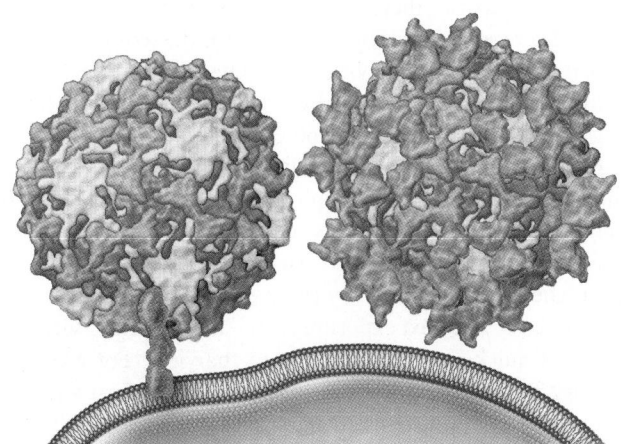

FIGURE 59–5 ■ (A) Self versus (B) non-self.

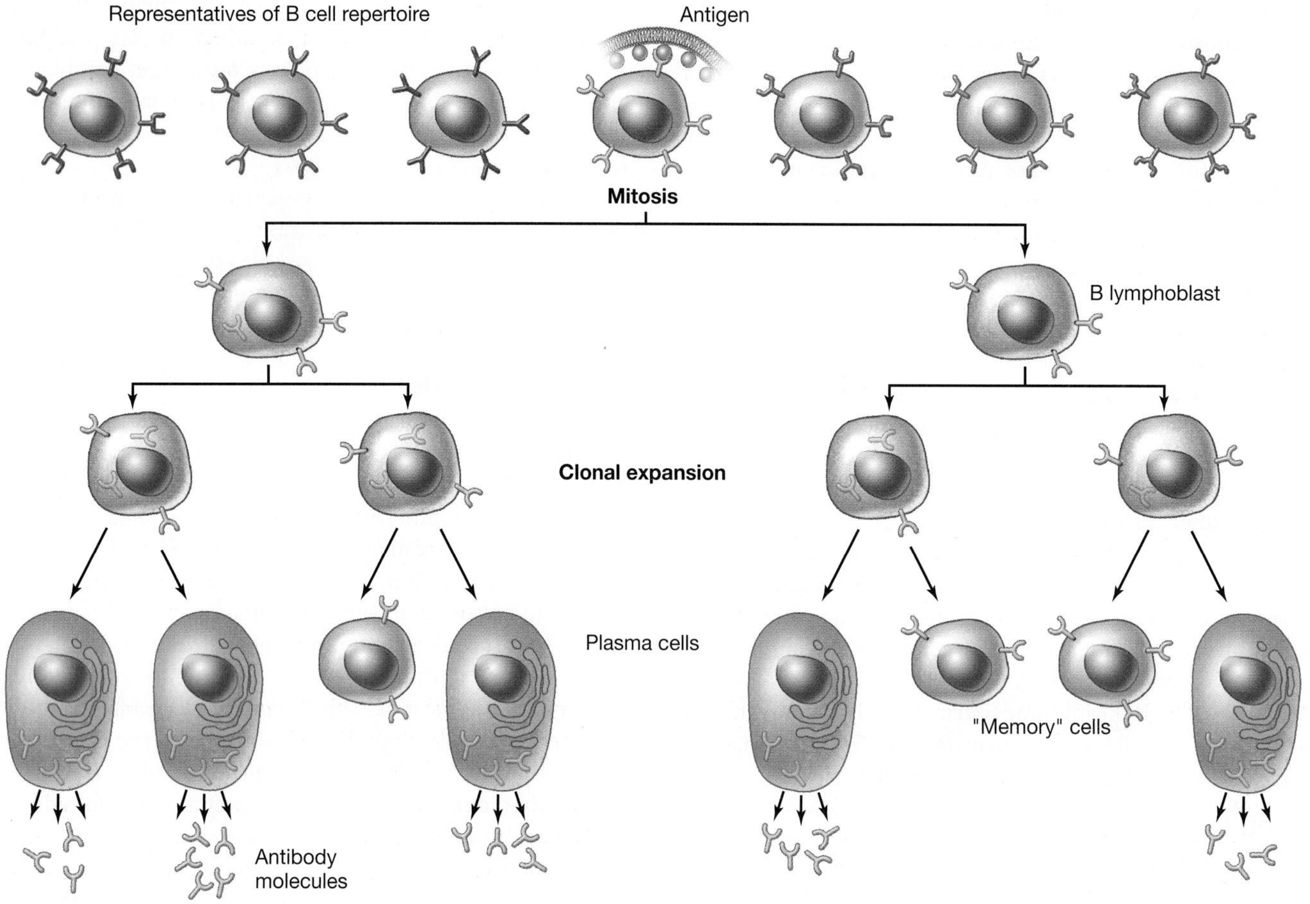

Representatives of B cell repertoire

Antigen

Mitosis

B lymphoblast

Clonal expansion

Plasma cells

"Memory" cells

Antibody molecules

FIGURE 59–6 ■ Immune cell differentiation from precursors.

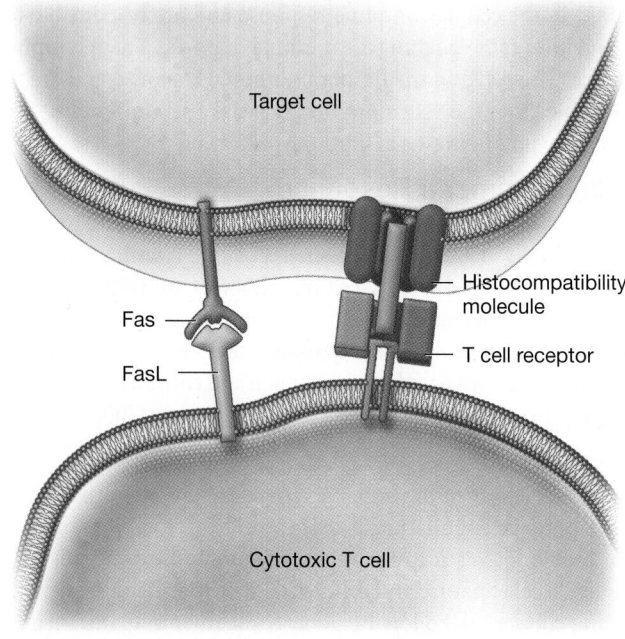

Target cell

Histocompatibility molecule

Fas

T cell receptor

FasL

Cytotoxic T cell

One method by which cytotoxic T cells induce their targets (e.g., virus-infected cells) to commit suicide (apoptosis)

FIGURE 59–7 ■ T cell.

of T cells are called the **cell-mediated immune response**. There are an extensive number of T-cell types. T cells are named by their function or by the identifying markers on the cell membrane (DeFranco et al., 2007). The most significant T cells and their role in immune function are discussed next.

T-Helper Cells **T-helper cells** are also called CD4 cells because of the CD4 receptors on the surface of this group of T cells. T-helper cells are divided into T-helper 1 and T-helper 2 cell lines. T-helper 1 cells help upregulate immune activity and produce chemicals called cytokines that stimulate cytotoxic cells to destroy mutant and cancer cells. T-helper 1 cells produce cytokines that are chemotactic (that is, they tell cells to come to the area of infection). CD4 receptors have been identified as the receptor that the human immunodeficiency virus (HIV) attaches to and uses to enter the T cell, thereby severely affecting immune function, which is discussed in detail in Chapter 60 ☺ (Sommer, 2007).

T-helper 2 cells stimulate B cells to make antibodies to specific antigens. This is accomplished through the release of chemicals such as interleukins and the antigen presentation process (DeFranco et al., 2007). Memory T cells function to retain a "chemical memory" of virus particles encountered by the memory cells. The next exposure to the "remembered" virus results in a quick immune response to the virus. For example, memory T cells are responsible for protection against virus infections such as rhinovirus, one group of cold viruses. The first exposure to a rhinovirus usually results in cold symptoms such as sore throat, sneezing, and cough. The memory T cells retain a memory of that specific rhinovirus which lasts for a lifetime. On second exposure to that same virus, the memory T cells are able to stimulate an immune response much more quickly, thus minimizing or preventing symptoms of infection. Frequent infections with rhinovirus occur because the virus mutates rapidly, creating a new virus antigen. Thus, the memory T cells must go through the process of developing a memory for each new rhinovirus. More than 200 rhinoviruses have been identified. Children have greater numbers of colds than adults because they have not been exposed to as many virus antigens as adults and subsequently have not developed the same immune memory as adults (Sommer, 2007).

Suppressor T Cells Suppressor T cells, also called CD8 cells, slow or stop the immune response. This downregulation is the primary role of suppressor T cells, and is an important part of regulation of the immune system because the ability to stop the production of antibodies and cell destruction is important once the threat of infection has been overcome (DeFranco et al., 2007).

Natural Killer Cells Natural killer cells, also referred to as "null cells," are types of T cells that lack CD4 or CD8 external receptors, but are able to directly kill cells or send cytokine messages to start the process of programmed cell death (apoptosis). Natural killer cells are usually directed to initiate cell death by T-helper 1 cells (Rote, 2006). Chart 59–2 describes lymphocyte function in greater detail.

CHART 59–2	**Lymphocyte Functions**
Lymphocyte	**Functions**
B cell	Antibody production.
Plasma cell	Antibody production, responsible for primary antibody response.
Memory cell	Antibody production, responsible for secondary antibody response.
T-cell lines	Regulation, stimulation, downregulation of immune function through the use of chemical mediators. Null cells and natural killer cells may destroy infected cells directly.
T-helper cells (CD4) T-helper 1 T-helper 2 Memory T-helper cells	Stimulate and upregulate immune function. Assist in antigen presentation. Activate B cells to make antibodies (T-helper 2); stimulate natural killer cells (T-helper 1); nonspecific immune memory function (memory T cells).
Suppressor T cells (CD8)	Can slow or downregulate immune function. Slow release of inflammatory cytokines.
Natural killer cells	T-cell line able to chemically kill infected cells and tumor cells.

Sources: DeFranco, A. L., Locksley, R., & Robertson, M. (2007). *Immunity: The immune response in infectious and inflammatory disease.* Sunderland, MA: Sinauer Associates; McCance, K., & Heuther, S. (2006). *Pathophysiology: The biological basis for disease in adults and children* (5th ed.). St. Louis: Mosby; Porth, C. (2007). *Essentials of pathophysiology* (7th ed.). Philadelphia: Lippincott Williams & Wilkins.

Cytokines and Lymphokines

Cytokines are chemical messages produced by cells to communicate with other cells in the body. Cytokines have a plethora of functions such as chemotaxis and opsonization. **Chemotaxis** is the movement of additional white blood cells to an area of inflammation in response to the release of chemical mediators by neutrophils, monocytes, and injured tissue. **Opsonization** is the chemical coating of an antigen or cell that makes that cell more attractive to phagocytes. Cytokines that are made by lymphocytes are called **lymphokines** and include interleukins and interferons. Other examples of cytokines are tumor necrosis factor, tissue factor, and growth inhibitory factor (DeFranco et al., 2007). A variety of cytokines and their functions are described in Chart 59–3 (p. 1872) (McCance & Heuther, 2006).

Interleukins

Interleukins are lymphokines, chemical mediators released by lymphocytes, that enable the cells of the immune system to communicate and coordinate the immune response. Interleukins are crucial to the immune response. Interleukin-1 and interleukin-6 are pro-inflammatory and stimulate the release of chemicals such as tumor necrosis factor and tissue factor that begin the inflammatory response, as discussed in Chapter 61 ✏. Interleukin-12 slows and helps stop the immune and inflammatory responses (Sommer, 2007).

Interferons

Interferons are proteins made and released by T cells when the invading organism is a virus. This group of lymphokines functions to protect other cells from viral attack. They inhibit the production of the virus within infected cells, prevent the spread of the virus to other cells, and enhance the activity of macrophages, natural killer cells, and cytotoxic T cells. Interferons also inhibit the growth of certain tumor cells. Interferons made by recombinant technology are used to treat a variety of disease states. One example of this is alpha interferon, which is used to slow the growth of new blood vessels in some cancerous vascular tumors (Rote, 2006).

Tumor Necrosis Factor

Tumor necrosis factor (TNF) is a small peptide that is produced by a variety of cells, including granulocytes and lymphocytes. TNF is critical in the stimulation of the initial inflammatory response, specifically the activity of macrophages and granulocytes. It also is important in telling cells to initiate programmed cell death or apoptosis when mutations occur. This function is important in inhibiting tumor development and growth because chronic inflammation has been implicated in the development of some types of cancerous tumors due to cell changes that occur with a long-term inflammatory response (DeFranco et al., 2007).

Tissue Factor

Tissue factor (TF) is another cytokine that is important in immune function and inflammation. Tissue factor can be released by a variety of injured tissue cells, macrophages, and platelets. The function of TF is to stimulate platelets to stick together and form the beginning of a clot. This is critical in stopping blood loss from injured blood vessels. Formation of a stable clot and initiation of the clotting cascade are important aspects of the inflammatory response, which is regulated by cells of the immune

| CHART 59–3 | Cytokines and Their Functions |

Cytokine	Functions
Tumor necrosis factor (TNF)	Stimulates immune and inflammatory responses. Is capable of killing cancer cells. Can activate macrophages and granulocytes. Is responsible in part for wasting seen in cancer. Can stimulate apoptosis.
Interleukin (IL)	
IL-1	Activates T cells, induces fever, is an inflammatory mediator, assists in upregulating immune function.
IL -2	Promotes T-cell growth and replication. Can activate T cells and natural killer cells.
IL-3 (multiple colony-stimulating factor)	Stimulates the proliferation of hematopoietic precursor cells.
IL-4	Stimulates growth of T cells, B cells, mast cells, eosinophils.
IL-5	Stimulates growth of B cells, eosinophils.
IL-6	Acts synergistically with IL-1 and TNF to increase inflammation. Stimulates growth of B cells and differentiation into plasma, memory cells. Can induce fever.
IL-7	Stimulates growth of T and B cells.
IL-8	Chemotactic factor for neutrophils and T cells.
IL-9	Some stimulation of precursor cells of the T-cell line and red blood cell.
IL-10	Stimulates B cells and antibody production. Slows cytokine release by T cells and natural killer cells.
IL-12	Stimulates gamma-interferon production. Promotes cell-mediated immune response.
IL-16	Chemotactic factor for T cells, monocytes, and eosinophils.
IL-17	Stimulates release of IL-6, IL-8, and granulocyte colony stimulating factor.
IL-18	Upregulates natural killer cell function. Stimulates the release of gamma Interferon.
Interferons	
Alpha-interferon	Can slow and inhibit viral replication. Also activates natural killer cells.
Beta-interferon	Blocks viral replication.
Gamma-interferon	Blocks viral replication, activates macrophages, can enhance natural killer cell function; differentiation of B cells.
Colony-stimulating factors	All colony-stimulating factors enhance differentiation and activation of white blood cell lines. Cells stimulated include macrophages and granulocytes. Erythropoietin stimulates differentiation and growth of red blood cells.

Sources: DeFranco, A. L., Locksley, R., & Robertson, M. (2007). *Immunity: The immune response in infectious and inflammatory disease.* Sunderland, MA: Sinauer Associates; McCance, K., & Heuther, S. (2006). *Pathophysiology: The biological basis for disease in adults and children* (5th ed.). St. Louis: Mosby; Porth, C. (2007). *Essentials of pathophysiology* (7th ed.). Philadelphia: Lippincott Williams & Wilkins.

system. Tissue factor is a very significant cytokine that contributes to the body's protective inflammatory response (Sommer, 2007). Chapter 61 ⊙ provides a detailed examination of the inflammatory process.

Complement Proteins and Function

Complement is a group of small proteins made in the liver and present in blood that can interact with cells and each other for a variety of functions. Complement proteins are important in the inflammatory and immune responses. Complement 3b is an opsonin or chemical that coats or attaches to an antigen or cell. After attachment the cell or antigen is especially attractive to neutrophils and macrophages. This stimulates the phagocytic cells to approach and consume the cell or antigen. Complement 3a and 5a are chemotactic and can chemically call phagocytic cells such as neutrophils as well as T cells and B cells to the area of infection (DeFranco et al., 2007).

Complement can be activated by immune complexes attached to cell membranes or antibodies attached to cell membranes. When this occurs, complement fragments form a complex either around an attached antibody or directly to re-

ceptors on the cell membrane or wall. This complex of complement is capable of directly lysing a cell wall and killing the organism or cell (Rote, 2006). Figure 59–8 ■ diagrams the classic complement pathway and the alternate pathway. Both pathways end in cell lysis or death.

Humoral Immune Response

The **humoral immune response** is defined as the antibodies or immunoglobulins and the B lymphocytes that produce them. Antibodies are proteins that bind to antigens and immobilize or destroy them. The attachment of the antibody to the antigen is called an immune complex. The immune complex helps stimulate the immune response and can provide long-term protection from bacterial, viral, and fungal antigens.

B Lymphocytes

B-lymphocyte cells (B cells) are white blood cells that differentiate in bone marrow and enter the blood (Figure 59–9 ■, p. 1874). B lymphocytes are responsible for the production of antibodies. **Antibodies**, which are also called **immunoglobulins**, are proteins made by B cells that are capable of attaching to antigens

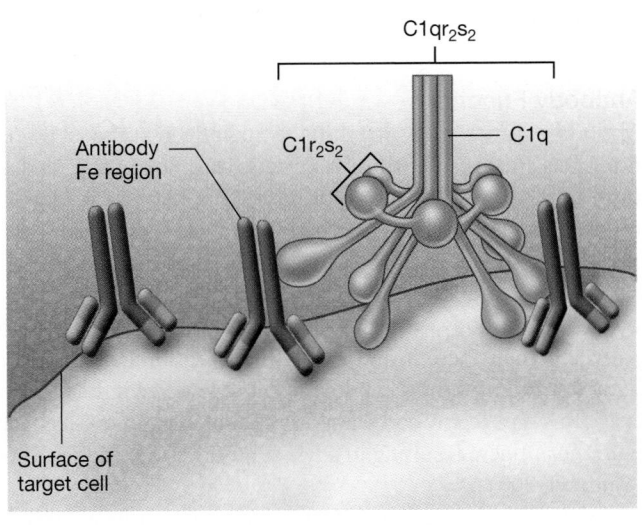

(a)

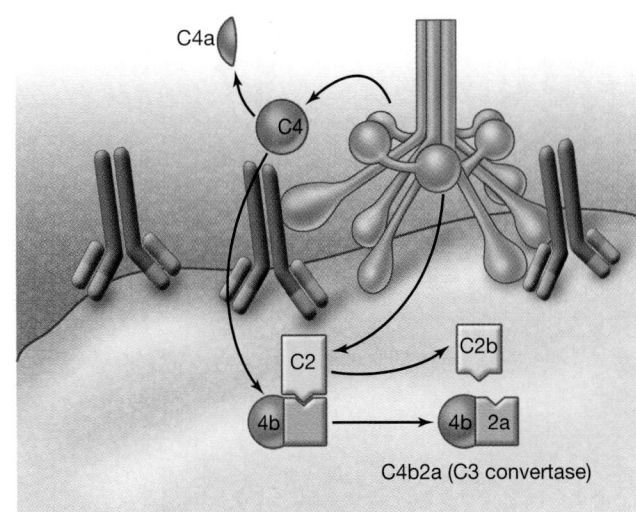

(b)

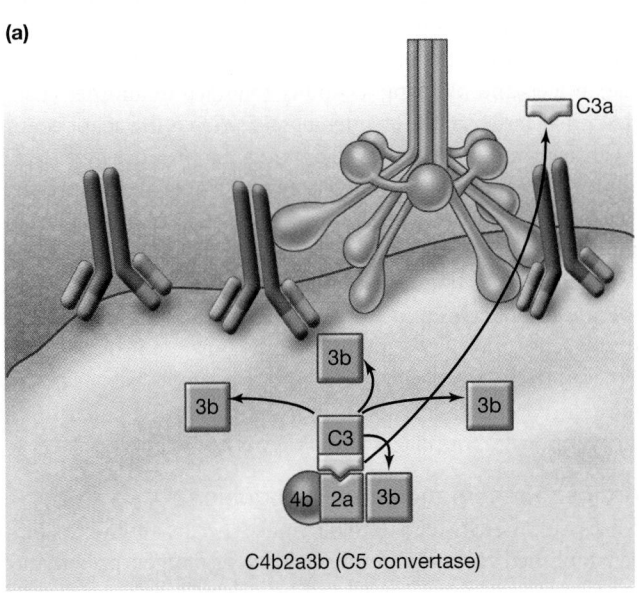

(c)

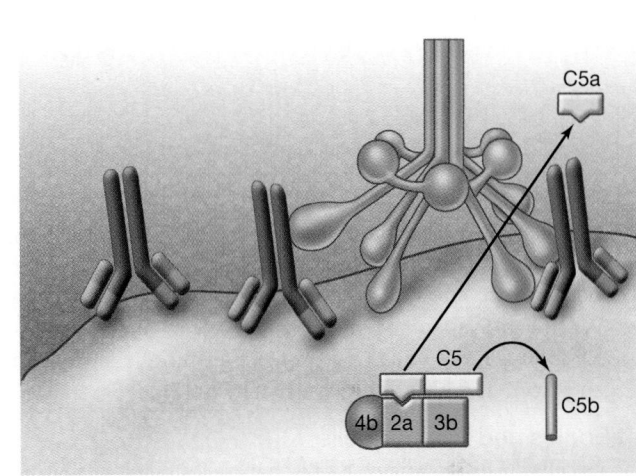

(d)

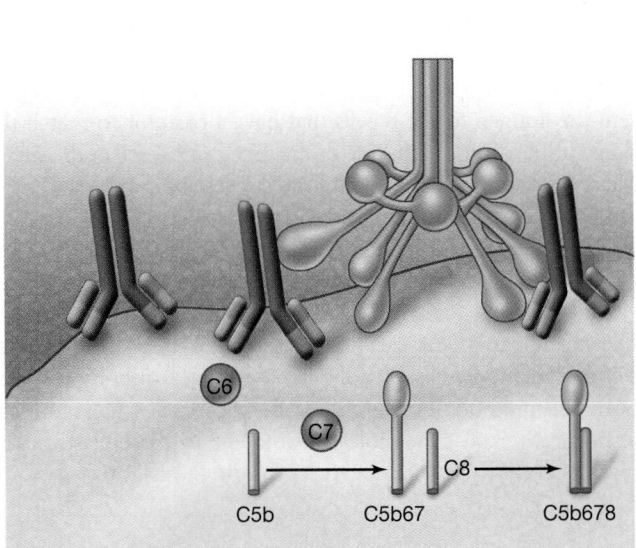

(e)

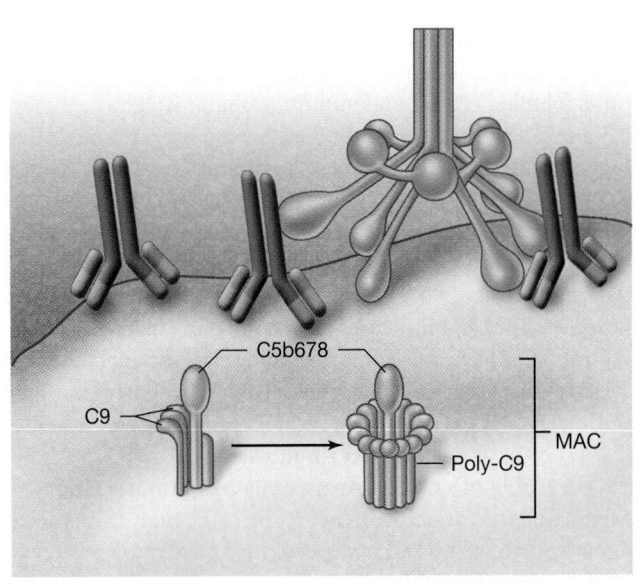

(f)

FIGURE 59–8 ■ Complement cascade.

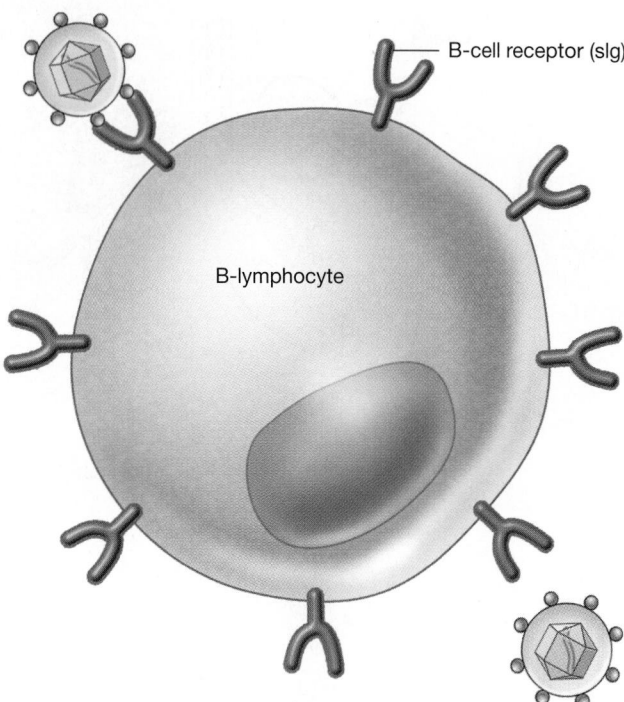

B-cell receptor (slg)

B-lymphocyte

FIGURE 59–9 ■ B cell.

and stimulating immune responses. B cells differentiate in the blood into either plasma B cells or memory B cells. B cells may be stimulated directly by some antigens or by T cells to make antibodies. Once stimulated, B cells make antibodies during their entire life span. Memory B cells can produce immunoglobulins more quickly and in greater numbers when an antigen is seen the second time (Sommer, 2007).

Antibodies and Plasma Cells

Plasma cells are differentiated B cells that are found in the plasma and are responsible for production of specific antibodies. Plasma cells produce the antibodies in response to a primary or initial exposure to an antigen. The most common groups of antibodies, also known as immunoglobulins, include immunoglobulin G (IgG), immunoglobulin A (IgA), immunoglobulin M (IgM), immunoglobulin D (IgD), and immunoglobulin E (IgE).

Some B cells produce antibodies that are secreted into saliva, lung, and intestinal tissue. These antibodies are usually of IgA and are referred to as secretory antibodies because they are found in secretions such as tears and saliva. Secretory antibodies provide immune defense at the portal of entry of a pathogen (DeFranco et al., 2007). Antibodies (immunoglobulins) have multiple shapes and functions as described in Chart 59–4.

Antibodies have one or more binding sites for attachment to antigens. The antibody is composed of a **fragment antigen binding (FAB) portion**, which is capable of being shaped to receive a specific antigen. **Deoxyribonucleic acid (DNA)** within B cells is capable of creating many millions of combinations of FAB portions of antibodies to help protect the body from the invasion by pathogens (DeFranco et al., 2007).

The **fragment crystalline (FC) portion** of the antibody is capable of attaching to the membrane of infected cells, mutant cells, or foreign pathogens (bacteria or viruses) and assisting macrophages to eliminate them (Rote, 2006). Figure 59–10 ■ (p. 1876) provides

a visual representation of an immunoglobulin and the FAB and FC binding sites.

Antibody Functions

Antibodies function by attaching to an antigen at the FAB portion. This creates an **antibody–antigen complex** (also called an **immune complex**) and is important in stimulating a strong immune response and destruction of the antigen. The antibody–antigen complex can attract other phagocytic cells such as neutrophils and macrophages to help eliminate the antigen. Each antibody is specifically shaped for only one type of antigen. When there is an exact fit between antigen and antibody, a strong antibody response results. However, if the fit is not exact, this type of antibody may not be able to bond as effectively with the antigen, resulting in a less profound immune response (Sommer, 2007).

Antibodies clustered around an antigen block its activity by neutralization, opsonization, agglutination, and precipitation. **Neutralization** is the process of changing the charge or shape of the antigen and blocking its ability to attach to another cell. As described earlier in the chapter, *opsonization* is the act of coating an antigen and making the cell or antigen more attractive to consume for phagocytic cells such as macrophages and neutrophils. Figure 59–11 ■ (p. 1876) demonstrates the formation of an immune complex that utilizes the process of opsonization. **Agglutination** is the surrounding and attaching of antibodies to the antigen and clumping together. Again, this stimulates the immune cells to locate the complex and consume it or destroy it. **Precipitation** occurs when an immune complex falls or precipitates out of circulation and is more easily found by neutrophils and monocytes for phagocytosis (DeFranco et al., 2007).

Antigen Presentation and Recognition

B cells must be activated or told to make specific antibodies; this is accomplished through the mechanism of antigen presentation. When a foreign antigen enters a host, the macrophages found in tissue, or monocytes found in blood, ingest the bacterium or virus and then digest the antigen. The macrophage expresses a portion of the digested antigen on its cell surface in the form of a small protein receptor with a part of the bacterial wall attached. T cells are often found near macrophages and can chemically bind to the receptor and accept the antigen onto their surface. T cells then present the antigen to the B cells that have a receptor to match the shape of the antigen. Linking of the T cell and B cell at the site of the antigen activates the B cell to make the appropriately shaped antibody to attach to the antigens (Rote, 2006). Figure 59–12 ■ (p. 1876) depicts the process of antigen presentation by a T cell to a B cell and the creation of antibodies.

Another mechanism of antigen recognition occurs when B cells are able to recognize antigens that may attach to surface receptors on the B cells and directly stimulate antibody production. This method of recognition often occurs during secondary response. It is also possible for antigens to directly stimulate plasma B cells by attaching to receptors on the cell surface (Sommer, 2007).

Memory B Cells

The first exposure to a specific antigen is known as a **primary immune response**. A primary immune response results in evidence of immunoglobulin production in 4 to 8 days after the initial ex-

CHART 59–4	**Immunoglobulins and Their Functions**	
Class of Immunoglobulin	**Primary Function**	**Structure**
IgG	Majority of circulating immunoglobulins are IgG. Capable of most immune functions, such as agglutination, opsonization, neutralization, activation of complement, precipitation. Can cross the placenta; major Ig found in neonatal blood.	IgG MHC Class I antigen-presenting protein
IgM	First antibody produced in primary immune response. This antibody is first produced during embryonic development.	CD4 T-cell receptor
IgA	Most commonly found in secretions such as saliva. Major function is to protect eyes, mouth, nose, gut, and lung from colonization and disease caused by viruses and bacteria. Secretory immunoglobulin, class. IgA2 most often found in lacrimal, saliva, gut, lung, nose secretions. Neutralizes bacterial and viral antigens.	
IgD	Least understood. Attaches to B cells and acts as an antigen. Present in small quantities in blood.	Monomer (see IgG)
IgE	Primary antibody in allergic responses. Least concentration of IgE in serum.	Monomer (see IgG)

Sources: DeFranco, A. L., Locksley, R., & Robertson, M. (2007). *Immunity: The immune response in infectious and inflammatory disease.* Sunderland, MA: Sinauer Associates; McCance, K., & Heuther, S. (2006). *Pathophysiology: The biological basis for disease in adults and children* (5th ed.). St. Louis: Mosby; Porth, C. (2007). *Essentials of pathophysiology* (7th ed.). Philadelphia: Lippincott Williams & Wilkins.

posure to an antigen. During this period some B cells differentiate into memory B cells that retain the ability to quickly recognize and produce antibodies to the antigen. The second time the host encounters the same antigen it produces antibodies in greater numbers, and more quickly than during the primary exposure. This stronger immune response is referred to as the **secondary immune response** and occurs in 1 to 3 days.

The presence of memory B cells often means the host will have a milder set of symptoms or no response to the pathogen. An example of a member B-cell response is primary and second exposure to cold or rhinovirus. During the first exposure to the antigen, cold and flu symptoms are at their peak for the first 4 to 5 days. The primary immune response requires 7 to 10 days to produce sufficient lymphokines and antibodies to eliminate the

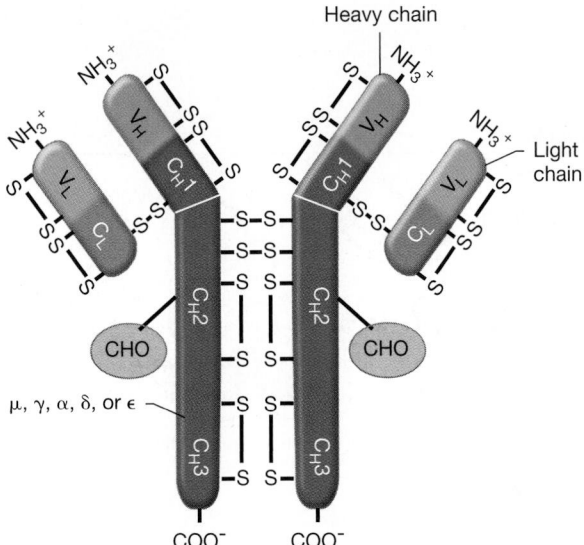

(a)

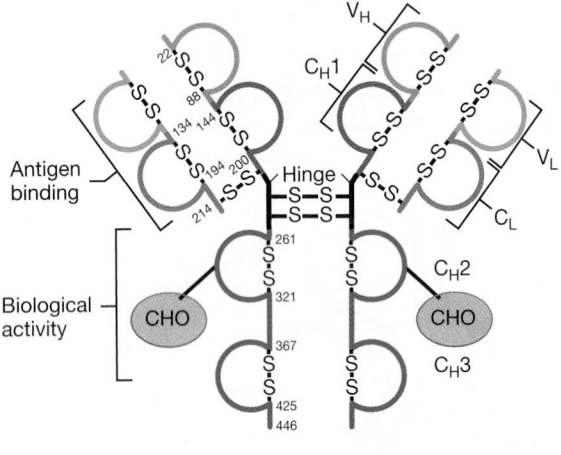

(b)

FIGURE 59–10 ■ Immunoglobulin with FAB and FC binding sites.

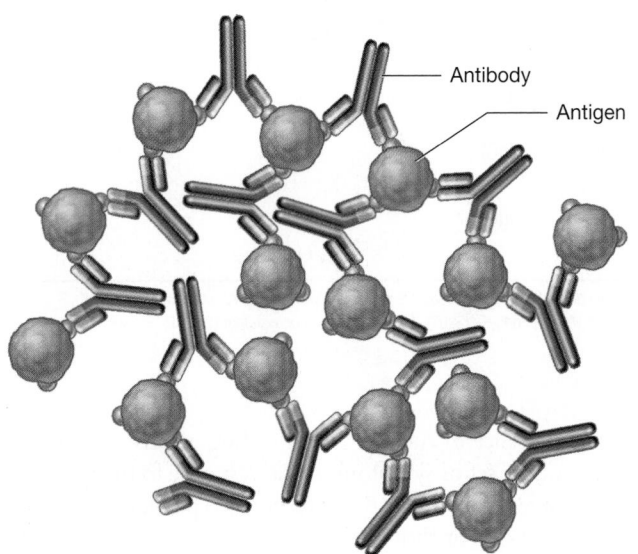

FIGURE 59–11 ■ Immune complex and the process of opsonization.

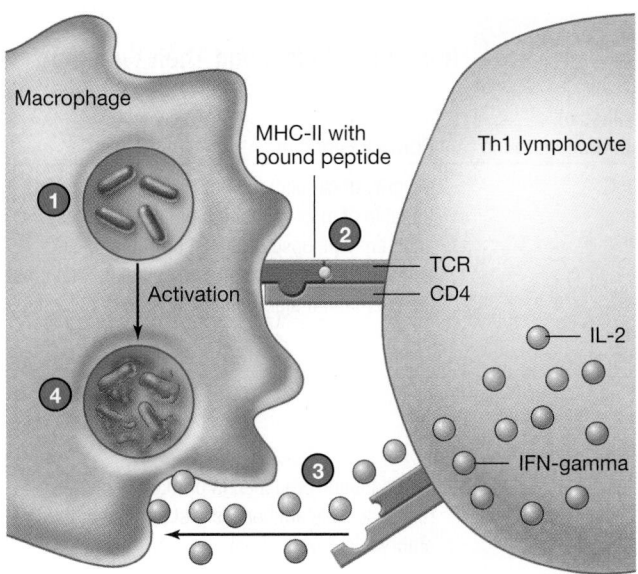

FIGURE 59–12 ■ Antigen presentation (sequential graphic).

virus and the symptoms that accompany it because the level of antibodies in the blood is lower with the primary response. The next exposure of the same rhinovirus activates memory B cells, and the production of antibodies specific to that antigen is quicker and greater in the secondary response. The consequence for the patient is mild or no cold symptoms (Figure 59–13 ■) (Porth & Sweeney, 2007).

Ongoing research regarding the body's production of antibodies in response to specific antigens has resulted in significant developments in the diagnosis and treatment of diseases that affect the immune system. Chart 59–5 discusses the history and development of monoclonal antibodies, which represent one application of these research advancements.

Immunizations

Immunization is a term often used interchangeably with *vaccination* or *inoculation* and involves the process of stimulating the immune system to create active immunity for protection against a disease. A **vaccine**, a preparation that contains an infectious agent or its components, is administered to stimulate the production of antibodies that can prevent infection or create resistance to infection from that agent (Rote, 2006).

Antigens used in vaccines to stimulate an immune response may be inactivated (whole-killed microorganisms or purified products derived from them), live-attenuated (live virus weakened through chemical or physical processes), or recombinant (artificially manufactured from segments of DNA from different sources). Vaccines against influenza, diphtheria, and tetanus use inactivated antigens. Attenuated vaccines include vaccines for measles, mumps, rubella, polio, yellow fever, and varicella. Genetically engineered recombinant antigens are currently being developed and are the basis for research in developing an HIV vaccine (Centers for Disease Control and Prevention [CDC], 2007b). Vaccines are most commonly administered by needle injections, but also can be given by mouth and by aerosol.

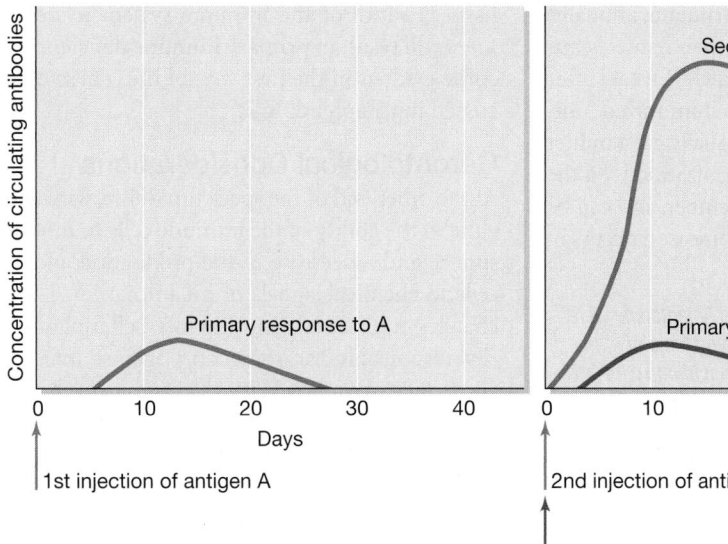
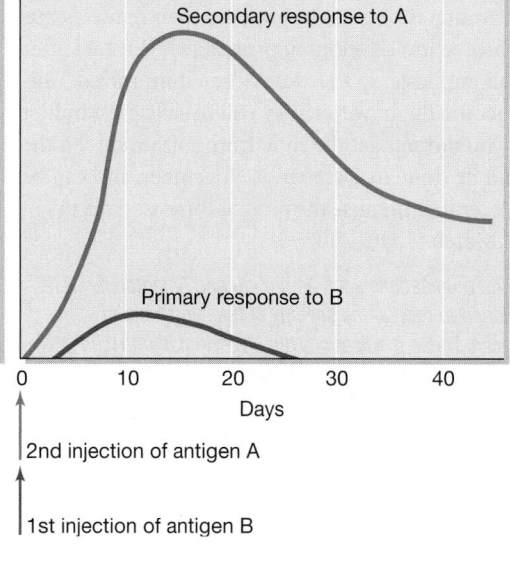

FIGURE 59–13 ■ Primary and secondary immune response curves.

CHART 59–5   Monoclonal Antibodies

When antibody production begins in response to an antigen, B cells become plasma cells and start to make antibodies. The normal antibody response includes variations in the antibodies produced because the multiple antigenic properties on the antigen cause a spectrum of B cells to proliferate. This results in more than one clone of the initial B cells, even though all the B cells were stimulated to proliferate by the same antigen. This is called the polyclonal response (Rote, 2006). However, in the 1970s researchers Kohler and Milstein (1975) developed a B-cell clone that produced a single antibody capable of binding with only one antigen called a monoclonal antibody. The monoclonal antibodies are antigen specific and can be produced in large quantities in a laboratory. Monoclonal antibodies are created by fusing antibody-producing B cells from the spleen of animals (usually mice) that have been injected with a specific antigen with rapidly growing plasma cells. One example of rapidly growing plasma cells is malignant myeloma cells. These are used because they proliferate rapidly and can live for a very long period of time in culture medium. This fusion process results in a hybridoma cell that produces a large quantity of monoclonal antibodies that are able to target a single antigen involved in a disease process (Dunne, 2007).

The development of monoclonal antibodies has had a profound effect on disease research, diagnosis, and treatment approaches. In cancer research, monoclonal antibodies are continually being developed to react against specific antigens on cancer cells and enhance the patient's immune response (Wilkes, 2005). They have been used extensively in cancer drug therapy to inhibit specific tumor growth factor (Franson, 2005). For example, Cetuximab is a monoclonal antibody used to treat metastatic colorectal cancer in combination with chemotherapy or when a patient is nonresponsive to chemotherapy treatment (Thomas, 2005; Wilson, Shannon, Shields, & Stang, 2007).

Monoclonal antibodies are also a vital part of early detection of viral infections. Monoclonal antibodies can be labeled with a fluorescent dye or enzyme and targeted for a specific viral pathogen, which allows visualization and identification of the pathogen with fluorescent microscopy (Dunne, 2007). Thus, monoclonal antibody technology enables the clinician to order tests for viral antigens to detect a disease early in its course and diagnose and treat it appropriately to realize the goal of improving patient outcomes (Rote, 2006).

National Guidelines for Immunization

All individuals should have their immunization status evaluated regularly. Recommended immunization schedules vary slightly by country. In the United States, the CDC conducts a national immunization program and publishes extensive information related to vaccines and recommended immunizations. The National Guidelines box summarizes immunizations for adults.

The CDC encourages annual immunization of the general population with the influenza vaccine, and strongly recommends it for adults 50 years and older, residents of long-term care facilities, individuals with chronic illnesses, immunosuppressed individuals, health care workers, and any other individuals coming in close contact with people at risk of contracting influenza. Inactive influenza vaccine has been used in the United States for many

NATIONAL GUIDELINES for Immunizations for Adults in the United States

Vaccines Needed by All Adults

1. Varicella (chickenpox) vaccine
2. Hepatitis B vaccines (adults at risk, i.e., health care workers, child care workers, military)
3. Measles-mumps-rubella (MMR) vaccine
4. Tetanus-diphtheria vaccine

Vaccines Needed for Those 50 Years of Age and Older

1. Influenza vaccine (for the flu) annually

Vaccines Needed for Those 65 Years of Age and Older

1. Pneumococcal vaccine (to prevent pneumonia caused by *Streptococcus pneumoniae*)

Vaccines Needed by All Health Care Workers

1. Influenza vaccine (for the flu) annually
2. Hepatitis B vaccine

Source: Centers for Disease Control and Prevention. (2007). *Immunizations.* Retrieved January 2, 2007, from http://www.cdc.gov/vaccines

years and is given annually because the flu virus mutates annually. The virus usually mutates in birds or pigs and then reinfects humans. Immune protection develops approximately 2 weeks after the immunization and lasts up to a year. Some immunized individuals will still get the flu; however, they will usually get a milder case than those who did not get the shot. Immunization with the flu vaccine should be done in October or November, and can be given as late as December because the peak of flu season occurs in January through March (CDC, 2007c).

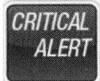 **CRITICAL ALERT** *Antiviral medications such as Tamiflu and Amantadine were developed to reduce the severity of the symptoms of influenza. These medications are given to patients with influenza to block viral infection and decrease the length of illness. Treatment of influenza is especially important for immunosuppressed patients or older adults who may not have a fully competent immune system (CDC, 2007c).*

Immunization with the pneumococcal vaccine to protect against *Streptococcus pneumoniae* diseases is strongly recommended by the CDC for individuals 65 years of age or older. Pneumococcal vaccine is also recommended by the CDC for individuals with high risk such as those who are immunocompromised, children under age 2, and children in day care situations. Pneumococcal infection results in serious disease such as pneumonia, bacteremia, meningitis, sinusitis, and otitis media. The CDC reports that pneumococcal disease kills more people in the United States each year than all other vaccine-preventable diseases combined (CDC, 2007d).

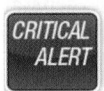 **CRITICAL ALERT** *The smallpox vaccine that many people received up to 50 years ago is now conferring only a percentage of the protection initially available. A bioterrorism attack using smallpox could potentially infect a large part of the population. As an individual ages, the cells that make the antibodies age as well and this can affect immune response to disease (DeFranco et al., 2007).*

Effects of Age on the Immune System

The major protection of the newborn against antigens occurs through the transfer of maternal IgG antibodies across the placenta during fetal development, especially during the last weeks of pregnancy (Rote, 2006). Hence, infants born prematurely may be significantly immune deficient. Immunoglobulin G antibodies remain active in the newborn for the first several months while the infant's production of immunoglobulins, specifically IgM, rises rapidly and attains adult levels by approximately 1 year of age (Sommer, 2007). Infant serum IgA levels are first detected approximately 2 weeks after birth and attain adult levels by 7 years of age. Further immune protection can be attained through the transfer of maternal IgA in the colostrum of milk during breast-feeding. Research has indicated that these antibodies provide local immunity for the intestinal system and decrease diarrheal infections in underdeveloped countries (Sommer, 2007).

The thymus is also a major contributor to immune development because it generates mature immunocompetent T lymphocytes during infancy and childhood. By puberty, when the mature immune cells are sequestered in the peripheral lymphoid tissues, the thymus atrophies and is replaced by adipose

tissue. Failure of the immune system to develop normally *in utero* will result in primary immune deficiencies that usually become evident in the first year of life. These deficiencies are discussed in Chapter 60 .

Gerontological Considerations

At the other end of the spectrum of life, with aging, there is a decline in the ability of the immune cells to mount an immune response and a decrease in the production and response of these cells to chemical signals of inflammation. The most significant changes occur in relationship to T-cell function, which is primarily responsible for protection against infections and tumors (Rote, 2006; Wojda & Witt, 2003). The number and percentage of T cells, both T-helper and suppressor T cells, decrease with age. Additionally, the ability of lymphocytes to produce interleukins is diminished as the body ages (Burns, 2004). The decline in T-cell numbers and function with aging results in greater susceptibility to infection. Influenza and pneumococcal pneumonia are two examples of diseases that most adults are relatively protected from until they reach age 55 to 60. After that time, the slower response of T cells and B cells can result in severe infections.

An additional effect of aging on the adult immune system is a delayed or decreased hypersensitivity reaction. When allergy testing is done in older adults, there may be a depressed ability to mount an inflammatory response to the antigen injected. This is referred to as **anergy**, and results from the diminished ability of the T-cell line to produce chemical mediators of inflammation. Individuals who show evidence of anergy are at greater risk of developing cancer and have higher rates of mortality in general (Sommer, 2007).

Aging also results in a decreased ability on the part of immune cells to identify self antigens, while at the same time there is an increase in the number of auto-antibodies produced. This results in higher incidences of autoimmune disease with aging (Rote, 2006; Wojda & Witt, 2003). Research also indicates that there is increased DNA mutation with aging that results in higher numbers of abnormal cells, and that the immune system fails to recognize and eliminate these problem cells. This in part accounts for the greater incidence of tumors and cancers in older adults (Camplejohn et al., 2003; Sommer, 2007). The Gerontological Considerations box summarizes the clinical effects of aging on the immune system.

 CRITICAL ALERT *Older adults may not demonstrate the classic symptoms of infection and inflammation such as fever. As a result of decreased immune function, older adults may become hypothermic when they have a systemic infection. The white blood cell count is usually elevated, but may not be as noticeable a response as that seen in a younger person. Symptoms such as altered level of consciousness and confusion should be carefully assessed and evaluated in any patient who is older and especially in patients from settings such as skilled facilities where the incidence of urinary tract infections may be higher (Porth, 2007).*

Genetic Implications

Nurses need an ongoing knowledge of the discoveries of genetic research to be able to identify and assess individuals at risk. Nurses also need an adequate understanding of the genetic research to be able to teach patients and families about the risk factors, tests, and

GERONTOLOGICAL CONSIDERATIONS of the Effects of Aging on the Immune System

Effect on Immune System	Clinical Signs
Decreased percentage of T cells	Risk of infection, tumor.
Decreased percentage of T-helper cells	Cannot initiate immune response as quickly.
Decreased percentage of suppressor T cells	Cannot downregulate immune system as quickly.
Decreased interleukin production	Slows inflammatory and immune responses to infection.
Decreased number of interleukin receptors on cells	Slows inflammatory and immune responses.
Delayed stimulation of T cells and B cells	Slows inflammatory response and may decrease ability to recognize cancer cells.
Decreased primary and secondary production of antibodies	Reduced response to infectious organisms, more severe infection, i.e., pneumonia.
Delayed hypersensitivity response	Decreased allergic response, increased severity of infections.
Increased auto-antibody production	More exacerbations of autoimmune disease.

Sources: Burns, E. A. (2004). Effects of aging on immune function. *Journal of Nutrition Health and Aging, 8*(1), 9–17; McCance, K., & Heuther, S. (2006). *Pathophysiology: The biological basis for disease in adults and children* (5th ed.). St. Louis: Mosby; Porth, C. (2007). *Essentials of pathophysiology* (7th ed.). Philadelphia: Lippincott Williams & Wilkins.

treatment of diseases with a familial or genetic association. Patients with high risk for inherited diseases such as cancer or immune abnormalities will benefit the most from this information.

DNA is the building block that forms genes. Genes are present in the nucleus of every cell and confer all of the inherited characteristics. Genes also regulate cell activity and determine how the cell develops and functions. The Human Genome Project identified and mapped all of the genes of the human body (Khoury, 2006). One result of this work has been a better understanding of the fundamental role that DNA and genes play in the development of the majority of diseases. Research has focused on discovering which genes are linked to the development of specific diseases such as immune disorders like asthma, systemic lupus erythematosus (SLE), and cancer. The major task ahead is to create the bridges from genomic discoveries to disease prevention and improved treatment (Tranin, 2006).

Alterations of specific genes on immune cells are a focus of ongoing immunologic genetic research. An example of this is the overproduction of IgE and leukotrienes and the development of asthma (Meurer, Lustig, & Jacob, 2006). Asthma is known to be a complex disorder with genetic and familial association. Specific genes are now being identified that have links to increased risk for developing asthma (Postma et al., 2005). Research has also linked variation in genotypes to how patients respond to common asthma medications such at albuterol, which supports the significance of genotyping in determining the most effective drug treatment to improve patient outcomes (U.S. Food and Drug Administration, 2005).

Currently genotyping is done at only a few research centers, but it is not unrealistic to envision this becoming a common aspect of the clinical work-up for patients with immune alterations (Steinke & Borish, 2006). DNA mutations and alterations in gene functioning have major ramifications for identifying and treating disease processes that affect the immune system and all other body systems. Genetics is discussed in Chapter 11 ✪.

ASSESSMENT OF THE IMMUNE SYSTEM

Immune function assessment begins with a thorough health history and physical examination because disorders of the immune system can affect any system in the body. Listening carefully to the patient's complaints about current and past medical problems provides valuable clues to immune function. It also gives direction for physical assessment and diagnostic testing that is completed in collaboration with the health care provider or other members of the health care team. Chart 59–6 outlines essential information about the immune system assessment.

▉ Patient History

A thorough assessment of a patient should include biographic data, demographic data, risk factors for illness, and focused

CHART 59–6 Key Criteria for Assessment of the Immune System

Assessment	Nursing Implications
Complete health history	Current complaint, prior diseases, immunizations, chronic disease, known immune disease, nutritional status, functional status.
Family health history	Genetic association with many diseases including some cancers, heart disease, some autoimmune diseases.
Social history	Abuse of alcohol or drugs, smoking, diet, sexual behaviors, and occupation can all impact immune function and likelihood of transmission of infectious diseases.
Medications	Drugs affect immune function. Drugs may interact with each other. Side effects may affect assessment (e.g., corticosteroids suppress immune function).
Physical Assessment	
Inspection	Skin and mucous membranes intact, examine all rashes, wounds, note any exudate.
Palpation	Palpate lymph nodes in neck, groin, axilla. Palpate abdomen and kidneys.
Percussion	Thorax, abdomen.
Auscultation	Lung sounds can give clue to infection. Auscultate for heart murmurs.

Sources: D'Amico, D., & Barbarito, C. (2007). *Health and physical assessment in nursing.* Upper Saddle River, NJ: Pearson Prentice Hall; DeFranco, A. L., Locksley, R., & Robertson, M. (2007). *Immunity: The immune response in infectious and inflammatory disease.* Sunderland, MA: Sinauer Associates; Porth, C. (2007). *Essentials of pathophysiology* (7th ed.). Philadelphia: Lippincott Williams & Wilkins.

inquiry into the patient's current problem. The most common complaints related to the immune system and lymphatic tissues involve infection, allergy response, enlarged lymph nodes, and lymphedema (Wilson & Giddens, 2005). Assessment should include recent exposure to any infectious diseases. Risk factors that impact immune function would include a genetic familial history of immune-related diseases as well as lifestyle choices and habits that increase exposure to communicable diseases. Sexually transmitted infections are discussed in Chapters 49 and 50 ☺. Substance abuse behaviors that may alter immune function are discussed in Chapter 16 ☺.

Inflammation is often the first step in stimulating the immune system. Indicators of inflammation should be assessed including questions about fever, malaise, swelling, redness, cough with or without pain, and decreased function of a limb or part of the body. Inquire about the presence of rashes, skin cracks, or open wounds with serous drainage, bleeding or pus that may indicate infection. Inquire if the patient is experiencing night sweats or cough with or without sputum. If sputum is present, what color is it? Various colors of sputum indicate infection with different types of organisms. For example, infections involving pseudomonas are usually a green color, whereas rust-colored sputum is associated with *Klebsiella* (Porth & Sweeney, 2007). It also is important to gain information about the duration and frequency of infections. Incurable or recurrent infections are often the first indicator of significant impaired immune function. An example of this is frequent and recurrent oral or vaginal candida infections, as seen in patients with HIV infection.

Pain

The integration of the immune system throughout the body's other systems means that alterations in immune function can present themselves in a variety of manifestations. Pain is one of the most common first complaints with immune abnormalities due to the presence of inflammation. For example, enlarged lymph nodes in the presence of viral or bacterial infection may be very tender and painful. Detailed assessment of pain is a vital aspect of the history and physical examination and should be quantified using a specific pain scale. Chapter 15 ☺ includes examples of pain assessment scales.

Past Medical History

Information gathered should include a history of childhood diseases, prior hospitalizations, and diagnostic and surgical procedures. Question the patient regarding a medical history of chronic disease such as hepatitis, diabetes, chronic obstructive pulmonary disease, or renal failure. This is significant because chronic diseases can impair immune function. Inquire about a history of diseases specifically related to immune disorders such as cancer or autoimmune diseases such as SLE or rheumatoid arthritis. Additionally, all patients should be assessed for allergies to medications, food, and environmental antigens such as pollen or pet dander (D'Amico & Barbarito, 2007).

It also is important to know if the patient has had surgeries that involved removing lymph nodes due to malignancy or trauma, or any organ transplant. Loss of lymph nodes will alter lymphatic drainage and decrease immune function. Organ transplant requires lifelong immunosuppressive medications that result in immune suppression and a significantly increased risk for contracting an infection. A history of any blood transfusions should also be obtained because blood products contain foreign antibodies that can alter normal immune response. Also, blood transfusions prior to 1985 were not screened for HIV. Subsequent screening has almost eliminated this risk (CDC, 2007a). Blood administration safety is discussed in extensive detail in Chapter 23 ☺.

Knowledge of the patient's immunization status also is important in preventing illness and promoting optimal health. Inquire about childhood diseases such as chicken pox, measles, mumps, whooping cough, or immunizations against these diseases, as well as a current tetanus vaccine, which must be updated every 10 years. Ask adult patients if they have received the annual influenza vaccine. Any adult with a history of pneumonia should receive the pneumococcus vaccine. Additionally, the CDC recommends that all adults over the age of 65 receive a pneumococcus vaccine if they have not already been immunized (CDC, 2007b). Inquire about past or present exposure to tuberculosis and the dates and results of tuberculin tests such as a tine test or purified protein derived (PPD) test, as well as any follow-up chest x-ray results. Obtain information on recent travel to another country or history of living in another country, especially developing countries, because a traveler is at risk of being exposed to multiple strains of resistant organisms (D'Amico & Barbarito, 2007).

Medication History

Medications can significantly affect the immune system. It is essential to obtain a complete list of all medications, including over-the-counter (OTC) medications, that the patient is currently taking. Common OTC medications such as nonsteroidal anti-inflammatory drugs (e.g., ibuprofen, cyclooxygenase-2 inhibitors, and aspirin) that are taken in large quantities can cause significant decreases in leukocytes and neutrophils. Prescription medications the patient is taking to treat ongoing medical problems can result in profound immune suppression. Drugs such as corticosteroids or cytotoxic agents such as cyclophosphamide are immunosuppressive and significantly increase the patient's susceptibility to infection. Antibiotics in large doses or administered over a prolonged period of time can also affect immune function and result in hemolytic anemia, leukopenia, and neutropenia as well as agranulocytosis (Shannon, Wilson, & Stang, 2004).

Interactions between various medications need to be considered before patients are treated with additional medications for the current complaint. Some medications, such as antibiotics, interfere with the action of others. Herbal supplements can also have significant drug interactions and patients should be questioned regarding herbal supplement use. Addition of new medications to the patient's treatment regime should prompt discussion with a consulting pharmacist to identify any possible medication interactions and an examination of laboratory values to identify possible immune alterations.

Family History

Many of the diseases that affect the immune system are related to specific gene alterations that predispose members of the same family to the development of similar immune disorders. Examples of this are certain types of malignancies such as breast cancer, autoimmune diseases such as SLE, and development of allergies (Porth & Sweeney, 2007). Inquire if any members of the patient's family have been diagnosed with cancer and what type, as well as any other diseases involving the immune system such as rheumatoid arthritis or allergic asthma. It is important to know if members of the patient's immediate family (parents, grandparents, siblings) are deceased and the cause of death. Genetic predisposition plays a critical role in the development of many diseases in addition to those that affect the immune system, such as heart disease, emphysema, and diabetes. This information helps identify the patient's risk factors for disease development and can direct the physical examination and diagnostic work-up.

Social History

It is important to ask about the patient's occupation. Exposure to certain environmental substances can effect the action of the immune system. For example, asbestos and coal dust are known to result in cell changes that can lead to cancerous tumor (Porth & Sweeney, 2007). Additionally, the risk of development of occupational allergies is directly related to the frequency of exposure to certain products, as exemplified by the increased incidence of latex allergies among individuals who have daily exposure to latex products (National Institute for Occupational Safety and Health, 2007). Issues of importance when attending to patients from various cultures or ethnic groups are discussed in the Cultural Considerations box.

Inquire about lifestyle habits such as smoking, alcohol and drug use, and sexual practices, all of which place the patient at an increased risk for development of diseases that impact immune function. Illicit injection drug use and multiple sexual partners are high-risk behaviors associated with transmission of infections of hepatitis and HIV, as discussed in Chapter 60 .

 Questions about lifestyle habits such as alcohol and drug use and sexual practices are sensitive. These issues should be addressed in a private setting, without other family or friends present. It is also helpful to ask sensitive questions toward the end of the patient history after the nurse has had an opportunity to establish rapport with the patient.

It is also important to obtain information related to the patient's social support system. The availability of family and friends to provide psychological and physical care during illness and as-

CULTURAL CONSIDERATIONS for Treating Patients from Various Cultures

Cultural factors also can impact the patient's concept of health, comfort with the medical exam, and choices of medical treatment. For some cultural groups decision making related to health care is not autonomous, and the patient may prefer that the head of the family or clan be present when the patient's diagnosis, treatment, or prognosis is discussed (Jarvis, 2004). Knowledge about the patient's cultural attitudes can facilitate taking the history and completing the physical examination. For example, concerns about modesty may be an issue during examination of lymph nodes in the breast and groin area for women in Asian, Hispanic, American Indian, or Alaskan Native cultural groups, and may be sensitively addressed by having a same-gender health care provider and covering the perineum during the exam (Wilson & Giddens, 2005).

sist the patient in managing medications and follow-up treatment is essential for compliance with the prescribed treatment regime. Diagnosis of diseases related to the immune system, such as cancer or HIV infection, are frequently devastating and provoke high anxiety related to the issue of dying. Chronic diseases, such as SLE or rheumatoid arthritis, can dramatically alter the patient's lifestyle and occupational choices. Nurses are in an ideal position to identify issues related to lack of social support and to provide resources and referrals to address this issue, in an effort to decrease the risk of depression and isolation that can result.

Physical Assessment

Lymphatic tissues and cells of the immune system are located throughout the body. The immune system affects every other body system. Often signs of immune abnormalities are subtle. Therefore, a thorough physical examination involves inspection, palpation, percussion, and auscultation of various body systems to identify any abnormal function. Careful examination and palpation of immune tissue, especially the lymph nodes, are particularly important because enlarged and painful lymph nodes may indicate infection, inflammation, or malignancy. Figure 59–2 ▪ (p. 1867) describes the location of lymph nodes and the tissues that are drained by part of the lymph system.

Inspection

Inspection is always the first step in a physical examination. Look globally at the patient. Does the patient look fatigued, feverish, or pale? Is the patient well nourished, thin, or obese? Fever indicates an acute infection. Fatigue and weight loss may be associated with chronic disease processes. Inadequate nutrition affects the ability of the immune cells to function normally and causes immunosuppression. Rapid and significant weight loss that is unintentional is a serious concern because it is a symptom of malignancy. An unintentional weight loss of 10 pounds or more in a month is also an indicator of a need for a nutritional consult. Optimal nutrition is essential for immune function. Loss of protein reserves results in atrophy of lymphoid tissue and decreased antibody and T-cell response. Decreased vitamin and mineral intake affects the proliferation and maturation of immune cells and suppresses immune function. Malnutrition lowers the body's resistance to disease and increases morbidity and mortality from infection (Scrimshaw, 2003; Urden, Stacy, & Lough, 2006). An extensive discussion on the importance of nutrition for body function can be found in Chapter 14 . General inspection also includes careful examination of the intactness of the skin and mucous membranes because they are the first line of defense in protecting the body from invasion by microorganisms.

Inspection should be directed to the area of complaint. For example, if the complaint is related to symptoms of a persistent cough and sore throat, inspect the mucous membranes of the throat and the lymph nodes of the neck (see Figure 59–2 ▪, p. 1867). Superficial lymph nodes should not be visible, thus the presence of edema, erythema, and red streaks is indicative of inflammation and infection (Wilson & Giddens, 2005).

Additionally, observe for edema of the extremities and at lymph node sites. Edema may be localized and related to a wound or infectious process that causes swelling in an extremity or related changes in normal circulatory flow. Areas of edema that are red and warm indicate inflammation. Note any signs of lymphedema, nonpitting edema at the site of lymph nodes that indicates inadequate drainage from lymphatic vessels and excessive accumulation of fluid in the interstitial spaces around the lymph vessels. This can occur for a variety of reasons including congenital abnormalities in the development of the lymphatic system (Milroy's disease), blocked lymphatic channels due to infection or malignancy, or surgical removal of lymph nodes related to trauma or prior malignancy. The presence of lymphedema should prompt questions related to the onset and duration of the swelling because this is a symptom associated with the development of malignancies (D'Amico & Barbarito, 2007).

Palpation

Palpate lymph nodes for size, tenderness, warmth, and mobility (see Figure 59–2 ■, p. 1867 for lymph node locations) and note if any are edematous. Ask the patient if it is painful to have the nodes palpated. Normally superficial lymph nodes are pain free and nonpalpable. Enlarged lymph nodes from acute infection are tender, slightly firm, and move freely. In contrast, malignancy is indicated when enlarged nodes are nontender, hard, asymmetrical, and nonmobile (attached to the underlying tissues) (Wilson & Giddens, 2005). If the nodes are enlarged or tender, focus assessment on the structures from which they drain. For example, if lymph nodes in the neck are bilaterally edematous, tender, firm, and freely movable, infection of the head and throat may be indicated. If the complaint is in the lower extremities, the groin lymph nodes should be palpated for edema and tenderness. Additionally, any edema in extremities should be palpated to determine the extent and level of pitting. A thorough examination also involves palpation of the abdomen, which contains a large number of immune tissues, for assessment of and pain or identification of a mass.

Percussion

Percussion is helpful in determining if there is inappropriate fluid or a mass in an organ, indicating disease. For example, percussion over the lung is done to determine if fluid is present that would change the normal resonant sound of the lung tissue to a dull sound, which may indicate infection. Kidneys are percussed to determine if there is tenderness in the area, indicating possible infection or tumor (Jarvis, 2004). Abnormalities in percussion sounds warrant further investigation and collaborative discussion with the health care provider for follow-up with more in-depth diagnostic testing of the body system involved.

Auscultation

Lung sounds such as coarse and fine crackles indicate fluid from infection or edema. Heart sounds such as valve sounds and murmurs give indications about the function of the organ. Cardiac valve dysfunction with murmurs is not uncommon in autoimmune diseases such as SLE or rheumatoid disease (Jarvis, 2004). Abdominal auscultation is done to assess bowel sounds. For example, a loss of bowel sounds may indicate an ileus or infarcted bowel.

Integumentary Assessment

Skin should be assessed with each evaluation of the patient. Normal skin is intact and free from areas of redness, swelling, rashes,

purpura, or lesions that may indicate inflammation, an allergic reaction, or infectious processes. Examine the skin and identify any nodules, lumps, or wounds that are present. Evaluate these abnormalities for symptoms of infection such as redness, inflammation, streaking lines, edema, or drainage. Signs of rash or petechiae indicate an allergic response or infection. A variety of autoimmune diseases have signs or symptoms seen on the skin. Scleroderma is one example of autoimmune disease that affects the quality of the skin. Patients with scleroderma often have firm, hard skin and may have a somewhat immobile facial expression. Chapter 60 ⊙ includes discussions of allergies and autoimmune diseases. Information on skin abnormalities is extensively discussed in Chapters 66 and 67 ⊙ .

While examining the skin, give special attention to bony prominences where redness can indicate the first stage of skin breakdown, and to skinfolds under the breast and in the groin where small cracks in the skin may go undetected. Inspect the mucous membranes, which should be pink, moist, and free of lesions.

 **CRITICAL ALERT** *A patient who is obese may have difficulty cleansing skinfolds especially on the back, the thighs, and under a pendulous abdomen. Skinfolds that are not cleaned regularly place the patient at increased risk for development of candidiasis (yeast) infection or the development of boils that can go undetected. The patient may also be embarrassed by lack of cleanliness and feel very uncomfortable with a skinfold examination. A caring and nonjudgmental attitude on the part of the nurse is vital in helping the patient feel accepted and building a therapeutic relationship.*

Neurological Assessment

The brain is protected from injury and invasion by the bones of the cranium. Protection from birth also includes the blood–brain barrier, which is the mechanism of tight connections between endothelial cells in blood vessels that prevent many particles from diffusing into the brain. The brain does not have lymph tissue, but protection is provided by lymph nodes in the neck (Rote, 2006). Examination of the head and neck involves inspection and palpation of the lymph nodes of the head located in front of and behind the ear and extending along the jaw and under the chin, the anterior and posterior neck, and the supraclavicular area. Palpation of the periauricular lymph nodes is done to assess lymph nodes that drain lymph fluid from the head (Figure 59–14 ■). The technique for palpation of the lymph nodes of the neck can be seen in Figure 59–15 ■. Swollen, tender, red nodes in these areas may reflect infection in the face, neck, or head.

Many autoimmune diseases have a neurological component. Physical examination of immune function in the neurological system includes assessment of the symmetry of the face. Examine the face for presence of facial droop or a facial expression that is frozen or not responsive to emotion. Disorders of the immune system that affect the neurological system include Guillain-Barré, myasthenia gravis, and cerebral vascular accident. Additionally, Bell's palsy also can present with an asymmetrical facial expression. Patients presenting with fever and stiffness of the neck should be assessed for meningitis. Extremities should be assessed for numbness, tingling, or unilateral or bilateral paralysis. Chapter 28 ⊙ provides information on neurological abnormalities and a description of a full neurological assessment.

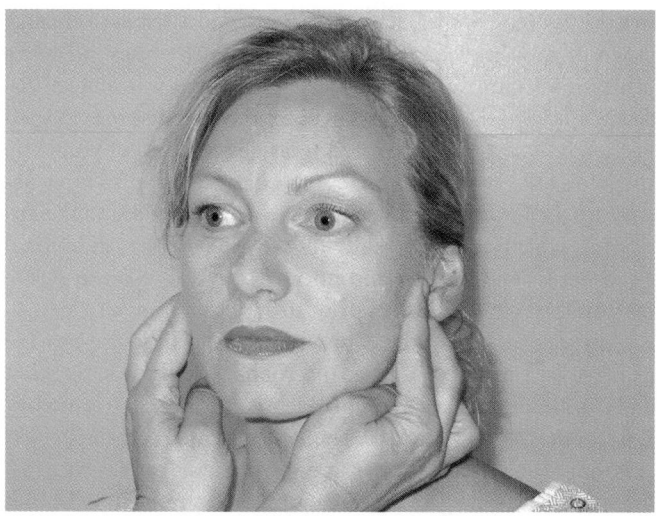

FIGURE 59–14 ■ Palpation of the periauricular lymph nodes.

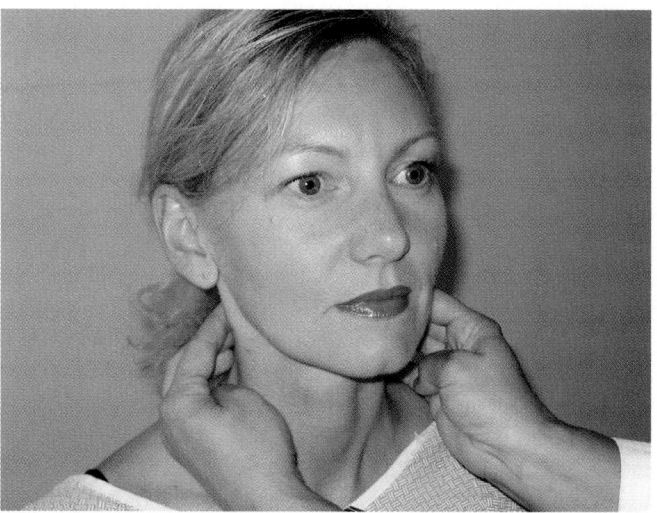

FIGURE 59–15 ■ Palpation of the posterior superficial cervical chain lymph nodes.

Cardiovascular Assessment

The heart and vascular system are closely associated with lymphatic vessels. A lymphatic vessel is located next to each combination of artery and vein. Chyle drains into the right atrium from the lymphatic and thoracic ducts. Chyle mixes with blood and is delivered from the heart into circulation. Protection is also provided by the presence of immune cells, including B cells, T cells, macrophages, neutrophils, and basophils. Immunoglobulin is also circulating in the blood. The vascular system allows rapid delivery of immune cells and chemicals to all areas of the body (Sommer, 2007). A functioning cardiovascular system is essential for proper immune function.

Assessment of immune function in the cardiovascular system itself primarily focuses on laboratory data and the clinical presentation of the patient. Elevated white blood cell counts often occur with inflammation from an ischemic cardiac event such as acute myocardial infarction or an infectious process such as endocarditis. See Unit 8 💿 for a full discussion of cardiac abnormalities.

Respiratory and Chest Assessment

The respiratory system utilizes several natural mechanisms of protection to support immune function. The upper airway contains the tonsils, which are made up primarily of lymphoid tissue and help trap and process antigens. The cough reflex helps remove debris from the bronchial airways. Ciliated cells in the trachea and airways move cells, debris, and bacteria toward the mouth and away from alveoli. Fixed macrophages are present in lung tissue to phagocytize bacterial cells and debris. The lungs also are rich in vascular tissue, and immune cells are present in circulation to help protect against debris, virus, and bacteria (Rote, 2006). Situations that damage the cilia and alter pulmonary tissue such as smoking or inhalation burn injuries place the patient at increased risk for infection. Medical treatment for acute respiratory failure that requires mechanical intubation bypasses all of the natural defense mechanisms and is one of the primary reasons that extubation as early as is safe for the patient is strongly recommended (Tablan, Anderson, Besser, Bridges, & Hajjeh, 2004).

Competent immune function is critical in the respiratory system because of the variety and quantity of microorganisms that the pulmonary tissues are exposed to on a daily basis. Lung sounds should be auscultated. Patients with infectious processes may have coarse or fine crackles or a friction rub of the pleura. A friction rub indicates inflammation of the pleura, which may be associated with infection (D'Amico & Barbarito, 2007). Patients who present with a complaint of pain with cough or difficulty breathing should be evaluated for elevated white blood cell counts. Because the lungs' ability to clear debris and bacteria is so important, the quality and quantity of secretions must be assessed. Secretions that are green, yellow, or brown should be evaluated by laboratory culture to detect an infectious process.

Assessment of the respiratory system and structures of the chest involves inspection and palpation of the nodes in the supraclavicular area, the axilla, and the breast. Figure 59–16 ■ demonstrates the appropriate hand position for examining supraclavicular lymph nodes. Palpation and detection of enlarged supraclavicular nodes are of particular concern because these nodes are at the end of a chain of ducts, such as the thoracic duct, that drain the upper abdomen, lungs, breasts, and

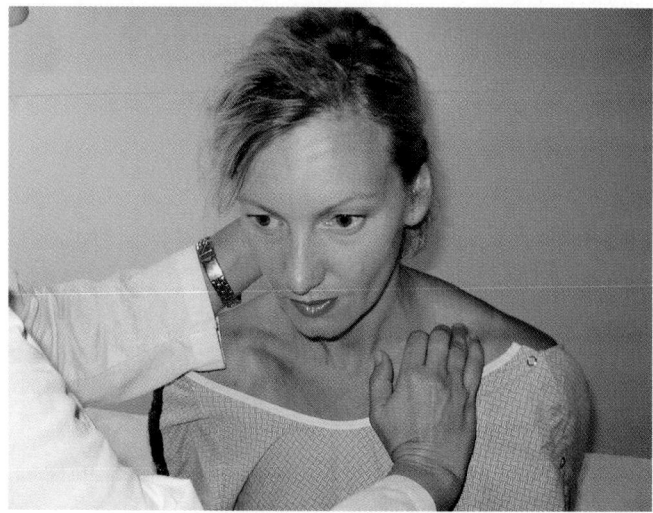

FIGURE 59–16 ■ Palpation of the supraclavicular lymph nodes.

arms and are often the site of metastatic disease (Wilson & Giddens, 2005).

The majority of the drainage from the breast flows into the axillary nodes. Palpation of axillary nodes is shown in Figure 59–17 ∎. Lymph nodes of the breast are located deep in the tissue and are rarely palpable. Axillary nodes that are enlarged, painful, and mobile indicate infection located in the breast or arm or systemic disease such as systemic syphilis. In contrast, axillary lymph nodes that are enlarged, painless, asymmetrical, and fixed to underlying tissue are indicative of malignant diseases such as breast cancer and Hodgkin's lymphoma (D'Amico & Barbarito, 2007).

Gastrointestinal Assessment

Immune function is supported through a variety of natural protective mechanisms within the gastrointestinal system (GI). The act of emesis can rid the stomach of toxins and bacteria. The stomach produces hydrochloric acid and maintains a pH of approximately 3.00. This is so acidic that only a few organisms can exist in the stomach. An example of one of the few organisms that can tolerate an acidic environment is *Helicobacter pylori*, which is the cause of many gastric ulcers. *H. pylori* can withstand the acidic environment and start to grow on the cell walls of the stomach. This growth is followed by acid secretion that further stresses the cells such that the cell walls in the stomach break down and an ulcer is formed (Rote, 2006). Gastric ulcers also may occur due to the secretion of additional acid as part of the stress response with illness. It is important to address this potential problem area.

 CRITICAL ALERT *A critical assessment of the protection of the entire gastrointestinal system is essential for all patients hospitalized for greater than a day or two. The stress of illness, as well as immobility, places the gastric mucosa at risk of degradation. The consequence of loss of protection can be GI bleed and/or stress ulcer. Proton pump inhibitors or H2-receptor blockers are necessary for many patients.*

The intestines have a rich vasculature. The vessels of the small and large intestine are responsible for absorption of large molecules of digestion. Large numbers of bacteria are always present in the intestines. Some bacteria are needed to assist in the breakdown of food molecules. The structure of the intestine offers protection for the body's internal environment from these bacteria. In addition, two-thirds of all fixed lymph tissue is located in the abdomen and is referred to as gut-associated lymphatic tissue (GALT) (Sommer, 2007). Specific clusters of lymph tissues are the Peyer's patches, which are not palpable, and the appendix, which produces pain in the right lower abdominal quadrant when inflamed and infected and can result in severe peritonitis if rupture occurs prior to surgical removal.

Accessory organs of the GI tract such as the liver also provide protection from antigens. Fixed macrophages in the liver filter out and consume bacteria and cellular debris. The liver also is responsible for the filtering of toxins. The spleen, located in the upper left abdominal quadrant, houses a large network of B and T lymphocytes and macrophages that filter antigens from the blood and it is important in immune function for fighting systemic infection.

Assessment of immune function of the GI system should include inspection, auscultation, percussion, and palpation of all four abdominal quadrants. Inspection assesses symmetry of the abdomen and quality of the skin. Lack of symmetry or taunt skin can indicate a mass or infection. Auscultation of abdomen occurs prior to percussing or palpating the abdomen, so that the presence or absence of bowel sounds or pain is not affected. Auscultation enables identification of bowel abnormalities, such as absent bowel sounds with paralytic ileus or mechanical obstruction. Percussion of the abdomen focuses on areas of tympany and dullness. Tympany usually indicates the presence of gas. Dullness is usually present over tissue or fecal material in the gastrointestinal tract and is also the sound with presence of a tumor. All four quadrants of the abdomen should be percussed. Chapter 44 🔗 demonstrates appropriate hand position for percussion of the abdomen. Areas of dullness should then be palpated for a mass. Pain upon palpation should be further assessed for quality, degree, duration, and other occurrences of the same pain. Pain can be related to infection or a disease process affecting the underlying tissue (Jarvis, 2004). Additional information on GI assessment can be found in Chapter 44 🔗 .

Genitourinary System

Organs of the genitourinary system provide natural immune protection for the body by several mechanisms. Mechanical flow of urine can wash debris from the urethra. The kidneys also filter out drug metabolites. Vaginal secretions contain immunoglobulins and other immune cells that can provide some protection from bacteria, fungi, and virus (Rote, 2006).

Immune assessment of the genitourinary system includes inspection, percussion, and palpation to identify the presence of infection or malignant tumors. External genitalia should be free from swelling and drainage. Skin should be intact and free from lesions and redness around the anus and upper inner thigh area. Percussion of the kidneys and bladder is not usually necessary unless the patient complains of specific flank pain, difficulty emptying the bladder, or an urge to urinate without being able to do so. Palpation of the bladder should be pain free and the bladder should be soft. Kidneys may be palpated by pressing one hand on the anterior surface of the abdomen below the ribs and pushing gently with the other hand from the back in the same

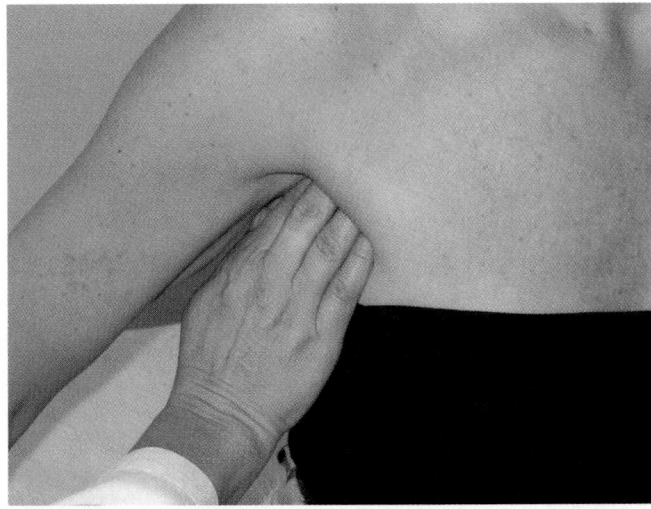

FIGURE 59–17 ∎ Palpation of axillary lymph nodes.

location below the ribs. Chapter 44 demonstrates palpation of the kidneys. Abnormalities of the genitourinary system are addressed in Chapter 47 .

Lymph nodes in the groin should also be inspected and palpated with either the genitourinary or musculoskeletal system exam. Figure 59–18 ■ demonstrates appropriate patient draping of the groin area and hand position for palpation during the inguinal lymph nodes examination. Normally, inguinal nodes are small and mobile and difficult to palpate. The superior and inferior inguinal lymph nodes receive drainage from the upper and lower leg, the vulva, and lower third of the vagina in females, and the penis and scrotal surface in males. Enlarged, tender, firm, and freely movable nodes indicate an infection or inflammatory process in any of these tissues and warrant further investigation. Additionally, assessment for the presence of lymphedema should be included.

Musculoskeletal Assessment

Musculoskeletal assessment that focuses on immune function should include inspection and palpation of joints and limbs for evidence of swelling, inflammation, or infection. Assess for the presence of pain with range of motion and any limitation of joint motion. Autoimmune diseases such as rheumatoid arthritis and SLE include joint pain and swelling as a significant symptom. An extensive discussion of musculoskeletal assessment can be found in Chapter 54 .

Common Laboratory and Diagnostic Exams of the Immune System

In addition to physical examination of immune tissues and various body systems, laboratory tests are required to evaluate the phagocytic, cellular, and antibody functions of the immune system. These tests are generally ordered when an abnormality such as an infection or a specific complaint related to an organ function is identified.

Laboratory Tests

An initial complete blood count (CBC) with manual differential is essential for identifying immune system abnormalities and providing a basis for determining the need for other forms of testing. Elevated total white blood counts (total WBC) can indi-

cate infection, inflammation, or in some cases blood disease such as leukemia. Low white blood cell counts indicate immunosuppression, as seen with various cancers or infections such as HIV and warrant full investigation. For example, a patient with symptoms of an undiagnosed HIV infection may have a low total WBC and a very low total lymphocytes count on the CBC differential. This would prompt the health care provider to follow up with further tests to determine the level of T lymphocytes called CD4 cells, and HIV antibody testing as described in Chapter 60 . Chapter 62 includes an in-depth discussion of the complete blood count.

White blood counts are differentiated into total lymphocytes, monocytes, neutrophils, bands (immature neutrophils), basophils, and eosinophils. All specific cell types are described as a percentage of total white cells. Neutrophils comprise approximately 70% of the total WBC and are the first cells on the scene of trauma, infection, or inflammation. Immature neutrophils are called bands. An increase in the number of bands in the serum circulation (>7%), indicates that the body is mounting a major inflammatory response, or fighting an infection, such as an abscess, because it is depleting the number of mature neutrophils and starting to use immature neutrophils that are less capable of ingesting antigens (Rote, 2006).

The CBC also includes information on platelets that are important in identifying immune abnormalities. Diseases such as systemic lupus erythematosis (SLE) may first be seen as thrombocytopenia on the CBC and prompt further testing. Another example is autoimmune thrombocytopenia, an autoimmune disease process in which the body identifies its own platelets as foreign and destroys them. Platelet abnormalities are of special concern because patients with platelet counts that are significantly decreased (<100,000 mm³) have an increased risk of bleeding. Decreased hemoglobin and hematocrit levels also occur in immune abnormalities. Anemia can result from autoimmune diseases. One of the first indications of a tumor can be decreased hemoglobin or hematocrit in the presence of no evidence of gross bleeding (Lefever-Kee, 2006). Abnormalities of lymphocyte counts on the CBC can be further evaluated by tests that examine specific T-cell and B-cell counts and immune function. This information is summarized in Chart 59–7 (p. 1886). Chapter 62 includes an in-depth discussion of laboratory data.

Immune Function Tests

Specific serum tests examine the function of the immune system. Erythrocyte sedimentation rate (also known as a "sedimentation rate" or "sed rate"), C-reactive protein, antinuclear antibody tests, anti-IgG, IgG levels, IgM levels, enzyme-linked immunosorbent assay, and Western blot are all examples of serum tests designed to look at one specific chemical or antigen and the body's response to it.

The erythrocyte sedimentation rate (ESR) is a serum test that is used to diagnose acute and chronic inflammation, as well as rheumatoid and autoimmune diseases. In the presence of inflammatory mediators, blood proteins are altered and red blood cells stick together and then fall out of solution when the blood sample is spun. This results in an elevated sedimentation rate. The test does not diagnose a specific disease, but is a sensitive and early indicator of a widespread inflammatory, autoimmune, or

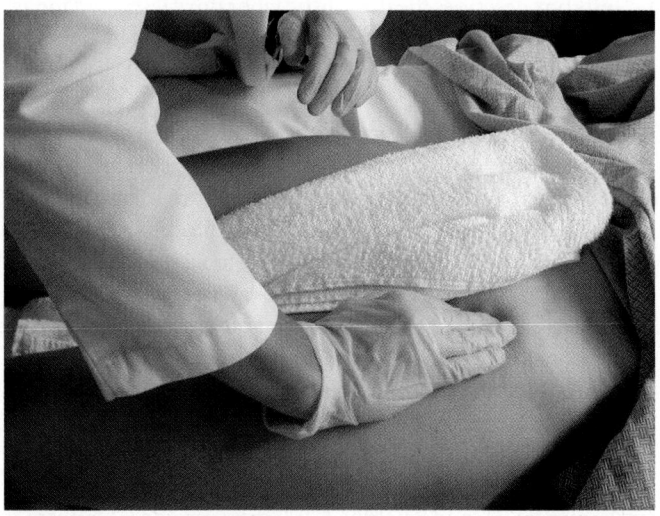

FIGURE 59–18 ■ Palpation of inguinal lymph nodes with draping.

CHART 59-7 Reading the White Blood Cells on a Complete Blood Count Differential

Reading the WBC Differential	Test Result Implications
Neutrophils (55–65% of WBC count)	Largest group of granulocytes, first on the scene. High counts of >67% of total WBC indicate inflammation or infection. Low counts may indicate systemic infection or abscess. If neutrophils are low and bands are very high, abscess or systemic infection is likely. Usually lives only about 72 hours.
Bands (immature neutrophils) (should be less than 10% of the total percentage of neutrophils)	Immature neutrophils with banded rather than segmented nuclei. An elevation in this count (more than 10% of total WBC count) may indicate a large bacterial infection such as an abscess, pneumonia, or sepsis.
Basophils (0.3–0.5% of WBC count)	Basophils are granulocytes that migrate out of circulation to become mast cells. Mast cells can release histamine in response to injury or cell death, a key first step in inflammation. Usually basophils comprise 0.75% of total WBC.
Eosinophils (1–3% of WBC count)	Eosinophils are granulocytes and comprise about 1–4% of total white blood cells. Eosinophils are elevated with allergies and parasite infestation.
Lymphocytes (20–30% of WBC count)	Lymphocytes are not usually more specifically identified. Lymphocytes usually comprise about 25–33% of total WBC. However, if very elevated, they may indicate infection or lymphoma. If very low, they may indicate infection or malignancy.
Monocytes (3–8% of WBC count)	Monocytes are nongranulocyte white blood cells that migrate out of circulation to become macrophages. Total monocytes are important for their potential to phagocytize cell debris, bacteria, virus, and fungal cells.

Sources: DeFranco, A. L., Locksley, R., & Robertson, M. (2007). *Immunity: The immune response in infectious and inflammatory disease.* Sunderland, MA: Sinauer Associates; McCance, K., & Heuther, S. (2006). *Pathophysiology: The biological basis for disease in adults and children* (5th ed.). St. Louis: Mosby; Porth, C. (2007). *Essentials of pathophysiology* (7th ed.). Philadelphia: Lippincott Williams & Wilkins.

malignant disorder. In SLE, for example, an ESR test is a standard part of a diagnostic work-up and is most often elevated. The ESR also is ordered when an autoimmune disease is suspected such as rheumatoid arthritis. A protein called rheumatoid factor is often present in the serum of patient's with rheumatoid disease in greater quantities than individuals without autoimmune diseases (Lefever-Kee, 2006).

A test often ordered in conjunction with the ESR is the C-reactive protein (CRP) test. CRP is a glycoprotein produced by the liver in response to acute inflammation. It is a more rapid and sensitive indicator of acute inflammation than the ESR and indicates the presence of inflammation but not the cause. CRP levels decline rapidly from serum when inflammation has subsided (Van Leeuwen, Kranpitz, & Smith, 2006). Increased levels of CRP can be found in immune-related diseases such as SLE, rheumatoid arthritis, Crohn's disease, and inflammatory bowel disease, but are not always consistently elevated for unknown reasons. The test has proven most helpful in diagnosis of acute flare-ups of inflammatory immune diseases and in monitoring response to therapy (Peng, 2005). Elevated levels are also found in acute bacterial infection, rheumatic fever, during the second half of pregnancy, and in acute myocardial infarction (Lefever-Kee, 2006). The major focus of recent research related to CRP has centered on its role in acute myocardial infarction. Chapter 40 ☺ contains an in-depth discussion to CRP as related to coronary artery disease.

Most immune function tests also look for the presence of an antibody to a specific antigen. Antigens are often destroyed by the time a test has been ordered or may be present in only small quantities or hidden inside cells. Antibody activity is much easier to measure and test. Diagnosis for specific autoimmune diseases such as SLE, scleroderma, or rheumatoid arthritis involves testing for a variety of antibodies. Antinuclear antibodies (ANAs) are immunoglobulins (IgG, IgM, IgA) that react with the nuclear portion of leukocytes, forming auto-antibodies against the host's DNA and ribonucleic acid (RNA). The presence of these antibodies is indicative of SLE and warrants further testing for anti-DNA antibodies, which are further diagnostic of SLE. Total ANA levels can also be elevated in scleroderma, rheumatoid arthritis, cirrhosis, leukemia, and malignancy (Porth & Sweeney, 2007; Van Leeuwen et al., 2006).

Other antibody tests evaluate infection with a specific bacterium or virus such as hepatitis or HIV. An example of this is the enzyme-linked immunosorbent assay (ELISA) and the Western blot tests, which detect the presence of antibodies created in response to infection with the HIV antigen. Many of the tests currently used to assess immune function utilize monoclonal antibodies as the mechanism to bind the auto-antibodies present in the patient's blood (Lefever-Kee, 2006). The Diagnostic Tests box describes the diagnostic laboratory tests used for assessment of the immune system and related nursing implications.

Computerized Axial Tomography

Immune system diseases can affect any body system. As a result computerized axial tomography (CT) scans are frequently used in the process of diagnosis of immune system abnormalities because they are able to provide detailed images of body structures. The CT scan uses a narrow x-ray beam that examines body sections from different angles and creates and a three-dimensional image of the organ or structure being studied. CT scans are 100 times more sensitive than two-dimensional x-rays and also show the shape, size, and sites of bleeding as well as mass effects in organs (Lefever-Kee, 2006). CT scans are most often used to identify areas of gross morphology and sites of possible tumors. Good-quality CT scans provide important information about organs and vascular function and enable identification of disease abnormalities.

DIAGNOSTIC TESTS to Assess Immune Function

Test and Normal Value	Expected Abnormality	Rationale for Abnormality

Blood count with differential
WBC count:
RBC:
  Males: 4.5–6 μL
  Females: 4–5 μL
HBG:
  Males: 13.5–18 g/dL
  Females: 12–16 g/dL
HCT:
  Males: 40–54%
  Females: 36–46%
WBC 5,000–10,000 μL
  Neutrophils: 55–65%
  Basophils: 0.3–0.5%
  Lymphocytes: 20–30%
  Monocytes: 3–8%
  Basophils: 0.3–0.5%
	RBC count, hemoglobin/hematocrit (HBG/HCT) are important in determining the presence of anemia, blood loss, and hydration status, and the number of red blood cells and white blood cells, including neutrophils, basophils, and monocytes.
	The differential white blood count (WBC) total percentages will equal 100%. The percentages vary depending on the type of disease process. For example, with acute bacterial infection the percentage of neutrophils will be elevated, whereas in acute allergy or parasite infection basophils will have an increased percentage.
		The blood count with differential is a routine part of hospital admission. Nursing assessment includes monitoring lab trends to determine the presence of a disease process and the effectiveness of treatment.

CD4 count 450–1,400/mm³	Total T-helper lymphocytes. Low numbers (<500) may indicate HIV or other immunodeficiencies.	A low CD4 is sensitive information and should not be shared casually.
Antinuclear antibodies (ANA): negative	Measures the number of antibodies made to parts of the patient's cells' nuclei. Indicates autoimmune disease.	Anticipate additional serum exams for immune function. Few autoimmune diseases are diagnosed with one serum exam.
Enzyme-linked immunosorbent assay (ELISA/ EIA): negative	Serum exams able to detect antibodies in blood. HIV is an example of an ELISA test.	It is important to know what antibody is being tested.
Western blot: negative	Another exam used to test for HIV. This exam is more sensitive to HIV. It is done if the initial ELISA for HIV is positive.	Western blot exams are also done for other immune related diseases.
Assays of IgG, IgA, IgM, IgD, IgE *Adult:* IgG: 650–1,700 mg/dL IgA: 770–400 mg/dL IgM: 40–350 mg/dL IgD: 0–8 mg/dL IgE: 1–120 mg/dL	Serum assays of level of IgG in the blood can help identify patients with deficiencies. IgG deficiency is relatively common.	Many immune diseases begin with multiple infections, fatigue, or vague symptoms. Immunoglobulin testing is an indication that immune function may be impaired. Care to reduce risk of infection is important.
Erythrocyte sedimentation rate (ESR or sed rate), Westergren method: *Males <50 years:* 0–15 mm/hour *Females <50 years:* 0–20 mm/hour	Test measures the time it takes red cells to precipitate out of serum. An increased rate implies inflammation, a common problem in many immune diseases.	Sed rate may be elevated in inflammatory diseases such as rheumatoid arthritis, chronic infection, cancer, and other immune problems. Care should be taken to assess patients for increased risk of infection.
C-reactive protein (CRP) Titer: >1:2	Measures acute inflammation 6–10 hours postinjury and tissue destruction. Nonspecific test for inflammation that rises early.	CRP may be elevated early in acute inflammatory process and tissue destruction related to bacterial infection, tissue ischemia, tissue necrosis, and flare-ups in autoimmune diseases.

Sources: Lefever-Kee, J. (2006). *Laboratory and diagnostic tests: Nursing implications* (6th ed.). Upper Saddle River, NJ: Pearson Prentice Hall; Van Leeuwen, A., Kranpitz, T., & Smith, L. (2006). *Davis's comprehensive handbook of laboratory and diagnostic tests with nursing implications* (2nd ed.). Philadelphia: F. A. Davis; Porth, C. (2007). *Essentials of pathophysiology* (7th ed.). Philadelphia: Lippincott Williams & Wilkins.

Specific CT tests may require a contrast agent to enhance the films and help identify small tumors or abnormalities. The nurses must have an understanding of why the test is ordered and any preparation of the patient that is required to ensure optimal testing. Patient teaching about the process is essential to alleviate fears about the unknown testing process, because all CT scans require the patient to lie still on the testing table. The CT scanner is shaped like a large donut and the testing table moves through the center hole of the structure. Feeling enclosed in the CT scanner can provoke anxiety in some patients. Patients may require sedation or the presence of the nurse to safely and successfully complete the exam.

Additional laboratory and diagnostic tests such as skin allergy testing and diagnostic testing for various autoimmune diseases,

HIV infection, and bone marrow biopsies are discussed in detail along with the specific disease processes in Chapter 60 ☺.

Health Promotion

Health promotion related to the immune system is focused on risk factor identification and management of allergies and infections. Education needs to include information on lifestyle choices and habits that increase the risk for communicable disease transmission. For example, there are more than 18 million cases of newly diagnosed sexually transmitted infections each year that are preventable with education and compliance with risk factor prevention such as condom use (CDC, 2006). Identification of genetic risk factors for allergies such as food allergies can prevent mild to life-threatening allergic reactions.

Immunization education is a critical element in disease prevention and can help save precious health care dollars spent on preventable infections. Immunization education is especially important for vulnerable populations such as infants and children because of their incompletely developed immune system, the elderly due to the slowing effects of aging on immune response, and individuals with suppressed immune response due to disease or medications.

■ Summary

A fully competent immune system is essential to protecting the human body from disease and disability. An alteration in the ability of the immune system to eliminate pathogens, distinguish self from non-self, or identify and eliminate the proliferation of mutant cells results in immune associate diseases. Immune tissues and cells are intricately associated with all body systems; therefore, a thorough assessment of immune function involves assessment of multiple body systems, as well as evaluation of cellular components of the immune system such as neutrophils and B and T lymphocytes and the development of specific antibodies. Abnormalities of the immune system can affect any system in the body, and they are frequently first evidenced by an inflammatory response. Chapters 60, 61, and 64 ☺ provide information on immune abnormalities including immune hypersensitivity responses, immune deficiency, inflammation, and cancer.

NCLEX® REVIEW

1. A patient is diagnosed with an immune deficiency disorder. The nurse realizes this patient is demonstrating a malfunction of which of the following body structures?
   1. Lymph nodes
   2. Spleen
   3. Bone marrow
   4. Adenoids

2. A patient is diagnosed with an autoimmune disorder. The nurse realizes this disease process was caused by:
   1. The body reacting to self receptors as an antigen.
   2. The body's ability to tolerate all self antigens.
   3. The body's ability to respond to non-self antigens.
   4. Adequate B and T cells that do not attack self antigens.

3. A patient is receiving a transfusion of plasma cells. The nurse realizes these cells will contribute to which of the following:
   1. Produce antibodies in response to exposure to an antigen
   2. Stop or slow the immune process
   3. Send messages to start the process of programmed cell death
   4. Stimulate cells to destroy cancer cells

4. A patient is diagnosed with liver cirrhosis. The nurse realizes that which of the following elements of immunity might be altered in this patient?
   1. Tumor necrosis factor
   2. Interferons
   3. Complement
   4. Interleukins

5. A patient tells the nurse that she does not want a flu shot because she doesn't want the live flu virus in her body. Which of the following should the nurse respond to this patient?
   1. The live flu virus is weakened so it won't cause the flu.
   2. The vaccine is made from killed flu organisms.
   3. The vaccine is made artificially so you won't get the flu from the shot.
   4. You can take the vaccine by mouth instead.

6. The nurse is caring for a patient with an infection. Which of the following explains how the patient's body will create antibodies to fight the infection?
   1. T-cell activation
   2. Antigen presentation
   3. Linking of T cells
   4. Linking of B cells

7. An elderly male doesn't understand why "just a little cold" developed into pneumonia. Which of the following should the nurse explain to this patient?
   1. Delayed hypersensitivity response
   2. Decreased primary and secondary production of antibodies
   3. Increased auto-antibody production
   4. Decreased percentage of suppressor T cells

8. A patient appears fatigued and tells the nurse he has no appetite even though he knows he can eat more because he's losing so much weight. Which of the following does this information suggest to the nurse?
   1. The patient has blocked lymph glands.
   2. The patient has an infection within an organ.
   3. The patient has a skin infection.
   4. The patient is at risk for malnutrition.

9. A patient is being assessed for rheumatoid arthritis. Which of the following diagnostic tests might be ordered to aid in this patient's diagnosis?
   1. Erythrocyte sedimentation rate
   2. Antinuclear antibodies
   3. Enzyme-linked immunosorbent assay
   4. Western blot test

Answers for review questions appear in Appendix D

KEY TERMS

acquired immunity *p.1869*
active acquired immunity *p.1869*
agglutination *p.1874*
anergy *p.1878*
antibody *p.1872*
antigen *p.1864*
antigen–antibody complex *p.1874*
apoptosis *p.1868*
B cells *p.1869*
B lymphocytes *p.1869*
cell-mediated immune response *p.1870*
chemotaxis *p.1871*
chyle *p.1865*
complement *p.1872*
cytokines *p.1871*
deoxyribonucleic acid (DNA) *p.1874*

fragment antigen binding (FAB)
   portion *p.1874*
fragment crystalline (FC) portion *p.1874*
human leukocyte antigens (HLAs) *p.1869*
humoral immune response *p.1872*
immune complex *p.1874*
immune tolerance *p.1864*
immunity *p.1864*
immunization *p.1876*
immunoglobulin *p.1872*
interferon *p.1871*
interleukin *p.1871*
lymph nodes *p.1866*
lymphatic system *p.1865*
lymphokines *p.1871*
natural immunity *p.1867*

neutralization *p.1874*
nongranulocyte *p.1865*
non-self antigen *p.1869*
opsonization *p.1871*
plasma cells *p.1874*
precipitation *p.1874*
primary immune response *p.1874*
secondary immune response *p.1875*
self antigen *p.1869*
T cells *p.1869*
T-helper cells *p.1870*
T lymphocyte *p.1869*
tissue factor (TF) *p.1871*
toll receptors *p.1868*
tumor necrosis factor (TNF) *p.1871*
vaccine *p.1876*

PEARSON
EXPLORE mynursingkit™

MyNursingKit is your one stop for online chapter review materials and resources. Prepare for success with additional NCLEX®-style practice questions, interactive assignments and activities, web links, animations and videos, and more!

Register your access code from the front of your book at
www.mynursingkit.com

REFERENCES

Burns, E. A. (2004). Effects of aging on immune function. *Journal of Nutrition Health and Aging, 8*(1), 9–17.

Camplejohn, R. S., Gilchrist, R., Easton, D., McKenzie-Edwards, E., Barnes, D. M., Eccles, D. M., et al. (2003). Apoptosis, ageing and cancer susceptibility. *British Journal of Cancer, 88*(4), 487–490.

Centers for Disease Control and Prevention. (2006). Sexually transmitted diseases treatment guidelines, 2006. *Morbidity and Mortality Weekly Reports, 55*(RR-11), 1–96. Retrieved July 21, 2008, from http://www.cdc.gov/std/treatment/2006/rr5511.pdf

Centers for Disease Control and Prevention. (2007a). *How safe is the blood supply?* Retrieved January 2, 2007, from http://www.cdc.gov/hiv/resources/qa/qa15.htm

Centers for Disease Control and Prevention. (2007b). *Immunizations.* Retrieved January 2, 2007, from http://www.cdc.gov/vaccines

Centers for Disease Control and Prevention. (2007c). *Key facts about flu.* Retrieved January 2, 2007, from http://www.cdc.gov/flu/keyfacts.htm

Centers for Disease Control and Prevention. (2007d). *Pneumococcal disease.* Retrieved January 2, 2007, from http://www.cdc.gov/vaccines/vpd-vac/pneumo/default.htm

D'Amico, D., & Barbarito, C. (2007). *Health and physical assessment in nursing.* Upper Saddle River, NJ: Pearson Prentice Hall.

DeFranco, A. L., Locksley, R., & Robertson, M. (2007). *Immunity: The immune response in infectious and inflammatory disease.* Sunderland, MA: Sinauer Associates.

Dillon, P. M. (2007). *Nursing health assessment: A critical thinking, case studies approach* (2nd ed.). Philadelphia: F. A. Davis.

Dunne, M. (2007). Infection, inflammation, and immunity. In C. M. Porth (Ed.), *Essentials of pathophysiology* (pp. 229–246). Philadelphia: Lippincott Williams & Wilkins.

Franson, P. (2005). Antivascular endothelial growth factor monoclonal antibody therapy: A promising paradigm in colorectal cancer. *Clinical Journal of Oncology Nursing, 9*(1), 55–60.

Jarvis, C. (2004). *Physical examination and health assessment* (4th ed.). St. Louis: W. B. Saunders.

Khoury, M. (2006). *The human genome project: "Gene sequencing and discovery are only the beginning."* Retrieved January 8, 2006, from

the Centers for Disease Control and Prevention website: http://www.cdc.gov/genomics/training/file/print/perspectives/AfterHGP.pdf

Kohler, G., & Milstein, C. (1975). Continuous cultures of fused cells secreting antibody of predefined specificity. *Nature, 256*, 495–497.

Lefever-Kee, J. (2006). *Laboratory and diagnostic tests: Nursing implications* (6th ed.). Upper Saddle River, NJ: Pearson Prentice Hall.

McCance, K., & Heuther, S. (2006). *Pathophysiology: The biological basis for disease in adults and children* (5th ed.). St. Louis: Mosby.

Meurer, J., Lustig, J., & Jacob, H. (2006). Genetic aspects of the etiology of asthma treatment. *Pediatric Clinics of North America, 53*(4), 715–725.

National Institute for Occupational Safety and Health. (2007). *Latex allergy: A prevention guide.* Retrieved July 21, 2008, from http://www.cdc.gov/niosh/98-113.html

Peng, S. (2005). C-reactive protein. *Medline Plus Medical Encyclopedia.* Retrieved January 4, 2007, from http://www.nlm.nih.gov/medlineplus/ency/article/003356.htm

Porth, C. (2007). *Essentials of pathophysiology* (7th ed.). Philadelphia: Lippincott Williams & Wilkins.

Porth, C., & Sweeney, K. (2007). Alterations in immune response. In C. M. Porth (Ed.), *Essentials of pathophysiology* (pp. 293–319). Philadelphia: Lippincott Williams & Wilkins.

Postma, K., Meyers, D., Jongepier, H., Howard, D., Kippelman, G., & Bleecker, E. (2005). Genomewide screen for pulmonary function in 200 families ascertained for asthma. *American Journal of Respiratory & Critical Care Medicine, 172*(4), 446–52.

Rote, N. (2006). Immunity. In K. L. McCance & S. E. Heuther (Eds.), *Pathophysiology: The biological basis for disease in adults & children* (5th ed., pp. 168–227). St. Louis: Mosby.

Scrimshaw, N. S. (2003). Historical concepts of interactions, synergism and antagonism between nutrition, and infection. *Journal of Nutrition, 133*(1), 316S–321S.

Shannon, M. T., Wilson, B. A., & Stang, C. L. (2004). *Health professional's drug guide.* Upper Saddle River, NJ: Pearson Prentice Hall.

Sommer, C. V. (2007). The immune response. In C. M. Porth (Ed.), *Essentials of pathophysiology* (pp. 134–149). Philadelphia: Lippincott Williams & Wilkins.

Steinke, J., & Borish, L. (2006). Genetics of allergic disease. *Medical Clinics of North America, 90*(1), 1–15.

Tablan, O., Anderson, L., Besser, R., Bridges, C., & Hajjeh, R. (2004). Guidelines for preventing health-care–associated pneumonia, 2003. *Morbidity and Mortality Weekly Reports, 53*(RR03), 1–36. Retrieved January 4, 2006, from http://www.cdc.gov/mmwr/preview/mmwrhtml/rr5303a1.htm

Thomas, M. (2005). Cetuximab: Adverse event profile and recommendations for toxicity management. *Clinical Journal of Oncology Nursing, 9*(3), 322–338.

Tranin, A. (2006). The bridge from genomic discoveries to disease prevention. *Oncology Nursing Forum, 334*, 891–910.

Twite, K., & Gaspard, K. (2007). Disorders of the white blood cells and lymphoid tissues. In C. M. Porth (Ed.), *Essentials of pathophysiology* (pp. 247–266). Philadelphia: Lippincott Williams & Wilkins.

Urden, L., Stacy, K., & Lough, M. (2006). *Thelan's critical care nursing: Diagnosis and management* (5th ed.). St. Louis: Mosby.

U.S. Food and Drug Administration. (2005). Genetics play role in response to asthma drug. *Food and Drug Administration Consumer Magazine, 39*(1), 36.

Van Leeuwen, A., Kranpitz, T., & Smith, L. (2006). *Davis's comprehensive handbook of laboratory and diagnostic tests with nursing implications* (2nd ed.). Philadelphia: F. A. Davis.

Wilkes, G. (2005). Therapeutic options in the management of colon cancer. *Clinical Journal of Oncology Nursing, 9*(1), 31–44.

Wilson, B. A., Shannon, M. T., Shields, K. M., & Strang, C. L. (2007). *Nurse's drug guide.* Upper Saddle River, NJ: Pearson Prentice Hall.

Wilson, S., & Giddens, J. (2005). *Health assessment for nursing practice* (3rd ed.). St. Louis: Elsevier Mosby.

Wojda, A., & Witt, M. (2003). Manifestations of aging at the cytogenetic level. *Journal of Applied Genetics, 44*(3), 383–399.

60

Caring for the Patient with Immune Response Disorders

Debra Brady
Kathy Yeates

With contributions by:
Kathleen Osborn

Outcome-Based Learning Objectives

After studying this chapter, the learner will be able to:

1. Differentiate the nursing management for patients with immune hypersensitivity responses and immune deficiencies.

2. Compare and contrast the immune hypersensitivity response related to allergy, autoimmune, and alloimmune disorders.

3. Compare and contrast the pathophysiology, clinical manifestations, and laboratory data for the human immunodeficiency virus (HIV) and acquired immune deficiency syndrome (AIDS).

4. Prioritize the nursing management of the patient with HIV/AIDS to decrease the incidence of opportunistic infections.

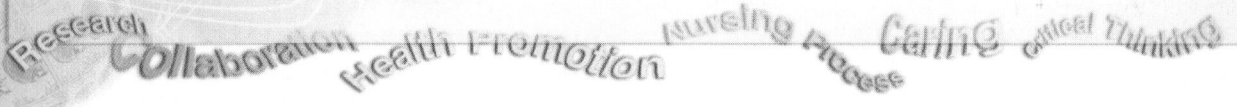

IMMUNE DISORDERS result from a loss of regulation of some aspect of the immune system. Immune disorders fall into two general categories: immune hypersensitivities and immune deficiencies. **Immune hypersensitivity** occurs when the immune system overresponds to an antigen, either from the environment, from the individual himself, or from another individual. Hypersensitivity disorders fall into three broad categories based on the type of triggering antigen, and include allergic, autoimmune, and alloimmune reactions. An **allergic response** occurs when the antigen is from the external environment, as opposed to an **autoimmune response**, which is triggered by a self-antigen. An **alloimmune response** occurs when the antigen is from another human. Within each of these categories are four specific mechanisms by which the immune system overresponds, referred to as **type-specific hypersensitivity reactions**.

Immune deficiencies occur when all or some part of the immune system fails to develop or is damaged through disease processes. The end result is an inability to mount an appropriate immune response. The two types of immune deficiencies are primary and secondary. **Primary immune deficiencies** result from genetic abnormalities. **Secondary immune deficiencies** occur for a variety of reasons including normal aging, malnutrition, malignancies, immunosuppressive drug therapy, and infections such as the human immunodeficiency virus (HIV).

◼ Immune Hypersensitivities: Allergic, Autoimmune, and Alloimmune Responses

An **immune hypersensitivity response** occurs when the immune system does not maintain self-tolerance, in other words, when it overreacts to the presence of a foreign antigen. This process also initiates the mechanisms of inflammation that result in destruction of healthy tissue. Hypersensitivity reactions can be categorized according to the type of antigen (allergy, autoimmune, alloimmune), the time sequence of the reaction (immediate or delayed), and the mechanism of immunologic response. When an antigen is environmental or external in origin it is referred to as an **allergy**. An example of this type of hypersensitivity reaction is "hay fever," or allergies to common weeds and pollen. In autoimmune reactions the body fails to recognize self-antigens and begins to destroy its own proteins. Multiple clinical disorders are associated with autoimmune diseases such as multiple sclerosis and systemic lupus erythematosus. An alloimmune response occurs when the immune system reacts against the antigens in or on the tissue from another individual, as seen with grafted tissue.

A hypersensitivity response that occurs within seconds to hours is categorized as an **immediate hypersensitivity reaction**.

An anaphylactic reaction is a prime example of this type of response. A **delayed hypersensitivity reaction** can take several hours to days, as exemplified by a contact dermatitis reaction. The way in which the immune system responds to an antigen and the time sequence of the reaction is determined by the mechanism of immunologic response. These are categorized as types I and IV and are discussed next.

Mechanism of Hypersensitivity Immune Response

Four distinct mechanisms or types of immunologic reactions are involved in allergic, autoimmune, and alloimmune reactions and can cause damage to body tissues: **type I (IgE-mediated allergic reactions)**, **type II (tissue-specific–mediated reactions)**, **type III (immune complex–mediated reactions)**, and **type IV (cell-mediated reactions)**. The type I, II, and III hypersensitivity responses involve antigen–antibody interactions and are known as immediate hypersensitivity reactions. The type IV response is an antigen–lymphocyte interaction and involves a delayed hypersensitivity reaction. Chart 60–1 provides an overview of these categories and specific clinical examples.

Type I IgE-Mediated Hypersensitivity

Type I IgE-mediated hypersensitivity, also known as anaphylactic hypersensitivity, is the most common of the hypersensitivity disorders and involves the production of antigen-specific IgE antibody after exposure to a foreign antigen or **allergen**. Examples include plant pollen, pet dander, foods, and drugs. **IgE antibodies** are produced by the plasma cells in response to the foreign antigen. The process of creating antibodies that match the antigen is called **sensitization**. The IgE antibodies connect to receptors on mast cells in the connective tissue. The process of sensitization may take only one exposure or several exposures to the allergen depending on the level of IgE production. This explains why many allergic responses take time to develop.

When a hypersensitivity reaction occurs, the allergen binds to IgE antibodies on the mast cell and causes degranulation of mast cells and release of histamine. **Histamine** causes smooth muscle contraction, vasodilatation, and increased vascular permeability

and primarily affects the skin, mucous membranes, and lung. The histamines are responsible for the clinical symptoms associated with type I reactions such as redness, itching, mucous production, and bronchial constriction. The reactions can be localized in tissue, or systemic as with an anaphylactic response. The severity of the clinical symptoms is dependent on the sensitivity of the individual, the amount of allergen exposure and mediator release, and the entry route of the allergen. For example, an injected allergen from an insect sting elicits a very rapid hypersensitivity response (Porth & Sweeney, 2007; Rote, 2006).

Type II Cytotoxic Specific Reaction

Type II hypersensitivity reactions involve **tissue-specific antigens**, which are proteins located in the cell membrane of some tissues such as blood, nerves, lungs, and kidneys. Type II reactions are mediated by IgG or IgM antibodies and occur when the immune system fails to recognize a host's self-antigen or antigens on donated red blood cells. IgG or IgM antibodies interact with the tissue-specific antigen on a target cell's plasma membrane to form antibody–antigen complexes. Type II reactions can occur in several ways. This explains the variety of clinical signs and symptoms observed in this type of reaction.

The hallmark of type II hypersensitivity reactions is that they are limited to those tissues or organs that have tissue-specific antigens. One example is Goodpasture's syndrome. Antibodies are formed against the tissue-specific antigen found in the basement membrane of the glomeruli in the kidneys and the alveoli in the lungs. The result is destruction of these tissues and the associated clinical symptoms of renal failure and lung damage. In myasthenia gravis the immune system fails to recognize the tissue-specific antigen on nerve ending receptor sites and binds to acetylcholine receptors on the muscle, causing faulty muscle enervation. Type II hypersensitivity reactions are responsible for Rh-hemolytic disease of the newborn and antibody–antigen reactions involving red blood cell (RBC) destruction such as incompatibility reactions in blood transfusions (Porth & Sweeney, 2007; Rote, 2006).

Blood Transfusion Reactions

Blood transfusion reactions are an example of a type II hypersensitivity antibody–antigen reaction that results in activation

---

CHART 60–1   Types of Immune Hypersensitivity Reactions

| TYPE I
IgE-Mediated Reaction | TYPE II
Tissue-Specific-
Mediated Reactions | TYPE III
Immune Complex-
Mediated Reactions | TYPE IV
Cell-Mediated Reactions |
|---|---|---|---|
| • Antibody–antigen mediated
• IgE production after exposure to an antigen
• Release of histamine and inflammatory mediators
• Clinical examples: allergy, anaphylaxis | • Antibody–antigen mediated
• Occurs at tissue-specific sites by interaction of antibody with tissue cell antigen
• Clinical examples: blood transfusion reaction, Goodpastures | • Antibody–antigen mediated
• Immune complexes form in circulation and travel to various tissues
• Clinical examples: serum sickness, SLE | • T-lymphocyte mediated
• Cytotoxic T cells attack and destroy cellular targets directly
• Clinical examples: latex allergies, PPD reactions |

Note: An antibody–antigen reaction is an immune complex reaction.

Sources: DeFranco, A. L., Locksley, R., & Robertson, M. (2007). *Immunity: The immune response in infectious and inflammatory disease.* Sunderland, MA: Sinauer Associates; Rote, N. (2006). Immunity. In K. L. McCance & S. E. Huether (Eds.), *Pathophysiology: The biological basis for disease in adults and children* (5th ed., pp. 168–227). St. Louis: Mosby; Sommer, C. (2007). The immune response. In C. M. Porth (ed.), *Essentials of pathophysiology* (pp. 247–268). St. Louis: Lippincott Williams & Wilkins.

of the complement cascade and initiation of a systemic inflammatory response. Inflammatory cascades and the systemic inflammatory response result in the lysis of target cells and are discussed in great detail in Chapter 61 ✐ . All RBCs have type-specific antigens on their surface except type O. The B lymphocytes produce antibodies specific to all other blood antigens. If the patient has type A blood, each blood cell is coated with antigen A and carries B antibodies. An individual with type B blood has B antigens on the surface of each red blood cell and carries A antibodies. If a patient with type A blood is erroneously given type B blood, the individual receives A antibodies that attach to the A antigen and form an immune complex (Figure 60–1 ■). This immune complex stimulates the complement cascade that produces lysis of the cell, resulting in cell death.

The major clinical problems with blood transfusion reactions relate to the stimulation of an overwhelming systemic inflammatory response and shock state. Oxygen carrying capacity is lost because the patient's own red blood cells are destroyed, as are the RBCs in the transfused blood. Additionally, the cellular debris following cell lysis contains large proteins that may block the tubules of the glomeruli in the kidney and can produce acute tubular necrosis (Rote, 2006).

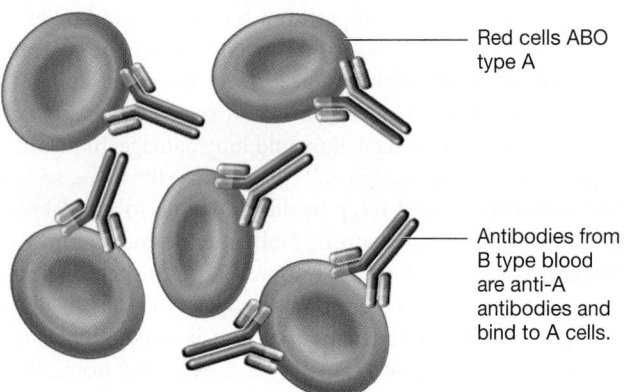

Red cells ABO type A

Antibodies from B type blood are anti-A antibodies and bind to A cells.

Step one transfusion reaction - ABO blood groups
Patient with A type blood received B type blood. B type blood has anti-A antibodies. These antibodies attach to the A type red cells.

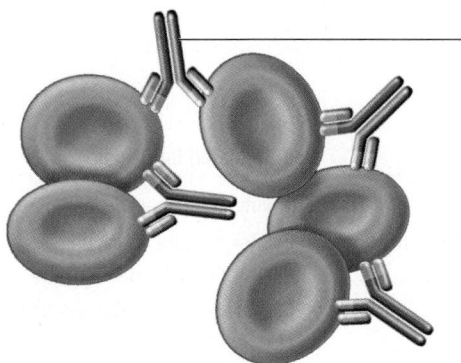

Type A red blood cells with antibodies from B type blood cross link and clump together. The immune system then sends phagocytes to ingest the clumped cells.

Step two transfusion reaction
Anti-A antibodies crosslink the cells together. This is agglutination. This makes it much easier for the immune system to send phagocytes to ingest the cells.
(From University of Michigan, Madison, 2002)

FIGURE 60–1 ■ Red blood cell immune complex.

The ABO blood antigen is only one example of many antibodies and antigens that blood is tested for prior to blood transfusion. Another important factor is the Rhesus (Rh) factor. This factor, along with the ABO factor, is the most significant because of the severity of the clinical response such as anaphylactic reaction and refractory shock. An extensive discussion of blood products, testing, and key safety factors in blood administration can be found in Chapter 23 ✐ .

Type III Immune Complex–Mediated Reaction

Type III hypersensitivity reactions also involve IgG and IgM antibody–antigen immune complexes. However, they differ from type II reactions because the antigen in type III reactions is soluble and released into circulation, instead of staying localized at a specific cell surface. The antigen can travel and deposit in extravascular tissue, such as joints, and then an antibody–antigen reaction can occur. In other instances, the antibody–antigen reaction can happen in the circulation, which results in the immune complex being deposited in tissue, such as the glomeruli. In either case, damage to the tissues results because the immune complex stimulates the complement cascade and the mediators of inflammation. Neutrophils attempt to phagocytize large immune complexes, and in the process lysosomal enzymes are released at the tissue site, further stimulating the inflammation process and damaging the surrounding tissues.

As a result of the mobility of the type III antigen–antibody complex, systemic or local responses also can occur although the reactions are not organ specific. Serum sickness is an example of a systemic response. Immune complexes are produced in the circulation in response to a foreign antigen and in response to some drugs such as sulfonamides and penicillin. The clinical symptoms of serum sickness include rash, fever, lymphadenopathy, arthralgias, and myalgias, and they result from the immune complexes being deposited in the walls of small blood vessels, kidneys, and joints throughout the body (Porth & Sweeney, 2007).

Type IV Cell-Mediated Reactions

Type IV reactions differ from the other three types of hypersensitivity reactions in that the response is delayed, instead of immediate, with onset 24 to 48 hours after antigen exposure. Secondly, the T cells of the immune system mediate these reactions, instead of antibodies. Type IV reactions occur as a result of an overreaction between normal cell-mediated mechanisms and an antigen that triggers the T cells to destroy the target cell directly or to release cells to produce lymphokines. The lymphokines activate phagocytic cells, especially macrophages at the inflammatory site. Examples of these types of reactions are seen with exposure to poison ivy, poison oak, and purified protein derivative (Rote, 2006).

Immune Hypersensitivity

The four mechanisms of immune response described above can be seen in all three categories of antigen reaction: allergic, autoimmune, and alloimmune. These categories account for the variety of clinical manifestations seen with hypersensitivity response.

Allergy Etiology and Epidemiology

The hallmark of allergy reactions is the IgE-mediated antibody–antigen response. An allergic reaction involves a type I hypersensitivity response in which an environmental antigen stimulates an overproduction of IgE antibodies that attach to mast cells. The interaction of these antibodies with an **allergen**, such as a type of environmental or foreign antigen, stimulates the release of histamine and proinflammatory mediators from mast cells. This release results in the irritating and uncomfortable symptoms associated with allergies including itching eyes, nose, and throat, cough, congestion, runny nose, watery eyes, and often bronchospasm. If the hypersensitivity reaction is severe, as with an anaphylactic reaction, the allergic response can be life threatening.

Allergic disease affects millions of people in the United States and the incidence is increasing on an annual basis (Asthma and Allergy Foundation of America, 2007). Evidence indicates that a large portion of this increased prevalence is among children who are developing allergic diseases in childhood (Brandtzaeg, 2007). Research has shown that the development of a food allergy in early childhood is associated with an increased risk of respiratory allergies (James, 2003; Wong, 2007). Current research is focused on risk factors that may be responsible, including those listed in the Risk Factors for Respiratory Allergies box. Studies to date have been disappointingly inconclusive (Bochner & Hamid, 2003; Halken, 2003; Zutavern & Brockow, 2006). Clear evidence of a single causative factor has not been identified and it is most probable that the occurrence of allergic diseases will be found to be a result of multiple factors (Asher et al., 2006; O'Connell, 2003).

The most consistent factor appears to be evidence of a genetic predisposition to hypersensitivity reactions. In the general population, the risk of developing an allergy is approximately 25%. This risk doubles when one parent has allergies (50% risk) and triples if both parents have allergies (75% risk) (Asthma and Allergy Foundation of America, 2007). The focus of allergy treatment is identification of the triggering allergen so that plans can be made to minimize or eliminate exposure to allergens and to manage symptoms.

Pathophysiology of Allergy Reactions

Normally, millions of IgE molecules of different specificities are attached to each mast cell. It is thought that individuals who are **atopic** (produce a hypersensitivity response) have a genetic predisposition to have greater than normal levels of IgE production (Dunne, 2007). With each reexposure to a triggering antigen, there is increased IgE production, increased mast cell degranulation, and increased release of histamine. The histamine causes vasodilation in local blood vessels. Additionally, endothelial cells pull apart and localized swelling occurs. This process can allow the allergen to enter the bloodstream. If this occurs a systemic

allergic response can result because basophils in the bloodstream also are stimulated to release histamine. This is the basis for an anaphylactic reaction (Rote, 2006).

Clinical Manifestations of Allergic Response

Clinical manifestations of the allergic response occur in tissues such as skin, mucous membranes, the lungs, and the gastrointestinal tract because they are highly vascular and have an abundance of mast cells as part of a fully competent immune system. There are a wide variety of allergic hypersensitivity reactions and clinical manifestations. Chart 60–2 (p. 1894) describes some of the common allergens and their associated symptoms.

Skin Allergies

Allergic responses are commonly manifested on the skin. This in fact is the basis for skin testing for allergies. A wheal and flare response is typical of a localized allergic response on the skin from exposure to an allergen, such as the resin of a star thistle plant, which binds with IgEs and causes immediate degranulation of the mast cells in the subcutaneous tissue. The clinical manifestation is a **wheal** or small, round, serous-filled raised blister, which is surrounded by a **flare** or round area of redness. This reaction occurs from the release of histamine, which causes local vasodilatation, redness, swelling, itching, and heat (Porth & Sweeney, 2007).

Other skin reactions, such as allergic contact dermatitis or a poison ivy reaction, are cell-mediated type IV delayed hypersensitivity reactions (Figure 60–2 ■, p. 1894). On first exposure the protein in poison ivy (which is the allergen), stimulates immune and memory T cells, which is an example of sensitization. A second contact with the poison ivy resin stimulates sensitized T cells. The reaction reaches maximum intensity in 24 to 72 hours and results in clinical symptoms of blistering vesicles and red, scaled areas (Rote, 2006).

Latex Allergy

Latex allergies can occur as both a type I allergic reaction or as a type IV cell-mediated reaction in response to contact with products containing natural latex. Type I reactions occur rapidly after exposure, usually within minutes. The release of IgE antibodies is responsible for the symptoms, which can include redness of the exposed skin, urticaria, asthma, itching, and conjunctivitis, which also may progress to anaphylactic shock (Rote, 2006). Exposure to the proteins that act as antigens in latex can occur through use of gloves on skin or IV catheters into the bloodstream. The antigens can also be inhaled through ventilator and handheld nebulizer tubing, and internal tissue can be exposed when surgical equipment and Foley catheters are used (Urden, Stacy, & Lough, 2006). Type I reactions can be life threatening because of their bronchial constrictive effect on the airway and vasodilation of blood vessels, which decreases perfusion pressure (American College of Allergy, Asthma and Immunology, 2007).

 **CRITICAL ALERT** *Latex reaction can occur during a surgical procedure. Symptoms of reaction in the anesthetized patient include flushing, facial edema, wheezing, bronchospasm, laryngeal edema, tachycardia, hypotension, and in extreme cases cardiac arrest.*

Latex reactions also can be a type IV delayed reaction, much like contact dermatitis, which present symptoms between 4 and 48 hours after exposure. Symptoms include dryness at the site of

RISK FACTORS for Respiratory Allergies

- Genetic predisposition
- Frequency of viral infections
- Increased use of antimicrobial cleansing products in the home
- Early childhood exposure to allergens
- Dietary factors
- Air pollution
- Immunizations

CHART 60–2   Common Allergens

Common Allergen	Characteristics	Symptoms
Pollen	Allergen is the dry pollen that is present in the air. Early spring: tree pollen (oak, elm, poplar) Early summer: rose pollen, grass pollen (Timothy, red-top) Early fall: weed pollen (ragweed)	Sneezing, runny nose, congestion, itching of the noses, eyes, ears, throat, and mouth
Animal dander	Allergen is the protein found in the saliva, dander, or urine of an animal with fur, not the "hair" of the animal.	Sneezing, itching, runny nose, swollen itchy eyes and throat
Dust mites	Allergen is the microscopic droppings of mites found in bedding, upholstery, carpets. Most common trigger of year-round allergies and asthma.	Congested or runny nose, sneezing (especially in the morning), itchy watery eyes, coughing, wheezing
Mold	Allergen is the spores that are disseminated by the fungi. Molds thrive in humid areas such as bathrooms and basements.	Sneezing, runny nose, congestion, itching of the noses, eyes, ears, throat, and mouth
Insect stings	Allergen is to the protein in the venom of the insect sting. Majority of sting reactions in the United States are caused by yellow jackets, honeybees, paper wasps, hornets, and fire ants.	Flushing, itching, hives, swelling at site of bite *Potential anaphylactic reaction:* light-headedness, feeling of impending doom, swelling in the throat, wheezing, severe bronchoconstriction, nausea, vomiting, drop in blood pressure, shock = medical emergency
Medications Common: antibiotics	Allergen is the protein in the medication or the substance with which the medication is made.	Rash, hives, general itching, tingling or itching of the mouth/pallet, potential anaphylactic reaction as described above
Food allergies Most common: nuts, fish, shellfish, milk, chicken eggs, kiwi, seeds	Allergen is to the protein in the food particle. Majority of reactions develop within the first hour. Generally, the longer it takes for symptoms to develop, the less severe the reaction.	Oral itching or tingling in the mouth/pallet, lip swelling, swelling of the face, generalized flushing, itching, nausea, vomiting, and potential anaphylactic reaction as described above

Sources: American Academy of Allergy, Asthma and Immunology. (2006). *Why is the incidence of allergy increasing?* Retrieved February 23, 2007, from https://www.aaaai.org/aadmc/inthenews/wypr/2006archive/increasing_allergies.html; American College of Allergy, Asthma and Immunology. (2007). *Be S.A.F.E.: Managing allergic emergencies.* Retrieved February 19, 2007, from http://www.acaai.org/public.

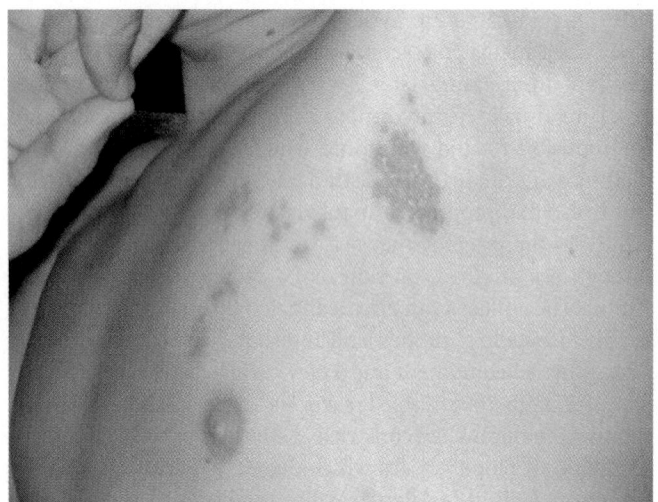

FIGURE 60–2 ■ Skin allergy type IV response.

exposure, itching, and cracking of the skin. These symptoms are followed by redness, swelling, and scabbing of the fissures and cracks in the skin. This usually occurs within a day or two of the initial symptoms. This type of reaction is often seen in health care workers who handle latex equipment and use latex gloves. All hospitals now provide latex-free gloves and most institutions provide latex-free disposable products of all kinds, such as IV tubing, blood tubing, ventilator equipment, and aerosol tubing. The increase in incidence of type IV latex reactions has coincided with the advent of standard precautions, which increased the use of gloves. Increased glove use has primarily been implicated as the foremost point of exposure for heath care workers. Estimates of the number of sensitized health care workers range from 8% to 17%. As with any antigen, the more often an individual is exposed to the antigen, the more likely the individual will become sensitized to that antigen. Powder in gloves has been removed in hospital settings to reduce the risk of aerosolized exposure to latex. These exposures can be dangerous to the sensitized individual and result in a life-threatening anaphylactic response (National Institute for Occupational Safety and Health [NIOSH], 2007).

Identifying individuals at risk for latex allergy is essential to preventing the allergic response. Factors such as working in any industry using latex or rubber components (health care workers, housekeepers, hairdressers) increases the risk, as does a history of hay fever or asthma, and/or allergies to certain foods such as bananas, avocado, kiwi, and strawberry. The proteins found in these foods have a similar structure to latex proteins and can trigger an allergic response. Patient populations with increased risk factors include those with neural tube defects such as myelomeningocele or spina bifida, those who require chronic bladder catheterization such as patients with spinal cord trauma or neurogenic bladders, and those who have had multiple surgeries. All of these factors involve multiple contacts with latex products, which enhance the risk of developing latex allergies. Any individual who is identified as part of the high-risk groups just listed or someone who can describe a contact dermatitis type reaction after exposure to latex should be considered at risk for a latex allergy (Ahmed, Sobczak, & Yunginger, 2003; NIOSH, 2007).

 Patients with neural tube deficits have a high risk of developing latex allergies (estimated 28% to 67% increased risk). They frequently also undergo multiple surgeries, which increase their risk factor. Latex-free products should always be used when caring for patients with neural tube deficits, even when prior latex allergy has not been identified (Urden et al., 2006).

As mentioned, latex-free products are now available and are to be used in all hospital settings with latex-sensitive individuals. These products are usually provided on special carts containing disposable equipment that is entirely latex free. The patient's room should have a latex allergy alert sign posted. Health care workers with latex sensitivity must stringently adhere to the same precautions. Powder-free and latex-free gloves must be used. In addition, special barrier creams are available to use on the hands for added protection. Symptoms of latex allergy need to be reported per agency protocol to the employee health center.

Food Allergies

Food allergy reactions most commonly involve mucous membranes and the gastrointestinal (GI) tract, but can quickly lead to an anaphylactic response. Food allergies are now the leading known cause of anaphylactic reactions treated in emergency departments in the United States. It is estimated that there are 30,000 food-related anaphylactic reactions that result in 150 to 200 deaths per year (Food Allergy & Anaphylaxis Network, 2006; Sampson, 2003). One example is the individual who is sensitive to peanuts. The peanut protein antigen attaches to the IgE antibody, causing the mast cells to degranulate and release histamine. The sensitive individual experiences early symptoms of allergy such as tracheal and oral itching, swelling, redness, nausea, and vomiting. The response can be limited to itching on the interior of the mouth and the GI tract, it or can be as profound as a severe anaphylactic reaction.

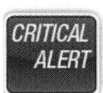 *One of the most common early symptoms of an allergic reaction is itching in the mouth and palate. It is important to assess this in individuals complaining of allergy symptoms or who are receiving a new drug such as an antibiotic or vaccine.*

Anaphylactic Reaction

Anaphylaxis can be a localized or systemic hypersensitivity response to an antigen that can quickly progress to a medical emergency if not recognized and treated appropriately. The continuum of symptoms in anaphylaxis can range from itching, erythema, vomiting, and breathing difficulties to severe laryngeal edema, respiratory distress, vascular collapse, shock, and death (Figure 60–3 ■, p. 1896)

Combinations of presenting symptoms may vary in an individual experiencing an anaphylactic reaction depending on the number of IgE antibodies on the mast cells, the number of mast cells that degranulate and release histamine, and the release of other proinflammatory mediators such as bradykinin and sero-

tonin. Symptoms of anaphylactic response are usually immediate (less than 30 minutes), although the oral route of allergen exposure can have a 2-hour delay. A secondary response or biphasic reaction is seen in approximately 20% of patients with anaphylaxis and can occur 4 to 8 hours after the initial remission of symptoms due to secondary mediators of inflammation such as bradykinin. In general, the anaphylactic reaction is more life threatening if the hypersensitivity response is immediate (Rote, 2006).

The result of a severe systemic anaphylactic reaction is a form of shock called *distributive shock* that results in massive vasodilatation, loss of blood pressure, and inadequate distribution of blood supply and oxygen to all body tissues. Chapter 61 ⊙ provides an in-depth description of distributive shock. Concurrent smooth muscle bronchoconstriction and laryngeal edema initially cause inspiratory and expiratory wheezing and difficulty breathing, which may progress to complete airway obstruction. Death can result from full circulatory collapse or severe bronchial constriction, or a combination of both. Nursing care focuses on early recognition of anaphylactic symptoms, airway management, and collaborative aggressive medication treatment to stem the continuum of anaphylactic response and prevent death.

 *Patients can be in extreme danger when breath sounds diminish after wheezing because the airways are completely constricted and no air is being inspired or expired due to edema.*

Treatment focuses on immediate administration of intramuscular adrenaline. Adrenaline's alpha-receptor agonist activity reverses vasodilation and decreases edema. Its beta-receptor activity relaxes smooth muscle thus dilating bronchioles, suppresses histamine release, and increases myocardial contractility. Administration of supplemental oxygen, establishment of intravenous (IV) access, and administration of IV fluid to support intravascular volume in patients with hypotension are also essential. Corticosteroids are a key aspect of ongoing drug therapy and work to control inflammatory mediators. Other medications that may be included in treatment are antihistamines and inotropic and antiarrhythmic agents.

Medical Management of the Allergic Hypersensitivity Response

The goal for successful medical treatment for individuals with allergic hypersensitivity is focused on avoidance of triggering allergens, prevention of a hypersensitivity response, and relief of allergy symptoms. Therefore, identifying the causative allergens is primary to effective management of allergic disease. This involves obtaining a thorough patient history and diagnostic studies, followed by creation of a drug therapy and treatment regime for allergy symptom management. For severe allergy problems this treatment plan may include allergy desensitization shots.

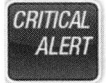 *A thorough history of allergies is essential prior to the start of any medications. Individuals with a family history of hypersensitivity response are at greater risk for allergic response. The nurse must be aware of a patient's allergies prior to administering any medication. This is especially crucial with IV medications, such as antibiotics, because the antigen is given directly into the bloodstream, bypassing the local response delay, and can result in stimulation of an immediate severe anaphylactic reaction.*

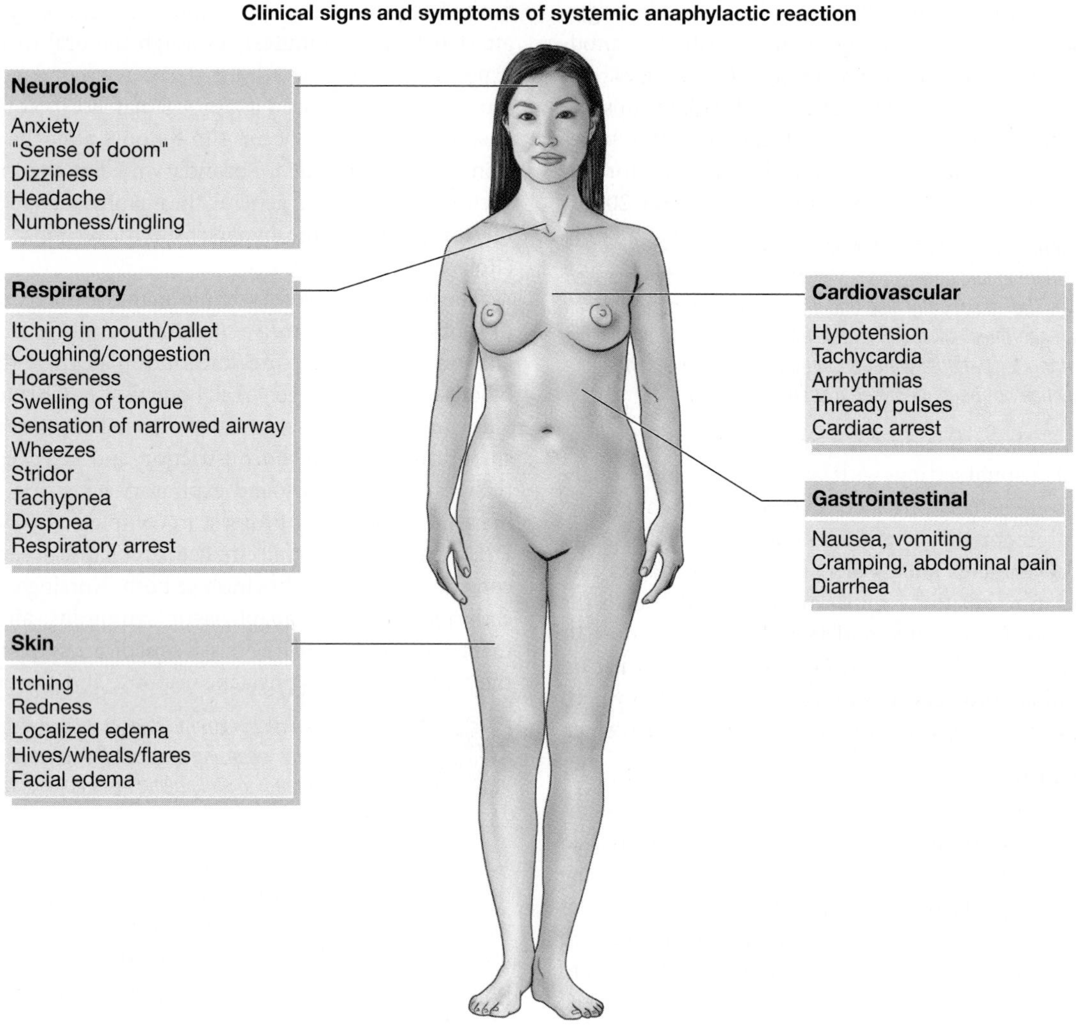

Clinical signs and symptoms of systemic anaphylactic reaction

Neurologic

Anxiety
"Sense of doom"
Dizziness
Headache
Numbness/tingling

Respiratory

Itching in mouth/pallet
Coughing/congestion
Hoarseness
Swelling of tongue
Sensation of narrowed airway
Wheezes
Stridor
Tachypnea
Dyspnea
Respiratory arrest

Cardiovascular

Hypotension
Tachycardia
Arrhythmias
Thready pulses
Cardiac arrest

Gastrointestinal

Nausea, vomiting
Cramping, abdominal pain
Diarrhea

Skin

Itching
Redness
Localized edema
Hives/wheals/flares
Facial edema

FIGURE 60–3 ■ Anaphylaxis symptoms.

Laboratory and Diagnostic Procedures

Allergy symptoms are very disruptive, uncomfortable, and can be expensive to treat. In the extreme they can be life threatening. Therefore, it is important to identify the specific triggering allergen(s) to which the atopic individual may be sensitized so that contact with the allergen can be avoided and a plan developed to treat the symptoms most effectively. Allergy testing includes blood and sputum laboratory tests to determine total IgE and allergen-specific IgE, as well as skin tests with small amounts of allergens to evaluate sensitivity.

Blood Tests

Initial laboratory tests to detect lymphocyte, eosinophil, and immunoglobulin abnormalities commonly include a complete blood count (CBC) with white blood cell differential (WBC). This provides a total lymphocyte and eosinophil count. The eosinophil count is usually elevated with type I hypersensitivity reactions and is one of the indicators used to confirm a diagnosis of allergy. Nasal smears, sputum, and bronchial secretions may also be tested for the presence of eosinophils, which indicate probable allergy.

Tests for measuring immunoglobulins include the radioimmunosorbent test (RIST), which measures circulating levels of total IgE. A more specific test is the radioallergosorbent test

(RAST), which provides a sensitive measurement of the specific IgE antibodies that are elevated in response to many allergens. Ongoing testing research has resulted in the development of a RAST that detects specific IgE antibody to approximately 15 allergens that evoke the large majority of pollen- and food-related allergic disorders (American Academy of Allergy, Asthma and Immunology, 2007).

The major advantage of RAST testing is the decreased risk of systemic reaction. However, it is more costly and results are not as readily available as with skin tests. Therefore, RASTs are generally reserved for individuals in which skin testing is not possible due to skin conditions that may interfere with the results, concerns about severe anaphylaxis, or because of medications that the individual is taking (American Academy of Allergy, Asthma and Immunology, 2007).

Skin Tests

Skin testing involves introducing small amounts of various allergens into the skin of allergic individuals through either intradermal injection or a scratch, or "prick test," technique on the individual's back. The scratch or prick test is the least sensitive of the two tests, but it also carries a lower risk of systemic reaction. It is performed by placing small drops of allergen onto the skin, then pricking through it to introduce the allergen. If the individual is sensitive to a specific allergen, IgE antibodies activate mast cells to degranulate, histamine is released, and a localized reaction is produced causing a wheal (swelling) and flare (redness) within 15 minutes. The diameter of the flare is usually indicative of the level of sensitivity to the allergen. Allergy medications may suppress skin reaction and result in a false-negative reading. Therefore, allergy medications including antihistamines and corticosteroids are generally held for 48 to 96 hours prior to allergy testing (American Academy of Allergy, Asthma, and Immunology, 2007).

The profound danger with skin testing is that in severely allergic individuals even a small amount of skin test allergen can cause a systemic anaphylactic response, which requires immediate and emergent attention. Therefore, skin testing should never be performed if the individual is experiencing respiratory abnormalities such as bronchospasm.

 Nursing care for the patient in the outpatient allergy testing clinic focuses on assessment for symptoms of anaphylactic response, respiratory assessment, airway management, and rapid treatment of anaphylactic emergency. Skin tests should never be undertaken if emergency equipment and medications to treat anaphylactic reaction are not available.

Pharmacologic Management of Allergies

Drug therapy is the primary focus of allergy management. The vast majority of allergies are mediated by an IgE interaction between an allergen and receptors on the IgE antibody that stimulate the release of histamine. The goal of medications that relieve allergy symptoms is to decrease histamine release and its effects on the mucosa, skin, and tissues. A wide variety of allergy medications are available. Health care providers may suggest over-the-counter (OTC) products or write specific drug prescriptions. Frequently, the medication the patient uses is determined by insurance coverage. The Pharmacology Summary of Medications to Treat Allergy Symptoms (p. 1898) describes common allergy medications for symptom management. Major categories of drugs that provide symptomatic relief include antihistamines, sympathomimetic and decongestant drugs, corticosteroids, mast cell stabilizers, and antipyretic drugs.

The wide variety of allergy medications available often leads to confusion regarding which medication to take to alleviate symptoms or how to dose the medications correctly. Therefore, a primary role for members of the health care team is providing patient education on the appropriate dosing of allergy medication and the potential adverse effects that can occur if medication directions are not followed.

Desensitization Immunotherapy

Desensitization, or giving "allergy shots," involves introducing small amounts of the triggering allergen to the sensitive individual in increasing amounts over a long period of time, with the goal of decreasing the severity of the allergic reaction. The exact mechanism of how desensitization occurs is not fully understood. It is thought that desensitization may work by inducing the production of blocking antibodies that bind with the allergen and neutralize it so that it cannot bind with IgE and degranulate mast cells. Desensitization injections also may stimulate the production of suppressor T lymphocytes, which suppress the production of IgE

and inhibit hypersensitivity (Rote, 2006). However, this form of treatment does have a significant risk of systemic anaphylaxis.

■ Nursing Management

Nursing care of patients with allergies is focused on helping patients and families identify and avoid allergy triggers, education about medication for symptom relief, and instruction regarding strategies to prevent a severe allergy hypersensitivity response. Nursing care also involves early recognition and emergent treatment of anaphylactic reaction. Application of the nursing process will facilitate a comprehensive approach to the assessment and care of the patient with allergies. The Nursing Process: Care Plan for the Patient with Anaphylactic Response feature (p. 1899) provides information and sample questions to be used in obtaining a thorough assessment and history of the allergies. Nursing diagnoses are developed from the assessment data. The care plan also provides detailed outcome goals and evaluation parameters, and the nursing interventions (with rationales) used to achieve these outcomes.

Health Promotion

The health care team can further promote patient health and safety by encouraging patients with a history of anaphylactic reactions to wear a medical alert bracelet or other form of medical identification tag that identifies allergies to medications, foods, or other substances. This type of ID alerts members of the health care providers to potential problems in the event of an emergency. Additionally, instructing patients with a history of anaphylactic reaction to carry a self-administered epinephrine kit to use in the event of an anaphylactic reaction is essential. Kits, such as the EpiPen (Figure 60–4 ■, p. 1903), are easy to use and can save lives in an anaphylactic emergency (American College of Allergy, Asthma and Immunology, 2007).

Collaborative care related to hypersensitivity response is focused on:

- Identifying allergens and preventing exposure and further reactions
- Appropriate use of allergy medications to relieve symptoms
- Prompt identification and treatment for patients experiencing anaphylactic response
- Follow-up care with an allergy specialist.

■ Collaborative Management

Optimal care of the patient with an allergic hypersensitivity response involves a collaborative approach among the health care provider, the nurse, and the pharmacist. Allergy diagnosis and development of an effective treatment plan are done by the health care provider. Nursing care involves extensive patient education on avoiding allergy triggers and teaching about allergy symptoms that require immediate medical attention. The nurse also educates the patient on medications, monitors the effectiveness of the treatment, and ensures that the patient's medical records reflect current allergy status. The pharmacist is an important member of the team who can advise patients about medication treatment options and provide extensive patient education on drug effects.

PHARMACOLOGY Summary of Medications to Treat Allergy Symptoms

Medication Category	Action	Application/Indication	Nursing Responsibility
Antihistamines			
First generation: • Diphenhydramine (Benadryl) • Clemastine (Tavist)	First-generation histamine receptor blocks the effects of histamine at H$_1$ receptors.	Treatment of allergies to provide symptomatic relief of itching eyes, nose, throat; runny nose; and watery eyes; and to decrease swelling. Used in combination with decongestants and for cold and sinus treatment.	Causes significant sedation. Monitor patient for drowsiness. Instruct patients to avoid alcohol and other Central nervous system (CNS) depressants when taking antihistamines to avoid cumulative effects of sedation.
Second generation: • Fexofenadine (Allegra) • Cetirizine (Zyrtec) • Desloratadine (Clarinex) • Loratadine (Claritin)	Less sedating. Longer half-life.		Second-generation antihistamines are contraindicated in patient with dysrhythmias because the drug prolongs the Q-T interval. Use with caution in patients with liver and/or renal impairment because these drugs are metabolized in the liver and excreted in the kidneys.
Intranasal Corticosteroids • Fluticasone (Flonase) • Beclomethasone (Beconase)	Applied directly to nasal mucosa. Does not have systemic side effects of steroids given orally or parenterally.	First-line treatment of allergic rhinitis to decrease local inflammation, swelling of tissues, and irritation of mucosa.	Instruct patient to clear nose, shake inhaler thoroughly, and assess for broken mucous membranes that will allow medication into bloodstream causing systemic effects prior to administration. May cause burning and dryness of nasal passages. Instruct patient to use preservative-free saline spray or petroleum jelly to decrease dryness.
Decongestants and Sympathomimetics • Pseudoephedrine (Sudafed, Actifed) PO • Phenylephrine (Neo-Synephrine, Sinex) Intranasal	Stimulates alpha-adrenergic receptors in the sympathetic nervous system, causing nasal passages to constrict.	Treatment of congestion. Dries mucous membranes and decreases drainage.	Assess for nasal excoriation and bleeding. Monitor the patient for psychosocial/emotional changes; may cause agitation. Monitor vital signs; can increase heart rate, and/or blood pressure. Oral sympathomimetics are contraindicated in patients with hypertension. Monitor blood glucose in patients who are diabetic because oral dose can increase glucose levels.

Sources: Adams, M., Josephson, D., & Holland, L. (2005). *Pharmacology for nurses: A pathophysiologic approach*. Upper Saddle River, NJ: Pearson Prentice Hall; Deglin, J., & Vallerand, A. (2007). *Davis's drug guide for nurses*. Philadelphia: F. A. Davis; Wilson, B. A., Shannon, M., Shields, K., & Stang, C. (2007). *Nurse's drug guide*. Upper Saddle River, NJ: Pearson Prentice Hall.

All members of the health care team have a role in identifying patients with allergies, providing appropriate education on allergy triggers and medications for symptom relief, and preventing anaphylactic response in multiple health care settings. Providing patient education to promote self-care regarding signs and symptoms of anaphylactic reaction is essential and is addressed in Chart 60–3 (p. 1904).

Research Topics Related to the Allergic Hypersensitivity Response

Research in the area of allergic hypersensitivity responses is multifaceted. The fact that allergies affect such a large section of the population makes identification of genetic and environmental factors that contribute to the development of allergies a major priority (see the Genetic Considerations box, p. 1904).

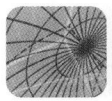

NURSING PROCESS: Patient Care Plan for Anaphylactic Response

Assessment of Airway and Gas Exchange

Subjective Data:

Are you allergic to any medications, food, or other substances?
Did you come in contact with something you are allergic to?
How much of the substance were you exposed to?
How long ago did you first notice itching or swelling or breathing changes?
Has this ever happened to you before?
Did you take anything to treat your allergies?

Objective Data:

Edema (e.g., face, eyes, tongue, extremities)
Work of breathing (e.g., increased rate, use of accessory muscles, gasping, loudness, grunt)
Lung sounds (e.g., strider, wheezes, absent breath sounds)
Oxygen saturation (e.g., <94% on room air)
Vital signs (HR > 100, RR > 22 < 8, SBP < 90, or mean arterial pressure [MAP] < 60)
Skin (e.g., red, rash, wheal and flare)

Nursing Assessment and Diagnoses	Outcomes and Evaluation Parameters	Planning and Interventions with *Rationales*
Nursing Diagnoses: *Ineffective Airway Clearance* related to bronchial and/or laryngeal spasm and edema *Alteration in Gas Exchange* related to bronchial and/or laryngeal spasm and edema	**Outcomes:** Clear airway. Adequate gas exchange. ***Evaluation Parameters:*** Patent airway. Even, unlabored respirations < 22/minute.	**Interventions and *Rationales:*** Assess for airway edema, stridor, wheezes, and decreased breath sounds. *Maintaining open airway is the highest priority.* Position for comfort, high semi-Fowler's. *Promotes lung expansion and respiratory effort.* Assess respiratory rate, pattern, work of breathing, chest wall movement. *Rapid, shallow respiratory rate and increased work of breathing indicate hypoxemia from airway obstruction and the need for ventilatory support.*
	Clear breath sounds.	Auscultate lungs for wheezes, stridor, decreasing or absent breath sounds. *Stridor indicates narrowing airway. Decreased breath sounds are ominous and indicate airway obstruction. Absence of breath sounds indicates complete airway obstruction.* Report respiratory distress to the health care provider. *Medical intervention may be indicated to prevent respiratory failure.*
	O$_2$ saturation > 94% on room air.	Administer humidified oxygen (O$_2$) as prescribed. *Supplemental O$_2$ increases the alveolar gas concentration and diffusion of O$_2$ to the cells and tissues of the body.*
	IV access available.	Establish intravenous (IV) access with large-bore IV. *To enable administration of emergency medications and fluid.*
	Emergency medications available and administered as prescribed.	Do not delay administration of emergency medications by non-IV route while establishing IV access. *Many emergency medications can be given S$_Q$ or IM if IV access is not available and are crucial for controlling airway edema and enabling gas exchange.* Administer medications as prescribed: subcutaneous epinephrine 1:1,000, 0.3–0.5 mL as ordered, repeat every 20–30 minutes as needed. *A potent bronchodilator and vasoconstrictor to counteract the effects of histamine.* Diphenhydramine (Benadryl) 50 mg IV or IM. *Blocks the bronchial constrictive effects of histamine released from mast cells.* Corticosteroid: Solu-Medrol 120 mg IV. *Blocks the proliferation of inflammatory mediators that increase airway obstruction.*
	No alteration in level of consciousness. Alert and oriented to person, place, and time. Pulse oximetry and ABGs within normal limits.	Assess for changes in level of consciousness (agitation, confusion, delirium, stupor, and coma). *Cerebral function is very sensitive to decreases in oxygenation, indicates tissue hypoxemia.* Frequent respiratory assessment, continuous monitoring of pulse oximetry, and arterial blood gases (ABGs). *Status can deteriorate quickly. A secondary or delayed response can also result from secondary mediators of inflammation such as bradykinin several hours after the initial incident.*

(continued)

NURSING PROCESS: Patient Care Plan for Anaphylactic Response—*Continued*

Nursing Assessment and Diagnoses	Outcomes and Evaluation Parameters	Planning and Interventions with *Rationales*
	Intubation equipment available and functioning.	Prepare for possible endotracheal intubation, gather intubation supplies, and collaborate with respiratory therapy (RT) for ventilator setup. *Intubation requires a team approach; gathering and checking equipment early prevents delay in intubation.* If intubation is required, collaborate with health care provider and RT to monitor ventilator and maintain ventilator settings. *To maximize oxygenation and ventilation, support cellular oxygenation, and prevent tissue hypoxemia and ischemia.* Assess respiratory function. *To verify bilateral breath sounds post intubation.*
	Endotracheal tube appropriately placed. Equal chest wall expansion and breath sounds. ABGs within normal limits. Transfer to the appropriate level of care.	Obtain chest x-ray postintubation. *To verify appropriate placement of endotracheal tube (ETT) in trachea 1–2 cm above the carina.* Test arterial blood gases (ABG). *To evaluate oxygenation.* Patients with severe anaphylactic response requiring intubation will be cared for in the intensive care unit (ICU) setting. The focus of care is controlling airway edema, normal ABGs, and extubation as soon as is safe for the patient.

Assessment of Cardiac Output

Subjective Data:
Do you feel dizzy or weak?
Have you fainted?

Objective Data:
Blood pressure (SBP < 90, mean arterial pressure (MAP) < 60)
Heart rate > 100
Are peripheral pulses present?
Is skin color pale or red or mottled?

Nursing Assessment and Diagnoses	Outcomes and Evaluation Parameters	Planning and Interventions with *Rationales*
Nursing Diagnosis: *Risk for Decreased Cardiac Output* related to vasodilation with anaphylactic shock	**Outcome:** Tissue perfusion maintained. ***Evaluation Parameters:*** Blood pressure and heart rate within normal limits, mean arterial pressure (MAP) >60 mmHg. (Chapter 25 ⊙ explains MAP)	**Interventions and *Rationales:*** Assess blood pressure, MAP, and heart rate frequently. Evaluate for a drop in blood pressure and increased heart rate (HR). *Indicates shock.* *Histamine and inflammatory mediators cause peripheral vasodilation, and capillary membrane permeability results in decreased volume of blood to the heart, drop in blood pressure, and decreased tissue perfusion. HR increases to try and meet cellular oxygen needs and compensate for tissue hypoxia.*
	Capillary refill < 3 seconds; skin pink, warm and dry; palpable peripheral pulses.	Assess peripheral perfusion for weak thready pulses, pale or mottled skin color, decreased skin temperature, slow capillary refill. *Indicates decreased blood flow in the capillaries, a sign of impaired tissue perfusion as shock progresses and cardiac output decreases.* Absence of circulatory failure. Report abnormal vital sign changes and assessment findings to the health care provider. *Medical intervention with IV fluids and medications may be immediately necessary to prevent circulatory failure.* Administer IV fluids. *To increase cardiac output and promote circulation and tissue perfusion.* Administer vasoactive IV medications (e.g., Levophed) as prescribed. *To vasoconstrict peripheral blood vessels, increase MAP > 60, support perfusion of vital central organs.*

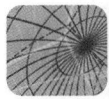

NURSING PROCESS: Patient Care Plan for Anaphylactic Response—*Continued*

Assessment of Pain and Anxiety

Subjective Data:

What is your pain level on the 1–10 scale, where a 1 is very little pain and 10 is the worst pain imaginable?

Are you feeling anxious?

Do you take pain or antianxiety medications routinely at home?

What helps when you have anxiety?

Do you have any medication allergies?

Do you have cultural or religious practices that impact your pain or anxiety?

Objective Data:

Facial grimaces with movement

Taut or anxious facial expression

Restlessness and irritability

Vital signs (HR > 100, BP > 140)

Nursing Assessment and Diagnoses	Outcomes and Evaluation Parameters	Planning and Interventions with *Rationales*
Nursing Diagnoses: *Pain* and *Anxiety* related to air hunger/hypoxia and emergency treatment procedures	**Outcomes:** Comfort level maintained. Anxiety controlled. **Evaluation Parameters:** Patient reports pain level < 3 or at acceptable level. States anxieties. Cooperative with emergency medical treatment. Premedicated for procedures as prescribed.	**Interventions and *Rationales*:** Assess pain and anxiety levels using an objective scale. *Increases consistency in quantifying pain.* Remain with patient, provide calm reassurance, and explain all treatments. *Air hunger is extremely frightening to the patient; anxiety will increase respiratory rate and oxygen demand and hinder patient's ability to cooperate with treatment.*
		Advocate for pain and sedation medications for intubation procedure if blood pressure is stable. *Endotracheal intubation is uncomfortable; anxiety increases sympathetic nervous system stimulation and oxygen demands.*
	Pain and anxiety assessed and treated while intubated.	Assess pain and anxiety while intubated using objective scales and alternative communication techniques (pointing to scale, writing board, and hand signs). *Endotracheal tube can cause pain at the back of the throat. Breathing through a small ETT can induce anxiety. Pain and anxiety will increase oxygen demands. The ETT prevents the patient from communicating verbally, but the nurse must still be able to address the patient's needs.* Administer medication as prescribed. *To maintain comfort and decrease anxiety.*

Nursing Assessment of Fluid/Volume Status

Subjective Data:

Do you feel dizzy, tired, or thirsty?

Objective Data:

Blood pressure (SBP < 90, MAP < 60 mmHg)

Heart rate > 100

Urine output < 30 mL/hr

Nursing Assessment and Diagnoses	Outcomes and Evaluation Parameters	Planning and Interventions with *Rationales*
Nursing Diagnosis: *Deficient Fluid Volume* related to anaphylactic shock	**Outcome:** Fluid volume and tissue perfusion maintained. **Evaluation Parameters:** Blood pressure normal. MAP > 60 mmHg.	**Interventions and *Rationales*:** Assess and continuously monitor blood pressure, MAP, HR, and urine output. *Anaphylactic shock results in vasodilation of blood vessels and decreased intravascular fluid volume that is clinically evident as decreased blood pressure, MAP, and urine output. Heart rate increases to compensate for decreased volume status. Patients with severe anaphylactic response and fluid volume deficits will need ICU level care.*
	Urine output = or > 30 mL/hr.	Place Foley catheter and monitor hourly urine output and fluid intake. *Decrease in blood pressure and MAP < 60 will decrease glomerular filtration rate and place patient at risk for prerenal failure. The kidneys receive 25% of the cardiac output. A urine output of less than 30 mL/hr indicates decreased perfusion to the kidneys and fluid volume deficit. Trending hourly fluid volume intake and output is essential with fluid resuscitation therapy.* Administer IV fluids as prescribed. *To increase intravascular volume and tissue perfusion.* Report decreased blood pressure, MAP, and urine output to the health care provider. *Medical intervention may be indicated to correct fluid volume deficit.*

(continued)

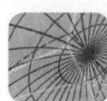

NURSING PROCESS: Patient Care Plan for Anaphylactic Response—*Continued*

Assessment of Potential Allergy Response

Subjective Data:

Do you have any allergies to medication, food, plants, animals, or other materials (such as latex)?

Do you have any history of previous allergy reactions such as rash, itching, tingling, or swelling in your mouth, or breathing difficulties?

Have you undergone allergy testing?

Does anyone in your family have allergies?

Do you take any allergy medications?

Objective Data:

Gather baseline data on:

Airway

Vital signs

Rash

Itching

Edema

Lung sounds

Nursing Assessment and Diagnoses	Outcomes and Evaluation Parameters	Planning and Interventions with *Rationales*
Nursing Diagnosis: *Risk for Injury* related to allergy hypersensitivity response	**Outcome:** Identification of allergy triggers and prevention of anaphylactic response. **Evaluation Parameters:** Allergies identified in patient's medical record.	**Interventions and *Rationales:*** Obtain a thorough patient and family allergy history at the time of admission and prior to administering new medications to the patient. *To prevent administering a medication or treatment, or using equipment to which the patient has an allergy. Safe nursing practice requires allergy assessment prior to medication administration.*
	Allergy triggers communicated to health care team and avoided.	Document patient allergies and inform other members of the health care team (health care provider, pharmacy, nursing staff). *To facilitate communication and prevent prescribing of medication or treatments or use of equipment to which the patient is allergic.* Follow agency protocol for placing allergy alerts in medical record, electronic patient database, the nursing Kardex (Rand), and on the patient's arm band. *To alert members of the health care team to the patient's allergies.*
	No allergy hypersensitivity reactions.	Assess for symptoms of hypersensitivity reaction when administering any medications to patient. *A history of allergy response increases the risk of future hypersensitivity responses.*

Assessment of the Patient's and Family's Education Needs Regarding Allergy Response

Subjective Data:

What causes your allergy symptoms?

How do you avoid triggering your allergies?

What can you do to alert health care providers about your allergies?

What should you carry with you if you have experienced an anaphylactic reaction?

Objective Data:

Verbalizes education needs

Identifies mode of receiving educational material

Participates in education discussion

Nursing Assessment and Diagnoses	Outcomes and Evaluation Parameters	Planning and Interventions with *Rationales*
Nursing Diagnosis: *Deficient Knowledge* regarding allergies and prevention of anaphylactic response	**Outcome:** Patient avoids allergy trigger and has no further anaphylactic reactions. **Evaluation Parameters:** Verbalizes understanding of allergy signs and symptoms, anaphylactic allergen triggers.	**Interventions and *Rationales:*** Assess the patient's and family's learning needs, readiness to learn, and preferred method of education (verbal, written, audiovisual). *To present information at a time and in a manner the patient and family can understand. Hypersensitivity reactions have a genetic link; therefore, families must be informed about potential hypersensitivity and how to prevent them.*
	Consistently follows plan to avoid allergy triggers.	Provide information on allergy management self-care as presented in Chart 60–3 (p. 1904), and assist the patient and family in developing a plan to eliminate exposure to the triggering allergen and decrease symptoms and progression of allergy sensitivity. *To promote self-care and help the patient and family eliminate allergy triggers.*
	Identifies symptoms of allergy response.	Instruct patient to monitor response to medications, foods, and insect stings by self-assessing for mouth/pallet itching, swelling, rash, itching of skin or eyes. *To identify symptoms of allergy response.*

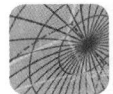

NURSING PROCESS: Patient Care Plan for Anaphylactic Response—*Continued*

Nursing Assessment and Diagnoses	Outcomes and Evaluation Parameters	Planning and Interventions with *Rationales*
	Seeks appropriate medical attention for allergy symptoms. Informs health care providers of allergy status.	Instruct patient to seek immediate medical attention for airway swelling or shortness of breath with exposure to triggering allergen. *Promotes seeking early medical treatment of potential life-threatening anaphylactic response.* Instruct patient to inform future health care providers of allergy and anaphylactic response. *Prevents future exposure to allergen and anaphylactic response.*
	Purchases and wears medical alert tag.	Instruct patient to purchase and wear a medic alert bracelet that lists the triggering allergen and history of anaphylactic response. *Alerts health care providers to allergen and anaphylactic response, especially in an emergency situation when patient may not be able to speak for herself.*
	Carries epinephrine self-medication emergency syringe.	If anaphylactic triggering allergen is an insect, plant, or food, instruct the patient to carry emergency epinephrine at all times. *To self-administer epinephrine for an anaphylactic reaction.*
	Keeps appointments and completes allergy testing if indicated.	Encourage follow-up appointments with primary care health care provider to determine need to see allergist and undergo IgE allergen-specific diagnostic testing. *To determine triggering allergens so that exposure to them can be eliminated.*

Sources: Adams, M., Josephson, D., & Holland, L. (2008). *Pharmacology for nurses: A pathophysiologic approach.* (2nd ed.) Upper Saddle River, NJ: Pearson Prentice Hall; American College of Allergy, Asthma and Immunology. (2007). *Be S.A.F.E.: Managing allergic emergencies.* Retrieved February 19, 2007, from http://www.acaai.org/public; Carpenito-Moyet, L. (2008). *Nursing care plans and documentation* (5th ed.). Philadelphia: Lippincott Williams & Wilkins.

A greater understanding of the association between allergies and the development of other pulmonary diseases also is a major priority. Additional areas of current medical and nursing research related to allergies are presented in the Research Opportunities and Clinical Impact box (p. 1905).

■ Autoimmune Hypersensitivity Response

The ability to differentiate self-antigens from foreign antigens is referred to as *immune tolerance.* Recognition of self-antigens is vital for normal immune function because it prevents the immune system from destroying the host. When the immune system fails to recognize self-antigens an autoimmune response occurs. This is the basis for **autoimmune diseases,** which can affect any tissue in the body. The triggering mechanisms for a breakdown of tolerance are varied among autoimmune diseases. In most instances, the exact mechanism that stimulates an autoimmune response is unknown, although several theories have been supported by research and multiple others are currently being investigated (Rote, 2006).

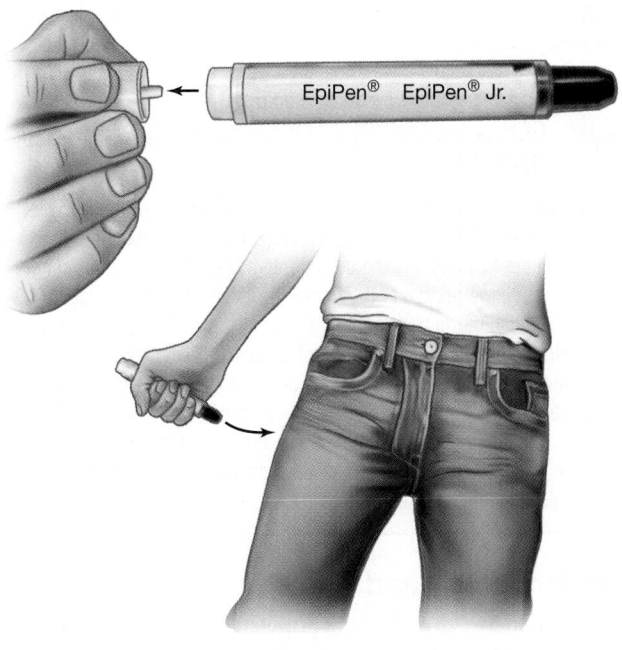

(b)

FIGURE 60–4 ■ EpiPen.

CHART 60–3 **Self-Care Allergy Management**

Allergens and Education Goal for Self-Care	Actions for Self-Care
Allergen: Pollen and mold *Goal:* Minimize exposure to pollens and molds.	• Remain inside on days when pollen counts are high. • Wear a mask when during high-exposure times (windy days, when grass is being cut). • Avoid contact with freshly cut grass, dry leaves, and weeds. • Avoid damp, moist structures like basements. • Clean showers and tubs several times a week. • Avoid sprays and perfumes.
Allergen: Dust mites and animal dander *Goals:* Reduce dust in the home, school, and work environment. Eliminate animal dander from home environment.	• Replace window coverings with pull shades. • Use hypoallergenic mattress and pillow. • Replace carpet with wood, tile, or linoleum. • Wash floor, dust, and vacuum several times a week. • Wear a mask when cleaning. • Minimize upholstered furniture, throw pillows/rugs, and tufted bedspreads. • Change air filter frequently on air conditioning/heating system. • Choose a pet that does not have fur or feathers such as fish or reptile.
Allergen: Insect stings *Goal:* Minimize exposure to insect venom.	• Quickly leave an area where bees, wasps, or yellow jackets are present. • Carefully check grass areas before sitting to avoid ants or other insects. • Carry an EpiPen when picnicking, hiking, or camping.
Allergen: Foods *Goal:* Eliminate foods from diet that may cause allergy symptoms.	• Identify specific foods to avoid by keeping an allergy food journal noting triggering foods and allergy symptoms. • Develop a list of foods to avoid and share this with anyone who cooks in the household. • Read labels when buying food and avoid allergy-triggering substances. • Ask questions regarding ingredients in food when eating out to avoid allergy triggers.
Allergen: Medication *Goal:* Avoid allergy-triggering medications.	• Make of list of medication allergies and inform any health care providers of allergies. • Wear a medical alert tag for history of anaphylactic medication response. • Review over the counter (OTC) medications with pharmacists to check for potential allergy.

Sources: American Academy of Allergy, Asthma and Immunology. (2006). *Why is the incidence of allergy increasing?* Retrieved February 23, 2007, from https://www.aaaai.org/aadmc/inthenews/wypr/2006archive/increasing_allergies.html; American College of Allergy, Asthma and Immunology. (2007). *Be S.A.F.E.: Managing allergic emergencies.* Retrieved February 19, 2007, from http://www.acaai.org/public.

GENETIC CONSIDERATIONS for the Allergic Hypersensitivity Response

The National Heart, Lung, and Blood Institute (NHLBI) of the National Institutes of Health is currently working on a study to examine the role of genetic factors in the development of lung disease including asthma. A large portion of the money spent on treating asthma is associated with the treatment of allergic asthma. The NHLBI study is working to define the distribution of abnormal genes seen in a number of lung diseases. The hope is that greater knowledge of genetic components of lung disease will lead to new clinical treatments. A second outcome for this study is a better understanding of the development of lung diseases such as allergic asthma (Steinke, Borish, & Rosenwasser, 2003).

Epidemiology and Etiology

Approximately 5% of the U.S. population is affected by autoimmune disorders (American Academy of Allergy, Asthma and Immunology, 2006). A genetic predisposition to autoimmune disease is supported by the association of various autoimmune abnormalities within family groups. The peak time of development of autoimmune disease is ages 15 to 45. Sex hormones appear to have some relationship to the frequency and manifestation of the autoimmune disease systemic lupus erythematosus because it occurs 10 times more frequently in women than men (Porth & Sweeney, 2007).

Pathophysiology of Autoimmune Diseases

Normally, immunologic tolerance is formed in humans during embryonic development. During this developmental period, some lymphocytes can be created that are not able to differentiate between self-antigens and non–self-antigens, referred to as autoreactive lymphocytes. To attain immune tolerance, the immune system must suppress or eliminate these autoreactive lymphocytes.

The loss of immune tolerance is the basis for all autoimmune diseases. Multiple mechanisms may be involved in the loss of tolerance, but in most instances the exact process is unknown. Research has centered on the following theories: (1) exposure to a previously sequestered antigen, (2) develop-

RESEARCH OPPORTUNITIES AND CLINICAL IMPACT RELATED TO THE ALLERGY HYPERSENSITIVITY RESPONSE

Research Area	Clinical Impact
Pursue development of new classes of allergy medication.	Decrease IgE stimulation and the inflammatory response; symptom control and improved functional ability.
Identify genetic factors associated with development of allergies.	Development of new therapies that more specifically target the allergy trigger and overproduction of IgE.
Identify environmental factors associated with development of allergies.	Development of new therapies that more specifically target the allergy trigger and overproduction of IgE.
Identify genetic and environmental links between allergies and the development of asthma.	Control of IgE stimulation to prevent development of asthma.
Determine pharmacologic action of herbal and complementary therapy in the treatment of allergy.	Identifying the effective or harmful action of herbal medications in treatment of allergy response to promote new treatments and deter use of unproven therapies.

ment of a neoantigen, (3) complications of an infectious disease, (4) emergence of a forbidden clone, and (5) alteration of a suppressor T cell (DeFranco, Locksley, & Robertson, 2007). Current research indicates that development of autoimmune disease is probably multifactorial and involves a combination of the multiple mechanisms described below, as well as the effect of an original insult, environmental influences, and genetic factors (Embry, 2004; Gomez-Peurta et al., 2005; Kuwabara, 2004). Chapter 59 🔗 provides a discussion about immune assessment.

Sequestered Antigens

Sequestered antigens are normal self-antigens found in cells that have not come in contact with the immunologic tissue during fetal development. Therefore, the immune system does not recognize it as a self-antigen. These are tissues that are not drained by the lymphatic system and therefore do not usually come in contact with immunologic cells. Examples of these include receptors on the cornea of the eye and the testicles. These are referred to as immunologic privileged sites. Although these tissues lack lymphatic tissues, they are vascular. Therefore, if trauma occurs immunologic cells will be delivered to the site. This can initiate an autoimmune response because the immune system has not recognized these antigens by previous exposure (Porth & Sweeney, 2007).

Neoantigens

Neoantigens are created by the developing fetal immune system while it is in the process of eliminating autoreactive lymphocytes. During the process of eliminating these autoreactive lymphocytes, pieces of the lymph receptors may not be destroyed. These small bits of immune garbage are neoantigens and they can hide in lymph tissues. They may attach at a later time to receptors on normal cells, triggering an autoimmune response (DeFranco et al., 2007).

Complications of Infectious Disease: Molecular Mimicry

When a foreign antigen invades the body and is destroyed by the immune system, small pieces of the cell wall of the bacterial or viral invader can remain in the circulation. If these foreign anti-

gen proteins attach to a normal cell, the complex makes the host cell look like the cell of the foreign antigen and this triggers the autoimmune response. Group A streptococcus bacteria are the most commonly studied bacteria that can initiate this response. An example of this is the streptococcal bacteria that attach to the cells of heart valves and stimulate the immune system to attack and destroy the heart valve tissue (Rote, 2006). Chapter 41 🔗 discusses the impact of this process on heart valve function.

Forbidden Clone

A clone is a second cell produced by replication of a cell. A *forbidden clone* is a mutant cell that is a type of autoreactive lymphocyte that should be eliminated. The theory about forbidden clones revolves around the concept that during normal embryonic development the original autoreactive lymphocyte is eliminated by the embryo's immune system, but a copy (clone) remains hidden (usually in lymphoid tissue). These cells can emerge at a later date and attach to self-antigens, thereby triggering an autoimmune response and destroying normal self-cells. This is an important area of research, because the exact triggering mechanisms of many autoimmune diseases, such as systemic lupus erythematosus or rheumatoid arthritis, are unknown (DeFranco et al., 2007).

Suppressor Cell Dysfunction

A major function of suppressor T cells is to control inappropriate immune responses. There are many different lines of suppressor T cells. If a single group of these T cells is dysfunctional, a tissue-specific autoimmune response can occur. If several lines of suppressor T cells are dysfunctional, generalized autoimmune disease can occur. An example of this is systemic lupus erythematosus (SLE). It is thought that T cell dysfunction is partly responsible for the large variety of autoantibodies seen in SLE because the T cells do not suppress the production of antibodies created by B cells against normal cells (DeFranco et al., 2007).

Superantigens

Normally, antigens ingested by macrophages are "presented" to T-helper cells to initiate the stimulation of B cells to make antibodies to that antigen. Chapter 59 🔗 discusses this concept in detail. Usually only a small number of T-helper cells are activated by one antigen. Some gram-positive bacteria such as Staphylococcus and Streptococcus can make chemicals called exotoxins that are capable of circumventing the normal antigen presentation process. Referred to as superantigens these exotoxins are capable of activating far greater numbers of T-helper cells. Toxic shock syndrome related to staphylococcus infection is one example of a superantigen-mediated disease (Porth & Sweeney, 2007). Chapter 49 includes an in-depth discussion of toxic shock syndrome.

Original Insult

The actual mechanism of some autoimmune responses is known to be the result of exposure to an identifiable insult, referred to an "original insult." For example, the allergy or type I hypersensitivity response is stimulated by the presence of a foreign protein such as pollen. The administration of certain drugs such as quinidine and methyldopa has been associated with an autoimmune lupus-like syndrome in susceptible elderly patients that dissipates when the medication is stopped (Rizzo & Gunta, 2007). In many autoimmune diseases, the original insult is not traceable. Research is examining areas such as viral infections, in which aspects of the viral particle remain on the plasma membrane of cells or are introduced permanently into the host's DNA (DeFranco et al., 2007).

Specific genetic markers may also play a role in autoimmune disease, as discussed in the Genetic Considerations for Autoimmune Disease box.

Clinical Manifestations

Autoimmune disorders can affect any tissue in the body, and are manifested in a variety of clinical symptoms depending on the system that is the target. The initiation of an autoimmune disorder is commonly associated with the onset of another illness or profound physical or psychological stressor, such as severe flu, pregnancy, or death of a significant other. It also is significant to note that once individuals have developed one autoimmune disorder, they are at increased risk for developing manifestations of other autoimmune diseases (Rote, 2006). Chart 60–4 lists the most common autoimmune disorders, target antigens, and symptoms.

Medical Management

Medical management involves determining the diagnosis, medication treatment plan, and symptom management for disease complications. The difficulty in differentiating autoimmune diseases is that many of them have multiple self-antigens and re-

---

GENETIC CONSIDERATIONS for Autoimmune Disease

Research indicates that genetic factors play a major part in autoimmune disease. Specific genetic markers have been associated with some autoimmune diseases, such as myasthenia gravis and SLE. Genetic markers, called **human leukocyte antigens (HLAs),** can be tested within families to determine if the individual tested is at risk for developing an autoimmune disease (Rizzo & Gunta, 2007). It is believed that an original insult in combination with genetic factors is responsible for stimulation of autoimmune response. Future research in this area is focusing on genome sequences that could contribute to the later development of autoimmune disease.

---

quire a significant number of tests prior to making a diagnosis with confidence.

Laboratory and Diagnostic Procedures

The focus of the diagnostic workup is serum tests. These tests include autoantibody testing, complement levels, and protein electrophoresis. **Autoantibody tests** evaluate the level of autoantibodies in the blood to specific self-antigens. One of the primary tests is the antinuclear antibody (ANA). This is a monoclonal antibody (see Chapter 59) that attaches to **autoantibodies** that are made in response to self-antigens from the nucleus. A positive ANA test indicates that autoantibodies to nuclear proteins are present and increases the likelihood of a diagnosis of autoimmune disease. For example, patients with SLE often have high levels of ANA and high levels of anti-DNA autoantibodies. A differential diagnosis of an autoimmune disease is usually based on cumulative evidence from several test results (see the Diagnostic Tests for Autoimmune Disease box, p. 1908) (Rote, 2006).

Drug Therapy

The wide variety of autoimmune disorders presents a challenge in drug therapy. The goals of drug therapy are to suppress the immune system in general and control symptoms related to specific self-antigens if possible. One of the mainstays of therapy is the use of **corticosteroids**, a class of drugs that decrease the inflammatory response and suppress immune activity by controlling T-cell response. As previously noted, T cells are responsible for the regulation of the immune system and stimulating B cells to produce antibodies. Decreasing T-cell stimulation of B cells and subsequent antibody production is essential to the control of autoimmune disease. Additional drugs such as cyclophosphamide (Cytoxan, a chemotherapy drug) are also used in autoimmune diseases such as SLE to control or moderate symptoms and decrease autoantibody activity. Cyclophosphamide acts to decrease antibody production by suppression of bone marrow activity, specifically B- and T-cell suppression (Adams, Josephson, & Holland, 2005). Other treatments to decrease autoantibody production include the use of monoclonal antibodies (Chapter 59) and **plasmapheresis**, which is discussed in Chart 60–5 (p. 1909).

Systemic Lupus Erythematosus

Systemic lupus erythematosus (SLE) is an example of a systemic type III hypersensitivity autoimmune disease characterized by damage to joints and soft organs as a result of the effects of autoantibodies and antibody–antigen activity (immune complex responses). Patients with SLE have symptoms as varied as joint pain, fever, malaise, recurrent infections, renal failure, and endocarditis with valve dysfunction. Cardiac valve disease is discussed in Chapter 41 . Renal failure is discussed in Chapter 47 .

Epidemiology and Etiology

The cause of SLE is unknown, but research indicates that the development of autoantibodies most likely results from a combination of factors including genetics, hormonal influences, immune abnormalities, and environmental factors (Rote, 2006). A genetic predisposition is clearly involved in that certain families show a larger number of SLE members than the population at large and there is evidence of SLE development in identical twins (Anaya, Tobon, Vega, & Castiblanco, 2006). It is possible that as many as

CHART 60–4	**Autoimmune Disorders by Body System**		
Disease/System	**Probable Antigen**	**Organ or Tissue**	**Symptoms**
Blood			
Immune thrombocytopenic purpura	Platelet surface	Blood	Bruising, purpura, bleeding
Antiphospholipid antibody syndrome	Platelet membrane phospholipids	Blood	Bleeding, purpura, bruising
Respiratory System			
Goodpasture's syndrome	Septal membrane of alveoli (basement membrane)	Lungs, alveoli	Shortness of breath, respiratory failure, decreased gas exchange
Renal System			
Immune complex glomerulonephritis	Various immune complexes	Glomeruli, kidney	Acute renal failure, inflammation, fever, pain
Goodpasture's disease	Glomeruli basement membrane	Glomeruli, kidney	Decreased renal function, anuria, oliguria, pain
Connective Tissue/Systemic Diseases			
Systemic lupus erythematosus	Antigens from DNA, organelles, cytoplasm, and possible extracellular sites	Joints, muscle, skin, kidney, heart, lung	Rash, joint pain, arthralgias, fatigue, fever, impaired renal function, increased risk of infection, heart valve disease
Rheumatoid arthritis	Immunoglobulin G, collagen	Joints	Pain and swelling in joints
Scleroderma	Nuclear antigens, immunoglobulin G	Multiple organs, including skin, joints	Hard, shiny painful skin, immobile masklike face
Endocrine System			
Graves' disease (hyperthyroidism)	TSH receptors on membrane of thyroid cells	Thyroid, metabolic	Myxedema, exophthalmos, increased metabolic rate
Insulin-dependent diabetes	Islet cells, insulin, receptors on pancreatic cells	Pancreas, metabolic	Hyperglycemia, polyuria, thirst, weight loss, ketosis
Addison's disease	Surface antigen on steroid producing cells in adrenal gland	Adrenal gland	Hypotension, fatigue
Primary myxedema	Microsomes	Thyroid	Orbital and facial edema, fatigue

Sources: DeFranco, A. L., Locksley, R., & Robertson, M. (2007). *Immunity: The immune response in infectious and inflammatory disease.* Sunderland, MA: Sinauer Associates; Rote, N. (2006). Immunity. In K. L. McCance & S. E. Huether (Eds.), *Pathophysiology: The biological basis for disease in adults and children* (5th ed., pp. 168–227). St. Louis: Mosby; Sommer, C. (2007). The immune response. In C. M. Porth (Ed.), *Essentials of pathophysiology* (pp. 247–268). St. Louis: Lippincott Williams & Wilkins.

four genes are involved in SLE development (Rizzo & Gunta, 2007). The disease is known to affect women more often than men and researchers are exploring the role of hormones in expression of SLE (National Institute of Arthritis and Musculoskeletal and Skin Diseases [NIAMSD], 2003) because the greatest incidence of the disease occurs in women ages 15 to 45.

Cultural factors may also play a role in SLE development because it occurs more frequently in African American, Hispanics, and Caucasians. Additionally, researchers have found that Hispanics and African Americans have a higher incidence of kidney damage and death rates when compared to Caucasians (NIAMSD, 2003).

Furthermore, environmental factors that may act as triggers for autoantibody production include ultraviolet light from the sun as well as interior lights, thermal burns, drugs, and possibly some viral triggers (Rizzo & Gunta, 2007; Medem, 2003). It has also been shown that drug-induced SLE syndrome can occur with exposure to certain medications such as procainamide, hydralazine, isoniazid, quinidine, methyldopa, and phenytoin (NIAMSD, 2003).

Pathophysiology

As mentioned earlier, the development of SLE is characterized by the formation of autoantibodies or antigen–antibody complexes that can damage a variety of tissues by identifying them as foreign cells and attempting to destroy them. This results from hyperactivity of B cells that are polyclonal and produce different types of autoantibodies (Rizzo & Gunta, 2007). Several autoantibodies have been identified in SLE including ANAs, such as anti-DNA, and antibodies against surface antigens on RBCs and platelets. Autoantibodies produced against these blood cells cause their destruction and lead to the clinical conditions of anemia and thrombocytopenia.

Clinical Manifestations

SLE may present with a variety of symptoms that do not point to a specific, easily identified disease process. This is what makes diagnosis of SLE very time consuming and challenging This difficulty in diagnosis is related to the potential number of autoantibodies and the wide range of organs that can be affected.

DIAGNOSTIC TESTS for Autoimmune Disease

Autoimmune Test	Expected Abnormality	Rationale for Abnormality
IgG levels	Measures levels of IgG in the blood. IgG is elevated in autoimmune diseases.	IgG levels are elevated in autoimmune diseases such as rheumatoid arthritis (RA) and Systemic Lupus Erythematosus (SLE). Individuals with autoimmune disease generally produce too many IgGs that can form antibody complexes with host cells and stimulate destruction of the host's cells.
Anti-IgG levels	Measures level of autoantibodies to IgG. Elevated levels of anti-IgG indicate the immune system is making antibodies to self proteins.	Patients with autoimmune disease such as RA often have elevated levels of anti-IgG antibodies. The immune system is responding to the rheumatoid factor and IgG complexes.
Antinuclear antibody (ANA)	Measures level of autoantibody to protein found in the cell nucleus. Elevated levels of ANA and specific patterns of staining indicate the body is making antibodies to self proteins. Individuals with negative tests do not have SLE or RA.	Patients capable of making antibodies to self proteins in elevated quantities are exhibiting signs of autoimmune disease.
Anti-DNA antibody (Tests for anti–double-strand DNA or anti–single-strand DNA)	Measures level of autoantibody to patient's own DNA. This is an enzyme-linked immunosorbent assay (ELISA)-type test. Positive tests indicate an individual is making IgG antibodies to the individual's own DNA. Individuals with negative tests do not have SLE or RA.	Patients with SLE and other collagen-associated autoimmune diseases make IgG antibodies that attack a variety of host or self proteins or markers.
Antiphospholipid antibody (Actually a group of antibodies including anticardiolipin antibodies)	Measure level of autoantibody to part of the cell wall. Platelet malfunction. Increased level of antiphospholipid antibodies indicates a risk of increased clotting. Increased levels are also see in SLE, RA, and antiphospholipid syndrome.	Patients with SLE, RA, and antiphospholipid syndrome have increased levels of the antiphospholipid antibody. The antibodies attach to phospholipids (one example is the IIB) on the platelet surface and stimulate clotting activity at the platelet level. Patients with SLE are at increased risk of clotting abnormalities such as thromboembolism.
Rheumatoid factor	Measures an autoantibody to the FC portion of IgG. These antibodies bind to synovial tissue and with complement stimulate phagocytosis of joint and bone tissue. High levels are found in patients with RA and Sjögren's syndrome.	Patients with autoimmune diseases such as RA, sarcoidosis, syphilis, and SLE, as well as viral infections, liver disease, and other chronic inflammatory diseases, all stimulate a positive test.
IgE antibodies (RAST)	A group of six respiratory and food allergies that promoted immediate allergic responses. RAST is radioallergosorbent. IgE in serum attaches to test antigens. Positive is 400% greater than normal IgE.	Patients with high IgE levels usually exhibit indications of allergic response. The individual capable of attaching IgE to test antigens will exhibit symptoms of allergy to triggers.
Erythrocyte sedimentation rate (ESR or sed rate)	Measures amount of settling of RBCs over 1 hour. Often first indicator of an acute inflammatory process or chronic inflammatory diseases.	Autoimmune diseases such as RA, inflammatory diseases, infections, carcinomas, and SLE all have increased sed rates. Chronic inflammation occurs in autoimmune disease when the host's immune system consumes or attacks cells that it views as non-self.
Complement 4 (C4) level	Level of C4 is decreased in patients with SLE and inborn C4 deficiency. Complement is a necessary part of a competent immune system.	Inborn C4 deficiency, SLE. Patients with inborn C4 deficiency do not make enough C4. In SLE and RA, patients make C4, but it is consumed in the phagocytic process of the immune system attacking self-antigens.
Total hemolytic complement (CH50)	CH50 is decreased in autoimmune diseases and increased in some carcinomas and acute inflammatory responses.	Patients with SLE, serum sickness, and severe RA are able to make adequate complement, but it is consumed in the autoimmune process of the host immune system inappropriately phagocytizing self cells such as collagen in joints and renal tubules.

DIAGNOSTIC TESTS for Autoimmune Disease—*Continued*

Autoimmune Test	Expected Abnormality	Rationale for Abnormality
Radioimmunoassay (ELISA/EIA for specific enzyme-linked diseases)	Positive results indicate autoimmune disease and are usually validated with second test.	ELISA tests allow labs to look for specific antibodies in autoimmune diseases such as Graves', Addison's, and HIV. A positive exam is repeated. A second positive triggers the next more sensitive test, i.e., Western blot for HIV.

Sources: Kee, J. L. (2005). *Laboratory and diagnostic tests with nursing implications* (7th ed.). Upper Saddle River, NJ: Pearson Prentice Hall; National Institute of Arthritis and Musculoskeletal and Skin Diseases. (2006). *Lupus: A patient care guide for nurses and other professionals* (3rd ed.). Retrieved September 2, 2008, from http://www.niams.nih.gov/hi/topics/lupus/lupusguide/chp7.htm; Van Leeuwen, A., Kranpitz, T., & Smith, L. (2006). *Laboratory and diagnostic tests with nursing implications* (2nd ed.). Philadelphia: F. A. Davis.

CHART 60–5 Plasmapheresis: A Treatment for Autoimmune Disease

Plasmapheresis refers to the technique of removing only the plasma portion of the blood. Plasmapheresis is usually a voluntary blood product donation process. The blood donor has her blood circulated through a machine that removes plasma and returns normal saline and RBCs back to the donor. Donated plasma contains clotting factors that can be used to help patients who have massive hemorrhage and are unable to clot their own blood effectively. The plasma also contains antibodies that are withdrawn during the pheresis process. Hence, plasmapheresis can also be used as a treatment in a number of autoimmune diseases. Plasmapheresis withdraws the immunoglobulins, immune complexes, and autoantibodies that are present in plasma, thereby decreasing the immune factors stimulating the autoimmune response.

Myasthenia gravis is an example of an autoimmune disease that can be treated with plasmapheresis. The process of filtering off the plasma also filters out large numbers of autoantibodies that are believed to be stimulating the myasthenia crisis. Plasmapheresis is usually only used to treat myasthenia crisis. Drug therapy remains the mainstay of therapy for patients not in crisis.

Plasmapheresis has also been indicated for patients with Guillain-Barré syndrome and rapidly progressing acute glomerulonephritis.

Nursing care of the patient receiving therapeutic plasma exchange or plasmapheresis includes patient education about the process of pheresis itself and the rationale that is applicable for treatment of the patient's specific disease process. The patient has a needle and catheter inserted into a vein and the blood is drawn from the vein and saline and red cells returned through the same catheter. Potential complications include hematoma at the needle insertion site, dizziness following donation, nausea, and hypotension. Specially trained nurses at major blood centers operate the pheresis machines and complete the treatment as ordered by the health care provider.

Sources: Porth, C., & Sweeney, K. (2007). Alterations in immune response. In C. M. Porth (Ed.), *Essentials of pathophysiology* (pp. 293–319). St. Louis: Lippincott Williams & Wilkins.

Laboratory tests to diagnose SLE are described in the Diagnostic Tests for Systemic Lupus Erythematosus box (p. 1910).

Symptoms often seen early in the disease include swollen joints, fatigue, unexplained fever, red rash (commonly a "butterfly" shape over the cheeks), arthritis, arthralgias, unexplained hair loss, photosensitivity, swollen lymph nodes, and edema in the legs or around the eyes. As the disease progresses, SLE can affect several organ systems. Although many patients have symptoms only in joints or skin, as many as 40% will have renal symptoms. Patients with SLE may develop nephritis or inflammation of the kidneys. The effect of this inflammation may temporarily or permanently reduce the ability of the kidney to filter nitrogenous wastes such as blood urea nitrogen and creatinine. Some patients with SLE will require short- or long-term hemodialysis related to the damage to their kidneys (Rote, 2006). Chapter 47 🔗 discusses hemodialysis.

Other organ systems that can become involved include the blood, blood vessels, lungs, or the neurological system. Anemia, leukopenia, and thrombocytopenia have all been noted in patients with SLE. These blood disorders are discussed in Chapter 63 🔗. Vasculitis and inflammation of blood vessels also occur in SLE. Swelling in blood vessels may affect the ability of blood to circulate and place the patient at risk for developing blood clots. Development of endocarditis, myocarditis, or pericarditis is also a potential risk for SLE patients. Valves may be damaged or destroyed in the patient with endocarditis. Patients with valve damage may present with chest pain or shortness of breath (Chapter 41 🔗).

Neurological manifestations of SLE include headache, memory loss, visual changes, changes in behavior, and stroke. The difficulty of evaluating neurological symptoms may be related to some of the side effects of medications used to treat the disease. Additionally, the stress of living with a complex disease such as SLE may add to some neurological symptoms (NIAMSD, 2003).

Medical Management

There is no cure for SLE; however, many patients have fewer exacerbations with adequate drug therapy. The key to therapy is reducing inflammation and immune response. Primary therapy for SLE is pharmacologic with the mainstay of therapy being corticosteroids. Drugs such as prednisone, dexamethasone, methylprednisolone, and hydrocortisone have all been used to treat SLE. Side effects have often interfered with patient compliance. Short-term side effects of corticosteroids include weight gain, increased appetite, edema, and emotional liability.

Patients with only joint pain and arthritis pain may be treated successfully with nonsteroidal anti-inflammatory drugs (NSAIDs) such as ibuprofen, naproxen, indomethacin, sulindac, piroxicam, and oxaprozin. These drugs reduce the pain, swelling, and immobility of joint arthralgias by blocking various chemicals of inflammation. To treat neurological symptoms, immunosuppressive drugs may be used. Drugs such as cyclophosphamide (Cytoxan) or azathioprine (Imuran) have been

DIAGNOSTIC TESTS for Systemic Lupus Erythematosus

Test	Expected Abnormality	Rationale for Abnormality
Antinuclear antibody (ANA) (a primary test for SLE)	Increased level of autoantibodies, usually IgG. Increased ANA in the serum indicates autoimmune activity. Specific staining patterns help differentiate SLE from other collagen diseases such as RA.	Autoantibodies to nuclear proteins increase because patients with SLE produce IgGs to a variety of self-antigens, including nuclear proteins. The immune system stimulates B cells to make antibodies to self proteins.
Anti-DNA antibody	Increased level of autoantibodies to patient's own DNA indicates a positive test.	The patient produces increased autoantibodies to own DNA because the T and B cells in patients with SLE are reacting to antigens that are normally viewed as self, in this case DNA.
Erythrocyte sedimentation rate (ESR or sed rate)	Elevated sed rate can indicate chronic inflammation. Elevated sed rate is often the first test done when patients are being worked up for general symptoms that could indicate autoimmune disease.	Sed rate is elevated in SLE because immune complexes continually stimulate the immune system, especially macrophages, to consume the IgG and the cell to which it is attached. This further stimulates inflammation.
Complement levels	Decreased due to presence of immune complexes that have used up complement factors.	Part of inflammation process related to abnormal antibody production.
Biopsy of skin and/or kidney	Changes in the kidney tissue.	Antibodies adversely affect the tissue.
Complete blood count (CBC)*	Decreased platelets, increased risk of bleeding and/or leukopenia.	Decreased platelets occur because immunoglobulins can attach to the antigens on the surface of the platelet and stimulate phagocytosis and activation of complement. Platelets can decrease in patients with SLE to less than 100,000 /mm^3 leading to development of bleeding abnormalities such as prolonged clotting time, purpura, petechiae, or oozing from invasive line insertion sites.
Chemistry panel (renal panel)*	Increased creatinine levels.	Increased creatinine indicating renal injury can occur in SLE because IgG attaches to renal cell surfaces, creating an immune complex that is then attacked by macrophages. This leads to decreased renal function at the tubular and cellular level and is evidenced by increasing creatinine levels.
Urinalysis*	The presence of protein and/or sodium in urine may indicate renal impairment.	Damage to the kidneys occurs with SLE when IgG attaches to renal tubule cells and this immune complex stimulates macrophages to phagocytize the renal cells leading to abnormal glomerular basement membrane function and the inability of the glomeruli to appropriately reabsorb sodium and proteins. Decreased renal function can eventually lead to renal failure, a major complication of SLE.

*This test is also a common laboratory abnormality seen in patients with complications related to SLE.

Sources: Kee, J. L. (2005). *Laboratory and diagnostic tests with nursing implications* (7th ed.). Upper Saddle River, NJ: Pearson Prentice Hall; National Institute of Arthritis and Musculoskeletal and Skin Diseases. (2006). *Lupus: A patient care guide for nurses and other professionals* (3rd ed.). Retrieved September 2, 2008, from http://www.niams.nih.gov/hi/topics/lupus/lupusguide/chp7.htm; Van Leeuwen, A., Kranpitz, T., & Smith, L. (2006). *Laboratory and diagnostic tests with nursing implications* (2nd ed.). Philadelphia: F. A. Davis.

used to decrease the action of some immune cells and block the growth of immune cells.

Another class of drugs used to treat SLE is antimalarial drugs. Hydroxychloroquine (Plaquenil), chloroquine (Aralen), and quinacrine (Atabrine) are all antimalarial drugs that have been effective in treating SLE. The exact mechanism of action for these drugs in SLE is unknown and research has centered on the effect of these drugs on suppressing immune function (DeFranco et al., 2007). When taken continuously, antimalarial drugs have been helpful in preventing "flares" or exacerbations of SLE.

Nursing Management

Nursing care of the patient with autoimmune disease focuses on educating patients and families regarding the disease process and medications, as well as providing interventions to promote symptom control and management. The goal of nursing care is to provide an individualized plan of care that promotes patient comfort and maximizes patient independence and self-care activities. The nursing process provides an excellent template for accomplishing this goal. An example of how the nursing process is applied in autoimmune disease is provided in the following discussion of SLE, with diagnoses for autoimmune diseases listed in Chart 60–6.

Nursing care of the patient with SLE presents numerous challenges. Attempts at diagnosis may be lengthy and difficult. Generalized and often vague symptoms of SLE can increase the patient's sense of loss of control and perception that health care professionals may not take them seriously. Flares of the disease may add to the patient's feelings of loss of control or depression.

Assessment

Nursing assessment begins with listening carefully to the patient's concerns and developing a supportive therapeutic relationship. The nursing assessment includes a thorough history of symptoms with focus on patient reports of fatigue, rashes, pain including headaches, and swollen joints. The history will guide the nurse in performing an in-depth physical examination of all systems because of the varied organs and tissues that can be affected by SLE.

Nursing Diagnoses

Common nursing diagnoses associated with SLE include:

- *Pain*
- *Fatigue*
- *Impaired Mobility*
- *Ineffective Tissue Perfusion*

CHART 60–6   **Nursing Diagnoses for Patients with Autoimmune Disease**

- *Deficient Knowledge* related to therapeutic regimen, self-care, and immunosuppressive medications
- *Deficient Knowledge* related to signs/symptoms of autoimmune disease exacerbation
- *Risk for Infection* related to immune suppression medications and alterations in immune function
- *Fatigue* related to autoimmune disease
- *Chronic Pain* related to autoimmune disease
- *Impaired Oral Mucous Membrane* related to immune suppression medications
- *Risk for Impaired Skin Integrity* related to immunosuppressive medications
- *Sexual Dysfunction* related to immunosuppressive medications and fatigue
- *Risk for Imbalanced Nutrition: Less Than Body Requirements* related to decreased appetite with chronic disease process
- *Risk for Activity Intolerance* and *Self-Care Deficit* related to disease exacerbation
- *Coping Ineffective,* related to chronic disease process lifestyle alteration and fatigue
- *Risk for Social Isolation* related to chronic fatigue, autoimmune disease exacerbations.

Sources: Carpenito-Moyet, L. (2008). *Nursing care plans and documentation* (5th ed.). Philadelphia: Lippincott Williams & Wilkins; National Institute of Arthritis and Musculoskeletal and Skin Diseases. (2006). *Lupus: A patient care guide for nurses and other professionals* (3rd ed.). Retrieved September 2, 2008, from http://www.niams.nih.gov/hi/topics/lupus/lupusguide/chp7.htm; University of California Davis Health System. (2001). *Living with your kidney transplant.* Sacramento: UC Davis Transplant Center.

- *Urinary Elimination Impaired*
- *Decreased Cardiac Output*
- *Coping. Readiness for enhanced coping ineffective*

Planning, Interventions, and Outcome and Evaluation Parameters

Planning nursing care of patients with SLE should focus on the specific problems the patient describes as well as assessment findings. Frequent reassessment to identify potential problems such as joint or renal impairment is done on an ongoing basis. Patient teaching regarding the importance of adhering to medication regimens, reporting side effects, and assisting the patient to identify flares of the disease early are vital nursing interventions. The remainder of nursing care centers around symptom control and psychosocial support. Outcome and evaluation parameters to determine the effectiveness of the treatment plan include symptom control, effective medication regime, and prevention of disease flares.

Health Promotion

It is important for individuals with SLE to understand the importance of obtaining regular health care, not just during disease flares. The patient needs to be taught to receive regular physical examinations, blood pressure checks, and laboratory work to enable the health care team to identify problems early and help prevent disease exacerbation. Annual gynecological and breast exams for women and prostate specific antigen (PSA) tests for men are recommended, as are annual influenza vaccines. An eye exam should also be done yearly if the patient is taking corticosteroids or antimalarial medications to screen for visual changes.

Learning to recognize the early warning signs of an SLE crisis is also vital in preventing it or reducing the intensity. Warning signs include increased fatigue, pain, rash, fever, abdominal discomfort, headache, and dizziness (NIAMSD, 2003). Maintaining a healthy lifestyle by eating well, exercising daily, and controlling stress is important in preventing SLE exacerbations. Developing an effective support system for emotional support, to improve coping skills, and to boost morale is an essential part of this process.

◼ Collaborative Management

Accurate diagnosis, early treatment, patient education on medications and disease management, and development of an individualized plan of care designed to empower the patient are critical for successful living with an autoimmune disease such as SLE. A team approach that involves health care providers or various specialties, nurses, and social workers is essential in creating an effective treatment plan that enables the patient to have a productive and rewarding life in spite of the devastating impact of an autoimmune disease.

Health care providers specifically manage the multiple phases of the diagnosis and medical treatment plan. This involves medication management, laboratory testing, and monitoring and treatment of disease progression. Nursing care, described earlier, includes symptom management, patient and education medications for symptom control, and education on early signs and symptoms of disease exacerbation. The social worker assists with home management, respite care for caregivers, and financial concerns.

Research Topics Related to the Autoimmune Hypersensitivity Response

Research related to the autoimmune hypersensitivity response is focused primarily on molecular genetic studies to determine genetic links in the development of allergic and autoimmune responses and advancement of new drug therapies to treat the diseases associated with these responses. As studies progress to clinical trials, nurses play a significant role in study coordination, gathering of data, and analysis of patient response to new treatments. Immunosuppressive drug therapy to treat autoimmune disease is an area of extensive research. There are multiple drug studies currently in the clinical trial phase that nurses are involved in coordinating (NHLBI, 2004b).

Research in autoimmune diseases also focuses on improving quality of life for patients with specific disease processes. For example, scleroderma is a systemic autoimmune disease that can result in the development of pulmonary fibrosis, the primary cause of mortality in these patients. Traditionally, treatment has focused on suppression of the immune system largely through the use of corticosteroids. Now a new approach using cyclophosphamide, which has been used to treat neoplasms of the immune system and SLE, is in clinical trials at 13 major university hospitals in the United States (NHLBI, 2004b).

Research in controlling the autoimmune hypersensitivity response also focuses on the development of monoclonal antibodies to treat specific diseases such as SLE. Additional information on current medical and nursing research related to autoimmune hypersensitivity is provided in the Research Opportunities and Clinical Impact box.

Alloimmune Hypersensitivity Response

The alloimmune response is a type of immune reaction in which the antigen, the host's immune system, responds to an antigen from another human or another species. This is the type of response that occurs when tissues or organs are transplanted. This is a normal immune response, because the immune system is reacting to foreign antigens. Therefore, matching the antigens between the donor and recipient of transplanted cells and suppressing the immune response are the key concepts in preventing organ and tissue transplant rejection.

Epidemiology and Etiology

The advancements in surgical technique and immunosuppressive medications have substantially improved the success of organ and tissue transplants. There is a growing shortage of available organs for transplant. Approximately 89,000 people in the United States are currently on the waiting list for an organ transplant, and another 4,000 are added annually (National Kidney Foundation, 2005). Organs that can currently be transplanted include the kidneys, liver, pancreas, heart, and lungs. Blood and numerous other body tissues including skin, bone, cartilage, corneas, veins, and bone marrow also can be transplanted. An autograph is a transplant of tissue or whole organ from one part of an animal to the same animal. Transplants between two identical twins are isographs. A transplant that occurs from one animal to another or one human being to another is called an allograft. When the graph occurs from a lower animal to a human it is a xenograft. The goal with any graft is to minimize the risk of alloimmune response that results in rejection of the transplanted tissue or organ (Rote, 2006).

Different mechanisms of hypersensitivity immune response are involved in alloimmune reactions. The type IV cell-mediated

---

RESEARCH OPPORTUNITIES AND CLINICAL IMPACT RELATED TO THE AUTOIMMUNE HYPERSENSITIVITY RESPONSE

Research Area	Clinical Impact
Development of monoclonal antibodies for treatment of autoimmune diseases	Control of autoimmune disease progression and clinical symptoms
Stem cell cloning to develop new methods for delivery of monoclonal antibodies	Improved drug therapy by reducing side effects of monoclonal antibody therapy
Identification of genetic factors that contribute to development of autoimmune diseases such as myasthenia gravis and Goodpasture's syndrome	Enable gene alteration to prevent and treat autoimmune disease
Identification of viral triggers of autoimmune dysfunction such as Epstein-Barr virus and autoimmune-associated migraine headaches	Prevention of disease progress and development of effective treatment
Identification of environmental triggers such as pesticides or radiation exposure that contribute to the development of autoimmune disease	Control of exposure to environment triggers to prevent altered immune function
Drug therapy for treatment of symptoms of autoimmune disease such as digital ulcers in scleroderma. For example, bosentan is an endothelin-1 antagonist that causes relaxation of the smooth muscle of the blood vessel and decreased pressures and is in current clinical trials in 21 U.S. test sites	New drug treatments to control pain and improve patient's quality of life. The bosentan study is evaluating improved blood flow and healing in finger ulcers of patients with scleroderma. Goal is a reduction of digital ulcers, improved healing of digital ulcers, and increased hand function (Korn & Seibold, 2004)

response is the type of alloimmune reaction involved in transplant rejection. The T cells are primarily responsible for this type of response. Antibody-mediated responses and complement also play a significant role in alloimmune reaction.

Pathophysiology

The antigen system primarily responsible for alloimmune reaction is the HLA system. There are six different HLA markers: HLA-A, HLA-B, HLA-C, HLA-D, HLA-DR, and HLA-DQ. These create identifying protein markers that are on cell surfaces throughout the body and differentiate self from non-self. Each of these markers is capable of creating multiple different gene subtype combinations that are the basis for HLA inheritance in families. Identical twins will have the same HLA markers; family members will have similar HLA markers. HLA matching is critical in organ transplant and is the ideal marker for genetic study of diseases (Rote, 2006).

To maximize the potential for graft acceptance, there must be a donor–recipient match between HLA subtypes. This match is vital because an organ that is transplanted (kidney, lung, or heart) is rich in donor vascular tissue, white blood cells, and lymphatic tissue, all of which carry HLA subtype antigens and, thus, are able to trigger an alloimmune response. An exact or extremely close HLA match is essential to prevent the host's immune system from reacting against the donor's graft. Tissues such as corneas, cartilage, and veins have minimum concentrations of immune tissue with specialized HLA antigens; therefore, only blood typing and crossmatching is required when matching a donor and recipient.

Graft Rejection

Host versus graft disease (HVGD) occurs when the recipient's immune system reacts against the foreign antigens on the cells of the graft. This can occur in allograft tissues or organs such as kidney, lung, and heart, and is classified as hyperacute, acute, and chronic. Type II and type IV hypersensitivity reactions occur in most types of rejection. The T cells involved in rejection are T-helper cells (CD4) and T-cytotoxic cells (CD8). Consequently, T-cell activity must be suppressed in order to prevent rejection. T-cell suppression is the primary target of immunosuppressive therapy for transplant recipients.

Hyperacute rejection is rare and occurs when the recipient has a preexisting antibody to the antigen in the graft tissue. The graft may turn white immediately or during the next several hours as vascular stasis occurs in the transplanted tissue. This is a result of the antigen–antibody complexes that stimulate the release of proinflammatory mediators and of complement. Complement, a primary mediator in the antigen–antibody reactions, attracts tissue-destroying neutrophils and macrophages, and stimulates the coagulation cascade, which results in coagulation in the microvasculature of the graft tissue (Rote, 2006). Hyperacute rejection occurs because of previous exposure to an antigen, such as with prior blood transfusions, organ transplants, or multiple pregnancies (Urden et al., 2006).

Acute graft rejection is a type IV cell-mediated immune response that occurs approximately 2 weeks to a month after transplant. This type of delayed hypersensitivity response occurs when the recipient's T cells are activated against the unmatched HLA antigens on the transplanted donor tissue. The result is destruction of the transplant tissue by T cells and inflammatory mediators. Immunosuppressive drugs may delay the response.

The symptoms exhibited during acute rejection are consistent with an inflammatory response and include fever, swelling, tenderness, and redness over the graft site. The result will be progressive organ failure evidenced in laboratory findings such as elevation in creatinine with kidney transplant rejection or increase in liver enzymes with liver transplant rejection. Acute rejection can be slowed or reversed with changes in immunotherapy treatment. Research to develop new and improved immunosuppressive drug therapies is ongoing (Food and Drug Administration [FDA], 2003b).

Chronic graft rejection occurs a few months to years after transplant and involves a slow progressive failure of the transplanted organ. Although improvements in immunotherapy have made significant strides in prevention or slowing of acute tissue rejection, chronic graft rejection continues to be a major problem. The exact mechanism of chronic graft rejection is not well understood. It is thought to involve T-cell-mediated cytotoxic cells and macrophages that damage the endothelial cell lining of blood vessels causing thickening and fibrosis of the microvasculature (Rote, 2006). Over time the organ slowly fails as evidenced by clinical symptoms and elevation of laboratory values that reflect organ function.

Graft Versus Host Disease

In **graft versus host disease (GVHD)** donor-grafted tissue contains functional immune cells that respond to the recipient's tissue antigens. As a result, the grafted tissue supersedes the immune function of the recipient and produces antibodies against the host tissue, initiates cytotoxic responses, and begins to attack tissue in the host. Patients who experience this type of immune reaction are usually severely immunocompromised.

GVHD is most often seen in bone marrow transplants (see Chapter 64 🔗 for a complete description of bone marrow transplant). This occurs because prior to bone marrow transplant, the host's immune system is reduced or eliminated by radiation and/or chemotherapy. When donor marrow is introduced, T lymphocytes in the donor marrow recognize that the recipient's HLA antigens are foreign and initiate an immune attack against cells rich in HLA antigens. Sites of initial GVHD symptoms include skin, liver, intestines, and, of course, the recipient's immune system cells. The response may be as mild as a rash on the skin or as severe as liver failure. GVHD can be prevented through the elimination or destruction of T cells in donated tissue with immunosuppressive therapy (Porth & Sweeney, 2007).

Clinical Manifestations

The clinical manifestations of alloimmune hypersensitivity response can occur through two different mechanisms. The most common mechanism is graft disease (HVGD) and involves the recipient's immune system reacting against the donor tissue. As discussed earlier, graft rejection is classified as hyperacute, acute, or chronic based on various symptoms and the amount of time that has elapsed since transplant. The second mechanism of alloimmune hypersensitivity response, GVHD, occurs when the immune cells in the donor's tissue mount a reaction against the host.

Medical Management

Medical management of the patient with alloimmune response is targeted at preventing graft rejection and early identification and suppression of immune activity that could lead to graft failure. As with other forms of autoimmune diseases, this involves depressing immune function. Immunosuppressive drug therapy is the focal point of alloimmune medical treatment.

Immunosuppressive Therapy

Immunosuppressive therapy will vary according to the type of organ or tissue being transplanted and institutional/health care provider protocols. For information on specific organ transplants, refer to the chapters related to the organ being transplanted such as heart, lungs, liver, and kidney. The goal of immunotherapy is to suppress the activity of the T-helper and T-cytotoxic cells and interfere with the secretion of interleukins (see Chapter 59 💿) that stimulate the inflammatory and immune response. Another focus of the treatment is to minimize the toxic effects of these drugs, which include nephrotoxicity, electrolyte abnormalities, hypertension, hepatoxicity, hyperglycemia, and the hematologic effects of leukopenia, thrombocytopenia, and anemia (Adams et al., 2005; Wilson, Shannon, Shields, & Stang, 2007). Therefore, patients must have frequent laboratory tests to evaluate blood chemistry, liver function, kidney function, and hematology cell production in order to monitor the effects of medication and allow for dose adjustments.

Initial immunotherapy begins prior to the transplantation procedure. High doses of immunosuppressive agents are used initially and for a short time after surgery. These doses are then tapered to maintenance levels. Common drugs used and the implications for nursing care are found in the Pharmacology Summary of Medications to treat Autoimmune and Immunosuppressive Drug Therapy feature. If rejection develops, high-dose steroids and antilymphocyte therapy such as monoclonal antibodies are frequently used.

Nursing Management

The goal of nursing management for the patient with alloimmune response is prevention of transplant rejection and promotion of optimal quality of life and independence. Nursing care of the patient with tissue transplant must focus on educating patients and families regarding the importance of immunosuppressive therapy including the side effects and precautions and also the signs and symptoms of transplant rejection. The nurse monitors for adherence to prescribed medications, and side effects of drug therapy such as alteration in renal and hepatic function, alteration in skin integrity, and possible opportunistic infection. The nursing process provides an excellent template to assess, treat, and evaluate patients with tissue transplant and subsequent alloimmune response. The Nursing Process: Care Plan for the Patient with an Organ Transplant feature (p. 1917) applies the nursing process to the most common nursing diagnosis associated with alloimmune response and graft rejection.

Collaborative Management

The essence of collaborative care is exemplified in the care of transplant patients. A strong multidisciplinary team approach and a committed family support system are essential to help prepare the patient for transplant and monitor the patient's medications, treatments, and follow-up care after transplant. Prior to transplant the patient is interviewed by a health care provider from the transplant team to determine appropriateness for transplant. An additional screening is done by a psychologist to determine if the patient is mentally prepared to receive a transplant and understand and comply with the required treatment regime. A pretransplant nurse coordinator is also involved, and is responsible for scheduling all of the required preliminary tests and appointments.

At the time of transplant and immediately following, other members of the multidisciplinary team become involved. These include a team of transplant surgeons and other health care provider specialties depending on any complicating factors. Transplant unit nurses care for the patient immediately after surgery and educate and prepare the patient and family for the responsibilities associated with discharge home. These include teaching about monitoring vital signs and preventing infection, medication administration and compliance, laboratory tests trending, and follow-up appointments.

The pharmacist also has a crucial role in medication education and working with the health care provider to tailor the medication treatment plan. Additionally, a dietitian provides teaching on nutritional needs and dietary restrictions specific for the organ being transplanted. For example, patients with renal transplant would receive teaching regarding a low-sodium diet. The social worker and discharge planner nurse assist in helping the family with financial concerns, arranging any home care needs, and connecting with community resources.

Post-transplant care involves the addition to the team of a post-transplant nurse coordinator. This nurse provides the patient and family with continual support and is the primary point of contact for them regarding questions, medications, any symptoms or complications, and follow-up appointments. The post-transplant coordinator functions as a very specialized case manager to triage any patient problems and determine what members of the transplant team the patient needs to see. Additionally, the patient continues to be followed on a regular basis by the transplant surgeon and several other members of the team to optimize successful transplant.

Research Topics Related to the Alloimmune Hypersensitivity Response

Research in the area of alloimmune hypersensitivity response is primarily focused on preventing transplant rejection. Areas of research involve development of new immunosuppressant medications with minimal side effects that promote optimal immune suppression and quality of life for the transplant patient. Information related to some of the current research in this area is presented in the Research Opportunities and Clinical Impact box (p. 1921).

Immunodeficiencies

Immune deficiencies occur when the immune system experiences abnormalities in function that result in a decreased or compromised ability to appropriately respond and protect the host from an antigenic attack. Primary immune deficiencies are the result of genetic abnormalities in the embryonic development of the immune system.

PHARMACOLOGY Summary of Medications to Treat Autoimmune and Immunosuppressive Drug Therapy

Drug	Action	Application/Indication	Nursing Responsibility
Nonsteroidal Anti-Inflammatory Drugs (NSAIDs) • Ibuprofen • Naproxen • Indomethacin • Sulindac • Piroxicam • Oxaprozin	Reduce the pain, swelling, and immobility of joint arthralgias by blocking release of prostaglandins and leukotrienes responsible for inflammation and pain.	Drug of choice for patients with autoimmune disease such as lupus with little or no organ involvement. Patients with serious organ involvement or disease flares will require steroid anti-inflammatory drugs and immunosuppressive medications.	Assess pain level. Various NSAIDs effect people differently and after a time they may develop a tolerance, requiring a change to a new drug in the class. Monitor for bleeding, GI upset, and decreased renal function. Instruct patient to take NSAIDs with food or milk to decrease GI symptoms. Salicylates (including ASA) are contraindicated in persons under age 19 due to Reye's syndrome.
Antimalarial Drugs • Hydroxychloroquine sulfate (Plaquenil) • Chloroquine (Aralen) • Quinacrine (Atabrine)	The exact mechanism of action for these drugs in SLE is unknown. They are effective in suppressing some immune function related to lupus and controlling mild inflammatory symptoms.	Low doses are used to manage mild symptoms of lupus including arthritis, skin rashes, mouth ulcers, fatigue, and fever. May enable reduction of total daily dose of corticosteroids.	Instruct the patient that medications may take several weeks to become effective in controlling symptoms. Monitor for vision changes; can cause retinal damage.
Glucocorticosteroids • Steroids: prednisone, dexamethasone, methylprednisolone, and hydrocortisone	Interfere with inflammatory response and antigen presentation. Block cytokine genes, thereby impairing synthesis of IL-1, -2, -3, and -6. Inhibit TNF.	Used to control exacerbations of autoimmune diseases. For transplant patients used in combination with calcineurin inhibitors such as cyclosporine, and antimetabolites and cytotoxic agents such as azathioprine as triple-drug immunosuppressive therapy to prevent transplant rejection.	Monitor laboratory tests: serum glucose, lipid levels. Administer insulin as prescribed. Monitor wound healing. Promote skin integrity (change position frequently, avoid adhesive tape). Provide patient education on diet and body changes: low-fat, low-cholesterol diet with low calories between meal snacks. Monitor changes in strength; provide a physical therapy consult as needed. Administer medication with food; collaborate with health care provider for orders for hydrochloric acid (H2) receptor blockers or antacids for gastric complaints. Monitor for signs and symptoms of infection. Instruct patient on techniques to avoid infection (perform hand hygiene frequently, avoid crowds and ill individuals).

(continued)

PHARMACOLOGY Summary of Medications to Treat Autoimmune and Immunosuppressive Drug Therapy—*Continued*

Drug	Action	Application/Indication	Nursing Responsibility
Calcineurin Inhibitor • Cyclosporine (Sandimmune and Neoral) • Tacrolimus (Prograf)	Reduce transcription of IL-2. Impair cytokines that are required for T-cell activation (more potent than cyclosporine).	The mainstay of immunosuppressive therapy; used as part of triple-drug immunosuppressive therapy to prevent transplant rejection. Now also commonly used to treat autoimmune diseases such as lupus.	Monitor and report abnormal laboratory tests: serum creatinine, BUN, potassium, serum transaminases, bilirubin, and glucose levels. Administer insulin as prescribed. Administer antiemetic and antidiarrhea agents as prescribed. Monitor and report serum cyclosporine trough levels and changes in neurological status for dose adjustments. Provide patient education on frequent oral care, such as dental cleaning every 6 months or more frequently if gingival hyperplasia occurs.
Antimetabolites • Azathioprine (AZA, Imuran) • Cyclophosphamide (Cytoxan) • Methotrexate (Rheumatrex) • Sirolimus (Rapamune) • Mycophenolate Mofetil (CellCept)	Inhibit aspects of lymphocyte replication, which decreases leukocytes. Inhibit proliferation of B- and T-cell lines. Decrease leukocytes. Selectively inhibit proliferation of B and T lymphocytes.	Used in combination with cyclosporine and steroids as triple-drug immunosuppressive therapy to prevent transplant rejection. Azathioprine is one of the most widely used immunosuppressive drugs for lupus. Cytoxan is reserved for treating lupus with kidney disease or other internal organ involvement. Rheumatrex is predominantly used for lupus arthritis. Sometimes used as an alternative to cyclophosphamide for lupus with kidney involvement.	Monitor and report symptoms of infection (hyper- or hypothermia, chills, malaise) and/or jaundice. Monitor and report abnormal labs: CBC, serum transaminases, and bilirubin. Monitor fluid intake and urine output daily. Assess gastrointestinal disturbances and administer antiemetics and antidiarrhea agents as ordered.
Monoclonal and Polyclonal Antibodies • Alemtuzumab (Campath) • Basiliximab (Simulect) • Daclizumab (Zenapax) • Infliximab (Remicade) • Muromonab-CD3 (Orthoclone OKT3) • Rituximab (Rituxan) • Lymphocyte immunoglobulin (Antithymocyte Globulin: Equine, Atgam)	Monoclonal antibody targeting CD3 receptor on T cells. Downregulates T-cell activity. A specific lymphocyte immunoglobulin that is a lymphocyte-selective immunosuppressant agent. Composed of sterile, purified, concentrated immunoglobulin G (IgG) from serum of horses immunized with human thymus lymphocytes. The immune globulin lymphocytes bind with the patient's antigen reactive T lymphocytes and decrease or alter killer T-cell function.	Organ and tissue transplant immune suppression. Used in combination with cyclosporine and corticosteroid therapy to prevent transplant rejection. To prevent or delay onset or to reverse acute renal allograft rejection.	Monitor and report fever, chills, nausea and vomiting, headache. Administer antiemetics and antipyretics as ordered. Monitor and report abnormalities in respiratory status (dyspnea, increased respiratory rate, decrease in pulse oximetry readings, abnormal breath sounds). Administer oxygen as ordered. Monitor pulse oxygen saturation and arterial blood gases (ABGs); report abnormalities. Monitor for signs/symptoms of infection.

Sources: Adams, M., Josephson, D., & Holland, L. (2008). *Pharmacology for nurses: A pathophysiologic approach.* (2nd ed.) Upper Saddle River, NJ: Pearson Prentice Hall; National Institute of Arthritis and Musculoskeletal and Skin Diseases. (2006). *Care of the lupus patient.* Retrieved February 19, 2007, from National Institute of Health website: http://www.niams.nih.gov/hi/topics/lupus/lupusguide/chp7.htm; University of California Davis Medical Center Transplant Center. (2001). *Living with your kidney transplant.* Sacramento: Author; University of California Davis Health System. (2003). *Atgam IV administration. Patient care standard A-7.* Sacramento: Author.

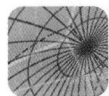

NURSING PROCESS: Patient Care Plan for Organ Transplants

Assessment of Knowledge Deficit

Subjective Data:

Do you have a way in which you best learn information (e.g., reading, watching a video on the subject, or having 1:1 instruction)?

Who in your family is going to help you at home with your medications, vital sign monitoring, and follow-up appointments?

Is this a good time to do some of your teaching or are you too tired or in pain?

Objective Data:

Patient is awake, alert, oriented.

Patient does not show signs of pain or discomfort (e.g., pain level assessed at tolerable for patient, VS stable).

Appropriate person from family is present.

Patient and family verbalize readiness to learn.

Nursing Assessment and Diagnoses	Outcomes and Evaluation Parameters	Planning and Interventions with *Rationales*
Nursing Diagnosis: *Deficient Knowledge* related to therapeutic regimen and self-care, immunosuppressive medications, signs/symptoms of transplant rejection, and discharge follow-up	**Outcomes:** Successful recovery without graft rejection or complications. Patient and family demonstrate self-care activities to prevent graft rejection. ***Evaluation Parameters:*** Participates in learning sessions and asks questions. Verbalizes education needs to reduce risk of graft rejection and maintain health. Develops plan to meet follow-up care needs and initiates lifestyle changes.	**Interventions and *Rationales*:** Assess patient's and family's level of understanding of information, participation in teaching sessions, initiation of self-care activities, and medication administration technique. Assess knowledge level and lifestyle expectations of patient and family. *To determine educational needs and clarify expectations.*
		Provide information via multiple modalities including written, video, presentations by transplant team, demonstration/return demonstration. *Provides individualized learning plan, enhances learning experience, and provides resources postdischarge.*
	Verbalizes understanding to notify transplant coordinator immediately for any health problems.	Instruct patient and family about the importance of adhering to medical treatment regime including follow-up appointments, frequent need for laboratory testing draws to assess effectiveness of immunosuppressive drug therapy. *To prevent complications of graft rejection or medication side effects.*
	Verbalizes rationale for and doses of specific immunotherapy medications and follow-up lab tests and appointments. Accurately self-doses all immunosuppressive therapy drugs prior to discharge. Demonstrates self-care by adhering to treatment regime including immunosuppressive drug therapy.	Review immunosuppressive medication doses, side effects, and administration schedule. *To provide information about why and how immunosuppressive drugs are administered.* Observe patient self-administering medications appropriately. *To assess appropriate medication administration.*
	Verbalizes signs and symptoms of transplant rejection.	Instruct about signs and symptoms of rejection: fatigue/general malaise, "flu-like" feeling, fever, sudden weight gain, delayed wound healing, pain in or around specific organ transplanted or changes in normal function. *To identify early signs of rejection.*
	Reports any symptoms of transplant rejection early to transplant coordinator.	Instruct to notify transplant coordinator immediately for any of the above symptoms. *To initiate prompt medical treatment.*

Assessment of Infection

Subjective Data:

Do you have any pain?

Do you have a temperature?

Are you having any "flu-like" symptoms (body aches, fatigue, cough, sore throat, stiff neck)?

Do you have any rashes?

Do you have any burning with urination?

Do you have any redness or tenderness anywhere?

Do you have any sores anywhere?

Do you have any unusual or foul-smelling drainage (e.g., from vagina, penis, rectum, ears)?

How long have the symptoms been going on?

What have you done to treat the symptoms?

Have you taken any over the counter (OTC), prescription, or herbal medications for symptom relief?

Objective Data:

Head-to-toe assessment with focus on the specific area of patient complaint; report any abnormal findings (e.g., abnormal vital signs, pain, "flu-like" symptoms, rashes, redness, discharge, sores, drainage, bloody stools, and urinary discomfort.

(continued)

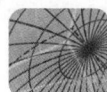

NURSING PROCESS: Patient Care Plan for Organ Transplants—*Continued*

Nursing Assessment and Diagnoses	Outcomes and Evaluation Parameters	Planning and Interventions with *Rationales*
Nursing Diagnosis: *Risk for Infection* related to immune suppression medications	**Outcome:** No infection. ***Evaluation Parameters:*** Patient and family verbalize understanding of signs/symptoms of infection and notify transplant coordinator immediately of any health problems.	**Interventions and *Rationales:*** Instruct patient and family to monitor and report any symptoms of infection. *To facilitate prompt medical treatment and minimize risk of rejection.* Instruct patient and family about signs and symptoms of infection: fever, chills, "flu-like" feeling, cough with or without sputum, sore throat, shortness of breath, rashes, burning with urination, foul discharge from penis, vagina, loose or bloody stools, any redness/tenderness or drainage from incision; swollen lymph nodes; any new or unusual pain, stiff neck, sores in mouth or on tongue. *To identify early signs/symptoms of infection, facilitate early medical treatment, and minimize risk of rejection.* Instruct to notify transplant coordinator immediately. *To initiate prompt medical treatment.*
	Patient and family demonstrate understanding of self-care by following plan to minimize infection risk.	Instruct patient and family on ways to minimize risk of infection including performing hand hygiene frequently, avoid crowded areas, and avoid contact with people who are sick. *To minimize exposure to infectious organisms.* Perform weekly self-exam to assess for swelling of lymph nodes. *To detect symptoms of infection early.* Drink 6–8 glasses of water a day and empty your bladder frequently, avoid bubble baths, urinate after sex, wear cotton crotch underwear. *To prevent urinary tract infections.* Wear a mask and gloves when working in the garden. *To avoid fungi and bacteria in soil.* Do not handle pet waste or litter box. *Cat litter can transmit infectious organisms.* Swim only in pools with chlorine. *Lakes and ponds have multiple infectious organisms.* Cook all meats thoroughly before eating and wash fruits/vegetables well. *To decrease bacteria.*
	Daily log completed and brought to follow-up appointments.	Instruct in self-care practices to monitor for complications and documenting in daily log: temperature, weight before breakfast, blood pressure, pulse, changes in medications, changes in health status. *To identify early signs of complications and provide trend information to transplant team.*
	Performs vital sign monitoring accurately and records information in daily log appropriately.	Observe patient taking own temperature, pulse, blood pressure, and weight and recording these prior to discharge. *To assess skill and ensure accuracy of readings and need for additional teaching.*

Assessment of Skin and Oral Mucosa

Subjective Data:

Do you have any red, sore, or open areas on your skin?

Do you have any redness or drainage from your surgical incision?

Do you have any sores in your mouth?

Are you able to bathe and do oral care daily?

Do you have acne?

Do you use a sun block?

Objective Data:

Assess:

Redness on pressure points (coccyx, heals, elbows)

Skin tears: around wound site, IV sites, lab draw sites where tape has been applied

Incision site: redness, drainage, foul odor, proximity of suture line, intact staples/sutures

Skinfolds, especially with patients who are obese: redness, breakdown

Oral membrane: open sores in mouth, white coating on tongue indicating possible candidiasis infection

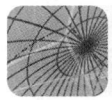

NURSING PROCESS: Patient Care Plan for Organ Transplants—*Continued*

Nursing Assessment and Diagnoses	Outcomes and Evaluation Parameters	Planning and Interventions with *Rationales*
Nursing Diagnosis: *High Risk for Impaired Skin Integrity* related to opportunistic infections	**Outcome:** Intact mucous membranes. ***Evaluation Parameters:*** Verbalizes importance of oral care. Practices self-care by performing oral care according to plan. Takes antibiotics prior to any dental work.	**Interventions and *Rationales:*** Inspect gums, mouth, and tongue daily and report abnormalities. *To facilitate appropriate medical treatment.* Provide frequent oral care. *To keep mucous membranes moist and promote patient comfort.* Instruct in importance of oral care; encourage frequent oral care during the day and regular dental checkups and inspection of gums, mouth, and tongue daily. *Immunosuppression increases risk of opportunistic infections. Medication side effects can cause hypertrophy of the gums.* Patient to inform dentist of immunosuppressed status. *To facilitate prescription of antibiotics prior to any dental work.* Patient to always take antibiotics prior to dental work. *To minimize risk of blood infection from dental work.*

Assessment of Post-Transplant Self-Care

Subjective Data:
Are you taking your medications, and are you able to keep your clinic appointments?
Are you able to eat a balanced, nutritious diet?
Have you gained or lost weight?
Are you easily fatigued or can you participate in daily light, low-impact exercise, such as walking?
Are you experiencing any sexual difficulties you would like to discuss?
Are you seeing family and friends regularly?
Are you planning to travel anywhere out of the area?

Objective Data:
Keeps follow-up lab and medical appointments
Weight (above or below goal weight)
Contacts transplant coordinator with travel plans

Nursing Assessment and Diagnoses	Outcomes and Evaluation Parameters	Planning and Interventions with *Rationales*
Nursing Diagnoses: *Activity intolerance, risk for* related to post-transplant status and necessity for lifelong immunosuppressive medication	**Outcome:** Intact skin and oral mucous membranes. ***Evaluation Parameters:*** No evidence of pressure ulcers, skin tears, or sores on mucous membranes. Verbalizes instructions for post-op wound care. Practices self-care by following post-op care instructions. Verbalizes importance of skin care. Practices self-care by performing skin care daily.	**Interventions and *Rationales:*** Assess for alteration in skin integrity and reposition frequently. *To promote skin integrity. Broken skin provides entry for bacteria.* Avoid the use of adhesive tape. *To minimize the risk of skin tears.* Instruct in postoperative home care: care of wound site, monitoring for redness and drainage. *Indicates infection.* Gently clean skin around incision daily with soap and water. *To decrease bacteria and risk of infection.* Do not apply lotion over wound. *Increases risk of infection.* Avoid heavy lifting/strenuous exercise. Do not lift more than 20 pounds for 6–8 weeks. *To prevent damaging suture/incision.* Get adequate rest and fluids. *To promote healing.* Discuss importance of bathing daily, using a mild soap, and applying lotion to dry skin. *To decrease bacteria on skin and, hence, risk of infection and to maintain skin integrity.* Discuss care of acne that can develop as a side effect of medication: no picking at acne, use of acne soap, use of over the counter (OTC) benzyl peroxide lotion in 5% or 10% if acne persists. *To maintain skin integrity and decrease risk of infection.* Instruct in necessity of treating skin carefully, avoiding strong sunlight, wearing sun block with an SPF of 15 or higher. *Steroid medications result in fragile skin that tears and burns easily. Broken skin provides entry for bacteria.* Assist as needed with oral care every 2–4 hours, keep mucous membranes moist, brush teeth with soft brush three times daily. *To maintain moist oral mucosa and decrease risk of infection. Brushing teeth removes the bacteria much more effectively than oral swabs.*

(continued)

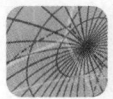

NURSING PROCESS: Patient Care Plan for Organ Transplants—*Continued*

Nursing Assessment and Diagnoses	Outcomes and Evaluation Parameters	Planning and Interventions with *Rationales*
		Assist as needed with lip care and application of lip balm. *To prevent drying and cracking and promote patient comfort.* Discuss and help problem solve difficulties with medication compliance and scheduling of appointments or laboratory tests. Provide referrals to collaborative services (dietary, social services, and transplant coordinator) as needed. *To promote compliance and optimal post-transplant care.*
		Discuss importance of selecting nutritious foods. Collaborate to create healthy menu options to make at home. *To promote healthy food choices and wound healing and maintain health.*
Imbalanced Nutrition: Less than Body Requirements related to decreased or inappropriate nutritional intake	Maintains optimal weight.	Determine optimal weight and plan to attain weight goal. *Medications can result in weight loss, or weight gain (especially prednisone, which stimulates appetite). Malnutrition impairs immune function; excessive weight places additional strain on all body organs.* Collaborate with dietitian if patient has special diet needs. *To promote optimal nutrition.*
	Lifestyle adapted to prevent transplant rejection and maintain optimal quality of life. Verbalizes and demonstrates lifestyle changes to adhere to medication and treatment regime, prevent infection, and promote optimal physical and mental health. Develops dietary plan and follows it at home.	Discuss importance of gradually increasing daily exercise and allowing rest periods between activities. *To promote increasing mobility and avoid excessive fatigue.* Collaborate with patient to develop a low-impact exercise plan that can be implemented when cleared by health care provider. *To encourage activity, promote overall health, decrease sedentary lifestyle, and prevent osteoporosis.*
Activity Intolerance related to postoperative transplant status	Practices self-care by participating in appropriate daily exercise.	Discuss risks of contact sports and strenuous exercises with new transplant. *To provide rationale for low-impact exercises and promote health.*
Risk for Sexual Dysfunction related to immunosuppressive medications and fatigue	Verbalizes concerns and questions regarding sexual function.	Offer information on possible sexual dysfunction related to immunosuppression medications and encourage discussion if patient has questions. *Medications can cause erectile dysfunction, decreased libido, and impaired orgasmic ability.*
Social Isolation related to decreased social interaction during transplant process, feelings of being "different"	Develops/maintains social support system.	Encourage family/friends to visit, call, and send cards and pictures. Encourage patient to phone and write notes to family/friends. *To decrease social isolation.*
Deficient Knowledge related to travel planning	Communicates travel plans, identifies transplant center closest to destination, and continues with scheduled medication regime.	Provide information on community resources including support groups/transplant clubs. *To provide support and guidance with problem solving.* Discuss importance of notifying transport team of travel plans. *To facilitate communication, plan for missed appointments, coordinate with transplant center at point of destination for any care needs.* Instruct patient to always hand-carry immunosuppressive medications if traveling by plane. *To avoid missing medication doses if luggage is lost.*

Sources: Carpenito-Moyet, L. (2008). *Nursing care plans and documentation* (5th ed.). Philadelphia: Lippincott Williams & Wilkins; Porth, C., & Sweeney, K. (2007). Alterations in immune response. In C. M. Porth (Ed.), *Essentials of pathophysiology* (pp. 293–319). St. Louis: Lippincott Williams & Wilkins.

Symptoms of primary deficiencies usually appear shortly after birth. Secondary immunodeficiency occurs when the immune system is damaged and unable to mount an appropriate immune response due to a variety of factors that range from normal aging to infections that eliminate immune cells and severely impair function as in HIV. The immunodeficiency section will briefly review the abnormalities related to primary immune deficiency and related disorders. The focus of this section will be on secondary immunodeficiencies and specifically the pathophysiology, clinical manifestations, and treatment of HIV.

Primary Immune Deficiencies

Primary immune deficiencies are categorized according to the type of immune cell that is genetically malformed or dysfunctional. These categories include phagocytic cell dysfunction, B-cell (humoral) deficiencies, T-cell (cell-mediated) deficiencies, and combined B-cell and T-cell deficiencies.

RESEARCH OPPORTUNITIES AND CLINICAL IMPACT RELATED TO THE ALLOIMMUNE HYPERSENSITIVITY RESPONSE

Research Area	Clinical Impact
Development of medications, such as monoclonal antibodies for use in preventing transplant rejection	Improved ability to transplant organs and reduce incidence of rejection
Identification of additional antibodies and markers to better match tissue and organs for transplant	Reduced transplant rejection through improved matching of host and recipient
Method of delivery of antirejection medication so that these medications are delivered directly to the transplant site rather than administered systemically	Reduced complications of systemic administration of antirejection drugs such as weight gain and increased risk of infection
Investigation into controlling immune cells through manipulation of newly identified cytokines	Regulation of the immune system to divert activity away from transplanted tissue, thus decreasing incidence of rejection
Trial of use of oral autoantigens to induce tolerance of transplanted pancreatic islet cells	Reduced transplant rejection of pancreatic islet cells in diabetic patients to improve quality of life and reduce comorbidities of diabetes
The role of B-cell deficiencies in reducing the risk of transplant rejection of pancreatic islet cells	Ability to better control and decrease B-cell activity to improve antirejection therapy for pancreatic transplant patients
Examination of HLA markers and the importance of a maximal match versus optimal match to prevent transplant rejection.	To better predict which transplants have higher risk of rejection and optimize antirejection drug therapy treatment.

Sources: American Academy of Allergy, Asthma and Immunology, http://www.acaai.org; Centers for Disease Control and Prevention, http://www.cdc.gov; DeFranco, A. L., Locksley, R., & Robertson, M. (2007). *Immunity: The immune response in infectious and inflammatory disease.* Sunderland, MA: Sinauer Associates.

Phagocytic Dysfunction

Several primary immune deficiencies have been identified related to abnormal function of phagocytic cells, most commonly neutrophils. For genetic reasons, neutrophils may not develop in adequate numbers or they may be dysfunctional. If an individual is unable to make an appropriate number of neutrophils, then she is unable to mount an adequate immune response. If the neutrophil DNA is dysfunctional, adequate numbers of neutrophils are unable to migrate and travel to the site of injury or infection and appropriately protect the host from foreign antigens (Rote, 2006).

B Cell (Humoral) Deficiencies

There are two different kinds of B-cell deficiencies. In the first group of disorders, B-cell precursors are unable to differentiate into plasma cells. This deficiency results in inadequate immunoglobulin levels (IgG, IgA, IgM, IgD, IgE) and recurrent infection. Immunoglobulins are discussed in Chapter 59 ⊙. The second type of B-cell disorder is the more serious one. In this disease, also known as Brutton's disease, the B cells are unable to differentiate into mature B cells. As a result no plasma cells can be found in circulation, and no immunoglobulins are produced causing major immune deficits including lack of immunologic memory (Rote, 2006).

T-Cell (Cell-Mediated) Deficiencies

The function of T cells is to regulate the immune response. T-cell deficiencies most commonly result in opportunistic infections. Therefore, these abnormalities do not commonly manifest themselves immediately after birth. This type of deficiency is suspected when an infant has repeated opportunistic infections such as candidiasis of the oral, vaginal, or rectal mucosa. There are a wide variety of T-cell-mediated deficiencies, which are differentiated by the type of T cells affected. One extreme example of T-cell-mediated dysfunction is the rare disorder called DiGeorge syndrome. In this disease the thymus does not develop properly and, therefore, T cells are unable to mature and appropriately stimulate an immune response to a foreign antigen. The result is susceptibility to opportunistic infections, symptoms of which begin to appear shortly after birth (Porth & Sweeney, 2007).

Combined B-Cell and T-Cell Deficiencies

Several variations of combined immunodeficiency syndrome have been identified and involve a mutation in one or more of the many genes that involve lymphocyte development and response. This results in low or absent levels of B lymphocytes and T lymphocytes in serum, as well as low or absent levels of IgG and IgA. Subsequently, the diseases that result from these deficiencies range from moderate to fatal in severity. The most severe form of congenital B- and T-cell deficiencies is severe combined immunodeficiency (SCID). This deficiency results from multiple genetic abnormalities that cause all white blood cell lines to fail to develop normally from a stem cell, leading to absence of all immune function. Infants with this genetic defect have failure to thrive, chronic diarrhea and multiple opportunistic infections that usually result in death before 2 years of age. More recently, bone marrow transplant has been used with success to treat infants identified with SCIDS at birth or within the first 3 months of life (Sommer, 2007). Bone marrow transplant is discussed in Chapter 64 ⊙.

Secondary Immune Deficiencies

Multiple factors contribute to secondary immune deficiencies; the most significant of these are listed in Chart 60–7 (p. 1922). Immunosuppressive therapy for treatment of autoimmune diseases and prevention of organ transplant rejection and also chemotherapy agents are the most prevalent medications that contribute to secondary immune deficiencies. Suppression of the

> **CHART 60–7 Common Causes of Secondary Immunodeficiency**
>
> - *Drug-induced immunodeficiency:* chemotherapy drugs, corticosteroids
> - *Age:* infants and older adults
> - *Malnutrition:* dietary deficiency, cirrhosis, cachexia
> - *Stress*
> - *Medical treatments:* surgery, anesthesia, radiation
> - *Injury:* trauma, burns
> - *Diseases:* AIDS, diabetes mellitus, chronic renal disease, malignancies, alcoholic cirrhosis, SLE

immune system places these patients at a high risk for **opportunistic infections (OIs)**, which are infections from microorganisms that are not usually considered pathogens, but cause disease if the immune system is impaired. Therefore, a primary focus of nursing care for patients who are immune suppressed is prevention of infection.

Other factors that can contribute to immune suppression are age and malnutrition. The effect of aging on the immune system is discussed in Chapter 59 ➋. Aging results in decreased thymus and T-cell functioning, which contribute to increased levels of autoimmune disease and malignancies in the older adult. Infants have decreased function because the immune system is still in the process of maturing.

Nutrition also plays a key role in immune function. Prolonged malnutrition with low protein intake contributes to decrease in lymphatic tissue, atrophy of the thymus gland, and altered cell-mediated immune response. Without appropriate nutritional intake, general cell function is impaired and increases the susceptibility to infection (Rote, 2006).

Major injuries such as trauma and burns destroy immune tissues such as the skin and can result in shock states that damage cell function. Medical treatment requiring surgery that removes immune organs such as the lymph nodes, the spleen, or the thymus also impairs immune response. Additionally, radiation suppresses immune function by destroying the lymph tissue directly or by causing atrophy of bone marrow function and depressing stem cell production of lymphocytes.

Numerous diseases significantly impact immune function by altering immune tissue or cells and leaving the individual susceptible to secondary infections. A primary example of the impact of disease on the immune system is evident in human immunodeficiency virus (HIV) infection, which is discussed in the remainder of the chapter.

Human Immunodeficiency Virus and Acquired Immunodeficiency Syndrome

Acquired immunodeficiency syndrome (AIDS) is the syndrome of opportunistic infections that occurs as the final stage of infection with the human immunodeficiency virus. AIDS was first recognized as a new disease entity in 1981, when previously healthy, young homosexual males in Los Angeles and New York were diagnosed with *Pneumocystis carinii* pneumonia (PCP) and a rare cancer, Kaposi's sarcoma. The diagnoses were extremely disturbing because these disease entities had previously

only been seen in individuals who were severely immunosuppressed, elderly, or debilitated, and indicated an unknown disease that caused profound immune impairment (Centers for Disease Control and Prevention [CDC], 1981a, 1981b).

During the course of the next few years, thousands of cases were primarily diagnosed among homosexual males and illicit injection drug users. Research, initially stymied because of the social stigma associated with homosexuality and illicit drug use, began to accelerate at a rapid rate as other population groups were diagnosed with AIDS. These individuals included hemophiliacs and other blood transfusion recipients, women through heterosexual contact with infected individuals, and finally infants of infected mothers. An understanding of the epidemic proportions of AIDS was beginning to dawn as cases were reported in multiple countries and almost all continents by the mid-1980s (CDC, 1995; Johnsen, 2003).

Etiology

The **human immunodeficiency virus (HIV)**, the virus that infects CD4 T cells and is the agent responsible for causing AIDS, was identified in 1984. It became apparent that AIDS was the most severe and final stage in a continuum of illnesses associated with HIV infection, which fatally impairs immune function. Subsequent research has identified two specific strains of HIV: HIV type 1 (HIV-1) and HIV type 2 (HIV-2). Virtually all of the cases in the United States are HIV-1. This strain is associated with acute and rapid progression from HIV infection to a diagnosis of AIDS. HIV-2 was identified in West Africa in 1986 and may have been present decades earlier. It is the dominant strain in Africa. HIV-2 involves a slower, milder progression to AIDS than HIV-1, with increased infectiousness at the end of the disease process. Both HIV-1 and HIV-2 have the same modes of transmission and are associated with the same opportunist infections (CDC, 1998).

Epidemiology

The severity of the HIV/AIDS epidemic has exceeded all initial predictions. As of December 2003, an estimated 20 million people worldwide had already died of AIDS, and another 38.6 million people, ages 15 to 45, were living with HIV/AIDS at the end of 2005 (United Nations Program on HIV/AIDS [UNAIDS], 2006). Of the 38.6 million people living with HIV/AIDS worldwide, 37 million are adults. Infected women comprise 47% of this population.

Resource-poor countries have been especially devastated by HIV/AIDS. Sub-Saharan Africa is home to 70% of the world's HIV/AIDS population and is the most affected region in the world (World Health Organization [WHO], 2007). This spread has primarily been attributed to heterosexual transmission, migration patterns, and limited condom use as well as significant mother-to-infant transmission. These factors have been fueled by poverty, lack of health care resources to diagnose HIV infection, lack of HIV prevention education, and limited access to antiretroviral treatment (Johnsen, 2003). The WHO's *AIDS Epidemic Update* estimates that in the year 2005 alone, there were 4.1 million people worldwide newly infected with HIV (13,000 new cases daily), and another 2.8 million deaths due to AIDS (UNAIDS, 2006). This represents a slight decline of about 10% since the peak HIV infection rate in the late 1990s. This is attributed to international efforts between 2001 and 2005 to provide antiretroviral therapy and prenatal screening, treatment, and education to pregnant women infected with HIV in resource-poor countries, specifically sub-Saharan African countries (UNAIDS, 2006).

In the United States, according to the CDC, as of December 2005, there was an estimated 1,039,000 to 1,185,000 people living with HIV infection, one-fourth of whom were unaware they were HIV positive. Approximately 40,000 new HIV infections are added to this number on an annual basis in the United States, half of which occur in people under 25 years of age. Seventy percent of new infections occur among men, and 30% among women (CDC, 2005c). The prevailing means of new HIV infection among men in the United States continues to be homosexual sex (60%), followed by injection of drugs with a contaminated needle (25%). New HIV infections in women in the United States continue to occur primarily through having unprotected heterosexual sex (75%), and approximately 25% are due to injection drug use with contaminated equipment (National Institute of Allergy and Infectious Diseases, 2004).

A cumulative total of 9,300 cases of AIDS have been reported in children ages 12 and under in the United States. Approximately 7% of these cases are attributed to exposure to infected blood products or tissue prior to 1985. The vast majority (about 91%) of cases are a result of prenatal exposure and infected mother-to-infant transmission (CDC, 2003a). The predominance of infected mother-to-infant transmission is consistent with global HIV/AIDS data for children, which estimates that 3 million children are now living with HIV/AIDS, the vast majority of whom are in resource-poor countries (WHO, 2002).

The face of HIV/AIDS is changing in the United States. Currently, 10% of the individuals diagnosed with HIV/AIDS are over 50 years of age. This percentage is expected to increase as effective antiretroviral medications increase life expectancy and the baby boom generation ages (Ress, 2003). HIV/AIDS in the United States also is changing in relationship to race and gender. There is an increase in the proportion of cases being reported among African Americans and Hispanics, as opposed to Caucasian males at the onset of the epidemic. More than half of new HIV infections occur among African Americans, though they represent only 13% of the population. Hispanics are also disproportionately represented (CDC, 2003a). Additionally, women account for an increasing proportion of AIDS cases. This is evidenced by the fact that from 1985 to 2002, the proportion of HIV/AIDS cases among women increased from 7% to 27% (National Institute of Allergy and Infectious Disease, 2004). It also is disturbing to note that women are diagnosed later and begin treatment at a later stage than men and, consequently, have higher morbidity and mortality rates (Branson et al., 2006).

The sad reality of HIV/AIDS infection in the 21st century is that in countries with limited economic resources it continues to be a devastating and rapidly fatal illness, predominantly affecting individuals 15 to 45 years of age in the prime of life and reproductive capacity. In economically stable countries, where there is access to antiretroviral treatment and public health resources, HIV/AIDS is transitioning to a chronic disease process that is involving an increased proportion of elderly, nonwhite, and female victims.

Transmission

While the devastation HIV can wreak is catastrophic, HIV transmission is limited to contact with infected body fluids that have lymphocytes that can harbor HIV. These fluids include blood, semen, vaginal secretions, and breast milk. There also must be a sufficient viral load and a susceptible host for transmission to occur. An infected individual with a high viral load (first months after initial infection, or during an AIDS illness) has an increased ability to transmit HIV. Additionally, prolonged or repeated exposure to infected fluids will greatly increase the risk of transmission (Rote, 2006).

It is important to understand that HIV is not spread through casual contact such as working with someone, shaking hands, hugging, dry kissing, or sharing eating utensils. Repeated studies have failed to demonstrate transmission of the virus through sweat, tears, saliva, urine, emesis, sputum, respiratory droplets, or feces. Studies on vector transmission by insects have also been negative (CDC, 2005c). The Risk Factors box lists the high risk factors associated with HIV transmission.

Sexual Transmission

The most common method of HIV transmission is through sexual contact with an HIV-infected partner. Sexual activity enables exposure to blood, semen, and vaginal secretions, which contain lymphocytes that harbor HIV. Breaks in the skin caused by sexual trauma, such as anal intercourse or the presence of genital lesions from other sexually transmitted infections (STIs), will increase the risk of infection.

The majority of reported HIV infections in the United States are in men who have sex with men, including homosexuals, bisexuals, and prison population groups (CDC, 2005c). The incidence of HIV infection among men who have sex with men declined in the 1990s due to intense AIDS awareness and education campaigns and an emphasis on safer sex practices. However, current data indicate an increased incidence of unsafe sexual practices, and rising HIV infection rates in some urban areas among men who have sex with men. Recent data from the CDC indicates that number of HIV/AIDS diagnoses among men who have sex with men increased 85% between 2003 and 2004 (CDC, 2005c). This may be attributed in part to the association between the knowledge of the benefits of antiretroviral therapy in deterring HIV progression to AIDS and a relapse in high-risk sexual behaviors. The National Guidelines box (p. 1924) lists CDC guidelines for antiretroviral therapy.

Heterosexual HIV transmission is the most common method of infection in developing countries such as Africa and Asia, where approximately 90% of all new HIV infections occur worldwide (Johnsen, 2003). The rate of infection among women is rising steadily. The majority of women do not engage in high-risk behavior and practice monogamy, but are being infected

RISK FACTORS for HIV Infection

- Unprotected sex (sex without a male or female condom) with an HIV-infected male or female
- Sharing of injection equipment
- Blood product recipient (especially prior to screening in 1985)
- Infants born to mothers with HIV infection

Sources: Centers for Disease Control and Prevention. (2007, July). *HIV and AIDS: Are you at risk?* Retrieved September 3, 2008, from http://www.cdc.gov/hiv/resources/brochures/at-risk.htm; Kirton, C. D., Talotta, D., & Zwolski, K. (Eds.). (2001). *Handbook of HIV/AIDS nursing.* St. Louis, Mosby; Shaw, J. K., & Mahoney, E. A. (Eds.). (2003). *HIV/AIDS nursing secrets.* Philadelphia: Hanley & Belfus.

NATIONAL GUIDELINES for Antiretroviral Therapy in HIV Infections

Population	Guideline	Summary
Adults and adolescents	*Guidelines for the Use of Antiretroviral Agents in HIV-1-Infected Adults and Adolescents* (2006)	Guidelines for treating HIV-infected adults and adolescents, including utilization of resistance testing, initiation of HIV treatment, preferred first-line regimens, adverse events to antiretroviral medications, managing treatment-experienced patients, and considerations for special populations.
Pregnant women and infants	*Recommendations for the Use of Antiretroviral Drugs in Pregnant HIV-1-Infected Women for Maternal Health and Interventions to Reduce Perinatal HIV-1 Transmission in the United States* (2006)	Guidelines for treating HIV-infected pregnant women and interventions to prevent perinatal transmission, including information on drug regimens, safety and toxicity of medications, delivery options, and care of infants born to HIV-infected mothers.
Pediatric	*Guidelines for the Use of Antiretroviral Agents in Pediatric HIV Infection* (2006)	Guidelines for treating HIV-infected infants, children, and adolescents, including clinical monitoring, initiation of treatment, pediatric-specific drug information, and managing complications.
Health care workers exposed to HIV on the job	*Updated U.S. Public Health Service Guidelines for the Management of Occupational Exposures to HIV and Recommendations for Postexposure Prophylaxis* (2005)	Guidelines for the procedures and prevention measures that should be followed when workers are exposed to HIV on the job.
HIV-infected individuals	*Guidelines for the Prevention of Opportunistic Infections in Persons Infected with Human Immunodeficiency Virus* (2002)	Public Health Service and Infectious Diseases Society of America guidelines for the prevention of opportunistic infections in persons infected with HIV.
HIV-positive adults, adolescents, and children with infections	*Treating Opportunistic Infections Among HIV-Infected Adults and Adolescents* (2004) *and Treating Opportunistic Infections Among HIV-Exposed and Infected Children* (2004)	Guidelines for treatment of infections in individuals who are HIV infected or HIV exposed.
Individuals with TB and HIV	*Treatment of Tuberculosis* (2003)	Guidelines for the treatment for and management of people with tuberculosis.
HIV-positive individuals and partners	*Incorporating HIV Prevention into the Medical Care of Persons Living with HIV* (2003)	Recommendations of the CDC, NIH, Health Resources and Services Administration, and the HIV Medicine Association of the Infectious Diseases Society of America, including risk screening, behavior interventions, partner counseling and referrals, legal issues, partner notification.
HIV testing in the general population	*Revised Recommendations for HIV Testing of Adults, Adolescents, and Pregnant Women in Health-Care Settings* (2006)	Recommendations on HIV testing procedures for health care providers working in hospital emergency departments, urgent care clinics, inpatient services, substance abuse treatment clinics, public health clinics, community clinics, correctional health care facilities, and primary care settings. Recommendation for general HIV screening, with ability to "opt-out" instead of screening only high-risk or symptomatic individuals.

Note: All of the guidelines listed in this chart are available from http://aidsinfo.nih.gov.

Source: Bartlett, J. G., & Lane, H. C. (2007). *Guidelines for the use of antiretroviral agents in HIV-1-infected adults and adolescents. Developed by the DHHS Panel on Antiretroviral Guidelines for Adults and Adolescents—A working group of the Office of AIDS Research Advisory Council.* Retrieved January 10, 2008, from http://aidsinfo.nih.gov/contentfiles/AdultandAdolescentGL.pdf.

through unsafe sex practices with their HIV-infected male partners (UNAIDS, 2006). HIV-infected male-to-female transmission occurs more frequently than infected female-to-male transmission. This occurs because the risk of infection is greater for the partner who receives the semen and has a prolonged exposure to contact with the HIV-infected fluid.

Contaminated Needle Transmission

A major factor in the spread of HIV has been transmission by sharing of injection equipment. Used needles contain only a small amount of blood, but this can be contaminated with HIV. Drug preparation equipment used in mixing drugs can also be contaminated. If individuals are consistently sharing needles and equipment, as is common with illicit drug use, the potential for repeated exposure exists, which increases the risk of transmission. Sharing equipment to inject drugs is the major means of transmission in Eastern and Central Europe, East Asia, and the Pacific Islands (UNAIDS, 2006).

Contaminated Blood Products

Blood products prior to 1985 were not screened for HIV antibodies. As a result HIV-contaminated blood has been the cause of 2% of the adult and 8% of the reported AIDS cases in the United States (CDC, 2006a). Since 1985, with the use of HIV antibody screening on all blood transfusion products, this risk has been significantly reduced. The blood supply in the United States is among the safest in the world. More recently, blood screening tests have become available to detect for the virus through DNA testing prior to the production of antibodies. The risk of infection (estimated to be 1 in 2,000,000 transfusions) does still exist because of the **window period**, the time between actual HIV infection and when the tests can detect the presence of the virus or antibodies to the virus in blood. The length of the window period is currently 12 to 16 days (American Red Cross, 2003). Further discussion on blood product testing can be found in Chapter 23 .

Perinatal Transmission

HIV infection can be transmitted from an infected mother to her infant during pregnancy, at the time of delivery through exposure to the mother's blood, or after birth via breast-feeding. Multiple factors influence this potential for transmission. Blood is a highly infectious substance and the fetus receives oxygen, nutrients, antibodies, and other substances via the placental circulation. HIV antibodies are transmitted from an HIV-infected mother to the infant via placental circulation. This is why infants born to HIV-infected mothers will test positive for HIV antibodies immediately after birth. However, transmission of the virus may not have occurred.

The process of HIV-infected mother-to-infant transmission is not clearly understood. Researchers currently believe that the placenta actually plays a protective role, creating a barrier to HIV transmission, and that 60% of HIV mother-to-infant transmissions may occur at the time of delivery (Anderson, 2004). It is known that the risk of HIV mother-to-infant transmission is significantly increased if the mother has a high amount of HIV in circulation, an advanced AIDS disease, and/or breast-feeds. Research has clearly indicated that treatment of the mother during pregnancy with antiretroviral therapy and a short-term treatment of the infant postdelivery substantially reduce the risk of HIV mother-to-infant transmission (Branson et al., 2006). It is estimated that without maternal antiretroviral treatments 14% to 40% of infants born to HIV-infected mothers would be infected (Averitt & Sowell, 2003). The rate of perinatal infection is related to the mother's access to health care and antiretroviral therapy. In economically poor countries such as South Africa, where there is limited antiretroviral treatment and health care, infection rates are among the highest (UNAIDS, 2006).

The mode of delivery for HIV-infected women is an area of ongoing research and clinical debate. Increasing evidence supports the theory that use of cesarean sections in clinical situations where there is prolonged labor, or rupture of membranes greater than 4 hours before delivery, or a high viral load may help prevent prenatal transmission (Averitt & Sowell, 2003). Others argue that for women who have undetectable viral loads or who are on antiviral medications and have received adequate prenatal care a vaginal delivery may be a viable option. The Public Health Service Task Force (2006) recommends scheduled cesarean section for HIV-1 RNA (viral load) > 1,000 copies/mL. Because a cesarean section is a surgical procedure and also may present risks to the mother and infant, the Public Health Service Task Force (2006) recommends that viral load levels be evaluated at 34 to 36 weeks' gestation to enable discussion between the mother and her clinician as to the optimal delivery mode. There is general consensus that a cesarean section helps minimize the risk of perinatal transmission when viral loads are high. However, more research is needed in relationship to the benefits of cesarean section in specific clinical situations before it is deemed the accepted mode of delivery for all HIV-infected women.

Transmission to Health Care Workers

Health care workers, especially laboratory technicians and nurses, have a very small but real risk of occupational exposure to HIV transmission through needlestick injuries and mucous membrane exposure of infected patient body fluids. The CDC (2001) estimates that the average risk of HIV infection following a cut exposure or needlestick exposure to HIV-infected blood is 0.3%. The key factors in HIV infection of health care workers has been exposure to a large volume of blood delivered by a deep puncture, or extended contact with infected bloody dressings to open cuts on the health workers' hands, arms, or face (NIOSH, 1999).

To address these issues, the CDC together with the Hospital Infection Control Practices Advisory Committee (HICPAC) developed and mandated standard precautions to reduce the risk of blood and body fluid exposure and transmission of pathogens. Additionally, the Needlestick Safety and Prevention Act became law in 2000 and it mandates the use of needleless devices by all health care facilities to protect against sharps injuries. The nurse needs to remain vigilant in the use of standard precautions when working with any blood and body fluids. Appropriate use of needle guards and needleless medication administration systems and disposal of sharps in designated containers are essential.

In the event of a blood or body fluid exposure, the CDC in *Management of Occupational Blood Exposures* (2001) recommends that specific steps be taken. These include immediately washing the exposed site with soap and water and repeated flushing of exposed mucous membranes with water. The process of determining the risk of exposure, HIV testing of the source of contamination, and baseline HIV testing of the health care worker should also occur immediately. To facilitate this process, most health care facilities require urgent reporting of blood exposure incidents to the health care workers' supervisors and follow-up with employee health services for treatment and any additional testing.

The CDC recommends that health care workers who have had a significant blood or body fluid exposure be offered antiretroviral medications postexposure because some data suggest that such prophylaxis may significantly reduce the risk of HIV infection. However, the adverse effects of antiretroviral therapy can be substantial and this must be considered when evaluating the exposure risk and use of prophylactic antiretroviral therapy. The course of antiretroviral therapy is 4 weeks and should be started immediately or within 72 hours of exposure to be maximally effective (CDC, 2005a).

Pathophysiology

HIV belongs to a class of viruses made up of ribonucleic acid (RNA). Every virus is an obligate parasite that requires a living cell as the host. RNA viruses also are called retroviruses because they must be transcribed back into DNA through the action of an enzyme called **reverse transcriptase** in order to reproduce. In the process of infection, the virus first enters a cell with a specific type of receptor found on the surface of some cells called a CD4 receptor. Lymphocytes, called **CD4+ T cells**, are T-helper cells that have more CD4 receptor sites than other types of cells; therefore, they are the primary targets of infection (Rote, 2006). HIV entering the host stimulates a humoral and cell-mediated response that activates the immune system and recruits CD4+ T cells to the area of infection in the blood. As a result HIV is able to infect many CD4+ T cells in a short period (Porth & Sweeney, 2007). Other cells such as monocytes, macrophages, astrocytes (cells in the brain), and

oligodendrocytes (cells in the central nervous system) also have CD4 receptors, which explains why HIV may infect these cells.

After the viral particle enters the cell, reverse transcriptase creates a DNA particle from the RNA. The DNA particle enters the nucleus and inserts itself into the host's DNA. HIV DNA can then direct proteins and enzymes to replicate the HIV portion and create more HIV particles. Figure 60–5 ■ describes this process. It is important to understand the viral replication process because medications to control HIV infection are directed at different aspects of HIV replication. The human immunodeficiency virus is devastating to the host's immune system, specifically the CD4+ T cells. As previously discussed under normal immune function in Chapter 59 ⊘, CD4+ T cells exist to help regulate the immune system. If an individual is unable to initiate an immune response because of the loss of T cells, even the most benign infection can be deadly.

HIV is a highly infective virus for several reasons. It replicates easily and rapidly and mutates frequently. These mutations make it extremely difficult to create a consistently effective drug or a vaccine because the shape of the HIV molecules changes frequently (Rote, 2006). Additionally, the normal number of CD4+ T cells is 800 to 1,200 microliter of blood, and competent T-helper cells live approximately 100 days. CD4+ T cells that

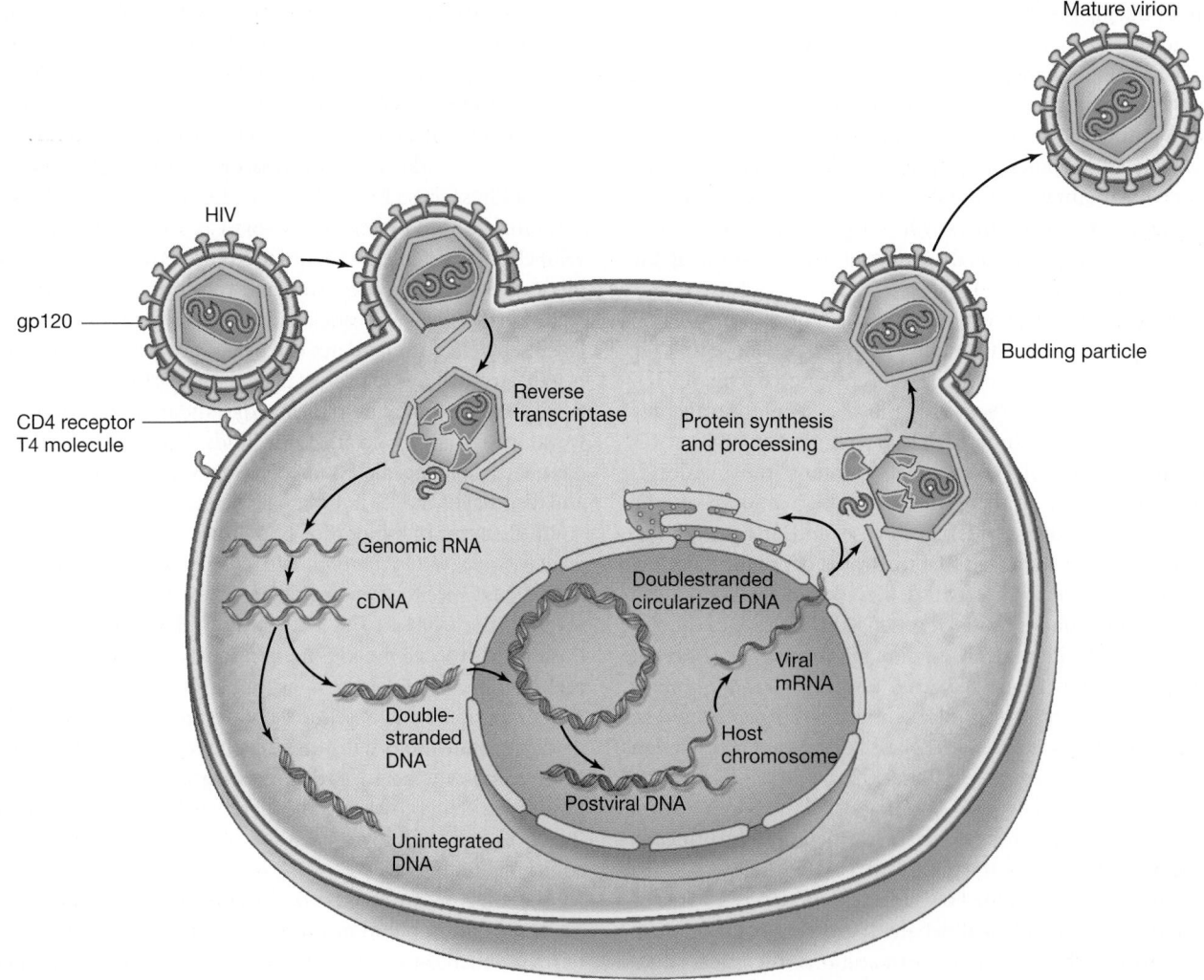

FIGURE 60–5 ■ HIV infecting CD4+ T cell.

have been infected with HIV are now known to live only 2 days (Fauci, 1996). It also is known that the infected host can adequately compensate for the loss of CD4+ T cells for several years. Research has shown the bone marrow to be capable of producing adequate cells despite the HIV infection destroying up to 1 billion CD4+ T cells per day for many years (Fauci, 1996).

Eventually, the immune system function and CD4+ T cells are overwhelmed by the virus and destroyed through several mechanisms. Every new HIV particle attaches to the cell membrane and buds outward as it breaks free of the host cell. When many HIV particles are released, holes develop in the plasma membrane. Cytoplasm and organelles can leak out, killing the cell. Lymphoid tissue also can house infected T cells and viral particles. Over time the degradation of the lymph system by HIV sheds additional virus into the blood. This has been shown to be a factor in the progression of the disease. Also, macrophages and monocytes can be infected with HIV. Macrophages become a reservoir for HIV because the molecule can replicate within the cell. Trauma, inflammation, and infection at the site of the macrophage can cause rupture of the macrophage and the release of HIV into surrounding tissue (DeFranco et al., 2007; Fauci, 1991). Additionally, as part of the normal immune response, antibodies to HIV attach to infected T-helper cells and stimulate the activation of the complement cascade. This results in the direct lysis of the cell membrane and death of the infected cell. Cell lysis by complement as explained in Chapters 59 and 63 ☺ also releases any completed viral particles into the host's system, further adding to the viral load.

Research is continuing to explore other mechanisms about how HIV destroys infected cells. Apoptosis or programmed cell death of infected cells is one theory currently being researched. Additionally, increased production of cytokines may be implicated in destruction of infected T-helper cells. Finally, superantigen and autoimmune responses also are being studied as possible mechanisms of cell destruction in HIV infection (DeFranco et al., 2007).

Stages of HIV/AIDS

The classification system of HIV infection and progression to AIDS was expanded and redefined by the CDC in 1993 to emphasize the significance of CD4+ T-cell counts as a marker of HIV-related immunosuppression. The subsequent classification system is based on two categories: clinical conditions associated with HIV infections and laboratory CD4+ T-cell counts. There are three major classifications that are differentiated by the clinical symptoms: A (asymptomatic), B (symptomatic, but not AIDS defining), and C (symptomatic AIDS indicator conditions). Three classifications also differentiate the CD4+ T-cell laboratory tests and are based on the declining number of CD4+ T cells per microliter of blood: category 1: >500 cells/µL; category 2: 200 to 400 cells/µL; and category 3: <200 cells/µL. Chart 60–8 (p. 1928) describes the CDC classification system. This classification system is important because it tracks the progression of the disease, helps determine the type and effectiveness of antiretroviral therapy, and determines if changes in therapy are required. It also provides clear definitions of AIDS diseases for research purposes, the results of which will facilitate more effective disease treatments.

Immediately following infection with HIV, the virus proliferates rapidly and the immune system begins to make antibodies against the virus. However, the viral replication of HIV increases more rapidly than the immune system is able to respond, resulting in a high **viral load** (the number of viral particles in a sample of blood). During the period of primary infection (1 to 3 weeks) the individual may by asymptomatic or display symptoms of **acute retroviral syndrome**, which is characterized by malaise, fever, lymphadenopathy, and skin rash. The fact that an infected individual can be asymptomatic or have only vague, flu-like symptoms makes early diagnosis of HIV infection difficult (Porth & Sweeney, 2007).

Additionally, the first months after infection encompass the "window period" in which the infected individual has not produced sufficient HIV antibodies that can be measured by an HIV antibody test. The window period usually lasts up to 3 months, but can extend to 6 months in some individuals. During the window period HIV antibody tests are negative, even in the presence of HIV infection. HIV antigen tests are now available that can detect the presence of viral particles as early as 2 weeks after infection; however, a window period still remains. These facts coupled with the initial high viral load are major contributing factors to the spread of HIV among those engaging in high-risk behaviors (Branson et al., 2006).

In the months following initial infection, proliferation of the virus, and stimulation of the immune responses, the viral load stabilizes. During this period of time, immune responses slow replication, but the virus is not completely eliminated. The infected individual in this first stage of HIV infection may show signs of an acute infection such as fatigue, fever, and generalized lymphadenopathy. It is during this time (usually between 3 weeks to 3 months after initial infection) that the individual converts to **HIV antibody positive status**, also referred to as *seropositive status*. This indicates that there is infection with HIV that is resulting in the production of HIV antibodies (Shaw, 2003). In some individuals conversion to HIV seropositive antibody status may take as long as 6 months. The individual may remain in category A, a relatively symptom-free stage for as long as 8 to 10 years, although the viral replication is active and will increase substantially as the immune system deteriorates (Porth & Sweeney, 2007).

Progression to category B HIV is defined by a transition from asymptomatic status to generalized symptoms. These symptoms may include but are not limited to fever of unknown origin, oral or vaginal candidiasis, herpes zoster, shingles, peripheral neuropathy, or pelvic inflammatory disease.

Category C is **AIDS indicator conditions**. A diagnosis of AIDS is made when the HIV-infected individual is diagnosed with an opportunistic infection or an AIDS defining cancer or when the CD4+ T-cell count falls below 200 cells/µL. Examples of AIDS defining diseases include PCP, toxoplasmosis, cytomegalovirus, non-Hodgkin's lymphoma, and Kaposi's sarcoma.

It is important that nurses understand the pathophysiology of HIV/AIDS and the specific stages of HIV disease and progression to AIDS because of the significant role nurses have in patient education about HIV/AIDS, transmission of the disease, and purpose of the prescribed medications. This knowledge base will also enable the nurse to identify issues and necessary nursing interventions specific to the different categories of HIV/AIDS. For example, an infected individual in category A

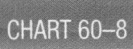

CHART 60–8 **Classification System for HIV Infection and Expanded AIDS Surveillance Case Definition for Adolescents and Adults**

Clinical Category A Asymptomatic, Acute HIV	Clinical Category B Symptomatic, But Not Category C Conditions	Clinical Category C AIDS-Defining Conditions
One or more of the conditions listed below in an adolescent (≥13 years) with documented HIV infection and no conditions in categories B or C: • Asymptomatic HIV infection • Persistent generalized lymphadenopathy • Acute HIV infection with accompanying illness (acute retroviral syndrome) or history of acute infection **CD4+ T-Cell Count Categories** A1 ≥ 500 cells/µL A2 ≥ 200–499 cells/µL A3 ≤ 200 cells/µL	Examples of conditions in category B include but are not limited to: • Candidiasis: oropharyngeal (thrush) • Candidiasis: vulvovaginal (persistent, frequent, or resistant to therapy) • Cervical dysplasia/cervical carcinoma *in situ* • Constitutional symptoms: persistent fever (38.5°C) or diarrhea lasting for more than 1 month • Hairy leukoplakia (oral) • Herpes zoster involving two distinct episodes, or more than 1 dermatome • Idiopathic thrombocytopenic purpura • Pelvic inflammatory disease • Peripheral neuropathy **CD4+ T-Cell Count Categories** B1 ≥ 500 cells/µL B2 ≥ 200–499 cells/µL B3 ≤ 200 cells/µL	• Candidiasis of bronchi, trachea, lungs, or esophagus • Cervical cancer (invasive) • Coccidioidomycosis • Cryptococcosis • Cryptosporidiosis with chronic diarrhea for more than 1 month • Cytomegalovirus disease (other than liver, spleen, or nodes) • Encephalopathy (HIV related) • Herpes simplex: chronic ulcers, bronchitis, pneumonitis, or esophagitis • Histoplasmosis • Isosporiasis with diarrhea for more than 1 month • Kaposi's sarcoma • Lymphoma: Burkitt's, immunoblastic, primary brain • *Mycobacterium avium* complex • *Mycobacterium tuberculosis* • *Pneumocystis carinii* pneumonia • Pneumonia (recurrent) • Wasting syndrome due to HIV **CD4+ T-Cell Count Categories** C1 ≥ 500 cells/µL C2 ≥ 200–499 cells/µL C3 ≤ 200 cells/µL

Note: As of January 1, 1993, individuals with category C conditions and those in categories A3 and B3 were considered to have AIDS.

Sources: Adapted from Centers for Disease Control and Prevention. (1993). Revised classification system for HIV infection and the expanded surveillance case definition of AIDS among adolescents and adults. *Morbidity and Mortality Weekly Report, 44* (RR-17). Retrieved February 23, 2007, from http://www.cdc.gov/mmwr/preview/mmwrhtml/00018871.htm; Centers for Disease Control and Prevention. (1999). Appendix: Revised surveillance case definition for HIV infection. *Morbidity and Mortality Weekly Report, 45* (RR-13), 29–31; Porth, C., & Sweeney, K. (2007). Alterations in immune response. In C. M. Porth (Ed.), *Essentials of pathophysiology* (pp. 293–319). St. Louis: Lippincott Williams & Wilkins.

with a latent infection will need educational information focused on avoiding transmitting the disease and new medications, whereas care for the individual with a declining CD4 count in category B will focus more on infection prevention, symptom management, and medication adherence.

Clinical Manifestations of HIV/AIDS

The clinical manifestations of HIV/AIDS are varied and may affect almost any organ in the body. Nurses need to understand the causes, signs and symptoms, diagnostic tests, and possible medical interventions in order to plan collaboratively for patient care. This will enable the nurse to provide appropriate nursing interventions and promote comfort measures that enhance the quality of life for patients with HIV/AIDS throughout the course of the disease. The specific clinical manifestations related to the opportunistic infections are outlined next.

Opportunistic Infections and Malignancies

Opportunistic infections (OI) occur in HIV-infected individuals as the virus destroys sufficient numbers of CD4+ T cells and the body is not able to protect itself. As CD4+ counts drop to <200 cells/µL the incidence of opportunistic infection accelerates rapidly. Malignancies occur due to impairment in the immune system's ability to recognize and destroy abnormal cells that are regulated, in part, by T-cell function.

Diseases associated with HIV/AIDS are a result of impairment of the immune system that leaves the HIV-infected individuals susceptible to OIs and malignancies. Diseases also can be the direct result of the effects of HIV on specific tissue, as seen in AIDS-related GI and neurological dysfunction. Chart 60–9 describes the clinical manifestations of the most common opportunistic diseases associated with HIV/AIDS, as well as the diagnostic tests and medical treatment the nurse needs to anticipate coordinating as part of collaborative care.

CHART 60–9   **HIV/AIDS: Common Opportunistic Diseases**

Clinical Manifestation by Body System	Possible Opportunistic Infection or Disease	Diagnostic Tests and Findings	Medical Treatment	Nursing Critical Assessments
Respiratory				
1. Increased respirations, nonproductive cough, dyspnea on exertion, adventitious breath sounds, increased, hypoxemia	1. *Pneumocystis carinii* pneumonia (PCP)	1. CD4 < 200 cells/μL Chest x-ray (bilateral patchy infiltrates), sputum culture or bronchoalveolar lavage (+ culture growth for PCP)	1. Antibiotic therapy (trimethoprim-sulfamethoxazole [TMP-SMZ]), bronchodilator therapy	1 & 2 & 3 Respiratory rate, work of breathing, auscultate breath sounds, pulse oximetry saturation, sputum color/amount, monitor arterial blood gases (ABGs), to determine need for oxygen and ventilation support
2. Dyspnea, productive cough, blood-tinged sputum 1 & 2 General body system: fever, night sweats, fatigue, weight loss are common to almost all respiratory opportunistic infections	2. *Mycobacterium tuberculosis* (TB)	2. TB skin test, chest x-ray, sputum for AFB stain and culture	2. Isoniazid (INH), ethambutol (Myambutol), rifampin (Rifadin), pyrazinamide	
3. Increasing shortness of breath eventually progressing to respiratory failure	3. Kaposi's sarcoma	3. Chest x-ray, bronchoscopy examination and biopsy	3. Chemotherapy, radiation, alpha-interferon to decrease tumor size	
Gastrointestinal (GI)				
1. Inflamed oral mucosa, GI pain/cramping, bloody diarrhea, weight loss	1. Cytomegalovirus (CMV)	1. Stool specimen for examination and culture, endoscopy exam, biopsy, and culture	1. Medications: foscarnet (Foscavir), ganciclovir (Cytovene), cidofovir (Vistide)	1 & 2 Daily fluid intake and output, diarrhea, daily weight, oral intake (calorie count) Laboratory tests: complete blood count (CBC), electrolytes, blood urea nitrogen (BUN), serum albumin and transferrin levels
2. Anorexia, diarrhea, nausea, vomiting, weight loss, abdominal pain	2. *Mycobacterium avium* complex (MAC)	2. Stool specimen and culture, small bowel biopsy with AFB stain and culture	2. Antibiotic treatment when T cells < 100 cells/μL clarithromycin, (Biaxin), azithromycin (Zithromax), ciprofloxacin (Cipro), rifampin (Rifadin)	
3. White patches in mouth, throat, tongue that bleeds if scraped, redness in oral cavity, → pain and difficulty swallowing, progressing to esophagus	3. Oral candidiasis	3. Microscope exam and culture of lesion scraping	3. Antifungals: Clotrimazole troches or Nystatin topical, po/IV fluconazole (Diflucan), clotrimazole (Lotrimin), itraconazole, amphotericin B (Fungizone)	3. Oral cavity, pain with swallowing, po intake ability
4. Anorexia, weight loss >10%, chronic diarrhea, fever >30 days unknown origin, chronic weakness, decreased muscle mass	4. HIV wasting (HIV causes changes to GI cells)	4. Rule out other causes: stool specimen and culture, endoscopy exam biopsy and culture	4. Symptom management • Diarrhea: octreotide acetate (Sandostatin) • Skin breakdown: barrier creams • Nutrition: appetite stimulant (Megestrol) • NV: antiemetic, Dronabinol • Oral nutritional supplement: Advera	4. Daily fluid I&O, diarrhea, daily weight, po intake (calorie count) Laboratory tests: CBC, electrolytes, BUN, serum albumin and transferrin levels

(continued)

| CHART 60–9 | **HIV/AIDS: Common Opportunistic Diseases—*Continued*** |

Neurological

1. Forgetfulness, decreased attention and concentration, progressive impaired motor function	1. HIV encephalopathy (virus causes dysfunction of neuro cells)	1. Rule out opportunistic infections or malignancy: cultures of blood, CSF; CT scan, MRI	1. Antiretroviral therapy, comfort measures, symptom management for any other clinical manifestations	1. Orientation, ability to remember medications, level of self-care with ADLs, gait, and risk of falling
2. Headaches, sensory and visual deficits, dizziness, aphasia, seizures, personality changes	2. Primary brain lymphoma	2. Tests listed above	2. Chemotherapy/ radiation	2. Same as above
3. Headache, decreased level of consciousness, fever, stiff neck, visual changes, seizures	3. Cryptococcal meningitis	3. CT scan, CSF analysis, serum antigen test	3. Antifungal medications: amphotericin B (Fungizone), fluconazole (Diflucan), flucytosine (Ancobon), itraconazole (Sporanox)	3. Level of consciousness, neurological function, symptoms of infection (fever, stiff neck, WBC)
4. Pain, numbness in extremities, general weakness, decreased deep tendon reflexes, impotence	4. HIV peripheral neuropathy (caused by HIV demyelinating disorder)	4. Rule out other potential causes by above tests	4. Neurontin for pain	4. Neurological function, pain, changes in sexual patterns

Skin

1. Nonblanching, flat or raised purple-brown lesions Progression of various shapes and sizes	1. Kaposi's sarcoma	1. Biopsy of lesion	1. Liquid nitrogen or cryotherapy to skin lesions, radiation of lesions, chemotherapy, alpha-interferon to decrease tumor size	1. Inspect skin for raised or flat purple-brown lesions of various sizes, pain or discomfort, changes in any other body system such GI and respiratory
2. Ulcer lesions of oral and nasal mucosa or ulcer lesions of the genital and perianal mucosa	2. Herpes simplex virus type 1 (HSV1) oral, herpes simplex virus type 2 (HSV2)	2. Viral culture	2. Antiviral medications: acyclovir (Zovirax), famciclovir (Famvir), valacyclovir (Valtrex), foscarnet (Foscavir)	2. Ask patient regarding pain/discomfort of mouth or perianal area. Inspect mucous membranes of the mouth, nose, and perianal area

Eyes

Visual changes: "seeing spots," unilateral visual loss → bilateral loss → blindness	Cytomegalovirus (CMV)	Ophthalmoscope examination	T-cell counts < 50 cells/μL = antiviral (ganciclovir or foscarnet), not curable infection, medication must be taken for life. Side effects of medications are significant and can interfere with HAART	Decreased vision ability, visual fields, presence of "spots," ability to read medication labels and identify drug and dose to take

CHART 60–9	**HIV/AIDS: Common Opportunistic Diseases—*Continued***

Female Genitalia/
Sexual Health

1. Genital itching, bleeding between menses, redness/swelling of external genitalia, white or yellow cheeselike discharge	1. Vaginal candidiasis	1. Microscopic examination and culture of lesion scraping	1. Antifungal medications: fluconazole (Diflucan), clotrimazole (Lotrimin), severe/incurable infection with above medications = amphotericin B (Fungizone)	1. Sexual health risk factors including multiple sex partners, unprotected sex, changes in genitalia or new discharge. Color of genitalia and presence of redness, vaginal discharge
2. Bleeding between menses or after intercourse; foul-smelling, blood-tinged vaginal discharge	2. Cervical intraepithelial neoplasia or cervical cancer	2. Cervical colposcopic examination and cone biopsy	2. Chemotherapy and radiation	2. Sexual health risk factors as above. Changes in menses bleeding or unusual vaginal discharge

Sources: Carpenito-Moyet, L. (2008). *Nursing care plans and documentation* (5th ed.). Philadelphia: Lippincott Williams & Wilkins; Corless, I. B., & Nicholas, P. K. (2003). Nursing care of patients with HIV/AIDS. In J. K. Shaw & E. A. Mahoney (Eds.), *HIV/AIDS nursing secrets* (pp. 33–39). Philadelphia: Hanley & Belfus; Crowe, S., Hoy, J., & Mills, J. (Eds.). (2002). *Management of the HIV-infected patient.* London: Taylor & Francis; Kirton, C. D., Talotta, D., & Zwolski, K. (Eds.). (2001). *Handbook of HIV/AIDS nursing.* St. Louis, Mosby; Porth, C., & Sweeney, K. (2007). Alterations in immune response. In C. M. Porth (Ed.), *Essentials of pathophysiology* (pp. 293–319). St. Louis: Lippincott Williams & Wilkins.

The last column lists critical assessment issues that need to be the focus of nursing assessment. This information provides more detail on specific AIDS-related diseases to enhance the nurse's understanding of these clinical manifestations.

Pneumocystis carinii Pneumonia

***Pneumocystis carinii* pneumonia (PCP)** is an opportunistic fungal respiratory infection that can develop in severely immunosuppressed individuals. In the early years of the AIDS epidemic, 75% of HIV-infected patients developed PCP at some point in their illness. Advances in disease understanding and treatment with prophylactic antibiotic therapy and corticosteroids have resulted in a decrease in the incidence of PCP. PCP is a fungal infection that proliferates in the alveoli causing bronchial consolidation. Chest x-ray results will indicate bilateral patchy infiltrates. PCP results in symptoms of acute respiratory failure with decreasing arterial oxygen levels to less than 70%, and increased work of breathing, which, if left untreated, will result in respiratory arrest and death (Judd & Mijch, 2002).

Mycobacterium Tuberculosis   *Mycobacterium tuberculosis* (TB) is another prevalent bacterial disease that is predominantly associated with infection, but also can be manifested in blood and cerebrospinal fluid (CSF). Unlike PCP respiratory infections, TB usually occurs early in continuum of HIV infection, often preceding a diagnosis of HIV infection. The CDC estimates that approximately 30% of TB cases among people ages 25 to 44 are occurring in HIV-infected individuals. Additionally, because the HIV infection impairs the immune system so severely, people infected with HIV and TB have a 100 times greater risk of developing active TB and becoming infectious, compared to people not infected with HIV (CDC, 2003b).

In patients who have TB, purified protein derivative (PPD), the laboratory test for detecting TB, will test positive early in HIV infections. As the immune system fails with progressing HIV disease, patients who have TB will usually have negative PPD tests because the appropriate immune response cannot be mounted to the PPD antigen. Conclusive diagnostic testing for TB is done by chest x-ray and acid-fast bacillus testing of sputum, blood, or CSF.

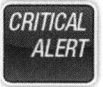 *Individuals who present with a persistent cough, night sweats, and fever should be tested for TB. If they have a positive TB test and the individual engages in high-risk behaviors, HIV testing should be discussed and encouraged.*

Hepatitis Virus B and C   Hepatitis virus B (HVB) and hepatitis virus C (HVC) are common opportunist infections in HIV-infected individuals because both are transmitted through shared body fluids such as blood, semen, and vaginal secretions, and high-risk behaviors promote the spread of both infections. Hepatitis is more easily transmitted because fewer hepatitis viral particles are required to initiate an infection than with HIV. Transmission by large or repeated exposures to contaminated blood by skin punctures is the most common mode of infection. Hence, the CDC estimates that 50% to 90% of HIV-positive injection drug users are also infected with HVC. Co-infection with HVC is present in approximately one-quarter of HIV-infected persons in the United States (CDC, 2005b).

The hepatitis virus affects liver function including metabolism of drugs, production of clotting factors, production of glucose and albumin, and filtering of waste, all of which contribute to the wasting syndrome in HIV. A combined HIV/HVB infection will increase morbidity and mortality due to the diminished function of both the immune system and the liver (CDC, 2005b). Therefore, the current U.S. Public Health Service/Infectious Diseases Society of America guidelines recommend HVB screening of all HIV-infected persons to promote early identification and treatment of HVB co-infection to reduce risk of chronic liver disease (Workowski & Berman, 2006).

***Mycobacterium Avium* Complex**   Another leading opportunistic infection is *Mycobacterium avium* complex (MAC), which includes a group of organisms (*M. avium, M. intracellulare*, and *M. scrofulaceum*). These organisms are usually found in food, water, and soil. They can cause respiratory infections, but most often are found in the GI tract, bone marrow, and lymph nodes. MAC infections are a major cause of severe weight loss and chronic diarrhea. Severe weight loss in persons with AIDS and a MAC infection is associated with T-cell counts less than 100 and high mortality rates.

In addition to MAC infections, other opportunistic pathogens such as cytomegalovirus (CMV) and candidiasis also affect the GI tract. CMV and MAC infections result in changes to the gastrointestinal lining that cause anorexia, chronic diarrhea, GI malabsorption, and significant weight loss. These are all symptoms of wasting syndrome, which is associated with a category C case definition of AIDS and is discussed next.

Wasting Syndrome   **Wasting syndrome**, one of the hallmark clinical manifestations of AIDS-related diseases, is defined as:

- A loss of lean body tissue from increased protein metabolism
- Changes in metabolic rates
- Anorexia and diarrhea.

Diagnostic criteria include chronic diarrhea for more than 30 days, weight loss of greater than 10% from baseline, and chronic weakness. Antiretroviral therapy and the production of lactic acid can be contributing causes (Bartlett, 2003). Tumor necrosis factor (TNF) and other cytokines have been implicated in research as a contributing factor that increases metabolic rate, anorexia, and metabolism of proteins. TNF and cytokines are described in detail in Chapter 59 . However, no conclusive studies have shown a direct effect from cytokine levels. Wasting syndrome is associated with severe debilitation in the advanced stages of AIDS.

Candidiasis   Candidiasis is a fungal opportunist infection that affects virtually all patients with AIDS. Oral candidiasis creates white patches in the mouth that can extend into the esophagus and stomach. This can make swallowing difficult and painful and significantly decrease oral intake due to discomfort. This places the patient at even greater risk for malnutrition and fluid and electrolyte imbalance. Also of concern is the fact that oral lesions can allow dissemination of the candidiasis into the bloodstream, causing a fungal sepsis that is life threatening.

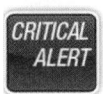 *Frequent and thorough oral assessment and care by the nurse is essential for the patient with oral candidiasis to maintain intact mucous membranes and prevent the spread of systemic infection by oral lesions.*

Candidiasis infection in skinfolds can lead to extensive skin breakdown. This is extremely uncomfortable for the patient and can lead to the development of a systemic fungal infection (see Figure 60–6 ■). Vaginal candidiasis in HIV-infected women is a frequent and recurrent problem. Women with AIDS also have a higher incidence of pelvic inflammatory disease (PID). The diagnosis and treatment of PID are discussed in Chapter 49 . As result of their immune-suppressed state, HIV-infected women with PID frequently require inpatient treatment with IV antibiotics.

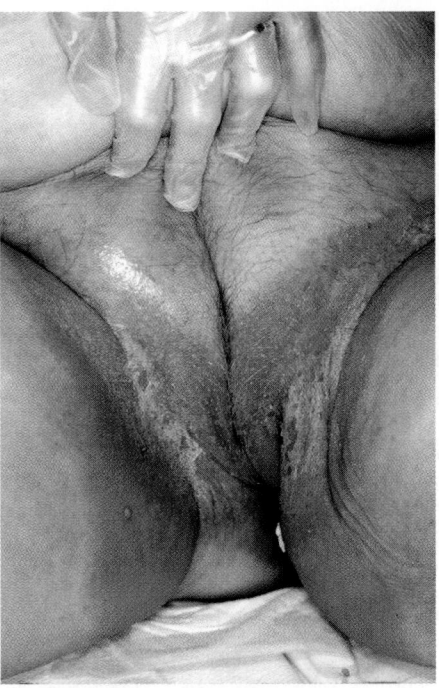

FIGURE 60–6 ■ Candidiasis in skinfolds.
Source: ISM/Phototake NYC

CRITICAL ALERT *Frequent and persistent vaginal candidiasis may be the first sign of HIV infection in a woman.*

Herpes Zoster and Herpes Simplex   Herpes zoster and herpes simplex viral infections are common in patients with HIV or AIDS. Herpes infections recur in any individual who has been infected because the virus remains in human DNA neurons. Stress, infections, and surgery can all stimulate a recurrence of shingles (herpes zoster) and/or cold sores (herpes simplex). For HIV-positive individuals, the risk of repeated exacerbations of herpes is increased due to the decreased ability to mount an immune response.

Other Infectious Organisms and Disease Processes
Opportunistic infections also are responsible for many of the neurological changes associated with AIDS. The majority of individuals with AIDS have neurological alterations at some point during the disease process. Cryptococcus is a fungus that causes a meningitis infection, mental changes, and seizures. TB and CMV infections are also implicated in neurological alteration. Additionally, CMV causes retinitis, which is the leading cause of blindness in patients with AIDS.

AIDS dementia complex is a major factor in decreased neurological function. Approximately 20% of patients with AIDS have the disorder (Brew, 2002). AIDS dementia is not caused by an opportunistic pathogen, but by actual changes to the neuro cells due to the HIV infection. The brain cells infected by HIV are predominantly the monocyte-macrophage CD4 cells. It is believed that HIV causes the release of chemicals that result in destruction of the cell and interfere with the neurotransmission needed for normal cerebral function (Porth & Sweeney, 2007). The clinical manifestations of these changes are a progressive decline in cognitive, motor, and behavioral functions. Initially memory deficits will occur, progressing to confusion, hallucinations, seizures, coma, and death.

Oncologic Manifestations

Patients with HIV/AIDS have an increased incidence of cancer. As cell-mediated immunity declines, malignant cells are not identified and destroyed internally, as they would be by an intact immune system. This leads to the development of the secondary cancers included in the CDC's classification of AIDS diseases: Kaposi's sarcoma, B-cell lymphoma (non-Hodgkin's), primary lymphoma of the brain, and invasive cervical carcinoma.

Kaposi's sarcoma is a malignancy involving the endothelial layer of the blood and lymphatic vessels and is the most common AIDS-related cancer. This is not surprising given the fact that lymphatic tissues are an integral part of the immune system where HIV infection resides and replicates. Raised or flat cutaneous lesions can appear anywhere on the body and are deep purple to brown and/or pink in color. The lesions can progress rapidly and cause extensive disfigurement, disruption in skin integrity, venous stasis, lymphedema, and pain. Lesions also can develop in internal organs rich in lymphatic tissue, such as the lining of the GI tract, and the lungs. This can lead to extensive tissue damage, organ failure, and death.

 Kaposi's sarcoma often develops on the face, resulting in extensive disfigurement and increasing feelings of social isolation and depression in the patient with AIDS. Nursing interventions are focused on addressing issues of altered body image and social isolation to maximize self-acceptance and support and decrease the risk of depression.

Lymphomas are malignancies of the lymphoid tissue that can be located anywhere in the body. The two lymphomas commonly associated with AIDS are non-Hodgkin's lymphoma and primary lymphoma of the brain. AIDS-related lymphomas differ from lymphomas found in the general population in that they are more aggressive tumors and tend to develop outside the lymph nodes, most commonly in the brain. Primary brain lymphoma is rapidly growing and is highly resistant to treatment. Common sites of non-Hodgkin's lymphomas are found in the bone marrow, liver, GI tract, mucous membranes, and the skin. Chemotherapy is frequently not successful in AIDS-associated non-Hodgkin's lymphoma because of prevalent immunosuppressive status and the complications that occur with opportunistic infections.

Invasive cervical carcinoma is a major complication for HIV-infected women. HIV-infected women have a 10 times greater prevalence of cervical dysplasia, which is a precursor lesion for cervical cancer, than women not infected with HIV (Kaplan, Masur, & Holmes, 2002). To promote early treatment and prevent the development of invasive cervical cancer, it is recommended that HIV-infected women have Papanicolaou (Pap) smears every 6 months and aggressive treatment with cone biopsy if pap smears are abnormal (see Chapter 49 ☺). To emphasize the importance of integrating gynecologic care into medical services for HIV-infected women, the CDC included invasive cervical cancer in the 1993 *Revised Classification System for HIV Infection*. HIV-infected women with cervical malignancy most commonly die of cervical cancer as opposed to other opportunistic diseases. Chapter 49 ☺ discusses STIs and the associated treatments.

Medical Management

There is no cure for HIV infection. Development of an HIV vaccine to prevent HIV infection or control HIV progression to AIDS has not been successful thus far. However, advancements in antiviral medication treatments have slowed the progression of HIV infection and have provided new opportunities and challenges for medical treatment of the patient with HIV/AIDS. Initial medical treatment involves identification of patients at risk, followed by diagnostic testing and counseling. Individuals who are positive for HIV infection may be started on antiretroviral therapy. Medical management also involves identification and treatment of OIs and symptom control that optimizes comfort and quality of life for the patient with HIV/AIDS.

Laboratory and Diagnostic Procedures

Tests that screen for HIV antibodies in the blood have a high degree of reliability and are used in diagnosing HIV infection. Testing for HIV antibodies also can be done on oral fluids and urine. The issue with antibody testing is the window period discussed earlier, in which infection is present, but antibodies are not detected by current test technology. The HIV antibody testing process described in the Diagnostic Tests box (p. 1934) produces highly accurate results that take 1 to 2 weeks to complete and involves pretest and post-test counseling.

Tests that determine the presence of a viral load (i.e., the number of copies of HIV antigens in a sample of blood) also have been developed. However, these tests are labor intensive and expensive and not used for routine HIV screening. The exception to this is the presence of clinical symptoms consistent with acute retroviral syndrome, which occurs during the window period where antibody testing will be negative (Bartlett & Lane, 2007). Viral load levels are routinely monitored on patients with confirmed HIV infection to determine antiretroviral medication needs.

In 2002 the FDA approved the OraQuick Rapid HIV-1 Antibody test and has subsequently approved three other rapid HIV tests that screen for HIV antibodies and return results in 15 to 60 minutes (CDC, 2006b). The benefit of this testing is that test results are immediately discussed with the individual, and he or she is informed that all positive tests are sent for confirmation by further antibody testing. The rapid HIV tests have a high degree of specificity (99%) and can be used in routine screening in emergency departments and labor and delivery suites.

Rapid HIV tests also have been studied as an outreach screening tool for high-risk groups such as those in chemical dependency programs, homeless shelters, gay youth drop-in centers, or prostitute support programs. The benefit of this type of screening is that it provides immediate results and increased rates of post-test counseling, which can potentially help prevent HIV transmission and initiate appropriate early treatment. The major disadvantage of rapid HIV testing is that there is a slightly higher rate of false-positive tests, and all positive tests must be confirmed with more HIV-sensitive and specific **Western blot (WB)** tests (Greenwald, Burstein, Pincus, & Branson, 2006).

HIV testing is confidential. Most states require written informed consent documentation prior to testing. However, in 2006 the CDC released revised recommendations for HIV testing of adults, adolescents, and pregnant women in health care settings that represents a radical departure from current testing practices, which focus on testing at-risk populations only.

DIAGNOSTIC TESTS for HIV and Patient Counseling

Test	Expected Abnormality	Rationale for Abnormality and Patient Counseling and Education
The following tests are for diagnostic screening of HIV antibodies:	CDC current recommendations call for HIV screening in all health care settings for adults, adolescents, and pregnant women once they are notified of testing, unless the individual declines (opt-out screening). This represents a change from HIV testing based on individuals with risk factors to HIV testing as a routine part of medical care. Many health care facilities are in the process of implementing these guidelines. Pretest counseling is not required in the current recommendations for acute care settings because the time-consuming nature of such counseling may decrease screening recommendation implementation. However, individuals being tested for HIV are often afraid to find out the test results. Providing a supportive open environment for counseling and education is an important aspect of nursing care.	*Screening Rationale:* Increase screening, foster earlier detection of HIV infection, identify and counsel persons with unrecognized HIV infection to enable treatment and reduce transmission of HIV. Routine screening as part of diagnostic work-up for illness can facilitate earlier diagnosis and treatment with HAART. *Pretest counseling:* • Establish a therapeutic relationship. • Inform of the benefits of testing. • Provide information about the test and testing procedures. Include the fact that all positive tests are confirmed with a second test. • Inform that obtaining results may require returning for a second visit, or may be available same day depending on the type of testing. • For individuals with identified risk factors, encourage annual screening. • Provide education regarding preventing of HIV transmission.
Enzyme immunoassay (EIA; previous test was the ELISA): Detects the presence of serum antibodies that bind to HIV antigens. Test requires two visits, testing, and then discussion of results/counseling process. Results take 2–3 days.	EIA results that are negative for antibodies are reported as negative tests. EIA tests that are positive are repeated. If the second EIA test is positive, a Western blot test is ordered.	*Rationale for EIA abnormality:* Positive antibodies indicate infection with HIV antigen that has caused the immune system to produce HIV antibodies. Negative test results do not need to be confirmed with a second test. Post-test counseling for the individual with risk factors who is HIV negative or who has an indeterminate test should include: • Discussion of risk behaviors and the possibility of false-negative tests during the window period. • If recent risk behaviors are identified, encourage follow-up testing at 3 weeks, 6 weeks, 3 months, and 6 months. • Reinforcement education regarding prevention of HIV transmission.
Western blot (WB) test: Antibody test with great sensitivity and specificity used to confirm presence of HIV antibodies. Results take 1–3 days.	Western blot results that are negative for antibodies are reported as negative tests; positive tests are reported as positive for HIV infection. Blood that tests positive is reported as HIV-antibody positive (seropositive) and confirms a diagnosis of HIV infection.	*Rationale for Western blot:* Confirms HIV antibodies. Has a lower false-positive rate than the EIA. Negative results indicate no infection with HIV antigen. Post-test counseling for the individual with an HIV-antibody positive test should include: • Provide emotional support. • Inform that test results indicate HIV infection, but that this does not necessarily indicate AIDS and further testing is needed. • Provide referrals and discuss options for treatment including antiretroviral treatment, HIV clinic referrals, and need for baseline testing on CD4+ T-cell counts and HIV viral load levels. • Discuss the variety of effective treatments to encourage hope. Discuss follow-up lab tests. • Determine the level of social support available. • Help the individual identify partners who need testing. • Provide information on HIV support groups and community resources. • Reinforce education information on prevention of HIV transmission.

DIAGNOSTIC TESTS for HIV and Patient Counseling—*Continued*

Test	Expected Abnormality	Rationale for Abnormality and Patient Counseling and Education
Rapid HIV antibody tests: Immunoassay screening tests for HIV antibodies that provide results in 10–60 minutes OraQuick (OraQuick Advance) rapid 1. HIV-1/HIV-2 antibody test 2. Reveal G2 rapid HIV-1 antibody test 3. Uni-Gold Recombigen HIV test 4. Multispot HIV-1/HIV-2 rapid test	All rapid HIV tests detect antibodies with sensitivities similar to EIAs, do not require instruments, and are interpreted visually. HIV antigens are fixed to the reagent strip; if HIV antibodies are present in the blood specimen, they affix to the antigen. The kit's colorimetric reagent binds to these antibody–antigen complexes to create a color change that is a visual indicator positive for antibodies. Results are available in approximately 20 minutes. A negative test requires no further confirmation test. A positive test is then confirmed by a Western blot test.	*Rationale for rapid HIV antibody tests:* Provides results in same visit as test to decrease rate of patients failing to return for confirmatory HIV test results, reduces barriers to early diagnosis of HIV, and increases access to treatment and prevention services. • Initially used predominately in community-based programs, and sex-worker outreach clinics for rapid identification of HIV, and in labor and delivery in acute care settings to minimize risk of perinatal transmission. Increased use in all health care settings encouraged as part of CDC recommendations to increase HIV screening (CDC, 2006c). • Inform patient that results will be available the same visit and that confirmatory testing is needed if the rapid test result is reactive. • Be supportive and prepared to give results along with counseling and referrals. • If result is negative inform patient that he/she is not infected, unless there was risk of exposure in the last 3 months. Then retesting is recommended at 3 and 6 months. • For positive results discuss confirmation testing with Western blot test. • Provide appropriate education and counseling based on initial test results as described above under EIA conventional testing.
Ongoing tests: CD4+ T cells and viral load tests are recommended at the time of initial HIV diagnosis to monitor the progression of HIV infection in seropositive patient and determine initiation or changes in antiretroviral therapy. *CD4+ T-cell count test:* Measures the total number of CD4 T-helper cells per microliter of blood.	CD4 low (<500 cells/µL) indicates decreased T-cell numbers and increased risk for opportunistic diseases.	*Rationale for CD4+ T-cell count test:* HIV attaches to CD4+ T cells, infecting them, destroying them, and decreasing the number of CD4+ cells, which impairs immune response; provides measurement of HIV progression to AIDS and effectiveness of HAART (p. 1937). • Provide patient with information on cell count levels, encourage follow-up lab tests and monitoring to determine treatment regime.
Viral load test: Done via polymerase chain reaction (PCR), HIV RNA, or bDNA tests to measure the actual amount of viral particles present in a blood sample.	Viral load levels of less than 10,000 copies/mL are considered "low" and copies greater than 100,000 are considered "high."	*Rationale for viral load test:* High levels indicate rapidly multiplying HIV, one marker of progression of HIV to AIDS; if patient on HAART indicates ineffective HAART treatment (p. 1937) due to drug resistance and/or lack of compliance with treatment regime. • HIV-infected individuals with viral load levels of less than 20,000 copies/mL have a low risk of disease progression. *Provide education on the following:* • Initial testing and follow-up testing: • Every 3–4 months in patients not on antiretroviral therapy. • Two to 8 weeks after initiation of antiretroviral therapy. • Every 3–4 months in patients on therapy. • When there is a decline in the clinical condition decisions need to be made to continue or change treatment.

Sources: Dybul, M., Fauci, A. S., Bartlett, J. G., Kaplan, J. E., & Pau, A. K. (2002). CDC Guidelines for Using Antiretroviral Agents Among HIV-Infected Adults and Adolescents Recommendations of the Panel on Clinical Practices for Treatment of HIV. Retrieved on September 5, 2008 from http://www.cdc.gov/mmwr/preview/mmwrhtml/rr5107a1.htm; Centers for Disease Control and Prevention. (2006c). Revised recommendations for HIV testing of adults, adolescents, and pregnant women in healthcare settings. *Morbidity and Mortality Weekly Report, 55*(RR-14), 1–17; Greenwald, J., Burstein, G., Pincus, J., & Branson, B. (2006). A rapid review of rapid HIV antibody tests. *Current Infectious Disease Reports, 8,* 125–131.

The revised CDC recommendations advocate HIV screening as a routine part of medical care for patients, similar to screening for other treatable conditions (CDC, 2006c). Individuals would be notified that testing will be performed unless the patient declines, a process that is referred to as opt-out screening. Persons at high risk for HIV should be screened annually. The guidelines also recommend that general consent for medical treatment be considered sufficient, and a separate written HIV testing consent not be required. Additionally, prevention counseling should not be required with diagnostic testing or HIV screening in health care settings. The ethical considerations surrounding HIV testing are discussed in the Ethical Issues box.

The rationale for the recommendations is that undiagnosed HIV-infected individuals frequently visit health care settings such as hospitals or acute care clinics years prior to a diagnosis, but are not tested for HIV in all health care settings. This results in a delay in effective antiretroviral treatment. Additionally, individuals aware of their positive HIV status significantly reduce sexual behavior that might transmit HIV, so early screening has the potential to substantially decrease the number of new HIV infections in the United States (Marks, Crepaz, Senterfitt, & Janssen, 2005). Routine prenatal HIV screening with streamlined counseling and consent procedures has substantially increased the number of pregnant women tested and contributed to significant declines in perinatal HIV transmission rates (CDC, 2002). This success has not been mirrored in the general population where HIV screening is rarely performed and the number of new HIV infections has remained stable at approximately 40,000 annually in the United States (Branson et al., 2006).

Furthermore, prevention efforts need to address each succeeding generation of adolescents ages 13 to 19 years. Forty-seven percent of high school students report they have had sexual intercourse at least once, and 37% indicated they did not use protection during their last sexual intercourse experience. This is despite the fact that 89% stated that they learned about HIV/AIDS in their high school curriculum (CDC, 2005d). It is estimated that over half of HIV-infected adolescents have not been tested and are not aware of their infected status (Branson et al., 2006). The goals of the recommendations are to increase HIV screening of patients, including pregnant women, in health care settings; promote early detection of HIV infection; identify and counsel HIV-infected individuals and connect them to clinical and prevention services; and further reduce HIV transmission in the United States.

Currently, testing is focused on high-risk individuals who self-identify the need for testing or are encouraged by health providers to be tested because of identified risk factors. Testing is funded and performed by the state public health departments. At the anonymous public testing site, the individual receives a test code, a name is not associated with the test results, and results do not become part of the medical record. Pretest and posttest counseling is available at testing sites or by phone (Corbett, 2004). Approximately 2.1 million tests are conducted annually in publicly funded testing and referral programs alone. However, the CDC reports that a large percentage of individuals, 60% to 70%, do not return for test results (CDC, 2006b). The recent development of rapid HIV tests with comparable sensitivity and the specificity of enzyme immunoassays (EIAs), which provide testing and results in the same visit, can help address this issue. Anonymous testing also can be done at home with HIV antibody test kits. However, home tests raise concerns about lack of availability of counseling and prevention education that are an integral part of HIV testing. Anonymous testing may be preferred by individuals who fear discrimination or placement of the test result in their medical record where insurance companies may have access to the information (Johnsen, 2003).

Counseling regarding HIV encompasses two components: provision of information and prevention counseling. Counseling should be presented in an open, nonjudgmental manner and in the language that the individual is best capable of understanding. Verbal as well as written information or audiovisual materials that the individual can take home and review should be included. The CDC's revised recommendations for HIV testing released in 2006 change some of the previous recommendations for prevention counseling for individuals who take rapid HIV tests in a health care setting. The recommendations indicate that prevention counseling should not be required with HIV diagnostic testing or as part of an HIV screening program in health care settings such as emergency departments, urgent care clinics, inpatient services, substance abuse treatment clinics, public health and community clinics, correctional facilities, and primary care settings (CDC, 2006b). This is an effort to remove barriers to HIV screening in busy health care settings. However, the CDC continues to support prevention counseling in all settings for persons at high risk for HIV and in nonmedical settings such as community-based organizations, outreach settings, or mobile vans (CDC, 2006b).

ETHICAL ISSUES Related to HIV Infection

A significant ethical issue that the nurse in the acute care setting may encounter when caring for a patient with a newly diagnosed HIV-positive antibody status is the issue of sexual or needle-sharing partners at high risk for HIV infection. The HIV-infected patient may be very hesitant, embarrassed, or fearful about disclosing an HIV-positive test result to partners. This creates an ethical dilemma in that it places partners at risk for undiagnosed HIV infection, limits their choices for testing and potential treatment if needed, and violates their rights to know their risk for infection.

The nurse must abide by the ethical principle of respect for autonomy and confidentiality, while at the same time encouraging the patient to employ the ethical principle of veracity (truthfulness) in informing partners. The nurse may encourage the patient in making this ethical choice by developing a therapeutic relationship, asking about support systems and partners, listening to concerns, reviewing benefits of early screening for partners, and obtaining a social service referral to access resources for partner notification. State legislation requires health departments to offer anonymous HIV partner notification services to newly reported HIV-infected persons. The HIV partner counseling services inform persons of their possible exposure, and offer counseling, testing, and referral services (CDC, 2003a).

The importance of notifying sexual and needle-sharing partners of their exposure to HIV is also enforced by Federal Ryan White CARE Reauthorization act of 1996, which requires health departments show "good faith" in notifying marriage partners of HIV-infected persons. The nurse can provide emotional support and obtain referral resources to help newly diagnosed HIV-infected patients and spouses communicate and address this difficult situation.

The CDC still recommends that patients in all settings receive information regarding HIV testing, HIV infection, and the meaning of results. Patients must be informed of the HIV screening in a face-to-face discussion or through written or audiovisual material. Information provided should include the testing process, the meaning of test results, ways HIV is transmitted and how to prevent it, and where to obtain further testing and services. Ongoing HIV counseling is vital for individuals who test positive for HIV. Overwhelming feelings of fear, anxiety, depression, and social isolation frequently occur with an HIV diagnosis. Nurses are in an optimal position to develop therapeutic relationships that support the HIV-positive patient, to review risk factors for transmitting HIV infection, and to encourage compliance with follow-up testing and antiretroviral therapy. Nurses also can help facilitate referrals to social services for assistance with financial concerns, and community and psychological support services.

Tests that monitor the progression of HIV infection include the CD4+ T-cell counts and viral load assay tests. CD4+ T-cell counts, as previously discussed, are essential in assessing for decreased immune function and the diagnosis of AIDS. Equally important are viral load tests such as the HIV RNA, polymerize chain reaction (qPCR), or the branched chain DNA (bDNA) tests, which measure the viral activity and are reported as the number of "copies" per milliliter. Viral load testing is done at the time of HIV diagnosis and as a baseline, and then every few weeks to months depending on the initiation or type of drug treatment therapy. Viral load levels of less than 10,000 copies/mL are considered "low" and copies greater than 100,000 are considered "high" (Corbett, 2004). HIV-infected individuals with HIV RNA levels of less than 20,000 copies/mL have a low risk of disease progression (Bartlett & Lane, 2007). As the HIV progresses the CD4+ T-cell counts decline and the viral load increases, resulting in susceptibility to OIs and malignancies.

Testing for HIV resistance to antiretroviral drugs in patients being treated for HIV infection is currently possible. This is an important tool in determining antiretroviral therapy. Genotyping and phenotyping assays are available. Genotyping assays detect drug resistance mutations present in reverse transcriptase and protease genes. Phenotyping assays measure the ability of the virus to grow in different antiretroviral drug concentrations. Information on drug resistance is important in identifying patients who are not responding to their antiretroviral medication regime and in guiding decisions regarding changes in therapy (Bartlett & Lane, 2007).

Antiretroviral Drug Therapy for HIV Infection

Antiretroviral drugs are pivotal in delaying the progression of HIV to AIDS. The goal of drug therapy is to decrease the viral load (HIV RNA level < 55,000 copies/mL), increase or maintain CD4+ T-cell counts at greater than 200 cells/mL (greater than 500 cells/µL preferred), and delay the onset of HIV symptoms and opportunistic infections. A variety of antiretroviral agents are now available for use in treatment.

The complexity of the medications involved and concerns about appropriate treatment for patients who are asymptomatic with low HIV RNA levels and an adequate CD4+ T-cell count has created some confusion on when to initiate antiretroviral therapy. Antiretroviral drugs have serious adverse effects and drug resistance can develop with prolonged use or nonadherence, requiring changes in therapy that limit future treatment options. To address these concerns, the U.S. Department of Health and Human Services published guidelines for the use of antiretroviral agents in HIV-1-infected adults and adolescents in July 2003, with subsequent revisions in 2006 (Bartlett & Lane, 2007). Viral load and CD4+ T-cell levels are essential parameters in deciding to initiate or change antiretroviral therapies. In general, treatment should be offered to persons who have HIV RNA levels > 55,000 copies/mL or <350 CD4+ T cells/µL.

Treatment for HIV involves combinations of various antiretroviral drugs that interfere with different aspects of the HIV replication cycle, and the treatment is referred to as **highly active antiretroviral drug therapy (HAART)**. Combination therapy has the greatest effect in controlling HIV proliferation and minimizing the development of drug resistance. Antiretroviral drugs are grouped according to the mechanism of action against HIV (see Figure 60–7 ■, p. 1938).

Nucleoside reverse transcriptase inhibitors are a group of drugs that prevent viral replication by blocking the attachment of the nucleoside to the replicated DNA molecule. The nonnucleoside reverse transcriptase inhibitors make up another group of drugs that also prevent viral replication, but through a different mechanism. These drugs prevent the bond between a nucleotide and the growing DNA molecule of HIV. An additional group of drugs, the protease inhibitors, stop the replication of new RNA by inhibiting the action of protease enzymes, which are responsible for the synthesis of reverse transcriptase. A more recent class of medication, fusion inhibitors, is also available and works by preventing HIV from binding to CD4+ T cells and infecting healthy cells. Chart 60–10 (p. 1939) provides additional information on specific medication and adverse effects that can be used in patient teaching.

Central to the treatment of HIV/AIDS is adherence to the prescribed antiviral medication regime. If antiviral medications are not taken properly or consistently, CD4+ T-cell counts will decrease and viral loads of HIV will significantly increase, leading to greater risk of opportunistic infection (Branson et al., 2006; Dybul et al., 2002; Kaplan et al., 2002). Furthermore, resistance to these medications can develop if the treatment regime is not followed (Branson et al., 2006; Little et al., 2002). Essential to creating strategies to improve adherence is a supportive therapeutic relationship between the patient and the provider, and a negotiated treatment plan that the patient commits to that considers his daily routines, meal schedules, and medication side effects (Bartlett & Lane, 2007).

The lack of adherence to medication treatment is a major concern in HIV treatment. The focal issue has been the complexity of dosing schedules, the volume of pills that the patient must manage, and the serious adverse effects of these medications, including fatigue, loss of appetite, diarrhea, and nausea and vomiting (Bartlett & Lane, 2007). Other issues that have been identified include socioeconomic factors such as homelessness, lack of insurance or finances, or lack of transportation to clinic appointments. Psychological factors also have been implicated including mental illness, poor coping skills, and failure to understand that self-care is a priority (especially for HIV-infected women balancing multiple caregiver roles) (Shaw & Mahoney, 2003).

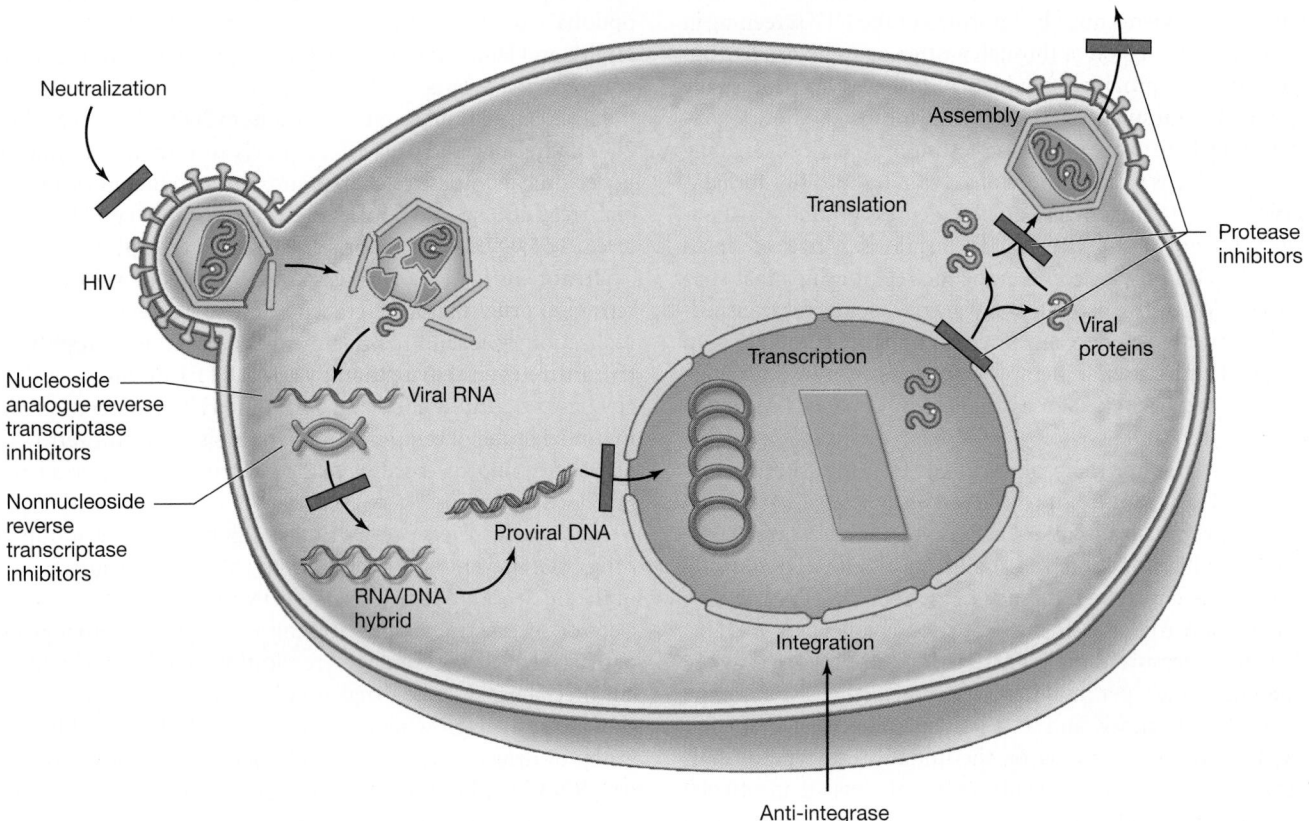

FIGURE 60–7 ■ HIV replication and targets of antiretroviral therapy.

Pharmaceutical companies have responded to these issues by developing combination antiviral medications to decrease the volume of pills patients must manage, and therefore simplifying medication schedules. Research is ongoing in this area. Another area of significant research involves antiretroviral therapy during pregnancy (Dabis, Bequet, & Ekouevi, 2005; Tasha, Kumwenda, & Gibbons, 2003). HIV-infected mother-to-fetus transmissions are responsible for more than 90% of HIV infection in children, and antiretroviral therapy during pregnancy has demonstrated significant declines in this transmission rate (Public Health Service Task Force, 2006).

Nurses play a pivotal role in medication adherence through extensive patient and family education and follow-up regarding medication side effects and concern. Additionally, nurses can facilitate the coordination and development of a patient-centered plan of care that addresses the socioeconomic, psychological, and physiological factors effecting medication adherence.

Treatment of Opportunistic Infections and Symptom Management

The medical treatment for opportunistic infections and symptom management was summarized earlier in Chart 60–9 (p. 1929). Drug therapy is the mainstay of treatment of opportunistic infections (OIs). The development of resistant organisms in an immunosuppressed individual is challenging and frequently involves treatment with new and innovative combinations of antibiotic therapy. Symptoms requiring treatment may be the result of antiretroviral drugs, treatment of opportunistic infection, or

proliferation of HIV resulting in greater loss of immune function. In addition to infection, commonly treated symptoms include diarrhea, anorexia and weight loss, skin breakdown, pain, and depression. Nurses have an essential role in ongoing assessment of the patient's response to treatment and facilitating symptom management in order to promote optimal patient outcomes.

◼ Nursing Management

The nursing care of the patient with AIDS involves multiple physical as well as psychological and social support issues. Because of the impairment to the immune system, any body organ can be the target of an opportunistic infection or cancer, making nursing care especially challenging. To date there is no cure for HIV. A diagnosis of HIV/AIDS is psychologically devastating to patients, the vast majority of whom are 15 to 45 years of age and have not previously confronted issues of mortality. HIV/AIDS also carries a social stigma that may result in rejection by family and friends and social isolation at a time when the patient faces issues of grief and fear of dying. Nurses have a primary role in addressing these needs, and providing skilled, compassionate nursing care that is respectful to the individual's values, culture, and right to make individual choices (American Nurses Association, 2004).

The nursing process provides a template to assess, treat, and evaluate patients with HIV/AIDS. Use of the nursing process will facilitate creation of individualized care plans that optimize symptom management, patient comfort, and family support.

CHART 60–10   HIV/AIDS Infection Antiretroviral Agents

Drug Therapy	Drug Action	Application/Indication	Nursing Responsibilities
Protease Inhibitors • Nelfinavir (Viracept) • Ritonavir (Norvir) (keep refrigerated) • Lopinavir and ritonavir (Kaletra) • Saquinavir (Fortovase) • Indinavir (Crixivan) (Take 1 hour before or 2 hours after eating.) • Amprenavir (Agenerase)	Stop the replication of new RNA by inhibiting the action of protease enzymes, which are responsible for the synthesis of reverse transcriptase.	One of the three categories of drugs that are combined to treat HIV and are referred to as HAART (p. 1937).	Monitor the patient for anemia, anorexia/nausea, diarrhea, headache, fever, malaise. Monitor labs: triglycerides, ALT, AST, alkaline phosphatase, CK and uric acid levels, thrombocytopenia. • Instruct patient to take with food due to bitter taste, and not to mix with juice because it increases the bitterness. • Inform patient of potential redistribution of body fat centrally (the "protease paunch"), facial atrophy, breast enlargement, "buffalo hump."
Non-Nucleoside Reverse Transcriptase Inhibitors • Delavirdine (Rescriptor) • Nevirapine (Viramune) • Efavirenz (Sustiva) (Not to be used during pregnancy or breast-feeding. Women of childbearing years need pregnancy test prior to taking drug.)	Prevent viral replication, but through a different mechanism than protease inhibitors. These drugs prevent the bond between a nucleotide and the growing DNA molecule of HIV.	One of the three categories of drugs that are combined to treat HIV and are referred to as HAART (p. 1937).	• Monitor patient for fatigue, rash, headache, painful peripheral neuropathy (reversible with lower doses), insomnia, nightmares (usually resolve in 2 weeks) retinal changes (eye exam recommended every 6–12 months). • Monitor for increase in ALT, AST, alkaline phosphatase. • Monitor creatinine levels of patient with renal insufficiency. • Instruct patient to maintain adequate hydration and not to take with antacids.
Nucleoside Reverse Transcriptase Inhibitors • Zidovudine (AZT, ZDT, Retrovir) (Take 1 hour before or 2 hours after meals.) • Lamivudine (3TC, Epivir) • Combivir (lamivudine and zidovudine combination) • Didanosine (ddI, Videx) (Take 1 hour before or 2 hours after meals. Two tablet doses, of which 1 is a buffer, must be chewed or dissolved to ensure adequate buffer for absorption.) • Stavudine (d4T, Zerit) • Zalcitabine (ddC, HIVID) • Tenofovir Disoproxil Fumarate (DF, Viread) • Adefovir dipivoxil (Preveon) • Abacavir (Ziagen) (Alcohol increases abacavir levels 41%. Some reported fatal hypersensitivity reactions.)	Prevent viral replication by blocking the attachment of the nucleoside to the replicated DNA molecule.	One of the three categories of drugs that are combined to treat HIV and are referred to as HAART (p. 1937).	• Monitor for bone marrow suppression: neutropenia, anemia, granulocytopenia. • Monitor ALT, AST. • Monitor creatinine clearance in patient with renal impairment. • Monitor for malaise, insomnia, nightmares (subside in about 2 weeks), painful peripheral neuropathy (reversible with lower medication doses), visual changes (eye exam recommended every 6–12 months), GI intolerance, and nausea/vomiting.

(continued)

CHART 60–10 HIV/AIDS Infection Antiretroviral Agents—*Continued*			
Drug Therapy	**Drug Action**	**Application/Indication**	**Nursing Responsibilities**
Fusion Inhibitor • Enfuvirtide (Fuzeon) (subcutaneous injection twice daily)	Interferes with entry of HIV-1 into host cells by inhibiting the fusion of the virus and cell membranes.	Treatment of advanced HIV disease with evidence of resistance to other therapies.	• Monitor for irritation at injection site, nausea, insomnia, peripheral neuropathy. • Instruct patient to keep medication refrigerated, reconstitute according to directions, rotate injection sites.

Sources: Adams, M., Josephson, D., & Holland, L. (2005). *Pharmacology for nurses: A pathophysiologic approach.* Upper Saddle River, NJ: Pearson Prentice Hall; Shaw, J. K., & Mahoney, E. A. (Eds.). (2003). *HIV/AIDS nursing secrets.* Philadelphia: Hanley & Belfus; Shannon, M., Shields, K., & Stang, C. (2007). *Nurse's drug guide.* Upper Saddle River, NJ: Pearson Prentice Hall.

Because of the complexity of HIV infection multiple nursing diagnoses apply. An extensive list of potentially applicable diagnoses is provided in Chart 60–11. Some of the most common nursing diagnoses that impact patients with HIV/AIDS, outcome goals, evaluation parameters, and appropriate nursing interventions are found in the Nursing Process: Care Plan for the Patient with HIV/AIDS. Alternative treatments for HIV/AIDS are addressed in the Complementary and Alternative Therapies box (p. 1947).

Treatment Choice Issues

Diagnosis of a disease process such as HIV/AIDS that has no cure is devastating. The highest prevalence of HIV infection is found in a very young population (15 to 45 years), the vast majority of whom have not faced issues of terminal illness or chronic treatment. This may prompt a desire to explore issues of spirituality, concepts of the soul, and life after death. It may result in feelings of overwhelming fear that result in a search for a higher power. The nurse needs to be sensitive to these issues and assess the patient's feelings regarding spiritual needs so that appropriate referrals can be made. The patient also may choose to explore alternative therapies. It is imperative that the nurse remain open minded about these options and respectful of the treatment choices that the patient makes.

Discharge Priorities

Due to the chronic nature of HIV/AIDS, the process of discharging a patient from the hospital is complex. The nurse must address the medication schedule, physical care needs, and emotional issues surrounding the diagnosis. If followed carefully, current treatments can prolong and give quality to the person's life. Additionally, caregiver considerations must be addressed. The Patient Teaching & Discharge Priorities box (p. 1947) and Chart 60–12 (p. 1948) outline the important information that is essential for patients with HIV/AIDS and their partners and caregivers that must be provided on discharge.

Ongoing Care

For patients who have been diagnosed with HIV/AIDS, collaborative care includes assessment of physical status as well as the knowledge level of the patient, partner, family, and friends in order to address education needs. The promotion of self-care, independence, and adherence to the prescribed treatment plan is the primary goal in the care of the patient with AIDS. With antiretroviral therapy, HIV infection is transitioning to a chronic disease. Many HIV-infected individuals are able to maintain home and work functions for several years and are regularly followed by their health care provider or an AIDS outreach clinic. As the disease progresses care needs increase and the patient becomes increasingly dependent on family and friends to provide support. Social workers, community support services, home care nurses, community health nurses, and hospice nurses are often able to provide complex in-home nursing care that enables patients to remain comfortable at home.

Nurses are pivotal in providing ongoing patient and family education and making appropriate referrals to a variety of community-based organizations that can also supply support such as meals, housekeeping, transportation, or shopping. They also have additional information on national resources that the patient or family can access. Such organizations include the National Association of People with AIDS, CDC National AIDS Hotline, and the National Association on HIV over Fifty. (For a discussion of AIDS in people over age 50, see the Gerontological Considerations box, p. 1948.) At the point where the patient's symptoms cannot be managed at home or a caregiver is not available, a transfer to skilled nursing care or an acute care facility is needed to ensure patient comfort.

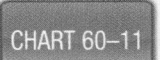

CHART 60–11 **Nursing Diagnoses for the Patient with HIV/AIDS**

• *Acute/Chronic Pain* related to opportunistic infections/malignancies

• *Impaired Skin Integrity* related to malnutrition, altered metabolic state, immobility, alerted sensation, skeletal prominence

• *Fatigue* related to malnutrition, hypermetabolic state with infection, fluid/electrolyte imbalance

• *Deficient Fluid Volume* related to copious diarrhea, profuse sweating, vomiting, hypermetabolic state, fever

• *Confusion* related to neurological opportunistic infections/malignancies and altered metabolic processes

• *Deficient Knowledge* related to disease, transmission, prognosis, treatment, and self-care

• *Ineffective Therapeutic Regimen Management* related to complexity of medications and socioeconomic limitations

• *Ineffective Coping* related to fear, grief, and despair with life-threatening disease process

• *Anxiety* related to anticipatory fear of physical decline and the dying process

Note: These are the most common potential nursing diagnoses for the patient with HIV/AIDS.

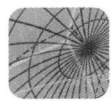

NURSING PROCESS: Patient Care Plan for HIV/AIDS

Assessment of Infection

Subjective Data:

Have you been running a temperature?

Have you had chills or periods of sweating?

Are you having any "flu-like" symptoms (body aches, fatigue, cough, sore-throat, stiff neck)?

Have you been coughing up any sputum? What color is it?

Have you noticed any rashes?

Do you have pain anywhere?

Do you have any burning with urination?

Do you have any redness or tenderness anywhere?

Do you have any sores anywhere?

Do you have any unusual or foul-smelling drainage (e.g., from vagina, penis, rectum, ears)?

How long have the symptoms been going on?

What have you done to treat the symptoms?

Have you taken any over the counter (OTC), prescription, or herbal medications for symptom relief?

Have you been taking your antiviral medications as prescribed?

Objective Data:

Abnormal vital signs (e.g., temp > 101 or < 97, HR >100, BP < 90 or MAP < 60)

Skin: rashes, wounds, sores, redness, heat, or edema

Oral cavity: sores, white patches, poor dental hygiene

Drainage: color, amount and foul smell from any wounds, incisions, mucous membranes

Urine: amber, cloudy, amount of time Foley catheter in place

Pain with palpation

Invasive lines/catheters: amount of time they have been in place, redness, drainage at insertion site

Laboratory Tests: CBC with differential to evaluate WBC count (neutrophils < 4,000 or

> 12,000/mm^3; bands > 10%

CD4 T-cell count: <500/cells/uL

HIV viral load count: >25,000 copies/mL

Cultures: blood, sputum, stool, urine, wound (+ for bacterial or viral pathogens)

Nursing Assessment and Diagnoses	Outcomes and Evaluation Parameters	Planning and Interventions with *Rationales*
Nursing Diagnosis: *Risk for Infection* related to immunodeficiency from HIV infection	**Outcome:** No infection. **Evaluation Parameters:** Vital signs within normal parameters. Alert and oriented. Clear lungs. Intact skin or mucous membrane without edema, pain, redness, or drainage. Wounds/incisions healing. No discomfort with urination. Invasive line and catheter sites are not red or draining. Symptoms of infection identified early and prompt treatment initiated.	**Interventions and *Rationales:*** Assess for symptoms of infection: fever, chills, diaphoresis; tachycardia, tachypnea, hypotension; decline in neurological status; dyspnea, cough, adventitious breath sounds; white patches in oral cavity or painful swallowing; redness, swelling, or drainage from wounds or vaginal or perianal area; open lesions on face, lips, or perianal area; urinary frequency, urgency, or burning sensation; pain in any location. *Promotes early detection of infection.* Notify health care provider of symptoms of infection. *Early detection and treatment help prevent progression to refractory sepsis. Infections increase patient mortality.*
	WBC within normal limits.	Monitor WBC count and differential. *Elevated or abnormally low WBC counts indicates possible infection.*
	Cultures negative for organisms.	Obtain cultures of blood, sputum, urine, wound drainage, skin lesions, mouth, and stool as ordered prior to the start of the first dose of antibiotic. *Assists in identifying infecting organisms and targeting appropriate treatment. Obtaining culture prior to starting antibiotics increases the potential to capture the organism in the culture. Do not delay the antibiotics if some cultures such as sputum cannot be obtained.*
	Medications given on time. Antibiotic therapy sensitive to infecting organism as evidenced by decreasing fever, WBC, and sputum production. Patient continues HAART regime. Health care providers and family perform hand hygiene frequently prior to and following patient contact.	Administer antimicrobial medications as prescribed. *Treats current infection or prevents additional opportunistic infections (OI).* Administer HAART as prescribed and stress adherence to medication regime. *Decreases rate of HIV replication and increases CD4 counts.* Prevent infection by washing hands before and after all patient contacts; instruct patient/family to perform hand hygiene frequently, especially after toileting, prior to eating or handling medications. *Reduces risk of OI cross-contamination.*
	Intake & output (I&O) balanced; patient maintaining or gaining weight.	Maintain fluid and nutritional intake; strict I&O, calorie count. *Dehydration and malnutrition impair immune function and wound healing.*

(continued)

NURSING PROCESS: Patient Care Plan for HIV/AIDS—*Continued*

Nursing Assessment and Diagnoses	Outcomes and Evaluation Parameters	Planning and Interventions with *Rationales*
	No new skin or mucous membrane breakdown.	Maintain skin and mucous membrane integrity with frequent turning and oral care every 2 hours. *Skin and mucous membranes are the first line of immune defense; lesions allow OI portal of entry.*
	Invasive lines and catheters secured. No invasive line or catheter-induced infections. Catheters and invasive lines removed promptly when no longer of benefit in patient treatment.	Maintain sterile technique during all invasive procedures (urinary catheterization, IV line placement). Perform meticulous care of any invasive lines or catheters; change out catheters according to agency policy.
	Patient performs activities of daily living (ADLs).	Maintain closed system for drains. Discontinue catheters/invasive lines as soon as possible. *Prevents hospital-acquired infections.* Anchor catheters/tubes (IV lines, urinary catheters) securely. *Reduces trauma to tissue and decreases risk of introducing pathogens from in and out movement of catheter.*
	Patient out of bed (OOB) and turned every 2 hours.	Assist with mobility, out of bed three or more times a day unless contraindicated or turning every 2 hours. *Prevents skin breakdown, deep venous thrombosis, constipation, and pulmonary stasis, which may increase length of hospitalization and infection risk.*
	Lungs clear.	Assist with inspirometer, coughing, and deep breathing every 1–2 hours when awake. *To prevent pulmonary stasis, which increases risk of OI.*
	Patient and family can verbally identify signs and symptoms of infection. Patient and family report early symptoms of infection to health care providers.	Instruct patient and family about signs and symptoms of infection and infection prevention and the need to report possible infection. *Enables early detection and treatment.*
	Patient environment is clean.	Maintain cleanliness/personal hygiene. Clean household surfaces with disinfectant. *Decreases presence of potentially infective organisms.*
	Has others handle pet cleanup.	Avoid handling animal waste or cleaning cages. *Infectious organisms such as CMV are in animal feces.*
	Uses recommendations for food handling.	Clean and cook foods thoroughly (scrub skins of fruits and vegetables, cook meat and eggs). *To eliminate pathogens.* Avoid exposure to others' body fluids and do not share eating utensils. *Patient/family teaching to minimize exposure to OI is essential to preventing infection.*

Assessment of Airway and Gas Exchange

Subjective Data:
Are you having difficulty breathing?
Have you been coughing?
What color is the sputum you are coughing up?

Objective Data:
Respiratory rate:
Use of substernal and/or intercostals muscles with inspiration/expiration
Unequal chest wall movement
Oxygen saturation:
Adventitious breath sounds: wheezes, fine or course crackles
Decreased level of consciousness (LOC) (lethargy→confusion→stupor)
Skin changes: mottled extremities, central cyanosis
Arterial Blood Gases (ABG)

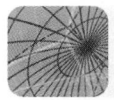

NURSING PROCESS: Patient Care Plan for HIV/AIDS—*Continued*

Nursing Assessment and Diagnoses	Outcomes and Evaluation Parameters	Planning and Interventions with *Rationales*
Nursing Diagnoses: *Ineffective Airway Clearance* related to (1) opportunistic pulmonary infection, increased bronchial secretions or (2) stasis of secretion from decreased ability to cough from general weakness	**Outcomes:** Clear airway. Adequate gas exchange. ***Evaluation Parameters:*** Respiratory rate 12–20 breaths/min. Unlabored breathing without use of accessory muscles.	**Interventions and *Rationales:*** Assess for rapid shallow respirations. *Indicates hypoxia and poor gas exchange.* Assess for use of accessory muscles. *Indicates increased work of breathing and progression to respiratory failure.* Assess for abnormal or absent breath sounds. *Indicates pulmonary infiltrates or consolidation that decreases gas exchange.*
Risk for Impaired Gas Exchange related to pulmonary secretions from opportunistic infections	Clear breath sounds. Alert and oriented. Skin is pink, warm. Normal ABG values. Pulse oximetry saturation > 94%. Appropriate medical treatment as needed. Patient cooperative with oxygen administration. Sputum culture obtained.	Assess for cough and sputum; note amount, color and consistency of sputum. *A yellow, green, or tan color indicates presence of infecting organism.* Assess level of consciousness (restless, confused, somnolence). *Altered level of consciousness is an early indicator of hypoxia and decreased perfusion to the brain.* Assess dusky, cyanotic skin color. *Indicates tissue hypoxia.* Monitor ABGs and pulse oximetry oxygen saturation. *To assess adequacy of gas exchange.* Report respiratory distress to health care provider. *Enables prompt initiation of appropriate medical treatment.* Administer humidified oxygen as prescribed. *Supplemental oxygen increases the alveolar gas concentration and diffusion of oxygen to the cells and tissues of the body. Humidification helps loosen secretions and promote airway clearance.*
	Antibiotic therapy sensitive to infecting organism as evidenced by decreasing fever, WBC, and sputum production. Patient able to cough and clear secretions.	Obtain sputum sample for culture. *To identify specific infecting organism so appropriate antibiotic is prescribed.* Administer antibiotic therapy as prescribed. *To treat infectious organism.* Maintain fluid intake of 3 L/day unless contraindicated. *To decrease viscosity of secretions.* Administer mucolytics and bronchodilators as prescribed. *To thin secretions and dilate airways, thus increasing gas exchange.*
	Patient verbalizes understanding and performs pulmonary self-care. Patient reports decreased breathing problems. Patient has energy to cough and clear secretions. Secretions cleared. Airway and ventilation maintained.	Maintain the head of the bed >30% at all times unless contraindicated. Instruct patient to turn, cough, deep breathe, and use the inspirometer every 1–2 hours when awake. *Facilitates breathing, increases gas exchange, and prevents atelectasis and pulmonary secretion stasis.* Encourage adequate rest periods. *Prevents excessive fatigue, which impairs ability to breathe.* Perform tracheal suctioning as needed. *Removes secretions if patient is unable to do so, clears airway, improves gas exchange.* Assist with endotracheal intubation; maintain ventilator settings as prescribed. *Maintains airway and gas exchange.*

Assessment of Nutrition

Subjective Data:

Do you have an appetite?

What are you eating and how often do you eat?

Are you losing weight?

Are you experiencing nausea or vomiting?

Are you having any difficulty chewing or swallowing?

Objective Data:

Daily weight

Laboratory tests: serum protein, albumin, transferrin levels, Hbg/Hct, electrolytes

Oral cavity: edema, white patches indicating *Candida* infection, open lesions, loose or decaying teeth

(continued)

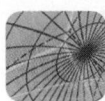

NURSING PROCESS: Patient Care Plan for HIV/AIDS—*Continued*

Nursing Assessment and Diagnoses	Outcomes and Evaluation Parameters	Planning and Interventions with *Rationales*
Nursing Diagnosis: *Imbalanced Nutrition: Less than Body Requirements* related to decreased oral intake associated with anorexia, nausea/vomiting, and impaired absorption and utilization of nutrients from effects of HIV infection	**Outcome:** Maintained or improved nutritional status. **Evaluation Parameters:** Gains weight. Adequate hydration. Normal electrolytes, albumin, hemoglobin/hematocrit, transferring levels.	**Interventions and *Rationales*:** Assess for significant weight loss or weight below normal for patient's height, weight, and age. *Indicates malnutrition.*
		Assess diet weight loss and diet history, food likes, dislikes, and intolerances. *Identifies education needs and allows for individual dietary plan.*
	Oral and esophageal opportunistic infections treated appropriately, as evidenced by no pain with swallowing, pink nonedematous mucous membranes. Laboratory values improving and trending toward normal ranges.	Assess and report abnormalities of oral cavity, mucous membranes, and swallowing. *To identify treatable OIs (oral candidiasis, esophagitis) that interfere with intake and facilitate medical treatment oral candidiasis.* Monitor fluid and electrolytes, serum protein, albumin, transferrin levels, hemoglobin/hematocrit energy level. *Low levels indicate inadequate intake/malnutrition, which places patient at increased risk for infection.*
	Intake of daily calories is nutritious and meets or exceeds body requirements.	Consult with dietician to determine patient's nutritional needs. *To obtain information on calorie needs and facilitate meal planning.* Monitor daily intake with calorie count. *To provide data on total daily calorie intake.* Consult with health care provider and dietitian on high-calorie supplements. *To increase calorie intake when larger volumes of food cannot be tolerated.*
	Patient and family use diet plan, report increased intake and weight is increased. Nutritious food available to patient.	Collaborate with patient/family to create a plan to increase intake: 1. Eat 6–7 small protein-rich foods. *To decrease nausea from feeling "over full" and to increase calorie intake.* 2. Select soft foods if patient has difficulty swallowing (eggs, ice cream, cooked vegetables, pureed meats). *To decrease swallowing pain.* 3. Rest prior to meals. *To conserve energy for eating.* 4. Hold liquids 1 hour prior to eating. *To reduce satiety.*
	Eats meals with others weekly.	5. Encourage patient to eat meals with family/friends. *To increase social interaction and provide encouragement to eat.* Assess need for community resources and consult social worker or community liaison regarding financial assistance if patient cannot afford food. *To provide resources on nutritious foods.*
	Decreased nausea and increased intake.	Administer prescribed medications: 1. Antiemetics. *To decrease nausea.* 2. Appetite stimulants (dronabinol, megestrol acetate). *To counteract anorexia effects of disease and medications.* 3. Cytokine inhibitors (thalidomide). *To improve appetite by suppressing TNF-α production (used only in cases of severe wasting syndrome).*
	Decrease in rate of weight loss.	Consult with health care provider and dietitian about enteral or parenteral nutrition if patient unable to gain weight. *Provides additional nutritional support (used with severe wasting syndrome).*

Assessment of Diarrhea

Subjective Data:

How many bowel movements are you having a day?
What is the consistency and color of the stool?
Are you taking any medications to stop diarrhea?
How many glasses of water/liquid are you drinking per day?
Are you experiencing abdominal pain or cramping?
Is the area around your rectum sore or bleeding?
What type of foods do you typically eat during the day?

Objective Data:

Vital signs (low BP, rapid HR may indicate dehydration)
Measurement of the number, volume, and consistency of bowel movements per day
Perianal area: red, excoriated
Skin turgor: tenting
Urine output: < 700 mL/day
Laboratory tests: abnormalities in electrolytes, phosphorus, magnesium, Hbg, RBCs
Stool culture: pathogens

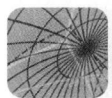

NURSING PROCESS: Patient Care Plan for HIV/AIDS—*Continued*

Nursing Assessment and Diagnoses	Outcomes and Evaluation Parameters	Planning and Interventions with *Rationales*
Nursing Diagnoses: *Bowel Incontinence* and *Diarrhea* related to HIV infection and/or opportunistic infections in the GI tract	**Outcome:** Normal bowel habits. ***Evaluation Parameters:*** One to two soft, formed stools/day. Fluid and electrolyte status maintained. Factors contributing to acute episodes of diarrhea identified and avoided. Weight increasing. Opportunistic infection treated appropriately as exhibited by decreasing incidence of diarrhea, normal stool cultures. Adequate fluid status maintained as evidenced by urine output > 700 mL/day, good skin turgor, stable blood pressure. Normal electrolytes, hemoglobin (Hgb), Red blood cells (RBC). Decreased abdominal cramping and acute episodes of diarrhea. Perianal skin intact. Patient and family use diet plan, report decreased episodes of diarrhea, and weight is increased.	**Interventions and *Rationales:*** Assess for frequency and volume of loose stools and for abdominal cramping. *To determine the amount of diarrhea, fluid volume loss, and level of abdominal discomfort.* Identify factors that cause and alleviate diarrhea. *To help individualize care and create an effective plan.* Weigh daily and document amount. *To trend weights as part of intervention assessment.* Obtain stool cultures. *Identifies opportunistic infections.* Administer antimicrobial therapy as prescribed. *To eliminate or control infecting organisms.* Instruct patient to have fluid intake of >3 L/day unless contraindicated. *To prevent hypovolemia.* Monitor and report abnormal laboratory values (potassium, sodium, calcium, phosphorus, magnesium, Hbg, RBCs). *Chronic diarrhea and small intestinal inflammation may impair electrolyte absorption and absorption of vitamins necessary for Hbg and RBC formation.* Administer anticholinergics, antispasmodics, and opioids as prescribed. *To decrease intestinal motility and spasms.* Assess for perianal excoriation. *To determine need for skin barrier creams or application of external drainage bag to protect skin.* Instruct patient/family in diet measures to decrease bowel hyperactivity. *To help rest bowel and possibly decrease diarrhea.* Eliminate bowel-irritating foods such as raw vegetables, nuts, and fried or fatty foods. *To reduce stimulation to the bowel.* Avoid coffee and nicotine. *Bowel stimulants.* Encourage nonspicy, bland diet (BRAT diet = bananas, rice, applesauce, toast). *Carbohydrates are easier to digest and cause less stimulation of the bowel.*

Assessment of Oral Mucous Membranes

Subjective Data:
Are you having any difficulty or pain with chewing and swallowing?
Do you have any sores in your mouth?
Are you brushing your teeth at least twice a day?
Do you use a lip balm to protect your lips?

Objective Data:
Oral cavity: edema, white patches, open lesions, loose or decaying teeth, purple lesions

Nursing Assessment and Diagnoses	Outcomes and Evaluation Parameters	Planning and Interventions with *Rationales*
Nursing Diagnosis: *Impaired Oral Mucous Membrane* related to immunologic deficit and presence of opportunistic infection/malignancy such as candidiasis, herpes, Kaposi's sarcoma; malnutrition and/or dehydration; side effects of drugs and chemotherapy; ineffective oral hygiene	**Outcome:** Integrity of mucous membranes maintained. ***Evaluation Parameters:*** Patient reports no oral discomfort. Mucous membranes pink, moist, intact.	**Interventions and *Rationales:*** Assess patient for oral pain and difficulty with chewing or swallowing. *Indicates problem in oral cavity that affects patient comfort and impacts oral intake.* Assess oral cavity for ulcerations, redness, white patches, especially on the side of the tongue. *Indicates probable oral candidiasis or progressing esophagitis.*

(continued)

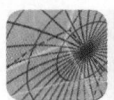

NURSING PROCESS: Patient Care Plan for HIV/AIDS—*Continued*

Nursing Assessment and Diagnoses	Outcomes and Evaluation Parameters	Planning and Interventions with *Rationales*
	Oral and esophageal opportunistic infections treated appropriately and effectively.	Report symptoms of candidiasis. *To initiate medical treatment.*
		Obtain cultures or oral lesions as prescribed. *To identify opportunistic pathogens and target medical treatment.*
	Identified dental problems treated appropriately.	Assess for swelling of gingiva, loose or decaying teeth. *Indicates poor oral hygiene; increases risk of infection from dental source.*
	Medications effective as evidenced by decreasing symptoms of infection.	Refer to dental consultation if necessary. *To treat oral decay.*
		Administer medications as prescribed: antifungals, antibiotics. *To treat infections.*
	Lips and surrounding skin intact.	Assess for cracks or fissures at corners of mouth and on lips. *Indicates sources of oral discomfort.*
	Tumors or growths in oral cavity treated appropriately as evidenced by decreased size of lesion and increased patient comfort.	Assess for purple lesions or tumors. *Indicates possible Kaposi's sarcoma or lymphoma.*
		Prepare patient for treatment with radiation, chemotherapy, and excision of lesions as prescribed. *To provide emotional support and coordinate care needs.*
	Patient reports decreasing oral discomfort, participates in oral care. Practices oral hygiene self-care instructions.	Assist with oral care every 2 hours. Rinse oral mucosa with saline and dilute hydrogen peroxide solution. *Decreases spread of lesions.*
		Use a soft toothbrush or sponge-tipped swab, nonabrasive toothpaste, and lip moisturizer.
		Brush teeth a minimum of twice a day. *Decreases acid formation from retained food, moistens mucous membranes, prevents infection, and promotes comfort.*
		Avoid lemon glycerin swabs and alcohol-based mouthwashes. *Acid irritates lesions and alcohol-based products dry mucous membranes.*
		Encourage use of commercial salivary product or hard candy or gum. *Neutralizes acids by increasing saliva flow and protects mucous membranes.*
		Instruct patient and family in aspects of oral hygiene. *To promote comfort and self-care.*
	Family/friends support oral hygiene self-care practices.	Collaborate with patient/family to plan menu that avoids salty, spicy, acidic, or abrasive foods. *To decrease aggravation of oral lesions.*
	Patient has decreased oral pain.	
	Moist pink mucous membranes.	Avoid extremely hot or cold foods. *Mucous membranes are sensitive to temperature extremes.*
		Instruct patient to have fluid intake of >2,500 mL/day if not contraindicated. *To maintain hydration and keep mucous membranes moist.*
		Encourage patient to avoid smoking. *To decrease drying and irritation to mucous membranes.*

Sources: Carpenito-Moyet, L. (2008). *Nursing care plans and documentation* (5th ed.). Philadelphia: Lippincott Williams & Wilkins; Corless, I. B., & Nicholas, P. K. (2003). Nursing care of patients with HIV/AIDS. In J. K. Shaw & E. A. Mahoney (Eds.), *HIV/AIDS nursing secrets* (pp. 33–39). Philadelphia: Hanley & Belfus; Porth, C., & Sweeney, K. (2007). Alterations in immune response. In C. M. Porth (Ed.), *Essentials of pathophysiology* (pp. 293–319). St. Louis: Lippincott Williams & Wilkins.

The HIV/AIDS epidemic means that nurses throughout all aspects of the health care system will be called on to care for patients with HIV infection. Foundational to nursing is providing care in a compassionate, committed, and nonjudgmental manner. Care for the patient with AIDS involves a wide spectrum of activities from a gentle touch that communicates compassion, to education on a complex medication regimen and multiple interventions to treat opportunistic infections and malignancies. Nurses also play a central role in providing emotional support to patients and families during the dying process and facilitating the discussions on end-of-life care. The complexity of HIV infection presents multiple care needs that nurses, using the nursing process, are well equipped to address. Nurses are an essential part of a collaborative care approach to optimizing treatment for the patient with AIDS.

Health Promotion

The primary mode of HIV/AIDS prevention is education and lifestyle modification for at-risk groups. Nurses, other health care providers, social workers, and community health educators, and schools play a central role in providing education about HIV/AIDS and infection prevention. Instructing individuals and communities on safer sex practices and ways to decrease disease transmission with injection drug use is essential. Chart 60–12 (p. 1948) provides a teaching guide for individuals and

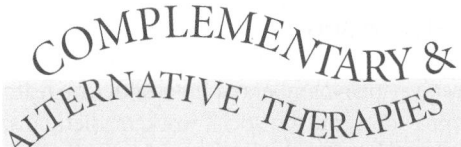

COMPLEMENTARY & ALTERNATIVE THERAPIES

for Patients with HIV/AIDS

THERE IS growing support among HIV-infected patients for the use of complementary and alternative treatments in symptom management. Alternative therapies focus on the interaction of the mind, body, and spirit and the concept of treating the whole person. Alternative therapies used in conjunction with traditional Western medicine therapies may improve the patient's overall well-being (Swanson et al., 2000). The four basic categories of alternative therapies are listed here along with examples of the therapies used most frequently:

1. *Nutritional therapies:* vegetarian or microbiotic diets, Chinese herb mixtures, vitamin C or beta-carotene substances

2. *Physical treatments:* acupressure, acupuncture, reflexology, therapeutic touch, crystals, and yoga

3. *Spiritual or psychological therapies:* humor, faith healing, guided imagery, hypnosis

4. *Biological therapies and drugs:* oxygen, zone, and urine therapy; non–FDA-approved drugs (*N*-acetylcysteine, pentoxifylline).

Source: Swanson, P., Harris, B., Holzmayer, V., Devare, S., Schochetman, G., and Hack J. (2000). Quantification of HIV-1 group M (subtypes A–G) and group O by the LCx HIV RNA quantitative assay. *Journal of Virological Methods, 89*(1, 2), 97–108.

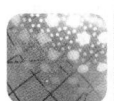

PATIENT TEACHING & DISCHARGE PRIORITIES for the HIV-Infected Individual with AIDS

Need	Teaching
Knowledge of disease process	Provide verbal and written instructions on ways HIV can be transmitted to avoid infecting other persons (unprotected sex, sharing of needles, exposing others to blood or body fluids).
Understanding of medications	Have patient administer medications on schedule and verbalize importance of compliance with HAART therapy to control disease progression and decrease risk of developing drug resistance.
	Teach the purpose, dose, and possible side effects of all medications to increase compliance and prevent over- or underdosing.
	Explain the importance of a follow-up laboratory appointment schedule to monitor medication effectiveness.
Prevention of opportunistic infections	Teach signs and symptoms of infection and strategies to avoid exposure to opportunistic infections.
	Encourage avoidance of people with communicable diseases such as colds or flu.
Reportable clinical manifestations	Instruct patient/family to report: • Symptoms of infection (fever, malaise, aching joints) • New or worsening rash or sores • Difficulty eating or swallowing • Nausea, vomiting, diarrhea that lasts for more than 2 days • New or worsening pain • Weight loss.
Ongoing care	Explain the purpose of clinic and laboratory follow-up appointments for ongoing monitoring of medication effectiveness and assessment of CD4+ T-cell and viral load counts.
	Provide schedule and contact information for appointments following discharge.
	Explain value of regular health screenings including checkups with monitoring of weight and dental care.
Family/support system	Assess availability of support system to provide emotional support, and assist with medications and transportation to appointments.
	Collaborate with discharge planner/case manager RN (if available) and assess discharge needs to home or extended care.
	Assess need for home assistive devices.
	Assess need for home health care provider.
Emotional adjustment of patient/family due to chronic nature of disease	Answer questions honestly.
	Encourage verbalization of feelings, fears.
	Discuss possibility of depression and encourage discussion of this with health care provider.

partners regarding practices to decrease HIV transmission risk that can be used by a variety of HIV/AIDS prevention educators.

It is important that HIV-infected patients and their families and friends understand the routes of transmission of HIV to prevent infection and alleviate fears of casual transmission. The information provided can address these issues and alleviate fears that may interfere with social support for the patient with HIV/AIDS.

Collaborative Management

A multidisciplinary collaborative approach to preventing HIV infection and transmission and providing treatment for patients with HIV/AIDS is essential. A variety of individuals using different educational approaches in varied settings can most effectively communicate the facts about HIV/AIDS. Effective treatment of individuals with HIV infection and AIDS requires

GERONTOLOGICAL CONSIDERATIONS Related to HIV/AIDS

In the United States, 10% of all reported AIDS cases occur in adults over 50 years of age. Older adults are at increased risk for contracting HIV/AIDS because of declining immune system function with aging. Additionally, AIDS is associated with youth, sexual activity, and IV drug use, factors that are generally not linked with the elderly population. Sexual contact is the most common form of HIV transmission, yet there is a prevalent misconception that older adults are not sexually active. Older adults are beyond childbearing years, so they often fail to use condoms when engaging in sexual activity. Additionally, older adults may have had a history of IV drug use that results in latent HIV infection. They also can be current IV drug users, but given the more conservative nature of their social group and the socially unacceptable nature of this addiction, this issue may be denied. As a consequence there is denial on the part of older adults and the health care community that this group is at risk for HIV infection, and the potential for misdiagnosis and subsequent failure to treat with antiretroviral therapy is significant (Ress, 2003).

Nurses must be aware that the older adult is also at risk for HIV/AIDS and assess the risk factors by means of a thorough nursing history. It is essential to advocate for the patient by asking the medical team about possible HIV antibody testing when a diagnosis is unclear and the patient has risk factors and symptoms consistent with an AIDS-related illness.

coordination between various members of the health care team such as health care providers, nurses, social workers, dietitians, and community workers at various levels of care from clinics, to home care, to acute care.

The health care provider is primarily responsible for diagnosis and development of the medical treatment plan. The role of the nurse is centered on providing emotional support and monitoring and managing disease symptoms. Nurses also provide education on medications and the importance of compliance with the medication regimen, ongoing laboratory tests and appointments, and minimizing the risk of opportunistic infections. Social workers offer assistance in addressing financial concerns, managing personal care needs, and accessing community referrals and social networks in the community and acute care setting. Dietitians also have a significant role in monitoring nutritional needs and developing specialized nutritional plans that may include supplements in light of HIV complications and wasting syndrome. For more on nutrition and how it affects patients with HIV/AIDS, see the Evidence-Based Practice feature.

Collaborative care of HIV-infected patients also involves extensive education of patients, family, and friends regarding antiretroviral medications and prevention of opportunistic infections as discussed earlier in Chart 60–9 (p. 1929). Collaborative care also involves identifying potential risk factors for HIV

CHART 60–12 **Patient and Partner Teaching Guide on Preventing HIV Transmission**

- Practice abstinence or mutual monogamy or limit the number of sexual partners.
- Do not have unprotected sex. Use latex condoms (animal skin condoms do not prevent HIV transmission). For latex allergies use female condoms that are latex free.
- Do not lubricate the condom with spermicidal agent nonoxynol-9 or use spermicidal agent nonoxynol-9 because this may increase vaginal tissue damage and the risk of HIV infection.
- Do not use oil-based sex lubricants because this can damage the condom. Water-based lubricants are safe to use.
- Do not reuse male or female condoms.
- Always use a condom with other methods of birth control. Cervical caps or diaphragms will decrease the risk of pregnancy, but not HIV transmission.
- Always use dental dams for oral female genital or anal stimulation.
- Avoid anal intercourse or manual anal intercourse "fisting" to prevent injury to tissues.
- Use safer sex practices, such as mutual masturbation, to decrease damage to mucous membranes.
- If entering a mutually exclusive monogamous relationship, both partners should undergo HIV testing. There is a window period of up to 6 months before HIV antibody testing is positive, so the above guidelines should be followed during the window period when HIV status is unknown.
- If you are HIV antibody positive, inform previous, current, and prospective sex partners and drug-using partners of your HIV status. Follow the above guidelines.

- If you are HIV antibody positive, inform health care providers of HIV status. Laws protect the confidentiality of this information. This information helps direct your medical treatment.
- If you are HIV antibody positive, do not share items that may be contaminated with blood such as needles, drug works, sex toys, razors, or toothbrushes.
- If you are HIV antibody positive, do not donate blood, plasma, sperm, or body organs.

GUIDELINES FOR SAFER USE OF INJECTION EQUIPMENT

If you use injection drugs, consider stopping and entering a treatment program. If you cannot make that choice, use the following guidelines to limit your risk of HIV and other disease transmission.

- Use sterile needles and syringes.
- Do not share your needles, syringes, or drug preparation equipment ("works").
- Access needle and syringe exchange programs, when available, to exchange used needles and syringes and obtain sterile ones.
- If injection equipment is shared, clean it thoroughly before use: Rinse the syringe and needle twice with tap water, fill the syringe with full-strength household bleach for 30 seconds, shake and squirt out, repeat bleaching process a second time, then rinse again twice with tap water.
- Do not share your drug preparation equipment. If it is shared, clean it thoroughly with bleach and water.
- Do not share your bleach or rinse water.

Sources: Centers for Disease Control and Prevention. (2007, July). *HIV and AIDS: Are you at risk?* Retrieved September 3, 2008, from http://www.cdc.gov/hiv/resources/brochures/at-risk.htm; Shaw, J. K., & Mahoney, E. A. (Eds.). (2003). *HIV/AIDS nursing secrets.* Philadelphia: Hanley & Belfus; Workowski, K. A., & Levine, W. C. (2002). Sexually transmitted diseases treatment guidelines. *Morbidity and Mortality Weekly Report, 51*(RR-06).

Healthy Nutrition and the Patient with HIV/AIDS

Clinical Problem

The relationship between nutrition and HIV/AIDS is complex and not fully understood. It is known, however, that healthy nutrition plays a role in alleviating common symptoms of HIV such as diarrhea, anorexia, sore mouth, and muscle wasting. There are many gaps in current knowledge about the impact of malnutrition on management and progression of HIV. It is known that HIV causes increased energy requirements, nutrient malabsorption and loss, complex metabolic alterations, and frequently a loss of appetite that culminates in weight loss and muscle wasting. The effect of HIV on nutritional status begins early in the course of infection, at times even before the patient is aware of being infected (Bogden et al., 2000).

Vitamins and minerals needed for the immune system to fight infections include A, B-complex, C, and E, and selenium and zinc. These substances are commonly found to be deficient in people living with HIV in all settings. In addition, deficiencies of antioxidant vitamins and minerals contribute to oxidative stress, which may accelerate immune cell death and increase the rate of HIV replication (Allard et al., 1998; Banki, Hutter, Goncharoff, & Perl, 1998).

Research Findings

Fawzi and colleagues (2004) conducted a study to evaluate the impact of micronutrient supplements (vitamin A alone, multivitamins including vitamin B-complex and vitamins C and E, and multivitamins plus vitamin A) on the risks of clinical disease progression, HIV-related complications, CD4+ cell counts, and viral load in HIV-positive women. The researchers followed 1,078 HIV-infected pregnant women over a 2-year period. The women were randomly assigned in blocks of 20 to receive a daily oral dose of one of four regimens of vitamins for the duration of the study.

The results of the study indicate that multivitamin supplementation with vitamin B-complex, vitamin C, and vitamin E significantly delayed the progression of disease among HIV-infected women, as reflected by the relative risk of progression to WHO stage 4 or death from AIDS-related causes. Supplementation with vitamin A alone had weaker effects that for the most part were not significantly different from those produced by placebo. The study also found that supplementation with multivitamins also reduced the incidence of complications including:

- Oral thrush
- Oral ulcers
- Difficulty swallowing
- Nausea
- Vomiting
- Diarrhea.

The researchers concluded that micronutrients may protect the integrity of oral and gastrointestinal epithelia and enhance local and systemic immunity.

Implications for Nursing Practice

This study clearly indicates the efficacy of vitamin supplements for HIV patients for retarding the progress of the disease. When teaching the patient and caregivers about the complex nutritional issues associated with the disease, the nurse needs to include information about the type, amount, and administration schedule of vitamins. It is essential that nurses stress the importance of a continued course of micronutrient supplements. These supplements are readily available and typically inexpensive, which makes it easier for patients to comply with the therapy.

Critical Thinking Questions

1. Which of the following interventions would be effective in increasing medication compliance for patients with HIV/AIDS?
   a. Education about the impact of the medication on disease progression
   b. Ease of availability and financial resources
   c. Caregiver compliance
   d. Show patient laboratory results that support stabilization of the disease

2. Which of the following clinical manifestations would you as the nurse assess for vitamin efficacy?
   a. Diminished or absent diarrhea
   b. Stabilization or increase in CD4+ counts
   c. Absence of candidiasis
   d. No painful swallowing

Answers to Critical Thinking Questions appear in Appendix D.

References

Allard, J. P., Aghdassi, E., Chau, J., et al. (1998). Effects of vitamin E and C supplementation on oxidative stress and viral load in HIV-infected subjects. *AIDS, 12,* 1653–1659.

Banki, K., Hutter, E., Goncharoff, N. J., & Perl, A. (1998). Molecular ordering in HIV-induced apoptosis. Oxidative stress, activation of caspases, and cell survival are regulated by transaldolase. *Journal of Biological Chemistry, 273*(19), 11944–11953.

Bogden, J. D., Kemp, F. W., Han, S., et al. (2000). Status of selected nutrients and progression of human immunodeficiency virus type 1 infection. *American Journal of Clinical Nutrition, 72*(3), 809–815.

Fawzi, W. W., Msamanga, G. I., Spiegelman, D., Wei, R., Kapiga, S., Villamor, E., et al. (2004). A randomized trial of multivitamin supplements and HIV disease progression and mortality. *New England Journal of Medicine, 351*(1), 23–32.

EVIDENCE-BASED PRACTICE

infection in patients who have not been diagnosed with HIV and patient knowledge of how HIV is transmitted. Key questions to determine the level of HIV infection risk are a vital aspect of assessment. It is also important to apply an understanding of HIV/AIDS epidemiology in identifying increasingly at-risk populations including women, non-Caucasians, and people over 50 years of age.

The complexity of HIV antiretroviral treatment, the psychologically devastating nature of the disease, and the various body systems that are affected by AIDS mandate a collaborative care approach to maximize patient treatment, and promote comfort and quality of life.

HIV key risk assessment questions to ask include the following: Have you had a blood transfusion of any type? If so, was it before 1985? Have you ever had a vaginal, anal, or oral sexual experience without a condom or barrier device? Have you ever had a sexually transmitted infection? Have you ever shared needles, syringes, or other injecting equipment with another person?

Research Topics Related to the Immune Deficiencies

Research related to immune deficiencies is multifaceted. Nurses are involved in many areas of study including coordinating clinical research sites, data collection, drug studies, and clinical outcomes research. The Research Opportunities and Clinical Impact box provides information on some of the current areas of medical and nursing research under investigation.

The development of a vaccine for HIV is a primary focus of continuing research related to HIV and AIDS. In 1987 The National Institute of Allergy and Infectious Diseases (NIAID) began the first clinical trial of an experimental vaccine. Since that time 23 potential vaccines and 10 adjuvants (substances that might enhance the vaccine's effects) have been tested. The development of a vaccine has been particularly challenging because

HIV mutates rapidly and lives within the cell and hides from antibodies. The NIAID began a phase II vaccine study in 1997 to determine if combining two experimental vaccines can safely stimulate an immune response. To accelerate vaccine development, in September 2003 the NIAID awarded $81 million to four companies researching different strategies for creating a vaccine. NIAID Director Anthony S. Fauci stated at the time of the awards, "A safe and effective HIV vaccine is critical to the control of HIV globally. These awards will speed the development of promising HIV vaccine candidates that are based on recent advances in HIV vaccine design and on the latest discoveries of HIV virology and immunology" (NIAID, 2003). There is a continual hope that at some point in the not-too-distant future, HIV infection will be preventable and AIDS a disease of the past.

RESEARCH OPPORTUNITIES AND CLINICAL IMPACT RELATED TO IMMUNE DEFICIENCIES

Research Area	Clinical Impact
Gene research to identify DNA factors associated with development of genetic immune deficiencies	Develop gene therapy that will help with prevention and treatment of genetic immune deficiencies.
	Provide information to promote informed decision making for couples in genetic counseling.
Development of a vaccine to protect against infection after exposure with HIV	Reduce active cases of HIV and AIDS through prevention with vaccine.
Epidemiologic studies that focus on areas of the world where the incidence of HIV is increasing and the risk factors noted in those areas	Reduce cases of HIV through education of populations at greatest risk worldwide.
Development of new classes of antiretroviral medications	Improve survival, slow progression of HIV infection, maximize development of antiretroviral medications.
Development of a DNA bank of genes, HIV genes, and enzyme codes	Promote research and development of better therapies and vaccines.
Clinical trials of patient compliance with a self-injectable medication (Enfuvirtide)	Provide new route of delivery of drug that may reduce side effects. However, an injectable form requires more extensive patient education.
Clinical trial of calcium carbonate to treat diarrhea in HIV patients receiving protease inhibitors	Reduce side effects and improve quality of life for patients taking multiple antiretroviral medications.
Clinical trials of high-dose combination therapy to extend life in advanced AIDS patients	Improve quality and delay further progression of disease for advanced AIDS patients, and decrease development of resistance.
Comparative studies on HIV viral loads, initiation of antiretroviral therapy, and development of drug resistance	Guide the appropriate initiation of antiretroviral therapy to help prevent development of drug resistance.
Study of adherence, quality of life, and satisfaction with combination drug therapy among patients with multiple years of HIV diagnosis	Improve teaching of medication therapy and increase compliance for newly diagnosed HIV patients starting therapy. Prevent drug resistance.
Comparative studies on viral loads and perinatal transmission for vaginal versus cesarean delivery modes	Develop clear guidelines on the safest method of delivery for HIV-infected pregnant women that also limits perinatal HIV transmission.
Comparative studies on effectiveness of complementary therapies for HIV disease progressive management	Provide new drug treatments to control pain and improve the patient's quality of life.

Clinical Preparation

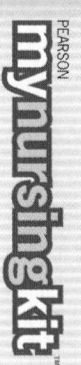

 Read

- History of Current Illness
- Past Medical History
- Physical Exam
- Admitting Medical Orders
- Laboratory Study Results

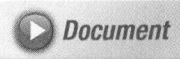 **Document**

- Summary of Hospitalization
- Pathophysiology Form
- Laboratory Values
- Laboratory Results Explanation

 **Apply**

- List of Potential Nursing Diagnoses
- Concept Map
- Critical Thinking Questions

Log on to MyNursingKit.com to download forms you will need and to complete further steps in the Clinical Preparation assignment.

HISTORY OF PRESENT ILLNESS

Mr. B is a 42-year-old Spanish-speaking, thin, anxious-appearing male in moderate discomfort due to abdominal pain that he first noticed 2 weeks ago and described as dull. He does not have a regular doctor and presented to the emergency department (ED) with abdominal pain. Patient requests a Spanish-speaking interpreter. He states, via an interpreter, that he has had increased abdominal pain during the past 5 days, has lost more than 20 pounds during the last 3 months, does not have an appetite, and is having increasing difficulty swallowing because of "sores" in his mouth. He has been unable to take solid foods for the past 3 days due to painful swallowing, and has taken very little juice or water during the past 24 hours. Denies nausea, vomiting.

He is being admitted by internal medicine to the medical–surgical unit. States he did not want to come to the doctor earlier because he does not have the money to pay the bill. Came to the ED today "because the pain was getting very bad, and I am afraid something is wrong with me." Upon admission to the floor, the patient is awake and alert. He states he is continuing to have pain in his abdomen despite medication.

Medical–Surgical History

No known allergies
Medications: none
Denies history of cancer or family history of cancer
Denies history of abdominal trauma or injuries, gastric reflux disease, hernia, or colitis
Positive history of fatigue, intermittent fever, chills, and night sweats during the past 6 months
Genital herpes onset age 19, intermittent recurrence, most recent occurrence 1 year prior
Surgeries: appendectomy at age 22 in Mexico

Social History

Immigrated to the United States 2 years prior, unmarried, lives with his brother and his brother's family; employed in lawn care and home maintenance business
Drinks 1–2 beers daily
Smokes 1/2 pack of cigarettes per day × 25 years
Prior IV drug use; none in the past 7 years
Intermittently sexually active with various partners

Physical Exam

Vital signs: BP 101/45, HR 108, RR 22, temp 36.8°C, oxygen saturation 95% on room air
Pain: 6/10
Neurological: alert and oriented × 3, worried expression on face, neurological exam normal, communicates with minimal English, primary language is Spanish

HEENT: oral mucous membranes are red and inflamed, multiple white lesions present on oral mucosa and extending to the posterior oral pharynx. Tonsils slightly enlarged, poor dental care, four teeth missing on anterior and left lateral upper jaw. Submandibular lymph nodes bilaterally enlarged and tender to palpations. Ears and eyes normal
Neck: cervical lymph nodes enlarged bilaterally, right greater than left, tender to palpation; full range of neck motion present
Respiratory: denies shortness of breath; unlabored respirations; equal chest wall expansion; no chest deformities evident or palpated; lungs clear
Cardiovascular: tachycardia with occasional irregular beat, S_1, S_2, no murmur, pulses palpable in all extremities, capillary refill WNL
GI/GU: abdomen slightly distended but soft, palpable mass lower quadrants, bowel sounds present in all quadrants, abdomen painful to light palpation in all quadrants, greatest area of pain in lower quadrants. Denies painful urination, normal size genitals, uncircumcised, no drainage from penis, with no evidence of lesions
Skin: intact, dry; poor skin turgor; no evidence of discoloration, rash, or bruising
12-lead ECG: showed sinus tachycardia, occasional PVCs and no other abnormalities
Abdominal CT: results indicate a pelvic mass in the retroperitoneal space above the bladder; size estimated at 20 cm by 15 cm

Admitting Medical Orders

Medical service
Consults: Surgical, Social Services, Oncology
Admit to medical–surgical floor with telemetry monitoring
Admitting diagnosis: abdominal pain, pelvic mass, r/o abdominal
  malignancy, oral and esophageal candidiasis
Allergies: none
Full code status
Strict I&O
Vital signs and oxygen saturation q4h
Daily weight
Diet: clear liquids
Ambulation ad-lib
Incentive spirometer q1–2h
Sequential compression devices (SCDs) to lower extremities when
  in bed
Call house officer: BP < 90 systolic or diastolic > 90; HR >120 and
  < 60, RR >30; temp > 38.2°C: oxygen saturation < 92%
IV: 0.9% saline with 20 mEq of KCl via infusion pump at 500 mL/hr
  × 1 liter, then decrease rate to 125 mL/hr
  Scheduled Medications
  Diflucan 200 mg po daily
  Protonix 40 mg po daily
  Nystatin 5 mL q6h, swish & swallow
  PRN Medications
  Morphine sulphate 2–4 mg IV push q2h prn for severe pain
  Vicodin 1–2 tabs (5/500) po q6h prn for moderate pain
  Ativan, 0.5 mg po q4h prn anxiety
  Zofran 4 mg IV q4h prn nausea

Ordered Laboratory Studies

CBC with differential on admission
Blood count daily
Complete metabolic panel (CMP), amylase, lipase, PO_4,
  PT/INR/PTT, UA, CD4 cell count
HIV antibody test (health care provider has completed consent for
  testing with patient and this is documented on chart)

Ordered Diagnostic Studies

12-lead ECG
Abdominal CT

LABORATORY STUDY RESULTS

Test	Day 1	Day 2	Day 3
Sodium	148 mEq/L	142 mEq/L	138 mEq/L
Potassium	2.9 mEq/L	3.9 mEq/L	4.2 mEq/L
Chloride	113 mEq/L	99 mEq/L	99 mEq/L
Venous carbon dioxide	22 mEq/L	25 mEq/L	25 mEq/L
Blood urea nitrogen (BUN)	42 mg/dL	22 mg/dL	19 mg/dL
Creatinine	1.1 mg/dL	0.9 mg/dL	0.7 mg/dL
Blood glucose	143 mg/dL	124 mg/dL	133 mg/dL
Calcium	7.9 mg/dL	7.8 mg/dL	7.9 mg/dL
Total protein	5.2 g/dL		
Amylase	72 units/L		
Lipase	27 units /L		
Magnesium	1.9 mEq/L	2.0 mEq/L	2.1 mEq/L
Phosphorus	3.1 mg/dL		
Albumin	2.9 g/dL	2.9	2.9
Alkaline phosphatase	225 units/L	197 units/L	192 units/L
Total bilirubin	1.2 mg/dL		
AST (SGOT)	64 units/L	99 units/L	104 units/L
ALT (SGPT)	52 units/L	80 units/L	92 units/L
WBC	1700/mm^3	1600/mm^3	1600/mm^3
Hemoglobin	10.1 g/dL	9.8 g/dL	9.8 g/dL
Hematocrit	30.2%	29.8%	29.8%
RBCs	4.0/mm^3	3.9/mm^3	3.9/mm^3
Neutrophils	88%		
Lymphocytes	2%		
Monocytes	3%		
Platelets	227,000/mm^3	208,000/mm^3	87,000/mm^3
PTT	34 seconds		
PT	13.1 seconds		
INR	1.22 seconds		
CEA		> 11 ng/mL	
CD4 count	170 cells/uL		
HIV antibody	Positive		
ABGs			
PO$_2$	92 mmHg		
Oxygen saturation	95%	94%	
pH	7.34		
PCO$_2$	39 mmHg		

CRITICAL THINKING QUESTIONS

1. What information was obtained that suggested the need for HIV testing?

2. Review the laboratory findings from the ED. Which ones are abnormal, what is the possible rationale for these abnormalities, and how are these abnormalities evidenced in physical assessment findings?

3. EIA and Western blot tests are ordered to confirm the diagnosis. The CD4 count results are 187 cells/μL. What is the rationale for ordering this test and what is the significance of the result?

4. Mr. B is HIV positive, but does he have AIDS according to the CDC guidelines?

5. What additional treatment should you anticipate for Mr. B based on his HIV test results and CD4 results?

Answers to Critical Thinking Questions appear in Appendix D.

NCLEX® REVIEW

1. The nursing management and collaborative care for patients with an immune hypersensitivity response differs from those who have immune deficiencies. When the nurse suspects the patient has developed an immune hypersensitivity response, the clinical picture may be based on which of the following characteristics?

1. The immune system loses self-tolerance and immune deficiencies result.

2. Hypersensitive reactions are determined by the type of antigen, the time sequence of the reaction, and the immunological response.

3. The primary mechanism of a hypersensitive response is a genetic disorder that occurred during the embryonic development of the immune system.

4. Hypersensitive responses are usually the result of opportunistic infections which activate a primary response from the T and B cells.

2. Which of the following describes processes that differentiate the immune hypersensitivity response resulting from an autoimmune mechanism from those resulting from an allergic or alloimmune mechanism?

1. The primary trigger for a hypersensitive reaction is a genetic defect.

2. The origin for an alloimmune reaction is from the host's DNA.

3. The trigger for an autoimmune response is a self-antigen.

4. Once activated, the hypersensitive response is identical regardless of trigger.

3. Which of the following differentiate the pathophysiology and clinical manifestations of Acquired Immune Deficiency Syndrome (AIDS) from Human Immunodeficiency Virus (HIV)? Select all that apply.

1. HIV is the end disease manifestation of AIDS.

2. AIDS is a syndrome of opportunistic infections that occurs as a final stage in patients infected with HIV.

3. HIV transmission is limited to contact with infected body fluids that have lymphocytes that can harbor HIV.

4. AIDS precedes HIV and allows for the progression of the virus' entry into the host's lymphocytes.

4. Nursing management of the HIV/AIDS patient to decrease the incidence of opportunistic infections may involve which of the following? Select all that apply.

1. Subjective assessment to promote the early detection of infection from any body region.

2. Start antibiotics prior to obtaining cultures to ensure the appropriate therapy is initiated in a timely manner.

3. Health care providers and family members wash hands before and after patient contact to reduce the risk of opportunistic infection cross-contamination.

4. Encourage hydration and maintenance of weight to support the immune system.

Answers for review questions appear in Appendix D

KEY TERMS

acquired immunodeficiency syndrome
    (AIDS) *p.1922*
acute graft rejection *p.1913*
acute retroviral syndrome *p.1927*
AIDS indicator conditions *p.1927*
allergen *p.1891*
allergic response *p.1890*
allergy *p.1890*
alloimmune response *p.1890*
anaphylaxis *p.1895*
atopic *p.1893*
autoantibodies *p.1906*
autoantibody tests *p.1906*
autoimmune diseases *p.1903*
autoimmune response *p.1890*
CD4+ T cells *p.1926*
chronic graft rejection *p.1913*
corticosteroids *p.1906*
delayed hypersensitivity reaction *p.1891*
desensitization *p.1897*
flare *p.1893*

graft versus host disease (GVHD) *p.1913*
highly active antiretroviral drug therapy
    (HAART) *p.1937*
histamine *p.1891*
HIV antibody positive status *p.1927*
host versus graft disease (HVGD) *p.1913*
human immunodeficiency virus
    (HIV) *p.1922*
human leukocyte antigen (HLA) *p.1906*
hyperacute rejection *p.1913*
IgE antibodies *p.1891*
immediate hypersensitivity reaction *p.1890*
immune deficiencies *p.1890*
immune hypersensitivity *p.1890*
immune hypersensitivity response *p.1890*
Kaposi's sarcoma *p.1933*
neoantigens *p.1905*
opportunistic infections (OIs) *p.1922*
plasmapheresis *p.1906*
Pneumocystis carinii pneumonia
    (PCP) *p.1931*

primary immune deficiency *p.1890*
reverse transcriptase *p.1926*
secondary immune deficiencies *p.1890*
sensitization *p.1891*
skin testing *p.1896*
systemic lupus erythematosus (SLE) *p.1906*
tissue-specific antigens *p.1891*
type-specific hypersensitivity
    reactions *p.1890*
type I (IgE-mediated) allergic
    reaction *p.1891*
type II (tissue-specific–mediated)
    hypersensitivity reaction *p.1891*
type III (immune complex–mediated)
    reaction *p.1891*
type IV (cell-mediated) hypersensitivity
    reaction *p.1891*
viral load *p.1927*
wasting syndrome *p.1932*
Western blot (WB) *p.1933*
wheal *p.1893*
window period *p.1925*

REFERENCES

Adams, M., Josephson, D., & Holland, L. (2008). *Pharmacology for nurses: A pathophysiologic approach.* (2nd ed.) Upper Saddle River, NJ: Pearson Prentice Hall.

Ahmed, D. D., Sobczak, S. C., & Yunginger, J. W. (2003). Occupational allergies caused by latex. *Immunology and Allergy Clinics of North America, 23*(2), 205–219.

Allard, J. P., Aghdassi, E., Chau, J., et al. (1998). Effects of vitamin E and C supplementation on oxidative stress and viral load in HIV-infected subjects. *AIDS, 12,* 1653–1659.

American Academy of Allergy, Asthma and Immunology. (2006). *Why is the incidence of allergy increasing?* Retrieved February 23, 2007, from https://www.aaaai.org/aadmc/inthenews/wypr/2006archive/increasing_allergies.html

American Academy of Allergy, Asthma and Immunology. (2007). *Tips to remember: What is allergy testing.* Retrieved February 16, 2007, from http://www.aaaai.org

American College of Allergy, Asthma and Immunology. (2007). *Be S.A.F.E.: Managing allergic emergencies.* Retrieved February 19, 2007, from http://www.acaai.org/public

American Nurses Association. (2004). *Position statement: AIDS/HIV Disease and socio-culturally diverse populations.* Retrieved January 19, 2004, from http://www.nursingworld.org/readroom/position/blood/bldvrs.htm

American Red Cross. (2003). *What happens to every blood donation.* Retrieved October 10, 2003, from http://www.redcross.org/services/biomed/blood/supply

Anderson, J. (Ed.). (2004). *A guide to the clinical care of women with HIV.* Retrieved February 23, 2007, from the Department of Health and Human Services Health Resources and Services Administration website: http://hab.hrsa.gov/publications/womencare05

Anaya, J., Tobon, G., Vega, P., & Castiblanco, J. (2006). Autoimmune disease aggregation in families with primary Sjogren's syndrome. *Journal of Rheumatology, 33*(11), 2227–2234.

Asher, M., Montefort, S., Bjorksten, B., Lai, C., Strachan, D., Weiland, S., et al. (2006). Worldwide time trends in the prevalence of symptoms of asthma, allergic rhinoconjunctivitis, and eczema in childhood: ISAAC phases one and three repeat multicountry cross-sectional surveys. *Lancet, 368*(9537), 733–748.

Asthma and Allergy Foundation of America. (2007). *Allergy facts and figures.* Retrieved February 19, 2007, from http://www.aafa.org

Averitt, S. A., & Sowell, R. L. (2003). Pregnancy and HIV/AIDS. In J. K. Shaw & E. A. Mahoney (Eds.), *HIV/AIDS nursing secrets* (pp. 133–143). Philadelphia: Hanley & Belfus.

Banki, K., Hutter, E., Gonchoroff, N. J., & Perl, A. (1998). Molecular ordering in HIV-induced apoptosis. Oxidative stress, activation of caspases, and cell survival are regulated by transaldolase. *Journal of Biological Chemistry, 273*(19), 11944–11953.

Bartlett, J. G. (2003). *Wasting [HIV] antibiotic guide.* Accessed December 25, 2003, from Johns Hopkins Division of Infectious Diseases website: http://hopkins-abxguide.org/terminals/diagnosis_terminal.cfm?id=622

Bartlett, J. G., & Lane, H. C. (2007). *Guidelines for the use of antiretroviral agents in HIV-1-infected adults and adolescents. Developed by the DHHS Panel on Antiretroviral Guidelines for Adults and Adolescents—A working group of the Office of AIDS Research Advisory Council.* Retrieved January 10, 2008, from http://aidsinfo.nih.gov/contentfiles/AdultandAdolescentGL.pdf

Bochner, B. S., & Hamid, Q. (2003). Advances in mechanisms of allergy. *Journal of Allergy and Clinical Immunology, 111*(3 Suppl.), S819–S823.

Bogden, J. D., Kemp, F. W., Han, S., et al. (2000). Status of selected nutrients and progression of human immunodeficiency virus type 1 infection. *American Journal of Clinical Nutrition, 72*(3), 809–815.

Brandtzaeg, P. (2007). Why we develop food allergies: Coached by breast milk and good bacteria, the immune system strives to learn the difference between food and pathogens before the first morsel crosses our lips. *American Scientist, 95*(1), 28.

Branson, B., Handsfield, H., Lampe, M., Janssen, R., Taylor, A., Lyss, S., & Clark, J. (2006). Revised recommendations for HIV testing of adults, adolescents, and pregnant women. *MMWR 55* (RR-14): 1-17 Retrieved on September 5, 2008 from http://www.cdc.gov/mmwr/pdf/rr/rr5514.pdf.

Brew, B. J. (2002). Neurological manifestations of HIV infection. In S. Crowe, J. Hoy, & J. Mills (Eds.), *Management of the HIV-infected patient.* London: Taylor & Francis.

Carpenito-Moyet, L. (2008). *Nursing care plans and documentation* (5th ed.). Philadelphia: Lippincott Williams & Wilkins.

Centers for Disease Control and Prevention. (1981a). Opportunistic infections and Kaposi's sarcoma in homosexual men. *Morbidity and Mortality Weekly Report, 30.* Retrieved September 22, 2003, from http://aids-info.net/micha/hiv/aids/cdc81.htm

Centers for Disease Control and Prevention. (1981b). Pneumocystis pneumonia—Los Angeles. *Morbidity and Mortality Weekly Report, 30,* 250. Retrieved September 22, 2003, from http://aids-info.net/micha/hiv/aids/cdc81.htm

Centers for Disease Control and Prevention. (1993). Revised classification system for HIV infection and the expanded surveillance case definition of AIDS among adolescents and adults. *Morbidity and Mortality Weekly Report, 44*(RR-17). Retrieved February 23, 2007, from http://www.cdc.gov/mmwr/preview/mmwrhtml/00018871.htm

Centers for Disease Control and Prevention. (1995). First 500,000 AIDS cases, United States, 1995. *Morbidity and Mortality Weekly Report, 44,* 46. Retrieved January 19, 2004, from http://www.thebody.com/cdc/mmnov24.html

Centers for Disease Control and Prevention. (1998). *Human immunodeficiency virus type 2.* Retrieved January 19, 2004, from http://www.cdc.gov/hiv/pubs/facts/hiv2.htm

Centers for Disease Control and Prevention. (2001). Appendix B: Management of occupational blood exposures. *Morbidity and Mortality Weekly Report, 50*(RR-11), 45–46. Retrieved February 27, 2007, from http://www.cdc.gov/mmwr/preview/mmwrhtml/rr5011a3.htm

Centers for Disease Control and Prevention. (2002). HIV testing among pregnant women in the United States and Canada 1998–2001. *Morbidity and Mortality Weekly Report 51,* 1013–1016. Retrieved February 27, 2006, from http://www.cdc.gov/search

Centers for Disease Control and Prevention. (2003a). *HIV partner counseling and referral services guidance.* Retrieved February 27, 2007, from http://www.cdc.gov/hiv/pubs/pcrs/pcrs-doc.htm

Centers for Disease Control and Prevention. (2003b). *TB education and training resource guide—TB and HIV/AIDS co-infection.* Retrieved February 23, 2007, from CDC National Prevention Information Network website: http://www.cdcnpin.org/scripts/tb/guide/co_inf.asp

Centers for Disease Control and Prevention. (2005a). Appendix B: Updated U.S. Public Health Service guidelines for management of occupational exposures to HIV and recommendations for postexposure prophylaxis. *Morbidity and Mortality Weekly Report, 54*(RR-09), 1–17. Retrieved February 25, 2006, from http://www.cdc.gov/mmwr/preview/mmwrhtml/rr5011a3.htm

Centers for Disease Control and Prevention. (2005b). *Co-infection with HIV and hepatitis C virus.* Retrieved February 23, 2007, from http:/ /www.cdc.gov/hiv/resources/factsheets/coinfection.htm

Centers for Disease Control and Prevention. (2005c). *HIV/AIDS update basic statistics.* Retrieved February 23, 2007, from http://www.cdc.gov/hiv/stats.htm

Centers for Disease Control and Prevention. (2005d). Youth risk behavior surveillance in the United States, 2005. CDC Surveillance Summaries, 2006. *Morbidity and Mortality Weekly Report, 55*(SS-5). Retrieved February 27, 2006, from http://www.cdc.gov/search

Centers for Disease Control and Prevention. (2006a). *How safe is the blood supply in the United States?* Retrieved February 23, 2007, from http://www.cdc.gov/hiv/resources/qa/qa15.htm

Centers for Disease Control and Prevention. (2006b). *Important updates on OraQuick procedures.* Retrieved February 23, 2007, from http:/ /www.cdc.gov/hiv/resources/qa/prevention.htm

Centers for Disease Control and Prevention. (2006c). Revised recommendations for HIV testing of adults, adolescents, and pregnant women in healthcare settings. *Morbidity and Mortality Weekly Report, 55*(RR-14), 1–17.

Corbett, J. V. (2004). *Laboratory tests and diagnostic procedures.* Upper Saddle River, NJ: Pearson Prentice Hall.

Corless, I. B., & Nicholas, P. K. (2003). Nursing care of patients with HIV/AIDS. In J. K. Shaw & E. A. Mahoney (Eds.), *HIV/AIDS nursing secrets* (pp. 33–39). Philadelphia: Hanley & Belfus.

Crowe, S., Hoy, J., & Mills, J. (Eds.). (2002). *Management of the HIV-infected patient.* London: Taylor & Francis.

Dabis, F., Bequet, L., Ekouevi, D., & ANRS 1201/1202 DITRAME PLUS Study Group. (2005). Field efficacy of zidovudine, lamivudine and single-dose nevirapine to prevent peripartum HIV transmission. *AIDS, 19*(3), 309–318.

DeFranco, A. L., Locksley, R., & Robertson, M. (2007). *Immunity: The immune response in infectious and inflammatory disease.* Sunderland, MA: Sinauer Associates.

Deglin, J., & Vallerand, A. (2007). *Davis's drug guide for nurses.* Philadelphia: F. A. Davis.

Dunne, M. (2007). Infection, inflammation, and immunity. In C. M. Porth (Ed.), *Essentials of pathophysiology* (pp. 229–246). St. Louis: Lippincott Williams & Wilkins.

Dybul, M., Fauci, A. S., Barlett, J. G., Kaplan, J. E., Pau, A. K., & Panel on Clinical Practices for Treatment of HIV. (2002). Guidelines for using antiretroviral agents among HIV-infected adults and adolescents. *Annals of Internal Medicine, 137*(5 Part 2), 381–433.

Embry, A. (2004). The multiple factors of multiple sclerosis: A Darwinian perspective. *Journal of Nutritional & Environmental Medicine, 14*(4), 307–317.

Fauci, A. S. (1991). Immunopathogenic mechanisms in human immunodeficiency virus infection. *Annals of Internal Medicine, 114,* 678–693.

Fauci, A. S. (1996). Immunological mechanisms of HIV infection. *Annals of Internal Medicine, 124,* 654.

Fawzi, W. W., Msamanga, G. I., Spiegelman, D., Wei, R., Kapiga, S., Villamor, E., et al. (2004). A randomized trial of multivitamin supplements and HIV disease progression and mortality. *New England Journal of Medicine, 351*(1), 23–32.

Food Allergy & Anaphylaxis Network. (2006). *Anaphylaxis.* Retrieved February 19, 2007, from http://www.foodallergy.org/anaphylaxis/index.html

Food and Drug Administration. (2003b). New regimen for kidney transplants. *FDA Consumer 37*(4), 1–4. Retrieved October 10, 2003, from http://www.fda.gov/FDAC/departs/2003/403_upd.html#kidney

Gomez-Peurta, J., Martin, H., Amigo, H., Aguirre, M., Camps, M., Cuardrado, M., et al. (2005). Long-term follow-up in 128 patients with primary antiphospholipid syndrome: Do they develop lupus? *Medicine, 84*(4), 225–230.

Greenwald, J., Burstein, G., Pincus, J., & Branson, B. (2006). A rapid review of rapid HIV antibody tests. *Current Infectious Disease Reports, 8,* 125–131. Hamilton, R. G., & Adkinson, N. F., Jr. (2003). Clinical laboratory assessment of IgE-dependent hypersensitivity. *Journal of Allergy and Clinical Immunology, 111*(2), 687–701.

Halken, S. (2003). Early sensitization and the development of allergic airway disease: Risk factors and predictors. *Pediatric Respiratory Review, 4*(2), 128–134.

James, J. M. (2003). Respiratory manifestations of food allergies. *Pediatrics, 111*(6), 1625–1631.

Johnsen, C. (2003). Epidemiology of HIV. In J .K. Shaw & E. A. Mahoney (Eds.), *HIV/AIDS nursing secrets* (pp. 1–8). Philadelphia: Hanley & Belfus.

Judd, F., & Mijch, A. (2002). In S. Crowe, J. Hoy, & J. Mills (Eds.), *Management of the HIV-infected patient.* London: Taylor & Francis.

Kaplan, J., Masur, H., & Holmes, K. (2002). Guidelines for prevention of opportunistic infections among HIV infected persons 2002. Recommendations of the U.S. Public Health Service and the Infectious Diseases Society of America. *Morbidity and Mortality Weekly Report, 51*(RR-8). Retrieved February 27, 2007, from http:/ /www.cdc.gov/mmwR/PDF/rr/rr5108.pdf

Kee, J. L. (2005). *Laboratory and diagnostic tests with nursing implications* (7th ed.). Upper Saddle River, NJ: Pearson Prentice Hall.

Korn, J., & Seibold, J. (2004). *RAPIDS-2: A randomized, double-blind, placebo-controlled, multi-center study to assess the effect of bosentan on healing and prevention of ischemic digital ulcers in patients with systemic sclerosis.* Retrieved January 19, 2004, from http:www.sctc-online.org/studies/rapids2.htm

Kuwabara, S. (2004). Guillain-Barré syndrome: Epidemiology, pathophysiology and management. *Drugs, 64*(6), 597–610.

Little, S. J., Holte, S., Routy, J. P., Daar, E. S., Markowitz, M., Collier, A. C., et al. (2002). Antiretroviral-drug resistance among patients recently infected with HIV. *New England Journal of Medicine, 347*(6), 438–439.

Marks, G., Crepaz, N., Senterfitt, J., & Janssen, R. (2005). Meta-analysis of high-risk sexual behavior in persons aware and unaware they are infected with HIV in the United States: Implications for HIV prevention programs. *Journal of Acquired Immune Deficiency Syndrome, 39*(138), 620–629.

Medem. (2003). *Care of the lupus patient.* Retrieved January 16, 2004, from http://www.medem.com/search

National Heart, Lung and Blood Institute. (2004b). *Scleroderma lung study.* Retrieved January 19, 2004, from http://sclerodemalungstudy.medsch.ucla.edu/title.htm

National Institute of Allergy and Infectious Diseases. (2003). *NIAID awards $81 million to HIV vaccine development.* Retrieved October 21, 2003, from http://www.niaid.nih.gov/newsroom/releases/HVDDTTeams2.htm

National Institute of Allergy and Infectious Diseases. (2003c). *NIAID initiative addresses primary immune deficiency diseases.* Retrieved September 22, 2003, from http://www.niaid.nih.gov/newsroom/releases/pirc.htm

National Institute of Allergy and Infectious Diseases. (2004). *Facts and figures: HIV/AIDS statistics.* Retrieved January 11, 2004, from http:/ /www.niaid.nih.gov/factssheets/aidsstat.htm

National Institute of Arthritis and Musculoskeletal and Skin Diseases. (2003). *Handout on health: Systemic lupus erythematosus.* Retrieved February 19, 2007, from National Institute of Health website: http://www.niams.nih.gov/hi/topics/lupus/slehandout/index.htm#Lupus_3

National Institute of Arthritis and Musculoskeletal and Skin Diseases. (2006). *Care of the lupus patient.* Retrieved February 19, 2007, from National Institute of Health website: http://www.niams.nih.gov/hi/topics/lupus/lupusguide/chp7.htm

National Institute for Occupational Safety and Health. (1999). *NIOSH alert: Preventing needlestick injuries in health care settings* (NIOSH Publication No. 2000-108). Retrieved October 10, 2003, from http:/ /www.cdc.gov/niosh/2000-108.html

National Institute for Occupational Safety and Health. (2007). *Latex allergy: A prevention guide* (NIOSH Publication No. 98-113). Retrieved February 16, 2007, from http://www.cdc.gov/niosh/98-113.html

National Kidney Foundation. (2005). *25 facts about organ donation and transplantation.* Retrieved February 23, 2007, from http://www.kidney.org

Needlestick Safety and Prevention Act. (2000). One Hundred Sixth Congress of the United States of America. Signed into law by President Clinton November 6, 2000. Retrieved October 10, 2003, from http://www.afscme.org/publications/2736.cfm

O'Connell, E. J. (2003). Pediatric allergy: A brief review of risk factors associated with developing allergic diseases in childhood. *Annals of Allergy Asthma Immunology, 90*(6 Suppl. 3), 53–58.

Porth, C., & Sweeney, K. (2007). Alterations in immune response. In C. M. Porth (Ed.), *Essentials of pathophysiology* (pp. 293–319). St. Louis: Lippincott Williams & Wilkins.

Public Health Service Task Force. (2006). *Recommendations for the use of antiretroviral drugs in pregnant HIV-1-infected women for maternal health and interventions to reduce perinatal HIV-1 transmission in the United States.* Retrieved February 23, 2007, from http://AIDSinfo.nih.gov

Ress, B. (2003). HIV disease and aging: The hidden epidemic. *Critical Care Nurse, 23*(5), 38–42.

Rizzo, D., & Gunta, K. (2007). In C. M. Porth (Ed.), *Essentials of pathophysiology* (pp. 1015–1045). St. Louis: Lippincott Williams & Wilkins.

Rote, N. (2006). Immunity. In K. L. McCance & S. E. Heuther (Eds.), *Pathophysiology: The biological basis for disease in adults and children* (5th ed., pp. 168–227). St. Louis: Mosby.

Sampson, H. (2003). Anaphylaxis and emergency treatment. *Pediatrics, 111*(6) ,1601–1608.

Shaw, J. K. (2003). Opportunistic infections. In J. K. Shaw & E. A. Mahoney (Eds.), *HIV/AIDS nursing secrets* (pp. 9–13). Philadelphia: Hanley & Belfus.

Shaw, J. K., & Mahoney, E. A. (Eds.). (2003). *HIV/AIDS nursing secrets.* Philadelphia: Hanley & Belfus.

Sommer, C. (2007). The immune response. In C. M. Porth (Ed.), *Essentials of pathophysiology* (pp. 247–268). St. Louis: Lippincott Williams & Wilkins.

Steinke, J. W., Borish, L., & Rosenwasser, L. J. (2003). Genetics of hypersensitivity. *Journal of Allergy and Clinical Immunology, 111*(2 Suppl.), S495–S501.

Tasha, T., Kumwenda, N., & Gibbons, A. (2003). Short postexposure prophylaxis in newborn babies to reduce mother-to-child transmission of HIV1: NVAZ randomized clinical trial. *Lancet, 362*(9391), 1171–1177.

United Nations Program on HIV/AIDS. (2006). *Report on the global AIDS epidemic: Executive summary.* Retrieved February 27, 2007, from http://www.unaids.org/en/hiv_data/2006GlobalReport/default.asp

Urden, L., Stacy, K., & Lough, M. (2006). *Thelan's critical care nursing: Diagnosis and management* (5th ed.). St. Louis: Mosby.

Van Leeuwen, A., Kranpitz, T., & Smith, L. (2006). *Laboratory and diagnostic tests with nursing implications* (2nd ed.). Philadelphia: F. A. Davis.

Wilson, B. A., Shannon, M., Shields, K., & Stang, C. (2007). *Nurse's drug guide.* Upper Saddle River, NJ: Pearson Prentice Hall.

Wong, G. (2007). Symptoms of asthma and atopic disorders in preschool children: Prevalence and risk factors. *Clinical and Experimental Allergy, 37*(2), 174–179.

Workowski, K., & Berman, S. M. (2006). Sexually transmitted diseases treatment guidelines 2006. *Morbidity and Mortality Weekly Report, 55*(RR-11), 76–78. Retrieved February 27, 2006, from http://www.guideline.gov

World Health Organization. (2007). *Global HIV prevalence has leveled off.* Retrieved January 6, 2009, from http://www.wpro.who.int/sites/hsi/ documents/epi_updates.htm

Zutavern, A., & Brockow, I. (2006). Timing of solid food introduction in relationship to atopic dermatitis and atopic sensitization: Results from a prospective birth cohort study. *Pediatrics, 117*(2), 401–412.

61

Caring for the Patient with Inflammatory Response, Shock, and Severe Sepsis

Renee Holleran

Outcome-Based Learning Objectives

After studying this chapter, the learner will be able to:

1. Compare and contrast the etiologies of anaphylactic, cardiogenic, hypovolemic, neurogenic, and septic shock.
2. Describe the cellular alterations that occur in shock.
3. Describe the body's response to shock.
4. Identify the factors that place a patient at risk of developing shock.
5. Discuss the emergency care of the patient in shock including identification of the underlying cause, management of the patient's airway, breathing, and circulation, and selected pharmacologic interventions.
6. Describe the acute care of the patient in shock, including oxygen management, circulatory management, nutritional management, skin care, and pain and sedation management.
7. Compare and contrast systemic inflammatory response syndrome (SIRS), sepsis, and severe sepsis based on the definitions used by the American College of Chest Physicians/Society of Critical Care Medicine.
8. Prioritize the treatment of the patient with SIRS and identify strategies to prevent the development of SIRS.
9. Understand the etiologies, epidemiology, and management of multiple organ dysfunction syndrome (MODS) as an end result of shock and severe sepsis.
10. Prioritize the treatment of the patient with MODS and identify strategies to prevent the development of MODS.

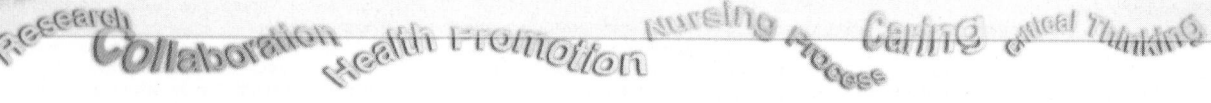

■ Shock

Shock has been described as the "rude unhinging" of the machinery of life. Shock in and of itself is not a disease, but a clinical manifestation of the body's inability to perfuse tissues adequately (McCance & Huether, 2006). Shock has multiple etiologies, including alterations in the circulating volume of blood or plasma in the body, alterations in the heart's capability to pump, and alterations in peripheral vascular resistance. Regardless of the cause of shock, the systemic response is detrimental and often leads to multiple organ dysfunction syndrome (MODS) and death. It is important to have an understanding about the causes of shock, so it can be prevented or rapidly recognized to prevent life-threatening complications.

Epidemiology

Explaining what shock was and how to treat it did not really begin until the late 19th and early 20th centuries. During World War I surgeons and physiologists thought that a toxin was released from traumatized tissues that caused shock. In 1964, shock was diagnosed when the patient had acute circulatory insufficiency that was characterized by a cardiac output inadequate to provide perfusion to major organs. Nurses and health care providers waited for specific clinical manifestations such as a systolic blood pressure less than 90 mmHg or an increase in heart rate before shock management began. Research was conducted to see how much volume needed to be lost before the patient was considered to be in "shock." Shock was looked at in "pieces" instead of as a systemic response to a particular insult to the body whether from an injury, disease, or infection (Grenvik, Ayres, Holbrook, & Shoemaker, 2000).

In recent years the definition and management of shock has been challenged. In 1992 and again in 2003, the American College of Chest Physicians and Society of Critical Care Medicine developed a consensus definition for sepsis and multiple organ failure. One of these definitions described **systemic inflammatory response syndrome (SIRS)**, a systemic response of the immune system that can be triggered by both infectious and noninfectious causes. Originally associated with sepsis, other researchers, particularly those who dealt with critically injured patients, recognized that SIRS is probably the first phase of shock (Ertel et al., 1995; Levy et al., 2003; Moore et al., 1996).

Mortality from shock is difficult to calculate because shock is generally not classified as a cause of death. Death usually results from multiple organ dysfunctions. For example, each year 660,000 to 750,000 people are hospitalized with an infectious process that causes sepsis, which leads to acute organ dysfunction (Micek, Shah, & Kollef, 2003). About 50% of these patients will die. Risk factors such as age, preexisting illness, and inappropriate antibiotic use can increase patient mortality (Martin et al., 2003). These risk factors are explained in more detail later in this chapter.

Etiology

The etiologies of shock have been classified in various ways. The most common classification is by the cause of the shock syndrome, for example, sepsis from infection is referred to as septic shock (McCance & Huether, 2006). Another classification is related to the amount of circulating volume in the body and how it is affected by the shock syndrome, for example, low-volume shock or absolute hypovolemia (Campbell, 2004; Chapman, 2003). This type of classification is outlined in Chart 61–1. The following subsections describe the etiology of shock based on the cause.

Anaphylactic Shock

Anaphylactic shock results from an antigen–antibody reaction. The body becomes hypersensitive to a specific agent such as a medication like penicillin. When this happens, vasodilatation of blood vessels occurs, causing pooling of blood. Because the blood has pooled in the periphery, perfusion to the tissues is markedly diminished or absent. In addition, other body systems will react to the toxin. In particular, the pulmonary system will respond with vasoconstriction, causing respiratory distress and potential respiratory arrest (McCance & Huether, 2006). Chart 61–2 lists causes of anaphylactic shock. Chapter 60 🔗 includes a more detailed discussion of anaphylaxis.

Cardiogenic Shock

When the heart is unable to pump effectively, cardiogenic shock will develop. Myocardial infarction is one of the most common causes of damage to the heart that may lead to the development of the heart's inability to function and eventually cause cardiogenic shock. Refer to Chapter 40 🔗 for a detailed description. Despite advances in technological care, the mortality rate of cardiogenic shock remains high. Chart 61–2 lists causes of cardiogenic shock.

CHART 61–1	Shock Syndromes
Shock Syndrome	**Etiology**
Low-volume shock (absolute hypovolemia)	Major loss of blood or circulating body fluid such as plasma.
High-space shock (relative hypovolemia)	Injury or toxin affects the blood vessels, which results in the redistribution of blood and fluid. For example, in spinal shock, damage to the sympathetic nervous system causes vasodilation and alteration in blood distribution.
Mechanical (obstructive) shock	A condition that slows or obstructs blood flow in or out of the heart. Examples include cardiac tamponade, tension pneumothorax, vena cava obstruction.

CHART 61–2	Causes of Specific Shock Syndromes
Shock Syndrome	**Causes**
Anaphylactic shock	Insect bites Medication allergies Food allergies Latex allergies Idiopathic reactions
Cardiogenic shock	Myocardial infarction Myocardial contusion Ruptured ventricles Ruptured papillary muscles Cardiomyopathy
Hypovolemic shock	Traumatic injury (abdominal trauma, chest trauma, orthopedic trauma) Gastrointestinal bleeding Vomiting and diarrhea Osmotic diuresis Diabetic ketoacidosis Thermal injuries
Neurogenic shock	Spinal cord or medulla trauma Anesthetic agents Severe emotional stress Severe pain
Septic shock	Bacterial infections Viral infections Immunosuppression Technology (indwelling urinary or intravenous catheters, feeding tubes) Antibiotic misuse

Hypovolemic Shock

Hypovolemic shock results from significant fluid loss that alters the amount of circulating volume in the body. Fluid loss can include loss of blood, plasma, or other body fluids. Hemorrhagic shock is the most common type of shock encountered when a person has suffered multiple system traumas. Hemorrhagic shock can also be the result of upper and lower gastrointestinal bleeding, ruptured aortic aneurysm, hemorrhagic pancreatitis, and long-bone fractures. Fluid loss that is not hemorrhagic can be caused by diarrhea, vomiting, and inadequate repletion of fluid losses as in heat stroke, burn wounds, and leaking of plasma into the interstitial or "third spacing," which can occur with intestinal obstruction, pancreatitis, and cirrhosis. Chapter 68 🔗 discusses "third spacing" of fluid.

The loss of intravascular volume causes a reduction in preload. *Preload* refers to the force that stretches the ventricles to an initial length. The resting force on the heart is determined by pressure in the ventricles at the end of diastole. Factors that affect preload include muscle fiber length, stretch, volume, and wall stress (Chapman, 2003). Because of these factors, blood volume returning to the heart is inadequate, which affects the amount of the blood returning to the circulation. When blood is lost, or unavailable because of sequestration, the ability to carry oxygen to the cells is also lost because of the decrease in hemoglobin. Chart 61–2 contains a summary of the most common causes of hypovolemic shock.

Neurogenic Shock

Neurogenic shock results from an imbalance between the sympathetic and parasympathetic stimulation of vascular smooth muscle, which results in vasodilation (McCance & Huether, 2006). The body's circulating blood volume generally remains unchanged. However, injury or medications that affect the spinal cord or medulla will cause an imbalance between the sympathetic and parasympathetic nervous systems. Because of this imbalance, clinical symptoms usually associated with shock are different. For example, the patient may be hypotensive, but not tachycardic. Chart 61–2 (p. 1957) contains a list of the causes of neurogenic shock. Chapter 32 includes an in-depth discussion of spinal cord injuries and neurogenic shock.

Septic Shock

Septic shock is defined as sepsis that is refractory to fluid resuscitation (McCance & Huether, 2006). Septic shock results in hypotension and perfusion abnormalities. Impaired perfusion will cause lactic acidosis, oliguria, and alterations in mental status. Septic shock occurs when an infectious agent or infection-induced mediator causes systemic decompensation. Because of the body's response to the mediators, there is decreased **systemic vascular resistance (SVR)** (arterial systolic pressure; normal SVR is 900 to 1,400 dyn·s/cm⁵), as well as maldistribution of the blood into the microcirculation, causing compromised tissue perfusion and cellular dysfunction (McCance & Huether, 2006; Society of Critical Care Medicine, 1999). Chapter 24 includes a detailed discussion regarding SVR. Despite advances in antibiotic and antiviral therapies, the cases of septic shock, particularly in hospitals, continue to rise. The mortality rate from septic shock is about 50% and increases when the patient has other comorbid risk factors such as immunosuppression, age, or preexisting diseases such as diabetes (Micek et al., 2003; Russell, 2006). Chart 61–2 (p. 1957) outlines the causes of septic shock.

In summary, there are multiple etiologies that may place the patient at risk for developing shock. It is important to be cognizant of any or all of these when a patient presents with symptoms that may indicate the initiation of the "rude unhinging of the machinery of life." Critical interventions must begin as early as possible to prevent irreversible shock, and death.

> **CRITICAL ALERT** *The primary treatment for all shock syndromes is early recognition of factors that may place the patient at risk for developing shock. Be aware of specific risk factors that may cause particular shock syndromes. For example, patients with an indwelling urinary catheter are at risk for becoming septic and predisposes them to septic shock.*

Pathophysiology

Shock is a syndrome that results from inadequate tissue perfusion. As previously discussed, there are multiple causes of shock that will produce alterations in circulating volume, alterations in cardiac pump function, or alterations in peripheral vascular resistance (PVR), resulting in impairment of cellular metabolism. This results in both impaired oxygen and glucose use.

The amount of oxygen available for tissue consumption per unit of time is defined as oxygen delivery (DO₂). The body generally does have some oxygen reserve available in order to respond to stress. However, if the patient has any preexisting illnesses or injury, this will strain the body and decrease or eliminate the additional oxygen cushion. The amount of oxygen extracted from the tissues for metabolism is known as oxygen consumption (VO₂). Oxygen consumption is calculated by determining the difference between the amounts of oxygen returned to the right side of the heart. It is dependent on the patient's cardiac output, hemoglobin concentration, and the arterial and venous oxygen saturation. When the patient has suffered an injury or illness that has caused an alteration in the blood flow for any of the above reasons, an oxygen debt will occur. This can be exaggerated by the patient's preexisting medical condition as well as by the patient's age, for example, the patient with chronic obstructive pulmonary disease whose oxygen level is lowered due to the disease process (Selfridge-Thomas, 1995).

Sodium moves from outside the cell to increase water into the cell. This causes potassium to exit the cell, thereby altering nervous, cardiovascular, and muscular cell function. These systems then become impaired. Additionally, water is drawn from the vascular space to compensate for water drawn into the cells, further reducing circulating blood volume. Cells will shift from aerobic to anaerobic metabolism to compensate for oxygen loss. This causes metabolic acidosis, which affects enzyme activities and cellular functions such as repair and division. Cellular damage causes enzymes to be released, which will destroy noninjured cells.

Glucose metabolism is impaired in a manner similar to that of oxygen metabolism. The result of this impaired metabolism is insulin resistance. This phenomenon has been observed in patients with sepsis and those who are critically ill or injured. The stress response that is initiated by an illness or injury triggers gluconeogenesis to supply glucose energy to heal. The liver and kidneys produce more glucose in response to epinephrine, norepinephrine, glucagons, and cortisol, which are part of the body's stress response (Cartwright, 2004). **Insulin resistance (IR)** has been described as unresponsiveness of anabolic processes to the normal effects of insulin and possibly tissue insensitivity to insulin. The severity of IR is thought to be the result of an increased production of serum cytokines (Ball, de Beer, Gomm, Hickman, & Collins, 2007; Zauner et al., 2007). Insulin resistance and glucose toxicity impair cellular growth metabolic processes. IR has been associated with multiple organ failure, nosocomial infections, and renal injury (Ball et al., 2007).

Overall the pathophysiology of sepsis has a profound effect on all of the body systems. This is well illustrated in Figure 61–1 ■. Because of inadequate tissue perfusion, the body turns to anaerobic metabolism to produce energy. In addition, other pathophysiological pathways are initiated that affect all body systems due to the release of toxins as well as the body's inability to effectively manage these toxins. If not stopped, these toxins will cause multiple organ failure and death.

As previously discussed and illustrated in Figure 61–1 ■, inadequate perfusion and a reduction in available oxygen will trigger cellular and systemic responses. Alteration in cellular metabolism causes alteration in ATP production, failure of the sodium-potassium pump, redistribution of cellular ions, and interstitial fluid shifts. Blisters or blebs develop on cell walls and eventually rupture, which will release cellular enzymes and cause further damage to other cells.

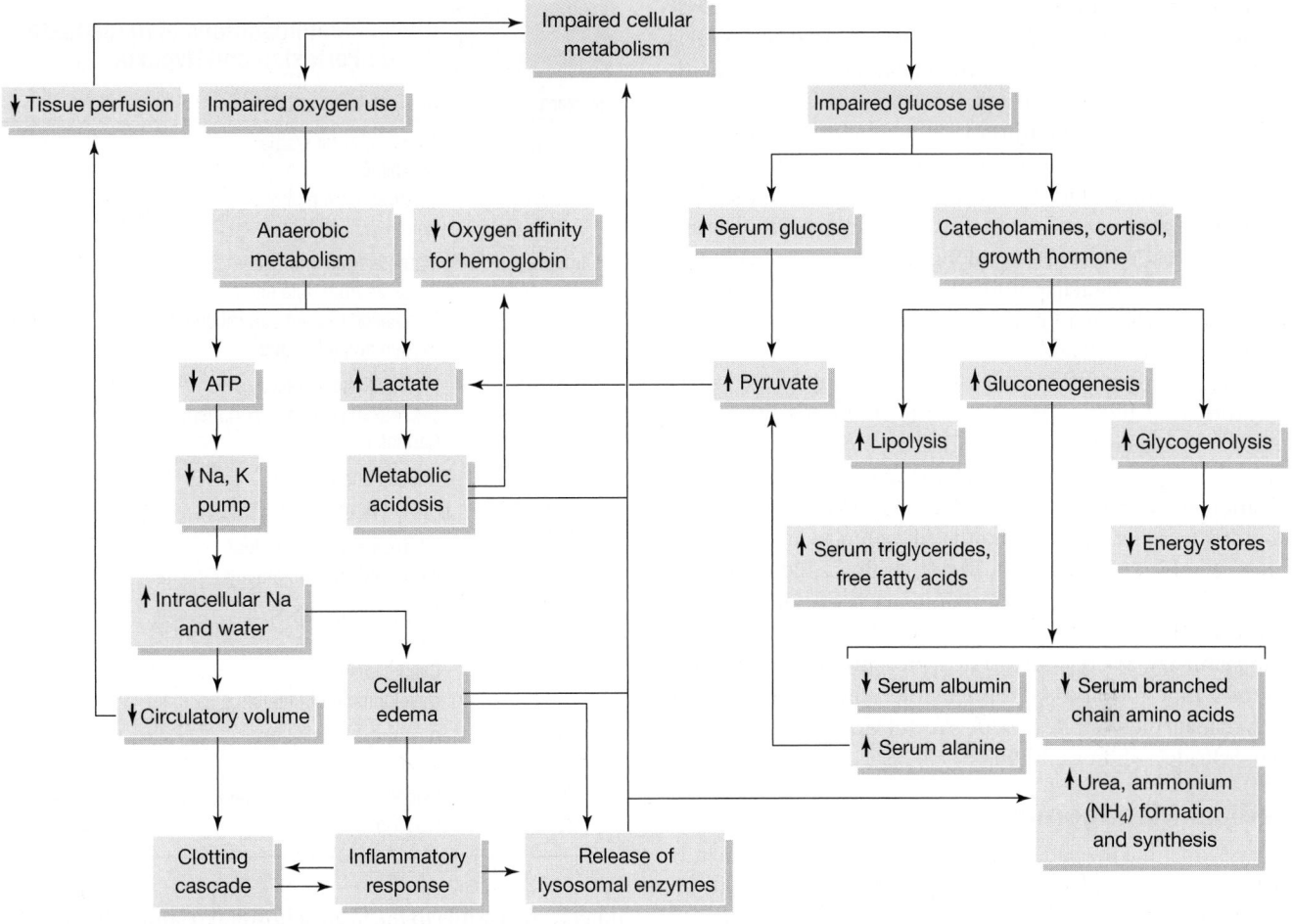

FIGURE 61–1 ■ A network of cascading events in response to inflammation.

Research continues to demonstrate that specific triggers such as infection, illness, and injury trigger a systemic inflammatory response syndrome (Johnson, Brunn, & Platt, 2004; Levy et al., 2003; Rangel-Frausto, 2005). In response, the immune system activates a complement cascade system that causes macrophages to respond. When macrophages respond to an "insult," they cause the release of substances that contribute to platelet aggregation causing clot formation, which "plugs" the vessel and at times causes vasodilation. Examples of these substances include cytokines, thromboxane, prostaglandins, and a slow-reacting substance of anaphylaxis. The end result is further tissue damage due to inadequate perfusion.

The brain is dependent on both oxygen and glucose. When either of these is not sufficient, an alteration in cerebral perfusion occurs. The patient will suffer an altered mental status, which will eventually lead to coma and even death.

Cardiac output declines because of an alteration in both preload and afterload. Afterload is the initial resistance that must be overcome by the ventricles in order to develop enough force to open the semilunar valves and propel the blood into the systemic and pulmonary systems. In addition, specific toxins such as myocardial depressant factor are released from damaged cardiac cells and a hypoperfused pancreas, causing further myocardial dysfunction and hypoxia. These result in cardiac dysrhythmia, which will further impair cardiac function. The pulmonary system suffers acute lung injury eventually leading to acute respiratory distress.

Urinary output is decreased because of the shift of sodium, which pulls water into the cells for conservation of fluid. Decreased blood flow to the kidneys impairs their ability to detoxify the toxic substances that result from anaerobic metabolism. Inadequate blood flow to the gastrointestinal (GI) tract causes the activation of circulating neutrophils that provoke multiple organ failure. The integumentary system responds by diverting blood from the skin. Pale, fragile skin affords little protection and places the patient at risk for hypothermia and further system disruptions.

A change in blood flow to the vital organs (brain, heart, and kidneys) triggers baroreceptors, which cause the release of catecholamines, increasing the heart rate and cardiac output and causing further vasoconstriction and tissue injury. See Chapter 21 ⊚ for an explanation of the normal regulation of blood pressure. Skeletal muscle, which is a major reservoir of amino acids, begins to break down and release these acids from their stores. Muscle weakness and eventual wasting result.

The "unhinging of the machinery of life" continues until irreversible changes and eventually death occur. What is unfortunate is that many of the interventions used for the treatment of shock actually contribute to the development of further complications such as third spacing, ischemia-reperfusion injury, ventilator-associated pneumonia (VAP), Multiple Organ Dysfunction Syndrome (MODS), and in some cases death. VAP is the most common hospital-acquired infection among patients who are mechanically ventilated.

Ischemia reperfusion injury is a multifactorial process that occurs when anaerobic metabolism is initiated by hypoperfusion and hypoxia that leads to an oxygen deficit in endothelial, parenchymal, or immune competent cells (Krau, 2007). The energy deficit that results from prolonged ischemia can lead to irreversible tissue damage through apoptosis or necrosis of parenchymal cells. In addition, reperfusion can also cause secondary tissue damage and organ dysfunction.

During the reperfusion phase, superoxide anions are generated from available oxygen. Superoxide anions are further reduced to hydrogen peroxide and hydroxyl ions, referred to as free oxygen radicals. These free oxygen radicals induce lipid peroxidation, membrane disintegration, and DNA damage, causing apoptosis and necrosis of endothelial, parenchymal, and immune cells (Kaszaki, Wolfard, Szalay, & Boros, 2006; Keel & Trentz, 2005). Ischemia-reperfusion injury is one of the major triggers of MODS (Krau, 2007).

In summary, as previously stated, prevention, early recognition of symptoms, and appropriate interventions are the primary management strategies for shock (McCance & Huether, 2006; Selfridge-Thomas, 1995).

Medical Management

The assessment of the patient who may be in shock must include a high index of suspicion because the body's initial ability to compensate may mask the clinical signs of shock. Patient risk factors such as significant injuries, catastrophic illness, age, and allergies must be quickly acknowledged. It is interesting that both the very young and aged share similar risk factors for developing shock including compromised immune systems due to age; fluid shifts; and an integumentary system that may not afford needed protection. Inadequate tissue perfusion and hypoxia will manifest itself in a variety of ways, as summarized in Chart 61–3.

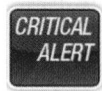 *Even though some specific clinical manifestations, such as hypotension and tachycardia, are associated with shock, physical fitness, preexisting illness, certain injuries (spinal cord trauma), and medications (beta-blockers) may mask the anticipated symptoms.*

The Emergency Period of Shock Care

The emergency period of care for the patient in shock begins as soon as the risk for shock has been identified. The primary goal of shock management is to identify the cause and intervene to prevent the pathophysiology that results from ischemic and anoxic cell injury (Arabi, Shirawi, Memish, Venkatesh, & Al-Shimemeri, 2003). The care of the patient will be directed at identifying and correcting the cause of the shock, maintaining oxygen perfusion, controlling active bleeding, supporting the patient's circulatory status, maintaining the patient's body temperature, managing pain, and providing emotional support.

Prehospital Care and Transport

Patients who are in shock have been identified as "load and go situations," which means that they must be transported as

System	Clinical Manifestation
CHART 61–3	**Clinical Manifestations of Inadequate Tissue Perfusion and Hypoxia**
Neurological	Altered mental status
	Irritability
	Seizures from hypoxia
	Coma
Pulmonary	Increased respirations
	Crackles from fluid shifts
	Decreased oxygen saturation despite an increase in oxygen administration
Cardiovascular	Increased heart rate
	Decreased or absent peripheral pulses
	Cardiac dysrhythmia
Gastrointestinal	Nausea and vomiting
	Absent bowel sounds
Genitourinary	Decreased urinary output
	Increased specific gravity
Integumentary	Cool clammy skin
	Mottling
	Cyanosis
	Development of decubiti
Musculoskeletal	Generalized weakness
	Wasting
	Inability to wean from ventilator due to muscle wasting

quickly as possible to the nearest hospital (Campbell, 2004; McSwain, Salomone, & Pons, 2007). The prehospital care provider needs to focus care on the critical interventions that need to be performed to save the patient's life while preparing for and initiating rapid transport (Figure 61–2 ■). A brief primary assess-

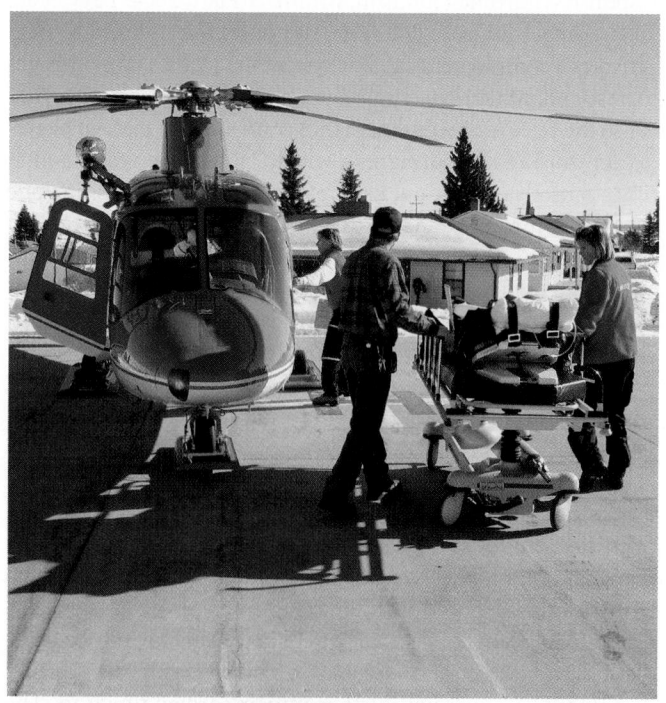

FIGURE 61–2 ■ Rapid transport for a patient in shock.

ment includes evaluating the patient's A = airway with cervical spine protection if trauma is suspected, B = breathing, C = circulation, D = disability, and performing E = exposure and environmental management. Only critical interventions such as airway management should be executed before transport. Additional interventions such as obtaining intravenous (IV) access, immobilization measures (such as the application of a traction splint), warming the patient, and performing a secondary assessment should be accomplished during transport (McSwain et al., 2007). Chapter 74  discusses the rapid primary and secondary assessment for the patient at risk for shock.

If an active source of blood or fluid loss is identified, it should be managed as much as possible before and during transport. (Fluid resuscitation is discussed in the next section.) Pelvic and long-bone fractures can cause enormous blood loss. Pneumatic antishock garments (PASGs), though controversial, may be of use for the patient in shock during transport. Chart 61–4 contains a summary of the indications and contraindications for use of PASGs in the prehospital setting (Campbell, 2004; McSwain et al., 2007). Another device that has been used to stabilize pelvic fractures is the trauma pelvic orthotic device (T-POD). It has been found to be effective in maintaining pelvic cross-sectional area and pelvic volume (Carrigan, Born, Fitzpatrick, & Reilly, 2004).

In summary, the prehospital care of the patient in shock involves early recognition of the risk of shock and rapid transport of the patient to definitive care. A primary assessment should be performed and critical interventions initiated. There should not be any additional delays in getting the patient to a center that can provide appropriate and life-saving care.

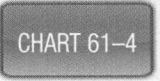 *The patient in shock should be rapidly transported to a facility that can provide the definitive care required. For example, a trauma patient in shock should be transported to a trauma center when possible.*

Emergency Department Care

The care of the patient in shock in the emergency department depends on a collaborative approach. It begins with performing a primary assessment and initiating critical interventions to support the patient's A = airway, B = breathing, and C = circulation. Interventions that were performed in the prehospital environment need to be reevaluated and considered when resuscitating

the patient, for example, how much fluid the patient received during transport. A secondary assessment is then performed including exposing the patient to identify any obvious signs of illness or injury that may be the source of the shock. An in-depth discussion of the primary and secondary assessments is contained in Chapter 74 . The Risk Factors box contains a summary of the most common risk factors for the development of shock.

The source of the clinical insult needs to be immediately identified. When there is no obvious indication, other pieces of patient history and risk factors must be considered, for example, the age of the patient or medications that the patient may be prescribed. For example, certain medications may place a patient at risk of shock, particularly septic shock. These include medications that cause immunosuppression and antibiotic and antiviral therapies. Additionally, the elderly and young are at greatest danger of developing shock because of changes in their immune system and body surface area related to age. An in-depth discussion of these differences and the potential risks the elderly pose are contained in Chapters 59 and 60 .

The pathophysiological changes initiated by the body's response to shock cause the patient to become hypoxic. Therefore, the patient will require airway and ventilatory support. This may be as simple as administering oxygen by 100% nonrebreather mask or it may require endotracheal intubation. A chest radiograph can reveal a possible infection or source of blood or other fluid loss or even an obstructive reason for shock such as a cardiac tamponade. Chapter 33  discusses respiratory assessment and management.

The patient's circulatory status needs to be assessed. Peripheral and central pulses should be palpated to determine perfusion. Remember, the body will divert blood from the periphery to enhance oxygenation of the brain, heart, and kidneys. The patient's skin will be pale, cold, and clammy. The patient will need to be kept warm by increasing the room temperature, covering with warm blankets, or using a commercial device to deliver heat. The skin is friable and at risk of additional injury so the patient should be handled and moved as gently as possible.

CHART 61–4 | **Indications and Contraindications for the Use of Pneumatic Antishock Garments with Shock**

Indications	Contraindications
Suspected pelvic fractures with hypotension	Penetrating thoracic trauma
Profound hypotension (systolic blood pressure less than 60 mmHg)	Stabilization of an isolated lower extremity fracture
Suspected intraperitoneal hemorrhage	Evisceration of abdominal organs
Suspected retroperitoneal hemorrhage	Impaled objects in the abdomen
	Pregnant abdomen
	Traumatic arrest

RISK FACTORS for the Development and Source of Shock

Indication	Source of Shock
Active bleeding anywhere on the body	Hemorrhage
Abdominal bruising	
Long-bone deformities	
Open fractures	
Amputations	
"Coffee-stain" emesis	
Penetrating trauma	
Purpura	Sepsis
Rashes	
Decubitus	
Gangrene	
Indwelling urinary catheters	
Indwelling IV ports	
Feeding tubes	
Burns	Hypovolemia
Dehydration	

A 12-lead ECG should be obtained to rule out myocardial injury as the source of shock. Prolonged ischemia related to hypotension can also place the patient at risk of a myocardial infarction. Chapter 38 ⊚ discusses the 12-lead ECG and Chapter 40 ⊚ discusses myocardial infarction. Blood studies are obtained to provide baseline assessment data, identify the physiological effects of the shock state, identify a source of infection, and evaluate the effects of specific treatments. Blood studies should include complete blood count (CBC) with a differential, serum electrolytes, whole blood glucose, blood urea nitrogen (BUN), serum creatinine, coagulation studies, liver function studies, and lactate levels. For the patient with suspected hemorrhagic shock, a type and screen or type and cross should be obtained.

When sepsis is suspected, specific laboratory tests should be performed to identify the source of the sepsis. Examples of these include blood cultures, urine cultures, cultures of any suspected wounds or appliances, and cerebrospinal fluid cultures. The Diagnostic Tests for Shock box contains a description of these tests. Additional radiography studies are required for diagnosis and may include computed tomography (CT) scans, magnetic resonance imaging (MRI), and angiography.

Because shock involves alterations in circulating volume, cardiac function, or peripheral vascular resistance (PVR), the primary purposes of circulatory resuscitation are as follows:

- Restore oxygen transport and cellular uptake of oxygen.
- Mitigate against oxygen debt accumulation and decrease the use of anaerobic metabolism to supply cellular energy.
- Restore pre-resuscitation oxygen deficit.
- Prevent the metabolic derangements that lead to SIRS and eventual MODS and eventually multiple organ system failure (MOSF). These complications are discussed later in the chapter.

What is important to remember is that circulatory resuscitation may involve both volume resuscitation as well us the use of va-

DIAGNOSTIC TESTS for Shock

Test	Expected Abnormality	Rationale for Abnormality
Complete blood count with a differential	Increased white blood cell count	An increased white blood cell count may indicate a stress response as well as an infection.
	Increase in neutrophils	An increase in neutrophils will help differentiate an infection as the cause of the shock.
Hemoglobin concentration	Decreased with fluid	Adequate hemoglobin is needed to ensure adequate oxygen delivery.
	Increased with fluid loss	
Platelet count	Increase in number of platelets	Platelets increase as a stress response.
Serum electrolyte levels	Decreased sodium levels	Movement of sodium into the cell displaces potassium from the cell.
	Increased potassium levels	
Whole blood glucose	Increased glucose levels	Glucose metabolism is impaired.
Blood urea nitrogen Creatinine	Increase in both	Renal dysfunction occurs.
Arterial blood gases	Respiratory alkalosis	Increase respirations to blow off CO_2 to decrease metabolic acidosis.
	Metabolic acidosis	Metabolic acidosis results from anaerobic metabolism.
	Hypoxia	Hypoxia results from inadequate tissue perfusion.
Serum lactate levels	Elevated	Reflect tissue perfusion. An increased level indicates inadequate tissue perfusion and anaerobic metabolism. A higher lactate level indicates a higher degree of shock and potential for death.
Coagulation studies PT and PTT	Prolonged	Due to cellular dysfunction and abnormal clotting cascade. More profound if disseminated intravascular coagulation (DIC) is present.
Blood cultures	Presence of bacteria	Blood cultures should not be used without a good reason. Patients who are febrile, elderly patients, IV drug abusers, and patients with neutropenia, prosthetic heart valves, or indwelling devices are examples of those who should have blood cultures drawn.
Urinalysis	Presence of white blood cells, bacteria, increased specific gravity	Identify source of infection. Indicates the level of the body's response to shock.
Gram stains	Specific sites recognized as a source of infection	Immediate test that would indicate the presence of bacteria from a specific source such as an indwelling urinary catheter.
Type and crossmatch		Identify specific blood type for infusion of blood and blood products.
Cardiac enzymes	Normal or abnormal	Identify myocardial injury as source of shock.

soactive medications to maintain adequate **end-organ perfusion**, the perfusion of the end organs such as the integumentary system.

Large-bore intravenous (IV) lines need to be inserted. Central IV access may be obtained with a catheter that will also allow the insertion of devices for hemodynamic monitoring. It is imperative to ensure aseptic technique to prevent the possibility of introducing infection and increasing the risk of sepsis. Chapter 22 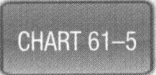 discusses the various types of intravenous catheters and their indications for use.

Fluid Resuscitation

During the last 20 years, the common methods once used for fluid resuscitation in shock have been challenged by research. Researchers have discovered many pertinent issues that must be considered when resuscitating the patient in shock. First, hypotension may actually be a protective mechanism, especially in the patient who has sustained a penetrating injury. Increasing a patient's blood pressure multiplies the chances that clots that have been formed will dislodge and, depending on the resuscitation fluid, dilutes circulating volume and in turn increases clotting time (Jacobs, 1994; Keel & Trentz, 2005; Kowalenko, Stern, Dronen, & Wang, 1992; Martin, Bicknell, Pepe, Burch, & Mattox, 1992). Chart 61–5 contains a summary of some of the complications of massive fluid resuscitation (Ackerman, 1994; Alexander, 1996; Edelman, White, Tyburski, & Wilson, 2007; Fernandes et al., 2007; Rueden & Dunham, 1994).

Fluids that are used for resuscitation include lactated Ringer's solution or normal saline. The type of fluid used will depend on the provider's preference, because at present the research has not clearly defined one more favorably over the other. The initial amount of fluid will range from 2 to 3 liters for an adult if the cause of the shock is unknown. If the patient has sustained blood loss, then administration of blood and blood products will be needed. Infusion therapy and blood administration are discussed in depth in Chapters 22 and 23 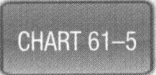, respectively. It is important to remember that patients who have sustained blood loss greater than 2 liters should not receive excessive fluid resuscitation from either colloids or crystalloids until surgical man-

---

CHART 61–5   Complications of Massive Fluid Resuscitation

- Hypothermia
- Coagulopathy
- Metabolic derangements
  - Acidosis
  - Hypocalcemia
  - Hypomagnesia
  - Hypophosphatemia
  - Hypokalemia
- Organ dysfunction and extravascular fluid shifts
- Adult respiratory distress syndrome
- Sepsis
- Acute renal failure
- Pneumonia
- Ventilator-assisted pneumonia
- Increased length of stay

---

agement of bleeding has been initiated because it dilutes the existing volume and further diminishes oxygen-carrying capacity. In contrast, a patient who is septic and hypotensive may require early fluid boluses to maintain a systolic blood pressure greater than 90 mmHg (Keel & Trentz, 2005; Russell, 2006).

Because of the complications of massive fluid resuscitation as noted in Chart 61–5, the effects of fluid resuscitation must be closely monitored. A urinary catheter should be inserted to measure urinary output. Adequate hydration in an adult should yield a urinary output of 30 to 50 mL/hr or 0.4 to 1.0 mL/kg of body weight. Adequate fluid resuscitation is also evaluated by a decrease in heart rate, presence and strength of the patient's central and peripheral pulses, patient's improving level of consciousness, and return of bowel sounds.

Hemodynamic monitoring can be used to monitor the effectiveness of resuscitation. This may include the insertion of a pulmonary artery catheter (PAC). However, any additional invasive procedures may leave the patient at risk of infection and sepsis. An in-depth discussion of the use of hemodynamic monitoring is included in Chapter 24 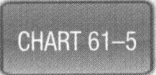.

Pharmacologic Support

Shock resuscitation may also include the need for pharmacologic support. Different medications may be used for different shock states. The purpose of the medication may be to augment blood flow to the brain, heart, and kidneys or to fight the infection that caused the sepsis leading to shock. The medications that are typically used in selected shock states are listed in the Pharmacological Summary feature (p. 1981) (Kline, 2002; McCaffery & Sinclair, 2006; Russell, 2006).

Pain Management

Pain management for the patient in shock is oftentimes neglected. One of the major reasons is that analgesics and sedation agents can cause hypotension and respiratory depression, furthering complications. However, research has adequately demonstrated the consequences of poor pain management, which include increased peripheral vascular resistance, increased consumption of myocardial oxygen, increased metabolic rate, increased levels of circulating stress hormones, hypercoagulability, decreased gastric motility, and hopelessness (Semonin Holleran, 2002). Pain management should never be neglected when providing care for the patient in shock.

Appropriate use of analgesics and sedative agents can only serve to support patients. Chapter 15 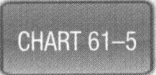 provides an in-depth discussion of the assessment and management of pain.

Additional Interventions

Depending on the cause of the shock, other interventions may be indicated. For example, the patient who has suffered a spinal cord injury will need to be appropriately immobilized during transport and in the emergency department. Chart 61–6 (p. 1964) contains a summary of additional interventions that may be indicated to manage shock based on the source of the clinical insult.

Acute Care Period of Shock

The unstable patient in shock will generally be admitted to the critical care unit. The care initiated will be continued including support of the patient's oxygenation and circulatory status.

NATIONAL GUIDELINES for the Initial Management of Sepsis

Initial Resuscitation	Guideline
Goal directed during the first 6 hours	Maintain with fluids and vasopressors: • Central venous: 8–12 mmHg • MAP > 65 mmHg • Urine output > 0.5 mL kg^{-1} hr^{-1} • Central venous (superior vena cava) or mixed venous oxygen saturation > 70%
Diagnosis	Appropriate cultures of suspected sources of infection.
Antibiotic therapy	Antibiotic therapy should be initiated within 1 hour of recognition of severe sepsis, after appropriate cultures are obtained. The antibiotic regimen should be reassessed every 48–72 hours on the basis of microbiological and clinical data with the aim of using the appropriate antibiotic to prevent the development of resistance and toxicity.
Source control	Drainage of abscesses. Debridement of necrotic tissue. Removal of infected devices.
Fluid therapy	Fluid resuscitation may consist of colloids or crystalloids. No evidence is available to support one over the other. Fluid challenge over 30 minutes of 500–1,000 mL monitoring vital signs and urinary output. May be repeated.
Vasopressors	When appropriate fluid challenge fails and there is a need to restore end-organ perfusion, therapy with vasopressors may be started. Norepinephrine or dopamine are preferably given through a central catheter. Arterial line should be placed for monitoring.
Inotropic therapy	Use in patients with low cardiac output despite adequate fluid resuscitation. Dobutamine may be used to increase cardiac output.
Steroids	IV stress dose corticosteroids are recommended only in patients with adequate volume replacement and who require vasopressors to maintain an adequate blood pressure.
Recombinant human activated protein C (rhAPC)	Recommended for patients who are at high risk of death and with no absolute contraindication related to bleeding risk or a relative contraindication that outweighs the risk of the treatment.
Mechanical ventilation of sepsis-induced acute lung Injury (ALI) and ARDS	Low tidal volume 6 mL/kg predicted based on body weight. Avoid high plateau pressures. To decrease days of mechanical ventilation and ICU length of stay, a conservative fluid strategy for patients with established ALI/ARDS who are not in shock. For patients with ALI/ARDS, application of at least a minimal amount of positive end-expiratory pressure. Use protocols for weaning.
Sedation, analgesia, neuromuscular blockade in sepsis	Protocols should be used to manage the patient and ensure adequate sedation and pain management, but avoid the consequences of immobility and too much medication.
Glucose control	Maintain blood glucose < 150 mg/dL after initial stabilization.
Bicarbonate therapy	Not recommended for treatment of hypoperfusion-induced lactic acidemia with pH > 7.15.
Deep venous thrombosis	Medical and mechanical treatment based on the severity of the patient's condition.
Stress ulcer prophylaxis	H$_2$ receptors have been found to be more effective in severe sepsis.
Consideration for limitation of support	Advance care planning and end-of-life issues must be considered and addressed.

Source: From Dellinger, R. P., Carlet, J. M., Masur, H., Gerlach, H., et al. (2008). Surviving Sepsis Campaign guidelines for management of severe sepsis and septic shock. *Critical Care Medicine,* 32(3), 858–873.

hand hygiene and the use of strict aseptic technique when managing any break in skin integrity such as wounds or invasive lines can help prevent infection. Patients who take steroids or other immunosuppressive medications must be taught how to recognize signs and symptoms of infection such as spiking a fever and chilling.

Nurses should also ensure the use of standard precautions, especially excellent hand hygiene, to prevent the transmission of microorganisms in the areas in which they work (Smith & McInnis, 2007).

Nursing care of the patient with sepsis is summarized in the Nursing Process: Patient Care Plan for Severe Sepsis (p. 1974).

CHART 61–8	Management of Severe Sepsis and Septic Shock

Intervention	Rationale
During the first 6 hours resuscitation is directed at: • Central venous pressure 8–12 mmHg • Mean arterial pressure (MAP) >65 mmHg • Urine output >0.5 mL/ kg/ hr • Central venous or mixed oxygen saturation >70%. Obtain vascular access. Aggressive fluid resuscitation of natural or artificial colloids or crystalloids may be used to achieve outlined parameters, vasopressors are used to maintain adequate perfusion and in some cases blood transfusions are done.	Goal-directed therapy has been shown to improve patient outcomes. Fluid resuscitation, use of vasopressors, and in some cases blood transfusions may be used to obtain the goals of adequate perfusion and oxygenation to compromised tissues.
Appropriate cultures of blood or any other potential infection site should be obtained before initiation of antibiotic therapy.	Diagnostic studies (e.g., blood cultures, radiographs, and CT exams) should be performed promptly to identify the source of the infection or causative agent organism. Sources such as abscesses need to be drained.
Antibiotic therapy is based on the patient history, underlying diseases, clinical syndrome, and susceptibility patterns in the patient's community and in the health care facility.	Failure to initiate appropriate antibiotic therapy promptly has adverse consequences. Inappropriate antibiotic therapy can lead to the development of a superinfection and the development of resistance.
Vasopressors should be started after an appropriate fluid challenge has failed. Vasopressors may also be indicated in the instance of a life-threatening hypotension along with fluid resuscitation.	Beyond a certain MAP, autoregulation in various vascular beds is lost. Vasopressors will be needed to maintain perfusion.
Provide inotropic support.	Supplements low cardiac output.
IV corticosteroids for 7 days in three or four divided doses are recommended in patient in septic shock, not responding to fluid replacement and vasopressor therapies.	Decreases stress response and may reverse shock states.
Use of recombinant human activated protein C is recommended in patients with a high risk of death such as patients who are in sepsis-induced organ failure, septic shock, or sepsis-induced respiratory distress. Patient must have a low risk of bleeding and the benefits of treatment must outweigh the risks.	The inflammatory response in severe sepsis is linked to procoagulant activity and endothelial activation. This drug has been shown in some cases to improve survival. It needs to be administered as early as possible.
Red blood cell administration should only be administered when hemoglobin decreases to < 7.0 g/dL.	Research has suggested that patients with severe sepsis can tolerate lower hemoglobin. Blood transfusions may actually worsen sepsis by initiating an additional inflammatory response.
Keep glucose < 150 mg/dL	Nutrition is important for the septic patient.
Mechanical ventilations should be closely monitored to prevent VAP, pulmonary injury, and adequate oxygenation.	Mechanical ventilation has been associated with multiple complications and an increased mortality. A weaning protocol should be in place and mechanically ventilated patients should undergo a spontaneous breathing test so that the patient can come off the ventilator as soon as possible.
Sedation, analgesia, and neuromuscular blockade should be goal driven.	Predetermined end points with the use of these medications prevent additional stress and harm to a compromised patient and also provide comfort and pain management.
Provide bicarbonate therapy for management of hypoperfusion-induced lactic acidemia.	There is no evidence to support this treatment.
Deep venous prophylaxis should be started to prevent the risk of emboli. This can be done with either low-dose unfractionated heparin or low-molecular-weight heparin. For patients with bleeding risk, mechanical devices should be used. In some patients, a combination of both may be required.	Prevents complications of deep vein thrombosis (DVT).
Stress ulcer prophylaxis should be initiated.	Stress ulcers cause additional complications in severe sepsis.
Consideration of limitation of support should be discussed with patient (when possible) and family. This should include: • Advanced care planning • Realistic goals of treatment • Withdrawal of support • Comfort care.	Aggressive management may not be in the patient's best interest. There may be no difference in outcome based on the cause of the severe sepsis and septic shock. Underlying quality of patient's life before the onset of severe sepsis and septic shock must be examined.

Source: From Dellinger, R. P., Carlet, J. M., Masur, H., Gerlach, H., et al. (2008). Surviving Sepsis Campaign guidelines for management of severe sepsis and septic shock. *Critical Care Medicine, 32*(3), 858–873.

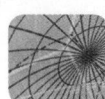

NURSING PROCESS: Patient Care Plan for Severe Sepsis

Assessment of Airway and Gas Exchange

Subjective Data:
Are you short of breath?
Are you getting enough air?
Do you breathe better sitting up?
Have you had a cough?
Are you coughing anything up and, if so, what color is it and how much?
Have you had a fever or chills?

Objective Data:
Work of breathing
Increased rate, use of accessory muscles, retractions
Lung sounds
Oxygen saturation
Skin color
Capillary refill

Nursing Assessment and Diagnoses	Outcomes and Evaluation Parameters	Planning and Interventions with *Rationales*
Nursing Diagnoses: *Gas Exchange, Impaired Risk for* related to inadequate tissue perfusion *Airway Clearance, Ineffective* related to altered mental status from inadequate tissue perfusion	**Outcome:** Adequate gas exchange. *Evaluation Parameters:* Normal arterial blood gases. Decreased respiratory rate because of a decreased need to compensate for metabolic acidosis; 12–20 breaths per minute. Adequate perfusion for the patient to become alert and oriented. Clear breath sounds.	**Interventions and *Rationales:*** Assess for symptoms of increased work of breathing, which indicate inadequate tissue perfusion: oxygen saturation, length of capillary refill, skin temperature, and color *to assess tissue perfusion.* Monitor ABGs and oxygen saturation to assess adequacy of gas exchange and level of shock state. *When the body responds to shock, it will divert blood from the periphery and direct it to the brain, lungs, and kidneys.* Monitor for changes in mental status such as restlessness and confusion. *Indicators of inadequate gas exchange with resultant cerebral hypoxia.* Observe for pallor and cyanosis, especially in the mucous membranes. *Indicators of inadequate gas exchange with resultant tissue hypoxia.* Administer 100% oxygen by nonrebreather mask. *To increase available oxygen and decrease tissue hypoxia.* Report respiratory distress and hypoxia to the health care provider. *Intubation and mechanical ventilation may be needed to deliver greater amounts of oxygen and maintain adequate tissue perfusion.*

Assessment of Fluid Volume Deficit

Subjective Data:
Are you thirsty?
How much fluid have you taken in?
What kind of fluids have you been drinking?
When was the last time you urinated?
Do you have any appetite?

Objective Data:
Decreased or absent peripheral pulses
Weak central pulses
Cool and clammy skin
Pale skin
Decreased or absent urinary output
Altered mental status
Alterations in vitals signs
Tachycardia, increased pulse pressure, decreased mean arterial pressure
Poor skin turgor

Nursing Assessment and Diagnoses	Outcomes and Evaluation Parameters	Planning and Interventions with *Rationales*
Nursing Diagnosis: *Fluid Volume, Deficient* related to alterations in circulating blood volume due to impaired vascular function from the effects of endotoxins on vasomotor tone	**Outcome:** Adequate circulating fluid volume. *Evaluation Parameters:* Adequate peripheral perfusion. Normal capillary refill time. Normal urinary output (minimum of 30 mL/hr). Improvement in mentation. Heart rate 60–100 beats per minute with normal sinus rhythm. Blood pressure systolic greater than 100 mmHg.	**Interventions and *Rationales:*** Insertion of large-bore intravenous catheters *to provide fluid resuscitation.* Insert central venous catheter *to measure pressure and monitor central pressure.* Insert a urinary catheter *to measure hourly urinary output. These measures help with assessment of adequacy of fluid resuscitation.* Monitor effectiveness of the use of prescribed vasopressors, *which are used to improve blood pressure and support circulation.* Monitor heart rate, blood pressure, and quality of central and peripheral pulses *to assess adequacy of fluid resuscitation.* Report signs of inadequate perfusion (e.g., hypotension, tachycardia, and low urinary output) to the health care provider *so that additional interventions such as administration of other vasopressor agents can be started to improve circulation.*

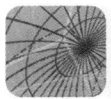

NURSING PROCESS: Patient Care Plan for Severe Sepsis—*Continued*

Assessment of Infection

Subjective Data:

Have you had an infection in the last 2 weeks?

How often do you urinate? Do you feel you completely empty your bladder with each urination?

Have you been running a fever?

Do you have a cough?

Do you have burning on urination?

Do you have a history of infections? If so, what kind? How were they treated?

Are you taking any medications such as steroids, antibiotics?

Have you had an organ transplant?

Have you recently traveled outside of the country? If you have, where? Were you told of possible diseases such as avian flu where you traveled?

Objective Data:

Fever	Presence of a urinary catheter
Chills	Feeding tube
Flushed skin	Decubitus
Presence of purpura, petechiae	Presence of wounds
Abscess	Urinary catheter?
Open wound	Feeding tube?
Burns	White blood count

Nursing Assessment and Diagnoses	Outcomes and Evaluation Parameters	Planning and Interventions with *Rationales*
Nursing Diagnoses: *Infection* related to a focus of infection	**Outcomes:** Identification of focus of infection. Infection resolved. ***Evaluation Parameters:*** Decrease or absence of fever. Removal of source of the infection, for example, draining of an abscess or removal of an invasive catheter. Normal white blood cell count and differential.	**Interventions and *Rationales:*** Measure and monitor the patient's body temperature using the most appropriate method. For example, rectal, esophageal, or bladder so the most accurate temperature is measured. *Effects of treatment can also be monitored.* Perform measures to decrease the patient's fever such as administration of an antipyretic or application of a cooling blanket. *To prevent side effects of fever such as dehydration.* Note the presence of a source of an infection, for example, urinary catheter, draining wound, rigid abdomen, and colored sputum. *To determine cause and infection site.* Obtain blood cultures by drawing blood from two sites. At least one should be drawn percutaneously and one drawn through each vascular access device unless the device was recently inserted to identify infectious agent. *To diagnose the presence of sepsis.* Obtain cultures from other sites such as urine, CSF, or other body fluids to identify source and infectious agents. *To identify source of infection.* Use aseptic technique when changing dressings or drawing blood from invasive lines *to prevent introduction of further sources of infection.* Perform hand hygiene frequently and use infection control measures when indicated *to prevent introduction of further sources of infection.* Instruct the patient's family about hand hygiene *to prevent further introduction of infection.* Report to the health care provider changes in temperature as prescribed *so appropriate interventions and medications can be given to manage a fever.* Administer antibiotics per health care provider's orders.

Assessment of Tissue Perfusion

Subjective Data:

Is it getting harder to breathe?

Are you more tired than before?

Is your chest hurting?

Are you having pain anywhere?

Objective Data:

Lung congestion	Abdominal distention and
Oxygen saturation	tenderness
Work of breathing	Bowel sounds
Central and peripheral pulses	Jaundice of eyes and skin
Cardiac rhythm	Enlarged liver
Urinary output	Muscle strength
Urine color	Mobility
Level of consciousness	

(continued)

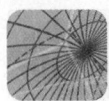

NURSING PROCESS: Patient Care Plan for Severe Sepsis—*Continued*

Nursing Assessment and Diagnoses	Outcomes and Evaluation Parameters	Planning and Interventions with *Rationales*
Nursing Diagnosis: *Tissue Perfusion, Ineffective* related to organ dysfunction	**Outcome:** Prevention of further organ failure and treatment instituted. **Evaluation Parameter:** Effective prevention of MODS.	**Interventions and *Rationales:*** Initiate prescribed treatments including fluid resuscitation and vasopressor and antibiotic administration. *To hemodynamically stabilize the patient and treat the cause of infection.* Carefully monitor intake and output. *To evaluate for adequate fluid resuscitation.* Turn and position patient frequently *to prevent skin breakdown and development of DVT.* Monitor for bleeding that may occur due to altered clotting mechanisms. *To prevent hemorrhage.* Prepare patient and family for end-of-life decisions. *To prepare the family for possible death.*

It is based on the management of the patient's airway and breathing to improve oxygenation and circulation. Circulatory support may include fluids as well as vasopressors to maintain a perfusing blood pressure and prevent additional complications.

Collaborative Management

The care of the patient with sepsis requires a multidisciplinary approach in order to increase the patient's chances of survival. The nurse plays an important role in the early recognition of the risk of sepsis occurring as well as recognizing its early signs when it does. Health care providers who participate in the management of the patient with sepsis include specialty health care providers such as a critical care intensivist, surgeons, and infectious disease specialists; nurses; pharmacists; and respiratory and physical therapists.

The health care providers who care for the patient with sepsis are responsible for identifying the cause of the sepsis. This may involve taking the person to surgery to drain an abscess or remove an injured organ. The intensivist is responsible for managing the patient's cardiovascular and pulmonary systems. Nurses are responsible for the continuous monitoring and administration of medications and fluids as well as the emotional and spiritual support of the patient and his family. Pharmacists participate in the evaluation of the appropriate antibiotics and vasoactive medications to fight the cause of the sepsis and maintain the patient's vital sign. Because many of these patients require intubation and mechanical ventilation, the respiratory therapist will assist in the management of the patient's oxygenation. Finally, the physical therapist will be responsible for supporting the nursing staff in providing range of motion (ROM) exercises for sedated patients and moving patients out of bed when possible to prevent further complications from immobility.

Multiple Organ Dysfunction Syndrome

Multiple organ dysfunction syndrome is the end result of severe sepsis. A critical injury or a disease process that initiates a mas-

sive systemic inflammatory response can also activate it. It does not require an infectious process to trigger it. Despite recognition of this disease process since the mid-1970s, mortality from MODS remains high, ranging from 60% to 100% (McCance & Huether, 2006).

Etiology

Multiple organ dysfunction syndrome (MODS) is a spectrum of organ dysfunction in a patient who has SIRS or septic complications. One or more organ systems may be involved (Bumbasirevic, Karamarkovic, Lesic, & Bumbasirevic, 2005; Gupta & Jonas, 2006). Triggers that can initiate MODS include multiple injuries, burns, hemorrhagic or hypovolemic shock, acute pancreatitis, acute respiratory distress syndrome (ARDS), and acute renal failure. Examples of patients who are at risk for the development of MODS include patients with chronic diseases; persons of advanced age; patients who have diabetes, cancer, pulmonary contusions, and widespread necrosis; and those with chronic infections who are being treated with immunosuppressant therapies. It remains a mystery why not all patients with these risk factors develop MODS. Research is now being directed at identifying biomarkers that place patients at greater risk of developing both sepsis and MODS (McCance & Huether, 2006).

Pathophysiology

Multiple organ dysfunction ranges from organ impairment to failure. MODS is classified into primary or early MODS and secondary or late MODS. In primary or early MODS, there is local and generalized hypoperfusion. This triggers both the inflammatory and stress responses discussed previously in this chapter. As a result, microphages and neutrophils are "primed or ready to fight" by cytokines and when any additional insult occurs, such as further tissue injury, the primed cells trigger an even greater response and start progressive organ dysfunction and secondary or late MODS.

Secondary or late MODS results from an excessive inflammatory response after a latent period following the initial insult that is manifested in organs distant from the original site of the injury (Krau, 2007; McCance & Huether, 2006). Just as in sepsis, three primary mechanisms are activated: the inflammatory response, coagulation, and fibrinolysis. It is the body's own defense mechanisms that ultimately contribute to organ compromise and failure (Krau, 2007).

The inflammatory response in MODS leads to hypermetabolism and maldistribution of blood flow. Maldistribution of blood results in tissue hypoxemia, further organ injury, and eventual cell death. Hypermetabolism that results from the stress response causes catabolism, further straining major organs such as the heart and eventually impeding cardiac output. Catabolism causes loss of lean muscle mass and depletion of oxygen and fuel supplies (McCance & Huether, 2006). Oxygen reserves are depleted in MODS because of the body's initial inflammatory response to the primary insult and resulting hypermetabolism. Myocardial depressant factor, which is secreted because of pancreatic hypoperfusion, causes further depression of the myocardium, thus contributing to further hypoxia.

Reperfusion injury, which results from the reestablishment of blood flow after ischemia, causes conversion of the enzyme xanthine dehydrogenase to xanthine oxidase to form oxygen free radicals with oxygen when hypoperfused tissues are reperfused. These oxygen radicals attack already damaged tissues. As discussed earlier in this chapter, reperfusion injury can lead to MODS (McCance & Huether, 2006). Figure 61–3 ■ (p. 1978) summarizes the pathophysiology of MODS. The treatment and management continues to challenge those who provide critical care and continues to be responsible for mortality that is generally the end result of MODS.

Clinical Manifestations and Diagnosis

The clinical manifestations of MODS depend on the area or areas of the body affected. Primary or early MODS is difficult to monitor. Examples of primary MODS in a trauma patient may include the primary cerebral edema seen in a head injury or ARDS that develops after a thoracic injury (Keel & Trentz, 2005). Secondary or late MODS has a specific pattern of injury that can be observed and measured. Several scoring systems exist that describe the progress of MODS. The sequential organ failure assessment (SOFA) score describes the degree of organ failure and how it changes over time. SOFA is summarized in Chart 61–9 (p. 1979). Secondary or late MODS generally evolves over 14 days to a period of weeks.

In summary, the clinical manifestations of MODS are the result of inflammatory mediator damage, tissue hypoxia, and hypermetabolism. The clinical manifestations of organ dysfunction are summarized in Chart 61–10 (p. 1979) (McCance & Huether, 2006).

Laboratory and Diagnostic Procedures

The laboratory and diagnostic tests used to evaluate MODS are specific to the organ systems that are failing. For example, hyperbilirubinemia and increased serum aspartate transaminase, serum alanine aminotransferase, lactic dehydrogenase, alkaline phosphatase, and ammonia levels are indicative of liver failure. Patchy infiltrates on a chest radiograph are seen with ARDS. Decreased or absent urinary output reflects renal failure. The Diagnostic Tests for MODS box (p. 1980) contains information on laboratory tests that are monitored in the patient with MODS.

Medical Management

The primary focus for the management of MODS is to prevent it from occurring. Rapid recognition of the source of infection or management of the cause of shock or sepsis is one way to decrease the risk of the secondary insult. Nosocomial infections from invasive lines or catheters as well as poor hand hygiene must also be managed. After the initial injury or infection has been treated, care is directed at controlling infection, providing adequate tissue oxygenation, restoring and maintaining vascular volume, and supporting individual organ function. Antibiotics must be chosen carefully and closely monitored (McCance & Huether, 2006). Because tissue hypoxia is a major problem, intubation and mechanical ventilation may be required. Oxygen saturation should be maintained between 88% and 92%. However, mechanical ventilation can lead to additional problems such as VAP, which may lead to the secondary assault triggering the onset of MODS.

Adequate volume resuscitation and vascular support need to be ongoing. Volume resuscitation decreases the risks of complications from hemoconcentrated blood due to shifts in interstitial spaces. Replacing and maintaining volume also improves the supply and demand imbalance that occurs with hypermetabolism. Vasopressors such as epinephrine or norepinephrine may be used to increase systemic vascular resistance and improve cardiac output and oxygenation. Any problem that increases oxygen demand such as fever needs to be managed. Excessive body temperatures may require cooling measures such as hypothermia blankets as well as medications such as acetaminophen. Patients may require analgesia and sedation to decrease pain and anxiety thus decreasing oxygen demand. Nutrition through enteral feeding helps maintain the gut barrier and reduces the translocation of bacteria, thus reducing the incidence of infection and other complications. Glucose levels are tightly controlled due to the effect of high glucose levels on tissue/organ function. Individual organs will require support and this management will be based on the organ or organ systems that have been affected.

■ Nursing Management

Nursing care for the patient with MODS includes early recognition of the risk factors for the development of MODS, and close monitoring of interventions initiated to treat the patients such as invasive lines and catheters. Meticulous skin care and aseptic technique must be used to insert and change any lines. The nurse should ensure that all who come in contact with the patient use meticulous hand hygiene and aseptic technique to prevent the risk of infection.

Frequent monitoring and assessment to trend changes in vital signs and clinical manifestations will provide the most reliable information about early signs of MODS. Nursing care needs to be focused on decreasing oxygen demand, which includes pain and anxiety management as well as spacing activity to allow for long periods of rest. The nurse should assess for signs of pain and anxiety and medicate as needed. Tachycardia related to pain and anxiety increases oxygen consumption due to the stress imposed on the body by pain. Positioning of the patient is important to prevent the complications that occur with immobility such as skin breakdown, pulmonary congestion, and pooling of blood and secretions. Hypermetabolism causes loss

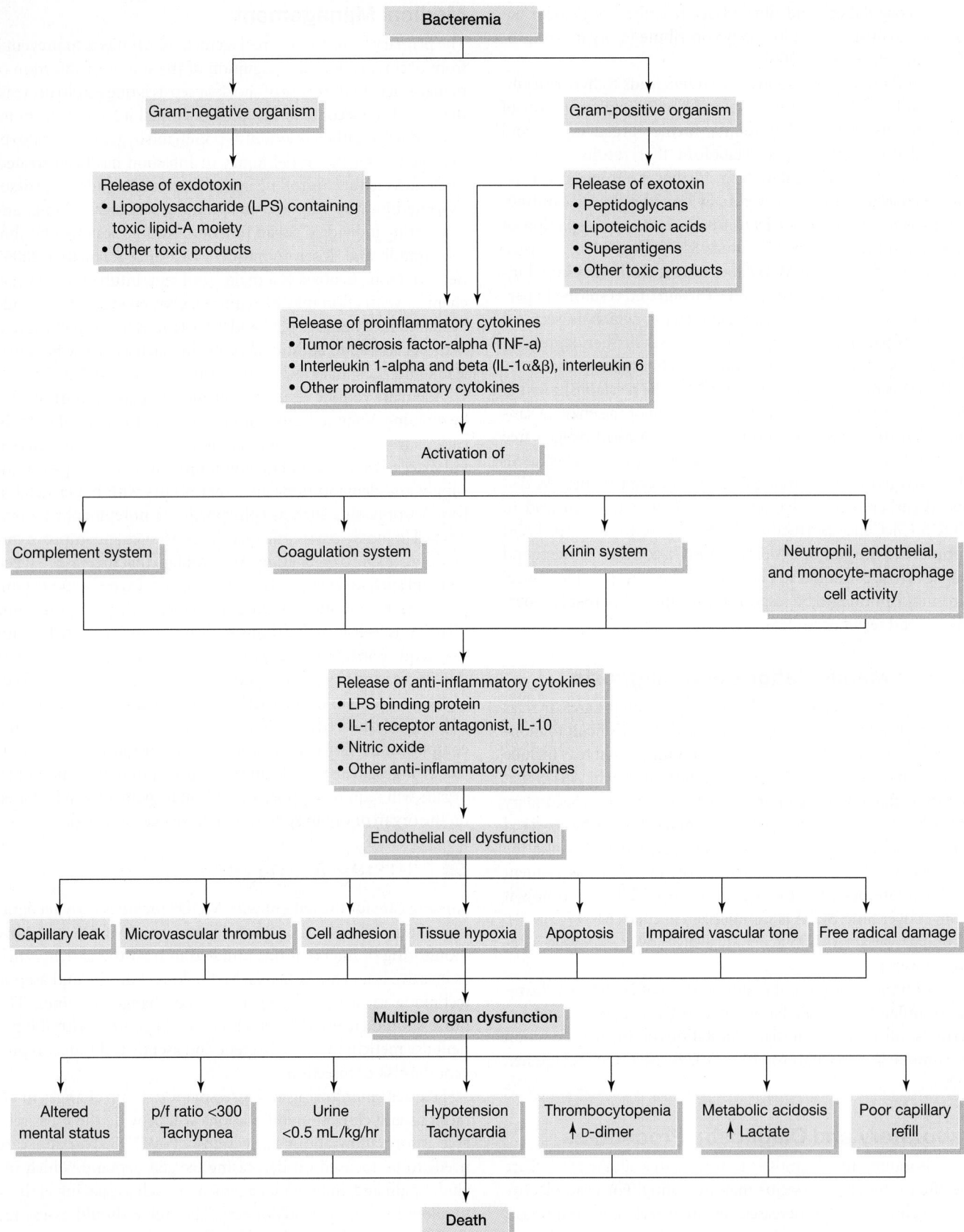

FIGURE 61–3 ■ Pathophysiology of MODS.

CHART 61–9   **Sequential Organ Failure Assessment (SOFA) Score**

	1	2	3	4
Respiration PaO$_2$/FiO$_2$(kP$_a$)	<53	<40	<26	<13
Coagulation platelets (10^3/μL)	<150	<100	<50	<20
Liver bilirubin (μmol/L)	20–32	33–101	102–204	>204
Cardiovascular Inotrope	MAP <70	Dopamine ≤ 5 μg/kg/min or dobutamine any dose	Dopamine >5 μg/kg/min or adrenaline < 0.1 μg/kg/min or noradrenalin < 0.1 μg/kg/min	Dopamine > 15 μg/kg/min or adrenaline > 0.1 or noradrenalin > 0.1
CNS		10–12	6–9	<6
GCS	13–14			
Renal Creatinine (μmol/L)	110–170	171–299	300–440	>440

Note: Key: MAP, mean arterial pressure; GCS, Glasgow Coma Scale.

CHART 61–10   **Clinical Manifestations of MODS**

PULMONARY

Dyspnea, patchy infiltrates, refractory hypoxemia, respiratory acidosis, and abnormal O$_2$ indices

Pulmonary hypertension

GASTROINTESTINAL

Abdominal distention and ascites

Intolerance of enteral feedings

Paralytic ileus

Gastrointestinal bleeding

Mucosal ulceration

Bacterial overgrowth in stool

LIVER

Increased bilirubin level

Increased liver enzymes

Increased serum ammonia level

Jaundice

Hepatomegaly

METABOLIC/NUTRITIONAL

Decreased lean body mass

Muscle wasting

Severe weight loss

Negative nitrogen balance

Hyperglycemia

Hypertriglyceridemia

Increased serum lactate levels

Decreased serum albumin

RENAL

Increased serum creatinine level and BUN

Oliguria, anuria, or polyuria related to acute tubular necrosis

CARDIOVASCULAR

HYPERDYNAMIC

Decreased:
   Pulmonary capillary wedge pressure
   Systemic vascular resistance
   Right atrial pressure

Increased:
   Oxygen consumption
   Cardiac output
   Cardiac index
   Heart rate

HYPODYNAMIC

Increased:
   Systemic vascular resistance
   Right atrial pressure
   Left ventricular stroke work index

Decreased:
   Oxygen delivery and consumption
   Cardiac output
   Cardiac index

CENTRAL NERVOUS SYSTEM

Lethargy

Altered level of consciousness

Fever

Hepatic encephalopathy

COAGULATION AND HEMATOLOGIC

Thrombocytopenia

Disseminated intravascular coagulation

IMMUNE

Infection

Decreased lymphocyte count

Anergy

Source: Adapted from McCance, K. L., & Huether, S. (2006). *Pathophysiology: The biologic basis for disease in adults and children* (5th ed.). St. Louis: Mosby.

DIAGNOSTIC TESTS for MODS

Test and Normal Values	Expected Abnormality	Rationale for Abnormality
Lactate level 1–2 mmol/L	4–5 mmol/L	Metabolic acidosis results from inadequate tissue perfusion and anaerobic metabolism.
D-dimer Negative	Positive	Indication of coagulopathy that is present in MODS.
Liver function tests	Increased	Liver is frequently one of the first organs to fail in MODS.
Arterial blood gases	pH acidosis PO_2 decreased	Acidosis and hypoxia result because of damage to the lungs and poor end-organ perfusion.

of muscle, so it is important to prevent additional loss of movement. Patients should receive active and passive ROM exercises to retain strength and joint motion.

Emotional support for both the patient and the family is essential. The high mortality rate associated with MODS points out the need to assist the family with preparing for difficult decisions about end of life. As discussed in Chapter 17 👁, the nurse needs to be aware of any religious or cultural needs related to death and dying.

Administration of vasopressors will place the patient at risk of injury to fingers, hands, toes, and feet due to peripheral vasoconstriction. Frequent assessment of peripheral circulation is needed. Additionally, fluid resuscitation and shunting of blood and nutrients can lead to edema. Therefore, skin impairment can occur and is another source of infection. Positioning and use of special beds may improve the risk of these complications.

Health Promotion

The primary emphasis in the treatment for shock is prevention. Early recognition of factors that place a patient at risk for the development of a shock syndrome may greatly reduce patient morbidity and mortality. See the Complementary & Alternative Therapies box (p. 1982) for a discussion of the use of T'ai Chi Chun to strengthen the immune system. Traumatic injury contributes to the risk for all types of shock because of organ system injury. Injury prevention strategies may add to decreasing the incidence of shock. Examples of injury prevention and control strategies can be found in the Emergency Nurses Association's Trauma Nursing Core Course (ENA, 2007). Examples include:

- Engineering and technologic interventions (e.g., high-mounted rear brake lights)
- Enforcement and legislative interventions (e.g., state seat belt and helmet laws)
- Placing children in properly fitted and located car seats
- Education and behavioral interventions (e.g., school- and hospital-based education programs).

Sepsis and septic shock have become a serious problem in the United States. Prevention strategies to reduce the incidence of septic shock include (Masur, 2003):

- Age-appropriate vaccinations
- Reduction of the incidence of antibiotic-resistant pathogens in ICUs

- Aseptic management of invasive lines
- Aseptic management of indwelling catheters, feeding tubes, and central lines
- Frequent hand hygiene (Hand hygiene has become a major quality indicator in hospitals, clinics, and any place patient care is given.)
- Efforts to limit antibiotic resistance through policies to prescribe them and surveillance of their use.

Chart 61–11 contains a summary of an action plan that is being implemented to combat antimicrobial resistance.

▉ Research

Research related to shock management is needed (1) to identify areas where practice could improve and (2) to evaluate and test selected interventions. Resuscitation end points and the identification of genetic markers that assist in the identification of patient's at risk to develop sepsis are needed (Gupta & Jonas, 2006). As pointed out earlier in this chapter, research continues to challenge how shock has been managed. The Research Opportunities and Clinical Impact Related to Shock Management box (p. 1983) provides a list of some of the research topics related to shock management that are under investigation. Keeping up with the constant changes in the literature is important to ensure that the patient is receiving the best and most effective care.

CHART 61–11 **Summary of Action Plan to Combat Antimicrobial Resistance**

- Conduct a national public health education campaign to promote appropriate antimicrobial use as a national health priority.
- Develop and facilitate the implementation of educational and behavioral interventions that will assist clinicians in appropriate antimicrobial prescribing.
- Evaluate the effectiveness (including cost effectiveness) of current and novel infection control practices for health care and extended care settings and in the community.
- Promote adherence to practices proven to be effective.
- Support demonstration projects to evaluate comprehensive strategies that use multiple interventions to promote appropriate drug use and reduce infection rates, in order to assess how interventions found effective in research studies can be applied routinely and most cost effectively on a large scale.

PHARMACOLOGY Summary of Medications to Treat Shock, Severe Sepsis, and MODS

Medication Category	Action	Application/Indication	Nursing Responsibility
Antibiotics			
Broad-spectrum antibiotics are used initially because the infectious agent is generally not known. Antibiotics should be chosen using the following guidelines: • What community the patient lives in or has come from • Epidemiology of sepsis in the hospital or community • Suspected agents: Fungi Gram-positive bacteria Highly resistant gram-negative bacilli Methicillin-resistant *Staphylococcus aureus* Vancomycin-resistant enterococcus Penicillin-resistant pneumococcus	Will depend on the type of antibiotic that is prescribed by the clinician.	Choice of antibiotic should be based on the epidemiology of sepsis in the hospital and the community. Identification of the site of source or site of infection will direct the type of antibiotic approved. Only one antibiotic at a time, or monotherapy, is recommended.	Assess history of drug allergies. Assess clinical manifestations of allergic reaction. Assess relief of clinical manifestations to determine drug effectiveness 48–72 hours after initiation of the antibiotic therapy.
Recombinant			
Human-Activated Protein C	*Antithrombotic:* Irreversible inactivation of Factors V and VIII. *Anti-inflammatory:* Reduces formation of TNF, IL-8, IL-6, and thrombin; limits the rolling of monocytes and neutrophils on injured endothelium. Also may reduce apoptosis. *Profibrinolytic:* Inhibits plasminogen activator inhibitor-1 (PA-1).	The following criteria should be used for the administration: • Severe sepsis of greater than 48 hours • High risk of death • Experienced medical care of the patient has not improved the condition • Static or deteriorating clinical condition • No evidence of: Morbid obesity Major surgery < 12 hours Intracranial surgery or stroke < 3 months Previous intracranial lesion Epidural congenital bleeding diathesis Gastrointestinal bleeding requiring intervention < 6 weeks Trauma with bleeding risk Pancreatitis Chronic renal failure Varices Cirrhosis Chronic jaundice or ascites Platelets < 30,000 × 10^6/L Antithrombotic medication Recent DVT or PE Hypercoagulable Immunocompromised	Assess history that may contradict the administration of this medication. Carefully assess any indications of bleeding or coagulation disorders. Carefully assess relief of clinical manifestations to determine drug effectiveness or worsening of the patient's condition.

(continued)

Medication Category	Action	Application/Indication	Nursing Responsibility
Corticosteroids			
Hydrocortisone Methylprednisone	Stimulates ACTH to increase cortisol. Stabilizes leukocyte lysosomal membrane. Inhibits phagocytosis and release of allergic substances. Reduces capillary dilation and permeability. Modifies immune response to various stimuli.	Treat adrenal insufficiency associated with septic shock. Treat inflammatory response related to spinal cord injury.	Assess relief of clinical manifestations. Carefully assess side effects: • Infection due to depressed immune response • Blood glucose • Gastric bleeding • Problems with wound healing.
Vasopressors			
Norepinephrine Dopamine Vasopressin	Reverse the vasodilation and reduced systemic vascular resistance. Promote alpha and beta sympathetic activity. Increase inotropy and chronotropy. Stimulate vasopressor receptors.	Vasopressors should not be used until appropriate fluid challenge fails to restore adequate blood pressure and organ perfusion. Vasopressin may be considered when fluid resuscitation and high-dose vasopressors have not worked.	Assess relief of clinical manifestations by monitoring MAP and urinary output. Assess the potential side effects of the medications such as peripheral vasoconstriction.
Insulin therapy	Inducts euglycemia, and anti-inflammatory effect. Protects endothelial and mitochondrial function.	Controls hyperglycemia, improves lipid levels, and has anti-inflammatory, anticoagulant, and anti-apoptic actions.	Assess patient glucose to maintain glucose level <150 mg/dL (8.3 mmol/L).
Recombinant			
Activated Coagulation Factor VII (rFVIIa)	Promotes coagulation.	Facilitates cell membrane binding.	Assess for bleeding.

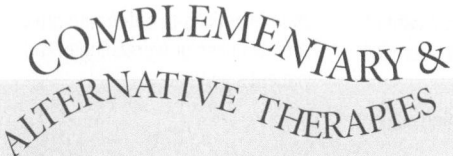

COMPLEMENTARY & ALTERNATIVE THERAPIES   T'ai Chi Chun

Description:
T'ai chi chun (TCC) is a CAM therapy that has multiple applications. Originating in Asia, TCC is a form of exercise that is used to improve balance, build muscle strength, and improve coordination. TCC uses a series of 20 slow, regular movements that many refer to as "moving meditation," and can be easily performed by older and medically compromised individuals.

Research Support:
A review of literature examined the quantity and quality of research evidence regarding the therapeutic benefits of Taiji, which is also known as tai chi chun (TCC). The research team examined more than 200 published reports, of which 17 controlled clinical trials met a high standard of methodological rigor. Evidence in these studies confirmed the following therapeutic benefits of TCC: improved quality of life, improved physical function including activity tolerance and cardiovascular function, improved pain management, improved balance, reduced risk of falls, enhanced immune response, and improved flexibility, strength, and kinesthetic sense. Researchers concluded that, according to preliminary research, TCC can be implemented in a variety of clinical populations (Klein & Adams, 2004).

A study conducted in Taiwan involved 37 middle-aged participants (14 men and 23 women) who engaged in 12 weeks of TCC exercises. Researchers investigated the effect of TCC on participants' functional mobility, beliefs about benefits of exercise on physical and psychological health, and immune regulation. Results showed that the participants experienced significant positive effects on functional mobility and beliefs about the health benefits of exercise after engaging in the 12 weeks of TCC. Immune system response was also positive: There was a significant decrease in monocyte count (although total white blood cell and red blood cell count did not change significantly); a significant increase in the ratio of T helper to suppressor cells (CD4:CD8); and a significant increase in CD4CD25 regulatory T cells (Yeh, Chuang, Lin, Hsiao, & Eng, 2006).

One paper discussed the results of a study that examined the effects of TCC on older adults' response and immunity to herpes zoster/shingles and varicella zoster virus. The study results showed that TCC improved health functioning and immunity to varicella zoster virus in older adults as compared to a control group (Irwin, Pike, & Oxman, 2004).

References
Irwin, M., Pike, J., & Oxman, M. (2004). Shingles immunity and health functioning in the elderly: T'ai chi chun as a behavioral treatment. *Evidence-Based Complementary and Alternative Medicine, 1*(3), 223–232.

Klein, P. J., & Adams, W. D. (2004). Comprehensive therapeutic benefits of Taiji: A critical review. *American Journal of Physical and Medical Rehabilitation, 83*(9), 735–745.

Yeh, S. H., Chuang, H., Lin, L. W., Hsiao, C. Y., & Eng, H. L. (2006). Regular t'ai chi chun exercise enhances functional mobility and CD4CD25 regulatory T cells. *British Journal of Sports Medicine, 40*(3), 239–243.

The death from sepsis that progresses to septic shock continues to increase each year. Research must be focused at multiple methods of prevention and management. Current research ideas and their clinical impact are discussed in the Research Opportunities and Clinical Impact Related to Sepsis, SIRS, and Severe Sepsis box (p. 1984).

Summary

Sepsis, severe sepsis, and septic shock continue to cost more human lives every year. Despite the creation of new medications, new methodologies to measure the effects of sepsis, and the increased admissions to critical care units, approximately 50% of the patients who succumb to septic shock will die. The health care costs are in the billions of dollars each year.

Nurses need to realize that in order to manage this grave problem, care must first focus on prevention strategies, and that when a septic syndrome has begun, the best evidenced-based treatments must be used to improve patient outcomes and stop unnecessary morbidity and mortality.

RESEARCH OPPORTUNITIES AND CLINICAL IMPACT RELATED TO SHOCK MANAGEMENT

Research Area	Clinical Impact
Physiological Research	
The role of apoptosis or programmed cell destruction in shock	Developing methods to intervene in the programmed destruction of cells
Role of heat-shock proteins in shock	Heat-shock proteins may play a role in the stress response initiated by the body in the shock state
Identity of specific markers that indicate a systemic shock response	Earlier diagnosis and identification of high risk patients
Development of an international definition of shock, SIRS, and sepsis	To standardize name and its significance related to research findings
Identification of the most appropriate solution for initial and continued fluid resuscitation: hypertonic saline, Ringer's lactate, or normal saline	Development of collaborative pathways for appropriate fluid resuscitation for the type of shock and nursing interventions to mediate the progression
Determination of whether fluid resuscitation should be controlled based on the source of the clinical insult. Theory that hypotensive may actually be a protective mechanism	
Hypothermia and minimal fluid resuscitation	Development of nursing guidelines for monitoring the patient's response to fluid resuscitation
Blood substitutes	
Recombinant hemoglobin solution	
Medications effective against bacteria and viruses without causing additional systemic damage, for example, ketolides, which bind to two sites on bacteria preventing the development of resistance	Antibiotic resistance is a growing problem, with an expanding number of resistant organisms occurring. Preventing resistance would help mitigate this issue.
Development of synthetic catecholamines to increase end-organ perfusion	Organ hypoperfusion causes complications and increase morbidity and mortality
Inhalation of nitric oxide (NO) inhibition by the use of methylene blue	NO has been found to increase in sepsis, which further contributes to vasodilation and decreased MAP
Staging of shock to guide clinical management	Development of nursing guidelines to monitor the stages of shock and progression of clinical manifestations
Development of guidelines for a universal approach to shock management so that better data can be collected about outcomes	Collaborative pathway for shock management
Shock monitoring: recent research questions the early use of invasive monitoring	Development of nursing guidelines for noninvasive monitoring
Use of extracorporeal membrane oxygenation therapy (ECMO)	ECMO can potentially remove mediators that initiate destructive cascades in such shock states as sepsis
Ethical Issues	
Identification of futile resuscitation parameters	Development of guidelines for the end points of resuscitation
Staging of shock and sepsis to identify irreversible futile resuscitation parameters	Development of nursing guidelines for withdrawal of support

RESEARCH OPPORTUNITIES AND CLINICAL IMPACT RELATED TO SEPSIS, SIRS, AND SEVERE SEPSIS

Research Area	Clinical Impact
Physiological Research	
Identification of how to implement guidelines for the management of severe sepsis and septic shock and measure patient outcomes	Implementation of a specific set of evidence-based guidelines should improve patient outcomes and control health care costs
Development of drugs that neutralize the inflammatory process	Drugs may be used to block the effects of specific toxins on the body
	Medications that neutralize the effects of the body's inflammatory response to infectious agents may improve the outcome of decompensated shock
Genetic studies that identify a person's predisposition to developing sepsis	Several gene polymorphisms have been associated with an increased susceptibility to sepsis
Vaccinations	Development of a vaccination that prevents SIRS when a patient has been exposed to an infectious agent
Ethical Issues	
Identification of end points that indicate that additional resuscitation would be futile	Development of guidelines for the end points of resuscitation
Development of guidelines for humane withdrawal of support	Development of nursing guidelines for withdrawal of support

Clinical Preparation

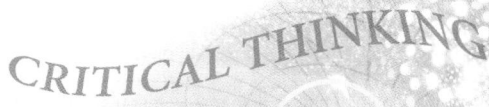

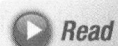 **Read**
- History of Current Illness
- Past Medical History
- Physical Exam
- Admitting Medical Orders
- Laboratory Study Results

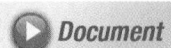 **Document**
- Summary of Hospitalization
- Pathophysiology Form
- Laboratory Values
- Laboratory Results Explanation

 **Apply**
- List of Potential Nursing Diagnoses
- Concept Map
- Critical Thinking Questions

Log on to MyNursingKit.com to download forms you will need and to complete further steps in the Clinical Preparation assignment.

HISTORY OF PRESENT ILLNESS

You are a nurse in a critical care unit and you have been notified that you will be receiving a new patient from the emergency department (ED). The ED nurse calls the following report: David is a 19-year-old college student who is brought to the ED by his friends. His friends said that he has been vomiting for the past 24 hours. This morning he was confused. The patient states that he does not feel well and has been "hot and cold." According to the patient's friends, there has been a recent outbreak of a viral infection on campus. They do not know what the name of the infection is, only that they had heard that it was occurring. The patient is awake and alert, but complaining of a headache. The ED nurse states that he has a petechial rash on his lower extremities and he has received a dose of ceftriaxone 2 grams intravenously.

His blood pressure is 100/70; heart rate 120; respiratory rate 28; his temperature is currently 100.8 orally.

Procedures Since Admission

Within a few hours of admission in the critical care unit, David's mental status begins to deteriorate. You notify the critical care resident and provide him with the following information. David's level of consciousness continued to deteriorate. The critical care resident elected to intubate David using sedation and neuromuscular blocking agents. David was placed on a ventilator. A second large-bore IV line was inserted to administer 2 liters of normal saline since David's blood pressure is staying around 90 systolic and his pulse is in the 130s to 150s. The resident also inserts an arterial line.

Medical–Surgical History

No known allergies
Taking no medications
No prior medical history other than normal childhood illnesses

Social History

David is a freshman at college; he is on the swimming team
States that he drinks beer on the weekend with his friends
Denies the use of illicit substances
Denies cigarette smoking

Physical Exam

Vital signs: BP 88/40; P 130; RR 36; T 104.0°F
Oxygen saturation: 90% on room air initially and then dropped to 86% on room air
HEENT: normal, braces on both upper and lower teeth
Heart: rapid rate; normal S_1, S_2
Lungs: bilateral basilar crackles
Abdomen: flat, soft nontender

Neurological exam: David is lethargic, but can be aroused with minimal stimulation. He is not able to answer simple questions, but will raise his arms and legs when asked. His pupils are 4 mm, equal, round and reactive. Complains of pain with neck movement
Skin: flushed and hot to the touch
Chest radiograph: basilar infiltrates
ECG: sinus tachycardia
Weight: 180 lbs (80 kg) Height 6'
Extremities: petechial rash on both lower extremities that does not blanch
DP and PT pulses 2+

Admitting Medical Orders

Medical ICU service
Floor: Medical Intensive Care Unit
Diagnosis: meningitis and septic shock
No known allergies

LABORATORY STUDY RESULTS

Test	Day 1	Day 2	Day 3
Sodium	141 mEq/L	139 mEq/L	138 mEq/L
Potassium	4.0 mEq/L	3.5 mEq/L	3.8 mEq/L
Chloride	100 mEq/L	113 mEq/L	113 mEq/L
Venous carbon dioxide	17 mEq/L	18 mEq/L	22 mEq/L
Calcium	6.6 mg/dL	7.0 mg/dL	8.6 mg/dL
Blood urea nitrogen	30 mg/dL	25 mg/dL	18 mg/dL
Creatinine	2.0 mg/dL	1.5 mg/dL	1.0 mg/dL
Blood glucose	150 mg/dL	138 mg/dL	120 mg/dL
Total Proteins	4.5 g/dL		
Magnesium	2.0 mg/dL	2.0 mg/dL	2.0 mg/dL
WBC	22, 000/mm³	10,000/mm³	10,500/mm³
Hemoglobin	14.0 gm/dL	13.4 gm/dL	14.7 gm/dL
Hematocrit	40.8%	38.7%	43.1%
RBC	4.69 m/mm³	4.49 m/mm³	4.97 m/mm³
Platelets	128 K/mm³	137 K/mm³	269 K/mm³
ABGs			
PO_2	78 mmHg	100 mmHg	150 mmHg
O_2 saturation	88%	94%	98%
pH	7.27	7.30	7.35
PCO_2	36.5 mmHg	30 mmHg	28 mmHg
HCO_3	24 mEq/L	22 mEq/L	24 mEq/L
CSF	Positive for group B streptococcus		
CT scan	Cerebral edema		
ELISA	Antiviral immunoglobulin		
INR	1.18	1.2	1.25
PTT	32 seconds	32.6 seconds	33 seconds
Sputum culture		Negative	
Nasopharyngeal culture		Positive for group B streptococcus	
CSF culture		Positive for group B streptococcus	
Latex agglutination	Certain antibodies in body fluids		
UA	Within normal limits		

Foley
NG tube to low wall suction
Bed rest
Intake and output
Isolation: respiratory isolation
Ventilator settings:
TV 480
RR: 16
Oxygen: 60%
Mode: Assist/control
Peep: 5
Vital signs: every 15 minutes until stable then every 1 hour
Neurological checks every 30 minutes
IV: lactated Ringer's at 100mL/hr. Maintain systolic blood pressure at 100 mmHg with normal saline fluid bolus of 500 mL × 1
NPO until further notice
Call house officer: pulse < 60 and > 100/minute; BP < 90 and > 160 systolic; temperature > 38.5; urine output < 30 mL/hr for 2 hours; respiratory rate > 30/minute; oxygen saturation <92%
Sequential compression devices (SCDs) to lower extremities

Scheduled Medications

Ceftriaxone 2 grams IV once a day
Lansoprazole 30 mg NG once a day
Levophed drip (4 mg/250 mL of normal saline) at 2–12 micrograms per kilogram to maintain a systolic blood pressure at 100 mmHg

PRN Medications

Fentanyl 20–50 micrograms IV q2h for sedation and analgesia
Ativan 2–4 milligrams IV q4h for sedation
Acetaminophen suppositories q4h for fever greater than 102°F

Ordered Laboratory Studies

STAT blood cultures were obtained in the emergency department
CSF studies: cell count, protein, glucose levels sent from the ED
Cultures: sputum, nasopharyngeal, cerebrospinal fluid (CSF)
Latex agglutination
Enzyme-linked immunosorbent assay (ELISA)
CBC, INR/PTT, Ca, Mg, phosphorous, electrolyte panel daily
UA

Ordered Diagnostic Studies

CT scan of head; repeat with changes
Lumbar puncture

CRITICAL THINKING QUESTIONS

1. Upon initial admission to the critical care unit, what complications should you assess David for?

2. How is meningitis transmitted and how can you protect yourself?

3. Why would a medication such as Levophed be started to maintain David's blood pressure?

Answers to Critical Thinking Questions appear in Appendix D

NCLEX® REVIEW

1. A patient is diagnosed as being in shock after starting a new medication. The nurse realizes this patient is most likely experiencing which of the following types of shock?
   1. Cardiogenic
   2. Anaphylactic
   3. Neurogenic
   4. Septic

2. A patient in shock is demonstrating signs of insulin resistance. The nurse realizes this is because of:
   1. The stress response.
   2. Undiagnosed diabetes mellitus.
   3. Excessive body weight.
   4. Undiagnosed metabolic syndrome.

3. A patient in shock is demonstrating an alteration in level of consciousness. The nurse realizes that this is most likely due to:
   1. Respiratory acidosis.
   2. Low circulating blood volume or hypoglycemia.
   3. Renal failure.
   4. Hypertension.

4. The nurse is triaging victims of a multi-vehicular collision. Which of the following patients would be the most prone to developing shock?
   1. 45-year-old male with a fractured femur
   2. 86-year-old female with abdominal injuries
   3. 55-year-old male with an injured arm and shoulder
   4. 38-year-old male with cervical spine injuries

5. A patient in shock has lost more than two liters of circulating blood volume. Which of the following should be provided to this patient?
   1. Normal saline
   2. Packed red blood cells
   3. Fresh frozen plasma
   4. Dextrose 5% and water

6. The nurse is providing care to a patient in shock with an alteration in tissue perfusion and an increased afterload. Which of the following should be provided to this patient?
   1. Dopamine hydrochloride
   2. Nitroprusside sodium
   3. Epinephrine
   4. Norepinephrine bitartrate

7. A patient is diagnosed with pancreatitis. The nurse realizes this patient is prone to developing:

1. Systemic inflammatory response syndrome.

2. Sepsis.

3. Septic shock.

4. Severe sepsis.

8. A patient with systemic inflammatory response is demonstrating a fluid volume deficit. Which of the following would indicate an adequate fluid status for this patient?

1. Urine output 0.25 mL/kg per hour

2. Oxygen saturation 65%

3. Mean arterial pressure 55 mm Hg

4. Central venous pressure 10 mm Hg

9. The nurse suspects a patient is demonstrating signs of a reperfusion injury. Which of the following can this lead to?

1. MODS

2. SIRS

3. Septic shock

4. ARDS

10. A patient has severe sepsis. Which of the following should the nurse do to detect the early signs of MODS?

1. Provide pain management

2. Maintain on strict bed rest

3. Reduce stress

4. Frequent assessment of vital signs and clinical status

Answers for review questions appear in Appendix D

KEY TERMS

end-organ perfusion *p.1963*
insulin resistance (IR) *p.1958*
ischemia reperfusion injury *p.1960*
multiple organ dysfunction syndrome
(MODS) *p.1976*

protein C *p.1970*
sepsis *p.1969*
septic shock *p.1958*
severe sepsis *p.1969*

systemic inflammatory response syndrome
(SIRS) *p.1956*
systemic vascular resistance *p.1958*

EXPLORE PEARSON **mynursingkit**™

MyNursingKit is your one stop for online chapter review materials and resources. Prepare for success with additional NCLEX®-style practice questions, interactive assignments and activities, web links, animations and videos, and more!

Register your access code from the front of your book at
www.mynursingkit.com

REFERENCES

Ackerman, M. (1994). The systemic inflammatory response, sepsis and multiple organ dysfunction. *Critical Care Nursing Clinics of North America, 6,* 243–250.

Alexander, D. (1996). New concepts in shock management. *Air Medical Journal, 15*(2), 85–91.

American College of Chest Physicians/Society of Critical Care Medicine Consensus Conference Committee. (1992). Definitions for sepsis and organ failure and guidelines for the use of innovative therapies in sepsis. *Critical Care Medicine, 20*(6), 864–874.

Arabi, Y., Shirawi, N. A., Memish, Z., Venkatesh, S., & Al-Shimemeri, A. (2003). Assessment of six mortality models in patients admitted with severe sepsis and septic shock to the intensive care unit: A prospective cohort study. *Critical Care, 7*(6), R116–R122.

Ball, C., de Beer, K., Gomm, A., Hickman, B., & Collins, P. (2007). Achieving tight glycaemic control. *Intensive and Critical Care Nursing, 23*(3), 137–144.

Bertolini, G., Luciani, D., & Bioli, G. (2007). Immunonutrition in septic patients: Philosophical view of the current situation. *Clinical Nutrition, 26,* 25–29.

Bochud, P., & Calandra, T. (2003). Pathogenesis of sepsis: New concepts and implications for future treatment. *British Medical Journal, 326*(1), 262–266.

Bumbasirevic, V., Karamarkovic, A., Lesic, A., & Bumbasirevic, M. (2005). Trauma-related sepsis and multiple organ failure: Current concepts in the diagnosis and management. *Current Orthopaedics, 19,* 314–321.

Campbell, J. E. (2004). *Basic trauma life support for paramedics and other advanced providers* (5th ed.). Upper Saddle River, NJ: Brady/Prentice Hall Health.

Carrigan, R. B., Born, C. T., Fitzpatrick, M. K., & Reilly, P. M. (2004). Temporary stabilization of pelvic fractures with the trauma pelvic orthotic device in the polytrauma patient. Poster Presentation at the American Association for the Surgery of Trauma Annual Meeting, Orlando, FL, September 2003; also presented at the 71st Annual meeting of the AAOS, San Francisco, March 2004.

Cartwright, M. M. (2004). The metabolic response to stress: A complex nutrition support management. *Critical Care Nursing Clinics of North America, 16,* 467–487.

Chapman, C. (2003). Shock emergencies. In L. Newberry (Ed.), *Sheehy's emergency nursing* (5th ed., pp. 505–515). St. Louis: Mosby.

Chettle, C. (2003, February 10). Sepsis. *NurseWeek.* Retrieved December 7, 2004, from http://www.nurseweek.com

Dellinger, R. P., Carlet, J. M., Masur, H., Gerlach, H., et al. (2008). Surviving Sepsis Campaign guidelines for management of severe sepsis and septic shock. *Critical Care Medicine, 32*(3), 858–873.

Edelman, D., White, M., Tyburski, J., & Wilson, R., (2007). Post-trauma hypotension: Should systolic blood pressure of 90–109 mmHg be included? *Shock, 27,* 134–138.

Emergency Nurses Association. (2007). *Trauma nursing core course.* Des Plaines, IL: Author. Retrieved from http://www.ena.org

Ertel, W., Keel, M., Bonaccio, M., Steckholzer, U., Gallati, H., Kenny, J. S., et al. (1995). Release of anti-inflammatory mediators after mechanical trauma correlates with severity of injury and clinical outcome. *Journal of Trauma, Injury, Infection and Critical Care, 39*(5), 879–887.

Fernandes, T., Pontieri, V., Loretti, A., Teixeira, D., Abatepaulo, F., Soriano, F., et al. (2007). Hypertonic saline solution increases the expression of heat shock protein 70 and improves lung

inflammation early after reperfusion in a rodent model of controlled hemorrhage. *Shock, 27,* 172–178.

Grenvik, A., Ayres, S., Holbrook, P., & Shoemaker, W. (Eds.). (2000). *Textbook of critical care* (4th ed.). Philadelphia: W. B. Saunders.

Gupta, S., & Jonas, M. (2006). Sepsis, septic shock and multiple organ failure. *Anesthesia and Intensive Care Medicine, 7,* 143–146.

Hollenberg, S., Ahrens, T., Annane, D., Astiz, M., Chalfin, D., Dasta, J., et al. (2004). Practice parameters for hemodynamic support of sepsis in adult patients: 2004 update. *Critical Care Medicine, 32*(9), 1928–1948.

Jacobs, L. (1994). Timing of fluid resuscitation in trauma. *New England Journal of Medicine, 331*(17), 1153–1154.

Johnson, G. B., Brunn, G. J., & Platt, J. L. (2004). Cutting edge: An endogenous pathway to systemic inflammatory response syndrome (SIRS)–like reactions through Toll-like receptor 4. *Journal of Immunology, 172,* 20–24.

Kaplow, R., & Hardin, S. R. (2007). *Critical care nursing: Synergy for optimal outcomes.* Boston: Jones and Bartlett.

Kaszaki, J., Wolfard, A., Szalay, L., & Boros, M. (2006). Pathophysiology of ischemia-reperfusion injury. *Transplantation Proceedings, 38,* 826–828.

Keel, M., & Trentz, O. (2005). Pathophysiology of polytrauma. *Injury, 36*(6), 691–709.

King, J. (2007). Sepsis in critical care. *Critical Care Clinics of North America, 19,* 77–86.

Kline, J. (2002). Shock. In J. Marx (Ed.) *Rosen's Emergency Medicine* (5th ed., pp. 33–47). St. Louis: Mosby.

Kowalenko, T., Stern, S., Dronen, S., & Wang, X. (1992). Improved outcome with hypotensive resuscitation of uncontrolled hemorrhagic shock in a swine model. *Journal of Trauma, 33*(3), 349–353.

Krau, S. D. (2007). Making sense of multiple organ dysfunction syndrome. *Critical care Nursing Clinics of North America 19,* 87–97.

Levy, M. M., Fink, M. P., Marshall, J. C., Abraham, E., Angus, D., Cook, D., et al. (2003). 2001 SCCM/ESICM/ACCP/ ATS/SIS International Sepsis Definition Conference. *Intensive Care Medicine, 29*(4), 530–538.

Martin, G. S., Mannino, D. M., Eaton, S., et al. (2003). The epidemiology of sepsis in the United States from 1979 through 2000. *New England Journal of Medicine, 348,* 1546–1554.

Martin, R., Bicknell, W., Pepe, P., Burch, J., & Mattox, K. (1992). Prospective evaluation of preoperative fluid resuscitation in hypotensive patients with penetrating truncal injury: A preliminary report. *Journal of Trauma, 33*(3), 354–362.

Masur, H. (2003). *Strategies to reduce the incidence of antibiotic-resistant pathogens in the ICU.* Retrieved December 10, 2003, from http://www.medscape.com

McCaffery, K., & Sinclair, J. (2006). Special considerations in pediatric intensive care. *Anaesthesia and Intensive Care Medicine, 7*(1), 22–28.

McCance, K. L., & Huether, S. (2006). *Pathophysiology: The biologic basis for disease in adults and children* (5th ed.). St. Louis: Mosby.

McSwain, N. E., Salomone, J. P., & Pons, P. (2007). *PHTLS: Prehospital trauma life support.* St. Louis: Mosby.

Micek, S. T., Shah, R. A., & Kollef, M. H. (2003). Management of severe sepsis: Integration of multiple pharmacologic interventions. *Pharmacotherapy, 23*(11), 1486–1496.

Miniño, A. M., Heron, M., & Smith, B. L. (2006, April 19). *Deaths: Preliminary data for 2004.* Retrieved September 6, 2008 from National Center for Health Statistics website: http://www.cdc.gov/nchs/products/pubs/pubd/hestats/prelimdeaths04/preliminarydeaths04.htm

Moore, F., Sauaua, A., Moore, E., Haenal, J., Burch, J. M., & Lezotte, D. C. (1996). Post injury multiple organ failure: A bimodal phenomenon. *Journal of Trauma, 40*(4), 501–512.

Mosenthal, A. C., & Murphy, P. A. (2003). Trauma care and palliative care: Time to integrate the two? *Journal of the American College of Surgeons, 197*(3), 509–516.

Porter, R. (1997). *The greatest benefit to mankind.* New York: W. W. Norton.

Porth, C. M. (2005). *Essentials of pathophysiology: Concepts of altered health states.* Philadelphia: Lippincott Williams & Wilkins.

Rangel-Frausto, M. S. (2005). Sepsis: Still going strong. *Archives of Medical Research, 36,* 672–681.

Reid, C. L., & Campbell, I. T. (2004). Nutritional and metabolic support in trauma, sepsis and critical illness. *Current Anaesthesia and Critical Care, 15,* 336–349.

Robertson, C. M., & Coppersmith, C. M. (2006). The systemic inflammatory response syndrome. *Microbes and Infection, 8,* 1382–1389.

Rueden, K., & Dunham, C. M. (1994). Sequelae of massive fluid resuscitation in trauma patients. *Critical Care Nursing Clinics of North America, 6,* 463–472.

Russell, J. A. (2006). Management of sepsis. *New England Journal of Medicine, 355*(16), 1699–1713.

Selfridge-Thomas, J. (1995). Shock. In S. Kitt, J. Selfridge-Thomas, J. Proehl, & J. Kaiser (Eds.), *Emergency nursing: A physiological approach* (2nd ed., pp. 37–53). Philadelphia: W. B. Saunders.

Semonin Holleran, R. (2002). The problem of pain in emergency care. *Nursing Clinics of North America, 37*(1), 67–78.

Smith, M. A., & McInnis, L. A. (2007). Antimicrobial resistance in critical care. *Critical Care Clinics of North America, 19,* 53–60.

Society of Critical Care Medicine. (1999). Practice parameters for hemodynamic support of sepsis in adult patients. *Critical Care Medicine, 27*(3), 639–660.

Spahn, D. R., Cerny, V., Coats, T. J., Duranteau, J., Fernandez-Mondejar, E., Gordini, G., et al. (2007). Management of bleeding following major trauma: A European guideline. *Critical Care, 11*(1). Retrieved April 21, 2007, from http://www.medscape.com/viewarticle/554058

Tazbir, J. (2004). Sepsis and the role of activated protein C. *Critical Care Nurse, 24*(6), 40–45.

Zauner, A., Nimmerrichter, P., Anderwald, C., Bischof, M., Schiefermeier, M., Ratheiser, K., et al. (2007). Severity of insulin resistance in critically ill medical patients. *Metabolism, 56,* 1–5.

Nursing Assessment of Patients with Hematologic Disorders

Janyce Cagan Agruss
Annita Watson

Outcome-Based Learning Objectives

After studying this chapter, the learner will be able to:

1. Explain how the hematologic system functions in an adult.
2. Describe the types, characteristics, and functions of blood cells.
3. Explain how the process of coagulation works in the event of an injury.
4. Describe appropriate nursing assessment/responsibilities related to the hematologic system in the adult patient.
5. Describe laboratory tests used to evaluate the hematologic system.
6. Distinguish between normal and abnormal test results for the hematologic system.
7. Discuss the meaning of "shift to the left."

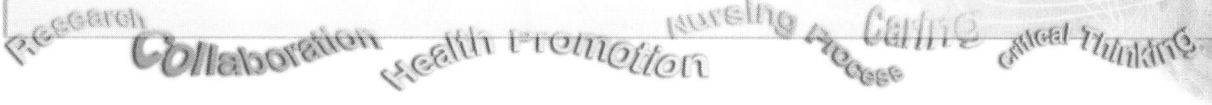

THE HEMATOLOGIC SYSTEM is a very complex body system. Just as cardiology is the study of the heart, **hematology** is the study of blood, and just as the tissue of the heart comprises the cardiovascular system, blood is the tissue that makes up the hematologic system. The hematologic system can have problems inherent to itself, but it can also be a valuable source of information that reflects problems in other organ systems. Whether the gathering of hematologic data is for the purpose of evaluating the hematologic system itself or assessing other body systems, the nurse has to understand the functions, structure, diagnostic tests, terminology, and nursing responsibilities that are pertinent and relevant to the hematologic system. The nurse gathers this information through the assessment process and is reliant on both subjective and objective data.

Subjective assessment is accomplished by interviewing the patient or someone accompanying the patient (e.g., family member, friend) to obtain data regarding the patient's illness or reason for being seen by the health care provider. Objective assessment is that obtained by means other than a patient interview, for example, laboratory tests, x-rays, vital signs. In an objective assessment, the data are retrievable without being dependent on the patient providing the information.

■ Anatomy and Physiology of the Hematologic System

The anatomy of the hematologic system can be understood best by describing its components. Most obvious is blood, comprised of a wide variety of cells and supportive fluids. Additionally, there are other organ systems that both contribute to the conceptual understanding as well as to the overall function of the hematologic system. These include the lymphatic system, the spleen (a lymphatic organ), the liver, and the reticuloendothelial/mononuclear phagocyte system.

To best understand the physiology of the hematologic system, the reader should understand that blood is considered to be a type of connective tissue with two important responsibilities. First, blood and its associated vessels and organs provide a transport system that delivers nutrition, oxygen, and secretory products such as hormones throughout the body, as well as wastes to the kidneys and liver for disposal. Second, the immunologic products of the hematologic system are critical to the defense of the body against infections and other foreign materials. In performing the two primary responsibilities related to being a transport system, blood also functions to maintain body temperature, control pH (to maintain a range of 6.8 to 7.4), remove toxins from the body, and regulate body fluid electrolytes. The contribution of each component of the hematologic system to these functions is discussed below.

Bone Marrow

Any discussion about the hematologic system should begin with the bone marrow. Bone marrow is the soft material found in the center of bones and it is the origin of all blood cells. Bone marrow, one of the largest organs of the body, makes up about 4% to 5% of a person's total body weight. It consists of islands of cellular components (red marrow) separated by fat (yellow marrow). The **stem cell**, the precursor cell of all blood components (red blood cells, white blood cells, and platelets), resides in the bone marrow. When the proper stimulating signal is received, the stem cells undergo a series of cell division and differentiation re-

Stem cell to erythrocyte

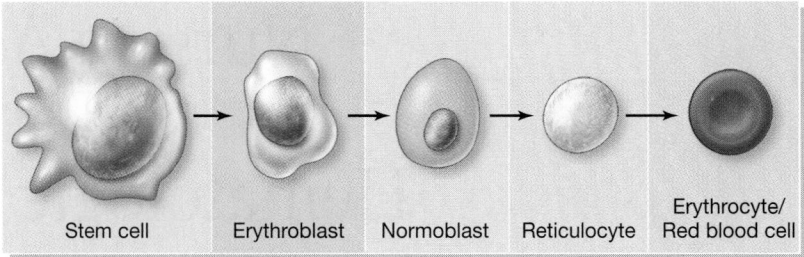

Stem cell   Erythroblast   Normoblast   Reticulocyte   Erythrocyte/ Red blood cell

FIGURE 62–1 ■ Stem cell to erythrocytes.

sulting in the release of mature or nearly mature cells into the systemic circulation as depicted in Figures 62–1 ■, 62–2 ■, and 62–3 ■. This process is called **hematopoiesis**. See Chapter 63 🔗 for a thorough discussion of hematopoiesis.

Stem cell to leukocytes

Stem cell   Myeloblast

Basophilic metamyelocyte   Basophil*

Eosinophilic metamyelocyte   Eosinophil*

Neutrophilic metamyelocyte   Band cell   Neutrophil*

Stem cell   Monoblast   Monocyte*

Stem cell   Lymphoblast   Lymphocyte*

*end product and mature form in a normal situation

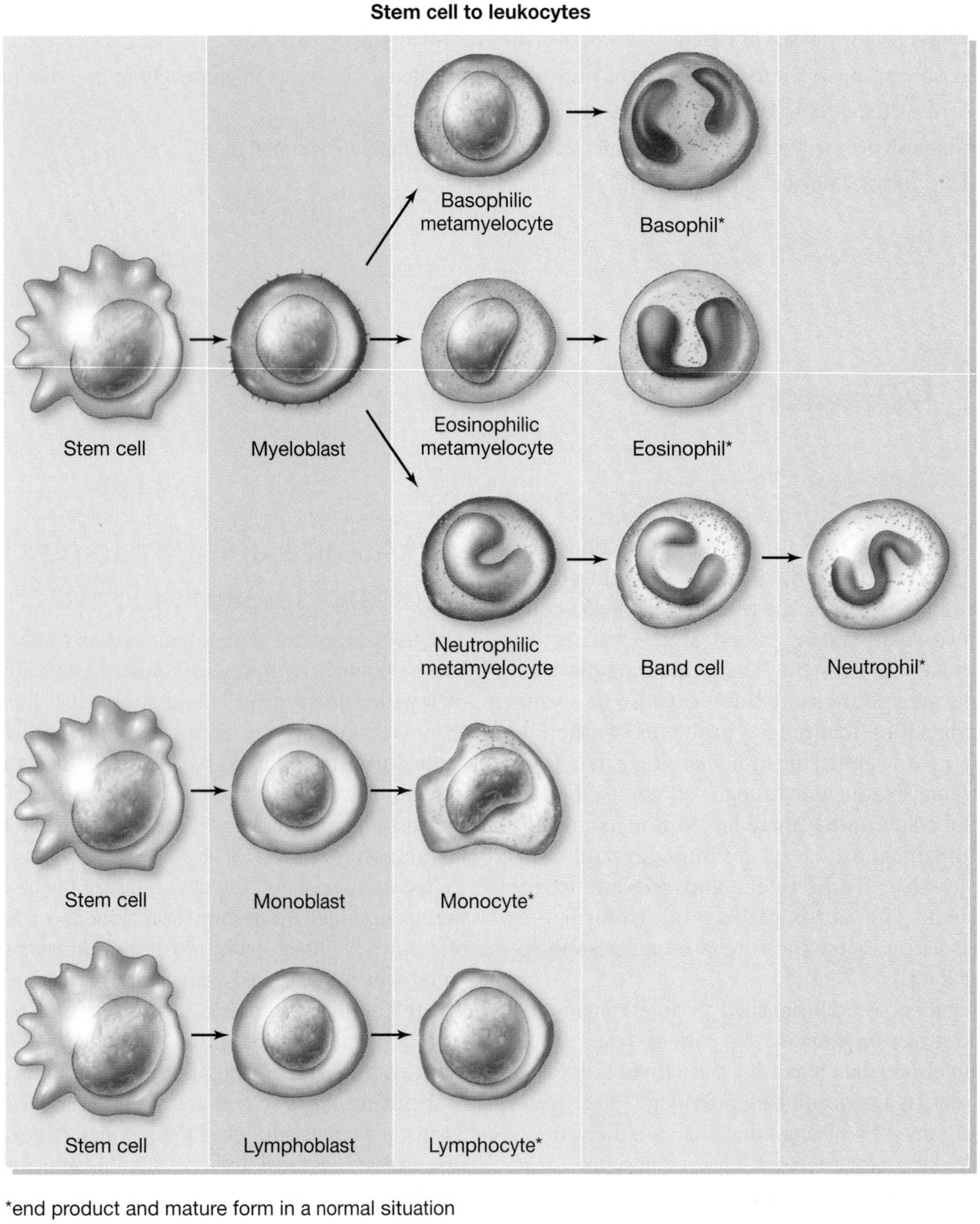

FIGURE 62–2 ■ Stem cell to leukocytes.

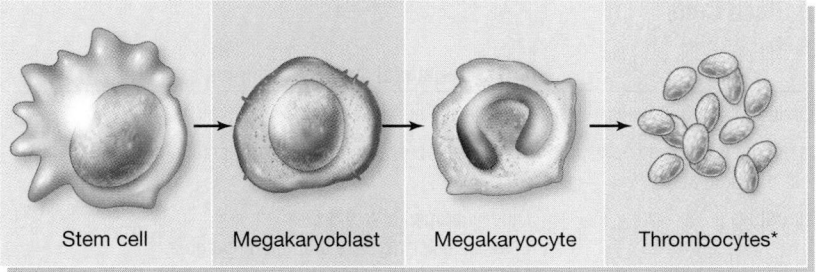

Stem cell to thrombocytes

Stem cell → Megakaryoblast → Megakaryocyte → Thrombocytes*

*end product and mature form in a normal situation

FIGURE 62–3 ■ Stem cell to thrombocytes (end product and mature form in a normal situation).

In children, all skeletal bones are involved in the production of stem cells. With aging, marrow activity decreases and usually is limited to the pelvis, ribs, sternum, and vertebrae. As a person ages, the proportion of red marrow diminishes and is replaced by yellow marrow (fat); however, in the healthy individual the fat can again be replaced by active (red) marrow if more blood cell production is required. In adults with diseases that cause bone marrow destruction, the liver and spleen also can produce blood cells by a process known as *extramedullary hematopoiesis.* Figure 62–4 ■ shows a picture of bone marrow. Nurses must always include bone marrow function when considering any disease related to the hematologic system.

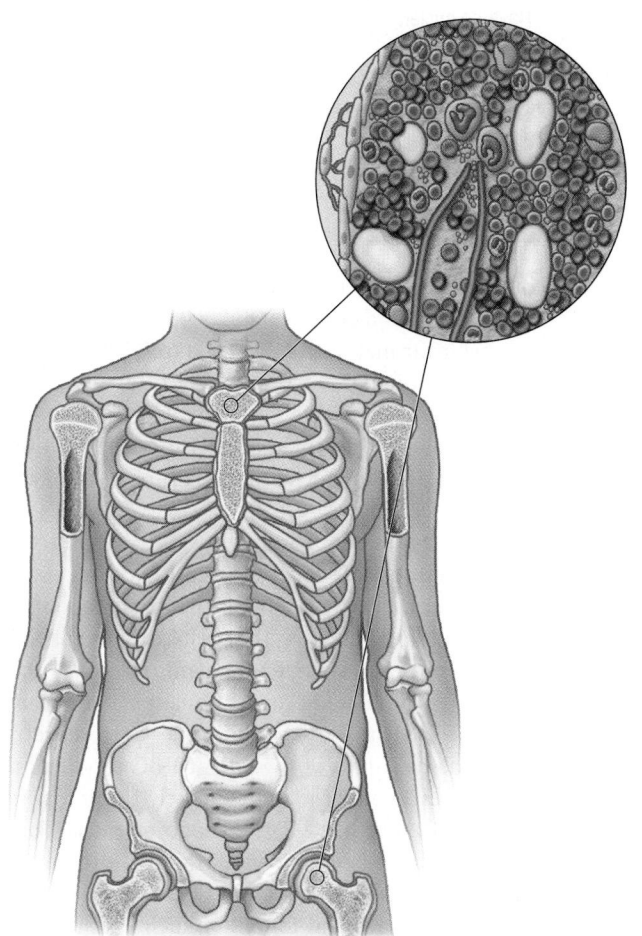

FIGURE 62–4 ■ Bone marrow.

Types of Blood Cells

Blood is a fluid tissue that has both function and structure. Blood contributes about 7% to the total body weight of a person with a volume (in an average-sized adult) of about 4 to 6 liters. It is composed of 55% plasma and 45% blood cells. **Plasma** is the straw-colored liquid in which the blood cells are suspended, and consists of approximately 90% water, with the remaining 10% being proteins, carbohydrates, electrolytes, and vitamins. A microscopic analysis of blood reveals a wide variety of blood cells that are broadly categorized into three major cell lines: **erythrocytes**, or **red blood cells (RBCs)**; **leukocytes**, or **white blood cells (WBCs)**; and **thrombocytes**, or **platelets**. Each cell line has its own characteristics and functions, as summarized in Chart 62–1 (p. 1992). Note that reticulocytes are immature red blood cells, typically composing about 1% of the red cells in the human body. Also note that *leukocyte* is a broad term applied to the various cells of the immune system, including granulocytes (basophils, eosinophils, and neutrophils), monocytes, and lymphocytes (T cells, B cells, and natural killer cells). Leukocytes are discussed below and in more detail in Chapters 59 ∞ and 60 ∞ .

Erythrocytes (Red Blood Cells)

Erythrocytes, or red blood cells, make up about 40% of the total blood volume. The RBC is produced in the bone marrow and its function is to become filled with hemoglobin, maintain the chemical integrity of hemoglobin, and carry and distribute hemoglobin to the body's tissues. **Hemoglobin** is an iron-containing protein in RBCs that transports oxygen around the body. When oxygen combines with hemoglobin, the resulting oxyhemoglobin is bright red.

The normal shape of the red blood cell, a biconcave disk, is the optimal shape to perform this function. A biconcave disk can best be described as a donut or lifesaver shape. The cell has a diameter of approximately 8 µm and is very flexible, thus, allowing it to pass easily through capillaries that may be as small as 2.8 µm. RBCs also have a very thin membrane, which allows the oxygen and carbon dioxide to easily diffuse. A photograph of RBCs is shown in Figure 62–5 ■ (p. 1992). Their disk shape allows for optimal filling by the hemoglobin and ideal transport to body tissues through the circulatory system. The shape also provides a large surface that facilitates the absorption and release of oxygen molecules. With age, RBCs become increasingly fragile and are damaged by passing through narrow capillaries.

Red blood cells are terminally differentiated; that is, they can never divide. They live about 120 days and then are ingested by phagocytic cells (those that engulf and ingest foreign particles, cell waste material, and bacteria) in the liver and spleen. They are eventually broken down by the spleen into the blood pigments bilirubin and iron. These components are then transported to the liver where the iron is recycled for use by new erythrocytes. The remainder of the heme portion of the molecule is degraded into bile pigments and excreted by the liver. Approximately 3 million RBCs die and are scavenged by the liver each second.

There are approximately 4.5 to 5.8 million erythrocytes per microliter of healthy blood (although there are variations between males and females and racial groups). In the laboratory

Characteristics and Functions of Blood Cells

	Function(s)	Characteristic(s) and/or Conditions
Erythrocytes	Transport oxygen and carbon dioxide to and from cells.	Lifesaver-shaped disk.
Reticulocytes	Synthesize hemoglobin after loss of the nucleus so new RBCs continue to be released into the circulation.	Immature, non-nucleated RBCs that contain RNA.
Leukocytes (WBCs)	Protect the body against foreign matter.	Different types of leukocytes. Leukocytosis: increase in the total number. Leukopenia: decrease in the total number.
Granulocytes:		Characterized by granules within their cytoplasm.
Neutrophils	The most abundant leukocyte, neutrophils may be increased or decreased in systemic infection. Work via phagocytosis.	Segmented neutrophil: nucleus has at least two lobes separated by a filament; this is the more mature version. Band neutrophil: nucleus without visible filament separating the lobes.
Eosinophils	Usually increased in allergic diseases.	Make up 3% of the leukocytes in adults. Cytoplasm contains larger round or oval granules.
Basophils	Function not exactly known, but may be present in hypersensitivity reactions.	Resemble neutrophils, except nucleus is indented. Least numerous of the leukocytes.
Monocytes/macrophages	Back up the neutrophils; may be increased in infections and/or hematologic disorders. Work via phagocytosis; they do cleanup work after neutrophils and may circulate for a longer period of time than the neutrophils.	Monocytes give rise to macrophages. Largest cell of normal blood.
Lymphocytes	Function to fight viral infection; may be increased or decreased in infectious illness.	T- and B-cell subsets.
Thrombocytes	Prevent blood loss by forming a platelet plug at the site of injury until a stable clot forms. May be increased in times of stress. May be decreased (thrombocytopenia) in bone marrow failure, autoimmune disease (idiopathic thrombocytopenia purpura), disseminated intravascular clotting (DIC)	Formed in the bone marrow. Have no nuclei.

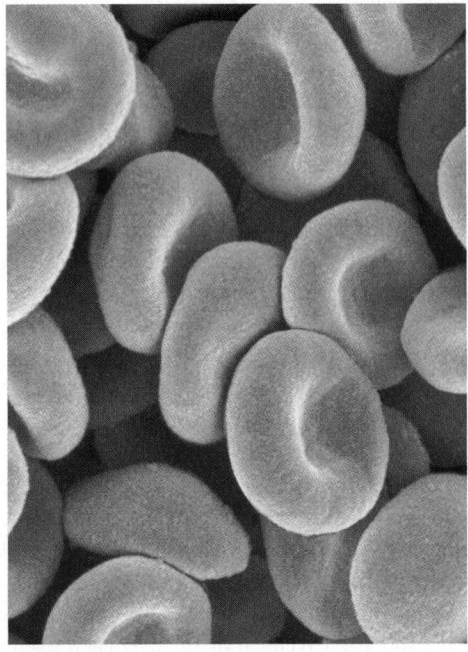

FIGURE 62–5 ■ Red blood cells (erythrocytes).
Source: © Micro Discovery/CORBIS All Rights Reserved

RBCs are counted as the total number of RBCs in 1 mm³ of blood. The typical red blood cell count is 4,600,000 to 6,200,000 per cubic millimeter for males and 4,500,000 to 5,100,000 cells per cubic millimeter for females. The number of RBCs is a measure of the blood's oxygen-carrying capacity. Hemoglobin accounts for approximately 95% of mature RBC composition. Immature erythrocytes have a nucleus, but mature erythrocytes have no nucleus.

The bone marrow releases immature forms of RBCs into circulation that are referred to as **reticulocytes**. Reticulocytes are juvenile RBCs produced by erythropoiesis that spend about 24 hours in the marrow before entering the peripheral circulation. They contain some nuclear material—remnants of RNA—that appears faintly blue (basophilic) in conventionally stained blood smears. When measured in the laboratory, the percentage of reticulocytes provides an index of the rate of RBC production. Normally reticulocytes account for approximately 1% of the circulating red blood cells (Porth, 2007). Reticulocytes persist for a few days in the circulation before forming the slightly smaller, mature red cell. The release of reticulocytes occurs as a normal response to an increased demand for RBCs, such as is the case with bleeding or possibly with disease.

In certain disorders such as sickle cell anemia the RBC has a different shape and is more rigid than normal cells, causing difficulty transporting hemoglobin to the tissues. Two major consequences occur when red blood cells sickle: hemolysis (destruction) of the sickled cells and vessel occlusion. The rigidity of the cells causes the obstruction of the microcirculation and ischemic injury to the tissues. This rigidity also makes the cells more prone to hemolysis or destruction while circulating through the spleen. The pain associated with sickle cell disease is due to vessel occlusion, resulting from ischemia. This can occur anywhere in the body (Porth, 2007). (See Chapter 63 🔗 to learn more about sickle cell anemia.)

Leukocytes (White Blood Cells)

As mentioned, the principal cells of the immune system are the leukocytes, or white blood cells. WBCs generally are not present, except in a very small amount, in the bloodstream unless they are needed for defense against an infecting organism. They remain in the bone marrow, lungs, liver, spleen, and lymph nodes as developing and mature cells. They are separated into two major categories: **granulocytes** (or polymorphonuclear leukocytes [PMN]) and agranulocytes. Granulocytes are further divided into neutrophils, basophils, and eosinophils as determined by their staining properties in the laboratory. Agranulocytes are made up of monocytes and lymphocytes. Leukocytes have longevity of a few hours to a few days. There are approximately 5,000 to 10,000 leukocytes per microliter of blood.

Lymphocytes

Leukocytes are composed of approximately 24% to 35% **lymphocytes**, whose purpose is to recognize and respond to foreign antigens. Lymphocytes that produce antibodies include the T cells, B cells, and natural killer cells.

Approximately 60% to 70% of blood lymphocytes are T cells and 10% to 20% are B cells. A commonly shared misconception holds that the "B" in B cells refers to bone marrow, since these cells arise from bone marrow tissue. In actuality, the "B" stands for "bursa of Fabricius," a gland in birds where the cells mature and the first such tissue found in vertebrates. Immature B cells are produced by the bone marrow and released into the bloodstream. Upon interacting with an antigen, or protein, the B cells become activated into plasma cells, which are responsible for the production of antibodies, or immunoglobulins. All antibodies formed by the plasma cell are programmed to recognize only one unique protein structure: the antigen that stimulated the original B cell. (See Chapter 60 🔗 on immune response disorders for further discussion.) The process, referred to as the **humoral immune response**, is the mechanism in which organisms gain immunity to previously encountered substances.

T cells (lymphocytes) complete their maturation in the thymus gland and function in the peripheral tissues to produce cell-mediated immunity, as well as aiding in antibody production. Both T-cell and B-cell activation are triggered by the recognition of the antigen by unique surface receptors.

Both T cells and B cells destroy antigens (a foreign substance that is not naturally present and should not be in the body) and produce "memory cells" and antibodies. Memory cells attack disease-causing organisms if there is a subsequent invasion. This second response is much quicker than the first, thus preventing symptoms of the disease from occurring (Porth, 2007).

Natural killer cells (NK cells) are a type of lymphocytes that are functionally distinct from T and B cells. Like cytotoxic T cells they contain granules filled with potent chemicals; however unlike cytotoxic T cells, they do not need to recognize a specific antigen before being activated. They are a major component of the innate immune system and play a major role in the rejection of tumors and cells infected by viruses.

Basophils

Basophils make up approximately 0.3% to 0.5% of the total white blood count. Along with the mast cells, basophils release heparin (anticoagulant) and histamine (vasodilator) and other inflammatory mediators into the bloodstream. They participate in the destruction of bacteria with lysozyme and strong oxidants and play an exceedingly important role in allergic reactions (Porth, 2007). An increased or higher percentage of basophils in the blood may indicate an inflammatory condition somewhere in the body.

Neutrophils

Neutrophils compose approximately 55% to 65% of leukocytes and because their nuclei are divided into three to five lobes they are typically referred to as polymorphonuclear leukocytes. Neutrophils are primarily responsible for maintaining a normal host defense against pathogens and are the first leukocytes to respond to organisms that invade the body. They act by carrying out the process of phagocytosis and also by releasing enzymes such as lysozyme that destroy certain bacteria. Neutrophils respond quicker to infection than do monocytes. However, when monocytes reach the site of infection they arrive in much larger numbers and, therefore, can phagocytize many more microbes than neutrophils are able to. They also clear up cellular debris after an infection. Chapters 59 🔗 and 60 🔗 discuss the immune response.

Eosinophils

Eosinophils comprise approximately 1% to 3% of the leukocytes. They liberate heparin, histamine, and serotonin in allergic reactions, intensifying an inflammatory response. The current belief is that they release enzymes or chemical mediators that detoxify agents associated with allergic reactions (Porth, 2007). An increased or higher than usual percentage of eosinophils in the blood may indicate a parasitic infection somewhere in the body. Eosinophils attach themselves to the parasite by special surface molecules and release hydrolytic enzymes and other substances that kill the parasite.

Monocytes and Tissue Macrophages

Monocytes and tissue macrophages arise from a common precursor in the bone marrow. **Monocytes** are the largest of the white blood cells and make up about 3% to 8% of the total leukocyte count. Monocytes and macrophages are a part of the **reticuloendothelial** (or mononuclear phagocytic) **system (RES)**, whose function is to engulf and digest microbes and other foreign substances. The RES also removes senescent cells from circulation, and provides phagocytic cells for both inflammatory and immune responses. Monocytes migrate from the blood to various tissues where they mature into macrophages. Macrophages, also known as scavengers, can either stay in one tissue or migrate from an organ via lymphoid tissues. Examples of tissue macrophages include Kupffer cells in the liver, alveolar macrophages in the lung, and microglial cells of the central nervous system. Macrophages are activated when their membrane comes in contact with an antigen. Once the microbe is ingested, the cell generates digestive enzymes and toxic oxygen and nitrogen products, thus killing the invading antigen.

The phagocytic white cells have a life span of about 2 to 4 months, which allows the macrophages to remain at the affected site longer, sometimes until the antigen is destroyed. The macrophage response time works in concert with that of the first responders, neutrophils, which can rapidly surround and identify sources of infection, but only live for approximately 12 hours (Dailey, 1998; McPherson & Pincus, 2006).

Thrombocytes (Platelets)

Thrombocytes, or platelets, are large cell fragments that are disk shaped and approximately 2 to 4 μm in diameter. They have many granules but no nucleus, and they live for 5 to 9 days. There are approximately 150,000 to 400,000 platelets per microliter of blood. The platelet membrane is covered with a glycocalyx, consisting of glycoproteins, glycosaminoglycans, and several coagulation factors absorbed from the plasma (Ross, 2003). Glycoproteins act as a receptor in platelet function. Specifically, glycoprotein IIb/IIIa binds fibrinogen and forms bridges between adjacent platelets when activated, a process referred to as *aggregation*. Platelet activation and its role in hemostasis are discussed below.

Figure 62–6 ■ shows a Wright-stained smear of normal blood in which normal blood cells are shown.

Lymphatic System

The **lymphatic system**, consisting of organs, ducts, and nodes, is responsible for removing excess fluid, proteins, and large particles from the interstitial (between cells) spaces back to the bloodstream. The ducts (called lymph vessels) are thin tubes, which run throughout the body in much the same way as blood vessels and with a similar structure to the capillary walls; however, instead of blood, they transport lymph fluid. Lymph fluid is formed from the natural diffusion of fluid across the semipermeable cell membranes of blood vessels and peripheral tissues into the interstitial space. The main functions of the lymphatic system are to:

- Collect and return interstitial fluid, and thus help maintain fluid balance.
- Defend the body against disease by producing lymphocytes.
- Absorb lipids from the intestine and transport them to the blood.

Essentially, the lymphatic system is the highway and delivery system of the body. Blood volume is maintained in every organ of the body as a result of the presence of lymph vessels. Lymph fluid is carried via the lymphatic system to every system in the body and then is returned to the circulatory system. Foreign objects such as bacteria and viruses also are carried through the body by the lymphatic system. When interstitial fluid volume rises, the increasing pressure drives the fluid into the lymphatic capillary walls. The walls of the capillaries are very permeable, allowing fluid to drain easily from the tissue into the lymphatic capillaries. The lymphatic capillaries, the entry point into the lymphatic vascular system, join to form the larger diameter lymphatic vessels, which ultimately drain into the subclavian veins of the neck. Once incorporated into the bloodstream, the lymphatic fluid can be appropriately processed by the liver, spleen, kidneys, and other organs.

Lymph nodes are small aggregates of lymphoid tissue located along the lymphatic vessels throughout the body. Each node processes lymph fluid from a discrete, adjacent anatomic site (Porth, 2007). The human body has hundreds of clusters of lymph nodes placed strategically in the axillae, groin, and along the great vessels of the neck, thorax, and abdomen. The functions of the lymph nodes include removing foreign material from lymph before it enters the bloodstream and acting as the center for proliferation of immune cells. The lymph nodes are encapsulated structures where the lymph or chyle is juxtaposed (in proximity) to capillary blood vessels. According to Swartz (2001), the lymph nodes function as filters and reservoirs, acting as incubators for white blood cells. White blood cells, particularly B cells and T cells, mature and proliferate in the lymph nodes as they gain exposure to antigens absorbed from the interstitial fluid. During times of infection, these nodes can become swollen and tender as active lymphocytes, phagocytes, and invading bacteria and viruses initiate inflammation and the immune response; hence, the term "swollen glands." Swollen glands can be palpated in the neck, axilla (armpit), or groin. There also are lymph nodes that cannot be palpated in the abdomen, pelvis, and chest. The lymph fluid distributes immune cells and other factors throughout the body.

The lymphatic system also contains certain hormones, protein, and gastrointestinal fat depending on the original location of the interstitial fluid. For instance, interstitial fluid, and consequently lymph fluid, surrounding the gastrointestinal tract is milky and turbid with a high percentage of fat. This lymphatic fluid is known as **chyle**. Microscopic evaluation of lymph fluid reveals a close resemblance to blood, but lymph fluid is much more dilute.

Spleen

The spleen is a large, ovoid secondary lymphoid organ located in the upper left corner of the abdominal cavity. It generally cannot be palpated because it is under the ribs. The spleen stores blood (20 to 40 mL of RBCs), removes old blood cells, and, as one of its primary roles, filters and destroys antigens before they

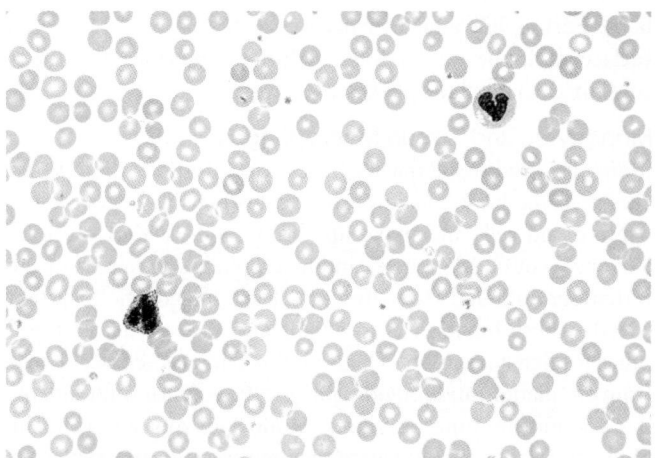

FIGURE 62–6 ■ Wright-stained smear of normal blood.
Source: © Visuals Unlimited/CORBIS All Rights Reserved

can enter the systemic circulation (Young, Gerson, & High, 2006). The spleen is able to remove defective or old erythrocytes from circulation. Most notably, the spleen is able to catabolize the hemoglobin released from decaying erythrocytes and return the iron component (heme) back to the bone marrow. Patients suffering from hematologic disorders that result in high turnover of erythrocytes frequently present with an enlarged spleen (splenomegaly). Additionally, the spleen stores approximately one-third of the total volume of platelets.

Liver

The liver is the largest visceral organ of the body that performs multiple functions. (See Chapter 46 ⊕ for further discussion on the physiology and associated disorders of the liver.) Briefly, the liver produces bile; metabolizes hormones and drugs; synthesizes proteins, glucose, and blood clotting factors; stores vitamins and minerals; changes ammonia produced by deamination of amino acids to urea; and converts fatty acids to ketones. As it relates to hematology, the liver stores blood and plays an important role in the clotting mechanism of blood (discussed below). The liver produces the coagulation factors that are necessary for fibrin clot formation, and the liver can produce anticoagulants so there is not too much clotting. Disorders of the liver are discussed in depth in Chapter 46 ⊕.

Normal Clotting Mechanism: Hemostasis

Hemostasis is defined as the stopping of blood flow. Under normal conditions hemostasis is regulated by a complex array of activators and inhibitors that maintain blood fluidity and prevent blood loss from the vascular space. The balance between the forces that cause blood to solidify or to remain fluid is very delicate and involves several interacting systems.

Intact blood vessels are central to moderating blood's tendency to clot. The endothelial cells of intact vessels prevent thrombus formation by secreting tissue plasminogen activator (t-PA) and by inactivating thrombin and adenosine diphosphate (ADP). Injury to vessels overwhelms these protective mechanisms and hemostasis occurs. A blood vessel must incur an injury in order for hemostasis to be initiated. Hemostasis then proceeds in two phases: primary and secondary hemostasis. Figure 62–7 ■ shows the normal sequencing of hemostasis, starting with the injury called the vascular phase.

Primary Hemostasis

Primary hemostasis is characterized by vascular contraction, platelet adhesion, and formation of a soft aggregate plug. It begins immediately after endothelial disruption. After the injury occurs there is an initial, temporary response of vasoconstriction. This is the body's adaptive mechanism that tries to stop or at least minimize blood loss following injury to a vessel. Vasoconstriction slows blood flow, enhancing platelet adhesion and activation. This vasoconstriction promotes the ability of platelets to gather at the site of injury. First, the platelet is attracted to the exposed subendothelial layer of collagen and adheres to it. To accomplish this, the platelet undergoes a shape change. Second, the platelets release ADP, which stimulates other platelets to stick together at the wound site, and then aggregation occurs. Aggregation occurs when the platelets adhere to each other to form a

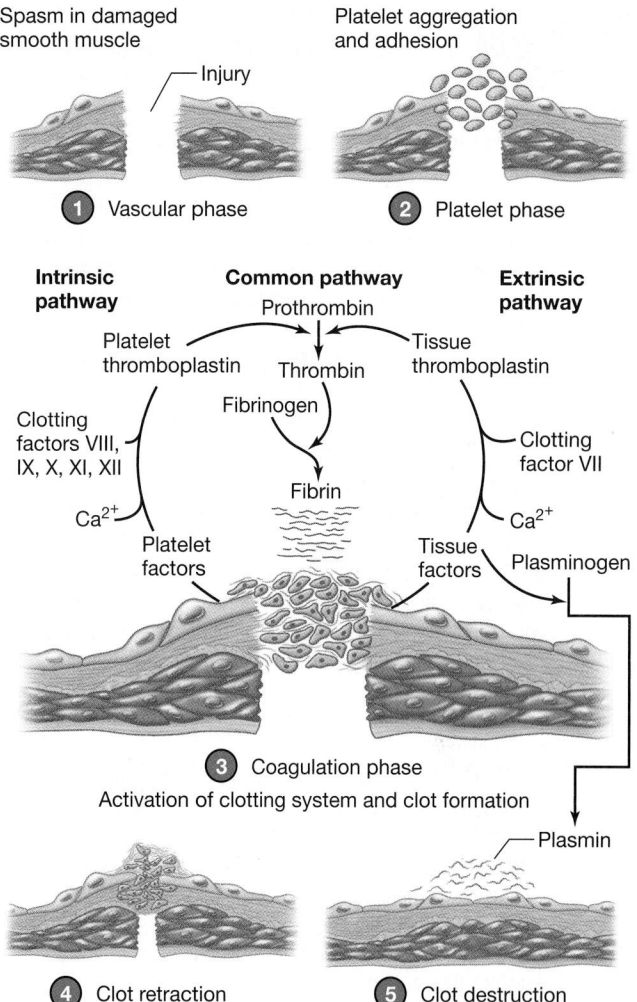

FIGURE 62–7 ■ Hemostasis progression.

beginning plug. Finally, coagulation occurs and fibrin forms around the platelet aggregate to initiate repair (Porth, 2007).

Primary hemostasis is short lived. The immediate postinjury vascular constriction abates quickly. If flow is allowed to increase, the soft plug could be sheared from the injured surface, possibly creating emboli.

Secondary Hemostasis

Secondary hemostasis is responsible for stabilizing the soft clot and maintaining vasoconstriction. This phase is initiated when the cascade system of coagulation is activated by substances released at the time of injury. Based on the type of stimulus or injury to the vessel, one of two clotting pathways is followed. These are referred to as intrinsic and extrinsic pathways, with the end result from either pathway being the conversion of prothrombin to thrombin. Thrombin is necessary for fibrinogen to be converted into fibrin, the stabilizing protein that anchors the fragile platelet plug to the site of injury; thereby, preventing further bleeding and allowing the injured vessel to heal. Primary and secondary hemostasis are summarized in Chart 62–2 (p. 1996).

Coagulation Factors and the Cascade System

Coagulation factors circulate in the plasma as cofactors or as procoagulants and, when activated, some of the components are

---

CHART 62–2 **Sequential Steps of Hemostasis**

A. Blood Vessel Spasm
1. Cutting a blood vessel causes a release of neural reflexes and humoral factors that result in muscle spasm.

B. Platelet Plug Formation
2. Platelets come in contact with the injured vessel wall, causing adhesion of the exposed edges of damaged blood vessels, forming a net with spiny processes protruding from their membranes.
3. Platelet aggregation occurs soon after adhesion, resulting in a platelet plug to stop the bleeding.
4. Platelet adhesion and aggregation stimulate the activation of the clotting cascade.

C. Blood Coagulation
5. Damaged tissues release tissue thromboplastin, which activates the first in a series of factors leading to the production of prothrombin activator.
6. Prothrombin activator converts prothrombin into thrombin, which, in turn, catalyzes a reaction that converts fibrinogen into fibrin. Fibrin forms a meshwork that cements the platelets and other blood components together. The amount of prothrombin activator formed is proportional to the amount of tissue damage.
7. Once a clot forms, it promotes still more clotting through a positive feedback system. Fibroblasts invade the area and produce fibers throughout the clots.
8. A clot that forms abnormally in a vessel is a thrombus; if it dislodges, it is an embolus.
9. Within 20–60 minutes after a clot has formed, clot retraction begins, causing the edges of the broken blood vessel to pull together, thus assisting with hemostasis.
10. Shortly after the formation of a clot, dissolution begins. Clots dissolve by fibrinolysis. The process involves the activation of plasmin by plasminogen, which then digests the fibrin strands of the clot. This allows blood flow to be reestablished and permanent tissue repair to take place.

---

needed for clot formation. The coagulation factors are generated in the liver cells, except for Factor VIII (or at least the von Willebrand's portion), which is produced in multiple organs, possibly the endothelial cells and megakaryocytes. The coagulation cascade system, as shown in Figure 62–8 ■, is the model typically referred to when describing the mechanism of coagulation.

Damaged tissue releases Factor III, which with the aid of Ca^{2+} will activate Factor VII, thus initiating the extrinsic mechanism. Factor XII from active platelets will activate Factor XI, thus initiating the intrinsic mechanism. Both active Factor VII and active Factor XI will promote cascade reactions, eventually activating Factor X. Active Factor X, along with Factor III, Factor V, Ca^{2+}, and platelet thromboplastic factor (PF_3), will activate prothrombin activator. Prothrombin activator converts prothrombin to thrombin. Thrombin converts fibrinogen to fibrin. Fibrin initially forms a loose mesh, but then Factor XIII causes the formation of covalent cross links, which convert fibrin to a dense aggregation of fibers. Platelets and RBCs become caught in this mesh of fibers, thus forming a blood clot.

As described above, coagulation is actually a cascade of events. In the normal scenario, one enzyme activates the following proenzyme until the mesh fibrin network is developed, established, and functioning, and a blood clot is formed and the bleeding stops.

Hereditary bleeding disorders, such as hemophilia, are caused by deficiencies in the factors involved in the coagulation cascade. Also, identification of the intrinsic versus the extrinsic pathway and what factors are involved in each of the pathways as described earlier is important because this information has implications for laboratory tests and medications that are ordered for patients.

History

Much of the evaluation of the hematologic system is based on a complete health history. When assessing a patient for hematopoietic system status it is important to be thorough and to consider presenting symptoms, chief complaint, and family history. Many hematologic conditions cause few symptoms, therefore, the use of extensive laboratory tests often is required to diagnose a hematologic disorder. Hematologic disorders are discussed in depth in Chapter 63 .

A thorough history will help the nurse identify symptoms related to abnormalities with the hematologic system as well as current or potential problems. Information learned from a thorough history and physical exam could help prevent undesirable responses to current therapies and treatment plans. The essential assessment is contingent on obtaining both subjective and objective data as previously defined.

Biographic and Demographic Data

Assessment of biographic and demographic data includes information regarding age, race, gender, and ethnicity, all of which can impact the susceptibility to some hematologic disorders. For example, African Americans have a higher incidence of sickle cell anemia than Caucasians, and a family history of coagulation disorders increases the risk for the individual. A patient may not know she has a "hematologic" problem, but she may know that she tends to have problems stopping bleeding.

Chief Complaint

The current issue is the focus of why the patient is being evaluated currently. Unless the patient already has some knowledge of his hematologic system from previous evaluations, he usually will not know that he has a hematologic problem. He will merely know that he does not feel well. From the questions asked during the history taking, nurses can begin to determine whether or not they think that the patient is having a problem that arises from the hematologic system.

The chief complaint tells the health care provider, in the patient's own words, what problem(s) she is currently experiencing. The chief complaint focuses the history-taking process and prioritizes treatment regimens. When the chief complaint is documented, the health care provider actually writes the words that the patient has used to describe the complaint. For example, the patient may state, "I always feel tired, no matter how early I go to bed" or "It is all I can do to get through the day."

It also is important to determine the patient's own perception of his health status in order to assist the patient with developing a plan for future health promotion. Risk factors such as smoking and alcohol intake should be assessed as should the

THE COAGULATION CASCADE

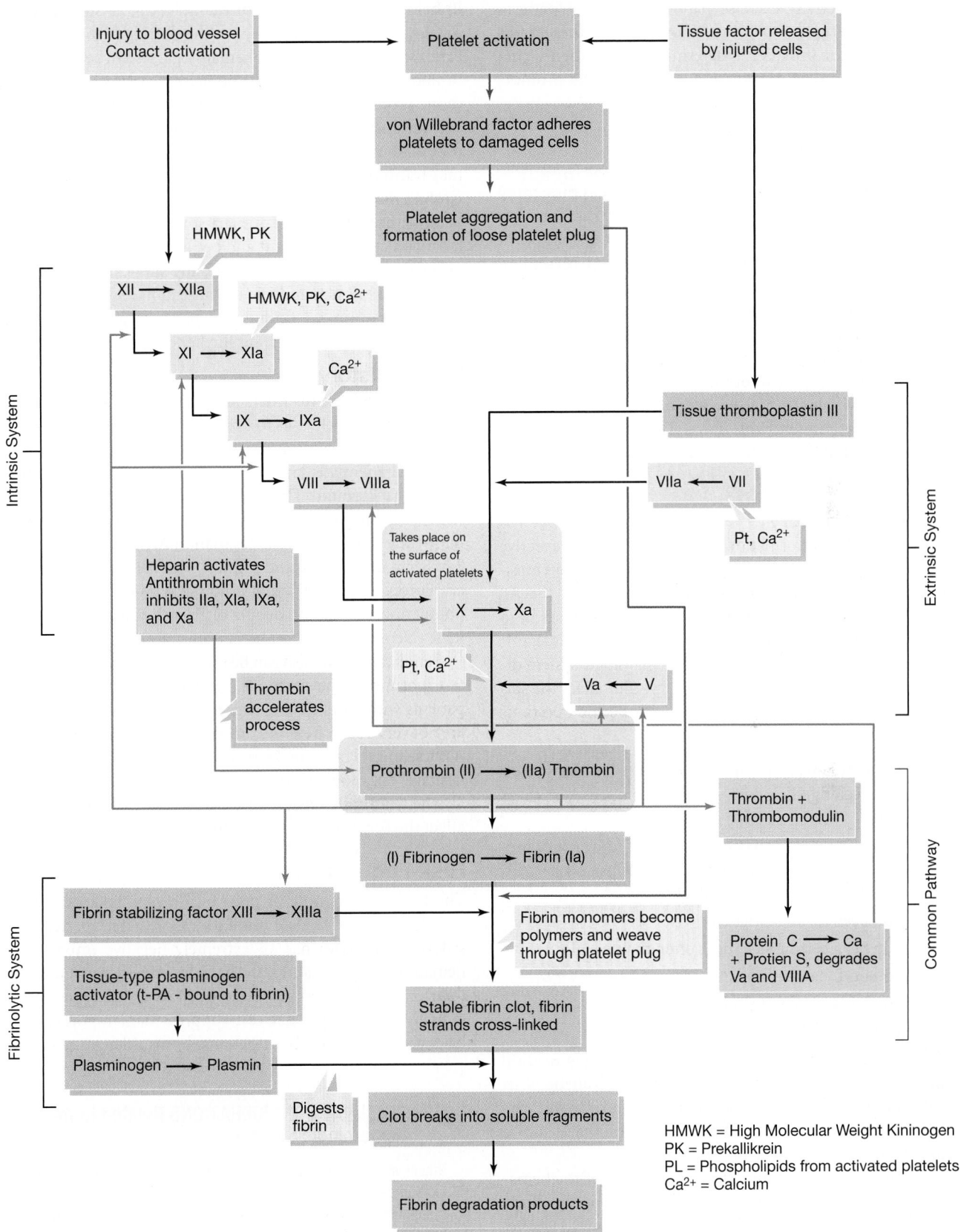

FIGURE 62–8 ■ Coagulation cascade.

patient's dietary history. Other assessment factors include elimination pattern, activity-exercise pattern, sleep–rest pattern, and cognitive-perceptual pattern. Knowledge of these areas helps the health care provider in determining the patient's current health status as well eliminating risk factors and promoting health restoration.

Presenting Symptoms

If patients are having problems with the erythrocyte, or RBC component, of their hematologic system, the usual presenting symptom is fatigue or weakness. The patient may say "I used to be able to make my bed in the morning after I got up, but now I am too tired to even do that." Another common presenting symptom of a hematologic problem is shortness of breath. In this situation patients may complain that they get tired and short of breath just walking around their own house.

If patients are having problems with the leukocytes, neutrophils, or WBC component of their hematologic system, they usually present with increasing episodes of illness and fevers. Finally, patients who present with unusual bleeding may be having problems with their platelets or thrombocytes or with their clotting mechanism.

Past Medical History

The history provides information from the patient's perspective and understanding. In assessing the patient, the nurse asks questions to determine what is happening to the patient, that is, what the patient is feeling and experiencing. In comparison to other systems (e.g., cardiovascular, nervous, reproductive), it is very unusual to ask questions about the hematologic system directly. Generally questions are asked that would reflect the status of the hematologic system. Several such specific questions are as follows:

1. Have you ever had any prior hematologic problems, such as anemia, bleeding disorders, and blood diseases such as leukemia?
2. What medicines have you been taking, including use of prescription and over-the-counter (OTC) drugs and herbals, many of which can interfere with clotting?
3. Have you been feeling fatigued?
4. Have you been getting sick more often than usual?
5. Have you been having fevers?
6. Have you had any bloody or black stools?
7. Have you ever vomited brown or red liquid?
8. Have you had surgery or a major injury requiring medical intervention, for example tumor removal, prosthetic heart valve placement, surgical excision of duodenum, and partial or total gastrectomy? Did anyone tell you that it took a long time to stop the bleeding?

   All of these procedures affect functioning of the hematologic system. For example, iron absorption occurs in the duodenum, and vitamin B_{12} is absorbed in the ileum. Wound healing complications and bleeding should be discussed as response to past surgeries and injuries.

9. Have you had your spleen removed?

These questions are suggestive of changes in the composition and characteristics of the blood cells.

Diseases that involve any of the hematologic organs will result in hematologic disorders. For example, cancer suppresses bone marrow, and liver disease impacts the clotting factors. Kidney disease also greatly impacts the hematologic system because it results in poor production of erythropoietin. Erythropoietin is a hormone produced by the kidney that promotes the differentiation and production of red blood cells in bone marrow. It starts the production of hemoglobin, the molecule within red blood cells that transports oxygen. Gastrointestinal (GI) disorders such as Crohn's disease also impact blood cell production and function because the GI tract is the primary source of the nutrients needed for blood cell development and because GI diseases carry a high propensity for bleeding. Similarly, any surgical manipulation of the component hematologic organs can have deleterious consequences. Assessment findings of previous gastrectomy, colectomy, or splenectomy warrant further diagnostic workup.

Family History

Many hematologic disorders have familial patterns. Genetic information offers clues as to possible hematologic problems that are known to be common in specific populations. For example, sickle cell anemia is known to be found in individuals with an African background. Thalassemia often can be found in patients with a Mediterranean background. Hemophilia is found more frequently in Caucasian males than in African American males. Tay-Sachs disease is found primarily in Jews of central and eastern European descent, and it is now also prevalent in non-Jewish populations, including people of French-Canadian/Cajun heritage (Nemours Foundation, 2008).

Familial patterns also can be the result of similar environmental exposure or behavior modeling within the family. For example, patients with families who engage in smoking, eat poor diets, or are not very active are more prone to engage in similar behaviors. A nurse should never make an assumption about patients' genetic heritage, but should always ask patients about their background.

The Cultural Considerations box discusses how culture can affect the function of the hematologic system.

Risk Factors

The traditional profile of poor health maintenance behaviors (smoking, excessive alcohol intake, poor dietary pattern, and a sedentary lifestyle) has an extremely negative impact on the hematologic system and is the basis for development of risk factors. Excessive alcohol use results in vitamin deficiencies and potentially GI damage that can suppress hematopoiesis. Poorly balanced diets also subject patients to insufficient quantities of

CULTURAL CONSIDERATIONS Related to the Hematologic System

Nurses should be prepared to care for diverse groups of people as the number of patients from other cultures entering the health care system increases. A great deal of variation is seen in the cultural habits of different demographic areas. Beliefs and values related to health, illness, and death, as well as daily habits, nutritional preferences, and health practices, may exist that are culturally important to patients and a part of their daily lives. For example, certain cultures only eat vegetarian foods, which can impact the amount of iron available to produce adequate RBCs.

iron, protein, vitamin B_{12}, and folate, all of which are critical in the production of blood cell lines.

Alterations in the hematologic system can come from a variety of sources including medications, diseases, behavior patterns, family history, and surgical interventions. Examples of risk factors associated with drugs and medications are given in the Risk Factors box. The presence of any of these risk factors places the patient at risk of hematologic system derangement. Many risk factors have only a temporary effect with the derangement subsiding once the risk factor is eliminated or resolved (e.g., temporary dietary deficiency), whereas others can result in permanent damage (bone marrow disease). When a patient presents with hematologic system risk factors, the interdisciplinary health team should provide appropriate assessment of existing alterations and education to prevent further damage.

Physical Examination

A complete physical examination is required to thoroughly assess the effects of hematologic system dysfunction. Because blood cells affect every major organ and body system, only a comprehensive examination can ensure that all possible derangements are identified. Generally, early indicators of hematologic derangement such as fatigue or bleeding can be identified during inspection. Although these signs can also be indicative of temporary and benign situations, keen health care providers will often act on these early indicators to progress toward more definitive diagnostic workups. If further physical examination, such as auscultation or palpation,

yields additional evidence of hematologic derangement, the health care provider would again move toward more definitive diagnostic tools such as laboratory and or radiologic assessments.

Inspection

Simple observation allows the health care provider to observe the patient's general appearance and exertional effort, both of which yield clues in an assessment of the hematologic system. Patients who are short of breath, fatigued, or exhibit poor stamina and poor mental acuity may be at risk of anemia or infection. Fever is a very serious sign that warrants prompt attention even in the absence of other clinical signs. For patients who are neutropenic (decreased neutrophil supply), oftentimes fever is the only observable indicator of infection in this very vulnerable population.

Skin

Changes in skin color often indicate erythrocyte disorders such as anemia (pale, loss of pallor), liver failure (yellow, jaundice), polycythemia vera (pink, flushed), or rapid breakdown of erythrocytes (brown, dark). Platelet and/or clotting derangements often produce tiny capillary bleeds manifesting as petechiae, purpura, or ecchymosis. The appearance of these skin changes, especially in the absence of recent identifiable injury, should be reported immediately so that a laboratory analysis can be performed. In patients with known hematologic deficiencies, assessment of the skin must be included during all routine assessments and whenever laboratory values or assessments of other body systems suggest hematologic derangement.

Head and Neck

The structures of the head, particularly the eyes and mouth, provide useful evidence in the evaluation of the patient with known, potential, or suspected hematologic derangement. Using a penlight, gloved hand, and tongue depressor, the nurse should thoroughly assess the gums, lips, tongue, and teeth. Symptoms warranting further collaboration and intervention include tenderness, increased or decreased saliva, inflammation, reddening, ulcerations, and bleeding. These symptoms are most worrisome in patients with neutropenia because they indicate signs of infection. See Chapter 64 🔗 for further discussion. Pernicious and iron deficiency anemia also produce a characteristic symptom of smooth tongue texture and pale gums.

With respect to the eyes, health care providers should assess the sclera for color and swelling. The appearance of yellow, jaundiced sclera warrants immediate reporting to the health care provider because this indicates an accumulation of bile pigment due to rapid or excessive hemolysis and also is a sign of liver disease. The neck should be inspected for signs of lymph node enlargement or tenderness, especially in the submaxillary, tonsillar, or supraclavicular regions.

Chest

Structures in the chest that yield clues to hematologic system health include the heart and the lymph nodes. The heart is a sensitive indicator of most abnormalities; for example, the heart rate will increase (tachycardia) in response to both infection and anemia. A widening pulse pressure is another compensatory mechanism to counteract inefficient oxygen delivery. The lymph nodes in the mediastinum or the axilla will become enlarged and tender in the presence of infection, lymphoma, and other metastatic cancers.

RISK FACTORS of Drugs and Medications

Many drugs have a deleterious effect on the hematologic system. Mechanisms of action include bone marrow suppression, which stunts the development of all three cell lines; suppression of the clotting cascade; and inflammatory process suppression, which affects WBC efficacy. Of particular concern are any drugs that are specifically termed as *myelosuppressive,* or suppressive of the bone marrow function. Drugs in this category, most notably chemotherapy drugs, will result in *pancytopenia,* or suppression of all three blood cell lines. Examples of more common drugs affecting blood function, specifically platelets, are salicylic acid (aspirin), clopidogrel (Plavix), eptifibatide (Integrilin), and ibuprofen (Advil).

Additionally, a patient can have an idiosyncratic reaction to any medication that may affect blood studies. For example, some individuals develop prolonged clotting times while taking antibiotics. Patients also may not understand the interactions when taking multiple medications or the impact of complementary drugs and/or diet. For example, when a patient is placed on warfarin, the amount of vitamin K taken needs to be minimized because it is an antidote for warfarin and will impact its ability to prolong clotting.

Social History

It is necessary to obtain a social history in order to identify potentially harmful habits and activities. For instance does the patient smoke and drink; if so how much and how often? Is he exposed to potentially traumatic events through his occupation and//or leisure activities? Does he live alone or with others, and if so, whom? These factors are important to determine as they may be risk factors which makes the patient more prone to homological disorders or complications from other disease factors.

CHART 62–3 **Use of Hematologic Testing to Determine Normal/Abnormal Conditions**

Body System	Normal Conditions	Abnormal Conditions
Hematologic	• CBC for work or school physicals • CBC for preoperative screening • CBC to monitor for side effects of medications	• Anemias/leukemias • RBC abnormalities • Infection
Gastrointestinal	• CBC for preoperative screening • CBC to monitor for side effects of medications	• Gastrointestinal bleeding • Appendicitis • Vitamin B_{12} deficiency
Cardiac	• CBC for preoperative screening	• Tachycardia-related anemia • Infection
Pulmonary	• CBC for preoperative screening	• Diffusing capacity of lung for carbon monoxide (D_LCO) • Infection
Renal	• CBC for preoperative screening	• Anemia • Infection
Musculoskeletal	• CBC for preoperative screening	• Infection

Abdomen

Abdominal tenderness is a general complaint, the appearance of which warrants a more detailed work-up. The first task is to isolate (if appropriate) the source of the tenderness, so as to identify which organ is involved. Enlarged spleens (splenomegaly) or livers (hepatomegaly) are general indicators of increased blood cell destruction, the cause of which must be identified. Additionally liver tenderness may be associated with clotting system abnormalities. Further blood studies are warranted whenever a complaint of abdominal tenderness is found.

Laboratory and Diagnostic Procedures

A variety of laboratory tests provide a thorough analysis of blood component status. Health care providers should evaluate laboratory tests not only for the relative quantity of components, but also for the size and character of each cell type. Most commonly, health care providers of any specialty rely on automated blood counts of peripheral cells (i.e., the complete blood count); however, microscopic evaluation of either peripheral blood or bone marrow aspirate yields additional information about size, character, and quality of blood cells. Chart 62–3 shows types of hematologic testing that can be conducted to determine normal and abnormal conditions.

Automated Blood Cell Analysis: Complete Blood Count

The automated blood count provides a highly accurate report of the number of blood cells (RBCs, WBCs, and platelets) in a given volume of peripheral blood. This section discusses each component of the complete blood count including normal/abnormal values and clinical implications. Chart 62–4 shows a listing of complete blood count (CBC) components and normal values. The normal values reflect the national standards for normal CBC values.

For further discussion, please refer to Chapter 63 🔗 on blood disorders and Chapter 60 🔗 on immune response disorders. Additionally, each of the disorder chapters discusses the laboratory values associated with the particular disorder.

Erythrocyte Evaluation

With regards to erythrocytes, the CBC provides a total number, morphologic analysis of blood cells, and hemoglobin analysis. The total RBC count is reported as RBC $\times 10^6/\mu L$ with normal values ranging from 3.6 to 5.2 depending on gender and ethnicity. Physiological increases in the RBC count occur with living in

CHART 62–4 **Complete Blood Count (CBC) Components and Normal Values**

Parameter	Normal Values
Red Blood Cell Indices	
Erythrocyte	*Men:* 4.6–6.2 $\times 10^6$ cells/mm^3 *Women:* 4.2–5.4 $\times 10^6$ cells/mm^3
Hemoglobin	*Men:* 13–18 g/dL *Women:* 12–16 g/dL
Hematocrit	*Men:* 45–54% *Women:* 36–46%
Mean corpuscular volume (MCV)	*Men:* 81–98 µmm^3 *Women:* 81–98 µmm^3
Mean corpuscular hemoglobin (MCH)	*Men:* 27–32 pg/dL *Women:* 27–32 pg/dL
Mean corpuscular hemoglobin concentration (MCHC)	*Men:* 32–36% *Women:* 32–36%
White Blood Cell Count Differential	
WBC count	4,500–11,000/µL
Polymorphonuclear neutrophils	1,800–7,800/µL (50–70%)
Band neutrophils	0–700/µL (0–10%)
Lymphocytes (MCV)	1,000–4,800/µL (15–45%)
Monocytes	0–800/µL (0–10%)
Eosinophils	0–450/µL (0–6%)
Basophils	0–200/µL (0–2%)
Platelet Function	
Platelets	150,000–400,000/µL

high altitude or after increased physical training, as a response to an increased need for oxygen. Pathologic reasons for an increase in the RBC count (polycythemia vera) are chronic obstructive lung disease and, in children with congenital heart disease who are cyanotic, as a response to chronic hypoxia. A decreased RBC count can be due to:

- Abnormal loss of erythrocytes (bleeding)
- Abnormal destruction of erythrocytes
- Lack of needed hormones and elements for production of erythrocytes
- Bone marrow suppression.

However, quantity alone is not a reliable indicator of red blood cell adequacy and function. For that reason, the RBC count is almost always evaluated in conjunction with hemoglobin analysis and morphologic indices (Corbett, 2008).

Recall that hemoglobin is the functional protein of the red blood cell that enables RBCs to carry out their primary function of oxygen transport. Hemoglobin (Hgb or Hb), measured in grams per deciliter, varies from 10 to 17 g/dL. Hemoglobin is reduced in cases of nutritional deficiency, bleeding, anemia, or hemodilution. Volume depletion (dehydration) or polycythemia vera, in turn, causes hemoglobin increases. The **hematocrit** value represents the percentage of hemoglobin in a given volume of whole blood that is occupied by packed RBCs, or the concentration of hemoglobin. However, this value is highly susceptible to fluid status changes such as dehydration; therefore, when making determinations about anemia, most clinicians tend to rely on hemoglobin. If a hematocrit value is not reported, it can be estimated by multiplying the hemoglobin by 3.

RBC indices reflect volume, color, and character of individual red blood cells, thus providing valuable data about the quality of these cells. The indices include these measurements: mean corpuscular volume, mean corpuscular hemoglobin, mean corpuscular hemoglobin concentration, and red cell distribution width.

The **mean corpuscular volume (MCV)** is a measure of the size of the RBCs. If the MCV is less than 78 μm^3, the erythrocytes are microcytic, or smaller than normal. This occurs with iron deficiency anemia, lead poisoning, and thalassemia major and minor. An MCV of greater than 100 μm^3 indicates that the erythrocytes are larger than normal (macrocytic). Macrocytic RBCs occur with liver disease, pernicious anemia, and folic acid deficiencies. The MCV can be used as a predictor of mortality in advanced cirrhosis. If the MCV is in the normal range the term *normocytic* is used. Anemia due to acute blood loss results in normocytic anemia (Corbett, 2008).

The **mean corpuscular hemoglobin (MCH)** measurement is the amount of Hgb present in one cell, whereas the **mean corpuscular hemoglobin concentration (MCHC)** is the proportion of each cell that is occupied by hemoglobin, indicating efficacy of interaction of the hemoglobin molecule with the erythrocyte. These two indices are discussed together because both are tests to determine whether the erythrocytes have a normal amount of Hgb (are normal color or *normochromic*), less Hgb (decreased color or *hypochromic*), or more Hgb (increased color or *hyperchromic*). Iron deficiency anemia is the most common cause of hypochromic anemia. Refer to Chapter 63  for further discussion of the clinical implications of variations in RBC indices.

The **red blood cell distribution width (RDW)** is a direct measurement of the homogeneity, or consistency, of red blood cell size. Immature cells are larger than mature cells and will result in RBC size variations. Additionally, the shape of red blood cells is highly influenced by the configuration of the hemoglobin molecule. Diseases such as sickle cell anemia and thalassemia, both diseases of hemoglobin, result in size variations. An increased RDW indicates a relatively heterogeneous population of red blood cells, indicating the presence of either abnormal or immature cells. The RDW is used to differentiate the various types of anemias.

The MCV, MCH, and MCHC measurements are primarily used in the classification of anemia. As discussed in Chapter 63 , *anemia* is a broad term applied to any situation resulting in a decrease in hemoglobin or erythrocytes. Anemia can be classified further (substantially) according to the underlying etiology, whether it is blood loss, iron deficiency anemia, or sickle cell anemia, for instance. These RBC indices are most useful in delineating the likely cause.

> **CRITICAL ALERT** *A drop in hemoglobin level below 10 or a serial decrease in hemoglobin on consecutive reports may indicate anemia and should be reported to the health care provider immediately.*

Leukocyte Evaluation

Leukocyte evaluation can be summarized by the white blood cell count value, which has a normal value of 4,500 to 10,000 cells per microliter. Normal values suggest that a patient has a sufficient number of cells to support host immune defense systems. However, the distribution of those WBCs is of significant clinical importance. White blood cells, or leukocytes, are a large heterogeneous group of cells, each with a unique role in host defenses as described earlier. Of these, the neutrophils are the first responder cells responsible for the initial detection of foreign antigens and initiation of the immune response cascade. However, the total neutrophil count is a summary value that combines immature (blasts), juvenile (bands), and fully mature stages of the neutrophils.

Only the fully mature neutrophils, and to some degree the juvenile subpopulations, are useful in defense. The bone marrow may be stimulated to release a large number of relatively immature cells and juvenile cells as a compensatory mechanism to combat severe infection. During this situation, the total WBC count increases, but the rise is due to the proliferation of juvenile cells. This phenomenon is termed a *shift to the left* and should be reported to the health care provider. In an otherwise healthy individual, this shift to the left may be an early sign of an otherwise undetected infection. If, however, the total WBC count remains within normal limits or even slightly below normal, and a shift to the left occurs, the patient may be left with insufficient host defenses. This can occur with bone marrow disease, immune system insufficiencies, or immunosuppressive therapies such as chemotherapy.

The **absolute neutrophil count (ANC)** is a useful measurement that reveals that proportion of the white blood cells that can be utilized in first response immune interactions. To calculate the ANC, add the bands to the neutrophils and multiply by the total WBC count. Values greater than 1,500 indicate normal immune defense. Some laboratories provide this number directly; however, it can be easily calculated from the white blood cell differential.

The WBC differential is a determination of each of the five types of WBCs in 100 WBCs. This is a separate test from the CBC and generally must be specifically ordered by the health care provider. In contrast to the automated CBC, the CBC with manual differential must be performed by a laboratory scientist who conducts a microscopic analysis of a blood smear. Bands and neutrophils (also called polymorphonuclear cells or stabs depending on the nomenclature used by the laboratory) are reported as a percentage of the total WBC count. See Chapters 60 and 64 on immunology and cancer, respectively, for further discussion.

 *ANC values below 1,000 indicate that the patient is at severe risk of infection and without sufficient defenses to prevent sepsis. Immediately assess the patient for signs of infection, initiate appropriate interventions, and report to the health care provider immediately.*

Platelet Evaluation

The platelet count is a useful indicator of bleeding risk because platelets are responsible for initiation of the clotting cascade. Fortunately, the platelet count requires little further calculation because its final value reported on the CBC can be used as an immediate indicator of platelet activity. Normal values range from 150,000 to 400,000. Increased platelet counts (thrombocytosis) occur with malignant tumors, especially if they are metastatic lesions, and with polycythemia vera and splenectomy. Low platelet counts (thrombocytopenia) may be idiopathic, related to cancer, due to an autoimmune disease, or the result of a viral infection. Low platelet counts are also common with acquired immunodeficiency disease (AIDS) (Corbett, 2008).

 *Platelet levels below 30,000 indicate that the patient may be at imminent risk of internal bleeding, especially cranial bleeds. In this event, report to the health care provider immediately and implement bleeding precautions.*

Coagulation Studies

As discussed when the clotting cascade was described earlier in the chapter, numerous components interact in a complex sequence of steps in response to endothelial injury (refer to Figure 62–8 ■, p. 1997). Insufficiencies in activity or supply in any of the components will result in abnormal bleeding. A variety of coagulation studies are utilized to identify individual insufficiencies. Chart 62–5 provides a description of each test and its normal values. Generally, longer time values indicate insufficient clotting factors or overactivity of clot-inhibiting therapy (such as heparin, Coumadin, or aspirin).

Bone Marrow Examination

Examination of the bone marrow may be required for several clinical scenarios, including these:

- Evaluation of unexplained peripheral blood cytopenias (decreased blood cell counts)
- Evaluation of unexplained excessive peripheral blood cell counts
- Evaluation of suspicious cells in the peripheral blood
- Staging or further analysis of leukemia or lymphoma
- Evaluation of fever of unknown origin
- Evaluation of patient iron stores when other tests are ambiguous.

Bone marrow aspiration removes a small amount of bone marrow *fluid* through a needle inserted into a bone. A bone marrow biopsy removes *bone* with the marrow inside and is obtained with a visual inspection of the marrow structure. Bone marrow samples are acquired by a health care provider using local anesthesia from the posterior superior iliac spine of the pelvis or the sternum.

Although there may be variations in technique among health care providers, if the biopsy is obtained from the iliac spine, the patient generally is placed into the lateral decubitus position with the top leg flexed and the lower leg straight. This position allows for optimal exposure of the iliac crest while providing stabilization with the lower leg. Oftentimes, nurses can assist the patient and health care provider in maintaining this optimal position.

Once the site is sterilized and anesthetized with local anesthetic, a small skin incision is made through which the bone marrow aspiration and biopsy needles are inserted. The bone marrow needle is comprised of an outer shell surrounding a stylet. Once the stylet has penetrated the marrow, it is removed and a syringe is attached to the shell allowing for aspiration of 2 to 3 mL of bone marrow. The bone marrow biopsy is done in much the same fashion with a specialized needle that is able to extract small amounts of bone. After the procedure, a small gauze square is applied with mild pressure to prevent bleeding. After the procedure patients should be assessed for pain and bleeding. Presence of either should be reported to the health care provider.

Bone marrow examination specifically evaluates the specimen for adequacy of volume and appropriate production of bone marrow cells. Specific results include:

- Evaluation of the adequacy of marrow development of each hematopoietic cell line.

CHART 62–5	**Coagulation Studies**	

Study	Measures	Normal Value
Prothrombin time (PT)	Extrinsic coagulation Factors I, II, V, VII, and X	12–15 seconds
Activated partial thromboplastin time (aPTT)	Intrinsic coagulation Factors I, II, V, VII, IX, X, XI, and XII	30–45 seconds
Bleeding time	Reflects platelet interaction and capillary constriction. A highly insensitive study, consequently use of this test is not favored	1–6 minutes
Thrombin time	Thrombin sufficiency	8–12 seconds
Fibrinogen	Fibrinogen sufficiency	200–400 mg/dL
Fibrin split products	Useful in detection of DIC. Reflects degree of fibrinolysis, which releases fibrin split products into bloodstream	<10 mg/dL

- Morphologic examinations of the cells to ensure that structures are consistent with normal cells.
- Infiltration of the bone marrow by inappropriate cells. Normally, only early precursors of blood cell lines should be observed in the marrow. Presence of other cells may indicate disease, most likely some type of malignancy.
- Fibrosis.

Gerontological Considerations

The effects of aging on the hematologic system currently are under study. It is thought, however, that the amount of red marrow and the number of stem cells decrease with aging, but the marrow is not completely depleted even in very old adults. The remaining stem cells retain their functional capacity to divide, but as they decrease in number they are gradually replaced by nonfunctional fat cells. This, in turn, potentially decreases the ability of the marrow to respond to the body's need for blood cells in the advent of injury or disease (Lichtman & Williams, 2001). The elderly patient is more vulnerable to possible problems with clotting, oxygen transport, and fighting infection, especially during periods of increased demand.

Laboratory parameters as they relate to the hematologic system of aging patients usually are not much different than those of a younger patient (Kane, Ouslander, & Abrass, 2004; McPherson & Pincus, 2006; Young et al., 2006). Although it is recognized that hemoglobin levels tend to decrease after middle age, more so in men than women (Guyton, 2006), aging changes do not usually occur with the WBC count or platelet count. It has been suggested that there may be some T-cell function loss and this may account for the poor response to immunizations in the elderly population (Young et al., 2006). The effect of anemia on the elderly is discussed in the Gerontological Considerations box.

Implications for Health Promotion

The hematologic system, without exception, affects every organ in the body. Its pivotal role dictates that its maintenance must be incorporated into any health promotion strategy. One need only review the risk factors of hematologic disorders to determine what health promotion activities should be taken. Individuals can do much to maintain and optimize the health of their hematologic system. Patients should be advised to examine their genetic history to determine whether there is any family history of bleeding disorders. Eating a well-balanced diet rich in iron, vitamin B_{12}, and proteins ensures that the bone marrow is supplied with the requisite building blocks for blood cells. Direct patient teaching by nurses or referral to a registered dietitian can be of tremendous benefit to patients trying to navigate a plethora of food choices. The effect of nutrition on the hematologic system is discussed in detail in Chapter 63 ⊘.

Exercise is critical for a healthy hematologic system both because it encourages production of blood cells from the marrow (resulting in reduced fatigue and shortness of breath) and it reduces the risk of cardiovascular disease. With increased exercise the patient is at decreased risk of coagulation disorders.

Excessive alcohol consumption damages the hematologic system on several fronts: (1) impaired nutrition, because beneficial calories are substituted with alcohol; (2) damage to the GI tract, resulting in bleeding and impaired absorption of vitamin B_{12}, iron, and folate; and (3) damage to the liver, resulting in decreased coagulation factors and erythrocyte processing. Nurses play a critical role in identifying opportunities to promote lifestyles that ensure the health of the hematologic system. Patients should be advised that diet may be a contributing factor for anemia. Refer to Chapter 63 ⊘ on blood disorders for additional information on health promotion.

Critical Thinking Related to the Hematologic System

It is imperative that the nurse become familiar with the components of the laboratory tests and other examination tests that are used to evaluate the hematologic system. The nurse must:

- Be able to explain the purpose of the tests to patients and/or their family.
- Be able to explain to the patients and/or their family why the hematologic system is being evaluated for a patient in a particular situation.
- Be able to identify normal and abnormal values of a complete blood count.
- Be able to differentiate normal versus abnormal laboratory values according to the reference ranges for the laboratory performing the test. These reference points must be available; if they are not provided on the laboratory report, the nurse can call the laboratory and ask for the normal reference ranges for that particular test.
- Identify situations where evaluation of the hematologic system would be appropriate or inappropriate.

Tracking laboratory values over a time period to determine trending in abnormalities is an essential nursing measure and requires critical thinking. An isolated abnormal finding may not be significant, but if the value continues to trend toward abnormality, it becomes significant.

The nurse must rely on critical thinking skills when interpreting patients' symptoms and assessment findings to determine possible and potential patient diagnoses and to consider the appropriate action(s) to take. Analysis of these data allows the nurse to make a diagnosis and then follow up with any required interventions. It is imperative that the nurse communicate and collaborate with other members of the health care team in developing and implementing a plan of care for patients with any hematologic findings outside of the normal range.

GERONTOLOGICAL CONSIDERATIONS Related to Anemia

If an elderly person is anemic, often it is due to disease processes, such as GI bleeding or malnutrition, in other systems as opposed to the hematologic system. Abnormal values in these areas need to be brought to the health care provider's attention because further evaluation may be necessary. Thinking that changes in these parameters are solely due to aging may result in an incorrect interpretation of the laboratory test, which could then lead to incorrect management of the problem. It often is the duration of the disease process, not the person's age, that results in illness, morbidity, and mortality.

Summary

As presented in this chapter, the hematologic system is deeply integrated with every body system. Thus, alterations in the hematologic organs or cells can manifest virtually anywhere and, conversely, damage in a peripheral organ can impact the function of the blood system. For these reasons a thorough knowledge of the anatomy and physiology of the hematologic system is a critical tool in the nurse's arsenal. Appropriate assessment skills, including physical examination and diagnostic study evaluation, should be core skills for all nurses.

NCLEX® REVIEW

1. As it relates to the hematologic system in the adult patient, the nurse understands that:
   1. The stem cell is a primitive cell located in the bone marrow that is the precursor of red blood cells, white blood cells, and platelets.
   2. The liver and spleen can produce blood cells during intramedullary hematopoiesis when disease has caused bone marrow destruction.
   3. The blood is considered to be a type of connective tissue with one primary function, to transport oxygen, hormones, and waste products.
   4. The proportion of yellow bone marrow diminishes and is permanently replaced by red bone marrow as the healthy patient ages.

2. The nurse educator is teaching a class of new nurses regarding the functions of the hematologic system in the adult. Which of the following statements made by one of the participants indicates the need for further instruction?
   1. "White blood cells usually remain in the bone marrow, lungs, liver, spleen, and lymph nodes, unless they are needed."
   2. "Immature reticulocytes will persist for several days in the circulation before becoming a small, mature red blood cell."
   3. "The cells of the reticuloendothelial system facilitate blood clotting and initiate the inflammatory and immune responses."
   4. "Erythrocytes are responsible for transporting, maintaining, and distributing hemoglobin to the body's tissues."

3. The nurse is planning the care of the patient who is newly diagnosed with anemia. The nurse anticipates performing which of the following laboratory tests to better classify the anemia?
   1. PT, aPTT, PLT
   2. HGB, HCT, ANC
   3. RBC, RDW, WBC
   4. MCH, MCV, MCHC

4. Which of the following laboratory test results should the nurse immediately report to the health care provider?
   1. HCT 28%
   2. PLT 400,000/μL
   3. WBC 10,000/μL
   4. MCH 30pg/dL

5. During shift report the nurse is told a patient's laboratory values indicate a shift to the left. The receiving nurse understands that this phenomenon indicates:
   1. The measurement of the proportion of white blood cells that are available for use in a first response immune reaction.
   2. An increase in the total white blood cell count because of the proliferation of juvenile band and immature blast cells.
   3. A quantitative method of indicating the efficacy of interaction between the hemoglobin molecule and the erythrocyte.
   4. That there are insufficiencies in either activity or supply in one or more of the components of the clotting cascade.

6. Which of the following statements describes the correct sequence of events within the normal hemostasis mechanism?
   1. Soft aggregate plug formation, vasoconstriction, fibrin conversion into fibrinogen, initiation of the intrinsic coagulation mechanism
   2. Vascular contraction, intrinsic adenosine diaphosphate release, prothrombin conversion into thrombin, fibrinogen conversion into fibrin
   3. Platelet adhesion, onset of primary hemostasis pathway, Factor XI activates Factor XII, initiation of the extrinsic coagulation mechanism
   4. Start of intrinsic clotting pathway, Factor III and Factor V release, platelet thromboplastic factor release, Factor X activates Factor XI

7. A patient presents to the primary care clinic complaining of increasingly worsening fatigue over the last two months. Which of the following questions should the nurse ask in order to better differentiate the source of the patient's complaint?
   1. "Are you allergic to shellfish or IV dye?"
   2. "Have you had your gallbladder removed?"
   3. "What medications are you currently taking?"
   4. "Is there a family history of heart disease?"

Answers for review questions appear in Appendix D

KEY TERMS

absolute neutrophil count (ANC) *p.2001*
basophil *p.1993*
chyle *p.1994*
eosinophil *p.1993*
erythrocyte *p.1991*
granulocyte *p.1993*
hematocrit *p.2001*
hematology *p.1989*
hematopoiesis *p.1990*
hemoglobin *p.1991*
hemostasis *p.1995*

humoral immune response *p.1993*
leukocyte *p.1991*
lymphatic system *p.1994*
lymphocyte *p.1993*
mean corpuscular hemoglobin
     (MCH) *p.2001*
mean corpuscular hemoglobin
     concentration (MCHC) *p.2001*
mean corpuscular volume (MCV) *p.2001*
monocyte *p.1993*
neutrophil *p.1993*

plasma *p.1991*
platelet *p.1991*
red blood cell (RBC) *p.1991*
red blood cell distribution width
     (RDW) *p.2001*
reticulocyte *p.1992*
reticuloendothelial system (RES) *p.1993*
stem cell *p.1990*
thrombocyte *p.1991*
white blood cell (WBC) *p.1991*

PEARSON
EXPLORE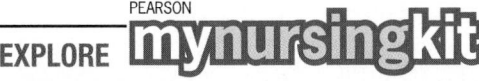

MyNursingKit is your one stop for online chapter review materials and resources. Prepare for success with additional NCLEX®-style practice questions, interactive assignments and activities, web links, animations and videos, and more!

Register your access code from the front of your book at
www.mynursingkit.com

REFERENCES

Corbett, J. V. (2008). *Laboratory tests and diagnostic procedures: With nursing diagnosis.* Upper Saddle River, NJ: Pearson Prentice Hall.

Dailey, J. (1998). *Blood.* Arlington, MA: Medical Consulting Group.

Department of Health and Human Services, Agency for Toxic Substances & Disease Registry. (2005). Top 20 hazardous substances. Retrieved October 10, 2008 from http://www.atsdr.cedc.gov/cxcx3.html

Guyton, A. C. (2006). *Textbook of medical physiology* (11th ed.). St. Louis: Elsevier.

Kane, R., Ouslander, J., & Abrass, I. (2004). *Essentials of clinical geriatrics* (5th ed.). New York: McGraw-Hill.

Lichtman, M. A., & Williams, W. J. (2001). Hematology in the aged. In E. Beutler, M. A. Lichtman, B. S. Coller, T. J. Kipps, & U. Seligsohn (Eds.), *Williams hematology* (6th ed.). St. Louis: Mosby.

McPherson, R., & Pincus, M. (2006). *Henry's clinical diagnosis and management by laboratory methods* (21st ed.). Philadelphia: W. B. Saunders.

Nemours Foundation. (2008). *Tay-Sachs disease.* Retrieved March 24, 2008, from http://www.kidshealth.org/parent/medical/genetic/tay_sachs.html

Porth, C. (2007). *Essentials of pathophysiology: Concepts of altered health states.* St. Louis: Lippincott Williams & Wilkins.

Ross, M. H. (2003). *Histology: A text and atlas* (4th ed., pp. 229–231). Philadelphia: Lippincott William & Wilkins.

Swartz, M. A. (2001). *Advanced Drug Delivery Reviews, 50*(1–2), 3–20.

Young, N., Gerson, S., & High, K. (2006). *Clinical hematology.* Philadelphia: Mosby.

63

Caring for the Patient with Blood Disorders

Kristine Abueg

Outcome-Based Learning Objectives

After studying this chapter, the learner will be able to:

1. Describe the physiology of hematopoiesis, thrombopoiesis, and hemostasis.

2. Explain the pathophysiological alterations in erythropoiesis, thrombopoiesis, and hemostasis that give rise to specific hematologic disorders.

3. Compare and contrast the causes, the therapeutic management, and clinical presentation of the various types of anemias and hemostasis disorders.

4. Analyze laboratory values, correlating to physical signs and symptoms, and distinguish between various hematologic disorders.

5. Explain appropriate nursing interventions for the management of thrombocytopenia.

6. Compare and contrast the hallmark clinical presentation of bleeding disorders versus clotting disorders.

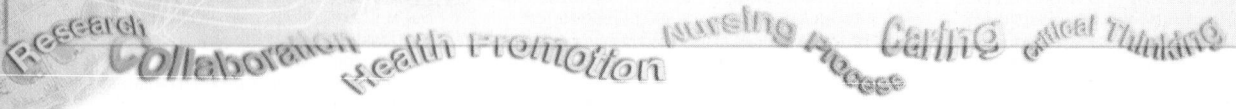

Hematology involves the study of blood and blood, or hematologic, disorders. Blood actually contains both plasma and blood cells (as explained in Chapter 62 ☺). Plasma, comprised of water, proteins, salts, lipids, glucose, and other organic compounds, makes up 55% of blood volume. Its main purpose is to act as a liquid transport system between tissues. Hematology, however, involves the study of the cellular components of blood, specifically erythrocytes (red blood cells), leukocytes (white blood cells), and thrombocytes (platelets). Normal function of the cellular components is described in Chapter 62 ☺. Hematologic disorders arise when the normal functioning of these cell lines is disrupted either by disease, genetics, or environmental factors. The study of hematology and blood disorders is best approached by a systematic review of different blood components. This chapter focuses specifically on two cell lines: thrombocytes and erythrocytes. Refer to Chapters 59 and 60 ☺ for an in-depth review of the nursing care of patients with leukocyte disorders.

Some hematologic disorders are chronic, resulting in the need for permanent lifestyle adjustments, whereas others are acute medical conditions requiring immediate medical attention. Chronic hematologic diseases include sickle cell disease, thalassemia, and hemophilia. Acute hematologic disorders include acute anemia, thrombocytopenia, and disseminated intravascular coagulation. These acute disorders usually are not independently occurring disease states, but serious side effects that result when another underlying disease process is present.

Most medical–surgical nurses are likely to care for patients with acute blood disorders, because most chronic diseases are well managed in the outpatient setting. However, patients with chronic hematologic disorders often are hospitalized for other illnesses such as infection, trauma, or cardiac problems. Physiological stressors can severely exacerbate chronic diseases potentially leading to "acute attacks." Such attacks, however, often can be prevented by diligent initial assessment paired with continual observation for deviation from the baseline. In the event an acute attack occurs, the nurse must ensure that immediate intervention and coordination with the interdisciplinary health team occur to prevent serious injury. For all of these reasons, it is critically important for the nurse to include any existing or potential hematologic disorder in a patient's care plan.

■ Hematopoiesis: Development of Blood Cells

Hematopoiesis is the process of blood cell development, beginning with the immature hematopoietic stem cell in the bone marrow and extending through to complete cellular maturation in the peripheral bloodstream. Problems that can occur during hematopoiesis account for many of the hematologic disorders discussed in this chapter; therefore, a review of the normal physiological processes involved in hematopoiesis is a useful foundation for the study of hematology.

As mentioned earlier, blood contains many specialized cell lines including erythrocytes (red blood cells), leukocytes (white blood cells), and platelets. Despite their variation in appearance and function, all of these cell types are generated from the hematopoietic stem cells. **Hematopoietic stem cells (HSCs)** reside largely in the spongy bone marrow of the femurs, hips, ribs, sternum, and other long bones, while a small volume of HSCs circulates in the peripheral blood. HSCs may be thought of as the common ancestor cell of all blood cell lines. Although HSCs eventually give rise to mature red blood cells (RBCs), platelets, and white blood cells (WBCs), they themselves do not possess the full capabilities of oxygen transportation, clotting, or immune response associated with their more mature progeny, the erythrocytes, platelets, and leukocytes. These *pluripotent* HSCs found in the bone marrow and the blood should not be confused with embryonic *totipotent* stem cells, which are found in developing embryos and can develop into any cell in the human body.

The goal of hematopoiesis is not only to produce large numbers of cells when needed, but also to produce well-differentiated cells. **Differentiation** is the process by which immature precursor cells (such as the hematopoietic stem cells) produce generations of increasingly more specialized cells, ultimately resulting in a fully functioning, mature cell (such as a mature erythrocyte or thrombocyte). Differentiation also is associated with increasing morphologic distinction, acquisition of a specialized cellular structure, and membrane proteins, and narrowing of the variety of blood cells that can be produced by a given cell. The hematopoietic cascade, as shown in Figure 63–1 ■, is a common and useful illustration of this process.

From the HSCs, the next level of specificity is the lymphoid or myeloid **progenitor cells**, or blood line–specific stem cells. The common lymphoid progenitor cell eventually gives rise to the lymphoid cells of the immune system, specifically the natural killer cells, the T cells, and the B cells. Refer to Chapter 60 ⊙ for a discussion of disorders related to these cell lines. The common **myeloid progenitor cell** further differentiates into the granulocyte-macrophage stem cell, the megakaryocytic stem cell, or the erythropoietic stem cell (proerythroblast). The granulocyte-macrophage stem cell will eventually give rise to the granulocytes (neutrophils, eosinophils, basophils) or the monocytes (monocytic cells of the immune system and macrophages). Immune system disorders related to these cell lines are discussed in Chapter 60 ⊙. Of interest to this chapter are the **megakaryocytic stem cells**, which eventually will develop the platelets, and the **erythropoietic stem cells (proerythroblasts)**, which will develop into mature erythrocytes or red blood cells.

The process of hematopoiesis is stimulated on an "as-needed basis." Cellular and chemical signals, generated when the body requires increased production of blood cells, interact with cells undergoing hematopoiesis, beginning with the HSCs. An HSC receives a chemical signal to produce a particular cell line, to self-replicate to increase available HSCs, or even to undergo apoptosis, programmed cell death. Conversely, the absence of these chemical signals or the presence of inhibitory signals is associated with decreased levels of hematopoiesis. This elegant system of feedback regulation ensures that energy reserves are allocated efficiently and not wasted on production of already abundant cells. Common types of chemical signals responsible for the regulation of hematopoiesis include soluble factors such as cytokines, direct cell-to-cell interaction, and contact with the extracellular matrix of the blood-forming organs. Specific signals include hormones such as erythropoietin in the case of RBC production, and thrombopoietin and interleukins in the case of platelet cell production.

Research has expanded our understanding about the complexity, variety, and intricate interplay that exists among these cellular and chemical signals. A major field of research is directed at understanding these signals in an effort to expand the production of small numbers of highly pluripotent HSCs for clinical transplantation and for other scientific studies. Currently, exogenous administration of hematopoiesis-stimulating chemicals is already a cornerstone of treatment for many diseases. Future treatment options will almost certainly evolve to incorporate medications derived from a growing understanding of these chemical signals. Specialized hematopoiesis of the RBC line (erythropoiesis) and platelet-forming cell lines (thrombopoiesis) are discussed later in the chapter as they relate to anemia and thrombocytopenia. As illustrated throughout this chapter, problems during hematopoiesis account for a large proportion of hematologic disorders. Successful hematopoiesis requires precise interaction and a delicate balance between numerous cells, chemical factors, and the physiological environment. Because hematopoiesis plays a pivotal role during the most primitive stages of embryonic and cellular development, even minor disruptions can have far-reaching amplified consequences. These consequences thus become the focus of hematology. This chapter builds on the pathophysiological foundation of hematopoiesis just outlined, highlighting alterations in the process that give rise to clinical disorders.

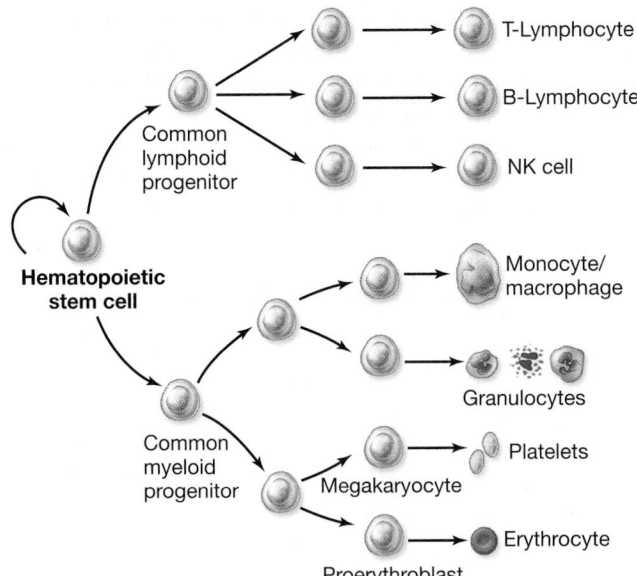

FIGURE 63–1 ■ The hematopoetic cascade.

Anemia

Anemia is defined as a decrease in the total body erythrocyte volume, usually measured by a decrease in hemoglobin protein, a decreased hematocrit, and/or a decreased RBC count. The primary function of the erythrocytes is the transportation of oxygen on the hemoglobin molecules; thus, insufficiencies in the erythrocytes translate into an inability to maintain sufficient oxygen delivery to the tissues.

Etiology and Classifications of Generalized Anemia

According to data published by the National Center for Health Statistics in 2002, iron deficiency anemia, the most common form of anemia, was responsible for 4,614 deaths in America. Comprehensive mortality and morbidity for all causes of anemia is difficult to ascertain for two reasons. First, anemia is considered to be widely underdiagnosed, because patients often fail to seek diagnostic evaluation for symptoms of fatigue and shortness of breath, both hallmark signs of anemia. Second, anemia is not a disease in and of itself, but rather a clinical side effect that results from some underlying pathologic disease process that often complicates a statistical tabulation. Anemia can be triggered either by (1) loss of blood volume, (2) altered production of erythrocytes (hypoproliferative disorders), or (3) altered (increased) destruction of red blood cells. The various underlying etiologies have unique clinical presentations, which trigger a differential diagnostic workup. After resolution of immediate life-threatening situations such as hypoxia or blood loss, treatment is tailored to address the primary hematologic disorder causing the anemia.

Normal Physiology of Red Blood Cell Development

A detailed overview of erythrocyte development, or erythropoiesis, is described next as a foundation for discussing various causes of anemia. Understanding the root causes of these diseases illuminates not only the cause, but also aids in patient education and the judicious application of treatment options.

Erythropoiesis

Erythropoiesis, the process of hematopoiesis of erythrocytes (red blood cells), is stimulated primarily by the presence of erythropoietin, which acts on HSCs to produce the myeloid progenitor cell, thus starting the cascade toward RBC production. **Erythropoietin** is a hormone produced by the juxtaglomerular cells of the kidneys during periods of **hypoxia**, or decreased blood oxygen levels. Erythropoietin production also is modulated by other factors including thyroid-stimulating hormone, adrenal cortical steroids, adrenocorticotropic hormone, and human growth hormone (HGH). All of these factors are produced during periods of increased growth and their promotion of erythropoietin ensures sufficient supplies of oxygen will be available to growing tissues.

As discussed earlier, hematopoiesis results in cellular differentiation. During erythropoiesis, the pluripotent hematopoietic stem cell undergoes increasing differentiation, producing first the myeloid stem cell, then the pronormoblast, then the basophilic normoblast, the polychromatophilic normoblast, the orthochromatic normoblast, and then the reticulocyte (Figure 63–2 ■). The reticulocyte, or juvenile erythrocyte, is morphologically identifiable by its distinct reticulum in the cytoplasm. The reticulocyte circulates for approximately 3 days in the bone marrow before being released into the peripheral bloodstream where, after approximately 24 hours of undergoing changes in its cytoplasm, the reticulocyte will mature into a fully developed erythrocyte. Note, however, that high levels of erythropoietin, which occurs, for example, during hypoxic states or infection, may stimulate early release of reticulocytes from the bone marrow into the peripheral bloodstream, which is reflected on a complete blood count.

At the end of its designated life span (approximately 120 days), the aging erythrocyte (*senescent* erythrocyte) begins to display cell surface proteins, which trigger phagocytosis in the reticuloendothelial system. As described in Chapter 59 ⊗ , the reticuloendothelial system is comprised of phagocytic cells in the lymph nodes, spleen, and liver that clear the body of waste. Circulating macrophages consume the senescent erythrocyte and the hemoglobin, recycling the precious iron molecule by transporting it back to the body's iron stores.

Dietary elements play a key role in RBC production. Deficiencies in any of these dietary elements can negatively affect erythropoiesis. RBC development is highly dependent on sufficient quantities of metals (iron, cobalt, and manganese), vitamins (B_{12}, B_6, C, E, folate, riboflavin, pantothenic acid, and thiamin), amino acids, and carbohydrates. Although cellular growth requires all of these elements, vitamin B_{12}, folate, and iron play particularly pivotal roles in erythropoiesis. Folate and vitamin B_{12} are required for the extensive DNA synthesis that occurs with erythropoiesis. All proliferating cells require iron,

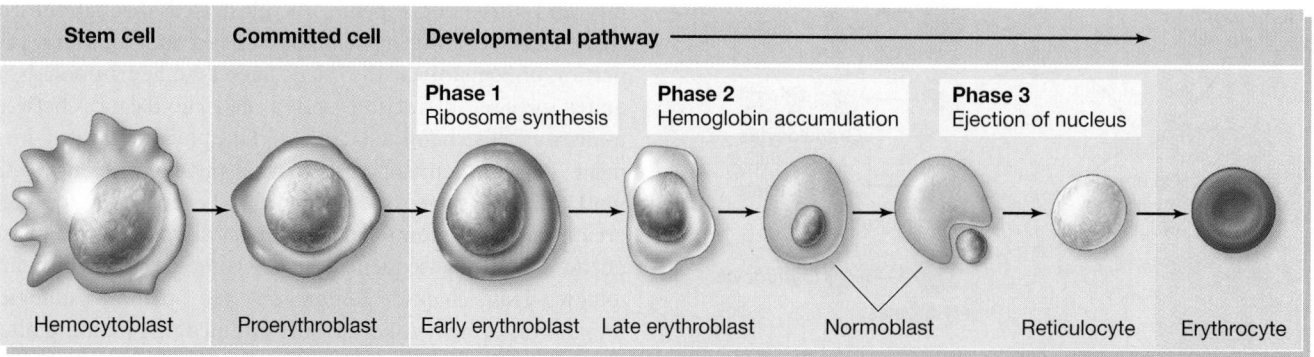

Stem cell	Committed cell	Developmental pathway ────────────────────►			
		Phase 1 Ribosome synthesis	**Phase 2** Hemoglobin accumulation	**Phase 3** Ejection of nucleus	
Hemocytoblast	Proerythroblast	Early erythroblast Late erythroblast	Normoblast	Reticulocyte	Erythrocyte

FIGURE 63–2 ■ Erythropoiesis.

but the iron requirements of erythroid cells in the late basophilic erythroblast through reticulocyte stages, when hemoglobin is synthesized and accumulates, are much greater than that for all other cell types (Koury & Ponka, 2004). Diseases such as megaloblastic anemia and iron deficiency anemia result when sufficient supplies do not exist to support erythropoiesis.

Hemoglobin Development

Hemoglobin is the core functional protein of the red blood cell, shuttling oxygen between tissues, allowing blood to transport 100 times more oxygen than could be transported in plasma alone. In erythropoiesis, hemoglobin first becomes detectable in the myeloid progenitor cell, with each subsequent cell generation gaining more and more hemoglobin molecule. Ultimately, the mature erythrocyte contains approximately 250 million hemoglobin molecules. Hemoglobin fulfills its oxygen-carrying function by binding iron to the four heme regions of the molecule. Closer observation of hemoglobin reveals that hemoglobin protein actually is comprised of four parts: two identical hemoglobin alpha chains and two identical hemoglobin beta chains. Iron binding is achieved when the hemoglobin alpha and beta chains form precise geometric configurations that allow iron to sit tightly in a lock-and-key style fit on the heme groups.

Healthy, functional hemoglobin conforms to one of two configurations. Which configuration it takes on depends on whether an O_2 molecule is bound to the heme, the pH of the environment, and the amount of a mediating chemical, 2,3-diphosphoglycerate. The combination of these factors varies in hypoxic states versus well-oxygenated states. This interaction is the foundation of the oxygen-release or oxygen-carrying mechanism of hemoglobin. An alteration to the geometric shape of hemoglobin is the underlying cause of many hematologic disorders such as thalassemia and sickle cell disease, which are discussed in detail later. The amount of hemoglobin in blood is a common clinical test used to diagnose disease. Although there are variations due to altitude, accepted values for hemoglobin for adult males are 13.8 to 18 g/dL, and for adult females 12 to 16 g/dL (g/dL = grams per deciliter).

Clinical Presentation of Generalized Anemia

Decreased erythrocyte volume results in **anemic hypoxia**, or decreased oxygen availability to the tissues specifically due to decreased concentration of functional hemoglobin or a reduced number of red blood cells. Anemic hypoxia should be distinguished from **hypoxic hypoxia**, in which oxygen deprivation occurs from defective oxygenation in the lungs, as caused by abnormal pulmonary function, airway obstruction, or a right-to-left shunt in the heart (Pearson, 2000). For the purposes of this chapter, anemic hypoxia will be referred to as hypoxia. The clinical presentation of the patient with anemia primarily is due to the effects of hypoxia.

Laboratory and Diagnostic Procedures

An assessment of the patient with anemia involves an analysis of laboratory studies. Common laboratory tests used in the diagnosis of anemia are the complete blood count (CBC) to detect hematologic alterations and arterial blood gases (ABGs) to detect acid–base disturbances used in the evaluation of hypoxia.

Complete Blood Count The complete blood count typically includes the following laboratory values pertinent to the study of red blood cells: hemoglobin (Hgb), hematocrit (Hct), red blood cells, reticulocyte mean corpuscle volume (MCV), and mean corpuscle hemoglobin (MCH). Normal values for these tests are summarized in Chart 63–1.

Hemoglobin values, as described in Chapter 62 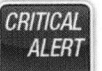, reflect the amount of hemoglobin protein measured in a volume of blood. Hemoglobin is decreased in cases of anemia of any etiology, hemorrhage, and hemodilution. Hemodilution occurs when excessive fluid (i.e., water and plasma) significantly dilutes a volume of blood, which can occur in situations such as water toxicity and excessive intravenous (IV) infusion. A significant drop in hemoglobin values (>3 g/dL) over a short time period (<24 hours) may indicate active bleeding.

CRITICAL ALERT *A significant drop in hemoglobin values (>3 g/dL over a short period of time [<24 hours]) should be reported immediately to the health care provider. This may indicate active blood loss. This finding is of particular concern if blood loss is not readily visible (i.e., from gums, emesis, or stool) suggesting internal bleeding. Patients should be immediately assessed for level of consciousness, lung sounds, and acute areas of pain.*

The hematocrit, as described in Chapter 62 , is the ratio of erythrocyte volume to a volume of whole blood, or the concentration of red blood cells. Hematocrit values follow the same pattern established by hemoglobin values: They decrease with excessive hydration (hemodilution), anemia, and hemorrhage.

The total RBC count reflects total volume of erythrocytes in a volume of blood. Total RBC values also tend to follow the directional patterns of hemoglobin and hematocrit. However, the total RBC value does not adequately indicate the quality or

---

CHART 63–1 Summary of Common Complete Blood Count Findings in Anemia

Lab Value	Normal Value	Expected Abnormality in Anemia	Rationale for Abnormality
Hemoglobin	*Women:* 12–16 g/dL *Men:* 13.5–18 g/dL	Decreased	Decreased hemoglobin production due to decreased erythrocyte production
Hematocrit	*Women:* 38–47% *Men:* 40–54%	Decreased	Decreased concentration of hemoglobin protein due to decreased erythrocyte production
Total RBC count	4.0–5.0 $10^6/\mu L$	Decreased	Reflects decreased total erythrocyte volume
Reticulocytes	0.5–1.5% of RBC count	Depends on etiology	Varies according to underlying etiology (acute or chronic, bone marrow involvement)

morphology of the erythrocytes. For these reasons, the morphologic RBC indices are often used in determination of anemia etiology, whereas the hemoglobin/hematocrit (H/H) ratio is more commonly used in the monitoring of anemia. Morphologic indices, as described in Chapter 62 , including MCV, MCH, MCHC (mean corpuscular hemoglobin concentration), and average concentration of hemoglobin in each red blood cell are useful tools in describing the blood cell structures characteristic of each type of anemia.

Reticulocytes reflect the number of juvenile erythrocytes present in peripheral blood. Reticulocytes increase in most types of sustained anemia as erythropoiesis accelerates as a compensatory mechanism. Decreases in reticulocytes are associated with bone marrow suppression or deficient production of erythrocytes. If a finding of decreased reticulocytes accompanies decreased total WBC count and decreased platelet count, a further examination including a bone marrow aspiration may be warranted in the work-up for leukemia, aplastic anemia, or some other life-threatening bone marrow failure.

CRITICAL ALERT *If decreased reticulocyte values accompany a global decrease in all cell lines (RBCs, WBCs, and platelets) the patient should be immediately assessed for bone marrow failure.*

Severity of Anemia

The severity of anemia symptoms generally is in direct proportion to the erythrocyte depletion as measured by the hemoglobin volume and hematocrit in the CBC. Delineating between severity states of anemia is somewhat arbitrary because a review of the literature reveals little agreement as to the exact hemoglobin values that constitute mild, moderate, or severe anemia states. Additionally, nurses should not rely solely on laboratory tests but must always incorporate physical and subjective findings when developing nursing interventions. Nonetheless, such delineation is a useful tool for discussion. Normal hemoglobin volume is defined at greater than 12 g/dL. Mild anemia is measured by a hemoglobin value of 10 to 12 g/dL. Moderate anemia is measured by a hemoglobin volume of 7 to 11 g/dL. Severe anemia is commonly defined by a hemoglobin volume of <7 g/dL and a hematocrit of less than 25%. Body system changes typically become more pronounced with increasing severity of anemia (Montoya, Wink, & Sole, 2002).

Physical Manifestations

The most common sign of anemia is generalized fatigue, as measured by patient self-report. The severity, pattern, and quality of fatigue are clinically significant findings that can contribute to the identification of an underlying etiology. In mild anemia, fatigue such as exertional dyspnea or lack of endurance may only manifest upon activity. With increasing severity of fatigue as hemoglobin levels drop, patients may report an inability to engage in activities of daily living (ADLs). Several fatigue severity scales that provide a rapid assessment of fatigue-related impairments have been validated in numerous research studies and are readily available for clinicians (Meek et al., 2000; Naschitz et al., 2004; Stouten, 2005). An example of one such fatigue scale, the Brief Fatigue Inventory, is shown in Figure 63–3 ■.

In addition to fatigue, physical manifestations of anemia can be grossly attributed to two major processes (Chart 63–2, p. 2012). The primary insult (hypoxia due to low erythrocyte volume) in-

flicts its own symptoms, whereas a secondary group of symptoms may arise from the body's attempt to compensate for the hypoxia. While every body system requires oxygen and, thus, is affected by anemia, the most notable evidence of hypoxia due to low erythrocyte volume can be observed in the cardiovascular system, the respiratory system, and in severe cases the neurological system (Lewis, Wallis, Leya, Hursting, & Kelton, 2003. Montoya et al., 2002):

1. **Cardiovascular system manifestations of anemia**—With mild anemia most patients may not report noticeable cardiovascular changes other than mildly increased fatigue. In moderate cases, the heart and vasculature system will attempt to compensate for decreased oxygen density by increasing the pulse rate (tachycardia). Sustained hypoxia or severe anemia can overcome the cardiovascular system, resulting in angina or even acute myocardial infarction.

2. **Respiratory system manifestations of anemia**—Anemic patients may present with varying degrees of respiratory difficulty. With mild cases of anemia, patients may experience exertional dyspnea or orthopnea.

3. **Neurological system manifestations of anemia**—Mild anemia typically does not result in neurological compromise. However, as hemoglobin levels drop and hypoxia increases (as in severe hemoglobin deficiency), patients may report headache, difficulty concentrating, vertigo, irritability, and eventually confusion.

Compensatory Mechanisms

In addition to the clinical presentation that results from hypoxia directly, nurses also must be aware of the manifestation of compensatory mechanisms. Biochemical detection of hypoxia in the bloodstream triggers a series of adaptive physiological compensatory mechanisms designed to slow organ damage. Despite the efficacy of these compensatory mechanisms, the reader should note that the oxygen requirements of tissues do not decrease over time. Hence, prolonged anemia and hypoxia can result in irreversible tissue damage if left unresolved. Immediately upon the detection of hypoxia, the body adapts with the following four processes:

1. **Decreased hemoglobin oxygen affinity**—Oxygen-starved, hypoxic peripheral tissues extract hemoglobin-bound oxygen from blood at high rates. Recall from the hemoglobin discussion earlier in the chapter that the configuration of the hemoglobin chains determines oxygen-binding capacity. Furthermore, the geometric configuration is driven by a number of environmental factors. Hypoxia creates an environment that causes the hemoglobin to form into an arrangement referred to as the **deoxyhemoglobin** configuration (Figure 63–4 ■, p. 2012).

   The result of this configuration is twofold. First, the heme iron atoms have a low binding affinity for oxygen, meaning that an oxygen (O_2) molecule is less likely to remain bound to the hemoglobin of an RBC. Secondly, the deoxyhemoglobin configuration stimulates the production of **2,3-diphosphoglycerate (2,3-DPG)**, which ultimately works to sustain the deoxyhemoglobin configuration. Both processes result in increased oxygen release to surrounding tissues. This process results in a *shift to the right*, a phrase used to summarize a graphical illustration of hemoglobin oxygen

Brief Fatigue Inventory

STUDY ID# _____   HOSPITAL # _____

Date: _____ / _____ / _____   Time: _____

Name: _____ _____ _____
           Last   First   Middle Initial

Throughout our lives, most of us have times when we feel very tired or fatigued. Have you felt unusually tired or fatigued in the past week?   Yes ☐   No ☐

1. Please rate your fatigue (weariness, tiredness) by circling the one number that best describes your fatigue right now.

0	1	2	3	4	5	6	7	8	9	10
No Fatigue										As bad as you can imagine

2. Please rate your fatigue (weariness, tiredness) by circling the one number that best describes your usual level of fatigue during the past 24 hours.

0	1	2	3	4	5	6	7	8	9	10
No Fatigue										As bad as you can imagine

3. Please rate your fatigue (weariness, tiredness) by circling the one number that best describes your worst level of fatigue during past 24 hours.

0	1	2	3	4	5	6	7	8	9	10
No Fatigue										As bad as you can imagine

4. Circle the one number that describes how, during the past 24 hours, fatigue has interfered with your:

A. General activity

0	1	2	3	4	5	6	7	8	9	10
Does not interfere										Completely Interferes

B. Mood

0	1	2	3	4	5	6	7	8	9	10
Does not interfere										Completely Interferes

C. Walking ability

0	1	2	3	4	5	6	7	8	9	10
Does not interfere										Completely Interferes

D. Normal work (includes both work outside the home and daily chores at home)

0	1	2	3	4	5	6	7	8	9	10
Does not interfere										Completely Interferes

E. Relations with other people

0	1	2	3	4	5	6	7	8	9	10
Does not interfere										Completely Interferes

F. Enjoyment of life

0	1	2	3	4	5	6	7	8	9	10
Does not interfere										Completely Interferes

FIGURE 63–3 ■ Brief Fatigue Inventory scale.

saturation as a function of oxygen partial pressure (Figure 63–5 ■, p. 2012). In cases of decreased hemoglobin oxygen affinity, any given partial pressure of oxygen is associated with less oxygen saturating the hemoglobin molecule. This translates to more unbound oxygen available to tissues, an effective short-term compensatory mechanism against hypoxia.

2. **Cardiovascular compensation**—In cases of severe anemia (measured by hemoglobin <7 g/dL), the resulting tissue hypoxia triggers cardiovascular compensation. First the cardiac output increases in an effort to circulate more blood. This increased heart rate is matched by a decrease in peripheral vasculature resistance to first allow blood to flow

---

CHART 63–2 **Common Signs of Anemia**

- Abnormal paleness or lack of color of the skin
- Increased heart rate (tachycardia)
- Increased respiratory rate (tachypnea)
- Breathlessness, or difficulty catching a breath (dyspnea)
- Lack of energy, or tiring easily (fatigue)
- Dizziness, or vertigo, especially when standing
- Headache
- Irritability
- Decreased hemoglobin, decreased hematocrit, decreased RBCs

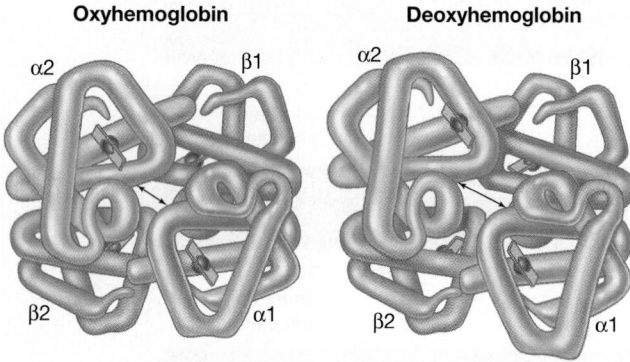

FIGURE 63–4 ■ Hemoglobin and deoxyhemoglobin, the oxygen transporter.

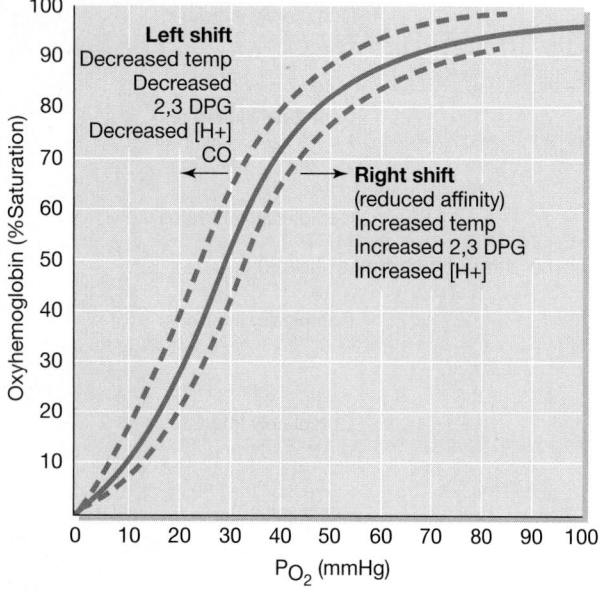

FIGURE 63–5 ■ Deoxyhemoglobin curve.

more quickly and then to reduce the oxygen demands of the heart muscle.

3. **Redistribution of blood flow**—Another compensatory mechanism is redistribution of blood flow. In hypoxic anemic states, the body selectively vasoconstricts blood vessels

to reroute oxygenated blood toward certain vital organs and away from less critical areas. Blood is shunted away from skin and toward the heart and brain and other critical organs. While this shunting preserves "critical organs" as long as possible, oxygen deprivation in the "less critical" organs can result in intermittent claudication and pain.

4. **Increased erythropoietin to stimulate RBC production**— Of interesting note, during the redistribution of blood flow, selective vasoconstriction shunts blood away from the kidneys, which are hardly noncritical organs. However, detection of hypoxia by the kidneys results in increased production of erythropoietin. Recall from the earlier discussion that erythropoietin is the critical cytokine that triggers erythropoiesis, which ultimately increases RBC mass. Thus, the shunting of blood away from the kidneys is an adaptive attempt at long-term resolution of anemia.

Care of the patient with anemia first requires resolution of hypoxia. Left unresolved, hypoxia can become a life-threatening medical emergency as critical organs are deprived of oxygen, instigating a cascade of cellular breakdown, tissue damage, organ failure, and possibly death. (See Chapter 35 ✐ for care of acute hypoxia.) If the hypoxia is associated with active and significant blood loss, an additional emergent priority is often the replacement of blood volume to attain erythrocyte levels sufficient to sustain oxygen delivery, as discussed later in the Anemia from Acute Blood Loss section.

In otherwise healthy patients without underlying hematologic disorders, these emergency interventions resolve not only the hypoxia, but the anemia as well. After stabilizing the cardiovascular, respiratory, and neurological risks of emergent hypoxia and blood loss, the focus shifts to determining the underlying cause of the anemia, usually via laboratory studies and a thorough history. Specific treatments and nursing interventions then are tailored to the underlying disease process. These specific treatments and nursing interventions are discussed later in relationship to each classification of anemia. However, some signs and symptoms and their correlating nursing interventions are common to all forms of anemia. These are discussed in the Nursing Process: Patient Care Plan for Generalized Anemia. When elderly patients are involved, the nurse should be aware of additional considerations, as outlined in the Gerontological Considerations box (p. 2015). The use of herbal supplements for the treatment of the fatigue that accompanies anemia is discussed in the Complementary and Alternative Therapies box (p. 2014).

Nursing Management

Nursing care for the patient presenting with anemia focuses on two goals: prevention of complications secondary to decreased oxygen-carrying capacity and thorough assessment to identify underlying etiologies. Decreased oxygen-carrying capacity carries the immediate risks associated with hypoxia: neurological and cardiac insults. Patients also frequently report activity intolerance and fatigue with sustained hypoxia, both of which must be addressed to prevent cardiovascular, respiratory, musculoskeletal, and digestive side effects.

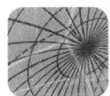

NURSING PROCESS: Patient Care Plan for Generalized Anemia

Assessment of Fatigue

Subjective Data:

Have you been short of breath? How long?

Do you have difficulty with energy throughout your day?

What makes it worse? What makes it better?

Do you have difficulty tolerating activity? Do you have difficulty with everyday chores?

Objective Data:

General: pallor, malaise, fatigue (preferably use validated scale)

Neurological: level of alertness, mental acuity

Respiratory: dyspnea, ventilation depth, tachypnea

Cardiovascular: tachycardia

Laboratory values: alterations to CBC

Nursing Assessment and Diagnoses	Outcomes and Evaluation Parameters	Planning and Interventions with *Rationales*
Nursing Diagnoses: *Activity Intolerance* related to decreased oxygen delivery to neuromuscular and cardiovascular systems	**Outcomes:** Free of shortness of breath. Able to perform ADLs. *Evaluation Parameters:* Patient self-report of lack of dyspnea upon exertion. Patient report of subjective decrease in bothersome fatigue effects as measured by fatigue scale scores. Unlabored respirations <24/min.	**Interventions and *Rationales:*** Assess normal activity pattern throughout day *in preparation for activity modification techniques (see below)*. Provide assistance with activities *to minimize shortness of breath.*
Self-Care Deficit related to fatigue and weakness impacting ability to participate in ADLs	**Outcome:** Patient reports appropriate self-care techniques. *Evaluation Parameters:* Patient/family verbalizes or demonstrates plan for accommodating self-care activities. Patient able to perform ADLs at a developmentally appropriate level. Patient demonstrates energy conservation techniques such as activity planning, appropriate exertion levels, and assistive devices as needed.	**Interventions and *Rationales:*** Modify activities to coincide with patient's biologic energy cycles. *Patients should maintain a minimum level of activity to prevent cardiovascular and muscoskeletal decompensation. However, patients may be discouraged by fatigue. Planning activities at points in the day with normally higher energy levels maintains patient participation in activity.*
Deficient Knowledge related to dietary causes, underlying etiologies, and patient self-management techniques	**Outcome:** Patient demonstrates knowledge of appropriate dietary modifications if indicated, lifestyle changes, and self-management techniques. *Evaluation Parameters:* Patient reports knowledge of diet modification (increased iron, folate, vitamin B_{12}) if appropriate. Patient demonstrates plan to incorporate appropriate activity level into daily care. Patient verbalizes understanding of underlying causes of anemia and fatigue.	**Interventions and *Rationales:*** Determine patient's previous knowledge of or skills related to his or her diagnosis and the influence on willingness to learn. *New information is assimilated into previous assumptions and facts and may involve negotiating, transforming, or stalling.* Provide developmentally appropriate patient education that addresses underlying disease process, diet modification, medications, and activity modification. *Symptoms of anemia may require long-term management that is optimized by patient compliance.*

Assessment of Hypoxia

Subjective Data:

Do you feel short of breath? Do you have chest pain?

Do other areas of your body ache? How often?

Do you feel dizzy?

Objective Data:

Dyspnea	Decreased hemoglobin and hematocrit
Decreased O_2 saturation	Dizziness
Tachycardia	Cyanosis
Tachypnea	Hepatomegaly/splenomegaly

(continued)

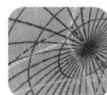

NURSING PROCESS: Patient Care Plan for Generalized Anemia—*Continued*

Nursing Assessment and Diagnoses	Outcomes and Evaluation Parameters	Planning and Interventions with *Rationales*
Nursing Diagnoses: *Impaired Gas exchange* related to insufficient hemoglobin oxygen delivery system, which can progress to cardiovascular, respiratory, neurological, and metabolic alterations	**Outcome:** Blood morphology and chemistry return to patient baseline. ***Evaluation Parameters:*** Hematocrit: • *Males:* 40.7–50.3% • *Females:* 36.1–44.3%. Hemoglobin: • *Males:* 13.8–17.2 g/dL • *Females:* 12.1–15.1 g/dL. RBC count: • *Males:* 4.7–6.1 million cells/µL • *Females:* 4.2–5.4 million cells/µL. ABG PaO_2: <90 ± 10. ABG pH: 7.35–7.45. Spot O_2 sat: <90% (depending on concurrent respiratory disease and age).	**Interventions and *Rationales:*** Monitor oxygen saturation levels and ABGs *as indicators of hypoxemia*. Administer supplemental oxygen when indicated *to maximize hemoglobin delivery of oxygen. However, use only when indicated by lab values. Hyperoxygenation suppresses erythropoiesis.* Administer blood transfusions for severe cases of anemia when ordered *to correct emergency deficiencies in oxygen delivery capacity.* Monitor for signs such as a falling hematocrit level, pain, pulmonary edema, fever, hypotension, hemolysis *as indicators of transfusion reactions (hemolysis and fluid overload).*
Risk of Injury: Falls related to weakness, dizziness, and possible compromised mental acuity	**Outcome:** Patient remains free of injury from falls. ***Evaluation Parameters:*** Patient experiences no injuries from falling. Environment is adjusted to minimize risk of falls. Patient verbalizes understanding of and demonstrates compliance with fall risk reduction plan.	**Interventions and *Rationales:*** Monitor for risk factors from falls such as unsteady gait, difficulty with transfers, orthopnea *to identify physiological and behavioral indicators of fall risk.* Adjust environment to minimize risk of falls by placing necessary items within reach of patient, positioning bed in low and locked position, frequent observation in an effort *to reduce additional risks of falls.* Reinforce patient instruction to call for assistance with ambulation if indicated *to avoid injury.* Assess vital signs (pulse, respirations, and BP) prior to ambulation *to identify possible need to alter mobility plan.*

Thorough assessments provide insight into the underlying etiology of anemia. Nurses are responsible for close monitoring of patient symptoms, alterations in laboratory values, and physical changes that may indicate the source of decreasing erythrocyte volume. Once these etiologies have been identified, the nurse, as part of the interdisciplinary health care team, is responsible for initiating interventions unique to that diagnosis.

The Nursing Process: Patient Care Plan for Generalized Anemia summarizes the interventions and rationales appropriate for patients presenting with initial signs and symptoms of anemia. This care plan is then enhanced with the nursing care indicated for specific underlying etiologies, which are discussed throughout the chapter.

COMPLEMENTARY & ALTERNATIVE THERAPIES

Herbal Supplements

Patients frequently seek out herbal supplements for the treatment of fatigue. The benefits of "energy boosters" are highly touted in the advertising for over-the-counter (OTC) preparations. Some patients who seek a more judicious integration of herbal and complementary medicine may enlist the care of a certified practitioner in complementary medicine, whereas others may rely solely on the advertising associated with OTC preparations.

Common herbs used for anemia include Spirulina, or blue-green algae (Mao, Van De Water, & Gershwin, 2000), alfalfa (*Medicago sativa*), dandelion (*Taraxacum officinale*) root or leaf, burdock (*Arctium lappa*), yellowdock (*Rumex crispus*), and dong quai (*Angelica sinensis*) (Blumenthal, 1999). If patients seek out homeopathic therapy, they may be prescribed ferrum phosphoricum or calcarea phosphorica. In addition to herbs, many patients may self-administer vitamins and minerals such as vitamin B_{12}, folic acid, and, most commonly, iron.

Many patients hold the common perception that herbs are natural and, therefore, inherently benign, however, many herbs can interact with traditionally prescribed medications or, if taken inappropriately, inflict untoward effects. The use of herbs, supplements, and vitamins should always be included and integrated into a thorough patient care plan.

References

Blumenthal, M. (1999). Twenty-seven major botanicals and their uses in the United States. In D. Eskinazi, M. Blumenthal, N. Farnsworth, & C. W. Riggins (Eds.), *Botanical medicine* (pp. 18–19). Larchmont, NY: Mary Ann Liebert.

Mao, T. K., Van De Water, J., & Gershwin, M. E. (2000). Effect of Spirulina on the secretion of cytokines from peripheral blood mononuclear cells. *Journal of Medicinal Food, 3*(3), 135–139.

GERONTOLOGICAL CONSIDERATIONS for Anemia

The frail elderly adult is at increased risk of anemia for several reasons ranging from the physiological changes associated with aging and the prevalence of comorbidities to nutritional deficiencies and sometimes the psychosocial consequences of aging. Agreement surrounding the prevalence of anemia in the older adult varies greatly, perhaps due to inconsistencies in the reporting of anemia. The most comprehensive study to date has been the third *National Health and Nutrition Examination Survey (NHANES) 1988–1994* (National Center for Health Statistics, 2008), which evaluated anemia in the community-dwelling adult. In persons 65 years and older, anemia was present in 11.0% of men and 10.2% of women, with the prevalence rising to more than 20% in people 85 years and older.

Nutritional deficiencies account for a large portion of anemia seen in older adults due in part to decreased appetite and difficulty in chewing. However, social processes such as meal preparation and financial constraints also may negatively impact an older adult's ability to consistently consume a well-balanced diet. Comorbidities such as cardiovascular disease, lung disease, cancer, and kidney failure can also negatively impact anemia by their effects on the organs of erythropoiesis, namely, the bone marrow and the erythropoietin-stimulating system of the kidneys. Perhaps most damaging to the effective treatment of anemia in the older adult is the unfortunate practice of dismissing patient reports of decreasing activity intolerance as a "normal part of aging." Although some decline in endurance and cardiovascular capacity may occur with age, symptoms such as ataxia, worsening angina, severe dyspnea, and certainly abnormal laboratory studies warrant further evaluation.

The consequences of anemia in the older adult have been associated with significant morbidities, further highlighting the need for vigilance. Anemia late in life has been correlated with increased rate of falls (Penninx et al., 2005), decreased muscle strength (Penninx et al., 2005), and a higher rate of hip fractures requiring surgery and increased length of stay (Dharmarajan, Pais, & Norkus, 2005). Tachycardia due to the compensatory mechanisms in sustained anemia also has been correlated with increased mortality. In chronic kidney failure in the older adult, sustained decreased hematocrit levels have been associated with left ventricular hypertrophy, increased morbidity and mortality, and poor quality of life (Lipschitz, 2003). The nurse plays a vital role in patient advocacy as part of providing adequate and unbiased care to the older adult.

Discharge Priorities

Management of anemia needs to continue after hospital discharge and may require long-term lifestyle and dietary change. It is essential that the patient and family be given the necessary information to make these changes. The Patient Teaching & Discharge Priorities box (p. 2016) outlines important information that should be conveyed to patients with generalized anemia.

Health Promotion

Treatment of anemia often involves lifestyle alterations to diet and activity level. Part of the assessment of the patient with anemia must include an evaluation of nutrition intake, especially iron, folate, vitamin B_{12}, and proteins because these are all required for erythropoiesis. Nurses play a critical role in helping patients identify dietary sources of these vital nutrients. The sections on iron deficiency anemia, folate deficiency anemia, and vitamin B_{12} anemia provide specific information about a diet that will provide these nutrients.

Activity level also must be addressed as part of a complete patient care plan. Anemia frequently is associated with fatigue and dyspnea, which may suppress a patient's ability to participate in ADLs or to maintain prior physical activity levels. However, mobility and exercise should be maintained to prevent cardiovascular and musculoskeletal deconditioning. If either of these two processes occurs, patients may run the risk of further exacerbating their fatigue and dyspnea. Nurses again play a pivotal role in assisting patients in identifying appropriate activity goals and incorporating activity into the daily patient care plan.

◾ Collaborative Management

Comprehensive care of the patient with anemia requires the collaboration of an interdisciplinary team including registered dieticians, physical and occupational therapists, respiratory therapists, pharmacists, health care providers, and nurses. Registered dieticians can provide excellent resources to patients on how to identify and treat dietary deficiencies that exacerbate anemia and how to conserve energy when preparing meals. Additionally, the scientific grounding of the registered dietician can help patients evaluate the numerous health benefits claimed in food advertising.

Respiratory therapists are identified experts in the diagnosis of hypoxia, especially in delineating anemic hypoxia from hypoxia of respiratory etiology. Their expertise is particularly valuable when evaluating the judicious use of oxygen therapy. Physical and occupational therapists play a key role in mobility preservation. Consultation with a physical and occupational therapist should be made early (within a few days of admission) so that exercise techniques can be incorporated early on before debilitating severe anemia takes hold. Some studies have even indicated that early mobility can actually act as a preventive measure, increasing the need for collaboration with physical and occupational therapists (Mock, 2004). The pharmacist's knowledge of pharmacokinetics and drug–drug and drug–food interactions is of tremendous benefit to a patient care plan and their guidance should be sought whenever medications are to be evaluated or prescribed.

Anemia from Acute Blood Loss

Anemia from acute blood loss describes the loss of RBC volume due to RBCs leaving the circulating vascular space. Anemia from blood loss comprises a heterogeneous group of disorders ranging from "slow bleeds" to rapid trauma. Appropriate care of these patients focuses on determination of the underlying cause, prevention of immediate cardiovascular and hematologic emergencies, and, if appropriate, attenuation of underlying disease.

Pathophysiology and Etiology

When discussing the mechanisms responsible for anemia due to blood loss, three parameters should be included: underlying cause, rapidity of onset, and volume lost. Underlying causes include obvious bleeding such as trauma or menorrhagia (excessive menstrual bleeding) as well as less visible causes such as disorders of the gastrointestinal mucosa, slow cranial bleeding, and internal hemorrhage. Nurses should not rely solely on visible blood as an indication of bleeding, and instead should be aware of the system clinical presentation of blood loss, as discussed later. Bleeding that

PATIENT TEACHING & DISCHARGE PRIORITIES for Generalized Anemia

Need	Teaching
Knowledge of dietary modifications	Of particular importance in iron deficiency anemia and megaloblastic anemias. Consult with registered dietitian to provide patient and family with effective tools and resources regarding meal planning, appropriate foods, and guidance on food label reading.
	Teach patients to eat frequent small meals to prevent fatigue.
Fatigue management	Reinforce teaching regarding daily fatigue scale.
	Teach patients to discuss results and trends of fatigue scale self-assessment with health care provider.
	Reinforce teaching regarding activity modification to maintain and preserve energy levels.
	Reinforce teaching that energy levels may decrease as a physiological response to disease process, and that asking for assistance and/or adjusting previous work/home activity schedules may be necessary.
	Suggest appropriate exercise activities for patient status including brief walks, chair exercises, bed exercises.
	Reinforce education regarding mobility as an effective means of prevention of cardiovascular and musculoskeletal deconditioning.
Understanding of medications	For iron supplementation, teach patients correct timing of administration and possible side effects (constipation). Reinforce key teaching points regarding hydration, constipation management, and iron absorption (see Chart 63–7, p. 2022).
	For hematopoietic growth factors, reinforce administration schedule for subcutaneous injections, which may include appointments with health care provider.
	Reinforce education regarding possible side effects of subcutaneous hematopoietic growth factors including bone pain and injection site soreness.
Disease prevention	Explain the need for maintenance of hemoglobin levels to ensure adequate oxygenation to tissues, thus decreasing risk of cardiac disease and infection.
Safety	Stress the importance of a medic alert bracelet to identify a heart problem to health care providers.
Reportable clinical manifestations	Instruct patient/family to report: • Change in exercise tolerance • Change in activity tolerance • Onset of new pain especially chest pain, headaches, or abdominal pain.

results from chronic conditions including Crohn's disease, diverticulitis, and rheumatoid arthritis frequently is associated with inflammation; this causes a functional iron deficiency and thus anemia. This syndrome is discussed in the Anemia of Chronic Disease section.

The rapidity of the blood loss impacts the body's ability to respond with compensatory mechanisms, which, in turn, relates to clinical presentation. With slow bleeds, which occur over the course of days to weeks, baroreceptors in the peripheral vascular system detect decreased pressure and respond by increasing plasma volume to preserve cardiovascular status. With this increase in volume, the heart and vascular system can generate enough blood pressure to maintain peripheral perfusion in the critical organs of the heart, lungs, brain, and kidneys. This process can result in a form of dilution anemia, in which the RBC mass is diluted by the increase in plasma volume. Hypoxia from this dilutional anemia is prevented by the compensatory mechanisms discussed earlier, including decreased hemoglobin oxygen affinity (shift to the right) and increased erythropoietin to stimulate RBC production. When the blood loss is rapid, occurring over the course of hours to days, total blood volume (including both RBCs and plasma) can decrease so severely as to cause hypovolemic shock. Hypovolemic shock is a medical emergency associated with high mortality and requires immediate emergency management interventions (see Chapter 61).

The third consideration is the total volume lost. With blood losses of up to 20% of total blood volume (Adamson, 2005), the compensatory mechanism of peripheral vasoconstriction initiates to shift blood flow to organs responsible for maintaining cardiovascular function and preventing hypoxia and hypovolemia. When blood loss becomes more pronounced, the body lacks sufficient circulating blood volume to support the vascular system or maintain adequate hydration and oxygenation of vital organs. The body's first attempt is to intensify cardiovascular compensatory mechanisms (tachycardia). However, with blood loss of at least 40% or more, all compensatory mechanisms become rapidly overwhelmed and symptoms of shock are imminent.

Clinical Presentation

Clinical presentation of the patient with blood loss is directly correlated to the *rapidity, location,* and *volume* of blood loss. Thorough assessment must include laboratory hematologic findings as well as cardiovascular measurements (pulse, blood pressure, and respiratory rate), integumentary signs (pallor, temperature, and diaphoresis), and renal and neurological changes. The action of multiple compensatory mechanisms may mask signs of anemia unless a multifaceted assessment is completed.

Physical Manifestations

Patients suspected of acute blood loss should be thoroughly monitored for changes in cardiovascular, integumentary, renal, and neurological status. These changes are summarized in the Nursing Process: Patient Care Plan for Generalized Anemia (p. 2013) and include tachycardia, tachypnea, decreased level of alertness, pallor, decreased urinary output, and diaphoresis. These start to become apparent with acute, rapid blood loss or when slow blood loss exceeds 20% of baseline. Additionally, bleeds of relatively small volume (i.e., less than 20%) into closed spaces can cause severe pain, swelling, tenderness, sudden changes in neurological status, and eventually death. Bleeding into the cranial vault, the pericardium, the pleural space, or musculoskeletal compartments is a medical emergency that requires prompt attention by the medical team. Please refer to specific chapters addressing these systems for a full discussion.

Bleeding into the gastrointestinal (GI) tract is often first detected via an observation of fecal occult blood, or hidden blood, in the stool. Fecal occult blood tests are cost-effective and rapid indicators of GI bleeding and, thus, are widely used as screening tools. **Melena**, or black tarry stools, appears when bacteria have had enough time to break down blood into component chemicals. In the case of lower GI bleeding, blood may not be in the colon long enough for bacterial breakdown; therefore, the presence of melena should not be the only indicator used to detect GI bleeding.

Alterations in Laboratory Values

For sudden blood loss, hematocrit values may not accurately indicate the severity of the problem because RBC mass is lost at the same rate as total blood volume; thus, the percentage of RBCs in the blood is unaffected. (Recall that hematocrit measures the percentage of RBCs in a volume of blood.) However, after 2 to 3 days when the body is able to initiate the compensatory mechanism of increasing plasma volume, RBCs become diluted, as reflected by decreasing erythrocyte, hemoglobin, and hematocrit values (Chart 63–3).

 CRITICAL ALERT *Any patient reporting with sudden pain in the abdominal area, retroperitoneal area, or musculoskeletal fascial compartments or a change in level of consciousness should be immediately assessed for blood pressure, pulse, and respiratory rate changes. These may indicate bleeding into a closed space, which requires immediate medical intervention. Do not rely on changes in laboratory values because these may not accurately reflect blood loss.*

Medical Management

The immediate goal of treatment for acute blood loss is prevention of cardiovascular collapse and hypoxia. Most patients presenting with slow bleeds also have normal kidney function, normal bone marrow function, and an adequate supply of iron. For these patients, the increased erythropoietin production is sufficient to compensate for lost RBCs; thus, additional treatment with blood products is unwarranted. Attention then turns to identification of the underlying disease process and attenuation of the blood loss. A thorough history will assist the clinician in identifying possible causes such as GI bleeding from intake of nonsteroidal inflammatory drugs (NSAIDs). Transfusion of red blood cells may be indicated for some patients to prevent cardiovascular system collapse. These patients are identified by a sudden decrease in hematocrit by more than 3%, significant observable hemorrhage, a hematocrit of <25%, or severe impending hypovolemia.

◾ Nursing Management

Nursing priorities in the care of patients suspected of acute blood loss are multifaceted, evolving with the degree of blood loss and stage of treatment. The first goal is careful observation for early indicators of blood loss, especially in patients who present with high-risk diagnoses. Postoperative patients are at particular risk

CHART 63–3	**Signs and Symptoms of Acute Blood Loss**			
% Blood Loss	**Approximate Volume in Adult (5,000 mL [79 kg])**	**Symptoms**	**Physical Syndrome**	**Measurable Signs**
<20	<1,000	Possible restlessness	Vasovagal reaction (peripheral vasoconstriction)	BP may be normal HR may be normal Urine output may be normal
20–30	1,000–1,500	Anxiety, dyspnea on exertion	Orthostatic hypotension, tachycardia on exertion	BP > 90 mmHg systolic HR 100–120 bpm RR > 24 Urine output 25–30 mL/hr
30–40	1,500–2,000	Syncope on sitting and standing	Orthostatic hypotension, tachcardia at rest	BP 70–90 systolic HR > 120 beats/min Cool, pale skin RR increased Urine output 5–15 mL/hr
40	>2,000	Confusion, shortness of breath	Shock	BP < 90 systolic HR > 140 beats/min Cold, clammy skin RR increased/hyperventilation Urine output minimal

Sources: Adapted from Gosch, S., Watts, D., & Kinnear, M. (2002). Management of gastrointestinal hemorrhage. *Postgraduate Medical Journal, 78*(915), 4; Green, B. T., & Rockey, D. C. (2003). Acute gastrointestinal bleeding. *Seminars in Gastrointestinal Disease, 14*(2), 44. Kasper, D. L., Fauci, A. S., Longo, D. L., Braunwald, E., Hauser, S. L., & Jameson, J. L. (Eds.), *Harrison's principles of internal medicine* (16th ed.). New York: McGraw-Hill.

of bleeding from new incisions (both internal and external) and should be carefully monitored for changes in level of consciousness, cardiovascular changes from baseline, excessive blood loss from incision sites, and reports of pain.

Other high-risk populations include but are not limited to patients presenting with abdominal pain of known or unknown etiology, patients with musculoskeletal trauma, and patients with deficient platelet function. Monitoring of these patients should involve comprehensive assessment of hematologic laboratory studies, trends in urine output, trends in cardiovascular indicators (blood pressure, pulse, and respirations), integumentary changes, pain descriptions, and musculoskeletal changes.

If transfusions are administered, nursing goals revolve around the safe administration of blood products and monitoring for signs and symptoms of fluid overload or a transfusion reaction, both of which are discussed later in this chapter in the section on transfusion therapy (also see Chapter 23 ☉). Once the source of the blood loss is identified, nursing interventions, including patient education, assessment, and treatment administration, become specific to the underlying disease process. Generally, once the source of blood loss is identified and resolved, no further treatment of anemia due to acute blood loss is warranted.

Iron Deficiency Anemia

Iron deficiency anemia (IDA) is the most common underlying cause of anemia worldwide. Although iron deficiency is more common in developing countries, a significant prevalence was observed in the United States during the early 1990s among certain populations, such as toddlers and females of childbearing age. One of the national *Healthy People 2010* objectives is to reduce iron deficiency in these vulnerable populations by 3% to 4% (U.S. Department of Health and Human Services, 2000).

Recall from the discussion on hematopoiesis that iron is required for the heme portion of the hemoglobin protein. Thus, erythrocyte production is slowed when iron-dependent hemoglobin supplies are depleted or insufficient. The erythrocytes that are produced are morphologically distinct because of their small size (**microcytic**) and pale color (**hypochromic**). Signs and symptoms of anemia appear when iron supplies are depleted to the point that the physiological needs of erythropoiesis cannot be met. Depletion of iron stores can be a result of a variety of underlying causes including dietary intake insufficiency,

blood loss, or malabsorption disorders. The responsibilities of the health care provider are to first address any immediate needs of anemia such as hypoxia, then to determine and correct the underlying cause of the iron deficiency.

Iron Metabolism

Alterations in iron metabolism have consequences in many forms of anemia, including iron deficiency anemia, anemia of chronic disease, thalassemia, and hemolytic spherocytosis. Estimates of total iron body stores in healthy adults vary from 2.5 to 4.5 grams in women, to 3.5 to 5.5 grams in men. International differences in body size and normal values account for the variation in commonly reported values.

Iron is distributed throughout the body in both active metabolic forms and storage forms. Hemoglobin typically houses 2,100 mg of iron, representing the most significant active metabolic form. Other active forms include myoglobin (200 mg); metabolic tissues of the liver, spleen, and bone marrow (150 mg); and the iron transportation system (3 mg). Iron also exists in two "storage forms" within cells, as **ferritin** (700 mg) and **hemosiderin** (300 mg). These storage forms are metabolically inactive, meaning they do not directly contribute to erythropoiesis, oxygen transport, or immune or neurological function; rather they act like iron reservoirs.

Approximately 1 mg of iron is lost on a daily basis from a variety of mechanisms, namely, via cell **desquamation**, or the shedding of the outer epidermal layer. To maintain bodily functions, the body requires about 25 mg daily, which is partially derived through dietary absorption (1 mg) via the intestines. However, the majority of the daily iron requirement is supplied from the storage forms (Koury & Ponka, 2004; Miret, Simpson, & McKie, 2003; Umbreit, 2005; Weiss, 2002). For this reason, serum ferritin is commonly included in the analysis of IDA.

As iron is consumed, it is absorbed via the intestinal cells of the duodenum and jejunum and immediately forms a complex with iron transport proteins, namely, **transferrin**, which delivers the iron molecule to the target cells (growing erythrocytes, placenta cells, liver cells, spleen, and bone marrow). The amount of transferrin-bound iron is commonly used for measurement of iron levels. Iron molecules that will not be immediately used for erythropoiesis are converted to the storage forms ferritin and hemosiderin (Chart 63–4).

The rate of intestinal cell absorption is regulated by physiological needs. Absorption *increases* with decreased iron stores,

| CHART 63–4 | **Key Chemicals of Iron Metabolism** |

Chemical	Function	Physiological Consequences
Ferritin	Storage form	Used as measurement of iron status. High ferritin level indicates adequate status.
Hemosiderin	Storage form	Measurement of iron status. High hemosiderin level indicates adequate status, although test is rarely performed due to prevalence of ferritin.
Transferrin	Delivers iron to target cell	High levels of iron-bound transferrin indicate adequate iron status.
Hepcidin	Hormone that regulates iron absorption	Inhibits iron absorption. Increases macrophage consumption of iron. Increases (stimulated by infection, inflammation, and malignancy) result in decreased iron available for erythropoiesis. Decreases cause iron overload.

detection of a low peripheral erythrocyte count, increased erythropoietic activity in the bone marrow (i.e., pregnancy, growth spurts), or hypoxemia. Conversely, intestinal iron absorption *decreases* in the presence of inflammation, a process that contributes to the "anemia of inflammation" or "anemia of chronic diseases" (Weiss, 2002). The body produces a variety of systemic signals (neurotransmitters, hormones, and cytokines) in response to these stimuli. **Hepcidin**, produced by the liver, has been identified as the key regulatory hormone of iron absorption, adjusting the rate of iron absorption in response to total iron body reservoirs. Although the exact molecular mechanism remains to be elucidated, an emerging current body of research suggests that these systemic signals act on the intestinal cells of the duodenum and jejunum to alter iron absorption through regulation of the iron transport proteins (Koury & Ponka, 2004; Miret et al., 2003).

Pathophysiology

Iron deficiency anemia results from a combination of one or more processes: (1) excess iron loss, (2) iron absorption abnormalities, (3) reallocation of iron stores, and (4) insufficient dietary intake. Excess iron loss, iron absorption abnormalities, and insufficient dietary intake are classified as **absolute iron deficiencies** indicating insufficient amounts of total body iron. Reallocation of iron stores is referred to as a **functional iron deficiency**, which is a condition in which there is a failure to supply enough iron to the bone marrow for erythropoiesis, despite adequate total body iron stores. Each of these etiologies is associated with some underlying behavioral or pathologic process:

1. **Excess iron loss**—Blood loss, and the iron housed in the hemoglobin, is the leading cause of iron deficiency (Ponka, 2001). Chronic blood loss is most commonly attributed to gastrointestinal bleeding. Causes of GI bleeding include peptic ulcer disease, diverticulitis, hemorrhoids, esophageal varices, tumors, steroids, small tears along the rectum, and use of NSAIDs (see Chapter 45 ⊙). Many of these processes can exist for long periods of time, evading detection by the patient and cumulatively allowing for a substantial loss of blood and iron. One milliliter of blood contains about 0.5 mg of iron. A steady blood loss of as little as 3 to 4 mL per day, which often goes undetected by the patient, results in 1.5 to 2 mg of lost iron daily. This loss places excess demand on daily iron needs, resulting in a negative iron balance. Menstrual bleeding, which typically results in 40 to 80 mL of daily blood loss, also is associated with iron deficiency anemia, in part explaining the prevalence of iron deficiency anemia (IDA) among women.

2. **Iron absorption abnormalities**—Iron absorption abnormalities refer to any clinical situation that decreases the rate of intestinal absorption. As discussed earlier, absorption relies on the intricate interplay between intestinal cells, systemic cell signals, the iron transport system, and the storage forms of iron. Gastrointestinal tract abnormalities, such as surgical manipulation, Crohn's disease, and celiac disease, reduce the intestinal wall surface available for iron absorption. Liver disease also can result in IDA because transferrin is synthesized in the liver and the storage forms (ferritin and hemosiderin) partially reside in the hepatic cells of the liver. Additionally, several studies are beginning to examine IDA that stems from genetic alterations in the iron transport proteins and intestinal absorption systemic signals, specifically hepcidin (Koury & Ponka, 2004; Miret et al., 2003; Umbreit, 2005; Weiss, 2002).

3. **Reallocation of iron stores**—Reallocation of iron stores refers to situations in which total body iron supplies are at normal levels, but the iron molecule is unavailable for erythropoiesis. In chronic inflammatory conditions, available iron is preferentially allocated to increased macrophage production. Again, hepcidin has been identified as the key hormone regulating macrophage consumption of iron. In fetal development, iron also is preferentially delivered to the developing fetus; however, maternal erythropoiesis may be impacted.

4. **Insufficient dietary intake**—When any of the preceding situations occurs, demand for iron can exceed iron intake. Initially, the storage forms act as buffers to adequately supply the active metabolic needs of the body. The efficiency of the storage forms means that early iron deficiency often is asymptomatic and therefore goes unreported by the patient. Hemoglobin and erythrocyte values are only mildly decreased, if at all. However, serum ferritin values may decrease from normal. Eventually, however, depletion of the storage forms can quickly outpace dietary intake, and the serum ferritin concentration falls. Erythropoiesis is impaired, producing pale (hypochromic), small (microcytic) erythrocytes. The decreased oxygen delivery capacity of these impaired erythrocytes results in the signs and symptoms of anemia.

Clinical Presentation

Iron deficiency anemia can have an insidious progression, often with no reportable symptoms despite falling iron stores. As iron depletion proceeds, IDA produces the signs common to all anemias and eventually manifests with morphologic, neurological, and integumentary symptoms unique to iron depletion. A laboratory analysis will reveal both qualitative and quantitative changes to RBC components. Oftentimes, IDA is first detected in the primary care setting during routine physicals or when patients seek evaluation for bothersome symptoms. The U.S. Preventive Services Task Force (2006) and the Centers for Disease Control and Prevention (CDC) (1998) have both issued national guidelines to assist practitioners in the early identification and treatment of these patients in an effort to prevent severe negative outcomes related to iron deficiency (see the National Guidelines box, p. 2020). In the acute care setting, iron deficiency most often presents as a consequence of bleeding, decreased oral intake, or chronic disease.

Physical Manifestations

Because the body's highly efficient iron storage system provides a rich reservoir for active metabolic needs, early IDA often does not produce bothersome symptoms. As with all anemia, the severity of the symptoms correlates to the degree of hemoglobin deficiency, which, in turn, correlates to volume of total iron body stores. As erythropoiesis becomes increasingly hampered, the patient may present with the general manifestations of anemia such as fatigue, pallor, shortness of breath, cold intolerance, headache, and activity intolerance. When iron stores fall critically low such that epithelial cell production is affected, the patient may present

---

NATIONAL GUIDELINES for Screening for Iron Deficiency Anemia

Source	Recommended Guideline
U.S. Preventive Services Task Force (2006) Centers for Disease Control and Prevention (1998)	*Recommendation:* Routine screening for iron deficiency anemia in asymptomatic pregnant women *Recommendation:* Routine iron supplementation for asymptomatic children ages 6 to 12 months who are at increased risk for iron deficiency anemia *Recommendation:* Periodic screening for anemia among high-risk populations of infants and preschool children, pregnant women, and nonpregnant women of childbearing age *Recommendation:* Universal iron supplementation to meet the iron requirements of pregnancy.

---

with symptoms uniquely indicative of IDA including pica (clay eating), glossitis (tongue inflammation), gastric atrophy, stomatitis, ice eating (pagophagia), and leg cramping (Montoya et al., 2002). Presentation of any of these symptoms beginning with mild activity intolerance warrants further evaluation of iron status.

Alterations in Laboratory Values

Laboratory tests in IDA reveal decreased erythrocytes common to all anemias. Hemoglobin and hematocrit levels also decrease in accordance with the severity of anemia. Additionally, low iron in the heme produces morphologically distinct erythrocytes. The MCV, MCHC, and MCH morphological indices are all decreased indicating a microcytic (small), hypochromic (light) cell suggestive of IDA. These erythrocyte changes are shown in Figure 63–6 ■.

Definitive diagnosis requires bone marrow aspiration revealing absent marrow stores of iron. However, other laboratory findings are sufficient to begin treatment of IDA, most notably low serum iron, serum ferritin, and serum transferrin and an elevated total iron binding capacity (TIBC). Serum iron levels fall as total body iron decreases; however, this value is highly sensitive to recent changes in diet. A decrease in serum ferritin is a more accurate indicator of iron stores. Serum transferrin (also referred to as TIBC) increases as a compensatory attempt to harvest more iron from the intestines, thus its value *increases* in IDA. These laboratory findings are summarized in the Diagnostic Tests box.

Medical Management

Treatment of iron deficiency anemia addresses three goals: alleviation of immediate distress caused by anemia, identification of the underlying etiology, and replacement of iron, if indicated. Immediate distress of anemia includes hypoxia and activity intolerance as discussed in the earlier section on generalized ane-

mia. A comprehensive patient assessment should include GI symptoms, menstrual patterns, or dietary changes because these will assist the practitioner in identifying the underlying etiology.

Because the majority of chronic blood loss is due to GI bleeding, a fecal occult stool is often ordered especially in the absence of adolescent growth spurts, menses, and pregnancy. A fecal occult stool test is an important and cost-effective first step in early detection of GI bleeding, particularly since melena (dark tarry stool) requires a relatively large blood loss of 50 to 75 mL from the intestinal tract. More invasive exploratory procedures may be indicated to first determine the source of the bleeding (cancerous tumors, polyps, ulcers), and also to stop hemorrhage if detected.

Dietary Modifications

Replacement of iron stores is first attempted with dietary alterations (Chapter 14). Dietary iron is consumed in one of two forms: **heme iron**, which is available in red meats and fish, and **nonheme iron**, which is available in vegetables, cereals, and fortified foods. A significant chemical difference exists between the two forms that impact their utility in dietary medication. Heme iron is considered readily **bioavailable**, meaning that its molecular configuration is readily used in erythropoiesis. More importantly perhaps, heme iron is much better absorbed (15% absorption rate) in the intestinal tract than nonheme iron (<5% absorption rate). Lastly, heme iron is rarely reduced by the presence of other substances in the intestinal tract. Nonheme iron absorption, however, is reduced by tannins (found in tea), calcium, polyphenols, and phytates (found in legumes and whole grains). Ascorbic acid is the only common food element known to increase nonheme iron bioavailability.

Consideration of bioavailability and food–food interactions should be included in patient education about dietary modifications (Grinder-Pederson, Bukhave, Jensen, Hojgaard, & Hansen, 2004; Hunt, 2003; Lopez & Martos, 2004; Umbreit, 2005). A major focus of nutrition research is the study of the interaction between various food groups and iron absorption.

Oral Iron Supplementation

Iron supplementation may be indicated if dietary modification alone is insufficient to correct iron stores, especially in severe cases of iron deficiency anemia (serum ferritin level that falls >10 from baseline). Supplemental iron is available in two forms: ferrous and ferric. Ferrous iron salts (ferrous fumarate, ferrous sulfate, and ferrous gluconate) are the best absorbed forms of iron supplements (Hoffman et al., 2000). For adults who are not pregnant, the CDC

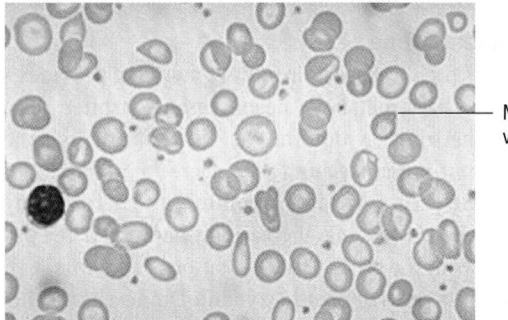

Microcytic RBC with light center

FIGURE 63–6 ■ Peripheral smear showing microcytic erthrocytes of IDA.
Source: Annita B. Watson

DIAGNOSTIC TESTS for Iron Deficiency Anemia

Test and Normal Values	Expected Abnormality in IDA	Rationale for Abnormality
Hemoglobin *Women:* 12–16 g/dL *Men:* 13.5–18 g/dL	Decreased	Early stages of IDA, hemoglobin will not be affected. In severe cases, low iron stores decrease hemoglobin production.
Hematocrit *Women:* 38–47% *Men:* 40–54%	Decreased	Decreased concentration of hemoglobin.
Serum Iron (Fe) *Women:* 63–140 µg/dL (11–25 µmol/L) *Men:* 75–150 µg/dL (13–27 µmol/L)	Decreased	Indicates decreased serum iron concentration. However, may be artificially increased by recent dietary ingestion or hemolytic states.
Serum ferritin 30–300 ng/mL *Average woman:* 49 *Average man:* 88	Decreased	Highly sensitive measurement of total body iron stores. The plasma ferritin value often falls to under 10% of its baseline level with significant iron deficiency.
Serum transferrin (also referred to as total iron binding capacity [TIBC]) 250–460 µg/dL	>8.5 µg/mL	Iron transport protein. Production is increased in response to low iron stores or increased iron needs.

CHART 63–5   **Common Oral Iron Supplement Formulations**

Generic Name	Tablet (mg) (Elemental Iron Content [mg])	Elixir Iron Content (mg in 5 mL)
Ferrous sulfate	325 mg (65 mg elemental iron)	300 mg (60 mg elemental iron)
	195 mg (39 mg elemental iron)	90 mg (18 mg elemental iron)
Extended-release ferrous sulfate	525 mg (105 mg elemental iron)	
Ferrous fumarate	325 mg (107 mg elemental iron)	
	195 mg (64 mg elemental iron)	100 mg (33 mg elemental iron)
Ferrous gluconate	325 mg (39 mg elemental iron)	300 mg (35 mg elemental iron)

Source: Adamson, J. W. (2005). Iron deficiency and other hypoproliferative anemias. In D. L. Kasper, A. S. Fauci, D. L. Longo, E. Braunwald, S. L. Hauser, & J. L. Jameson (Eds.), *Harrison's principles of internal medicine* (16th ed., pp. 587–593). New York: McGraw-Hill.

recommends taking 50 to 60 mg of oral elemental iron (the approximate amount of elemental iron in one 300-mg tablet of ferrous sulfate) twice daily for 3 months for the therapeutic treatment of IDA. **Elemental iron** is the amount of iron in a supplement that is available for absorption (Chart 63–5).

Iron supplements can cause several gastrointestinal side effects, including constipation and upper epigastric pain, which contribute to patient noncompliance. Patient education should include techniques that can avoid such complications and also enhance iron absorption (see Chart 63–6). Switching to milder oral preparation such as ferrous gluconate tablets (325 mg with 39 mg of elemental iron) of carbonyl iron (Ircon) may be indicated if these techniques continue to prove unsuccessful.

Response to oral iron supplementation may be measured by an increase in peripheral reticulocytes as soon as 4 days after initiation of therapy, and by a rise in hemoglobin, hematocrit, and serum ferritin within 2 to 3 weeks. Patients should be advised to continue therapy for 2 to 3 months to fully restore depleted iron storage reservoirs (National Institutes of Health, 2005).

Parenteral Iron Supplementation

Parenteral iron supplementation may be indicated for patients who require more rapid correction of depleted iron stores or pa-

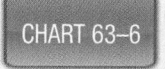**CHART 63–6**   **Patient Education Regarding Oral Iron Supplements**

- Supplemental iron tablets should be taken 3 to 4 times daily per your health care provider's prescription.
- Some patients experience heartburn, nausea, or constipation when taking iron supplements. To help avoid these side effects, take iron tablets with a snack or full meal and at least 8 ounces of fluids.
- Do not lie down for at least 1 hour after taking iron pills.
- Your health care provider may prescribe a stool softener for you to help with constipation.
- Taking iron tablets with vitamin C (i.e., orange juice, strawberries) will help your body better absorb the iron.

tients with chronic kidney disease. However, significant side effect profiles of parenteral preparations have been reported including nausea, congestive heart failure, anaphylaxis, liver necrosis, and severe headache. Aronoff (2004) published a comprehensive meta-analysis of the literature surrounding parenteral IV therapy and found that rates of side effects such as anaphylaxis and infection were related to dose size and method of administration. Nonetheless, he also concluded that to be judged safe, IV iron therapy must show hematologic benefit (such as an increase in hemoglobin, decrease in erythropoietin dose, or both) without risking an increase in mortality or morbidity. A number of different IV preparations are currently available and each carries with it specific administration recommendations. Monitoring and test dose guidelines are listed in Chart 63–7.

 During any administration of IV iron supplementation, if the patient reports any signs and symptoms of hypersensitivity or allergic reaction, stop the infusion, stay with the patient, monitor the airway, and call the health care provider immediately.

Nursing Management

Nursing care of the patient with iron deficiency anemia focuses on management of symptomatic hypoxia consistent with all anemias. This includes providing patient education regarding prevention, detection, and management of iron deficiency and monitoring of possible complications from iron supplementation. Management of hypoxia related to anemia is a collaborative process and is addressed in the Nursing Process: Patient Care Plan for Generalized Anemia feature presented earlier in the chapter (p. 2013). Once IDA has been identified, nurses must provide patient education that can prevent recurrence. Because chronic GI blood loss is a major culprit, patients should be taught about the risk factors for GI bleed and early signs and symptoms (see Chapter 45).

Nursing care also must focus on promotion of safe and effective iron supplementation. As discussed earlier, the efficacy of oral and IV iron supplementation is dependent on a variety of factors including timing of administration and management of bothersome side effects. To prevent noncompliance, patients should be advised about these risks prior to beginning iron supplementation and taught the management techniques listed in Chart 63–6 (p. 2021). Particularly with regard to oral supplementation, nurses should perform thorough abdominal assessments for heartburn and constipation. Encouraging proper positioning (high Fowler's or sitting), mobilization, and fluid intake will help minimize the occurrence of digestive problems. Patient education also should include dietary recommendations that will reinforce postdischarge behavior. Although a registered dietitian should be consulted whenever providing dietary recommendations, nurses should also reinforce dietary teaching whenever possible.

Collaborative Management

The comprehensive care of the patient with IDA benefits from the collaboration of nurses, pharmacists, and registered dietitians. Pharmacists should be consulted to prevent drug–drug and drug–food interactions that may inhibit iron absorption. In the acute care setting, registered dietitians coordinate inpatient meal planning to ensure that sufficient quantities of iron are supplied. Their planning efforts, however, require nursing staff to accurately assess and document patient intake of meals and snacks. Oftentimes, dietary intake is negatively impacted by financial and social limits such as shopping and meal preparation challenges. Long-term comprehensive care must then involve social workers and discharge planners who can assist the family with financial concerns and identification of community resources.

Anemia of Chronic Disease

Anemia is a common consequence of chronic diseases. The most common chronic diseases associated with anemia are cancer, chronic kidney failure, autoimmune disorders, and infectious diseases such as acquired immunodeficiency syndrome (AIDS). The prevalence of anemia of chronic disease (ACD) varies significantly depending on the underlying chronic disease and tends to increase with severity of the disease and age of the patient. Weiss and Gordeuk (2005) published a meta-analysis of anemia and chronic disease and reported prevalence ranges from 8% to 95%. In rheumatoid arthritis, anemia is the most common nonmusculoskeletal side effect, reported in 30% to 60% of patients. In cancer, anemia is reported in 30% to 90% of patients (Knight, Wade, & Balducci, 2004), and estimates in chronic kidney disease report a prevalence as high as 80% (National Kidney Foundation [NKF], 2001).

Recognition of ACD contributes to difficulties in statistical analysis. Fatigue and general malaise indicative of anemia are

CHART 63–7	**Recommendation for Parenteral Infusion of Iron Supplementation**		
Name (Generic and Trade)	**Comments**	**Test Dose**	**Infusion Guidelines**
Iron dextran injection (INFeD, DexFerrum)	Appropriate for single-dose administration. Intramuscular route available.	25 mg slow IV push, then 1 hour monitoring required on first infusion	100 mg over 2–5 minutes IV push *OR* Dilute dose in 250–1,000 mL 0.9%NS over 1–6 hours
Sodium ferric gluconate in sucrose (Ferrlecit)	Recommendation by National Kidney Foundation for 125 mg repeated in 8 doses Suggested as alternative for patients hypersensitive to iron dextran	Not required; at health care provider's discretion 25 mg IV slow push or 25 mg in 50 mL of NS IV over 60 minutes	100 mg over 2–5 minutes IV push *OR* Dilute dose in 250–1.000 mL 0.9%NS over 1–6 hours
Iron sucrose injection (Venofer)		Not required; at health care provider's discretion 25 mg IV slow push	100 mg IV over 5 minutes *OR* Dilute dose in 100 mL 0.9%NS over 15 minutes

sometimes dismissed by health care providers as psychosocial consequences of chronic disease. However, numerous studies report decreased side effects and increased quality of life and survival rates when hemoglobin levels are vigilantly monitored and maintained at therapeutic levels above 10 g/dL, the criteria recommended by both the National Kidney Foundation's Kidney Disease Outcomes Quality Initiative (KDOQI) (National Kidney Foundation, 2001) and the National Comprehensive Cancer Network's clinical practice guidelines (Gillespie, 2003; National Comprehensive Cancer Network, 2008; Weiss & Gordeuk, 2005).

Pathophysiology

As mentioned earlier, anemia results from the inflammatory or infectious processes of chronic diseases including chronic kidney disease, cancer, rheumatoid arthritis, and chronic inflammatory bowel disease. Chemical signals produced by invading bacteria or a virus, a tumor, or the body itself attack erythropoietic cells and organs to negatively impact erythrocyte production and iron metabolism through a variety of mechanisms. These mechanisms can be categorized as follows:

1. **Decrease in iron absorption**—Iron availability is diminished by a decrease in the rate of intestinal iron absorption. Chronic disease also can trigger decreased appetite, further diminishing iron absorption. This process contributes to absolute iron deficiency.

2. **Diversion to macrophages**—As the body attempts to fight infection, cytokines divert available iron to the production of macrophages characteristic of chronic disease, resulting in a functional iron deficiency.

3. **Increased hemolysis of erythrocytes**—An increase in RBC hemolysis is stimulated by cytokines produced during inflammation and infection. Circulating macrophages then scavenge the liberated iron, again contributing to a decrease in circulating erythrocytes and functional iron deficiency.

4. **Decreased erythropoietin production and response**—Erythropoiesis also is impacted by a blunting of erythropoietin in chronic kidney disease or secondary to malignancy or infection. These diseases result in decreased production of erythropoietin and in the desensitization of the myeloid progenitor cell to the stimulating effects of erythropoietin. As a result, erythropoiesis rates fail to increase to meet the

increased physiological demands imposed by disease and infection.

5. **Impaired erythropoiesis in the bone marrow**—Malignant tumors and infections first deplete iron and vitamin supplies and then crowd the bone marrow, leaving few resources for erythropoiesis. They also trigger apoptosis of the myeloid progenitor cells.

The simultaneous actions of these mechanisms ultimately result in measurable decreases in erythrocytes, hemoglobin, and hematocrit, along with hypoxia, activity intolerance, and fatigue.

Clinical Presentation

The physical signs and symptoms associated with ACD generally are indistinguishable from these associated with generalized anemia because both result directly from decreased circulating erythrocytes. Anemia also can exacerbate symptoms unique to the underlying disease process. In both cancer and chronic kidney disease, hematocrit and hemoglobin levels maintained below 10 mg/dL for more than 6 weeks are associated with increased myelosuppression, infection, left ventricular hypertrophy, and congestive heart failure. Cognitive and emotional complications include headaches, loss of concentration, depression, and impaired memory (Balducci, 2004; Gillespie, 2003; Ouellette, 2005).

Alterations in Laboratory Values

Anemia of chronic disease is distinguished by its etiology (association with an underlying chronic disease process) and its presentation in laboratory studies. ACD generally presents as mild anemia with hemoglobin levels typically between 8 and 9.5 g/dL. The CBC will show decreased total erythrocytes and decreased reticulocytes, indicating diminished erythropoiesis. The morphology of erythrocytes and iron status laboratory values will vary between ACD with absolute iron deficiency and ACD with functional iron deficiency. Typically, erythrocytes in ACD present first as normochromic and normocytic, then with increasing iron depletion progress to hypochromic and hypocytic, reflected by the MCHC, MCV, and MCH morphology indices. Ferritin levels in ACD with functional iron deficiency are increased, but decrease from baseline with absolute iron deficiency. Transferrin levels are decreased in all iron deficiency stages of ACD. These laboratory trends are summarized in Chart 63–8.

CHART 63–8	**Laboratory Value Trends in Anemia with Chronic Disease and Variations for Iron Status**	
	ACD with Functional Iron Deficiency	**ACD with Absolute Iron Deficiency**
Complete blood count: hemoglobin	Decreased: Hgb < 10	Decreased
Complete blood count: hematocrit	Decreased	Decreased
Complete blood count: RBCs	Decreased	Decreased
Complete blood count: reticulocytes	Normal or decreased	Decreased
Morphology studies	Normochromic, normocytic; MCHC, MCV, MCH normal	Hypchromic, hypocytic; mean corpuscular hemoglobin concentration (MCHC), mean corpuscular volume (MCV), mean corpuscular hemoglobin (MCH) decreased
Iron studies: ferritin	Normal or increased	Decreased
Iron studies: transferrin	Decreased	Decreased
Iron studies: total body iron	Normal	Decreased

Medical Management

The goal of therapy in ACD is maintenance of hemoglobin and hematocrit at sufficient levels to promote disease healing and prevent systemic complications. The target range for hemoglobin and hematocrit are Hgb 11 g/dL (Hct 33%) to Hgb 12 g/dL (Hct 36%) as prescribed by the National Anemia Action Council, National Comprehensive Cancer Network, and NKF practice guidelines. Maintenance of hemoglobin and hematocrit values at these ranges has been correlated with decreased mortality and morbidity (National Anemia Action Council, 2008; National Comprehensive Cancer Network, 2008; National Kidney Foundation NKF, 2001).

The ultimate resolution of anemia in chronic disease, however, can be accomplished only with resolution of the underlying disease, such as cancer, chronic inflammation, or chronic kidney disease. Unfortunately, most of these diseases currently do not enjoy definitive options for permanent cure, implying that management of anemia becomes a lifelong challenge. Three primary options are implemented to maintain optimal hemoglobin and hematocrit values: blood transfusion, iron supplementation, and exogenous application of erythropoietin. Each option along with indications and monitoring guidelines is discussed next.

The judicious use of blood transfusion is an option in correcting acute anemia associated with chronic disease. Blood transfusion is reserved for patients with severe anemia (Hgb <8) or with obvious signs of bleeding such as visible loss of blood or a significant drop in hemoglobin/hematocrit in a relatively short period of time. The risks of blood transfusion, especially repeated transfusions over the course of many months to years, may outweigh the benefits to the patient. Repeated blood transfusions place the patient at risk for fluid overload and iron overload. Patients also can become sensitized to the proteins found in donated blood, increasing their risk for transfusion-related allergic reactions. See Chapter 23 🔘 for a complete discussion of transfusion-related side effects.

Iron supplementation for ACD is reserved for patients with absolute iron deficiency. When ferritin levels indicate sufficient iron stores (greater than 100 ng/mL), as is the case in functional iron deficiency, with iron supplementation the patient is exposed to the possible effects of iron overload including tissue damage and acute cardiovascular events. When ferritin and transferrin levels show iron depletion, iron supplementation has shown some benefit in maintaining hemoglobin levels at the target range of <10. Iron supplementation may also be indicated for patients being treated with erythropoietic agents.

Erythropoietic agents are medications composed of the exogenous forms of erythropoietin, the primary stimulating hormone of erythropoiesis produced in the kidneys. The use of erythropoietic agents for the correction of ACD is reserved for patients with chronic kidney disease and patients undergoing chemotherapy or immunosuppressive therapy. These medications work much the same way that natural erythropoietin does, by stimulating differentiation and proliferation of the hematopoietic cascade. In chronic disease, erythropoietic agents also have been found to preferentially stimulate iron absorption by the erythroid progenitor cell over macrophages. Guidelines for use vary among diseases; refer to the chapters on kidney failure (Chapter 47 🔘) and cancer (Chapter 64 🔘) for guidelines.

■ Nursing Management

Anemia complicates an already difficult diagnosis of chronic disease. Conversely, prevention, detection, and early treatment of anemia can improve the patient's quality of life and clinical outcomes. Nurses play a key role in recognizing early signs of anemia, especially in the acute hospitalized patient. Nursing priorities for the care of the patient with any chronic disease should include assessment of activity tolerance and assessment of integumentary signs such as pallor, respiratory difficulty, and cognition, as described in the Nursing Process: Patient Care Plan for Generalized Anemia feature presented earlier in the chapter (p. 2013). Detection of any such signs indicates the need for immediate implementation of nursing interventions to reduce risk of falls and hypoxia.

Frequent analyses of laboratory values also assist the nurse in detecting underlying bleeding and/or iron deficiency. Patient education and establishment of the therapeutic patient–nurse relationship is particularly important for these patients who may be experiencing depression and exhaustion already brought on by their underlying disease process. Patient education priorities include proper medication administration, increasing awareness of side effects of therapy, safety interventions, and signs and symptoms of worsening anemia.

Megaloblastic Anemias: Folate Deficiency, Vitamin B_{12} Deficiency, and Pernicious Anemias

Megaloblastic anemia results from impaired DNA synthesis of the erythrocyte RBC precursors. The impaired DNA synthesis results in production of large, immature red blood cells termed **megaloblasts**. Due to their immaturity and large size, these megaloblasts are often sequestered in the bone marrow rather than released into the periphery. If released into the peripheral bloodstream, megaloblasts are subject to an increased rate of hemolysis due to structural defects in their membranes. Both processes—bone marrow sequestration and increased hemolysis—result in a decreased total RBC count, or anemia. Most commonly, megaloblastic anemia is caused by deficient dietary intake of folic acid or vitamin B_{12} (cobalamin) or by malabsorption of vitamin B_{12} (pernicious anemia). These processes account for the vast majority of megaloblastic anemias; however, other causes have been implicated, as summarized in Chart 63–9.

Etiology and Pathophysiology

The exact chemical roles of vitamin B_{12} and folate in erythropoiesis are still under investigation, although a great deal of research is being focused on the subject. What is known, however, is that **folate** plays a critical role in the biochemical reactions involved in cell development, especially erythropoiesis. Folate is the natural form, whereas folic acid is the synthetic form found in supplements and fortified food. Laboratory studies show that an absence of folate suppresses the proliferation of maturing erythrocytes. Furthermore, it also is known that folate is absorbed as an inactive dietary form and must be converted to an active form before being used in DNA synthesis.

Vitamin B_{12} (cobalamin), an essential nutrient found in animal proteins, is responsible for this conversion of inactive folate

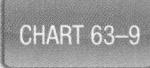

CHART 63–9   Common Causes of Megaloblastic Anemia

Major Causes

- Insufficient dietary intake of folic acid
- Insufficient dietary intake of vitamin B_{12} (cobalamin)
- Deficiencies in gastric intrinsic factor leading to malabsorption of vitamin B_{12} (pernicious anemia)

Other Causes

- Intestinal malabsorption due to chronic GI inflammatory processes or surgical shortening
- General malnutrition
- Liver disease
- Chronic hemolytic anemias
- Anticonvulsant medications such as phenytoin that interfere with folate absorption
- Drugs that have antifolate activity including methotrexate and trimethoprim
- Chemotherapies with DNA suppression activity
- Alcohol abuse

to active folate. This inextricable relationship is the reason vitamin B_{12} deficiency and folate deficiency have similar clinical presentations and often occur simultaneously. Once absorbed, vitamin B_{12} and folate are either transported directly to the bone marrow for erythropoiesis or stored in the liver and, to a small degree, in the pancreas.

Vitamin B_{12} requires the action of gastric **intrinsic factor** (**IF**) before being absorbed into the intestinal mucosa and bloodstream. Intrinsic factor is a substance secreted by the gastric parietal mucosa. Megaloblastic anemias that result from deficiencies in IF are termed **pernicious anemias**.

Clinical Presentation

Folate deficiency anemia, vitamin B_{12} deficiency anemia, and pernicious anemia typically progress slowly with symptoms manifesting gradually over years and months rather than days. In addition to the clinical signs common to all anemias, megaloblastic anemias also present with characteristic signs and symptoms and laboratory test results.

Physical Manifestations

The Nursing Process: Patient Care Plan for Generalized Anemia (see feature earlier in chapter, p. 2013) delineates the most common signs of anemia including fatigue, activity intolerance, exertional dyspnea, tachycardia, and hypoxia. Although this chapter focuses on the pivotal role of vitamin B_{12} and folate in erythropoiesis, both substances also are required for *all* DNA synthesis. In the absence of sufficient folate and vitamin B_{12} (either from dietary insufficiency or pernicious anemia), the patient can manifest gastrointestinal and integumentary signs and symptoms. These result from the absence of these vitamins in the production of epithelial cells. GI symptoms include a swollen and sore tongue (classically described as "smooth and beefy red"), anorexia, and nausea. Integumentary signs include hyperpigmentation over the hands and knuckles. Neurological symptoms

occurring with vitamin B_{12} deficiencies include peripheral neuropathy, unsteadiness, lack of coordination, ataxia, confusion, and memory loss. Reflexes may also be diminished, and a positive Babinski's sign may be observed. (Refer to Chapter 28 🔗 for a discussion neurological assessment.) These result from loss of myelination of nerve cells, of which vitamin B_{12} plays a critical role. Unfortunately, these symptoms often are permanent and irreversible.

Folate deficiency is clinically indistinguishable from vitamin B_{12} deficiency with the exception of neurological insults, which are not common in folate deficiency. Because nervous system findings are atypical, their appearance is clinically significant and warrants analysis for vitamin B_{12} deficiency or overlying neurological disease processes. The most common problem specifically associated with folate deficiency is neural tube defects, such as spina bifida, in newborns of mothers who had inadequate folate intake during pregnancy. Folate deficiency has also been linked to increased homocysteine (an amino acid found in the blood) levels, which in turn increases risk of cardiovascular disease and thrombosis. See Chapter 40 🔗 for a complete discussion of homocysteine and cardiovascular disease.

Alterations in Laboratory Values

Megaloblastic anemias result in changes to the CBC and RBC morphological studies. The hallmark diagnostic finding indicating megaloblastic anemia is macrocytosis or MCV (typically over 110 μm^3). Patients present with the decreased hemoglobin value typical of anemia as well as decreased reticulocytes count. Increased hemolysis can result in decreased erythrocyte levels. To specifically diagnosis megaloblastic anemia and its etiology, vitamin B_{12} and/or folate levels may need to be evaluated. An analysis of vitamin B_{12} and folate levels assists in establishing a definitive diagnosis. A serum vitamin B_{12} level of <100 pg/mL and a serum folate level of <5 ng/mL is diagnostic of vitamin B_{12} and folate deficiency, respectively.

The next task then is to determine the cause of the vitamin B_{12} and/or folate deficiency. A thorough nutritional history assists in isolating dietary causes; however, problems with absorption can be identified using a **Schilling test**. The patient is first given an *oral* dose of radioactively labeled vitamin B_{12}, and a 24-hour urine collection is measured for vitamin B_{12} excretion. Normally urinary excretion is at least 8% to 40% of total radioactively labeled vitamin B_{12}, indicating that the substance was absorbed and metabolized. If urinary excretion is lower than 8%, this may indicate an inability to absorb vitamin B_{12}, and a second stage of the test is performed. In this stage, the patient again is given an oral dose of radiolabeled vitamin B_{12}, but now with a parenteral dose of intrinsic factor. A 24-hour urine collection is repeated and results are compared with the first urine collection results. An increase in urinary excretion of radiolabeled vitamin B_{12} with the addition of IF suggests pernicious anemia.

Analysis then turns to identifying the cause of pernicious anemia. Radiologic examinations, histories, endoscopies, and occasionally surgical exploration may reveal conditions such as celiac disease, tropical sprue, gastric shortening, Crohn's disease, blind loops, and diverticuli, all of which contribute to decreased intestinal production of intrinsic factor. Another diagnostic exam involves the insertion of a nasogastric tube to measure gastric acid secretion. Insufficiencies in gastric acids point to gastric parietal cell problems, which also contribute to insufficient IF and vitamin B_{12} malabsorption.

Medical Management

The first task of medical management is to remove or alter any contributing factors to folate and/or vitamin B_{12} deficiency such as suppressive medication regimes. Dietary causes of both folate and vitamin B_{12} deficiency can be effectively treated with counseling, diet modifications, or vitamin supplementation. Recommended doses of folate supplements start with daily oral administration of 1 mg of folic acid for 4 months, and maintenance with 0.4 mg in a multivitamin for patients with an underlying cause or inadequate diet. Folate deficiencies due to malabsorptive processes require treatment of the underlying cause. Intravenous folate should always be considered in the management of alcoholism to help minimize some of the painful side effects of recovery.

Vitamin B_{12} supplementation usually is achieved via dietary modifications rather than pill form. The latest Recommended Dietary Allowance (RDA) for vitamin B_{12} is 2.4 mcg/day for persons aged 14 to 70 years; the average diet in the United States contains about 5 mcg daily. The prevalence of foods fortified with vitamin B_{12} means that increased intake can be readily achieved. However, the assistance of a registered dietitian is extremely valuable to ensure proper intake of recommended doses (see the Collaborative Management section that follows).

Vitamin B_{12} deficiency in the patient with absorption problems usually is managed with parental supplementation of the vitamin. The treatment schedule begins with parenteral 1,000 mcg vitamin B_{12}, followed by 1,000 mcg intramuscularly once a month for the rest of the patient's life. The efficacy of this approach is well documented. Patients report increased strength and stamina soon after institution of regular doses. Blood cell morphology begins to show normal red blood cells within hours of treatments with subsequent remission of the anemia during the next several weeks (Babior, 2000).

Oral supplementation has been available since 1968, however, it is not widely used for two reasons: for fear of noncompliance and a lack of understanding of alternate biochemical pathways for vitamin B_{12} absorption. However, there is growing evidence that oral administration may be just as effective as parenteral administration given appropriate doses (Nilsson et al., 2005; Nyholm et al., 2003).

◼ Nursing Management

Nurses caring for the patient with megaloblastic anemias have the following priorities:

- *Continued assessment for signs and symptoms of hypoxic distress in severe cases.* The Nursing Process: Patient Care Plan for Generalized Anemia (see feature earlier in chapter, p. 2013) provides assessment guidelines and nursing interventions appropriate for use in megaloblastic anemia.
- *Prevention of mechanical injury from neurological changes.* In addition to the harm caused by hypoxia, these patients are at increased risk of falls and injury secondary to ataxia and lack of balance coordination. Patients with peripheral neuropathy secondary to vitamin B_{12} deficiency have diminished periph-

eral sensations, which increase their risk of injury. Nurses must include an assessment of progressive nerve damage and sensation and most importantly ensure the patient's environment is safe so as to limit injury.

- *Identification of high-risk populations.* Because vitamin B_{12} primarily is found in meats, vegetarians, especially vegans, are at particularly higher risk for vitamin B_{12} deficiency. The rate of folate deficiency is also particularly a concern in women of childbearing age and in the elderly. With this knowledge in hand, nurses may emphasize assessment of dietary histories and patient education to target these high-risk groups.
- *Patient education and reinforcement regarding dietary modifications and/or supplementation.* Patient education regarding dietary modifications is discussed in the next section. For patients requiring supplementation, nursing reinforcement and encouragement can be pivotal to ensuring compliance with a lifelong regime. Nurses should assess patients for compliance, efficacy, and safety of the intramuscular vitamin B_{12} injections and provide feedback as to its action. This can be accomplished by reviewing hematologic studies with the patient and indicating improvements when indicated.
- *Collaboration with the interdisciplinary team.* Collaboration with the health care team is important to ensure a comprehensive multifaceted approach to correction of underlying causes.

◼ Collaborative Management

A major discharge priority for patients with megaloblastic anemia is verbalization of an understanding of dietary modifications and, if indicated, safe performance of medication self-administration techniques. To accomplish these goals, the nurse should collaborate with the health care provider, the registered dietitian, the pharmacist, and the discharge planner.

Dietitians play a critical role in providing accurate and appropriate patient education. Patients can become easily confused with food labels, such as "excellent" or "good" designed for advertising purposes. Handouts and food plans should be provided for clarification. Charts 63–10 and 63–11 (p. 2028) summarize selected food sources of vitamin B_{12} and folate, respectively. Information such as this, when discussed with a dietitian and patient, can help address concerns about adequate food sources. Family members should always be included in the patient education plan, both for support, but also to identify family members' risk of nutritional deficiency and to address familial behavioral patterns such as meal planning habits.

Collaboration with the pharmacist also should not be overlooked. A number of drugs can interfere with vitamin B_{12} or folate absorption and metabolism. The pharmacist is able to monitor drug regimens to prevent such deleterious drug–food interactions. Additionally, the pharmacist can provide materials to help with the administration of parenteral supplements.

Hemoglobinopathies

Hemoglobinopathy is a term used to describe a class of red blood cell disorders characterized by abnormal hemoglobin, which can

CHART 63–10   Selected Food Sources of Vitamin B_{12}

Food	Micrograms per Serving	Percent Daily Value
Mollusks, clam, mixed species, cooked, 3 ounces	84.1	1400
Liver, beef, braised, 1 slice	47.9	780
Fortified breakfast cereals (100% fortified), 3/4 cup	6.0	100
Trout, rainbow, wild, cooked, 3 ounces	5.4	90
Salmon, sockeye, cooked, 3 ounces	4.9	80
Trout, rainbow, farmed, cooked, 3 ounces	4.2	50
Beef, top sirloin, lean, choice, broiled, 3 ounces	2.4	40
Fast-food cheeseburger, regular, double patty and bun, 1 sandwich	1.9	30
Fast-food taco, 1 large	1.6	25
Fortified breakfast cereals (25% fortified), 3/4 cup	1.5	25
Yogurt, plain, skim, with 13 grams protein per cup, 1 cup	1.4	25
Haddock, cooked, 3 ounces	1.2	20
Clams, breaded and fried, 3/4 cup	1.1	20
Tuna, white, canned in water, drained solids, 3 ounces	1.0	15
Milk, 1 cup	0.9	15
Pork, cured, ham, lean only, canned, roasted, 3 ounces	0.6	10
Egg, whole, hard boiled, 1	0.6	10
American pasteurized cheese food, 1 ounce	0.3	6
Chicken, breast, meat only, roasted, 1/2 breast	0.3	6

Source: U.S. Department of Agriculture, Agricultural Research Service. (2003). *USDA nutrient database for standard reference, release 16.* Retrieved February 1, 2006, from the Nutrient Data Laboratory website: http://www.nal.usda.gov/fnic/cgi-bin/nut_search.pl.

result in a variety of clinical problems including hypoxia, accelerated RBC destruction, and decreased RBC production. All of these diseases result from genetic mutations in the coding sequences controlling the component hemoglobin chains. Classification of these diseases is often based on the type of genetic alteration (either point mutation, base pair, or deletion). They also are commonly classified on the basis of the molecular and chemical effect of the alteration. Alterations include decreased oxygen-binding capacity and structural defects that decrease the life span.

As with most genetic disorders, the severity of clinical symptoms depends on the role of the gene involved and on the inheritance pattern, with homozygous patients frequently presenting with severe debilitating disease, whereas heterozygous patients can often live asymptomatically unless presented with acute illness or environmental stress. More than 800 distinct diseases have been attributed to hemoglobinopathy, of which thalassemia and sickle cell disease are the most prominent. Both of these diseases are discussed in the following sections.

Thalassemia

The term **thalassemia** refers to a group of hematologic disorders characterized by the genetic inheritance of a mutated hemoglobin-coding gene that appears most frequently in persons of Southeast Asian, African, and Mediterranean descent. The hallmark characteristic of thalassemia is a structural change in the hemoglobin molecule that subjects affected red blood cells to increased rates of hemolysis. The thalassemias are

chronic disease states that are usually detected during infancy or adolescence. Cure of these anemias is not the goal for the acute care nurse. The focus instead becomes prevention of disease complications and treatment of symptom exacerbation.

Pathophysiology

Recall from the earlier discussion on hemoglobin synthesis that oxygen binding occurs when alpha and beta chains form precise geometric configurations that allows iron to sit tightly in a lock-and-key style fit on the heme groups. Thalassemia arises when the alpha and beta chains are of unequal proportions, which ultimately reduces the rate of RBC maturation in the bone marrow. Cells that do survive bone marrow development and enter the bloodstream are recognized in the spleen as structurally abnormal and are subject to higher rates of hemolysis.

The thalassemias are broadly divided into two groups: alpha thalassemia or beta thalassemia, depending on the type of inherited gene mutation. Beta thalassemia results from reduced beta chains, whereas the alpha thalassemias result from reduced alpha chains. Diseases are also characterized by their gene inheritance pattern: homozygous carriers, defining the inheritance of two defective genes, or heterozygous carriers, defining the inheritance of only one defective gene. Each combination of gene inheritance is associated with distinct clinical features.

Clinical Presentation

Alpha thalassemias are generally milder than the beta thalassemias and often present without symptoms or very mild

CHART 63–11 Selected Food Sources of Folate and Folic Acid

Food	Micrograms per Serving	Percent Daily Value as Developed by the Food and Drug Administraton
Breakfast cereals fortified with 100% of the DV (fortified with folic acid) 3/4 cup*	400	100
Beef liver, cooked, braised, 3 ounces	185	45
Cowpeas (blackeyed), immature, cooked, boiled, 1/2 cup	105	25
Breakfast cereals, fortified with 25% of the Daily Value 3/4 cup*	100	25
Spinach, frozen, cooked, boiled, 1/2 cup	100	25
Great Northern beans, boiled, 1/2 cup	90	20
Asparagus, boiled, 4 spears	85	20
Rice, white, long-grain, parboiled, enriched, cooked, 1/2 cup*	65	15
Vegetarian baked beans, canned, 1 cup	60	15
Spinach, raw, 1 cup	60	15
Green peas, frozen, boiled, 1/2 cup	50	15
Broccoli, chopped, frozen, cooked, 1/2 cup	50	15
Egg noodles, cooked, enriched, 1/2 cup*	50	15
Broccoli, raw, 2 spears (each 5 inches long)	45	10
Avocado, raw, all varieties, sliced, 1/2 cup sliced	45	10
Peanuts, all types, dry roasted, 1 ounce	40	10
Lettuce, Romaine, shredded, 1/2 cup	40	10
Wheat germ, crude, 2 tablespoons	40	10
Tomato juice, canned, 6 ounces	35	10
Orange juice, chilled, includes concentrate, 3/4 cup	35	10
Turnip greens, frozen, cooked, boiled, 1/2 cup	30	8
Orange, all commercial varieties, fresh, 1 small	30	8
Bread, white, 1 slice*	25	6
Bread, whole wheat, 1 slice*	25	6
Egg, whole, raw, fresh, 1 large	25	6
Cantaloupe, raw,1/4 medium	25	6
Papaya, raw, 1/2 cup cubes	25	6
Banana, raw, 1 medium	20	6

*Items marked with an (*) are fortified with folic acid as part of the Folate Fortification Program.

Source: U.S. Department of Agriculture, Agricultural Research Service. (2003). *USDA nutrient database for standard reference, release 16.* Retrieved February 1, 2006, from the Nutrient Data Laboratory website: http://www.nal.usda.gov/fnic/cgi-bin/nut_search.pl.

symptoms that respond well to supportive care when indicated. The severity of symptoms in patients with beta thalassemias depends heavily on the inheritance pattern (see the Genetic Considerations box). The term *beta-thalassemia minor* describes the inheritance of only one defective gene and one normal gene (heterozygous), whereas the term *beta-thalassemia major* is used for the inheritance of two defective genes (homozygous).

GENETIC CONSIDERATIONS for Thalassemia

Persons of Southeast Asia, Africa, and Mediterranean descent bear a genetic predisposition to thalassemia. Patients with alpha-thalassemia and beta-thalassemia minor are often asymptomatic and not identified; however, patients with beta-thalassemia major usually require transfusions beginning early in life (Forget, 2000).

Beta-thalassemia minor patients are able to produce small amounts of normal hemoglobin and, thus, are frequently asymptomatic due to long-term physiological adaptation. These patients are carriers for the genetic trait; therefore, genetic counseling may be offered for patients of reproductive age. Beta-thalassemia major (also called Cooley's anemia) results from complete lack of the beta protein in the hemoglobin chain manifesting as severe, life-threatening anemia. Symptoms that result from the increased rate of hemolysis include jaundice, hepatomegaly (enlarged liver), and splenomegaly (enlarged spleen). Pronounced pallor, tachycardia, and lethargy result from a critical lack of oxygen-binding capacity. The bone marrow is constantly in a state of increased erythropoiesis in an attempt to compensate for hemolysis and hypoxia, resulting in bone marrow expansion, recognized as thickening of facial bones and abnormal skeletal growth (Forget, 2000). The physiological demands imposed by beta-thalassemia major often can be so serious that many children who acquire the disease do not survive into adulthood. *3Beta-thalassemia intermedia* was a term coined by Sturgeon and colleagues in 1955 to describe a small group of patients who do not fit neatly into either the beta-thalassemia major or beta-thalassemia minor paradigms. These patients are hematologically too severe to be called "minor" and too mild to be called "major." These individuals are homozygous for thalassemia genes, but maintain hemoglobin levels of 7 to 10 g/dL without regular transfusions.

Alterations in laboratory values for thalassemia patients depend again on the form of the inherited mutation and the inheritance pattern. In addition to alterations in hemoglobin and red blood cells, clinicians should monitor for alterations in bilirubin, which provide indications of hemolytic effects in the liver. Chart 63–12 summarizes the changes in laboratory values and clinical symptoms relative to the type of thalassemia (Benz, 2003).

In addition to clinical presentation directly related to thalassemia, the constant need for transfusion to maintain adequate RBCs often results in transfusion-related complications and iron overload, as discussed next. Excessive iron comes from the patient's own hemolyzed red blood and the transfused blood, as well as increased iron absorption from food as a compensatory mechanism to combat anemia. The excess iron is stored in the spleen, liver, endocrine organs, and heart causing splenomegaly, hepatomegaly, cirrhosis, hormone imbalances, and cardiomyopathy, which can all eventually become fatal.

Medical Management

Patients with alpha thalassemias and beta-thalassemia minor are usually asymptomatic and usually do not require medical intervention. Patients with thalassemia major, however, often require frequent transfusions of packed RBCs to correct falling hematocrit and hemoglobin levels that result from rampant hemolysis. Transfusion doses are titrated to maintain therapeutic hemoglobin levels between 7 and 10 g/dL or to correct severe symptoms.

However, the leading cause of death among patients with thalassemia has shifted from hemoglobin-deficient anemia to iron overload associated with chronic blood transfusion therapy (Vichinsky, 2005). Thus, iron levels must be carefully monitored to prevent iron overload. Two common methods used to monitor iron are the serum ferritin test and liver biopsy. Iron chelation therapy with drugs such as desferrioxamine (Desferal) is administered intravenously or subcutaneously in an effort to bind and neutralize excessive iron from patients' bodies. Hydration and oxygenation complement transfusion and chelation

therapy in an effort to rid the body of excess erythrocyte waste and maintain oxygen levels (Hoffbrand, 2005; Vichinsky, 2005).

◼ Nursing Management

Nursing assessment of patients with thalassemia focuses on the hemolytic and hypoxic effects manifested in the integumentary, gastrointestinal, lymphatic, and cardiovascular systems. Patients should be observed for jaundice in the skin and eyes due to RBC destruction, and pallor from hemoglobin-deficient anemia. Abdominal pain and liver and spleen tenderness are indicators of thalassemia and should be included in a comprehensive assessment. Cardiovascular signs and symptoms of activity intolerance and hypoxia should also be assessed as indicators of both hemoglobin deficiency and iron accumulation in the cardiac muscle.

Nursing interventions based on the preceding assessments should prioritize activity alterations, pain management, and collaboration with the multidisciplinary team. The Nursing Process: Patient Care Plan for Generalized Anemia (see feature earlier in chapter, p. 2013) should be implemented in the care of these patients. If transfusion therapy is warranted, the nurse plays a critical role in managing the administration of blood products including assessing for signs of a transfusion reaction such as fluid overload, fever, and anaphylaxis.

Sickle Cell Disease

Sickle cell anemia is perhaps the most well known of the chronic erythrocyte disorders. In the United States it is estimated that more than 70,000 people suffer from sickle cell disease with about 1,000 babies born annually with the disease. Sickle cell occurs most frequently in African Americans and Hispanic Americans. About 1 in every 500 African Americans has sickle cell disease. It also affects people of Arabian, Greek, Maltese, Italian, Sardinian, Turkish, and Indian ancestry (see the Genetic Considerations box, p. 2030). **Sickle cell anemia** is the term given to a group of genetically based RBC diseases all characterized by misshapen "sickle-shaped" red blood cells. The source of the sickling is a malfunctioning hemoglobin molecule that twists the entire RBC from a soft, pliable, round donut shape into a long, hard, sticky elongated cell (Figure 63–7 ◼, p. 2030).

Pathophysiology

Patients with sickle cell anemia acquire the sickle hemoglobin (HbS), a mutated version of the normal form of hemoglobin A.

CHART 63–12	**Laboratory Values and Clinical Presentation of the Thalassemias**			
	Alpha Thalassemia	**Beta-Thalassemia Minor**	**Beta-Thalassemia Intermedia**	**Beta-Thalassemia Major**
Hemoglobin	Normal	>10 g/dL (normal)	7–10 g/dL	<7 g/dL
Red blood cell appearance	Microcytic and Hypochromic			
Red blood cells		Usually normal	Usually normal or decreased	Severely decreased
Jaundice	Usually absent	Usually absent	Usually absent or mild	Severe
Splenomegaly	Usually absent	Usually absent	Usually absent or mild	Severe
Skeletal changes	Absent	Usually absent	Usually absent or mild	Severe

MyNursingKit Animation: Metabolic: Sickle-Cell Anemia—Etiology and Pathophysiology

GENETIC CONSIDERATIONS for Sickle Cell Disease

Sickle cell disease is acquired through genetic inheritance in families of African American, Hispanic American, Arabian, Greek, Italian, Sardinian, Maltese, Turkish, and Indian ancestry. Patients who inherit the sickle cell gene from one parent (heterozygous HbS/HbA) usually do not exhibit symptoms and are termed sickle cell carriers. Patients who inherit the sickle cell gene from both parents (homozygous) are subject to severe sickle cell crises. Because both homozygous and heterozygous patients can pass their genes onto their children, sickle cell carriers typically undergo some type of genetic counseling prior to childbearing (Armandola, 2002, Ramsey et al., 2001).

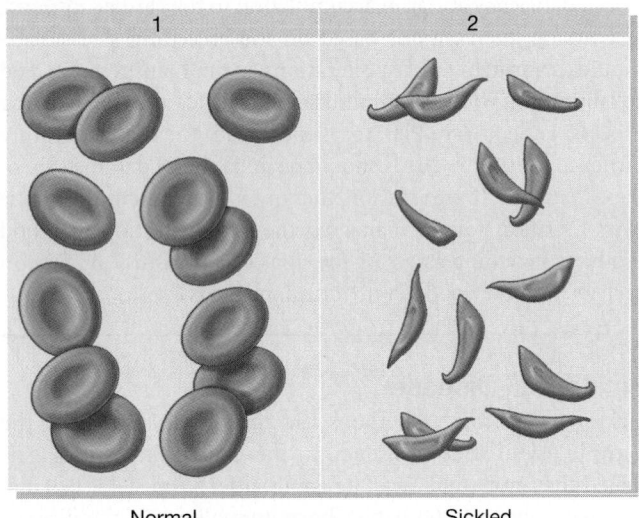

1	2
Normal	Sickled

FIGURE 63–7 ■ Red blood cells from sickle cell anemia.

Recall from the discussion on hemoglobin development and function earlier in the chapter that oxygen binding results in a geometric alteration of the hemoglobin molecule. In normal hemoglobin the oxygenated state and the deoxygenated state coexist without deleterious side effects. HbS, however, causes affected cells to transform into a rigid, elongated sickle shape upon release of the oxygen molecule, rather than the normal, flexible round configuration. Under normal circumstances, deoxygenated sickled cells make up only a small proportion of total blood volume, with minimal physical effects. However, any stress that results in oxygen deprivation increases the proportion of sickled cells.

Sickle cells possess "sticky membranes" and unusual shapes that occlude small blood vessels (a condition called *erythrostasis*), which serve to further potentiate oxygen deprivation. Sickled cells also are trapped by the spleen, further reducing circulating red blood cells and contributing to hypoxia. Initially, the hypoxia will stimulate increased erythropoiesis, thus reversing the cycle. However, if the hypoxia becomes extreme, widespread vessel occlusion leads to a syndrome termed *sickle cell crisis*. These crisis states are responsible for the severe pain of sickle cell disease. Pain, in turn, increases the demand for oxygen, hinders mobility and respiration, and taxes the cardiovascular system. Together the sequence of events escalates into a cycle of deoxygenation and RBC sickling. Gone unchecked, the resultant thrombosis and acidosis progress to organ failure and eventually death.

Crisis Syndromes of Sickled Red Blood Cells The following critical situations may be seen in patients with sickle cell anemia:

- **Vaso-occlusive crisis**—Vaso-occlusive crisis is the occlusion of small vessels by long, hard chains of stacked sickled cells. This occlusion prevents oxygenation of surrounding tissues and tissue downstream of the occlusion. Oxygen deprivation in arterial vessels causes ischemic attacks and infarction. Oxygen deprivation to venous vessels leads to swollen, tender tissues as a result of the buildup of fluids and wastes. Both arterial and venous occlusions are hallmarked by severe pain.

- **Sequestration crisis**—Sequestration crisis occurs when sickled RBCs overwhelm and clog the spleen. As a result, circulating blood volume decreases, manifesting as decreased blood pressure, which in turn stagnates blood flow and causes deoxygenation. Sequestration crisis manifests as a painful, tender, grossly enlarged spleen.

- **Aplastic crisis**—The large numbers of RBCs destroyed in the spleen by sickle cell anemia places an extraordinarily high demand on the amount of bone marrow available to replenish available circulating erythrocytes into the bloodstream. This extraordinary demand overwhelms the bone marrow regulatory feedback mechanism, resulting in complete bone marrow shutdown, akin to a system overload. This complete bone marrow shutdown is referred to as aplastic crisis. As a result of aplastic crisis, reticulocytes (juvenile RBCs) are not produced, causing a severe drop in hemoglobin, up to 1 g/dL per day manifesting in severe lethargy, malaise, and deoxygenation.

- **Hyperhemolytic crisis**—Hyperhemolytic crisis is a rare complication. As the name implies, hyperhemolytic crisis is hallmarked by a massive increase in RBC destruction. Like aplastic crisis, hemoglobin rates drop rapidly. However, if the bone marrow is still intact, reticulocyte production is increased.

Clinical Presentation

The extent and severity of the disease depends on two criteria: the inheritance pattern (homozygous for HbS or heterozygous HbS/HbA) and the presence of deoxygenating triggering factors. Patients who are heterozygous HbS/HbA (termed sickle cell carriers) often live asymptomatic lives because the normal hemoglobin produced by HbA sufficiently prevents sickling crisis. Homozygous patients also usually live asymptomatic lives unless subjected to stressors such as infection, pain, blood loss, or high altitudes. Sickle cell crisis appears when the patient is subjected to such stressors or prolonged hypoxia. Peripheral tissue and organ damage become more apparent, and oxygen deprivation and blood stagnation increase with prolonged sickle cell crisis. Although every body system eventually can become affected, certain signs and symptoms are most frequently observed. These are:

- Persistent, usually painful, erection of the penis due to veno-occlusion causes both severe pain and embarrassment for male patients.

- Acute renal failure results primarily from arterial occlusion in the renal capillaries, which, in turn, leads to focal areas of hemorrhage or necrosis. Additionally, myoglobin and RBC waste products from extremely high RBC destruction can overload renal tubules, causing renal failure.

- Acute chest syndrome (ACS) results from a variety of causes. Causes directly pertaining to sickle cell crisis include pulmonary tissue infarction due to capillary occlusion and hypoventilation secondary to rib/sternal bone infarction. Treatment of sickle cell crisis can also exacerbate acute chest syndrome. Examples include hypoventilation secondary to narcotic administration and pulmonary edema induced by narcotics or fluid overload. Regardless of the cause, the resultant hypoxia severely increases hemoglobin sickling, making the appearance of ACS an ominous sign in the sickle cell patient. See Chapters 33, 34, and 36 🔗 for complete discussion of ACS.

- Splenomegaly (enlarged spleen) results from splenic sequestration.

- Avascular necrosis (AVN), also known as ischemic necrosis, osteonecrosis, or aseptic necrosis of the large joints, results from interruption of the arterial supply of the femoral head. Patients with AVN have severe chronic joint pain, decreased weight-bearing ability, and joint malformation.

- Hemolytic anemia, or acute anemia caused by the accelerated breakdown of red blood cells, is characterized by splenomegaly, jaundice, and decreased urine output. Hemolytic anemia is discussed in greater detail later in this chapter.

As the microvasculature becomes increasingly occluded, major organs begin to suffer irreversible damage from hypoxia and thrombosis. Evidence of organ failure includes decreased level of consciousness (decreased cerebral tissue perfusion), decreased urine output and increased serum creatinine (decreased renal tissue perfusion), chest pain (decreased cardiopulmonary tissue perfusion), and abdominal pain (decreased liver, colon, and spleen perfusion).

Alterations in Laboratory Values

Laboratory studies analyzing RBC morphology are used to monitor for the prevalence of sickle cell hemoglobin. Hemoglobin electrophoresis analysis can reveal the presence of HbS in patients with sickle cell disease. Slide smears of peripheral blood samples can reveal partially or completely sickled cells with the proportion of sickled cells to normal cells increasing during crisis states. Hemoglobin values will be normal in patients with the sickle cell trait, but decreased below 7 g/dL during deoxygenation states or in homozygous patients. As sickling progresses the patient also will display evidence of increasing RBC breakdown manifested by decreased RBCs and increased bilirubin.

Medical Management

The cornerstone of sickle cell disease management is prevention of sickle cell crisis by ensuring adequate oxygenation via avoidance of triggering events at all times. Because patients are usually diagnosed as children, prevention of sickle cell crisis states should always involve collaboration with the parent. Any patient presenting to the acute care setting with a known history of sickle cell disease warrants particular attention to oxygenation and hydration status. In the unfortunate event that sickle cell crisis develops, supportive care must be implemented to prevent severe pain, organ failure, and death.

Treatments should include administration and monitoring of supplemental oxygen, analgesics for vaso-occlusive crisis, hydration, and, if indicated, blood cell transfusions to reverse hypoxia. Pharmacologic treatments to prevent sickle cell crisis are

currently being researched. Avenues for investigation include drugs such as hydroxyurea, butyrate, and arginine that stimulate the body to make normal types of hemoglobin, drugs to increase oxygenation to small blood vessels (Poloxamer 188, Flocor), drugs that make sickled cell membranes less "sticky," and gene therapies (Armandola, 2002; Marlowe & Chicella, 2002; Solovey, Solovey, Harkness, & Hebbel, 2001; Wang et al., 2002). Complementary and alternative therapy options are presented in the box on page 2034.

Nursing Management

Prevention of sickle cell crisis is a primary goal for any patient admitted with sickle cell disease, regardless of the primary admitting diagnosis. Situations that are most likely to cause HbS chains to sickle and stack include dehydration, blood stagnation, decreased pH (acidosis), and decreased PaO_2. Disease management thus focuses on:

- Maintenance of adequate hydration
- Maintenance of oxygenation to prevent acidosis and decreased PaO_2
- Prevention of hypercoagulability.

Effective management of these patients involves first identifying high-risk factors and then implementing effective preventive nursing and medical interventions. In the event that sickle cell crisis occurs, the medical team must quickly mobilize to treat pain and eliminate the triggering factors. Finally, all patients with sickle cell disease must be regularly assessed for evidence of organ and tissue dysfunction. In addition to the Nursing Process: Patient Care Plan for Generalized Anemia presented earlier (p. 2013), the Nursing Process: Patient Care Plan (p. 2032) for Sickle Cell Disease outlines specific nursing interventions aimed at preventing these sickling crisis states, addressing sickle cell crisis, and continued assessment of long-term sequelae.

Collaborative Management

Nursing collaboration with the multidisciplinary team is an effective means to address the multifactorial, complex needs of the patient with sickle cell disease. Interdisciplinary team members should include pharmacists, physical and occupational therapists, respiratory therapists, medical specialists such as hematologists, and the patient's primary health care provider.

Because pain is a major factor in sickle cell crisis, analgesia is certain to play a role in the acute hospitalization. Pharmacologic expertise can help ensure that appropriate and effective options are readily available and implemented (Buchanan, Woodward, & Reed, 2005). Emerging trends in the management of sickle cell disease suggest that nonpharmacologic interventions and long-term physical exercise plans can help prevent many of the complications related to sickle cell disease.

Physical, occupational, and rehabilitation therapists can provide assistance both in the acute care setting, but more importantly can provide patient education and referrals in preparation for discharge (see the Patient Teaching & Discharge Priorities box, p. 2034) (Bodhise, Dejoie, Brandon, Simpkins, & Ballas, 2004; Ramsey et al., 2001). Respiratory therapy, particularly during

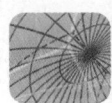

NURSING PROCESS: Patient Care Plan for Sickle Cell Disease

Assessment of Tissue Perfusion

Subjective Data:

Have you been short of breath?

Are you dizzy?

Are you having chest pain?

Have you had any nausea or vomiting or abdominal pain?

Do any of your extremities hurt?

Objective Data:

Integumentary: skin temperature cool, pale

Pulses: diminished, weak peripheral pulses

Renal: decreased urinary output, concentrated

Cerebral: restless, anxious, decreased level of alertness

Cardiopulmonary: tachypnea, tachycardia, angina, oxygen saturation decreased

Gastrointestinal: pain and tenderness with or without palpation

Laboratory values: hemoglobin <7, positive HbS, RBCs decreased, bilirubin elevated

Nursing Assessment and Diagnoses	Outcomes and Evaluation Parameters	Planning and Interventions with *Rationales*
Nursing Diagnosis: *Risk for Ineffective Tissue Perfusion: Cerebral, Renal, Cardiopulmonary, and Abdominal Organ* related to vaso-occlusive crisis	**Outcome:** Free of injury due to peripheral hypoxia. **Evaluation Parameters:** Cerebral: Patient remains alert and oriented. Cerebral: Pupil response remains unchanged from baseline. Cerebral: Gross reflex assessment remains unchanged from baseline. Renal: Urinary output remains adequate for patient (at least 30 mL/hr for nondialysis patients). Renal: Electrolyte blood studies and urinalysis remain within normal limits. Renal: Patient remains free of edema. Cardiopulmonary: Peripheral pulses remain intact compared to baseline. Cardiopulmonary: Patient remains free of chest pain. Cardiopulmonary: Lung and chest auscultation do not reveal adventitious or irregular sounds. Cardiopulmonary: Oxygenation status remains within normal limits as measured by spot O_2 saturation above 90% or within normal baseline parameters for patient and ABGs pH 7.3–7.5, $PaCO_2$ 35–45 mmHg. Abdominal: Gastric motility remains intact. Abdominal: Patient remains free of nausea, vomiting, severe cramping, and diarrhea.	**Interventions and *Rationales:*** Frequently monitor neurological signs including level of consciousness, Glasgow Coma Scale, papillary changes, and cranial nerves *to detect changes in level of consciousness and nerve damage*. Assess for signs of edema, urine output (color, amount) *as indicators of renal function*. Monitor blood studies (renal function tests, electrolytes) and urine tests (creatinine, protein) *as indicators of renal function*. Encourage oral fluid intake and administer intravenous fluid (as ordered) *to maintain fluid balance, hydration, and renal cell perfusion*. Administer hypotonic fluids such as dextrose 5% in water or in 0.45% normal saline. *Hypotonic fluids entering RBCs will reduce tendency of hemoglobin to crystallize into sickle shape and will promote dilution of already sickled cells and occluded vessels*. Report changes and trends in renal output and renal lab studies immediately to health care provider *to ensure timely interventions are implemented*. Assess peripheral pulses *as indicators of peripheral tissue perfusion*. Assess cardiac sounds *to detect irregular heart rhythms*. Assess jugular vein distention and peripheral edema *as indicators of cardiac muscle status*. Encourage patient to avoid strenuous activity to *decrease cardiac workload and oxygen demands*. Assess for adventitious or diminished breath sounds. *Indicates decreased gas exchange and hypoxia*. Monitor respiratory rate and depth *to assess for respiratory distress*. Collaborate with respiratory therapist to administer high-flow oxygen therapy as ordered *to maximize oxygen availability in peripheral tissues*. Collaborate with health care provider to obtain ABGs when spot O_2 sat falls below 80% *as a more accurate analysis of acid–base balance*. Provide incentive spirometry every hour *to prevent atelectasis and acute chest syndrome*. Collaborate with health care provider for administration of oxygen for spot O_2 states of less than 80% *to prevent acidosis. However, do not administer O_2 for patients who are not hypoxic, because this may suppress bone marrow production of RBCs*. Assess for abdominal pain and tenderness *as indicators of gastric perfusion*. Perform abdominal auscultation *as indicators of gastric perfusion*. Monitor for nausea, appetite, vomiting, and diarrhea *as indicators of gastric function*. Offer small frequent meals *to minimize distention*.

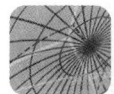

NURSING PROCESS: Patient Care Plan for Sickle Cell Disease—*Continued*

Assessment of Pain of Sickle Cell Disease

Subjective Data:
Are you feeling any pain? If so, where?
What makes it worse? What makes it better?
Can you describe it?
How have you treated sickle cell pain in the past?

Objective Data:
General: pallor, malaise, fatigue
Fever: assess for possible sites of infection
Neurological: level of consciousness (ominous sign of intracranial bleeding)
Lung sounds: crackles, diminished lung sounds
Respiratory: cough, dyspnea, ventilation depth
Cardiovascular: poor capillary refill, tachycardia, hypotension
Pain: location, quality, onset, and alleviating factors
Abdominal: painful, swollen left upper quadrant
Genitourinary: priapism
Neuromuscular: painful swollen joints, especially hips
Renal: renal lab values, urinary output volume and character
Lab values: hemoglobin (presence of sickle cell disease) A2 and F hemoglobin
Full blood count (FBC) to detect anemia, and reticulocyte count

Nursing Assessment and Diagnoses	Outcomes and Evaluation Parameters	Planning and Interventions with *Rationales*
Nursing Diagnosis: *Pain* related to vaso-occlusive crisis	**Outcomes:** Maintenance of adequate oxygenation and acid–base balance. Maintenance of comfort level. ***Evaluation Parameters:*** Able to communicate pain level and therapies that help alleviate it. Pain reduced and/or absent as evidenced by patient report and no pain behaviors: grimacing. Nonpharmacologic method of control is effective as evidenced by patient report and no pain behaviors. Reports satisfaction with pain management program.	**Interventions and *Rationales:*** Collaborate with patient to determine preferred pain control modalities. *Patients with chronic sickle cell disease are most familiar with personalized effective treatment options. Collaboration also promotes trust and therapeutic relationships.* Assess pain including rating and character frequently and reassess after any pain intervention *to provide early detection of pain and to measure effectiveness of interventions.* Administer pain medication on fixed schedule *to maintain consistent blood levels.* Administer RBCs per health care provider order in specific situations such as symptomatic anemia, a hematocrit reading 7 points below baseline, orthostasis, and a reticulocyte count of zero. *RBC transfusions provide nonsickled oxygen-carrying hemoglobin, increase oxygenation, and treat aplastic crisis.* Monitor for signs such as a falling hematocrit level, pain, pulmonary edema, fever, hypotension, and hemolysis *as indicators of transfusion reactions (hemolysis and fluid overload).*

acute chest syndrome, can help mitigate hypoxia and pain via the application of oxygen therapy. Finally, the patient's primary health care provider may benefit from consultation with a hematologist who specializes in sickle cell disease. The Evidence-Based Practice feature (p. 2035) discusses other interventions that can be used with patients who have sickle cell disease.

Hemolytic Anemias

Hemolytic anemia is a term applied to wide range of diseases characterized by increased RBC destruction, or hemolysis. Hemolysis begins in the peripheral bloodstream with the recognition by phagocytes of dying or damaged red blood cells. The spleen, liver, and reticuloendothelial system then completes degradation. Normally, the rate of hemolysis is balanced by the rate of erythropoiesis, thus maintaining a consistent volume of oxygen-carrying red blood cells in the peripheral circulation.

Infection, toxins, certain medications, injury, and other environmental stressors can all trigger minor increases in hemolysis, which then result in a decrease in circulating red blood cells, triggering hypoxia. In healthy patients, this hypoxia stimulates increased erythropoietin production, accelerated erythropoiesis, and compensation of hypoxia. Clinically significant hypoxia, characterizing hemolytic anemia, results when the hemolysis persists or is so extensive that erythropoiesis cannot sufficiently compensate. Hemolytic anemia should be distinguished from anemia due to bone marrow disorders (Chart 63–13, p. 2035). In the latter, clinically significant hypoxia results from sluggish erythropoiesis; this cannot compensate for normal hemolysis.

Pathophysiology

Several pathophysiological processes can ultimately result in the anemia of hemolytic etiology just described. Commonly, causes of hemolytic anemia are grouped according to such processes. Certain causes are due to intrinsic defects in the erythrocyte, which decreases its ability to survive the normal RBC life span of 120 days. Deficiencies in metabolic, protective enzymes are the

PATIENT TEACHING & DISCHARGE PRIORITIES for Sickle Cell Anemia

Need	Teaching
Disease process	Discuss cause of disease.
Patient/family	Discuss triggers and risks of sickle cell crisis.
Prevention/management of sickle cell crisis	Discuss activities/scenarios that can exacerbate hypoxic state emphasizing oxygenation and hydration.
Patient/family	Teach family to recognize key physical symptoms of sickle cell crisis.
	Discuss appropriate use of oxygenation.
	Discuss appropriate use of pain medication to control pain.
Pharmacologic management	Discuss appropriate use of pharmacologic treatments including side effects and recommended dosing schedule.
Patient/family	Consult with pharmacist for drug-specific teaching.
Nutrition	Discuss role of balanced nutrition emphasizing need for key elements: vitamin B_{12}, folate, and iron.
Patient/family	Refer patient to dietitian for assistance in meal planning.
Physical exercise	Discuss and explore appropriate physical exercise options that would maintain muscle/bone/cardiovascular strength but limits risks of hypoxia.
Patient/family	Refer patient/family to physical, rehabilitation, and occupational therapy for outpatient consultation.

COMPLEMENTARY & ALTERNATIVE THERAPIES

Multiple Therapies

Description:

Several CAM therapies may be appropriate and effective for a specific ailment. For example, there are several CAM therapies that may be effective for sickle cell anemia.

Research Support:

Oxidation plays a significant role in the pathophysiology of sickle cell anemia. Studies have shown in-vitro antioxidant actions from aged garlic extract. One subsequent study examined the antioxidant effect of AGE on sickled red blood cells (RBCs). Study participants included 5 patients with sickle cell anemia (two men and three women, aged 24 to 58) who received a dose of 5 mL AGE daily. Whole blood samples collected from the participants at baseline and after the 4-week treatment period were analyzed for Heinz bodies. Results showed that, in all patients, there was a decrease in the number of Heinz bodies, which suggests that AGE has a significant antioxidant activity on sickled RBCs (Takasu, Uykimpang, Sunga, Amagase, & Niihara, 2006).

A Johns Hopkins University study identified CAM therapies that families of children with sickle cell anemia use and their interest in CAM. The study involved a telephone survey of 57 parents of children with sickle cell anemia. Study results were as follows:

- 54% used CAM therapies.
- 42% used bioenergetic therapies (prayer, spiritual, and energy healing).
- 28% used CAM that related to lifestyle, mind, and body (relaxation techniques, exercise, imagery, and diet).
- 12% used biochemical therapies (herbal medicines, megavitamins, and folk remedies).
- 5% used biomechanical therapy (massage).
- 83% felt that CAM was helpful.

Researchers concluded that use of CAM therapies, especially prayer, relaxation techniques, and spiritual healing is common for children with sickle-cell anemia (Sibinga, Shindell, Casella, Duggan, & Wilson, 2006).

Another study examined Qigong (pronounced "CHEE-kung") therapy, which is a form of energy healing, on breast cancer patients undergoing chemotherapy. White blood cells, platelets, and hemoglobin were measured in blood samples obtained from the study participants. The study involved 67 women, 32 in the experiment group who received a 21-day qigong therapy, and 35 in the control group who received no therapy. Researchers measured patients' blood counts the day before chemotherapy and during chemotherapy on days 8, 15, and 22. The 3-week qigong therapy resulted in significant differences in white blood cells, platelets, and hemoglobin between the experiment and control groups. Although researchers concluded that qigong therapy may improve blood counts in breast cancer patients undergoing chemotherapy, they recommended that more studies be conducted on Qigong before it can be introduced in clinical nursing practice (Yeh, Lee, Chen, & Chao, 2006).

References

Sibinga, E. M., Shindell, D. L., Casella, J. F., Duggan, A. K., & Wilson, M. H. (2006). Pediatric patients with sickle cell disease: Use of complementary and alternative therapies. *Journal of Alternative and Complementary Medicine, 12*(3), 291–298.

Takasu, J., Uykimpang, R., Sunga, M. A., Amagase, H., & Niihara, Y. (2006, March). Aged garlic extract is a potential therapy for sickle-cell anemia. *Journal of Nutrition, 136*(3 Suppl), 803S–805S.

Yeh, M. L., Lee, T. I., Chen, H. H., & Chao, T. Y. (2006, March-April). The influences of Chan-Chuang qi-gong therapy on complete blood cell counts in breast cancer patients treated with chemotherapy. *Cancer Nursing, 29*(2), 149–155.

Sickle Cell Crisis

Clinical Problem

Painful sickle cell crisis is not only a dreaded consequence of the disease but also presents a host of medical management problems to the health care team. Uncontrolled sickle cell crisis places the patient at risk of stroke, heart attack, and organ ischemia, as well as unrelenting pain. Numerous interventions have traditionally been applied in an attempt to control pain and increase oxygenation, thus reversing erythrocyte sickling and decreasing blood viscosity. Nurses and health care providers should be armed with treatment options that have demonstrated rapid effectiveness so that pain is relieved and to minimize the risk of long-term organ damage.

Research Findings

Two meta-analyses (Lottenberg & Hassell, 2005; Mehta, Afenyi-Annan, Byrns, & Lottenberg, 2006) specifically weighed the evidence regarding commonly implemented interventions used to treat painful sickle cell crisis including pharmacologic pain management, incentive spirometry, and hydration with IV fluid. With regard to oxygenation, both reports cite a randomized controlled study (38 hospitalizations) examining the impact of incentive spirometry. Each patient in the spirometry group took 10 maximal inspirations using an incentive spirometer every 2 hours while awake until the chest pain subsided. Of the 19 patients assigned to the spirometry group, only 1 developed pulmonary complications compared to 8 patients assigned to the nonspirometry group. Pulmonary complications included atelectasis, thoracic bone infarction, and infiltration.

Implications for Nursing Practice

These studies clearly provide strong evidence supporting incentive spirometry (IS) to reduce the risk of severe pulmonary complications during sickle cell crisis. Nurses play a very crucial role in providing education about the appropriate use of the incentive spirometer. Patients should be taught to use IS frequently and to maximal volume.

Nurses should include IS observation as part of their regular assessment and documentation. Barriers to effective incentive spirometry include pain, short duration of inspiration, and frustration since beneficial effects may take many days to appear. Nurses should assess for pain in relationship to IS and provide adequate pain management to ensure full chest expansion.

Encouragement and progress tracking should also be offered frequently as a motivational factor. Nurses can enlist family members in these motivational efforts by teaching them to read and report the intake volume of the incentive spirometry to the patient. When appropriate, chest auscultation results and general assessment observations should also be shared with patients to ensure them that their incentive spirometry efforts are in fact effective. Changes in IS volumes should be reported immediately, especially in connection with chest pain and changes in oxygenation.

Critical Thinking Questions

1. Identify the common barriers to effective incentive spirometry in the patient with sickle cell disease.

2. Discuss nursing measures that would increase the use of incentive spirometry in the patient with sickle cell disease.

3. List critical elements that should be included in a respiratory assessment of a patient experiencing sickle cell crisis.

Answers to Critical Thinking Questions appear in Appendix D.

References

Lottenberg, R., & Hassell, K. L. (2005). An evidence-based approach to the treatment of adults with sickle cell disease. *ASH Education Book*, pp. 58–65.

Mehta, S. R., Afenyi-Annan, A., Byrns, P.J., & Lottenberg, R. (2006). Opportunities to improve outcomes in sickle cell disease. *American Family Physician, 74*(2), 313–314.

EVIDENCE-BASED PRACTICE

CHART 63–13   **Differences in Hemolysis in Hemolytic Anemia and Bone Marrow Disorders**

Normal Hemolysis and Bone Marrow Function	Hemolytic Anemia	Anemia Due to Bone Marrow Disorders
Hemolysis matched by erythropoiesis	Increased hemolysis, normal erythropoiesis	Normal hemolysis, decreased erythropoiesis

---

first intrinsic cause of hemolytic anemia. The most common defect of this type is glucose-6-phosphate dehydrogenase deficiency. A second intrinsic defect results from fragility and instability in the membrane structure, which is the hallmark of hereditary spherocytosis. A third type of intrinsic defect, which results in increased hemolysis, is the hemoglobinopathies, such as those that occur in sickle cell anemia and thalassemia. However, the primary clinical effects are more closely attributed to hemoglobin rather than hemolysis and were thus discussed separately.

Extrinsic causes include situations where the red blood cell is structurally and chemically normal but an unfavorable external environment leads to increased hemolysis. These types of causes include infections, certain medications, autoimmune processes, toxins, and malignancies. Hemolytic anemias from these extrinsic causes are classically grouped together as the acquired hemolytic anemias. The hemolytic anemias also are commonly classified as being intravascular or extravascular, referring to the primary site of hemolysis. In intravascular hemolysis, damaged RBCs are destroyed in the peripheral circulation, and are associated most commonly with mechanical trauma and toxins. In extravascular hemolysis the primary site of destruction is in the spleen and liver. Normally, a red blood cell has enough flexibility to maneuver through the spleen and liver several times throughout the course of its life span. However, membrane defects (including antibody binding) cause some red blood cells to get trapped and eventually become phagocytosed and destroyed. The clinical signs and symptoms, pathophysiology, and treatment unique to each of the underlying etiologies are discussed on the next page.

Clinical Presentation

In addition to unique signs and symptoms associated with individual disease processes, the hemolytic anemias share common physical findings. Consistent with hypoxia of anemias, the patient may complain of fatigue, activity intolerance, and shortness of breath. Severity of hypoxic symptoms correlates with severity of hemolysis. Patients with chronic disorders such as enzyme deficiencies may present only with hypoxic symptoms during periods of acute exacerbation. Jaundice, hemoglobinuria (red-brown urine), splenomegaly, and hepatomegaly (particularly in combination with poor liver function) are additional indicators of persistent hemolysis. Decreased, concentrated urine output is an indication of acute renal failure due to occlusion by lysed red blood cells and is an emergent sign requiring immediate intervention.

Alterations in Laboratory Values

Although the initial cause may vary, hemolytic anemias share some common trends in laboratory studies. Early stages of hemolytic anemia may reveal reticulocytosis (elevated reticulocyte count) in response to accelerated erythropoiesis. RBC counts will be decreased according to the severity of the hemolysis. Plasma haptoglobin levels also may be decreased (especially in intravascular hemolytic anemias) as liberated globin from lysed red blood cells binds all available haptoglobin. As haptoglobin molecules become overwhelmed, a large portion of the hemolyzed hemoglobin is excreted as unconjugated bilirubin. The level of unconjugated bilirubin in hemolysis is typically 70 to 85 μmol/L (4 to 5 mg/dL), or higher if liver function is impaired. If the marrow cannot compensate to replace the RBCs (as indicated by a *decreased* reticulocyte count), the anemia will worsen. Other indicators supporting a diagnosis of hemolytic anemia are increased lactate dehydrogenase (LDH), and serum AST (SGOT) both due to accelerated RBC destruction (Chart 63–14) (Bunn & Rosse, 2003).

Medical Management

The first goal in the emergent management of the patient presenting with symptomatic hemolytic anemia is the stabilization of oxygenation status. Oxygen is administered to prevent critical organ hypoxia, however, administration should be carefully titrated to prevent suppression of erythropoiesis. Intravenous infusions serve to both maintain fluid volume for cardiovascular status and to preserve renal function by flushing the body of excess waste and unconjugated bilirubin. Another goal is the amelioration of rampant hemolysis. If appropriate, triggering agents such as drugs or toxins should be immediately removed. If the cause is extravascular and the patient presents with splenomegaly, a splenectomy, or surgical removal of the spleen, may be indicated (Dhaliwal, Cornnett, & Tierney, 2004). Splenectomy, however, usually is only indicated for certain forms of hemolytic anemia without identifiable triggering agents or in severe cases of acquired hemolytic anemia.

Once the patient is stabilized and risk of imminent organ failure has subsided, attention turns to identification of the underlying pathophysiological process. A CBC and RBC morphology can help rule out or point to bone marrow involvement. Liver function tests can assist in distinguishing hemolytic anemia from nonhematologic causes such as liver failure. A thorough patient history that emphasizes family history and possible toxin and drug exposure also provides important diagnostic clues.

■ Nursing Management

Nursing care of the patient with hemolytic anemia has three main goals: avoidance of triggering factors in susceptible patients and prevention and treatment of complications. High-risk patients such as those with enzyme deficiencies, membrane deficiencies, hemoglobinopathies, or patients with a history of autoimmune hemolytic anemia may initially arrive into the acute care setting without symptoms of rampant hemolysis. To minimize risk of hemolysis, the nurse should carefully review patient histories to identify high-risk persons.

Once identified, collaboration with the interdisciplinary team can help ensure that potential triggering agents are removed from the environment, if appropriate. These high-risk patients should be monitored closely for signs of generalized anemia including increasing fatigue, activity intolerance, and hypoxia, as described earlier in the Nursing Process: Patient Care Plan for Generalized Anemia (p. 2013). Assessments revealing decreased urinary output, hemoglobinuria, left flank pain (from splenomegaly), and fever suggest hemolytic anemia in particular. Analysis of laboratory values revealing reticulocytosis, decreased RBCs, increased bilirubin, and increased lactate dehydrogenase will further confirm hemolytic anemia.

Nursing interventions should then focus on minimizing the effects of blood cell hemolysis. The patient is at high risk for renal failure, thus, the nurse should prioritize interventions to maintain renal blood flow. These include encouraging oral intake and administration of IV fluid and blood component therapy as ordered. Frequent monitoring of urinary output, skin turgor, peripheral edema, and lung sounds will assist the nurse in determining fluid needs. Uncomfortable itching from excessive bilirubin, decreased oxygenation, and activity intolerance all increase the patient's risk for skin breakdown. Nurses should implement aggressive wound prevention protocols such as frequent turning, alleviation of pressure, and frequent skin lubrication to prevent skin breakdown. A third high-risk area of concern is pain related to splenomegaly and intravascular occlusion from lysed

---

CHART 63–14 **Signs and Symptoms of Hemolytic Anemia**

Physical Assessment	Laboratory Values
• Fatigue	• Reticulocytes: increased (reticulocytes decrease in severe hemolytic anemia or with failing bone marrow)
• Activity intolerance	
• Shortness of breath	
• Tachycardia	• Red blood cells: decreased
• Tachypnea	• Serum erythropoietin: increased
• Jaundice (severe cases)	
• Hemoglobinuria (severe cases)	• Serum haptoglobin: decreased
• Decreased urine output	• Unconjugated bilirubin: increased
• Splenomegaly	
• Hepatomegaly	• Lactate dehydrogenase: increased
	• Serum AST: increased

red blood cells. The nurse must perform frequent pain assessments and offer comfort measures, antipyretics, and analgesics (as ordered) to minimize increasing pain.

Glucose-6-Phosphate Dehydrogenase Deficiency

Glucose-6-phosphate dehydrogenase (G6PD) deficiency is the most common enzyme deficiency contributing to hemolytic anemia. Deficiencies in the enzyme are genetically encoded and relatively common especially in persons of African American and Mediterranean descent. Pyruvate kinase deficiency also results in hemolytic anemia, but occurs less frequently. Enzymatic deficiencies in erythrocytes increase the red blood cell's sensitivity and susceptibility to oxidative stress. Normal metabolism is associated with oxidative stress and produces an accumulation of free radicals and other substances that can disrupt function and growth. Enzymes such as G6PD and pyruvate kinase neutralize such free radicals, thus protecting the RBCs. Free radical accumulation is accelerated by a variety of situations that cause oxidative problems including exposure to certain drugs (malarial drugs, sulfonamides, nitrofurantoins, and chloramphenicol), dehydration, sepsis, and diabetic ketoacidosis. Therapeutic management involves removal of the triggering agent and supportive care until the hemolysis subsides. Due to the relatively high occurrence in certain ethnic groups, susceptible patients should be screened for G6PD deficiency before being administered oxidant drugs. Once a patient has been diagnosed and triggering agents identified, most patients with G6PD can live asymptomatically.

Hereditary Spherocytosis

Another cause of hemolytic anemia is defects in the red blood cell membrane. The RBC membrane is a specialized lattice structure of proteins arranged to produce strength, resilience, elasticity, and durability as the red blood cell navigates the peripheral bloodstream. Survival of the 120-day life span of the RBC is highly enhanced by this strong exoskeleton. Genetic disorders including hereditary spherocytosis, hereditary elliptocytosis, hereditary pyropoikilocytosis, and hereditary stomatocytosis all encode proteins that weaken the lattice structure and produce malformed erythrocyte membranes. For example, in **hereditary spherocytosis (HS)**, RBCs lack spectrin, a key membrane protein, which then forces the RBCs into an unstable spherical shape rather than the normal, more stable concave form. HS is a genetic disorder appearing in individuals of northern European descent, affecting approximately 1 in 1,000 to 2,500 patients. The mutated spherical shape of HS cells increases their rate of splenic destruction, resulting in higher rates of hemolysis. Figure 63–8 ■ shows grouped RBCs shown in profile and normal RBCs compared to a sickle RBC (Gallagher, 2005).

Clinical Presentation

Clinical presentation of HS varies with disease severity and inheritance pattern. Autosomal dominant forms and homozygous gene patterns produce persistent anemia, jaundice, and splenomegaly beginning early in life, thus, patients are frequently diagnosed as children. Heterozygous gene patterns can produce carrier states, in which patients are able to develop sufficient compensatory mechanisms and remain asymptomatic. Pallor, activity intolerance, and hypoxia may appear only when

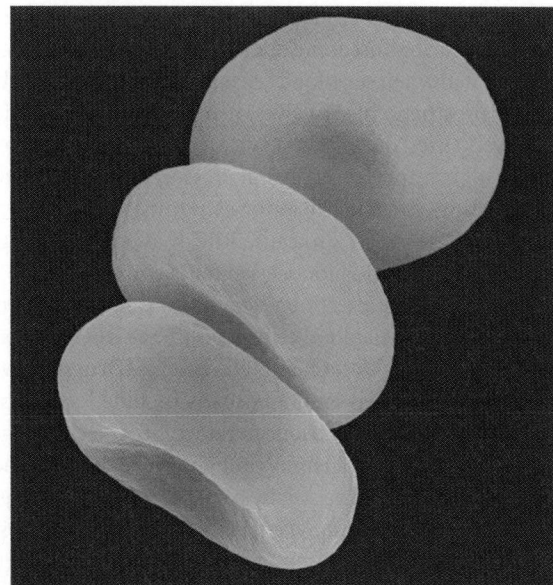

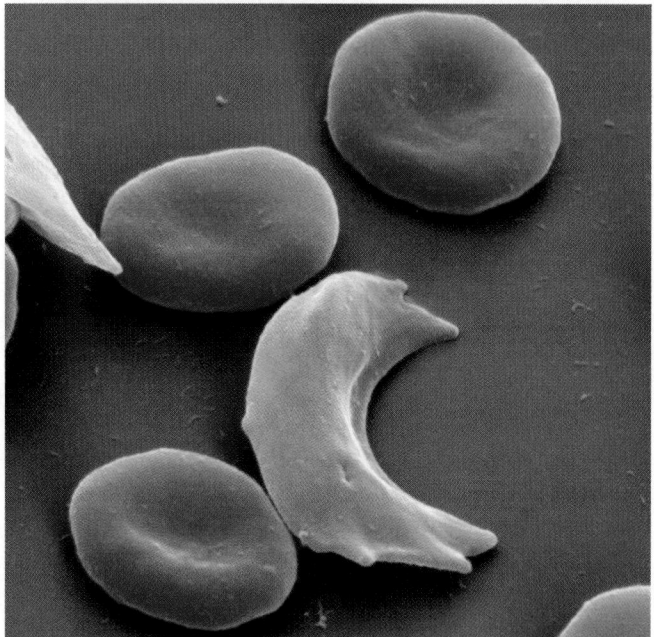

FIGURE 63–8 ■ (top) RBCs in profile, forming rouleaux and (bottom) Normal RBCs compared to a sickled RBC.
Source: (top) © Visuals Unlimited/CORBIS All Rights Reserved; (bottom) Oliver Meckes & Nicole Ottawa/Photo Researchers, Inc.

erythropoiesis is unable to compensate for hemolysis, such as occurs in severe infections, the presence of certain toxins, renal involvement, or bone marrow involvement. Rampant hemolysis of HS red blood cells will be indicated by splenomegaly and jaundice. These may be accompanied by biliary disease and cholecystitis.

Acquired Hemolytic Anemias

Acquired hemolytic anemias develop when an unfavorable external environment leads to increased hemolysis of structurally and chemically normal red blood cells. Such an environment can be mediated by three distinct pathophysiological processes: mechanical causes, infectious agents and toxins, and autoimmune reactions. Mechanical causes of hemolytic anemia describe any situation where normal red blood cells are subjected to extreme or repeated shearing forces, heat, or osmotic attack. Such forces can be generated when red blood cells are exposed to foreign bodies such as prosthetic heart valves, hemodialysis filters, shunts, and cell savers (used during surgery). Mechanical trauma such as prolonged high-impact exercise or pressure also can result in RBC destruction, particularly in the extremities. Prolonged heat exposure above 49°C can also cause RBC lysis, underscoring the potential dangers behind blood-warming devices.

Certain toxins and infectious agents also can cause chemical reactions within the red blood cell, or within the RBC membrane causing premature lysis and hemolytic anemia. Drugs known to contribute to shortened RBC life spans include lead, copper, interferon-alpha, nitrites, dapsonea, and arsenic. Infectious agents cause acquired hemolytic anemia through several different mechanisms including direct invasion by parasites (malaria), release of bacterial toxins (*Clostridium perfringens* and *Haemophilus influenzae* type B), and promotion of splenic sequestration.

Immune-mediated hemolytic anemia is one of the most common causes of acquired hemolytic anemia, and is further divided into autoimmune hemolytic anemia and alloimmune hemolytic anemia. **Autoimmune hemolytic anemia** describes any situation where the patient's own healthy immune system generates antibodies against proteins on his or her own red blood cells (autoantibodies). These autoantibodies are generally divided into two types, warm antibody hemolytic anemia and cold antibody hemolytic anemia. In the warm antibody type, the autoantibodies attach to and destroy red blood cells at temperatures equal to or in excess of normal body temperature. In the cold antibody type, the autoantibodies become most active and attach red blood cells only at temperatures well below normal body temperature. The warm antibody hemolytic anemia accounts for more than 80% of all disease cases. In either type of anemia, the mechanisms that trigger the generation of autoantobodies remain unclear. Possible causes include alteration to immune system development or stimulation by the microbial infections. Alloimmune hemolytic anemia occurs most commonly after prolonged exposure to donated RBC transfusion or after pregnancy. Other causes include malignancy, drugs, autoimmune disorders, systemic lupus erythematosus, and viral infection.

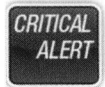 *Correct crossmatching of blood involves ensuring that the RBC antibodies from donors will not stimulate autoimmune reactions in the recipient. Nurses must very carefully monitor blood cell transfusions checking for correct crossmatch prior to infusion and watching extremely closely for signs and symptoms of hemolytic anemia.*

Treatment must first address identification and removal of triggering agents. If immune-mediated reactions are suspected, Coombs' test will be ordered. Coombs' test detects the presence of circulating antibodies against RBC surface proteins. The presence of any antibodies is an abnormal result indicative of immune-mediated hemolytic anemia. Any of the alterations to laboratory values listed earlier in Chart 63–14 (p. 2036) also will support a diagnosis of hemolytic anemia.

Supportive care should focus on mitigating the immune response by use of immunosuppressive agents and corticosteroids. If mechanical forces are suspected, peripheral blood smears will reveal ruptured blood cells. Treatment for these cases is tailored

to the unique trauma involved. Nursing management is consistent with that presented earlier for hemolytic anemia and generalized anemia. Additionally, nurses should include an assessment for hemolytic anemia whenever a patient presents with history of the risk factors presented above. The Pharmacology Summary feature for anemia lists medications used to treat this disorder and their actions, applications, and nursing responsibilities.

Hemostasis: Regulation of Bleeding and Thrombosis

Hemostasis is the critical biologic process that mitigates blood loss due to injury to any blood vessel. Hemostasis is achieved via very complex and tightly controlled interactions among regulatory mechanisms, cellular components, vessel structures, hormones, plasma proteins, and other chemicals. Although it may appear that hemostasis would only be activated occasionally (i.e., with visible injuries), in actuality the microvasculature is constantly subjected to "mini-traumas" from normal changes in blood pressure and seemingly insignificant physical contact with the environment. Failure of any of the hemostasis mechanisms leads to abnormal clotting, abnormal bleeding, or in some cases both. A review of the normal processes of hemostasis assists the health care provider in understanding diseases that result from deviations in normal hemostasis.

Hemostasis Concepts

The process of hemostasis is a very tightly regulated and elaborate system of interacting proteins, cellular components, and chemical reactions. A discussion of some of the key concepts involved in hemostasis is a useful introduction to the chemical pathways that utilize them.

Cascades

The term *cascade* is an appropriate and important concept throughout hemostasis. In the absence of injury, the chemical components of hemostasis (factors, protein receptors) normally exist in an "inactivated" state in the bloodstream or on cell surfaces. However, injury sets off a chain of events that activates these chemical components. This activation process proceeds in a very specific sequence in which the activation of one chemical component in turn triggers the activation of the next chemical component. For instance, tissue factor transforms Factor VII into Factor VIIa. When Factor VIIa reaches sufficient quantities, it triggers the activation of Factor X into Factor Xa. Each step in the cascade can only proceed if the prior step produced sufficient quantities of activated factors. This concept helps to explain the bleeding (or insufficient clotting) tendencies that accompany certain diseases, such as liver failure, hemophilia, and von Willebrand's disease, which result in insufficient production of factors.

Factors

Factors are proteins present in the bloodstream that, when activated, help facilitate the next step of the coagulation cascade. Most factors are synthesized in the liver in a chemically inactive form. When the chemically inactive form comes into contact with its very specific catalyst, chemical and structural changes occur that convert the inactive form to the active form. Classically, the suffix *a* has been used to designate the active form of

PHARMACOLOGY Summary of Medications to Treat Anemia

Medicine Category	Action	Application/Indication	Nursing Responsibility
Erythropoietic agents	Provides exogenous source of erythropoietin, which stimulates differentiation and proliferation of the hematopoetic cascade. Also, stimulates iron absorption by the erythroid progenitor cells.	Anemia of chronic disease, renal failure, or cancer. Indicated with hemoglobin less than 20.	Assessment of laboratory values to assess efficacy of treatment. Assessment of side effects such as bone pain related to therapy. Patient education regarding self-administration techniques, if appropriate.
Oral iron supplementation	Provides additional iron supply to increase amount of elemental iron available for hemoglobin synthesis.	Iron deficiency anemia when dietary modification is insufficient.	Assessment of drug allergy history prior to administration. Assessment of clinical manifestations of complications such as upper epigastric pain, constipation. Patient education regarding techniques to enhance iron supplement absorption and prevent or treat constipation.
Parenteral iron supplementation	Stimulates release of iron from plasma, which replenishes depleted iron stores in bone marrow.	Severe iron deficiency anemia requiring rapid correction or for patients with chronic kidney disease.	Assessment of drug allergy history. Patient education regarding infusion procedure and potential/expected reactions. Monitoring for signs and symptoms of hypersensitivity and anaphylaxis during and after infusion.
Vitamin supplementation: folates and vitamin B_{12}	Corrects deficiency in key elements required for hemoglobin synthesis.	Serum vitamin B_{12} level less than 100 pg/mL and serum folate level less than 5 ng/mL.	Patient education regarding necessity for vitamin supplementation. Referral to dietary consult to identify additional sources of bioavailable vitamins in foods. Assessment of vitamin therapy efficacy such as patient report of energy.

the factor from the inactive form, and roman numerals used as a consistent label for all factors. Once in the active form, the factor can now act as a very specific catalyst for the activation of the next step of the cascade. Deficiencies in any of the clotting factors either from liver disease, vitamin K deficiency, or genetic causes manifests as a disorder of hemostasis. Chart 63–15 (p. 2040) lists the major factors central to hemostasis. The role of each factor is addressed in the discussion about the clotting cascades.

Hemostasis Pathways

Maintenance of normal blood flow requires hemostasis mechanisms to accomplish four critical goals: (1) recognition of the injury, (2) clot formation, (3) cessation of bleeding, and (4) clot lysis. Injuries to blood vessels are detected simultaneously by a number of body systems including the autonomic nervous system (which controls pain and vasoconstriction) and the hematologic system. Vasoconstriction in the target area serves to reduce the chance of blood loss from the injured site. More importantly perhaps, the mechanical (squeezing) action also helps to release chemicals that initiate clot formation. The clot begins as a soft, pliable plug that typically is used to slow minor bleeding (pri-

mary hemostasis), but then it progresses to a strong meshlike cover, encasing the injured vessel while it heals (secondary hemostasis). Once the injured vessel is healed, the clot must be removed in order to maintain a smooth surface on the blood vessel. The following section describes the hemostasis pathways beginning with formation of the soft plug (mediated by platelets), continuing onto the formation of the meshlike cover (accomplished via the clotting cascade), and finally termination of the clot (a process termed fibrinolysis). Figure 63–9 ■ (p. 2040) provides a graphic illustration of the stages of hemostasis.

Platelet Plug Formation: Primary Hemostasis

Under normal circumstances, circulating platelets neither stick to each other or to vessel walls. When injury to a vessel occurs, injured blood vessels interact with circulating platelets, ultimately leading to the formation of a clump of platelets, called the soft platelet plug, in a process known as *primary hemostasis*. The catalyst for primary hemostasis is the release of substances from the exposed subendothelial layer that interact with protein receptors on platelet's surfaces, inducing chemical and configurational changes, a process termed *activation*.

CHART 63–15	Major Factors Central to Hemostasis	
Factor	**Also Known As**	**Clotting Cascade Pathway***
I	Fibrinogen	Both
II	Prothrombin	Both
III	Tissue factor	Tissue factor (extrinsic)
IV	Calcium	Both
V	Proaccelerin	Both
VI	Accelerin	Both
VII	Proconvertin, cothromboplastin	Tissue factor (extrinsic)
VIII	Antihemophilic factor A	Contact activation (intrinsic)
IX	Christmas factor	Contact activation (intrinsic)
X	Stuart–Power factor	Both (common pathway)
XI	Plasma thromboplastin	Contact activation (intrinsic)
XII	Hegman factor	Contact activation (intrinsic)
XIII	Fibrin stabilizing factor	Both

*Refer to discussion on clotting cascade in the text.

Sources: Moran, T., & Viele, C. (2005). Normal clotting. *Seminars in Oncology Nursing, 21*(4), 1–11; Porth, C. M. (2007). *Essentials of pathophysiology: concepts of altered health states* (2nd ed.). Philadelphia: Lippincott Williams & Wilkins.

Once activated individual platelets undergo geometric and chemical changes that allow them to form a soft platelet plug. Formation of the platelet plug occurs rapidly via four distinct actions:

1. **Adhesion**—Adhesion refers to the sticking of platelets onto the injured vessel wall. Adhesion is initiated when von Willebrand's factor forms a bridge between exposed collagen from the subendothelial layer of the vessel wall and proteins (glycoprotein Ib) on the platelet surface. Patients afflicted with von Willebrand's disease lack sufficient quantities of the factor and can suffer uncontrolled bleeding.

2. **Aggregation**—On activated platelets, protein receptors (specifically IIb and IIa) seek out and bind to neighboring platelet membranes. Additionally, activated platelets adhere to fibrinogen, a chemical secreted into the bloodstream by the liver. Fibrinogen has the ability to form fibrous meshlike networks between platelets.

3. **Secretion**—The third function of activated platelets is the secretion of substances (a process called degranulation). Adenosine diphosphate (ADP) and serotonin recruit additional platelets to the site of injury and also stimulate more vasoconstriction. Other substances, including fibronectin, thromboxane A_2, thrombospondin, arachidonic acid, and platelet Factor V, stimulate the platelet membrane to form pseudopods (elongated shapes) and interact with fibrinogen, which help to stabilize the platelet plug. This soft platelet plug can form within seconds in the individual not lacking any of the required chemical factors. Its primary goal is the immediate abatement of minor bleeding; however, the temporary plug can be easily sheared off unless stabilized. Intracellular calcium, which is required for factor activation in the clotting cascade, also is released from the platelets.

4. **Assembly**—Finally activated platelet cell surfaces promote the assembly of enzymes necessary for the initiation of the

Normal

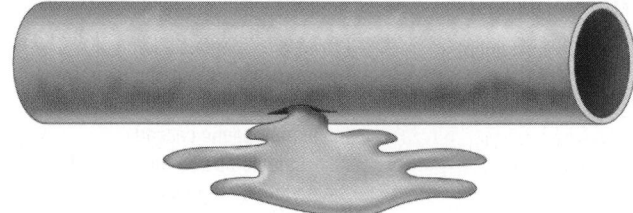
1 Bleeding starts

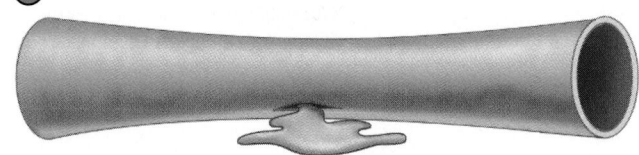
2 Vasoconstriction

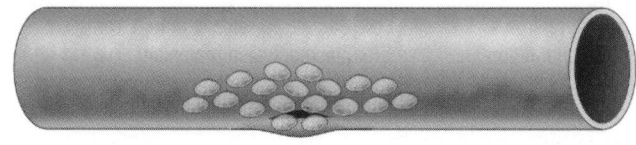
3 Soft platelet plug - primary hemostasis

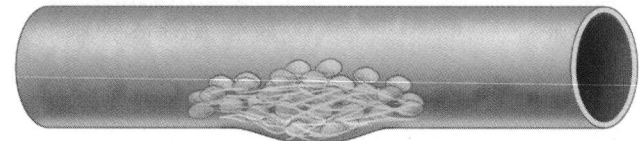
4 Fibrin clot formation - secondary hemostasis

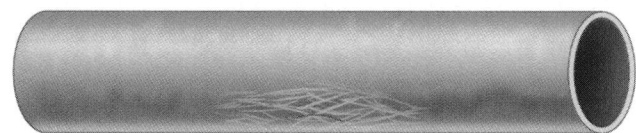
5 Clot lysis

FIGURE 63–9 ■ Stages of hemostasis.

clotting cascade. For example, von Willebrand's factor bound to the platelet can also bind coagulation factor VIII, a component of the clotting cascade (discussed next).

Clotting Cascade: Secondary Hemostasis

While vasoconstriction and platelets act rapidly to minimize blood loss, sustained turbulent blood flow at the site of injury can shear the platelet plug. The clotting cascade describes the sequential activation of factors ultimately leading to the formation of a fibrin sheath, which stabilizes the platelet plug. Rather than being a single cascade of events, the term *clotting cascade* actually describes two distinct series of events: the contact activation (or intrinsic) pathway and the tissue factor (or extrinsic) pathway. If successful, each pathway results in the activation of Factor X to Factor Xa, which begins the final stage of clotting, the common pathway.

The molecular mechanisms underlying the clotting cascade have been the focus of intense research for several years, most likely due to the role of clotting and hemostasis in diseases such as cardiovascular disorders, thrombosis, and stroke. Scientific advancements have reshaped the classic understanding of and terminology used with the clotting cascade process. Traditionally, it was thought that the two pathways acted independently to form the fibrin net. Now, however, it is widely recognized that deficiencies in one pathway cannot be compensated for by the other pathway, suggesting some degree of interaction. Second, the terms *intrinsic pathway* and *extrinsic pathway* have been replaced by the terms *contact activation* and *tissue factor*, respectively, describing the discovery of the initiating events of each pathway.

Contact Activation: The Intrinsic Pathway

The contact activation pathway describes the clotting cascade branch initiated by the contact between circulating plasma proteins and the negatively charged surface of the injured subendothelial layer. Figure 63–10 ■ describes the activation steps. Hageman factor (Factor XII) sets off the cascade by contacting the subendothelial layer, which causes it to become Factor XIIa (activated factor), setting off the series of activations culminating with Factor VIIa, which then leads to the common pathway (Hoffman & Monroe, 2005).

Tissue Factor: The Extrinsic Pathway

The extrinsic pathway describes the branch of the clotting cascade pathway initiated by tissue factor (TF) also called tissue thromboplastin, a substance released from injured cells of the subendothelial layers. In the presence of calcium and lipids released from platelets, tissue factor first activates Factor VII into Factor VIIa. Then tissue factor interacts with the newly activated Factor VIIa to activate Factor X into Factor Xa, the beginning step of the common pathway (Figure 63–11 ■).

The Common Pathway

Both the contact activation and tissue factor pathways converge with the activation of Factor X into Factor Xa (Figure 63–12 ■, p. 2042). In the presence of calcium and lipids from activated platelets, Factor Xa converts prothrombin (Factor II) to throm-

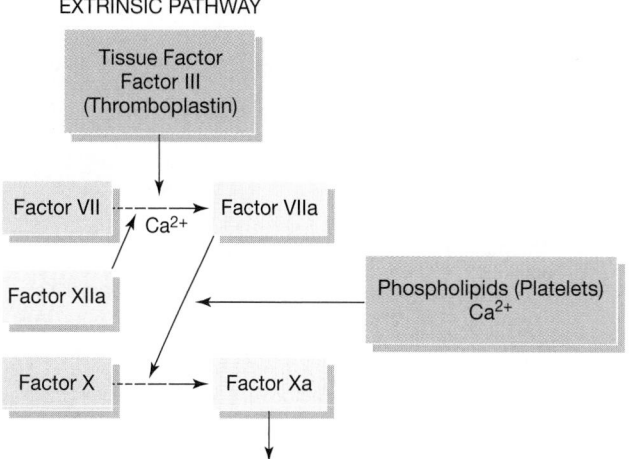

EXTRINSIC PATHWAY

FIGURE 63–11 ■ The tissue factor activation (extrinsic) pathway.

bin (Factor IIa). Thrombin is an extremely powerful component in coagulation, playing three main roles. First, thrombin interacts and amplifies the contact activation (intrinsic) and tissue factor (extrinsic) pathways to form a positive feedback loop ensuring that coagulation continues. Second, thrombin interacts with fibrinogen to make fibrin strands (polymers). Last, thrombin also activates fibrin stabilizing factor (Factor XIII). In the presence of calcium, again released from platelets, Factor XIIIa and the fibrin strands weave through the platelet plug, forming a strong mesh (termed the fibrin mesh) and effectively sealing the site of injury and halting bleeding.

Termination of Clotting

The processes of platelet plug formation (primary hemostasis) and coagulation (secondary hemostasis) ultimately result in the formation of a fibrin mesh that effectively halts bleeding. However, left unchecked, continued fibrin formation can lead to vessel occlusion by expanding clots, thrombosis, blood stasis, and embolism. These molecular processes are the underlying causes behind serious diseases such as embolic stroke, cardiovascular disease, and deep venous thrombosis (DVT). To prevent such damage and to maintain smooth, adequate blood flow, hemostasis must include a process to regulate and eventually terminate clotting when no longer required. This termination phase of coagulation hinges on the action of three inhibitors: antithrombin, tissue factor pathway inhibitor, and protein C.

Antithrombin is a naturally occurring protein circulating in the bloodstream that neutralizes the actions of thrombin and activated Factors Xa, XIa, XIIa, and IXa. As injuries heal and vasoconstriction begins to subside, blood flow begins to return to normal levels, bringing antithrombin to the site of coagulation. Antithrombin is a key target in the pharmacologic treatment of thrombosis, because its activity is significantly accelerated by the anticoagulant heparin (Bajaj, Birktoft, & Steer, 2001).

Tissue factor pathway inhibitor (TFPI) neutralizes Factor X, halting progression of the common pathway and production of thrombin. Increased TFPI levels have been observed in the presence of heparin and low-molecular-weight heparin, and new drug therapies that enhance the action of TFPI are currently being developed (Bajaj et al., 2001).

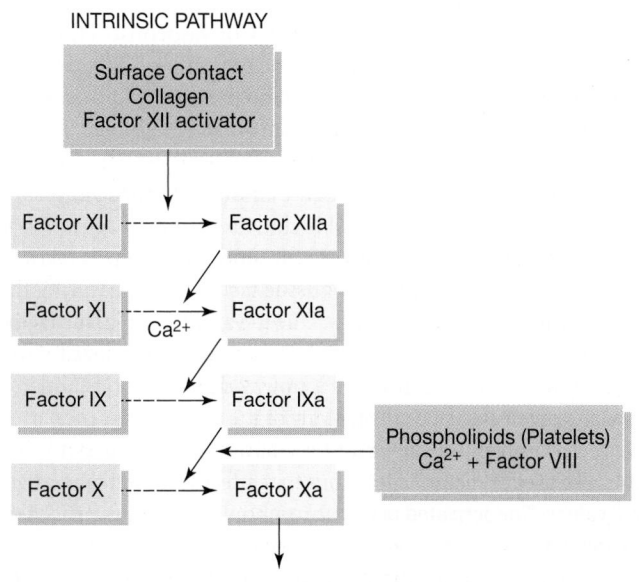

INTRINSIC PATHWAY

FIGURE 63–10 ■ The contact activation (intrinsic) pathway.

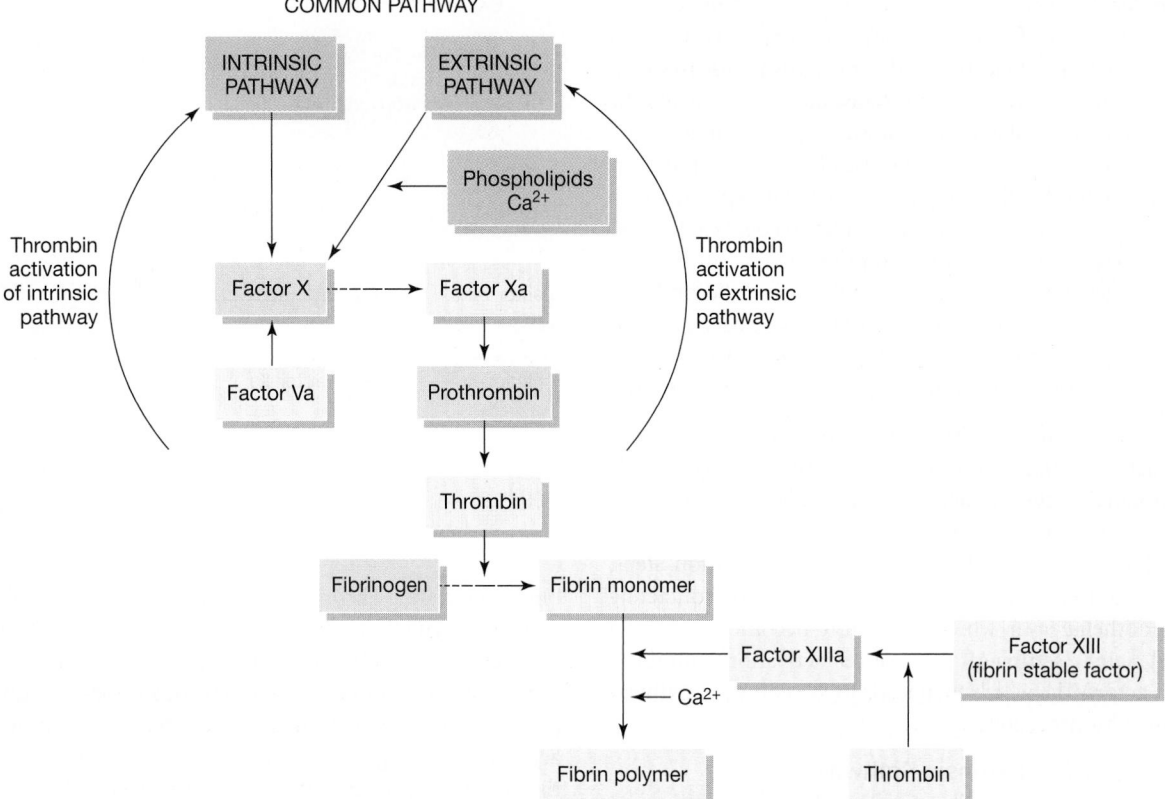

FIGURE 63–12 ■ The common pathway.

Activated protein C neutralizes Factor V of the tissue factor (extrinsic) pathway and Factor VIII of the contact activation (intrinsic) pathway. The activation of protein C occurs with the binding of thrombin to the subendothelial layer of the vessel wall; thus, accelerated thrombin production results in accelerated protein C activation and an effective braking mechanism for coagulation. Activated protein C therapy plays an important role in the therapeutic management of thrombosis especially in the management of septic shock (Chapter 61 🔗).

Additional chemicals such as nitric oxide, prostacyclin, and thromboxane also limit excessive contributions to coagulation control by limiting platelet aggregation, activation, adhesion, and vasoconstriction. Activation of these components is the target of many anti-inflammatory drugs including non-steroidal anti-inflammatory drugs (NSAIDs), aspirin, and Cox-1 inhibitors.

Fibrinolysis: Clot Elimination

Once the endothelial layers of the blood vessel membrane have healed, the fibrin clot should be removed to optimize blood flow. The last phase of hemostasis is fibrinolysis, or the dissolution of the fibrin strands. Tissue plasminogen activator (t-PA), released by the endothelial cells during coagulation, and urokinase cause the activation of plasminogen to plasmin. Plasmin is a powerful enzyme that first digests fibrin strands into fibrin degradation products (FDPs), themselves extremely powerful promoters of fibrinolysis. FDPs are able to inhibit thrombin activity to slow clot formation and to accelerate plasmin production. As with most of the chemical elements in the coagulation cascade, medical research has developed drug treatments that exploit the natural activity of t-PA and urokinase in the management of thrombosis.

Laboratory and Diagnostic Procedures

Several blood tests are available to measure the efficacy of platelet plug formation (primary hemostasis), coagulation (secondary hemostasis), and fibrinolysis. The platelet count, usually part of the CBC, describes the number of circulating platelets in a volume of blood. Normal values range from 150,000 to 400,000 per microliter of blood. Values of less than 150,000 define thrombocytopenia and imply impaired clotting by platelets. However, spontaneous bleeding rarely occurs at levels above 50,000. Values greater than 400,000 are labeled thrombocytosis and imply excessive platelet clotting.

Bleeding time measures the efficacy of vasoconstriction and platelet response. In the bleeding time test, a blood pressure cuff is inflated around the arm to a specific pressure and then small incisions are made in the patient's arm. Normally, clot formation begins within 3 to 7 minutes.

Clotting time studies measure the amount of time required for a volume of blood to form a stable clot. Prothrombin time (PT) is measured in seconds and reflects the amount of time it takes to form a clot after the addition of tissue factor, thus measuring the tissue factor (extrinsic) pathway. Due to variations in tissue factor batches among laboratories, the International Normalized Ratio (INR) value was developed and is now widely used as a standardized interpretation of the test. Many of the components measured by the prothrombin time require vitamin K for their synthesis, thus diseases or dietary alterations that affect vitamin K also affect PT values. The activated partial thromboplastin time (aPTT), also expressed in seconds, measures the efficacy of the contact activation (intrinsic) pathway in clot formation. The normal values for these tests are listed in Chart 63–16.

CHART 63–16	Blood Tests/Values Indicative of Hemostasis	
Lab Value	**Normal Value**	**Rationale**
Platelets	150,000–400,000/mm³	Measures number of platelets in volume of blood. Reduction indicates thrombocytopenia.
Bleeding time	<12 minutes	Measures primary hemostasis efficacy.
Prothrombin time (PT)	10–20 seconds (significant variation in normal values between laboratories)	Measures efficacy of extrinsic pathway. Increased values indicate thrombotic tendencies. Reduction indicates bleeding tendencies.
International Normalized Ratio (INR)	0.8–1.2 INR	Used in conjunction with PT. Elevated in Coumadin therapy.
Partial thromboplastin time (aPTT)	Varies (compare with control); 35–45 seconds	Measures efficacy of intrinsic pathway. Increased values indicate thrombotic tendencies. Reduction indicates bleeding tendencies.
Fibrin degradation products (FDP)	<10 µg/mL	Measures efficacy of fibrinolytic system.
D-dimer	<0.5 mg/L	Measures efficacy of fibrinolytic system.

Fibrin degradation products (FDPs), especially D-dimer, measure the volume of these powerful fibrinolysis activators. Values are increased during sepsis, disseminated intravascular coagulation (or any coagulation event), and pregnancy.

Disorders of Hemostasis

When the tight regulation of hemostasis is disrupted by disease, drugs, or environmental factors, the affected patient can present with abnormal bleeding, abnormal clotting, or in some cases both. Like all blood disorders, disorders of hemostasis can be either acquired (as in response to sepsis or bone marrow suppression therapy) or chronic (as in genetic disorders of hemophilia and von Willebrand's disease). Disorders of hemostasis also can be categorized according to the deficient or errant component. Disorders of the platelet and vessel wall can be categorized as disorders of primary hemostasis and include thrombocytopenia, hemolytic uremic syndrome, and von Willebrand's disease. Disorders involving factor deficiencies affecting coagulation can be categorized as secondary hemostasis disorders and include liver disease, vitamin K deficiency, and hemophilia.

Disorders of Primary Hemostasis

Disorders of primary hemostasis include any problems affecting platelets or platelet interaction with the subendothelial vessel layer. All of these disorders result in prolonged bleeding times, resulting from slowed platelet plug formation. Qualitative problems or reduction of platelets from normal values are classified as the various thrombocytopenias and represent a significant portion of all disorders of hemostasis. Diseases resulting from abnormal interaction between the subendothelial layer of the vessel, although less common, also result in abnormal bleeding times and describe any disease process that affects platelet aggregation, adhesion, or secretion. Hemolytic uremic syndrome and von Willebrand's disease are discussed below as exemplars of this class of primary hemostasis disorders.

Thrombocytopenia

Thrombocytopenia is defined as a decrease in the number of circulating platelets from the normal value of 150,000/µL. Although significant, spontaneous bleeding usually is not observed until levels fall below 50,000/µL. It is one of the most common hematologic problems experienced by patients and warrants a thorough understanding by nurses and other health care providers. The causes of thrombocytopenia are numerous but, like most hematologic disorders, can be divided into two broad categories: thrombocytopenia due to impaired or suppressed production of platelets and thrombocytopenia due to accelerated destruction of platelets. The major patient care issue associated with thrombocytopenia is an increased tendency for bleeding.

Normal Physiology of Platelets

An understanding of the normal physiology of platelet development provides an effective foundation for a discussion about platelet disorders. Platelets are not cells with independently functioning nuclei and cytoplasmic structures like white blood cells and red blood cells; rather, they are shed fragments of the megakaryocyte. Platelet development proceeds in much the same fashion as that of red blood cells and white blood cells. Recall from the discussion at the beginning of the chapter about hematopoiesis that all cellular elements of the blood arise in the bone marrow from the hematopoeitic stem cell before undergoing differentiation, maturation, and release into the peripheral bloodstream (see Figure 63–1, p. 2007).

The complete pathway from HSC to fully mature platelet release into the periphery is called *thrombopoiesis*. The primary regulating substance in thrombopoiesis is thought to be the hormone **thrombopoietin**, produced by the liver and kidneys. Thrombopoietin directs the HSC to produce the megakaryocyte, the precursor to fully functioning platelets. Thrombopoietin additionally stimulates the megakaryocyte to undergo mitosis and reproduce itself (thus exponentially increasing the potential for platelet quantities), and most importantly triggers the fragmentation of the megakaryocyte into small particles. These particles are platelets, which are then released into the periphery and generally survive an 8- to 12-day life span. Senescent (aging) platelets begin to express cell surface proteins, which trigger its destruction by macrophages in the spleen and reticuloendothelial system. Alterations to thrombopoiesis can have deleterious effects on hemostasis ranging from increased bleeding to increased thrombosis.

Pathophysiology of Thrombocytopenia

Thrombocytopenia has been attributed to several underlying causes, which can be broadly divided into suppressed production or accelerated destruction. The pathophysiology of each class and representative disease processes are discussed below.

Impaired Production of Platelets A number of disease processes as well as environmental factors impede thrombopoiesis and result in thrombocytopenia. Diseases such as leukemia, lymphoma, multiple myeloma, metastatic cancers, and aplastic anemia are associated with global suppression of hematopoiesis, which will thus include suppressed platelet production. Additionally, most of the treatment approaches (chemotherapy and radiation) used in cancer and other bone marrow diseases independently suppress thrombopoiesis. Exposures to viruses have resulted in selective suppression of the megakaryocyte and include human immunodeficiency virus (HIV), Epstein–Barr, rubella, and mumps exposure. A third mechanism for impaired platelet production is liver disease resulting in insufficient quantities of thrombopoietin, vitamin B_{12}, and vitamin K (Rios, Sangro, Herrero, Quiroga, & Prieto, 2005). Finally, exposure to certain drugs, especially large quantities of alcohol and thiazide diuretics, can suppress megakaryocyte production.

Accelerated Destruction of Platelets Thrombocytopenia due to accelerated destruction can be subdivided into two categories: autoimmune causes and nonautoimmune causes. Autoimmune-accelerated destruction of platelets describes any situation in which the patient appropriately develops antibodies against invading pathogens, which then inappropriately attach to surface proteins of circulating platelets. When these antibody-bound platelets reach the spleen they are prematurely removed, causing thrombocytopenia. This autoimmune response has been observed following exposure to systemic lupus erythematosus, rheumatoid arthritis, HIV, and excessive transfusions, as well as certain drugs including depakote and heparin (Davoren & Aster, 2006; Gesundheit, Kirby, Lau, Koren, & Abdelhaleem, 2002).

Nonautoimmune processes contributing to early platelet destruction include exposure to prosthetic heart valves, thrombotic thrombocytopenic purpura (TTP), sepsis, and hemolytic uremic syndrome. In these situations, the thrombocytopenia can be attributed to increased utilization of platelets by the underlying disease process. As the platelets (appropriately) respond to vessel damage caused by these processes, they are removed from circulation, manifesting as a decreased platelet count.

Clinical Presentation

A diagnosis of thrombocytopenia often is made after observation of active bleeding, underscoring the need for vigilant assessment. Figure 63–13 ■ provides a graphical representation of bleeding sites throughout the body. Increased bleeding and a decreased platelet count are the primary diagnostic indicators of thrombocytopenia.

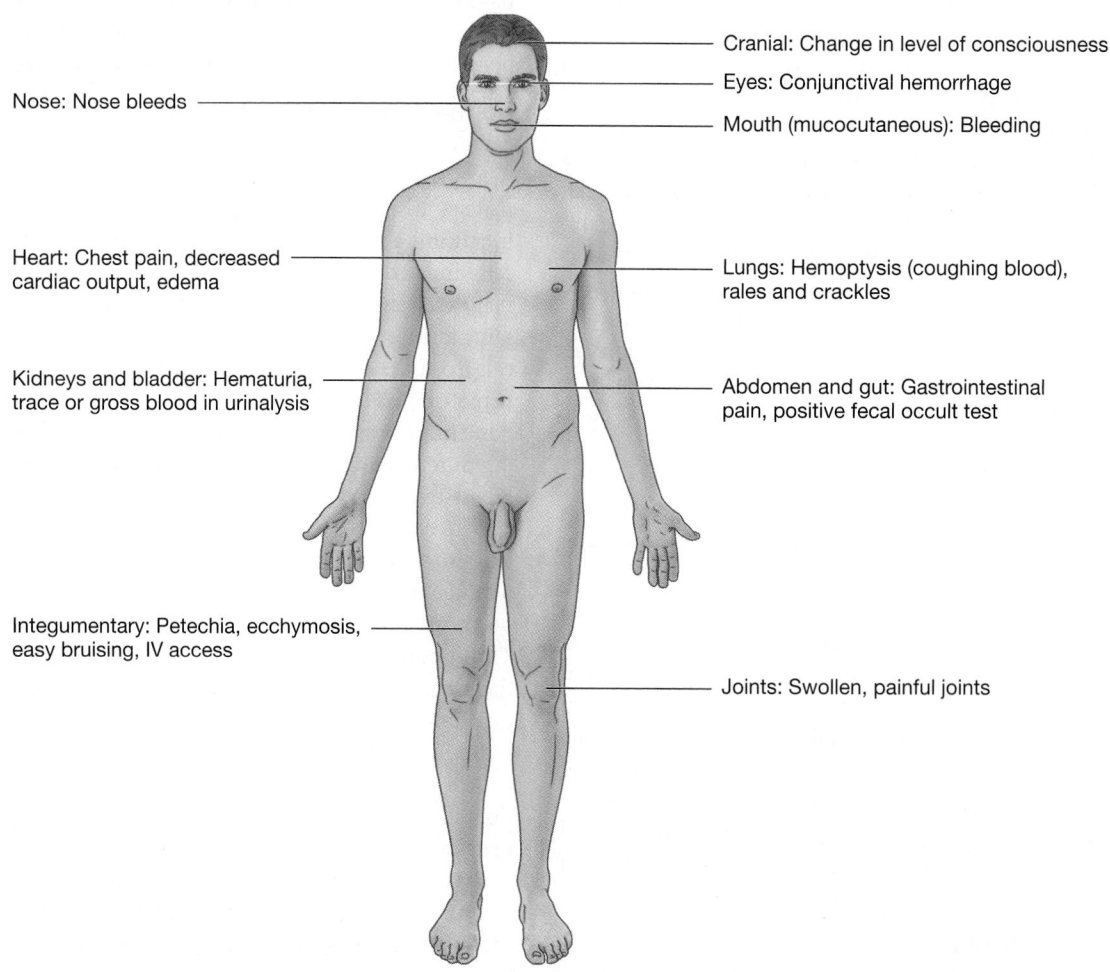

FIGURE 63–13 ■ Assessment of bleeding sites.

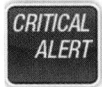 *Patients who present with platelet counts of less than 20,000 μL are at imminent risk of internal bleeding. A drop in the platelet count below this level should be immediately reported to the health care provider as part of a comprehensive assessment including neurological, respiratory, cardiovascular, and abdominal symptoms. Prepare for possible platelet transfusion.*

Physical Manifestations The primary physical manifestations of thrombocytopenia are the appearance of mucosal and cutaneous bleeding, and prolonged bleeding after invasive procedures. Degree of symptom severity correlates with platelet count. Below 100,000/mm³ patients may experience prolonged bleeding after surgery or any invasive procedure such as IV catheterization or dental treatments. Patients do not typically present with mucosal or cutaneous bleeding until platelet values reach 50,000/mm³ or lower. Mucosal bleeding can be observed in the gums especially following aggressive brushing or flossing, in the urinary tract, or from the nares. Patients also may report blood-tinged sputum after coughing or blood in the stool. Cutaneous bleeding appears as discoloration of the skin and can often be mistaken for rash. Cutaneous bleeding can be described as a continuum from small pinpoint lesions (petechiae), to larger group patches (purpura), to ecchymosis, or large (centimeters) patches of active bleeding into the skin.

At 20,000/mm³ the patient is considered at risk for spontaneous bleeding. Although anemia due to acute blood loss should be addressed, a greater concern is bleeding into closed spaces such as the cranium, pleural space, pericardial space, or abdomen. At critically low platelet values, patients should be frequently assessed for changes in level of consciousness, respiratory status, cardiovascular status, or abdominal pain.

Alterations in Laboratory Values Thrombocytopenia is a disease of primary hemostasis reflected in the platelet count and bleeding time. PT, aPTT, and INR are of little diagnostic value in the evaluation of thrombocytopenia because they focus on secondary hemostasis.

Medical Management

Management of thrombocytopenia must address any underlying etiology. If the thrombocytopenia results from impaired production due to bone marrow suppression, a watchful waiting approach and protective measures usually are the first line of management. Exogenous thrombopoietin to stimulate platelet production currently is in investigational stages. Platelet transfusion may be administered in these populations. If the thrombocytopenia is attributable to accelerated destruction of platelets, the causative factors must be identified and addressed. Drug-induced thrombocytopenia can be addressed by cessation of the offending drug. In immune-mediated accelerated destruction, immunosuppressive treatment may be initiated to reduce antibody production. Options may include corticosteroids, splenectomy, and IV immunoglobulin. Specific treatments for immune-mediated thrombocytopenia and heparin-induced thrombocytopenia are addressed later.

Nursing Management

Nurses in a variety of clinical settings must be familiar with the risks, early signs, and management of these diseases because they can occur as a side effect of a vast array of diseases and treatments. Oftentimes, thrombocytopenia is first detected by astute nursing observation and assessment, followed up by effective collaboration. Nursing interventions implemented for the patient with thrombocytopenia focus on early detection, risk reduction, management of medical interventions, and patient education. Common bleeding precautions used to minimize risk of bleeding in high-risk patients are listed in Chart 63–17. The Nursing Process: Patient Care Plan for Thrombocytopenia and Bleeding Disorders (p. 2046) outlines appropriate care for patients with thrombocytopenia and bleeding disorders. Teaching for patients with bleeding disorders is addressed in the Patient Teaching & Discharge Priorities box (p. 2047).

Collaborative Management

Patients who have thrombocytopenia require the coordinated efforts of a multidisciplinary team to prevent exacerbation of injury and to optimize recovery. Pharmacists play a key role in the management of thrombocytopenia due to their expertise in drug side effect profiles and drug–drug interactions. Their guidance can assist the multidisciplinary team to identify drugs that might exacerbate thrombocytopenia and, moreover, to find alternative treatments with the same efficacy but with decreased deleterious side effects.

Especially in cases of bone marrow suppression, optimal nutrition plays a key role in patients' recovery from thrombocytopenia. Many patients with thrombocytopenia suffer from decreased appetite, which can result in severe nutritional deficits, or fear of oral cavity injury (and bleeding) from chewing or swallowing. Registered dietitians can develop nutrition plans that both maximize key nutrients and minimize further injury to the oral mucosa.

Immune Thrombocytopenia Purpura

Immune thrombocytopenic purpura (ITP) (previously referred to as idiopathic thrombocytopenic purpura) is an autoimmune

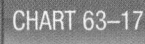 **CHART 63–17** **Bleeding Precautions**

Although exact bleeding precautions vary among clinical sites, the following measures are widely implemented to minimize the risk of injury to patients:

- Avoid intramuscular and subcutaneous injections.
- Hold firm pressure to venipuncture sites for a minimum of 5 minutes.
- Minimize venipunctures and invasive procedures.
- Provide a soft toothbrush or tooth sponges for mouth care.
- Avoid rectal suppositories, thermometers, enemas, and other rectal/vaginal manipulation.
- Prevent constipation and straining with stools.
- Use electric razor only.
- Maintain a safe environment to avoid injury.
- Assist with ADLs and ambulation as necessary to avoid injury.
- Avoid medications with antiplatelet activity (e.g., aspirin and aspirin-containing products, NSAIDs).

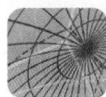

NURSING PROCESS: Patient Care Plan for Thrombocytopenia and Bleeding Disorders

Assessment of Abnormal Bleeding

Subjective Data:

Do you have any history of disease?

Do you have recent history of exposure to viruses such as measles, mumps, varicella, rubella?

Are you currently being treated with any medications? If so, which?

Do you take any OTC drugs, herbs, or street drugs?

How much alcohol do you drink on a daily basis?

Have you noticed any increased bleeding?

Objective Data:

Skin: petechiae, ecchymosis

Mucosa: color, tenderness, increased bleeding

Conjunctivae: bleeding

Urine: color

Neurological: level of consciousness (ominous sign of intracranial bleeding)

Lung sounds: crackles, diminished lung sounds

Abdominal: painful, swollen

Laboratory values: platelets less than 100,000/μL; compare to previously recorded studies

Nursing Assessment and Diagnoses	Outcomes and Evaluation Parameters	Planning and Interventions with *Rationales*
Nursing Diagnoses: *Risk for Injury* related to increased intracranial pressure, abdominal bleeding, pericardial bleeding, and/or bleeding into pleural space	**Outcome:** Free of injury due to bleeding. **Evaluation Parameters:** Laboratory: Hemoglobin values remain within normal limits. Laboratory: Platelet, APTT, PT, and INR values remain within normal limits. Vital signs: Vital signs remain within baseline normal limits for patient.	**Interventions and *Rationales:*** Frequently monitor laboratory values for signs of precipitous decrease in hemoglobin *to detect changes in level of circulating red blood cells.* Frequently monitor laboratory values for signs of increased bleeding times *to detect tendencies to bleed.* Assess vital signs especially blood pressure *as indicators of vascular space volume. In the event of bleeding, blood volume leaves vascular space.* Report critical values immediately *because health care provider may wish to initiate blood product transfusion.*
	Cerebral: Patient remains alert and well oriented. Cerebral: Pupils remain equal, round, and reactive to light. Cerebral: Gross reflex assessment remains unchanged from baseline. Abdominal: Patient denies abdominal pain. Abdominal: Bowel sounds at baseline or present in all four quadrants.	Frequently monitor neurological signs including level of Glasgow Coma Scale, papillary changes, and cranial nerves *to detect changes in level of consciousness and nerve damage.* Monitor restlessness, and confusion *as indicators of increased intracranial pressure and/or decreased oxygenation due to bleeding.* Frequently assess (inspection, auscultation, palpation, percussion) abdominal status and seek patient report of abdominal pain *to detect signs of bleeding into abdominal cavity and hypoxia in abdominal structures due to blood loss.*
	Patient denies chest pain, shortness of breath.	Assess abdomen for pain, tenderness, distention *as indicators of internal abdominal bleeding.* Assess for adventitious or diminished breath sounds. *Indicates decreased gas exchange and hypoxia.* Monitor respiratory rate and depth *to assess for respiratory distress.*
	Urine color clear. Free of blood in stool.	Frequently assess urine and stool color. *Possible early indicator of systemic internal bleeding. Detection of early signs allows for timely administration of platelet transfusion.*
Impaired Skin Integrity related to abnormal bleeding into cutaneous areas and mucosal surfaces	**Outcome:** Free of serious injury due to internal bleeding. **Evaluation Parameters:** Alert and oriented. Clear breath sounds and absence of respiratory distress. Free of reports of abdominal pain. Lab values (platelet/Hct/Hgb) within normal limits for patient. Free of petechiae, ecchymosis, hematuria. Blood pressure within normal limits. **Outcome:** Minimal or no bleeding observed. **Evaluation Parameters:** Free of petechiae, ecchymosis. Free of bleeding from gums, mucosa, and catheter sites. Urine color clear. Free of blood in stool.	**Interventions and *Rationales:*** Frequently assess skin, mucosa membrane for evidence of color change, tenderness, and bleeding. *For clinical manifestations of bleeding.* Frequently assess urine and stool color. *Possible early indicator of systemic internal bleeding. Detection of early signs allows for timely administration of platelet transfusion.* Monitor respiratory rate and depth *to assess for respiratory distress.* Assess abdomen for pain, tenderness, distention *as indicators of internal abdominal bleeding.* Assess vital signs, especially blood pressure *as indicators of vascular space volume. In the event of bleeding, blood volume leaves vascular space.*

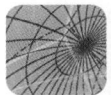

NURSING PROCESS: Patient Care Plan for Thrombocytopenia and Bleeding Disorders—*Continued*

Assessment of Patient Self-Management

Subjective Data:

What do you understand about thrombocytopenia?

Do you have any particular fears about thrombocytopenia?

What signs and symptoms might you observe that cause you concern?

Objective Data:

Skin color and condition, absence of petechiae

Mucosa membrane color

Urine and stool color

Cognition

Level of agitation and restlessness

Comprehension

Vital signs within normal values

Lab values: platelets less than 100,000/mm³; compare to previously recorded studies

Verbalization of condition

Nursing Assessment and Diagnoses	Outcomes and Evaluation Parameters	Planning and Interventions with *Rationales*
Nursing Diagnosis: *Deficient Knowledge related to management of thrombocytopenia*	**Outcome:** Patient and family verbalize understanding of required skills and knowledge required in the management of thrombocytopenia. ***Evaluation Parameters:*** Patient verbalizes understanding of bleeding precautions including avoidance of contact sports, use of razors, oral care. Patient reports signs and symptoms that warrant immediate attention by health care provider. Patient reports understanding of medications that should be avoided including aspirin and other drugs specific to patient's history.	**Interventions and *Rationales:*** Frequently reinforce patient education regarding bleeding precautions *to minimize risk of injury.* Educate patient and family about tests and procedures *to increase understanding of disease process.* Educate patient and family concerning the disease, treatment, and potential complications *to increase understanding of disease process.* Collaborate with multidisciplinary team to *reinforce pharmaceutical, nutritional, and rehabilitation/educational interventions.*

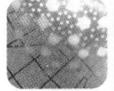

PATIENT TEACHING & DISCHARGE PRIORITIES for Generalized Bleeding Disorders

Need	Teaching Objective
Disease process	Discuss cause of disease.
Patient/family	Assist patient/family in recognition of cutaneous, GI, and genitourinary tract bleeding.
	Refer patient/family to appropriate support groups.
Pharmacologic management	Practice and discuss self-administration of blood factors or supplementation as ordered.
Patient/family	Consult with pharmacist for drug-specific teaching.
Nutrition	Discuss role of balanced nutrition emphasizing need for key elements: vitamin B$_{12}$, folate, and iron.
Patient/family	Discuss need to reduce exposure to alcohol and thiazide medications.
	Refer patient to dietitian for assistance in meal planning.
Physical exercise	Discuss and explore appropriate physical exercise options that would maintain muscle/bone/cardiovascular strength but limits risks of trauma.
Patient/family	Refer patient/family to physical, rehabilitation, and occupational therapy for outpatient consultation.
Safety	Discuss need to avoid sharp objects or sports that would cause injury.
Patient/family	Advise use of electric razors.
	Advise evaluation of home setting to eliminate sharp corners or fall hazards.
	Advise patient/family to alert dentists and other medical professionals to bleeding risks.
	Discuss signs and symptoms that require emergency intervention.

disease marked by a decrease in the number of platelets due to destruction by antibodies produced against a patient's own platelets. It is the most common of the immune-mediated thrombocytopenias. There are two distinct forms of ITP: an acute form, which affects primarily children and neonates and is usually self-limiting, and a chronic form, which lasts more than 6 months and affects primarily adults (Stasi & Provan, 2004). The following discussion will primarily address chronic forms of ITP.

Pathophysiology

Chronic forms of ITP can be subdivided into two categories: *secondary* and *primary*. Secondary immune thrombocytopenic purpura refers to the appropriate development of antibodies against invading pathogens or drugs, which then inappropriately cross-react against platelets causing their destruction. In primary ITP, antibodies against platelet surface proteins also are observed but occur in the absence of viral, bacterial, or drug exposure. The molecular mechanisms that give rise to either type of ITP are not clearly elucidated and are a focus of current research studies.

Clinical Presentation

The physical manifestations of ITP are similar to those presented earlier in the discussion about thrombocytopenia. Primary ITP can be distinguished from secondary ITP by the absence of recent infection or drug exposure. Additionally, splenomegaly usually is only observed in secondary forms. Laboratory values will reveal decreased platelet levels and perhaps anemia (due to bleeding).

Medical Management

Management of ITP has two primary goals: removal of the triggering event (if identifiable) and abatement of the immune response. In cases of secondary ITP, the underlying disease process must be treated and resolved so that the body is rid of the invading antigen responsible for antibody production. In the case of drug-induced ITP, immediate cessation of the drug is warranted.

Attention then turns to abatement of the immune response, which usually is attempted with immunosuppressive therapy. Steroids such as prednisone are the first choice in asymptomatic patients with decreased platelet counts of less than 50,000/mm³. If steroids prove ineffective, or major bleeding occurs, intravenous immunoglobulin (IVIG) is administered. IVIG has been associated with significant rates of hypersensitivity reactions and thus administration should be monitored closely. Splenectomy will be considered if patients continue to require significant doses of steroids or immunosuppressive therapy after several months (Cines & Blanchette, 2002; Stasi & Provan, 2004). The Nursing Process: Patient Care Plan for Thrombocytopenia and Bleeding Disorders (p. 2046) is appropriate for use in the patient with ITP.

Heparin-Induced Thrombocytopenia

Heparin-induced thrombocytopenia (HIT) is an example of drug-induced, immune-mediated thrombocytopenia. Although the frequency of HIT is relatively rare, 3% of patients treated with unfractionated heparin form thrombosis and 0.5% of patients exposed to diluted heparin flushes for IV therapy management experience thrombocytopenia (Rice, Nguyen, & Vann, 2002). Its incidence is steadily increasing, which is thought to be due to the ubiquitous use of heparin for DVT, pulmonary embolism, acute myocardial infarction, and IV catheter maintenance. Heparin-induced thrombocytopenia occurs most frequently in patients undergoing cardiovascular or orthopedic surgeries, because heparin is widely utilized to prevent thrombosis in these high-risk populations.

Pathophysiology

Patients on heparin therapy (including intermittent IV catheter flushes) can develop antibodies to heparin that cross-react against their own platelets. Specifically, heparin can induce the production of the antiheparin platelet factor 4 (AHPF4) antibody. This antibody causes two reactions. First, as with the autoimmune-mediated thrombocytopenia, these antibodies recognize and bind to platelets, a process that causes their accelerated destruction in the spleen. Second, and perhaps more significantly, when the AHPF4 antibody binds to platelets, it can induce platelet activation thus initiating the clotting cascade, coagulation, and, possibly, thrombosis (Lewis et al., 2003).

Clinical Presentation

A decrease in platelet count, particularly following heparin therapy often is the only indication of HIT. The onset of thrombocytopenia or a drop from baseline values typically occurs within 5 to 14 days after starting heparin therapy. Platelet counts of 80,000 to 100,000/mm³ or counts that drop by 30% or more suggest thrombocytopenia. Initially, the patient may not present with thrombotic complications such as DVT or thrombosis, despite the presence of HIT. However, thrombosis eventually does occur in approximately 35% to 75% of patients with HIT. HIT-related thrombosis leads to DVT, stroke, and cardiac events, which, in turn, carry amputation rates as high as 20% and mortality of 30% to 50% (Hirsh, Heddel, & Kelton, 2004; Warkentin & Kelton, 1996).

Medical Management

HIT can be extremely difficult to manage (1) because of its insidious presentation, (2) because heparin is normally the drug of choice for the management of thrombosis, and (3) because cessation of heparin therapy alone has proven to be an ineffective approach. Diligent observation and early intervention with appropriate drug therapies are the cornerstones of treatment for HIT. Baseline platelet levels should be measured and frequently monitored for all patients who have been recently exposed to all forms of heparin including low-molecular-weight heparin, unfractionated heparin, and heparin flushes. Patients receiving unfractionated heparin warrant even greater monitoring. Although abnormal bleeding can be observed in HIT, the absence of abnormal bleeding should not be ruled out with HIT. Clinical diagnosis of HIT is made on the basis of reduction of the platelet count, correlation with heparin administration, and when other causes (drugs, viruses, and bone marrow involvement) have been excluded (Rice et al., 2002). Laboratory tests also are available that can detect the presence of the anti-heparin platelet factor 4 (AHPF4) antibody.

Once HIT is suspected, heparin therapy (including catheter flushes and low-molecular-weight heparin) should be stopped immediately. A nonheparin anticoagulant such as direct thrombin inhibitors (lepirudin, argatroban, or bivalirudin) often is recommended as a first-line defense followed by warfarin therapy if existing thrombosis is suspected. Direct thrombin inhibitors carry similar risks to bleeding as do other anticoagulants and should be monitored using aPTT and INR.

■ Nursing Management

Nurses play a key role in the prevention and management of HIT. Nurses should carefully monitor the platelet counts of any patient receiving any form of heparin treatment. The rise of HIT has made the prophylactic use of heparin flushes to maintain IV catheter patency a controversial issue, especially in light of the prevalence of alternatives. Alternative options to maintain catheter patency include positive pressure valves, valved vascular access devices, use of normal saline for flushing, and specially coated central lines. Further epidemiologic research is needed in this area to develop national guidelines (Rosenthal, 2003).

If HIT is suspected, the nurse's responsibilities include the careful administration of antithrombotic therapy, monitoring of appropriate laboratory values, and assessment of bleeding risk. If bleeding also is suspected, the nurse should implement appropriate care plans to prevent anemia, hemorrhage, or injury. The Nursing Process: Patient Care Plan for Thrombocytopenia and Bleeding Disorders (p. 2046) provides details

appropriate for use in this population. Other therapies for HIT are discussed in the Evidence-Based Practice box.

von Willebrand's Disease

Von Willebrand's disease (vWD), the most common inherited bleeding disorder, affects 1% to 2% of the international population. vWD results from mutations in the essential clotting factor, von Willebrand's factor (vWF), which plays key roles in both primary and secondary hemostasis. Clinical presentation of vWD depends on the extent and location of the genetic mutation (see the Genetic Considerations box, p. 2050) and varies widely, but vWD is most commonly associated with mucosal and cutaneous bleeding and prolonged bleeding times. Emerging epidemiologic studies reveal that the prevalence of the disease is underestimated and that many cases, especially in women, go widely undiagnosed with symptoms often being attributed to idiopathic menorrhagia (prolonged menstrual bleeding) (Lukes, Kadir, Peyvandi, & Koudies, 2005).

Heparin-Induced Thromboctyopenia

Clinical Problem

Intravenous therapies are a crucial component of most hospitalized patient treatments, which underscores the importance of maintaining patent IV access. Nurses have traditionally maintained IV access with a combination of regular site assessment and manual instillation of a flush solution into the IV catheter site. Without proper nursing maintenance, IV access sites can easily become occluded due to the body's natural tendency to form fibrin sheaths over any foreign object. This normally beneficial mechanism has evolved to isolate harmful pathogens; however, the fibrin sheath formation also blocks the indwelling end of the intravenous catheter. This blockage, in turn, prevents instillation of medications and blood withdrawal, thus requiring the instillation of a new IV access site, possible patient discomfort or injury related to installation, and delay in treatment.

For many years, heparinized saline flushes have been used to prevent fibrin clot formation. However, mounting evidence has revealed a growing incidence of heparin-induced thrombocytopenia (HIT). In HIT, exposure to heparin appropriately stimulates antibody formation against the heparin molecule. However, the same antibody formed against heparin has also shown efficacy activity against platelets. HIT is the depletion of platelets as a result of an autoimmune activity. Nursing practice must incorporate techniques that have shown efficacy in preserving IV access but that do not place the patient at additional risk of injury.

Research Findings

A number of studies are beginning to evaluate the efficacy of heparinized saline flushes against plain saline flushes in the maintenance of IV access. In a large study, 361 IV lock sites were assigned to either saline or heparin use exclusively. Sites were flushed every 12 hours with either 3 mL of normal saline or 3 mL of a diluted (10 units/mL) solution of heparin. At the conclusion of the study, there was no statistically significant difference in incidence of extravasation, phlebitis, clotting, or blood return between either group.

A similar study at the Mayo Clinic was conducted in the obstetric population, who are particularly prone to clotting disorders due to hematologic changes in pregnancy. In this study of 73 patients, results indicate no statistically significant differences in IV lock patency or in

phlebitis between heparin or normal saline flushes. Similar results appear in arterial line maintenance. Sixty-five patients in a New Zealand intensive care unit were randomly assigned to receive either normal saline (NS) or heparinized saline (HS) (3 mL/hr as a continuous flush) to maintain their arterial lines needed for monitoring and blood sampling. Each patient's nurse was asked to score the function of the line at the end of each nursing shift. At the conclusion of the study, nursing assessment of line function revealed no difference between flush solutions.

Implications for Nursing Practice

The studies discussed here provide evidence for limiting of patient exposure to heparin in IV access flushes. The primary goal of routine flushes is to ensure patency and delivery of medications and therapies. Clearly, this goal can be achieved via the use of saline without the additional exposure to potentially life-threatening heparin-induced thrombocytopenia. For patients who do not show evidence of IV line occlusion, nurses should collaborate with their interdisciplinary team to limit flush solutions to saline only.

Critical Thinking Questions

1. Which nursing actions are most effective in preservation of intravenous line patency?

2. What are the benefits and risks of heparinized flush solutions?

Answers to Critical Thinking Questions appear in Appendix D.

References

Fujita, T., Namiki, T., Suzuki, T., Yamamoto, E. (2006). Normal saline flushing for maintenance of peripheral intravenous sites. *Journal of Clinical Nursing, 15*(1):103–104.

Niesen, K. M., Harris, D. Y., Parkin, L. S., Henn, L. T. (2003). The effects of heparin versus normal saline for maintenance of peripheral intravenous locks in pregnant women. *Journal of Obstetrics and Gynecology, 32*(4):503–508.

Whitta, R. K., Hall, K. F., Bennetts, T. M., Welman, L., & Rawlins, P. (2006). Comparison of normal or heparinised saline flushing on function of arterial lines. *Critical Care Resuscitation, 8*(3):205–208.

EVIDENCE-BASED PRACTICE

GENETIC CONSIDERATIONS for Hemophilia

Hemophilia results from inheritance of defective genes controlling the clotting system. Because hemophilia is an X-linked genetic disorder, the severity of the disease depends on whether the patient received one or two defective copies from each parent, and whether the patient is male or female. Males only bear one X chromosome, passed from the mother, implying that one copy of the mutated hemophilia gene will result in the disease. However, females, bearing two X chromosomes need to inherit two mutated versions to display the disease.

Pathophysiology

The von Willebrand's factor protein plays two roles in clot formation. In primary hemostasis, vWF acts as a binding bridge between platelets and the damaged subendothelium at the site of vascular injury. In secondary hemostasis, vWF protects Factor VIII, which is important in the contact activation (intrinsic) pathway, from degradation and delivers it to the site of injury.

vWD describes not only one distinct disease, but a heterogeneous group of disorders all involving disturbances in the vWD gene. The normal vWD gene is a very large, complex structure, usually producing a mature protein of more than 2,050 amino acids. Disturbances to this protein sequence can result in structurally abnormal vWF, too little vWF (most common), or too much vWF, accounting for more than 40 different variations of vWD. Insufficiencies in patients with vWD cause delayed platelet plug formation, prolonged bleeding times, and impaired fibrin clot formation. Alternately, excess production of vWF can lead to thrombosis.

Clinical Presentation

The severity of von Willebrand's disease varies widely depending on the extent and location of the genetic derangement. The exact genetic derangements have yet to be elucidated, but it is apparent to clinicians that patients can present with a wide variation of bleeding tendencies. In an attempt to classify vWD according to disease severity, the International Society on Thrombosis and Hemostasis proposed a simplified classification of vWD (Sadler, 1994), which has since been adopted by both researchers and clinicians worldwide. The classification system is based on the amount and characteristics of detectable vWF in the bloodstream by laboratory tests and on clinical presentation. Chart 63–18 describes the variations in clinical presentation of each classification of vWD.

As suggested in Chart 63–18, some patients may appear generally asymptomatic with only mildly increased bleeding tendencies, whereas others (type 3) with the most severe forms experience joint bleeding and hemorrhage. Fortunately, type 3 vWD requires inheritance of two copies of the mutated von Willebrand's gene, making it the rarest form of the disease. Other indicators of vWD include prolonged bleeding after minor cuts, bleeding from the gums, and mucocutaneous bleeding (petechiae, ecchymosis).

vWD will manifest as prolonged bleeding times and a reduction of vWF in the blood. The vWF quantity is directly measured by using an ELISA test that can provide a quantitative measurement. Platelet count will appear normal. PT, aPTT, and INR should also be normal.

CHART 63–18	Classifications of von Willebrand Disease
Classification	**Clinical Presentation**
Type 1	Partial quantitative deficiency of vWF Mildly decreased clotting ability
Type 2A	Qualitative defect Mildly dysfunctional ability of vWF to bind platelets Primary hemostasis defect affecting platelet plug formation
Type 2B	Qualitative defect Moderately dysfunctional ability of vWF to bind platelets Primary hemostasis defect affecting platelet plug formation
2M	Qualitative defect Severely dysfunctional or absent ability of vWF to bind to platelets Primary hemostasis defect affecting platelet plug formation
2N	Qualitative defect Mildly dysfunctional ability of vWF to bind to Factor VIII Secondary hemostasis defect affects fibrin clot formation
3	Severe or total deficiency of vWF affecting both platelet plug formation and fibrin sheath formation Patients can present with chronic mucosal and cutaneous bleeding, and/or joint bleeding Sometimes misdiagnosed as hemophilia

Source: Sadler, J. E. (1994). A revised classification of von Willebrand disease. For the Subcommittee on von Willebrand factor of the Scientific and Standardization Committee of the International Society on Thrombosis and Haemostasis. *Thrombosis and Haemostasis, 71*(4), 520–525.

Medical Management

Treatment for von Willebrand's disease is based on the current presenting symptom. In the event of problematic uncontrolled bleeding or as prophylaxis prior to invasive procedures, the patient can be treated with replacement of the deficient vWF. Desmopressin vasopressin analog (DDAVP), a synthetic hormone usually given by injection or nasal spray, induces production of vWF and subsequent increase in Factor VIII levels. DDAVP is administered at a dose of 0.3 µg/kg, with effects starting within 30 to 60 minutes and lasting for several hours. Because it is a synthetic hormone, hypersensitivity reactions including tachycardia, headache, and facial flushing are potential side effects of infusion.

Replacement therapy, the second option, is the injection of a concentrate of vWF and Factor VIII extracted either with fresh frozen plasma (FFP) or cryoprecipitate. However, very large volumes of FFP or cryoprecipitate are required to sufficiently replace vWF and Factor VIII, predisposing the patient to fluid overload and transfusion reactions. For these reasons, replacement therapy is reserved for those patients who cannot tolerate DDAVP or those with emergent bleeding in type 3 disease. Commercially prepared concentrations of vWF currently are in clinical trials as low-volume alternatives to FFP and cryoprecipitate infusions.

 Nursing Management

As with other bleeding disorders, nursing responsibilities for patients with von Willebrand's disease include implementation of bleeding precautions, environmental risk reduction, and diligent assessment. Although platelet values tend to be normal in these patients, patients with severe disease can present with prolonged bleeding times (aPTT). The Nursing Process: Patient Care Plan for Thrombocytopenia and Bleeding Disorders, presented earlier in the chapter (p. 2046), is appropriate for use in these patients because it outlines physiological assessments and nursing interventions that can be applied in vWF. Because von Willebrand's disease is a chronic lifelong condition, discharge priorities for these patients emphasize education, which reinforces prevention of injury.

Disorders of Secondary Hemostasis

Disorders of secondary hemostasis refer to any disease process that disrupts the formation of the fibrin sheath via errors in the tissue factor (extrinsic) pathway or the contact activation (intrinsic) pathway. The most common cause of these disorders is deficiencies in quantity or quality of the clotting factors. Whereas disorders of primary hemostasis usually appear within minutes of injury and in superficial sites (mucosa, integumentary), bleeding associated with disorders of secondary hemostasis can occur days to weeks after injury and in the deep subcutaneous layers, the muscles, and the joints. Several disorders of secondary hemostasis have been identified; however, the most common are vitamin K deficiency and hemophilia, which is discussed next.

Hemophilia

Hemophilia is perhaps the most well-known disease of hemostasis and affected approximately 18,000 persons (primarily male) in the United States as of 2005. **Hemophilia** is a chronic condition that arises from the inheritance of mutated genes controlling Factor VIII or Factor IX. Characteristic presenting symptoms are uncontrolled bleeding particularly into large muscle groups and joints.

Pathophysiology

Patients with hemophilia inherit mutated copies of the genes controlling clotting factors VIII or clotting factor IX. Recall from the discussion on normal hemostasis above that both Factor VIII and Factor IX are required in the contact activation (intrinsic) pathway for the eventual activation of Factor X, leading to the common pathway and the conversion of fibrinogen to fibrin. Therefore, the lack of either of these factors may significantly alter formation of the fibrin sheath, clot formation, and, ultimately, clinical bleeding. Patients with hemophilia who inherit altered clotting factor VIII are considered to have hemophilia A, whereas inheritance of altered clotting factor IX is referred to as hemophilia B. Both diseases are recessive X-linked genetic disorders with implications for gender-based inheritance.

Clinical Presentation

The severity of hemophilia is related to the amount of clotting factor in the blood and is graded on a continuum from mild to severe. Mild hemophilia is characterized by insufficient clotting factor. The clinical presentation of each, hemophilia A and hemophilia B, is identical, with differentiation relying on chemical assays of blood samples.

Physical Manifestations
The hallmark clinical presentation of hemophilia is prolonged bleeding and an inability to form clots in response to injury, both of which can appear and persist for days to weeks. For patients with severe disease completely lacking any Factor VIII or Factor IX, such bleeding can have serious life-threatening consequences. Distinguished from disease of primary hemostasis, which causes increased bruising and superficial hemorrhages in the integumentary (petechiae), patients with hemophilia typically suffer from bleeding deep in the tissues. Typical bleeding sites include joints and organs. If left uncontrolled the internal bleeding can cause severe pressure on closed compartments.

Serious consequences of internal bleeding into closed spaces include increased intracranial pressure, hemiarthrosis (bleeding into the joints) leading to compartment syndrome, and oropharyngeal bleeding (into the esophagus). The eventual sequelae following each of these situations can cause lifetime disability. Increased intracranial pressure can cause ischemia and brain tissue damage. Bleeding into the joints predisposes the patient to arthritis, synovial tissue damage, and joint malformation. Oropharyngeal bleeding may occlude the airway so severely as to require intubation.

Alterations in Laboratory Values
Although the clinical presentations of hemophilia A and hemophilia B are identical, treatment options vary; thus, laboratory analysis is critical in developing an effective care plan. Patients with hemophilia have usually been diagnosed as children, prior to admission to the acute care setting. For patients known to have hemophilia, diagnostic tests such as the CBC are used to determine degree of blood loss. Bleeding and clotting studies, a platelet count, bleeding time, PT, aPTT, and INR are indicated for any patient suspected of having hemophilia. Because Factor VIII and Factor IX are disorders of the intrinsic pathway, the patient typically will have a prolonged aPTT with all other tests normal. Specific assays that detect blood levels of Factor VIII and Factor IX are used to distinguish between the two forms of hemophilia.

Medical Management

Medical management of hemophilia revolves around *factor replacement therapy*, or the administration of exogenous (donated or manufactured) Factor VIII and Factor IX. (See the Pharmacology Summary in the chapter for medications used to treat clotting disorders, p. 2054.) Previously, factor replacement therapy was achieved via fresh frozen plasma; however, possible exposure to viruses and risk of volume overload combined with the availability of commercially prepared factors has decreased the use of FFP. For mild episodes or as prophylaxis prior to procedures, DDAVP has become the treatment of choice. DDAVP stimulates the temporary production of Factor VIII.

In the event of bleeding, antifibrinolytics are sometimes used. These medications slow the fibrinolytic system, thus extending the effect of already-formed fibrin sheaths and slowing the inhibitory effects of fibrin degradation products. However, these medications have only shown significant clinical efficacy in mucosal and oral bleeding. Another principle of hemophilia treatment is the prevention of deleterious sequelae and further injury. Toward that goal, aspirin and other platelet interfering drugs are avoided.

Nursing Management

For the nurse caring for the hospitalized patient with hemophilia, cure is not the goal. Instead disease management focuses on reduction of environmental factors that increase risk and on management of the administration of the replacement factors. Bleeding precautions as shown earlier in Chart 63–17 (p. 2045) should be initiated with particular emphasis on maintaining a safe environment. Nursing problems applicable to the care of the patient with hemophilia include risk for injury (addressed with implementation of the Nursing Process: Patient Care Plan given earlier in the chapter, p. 2046), pain due to hemiarthrosis, and the need for patient education. Pain should be assessed regularly including pain level and quality. Analgesics should be administered to manage pain.

Complex Disease of the Clotting Cascade: Disseminated Intravascular Coagulation

Disseminated intravascular coagulation (DIC) is triggered by an injury or event leading to persistent activation of the clotting cascade. It manifests as widespread clot formation and thrombosis. Situations that are known to trigger DIC include sepsis, trauma (including surgery), malignancy, toxin exposure, and obstetric complications. Under normal circumstances, the clotting pathways act only transiently until vessel damage is healed. But the aforementioned situations can cause such widespread, persistent endothelial injury that the clotting pathways are required to respond with equal perseverance to seal off injured blood vessels. Eventually, this situation leads to two phenomena—the depletion of the clotting factors and the activation of the fibrinolytic system—that lead to uncontrolled bleeding. The complexity of the pathology and the simultaneous appearance of bleeding and massive thrombosis make DIC a very challenging clinical problem.

Pathophysiology

DIC is commonly associated with sepsis, trauma, cancer, or obstetric emergencies (Figure 63–14 ■). Sepsis and trauma both appear to cause DIC by widespread release of coagulation-promoting cytokines or intracellular chemical signals. In sepsis, these cytokines are released by the body in response to systemic infections with gram-negative or gram-positive bacteria and, in some cases, viruses. In severe trauma multiple mechanisms lead to DIC including endothelial damage and widespread hemolysis, which cause cytokines to be released in much the same manner as sepsis. In cancer, malignant tumors release tissue factor and other coagulation-promoting chemicals, ultimately leading to thrombosis. In obstetric emergencies, release of placental fluid or massive blood loss during childbirth is responsible for initiation of the clotting pathways.

Emerging research reveals that following initial injury by any of the mechanisms listed above, DIC appears to follow a specific sequence of molecular events (Levi, 2005). First, all of the above mechanisms cause endothelial layer damage, which in turn causes massive release of tissue factor, initiating the tissue factor (extrinsic pathway) branch of the clotting cascade. The persistence of the injury results in prolonged activation of the clotting cascade. Second, thrombin production is greatly amplified. Recall that thrombin is an extremely power-

ful promoter of coagulation. Studies show that abnormal thrombin amplification is caused by defects in the regulators that normally inhibit thrombin (antithrombin, tissue factor pathway inhibitor, and protein C). The cause and nature of theses defects are still under investigation.

These derangements cause widespread coagulation fibrin deposits and thrombosis in the microvasculature. The thrombosis occludes small vessels leading to cyanosis, tissue hypoxia, and necrosis. Eventually blood flow begins to affect the microvasculature of organs, especially the kidneys, lungs, and heart. As coagulation proceeds unchecked, the body's supply of clotting components is exhausted and eventually depleted.

Clinical Presentation

As suggested by the pathophysiology just discussed, DIC presents with paradoxical widespread thrombosis and bleeding. Laboratory values reveal prolonged clotting times and consumption of coagulation factors.

Physical Manifestations

Bleeding, although a later consequence of DIC, often is the first and most obvious sign detected. It frequently is manifested at mucocutaneous sites and as prolonged oozing from puncture

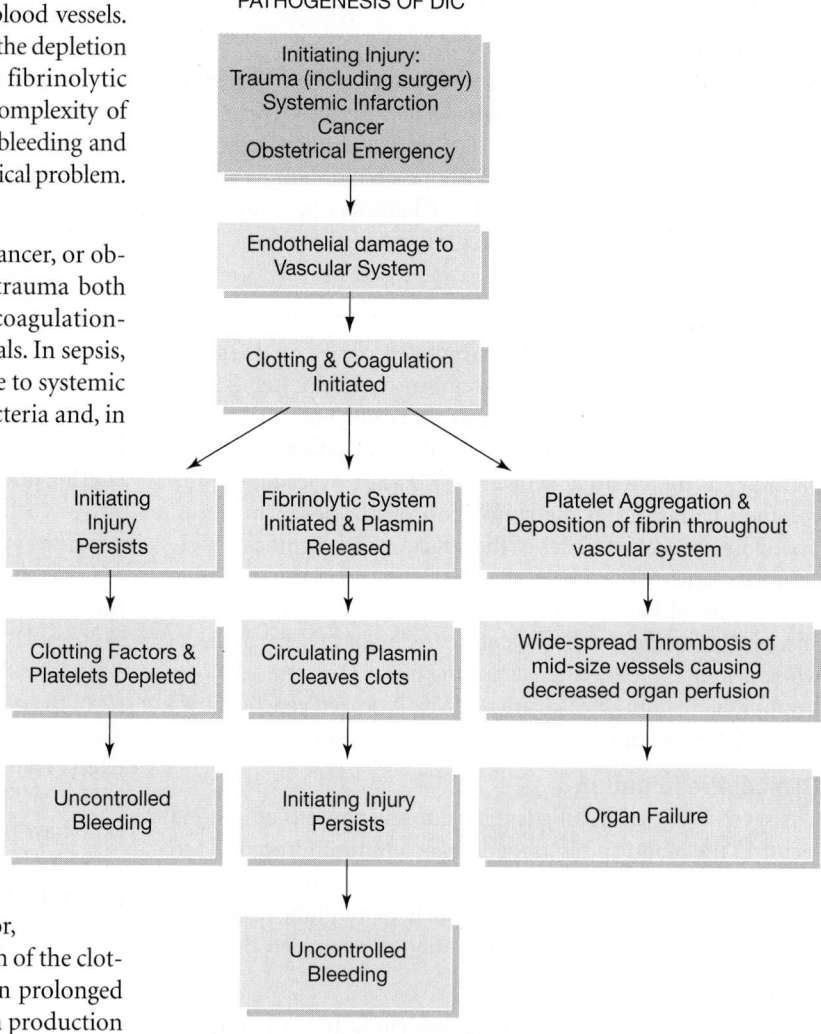

PATHOGENESIS OF DIC

FIGURE 63–14 ■ Pathogenesis of DIC.

sites. Figure 63–13 ■ (p. 2044) illustrates common bleeding sites. As DIC progresses, bleeding in gastrointestinal (GI) tract, central nervous system (CNS), heart, and genitourinary tract can occur. These are manifested as melena, a change in level of consciousness (hemorrhagic stroke), chest pain and shortness of breath, and hematuria, respectively. Extreme hypotension, tachycardia, a decreased level of consciousness, and critically low urine output (<30 mL/hr) all indicate hemodynamic shock due to blood loss.

Thrombosis can be more difficult to observe. Mild cyanosis, parasthesia (numbness), pain, and weakened pulses especially in the extremities are all indicators of microvasculature thrombosis. As the thrombi spread to affect the organs, patients can present with decreased level of consciousness (ischemic stroke), abdominal pain from GI tract occlusion, decreased urinary output (poor renal perfusion), chest pain (cardiac), and respiratory difficulty (lung). Note that many of the signs indicative of thrombosis also are indicators of bleeding. The similarity stems from the tissue hypoxia that can result from bleeding (anemia due to acute blood loss) and thrombosis (lack of circulation, hence lack of oxygenation). Clinical indicators of DIC are summarized in Chart 63–19.

Alterations in Laboratory Values

Chart 63–20 outlines the expected changes in laboratory values in the patient with DIC, which primarily reflect the consumption of clotting factors. As a result, platelet counts and fibrinogen and clotting factor titers are decreased, leading to prolonged PT, aPTT, and INR. The D-dimer test indicates excessive fibrinolysis, the end point of excessive activation of the clotting pathways.

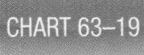
CHART 63–19 **Clinical Indicators of Disseminated Intravascular Coagulation**

HISTORY
- Sepsis
- Trauma
- Blood transfusion
- Liver dysfunction
- Malignancy
- Recent pregnancy (retained placenta)

SIGNS
- Bleeding from mucosa
- Bleeding from catheter sights
- Petechiae, ecchymosis, and purpura
- Decreased sensation in extremities
- Extremities cool to the touch
- Altered level of consciousness
- Hemoptysis

SYMPTOMS
- Pain described as swelling, sharp
- Shortness of breath/tachypnea
- Fatigue
- Hypotension
- Tachycardia

CHART 63–20 **Expected Changes in Laboratory Values in the Patient with Disseminated Intravascular Coagulation**

Platelet Count	Decreased (<100,000 μL)
PT, aPTT	Prolonged
INR	Increased
Fibrinogen	Decreased
Clotting Factors: V, VIII, X, XIII	Decreased
Fibrin degradation products and D-dimer	Positive* (most sensitive)
Clotting inhibitors: antithrombin III and protein C	Decreased

*D-dimers and FDP can become elevated whenever the coagulation and fibrinolytic systems are activated. This occurs in a variety of conditions, and therefore the tests are not specific for any one diagnosis.

Medical Management

Complete removal of the underlying injury is required for the total resolution of DIC. All other treatments are used to mitigate the damage of thrombosis or bleeding until the sepsis, trauma, cancer, or obstetric emergency subsides. The cornerstone principle that guides treatment options is the cessation of rampant coagulation pathways. Common treatments include the following:

- **Anticoagulant therapy**—Anticoagulants such as unfractionated or low-molecular-weight heparin can prevent the formation of new thrombi. Low doses are titrated carefully and monitored to prevent exacerbation of possible bleeding in DIC. New anticoagulants that specifically target thrombin (thrombin inhibitors) currently are being studied for their potential use in DIC.

- **Replacement therapy**—Patients at risk of hemodynamic collapse from excessive bleeding may be candidates for transfusion of platelets, FFP, or concentrations of coagulation factors. The use of these treatments is reserved for patients at imminent risk due to depletion of clotting factors, because inappropriate use may exacerbate development of thrombosis (Levi, de Jonge, & van der Poll, 2006).

- **Restoration of anticoagulant (antithrombin) pathways**—Administration of antithrombin agents is a relatively new therapy approach that shows significant promise. Examples of antithromobin therapies include activated protein C and antithrombin concentrations (Levi, de Jonge, & van der Poll, 2004).

Drugs used to treat DIC and other clotting disorders are shown in the Pharmacology Summary of Medications to Treat Clotting Disorders.

■ Nursing Management

DIC should be considered a medical emergency with emphasis on circulation and oxygenation, especially with respect to major organs such as heart, lungs, CNS, and kidneys. The most effective nursing intervention is anticipation of DIC in any patient with infection, trauma (including large surgeries such as GI surgeries), cancer, or obstetric emergency. Diligent assessment for

PHARMACOLOGY Summary of Medications to Treat Clotting Disorders

Medicine Category	Action	Application/Indication	Nursing Responsibility
Immune suppressive medications: Steroids Intravenous immunoglobulin	Suppression of immune response including autoimmune response.	Autoimmune thrombocytopenia (idiopathic and heparin induced) in asymptomatic patients with decreased platelet counts less than 50,000/mm³. IVIG is indicated in patients for whom steroids have proven ineffective or who have significant bleeding due to lack of platelet activity.	Assessment of laboratory values to monitor efficacy. Assessment of and patient education regarding signs and symptoms of infection since steroids will reduce immune system protection. Assessment of serum glucose levels secondary to steroid elevation. Assessment and patient education regarding mood shifts.
Clotting factor replacement therapy: Indirectly via hormone stimulation Desmopressin (DDAVP) Direct factor replacement	Induces production of deficient clotting factors (DDAVP induces production of von Willebrand's factor). Immediately replenishes deficient or depleted stores of clotting factors.	von Willebrand's disease, hemophilia, disease with uncontrolled bleeding or prophylaxis prior to invasive procedures. Direct factor replacement therapy is reserved for patients who cannot tolerate DDAVP.	DDAVP has potent antidiuretic effects, thus fluid intake should be adjusted downward to decrease the potential occurrence of water intoxication and hyponatremia. Assessment of serum electrolytes, neurological status, cardiovascular status, urinary output, and edema are to be closely monitored. Assessment of immune-mediated hypersensitivity reaction (Micromedex, 2006).

early indicators of DIC should include laboratory analysis, mucocutaneous bleeding, neurological function, and peripheral circulation. Normal findings should be documented as a baseline comparison against continual assessments. Abnormal findings should also be documented and require immediate collaboration with the health care provider.

Once DIC is suspected, attention then turns to mitigating any life-threatening sequelae. Priorities of care include implementation of bleeding precautions, maintenance of fluid balance, maintenance of acid–base balance and oxygenation, maintenance of skin integrity, and psychosocial support. Bleeding precautions were listed earlier in Chart 63–17 (p. 2045). Fluid balance derangements, which occur as a result of bleeding as well as thrombotic occlusion of the cardiovascular and renal systems, are assessed by measurement of urine output, skin turgor, and blood pressure. Oxygenation (hypoxia) problems also occur due to microvasculature occlusion and are indicated via changes in level of consciousness, cyanosis, reports of pain, and analysis of ABGs. Supplemental oxygen often is administered to prevent severe acidosis.

Attention should be paid to maintenance of skin integrity because the patient is at high risk of breakdown due to ischemia and bleeding and because additional wounds can trigger additional activation of the clotting pathways.

Emotional support also should be provided to the patient and family. DIC occurs as a serious consequence of an already existing disease process. Family and patient coping strategies may have already been exhausted by the initial injury or infection, and the addition of DIC and its treatment can cause extreme stress, especially since a diagnosis of DIC often requires transfer to an intensive care unit. Nursing assessment should always include coping ability and patients' stated fears or concerns. Nurses

should seek the collaboration of social workers, chaplains, and other professionals to assist both the patient and family.

DIC requires the application of multiple nursing skills including the administration and monitoring of transfusion therapy, oxygen therapy, and anticoagulant therapy. Monitoring of transfusion therapy should include the basic skills outlined in Chapter 22 ✑. Oxygen therapy is used to prevent acid–base derangement and correct hypoxia due to insufficient tissue perfusion. However, oxygen therapy must be closely monitored via oxygenation saturation and ABG levels. Additionally, oxygen therapy can dry delicate mucosal tissue, thus reinforcing the need for careful skin assessment. Anticoagulant therapy is usually addressed with heparin infusions, which require careful monitoring of laboratory values (aPTT, INR) and signs and symptoms of bleeding.

Aplastic Anemia

Aplastic anemia is a relatively rare disorder characterized by severe pancytopenia (low or absent red blood cells, white blood cells, and platelets) in both the periphery and bone marrow. Incidence rates are less than 2 persons per million in the United States; however, rates are higher in patients of Asian or European descent (Mayo Clinic, 2007). The severe depletion of defensive immune cells, oxygen-carrying red blood cells, and clotting platelets is a life-threatening condition for patients requiring the urgent implementation of protective interventions.

Pathophysiology

Aplastic anemia is thought to be caused by damage to the HSCs, resulting in their inability to reproduce and differentiate. In many cases, the cause of the damage is often unknown (idiopathic); in other cases, aplastic anemia results from toxic exposure, infectious processes, or in relationship to another disease process (Sleijfer & Lugtenburg, 2003). Toxins known to cause aplastic anemia include benzene, certain insecticides, kerosene, and heavy metals. Infections associated with aplastic anemia include Epstein–Barr virus, HIV, and cytomegaloviruses. Unfortunately, some therapeutic medications also may cause the pancytopenia of aplastic anemia. These drugs include chloramphenicol, certain antiepileptics, chemotherapeutic agents, and psychotropics (especially clozapine) (Bakhshi & Abella, 2008).

The diversity of the causes implies that the underlying mechanism may be equally diverse. Molecular research has shown that in most acquired diseases, the suppression of the hematopoetic stem cell is mediated by T cells that induce apoptosis (cell death) of the HSC. However, the mechanism that causes these T cells to attack the HSC is unknown and under investigation. Drug-induced aplastic anemia has been associated with deficiency in a protein responsible for removing drug metabolites from cells; hence, affected cells may have abnormally high intracellular levels of drugs that interfere with cell function. Congenital aplastic anemia may result from chromosomal abnormalities causing early HSC death.

Clinical Presentation

Regardless of the underlying cause, the hallmark sign of aplastic anemia is pancytopenia and the absence of HSCs from the bone marrow. Patients commonly will present with evidence of mucocutaneous bleeding, easy bruising, and oozing from puncture sites due to thrombocytopenia, and hypoxia due to severe anemia. Patients may report frequent infections due to WBC depletion. Laboratory analyses will reveal correlating laboratory values such as depressed platelet, WBC, and RBC counts. Peripheral blood smears will reveal lack of reticulocytes as well. Measures of increased iron stores, increased serum ferritin, and increased serum ferritin will reveal excess iron since the vital element is not being used for RBC production. Aplastic anemia is definitively diagnosed with a bone marrow aspiration study that reveals a hypocellular marrow space that is often replaced with fatty deposits.

Medical Management

Stem cell transplant is the curative treatment for aplastic anemia. Transfusion with donated stem cells will presumably repopulate the hypocellular bone marrow with healthy hematopoietic stem cells, which will then produce fully functioning red blood cells, white blood cells, and platelets. Immunosuppressive therapy is another common approach to aplastic anemia, particularly in patients who are not candidates for stem cell transplantation. Immunosuppressive agents such as antithymocyte globulin (ATG) and cyclosporine A (CsA) depress T-cell action on the HSCs. Blood transfusions with packed RBCs and platelets are administered to replace much needed blood elements. Prophylactic antibiotics and antifungals may be ordered to protect the severely neutropenic patient. Iron chelation therapy may be administered to reduce excess iron stores.

Nursing Management

The patient with aplastic anemia benefits from nursing interventions designed for anemia, thrombocytopenia, and infection prevention. A common cause of death among these patients is death due to infection, thus prevention is a priority. Careful hand hygiene should be both stringently practiced and enforced, and also taught to the patient. All instruments and items that come in contact with the patient should be cleansed before and after each use.

The patient should be frequently assessed for signs of infection including general malaise, oozing or inflammation around puncture sites, cough, or pain. Bleeding due to thrombocytopenia and hypoxia due to anemia also are results of pancytopenia of aplastic anemia. The Nursing Process: Patient Care Plans for generalized anemia and thrombocytopenia (pp. 2013 and 2046) describe appropriate nursing interventions for use in this population.

Research

Research is essential to improve the care, quality of life, and survival of patients with hematologic disorders. The goal of research is to identify areas where practice could improve and evaluate and test methods for these improvements. The research topics related to hematologic disorders are listed in the Research Opportunities and Clinical Impact box (p. 2056). The list provides both medical and nursing research topics still under investigation. Electronic databases are a source for finding specific studies related to these topics.

Summary

Hematologic disorders comprise a broad class of diseases affecting the cells and components of the blood. The functions performed by the cells of the bloodstream include oxygen transportation, hemodynamic stability, and response to injury, all of which are necessary to adequate functioning of body systems.

Although some diseases of the hematologic system are chronic, acute illnesses including infection and surgery as well as many common medications can alter the functioning of the blood. Derangements in the hematologic system affect not only the blood system, but every system in the body including vital organ function. For these reasons, assessment of hematologic functioning is required for every patient regardless of admitting diagnosis. Nurses should include signs and symptoms of hypoxia, oxygenation, and bleeding as part of every assessment and seek consultation as necessary.

RESEARCH OPPORTUNITIES AND CLINICAL IMPACT RELATED TO BLEEDING DISORDERS

Research Area	Clinical Impact
Physiology	
• Manipulation of cellular signaling pathways (biotherapy) to promote normal hematopoiesis or to suppress abnormal hematopoiesis	Establish effective methods of treatment and ultimately cure for certain hematologic disorders that result from altered hematopoiesis. Results of molecular science are the first step in drug development for clinical trials.
• Discovery and elucidation of the mechanisms that control clotting	Development of treatment protocols to prevent thrombotic disease.
Emerging Treatment Protocols (in Clinical Trials)	
• Cord blood infusion for treatment of diseases of hematopoiesis	Cord blood banking is an emerging option for parents. These studies evaluate efficacy, cost, and quality of life to determine if cord blood transfusion will become a recommended option for high-risk families.
• Bone marrow transplant	Bone marrow transplant is currently the only definitive cure for most chronic hematologic disorders. However, risks are substantial. This research develops safe and effective protocols.
• Novel applications of existing protocols	
• Manipulation of clotting factors to treat thrombotic diseases such as cardiovascular disorders, stroke, and DVT	Drugs and treatment protocols in current clinical trials increase our understanding of both chronic and acute diseases and help establish effective treatments.
	The efficacy of oral vitamin B_{12} supplementation compared to parenteral. Oral supplementation is cheaper and generates much less patient anxiety. Several trials are being conducted to quantitatively and qualitatively measure efficacy.
Quality-of-Life (QOL) Research	
• Evaluation of QOL for adult patients with chronic hematologic disease compared to other diseases	Establish domains of QOL.
	Benchmarks QOL in hematology against other diseases with well-understood QOL implications.
• Evaluation of QOL across the life span for aging patients with hematologic disorders	As care advances, the average life span of patients with chronic hematologic disorders increases with implications for physiological, social, and medical implications.
Complementary/Alternative Approach	
Guided imagery and other nonpharmaceutical techniques to manage sickle cell pain	Studies impact of complementary approaches on disease management and experience.

Clinical Preparation

CRITICAL THINKING

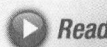 **Read**

- History of Current Illness
- Past Medical History
- Physical Exam
- Admitting Medical Orders
- Laboratory Study Results

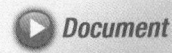 **Document**

- Summary of Hospitalization
- Pathophysiology Form
- Laboratory Values
- Laboratory Results Explanation

 **Apply**

- List of Potential Nursing Diagnoses
- Concept Map
- Critical Thinking Questions

Log on to MyNursingKit.com to download forms you will need and to complete further steps in the Clinical Preparation assignment.

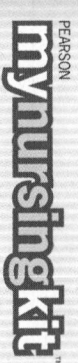

HISTORY OF PRESENT ILLNESS

Patient JS is a 60-year-old female being treated on your unit. She was admitted from the emergency department (ED) with a diagnosis of gastrointestinal bleeding in the lower GI tract. JS reports that she noticed changes in the color, odor, and consistency of her bowel movements 2 days before being seen in the emergency department. In the ED a fecal occult stool test was positive for blood. She denies any change in her diet. She denies any travel. Ms. JS has not had any major surgery or major procedures since her admission.

Medical–Surgical History

Her past medical history is unremarkable except for well-controlled non–insulin-dependent type 2 diabetes. She has no prior history of chronic GI inflammatory processes.

Social History

Ms. JS is widowed and lives by herself. She has no close relatives in the area. Ms. JS reports only drinking alcohol occasionally (defined as 1 to 2 glasses of wine per month) and a history of smoking 1 pack per day times 10 years, although she reports quitting more than 15 years ago.

Physical Exam

When you assess Ms. JS she is alert and well oriented to person, place, time, and purpose. You perform a head-to-toe physical assessment, which results in the following findings:

- Cranial nerves intact
- Small conjunctival hemorrhage in the left eye; patient reports it appeared 1 week ago
- Mild pallor noted in skin tone
- Oral mucosa clear; however, gums appear slightly pink; patient reports she noticed faint pink streaks when she brushes her teeth
- Lung sounds clear, heart sounds clear
- Vital signs: 38.2°C, BP 120/80, pulse 82 beats per minute, respirations 16
- You notice that she has shortness of breath when moving from lying to sitting and requires your assistance when moving from sitting to standing. She reports that her fatigue has been increasing during the past few weeks. She is reporting less energy throughout the day. As you continue, you notice that her peripheral pulses are intact, although you note that her extremities are cool, pale. She has small petechiae on her forearms and you notice that her IV site is oozing small amounts of blood.

Admitting Medical Orders

Admit to general medical unit

Diagnosis: gastrointestinal bleeding in the lower GI tract; rule out anemia
Allergies: none noted
Vital signs and O$_2$ sats q4h
Activity: ambulate with assistance
Diet: soft diet, except when NPO prior to colonoscopy (after midnight)
Call house officer: HR < 60 or >120, systolic blood pressure < 90 or > 160, RR < 12 or > 30, temperature > 38.5°C
IVs: normal saline via IV infusion at 125 mL/hr
Intake and output q shift

Scheduled Medications

Potassium 10 mEq IV × 3 doses over 1 hour each; recheck serum potassium 1 hour following replacement
Metformin HCl tablet 500 mg 2 times daily with food

PRN Medications

None noted

Ordered Laboratory Studies

CBC, Chem 7, and reticulocytes daily
Stools for occult blood daily

Ordered Diagnostic Studies

Accu-Cheks q ac and at bedtime
Colonoscopy in a.m.

LABORATORY STUDY RESULTS

Test	On Admission	Day 1	Day 2
Hematocrit	35 g/dL	36 g/dL	38 g/dL
Hemoglobin	11%	12%	12.5%
Reticulocytes	0.45%	0.45%	0.43%
Platelets	75,000 µL	75,000 µL	70,000 µL
Sodium	135 mEq/L	140 mEq/L	140 mEq/L
Potassium	3.0 mEq/L	3.5 mEq/L	3.5 mEq/L
Chloride	95 mEq/L	100 mEq/L	100 mEq/L
CO_2	22 mEq/L	24 mEq/L	25 mEq/L
Serum glucose	110 mg/dL	114 mg/dL	115 mg/dL
Occult stool test	Positive	Positive	Positive

CRITICAL THINKING QUESTIONS

1. What syndromes do the lab values reflect?
2. Is the bone marrow attempting to compensate? Which laboratory value reflects bone marrow?
3. Which signs or symptoms correlate with and can be accounted for by the platelet count?
4. Which signs or symptoms can be correlated to the hemoglobin and hematocrit?
5. Which protective mechanisms should the nurse employ? Why would the nurse implement them?

Answers to Critical Thinking Questions appear in Appendix D.

NCLEX® REVIEW

1. A patient sustained multiple fractures to both femurs and several ribs. The nurse realizes this patient is at risk for developing:
   1. Infection.
   2. Low platelet count.
   3. Reduction in hematopoetic stem cells.
   4. Reduction in red blood cells.

2. A patient has missed receiving a vitamin B_{12} injection for two months. The nurse realizes this patient is at risk for developing:
   1. Reduced red blood cell production.
   2. Reduced white blood cell production.
   3. Reduced platelet production.
   4. Increased red blood cell destruction.

3. While conducting a physical examination, the nurse suspects a patient is experiencing iron deficiency anemia. Which of the following did the nurse assess in this patient?
   1. Fatigue
   2. Fever
   3. Tachycardia
   4. Glossitis

4. A patient with anemia due to acute blood loss has a normal hematocrit level. The nurse realizes this is due to:
   1. A compensatory mechanism.
   2. RBC mass being lost at the same rate as total blood volume.
   3. An increase in plasma volume.
   4. Diluted RBC volume.

5. The nurse is caring for a patient with thrombocytopenia. Which of the following should be included in this patient's care?
   1. Monitor volume of urine output
   2. Nutrition consult for high protein diet
   3. Encourage increased activity
   4. Frequent skin and oral mucosa assessment

6. A patient with hemophilia is in the emergency department being evaluated after being in a motor vehicle accident. The nurse realizes that this patient's injuries will be:
   1. Immediate.
   2. Minimal.
   3. Persistent and last for days or weeks.
   4. Superficial.

Answers for review questions appear in Appendix D

KEY TERMS

2,3-diphosphoglycerate (2,3-DPG) *p.2010*
absolute iron deficiency *p.2019*
anemia *p.2008*
anemic hypoxia *p.2009*
aplastic anemia *p.2054*
autoimmune hemolytic anemia *p.2038*
bioavailable *p.2020*
deoxyhemoglobin *p.2010*
desquamation *p.2018*
differentiation *p.2007*
elemental iron *p.2021*
erythropoiesis *p.2008*
erythropoietic stem cells
    (proerythroblast) *p.2007*
erythropoietin *p.2008*
ferritin *p.2018*
folate *p.2024*
functional iron deficiency *p.2019*
glucose-6-phosphate dehydrogenase (G6PD)
    deficiency *p.2037*

hematology *p.2006*
hematopoiesis *p.2006*
hematopoietic stem cell (HSC) *p.2007*
heme iron *p.2020*
hemoglobin *p.2009*
hemoglobinopathies *p.2026*
hemolytic anemia *p.2033*
hemophilia *p.2051*
hemosiderin *p.2018*
hemostasis *p.2038*
heparin-induced thrombocytopenia
    (HIT) *p.2048*
hepcidin *p.2019*
hereditary spherocytosis (HS) *p.2037*
hypochromic *p.2018*
hypoxia *p.2008*
hypoxic hypoxia *p.2009*
intrinsic factor (IF) *p.2025*

iron deficiency anemia (IDA) *p.2018*
megakaryocytic stem cells *p.2007*
megaloblast *p.2024*
megaloblastic anemia *p.2024*
melena *p.2017*
microcytic *p.2018*
myeloid progenitor cell *p.2007*
nonheme iron *p.2020*
pernicious anemia *p.2025*
progenitor cells *p.2007*
Schilling test *p.2025*
sickle cell anemia *p.2029*
thalassemia *p.2027*
thrombopoietin *p.2043*
transferrin *p.2018*
vitamin B_{12} (cobalamin) *p.2024*
von Willebrand's disease *p.2049*

EXPLORE **PEARSON mynursingkit**™

MyNursingKit is your one stop for online chapter review materials and resources. Prepare for success with additional NCLEX®-style practice questions, interactive assignments and activities, web links, animations and videos, and more!

Register your access code from the front of your book at
www.mynursingkit.com

REFERENCES

Adamson, J. W. (2005). Iron deficiency and other hypoproliferative anemias. In D. L. Kasper, A. S. Fauci, D. L. Longo, E. Braunwald, S. L. Hauser, & J. L. Jameson (Eds.), *Harrison's principles of internal medicine* (16th ed., pp. 587–593). New York: McGraw-Hill.

Aronoff, G. (2004). Safety of intravenous iron in clinical practice: Implications for anemia management protocols. *Journal of the American Society of Nephrology, 15,* 99–106.

Armandola, E. A. (2002). Management of sickle cell anemia: New approaches. Paper presented at the *7th Congress of the European Hematology Association,* Florence, Italy.

Babior, B. M. (2000). The megaloblastic anemias. In E. Beutler, A. Lichtman, B. S. Coller, T. J. Kipps, U. Seligsohn, et al. (Eds.), *Williams' hematology* (6th ed.). New York: McGraw-Hill.

Bajaj, M., Birktoft, J., & Steer, S. (2001). Structure and biology of tissue factor pathway inhibitor. *Thrombosis and Hemostasis, 86,* 959–972.

Bakhshi, S., & Abella, E. (2008). Aplastic anemia. *Emedicine,* Retrieved October 19, 2008 from http://www.emedicine.com/MED/topic162.htm

Balducci, L. (2004). Anemia, cancer, and aging, *Cancer Control, 10*(6), 478–486.

Benz, E. J. (2003). Thalassemia syndromes. In D. L. Kasper, A. S. Fauci, D. L. Longo, E. Braunwald, S. L. Hauser, & J. L. Jameson (Eds.), *Harrison's principles of internal medicine* (16th ed., pp. 594–601). New York: McGraw-Hill.

Blumenthal, M. (1999).Twenty-seven major botanicals and their uses in the United States. In D. Eskinazi, M. Blumenthal, N. Farnsworth, & C. W. Riggins (Eds.), *Botanical medicine* (pp. 18–19). Larchmont, NY: Mary Ann Liebert.

Bodhise, P. B., Dejoie, M., Brandon, Z., Simpkins, S., & Ballas, S. K. (2004). Non-pharmacologic management of sickle cell pain. *Hematology, 9*(3), 235–237.

Buchanan, I. D., Woodward, M., & Reed, G. W. (2005). Opioid selection during sickle cell pain crisis and its impact of development of acute chest syndrome. *Pediatric Blood Cancer, 45*(5), 716–724.

Bunn H. F., Rosse W. (2003). *Hemolytic anemias and acute blood loss, Harrison's Principles of Internal Medicine,* 15th edition, Japanese translation. Edited by Braunwald E. Fauci, A. S., Kasper, D. L., Hauser, S. L., Longo, D. L., Jameson, J. L. Tokyo: Medical Sciences International, 2003, pp 704–16.

Centers for Disease Control and Prevention. (1998). Recommendations to prevent and control iron deficiency in the United States. *Morbidity and Mortality Weekly Reports, 47,* 1–29.

Cines, D. B., & Blanchette, V. S. (2002). Immune thrombocytopenia purpura. *New England Journal of Medicine, 346*(13), 995–1008.

Davoren, A., & Aster, R. H. (2006). Heparin-induced thrombocytopenia and thrombosis. *American Journal of Hematology, 81*(1), 36–44.

Dhaliwal, D. G., Cornnett, P. T., & Tierney, L. M. (2004). Hemolytic anemias. *American Family Physician, 69*(11), 2599–2606.

Dharmarajan, T. S., Pais, W., & Norkus, E. P. (2005). Does anemia matter? Anemia, morbidity, and mortality in older adults: Need for greater recognition. *Geriatrics, 60,* 22–29.

Forget, B. G. (2000). Thalassemia syndromes. In R. Hoffman et al. (Eds.), *Hematology: Basic principles and practice* (3rd ed., pp. 485–510). New York: Churchill Livingstone.

Fujita, T., Namiki, T., Suzuki, T., & Yamamoto, E. (2006). Normal saline flushing for maintenance of peripheral intravenous sites. *Journal of Clinical Nursing, 15*(1), 103–104.

Gallagher, P. G. (2005). Red cell membrane disorders. *Hematology, 2005*(1), 13–18.

Gesundheit, B., Kirby, M., Lau, W., Koren, G., & Abdelhaleem, M. (2002). Thrombocytopenia and megakaryocyte dysplasia: An adverse effect of valproic acid treatment. *Journal of Pediatric Hematology and Oncology, 24*(7), 589–590.

Gillespie, T. (2003). Anemia in cancer: Therapeutic implications and interventions. *Cancer Nursing, 26*(2), 119–128.

Grinder-Pedersen, L., Bukhave, K., Jensen, M., Hojgaard, L., & Hansen, M. (2004). Calcium-fortified foods do not inhibit nonheme-iron absorption from a whole diet consumed over a 4-day period. *American Journal of Clinical Nutrition, 80*(2), 404–409.

Hirsh, J., Heddel, N., & Kelton, J. G. (2004). Treatment of heparin-induced thrombocytopenia: A critical review. *Archives of Internal Medicine, 164*(4), 361–369.

Hoffbrand, V. A. (2005). Deferiprone therapy for transfusional iron overload. *Best Practice & Research: Clinical Haematology, 18*(2), 299–317.

Hoffman, M. M., & Monroe, D. M. (2005). Rethinking the coagulation cascade. *Current Hematology Reports, 4*(5), 391–396.

Hoffman, R., Benz, E., Shattil, S., Furie, B., Cohen, H., Silberstein, L., et al. (2000). Disorders of iron metabolism: Iron deficiency and overload. In R. Hoffman et al. (Eds.), *Hematology: Basic principles and practice* (3rd ed., Chap. 26). New York: Churchill Livingstone.

Hunt, J. R. (2003). Bioavailability of iron, zinc, and other trace minerals from vegetarian diets. *American Journal of Clinical Nutrition, 78*(3), 633.

Knight, K., Wade, S., & Balducci, L. (2004). Prevalence and outcomes of anemia in cancer: A systematic review of the literature. *American Journal of Medicine, 5*(116), 11S–26S.

Koury, M. J., & Ponka, P. (2004). New insights into erythropoeisis: The roles of folate, vitamin B_{12} and iron. *Annual Review of Nutrition, 24,* 105–131.

Levi, M. (2005). Disseminated intravascular coagulation: what's new? (2005). *Critical Care Clinics, 21*(3), 449–467.

Levi, M., de Jonge, E., & van der Poll, T. (2004). New treatment strategies for disseminated intravascular coagulation based on current understanding of the pathophysiology. *Annals of Medicine, 36*(1), 41–49.

Levi, M., de Jonge, E., & van der Poll, T. (2006). Plasma and plasma components in the management of disseminated intravascular coagulation. *Best Practice and Research: Clinical Haematology, 19*(1), 127–142.

Lewis, B. E., Wallis, D. E., Leya, F., Hursting, M. J., & Kelton, J. G. (2003). Argatroban anticoagulation in patients with heparin-induced thrombocytopenia. *Archives of Internal Medicine,163,* 1849–1856.

Lipschitz, D. (2003). Medical and functional consequences of anemia in the elderly. *Journal of the American Geriatrics Society, 51*(Suppl. 3), S10–S13.

Lopez, M. A., & Martos, F. C. (2004). Iron availability: An updated review. *International Journal of Food Science and Nutrition, 55*(8), 597–606.

Lottenberg, R., & Hassell, K. L. (2005). An evidence-based approach to the treatment of adults with sickle cell disease. *ASH Education Book, 58*–65.

Lukes, A. S., Kadir, R. A., Peyvandi, F., & Kouides, P. A. (2005). Disorders of hemostasis and excessive menstrual bleeding: Prevalence and clinical impact. *Fertility and Sterility, 84*(5), 1338–1344.

Mao, T. K., Van De Water, J., & Gershwin, M. E. (2000). Effect of spirulina on the secretion of cytokines from peripheral blood mononuclear cells. *Journal of Medicinal Food, 3*(3), 135–139.

Marlowe, K. F., & Chicella, M. F. (2002). Treatment of sickle cell pain. *Pharmacotherapy, 22*(4), 484–491.

Mayo Clinic. (2007). *Myelodysplastic syndromes.* Retrieved October 20, 2008, from http://www.mayoclinic.com/print/myelodysplastic-syndromes/DS00446/DSECTION+all...

Meek, P. S., Nail, L. M., Baresvil, A., Schwartz, A. L., Stephen, S., Whitmer, K., et al. (2000). Psychometric testing of fatigue instruments for use with cancer patients. *Nursing Research, 49*(4), 181–190.

Mehta, S. R., Afenyi-Annan, A., Byrns, P. J., & Lottenberg, R. (2006). Opportunities to improve outcomes in sickle cell disease. *American Family Physician, 74*(2), 313–314.

Micromedex. (2006). University of Minnesota Libraries. Retrieved October 19, 2008 from http://www.biomed.lib.umn.edu/help/guides/micromedex

Miret, S., Simpson, R. J., & McKie, A. T. (2003). Physiology and molecular biology of dietary iron absorption. *Annual Reviews in Nutrition, 23*, 283–301.

Mock, V. (2004). Evidence-based treatment for cancer-related fatigue. *Journal of the National Cancer Institute Monographs, 32*, 112–118.

Montoya, V. L., Wink, D., & Sole, M. L. (2002). Adult anemia: Determine clinical significance. *Nurse Practitioner, 27*(3), 38–53.

Naschitz, J. E., Rozenbaum, M., Shaviv, N., Fields, M., Enis, S., Babich, J. P., et al. (2004, January 1). The feeling of fatigue: Fatigue severity by unidimensional versus composite questionnaires. *Behavioral Medicine.*

National Anemia Action Council. (2008). *Iron Deficiency Anemia.* Retrieved October 20, 2008, from http://www.anemia.org/patients/information-handourts/iron-deficiency/

National Center for Health Statistics. (2008). *National Health and Nutrition Examination Survey.* Retrieved September 30, 2008, from http://www.cdc.gov/nchs/nhanes.htm

National Comprehensive Cancer Network. (2008). Cancer and Chemotherapy-Induced Anemia, V.3.2009. Retrieved October 20, 2008, from www.nccn.org

National Institutes of Health, Office of Dietary Supplements. (2005). *Dietary supplement fact sheet: Iron.* Retrieved February 11, 2006, from http://ods.od.nih.gov/factsheets/iron.asp

National Kidney Foundation. (2001). KDOQI clinical practice guidelines for anemia of chronic kidney disease: Update 2000. *American Journal of Kidney Disease, 37*, S182–S238.

Niesen, K. M., Harris, D. Y., Parkin, L. S., & Henn, L. T. (2003). The effects of heparin versus normal saline for maintenance of peripheral intravenous locks in pregnant women. *Journal of Obstetrics and Gynecology, 32*(4), 503–508.

Nilsson, M., Norberg, B. M., Hultdin, J., Sandstrom, H., Westman, G., & Lokk, J. (2005). Medical intelligence in Sweden. Vitamin B_{12}: Oral compared with parenteral? *Journal of Postgraduate Medicine, 81*(953), 191–193.

Nyholm, E., Turpin, P., Swain, D., Cunningham, B., Daly, S., Nightingale, P. et al. (2003). Oral vitamin B_{12} can change our practice. *Journal of Postgraduate Medicine, 79*(930), 218 – 219.

Ouellette, D. R. (2005). The impact of anemia in patients with respiratory failure. *Chest 128*, 576S–582S.

Pearson, D. J. (2000). Pathophysiology and clinical effects of chronic hypoxia. *Respiratory Care, 45*(1), 39–51.

Penninx, B. J., Pahor, M., Cesari, M., Corsi, A. M., et al. (2004). Anemia is associated with disability and decreased physical performance and muscle strength in the elderly. *Journal of the American Geriatrics Society, 52*(5), 719.

Penninx, B. J., Pluijm, S. M. F., Lips, P., Woodman, M., Miedema, K., Guralnik, J. K. et al. (2005). Late-life anemia is associated with increased risk of recurrent falls. *Journal of the American Geriatrics Society, 53*(12), 2106–2111.

Ponka, P. (2001). Iron deficiency. In R. E. Rakel & E. T. Bope (Eds.), *Conn's current therapy* (pp. 369–376). London: Saunders.

Ramsey, L. T., Woods, K. F., Callahan, L. A., Mensah, G. A., Barbeau, P., & Gutin, B. (2001). Quality of life improvement for patients with sickle cell disease. *American Journal of Hematology, 66*(2), 155–156.

Rice, L., Nguyen, P. H., & Vann, A. R. (2002). Preventing complications in heparin-induced thrombocytopenias: Alternative anticoagulants are improving patient outcomes. *Postgraduate Medicine, 112*(3).

Rios, R., Sangro, B., Herrero, I., Quiroga, J., & Prieto, J. (2005). The role of thrombopoietin in the thrombocytopenia of patients with liver cirrhosis. *American Journal of Gastroenterology, 100*(6), 1311–1316.

Rosenthal, K. (2003). Consider alternative technologies to maintain vascular access devices. *Nursing Management, 34*(8), 53–56.

Sadler, J. E. (1994). A revised classification of von Willebrand disease. For the Subcommittee on von Willebrand factor of the Scientific and Standardization Committee of the International Society on Thrombosis and Haemostasis. *Thrombosis and Haemostasis, 71*(4), 520–525.

Sleijfer, S., & Lugtenburg, P. J. (2003). Aplastic anemia: a review. *Netherlands Journal of Medicine, 61*(5), 157–163.

Solovey, A. A., Solovey, A. N., Harkness, J., & Hebbel, R. P. (2001). Modulation of endothelial cell activation in sickle cell disease: A pilot study. *Blood, 97*, 1937–1941.

Stasi, R. S., & Provan, D. (2004). Management of immune thrombocytopenic purpura in adults. *Mayo Clinic Proceedings, 79*, 504–522.

Stouten, B. (2005). Identification of ambiguities in the 1994 chronic fatigue syndrome research case definition and recommendations for resolution. *BMC Health Services Research, 5*, 37.

Sturgeon, P., Itano, H. A., et al. (1955). Genetic and biochemical studies of intermediate types of Cooley's anemia. *British Journal of Haematology, 1*, 264.

Umbreit, J. (2005). Iron deficiency anemia: A concise review. *American Journal of Hematology, 78*, 225–231.

U.S. Department of Health and Human Services. (2000). *Healthy people 2010: Understanding and improving health and objectives for improving health* (2nd ed., 2 volumes). Washington, DC: Author.

U.S. Preventive Services Task Force. (2006). Screening for iron deficiency anemia, including iron supplementations for children and pregnant women: recommendation statement. *American Family Physician.* Retrieved October 17, 2008, from http://www.aafp.org/afp/20060901/us.html

Vichinsky, E. (2005). *Treating thalassemia.* Retrieved March 5, 2006, from Northern California Comprehensive Thalassemia Center website: http://www.thalassemia.com

Wang, W. C., Helms, R. W., Lynn, H. S., et al. (2002). Effect of hydroxyurea on growth in children with sickle cell anemia: Results of the HUG-KIDS study. *Journal of Pediatrics, 140*(2), 225–229.

Warkentin, T. E., & Kelton, J. G. (1996). A 14-year study of heparin-induced thrombocytopenia. *American Journal of Medicine, 101*(5), 502–507.

Weiss, G. (2002). Pathogenesis and treatment of anaemia of chronic disease. *Blood Reviews, 16*, 87–96.

Weiss, G., & Gordeuk, V. R. (2005). Benefits and risks of iron therapy for chronic anaemias. *European Journal of Clinical Investigation, 35*, 36S–45S.

Whitta, R. K., Hall, K. F., Bennetts, T. M., Welman L., & Rawlins, P. (2006). Comparison of normal or heparinised saline flushing on function of arterial lines. *Critical Care Resuscitation, 8*(3), 205–208.

Caring for the Patient with Cancer

Dawn Lambie

Outcome-Based Learning Objectives

After studying this chapter, the learner will be able to:

1. Identify the prevalence and incidence of cancer, list the common risk factors, and describe the correlation to development of malignancy.

2. Discuss the pathophysiology of cancer.

3. Compare and contrast the five common types of solid tumor cancer (prostate, breast, colorectal, lung, and brain) and cancers of the hematopoietic and lymphatic system.

4. Develop a detailed nursing plan of care for patients with cancer of the prostate, breast, colon or rectum, lung, brain, hematopoietic system, and lymphatic system.

5. Describe current treatment approaches to fatigue, nutrition, and pain and the importance of improving quality of life for patients with cancer.

6. Discuss the rationale for treatment modalities such as surgery, radiation therapy, chemotherapy, biotherapy, and transplantation.

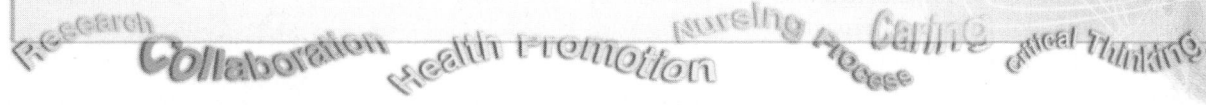

Research   Collaboration   Health Promotion   Nursing Process   Caring   Critical Thinking

FEW WORDS evoke an emotional response as dramatic as the word **cancer**. The impacts, both physiologically and psychologically, cause considerable changes in the lifestyles of both patients and families. The diagnosis of cancer in a family member will change the emotional status, finances, division of responsibility, and social activities of the entire family (Kaye, 1993). Nurses need to be aware of their own feelings and attitudes toward cancer and cancer care in order to be supportive of patients and their families.

For the past two centuries nurses have dedicated their lives to changing the experience of illness, leading to changes in nursing practice (Lynaugh, 2001). Leaders in cancer nursing have directed their efforts toward prevention, detection, education, and the creation of a specialty within nursing that embraces the whole of the human being who has cancer. Sadly, society continues to perceive malignancy as incurable with accompanied dread and hopelessness. Of critical importance is the role of nursing in the continued development of cancer screening, detection, and prevention programs. These programs have already demonstrated improved survival rates and quality of life for patients undergoing cancer treatment.

Following the first National Cancer Nursing Research Conference in 1973, oncology nurses identified the need to form a national organization to support their profession. Cancer nursing was first recognized as a subspecialty in the nursing profession in the year 1975 with the incorporation of the Oncology Nursing Society (ONS). Since its inception, ONS has grown to a membership of more than 30,000 registered nurses and other health care providers. The organization is dedicated to maintaining excellence in patient care, education, research, and administration in oncology nursing (ONS, n.d.). To be an effective oncology nurse, a nurse must possess a broad base of knowledge about the pathophysiology and psychosocial aspects of the disease and its treatment. Patients rely on nurses for support and assistance throughout all phases of their illness, from diagnosis to end-of-life care.

Epidemiology

When studying cancer, the outcome for therapeutic research is to discover a cure. In contrast, the outcome of epidemiological research is to prevent cancer (Schulmeister, 2001a). Understanding basic epidemiologic terminology will help the nurse reach a sound interpretation of literature about cancer and its causes. In addition, this knowledge will assist the nurse in identification of target population groups for education, prevention, and screening programs.

Incidence is the number of newly diagnosed cases of cancer in a specific time period in a defined population. It will be expressed as a rate per 100,000 persons, allowing for comparison between different populations. For example, when evaluating the number of estimated breast cancer cases in Minnesota for the year 2005 (3,240) and the number in California (19,790), researchers must consider the state's population or the numbers are meaningless (American Cancer Society [ACS], 2007).

Prevalence is the measurement of all cancer cases at a designated point in time. The number is divided by the total population living at the time. The prevalence rate is very useful when planning the creation of health care facilities, determining necessary manpower, and designing and implementing screening programs (Schulmeister, 2001a).

Mortality is the number of deaths from cancer in a specific period of time and within an identified population. The total number of persons dying of cancer is divided by the total population living at that time. Since 1930 the United States has been collecting mortality data. The 2007 estimated number of cancer deaths in the United States is 559,650 persons (ACS, 2007). Death certificates typically identify a single cause of death, leading to inaccuracy in the reporting of cancer deaths. Mortality figures are very useful in determining the impact of treatment, whereas incidence figures are more helpful when determining the cause of cancer.

Survival is the observation of persons with cancer over time and the likelihood of their dying over several time periods. This information is the link between incidence and mortality data, providing useful measures of the end result of treatment. In addition, survival information may provide evidence of improvement over time in the management of cancer.

Cancer Statistics

As mentioned, the ACS has estimated that approximately 559,650 Americans will die from cancer in the year 2007, resulting in 1,533 deaths per day (ACS, 2007). Refer to Chart 64–1 for details. The total number of cancer deaths continues to rise due to an aging and expanding population. Figure 64–1 ■ represents the number of cancer cases and deaths according to site and gender. This information is important for nurses to understand in order to develop and implement patient education regarding cancer prevention.

■ Etiology and Pathophysiology

Cancer is not an unruly growth of immature cells, but rather a logical, coordinated process in which normal cells undergo changes and develop special functions. An understanding of the morphology and biochemistry of the normal cell is crucial in building an appreciation of the disease itself.

Proliferative Growth Patterns

Cancer cells do not have the usual limitations on cell proliferation placed by the host. Proliferation and cancer are not always synonymous terms. Proliferation does not always insinuate the presence of

CHART 64–1 ■ **Estimated Cancer Cases and Cancer Deaths**

Estimated Cancer Cases			Estimated Cancer Deaths*		
Total	Female	Male	Total	Female	Male
1,444,920	678,060	766,860	559,650	270,100	289,550

*Estimated number of cancer deaths expected in the United States was determined using underlying cause-of-death data from death certificates as reported to the National Center for Health Statistics.

Source: American Cancer Society. (2007). *Cancer facts and figures 2007.* Atlanta, Georgia. Retrieved from http://www.cancer.org/docroot/STT/content/ STT_1x_Cancer_Facts__Figures_2007.asp.

Estimated number of new cancer cases (10 leading sites by gender), U.S. 2007

Female		Male	
Breast	26%	Prostate	29%
Lung and bronchus	15%	Lung and bronchus	15%
Colon and rectum	11%	Colon and rectum	10%
Uterine corpus	6%	Urinary bladder	7%
Non-Hodgkin's lymphoma	4%	Melanoma of the skin	4%
Melanoma of the skin	4%	Non-Hodgkin's lymphoma	4%
Thyroid	4%	Kidney/renal pelvis	4%
Ovary	3%	Oral cavity/pharynx	3%
Kidney and renal pelvis	3%	Leukemia	3%
Leukemia	3%	Pancreas	2%
Other	21%	Other	19%

Estimated number of new cancer deaths (10 leading sites by gender), U.S. 2007

Female		Male	
Lung and bronchus	26%	Lung and bronchus	31%
Breast	15%	Prostate	9%
Colon and rectum	10%	Colon and rectum	9%
Pancreas	6%	Pancreas	6%
Ovary	6%	Esophagus	4%
Leukemia	4%	Leukemia	4%
Non-Hodgkin's lymphoma	3%	Liver/intrahepatic bile duct	4%
Uterine corpus	3%	Non-Hodgkin's lymphoma	3%
Brain/CNS	2%	Urinary bladder	3%
Liver and hepatic duct	2%	Kidney and renal pelvis	3%
Other	23%	Other	24%

FIGURE 64–1 ■ Epidemiology of cancer.

CHART 64–2	**Terms of Proliferative Growth Patterns**	
Types of Cellular Change	**Definition**	**Example**
Hypertrophy	Increase in cell size	Increase in muscle cell size
Hyperplasia	Increase in cell number	Breast epithelium during pregnancy
Metaplasia	Replacement of one adult cell type by a different adult cell type	Replacement of columnar epithelium of respiratory tract by squamous epithelium
Anaplasia	Reverse cellular development with more primitive cell type	Irreversible changes to an accompanying cancer
Neoplasia	Abnormal cellular changes and growth of new tissue	Malignancies
Dysplasia	Abnormal growth of cells that vary in size, shape or organization of cells or tissues	Precancerous changes in cervical cells

cancer. Abnormal cellular growth is known as *nonneoplastic* and *neoplastic*. The terms are summarized in Chart 64–2.

Nonneoplastic Growth Patterns

There are four common nonneoplastic growth patterns: hypertrophy, hyperplasia, metaplasia, and dysplasia (Pfeifer, 2001). They are not neoplastic conditions, but may precede the development of cancer. Hypertrophy refers to an increase in a cell's size. Situations that create hypertrophy include increased workload, stimulation by hormones, and compensation from loss of other tissue. Hyperplasia refers to an increase in tissue mass due to a reversible increase in the number of cells of a certain tissue type. This is a normal physiological response in times of rapid growth and development such as pregnancy and adolescence. Abnormality occurs when the volume of cells produced is larger than the physiological demand. Metaplasia occurs when one mature cell type is substituted for another type not typically found in the involved tissue. A stimulus such as inflammation, vitamin deficiencies, irritation, and chemical agents can induce metaplasia. If the stimulus is removed, the process is reversible. Otherwise it will progress to dysplasia, which occurs when there are alterations in normal mature cells. These alterations can include variation from normal cell size, shape, or organization or replacement of one mature cell type with a less mature cell type. External stimuli are the usual impetus for creating dysplasia, but if removed the process may be reversible. These can include radiation, inflammation, toxic chemicals, and chronic irritation.

An irreversible change in the structure of an adult cell that deteriorates to a more immature level is known as *anaplasia*. This type of cellular change is the classic finding of cancer. Anaplastic cells no longer have the ability to implement their unique functions and overall are chaotic in their nature.

Neoplastic Growth Patterns

The term **neoplasm** means "new growth." Inherent in this definition is the understanding that there is an abnormal tissue mass that goes beyond the normal cell boundaries and results in the inability of the cell to perform its normal function. Neoplasms can be destructive to the host because they occupy space and battle for nutrients crucial to maintain its life. There are two categories of neoplasm: benign and malignant. Papillomas and warts are examples of benign neoplasms. Malignant neoplasms, referred to as cancer, have the potential to destroy the host and include solid tumors and leukemias. Refer to Chart 64–3 for a comparison between benign and malignant tumors.

CHART 64–3	**Differences Between Benign and Malignant Neoplasms**
Benign	**Malignant**
Usually slow growing, expansive	May proliferate rapidly or grow slowly, infiltrative patterns
Localized or encapsulated	Spread (metastasize) throughout the body invading nearby tissue
Fibrous capsule	No enclosing capsule
Rarely recur after removal	May recur even after treatment
Usually regular in shape	Irregular shape with poorly defined border
Well differentiated	Poorly differentiated
Slight vascularity	Moderate to significant vascularity

Sources: Erickson, J. (2003). Cancer. In W. Phipps, F. Monahan, J. Sands, J. Marek, & M. Neighbors (Eds.), *Medical–surgical nursing health and illness perspectives* (7th ed.). St. Louis: Mosby; Otto, S. (2001c). *Oncology nursing* (4th ed.). St. Louis: Mosby.

Characteristics of a Cancer Cell

Metabolism for normal cells is achieved through aerobic glycolysis, in which oxygen is the crucial element in maintenance of cellular activity. Malignant cells utilize higher rates of aerobic glycolysis with a resulting decrease in oxygen needed for survival. This difference in metabolism may be due to differences in intracellular enzyme structure and quantity (Volker, 1994).

Cancer cells differ according to the cell type from which they derive. It is incorrect to apply a standard definition to all cancer cells (McNance & Roberts, 2002). Some tumors may retain useful functions and closely resemble normal tissue, whereas others are chaotic enough that the tissue of origin cannot be determined. Certain cellular characteristics that are typical features of cancerous tissue include local increase in number of cells, loss of normal arrangement of cells, dissimilarity of cell shape and size, increase in nuclear size and total DNA seen by an increase in the density of staining, increase in mitotic activity, and abnormal mitoses and chromosomes.

Cancer cells are chaotic cells with significant cellular proliferation and assorted sizes and shapes. *Progression* is a term used to explain the unorganized dividing of cells and the invasion and destruction of nearby tissue. It is important to understand that progression refers to an increase of abnormal biologic properties, not always a progression in tumor size. The increase in biologic activities is related to the tumor's malignant capabilities or its lack of differentiation. Therefore, cancer can be considered an aberrant cell mass.

Tumor Growth

Malignant tumors grow in an uninhibited way and do not adhere to the normal process of cell reproduction (Volker, 1994). As the body loses cells or increases tissue function demands, there is a natural increase in the number of cells and cell replacement. Cell development approximates cell destruction (Pfeifer, 2001). Cancer cells do not reproduce faster than normal cells; in fact, many are slow growing compared to regular cells. Examples of this unique process include cells of the bone marrow and those located in the epithelial lining. All tumors contain cells that ignore the restraints typical of proliferation, but not all cancer cells proliferate indefinitely. This erratic behavior results in cell growth beyond normal margins and an increase in pressure on surrounding organs. In addition, cells may be noted to actually invade surrounding tissues and structures.

Carcinogenesis

Carcinogenesis is defined as the process of tumor development (McNance & Roberts, 2002). Normal cells are altered, resulting in the development of cancerous cells. It is a multistep process that is in constant unrest and is influenced by a variety of forces. A carcinogen (initiating agent) is a chemical, biologic, or physical agent with the potential of changing the molecular structure of the genetic component (DNA) of a cell. The transformation of the cell is due to direct contact with the carcinogen, and the result is permanent and irreversible. A co-carcinogen (promoting agent) changes the expression of the genetic information of the cell that assists in cellular transformation. Examples of co-carcinogens include hormones, drugs, and plant products. A complete carcinogen (e.g., radiation) is capable of performing functions of both an initiating agent and promoting agent. Anticarcinogens (reversing factors) are substances found in most diets, vitamins C, A, and E, and selenium. These substances may interfere with the effects of initiating agents and prevent cancerous growths.

Scientists have yet to definitively prove that the first event in carcinogenesis is a mutation, but regardless of the cause, there is an irreversible alteration in the genetic code of cells (Erickson, 2003). A number of theories have been proposed to explain the development of cancer, but no single idea has been accepted, which answers why a cause for most human cancers has yet to be determined (Pfeifer, 2001). Many of the theories of carcinogenesis discuss three common stages: initiation, promotion, and progression. In 1947 the Berenblum theory attempted to explain the first two stages, but over time the third stage of progression was proposed to further explain the complex phenomena of cancer development (Pfeifer, 2001). Figure 64–2 ■ illustrates the stages of initiation, promotion, and progression. This theory suggests that the process of changing a normal cell into a cancer cell involves three stages where all activity occurs in the cell's DNA.

In the first stage, initiation, a carcinogen alters a particular gene, resulting in damaged DNA. The three possible outcomes of this transformation include:

- Repair of the gene with no cancer development
- The occurrence of permanent changes, but there is no cancer development unless the cell is exposed to a co-carcinogen later

- Transformation into a cancer cell if the initiating agent is a complete carcinogen.

An oncogene is a slightly altered form of a normal gene that is responsible for cell growth and repair and has been associated with the development of cancer when activated (McNance & Roberts, 2002). Tumor suppressor genes hinder cellular growth, thus causing cellular death. An example of this is the p53 tumor suppressor gene on chromosome 17. This gene prohibits cells with DNA damage from multiplying. Mutations to the p53 gene have been identified in half of all human cancers (Erickson, 2003).

In promotion, the second stage, co-carcinogens produce either reversible or irreversible destruction to the proliferative mechanism of the cell (Pfeifer, 2001). Cancerous cell formation occurs with irreversible cell damage. Progression, the final stage, involves morphologic changes within cells that begin to demon-

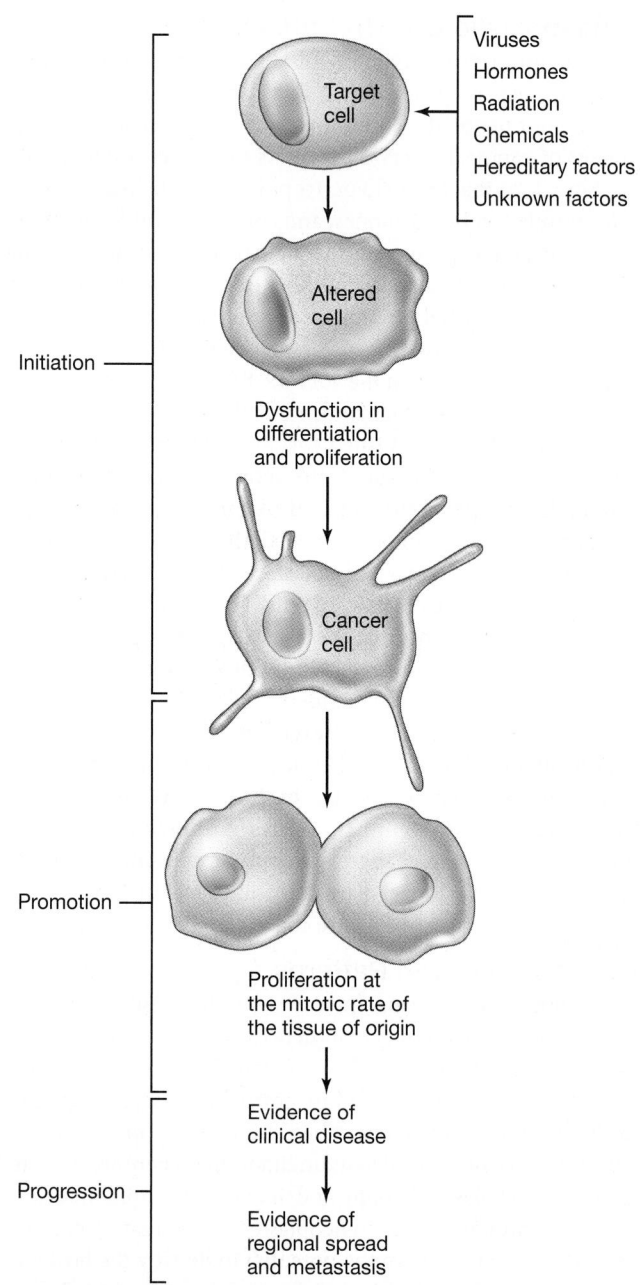

FIGURE 64–2 ■ Cellular changes with cancer.

strate malignancy and the evolution of metastatic potential. This last stage is irreversible.

In humans, the process of carcinogenesis is much more complex than any laboratory model and frequently occupies many years of an individual's life (Pfeifer, 2001). Distinguishing among the three phases is difficult because of the presence of the latent period. Occurring between the initial exposure to a carcinogen and the evidence of detectable malignancy, this period is void of specific clinical or subjective findings. Adding to the

difficulty in determining the beginning and end of the stages is the absence of tests to detect latent transformed cells. This explains why it impossible to predict whether the risk of cancer exists in subsets of a population group.

Tumor Nomenclature

Tumors receive their names according to the originating tissue type as seen in Chart 64–4. The identification of the tissue is often difficult due to a variety of cell types within one malignancy.

CHART 64–4 Nomenclature and Classification of Neoplasms

Tissue of Origin	Malignant Tumor	Benign Tumor
Epithelial		
Squamous cells	Squamous cell carcinoma	Squamous cell papilloma
Basal cells	Basal cell carcinoma	No benign tumor for this type of cell
Liver cells	Hepatocellular carcinoma	Hepatocellular adenoma
Melanocytes	Malignant melanoma	Nevus
Renal epithelium	Renal cell carcinoma	Renal tubular adenoma
Glands	Adenocarcinoma	Adenoma
Endothelial/Related Tissue		
Lymphoid tissue	Lymphatic leukemia	No benign tumor for this type of cell
	Malignant lymphoma	No benign tumor for this type of cell
	Reticular cell sarcoma	No benign tumor for this type of cell
Bone marrow	Multiple myeloma	No benign tumor for this type of cell
	Leukemia	No benign tumor for this type of cell
	Ewing's sarcoma	No benign tumor for this type of cell
	Lymphosarcoma	No benign tumor for this type of cell
Lymph vessels	Lymphangiosarcoma	Lymphangioma
Mesothelium	Malignant mesothelioma	No benign tumor for this type of cell
Meninges	Malignant meningioma	Meningioma
Neural and Retinal Tissue		
Nerve fibers and sheaths	Neurofibrosarcoma	Neurilemoma, neurofibroma
	Neurogenic sarcoma	No benign tumor for this type of cell
Nerve cells	Neuroblastoma	Ganglioneuroma
	Spongioblastoma	Glioma
Muscle Tissue		
Smooth muscle	Leiomyosarcoma	Leiomyoma
Striated muscle	Rhabdomyosarcoma	Rhabdomyoma
Connective Tissue		
Fibrous tissue	Fibrosarcoma	Fibroma
Embryonic fibrous tissue	Myxosarcoma	Myxoma
Fat	Liposarcoma	Lipoma
Bone	Osteogenic sarcoma	Osteoma
Cartilage	Chondrosarcoma	Chondroma
Synovial membrane	Synovial sarcoma	Synovioma
Other		
Placenta	Chorion-epithelioma	Hydatidiform mole
	Embryonal carcinoma	Dermoid cyst
	Embryonal sarcoma	No benign tumor for this type of cell
	Teratocarcinoma	No benign tumor for this type of cell

Sources: Adapted from McNance, K., & Roberts, L. (2002). Biology of cancer. In K. McNance & S. Huether (Eds.), *Pathophysiology: The biological basis for disease in adult and children* (4th ed.). St. Louis: Mosby; Otto, S. (2001c). *Oncology nursing* (4th ed.). St. Louis: Mosby.

Within a cluster of neoplastic cells there may be benign cells as well, making identification even more difficult (Erickson, 2003). Tumors are classified according to the following: cell type, originating tissue, malignant or benign, degree of differentiation, site, and function (McNance & Roberts, 2002).

The degree of differentiation refers to the cell's maturity. Undifferentiated tumors are those that have completely lost identity with the tissue of origin. Well and moderately differentiated tumors possess cells that continue to demonstrate the tissue of origin.

Histogenetic Classification

The suffix *oma*, Greek for "tumor," is used for both benign and malignant tumors. **Benign** tumors are those whose prefix designates specific tissue, whereas **malignant** tumors use the root *carcin* (epithelial tissue) and *sarc* (connective tissue) In addition, other cancer types include lymphomas (lymphatic system), gliomas (glial cells of the central nervous system), and leukemias (blood-forming organs, usually bone marrow). Examples of benign tumors are fibromas and adenomas, which are located in fibrous and glandular tissue. The only exceptions to this are melanoma and hepatomas. Melanomas are malignancies of the melanocytes and hepatomas are malignancies of the liver. Specific connective tissue sarcomas use several different prefixes depicting the anatomic location of the tumor (Pfeifer, 2001). These include:

- *Osteo-* (bone)
- *Chondro-* (cartilage)
- *Lipo-* (fat)
- *Rhabdo-* (skeletal muscle)
- *Leiomyo-* (smooth muscle).

Preinvasive epithelial tumors with glandular or squamous cell origins are called **carcinoma *in situ*.** They typically occur in the cervix, skin, oral cavity, bronchus, and esophagus. Carcinoma *in situ* neoplasms have not invaded the basement membrane of the epithelial site, thus the surrounding tissues are left untouched by malignant cells (McNance & Roberts, 2002).

Classifying Degree of Malignancy

Examination of tumor tissue under the microscope is the only way to classify, or grade, the degree of malignancy. Four grades are used as a standardized method of communicating the appearance of the cells and their potential for spread and growth. Using a standardized language allows practitioners to determine treatment options while providing prognostic information. A grade 1 tumor is small in size, more differentiated, and the least malignant. Grade 4 tumors are those with cells that appear more abnormal, are usually very aggressive in nature, and are considered to have a high degree of malignancy.

Staging is the portion of the classification system that describes the extent of the tumor and evidence of metastasis throughout the body. The TNM system is used to describe the presence and extent of local, regional, and distant disease. *T* refers to primary tumor size, *N* refers to the absence or presence of regional lymph nodes, and *M* refers to absence or presence of distant metastases. It is important to understand that not all malignancies will have similar degrees of grading and classification; ultimately, the labels will be determined by the pathologist upon

examining the tissue specimens. Details of the classification system are found in Chart 64–5.

Route of Tumor Spread

Cells that are experiencing the transformation process have abnormal or decreased anchorage. Anchorage independence is the inability of the cell to maintain cellular or extracellular matrix attachments. Cancer cells do not require a surface on which to attach and multiply. Missing this cellular characteristic that inhibits proliferation will result in cancerous cell growth in new regions, or metastases (McNance & Roberts 2002).

Cancer may invade local tissues or spread to distant areas by hematogenous or lymphatic routes. As tumors grow locally, their cells extend to and invade lymph nodes found in the same anatomic region resulting in distant metastases. Some tumors are known to metastasize to distant organs prior to or during involvement with local lymph nodes (Pfeifer, 2001).

Direct

Direct spread is the ability of a tumor to invade and eradicate adjoining tissue (Groenwald, Frogge, Goodman, & Yarbro, 1997). The following enhances this process:

- Tumor angiogenesis factor stimulates new capillary growth, which allows for continued tumor growth due to adequate nutrition and oxygen. Once a tumor reaches 2 mm^3 in size, it requires additional blood supply to grow. The new vascular growth provides not only the essential elements for growth but also a route for tumor cells to leave the primary site (Merkle & Loescher, 2005).

CHART 64–5 **TNM System of Tumor Classification and Staging**

Primary Tumor Size (T)

T0	No evidence of a primary tumor or lesion
Tis	Carcinoma *in situ*
T1	Lesion contained in organ of origin
T2	Localized lesion with deep growth into adjacent structures
T3	Advanced lesion limited to a region of the original organ
T4	Advanced lesion spreading into adjacent organs

Regional Lymph Nodes (N)

N0	No evidence of disease in lymph nodes
N1	Evidence of disease in regional lymph nodes but not likely metastatic
N2, 3, 4	Increasing involvement of regional lymph nodes

Anatomic Extent of Metastasis (M)

M0	No evidence of metastasis
M1, 2, 3	Worsening degrees of metastatic involvement, including distant lymph nodes and functional impairment

Sources: Erickson, J. (2003). Cancer. In W. Phipps, F. Monahan, J. Sands, J. Marek, & M. Neighbors (Eds.), *Medical–surgical nursing health and illness perspectives* (7th ed.). St. Louis: Mosby; McNance, K., & Roberts, L. (2002). Biology of cancer. In K. McNance & S. Huether (Eds.), *Pathophysiology: The biological basis for disease in adult and children* (4th ed.). St. Louis: Mosby; Pfeifer, K. A. (2001). Pathophysiology. In S. Otto (Ed.), *Oncology nursing* (4th ed.). St. Louis: Mosby.

- Mechanical pressure and increased rate of tumor growth occur when intratumor pressure causes finger-like projections to be pushed into adjacent tissue. Uncontrolled tumor growth creates expanding masses that apply pressure on local tissues.
- Cell motility and loss of cellular adhesiveness promote tumor cell distribution due to the slippery nature of the cancer cell, which enhances movement.
- Tumor-secreted enzymes may be associated with the degree to which cells have the potential to invade surrounding tissues and destroy the normal tissue barriers. An example of this is plasminogen activator.

Serosal seeding is another mechanism by which tumor cells demonstrate direct spreading (Groenwald et al. 1997). Embolization of tumor cells occurs after malignant cells invade local tissues and infiltrate body cavities. These cells then attach themselves to the serosal surface of organs within the involved cavity. The most common site for serosal seeding to occur is the lung and ovary. Penetration of the parenchyma of the organ is unlikely to occur despite the presence of tumor cells within the surface of organs in the pleural and peritoneal cavities.

Surgical instrumentation has been shown to participate in the direct spread of cancerous cells by the contamination of normal cells during surgical procedures (Volker, 1992). As needles are withdrawn during biopsies, seeding of malignant cells may occur, or manipulation of a tumor during the operative procedure may release cells into the vascular supply and into the circulation.

Metastatic

Metastasis is defined as the spread of cancerous cells from a primary site of origin to a distant site (McNance & Roberts, 2002). Of extreme importance is to recognize the effect of metastasis and that a benign tumor does not exhibit this type of behavior. The capability of malignant cells to travel to distant sites and begin invasion into adjacent tissues is very powerful and oftentimes deadly. Chart 64–6 lists the four most common cancers and their metastatic sites.

French physician Joseph Claude Recamier was the first to use the term *metastasis* in 1829 (Hawkins, 2001). Previously, researchers thought that tumors spread by direct extension and invading lymph nodes. At that time, it was thought that distant metastasis was caused by new tumor growth unrelated to the primary tumor. Recamier was the first physician to prove metastasis was caused by malignant cells separating from the primary tumor and traveling through the bloodstream and lymphatic circulation to distant anatomic locations (Liotta, 1992).

Approximately 50% to 60% of patients diagnosed with solid tumors are discovered to have metastatic disease. Some patients will have clinically detectable metastasis, whereas others will have micrometastases or clinically undetectable disease (Liotta & Kohn, 1990). Prognosis is dramatically worsened if evidence of metastasis is present at the time of diagnosis.

The metastatic process, although commonly evident clinically, is a unique, intricate series of events. A cancer cell released from a primary tumor with the mission to establish residency in a distant anatomic site has a long and difficult task in order to survive. It is believed that only 1 in 10,000 tumor cells that separate from the primary tumor are able to endure long enough to begin the metastatic process (Liotta, 1992).

Understanding the mechanism of metastasis is important to increase our appreciation of metastatic patterns; however, metastasis is known to be unpredictable in nature. Mechanisms of metastasis include (1) angiogenesis, (2) migration, (3) cell attachment, (4) cell invasion, and (5) growth factors.

Angiogenesis is the creation of new blood vessels due to migration and proliferation of endothelial cells from existing blood vessels. Although angiogenesis is a favorable occurrence in wound healing, ovulation, and embryogenesis, it is not so favorable in the development of malignancies. Vascular endothelial growth factor (VEGF) is an essential component for the growth and proliferation of cancer cells. New blood vessels provide nutrients, protein growth factors, and oxygen to the tumor mass. With the development of angiogenesis inhibitors (e.g., Avastin), this vital process for tumor growth can be slowed or stopped, affording patients better treatment options (Viele, 2005).

Because vessels created by angiogenesis tend to have permeable walls, malignant cells enter easily, allowing access to the circulatory and lymphatic systems (migration). Tumor masses produce motility factors that enable cells to move with more ease throughout the circulatory and lymphatic systems. Once in the circulation, cancer cells cluster in the first vascular bed distal to the original site. After blood circulates through the heart, the pulmonary vascular bed is the first encountered by the cancerous cells. Intestines drain their blood supply into the liver, thus exposing it to malignant cells. Understandably, the most common site of metastasis is the lung followed by the liver.

Another common vehicle for the transportation of malignant cells is the lymphatic system. Tumor emboli, which form as a result of circulating tumor cells, are trapped in lymph nodes. Not all lymph nodes will be hosts for these deadly cells; in fact, cancerous cells will bypass several lymph nodes before settling into a distant nodal site. This is known as "skip" metastasis (Hawkins, 2001).

Normally, cells adhere to one another and to the extracellular matrix (ECM). When discussing cell attachment, the nurse must understand that tumor cells form temporary attachments to ECM components and to other cells not part of their origin. Cell-to-cell adhesion is altered resulting in tumor cells attaching themselves to cells of a different origin. For example, breast cancer metastasizing to the bone occurs when a breast tissue cell relocates to the bone. This form of cell attachment is assisted by cell surface receptors such as CD44. The next type of cellular attachment is adhesion to the ECM, which promotes cellular growth and endurance. As discussed earlier, anchorage dependence is necessary for cells to attach to surfaces that nurture their proliferation.

CHART 64–6	Common Sites of Metastases of the Four Most Frequently Occurring Cancers

Origin	Site of Metastasis
Breast	Bone, lung, liver, brain, lymph nodes
Prostate	Bone, lung, liver, bowel, kidney, lymph nodes
Lung	Bone, liver, kidney, brain, bone marrow, lymph nodes
Colon	Lung, liver, brain, lymph nodes

Cell invasion is essential for the metastatic process. As a result, tumor cells drift from physical barriers into a vessel (intravasation) or out of a vessel (extravasation). Cancer cells are able to reach normal tissue despite numerous mechanical barriers with the assistance of tumor cell invasion. Basement membrane invasion occurs when cancer cells leave the primary tumor, penetrate into the blood or lymphatic vessels, and exit from the vasculature.

Growth factors contribute substantially to the metastatic process. Angiogenesis is potentiated or impeded by growth factors. In addition, tumor proliferation produces a decreased reliance on exogenous growth factors. The existence of growth factors at the metastatic site is imperative for continued growth of cancerous cells. Chart 64–7 illustrates various growth factors known to stimulate cancerous development.

The phenomenon of metastasis is uniquely complex as it navigates through normal body controls and regulatory functions. The process oftentimes is associated with worsened prognosis and increased mortality. Understanding the metastatic process will assist researchers in discovering and developing new and more effective treatment options.

CHART 64–7 Correlation of Growth Factors and Cancers

Growth Factor	Location of Cancer Cell Stimulation
Epidermal growth factor	Prostate Anal
Epidermal growth factor • Amphiregulin	Breast
Epidermal growth factor • Insulin-like growth factor	Breast Prostate Colon
Fibroblast growth factor	Breast Prostate Thyroid Bladder
Platelet-derived growth factor	Melanoma
Transforming growth factor	Colorectal

Health Promotion: Prevention, Screening, and Detection

Surviving cancer is, in part, a result of improved therapies and earlier detection. The 5-year survival rate has improved from 50% in 1975–1977 to 66% in 1996–2002 (ACS, 2007). Represented in these statistics are those people who are living 5 years after diagnosis, including those who are disease free, in remission, or under treatment with evidence of disease.

Regularly scheduled screening appointments may result in earlier detection of cancers of the breast, colon, rectum, cervix, prostate, testis, oral cavity, and skin. Earlier detection allows for diagnosis at an early stage of tumor development, which may lead to a more positive outcome for the patient (Gullatte & Otto, 2001). In 1999, the American Cancer Society set goals that would significantly lower cancer incidence and mortality rates and improve quality of life of cancer survivors by 2015 (see the National Guidelines box). One example of efforts aimed at accomplishing these goals is the collaborative work with the American Heart Association and American Diabetes Association called "Everyday Choices for a Healthier Life." These three organizations are examining tobacco use, obesity, physical inactivity, and underutilization of effective screening tests.

Nurses are becoming more involved with cancer detection and screening programs, however, assisting individuals in selecting the appropriate cancer prevention and detection options can only be done once the nurse understands the principles of each (Mahon, 2000).

Nurses play a crucial role in educating the public about cancer prevention, risk factors, and early detection. By teaching members of our society strategies to prevent cancer, how to reduce the risk of developing a malignancy, and the important tests used for early detection when the disease is easier to treat, nurses may begin to reduce the fear associated with cancer that is often portrayed in the media. It is unknown whether individuals will consider adapting behaviors and practices with ongoing health education. Influencing factors include perceived susceptibility, cost of behavior changes, and the actual health message delivered (Erickson, 2003).

Barriers exist that prevent the success of cancer screening programs. Those that are associated with health care providers

NATIONAL GUIDELINES 2015 American Cancer Society (ACS) Goals and Objectives for 2015

Goals

Age-adjusted mortality rates reduced by 50%.

Age-adjusted incidence rates reduced by 25%.

Measurable improvement in the quality of life from the time of diagnosis through the balance of life.

Objectives

Proportion of adults who use tobacco products reduced to 12%.

Proportion of youth who use tobacco products reduced to 10%.

Proportion of persons who follow the ACS guidelines for consumption of fruits and vegetables increased to 75%.

Proportion of adults who follow the ACS guidelines for appropriate level of physical activity increased to 90%.

Proportion of youth who follow the ACS guidelines for appropriate level of physical activity increased to 60%.

Proportion of school districts that provide school health education increased to 50%.

Proportion of all persons who use at least two or more protective measures to reduce the risk of skin cancer increased to 75%.

Proportion of women (ages 40 or older) who have ACS recommended breast screening increased to 90%.

Proportion of persons (ages 50 or older) who have ACS recommended colorectal screening increased to 75%.

Proportion of men (ages 50 or older) who follow ACS recommended guidelines for prostate cancer increased to 90%.

include the lack of time and expertise needed to integrate inclusive cancer screening programs. Those barriers experienced by patients include lack of transportation, poor financial status, or no support to access the screening programs. Our health care system struggles with the lack of resources to support a comprehensive screening program. Diverse populations are experiencing additional barriers to cancer screening programs. Access to screening programs is less common for those who are poor or less educated, those for whom English is a second language, and for certain minority groups. Creating and implementing cancer screening programs mandates the nurse to be open to a variety of issues that may impact the program's success.

The U.S. Department of Health and Human Services' *Healthy People 2010* objectives discuss goals related to increasing the quality of life, increasing the number of healthy years, and to eliminating health inequalities (see the National Guidelines box). Cancer is identified as the third area of focus out of 28. The overall goal for cancer care is to reduce the number of cases along with the disability, illness, and death associated with the disease. Suggestions for reaching these reductions include (1) smoking cessation, (2) diet modification, (3) early detection via screening programs, and (4) current cancer treatment options. To impact the morbidity and mortality associated with cancer, early diagnosis and treatment are pivotal.

Definitions

To develop sound cancer prevention and early detection programs, an understanding of the terminology used is essential. With this knowledge, nurses can assist individuals in making appropriate choices of cancer prevention and early detection strategies.

Cancer Screening

Cancer screening is the use of tests to discover cancer in someone who does not have signs or symptoms of the cancer (Mahon, 2000). An analogy would be the use of cheesecloth when straining a sauce during the preparation of a gourmet meal. The cheesecloth catches solid pieces of ingredients used to flavor the sauce but possibly undesirable to eat. These solid pieces are similar to signs of possible cancer that need to be evaluated carefully before being considered innocent or useful. A positive cancer-screening test does not indicate a definitive diagnosis of cancer; rather, it indicates that more testing needs to be done. The term *early detection* is used interchangeably with *cancer screening*.

Cancer Prevention

Cancer prevention consists of three levels. Fist, primary prevention refers to preventing diseases via immunizations and avoidance of known carcinogens. This form of prevention reduces the risk of developing cancer (e.g., educating youth regarding effects of tobacco use) with the understanding that there is no guarantee an individual will not show signs of malignancy in the future. Secondary prevention involves early detection and treatment of subclinical disease in those individuals without signs or symptoms of a malignancy. Examples include Pap smears and mammograms. Tertiary prevention is the management of a disease with the hopes to prevent progression, recurrence, or complications. Examples include monitoring for recurrence with the use of tumor markers and detecting second primary tumors early in those who are long-term survivors.

Screened Individual

Individuals who are undergoing cancer screening tests are not considered patients. Only when an abnormal screening test is discovered is the individual considered a patient. An easily understood example is that of women who routinely undergo clinical breast exams and mammography. Women with negative results are not labeled as patients. Wellness is the main focus of all cancer prevention levels.

Target Population

The target population identifies those individuals who possess characteristics that make them suitable for screening. Oncology experts believe the following characteristics are typical of a target population: (1) gender, (2) family history, (3) presence of risk factors, (4) ethnicity, and (5) age (Clark & Reintgen, 1996).

Being aware of these characteristics is important so the nurse can accurately educate the patient and family regarding the importance of recommended screening tests. Having an appreciation of the cultural beliefs and practices that influence a person's decision to be screened for cancer will give the nurse insight into how the individual approaches her health and wellness. The Cultural Considerations box (p. 2070) illustrates a few examples of how culture affects health practices.

Risk Factors

Assessing cancer risk is a common and crucial thread in all three levels of cancer prevention. Making appropriate screening

---

NATIONAL GUIDELINES *Healthy People 2010* **Cancer Goals**

GOAL: Reduce the number of new cancer cases as well as the illness, disability, and death caused by cancer.

Overall cancer deaths	Melanoma deaths
Lung cancer deaths	Sun exposure and skin cancer
Breast cancer deaths	Provider counseling about cancer prevention
Cervical cancer deaths	Pap tests
Colorectal cancer deaths	Colorectal cancer screening
Oropharyngeal cancer deaths	Mammograms
Prostate cancer deaths	Statewide cancer registries
	Cancer survival

Source: U.S. Department of Health and Human Services. (2000). *Healthy people 2010: Understanding and improving health.* Retrieved February 5, 2008, from http://www.healthypeople.gov.

CULTURAL CONSIDERATIONS Related to Health Practices

Temporal orientation (perceived importance of detecting health problems early) and perceptions of internal control and physical space in both African American and Caucasian women affect incidence of screening for mammograms. African American women have an increased sense of fatalism related to breast cancer. This belief about the inevitability of dying from the disease prevents them from undergoing regular mammogram screening (Russell, Perkins, Zollinger, & Champion, 2006).

The leading cause of death among Korean persons is cancer, with breast cancer being the most common cancer in Korean women (7.1% of all cancer diagnoses). The mortality rate for females has increased by 280% since 1983. Due to these staggering numbers, mammogram screening is recommended beginning at the age of 30 for Korean women, which is a decade earlier than for American women (Ham, 2006).

Greek women experience an increase in fatigue while undergoing adjuvant radiotherapy for breast cancer. Initially, the patient's fatigue is felt to be minimal but gradually increases to the point where the patient has significant changes in their health status. One known intervention to reduce the effect of fatigue is to participate in exercise activities. Because exercise is not a common behavior of many Greek women, nurses are asked to explore culturally appropriate alternatives (Lavdaniti et al., 2006).

Breast and cervical cancer screening is low among Chinese, Japanese, and Vietnamese American women. Given that Asian Americans have a high rate of liver and stomach cancer combined with infrequent screening practices for breast and cervical cancer, nurses have an opportunity to assist with health promotion and education (Lee-Lin & Menon, 2005).

Filipino women typically demonstrate avoidance when dealing with a cancer diagnosis. Several factors improve their willingness to participate in screening activities: supportive family members, suggestions from familiar health care providers, health insurance, and personal attributes (physical symptoms, family history, past diagnosis, and health literacy) (Wu & Bancroft, 2006).

RISK FACTORS for Cancer

Exogenous	Endogenous
Drugs and chemicals: Environmental and occupational factors influence the number of chemicals and drugs proven to be carcinogenic.	*Age:* Incidence increases with age.
Lifestyle behaviors: Tobacco is most deadly carcinogen.	*Genetic predisposition:* Occasional genetic link.
Nutrition: Diets low in fiber and high in fat.	*Hormones:* Influence the process of carcinogenesis.
Sexual activity: Women who engage in sex with multiple partners and begin relations early in life have increased risk of cancer.	*Immune dysfunction:* Immunocompetence is essential for identification of antigens (malignant cells).
Alcohol: Large consumptions of ethyl alcohol are linked to certain cancers of the head and neck.	
Radiation: Ionizing and ultraviolet radiation can cause cancer; the effects of EMFs, if any, are unknown.	
Viruses: Several different cancers have been linked to viruses.	
Psychosocial: Stress and the relationship to neoplasms are still being investigated.	

factors include age, genetic background (see the Genetic Considerations box), and immune competence. Exogenous factors include tobacco, radiation, diet, chemicals, and infections.

Age

As we age, the likelihood of developing a malignancy increases. Up to age 39 the probability is between 1% and 2%, and from ages 40 to 61 the chance increases to 8% to 9%. Men have demonstrated a higher incidence of cancer (33%) between the ages of 60 and 79 as compared to women (22%) (Erickson, 2003). The lifetime incidence of cancer is higher for men (43.39%) than for women (38.25%). Because of breast cancer, a woman's chance of developing cancer by the age of 60 is slightly increased (Jemail, Thomas, Murrey, & Thun, 2002).

The concept of aging as it relates to cancer development can be incorporated into the discussion of other risk factors, but to truly understand the impact of the aging process attention must be given to the theories that attempt to explain the changes. First, over time we are repeatedly exposed to a cumulative increase in the number of carcinogens, which increases the chance of a malignancy emerging. Next, cells that have aged may be less tolerant of the genetic abnormalities that occur with cancer and unable to initiate damage repair. Finally, as we age our immune system does not function as efficiently, thus opening the door for abnormal cellular growth associated with cancer formation.

Hormones

Cancer of the brain, breast, endometrium, and prostate occur in target tissues, or those that are hormone responsive. Hormones have not been proven to have a direct carcinogenic effect.

recommendations is extremely difficult if there has not been an accurate and complete assessment of cancer risk (Mahon, 2000). A screening program should incorporate an education portion that includes a discussion of the seven warning signs of cancer (Chart 64–8).

Nurses are responsible for assessing patients for the seven warning signs of cancer and alerting the health care provider or encouraging the patient to seek medical evaluation.
Ongoing education about the seven warning signs of cancer is essential in order for patients and their families to understand the importance of recognizing unusual symptoms and seeking early medical attention.

The presence of interacting cellular, genetic, immunologic, and environmental forces, potentially creating malignancy, is frequently referred to as *risk factors.* Risk factors are categorized according to whether they originate from outside the host (exogenous) or within the host (endogenous) (see the Risk Factors box). Both endogenous and exogenous risk factors cause cancer by damaging the genes that regulate normal cell growth or by perpetuating the growth of existing abnormal cells. Endogenous

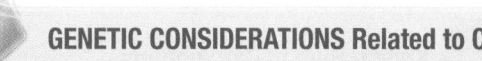

| CHART 64–8 | Seven Warning Signs of Cancer |

C: hange in bowel or bladder habits

A: sore that does not heal

U: nusual bleeding or discharge from any body orifice

T: hickening or a lump in the breast or elsewhere

I: ndigestion or difficulty swallowing

O: bvious change in a wart or mole

N: agging cough or hoarseness

Rather, they support carcinogenesis by preparing target tissues so they are ripe for the carcinogen insult, by permitting the carcinogenesis to continue, or by modifying the growth of an established tumor. The duration in which tissue has been exposed to a hormone may influence carcinogenesis.

Immune Dysfunction

Our immune system is an intricate network of surveillance that controls the proliferation of potential cancer cells. The immune system screens the human body for these cells and activates forces to eliminate them before a tumor can be developed. Humoral factors are those that produce antibodies in the battle against cancer cells, where cellular factors include sensitized lymphocytes and macrophages. Frequently, cancer cells contain antigens that are different from the person's own antigens, which results in destruction by the immune system. The normal immune system is able to detect and destroy approximately 10 million cancer cells at one time. Tumors that replicate faster than the rate at which the normal immune system can work will continue to grow unrestrained. Today's diagnostic capabilities require a mass measuring only 1 cm in diameter for recognition. Regrettably, a tumor that is 1 cm contains at least 1 billion cells.

Most often cancers occur in individuals whose immune system is impaired due to malnutrition, chronic disease, advancing age, and stress. People with immunodeficiency states are more susceptible to developing malignancy than those whose immune system is intact. See Chapter 60 🔗 for a discussion of the immune system.

Drugs and Chemicals

Millions of chemicals have been registered with the Chemical Abstracts Service and more than 50,000 are predicted to be used regularly in business and industry. Despite acknowledging the importance of monitoring and regulating these substances, less than 1,000 chemicals or exposures have been examined to determine their role in the development of cancer (Stellman & Stellman, 1996). Great effort has been given to publishing and organizing data on cancer risk attributed to chemical carcinogens.

Chemical carcinogens are those that contain compounds or elements that alter DNA. An awareness of the relationship between chemical exposures and disease began as early as the 1700s (Pfeifer, 2001). Men employed as chimney sweeps developed an increased incidence of scrotal cancer, likely due to the continued exposure to coal burned as fuel. Although it is easy to attribute chemical carcinogens to occupational exposure, the vastness of

GENETIC CONSIDERATIONS Related to Cancer

The understanding of the link between genetics and the development of cancer is partly due to the worldwide Human Genome Project, which began in 1990. The project sought to locate, map, and sequence more than 100,000 genes that make up the human genome. Little has been linked to genetic factors (10%), but significant incidence is demonstrated among racial groups. The highest prevalence and mortality rates are seen in African Americans. Hispanics and Asian/Pacific Islanders have a 40% lower incidence, and American Indians a 50% lower incidence than African Americans.

There are three main categories of genetic cancer. First, inherited cancer syndromes typically are autosomal dominant and possess many different genes that regulate cell growth and gene repair. Diagnosis is usually done at an early age and the syndromes frequently are associated with multiple primary tumors. An example is the breast/ovarian cancer syndrome in which chromosome 17 houses a mutated tumor suppressor gene (BRCA1). The risk of developing breast and ovarian cancer is significantly increased if a female carries BRCA1. Next, a group of genetic disorders that are typically nonmalignant have been known to predispose a person to developing malignancy. For example, the presence of ataxia-telangiectasia can be correlated to the development of breast cancer and leukemia. Finally, familial "clustering" occurs when there is an increased prevalence of cancer than would be expected statistically; however, the specific genetic factors have yet to be determined. Breast cancer is the most common example of a cancer that appears to cluster in families.

Sources: American Cancer Society. (ND). *Risk factors.* Retrieved on September 22, 2008, from http://www.cancer.org/downloads/AA/CancerAtlas02.pdf; Erickson, J. (2003). Cancer. In W. Phipps, F. Monahan, J. Sands, J. Marek, & M. Neighbors (Eds.), *Medical–surgical nursing health and illness perspectives* (7th ed.). St. Louis: Mosby.

---

environmental exposures must be understood. The Occupational Safety and Health Act of 1970 authorized the Occupational Safety and Health Administration (OSHA) to impose restrictions on the amount of exposure to known carcinogens. Threshold limit values (TLVs), or the maximum allowable exposure, are difficult to determine because identification of carcinogens in the environment and workplace is very time consuming (Erickson, 2003). The U.S. Department of Health and Human Services publishes a list of known human carcinogens biannually. The *Tenth Report*, published in 2002, identifies new or changed carcinogens from previous reports. The *Tenth Report* list of carcinogens known to affect humans is shown in Chart 64–9 (p. 2072).

Drugs used for therapeutic purposes also have been known to be carcinogenic. In the 1970s the agent diethylstilbestrol (DES) was administered to prevent spontaneous abortion, but a link was discovered between its use and vaginal cancer. The relationship between cancer and drug therapy is dynamic, as can be seen in the carcinogenic history of oral contraceptives. Initially, birth control pills were identified to have a carcinogenic potential for breast cancer. Recently, it has been determined they have a protective effect against ovarian and endometrial malignancies (Erickson, 2003).

Agents used to combat cancer have also been known to increase the risk of causing secondary malignancies. Years after receiving agents such as chlorambucil and cyclophosphamide, people have experienced a notable increased likelihood of developing leukemia. Individuals who require immunosuppressive

CHART 64–9	**Known Human Carcinogens**
Aflatoxins	Estrogens
Alcohol	Ethylene oxide
4-Aminobiphenyl	Lead chromate
Analgesic mixtures with phenacetin	Melphalan
Arsenic compounds	Methoxsalen with ultraviolet A therapy
Asbestos	Mineral oils
Azathioprine	Mustard gas
Benzene	2-Naphthylamine
Benzidine	Nickel compounds
Beryllium and its compounds	Radon
1,3-Butadiene	Silica
1,4-Butanediol dimenthylsulfonate (Myleran)	Smokeless tobacco
Cadmium and its compounds	Solar radiation, exposure to sunlamps and sun beds
CCNU, methyl	Soots
Chlorambucil	Strong inorganic acid mists with sulfuric acid
Chloromethyl methyl ether	Tamoxifen
Chromium hexavalent compounds	2,3,7,8-Tetrachlorodibenzo-*p*-dioxin (dioxin)
Coal tar	Thiotepa
Coke over emissions	Thorium dioxide
Cyclophosphamide	Tobacco smoking
Cyclosporin A	Vinyl chloride
Diethylstilbestrol	Ultraviolet radiation, broad-spectrum UV radiation
Dyes metabolized to benzidine	Wood dust
Environmental tobacco smoke	
Erionite	

Source: Adapted from U.S. Department of Health and Human Services, Public Health Service, National Toxicology Program. (2002, December). *Report on carcinogens* (10th ed.). Washington, DC: Author.

agents to prevent transplant rejection are known to demonstrate higher incidence of the development of secondary malignancies (Antin, 2002).

Tobacco

Cigarettes are responsible for killing more Americans (440,000 predicted in 2006) than alcohol, vehicle crashes, suicide, AIDS, homicide, and illegal drugs combined (ACS, 2006a). Tobacco from pipes, cigars, cigarettes, and second-hand smoke has been reported to cause 87% of all lung cancers. Current reports indicate lung cancer as the leading cause of cancer-related deaths in both males and females and accounts for 13% of new cancer diagnoses (ACS, 2006a). Exposure to tobacco through passive means (exhaled smoke) appears to increase the risk of lung cancer in nonsmokers who live with smokers (Gullatte & Otto, 2001).

The carcinogenic effect of tobacco is demonstrated in several different agents that promote the growth of malignant cells over time. There appears to be a direct relationship between the numbers of years smoking, number of cigarettes smoked per day, and the age when smoking began. Choosing to indulge in smokeless tobacco is not without risk. The use of chewing tobacco places a person at higher risk for developing head and neck cancer. By eliminating smoking as a lifestyle choice, a person can live longer and reduce the risk of lung cancer by approximately 50% (Erickson, 2003). Other health-related issues are positively affected by smoking cessation, such as a reduction in the risk of cardiac disease and complications from pregnancy.

Approximately one in every five Americans is addicted to tobacco products (ACS, 2006a). According to the ACS, there has been a dramatic increase in successful quit attempts in those who seek assistance with cessation. However, with inadequate health insurance coverage and the cost of treatment programs, many individuals remain addicted to tobacco products. In 2007, the Centers for Disease Control and Prevention's (CDC's) *Morbidity and Mortality Weekly Report* concluded that there continues to be a need for states to assist with funding of smoking cessation and counseling programs (CDC, 2007). Thirty-four states provide some type of coverage to assist those who wish to quit using tobacco products, including over-the-counter (OTC) products, prescription drugs, or counseling services. Seventeen states offer no tobacco treatment coverage services.

The past several years have seen a unique twist on the effect of publicity associated with tobacco use. Smoking cessation campaigns across the country have been more common in the last few years. *Healthy People 2010* objectives for tobacco use are listed in the National Guidelines box. The ACS has identified school health education as critical to the effort to assist young people in developing and maintaining health practices that reduce cancer risk. Litigation by lung cancer victims or families against tobacco companies has increased the attention paid to a behavior our society appears to be identifying as dangerous and life threatening.

Nutrition and Physical Activity

Approximately 20% of all cancer deaths are attributed to nutrition and physical activity factors (ACS, 2007). The association between food and the incidence of cancer is becoming more known and publicized. The link between high-fat foods and an increase in the development of colon, breast, and prostate cancers has been known for almost a decade (Holmes et al., 1999). The most current relationship between body weight and the development of cancer identifies an alarming rate of obesity and overweight among adolescents 12 to 19 years of age (ACS, 2007). In the past 20 years, the prevalence of obesity in African American girls has tripled. Overall, two-thirds of U.S. adults (20 years and older) are overweight or obese.

Diets high in fiber content appear to provide a protection against colon cancer. The exact mechanism of protection remains unknown, but fiber is known to reduce the concentration of fecal bile acids, dilute colon contents, and decrease colon transit time, which is helpful in decreasing the time colonic contents are exposed to carcinogens (Ziegler, Devesa, & Fravmeni, 1991). Rich sources of dietary fiber include fruits, vegetables, legumes, and whole-grain breads and cereals. Foods with vitamins C and D, beta-carotene, and selenium seem to repair cellular damage due to free radicals, which are known to destroy the genetic makeup of cells, thus creating a cellular environment that resists malignancy development.

Maintaining regular physical activity reduces the risk of deaths due to coronary heart disease and also reduces the risk of

NATIONAL GUIDELINES *Healthy People 2010* Tobacco Use Goals

Reduce coronary heart disease deaths.

Reduce lung cancer deaths.

Reduce chronic obstructive pulmonary disease (COPD) deaths.

Reduce cigarette smoking in those 18 years of age and older.

Reduce cigarette smoking in males.

Reduce cigarette smoking in females.

Reduce smoking initiation.

Increase smoking cessation attempts.

Increase smoking cessation during pregnancy.

Reduce children's exposure to smoke at home.

Reduce smokeless tobacco use in males 12 to 17 years of age.

Reduce smokeless tobacco use in males 18 to 24 years of age.

Increase number of school districts providing tobacco-free environments.

Increase number of school districts providing antismoking education in middle school.

Increase number of school districts providing antismoking education in high school.

Increase number of worksite policies banning smoking.

Increase number of states with clean indoor air laws for private workplaces, public workplaces, restaurants, public transportation, hospitals, day care centers, and grocery stores.

Increase number of states with youth tobacco laws.

Increase number of states with plans to reduce tobacco use.

Reduce oral cancer deaths in males 45 to 74 years of age.

Reduce oral cancer deaths in females 45 to 74 years of age.

Reduce stroke deaths.

Change the average age at first use of cigarettes, alcohol, and marijuana at 12 to 17 years of age.

Reduce the use of alcohol in the past month in those 12 to 20 years of age.

Reduce the use of marijuana in the past month in those 12 to 25 years of age.

Reduce the use of cocaine in the past month in those 12 to 25 years of age.

Increase high school seniors' perception of disapproval of heavy alcohol use, occasional marijuana use, cocaine use once or twice, and smoking one or more packs of cigarettes a day.

Increase high school seniors' perception of harm due to heavy alcohol use, regular marijuana use, cocaine use once or twice, smoking one or more packs of cigarettes a day, and use of smokeless tobacco regularly.

Increase tobacco excise tax for cigarettes and smokeless tobacco.

Increase number of states with preemptive clean indoor air laws.

Increase number of states with cigarette vending machine laws.

Source: Adapted from U.S. Department of Health and Human Services. (2000). *Healthy people 2010: Understanding and improving health.* Retrieved February 5, 2008, from http://www.healthypeople.gov.

---

stroke, colon cancer, breast cancer, diabetes, and hypertension (Erye et al., 2004). By keeping physically fit, people tend to control their weight better, which reduces the risk of developing cancer related to excess weight. The ACS publishes guidelines for nutrition and physical activity for cancer prevention that aims at assisting in identifying important healthy behaviors (ACS, 2004).

Sexual Activity

Never before has the correlation between sexual practices and cancer risk been more obvious and concerning. The development of genital cancer is strongly related to sexual practices. In fact, studies have identified an association between sexual activities and AIDS and cancers of the cervix, vagina, and vulva (Gullatte & Otto, 2001). Sexually transmitted infections (STIs), beginning sexual activity at a young age, multiple sexual partners, and high-risk sexual partners all have been implicated in the development of cervical cancer. Viruses, such as herpes simplex virus (HSV) and human papillomavirus (HPV), have also been known to increase the incidence of cervical cancer.

Penile cancer, although rare (1 in 100,000 men), is more common in men who are uncircumcised, infected with HPV, and use tobacco. It is speculated that males who are uncircumcised may be prone to more incidence of smegma, which leads to irritation and inflammation of the penis (ACS, 2006b). Exposure to HPV from multiple sexual partners, sexual intercourse at a young age, and unprotected sex will make a person more likely to develop malignancy. Smoking creates harmful chemicals that are absorbed into the bloodstream and disseminated throughout the body, resulting in damage to the DNA of cells. Cells of penile tissue are not immune to this destructive process. Chapter 50 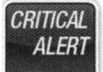 presents a more detailed discussion of this rare but devastating cancer.

> **CRITICAL ALERT** *It is important to assess patients for risky lifestyle practices that increase their chances of developing cancer. Educating patients and their families about smoking cessation, limiting the use of alcohol, and safe sexual practices as they relate to the incidence of developing cancer (and other diseases) may contribute to changing or preventing undesirable lifestyle practices.*

Alcohol

Ethyl alcohol consumption is known to cause cancers of the oral cavity, pharynx, larynx, esophagus, liver, and breast (ACS, 2008a). Men should refrain from consuming more than 2 drinks per day and women 1 drink per day. When combined with tobacco use, alcohol is the leading etiologic factor in developing squamous cell carcinoma of the oral cavity, larynx, and esophagus. It is quite possible alcohol may behave like a co-carcinogen or have a synergistic effect with tobacco (Sigler & Schuring, 1993).

Radiation

Waves and particles of energy, or **radiation**, are known to cause cancer. Radiation has the potential to be a complete carcinogen, thus possessing both initiating and promoting properties. Ionizing radiation has electromagnetic waves that are powerful enough to remove electrons from molecules, thereby weakening the cell by altering its biochemical behavior. Radiation causes mutation of the cell's DNA, which can weaken the cells' defense against a carcinogen or cause cell death. These changes take only seconds, whereas the development of a malignancy may take years. The degree of damage to the cells is related to the dose of radiation received.

Historically, radiation exposure was first recognized after the invention of the x-ray in 1895. People working with x-ray generators were noted to have skin reactions resulting in a skin sore, which led to the first radiation-caused cancer diagnosed in 1902 (ACS, 2003). In 1911, leukemia was first reported among radiation workers.

Ionizing radiation includes x-rays, gamma rays, cosmic rays, and radioactive materials such as alpha particles, beta rays, and protons. Even though each form of radiation has different energy levels, all are capable of causing cellular destruction. The three types of ionizing radiation are natural background radiation, nonmedical synthetic radiation, and medical radiation. Natural background radiation is present in cosmic rays from the solar system and radioactive elements found in the soil. This form of radiation is the major contributor to worldwide radiation exposure. Nonmedical synthetic radiation was created by aboveground nuclear weapons testing usually done prior to 1962 and some commercial and occupational sources. Medical radiation is found in diagnostic x-rays and radiation therapy. Radiation therapy is used to treat certain forms of cancer and involves the use of doses that are thousand of times higher than those of x-rays (ACS, 2003). The amount of exposure during radiographic examinations depends on the machine used and the capability of the technician. Although the amount of exposure to the average hospital nurse who may assist a patient during an x-ray is slight, nurses need to step away from the area close to the x-ray machine (Erickson, 2003).

Exposure to high-dose ionizing radiation can cause a variety of problems including leukemia, bone cancer, leukopenia, and damage to the reproductive cells. The thyroid gland and the bone marrow are most sensitive to radiation, whereas the kidney, ovaries, and bladder are least sensitive. Health care employees whose job involves exposure to radiation must wear film badges. These badges absorb radiation on a photographic film and are developed each month to determine the amount of cumulative radiation exposure. Individuals who are pregnant are usually not assigned to departments that require exposure to radiation due to the susceptibility of the fetus to the negative effects of radiation. Ultraviolet radiation is comprised of electromagnetic waves that are less powerful, but still able to produce carcinogenic effects (Erickson, 2003).

Ultraviolet radiation is present in the form of sunlight and industrial sources such as welding arcs and germicidal lights (Pfeifer, 2001). Despite the vast amount of documentation linking sunlight to the development of skin cancer, many still place the importance of tanned skin above the consequence of having cancer. Ultraviolet light is able to penetrate tissues, which results in the skin being potentially defenseless. Those at greatest risk for acquiring either basal or squamous cell cancer of the skin and melanoma are fair-skinned Caucasian individuals and outdoor workers.

Detecting skin cancers early is pivotal to decreasing mortality rates and the extent of surgical interventions. Areas such as the nose, cheek, and ears are common sites for basal and squamous cell cancers to appear. These tumors appear as waxlike, pale nodules or scaly, reddened patches. Melanomas have the appearance

of moles and erupt anywhere throughout the body. The uniqueness of melanomas is that they have the tendency to change color, shape, and size while forming localized ulcerations that may bleed. Pictures that assist the reader in better understanding how these tumors appear are found in Chapter 66 🔗. Chart 64–10 lists the warning signs of melanoma.

Radon, a colorless and odorless radioactive gas, is released when uranium decays. It is contained in soil and rocks and is located in underground mines and basements. The carcinogenic risk of radon is approximately the same as that associated with breathing second-hand smoke. According to the ACS, most radon-induced cancers are lung cancers and occur more commonly in those who smoke.

Electromagnetic fields (EMFs) are low-frequency energy fields associated with electrical power lines, household appliances, and facilities that produce electricity. Society continues to focus on the cancer risk associated with EMFs despite no scientific evidence to support the concern. Literature has identified no form of electromagnetic energy at frequency levels below that of ionizing radiation and ultraviolet radiation as a cause of cancer (Heath, 1996).

Viruses

Only recently has the relationship between viruses and cancer development in humans been established. Viruses are believed to infect the host DNA, which changes the portion that regulates normal cell proliferation and repair (proto-oncogene). In addition, cell mutation is initiated (Groenwald et al., 1997). Cancer is produced only after a prolonged incubation or latency period (usually years), which makes it very difficult for researchers to connect a viral exposure with a specific cancer (Malin, 2005). Viral carcinogens can be either slow acting or fast acting, but all are tissue specific. Slow-acting viral carcinogens include adenoviruses and herpes viruses. Human T-cell leukemia/lymphoma virus (HTLV) is an example of a fast-acting carcinogen. People are particularly vulnerable to viral carcinogens as they advance in age or their immune system begins to function inadequately.

The relationship between certain viruses and the incidence of cancer has been demonstrated in the literature. The hepatitis B virus has been linked to malignancy of the liver, and the Epstein–Barr virus (EBV) has been known to increase the incidence of developing nasopharyngeal cancer. The human papillomavirus is associated with cancer of the genitalia, especially in women. It is strongly suspected that HPV is also linked to cervical cancer. Kaposi's sarcoma is known to be caused by the presence of the cytomegaloviruses (CMVs), which are frequently seen in patients with the HIV virus.

Psychosocial

How a person's state of mind affects his immune and hormonal systems has not yet been determined, nor is it easily explained.

CHART 64–10	Warning Signs of Melanoma: The "ABCD Rule"
A is for	asymmetry
B is for	border irregularity
C is for	change in color or pigmentation
D is for	diameter greater than 6 mm

It has been suggested that stressors such as death of a loved one, life changes, and personality variables may have a relationship in the development of cancer. Most reports of the link between the mind and cancer are subjective and more research needs to be done to explain how the relationship works (Erickson, 2003).

Diagnosing Cancer

Cancer treatment decisions are based on the results of accurate diagnostic findings performed by a multidisciplinary team. A person with cancer typically undergoes a battery of tests to determine the location, extent, and tumor type of the malignancy. Diagnostic modalities need to be individualized to the patient and may include a thorough history and physical, appropriate imaging tests, invasive procedures, laboratory studies, and pathology examination of tissue or blood. New diagnostic techniques have provided the opportunity for the development of sophisticated plans of treatment that positively affect patient survival. Once diagnosis is confirmed, further diagnostic studies may be necessary to stage the cancer, which will define an appropriate treatment plan.

The nurse needs to prepare the patient and family for each test and procedure. This includes explaining the rationale for the test and any preparation the patient needs to complete prior to the diagnostic procedure. Preparation examples include eliminating food and drink for a certain number of hours prior to testing (NPO) and administering bowel-cleansing agents such as enemas or oral preparations. Providing emotional support during a time when patients and families experience a tremendous amount of anxiety is crucial. Even though the term *cancer* may not have been discussed with the patient, he and family members may be experiencing an overriding fear about what the possibilities may be. During the diagnostic phase, it is critical for the nurse to offer ongoing support to patients and their families.

History and Physical

Early detection of cancer can be done through screening and is how some patients discover their diagnosis. In contrast, other patients end up in the health care provider's office after noticing unusual symptoms or after a wellness examination during which suspicious symptoms were detected (Alexander, 2001). Nurses perform a comprehensive health history and systems assessment that can be combined with the history and physical done by the health care provider. The information obtained by both disciplines provides a holistic view of the patient's health condition and needs. Listening to patients report their health history provides a perfect opportunity to identify risk factors pertinent to the individual and may elevate the suspicion of malignancy. Further diagnostic evaluation will be determined based on the assessment findings that identify potential diagnoses. The Diagnostic Tests box illustrates the tests done to evaluate for cancer, monitor treatment success and effects, and determine recurrence of disease.

DIAGNOSTIC TESTS for Cancer

Test	Expected Abnormality	Rationale for Abnormality
Serum chemistries and liver function tests	Elevated/lowered sodium, elevated potassium, elevated creatinine and BUN, elevated liver function tests.	Assess for abnormality of liver, kidney, or bone related to malignancy or treatment.
Complete blood count (CBC)	Lowered WBC, platelets, RBC, Hgb, and Hct. May have elevated WBC with leukemia.	Assess for treatment toxicity or bone marrow function.
Hemocult test	Positive (blue color) result indicates need for further diagnostic studies.	Assess for presence of blood in stool for screening purposes.
Bone marrow biopsy (aspiration)	Abnormal numbers, size, and shape of WBC, RBC, and megakaryocytes.	Assess for hematologic abnormalities.
Pap smear	Abnormal-appearing cervical cells, precancerous or malignant.	Assess for premalignant changes and cervical cancer.
Urine protein immunoelectrophoresis	Increased levels of heavy-chain M proteins (Bence-Jones proteins).	Assess urine protein and immunoglobulin levels seen in multiple myeloma.
Serum protein immunoelectrophoresis	Increased levels of heavy-chain M proteins.	Assess serum protein and immunoglobulin levels seen in multiple myeloma.
Urine catecholamines	Increased levels of epinephrine, norepinephrine, metanephrine, and vanillylmandelic.	Assess for neuroblastoma and pheochromocytoma.
CA125 (antigen, tumor marker)	Elevated in ovarian cancer and nonmalignant conditions that cause inflammation of the pleura (e.g., endometriosis, PID, pancreatitis).	Assess response to treatment in ovarian, pancreatic, breast, colon, lung, and liver cancer.
CA19-9 (tumor marker)	Elevated in colorectal, pancreatic, stomach, and bile duct cancer.	Assess response to treatment in pancreatic, colorectal, and gastric cancer.
CA27-29 (tumor marker)	Elevated in breast cancer. Occasionally elevated in cancer of the colon, stomach, kidney, lung, pancreas, ovary, uterus, and liver.	Assess response to treatment of breast cancer.

(continued)

Test	Expected Abnormality	Rationale for Abnormality
CA72-4 (tumor marker)	Elevated in ovarian, colorectal, and gastric cancer.	Assess response to treatment of ovarian, colorectal, and gastric cancer.
PSA (prostate-specific antigen, tumor marker)	Elevated in prostate cancer and benign prostate enlargement.	Assess response to treatment of prostate cancer. Also used for screening at-risk persons.
CEA (carcinoembryonic antigen, tumor marker)	Elevated in breast, colorectal, and lung cancer.	Assess response to treatment of breast, colorectal, and lung cancer.
HCG (human chorionic gonadotropin, tumor marker)	Elevated in germ cell cancers (ovarian and testicular) and pregnancy.	Assess response to treatment of testicular and certain ovarian cancer.
AFP (α-fetoprotein)	Elevated in liver and germ cell cancer, benign liver disease, and pregnancy.	Assess response to treatment of testicular, liver, and certain ovarian cancers.
Lactate dehydrogenase (LDH)	Elevated in most cancers.	Most helpful in monitoring treatment effect.
Neuron-specific enolase (NSE)	Elevated in lung, thyroid, kidney, testicle, and pancreatic cancer, neuroblastoma, Wilms' tumor, and melanoma.	Most helpful in small cell lung cancer (SCLC) and neuroblastoma to assess response to treatment.
IMAGING STUDIES		Least invasive diagnostic studies performed first.
Radiographic: x-ray, CT scan, mammogram, barium swallow/enema, IVP	Detects abnormal masses in abdomen, chest, pelvis, and breast.	Performed during initial diagnostic work-up and to monitor effectiveness of treatment.
Ultrasonic studies	Used to detect tumors in peritoneal space, pelvis, abdomen, prostate, and breast.	Echoes of high-frequency sound waves to visualize internal structures are helpful in distinguishing between benign cysts and malignancies. Some techniques involve inserting an ultrasound wand into a body cavity (e.g., rectum) to visualize surrounding organs (e.g., prostate).
Magnetic resonance imaging (MRI)	Detects tumors in the brain, chest, and abdomen.	Use of a magnetic field and radio-frequency waves to align hydrogen nuclei in tissues.
Nuclear medicine scans	Common organs evaluated include the brain, thyroid, and liver.	Radioactive isotopes are injected or ingested and then traced to the tissues where the isotope is attracted. Monoclonal antibodies are occasionally used to tag antigens known to be associated with malignancies. Organs with disease frequently show signs of increased or abnormal uptake of the material.
Positron emission tomography (PET)		Study glucose metabolism in body tissues and differentiate the rates of tissue metabolism. Images are obtained by detection of positron emissions from radionuclides. Tumors have more rapid rates of glycolysis compared to the tissue of origin. Gamma camera tomography maps structures and identifies malignancies.
INVASIVE DIAGNOSTIC STUDIES		
Pathology		Cells are obtained via surgical incision, biopsy, or cytologic examination techniques. These cells are examined for malignancy and, if positive, graded, which assists the health care provider in prescribing an appropriate plan of care.
Biopsy	Detects presence of abnormal tissue cells obtained from site of suspicious growth.	See above.
Endoscopy		Hollow metal tubes equipped with a light are used to visualize body cavities for diagnostic and therapeutic purposes. These tubes, known as scopes, are instruments named for the body area they visualize. Direct visualization provides the health care provider the opportunity to examine the anatomic location and obtain samples of tissue or secretions that can be used to diagnose malignancy.

Sources: Akhurst, T., & Larson, S. (1999). Position emission tomography imaging of colorectal cancer. *Seminar in Oncology, 577*(26); Alexander, J. (2001). Diagnosis and staging. In S. Otto (Ed.), *Oncology nursing* (4th ed.). St. Louis: Mosby; Erickson, J. (2003). Cancer. In W. Phipps, F. Monahan, J. Sands, J. Marek, & M. Neighbors (Eds.), *Medical–surgical nursing health and illness perspectives* (7th ed.). St. Louis: Mosby; Fischbach, F., & Dunning, M. (Eds.). (2006). *Nurses' quick reference to common laboratory and diagnostic tests.* Philadelphia: Lippincott Williams & Wilkins; Omerod, K. (2005). Diagnostic evaluation, classification, and staging. In C. H. Yarbro, M. H. Frogge, & M. Goodman (Eds.), *Cancer nursing: Principles and practice* (6th ed.). Sudbury, MA: Jones and Bartlett.

CHART 64–11   Endoscopic Instruments and Their Anatomic Use

Instrument	Anatomic Location
Bronchoscope	Bronchus
Gastroscope	Stomach
Colonoscope	Colon
Proctoscope	Anus and sigmoid colon
Laparoscope	Abdominal structures: • Liver • Diaphragm • Peritoneum • Gastrointestinal structures • Genitourinary structures • Gynecologic structures

Chart 64–11 explains the names of instruments and associated anatomic locations used during endoscopic procedures. In addition, the reader should review Chapter 59 ⊘, which discusses the use of monoclonal antibodies in the patient with an altered immune system, and Chapter 49 ⊘, which explains the Pap smear in more detail.

Commonly Occurring Cancers

Nurses who care for patients with cancer are asked to develop a knowledge base that is extensive and ever changing. Discoveries that change the diagnosis, treatment, and prognosis of this devastating disease are continuous. This fluidity demands that nurses continue to quest for more information to assist them in developing their nursing practice. Chart 64–12 (p. 2078) presents general information, clinical findings, diagnostic techniques, prognosis, and treatment modalities to assist the nurse in gaining a better understanding of the commonly occurring cancers. A more in-depth discussion of the current diagnostic studies and treatment modalities is presented later in this chapter.

Cancers of the Hematopoietic and Lymphatic Systems

Cancers of the hematopoietic and lymphatic systems are very complex and challenging disorders that are full of potentially life-threatening complications. Developing an understanding of the immune and hematologic system will assist the nurse in becoming confident when caring for patients with these disorders. Cancers occurring in the hematopoietic and lymphatic system include leukemia, lymphoma, and multiple myeloma. Due to the rare incidence of multiple myeloma, this discussion will concentrate on leukemia and lymphoma. Leukemias are classified as either acute (aggressive with severe symptoms) or chronic (slowly progressing with fewer symptoms).

The type of leukemia depends on the stem cell line affected: lymphoid or myeloid. The factors that control the organized differentiation and maturation of blood cells are absent. This disorganization results in the halting of maturation of specific cell lines, allowing for immature cells to replicate and accumulate in the bone marrow. When too many immature cells accumulate in the bone marrow, other normal cell lines are prevented from maturing and developing. Patients with leukemia will experience symptoms associated with "crowding out" of the bone marrow cells, such as platelets, red blood cells (RBCs), and white blood cells (WBCs). This will be recognized when the nurse assesses the laboratory data for a reduction in platelets, RBCs (including hemoglobin and hematocrit), and WBCs. It is important to remember that a patient with leukemia may have an abnormally high WBC count, however, the effectiveness of these cells is compromised. Nurses must be aware that patients with leukemia will have multiple laboratory abnormalities and their assessment should evaluate for signs of infection, bleeding, and anemia.

Cancers of the lymphatic system (**lymphomas**) involve organs and tissues such as the lymph nodes, spleen, thymus, bone marrow, blood, and lymph. From interstitial fluid comes lymph, which flows through lymphatic vessels and eventually into the circulatory system via the thoracic duct. Particulate is filtered through lymph nodes located in a variety of places throughout the human body. Lymphocytes originate in the bone marrow and develop into several different types of mature lymphocytes. The cells are susceptible to malignant transformation at any point during maturation and differentiation. Malignant lymphomas are grouped according to the characteristics of the lymphocyte, such as Hodgkin's disease and non-Hodgkin's disease (see Chart 64–12, p. 2078).

Cancer Treatment Modalities

Multiple treatment modalities are available to patients diagnosed with cancer. Each modality has certain risks, side effects, and chances for success. The nurse can assist the patient and family in obtaining information regarding treatment options so they are able to make an informed decision about their plan of care.

Surgery

Surgical approaches to cancer have existed for centuries. In 1809 Ephraim MacDowell demonstrated modern surgical approaches when he excised a 22-pound ovarian tumor from a woman who lived an additional 30 years. He performed 12 more ovarian resections which became a hallmark in the advancement of elective surgery for cancer (Hill, 1979). Surgical efforts built on the work of surgeons like MacDowell, but in the 1950s it was noted the mortality rates associated with radical procedures were not improving. The evidence was mounting to evaluate the benefit of surgery alone as treatment for all tumors.

Surgeries in patients with cancer are performed to establish a diagnosis and treat the disease. A histologic diagnosis is pivotal in establishing a definitive diagnosis of cancer along with a staging of the tumor, which determines the extent and type of the cancer. Understanding the diagnosis will allow the health care team to design a plan of care unique to each individual and his or her disease. Diagnosis is accomplished by obtaining tissue samples from an incisional biopsy, excisional biopsy, needle biopsy, or endoscopy. A **biopsy** is a procedure in which a portion of tissue is examined for the presence of abnormal cells. The technique used depends on the tumor's location, size, and growth characteristics.

| CHART 64–12 | **Commonly Occurring Cancers** | | | | |

Cancer	Clinical Findings	Diagnostic Technique	Prognosis	Treatment
Breast	Noninvasive (carcinoma *in situ*): confined to the ducts and or lobules Invasive (infiltrating): cancerous cells penetrate tissue outside of ducts (80%) or lobules (10%) Inflammatory: swelling, erythema, and invasion of dermal lymphatics.	Mass: hard, irregular, nontender Thick breast or axilla Nipple discharge Nipple retraction or inversion Dimpling or puckering of skin Changes in size, shape, and texture of breast	Mammogram Self-breast exam Biopsy, fine-needle or core needle Pathology testing: cytologic or histologic	Tumor size and presence of lymph node(s) have important role in predicting survival. Presence of hormone receptors has negative impact on survival. There remain percentages (20%) of those who develop recurrence.	Surgery: • Lumpectomy • Mastectomy • Breast reconstruction Radiotherapy: external beam Chemotherapy: • Adjuvant • Hormonal High-dose chemotherapy with transplantation (for advanced cancer)
Colon and rectum	Majority are adenocarcinomas Rectum: 40–50% Descending sigmoid colon: 20–35% Cecum and ascending colon: 16% Transverse colon: 8%	Changes in bowel habits Blood in stool Flatulence Indigestion Weight loss Fatigue	Barium enema Colonoscopy	Distant metastases negatively impact survival. Once treatment is completed, follow-up treatment is advised (physical examination, colonoscopy, CEA levels).	Surgery: colon resection with temporary or permanent colostomy Chemotherapy Radiotherapy for involvement in the perineum or viscera
Prostate	Adenocarcinomas (95%) Endogenous hormones and environmental factors may be causative factors	*Early:* Painful urination Frequency Hematuria *Late:* Pain (bone, joint, back) Fatigue Weight loss	Prostate-specific antigen (PSA) Direct rectal examination (DRE) Transrectal ultrasound (TRUS) Biopsy	Transitional zone involvement is less aggressive. Metastatic disease negatively impacts survival.	Surgery: radical prostatectomy Radiotherapy: external beam or brachytherapy Cryotherapy Chemotherapy Expectant management ("watchful waiting")
Brain and CNS • Brain • Spinal cord	Intracerebral: brain, neuroglia, neurons, cells of blood vessels of connective tissue Extracerebral: meningiomas, acoustic nerve, pituitary, and pineal gland Classification between benign and malignant is not differentiated because surgical accessibility dictates prognosis Astrocytoma (>50%) Glioblastoma multiforme (20%)	*Early:* Headache Seizures Nausea Vomiting *Late:* Impaired cognitive skills Short-term memory loss Difficulty with speech Sensory and motor defects Visual changes Personality changes Loss of sphincter control	Complete physical and neurologic examination MRI PET Single-photon emission computed tomography (SPECT) Magnetic resonance spectroscopy (MRS) Biopsy	Prognosis is poor related to accessibility difficulties. Glioblastomas have poorest prognosis.	Surgery with or without placement of wafers impregnated with chemotherapy Radiotherapy: intraoperative with radioactive seeds Intraoperative Hyperthermia Radiosurgery Stereotactic therapy: gamma knife, linear accelerator, and heavy beam particles Photodynamic therapy Chemotherapy

| CHART 64–12 | **Commonly Occurring Cancers—*Continued*** |

Cancer	Clinical Findings	Diagnostic Technique	Prognosis	Treatment
Lung	Small cell anaplastic carcinoma Non–small cell: squamous cell carcinoma Adenocarcinomas Large cell anaplastic carcinoma Mixed cell types	Change in cough Chest pain Respiratory ailments not treated with antibiotics Dyspnea Wheezing Hemoptysis Weight loss Fatigue Dysphagia	History and physical examination Chest x-ray (anterior, posterior, lateral) CAT scan MRI CBC with differential Platelet count Chemistry panel Bronchoscopy	Prognosis for 5-year survival after surgical resection is best in patients who have carcinoma *in situ.* Prognosis for 5-year survival after surgical resection is worst for those patients who have cancer that has invaded the lymph nodes or other distant organs or structures.	Surgery Laser therapy (used for relief of complications associated with endobronchial lesions) Radiotherapy: external beam Brachytherapy Chemotherapy
Multiple myeloma	Most common in African Americans, males, age 70 Malignancy of B cell Immunodeficiency due to depressed antibody-mediated immunity	Findings are related to excess of Bence-Jones proteins. Infections: • Pneumonia • Urinary Tract Infection (UTI) • Systemic Skeletal: • Pain worse with movement • Hypercalcemia • Pathologic fractures • Vertebral collapse Renal failure: • Proteinuria • Obstructed distal and proximal tubules • Hyperuricemia Blood/bone marrow dysfunction: • Anemia • Hyperviscosity • Coagulation disorders Neurologic: • Spinal cord compression • Peripheral neuropathy	1. Serum electrophoresis to determine Bence-Jones proteins. 2. Serum immunoglobulin electrophoresis 3. Bone marrow biopsy: increase in abnormal, atypical, immature B cells. 4. Radiographic: osteolytic lesions in bones	1. Incurable, sometimes treatable 2. 1/3 patients do not respond to therapy and die within weeks of diagnosis.	Chemotherapy Corticosteroids Immunotherapy Bone marrow transplant (autologous) Radiation therapy

(continued)

| CHART 64–12 | **Commonly Occurring Cancers—*Continued*** |

Cancer		Clinical Findings	Diagnostic Technique	Prognosis	Treatment
Leukemias					
Acute lymphocytic leukemia (ALL)	Most common in children *Etiology:* Radiation Chemicals Drugs Viruses	*Anemia:* Malaise Fatigue *Neutropenia:* Fever Bone pain Thrombocytopenia: Bleeding Bruising CNS involvement (10%) due to meningeal infiltrates	Peripheral blood smear: • CBC with differential • Bone marrow biopsy	Complete remission: 80–90% Cure: 30–40% Children achieve cure at rate of 60–85%	Chemotherapy: • Induction therapy to achieve remission • CNS treatment if needed • Postremission therapy Bone marrow or stem cell transplantation
Acute myeloid leukemia (AML)	*Etiology:* Radiation Chemicals Drugs Viruses Certain genetic disorders increase incidence of acquiring AML	*Anemia:* Malaise Fatigue *Neutropenia:* Fever Bone pain *Thrombocytopenia:* Bleeding Bruising Anemia is usually present when health care provider sees patient for the first time. Recurrent infections not resolved with antibiotics.	Peripheral blood smear: • CBC with differential • Bone marrow biopsy	Patients over 70 years of age are intolerant of induction therapy. WBCs > 100,000/mm^3 related to increased mortality during first week of therapy.	Chemotherapy: • Induction therapy to achieve remission • Postremission therapy Biotherapy: monoclonal antibodies Bone marrow or stem cell transplantation
Chronic lymphocytic leukemia	B-cell lymphocytes undergo a malignant transformation Few cases are of the T-cell line	25% of patients are symptom free Evidence of disease found on routine examination and laboratory work Frequent respiratory and skin infections	Peripheral blood smear: • CBC with differential • Flow cytometry to evaluate immunophenotype of cells • Bone marrow biopsy (for prognostic information)	Survival is often determined by the severity of disease when diagnosed. No pattern of predictability of disease course.	Often difficult to decide when to begin treatment. Treatment is aimed at alleviating symptoms, not cure. Treatment for complications: • Antibiotics • IV immunoglobulin Chemotherapy Splenectomy or radiotherapy (rarely done) Bone marrow or stem cell transplantation

CHART 64–12	**Commonly Occurring Cancers—*Continued***				
Cancer		**Clinical Findings**	**Diagnostic Technique**	**Prognosis**	**Treatment**
Chronic myeloid leukemia	Myeloproliferative disorder Presence of Philadelphia chromosome Three stages: 1. Chronic 2. Accelerated 3. Blast crisis	*Chronic Phase:* Fatigue Pallor Dyspnea Anemia Night sweats Weight loss Sternum pain *Accelerated:* Chronic symptoms recur after treatment. *Blast crisis:* Aggressive and terminal phase that includes above symptoms with increased severity.	Peripheral blood smear: • CBC with differential • Bone marrow biopsy	Chronic phase lasts 3–4 years. Once blast crisis occurs, median survival is <6 months. 85% of patients die during blast crisis due to complications such as bleeding and infections.	Chemotherapy Biotherapy: interferon Bone marrow or stem cell transplantation
Lymphomas					
Non-Hodgkin's disease	Similar to Hodgkin's disease, but without the Reed-Sternberg cell *Etiology:* Infections Autoimmune disorders Environmental factors Typically female, Caucasian, and approximately 55 years of age	Painless lymphadenopathy (cervical or supraclavicular region) As disease worsens swelling and obstructive symptoms occur	Lymph node biopsy Chest x-ray Bone marrow biopsy Serum blood analysis: • Hepatitis B and C • CBC with differential • Chemistries	Indolent disease has most favorable prognosis. Highly aggressive disease requires high-dose therapy that increases risk of life-threatening complications.	Chemotherapy Biotherapy: monoclonal antibodies Bone marrow or stem cell transplantation
Hodgkin's disease	Presence of Reed-Sternberg cells *Etiology:* Viral exposure Epstein–Barr virus most common Woodworking Most common in young adults, age 26–31 years Occasional peak in prevalence at age 60 years	Lymphadenopathy: Cervical Supraclavicular Mediastinal Fever Night sweats Weight loss	Lymph node biopsy Staging laparotomy if receiving radiation Chest x-ray Bone marrow biopsy Serum blood analysis: • CBC with differential • Chemistries	If early stage, 20-year survival is near 80%. If receiving salvage therapy after relapse, survival is 80–95%.	Radiotherapy Chemotherapy Bone marrow or stem cell transplantation

Sources: Crane-Okada, R. (2001). Breast cancers. In S. Otto (Ed.), *Oncology nursing* (4th ed.). St. Louis: Mosby; Daniel, B. (2001). Malignant lymphoma. In S. Otto (Ed.), *Oncology nursing* (4th ed.). St. Louis: Mosby; Iovino, C., & Camacho, L. (2003). Acute myeloid leukemia: A classification and treatment update. *Clinical Journal of Oncology Nursing, 7*(5), 535–540; O'Rourke, M. (2001). Genitourinary cancers. In S. Otto (Ed.), *Oncology nursing* (4th ed.). St. Louis: Mosby; Ososki, R. (2001). Leukemia. In S. Otto (Ed.), *Oncology nursing* (4th ed.). St. Louis: Mosby.

Typically, a biopsy is done first followed by a period of approximately 2 weeks before additional surgery. This delay allows the patient and family time to adjust to the diagnosis and begin making decisions about treatment options (Pfeifer, 2001).

Primary Treatment

Primary treatment for cancer involves the removal of a malignancy and a margin of surrounding normal tissue. Reducing the amount of total body tumor burden and improving the survival rate is the goal of this surgical approach. Wide excision (en bloc dissection) approaches are used to remove the primary tumor along with regional lymph nodes, intervening lymphatic channels, and involved adjacent structures. Examples of wide excisions are radical neck dissection, radical mastectomy, and abdominal-perineal resection. Local excision is used for skin cancers and consists of the simple excision of a tumor and a small amount of surrounding tissue.

It is important for the patient to be taught the benefits and burdens of undergoing surgery for cancer. The patient and family need to be taught the potential complications, the expected length of recovery, and the degree of disfigurement associated with the procedure. In addition, the benefits of other treatment options, such as chemotherapy, radiotherapy, and conservative surgical approaches need to be presented. When given this type of information, patients can make informed decisions about the type of treatment they wish to receive.

Adjuvant Treatment

Adjuvant treatment is aimed at improving outcomes by providing additional cancer therapy. Cytoreductive therapy (debulking) is surgery used to remove a large tumor burden, which will reduce the quantity of cancer cells. Then other therapies are used on the remaining tumor burden. Occasionally, prophylactic surgery will be performed on diseased organs that have a high incidence of developing a subsequent cancer. An example of this adjuvant approach is a colectomy for a patient with ulcerative colitis because the incidence of developing colon cancer when ulcerative colitis is present is about 40% (DeVita, Hellman, & Rosenberg, 1997).

Salvage Treatment

Salvage treatment is an extensive surgical approach that is used when there has been local recurrence since prior surgery. An example of this technique would be mastectomy after breast conservation done by lumpectomy and radiation therapy (Szopa, 2005).

Palliative Treatment

Palliative surgery is a useful therapy for those patients with advanced disease. The purpose of the surgical procedure is to reduce disease or treatment-related symptoms, when a cure is not possible. Prior to recommending palliative surgery, the surgeon will consider the rate of tumor growth, the projected life expectancy, and the expected treatment outcomes. The goals of palliative surgery are to alleviate suffering and prevent the occurrence of symptoms if the patient decides to forego other treatments.

Combination Treatment

Combination treatment involves several different treatment modalities to minimize the change in the patient's appearance and functional ability. By using chemotherapy, radiation therapy, or biotherapy during the preoperative, intraoperative, or postoperative periods, tumor resectability will improve as well as the overall treatment outcomes (Pfeifer, 2001).

Reconstructive Treatment

Patients who undergo surgical procedures that leave a deficit in function or appearance may be candidates for reconstructive surgery. The goal of this treatment option is to improve function or obtain a more acceptable cosmetic effect. Discussions about possible reconstructive surgery will occur prior to the primary surgery so the patient can make a fully informed decision. Cancers of the breast, skin, and head and neck are the most commonly indicated for reconstructive surgery (Rokita, 2004).

Preoperative Care

Planning care for the surgical oncology patient should be considered comparable to the nursing care expected for any surgical patient. However, an awareness of the problems and complications exclusive to those diagnosed with cancer is essential for the nurse to provide compassionate holistic care. The health care team will assess the patient's emotional and physical status in order to predict how well she will tolerate surgery and the recovery period. The patient's functional status may be evaluated using several validated scales, such as the Karnofsky Performance Scale, Eastern Cooperative Oncology Group (ECOG) scale, and the World Health Organization scale. Chart 64–13 explains the scoring indicators included in the Karnofsky Performance Scale, which is one of the hallmark tools used in cancer treatment. These scales reflect the ability of the patient to care for self and carry out normal activities. This information will assist the health care team in developing a comprehensive plan that will maximize the patient's recovery capability (Erickson, 2003).

The presence of other medical problems, such as heart disease or lung disease, may complicate postoperative recovery. In addition, physical debilitation due to advanced disease or type of symptoms present requires special attention. Improving the patient's physical well-being includes treating symptoms such as pain, malnutrition, fatigue, insomnia, depression, and headaches. Managing a patient's symptoms in the preoperative period will affect the patient's response to surgery and recovery. The nurse needs to identify comorbidities and other symptoms prior to surgery and individualize the postoperative plan of care as needed.

During the preoperative period the nurse focuses on assessment and intervention by becoming more familiar with the patient's knowledge and adaptation of his situation. By knowing the purpose of the surgical procedure, the nurse can better understand behaviors exhibited by the patient. For instance, behaviors demonstrated by patients who recently were diagnosed with cancer are different than those by patients with metastatic disease who undergo palliative surgery for relief from spinal cord compression. The nurse must understand what kind of surgery will be performed in order to plan for appropriate preoperative preparation such as bowel preparation or nutritional support. Knowing which procedure will be performed will also alert the nurse to the location and size of the surgical incision and what type of indwelling device may be needed during the postopera-

CHART 64–13	**Karnofsky Performance Scale**
100	Normal; no complaints; no evidence of disease
90	Ability to carry on normal activity; minor signs or symptoms of disease
80	Normal activity with effort; some signs or symptoms of disease
70	Ability to care for self; inability to do normal activity or do active work
60	Occasional assistance necessary, but ability to care for most needs
50	Considerable assistance and frequent medical care necessary
40	Disabled; special care and assistance necessary
30	Severely disabled; indication for hospitalization although death not imminent
20	Very sick; hospitalization necessary; active supportive treatment necessary
10	Moribund; fatal processes progressing rapidly
0	Death

tive period. With this information the nurse can engage each patient in teaching that is customized for her or his situation.

The diagnosis of cancer has a dramatic impact on patients and their loved ones. Many feel hopeless, powerless, and depressed. Oftentimes patients will be apprehensive about the upcoming surgery, demonstrating anger, anxiety, and perhaps panic (Pfeifer, 2001). The nurse develops a therapeutic relationship with the patient and her significant others by maintaining an open, honest, and caring approach to communication. A trusting relationship can assist the patient in maintaining a realistic sense of hope.

Age and physical status play an important role in accepting the diagnosis of cancer and postoperative recovery and rehabilitation (Erickson, 2003). Those in early adulthood to middle age typically have more physical endurance; however, they may have many emotional concerns. This is the most productive time in their lives for their careers, education, child rearing, and sexual activity. Some may fear a loss of job security, financial independence, and reproductive ability, role adjustment, and disfigurement. Elderly patients may fear burdening their family, both physically and financially, and suddenly are faced with recognizing their own mortality. It is important for nurses to use a caring approach when listening to the patients' concerns and support them with information and resources appropriate for their needs.

◼ Nursing Management

Postoperative nursing care of the oncology patient varies according to the type of cancer, type of surgery performed, previous therapies, and comorbidities. A comprehensive plan of care encompasses the patient's physical and psychological needs and can be found in Chapters 25 ☞ to 27 ☞ where care of the surgical patient is presented. The oncology nurse knows that patients have unique medical and emotional needs that require an understanding of the overall management of the cancer patient.

Radiation Therapy

Radiation therapy is the use of ionizing rays or particles to treat cancer. More than 50% of all patients with cancer will be treated with radiation therapy during the course of their illness. The use of radiation in the treatment of disease, or radiotherapy, has been used since 1895 when radium, radioactivity, and x-rays were discovered. In 1898 the first successful radiation therapy treatment for cancer was used. Unfortunately, a host of complications occurred due to the delivery of large doses in a single treatment. During the early and mid-1900s, scientists studied the effects of radiation on tissues. Results of these studies were responsible for the inception of fractionalization, or dividing of the total dose of radiation into several small doses. During the 1950s several discoveries aided the advancement of radiotherapy including the use of vacuum tubes, which allow for higher energy to be delivered to deeper tissues, and linear accelerators, which provided deeper penetration with less scatter to normal tissues (Iwamoto, 2001).

Radiation is a localized treatment that can be used alone or in combination with other treatments such as chemotherapy and surgery. Prescribing radiation therapy in the treatment of cancer serves several purpose: to make a curative attempt to eradicate the disease; to control metastatic activity, allowing the patient relief of symptoms; to prevent microscopic disease asso-

ciated with specific primary tumors; and to improve a patient's quality of life by relieving or reducing symptoms seen with advanced cancer (Sitton, 1997). Chart 64–14 illustrates the symptoms of advancing disease targeted by radiation therapy.

Ionizing radiation destroys the ability of cancer cells to multiply and grow. This is accomplished by delivering energy potent enough to break the chemical bonds in molecules, leading to cellular damage or death. The nucleolus of a cell is penetrated by the ionizing rays or particles and interacts with its water content to form hydroxyl (free) radicals. The cells' DNA is then damaged, which results in the disruption of chromosomal strands. Cellular death depends on the ability of the chromosomal damage to repair itself (Iwamoto, 2001).

Therapeutic radiation includes electromagnetic and particulate. Electromagnetic sources are x-rays and gamma rays (energy rays without mass). Machines are the delivery mechanism for x-rays, whereas radioactive materials are responsible for emitting gamma rays. Electromagnetic sources penetrate deep into tissue layers before releasing their energy and causing cellular damage. Particulate radiation contains mass, which prohibits it from penetrating into deep tissue, but delivers energy into the cells close to the surface (Erickson, 2003).

The health care provider will determine the radiosensitivity of the cancer cells, or target tissue, prior to prescribing the course of radiation therapy. *Radiosensitivity* is the measurement of potential

CHART 64–14	Symptoms Relieved by Radiation Therapy	
Symptom	**Etiology**

Hemorrhage
  Fatigue
  Weakness
  Pallor
  Lowered blood pressure (BP),
  elevated heart rate (HR)
	Primary tumor

Pain	Bone metastasis

Vascular obstruction
  Alterations in pulses
  Cool, discolored skin
	Primary tumor

Gastrointestinal obstruction
  Abdominal pain
  Nausea and vomiting
  Absent bowel sounds
	Primary tumor

Kidney and ureter obstruction
  Flank pain
  Lower abdominal pain
  Difficulty urinating
	Primary tumor

Tracheal obstruction
  Dyspnea
  Reduced oxygen saturation
	Primary tumor

Spinal cord compression
  Numbness, tingling
  Difficulty moving
	Primary tumor

Neurological symptoms
  Headache
  Seizures
  Impaired speech
	Brain metastasis

susceptibly of cells to ionizing radiation and how rapidly destruction will occur. Rapidly dividing cells, either benign or malignant, are more sensitive (e.g., mucosa). Those cells that are slow to divide or nondividing are radioresistant (e.g., muscle or neurons) (Sitton, 2005). Because all body tissue has a degree of radiosensitivity, nurses caring for patients with cancer must understand how various tumor types will respond to radiation therapy. Chart 64–15 reviews the effect of radiotherapy on specific tumor types.

A health care provider trained in radiation oncology (radiation oncologist) will determine the maximum radiation dose possible that will not harm normal tissues surrounding the target area. Various factors are considered when calculating the dose for any given patient: patient's age, tumor size and stage, evidence of metastasis, and overall prognosis if radiation therapy is used as part of the treatment plan (Erickson, 2003). The total dose of radiation is divided into smaller doses (fractionalization) and delivered daily for several weeks. The rationale for the fractionalization is to maximize malignant cell kill, which occurs when cells enter mitosis, and to minimize damage to surrounding tissue and allow for repair to begin.

Administration of Radiation Therapy

Radiotherapy can be delivered in several ways. Teletherapy (external-beam) requires the use of a machine at a predetermined distance from the body. Brachytherapy (internal radiation) is performed using a sealed radioactive source placed in or near the malignancy. Occasionally, radioactive materials are delivered systemically via the oral or intravenous route. The most common cancer treated in this manner is that of the thyroid.

External Radiation Therapy

External radiation therapy can be used alone or with surgery to better enhance the patient's chance of survival. Typically, when radiation is used alone, it is done so with the intent of achieving cure. Cancers that are known to respond to radiation alone include cancer of the prostate, uterus, cervix, pelvis, skin, oral cavity, and early Hodgkin's disease. When radiation is used in combination with surgery, the goal is either cure or palliation of distressing symptoms. Those cancers that can be cured with both therapies include head and neck, breast, uterus, bladder, testes, and bone.

For patients who undergo both surgery and radiation and are anticipating a curative outcome, administration of radiation may be done before or after surgery. Advantages of preoperative radiation include decreasing tumor size, which increases the likelihood of successful removal of the entire mass, obliteration of cancerous cells beyond the surgical field, and elimination of lymph nodes where malignancy could form. Nurses who care for patients receiving preoperative radiation therapy will need to pay special attention to wound healing because there will be delays in normal tissue repair due to the side effects of the therapy.

The delivery of postoperative radiation therapy is intended for the elimination of residual tumor and subclinical disease. Although higher doses may be delivered, treatment is delayed until postoperative wound healing is finished.

Prior to any radiation therapy beginning, the patient will need to undergo the treatment-planning phase. The purpose of this phase of treatment is to ensure the best way to deliver the treatments needed. After a radiation oncologist examines the patient, localization of the tumor will begin. A simulator machine is used to localize the tumor, and the anatomic area that will receive radiation (port) will be marked with either ink or permanent tattoos. Figure 64–3 ■ illustrates a simulator used in the treatment-planning phase and a linear accelerator, which delivers the radiotherapy. Precise identification of the area that will receive the radiation is critical to minimize tissue damage. Other examination procedures, such as computed tomography (CT) scans, magnetic resonance imaging (MRI), intravenous pyelogram (IVP) or barium enemas, may be used depending on the area being treated (Iwamoto, 2001).

Ports, or their position, may be changed on different days to ensure the delivery of safe and optimal radiation therapy. During treatment the patient may find himself in difficult and uncomfortable positions' however, immobilization is pivotal for accurate delivery of radiation. Devices to assist with immobilization or positioning may be necessary and are made specifically for each patient. Figure 64–4 ■ shows immobilizers used to assist with positioning. Certain patient populations, such as children and the elderly, may require special molds, casts, boards, or belts to help them maintain proper positioning. The nurse educates patients that the planning phase may take several hours and encourages them to request pain medication as needed to promote comfort (Erickson, 2003).

Patients receiving external radiation therapy should expect to receive treatments daily (weekends excluded) for several weeks. The actual treatment takes approximately 5 minutes; however, more time is taken to properly position the patient. For those patients receiving palliative radiotherapy, fewer treatments will be given at higher doses. Total body irradiation is delivered to those patients who have leukemia and are preparing for bone marrow transplantation due to the multiple areas that may be harboring leukemic cells.

Several unique approaches to external radiotherapy are being used for specific cancers. Chart 64–16 (p. 2086) identifies the various approaches available.

CHART 64–15	**Effect of Radiotherapy on Tumor Types**	
Tumor Type	**Effect**	**Dose**
Leukemia Lymphoma Myeloma Seminoma Dysgerminoma	Highly effective	Modest
Squamous cell of oral cavity, esophagus, cervix, vagina, bladder, skin	Moderate/highly effective	High
Vasculature and connective tissue of all tumors, astrocytomas	Moderately effective	High
Tumors of bone and cartilage, renal cell, hepatomas, pancreatic cancer, salivary gland tumors, tumors of muscle, brain, and spinal cord	Fairly ineffective	High Beyond normal tissue tolerance

Sources: Erickson, J. (2003). Cancer. In W. Phipps, F. Monahan, J. Sands, J. Marek, & M. Neighbors (Eds.), *Medical–surgical nursing health and illness perspectives* (7th ed.). St. Louis: Mosby; Iwamoto, R. (2001). Radiation therapy. In S. Otto (Ed.), *Oncology nursing* (4th ed.). St. Louis: Mosby.

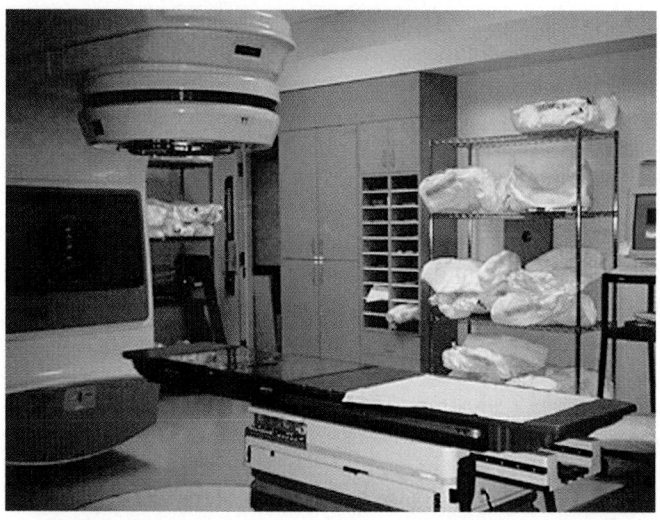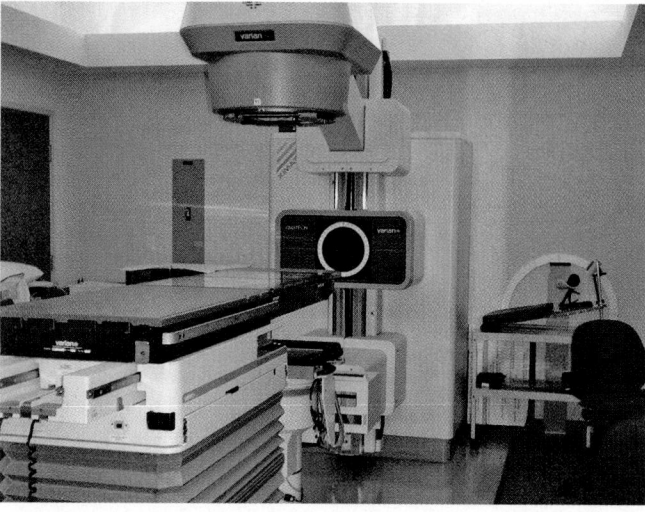

FIGURE 64–3 ■ Accelerator and simulator for radiation therapy. (Roseville Radiation Center)

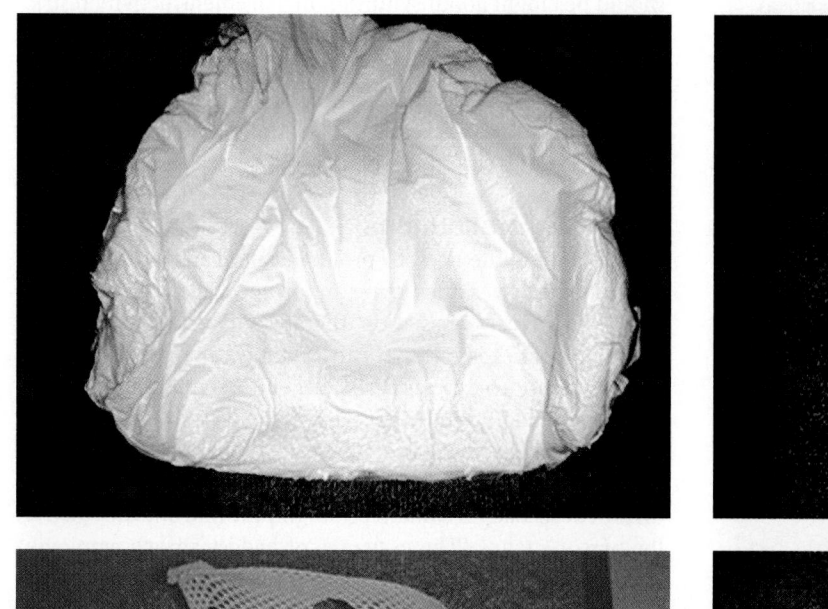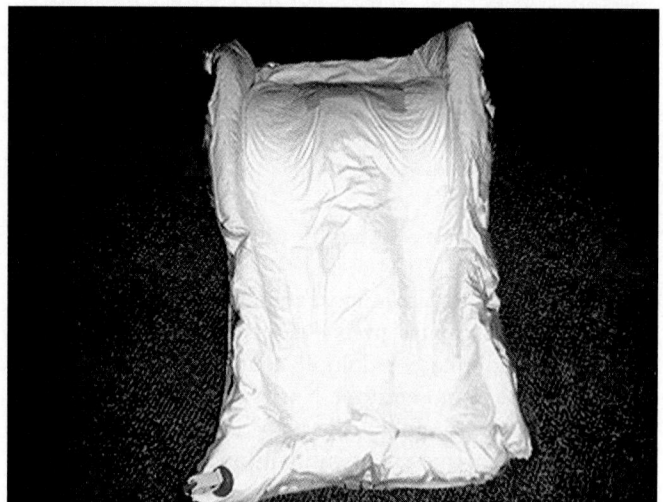

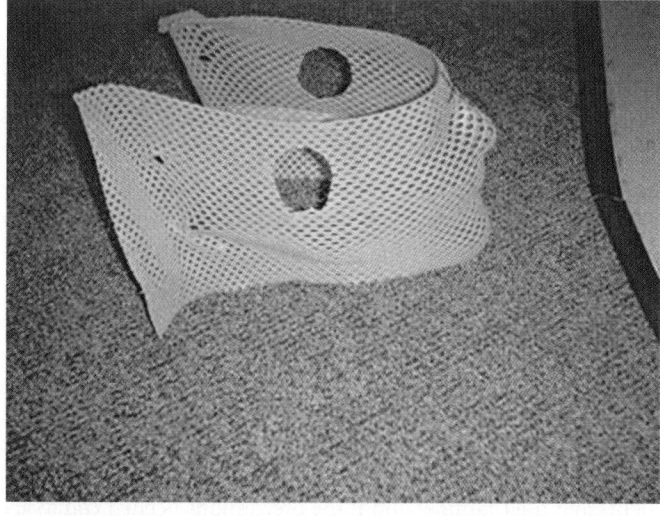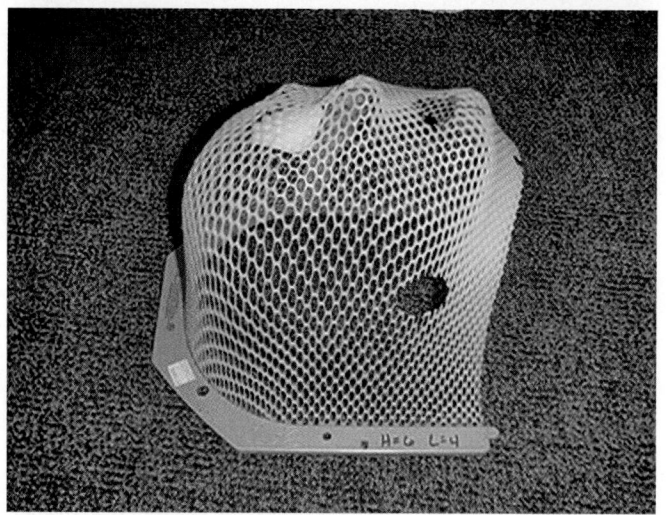

FIGURE 64–4 ■ Immobilizers for radiation therapy. (Roseville Radiation Center)

Photodynamic Therapy

An innovative approach to cancer treatment is photodynamic therapy (PDT) (Levy, 1994). Cancers of the skin, lung, esophagus, superficial bladder, and head and neck are currently the focus of this unique treatment. In addition, PDT has been used for purging bone marrow prior to autologous donor transplantation for leukemia and lymphoma (Overholt, Panjehpour, & Haydeck, 1999). PDT uses light-sensitive molecules (photosensitizers) that form oxygen radicals after exposure to light. Cellular damage or death is a

| CHART 64–16 | Unique Approaches in Radiation Therapy |

Approach	Purpose
Intraoperative radiation therapy (IORT)	Control of local recurrence by directly visualizing and treating tumors.
Radiosensitizers	Medication used to enhance the effect of radiation.
Radiopharmaceuticals	Intravenous delivery of radioactive substances to treat pain from multiple osteoblastic bony metastases.
Stereotactic external-beam irradiation	Three-dimensional beam distribution, which provides high-dose treatment for small intracranial volumes. Treatment in other body areas is currently being done.

Sources: Blomgren, H., Lax, I., Goranson, H., Kraepelien, T., Nilsson, B., Naslund, I., Svanstrom, R., Tilikidis, A., et al. (1998). Radiosurgery for tumors in the body: Clinical experience using a new method. *Journal of Radiosurgery, 1*(1); Brunner, D. (1990). Report on the Radiation Oncology Nursing Subcommittee of the American College of Radiation Task Force on Standards Development. *Oncology, 4*(80); Campbell, C., & Iwamoto, R. (1992). Intraoperative radiation therapy. *Today's OR Nurse, 14*(1); Larson, D. (1998). Stereotactic external-beam irradiation. In C. Perez & L. Brady (Eds.), *Principles and practices of radiation oncology* (3rd ed.). Philadelphia: Lippincott Williams & Wilkins; Noll, L., & Riese, N. (1997). Chemical modifiers of radiation therapy. In K. Dow et al. (Eds.), *Nursing care in radiation oncology* (2nd ed.). Philadelphia: W. B. Saunders.

result of the radicals altering the DNA, cytoplasm, and cell membrane.

Porfimer sodium is the most commonly used photosensitizer. A laser treatment is given 48 hours after administration of the agent. Tumor masses require 48 hours to acquire a sufficient quantity of the photosensitizer. Nurses caring for those receiving PDT must be careful to educate patients and their families regarding the extreme photosensitivity and precautions necessary to prevent skin damage from sources such as examination lights and sunlight.

Internal Radiation Therapy

Brachytherapy (internal radiation therapy) uses sealed radioactive sources (implants) that are placed into or on a tumor. The term *brachytherapy* means "near treatment." This approach allows for a high concentration of radiation to be delivered to a specific site in a short period of time. The major disadvantages include the need to access the tumor by invasive procedures and the skill required of personnel administering this unique therapy (Hoskin & Coyle, 2005). Brachytherapy may also be used in combination with external radiation therapy to enhance the overall effect on the tumor. A high dose of radiation can be delivered to a small malignant mass while very little is delivered to adjacent tissues. The therapy can be received over a period of several days using a low dose rate (LDR) or over a few minutes using a high dose rate (HDR) (Flynn, 2005). Cancers of the prostate, brain, tongue, lips, lung, breast, esophagus, vagina, cervix, endometrium, rectum, and bladder may be treated with brachytherapy.

Placement of implants into the body cavity or structure is done via special applicators. Radioactive material contained in applicators such as ribbons, wires, seeds, capsules, needles, or tubes is encapsulated to prevent body fluids from becoming contaminated. Placement occurs away from the nursing unit, in the operating room, treatment room, or radiation department. After placement of the applicator, the patient returns to her hospital room and the radioactive isotope is inserted. This approach, called afterloading, is used to minimize the unnecessary risk of exposure of hospital employees to the radioactive material. The implant is left in place anywhere from a few hours to several days, during which the patient remains hospitalized.

The technique of HDR brachytherapy is another approach used to deliver radiotherapy. It involves positioning of the applicator into the cavity of a tumor, then loading the applicator with pellets or tubes with a wire by remote control. The applicator is unloaded at the end of the treatment, which lasts minutes. Figure 64–5 ■ illustrates the use of the applicator as used for prostate cancer. The HDR technique is done weekly for several weeks and does not necessitate hospitalization (Erickson, 2003).

Educating patients and their families about the implant, including the process, effects, and strategies to manage its effects, is an important role of the nurse. Prior to implantation, patients should be taught about symptom management, activity restrictions while the implant is in place, what causes current symptoms, and how the implant could change those symptoms. Once the implant is in place, patients need to be informed about when to notify the health care provider and potential side effects of the treatment along with the customary management.

Radiation Precautions

Understanding the need to protect health care providers from the risk of injury is of extreme importance when discussing patients who receive radiation therapy. Adhering to radiation safety guidelines is necessary to minimize the risk of occupational radiation exposure. Placement of internal radiation sources should be done in specially designed rooms that prevent leakage of radioactivity. Individuals working in these areas must wear a personal monitor (e.g., film badge) to measure their radiation dose. Badges contain photographic film and are worn on the person's trunk. The exchange of badges among employees should never be done because it prevents accurate determination of the amount of exposure to a specific individual. Each month badges are read for the amount of exposure and a new one is provided to the employee (Sitton, 2005).

Planning is extremely important when caring for a patient who receives radiation sources that emit gamma rays because they expose the caregivers over a varying period of time. Providers need to limit time exposed to these patients to prevent injury to themselves and others. Danger of exposure is reduced as the radioactive substance reaches its half-life or the point in time when half of the radioactivity has dissolved. Essential considerations in minimizing exposure to radiation are time, distance, and shielding. Chart 64–17 (p. 2088) explains these principles and related nursing responsibilities.

Nursing personnel also have the opportunity to educate patients and their families about the precautions needed and to alleviate fears associated with radiation therapy. Nurses need to recognize their own fears or concerns so they can develop and implement an effective plan of care for their patients. Attending in-services or educational sessions about radiation safety practices combined with a skills laboratory for practicing appropriate patient care activities will help clarify misconceptions and assist the nurse in providing comprehensive quality care. National and

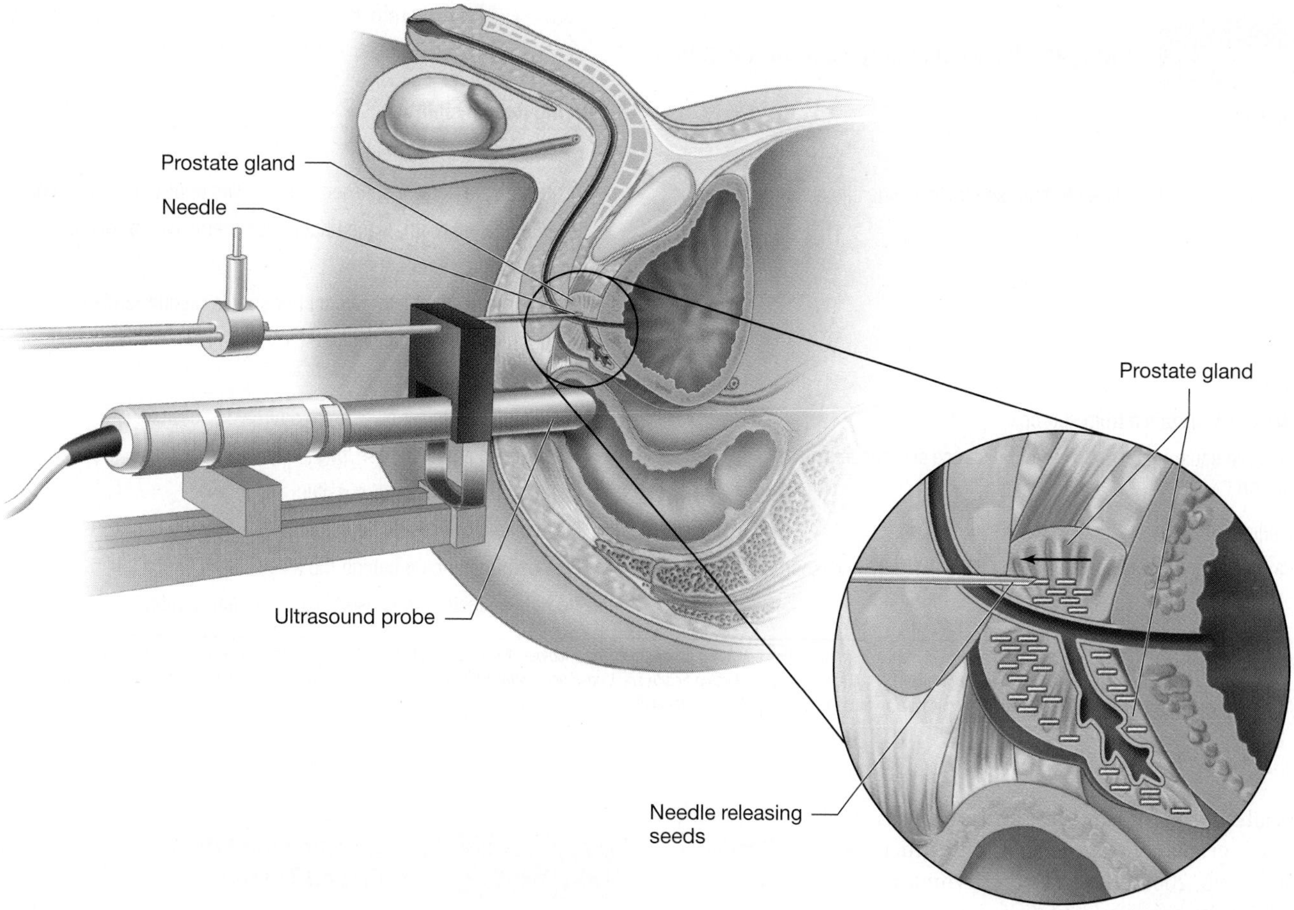

FIGURE 64–5 ■ Brachytherapy applicator.

state regulations mandate the monitoring of radiation levels, which provides for a safe workplace (Sedhom & Yanni, 1985).

Radiation Side Effects

Nurses play an important role in assessing, planning, implementing, and evaluating outcomes used to prevent or minimize the side effects associated with radiotherapy. Collaborating with the radiation oncology team allows for an opportunity to provide continuity and quality patient care, which will maximize efforts aimed at relief of side effects. Radiation therapy is a localized treatment that produces site-specific and general side effects that can be distressing to the patient and their loved ones.

Side effects experienced by most radiation therapy patients include skin changes, loss of appetite, fatigue, and bone marrow suppression. Radiation alters capillary blood flow leading to detectable skin changes. Skin reactions may occur within 2 weeks of beginning treatment. Erythema may be noted to range from mild, light pink to deep and dusky red (Sitton, 1997). Desquamation, first dry then moist, may occur in some patients. Moist desquamation is known to cause the epidermal layers of the skin to slough, leaving an area that is raw, painful, and draining serous exudate. Patients who have skinfolds, particularly in the axilla or groin, are more likely to develop skin reactions that progress to moist desquamation. There are ways to help minimize problems caused by skin changes associated with radiation therapy. These patients need education focused on maintaining good hygiene and when to alert their health care provider for signs of skin infection.

CRITICAL ALERT *Assessing the patient's skin during the course of radiotherapy for signs of reactions (redness, erythema, and desquamation) is essential. Pay particular attention to areas with skinfolds, such as the axilla and groin. The nurse should report signs of skin breakdown to the health care provider so possible treatment can be initiated. If skin reactions are minimized, the patient will experience less suffering, fewer (if any) complications, and be more likely to continue with the therapy.*

Anorexia, or loss of appetite, can be due to the cancer or the prescribed treatment. Although it is not completely clear what causes anorexia, contributing factors include inactivity, medications, and altered ingestion and digestion of food. Another explanation for anorexia could be found in the release of tumor necrosis factor (TNF) and interleukin-1 (IL-1). These **cytokines**, which have an appetite-suppressing effect, are released from macrophages while attempting to defeat a cancer. Loss of appetite usually peaks 4 weeks into treatment and subsides shortly after treatment ends. If anorexia persists, weight loss may occur resulting in the development of fatigue (Iwamoto, 2001). Refer to the upcoming Nursing Process: Care Plan for Cancer feature (p. 2089) for detailed nursing interventions and expected outcomes related to anorexia.

Many patients who receive radiotherapy experience fatigue. The exact causative mechanism is unknown, although it is thought to be due to the result of tumor breakdown, which releases by-products into the bloodstream (Sitton, 1997). Another explanation for the development of fatigue is the increase in basal metabolic rate consuming the body's energy stores. Fatigue

CHART 64–17	**Principles for Minimizing Radiation Exposure**
Principle	**Nursing Responsibilities**
Time • Exposure directly related to time spent within specific distance of source	• Minimize time in proximity. • Organize care activities; assemble supplies prior to entering room. • Prior to leaving room, place patient care items within reach. • Rotate staff assignments. • One-half hour of patient contact per shift is recommended. • Encourage self-care activities.
Distance • Maximize distance from source. • Inverse square law: doubling the distance decreases exposure by one-fourth	• Private room required. • Perform duties as far away from source as possible. • Never touch a source; use long-handled forceps. • Visit from the doorway if possible.
Shielding • Type of shielding and its thickness depends on type of source	• Place shield at bedside if needed. • Provide nursing care behind the shield. • Do not use lead aprons used in x-ray departments.

Sources: Dunne-Daly, C. (1997). Principles of brachytherapy. In K. Dow et al. (Eds.), *Nursing care in radiation oncology* (7th ed.). Philadelphia: W. B. Saunders; Erickson, J. (2003). Cancer. In W. Phipps, F. Monahan, J. Sands, J. Marek, & M. Neighbors (Eds.), *Medical–surgical nursing health and illness perspectives* (7th ed.). St. Louis: Mosby; Sitton, E. (1998). Managing side effects of skin changes and fatigue. In K. Dow et al. (Eds.), *Nursing care in radiation oncology* (7th ed.). Philadelphia: W. B. Saunders.

typically begins during the third or fourth week of treatment and will gradually wane once the treatment is over (Bender & Rosenzweig, 2004). Several other symptoms resulting from the alteration in energy production compound the effect of fatigue on cancer patients. These include pain, anorexia, infection, dyspnea, anemia, and depression.

The loss of energy and feeling of tiredness tend to be cumulative and have a significant impact on patients' quality of life. Patient education regarding the side effects of radiation begins before treatment and needs to continue once it is over. Teaching patients that side effects should be expected may decrease their fear that treatment is ineffective. Nursing care needs to be designed with energy conservation in mind. Clustering patient care activities together will allow for prolonged periods of rest for patients who are experiencing fatigue. Teaching patients and their caregivers these principles will assist the patient in coping with the tiredness experienced with fatigue while at home.

Bone marrow suppression occurs due to the prevalence of bone marrow being affected in nearly every treatment port. The common areas include pelvis, sternum, ribs, spine, metaphyses of long bones, and the skull (Iwamoto, 2001). The nursing care required is complex and challenging. Complete blood counts (CBCs) should be monitored at regular intervals during therapy or more frequently if concerning symptoms occur such as infection, bleeding, and fatigue. Providing patient and family education about precautions for neutropenia, thrombocytopenia, and anemia is essential and frequently requires reinforcement throughout the radiotherapy course.

The nurse plays a valuable role in helping the patient cope with side effects produced by radiotherapy. It also is important to recognize how the side effects will impact the patient's quality of life and how socialization may be difficult if not impossible. Many side effects are specific to the area where radiation is delivered. Site specific side effects are found in Chart 64–18.

CHART 64–18	**Site-Specific Side Effects of Radiation Therapy**
Site	**Side Effects**
Head and Neck	Stomatitis (irritation of the oral mucosa): • *Mild:* generalized erythema, few ulcerations, and small white patches • *Severe:* convergent ulcerations with bleeding and white patches covering >25% of oral cavity Xerostomia (dryness of the mouth) Tooth decay and caries Osteoradionecrosis Hypopituitarism Taste changes
Chest	Esophagitis Cough Radiation pneumonitis Lung fibrosis
Abdomen	Gastritis Nausea and vomiting
Pelvis	Diarrhea Cystitis Erectile dysfunction Vaginal stenosis Ovarian failure Cessation of spermatogenesis
Brain	Cerebral edema Alopecia Changes in hair texture and color

Nursing Management

A comprehensive plan of care will encompass the patient's physical and psychological needs. The Nursing Process: Care Plan for Cancer feature identifies the appropriate nursing diagnosis and pro- vides a detailed plan of care for the oncology patient. The nursing management sections for the patient receiving chemotherapy and biotherapy provide details pertinent to those patients receiving cancer-related treatments, including radiation therapy.

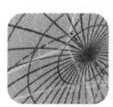

NURSING PROCESS: Patient Care Plan for Cancer

Assessment of Infection

Subjective Data:
Have you had fevers, chills, or body aches?
Have you noticed drainage from your skin?
Have you noticed changes in your urine odor?
Have you experienced painful urination?

Objective Data:
Signs of infection (e.g., dysuria, foul-smelling urine, elevated temperature, exudate from skin breakdown, elevated white blood count (WBC) count)

Nursing Assessment and Diagnoses	Outcomes and Evaluation Parameters	Planning and Interventions with *Rationales*
Nursing Diagnosis: *Risk for Infection* related to skin reactions, skin breakdown, multiple invasive lines, and myelosuppression	**Outcome:** No evidence of infection. *Evaluation Parameters:* Skin integrity is maintained. Urine appearance is clear, yellow, and possess no foul odor. Invasive lines are free from signs of infection. Patient demonstrates appropriate self-care behaviors.	**Interventions and *Rationales:*** Perform hand hygiene before and after working with patient. *Prevents spread of infection.* Monitor and record vital signs. *Elevated temperature and heart rate may indicate infection.* Assess for signs of infection and notify health care provider immediately: • Increased WBCs • Changes in temperature; >101°F (38.3°C) • Presence of chills, diaphoresis • Presence of myalgias • Cough, with or without sputum • Purulent drainage from site of skin reactions, intravenous site, or invasive line sites • Pain with urination, frequency with urination, foul-smelling urine • Mental status changes • Diarrhea. *Identifies need for prompt treatment.* Obtain cultures and sensitivities prior to administering antibiotic therapy. *Identifies organism responsible for infection, which directs appropriate treatment.* Administer antibiotics, antifungals, and antivirals as prescribed. Note presence of drug allergy. *Treatment of infection and prevention of drug reaction.* Initiate measures to reduce infection: • Private room if absolute neutrophil count (ANC) < 1,000/mm³ • Avoid contact with those who have known or recent infection or recent vaccination. • Hand hygiene • Avoid rectal or vaginal procedures (temperatures, examinations, medications). • Administer stool softeners to prevent straining • Meticulous hygiene • Avoid use of straight-edge razor. • Avoid raw meat and fish, fresh fruit and vegetables, fresh flowers and plants. • Provide clean liquids daily (e.g., denture cleaning solution, respiratory equipment fluid, drinking water). • Change solutions per protocol. • Avoid intramuscular injections. • Use strict aseptic technique when inserting medical devices (e.g., urinary catheters). *Infection control practice.* Instruct patient and family about infection prevention measures. *Reduces the risk of infection and encourages good infection control practices.*

(continued)

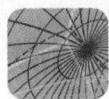

NURSING PROCESS: Patient Care Plan for Cancer—*Continued*

Assessment of Tissue Perfusion and Cardiac Output

Subjective Data:
Are you feeling breathless with minimal exertion?
Are you having chest discomfort?
Have you noticed weight gain or swelling?
Have you experienced feeling cold?

Objective Data:
Poor-quality pulses
Weight gain and edema
Increased respiratory rate
Presence of crackles in lungs

Nursing Assessment and Diagnoses	Outcomes and Evaluation Parameters	Planning and Interventions with *Rationales*
Nursing Diagnoses: *Ineffective Tissue Perfusion* and *Decreased Cardiac Output* related to chemotherapy induced cardiac toxicity and capillary leak syndrome	**Outcome:** Normal tissue perfusion and cardiac output. ***Evaluation Parameters:*** Adequate peripheral perfusion as evidenced by: • Extremity pulses present by palpation and/or ultrasound • Capillary refill < 2 seconds on distal extremities • Color and temperature normal to extremities. Adequate urinary output evidenced by 30 mL/hr. Normal neurological function. No evidence of heart failure.	**Interventions and *Rationales:*** Evaluate baseline cardiac studies (e.g., echocardiogram, ECG, MUGA scan). *Provides baseline cardiac function to allow for future comparison.* Calculate and document cumulative dose of chemotherapeutic agents, if appropriate. *Provides ongoing information regarding maximum lifetime dosage.* Assess for signs of congestive heart failure and report to health care provider: • Dyspnea • Tachycardia • Distended neck veins • Pedal edema • Crackles • Nonproductive cough • Extra heart tones (S_3) • Hepatomegaly. *Allows for prompt treatment.* Monitor vital signs for changes, and report to health care provider, such as: • Tachycardia • Tachypnea • Hypotension or hypertension. *Allows for prompt treatment.* Assess for syncope, dizziness, and weakness. *Indicates inadequate perfusion.* Monitor serum electrolytes. *Provides additional sources for alteration in cardiac function.* Administer medications to support cardiac function. (e.g., diuretics, inotropic agents, vasodilators, oxygen). *Maximizes cardiac function.* Position flat or with legs elevated. *Maximizes blood return to heart.* Encourage patient to adhere to dietary modifications (e.g., fluid restriction, sodium restriction, no alcohol, no tobacco). *Maximize cardiac function.* Instruct patient and family that cardiac effects may be irreversible. *Allows for time to consider lifestyle changes.* Collaborate with oncologist for reduced dosing of chemotherapy if ejection fraction is <55%. *Minimizes exposure to toxic effect of antineoplastic agents.* Monitor peripheral perfusion by assessing: • Capillary refill (<3.0 seconds) • Pulses present and strong throughout • Skin dry, color pink, and temperature warm. *Provides information about the quality of circulation.* Monitor urinary output for normal (> 30 mL/hr). Report abnormal findings to health care provider. *Indicates adequate renal perfusion and allows for prompt treatment if necessary.* Monitor neurological status and report abnormalities to health care provider. *Indicates possible perfusion abnormalities and need for prompt intervention.*

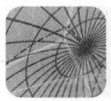

NURSING PROCESS: Patient Care Plan for Cancer—*Continued*

Assessment of Gas Exchange and Airway Clearance

Subjective Data:
Are you able to do your normal activities without breathlessness or fatigue?
Have you noticed a productive cough? If so, describe your sputum.

Objective Data:
Abnormal arterial blood gases (ABGs) and oxygen saturation
Abnormal lung sounds, rate and depth of respirations
Changes in amount and characteristics of sputum
Changes in mental status

Nursing Assessment and Diagnoses	Outcomes and Evaluation Parameters	Planning and Interventions with *Rationales*
Nursing Diagnoses: *Risk for Impaired Gas Exchange* and *Ineffective Airway Clearance* related to chemotherapy, biotherapy, and transplant-induced pulmonary toxicity	**Outcome:** Adequate gas exchange and airway clearance. ***Evaluation Parameters:*** Normal ABGs. No dyspnea: unlabored respirations < 24/minute. Normal neurological status. Normal breath sounds. No signs of impaired tissue oxygenation. Oxygen saturation is within normal limits.	**Interventions and *Rationales:*** Assess for adventitious or diminished breath sounds. *Indicates decreased gas exchange.* Note depth, rate, rhythm, and effort of respiration. *Assesses for respiratory distress or increased work of breathing.* Note presence of cough, amount, color, and consistency of sputum. *Assesses for development of respiratory infections or pulmonary edema.* Monitor ABGs and oxygen saturation via pulse oximetry. *Determines adequacy of gas exchange.* Monitor restlessness and confusion. *Indicators of inadequate gas exchange with resultant brain hypoxia.* Assess skin and mucous membranes for color (dusky, ashen, or cyanotic). *Indicators of tissue hypoxia and need for prompt intervention.* Instruct patient to cough and deep breathe. *Promotes gas exchange.* Administer humidified oxygen therapy as prescribed. *Promotes airway clearance.* Monitor for complaints of chest pain and report to health care provider. *May indicate acute pulmonary event such as pulmonary embolism, pleural effusion, or pneumothorax.* Instruct patient and family about symptoms of pulmonary toxicity and to report findings to health care provider. *Allows for prompt intervention.* Instruct patient and family regarding possibility of irreversible pulmonary effects. *Allows patient to consider initiating lifestyle changes consistent with pulmonary function.*

Assessment of Bleeding

Subjective Data:
Have you noticed unusual bruising?
Have you noticed any blood in your urine or stools?
Have you experienced dizziness or light-headedness?

Objective Data:
Blood studies (platelets, hemoglobin, and hematocrit) lowered
Oozing from venipunctures
Unusual amount of bruising
Bleeding gums after oral hygiene
Hematuria and guaiac-positive stools
Change in mental status or behavior
Change in vital signs

Nursing Assessment and Diagnoses	Outcomes and Evaluation Parameters	Planning and Interventions with *Rationales*
Nursing Diagnosis: *Potential for Deficient Fluid Volume* related to bone marrow suppression, hepatotoxicity, hepatic Veno Occlusive Disease (VOD), and hematologic laboratory abnormality induced by cancer treatments	**Outcome:** No evidence of bleeding. ***Evaluation Parameters:*** Platelet count will be within normal limits. Hemoglobin and hematocrit will be within normal limits. Hemodynamic status will be maintained. Patient will demonstrate appropriate self-care behaviors.	**Interventions and *Rationales:*** Monitor platelet counts and report a count of <50,000/mm^3 to health care provider. *Identifies need for prompt treatment.* Monitor liver function tests and coagulation studies. *Identifies need for prompt treatment.*

(continued)

NURSING PROCESS: Patient Care Plan for Cancer—*Continued*

Nursing Assessment and Diagnoses	Outcomes and Evaluation Parameters	Planning and Interventions with *Rationales*
		Assess for bleeding and report findings to the health care provider: • Decrease in hemoglobin and hematocrit • Prolonged bleeding or oozing from invasive procedures, venipunctures, cuts, or scratches • Presence of petechiae or ecchymosis • Presence of frank or occult blood in emesis, stool, or sputum • Presence of blood from any body orifice • Change in mental status • Change in vital signs (e.g., ↑ heart rate, ↓ BP) • Skin color pale, temperature cool. *Early detection aids in early treatment.* Perform venipunctures once daily for all laboratory tests. *Minimizes the risk of bleeding.* Avoid taking rectal temperatures; avoid use of suppositories or enemas. *Minimizes the risk of bleeding.* Apply direct pressure to injection and venipuncture sites for a minimum of 5 minutes. *Minimizes bleeding.* Instruct patient regarding ways to minimize the risk of bleeding: • Perform oral hygiene with soft toothbrush or toothettes. • Avoid use of commercial mouthwashes. • Avoid straight–edge razors. • File nails with emery board. • Avoid foods that are difficult to chew. *Provides for appropriate self-care behaviors.*

Assessment of Fluid Volume Status

Subjective Data:
How frequent (if any) are your diarrhea episodes?
Are you able to consume fluids?
Do you feel dizzy or light-headed when you change positions?
Are there any remedies that have helped?
Have you noticed an increase in your weight?
Do you become breathless?

Objective Data:
Poor skin turgor, dry mucous membranes
Elevated heart rate with position changes
Output exceeds intake
Multiple diarrhea episodes
Presence of edema and weight gain
Crackles in lungs

Nursing Assessment and Diagnoses	Outcomes and Evaluation Parameters	Planning and Interventions with *Rationales*
Nursing Diagnoses: *Risk for Deficient Fluid Volume* related to nausea, vomiting, diarrhea (due to pelvic radiation & cancer), hepatic VOD, and capillary leak syndrome *Risk for Excess Fluid Volume* related to hepatic VOD	**Outcomes:** Adequate hydration. Absence of skin breakdown. Normal electrolytes. ***Evaluation Parameters:*** Normal serum electrolytes. Skin surrounding anus remains intact. Cessation of diarrhea episodes. No evidence of dehydration or fluid overload. Absence of skin breakdown. Normal electrolytes.	**Interventions and *Rationales:*** Assess bowel pattern. *Determines baseline.* Record frequency of diarrhea and vomiting episodes. *Indicates degree of fluid loss.* Establish and maintain IV access. *Allows for fluid volume replacement if needed.* Administer IV fluids per protocol. *Determines need for fluid administration or restriction and prevents dehydration.* Record accurate intake and output. *Determines adequacy of fluid volume replacement.* Monitor daily weights using the same scale and with the same clothing. *Indicates fluid retention or loss.* Monitor serum electrolyte values, hemoglobin and hematocrit, liver function tests, and coagulation studies and notify health care provider of critical abnormalities. *To monitor hematologic changes associated with fluid changes.* Monitor for presence of edema. *Indicates fluid retention.* Measure abdominal girth daily and apply landmark indicators to abdomen. *Indicates presence of accumulating ascites and allows for accuracy and consistency in measurements.*

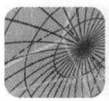

NURSING PROCESS: Patient Care Plan for Cancer—*Continued*

Nursing Assessment and Diagnoses	Outcomes and Evaluation Parameters	Planning and Interventions with *Rationales*
		Restrict sodium and water intake. *Prevents fluid retention in extracellular spaces.*
		Monitor lung sounds. *Evaluates for fluid accumulation in lung, which may require prompt treatment.*
		Place patient in semi-Fowler's position to avoid the patient lying flat. *Allows for optimal ventilation in the presence of ascites.*
		Assess for excoriation of skin surrounding anus. *Identifies need for interventions.*
		Instruct patient to cleanse area frequently. *Prevents skin breakdown.*
		Instruct patient to notify health care provider if skin breakdown occurs. *Allows for prompt treatment.*
		Administer antidiarrhea medication per protocol. *Reduces frequency of diarrhea episodes.*
		Instruct patient to use low-residue diet and limit fat content. *Reduces amount of diarrhea.*

Assessment of Skin Integrity and Oral Mucous Membranes

Subjective Data:
Have you noticed pain in your mouth?
Have you noticed sores in your mouth?
Have you noticed areas of skin breakdown?
Have you noticed hair loss?
Do you have pain, drainage, or swelling in area of skin breakdown?

Objective Data:
Presence of mouth sores
Reports of pain in mouth with citrus drinks
Poor oral intake
Presence of skin breakdown and hair loss
Presence of skin redness
Signs of pain or infection

Nursing Assessment and Diagnoses	Outcomes and Evaluation Parameters	Planning and Interventions with *Rationales*
Nursing Diagnosis: *Impaired Skin Integrity* related to alopecia, stomatitis, xerostomia, skin reactions due to radiation therapy, invasive procedures and lines, biotherapy-induced dry desquamation, rashes, and pruritus, edema, cancer diagnosis and treatment	**Outcomes:** Maintain or restore skin integrity. Cope with hair loss. Mucous membranes are intact. ***Evaluation Parameters:*** Minimal skin changes noted. Appropriate self-care behaviors are demonstrated. Skin infections are absent. Social interaction is maintained. Intact oral mucous membranes are maintained. Nutritional status is maintained. Patient is not suffering. Skin integrity is maintained or restored.	**Interventions and *Rationales:*** Inspect oral cavity daily. *Provides information needed to determine if treatment is necessary.* Instruct patient regarding proper oral care: • Brush and floss teeth as tolerated. • Use moistening gauze or toothettes instead of toothbrush if needed, for instance, if platelet count is low (<40,000/mm³). • Rinse with normal saline four times per day. • Avoid commercial mouthwashes. • Cleanse mouth before and after meals. *Prevents trauma and maintains oral hygiene.* Administer cytoprotectives as ordered (e.g., Ethyol). *Promotes comfort and reduces incidence of mucous membrane breakdown.* Provide bland and soft diet. *Allows for ease of chewing and swallowing and reduces discomfort.* Administer saliva substitutes and moisten food as needed. *Allows for ease of swallowing.* Instruct patient to report signs of stomatitis: • Burning • Pain • Areas of redness • Open lesions on the lips • Pain with swallowing • Intolerance to temperature extremes. *Identifies beginning stages of mucous membrane breakdown and facilitates prompt treatment.*

(continued)

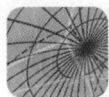

NURSING PROCESS: Patient Care Plan for Cancer—*Continued*

Nursing Assessment and Diagnoses	Outcomes and Evaluation Parameters	Planning and Interventions with *Rationales*
		Assist in oral hygiene during mild stomatitis: • Normal saline rinses every 2 hours, every 6 hours during sleep. • Use soft toothbrush or toothette. • Avoid use of dentures except for meals. • Maintain proper fit of dentures. • Moisten lips with lubricating ointment. • Avoid eating foods that are spicy, those with temperature extremes, and those that are difficult to chew. *Promotes hygiene, minimizes trauma, and provides for comfort.* Assist in oral hygiene during severe stomatitis: • Discontinue use of dentures. • Rinse with prescribed agent or irrigate oral cavity with mixture of saline, anti-*Candida* agent (Mycostatin), and topical anesthetic agent. • Position patient properly for irrigations. • Provide oral suction device. • Use gauze or toothette with irrigation solution for cleansing. • Lubricate lips. *Promotes hygiene and comfort.* Assess patient's ability to chew, swallow, and presence of gag reflex. *Identifies risk for aspiration.* Encourage use of pureed diet or liquid diet. *Promotes comfort and maintains nutrition.* Monitor for signs of infection and notify health care provider immediately. *Facilitates prompt treatment.* Obtain tissue cultures as needed. *Provides evidence of infection.* Administer analgesics, topical and systemic, as prescribed. *Promotes comfort.* Discuss patterns of hair loss and regrowth with patient and family. *Provides information so preparations for loss can begin and provides an understanding of the temporary nature of alopecia.* Encourage expression of concerns related to hair loss. *Facilitates coping.* Reduce or prevent hair loss: • Cut long hair prior to treatment. • Use mild shampoo, conditioner in small amounts. • Gently pat hair dry. • Avoid electric curlers, curling irons, dryers, clips, barrettes, hair sprays, hair dyes, or other hair chemicals. • Avoid excessive brushing or combing; use wide-tooth comb. • Use scalp tourniquets or hypothermia as appropriate. *Prevents hair loss as long as possible by decreasing the uptake of chemotherapy. Also maintains presence of hair as long as possible by reducing weight and manipulation.* Encourage patient to avoid actions that traumatize the scalp: • Keep scalp lubricated to reduce itching (use vitamins A and D). • Use sunscreen or hat when exposed to ultraviolet rays. *Prevents breakdown of the skin.* Offer ways to cope with hair loss: • Obtain wigs or hairpieces prior to hair loss. • Take photograph of hair loss to wig shop to improve matching of hair color. • Contact American Cancer Society for available resources. • Wear scarf, hat, or other device as needed. *Reduces changes in appearance.* Assess skin integrity. *Provides baseline information.*

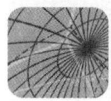

NURSING PROCESS: Patient Care Plan for Cancer—*Continued*

Nursing Assessment and Diagnoses	Outcomes and Evaluation Parameters	Planning and Interventions with *Rationales*
		Instruct patient regarding skin care of area within treatment field: • Cleanse with lukewarm water. • Avoid use of soap, powders, deodorants, and fragrances. • Avoid shaving. • Keep skinfolds dry and clean. • Use devices to protect skin from sun, heat, and cold. • Avoid use of restrictive or tight-fitting clothing. • Avoid use of tape. • Avoid massaging, vigorous rubbing, or scratching. *Minimizes skin trauma and provides protection.* Instruct patient regarding skin care if dry desquamation occurs: • Cleanse with lukewarm water. • Avoid use of soap, powders, deodorants, cosmetics, ointments, and fragrances. • Avoid shaving. • Avoid rubbing or scratching. • Avoid hyperthermia or hypothermia treatments. • Avoid use of adhesive tapes. • Avoid exposure to sunlight or cold weather conditions. • Avoid use of restrictive clothing; use of cotton materials is preferred. • Apply hydrophilic moisturizing lotion or ointment two to three times per day (e.g., vitamins A and D ointment or Aquaphor). *Prevents further skin damage and drying and aids in healing.* Instruct patient regarding skin care if moist desquamation occurs: • Notify health care provider if blistering occurs. • Keep blisters intact. • Avoid frequent cleansing of the area. • Apply saline irrigations or cold compresses three to four times per day. • Apply dressings as prescribed (e.g., Vigilon). • Apply zinc oxide or silver sulfadiazine with nonstick dressing if radiation treatments are being held. • If area is draining, apply thin layer of gauze. *Provides for healing, decreases inflammation, and prevents infection.* Administer antihistamines per protocol. *Relieves itching associated with pruritus.* Apply cold towels to affected area. *Relieves itching associated with pruritus.* Instruct patient to maintain room humidity between 30% and 40%. *Relieves itching associated with pruritus.*

Assessment of Fatigue

Subjective Data:

Do you feel unusually tired?

Do you perform your normal activities?

Do you have difficulty performing your normal activities?

How many hours per night do you sleep?

How is your appetite?

Do you have help at home?

Objective Data:

Monitor hemoglobin, hematocrit, RBCs, electrolytes

Adequate nutritional intake

Presence of pain or edema

Monitor energy expenditure

(continued)

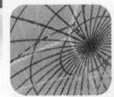

Nursing Assessment and Diagnoses	Outcomes and Evaluation Parameters	Planning and Interventions with *Rationales*
Nursing Diagnosis: *Activity Intolerance* related to fatigue, bone marrow suppression, anorexia, and hepatotoxicity	**Outcome:** Able to perform activities of daily living (ADLs). ***Evaluation Parameters:*** Maintain ADLs and minimize fatigue. Serum laboratory studies within normal limits. Adequate energy levels are maintained. Patient shows no evidence of suffering or discomfort. Adequate diet with recommended calorie and protein intake is maintained.	**Interventions and *Rationales:*** Encourage frequent rest periods. *Energy is conserved and replenished.* Encourage more sleep hours at night. *Restores energy levels.* Encourage patient to reorganize daily schedule of activities and seek assistance with shopping, cooking, housework, etc. *To minimize energy expenditure.* Encourage a temporary decrease in work hours. *Decreases physical and psychological stress and provides for rest.* Assess nutritional intake for adequate protein and calorie intake. *Provides source of energy.* Administer blood products per protocol. *Provides adequate oxygen availability, which will decrease fatigue.* Monitor fluid and electrolyte balance. *Provides information regarding nerve transmission and muscle function.* Assess for sources of discomfort and suffering. *Minimizes energy expenditure.*

Assessment of Nutrition

Subjective Data:

How has your appetite been?

Have you lost weight?

Have you been able to perform your normal activities?

Objective Data:

Weight loss

Decreased albumin and prealbumin levels

Poor dietary intake per calorie count and clinical nutrition consult

Nursing Assessment and Diagnoses	Outcomes and Evaluation Parameters	Planning and Interventions with *Rationales*
Nursing Diagnosis: *Imbalanced Nutrition: Less Than Body Requirements* related to chemotherapy and biotherapy-induced nausea, vomiting, hepatotoxicity, anorexia, and effects of pre- and post-transplant treatment	**Outcome:** Adequate nutritional status and maintenance of body weight. ***Evaluation Parameters:*** Patient experiences fewer episodes of nausea and vomiting. Adequate calorie intake maintained. Serum laboratory studies within normal limits. Adequate energy levels are maintained. Prescribed diet is tolerated.	**Interventions and *Rationales:*** Monitor accurate intake and output and record. *Indicates trends in intake pattern.* Perform nutritional assessment: • Calorie count • Ability to swallow • Food preferences • Patterns and behaviors related to eating • Ethnic and cultural preferences. *Indicates adequacy of nutrition.* Monitor serum albumin, prealbumin, glucose, magnesium, sodium, and iron. *Assesses adequacy of nutritional intake.* Assess for signs of malnutrition: • Muscle wasting • Edema • Changes in hair condition • Changes in skin. *Indicates adequacy of nutrition.* Consult nutritionist to determine appropriate needs for individual. *Assists in establishing or maintaining adequate nutrition.* Provide meticulous oral care. *Prevents infection and promotes appetite.* Administer antiemetics and appetite stimulants per orders. *Assists in improving appetite by reducing nausea and vomiting.* Encourage small frequent meals that are high in calories and protein. *Such meals are more suitable for digestion, better tolerated.* Encourage adequate fluid intake, limiting fluids during mealtime. *Prevents the development of satiety.* Increase activity level as tolerated. *Activity stimulates the appetite.* Provide environment suitable for eating: • Pain free • Relaxed environment • Presentation of food tray. *To increase appetite.* Monitor tube feedings or IV total parenteral nutrition per protocol. *Determines tolerance of nutritional delivery system.*

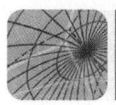
Nursing Assessment and Diagnoses	Outcomes and Evaluation Parameters	Planning and Interventions with *Rationales*
		Administer cytoprotectives as ordered (e.g., Ethyol). *Promotes comfort and improved nutrition by preventing dry mouth.* Provide discharge teaching to patient and family regarding nutritional needs. *Maintains nutritional status at home.*

Assessment of Pain

Subjective Data:
Are you experiencing pain?
If so, describe the quality, intensity, provoking factors, etc.
Rate pain on scale of 1–10.

Objective Data:
Unwilling to participate in care
Facial grimacing
Guarding or protecting of painful site
Using increasing doses of pain medication

Nursing Assessment and Diagnoses	Outcomes and Evaluation Parameters	Planning and Interventions with *Rationales*
Nursing Diagnosis: *Pain* related to skin reactions, cough from chest radiation, chemotherapy-induced pancreatitis, chemotherapy- and biotherapy-induced peripheral neuropathy and bone pain, mucositis, invasive procedures, and disease process	**Outcome:** Pain is controlled. ***Evaluation Parameters:*** Patient verbalizes pain level and previous interventions that were successful in alleviating pain. Pain is reduced or absent as evidenced by patient denying presence or by nonverbal behaviors: no facial grimacing, restlessness, etc. Patient reports complementary strategies of pain control are effective.	**Interventions and *Rationales:*** Assess pain using pain scale (0–10) to quantify pain level. *Provides consistency for evaluating pain.* Assess discomfort characteristics: • Location • Quality • Frequency • Duration • Alleviating therapies. *Provides baseline for assessing change.* Assess other factors contributing to pain: • Fear • Fatigue • Anger • Anxiety. *Provides data about factors that decrease the patient's tolerance to pain.* Ensure adequate fluid intake. *Minimizes frequency and intensity of cough.* Instruct patient to avoid irritants such as smoke. *Minimizes cough.* Instruct patient regarding the use of humidification in the air. *Minimizes cough.* Administer analgesics according to protocol. *Provides pain relief.* Monitor for side effects of analgesics and treat accordingly. *Ensures tolerance of analgesics.* Encourage use of pureed diet or liquid diet. *Promotes comfort and maintains nutrition.* Monitor for signs of infection and notify health care provider immediately. *Facilitates prompt treatment.* Administer analgesics prior to a procedure or treatment that may cause discomfort. *Controls increased pain level related to procedures and treatments.* Instruct patient to notify nurse when pain is not relieved or when pain begins to occur again. *Indicates need for additional pain management therapies or the administration of analgesics earlier in the pain cycle.* Collaborate with the patient and the multidisciplinary team when changes in pain management are necessary. *Increases the patient's sense of control and allows for agreement and input from all team members.* Instruct patient and family about complementary strategies to relieve pain and discomfort: • Guided imagery • Relaxation techniques • Distraction • Cutaneous stimulation. *Helps reduce anxiety and promotes relaxation.*

(continued)

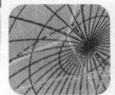

Assessment of Body Image Disturbance

Subjective Data:
What feelings do you have about the change in your appearance?
Have you been participating in your care and normal activities?
Have you been socializing?

Objective Data:
Isolating behaviors
Avoidance
Not involved with personal care

Nursing Assessment and Diagnoses	Outcomes and Evaluation Parameters	Planning and Interventions with *Rationales*
Nursing Diagnosis: *Disturbed Body Image* related to skin reactions, alopecia, long-term venous access devices, decreased sexual function, role changes, and other cancer treatments	**Outcomes:** Social integration Normal social interactions and acceptance of body image changes ***Evaluation Parameters:*** Participates in self-care activities. Demonstrates interest in appearance. Resumes or continues interactions with others in established social network. Explores alternative ways of expressing concern and affection with partner.	**Interventions and *Rationales:*** Assess patient's feelings about body image and level of self-esteem. Validate concerns. *Provides baseline for evaluating changes and determining effectiveness of interventions.* Advocate for participation in activities and decision making. *Facilitates a sense of control.* Encourage patient to verbalize concerns. *Begins coping process.* Provide personalized care. *Prevents depersonalization.* Discuss patterns of hair loss and regrowth with patient and family. *Provides information so preparations for loss can begin and provides an understanding of the temporary nature of alopecia.* Assist in self-care when fatigue, nausea, vomiting, or other distressing symptoms occur. *Improves self-esteem by ensuring physical well-being.* Help patient in selecting cosmetic devices that increase sense of attractiveness. *Promotes positive body image.* Offer ways to cope with hair loss: • Obtain wigs or hairpieces prior to hair loss. • Take photograph of hair to wig shop to improve matching of hair color. • Contact American Cancer Society for available resources. • Wear scarf, hat, or other device as needed. *Reduces changes in appearance.* Encourage dialogue between patient and partner regarding sexual function and alternatives. *Allows for affection and acceptance.*

Assessment of Urinary Elimination

Subjective Data:
Do you have difficulty urinating?
What is the color of your urine?
Do you have pain upon urination?
What is your typical fluid intake throughout the day?

Objective Data:
Presence of hematuria
Foul-smelling urine
Presence of fever
Complaints of pain with urination

Nursing Assessment and Diagnoses	Outcomes and Evaluation Parameters	Planning and Interventions with *Rationales*
Nursing Diagnosis: *Impaired Urinary Elimination* related to radiation therapy	**Outcomes:** Minimize cystitis. Able to urinate normally. ***Evaluation Parameters:*** Laboratory studies within normal limits. No evidence of discomfort or suffering. Adequate fluid intake maintained. Normal urinary patterns.	**Interventions and *Rationales:*** Assess for hematuria. *Indicates possible infection or cystitis.* Monitor fluid intake and encourage adequate intake. *Decreases incidence of cystitis.* Monitor for signs of urinary tract infection. *Promotes prompt treatment.* Obtain urine analysis and culture. *Evaluates for infection.* Assess for pain with urination. *Determines presence of symptoms needing further treatment.* Administer antibiotics, bladder analgesics, and antispasmodics as ordered. *To treat infection and pain.* Evaluate patient's understanding of cause of cystitis and measures to relieve symptoms. *Provides evidence of need for education.*

Assessment for Impaired Swallowing

Subjective Data:
Have you had difficulty swallowing?
Do you have pain with swallowing?

Objective Data:
Reports of pain with swallowing
Inability to swallow bolus of food or fluids
Refusing food or fluids

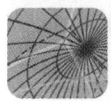

NURSING PROCESS: Patient Care Plan for Cancer—*Continued*

Nursing Assessment and Diagnoses	Outcomes and Evaluation Parameters	Planning and Interventions with *Rationales*
Nursing Diagnosis: *Risk for Impaired Swallowing* related to esophagitis or pharyngitis	**Outcome:** No difficulties with swallowing. **Evaluation Parameters:** Adequate nutritional status is maintained. Adequate pain management is maintained. Full course of radiation therapy is completed.	**Interventions and *Rationales:*** Instruct patient to follow a soft, bland, or liquid diet that is high in protein and calories. *Facilitates swallowing and promotes adequate nutritional intake.* Administer anesthetic and coating mouth rinses prior to eating. *Relieves discomfort associated with swallowing.* Administer analgesics per protocol. *Relieves discomfort associated with swallowing and allows for patient to continue with therapy.*

Assessment of Sexual Dysfunction

Subjective Data:
Are you satisfied with your sexual functioning?
Are you experiencing difficulty with sexual function?

Objective Data:
Minimal communication between patient and partner
Lack of touching and closeness between patient and partner

Nursing Assessment and Diagnoses	Outcomes and Evaluation Parameters	Planning and Interventions with *Rationales*
Nursing Diagnoses: *Risk for Sexual Dysfunction* related to radiation therapy of the pelvis *Altered Sexuality Patterns* related to late effects of transplantation	**Outcome:** Maintains sexual functioning as desired. **Evaluation Parameters:** Patient and partner understand rationale for treatment. Patient and partner maintain effective communication. Sexual functioning is improved.	**Interventions and *Rationales:*** Assess level of dysfunction via patient interview. *Determines baseline and need for interventions.* Encourage patient to discuss concerns with partner. *Facilitates effective communication.* Facilitate consultation with urologist as needed, including patient education regarding rationale. *Provides treatment and education.* Monitor for symptoms that affect libido. *Allows for treatment and understanding of changes.* Assess for fear, anxiety, diminished self-image, and depression. *Indicates need for resources for coping.* Facilitate communication about sexual issues. *Promotes open communication between patient and partner.* Instruct patient on hygiene and contraceptive measures. *Prevents infections and pregnancy.*

Assessment of Growth and Development

Subjective Data:
Parents report delayed progress in school.
Appears to be of short stature.

Objective Data:
Height and weight lower than normal
Motor abilities abnormal
Cognitive testing abnormal

Nursing Assessment and Diagnoses	Outcomes and Evaluation Parameters	Planning and Interventions with *Rationales*
Nursing Diagnosis: *Delayed Growth and Development* related to late effects of transplantation in children	**Outcome:** Normalized growth and development. **Evaluation Parameters:** Growth patterns are normal according to standardized charts. Educational needs are being met. Identifies need to access support systems. Actively participates in recovery.	**Interventions and *Rationales:*** Monitor patient's growth according to standard charts. *Helps determine if growth patterns are impaired.* Evaluate normal growth and development behaviors consistent with the patient's age. *Indicates need for possible treatment.* Monitor for learning disabilities. *Indicates need for special educational resources.* Administer growth hormone per protocol. *Assists in normalizing growth and development patterns.* Provide educational and emotional resources to patient and family. *Improves coping and ability to function with deficits.*

Assessment of Coping

Subjective Data:
Do you feel saddened?
Have you been withdrawing from your normal activities and routines?
Have you been sleeping well? If not, why?
Do you have a support system that comforts you?

Objective Data:
Withdrawn behavior
Unwilling to participate in care
Insomnia
Frequent episodes of crying, anger, aggressive behavior

(continued)

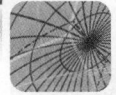

Nursing Assessment and Diagnoses	Outcomes and Evaluation Parameters	Planning and Interventions with *Rationales*
Nursing Diagnosis: *Ineffective Coping* related to alopecia, fatigue, biotherapy-induced depression, anxiety, transplant process, role changes, lifestyle changes, diagnosis of cancer	**Outcome:** Patient will demonstrate effective coping skills. ***Evaluation Parameters:*** Demonstrates effective coping strategies for living with cancer. Identifies need to access support systems. Actively participates in recovery.	**Interventions and *Rationales:*** Assess patient's and family's understanding of diagnosis, recommended treatment, and prognosis. *Provides information about need for further teaching if not consistent with actual diagnosis, treatment, or prognosis.* Encourage patient to express feelings. *Effective coping strategy.* Monitor aggressive behaviors. *May indicate ineffective coping.* Assess patient's and family's support systems. *Indicates need for recommendations.* Consult psychiatrist, psychologist, or spiritual counselor. *Provides expertise that will evaluate for effective coping and make recommendations for assistance.* Encourage family to use memory prompts with patient for orientation in regard to time, date, and location. *Allows for reorientation and participation in care.*

Assessment of Knowledge

Subjective Data:

What have you been told about your disease and treatment?
How would you manage side effects of treatment?
What symptoms would you contact your health care provider for?

Objective Data:

Assess understanding of diagnosis and recommended treatments.
Assess understanding of potential side effects and related remedies.

Nursing Assessment and Diagnoses	Outcomes and Evaluation Parameters	Planning and Interventions with *Rationales*
Nursing Diagnosis: *Deficient Knowledge* related to radiation therapy, chemotherapy, biotherapy side effects, and self-care needs	**Outcome:** Understand the use of radiation therapy for cancer and the self-care behaviors necessary to manage side effects. ***Evaluation Parameters:*** Patient verbalizes an understanding of the purpose for therapy, side effects, and measures used to minimize side effects, and protective measures. Patient demonstrates appropriate self-care behaviors. Patient understands the use of biotherapy and chemotherapy for cancer and the self-care behaviors necessary to manage side effects. Patient understands the use of transplantation for cancer and the self-care behaviors necessary to manage side effects. Patient demonstrates appropriate self-care behaviors.	**Interventions and *Rationales:*** Assess patient's expectations and concerns about therapy. *Determines baseline knowledge.* Instruct patient and family about: • The purpose of using radiation therapy to treat cancer • Routines such as consultation, simulation, treatment schedules, routine appointments, and follow-up • Expected length of each visit • Appearance of equipment and environment. *Decreases anxiety associated with treatment.* Instruct patient and family about the effects and side effects associated with radiation therapy. *Decreases anxiety associated with treatment.* Instruct patient and family about measures used to minimize side effects. *Provides for less distress associated with treatment, which maximizes chance of patient continuing with therapy.* Instruct patient and family about visiting restrictions and isolation requirements associated with internal radiation therapy. *Provides for an understanding of the need to protect others.* Instruct patient and family about: • The purpose of using chemotherapy and biotherapy, and transplantation to treat cancer • Routines such as appointments and follow-up treatments • Expected length of each visit • Appearance of infusion equipment and vascular access devices. *Decreases anxiety associated with treatment.* Assess patient's expectations and concerns about transplantation. *Determines baseline knowledge.* Instruct patient and family about the effect and side effects associated with transplantation and associated conditioning. *Decreases anxiety associated with treatment.* Instruct patient and family about measures used to minimize side effects. *Provides for less distress associated with treatment, which maximizes chance of patient continuing with therapy.*

Sources: Bender, C., & Rosenzweig, M. (2004). Cancer. In S. Lewis, M. Heitkemper, & S. Dirksen (Eds.), *Medical–surgical nursing assessment and management of clinical problems* (6th ed.). St. Louis: Mosby; Iwamoto, R. (2001). Radiation therapy. In S. Otto (Ed.), *Oncology nursing* (4th ed.). St. Louis: Mosby; Keller, C. (2001). Bone marrow and stem cell transplantation. In S. Otto (Ed.), *Oncology nursing* (4th ed.). St. Louis: Mosby; Oncology Nursing Society. (2001). *Chemotherapy and biotherapy guidelines and recommendations for practice.* Pittsburgh: Author; Rokita, S. (2004). Oncology: Nursing management in cancer care. In S. Smeltzer & B. Bare (Eds.), *Brunner & Suddarth's textbook of medical–surgical nursing* (10th ed.). Philadelphia: Lippincott Williams & Wilkins; Wikle-Shapiro, T. (1998). Nursing implications of bone marrow and stem cell transplantation. In J. K. Itano & K. N. Taoka (Eds.), *Core curriculum for oncology nursing* (3rd ed.). Philadelphia: W. B. Saunders.

Chemotherapy

Chemotherapy is defined as the systemic administration of cytotoxic drugs to treat cancer. In one form or another, this systemic therapy has been present for centuries. Current practice can be linked to the early 1900s when studies were conducted using laboratory rodents to determine the effectiveness of potential cancer chemotherapeutic agents (DeVita, 1997). During World War I and World War II soldiers were exposed to mustard gas, which was discovered to cause bone marrow and lymphoid suppression. This discovery led to the use of mustard agents in the treatment of Hodgkin's and other lymphomas for the first time in 1940. The use of chemotherapy became a standard of practice in the treatment of cancer in the 1970s (Grever & Chabner, 1997).

It was estimated that there would be 1,437,180 new cases of cancer diagnosed in 2008 (ACS, 2008b) and half of these would be treated with systemic chemotherapy. Given the prevalence of cancer, nurses need to understand the purpose of administering chemotherapy and how it is used. The primary reasons for prescribing chemotherapy are to prevent tumor cells from multiplying, spreading to adjacent tissues, or developing metastasis (Otto, 2001a). Therapy aims to provide a cure, control spread of the disease, or palliate signs of suffering. Chemotherapy may be used in several different ways, and oncologists prescribe treatment for patients with specific goals in mind. Chart 64–19 explains the five different ways of using chemotherapy and their purposes. Improvement in overall survival rate and increased periods of disease-free intervals can be attributed to the ongoing development of chemotherapy approaches to cancer treatment. The past five decades have been exciting for those caring for patients with cancer due to the dynamic state of chemotherapy research and the subsequent development of a host of new agents.

Principles of Chemotherapy

Every time a malignancy is exposed to a chemotherapeutic agent, a percentage of tumor cells are destroyed. The aim is destruction of as many cells as possible, up to 99% depending on the dose. Completely eradicating all tumor cells is virtually impossible, but the hope is to leave as few cells as possible so the body's immune system can finish the job. Chemotherapy is thought to kill a fixed percentage of the total number of cancer cells. This cell-kill hypothesis, shown in Figure 64–6 ■, suggests that if a drug has a 90% cell-kill rate and the tumor has 1,000 cells, at the end of the first treatment there would only be 100 cancerous cells remaining. The next treatment would leave the

number of cells at 10, thus the reason for scheduling chemotherapy in multiple courses over a period of time.

Both cancerous cells and normal cells replicate via the various phases in the cell cycle. The cell cycle time is that time necessary for one tissue cell to divide and reproduce two identical daughter cells. The cycle for any cell has four phases each with its own important role. These include the G_1 phase, in which RNA and protein synthesis occur; the S phase, in which DNA synthesis occurs; the G_2 phase, which is the premitotic phase in which DNA synthesis is completed and mitotic spindles form; and finally mitosis (M phase) is the phase in which cell division occurs. Phase G_0, which is the resting or dormant phase, occurs after mitosis and prior to the G_1 phase (McNance & Roberts, 2002). These G_1 cells are particularly dangerous because they are not actively dividing but have the potential to replicate. Chemotherapeutic agents are meant to interrupt the cell replication at pivotal points within the cycle and are more effective when targeting cells that are actively dividing.

Because the goal of chemotherapy is to reduce the number of malignant cells present in both the primary and metastatic

The cell kill hypothesis

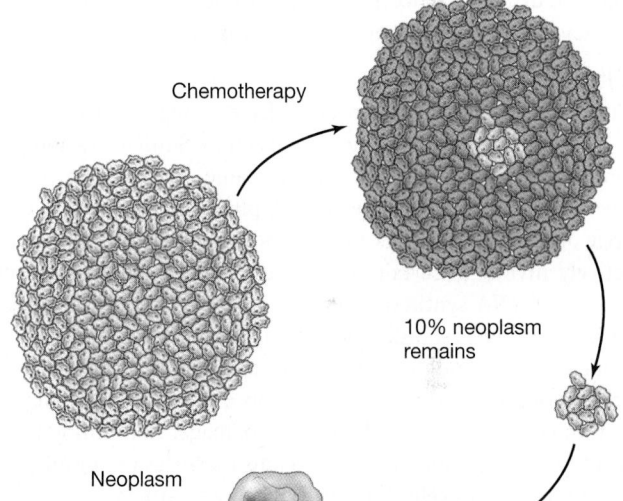

FIGURE 64–6 ■ Cell-kill hypothesis.

CHART 64–19	**Uses of Chemotherapeutic Agents in Treating Cancer**		
Type of Therapy	**Use**	**Purpose**
Adjuvant	Used in combination with other cancer treatment modalities	To treat micrometastasis
Neoadjuvant	Used prior to surgical resection of tumor	To shrink tumor in order to maximize surgical resection capabilities
Primary	Used for localized cancer when other treatment options are not as effective	To maximize chance of cure or disease control
Induction	Used for cancers for which other alternatives do not exist	To maximize chance of cure or disease control
Combination	Use of two or more chemotherapeutic agents	To allow each medication to enhance the effect of the other or to act synergistically with it

tumor site, it is important to discuss the factors that determine the response of cancer cells to chemotherapy. First, the mitotic rate of the tumor affects the response of chemotherapy due to the rapid proliferation of cancerous cells. The more rapid the mitotic rate, the greater the response to chemotherapy. Tumor size affects response because the smaller number of cancer cells correlates to an improved response to treatment. In addition, when the tumor cells are young, a larger percentage of proliferating cells is more vulnerable to chemotherapy.

Certain anatomic sites offer a protected climate from the effects of chemotherapy. Few agents, such as nitrosoureas and bleomycin, cross the blood–brain barrier lending the brain protection from the effects of chemotherapy. The presence of resistant tumor cells reduces the likelihood of chemotherapy producing a positive effect. This is accomplished when mutation of cancer cells results in variant cells resistant to chemotherapy and when certain cancer cells are unable to convert the drug to an active form (Bender & Rosenzweig, 2004).

The majority of chemotherapeutic agents are most effective when working against dividing cells, not those in a resting phase as seen in G_0. As the tumor grows, more cells become inactive and convert to the resting phase. The presence of noncycling cells and drug resistance are the main difficulties encountered in the development of chemotherapeutic agents.

Classification

Chemotherapeutic drugs are classified or categorized according to their structure and mechanism of action. Similarities and differences exist between agents in the same classification. Those agents that act during a specific cell phase are classified as cell-cycle phase-specific drugs and are known to destroy cells that are actively dividing. Certain agents act on the S phase affecting DNA and RNA synthesis, whereas others act on the M phase, which terminates spindle formation. Chemotherapeutic agents that are active throughout the entire cell cycle are called cell-cycle phase-nonspecific drugs. These agents exert a longer acting effect on cells, leading to cell death or damage. Combining these two types of chemotherapeutic agents increases the number of susceptible tumor cells destroyed during a treatment period and reduces the adverse affects on normal cells, which affords the patient the possibility of achieving an improved response to treatment (Rokita, 2004). The Pharmacology Summary lists common antineoplastic (and biotherapy) agents used to treat cancer along with their common side effects and the related nursing interventions. This list is not meant to be comprehensive; rather, it gives an overview of information the nurse needs when planning care for a patient with cancer.

Administration and Safe Handling

Chemotherapeutic drugs are administered in a variety of locations and by a variety of routes. These agents can be given to patients who are in the hospital, in an outpatient infusion center, or in the home. Depending on the type of agent used, they may be given by the following routes: oral, intravenous, intramuscular, subcutaneous, arterial, intracavitary, and intrathecal. An oncology nurse knows, through experience and training, that the route is determined by the drug used, dose, type, location, and extent of tumor. Special education and training are essential in order to develop a safe practice for administering chemotherapy. The Oncology Nurses Society (ONS), together with OSHA,

has developed guidelines for the administration and handling of chemotherapy and biotherapy (Occupational Safety and Health Administration, Office of Occupational Medicine, 1995).

Safety Concerns

With the development of numerous chemotherapeutic agents in recent years came a heightened awareness of the hazards associated with those agents. Exposure to these agents can occur by inhalation, absorption, or digestion. Those handling chemotherapeutic agents need to be given training regarding the hazards and how to implement safeguards that will protect themselves and others. Hospitals and regulatory agencies recognize the risk to health care professionals and have developed precautions for those involved in the preparation, administration, and disposal of chemotherapeutic agents (Otto, 2001a). Chart 64–20 (p. 2109) lists the common precautions that should be taken by those caring for the patient receiving chemotherapy, including suggestions that would apply in home care settings. Typically nurses do not prepare chemotherapy agents, however, it is important to understand the safety precautions implemented by others to appreciate the seriousness of agents they will be asked to administer. Education of all staff is an ongoing process that should include a discussion of unique patient care situations, introduction of new equipment, and reproductive issues (Singleton & Connor, 1999).

Dose Calculations

Chemotherapeutic agents are dosed based on the body surface area (BSA) in adults and children. Pharmacists who prepare chemotherapy agents use equations to determine the appropriate dose for a patient based on his height and weight. To maintain accurate dosing, it is crucial for the nurse to monitor weight changes throughout the course of chemotherapy and communicate this information to the pharmacist. A patient's weight frequently changes throughout treatment due to drug-induced side effects such as nausea, vomiting, anorexia, and fatigue. Other factors that are considered when determining the dose of chemotherapy agents include renal function and other comorbidities (e.g., chronic obstructive pulmonary disease, heart failure, and renal failure).

Administration

The oncologist prescribing chemotherapy selects a route of administration that will deliver the optimal amount of drug to the tumor. A variety of methods are used to meet this goal. Chart 64–21 (p. 2110) explains the routes of administration along with specific nursing concerns for each. The nurse should understand the decision to use a specific delivery method and route is based on the pharmacokinetics of the drug to be used, as well as, characteristics of the patient and the cancer (Erickson, 2003).

Oral and intravenous (IV) routes are the most commonly used. All delivery methods have associated inherent risks. Intravenously administered agents pose particular concern associated with the risk of irritation to the vessel wall and extravasation (leaking of drug into tissue surrounding infusion site) causing local tissue damage. Chemotherapeutic drugs that cause severe local tissue breakdown and necrosis are called *vesicants* (Bender & Rosenzweig, 2004). Nurses need to be alert to symptoms common with extravasation such as pain, swelling, redness, and appearance of vesicles on the skin.

PHARMACOLOGY Summary of Medications for Cancer Treatment

Medication Category	Action	Application/Indications	Nursing Responsibility
Biotherapy Agents			
Interferons: • α-Interferon • β-Interferon • γ-Interferon	Antiviral and antitumor properties. Stimulate immune system or stop tumor growth. Enhance lymphocyte and antibody production. Assist with destruction of macrophages and natural killer cells. Inhibit cell replication by increasing phases of cell cycle. Mediate function of other cytokines (e.g., IL-2, TNF).	α-Interferon approved for use in hairy-cell leukemia, Kaposi's sarcoma, CML, high-grade non-Hodgkin's lymphoma, and melanoma. β-Interferon, γ-interferon approved for use in a variety of nonmalignant diseases.	Monitor for depression. Notify health care provider for possible consultation to social services and/or psychiatry. Monitor for flu-like symptoms (e.g., fevers, chills, malaise, headache, anorexia). Monitor for evidence of dehydration (e.g., concentrated urine, poor skin turgor, dry mucous membranes). Monitor electrolytes. Monitor for signs of infection (e.g., fever, increased sputum, dyspnea, urgency, and frequency). Implement neutropenic precautions as necessary. Implement safety precautions during activity. Administer antidiarrheals.
Interleukins	Produced by lymphocytes and monocytes. Known as lymphokines and monokines. Stimulate the proliferation of T lymphocytes and activation of natural killer cells. Stimulate the release of other cytokines (e.g., TNF, γ-interferon).	Most ILs are under investigation for use in the clinical setting. IL-2 is currently being used for the following conditions: • Metastatic renal cell carcinoma • Advanced metastatic melanoma • AML • Non-Hodgkin's lymphoma	Monitor for severe flu-like symptoms (e.g., fevers, chills, rigors, malaise, headache, anorexia). Monitor for capillary leak syndrome (e.g., generalized edema, decreased urine output, hypotension). Monitor for evidence of dehydration (e.g., concentrated urine, poor skin turgor, dry mucous membranes). Monitor electrolytes. Monitor for signs of infection (e.g., fever, increased sputum, dyspnea, urgency, and frequency). Implement neutropenic precautions as necessary. Implement safety precautions during activity. Administer antidiarrheals.
Granulocyte colony-stimulating factor: • Neupogen	Promote proliferation and differentiation of neutrophils. Enhance functional properties of mature neutrophils. Stimulate granulocyte and macrophage proliferation. Enhances functional properties of mature granulocytes and macrophages.	Used to treat or prevent severe thrombocytopenia and to reduce the need for platelet transfusions. Used after induction therapy in AML. Used after allogeneic and autologous bone marrow transplant (BMT).	Monitor for flu-like symptoms (e.g., fevers, chills, malaise, headache, anorexia). Monitor for bone pain and administer analgesics as needed. Monitor skin for development of rashes. Monitor for hypertension. Monitor for signs of decreased cardiac output or inadequate tissue perfusion (e.g., diaphoresis, pale color, poor-quality pulses, chest pain, edema, crackles, decreased urine output).
Granulocyte macrophage colony-stimulating factor: • Leukine	Stimulate growth and differentiation of stem cells in bone marrow to increase RBC production. Secreted by the kidney.	Used to treat chronic anemia associated with end-stage renal disease and anemia associated with cancer and HIV treatment.	
Hematopoietic growth factors: • Erythropoietin (Epogen) • Oprelvekin (Neumega)	Stimulate growth and development of platelets.	Used in acute promyelocytic leukemia, which is an extremely rare form of leukemia.	

(continued)

PHARMACOLOGY Summary of Medications for Cancer Treatment—*Continued*

Medication Category	Action	Application/Indications	Nursing Responsibility
Monoclonal Antibodies (MAbs): • Cetuximab (Erbitux) • Gemtuzumab ozogamicin (Mylotarg) • Ibritumomab tiuxetan (Zevalin) • Rituximab (Rituxan) • Trastuzumab (Herceptin) **Angiogenesis inhibitor (VEGF):** • Bevacizumab (Avastin)	Produced by injecting mice with tumor cells that act as antigens and obtaining antibodies from their spleens. Antibody cells are combined with cancer cells to produce more antibodies (hybridoma). Unconjugated: directly attack tumor cells; conjugated: attached to other agents (radioisotopes, toxins, chemotherapy). Aid in diagnostic evaluation by combining with a radioactive substance (radioimmunodetection).	For use in detecting and treating ovarian, breast, pancreatic, gastric, esophageal, and colorectal cancers. Used in purging tumor cells from bone marrow and peripheral blood prior to bone marrow transplantation. Treatment of cancers: • Non-Hodgkin's lymphoma • Metastatic breast cancer that overexpresses the HER2 oncogene (known to be associated with aggressive disease and decreased survival) • Leukemia (used in prevention of graft versus host disease (GVHD) after transplantation) • Metastatic colorectal cancer	Monitor CBC and differential. Monitor for signs of bleeding (e.g., bruising, bloody stool/urine, hypotension, tachycardia). Monitor for signs of infection (e.g., fever, increased sputum, dyspnea, urgency, and frequency). Implement neutropenic precautions as necessary. Monitor for signs of hypersensitivity reaction (changes in BP, rash, edema, facial flushing, dyspnea). Monitor for evidence of dehydration (e.g., concentrated urine, poor skin turgor, dry mucous membranes). Monitor electrolytes. Administer antiemetics as needed. Administer antidiarrheals as needed. Monitor for signs of decreased cardiac output or inadequate tissue perfusion (e.g., diaphoresis, pale color, poor-quality pulses, chest pain, edema, crackles, decreased urine output). Monitor renal function tests (e.g., creatinine, BUN, creatinine clearance). Encourage the use of oral saline rinses and avoiding the use of mouthwashes. Provide list of community resources for wigs, hats, caps, etc. Instruct patient about reproductive issues and provide resources as needed.
Antineoplastic Agents Alkylating agents: • Busulfan • Carboplatin • Chlorambucil • Cisplatin • Cyclophosphamide • Dacarbazine • Ifosfamide • Melphalan • Nitrogen mustard	Disrupt DNA replication and RNA transcription by cross-linking DNA strands. Cell cycle nonspecific.	Ovarian, breast, lung, testicular, and head and neck cancer. Multiple myeloma, leukemias, lymphoma, sarcoma.	Monitor CBC and differential. Monitor for signs of bleeding (e.g., bruising, bloody stool/urine, hypotension, tachycardia). Monitor for signs of infection (e.g., fever, increased sputum, dyspnea, urgency, and frequency). Implement neutropenic precautions as necessary. Monitor for evidence of dehydration (e.g., concentrated urine, poor skin turgor, dry mucous membranes). Monitor electrolytes. Administer antiemetics as needed. Administer antidiarrheals as needed. Encourage the use of oral saline rinses and avoiding the use of mouthwashes. Provide list of community resources for wigs, hats, caps, etc. Monitor for signs of seizures and implement seizure precautions. Monitor renal function tests (e.g., creatinine, BUN, creatinine clearance). Instruct patient to drink plenty of fluids prior to and during treatment. Administer bladder protectant as needed (Mesna). Instruct patient about reproductive issues and provide resources as needed.

PHARMACOLOGY Summary of Medications for Cancer Treatment—*Continued*

Medication Category	Action	Application/Indications	Nursing Responsibility
Nitrosoureas: • Carmustine (BCNU) • Lomustine (CCNU) • Semustine (methyl-CCNU) • Streptozocin	Block enzymes needed for synthesis of purine, resulting in immediate cell death. Similar actions to alkylating agents; cross blood–brain barrier. Cell cycle nonspecific.	Lymphomas, multiple myeloma, CNS tumors, malignant melanoma, pancreatic cancer.	Monitor CBC and differential. Monitor for signs of bleeding (e.g., bruising, bloody stool/urine, hypotension, tachycardia). Monitor for signs of infection (e.g., fever, increased sputum, dyspnea, urgency, and frequency). Implement neutropenic precautions as necessary. Monitor for evidence of dehydration (e.g., concentrated urine, poor skin turgor, dry mucous membranes). Monitor electrolytes. Administer antiemetics as needed. Instruct patient to drink plenty of fluids prior to treatment. Administer bladder protectant as needed (Mesna). Monitor renal function tests (e.g., creatinine, BUN, creatinine clearance). Monitor serum osmolarity and electrolytes. Monitor dyspnea and cough.
Antimetabolites: • Methotrexate (MTX) • Cytarabine (Ara-C) • Fluorouracil (5-FU) • Gemcitabine (Gemzar) • Hydroxyurea • Deoxycoformycin (pentostatin) • Capecitabine (Xeloda)	Hinder the synthesis of DNA by blocking the use of necessary enzymes. Cell cycle phase-specific (S phase).	Leukemias, lymphomas, myelodysplasia syndrome, breast and colon cancer.	Monitor CBC and differential. Monitor for signs of bleeding (e.g., bruising, bloody stool/urine, hypotension, tachycardia). Monitor for signs of infection (e.g., fever, increased sputum, dyspnea, urgency, and frequency). Implement neutropenic precautions as necessary. Monitor for evidence of dehydration (e.g., concentrated urine, poor skin turgor, dry mucous membranes). Monitor break in skin integrity (e.g., rashes, blistering on palms and feet). Monitor liver and renal function and electrolytes. Administer antiemetics as needed. Instruct patient to drink plenty of fluids prior to treatment. Encourage the use of saline rinses and avoiding the use of mouthwashes. Provide ice water during drug administration. Administer analgesics as needed. Provide list of community resources for wigs, hats, caps, etc. Encourage use of sunscreen year-round.

MyNursingkit | Animation: Drugs Methotrexate

(continued)

PHARMACOLOGY Summary of Medications for Cancer Treatment—*Continued*

Medication Category	Action	Application/Indications	Nursing Responsibility
Antitumor antibiotics: • Bleomycin • Daunorubicin • Doxorubicin (Adriamycin) • Mitoxantrone	Interfere with function and synthesis of nucleic acids, resulting in disruption of RNA and DNA replication. Cell cycle nonspecific.	Various solid tumors. Lymphomas and acute lymphocytic leukemia.	For vesicants: IV push over 6–10 minutes, flushing with 75–100 mL solution. Monitor CBC and differential. Monitor for signs of bleeding (e.g., bruising, bloody stool/urine, hypotension, tachycardia). Monitor for signs of infection (e.g., fever, increased sputum, dyspnea, urgency, and frequency). Implement neutropenic precautions as necessary. Monitor for evidence of dehydration (e.g., concentrated urine, poor skin turgor, dry mucous membranes). Monitor electrolytes. Administer antiemetics as needed. Encourage the use of saline rinses and avoiding the use of mouthwashes. Provide ice water during drug administration. Administer analgesics as needed. Administer appetite stimulants as needed. Monitor for signs of decreased cardiac output or inadequate tissue perfusion (e.g., diaphoresis, pale color, poor-quality pulses, chest pain, edema, crackles, decreased urine output). Monitor for cough and dyspnea. Instruct patient about potential darkening of previously irradiated areas. Provide list of community resources for wigs, hats, caps, etc.
Plant alkaloids (Taxane): • Paclitaxel (Taxol) • Docetaxel (Taxotere)	Stabilize microtubule, which interferes with cell division. Cell cycle phase-specific (G_2 and M phase).	Breast, non–small cell lung, ovarian, and head and neck cancer.	For vesicants: IV push over 6–10 minutes, flushing with 75–100 mL solution. Premedicate with diphenhydramine, cimetidine, and dexamethasone. Monitor for signs of hypersensitivity reaction (changes in BP, rash, edema, facial flushing, dyspnea). Monitor neurological status (motor weakness, paresthesia). Provide list of community resources for wigs, hats, caps, etc. Monitor CBC and differential. Monitor for signs of bleeding (e.g., bruising, bloody stool/urine, hypotension, tachycardia). Monitor for signs of infection (e.g., fever, increased sputum, dyspnea, urgency, and frequency). Implement neutropenic precautions as necessary. Instruct patient to allow for frequent rest periods and to cluster activities as possible. Administer analgesics as needed. Monitor for signs of decreased cardiac output or inadequate tissue perfusion (e.g., diaphoresis, pale color, poor-quality pulses, chest pain, edema, crackles, decreased urine output).

PHARMACOLOGY Summary of Medications for Cancer Treatment—*Continued*

Medication Category	Action	Application/Indications	Nursing Responsibility
Plant alkaloids (vinca alkaloids): • Vinorelbine (Navelbine) • Vincristine • Vinblastine	Inhibit mitosis, resulting in immediate cell death (cytocidal). Cell cycle phase-specific (M phase).	Breast, testicular, small-cell lung, ovarian, and head and neck cancers. Lymphomas, acute lymphocytic leukemia (ALL), Chronic Myelogenous leukemia (CML).	For vesicants: IV push over 6–10 minutes, flushing with 75–100 mL solution. Monitor for local skin changes. Monitor CBC and differential. Monitor for signs of bleeding (e.g., bruising, bloody stool/urine, hypotension, tachycardia). Monitor for signs of infection (e.g., fever, increased sputum, dyspnea, urgency, and frequency). Implement neutropenic precautions as necessary. Monitor neurological status (motor weakness, paresthesia). Monitor liver function tests. Administer laxatives, stool softeners. Administer analgesics as needed. Provide list of community resources for wigs, hats, caps, etc.
Plant alkaloids (camptothecins): • Irinotecan • Topotecan	Alter DNA structure by inhibiting topoisomerase I. Cell cycle phase-specific (S phase).	Colorectal, non–small cell lung, and ovarian cancer. ALL.	Monitor CBC and differential. Monitor for signs of bleeding (e.g., bruising, bloody stool/urine, hypotension, tachycardia). Monitor for signs of infection (e.g., fever, increased sputum, dyspnea, urgency, and frequency). Implement neutropenic precautions as necessary. Administer atropine as needed to reduce cholinergic-induced diarrhea. Monitor for signs of dehydration (e.g., concentrated urine, poor skin turgor, dry mucous membranes). Provide list of community resources for wigs, hats, caps, etc.
Plant alkaloids (epipodophyllotoxins): • Etoposide (VP-16) • Teniposide (VM-26)	Irreversible blocking of cells during premitotic phases, resulting in destruction of DNA strands. Interferes with topoisomerase II enzyme reaction. Cell cycle phase-specific (late G_2 and S phase).	Breast, testicular, and small-cell lung cancer. Lymphomas, ALL, and multiple myeloma.	Monitor CBC and differential. Monitor for signs of bleeding (e.g., bruising, bloody stool/urine, hypotension, tachycardia). Monitor for signs of infection (e.g., fever, increased sputum, dyspnea, urgency, and frequency). Implement neutropenic precautions as necessary. Monitor for evidence of dehydration (e.g., concentrated urine, poor skin turgor, dry mucous membranes). Monitor electrolytes. Administer antiemetics as needed. Monitor blood pressure throughout infusion. Monitor for signs of anaphylaxis (changes in BP, rash, edema, facial flushing). Provide list of community resources for wigs, hats, caps, etc.

(continued)

Medication Category	Action	Application/Indications	Nursing Responsibility
Hormonal Therapy Glucocorticoids: • Prednisone • Hydrocortisone • Solu-Medrol • Dexamethasone Estrogens: • Diethylstilbestrol (DES) • Estramustine (Emcyt) • Estradiol (Estrace) Antiestrogens: • Tamoxifen Estrogen receptor antagonists: • Fulvestrant (Faslodex) Nonsteroidal aromatase inhibitors: • Anastrozole (Arimidex) Steroidal aromatase inhibitors: • Exemestane (Aromasin) Luteinizing hormone-releasing hormone (LHRH) analog • Leuprolide (Lupron) Nonsteroid antiestrogen: • Bicalutamide (Casodex) • Flutamide (Eulexin)	Interfere with proteins and hormone receptors throughout the cell cycle. Cell cycle nonspecific.	Prostate, breast, and endometrial cancers.	Monitor CBC and differential. Monitor for signs of infection (e.g., fever, increased sputum, dyspnea, urgency, and frequency). Implement neutropenic precautions as necessary. Monitor blood pressure. Instruct the patient to lower sodium intake. Instruct the patient to observe for swelling in the ankles, lower extremities, and hands. Instruct the patient to avoid discontinuing medication unless advised by health care provider. Instruct patient about signs of feminization and masculinization.
Miscellaneous: • Asparaginase (Elspar) • Bortezomib (Velcade) • Hydroxyurea • Imatinib mesylate (Gleevec)	Inhibit protein synthesis. Inhibit chymotrypsin-like activity of 25S proteasome. Act on S phase as an antimetabolite. Inhibit proliferation and induce apoptosis.	ALL. Multiple myeloma. Chronic myelogenous leukemia, melanoma, and head and neck cancer. Chronic myelogenous leukemia in blast crisis or chronic phase with failure of interferon.	Monitor CBC and differential. Monitor for signs of bleeding (e.g., bruising, bloody stool/urine, hypotension, tachycardia). Monitor for signs of infection (e.g., fever, increased sputum, dyspnea, urgency, and frequency). Implement neutropenic precautions as necessary. Monitor for evidence of dehydration (e.g., concentrated urine, poor skin turgor, dry mucous membranes). Monitor electrolytes. Monitor for signs of hypersensitivity reaction (changes in BP, rash, edema, facial flushing, dyspnea). Administer antiemetics as needed. Administer analgesics as needed (e.g., nonopioids for neuropathic pain). Administer laxatives as needed. Monitor level of sedation and implement safety measures as needed. Encourage the use of saline rinses and avoiding the use of mouthwashes. Provide ice water during drug administration.

Sources: Bender, C., & Rosenzweig, M. (2004). Cancer. In S. Lewis, M. Heitkemper, & S. Dirksen (Eds.), *Medical–surgical nursing assessment and management of clinical problems* (6th ed.). St. Louis: Mosby; Rokita, S. (2004). Oncology: Nursing management in cancer care. In S. Smeltzer & B. Bare (Eds.), *Brunner & Suddarth's textbook of medical–surgical nursing* (10th ed.). Philadelphia: Lippincott Williams & Wilkins; Viele, C. (2005). Keys to unlock cancer: Targeted therapy. *Oncology Nursing Forum, 32*(5).

CHART 64–20	**Safe Handling of Chemotherapeutic Drugs**

Drug Preparation

Prepare in a biological safety cabinet (BSC):

- Vented system to outside environment
- Provide vertical laminar airflow to carry contaminated air away from BSC operator
- Blower that operates continuously
- Located in low traffic area
- Used only with trained individuals.

Handwashing prior to donning personal protective equipment (PPE).

Wear appropriate (PPE):

- Gloves that are powder free with long cuffs (change every 30 minutes)
- Gowns
- Face shields or goggles
- PPE should be replaced if torn, punctured, or soiled.

Use plastic-backed sterile absorbent pad on work surface.

Maintain sterile technique.

Use appropriate technique when opening ampules.

When reconstituting drugs in vials, use dispensing pins with venting devices to avoid aerosolization.

Use tubing and syringes with Luer-lock fittings.

Avoid overfilling of syringes.

Prime all tubing with normal saline or dextrose prior to adding cytotoxic drug.

Label each container "Cytotoxic Drug."

Place container in sealed bag before transport.

Dispose of all material that has come into contact with cytotoxic drug into appropriate receptacle.

Drug Administration

Explain to patient that protective wear minimizes the exposure of health care providers to the harmful effects of chemotherapeutic drugs.

Wear appropriate PPE.

Implement High Alert Medication Safety practice.

Administer drugs in a safe and unhurried environment, working at eye level.

Use Luer-lock fittings on all intravenous tubing, needles, and syringes used for delivery of cytotoxic drugs.

Place disposable, absorbent, plastic-backed pad under work area to collect droplets of the drug.

Implement standard precautions when handing the blood, vomitus, or excreta of a patient who has received cytotoxic drugs within the last 48 hours.

Disposal of Supplies and Drugs

Do not recap needles or break syringes.

Placed all used supplies in a leak proof, puncture proof, labeled container.

Keep containers in all areas where preparation and administration of cytotoxic drugs occur.

Environmental service personnel trained in safe handling procedures should remove containers.

Personnel should wear appropriate PPE.

Containers should be disposed of according to regulations of hazardous wastes.

In home situations:

- Place containers in an area away from children and pets until retrieved by appropriate agency.
- Check county and state regulations.

Arrange with medical supply company, health care provider's office, or private waste management company for proper disposal.

Sources: Occupational Safety and Health Administration, Office of Occupational Medicine. (1995). *Controlling occupational exposure to hazardous CPL2-2.20B CH-4.* Washington, DC: U.S. Department of Labor; Singleton, L., & Connor, T. (1999). An evaluation of the permeability of chemotherapy gloves to three cancer chemotherapy drugs. *Oncology Nursing Forum, 26*(4); The Joint Commision, (2008). *High Alert Medication: Strategies for Improving Safety,* Joint Commission Resources.

Agency policy will identify nursing actions required once symptoms of extravasation have been recognized. Oftentimes IV drugs are delivered via central vascular access devices. Refer to Chapter 22 🔗 for detailed information on these types of devices along with the nursing implications.

Chemotherapy Side Effects and Toxicities

Chemotherapy produces effects on both normal cells and cancer cells. Side effects or toxic effects are the result of the destruction of normal cells that produce specific signs and symptoms and are classified as acute, delayed, or chronic. Chart 64–22 (p. 2112) lists the effects found in each category (Bender & Rosenzweig, 2004). Cells with rapid growth rates are more susceptible to damage, resulting in noticeable signs and symptoms. Examples of cells affected by this process are epithelium, bone marrow, hair follicles, and sperm. The body will respond to the products of cellular destruction by demonstrating fatigue, anorexia, and taste alterations.

Gastrointestinal System Effects

Nausea and vomiting are the most common gastrointestinal (GI) side effects. Within 1 hour of therapy commencing the patient may experience vomiting that may last up to 24 hours or more. Drugs that can reduce or eliminate nausea and vomiting are an essential part of the treatment plan for patients receiving chemotherapeutic agents and may be given prior to therapy starting and for several days after it ends. Antiemetics include serotonin blockers, which block serotonin receptors located in the GI tract and chemoreceptor trigger zone (CTZ) in the medulla, dopaminergic blockers that block dopamine receptors of the CTZ, phenothiazines, sedatives, corticosteroids, and histamines. The latter four agents are commonly used in combination with serotonin blockers when patients receive chemotherapeutic drugs that have increased emetic potential (Bremerkamp, 2000).

Nurses are responsible for being aware of the types of drugs their patients are receiving so they can anticipate what interventions may be needed to relieve suffering from nausea and vomiting. Some patients will require antiemetic therapy for several days after chemotherapy and need to be encouraged to comply with their prescribed medication regime to lessen the emetic effects of the chemotherapy. Other interventions such as relaxation techniques, guided imagery, and altering the patient's diet may also assist in reducing nausea and vomiting.

CHART 64–21	**Routes of Administration**

Route		Nursing Implications
Oral	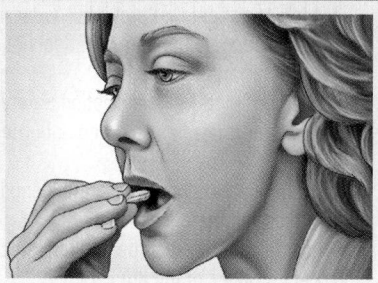	• Educate the patient about the significance of complying with prescribed schedule, optimal dosing, and patient safety. • Devise educational strategies such as individualized medication sheets to reinforce information. • Educate the patient about strategies to reduce potential for side effects (e.g., taking drugs with emetic potential with meals, taking drugs that require adequate fluid intake early in the day). • Coordinate educational sessions with oncologist and pharmacist since nurses may have minimal patient contact.
Subcutaneous	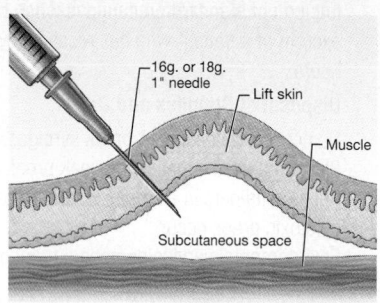	• Educate the patient and/or caregiver to give injections and allow for return demonstration. • Encourage patient to rotate injection sites and keep written log.
Intramuscular	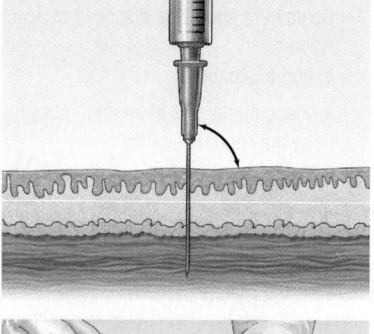	Same as subcutaneous.
Intravenous (may be given via central venous catheters or peripheral venous access) • Push • Piggyback • Side-arm • Infusion	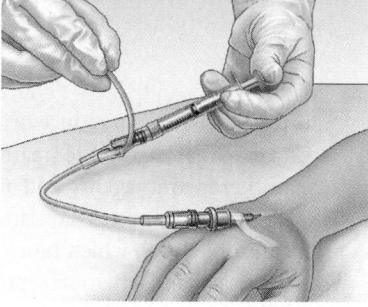 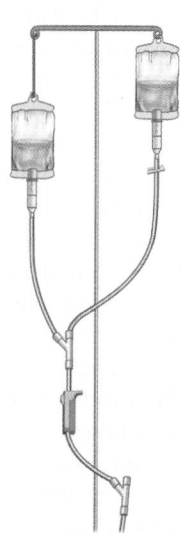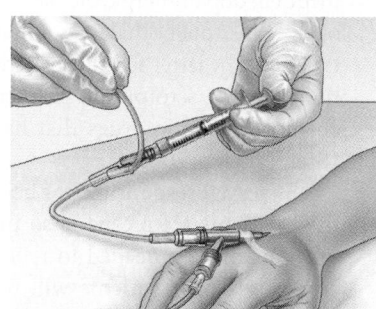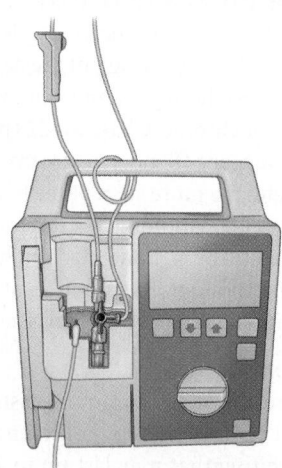	• Administered directly into vein via a syringe. • Administered using a secondary bag and tubing while primary infusion is running concurrently. • Administered into the side port of a running IV infusion. • Drug is added to appropriate size IV bag. • All medications administered via the IV route should have the blood return of the vein evaluated at regular intervals during the infusion (as determined by agency policy).

Labels in Subcutaneous figure: 16g. or 18g. 1" needle; Lift skin; Muscle; Subcutaneous space

| CHART 64–21 | **Routes of Administration—*Continued*** |

Route	Nursing Implications
Topical 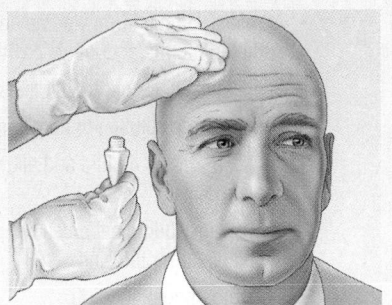	• Educate the patient to cover surface area with thin layer of medication, then wear loose-fitting clothing. • Wear gloves during application and perform hand hygiene after procedure. • Educate the patient to avoid touching the medication.
Intracavitary 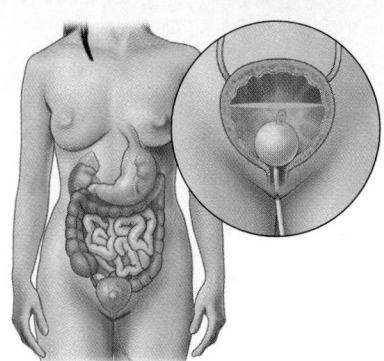	• Instill medication into either the bladder (via a catheter) or the pleural cavity (via a chest tube). • Administer premedication to reduce local irritation.
Intrathecal 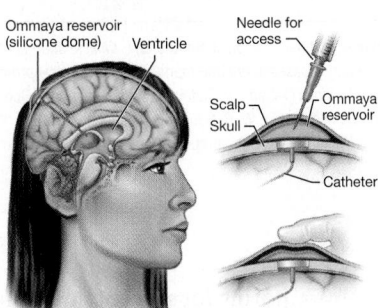	• An Ommaya reservoir, which is subcutaneously implanted, is used to gain access to ventricular cerebrospinal fluid (CSF). • Used to treat cancers that metastasize to central nervous system (CNS) (breast, lung, GI, leukemia, and lymphoma). • Does not depend on diffusion to move drug into CSF. • May last months to years without complications. • Sterile technique used throughout procedure. • Usually administered by a health care provider. • Evaluate for neurotoxicities.
Intra-arterial 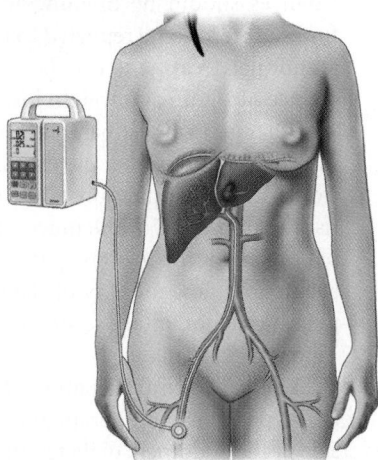	• Catheter placement into artery near inoperable tumor (liver, bladder, brain, head and neck, cervix, and bone). • Use infusion pump. • Monitor vital signs, color and temperature of extremity, and signs of local bleeding throughout therapy. • Monitor appropriate laboratory studies (e.g., liver function tests) for organ toxicity. • Educate patient about the care of the catheter and pump if to be used at home.

(continued)

CHART 64–21	Routes of Administration—*Continued*

Route	Nursing Implications
Intraperitoneal 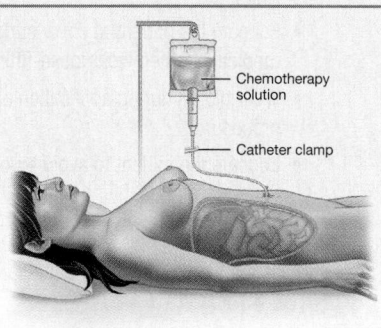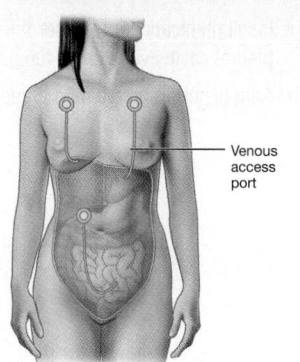	• Administration of drug via implantable port or external suprapubic catheter into the abdominal cavity. • Used typically for peritoneal metastases due to ovarian cancer. • Heat infusate solution to body temperature prior to infusing. • Infuse 1–2 liters of fluid and allow to "dwell" for 1–4 hours before draining. • Monitor for abdominal pressure, pain, fever, and electrolyte imbalance after infusing. • Measure abdominal girth.

Sources: Barber, F., & Fabugais-Nazario, L. (2003). What's old is new again: Patients receiving hepatic arterial infusion chemotherapy. *Clinical Journal of Oncology Nursing, 7*(6); Bender, C., & Rosenzweig, M. (2004). Cancer. In S. Lewis, M. Heitkemper, & S. Dirksen (Eds.), *Medical–surgical nursing assessment and management of clinical problems* (6th ed.). St. Louis: Mosby; Booker, M. (1996a). Arterial therapy. In M. Booker & D. Ignatavicius (Eds.), *Infusion therapy techniques and medications* (1st ed.). Philadelphia: W. B. Saunders; Booker, M. (1996b). Central nervous system therapy. In M. Booker & D. Ignatavicius (Eds.), *Infusion therapy techniques and medications* (1st ed.). Philadelphia: W. B. Saunders; Hartigan, K. (2003). Patient education: The cornerstone of successful oral chemotherapy treatment. *Clinical Journal of Oncology Nursing, 7*(6); Markam, M., & Walker, J. (2006). Intraperitoneal chemotherapy of ovarian cancer: A review with a focus on practical aspects of treatment. *Journal of Clinical Oncology, 24*(6).

CHART 64–22	Classification of Chemotherapy Toxicities

Classification	Toxicity
Acute	Vomiting Allergic reactions Cardiac arrhythmias
Delayed	Mucositis: • Mouth sores • Gastritis • Diarrhea Alopecia Bone marrow suppression
Chronic	Cardiac damage: • Reduced contractility Pulmonary damage: • Fibrosis and scarring Hepatic damage: • Elevated liver enzyme tests Renal damage: • Elevated creatinine and BUN

Monitoring for signs of fluid volume deficit and electrolyte imbalances should be ongoing nursing actions, and abnormal findings need to be reported to the health care provider so that additional treatment can be started in order to reduce the chance of significant weight loss and malnutrition.

Other gastrointestinal (GI) toxicities are due to the rapid rate of proliferation of the cells that line the GI tract. These include stomatitis (inflammation of the oral cavity), anorexia, mucositis (inflammation of the mucosal lining), and diarrhea. Constipation can occur in some patients receiving chemotherapeutic agents that slow motility of the large intestine and may be due to reduced food intake secondary to persistent nausea and vomiting (ONS, 2001).

Pancreatitis (inflammation of the pancreas) occurs with certain types of chemotherapeutic agents, radiotherapy to the left side of the abdomen, diabetes, tumor lysis syndrome (TLS), and the presence of intrahepatic catheters (ONS, 2001). Common signs and symptoms include abdominal pain, fever, tachycardia, and nausea and vomiting. When a patient is suspected of having pancreatitis, the nurse should review laboratory data for elevated serum amylase and lipase and hypoglycemia. Pancreatitis, if not successfully treated, can put the patient at risk for developing shock leading to possible death. Nurses administering chemotherapy agents known to cause pancreatitis should be alert to potential signs and symptoms and collaborate with the oncologist to begin prompt treatment.

Although not real common, hepatotoxicity occurs due to the direct toxic effect to the liver as a result of the metabolism of antineoplastic drugs. The likelihood of developing liver dysfunction related to chemotherapy is increased if the patient has a history of prior infections or damage (cirrhosis, hepatitis), cancer of the liver, radiotherapy to the right side of the abdomen, history of alcoholism, intrahepatic chemotherapy, and advancing age (Ludwig et al., 1999). Clinical findings associated with hepatotoxicity are those consistent with liver dysfunction, including jaundice, ascites, fatigue, malaise, anorexia, nausea and vomiting, right upper quadrant pain, dark orange urine, and bleeding tendencies. In addition, laboratory data used to determine hepatic function such as liver function tests and coagulation studies will be abnormal.

Genitourinary System Effects

A few chemotherapy agents damage kidneys due to the accumulation of end products after cell lysis and the direct effect during excretion. Chemotherapy can cause tumors to undergo rapid cell lysis, which causes an increase in uric acid production and urinary excretion resulting in kidney damage. In addition, the release of intracellular contents in the circulation causes increased levels of serum potassium and phosphates and decreased levels of serum calcium. Nurses need to be aware of the renal effect of the chemotherapy agent being administered and monitor serum blood urea nitrogen (BUN), creatinine, electrolytes, and creatinine clearance. Abnormal findings need to be reported to the health care provider so adjustments in drug dosing can be considered. Prevention of uric acid crystals can be accomplished by ensuring adequate hydration, alkalinization of the urine, and administering drugs aimed at reducing serum uric acid.

Hemorrhagic cystitis is bladder mucosal damage occurring as a result of inflammation and irritation from the metabolism of by-products of chemotherapeutic agents. The development of hemorrhagic cystitis is associated with administration of certain alkylating agents and prior radiotherapy to the pelvis or bladder. Nurses need to be alert to the few, but important, signs and symptoms that may produce suffering for most of these patients. These include dysuria, frequency, nocturia, oliguria, and hematuria.

Cardiopulmonary System Effects

Certain chemotherapeutic agents have toxic effects on the cardiopulmonary system that may produce permanent functional changes for the patient. Patients who are to receive antitumor antibiotics should have a cardiac evaluation prior to treatment to determine baseline cardiac function. During therapy the nurse needs to monitor for heart failure and signs of decreased cardiac output. A decrease in pulmonary function is a lifelong effect associated with long-term chemotherapy. Nurses need to evaluate the patient for changes in pulmonary function, including pulmonary function tests (Rokita, 2004).

Hematopoietic System Effects

The majority of chemotherapy agents cause a disruption in the normal functioning of the immune system. *Myelosuppression* is the term used to define a depression of bone marrow function. WBCs, RBCs, and platelets are susceptible to bone marrow suppression from chemotherapy. Neutropenia (reduced neu-

trophils) and thrombocytopenia (reduced platelets) along with the presence of anemia (reduced hemoglobin and hematocrit) are the main factors that limit the doses of chemotherapy given to a patient (Rokita, 2004).

Neutropenia is defined as a reduction in the number of circulating neutrophils, whereas leukopenia is defined as a reduction in the number of circulating WBCs. The importance of monitoring the neutrophils in those patients receiving chemotherapy lies in their ability to protect the host from bacterial invasion. Assessing the laboratory data includes monitoring the WBC count and calculating the **absolute neutrophil count (ANC)**. Calculation of the ANC is done by multiplying the WBC by the total percentage of neutrophils (polys and bands):

Example:

Laboratory result: WBC = 1,600 polys = 48%; bands = 5%

Calculation: Polys (48%) + bands (5%) = 53%

WBC (1,600) × polys and bands (53%) = 848.

An ANC of less than 500 is considered to put the patient at severe risk of infection (Otto, 2001a). It is important for the nurse to understand that neutropenia can occur when the total WBC is within normal range; therefore, knowing the ANC allows a correct assessment of the neutrophil status.

The term **nadir** refers to the point at which the lowest blood count is reached. Oncology nurses understand that when a patient receives chemotherapy, the nadir occurs approximately 7 to 10 days after treatment, at which point the patient is most susceptible to infection. Providing ongoing patient education regarding the signs of infection and when to report findings to the health care provider is critical. A detailed discussion of nursing management of patients experiencing side effects from chemotherapy is found in the Nursing Process: Care Plan for Cancer feature earlier in this chapter (p. 2089).

 When caring for patients receiving chemotherapy or biotherapy, the nurse should evaluate the laboratory data to determine the presence of anemia, thrombocytopenia, and neutropenia. Calculation of the ANC will provide the most accurate picture of the patient's risk for infection. The nurse should notify the health care provider immediately if the patient demonstrates signs of infection.

The availability of drugs used to stimulate the bone marrow has allowed patients to continue with chemotherapy despite the associated side effects. Granulocyte colony-stimulating factor (G-CSF) and granulocyte-macrophage colony-stimulating factor (GM-CSF) stimulate the bone marrow to produce WBCs at a more rapid pace in order to reduce the duration of neutropenia. Erythropoietin (Epogen, Procrit) is used to increase the production of RBCs, thus playing a pivotal role in preventing the anemia-induced symptoms associated with chemotherapy. The benefit of administering these agents is a reduction of the incidence of infection that allows for continuing the prescribed chemotherapeutic drug regime.

Reproductive System Effects

Both testicular and ovarian functions can be affected by antineoplastic drug therapy. Sterility and early menopause are risks a patient needs to be aware of prior to receiving chemotherapy. Males may experience an absence of spermatozoa that can be either permanent or temporary. Men should be offered the option to bank sperm prior to the start of treatment to prevent damage to sperm or sterility. Education for both patients and their partners about the potential risk to reproductive functions and appropriate protection behaviors (e.g., reliable birth control) should be provided prior to beginning therapy (Rokita, 2004).

Neurological System Effects

Neurological effects are usually reversible and disappear after completion of chemotherapy treatments. Toxicities can arise as direct or indirect damage to the central nervous system (CNS), peripheral nervous system, cranial nerves, or a combination of the three. Peripheral neuropathies, loss of reflexes, hearing loss due to damage of the acoustic nerve, and paralytic ileus are examples of the more commonly occurring effects. The nurse needs to educate the patient and family about the importance of patient safety, detection of signs and symptoms, when to notify the health care provider of evidence of toxicity, and referrals for coping strategies.

General Effects

The incidence of fatigue has been identified in research frequently enough to consider it as a major concern in cancer symptom management (Nail, 2004). Fatigue is one of the many side effects seen during cancer therapy that can affect a person's ability to function. Several factors contribute to the degree of fatigue experienced by patients receiving chemotherapy. These include immobility, malnutrition, stress, lack of sleep, anemia, hypoxia, infection or febrile states, pain, and multiple cancer therapies (e.g., biotherapy, chemotherapy, radiation therapy, and surgery). The nurse needs to encourage patients to balance activity and rest, optimize nutritional intake, and consider physical therapy consultation if necessary.

◼ Nursing Management

Managing patients with cancer undergoing chemotherapy is complex and challenging. Nurses must be able to perform assessments that include the immune status, pain control, hemodynamic stability, and emotional coping. The ability to differentiate between toxic effects (e.g., heart failure), which can be irreversible, and expected side effects (nausea and vomiting), most of which can be managed successfully with other drugs, is one of the unique features of an oncology assessment.

The Nursing Process: Care Plan for Cancer feature earlier in this chapter (p. 2089) identifies the appropriate nursing diagnosis and provides a detailed plan of care for the oncology patient regardless of the type of treatment being given.

◼ Collaborative Management

The use of a multidisciplinary oncology team that effectively collaborates to achieve quality patient care is essential. The diagnosis of cancer holds many emotions and experiences for both the patient and family. A plan of care needs to consider the patient's ability to tolerate diagnostic efforts, treatment recommendations, and long-term recovery. Depending on multiple

variables, cancer tends to be a disease that is chronic in nature. Patients will demonstrate signs and symptoms relative to where they are in their disease trajectory and treatment plan. Each member of the team (health care providers, nurses, physical therapists, occupational therapists, speech therapists, social workers, psychiatrists/psychologists, pharmacists, and spiritual counselors) provides an expertise that will afford the patient and family the opportunity to optimize their quality of life throughout each phase of their disease.

Biotherapy

Biotherapy (biologic therapy) is known as treatment with agents whose origin, mostly mammal, is from biological sources and/or affecting biological responses (Oldham, 1991). Historically, cancer treatment has included surgery, radiotherapy, and chemotherapy, or a combination of all three therapies. Biotherapy has emerged since the 1980s as another treatment option for cancer patients receiving high-dose chemotherapy and transplantation. Nurses caring for patients receiving biotherapy need to possess an understanding of the immune system before they can begin to comprehend the rationale behind this unique treatment modality and the primary agents currently used. Refer to Chapters 59 ◔ and 60 ◔ for a review of the immune system. Although the mechanism of action varies with each type of biologic response modifier (BRM), the goal is the same: to destroy or halt the malignant growth of a tumor. A therapeutic effect is accomplished by altering the immunologic relationship between the tumor and the host (patient) (Rokita, 2004). Direct antitumor effects, restoration, augmentation, or modulation of host immune system mechanisms, and disrupting tumor cells' ability to metastasize or differentiate may affect host and tumor response. In addition, these agents, specifically monoclonal antibodies (MAbs), are used in diagnosing cancer by using low-dose radioisotopes tagged to MAbs that can detect tumors using special scanning equipment (Gale, 2005).

The popularity of biotherapy research has led to the development of nonspecific immunomodulating agents and new agents that include monoclonal antibodies, hematopoietic growth factors, interferons (INF), and interleukins. The latter three agents are part of a group of agents called cytokines, which are protein products from cells that function as cell regulators to enhance the production and functioning of the immune system. For example, lymphokines are products of lymphocytes and monokines are products of monocytes; interleukins are proteins that act as messengers between cells. Cytokines are described in Chapter 60 ◔. Nonspecific agents surfaced when early research identified Bacille-Calmette-Guerin (BCG) and *Corynebacterium parvum*. When injected into humans these agents work as antigens that stimulate the immune response, which should destroy malignant cells. Very positive outcomes have been demonstrated with multiple trials on animal and human models. BCG is known to be effective as a treatment for localized bladder cancer and appears to have promise in the treatment for malignant melanoma.

The Pharmacology Summary chart presented earlier (p. 2103) in this chapter lists biotherapy (and chemotherapy) agents along with specific clinical indicators, administration information, and side effects. Only agents approved for use by the Food and Drug Administration (FDA) are discussed; however, it is important to realize that multiple agents are under investigation that may be determined to be beneficial for use in patients with cancer in the future.

Side effects discussed in this chapter are those generally common to all agents. When administering biotherapy agents it is the responsibility of the nurse to know the specific agent being given and become familiar with side effects specific to that drug. If side effects are not treated successfully or become too burdensome to the patient, the therapy may be dose limiting. Other concerns when administering biologic therapy include safe handling of the drugs (determined by agency policy), rate of administration, and length of time stable once reconstituted according to the manufacturer's package insert, the need for special infusion filters or equipment, and the compatibility with other medications.

Oncology nurses are becoming more familiar with administering BRMs as more agents become available for commercial use. Nurses caring for patients receiving biotherapy need to be familiar with many unique details and should be comfortable and excited with a field of cancer treatment that is rapidly changing. Nurses must have the motivation to expand their knowledge and understanding of new treatment options for cancer patients because new discoveries are frequently being made. Nurses should gain much satisfaction from being involved with developing new standards of care and mentoring new nurses in the field of cancer nursing.

■ Nursing Management

Biotherapy agents differ from chemotherapeutic agents in action and toxicity patterns, but at the same time share many of the same side effects. Nurses can use their knowledge of chemotherapy-induced side effects to assist them in planning care for those patients receiving biotherapy. A comprehensive plan of care encompasses the patient's physical and psychological needs (refer to the Nursing Process: Care Plan for Cancer, p. 2089).

Transplantation: Bone Marrow and Peripheral Blood Stem Cell

Survival rates for cancer patients have improved due to treatments such as surgery, radiotherapy, and chemotherapy. Despite this promising outcome, many cancers that initially respond to therapy tend to reappear. **Bone marrow transplantation (BMT)** offers patients the ability to receive intensive chemotherapy or radiation therapy when resistance to or failure of standard treatment occurs (Bender & Rosenzweig, 2004). BMT is the transfer of hematopoietic cells from the bone marrow of one person into another person and has been used to treat a variety of diseases. Another option, **peripheral blood stem cell (PBSC) transplantation**, is becoming more widely used in lieu of the traditional bone marrow transplantation. Long-term survival is improved with both forms of treatment, making transplantation one of the most promising cancer therapies.

Transplantation has been performed for more than a century, but only since the mid-1960s have the chances of survival really improved. In the 19th century bone marrow was fed or injected into patients with grim results; however, significant progress has been made with the discovery of human leukocyte antigen (HLA) typing (discussed in Chapter 60 ☺), antirejection medications, and antibiotics.

Indications for Transplantation

The majority of transplants are performed for malignant disorders, although success has been demonstrated for use in patients with nonmalignant diseases (Keller, 2001). Several factors determine the type of transplant that will provide the best chances for survival. These include type and stage of disease, patient's age and performance status, and donor availability.

Types of Bone Marrow Transplantation

The types of BMT are based on the where the donor cells originate (see Chart 64–23). **Autologous BMT**, which comes from the recipient, is used for disorders where the patient's bone marrow has adequate stem cells that can produce functioning erythrocytes, leukocytes, and platelets. The patient's own bone marrow or stem cells are harvested and placed into frozen storage to be reinfused into the patient when the conditioning regime (chemotherapy or radiation with chemotherapy) is completed (Keller, 2001). In the past decade more autologous BMTs have been performed, typically for hematologic malignancies. **Allogeneic bone marrow**, which is from a histocompatible donor, is used for patients with hematologic malignancies, marrow failure, severe combined immunodeficiency syndrome (SCIDS), and certain inherited metabolic disorders. The majority of allogeneic transplants are done for acute myelogenous leukemia (AML), acute lymphocytic leukemia (ALL), and chronic myelogenous leukemia (CML).

Sources of Transplantation

In 1987 the National Marrow Donor Program (NMDP) was established to allow for easier access to unrelated donors. The registry contains more than 4 million individuals who have had tissue typing and expressed a desire to donate bone marrow. In 1999 the NMDP established a central registry of cord blood banks so that transplant centers could search for these donors more easily. When a donor is chosen they do not know who will be the recipient nor does the recipient know who has made such a generous donation.

Peripheral Blood Stem Cells

Traditionally, stem cells have been harvested from within the bone marrow cavity. The use of stem cells in peripherally circulating blood was first performed in the late 1950s (Santos, 2000). It has become more common since effectiveness was demonstrated in 1986 (Voss, Armitage, & Kessinger, 1993). Currently,

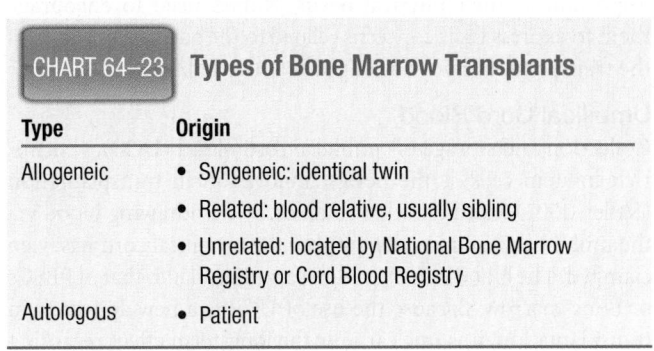

CHART 64–23	Types of Bone Marrow Transplants
Type	**Origin**
Allogeneic	• Syngeneic: identical twin
	• Related: blood relative, usually sibling
	• Unrelated: located by National Bone Marrow Registry or Cord Blood Registry
Autologous	• Patient

the use of PBSC transplantation for hematopoietic support following high-dose chemotherapy is the standard of practice for several malignant and nonmalignant diseases.

Autologous PBSC collection involves two phases: mobilization and apheresis. Mobilization involves stimulating the production of PBSCs with the administration of G-CSF or GM-CSF, possibly with chemotherapy. Apheresis is the collection of PBSCs through a double-lumen central venous catheter that is placed into the patient. Blood is run through a cell separator that is programmed to collect either lymphocytes or low-density leukocytes and return other blood components to the patient. Apheresis usually takes one to three sessions each lasting 3 to 4 hours. When the collection is completed the stem cells are placed into a blood bag and cryopreserved and remain frozen at −196°C until needed for transplantation.

Allogeneic PBSC collection involves the same phases as discussed for autologous transplantation. The donor receives G-CSF for approximately 4 to 5 days, which is adequate for mobilization. Side effects that may be experienced by the donor include bone pain, headache, fatigue, nausea, and insomnia (VanBurik & Weisdorf, 1999). Apheresis is usually done via a peripheral line inserted into the antecubital veins using the cell separator. Nurses need to instruct the donor about the importance of keeping follow-up doctor appointments since the most significant side effect is a drop in platelet count of up to 50%, which places the donor at risk for bleeding.

Bone Marrow Harvesting

The process of obtaining bone marrow for transplantation is called harvesting. For an autologous donor the procedure would occur in the operating room, likely under general anesthesia. Multiple punctures are made in the posterior or anterior iliac crest to obtain the necessary amount (500 to 700 mL) of marrow needed for transplant. Once the marrow is obtained it is mixed with heparin, filtered to remove bone fragments and fat, and placed into a blood bag. At this point, the bone marrow is purged, which is the process of removing any remaining malignant cells from the marrow. Once the purging step is completed, the marrow is placed into a blood bag and frozen just like PBSCs.

Allogeneic bone marrow harvesting involves the same process as autologous harvesting, minus the purging. After the marrow is harvested from the donor, it is immediately transfused into the recipient. Nursing care of the donor includes routine postoperative care. In addition, donors need to be informed that they may expect pain at the donor sites for approximately 1 week. This pain is usually remedied by nonnarcotic analgesics. The psychological and emotional needs of donors are equally as important as their physical needs. Nurses need to encourage them to express their concerns related to the success or failure of the transplant and provide support as needed.

Umbilical Cord Blood

Collection and storage of umbilical cord blood (UCB), which is rich in stem cells, is the newest innovation in transplantation (Keller, 2001). Cord blood is obtained by withdrawing blood via the umbilical vein immediately after the umbilical cord has been clamped. The blood is then cryopreserved similar to that of PBSCs or bone marrow. Because the use of UCB is a new approach in transplantation, it is unclear how the long-term effect regarding

relapse of the disease rate will be demonstrated. In addition, there are ethical issues specific to the use of UCB such as the timing of consent and identifying links between mother and baby, which may be the focus of clinical, ethical, and regulatory scrutiny.

The Transplantation Process

Selection of the appropriate donor and recipient is crucial so graft rejection and other serious complications are avoided. Criteria for the selection of a marrow or stem cell donor are few, but very important. First, histocompatibility as measured by HLA and mixed lymphocyte culture (MLC) testing must be determined. The donor's health status is evaluated to minimize the risks associated with donating and to prevent infecting the recipient with diseases such as hepatitis and HIV. Next, the donor's psychosocial profile is evaluated in an attempt to predict her attitudes and feelings toward the procedure and unknown outcomes. Finally, the donor's age is taken into consideration due to the amount of marrow needed for transplantation. Younger donors tend to be smaller in size, which limits the amount of marrow available for harvest (Keller, 2001).

A multidisciplinary approach is needed to evaluate the patient prior to receiving either bone marrow or stem cells. The pretransplant management consists of a detailed evaluation, including laboratory tests, procedures, and consultations, that is performed to determine the recipient's physical and psychosocial status (Anderson-Reitz, 2004). It is important to remember people embraced by the patient such as family and friends, all of whom may be asked to provide assistance during the transplantation process and recovery.

Once the initial evaluation is complete, the patient will undergo conditioning, which is the process of preparing the patient to receive bone marrow or stem cells. Conditioning serves three vital purposes: to eliminate malignant disease, to kill the current immunologic state, and to develop space in the marrow cavity for the transplanted stem cells as they begin reproducing. The regime will consist of high dose chemotherapy (HDCT) with or without radiotherapy and will result in severe myelosuppression. With conditioning complete, the bone marrow or stem cells may be infused. An autologous transplant is done by rapid IV push using syringes or by hanging the bag of cells and infusing over 20 to 30 minutes. During the procedure patients may experience mild dyspnea from the volume being infused and nausea and vomiting from the preservatives contained in the solution. Allogeneic marrow or stem cells are infused slowly over 1 to 5 hours. Patients may experience side effects similar to those seen in a blood transfusion, as discussed in Chapter 23 (Keller, 2001).

Establishment of new bone marrow is referred to as **engraftment** (Rokita 2004). The time required for complete engraftment depends on the source of the stem cells. Typically, bone marrow engrafts within 3 weeks, whereas stem cells take 11 to 16 days and cord blood takes 26 to 42 days. Of utmost concern is the pancytopenia and immunosuppression experienced during the immediate period post-transplant. Nurses must be very diligent at monitoring post-transplant patients for signs of infection and bleeding.

Bone marrow transplantation nursing has evolved with the development of transplantation approaches and therapies. The complexity of this field of nursing is evident in the challenging needs of the acute care patient. Because the age of BMT patients can cross the life span, the nurse must possess skills for managing infants as well as older adults (Wingard, 2007).

Complications of Transplantation

Patients who become transplant recipients are at risk for life-threatening complications, primarily due to the effects of the conditioning regime. Complications associated with the conditioning regime are numerous and can include bleeding, infection, nausea and vomiting, diarrhea, mucositis, and graft-versus-host disease (GVHD) (Anderson-Reitz, 2004). Several months to several years after transplant, the patient may experience late effects such as chronic GVHD, avascular necrosis, osteoporosis, cataracts, gonadal dysfunction, growth failure, hypothyroidism, secondary malignancies, need for revaccinations, and changes in quality of life.

Nurses who care for those patients undergoing transplantation need to be aware of the signs of graft failure and GVHD. Graft failure (rejection) occurs very rarely, but its significance requires nurses to be astute in their ability to assess patients for signs of infection and bleeding. Graft rejection is confirmed by serial bone marrow biopsies and will require the patient to undergo another transplant or death will be the result. GVHD occurs after allogeneic transplants and is the result of an immune-mediated reaction of the new stem cells reacting to the body of the recipient.

◼ Nursing Management

Transplant centers have begun to develop unique care models due to competition among health care institutions, a desire to improve outcomes, and the need to decrease costs (Schmit-Pokorny, Franco, Frappier, & Vyhlidal, 2003). Involving the patient and family members in all aspects of care has created an environment that is more personal and individualized while reducing costs and rehospitalizations. The nurse has the opportunity to assist the patient in becoming more confident and competent in self-care. Caring for patients receiving transplantation is complex and challenging, requiring a systematic approach to assessment along with the ability to remain flexible when implementing a plan of care. The patient's condition changes day to day and even hour to hour, requiring the nurse to adapt to these variations quickly and competently. A comprehensive plan of care will encompass the patient's physical and psychological needs (refer to the Nursing Process: Care Plan for Cancer earlier, p. 2089).

◼ Cancer Emergencies

Oncologic emergencies occur as a result of the disease process or side effects of treatment. On occasion, patients will present to their health care provider with a variety of distressing complaints and it is determined by evaluation that the patient has a malignancy. Regardless of the cause of the emergency, catastrophic results can occur if prompt and effective interventions are not initiated (Woodard & Hogan, 1996). The two main categories of emergencies are structural and metabolic in addition to hypersensitivity (anaphylaxis) and tumor lysis syndrome (My-

ers, 2001). Chart 64–24 (p. 2118) presents the important emergencies along with a definition, clinical findings, and treatment options. Oncology nurses understand the importance of continuously monitoring their patients for both subtle and obvious changes that may indicate the development of these potential life-threatening emergencies.

◼ Living with Cancer: Supportive Therapies and Symptom Management

The diagnosis of cancer does not have to be equated with miserable suffering and death. During the past 30 years a person's chance of surviving cancer has improved due to multiple factors: (1) a better understanding of the disease, (2) changes in dose-limiting treatment toxicities, (3) new targeted therapies, (4) improved screening and early detection programs, (5) evidenced-based practice, (6) improved supportive interventions, and (7) changes in sociocultural factors (Dow & Loerzel, 2004). Although these factors have given patients with cancer an improved chance of survival, patients also may need to live with a variety of symptoms or complications that have the potential to be distressing. Nurses caring for cancer patients need to be aware of the potential problems, perform accurate assessments, and determine appropriate nursing interventions to alleviate any suffering or distress.

It is not uncommon for patients to consider the use of complementary and alternative medicine (CAM) therapies throughout the course of cancer treatment (Fouladbakhsh, Stommel, Given, & Given, 2005). For example, the use of pomegranate juice by patients with cancer is discussed in the Complementary and Alternative Therapies box (p. 2119). Oftentimes patients choose not to reveal these practices to their health care providers. Of particular importance is determining the use of herbal and vitamin supplements that may interact negatively with concurrent use of traditional treatment options. Nurses need to provide education regarding the use of CAM while respecting an individual's right to make decisions.

Patients face multiple challenges throughout their cancer experience. One of the most difficult issues (for patients and nurses) is the ethics of cancer care. Ethical issues are common in oncology nursing, as evidenced by the examples listed in the Ethical Issues box (p. 2120). Nurses have opportunities to develop relationships with their patients who have cancer and their families as they go through diagnosis and treatment. This relationship provides the nurse with an understanding of the goals and values the patient possesses as they relate to their cancer experience. Collaborating with the multidisciplinary team is important to determine a plan of care that honors and respects these goals and values.

Nutrition

The nutritional status of cancer patients can be altered in a variety of ways. Emotional stress from impaired nutritional intake coupled with the metabolic demand of cancer and its treatment can have a profound effect on the patient. Nurses cannot ignore how eating can be a part of one's social presence and often is a source of enjoyment (Schulmeister, 2001b).

CHART 64–24	**Oncologic Emergencies**

Emergency	Findings	Treatment
Metabolic		
Disseminated intravascular coagulation (DIC) (see Chapter 63 ☺)	Signs of bleeding and clotting	• Elimination of triggering event • Supportive measures (transfusion of blood products)
Hypercalcemia: serum calcium levels >9–11 mg/dL	Lethargy Altered mental status Nausea and vomiting Anorexia Polydipsia Constipation	• Hydration • Diuresis to enhance the excretion of calcium • Pharmacology: bisphosphonates (inhibit the action of osteoclasts) • Increased mobilization
Malignant pleural effusion; accumulation of fluid in the pleural cavity	Dyspnea at rest or activity Cough (nonproductive) Chest pain Malaise Weight loss Fear of suffocation, anxiety	• Radiation or chemotherapy aimed at the primary tumor • Insertion of chest tube with drainage capability • Pleurodesis
Sepsis (see Chapter 61 ☺)	Fever Chills Changes in blood pressure Rapid respiratory rate Mental cloudiness	• Recognition of impending shock is key • Infection control practices • Private rooms • Hemodynamic monitoring while in the intensive care unit (ICU) • Antibiotic therapy
Syndrome of inappropriate antidiuretic hormone (SIADH): endocrine paraneoplastic syndrome causing water imbalance (see Chapter 52 ☺)	Hyponatremia Decreased serum osmolality Water retention Increased urine osmolality Normal skin turgor Normal blood pressure	• Treat underlying cause • Fluid restriction • Diuretic therapy
Hypersensitivity reaction (anaphylaxis): immunologic response to foreign substance or antigen; may be life threatening	Occurs within minutes of receiving certain chemotherapy agents Dyspnea Agitation Hypotension Laryngeal edema and spasm	• Prevention is the key • Careful monitoring of blood pressure, pulse, and oxygen saturation during infusion • Emergency equipment needs to be available
Tumor lysis syndrome: rapid lysis of malignant cells resulting in renal (e.g., acidosis), electrolyte (e.g., hyperuricemia, hyperkalemia), cardiac, and neurologic complications	Nausea and vomiting Edema Flank pain Hematuria Changes in blood pressure Lethargy Muscle twitching and weakness	• Prevention is the key • Pretreatment hydration • Pharmacologic therapy (diuretics, xanthine oxidase inhibitors, sodium bicarbonate) • Supportive measures for potential organ failure
Structural		
Increased intracranial pressure: volume of the brain, CSF, and cerebral blood volume increase (see Chapter 31 ☺)	Signs and symptoms of increased intracranial pressure	• Pharmacologic therapy (osmotic diuretics, corticosteroids, anticonvulsants) • Surgery to relieve pressure and evacuate fluid • Radiation and chemotherapy to shrink tumor bulk
Spinal cord compression: malignancy that invades the epidural space and cauda equina (see Chapter 32 ☺)	Signs and symptoms of cord compression are specific to the area of the cord being compressed	• Pharmacologic therapy (corticosteroids) • Radiation therapy to reduce tumor bulk • Surgery when bony instability occurs
Superior vena cava syndrome: obstruction of venous flow through the vena cava resulting in compression of intrathoracic structures, vascular congestion, and venous hypertension	Dyspnea Cough Feeling of fullness in the head Chest pain	• Pharmacologic therapy (fibrinolytic therapy) • Radiation therapy to reduce tumor bulk • Chemotherapy for specific cell types • Surgery (stents or bypass)

CHART 64–24	Oncologic Emergencies—*Continued*	
Emergency	**Findings**	**Treatment**
Cardiac tamponade: compression of the cardiac muscle by malignant fluid accumulation within the pericardial sac (see Chapter 42 🔗)	Dyspnea Chest pain Tachycardia Cough	• Pharmacologic therapy (diuretics, corticosteroids, NSAIDS) • Removal of fluid via pericardiocentesis, pericardiotomy, pericardiectomy

Sources: Bender, C., & Rosenzweig, M. (2004). Cancer. In S. Lewis, M. Heitkemper, & S. Dirksen (Eds.), *Medical–surgical nursing assessment and management of clinical problems* (6th ed.). St. Louis: Mosby; Myers, J. (2001). Oncologic complications. In S. Otto (Ed.), *Oncology nursing* (4th ed.). St. Louis: Mosby; Woodard, W., & Hogan, D. (1996). Oncologic emergencies: Implications for nurses. *Journal of Intravenous Nursing, 19*(2).

Weight loss in patients with cancer is likely to result in poor clinical and psychological outcomes (Dell, 2002). The nurse can recognize the syndrome of cancer cachexia by the presence of anorexia, weight loss, muscle and adipose tissue wasting, hyperlipidemia, and other metabolic derangements. It is present in 80% of those who die of cancer (Cunningham, 2004). Figure 64–7 ■ (p. 2120) illustrates how profoundly cachexia affects the human body. Cachexia is the result of altered absorption and changes in metabolism, such as protein, fat, and carbohydrates (National Cancer Institute, 2003). It is important for the nurse to remember that cachexia can be present in patients who have adequate caloric and protein intake but are failing to absorb the necessary nutrients.

For those patients receiving chemotherapy, inadequate nutrition is of utmost concern. One of the most dreaded side effects of chemotherapy is nausea and vomiting. Uncontrolled nausea and vomiting can eventually result in cachexia preceded by anorexia and weight loss (Finley, 2003b). Oncology nurses are vital in ensuring that the nutritional needs of these patients are being met. Recognizing the early signs of cachexia and implementing effective interventions is key in slowing or reversing the progression of cachexia syndrome.

Nutritional screening is the process of evaluating patients for the risk of developing malnutrition. The goal of screening is to identify patients at risk, prevent or treat malnutrition early, and individualize the nutritional plan of care (McMahon, 2003). Working together with a nutritionist, the nurse can perform an effective nutritional screening evaluation by determining food intake, presence of symptoms, functional status (Karnofsky Performance Scale), weight, physical assessment, and laboratory data analysis. Chart 64–25 (p. 2121) lists the signs and symptoms along with laboratory data that can be used to determine malnutrition. The nurse/nutritionist needs to use sensitivity when discussing issues associated with dietary habits because many patients are hesitant to discuss their nutritional habits.

Nutritional Support

Once the need for nutritional support has been determined, the method of delivery is the next decision to be made. For those patients with mild anorexia, nutritional counseling may be adequate, whereas those patients with severe anorexia or cachexia may require parenteral nutritional support. Oral nutrition is the preferred route, but those patients with mechanical inability to

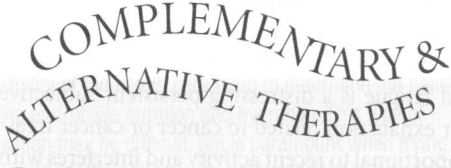

COMPLEMENTARY & ALTERNATIVE THERAPIES   Pomegranate Juice

Description:
Studies have shown that plant phytochemicals may prevent cancer due to antioxidants and nutrients (Pantuck et al., 2006). The pomegranate (*Punica granatum*) fruit has been shown to have high levels of antioxidants and other nutrients. The level of interest and research on pomegranate has surged over the last decade. The pomegranate fruit is comprised of the following components, each of which have pharmacologic activity: seed, juice, peel, leaf, flower, bark, and roots. The most notable therapeutic properties of pomegranate are antioxidant and anticancer activities, including interference with tumor cell proliferation, cell cycle, invasion, and angiogenesis (Lansky & Newman, 2007).

Research Support:
One study examined the effects of pomegranate juice on the levels of prostate-specific antigen (PSA) in men with prostate cancer and a rising PSA following conventional therapy. Patients consumed 8 oz of pomegranate juice daily. Results showed that mean PSA doubling time significantly increased with pomegranate juice consumption, from a mean of 15 months at baseline to 54 months post-treatment. Researchers concluded that the positive results from this study indicate that further testing is needed in a placebo-controlled study (Pantuck et al., 2006).

Another study examined the effect of pomegranate juice on inflammatory cell signaling proteins in patients with colon cancer. The study used pomegranate juice with a concentration of 50 mg/L. Results showed that the pomegranate juice significantly suppressed inflammatory cell signaling proteins by 79% (Adams et al., 2006).

References
Adams, L. S., Seeram, N. P., Aggarwal, B. B., Takada, Y., Sand, D., & Heber, D. (2006). Pomegranate juice, total pomegranate ellagitannins, and punicalagin suppress inflammatory cell signaling in colon cancer cells. *Journal of Agricultural and Food Chemistry, 54*(3), 980–985.

Lansky, E. P., & Newman, R. A. (2007). *Punica granatum* (pomegranate) and its potential for prevention and treatment of inflammation and cancer. *Journal of Ethnopharmacology, 109*(2), 177–206.

Pantuck, A. J., Leppert, J. T., Zomorodian, N., Aronson, W., Hong, J., Barnard, R. J., et al. (2006). Phase II study of pomegranate juice for men with rising prostate-specific antigen following surgery or radiation for prostate cancer. *Clinical Cancer Research, 12*(13), 4018–4026.

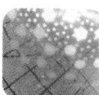

PATIENT TEACHING & DISCHARGE PRIORITIES for Cancer

Need	Teaching
Treatment side effects and toxicities: Patient/family Family/support system Setting	Instruct patient regarding proper oral care: • Brush and floss teeth as tolerated. • Use moistening gauze or toothettes instead of toothbrush if needed, for instance, if platelet count is low ($<$40,000/mm^3). • Rinse with normal saline four times per day. • Avoid commercial mouthwashes. • Cleanse mouth before and after meals. Instruct patient to report signs of stomatitis: • Burning • Pain • Areas of redness • Open lesions on the lips • Pain with swallowing • Intolerance to temperature extremes. Take antiemetics and appetite stimulants per orders. Suggest small frequent meals that are high in calories and protein. Encourage adequate fluid intake limiting fluids during mealtime. Monitor for signs of infection and notify health care provider immediately. Avoid contact with those who have known or recent infection or recent vaccination. Avoid raw meat and fish, fresh fruit and vegetables, fresh flowers and plants. Avoid use of straight edge razor. Instruct patient regarding ways to minimize the risk of bleeding: • Perform oral hygiene with soft toothbrush or toothettes • Avoid use of commercial mouthwashes • Avoid straight-edge razors • File nails with emery board • Avoid foods that are difficult to chew Encourage frequent rest periods. Encourage more sleep hours at night. Encourage patient to reorganize daily schedule of activities and seek assistance with shopping, cooking, housework, etc. Encourage a temporary decrease in work hours. Assess availability, knowledge, and compliance with treatment regimen. Assess respite needs and resources. Assess discharge placement needs: • Home • Hospice • Extended care facility. Assess the home environment for needed assistive devices. Assess the need for professional home health. Assess the need for follow-up appointments.
In-home treatments: Patient/family Family/support system Setting	Instruct patient and family on how to operate and troubleshoot infusion equipment. Instruct patient and family on how to care for an implantable infusion device. Instruct patient and family on the proper storage of medications and solutions. Assess availability, knowledge, and compliance with treatment regimen. Assess respite needs and resources. Assess home environment for risk factors. Assess home environment for needed assistive devices. Assess the need for professional home health. Assess the need for follow-up appointments.

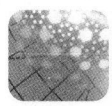

PATIENT TEACHING & DISCHARGE PRIORITIES for Cancer—*Continued*

Need	Teaching

Coping:
  Patient/family
  Family/support system
  Setting
	Instruct patient to consider participating in activities and decision making.

	Encourage patient to verbalize concerns.
	Instruct about patterns of hair loss and regrowth.
	Encourage patient to view venous access device.
	Encourage patient in selecting cosmetic devices that increase sense of attractiveness.
	Offer ways to cope with hair loss: • Obtain wigs or hairpieces prior to hair loss • Take photograph of hair loss to wig shop to improve matching of hair color • Contact American Cancer Society for available resources • Wear scarf, hat, or other device as needed
	Encourage dialogue between patient and partner regarding sexual function and alternatives.
	Assess the need for professional home health.
	Assess the need for follow-up appointments.

RESEARCH OPPORTUNITIES AND CLINICAL IMPACT RELATED TO CANCER

Research Area	Clinical Impact
Physiological Research	
Photodynamic therapy for treatment of esophageal and lung cancer	Provides additional treatment options.
Effects of handling chemotherapy on the person administering the medication, offspring	Increases awareness of hazards associated with administration of chemotherapy.
Use of new interleukins as antitumor and myeloprotective agents	Provides additional treatment options and prevention of life-threatening toxicities.
Use of new interferons to treat the severity of GVHD and other cancers	Decreases incidence of metastasis.
Use of gene therapy for advanced cancers and prevention of myelosuppression	
Determining the benefit/risk ratio and efficacy of chemotherapeutic chronotherapy	
Use of drugs to prevent the development of blood vessels (antiangiogenesis therapy) in cancer treatment	
Symptom and Toxicity Management	
Evaluation of postoperative symptoms in those with lung cancer	Relieves distressing symptoms to increase healing and recovery.
Use of virtual reality interventions for chemotherapy symptoms	Relieves distressing symptoms to aid in recovery and treatment tolerance.
Innovative approaches to symptom management (cluster intervention, neutropenic protocols, fatigue guidelines, mucositis standard of care)	Increases awareness of unique symptoms and appropriate treatments to relieve suffering.
Causes of fatigue and solutions	Provides information to assist in the development of individualized nursing care plan.
Skin care for patients receiving radiotherapy	
Association between treatment and disease-related symptoms and activity	Increases awareness of need for pain control and availability of treatment modalities.
Symptoms at the end of life	
Association between patient's perceptions of treatment toxicities and ability to care for self	
Nursing pain management of inpatients and outpatients	

RESEARCH OPPORTUNITIES AND CLINICAL IMPACT RELATED TO CANCER—*Continued*

Research Area	Clinical Impact
Psychosocial and Emotional Issues	
Coping with disease and treatment	Improves psychological interventions to augment coping.
Coping of caregivers and families of patients with cancer	Provides insight into how patients make decisions regarding treatment so appropriate and effective communication can be implemented.
Decision making after cancer testing (BRCA genetic testing)	
The role of caring and the meaning of illness	Highlights importance of caring.
Quality of life	Impact of the disease and treatment.
Quality of life and influencing factors	Impact on vocation.
Employment behaviors in patients with treatment-related symptoms	Importance of family members' involvement in caregiving.
Delivery of care by family members	Importance of ascertaining patients' end-of-life choices and advocating appropriately.
Preferred versus actual location of death	
Cultural Diversity	
Symptom management in various cultural groups	Improves understanding of cultural differences in cancer management.
Participation of various cultural groups as subjects in cancer research efforts	
Use of specific treatment regimes in various cultural groups	
Decision making in various cultural groups	
Evaluating cancer risk behaviors and emotional status in various cultural groups	
End-of-life issues and ethnicity	
Prevention/Detection/Screening	
Tertiary chemoprevention to reduce the risk of cancer in those who are highly susceptible	Reduces risk of developing cancer.
Health and risk behaviors in childhood cancer survivors	Improves understanding of behaviors and allows for the development of screening programs to meet patients' needs.
Mammography decision making in women with family history of breast cancer	Allows for improved prevention and screening programs.
Disclosure of breast symptoms	
Use of telephone counseling in rural areas	
Changing health beliefs in those at risk for colon cancer	
Womens' perceptions of their risk of developing breast cancer	
Communicating breast cancer risk among family members	

(Rokita, 2004). Clinical trials can involve four phases, as described in Chart 64–29, each having a specific goal regarding research outcomes.

Oncology nurses have the unique opportunity to participate in many aspects of research efforts including obtaining informed consent, developing and implementing educational sessions for patients and their families, administering treatments under investigation, and collecting pertinent data (Gullatte & Otto, 2001). Being a patient advocate throughout all phases of clinical trials is also the role of the nurse and the health care team.

CHART 64–29	**Phases of Clinical Trials**

Phase	Details
Phase I	Determine optimal dosing, scheduling, and toxicity.
Phase II	Further defines toxicities. Determines effectiveness related to specific tumor types. Participants usually include those who have not responded to standard treatments.
Phase III	Establish the effectiveness of new medications or procedures. Comparisons are made to conventional therapy. Nurses are involved with: • Identification of subjects • Obtaining informed consent • Educating subjects • Monitoring and assisting with compliance • Documenting subject responses.
Phase IV	Further investigation of new uses, dosing schedules, and toxicities.

Clinical Preparation

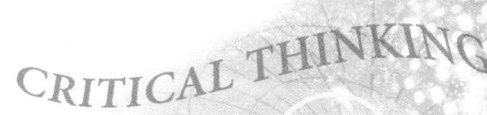

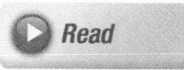

- History of Current Illness
- Past Medical History
- Physical Exam
- Admitting Medical Orders
- Laboratory Study Results

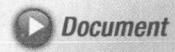

- Summary of Hospitalization
- Pathophysiology Form
- Laboratory Values
- Laboratory Results Explanation

- List of Potential Nursing Diagnoses
- Concept Map
- Critical Thinking Questions

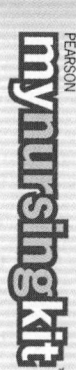

*Log on to MyNursingKit.com to download forms you will need and to complete further steps in the Clinical Preparation assignment.

HISTORY OF PRESENT ILLNESS

Mrs. S. is a 43-year-old female presenting to the Emergency Department (ED) for back pain. She was evaluated and discharged home with a prescription for a nonsteroidal anti-inflammatory drug (NSAID) and asked to follow up in the physical therapy department in 2 days. The following evening she again presented to the ED for worsening back pain along with numbness in her right buttocks. She appears well nourished, slightly pale, in obvious discomfort. While you assist her to the restroom you notice slight right foot drop and the appearance of dyspnea. Upon returning to the bed she is obviously dyspneic with a respiratory rate of 28. Oxygen saturation is 89% on room air. Lung sounds are diminished on the right side; otherwise, wheezes heard throughout. She admits to occasional productive cough. The results of a chest x-ray suggest lung cancer.

She is scheduled for a CT scan and while she is being moved from the gurney to the CT scan table, she cries out in pain while holding her right leg. The CT scan suggests a malignancy. Additional x-rays discover she has a fractured right hip. You're the nurse caring for Mrs. S. and you have received report from the nurse from surgery. Upon arrival to the floor Mrs. S. is awake, crying, groaning, and complaining of pain in her right hip area. You note on her laboratory data that her hematocrit is 22% and per order administer 2 units of packed red blood cells.

Medical–Surgical History

Allergies: none

Medical problems: hypothyroidism, depression

Medications: Prozac, Synthroid, and Motrin

Surgical history: appendectomy at the age of 13, C-section for two children

Social History

Married with two children (boys age 12 and 20)

Smokes 1.5 packs/day for 28 years

Occasional alcohol use

Physical Exam

Vital signs: BP 148/89, HR 128, RR 24, T 38.0°C

HEENT: WNL, oropharynx clear

Neck: supple, no lymphadenopathy

Lungs: diminished with wheezes throughout

Cardiovascular: JVP not elevated; normal S_1 and S_2; regular rate and tachycardic, no significant murmur, rub, or gallop; carotids 2+ without bruits

Abdomen: soft, nontender, nondistended, normoactive bowel sounds

Extremities: no edema, complaining of severe pain in her right hip

Neurological: normal, alert, and oriented × 4

Admitting Medical Orders

Ortho service

Oncology consultation

Admit to surgical floor

Diagnosis: status postrepair of fractured right hip; rule out cancer

No known allergies

Vital signs and oxygen saturation q4h

Bed rest with immobilization of right leg

Clear liquids when tolerated

I&O

Foley

Dry sterile dressing to right hip, change prn

Oxygen 1–2 L per nasal cannula as needed to maintain oxygen saturation > 90%

Call house officer: pulse < 60 and > 130/minute; BP < 90 and > 160 systolic; temperature > 38.5; urine output < 30 mL/hr for 2 hours; respiratory rate > 30/minute; oxygen saturation < 92%

Sequential compression devices (SCDs) to lower extremities

Intravenous line with 0.9% normal saline at 125 mL/hr; routine venous access device care

Neurovascular assessments to right lower extremity every 2 hours

Code status: full

Transfuse 2 units red blood cells if HCT< 24%. CBC after 2 units

Scheduled Medications

Prozac 20 mg oral every a.m.

Synthroid 0.25 mcg oral every a.m.

Duragesic patch 50 mcg; change every 72 hours

PRN Medications

Morphine sulfate PCA: 1 mg incremental dose q10min. If pain not well controlled, give morphine sulfate bolus 1–5 mg IV × 1

Tylenol 650 mg oral q4–6h as needed for pain or fever

Ativan 1–2 mg oral or IV q8h as needed for anxiety

Zofran 8 mg oral q8h as needed for nausea

Benadryl 25 mg oral q6h for itching or for sleep

Milk of Magnesia 30 mL po q4h prn constipation

Ordered Laboratory Studies

Chemistry, on admission

CBC with differential

Ordered Diagnostic Studies

Chest x-ray

12-lead ECG

CT scan of chest and spine

X-ray of right hip

LABORATORY STUDIES RESULTS

Test	Emergency Department	Postop Day 1	After Blood Transfusion
Chemistry			
Sodium	138 mEq/L		
Potassium	4.2 mEq/L		
Chloride	98 mEq/L		
Carbon dioxide	26 mEq/L		
Blood urea nitrogen (BUN)	12 mg/dL		
Creatinine	0.8 mg/dL		
Blood glucose	110 mg/dL		
Hematology			
White blood cells	11,000/mm³	12,000/mm³	20,000/mm³
Bands	4%		
Segmented neutrophils	48%		
Hemoglobin	8.6/g/dL	8.0/g/dL	9.0/g/dL
Hematocrit	26%	22%	27%
Red blood cells	4.1/mm³	3.7/mm³	3.6/mm³
Platelets	150,000/mm³	148,000/mm³	127,000/mm³

CRITICAL THINKING QUESTIONS

1. What critical assessments need to be made?

2. How can the nurse accurately determine the patient's risk for infection?

3. What nursing measures are appropriate related to infection?

4. What risk factor(s) put Mrs. S. at risk for developing lung cancer?

Answers to Critical Thinking Questions appear in Appendix D.

NCLEX® REVIEW

1. A patient tells the nurse that she doesn't want to "get cancer." Which of the following should the nurse instruct this patient?

1. There is nothing that you can do to prevent the onset of cancer.

2. Instruct in the avoidance of tobacco, excessive alcohol, and a high fat diet.

3. Avoid all types of stress.

4. The chance of developing cancer decreases with age.

2. A patient with cancer asks how a tumor can grow within an organ. The nurse explains how a blood supply is formed or the concept of:

1. Cell attachment.

2. Cell invasion.

3. Angiogenesis.

4. Migration.

3. An elderly male patient was told that he most likely has cancer and the treatment at this time will be "watch and wait." The nurse realizes this patient most likely is experiencing which type of cancer?

1. Melanoma

2. Prostate

3. Brain

4. Colon

4. The nurse is planning care for a patient with cancer. Which of the following should be included to reduce the risk of infection for this patient?

1. Measure rectal temperature every 4 hours.

2. Encourage a diet high in fresh fruit and vegetables.

3. Use strict aseptic technique when caring for venous access devices.

4. Provide intramuscular pain medications.

5. A patient receiving radiation therapy for cancer is demonstrating signs of fatigue. Which of the following can the nurse do to assist this patient?

1. Cluster care activities to increase rest periods.

2. Restrict calories.

3. Discuss activities to increase energy.

4. Review strategies to overcome fatigue over the long term.

6. A patient with cancer is scheduled to receive biotherapy. The nurse realizes the intention for this treatment is to:

1. Eliminate the need for surgery.

2. Reduce the negative impact of chemotherapy.

3. Alter the immunological relationship between the tumor and the patient.

4. Increase the patient's appetite.

Answers for review questions appear in Appendix D

KEY TERMS

absolute neutrophil count (ANC) *p.2113*
allogeneic bone marrow *p.2115*
anorexia *p.2087*
autologous BMT *p.2115*
benign *p.2066*
biopsy *p.2077*
biotherapy *p.2114*
bone marrow transplantation *p.2115*
cancer *p.2061*

carcinogenesis *p.2064*
carcinoma in situ *p.2066*
cytokines *p.2087*
engraftment *p.2116*
incidence *p.2061*
lymphoma *p.2077*
malignant *p.2066*
metastasis *p.2067*
mortality *p.2062*

nadir *p.2113*
neoplasm *p.2063*
palliative *p.2082*
peripheral blood stem cell (PBSC)
    transplantation *p.2115*
prevalence *p.2062*
radiation *p.2073*
staging *p.2066*
survival *p.2062*

EXPLORE PEARSON **mynursingkit**™

MyNursingKit is your one stop for online chapter review materials and resources. Prepare for success with additional NCLEX®-style practice questions, interactive assignments and activities, web links, animations and videos, and more!

Register your access code from the front of your book at
www.mynursingkit.com

REFERENCES

Akhurst, T., & Larson, S. (1999). Position emission tomography imaging of colorectal cancer. *Seminar in Oncology, 577*(26).

Alexander, J. (2001). Diagnosis and staging. In S. Otto (Ed.), *Oncology nursing* (4th ed.). St. Louis: Mosby.

American Cancer Society. (2001). *American Cancer Society supports closing gap between effective smoking cessation efforts and health care coverage.* Retrieved from http://www.cancer.org/docroot/MED/content/MED_2_1x_American_Cancer_Society_Supports_Closing_Gap_Between_Effective_Smoking_Cessation_Efforts_and_Health_Care_Coverage.asp

American Cancer Society. (2003). *Radiation exposure and cancer.* Retrieved from http://www.cancer.org/docroot/PED/content/PED_1_3X_Radiation_Exposure_and_Cancer.asp?sitearea=PED

American Cancer Society. (2004). *Cancer prevention and early detection facts and figures.* Retrieved on September 22, 2008, from http://www.cancer.org/downloads/STT/CPED2004PWSecured.pdf

American Cancer Society. (2006a). *Cigarette smoking.* Retrieved from http://www.cancer.org/docroot/PED/content/PED_10_2X_Cigarette_Smoking.asp

American Cancer Society. (2006b). *Do we know what causes penile cancer?* Retrieved from http://www.cancer.org/docroot/CRI/content/CRI_2_4_2X_Do_we_know_what_causes_penile_cancer_35.asp?sitearea=

American Cancer Society. (2007). *Cancer facts and figures 2007.* Retrieved from http://www.cancer.org/docroot/STT/content/STT_1x_Cancer_Facts__Figures_2007.asp

American Cancer Society. (2008a). *Seven Steps To Reduce Your Cancer Risk.* Retrieved on September 22, 2008 from http://www.cancer.org/docroot/COM/content/div_NE/COM_1_1x_Seven_Steps_To_Take_To_Prevent_Cancer.asp?sitearea=COM

American Cancer Society. (2008b). *Cancer facts and figures 2008.* Retrieved on September 22, 2008 from http://www.cancer.org/downloads/STT/2008CAFFfinalsecured.pdf

American Cancer Society. (ND). *Risk factors.* Retrieved on September 22, 2008, from http://www.cancer.org/downloads/AA/CancerAtlas02.pdf

Anderson-Reitz, L. (2004). Supportive care of the hematopoietic stem cell transplant patient. *Oncology Supportive Care, 2*(3).

Andrykowski, M., et al. (1998). Off-treatment fatigue in breast cancer survivors: A controlled comparison. *Journal of Behavior Medicine, 21*(1).

Antin, J. (2002). Long-term care after hematopoietic cell transplantation in adults. *New England Journal of Medicine, 347*(1), 36–42.

Ashby, V., & Dalton, J. (2000). Pain assessment and management in people with cancer. In B. Nevidjon & K. Sowers (Eds.), *A nurse's guide to cancer care.* Philadelphia: Lippincott Williams & Wilkins.

Barber, F., & Fabugais-Nazario, L. (2003). What's old is new again: Patients receiving hepatic arterial infusion chemotherapy. *Clinical Journal of Oncology Nursing, 7*(6).

Barnett, M. (2001). Fatigue. In S. Otto (Ed.), *Oncology nursing* (4th ed.). St. Louis: Mosby.

Bender, C., & Rosenzweig, M. (2004). Cancer. In S. Lewis, M. Heitkemper, & S. Dirksen (Eds.), *Medical–surgical nursing assessment and management of clinical problems* (6th ed.). St. Louis: Mosby.

Blesch, K. (1991). Correlates of fatigue in people with breast and lung cancer. *Oncology Nursing Forum, 18*(1), 81.

Blomgren, H., Lax, I., Goranson, H., Kraepelien, T., Nilsson, B., Naslund, I., et al. (1998). Radiosurgery for tumors in the body: Clinical experience using a new method. *Journal of Radiosurgery, 1*(1).

Booker, M. (1996a). Arterial therapy. In M. Booker & D. Ignatavicius (Eds.), *Infusion therapy techniques and medications* (1st ed.). Philadelphia: W. B. Saunders.

Booker, M. (1996b). Central nervous system therapy. In M. Booker & D. Ignatavicius (Eds.), *Infusion therapy techniques and medications* (1st ed.). Philadelphia: W. B. Saunders.

Bower, J., et al. (2000). Fatigue in breast cancer survivors: Occurrence, correlates, and impact on quality of life. *Journal of Clinical Oncology, 18*(4).

Bremerkamp, M. (2000). Mechanisms of action of 5-HT3 receptor antagonists: Clinical overview and nursing implications. *Clinical Journal of Oncology Nursing, 4*(5).

Brunner, D. (1990). Report on the Radiation Oncology Nursing Subcommittee of the American College of Radiation Task Force on Standards Development. *Oncology, 4*(80).

Campbell, C., & Iwamoto, R. (1992). Intraoperative radiation therapy. *Today's OR Nurse, 14*(1).

Centers for Disease Control and Prevention. (2007). *State and community resources.* Retrieved on January 13, 2007, from http://www.cdc.gov/tobacco/tobacco_control_programs/stateandcommunity/index.htm

Clark, R. A., & Reintgen, D. S. (1996). Principles of cancer screening. In D. S. Reintgen & R. A. Clark (Eds.), *Cancer screening.* St. Louis: Mosby.

Crane-Okada, R. (2001). Breast cancers. In S. Otto (Ed.), *Oncology nursing* (4th ed.). St. Louis: Mosby.

Cunningham, R. (2004). Anorexia-cachexia syndrome. In C. H. Yarbro, M. H. Frogge, & M. Goodman (Eds.), *Cancer symptom management* (3rd ed.). Sudbury, MA: Jones and Bartlett.

Daniel, B. (2001). Malignant lymphoma. In S. Otto (Ed.), *Oncology nursing* (4th ed.). St. Louis: Mosby.

Dell, D. (2002). Cachexia in patients with advanced cancer. *Clinical Journal of Oncology Nursing, 6*(4), 235–238.

DeVita, V. T., Jr. (1997). Principles of cancer management: Chemotherapy. In V. T. DeVita, Jr., S. Hellman, & S. A. Rosenberg (Eds.), *Cancer: Principles and practice of oncology* (5th ed.). Philadelphia: Lippincott Williams & Wilkins.

DeVita, V. T., Jr., Hellman, S., & Rosenberg, S. A. (Eds.). (1997). *Cancer: Principles and practice of oncology* (5th ed.). Philadelphia: Lippincott Williams & Wilkins.

Donovan, H., & Ward, S. (2005). Representation of fatigue in women receiving chemotherapy for gynecologic cancers. *Oncology Nursing Forum, 32*(1).

Dow, K., Ferrell, B., Haberman, M., & Eaton, L. (1999). The meaning of quality of life in cancer survivorship. *Oncology Nursing Forum, 26*(3), 519–528.

Dow, K., & Loerzel, V. (2004). Cancer survivorship: A critical aspect of care. In C. H. Yarbro, M. H. Frogge, & M. Goodman (Eds.), *Cancer symptom management* (3rd ed.). Sudbury, MA: Jones and Bartlett.

Dunne-Daly, C. (1997). Principles of brachytherapy. In K. Dow et al. (Eds.), *Nursing care in radiation oncology* (7th ed.). Philadelphia: W. B. Saunders.

Erickson, J. (2003). Cancer. In W. Phipps, F. Monahan, J. Sands, J. Marek, & M. Neighbors (Eds.), *Medical–surgical nursing health and illness perspectives* (7th ed.). St. Louis: Mosby.

Ersek, M. (2003). Artificial nutrition and hydration. *Journal of Hospice and Palliative Care Nursing, 5*(4), 221–230.

Ersek, M., Ferrell, B., Dow, K., & Melancon, C. (1997). Quality of life in women with ovarian cancer. *Western Journal of Nursing Research, 19*(2), 334–350.

Erye, H., Kahn, R., Robertson, R., & Committee AAACW. (2004). Preventing cancer, cardiovascular disease, and diabetes: A common agenda for the American Cancer Society, the American Diabetes Association, and the American Heart Association. *CA—Cancer Journal for Clinicians, 54* (4).

Ferrell, B., & Dow, K. (1997). Quality of life among long-term cancer survivors. *Oncology, 11*(3), 565–568.

Ferrell, B., Dow, K., Leigh, S., Ly, J., & Gulasekaram, P. (1995). Quality of life in long-term cancer survivors. *Oncology Nursing Forum, 22*(5), 915–922.

Ferrell, B., Grant, M., Funk, B., Otis-Green, S., & Garcia, N. (1998a). Quality of life in breast cancer. Part II: Psychological and spiritual well-being. *Cancer Nursing, 21*(1), 1–9.

Ferrell, B., Grant, M., Funk, B., Otis-Green, S., Garcia, N. (1998b). Quality of life in breast cancer survivors: Implications for developing support services. *Oncology Nursing Forum, 25*(4), 887–895.

Finley, J. (2003a). Detection and management of cachexia in cancer patients. *Advanced Studies in Nursing, 1*(1), 8–12.

Finley, J. (2003b). Management of cancer cachexia and chemotherapy associated nausea and vomiting. *Advanced Studies in Nursing, 1*(1), 7.

Fischbach, F., & Dunning, M. (Eds.). (2006). *Nurses' quick reference to common laboratory and diagnostic tests.* Philadelphia: Lippincott Williams & Wilkins.

Flynn, A. (2005). Isotopes and delivery systems for brachytherapy. In P. Hoskin & C. Coyle (Eds.), *Radiotherapy in practice brachytherapy.* New York: Oxford University Press.

Fouladbakhsh, J., Stommel, M., Given, B., & Given, C. (2005). Predictors of use of complementary and alternative therapies among patients with cancer. *Oncology Nursing Forum, 32*(6).

Gale, C. (2005). Nursing implications of biotherapy and molecular targeted therapy. In J. Itano & K. Taoka (Eds.), *Core curriculum for oncology nursing* (4th ed.). St. Louis: W. B. Saunders.

Ganz, P., Coscarelli, A., Fred, C., Kahn, B., Polinsky, M., & Peterson, L. (1996). Breast cancer survivors: Psychosocial concerns and quality of life. *Breast Cancer Research and Treatment, 38*(1), 183–199.

Given, C., Given, B., Azzouoz, F., Kozachik, S., & Stommel, M. (2001). Predictors of pain and fatigue in the year following diagnosis among elderly cancer patients. *Journal of Pain and Symptom Management, 1*(2), 456–466.

Grever, M., & Chabner, B. (1997). Cancer drug discovery and development. In V. T. DeVita, Jr., S. Hellman, & S. A. Rosenberg (Eds.), *Cancer: Principles and practice of oncology* (5th ed.). Philadelphia: Lippincott Williams & Wilkins.

Groenwald, S., Frogge, M. H., Goodman, M., & Yarbro, C. H. (Eds.). (1997). *Cancer nursing: Principles and practice* (4th ed.). Sudbury: Jones and Bartlett.

Gullatte, M., & Otto, S. (2001). Cancer clinical trials. In S. Otto (Ed.), *Oncology nursing* (4th ed.). St. Louis: Mosby.

Ham, O. (2006). Factors affecting mammography behavior and intention among Korean women. *Oncology Nursing Forum, 33*(1).

Hartigan, K. (2003). Patient education: The cornerstone of successful oral chemotherapy treatment. *Clinical Journal of Oncology Nursing, 7*(6).

Hawkins, R. (2001). Mastering the intricate maze of metastasis. *Oncology Nursing Forum, 28*(6), 959–965.

Heath, C. W. (1996). Electromagnetic field exposure and cancer: A review of epidemiologic evidence. *CA—A Cancer Journal for Clinicians, 46*(29).

Hill, G. (1979). Historical milestones in cancer surgery. *Seminar of Oncology, 6*(409).

Holmes, M. D., Hunter, D. J., Colditz, G. A., Stampfer, M. J., Hankinson, S. E., Speizer, F. E., et al. (1999). Association of dietary intake of fat and fatty acids with the risk of breast cancer. *Journal of the American Medical Association, 281*(10).

Hoskin, P., & Coyle, C. (2005). Introduction. In P. Hoskin & C. Coyle (Eds.), *Radiotherapy in practice brachytherapy.* New York: Oxford University Press.

Iovino, C., & Camacho, L. (2003). Acute myeloid leukemia: A classification and treatment update. *Clinical Journal of Oncology Nursing, 7*(5), 535–540.

Iwamoto, R. (2001). Radiation therapy. In S. Otto (Ed.), *Oncology nursing* (4th ed.). St. Louis: Mosby.

Jemail, A., Thomas, A., Murrey, T., & Thun, M. (2002). Cancer statistics, 2002. *CA—A Cancer Journal for Clinicians, 52*(1), 23–47.

Kalman, D., & Villani, L. (1997). Nutritional aspects of cancer related fatigue. *Journal of the American Dietetic Association, 97*, 650.

Kaye, J. (1993). Psychological distress in cancer patients and their spouses. *Journal of Cancer Education, 8*(47).

Keller, C. (2001). Bone marrow and stem cell transplantation. In S. Otto (Ed.), *Oncology nursing* (4th ed.). St. Louis: Mosby.

Kinsella, K., & Velkoff, V. (2001). *An aging world: 2001* (NIH publication no. P95/01-1). Washington, DC: U.S. Government Printing Office.

Larson, D. (1998). Stereotactic external-beam irradiation. In C. Perez & L. Brady (Eds.), *Principles and practices of radiation oncology* (3rd ed.). Philadelphia: Lippincott Williams & Wilkins.

Lavdaniti, M., Patiraki, E., Dafni, U., Katapodi, M., Papathanasoglou, E., & Sotiropoulou, A. (2006). Prospective assessment of fatigue and health status in Greek patients with breast cancer undergoing adjuvant radiotherapy. *Oncology Nursing Forum, 33*(3).

Lee-Lin, F., & Menon, U. (2005). Breast and cervical cancer screening practices and interventions among Chinese, Japanese, and Vietnamese Americans. *Oncology Nursing Forum, 32*(5).

Levy, J. (1994). Photosensitizers in photodynamic therapy. *Seminars in Oncology,* (21)4.

Liotta, L. A. (1992). Cancer cell invasion and metastasis. *Scientific American, 266*(2), 54–63.

Liotta, L. A., & Kohn, E. (1990). Cancer invasion and metastasis. *Journal of the American Medical Association, 263,* 1123–1126.

Ludwig, R., Weirich, A., Abel, U., Hofmann, W., Graf, N., & Tournade, M. (1999). Hepatotoxicity in patients treated according to Nephroblastoma Trial and Study SIOP-9/GPOH. *Journal of Medical and Pediatric Oncology, 33*(5).

Lynaugh, J. (2001). Forward. In J. Johnson, S. Baird, & L. Hilderley (Eds.), *It took courage, compassion, and curiosity: Recollections and writings of leaders in cancer nursing: 1890–1970* (1st ed.). Pittsburgh: Oncology Nursing Society.

Lynn, D. (1994). *Myself resolved an artist's experience with lymphoma.* Philadelphia: Meniscus Health Care Communications.

Mahon, S. M. (2000). Principles of cancer detection and early prevention. *Clinical Journal of Oncology Nursing, 4*(4), 169–176.

Malin, A. (2005) Epidemiology. In C. H. Yarbro, M. H. Frogge, & M. Goodman (Eds.), *Cancer nursing: Principles and practice* (6th ed.). Sudbury, MA: Jones and Bartlett.

Markam, M., & Walker, J. (2006). Intraperitoneal chemotherapy of ovarian cancer: A review with a focus on practical aspects of treatment. *Journal of Clinical Oncology, 24*(6).

McMahon, K. (2003). Components of nutritional screening and assessment. In *Oncology Nursing Society 2003 annual congress symposium highlights* (pp. 5–6). Pittsburgh: Author.

McNance, K., & Roberts, L. (2002). Biology of cancer. In K. McNance & S. Huetter (Eds.), *Pathophysiology: The biological basis for disease in adult and children* (4th ed.). St. Louis: Mosby.

Mellon, S. (2002). Comparisons between cancer survivors and family members on meaning of the illness and family quality of life. *Oncology Nursing Forum, 29*(7), 1117–1125.

Merkle, C., & Loescher, L. (2005) Biology of cancer. In C. H. Yarbro, M. H. Frogge, & M. Goodman (Eds.), *Cancer nursing: Principles and practice* (6th ed.). Sudbury, MA: Jones and Bartlett.

Miaskowski, C., & Lee, K. (1999). Pain, fatigue, and sleep disturbances in oncology outpatients receiving radiation therapy for bone metastasis: A pilot study. *Journal of Pain Symptom Management, 17*(3), 320.

Mock, V. (2003). Clinical excellence through evidenced-based practice: Fatigue management as a model. *Oncology Nursing Forum, 30*(4).

Murphy, M. (2001a). Cancers of the brain and central nervous system. In S. Otto (Ed.), *Oncology nursing* (4th ed.). St. Louis: Mosby.

Murphy, M. (2001b). Colorectal cancers. In S. Otto (Ed.), *Oncology nursing* (4th ed.). St. Louis: Mosby.

Muss, H. (2001). Older age—not a barrier to cancer treatment. *New England Journal of Medicine, 345*(15), 1128–1129.

Myers, J. (2001). Oncologic complications. In S. Otto (Ed.), *Oncology nursing* (4th ed.). St. Louis: Mosby.

Nail, L. (2004). Fatigue. In C. H. Yarbro, M. H. Frogge, & M. Goodman (Eds.), *Cancer symptom management* (3rd ed.). Sudbury, MA: Jones and Bartlett.

Nail, L., & Jones, L. (1995). Fatigue side effects and treatment and quality of life. *Quality of Life Research, 4*(1), 8.

National Cancer Institute. (2003). *Nutrition.* Retrieved from http://www.cancer.gov

National Comprehensive Cancer Network. (2003). Cancer-related fatigue: Clinical practice guidelines in oncology. *Journal of the National Comprehensive Cancer Network, 1*(1).

National Comprehensive Cancer Network. (2006). *Cancer-related fatigue: Clinical practice guidelines in oncology.*

Nelson-Marten, P., & Glover, J. (2005). Selected ethical issues in cancer care. In J. K. Itano & K. N. Taoka (Eds.), *Core curriculum for oncology nursing* (4th ed.). Philadelphia: W. B. Saunders.

Noll, L., & Riese, N. (1997). Chemical modifiers of radiation therapy. In K. Dow et al. (Eds.), *Nursing care in radiation oncology* (2nd ed.). Philadelphia: W. B. Saunders.

Occupational Safety and Health Administration, Office of Occupational Medicine. (1995). *Controlling occupational exposure to hazardous CPL2-2.20B CH-4.* Washington, DC: U.S. Department of Labor.

Oldham, R. (1991). Biotherapy: General principles. In R. K. Oldham (Ed.), *Principles of cancer biotherapy* (2nd ed.). New York: Marcel Dekker.

Omerod, K. (2005). Diagnostic evaluation, classification, and staging. In C. H. Yarbro, M. H. Frogge, & M. Goodman (Eds.), *Cancer nursing: Principles and practice* (6th ed.). Sudbury, MA: Jones and Bartlett.

Oncology Nursing Society. (2001). *Chemotherapy and biotherapy guidelines and recommendations for practice.* Pittsburgh: Author.

Oncology Nursing Society (2006). *Cancer pain management position statement.* Pittsburgh: Author.

Oncology Nursing Society, Vision, Mission, Core Values (ND). Retrieved September 22, 2008 from http://www.ons.org/about/corevalues.shtml.

Oncology Nursing Society & Geriatric Oncology Consortium (2004). *Oncology Nursing Society and Geriatric Oncology Consortium joint position on cancer care in the older adult.* Pittsburgh: Oncology Nursing Society.

O'Rourke, M. (2001). Genitourinary cancers. In S. Otto (Ed.), *Oncology nursing* (4th ed.). St. Louis: Mosby.

Ososki, R. (2001). Leukemia. In S. Otto (Ed.), *Oncology nursing* (4th ed.). St. Louis: Mosby.

Otto, S. (2001a). Chemotherapy. In S. Otto (Ed.), *Oncology nursing* (4th ed.). St. Louis: Mosby.

Otto, S. (2001b). Lung Cancers. In S. Otto (Ed.), *Oncology nursing* (4th ed.). St. Louis: Mosby.

Otto, S. (2001c). *Oncology nursing* (4th ed.). St. Louis: Mosby.

Overholt, B., Panjehpour, M., & Haydeck, J. (1999). Photodynamic therapy for Barrett's esophagus: Follow-up in 100 patients. *Gastrointestinal Endoscopy, 49*(1).

Park, C., & Folkman, S. (1997). Meaning in the context of stress and coping. *Review of General Psychology, 1,* 115–144.

Pfeifer, K. A. (2001). Pathophysiology. In S. Otto (Ed.), *Oncology nursing* (4th ed.). St. Louis: Mosby.

Piper, B., Dibble, S., Dodd, M., Weiss, M., Slaughter, R., & Paul, S. (1987). The revised Piper Fatigue Scale: Psychometric evaluation in women with breast cancer. *Oncology Nursing Forum, 25*(3).

Piper, B., Dibble, S., Dodd M., Weiss, M., Slaughter, R., Paul, S. (1998) The revised Piper Fatigue Scale: psychometric evaluation in women with breast cancer. *Oncology Nursing Forum. 25*(4):677–684.

Ponto, J., Frost, M., Thompson, R., Allers, T., Will, T., Zahasky, K., et al. (2003). Stories of breast cancer through art. *Oncology Nursing Forum, 30*(6), 1007–1113.

Rokita, S. (2004). Oncology: Nursing management in cancer care. In S. Smeltzer & B. Bare (Eds.), *Brunner & Suddarth's textbook of medical–surgical nursing* (10th ed.). Philadelphia: Lippincott Williams & Wilkins.

Russell, K., Perkins, S., Zollinger, T., & Champion, V. (2006). Sociocultural context of mammogram screening. *Oncology Nursing Forum, 33*(1).

Santos, G. (2000). Historical background to hematopoietic stem cell transplantation. In K. Atkinson (Ed.), *Clinical bone marrow and blood stem transplantation.* New York: Cambridge University Press.

Schmit-Pokorny, K., Franco, T., Frappier, B., Vyhlidal, R. (2003). The cooperative care model: an innovative approach to deliver blood and marrow stem cell transplant care. *Clinical Journal of Oncology Nursing, 7*(5).

Schulmeister, L. (2001a). Epidemiology. In S. Otto (Ed.), *Oncology nursing* (4th ed.). St. Louis: Mosby.

Schulmeister, L. (2001b). Nutrition. In S. Otto (Ed.), *Oncology nursing* (4th ed.). St. Louis: Mosby.

Sedhom, L., Yanni, M. (1985). Radiation therapy and nurses' fears of radiation exposure. *Cancer Nursing, 8*(129).

Shell, J., & Kirsch, S. (2001). Psychosocial issues, outcomes, and quality of life. In S. Otto (Ed.), *Oncology nursing* (4th ed.). St. Louis: Mosby.

Sigler, B., & Schuring, L. (1993). *Ear, nose, and throat disorders* (Mosby's Clinical Nursing Series), St. Louis: Mosby.

Singleton, L., & Connor, T. (1999). An evaluation of the permeability of chemotherapy gloves to three cancer chemotherapy drugs. *Oncology Nursing Forum, 26*(4).

Sitton, E. (1997) Managing side effects of skin changes and fatigue. In K. Dow et al. (Eds.), *Nursing care in radiation oncology.* (7th ed.). Philadelphia: W. B. Saunders.

Sitton, E. (2005). Nursing implications of radiation therapy. In J. K. Itano & K. N. Taoka (Eds.), *Core curriculum for oncology nursing* (4th ed.). Philadelphia: W. B. Saunders.

Spross, J., McGuire, D., & Schmitt, R. (1990a). Oncology Nursing Society position paper on cancer pain. Part I. Scope of nursing practice regarding cancer pain, ethics, and practice. *Oncology Nursing Forum, 17*(3), 595.

Spross, J., McGuire, D., & Schmitt, R. (1990b). Oncology Nursing Society position paper on cancer pain. Part II. Education, research, and list of cancer management resources. *Oncology Nursing Forum, 17*(4), 751.

Spross, J., McGuire, D., & Schmitt, R. (1990c). Oncology Nursing Society position paper on cancer pain. Part III. Nursing administration, pediatric cancer pain and appendices. *Oncology Nursing Forum, 17*(5), 943.

Stellman, J. M., & Stellman, S. D. (1996). Cancer and the workplace. *CA—A Cancer Journal for Clinicians, 46*(2).

Sura, W., Murphy, S., & Gonzales, I. (2006). Level of fatigue in women receiving dose-dense versus standard chemotherapy for breast cancer: A pilot study. *Oncology Nursing Forum, 33*(5).

Swenson, C. (2001). Pain management. In S. Otto (Ed.), *Oncology nursing* (4th ed.). St. Louis: Mosby.

Szopa, T. (2005). Nursing implications of surgical treatment. In J. K. Itano & K. N. Taoka (Eds.), *Core curriculum for oncology nursing* (4th ed.). Philadelphia: W. B. Saunders.

U.S. Department of Health and Human Services. (2000). *Healthy people 2010: Understanding and improving health.* Washington, DC: Author.

U.S. Department of Health and Human Services, Public Health Service, National Toxicology Program. (2002, December). *Report on carcinogens* (10th ed.). Washington, DC: Author.

VanBurik, J., & Weisdorf, D. (1999). Infections in recipients of blood and marrow transplantation. *Hematology Oncology Clinics of North America, 13*(5).

Viele, C. (2005). Keys to unlock cancer: Targeted therapy. *Oncology Nursing Forum, 32*(5).

Volker, D. L. (1992). Pathophysiology of cancer. In J. C. Clark & R .F. McGee (Eds.), *Core curriculum for oncology nursing* (2nd ed.). Philadelphia: W. B. Saunders.

Volker, D. (1994). Neoplasia. In P. Beare & J. Myers (Eds.), *Principles and practice of adult health nursing* (2nd ed.). St. Louis: Mosby.

Voss, J., Armitage, J., & Kessinger, A. (1993). High dose chemotherapy and autologous transplant with peripheral blood stem cells. *Oncology, 7*(8).

Wikle-Shapiro, T. (1998). Nursing implications of bone marrow and stem cell transplantation. In J. K. Itano & K. N. Taoka (Eds.), *Core curriculum for oncology nursing* (3rd ed.). Philadelphia: W. B. Saunders.

Wingard, J. (2007). Bone marrow to blood stem cells past, present, future. In S. Ezzone and K. Schmit-Pokorny (Eds.), *Blood and bone marrow stem cell transplantation: Principles, practice, and nursing insights* (3rd ed.). Sudbury, MA: James and Bartlett.

Winningham, M., Nail, L., Burke, M., Brophy, L., Cimprich, B., & Jones, L. (1994). Fatigue and the cancer experience. *Oncology Nursing Forum, 21*(1), 23–36.

Woodard, W., & Hogan, D. (1996). Oncologic emergencies: Implications for nurses. *Journal of Intravenous Nursing, 19*(2).

Wu, T., & Bancroft, J. (2006). Filipino American women's perceptions and experiences with breast cancer screening. *Oncology Nursing Forum, 33*(4).

Zebrack, B. (2000). Quality of life of long-term survivors of leukemia and lymphoma. *Journal of Psychosocial Oncology, 18*(4), 39–59.

Ziegler, R. G., Devesa, S. S., & Fravmeni, J. F., Jr. (1991). Epidemiologic patterns of colorectal cancer. In V. T. DeVita, Jr., S. Hellman, & S. A. Rosenberg (Eds.), *Important advances in oncology.* Philadelphia: Lippincott Williams & Wilkins.

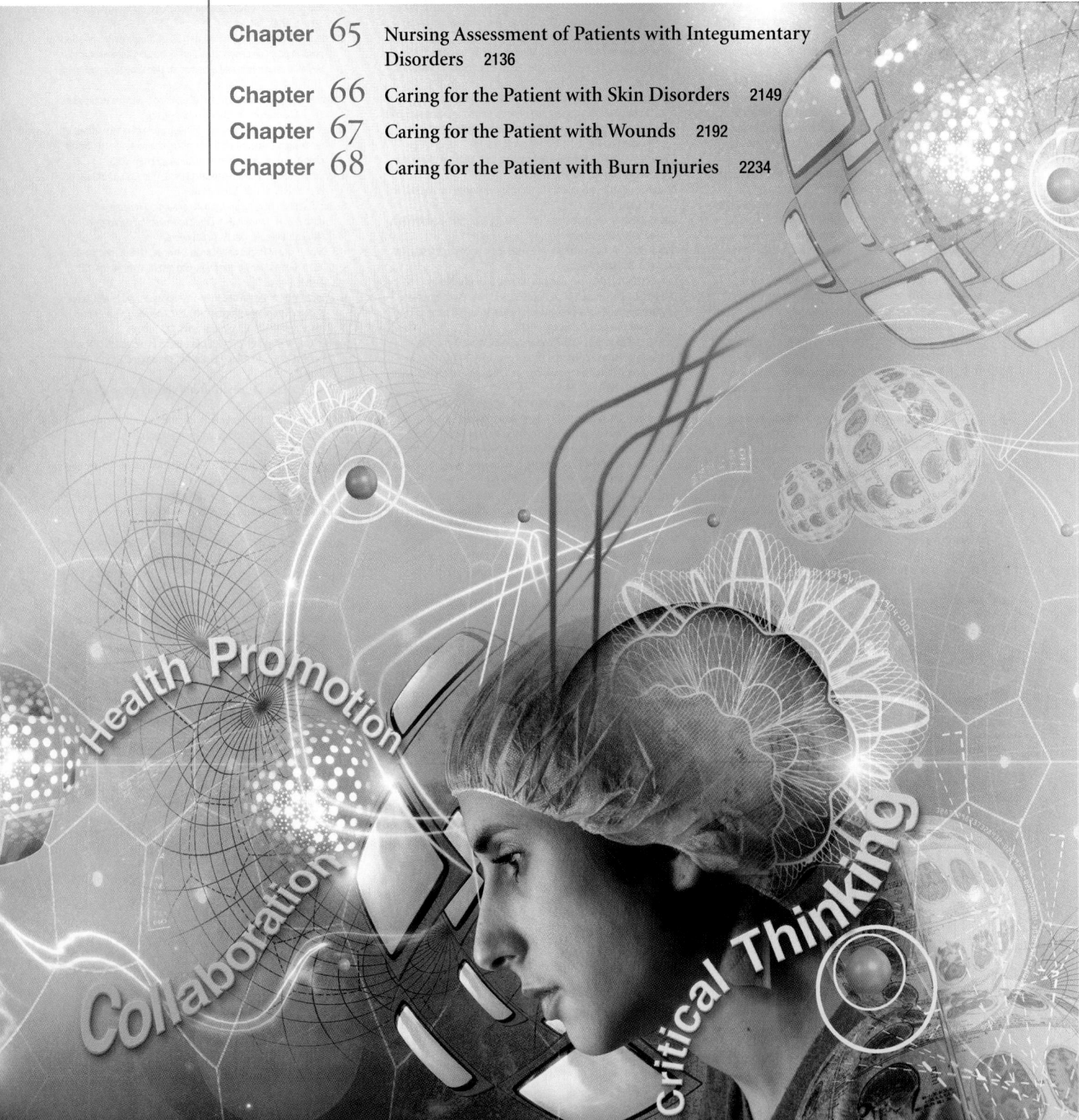

Health Promotion

Collaboration

Critical Thinking

Profiles in Nursing

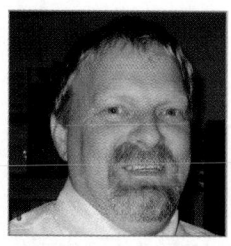

LEN My name is Len and I am the nurse manager in the Burn Intensive Care Unit (ICU) at a major teaching hospital. Although the Burn ICU specializes in the care of victims of traumatic burn injuries, we provide expert, cutting-edge care for a wide variety of other injuries and illnesses as well. Besides burn injuries, our patients are a diverse mix of people with trauma, chronic illnesses, and complex wounds.

After graduating from nursing school, I worked in a Burn Unit that also provided wound care services. I remember looking helplessly into the faces of patients with diabetes, while trying desperately to save their lower extremities from amputation. The stories they told of their cultural practices and traditions taught me valuable lessons about human compassion. I also learned that the physiological effects of their diabetes were further complicated by cultural and social gaps between native cultures and Western medicine. I developed a passion for helping those who desperately needed specialized interventions and I knew I wanted to devote my career to delivering care to a diverse population of people needing treatment for burns, complex wounds, and devastating illnesses.

The needs of burn patients and their families are even more complex than most people can possibly imagine. Teamwork and collaboration are absolutely essential for these patients to live and function. Every member of the burn team must be an expert in his or her own discipline. Health care professionals involved in the care of burn patients include burn surgeons, plastic reconstructive surgeons, pulmonologists, infectious disease experts, psychiatrists, cardiologists, ophthalmologists, respiratory therapists, physical and occupational therapists, laboratory specialists, pharmacists, dietitians, social workers, chaplains, and, of course, nurses. Burn nurses coordinate the care and implement the interventions ordered by the specialists. The role of the professional nurse does not rest with monitoring the patient's ventilator, cardiac monitor, hemodynamic status, emotional state, and pain level. We also perform daily dressing changes on large wounds and fragile skin grafts that can take up to 3 hours.

Burn patients often require very large quantities of IV fluids to prevent rapid and sudden cardiovascular collapse and hypovolemic shock. The process of infusing these large quantities of fluids is known as fluid resuscitation and is totally managed by the burn nurse. As many as three nurses, a surgeon, and a respiratory therapist may be required initially to admit and stabilize the victim of a large burn injury.

Caring about the welfare of your patients is what separates a technical nurse from a truly professional one who is committed to the profession. Due to the devastating nature of burn injuries, it is imperative for nurses to use a caring approach. A case comes to mind of a woman whose life was changed in a quick second. While getting dressed one morning, she was applying hairspray while evidently smoking a cigarette. The aerosolized hairspray ignited and she suffered full-thickness burns over a large portion of her body. After stabilization, she went to surgery to have her burns skin grafted. Our burn surgeon did such a remarkable job of placing a perfect graft over her severely damaged face. I spent 12 tedious hours with a scalpel, cotton swabs, ointment, and rolled gauze keeping serous fluid and blood from collecting under the skin graft. If fluid were allowed to collect, those portions of the graft would die due to a lack of blood supply. In spite of her injuries, I could see she was a beautiful woman whose physical appearance would now depend on me over the next few hours to make certain the skin would successfully attach. Times like these are a true test of one's commitment to others. It would have been easy to do an adequate job on this complete stranger by assessing and rolling the graft three or four times an hour. In this case, however, the fluid was collecting far too frequently. Although this woman was unknown to me, I did not see a stranger that night. I saw someone's wife and a child's mother lying in a bed on life support and placing a large portion of her future into the hands of someone she had never before met. Though I became fatigued, I stayed there never far from her face just to make sure the grafts were safe. I cannot remember whether I ate or drank much fluid that night while residing in her hot 90-degree room wrapped in a surgical gown and gloves.

Being a burn nurse is more than simply having good critical care skills, doing wound care, and managing the infusion of 30 liters of fluid into a person during a 24-hour period. It requires practicing with compassion in extreme circumstances, and accepting that the best you have to offer may not be enough. Despite the many emotionally trying circumstances I often encounter in the Burn ICU, I am more committed than ever to delivering care to a diverse population of people.

> "Caring about the welfare of your patients is what separates a technical nurse from a truly professional one who is committed to the profession."

65

Nursing Assessment of Patients with Integumentary Disorders

Peggy Ellis
Teri A. Murray
Kathleen Osborn

Outcome-Based Learning Objectives

After studying this chapter, the learner will be able to:

1. Discuss the structure and function of the skin.
2. Obtain a health history relative to assessment of the skin, hair, and nails.
3. Collect subjective and objective data relative to assessment of the skin, hair, and nails.
4. Utilize correct techniques of physical exam when assessing the skin, hair, and nails.
5. Distinguish between normal and abnormal assessment findings in the skin, hair, and nails.
6. Describe skin lesions by morphologic classification.
7. Identify biologic and cultural variations in assessment of the skin.

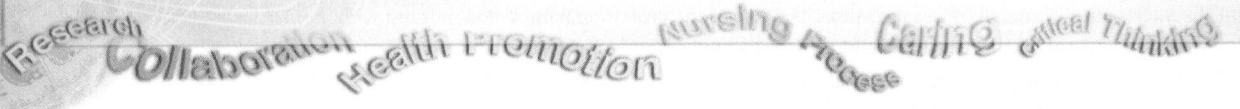

THE INTEGUMENTARY system is composed of the skin, hair, nails, and glands. The skin is the most visible organ of the body and accounts for about 7% of the body weight. It is composed of three layers: the epidermis, dermis, and subcutaneous tissue described later (Porth, 2007). The epidermal appendages of the skin include the hair, nails, sebaceous glands, and the eccrine and apocrine sweat glands. The skin is pliable, is able to withstand insults from external agents, and has a remarkable ability to heal. Additionally, through the sense of touch, it enables individuals to perceive the world around them, and its changes in color reflect emotional reactions to the environment. It is critical that the nurse be able to recognize and identify skin abnormalities. Assessment of the skin and its appendages requires a thorough understanding of the structure and function of the integumentary system and knowledge of normal and abnormal findings.

Anatomy and Physiology of the Skin

The skin is the largest organ of the body whose primary function is to provide a protective barrier to the vital organs, and it prevents harmful organisms from entering the body. It protects underlying tissues and structures from microorganisms, chemical injury, or trauma, and it guards against excessive exposure to ultraviolet rays from the sun. Other functions of the skin include:

- Retards the loss of body heat and fluids
- Assists in the control of body temperature
- Contains the sensory receptors that allow an individual to feel heat, cold, pressure, and pain
- Contains immune systems cells
- Functions as a excretory organ (sweat glands)
- Functions as a synthesizer of vitamin D (sunlight reacts with cholesterol)
- Determines identity (race, fingerprints)
- Stores blood and fats
- Reflects emotion through color changes.

The skin also manifests diseases or injury. For example, rashes may be associated with systemic diseases such as lupus erythematosus and jaundice associated with liver disease (Porth, 2007). Redness and swelling are associated with injuries such as fractures and internal bleeding.

Skin Layers

There are three anatomical layers of the skin: the epidermis, dermis, and subcutaneous tissue (Figure 65–1 ■). Each layer is described next.

Epidermis

The epidermis is the thin, avascular outer layer that is nourished by the blood vessels from the dermis. Four distinct cell types are contained in the epidermis: keratinocytes, melanocytes, Merkel's cells, and Langerhans' cells. *Keratinocytes* are the most numerous cells of the epidermis; and as they mature they move to the surface, die, and thereby form the outermost surface of the skin (stratum corneum). These cells produce keratin, which provides the major protective barrier. The maturation and death of keratinocytes occur approximately every 4 weeks. If the process occurs too quickly, the skin appears thin and may break down more easily. If old cells have not sloughed before the formation of new cells, the skin appears thickened and scaly. *Melanocytes* are the pigment-producing cells. Pigment granules (melanin), which are black or brown, give the skin and hair its color. The more melanin an individual has, the darker the skin and hair. The primary function of melanocytes is to protect the skin from ultraviolet rays. *Merkel's cells* provide sensory information, and *Langerhans' cells* are macrophages of the immune system that arise from the bone marrow and migrate to the epidermis. These cells recognize a foreign antigen and bind it to their surface, process it, and then migrate with the antigen back to the lymphatic vessels and into the regional lymph nodes. The epidermis also contains sweat glands and sebaceous glands.

Dermis

A basement membrane connects the epidermis to the dermis. This is the layer involved in blister formation. The dermis, composed of fibrous connective tissue, contains the blood vessels, hair follicles, nerve endings, sweat glands, and sebaceous glands. It separates the epidermis from the subcutaneous tissue and provides nutrition for the epidermis. The dermis is composed of

two layers: the papillary dermis and the reticular dermis. The papillary dermis is the superficial layer, consisting of collagen fibers and ground substances (a viscid gel that is rich in mucopolysaccharides) that lie adjunct to the epidermis. This layer is densely covered by dermal papillae that contain capillary venules that nourish the epidermal layer. Lymph vessels and nerve endings are also found in this layer. The reticular dermis, the thicker layer, is composed of a complex meshwork of three-dimensional collagen bundles interconnected with large elastic fibers and ground substance. The reticular dermis also contains dermal dendrocytes, which have phagocytic properties that participate in immune function of the skin. The specific immune cells found in dermis include T cells, mast cells, and fibroblasts (Porth, 2007). The T cells provide a delayed-type hypersensitivity that is described in Chapter 60 ⬡.

Subcutaneous Tissue

Subcutaneous tissue, made up of loose connective tissue and fat cells, functions to lend support to the vascular and neural structures that supply the outer layer of skin. Because of the presence of the eccrine glands and deep hair follicles, and several skin diseases that extend into this layer, it is considered part of the skin (Porth, 2007).

Blood and Lymph Supply, Sebaceous Glands, and Innervation

The arterial vessels that nourish the skin are located between the papillary and reticular layers of the dermis and between the dermis and the subcutaneous tissue layer. Blood returns via small veins that accompany the subcutaneous vessels. The lymphatic system is located in the dermis and helps combat skin infections. The majority of the vessels are under sympathetic nervous system control. The sympathetic nervous system also controls the arrector pili muscles that cause elevation of the hair on the arms and dimpling of the skin (goose bumps). The dermis contains a rich supply of sensory neurons. The receptors for touch, pressure, heat, cold, and pain are in the dermis (Porth, 2007).

■ Gerontological Considerations

Several physiological changes occur in the skin with the aging process. Both the epidermis and the dermis thin; there is a reduction in subcutaneous tissue and collagen, and a thickening of the blood vessels. In addition, the number of melanocytes, Merkel's cells, and Langerhans' cells decreases. This results in color changes and decreased resistance to organisms. The keratinocytes actually shrink, although the amount of dead keratinized cells on the skin surface increases. These changes result in thinner skin with less padding, making it more susceptible to breakdown from trauma. There is a decrease in hormonally induced sebaceous gland activity. Therefore, older individuals have drier, more scaly skin, especially in the winter months when there is an increased need for home heating. Finally, there is less hair and nail growth, and hair permanently loses pigment with the aging process (Porth, 2007). Graying may begin as early as in the third decade of life and is caused by reduced melanin production in the hair follicles. Genetic factors tend to determine the age of the onset of graying. Chapter 66 ⬡ includes an in-depth discussion of age-related skin diseases.

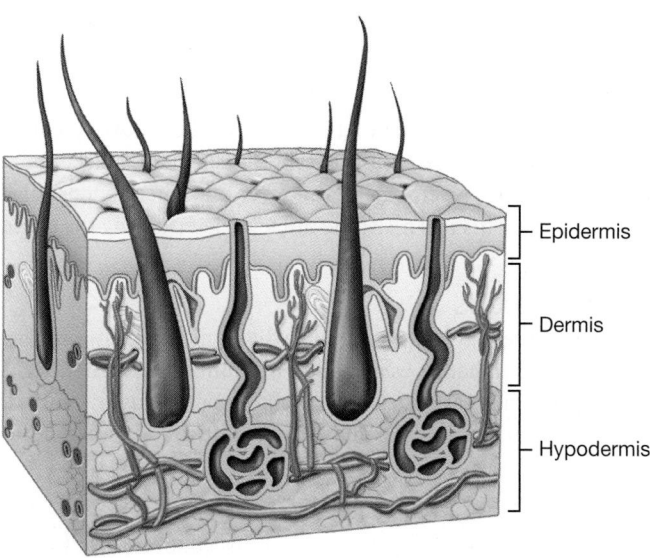

FIGURE 65–1 ■ Skin layers.

- Epidermis

- Dermis

- Hypodermis

Physiological Impact of Ultraviolet Rays

The sun's rays are measured in wavelengths that range from 290 nanometers in the ultraviolet (UV) range to 2,500 nanometers in the infrared range. There are three types of ultraviolet rays: ultraviolet A (UVA), ultraviolet B (UVB), and ultraviolet C (UVC). The UVB rays are primarily responsible for sunburn and the cumulative damage to the skin from the sun (Porth, 2007). UVA rays produce elastic skin and actinic skin damage. Exposure to UV radiation causes sunburn and skin cancer and accelerates skin aging. A growing concern is that UV radiation can reduce the effectiveness of the human immune system, thereby enhancing the risk of infection and limiting the efficacy of immunization against disease (World Health Organization, 2001). Chapter 66 🌐 includes an in-depth discussion of sun-related skin diseases.

> **CRITICAL ALERT**
>
> *A common belief is that only fair-skinned people need to be concerned about overexposure to the sun. It is true that darker skin has more protective pigment, although the skin is still susceptible to the damaging effects of ultraviolet (UV) radiation. The incidence of skin cancers is lower in dark-skinned people; nevertheless, skin cancers occur and are often detected among them at a later, more dangerous stage. The risk of other UV-related health effects, such as eye damage, premature aging of the skin, and immunosuppression, also occurs in dark-skinned people.*
>
> (World Health Organization, 2001).

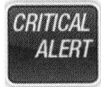 # History

The health history, the major subjective source of data, provides valuable insights into the patient's past and current health status. The health history is composed of several components that provide structure for data collection and an organized record of the patient's response to skin problems. The components of the history are outlined next.

Biographic and Demographic Data

Biographic and demographic data include data such as the patient's name, address, telephone number, social security number, contact person, age, gender, race or ethnic origin, marital status, birthplace, occupation, level of education, and religious affiliation. This information is critical in identifying one patient's record from another's, and it provides a general overview of the person's communication abilities, reliability as a historian, and general personal attributes. Biographic and demographic information is needed for epidemiologic comparisons. For example, the incidence or prevalence of a particular health condition may be attributed to a certain geographic locale, a racial or ethnic group, or a specific gender. It is important to date the history so that, if the patient's condition changes, events can be correlated chronologically. Examples of biographic and demographic data that may be significant to assessment of the skin include environmental or occupational toxins, neighborhood waste, or landfills. Environmental toxins include overexposure to frost, wind, and ultraviolet rays from the sun. Neighborhood waste and landfills could involve exposure to arsenic, creosote, coal tar, and/or petroleum products. Environmental toxins, neighborhood waste, and landfills are risk factors for skin cancer. Finally the nurse also should inquire about travel to different environments such as camping or travel to rural areas of the world.

Chief Complaint

The assessment begins with identifying the patient's current issue or the reason for seeking health care, which is referred to as the chief complaint. When a patient is admitted, the nurse begins the interview by asking the patient what he considers the most current and acute health issue. It is typically best elicited by the nurse's asking "What brought you here?" It is generally a concise statement in the patient's own words indicating his rationale for seeking health care. Examples of chief complaints are "I have had a rash for 3 days"; "I've noticed discolorations on my legs and arms for 2 weeks"; "My hair has been thinning for 6 months"; "I think I have a fungal infection in my cuticle."

Presenting Symptoms

The presenting symptoms detail the chronology of each symptom, how it developed, and what events surrounded the symptoms. In the skin, the presenting symptoms may be changes in the condition of the patient's skin, such as dryness, pruritus, sores, and lumps; changes in a mole or a wart; skin lesions; or changes in skin color or texture. When obtaining information from the patient related to the presenting symptoms, the nurse should question the patient about his perception of the cause as well as what measures the patient may have already taken to remedy the condition.

Past Medical History

The past medical history can be of great value in assessing the current problem. The purpose in obtaining information about the past medical history is to identify the patient's entire past relevant health problems. Past illnesses could possibly have some effect on the patient's current health. The nurse would ask the patient about previous skin conditions, allergic reactions, unusual sensations, history of allergies, and other diseases that may affect the condition of the skin. A disease such as systemic lupus erythematosus causes a butterfly rash on the face. Use of chemotherapeutic agents to treat cancer may cause hair loss. Cancer, heart disease, liver disease, and anemia can cause changes in the nails such as grooves, ridges, and discolorations.

Childhood Illnesses

Inquire whether the patient has had any of the following childhood illnesses: measles, mumps, whooping cough, chickenpox, smallpox, scarlet fever, rheumatic fever, diphtheria, acne, and poliomyelitis. This will assist the nurse in determining the cause of any residual scarring.

Immunizations

The nurse needs to inquire about what childhood immunizations the patient had as well as adult immunizations. Ask the patient specifically about polio, diphtheria, pertussis, human papillomavirus (HPV), tetanus toxoid, influenza, last tuberculin skin test, and any skin reactions to the immunizations.

Previous Illnesses

The nursing assessment includes questions about major illnesses such as diabetes, cardiovascular disease, and infectious diseases. Patients with diabetes are prone to skin breakdown and delayed wound healing (Chapters 53 and 67 ⊚). Patients with cardiovascular disease may have clubbed nail beds (Chapter 37 ⊚). Infectious diseases such as cellulitis have skin manifestations, which assist with the diagnosis.

Medications

Inquire about medications taken regularly (names, dosages, frequency, reason for taking, side effects) and whether the patient complies with the medication regimen. Inquire about over-the-counter medication use; include herbal medications, vitamins, and any home remedies as well. Drugs may produce skin eruptions, decrease or increase sunlight sensitivity, and cause hyperpigmentation.

Allergies

Inquire about allergies to medications, foods, and environmental allergens. Have the patient describe what clinical skin manifestations occur when she experiences an allergic reaction as well as what makes the reaction subside.

■ Health Assessment

The current health status is the general state of health as perceived by the patient. A question to elicit this information might be "Over your lifetime, have you had ongoing skin problems?" The nurse needs to identify risk factors that impact the skin such as sun exposure and the use of cigarettes. The nurse must assess the amount of time spent in the sun as well as other risk factors associated with the development of skin cancer. These risk factors are outlined in the Risk Factors box. Other significant habits and lifestyles are assessed during the health history outlined next.

Social History

Social history includes use of alcohol or street drugs that can have adverse effects on the conditions of the patient's skin. Drugs and alcohol can have a pathologic effect on a patient's skin. This effect may result from the direct toxic effect or from personal neglect, environmental factors, and/or poor nutrition. The presence of certain cutaneous lesions in a patient should prompt an investigation into the patient's drinking and drug habits. The nurse should inquire about the patient's skin care habits and routine, use of special cleansing agents or soaps, use

---

RISK FACTORS Associated with Skin Cancer

- Age 50 or older
- Male gender
- Family history of skin cancer
- Fair complexion with light-colored hair or eyes
- Precancerous lesions
- Geographic location such as high altitude or near the equator
- Exposure to certain elements such as radium, isotopes, x-rays
- Exposure to coal, tar, creosote, and petroleum products
- Extended exposure to sunlight
- Repeated skin trauma or irritation
- Tendency to burn easily
- History of severe and/or multiple sunburns as a child.

---

of cosmetics or other dermatologic products, sun exposure patterns, use of sunscreen and sunblock, and exposure to stressors.

If suspected due to the presence of cutaneous lesion, the nurse needs to inquire about skin popping. Skin popping is a technique used by individuals to administer illicit drugs. The technique, also called "subcutaneous" or "subQ," involves injecting of the drug between skin and fat layers. Skin popping is used for several reasons including:

- Individuals not wanting to inject right into a vein
- Individuals finding it too difficult to hit the vein
- Because drugs absorb more slowly
- Less of a "rush," but the effects of the drug may last longer
- Trying to keep from getting dope sick
- To reduce the risk of drug overdose
- Individuals not having veins left to shoot the drug into. (Public Health; Seattle & King County, 2008)

Skin popping is a significant risk factor in skin and soft tissue infections, which are common among injection drug users (IDUs). There is an increased incidence of *Staphylococcus aureus* skin infections among IDUs. Additionally, outbreaks of uncommon infections including tetanus, wound botulism, and a sepsis/myonecrosis syndrome due to *Clostridium* species have been seen with IDUs (Brown & Ebright, 2002).

Occupation

This is the description of the patient's usual work. The nurse inquires about the patient's work conditions and hours, duration of employment, and any occupational exposure to irritants, pollutants, or allergens, and frequent sun exposure. Skin neoplasms do result from occupational or environmental agents. For example, individuals that work in the sun have an increased risk for the development of skin cancer.

Cultural Considerations

The nurse would inquire about any cultural habits or practices that may affect the patient's skin. This would include any culture-related dietary habits as well. For example, in Southeast Asia, there is a custom of scraping the skin when a person is sick, causing bruising and open sores. This is thought to aid in the healing process.

Environment

The nurse should inquire of the patient about environmental exposure to chemicals, toxins, animals, outdoors, paint, aerosols, petroleum products, and tar. These products can irritate the skin, causing rashes and skin breakdown.

Habits

In addition to social habits mentioned earlier the nurse should inquire about the patient's sleep patterns and whether there have been any recent changes. The nurse should ask specifically whether the patient experiences symptoms such as itching at night or night sweats. Ask the patient whether he bites or chews the nails or picks at the skin. These habits may cause a loss of skin integrity and increase the risk of a skin infection.

Exercise

The nurse should inquire about the patient's exercise habits. Does the patient exercise on a regular basis? What are the recreational activities of the patient? Do the recreational activities expose the patient to excessive weather elements, such as wind, cold, heat, or sun? Does the individual work out at community gyms? There may be a risk for contracting fungal infections or community acquired methicillin-resistant *Staphylococcus aureus* (MRSA) from the equipment or showers. Caution the patient not to share towels and to cover and protect any open areas on the skin. Ask the patient how much and how easily she perspires. Profuse, out of the ordinary perspiration may be indicative of a systemic disorder. Obesity is one cause of excessive perspiration.

Nutrition

The nurse would assess the patient's dietary pattern to see whether the patient eats well-balanced, nutritious meals. The history should focus on the patient's overall eating habits and use of chocolate, caffeine, sweets, and carbonated beverages. Inquire about recent changes in diet. Dietary changes may cause rashes and other skin reactions.

Physical Examination

When conducting a physical examination of the skin, the nurse must be cognizant of age-related changes. What is normal for a young person will be changed or absent in the elderly population. Certain skin changes related to the aging process are not in and or themselves pathologic. Therefore, the nurse also must possess the knowledge of normal versus abnormal for each age group when assessing the skin. Pathologic changes are outlined in detail in Chapter 66 .

Inspection

When conducting the physical assessment of the skin, the nurse must be aware of ethnic variations related to skin color and texture, mucous membrane coloring, and hair texture. The nurse must perform a thorough physical examination in a well-lit room, preferably in indirect natural daylight. To examine the skin properly, the nurse must take a brief but careful look at the patient's entire body and examine specific areas of concern in detail. A small magnifying glass and a centimeter ruler or tape are required when assessing lesions. The assessment should proceed in an orderly fashion, beginning with an examination of the most frequently exposed areas such as the face, hands, arms, legs, and feet. Along with the skin, the nurse would also examine the appendages, hair, scalp, and nails.

Inspection of the Skin

The nurse inspects the skin while the patient is in a sitting or lying position with all clothes removed except an examination or hospital gown. The nurse inspects the skin for color, temperature, thickness, moisture, texture, turgor, edema, and lesions. Special attention needs to be paid to pressure points, especially in the elderly population. If the patient has tubes and or stomas, the adjunct skin should be assessed for breakdown and rashes. The nurse needs to be aware of ethnic differences, especially in the darker skinned populations, when conducting an assessment.

 CRITICAL ALERT *Ethnic considerations: The best areas to assess pallor, cyanosis, and jaundice are oral mucous membranes and conjunctiva in dark-skinned people.*

Color

Skin color varies from person to person depending on the ethnicity and race of the person. Melanin, carotene, the level of oxygen in the blood, and the amount of sun exposure will all influence the color of the patient's skin. Dark skin contains more melanin than does fair skin. Asians have more carotene pigments, which gives the skin the yellow hue. In addition, skin color will vary from body part to body part. Usually, the most frequently exposed areas are noticeably different from the unexposed areas. The difference may be due to the more frequent exposure from the sun, wind, and other environmental elements on exposed skin. Normal skin color ranges from a whitish pink to a dark chocolate brown, depending on race. When evaluating skin color changes, the nurse must be cognizant of variations in skin color based on the patient's racial background, as presented in the Cultural Considerations box. When assessing for color changes, the nurse should give consideration to the room's lighting and temperature as well as the position of the patient. For example, is there a color change when the patient's leg is in a dependent position?

Palpation

Palpation is examination of the skin through the use of touch. Generally, the nurse will inspect and palpate simultaneously. When palpating the skin, the nurse assesses the skin temperature, texture, thickness, moisture, turgor, edema, and lesions. The presence or absence of a pulse needs to be determined, as it may indicate a diminished blood supply to the area.

Temperature

Using the dorsal surface of the hand, which is most sensitive to temperature, the nurse first palpates the forehead and proceeds in a systematic fashion downward, being certain to include the hands and feet. The nurse should always make side-to-side comparisons. Assess for bilateral symmetry by palpating similar areas simultaneously, using both the right and left hand. For example, are both hands the same temperature, or is one warmer or cooler than the other? Normal skin temperature ranges from slightly warm to slightly cool. This may fluctuate depending on the temperature of the patient's environment. Skin temperature will be increased with any condition that increases blood flow to the area. For example, localized skin temperature could be increased due to tissue injury, trauma, or infection. Occasionally, the temperature is slightly cooler in a person's hands and feet, but the temperature should be similar on both sides. A difference in temperature bilaterally warrants further investigation and could be indicative of vascular problems or infection.

Generalized skin temperature increases may occur in systemic infections, fever, or metabolic disorders such as hyperthyroidism. Conversely, temperature to the skin is decreased when blood flow to the skin is diminished. Conditions that may cause a decrease in local skin temperature result from diminished blood supply to the area, vasoconstriction, occlusion, or peripheral arterial insufficiency. Generalized skin temperature decreases may occur when the environment is cool and in the presence of metabolic disorders such as hypothyroidism.

CULTURAL CONSIDERATIONS for Assessing Skin Color Changes

Skin Color Variation	Description of Variation	Appearance in Light Skin	Appearance in Dark Skin
Carotenemia	A yellowish discoloration of skin that differs from jaundice because it does not involve the sclera or mucous membranes. It is often associated with a high intake of foods with carotene (sweet potatoes, squash, and carrots).	A yellowish stain in the skin.	May be difficult to assess.
Cyanosis	A bluish-gray discoloration of the skin that is often caused by decreased perfusion of the tissues with oxygenated blood.	Bluish tinge notably in skin, lower eyelid, mucous membranes, lips, earlobes, soles of the feet, and palms.	Ashen-gray discoloration of the skin, mucous membranes, lips, and tongue.
Ecchymosis	Purplish, blue, and black marks that are usually caused by trauma. Ecchymosis occurs due to the extravasation of blood. Over time the discoloration fades to greenish-brown and then yellow as the blood is reabsorbed into the vascular system.	Purplish, blue-black areas may be seen anywhere on the skin.	Purplish, blue-black areas on the skin may be difficult to see in poor lighting.
Erythema	A reddish discoloration of the skin that is caused by dilation of the capillaries. This is usually due to local irritation or inflammation, embarrassment (blushing), heat, or fever.	Redness that can be seen anywhere on the body. It may be generalized or localized.	Redness that appears on the body but is difficult to see unless in a well-lit area.
Hyperpigmentation	Hyperpigmentation can be in a specific or a general area. It results from changes in the distribution of melanin. It is often seen in pregnancy (linea nigra); persons of color are often born with dark discolorations located on the lower back and buttocks, called mongolian spots. Both linea nigra and mongolian spots disappear over time or when the pregnancy is over.	Spots or lines that appear darker than the general skin.	Spots or lines that appear darker than the general skin.
Jaundice	A yellowish discoloration of the skin, sclera, and mucous membranes that is often associated with increased amounts of bilirubin in the blood. Some newborns are born with pathologic jaundice, in which skin color changes are noted within the first 24 hours of life. Jaundice is generally caused by disorders that cause an increase in the serum bilirubin level.	A yellow staining noticeable in the skin, hard palate, sclera, palms, and soles of the feet.	Can be seen in the hard palate, sclera, palms, and soles of the feet.
Pallor	Paleness of the skin that occurs when the red-pink tones from the oxygenated hemoglobin in the blood are lost. The skin takes on the appearance of collagen (connective tissue), which is almost white.	Loss of rosy glow in the skin.	Ashen appearance. The skin will lack red tones, which normally give dark skin a luster or a glow. Pallor can best be seen in the palpebral conjunctiva, the preferred site for assessment of pallor related to anemia.
Petechiae	Pinpoint purpuric lesions of the skin.	Pinpoint purpuric lesions can be seen on the skin.	May be difficult to see except in good lighting.
Vitiligo	The absence of pigmentation in a circumscribed area.	May be difficult to see except in good lighting.	A circumscribed area or areas with loss of pigmentation.

Source: Halder, R. M. & Nootheti, P. K. (2003). Ethnic skin disorders overview. *Journal of the American Academy of Dermatology 48* (6 Supplement): S143–S148.

Texture

The texture of the skin ranges from smooth and soft to rough and hard. The nurse should use the palmar surface of the fingers and finger pads when palpating for texture. Normal skin texture is smooth, soft, and even. The texture may be rougher in exposed areas or areas of pressure, such as the elbows, palms, and soles of the feet. Conditions such as hyperthyroidism will alter the texture of the skin. Hyperthyroidism usually causes the skin to be smooth with a velvet-like texture. Hypothyroidism causes the skin to be rough and scaly. The skin of the elderly has an increased incidence of scaling as well.

Thickness

The skin should be thin and firm over most parts of the body. Normally, it is thicker on the palms, soles of the feet, elbows, and knees and thinner over the eyelids. Skin thickness varies with age or illness, as in the thin, fragile skin of the elderly or the patient who is severely emaciated. Very thin skin with a shiny appearance

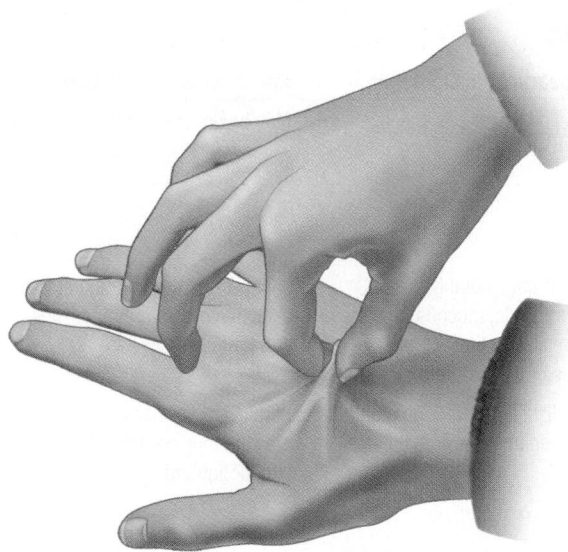

FIGURE 65–2 ■ Skin turgor.

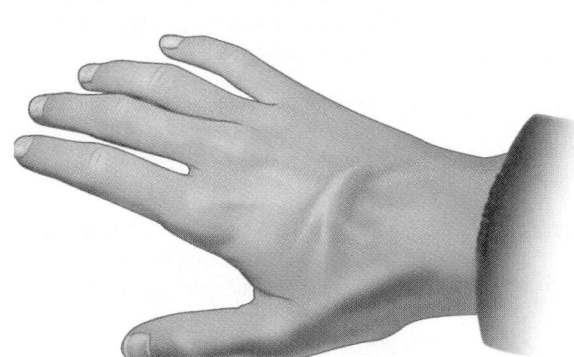

is often indicative of impaired circulation. An individual's occupation may affect the thickness of the skin due to callous formation.

Moisture

The nurse will assess for moisture using the dorsal surface of the hand. The dorsal surface is generally drier, and using it will help to avoid confusion of the moisture on the patient's skin with that on the nurse's hand. Moisture on the skin does vary from one body part to another. The soles of the feet, the palms of the hands, and the intertriginous areas (where two surfaces are close together) contain more moisture than other parts. There should be minimal perspiration on the patient's skin unless he has just engaged in vigorous exercise, the environmental temperature is warm, or the patient has an elevated body temperature. The skin regulates body temperature by producing perspiration that evaporates, thus cooling the skin when the body temperature increases. The skin is normally drier in winter months when it is cooler and humidity is low. Dehydration will cause the skin to be drier. Medical disorders that cause dryness include myxedema and nephritis.

Turgor

Turgor refers to the elasticity and mobility of the skin. Elasticity is described as the resiliency of the skin: its ability to return to a normal position and shape. Mobility is the skin's ability to be lifted. To assess turgor, the nurse would grasp a fold of the patient's skin using the forefinger and thumb (Figure 65–2 ■). The nurse notes how rapidly the skin returns to its normal shape. Normal, healthy skin returns rapidly to its previous shape. When turgor is decreased, the skin fold holds its pinch formation before returning to its normal shape. Loss of turgor is associated with dehydration and aging. As individuals age, the skin normally loses its elasticity. The chest wall is ideal to assess turgor because it is not subject to the age-related changes associated with loss of elasticity. Increased skin turgor makes it difficult or impossible to pinch up the skin. It may be produced by conditions such as scleroderma, which causes the underlying connective tissue to become hard and immobile.

Edema

Edema is caused by the accumulation of fluid in the intercellular spaces. Edema makes the skin appear puffy and tight. Edema is often noted in dependent areas such as the hands, feet, and sacral area. To assess for edema, the nurse would palpate the patient's skin with the pads of the finger. Normally the skin surface stays smooth. If the pressure leaves an indentation in the skin, "pitting" edema is present. Pitting edema is generally evaluated on a 4-point scale, but varies among examiners:

- 1 + Mild pitting in which there is slight indentation, no obvious swelling of the leg
- 2 + Moderate pitting in which the indentation rapidly subsides
- 3 + Deep pitting in which the indentation lasts a short time
- 4 + Very deep pitting in which the indentation lasts a long time (Figure 65–3 ■).

Because measuring edema varies among examiners, some nurses prefer to record edema in terms of time duration of the

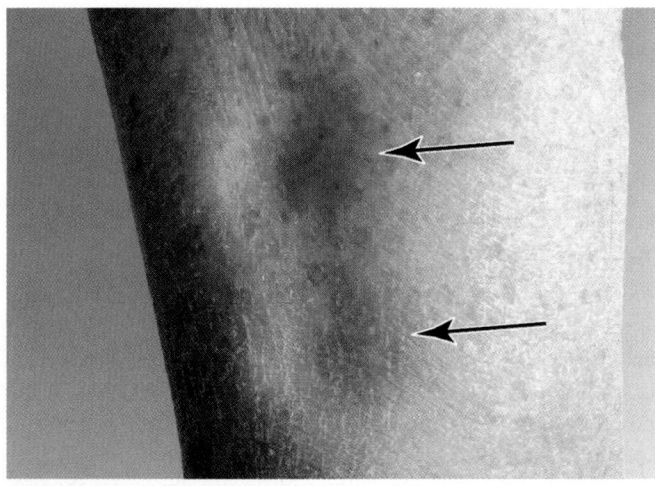

FIGURE 65–3 ■ Pitting edema.
Source: Medical-On-Line Ltd.

indentation. For example, the pitting edema lasts between 15 and 30 seconds before the skin returns to normal.

Lesions

When the nurse assesses the skin, careful attention should be paid to the presence of lesions. Lesions must be assessed using two of the techniques of examination, inspection and palpation. The nurse should use a magnification glass in order to evaluate skin lesions accurately. Lesions should be described according to distribution, location, configuration, and the presence of exudate.

Distribution and Location

Distribution of the lesions on the skin is described according to location or body region affected. Lesions may be confined to one small area (localized), confined to an entire area such as the chest (regional), or spread over the entire body (generalized). The nurse notes whether the lesions are distributed symmetrically or asymmetrically. Noting the characteristic pattern of lesions can provide additional clues in the diagnosis of a specific skin condition.

Configuration or Pattern of Arrangement

The nurse must also note the configuration of the lesions. **Configuration** refers to the pattern of arrangement or position of the lesions. The nurse should assess how lesions are patterned on the body. Are they **discrete lesions** (individual or separate), congruent (running together), grouped in a characteristic pattern, **linear lesions** (forming a line), and/or arciform lesions (arc-shaped) lesions? For example, ringworm or tinea corporis has an annular or circular configuration.

Types of Lesions

The lesion should be further examined for color, size, shape, texture, firmness, discharge, and morphologic classification. The **morphologic classification** of the skin is described in terms of type of lesion (primary, secondary, or vascular), size, shape or configuration, color, texture, elevation or depression, and pedunculation. If the lesion has drainage, the drainage is described in terms of color, odor, amount, and consistency. A **primary lesion** occurs as an initial reaction to a pathologic condition (Chart 65–1). A **secondary lesion** results from a change in the primary lesion or external trauma to the primary lesion (Chart 65–2, p. 2144). **Vascular lesions** appear as red- or purple-pigmented lesions (Chart 65–3, p. 2144). They are generally indicative of conditions that cause bleeding (petechiae and ecchymosis) or liver disease (spider angioma), or may be due to benign conditions such as telangiectasia. Determining whether the lesions blanch will help identify the type of lesion. Pectechie and ecchymosis will not blanch, whereas telangiectases will blanch.

Lesions should be measured with a small, clear, flexible ruler or tape measure. Lesion size is described in centimeters, and all dimensions should be measured (length, width, and depth). The color of individual lesions also is documented. The color of the lesion may be well circumscribed (confined to the lesion) or may be more diffuse, where the borders are not clearly defined. For example, **ecchymosis** is initially dark red or purple but gradually fades to yellowish green before it disappears.

While wearing gloves, the nurse also palpates the lesions to determine the texture or firmness. Additionally, the pattern of how the lesions appear on various areas of the body is assessed. For example, are they clustered in one area, or are they diffusely spread all over the body? It is important to ask the patient about the presence of itching and pain associated with lesions. The

CHART 65–1	Primary Skin Lesions		
Primary Lesion	**Description**	**Pain/Itching**	**Examples**
Abscess	A pus-filled nodule.	Localized tenderness. Typically intensity increases as size increases.	An infected wound that forms a pocket of pus under the skin surface.
Bulla	A vesicle or blister usually about 1 centimeter in diameter.	Itching and pain present.	Sunburn, poison oak, poison ivy.
Cyst	A palpable fluid-filled or solid subcutaneous sac.	Typically not painful.	Sebaceous cyst.
Furuncle	A pus-filled lesion usually greater than 0.5 centimeter.	Tender, depends on size.	Boil.
Macule	A flat, nonpalpable circumscribed area of a change in skin color.	Not painful.	Freckles, purpura.
Nodule	A well-circumscribed, firm, palpable lesion deeper within the dermis than a papule.	Not painful.	Sarcoma, subcutaneous nodules.
Papule	A solid, elevated, circumscribed mass that is generally less than 1 centimeter in diameter.	Not painful.	Wart.
Patch	A macule larger than 1 centimeter.	Not painful.	Vitiligo, port-wine stain.
Plaque	Very similar to a papule but greater than 1 centimeter in diameter.	Painful.	Psoriasis, discoid lupus erythematosus.
Pustule	A pus-filled vesicle or bulla.	May be tender.	Acne, impetigo.
Tumor	A solid mass generally larger than 1 centimeter.	Not painful.	Fibroma, lipoma.
Wheal	A circumscribed irregularly shaped elevation of the skin caused by cutaneous edema.	May or may not be tender.	Urticaria.

CHART 65–2	**Secondary Skin Lesions**		
Secondary Lesion	**Description**	**Pain/Itching**	**Examples**
Atrophy	Thinning of the skin resulting from wasting of the dermis. There is a depression in the dermis. The skin is translucent and paper-like.	Not painful.	Striae, normal aging skin.
Crust	A dried serum or blood exudate as found on the surface of an abrasion or excoriation. The size and color vary.	Crust is not tender, but wound underneath may still be tender depending on stage of healing.	Scab, healing fever blister.
Erosion	An absence of the superficial dermis. The lesion is moist and glistening.	Tender.	Syphilitic chancre.
Excoriation	The loss of superficial tissue.	Slight tenderness.	Abrasion, scratch.
Fissure	A linear crack or break from the epidermis to the dermis.	Slight tenderness depending on size and location.	Athlete's foot; chapped, cracked lips as seen in severe dehydration.
Lichenification	Rough, thickened epidermis with increased visibility of the superficial skin markings.		Chronic dermatitis.
Scale	An abundance of dry or oily keratinized cells. Color or size may vary.		Exfoliative dermatitis.
Ulcer	Destruction of the skin beneath the epidermis.	May or not be tender, depending on size, location, depth, and whether acute or chronic.	An open sore sometimes on the leg, as with peripheral vascular disease.
Scar (cicatrix)	Fibrous tissue replacing the injured dermis.	Not painful depending on stage of healing.	Healed wound or surgical wound.
Keloid	An overproduction of scar tissue that extends laterally beyond the initial wound that is usually raised and smooth in appearance. Has a high incidence of occurrence in dark-skinned races and in children.	May or may not be tender. May itch.	Healed wound or surgical wound that is larger than the original wound size.
Hypertrophy	An overproduction of scar tissue that does not extend beyond the initial wound. It has a raised thickened appearance.	May or may not be tender. May itch.	Healed wound or surgical incision that has a thickened appearance.

CHART 65–3	**Vascular Lesions**	
Lesion	**Description**	**Cause**
Cherry angioma	A distinct, benign vascular lesion 0.5–5 millimeters in diameter. A firm, deep-red papule.	Generally found on most people after age 30, and the incidence increases with age.
Ecchymosis	Red-purple nonblanchable discoloration of variable size.	Vascular wall destruction, trauma, vasculitis.
Petechiae	Red-purple nonblanchable discoloration less than 0.5 centimeter in diameter.	Intravascular defects, infection.
Purpura	Red-purple discoloration greater than 0.5 centimeter in diameter.	Intravascular defects, infection.
Spider angioma	Red central body with radiating spider-like legs that blanches with pressure to the central body.	Liver disease, vitamin B deficiency, idiopathic.
Telangiectasia	Fine, irregular red lines.	Dilation of capillaries.
Venous star	Bluish spider irregularly shaped with linear lines.	Increased pressure in superficial veins.

length of time that lesions have been present and the precipitating factors that caused them to occur, are also assessed.

If palpation is not adequate to arrive at a diagnosis, **diascopy** is used to examine superficial skin lesions with a diascope. A diascope, a high-powered spotting scope for straight or angled viewing, is often used to observe color changes of a lesion.

Inspection of the Lips

Assessment of lips includes confirming that they are symmetrical, smooth, pink, moist, and without lesions. Systemic dehydration may be manifested in dry, scaling, cracking lips. Herpes viral infections and skin cancer are disorders common to the lips. Herpes presents with vesicle on the lip that extends onto the skin. Skin cancers most commonly occur on the lower lip or the underside of the tongue (D'Amico & Barbarito, 2007). Cancer is suspected when there is an open area (sore) that does not heal. The nurse needs to inquire about a history of heavy cigarette, pipe, and cigar smoking; chewing tobacco use; and alcohol intake, as these are risk factors for the development of oral cancer.

Inspection of the Hair

Hair color is created by the production of melanin. Hair color varies from pale or platinum to dark black and is dictated by the genetic background and ethnic origin. Hair texture may be very fine to course and curly to straight. Normal hair in the absence of disease should have a vibrant appearance with a natural gloss. The normal texture of the hair may be changed due to environmental conditions and harsh treatment with colors, dyes, blowdrying, and permanent waving.

The hair should be evenly distributed on the head. **Alopecia**, loss of hair, can be a result of familial patterns of baldness, disease, medications, or a pathologic condition. Diffuse hair loss may be caused by hormonal changes, systemic infections, and reaction to chemicals or medications. Patchy hair loss can be caused by scalp infections such as ringworm, burn injuries, and trauma, and from permanent waving or other harsh chemical treatments.

The scalp should be assessed for lesions. When assessing the nurse should don gloves and separate the patient's hair into small sections and lift it. The nurse inspects the scalp for lesions, pest infestations such as lice, and dandruff.

Inspection of and Palpation of the Nails

The nurse inspects and palpates the patient's nails. The nail surface is normally slightly curved with the posterior and lateral folds smooth and rounded. The nail edges should be smooth, rounded, and clean. The normal nail bed angle is 160 degrees. The nail base is firm to palpation. A nail bed with greater than 160-degree angle suggests a clubbed nail. Clubbing of nails indicates a state of chronic hypoxia and is often seen with congenital and adult heart disease and chronic obstructive pulmonary disease.

The surface of the nail should be smooth and nonbrittle, with no splitting. Pits, transverse grooves, or lines may indicate a nutritional deficiency (Figure 65–4 ■). Patients with arterial insufficiency may have thickened, ridged nails.

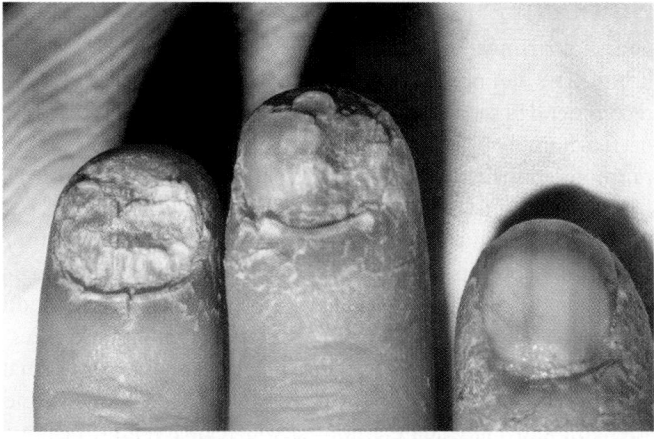

FIGURE 65–4 ■ Fingernails with pits, grooves, and lines.
Source: From Neil S. Prose, K. G. Abson, and R. K. Scher. Internat. J. Dermat. 31: 453, (1992)

The nail plate is translucent and the nurse should expect to see a pink nail bed. Dark-skinned patients may have brownish, pigmented areas or linear bands along the nail edge. The nurse palpates the nail bed to determine capillary refill. To assess capillary refill, the nurse would depress the nail edge to blanch and then release, noting the return of color. Capillary refill is usually documented as brisk, which is a normal response. However, it may have a sluggish return to color for patients with cardiovascular or respiratory disease and low hemoglobin.

■ Genetic Implications

The family history informs the nurse about the general health of the patient's blood relatives and spouse. This information allows the nurse to identify any illnesses that have a genetic, familial, or environmental link as well as implications for the patient's current and future health problems. The blood relatives include the maternal and paternal grandparents, parents, siblings, aunts, uncles, and children. Inquire about diseases that demonstrate genetic or familial tendencies. Familial tendencies have not been identified as genetic disorders but have been found in family clusters. Usually the information obtained about the family is documented in a genogram. The family genogram is an effective way to document a large amount of data obtained from the family history. Any family history of allergic disorders or conditions such as asthma, hay fever, skin cancer, melanoma, psoriasis, eczema, or infestations of lice or scabies should be solicited from the patient as well as familial hair loss patterns.

■ Critical Thinking Related to Skin Assessment

Critical thinking is essential in order to prioritize the most significant clinical manifestations that need further investigation. Skin disorders can be as benign as slight sunburn to life-threatening disorders such as necrotizing fasciitis. It is imperative that the nurse be able to distinguish normal from abnormal, benign from serious. The nurse must rely on critical thinking skills in interpreting the patient's symptoms and assessment findings to determine possible and potential patient diagnoses and to consider the appropriate actions to take. Analysis of this data allows the nurse to make a diagnosis and then follow up with an intervention. It is imperative that the nurse communicate and collaborate with other members of the health care team in developing and implementing a plan of care.

Regardless of the health problem, each symptom identified should be thoroughly described in order for the nurse to gain a full understanding. The nurse will ask the patient, "Tell me more about the problem," or "How did it start?" The patient will usually proceed with a discourse about the symptoms. The nurse uses skillful interview techniques to explore and investigate each symptom further. Any symptom analysis would be incomplete without a thorough description of symptom characteristics (Chart 65–4, p. 2146).

Symptoms related to skin conditions include itching, drainage, color changes, changes in moles or warts, or a lesion that does not heal. The nurse should inquire whether the onset was gradual or sudden and about the length of time the problem has persisted. If

CHART 65–4 Skin Disorder Analysis Criteria

SYMPTOM ANALYSIS

Onset

- When did it first occur?
- Did it occur gradually or suddenly?
- What are the precipitating factors?
- How long does it last?
- Is it continuous or is it intermittent?
- Is there a pattern of remission or exacerbation?

Location

- Where is it located?
- Does it radiate?

Timing

- When does it occur?
- How long does it last?
- How often does it occur?
- Is there a particular setting in which it occurs?

Quality

- How would you describe the symptom?
- How does the symptom rate on a scale of 1–10, with 10 being the most extreme?
- Is the symptom getting better or worse?

Quantity

- What is the frequency of occurrence?
- What is the extent of its occurrence?
- Does it occur in a specific setting?

Aggravating Factors

- What makes it worse?

Alleviating Factors

- What makes it go away?
- What makes it better?

Associated Phenomena

- What else happens when you experience the symptom?
- What treatments have you tried including prescription, over-the-counter, and herbal medications and remedies?

the condition were a rash, the nurse would question the patient to determine whether it is progressive and spreading. Exploring precipitating factors would provide critical clues such as whether a change in skin care products, new cologne, or a new house pet precipitated the condition. Associated symptoms would be whether the patient had a recent viral illness, had a high fever, or had exposure to increased physical or psychological stress.

◼ Implications for Health Promotion

Health promotion for the skin primarily focuses on protection and early treatment. Protecting the skin will help prevent breakdown and early treatment may prevent complications. Patient teaching must include information about the risk factors that cause the various integumentary abnormalities. When assessing the patient, it is essential for the nurse to identify high-risk behaviors such as sun exposure that require education. Correct use of sunscreens and limited exposure to the sun need to be stressed. An in-depth discussion of sun protection is included in Chapter 66 .

CRITICAL ALERT *It is important for the nurse to stress that most sunscreens must be applied 15 to 30 minutes prior to sun exposure. Additionally, sunscreens need to be reapplied after swimming or excessive perspiration.*

Adequate rest balanced with a healthy exercise program has many beneficial effects. Rest is restorative to the body, and lack of it is often manifested in the color of the skin. For example, dark circles under the eyes are a common manifestation of lack of sleep. Exercise causes vasodilation, typically manifested on the skin as a "healthy glow." Increased circulation also promotes wound healing and prevents the occurrence of wound infections. Education about overexposure to heat, cold, and sun will prevent skin breakdown. The National Guidelines feature outlines safe skin care.

Hygiene

The skin and hair need to be cleansed regularly to prevent bacterial buildup, remove excess oil, and prevent odor. Education about skin hygiene needs to be tailored to match the skin type. For example, oily skin needs a cleanser that promotes drying, whereas dry skin needs a more gentle cleanser that prevents drying. The skin should be washed gently so as not to cause irritation and breakdown. If any irritation occurs, the individual must be instructed to stop using the product and try another one. Soaps tend to be more alkaline, thereby neutralizing the normal skin pH of 4.2 to 5.6. This may promote bacterial growth and increase the risk for infection. If this is occurring, the patient must be instructed to try other cleansers.

The elder population needs to use gentle, less drying cleansers and shampoos because skin and scalp dry out with age. Moisturizers are typically helpful for dry skin and scalp in preventing scaling and pruritus. Individuals may need to try different products in order to find the one that is best tailored for their skin type. Chapter 66 discusses the specific skin disorders.

Nutrition

Nutritional intake has a major impact on skin, hair, and nail health. The diet needs to be well balanced and include the daily recommended servings of each food group. The skin specifically needs vitamins A, B, C, and K. Vitamin A and C are needed to promote epithelialization and normal rate of wound healing. Lack of vitamin C is also associated with bleeding gums, petechiae, and purpura. The B complex vitamins are essential for normal metabolic processes and preventing certain dermatologic conditions such as seborrhea. Lack of vitamin K delays blood clotting and therefore can increase the risk of bruising and excessive bleeding with injuries. Protein intake is essential for normal cell growth and collagen formation, which increase wound strength, and inadequate amounts will retard wound healing. Chapter 14 contains an in-depth discussion of normal nutritional intake and the associated side effects of malnutrition.

NATIONAL GUIDELINES for Safe Skin Care

National Organization	Recommendation
American Cancer Society	Monthly skin self-examination for all adults.
	Health care provider skin examination every 3 years in persons aged 20–39 and annually in persons over 40.
	Education of patients concerning sun avoidance and use of sunscreen.
	Avoidance of artificial tanning devices.
American Academy of Family Physicians	Complete skin examination for adolescents and adults with increased recreational or occupational exposure to sunlight, a family or personal history of skin cancer, or evidence of precursor lesions.
	Skin protection from ultraviolet light for all persons with increased exposure to sunlight.
American Academy of Dermatology	Regular screening visits for skin cancer and patient education concerning periodic skin self-examination.
	Education of patients concerning sun avoidance and use of sunscreen.
	Avoidance of artificial tanning devices.
American Medical Association	Education of patients concerning sun avoidance and use of sunscreen.
	Avoidance of artificial tanning devices.
Canadian Task Force	Avoidance of sun exposure and use of protective clothing.
National Institutes of Health Consensus Panel	Regular screening visits for skin cancer and patient education concerning periodic skin self-examination.
	Avoidance of artificial tanning devices.

Source: U.S. Preventive Services Task Force. (1996). *Guide to clinical preventive services* (2nd ed.). Alexandria, VA: International Medical Publishing.

◼ Conclusion

It is essential to conduct a thorough, complete health history and an accurate assessment of the skin and the epidermal appendages to distinguish between normal and abnormal findings. As described earlier, many systemic diseases are manifested through the skin, hair, and nails. The nurse needs to possess the knowledge and skills necessary to evaluate each of these areas critically and utilize findings to help determine a nursing diagnosis. The National Guidelines box provides guidelines set forth by national organizations regarding safe skin care.

NCLEX® REVIEW

1. A patient tells the nurse that she "avoids the sun." The nurse realizes this patient could be at risk for developing:
   1. Hypothermia.
   2. Dehydration.
   3. Hypercholesterolemia.
   4. Vitamin D deficiency.

2. During an assessment, the nurse asks a patient if he has been to any foreign countries. This information would be applicable to which of the following categories of the health history?
   1. Past medical history
   2. Chief complaint
   3. Biographic and demographic data
   4. Previous illnesses

3. A 25-year-old patient is admitted with severe cutaneous skin lesions. Which area of the assessment should the nurse focus first?
   1. Culture
   2. Occupation
   3. Habits
   4. Social history

4. The nurse is preparing to examine a patient's skin. Which of the following should the nurse do when conducting this assessment?
   1. Wear sterile gloves.
   2. Assess least frequently exposed areas first.
   3. Inspect and palpate the skin at the same time.
   4. Ask the patient to stand up for the assessment.

5. The nurse assesses a patient's nails to be at a 160 degree angle with a smooth surface. These findings would be indicative of:
   1. Chronic hypoxia.
   2. COPD.
   3. A nutritional deficiency.
   4. Normal findings.

6. An African American patient has an overproduction of scar tissue along the site of a total hip replacement. The nurse realizes this scar would be considered a:
   1. Scale.
   2. Cherry angioma.
   3. Keloid.
   4. Fissure.

7. While assessing the skin of an African American patient, the nurse notes the absence of pigmentation along the right lateral thoracic region. This finding would be documented as:
   1. Jaundice.
   2. Pallor.
   3. Petechiae.
   4. Vitiligo.

Answers for review questions appear in Appendix D

KEY TERMS

alopecia *p.2145*
configuration *p.2143*
diascopy *p.2144*
discrete lesion *p.2143*
distribution *p.2143*

ecchymosis *p.2143*
edema *p.2142*
linear lesion *p.2143*
morphologic classification *p.2143*

primary lesion *p.2143*
secondary lesion *p.2143*
turgor *p.2142*
vascular lesion *p.2143*

PEARSON
EXPLORE mynursingkit™

MyNursingKit is your one stop for online chapter review materials and resources. Prepare for success with additional NCLEX®-style practice questions, interactive assignments and activities, web links, animations and videos, and more!

Register your access code from the front of your book at
www.mynursingkit.com

REFERENCES

Brown, P. D., & Ebright, J. R. (2002). Skin and soft tissue infections in injection drug users. *Current Infectious Disease Reports, 4*(5), 415–419. Retrieved November 12, 2007, from http://opioids.com/skin-popping/index.html

D'Amico, D., & Barbarito, C. (2007). *Health and physical assessment in nursing.* Upper Saddle River, NJ: Pearson Prentice Hall.

Porth, C. (2007). *Essentials of pathophysiology.* Philadelphia: Lippincott Williams & Wilkins.

Public Health: Seattle & King County. (2008). *HIV/AIDS Program: Muscling and skin popping.* Retrieved August 29, 2008, from http://www.metrokc.gov/health/apu/harmred/muscling.htm

U.S. Preventive Services Task Force. (1996). *Guide to clinical preventive services* (2nd ed.). Alexandria, VA: International Medical Publishing.

World Health Organization. (2001). *Protecting children from ultraviolet radiation.* Retrieved November 10, 2007, from http://www.who.int/mediacentre/factsheets/fs261/en/

Caring for the Patient with Skin Disorders

Peggy Ellis
Teri A. Murray
With contributions by: John M. Osborn

Outcome-Based Learning Objectives

After studying this chapter, the learner will be able to:

1. Differentiate the etiology, pathophysiology, and interventions for infections of the skin.
2. Identify preventive measures for skin disorders.
3. Identify the impact of the environment on the skin.
4. Describe the signs and symptoms, diagnostic tests, and treatment of skin disorders.
5. Develop a nursing plan of care for a patient with a skin disorder.
6. Differentiate the psychological and physical implications for the patient with a skin disorder.
7. Describe the effects of aging on the skin.

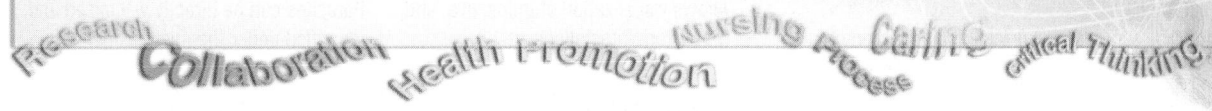

Research Collaboration Health Promotion Nursing Process Caring Critical Thinking

THE SKIN is the largest organ system of the body and serves as the protective barrier against the external environment including infectious agents. It is responsible for helping to regulate body temperature and contains receptors for sensation. The skin helps define cultural and ethnic backgrounds and helps define one's self-image. The skin also can be helpful when expressing emotion.

Disorders of the skin are a common reason for visiting the health care provider. The skin is often a mirror to the rest of the body. The patient may often complain of a rash, itching, or an unusual lesion. There can be disorders of only the skin or systemic disorders that are reflected in the skin. Certain disorders of the skin are treated with medication and/or nonpharmacologic measures, whereas others require surgical intervention.

Skin disorders are usually diagnosed by evaluating the history of onset of symptoms and precipitating factors, including systemic diseases, and performing a physical examination. Most skin disorders have distinct, recognizable lesions that assist with the diagnosis. However, if the abnormality is uncertain, it is cultured, scraped, or biopsied and microscopically examined to identify the diagnosis. The Diagnostic Tests box (p. 2150) describes the common laboratory and diagnostic tests and abnormalities associated with skin disorders.

Nails

Toenails and fingernails are considered a part of the skin and need to be assessed for abnormalities. The nails reflect nutritional status and general health as well as the presence of systemic disorders and exposure to toxic agents. Careful assessment is an important part of diagnosing both local and systemic disorders. Systemic disorders often cause changes in the shape or contour of the nail. Chart 66–1 (p. 2151) provides an overview of nail abnormalities related to systemic disease.

Brittle Nails

Brittle nails are defined as nails in which the distal plate splits, leading to peeling of the distal portion of the nail. Brittle nails are excessively ridged and dry. Usual water content of the nail is about 18%, whereas brittle nails have a water content of only about 16% (Singh, Haneef, & Uday, 2005). This is caused by prolonged immersion in water, dry skin with dryness of the nail plate, or chemical or mechanical trauma that leads to nail dehydration (Chart 66–2, p. 2151), presents other causes (Fawcett, Linford, & Stulberg, 2004). When brittle nails are noted, a thorough history and physical should be performed to help determine the cause. Note the specific nails that are involved and the changes in the nail plate.

DIAGNOSTIC TESTS for Skin Disorders

Test	Expected Abnormality	Rationale for Abnormality
Biopsy: Surgically removing all or part of the lesion for inspection under the microscope. Can be excisional, punch, shave, or immunofluorescent.	Identification of microorganisms or cell type. Can identify cancer cells, inflammatory reactions, and other types of cell abnormalities.	Enables examination of cells for identification of type, or malignant vs. benign. Helps with diagnosis and proper treatment.
Potassium hydroxide smear: A sample of the lesion is taken, wet with a solution of potassium hydroxide, and placed on a slide for examination.	Potassium hydroxide clears off debris and bacteria so that fungi can be identified.	Able to diagnose whether fungi are the cause of a skin disorder.
Tzanck smear: Scraping of lesion is taken and placed on slide. The material is stained with Giemsa, Wright's, or Sedi stain to identify multinucleated giant cells or atypical keratinocytes.	Demonstrates the presence of multinucleated giant cells, which indicates herpes simplex virus or varicella-zoster virus.	Not a very accurate test but can help to diagnose the presence of herpes simplex virus.
Culture: Sample of lesion is placed in a culture medium to allow growth of organism.	The microorganism will grow on the culture medium and can be identified.	Proper identification of the causative organism can allow for effective treatment.
Immunofluorescent studies: Tissue samples are stained for antibodies and examined under a fluorescence microscope.	Will detect immune complexes and the presence of immunoglobulins in immunologically mediated disorders.	Identifies immunologically mediated dermatitis.
Wood's lamp: "Black" light that can be shone on a rash to produce fluorescence.	Tinea will fluoresce green under a Wood's light. Other fungi may fluoresce yellow to orange.	Helps identify fungi that are the causative agent.
Polymerase chain reaction (PCR): Method of identifying the DNA in the pathogen.	Identifies mutations in DNA related to antigen–antibody reactions.	Allows the recognition of bacteria and viruses, especially those difficult to identify through a culture. Can also identify genetic disorders.
Skin scrapings: Cells can be scraped off the lesions and placed on a slide.	Allows visualization of mites, ova, and feces from infestations.	Parasites can be directly visualized and identified under the microscope.
Patch test: Suspected allergens are applied to the skin of the back or arm for 48 hours to see whether there is a reaction.	If the patient has an allergy to the substance applied to the skin, wheals and flare reactions will be evident.	Determines whether dermatitis is allergic or irritant, and identifies the allergen.

Treatment of Brittle Nails

If the hands must be immersed in water, it is important to wear gloves. The hands and nails can be massaged daily with lubricants or oils after soaking in lukewarm water for 15 minutes. Keep the nails well groomed and avoid using them as tools to scrape or pry. Systemic treatment with biotin has been found to improve the nails. Biotin is a component of the vitamin B complex that helps maintain healthy muscle, hair, and skin by stimulating keratinization. Patients who are given oral biotin at a dosage of 2.5 milligrams a day have shown improvement of nail strength over 3 to 6 months. Biotin is well tolerated with very few side effects. Therefore, it is a reasonable choice when other treatment measures fail (Scher, Fleckman, Tulumbas, McCollam, & Enfanto, 2003).

Nail Infections

The most common infection of the nail is onychomycosis, or tinea unguium, which is a chronic fungal infection under the nail. It usually occurs in the toenails but can occur in the fingernails as well. It commonly leads to deformed, cracked nails that initially become white or silvery and then turn yellow or brown. The nail beds are thickened but usually are not uncomfortable or painful. The infection can spread to other nails and is diagnosed through cultures and microscopy. This condition is difficult to treat and is typically slowly responsive to the oral and topical antifungal medications. The nail may eventually have to be surgically removed in order to clear up the infection.

Paronychia is an acute or chronic infection of the folds of tissue around the nail or the cuticle that usually begins after minor trauma. The causative organism is most frequently *Streptococcus* or *Staphylococcus*, but it can also be related to a fungus. In acute paronychia, an abscess may develop that requires surgical drainage for relief of pain. In chronic paronychia, the infection develops more slowly with progressive tenderness and swelling around the cuticle. Treatment involves the application of hot compresses and topical antibiotics.

Nail Trauma or Loss

Nail trauma can lead to disorders such as subungal hematoma and pincer nail. Trauma to the nail or nail bed may result in

CHART 66–1 **Nail Abnormalities Related to Systemic Disease**

Nail Abnormality	Description	Disease
Beau's lines	Transverse furrows on fingernails.	Stress. Acute severe illness. Nutritional disorders. Circulation disorders. Abnormal metabolic states.
Spoon nails (koilonychia)	Nails are concave like a saucer. Nail plate is thinned.	Hypochromic anemia. Rheumatic fever. Syphilis.
Nail pitting	Thickened nail plate with small pits.	Psoriasis.
Nail clubbing	Flattened nail plate. Bulbous distal phalanx. Increased angle between nail and dorsal surface of finger.	Chronic hypoxia. Heart disease. Pulmonary disease. Cystic fibrosis. Bronchogenic carcinoma.
Mees' lines	White, transverse line.	Poisoning. Acute illness.
Lindsay's nails	Proximal portion of nail is white while distal portion is red or pink.	Chronic renal disease. Azotemia.
Terry's nails	White nail beds with distal band of reddish brown.	Cirrhosis. Hypoalbuminemia. Congestive heart failure. Diabetes type II.

CHART 66–2 **Causes of Brittle Nails**

Occupational Causes	Physical Causes
Chemicals such as acetone	Aging
Typing	Atherosclerosis
Playing a musical instrument	Poor nutrition with deficiencies in vitamins A, B_6, and C
Grasping	Chronic renal failure
Prying	Cardiovascular disease
Scraping	Raynaud's disease
Frequent hand washing	Thyroid disease
	Psoriasis
	Eczema
	Onychomycosis
	Warts
	Squamous cell or basal cell carcinoma

changes in the size, shape, or color of the nail. A subungal hematoma is usually related to trauma to the nail that causes bleeding and bruising under the nail. This typically leads to separation of the nail plate. The blood will cause a dark discoloration that will remain until the nail plate grows out. It may be necessary to puncture the nail to relieve the excess pressure caused by the blood building up under the nail. Pincer nail usually affects the toenail and is evidenced by the lateral edges of the nail curling in and under it, leading to a tube-like appearance of the nail. It is usually caused by pointed-toed shoes or high heels that squeeze the toes together. If the pincer nail causes pain, the nail may need to be surgically removed.

An ingrown nail occurs when the corners of the nail plate grow into the lateral nail fold and dermis. It is usually due to poorly fitting shoes, improper nail trimming, or trauma. The individual experiences pain, redness, and swelling, and an infection may develop leading to an abscess. This condition can be prevented by wearing proper fitting shoes and trimming the nails straight across. Treatment options depend on the severity of the symptoms. Soaking the nail, along with systemic and/or topical antibiotics, may be used. A cotton wick can be inserted into the lateral nail groove to allow for drainage and relief of pressure. If these strategies are unsuccessful, or if the symptoms are more severe, a wedge resection of the corner of the nail can be performed with removal of the lateral one-fourth of the nail. Removal of the lateral nail matrix may be necessary to create a new lateral nail fold and prevent the recurrence of an ingrown nail.

■ Hair

Hair disorders include too much hair, known as hirsutism, or not enough hair, known as alopecia. **Hirsutism** is defined as the excessive growth of hair and is caused by an increased testosterone level, Cushing's syndrome, carcinoma of the adrenal gland, testicular tumors, or acromegaly. This condition occurs more commonly in women. The increase in hormones stimulates the hair follicle to grow, especially on the lip, chin, chest, areola, abdomen, lower back, buttock, inner thighs, and external genitalia. The treatment consists of diagnosing and treating the underlying cause.

Alopecia is defined as the loss of hair that can occur in men and women at any age. One of the most common forms of alopecia is **androgenetic alopecia**, also known as male pattern baldness. Androgenetic alopecia is a physiological baldness in which androgen levels are normal; however, there is a genetic predisposition to balding. In men, it usually begins with bitemporal thinning of the hair and progresses to the frontal area, whereas in women the pattern is central thinning. The degree of baldness and the age of onset are determined by the inheritance of several genes. The hair shafts gradually shrink until they become finer and thinner. It is not related to any serious health problems but can be psychologically disturbing. Certain topical medications can be applied to the scalp, but their effectiveness is variable. The two medications that have been found to be the most effective are finasteride and minoxidil. Finasteride blocks the conversion of testosterone to 5-alpha dihydrotestosterone (DHT). DHT is needed for the development of androgenetic alopecia. Minoxidil is a vasodilator applied topically that leads to enhanced hair growth due to the increased blood flow. These medications must be used for 4 to 12 months before effectiveness can be evaluated (Stough et al., 2005).

Androgenic alopecia occurs in women and is recognized as a symptom of polycystic ovary syndrome. Chapter 49 ⊘ discusses polycystic ovary syndrome. It is related to excessive androgen production that causes a decrease in size of the hair follicles leading to hair loss in central and frontal areas. Hair loss also can be related to systemic medications; for example, many of the chemotherapeutic agents used for treating cancer can lead to hair loss. Systemic diseases related to hair loss include hypothyroidism, insulin resistance, and cardiovascular disease.

Alopecia also is associated with high levels of anxiety and depression, low self-esteem, poor quality of life, and poor body image. Hair is closely related to an individual's identity and attractiveness. Visits to psychologists/psychiatrists may be beneficial in helping patients deal with problems associated with alopecia (Hunt & McHale, 2005).

Skin

The skin is affected by health and healthy lifestyle choices. When teaching patients and families about how to maintain healthy skin, it is essential to discuss the importance of adequate nutrition. The skin needs protein, vitamin C, iron, and zinc to be healthy. Protein and vitamin deficiencies, along with obesity, can decrease the skin's ability to regenerate and affect the circulation to the skin, leading to skin lesions and delayed wound healing. Water is important to maintain elasticity in the skin. Approximately 64 ounces of water is needed daily to keep the skin well hydrated. Regular exercise helps maintain adequate circulation, providing oxygen and nutrients to the skin. Regular bathing keeps the excess bacteria and oils in check so that the skin can remain healthy. However, bathing more frequently than necessary should be avoided because it can cause dryness of the skin. The patient should be asked about bathing practices, including the type of cleanser used and the frequency of bathing. If the skin is dry, emollient cream or lotion should be applied immediately after bathing to maintain hydration. The skin should be inspected monthly for new growths or changes in skin lesions. (See Chapter 65 @ for skin assessment.) Racial differences in skin may account for changes in skin response to daily care and environmental irritants, as seen in the Cultural Considerations box.

Sunlight

The sun, along with other pollutants in the air, can irritate and damage the skin, with most of the damage occurring before the age of 18. Nearly 80% of this damage can be prevented if sunscreen is applied properly in those first 18 years of life (Samuel, Brooke, Hollis, & Griffiths, 2005). Recognizable changes occur with years of exposure to ultraviolet radiation due to repetitive tanning and sunburning. The potential for sunburn varies with skin type. Chart 66–3 lists the common descriptions of skin types and their potential for sunburn. The superficial dermis that is damaged by the sun demonstrates a breakdown of collagen and an accumulation of abnormal elastin, which lead to wrinkling and lack of resilience in the skin. When the sun damages the skin, DNA production is impaired. DNA is needed for maintenance of the genetic integrity of the skin. Therefore, impaired DNA production can lead to skin cancer and immune suppression. Sunlight also is considered a major cause of skin cancer, especially when the skin is repeatedly sunburned. Various skin cancers are discussed in this chapter. The prevention of skin cancer is an objective of *Healthy People 2010* (U.S. Department of Health and Human Services, 2000). The National Guidelines box lists the Centers for Disease Control and Prevention's guidelines related to skin cancer and protection of the skin from the sun.

Health Promotion Related to Sun Protection

The best way to avoid the damage created by the sun is to avoid the sun, wear sunscreen, or wear protective clothing when in the sun. The amount of time in the sun at midday should be limited. Sunscreens should contain avobenzne, dioxybenzone, oxybenzone, titanium dioxide, or zinc oxide for the best protection from both ultraviolet A (UVA) and ultraviolet B (UVB) rays. A sun protection factor (SPF) rates sunscreens. The higher the SPF rating the sunscreen has, the greater the protection. The current recommendation is an SPF of 15 (CDC, 2006b). Generous layers of sunscreen should be applied with special attention paid to areas often neglected such as the neck, temples, and ears. Sunscreen can be diluted or rinsed off completely by sweat, water immersion, or rubbing. Therefore, it should be applied often. The United Kingdom has begun a campaign to reduce exposure to sunlight and prevent sunburn. Part of that effort is the SunSmart program. Chart 66–4 outlines the basis of SunSmart and can be used for patient education (Affleck, 2005; Cancer Research UK, 2003).

 CRITICAL ALERT *When spending time in the sun, it is important to use a sunscreen with a sun protection factor (SPF) of 15 to 30 and to reapply it often. Sunscreen should be applied 30 minutes prior to sun exposure.*

 CULTURAL CONSIDERATIONS for Racial Differences in Skin

Physiological skin differences among racial and ethnic groups include:

- African Americans have increased lipid content.
- African Americans have increased thickness of the stratum corneum and increased spontaneous desquamation.
- Water content of the skin is greater in Hispanics and less in Caucasians.
- An increase in melanin decreases sun damage.

The three most common disorders in darkly pigmented skin are:

- Acne
- Eczema
- Pigmentary disorders.

Source: From Halder, R. M., & Nootheti, P. K. (2003). Ethnic skin disorders overview. *Journal of the American Academy of Dermatology, 48* (Suppl. 6), S143–S148.

CHART 66–3	**Common Descriptions of Skin Types for Anticipating Sunburn**

Type	Description
Type I	Always burns, never tans
Type II	Burns easily, tans minimally
Type III	Burns moderately, tans gradually
Type IV	Burns minimally, tans well
Type V	Rarely burns, tans profusely
Type VI	Never burns, deeply pigmented

CHART 66–4	**SunSmart Program**

There are five points to the SunSmart program. To help remember the five points, think *SMART*:

- *S*tay in the shade 11 a.m.–3 p.m.
- *M*ake sure you never burn.
- *A*lways cover up.
- *R*emember to take extra care with children.
- *T*hen use factor 15+ sunscreen.

Sources: Affleck, P. (2005). Sun exposure and health. *Nursing Standard, 19*(47), 50–54; and Cancer Research UK. (2003). Cancer Research UK gets SunSmart with the big screen. Retrieved September 8, 2008 from http://info.cancerresearchuk.org/news/archive/pressreleases/2003/may/216205.

NATIONAL GUIDELINES for Skin Cancer Prevention

- Minimize exposure to the sun during peak hours of 10 a.m. to 4 p.m.
- Seek shade from the sun.
- Wear clothes and wide-brimmed hats that protect the skin and face.
- Wear wraparound sunglasses that block close to 100% of ultraviolet (UV) rays.
- Use a broad-spectrum sunscreen that blocks both ultraviolet A (UVA) and ultraviolet B (UVB) rays and has a sun protection factor (SPF) of at least 15 or higher. Apply generously 30 minutes before going outside, and reapply after swimming, exercising, or sweating.
- Avoid using sun lamps and tanning beds. They are also sources of UV radiation.

Source: Centers for Disease Control and Prevention (CDC). (2006b). *Health topics: Skin cancer school health guidelines.* Retrieved December 12, 2007, from http://www.cdc.gov/healthyyouth/skincancer/guidelines/summary.htm#top.

Nonmalignant Disorders Related to Sun Exposure

Exposure to the sun leads to damaged, abnormal skin cells that can be premalignant. Lesions related to these disorders are generally found on areas of the skin exposed to the sun. Photodermatitis and actinic keratosis are both skin disorders related to skin exposure to the sun.

Etiology, Epidemiology, and Pathophysiology of Photodermatitis

Photodermatitis is an inflammatory adverse reaction to sunlight. It is a common hypersensitivity to sun in which the individual sunburns more easily than usual or develops papular or vesicular lesions with exposure to the sun. It can occur in all ages and races but is more common in young women. This condition can be a true immunologic reaction that can be genetically determined. It also may occur because of the use of certain medications, in association with certain diseases, or with the use of contact agents that increase photosensitivity, such as those listed in Chart 66–5.

Clinical Manifestations of Photodermatitis

Clinically, patients develop an erythematous, papular rash that burns and itches. The rash may become vesicular with oozing and edema. It is accompanied by systemic symptoms such as

CHART 66–5	**Agents Associated with Photosensitivity**

Amiodarone	NSAIDs
Antipsychotic agents	Oral contraceptives
Barbiturates	Phenothiazines
Benzodiazepines	Phenylbutazone
Carbamazepine	Piroxicam
Chlorothiazide	Promethazine
Coal tar	Protriptyline
Dacarbazine	Psoralens
5-Fluorouracil	Quinidine/quinine
Furosemide	Retinoids
Griseofulvin	Simvastatin
Hypoglycemic agents	Sulfonamides
Ketoprofen	Sulfonylureas
Lomefloxacin	Sulindac
Methotrexate	Tetracyclines
Mitomycin C	Thiazides
Nalidixic acid	Tricyclics

pain, fever, malaise, chills, headache, and nausea. The rash occurs on areas exposed to the sun and persists for 7 to 10 days. Treatment consists of protection from the sun and management of the clinical manifestations.

Etiology, Epidemiology, Clinical Manifestations, and Treatment of Actinic Keratosis

Actinic keratosis lesions occur commonly after age 40 and are found on sun-exposed areas of the head, neck, arms, legs, tops of ears, and dorsal hands. **Actinic keratosis** lesions begin as hyperemic, poorly defined lesions and develop into scaly, rough, skin-colored macules with rough surfaces. Actinic keratosis is considered a premalignant lesion that may develop into squamous cell carcinoma. These lesions can be treated with topical 5-fluorouracil cream or solution, cryosurgery, or liquid nitrogen. They can also be treated with Aldara, which is thought to stimulate the immune system to remove these precancerous lesions. The patients will need instructions about sun protection measures for the remainder of their lives.

Etiology, Epidemiology, and Pathophysiology of Contact Dermatitis

Contact dermatitis is an inflammation of the skin related to exposure to an irritant or allergen in the environment. Irritant contact dermatitis is caused by a substance that is irritating to the skin but not due to an allergy. Allergic contact dermatitis is a type IV cell-mediated immune reaction that occurs after contact with an allergen. Cell-mediated immune reactions are mediated by T lymphocytes, which lead to destruction of the allergen (see Chapter 60). It may take several exposures before a reaction occurs. One of the most common types of allergic contact dermatitis is poison ivy or poison oak. It is difficult to distinguish between allergic or irritant reactions; however, an irritant reaction usually does not spread beyond the area of contact. The intensity of the skin reaction depends on the degree of sensitivity and the concentration and quantity of the exposure to the antigen. At first the dermatitis is usually confined to the area of direct exposure but may spread beyond that area.

CRITICAL ALERT *Poison ivy is a green plant with leaves arranged in threes, with one at the end and the other two opposing each other. It grows as a climbing vine on trees and poles or fences and bricks. It may have green flowers and white berries.*

Diagnosis, Clinical Manifestations, and Treatment of Contact Dermatitis

In the acute phase, the symptoms include edema, erythema (redness of the skin due to congestion of capillaries in the lower layers of the skin), vesicles, itching, and papules. If it continues into a chronic phase, the skin becomes dry, thickened, and may develop **fissures** (linear cracks or furrows in the continuity of the epidermis). The diagnosis usually requires the history of possible exposure and development of the rash, and physical examination. Patch testing can be done if necessary to determine the identity of the offending agent. Treatment includes stopping the exposure to the allergen or irritating agent. Future exposures to the causative agent should be avoided. The inflammatory process is treated using a mid- to high-potency topical corticosteroid. If the dermatitis is severe, oral steroids may be used. The itching should be treated with antihistamines. The Pharmacology Summary feature (p. 2181) presents medications used to treat skin disorders, including corticosteroids and antihistamines. Patients should be instructed not to scratch because scratching will increase the itching sensation and may cause a secondary infection.

Etiology, Epidemiology, Pathophysiology, and Clinical Manifestations of Urticaria

Urticaria, or hives, are raised, erythematous, intensely pruritic plaques or wheals that are surrounded by a white halo. These lesions vary in size and distribution and commonly occur as an allergic reaction to medications, foods, or insect bites. They also can be related to infections such as viral hepatitis, sinusitis, gingivitis, or cystitis. Aggravating factors include chemical irritants, fever, alcohol, exercise, and emotional stress. Histamine, the most common mediator of this reaction, is released by mast cells as a part of the immune response to allergens. Histamine causes an increased permeability of the microvessels of the skin, leading to a leakage of fluid into the tissues, causing edema at the site, and stimulating the itch receptors in the skin. The rash related to urticaria does not usually appear in the mucous membranes, the palms of the hands, the soles of the feet, or the axilla. Urticaria has several clinical variations outlined in Chart 66–6.

Urticaria is diagnosed by history of the exposure to possible causative agents and appearance of the lesion. Causative factors need to be identified and avoided. Most cases resolve spontaneously, but antihistamines may be given to block the action of histamine. See the Pharmacology Summary feature (p. 2181). Itching can be relieved with cold compresses or cool, colloid-type baths (Aveeno). It may be helpful to decrease stress, to avoid hot showers, and to exercise.

Etiology, Epidemiology, and Pathophysiology of Atopic Dermatitis

Atopic dermatitis, also known as eczema, is a chronic, inflammatory skin disorder characterized by dry skin related to water loss in the epidermis and decreased skin lipid levels. It can occur at any age but is more common in children. It generally cycles through periods of acute flare-ups and remissions. It can be

CHART 66–6 Urticarial Variants

Variant	Duration	Causes
Acute	Lasts less than 6 weeks.	Food, drinks, medications, pollen, chemicals.
Chronic	Affects mostly adults. Lasts more than 2 months.	Cause is difficult to determine. May be related to underlying disease such as cancer, hepatitis, collagen disease, or Graves' disease.
Cold	Lasts 30 to 60 minutes.	Induced by exposure to cold surfaces, air, or water.
Physical urticaria	Intermittent. Lasts 1 to 2 hours.	Induced by things that increase body temperature such as showers, exercise, fever, and stress.

caused by irritants in the environment, or it can have an immunologic cause. Patients with atopic dermatitis often have a familial predisposition, including a family history of asthma or hay fever. Environmentally, it is aggravated by contact with allergens, perspiration, excessive heat, dry air, emotional stress, and rough clothing. Children often outgrow atopic dermatitis; however, it can become chronic into adulthood.

Clinical Manifestations and Diagnosis of Atopic Dermatitis

Atopic dermatitis is characterized by severe itching. The lesions are irregular, red papular patches that are weepy, shiny, or thickened. The lesions also may be plaques that are scaly and crusted. The characteristic distribution is on the face, the neck, the upper trunk, and the bends of the elbows and knees. The lesions can develop a secondary *Staphylococcus aureus* infection due to skin trauma and breakdown from scratching. It is diagnosed by history, including possible triggers for flare-ups, and physical examination to note the appearance and distribution of the lesions. Laboratory tests are not usually required; however, immunoglobin E (IgE) levels may be elevated, indicating an immune reaction. Allergy testing may be done to determine whether an allergic process is instrumental in causing the problem.

Medical Management of Atopic Dermatitis

Treatment involves controlling the aggravating factors and treating the rash. It is important to moisturize the skin to maintain the skin barrier. Bathing should be held to a minimum; however, when bathing, the patient should use tepid water and mild, unscented soap such as Cetaphil or Dove. To prevent itching and lubricate the skin, a thick, greasy moisturizer should be used at least once a day after bathing. Clothing should be soft, light, and preferably made of cotton or some natural, soft fiber. New clothes should be laundered before wearing to wash out any irritating chemicals. Any activity that causes perspiring should be avoided. Once a rash develops, the patient may be placed on a course of topical or oral corticosteroids to reduce inflammation and itching. Urea creams or nonsteroidal anti-inflammatory ointments are effective for hydrating the skin and decreasing itching. Oral antihistamines also may help decrease itching. See the Pharmacology Summary feature (p. 2181). If lesions are wet or crusted,

COMPLEMENTARY & ALTERNATIVE THERAPIES
Traditional Chinese Herbal Medicine

Description:

Atopic eczema may benefit from Chinese herbal medicines (Tse, 2003). These herbal medicines are part of an ancient medical tradition in China, otherwise known as traditional Chinese medicine (TCM). TCM is comprised of not only herbal medicines, but also acupuncture and related physical therapies, and general nutritional and life style guidelines. TCM is often performed in conjunction with conventional, or orthodox, medicine (OM) in China and other areas of Asia. In 1992, a randomized clinical trial of the use of 10 TCM herbs for atopic eczema was published and showed some benefit in treating atopic eczema. However, herbal TCM is still regarded with skepticism, as some TCM herbs provided by practitioners in the West have strayed from the standards of true TCM, and have caused liver and kidney toxicity. Some herbs have even been adulterated with pharmaceutical (OM) drugs. This has resulted in giving herbal TCM a poor reputation and recognition. These problems can be blamed on a lack of professional regulation, practitioner qualification, herbal product standards, and evidence-based clinical studies (Chan, 2005).

Research Support:

An Australian study assessed CAM use in patients with acne, psoriasis, or atopic eczema, as well as the patients' attitudes about CAM. The study involved interviewing 26 patients with acne, 29 patients with psoriasis, and 7 patients with atopic eczema. Results of these interviews showed that CAM therapy use was common, and patients had a tendency to value CAM over conventional therapies because they perceived that CAM therapies had less potential for adverse effects. Researchers concluded that, due to the extensive use of CAM therapies by patients with skin conditions, practitioners should be aware of this and alert for any implications and interactions (Magin, Adams, Heading, Pond, & Smith, 2006).

A literature review of studies was conducted in 2004 on the use of herbal TCM in treating atopic eczema. Four randomized controlled trials met the researchers' inclusion criteria. These trials showed that herbal TCM may be effective in the treatment of atopic eczema; however, researchers recommended further well-designed, larger-scale trials (Zhang et al., 2004).

References

Chan, K. (2005). Chinese medicinal materials and their interface with Western medical concepts. *Journal of Ethnopharmacology, 96*(1–2), 1–18.

Magin, P. J., Adams, J., Heading, G. S., Pond, D. C., & Smith, W. (2006). Complementary and alternative medicine therapies in acne, psoriasis, and atopic eczema: Results of a qualitative study of patients' experiences and perceptions. *Journal of Alternative and Complementary Medicine, 12*(5), 451–457.

Tse, T. W. (2003). Use of common Chinese herbs in the treatment of psoriasis. *Clinical and Experimental Dermatology, 28*(5), 469–475.

Zhang, W., Leonard, T., Bath-Hextall, F., Chambers, C. A., Lee. C., Humphreys, R., et al. (2004). Chinese herbal medicine for atopic eczema. *Cochrane Database of Systematic Reviews, 18*(4), CD002291.

soaking in Burrow's solution or colloidal oatmeal such as Aveeno may be helpful. Antibiotics may be needed to prevent or treat secondary skin infections. Alternative therapies such as traditional Chinese herbal medicine, as discussed in the Complementary and Alternative Therapies box, may be helpful as well.

Etiology, Epidemiology, and Pathophysiology of Skin Reaction to Medications

Skin reactions occur commonly as an allergic reaction to a medication. They can occur rapidly, as in an immediate-type hypersensitivity after exposure to the drug, or can take a few days to develop, as in a delayed hypersensitivity reaction (see Chapter 60 ☉). Allergic medication reactions are due to the function of the T cell that recognizes the medication as a foreign substance and reacts to it. This reaction usually requires a previous exposure to the medication so that the body can develop an immune response. Urticarial and maculopapular skin reactions occur most commonly with amoxicillin, trimethoprim-sulfamethoxazole, and ampicillin or penicillin. Medications such as phenolphthalein, pyrazolone derivatives, tetracyclines, nonsteroidal anti-inflammatory drugs (NSAIDs), barbiturates, and trimethoprim-sulfamethoxazole are more commonly related to fixed medication eruptions, which are rashes appearing in the same sites after each ingestion of the medication.

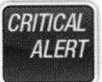 **CRITICAL ALERT** *Adverse medication events in the elderly can be life threatening. Approximately 27.6% of all adverse medication events and 42.2% of life-threatening or fatal adverse medication events have been found to be preventable. These errors occurred more commonly with cardiovascular drugs and usually in the prescribing phase (60.8%) or in patient adherence (21.2%) (Gurwitz et al., 2003).*

Clinical Manifestations of Skin Reaction to Medications

The most common manifestations of an allergic skin reaction to medications are erythema, pruritus, and urticaria. The lesions are usually maculopapular occurring in a symmetrical, generalized distribution that spares the face. Fever and other systemic symptoms may accompany the rash. It is important to obtain a detailed history from the patient to identify whether a rash similar to this has occurred before and what medications the patient was taking with the prior rash as well as currently. Patients may not relate the rash to the use of a certain medication, so a specific and detailed assessment is important.

Medical Management of Skin Reaction to Medications

Treatment involves stopping the offending agent. Patients should be warned that it might take a few weeks for the rash to disappear even after stopping the medication. Antihistamines are helpful in slowing the immune response responsible for the rash and the itching, and thus promote healing. Systemic corticosteroids may be indicated if the reaction is widespread or severe. See the Pharmacology Summary feature (p. 2181). Colloidal baths are helpful to soothe extreme itching.

Skin Changes Related to Tobacco Smoking

Smoking has a negative effect on the skin, causing it to age prematurely. Smoking leads to vasoconstriction, which decreases blood supply and nutrients to the skin, and it breaks down the elastin in the skin, leading to wrinkles. There is evidence that facial wrinkling is associated with the number of pack-years smoked (Patel et al., 2006).

Skin Changes Related to Cultural Practices

Cultural practices can affect the health of the skin. For example, pomade acne is common in African Americans and Hispanics. This disorder is a form of acne caused by the use of grooming products on the scalp spreading to the forehead. These grooming agents contain substances that can lead to acne, such as lanolins and isopropyl myristate. Capsaicin-induced dermatitis is seen in Hispanic people. This condition, caused by handling hot chili peppers with bare hands, leads to erythema, burning pain, and irritation (Halder & Nootheti, 2003).

Some alternative medicine practices lead to the formation of dermatologic lesions. Coin rubbing is an Asian practice done to relieve symptoms of the flu, fever, and headaches. In this practice, a coin or a similar object is used to scrape the skin, causing ecchymotic streaks. The scraping usually occurs between the ribs, along the inner aspects of both arms, and along both sides of the spine. Cupping, another cultural practice that is done to treat pain, involves soaking a cotton ball in alcohol and igniting it. The cotton ball is then placed in a cup or jar, which is then inverted and placed on the skin. Once placed on the skin, the flame goes out and a vacuum is created. This vacuum pulls the skin into the cup or jar, leading to circular, ecchymotic, painful burns usually done symmetrically in rows of two to four cups. Moxibustion is a cultural practice that involves igniting dry weeds or incense-like material and applying the lit tip to acupuncture sites. It is used to treat a variety of disorders. It may be confused with abuse and should be considered when assessing skin disorders.

Skin Changes Related to Tattoos

Tattoos are pictures and words applied anywhere on the body, including permanent makeup applied to the eyes and lips. A tattoo is defined as a permanent mark or design made on skin by inserting ink or dye via a needle into the dermal layer of the skin with repeated punctures. The needle is connected to a small machine with tubes containing dye that apply repeated piercing to the skin, much like the action of a sewing machine. The process, which can take several hours for a large tattoo, causes a small amount of bleeding and minor to potentially significant pain. Tattooing is an increasingly popular practice; however, it is not without health risks. The skin integrity is altered, which means the individual is susceptible to skin reactions and infections. The most common infections following tattooing are caused by *Staphylococcus aureus*, which may be a result of poor hygiene on the part of either the provider or the customer, during and after the procedure. There is increased risk for potentially serious antibiotic-resistant skin infections such as community acquired methicillin-resistant *Staphylococcus aureus* with unlicensed tattoo artists who do not follow proper infection control procedures (CDC, 2006a; MayoClinic.com, 2008). Typical signs and symptoms of an infection include redness, warmth, swelling, and a pus-like drainage. Some antibiotic-resistant skin infections can lead to pneumonia, bloodstream infections, and necrotizing fasciitis.

Some degree of bleeding is inevitable during the tattooing process; therefore, the transmission of bloodborne pathogens is possible. If the equipment used to create the tattoo is contaminated with the blood of an infected person, it is possible to contract a number of serious bloodborne diseases. Bloodborne pathogen transmission is associated with the reuse of tattoo needles without proper and adequate sterilization. It is also possible that the electric equipment itself may be contaminated. Infection with hepatitis B virus is a well-documented post-tattoo complication. Other infections include hepatitis C, tetanus, tuberculosis, and the human immunodeficiency virus, the virus that causes AIDS (MayoClinic.com, 2008).

 Instructions to individuals who are planning to have either a tattoo or body piercing need to include having to question the health standards of the establishment. Many local health departments have sanitation guidelines for tattoo and body piercing establishments.

Tattoo dyes can cause allergic skin reactions, resulting in an itchy rash at the tattoo site. Red ink is most commonly associated with allergic reactions, although any color of ink may cause an allergic reaction in sensitive patients. Some allergic reactions may take years to develop; therefore, patients should be queried about old tattoos as well as newer ones during assessment. Additionally, granulomas may form around the tattoo ink, especially the red ink. Tattooing can also cause keloid scar formation if the individual is prone to them (MayoClinic.com, 2008). Tattoo ink is not regulated by the Food and Drug Administration and may contain heavy metals: alcohols, ethylene glycol (automobile antifreeze), formaldehyde, glutaraldehyde, ferrocyanides, aluminum, mercury, cadmium, cobalt, chromium, and lead. Tattoo "inks" may also be homemade and therefore may be composed of any number of potential toxins and/or allergens (County of Kern: Department of Health Services, 2007).

Due to the makeup of the dye or ink, there may be a reaction during a magnetic resonance imaging (MRI) scan. Although it happens rarely, tattoos or permanent makeup may cause swelling or burning in the affected areas during the MRI exam. In some cases, when the scan is in the immediate area of the dye such as the eye, tattoo pigments may interfere with the quality of the image (MayoClinic.com, 2008).

Care of the tattoo includes regular cleaning with soap and water and applying moisturizer. The sun should be avoided for the first few weeks after application. Tattoos may take up to several days to heal. The individual needs to be instructed not to pick at a scab, which increases the risk of infection, can damage the design, and increases the risk of scar formation.

Tattoo removal is possible, although complete removal is difficult and skin color variations and scarring are likely to remain. Methods of removal include:

- Laser surgery is the most effective way to reduce the appearance of a tattoo. Pulses of laser light pass through the top layer of skin, and the energy of the light is absorbed by the pigment in the tattoo. This process creates a very low grade of inflammation and allows the body to shed small areas of altered pigment. It requires repeated treatments over time to lighten the tattoo, and the treatment might not completely erase it.

- Dermabrasion uses a sanding process to remove the outer layer of skin and lighten the tattoo.

- Surgical removal involves cutting out the tattoo and surgically closing the open area, leaving a scar.

Skin Changes Related to Body Piercing

Body piercing involves creating a hole in a body part for the purpose of inserting jewelry. The most common body piercing areas are the lobe and other areas of the ear, nose, eyebrow, lip, tongue, and naval. Body piercing has risks similar to those of tattoos, although due to improvements in safety procedures and equipment, the popular practice of earlobe piercing is viewed as generally less risky than other body piercing. A single-use, sterilized ear piercing device or an ear piercing gun with sterilized, disposable cartridges may be safest (MayoClinic.com, 2008). Some practitioners use a reusable piercing gun for these types of piercing, which is difficult to sterilize and can more easily damage the skin. The most common infections associated with "gun"-type ear piercing are *Staphylococcus aureus* and *Pseudomonas aeruginosa* (County of Kern: Department of Health Services, 2007). In addition, any time the skin is punctured, there are risks including:

- Bloodborne diseases may occur if the equipment used to do the piercing is contaminated with the blood of an infected person. There is a risk for contracting hepatitis C, hepatitis B, tetanus, tuberculosis, and HIV.
- Allergic reactions may occur if the jewelry is made of nickel or brass.
- Oral complications that may occur with jewelry worn in tongue piercing include infection, chipped and cracked teeth, and damaged gums.
- Skin infection clinical manifestations include redness, swelling, pain, and a pus-like discharge.
- Infections from piercing in the upper ear cartilage are especially serious. Antibiotics are often ineffective. Because cartilage does not have its own blood supply, the drug cannot reach the infection site. Such infection can lead to cartilage damage and serious, permanent ear deformity.
- Body piercing can cause scarring, and if the individual is susceptible, piercing can cause keloid scar formation, discussed later.

Postprocedure care for the pierced area depends on the body part pierced. Oral piercing (tongue or lip) includes instructing the individual to rinse the mouth with an antibacterial, alcohol-free mouth rinse for 30 to 60 seconds after meals until the piercing heals. A new soft-bristled toothbrush should be used to avoid introducing bacteria into the mouth. Piercings of the nose, ears, eyebrow, and navel need to be cleaned gently with warm water and an antibiotic cleanser to remove any crusting. The jewelry should be gently turned back and forth to work the cleanser around the opening. Avoid alcohol and peroxide, as they can dry the skin; and ointments should not be applied, as they keep oxygen from reaching the piercing and can leave a sticky residue (MayoClinic.com, 2008). The piercing site will heal over without the jewelry in place.

Health Promotion Related to Tattoos and Skin Piercing

There are no licensing laws or regulations governing tattooing and piercing; therefore, individuals must protect themselves by being better informed about the entire process. Certain inherent risks, described earlier, are associated with body piercing and tattooing; however, being informed about the following will improve safety:

- Discuss the sterilization techniques by inquiring about the use of an autoclave; request to see it in operation. If none is used, go elsewhere.
- Discuss the sterilization of jewelry and instruments such as sterilization of ink pouches with intact color-change seals. If possible, ask to see the packaged sterilized instruments.
- Ask whether excess tattoo ink is being poured back into the main supply.
- Follow all after-care instructions and report complications including redness, swelling, pain, or discharge to a health care provider immediately.

■ Scar Formation

When patients have a full-thickness injury, healing occurs replacing the injured tissue with connective tissue forming a scar. Wounds heal in three phases: the inflammatory phase, which prepares the wound for healing; the proliferative phase during which new tissue builds to fill in the wound space; and the remodeling phase when the scar strengthens. Phases of wound healing are discussed in detail in Chapter 67 ☺. Scars can be small and asymptomatic or large with restricted function such as occurs with a hypertrophic or keloid scar formation. Abnormal scar formation includes hypertrophic and keloid scar formation.

Hypertrophic and Keloid Scar Formation

Hypertrophic and keloid scar formation is an abnormal, excessive development of connective tissue or collagen. The cause of the development of these scars is unclear, but they seem to occur in genetically predisposed individuals. They occur more frequently when the injury occurs over the sternum, anterior chest, shoulder, upper lip, earlobe, and neck. It is believed that keloid formation arises more in African Americans, Asians, and children. Chart 66–7 compares the appearance of hypertrophic scars and keloid scars. Both scars are identified by observation and a history of trauma. If the patient has a history of keloid

CHART 66–7	Comparison of Hypertrophic and Keloid Scars	
Hypertrophic Scars	**Keloid Scars**
Begin as red, firm lesions.	Begin as pink, firm, rubbery plaque with telangiectasia.
Skin is shiny and stretched with smooth, dome-shaped surface.	Smooth, irregularly shaped, and hyperpigmented.
May be itchy and tender.	May be tender or painful, pruritic, or burning.
Usually contained within the area of injury.	Claw-like edge that extends outside the area of injury.
Resolve spontaneously without treatment in 6 to 18 months.	Resistant to therapy; may enlarge over time.

scar formation, it may be helpful to apply pressure dressings to the injury site for 8 hours a day for 4 to 6 months to decrease the scar hypertrophy and prevent decreased range of motion. Corticosteroids injected into the scar lesion may be beneficial. Surgical excision of the scar can be done but the abnormal scarring may reoccur. Referral to a plastic surgeon or dermatologist may be indicated. Chapter 68 discusses keloid scar formation with burn scars and contains graphics of the scar formation.

General Skin Lesions and Disorders

Skin disorders may result in a variety of skin lesions with multiple configurations and signs and symptoms. Skin disorders can be benign or malignant, due to infectious agents, and/or from infestations by insects. It is important for the nurse to assess these lesions, their characteristics, location, exudates, and distribution on the body. Appearance of new skin lesions occurs as a part of the aging process. Skin lesions common among the elderly are outlined in the Gerontological Considerations box.

Benign Skin Disorders

Benign skin disorders include those that are not carcinogenic. Most often these disorders are painless and asymptomatic. Any abnormal growth on the skin is of concern to a patient; therefore, it is essential that the nurse thoroughly evaluate and report skin changes. Common benign skin disorders are discussed next.

Moles or Nevi

Moles or **nevi** are common skin lesions that appear on almost everyone in almost any location but are more common in sun-exposed areas. They can be present at birth or can be acquired as an individual grows, although new ones usually do not appear after age 40. Moles are usually asymptomatic but can be irritated by clothing or trauma. The various types of moles are described in Chart 66–8. Moles are generally considered harmless but may become malignant and need to be evaluated periodically. Changes in color, diameter, or the border of the mole need to be reported to the health care provider, as these changes could indicate a premalignant or malignant change.

Skin Tags

Skin tags are common flesh-colored or brown papules that grow on a thick stalk. They are about 1 to 10 millimeters in diameter and most frequently develop on the neck, axillae, groin, eyelids, or in skin fold areas. They are usually asymptomatic unless they

---

GERONTOLOGICAL CONSIDERATIONS
for Skin Lesions

Skin Lesion	Description
Skin tags	Soft, brown, flesh-colored papules
Keratosis	Horny or abnormal growth of keratinocytes
Lentigines	Well-bordered brown to black macules commonly called liver spots
Vascular lesions	Vascular tumors with chronically dilated blood vessels

---

CHART 66–8 **Types of Moles or Nevi**

Type of Mole or Nevus	Description
Junctional	Flat or slightly raised, brown-tan papule, less than 6 millimeters in diameter. Usually occurs at the dermal–epidermal junction.
Compound	Slightly to markedly raised, pigmented papule. Symmetrical with irregular border and smooth or slightly papillary surface. Center more pigmented than border.
Intradermal	Elevated, fleshy papule. Pale or flesh colored with pigmented flecks. May have coarse, dark hairs growing from it.
Halo nevus	Mole surrounded by a ring of hypopigmentation. Usually disappears over several months with halo repigmenting.
Blue nevus	Solitary, bluish macula or papule usually located on the head, neck, or buttocks. Enlarges slowly and persists for 10 to 15 years.
Becker's nevus	Usually occurs on the shoulder, submammary area, or back. Consists of a brown macule or patch of hair. Irregular, sharply demarcated border. Varies in size but can be quite large.

---

are irritated by clothing or jewelry, which may cause bleeding and tenderness. Skin tags are benign and may last indefinitely without problems. They do not require treatment; however, if desired they can be removed by simple scissor excision.

Lipoma

A **lipoma** is a nodule of fat tissue that is usually benign and is identified as a soft, freely mobile growth under the skin. It is slow growing and may vary in size from 1 to several centimeters in diameter. It is most commonly located on the shoulders, legs, arms, buttocks, and back but can occur anywhere on the body. Treatment is not necessary; however, if the lesion is cosmetically bothersome to the patient, it can be surgically excised.

Epidermal Cyst

An epidermal cyst is a capsule filled with keratin that appears spontaneously in areas of friction or on hair-bearing areas, but it commonly occurs on the face, postauricular fold, posterior neck, and trunk. Occluded **pilosebaceous follicles** (sebaceous cyst containing hair follicles) probably form the wall of the cyst. A cyst is freely movable but firm and tense feeling. It is dome shaped and pale, ranging in size from 0.5 to 5 centimeters, with a central opening that drains a pasty, malodorous material made up of necrotic keratin. It generally does not cause complications but can become infected; therefore, it may need antibiotics and in some instances may require surgical removal.

Hyperpigmentation of the Skin

This category of skin disorders involves an increase in normal skin colors. It occurs because of increased or abnormally distributed melanin. It may be diffuse or limited to a specific space. Typically the major concern to the patient is the cosmetic effect.

Café-au-Lait Spots

Café-au-lait spots are asymptomatic tan macules that have smooth borders and vary in diameter from 0.5 to 20 centimeters. They are generally considered to be benign but can indicate the presence of neurofibromatosis if there are six or more spots. No treatment is necessary, but they can be eliminated with laser or bleaching agents if they are cosmetically undesirable.

Liver Spots (Solar Lentigo)

Solar lentigo, commonly referred to as an age spot or liver spot, refers to lesions that develop due to a familial tendency and chronic sun exposure in Caucasians over age 60. They are macules that are darker and larger than freckles and do not fade during winter. They occur in sun-exposed areas such as the backs of the hands, forearms, shoulders, and forehead. Their color is uniform with sharply demarcated borders. The lesions are usually asymptomatic but may be of cosmetic concern. The best treatment is prevention through the limitation of exposure to sunlight and the application of sunscreen. Bleaching creams are available that can be applied topically and will slowly fade the spots. Cosmetic resurfacing of the skin through the use of lasers or liquid nitrogen application can also decrease the pigmentation.

Hypopigmentation of the Skin

Hypopigmentation of the skin is a decrease in melanin that can be hereditary or acquired. There are diseases of the skin that lead to a loss of melanin causing a pale or gray appearance to the skin. One of the most common disorders leading to hypopigmentation is vitiligo.

Vitiligo

Vitiligo is a localized loss of melanocytes from the skin and hair creating white patches of skin (Figure 66–1 ■). The cause is unknown but may be related to an autoimmune disorder and inhibition of melanogenesis. It occurs spontaneously after emotional or physical stress or may be related to trauma. Vitiligo progresses slowly over years with new patches of hypopigmentation occurring throughout life. The white macules can occur in a symmetrical pattern or can be segmental, limited to one seg-

ment of the body. The most common sites are the backs of the hands, face, body folds, axillae, and genitalia. Vitiligo causes no discomfort and is purely of cosmetic concern. Spontaneous repigmentation can occur but is usually spotty. The white areas can be covered with dyes and cosmetics to minimize the color irregularities. Sunless self-tanning agents may also be helpful by darkening the skin through staining. If the lesions are in sun-exposed areas, sunscreens should be used because of the higher risk of sunburn. Topical corticosteroids may be used to treat inflammation associated with the areas of hypopigmentation. See the Pharmacology Summary feature (p. 2181).

Acne Vulgaris

Acne vulgaris is a skin condition that occurs most frequently during the teenage years at varying levels of severity. It is caused by obstruction of a hair follicle due to overgrowth of sebum and keratin debris, an overproduction of oil due to enlarged oil glands, and bacteria known as *P. acnes* (Gorgos, 2006). These substances provide a good medium for bacterial growth, especially *Propionibacterium acnes* (*P. acnes*). *P. acnes* contain lipases that result in the breakdown of free fatty acids. Free fatty acids irritate the skin and cause a foreign body reaction leading to inflammation. The characteristic skin lesion, known as a comedo, is typically located on the face, chest, and back (Figure 66–2 ■).

Acne is defined by type and severity. There are three types of acne: comedonal, papulopustular, and nodulocystic. Comedonal acne is defined as noninflammatory with whiteheads or closed comedos, and blackheads or open comedos. Whiteheads, or closed comedos, occur when the opening to the skin is closed, and they look like tiny flesh-colored bumps. Blackheads, or open comedos, occur when the opening to the skin is open but capped with blackened skin debris, giving them a black appearance. Papulopustular acne is inflammatory with small papules and pustules that contain a central core of purulent material. Nodulocystic acne is inflammatory with a lesion or cyst greater than 5 millimeters in diameter. These cysts can be localized or can form tracts under the skin with abscesses. Nodulocystic acne is a serious problem requiring aggressive treatment. The severity of acne is rated as mild, moderate, and severe. Mild acne is defined

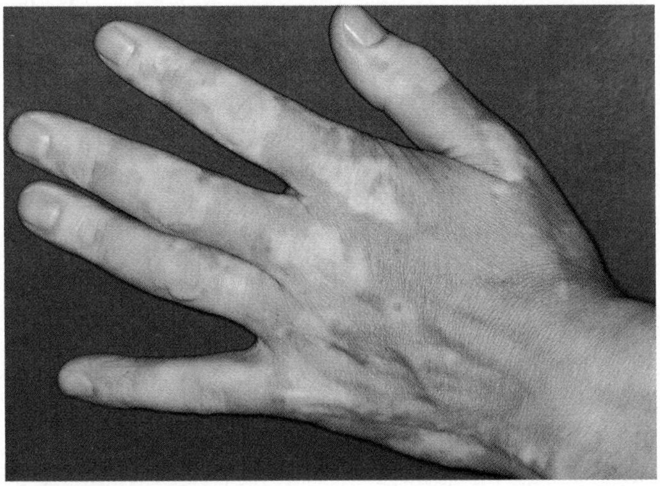

FIGURE 66–1 ■ Vitiligo.
Source: ISM/Phototake NYC

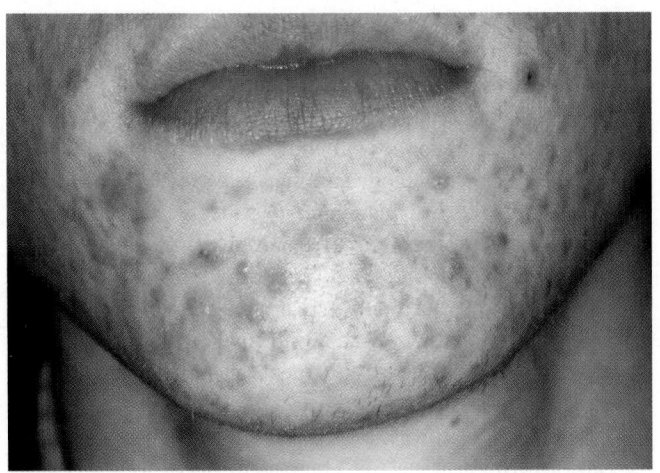

FIGURE 66–2 ■ Acne vulgaris.
Source: Dr. P. Marazzi/Photo Researchers, Inc.

as open and closed comedos and noninflamed lesions. Moderate acne is defined as open and closed comedos with some pustules and inflamed lesions. Severe acne is defined as open and closed comedos, and lesions that are inflamed and pustular. There are also nodules and significant scarring (Layton, Buchanan, & Courtenay, 2006).

Several factors have been identified as contributors to acne. Androgens play a role in the development of acne by stimulating the production of sebum, leading to obstruction of hair follicles and allowing for bacterial growth. However, estrogens can suppress the production of sebum. There is a genetic predisposition to acne as well as a link between stress and acne formation. There have, however, been no connections found between makeup use or diet and acne, which were once thought to be true. Men usually have more severe disease than women, but acne in women may persist into adulthood.

Treatment of choice for acne is based on the type and severity of the acne, the patient's skin type, and the presence or potential for scarring. Treatment will take about 6 to 8 weeks to see improvement. Nonpharmacologic approaches to therapy involve good hygiene that includes washing the face with soap and water. The patient should avoid topical exposure to oils and greases. Hats, sweatbands, and shirt collars can contribute to the collection of oil on the forehead, neck, and back and can contribute to an outbreak. Mild acne requires only topical agents such as benzoyl peroxide, salicylic acid, and azelaic acid that serve to help unblock the pores. These medications have bactericidal qualities that reduce the number of *P. acnes* and act to break down the keratin. Topical retinoids, such as Retin-A, are comedolytic agents that work as anti-inflammatory agents and normalize the abnormal growth of keratins. Oral contraceptives may be helpful for young women because they will decrease circulating androgens.

For moderate acne, a topical antibiotic should be added to the topical cleansing agent. Topical antibiotics decrease the numbers of *P. acnes* in sebaceous follicles and help to decrease inflammation. Once pustules or papules have developed, an oral antibiotic might be helpful. The antibiotic of choice is tetracycline at a dose of 500 milligrams twice daily. Erythromycin, doxycycline, and minocycline have also been shown to be effective. For severe acne, isotretinoin (Accutane) may be used. Accutane is an oral retinoid that decreases sebaceous gland activity and prevents the development of new comedos. Accutane has numerous side effects such as nosebleeds; inflammation of the lips and eyes; pain and stiffness in muscles, bones, and joints; and elevated triglyceride levels. Therefore, its use should be monitored carefully. It should never be used in pregnant women due to the major teratogenic effects. See the Pharmacology Summary feature (p. 2181). Finally, patients should be instructed not to squeeze, rub, or pick at comedos because doing so may result in scarring.

Lasers and light treatments have been used to treat acne. Lasers damage oil glands by using heat. Light treatments in the form of photodynamic therapy treat the overactive oil glands and the *P. acnes* bacteria. Both of these treatments are effective in reducing the oil production, leading to improved acne (Gorgos, 2006).

Nurses need to educate patients about the contributing factors and treatment for acne. The patient needs to understand that treatment is slow and that it will take 6 to 8 weeks to see the effects of any treatment regimen. The effects and side effects of all medications should be explained. The patient may require emotional support to deal with the psychological effects of acne because the lesions and scarring may have a negative effect on the patient's self-esteem and quality of life.

Psoriasis

Psoriasis is a chronic, noncontagious inflammatory skin disorder that affects over 4 million people in the United States (Figure 66–3 ■). Its exact cause is unknown, but there is a genetic tendency and evidence of an immune response that involves T-cell activation by an antigen stimulating the inflammatory process. The disease is chronic and incurable with exacerbations and remissions. Certain trigger factors cause an exacerbation, and these include stress, infection, medications such as beta-adrenergic blockers, smoking, and high alcohol consumption (Young, 2005). There are many types of psoriasis but chronic plaque psoriasis is the most common (Chart 66–9).

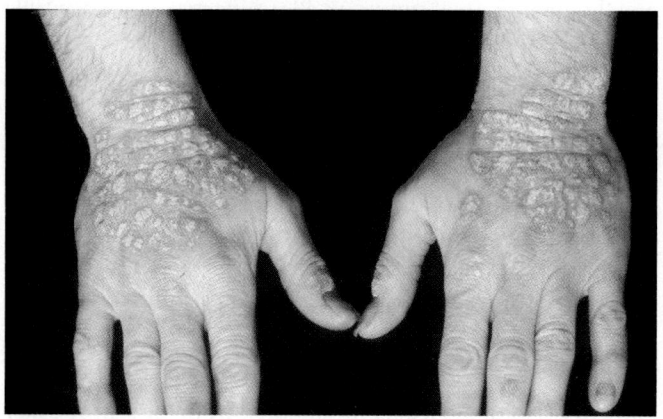

FIGURE 66–3 ■ Psoriasis.
Source: NMSB/Custom Medical Stock Photo, Inc.

CHART 66–9	Types of Psoriasis
Type	**Description**
Plaque	Red, scaly papules that coalesce. Lesions are well demarcated and symmetrical. Scale is adherent and silvery white with bleeding when removed.
Guttate	Associated with a sudden appearance of scaly papules that are "drop-like" and generally appear on the trunk.
Localized pustular	Discrete, small, sterile pustules that do not rupture but turn brown and scaly.
Generalized pustular	Erythema with sterile, generalized pustules over much of the body. Associated with systemic symptoms such as fever, chills, and leukocytosis.
Erythrodermic	Exfoliates with red skin all over body. There may be skin peeling with fluid balance problems. Very serious disease.
Nail psoriasis	Pitting of nails with separating of the nail from the nail bed. Nail plate may turn yellow.
Scalp psoriasis	Erythematous, scaly plaques that occur on the scalp or near the hairline. Usually is limited to the scalp.

The lesions of psoriasis are erythematous papules and plaques with silver-white scales that are sharply demarcated. They are the result of hyperproliferation of keratinocytes. A variety of sizes of lesions can coalesce into very large plaques. These lesions usually occur on the extensor surfaces of the knees and elbows, the scalp, the lower back, genitalia, or nails but can occur anywhere on the body. Some individuals experience pain and swelling in the joints that is associated with psoriasis called psoriatic arthritis.

Psoriasis is diagnosed by history of lesion development, trigger factors, family history, and physical examination. The appearance and distribution of the lesions can be enough to provide a diagnosis; however, skin biopsy can be done if there is question. The first line of treatment is topical agents such as emollient creams or ointments that can be used to prevent cracking and fissuring of the skin. Emollients help to moisturize the skin, easing itching and scaling. Corticosteroids are used to decrease inflammation; but the relief they provide is temporary, so they are best used in cycles for 7 to 10 days with rest periods in between. Vitamin D_3 analogue creams can be used directly on a plaque to control irritation and erythema. Coal tar preparations can be effective in resolving the lesions, although the exact mechanism of action is unknown. Phototherapy is effective when the psoriasis affects more than 30% of the body. Ultraviolet B is given three to five times weekly with exposures intense enough to cause erythema. Clearing of the lesions takes an average of 7 weeks. Phototherapy can also be used in conjunction with other medications. Most commonly used is ultraviolet A (UVA) with a photosensitizing medication such as psoralen. Psoralen is given prior to the exposure to ultraviolet light (UV). It inhibits DNA synthesis after activation with UVA, decreasing cellular proliferation. Systemic therapy is used in patients who are very uncomfortable or who have psoriasis affecting a large portion of the body. Methotrexate, a commonly used systemic medication, acts to prevent hyperkeratinization by suppressing proliferating cells or psoratic epidermal cell reproduction. Cyclosporine, an immunosuppressive drug that suppresses the growth of T cells, is used for severe inflammatory psoriasis. Etanercept is an example of biologic agents that have been used recently as a treatment for psoriasis. These medications interfere with the immunologic process, that has been found to be involved in psoriasis, with relative safety. They have been found to improve the skin lesions of psoriasis.

The psychological implications of psoriasis are great. It is a disfiguring disease that can result in low self-esteem, poor self-perception, depression, and anxiety. It can affect an individual's business, social, and sexual relationships. It may also cause problems with working due to the time off work for treatment, resulting in job loss and decreased income. Nurses need to be aware of not only the physical needs of the patient with psoriasis but also the emotional needs.

Seborrheic Keratosis

Seborrheic keratosis is a benign epidermal lesion seen predominantly in the middle-aged and elderly population. The exact cause is unknown, but it appears to be related to sun exposure. There are usually no associated symptoms, but the lesions can be irritated by clothing or jewelry. The lesions of seborrheic keratosis are warty, dirty yellow to black papules with sharp margins.

They can also be flat, and the color can vary from white to pink to black within the lesion. They have a "stuck on" appearance with a waxy feel, and they tend to occur more commonly on the back, central chest, face, and scalp. A sudden onset of numerous seborrheic keratoses, known as the Leser-Trélat sign, is often associated with the presence of an internal malignancy.

Diagnosis is made on the basis of history of sun exposure and lesion appearance, and physical examination of the lesions. The lesions will continue to grow and new lesions will continue to appear. No treatment is usually necessary, although they can be surgically removed for cosmetic or diagnostic reasons.

Dermatofibroma

Dermatofibromas are common, asymptomatic, benign, firm tan or brown papules occurring more frequently in middle-aged women. They are more commonly seen on the legs, elbows, or lateral trunk, often at the site of a previous trauma such as an insect bite. They characteristically dimple when pinched between the thumb and forefinger. Diagnosis is usually based on history of the symptoms and physical examination of the lesion. Treatment is not necessary, but dermatofibromas may be surgically removed for cosmetic reasons.

Genetic Disorder: Neurofibromatosis

Neurofibromatosis is an autosomal dominant inherited disorder; however, this condition also may arise spontaneously, without a previous family history. There are two types of neurofibromatosis. Type 1 is the most common and is known as von Recklinghausen's disease. It is characterized by multiple hyperpigmented macules; neurofibromatosis; and small, multiple, palpable, pedunculated, mobile, and pigmented nodules. These lesions become apparent after the first decade of life and are disfiguring. People with type 1 also have other associated disorders such as scoliosis and erosive bone defects. Type 2 neurofibromatosis is characterized by tumors of the eighth cranial or acoustic nerve. Symptoms associated with type 2 include headaches, hearing loss, impaired balance, facial pain, and tinnitus. This condition is often accompanied by intracranial or intraspinal tumors.

Neurofibromatosis is diagnosed by history of symptoms and physical examination. Magnetic resonance imaging may be necessary to detect tumors in the brain or spinal cord. The severity of the disease is variable. Disfigurement caused by tumors and nodules on the skin can be corrected with plastic surgery. Tumors of the spinal cord and brain can be treated surgically as well. The care of these patients is multidisciplinary, requiring visits to several specialists. Patients may need to see specialists such as an ophthalmologist for optic gliomas, a neurologist for neurofibromatosis, a dermatologist for nodules on the skin, or an orthopedist for osseous lesions. The patient must be followed closely for problems related to the formation of tumors. First-degree relatives should be screened for the presence of the disease, and genetic counseling is recommended to avoid passing the disease to future generations.

Malignant Conditions of the Skin

Skin cancer is the most common form of cancer occurring in the United States (CDC, 2002). Exposure to the sun's ultraviolet rays is a direct contributing factor in the development of skin cancer.

Individuals at the highest risk for skin cancer include those with fair or light skin color, those with a family history or personal history of skin cancer, individuals with chronic sun exposure, those with intermittent but intense exposure to the sun, those with sunburns early in life, and those with a large number of moles or freckles indicating sun sensitivity and sun damage. There are three types of skin cancer: The most common type is basal cell carcinoma, followed by squamous cell carcinoma, and then malignant melanoma.

Basal Cell Carcinoma

Basal cell carcinoma is more common in Caucasian people and not as common in African Americans. It is usually nonmetastasizing and occurs most frequently on the head and neck, where there is the greatest sun exposure. There are different types of basal cell carcinoma. The most common is nodular, which appears as a smooth skin-colored nodule. It is dome shaped with a rolled edge. It may have an overlying dilation of vessels seen just beneath the skin surface. The second most common type of basal cell carcinoma is superficial basal cell carcinoma. It is usually seen on the chest and back and is described as a flat, nonpalpable, erythematous plaque with distinct borders. It is often difficult to distinguish because it looks like many other skin lesions. Figure 66–4 ■ is an example of a basal cell carcinoma.

Squamous Cell Carcinoma

Squamous cell carcinoma consists of tumors of the outer epidermis that occur with frequent exposure to the sun and can be relatively aggressive when spreading. There are two types of squamous cell carcinoma: intraepidermal, which remains in the epidermis for a long time but can eventually spread to area lymph nodes and become invasive, which can be either slow or rapid growing. Squamous cell carcinoma is described as a small, red, scaling lesion sitting on an elevated base with an irregular border that may itch or be a nonhealing lesion after minor trauma. Squamous cell carcinoma develops from precancerous lesions and can metastasize through the lymphatic system to regional lymph nodes. Figure 66–5 ■ is an example of a squamous cell carcinoma.

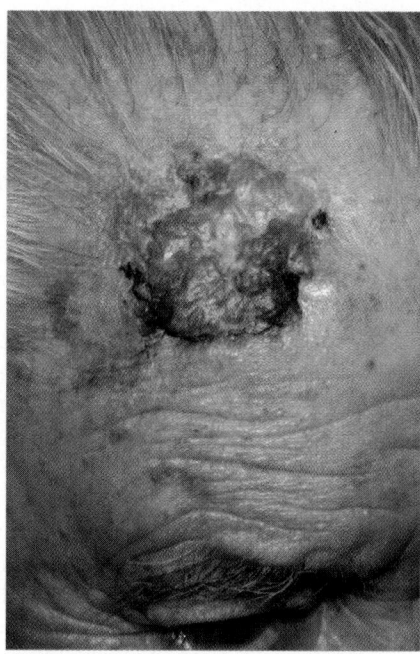

FIGURE 66–5 ■ Squamous cell carcinoma.
Source: Visuals Unlimited

Malignant Melanoma

The incidence of melanoma has more than tripled in the Caucasian population in the United States in the last 20 years. Malignant melanoma currently is the seventh most common cancer in the United States (Jemal et al., 2006; Swetter, 2008). Malignant melanoma is a skin cancer that originates from melanocytes. Early detection with early intervention is usually curative. Because of the aggressive and invasive nature of malignant melanoma, the prognosis is poor when it is diagnosed in the later stages. It is recommended that all individuals examine their skin and know the risk factors of malignant melanoma, as presented in the Risk Factors box.

Malignant melanoma is the most dangerous skin cancer because it is a rapidly growing invasive tumor that can metastasize to almost any organ in the body and result in death. It is a tumor involving melanocytes that is related to sun exposure. Fair-skinned people who sunburn easily and freckle are at the greatest risk. Severe, blistering sunburns in early childhood and intense sun exposure increase the susceptibility to melanoma. It appears as a changing or unusual mole with an irregular border, an uneven surface, and that has a varied size and shape (see the Risk Factors box). The color varies with combinations of brown, black, blue, gray, red, and white. It may be tender and will sometimes ulcerate and bleed. The four types of malignant melanoma are outlined in Chart 66–10. Because malignant melanoma is rapidly progressing, it is important to stage the disease in order to determine the best treatment option. In stage I the lesion is less than 1 millimeter thick with no evidence of tumor growth into lymph nodes. A stage II lesion is thicker than 1 millimeter with lymph nodes that are not enlarged, but there may be metastasis to other organs and lymph nodes. Stage III indicates there has been metastasis to distant organs. There is lymph node enlargement near the melanoma site, and there are

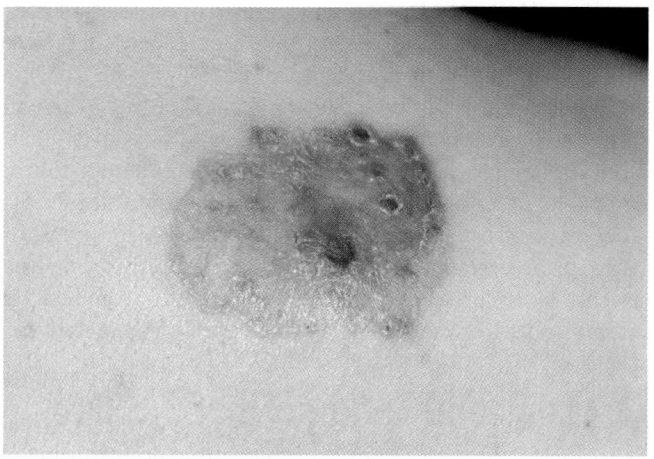

FIGURE 66–4 ■ Basal cell carcinoma.
Source: Phototake NYC

RISK FACTORS for Malignant Melanoma

Patient at high risk for malignant melanoma:

- Has a large number of typical moles.
- Has an increased number of atypical moles.
- Burns easily from exposure to the sun, freckles from sun exposure, or has difficulty tanning.
- Has a family history of malignant melanoma.
- Has previously been diagnosed with malignant melanoma.

The ABCDs of Malignant Melanoma

A   *Asymmetry.*   Early melanoma is asymmetrical, as opposed to the typical mole that is symmetrical.

B   *Border.*   Melanomas have irregular borders, whereas most moles have clearly delineated edges.

C   *Color.*   Melanomas are usually variegated and are in shades of brown, tan, blue/black, or a combinations of colors. Typical moles tend to be uniform in color.

D   *Diameter.*   Melanomas are often larger than 6 millimeters in diameter. The typical mole is generally less than 6 millimeters in diameter (the approximate size of a pencil eraser).

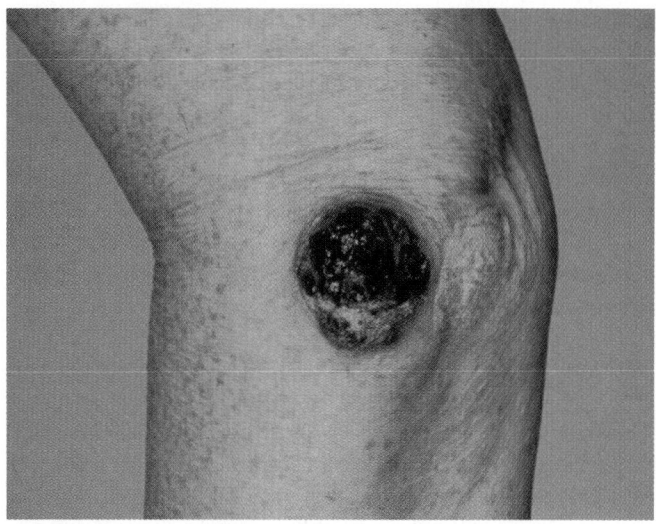

FIGURE 66–6 ■ Malignant melanoma.
Source: Biophoto Associates/Science Source

CHART 66–10 **Types of Melanoma**	
Type	**Description**
Superficial spreading	Makes up 50% of the cases of melanoma. Occurs in younger adults. It looks like a nevus with a raised edge and lateral growth. It may be ulcerated and bleeding.
Nodular melanoma	Makes up 20–25% of all cases and usually occurs in young adults. Raised, dome-shaped lesion. It is usually a uniform blue-black color. It resembles blood blisters. It rapidly invades the dermis.
Lentigo melanoma	Makes up 15% of all cases and occurs in older adults. Slow-growing, flat nevus. Grows horizontally and radially.
Acral lentiginous melanoma	Least common form making up less than 10% of all cases. Occurs on the palms of the hands, soles of the feet, nail beds, and mucous membranes.

CHART 66–11   **Assessing for Skin Cancer**
The ABCD Method
A = Asymmetry
B = Border irregularity
C = Color variation
D = Diameter greater than the size of a pencil eraser
The Seven-Point Checklist
One or more major signs or three or four minor signs without a major sign can indicate a need to biopsy.
Major Signs
Change in size
Change in shape
Change in color
Minor Signs
Inflammation
Crusting or bleeding
Sensory changes

positive lymph nodes away from the original tumor site. Stage IV is generally widespread and incurable (Demierre, Allten, & Brown, 2005). Figure 66–6 ■ is an example of a malignant melanoma.

Assessment of Skin Cancer

Skin cancer is often asymptomatic; therefore, it is important to assess the skin frequently for changes in moles or new growths. One of the most common methods used to evaluate changes in skin lesions is the ABCD rule. Another common guideline for assessment is the seven-point checklist used for melanoma. Chart 66–11 describes both of these methods of skin evaluation. These guidelines have been found to have less than desirable di-

agnostic accuracy, especially when used for skin cancers other than melanoma; so other modalities are being evaluated for use such as total-body photography, color histogram analysis, and skin surface microscopy. The most accurate way to diagnose skin cancer is through biopsy.

Medical Management of Skin Cancer

All skin cancers should be surgically removed with the intent to cure the cancer. Basal cell and squamous cell cancer can be removed with surgical excision, chemosurgery, radiation, or curettage. Melanoma also needs surgical excision; however, it is important to go through a process of staging melanoma so that appropriate treatment can be planned. Diagnostic procedures such as chest x-ray, ultrasound, computed tomography (CT), magnetic resonance imaging (MRI), lymphoscintigraphy, and positron-emission tomography (PET) are used to detect metastasis. Melanoma is treated with deep and wide surgical excision to remove the entire tumor so that the margins are clear of melanoma cells. For stages I and II, this may be all the treatment that is necessary. For stages III and IV, when the disease has become systemic, immunotherapy, chemotherapy, or radiation therapy may be used along with regional lymph node dissection. Frequent and regular follow-up examinations should be done. An in-depth description of the diagnosis and treatment of malignant melanomas is given in Chapter 64 .

Skin Infections

The skin is subject to infections caused by bacteria, viruses, or fungi. Normally the skin's flora, sebum, and immune responses help prevent infection. However, depending on the virulence of the organism and the strength of the individual's resistance, infections may occur.

Bacterial Infections

Bacteria are normally present on the skin and are not considered pathogenic. However, if they invade the skin or if the resistance of the patient is low, they can result in superficial or systemic infection. Certain organisms that are not normally on the skin also can cause infection if they invade the skin.

Cellulitis and **erysipelas** are both infections of the dermis and subcutaneous tissue layers due to a break in the skin. Cellulitis, characterized by erythema, edema, and pain, is usually caused by staphylococcus or streptococcus infections. Erysipelas is an acute, inflammatory, superficial form of cellulitis resulting from *Staphylococcus aureus* (most common) or group A beta-hemolytic streptococcus and involving the lymph system. In erysipelas, one or more well-defined lesions are bright red, tender, and warm to touch with lymphatic involvement causing a red streak along the skin leading away from the primary lesion. Associated symptoms may include fever, chills, headache, and vomiting. Due to a loss of skin integrity, patients with surgical wounds or trauma sites are susceptible to the development of these infections. The most common areas are the lower extremities, face, ears, and buttocks; however, other areas on the body can be affected as well.

Individuals with a compromised immune system have an increased susceptibility to cellulitis. In cellulitis, the skin becomes erythematous, swollen, tender, and tight over the infected area, and there is an indefinite border. There may be vesicles, blisters, or abscesses. Regional lymphadenopathy may occur in both cellulitis and erysipelas.

Diagnostic blood studies reveal mild leukocytosis with a left shift or an elevation in neutrophils, and a wound culture will identify the causative organism. Treatment involves resting the affected site with elevation if possible. Antibiotics sensitive for the causative organism are indicated. Pain medication or soaking with cool Burrow's solution can help relieve the tension and pain. Without treatment, cellulitis or erysipelas may spread to the bloodstream causing septicemia. The diagnosis, treatment, and prognosis of septicemia are described in Chapter 61 .

Impetigo

Impetigo is a common skin infection caused by *Staphylococcus aureus* and/or group A beta-hemolytic streptococcus. It is a contagious, rapidly spreading infection that may occur after a minor skin injury such as an insect bite. It is usually transferred from individual to individual by direct contact and is more common in children and infants.

There are two types of impetigo: bullous and nonbullous. Bullous impetigo is characterized by a thin-roofed bulla or vesicle on an erythematous base. The bulla or vesicle collapses and drains a honey-colored crust, which dries and develops a "stuck on" appearance. Nonbullous impetigo results in vesicles or pustules on an erythematous base that also rupture, leading to a superficial honey-colored crust. Both types may develop satellite lesions. Lesions may itch or may be slightly tender.

Cultures of the lesions are not commonly done but may help in assessing antibiotic sensitivity. Treatment involves removal of crusts by soaking in warm tap water and washing with gentle antibacterial soap such as Dial or Hibiclens. Topical antibiotics such as Bactroban may be helpful, but if the infection is widespread, an oral antibiotic may be indicated. The patient should avoid contact with others and sharing towels or sheets.

Folliculitis

Folliculitis is inflammation of hair follicles that is commonly caused by *Staphylococcus* but may also be caused by trauma or *Pseudomonas aeruginosa*, which is a gram-negative organism frequently associated with nosocomial infections or infections originating in the hospital. Common causes include tight clothing, curly hair that grows back into the skin, and shaving too closely on a regular basis, leading to ingrown hairs or hairs that reenter the skin as they grow. African Americans are particularly susceptible to folliculitis due to ingrown hairs because of their curly hair. Folliculitis due to *Pseudomonas aeruginosa* is related to the use of hot tubs, whirlpools, or exposure to contaminated water. The desquamated skin cells in the water provide a good medium for bacterial growth, and free chlorine levels are decreased by the large number of people in the pool or hot tub (CDC, 2000). Folliculitis due to *Pseudomonas* is not spread from person to person but is usually due to inadequate care of the pool or tub. The *Pseudomonas* invades the hair follicle pores after superhydration of the skin by the contaminated water. Symptoms will occur 1 to 5 days after exposure to the contaminated water.

Folliculitis presents as circular papules and pustules associated with the hair follicles and surrounded by an area of erythema. They may itch and are usually located in areas of tight clothing, bathing suits, or any place where hair grows. With *Pseudomonas* folliculitis, symptoms may also include low-grade fever, sore throat, and lymphadenopathy. Folliculitis is diagnosed by history of lesion development and exposure to contaminated water, and physical exam. The lesions may be cultured to diagnose the causative organism and identify antibiotic sensitivities.

Treatment involves administration of antibiotics and other nonpharmacologic measures. If the folliculitis is limited and superficial, topical antibiotics such as Bactroban may be effective. For more involved infections, antibiotics are prescribed such as dicloxacillin when the causative agent is *Staphylococcus,* or Cipro when the causative agent is *Pseudomonas.* The affected area should be cleansed with antibacterial soap twice daily. The application of warm compresses may be helpful to soothe any itching or burning of the skin. If the folliculitis is due to ingrown hairs, the patient should be instructed to refrain from shaving until the infection is resolved. Once shaving is resumed, the patient should be instructed to shave every few days rather than daily, using a thick shaving gel to hydrate the skin. The patient should use a fresh razor blade with each shave, avoid shaving too close, and shave in the direction of hair growth. Using an electric razor instead of a straightedge blade may be helpful. Any hair tips that are beginning to grow back into the skin can be straightened out using a sterile needle or a clean soft-bristled toothbrush in a circular motion. Shaving should be followed with the use of a moisturizing lotion. Pseudomonas folliculitis is usually self-limiting.

Furuncles and Carbuncles

Furuncles and carbuncles are abscesses that develop when the infection from folliculitis becomes deeper and involves more follicles. These lesions develop when a sebaceous gland is obstructed causing a deep inflammatory reaction and infection from *Staphylococcus*. A **furuncle** is defined as a boil or a walled-off, deep, painful, firm mass that contains pus (Figure 66–7 ■). It is usually 1 to 5 centimeters in diameter. A carbuncle is a larger abscess that interconnects several hair follicles. It is about 3 to 10 centimeters in diameter and is extremely painful. A **carbuncle** will drain pus from multiple follicles, leaving crater-like nodules, and may be associated with fever and chills. Furuncles and carbuncles can occur any place where there is hair but may be more common in areas of increased friction or perspiration such as under the belt, in the groin, or in the axillae.

Furuncles and carbuncles are diagnosed by physical examination. The drainage may be cultured to help define the most effective treatment. The treatment includes incision and drainage of the abscess and warm compresses to help relieve the discomfort. Antibiotic ointments such as Bactroban or Neosporin may be used. Systemic antibiotics such as dicloxacillin or erythromycin also may be used.

Viral Infections

Viruses are intracellular pathogens that invade live cells. They contain either DNA or RNA and require host cell genetic material to replicate. They can destroy the cell during the process of entering the cell and replicating, or by causing an immune response causing cell destruction. The various types of viral infections of the skin are outlined next.

Herpes Simplex Type 1 and Type 2

Two different but similar virus types can cause herpes simplex viral infections: type 1 and type 2. Herpes simplex type 1 is found in oral lesions or cold sores, and lesions of the eye or brain that are nongenital in nature. Herpes simplex type 2 is genital and sexually transmitted. With oral–genital sexual contact, both type 1 and type 2 can present as oral. Herpes simplex is caused by a herpes virus that lives in a nerve root. It will remain asymptomatic until something triggers an outbreak. Exposure to the sun, stress, and fever are common triggers.

The lesions of herpes simplex are vesicles that are on an erythematous base and appear in groups. They are preceded by burning, stinging, or pain a few hours before the lesions erupt. The lesions may last for 2 to 6 weeks after which a second eruption may occur but be less severe. The lesions contain the live virus that can be transmitted to others through direct contact with infected lesions or genital secretions. Herpes simplex can be spread by kissing, poor hand hygiene, oral intercourse, or other sexual contact.

Diagnosis of herpes simplex is made through the evaluation of symptoms and the physical appearance of the lesions. The virus can be identified through a Tzanck smear or culture of the lesions (see the Diagnostic Tests box for skin disorders, p. 2150). The infection cannot be cured but the symptoms can be treated. Topical antiviral agents can be used to speed healing. Oral antiviral agents are available and can suppress the infection or decrease the severity if given at the onset of signs and symptoms. See the Pharmacology Summary feature (p. 2181).

Herpes Zoster

Herpes zoster is a viral infection often referred to as **shingles**. It occurs because of the reactivation of latent varicella-zoster virus, or the virus that causes chickenpox. After having the chickenpox, this virus remains dormant in the dorsal root and cranial nerve ganglia, and becomes activated usually when a person is immunocompromised due to age or some other disease process such as AIDS, Hodgkin's disease, and some cancers.

The lesions of herpes zoster are erythematous vesicles scattered over the skin surface along one or two adjacent dermatomes (Figure 66–8 ■). The vesicles occur in clusters of

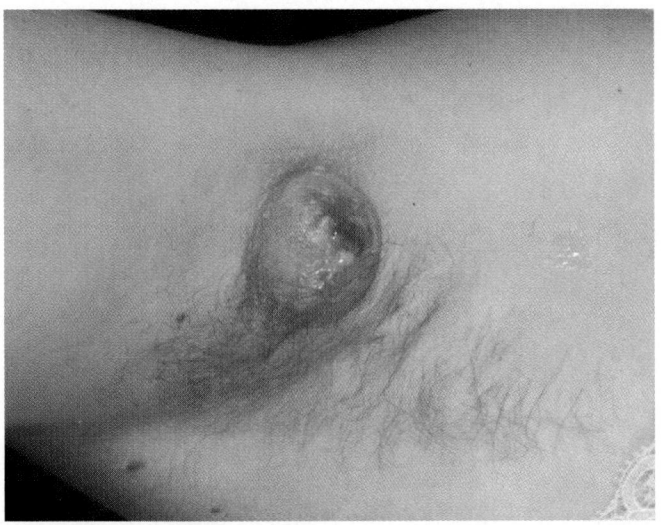

FIGURE 66–7 ■ Furuncles and carbuncles.
Source: NMSB/Custom Medical Stock Photo, Inc.

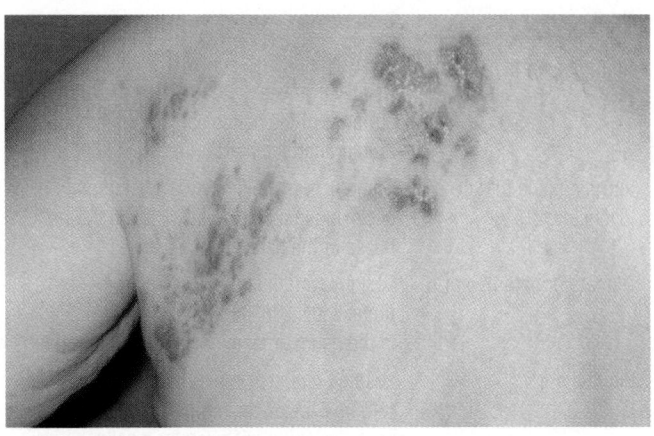

FIGURE 66–8 ■ Herpes zoster.
Source: Bart's Medical Library/Phototake NYC

various sizes and, with time, become cloudy with purulent fluid. The lesions are preceded by pain, itching, or burning in the area. The patient may also experience fever, headache, and malaise prior to the eruption of the lesions. The lesions are tender with a thoracic distribution being the most common. Lesions may also occur on the face, on the neck, and in the eye along the dermatomes of cranial nerves. A common complication is postherpetic neuralgia, which is pain for weeks, to months, and sometimes for a lifetime, after the lesions resolve. The pain is described as itching, burning, sharp, and shooting and may be severe enough to incapacitate the patient. Pain may be severe enough to cause the patient to avoid anything that touches the area, even clothing.

Herpes zoster is diagnosed by physical assessment and history. The lesions can be cultured but the virus is not easily isolated. Polymerase chain reaction (PCR), which directly identifies the virus, may be used for diagnosis. Treatment is aimed at shortening the course of herpes zoster and preventing or alleviating pain. Systemic antiviral agents are used such as acyclovir or famciclovir. See the Pharmacology Summary feature (p. 2181). Treatment can also include nerve blocks, tricyclic antidepressants, or anticonvulsants to help alleviate pain. However, there is no cure, so herpes zoster can reemerge.

Warts

Warts, or **verrucae**, are viral epidermal eruptions caused by human papillomavirus. They are benign and occur most commonly on the hands and feet. They usually are self-limiting and disappear spontaneously in months or years. However, some people prefer to be treated because the appearance of warts may be cosmetically undesirable, and warts on the sole of the foot may be painful. There are many different types of warts (Chart 66–12). The virus causing warts can be transmitted by contact when there are small breaks in the skin. Anal or genital warts are sexually transmitted. Nongenital warts are usually not precancerous; however, genital warts can increase the risk for cervical cancer (see Chapter 49 ☺).

Warts are small, hyperkeratotic flesh-colored papules that are flat or dome shaped with black dots on the surface usually seen on the extremities, especially the hands. The black dots are thrombosed capillaries. Warts can occur singly or in groups and have a rough surface. Warts are usually asymptomatic but can be tender or irritated by clothing. Plantar warts are usually tender. Plantar warts occur on weight-bearing areas where they are pushed into the skin making them appear level with the skin surface. Genital warts appear in the anogenital region and have a light-colored surface and cauliflower appearance. They are diagnosed by physical examination and history. Treatment is difficult and usually requires multiple visits to the health care provider's office. Usual treatment consists of the application of salicylic acid, use of cryotherapy or freezing of the wart, topical immunotherapy, or intralesional bleomycin. Recently, the use of duct tape to occlude the wart has been found to be effective. Duct tape is applied to the site so that the wart is completely occluded and is left in place for 2 months. The use of duct tape has been reported to be as effective as cryotherapy (Abernethy et al., 2006).

Fungal Infections

Fungi may be multicellular or monocellular but are larger than bacteria. They live on dead keratinized cells of the epidermis. Some types are considered part of the normal skin flora, but they can cause uncomfortable infections in the skin. The various fungi that affect the skin and mucus membranes are discussed next.

Candidiasis

Candidiasis is a common infection caused by the *Candida* species of fungus (Figure 66–9 ■). This organism normally lives in the gastrointestinal tract, mouth, and vagina, and causes no harm because it is kept in control by intact skin, intact immune system, and secretions from other microorganisms that live on the skin. When the immune system is depressed, *Candida* can cause the development of opportunistic infections. It can occur with tissue damage, removal of competing organisms such as occurs with antibiotic administration, increase in glucose levels as in diabetes, or a warm, moist environment such as in skin folds. Skin candidiasis is especially prevalent in the very young, such as infants, and the very old and debilitated. The presence of predisposing factors such as wet clothing, obesity, or hyperglycemia

CHART 66–12	**Types of Warts**
Type	**Description**
Common wart	Flesh-toned or gray-brown, scaly papules. Usually involves the dorsal and palmar surfaces of the hands and fingers and the area around the nails.
Verruca plana (flat or juvenile wart)	Smooth, flat, or slightly elevated papule, occurring in multiples. Located on the face, backs of the hands, and shins.
Digitate or filiform warts	Lesions with multiple finger-like projections. Usually a single lesion located in the beard area, eyelids, neck, or scalp.
Plantar wart	Located on the plantar surface of the foot in pressure areas. Usually a single lesion that is tender. Often mistaken for a callus.

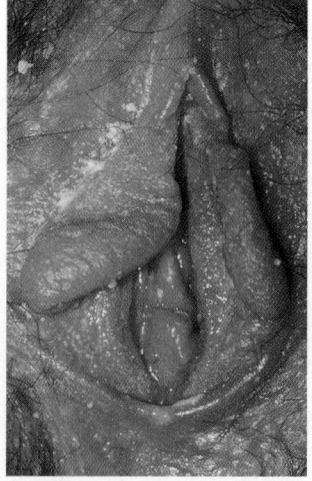

FIGURE 66–9 ■ Candidiasis.
Source: Custom Medical Stock Photo, Inc.

promotes the development of the rash. Most commonly it is seen in the perineal area, under the breasts, on the oral mucous membranes, in the vagina, and on the head of the penis. It can enter the bloodstream and infect major organs as well.

The lesions of candidiasis are pustules that peel away, leaving an erythematous, macerated patch covered by a gray-white membranous plaque with a sharply defined border. The rash appears shiny, moist, and inflamed; generally itches; and is painful. It develops satellite lesions or pustules outside the main rash area.

Candidiasis is diagnosed by history of symptoms, immunosuppression, or antibiotic use, and physical examination. A wet smear with potassium hydroxide can be used to identify the spores under the microscope (see the Diagnostic Tests box for skin disorders, p. 2150). Treatment involves the application of antifungal creams such as miconazole or ketoconazole. Cool compresses with water or Burrow's solution may help promote dryness and relief from itching and soreness. Keeping the skin dry and wearing loose, absorbent clothing help to eliminate predisposing factors. Topical agents such as Mycostatin are available in powders, vaginal suppositories, or suspensions to swish in the mouth. If the candidiasis is systemic, oral or intravenous antifungal agents can be given. See the Pharmacology Summary feature (p. 2181).

Tinea

Tinea is referred to as ringworm by the general public. However, there are many different types, and the manifestations vary with the location, duration, and pathogen involved. It commonly occurs in immunocompromised individuals but has other predisposing factors such as crowded conditions, poor hygiene, or wearing tight clothing. Tinea is diagnosed by history of signs and symptoms, and physical examination of the lesions. It is also important to do a potassium hydroxide wet mount preparation because the presence of fungal hyphae can be seen on the slide and are diagnostic (see the earlier Diagnostic Tests box on p. 2150 for skin disorders). Tinea can be treated with oral and topical antifungal agents. Usually topical agents are enough but if the infection is widespread, chronic, or the patient is immunocompromised, oral medications may be needed. See the Pharmacology Summary feature (p. 2181). The types of tinea include tinea pedis, tinea corporis, tinea capitis, and tinea cruris.

Tinea Pedis

Tinea pedis is a **dermatophyte** infection of the foot commonly referred to as "athlete's foot." It usually involves the web between the fourth and fifth toes but may occur between any of the toes and the plantar or dorsal surface of the foot. It occurs most commonly in postpubescent adolescents and adults. The infection is predisposed by the wearing of tight shoes that promote warmth and perspiration, poor hygiene, or repeated exposure to fungal organisms on locker room floors. The lesions are circular and scaly with central clearing. In the toe webs, the skin appears scaly, fissured, and macerated. The patient complains of itching and tenderness in the area.

Tinea Corporis

Tinea corporis is infection of the trunk and limbs. It occurs more commonly in warm climates and can occur at any age. The lesions are round, annular, scaly patches. They can also appear as papules, pustules, and vesicles that are inflamed and red. The lesions are multiple but uniform in appearance and are usually evident on exposed areas of the body. The lesions may be mildly pruritic but are often asymptomatic.

Tinea Cruris

Tinea cruris, also known as "jock itch," is a fungal infection of the groin and occurs almost exclusively in adult males. It is related to a warm, moist environment and obesity. The lesions are circular, beginning in the crural fold, and are erythematous or slightly brown in the center. The edge is raised, slightly scaly, and well defined. It is usually asymptomatic but may be pruritic.

Tinea Capitis

Tinea of the scalp and hair follicle is a contagious infection transmitted by personal contact. It can be spread through combs, animals, hats, blankets, telephones, and theater seats. It is more common in children and African Americans. The lesions usually appear as patchy, circular areas of hair loss. There may be visible stubs of broken off hairs within the patch of hair loss, and there may also be inflammation and scaling on the scalp. The rash may consist of fine white scales on the scalp with the appearance of dandruff or may have pustules or scabbed areas without scaling or hair loss. Tinea capitis may be associated with fever, occipital adenopathy, and leukocytosis.

◼ Infestations and Insect Bites

The skin can be invaded by insects, ticks, or parasites. Typically there is a single lesion on the skin; however, the lesion depends on the causative agent.

Bees and Wasps

The most common types of insect stings are those of honeybees followed by those of wasps. The honeybee's stinger remains embedded in the skin, whereas other species of bees and wasps leave nothing behind. Initially there is a sharp, painful sting that lasts only a few minutes. It is typically followed by mild burning and a raised white wheal with a red center that resolves in a few days.

Bee and wasp stings are dangerous only if there is a toxic systemic reaction or an allergic anaphylactic reaction. Dangerous reactions occur more commonly in adults over age 40. The symptoms of a toxic reaction include vomiting, diarrhea, headache, fever, muscle spasm, and loss of consciousness. The most severe reaction is an anaphylactic reaction, which involves itching, hives, shortness of breath, wheezing, nausea, abdominal cramps, and may lead to respiratory arrest and death. These reactions occur within minutes to hours of the sting, although allergic reactions can be delayed, occurring up to a week after the sting. Severe generalized reactions are treated with epinephrine and oral or intramuscular antihistamines, and require treatment in an emergency department. If it is a localized, nonallergic reaction, apply ice and give oral antihistamines to prevent spreading of the venom. See the Pharmacology Summary feature (p. 2181) in this chapter.

 *Bee and wasp stings can result in a local reaction or a systemic anaphylactic reaction. For a local reaction, apply ice, compress the site with a tight bandage, and elevate the site. Antihistamines can be given for itching. For a systemic anaphylactic reaction, give intramuscular (IM) epinephrine; beta-2 adrenergic agonist inhalers for bronchospasm, such as albuterol; and antihistamines.*

Ticks

Ticks can be bearers of diseases such as Lyme disease and Rocky Mountain spotted fever. They are very small and embed their heads in the skin to obtain blood. They can enlarge to many times their normal size while they are eating and leave toxins and microorganisms behind. Initially the tick bite leaves a local reaction involving pain, erythema, a papule, and itching. The tick should be removed totally intact if possible. If the head is left behind, a nodule may remain requiring excision. The best approach is prevention of the tick bite by wearing protective clothing, tucking the pants into the socks, and wearing closed-toed shoes.

Ticks can be removed by grasping them as closely as possible to the skin with forceps and pulling upward. Do not squeeze the tick, or apply hot matches or nail polish. Then clean the wound with soap and water or a mild disinfectant. Instruct the patient to report any fever or unusual rash to the health care provider.

Pediculosis

Pediculosis is the infestation of the skin by lice. Lice are highly contagious parasites that survive by sucking blood. There are three types of lice: pediculosis capitis or head lice; pediculosis corporis or body lice; and pediculosis pubis or pubic lice. The female lice reproduce frequently, producing hundreds of **nits**, or eggs, that attach to the hair shaft. The nits hatch into lice that continue to reproduce. Lice secrete toxic saliva that causes trauma and releases toxins leading to itching and dermatitis. Lice are spread by personal contact through combs, brushes, sexual activity, and shared clothing and bed linens.

The major symptom of lice infestation is itching. In the scalp, the nits can be seen as yellow, oval specks attached to the hair shaft. There is extreme pruritus around the back and sides of the scalp. On the body, the lesion is a pinpoint red macule, papule, or wheal with a hemorrhagic puncture site. The center can crust and become infected. The pubic louse or "crab," as it is commonly referred to, is seen on pubic hair. Lice are diagnosed through physical examination and culture. The ova of lice will fluoresce under an ultraviolet light or Wood's lamp.

Treatment involves good hygiene and avoiding the sharing of hats, combs, or clothes. Lindane shampoo, pyrethrins, or permethrin can be used for head lice. Corticosteroid lotions or creams can be used for body lice to help relieve itching. Antihistamines are also helpful for preventing itching.

Scabies

Scabies, caused by a parasite called *Sarcoptes scabiei*, is commonly found in underdeveloped countries and areas where there is overcrowding and poor hygiene. It is contagious and transmitted by close personal contact, clothing, and bedding. The female mite tunnels into the skin, creating a burrow and depositing eggs. The eggs can sometimes be seen at the end of the burrows as tiny maculopapular dots. Intense itching that worsens at night is the primary symptom. The mite can enter the skin and travel all over the body so the itching is generalized. Lesions that are papular, vesicular, or linear occur in the wrists, web spaces of the hands, sides of the hands and feet, genital area, warm intertriginous regions, and abdomen.

Scabies is diagnosed by physical examination with identification of the mites, or burrows. Mites can be seen under a microscope after an application of mineral oil or potassium hydroxide. Treatment consists of the application of scabicide preparations such as permethrin cream or Lindane. The lotion or cream is applied to the entire skin surface including under the nails and in the umbilicus. The medication is left on for 6 hours then washed off. All contacts must be treated. Clothing and bedding should be washed and dried in a hot dryer.

■ Pressure Ulcers

Pressure ulcers are defined by the National Pressure Ulcer Advisory Panel (NPUAP) (1992) as "localized areas of tissue necrosis that develop when soft tissue is compressed between a bony prominence and an external surface for a prolonged period of time." These wounds are also referred to as decubitus ulcers or bedsores, but pressure is an important factor in their development so the term *pressure ulcer* is more appropriate. The incidence of pressure ulcer occurrence has been used to indicate quality of patient care because most are preventable. The reported incidence of pressure ulcer development in acute care settings ranges from 0.4% to 38% (Reddy, Gill, & Rochon, 2006). Pressure ulcers can occur at any age, in any socioeconomic or ethnic group, and more commonly occur on the heels and in the sacrococcygeal area. A complete description of pressure ulcer management is included in Chapter 67 .

■ Common Treatment of Skin Disorders

Common treatments for skin disorders involve creams and lotions, wet dressings, and corticosteroids. There is an old saying related to the treatment of skin disorders that "if it is dry, wet it, and if it is wet, dry it." Dry skin diseases are those that have lost water, lipids, and proteins, and they are treated with creams and lotions. Wet skin disorders are usually inflammatory disorders that are draining. When serum and exudates drain, they take lipids and proteins with them. These disorders are treated with wet compresses to suppress the inflammation and débride the wound.

Creams and lotions are used to restore the water and lipids to the skin. Creams are thicker than lotions and are more lubricating. Creams are slightly greasy in texture and best used in intertriginous areas. Ointments have a texture similar to that of petroleum jelly. They have a greater penetration in the skin than creams; therefore, they may be too occlusive for rashes with exudate or in intertriginous areas. Medications with urea or lactic acid are excellent lubricators and very effective in rehydrating the skin.

Wet dressings or compresses are used to decrease inflammation and débride draining skin lesions. Burrow's solution, acetic acid, or silver nitrate creams are often used for wet dressings. Chart 66–13 is a description of the techniques for the application of wet dressings.

Corticosteroids may be used topically or systemically. They are used because of their anti-inflammatory properties. Steroids are known to decrease the formation of several potent inflammatory mediators and to decrease vascular permeability. Topi-

CHART 66–13   Technique for Application of Wet Dressings

1. Use clean, soft cloth or the dressing type ordered by the health care provider. Gauze pads, wraparound gauze, cotton cloths, or clean old T-shirts may be used.

2. Fold the cloth so there are at least four to eight layers, and cut to fit an area slightly larger than the area to be treated.

3. Wet the dressings, if necessary, by immersing them in the solution, and wring them out to the point of being wet but not dripping. Solution should be room temperature.

4. Place the compresses on the affected area and smooth them out. Leave them in place for 30 minutes to 1 hour. Do not pour solution on a wet dressing to keep it wet. Remove the compress and replace it with a new one.

5. Dressings are left in place for 30 minutes. Dressings may be used two to four times a day or continuously. Discontinue use of the wet compresses when the skin becomes dry.

---

cal preparations are available in low, mid, and high potency. The strength needed depends on the disorder and the location on the body. Chapter 67 includes a complete description of products used to treat pressure ulcers.

Nursing Management

Nursing care for patients with skin disorders involves skills in multilevel assessment, clinical decision making, and critical thinking. Knowledge about the varied treatment strategies provides a basis for safe, quality nursing care. The nurse will need to collaborate with other members of the health care team to treat the whole patient and address the wide variety of needs the patient may have. The nursing process provides a framework for nursing management.

Assessment

The focus of nursing care is to prevent problems or recognize complications early so they can be successfully treated. The nurse must assess the patient frequently, noting changes in skin color, texture, wound size, drainage, and temperature. Analysis of the data collected during assessment will provide a basis for determining a treatment plan and assessing response to treatment. Patients with skin disorders may develop problems with hydration, fluid balance, or nutrition. Fluid loss through wounds leads to dehydration and electrolyte imbalances. The skin also provides protection against infection; so when its barrier is broken, infection becomes more likely. It is very important to assess for signs of infection both in the wound and systemically. Clinical manifestations of infection include fever, increased redness or drainage, increased pain, changes in odor or color of drainage, increased white blood cell count, and increased tissue erosion. If the infecting organism is contagious, such as occurs with *Staphylococcus,* isolation procedures may be needed (see Chapter 20).

Psychological assessment needs to be uppermost in the mind of the nurse as care is given to patients with skin disorders. The appearance of the skin affects self-esteem and body image. Skin disorders can cause the patient to withdraw from social situations. Society can be unkind to people that have scars or rashes with an unpleasant appearance. Some individuals may withdraw from the patient, fearing the disorder is contagious. Patients should be provided with an open, supportive environment in which they are comfortable voicing their concerns.

Nursing Diagnoses

The following nursing diagnoses are related to the patient with skin disorders:

- *Impaired Skin Integrity* related to epithelial skin disorder
- *Risk for Infection* related to loss of skin integrity
- *Acute Pain* related to skin disorder and exposed nerve endings
- *Fear* and *Anxiety* related to changes in health status/role functioning; situational crisis
- *Disturbed Body Image* related to disorder.

Planning

A collaborative and comprehensive approach to care will optimize the recovery process. The plan uses the assessment data to prioritize care. First, the cause must be identified and removed if possible. For example, if a rash occurs after administration of an antibiotic, the nurse must notify the health care provider and have the medication changed. Depending on the nature and extent of the skin disorder, dieticians, case managers, social workers, consultative health care providers (cardiovascular, infectious diseases, surgeons, and plastic surgeons), nursing staff, and ancillary staff should be part of the plan of care, as all play a role in the treatment.

Outcome and Evaluation Parameters

The outcome for patients with skin disorders is to heal without scarring or loss of function. The outcome goals are to promote the patient's recovery, provide support, and manage the disorder to prevent complications. The evaluation parameters include healed skin and no evidence of a systemic complication. The skin integrity will be intact and the clinical manifestations of infection will be absent. The patient will resume previous level of performing activities of daily living.

Interventions and Rationales

Interventions are based on the type of skin disorder. Once the cause has been removed the treatment begins. The involved area must have effective wound care and appropriate selection of dressing, if necessary. If the involved area is in the perineum, the nurse must make every effort to prevent urine and fecal contamination. The area needs to be kept clean and dry. Wound care, dressing, and skin barriers are described in depth in Chapter 67 .

Nutrition is essential for wound healing to occur. The nurse must assess the amount and type of food intake and intervene if lack of appetite persists. Hydration is also important for wound healing. Therefore, assessing fluid intake is essential, encouraging the patient to take in an adequate amount of fluid, and if necessary obtaining a health care provider's order for intravenous fluids.

If an infection occurs, treatment needs to be tailored to the clinical manifestations. For example, the patient may need antibiotics or antifungal medications to treat the cause. If fever is present, antipyretics and cooling measures may be necessary. Finally, if the organism is communicable, the patient will need isolation.

Evaluation

A plan for care of the patient with skin disorders should be reevaluated regularly to ensure that the plan is still effective. Any change in the patient's condition could have a negative impact on the wound healing process and the effectiveness of the plan of care. In a long-term care setting, reevaluation should be done regularly and documented. Interventions and plans of care need changing if the current treatment plan is unsuccessful. Evaluation criteria of progress would be a decrease in the size and depth of the involved area. If this healing is not occurring, then the area needs to be assessed as to why it is not, such as for infection or decreased tissue perfusion.

Collaborative Management

A collaborative approach to the management of patients with skin disorders is essential. Skin disorders have many facets that influence the patient both physically and emotionally. A multidisciplinary team that includes health care providers, nurses, psychologists/psychiatrists, occupational therapists, physical therapists, nutritionists, and pharmacists is necessary to help the patient recover. Health care provider care is discussed throughout this chapter and may include medical care as well as surgical care. In addition, psychiatric care may be needed to assist with adjustment to alterations in appearance related to the skin disorder. The occupational therapist can assist the patient to return to work or function to meet everyday needs. The physical therapist can help keep muscles strong and address the limitations of movement that may occur with scar formation. Patients with skin disorders often lose electrolytes and have increased metabolic demands that lead to weight loss and increased nutritional needs. These needs can be addressed by a nutritionist. The pharmacist will be concerned with the medications and their interactions and effectiveness. The pharmacist can assist with educating the patient about medication management and the possible side effects. The nurse's role is addressed with the specific disorders throughout this chapter. The nurse serves as the team leader to facilitate communication between members of the team and as the patient advocate.

Discharge Priorities

Most patients with dermatologic disorders are cared for at home. Discharge planning begins with the diagnosis of the condition. Patient teaching aimed at self-care is an important part of planning for discharge. The Patient Teaching & Discharge Priorities box outlines specific discharge priorities.

Life-Threatening Skin Disorders

With prompt and appropriate treatment, most skin disorders are manageable with a minimum of side effects or lifelong sequelae. However, certain skin disorders can cause major physical disfigurement, have disfiguring sequelae, and in some instances are life threatening. These conditions begin as a skin disorder and then progress to multiple organ involvement, thereby becoming life threatening. Necrotizing fasciitis, Stevens–Johnson syndrome, and toxic epidermal necrolysis are the most common life-threatening skin disorders.

Necrotizing Fasciitis

Necrotizing fasciitis (NF), first described in 1848, is an infection of the superficial fascia or the connective tissue surrounding muscle and subcutaneous tissue, leading to fascial necrosis. It is commonly referred to as the "flesh-eating bacteria." Although relatively uncommon, it is significant because of the difficulty in recognizing it and the rapidity with which it spreads and can become fatal. This infection can occur at any age or in any location and is not specific to gender. Approximately one-half of the cases occur in young previously healthy patients (CDC, 2008). NF also occurs with a variety of conditions from simple minor injuries to complicated major surgeries or trauma. The very young and very old are at increased risk, as are those with diabetes mellitus, atherosclerosis, chronic renal failure, obesity, immunosuppression, malnutrition, illicit drug injections, alcoholism, and peripheral vascular disease. The Risk Factors box identifies those at risk for necrotizing fasciitis.

There are three types of necrotizing fasciitis (NF). Type 1 is polymicrobial and related to mixed aerobic or anaerobic bac-

---

RISK FACTORS for Necrotizing Fasciitis

Age: very young and very old

Individuals with throat or skin infections

Individuals with chronic illnesses such as:
- Cancer
- Diabetes
- Renal failure on dialysis.

People using steroids

Obesity

Poor nutrition or malnutrition

Immunosupression

Needle puncture site with illicit drug use

Frostbite

Chronic venous leg ulcers

Open bone fractures

Insect bites

Childbirth

Surgical wounds

Trauma

AIDS

Major burns

Prolonged antibiotic therapy

Alcoholics

Peripheral vascular disease

Multiple myeloma

Hypertension

Skin biopsy

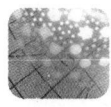

PATIENT TEACHING & DISCHARGE PRIORITIES for Skin Disorders

Need	Teaching
Wound Care	Evaluate for signs of infection such as increased redness, drainage, fever, or foul odor.
Patient/family	Perform cleaning of wounds and dressing changes as ordered by the health care provider.
	Perform hand hygiene and wear gloves while performing dressing changes.
	Avoid scratching healed areas.
	Keep unaffected skin clean and well hydrated.
	Avoid exposure to the sun.
	Wear loose-fitting, soft clothing.
Family/support system	Assess knowledge of illness:
	• Teach actions to decrease risk of infection.
	• Teach signs and symptoms that should be reported to the health care provider.
	Assess compliance with treatment:
	• Provide written instructions.
	• Assess the patient/family's abilities to provide care at home.
Setting	Assess effectiveness of available support systems.
	Assess discharge placement needs:
	• Home
	• Rehabilitation facility
	• Extended care facility.
	Assess home environment for need for assistive devices and safety.
	Assess need for professional home health needs.
	Assess abilities to obtain food, medications, and supplies.
Nutrition	Maintain a high-calorie, high-protein, well-balanced diet.
Patient/family	Include vitamin C, iron, and zinc in the diet.
Family/support system	Assess appetite and weight loss.
Setting	Avoid foods that cause hypersensitivity reactions.
	Teach foods to include and avoid in the diet.
	Assess financial resources.
Psychological Adjustment	Encourage verbalizations of feelings and fears.
Patient/family	Encourage positive reinforcement rather than rejection from the family.
Setting	Answer questions honestly.
	Encourage participation in support groups for the patient's specific disorder.
Pruritus	Avoid things that are irritating or intensify itching such as excessive bathing.
Patient/family	Application of cold or emollient lotion to rehydrate the skin.
Setting	Recommend baths with cornstarch or oatmeal.
	Proper application and use of prescribed medications.
	Wear nonrestrictive, light clothing.
	Assess temperature and humidity.
Pain	Assess pain level and report increases in pain.
Patient/family	Assess effectiveness of pain medications.
Setting	Assess patient/family knowledge of pain medication and side effects.
	Assess environment for safety.

teria such as *Clostridium, Pseudomonas aeruginosa, Staphylococcus aureus, Bacteroides fragilis, Escherichia coli*, and *Klebsiella pneumoniae*. Type 2 is monomicrobial and caused by group A streptococci. Type 3 is caused by gas gangrene or clostridial myonecrosis. A variant of type 1 NF is caused by saltwater contaminated with *Vibrio* species. Sometimes group A streptococci are found in combination with *Staphylococcus aureus* or *Staphylococcus epidermidis* in type 2. Group A streptococci are normally found in the throat and on the skin. These organisms can be transmitted through coughing or sneezing, or through direct contact with secretions. Transmission can also occur through contact with infected wounds or sores on the skin. Entry through the skin can occur when there is a surgical wound or a small cut. Contaminated hands can carry the organism as well.

Pathophysiology of Necrotizing Fasciitis

Once a break in the skin occurs and is contaminated, the organisms spread from the subcutaneous tissue along the superficial and deep fascia, facilitated by bacterial enzymes and toxins, which continue to break down tissue. The infection causes:

- Tissue ischemia
- Superficial nerve damage
- Vascular thrombosis and occlusion
- Tissue liquification necrosis
- Septicemia when systemic toxicity occurs.

Certain strains of NF cause the development of streptococcal pyrogenic exotoxins A, B, and C. These exotoxins, along with streptococcal superantigen, stimulate the release of cytokines and produce hypotension (CDC, 2008). This leads to occlusion and interruption of vessels that supply the skin. The ischemia produces bullae formation, ulceration, and necrosis of the skin.

Clinical Manifestations of Necrotizing Fasciitis

Necrotizing fasciitis (NF) is difficult to diagnose because the symptoms are many and varied. One way of tracking the course of the disease is through the progression of the symptoms and laboratory findings. The symptoms usually begin about 1 week after the initiating event and can be divided into three stages: early, advanced, and critical (Chart 66–14). The early symptoms begin in the first 24 to 48 hours. The most common parts of the body affected include the extremities, the perineum, and the truncal areas, but NF can be found anywhere on the body (Hasham, Matteucci, Stanley, & Hart, 2005). The wound site looks essentially normal with wound margins not obvious, but the patient experiences flu-like symptoms, localized pain, erythema, and swelling. It is easy to misdiagnose the infection at this stage because the symptoms are vague and fit with many other problems. The hallmark sign is pain beyond what would be expected for the extent of the injury.

The second stage, known as the advanced stage, occurs within 2 to 4 days. During this phase, the early symptoms worsen. The skin becomes swollen and tight, a dusky blue color develops, and fluid-filled blisters or bullae develop. This occurs because of ischemia and progressive thrombosis (Wong & Wang, 2005). The texture of the wound has been described as "wet wood." The skin becomes thin and hyperesthetic or anesthetic because of destruction to cutaneous nerves. This lack of sensation is a sign that the patient is not experiencing cellulitis.

The third, or critical, stage occurs within 4 to 5 days. During this stage, the bluish-colored areas become gangrenous. The skin begins to slough, and septic shock can occur leading to hypotension, high fever, delirium, loss of consciousness, pain, liver failure, renal failure, and eventually death. Without systemic complications the mortality rate for NF can be as high as 25%, although it increases to as high as 76% when sepsis and renal failure occur (Wong & Wang, 2005). Figure 66–10 ■ is an example of advanced necrotizing fasciitis.

Diagnosis of Necrotizing Fasciitis

Necrotizing fasciitis should be diagnosed early so that treatment can begin as soon as possible. The chance of the patient's surviving is better with an early diagnosis. Diagnosis is made based on

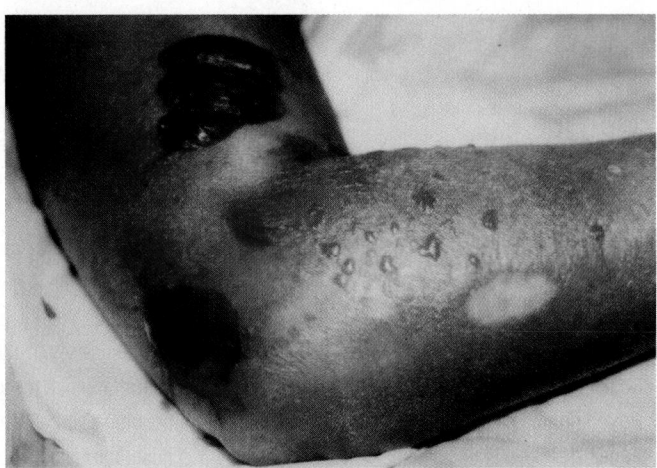

FIGURE 66–10 ■ Advanced necrotizing fasciitis.
Source: Courtesy of Donals E. Lon, B. Demers, A. E. Simor, H. Vellend, P. N. Schlievert, S. Byrne, F. Jamieson, S. Walmsely. *CID* 1:792-800, (1993)

CHART 66–14	**Signs and Symptoms of Necrotizing Fasciitis**	
Early Stage **First 24–48 hours**	**Advanced Stage** **2nd–4th Day**	**Critical Stage** **4th–5th Day**
Flu-like symptoms such as fever, chills, myalgia, nausea, vomiting, and diarrhea. Abrupt localized pain beyond what would be expected. Patchy discoloration of skin that is violaceous to erythematous without defined borders. Nonpitting edema outside the area of discoloration. Skin is essentially normal in appearance.	Skin swollen and tight and erythema is noted. Area becomes dusky blue in color. Blisters or bullae filled with purplish, foul-smelling, thin, watery fluid. Skin has paper-like appearance. There may be palpable crepitation due to the presence of gas. Spread of the infection—increasing wound size. Increased leukocytes. Decreased sodium.	Skin sloughs. Gangrene develops. Hypotension. Delirium. Loss of consciousness. Liver failure. Renal failure. Fever. Acute respiratory distress syndrome (ARDS). Coagulopathy. Fascia appears gray to grayish green. Elevated heart rate. Tissue necrosis.

signs and symptoms and laboratory testing. The problem is that often it is difficult to make a differential diagnosis because the signs and symptoms of NF are similar to those of other conditions. It is generally believed that if the following symptoms are present, NF should be suspected:

- Rapid progression of wound size
- Poor response to therapeutic interventions
- Blistering necrosis
- Cyanosis
- Extreme local tenderness
- High temperature
- Tachycardia
- Hypotension
- Altered level of consciousness.

Laboratory findings include leukocytosis with an elevated number of neutrophils and bands. The creatine phosphokinase (CPK) levels will be elevated due to muscle damage. If there is renal damage, the blood urea nitrogen (BUN) and creatinine will be elevated. There may also be some electrolyte imbalances and anemia. However, a complete blood count, electrolyte levels, a sedimentation rate, and C-reactive protein level may look similar to those of cellulitis. Blood and wound cultures should demonstrate the presence of group A streptococcus or other organisms known to be involved in the development of necrotiz-

ing fasciitis. Computed tomography (CT) and magnetic resonance imaging (MRI) scans can help to define the extent of the fasciitis and may show gas in the subcutaneous tissues produced by the bacteria and deep fascia thickening. The Diagnostic Tests box presents the laboratory and diagnostic tests and abnormalities associated with necrotizing fasciitis. Surgeons may prefer to biopsy or may take the patient to surgery to assess the fascia directly. When directly assessed, there will be lack of bleeding in the fascia and the presence of foul-smelling pus (Wong & Wang, 2005).

Medical Management of Necrotizing Fasciitis

The best chance for survival occurs with early diagnosis and beginning treatment as soon as possible. Because of the complexity of the disease, a team approach is essential when managing the patient. Typically patients are placed in a surgical intensive care unit to monitor hemodynamic factors and provide frequent wound care. The treatment for necrotizing fasciitis is three pronged: antibiotics, surgical débridement, and supportive care. Treatment begins with the early administration of broad-spectrum antibiotics and intensive surgical débridement. Broad-spectrum antibiotics are started initially; however, once the culture results have returned, an antibiotic that targets the organism is preferred. The most common antibiotic is benzylpenicillin, given intravenously in large doses. Penicillin by itself may not be successful, so the addition of clinidamycin is helpful in producing a favorable outcome. Metronidazole and third-generation cephalosporin

DIAGNOSTIC TESTS for Necrotizing Fasciitis

Test	Expected Abnormality	Rationale for Abnormality
White blood count (WBC) with differential	Elevated with an elevated number of bands signifying left shift.	Due to acute infectious process.
Creatine phosphokinase (CPK)	Elevated.	Released from muscle cells when damaged.
Blood urea nitrogen (BUN) and creatinine	Elevated.	Will occur if there is renal damage. Also some antibiotics can affect renal function.
Red blood count (RBC), hemoglobin, hematocrit	Decreased.	Demonstrates anemia due to bleeding and possibly renal failure.
Blood and wound cultures	Growth of causative organism: usually group A streptococcus.	Demonstrates organisms involved.
Serum sodium	Decreased.	Due to wound infection and leakage.
Computed tomography (CT) and magnetic resonance imaging (MRI)	Demonstrates extent of fasciitis and gas in subcutaneous tissues.	Can show breakdown of tissue. Organisms responsible produce gas. Will assist in directing rapid surgical débridement.
T2-weighted MRI	Shows well-defined regions of high signal intensity in the deep tissues.	Will assist in directing rapid surgical débridement.
Excisional deep skin biopsy Cultures of the affected tissue Gram staining of the exudates	Helpful in diagnosing and identifying the causative organisms. May provide a clue as to whether a type 1 or type 2 infection is present.	The type influences the antibiotic therapy.
Histologic findings	A dense infiltration of neutrophils may be observed in deeper parts of the subcutaneous tissue and fascia. Subcutaneous fat necrosis and vasculitis are also evident. Eccrine glands and ducts may be necrotic. Alcian blue or periodic acid-Schiff (PAS) staining with diastase may show clusters of bacteria and fungi.	Sections show superficial fascial necrosis with blood vessels occluded by thrombi.

antibiotics have also been useful. Some health care providers may opt to use intravenous immunoglobulin (IVIG) with severe streptococcal infections associated with NF. The use of intravenous immunoglobulin may be a useful adjunct treatment to increase the immune response.

Early surgical débridement is necessary to remove all necrotic tissue and prevent the spread of the infection. Initially the patient is taken to surgery as often as every 12 to 24 hours, where débridement is done until clear margins are obtained. This regimen is continued until tissue necrosis stops and fresh viable tissue begins to grow. It may be necessary surgically to excise organs and amputate involved limbs to remove irreversible necrosis and gangrene or because of overwhelming toxicity. Prompt surgery increases the likelihood of survival.

Skin grafting is typically required to close the full-thickness injuries. Chapter 68 has a complete description of the various skin grafting techniques.

Supportive therapies may include high-calorie diet, hyperbaric oxygen therapy, and the application of a vacuum assisted closure device. Because patients with necrotizing fasciitis are breaking down tissue and have a high metabolic state, extra calories are required. A description of hypermetabolic state is included in Chapter 68 .

A vacuum assisted closure device (wound VAC) is typically applied to the wound after débridement when clear edges have been obtained. This device does three things to improve wound healing:

- It creates a negative pressure in the wound by applying suction. The suction drains interstitial edema fluid, thus decreasing pressure on capillaries and improving perfusion.

- The negative pressure also provides a mechanical stretch/distortion of the cells in the wound bed, which stimulates production of granulation tissue.

- The suction removes stagnant fluid in the wound, thus decreasing the bacterial burden in the healing wound bed.

Vacuum assisted closure is discussed in detail in Chapter 67 .

Streptococcal toxic shock syndrome, which is characterized by hypotension and multiorgan failure, can lead to death. Therefore, fluid resuscitation and hemodynamic monitoring are required. The management of shock is discussed in detail in Chapter 61 .

Nursing Management

Nursing care for patients with necrotizing fasciitis requires excellent assessment, clinical decision making, and critical thinking skills. Nurses need to be aware of the possibility of necrotizing fasciitis, even with the smallest of traumatic injuries. It is important to recognize those patients at risk (see the Risk Factors box for necrotizing fasciitis, p. 2170) and to alert the health care provider when warranted.

The usual infection control precautions are important, such as hand hygiene to prevent the chances of spreading the bacteria. The patient should be in a private room and under contact isolation (see Chapter 20). It is important to assess the patient's status regularly. The nurse should check vital signs, oxy-

gen saturations, intake and output, and laboratory values frequently and report abnormalities to the health care provider. The possibility of septic shock or fluid imbalances should be monitored. The wound is assessed for expansion of the erythema, changes in edema, changes in color, and drainage.

Pain is an important issue in the patient with necrotizing fasciitis. Pain may be difficult to monitor because it often seems out of proportion to the patient's injury. It is important to assess the pain because it is an indication of the pathologic process. Therefore, changes in pain need to be reported to the health care provider, and pain should be treated accordingly. The dressing changes are long, complex, and very painful, requiring premedication. The usual pain medication is morphine sulfate; however, alternative therapies such as imagery and music therapy may be helpful as well. The nurse is responsible for monitoring the administration of medications and assessing for side effects or signs of toxicity. Chapter 15 provides a complete description of the pain management protocol.

 Remember that pain is a subjective experience and may be more or less than is typical for other patients with a similar diagnosis. Assess pain carefully using a pain scale.

Nutritional needs of the patient are a concern to promote wound healing. Because of the infection, pain, and wound healing, the patient's calorie needs are increased. The patient with necrotizing fasciitis requires two to three times the normal amounts of calories and protein for healing. Supplements may also be required for wound healing such as vitamin C, vitamin E, and iron. The nutritionist should be consulted, and if the patient can eat, frequent, high-calorie meals are indicated. To increase compliance with nutritional intake, the patient's likes, dislikes, and cultural needs must be considered. If the patient is not able to eat, total parenteral nutrition (TPN) or enteral feeding may be indicated. The nurse also must monitor the administration of parenteral or enteral nutrition.

A fluid balance chart is needed to keep track of urine output and intravenous and oral intake. The patient should be assessed for signs of fluid imbalance such as crackles in the lungs, edema in dependent areas, or decreased urine output. Any abnormalities should be reported to the health care provider.

Wound care of the affected skin is important. The patient's wounds are assessed frequently for any changes such as in drainage, color, odor, or increasing size. Unaffected skin is assessed as well. Evaluation of pressure areas and maintenance of skin integrity in unaffected skin are essential parts of the assessment. The patient is repositioned at least every 2 hours and assessed for signs of skin breakdown. Wound care and dressing changes are complicated procedures requiring planning and the support of the patient. Strict sterile technique is used.

The patient with necrotizing fasciitis has many psychological needs. There is frequently a long hospital stay followed by months of rehabilitation. The interruption in skin integrity leads to an altered body image, threatens the patient's self-esteem, and may lead to extreme anxiety and grief. The physical appearance, along with the fact that the patient is often in isolation, may affect the number of visitors, leading to depression and social isolation. The prolonged illness may have a financial impact, especially if the patient is the main wage earner of the family. Additionally, disabilities after recovery may keep the patient from returning to work. The patient should be encouraged to voice concerns and feelings, and a mental health specialist should be consulted.

Application of the nursing process will facilitate a comprehensive, holistic approach to the patient. The assessment data, which include sample questions specific to skin disorders, are found in the Nursing Process: Patient Care Plan feature. This care plan applies the nursing process to the relevant nursing diagnoses and provides a comprehensive care plan for the patient with necrotizing fasciitis.

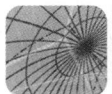

NURSING PROCESS: Patient Care Plan for Necrotizing Fasciitis

Assessment of Skin Integrity

Subjective Data:
Where are the lesions located?
Are there any associated symptoms?
How long have the lesions been present?
Is there any drainage? If so, what color and consistency?
Do you have any chronic health problems?
Has there been any recent exposure to drugs, environmental or occupational toxins, or people with similar skin conditions?

Objective Data:
Skin color
Presence of drainage: color, consistency, odor
Pattern of the lesions
Skin temperature around the lesions

Nursing Assessment and Diagnoses	Outcomes and Evaluation Parameters	Planning and Interventions with *Rationales*
Nursing Diagnosis: *Impaired Skin Integrity* related to skin lesions	**Outcomes:** No signs of infection or worsening of infection. **Evaluation Parameters:** Skin will not have drainage, or drainage will not be yellow or green with a foul odor. Skin color will be pink; no blue or gray. Wound will show signs of healing.	**Interventions and *Rationales:*** Assess skin for drainage, warmth, and redness. *Indicates presence of infection.* Assess skin lesions for changes. *Indicates progression or healing of skin disorder.* Implement an individualized treatment plan for site of skin impairment. Use aseptic technique. *Treatment should be implemented according to patient needs and to prevent infection.* Remove or control impediments to wound healing. Reposition every 2 hours, and assess for signs of skin breakdown. *Wound healing can be delayed if impediments are not relieved.* Teach patient care of skin wounds. *It is important for the patient to understand and comply with care.* Patient should be placed in a private room with contact isolation. *To decrease the chance of infection.*

Assessment of Fluid Status

Subjective Data:
Are you having any difficulty breathing?
Do you have edema?
Do you have any chronic health problems?

Objective Data:
Lung sounds
Presence of edema in ankles, in dependent areas, or around lesions
Vital signs

Nursing Assessment and Diagnoses	Outcomes and Evaluation Parameters	Planning and Interventions with *Rationales*
Nursing Diagnosis: *Risk for Imbalanced Fluid Volume* related to fluid loss	**Outcome:** Adequate fluid balance. **Evaluation Parameters:** Lung sounds will be clear with a normal respiratory rate. Urine output will be within 1,000 milliliters of intake. Extremities and wounds will not be edematous. Laboratory values, such as electrolytes, will be within normal range.	**Interventions and *Rationales:*** Assess the patient's preoperative status. *Awareness of preexisting fluid overload or dehydration can prevent fluid problems postoperatively.* Monitor vital signs. *Vital signs, such as increased pulse or respiration, can indicate fluid volume overload or dehydration.* Monitor intake and output of fluids. *Can help monitor fluid status. Intake should be within 1,000 milliliters of output for 24 hours.* Assess for signs of edema in dependent areas or around lesions. Weigh patient at least weekly. Monitor fluid status. *Can indicate fluid retention.* Assess electrolyte levels. *Electrolytes can be altered with fluid overload or dehydration and can cause problems.*

(continued)

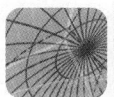

NURSING PROCESS: Patient Care Plan for Necrotizing Fasciitis—*Continued*

Assessment of Physical Mobility

Subjective Data:
How active are you physically?
Has your activity level changed with your skin problems? How?
What limits your activity?

Objective Data:
Assess range of motion of all extremities.
Assess patient's strength.
Assess oxygen saturation levels.

Nursing Assessment and Diagnoses	Outcomes and Evaluation Parameters	Planning and Interventions with *Rationales*
Nursing Diagnosis: *Impaired Physical Mobility* related to discomfort	**Outcome:** Patient is mobile and independent. **Evaluation Parameters:** Physical activity is increased as the patient's condition allows. Patient verbalizes a feeling of increased strength and ability to move. Patient is able to perform activities of daily living.	**Interventions and *Rationales*:** Assess mobility skills. *Provides a baseline and makes nurse aware of opportunities for improvement.* Monitor patient's ability to tolerate activity. *Provides information about problems that might inhibit activity.* Treat pain before activity. *Pain limits mobility.* If patient is immobile, perform passive range of motion or any activity that is not contraindicated. *Helps to maintain joint mobility and increase circulation.* Help patient to achieve mobility and independence as soon as possible. *Early mobilization can help prevent complications related to immobility.*

Assessment of Pain

Subjective Data:
Using a scale of 1–10, with 1 being very little pain and 10 being the worst imaginable pain, what is your pain level?
What is your experience with pain?
Do you routinely take pain medication at home? If so, how much and what kind? What kind of pain do you experience at home?
Are you allergic to any pain medication?
Do you have any cultural or religious beliefs that impact your pain control?
Where is your pain located?
Can you describe what type of pain you are having?
Does your pain radiate or stay in one place?
Is your pain constant or intermittent?
What brings your pain on or relieves it?

Objective Data:
Grimacing with movement
Restlessness and irritability
Taut facial expression
Watch how the patient moves
Vital signs
Check skin for diaphoresis and pallor
Clenched teeth

Nursing Assessment and Diagnoses	Outcomes and Evaluation Parameters	Planning and Interventions with *Rationales*
Nursing Diagnosis: *Acute Pain* related to exposed nerve endings	**Outcome:** Adequate pain control. **Evaluation Parameters:** Patient reports pain before it becomes unbearable. Patient reports pain relief. Pain decreases, requiring less medication. Patient is able to perform activities without pain.	**Interventions and *Rationales*:** Assess severity and quality of pain frequently. *Helps to determine cause and presence of pain so it can be relieved.* Explore need for medications to relieve pain. *Pharmacologic interventions should be used when needed to relieve pain.* Discuss patient's fears of unrelieved pain, overdose, or addiction. *The patient's concerns may prevent reporting of pain.* Review patient records to determine effectiveness of medications for pain relief. *Systematic tracking of pain relief will help identify and improve problems with pain management.* Support the patient's use of nonpharmacologic interventions for pain relief. *Nonpharmacologic interventions can be effective as a supplement to pharmacologic interventions.* Plan care and activities around periods of pain. *Pain diminishes ability to be active.*

Assessment of Body Image Disturbance

Subjective Data:
How has your lifestyle changed since the skin disorder started?
Do you have negative feelings about your body or your appearance?
Do you fear rejection by others?

Objective Data:
Is there an actual change in the appearance of the patient?
Is the patient hiding from or avoiding others?

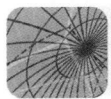

NURSING PROCESS: Patient Care Plan for Necrotizing Fasciitis—*Continued*

Nursing Assessment and Diagnoses	Outcomes and Evaluation Parameters	Planning and Interventions with *Rationales*
Nursing Diagnosis: *Disturbed Body Image* related to illness	**Outcome:** Patient accepts or is satisfied with body image. ***Evaluation Parameters:*** Patient states acceptance of body changes. Patient returns to previous social involvement.	**Interventions and *Rationales:*** Acknowledge the patient's feelings related to changes in body image. *Changes in body image may lead to a variety of reactions. Patients should feel supported and able to express their feelings.* Allow the patient to explore the changes gradually. *Patient should be able to explore the changes when ready.* Encourage the patient to be involved in the decision making and accept inadequacies and strengths. *When patients have a say in their care, they are more likely to adapt to changes.* Assess the influence of cultural beliefs, norms, and perceptions on body image. *The patient's body image is influenced by culture and the norms of that social context.*

Assessment of Sleep Pattern

Subjective Data:
How are you sleeping?
Do you have trouble falling asleep?
Do you wake up in the middle of the night?
What keeps you from sleeping?
What are your bedtime rituals?

Objective Data:
Observe patient sleeping.
Assess environment for noises, temperature, lighting, or disturbances.

Nursing Assessment and Diagnoses	Outcomes and Evaluation Parameters	Planning and Interventions with *Rationales*
Nursing Diagnosis: *Readiness for Enhanced Sleep* related to pain and anxiety	**Outcomes:** Patient falls asleep and sleeps without interruption. ***Evaluation Parameters:*** Patient sleeps throughout night. Patient verbalizes a feeling of not being fatigued.	**Interventions and *Rationales:*** Assess patient's sleep patterns and bedtime rituals. Sleep patterns are individual. *Sleep can be enhanced by adhering to usual rituals when possible.* Determine current level of anxiety or pain. *Anxiety and pain prevent sleep.* Provide measures before bedtime to assist with sleep. *Simple interventions such as warm milk or a back massage can help induce sleep.* Keep environment quiet and interruptions at a minimum. *Noise can interfere with sleep.* Plan for long periods of uninterrupted sleep. Discourage long naps during the day. *Can interfere with prolonged good sleep.*

Assessment of Ineffective Protection

Subjective Data:
Is there pain in the lesions or skin, and has it changed?
Has the appearance of the skin lesions changed?
How have you been caring for the skin lesions?
What has your diet been like?
Have you been sleeping well?
Have you been following the prescribed treatment such as medications and wound care?

Objective Data:
Inspect skin lesions for redness, warmth, and drainage
Vital signs
Signs of infections other than on the skin
Age

Nursing Assessment and Diagnoses	Outcomes and Evaluation Parameters	Planning and Interventions with *Rationales*
Nursing Diagnosis: *Ineffective Protection* related to interrupted skin integrity	**Outcome:** Patient is free of any new signs of infection. ***Evaluation Parameters:*** Patient verbalizes precautions to prevent infection. Patient eats a well-balanced diet. Patient performs proper wound care.	**Interventions and *Rationales:*** Monitor vital signs. *Vital signs can demonstrate signs of infection.* Assess nutritional status. *Nutrition is important for supporting the immune system.* Assess for signs of new or worsening infection. *Infection should be identified early, and treatment initiated to decrease the chances of mortality or complications.* Implement interventions to prevent the spread of infection. *Infection is easily spread from one patient to another or one site to another if infection control measures are not observed.* Teach the patient and family about precautions to take to avoid infection. *Reduce the risk of infection from visitors.*

(continued)

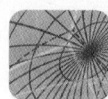

NURSING PROCESS: Patient Care Plan for Necrotizing Fasciitis—*Continued*

Assessment of Nutrition

Subjective Data:
How is your appetite?
Do you have sores in your mouth?
What kinds of foods are you eating?
What kinds of foods do you like or dislike?
Are there any cultural practices that would influence your diet?

Objective Data:
Assess nutritional status.
Assess 24-hour food intake.
Assess for sores in the mouth.

Nursing Assessment and Diagnoses	Outcomes and Evaluation Parameters	Planning and Interventions with *Rationales*
Nursing Diagnosis: *Imbalanced Nutrition: Less than Body Requirements*	**Outcome:** Patient will have an adequate intake to meet the body's needs for repair. **Evaluation Parameters:** Patient eats most of the food served. Weight will be improved or maintained at a healthy level.	**Interventions and *Rationales:*** Monitor food intake. *Food intake needs to be adequate for healing.* Serve small amounts of high-calorie, high-protein food every 2 hours. *Patient is more likely to eat small amounts more frequently than large amounts less often.* Provide a well-balanced diet with foods the patient likes. *Patient will be more likely to eat.* Consult with a dietician. Assess the need for parenteral or enteral feedings. *If the patient is unable to eat enough food orally to keep up with the body's demands, other avenues may need to be explored and utilized.*

Assessment of Social Isolation

Subjective Data:
Is there anyone depending on you for care at home?
Are you the breadwinner for the family?
Can your loved ones visit you?

Objective Data:
Loved ones are visiting.

Nursing Assessment and Diagnoses	Outcomes and Evaluation Parameters	Planning and Interventions with *Rationales*
Nursing Diagnosis: *Social Isolation* due to prolonged illness	**Outcomes:** Patient will have a plan for care of others who are dependent. Patient will have plan for care of self at home. **Evaluation Parameter:** Patient returns to previous life roles.	**Intervention and *Rationale:*** Consult social worker or case manager. *Allows for plans to be made for needed care and decreased anxiety in patient.*

■ Collaborative Management

The care for a patient with necrotizing fasciitis is multidimensional and multidisciplinary, requiring the nurse to serve as the team coordinator and patient advocate. The goals are to assure that the patient receives high-quality care and has an understanding about the disease process and treatment. These patients require intensive nursing and medical management, along with the expertise of the physical and occupational therapists, psychologists/psychiatrists, pharmacists, and nutritionists. To ensure complete closure and prevention of infection, wound care is managed by both the nurses and the health care providers. The initial medical team needs to include a surgeon, an infectious disease specialist, a pathologist, and a microbiologist. The remainder of the team members depends on the severity and location of the wound and may include an urologist; a specialist in plastic surgery; or an ear, nose, and throat (ENT) surgeon in cases of infections of the cervical area. The members of the nursing team depend on the severity of the wound and the hemodynamic stability of the patient. Nurses knowledgeable in wound care are essential, and critical care nurses may be needed to monitor and maintain the hemodynamic parameters.

As the wound heals, the scar formation causes contracture formation, which, depending on the site of the wound, may decrease joint range of motion. Physical therapy is initiated as soon as possible and continues after hospital discharge to maintain and increase range of motion in the joints. When contracture formation is severe, the surgeon needs to release the contractures surgically.

The pharmacist assists the medical team with pain and infection control management. The infection must be controlled to prevent further tissue and organ loss. The antibiotics are monitored by the nurses, health care providers, and pharmacists to ensure sensitivity to the organisms. Pain management is a major concern for this patient. During dressing changes, the use of conscious sedation is frequently required due to the severity of the pain. Additionally, ongoing pain management between the dressing changes is necessary to ensure patient comfort. Because of the longevity of the hospitalization, the pain management protocols require frequent adjustment. The pharmacist is an essential part of this process.

The disabilities experienced by the patient may lead to changes in lifestyle and occupation. Often the patient is unable to return to the previous profession due to physical limitations. Family dynamics and role function often change at least temporarily and perhaps permanently depending on the degree of disability. The occupational therapist, social worker, and psychologist/psychiatrist all assist the patient with physical and psychological adjustments after discharge.

Finally, the nutritionist must develop a comprehensive plan for nutrition for enhancing wound healing, regaining strength, and preventing complications. The dietician works with the health care team from the time of admission through discharge to ensure proper nutritional support.

Health Promotion

Because necrotizing fasciitis can occur at any age or location and is not specific to gender, it is imperative to educate patients, families, and the general public about the risk factors (see the earlier Risk Factors box for necrotizing fasciitis, p. 2170) and how to avoid them. As stated earlier, about one-half of the cases occur in young previously healthy patients; therefore, avoiding behaviors such as skin popping (Chapter 65 ☻) will decrease the risk. If the individual has already contracted the disease once, education needs to include avoiding being reexposed. Patients need to be told to seek medical help for wounds that are not healing or appear infected.

Stevens–Johnson Syndrome

Stevens–Johnson syndrome (SJS) is a severe, acute, self-limiting skin reaction to infection or certain medications. It affects the epidermal layer of the skin and mucous membranes. SJS usually begins with flu-like symptoms or symptoms of an upper respiratory infection and progresses to mucosal erosions and erythematous skin macules that blister and cause denudation or skin detachment. The incidence is approximately 4 to 7 cases per million inhabitants per year, and SJS occurs most commonly in children and young adults (Khalili & Bahna, 2006).

Etiology of Stevens–Johnson Syndrome

The cause of Stevens–Johnson syndrome (SJS) is most commonly an adverse reaction to medication or an infection. In children the cause is usually infection, whereas in adults the cause is typically drugs or malignancy (Hockett, 2004). The most common medications leading to SJS are sulfonamides, beta-lactam antibiotics, penicillin, anticonvulsants, some nonsteroidal anti-inflammatory medications, and allopurinol. The most common infections implicated as a cause include herpes simplex virus and *Mycoplasma pneumoniae*. HIV infection, cancer, or the presence of an autoimmune disorder increases the risk of developing SJS. Symptoms generally appear within 14 days of exposure to the causative agent (Hockett, 2004).

The triggering mechanism for SJS is unclear, but the pathophysiology is immunologic with a cell-mediated cytotoxic reaction against epidermal cells. Cell destruction is thought to be caused by a cytokine such as tumor necrosis factor (Hockett, 2004; Khalili & Bahna, 2006). Immune complexes made up of the drug metabolites and antibodies develop and become trapped in the microvasculature of the skin (Letko et al., 2005). They are attacked by lymphocytes and macrophages, leading to destruction and necrosis of the epidermis (Tsang, Tsang, & Wong, 2004).

Diagnosis and Clinical Manifestations of Stevens–Johnson Syndrome

The diagnostic criteria of SJS are defined differently by different authors. There is no universally accepted definition. However, SJS generally begins with flu-like symptoms such as headache, rhinorrhea, cough, and body aches. Target skin lesions are present and are described as having a bright-pink or red inner ring, a ring of lighter pink, and then a ring of dark pink. These lesions are concentric macular exanthemas that focus on the face, neck, and extremities, which then become blisters that grow together and break open such as might be seen in burns (Hockett, 2004). The lesions are found on less than 20% of body surface area in the first 48 hours and result in skin detachment (Letko et al., 2005). SJS is diagnosed by skin biopsy and immunofluorescent studies that demonstrate the presence of immunoglobulin M (IgM) and C3 deposits in the vascular walls. Letko et al. (2005) defined SJS by the following: (1) involvement of at least two mucous membranes, (2) presence of target lesions with sudden epidermal detachment, (3) fever, (4) skin biopsy compatible with erythema multiforme and Stevens–Johnson syndrome, (5) positive Nikolsky's sign, and (6) involvement of less than 20% of the total body surface area. Nikolsky's sign can be assessed by applying slight thumb pressure that leads to separation of the epidermis from the dermis when the thumb slides laterally on the skin (Hockett, 2004). At least 61% of patients with SJS have mucous membrane involvement with the mouth, eyes, skin, genitalia, esophagus, and respiratory tract affected. Ocular involvement occurs in 39% of all patients with SJS (Forman, Koren, & Shear, 2002). The mucosal lesions are painful and have a crusted surface. They may lead to blindness or impaired nutrition.

SJS is often misdiagnosed because the first symptoms can be attributed to the flu or an upper respiratory infection and are vague, such as fever, cough, headache, fatigue, sore throat, and malaise. Approximately 1 to 3 days after these symptoms, the target lesions appear and are concentric, quickly becoming confluent blisters. Within hours the skin becomes painful and Nikolsky's sign may be positive.

Medical Management of Stevens–Johnson Syndrome

Mortality rates for SJS are 1% to 5% (Khalili & Bahna, 2006). Early diagnosis and withdrawal of the causative agent are essential to decrease morbidity and mortality. There is no universally accepted treatment other than supportive care. Treatment with glucocorticoids is controversial. Some studies have suggested that glucocorticoids lead to increased morbidity and mortality, whereas others report that short-term use of glucocorticoids in high doses improves outcomes (Letko et al., 2005). The use of intravenous immunoglobulin (IVIG) has shown some success and improved outcomes; however, more research is needed (Khalili & Bahna, 2006). Intravenous fluid replacement similar to that initiated with the treatment of burns must be started to prevent dehydration and treat electrolyte loss through skin lesions (see Chapter 68 ☻). Often these patients are taken to burn units for care. Total parenteral nutrition (TPN) is necessary to treat protein loss that occurs with skin detachment and to help prevent stress ulcers. Prevention of infection is important. Prophylactic antibiotics are generally unnecessary but careful aseptic technique is needed.

Skin cultures may be taken every 48 hours to aid in the decision to start antibiotics if necessary. Dressings are used to protect the epidermis but tape should be avoided. Dressings consist of gauze with petrolatum or silver nitrate. Biologic skin covers such as cadaveric allografts may also be used. Topical anesthetics and systemic pain medication may be needed to decrease pain related to dressing changes. Emotional and psychiatric support is essential.

Toxic Epidermal Necrolysis

Toxic epidermal necrolysis (TEN) is a part of the same syndrome of diseases as is Stevens–Johnson syndrome, described earlier. It is a more severe form of the disorder and is life threatening with more extensive skin detachment. Although the disorder is rare, occurring in only 1 person per million, it can have mortality rates of 40% (Klein, 2006). It generally occurs in people between the ages of 46 and 63 but can occur at any age. It more commonly affects women. The causes are the same as those for Stevens–Johnson syndrome with the most common being an adverse reaction to drugs such as sulfonamide antibiotics, anticonvulsant agents, and allopurinol. The pathophysiology is unknown; however, it is thought to be related to an immune response that is cell mediated by the T lymphocytes. Skin lesions have been found to have macrophage infiltration of the dermis and epidermis with tumor necrosis factor in the epidermis (Letko et al., 2005).

Diagnosis and Clinical Manifestations of Toxic Epidermal Necrolysis

TEN is diagnosed by skin biopsy and immunofluorescent studies. The criteria for defining TEN include the following: (1) involvement of at least two mucous membranes, (2) loss of confluent sheets of epidermis leaving an exposed dermis, (3) fever, (4) erosions of more than 30% of the total body surface area, and (5) skin biopsy compatible with TEN. There is also a positive Nikolsky's sign. Like SJS, TEN begins with symptoms of an upper respiratory infection. Approximately 2 to 3 days after the respiratory symptoms, the epidermis blisters and begins splitting and sloughing from the dermis. There are no target lesions, but there are large areas of epidermal sloughing with a dark-red, oozing dermis. These areas are painful and tender. Mucous membranes are also affected. Once diagnosed, patients with TEN can be assessed to predict mortality. The SCORTEN scoring system is used for that purpose. It gives points to 7 parameters, which are added to result in a score between 0 and 7. A score of 0 to 1 is related to a mortality of 3.2%, whereas a score of 5 or more predicts a mortality of at least 90%. The SCORTEN should be performed during the first 24 hours after hospital admission and again on day 3 of hospitalization. The ability to predict mortality can be useful in discussing the patient's condition with family members and in evaluating the effectiveness of new treatments (Guegan, Bastuji-Garin, Poszepczynska-Guigne, Roujeau, & Revuz, 2006).

Medical Management of Toxic Epidermal Necrolysis

Early diagnosis and withdrawal of offending agents are important in decreasing mortality. To achieve the best outcomes, treatment should occur in a burn unit or intensive care unit for patients with TEN. There is no definitive treatment, so the care provided is mostly supportive and symptomatic. The development of an in-

fection or sepsis increases the risk of mortality. Treatment goals are the same as for SJS. Intravenous fluid replacement is needed to prevent dehydration and treat electrolyte losses. TPN is needed to supply badly needed nutrients for growth and repair and to address the protein loss that occurs with the hypermetabolic state. The hypermetabolic state is described in Chapter 68 ©. Wounds are generally débrided in the operating room, and biologic dressings, such as homografts and xenografts, are used to decrease the chance of infection, reduce pain, prevent fluid loss, and control body temperature. Reepithelialization begins about 18 days after the development of the first symptoms. As with SJS, treatment with corticosteroids is controversial.

■ Nursing Management for Stevens–Johnson Syndrome and Toxic Epidermal Necrolysis

Like necrotizing fasciitis, nursing care for Stevens–Johnson syndrome and toxic epidermal necrolysis requires knowledgeable assessment skills and critical thinking. Nurses need to be cognizant of the possible development of these conditions. At the first signs of a drug reaction, the health care provider must be alerted and the offending agent stopped immediately. Once either of these conditions develops, it is best managed in a burn unit using a multidisciplinary approach with the nurse as the gatekeeper. The nursing process provides the framework to manage these patients.

Assessment

The extent of total body surface area involvement determines the systemic impact for both Stevens–Johnson syndrome and toxic epidermal necrolysis. The nurse needs to assess the amount of skin involved by using a standard measurement such as the rule of nines described in Chapter 68 ©. Fluid loss is not as severe as that seen in burn patients but can be significant, especially if the mucous membranes are involved in areas that cannot be observed, such as the lungs and gastrointestinal tract. Fluid status needs ongoing assessment by monitoring vital signs, urine output, central venous pressure, and cardiac output if a Swan-Ganz catheter is in place. The hemoglobin (Hgb) and hematocrit (HCT) also need to be assessed frequently because they both increase with the loss of intravascular volume; and in the presence of inadequate fluid resuscitation, the Hgb and HCT become abnormally elevated. Chapter 68 © includes a complete description of fluid management. The patient should be assessed for involvement of mucous membranes. The eyes should be assessed daily for involvement and daily eyedrops may be needed.

Nursing Diagnoses

The nursing diagnoses for patients with Stevens–Johnson syndrome or toxic epidermal necrolysis include:

- *Deficient Fluid Volume* related to increased capillary permeability, increased intravascular hydrostatic pressure, and increased evaporative loss
- *Risk for Imbalanced Fluid Volume* related to excessive IV fluid administration and diminished organ capacity for excessive volume load

PHARMACOLOGY Summary of Medications Used to Treat Skin Disorders

Medication Category	Action	Application/Indication	Nursing Responsibility
Topical corticosteroids: • Betamethasone (Diprolene) • Fluocinonide (Lidex) • Mometasone (Elocon)	Inhibits inflammatory process leading to vasoconstriction of dilated vessels.	Used for inflammatory and pruritic conditions, and hyperplastic and infiltrative disorders. This includes conditions such as atopic and allergic dermatitis, hypertrophic scars, and psoriasis.	Should be applied in a thin layer and rubbed in thoroughly on wet skin. Areas of the body with thin skin, such as the face, or intertriginous areas are more susceptible to side effects. Some infections may be made worse by corticosteroids.
Antiacne medications: • Benzoyl peroxide (Benoxyl 10)	Broad-spectrum bacteriostatic activity against *P. acnes* with anti-inflammatory actions as well.	Decreases inflammation and is keratolytic. It is rubbed into the acne lesions once or twice daily.	Patients should be taught how to use it and the side effects. May irritate the skin. Use should start slow and be gradually increased. Can be irritating to the skin. Produces phototoxicity.
• Retinoic acid/tretinoin	Keratolytic agent used to increase cell turnover and prevent comedos. Reduces inflammation.	Used as a cream, gel, or solution, and applied topically. Applied sparingly at bedtime. Avoid using around nose, eyes, or mouth.	May aggravate acne during the first 2–4 weeks of therapy until the skin becomes acclimated.
• Antibacterial agents such as erythromycin and tetracycline	Antibacterial agents effective against *P. acnes*. Reduces inflammation.	Taken orally or topically. Is used orally for deep acne.	There is no toxicity with topical use. Monitor for allergic reactions with oral use.
Antifungal agents: • Miconazole (Lotrimin) • Nystatin (Mycostatin) • Ketoconazole (Nizoral)	Kills or inhibits the growth of fungi.	Applied topically. Each drug is specific to a particular organism. Applied sparingly once or twice daily.	Monitor for side effects or allergies. Thoroughly rub the drug into the skin. Do not use with occlusive coverings unless prescribed by the health care provider. Keep areas clean and dry.
Antihistamines: • Diphenhydramine (Benadryl) • Loratadine (Claritin) • Fexofenadine (Allegra)	Blocks histamine leading to vasoconstriction and decreased capillary permeability. Decreased itching and edema.	Decreases itching and signs of urticaria. Taken orally.	May cause drowsiness and dryness of the mouth. Some are nonsedating.
Antiviral: Acyclovir (Zorivax)	Inhibits the growth of herpes virus.	Effective against herpes simplex 1 and 2, varicella-zoster, herpes zoster, Epstein–Barr virus, and cytomegalovirus. Given topically or orally.	Monitor for effectiveness of the drug. Monitor for side effects. Prevent spread of infection. Encourage adequate fluid intake. Inform patient that this drug is not a cure for herpes.

- *Ineffective Tissue Perfusion* related to constricting edema formation and circumferential wounds
- *Impaired Gas Exchange* related to lung involvement and fatigue
- *Impaired Skin Integrity* related to epithelial skin loss
- *Risk for Infection* related to loss of skin integrity and impaired nonspecific and specific immunity
- *Acute Pain* related to burn injury and exposed nerve endings
- *Imbalanced Nutrition: Less than Body Requirements* related to hypermetabolic demands of disorder, decreased appetite, immobility, pain, nausea/vomiting, and depression
- *Fear* and *Anxiety* related to changes in health status/role functioning; situational crisis
- *Ineffective Thermoregulation* related to epithelial skin loss

- *Disturbed Body Image* related to loss of skin and potential loss of function.

Planning

A collaborative and comprehensive approach to care will optimize the recovery process. The plan uses the assessment data to prioritize care. First, the cause must be identified and removed if possible. Depending on the nature and extent of the disorder, dieticians, case managers, social workers, consultative health care providers (cardiovascular, infectious diseases, surgeons, and plastic surgeons), nursing staff, and ancillary staff should be part of the plan of care, as all play a role in the prevention and treatment. Stevens–Johnson syndrome and toxic epidermal necrolysis disorders can be life threatening; therefore, it is essential that the plan be correctly prioritized. As always, protection of airway and maintenance of normal oxygen levels are the first priority. Due to fluid shifts, it also is essential to monitor the patient's hemodynamic status and electrolyte levels. Infection prevention is another critical priority for these patients due to loss of skin integrity.

Outcomes and Evaluation Parameters

The immediate outcome is to stabilize the patient's airway, hemodynamic status, fluids and electrolytes, and pain control. Until the skin can be replaced, another critical outcome is infection prevention, which is manifested by absence of fever, increased white blood count, and clinical manifestations of wound infection, discussed earlier. The long-term outcome for patients with Stevens–Johnson syndrome and toxic epidermal necrolysis is to heal without scarring or loss of function, as manifested by a return to previous level of functioning.

Interventions and Rationales

Initial nursing interventions include managing the patient's airway, and monitoring and intervening to maintain a normal hemodynamic status. Ventilator support may be necessary, especially if the mucous membranes of the lung are involved. Pneumonia may occur related to mucus retention and sloughing of the tracheobronchial mucosa. Adequate oxygenation should be maintained through frequent respiratory assessment and delivery of oxygen when necessary (Hockett, 2004). A complete description of nursing management of the ventilated patient can be found in Chapter 36 ⊕.

The fluid shifts out of the intravascular space into the interstitial space with these types of disorders, thereby decreasing the circulating blood volume. Fluid replacement and monitoring of urine output and electrolyte balance are critical to survival. As described earlier, the nurse must closely assess the patient's individual response to fluid replacement to maintain hemodynamic stability. A complete description of fluid replacement for patients who have loss of skin integrity is included in Chapter 68 ⊕. Hemodynamic monitoring is found in Chapter 24 ⊕.

Due to exposed nerve endings, these disorders are very painful. Pain management is an ongoing issue that requires frequent reassessment. Augmenting pain medications during dressing changes and any other painful procedures is essential and will promote healing. Dressing changes can be long and involved, as well as painful. Patients are given continuous morphine infusions by patient-controlled analgesia (PCA) pumps. Nurses need to monitor for breakthrough pain and give medication as needed.

The patient needs to be protected from infection until skin integrity has occurred. Skin and mucous membrane care should be meticulous to avoid infection. Strict aseptic technique is mandatory when performing skin assessment and dressing changes. The patient should be placed in a private room and closely monitored for the presence of infection by daily blood and wound cultures. Oral lesions can be treated with mouthwashes and topical anesthetics. Gastrointestinal involvement may be mild or severe requiring nasogastric intubation or parenteral nutrition. If the eyes are affected, medication to prevent infection may be necessary, and direct light and brightly lit rooms should be avoided because of photophobia.

Typically there is no scarring or contractures. However, physical therapy and range-of-motion exercises are essential to pre-

serve joint function. Psychological support is very important in the nursing care of patients experiencing Stevens–Johnson syndrome or toxic epidermal necrolysis. These diseases are severe, life threatening, and progress rapidly. The patient can become almost unrecognizable overnight. Counseling and spiritual support should be made available to the patient and family members.

Due to the hypermetabolic state and the increased need for calories for wound healing, nutrition also is a priority. Early consultation with a dietician to establish calorie, protein, carbohydrate, and nutrient needs will help prevent a malnourished state. Nursing care includes recording accurate intake and output, and a calorie count every shift. Maintain oral hygiene and monitor the gastrointestinal tract for bowel sounds and distention. If enteral feeding is being done, tube placement and function are monitored as well as the patient's tolerance of the prescribed diet. Daily weight measurement and laboratory values such as total protein levels, complete blood count, glucose, iron, and prealbumin, as well as wound healing, are also measures of adequate nutrition.

Evaluation

A plan for care of the patient with Stevens–Johnson syndrome or toxic epidermal necrolysis must be reevaluated regularly to ensure that the plan is still effective. Any change in the patient's condition could have a negative impact on the wound healing process and the effectiveness of the plan of care. Evaluation criteria of progress would be a decrease in the size and depth of the involved area. If this healing is not occurring, then the area needs to be assessed as to why it is not, such as for infection or decreased tissue perfusion.

◾ Cosmetic Surgical Procedures

Cosmetic surgery is done to enhance the attractiveness of certain normal features related to the skin and its underlying structures. This surgery includes reshaping of the nose, body contouring, breast surgery, and facial rejuvenation for the aging process such as resurfacing or tightening of the skin. Reconstructive surgery is performed in those who may have deformities related to cancer, congenital abnormalities, disease, and structural and/or traumatic injuries that result in functional disabilities or abnormal appearance. Congenital deformities include prominent ears, cleft lip and palate deformities, and congenital nevi.

Cosmetic surgery is individualized depending on one's race or ethnicity. For example, darker skinned non-Caucasian individuals present a unique set of needs separate from those of Caucasians. The Cultural Considerations box outlines concerns related to ethnic skin and cosmetic surgery. Today, many surgical procedures can be done to correct skin-related problems for all ethnic groups, and a number of them are discussed next.

Blepharoplasty

Blepharoplasty is a surgical procedure performed to remove the excess skin and fat and occasionally a portion of the orbicularis oculi muscle around the eye. With aging, the relocation of fat, loss of skin elasticity, and excess muscle around the eye can interfere with vision or cause an unwanted appearance. A blepharoplasty can be done alone or along with a face-lift or brow lift (Figure 66–12 ◾, p. 2184). Local anesthetic and conscious sedation is usually enough to allow the procedure to be performed. There is some swelling and bruising at the site that will subside in about 10 to 14 days. Complications are unusual but include bleeding, hematoma formation, epidermal inclusion cysts of the incisions, ectropion, infection, and asymmetry.

Rhinoplasty

Rhinoplasty is the surgical alteration of nasal structures, which usually includes the bone and cartilage. It is performed for cosmetic reasons and is often done at the same time as surgical procedures to correct functional problems associated with the obstruction of the nasal passages. Rhinoplasty also is performed for reconstructive conditions such as abnormalities associated with cleft lip and palate deformities or nasal trauma. Rhinoplasty is considered one of the most difficult surgical procedures a plastic surgeon performs. It requires consideration of a myriad of anatomic factors as well as psychological and ethnic factors.

Rhinoplasty can be performed under local or general anesthesia. Topical and injectable vasoconstrictors and anesthetic agents are used. The patient may or may not be hospitalized. The nose will be packed postoperatively for a few days to prevent bleeding and support the nasal structures, and an exterior nasal splint is applied for about a week to a week and a half. There is swelling and periorbital bruising that takes about 2 weeks to subside. However, it takes up to a year for all swelling and sensation to stabilize and to appreciate the final result. This procedure has an increased incidence of needing a secondary procedure to achieve the best result, which is usually done after a year. Figure 66–11 ■ is an example of before and after a rhinoplasty.

Preoperatively, it is important to assess the patient's motivation and desires. An assessment should be made of what the patient's expectations are for the procedure and whether these can be met considering the patient's unique anatomy. Some surgeons perform computer imaging to allow the patient to visualize the results of the surgery preoperatively (Tysome & Sharp, 2006). It is also important to note anything in the patient's history that could affect the outcomes of the surgery. Prior nasal trauma or surgery, sinus or allergy disease, systemic illnesses, medication abuse, respiratory impairments, and emotional stability are examples of factors that need to be evaluated. The surgeon also should consider the ethnicity of the patient. The noses of many African American, Hispanic, and Asian patients may look different from the noses of other nationalities and will require individualized approaches and goals for surgery.

Postoperative complications from rhinoplasty are rare but may include epistaxis, infection, prolonged edema, nasal airway obstruction, and an unsatisfactory cosmetic result. Rhinoplasty is commonly performed and is considered safe and effective.

Rhytidectomy

Rhytidectomy is surgery on the skin to eliminate wrinkles and improve the appearance of the face. It is also referred to as "facial rejuvenation" or "face-lift." The purpose of a rhytidectomy is to set back the signs of aging by approximately 10 years or more. The patient will continue to look younger by approximately 10 years for the rest of her life, even as aging progresses. The Gerontological Considerations box outlines the normal facial changes caused by aging. The rhytidectomy is becoming more common with people wanting natural-looking results because physical appearance is important in how individuals are perceived by others. Appearance also is linked to body image, self-esteem, and confidence. The lines on the face help communicate feelings that occur when interacting with others. Therefore, a youthful appearance may affect an individual in social and professional arenas. Surgery cannot reverse all the effects of aging, but it can reposition tissues and redistribute volume to create a more youthful and rested appearance.

Several anatomic areas can be improved as a part of the rhytidectomy, including the forehead and eyebrows, nasolabial

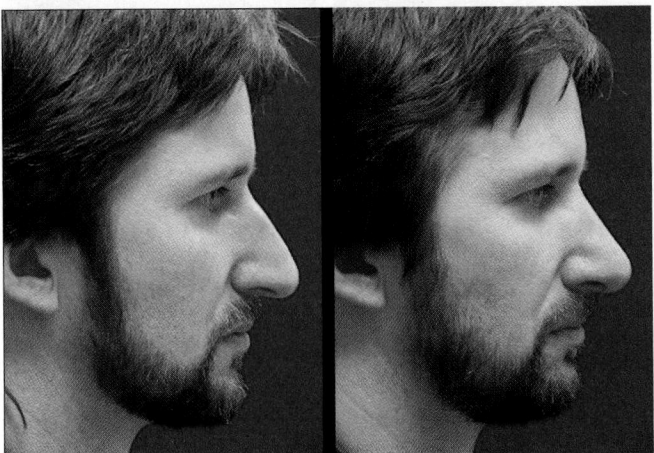

FIGURE 66–11 ■ Before and after a rhinoplasty.
Source: Michael Bermant, MD, Board Certified, American Board of Plastic Surgery/ http://www. plasticsurgery4u.com

folds, jowls, skin and the platyoma muscle of the neck, and malar fat pads. It is important for the surgeon to identify what the patient's expectations are and to discuss what can and cannot be accomplished, so that the expectations are realistic.

Rhytidectomy can be performed with either local anesthesia and conscious sedation, or general anesthesia. The incisions are made at or within the hairlines, behind the ears, or in natural skin creases so that the scars are less noticeable. Typically this procedure is done on an outpatient basis, although in some instances a surgeon may opt to keep a patient hospitalized the first night. There may be drains and padded dressings to protect the face, and swelling of the face and eyelids is present postoperatively, being the most severe at about the second postoperative day. Complications are rare but may include hematoma, infection, asymmetry, skin necrosis, transient facial weakness, and permanent loss of sensation. With makeup, patients are usually presentable in about 1 to 2 weeks. Figure 66–12 ■ demonstrates before and after pictures.

Dermabrasion

Dermabrasion is the process of removing the epidermis and the outer portion of the dermis, creating a partial thickness skin loss. The purpose of this procedure is to allow new skin to regenerate into a smoother surface. See Chapter 68 ⊚ for a complete description of a partial thickness injury. Dermabrasion is used to improve scars, fine wrinkles, sun spots, and areas of hyperpigmentation. A diamond fraise cylinder that has abrasive properties is used to perform the procedure, thus allowing for regrowth of new skin over the abraded area. This procedure is generally limited to use on the face, and either local or general anesthesia is necessary. An open wound is created, which eventually heals in about 7 to 14 days depending on the depth of the abrasion. The patient may need to apply an emollient during this time. Complications include infection, changes in skin color, and scarring. Patients have generally reported being very satisfied with the outcome of the procedure when it has been realistically presented preoperatively.

Microdermabrasion

Microdermabrasion is a skin-freshening technique that helps repair skin that has been damaged by the sun and the effects of aging. The purpose of the procedure is much the same as dermabrasion, just not as deep, and is used to improve scars, fine wrinkles, and hyperpigmentation. The back of the hands and the face are the common areas that benefit from this procedure. A plastic surgeon or esthetician uses a device like a fine sandblaster to spray tiny crystals across the skin, mixing gentle abrasion with suction to remove the dead outer layer of skin. More than one treatment may be needed to reduce or remove fine wrinkles and unwanted pigmentation. No anesthesia is necessary, although the patient may describe a feeling of warmth and throbbing afterward. The skin remains reddened and dry for approximately 4 to 5 days. The patient is instructed to use moisturizers, and long-term use of sunscreens is necessary because the abraded area is more sensitive to burning. If performed properly, complications from this procedure are extremely rare.

Laser

The laser has been used for treating wrinkles, acne, nevi, seborrheic keratosis, actinic keratosis, hemangiomas, tattoos, scars, and unwanted hair. There are many different types of lasers, but the basic principle is that a laser light generates heat that is absorbed into the skin. Different types of tissue will absorb only specific laser wavelengths; thus, the choice of the laser depends on the type of tissue being treated and the problem. The laser beam focused on the skin quickly heats and leads to resurfacing of only the area being treated. Most lasers are used in private offices and small surgical suites under no anesthesia or only local anesthesia. However, the deeper procedures involving greater surface areas may need general anesthesia.

Preoperative preparation of the patient involves detailed teaching about what is involved and what can be expected from the treatments. Depending on the type of laser used, the condition being treated, and the depth of the treatment, treatments may include up to 3 to 5 sessions occurring biweekly or monthly.

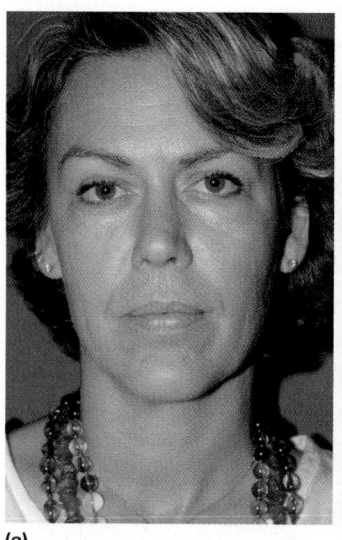
(a)

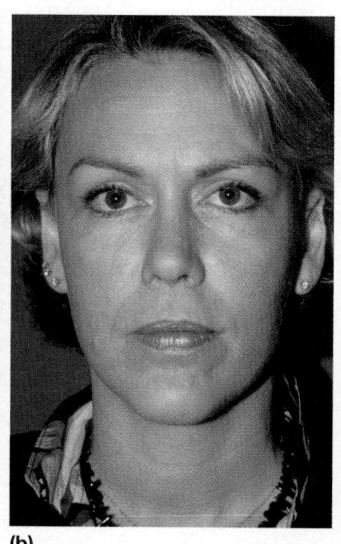
(b)

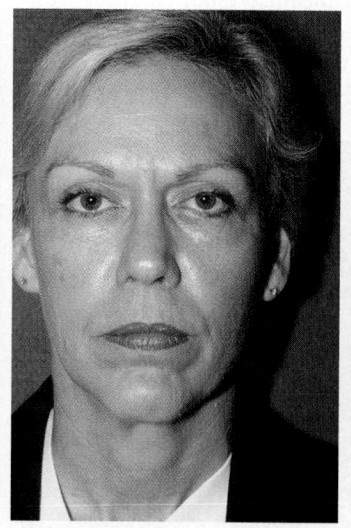
(c)

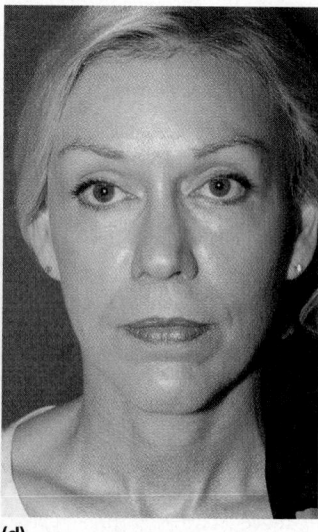
(d)

FIGURE 66–12 ■ Same patient, different ages. A and B: Age 40 years, before and after rhytidectomy and blepharoplasty: C and D: Age 54 years, before and afer rhytidectomy and brow lift.
Source: Courtesy of John M. Osborn MD, FACS, Plastic Surgery Center, Sacramento, CA

Improvement occurs on a continuous basis for up to 6 months after the treatments have been completed. After the procedure, there will be mild to severe localized erythema and swelling at the site of the treatment. Again, depending on the depth of the treatment area, there may be mild to moderate discomfort with the skin feeling dry and tingly for up to a few months. Complications postoperatively are rare but include permanent erythema, edema, acne formation, contact dermatitis, pruritus, infections, and pigmentary alterations.

Injectable Tissue Fillers

As a result of the aging process, a loss of facial fullness and the development of wrinkles occur. A nonsurgical treatment to soften these facial lines and help restore volume and facial contours is injectable fillers. These fillers also are used to treat scars, sun-damaged skin, and thin lips. Outlined here are the different types of tissue fillers on the market:

- Collagen is a natural protein that supports the skin. The two sources are human and bovine collagen. Bovine collagen requires prior allergy testing. The results may last 2 to 4 months.
- Hyaluronic acid is a natural substance found in human bodies. It is used to enhance lips and fill facial creases such as nasolabial folds. It may also be appropriate for some surface wrinkles and concave scars. The results may last 6 months or longer.
- Hydroxyapatite is a mineral-like compound found naturally in human bones, suspended in a gel-like formulation. It is the heaviest of facial fillers and is recommended to fill deeper creases such as nasolabial folds, marionette lines, and frown lines, as well as to enhance fullness of the cheeks and other facial contours.
- Human fat, harvested from the patient's own body, can be injected to enhance facial fullness, fill deep creases, and build up shallow contours. Fat injection requires a more extensive procedure than injection of other fillers because it uses liposuction techniques to extract the fat used for injection. Treatment can last up to a year or more in some cases, and results are highly variable. Fat can be stored for future treatment, although the results from the use of preserved fat are not as favorable.

All tissue fillers except fat are injected by either the health care provider or a specially trained nurse. Fat injections are done solely by the health care provider because the fat needs to be harvested by liposuction. Prior to the injection, the site is cleaned by an antibacterial agent, and icing or a topical numbing agent may be offered to make patients more comfortable. Some tissue fillers contain an anesthetic agent. In other cases, local anesthetic may be administered to the treatment site.

Complications from fillers are uncommon, and the risks vary depending on the specific filler used and the relative permanence of the filler substance. Complications outlined by the American Society of Plastic Surgeons (ASPS) (2007) include:

- Infection at the injection site
- Development of nodules that may require surgical excision
- Acne-like skin eruptions
- Antibody reaction to filler material that may reduce the effectiveness of future injections
- Facial asymmetry
- Bleeding, bruising, and swelling
- Temporary paralysis of other muscle groups or other unintended effects due to migration of the filler material from the original site
- Skin necrosis
- Skin rash, itching, and swelling
- Skin redness
- Skin sensitivity
- Under- or overcorrection of defects.

Botulinum Injections

Botulinum toxin type A (Botox) is purified protein complex derived from bacterium *Clostridium botulinum*. Once injected into the muscle, it blocks the release of chemical acetylcholine, thereby temporarily paralyzing the muscles (ASPS, 2007). It is currently being used as a safe and effective cosmetic agent to temporarily improve frown lines between the eyebrows (glabellar lines), forehead creases, laugh-line wrinkles near the eyes, and thick bands in the neck. Botox also can be used to combat migraine headaches and to treat hyperhidrosis (excessive perspiration). A new and still evolving role for Botox is that of a pain reliever for mastectomy patients. Women injected with Botox in the pectoral muscles following the surgical removal of their breast experienced significantly less pain and shorter hospital stays (ASPS, 2007).

Liposuction

Liposuction, is a form of body sculpting or body contouring. It is one of the most common cosmetic surgeries performed. Depending on the elasticity of the skin, it can be performed on anyone after the age of 16. Older patients with less elasticity are not as good candidates as younger patients and need to be realistic about their expectations. The purpose of liposuction is to remove subcutaneous fat in diet-resistant areas of the body that are out of proportion. Liposuction is not viewed as a treatment for obesity but can help contour the body of someone with normal body weight and good skin tone but localized areas of fat accumulation. Patients need to be evaluated and instructed so that unrealistic expectations will not be an issue.

Tumescent liposuction involves infiltrating diluted lidocaine and epinephrine into the subcutaneous tissue to provide anesthesia prior to the actual liposuction. Therefore, general anesthesia is not required but may be used along with the infiltrate at the discretion of the patient or the health care provider (Kucera et al., 2006). Tumescent liposuction allows for the aspiration of a higher amount of fat and a smaller amount of blood (Coldiron et al., 2006). Prior to the procedure, the areas to be removed are marked while the patient is in an upright position, because fat tends to shift when the patient is horizontal and sedated. The diluted mixture of lidocaine and epinephrine is injected into the site to provide anesthesia, cause vasoconstriction, and allow for greater volumes of fat to be aspirated. A small cannula is then inserted through a 2- to 10-millimeter incision and advanced throughout the fat using back-and-forth movements. The fat is mechanically broken up, and tunnels are created. The loosened fat is then removed using suction. The average amount suctioned is between

2 and 3 liters, although any amount up to 10 liters may be aspirated. Any patient who has over 5 liters aspirated should remain in an overnight care facility for observation of vascular complications and hemodynamic compromise. The risk of complications from this procedure is relatively small. The most common complications include contour irregularities, the development of a hematoma or seroma, transient numbness, asymmetry, and persistent postoperative edema (Coldiron et al., 2006).

Postoperatively, patients are usually discharged home once they are stable. Compression dressings are worn over the areas treated to compress the tunnels created by the cannula, to ensure a more even result, to prevent fluid from collecting in the tunnels, and to increase patient comfort. Recovery is rapid with most discomfort resolved within 5 days, although the compression dressings are used from 1 to 6 weeks postoperatively.

Patients are generally satisfied with the results and are able to maintain the fat loss. With weight gain, some fat buildup in the treated areas will occur, but the gain will be in the same proportion as the gain in the rest of the body. Fat cells enlarge with weight gain and do not multiply.

Abdominoplasty

An abdominoplasty is performed to remove excess skin and fat from the lower abdomen and to tighten the muscles of the abdominal cavity. Usually as a result of pregnancy, but also as a result of obesity and the accumulation of intra-abdominal fat, the rectus abdominis muscles separate in the midline, causing a weakness in the muscular support of the abdominal contents. The surgery consists of making an incision across the lower abdomen just above the symphysis pubis out to and sometimes beyond the anterior iliac crest. The skin and adipose tissue are undermined over the abdominal muscles to the level of the lower sternum and the medial ribs, creating a skin and fat flap. The umbilical stalk is left intact but separated from the surrounding skin during the dissection. The muscles are then plicated (sewn together) in the midline to tighten the abdominal musculature and support the abdominal contents. The overlying skin and fat are then redraped inferiorly, and the excess skin and fat are excised. The umbilicus is then reattached through a new hole created in the skin above it, and the skin inferiorly is closed, leaving a scar across the lower abdomen and around the umbilicus.

Panniculectomy

A panniculectomy is the surgical excision of just excess skin and fat that hang over the pubic area as a skin apron, most commonly following excessive weight loss. With this procedure there is no undermining of the skin and fat and no plication of the muscles, as described for the abdominoplasty. It is usually performed to reduce strain on the back and to prevent intertrigo rashes that form under the apron between the skin layers. With the increasing popularity of bariatric surgical procedures, this procedure is becoming more common; and because it is usually performed for functional versus cosmetic reasons, it is usually covered financially by insurance carriers. Bariatric surgery is described in detail in Chapter 14 ☺.

Nursing Management

Dermatologic surgery is generally an elective procedure that may be done in the outpatient setting or as an inpatient, depending on the patient and the procedure. The patient has generally had several discussions with the health care provider about the procedure, its possible complications, and the patient's expectations. The needs of the patient, however, are very much like the needs of any patient undergoing surgery. Chapters 25, 26, and 27 ☺ discuss the preoperative, intraoperative, and postoperative needs of the patient.

Immediately after surgery, the patient will be monitored in a postanesthesia care unit (PACU) for complications related to the surgery and anesthesia. Chapters 26 and 27 ☺ discuss patient care in the PACU. Depending on the type of surgery, there may be a pressure dressing to prevent bleeding and decrease edema. The nurse will need to check the dressings frequently for bleeding and to monitor the patient for signs of hemorrhage, such as increased pulse rate, decreased blood pressure, or changes in level of consciousness. The patient also may have drains in place that the nurse will need to monitor for amount and color of drainage. The patient needs to be kept comfortable. This may require special positioning and pain medication.

The patient should be instructed not to remove scabs, and the incisions should be kept clean and dry. Any redness, increased warmth, or drainage should be reported to the surgeon. The patient will need teaching about treatments or care of the incision at home.

Postoperative care for the abdominoplasty or panniculectomy includes instructing the patient to minimize tension on the suture line by sleeping in a semi-Fowler's position, not lifting heavy objects, and avoiding strenuous exercise. Instruct the patient not to smoke tobacco, as it constricts blood vessels, which diminishes the blood supply needed for wound healing. It is essential to teach pain management techniques such as splinting the wound when coughing, walking in a hunched over position, and consistent use of pain medications. It also is important to discuss the clinical manifestations of wound infection, which include wound separation, drainage, redness, increased pain, and fever. The nurse must stress to the patient what signs and symptoms need to be reported to the surgeon.

Health Promotion

The patient undergoing cosmetic surgery and the patient's family will need teaching related to the type and extent of surgery. Specific instructions should be given related to the type of incision, length of surgery, length of recovery, and possible complications. Although the surgeon will generally provide the patient with this information, is it important that the nurse reinforce and clarify that the patient understands the information. The patient needs to be aware of any postoperative limitations or special care needs.

There may be special preoperative preparations. For example, rhytidectomy patients need to be instructed to wash their hair and face with antibacterial soap several times to decrease the bacterial count. The patient should be instructed not to ingest aspirin, ibuprofen, or other platelet coating drugs for at least 2 weeks before and after surgery because of the increased risk of bleeding. The patient will need a physical examination and routine diagnostic laboratory tests prior to surgery to assess physical readiness for anesthesia. Chapter 25 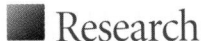 discusses preoperative instructions in detail. The patient should be prepared psychologically for postoperative edema and discoloration. Due to this bruising and edema, the true effects of the surgery cannot be evaluated for several weeks.

Research

Research opportunities exist related to skin disorders and cosmetic surgery. The goals of research are to identify effective means of caring for patients with skin problems and to support patients psychologically who have experienced changes in appearance. The research topics related to skin disorders are identified in the Research Opportunities and Clinical Impact box.

RESEARCH OPPORTUNITIES AND CLINICAL IMPACT RELATED TO SKIN DISORDERS AND COSMETIC SURGERY

Research Area	Clinical Impact
Effects of various moisturizers on the skin.	Keeping the skin intact and avoiding dryness.
Mechanisms to diagnose skin cancer accurately.	Early detection and treatment.
Treatment for common skin conditions.	Many skin conditions do not have adequate treatment available for cure or control.
Lifestyle outcomes of cosmetic surgery. Social and psychological implications of cosmetic surgery.	There is a need to determine whether cosmetic surgery makes a difference in lifestyle and body image.
Risk factors for herpes zoster.	More information is needed about who might be at risk other than those who are immunocompromised.
The effects of cosmetic surgery on the ethnic population.	Most research related to cosmetic surgery has been done with the Caucasian population. How does ethnic skin respond?
Define epidemiology with necrotizing fasciitis using population-based studies. Factors that help predict who might develop necrotizing fasciitis.	Identify those with the greatest risk for acquiring necrotizing fasciitis.
Testing of computer health care provider's orders. Interventions to improve patient understanding of and compliance with medication dosage and administration.	There is a need to decrease medication errors.
The role of nonsteroidal anti-inflammatory drugs (NSAIDs) in the development of necrotizing fasciitis.	Clarifies whether NSAIDs aggravate or initiate the development of necrotizing fasciitis.

Clinical Preparation

 **Read**

- History of Current Illness
- Past Medical History
- Physical Exam
- Admitting Medical Orders
- Laboratory Study Results

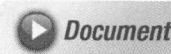 **Document**

- Summary of Hospitalization
- Pathophysiology Form
- Laboratory Values
- Laboratory Results Explanation

 **Apply**

- List of Potential Nursing Diagnoses
- Concept Map
- Critical Thinking Questions

Log on to MyNursingKit.com to download forms you will need and to complete further steps in the Clinical Preparation assignment.

HISTORY OF PRESENT ILLNESS

Mr. Tatum is a 47-year-old white male who was admitted to the hospital with necrotizing fasciitis located in a wound in his right lower leg. He reports being hit on the lower leg with a log while he was chopping wood about 7 days ago. At the time of the injury, he removed several splinters. Following the injury the pain increased to the point that it became difficult for him to walk. He noted that there was increased swelling and a mottled appearance where the splinters were, and that the wound had doubled in size in the last 2 days. He brought himself to the emergency department for an evaluation of the leg and to rule out a fracture. No fracture was found, however the assessment revealed a cellulitis with a hard "woody" texture to the wound. He was admitted for further wound evaluation.

Upon admission Mr. Tatum was taken to surgery for a debridement and culture of his wound. The culture showed group A streptococcus. He is scheduled for a second debridement in 12 hours. The surgical debridement will continue until clear borders are obtained. Application of a vacuum-assisted closure device was done in surgery.

Medical–Surgical History

Mr. Tatum has been in relatively good health. Lately he has had some problems with tendonitis in the left elbow and was on Naprosyn. No other chronic health problems. He was on no medications prior to admission other than Naprosyn.

Social History

Mr. Tatum lives in the country but works as a mechanic at the local steel plant.

He reports that he drinks approximately 6 beers per week, mostly on the weekend. He does not use illicit drugs. He smokes about 1 pack of cigarettes per day.

Physical Exam

Vital signs; BP 120/76; P 96; RR 16; T 99.4°F
Oxygen sat 93% on room air
HEENT: normal but poor dentition
Heart: regular rate and rhythm; normal S_1, S_2
Lungs: clear to auscultation in all fields
Abdomen: obese, soft, nontender
Normal neuro exam
No rash
Chest x-ray: clear
ECG: WNL
Weight: 210 lbs (95.4 kg); height: 6'1"
Extremities: left leg appears normal with good color, no edema, dorsalis pedis and posterior tibial pulses 2+ bilaterally
Anterior right lower leg has wound approximately 5 inches in diameter about mid-shin. The area around the wound is erythemic with bluish patches and bullae draining clear watery liquid. The wound is surrounded by nonpitting edema from the knee to the ankle. Area around wound is very tender to touch.

Admitting Medical Orders

Plastic Surgery Service
Surgical floor

Diagnosis: necrotizing fasciitis of right leg
Allergic to codeine
Oxygen at 2–3 liters nasal cannula, keep oxygen saturation ≥ 92%
Bed rest with bathroom privileges
Vital signs and O_2 saturation levels q2h
Call house officer: pulse < 60 and > 110/minute; BP < 90 and > 130 systolic; temperature > 38.5°C; urine output < 30 mL/hr for 2 hours; respiratory rate > 30/minute; oxygen saturation < 92%
Sequential compression device (SCD) to lower left extremity
Incentive spirometer every 2 hours while awake
Foley
I&O
NPO after midnight for OR
Calorie count
IV: D5 lactated Ringer's at 100 mL/hr
Contact isolation
Wound VAC to right lower leg with 125 mmHg of continuous suction

Scheduled Medications

Clindamycin 900 mg IV q8h
Ampicillin 1.0 gm IV q6h

Gentamicin 90 mg IV three times per day
Famotidine 20 mg IV twice daily
Naprosyn 500 mg po twice/day (when taking po)

PRN Medications

Morphine sulfate via patient-controlled analgesia: concentration:
1 mg/mL Basal rate 1 mg/hr; incremental: 1 mg;
6-minute lock-out
Phenergan 25 mg IV q6h prn nausea
Triazolam 0.125–0.25 mg po q noc, prn sleep (when taking po)
Ativan 0.5–2 mg IV q6–8h prn anxiety

Milk of Magnesia 30 mL po daily prn constipation (when taking po)
Tylenol 650 mg po/PR prn q4h for fever > 38.5°C

Ordered Laboratory Studies

STAT wound culture (done in OR)
CBC, Chem 20 panel, CK now
Daily: CBC, PT-INR/PTT, Ca, Mg, phosphorus, Chem 7 panel
Blood culture every 24 hours prn temp > 38.5°C

Ordered Diagnostic Studies

ECG
CT scan of right leg

LABORATORY STUDY RESULTS

Test	Day 1	Day 2	Day 3
White blood cells (WBCs)	18,000/mm³	22,000/mm³	28,000/mm³
Neutrophils	80%	88%	96%
Hemoglobin	12 g/dL	11 g/dL	10 g/dL
Hematocrit	36%	33%	30%
Red blood cells (RBCs)	4.5/mm³	4.1/mm³	3.8/mm³
Platelets	250,000/mm³	400,000/mm³	540,000/mm³
Sodium	136 mEq/L	138 mEq/L	139 mEq/L
Potassium	4.0 mEq/L	4.8 mEq/L	5.0 mEq/L
Chloride	96 mEq/L	97 mEq/L	101 mEq/L
Carbon dioxide	30		
Magnesium	1.8 mEq/L		
Phosphorus	4 mg/dL		
Blood urea nitrogen (BUN)	22 mg/dL	34 mg/dL	49 mg/dL
Creatinine	1 mg/dL	1.3 mg/dL	1.7 mg/dL
Glucose	198 mg/dL	192 mg/dL	160 mg/dL
Calcium	9.2 mg/dL		
Total protein	5.2 g/dL		
Albumin	3.6 g/dL		
Alkaline phosphatase	105 units/L		
Aspartate aminotransferase (AST)	38 units/L		
Total bilirubin	1.1 mg/dL		
Creatine kinase	280 units/L		
PTT	32 seconds		
PT	9.6 seconds		
INR	1.2		
Wound culture	Group A beta-hemolytic streptococcus		
CT scan	Asymmetric fascial thickening with gas tracking along the fascial planes		

CRITICAL THINKING QUESTIONS

1. What complications should you assess for in Mr. Tatum and why?

2. How is Mr. Tatum's necrotizing fasciitis transmitted and how can you protect the other patients you are caring for?

3. Mr. Tatum is concerned about his leg and asks you whether it will ever be back to normal. How should you respond?

Answers to Critical Thinking Questions appear in Appendix D.

NCLEX® REVIEW

1. The nurse is instructing a patient to reduce bathing and use a mild unscented soap. These interventions are appropriate for which of the following skin disorders?
   1. Atopic dermatitis
   2. Poison ivy
   3. Urticaria
   4. Contact dermatitis

2. The nurse is instructing a patient with a skin disorder on nutrition. Which of the following should be included in this instruction?
   1. Restrict calories.
   2. Eat foods high in vitamin C, iron, and zinc.
   3. Limit high-water content foods.
   4. Limit fatty foods.

3. A patient asks what she could do to make sure her teenage daughter doesn't develop skin cancer. Which of the following should the nurse instruct this patient?
   1. Eat a well-balanced diet.
   2. Maintain a normal weight for height.
   3. Take a daily multivitamin.
   4. Instruct in the use of sunscreen.

4. A patient with a skin disorder is prescribed a topical corticosteroid. Which of the following should the nurse instruct this patient about the use of this medication?
   1. Rub the medication into wet skin thoroughly.
   2. Apply a thick layer of the medication and allow it to air dry.
   3. Stay out of the sun when you use this medication.
   4. It may cause drowsiness.

5. A patient has been admitted to the hospital with a skin disorder. Which of the following should the nurse include in the assessment of this patient?
   1. Signs of infection
   2. Employment history
   3. Social activities
   4. Neurological status

6. A patient tells the nurse that she "doesn't socialize much in the summer" because she needs to wear long sleeves to cover the psoriasis on her arms. Which of the following should the nurse respond to this patient?
   1. That's too bad.
   2. You probably like the winter much better.
   3. There are light materials that you could wear to protect your arms while still enjoying the summer activities.
   4. I would go out anyway.

7. A patient tells the nurse that as she gets older, it seems like her face is getting longer. Which of the following should the nurse respond to this patient?
   1. It is a sign of disease.
   2. This is a normal part of aging.
   3. It happens because of exposure to smoke.
   4. It happens because of sun exposure.

Answers for review questions appear in Appendix D

KEY TERMS

acne vulgaris *p.2159*
actinic keratosis *p.2153*
androgenetic alopecia *p.2151*
androgenic alopecia *p.2151*
atopic dermatitis *p.2154*
blepharoplasty *p.2182*
café-au-lait spot *p.2159*
candidiasis *p.2166*
carbuncle *p.2165*
cellulitis *p.2164*
contact dermatitis *p.2153*
dermabrasion *p.2184*
dermatofibromas *p.2161*
dermatophyte *p.2167*

erysipelas *p.2164*
fissure *p.2154*
folliculitis *p.2164*
furuncle *p.2165*
hirsutism *p.2151*
impetigo *p.2164*
lipoma *p.2158*
liposuction *p.2185*
necrotizing fasciitis (NF) *p.2170*
neurofibromatosis *p.2161*
nevi *p.2158*
nits *p.2168*
paronychia *p.2150*
pediculosis *p.2168*

photodermatitis *p.2153*
pilosebaceous follicles *p.2158*
psoriasis *p.2160*
rhinoplasty *p.2183*
rhytidectomy *p.2183*
scabies *p.2168*
seborrheic keratosis *p.2161*
shingles *p.2165*
solar lentigo *p.2159*
Stevens-Johnson syndrome (SJS) *p.2179*
toxic epidermal necrolysis (TEN) *p.2180*
urticaria *p.2154*
verrucae *p.2166*
vitiligo *p.2159*

REFERENCES

Abernethy, H., Cho, C., DeLanoy, A., Khan, O., Kerns, J. W., & Knight, K. (2006). What nonpharmacological treatments are effective against common nongenital warts? *Journal of Family Practice, 55*(9), 801–802.

Affleck, P. (2005). Sun exposure and health. *Nursing Standard, 19*(47), 50–54.

American Society of Plastic Surgeons (ASPS). (2007). *Injectable fillers.* Retrieved January 5, 2008, from http://plasticsurgery.org/patients_consumers/procedures/InjectableFillers.cfm?gclid=CKPEo4_V35ACFRdPagodPzD0WQ

Cancer Research UK. (2003). *Cancer Research UK gets SunSmart with the big screen.* Retrieved September 8, 2008, from http://info.cancerresearchuk.org/news/archive/pressreleases/2003/may/216205

Centers for Disease Control and Prevention (CDC). (2000). *Pseudomonas dermatitis/folliculitis associated with pools and hot tubs—Colorado and Maine, 1999–2000. Morbidity and Mortality Weekly Report, 49*(48), 1087–1091. Retrieved September 3, 2008, from http://www.cdc.gov/mmwr/preview/mmwrhtml/mm4948a2.htm

Centers for Disease Control and Prevention (CDC). (2002). *Skin cancer: Preventing America's most common cancer, fact sheet 2002.* Retrieved February 18, 2004, from http://www.cdc.gov/HealthyYouth/skincancer/pdf/facts.pdf

Centers for Disease Control and Prevention (CDC). (2006a). *Methicillin-resistant Staphylococcus aureus skin infections among tattoo recipients—Ohio, Kentucky, and Vermont, 2004–2005.* Retrieved December 12, 2007, from http://www.cdc.gov/mmwr/preview/mmwrhtml/mm5524a3.htm

Centers for Disease Control and Prevention (CDC). (2006b). *Health topics: Skin cancer school health guidelines.* Retrieved December 12, 2007, from http://www.cdc.gov/healthyyouth/skincancer/guidelines/summary.htm#top

Centers for Disease Control and Prevention (CDC). (2008). *Division of bacterial and mycotic diseases. Group A streptococcal (GAS) disease.* Retrieved August 30, 2008, from http://www.cdc.gov/ncidod/dbmd/diseaseinfo/groupastreptococcal_g.htm

Coldiron, B., Coleman, W. P., Cox, S. E., Jacob, C., Lawrence, N., Kaminer, M., et al. (2006). ASDS guidelines of care for tumescent liposuction. *Dermatologic Surgery, 32*, 709–716.

County of Kern: Department of Health Services. (2007). *Complications associated with body piercing and tattooing.* Retrieved December 12, 2007, from http://www.co.kern.ca.us/health/tattooing513.asp

Demierre, M., Allten, S., & Brown, J. (2005). New treatments for melanoma. *Dermatology Nursing, 17*(4), 287–295.

Fawcett, R. S., Linford, S., & Stulberg, D. L. (2004). Nail abnormalities: Clues to systemic disease. *American Family Physician, 69*, 1417–1424.

Forman, R., Koren, G., & Shear, N. H. (2002). Erythema multiforme, Stevens–Johnson syndrome and toxic epidermal necrolysis in children: A review of 10 years' experience. *Drug Safety, 25*(13), 965–972.

Gorgos, D. (2006). Dermatology nursing news: Skin update. *Dermatology Nursing, 18*(1): 89–92, 95–98, 107.

Guegan, S., Bastuji-Garin, S., Poszepczynska-Guigne, E., Roujeau, J., & Revuz, J. (2006). Performance of the SCORTEN during the first five days of hospitalization to predict the prognosis of epidermal necrolysis. *Journal of Investigative Dermatology, 126*(2), 272–276.

Gurwitz, J. H., Field, T. S., Harrold, L. R., Rothschild, J., Debellis, K., Seger, A. C., et al. (2003). Incidence and preventability of adverse drug events among older persons in the ambulatory setting. *JAMA, 289*, 1107–1116.

Halder, R. M., & Nootheti, P. K. (2003). Ethnic skin disorders overview. *Journal of the American Academy of Dermatology, 48*(Suppl. 6), S143–S148.

Hasham S., Matteucci, P., Stanley, P. R., & Hart, N. B. (2005). Necrotizing fasciitis. *British Medical Journal, 330*(9), 830–833.

Hockett, K. C. (2004). Stevens–Johnson syndrome and toxic epidermal necrolysis: Oncologic considerations. *Clinical Journal of Oncology Nursing, 8*(1), 27–30.

Hunt, N., & McHale, S. (2005). The psychological impact of alopecia. *British Medical Journal, 331*(7522), 951–953.

Jemal, A., Siegel, R., Ward, E., Murray, T., Xu, J., Smigal, C., et al. (2006). Cancer statistics, 2006. *CA: A Cancer Journal for Clinicians, 56*(2), 106–130. Retrieved September 4, 2008, from http://caonline.amcancersoc.org/cgi/content/full/56/2/106

Khalili, B., & Bahna, S. L. (2006). Pathogenesis and recent therapeutic trends in Stevens–Johnson syndrome and toxic epidermal necrolysis. *Annals of Allergy, Asthma, & Immunology, 97*, 272–281.

Klein, P. A. (2006). Stevens-Johnson Syndrome and Toxic Epidermal Necrolysis. *eMedicine.* Retrieved September 8, 2008 from http://www.emedicine.com/derm/TOPIC405.HTM

Kucera, I. J., Lambert, T. J., Klein, J. A., Watkins, R. G., Hoover, J. M., & Kaye, A. D. (2006). Liposuction: Contemporary issues for the anesthesiologist. *Journal of Clinical Anesthesia, 18*(5), 379–387.

Layton, A., Buchanan, P., & Courtenay, M. (2006). Continuing professional development. Treatment of acne vulgaris. *Primary Health Care, 16*(4), 41–49.

Letko, E., Papliodis, E. N., Papliodis, G. N., Daoud, Y. J., Ahmed, A. R., & Foster, C. S. (2005). Stevens–Johnson syndrome and toxic epidermal necrolysis: A review of the literature. *Annals of Allergy, Asthma, & Immunology, 94*(4), 419–436.

MayoClinic.com. (2008). *Tattoos: Risks and precautions to know first.* Retrieved August 30, 2008, from http://www.mayoclinic.com/health/tattoos-and-piercings/MC00020

National Pressure Ulcer Advisory Panel (NPUAP). (1992). *Statement on pressure ulcer prevention.* Retrieved September 8, 2008, from http://www.npuap.org/positn1.htm

Patel, B. D., Loo, W. J., Tasker, A. D., Screaton, N. J., Burrows, N. P., Silverman, E. K., et al. (2006). Smoking related COPD and facial wrinkling: Is there a common susceptibility? *Thorax, 61*(7), 568–671.

Reddy, M., Gill, S. S., & Rochon, P. A. (2006). Preventing pressure ulcers: A systematic review. *Journal of the American Medical Association, 296*(8), 974–984.

Samuel, M., Brooke, R. C. C., Hollis, S., & Griffiths, C. E. M. (2005). Interventions for photodamaged skin. *The Cochrane Database of Systematic Reviews*, Issue 1. Retrieved August 30, 2008, from http://www.cochrane.org/reviews/en/ab001782.html

Scher, R. K., Fleckman, P., Tulumbas, B., McCollam, L., & Enfanto, P. (2003). Brittle nail syndrome: Treatment options and the role of the nurse. *Dermatology Nursing, 15*(1), 15–24.

Singh, G., Haneef, N. A., & Uday, A. (2005). Nail changes and disorders among the elderly. *Indian Journal of Dermatology, Venereology, and Leprology, 71*(6), 386–392.

Stough, D., Stenn, K., Haber, R., Parsley, W. M., Vogel, J. E., Whiting, D. A., et al. (2005). Psychological effect, pathophysiology, and management of androgenetic alopecia in men. *Mayo Clinic Proceedings, 80*(10), 1316–1322.

Swetter, S. (2008). Malignant melanoma. *eMedicine from Web MD.* Retrieved August 30, 2008, from http://www.emedicine.com/derm/topic257.htm

Tsang, M. O., Tsang, K. Y., & Wong, W. (2004). The use of recombinant human epidermal growth factor (rhEGF) in a gentleman with drug-induced Steven Johnson syndrome. *Dermatology Online Journal, 10*(1), 25. Retrieved September 4, 2008, from http://dermatology.cdlib.org/101/correspondence/TEN/tsang.html

Tysome, J. R., & Sharp, H. R. (2006). Current trends in photographic imaging for rhinoplasty surgery. *The Internet Journal of Otorhinolaryngology, 5*(2). Retrieved August 30, 2008, from http://www.ispub.com/ostia/index.php?xmlFilePath=journals/ijorl/vol5n2/imaging.xml

U.S. Department of Health and Human Services (DHHS). (2000). *Healthy People 2010 understanding and improving health.* Washington, DC: Author.

Wong, C., & Wang, Y. (2005). The diagnosis of necrotizing fasciitis. *Current Opinion in Infectious Disease, 18*(2), 101–106.

Young, M. (2005). The psychological and social burdens of psoriasis. *Dermatology Nursing, 17*(1), 15–19.

Zhang, W., Leonard, R., Bath-Hextall, F., Chambers, C. A., Lee, C., Humphreys, R., et al. (2004). Chinese herbal medicine for atopic eczema. *The Cochrane Database of Systematic Reviews.* Issue 4. Retrieved August 30, 2008, from http://www.cochrane.org/reviews/en/ab002291.html

Harold Engle
Kathleen Osborn

With contributions by:
Jan Clark

Outcome-Based Learning Objectives

After studying this chapter, the learner will be able to:

1. Compare and contrast the clinical manifestations of the three phases of wound healing.
2. Describe wound characteristics and nursing documentation that are required in a periodic wound assessment.
3. Describe key factors that are relative to the prevention of pressure ulcers.
4. Compare and contrast wound classifications and respective treatments.
5. Evaluate therapies and their benefits with respect to wound healing.
6. Understand the psychosocial and liability factors pertaining to wound care.
7. Describe how research in wound care will lead to better efficiency and outcomes with evidence-based practice.

Research   Collaboration   Health Promotion   Nursing Process   Caring   Critical Thinking

WHAT IS the largest organ of the human body? The skin is the largest organ of the human body and functions to protect internal organs from insults such as infection and injury. These insults may be as minor as a bump or bruise or as major as a life-threatening infection or trauma. Whether the injury is caused by a surgeon's scalpel, trauma from a bullet or stab wound, or tissue damage from a myocardial infarction, the repair process is similar. The primary objective of the wound healing process is to restore skin integrity and structural continuity of the injured area (Porth, 2007).

Skin is an organ of the integumentary system that is comprised of three layers of tissue: epidermis, dermis, and subcutaneous tissue. Each layer has a different composition and function. The outermost layer of skin is the epidermis. It contains melanocytes for pigmentation, Langerhans' cells as part of the immune system, sensory nerves, and keratinocytes. The main function of the epidermis is protection and sensation. The dermis, the thickest layer of the skin, contains the microvascular system along with hair follicles, sweat glands, lymph vessels, sebaceous (oil) glands, and nerve endings. It is constructed of collagen, a protein made from fibroblasts. It is also comprised of elastin, which makes the skin flexible and elastic. The main functions of the dermis are thermoregulation and blood supply to the epidermis. The last layer of the skin, the subcutaneous fat

layer (also known as hypodermis), is comprised of stored fat cells. It is an avascular layer as well. Its main function is insulation and protection of the underlying organs (Porth, 2007). Chapter 65 🌐 discusses the anatomy of the skin in detail.

Physiology of Wound Healing

What happens when the skin is compromised by an injury? Once tissue injury has occurred, the primary objective is to restore tissue integrity through the healing process. There are three phases of wound healing: homeostasis/inflammation, proliferation, and remodeling (Figure 67–1 ■). These phases represent a cascade of events that overlap and are dependent on one another. Each phase contributes to the desired result of healing the wound. Any disruption or absence of a phase can result in a delayed or prolonged healing. Each phase is discussed next.

Phase One: Homeostasis/Inflammatory Phase

Homeostasis is the tendency of the human body to maintain stability, and maintaining stability is the first reaction when a wound occurs. Injury to the epidermis, dermis, and subcutaneous tissue causes blood cells to spill into the wound, and the first step toward homeostasis is to get the bleeding stopped. A vasoconstric-

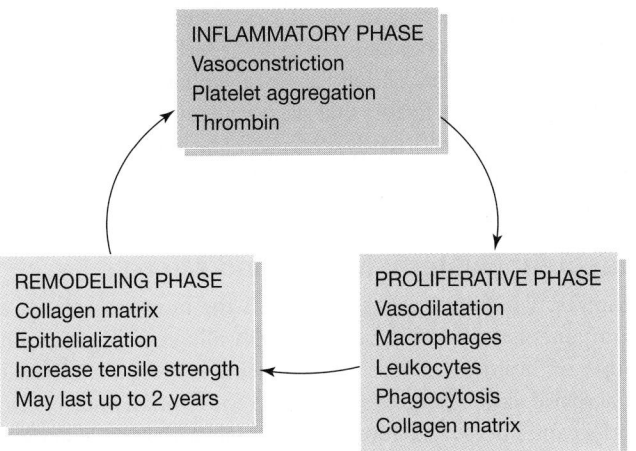

INFLAMMATORY PHASE
Vasoconstriction
Platelet aggregation
Thrombin

REMODELING PHASE
Collagen matrix
Epithelialization
Increase tensile strength
May last up to 2 years

PROLIFERATIVE PHASE
Vasodilatation
Macrophages
Leukocytes
Phagocytosis
Collagen matrix

FIGURE 67–1 ■ Phases of wound healing.

tive substance is released by the platelets that assist in this process. Coagulation factors, which promote platelet aggregation in the endothelium of the injured vessel at the site of injury, are also released. The bleeding is usually stopped by a thrombus formation. Thrombus formation is discussed in detail in Chapter 62 .

The next step in regaining homeostasis is the secretion of **growth factors**, which are a group of extracellular polypeptides (secreted by platelets and macrophages) that affect cell growth, reproduction, movement, and function. Growth factors recruit the necessary cells to synthesize and regulate the wound repair. Scientists have identified several of these growth factors and their effects on the wound repair process: for example, platelet-activating factor (PAF), which induces platelet aggregation (Porth, 2007), and epidermal growth factor (EGF), which may have an important part in wound healing by stimulating keratinocyte proliferation and migration of cells (Gibbs et al., 2000). The keratinocyte growth factor impacts the remodeling process by stabilizing epidermal turnover and barrier function (Gibbs et al., 2000).

The **inflammatory phase** of wound healing begins at the time of the injury or surgery. The purpose of this critical phase is to prepare the site for growth of new tissue. This phase of wound healing cleans the wound in preparation for closure. In a clean acute wound, the inflammatory phase lasts approximately 3 to 5 days, but in a wound complicated by infection or necrosis, the inflammatory phase is prolonged and wound healing is delayed (Waldrop & Doughty, 2000). Within hours after injury, histamines are released from mast cells, causing local vasodilation and increased capillary permeability. This allows leakage of serous fluid into the injured site, which results in erythema, edema, and the production of exudates.

Prostaglandin, which is released during the inflammatory phase, is a long-chain fatty acid that regulates platelet aggregation and controls inflammation and vascular permeability. The inflammatory phase is characterized by the presence of granulocytes, macrophages, and lymphocytes, which are attracted to the injured site by the complement factors and antigens. These cells, called **phagocytes**, perform **phagocytosis**, the process of absorbing and enzymatically degrading foreign matter and devitalized tissue, thus preparing the wound for closure. The by-product of phagocytosis is exudate. Exudate, or drainage

from the wound, is usually at its peak during the inflammatory phase. Note that the drainage from the wound during the inflammatory phase does not indicate infection in the wound; it is the body's normal response to injury.

Suppression of the inflammatory phase can contribute to a delay in wound healing. Radiation therapy can suppress the inflammatory phase by causing depletion of the neutrophils and macrophages, which release the growth factors. Malnutrition, dehydration, and chronic steroid use also can suppress the inflammatory phase. Chronic use of steroids specifically results in decreased production of histamines, suppressing the inflammatory response.

Phase Two: Proliferation

The proliferative phase is the next phase in the healing process. Reconstruction occurs at this phase. It can last up to 3 weeks after the inflammatory phase in a normal, healthy person. Growth factors described earlier originating from injured vessels stimulate the formation of vascular buds and regrowth of vascular loops. Stimulated endothelial cells multiply and form tubular structures differentiating into arterioles or venules, a process referred to as **angiogenesis**. These new blood vessels can begin to form in a wound within 3 days of injury, provided there is sufficient blood circulation to the wound bed.

Simultaneously, in the process of revascularization, connective tissue begins to form at the wound margins. **Fibroblasts** are the small cells that migrate along the fibrin network to produce the connective tissue and collagen fibers. **Collagen synthesis** is the multistep process in which fibrin proteins form a matrix to support the newly forming tissue. Collagen synthesis is dependent on adequate amounts of vitamin C, iron, and copper in the diet. The newly formed collagen fibers are not organized in the same tension contours as in healthy tissue, thus decreasing the tensile strength and elasticity in a repaired wound. Collagen fibers in scar tissue actually have a disorganized appearance (Christian, Talavera, Stadelmann, Slenkovich, & Downey, 2006). The end result is that scar tissue never has the same tensile strength as normal tissue.

Due to angiogenesis, granulation tissue develops. **Granulation tissue**, aptly named for the recognizable tiny, round, granule-like nodules, is a highly vascular connective tissue that contains newly formed capillaries, proliferating fibroblasts, and residual inflammatory cells (Porth, 2007). Granulation tissue appears beefy red and moist because of the dense revascularization process. Granulation tissue gradually fills the defect of the wound. If granulation tissue is slow to form, one can presume that there is an insufficient blood supply, there is a wound infection, or one of the growth factors necessary for revascularization is deficient, all of which interrupt the normal rate of wound healing. This part of the proliferative phase begins about 3 days after initial injury and may overlap with the inflammatory phase.

Epithelialization is the process by which the wound closes from its margins, covering the defect with a layer of new skin. This is accomplished by cell migration from the wound edges over granulation tissue. The wound bed must be moist and well perfused with blood in order for epithelialization to occur. Epithelialization, usually first seen at the wound margins, appears as a small pink or pearl-like area. Islands of epithelial cells can

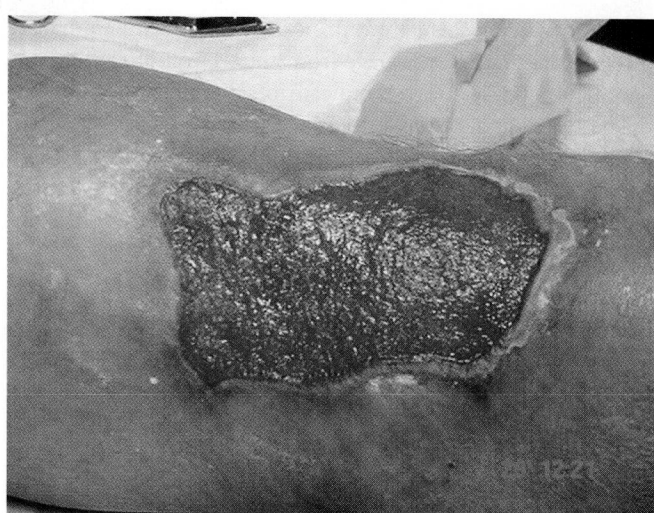

FIGURE 67–2 ■ Granulation and epithelialization tissue.
Source: Courtesy of Harold Engle

appear within the wound defect on the surface of the granulation. This new skin is quite fragile and must be protected from injury. A moist environment encourages the migration of these cells across the wound surface from all directions. Granulation and epithelialization, if not interrupted, continue to develop for up to about 14 to 21 days (Figure 67–2 ■).

 Partial thickness wounds (e.g., skin tears, abrasions) do not require granulation to heal because epithelial cells are able to migrate across the wound, rebuilding dermis.

Full-thickness wounds require granulation to fill the defect caused by the wound. This is not regenerated tissue but scar tissue.

Phase Three: Remodeling

Remodeling, the third and final phase of wound healing, occurs after the wound is closed. It begins about 3 weeks after the injury and can still be in progress from 6 months to 2 years later. During this phase the scar changes and matures. The bulk decreases and the color changes from pink to pearly white. The incisional strength builds, and by the end of 8 weeks it is about 70% of its original strength. During remodeling collagen fibers are partially broken down by enzymes and reconfigured. Contraction due to the myofibroblasts can cause collagen fibers to become taut; scar tissue shrinks and cutaneous tissue becomes smaller. Tension lines are frequently visible on the cutaneous surface (outer skin) of scar tissue. Healed wounds achieve only part of the original tensile strength and therefore are at a greater risk of future breakdown. The remodeling phase leaves the affected area with only 65% to 80% of its original tissue strength, and the affected area will be more prone to reinjury in the future. The remodeling phase may last up to 2 years.

 The nurse needs to teach the patient that the scar tissue will never reach its preinjury strength. Therefore, it is essential to protect it from trauma and overexposure to the sun to prevent future skin breakdown.

■ Wound Healing Assessment

There are many factors that influence the wound healing process or lack thereof. A wound develops as a result of some type of insult or injury. The body has a normal process for wound heal-

ing, as described earlier in the phases of healing. Many factors play a role in the progression or lack thereof in wound healing. These factors are critical elements for the phases of wound healing to proceed. Any factors that are not adequate will delay healing until they are sufficiently corrected. The nurse must be aware of the risk factors that may impact the rate of wound healing when assessing patients.

Vascular System: Macro and Micro

The vascular component to healing is the most essential of all components; without it, no phase of healing can begin and no hope of healing can occur. The vascular system consists of macrocirculation (large vessels such as the femoral or carotid arteries) and microcirculation (small vessels such as capillary beds or superficial artery systems). The vascular system is essential to deliver the clotting factors, oxygen, leukocytes, macrophages, prostaglandins, and growth factors that contribute to the healing process. Without adequate circulation, a wound will not heal. There are multiple tests that can determine circulation. Macrocirculation of the lower extremities can be tested by performing an ankle-brachial index (ABI). The measurement is a ratio of ankle systolic pressure to brachial systolic pressure. Normally, the ankle systolic pressure is at or slightly higher than the brachial systolic pressure. A ratio of less than 0.9 is indicative of circulatory disease in the lower extremities. The ABI is a noninvasive, inexpensive tool to determine whether additional testing for circulatory disease is warranted. Chapter 43 ⊕ further describes the ABI.

Other noninvasive tools to test circulation are Doppler studies that utilize ultrasound to test arterial blood flow and estimate arterial circumference and/or occlusion. An invasive study for circulatory evaluation is a femoral angiogram, whereby a catheter is inserted into the femoral artery and pictures are taken with enhancement by a dye that reveals actual blood flow and determines a percentage of blockages, if any. A procedure to restore circulatory flow to the lower extremities can be performed that utilizes a blade that cuts through the plaque and a vacuum suction to remove the plaque.

Microcirculation can be evaluated as well. Microcirculation involves the capillary beds that actually "feed" the wound area itself. A test, best known as a transcutaneous oxygen measurement (TCOM), can evaluate the tissue at a depth of one-fourth inch. The test utilizes an electrode that is heated to vasodilate the capillary bed. A solution is used as the medium for the diffusion of gases, including oxygen, and a measurement of the partial pressure of oxygen is recorded. Chart 67–1 notes the areas and partial pressures one expects to see for adequate circulation to heal.

Venous System

The venous system is also a component of and a factor in the wound healing process. The venous system returns the deoxygenated blood to the heart. The dilation of the venous system due to incompetent valves causes edema. The edema compresses the tissue and thus compresses the capillary beds and decreases circulation. Due to changes in capillary permeability in the edematous areas, fluid leaks into the local tissues. Infection then can set in as bacteria on the skin invade the area and are attracted to the fluid-filled medium.

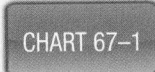

CHART 67–1	**Transcutaneous Oxygen Measurement (TCOM)**

PO₂

PO_2

Chest 60–80 mmHg (reference lead).

Extremity 30–40 mmHg (desired).

If extremity < 30 mmHg, apply 100% O_2 and measure response.

If response increases PO_2 in mmHg, patient is possible candidate for hyperbaric oxygen therapy.

CHART 67–2	**Systemic and Situational Factors Impacting Wound Healing**

Smoking	Incontinence
Age 75 or over	Diaphoresis
Inadequate nutrition	Paralysis
Low albumin/protein	Neurological disease
Anemia	Immunosuppression
Dehydration	Infection
Immobility	Dementia
Edema	Cancer
Spasticity	Kidney disease
Contractures	Lung disease
Emphysema	Dermatologic conditions
Heart disease	Impaired circulation
Emaciation/cachexia	Obesity
Diminished sensation	Diabetes
Steroid use	Present pressure ulcers
Stress	Uncontrolled pain

A simple and noninvasive clue that there is venous insufficiency besides edema is the presence of hemosiderin staining (Figure 67–3 ■). Hemosiderin staining is a direct result of red blood cells that are "trapped" in the interstitial tissues and the breakdown of heme, or iron, into the tissue itself. Venous Doppler tests using ultrasound measure venous congestion and regurgitation (a direct result of incompetent valves) and can accurately detect venous insufficiency. Chapter 43 ⊕ discusses peripheral vascular disease.

■ Risk Factors That Impact Wound Healing

Many important factors can cause a delay in wound healing. Some are directly controlled by the patient, whereas others have an effect that is less easily controlled by the patient. The following factors will be discussed: nutrition and hydration, infection, comorbid conditions, medications, stress, glucose control and diabetic management, smoking, and gerontological considerations. Chart 67–2 outlines systemic and situational factors impacting wound healing.

Nutrition and Hydration

Nutrition is one of the most understated and undervalued components of and factors in wound healing. Nutrients are essential for normal healing because malnutrition interrupts the rate of normal tissue repair. The diet must be high in protein and calories with vitamin and nutritional supplements. Proteins are the building blocks of collagen, a cellular matrix that forms the basis of tissue granulation. Micronutrients, those that are needed in small amounts, include the fat soluble vitamins A, D, E, and K and the water soluble vitamins C and the B family. Vitamins such as A, D, E, and K play a role in the wound healing process as cofactors, antioxidants, antiplatelet properties, cell membrane stability, and in other vital functions. Supplemental vitamins and nutritional supplements should be monitored.

Supplements that are high in proteins and vitamins can assist in replacing low levels of albumin and aid in the formation of collagen to "fill" the wound to a level depth. Supplemental amino acids include arginine, glutamine, and hydroxy-methyl butyrate (HMB). A therapeutic nutrition drink is available that contains all three amino acids; it is called Juven (Ross Products, Abbott Laboratories).

The need for nutrients continues throughout the healing process. Using every opportunity to get patients to take in nutrients can be a nursing challenge. A comprehensive nutritional assessment should be done for nonhealing and chronic wounds. Chart 67–3 (p. 2196) outlines the specific vitamins and nutrients and their roles in the wound healing process. Diagnostic tests to check protein levels are albumin and more recently prealbumin tests. Prealbumin helps to determine whether the decrease in albumin is due to dietary intake or some organic issue independent of dietary intake. Chapter 14 ⊕ includes a discussion of albumin and prealbumin.

> **CRITICAL ALERT**
> *If prescribed diet allows, offer medications with one of the canned nourishment supplements or Instant Breakfast mixes. The opportunity to offer calorie-laden fluids can be helpful to those patients who have difficulty consuming enough calories.*

Maintaining adequate hydration assists in healing and decreases the risk of development of additional wounds. Proper hydration is often overlooked after intravenous fluids are discontinued. Offering patients fluids on a regular basis assists in

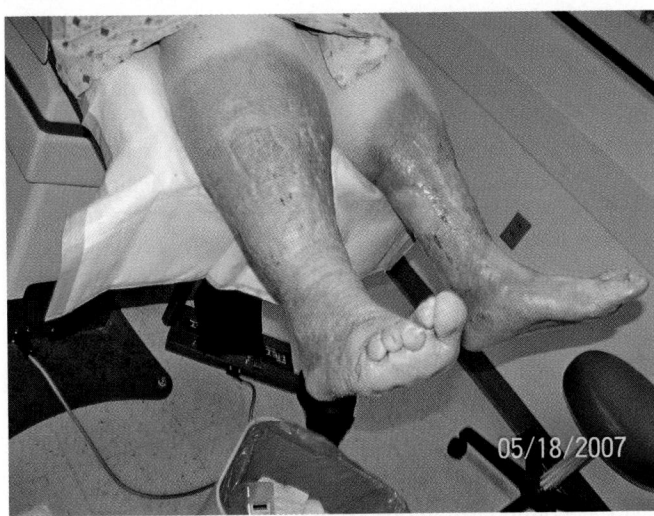

FIGURE 67–3 ■ Hemosiderin stain.
Source: Courtesy of Harold Engle

CHART 67–3 **Essential Vitamins and Nutrients for Wound Healing**

Vitamin and Nutrients	Function in Wound Healing
Vitamin A	Stimulant for onset of wound healing process. Stimulant of epithelialization and fibroblast deposition of collagen.
B vitamins (B$_6$, B$_{12}$)	Critical to metabolism and to synthesis of protein, fat, and carbohydrate, but no reported benefits of vitamin B specific to wound healing.
Vitamin C	Collagen synthesis, capillary wall integrity, fibroblast function, and immunologic function.
Vitamin E	By fighting oxidative damage, it can be effective in reducing infection risk, but daily levels in excess of 100 international units retard healing.
Vitamin K	Essential for blood clotting (coagulation).
Iron	Excessive consumption could result in bacterial proliferation.
Zinc	Essential for protein synthesis and collagen formation. Necessary for formation of T lymphocytes, supporting immunity. Deficiency leads to decreased epithelialization and fibroblast proliferation.
Copper	Cofactor for connective tissue production. Collagen cross-linking.
Arginine (amino acid)	Produces nitric oxide, which is essential for collagen accumulation and angiogenesis, and enhances immunity.
Glutamine (amino acid)	Critical role in preserving nitrogen balance, protein synthesis, cellular structure, and metabolism. Source for cellular respiration.

maintaining hydration. Intake and output must be documented in order to monitor hydration status. Fluid intake should be measured every 24 hours if inadequate hydration is suspected. Chapter 14 includes a complete description of nutritional requirements.

Infection

Infection, the process of organisms invading and destroying cells, can also determine the rate of wound healing or lack thereof. Wounds can be contaminated, colonized, and infected. Contamination is the presence of bacteria on the wound surface with no multiplication of the bacteria. Colonization is the presence of bacteria that are multiplying on the wound surface but are not invading tissue. Infection means the bacteria are invading viable tissue. The presence of bacteria in pus, slough, or necrotic tissue does not mean the tissue is infected (McGuckin, Goldman, Bolton, & Salcido, 2003). Three basic elements must exist for a clinical definition of infection (Gardner & Frantz, 2004):

- Microorganisms must be present in viable tissue.
- Microorganisms must multiply enough to impair healing or cause injury.
- Invading microorganisms must produce a host response or tissue injury.

It is generally accepted that clinical infection in acute wounds has been correlated with tissue levels greater than 10^5 organisms per gram. To diagnose infection, laboratory microbiologic results must be evaluated in conjunction with local clinical findings. It is important to recognize the classic signs and symptoms of infection: erythema, heat, edema, pain, and purulent exudate. These symptoms are the host's response to invading organisms. These symptoms are reliable indicators of infection in acute wounds.

Infection requires the body to "fight" infection with white blood cells, macrophages, and leukocytes, and the attention to healing becomes secondary as the body focuses on the immediate problem of the infection at hand. Infection also leaves *bioburden*, or waste, that must then be disposed of before collagen synthesis and granulation can occur. Microorganisms such as methicillin-resistant *Staphylococcus aureus* (MRSA) and *Klebsiella pneumoniae* with a resistant erythromycin sensitive beta lactamase (ESBL) strain are now invading wounds. These multidrug-resistant strains require multiple antibiotics with long durations.

The tissue injury produced by microorganisms is more likely found in chronic wounds. These symptoms include delayed healing, friable granulation tissue that bleeds easily, discoloration, unexpected pain/tenderness, wound breakdown, and abnormal smell (Cutting & White, 2005; Gardner & Frantz, 2004). Nursing management includes obtaining a culture when ordered by the health care provider. It is important to know the proper procedure: Cleanse the wound thoroughly with saline; and then with the sterile culturette swab, apply pressure and roll the swab over and over a 1 centimeter square. The portion of the wound to be cultured can be anywhere within the wound bed; choose a spot where tissue fluid can be expressed by pressing with the swab. The purpose is to take a culture of the tissue fluid, not of the exudate on top of the wound. Tissue biopsy is the gold standard to determine infection, but this is not done by nurses and is not readily available in all institutions. The Diagnostic Tests box outlines laboratory and diagnostic findings related to wound healing.

Comorbidities

Comorbidities, which are concurrent disease processes, also affect the wound healing process. For example, diabetes, a disorder characterized by the inability to store glucose and thus the

DIAGNOSTIC TESTS Related to Wound Healing

Test and *Normal Values*	Expected Abnormality	Treatment
White blood cells (WBC): 4,500–11,000/mm³	Increased with inflammation and acute infection. Decreased with thrombocytopenia, cancers, anemias, or liver disease.	Diagnose and track infection. WBC alone does not tell health care providers anything without differential.
Platelets: 150,000–400,000/mm³	Increased with inflammation and infection. Indication of concealed bleeding (i.e., gastrointestinal [GI]).	Basic element of coagulation. Decreased count can drive treatment.
Red blood cells (RBC): *Female: 4–5.5 million/mm³* *Male: 4.5–6.2 million/mm³*	May be decreased due to bleeding from the wound. Menses in women. Renal disease. Decrease might indicate depleted blood volume. Chronic infections.	Monitor for need for medications or blood administration to increase value.
Hemoglobin (Hgb): *Female: 12–15 g/dL* *Male: 14–16.5 g/dL*	May be decreased due to bleeding from the wound, hypoxia, anemias, or overhydration. Some prescription medications can decrease count.	Monitor with hematocrit for need for medications or blood administration to increase value.
Hematocrit (HCT): *Female: 35–47%* *Male: 42–52%*	May be decreased due to bleeding from the wound.	Monitor for need for medications or blood administration to increase value.
Total proteins: 6.3–8.3 g/dL	May be decreased with malnutrition. Decrease indicates immunosuppression.	Monitor need for nutritional supplements.
Serum albumin: 3.5–5.5 g/dL	May be decreased with malnutrition injury because albumin catabolism increases as a result of injury.	Monitor need for nutritional supplements. Half-life is 21 days; easily influenced by medications and fluid status.
Serum prealbumin: 16–40 mg/dL	Reflects immune and inflammatory status.	Current protein status.
Wound culture and sensitivity: *Negative*	Will be positive if there is contamination, colonization, or infection.	Assess for wound infection and which antibiotic will be effective in treating it.

Source: Adapted from Corbett, J. V. (2004). *Laboratory tests and diagnostic procedures with nursing diagnoses* (6th ed.). Upper Saddle River, NJ: Pearson Prentice Hall.

occurrence of elevated blood glucose levels, is the single most prevalent comorbidity in patients requiring chronic wound care. Diabetes causes neuropathy, or decreased sensation. (See the discussion on wound healing and diabetes later in this chapter.) Diabetes also interferes with the immune system and circulation by the hardening of the vessels and capillary beds. This hardening is the process whereby the vessel and capillary beds are infiltrated by fatty deposits that accumulate, cause localized damage to the endothelial lining of the vessel, and cause it to scar over repeated damage and healing.

Hypertension and atherosclerotic disease also cause problems with circulation and edema that compromise wound healing. Autoimmune disorders such as lupus or scleroderma decrease the body's ability to fight off infection; and when a wound is found in patients with these disorders, the delayed healing due to decreased immunity is evident.

Medications

Some medications can affect the wound healing process. Steroids decrease the immune system by delaying white blood cell migration and fibroblasts, thus impacting the inflammatory phase of wound healing. The ground matrix, collagen synthesis, regeneration of blood vessels, and epithelialization are also significantly delayed due to steroid use. One area of research now in progress is in the use of retinoids, vitamin A, to combat these effects. Retinoids have been shown in some trials to combat the ill effects of steroids directly and potentially reverse some of their adverse effects (Wicke et al., 2000). Chemotherapy drugs, specifically methotrexate, can delay the wound healing process by decreasing the immune system as well as by bone marrow suppression and anemia. Communication with patients is crucial to develop a realistic plan of care. The medications they take are a necessity; therefore, the plan of care must include educating the patient that the process of wound healing will be delayed. Realistic timelines should be provided, as these will help decrease anxiety.

Stress

Stress causes a release of hormones, including glucocorticoids, which reduces the production of cytokines, an essential component of the inflammatory process. The glucocorticoids also alter leukocyte movement. Reduction in these two factors causes immunosuppression. Because wound healing begins with inflammation, if this phase becomes suppressed, there is a delay in wound healing. Previous research has demonstrated that stress was associated with a 25% to 40% delay in wound closure across the models tested (Marucha, 2005). Stress also causes catecholamine release, which in turn causes vasoconstriction that will reduce perfusion and oxygenation to subcutaneous tissue and wounds.

Minimizing the patient's level of stress will promote the progression of wound healing. Pain and noise are common stressors for hospitalized patients. When pain is present, energy is spent in enduring the pain and not in healing the wound. Control of pain with analgesics and diversional activities will help decrease stress.

Manipulation of the patient's environment will reduce external stressors. Nurses are in a unique position to control the patient's environment. The nurse needs to be sensitive to the environmental noise and mitigate it when possible. Chapter 12 ⊘ provides an in-depth discussion of the impact of stress on the human body. The impact of stress on the immune system is discussed in Chapters 59 and 60 ⊘.

Glucose Control and Diabetic Management

Glucose control is essential for normal healing. High levels of glucose impair wound healing, and it is important to control the blood sugar very early in wound care to maximize wound healing potential. For example, high glucose levels result in altered leukocyte functioning and increased risk of infection. Monitoring the daily blood glucose levels and HgA1c values is important and helps to educate the patient about the need for glucose control. Recommended HgA1c value is 6.5% (Frykberg, 2002). This roughly estimates a blood glucose level of 120 mg/dL. Optimal glucose control is currently 70 to 110 mg/dL. Assess the patient's knowledge of diabetes and glucose control, and reinforce areas where it is lacking. If necessary, a consultation with a diabetes educator can refresh the patient's knowledge and address knowledge deficits about the disease. Diabetes education classes provide a foundation for the beginning of a lifetime of disease management. High levels of glucose impair wound healing, and it is important to control the blood sugar very early in wound care management. Careful monitoring and blood sugar should extend beyond wound healing and into the remodeling phase.

Smoking

The association between cigarette smoking and delayed wound healing is a common phenomenon in the clinical setting. The effects of nicotine, carbon monoxide, and hydrogen cyanide contained in cigarettes are the culprits that impact the normal rate of wound healing. Nicotine has the following effects on the tissues, which result in delayed wound healing:

- It is a vasoconstrictor that reduces blood flow to the skin, resulting in a loss of oxygen and nutrients, ischemia, and impaired healing of injured tissue.

- It increases platelet aggregation, thereby increasing the risk of thrombotic microvascular occlusion and tissue ischemia.

- It reduces the proliferation of red blood cells, fibroblasts, and macrophages.

Carbon monoxide decreases oxygen transport and slows metabolism. Finally, hydrogen cyanide inhibits the enzyme systems necessary for oxidative metabolism and oxygen transport at the cellular level. The overall effect of smoking on wound healing is a slower healing process. Open wounds are at an increased risk for wound infection and increased scar formation. Patients should be advised to stop smoking prior to elective surgery or when recovering from wounds resulting from trauma, disease, or emergent surgery. The nurse needs to assess the patient for the clinical manifestations of delayed wound healing and report them to the health care provider.

Gerontological Considerations and Comorbidities

Age-related changes in skin occur normally. **Rete pegs** (or epidermal ridges) are protrusions in the fifth layer of the epidermis that extend down into the dermis to help anchor the epidermis to the dermis. In the elderly (as in neonates), the ridges are flatter, failing to anchor the epidermis and making it easier for the epidermis to slide away from the dermis, resulting in skin tears (Figure 67–8 ■, p. 2203). Additionally, sweat glands decrease production, which results in drier skin. The increased incidence of **xerosis** (a skin condition characterized dry, pruritic, cracked, or fissured skin with scaling and flaking) in persons over the age of 60 can be attributed to (1) a decrease in the lipid component of skin, (2) a loss in water retention, and (3) frequent fragranced baths and showering (Norman, 2003). There is decreased dermal thickness causing thinning of the skin, especially along lower legs and forearms, as evidenced by the prominence of skin tears on extremities. Fewer collagen and elastin fibers cause less elasticity (recoil) in the skin. The skin is less effective as a barrier against water loss and bruising. There is a natural loss of thermal regulation, tactile sensitivity, and pain perception. **Senile purpura**, another age-related change, is a type of hemorrhaging under the skin due to thinner, more fragile blood vessels. Senile purpura often occurs at the site of skin tears. All of these factors place an elderly person at higher risk of dehydration, skin tears, burns, and traumatic injury. In addition, wound healing is prolonged in older adults for the following reasons:

- Re-epithelialization takes almost twice as long.

- The rate of wound dehiscence is greater in older adults and thought to be due to the decreased tensile strength of the wound.

- A greater number of comorbidities results in prolonged wound healing. Healing may be prolonged by conditions that result in poor cardiac output or low oxygen-carrying capacity such as heart failure. Diabetes, peripheral vascular disease, and poor nutrition all result in longer healing times in any age population.

Careful attention to aged skin is good prevention. Emollient skin care products help the skin retain moisture. Protect arms and legs from sun and trauma with clothing. Consistent use of sunscreen also is beneficial to prevent skin breakdown. A review of medications that may affect skin is in order. Gentle cleansing and physical assistance are essential.

Preinjury Status

All of the factors described earlier impact the wound healing process. When a patient is admitted, it is essential to assess the physical and emotional status. Lifestyles and habits that will impact healing such as smoking and poor nutrition must be identified. Both physiological and psychological factors alter the rate of wound healing as well as morbidity and mortality. The longer the illness existed before surgery or trauma, and preinjury nutritional status both contribute to rate of wound healing and risk of infection.

Classification of Wounds and Treatment

Several classifications for wounds exist. This chapter covers the most common types of wounds: diabetic, venous, arterial, vasculitic, traumatic, cancer, and pressure wounds. They all come from different origins, and their plans of treatment vary based on wound type. Wound classifications are helpful when documenting wound assessment and care because they tell a history of the wound. For example, identifying a wound as chronic or acute provides an immediate awareness of the direction that wound care should follow and expectations of the healing process. **Chronic wounds** are defined as wounds that do not follow the expected sequence of repair in a timely and uncomplicated manner. **Acute wounds** are recent wounds that are either traumatic or iatrogenic in etiology. Examples of **traumatic wounds** are abrasions, blisters, cuts, bites, stab wounds, gunshot wounds, and burn injuries. **Iatrogenic wounds** include intravenous (IV) puncture sites, incisions, radiation-induced skin damage, and grafts. Acute wounds progress through the stages of wound healing normally.

Chronic wounds generally occur due to inadequate blood supply in the tissue, repeated prolonged insults to the tissue, and disruptive underlying pathologic processes. The wound healing cascade is interrupted at some point by systemic deficiencies or extrinsic insults. Examples of chronic wounds are pressure ulcers, diabetic ulcers, vascular ulcers, and fungating tumors. Wounds that do not respond to appropriate treatment within 6 weeks are considered chronic in nature and should be referred to a wound specialist.

The type of wound determines the basic plan of care and treatment for that wound, but keep in mind that everyone responds differently to treatment and that the plan must be individualized. Wound care is not just a science but an art, and "thinking outside the box" has led to a great many strides in aggressive wound care therapy. Described next are classifications to describe further the extent of damage and current phase of healing, including diabetic, venous, arterial, vasculitic, traumatic, pressure, pyoderma gangrenosum, cancer, pressure, fungal, partial thickness and full-thickness wounds, and skin tears.

Diabetic Wounds

Diabetic ulcers are the most common form of chronic ulcer seen in outpatient and inpatient settings (Frykberg, 2002). The most frequent areas to find a diabetic ulcer are on the plantar surface of the foot or toe/metatarsal head (Figure 67–4 ■). The mitigating factors that promote development of a wound in a patient with diabetes are neuropathy, macro/microvascular changes, and a slow, decreased immune response. Neuropathy is decreased or absent sensation in an area due to elevated blood glucose levels that over time affect the myelin sheath surrounding the nerves and degrade the sheath, exposing the nerves. The nerves then die over time without the

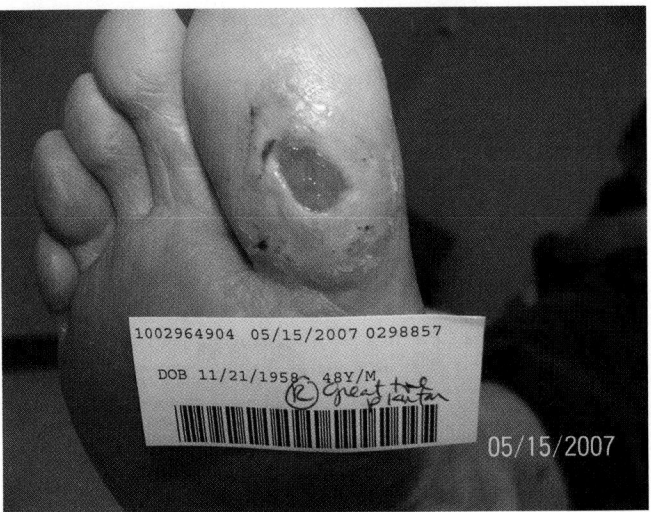

FIGURE 67–4 ■ Diabetic plantar ulcer.
Source: Courtesy of Harold Engle

myelin sheath to protect them from the body's own immune response.

Macro- and microvascular changes are due to elevated blood glucose levels that over time cause fatty deposits to stick to the endothelial lining of vessels and cause narrowing and then blockage of circulation (Porth, 2007). The immune response is also delayed in a patient with diabetes. Although the exact cause is unknown, it has been well documented that a slow response to a wound or infection, and thus slow-to-develop outward signs of a problem, causes a delay in the wound healing process and a delay in alerting the patient with diabetes that a problem is occurring. Delay in seeking care causes a delay in treatment (Shah & Hux, 2003).

Diabetic wounds usually appear on the feet but also may occur in other places on the body. These wounds are typically caused by traumatic injury to the foot because the patient with diabetes suffers from neuropathy, which may result in little or no sensation in the feet. Not being aware of the injury, the patient may continue to traumatize the wound by walking. Two reliable methods of classifying diabetic wounds exist. The original Wagner Ulcer Grade Classification System has been modified to take into account ischemia and infection along with depth of penetration (Chart 67–4). In this system ulcers graded with low scores are less complex. Higher scores indicate more complex ulcers that may require surgical intervention. Wagner's classification system is the

---

CHART 67–4   Wagner Ulcer Grade Classifications

A. **Grade 1:** Superficial diabetic ulcer

B. **Grade 2:** Ulcer extension
1. Involves ligament, tendon, joint capsule, or fascia
2. No abscess or osteomyelitis

C. **Grade 3:** Deep ulcer with abscess or osteomyelitis

D. **Grade 4:** Gangrene to portion of forefoot

E. **Grade 5:** Extensive gangrene of foot

most widely used to describe the natural history of the dysvascular foot, even though evidence of its validity and reliability are lacking (Smith, 2002). Smith (2002) proposes that the University of Texas Wound Classification System—known as the Size (Area and Depth), Sepsis, Arteriopathy, and Denervation (S[AD]SAD) classification system—will become the standard with a detailed breakdown regarding vascularity and infection. The University of Texas classification system for diabetic wounds is in Chart 67–5. New wound care products such as tissue engineered grafts and ointment containing platelet-derived growth factors (Regranex) have been effective treatments. Offloading (relieving the pressure from a specific site) still remains the most likely method of ensuring a plantar or heel ulcer will heal (Steinberg, 2004).

Medical Management

After reviewing the factors affecting a diabetic wound, a plan of care is developed that involves diagnostic studies to evaluate the extent of those factors. A test to check for neuropathy is called the loss of protective sensation (LOPS) test. LOPS uses a monofilament called 5.07 Semmes-Weinstein nylon monofilament, which measures sensation in eight areas in order to determine the extent of neuropathy (Wood et al., 2005). LOPS, arterial Doppler studies to check circulation, cultures of the wound, and basic chemistry and differentials are evaluated to correct any of those factors if possible. Differentials show the various types of immune cells that are present in the body. The main focus is on the percent of neutrophils, because the percentage goes up when an acute reaction occurs in response to infection. Neutrophils, also called PMNs or polymorphonuclear leukocytes, respond to inflammation and have phagocytic (microorganism-killing) properties. The other types of immune cells are eosinophils, which respond to parasitic infections and allergic reactions, and basophils, which respond to leukemia and myelo diseases of the muscle (Porth, 2007). One serious result of a diabetic wound is bone infection, or osteomyelitis. A diagnostic test such as magnetic resonance imaging (MRI), computed tomography (CT), bone scan, or indium scan (tagged white blood cells with indium, a radioactive material) can determine the presence of a bone infection. A biopsy of the bone can be performed as well. A biopsy can be read by a pathologist, and the shape or morphology of the tissue can be determined to be present with infection or not. If aggressive therapy and advance treatment modalities such as hyperbarics (100% oxygen under pressure) are not successful, an amputation may be necessary to protect the patient from an infection that spreads throughout the entire limb, body, and bloodstream. Offloading, the process of relieving pressure, should be accomplished, particularly in the plantar areas, so that compression of the microcirculation due to pressure does not occur. (See the discussion on offloading in the Wound Management section later in this chapter.)

Venous Ulcers

Venous ulcers are another type of chronic wound. Most venous ulcers are on the lower extremities and the pretibial area but can occur almost anywhere on the leg. One recent contributor to the number of venous ulcers that are now observed relates to the vein harvesting for coronary artery bypass grafting. Pregnancy and occupation can also lead to venous congestion and the development of venous ulcers. Venous ulcers are not well defined in their margins from an assessment standpoint. They are accompanied by edema and often hemosiderin staining. **Hemosiderin staining** occurs when the heme part of the red blood cell is deposited in the tissues as red blood cells get trapped and accumulate due to venous congestion (Figure 67–3 ■, p. 2195). As the red blood cell dies, the heme is deposited, and the staining color of brownish hue results. When venous congestion occurs in the lower extremities, the veins are stretched like a rubber band. Over time, the constant stretching of the veins decreases their elasticity (the ability for a rubber band to retract to its original position and shape). There are valves in the veins that open and close and allow venous return to the heart. If the veins become inelastic over time, the valves become incompetent or "leaky" and regurgitate the fluid, allowing pooling of the fluid in the lower extremities. The venous congestion, or edema, now compresses the capillary beds and constricts the fluid's flow in the dermis to feed the skin. If an injury occurs or the fluid accumulates so much that it leaks through the skin pores, bacteria can set in and an ulcer develops.

CHART 67–5	**University of Texas Classification System for Diabetic Wounds**			
Stage	**Grade 0**	**Grade I**	**Grade II**	**Grade III**
A	Preulcerative or postulcerative lesion completely epithelialized	Superficial wound not involving tendon, capsule, or bone	Wound penetrating to tendon or capsule	Wound penetrating to bone or joint
B	Preulcerative or postulcerative lesion completely epithelialized with infection	Superficial wound not involving tendon, capsule, or bone with presence of infection	Wound penetrating to tendon or capsule with presence of infection	Wound penetrating to bone or joint with presence of infection
C	Preulcerative or postulcerative lesion completely epithelialized with ischemia	Superficial wound not involving tendon, capsule, or bone with presence of ischemia	Wound penetrating to tendon or capsule with presence of ischemia	Wound penetrating to bone or joint with presence of ischemia
D	Preulcerative or postulcerative lesion completely epithelialized with infection and ischemia	Superficial wound not involving tendon, capsule, or bone with presence of infection and ischemia	Wound penetrating to tendon or capsule with presence of infection and ischemia	Wound penetrating to bone or joint with presence of infection and ischemia

Source: From Lavery, L. A., Armstrong, D. G., & Harkless, L. B. (1996). Classification of diabetic foot ulcerations. *Journal of Foot and Ankle Surgery, 35*(6), 528.

The decreased circulation does not allow the normal healing process to occur, as the platelets, growth factors, and leukocytes can no longer reach the area of insult and the ulcer becomes worse.

Medical Management

The treatment for the patient is to decrease the edema by compression. Compression therapy will allow pressure to be increased to the lower extremity to promote venous return and decrease venous congestion, allowing the capillary beds at the level of the wound to open and the healing process to occur. The patient should be instructed that the venous congestion is chronic and that, most often, the patient will have to undergo compression therapy of some type for the rest of his life to prevent further ulcers and associated complications. Compression can be achieved by the use of compression stockings, wraps, or a compression pump. One caution before using compression as treatment is to make sure the patient has adequate arterial circulation and no deep venous thrombosis. Performing venous and arterial Doppler ultrasounds can determine flow and presence or lack thereof of a deep venous thrombosis. Another caution is that compression therapy can lead to an increase in the patient's preload volume, and those patients with concurrent cardiac maladies such as heart failure and low ejection fractions may not tolerate the additional volume. These patients must see their cardiologist, and an adjustment on their diuretic therapy may need to occur. In addition to compression therapy, the wound may need to be débrided to allow the healing phases to begin.

Arterial Ulcers

Arterial wounds may perhaps take the longest to heal. They are often located on the malleolar area of the lower extremity (Figure 67–5 ■). They present with a "punched out" appearance with well-defined margins, unlike the venous ulcer. Associated assessment reveals poor palpable pulses and a Doppler may be needed to auscultate the pulse. The lower extremity is cool to the touch, discolored, and hair loss may be evident. Chart 67–6 presents a comparison of arterial and venous ulcers.

Medical Management

An arterial ulcer requires surgical intervention to restore the blood flow. A débridement of the wound should not occur until circulation is restored, because the wound cannot heal at all and a débridement, especially of protective dead skin, can actu-

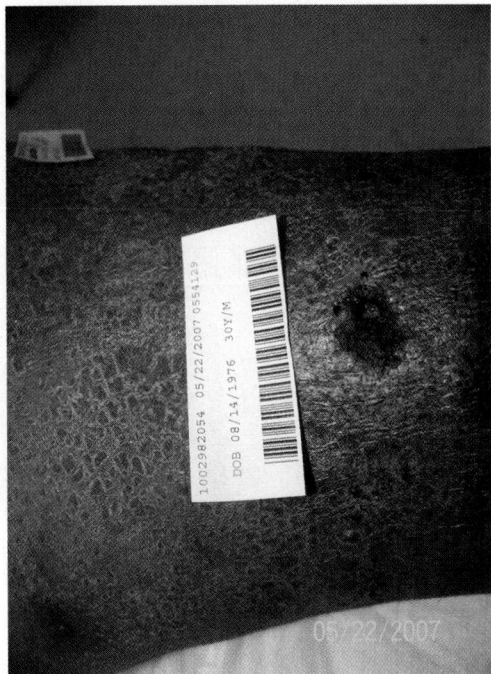

FIGURE 67–5 ■ Arterial ulcer.
Source: Courtesy of Harold Engle

ally worsen the ulcer. With arterial circulation restored, the process of débridement and wound healing can occur, over time.

Vasculitic Ulcers

Vasculitis is the inflammation of the vascular bed system at the micro and possibly macro level that is extremely painful (Figure 67–6 ■, p. 2202). Vasculitic ulcers are associated with collagen vascular disorders such as systemic lupus erythematosus (SLE) or rheumatoid arthritis. They can also occur in patients with other associated vasculitic conditions such as polyarteritis, livedo vasculitis, and Takayasu's disease. Vasculitic ulcers usually present as a small ulcer noted on the leg that appears at first to be benign and inconsequential but takes a long time to make any progress in healing. (Hiok, 1997). These ulcers are more prevalent in females. Vasculitic ulcers are some of the most painful ulcers that a patient can develop.

CHART 67–6	Differing Characteristics of Arterial and Venous Ulcers	
Characteristic	**Arterial Insufficiency Ulcer**	**Venous Stasis Ulcer**
Location	Distal aspect of extremity (toe tips), pressure points on foot	Medial malleolus Distal and lateral aspects
Size and shape	Deep, small craters with well-defined margins	Normally limited to dermis; shallow subcutaneous tissue with irregular margins Can be "pinholes" through which serous fluid leaks
Wound bed	Pale or necrotic	Red or yellow slough, adhering or loose
Volume of exudate	Minimal	Normally large amount
Periwound skin appearance	Pale in color and faint erythema can be seen	Macerated, crusted, or scaling
Pain	Cramping or constant deep-aching pain	Variable; dull, aching, intermittent burning, etc.

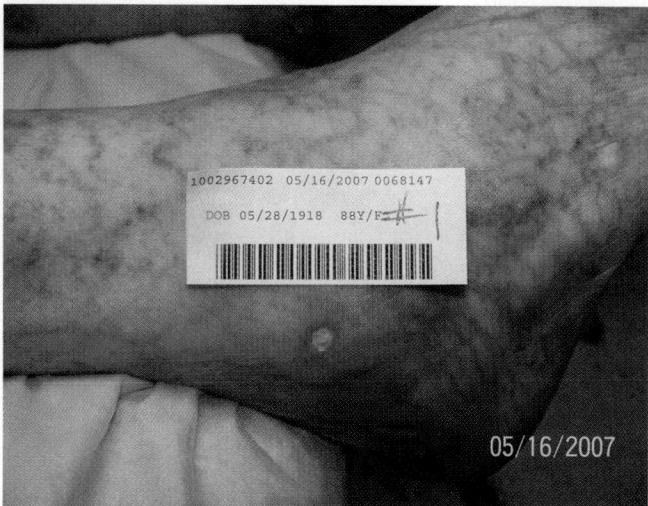

FIGURE 67–6 ■ Vasculitis.
Source: Courtesy of Harold Engle

Medical Management

A biopsy can be taken to confirm the diagnosis of a vasculitic ulcer because the pathogenesis of the process is not fully known. Medications such as pentoxifylline, dapsone, calcium channel blockers, and corticosteroids have been used in the treatment of the ulcer.

Traumatic Wounds

Traumatic wounds develop from some type of blunt or sharp trauma. Adequate cleaning and removal of foreign debris are the most important steps in the healing of these wounds because infection causes a delay in the healing process. Comorbidities such as diabetes, heart failure, and autoimmune disorders may contribute to the severity and response to the healing process of these wounds.

Medical Management

Prophylactic antibiotic therapy can assist in the progress of healing. If an affected area is down to exposed bone, osteomyelitis is a risk. Skin grafts and flaps may be required to cover any areas of missing tissue that cannot be replaced. The patient and family must be educated on signs and symptoms of infection, dehiscence, or evisceration, discussed later in the chapter.

Pyoderma Gangrenosum

Pyoderma gangrenosum is an uncommon dermatosis that can be diagnosed with a biopsy of the affected skin. It presents as small red bumps that may look like an insect bite. The reddened areas open up over time as sores and have a reddish-purple hue around the margins. They most often occur on the legs but may affect other areas of the body as well. Pyoderma gangrenosum is rare and treatable but also may return in the future. Treatment may include a combination of corticosteroids and immunosuppressants in addition to good general wound care (MayoClinic.com, 2006).

Cancer

Wounds that have been identified as unable to heal over an extended period of time (months to years) and not classified as another type of wound may be suspected as cancerous (Figure 67–7 ■). A biopsy of the wound can confirm this suspicion. Usu-

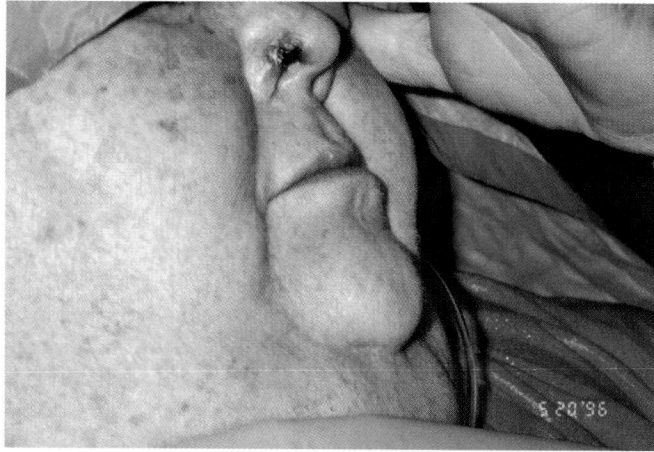

FIGURE 67–7 ■ Cancer lesion.
Source: Jan Clark

ally, the wound has irregular margins, irregular hues of color, and the skin in the affected area may be friable and unhealthy in general appearance.

Medical Management

Removal of the affected cancerous lesions via surgery is the treatment of choice along with possibly immunosuppressants or radiation therapy, depending on severity. The patient should be instructed to inspect her skin vigilantly on a routine basis, have a caregiver inspect the hard-to-visualize areas of the body, and report any suspicious-looking areas to her primary health care provider or dermatologist.

Partial Thickness or Full-Thickness Wound Depths

The current discussion among wound care experts is that staging pressure ulcers should give way to a simpler method of describing injury that is appropriate for all wounds, including pressure ulcers: A wound is either a partial thickness or a full-thickness injury. Partial thickness wounds involve only the skin layers of the epidermis and/or part of the dermis. These wounds are shallow and appear bright pink to red. When they involve the dermis, the wounds may be pale pink with islets of red basement membrane. The **basement membrane** is a thin, acellular layer between the dermis and epidermis. It acts as scaffolding for the epidermis. Blood supply and nutrients reach the epidermis by passing through the basement membrane. Wound healing with partial thickness injuries occurs primarily by epithelialization, which is the migration of epithelial cells from the edges of the wound and from the base of hair follicles, sweat glands, and sebaceous glands. This process continues until the wound is healed.

Full-thickness wounds involve both the epidermis and the dermis and may extend into the subcutaneous tissue, fascia, muscle, and bone. Repair of full-thickness injuries occurs by granulation and wound contraction or with sutures or skin grafts. Chapter 68 ☜ includes a diagram of partial versus full-thickness wound depth.

Medical Management

Partial thickness and full-thickness wounds require an assessment of all factors of wound healing for any deficiencies. Débridement is essential to stimulate the phases of healing and to keep the wound acute so that the body responds to those chemical signals. Prevention of infection and decreasing bioburden will also speed up the healing process. Finally, the proper choice of dressing to maintain an optimal healing environment will facilitate healing as well.

With proper wound management, partial thickness injuries involving only the superficial dermis heal spontaneously in about 2 weeks, and they usually cause no cosmetic or functional impairment. Partial thickness wounds involving the deep dermis heal spontaneously, but may require a prolonged period (greater than 21 days) to do so. These wounds may result in some scar or contracture formation. Closure of full-thickness injuries occurs by granulation, epithelial migration, contracture, and/or surgical intervention.

Skin Tear Classifications

Skin tears (Figure 67–8 ■) are common in elderly patients whose skin has become fragile and thin. Payne-Martin Classification for Skin Tears provides health care providers with a means to enhance documentation and track outcomes of care. It improves assessment, prevention, and treatment of skin tears. The system uses three categories based on the amount of tissue lost (Chart 67–7).

Nurses should recognize patients at risk for skin tears. Some factors to be considered are age, condition of skin, use of steroids, unsteady balance and gait, easy bruising, and vision impairment. Prevention of skin tears includes avoiding use of harsh soaps and alcohol-based cleansers; using a patting motion to clean and dry skin; avoiding scrubbing skin; applying moisturizers; and adding padding to wheelchair arms, bed rails, and other objects that can do harm. Consider long sleeve clothing, long socks with the toes cut out, or commercial arm protectors to protect upper extremities. Educate staff, family, and caregivers to use caution in repositioning those patients at risk.

Nurses need to take special care when removing tape from patients' skin that is at high risk for skin tears. Hold the skin down as the tape is being pulled off. Best of all, do not use tape on the skin, but bandage and put the tape on the bandage.

Medical Management

Treatment of skin tears should include irrigating the tear with saline and trying to reposition any skin flap back in place. Skin flaps that are kept moist are more likely to adhere and heal. Use of adhesive tapes or transparent films can result in additional skin tears. Steri-Strips stay in place but become crusted with dry blood and can harbor pathogens. Preferred dressings should be nonadherent such as foam, hydrogel sheets, and alginates that are absorbent and become gel like. Some health care providers handling wound care have had success with zinc-impregnated gauze wraps secured with an elastic-like tape, such as Coban, on the zinc wrap itself and not stretched tight. These dressings can be left for several days without being changed if the wound drainage is minimal.

Telfa dressings are also widely utilized for skin tears. Telfa is a nonstick application that protects the wound from outside injury or infection, has some absorptive properties, and allows the dressing to be removed without further damage to the skin.

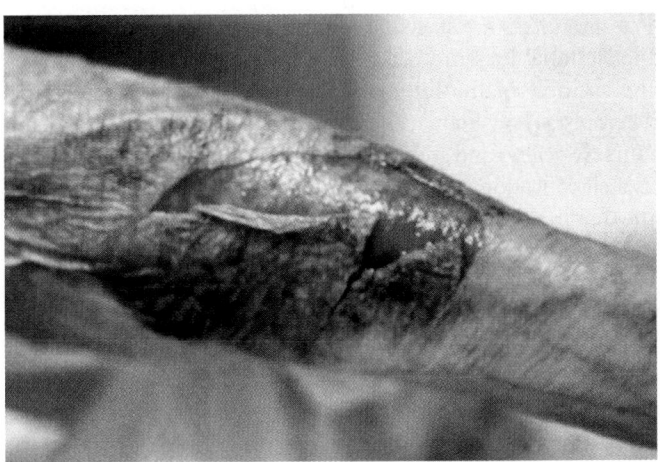

FIGURE 67–8 ■ Skin tear.
Source: Jan Clark

CHART 67–7	Payne-Martin Classification and Treatment for Skin Tears
Category	**Description**
Category I:	Skin tear without tissue loss. A. Linear type: epidermis and dermis pulled apart as if an incision has been made. B. Flap type: epidermal flap completely covers the dermis to within 1 millimeter of the wound margin.
Category II:	Skin tear with partial tissue loss. A. Scant tissue loss: a loss of 25% or less of the epidermal flap. B. Moderate to large tissue loss: loss of more than 25% of the epidermal flap.
Category III:	Skin tear with complete tissue loss. No epidermal flap: black (necrosis), yellow drainage, pink or red granulation tissue completely exposed.
Treatment	
Appropriate skin tear treatment Little or no bleeding	Adhesive dressings or tapes should never be used to secure dressings onto fragile skin. A moisture barrier applied to periwound skin will help protect it and prevent further trauma. A gauze bandage wrapped around the extremity should be secured with tape onto the bandage, not the skin. Hydrogel sheet dressings or foam. Foam dressings.
Moderate bleeding	Zinc-impregnated gauze and cotton Webril wrapped around extremity, secured with Coban on bandage; none of it should be wrapped tightly.

Pressure Ulcers

Pressure ulcers develop when pressure causes decreased circulation to an area. The compression interferes with the tissue blood supply, leading to vascular insufficiency, tissue anoxia, and cell death, resulting in tissue necrosis. According to the National Pressure Ulcer Advisory Panel (NPUAP) (2007b), "A **pressure ulcer** is localized injury to the skin and/or underlying tissue usually over a bony prominence, as a result of pressure, or pressure in combination with shear and/or friction." Pressure ulcers are often related to the elderly, but that is not the only at-risk population for the disease. Patients with paraplegia, those with quadriplegia, those who have had strokes, patients with depression, and anyone who is not moving or will not move to relieve pressure off an affected area can develop a pressure ulcer. The most common areas of where pressure develops are those areas when lying in a bed or sitting in a chair or wheelchair that come in contact with the surface. Heels, sacral areas, ischial areas, and the lower back are the most common areas. Other areas include the elbows, the occiput of the head, the spine, and even the ears. The ears can develop pressure ulcers as a result of long-term oxygen use with a nasal cannula. The nasal cannula is held in position behind the ears, and time can cause that area to develop a pressure ulcer.

Etiology of Pressure Ulcers

Pressure ulcers occur when pressure, due to the compression of the skin between bone and another surface over time, impedes blood flow causing tissue ischemia leading to necrosis and ulcer formation. There can be deep internal pressure causing deep internal tissue damage with no evident epidermal damage, or the pressure can be evident first in the epidermal tissue. Pressure ulcers are caused by intrinsic and extrinsic factors. Intrinsic factors are defined as the internal conditions that exist related to the patient's physical or mental health such as nutritional status, mobility, incontinence, age, and skin condition. Extrinsic factors are derived from the environment such as skin hygiene, medication, shear, and friction. Shear occurs as the skeleton moves against the muscles and other internal structures, causing the tissues to be pulled in opposite directions. This causes the bone to rub against the internal structures and distorts the shape of the capillaries, causing them to be occluded and contributing to the formation of a pressure ulcer. Friction occurs when the body moves against an unyielding surface causing the epidermis to be stripped away and ulcers to form (Baranoski, 2006). Common sites for pressure ulcers are seen in Chart 67–8.

CHART 67–8	Common Sites for Pressure Ulcers

Patient Position	Pressure Ulcer Sites
Supine	Scapula, occiput, sacrum, heels
Lateral	Ear, shoulder, trochanter, medial knee, malleolus, foot edge
Prone	Nose, forehead, chest, iliac crests, foot edge, toes

Risk Factors for Pressure Ulcer Development

Risk factors have been identified that make a patient more prone to the development of a pressure ulcer. Risk assessment requires the evaluation of the presence of those factors. Patients who have restricted activity, as would occur with quadriplegia, strokes, and fractured hips, are at risk. Not only are these patients inactive, but they also may have decreased sensation preventing them from feeling the pain associated with the development of a pressure ulcer. Patients with poor nutrition are more susceptible. Patients who are very thin or have decreased protein in the diet have skin that is more likely to ulcerate. Patients who have urinary or fecal incontinence or are exposed to other types of moisture such as perspiration, wound drainage, or emesis are more prone to ulcers. Moisture causes a weakening of the cell wall of skin cells and changes the protective pH of the skin, making the skin more susceptible to skin breakdown (Arnold, 2003). The existence of a comorbid condition such as diabetes mellitus, hypertension, respiratory disease, or vascular disease also increases the risk for pressure ulcers.

Pressure Ulcer Staging

Pressure ulcers are staged according to depth of injury. In 1994 the National Pressure Ulcer Advisory Panel (NPUAP) followed the example of the International Association of Enterostomal Therapists (now known as the Wound, Ostomy and Continence Nurses Society) and adopted Shea's descriptions of pressure sores as a classification system of staging pressure ulcers according to the depth of tissue involved. A staging classification system was developed to allow for consistency in the assessment and description of these wounds; however, it should be noted that a wound that is necrotic and covered with eschar cannot be staged because the depth cannot be measured. The National Guidelines box outlines the NPUAP's four stages of pressure ulcers (2007b). In 1992 these stages were incorporated into the clinical practice guidelines for prevention and treatment of pressure ulcers by the Agency for Health Care Policy and Research (AHCPR) (which is now the Agency for Healthcare Research and Quality, or AHRQ). Stage I pressure ulcers were redefined in 1997 to reflect the new knowledge of accumulated clinical experience. The new definition included more subtle skin changes detected by skilled wound/skin assessments, such as skin temperature, tissue consistency, and color inconsistencies of dark skin tones. In 2002, NPAUP proposed a new description, *deep tissue injury* (DTI) to describe the purple ecchymotic injury seen in intact skin that indicates pressure-related injury to subcutaneous tissues, which may develop into a Stage III or IV pressure ulcer even with optimal treatment. Staging describes the tissue involved in a pressure ulcer, but it alone does not provide a basis for determining topical treatment of wounds. Only pressure ulcers can be staged with this classification system (Figure 67–9 ■, p. 2206). Skin tears, diabetic ulcers, surgical wounds, and burn injuries each have their own classification system. Once the ulcer begins to heal, it is not appropriate to use the staging in a reverse order to describe healing. Once an ulcer has reached a certain stage, such as Stage IV, it is always considered a Stage IV ulcer.

Scales for Predicting Pressure Score Risk

Several risk assessment tools exist to determine the probability of pressure ulcer development. They include the Gosnell, Nor-

NATIONAL GUIDELINES for Pressure Ulcer Staging from the National Pressure Ulcer Advisory Panel

Stage of Wound	Guideline
Deep tissue injury (DTI)	Deep tissue injury is a new stage that is characterized by purple or maroon tissue over bony prominence areas from pressure or shear with intact skin. It often feels "boggy" (soft) or indurated (hard). It should be classified as a DTI, and close monitoring for further deterioration should be performed.
Stage I	Intact skin with nonblanchable area of redness. A keynote for other clues, especially for those with darker skin tones, is any change in color, warmth, edema, or pain over a bony prominence area of pressure.
Stage II	Classified most often as an open or fluid-filled blister. Partial thickness avulsion of skin into dermis layer and may present as a shallow open ulcer.
Stage III	Involves full-thickness loss in which the hypodermis or subcutaneous fat layer may be exposed. It may be shallow or deep, depending on the amount of hypodermis tissue.
Stage IV	Full-thickness wound with exposed tendon, muscle, and/or bone. Most often has slough (dead cells) or eschar (dead tissue). Assessment for undermining and tunneling is prudent as they most often accompany this stage of wound. Again, one cannot use depth to determine the stage because certain anatomic locations may have less depth to tendon, muscle, and/or bone.
Unstageable	Eschar and/or slough that covers the wound area cannot be staged because the underlying tissue cannot be assessed. It is therefore classified as unstageable until the eschar is removed, and then the wound should be documented related to its defining characteristics.

Source: National Pressure Ulcer Advisory Panel (NPUAP). (2007b). Updated staging system. Pressure ulcers stages revised by NPUAP. Retrieved September 1, 2007, from http://www.npuap.org/pr2. htm. "Reproduction of the National Pressure Ulcer Advisory Panel (NPUAP) materials in this document does not imply endorsement by the NPUAP of any products, organizations, companies, or any statements made by any organization or company."

ton, Braden Scale, and other versions developed for specific institutions or populations or for items considered such as concurrent pressure ulcer, comorbidities, age, and continence issues. The Braden Scale for Predicting Pressure Sore Risk is the most widely used and most clinically validated tool that allows nurses and other health care providers to score a patient's level of risk for developing pressure ulcers reliably (Figure 67–10 ■, p. 2207). There are institutional variations of the Braden scale to serve special populations such as in pediatric and intensive care units. The scale consists of six categories with subscales: sensory perception, moisture, activity, mobility, nutrition, and friction and shear. Each category and subscale condition needs to have a score assigned to it for an individual patient. The first category is sensory perception. The patient can be awake and alert with no impairment, partially paralyzed or in a coma and totally unresponsive, and anywhere in between. The nurse decides where on that range the patient is closest. The moisture score pertains to perspiration as well urinary and fecal incontinence. Activity refers to bed rest, up to chair, ambulate, and up ad lib. The subscales of nutrition are given very specific parameters. Some institutions have substituted prealbumin values in some of the ranges. Each category is assigned a score of 1 to 4 with the exception of friction and shear. The scores are assigned and added up. Lower scores indicate higher risk of pressure ulcer development. The highest score is 23 and the lowest is 6. A score of 18 or lower indicates a risk for pressure ulcer development. The nurse can look at the subscales and identify specific risks and implement prevention interventions.

A second widely used scale to predict the risk for pressure ulcer development is the Norton Scale (Figure 67–11 ■, p. 2208). It was originally developed in 1960, was subsequently modified, and is still being used (Halek & Mayer, 2002). The modified Norton Scale uses a point system to assess the patient's physical con-

dition, mental condition, activity, mobility, and incontinence. Points are assigned to each area based on the nurse's assessment. Higher points are assigned to higher function. Therefore, a score of 25 or less places a patient at risk for pressure ulcers. The lower the score, the higher the risk for the development of a pressure ulcer. The risk is identified as: low (25–24 points); medium (23–19 points); high (18–14 points); and very high (13–9 points).

Pressure ulcer prevention interventions should be outlined in the institution's policy and procedure manual and be based on the recommendations of the nationally accepted standards of care for pressure ulcers: the Agency for Health Care Policy and Research (AHCPR) Publication No. 92-0047, *Pressure Ulcers in Adults: Prediction and Prevention* (1992), and Publication No. 95-0652, *Treatment of Pressure Ulcers in Adults* (1994). The subsequently published Wound, Ostomy and Continence Nurses Society's (WOCN) *Guideline for Prevention and Management of Pressure Ulcers* (2003) is a secondary review of the literature and an establishment of a level of evidence rating. It supports the findings and recommendations of the original AHCPR guidelines, with the agency now known as the Agency for Healthcare Research and Quality (AHRQ).

Medical Management

Prevention is the key to pressure ulcers, and education of the patient and family/caregiver can provide the patient with the ability to prevent or at least minimize the development in the future. Once a pressure ulcer develops, the goals of treatment are to maintain or improve oxygenation to the area, prevent infection, and promote healing. Many products may be used to treat pressure ulcers. Some work by absorbing exudate and keeping the skin dry; some products débride the wound, whereas others are used for protection and insulation of the wound. Treatment decisions are generally guided by the stage of the ulcer. For Stage I

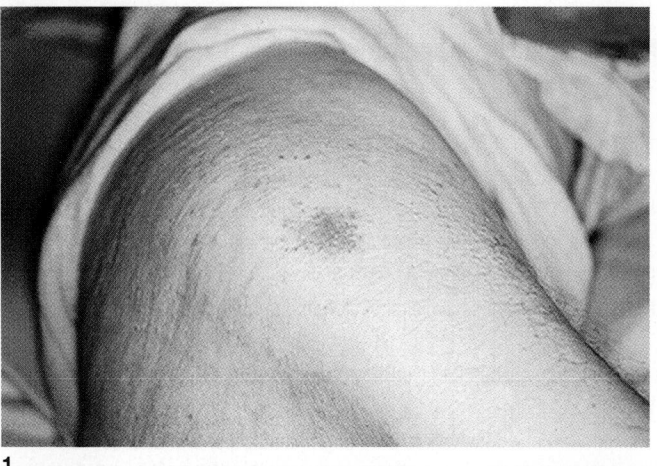

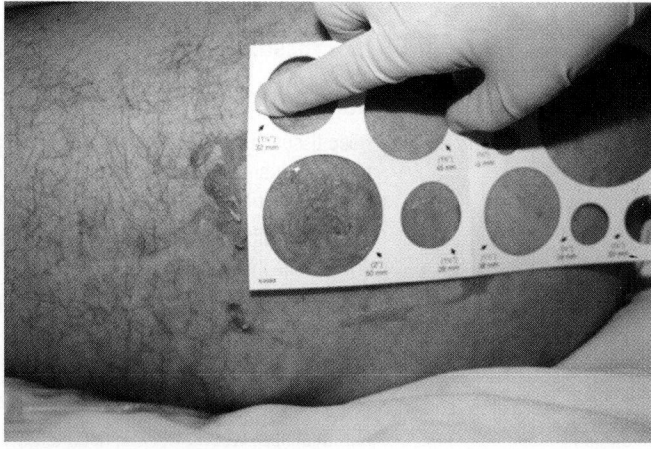

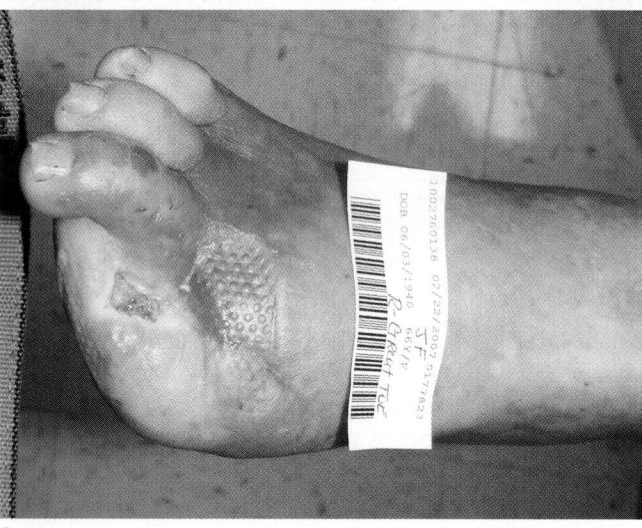

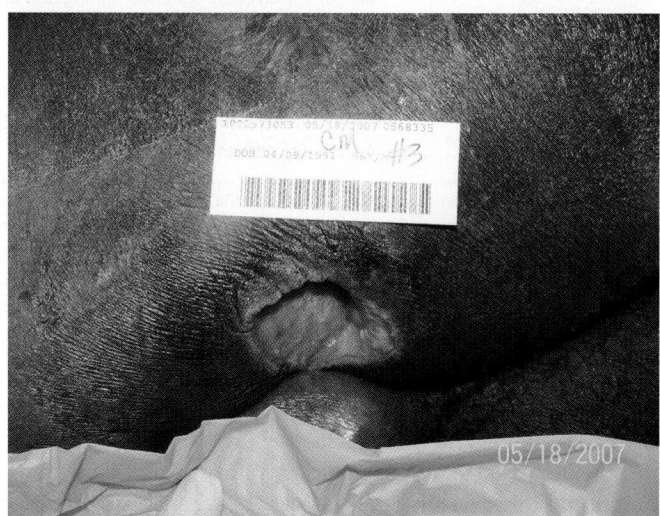

FIGURE 67–9 ■ Four stages of pressure ulcers.
Source: 1, 3, 4: Courtesy of Harold Engle; 2: Jan Clark

ulcers, frequent turning and removal of pressure should be done to prevent progression of the ulcer. Stage II and Stage III ulcers need a moist healing environment. Stage IV wounds maybe require débridement either surgically or mechanically through dressings or enzymes. Normal saline, hydrogen peroxide, or other commercial cleansers can be used to clean the ulcer. Minimal pressure should be used during cleaning to avoid trauma to the tissues in the wound bed. Topical dressings may be used to protect the wound and keep it moist and insulated. It may be necessary to pack the wound to fill dead space and tunnels. Adjunct therapies such as hyperbaric oxygen, application of growth factor, biosynthetic agents, and negative pressure therapy may be used, which are discussed later in this chapter.

■ Nursing Management

Once a pressure ulcer develops, the nurse is responsible for assessing the wound at periodic intervals for improvement and response to treatment. The nursing process provides a framework for the management of patients with pressure ulcers. An assessment of pressure ulcers starts with accurate documentation. The Centers for Medicare & Medicaid Services (CMS) is changing how one codes a pressure ulcer. A pressure ulcer will now be

coded as community acquired (outside of the area one is working) or hospital acquired (developed in the area in which one is working). CMS will not reimburse for hospital acquired pressure ulcers, and documentation is the key on admission of the patient.

Assessment

An in-depth assessment can identify patients at risk, and actions can be taken to prevent the development of a pressure ulcer. The National Institute for Health and Clinical Excellence (NICE, 2005) supports that the skin should be inspected daily to observe for any changes in skin condition. The nurse must assess and document the location of the wound because that can provide clues about the cause of the ulcer. A wound on the ischial tuberosity would suggest pressure during sitting, whereas a wound over the sacrococcygeal area indicates shear along with pressure (Arnold, 2003). The size of the wound should be assessed and documented with the patient in the same position each time. The wound's greatest length, greatest width, and depth at the deepest point should be noted. It is important to identify any sinus tracts or undermining, and the presence of any foreign bodies in the wound. The "red, yellow, black" system (see the Wound Assessment section later in this

Braden Risk Assessment Scale

NOTE: Bed and chairbound individuals or those with impaired ability to reposition should be assessed upon admission for their risk of developing pressure ulcers. Patients with established pressure ulcers should be reassessed periodically.

Patient Name: _____ Room Number: _____ Date: _____

Sensory Perception	**1. Completely Limited**	**2. Very Limited**	**3. Slightly Limited**	**4. No Impairment**	Indicate Appropriate Numbers Below
Ability to respond meaningfully to pressure-related discomfort	Unresponsive (does not moan, flinch or grasp) to painful stimuli, due to diminished level of consciousness or sedation. OR limited ability to feel pain over most of body surface.	Responds only to painful stimuli. Cannot communicate discomfort except by moaning or restlessness. OR has a sensory impairment which limits the ability to feel pain or discomfort over 1/2 of body.	Responds to verbal commands, but cannot always communicate discomfort or need to be turned. OR has some sensory impairment which limits ability to feel pain or discomfort in 1 or 2 extremities.	Responds to verbal commands. Has no sensory deficit which would limit ability to feel or voice pain or discomfort.	
Moisture	**1. Constantly Moist**	**2. Very Moist**	**3. Occasionally Moist**	**4. Rarely Moist**	
Degree to which skin is exposed to moisture	Skin is kept moist almost constantly by perspiration, urine, etc. Dampness is detected every time patient is moved or turned.	Skin is often, but not always, moist. Linen must be changed at least once a shift.	Skin is occasionally moist, requiring an extra linen change approximately once a day.	Skin is usually dry. Linen only requires changing at routine intervals.	
Activity	**1. Bedfast**	**2. Chairfast**	**3. Walks Occasionally**	**4. Walks Frequently**	
Degree of physical activity	Confined to bed.	Ability to walk severely limited or non-existent. Cannot bear own weight and/or must be assisted into chair or wheelchair.	Walks occasionally during day, but for very short distances, with or without assistance. Spends majority of each shift in bed or chair.	Walks outside the room at least twice a day and inside room at least once every 2 hours during waking hours.	
Mobility	**1. Completely Immobile**	**2. Very Limited**	**3. Slightly Limited**	**4. No Limitations**	
Ability to change and control body position	Does not make even slight changes in body or extremity position without assistance.	Makes occasional slight changes in body or extremity position but unable to make frequent or significant changes independently.	Makes frequent though slight changes in body or extremity position independently.	Makes major and frequent changes in position without assistance.	
Nutrition	**1. Very Poor**	**2. Probably Inadequate**	**3. Adequate**	**4. Excellent**	
Usual food intake pattern	Never eats a complete meal. Rarely eats more than 1/3 of any food offered. Eats 2 servings or less of protein (meat or dairy products) per day. Takes fluids poorly. Does not take a liquid dietary supplement. OR is NPO and/or maintained on clear liquids or I.V.'s for more than 5 days.	Rarely eats a complete meal and generally eats only about 1/2 of any food offered. Protein intake includes only 3 servings of meat or dairy products per day. Occasionally will take a dietary supplement. OR receives less than optimum amount of liquid diet or tube feeding.	Eats over half of most meals. Eats a total of 4 servings of protein (meat, dairy products) each day. Occasionally will refuse a meal, but will usually take a supplement if offered. OR is on a tube feeding or TPN regimen which probably meets most of nutritional needs.	Eats most of every meal. Never refuses a meal. Usually eats a total of 4 or more servings of meat and dairy products. Occasionally eats between meals. Does not require supplementation.	
Friction and Shear	**1. Problem**	**2. Potential Problem**	**3. No Apparent Problem**		
	Requires moderate to maximum assistance in moving. Complete lifting without sliding against sheets is impossible. Frequently slides down in bed or chair, requiring frequent repositioning with maximum assistance. Spasticity, contractures or agitation lead to almost constant friction.	Moves feebly or requires minimum assistance. During a move, skin probably slides to some extent against sheets, chair restraints, or other devices. Maintains relatively good position in chair or bed most of the time, but occasionally slides down.	Moves in bed and in chair independently and has sufficient muscle strength to lift up completely during move. Maintains good position in bed or chair at all times.		

NOTE: Patients with a total score of 16 or less are considered to be at risk of developing pressure ulcers.
(15 or 16 = low risk; 13 or 14 = moderate risk; 12 or less = high risk)

Total Score:

© Copyright Barbara Braden and Nancy Bergstrom, 1988

FIGURE 67–10 ■ Braden Risk Assessment Scale.
Source: Barbara Braden and Nancy Bergstrom.

The Norton Scale

NOTE: Scores of 14 or less rate the patient as 'at risk'

	Physical Condition		Mental Condition		Activity		Mobility		Incontinence		Total Score
	Good	1	Alert	1	Ambulant	1	Full	1	Not	1	
	Fair	2	Apathetic	2	Walk/help	2	Slightly	2	Occasional	2	
	Poor	3	Confused	3	Chairbound	3	Limited	3	Usually-urine	3	
	Very bad	4	Stupor	4	Bedridden	4	Very limited, Immobile	4	Doubly	4	
Name: Date:											
Name: Date:											
Name: Date:											
Name: Date:											
Name: Date:											
Name: Date:											
Name: Date:											
Name: Date:											

FIGURE 67–11 ■ Norton Scale.

Source: Doreen Norton, Rhoda McLaren, and A. N. Exton-Smith, *An Investigation of Geriatric Nursing Problems in Hospital,* copyright National Corporation for the Care of Old People (now Centre for Policy on Ageing), London, 1962.

chapter) is often used to describe the wound bed with black indicating eschar, yellow indicating subcutaneous tissue or devitalizing necrotic tissue, and red indicating the presence of muscle or granulation tissue (Arnold, 2003). The color of the wound bed can provide information about the vascular supply, presence of infection, nutritional status, and presence of healthy versus necrotic tissue. The presence of exudates should be noted, paying particular attention to the amount, color, consistency, and odor. The characteristics of the exudates can provide clues to the presence and type of infection. The presence of pain both during dressing changes and separate from dressing changes should be noted. Periwound description, drainage, presence of infection, and tissue type (eschar, slough, and granulation) are also to be recorded. Record a concise history with comorbidities, past treatments, pain scale, and any psychosocial aspects that impact the plan of care. Risk scales such as the Braden scale or Norton Scale should be performed to identify those at risk. Interventions will be derived from the risk score.

Newer technology includes pressure mapping, which is a form of computerized technology that allows for the assessment of areas of increased pressure. A thin mattress or sensor pad is placed under the patient and is connected to a computer screen. The screen then shows the patient's pressure points (Hanson, Langemo, Anderson, Hunter, & Thompson, 2006). This allows the nurse to identify patient positions that may increase the risk of the development of pressure ulcers and to evaluate the use of a variety of support surfaces.

Nursing Diagnoses

The following nursing diagnoses are related to pressure ulcers:

- *Risk for Infection*
- *Impaired Tissue Integrity*
- *Ineffective Tissue Perfusion*
- *Disturbed Body Image.*

Planning

A collaborative and comprehensive approach to wound care is essential. Many hospitals have wound care protocols, and others have wound care nurses or teams designed specifically to accomplish the task of leading the plan of care. Dieticians, case managers, social workers, consultative health care providers (cardiovascular, infectious diseases, surgeons, and plastic surgeons), nursing staff, and ancillary staff should be part of the plan of care, as all play a role in the prevention and treatment of pressure ulcers. The plan must focus on alleviating pressure, treatment of existing ulcer with sound wound care, education, nutrition, rehydration, mobility, and bed support surfaces (if applicable). Here are some examples of interventions as they relate to the Braden scale scores:

Low Risk (15–18)

1. Keep skin clean and dry.
2. Use moisturizer on dry skin.
3. Do not massage bony prominences.
4. Protect skin from moisture; use underpads and briefs.
5. Use skin-protecting ointments (Aloe Vesta or equivalent) to protect skin exposed to urine, stool, or wound drainage.
6. Decrease friction and shear.
7. Increase mobility and activity as tolerated.
8. Assess skin daily.

Moderate Risk (13–14)

1. ALL OF THE ABOVE+
2. Wound care coordinator evaluation.
3. Use lift pads/trapeze (trapeze requires health care provider's order) to minimize friction and shear.
4. Consider a pressure reduction device on the beds and chair.
5. Consider utilizing a turning schedule.
6. Encourage proper dietary intake, and consider a dietician consult.
7. If bed- or chair-bound, reposition the patient every 1 to 2 hours.
8. Protect heels and elbows; elevate heels off the bed surface, and use pillows between knees.
9. Increase mobility and activity in patients that are bed- or chair-bound.

High Risk (10–12)

1. ALL OF THE ABOVE +
2. Consult dietitian and wound care coordinator evaluation (must enter as consult evaluations in computer).
3. Elevate head of bed only as necessary for meals, treatments, and as medically necessary.
4. Obtain order from health care provider for pressure reduction/relief therapeutic bed.

Note: Low air loss beds do not substitute for turning.

Very High Risk (9 or below)

1. ALL OF THE ABOVE+
2. Obtain order from health care provider for pressure relief therapeutic bed.

A head-to-toe assessment can determine areas where pressure ulcers are already developed or at-risk areas. Bed support services can reduce or relieve pressure as can gel cushions for wheelchairs. Pressure mapping, as described earlier, can determine a patient's "hot areas" where pressure in a wheelchair is the most intense, and a special wheelchair pad can be customized to redistribute the pressure to other areas of less concern.

Outcomes and Evaluation Parameters

In an acute care setting in which an average length of stay is 4 to 5 days, one will not see great improvement of a pressure ulcer in regard to dimensions. However, changes in the amount of drainage, the size and appearance of the periwound area, and the clinical manifestations of infection are noticeable in this time frame. At a minimum, one should not see regression of the pressure ulcer.

The National Pressure Ulcer Advisory Panel (NPUAP) developed a tool to document healing of the pressure ulcer. This tool, known as the Pressure Ulcer Scale for Healing (or PUSH) tool, requires assessing and scoring of the ulcer based on three elements: length times width, exudate amount, and tissue type. The scores are summed and graphed over time so that changes in the ulcer can be monitored. If the score goes down, the wound is healing; and if the score goes up. the wound is deteriorating (NPUAP, 1998). Other methods for evaluation may be similar to the PUSH tool in looking at other factors in healing. An example of the PUSH tool is shown in Chart 67–9 (p. 2210) (NPUAP, 2007a).

Interventions and Rationales

The first intervention is to relieve the pressure. It may be as easily accomplished as using pillows to offload, turning at least every 2 hours or less, or as concrete as pressure reduction or relief devices such as the bed support surfaces. It may require an offloading device such as a shoe or sometimes a total contact cast. The rationale for this first intervention is obvious, as the source of the ulcer was the pressure. Next the existing pressure ulcer must be treated with good wound care and an appropriate selection of dressings. An appropriate dressing promotes the optimum wound environment and serves as protection from outside insult. Dressings are described in detail in the Wound Management section later in this chapter.

The nurse must also assess for incontinence with regard to the specific area around the perineum. Incontinence causes the skin to break down. Acids from the urine and/or stool, along with a warm, moist environment, can be an enhancement for fungal and yeast growth. Moisture barrier and antifungal/antiyeast creams protect and promote good healthy skin in an environment where incontinence occurs. One may also consider an indwelling catheter or a diverting colostomy to remove the incontinence from an existing pressure ulcer.

Nutrition supplementation is an essential intervention. Protein is the building block for collagen synthesis, interstitial fluid balance, granulation, and epithelialization. Vitamins and minerals support the chemical agents of healing as cofactors. Vitamins also have antioxidant properties to prevent free radical formation and ensure healthy skin reproduction. ProMod or other supplements can be added to gastrostomy feedings or as dietary supplements on trays. The patient should have an intake of sufficient calories and protein to prevent weight loss and maintain normal prealbumin levels.

Baths should be given only when needed to avoid drying out the skin. When bathing, use gentle cleansers with warm, not hot,

CHART 67–9 **NPUAP PUSH Tool**

Observe and measure the pressure ulcer. Categorize the ulcer with respect to surface area, exudate, and type of wound tissue. Record a sub-score for each of these ulcer characteristics. Add the sub-scores to obtain the total score. A comparison of total scores measured over time provides an indication of the improvement or deterioration in pressure ulcer healing.

Length × Width	0	1	2	3	4	5	Sub-score
	0 cm²	<0.3 cm²	0.3–0.6 cm²	0.7–1.0 cm²	1.1–2.0 cm²	2.1–3.0 cm²	
		6	**7**	**8**	**9**	**10**	
		3.1–4.0 cm²	4.1–8.0 cm²	8.1–12.0 cm²	12.1–24.0 cm²	>24.0 cm²	
Exudate Amount	0	1 Light	2 Moderate	3 Heavy			Sub-score
	None						
Tissue Type	0	1	2	3	4		Sub-score
	Closed	Epithelial Tissue	Granulation Tissue	Slough	Necrotic Tissue		
							Total Score

Source: National Pressure Ulcer Advisory Panel (NPUAP). (2007a). Updated staging system. Retrieved October 1, 2007, from http://www.npuap.org/push3-0.htm. "Reproduction of the National Pressure Ulcer Advisory Panel (NPUAP) materials in this document does not imply endorsement by the NPUAP of any products, organizations, companies, or any statements made by any organization or company."

water. The skin should be kept well hydrated with nonalcohol moisturizers used for dry skin. Friction during bathing and massage over bony prominences should be avoided because it can cause additional tissue damage. It is important to use proper positioning and to use techniques to avoid friction when moving the patient. Friction can also be avoided by using cornstarch. If incontinence occurs, the skin should be cleansed at the time of soiling, a topical moisture barrier should be applied, and absorbent underpads or briefs should be used to provide a quick drying surface.

Positioning is important in the prevention of pressure ulcers. The goal is to get the patient mobile and active as soon as possible; however, when mobility is physically impossible, the patient's position should be changed a minimum of every 2 hours. A sufficient number of people should be available to move the patient so that shearing and friction during movement can be avoided. Assistive devices such as transfer boards or mechanical lifts may be helpful to minimize tissue injury during movement. The "rule of 30" is used for positioning. This rule states that the head of the bed should be elevated 30 degrees or less and the body placed in a 30-degree laterally inclined position when placed on either side. These positions avoid pressure directly over the trochanter and promote improved circulation to the skin over the sacrum and ischial tuberosities (Black et al., 2007). Pillows or foam wedges may be used to keep the patient properly positioned. The prone position may also be used if the patient is able to tolerate it. Attention should be focused on maintaining proper alignment so that functional ability can be maintained.

Education is the main key to keeping the plan of treatment on the right track postdischarge. The next level of care must be communicated too as far as the plan of care and past failures and successes. The family must be active participants if the patient is being discharged home. Home health help may be needed to continue support and evaluation as well as continued education. The patient and family must know how to prevent further pressure ulcers from developing as well as early intervention and the resources available to them. Education is essential for the future success of the patient with pressure ulcers, as most often the conditions are chronic and the environment for continued deterioration still exists.

Evaluation

A plan for care of pressure ulcers should be reevaluated regularly to make sure the plan is still effective. Any change in the patient's condition could have a negative impact on the wound healing process, and reevaluation of effectiveness of the plan of care should occur. In a long-term care setting, reevaluation should be done weekly and documented, and interventions and plans of care changed if the current treatment plan is unsuccessful. An evaluation criterion of progress would be a decrease in the size and depth of the wound. If this is not occurring, then the wound needs to be assessed as to why the healing is not occurring, such as the presence of infection or decreased tissue perfusion.

◼ Collaborative Management

Collaborative management involves the use of an interdisciplinary team to assist in correcting or optimizing the influential factors involved in wound healing. A health care provider may consult a wound care center and wound care specialist to collaborate. A general or plastic surgeon may be needed for an incision and drainage (I&D), débridement, flap, or other surgical procedure. A registered dietician (RD) may be required to evaluate nutritional status and offer suggestions. A physical therapist may be needed to increase mobility and alleviate pressure from immobility. A pedorthist may be needed to develop specialized footwear and offloading devices to alleviate pressure to wound area. A vascular specialist may be needed to restore circulation to the wound area. An infectious disease health care provider may be needed to follow the patient with an infected wound and provide antibiotic coverage that is appropriate. A social worker or case manager may be needed to ensure that proper wound care follow-up at home is performed and that the patient has that necessary social support system to be at home. Home health care may be needed for advanced wound care and continued evaluation. There could be many disciplines involved in a patient's care to heal a wound, and communication and a good plan of care are necessary to coordinate all the aspects of healing.

Health Promotion

Pressure ulcers occur in 10% to 17% of all hospitalized patients and 20% to 40% of all nursing home patients (Pressure Ulcers, 2005). These figures are important because they forecast the anticipated number of persons needed in health care jobs to take care of the patients with these wounds. The figures also forecast the expense of treating and healing the pressure ulcers. In 2010 the National Pressure Ulcer Advisory Panel (NPUAP) will publish new findings about the rate of pressure ulcer development in conjunction with *Healthy People 2010*, the U.S. Department of Health and Human Services (2000) blueprint for national health goals. One of the many objectives of this federal initiative is to reduce the incidence of pressure ulcers by 50% by the year 2010. With the increased attention of regulatory agencies, pressure ulcer prevention should be of great concern to the nurse.

The goals of the nurse are to identify and teach other caregivers to identify those at risk of developing pressure ulcers and implement prevention. If pressure ulcers should develop, then treatment should reflect good healing rates and efficient expenditures. The institution or agency is expected to achieve implementation of prevention and treatment through the education of its staff. Nursing is actually graded in a report card by the American Nurses Association (ANA) on how successfully pressure ulcers are being prevented and treated. Nurse-sensitive outcome indicators have been established by the ANA to help demonstrate nursing's unique contributions to health care. ANA instituted the Nursing Care Report Card for Acute Care in which 10 specific quality indicators of nursing were developed and defined. One of these indicators is the maintenance of skin integrity. The ANA Safety and Quality Indicator Project national database is growing through participating acute care institutions and is beginning to show evidence that nursing does indeed impact health outcomes (Duffy & Korniewicz, 2000).

Interventions are where the nurse can make a difference with attentive care, expert skills, and critical judgment. Above all things, it is essential that pressure is relieved from the pressure ulcer in order to have healing begin. The cause of the ulcer must be removed to see improvement.

◼ Wound Assessment

Wound assessment requires the use of four of the five senses. Palpation can determine softness (maceration), hardness (induration), or edema. Olfaction can determine infection and dead/slough tissue. Inspection can determine periwound condition, size, and drainage. Auditory sense requires active listening to the patient with regard to pertinent history, past failures/successes for healing, and pain.

Measurement

A wound must be objectively assessed to determine a baseline and effectiveness of a plan of care. Measurements can be made from a head-to-toe reference or longest length and perpendicular width. Either way, the main function of measurements is consistency from a reference standpoint. A wound should be measured for length, width, and depth. The wound is usually measured in centimeters. The depth measurement should be directly perpendicular to the patient's skin and down into the wound and not a measurement parallel to the patient's body. Again, subsequent measurements should use the same point of reference to denote progress or regression adequately. The surface area of the wound is the length multiplied by the width in centimeters squared (cm^2). The volume is the length multiplied by the width and the depth in centimeters cubed (cm^3). A wound routinely heals by decreasing depth first and then contraction by decreasing length and width. That being said, a combination of changes can occur in any dimension, and the volume changes most accurately capture and note wound progression/ regression.

Additional measurements refer to how the wound is shaped underneath the skin surface. A sinus tract is an area, sometimes referred to as a tunnel, where there is nonhealed detached tissue under intact skin. These areas tend to become infected and may develop abscesses if the opening is sealed, blocking drainage. Sinus tracts are measured in centimeters. Referring to location, the area of tunneling is defined on a clock face with 12 o'clock being the head of the body. For example, if a wound located on the anterior aspect of the leg has tunneling on the medial side of the left leg, the measurement would be *x* amount of centimeters at the 9 o'clock position. There is also a measurement for undermining. Undermining is like a cliff without tissue below and more broad, and is measured from each point or side using the clock-face method (Figure 67–12 ◼).

Location

The correct assessment and documentation of the location of the wound is necessary for consistency and accuracy in follow-up of the wound care. There may also be some additional areas of breakdown, and there should be no confusion as to the number

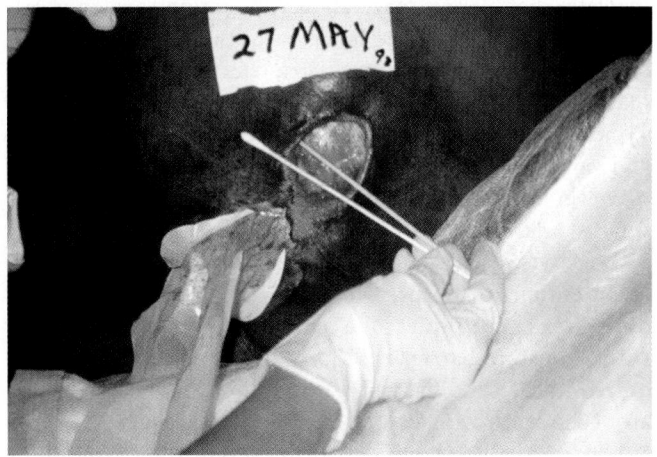

FIGURE 67–12 ◼   Undermining.
Source: Jan Clark

and locations of the wounds so that consistent and accurate documentation can occur. Using words such as *medial, lateral, proximal, distal,* and other anatomic location definitions will give clear and concise information.

Wound Drainage

A wound may have many different types of drainage. The drainage may be sanguineous (bloody), serosanguineous (bloody with plasma fluid), serous (plasma only), or purulent (infected). Sanguineous drainage occurs when there is acute trauma to the vascular bed. It may be a result of further insult either due to environmental causes such as hitting the wound area on a foreign object, or from insult due to intentional causes such as a sharps débridement. Serosanguineous drainage is more related to overall edema leading to capillary weakness and leakage. Serous drainage may occur when edema has forced fluid to move from the intravascular department into the tissue and then leakage through the wound bed. Purulent drainage is a sign of infection and indicates the need for antibiotic therapy and/or silver dressing treatment. The amount and type of drainage are documented in the patient's record at regular intervals.

Bioburden

Bioburden is when foreign material, collagen debris, and other biofilms and breakdown from bacterial load and injury cause a delay in the wound healing process and a decrease in biochemical response to healing. Bioburden may be controlled with a combination of irrigation with a syringe, anti-infective agents, or surfactant cleansers.

Periwound Assessment

The periwound area is defined as the area surrounding the wound base circumferentially. The periwound area is a very important indicator of how severe the wound is and of progression or regression of wound closure. The periwound area may be reddened around the wound base. The reddened area indicates that an acute inflammatory process is occurring that may be due to further injury underlying the skin around the wound or infection. If the periwound area is "boggy" or soft, it indicates that there is maceration. Maceration is when excessive moisture destroys the skin's integrity and leaves the skin layers suboptimal. A hardened area referred to as induration indicates tissue that is edematous, infected, injured, or dead. Typically the induration area is opened to relieve the pressure and remove any dead tissue that may exist. The periwound area may also have a yeast or fungal infection due to use of intravenous, oral, or local antibiotic use.

Effective wound management requires one to pay particular attention to the periwound area. Creams that contain dimethicone can protect the periwound area from drainage with a moisture-barrier effect. A moisture product may be required for dry and flaky periwound skin that may be under an occlusive dressing. Antifungal and yeast creams may be applied to the periwound areas to prevent these conditions that commonly occur after chronic antibiotic use and in dark, moist areas. Some lotions can contain lidocaine, an anesthetic to control pain, or hyaluronic acid to control redness and inflammation.

Wound Descriptions

Describing the appearance of the wound helps determine prognosis and treatment plan. One system of wound description is the red, yellow, black system. Red identifies a beefy-red to pink granular bed and identifies the most common treatment for the wound stage based on that wound bed. The yellow stage identifies a wound with fibrin or slough and a plan of treatment designed for that stage of the wound bed. The black stage is when the wound bed has eschar, and a plan of treatment is designed for that stage as well. It is simple to use because the color system is easily identifiable and easily treatable with a set of guidelines to follow for treatment as described in the next section.

◼ Wound Management

It is essential that the health care team remember that dressings assist in the body's overall ability to heal itself. They are not intended to be a substitute to identifying and treating the underlying causes of a wound. They simply promote an optimal environment for wound healing progression to occur.

Healing can occur by three methods: primary, secondary, or tertiary intention. **Primary intention** is a closure by sutures, stitches, Steri-Strips, or staples. It is utilized when healing is expected within 10 days and new tissue formation is minimally required. **Secondary intention** is a wound that is allowed to remain open to granulate in and contract. Many traumatic and postsurgical wounds are treated in this manner. **Tertiary or third intention** is a delayed closure to allow for drainage of fluid, contamination control, and/or a plan for surgical intervention at a later date (Smith & Nephew Clinical Staff, 2001).

Physiological local wound environment means that through appropriate topical therapies a wound will ultimately return to the characteristics of healthy or normal functioning (Rolstad, Ovington, & Harris, 2000). Principles of topical therapy are derived from scientific studies of the wound healing process and evidence-based practice. These principles are described in this section.

Offloading

Offloading is a very important factor that influences the wound healing process. Offloading is the process of relieving pressure on a bony prominence, callus, or wound. Standing places 50% of one's body weight on each leg. Walking, dependent on the speed, can equal one to one and one-half times the body weight on an affected area. Offloading devices such as boots, wheelchair cushions, splints, and total contact casting can redistribute pressure or relieve pressure entirely, depending on the device. Turning a patient every 2 hours and floating a patient's heels off the bed on pillows are also forms of offloading. The object is to relieve the pressure that causes a decrease in circulation by compression of the capillary beds and localized tissue destruction. The affected area will form a hardened area called a callus to protect the area from further damage (Martin, Oldani, & Claxton, 2005).

Remove Necrotic Tissue and Foreign Bodies or Particles

Foreign bodies or particles in a wound may be there because of trauma (splinters, glass, and grass). When the wound is cleaned, efforts are made to flush out any loose debris. Hydrogen peroxide may be helpful to clean the initial trauma-induced wound; but after its initial use, refrain from cleansing the wound with hydrogen peroxide because when used in full strength it is toxic to the new fibroblasts that are trying to rebuild the wound. The foreign body may be a suture or staple in a wound that has healed over, and now the wound is reopening because the suture or staple may be working its way to the surface of the skin.

Necrotic tissue is devitalized tissue that ranges from the yellow fibrinous slough to a thick, leathery-like dark brown or black scab-like wound, referred to as eschar. Chapter 68 ⊚ discusses burn eschar. Débridement of necrotic tissue is very important because it harbors bacteria. One exception to the rule is eschar covering ischemic wounds, such as dry gangrenous toes. The eschar in an ischemic wound serves as protection against infection, and there is little chance of adequate microcirculation being able to help heal the wound if débrided. The consensus for treatment is painting the ischemic wound with an antiseptic solution such as povidone-iodine and covering it with dry dressings (Drosou, Falabella, & Kirsner, 2003).

Four methods of débridement are sharp, mechanical, enzymatic, and autolytic (Chart 67–10). Sharp débridement is done with scalpel, scissors, or nippers. Anesthetics or the operating room may be required depending on wound size and depth. Mechanical débridement is the dislodging of necrotic tissue, which is accomplished in several ways, including:

- Wet-to-dry dressings are used for mechanical débridement: The slough adheres to the dressing as it dries and is pulled off when the dressing is removed.
- The whirlpool method of débridement also is a mechanical débridement method. It is currently out of favor because of the increased risk of infection and has been replaced with pulse lavage (Vaughn, 2002).
- Pulse lavage is an electrically powered device that emits a regular, automatic interruption of fluid flow with a handheld device. The most common irrigant is saline.

Enzymatic débridement is chemically induced by prescriptive ointments that contain papain urea or collegenase, which penetrates the slough and eschar causing them to soften and "melt down." Once softened, the slough and eschar are mechanically débrided.

Autolytic débridement is allowing the body to utilize the phagocytes to destroy the necrotic tissue. This is often a preferred method of débridement for those persons for whom daily (or more frequent) dressing changes would be a hardship; that is, patients who are critically ill that cannot be turned. Autolytic débridement is a slow and nonaggressive treatment. Occlusive dressings are often used to soften eschar before sharp débridement to avoid débridement of viable tissue. Occlusive dressings are contraindicated on infected wounds.

CHART 67–10 Débridement Methods		
Method	**Advantages**	**Disadvantages**
Sharp Necrotic tissue removed with scalpel, nippers, or scissors.	Can be used on wound with any amount of slough or eschar. Treatment is swift.	Performed by only skilled nurses or health care providers. Patient may experience pain. May require local anesthetic. May require surgical time procedure (known as incision and drainage).
Autolytic Example: Occlusive dressings, such as transparent film, or hydrocolloids cause physiological "melting" of the necrotic tissue by phagocytes.	Pain free. Can be used on any wounds with slough or eschar. Often preferred for patients who are in the intensive care unit (ICU) and may not be able to tolerate the multiple dressing changes necessary after sharp débridement. Transparent films and wound gel are easy methods to use to achieve autolytic débridement.	Requires more time than sharp or enzymatic methods. Cannot use for infected wounds.
Enzymatic Examples: Accuzyme (papain). Panifil. Xenoderm. Urea active ingredient causing disintegration of slough and eschar.	Faster than autolytic, normally. Usually pain free. Can use for infected wounds. Tissue specific.	Patient may be sensitive to active ingredient. Educate patient that method will increase exudate production. Exudate management.
Mechanical Examples: Wet-to-dry dressing is classic example: the pulling away of tissue that has adhered to the dry dressing. Pulse lavage using high-pressure water streams to dislodge necrotic tissue.	Can be used for infected wounds. Removes loose devitalized tissue.	May be painful. Not tissue specific (removes good granulation tissue with necrotic tissue).

Obliterate Dead Space

Dead space refers to tissue destruction under intact surface tissue, such as tunneling or sinus tract formation. Dead space areas provide a fluid medium and a desirable environment for pathogen growth. The nurse needs to probe margins of the wound to identify any tracts, undermining, or tunneling. These areas need to be packed with a retrievable material to prevent the tract from closing prematurely and forming an abscess. Pack these areas with one piece of dressing to obliterate the dead space, always leaving a tail of the packing material to prevent granulation tissue closing over the wound that has packing in it. Always document the size and shape, and direction of the sinus tract or tunnel and how much dressing it took to pack the wound. There is always the possibility of packing material being left in the wound.

 Always use a continuous piece of dressing for packing the wound rather than several small pieces because they might get inadvertently left in the track—especially deep wounds with sinus tracts.

Absorb Excess Exudate

Large amounts of exudates may macerate wound margins. Bacterial toxins in the exudate may inhibit the wound healing process (White & Cutting, 2006). A highly exudating wound also may be infected. Measures to protect the intact periwound skin include using liquid skin barriers, moisture barriers, and absorbent dressings. Dressings past their absorbent capacity should be changed promptly.

Provide Thermal Insulation and Protection

Wounds need to be kept at the body's core temperature. When the temperature of the wound is lowered, leukocyte mobility is impaired, and phagocytic efficiency and affinity of hemoglobin for oxygen are reduced (Enoch & Harding, 2003). These conditions slow wound healing. Therefore, dressing changes need to be done quickly because leaving wounds open without dressings can slow blood flow to the wound and delay epidermal migration due to reduced temperatures. Cleansing a wound can reduce the local tissue temperatures for up to 40 minutes. Mitosis and leukocyte activity can be delayed for up to 3 hours after cleansing. If a dressing change is interrupted, cover the wound with sterile gauze to help slow down temperature reduction in the wound and to protect it from airborne organisms. Protect the healing wound from trauma such as wheelchair legs, furniture, pets, and or other objects that may harm the wound. New trauma disrupts newly formed vessels, connective tissue, and epidermis.

Maintain a Moist Wound Surface

Keeping the wound bed moist prevents desiccation and cell death. It facilitates epithelial migration promotes angiogenesis, and connective tissue synthesis. Additionally, moist wound beds are less painful. Three investigations in the mid-20th century showed that "moist wound healing" was achieved by covering the experimental wounds with an occlusive membrane consisting of thin plastic film. Starting in 1958 with Odland observing that a blister healed faster if it were left unbroken, the idea that dressings were pharmacologic agents was taken

seriously (Odland, 1958). In 1962 Winter showed that occlusion of wounds with a polyethylene film more than doubled the wound healing rate in domestic pigs (Winter, 1962). Hinman and Maiback established the beneficial effect of occlusion on resurfacing of experimental wounds in normal human subjects (Hinman & Maibach, 1963). These principles still hold true today.

A moist wound environment created by occlusive dressings facilitates granulation tissue development through increased gel-matrix secretion, new blood vessel growth, collagen secretion, fibroblast proliferation, and epidermal migration (Smith, 2002). Benefits of moist wound healing are faster epidermal resurfacing and fewer infections.

Protection from maceration of the periwound skin is part of the delicate balance of moist wound healing (Clark, 2002). A variety of products described later support this concept. Products that add moisture, protect from moisture, absorb moisture, and maintain moisture are all available to the health care provider for promotion of optimal wound healing. Moist wound healing is not a new concept, but has been slow to become the automatic choice of health care providers. Moist wound healing has, however, become the mantra of specialists trained in wound care management. These specialists recognize the benefits of occlusive dressings that facilitate moist wound healing. Chart 67–11 outlines dressing categories, characteristics, and uses.

Wound Cleansers

Wound cleansing is a controversial topic within the ranks of wound care experts. Antiseptics such as hydrogen peroxide, povidone-iodine, acetic acid, and Dakin's solution, which can kill bacteria, can also be cytotoxic to white blood cells and fibroblasts. Removing bacteria from the wound bed can be done with normal saline at pressure between 4 and 15 pounds per square inch (psi). Above 15 pounds per square inch the pressure tends to drive bacteria into the tissue. Many commercial cleansers may inhibit the viability and phagocytic activity of leukocytes unless they are diluted due to toxic ingredients. Commercial wound cleansers contain surfactants and preservatives, and many come with a built-in sprayer achieving a desirable pounds per square inch pressure. An accepted rule of using saline as a cleanser is that after sterile saline is opened, it is good for only 24 hours; then it should be discarded. Saline kept refrigerated may be safe longer than 24 hours, but it is always a good idea to check labels or ask the manufacturer. Water is acceptable as a wound cleanser as long as it is free from contaminants. Some wound cleansers that are promoted as killing bacteria are not toxic to tissues; for example, Techni-Care Surgical Scrub (Care-Tech Laboratories, Inc.).

 *Skin cleansers should never be used on wounds. Skin cleansers are formulated to break chemical bonds that bind fecal matter to the skin; they are not suitable for the delicate tissue of a wound bed.*

Wound Care Products

Nurses may choose from several different types of dressings for wound management. The factors in making a decision on a

CHART 67–11 **Dressing Categories, Characteristics, and Uses**

Dressing Category and Description	Brand Names	Indications for Use	Advantages	Disadvantages
Transparent Films Primary or secondary dressings. Polyurethane with a porous adhesive layer that allows oxygen to pass through the membrane and moisture vapor to escape.	Opsite Bioclusive CarraFilm Polyskin Tegaderm UniFlex	Partial thickness wounds. Stages I and II pressure ulcers. Donor sites. Superficial burns.	Wound visible. Promotes autolytic débridement. Reduces friction. Pain reduction. Waterproof. Conformable.	Nonabsorptive. Fluid retention properties may lead to maceration or increased risk of fungal infection. May be difficult to apply for some persons. Contraindicated for infected wounds and sensitive or fragile skin.
Hydrogels Primary or secondary dressings. Amorphous or sheet design. Nonadherent, water or glycerin based.	Sheets: ClearSite Vigilon Elasto-Gel XCell Gels: DuoDerm gel Carrasyn Curasol gel Hypergel	Painful wounds. Skin tears. Radiation burns. Donor sites. Necrotic wounds. Partial or full-thickness wounds. Stages II–IV pressure ulcers. Wound edges. Neuropathic (diabetic) ulcers.	Nonadherent. Moisture retentive. Encourages autolytic débridement. Keeps wound edges supple. Pain reduction. Easy to apply and remove.	May macerate. Little absorption. Sheet dressing can dehydrate. Gels require secondary dressing. Sheets require tape or bandage to keep in place or may come with adhesive border. (Do not use the adhesive border on fragile skin; cut it away and secure with bandage.)
Hydrocolloids Primary dressings. Hydrophilic colloid particles bound to polyurethane foam; impermeable to bacteria.	DuoDerm CGF DuoDerm, thin Restore SignaDress Tegasorb Nu-Derm Cutinova Hydro	Partial thickness wounds. Stages II and III pressure ulcers.	Enhances autolytic débridement. Self-adherent, but not to wound. Pain reduction. Good for 2–5 days. Waterproof. Moisture retentive. Thermal insulation.	Minimal absorption. Some with aggressive adhesive. Contraindicated for infected wounds. Characteristic odor may be confused with infection.
Foams Primary dressings. Hydrophilic polyurethane.	3M Allevyn PolyMem Tielle Hydrasorb Lyofoam Mepilex	Venous stasis ulcers (can use under compression wraps). Tracheostomy. Draining wounds. Dermal wounds. Surgical incisions. Skin tears. Neuropathic (diabetic) ulcers.	Absorptive. Cushioning. Thermal insulation. Easy to apply and remove. Nonocclusive. Nonadherent.	May require secondary dressing or tape to secure. May macerate periwound skin if not changed appropriately. Not for dry, nondraining wounds.
Alginates Highly absorptive dressing of brown seaweed fibers; forms a soft gel when mixed with wound fluid. Available in ropes or sheets.	Kaltostat Sorbsan Algiderm Carrasorb Comfeel Seasorb	Highly exudative, draining wounds. Incisions. Venous stasis ulcers. Dermal wounds. Stages III and IV pressure ulcers. Tunneling or undermined areas. Split-thickness skin grafts.	Nonadherent. Can be used on infected wounds. Hemostatic properties for minor bleeding. Reduced frequency of dressing changes.	Requires secondary dressing. Contraindicated for wounds with exposed tendons, bone due to possible desiccation.
Composite Combination of products that provide multiple functions (i.e., bacterial barrier, absorption layer, and adhesive border). It can be any combination of dressings.	Primapore Versiva Viasorb Alldress	Surgical incisions. Stages II–IV pressure ulcers. Partial or full-thickness wounds.	Multiple sizes and shapes. Easy to apply. Usually absorbent. Check insert instructions for each brand dressing.	Adhesive borders may limit use due to fragile skin. Does not necessarily provide moist wound healing. Check insert instructions for each brand dressing.

(continued)

CHART 67–11	Dressing Categories, Characteristics, and Uses—*Continued*			
Dressing Category and Description	**Brand Names**	**Indications for Use**	**Advantages**	**Disadvantages**
Silver dressings	Aquacel Ag Acticoat Biostep Ag Silverlon Prisma Silversorb Maxsorb Ag Silverfoam (for wound VAC)	Silver is used as an antimicrobial in its ionic form, Ag⁺. It may be used in a gel form to provide moisture, an absorbent form like a foam or alginate, or with a collagen product. The wound VAC has a foam with silver in it as well now.	Can be used in multiple different types of dressings. Bacteriocidal to methicillin-resistant *Staphylococcus aureus* (MRSA) and vancomycin-resistant enterococcus (VRE) infections. Useful for prophylaxis as well.	Some studies show that too much silver may be inhibitory to healthy epithelialization. Further studies are underway.
Collagens	Biostep Collagenase Puracol Fibracol, SkinTemp Promogran	Collagens are used to provide collagen to the wound bed after the body denatures the initial injured collagen. Collagen is the protein matrix that is the major part of the extracellular matrix (ECM) and provides stability and tensile strength.	It is used to speed up the healing process by filling in the wound bed faster than the body could on its own. Some forms now also control the amount of matrix metalloproteinases (MMPs) and therefore prevent the body from breaking down the new collagen bed.	Timing, initially, the wound bed will have MMPs that denature the injured collagen, so it can be replaced with healthy collagen. In acute wounds, collagen may not be indicated. In chronic wounds, the amound of MMPs should be controlled to allow the dressing to be assimilated into the wound bed without denaturing by MMPs.

particular product are protection, degree of drainage or lack thereof, antimicrobial activity, biochemical needs, collagen requirements, and pain relief. As the wound treatment plan continues, it may be necessary to switch dressing types based on the needs for that wound bed at the time of assessment. The same dressing will most often not be required the entire treatment of the wound. It is very important to understand that despite algorithms and protocols, what drives choices for dressings is a skilled assessment of the wound on which to base decisions about dressings. The wound is viable and changing; flexibility regarding the type of dressings used is necessary to continue to show improvement in the wound. Moist wound healing is a delicate balance of moisture—keeping the wound bed moist and the periwound skin dry and intact. Basic, good wound care is pretty simple: If a wound is dry, add moisture; if a wound is wet, use an absorbent dressing; and always protect the periwound skin.

The most common type of dressings are presented next with the understanding that there are many different variations in size, brand, and combinations to provide a highly individualized plan of treatment that is cost effective, convenient, and outcome driven. See Chart 67–11 for a summary of common dressing categories, characteristics, and uses.

Moisture Retentive Dressings

The goals of moisture retentive dressings, occlusive dressings, or semiocclusive dressings are all the same: maintaining a moist wound environment. There are hydrogels, calcium alginates, silver dressings, collagens, foams, polyurethane films, hydrocolloids, contact layers, composites, and combinations, all of which are described here. Generally these dressings are painless, reduce the need for multiple dressing changes daily, and result in faster heal-

ing rates. On the cellular level, cells desiccate without moisture and cannot do their job of building tissue to fill in and cover a wound. Moist wound healing is facilitated by moisture retentive dressings.

 **CRITICAL ALERT** *To the patient who tells the nurse that he leaves the dressing off at night so the wound can get air, the nurse needs to explain that the wound gets oxygen from the blood supply, not from the ambient air. Do not let the wound dry out.*

Hydrogels

Hydrogels are made of a saline base. They provide moisture to the wound bed that is required for epithelialization to occur as the cells migrate across the wound bed. Hydrogels can come in a tube of gel, in sheets, or impregnated in a gauze pad. Hydrogels are used for wounds that are dry and require moisture. They are not intended for wounds with excess drainage. A caution with this dressing is that maceration, the tendency for the periwound area of good skin to get wet and soft and potentially break down, can occur. Close supervision of the wound's progress and astute assessment are required.

Alginates

Alginates are composed of algae or seaweed. These dressing can absorb at least about five to ten times their surface area of drainage. In chronic wounds, the chemical's matrix metalloproteinases, or MMPs, are out of ratio for wound healing to occur. MMPs degrade collagen and denature it. As a reminder, collagen is the scaffold whereby tissue growth occurs. A certain amount of MMPs are necessary to control other biochemical signals and degrade collagen that is injured. Alginates absorb the excess wound drainage to inactivate some MMPs as well as prevent against maceration, as described earlier.

Silver Dressings

Silver in its ionic form is a natural bactericidal agent, even against the most resistant bacterial strains such as MRSA (methicillin-resistant *Staphylococcus aureus*) and VRE (vancomycin-resistant enterococcus). Silver, when in contact with the bacteria, interferes with bacterial cell DNA, bacterial enzymes, and proteins in the cell wall to create its bactericidal effect. Silver has been used since the late 1800s for its antimicrobial activity. It can be found in gels, alginates, saturated gauze, metallic nylon, and other media to deliver the silver cation Ag^+. Some silver dressings require saline to be activated and some do not. There is a debate as to how much silver is effective and whether larger than required amounts of silver can be harmful and destructive. The main focus, however, should be the rate at which the silver is deposited into the wound bed and the wound bed's characteristics. Silver will kill only the surface bacteria it comes in contact with, and oral antibiotic therapy should continue.

Collagens

Collagen dressings are also utilized for wound care treatment. Native collagen that is stable and can resist early degradation by MMPs can provide an extracellular matrix (ECM) that allows wound healing to continue. Extracellular matrix is the matrix of native collagen, connective tissue, and basement membrane that forms the foundation or scaffold on which the epithelial tissue is embedded. There are many different types of collagen dressings. Characteristics such as size, depth, shape, drainage, or lack thereof, infection, and bioburden, all factor into selecting the right type of collagen medium to utilize (Nataraj et al., 2007).

Foams

A foam dressing is made of a spongy material that is highly absorptive as compared to its surface area. It is also soft and pliable so that it can conform to any environment. Foams can be used in two ways. One use is for absorption. They can be used alone or in combination with an alginate to "wick" away excess moisture and prevent maceration. They can also be utilized for protection as a barrier against foreign insult. For example, a patient in a wheelchair with a lower leg wound is prone to further trauma due to hitting the wound on the wheelchair with transfers. The foam then provides a cushion for the insult and protects the already compromised wound bed from further damage. It can also be utilized to protect from friction and shear forces from surfaces and contact with other body parts.

Transparent Films

Transparent films are made of a clear sticky wrap much like the plastic wrap used for storage of food with glue on one side. Transparent films can be used to visualize a wound bed and for an occlusive dressing. It should be noted however, that on elderly patients with frail skin, another option should be considered. This film tends to stick and protect so well that when it is time to remove it, it can cause further damage by clinging to and separating the skin during its removal. Transparent films are excellent, however, for protection from incontinence and foreign contact getting to the wound bed and can allow the wound dressing to remain intact for a greater duration.

Gauze

Gauze is the most widely used dressing and may be wrongly alluded to as a standard of care (Ovington, 2002). Research has shown that wet-to-dry dressings and gauze are commonly ordered for wounds in which there is scant evidence to support their use, such as with open surgical wounds healing by secondary intention (Armstrong & Price, 2004). Wet-to-dry dressings consist of saline-moistened gauze placed inside or on a wound bed, covered with dry gauze, and secured. When the moistened gauze dries, it adheres to the wound. When it is removed, it pulls away good tissue along with the necrotic tissue and debris. This is nonselective débridement, and there is a high risk for reinjury of the wound bed. Plus, it is usually painful.

Wet-to-moist or moist gauze dressings are saline-moistened gauze placed in the wound and kept moist until removed. This may require rewetting the gauze, but generally it means that the dressing is changed before it dries out, which in reality may or may not happen. More frequent dressing changes may mean more pain for the patient, more work for an elderly caregiver spouse, and more expense for a home health nurse or hospital staff nurse.

Negative Pressure Therapy

Negative pressure therapy is a dressing that uses a vacuum or negative pressure to assist in drainage collection and promotion of granulation and angiogenesis. Wound vacuum assisted closure (VAC) is a system that uses controlled negative pressure (vacuum) to help promote wound healing (Figure 67–13 ■, p. 2218). This therapy helps remove infectious materials and other fluids from the wound. The wound VAC system consists of a computer-controlled therapy unit, canister, sterile plastic tubing, foam dressing, and a clear VAC drape dressing. The foam dressing is gently packed into the open wound bed, taking care not to leave any on normal skin. A tube is then connected to the foam at one end and the VAC control unit at the other end. Once the foam is in place, it is sealed with a clear drape that is similar to a large bandage. Suction is applied and infectious materials and other fluids from the wound are pulled through the tube and into the canister. The wound VAC works best in a clean, granular bed; and débridement and infection control should be accomplished first before a wound VAC is applied. It is changed every 2 to 3 days.

Wound VAC negative pressure wound therapy (NPWT) can be prescribed for many chronic and traumatic wound patients in the hospital, in the extended care facility, and in the home. The negative pressure and drainage system (1) promotes granulation tissue formation through the promotion of wound healing (Argenta & Morykwas, 1997; Joseph et al., 2000); (2) uniformly draws wounds closed by applying controlled, localized negative pressure; (3) removes interstitial fluid allowing tissue decompression; (4) removes infectious materials; and (5) provides a closed, moist wound healing environment. Wound VAC is used in the hospital setting, in the extended care facility, and at home for the following conditions:

- Chronic open wounds (diabetic and pressure ulcers)
- Acute and traumatic wounds
- Meshed grafts
- Subacute wounds (i.e., dehisced incisions)
- Skin grafts and flaps. (MedTech1.com, 2005)

Nursing care includes maintaining and documenting the negative pressure level, changing the foam per the health care provider's order, and assessing wound healing.

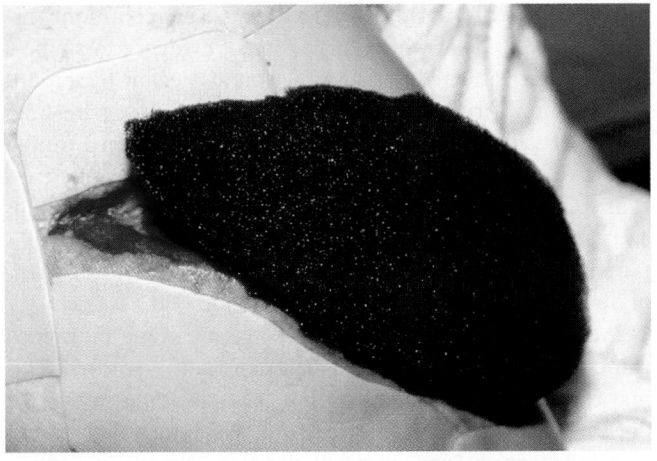

1.

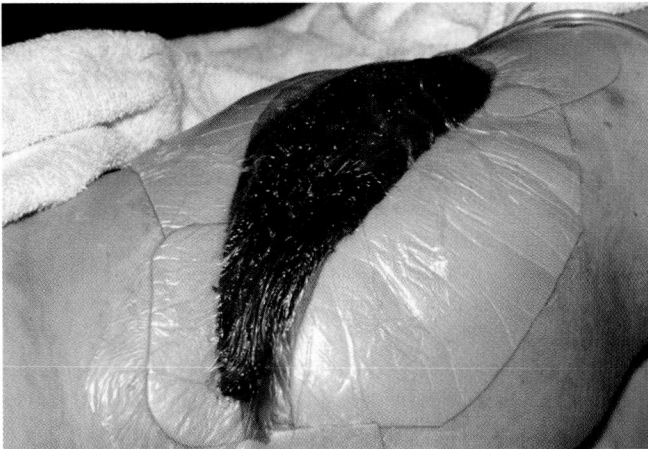

3.

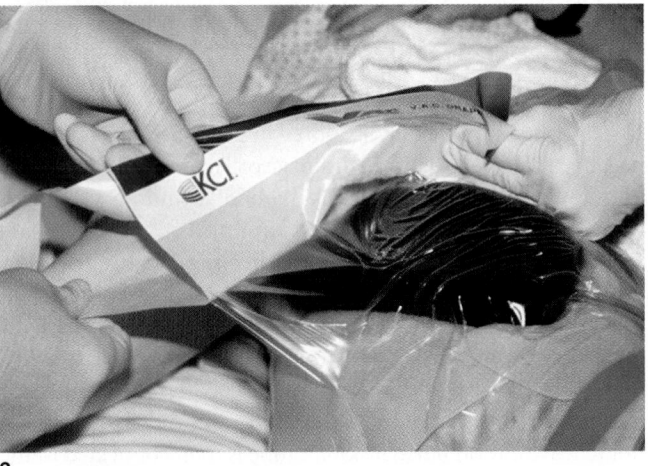

2.

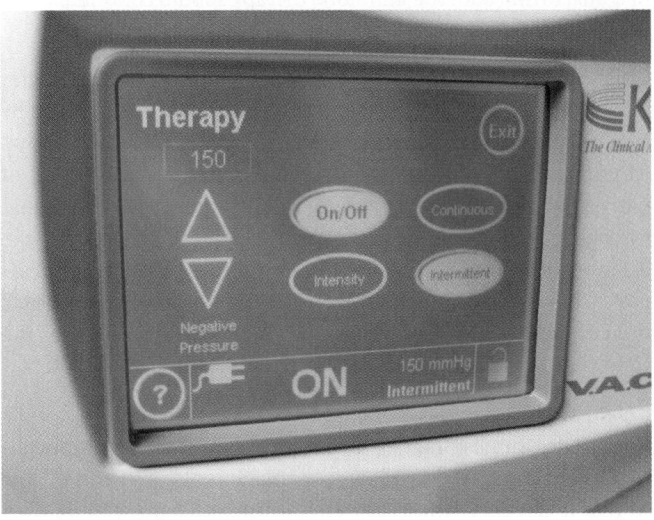

4.

FIGURE 67–13 ■ Wound vacuum assisted closure (VAC).
Source: 1, 2: Jan Clark; 3, 4: Cheryl Wraa

Adjuvant Therapy

There are adjuvant treatments one could consider in a plan of care to promote the healing process. These treatments are used in conjunction with good wound care and identification of the causative factors that relate to wound healing or lack thereof. One such treatment is the use of skin grafts or flaps to close or fill in a wound. A skin graft requires an area of the patient's healthy skin on the body (usually from the lower extremity thigh area) to be excised and placed over the wound area and sutured or stapled in to affix the graft. Of note, the wound should be a clean (free of infection and debris), granulating wound that is ready to accept the graft. One must also consider the patient's vascular and nutritional status to ensure graft survival and take. Pressure must not be applied to the affected area, and that may require a pressure relief device like a "sand bed," which is made of silicone beads that are heated and effectively move under the patient so that no pressure is applied to the affected area. Skin grafting is described in detail in Chapter 68 .

Tissue Grafts

Another adjuvant treatment is the use of tissue grafts. These grafts can be derived from human tissue or from animal tissue.

They contain collagen and/or fibroblasts and keratinocytes, the major components of the dermal and epidermal layers of skin. These applications are placed directly to the wound bed and affixed or anchored so that the graft stays in place. The benefit of this graft over a skin graft is that there is no donor site required to heal, no requirement of anesthesia or invasive surgery, and it is minimally invasive. Tissue grafts can also be performed repetitively to get the intended result.

Whirlpool Therapy

Whirlpool therapy is another adjuvant treatment. A whirlpool is a tub that has circulating water to remove debris and bioburden in the wound to promote wound healing. It is often performed daily and can be found in many inpatient and outpatient physical therapy departments. One side effect of whirlpool use is infection (Vaughn, 2002).

Hyperbaric Oxygen Therapy

Hyperbaric oxygen therapy is also an adjuvant treatment. **Hyperbaric oxygen therapy (HBOT)** refers to intermittent treatment of the entire body with 100% oxygen at 20 times greater than normal atmospheric pressures. HBOT has been used to improve wound healing in patients with compromised oxygenation and/or perfusion because it stimulates the growth of new blood vessels in areas with reduced circulation and arterial blockage (Cranton, 2005). Patients are placed in either chambers that can be individual or large, room-like chambers that can accommodate several people at one time. The patient breathes in this oxygen under pressure in a chamber. The oxygen under pressure forces the oxygen into the plasma surrounding the red blood cells to "supersaturate" the patient with oxygen. Its benefits are increased tissue oxygen levels, angiogenesis (new blood vessel formation), antibacterial activity (oxygen kills anaerobic bacteria and its toxins), enhanced leukocyte killing (T-cell formation), and prevention of reperfusion injury. There are about 14 approved diagnoses accepted by the Centers for Medicare & Medicaid Services (CMS) for hyperbaric oxygen therapy. One example is that patients who have diabetic wounds at a depth of Wagner Grade 3, failed conventional wound therapy for 30 days, and had vascular and glucose optimization can receive hyperbaric therapy. Patients with osteomyelitis and patients at risk of failing a surgical flap can receive hyperbaric oxygen therapy as well. HBOT also is used to treat extensive wounds such as burn injuries, infected wounds, and wounds in patients who are at high risk for delayed healing. Wherever blood flow and oxygen delivery to vital organs are reduced, function and healing can potentially be aided with HBOT. Recently HBOT has been used for treatment of chronic degenerative health problems related to atherosclerosis, stroke, peripheral vascular disease, diabetic ulcers, wound healing, cerebral palsy, brain injury, multiple sclerosis, macular degeneration, and many other disorders (Cranton, 2005).

There must be a trained hyperbaric technician and health care provider that supervise the hyperbaric treatment as well. Special precautions muse be taken with regard to fire hazards when considering oxygen under pressure. The treatment lasts about 2 hours and is given daily for anywhere from 20 to 60 treatments. There are rare side effects of hyperbaric oxygen therapy, such as oxygen toxicity seizures, eardrum rupture, pneumothorax, hypoglycemia in patients with diabetes, and temporary visual changes; but because these effects can be potentially serious, constant supervision is required, as stated earlier (Undersea & Hyperbaric Medical Society, 2007).

Electrical Stimulation

Electrical stimulation (ES) is the use of electrical current to stimulate cellular processes. The literature remains unclear as to the exact "dosage" (Sussman, 1998). Benefits are reported to be an antibacterial effect, increased blood flow, cell proliferation, edema reduction, and autolytic débridement facilitation.

Normothermia (Radiant Heat)

Radiant heat is believed to increase blood flow through vasodilation, thereby promoting cell proliferation. New methods of delivering the radiant heat have been developed. The system consists of a power supply, control unit, warming insert, and dressing that supports the warming insert and protects the wound. The system maintains appropriate levels of temperature and moisture in and around the wound.

Specialty Support Surfaces

Specialty support surfaces are mattresses or overlays that provide pressure reduction or pressure relief. Pressure reduction and pressure relief are based on the principle of decreasing interface pressure. The pressure between a bony prominence and surface such as a hospital bed or seating surface is **interface pressure**. Decreasing interface pressure decreases pressure on capillaries. Ischemia results when capillaries are occluded, shutting down oxygen and nutrients necessary for cellular viability. Cellular death results in tissue necrosis—pressure ulcers. On admission to the hospital, nursing assessment of the patient includes pressure ulcer risk. Ideally a primary part of the care plan is selection of an appropriate surface (Coats-Bennett, 2002). To be able to make decisions about which specialty support surface will most benefit the patient requires an in-depth understanding not only of the specialty support surface performance but also of the patient's condition. An assessment of the patient should include risk for skin breakdown, location of present ulcers or wounds, sensory perception, mobility status, chronic illness, nutritional status, moisture and continence issues, and the patient's ability to be repositioned due to procedures, surgeries, hardware (e.g., fixators), and hemodynamic stability.

A "gatekeeper" is essential to provide the patient with the correct support surface and to control costs. Frequently that position is filled by the wound ostomy continence nurse or someone else who has had extensive education about specialty support surfaces and an understanding of the Centers for Medicare & Medicaid Services (CMS) categories for reimbursement purposes. Detailed descriptions of a patient's wound, activity level, and state of health are important documentation in obtaining reimbursement for specialty support surface. Evidence-based decision tools to select appropriate specialty surfaces are helpful and can be formulated specific to institutions and the products they use (Warren, Yoder, Young-McCaughan, 1999). In addition to the specialty support surfaces, institutions and home health services can utilize overlays of gel, foam, or air for pressure reduction. Other specialty support surfaces facilitate pulmonary rescue of patients and support bariatric patients.

Pressure Reduction and Pressure Relief

Standard hospital mattresses have interface pressures of approximately 100 mmHg. Without frequent repositioning, healthy individuals can experience occluded capillaries. Pressure reduction surfaces can lower interface pressure, but will not consistently lower interface pressure below 32 mmHg, which is capillary closing pressure (Coats-Bennett, 2002). Pressure relief products vary in interface pressure. Many are dynamic, so that the interface pressure is constantly changing to ensure that pressure load is distributed.

Therapeutic Mattress Replacements

Therapeutic mattress replacements (TMR) are called so because they replace the standard hospital mattress. They are made of various layers, usually with a 4- to 6-inch layer of high-density foam. TMRs can include layers of air or gel. They are covered by waterproof covers, which help reduce pressure, friction, and shear.

CHART 67–12 Skin Breakdown Protection Overlays

Overlay	Description	Use
Foam	Construction of a foam overlay's height, density, and indention load deflection (ILD) produces the characteristics to evaluate for effective pressure reduction. Base height should be measured from the base of the overlay to the lowest point of convolution in an "egg-crate" foam construction. To provide pressure relief, 4 inches or more of height is necessary.	At risk for pressure ulcers Stages I and II pressure ulcers
Gel	Gel overlays are filled with silicon elastomer, silicon, polyvinyl chloride, or similar gel materials. They help reduce friction. The gel is displaced by the patient's body weight and provides flotation.	At-risk patients Stages I and II pressure ulcers
Air	Powered air overlays are considered dynamic (air is in motion). Air overlays consist of air cells that are inflated and produce consistent pressure reduction. Alternating air overlays consist of air cells constantly deflated and inflated, effectively reducing the effects of pressure duration by changing pressure distribution. Some of these are designed so the airflow moves quickly into small chambers so the effect is pulsating. Nonpowered air overlays are static (no air motion). Static air overlays have connecting air cells that conform to body weight to displace pressure load.	At-risk patients Stages I, II, III, and IV pressure ulcers Burns Surgical flaps
Water	Water-filled overlays are vinyl mattresses filled with water. The patient should displace the water without bottoming out, effectively floating the patient.	At-risk patients Stages I, II, and III pressure ulcers

Overlays are to be placed on top of a TMR or standard hospital mattress. Overlays can be powered or nonpowered. Nonpowered overlays are static air, foam, water, or gel filled. Powered overlays may provide alternating pressure or low air loss. They differ widely in pressure reduction: the ability to support the patient and redistribute pressure load. Chart 67–12 summarizes the various overlays available.

Pressure Relief

Two types of pressure relief are low air loss therapy and air fluidized therapy.

In *low air loss therapy*, low air loss overlays sit on top of the standard or therapeutic mattress replacement, or as a mattress that replaces the mattress on the frame. A pump is connected to the mattress or overlay, attached to the foot of the bed, and plugged in to electricity. Some models feature a short-term battery to keep the mattress from deflating. Low air loss mattresses arriving within a special frame are considered "air support systems." A series of pillows are inflated with air in continuous motion, to specific patient measurements of weight and height. Therapy provided by low air loss beds includes maintaining capillary blood flow, eliminating shear and friction, and reducing moisture. NEVER place a patient with spinal injury on a low air loss mattress until the injury has been radiologically cleared or the neurosurgeon or orthopedic surgeon orders it. (Each institution needs to have a specific policy.) The potential for further injury exists because the "air bed" does not support the spine.

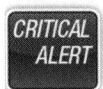 **CRITICAL ALERT** *Do not diminish the pressure-relieving effects of the low air loss surface by using extra layers of sheets or pads. Extra padding increases pressure. Use only the pads recommended by the bed manufacturer.*

Air fluidized therapy utilizes a high rate of airflow to fluidize fine particulate material to produce a support medium that has characteristics similar to liquid. The support system does not utilize a mattress; the fluidized particulate matter is contained within a sheet that conforms around the patient's body. One-third of the body is floating and the rest is enveloped within the sheet of constantly moving matter. Indications for these beds are surgical flaps and grafts and in some cases intractable pain. Pain relief occurs because the fluidized air relieves pressure on painful areas as well as bony prominences or surgical flaps/grafts.

Bariatric Systems

Patients weighing more than 500 pounds or having a body mass index above 40 should be considered for placement on a bariatric system for safety reasons. Bariatric systems utilize a reinforced frame to support body mass. Most can be converted to a chair position. Some systems provide a wider area to help support and facilitate the repositioning of patients. Low air loss mattresses are available on bariatric systems. Newer models can make full-body lateral rotation turns with the low air loss surface.

Kinetic or Oscillation Therapy

Pulmonary rescue is another function of a specialty support surface. These special frames actually turn patients to mobilize the secretions in their lungs. Overlays can systematically deflate and inflate on opposite sides to create a shift in the patient's chest, although the turn is not as significant as that of a turning frame. The frames now come with controls to turn patients in incremental degrees, and to select turning positions and time involved in each turn. Certain models have incorporated a low air loss support surface into the frame. They also usually come with scales for weighing patients. In addition, options for percussion and or/gentle pulsation modes to aid in pulmonary toilet and enhance circulation are available. Long periods of the turning mechanism being turned off require reevaluation of the bed's impact on the patient, and other options should be considered (Coats-Bennett, 2002). Most importantly, it must be understood that these "turning" beds do not replace the need for repositioning patients or protecting heels to prevent pressure ulcers.

Summary

Pressure reduction surfaces include therapeutic mattress replacements, 4-inch foam overlays, static air, gel, water, and dynamic air overlays. Pressure relief surfaces include low air loss and air fluidized surfaces. Kinetic or "turning beds" are used for pulmonary rescue. Bariatric beds are for patients who are obese. These must be considered therapy and documented as such with

COMPLEMENTARY & ALTERNATIVE THERAPIES

Horse Chestnut Seed Extract

Description:

The horse chestnut is the fruit of the horse chestnut tree (*Aesculus hippocastanum* L.). A medicinal extract, horse chestnut seed extract (HCSE), is prepared from the seed of the fruit. HCSE is commonly used in Europe for chronic venous insufficiency (CVI). CVI is a condition that includes symptoms such as leg swelling, varicose veins, leg pain, itching, and skin ulcers.

Research Support:

A literature review was conducted to evaluate the efficacy and safety of oral HCSE for the treatment of CVI. Researchers sought randomized controlled trials that compared use of oral HCSE single preparations with placebo in people with CVI. Researchers excluded trials if the HCSE was one of several active components in a combination preparation, or as a part of a combination treatment. Study results showed that HCSE treatment improved CVI-related signs and symptoms compared to placebo, and that there were only mild and infrequent adverse effects associated with HCSE treatment. Although researchers concluded that HCSE may be effective as a safe short-term treatment for CVI, they felt that more rigorous trials are needed to confirm its efficacy (Pittler & Ernst, 2006).

In an Australian prospective triple–blind randomized placebo-controlled trial, 54 patients with venous leg ulcers from a large South Australian community nursing service were randomly allocated to receive horse chestnut seed extract (n=27) or placebo (n=27) for 12 weeks. Ulcers were assessed at weeks 0, 4, 8 and 12 utilizing a wound assessment tool and the Alfred/Medseed Wound Imaging System. The difference between groups in the number of healed leg ulcers and change in wound surface area, depth, volume, pain and exudate was not statistically significant. However, horse chestnut seed extract did have a significant effect on the percentage of wound slough over time and on the number of dressing changes at week 12. Even though horse chestnut seed extract is likely to attenuate the pathogenesis of venous insufficiency and, in turn, facilitate venous ulcer healing, the current study did not statistically support such a claim. However, taking into account the small sample and insufficient power of the trial, and the significant improvement in wound slough and visit frequency, it appears that it may be useful in the management of venous leg ulcers (Leach, Pinocombe, & Foster, 2006a).

Another study assessed the cost-effectiveness of using HCSE for venous ulcer treatment versus conventional therapy, which involves dressings and compression, alone. The randomized, placebo-controlled study, which was conducted for 12 weeks in South Australia, involved 54 patients with venous ulcers. Researchers compiled the cost of HCSE in addition to dressing materials, travel, staff salaries, and infrastructure for each patient when comparing HCSE treatment to conventional treatment. Results showed that HCSE therapy combined with conventional therapy was more cost effective than conventional therapy alone considering only dressing materials costs per patient. Researchers pointed out that the total cost of wound care is significantly impacted by dressing change frequency. They concluded that the use of HCSE in venous ulcer treatment may enhance clinical efficiency due to less frequent nursing visits (Leach, Pinocombe, & Foster, 2006a).

References

Leach, M. J., Pincombe, J., & Foster, G. (2006a). Clinical efficacy of horse chestnut seed extract in the treatment of venous ulceration. *Journal of Wound Care, 15*(4), 159–167.

Leach, M. J., Pincombe, J., & Foster, G. (2006b). Using horse chestnut seed extract in the treatment of venous leg ulcers: A cost–benefit analysis. *Ostomy Wound Management, 52*(4), 68–70, 72–74, 76–78.

Pittler, M. H., & Ernst, E. (2006). Horse chestnut seed extract for chronic venous insufficiency. *Cochrane Database of Systematic Reviews, 25*(1), CD003230.

---

observed outcomes and achieved goals. They should be used in conjunction with optimal nutrition, appropriate positioning, optimal transferring and turning techniques, and routine skilled nursing care and assessments. Support surfaces should be changed to reflect the goals and objectives of the patient's current plan of care (Coats-Bennett, 2002).

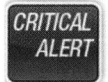 **CRITICAL ALERT** *It is essential to debunk the myth that once a patient is on a specialty support surface she does not need to be repositioned. Manufacturers of specialty beds and wound care experts agree that nurses need to reposition patients on specialty beds frequently.*

■ Complementary and Alternative Therapies

The use of complementary and/or alternative therapies may be attractive to patients for wound healing, especially of nonhealing chronic wounds. Alternative medicine products may include honey, aloe, chamomile, calendula, and tea tree oil. A number of over-the-counter topical and ingestible agents promote wound healing, decrease scar formation, and prevent bruising. These agents are frequently less costly and more accessible than prescription pharmaceutical agents and dressings. One example of a topical agent is ordinary honey. It has successfully healed chronic wounds in patients who have failed to get closure with other methods. The Complementary and Alternative Therapies feature outlines the use of horse chestnut seed extract for the treatment of chronic venous insufficiency.

■ Management of Drains

Care of surgical drains and tubes in postoperative patients is important in order to avoid complications. Nurses in home health and in long-term acute care facilities must learn to manage drains and tubes because of shorter lengths of stay in acute care facilities. To care for the postoperative patient with drains, the nurse must know the type, purpose, and location of the surgical drain, proper management strategies, potential problems, and how to troubleshoot complications. The nurse also must ensure that the system is securely stabilized and assess patency on a regular basis. Because drains are removed when they are no longer needed, monitoring the amount of drainage is important in order to determine the length of time the drain needs to stay in place. If the tube or drain is not draining fluid, there may be a problem with the system. The nurse should make a systematic check from where the drain leaves the patient's body to the collection device to check for kinks, blood clots, or mucous or tissue shreds. Milking the tube away from the patient can be done to sustain patency of the tube. Any significant change in amount or character of drainage must be reported to the health care provider.

Nurses need to protect the skin from any drainage or leakage to prevent irritation. Dry gauze dressings can be used to help lift the drainage tube away from the skin and help stabilize the device. Stabilizers such as the Hollister Drain Tube Attachment Device keep drains and tubes from migrating in and out of the exit site. Constant friction due to migration of the tube causes the space around the tube to enlarge, allowing more movement of the tube and more leakage around the tube. With more moisture and friction, hypergranulation can occur. **Hypergranulation** is the formation of soft, pink, fleshy projections in the open area, which is the body's attempt to heal the enlarged track. Silver nitrate sticks are often used to burn down this tissue because it creates more moisture and causes pain in some instances. Moisture barriers can be used to protect the skin from breakdown if there is leakage from in or around the drain insertion site.

Preventing complications should be the goal of drain/tube management. Therefore, the nurse should consistently use hand hygiene before and after patient care, use aseptic techniques when cleaning and dressing surgical drains/tubes, and dispose properly of drainage containers and drains when removed. Skin around the drain needs to be kept clean and dry.

Surgical drains are often indicated for decompression in areas with a significant amount of fluid accumulation, fistulas, infected tissue, and potential dead space. Two types of drains are used: active or passive.

Active Drains

Active drains are low-pressure suction devices that are constantly removing fluids via a closed drainage system. The drain is attached to a collapsible reservoir that exerts negative pressure to pull fluids from the wound bed. Active drain advantages include minimal tissue trauma, accurate drainage measurements, and the closed system decreases infection risk. Examples of common active drains are Jackson–Pratt and Hemovac (Figures 67–14A, 67–15 and 67–16 ■).

Nursing interventions for active drains include:

- Keep the drain tubing straight without kinks.
- Keep the reservoir compressed (a collapsed position) to maintain the negative pressure.

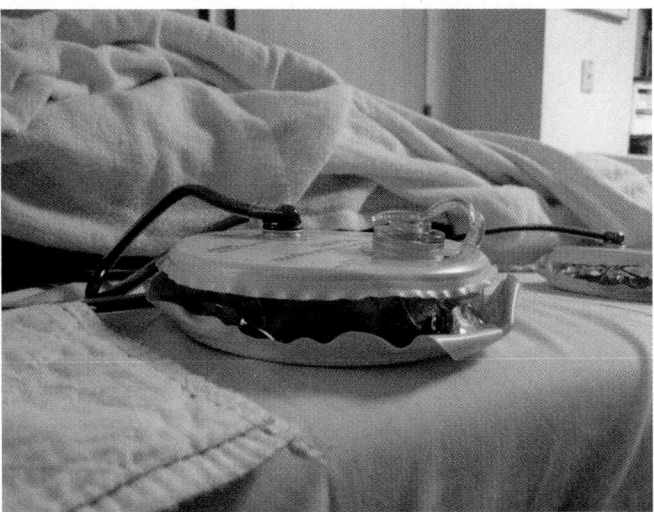

FIGURE 67–15 ■ Hemovac drain.
Source: Cheryl Wraa

- For optimal function, the reservoir should be emptied before it is half full.
- Unclog blood or tissue shreds from the drain tubing by milking or stripping toward the reservoir.
- Document amount and color of drainage.

Wounds initially have sanguineous or serosanguineous drainage. As the wound heals, there is less amount of drainage, and it becomes more serous.

Passive Drains

Passive drains are made of soft, flat, flexible material and are usually placed in a stab wound near an incision site. Pus, blood, necrotic debris, and fluids interfere with wound healing and can provide a milieu for pathogens. Passive drains provide a conduit that functions by gravity for the removal of this drainage, which may be too viscous for the active drains. An example of a common passive drain is a Penrose drain (Figure 67–14B ■).

The drain is typically sutured to secure it and keep it from migrating in or out of the wound. Flat gauze sponges or fenestrated sponges are used at the end of the drain to absorb the exudates. They are removed and new ones applied when the dressing be-

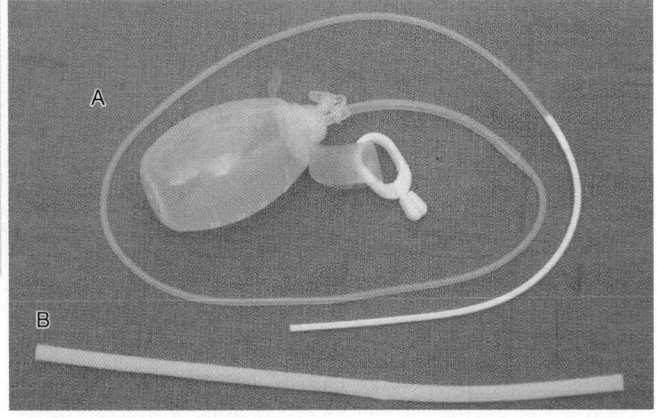

FIGURE 67–14 ■ A Jackson–Pratt and B Penrose drain.
Source: Courtesy of John M. Osborn, M. D., FACS, Sacramento, CA Plastic Surgery Center

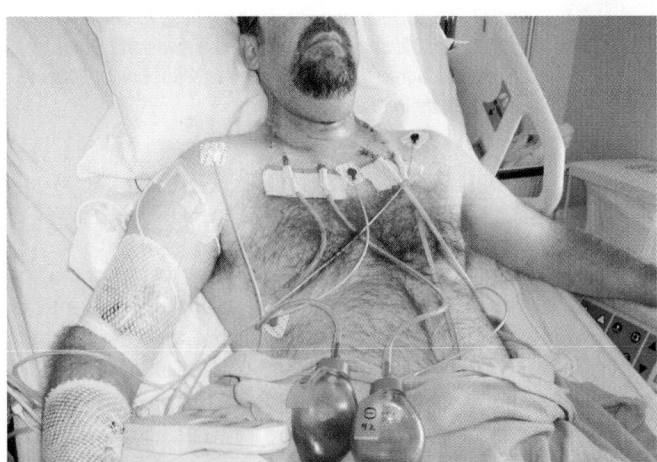

FIGURE 67–16 ■ Jackson-Pratt drain with serosanguineous drainage.
Source: Ann E. F. Sievers, RN

comes saturated, as these dressings may become wet with irritants to the skin. Care must be taken not to pull the drain out of the wound inadvertently during the dressing change. The nurse must protect the skin with a moisture barrier and frequently check the dressing to assess need for replacement.

Percutaneous Drainage Catheters

Interventional radiologists implant a percutaneous drainage catheter to allow drainage from sites where fluid collection may be infected, or to collect the fluid for laboratory studies to determine the nature of the fluid. The catheter is connected to a dependent drainage system such as a urinary leg bag. Placement sites include the biliary, peritoneal cavity, groin, breast, or anywhere infection is suspected.

Nursing care includes assessment for patency and irrigation of the catheter to maintain patency. Aseptic technique is used, and a health care provider's order is needed for the irrigation procedure, which includes the frequency and volume of irrigating solution to be used. Forceful instillation of fluid and forceful aspiration are never used. Accurate documentation is required regarding the color, amount, and consistency of fluid and the patient's tolerance of the procedure. Sterile dressings are used to cover the percutaneous site.

Impaired Wound Healing

Impaired wound healing is defined as the disruption of the normal biochemical repair or regeneration process. Abnormalities may be manifested in a number of ways, described next. If healing is occurring at a normal rate, the wound edges of an incision should not separate after the first 24 hours. Assessing the wound edges will give the nurse information about the healing process. If the edges are separated or there is serous or serosanguineous drainage, the nurse needs to assess the wound frequently for signs of impaired wound healing.

Dehiscence

Wound dehiscence is the separation of sutures or staples along the incision in a previously closed wound (Figure 67–17 ■). Dehiscence can be caused by infection or tension on the skin pulled together tightly with sutures or staples. Patients that are obese and patients on steroids are at a higher risk for the development of dehiscence. A sign of impending dehiscence is the leakage of serous or serosanguineous fluid from the incision for several days after injury or surgery. This indicates that collagen is not being properly formed and the tensile strength of the wound is impaired. If there is serosanguineous drainage, it should be absorbed by a sterile cover dressing. The characteristics of wound dehiscence drainage (amount, color, and odor), along with the length of the separation, should be reported to the surgeon emergently. The patient may need to return to surgery for wound closure, or the wound may need to be packed with dressings. To prevent maceration or irritation of the normal skin adjacent to the wound edges, liquid skin barriers or moisture barriers should be applied to the periwound skin with each dressing change.

Evisceration

Wound evisceration is defined as the protrusion of organs from a wound site (Figure 67–18 ■). It typically occurs following a wound dehiscence. The nurse needs to cover the organs with a sterile saline-moistened dressing and call the surgeon emergently. The patient will need to return to surgery for repair of the evisceration.

Hematoma and Seroma Formation

Hematoma is defined as an area of swelling or a mass of blood confined to an organ, tissue, or space due to a broken blood vessel. Due to the abnormal collection of blood in the tissues, hematomas are typically painful. It is the increased pain in the area when it should be decreasing that often leads to the diagnosis of hematoma. A hematoma can become infected and large enough to split the skin open and cause drainage. The treatment consists of cold compresses for the first 24 hours to decrease bleeding, elevation of the affected area, and, if large enough, aspiration is necessary. Antibiotics may be necessary if the hematoma becomes infected. The nurse needs to report the presence of a hematoma to the health care provider and do serial assessments to assess changes in the size. The wound will not completely heal until the hematoma has dissolved.

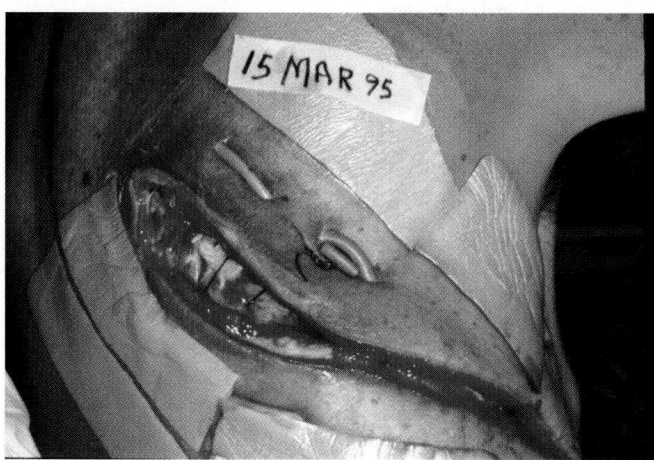

FIGURE 67–17 ■ Wound dehiscence.
Source: Jan Clark

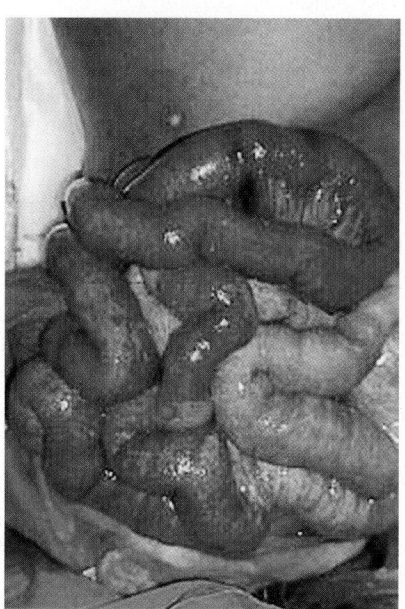

FIGURE 67–18 ■ Wound evisceration.
Source: Jan Clark

A **seroma** is the same as a hematoma except that instead of a collection of blood it is a collection of serous fluid. Its presence impacts wound healing; therefore, the typical treatment is aspiration or incision, and drainage procedure with postprocedure packing and secondary intention closure.

Literature suggests that patients that are obese are more prone to hematoma and seroma formation. Donor-site infections, donor-site seromas, and hernias also occur more frequently in patients that are obese. The large pannus predisposes patients to fluid accumulation, creating an environment conducive to seroma formation, infection, and wound edge separation or dehiscence (Wilson & Clark, 2004).

■ Nursing Management

Use of the nursing process guides the management of wounds. Beginning with a thorough nursing assessment of the wound is important in making decisions about treatment and goals because of the viable and changing nature of a wound. The treatment plan may need to be changed to facilitate these changes in the wound (Ovington, 2002). Typically guided by the health care provider's orders, the nurse is responsible for daily management of the wound. Therefore, the nurse is in a unique position to detect changes in the wound environment that indicate complications. Reporting these changes could prevent problems that may become life threatening. The nurse is in a pivotal position as a patient advocate to facilitate management by all the members of the health care team.

Assessment

Nurses are required to do routine scheduled and interventional assessments of their patients in all settings: acute and long-term acute care, home health, and nurse-managed clinic visits. The assessment becomes a written record of subjective and objective data. A systematic approach ensures a continuity of documentation and an accurate history of interventions and results. Assessment tools such as the Braden scale (p. 2207) are a reliable resource for the nursing documentation because of the succinct terminology. For example, assessment tools provide scores, numbers, and categories or indications of the acuity of a condition and specifically identify areas for intervention.

Skin Assessments

Skin assessments are different from wound assessments. Basic skin assessment should include observation of the entire body, checking temperature, color, moisture, turgor, and integrity. Chart 67–13 combines the elements of basic and comprehensive skin assessments as developed by Baranoski and Ayello (2004). Maintaining skin integrity in special populations—that is, the aged with frail skin, who have chronic diseases, or those who are immunosuppressed—can be a challenge. Routine assessments,

CHART 67–13	Basic and Comprehensive Skin Assessment Elements			
Basic Skin Assessment	**Characteristics**	**Comprehensive Skin Assessment**	**Characteristics**	
Temperature	Normally warm to touch. Warmer than normal could signal inflammation. Cooler than normal could signal poor vascularization.	Inspection	Normally smooth, slightly moist, and same general tone throughout. Tone: Melanocytes provide ranges from light ivory, light to deep brown, black, yellow to olive, light pink to dark ruddy pink or red.	
Color	Intensity: paleness. Normal color tones. Hyperpigmentation or hypopigmentation reflecting blood flow or melanin deposits.	Palpation	Moisture: perspiration. Edema: eyes, extremities, sacrum. Tenderness. Turgor, elasticity. Texture.	
Moisture	Dry or moist to touch. Hyperkeratosis (flaking, scales). Eczema. Dermatitis, psoriasis, rashes. Edema.	Olfaction	Normal body odor. Absence of pungent odor. Poor hygiene. Odor may indicate presence of bacteria or infection.	
Turgor	Normally returns quickly to its original state. Slow return to original shape: dehydration or effect of aging.	Hair and Nails	Hair: • Hirsutism: excessive body hair • Alopecia: hair loss. Nails: • Color, shape, contour • Clubbing, texture thickness.	
Integrity	No breakdown. Type of skin injury (record appropriate classification system to identify injury).	Skin Alterations	Previous scars. Graft sites. Healed ulcer sites. Piercings.	

Source: Baranoski, S., & Ayello, E. (Eds.). (2004). *Wound care essentials: Practice principles.* Philadelphia: Lippincott Williams & Wilkins.

preventive interventions, and maintenance hydration are key elements of maintaining skin integrity.

Wound Assessments

Fresh postoperative wounds do not require the intense scrutiny of historical data like a chronic wound does because these data are available in the chart, but a systematic approach to assess wound characteristics is still useful. Initial chronic wound assessments should include the patient's immune status, allergies, blood glucose levels, hydration, nutrition, latest blood albumin levels, oxygen and vascular supply, social history, habits (e.g., smoking), a review of current medications, and if possible the patient's history of wound (etiology, age of wound, treatments thus far). These factors give the health care provider clues about why a chronic wound is not healing.

Measuring and tracking wound size is an outcomes approach to intervention. Special products are available to assist in proper measurement techniques. Length, width, and depth of the wound are standard measurements. Special measuring instruments, such as Puritan DM Stick (Puritan Medical Products Co., LLC), a sterile foam-tipped plastic swab marked in millimeters, safely and comfortably give accurate, consistent measurements. Tracing graphs of transparent film, such as E-Z Graph System of wound assessment (E.S. Graph of Victoria, Inc.), enable health care providers to outline the shape of the wound and show progress of the wound surface contracture. These tracings offer a great psychological boost to patients whose wounds are healing by millimeters, when they can see progress as compared to original wound size. Several measurement tools are available that graph or assign scores to the progress of the wound. Many institutions and agencies have protocols to include these tracking tools (Chart 67–14, p. 2226).

Nursing Diagnoses

The following nursing diagnoses are related to wound healing:

- *Risk for Infection*
- *Impaired Tissue Integrity*
- *Ineffective Tissue Perfusion, peripheral*
- *Disturbed Body Image.*

Planning

A plan for care is identified by the type of wound and the factors that coexist to impede the healing process. The plan of care should be individualized, and the patient and family should be involved in the planning process. The patient and family must agree to the plan of care and the interventions because they are responsible for the accurate and complete implementation of the plan overall. The plan will include diagnostic studies to follow up on factors that may or may not impede progress. All the information must be gleaned so that a correct and meaningful treatment plan is pursued.

Outcomes and Evaluation Parameters

The outcomes of interventions provide a basis for performance evaluation. By combining assessment skills and reviewing collected data, nurses are prepared to do an evaluation of the pa-

tient's overall condition. Connecting the specialized pieces such as wound assessment, respiratory assessment, and vascular assessment with integrated interventional data can result in an evaluation that is specific; for example, poor perfusion is contributing to slow wound healing and subsequent increased risk for infection.

The outcome or goal for the patient must be identified after all the diagnostic data are considered. The outcome may be driven by the goal of healing, the goal of preventing further damage, or even amputation. The outcome is directly related to how the plan of care impacts the factors that impede healing and the interventions to promote the most optimal environment. A good wound care plan addresses all the factors in wound healing to allow the body to heal itself. The wound will heal if all the factors that affect wound healing are addressed.

Evaluation parameters would include the clinical manifestations of effective wound healing. The wound is getting smaller in diameter as well as in depth. There is an absence of drainage, odor, and normal white blood count. The patient would be experiencing less pain and tenderness. Complete wound closure is the final evaluation parameter.

Interventions and Rationales

Nursing interventions are aimed at prevention of wound complications and promotion of healing. Interventions are developed based on assessment and diagnostic results. Wound management needs to follow the four principles of wound management. Débridement (see Chart 67–10, p. 2213) by any method will cause the body to respond to its signals through the phases of wound healing. For example, débridement will send signals that trigger platelet aggregation, MMP (matrix metalloproteinases) to denature harmed collagen, leukocytosis and phagocytosis to clean up the environment, and growth factors to heal the wound with new collagen synthesis. Dressings can be applied to provide moisture for epithelial migration in a dry wound or moisture retention and absorption to prevent maceration and further collagen damage in a wet wound. Silver can be applied as an antimicrobial agent. Offloading devices such as specialized shoes, splints, wheelchair cushions, or bed surfaces will alleviate pressure and restore circulation for healing. Nutrition should be addressed and supplements given to assist in correcting any deficiencies. Vascular status should be addressed and corrected if possible. Bioburden and infection must be controlled. Perineal care of the incontinent patient will help prevent skin breakdown. Keeping skin dry decreases friction and prevents breakdown from abrasive force. With microabrasions the skin has reduced barrier capability, allowing permeability to irritating substances and proliferation of bacteria and fungal infections. Protect the skin from wetness and fecal irritants by using moisture barriers on a regular basis on anyone who cannot get up and go to the bathroom on his own. Most soap leaves a difficult-to-rinse residue and has high pH levels that interfere with the skin's protective acid mantle. Soap can be irritating and strip the natural lubricant from skin. Skin cleansers should have nonionic surfactants that do not strip natural body oil. Skin cleansers can be any combination of products: antibacterial; 3-in-1 products for cleansing, moisturizing, and protecting; and pH balanced. Moisture barriers protect the skin from too much moisture (incontinence, perspiration). Many types and brands

| CHART 67–14 | **Wound Assessment Guidelines** |

Wound Characteristic	Descriptors	Assessment Verbiage
Location	Upper/lower extremities Lateral/medial Left/right Midline Central Dorsal/plantar	Use anatomic location, such as malleolar or occipital. Describe proximity to other wounds consistently. Number wounds if more than one. Identify wound by classification and/or location. Example: "#1 skin tear, right upper extremity."
Size	length, width, and depth in centimeters	Always measure in centimeters; never estimate size by comparison; i.e., a quarter, the size of an orange.
Tracks	Centimeters and direction	Use a clock face as a frame of reference with 12 o'clock being toward the head. Example: "3-centimeter track at 2 o'clock."
Undermining	Centimeters and location	Example: "Undermining from 11 to 2 o'clock, from 1 to 1.5 centimeters."
Color	Red, yellow, black	Use percentages and shades of color. Example: "Pale red 60%, yellow 25%, black 15%."
Tissue	Granulation Epithelialization Necrotic Slough Eschar	Use descriptors: "Thick black eschar with 0.3-centimeter rim of pink tissue." "Beefy red granulation." "Pink epithelial tissue migrating toward center from 3 to 5 o'clock."
Exudate/drainage	Serous Sanguineous Serosanguineous Purulent	Use color and amount in descriptions: "Moderate serosanguineous, pink-tinged." "Minimal sanguineous, dark red." "Foam dressing saturated to edges of dressing and accumulation of exudates under dressing." (This might indicate increased drainage [infection?] or just a need for a more absorbent dressing.)
Odor	Subjective and difficult to quantify Indicate presence or not, foul	Remember that moisture retentive dressings also retain wound odor. When trying to control odor, description of presence of odor can measure outcomes: "Odor in room." "Odor at bedside." "Odor when dressing removed."
Wound margins	Rolled With epithelial tissue Defined, well demarcated Nondefined or nondemarcated	Describe margin appearance.
Periwound		
Erythema	Presence or not Intensity (color)	Use a marker pen on the skin to outline presence of suspicious erythema that might indicate infection/cellulitis.
Induration	Presence or not	May describe as increasing or resolving.
Maceration	Presence or not Extent in centimeters	Tissue maceration occurs when wound drainage or dressing moisture drowns cells. When the offending reason is contained or removed, the condition is repaired autolytically: The macerated tissue sloughs off and new skin has been generated.
Intervention and Tolerance		
Pain	Scale of 0–10	Clarify pain: "Tender when probed." "Premedicated with. . . ." "Pain subsided after packing completed."
Tolerance of procedure	Cleaning Packing Débridement	May overlap with pain assessment. A record here determines whether the patient needs premedication. Or does pain occur only during probing and packing and then subside?

of moisture barriers, body cleansers, and moisturizers are available. Emollients help keep moisture in the skin. Moisturizers add moisture to skin.

When a patient has a factor that impedes healing that cannot be corrected, the patient may be placed in conservative care and treated to prevent any further deterioration. Sometimes an amputation may be required to save the patient's life. It is not an easy decision, and the patient, family, and health care providers should come to an agreement that preservation of life overrides preservation of limb.

Evaluation

A wound and its environment and contributing factors determine the plan of care. The plan and treatment are altered in response to the assessment results of the wound, the periwound area, and any factors impeding its progress in healing. For instance, a wound may initially be draining a large amount of fluid and require an alginate. Once the drainage has decreased to a minimum, the wound bed may become dry and then require a moisture dressing such as a hydrogel to facilitate epidermal cell migration. Daily wound evaluation and documentation are indicated until there is complete wound closure. At this point the patient may also have returned to activities of daily living and so requires an offloading device. Education about protecting the newly healed wound until it matures is essential, or wound breakdown will occur.

Nursing Documentation

Nursing documentation in the patient's record must be accurate and complete in documenting the assessment, interventions, and outcomes, as well as the patient's responses to treatment. For example, wound characteristics noted after an assessment must be descriptive enough for someone who has not seen the wound to get a good mental picture. Note whether there has been a measurable outcome; that is, decrease in size, decreased drainage, increased epithelial tissue. The documentation needs to include what was used to clean the wound (saline or wound cleanser), type of dressing used and amount, and how the dressing was secured if necessary. Note significant changes that might indicate infection, and report them to the health care provider. Wound documentation also should include a patient's emotional response toward the wound and participation in wound care management. Specific to documentation of wound care, the following items should be part of the record:

- Be specific with date and time.
- Was the wound present on admission? This can be ascertained only if a head-to-toe inspection of the skin is done by the nurse.
- Record the name and score of any risk assessment tool that is used.
- How long has the patient had the wound?
- What is the specific location of the wound?
- What are the wound's surface dimensions and depth?
- What types of dressings were used and how much?
- Note changes in quantity and odor of exudates/drainage.
- What is the condition of skin surrounding the wound?
- What support surface is the patient on? Remember that specialty support surfaces are therapeutic treatment and

should be acknowledged in interventions/assessment and documentation.

- Is there progress or deterioration of the wound?
- What are the patient's and family/caregiver's reactions to the wound? Do they participate in wound care? Are their expectations reasonable?

It is necessary for the records to reflect the health care provider's orders requiring specific dressing type, frequency of dressing changes, dressing amounts used, and expected length of need. The record must reflect a diagnosis with wound description and classification if applicable. Each wound should be described separately and evaluation of wound is required monthly. Documentation can make the difference in whether treatment and/or supplies are reimbursed.

■ Collaborative Management

The primary aim of clinical management for wound healing is expedient closure of the wound with no complications. The interdisciplinary team members including the primary health care provider, certified wound care specialist nurse, nutritionist, hospitalist, vascular surgeon and/or oncologist, pharmacist, and the nurse should be included in the wound care plan. Typically wounds are not an isolated problem for most patients. The patient's comorbidities must continue to be treated. In the acute setting, the wound is often not the admitting diagnosis. Traumatic wound treatment is begun on admission in the emergency department. Frequently the certified wound care nurse is called for these wounds by surgeons to provide continuing care of the wound. If the patient is admitted with a chronic wound, the certified wound care nurse should be notified; an assessment of wound will be made; the admitting or referring health care provider will be notified of recommended treatment; orders will be obtained; and staff nurses will institute them. Staff nurses doing admission assessments need to remove existing dressings and assess, document, and report the presence of wounds. Most hospitals ensure that a nutritionist sees a patient within 24 hours of admission. Nutritionists will make recommendations for dietary considerations such as calorie intake, supplements, and vitamins, and place them in the chart. Nurses are expected to monitor intake. Plastic or vascular surgeons may be consulted for nonhealing chronic wounds as well as traumatic injuries. They may be called to perform sharp débridement. Dermatologists may be consulted for other skin issues such as rashes. Podiatrists may be consulted for foot and diabetic wounds. Endocrinologists may be consulted to control diabetes. Pharmacists may be depended on to advise about medications that will slow down wound healing and the timing for tests for antibiotic efficacy with peaks and troughs. Blood samples are drawn at specific intervals before and after antibiotic administration and sent to the laboratory to determine the amount of antibiotic in the system. This can determine whether the amount of antibiotic should be adjusted for efficacy. Respiratory therapists ensure that the patient's oxygenation is optimal. Physical therapists may do wound care in some settings. Physical therapists need to be informed about wounds so dressings and drains are free of tension. Some treatment/therapies may be covered by different services in different settings such as Unna's boot (Chapter 43 ⊛) for venous stasis ulcers or application of plaster casts to take the pressure off of diabetic wounds. A growing trend is the service of the hospitalist, a health care provider that specializes in coordinating and communicating the care of patients while in the hospital with the primary care health care provider and all other services consulted. A collaborative team approach ensures that all aspects of the wound healing process are being guided by people that are knowledgeable in each aspect of care.

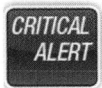 **CRITICAL ALERT** *Most chronic wounds are not emergencies (unless sepsis is present). Remember that saline and gauze are the safe universal dressing and that pressure relief is essential in preventing ulcer formation.*

All these individuals may or may not actually meet to discuss a patient's care. Charting by all of the individuals is ideally read as each comes to assess and treat the patient. Nurses have an obligation to read the notes to become informed of patient status. In home health, communication of patient status to the health care provider is of paramount importance, because the home health nurse may be the only one doing a physical assessment for long periods of time. Accurate descriptions of existing wounds are valuable to the health care providers making decisions regarding patient care.

Health Promotion

Education of the patient or caregiver regarding decisions and goals of treatment has been found to be an important factor in successful wound healing. Tenets of an effective teaching plan include:

- Wound care
- Infection prevention/assessment
- Nutrition
- Lifestyles and habits that prevent or slow wound healing
- Prevention of wound breakdown
- Follow-up care.

Each of these factors must be taught to the patient and family/caregivers in a logical, understandable fashion. For example, a written plan and return demonstrations from the patient/family help facilitate teaching.

Identifying the patient's needs for discharge begins on admission to the health care setting. The process includes assessment, identification of continuing care needs, planning, and implementing a plan that will meet those determined needs. Today it is a common practice to send patients home before wounds have completely healed and to have their care continued at home and in the outpatient clinic setting. A variety of health care professionals can be involved with the process, as described earlier, but the nurse is the pivotal figure in establishing a comprehensive discharge plan. Developing a complete plan of care and providing a manner in which routine reevaluation and modification of the plan can occur will facilitate the process until wound closure has occurred. Nurses must educate patients and family/caregivers about all aspects of the wound care. Concise written instructions beginning with a statement about hand hygiene should be given to the patient or caregiver. Return demonstration ensures that the patient and caregiver understand the procedures. If the patient is to be discharged with a drain in place, the patient should know the purpose of the drain, expected output, drain care and emptying, how to troubleshoot, whom to contact for questions, and whom to contact for an emergency.

Discharge Planning

Patients and their family need to be actively involved in the discharge planning process. The nurse must evaluate the knowledge and willingness to participate in the wound care and then develop instructions and guidelines for the patient and caregiver. If barriers exist that will affect their ability to provide effective care, an alternative plan must be instituted. For example, recognizing cultural influences and family roles is essential, so the teaching can be individualized and meaningful. An assessment of resources and transportation also is an essential component of the plan. The nurse needs to evaluate the patient and family's ability to afford and obtain the necessary supplies for the wound care. State and federal resources may need to be sought to provide the necessary equipment and supplies. The Patient Teaching & Discharge Priorities box describes the necessary components of the discharge teaching plan.

▇ Psychological Considerations

Acute and chronic wounds affect quality of life. Patients often experience depression, isolation, and financial burdens caused by wounds. Cultural issues may create misunderstanding or "compliance" issues. Nurses are often first aware and most aware of these conditions. Assessing the meaning and significance of the wound to the patient and family or caregiver is often overlooked. Frequently pain is associated with wounds and body image may be disturbed. Pain occurs due to the nerve endings being exposed, and some of the interventions utilized to heal the wound can cause varying degrees of pain. As with all assessment of pain, it is what the patient states it is as far as severity, character, duration, and tolerance level. Medications can be prescribed to alleviate the pain. Nonnarcotic medications such as nonsteroidal anti-inflammatories (NSAIDs) can alleviate pain and decrease inflammation. Narcotic medications such as opioid or opioid derivatives can be given. One should consider adequate pain coverage before dressing changes, changes in position, or mobility. Controlling pain can help patients to be more compliant with the treatment plan and willing to investigate other treatment modalities if their pain is sufficiently controlled to a tolerance level that they can withstand. Pain can be assessed on a number scale, facial scale, vital sign assessment, or combinations of such scales. Chapter 15 ⊛ includes an in-depth discussion of pain management.

Depression can occur when a patient has a wound. It may affect the way she sees herself or the way she perceives that others see her, especially if the wound is easily visible. Not only does the patient have an emotional response to her wound, but almost everyone the patient encounters has an emotional response to her wound. Wounds are perceived as unpleasant, disgusting, scary, and a nuisance. Depression may affect the patient's ability to perform the daily activities he desires to do, and it may limit patient independence. It can be very costly for the treatments and medications. The patient may have to wear some special type of shoe or device that makes her self-conscious.

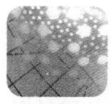

PATIENT TEACHING & DISCHARGE PRIORITIES for the Management of Wounds

Need	Teaching
WOUND CARE Patient/family Family/support system Setting	Perform daily cleansing and dressing changes: • How often to change the dressing • Type of dressing and solutions. Elevate areas where edema formation occurs. Avoid sunlight, as it can cause, among other things, healed wounds to discolor or darken permanently: • Avoid overexposure to sun. • Use sunscreen products when exposed to sunlight. • Use clothing and hats for added protection. Avoid exposure to extreme temperatures and harsh chemicals. Wear loose-fitting, soft clothing. Assess availability of, knowledge of, and compliance with treatment regimen. Have family perform return demonstration. Assess discharge placement needs: • Home • Rehabilitation facility • Extended care facility. Assess need for professional home health needs. Assess need for follow-up appointments.
WOUND INFECTION Patient/family Family/support system Setting	Assess for infection of open wounds and healed wound breakdown with each dressing change, and report as necessary. Signs and symptoms include: • Odor and exudate • Fever • Increased drainage • Swelling • Lack of wound closure • Increased pain. Teach minimization of risk factors for infection: • Hand hygiene • Clean technique with dressing changes. Explain signs and symptoms that require medical attention. Assess environment for risk factors that increase the risk of infection.
NUTRITION Patient/family Setting	Maintain a high-calorie, high-protein diet. Continue taking vitamins and mineral supplements as ordered. Observe for appetite and weight loss, and food intolerance. Assess financial resources. Home. Rehabilitation center.
PAIN MANAGEMENT Patient/family Setting	Assess pain level and report any increase in pain. Assess effectiveness of pharmacologic interventions. Wean patient off pain medication when pain lessens. Report a sudden increase in pain. Assess environment for safety and promotion of therapeutic needs.

MyNursingKit | Video: Infection Control: Dressing Change—Clean Technique

The nurse needs to assess the patient for her feelings about her wound and associated treatment. Empathize with the patient, and try to devise a plan that is least intrusive and yet realistic. A nurse can address the concerns by providing privacy during dressing changes; factual explanation of the wound to patient and family or caregiver; frank discussions with the patient and caregiver about how the wound is affecting them; scheduling wound care at the best time for the patient; and applying appro-

priate dressings and performing timely dressing changes. Instruct the patient on what can or will happen if treatment is not followed according to the individualized plan. Patients want to be informed and want honest feedback but need some compassion with the delivery of their care. Educational sites on the Internet for them to visit as well as support groups may be helpful. The wound affects one's daily lifestyle and thus cannot help but be a nuisance and a factor in the way that the patient feels about himself and how others perceive him to be. An individual who has had a recent amputation, has a whole new set of restrictions and adaptations to overcome. The patient will need education to prevent further insults from occurring to preserve the best way of life he can expect. Document the patient's response to the wound. Chapter 13 ⊕ includes an in-depth discussion of the psychosocial aspects of nursing.

Ethical Issues

Treatment of wounds can also lead to a discussion about aggressive versus conservative care. For example, what is the appropriate care for a nursing home resident patient who has previously had multiple strokes and is now aphasic and bedbound? A sacral pressure ulcer develops and eschar is observable. The patient is debilitated and has failure to thrive. Is aggressive treatment of the wound with surgical intervention appropriate? Does the patient have the ability to heal if surgical intervention is performed? Can the patient even be cleared for surgery safely? These are all questions that must be asked and considered before developing a treatment plan. The patient may not be a candidate for aggressive care, and a conservative approach may be the ethical and prudent action. The goal may be to prevent the further deterioration of the wound. Obviously, a collaborative approach among the health care team, patient, and family must occur to make a decision on what ultimate goal or outcome is desired. As hard as it is at times as health care professionals, sometimes the best plan is not the most aggressive but the most realistic plan that requires acceptance. Decisions for care and the degree of aggressiveness or lack thereof, must be consistent with the patient's overall physiological status and well as the patient's and family's goals. Those goals may be complete restoration, ability to function, or provision of comfort. Caregivers experience a myriad range of emotions. Balancing the needs of the patient with that of the caregiver can be a difficult role. As the nurse it is important to understand that the health-related quality of life is the patient's perception of well-being and not an evaluation of clinical status.

■ Research

Research is essential in order to continue improving wound care, complication rates, healing time, and scar formation. The goal of research is to identify areas in which practice needs to be improved and then to evaluate and test methods in these areas. The Research Opportunities and Clinical Impact box related to wound healing provides a list of both medical and nursing research topics still under investigation. Electronic databases are a source for finding specific studies related to these topics.

■ Liability

It is essential that the nurse understands how the regulatory and accrediting bodies such as the Joint Commission assess individual wound interventions and their effectiveness. These regulatory bodies monitor what nurses do as individuals and what they accomplish aggregately within an institution. Hospitals must have quality assurance records regarding pressure ulcer incidence and measures for reduction.

The development of wounds, in particular pressure ulcers, has led to a lot of controversy over quality of care and thus liability. Pressure ulcers, for the most part, are preventable. Prevention requires a plan of action that is individualized and vigilant. As a result of so many preventable ulcers that have developed over the years, the U.S. government has taken steps to try to ensure that all necessary action be taken to prevent pressure ulcers from developing due to negligence. A federal tag, called F-tag 314, requires long-term care facilities (nursing homes) to comply with certain regulations concerning prevention and treatment of pressure ulcers in the long-term care setting. The long-term care facility must assess those at risk for development of a pressure ulcer, follow certain preventative guidelines, demonstrate compliance with those guidelines, and, if the patient still develops a pressure ulcer, show appropriate intervention. The patient must then be monitored for progress and the plan of care altered if the plan fails to achieve the desired result of healing. The Centers for

RESEARCH OPPORTUNITIES AND CLINICAL IMPACT RELATED TO WOUND HEALING

Research Area	Clinical Impact
Wound healing dressings that promote faster healing.	Prevent infection.
Wound healing cleansers.	Prevent infection.
Topical hyperbaric oxygen treatment.	Increase healing rates.
Dietary factors that impact wound healing.	Increase healing rates.
The nature of pain induced by direct tissue injury.	Patient comfort and increased wound healing.
Nursing pain management.	
Pain and anxiety measurement and management during procedures.	
Mechanisms to prevent scar formation.	Improve wound appearance and prevent contracture formation.
Prevention of hypertrophic and keloid scar formation.	Improve wound appearance and prevent contracture formation.
Techniques to increase tensile strength and reduce wound breakdown.	Improve techniques to increase wound healing and prevent scarring.
Role of growth factors in wound healing.	Improve techniques to increase wound healing.

Silver as an Antimicrobial Agent

Clinical Problem

Infection is a common complication for a patient with a wound, especially a chronic wound. Prophylactic antibiotic use has allowed more resistant bacterial organisms to proliferate. Because wounds that are chronic may now be colonized with bacteria, deciding when and how to treat can be a complicated decision. Silver is a product that has come into wide use as a local antimicrobial agent, and the evidence surrounding its effectiveness, how much to use, and in what medium has been the subject of great debate in wound care.

Research Findings

Ip, Lui, Poon, Lung, and Burd (2006) performed a study that utilized an agar medium and various types of microorganisms such as methicillin-resistant *Staphylococcus aureus* (MRSA) and vancomycin-resistant enterococcus (VRE), as well as other microbes. Different silver dressings were applied. The result revealed that those with a higher concentration of ionic silver had a quicker and broader bacteriocidal effect. It was noted, however, that too much silver could potentially damage tissue and kill keratinocytes and fibroblasts. The most important factors relative to antimicrobial effectiveness are the bioavailability concentration and rate of delivery to the tissue. Indeed, different concentrations of silver ions could be used depending on intended desire. Prophylactic treatment could contain fewer silver ions than treatment of an active infection. The goal is to deliver the minimum amount of silver ions to perform the intended outcome.

Implications for Nursing Practice

It appears that silver is an important part of antimicrobial activity for a wound to prevent infection or treat an active infection. Silver should be treated as any other drug and utilized appropriately to the individual situation and only for its intended use. Silver is relatively cheap, abundant, and highly effective against resistant microorganisms. Its success has been repeatedly demonstrated and makes it a useful tool in wound care.

Critical Thinking Questions

1. What are some goals for the use of silver as it relates to wound care?

2. Ionic silver (Ag^+) is the effective chemical against bacteria. What would happen if it were to meet the chloride ion (Cl^-) *in situ* (in its environment in the wound)?

3. Identify other nursing measures to prevent infection in a wound.

Answers to Critical Thinking Questions appear in Appendix D.

Reference

Ip, M., Lui, S., Poon, V., Lung, I., & Burd, A. (2006). Antimicrobial activities of silver dressings: An *in vitro* comparison. *Journal of Medical Microbiology, 55,* 59–63.

EVIDENCE-BASED PRACTICE

Medicare & Medicaid Services (CMS) guidelines for October 2008 will not pay for treatment of a pressure ulcer that develops during the hospital stay. A hospital acquired pressure ulcer will have its own diagnosis-related group (DRG) code, and it will be differentiated from a community acquired DRG code. The statistics of the hospitals will be available to the public in the near future. CMS ultimately will not pay for the continuation of care for the patient with a hospital acquired pressure or decubitus ulcer, and the hospital will be responsible for all care of that patient related to that ulcer going forward. The hospital will bear the financial responsibility for the care of that patient's pressure ulcer even if the patient is no longer physically in that hospital. Documentation by health care providers and nursing staff will be pivotal in establishing whether the pressure ulcer was present on admission (POA).

■ Summary

Many recent advancements have been made with regard to wound care treatment. For example, living tissue dressing applications such as Apligraf have decreased the recovery time of healing effectively. Other xenografts (from a nonhuman animal source) such as Primatrix and Oasis have been developed as rich collagen sources to "fill in" a wound and again speed up the healing process. Ultraviolet light therapy and ultrasound therapy are being utilized to control bioburden and promote the healing process as well. The future may hold many significant advances with gene therapy and alteration/replication. Research and advancements will occur in wound therapy and healing; but the factors required for a wound to heal will not change, and the body will "heal thyself" as long as those factors required are present.

NCLEX® REVIEW

1. A patient with poor circulation has a leg wound. The nurse realizes that which phase of the wound healing process could be compromised in this patient?

    1. Homeostasis

    2. Inflammatory

    3. Proliferation

    4. Remodeling

2. A patient has been diagnosed with a tunneling wound. The nurse would document the size of the wound:

    1. In inches.

    2. In centimeters squared.

    3. Using the clock face method.

    4. In centimeters cubed.

3. A patient, prone to pressure ulcer development, is unable to move independently in bed. Which of the following should the nurse to do assist this patient?

1. Move the patient's limbs every hour.

2. Use the rule of 30 to reposition the patient every two hours.

3. Minimize the use of assistive devices to move the patient.

4. Avoid the use of foam wedges.

4. A patient has a category II skin tear on her forearm. Which of the following would be appropriate to care for this wound?

1. Use compression therapy.

2. Plan for surgical intervention.

3. Apply a moisture barrier and secure with gauze.

4. Plan for debridement of the wound.

5. A critically ill patient needs to have a leg wound debrided. The nurse realizes that the best approach to use for this patient wound be:

1. Autolytic debridement.

2. Sharp debridement.

3. Mechanical debridement.

4. Enzymatic debridement.

6. A patient with a leg wound tells the nurse that she's ugly and is not really sure if she wants to take care of the wound when she goes home. Which of the following should the nurse say in response to this patient?

1. It's not that bad.

2. Tell me why you think the wound is ugly.

3. I have to agree with you.

4. Maybe you can stay in the hospital until it's healed.

7. A patient with a wound has a poor appetite. The nurse realizes this will impact the patient's:

1. Risk of infection.

2. Healing rate.

3. Wound appearance.

4. Comfort level.

Answers for review questions appear in Appendix D

KEY TERMS

acute wounds *p.2199*
angiogenesis *p.2193*
basement membrane *p.2202*
chronic wounds *p.2199*
collagen synthesis *p.2193*
epithelialization *p.2193*
fibroblasts *p.2193*
granulation tissue *p.2193*
growth factors *p.2193*
hematoma *p.2223*
hemosiderin staining *p.2200*

homeostasis *p.2192*
hyperbaric oxygen therapy (HBOT) *p.2218*
hypergranulation *p.2222*
iatrogenic wounds *p.2199*
impaired wound healing *p.2223*
inflammatory phase *p.2193*
interface pressure *p.2219*
phagocytes *p.2193*
phagocytosis *p.2193*
pressure ulcer *p.2204*
primary intention *p.2212*

prostaglandin *p.2193*
remodeling *p.2194*
rete pegs *p.2198*
secondary intention *p.2212*
senile purpura *p.2198*
seroma *p.2224*
tertiary or third intention *p.2212*
traumatic wounds *p.2199*
wound dehiscence *p.2223*
wound evisceration *p.2223*
xerosis *p.2198*

EXPLORE PEARSON mynursingkit™

MyNursingKit is your one stop for online chapter review materials and resources. Prepare for success with additional NCLEX®-style practice questions, interactive assignments and activities, web links, animations and videos, and more!

Register your access code from the front of your book at
www.mynursingkit.com

REFERENCES

Agency for Health Care Policy and Research (AHCPR). (1992). *Pressure ulcers in adults: Prediction and prevention* (Publication No. 92-0047). Rockville, MD: Author. Retrieved September 11, 2008, from http://www.ncbi.nlm.nih.gov/books/bv.fcgi?rid=hstat2.chapter.4409

Agency for Health Care Policy and Research (AHCPR). (1994). *Treatment of pressure ulcers in adults* (Publication No. 95-0652). Rockville, MD: Author. Retrieved September 11, 2008, from http://www.ncbi.nlm.nih.gov/books/bv.fcgi?rid=hstat2.chapter.5124

Argenta, L. C., & Morykwas, M. J. (1997). Vacuum assisted closure: A new method for wound control and treatment: Clinical experience. *Annals of Plastic Surgery, 38*(6), 563–577.

Armstrong, M. H., & Price, P. (2004). Wet-to-dry gauze dressings: Fact and fiction. *Wounds, 16*(2), 56–62.

Arnold, M. C. (2003). Pressure ulcer prevention and management: The current evidence for care. *AANC Clinical Issues: Advanced Practice in Acute Critical Care, 14*(4), 411–428.

Baranoski, S. (2006). Raising awareness of pressure ulcer prevention and treatment. *Advances in Skin and Wound Care, 19*(7), 398–405.

Baranoski, S., & Ayello, E. (Eds.). (2004). *Wound care essentials: Practice principles.* Philadelphia: Lippincott Williams & Wilkins.

Black, P. et al., (2007). National pressure ulcer advisory panel's updated pressure ulcer staging system. Medscape Nurses from web MD.

Retrieved on September 13, 2008, from http://www.medscape.com/viewarticle/563159

Christian, P., Talavera, F., Stadelmann, W., Slenkovich, N., & Downey, S. (2006). Wound healing, growth factors. *eMedicine.* Retrieved September 7, 2008, from http://www.emedicine.com/plastic/topic457.htm

Clark, J. J. (2002). Wound repair and factors influencing healing. *Critical Care Nursing Quarterly, 25*(1), 1–12.

Coats-Bennett, U. (2002). Use of support surfaces in the ICU. *Critical Care Nursing Quarterly, 25*(1), 22–32.

Corbett, J. V. (2004). *Laboratory tests and diagnostic procedures with nursing diagnoses* (6th ed.). Upper Saddle River, NJ: Pearson Prentice Hall.

Cranton, E. M. (2005). *Hyperbaric oxygen therapy.* Retrieved September 13, 2008, from http://drcranton.com/hbo.htm

Cutting, K. F., & White, R. J. (2005). Criteria for identifying wound infection—Revisited. *Ostomy Wound Management, 51*(1), 28–34.

Drosou, A., Falabella, A., & Kirsner, R. (2003). Antiseptics on wounds: An area of controversy (Part one). *Wounds.* Retrieved October 29, 2007, from http://www.woundsresearch.com/article/1586

Duffy, J., & Korniewicz, D. (2000). Outcomes measurement using the ANA safety and quality indicators. *Nursing World.* Retrieved October 29, 2007, from http://nursingworld.org/mods/archive/mod72/ceomfull.htm

Enoch, S., & Harding, K. (2003). Wound bed preparation: The science behind the removal of barriers to healing (Part two). *Wounds.* Retrieved October 29, 2007, from http://www.woundsresearch.com/article/1798

Frykberg, R. G. (2002). Diabetic foot ulcers: Pathogenesis and management. *American Family Physician, 66*(9), 1655–1662.

Gardner, S. E., & Frantz, R. A. (2004). Wound bioburden. In S. Baranoski & E. A. Ayello (Eds.), *Wound care essentials: Practice principles* (pp. 91–116). Philadelphia: Lippincott Williams & Wilkins.

Gibbs, S., Silva Pinto, A. N., Murli, S., Huber, M., Hohl, D., & Ponec, M. (2000). Epidermal growth factor and keratinocyte grow factor differentially regulate epidermal migration, growth and differentiation. *Wound Repair Regeneration, 8*(3), 192–203.

Halek, M., & Mayer, H. (2002). Predictive validity of the original and expanded Norton Scale in geriatric nursing. *Pflege, 15*(6), 309–317.

Hanson, D., Langemo, D., Anderson, J., Hunter, S., & Thompson, P. (2006). Pressure mapping: Seeing the invisible. *Advances in Skin and Wound Care, 19*(8), 432–434.

Hinman, C. D., & Maibach, H. (1963). Effect of air exposure and occlusion on experimental human skin wounds. *Nature, 200,* 377–378.

Hiok, T. L. (1997). *Leg ulcers: A multidisciplinary approach.* Retrieved September 1, 2007, from http://www.nsc.gov.sg/cgi-bin/WB_ContentGen.pl?id=242&gid=49

Ip, M., Lui, S., Poon, V., Lung, I., & Burd, A. (2006). Antimicrobial activities of silver dressings: An *in vitro* comparison. *Journal of Medical Microbiology, 55,* 59–63.

Joseph, E., Hamori, C. A., Bergman, S., Roaf, E., Swann, N. F., & Anastasi, G. W. (2000). A prospective randomized trial of vacuum assisted closure versus standard therapy of chronic nonhealing wounds. *Wounds, 12*(3), 60–67.

Lavery, L. A., Armstrong, D. G., & Harkless, L. B. (1996). Classification of diabetic foot ulcerations. *Journal of Foot and Ankle Surgery, 35*(6), 528.

Leach, M. J., et al. (2006a). Clinical efficacy of horse chestnut seed extract in the treatment of venous ulceration. *Journal of Wound Care, 15*(4), 159–167.

Leach, M. J., et al. (2006b). Using horse chestnut seed extract in the treatment of venous leg ulcers: A cost–benefit analysis. *Ostomy Wound Management, 52*(4), 68–70, 72–74, 76–78.

Martin, N., Oldani, T., & Claxton, M. (2005). A guide to offloading the diabetic foot. *Podiatry Today, 9*(18), 67–74.

Marucha, P. T. (2005). *Modulation of inflammation by stress and psychosocial factors.* Retrieved August 6, 2005, from http://medicine.osu.edu/mindbody/project_2.html

MayoClinic.com. (2006). *Pyoderma gangrenosum.* Retrieved September 1, 2007, from http://www.mayoclinic.com/health/pyoderma-gangrenosum/DS00723

McGuckin, M., Goldman, R., Bolton, L., & Salcido, R. (2003). The clinical relevance of microbiology in acute and chronic wounds. *Advances in Skin & Wound Care, 16,* 12–25.

MedTech1.com. (2005). *What is V.A.C.® therapy?* Retrieved December 14, 2006, from http://www.medtech1.com/companies/kci.cfm

Nataraj, C., Ritter, G., Dumas, S., Helfer, F., Brunelle, J., & Sander, T. W. (2007). Extracellular wound matrices: Novel stabilization and sterilization method for collagen-based biologic wound dressings. *Wounds.* Retrieved September 1, 2007, from http://www.woundsresearch.com/article/7374

National Institute for Health and Clinical Excellence (NICE). (2005). *Pressure ulcer management.* Retrieved September 11, 2008, from http://www.nice.org.uk/CG029

National Pressure Ulcer Advisory Panel (NPUAP). (1998). *Instructions for using the PUSH tool.* Retrieved September 13, 2008 from http://www.npuap.org/pushinstr.htm

National Pressure Ulcer Advisory Panel (NPUAP). (2007a). *Updated staging system.* Retrieved October 1, 2007, from http://www.npuap.org/push3-0.htm

National Pressure Ulcer Advisory Panel (NPUAP). (2007b). *Updated staging system. Pressure ulcer stages revised by NPUAP.* Retrieved September 1, 2007, from http://www.npuap.org/pr2.htm

Norman, D. (2003). The effects of stress on wound healing and leg ulceration. *British Journal of Nursing, 12*(21), 1256–1263.

Odland, G. (1958). The fine structure of the interrelationship of cells in the human epidermis. *Journal of Biophysical, Biochemistry and Cytology, 4,* 529–535.

Ovington, L. (2002). General principles of wound care. In P. J. Sheffield, A. P. S. Smith, & C. E. Fife (Eds.), *Wound care practice* (pp. 159–187). Flagstaff, AZ: Best Publishing.

Pittler, M. H., & Ernst, E. (2006). Horse chestnut seed extract for chronic venous insufficiency. *Cochrane Database of Systematic Reviews, 25*(1), CD003230.

Porth, C. (2007). *Essentials of pathophysiology* (2nd ed.). Philadelphia: Lippincott Williams & Wilkins.

Pressure ulcers. (2005). *Professional guide to diseases* (8th ed.). Retrieved October 24, 2007, from http://www.wrongdiagnosis.com/b/bedsores/book-diseases-7a.htm

Rolstad, B. S., Ovington, L. G., & Harris, A. (2000). Principles of wound management. In R. A. Bryant (Ed.), *Acute and chronic wounds: Nursing management* (2nd ed., pp. 85–124). St. Louis: Mosby.

Shah, B. R., & Hux, J. E. (2003). Quantifying the risk of infectious diseases for people with diabetes. *Diabetes Care.* Retrieved September 1, 2007, from http://care.diabetesjournals.org/cgi/content/abstract/26/2/510

Smith, A. P. S. (2002). Etiology of the problem wound. In P. J. Sheffield, A. P. S. Smith, & C. E. Fife (Eds.), *Wound care practice* (pp. 3–48). Flagstaff, AZ: Best Publishing.

Smith & Nephew Clinical Staff. (2001). *Treatment options for surgical wounds.* Retrieved September 13, 2008, from http://wound.smith-nephew.com/au/node.asp?NodeId=3746

Steinberg, J. S. (2004). Understanding growth factors and matrix metalloproteinases in the diabetic foot wound. *Wounds, 16*(Suppl. B), 13S–24S.

Sussman, C. (1998). *Electrical stimulation.* Retrieved October 1, 2007, from http://www.medicaledu.com/estim.htm

Undersea & Hyperbaric Medical Society. (2007). *Indications for hyperbaric oxygen therapy.* Retrieved October 1, 2007, from http://www.uhms.org/Default.aspx?tabid=270

U.S. Department of Health and Human Services (DHHS). (2000). *Healthy People 2010 understanding and improving health.* Washington, DC: Author.

Vaughn, M. (2002). Physical therapeutic modalities in wound healing. In P. J. Sheffield, A. P. S. Smith, & C. E. Fife (Eds.), *Wound care practice* (pp. 159–187). Flagstaff, AZ: Best Publishing.

Waldrop, J., & Doughty, D. (2000). Wound-healing physiology. In R. A. Bryant (Ed.), *Acute and chronic wounds: Nursing management* (2nd ed., pp. 17–40). St. Louis: Mosby.

Warren, J. B., Yoder, L. H., & Young-McCaughan, S. (1999). Development of a decision tree for support surfaces: A tool for nursing. *MEDSURG Nursing, 8*(4), 239–248.

White, R., & Cutting, K. (2006). *Modern exudate management: A review of wound treatments.* Retrieved October 1, 2007, from http://www.worldwidewounds.com/2006/september/White/Modern-Exudate-Mgt.html

Wicke, C., Halliday, B., Allen, D., Roche, N. S., Scheuenstuhl, H., Spencer, M., et al. (2000). Effects of steroids and retinoids on wound healing. *Archives of Surgery, 135,* 1265–1270.

Wilson, J. A., & Clark, J. J. (2004). Obesity: Impediment to postsurgical wound healing. *Advances in Skin & Wound Care, 17*(8), 426–435.

Winter, G. D. (1962). Formation of scab and the rate of epithelialization of superficial wounds in the skin of the young domestic pig. *Nature, 193,* 293–294.

Wood, W. A., et al. (2005). Testing for loss of protective sensation in patients with foot ulceration: A cross-sectional study. *Journal of the American Podiatric Medical Association, 95,* 469–474.

Wound, Ostomy, and Continence Nurses Society (WOCN). (2003). *Guideline for prevention and management of pressure ulcers.* Glenview, IL: Author. Retrieved September 11, 2008, from http://www.guideline.gov/summary/summary.aspx?doc_id=3860

Caring for the Patient with Burn Injuries

Kathleen Osborn

Outcome-Based Learning Objectives

After studying this chapter, the learner will be able to:

1. Differentiate between the three classifications of burn injury: mild, moderate, and major.

2. Compare and contrast the causes, incidence, prevalence, types, and prevention of burn injuries.

3. Describe the pathophysiological response of burn injury at the tissue and organ level.

4. Compare and contrast the three periods of burn care.

5. Describe the significance and components of burn severity assessment including size and depth of injury, impact of patient's age on injury, part of the body burned, and past medical history.

6. Describe the components of a comprehensive burn treatment plan for each of the three periods of burn care including fluid resuscitation, pain management, wound care, surgical management, contracture prevention, nutritional needs, and emotional adjustment.

7. Describe the discharge teaching needed to facilitate an optimal recovery and return to society.

8. Identify the potential complications associated with each period of burn injury.

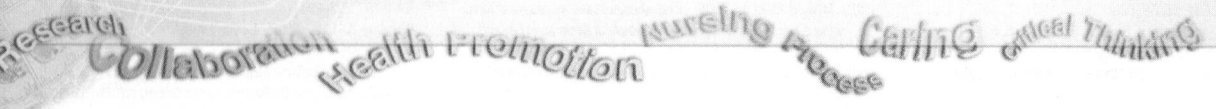

BURN INJURIES are a traumatic, dehumanizing injury that can be fatal, disfiguring, and incapacitating. Burns cause a loss of skin integrity that ranges from a minor superficial injury to a deep full-thickness injury that extends into the underlying structures and organs. As noted in National Guidelines box, according to the American Burn Association (ABA), burns are classified as minor, moderate, or major. All three categories of injury may cause a systemic response; but the deeper and more extensive the injuries are, the greater and more serious the systemic reaction becomes.

Epidemiology

The incidence of burn injuries has been declining in the last 50 years, although the United States (U. S.) remains one of the leading countries in the developed world in the number of fire- and burn-related fatalities. Burn injuries are second only to motor vehicle crashes as the leading cause of accidental death in the U. S. (Burn Survivor Resource Center, 2002b). According to the American Burn Association, each year in the U. S., 1.1 million burn injuries require medical attention, and approximately 45,000 of these require hospitalization (National Institutes of General Medical Sciences, 2006). Approximately 4,500 people die each year from burn injuries, and up to 10,000 people in the U. S. die every year of burn-related infections. Pneumonia is the most common infection among hospitalized patients with burns (Murray, 2008). Fire departments respond to fires every 15 seconds, and residential fires occur every 60 seconds (Burnsurgery.org, 2004).

For fire-related injuries, the home is the most common site, accounting for the majority of all fire-related deaths. Cigarettes are a leading cause of fatal homes fires. Annually between 900 and 1,000 people die from fires started by cigarettes, and an additional 2,500 to 3,000 are injured. The cost of human life and property damage is in the billions of dollars each year from cigarette-related fires.

The decline in the death rate from burn injuries is mostly attributed to early excision and closure of the burn wound. Additional reasons for improved survival rates are improved resuscitation, control of infection, and support of the hypermetabolic response. The mortality rate for burns is highest in the very young and in the elderly population. (Reasons for this are discussed later in this chapter.)

Etiology

Burn injuries occur when there is direct or indirect contact with a heat source. No matter what the causative factor, burn injury results in a loss of skin integrity. Depending on the cause and extent of the injury, there can be both localized and systemic

NATIONAL GUIDELINES for the Classification of Burn Injury

Minor Burn Injury	Moderate Burn Injury	Major Burn Injury
Excludes:	Excludes:	Includes:
Electrical injury	Electrical injury	All electrical injuries
Complicated injuries (multiple trauma)	Inhalation injury	Inhalation injury
High-risk patients such as older adults and those with chronic illnesses.	Complicated injuries (multiple trauma)	Complicated injuries (multiple trauma)
Includes:	High-risk patients such as older adults and those with chronic illnesses.	High-risk patients such as older adults and those with chronic illnesses
Partial-thickness injuries < 15% of total body surface area (TBSA) in adults	Includes:	All burns involving ears, eyes, face, hands, feet, and perineum
Full-thickness injuries < 2% of TBSA not involving ears, eyes, face, hands, feet, and perineum.	Partial-thickness injuries 15–25% of total body surface area in adults	Partial-thickness injuries > 25% of total body surface area in adults
	Full-thickness injuries 10% of TBSA not involving ears, eyes, face, hands, feet, and perineum.	Full-thickness injuries 10% or greater of TBSA.

Source: American Burn Association. http://www.ameriburn.org/

tissue damage. Inhaling smoke causes injury to the lungs, referred to as **inhalation injury**. Management of burns is standard regardless of the cause except for inhalation and electrical burns. The unique aspects of inhalation and electrical burn injuries are outlined later, as they involve more than just trauma to the skin.

Types of Burn Injury

Burns occur as a result of exposure to fire (thermal); direct contact with electricity, radiation, or chemicals; and scalds. It is important to know how the patient was burned because each type of burn injury has unique treatments, morbidity and mortality statistics, and sequelae. Chart 68–1 outlines the various types of injury and the associated causes.

Thermal Burns

Thermal burns from flames are the most common type of burn injury. These injuries occur when heat is transferred to the body from an external source; for example, flames from a fire. The depth of the injury is related to the length of exposure and the temperature of the heat source.

Scald Burns

Scald burns are a type of thermal injury that occurs from contact with hot foods or liquids, including steam. The severity of the burn is related to the temperature of the hot liquid and the length of time it is in contact with the body. At 120°F (48°C), skin requires 5 minutes for a full-thickness burn to occur. When the temperature of the liquid is 140°F (60°C), it takes only 5 seconds or less for the a serious burn. Coffee, tea, and other hot drinks are usually served at 160° to 180°F (71° to 82°C).

Electrical Burns

Electrical burns tend to be deeper than most burn injuries. The depth and severity of the injury depends on the amount of voltage, the length of exposure, the type of current, the pathway of flow, and the local tissue resistance. It is difficult to assess the extent of damage accurately for two reasons. First, much of the damage occurs internally due to the electrical current traversing along the tendons and vessels as it flows through the body, creating deep wounds that often extend into the subcutaneous tissue and muscle fascia (Cancio et al., 2005). Second, the destructive process initiated at the time of injury continues for weeks afterward. At the time of contact, the electrical flow follows the path of least resistance through the body, which is typically along muscles, long bones, blood vessels, and nerves. The entry and exit sites give a clue as to how much damage has been sustained. For example, if the entry wound is the hand and the exit is the bottom of the foot, the current traveled through most of the major organs. If the entry/exit was hand to shoulder, then just the arm sustained injury. Figure 68–1 ■ (p. 2236) is an example of tissue damage from an electrical injury. The damage to the skin appears deceptively small as compared to the damage that is sustained by internal muscle, fat, and fascia along the path of electrical flow. When deep muscle injury has occurred, myoglobin is released into the circulation from the muscle tissue. It is transported to the kidneys where it can block the renal tubules due to its large size, causing acute tubular necrosis.

CHART 68–1	Causes of Burn Injuries

Type of Injury	Cause
Thermal	Flame, flash injuries (explosion), contact with hot metal and hot, sticky tar
Electrical	Contact with electrical current, sparks or electrical arcing, alternating current, direct current, high-voltage lines, and lightning
Radiation	Overexposure to sunlight, radiation treatment for cancer
Chemical	Contact with strong acids, alkalis, or an organic compound
Scalds	Steam, hot liquids
Inhalation	Exposure of upper airway to intense heat, flames, and smoke Exposure of lung parenchyma to chemicals, steam, or aspiration of hot liquids
Nuclear	Nuclear power plant accidents

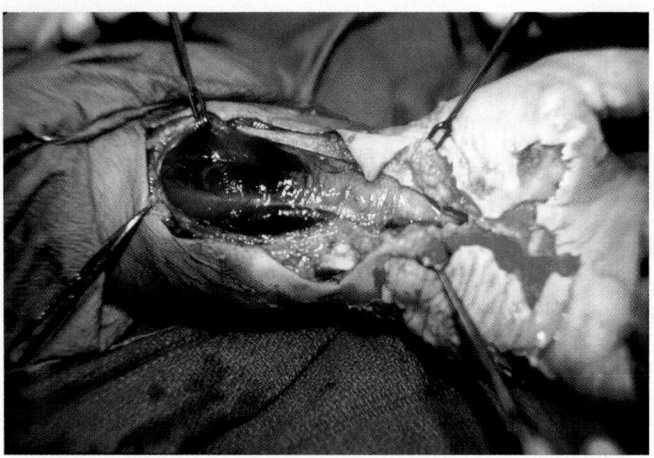

FIGURE 68–1 ■ Black muscle from electrical injury.
Source: Courtesy of: John M. Osborn, M.D., FACS, Sacramento, CA Plastic Surgery Center

Additionally, at the time of the injury, contact with the electrical current can cause tetanic muscle contractions that can be strong enough to cause fractures of long bones and vertebrae. These tetanic contractions also can occur in the respiratory muscles and cardiac muscles, causing suffocation and disruption of the cardiac conduction system resulting in dysrhythmias and cardiac arrest. Delayed neurological changes and cataract formation also may occur (Benson, Sidor, Schwartz, Desposito, & Hostetler, 2006).

Radiation Burns

Radiation burns are usually a result of overexposure to the sun or are associated with radiation treatment for cancer. Radiation injury also may occur from industrial accidents such as at nuclear power plants. Tissue damage occurs from the transfer of radiant energy to the body, which stimulates reactions with body chemicals resulting in cell death. The cells most susceptible to injury are those that divide rapidly such as bone marrow, skin, and the gastrointestinal tract. The depth of the injury depends on how close the individual was to the source as well as the length of time to exposure. Typically radiation injuries involve only the epithelial layer of skin (Wolf & Herndon, 2000).

Chemical Burns

Chemical burns occur when the skin is in contact with caustic chemical compounds such as strong acids, alkalis, or organic compounds. There are common household chemicals that cause burns such as bleach, boric acid, creosote, paint thinner, and plumbing pipe decloggers such as Drano or Liquid-Plumr. In the workplace occupational agents such as liquid concrete in the road construction and paving industry are also the source of chemical burns (Burn Survivor Resource Center, 2002a). The depth of the injury from a chemical is directly related to the length of exposure. Liberal washing of the skin and removing clothing and jewelry as quickly as possible will limit the depth of the injury (Surgical-tutor.org.uk, 2006). Emergency treatment of chemical burns is discussed later in this chapter.

Inhalation Injury

Inhalation injuries occur in 20% to 30% of patients admitted to burn centers (Lucile Packard Children's Hospital at Stanford, 2008). These injuries resulting from inhalation of heated air and smoke present a unique set of problems, one of which is difficulty in diagnosing the full extent of the injury. There is a set of criteria used to evaluate for the presence of an inhalation injury, which includes that the injury occurred in an enclosed area; there are burns of the face and neck; and there are singed nasal hairs, a hoarse, dry cough, bloody/sooty sputum, and labored respirations. Additionally, there may be edema, blisters, and ulcerations along the mucosal lining of the oropharynx and larynx. The edema continues to increase for 24 to 48 hours after the injury; thus, close monitoring for pulmonary complications, including acute respiratory distress syndrome (Chapter 36), is essential. Smoke inhalation in addition to cutaneous external burn injuries results in increased morbidity and mortality as compared to external injuries alone (Demling, 2005). The majority of deaths from burn injuries are due to smoke inhalation rather than to surface burns. Associated smoke inhalation injuries increase mortality rate by 77% when combined with cutaneous injuries (Mandel & Hales, 2008).

Nursing care includes vigorous pulmonary toilet, continuous monitoring of oxygen saturation levels, daily chest radiographs, and an early assessment of the need for intubation and mechanical ventilation. Respiratory distress may or may not develop, but evidence of it needs to be part of an ongoing assessment. Due to the edema from the injury, ongoing assessment for airway obstruction is essential. Signs of airway obstruction include:

- Stridor
- Use of accessory muscles
- Respiratory distress
- Hypoxia
- Deep burns of the face and neck
- Blister or edema of the oropharynx. (Mandel & Hales, 2008)

 *Continuous monitoring of arterial blood gases (ABGs) is necessary to assess the need for intubation and ventilatory support. Have necessary supplies ready for emergent intubation with inhalation injuries.*

Health Promotion

The decline in burn injuries in the U. S. is due in part to the focus on injury prevention. High-risk populations have been identified, as listed in the Risk Factors box, and prevention programs have been established to increase knowledge of burn prevention. Firefighters and health care workers teach burn prevention to various populations in multiple settings. These education programs include information about teaching children and adults caring for them that if clothing catches fire, the person needs to "stop, drop, and roll," as this will assist in putting the flames out. Wrapping the victim in a blanket, coat, or sheet also will help extinguish the flames because the oxygen needed to sustain the flame is cut off. Applying copious cool water immediately after the injury helps decrease the severity of the burn. The older adult population is the most susceptible to burns caused by clothing catching fire while cooking or smoking; therefore, education programs about burn prevention also need to target this population.

The nurse is in a pivotal position to collaborate with other disciplines to develop prevention programs in local communities. The majority of fires are started in the home through igno-

RISK FACTORS for Burn Injuries

Population	Risk
Older adults	Clothing catching fire while cooking or smoking
	Living in apartments above the first floor
Infants and children	Matches and cigarette lighters
	Sun exposure
	Electrical outlets
	Clothing
	Scald injuries
	Microwave ovens
	Kitchen stoves
	Fireplaces
	Chemicals
	Fireworks
Young adults	Motor vehicle crashes
	Stun guns
	Sun exposure
	Methamphetamine laboratories
	Fireworks
	Taser
Firefighters	Exposure to all types of fires while in the line of duty

rance and carelessness. Children playing with matches and cigarette lighters account for approximately 35% of all burn injuries (Lucile Packard Children's Hospital at Stanford, 2008). Prevention education focuses on keeping children safe by keeping matches and lighters out of reach. Parents also need to be taught that uncovered electrical outlets in homes pose a threat to small children. Plastic plugs need to be inserted in every plug within reach of a child.

Scald burns from hot tap water are totally preventable. The ABA recommends the following simple safety tips to decrease the risk of scald burns:

- Set home water heaters no higher than 120°F.
- Provide constant adult supervision of young children or those who may have difficulty removing themselves from hot water on their own.
- Fill the bathtub to the desired level before getting in. Run cold water first, then hot.
- Mix tub water thoroughly and check the temperature with one's elbow before getting in the water.
- Install antiscald temperature devices that stop or interrupt the flow of water when the temperature reaches a predetermined level.
- Cook on back burners when children are present.
- Keep children out of cooking areas when hot food or liquids are being transported.
- Place hot items in the center of the table during mealtime.
- Never drink or carry hot liquids while carrying a child.

The focus of chemical burn prevention is, first, keeping chemicals in a safe place and, second, knowing how to neutral-

ize them when they occur. All home chemicals need to be locked away from children. If contact occurs, copious amounts of water irrigation will decrease the severity of the burn.

Radiation burns typically are not deep injuries, but repeated exposure increases the risk of skin cancer. The goal for the prevention of radiation burns is to educate the public to limit exposure to sun, wear protective clothing and sunscreen when exposed to the sun, and avoid the use of artificial sources of ultraviolet light (tanning booths, sunlamps, and tanning beds). The amount of protection offered by a sunscreen is referred to as the sun protection factor (SPF). The higher the SPF number, the greater the protection. Protection from the sun offered by sunscreens may be classified as follows:

- Minimal: SPF 2 to 11
- Moderate: SPF 12 through 29
- High: SPF 30+. (Some sunscreens claim SPFs higher than 30, although the added protection at such higher levels is insignificant.) (Centers for Disease Control and Prevention, 2006).

In the industrial setting, the most effective means of preventing exposure to radiation is proper maintenance of equipment, education of employees who work near equipment, and regularly scheduled safety checks.

Approximately three-fifths of burn injuries occur in homes where there are no smoke detectors or the smoke detectors are nonfunctioning; thus, the education focus has centered on installation and periodic checking of smoke detectors. The Centers for Disease Control and Prevention (CDC) gives funding to state health departments to provide the Smoke Alarm Installation and Fire Safety Education (SAIFE) program in high-risk homes in 16 states. The programs use local fire department contractors to canvass neighborhoods, installing long-lasting lithium-battery-powered smoke alarms and providing general fire safety education and a 6-month battery checkup (Ballesteros, Jackson, & Martin, 2005). Additionally, most cities in the United States have fire departments that will install smoke detectors free of charge for older adults.

One goal of the Federal Emergency Management Agency (FEMA) focuses on decreasing residential fire deaths by increasing awareness of hazards in the home and the need for smoke detectors and a fire extinguisher. The National Guidelines box (p. 2238) outlines the national guidelines for fire prevention set forth by FEMA.

Lawmakers' role in fire prevention is multifaceted. First, laws requiring public buildings to have protective measures in place such as fire-retardant fabrics, proper egress routes, smoke detectors, and sprinkler systems must be enforced. Second, the government must enforce laws requiring proper labeling of not only flammable products but also toxic chemicals and their associated antidotes.

On a national level, the ABA has succeeded in getting key pieces of legislation passed. Additional funding for burn centers was approved as part of bioterrorism legislation in the event of a bioterrorist act against the United States (ABA, 2002). Representatives of the ABA testified before a congressional committee and were successful in passing a law to increase the flammability standards for clothing worn by children up to age 7 (HR 4896 and S 2188). Legislation on "safe cigarettes" is another issue that

NATIONAL GUIDELINES for Fire Prevention

Guideline	Prevention Measures
Smoke alarms	Working smoke alarms can double the chances of survival.
	Every home needs at least one smoke alarm.
	Test it monthly, keep it free of dust, and replace the battery at least once a year.
	Smoke alarms themselves should be replaced after 10 years of service, or as recommended by the manufacturer.
Electrical fires	Never overload circuits or extension cords. Do not place cords and wires under rugs, over nails, or in high-traffic areas.
	Immediately shut off and unplug appliances that sputter, spark, or emit an unusual smell.
	Have appliances professionally repaired or replaced.
Appliances	When using appliances, follow the manufacturer's safety precautions.
	Overheating, unusual smells, shorts, and sparks are all warning signs that appliances need to be shut off and then repaired or replaced.
	Unplug appliances when not in use.
	Use safety caps to cover all unused outlets, especially if there are small children in the home.
Alternate heaters	Portable heaters need their space.
	Keep anything combustible at least 3 feet away.
	Keep fire in the fireplace.
	Use fire screens and have chimneys cleaned annually. The creosote buildup can ignite a chimney fire that could easily spread.
	Kerosene heaters should be used only where approved by authorities.
	Never use gasoline or camp stove fuel.
	Refuel outside and only after the heater has cooled.
Affordable home fire safety sprinklers	When home fire sprinklers are used with working smoke alarms, the chances of surviving a fire are greatly increased.
	Sprinklers are affordable; they can increase property value and lower insurance rates.
Escape plan	Practice an escape plan from every room in the house.
	Caution everyone to stay low to the floor when escaping from fire and never to open doors that are hot.
	Select a location where everyone can meet after escaping the house.
	Keep window escape ladders on any floor above the main level.
	Get out and then call for help.
Caring for children	Children under age 5 are naturally curious about fire.
	Many play with matches and lighters.
	Children set over 20,000 house fires every year.
	Take the mystery out of fire play by teaching children that fire is a tool, not a toy.
	Check labels on clothing for young children to ensure that the fabrics are fire retardant.
Caring for older people	Every year more than 1,200 senior citizens die in fires.
	Many of these fire deaths could have been prevented.
	Seniors are especially vulnerable because many live alone and cannot respond quickly.
Smoking precautions	Careless smoking is the leading cause of fire deaths and the second leading cause of injuries among people age 65 and older.
	Cigarettes continue to burn when they are not properly extinguished.
	When a resting cigarette is accidentally knocked over, it can smolder for hours before a flare-up occurs.
	Put cigarette or cigar out at the first sign of feeling drowsy while watching television or reading.
	Use deep ashtrays and put cigarette all the way out.
	Never smoke in bed.
	Do not walk away from lit cigarettes and other smoking materials.
	Do not put ashtrays on the arms of sofas or chairs.

Source: U.S. Fire Administration. (2006). *Working together for home fire safety.* Retrieved October 5, 2006, from http://www.usfa.fema.gov/downloads/pdf/fswy11.pdf

the ABA has actively lobbied for changes. A fire-safe cigarette, which would require manufactures to institute small design changes, has significantly less propensity to ignite furniture and mattresses. The ABA supports legislation that would require manufacturers to institute these changes (HR 4607 and S 2317).

Pathophysiology of Tissue Injury

As discussed earlier, burn injuries are caused when tissue is exposed to thermal, electrical, radiation, or chemical energy. The tissue injury resulting from these agents causes coagulation of cellular protein. The amount of tissue damage is related to the length of exposure and the temperature of the offending agent. As the temperature increases, cellular functions become impaired. Cell membranes are disrupted when exposed to temperatures between 40° and 44°C (104° and 110°F). Exposure of tissue to 60°C (140°F) for longer than 1 second will cause a **partial-thickness injury** (epidermis and part of the dermis). A **full-thickness injury** (epidermis and dermis) will occur with temperatures greater than 70°C (158°F) (Flynn, 2002). Full-thickness versus partial-thickness injury is described later in this chapter.

Tissue Injury

When thermal damage occurs on the skin surface, three distinct zones of injury are created. These zones relate to the level of damage in a given area. The center of the wound, referred to as the **zone of coagulation**, is the area where there is the greatest amount of injury to the tissue. If all the layers of the skin have been destroyed, this area contains denatured protein and coagulated nonfunctioning blood vessels. The appearance of the tissue is white or pearly gray and has a leather-like texture. Nerve endings have been destroyed; therefore, there is no sensation in this area. If all the layers of the skin are not destroyed, the zone of coagulation appears red and is very painful. With both types of injury, there is edema formation in the surrounding area because of the release of vasoactive mediators such as histamines, serotonin, interleukin-1, and prostaglandins from the injured cells (Demling, 2005). An in-depth discussion of the effect of vasoactive mediators is covered in Chapter 61 ⊕.

Surrounding the zone of coagulation is an area of potentially viable but injured cells referred to as the **zone of stasis**. The mi-

crovasculature in this area is clogged with heat-injured erythrocytes. Vasoactive mediators from these injured cells cause edema formation, further impairing blood flow to the area. This decrease in blood flow to the area continues for approximately 16 to 24 hours after the injury. Survival and recovery of the cells in the zone of stasis depend on prompt and appropriate wound care, edema control, and systemic fluid resuscitation. These interventions decrease the incidence of cellular dehydration, ischemia, and infection. If prompt measures are not instituted, these extremely vulnerable cells die, becoming part of the zone of coagulation. The tissue in this area initially appears moist, red, and blanches with pressure because of the presence of viable capillaries.

In the outermost portion of the injured area, there is minor cell damage; this area is referred to as the **zone of hyperemia**. Once again, due to the vasoactive mediators, there is prominent blood flow to this area. This blood contains the nutrients needed to support the zone of stasis, and it contains the necessary mediators to continue the inflammatory process within the zones of stasis and coagulation. Like the zone of stasis, the zone of hyperemia has viable capillaries and, therefore, will blanch with pressure (Oliver, Spain, & Stadelmann, 2005). Tissue in this area appears pink and moist. Complete healing of this area is expected, unless there is additional insult such as infection or profound tissue inflammation (Figure 68–2 ■).

Systemic Injury

Burn injuries, depending on the size and depth, potentially could impact every organ system in the body. Immediately after a burn injury, fluid begins to shift from the intracellular and intravascular compartment into the interstitial space. This is

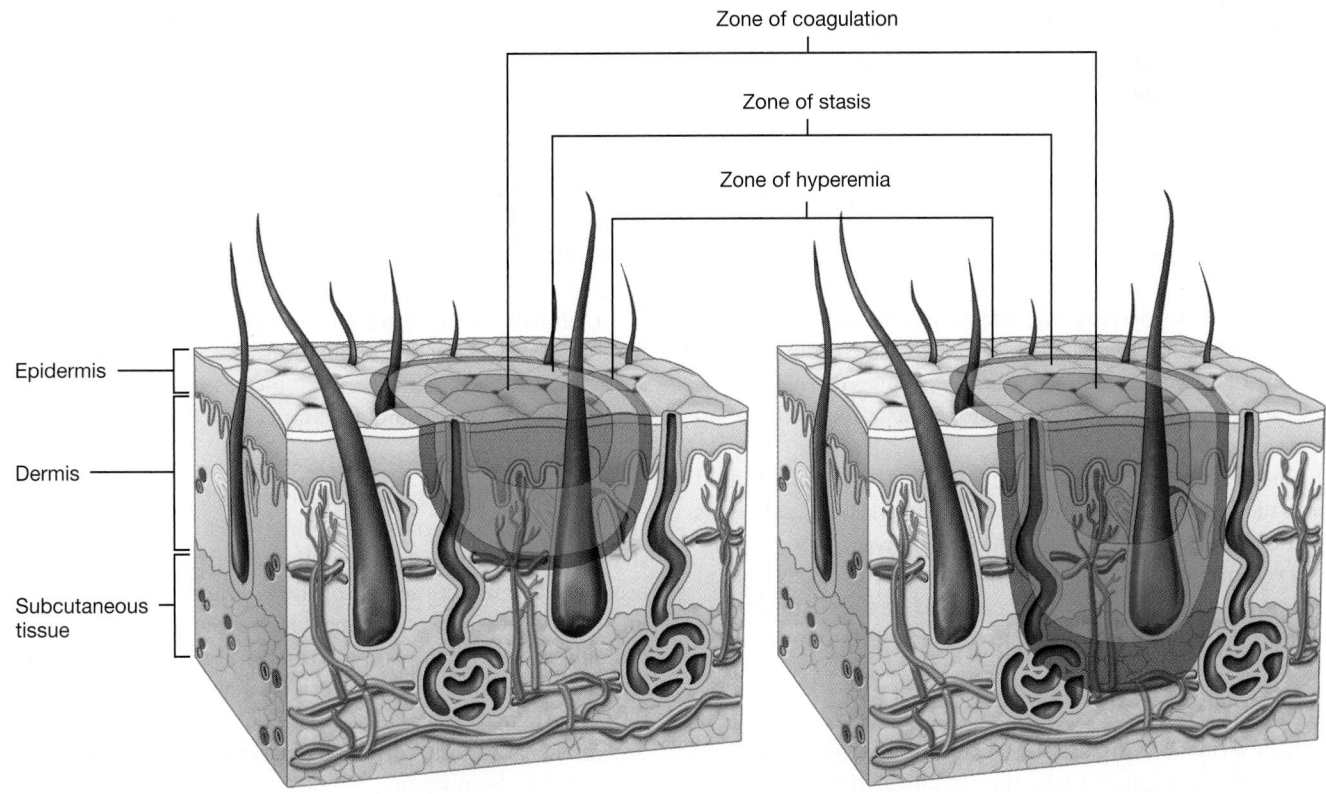

FIGURE 68–2 ■ Three zones of injury.

commonly referred to as "third spacing" of fluid and, if left untreated, will lead to burn shock. Additionally, edema develops in unburned tissues and organs distant from the site of injury when the burn size exceeds 20% total body surface area (Ahrns, 2004). Burn shock is the pathophysiological mechanism that underlies most of the systemic effects of a burn injury on the tissues and organs of the body. Burn shock occurs because of a loss of intravascular fluid and, thus, circulating blood volume. This loss of fluid occurs for two reasons; First, fluid is lost to the environment through the wound (insensible loss), and second, fluid is lost due to movement from the intravascular space into the interstitial space (Oliver et al., 2005).

Pathphysiologically, what is occurring is that at the time of the injury there is a release of an excessive amount of the Hageman factor (factor XII), which initiates and activates the inflammatory cascade (Porth, 2007). Proinflammatory mediators such as histamines, arachidonic acid metabolites, prostaglandins, bradykinin, and catecholamines are released from the injured tissue (Porth, 2007; Wolf & Herndon, 2000). These mediators cause arteriolar and venular dilation, which results in increased capillary permeability and, thus, leaking of fluid, electrolytes, and protein out of the intravascular space into the interstitial space causing interstitial edema. This leaking is due to changes in the osmotic pressure within the injured tissue. Because of oncotic changes, fluid moves with the protein that is leaving the vascular space, further increasing the edema formation in the wound. The outcome is a dramatic outpouring of fluids, electrolytes, and proteins into the third space, resulting in the decrease in circulating blood volume and consequently a decreased cardiac output. The development of shock is due to loss of the circulating blood volume, causing an intravascular hypovolemic state. The end result is decreased oxygen and nutrients to the tissues. Both localized and systemic edema occur because of the fluid shifts. This process of fluid movement begins at the time of injury, peaks in 12 to 24 hours after the injury, but will continue for 48 to 72 hours until the vascular permeability is at least partially reestablished and the leaking ceases.

The edema formation occurring during burn shock impairs peripheral circulation and results in tissue necrosis of the underlying tissues. Therefore, treatment during this initial period of fluid shifting focuses on aggressive fluid resuscitation for the hypovolemia, maintaining normal oxygen levels, and blocking the mediators to decrease the edema formation. These treatments will help prevent the conversion of the zone of stasis to the zone of coagulation. Because fluid continues to leak even after capillary integrity is restored, fluid resuscitation continues to be monitored closely.

What is unique to the patient with burns is that very little fluid leaves the body. Therefore, when the fluid stops leaking and begins to return to the vascular space, a marked increase in the intravascular volume occurs. When this process begins, fluid resuscitation needs to be adjusted so as not to cause fluid overload. Fluid resuscitation and monitoring are discussed later in this chapter.

Organ Injury

Virtually all systems in the body are affected in a major burn injury because the mediators leave the confines of the local tissue injury through the circulation and travel to remote organs causing injury (Oliver et al., 2005). Under normal conditions these medi-

ators are efficient and immune protective, but in the case of major trauma such as burn injury, they become poorly regulated, causing overwhelming inflammation and coagulation, and fibrinolysis can ensue, which can constantly be reactivated (Porth, 2007).

Cardiac Response

The initial hypovolemic state of burn shock significantly alters cardiovascular function with burns of greater than 40% total body surface area. One reason for this alteration is the loss of circulating blood volume, which decreases cardiac output and results in a loss of nutrients and oxygen delivered to the tissues. The second mechanism that impacts cardiac output is stimulation of the sympathetic nervous system (flight or fight), which causes the release of catecholamines (epinephrine and norepinephrine). These catecholamines cause vasoconstriction and an increase in systemic vascular resistance, which increases cardiac workload. Release of tumor necrosis factor, an inflammatory mediator, has a significant negative inotropic effect causing myocardial depression. The effect of this mediator goes on even after adequate fluid resuscitation (Porth, 2005). Due to these combined effects, heart failure is a major risk factor when attempting to achieve homeostasis in the early phase of burn care. This is especially true in the elderly population.

The cardiac conduction system also may be affected by increased serum potassium levels. Cell damage causes the release of intracellular potassium, which may cause hyperkalemia. Increased levels of potassium cause changes in the myocardial action potential, resulting in abnormalities in the cardiac conduction system. These abnormalities increase the risk of ventricular dysrhythmias and cardiac arrest. The Diagnostic Tests box describes the laboratory and diagnostic tests and the initial and later abnormalities associated with burn injuries.

Pulmonary Response

Increased pulmonary vascular resistance created by the release of the mediators such as serotonin, impacts pulmonary function, even in the absence of inhalation injury. This increased resistance also is compounded by the increase in systemic vascular resistance. Pulmonary edema, therefore, occurs because of increased capillary pressure combined with the vasoconstriction of the microcirculation. If left-sided heart failure also is present, this further increases capillary pressure and impacts oxygen exchange.

In summary, both the heart and lungs are affected by the proinflammatory mediators on a microvascular level. These changes are marked by a loss of fluid volume, increased vascular resistance, and finally a decreased cardiac output (Wolf & Herndon, 2000).

Gastrointestinal Response

With activation of the sympathetic nervous system, there is an increase in circulating catecholamines, which causes blood to be shunted away from the gastrointestinal (GI) organs. This results in decreased gut motility and absorption of nutrients. When a burn injury occurs, there is a subsequent increase in metabolism, which can rapidly deplete body stores. With the loss of motility, which is referred to as a *paralytic ileus*, nutrients may not progress through the GI tract and be absorbed. This lack of motility leads to gastric distention, nausea, and vomiting. A paralytic ileus is an indication to withhold administration of enteral feedings, further compromising the nutritional state. There is some evidence that early administration of enteral feedings actually decreases the incidence of

DIAGNOSTIC TESTS for Burn Injuries

Test	Initial Expected Abnormality	Later Expected Abnormality	Rationale for Abnormality
Potassium level	Increased.	Decreased after burn shock; fluid shifts back to intracellular and intravascular spaces.	Increased due to cell lysis and fluid shifts to extracellular spaces. Decreases with fluid resuscitation.
Sodium level	Increased.	Normalizes with fluid replacement. Will decrease with repeated Hubbard tank treatments.	Due to dehydration and then decreased with fluid shifts.
Hematocrit (HCT)	For the first 12–48 hours after the burn injury, there is an increase in the hematocrit due to hemoconcentration related to intravascular fluid volume loss.	Decreased with adequate hydration due to cell destruction from injury. Once fluid balance has been reestablished, a lower and more accurate hematocrit reading occurs.	Red blood cells are lost both directly in the burn and as a result of increased fragility. Circulating red blood cell mass becomes trapped and destroyed within the burn wound at the time of injury. Erythrocyte losses continue to occur for several days after the injury.
Hemoglobin (Hgb)	Increased due to hemoconcentration.	Decreased with adequate hydration due to cell destruction from injury.	Red blood cells are lost both directly in the burn and as a result of increased fragility. Circulating red blood cell mass becomes trapped and destroyed within the burn wound at the time of injury. Erythrocyte losses continue to occur for several days after the injury.
Platelets	Decreased due to dilution and consumption.	Normal if bone marrow manufactures enough. May be increased in the presence of infection.	Dilution and consumption immediately after a burn injury cause an abnormal decrease both in the platelet count and in clotting factors. It is believed that a large number of platelets are utilized to stabilize the vasculature in and around the burned area.
White blood cells (WBC)	Granulocytes continue to increase for the first 24 hours after the injury, and then the count begins to fall.	Increased with infection and decreased in immunodeficient states.	This increase is due to mobilization of preexisting stores. The decrease in the granulocyte level is due in part to the dilutional effects of fluid replacement therapy, and due to concentration in the injured areas.
Creatinine/blood urea nitrogen (BUN)	Normal to increased depending on fluid replacement.	Low if malnourished. Increased in presence of renal insufficiency.	Increases seen with electrical burns where extensive tissue damage is suspected.
Blood glucose; nondiabetic	Increased.	Increased or decreased depending on nutritional replacement.	Due to stress response and changes that occur with fluid resuscitation and type of nutritional replacement.
Total protein	Decreased.	Increased or decreased depending on nutritional status.	Fluid shifts cause a decrease, and nutritional replacement will increase it.
Prealbumin	Decreased.	Increased or decreased depending on nutritional status.	Massive inflammation causes a decrease, and nutritional replacement will increase it.
Creatine kinase (CK) level	Elevated.	Returns to normal after 48 hours.	Electrical burns due to extensive tissue damage.
Urine specific gravity	Elevated.	Decreased to normal levels with rehydration.	Dehydration.

paralytic ileus and helps maintain mucosal integrity (Chen, Xie, & Jiang, 2001). This issue of whether or not to administer enteral feedings remains a topic of research.

Blood flow to the GI tract immediately after burn injury also is affected by the release of angiotension II, a potent vasoconstrictor. This substance, which is released in response to low systemic fluid volume, has a direct vasoconstrictive effect on the splanchnic vasculature smooth muscle, causing ischemia to the gut (Tadros, Traber, Heggers, & Herndon, 2000, 2003). This ischemia causes intestinal mucosal atrophy and an increased permeability of the mucosa molecules (Yamamoto et al., 2001). Bacteria that are normal in the GI tract are held there by the mucosa. In burn injuries and burn wound sepsis, GI mucosal atrophy causes movement of intraluminal bacteria to extraluminal sites, referred to as *bacterial translocation* (Yamamoto et al., 2001). Bacterial translocation is thought to be one of the mechanisms that cause systemic sepsis and multisystem organ failure (Menchaca-Diaz et al., 2003). Research continues to investigate how to decrease the rate of bacterial translocation. Glutamine, a dietary supplement, has demonstrated to partially reverse gut atrophy and integrity. Glutamine administration decreases the incidence of gram-negative bacteremia and improves mortality rates (Tadros et al., 2003; Wischmeyer et al., 2001). Early enteral feedings appear to prevent or at least slow down mucosal atrophy (Chen et al., 2001).

Patients with severe burn injuries experience stress gastritis within 72 hours. Gastrointestinal (GI) erosions can occur within 5 hours of injury in 80% of all patients with severe burns. These erosions cause only minor upper bleeding, but within 72 hours this minor bleeding may progress to frank GI ulcerations (Curling's ulcer), resulting in major hemorrhage. This sequence of events was frequently seen in the patients when no ulcer prophylaxis (either antacids or H_2-receptor antagonists) was used (Fadaak, 2000).

Renal Response

The hypovolemia that occurs as a result of fluid shifts causes a decrease in renal blood flow and filtration rates. Therefore, abnormal increases in renal function studies (blood urea nitrogen [BUN] and creatinine), coupled with a marked decrease in or no urine output, may be seen during the early resuscitation phase (see the earlier Diagnostic Tests box, p. 2241). The kidney is able to recover if fluid resuscitation is initiated quickly and adequately.

After a major burn injury, the dead or damaged erythrocytes release large amounts of hemoglobin. If the burn extends deep enough to cause muscle injury, myoglobin also may be released into the bloodstream, such as seen with electrical injuries. Under normal circumstances, both of these substances are conjugated by haptoglobin and transferred to the liver. But if large amounts are released at once, the liver is unable to handle the increased load, and these substances are excreted in the urine. Myoglobin and hemoglobin will damage the renal tubules and promote renal failure. There is a higher risk for renal failure when any of the following is also present: dehydration, acidosis, massive presence of necrotic tissues after third- and fourth-degree electrical and chemical burns, hypercatabolic state, and/or shock.

Immune Response

The three major functions of the normal mature immune system are defense, homeostasis, and surveillance. The defense function provides the body with the ability to fight infection, while the homeostatic function controls the activities of the defense system. Finally, the surveillance function recognizes foreign materials.

The body's first line of defense, the skin, is destroyed with a burn injury. As discussed earlier, these injuries trigger the inflammatory response, causing the release of proinflammatory mediators, which induce localized vasodilation and increased capillary permeability. As a result, venous stasis and microthrombi occur at the injury site. The hypovolemia that occurs immediately after a burn injury causes an increase in blood viscosity, which results in sluggish blood flow to the wound bed. This results in a decreased delivery of oxygen, antibodies, and nutrients, which retards wound healing and increases the risk of

infection. A second manifestation of mediators, such as tumor necrosis factor and interleukin, is impairment of the function of lymphocytes, macrophages, and neutrophils, causing a decreased ability to fight infection. See Chapter 59 for a complete description of the immune system.

The protein that is lost due to third spacing from capillary leaking impairs both the cell-mediated and humoral immune systems. The humoral immune response needs B cells to produce antibodies and immunoglobulins. In the patient with burns, the serum levels of immunoglobulins are decreased, therefore diminishing the normal immune response. A decrease in the production of T cells negatively impacts cell-mediated cytotoxic activity. The decreased function of both cell-mediated and humoral immune responses creates a state of immunodeficiency and increases the risk of the development of opportunistic infections and death despite aggressive antimicrobial therapy.

A final insult to the immune system may occur because of the relationship between nutrition and immunocompetence. When the burn injury occurs, a hypermetabolic state is created, which places the victim at high risk for malnutrition (Pereira, Murphy, & Herndon, 2005). Without adequate calories, proteins, and trace elements, there is a decrease in the function of the immune system and, therefore, susceptibility to infection increases.

Integumentary Response

The skin protects against infection, prevents loss of body heat, helps control body temperature, functions as an excretory organ (sweat glands), is a sensory organ, and produces vitamin D when sunlight reacts with cholesterol. Finally, it determines identity; that is, race and fingerprints. Burn injuries cause a transient and, in some cases, permanent loss of many of these functions. With partial-thickness injuries, enough of the substructures of the skin remain intact to regenerate function. However, with full-thickness injuries, many functions such as hair growth, perspiration, and sensory functions are permanently lost.

The overall thickness of the skin varies depending on the part of the body it covers. For example, the skin on the back tends to be thicker than the skin on the inner aspect of the arms. Therefore, similar temperatures produce different depths of injury depending on the part of the body burned.

Multisystem Dysfunction

In major burn injuries, proinflammatory mediators, such as cytokines, are released in a chaotic, repeatedly reactivated fashion. This causes a continual reactivation of the inflammatory response, which in turn causes distant and multiorgan involvement leading to dysfunction and death (Gosian & Gamilli, 2005; Porth, 2007). Chapter 61 discusses in detail the sequence of events that causes multiorgan involvement and dysfunction.

Periods of Burn Injury Management

Three distinct periods of care for the acute burn injury have been identified: the emergency or resuscitative period, the acute period, and finally the rehabilitative phase. Each phase has different goals and priorities, even though these stages tend to overlap. In order for the patient to have optimal physical as well as emotional healing, each stage of care requires a multidisciplinary team of health care providers with specialized training. The goals and treatments of each phase or period are described next.

Emergency Phase

The emergency period of burn care begins at the time of the injury and lasts for the first 2 to 3 days. The goal during this phase is to resolve the immediate insult by certain means, which include maintaining an airway and oxygen levels, treating concurrent injuries, correcting the fluid imbalance, preventing wound infection, conserving body heat, relieving pain, and providing emotional support.

Prehospital Care and Transport

The focus of treatment at the scene of the injury is first to ensure the safety of the rescuers and then to remove the victim from the burn source. An initial assessment is required to determine vital signs and the severity of the burn and other injuries. This assessment follows the ABCDEF format: A = airway, B = breathing, C = circulation, D = disability, neurological deficit, E = exposure and evaluation, and F = fluid resuscitation. Any smoldering clothing and restrictive jewelry must be removed to decrease the depth of the injury. Burn victims are unlikely to develop shock in the first 30 minutes; therefore, after airway stabilization the patient can be transported to a local emergency department or directly to a burn center. If the patient is less than 60 minutes away from a hospital, the American Burn Association teaches that intravenous line insertion is not necessary at the scene of the accident.

Application of clean normal saline-soaked towels helps with cooling the burned skin, often is effective for pain relief, and may limit the extent of burn damage. These cold soaks must be used cautiously; limit them to 5% to 10% of the body surface at any one time, and limit them in time to prevent systemic hypothermia. Ice is not used because it may cause further injury to the skin and exacerbate hypothermia. The burning process generally stops after 5 minutes of water cooling, and any further cooling only contributes to hypothermia. For patient comfort the burn should be covered with clean, dry blankets.

Chemical burns require copious irrigation with water for at least 20 minutes to reduce the concentration of chemicals and, thus, the depth of the injury. If the chemical is in the eyes, contact lenses must be removed, and the eyes are irrigated with copious amounts of water. A minimum of 2 liters of fluid is used for each eye, and irrigation may be needed for several hours after the injury (EmedicineHealth, 2006).

No oils or salves should be applied to any type of burn injury. If the patient has not had tetanus toxoid in the last 5 years, it is administered early, often in the field. If the patient has never received tetanus or has not had a booster in the last 10 years, tetanus immunoglobulin is given. Due to a loss of skin integrity, body temperature drops; therefore, the patient should be covered with clean blankets before transfer.

Emergency Department Care

Once the patient reaches the emergency department (ED), a rapid and thorough initial assessment is done, beginning with the respiratory and cardiovascular systems. As always, the first priority is to assess the patency of the patient's airway and the adequacy of gas exchange. If the burns occurred on the face and neck, massive airway edema can cause airway obstruction and death. An assessment for heat or smoke inhalation is done emergently, as these agents can cause damage to the airways and lung parenchyma. The nasal passages and oral airway are assessed for soot. If respiratory distress is present and/or there are burns of the face and neck, nasotracheal or endotracheal intubation is indicated within 1 to 2 hours after the injury, before swelling further compromises the airway (McCall & Cahill, 2005). After intubation, the need for oxygen and ventilatory support is assessed and instituted. Ongoing monitoring of arterial blood gases and oxygen saturation levels determines the effectiveness of the interventions. The nurse is responsible for monitoring the patient's airway and assessing the adequacy of gas exchange. An in-depth discussion of respiratory assessment, intubation, and mechanical ventilation is in Chapters 33 😊 and 36 😊.

An assessment of the cardiovascular system is essential because it provides information regarding fluid volume status and the potential for the development of shock. A 12-lead electrocardiogram (ECG) is necessary to detect myocardial ischemic changes and cardiac dysrhythmias, especially with electrical injuries. The carotid and peripheral pulses are assessed for rate and quality. The skin is inspected for color, sensation, and capillary refill. Finally, the blood pressure and apical pulse are assessed. Due to the progressive nature of fluid volume loss, these assessments must be performed on a frequent and ongoing basis.

Concurrent with airway management and cardiovascular assessment, it is essential to place large-bore intravenous (IV) catheters. Most health care providers believe that shortening the time from injury to IV insertion and beginning of fluid resuscitation will decrease the mortality rate. The best insertion site is through nonburned tissue, if possible. If there is no nonburned area for intravenous access, then placement through burned tissue is necessary and justifiable, given the risk for the development of hypovolemic shock. This is done as early as possible while the nonviable tissue (**eschar**) is still sterile (Figure 68–3 ■). Placement of an indwelling urinary catheter also is necessary, as urine output is considered the most reliable indicator of fluid status.

In burn injuries greater than 20% of total body surface area (TBSA), the patient is prone to nausea and vomiting because of a loss of blood flow to the gastrointestinal tract, as discussed earlier in this chapter. Due to the risk of aspiration, oral fluids are withheld, and a nasogastric tube may be inserted to prevent abdominal distention and vomiting. The next priority during the emergency period is to assess for any concurrent injuries. Life-threatening injuries such as pneumothorax, spinal cord, or acute

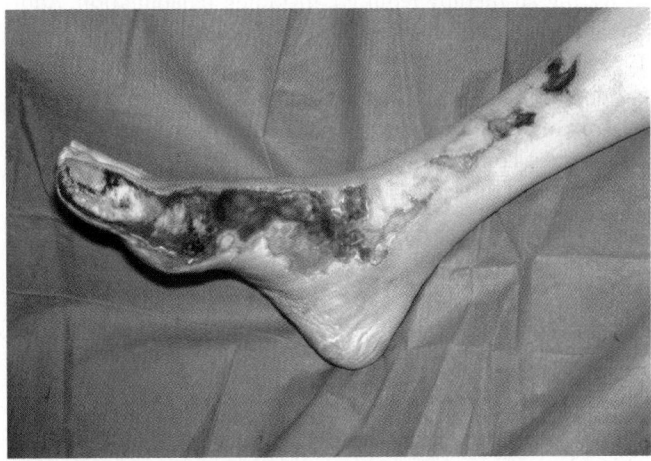

FIGURE 68–3 ■ Eschar.
Source: Courtesy of: John M. Osborn, M.D., FACS, Sacramento, CA Plastic Surgery Center

brain injuries need to be stabilized and treated. Final treatment of concurrent injuries, such as surgery, is typically delayed if possible until the patient is hemodynamically stable.

The loss of skin integrity decreases the patient's ability to retain and maintain body heat. When body temperature decreases, shivering occurs as a compensatory mechanism to increase body heat. This shivering increases oxygen and metabolic needs, and must be avoided. Burn wounds are covered with dressings, blankets are applied, and the room temperature is elevated to increase and maintain body temperature.

Blood studies are obtained to provide baseline data and to assist in identifying preexisting conditions. For patients with 30% or greater TBSA, the blood studies should include a complete blood count, serum electrolytes, blood glucose, blood urea nitrogen (BUN), serum creatinine, and coagulation studies. If substance abuse is suspected or if there is an altered level of consciousness in the absence of a head injury, a toxicology screen is indicated. If inhalation injury is suspected or the patient is in respiratory distress, arterial blood gases and a chest x-ray are necessary. In the case of electrical burns where extensive tissue damage is suspected, serum creatine kinase (CK), blood urea nitrogen, and creatinine levels should be evaluated, typically on an ongoing basis (see the Diagnostic Tests box, p. 2241). To diagnose any concurrent injuries, x-rays and scans need be completed where indicated.

Burns are a life-threatening, disfiguring injury that has a major emotional impact on both the patient and family. Thus, emotional support is essential in all stages of burn recovery and must begin in the emergency period.

Prevention of wound infection is a critical concern from the time of injury to final wound closure. Therefore, once the patient has been stabilized, the focus of care shifts to the assessment of burn size and depth. Burns are categorized as minor, moderate, or major (see the National Guidelines box for the ABA's classification of burn injury, p. 2235), and a determination is made as to whether the patient requires hospitalization. If hospitalization is indicated, then the decision needs to be made as to whether to admit the patient to a medical–surgical floor or to a specialized burn center.

Burn Center Criteria

In order to qualify as a burn center, the unit must be capable of delivering all therapy required, including rehabilitation. Additionally, the center must provide training and conduct research. Typically burn centers are associated with university hospitals and/or hospitals with 500 or more beds. Burn centers provide treatment for minor, moderate, and major burn injuries. A burn center must contain a minimum of six beds and have a designated medical director who is board certified in general or plastic surgery, with one additional year of specialized training in burn care. Besides specially trained nurses, the center must also employ licensed physical therapists, occupational therapists, and licensed dieticians with previous experience in burn care (Demling, DeSanti, & Orgill, 2004). Most major burn centers also have social workers, clergy, child life specialists, and psychologists. Each member of the team must understand the critical aspects of wound care, infection control, and the psychological and rehabilitative needs of the patient with burns. Transfer of any patient, whether it is from the field or the ED,

must be coordinated with the burn center health care provider. All pertinent information regarding injuries, hemodynamic status, fluid resuscitation, and treatments must be reported to the burn center staff.

The American Burn Association and the American College of Surgeons have established these criteria for admission to a burn center:

1. Partial-thickness and full-thickness burns greater than 10% body surface area (BSA) in patients under 10 years or over 50 years of age.
2. Partial-thickness and full-thickness burns greater than 20% BSA in other age groups.
3. Partial-thickness and full-thickness burns involving the face, hands, eyes, ears, feet, genitalia, perineum, or those that involve skin overlying major joints.
4. Full-thickness burns greater than 5% TBSA in any age group.
5. Electrical burns, including lightning injury (significant volumes of tissue beneath the surface may be injured and result in acute renal failure and other complications).
6. Significant chemical burns.
7. Inhalation injury.
8. Burn injury in patients with preexisting illness that could complicate management, prolong recovery, or affect mortality.
9. Any patient with burns in whom concomitant trauma poses an increased risk of morbidity or mortality may be treated initially at a trauma center until stable before being transferred to a burn center.
10. Children with burns seen in hospitals without qualified personnel or equipment for their care should be transferred to a burn center with these capabilities.
11. Burn injury in patients who will require special social and emotional or long-term rehabilitative support, including cases involving suspected child abuse and neglect. (Demling & DeSanti, 2006b)

Admission to a Burn Center

If the patient meets the criteria listed, admission to a burn center is indicated. During the admission process, both the local and systemic effects of the burn injury are quickly assessed and treated. The admission process begins with airway management, hemodynamic stabilization, and an assessment of the burn size and depth. After an in-depth assessment, a comprehensive treatment plan is instituted that provides the care needed to ensure an optimal recovery. The nurse is pivotal in coordinating the admission process and the treatment plan.

Admission Assessment

The admission assessment of a patient following a burn injury needs to include the history of the event that caused the injury, the time the injury occurred, the causative agent and the duration of exposure, where the injury occurred (e.g., enclosed space), any concurrent injuries, and any on-the-scene first aid treatments.

This assessment is vital because portions of the treatment plan depend on this information. For example, fluid resuscitation calculations are based on the time of the injury as opposed to the time of admission to the hospital. The causative agent is especially important with chemical burns such as from strong acids or alkaline agents, which may require neutralization to stop the ongoing burning effect. If the injury occurred in an enclosed area, such as a house, there also may be inhalation injuries that require special consideration and treatment. Concurrent injuries, such as fractures, often are associated with burns and require a treatment plan for stabilization. Finally, first aid treatments and home remedies applied prior to arrival at the hospital need to be documented and reported to the health care team.

Clinical Manifestations and Determinants of Burn Wound Severity

In order to treat a burn injury adequately, its severity must be evaluated using the following five factors: the size of the injury, the depth of injury, the age of the patient, past medical history, and the part of the body burned. Each of these factors impacts the treatment plan as well as the morbidity and mortality for a given patient.

Burn Size

When estimating burn size, it is expressed as a percent of total body surface area. Two common formulas are used to estimate percent of body burned. The first formula is the **rule of nines** that divides the body into seven areas, which each represent 9% or multiples of 9% of the body surface area. For an adult, the head and neck are 9%, the arms are 9% each, the lower extremities are 18% each, the trunk is a total of 36% (18% anterior, 18% posterior), and the perineum is 1%. Thus, the total = 100%. Age and growth and development are factors in determining the distribution of the body surface area. Figure 68–4 ■ outlines the rule of nines for both adults and children. The rule of nines is an easy-to-remember general estimate of body surface area and is considered adequate for the prehospital and emergency care periods.

The second formula is the **Lund-Browder formula** (Figure 68–5 ■, p. 2246). This formula divides the body into smaller percentage areas and is considered more accurate, especially for children and infants. The formula determines surface area measurements for each body part according to the age of the patient.

When a patient is admitted, the affected areas are shaded in on a chart using either the rule of nines or the Lund-Browder formula. The total body surface area (TBSA) involved in the burn injury is then calculated. Most burn centers total the partial-thickness and full-thickness injuries separately. The totaled sum of body surface burned is used when calculating fluid resuscitation needs, as well as metabolic and immunologic responses. The TBSA also is a critical determinant of overall morbidity and mortality (Osborn, 2003).

Burn Depth

The depth of a burn injury is an important predictor of morbidity and mortality as well as of surgical management and functional and cosmetic outcomes (Osborn, 2003). There are a number of accepted terms used to refer to the depth of the injury. Burn depth is expressed in terms of full-thickness and partial-thickness, and/or first, second, third, and fourth degrees. First- and second-degree burns are partial-thickness injuries, which result in partial destruction of the skin layers. Enough epithelial cells, hair follicles, and sweat glands remain intact to provide a new epidermis.

Partial-thickness injuries involving only the superficial dermis (first degree), heal spontaneously in about 2 weeks and usually cause no cosmetic or functional impairment. Partial-thickness wounds involving the deep dermis (second degree), heal spontaneously, but may require a prolonged period (greater than 21 days) to do so, and may result in some scar or contracture formation (Figure 68–6 ■, p. 2246). Infection, trauma, and a decreased blood supply increase the risk of a partial-thickness injury converting to a full-thickness injury.

Full-thickness injuries (third degree) result in the destruction of all skin layers, and there may be destruction of subcutaneous tissue, muscles, and bones (Figure 68–7 ■, p. 2247). Some health care providers refer to burns that involve muscles and bones as fourth-degree injuries. Full-thickness burns have no sensation to pain on light touch due to the destruction of the pain and touch receptors. Closure of the wound occurs by granulation, epithelial migration, contracture, and/or surgical intervention. (See the discussion of wound management later in this chapter.) Figure 68–8 ■ (p. 2247) demonstrates the difference in skin depth between a partial-thickness and a full-thickness injury.

The differential diagnosis of burn depth is based on the cause of the injury, the appearance of the wound, and the presence or absence of sensation in the area. Chart 68–2 (p. 2248) provides guidelines for helping make the determination between partial-thickness and full-thickness injury.

An assessment of the pattern of the burn injury during the emergency period also is essential. If the injury is circumferential (involving the entire circumference of an area), there is an increased risk for diminished blood supply to the area distal to the injury. (See the treatment of circumferential injuries later in this chapter.)

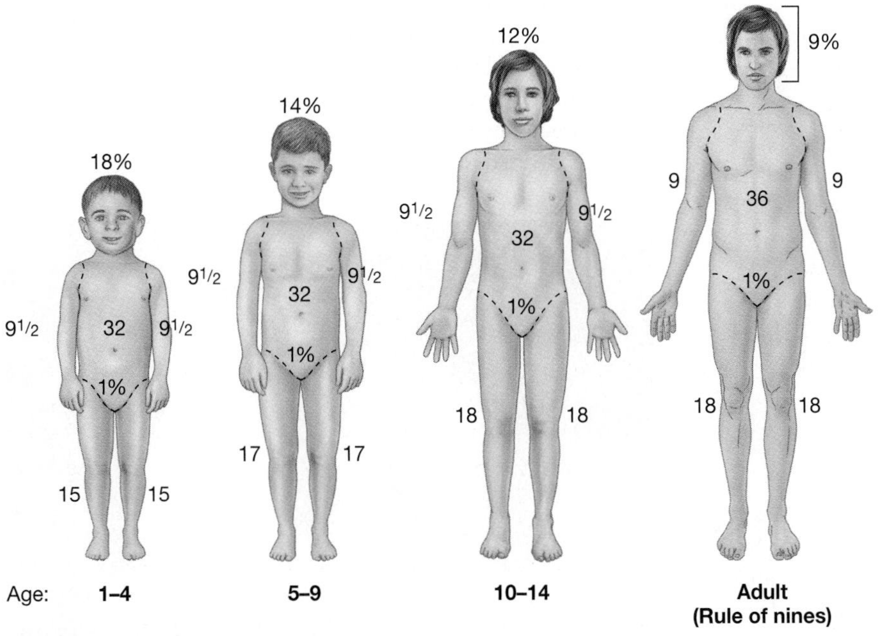

FIGURE 68–4 ■ Rule of nines.

Area	Age (years)					% 1°	% 2°	% 3°	% Total
	0–1	1–4	5–9	10–15	Adult				
Head	19	17	13	10	7				
Neck	2	2	2	2	2				
Ant. trunk	13	13	13	13	13				
Post. trunk	13	13	13	13	13				
R. buttock	2½	2½	2½	2½	2½				
L. buttock	2½	2½	2½	2½	2½				
Genitalia	1	1	1	1	1				
R.U. arm	4	4	4	4	4				
L.U. arm	4	4	4	4	4				
R.L. arm	3	3	3	3	3				
L.L. arm	3	3	3	3	3				
R. hand	2½	2½	2½	2½	2½				
L. hand	2½	2½	2½	2½	2½				
R. thigh	5½	6½	8½	8½	9½				
L. thigh	5½	6½	8½	8½	9½				
R. leg	5	5	5½	6	7				
L. leg	5	5	5½	6	7				
R. foot	3½	3½	3½	3½	3½				
L. foot	3½	3½	3½	3½	3½				
					Total				

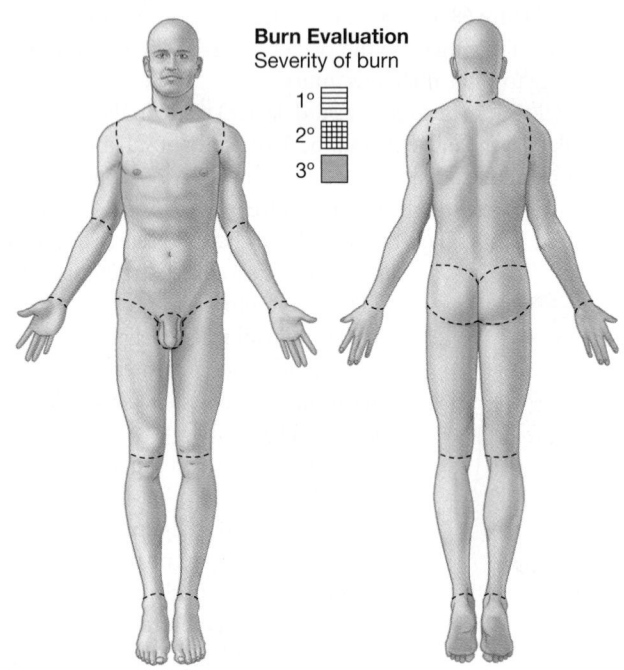

Burn Evaluation
Severity of burn

1° ▦
2° ▦
3° ▦

FIGURE 68–5 ■ Lund-Browder formula.

Age

The very young and the elderly have higher mortality rates than a young adult with the same percentage of burn injury. In the younger population (usually under 2 years of age), there are two specific reasons for increased mortality. First, infants and young children have an immature immune system with a weak antibody response to infection and tend to die of septicemia. Second, the very young have a greater proportion of body surface area per amount of body mass. As a result, there is a higher risk for fluid volume loss, requiring greater fluid resuscitation for total percent burn as compared to adults. Therefore, there is an increased risk for the development of hypovolemic shock.

In the older population (over 60 years of age), burns tend to exacerbate previous medical problems such as cardiovascular disease, renal insufficiency, diabetes, and chronic obstructive pulmonary disease. This population tends to have decreased physiological reserves, which are needed to respond to the stress of a burn injury; therefore, older adults are at a higher risk for shock and multisystem organ failure. Additionally, the older population tends to heal more slowly, resulting in a greater risk for the development of infection and pneumonia.

Past Medical History

Cardiac, respiratory, renal, and endocrine diseases and/or a history of substance abuse decreases the rate of survival of a major burn injury at any age. The added insult of a burn injury exacerbates these preexisting conditions and increases morbidity and mortality.

Part of Body Burned

The area of the body affected by burns is significant due to the associated side effects and the potential for cosmetic and functional deformities. For example, burns of the head, neck, and chest tend to have pulmonary complications and are considered more serious than a burn of the same size on the lower leg. Burn injuries occurring in the perineum and upper thighs are more prone to infections due to local contamination. For cosmetic as well as functional reasons, burns of the face, neck, and hands require special treatment for both physical as well as psychological reasons.

In summary, many health care providers believe as a general rule of prognosis that if the age of the patient and the percentage of burn add up to more than 100, there is little chance of survival. Adding any prior chronic medical problems to this situation decreases the chances of survival even further. The single most powerful factor in predicting mortality from fire is smoke inhalation, which is covered in this chapter.

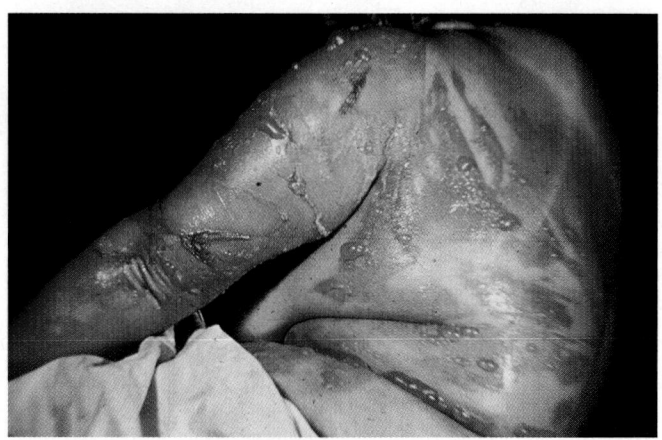

FIGURE 68–6 ■ Partial-thickness injury.
Source: Courtesy of: John M. Osborn, M.D., FACS, Sacramento, CA Plastic Surgery Center

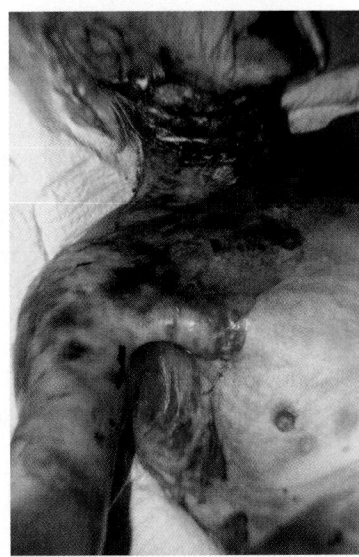

FIGURE 68–7 ■ Full-thickness injury.
Source: Courtesy of: John M. Osborn, M.D., FACS, Sacramento, CA Plastic Surgery Center

Laboratory and Diagnostic Evaluation

Tissue and cell destruction, and fluid and electrolyte shifts, cause many hematologic changes following a burn injury. The most radical changes occur in the first 24 to 48 hours after the injury. Therefore, careful monitoring of laboratory values is critical during this hemodynamic stabilization period, although careful monitoring of laboratory data must continue throughout all phases of burn recovery. Hematologic response to burn injury is discussed next and outlined in the earlier Diagnostic Tests box (p. 2241).

Red Blood Cells

Red blood cells are lost both directly in the burn and as a result of increased fragility. Circulating red blood cell mass becomes

trapped and destroyed within the burn wound at the time of injury. The cell loss is not only due to direct heat damage because erythrocyte losses continue to occur for several days after the injury. What is somewhat misleading is that in the first 12 to 48 hours after the burn injury there is an increase in the hematocrit. This increase is not due to an increase in erythrocytes but instead is the result of hemoconcentration related to intravascular fluid volume loss. Once fluid balance has been reestablished, a lower and more accurate hematocrit reading occurs. Red blood cell production is dependent on adequate iron stores and normal metabolism. Circulating levels of iron are depressed after burn injury, which may explain why erythrocyte production is decreased despite normal production of erythropoietin from the kidney.

Leukocytes

Immediately after the burn injury there is an increase in granulocytes, which constitute 60% to 80% of the total number of normal blood leukocytes (white blood cells). This increase is not due to an increased production but rather is from mobilization of preexisting stores. The granulocytes continue to increase for the first 24 hours after the injury, and then the count begins to fall. The decrease in the granulocyte level is due in part to the dilutional effects of fluid replacement therapy and because the granulocytes have concentrated in the injured areas. Within 48 hours after the injury, stores of granulocytes are depleted, and the patient is dependent on the bone marrow for the production of new cells. Infection and septicemia are factors that stimulate the production of granulocytes.

Platelets

Dilution and consumption of platelets immediately after a burn injury cause an abnormal decrease both in the platelet count and in clotting factors. In addition, it is believed that a large

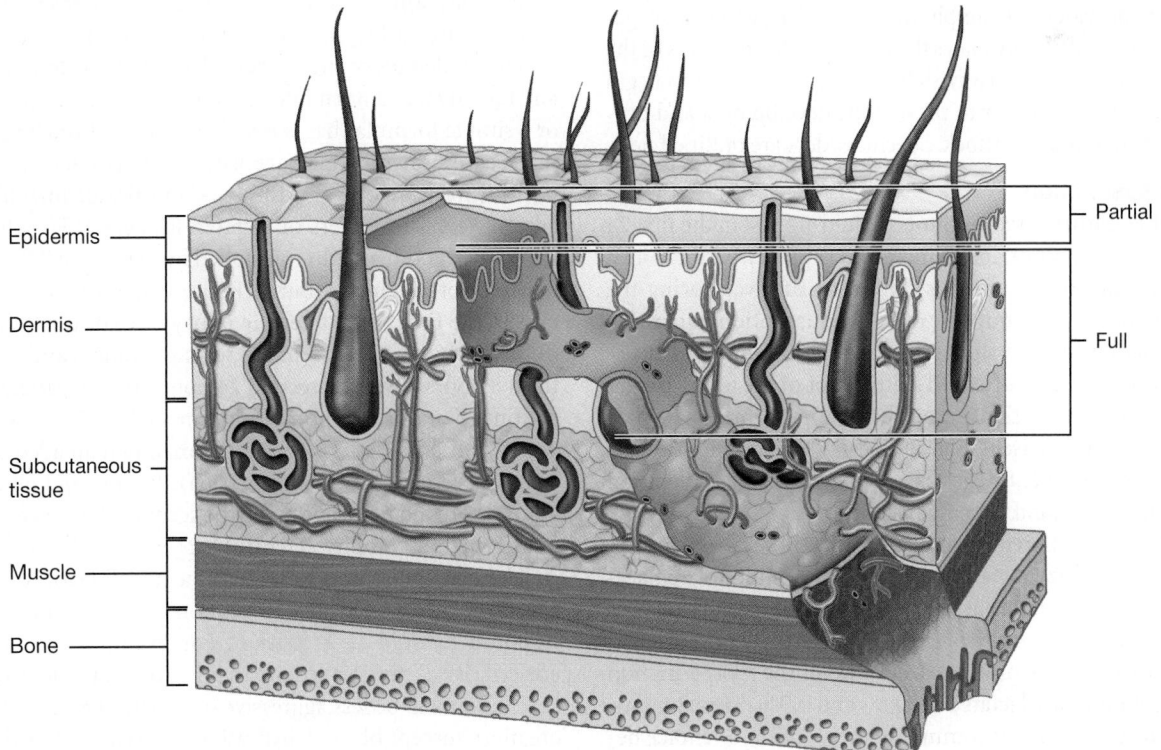

FIGURE 68–8 ■ Skin layers of partial-thickness versus full-thickness injury.

CHART 68–2	**Determination of Burn Depth**		
	Superficial Injury	**Partial-thickness Injury**	**Full-Thickness Injury**
Skin Depth	Epidermis	Epidermis and most of the dermis Base structures of sebaceous and sweat glands intact	Epidermis, dermis, and may include subcutaneous tissue, muscle, and bones
Skin Appearance	Red, may have local edema Blanches with pressure	Pink or dark-pink May appear dull, white, tan, or cherry Blanches with pressure	Dark red, white, charred black, gray Pearl, dark tan, waxy No blanching Charred blood vessels visible
Pain	Increased sensitivity	Increased sensitivity	Absent: nerve endings destroyed
Blister Formation	None	Large, thick walled, and will increase in size	Usually none or, if present, thin walled and will not increase in size
Texture	Slightly firm if edema present	Firm due to edema	Dry and leather like
Possible Causes	Sun Ultraviolet light Flash flame	Hot liquids or solids Flash or direct flame to clothing Chemicals Ultraviolet light	Hot liquids or solids Flame Chemicals Electrical contact
Healing Time	2–5 days No scarring	5–35 days No grafting unless converts to full-thickness injury	Little to no healing potential Requires grafting

number of platelets are utilized to stabilize the vasculature in and around the burned area. The bone marrow does not store platelets, and therefore, increased production is necessary to meet the needs of the body. It is not uncommon to replace platelets during the first 36 hours after the injury.

Medical Management

Survival following a burn injury is dependent on an in-depth, timely assessment and the development of a treatment plan. The health care provider will supply the orders for patient management, and the nurse coordinates the plan with the members of the health care team. After airway stabilization, it is critical to begin fluid resuscitation in order to prevent the development and progression of hypovolemic shock. Specific orders are outlined next.

Fluid Resuscitation

As described earlier, large amounts of fluid are lost in the first 24 to 48 hours after injury due to increased capillary permeability. Therefore, fluid replacement is critical to survival during the emergency period. The purpose of fluid resuscitation is to maintain circulating blood volume and cardiac output, which become compromised due to fluid shifting out of the intravascular space into the interstitial space. The goal is to prevent hypovolemic shock, tissue ischemia, and death. The amount of fluid needed for replacement depends on the size of injury, depth of burn, patient's age, and past medical history.

A number of different formulas have been devised in an attempt to standardize the amount and type of fluid for replacement. All of the formulas use either crystalloids or colloids or a combination of both. A crystalloid is an electrolyte solution that may be either isotonic or hypertonic. Two of the most common isotonic solutions are lactated Ringer's and 0.9% normal saline. Lactated Ringer's is most commonly the solution of choice because it most closely mimics the body's extracellular fluid. Crystalloid solutions typically are used in the first 12 hours until

capillary permeability begins to stabilize. Once the capillary leaking has slowed, some formulas give colloid products such as fresh frozen plasma, dextran, and albumin. These hypertonic solutions not only provide volume but also generate an osmotic pressure, which pulls fluid back from the interstitial space into the intravascular space. Fresh frozen plasma also restores lost clotting factors, and red blood cell replacement is indicated if a significant change has occurred in the hemoglobin and hematocrit levels. Some formulas also give 5% dextrose solution for maintenance and replacement of insensible losses.

The guidelines of the Advanced Trauma Life Support course and the Advanced Burn Life Support course recommend the use of a simple formula that is readily available at the hospital. The most common formulas are listed in Chart 68–3. Generally, health care providers use the Parkland/Baxter formula, which administers 4 milliliters of lactated Ringer's (LR) solution per kilogram of body weight multiplied by percent of TBSA of burn (4 mL/kg of weight × % burn). Because most of the fluid loss occurs in the first hours after the injury, 50% of the fluid is given in the first 8 hours, 25% in the second 8 hours, and 25% in the third 8 hours. Over the second 24 hours, the LR generally is discontinued and a hypotonic solution such as 5% dextrose and water with potassium is titrated to maintain an adequate urine output (Demling & DeSanti, 2006a). Plasma and albumin are administered in boluses during the second 24 hours to maintain hemodynamic stability (Flynn, 2002).

These formulas were designed as a guideline for fluid administration. Each patient has to be monitored individually for his response to fluid resuscitation. For example, due to the increased risk of diminished organ function in the elderly, fluid resuscitation will be less aggressive than with the very young who are more susceptible to dehydration. Therefore, all patients with burn injuries require close monitoring for adequacy of fluid replacement and organ perfusion.

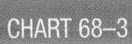

CHART 68–3 Fluid Replacement Formulas for Burn Injuries

Parkland/Baxter Formula

First 24 hours:

4 mL/kg × % total body surface area (TBSA) of lactated Ringer's

1/2 given in first 8 hours, 1/4 in second 8 hours, 1/4 in third 8 hours

Second 24 hours:

Dextrose and water, plus potassium

Colloid: 20–60% of calculated plasma volume (0.35–0.5 mL/kg × % TBSA)

Consensus Formula

First 24 hours:

2–4 mL/kg × % TBSA of lactated Ringer's

1/2 given in first 8 hours, 1/4 in second 8 hours, 1/4 in third 8 hours

Second 24 hours:

0.3–0.5 mL/kg × % TBSA of colloid solution

Electrolyte-free solution to maintain urine output

Brooke Army Formula

First 24 hours:

1.5 mL/kg × % TBSA of lactated Ringer's

0.5 mL/kg × % TBSA of colloid solution

1/2 given in first 8 hours, 1/4 in second 8 hours, 1/4 in third 8 hours

Second 24 hours:

0.5–0.75 mL/kg × % TBSA of lactated Ringer's

2,000 mL of dextrose and water

Evans Formula

First 24 hours:

1 mL/kg × % TBSA of 0.9 normal saline

1 mL/kg × % TBSA of colloid solution

1/2 given in first 8 hours, 1/4 in second 8 hours, 1/4 in third 8 hours

Second 24 hours:

0.5 mL/kg × % TBSA of 0.9 normal saline

2,000 mL of dextrose and water

Fluid Resuscitation Assessment End points are objective criteria that define a measured outcome or goal of treatment. If end points are not achieved, resuscitation measures must be adjusted and reassessed. End points are important with burn resuscitation because then fluids are titrated using objective data instead of being only formula driven (Ahrns, 2004). Therefore, assessing normal organ function provides a means of monitoring fluid replacement. Fluid resuscitation end points include:

- **Mentation**—Orientation and level of consciousness are sensitive to changes in oxygen delivery because the brain needs constant blood for normal function. Deficient fluid resuscitation resulting in inadequate oxygen delivery to the brain can cause agitation, restlessness, confusion, and even stupor. In the absence of head trauma, a well-hydrated patient should be alert and oriented.

- **Skin color and temperature**—Vasoconstriction caused by intravascular depletion is manifested by cool, pale, and clammy skin or mottled skin with advanced shock. Additionally, due to loss of skin and subsequent temperature regulation, core body temperature may be decreased.

- **Heart rate**—Tachycardia, a heart rate greater than 100 beats per minute, is a better indicator of hypovolemia and with hydration will return to the upper limits of normal for the age range.

- **Blood pressure**—The blood pressure (BP) tends to be a poor indicator of perfusion in the very early stage because pronounced catecholamine release results in an increased systemic vascular resistance (SVR), causing normal BP to be maintained even in the presence of hypovolemia.

- **Urine output**—Most health care providers agree that the urine output is the best gauge of adequate hydration and in an adult it should be 0.5 to 1 mL/kg of body weight per hour (Demling & DeSanti, 2006a). Typically, a minimum urine output of 30 mL/hr is the gauge.

- **Specific gravity**—Specific gravity, which is also monitored on an hourly basis, becomes elevated (>1.025) with dehydration and decreases as fluid is replaced.

- **Central venous pressure (CVP)**—A CVP of between 4 and 12 indicates adequate fluid volume (Ahrns, 2004).

- **Hemoconcentration factors**—Hemoglobin (Hgb) and hematocrit (HCT) increase with the loss of intravascular volume; and in the presence of inadequate fluid resuscitation, the Hgb and HCT become abnormally elevated. The level of these values is proportional to the level of fluid volume. As fluid returns to the intravascular space, the Hgb and HCT levels will return to normal and typically become abnormally low due to cell destruction (see the Diagnostic Tests box, p. 2241). Overhydration will give false low readings.

- **Gastrointestinal function**—Normal gastrointestinal function is inferred by the return of bowel sounds.

 A hemoglobin (Hgb) of > 20 g/dL and/or a hematocrit (HCT) of > 60% is an indication that fluid resuscitation is inadequate and needs to be increased. The Hgb and HCT are not the best indicators of fluid balance because many blood cells are destroyed with the initial tissue injury. Use other indicators of fluid balance, such as heart rate, central venous pressure (CVP), and blood pressure (BP), because they are more reflective of the adequacy of hydration.

Pain Management

Pain management is a complex issue for a burn victim in that pain varies in character and intensity throughout all phases of burn treatment. Pain is related to tissue injury and the healing process and is complicated by fear, anxiety, depression, and the chronicity of the injury. The goal of pain management is to provide maximal comfort on an ongoing basis. To accomplish this, it is necessary to establish a partnership with the patient regarding how to manage pain relief.

Once fluid resuscitation has begun, narcotic analgesics are administered intravenously to help control pain. For effective pain management, interventions must be evaluated and modified on an ongoing basis. Pain causes an activation of the sympathetic nervous system, causing vasoconstriction, which decreases blood flow to the wound and delays healing.

If pain is not managed appropriately at the outset of the injury, then long-term pain management issues may ensue. The main tenets of pain management for patients with burns are:

- Analgesics are more effective if given on a scheduled basis rather than only as requested by the patient.
- Intramuscular (IM) injections are not used during the emergency period because of poor absorption.
- IM injections are avoided in children, because they fear the injection as much as the pain.
- Bowel management begins with narcotic pain management.
- Doses of medication should be modified as the clinical situation dictates (e.g., dressing changes).
- Anxiety needs to be treated for effective pain management.
- Pain management must be individualized to the patient with consideration being given to the time since the injury, patient's age, percentage burn, or burn depth.

A comprehensive approach to pain management includes assessing the pain level, anticipating prophylactic analgesic needs, and administering narcotics as ordered. In the event that the patient cannot verbalize or assist in the assessment of pain relief, there are physiological responses that must be assessed on a regular basis. These include increased heart rate, diaphoresis, increased agitation, grimacing, and rhythmic movement or lack of movement (Flynn, 2002).

In the beginning acute stages of burn injury, the most commonly used agents are opioids such as morphine sulfate, fentanyl, and codeine. Small, frequent doses on a non–pain-contingent schedule are indicated for the continuous pain or background pain that is associated with loss of skin integrity. Procedural pain such as dressing changes are best managed by additional intravenous opioids. Patients typically report excruciating pain with dressing changes, especially with partial-thickness injuries. As the burn injury heals, less potent drugs are indicated such as nonsteroidal analgesics. The length of time required to treat burn injuries necessitates a comprehensive interdisciplinary team approach that is essential for maximizing a patient's functional outcome while minimizing psychological distress. Adequate management of pain requires that the plan be reevaluated frequently. Chapter 15  provides an in-depth discussion of pain management principles.

Alternative Therapies for Pain Management   It is essential to allow the patient to verbalize the pain experience and explore alternative therapies for pain relief. These therapies include guided imagery, hypnosis, and music and are used as an adjunct to medication. The Complementary and Alternative Therapies box details music therapy's use in the management of pain.

CRITICAL ALERT   *Assess adequacy of pain management for dressing changes daily. Secure health care provider's orders for more medication, and have these orders available as backup if needed. Be sensitive to cultural diversity in response to pain and medicate accordingly.*

COMPLEMENTARY & ALTERNATIVE THERAPIES   Music

Description:

Pain management is a vital issue in burn care. Research has shown that the experience of pain affects both the body and the mind. Therefore, nurses must use a holistic view of pain management and healing when caring for patients with burns. In addition to the use of cognitive, behavioral, and pharmacologic interventions for pain management, nurses should consider the use of music as an intervention. Research has shown that music is helpful for pain management. Music provides a simple, inexpensive intervention that the nurse can easily adapt to the individual needs of patients with burns (Prensner, Yowler, Smith, Steele, & Fratianne, 2001).

Research Support:

A Korean study assessed whether music therapy could affect anxiety and pain for patients undergoing burn dressing changes. The study involved 32 adult patients with burns, 15 of whom received the routine burn dressing changes (the control group) and 17 of whom listened to self-selected music through headphones during burn dressing changes for 3 days (the experimental group). Participants in the experimental (music) group completed the State Anxiety Inventory and a self-report of pain scores before and after burn dressing changes. Results showed that the participants who received music therapy reported significant reductions in both anxiety and pain before and after burn dressing changes as compared to participants who did not receive music therapy. Researchers concluded that music therapy with self-selected music is a valuable intervention for the treatment of pain and anxiety in patients undergoing burn dressing changes (Son & Kim, 2006).

Another study assessed the effect of music therapy on 14 randomly selected pediatric burn patients. The experimental group listened to live music and the control group received verbal interaction only. Psychological, behavioral, and physiological outcomes were reported using the Wong Baker FACES Pain Rating Scale, the Fear Thermometer, the Nursing Assessment of Pain Index, heart rate, and respiration rate. Although the results of the study were mixed and inconclusive, researchers recorded improved pain and anxiety through anecdotal reports from the experimental group. Based on these results, researchers stated that further study is needed in order to recommend use of music therapy for patients with burns (Whitehead-Pleaux, Baryza, & Sheridan, 2006).

References

Prensner, J. D., Yowler, C. J., Smith, L. F., Steele, A. L., & Fratianne, R. B. (2001, January-February). Music therapy for assistance with pain and anxiety management in burn treatment. *Journal of Burn Care and Rehabilitation, 22*(1), 82–88.

Son, J. T., & Kim, S. H. (2006). The effects of self-selected music on anxiety and pain during burn dressing changes. *Taehan Kanho Hakhoe Chi, 36*(1), 159–168.

Whitehead-Pleaux, A. M., Baryza, M. J., & Sheridan, R. L. (2006). The effects of music therapy on pediatric patients' pain and anxiety during donor site dressing change. *Journal of Music Therapy, 43*(2), 136–153.

Nursing Management

The nursing care needs of the newly admitted patient with burns are complex and multifaceted. Use of the nursing process will facilitate a comprehensive approach to patient assessment and care. The Nursing Process: Patient Care Plan feature applies the nursing process to the applicable nursing diagnoses and provides a comprehensive care plan for a patient with burns during the emergency period.

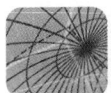 **NURSING PROCESS: Patient Care Plan for the Emergency Period**

Assessment of Fluid Volume Loss

Subjective Data:

Do you know where you are?

Tell me your name.

Are you feeling light-headed or dizzy?

Are you feeling thirsty?

Objective Data:

Blood pressure

Cardiac output

Urine output

Hemoglobin and hematocrit

Nursing Assessment and Diagnoses	Outcomes and Evaluation Parameters	Planning and Interventions with *Rationales*
Nursing Diagnosis: *Deficient Fluid Volume* related to increased capillary permeability, increased intravascular hydrostatic pressure, and increased evaporative loss	**Outcomes:** Adequate intravascular volume. Fluid and electrolytes within normal limits. No signs and symptoms of hypovolemic shock. Mental alertness and cognitive orientation. ***Evaluation Parameters:*** Normal vital signs. Normal serum electrolytes, hemoglobin, and hematocrit. Urine specific gravity between 1.010 and 1.020. Urine output at 0.5 mL/kg per hour.	**Interventions and *Rationales:*** Insert large-bore intravenous (IV) catheter through nonburned tissue per order. *To facilitate fluid replacement.* Administer and titrate IV fluids per ordered formulas and parameters. *To replace lost volume.* Record amount of IV fluid infused. *To monitor fluid replacement.* Assess vital signs and urine output at least hourly until stable and then per health care provider's order/unit policy. *To assess adequacy of fluid replacement.* Monitor central venous pressure (CVP) and pulmonary artery wedge pressure (PAWP) if possible. *To assess adequacy of fluid replacement and cardiac output.* Monitor arterial blood gases (ABGs). *To assess acid–base balance and presence of shock.* Obtain baseline weight if possible and monitor regularly. *To monitor adequacy of nutritional replacement.* Test all stools and emesis for blood. *To monitor for blood loss from stress ulcers.* Maintain a heated environment. *To prevent loss of body heat due to loss of skin integrity.* Monitor serum electrolytes, hemoglobin, and hematocrit, and report critical abnormalities to the health care provider. *To monitor hematologic changes associated with fluid loss and tissue destruction.* Monitor for blood loss from burns or other injuries. *To assess need for blood replacement therapy.* Assess orientation frequently and regularly. *Monitor adequacy of fluid replacement and presence of associated head injury.* Provide oral fluids, if patient is able to drink. *Encourage fluid intake to replace lost fluid.*

Assessment of Excess Fluid

Subjective Data:

Do you feel short of breath?

Do you have a cough?

Objective Data:

Congested lungs

Increased heart rate

Increased blood pressure

Increased CVP

Increased PAWP

Increased rate and depth of respirations

Increased weight

Nursing Assessment and Diagnoses	Outcomes and Evaluation Parameters	Planning and Interventions with *Rationales*
Nursing Diagnosis: *Risk for Imbalanced Fluid Volume* related to excessive IV fluid administration and diminished organ capacity for excessive volume load	**Outcome:** Adequate hydration with no evidence of fluid overload. ***Evaluation Parameters:*** Normal vital signs. Normal CVP, PAWP. Normal ABGs, electrolytes. Vesicular lung sounds clear. No dyspnea. No increase in body weight. Normal urine output and specific gravity.	**Interventions and *Rationales:*** Assess body weight if possible. *Monitor for excess fluid buildup.* Assess urine output and specific gravity. *Monitor hydration status.* Assess arterial blood gases (ABGs) and electrolytes. *To assess acid–base balance, severity of shock state, and electrolyte changes due to fluid shifts.* Monitor intake and output hourly. *To assess rate of fluid replacement.* Monitor lung sound. *To assess for fluid build-up.*

(continued)

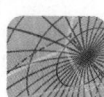

NURSING PROCESS: Patient Care Plan for the Emergency Period—*Continued*

Assessment of Tissue Perfusion

Subjective Data:
Can you feel me touch your fingers and toes?
Can you move your fingers and toes?
Where are you having pain?

Objective Data:
Nail bed color and capillary refill
Temperature of fingers and toes
Peripheral pulses

Nursing Assessment and Diagnoses	Outcomes and Evaluation Parameters	Planning and Interventions with *Rationales*
Nursing Diagnosis: *Ineffective Peripheral Tissue Perfusion* related to constricting edema formation and circumferential burns	**Outcome:** Adequate peripheral tissue perfusion. **Evaluation Parameters:** Extremity pulses present by palpation and/or ultrasound. Capillary refill < 3 seconds on distal extremities. Absence of numbness or tingling. Absence of increased pain.	**Interventions and *Rationales:*** Remove constricting clothing, jewelry, and dressings. *To promote tissue perfusion.* Elevate affected extremities above the heart. *To reduce edema formation.* Monitor arterial pulses by palpation and/or ultrasound every hour during the first 24–48 hours. *To assess perfusion status during edema formation.* Assess pain and capillary permeability on both burned and unburned areas. *To assess the impact of edema formation.* Assess for numbness or tingling. *To assess perfusion status during edema formation.* If pulses diminish or become absent, if pain increases, or if capillary refill slows, notify the health care provider immediately. *These are indications of a loss of perfusion and need medical intervention to prevent necrosis formation.* If indicated, prepare patient for escharotomy. *To prevent loss of affected extremity or prevent respiratory depression.*

Assessment of Airway and Gas Exchange

Subjective Data:
How did you get burned?
Did the injury occur in an enclosed space?
Do you have any preexisting health problems such as heart, lung, or kidney disease?

Objective Data:
Lung sounds
Oxygen saturation
Work of breathing; e.g., gasping, increased rate, loudness
Vital signs
Skin and nail bed color

Nursing Assessment and Diagnoses	Outcomes and Evaluation Parameters	Planning and Interventions with *Rationales*
Nursing Diagnoses: *Impaired Gas Exchange* related to inhalation injury and fatigue. *Ineffective Airway Clearance* related to tracheal edema	**Outcome:** Adequate gas exchange. **Evaluation Parameters:** Normal arterial blood gases. Free of dyspnea: unlabored respirations < 24/minute. Alert and oriented. Clear breath sounds. No restlessness, cyanosis, or fatigue. Oxygen saturation is within normal limits.	**Interventions and *Rationales:*** Assess for adventitious or diminished breath sounds. *Indicates decreased gas exchange.* Note presence of cough, and amount, color, and consistency of sputum. *Assessing for inhalation injury.* Monitor ABGs and oxygen saturation. *To assess adequacy of gas exchange and level of shock state.* Monitor respiratory rate and depth. *To assess for respiratory distress.* Monitor restlessness and confusion. *Indicators of inadequate gas exchange with resultant brain hypoxia.* Observe for cyanosis, especially in the mucous membranes. *Indicators of inadequate gas exchange with resultant tissue hypoxia.* Turn, cough, deep breathe, elevate head of bed, and instruct on use of incentive spirometry. *Measures to promote gas exchange.* Administer humidified oxygen as prescribed. *To loosen secretions and promote airway clearance.* Report respiratory distress to the health care provider. *Medical intervention may be indicated to prevent respiratory failure.* Assess need for suctioning and/or endotracheal intubation. *To maintain adequate gas exchange.*

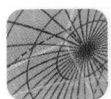

NURSING PROCESS: Patient Care Plan for the Emergency Period—*Continued*

Assessment of Skin Integrity

Subjective Data:
Where are you having pain?

Objective Data:
Percent total body surface area burn using standardized measurement scales
Depth of injury

Nursing Assessment and Diagnoses	Outcomes and Evaluation Parameters	Planning and Interventions with *Rationales*
Nursing Diagnosis: *Impaired Skin Integrity* related to epithelial skin loss	**Outcome:** Normal wound healing to reestablish skin integrity. ***Evaluation Parameters:*** Burn wounds will heal spontaneously or by surgical closure as evidenced by no open wound, no drainage, and no odor. Absence of clinical manifestations of wound infection.	**Interventions and *Rationales:*** Assess extent of total body surface area (TBSA) of burn. Cleanse and débride wound. *Determines treatment and prognosis.* Assess wound for depth, location, and dimensions. *Determines treatment and prognosis.* Elevate affected areas. *To decrease edema.* Position therapeutically. *To prevent contracture formation.* Apply antibiotic cream and/or dressing per health care provider's order. *To prevent infection.* Clean, débride wounds daily, and assess for separation of eschar and evidence of granulation tissue. *Preparation for skin grafting.* Assess for presence or absence of granulation tissue and necrotic tissue. *Assess wound status for grafting.* Assess for infection (see *Risk for Infection* nursing diagnosis). *To prevent occurrence and spread of infection.* Establish a skin breakdown prevention plan. Monitor blood glucose. White blood count (WBC) daily. *Infection assessment.* Monitor donor sites for infection. *May convert site to a full-thickness injury.* Administer vitamins and minerals per order. *To promote wound healing.*

Assessment for Infection

Subjective Data:
Is your pain increasing?
Do you feel weaker?

Objective Data:
Previously healed wounds are breaking down
Open wounds not healing
Partial-thickness injuries/donor sites converting to full-thickness injuries
Increased odor and drainage from wound sites
Wound cultures positive for organisms
Fever
Increased WBC

Nursing Assessment and Diagnoses	Outcomes and Evaluation Parameters	Planning and Interventions with *Rationales*
Nursing Diagnosis: *Risk for Infection* related to loss of skin integrity and impaired nonspecific and specific immunity	**Outcome:** Effective infection prevention. ***Evaluation Parameters:*** Burn will not be colonized by organisms. Healing and re-epithelialization as noted by wound closure. Skin integrity will be restored.	**Interventions and *Rationales:*** Cleanse and shave wound per protocol. *To prevent contamination from surrounding tissue and hair.* Assess for infection and document with each dressing change. *To prevent spread of infection.* Assess for drainage: exudate, color, odor, and amount. *Factors that indicate infection.* Assess for undermining or sinus tract formation. *Indicates infection.* Use strict aseptic technique. *To prevent infection.* Notify health care provider of presence of infection or wound enlargement. *To facilitate medical intervention.* Monitor serum WBC daily. *Increased WBC indicates presence of infection.* Maintain nutritional therapies. *Malnutrition increases the risk of infection.* Monitor and record temperature hourly. *Indicates infection.* Culture wounds and body secretions per protocol. *To assess for infection.*

(continued)

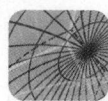

NURSING PROCESS: Patient Care Plan for the Emergency Period—*Continued*

Assessment of Nutritional Status

Subjective Data:

How is your appetite?

What can be done to help improve it?

Do you understand the importance of maintaining adequate nutrition?

Do you feel nauseated?

What kinds of food do you enjoy?

Objective Data:

Presence of bowel sounds

Calorie count

Prealbumin level

Weight changes

Nursing Assessment and Diagnoses	Outcomes and Evaluation Parameters	Planning and Interventions with *Rationales*
Nursing Diagnosis: *Imbalanced Nutrition: Less than Body Requirements* related to hypermetabolic demands of burn injury, decreased appetite, immobility, pain, nausea/vomiting, and depression	**Outcome:** Adequate nutrition maintained. **Evaluation Parameters:** Adequate calorie and nutrient intake maintained. Tolerates prescribed diet. Nutritional laboratory values within normal limits. Regular bowel pattern. Maintains preinjury body weight (+ or − 10%). Gastric pH > 5. Stool and gastric aspirate are negative for blood. Fluid and electrolyte balance is normal. Progressive wound healing. Free of complications. Adequate energy levels.	**Interventions and *Rationales:*** Record accurate intake and output, and calorie count every shift. *Indicates adequacy of nutrition.* Maintain oral hygiene. *Helps promote appetite and prevents infection.* Monitor gastrointestinal tract for bowel sounds and distention. *Assesses normal digestive process.* Monitor feeding tube placement and function. *To prevent complications such as aspiration.* Administer enteral tube feedings at prescribed rate and concentration. *To maintain nutrition.* Monitor for residual formula by aspiration per health care provider's order. *To assess tolerance and absorption of feedings.* Monitor weight daily. *Indicates adequacy of nutrition.* Consult nutritionist to establish calorie, protein, carbohydrate, and nutrient needs. *To maintain nutrition.* Allow patient to select desired foods. *To promote appetite.* Involve family in meal planning. *To assess patient's likes and dislikes.* Provide high-calorie, high-protein, high-carbohydrate diet, including snacks. *To augment between meal calorie intake.* Avoid painful procedures near mealtime and make the environment pleasant for eating. *To increase appetite.* Monitor laboratory values; i.e., total protein levels, complete blood count, glucose, iron, and prealbumin. *To ensure adequacy of nutrition.* Monitor elimination patterns. *To assess gastrointestinal (GI) function.* Monitor wound healing progress. *Wound healing progress is impacted by nutritional status.* Monitor pH and guaiac tests on gastric aspirate and stools. *To assess for GI bleeding.* Administer antacids, stool softeners, laxatives, and antiulcer agents per health care provider orders. *To prevent GI bleeding.* Assess dietary patterns in culturally diverse populations. *To tailor diet to foods of a particular culture.*

Assessment of Pain

Subjective Data:

What is your pain level using the 0–10 scale? A 1 is very little pain and a 10 is the worst imaginable pain.

What is your experience with pain?

Do you routinely take pain medications at home; if so, what for and what kind?

Are you allergic to any pain medication?

Do you have any cultural or religious beliefs that impact your pain control?

Objective Data:

Grimacing on movement

Restlessness and irritability

Taut facial expression

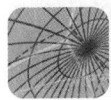

NURSING PROCESS: Patient Care Plan for the Emergency Period—*Continued*

Nursing Assessment and Diagnoses	Outcomes and Evaluation Parameters	Planning and Interventions with *Rationales*
Nursing Diagnosis: *Acute Pain* related to burn injury and exposed nerve endings	**Outcome:** Comfort level maintained. **Evaluation Parameters:** Able to communicate pain level and therapies that help alleviate it. Pain reduced and/or absent as evidenced by patient report and no pain behaviors: grimacing. Nonpharmacologic method of control is effective as evidenced by patient report and no pain behaviors. Reports satisfaction with pain management program.	**Interventions and *Rationales:*** Use pain scale (0–10) to quantify pain level. *Quantifying pain increases consistency.* Instruct patient to inform nurse if pain is not relieved. *Indicates need to change pain management plan.* Assess cultural and religious impact on patient's responses. *Different cultures and religions respond differently to pain.* Correct misconceptions about risk of addiction and overdose. *To decrease anxiety related to medication addiction.* Explain, prepare, and medicate patient for painful procedures (dressing change) and anticipated discomforts. *To control increased pain level related to procedure.* Provide a supportive environment wherein patient is able to express pain level. *Opens communication and facilitates pain management.* Use pain control measures before pain becomes severe. *This increases comfort and decreases need for medication.* Teach nonpharmacologic method of control; i.e., guided imagery and massage, and breathing exercises. *These measures augment pain relief.* Cover wounds. *Covering areas where there is no skin decreases the pain.* Elevate affected areas. *Elevation decreases edema formation, which can be painful.* Provide rest periods between procedures to assist with coping with ongoing pain. *Decreases the fatigue related to long-term pain.* Revise pain management plan as wounds heal and pain decreases. *To prevent overmedication.* Plan diversional activities. *To augment pain-relief measures.*

Assessment of Fear and Anxiety

Subjective Data:
Tell me what you are feeling about your injuries.
Who are the people in your life that are your support system?
How have you handled fearful situations in the past?

Objective Data:
Facial expressions
Mood
Verbalization of fear regarding injury, impact on family, and future

Nursing Assessment and Diagnoses	Outcomes and Evaluation Parameters	Planning and Interventions with *Rationales*
Nursing Diagnoses: *Fear* and *Anxiety* related to changes in health status/role functioning; situational crisis	**Outcome:** Anxiety level minimized. **Evaluation Parameters:** Verbalizes anxious feelings. Verbalizes what relieves anxiety. Anxiety relieved by consistently demonstrating aggression and anxiety control, coping, impulse control, self-mutilation restraint, and substantially effective social interaction skills. Verbalizes absence of sensory perceptual disorders. Verbalizes absence of physical manifestations of anxiety. Behavioral manifestations of anxiety absent.	**Interventions and *Rationales:*** Assess and document level of anxiety. *To track trends in anxiety levels.* Explore with the patient/family techniques to reduce anxiety. *This gives the patient a sense of control and opens communication about the subject.* Provide factual information concerning diagnosis, treatment, disfigurement, disabilities, and prognosis. *Truthful explanations increase trust and potentially decrease anxiety.* Explain all procedures and allow time for mental preparation. *This decreases fear and anxiety of the unknown.* Explore with patient effective ways to minimize anxiety. *This gives the patient a sense of control.* Instruct patient on use of relaxation techniques. *To relieve anxiety.* Assess need for and administer antianxiety and pain medication. *If alternative measures are not effective, may need antianxiety agents.* Assist patient/family in setting realistic goals for progress. *Indicates effectiveness of emotional adjustment.* Consider psychiatric counseling for patients/families who exhibit inability to accept situation. *Provide an ongoing plan and interventions to promote long-term relief from anxiety.*

(continued)

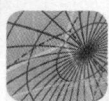

Assessment for Temperature Regulation

Subjective Data:
Do you feel cold/too warm?

Objective Data:

Body temperature   Shivering   Dusky nail beds

Nursing Assessment and Diagnoses	Outcomes and Evaluation Parameters	Planning and Interventions with *Rationales*
Nursing Diagnosis: *Ineffective Thermoregulation* related to epithelial skin loss	**Outcome:** Normal thermoregulation maintained. ***Evaluation Parameter:*** Body temperature maintained between 37.5° and 38.7°C (99.5°–101.5°F).	**Interventions and *Rationales:*** Minimize heat loss by covering patient with dressing and blankets. *To decrease heat loss due to a lack of skin integrity.* Apply heat lamps and radiant heat shields. *To decrease heat loss due to a lack of skin integrity.* Keep room temperature elevated, especially during dressing changes. *To decrease heat loss due to a lack of skin integrity.* Monitor rectal and core temperatures as per orders and report changes. *To assess effectiveness of interventions.*

Assessment of Patient Perception of Environment and Injury

Subjective Data:
What questions do you have about your injury and the necessary therapy for healing?
Have you been in situations in your life in which you feel you have very little control?
How do you typically cope with situations in which you are not in control?

Objective Data:
Compliance with treatments

Nursing Assessment and Diagnoses	Outcomes and Evaluation Parameters	Planning and Interventions with *Rationales*
Nursing Diagnosis: *Powerlessness* related to foreign environment and critical injury	**Outcome:** Realistic perception of control. ***Evaluation Parameters:*** Verbalizes realistic perception of abilities to perform. Identifies health outcome priorities. Verbalizes powerlessness. Identifies actions that are within his control. Verbalizes ability to perform necessary actions. Reports adequate support from staff and family.	**Interventions and *Rationales:*** Determine knowledge of health and injury. *Determines where to begin teaching.* Discuss realistic options for self-care. *Gives patient hope and realistic view of limitations.* Reinforce personal strengths. *Decreases sense of powerlessness.* Encourage verbalization of feeling of powerlessness. *Opens communication.* Assist patient to increase independence when realistic. *Decreases powerlessness.* Allow control over surroundings and schedule when possible. *Decreases powerlessness.* Keep items within reach. *Decreases powerlessness.* Set short-term realistic goals. *Decreases powerlessness.* Explore patient's support mechanisms: family, church, and friends. *Needed as a source of support.*

Assessment of Patient and Family Knowledge of Injury

Subjective Data:
What do you understand about your injury?
Do you have questions about the injury/treatment program?
What would you like me to tell you about your injury?

Objective Data:
Patient/family verbalizes knowledge of seriousness of injury and prognosis.

Nursing Assessment and Diagnoses	Outcomes and Evaluation Parameters	Planning and Interventions with *Rationales*
Nursing Diagnosis: *Deficient Knowledge* regarding burn resuscitation	**Outcome:** Adequate knowledge of treatment regimen. ***Evaluation Parameter:*** Patient and family will verbalize understanding of treatments and care.	**Interventions and *Rationales:*** Assess patient/family's readiness and ability to learn, and individual learning needs. *The person must be psychologically ready to learn.* Determine level of existing knowledge. *Begin the teaching where existing knowledge ends.* Provide factual information about diagnosis, treatments, and prognosis. *To increase knowledge and understanding.* Explain all procedures in simple, concise language—allowing for questions. *Increases understanding.* Encourage questions. *Keeps open communication and augments understanding.* Ongoing education of treatment plan and rationale. *Ongoing education is necessary as situation and condition change.* Document response to teaching. *Assists health care team when implementing a teaching plan.*

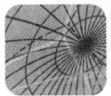

NURSING PROCESS: Patient Care Plan for the Emergency Period—*Continued*

Assessment of Psychological Adjustment to Scarring and Contractures

Subjective Data:
What impact does the change in your physical appearance have on your life?
How do you plan to cope with these changes?

Objective Data:
Does patient look at burn wounds?
Does patient ask questions about the wounds?
Is patient's perception realistic regarding body image changes?
Are the patient/family willing to learn and participate in the required care after hospital discharge?

Nursing Assessment and Diagnoses	Outcomes and Evaluation Parameters	Planning and Interventions with *Rationales*
Nursing Diagnoses: *Disturbed Body Image* related to scar formation and functional loss *Risk for Complicated Grieving* related to body image change, risk of family role change, and possible occupational change	**Outcome:** Acceptance of body image changes. ***Evaluation Parameters:*** Patient verbalizes understanding of body changes. Patient verbalizes acceptance of self.	**Interventions and *Rationales:*** Assess patient's level of anxiety and knowledge related to body image changes. *Body image changes occur as healing progresses.* Encourage discussion of meaning of loss. *Increases adjustment.* Observe interaction with significant people. *Indication of adjustment.* Assess for signs of grieving. *Indication of adjustment.* Establish therapeutic environment with an atmosphere of acceptance. *Increases adjustment.* Explain expected appearance. *Increases adjustment.* Offer mirror for viewing of facial burns. *Assesses adjustment.* Be realistic and positive during explanations. *Increases adjustment.* Plan family involvement during teaching. *Increases adjustment.* Set realistic goals for future. *Increases trust and is reality based.*

Source: Wilkinson, J. M. (2009). *Nursing diagnosis handbook; with interventions and outcomes* (8th ed.). Upper Saddle River, NJ: Prentice Hall.

■ Collaborative Management

To achieve optimal recovery and return to society, patients with burns need a multidisciplinary team approach, including health care providers, nurses, physical and occupational therapists, social workers, psychologists/psychiatrists, and dieticians. To ensure complete closure and prevention of infection, wound care is managed by both the nurses and the health care providers. As the burn scar heals, it continues to contract, thereby decreasing range of motion in the surrounding area. Physical therapy is begun within a few days after admission and continues for at least a year after hospital discharge. Ongoing physical therapy will help increase range of motion in the joints. When contracture formation is severe, the surgeon needs to release the contractures surgically. Due to the scarring and contractures, it may not be possible for the patient to return to her previous profession. The occupational therapist assists the patient with exercises that will enhance fine motor movements, while the social worker and a psychologist/psychiatrist are used to help the patient adjust to body image changes and perhaps loss of profession. Family dynamics often are impacted by the prolonged hospitalization and change in role function within the family structure. The psychologist/psychiatrist also assists the patient with the adjustments of these changes. Finally, a comprehensive plan for nutrition is important for enhancing wound healing, regaining strength, and preventing complications. The dietician works with the health care team from the time of admission through discharge to ensure proper nutritional support.

Acute Phase

The acute period of burn management begins when the patient is hemodynamically stable and ends with closure of the burn wounds. The goals of treatment during this period include wound cleansing and healing; pain relief; preserving body heat; preventing infection; promoting nutrition; and splinting, positioning, and exercising affected joints.

Wound Care

After airway and hemodynamic stabilization, wound care is the next priority. Infection is the most serious threat to further tissue injury and the development of sepsis; therefore, survival may be dependent on preventing wound contamination. Nurses generally coordinate and perform wound care; thus, nursing assessment and interventions are critical. Care of the wound includes cleansing, débridement, shaving, culturing, assessment for infection and adequate circulation, and applying topical antibiotics. These aspects of wound care are discussed next.

Cleansing

Cleansing of the burn wound at the time of admission may be accomplished by a number of methods depending on the preference of the health care provider, available equipment, and the stability of the patient. The purpose of the cleansing is to remove debris from the wound, eliminate dead tissue, and prevent further destruction of viable tissue by infection. For the cleansing process, the patient may be submerged in a Hubbard tank, hosed over a spray table, placed in a shower, or washed at the bedside. The advantage of using a Hubbard tank is that the patient can be totally submerged in the water, which helps remove topical antibiotics and dead tissue (eschar), and facilitates range-of-motion exercises. Submersion in a Hubbard tank is typically limited to 30 minutes or less because submersion in water leaches sodium from the open wound, causes heat loss, and is very painful. Whichever method is used, the wound is washed with gauze and a mild bacteriostatic soap such as chlorhexidine gluconate (Hibiclens) or any noncytotoxic cleansing agent. Removal of blisters is controversial; most health care providers believe that if blisters are intact they should be left in place, but if they are open the loose tissue should be removed. Washing of open wounds is a painful process; therefore, it is imperative that the patient be premedicated prior to dressing changes. Heat shields, warm blankets, and increased room temperature are methods used to help maintain body temperature during dressing changes.

Wound Débridement

The purpose of wound débridement is to remove loose tissue, wound debris, and eschar (nonviable tissue) in order to prepare the wound for closure. In Figure 68–9 ■ the white tissue is dead eschar, which needs to be débrided before the wound is ready for grafting. Débridement of a burn wound can be accomplished by three methods: mechanically, chemically, and surgically. Mechanical débridement is accomplished by using wet-to-dry dressings. Mechanical débridement is done by manually cutting the dead tissue with scissors and forceps, as well as with hydrotherapy. During daily dressing changes, nurses use scissors and forceps to remove and cut away the dead tissue. Use of the Hubbard tank, a spray table, and/or the shower gradually softens the dead tissue, which facilitates easier removal. Chemical removal of eschar is accomplished by the use of commercially prepared enzymatic or fibrinolytic agents that digest necrotic tissue, such as Elase (Parke-Davis Division of Warner-Lambert Co., Morris Plains, New Jersey). This agent is a combination of two lytic enzymes in a petroleum base. Enzymatic débridement agents must be applied only within the open wound and must be discontinued once the eschar is gone and granulation tissue

is present. More extensive wound débridement is done in surgery by excising the burn wound. The techniques used to remove eschar are discussed in the Surgical Management section later in this chapter.

Shaving, Culturing, and Photographs

With the exception of the eyebrows, body hair is shaved within the wound itself and up to 2.5 centimeters from the periphery of the wound. This is done to avoid wound contamination because hair attracts and shelters bacteria. Wound culturing is typically done on admission to obtain baseline information and is repeated approximately every 7 days unless the wounds become symptomatic with exudate and odor. Culturing protocols are specific to site and health care provider. Photographs are taken on admission to provide baseline data and then repeated periodically throughout the healing process.

Escharotomies

During the initial phase of management, a surgical intervention may be required to maintain adequate circulation to the underlying tissues. Burn-induced changes in capillary permeability and the infusion of large volumes of crystalloid solutions to maintain vascular volume, cause edema to form beneath the inelastic eschar. If a full-thickness injury involves an entire circumferential area, the edema creates a tourniquet-like effect and diminishes or completely cuts off circulation distal to the injury site. If left untreated, there is a high risk for tissue necrosis and in some instances total loss of the tissue including limbs. Doppler ultrasound signals are often used to assess perfusion in the involved areas. Loss of ultrasound signals is an indication for an escharotomy. Incisions or **escharotomies** are made through the burn tissue to relieve the constricting effects of the edema. These incisions should extend the entire length of a full-thickness injury, including joints, to ensure release of neural and vascular compression (Figure 68–10 ■). The incisions penetrate the eschar and immediate subadjacent connective tissue to permit expansion of the edematous underlying tissue. Frequent monitoring of the circulation distal to the escharotomy site is part of the ongoing nursing assessment and includes pulses, tissue color including paleness and cyanosis, sensation, increased pain, capillary refill, and decreased temperature. Often it is necessary to monitor circulation every 15 to 20 minutes. If distal blood flow does not improve, a second escharotomy is needed.

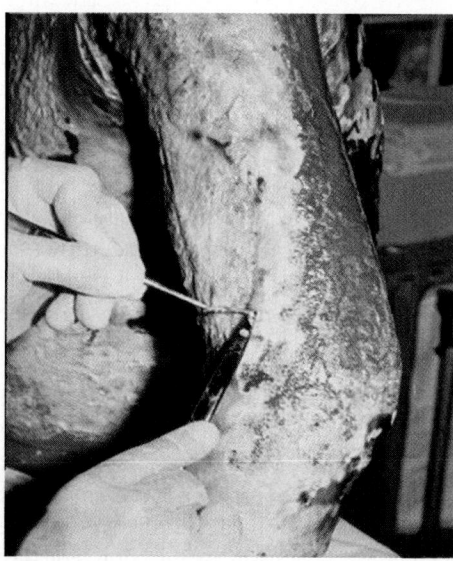

FIGURE 68–9 ■ Débridement of eschar.
Source: Courtesy of: Robert M. Faggella, Jr. M.D., FACS Sacramento, CA

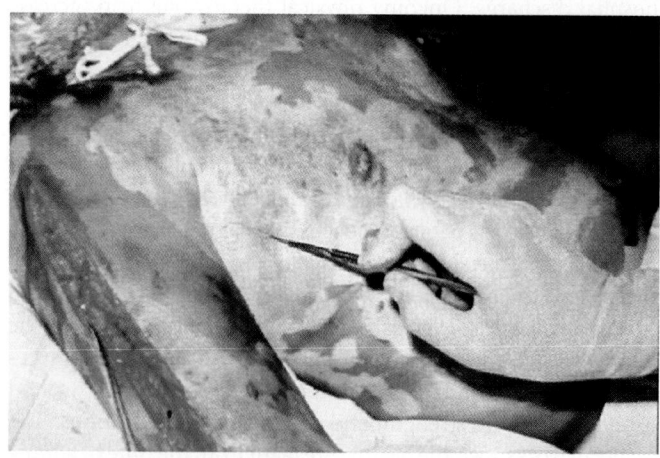

FIGURE 68–10 ■ Escharotomy.
Source: Courtesy of: Robert M. Faggella, Jr. M.D., FACS Sacramento, CA

Typically, no anesthesia is required because full-thickness injuries have limited or no sensation, and generally blood loss is minimal and is readily controlled with pressure.

Circumferential burns of the neck and chest may occlude the airway and decrease chest expansion and pulmonary function, resulting in respiratory distress. A chest escharotomy may be needed to restore a patent airway and effective ventilation. Monitoring respiratory effort is a critical part of the initial nursing assessment and includes respiratory rate, oxygen saturations, arterial blood gases, cyanosis, lung sounds, and shortness of breath (see Chapter 33 🌐 for complete respiratory assessment). Mechanical ventilation may be necessary due to low tidal volumes.

In Figure 68–11 ■, the broken lines are the preferred sites for escharotomy incisions. The solid segments emphasize the importance of extending the incisions across joints with a full-thickness injury.

Fasciotomy

On rare occasions an incision of the muscle fascia beneath the burned tissue is required to restore circulation in a burned limb. This procedure is required for very deep burns involving the fas-

cia and muscle, for associated traumatic limb injuries, and for high-voltage electrical injury. Stony, hard edema of the muscle compartments and absence of peripheral pulses distal to the site of the electrical contact should prompt immediate fasciotomy and exploration of the muscle compartments. The circulation can be assessed with a Doppler ultrasound.

 Assessment of pulses, capillary refill, and color of the area distal to the escharotomy is critical. Any changes in the circulatory status need to be reported to the health care provider immediately. If an escharotomy is done in the chest area, close monitoring of lung sounds is essential to assess gas exchange. Until the swelling subsides, the need for repeated escharotomies continues.

Application of Topical Antibiotics/Dressing

The use of topical antibiotics started in the late 1940s when infection was the leading cause of death in patients with burns. The overall objective for the use of these agents is to prevent infection and to penetrate the burn wound. The penetrating action helps the burn tissue (eschar) separate from the deep viable tissue, and the antimicrobial action of the topical agents assists in preventing infection. These agents are usually applied once or twice daily after the wound has been cleaned and débrided. The Pharmacology Summary feature (p. 2260) outlines the most commonly used agents. Silver sulfadiazine appears to be the most frequently used medication in the United States, although a number of health care providers use a combination of drugs to maximize antimicrobial protection and minimize the associated side effects (Murphy, Lee, & Herndon, 2003).

Two techniques are commonly used for antibiotic application. First, with the open method, the antibiotic cream is applied directly to the wound with a gloved hand, and the wound is left open to air. Ointment is reapplied as necessary to ensure constant coverage. This method is used most frequently for the face and ears. The advantages are better visualization of the wound, easier mobility and joint range of motion (ROM), cost, and simplicity of wound care.

Disadvantages include an increased risk of hypothermia with extensive injuries and easy removal of the ointment with patient activity. The second method is referred to as the closed method, whereby either the antibiotic cream is applied directly to the wound with a gloved hand and then covered with a dry gauze dressing, or the dressing itself is impregnated with the cream and then applied to the wound. Even though there is less mobility with the closed method, the advantage is less heat and fluid loss from the wound surface.

Special Care Sites

For burns in and around the eye, special care must be taken because the skin is very thin and delicate. When cleansing and applying topical antibiotics to this area, care must be taken to keep the cleanser as well as the antibiotic cream out of the eye itself to help prevent conjunctivitis. The nose is another area where special consideration is needed because full-thickness burns of the nose could lead to a loss of tissue and cartilage. Débridement and cleansing must be gentle, and any nasal tubes should be monitored for placement to prevent erosion of nasal tissue. Burns of the ears also require special attention because the skin overlying the external ear, the auricle, is thin and prone to infection. This area must be cleaned gently and inspected frequently for infection. Pillows and gauze dressing beneath the head are contraindicated for burns

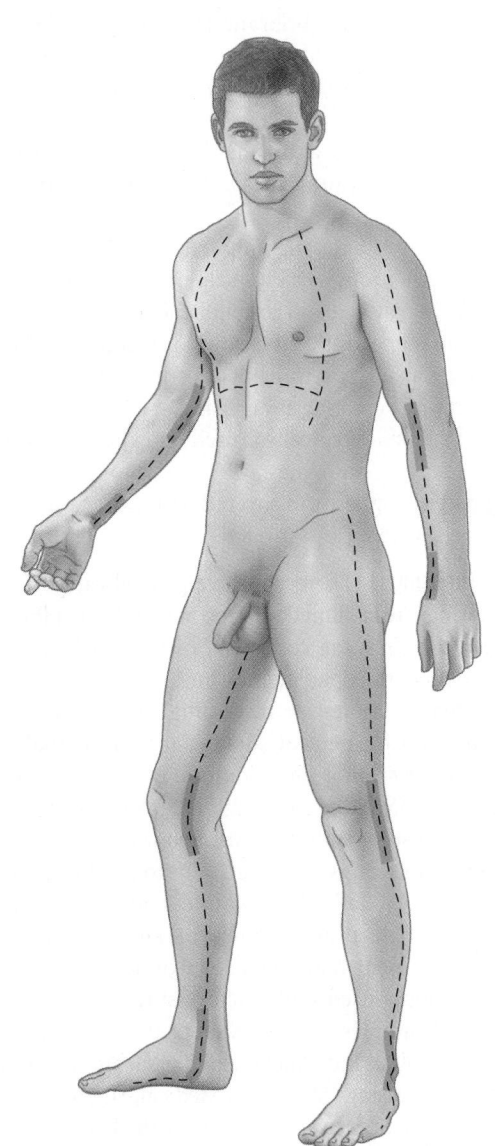

FIGURE 68–11 ■ Common escharotomy sites.

PHARMACOLOGY Summary of Topical Medications for Burns

Medication Category	Action	Application/Indication	Nursing Responsibility
Silver sulfadiazine (Silvadene)	Broad-spectrum antimicrobial with limited penetration ability.	Deep partial- to full-thickness burns. Wound infection.	Apply 1/4 inch thick using either open or closed dressing method, 2–3 times daily. Discontinue when eschar is gone. Not painful—soothing.
Silver nitrate	Broad-spectrum antimicrobial; poorly penetrates eschar.	Deep partial- to full-thickness burns. Wound infection.	Apply using either open or closed dressing method. Will turn wound black and is painful.
Mafenide Acetate (Sulfamylon)	Bacteriostatic for gram-positive and gram-negative organisms; penetrates thick eschar and cartilage.	Deep partial- to full-thickness burns. Wound infection.	Apply 1/4 inch thick using either open or closed dressing method, 2–3 times daily. Painful.
Petroleum- and mineral-based antimicrobials (Neosporin, Bacitracin)	Mild bactericidal for gram-positive and gram-negative organisms; poor penetration.	Partial-thickness burns.	Maintain adequate layer to prevent wound drying.

of the ear because the external pressure could decrease circulation and lead to pressure necrosis. Burns of the fingers and toes require individual dressing to each digit to help prevent web space contracture formation. Finally, deep burns where bone and tendons are exposed, must be kept moist until complete wound coverage is achieved. This requires the use of moist dressings that must be changed every 4 to 8 hours.

Temporary Dressings

Biologic, biosynthetic, synthetic, and composite dressings are useful as temporary coverings for burn wounds. The agent selected for use is determined by the condition of the wound, the inherent properties of each agent, and the goals of treatment. Chart 68–4 outlines the common agents, their indications for use, and the associated nursing care.

Biologic Dressings Biologic dressings include **heterografts** such as pigskin or allografts obtained from living or deceased humans. Heterografts are usually impregnated with silver nitrate to retard bacterial infection. Both of these dressings mimic human skin and are used for several purposes, including (1) covering clean superficial or partial-thickness wounds, (2) protecting granulation tissue or excised ungrafted wounds, (3) preventing fluid and temperature losses, and (4) testing the receptivity of the wound for **autografting** (patient's own skin). As seen in Figure 68–12 ■, pigskin (black) is being used when there is not enough of the patient's own skin to cover the wound. **Allografts,** skin harvested from human cadavers, are stored in skin banks located throughout the United States. Typically an allograft is rejected within 14 to 21 days following application. During the dressing, the nurse assesses, trims, and removes the biologic dressings where healing has occurred.

Biosynthetic Dressings **Biosynthetic dressings** are a combination of biologic and synthetic materials and are effective as temporary covering for a variety wounds. One of the more common biosynthetic dressings is Biobrane (Dow B. Hickman Pharmaceuticals, Inc., Sugar Land, Texas), which has been effective in the treatment of superficial partial-thickness burns such as scalds and as a donor-site dressing. A **donor site** is the

area on the body where the skin is surgically harvested to use for covering burn wounds. Biobrane (Figure 68–13 ■) is a semitransparent dressing that is typically soaked in 0.9 normal saline and stretched over the wound and secured with staples, tape, and/or Steri-Strips. Once applied the patient is able to use the involved area such as hands for performing activities of daily living. As the wound heals, the Biobrane loosens and is trimmed away.

A second biosynthetic dressing that is more commonly used in the United Kingdom is calcium alginate. This product is manufactured from seaweed and contains calcium, which reacts with the sodium in the wound and creates a protective gel. This dressing is able to absorb as much as 20 times its own weight in wound fluid while creating a warm, moist environment for healing. Calcium alginate typically is used for exudative wounds and for split-thickness donor sites. After the wound is irrigated, calcium alginate is applied and covered with a dressing. The dressing is changed when it is saturated.

Synthetic Dressings There are three general categories of synthetic dressings: thin filmed, composite, and nonadherent. The thin-filmed dressings are composed of polyethylene and, when applied, provide a transparent, moisture-retentive, waterproof environment that promotes wound healing. These dressings are useful only for the treatment of superficial, clean partial-thickness burns and to cover donor sites. Commonly used products are OpSite, Tegaderm (3M, Medical Division, St. Paul, Minnesota), and Bioclusive (Johnson & Johnson, Arlington, Texas).

Composite dressings (Lyofoam) are foam dressings used in the treatment of exudative burn wounds and graft sites. One layer of the dressing wicks away exudate while another layer maintains a moist environment that facilitates wound healing. The third type of commonly used synthetic dressing is nonadherent fine mesh gauze. Examples of nonadherent dressing include Xeroform gauze (Kendall Inc., Mansfield, Massachusetts) and Scarlet Red ointment dressing (Sherwood Medical, St. Louis, Missouri). These products are to cover clean partial-thickness wounds, new split-thickness skin grafts, and donor sites. The dressings are applied directly over the wound and then changed if they fall off. If

CHART 68–4   Temporary Coverings for Burn Wounds

Covering	Description	Indications/Uses	Nursing Care
Biologic Dressings			
Xenograft (heterograft)	Porcine (pigskin).	Clean partial-thickness injuries. Débrided full-thickness injuries.	Left covered with gauze dressings may be used for the first 24 hours.
Allograft (homograft)	Human cadaver skin harvested within 24 hours of death and preserved by refrigeration and cryopreservation.	Protect excised wounds and test for receptivity of wound bed for autograft.	Left covered with gauze dressings are used to protect site and absorb drainage.
Biosynthetic Dressings			
Biobrane	Collagen-embedded nylon fabric partially bonded to a silicone film.	Partial-thickness injuries. Secured to wound with staples, Steri-Strips, or gauze. Will adhere to wound.	Remove dressing once Biobrane has adhered to wound—left open to air. Trimmed away as wound healing occurs.
Calcium alginate	From alginates found in brown seaweed.	Exudative wounds. Split-thickness donor sites.	Applied to wound after irrigation and covered with absorbent dressing. Changed when cover dressing is saturated.
Synthetic Dressings			
Thin-filmed dressings: OpSite Tegaderm Bioclusive	Semipermeable, adherent polyurethane film dressings.	Protect and facilitate healing in small, clean partial-thickness burns. Cover partial-thickness donor sites.	Dressing needs to have intact skin margins to adhere to the dressing. Does not need dressing over the top unless draining exudate. Remove when wound healed.
Composite dressings: Lyofoam	Polymeric dressings designed to provide moisture-retentive, absorbent, insulating environment.	Cover moderate to highly exudative wounds.	Placed directly over exudative wounds and covered with absorbent dressing. Dressing change frequency depends on amount of exudate.
Nonadherent dressings: Xeroform	Fine mesh gauze impregnated with 3% bismuth tribromophenate. Mild antimicrobial.	Clean partial-thickness wounds. Provides protective barrier, and promotes epithelial growth.	Monitor for and maintain adherence to wounds: Change if nonadherent. Monitor for infection.
Scarlet Red	Fine mesh gauze impregnated with lanolin, olive oil, petrolatum, and red dye.	Promotes epithelial development and protects wound.	Applied to clean partial-thickness injury. Applied in surgery to donor sites.

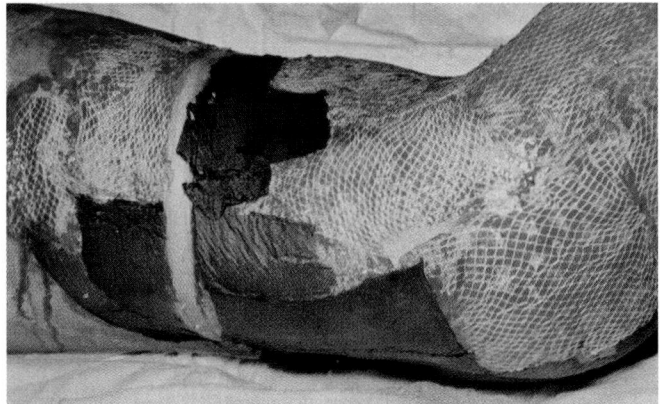

FIGURE 68–12 ■ Black pigskin and meshed skin grafts.
Source: Courtesy of: Robert M. Faggella, Jr. M.D., FACS Sacramento, CA

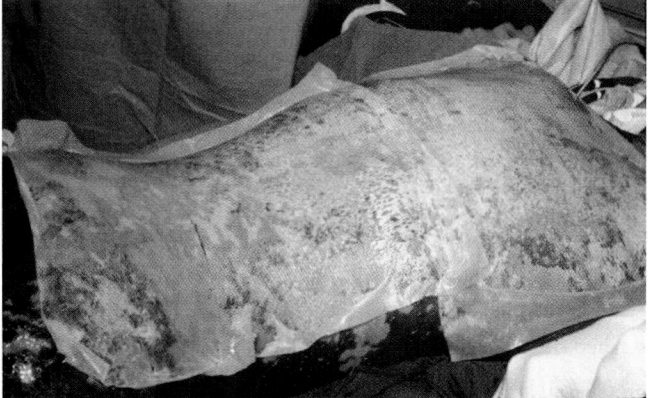

FIGURE 68–13 ■ Application of Biobrane.
Source: Courtesy of: UC Davis, University of California

used for donor-site covering, they are covered with an outer dressing, which typically remains in place for 24 hours. Once the outer dressing is removed, the fine mesh gauze remains in place for 5 to 7 days and is allowed to dry out and loosen as healing oc-

curs. If used for skin grafting, a single layer is applied over the graft site and then reinforced with several layers of coarse mesh gauze and left in place for 5 to 7 days. See Chart 68–4 for a summary of the temporary coverings for burn wounds.

Infection Assessment

Early recognition of a wound infection is critical in limiting morbidity and mortality. Due to immunosuppression and open wounds, the patient with burns is at a high risk for the development of an infection. Wound infection is defined as the presence of bacteria, fungi, or viruses in or around the open wound. The nursing management plan to prevent infection includes (1) vigilant monitoring for signs and symptoms of infection and sepsis, (2) maintaining a hygienic environment to reduce the presence of microorganisms, (3) use of aseptic technique for wound care and invasive procedures, and (4) timely administration of both systemic and topical antibiotics. Daily assessment of the wound is primarily a nursing responsibility. When dressings are removed, the wound is assessed for changes in wound exudate (color, odor, and amount), signs of cellulitis (inflammation/erythema of surrounding tissue), increased wound pain, and loss of previously healed skin.

If infection goes undetected or untreated, it can progress to a deeper wound infection leading to sepsis. Infection also can convert a partial-thickness injury to a full-thickness injury. Characteristics of an invasive infection include focal, dark, red, brown, or black discoloration in the eschar; rapid conversion (necrosis) of an area of partial-thickness injury to full-thickness injury; early, rapid separation of the eschar (fungal infection characteristic); and hemorrhagic fat necrosis.

The prevention of the introduction of exogenous organisms, which cause infection, requires strict adherence to standard precautions and adherence to strict aseptic technique. The nurse must assess all personnel and visitors entering the patient's room for the presence of infection. A sign should be placed on the patient's door indicating the need not to enter if the visitor is sick.

Hyperbaric Oxygen Therapy

Hyperbaric oxygen therapy (HBO) is a means of providing additional oxygen to the body tissues by placing the patient's entire body under increased atmospheric pressure in a closely monitored airtight chamber. During HBO therapy, the patient breathes 100% oxygen for a predetermined period of time. Hyperbaric oxygen therapy has been used for split-thickness skin graft acceptance, flap survival and salvage, wound re-epithelialization, and acute thermal burns. Research continues on the impact of HBO on wound healing to try to take advantage of the angiogenic properties of increasing oxygen gradients resulting from hyperbaric therapy (Neumeister, 2005).

Surgical Management

The surgical management of burn injuries is a complex process involving a sequence of carefully planned surgical stages. The process begins with surgical débridement of damaged tissue, followed by wound closure using a number of techniques described next.

Burn Wound Excision

Historically, treatment for full-thickness injuries involved waiting for the eschar to separate over time with cleansing and débridement. Then the patient was taken to surgery for grafting to close the open wound. This method of treatment was associated with frequent wound infections, prolonged, painful daily débridement and dressing changes, and lengthened hospital stays. Since the late 1970s surgical techniques have been developed to excise eschar, allowing early closure of the burn wound. Early surgical débridement and grafting have decreased the length of hospital stay, decreased the number of septic episodes, and improved survival rates.

Two types of excision are used for burn wounds: tangential excision and fascial excision. Tangential excision, the most frequently used procedure, involves sequential removal of thin layers of eschar until viable dermis or subcutaneous fat is exposed. The depth of the excision is determined by the appearance of healthy tissue and bleeding from dermal or subcutaneous beds. The goal is to create a clean living wound bed with circulation to support graft adherence. The advantage of the tangential excision is decreased risk of infection due to early closure and better preservation of surrounding tissues and body contours, thus, resulting in a better cosmetic result. The disadvantage is that blood loss may be considerable if large surface areas are tangentially excised.

Fascial excision involves removal of eschar and the underlying subcutaneous tissue to the level of the muscle fascia. This technique is usually reserved for patients with very deep, life-threatening burns, typically from electrical injury. The advantages of this technique are that there is less blood loss, it provides a viable graft bed, and less time is required for surgery. The disadvantages include an unsightly cosmetic deformity, loss of superficial nerves, near complete cutaneous denervation, and a high incidence of distal edema when the excision is superficial.

Burn Wound Closure

Burn wounds are usually closed with cutaneous autografts (patient's own skin). Split-thickness skin grafts and occasionally full-thickness skin grafts can be used to accomplish closure. The skin grafts are harvested from the patient's healthy tissue (donor site) and applied to the burn wound.

Harvesting of Skin Harvesting of skin is accomplished by two methods, and the choice of which to use depends on the desired depth of graft. **Full-thickness skin grafts** are removed surgically by excising the entire thickness of the donor skin to the level of the subcutaneous tissue, typically 0.025 to 0.3 inch thick. Donor sites need to be closed by either sutures or split-thickness skin grafts, and therefore, full-thickness grafts are limited to the repair of small wounds or defects. The advantage of this technique is that it permits the transfer of the entire dermal layer, resulting in greater durability and less wound contracture than the split-thickness grafts. Full-thickness skin grafts are used most frequently for areas that require thicker skin to prevent breakdown, such as the palm of the hand, the bottom of the foot, and over joints. Full-thickness grafts also are used for facial defects because there is less contracture formation and a better cosmetic result.

The more common method used for covering a burn wound is a **split-thickness skin graft**, which is a partial layer of skin, including the epidermis and part of the dermis. The skin is harvested from the patient's donor site with a surgical instrument called a dermatome. The dermatome is guarded, making it easier to control the thickness of the harvested skin, which is usually 0.008 to 0.0012 inch thick (Figure 68–14 ■).

When the skin has been harvested, it can be used as either a sheet skin graft or a **meshed skin graft**. Meshing a graft means cutting holes in the harvested skin, which allows it to be stretched over a greater surface area. To mesh the graft, the harvested skin is placed on a plastic template and guided through a

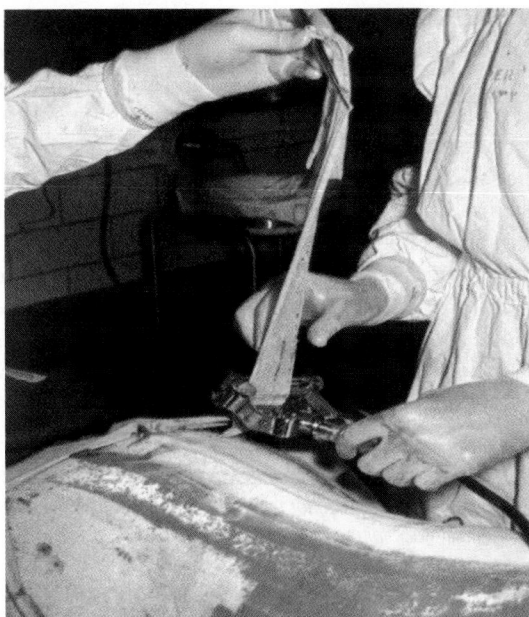

FIGURE 68–14 ■ Dermatome harvesting skin.
Source: Courtesy of: Robert M. Faggella, Jr. M.D., FACS Sacramento, CA

mechanical meshing apparatus, thereby cutting the diamond-shaped pattern of holes (Figure 68–15 ■). The meshed skin graft can be increased from two to nine times its original size, depending on the size of the holes. Skin grafts expanded beyond four times, referred to as 4:1, their original size require longer healing time, have a greater propensity for scar formation, and are usually used only for patients with massive injuries and limited donor sites. The holes in the graft will close over time by epithelialization from the skin edge. With meshed split-thickness skin grafts, there is less of a concern of blood and serous fluid collecting under the grafted area, increasing the percentage of graft adherence. The disadvantage of this method is that the epithelial scar formation from these meshed grafts is in the shape of a diamond, producing a characteristic checkerboard appearance.

Split-thickness grafts that have not been meshed are referred to as **sheet skin grafts** (Figure 68–16 ■). Sheet grafts provide a better cosmetic and functional result and should be used when adequate donor sites are available. Priority areas for using sheet grafts, if the burn is small, include the head, face, hands, neck, upper torso in women, and joint surfaces for growing children. A disadvantage of sheet grafts as compared to meshed grafts is that when blood, bacteria, and serous drainage collect under the graft, the graft has difficulty adhering to the wound surface. Both sheet and meshed skin grafts initially adhere to the wound by means of surface tension and later because of fibrin formation. Within 48 hours, circulation begins to occur, as evidenced by an increasing pink or red color on the graft surface. Depending on the preference of the surgeon, grafts may be sutured or stapled in place. Loss of the skin graft may occur for several reasons. First, hematoma or seroma formation beneath the graft will prevent it from adhering to the wound surface. During the first few days following surgery, the sheet grafts must be examined frequently so that subgraft hematoma or seroma formation can be removed either by needle aspiration, incising the graft to express blood and fluid, or by physically pulling a hematoma through an incision with forceps. Fluid

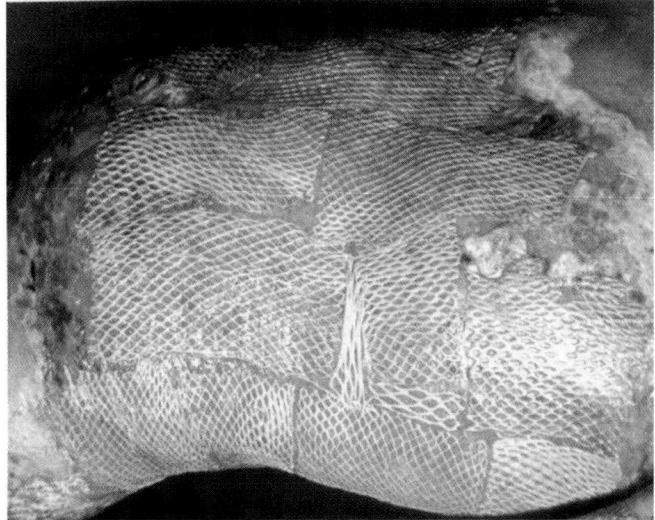

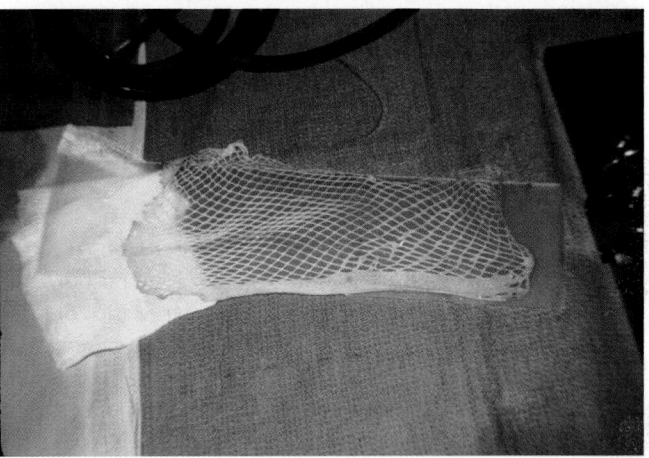

FIGURE 68–15 ■ 3:1 meshed skin graft.
Source: (top): Courtesy of: Robert M. Faggella, Jr. M.D., FACS Sacramento, CA; (bottom): Courtesy of: John M. Osborn, M.D., FACS, Sacramento, CA Plastic Surgery Center

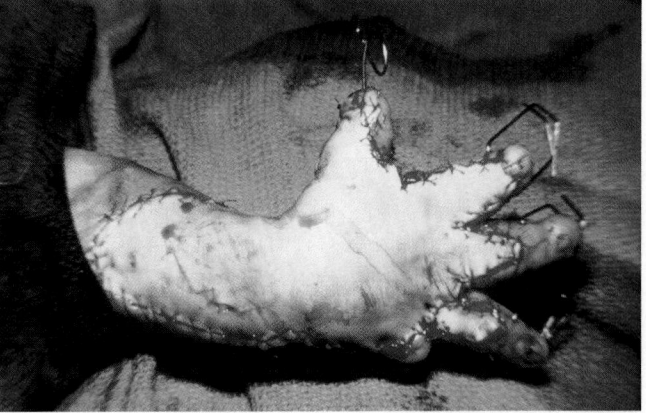

FIGURE 68–16 ■ Sheet skin grafts.
Source: Courtesy of: John M. Osborn, M.D., FACS, Sacramento, CA Plastic Surgery Center

collecting under the graft can be rolled to the side with cotton-tipped applicators.

Second, persistent motion of the grafts will prevent vascular connections and graft adherence; therefore, the grafted area must remain immobilized. Splinting of the grafted area ensures immobilization of the graft for the first few days. Normal movement may be resumed at approximately 5 days, depending on the area involved and the health care provider's preference. Finally, an infection in the grafted area will create exudate under the graft and prevent graft adherence. The wound surface should be meticulously clean and free of infection at the time of graft application. All health care personnel must use strict aseptic technique when caring for the skin grafts.

Cultured epithelial autografting (CEA) is a method to obtain the patient's own skin when there is limited donor-site availability. Once a patient has been identified as a candidate, skin biopsies (usually 2 to 3 centimeters long by 1 centimeter wide) are taken from nonburned tissue and sent to a commercial site where they are cultivated in a medium of epidermal growth factor. This tissue is grown for 18 to 25 days to where it expands to 10,000 times its original size. The cultured grafts are returned to the burn center and applied surgically using the same procedure as for split-thickness skin grafts. Enough CEA to cover an entire body can be grown in 24 days; however, there continue to be limitations to its use. The skin has no dermal layer; therefore, it is thin and friable, resulting in breakdown and contracture formation (Supp, Neely, Supp, Warden, & Boyce, 2005).

Donor-Site Care When skin is harvested from a donor site, a superficial partial-thickness wound is created (Figure 68–17 ■). Healing occurs by epithelial migration in about 10 to 14 days. Donor sites can be reused approximately three to four times with a 10- to 14-day healing period between each use. As much as the size of the injury permits, the donor-site skin should be selected to match the recipient-site skin in texture and color.

The focus of care for the donor sites in the postoperative period is preventing infection. If the site becomes infected, it may convert from a partial-thickness to a full-thickness injury, which then must be grafted. Several dressing options are available for donor sites in the postoperative period. Currently, Vaseline gauze with bismuth; antibacterial polyurethane film; and silver-impregnated mesh are common donor-site dressings. A more traditional approach to donor-site care has been to use a dry fine mesh gauze or gauze impregnated with petrolatum or antimicrobial agents (i.e., Xeroform) to cover the donor site. The choice of donor-site dressing is made by the health care provider. See Chart 68–4 (p. 2261) for a description of the agents used to cover donor sites. As the donor site heals, it dries out (scab formation) and the dressing separates from the wound. The healing process takes about 10 to 14 days. The primary nursing goals are to allow airflow around the donor site to assist in the drying process and prevention of infection.

Donor sites may have a tendency to form hypertrophic scarring, especially in dark-skinned or very fair people. A single harvest from an individual area usually does not cause scarring; however, repeated harvesting from the same site increases the risk of scarring. After the donor site has healed, it requires the same long-term care as do burn wounds, such as avoiding the sun and use of moisturizing creams. Some health care providers use pressure garments to reduce donor-site hypertrophy.

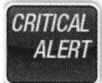

Nurses are primarily responsible for prevention of infection in a donor site. Early detection and reporting will help prevent conversion of a donor site from a partial-thickness to a full-thickness injury.

Alternative Skin Covering In patients with large burn injuries, there is a limited amount of unburned skin suitable as a donor site; therefore, available donor sites need to be used repeatedly. Several products that are currently available provide a deep dermal layer covering of the burn wound, which then can be covered with an ultra-thin split-thickness skin graft. Ultra-thin donor sites heal faster, complications are minimized, and they are ready for reuse sooner where repeated autograft harvesting is necessary. AlloDerm and Integra (Integra Life Sciences Corporation, Plainsboro, New Jersey) are two products currently in use. AlloDerm is an acellular, nonimmunogenic dermal substitute derived from human cadaver skin (Livesey et al., 1995). This product is meshed and applied to a full-thickness injury after it has been excised of dead tissue. A thin split-thickness skin graft is placed over the AlloDerm during the same surgical procedure. AlloDerm is useful for wounds extending over joints where a thicker layer of skin will help prevent contractures, thereby increasing range of motion. Integra is a two-layered skin substitute composed of an internal layer of collagen net and an external layer of silicone. After wound débridement, Integra is placed into the wound. It takes the dermal layer 2 to 3 weeks to become vascularized; then the outer layer is removed and an ultra-thin split-thickness skin graft is applied (Figure 68–18 ■).

If replacement of normal functioning skin is the goal for skin substitutes, then there is no perfect skin substitute. Each of these products has limitations and all are expensive to use. Further

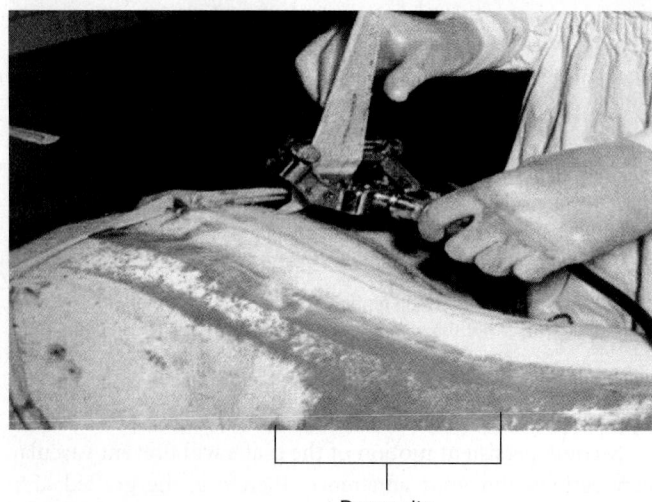

Donor site

FIGURE 68–17 ■ Donor site.
Source: Courtesy of: Robert Fagella, Jr. MD FACS, Sacramento, CA

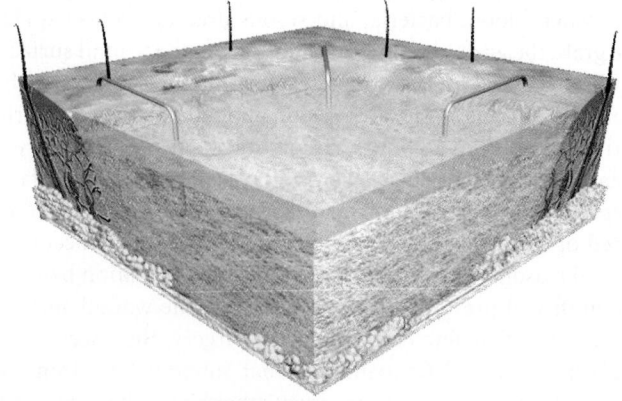

FIGURE 68–18 ■ Integra.
Source: Courtesy of: Johnson and Johnson Wound Management a Division of Ethicon, Inc.

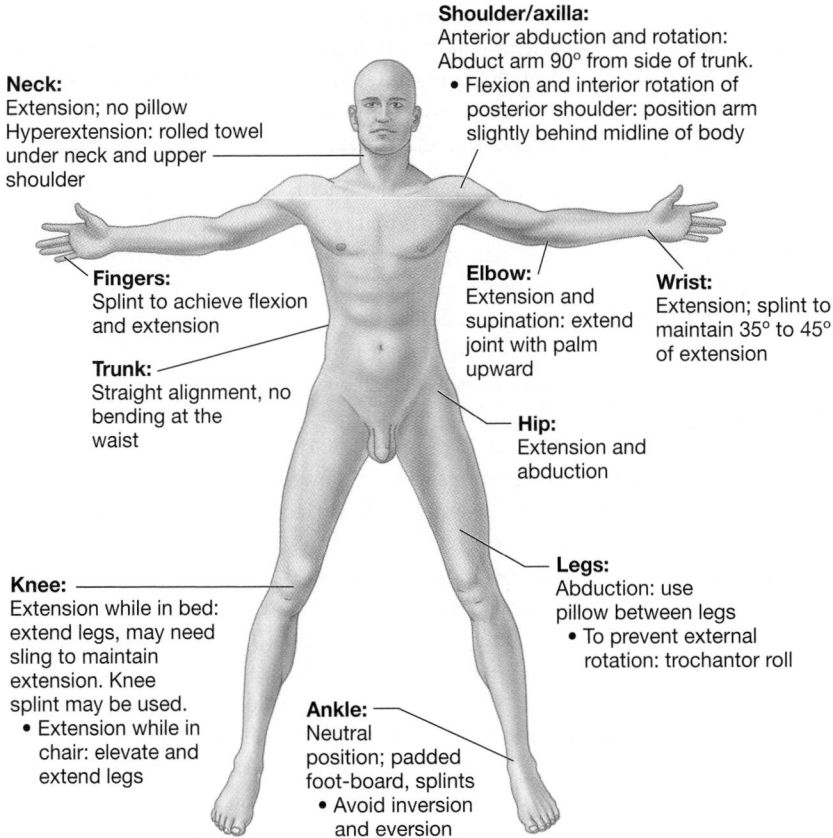

Neck:
Extension; no pillow
Hyperextension: rolled towel under neck and upper shoulder

Shoulder/axilla:
Anterior abduction and rotation:
Abduct arm 90° from side of trunk.
• Flexion and interior rotation of posterior shoulder: position arm slightly behind midline of body

Fingers:
Splint to achieve flexion and extension

Elbow:
Extension and supination: extend joint with palm upward

Wrist:
Extension; splint to maintain 35° to 45° of extension

Trunk:
Straight alignment, no bending at the waist

Hip:
Extension and abduction

Knee:
Extension while in bed: extend legs, may need sling to maintain extension. Knee splint may be used.
• Extension while in chair: elevate and extend legs

Legs:
Abduction: use pillow between legs
• To prevent external rotation: trochantor roll

Ankle:
Neutral position; padded foot-board, splints
• Avoid inversion and eversion

FIGURE 68–19 ■ Common anticontracture positions.

evaluation and testing are needed to improve efficacy and bring down the cost of the products.

Promoting and Maintaining Normal Mobility

As wound healing progresses, the need for promoting and maintaining mobility increases and changes. The goal of therapy is to regain strength, endurance, and joint mobility in order to achieve optimal functioning. Therapeutic positioning, splinting, and range-of-motion exercises are essential in meeting this goal and cannot be overemphasized. It is essential that the family be actively involved because the program needs to continue after discharge for at least a year.

Positioning

From the day of admission, therapeutic positioning is used to protect the patient's wounds, decrease edema, and counteract scar contraction. The anatomic sites where contracture formation is a risk must be identified in the early stages and anticontracture measures instituted to counter scar contraction. Involved extremities are placed in a functional position, and joints are typically placed in extension. Figure 68–19 ■ demonstrates the correct therapeutic anticontracture positions. Pillows, ropes, gauze rolls, linen, and pulleys are used to accomplish these positions. Finally, frequent position change is necessary to prevent skin pressure and breakdown. Beds with special mattresses and pressure-reducing capabilities are frequently used to prevent skin breakdown.

Splinting

Splinting begins as soon as possible after the injury for several reasons, including protection of joints and skin grafts, anatomic positioning to prevent contracture formation, and maintenance and

elongation of scar length. Ideally, splints should be made of a material that allows them to be reshaped as edema decreases and the burn scar changes and heals (Figure 68–20 ■). If the patient experiences pain, sensory impairments, or wound breakdown, the splint is removed and redesigned to prevent these complications. Padding of the splints decreases the occurrence of skin breakdown. Simple everyday items such as high-top shoes can be used for splinting purposes, and serial casting (e.g., removed and replaced as contour extremity changes) also can serve to maintain normal positioning of affected areas.

Exercise Program

An active, progressive exercise program is essential to prevent permanent burn scars from forming contractures and to maintain normal range of motion (ROM) in affected joints. Exercise increases circulation and pulmonary function, decreases edema formation, offsets some of the manifestations of immobilization, and allows for the preservation of functional motor skills. The exercise program begins on the day of admission and continues until the scars have matured. Exercise is very difficult in the beginning due to pain, edema, and loss of tissue elasticity. The health care team must assist the patient in understanding the importance of exercise despite painful limitations imposed by the injury.

Varying levels of physical assistance are required depending on the extent of the injury and the motivation of the patient. If, for example, weakness prevents true ROM, assistance is provided to help the patient complete the motion. This is referred to as active–assistive exercise and is frequently used with patients that are burn injured. The active component provides the same benefits as active ROM exercises, and the assistive component facilitates complete, properly directed motion. Passive ROM exercises are used for patients who are unable to move on their own. They also may be used to assess motion, maintain and mobilize joints and soft tissue, and minimize contracture formation.

The patient's ability to ambulate is affected by strength, endurance, pain, edema, and contracture formation. A progressive ambulation program is essential to prevent contracture formation

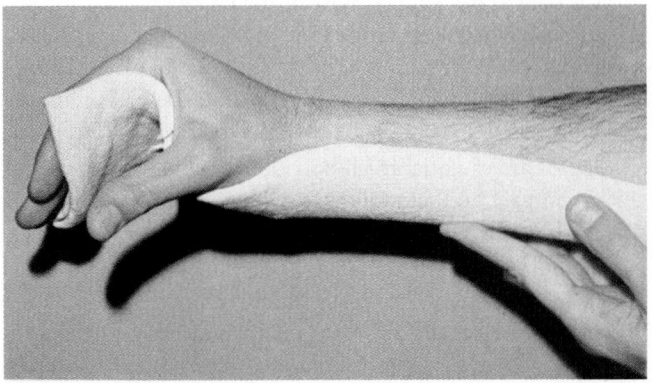

FIGURE 68–20 ■ Arm splint.
Source: Courtesy of: Robert M. Faggella, Jr. M.D., FACS Sacramento, CA

and needs to begin as soon as the patient is able to tolerate it. Initially the program begins with sitting, followed by standing and pivoting, and gradually ambulating. Prior to getting the patient out of bed, some type of elastic dressing or pressure garment is applied to prevent orthostatic hypotension, venous stasis, and edema formation.

Nutritional Requirements

Nutrients are essential for normal healing, and inadequate nutrition has a negative impact on the immune response, wound healing, metabolic function, and survival. The key cause of ineffective wound healing is malnutrition (Greenhalgh, 2005). At the time of the burn injury, patients experience extreme metabolic stress that is proportional to the size of the injury. After a burn injury, the resting energy expenditure (REE) increases by as much as 50% to 150% higher than that of the average trauma patient (Demling et al., 2004). This hypermetabolic response and the mobilization of glucose are necessary for wound healing. Without adequate glucose, excessive protein catabolism occurs (Demling et al., 2004; Pereira et al., 2005). Thus, early and adequate nutritional interventions are critical to the survival of the patient with burns. The hypermetabolic state tends to decrease in the weeks following the injury, but the metabolic rate does not return to normal until the wound is completely healed.

The goal of a nutritional replacement program during the acute phase is to provide adequate calories to promote wound healing (Greenhalgh, 2005). A number of formulas are used to estimate amount of calories needed to accomplish this goal. One generally accepted formula is (25 kilocalories X kilograms of body weight) + (40 kilocalories × % TBSA burn). It is not unusual for caloric needs to exceed 5,000 calories per day. The goal is to have the patient not lose more than 10% of his preburn weight. Calorie requirements need to be recalculated frequently because nutritional needs change with the healing process and changes in the hypermetabolic state. Specific nutrients needed for tissue repair include proteins, carbohydrates, lipids, and vitamins and trace minerals.

1. Proteins are needed for collagen synthesis, for wound remodeling, and for normal immune response. Protein loss, the stress of the injury, and tissue destruction all contribute negative nitrogen. There are differing opinions on the exact amount of protein needed to prevent proteolysis of lean body mass. The formulas used to calculate protein replacement generally estimate up to 2 grams of protein per kilogram per day (Greenhalgh, 2005).

2. Carbohydrates supply most of the energy needed for cell function and the immune response. Most practitioners believe that nonprotein energy intake should be primarily carbohydrates, with exogenous insulin added as clinically indicated to prevent hyperglycemia (Hart et al., 2001).

3. Lipids are essential in all nutritional regimens, but due to the impact on the immune system, many burn centers use no lipids at all (Borde, Bernier, & Garrel, 2002).

4. Vitamins and trace minerals are an integral part of the immune response, protein synthesis, and cell repair. They stimulate epithelialization, capillary budding and strength, and collagen formation, and are cofactors in enzymatic reactions (Greenhalgh, 2005). The exact vitamin and mineral requirements for optimal healing differ between patients,

although there are general guidelines for replacement. Patients with major burn injuries typically receive a multivitamin, 10,000 units of vitamin A, and 200 milligrams of zinc once per day, and 500 milligrams of ascorbic acid twice per day, depending on the health care provider's preference.

Whenever possible, patients with burns are encouraged to use the oral route for nutritional replacement. It is not uncommon, however, for patients to have difficulty consuming sufficient calories and protein by mouth. When this occurs it is essential to meet the metabolic demand with additional supplements. Meals are supplemented with high-calorie (1 to 1.5 calorie/mL) snacks. The enteral route is preferred because it maintains the structural and functional integrity of the gastrointestinal tract (Andel, Kamolz, Horauf, & Zimpfer, 2003). Many burn centers institute early enteral feedings within 24 hours of admission for any burn greater than 40% total body surface area. Early feeding is believed to improve the gastrointestinal, immunologic, nutritional, and metabolic responses to the burn injury. Enteral feedings instituted before 18 hours after the injury have shown a significantly decreased mortality rate (Gottschlich et al., 2002). Typically the enteral feedings are trickled very slowly via a feeding tube, and patients are monitored closely for aspiration.

Regular monitoring of laboratory values related to adequacy of intake is essential. Total protein levels, complete blood count (CBC), glucose, iron, and prealbumin all indicate adequacy of nutrition. There is a complete discussion of nutritional replacement and monitoring provided in Chapter 14 ⊙ .

■ Nursing Management

The aim of nursing care during the acute phase is to ensure optimal healing and prevent complications. Use of the nursing process will facilitate a comprehensive approach to patient assessment and care. The Nursing Process: Patient Care Plan feature applies the pertinent nursing diagnoses and provides a comprehensive care plan for a patient with burns during the acute period.

■ Collaborative Management

A collaborative care approach is optimal for management of patients with burn injuries. Utilizing a multidisciplinary team approach that includes health care providers, nurses, physical and occupational therapists, psychologists/psychiatrists, and a pharmacist will facilitate the best possible quality of life for the patient and the family. The occupational therapist helps facilitate realistic occupational goals, while the physical therapist assists in the rehabilitation of affected areas to prevent contracture formation. In addition to the nursing care described earlier (p. 2251) and in the Nursing Process: Patient Care Plan for the Acute Phase feature, the nurse plays a pivotal role in coordinating the efforts of the health care team.

Rehabilitative Phase

The rehabilitative phase typically begins when there is less than 20% open wound and the patient is functioning at the highest possible level since admission. Depending on the size of the injury, the rehabilitative phase may begin as early as 2 weeks or as

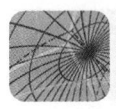

Assessment of Fatigue and Ability to Perform Activities

Subjective Data:
Do you feel fatigued after physical activities?
Do you feel like you are gaining or losing strength as your burns heal?

Objective Data:
Heart rate, blood pressure, and respiratory rate increase with activity.
Strength and endurance change as burn wounds heal.
Ability to perform activities of daily living.

Nursing Assessment and Diagnoses	Outcomes and Evaluation Parameters	Planning and Interventions with *Rationales*
Nursing Diagnosis: *Activity Intolerance* related to severity of injury	**Outcomes:** Increased endurance and energy conservation. ***Evaluation Parameters:*** Patient reports improvement in fatigue levels. Patient demonstrates more daytime wakefulness. Patient demonstrates ability to pace activities to conserve energy. Tolerates usual activities. Recognizes energy limitations. Balances activity with rest. Endurance level adequate for activity.	**Interventions and *Rationales:*** Discuss with patient/family the relationship of burn injury to fatigue. *As wounds heal and nutritional state stabilizes, energy will increase.* Assess emotional, spiritual, and physical responses to activity. *To institute changes to plan if necessary.* Evaluate patient's motivation and desire to increase activity. *To institute changes to plan if necessary.* Determine causes of fatigue. *To modify plan if necessary.* Monitor cardiorespiratory response to activity. *To assess appropriateness of activity level.* Monitor oxygen saturation response to activity. *To assess appropriateness of activity level.* Pace daily activities to conserve energy. *Prevent overexertion.* Ensure adequate nutritional support. *To increase strength and endurance.* Ensure sleep and rest period, record hours of sleep on record. *To increase strength and endurance.* Consult with physical therapist and occupational therapist to develop exercise program. *A progressive program to sustain progress.* Establish a conditioning program with patient-centered goals. *To increase compliance.*

Assessment of Mobility

Subjective Data:
How far are you able to ambulate?
Do you feel any change in the range of motion in the affected areas with exercise?
What is your understanding of the need for and importance of daily exercise?

Objective Data:
Range of motion in affected areas
Ability to perform active exercises
Wound healing progress
Patient/family's knowledge of need for continued exercise and splinting of affected areas

Nursing Assessment and Diagnoses	Outcomes and Evaluation Parameters	Planning and Interventions with *Rationales*
Nursing Diagnosis: *Impaired Physical Mobility* related to burn wounds and contracture formation	**Outcome:** Joint movement normal for injury level. ***Evaluation Parameters:*** Patient verbalizes understanding of restricted activity. Patient maintains strength and position of function in all affected areas. No contracture formation.	**Interventions and *Rationales:*** Consult with physical therapist and occupational therapist to formulate a plan for maintaining and increasing mobility. *A progressive program is necessary to sustain progress and prevent contracture formation.* Perform active and passive range-of-motion (ROM) exercises every 2 hours. *To prevent contracture formation.* Apply splints as prescribed. Maintain antideformity positions and reposition hourly (Figure 68–19 ■, p. 2265). *To prevent contracture formation.* Elevate affected extremities. *To decrease edema.* Maintain limbs in functional alignment. *To prevent contracture formation.* Anticipate need for analgesia. *To increase mobility.* Ambulate when stable. *Essential to begin activity program to increase endurance and decrease contracture formation.* Assess for loss of ROM and muscle atrophy related to immobility. *High risk for contracture formation.* Educate patient/family regarding rationale for imposed activity restrictions; i.e., recent skin grafting. *To prevent loss of skin graft.* Provide diversional activities to increase compliance with immobility. *To prevent loss of skin graft.*

(continued)

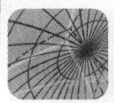

Assessment of Ability to Perform Activities of Daily Living

Subjective Data:
To what extent are you able to take care of your physical needs?
Is this ability increasing as your wounds heal?
Do you have people that can help you after you are discharged?

Objective Data:
Ability to perform activities of daily living
Psychological motivation to function independently

Nursing Assessment and Diagnoses	Outcomes and Evaluation Parameters	Planning and Interventions with *Rationales*
Nursing Diagnosis: *Readiness for Enhanced Self-Care* related to wounds and activity intolerance	**Outcome:** Increasing ability to perform activities of daily living. **Evaluation Parameters:** Verbalizes increased sense of control. Demonstrates self-care activities within limits of functional ability. Accepts assistance when needed. Progressively increases mobility.	**Interventions and *Rationales:*** Consult with occupational therapist regarding need for assistive devices. *These will increase self-care ability.* Ensure patient has adequate time to perform tasks at own pace. *Patients are slow and tentative in the beginning.* Increase self-care activities as soon as possible. Ensure patient participation in planning care. *To decrease powerlessness and increase self-confidence.* Monitor for changes in functional abilities. *To monitor progress.* Instruct patient/family on alternative ways to perform activities of daily living. *To increase patient/family involvement.*

Assessment of Patient and Family Coping Skills

Subjective Data:
What skills have you used in the past to cope with stressful situations?
What people in your life do you use for emotional support?
Tell me your perception of your injuries.
Tell me your perception of your limitations.

Objective Data:
Willingness to be compliant with therapy.
Determine patient's level of independence.
Assess effectiveness of support systems.

Nursing Assessment and Diagnoses	Outcomes and Evaluation Parameters	Planning and Interventions with *Rationales*
Nursing Diagnoses: *Readiness for Enhanced Individual Coping* related to situational crisis, inadequate support systems, and unrealistic perceptions of recovery	**Outcome:** Effective coping. **Evaluation Parameters:** Patient/family: Verbalize feelings. Identify and utilize effective coping strategies, appropriate for injury status. Identify ineffective coping strategies and patterns. Seek information about injury, treatment, and prognosis. Employ behaviors to reduce stress. Report decrease in negative feelings. Demonstrate impulse control. Demonstrate normal information processing. Recognize support systems. Employ behaviors to reduce stress. Report decrease in negative feelings.	**Interventions and *Rationales:*** Assess and determine degree of impairment. *To assist in the development of a plan to promote coping.* Determine past coping skills. *To assist in the development of a plan to promote coping.* Assess current coping skills. *To assist in the development of a plan to promote coping.* Explore with patient feelings about injury, and explore previous methods of dealing with life problems. *Assessment will assist in augmenting patient's ability to cope, or it will determine need for intervention.* Identify patient's view of injury and its congruence to view of health care team. *To assess patient's perception of reality.* Monitor aggressive behaviors. *A sign of ineffective coping and that intervention is needed.* Identify patient/family's view of condition and how it relates to actual condition. *Assessment of how realistic their perceptions are. Determines where intervention is needed.* Assess patient/family's support systems. *May be used as a source of support.* Evaluate impact on patient/family's life situation. *Loss of previous life function impacts coping.* Determine risk for self-harm. *Severe alterations in body image and functional level place the patient at a high risk for self-harm.* Provide factual information about diagnosis, treatments, and prognosis. *Realistic, factual information is essential to augment adjustment.* Encourage verbalization of fears and let patient know these reactions are normal. *To enhance open, factual communication.* Explain procedures. *To increase knowledge and decrease fear of unknown.* Assist patient in dealing with changes in body image, and appraise adjustment. *To enhance adjustment.* Discuss future treatment options for changes in body image. *To increase knowledge and decrease fear of unknown.* Encourage family and friends to participate in care. *Enhances adjustment of significant others.* Consult psychologist if necessary. *To enhance adjustment.*

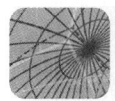

NURSING PROCESS: Patient Care Plan for the Acute Period—*Continued*

Nursing Assessment and Diagnoses	Outcomes and Evaluation Parameters	Planning and Interventions with *Rationales*
Deficient Fluid Volume due to evaporative loss	See the earlier Nursing Process: Patient Care Plan for the emergency period of care for the information pertinent to each of the nursing diagnoses in the left column (p. 2251).	
Impaired Skin Integrity related to burn wounds		
Risk for Infection related to loss of skin integrity and impaired nonspecific and specific immunity		
Ineffective Thermoregulation related to loss of skin integrity		
Acute Pain related to burn injury and exposed nerve endings		
Imbalanced Nutrition: Less than Body Requirements related to hypermetabolic demands of burn injury		
Fear and *Anxiety* related to changes in health status/role functioning; situational crisis		
Deficient Knowledge related to burn wound care and treatment, disfigurement, and functional loss		
Disturbed Body Image related to scar formation and functional loss		
Risk for Complicated Grieving related to body image change, risk of family role change, and possible occupational change		

Source: Wilkinson, J. M. (2009). *Nursing diagnosis handbook; with interventions and outcomes* (8th ed.). Upper Saddle River, NJ: Prentice Hall.

long as several years after the burn injury. During the rehabilitative phase, the patient with burns has stabilized physically and frequently is more aware of the long-term ramifications of her injury. Emphasis is placed on physical and psychological restorative therapy. Treatment aims include physical therapy to increase strength, endurance, function, and ROM; ongoing functional and cosmetic reconstruction; and psychological preparation for the patient's return to society. Pain management and nutrition are still concerns during the rehabilitative phase. Discharge planning and occupational preparation also are addressed during the rehabilitative phase.

Scar and Contracture Formation

With newly healed skin of partial-thickness wounds, there is minimal scar formation because the epidermis does not thicken. Frequently patients complain of dryness and itching in the newly healed areas, which are treated with frequent application of lotions and in more severe cases oral medication such as diphenhydramine hydrochloride (Benadryl). With a full-thickness injury, the dermal layer of skin has been affected, and the skin is repaired through scar formation. During the healing process, hypertrophic scars and contractures can form. **Hypertrophic scar** (Figure 68–21 ■) formation is defined as an overgrowth of dermal tissue that remains within the boundaries of the wound. There is a higher risk of hypertrophic scar formation in areas of stress and movement such as the hands, chest, and legs. If the hypertrophic scar extends beyond the wound

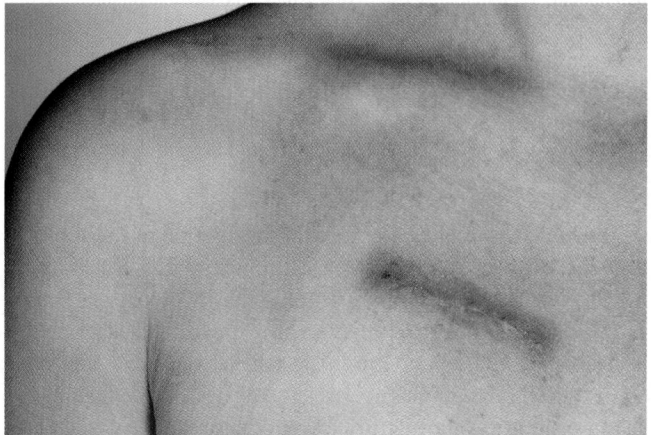

FIGURE 68–21 ■ Hypertrophic scar.
Source: Bart's Medical Library/Phototake NYC

edges, it is referred to as a **keloid scar** (Figure 68–22 ■, p. 2270). Certain areas of the body that are more prone to keloid formation include the chest, the presternal area, and the shoulders and deltoid region. Once keloid scars have formed, there is limited treatment available. Current treatments that have experienced some success are injecting steroids into the scar and laser therapy. There is a genetic predisposition for the development of keloid scarring, which is discussed in the Genetic Considerations box (p. 2270).

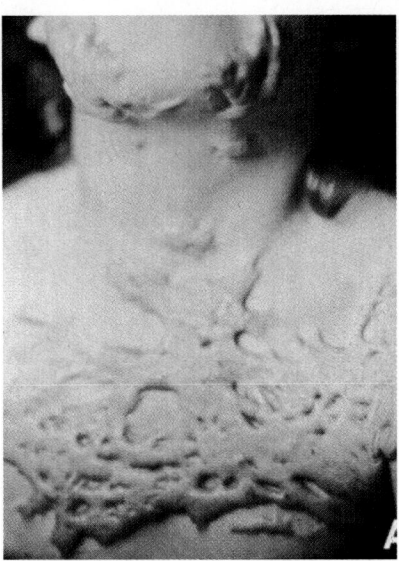

FIGURE 68–22 ■ Keloid scar.
Source: Courtesy of: Robert M. Faggella, Jr. M.D., FACS Sacramento, CA

GENETIC CONSIDERATIONS for Keloid Scar Formation

There is a genetic predisposition for the development of keloid scar formation in the African American race. African Americans have approximately a 15 times greater incidence of keloid formation.

Source: Tuan, T., et al. (2003). Increased plasminogen activator inhibitor-1 in keloid fibroblasts may account for their elevated collagen accumulation in fibrin gel cultures. *American Journal of Pathology, 162*(5), 1579–1589.

During the healing process of full-thickness injuries, the burn scar shrinks and becomes inelastic, resulting in contracture of the wound. A contracture (Figure 68–23 ■) is defined as a permanent shortening of connective tissue. Once formed, contractures resist stretching, limiting body motion and flexibility. Splinting, exercise, and constant pressure help prevent the formation and progression of contractures.

Exercise Program

As the burn wound heals, continual contraction of the scar creates the majority of the chronic problems. This contraction process causes a decrease in function in the involved area. Beginning rehabilitation on admission to a treatment center helps prevent contractures and diminishes the need for reconstructive surgery. Several therapies are used by the health care team to assist in preventing contracture formation, described earlier. The exercise program includes promotion of functional skills, stretching exercises, and scar massage.

Functional Skills

Functional skills are defined as the specific motor abilities necessary to perform activities of daily living (ADL) in order to function independently. In the beginning, exercises should focus on basic activities including ambulating, hygiene, and self-feeding. During the rehabilitative phase, exercise programs need to be expanded to include the specific skills needed for functioning in the home and the job environment.

All exercise programs are progressive in order to increase the patient's strength and endurance. Protein catabolism associated

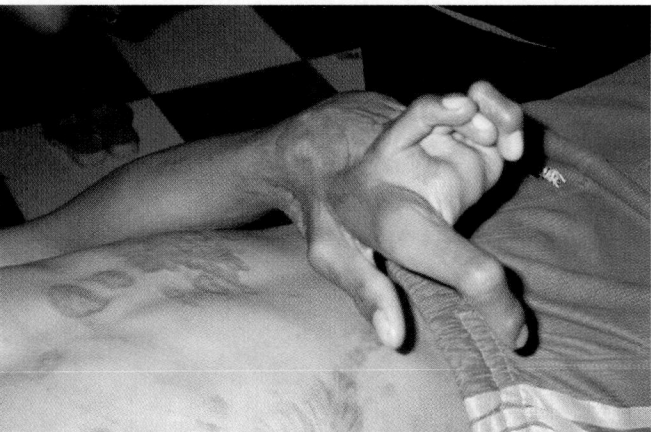

FIGURE 68–23 ■ Contracture formation.
Source: Courtesy of Kathleen Osborn

with the burn injuries as well as days of immobility lead to a decrease in muscle mass and strength. It is important to remember that endurance and conditioning underlie the success of any exercise program. Exercise programs need to be at regular intervals throughout the day and followed by periods of rest. It is the repetitive nature of the programs that builds strength and endurance and prevents contracture formation. Range-of-motion exercises are omitted for 3 to 7 days after skin grafting.

Stretching Exercises

Stretching exercises are used to elongate shortened soft tissue. The fundamental goal of a stretching program is to increase ROM. Stretching can be a passive or an active activity, although patients must learn to perform self-stretching exercises as they prepare for discharge. Stretching is done primarily after wound closure during the rehabilitative phase. The stretch should be gentle, slow, and sustained. Blanching of the scar represents appropriate stretch. Immediately after a stretching session, positioning and splinting are used effectively to maintain the elongation of the tissue.

Scar Massage

Completely healed burn wounds are massaged with oil or lotion to break down hardened areas, increase circulation, decrease hypertrophy, possibly increase range of motion, and improve appearance. Massage is performed one to four times daily. Patients and families are taught to continue scar massage after discharge.

Pressure Dressing and Garments

The use of pressure dressings and garments to decrease hypertrophic scar formation and increase wound pliability is a widely accepted practice (Figure 68–24 ■) (O'Brien, Weinstock-Zlotnick, Sanchez, Gorga, & Yurt, 2005). It is believed that the pressure from the garments causes ischemia, thereby decreasing collagen production, which thickens scars. In general, wounds that require more than 14 days to heal will scar and therefore should be placed in pressure garments. Elastic bandages are used initially for wound compression and edema formation. During the rehabilitative phase before hypertrophy begins, patients are measured for custom-fit elastic garments that provide three-dimensional pressure on all affected areas (Burn Survivors Throughout the World, 2006). In order to be effective, the pressure exerted by the garment must exceed capillary pressure (25 mmHg). Pressure garments are worn continuously (23 hours per day) for several months and/or years, depending on the hy-

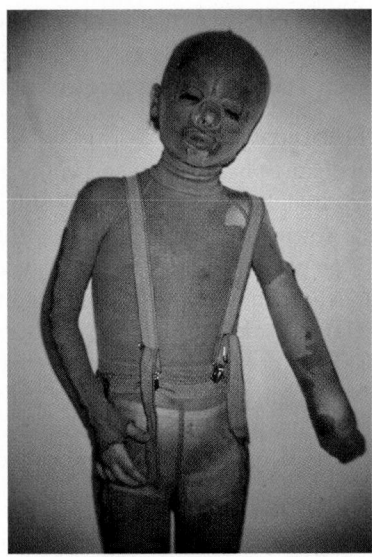

FIGURE 68–24 ■ Compression garment.
Source: Courtesy of: John M. Osborn, M.D., FACS, Sacramento, CA Plastic Surgery Center

pertrophic scarring. Even though the garments reduce scar formation, patient compliance—especially in the hot weather—has long been an issue. Patient teaching needs to stress the benefits of the garments in an effort to increase compliance. Periodic refitting is necessary to ensure proper fit and pressure.

Functional and Cosmetic Reconstruction

Once burn scars have healed, certain surgical options are available to improve function and cosmetic appearance. Typically, reconstruction begins after the scar has matured, which takes about a year. However, surgery may be indicated earlier if there is a serious functional impairment. Surgical intervention includes both scar excision and/or scar realignment. Small hypertrophic scars can be completely excised in one surgery. Larger hypertrophic areas need serial surgeries to remove the scar segmentally, one portion at a time.

Scar realignment is a technique used when the scar develops in a different direction than the normal tissue. Abnormal scar alignment causes excessive wound contracture and decreased ROM in the area. Scars can be surgically reoriented to increase ROM and decrease the visibility of the scar. A Z-plasty is a common method utilized for scar realignment (Figure 68–25 ■).

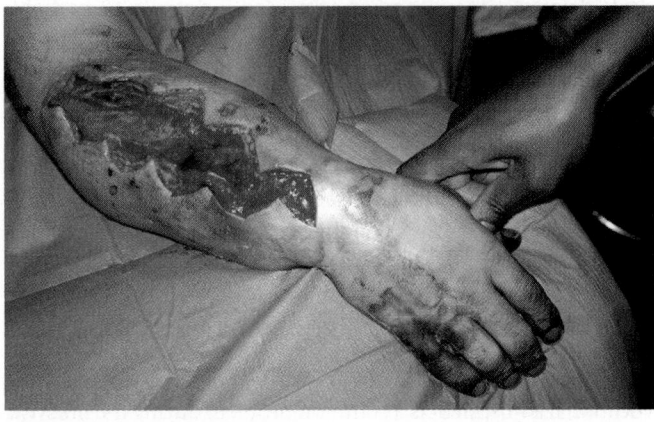

FIGURE 68–25 ■ Z-plasty.
Source: Courtesy of: John M. Osborn, M.D., FACS, Sacramento, CA Plastic Surgery Center

Psychological Recovery

Burn injuries that cause scarring, regardless of size, alter patients' perceptions of body image. The preinjury coping mechanisms have a major impact on how a patient copes following a burn injury. Some of the most common preinjury disorders found in people that are burn injured include depression, antisocial behavior, personality disorder, organic brain syndrome, and alcohol and drug abuse. Patients with preexisting psychiatric issues are at a higher risk for self-inflicted burns either as attempted suicide or self-mutilation (Erzurum & Varcellotti, 1999; Mabrouk, Mahmod, Massoud, Magdy, & Sayed, 1999). Research supports that there is a higher incidence of psychological maladjustment among people who sustain burn trauma than in people who sustain other types of trauma (Fauerbach, Lawrence, Munster, Palombo, & Richter, 1999).

During the healing process, a number of psychological reactions occur. In the beginning stages of treatment during the emergency period, patients often use withdrawal and denial as coping mechanisms. These patients tend to keep their eyes closed, remain immobile, and have little interaction with family and staff. Regression also is a common reaction in the patient that is burn injured, manifested by child-like behaviors such as dependence and temper tantrums. Other psychological reactions during the healing process include anger, hostility, depression, and anxiety. These reactions are manifested in a number of ways including restlessness, agitation, sleep disturbances, hostility toward staff and family, and self-degradation. Recently, post-traumatic stress disorder is being diagnosed with increasing frequency in patients with burns after discharge from the acute care setting (Van Loey & Van Son, 2003; Yu & Dimsdale, 1999). The Ethical Issues box (p. 2272) discusses some of the dilemmas that burn victims and their families, as well as the health care team grapple with while recovering from the burn injuries.

Grief is a natural and frequent reaction to burn injuries. Besides the change in body image, other contributing factors to the grief reaction include loss of physical functioning, potential changes in vocation, and separation from home and family. The patient that is burn injured must be given an opportunity to express concerns and feelings about the body image change and be reassured that this grieving process is normal and will eventually dissipate. The nurse's role is to be an active, nonjudgmental listener, allowing the patient time to express feelings and grieve the loss of former self. The nurse must answer questions honestly, acknowledge the patient's difficulty with coping, and encourage positive behaviors. Patients typically cope better if they are kept informed of planned treatments and surgeries. It is anxiety producing to be faced with unexpected events, especially when the patient has had to give up most of his independence. As wounds heal, the patient must resume control of as many activities and functions as is possible.

Measures to assist the patient in coping with grief and loss include resuming activities of daily living and socializing with family and friends. These activities enhance self-efficacy and worth, and give the patient more control. Additionally, a combination of psychotherapy and pharmacologic treatments often are effective in promoting adjustment. Burn support groups have also been effective in promoting adjustment to the disfigurement and reentrance into society.

ETHICAL ISSUES In the Treatment of Burn Injuries

There are a multitude of ethical issues related to the resuscitation, care, and rehabilitation of burn victims and their families. A comprehensive team approach is needed to achieve the most effective outcome. Initially burn injuries may be life threatening. Therefore, decisions must be made about the extent of resuscitation, especially with a massive injury; when to withhold or withdraw care; quality of life, both immediate and long term; and achieving a dignified and comfortable death in the case of futility. These issues are evaluated by the team and presented to the patient and family for their decision. The nursing role is to advocate for the patient, be supportive of the decision, and provide the family with factual, realistic data about the patient's condition and medical interventions.

Ethical dilemmas may arise for the nurse when it is difficult to support the decision for personal and/or professional reasons. One example would be an elderly patient who has sustained an injury that is not survivable due to age and past medical history. The family has made the decision that it wants everything done for this patient. The nurse is aware that this decision is going to cause a great deal of suffering for this patient with little hope of survival. In this case the nurse is obliged to treat this patient with the hope of survival. The dilemma for the nurse may be the conflict between being a patient advocate, supporting the family's decision, and dealing with one's own personal belief system. This is typically a very difficult ethical dilemma for the health care team. Team conferences typically occur to discuss a team approach to care and a plan to provide consistency in the approach to patient care.

Specific ethical issues for patients that are burn injured and their families include:

- Quality of life after the injury, both immediate and long term
- Extent of resuscitation after a massive injury
- When to withhold or withdraw care
- Body image adjustment
- Dignified and comfortable death
- Psychological adjustment
- Considerations of futility
- Nonmaleficence
- Financial costs.

Sensitivity to the patient's spiritual beliefs also is an essential part of the psychological recovery. A person's faith often will help guide her in life especially when a crisis has occurred, such as burn injury. The health care team needs to evaluate the need for spiritual guidance and support with each individual patient and then follow through with providing a spiritual guidance counselor of the patient's choice (priest, minister, rabbi, etc.).

Pain Management

Pain is markedly decreased with closure of the wound. Small areas of open wound may still need dressing changes that are painful, and newly healed skin is sensitive. In addition, the exercise therapies are often painful due to stiff, noncompliant skin in the affected areas. Therefore, pain management is still an issue and needs to be evaluated individually and on an ongoing basis. Along with diversional activities and relaxation techniques, oral analgesics typically relieve the pain experienced in the rehabili-

tative phase. Patient report of the absence of symptoms and/or an assessment of lack of pain behaviors, such as guarding, is necessary to assess when tailoring pain management therapies.

Nutritional Requirements

During the rehabilitative phase, the negative nitrogen balance and anorexia have resolved. Because the wound is still healing, high-calorie and high-protein diets are necessary. A nutritionist can assist with a nutrition plan to ensure adequate daily caloric intake. Promotion of independent eating also is important. If it is functionally difficult for the patient to eat due to involvement of hands, occupational therapy is needed to obtain devices that will facilitate self-feeding. Finally, in preparation for discharge, the patient and family need instructions about meal planning and the reporting of difficulties such as cachexia, weight loss, and food intolerance.

Discharge Priorities

Discharge planning is a complex process that begins when the patient is admitted to the hospital. An organized comprehensive plan of care with both short-term and long-term goals will ensure the highest level of recovery. As healing progresses, the patient and family need to be prepared for discharge. The ultimate goal is to return the patient to as close as is reasonably possible to the preinjury state.

Discharge planning requires a team approach with each member contributing from his or her area of expertise. In order to institute a realistic plan and ensure compliance, the patient and family have to be active, participating members of the team. Teaching is essential in order to prepare the patient and family for self care. Nurses play a key role in the implementation of the teaching plan because they coordinate and evaluate patient needs on an ongoing basis.

Health Promotion

To augment understanding, an organized, comprehensive teaching plan is necessary. The Patient Teaching & Discharge Priorities box outlines the necessary components of the discharge teaching plan, which includes wound care, infection assessment, nutrition, pain management, sexuality issues, scar and contracture prevention, psychological adaptation, and vocational rehabilitation.

Major burn wounds take 12 to 18 months to heal completely. Discharge instructions include care of both the open and healed wounds. Normal manifestations of newly healed wounds include dryness, itching, and an increased sensitivity to sunlight. Specific instructions need to stress how to assess the wound for complications such as newly formed open areas, blister formation, and signs and symptoms of infection. The instructions also need to include when and why it is necessary to notify the health care provider of complications. Discharge teaching plays a major role in preventing excessive scar and contracture formation. Teaching regarding ongoing pain management, sexuality issues, and emotional adaptation are all critical to ensure an optimal recovery. Comprehensive instructions are outlined in the Patient Teaching & Discharge Priorities box.

Occupational Recovery

Vocational adjustment is a common problem during the first year after discharge from the hospital. Often the patient has an extended recovery time after hospitalization before he is physically

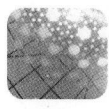

PATIENT TEACHING & DISCHARGE PRIORITIES for Burn Management

Need	Teaching
WOUND CARE	Perform daily cleansing and dressing changes for open areas.
	Elevate areas where edema formation occurs.
Patient/family/support system	Avoid scratching the healed areas, as this could cause breakdown: • Encourage liberal use of emollient lotions for dryness and flaking. • Use diphenhydramine hydrochloride (Benadryl) for pruritus (itching). • Keep fingernails short and use gloves when sleeping.
	Avoid sunlight, as it can cause, among other things, healed wounds to discolor or darken permanently: • Avoid overexposure to sun. • Use sunscreen products when exposed to sunlight. • Use clothing and hats for added protection.
	Avoid exposure to extreme temperatures and harsh chemicals.
	Wear loose-fitting, soft clothing.
Setting	Assess availability of, knowledge of, and compliance with treatment regimen.
	Assess respite needs and resources.
	Assess discharge placement needs: • Home • Rehabilitation facility • Extended care facility.
	Assess home environment for need for assistive devices.
	Assess for professional home health needs.
	Assess need for follow-up appointments.
WOUND INFECTION	Assess for infection of open wounds and healed wound breakdown with each dressing change, and report as necessary.
Patient/family/support system	Signs and symptoms include: • Odor and exudate • Fever • Increased drainage • Swelling • Lack of wound closure.
	Apply antibiotic ointments as prescribed.
	Teach minimization of risk factors for infection.
Setting	Explain signs and symptoms that require medical attention.
	Assess environment for risk factors.
NUTRITION	Maintain a high-calorie, high-protein diet.
Patient/family/support system	Continue taking vitamins and mineral supplements as ordered.
Setting	Observe for appetite and weight loss, and food intolerance.
	Taper calorie intake once preinjury or ideal weight has been achieved to prevent excessive weight gain.
	With professional guidance, institute an exercise program; i.e., physical therapist.
	Assess financial resources.
PAIN MANAGEMENT	Assess pain level and report any increase in pain.
Patient/family/support system	Assess effectiveness of pharmacologic interventions.
Setting	Wean patient off pain medication when pain lessens.
	Assess environment for safety and promotion of therapeutic needs.
SEXUALITY	Answer questions about sexual potential.
Patient/partner	Encourage both partners to express fears and concerns.
Setting	Encourage privacy and a familiar environment.

(continued)

PATIENT TEACHING & DISCHARGE PRIORITIES for Burn Management—*Continued*

Need	Teaching
SCAR FORMATION PREVENTION AND EXERCISE PROGRAM Patient/family/support system Setting	Stress and assess compliance with wearing of pressure garments 23 hours a day. • If pressure garment is too loose, it is ineffective; discontinue use and will need new garment. • If it is too tight, it can cause numbness, tingling, and skin breakdown; discontinue use and will need new garment. • Need two sets. Ace wraps need to be worn per health care provider's order, usually when out of bed. Progressive passive and active range-of-motion (ROM) exercises. Progressive stretching and ambulation. Progressive exercise program to increase overall stamina (walking). Referral to physical therapy for development of an exercise program.
EMOTIONAL ADJUSTMENT Patient/family/support system Setting	Answer questions honestly. Encourage verbalization of frustrations and anger. Encourage positive reinforcement from the family. Encourage independent functioning as soon as possible. Stress that it is not uncommon to feel a letdown after discharge. Encourage participation in a burn support group.
OCCUPATIONAL RECOVERY Patient/family/support system Setting	Referral to the local office of the state labor and industry board for vocational counseling. Referral to vocational interest, aptitude, and psychological testing to determine areas of interest. Provide realistic plan, patient and family education, and engage an employer in the process.

and emotionally ready to return to work. Additionally, due to disfigurement and functional limitations, the patient may be unable to resume his previous job/profession. Therefore, the patient may need a referral to the local office of the state labor and industry board for information on job retraining programs. For many patients, vocational interest, aptitude, and psychological testing may be necessary to determine areas of occupational interest. Successful reentry into the work environment depends on a realistic plan, patient and family education, and engaging an employer in the process.

◼ Nursing Management

The aim of nursing care during the rehabilitative phase is to prepare the patient both physically and psychologically to return home and to work. Use of the nursing process will provide a comprehensive approach to achieve these goals.

Nursing Diagnoses

A number of nursing diagnoses may be applicable in the rehabilitative phase. The most significant diagnoses for the patient that is burn injured include:

- *Acute Pain*
- *Impaired Skin Integrity*
- *Impaired Physical Mobility*
- *Activity Intolerance*
- *Deficient Knowledge related to injuries and limitations*
- *Disturbed Body Image*
- *Fear* and *Anxiety*

- *Readiness for Enhanced Self-Care*
- *Readiness for Enhanced Nutrition.*

These diagnoses depend on the degree of disfigurement and loss of functional capacity, as well as the home environment and support systems. The patient's personal coping skills and ability to adapt to the change in body image also impact applicable nursing diagnoses. Additional diagnoses related to the rehabilitative phase include:

- *Social Isolation* related to disfigurement and loss of function
- *Readiness for Enhanced Family Processes* related to risk of role change and loss of earning capacity
- *Readiness for Enhanced Individual Coping* related to ongoing maladjustment to burn injury
- *Risk for Complicated Grieving* related to ongoing realization of extent of injury
- *Noncompliance* related to wearing the elastic garments and continued need for physical therapy
- *Disturbed Sensory Perception* related to sensory overload/deprivation and sleep pattern disturbance
- *Impaired Home Maintenance* related to unavailable support system.

◼ Collaborative Management

In the rehabilitative phase, the need to collaborate with all of the health care specialties continues. As the patient is prepared for discharge, each aspect of the physical and psychological needs is evaluated, and a plan is put in place to address them all. As is consistent with the entire hospital stay, the nurses coordinate the health care team to ensure that all aspects of care are addressed. The length of time that physical therapy and occupational therapy continue on an outpatient basis depends of the size and area of injury. The psychosocial needs of returning to society, family, and hopefully occupation are addressed by psychologists/psychiatrists prior to discharge as well as on an ongoing basis after discharge. Because the hypermetabolic state continues until all the wounds are healed, the need for dietary consultation continues. Finally, the surgeons begin the reconstructive process that may continue for months or years, depending on the extent of the injury.

Complications of Burn Injuries

It is a generally believed that complications are a "rule" rather than an exception for patients that are burn injured. Burn injuries should never be viewed in isolation because of their profound effect on multiorgan systems. The most common complications that lead to increased mortality include wound infection, nosocomial pneumonia, sepsis, acute renal failure, gastrointestinal ulcers, and respiratory failure. Certain complications occur more frequently in a given period or phase of burn treatment. Chart 68–5 outlines the complications specific to each period of burn management.

Gerontological Considerations

The incidence of burn injuries is less in the adult population under age 60, but the mortality rates continue to be higher than in the younger population (U.S. Library of Medicine and the National Institutes of Health, 2006). One-third of all persons who die in home fires are adults older than age 65. There is a greater incidence of inhalation injury in the elder adults because of their inability to escape the fire. Elderly patients with burns suffer from greater morbidity and mortality than do younger patients with similar burn extents (Redlick et al., 2002). In addition, the elderly often delay seeking medical care for burn injuries, which predisposes them to complications such as cellulitis and infec-

tion. With the onset of early wound excision and grafting, the mortality rates have declined in the last three decades. It is a general belief that the elderly survivors of burn injuries have decreased functional recovery. In addition elderly people tend to have other conditions that impact their recovery. See Evidence-Based Practice box on page 2277.

Each period of burn recovery is prolonged in the elderly. This is due in part to diminished reserve capacity of organ systems. For example, wound healing is delayed because of diminished host resistance and impaired cell-mediated and humoral immunity. Therefore, older adults have a decreased ability to fight infections and are more prone to sepsis. Once wounds are healed, there is a decreased tensile strength; thus, they break down and reopen easily.

Special nursing care considerations for the elderly include a careful assessment of the cardiovascular and pulmonary systems during early fluid resuscitation. This population is more prone to the development of pulmonary edema and heart failure. Monitoring of heart rate, blood pressure, and breath sounds on a frequent and ongoing basis is critical during rapid fluid administration to detect early signs and symptoms of heart failure. Mobilizing the patient as early as possible to maintain pulmonary function and promote independence also is an important aspect of care. Strict asepsis is critical because of the diminished immune response and increased susceptibility to infection. Finally, consistent attention to the nutritional intake of an elderly person is essential in that it impacts wound healing and survival.

Research

Research is essential to improve the care, quality of life, and survival of patients with burn injuries. The goal of research is to identify areas where practice could improve and evaluate and test methods for these improvements. The research topics related to burn injuries are included in the Research Opportunities and Clinical Impact box (p. 2276). The list provides both medical and nursing research topics still under investigation. Electronic databases are a source for finding specific studies related to these topics.

CHART 68–5	**Complications of Burn Injuries**	
Emergency Phase	**Acute Phase**	**Rehabilitative Phase**
Immunosuppression: both humoral and cell mediated.	Wound infection.	Scarring and contracture formation.
Sepsis: highest incidence in burns greater than 40%.	Psychological problems; grieving process; patients fear both death and survival.	Psychological problems.
Bacterial translocation from the gut.		Loss of function and deformities.
Pneumonia and acute respiratory distress syndrome (ARDS), especially if an inhalation injury has occurred.		Normal grieving process switches to a focus on what are realistic future goals in terms of function and interpersonal issues.
Renal and heart failure from shock.		
Stress ulcers: rare due to medications and early tube feedings.		
Psychological problems.		
Normal grieving begins: denial.		

RESEARCH OPPORTUNITIES AND CLINICAL IMPACT RELATED TO BURN INJURY MANAGEMENT

Research Area	Clinical Impact
Physiological Research	Mediating the shock state and potentially decreasing the mortality rate.
Drugs to reverse the release of natural dilators to prevent the shunting of blood from the vascular system.	
Fluid resuscitation techniques: high-concentration salt mixtures and high molecular weight salt mixtures instead of balanced salt mixtures for larger burn injury resuscitation.	
Hyperdynamic resuscitation and role of serum lactate in severely burned patients.	
Complex multiorgan response to burn injuries.	
High-frequency percussive ventilation for the treatment of inhalation injuries.	Prevent respiratory failure.
Direct instillation of combined aerosolized medications and hormones into the lungs of inhalation injury patients to decrease airway damage.	
Selective decontamination of the gastrointestinal (GI) tract to decrease wound infections and pneumonia.	Prevent systemic infection.
Early feeding of patients with burns to prevent translocation of bacteria to the bloodstream, causing sepsis.	
Use of glutamine supplements and the hypermetabolic response.	Augment wound healing.
Pain Management	Patient comfort and increased wound healing.
The nature of pain induced by direct tissue injury.	
Nursing pain management.	
Brief cognitive interventions for burn pain.	
Rapid induction analgesia for the alleviation of procedural pain during burn care.	
Relationship of itch to pain.	
Factors predicting hypnotic analgesia in patients with clinical burns.	
Pain and anxiety measurement and management during procedures.	
Emotional and Psychological Research	Assess factors that influence compliance and acceptance of burn injury and permanent scarring.
Predictors of post-traumatic stress syndrome and distress following acute burn injuries.	
Anxiety: current practices in assessment and treatment of anxiety in patients with burns.	Impact on vocation.
Chronic sorrow.	
Self-blame, compliance, and distress among patients with burns.	Impact on long-term adjustments to changes in body image.
Return to vocational stability.	
Massage therapy to reduce anxiety and cortisol levels.	Improve psychological interventions to augment coping.
Music influencing postprocedural recall.	
Factors that enhance positive long-term psychological adaptation.	
Family characteristics that augment psychological adaptation.	
Sexuality after burn injury.	
Burn Wound Research	Improve techniques to increase wound healing and prevent scarring.
The nature of fabric flammability and its effect on human skin.	
Living skin grafts (cultured autografts) used with Integra, for permanent burn wound closure.	
Treatment of pruritus and burn wounds.	
Hypnosis and burn wound healing.	
Massage therapy and itching.	
Comparative study of burn wound cellulitis treatments.	
Use of Integra artificial skin in preventing skin contractures to joints of burn wounds.	
Burn size estimation using direct template drawings.	
Use of music during wound débridement.	
Direct measurement of cutaneous pressures generated by pressure garments.	
Techniques to increase tensile strength and reduce wound breakdown.	
Regulation and secretion of human growth factors used to modulate the hypermetabolic response to burn, and augment wound and donor-site healing.	

Diabetes and Burns

Clinical Problem

Treating patients with diabetes for any other disease or disorder is associated with an increased risk for complications. For example, peripheral neurological impairments associated with diabetes result in a decrease in protective sensation and tissue vascularity. The lack of vascularity results in slowing the rate of wound closure, thereby increasing the risk for infection. Nurses need to understand and apply evidence-based findings when caring for patients with diabetes that are burn injured in order to prevent infection and promote wound healing.

Research Findings

Kowal-Vern & Latenser (2004) conducted a research study to determine the demographic characteristics of patients with diabetes that sustain burns and their rate of community-acquired and nosocomial infections. A 46-month retrospective chart and patient registry review was completed comparing patients with diabetes that have sustained burn injuries with patients without diabetes that have had such injuries. The infection rate, patient's age, mechanism of injury, time of year injuries occurred, time from injury to treatment, and complications were all evaluated. Adult patients with diabetes had a significant increase in community-acquired burn wound cellulitis and sepsis as compared to the population that was nondiabetic. The most common organisms in diabetic burn infections were *Streptococcus, Proteus, Pseudomonas, Candida* species, and methicillin-resistant *Staphylococcus aureus* (MRSA). Only 38% of the patients with burns presented for treatment promptly. Based on the study's findings, the researchers concluded that peripheral neuropathy may have precipitated the injury and delayed medical treatment in lower extremity burns of patients with diabetes. The researchers also concluded that there was an increased risk of nosocomial infections, which prolong hospitalization.

Implications for Nursing Practice

This study clearly indicates a need for nurses to educate patients with diabetes about the potential for burn injuries, the need for immediate medical treatment, and the possible complications of burn injuries. Additionally, nurses need to understand that when caring for patients with burns there is a significantly increased risk for wound infection and sepsis. Ongoing nursing assessment of the burn wound for infection needs to be rigorous with the understanding of the risk for patients that have diabetes. The nurse needs to understand the importance of reporting the first signs of infection so that treatment can be instituted as soon as possible.

Critical Thinking Questions

1. In order of priority, what are the most important points that would be included in an education plan for patients with diabetes and their families?

2. Compile a list of high-risk environmental and patient factors that would increase the risk of burn injuries.

3. Identify nursing measures that would decrease the risk of infection for patients with diabetes.

Reference

Kowal-Vern, A., & Latenser, B. A. (2004). Infections in diabetic burn patients. *Diabetes Care, 27*(10), 229–233.

Answers to Critical Thinking Questions appear in Appendix D.

EVIDENCE-BASED PRACTICE

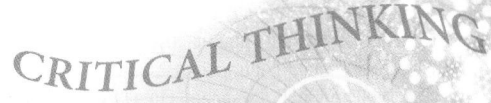

Clinical Preparation

CRITICAL THINKING

 Read

- History of Current Illness
- Past Medical History
- Physical Exam
- Admitting Medical Orders
- Laboratory Study Results

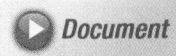 **Document**

- Summary of Hospitalization
- Pathophysiology Form
- Laboratory Values
- Laboratory Results Explanation

 **Apply**

- List of Potential Nursing Diagnoses
- Concept Map
- Critical Thinking Questions

*Log on to MyNursingKit.com to download forms you will need and to complete further steps in the Clinical Preparation assignment.

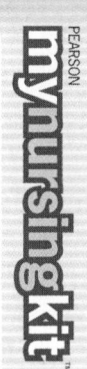

HISTORY OF PRESENT ILLNESS

As the on-coming nurse in a major burn center, you are receiving report about Mrs. X, a 60-year-old housewife who was admitted to the hospital following a fire that occurred in her home. A neighbor noted the smoke coming from the house and called 911 for emergency assistance. The firefighters had to carry Mrs. X from the burning house because she was unconscious. Despite resuscitative efforts, Mrs. X's husband was declared dead at the scene of the fire. Mrs. X's two grown children have been notified of the accident and are currently in the waiting room. This is the patient's hospital day 2. A large-bore triple lumen subclavian catheter was placed, and lactated Ringer's solution is infusing using the Brooke Army Formula guidelines. A Foley catheter was inserted, and her urine output is being monitored hourly and has been at least 30 mL/hr. A femoral arterial line was placed and has a good wave form. She is being medicated for pain with moderate relief.

Her last vital signs were temperature: 39°C, pulse: 126 beats per minute, respiratory rate: 16/minute, and BP: 104/80. A nasogastric (NG) tube was placed in order to decompress the stomach if nausea and vomiting should occur and for medication instillation. The patient denies nausea and she is tolerating NG medications. Her abdomen is soft with hypoactive bowel sounds noted in all four quadrants. She has not had a bowel movement since admission.

Medical–Surgical History
No known allergies
Hypertension
Myocardial infarction 2 years ago
Non–insulin-dependent diabetes
Atrial fibrillation
Depression
Two live births via vaginal delivery
Medications: Digoxin, Captopril, Paxil, and Glipizide

Social History
Was living independently with husband up to time of the fire
Two grown children
One son lives in local area
No tobacco use

Physical Exam
27% total body surface area burned
Approximately 12% is full-thickness injury, primarily on left arm and leg
Left arm and leg: circumferential injuries that required escharotomies
Remainder of burn wounds are on face and chest
Following escharotomies, pulses present in both left arm and leg, and patient able to wiggle toes on command
Restless, anxious, and complaining of severe pain
Moving all four extremities equally, on command
Pupils respond to light equally at 4 millimeters
Apical pulse: can be heard at the apex; peripheral pulses: +4 (0–4 scale) and slightly irregular, no extra heart sounds
Cardiac monitor: sinus tachycardia with occasional premature ventricular contractions
Capillary refill < 3 seconds in all extremities
Inhalation injury: currently intubated on ventilatory support with 50% oxygen
Lungs: wheezes and diminished breath sounds in bilateral bases; suctioned every hour for carbon-stained thick mucus
Oxygen sat 94–96%

Admitting Medical Orders
Burn service
Admit to burn intensive care unit
No known allergies

Diagnosis
27% burn injury

Orders
Vital signs, oxygen saturation, and urine output every hour
Foley

AccuCheck before meals and at bedtime
IV lactated Ringer's solution 180 mL/hr
Hubbard tank and dressing change with Silvadene daily
Bed rest
Strict I&O
Elevate left arm and left leg on 2 pillows each
HOB 30 degrees
PT/OT daily
NG feeding: replete at 5 mL/hr
Check residual q4h, stop feeding for 1 hour if > 100 milliliters
Ventilator: FIO$_2$ at 50%, TV: 700, Rate: 10, Peep: 5, PS/PC: 18/22
Suction prn
Daily weight
Call house officer: Pulse < 60 & > 110/minute; BP < 90 & > 130 systolic; temperature > 38.5; urine output < 30 mL/hr for 2 hours; respiratory rate > 30/minute; oxygen saturation < 92%

Scheduled Medications
MVI 1 NG daily
Folic acid 1 mg NG daily
Vitamin A 20,000 units NG daily
Zinc 220 mg NG daily
Thiamine 100 mg NG daily
Pepcid 20 mg IV q12h
Cefataxime 1 g IV q8h
Digoxin 0.25 mg IV daily
Captopril 25 mg NG 3 × daily, hold for SBP < 100
Paxil 30 mg NG daily
Glipizide SR 10 mg NG daily
Tobramycin 5 mg/kg on call to OR

PRN Medications
Tylenol 650 mg q6h NG/PR prn pain and temp > 101.5
Benadryl 50 mg IV/NG q6h prn itching and insomnia
Fentanyl 50–150 mcg IV prn dressing change
Phenergan 25 mg IV q6h prn nausea and vomiting
Versed 2–4 mg IV prn dressing change
Morphine sulfate drip 1 mg/mL at 1–7 mg/hr titrate to effect
Versed drip 0.5 mg/mL at 0.5–3 mg/hr titrate to effect for agitation/anxiety

Laboratory Studies
ABG, CBC, Chemistry 7 daily
Type and cross for 4 units of packed red blood cells
Blood, sputum, and urine culture

Diagnostic Studies
Chest x-ray daily

LABORATORY STUDY RESULTS

Test	Day 1	Day 2	Day 3
Sodium	138 mEq/L	148 mEq/L	135 mEq/L
Potassium	4.8 mEq/L	5.8 mEq/L	5 mEq/L
Chloride	103 mEq/L	110 mEq/L	108 mEq/L
Carbon dioxide (CO_2)	28 mg/dL	31 mg/dL	25 mg/dL
Blood urea nitrogen (BUN)	10 mg/dL	10 mg/dL	9 mg/dL
Creatinine	1.1 mg/dL	1.3 mg/dL	1.8 mg/dL
Blood glucose	141 mg/dL	135 mg/dL	132 mg/dL
Calcium	8.6 mg/dL	9 mg/dL	9 mg/dL
Magnesium	1.9 mg/dL	1.9 mg/dL	2 mg/dL
Phosphorus	2.2 mg/dL	3.4 mg/dL	3.8 mg/dL
Albumin	2.7 g/dL	2.27 g/dL	1.97 g/dL
White blood cells (WBC)	15,800/mm³	9,900/mm³	4,600/mm³
Red blood cells (RBC)	6.9/mm³	5.88/mm³	4.73/mm³
Hemoglobin (Hgb)	19.3/mm³	18.2/mm³	14.7/mm³
Hematocrit (HCT)	56.6%	54.1%	43.5%
Platelets	188,000/mm³	180,000/mm³	149,000/mm³
International normalized ratio (INR)	0.8		
Arterial blood gases (ABGs)			
PO_2	135 mmHg	96 mmHg	94 mmHg
Oxygen saturation	98%	99%	97%
pH	7.31	7.37	7.39
PCO_2	52 mmHg	49 mmHg	44 mmHg
HCO_3	26 mEq/L	28 mEq/L	26 mEq/L

CRITICAL THINKING QUESTIONS

1. Besides burn wound assessment and fluid resuscitation needs, what other priorities would be essential to assess Mrs. X for?

2. What is the rationale for performing an escharotomy, and what clinical manifestations would result if an escharotomy were not done?

3. What impact does diabetes have on Mrs. X's prognosis?

4. What impact does fluid resuscitation have on Mrs. X's sodium, chloride, hemoglobin, and hematocrit levels?

Answers to Critical Thinking Questions appear in Appendix D.

NCLEX® REVIEW

1. The nurse is assessing the patient with an electrical burn. It is noted that the patient has a 1% partial-thickness burn to the left foot and a 2% full-thickness burn to the right shoulder, where they contacted the electrical source. The patient is awake, alert and oriented. Vital signs are HR 97 with frequent ectopy, BP 136/75, RR 22, SpO₂ 94% on room air. The nurse knows that this patient's injuries should be classified as a:

   1. Minor burn injury.
   2. Moderate burn injury.
   3. Major burn injury.
   4. Medium burn injury.

2. A nurse is teaching a class on injury prevention to a group of new mothers. Which of the following statements made by one of the participants indicates the need for further instruction regarding burn injury prevention?

   1. "Every house should have at least one clean working smoke detector."
   2. "SPF 30+ can help reduce the likelihood of getting a radiation burn."
   3. "Make sure all children's sleepwear is made from fire retardant fabrics."
   4. "Liquid at 140° F requires five minutes to cause a full-thickness burn."

3. It is important to understand the pathophysiological changes that occur in the severely burned patient. When the student nurse inquires about these changes, the most appropriate response by the nurse would be:

1. "With bacterial translocation the gastrointestinal mucosal atrophy that occurs causes intraluminal bacteria to migrate to extraluminal sites."

2. "Decreased cardiac output can occur early after a burn because stimulation of the parasympathetic nervous system causes vasoconstriction."

3. "Hepatic failure ensues when damaged erythrocytes and muscle tissue cause the excess release of hemoglobin and myoglobin, respectively."

4. "It is not uncommon to transfuse leukocytes within the first two days because granulocyte stores and circulating iron stores are depleted."

4. Upon admission to the burn unit the patient with a 35% TBSA thermal burn begins to undergo intensive wound care and physical therapy. Pain control and topical antimicrobial medications are also important. The nurse understands the patient is in which period of burn care?

1. The resuscitative period
2. The acute care period
3. The emergency period
4. The rehabilitative period

5. Four victims of a house fire arrive in the emergency department. Based on what you know about burn severity assessment, which of the following patients should the nurse see first?

1. A 35-year-old with a history of migraines and 40% TBSA full-thickness thermal burns to the neck, left upper extremity and circumferentially around the chest. Vital signs are HR 116, BP 90/68, RR 26 and shallow, SpO$_2$ 90%.

2. A 70-year-old with a history of diabetes and 14% TBSA partial-thickness thermal burns to the back and right shoulder and 1% TBSA full-thickness burn to the right arm. Vital signs are HR 88, BP 130/75, RR 22 and regular, SpO$_2$ 98%.

3. A 12-year-old with a history of astigmatism and 20% TBSA partial-thickness thermal burns to the anterior left lower extremity, left foot and abdomen. Vital signs are HR 80, BP 110/65, RR 24 and regular, SpO$_2$ 100%.

4. A 44-year-old with a history of hypertension and 8% TBSA full-thickness thermal burns to the right upper extremity and 15% TBSA partial-thickness burns to the abdomen and anterior chest. Vital signs are HR 98, BP 148/92, RR 22 and regular, SpO$_2$ 98%.

6. Which of the following nursing diagnoses is most important during the emergency period of burn care?

1. Altered skin integrity related to epithelial skin loss
2. Fluid volume deficit related to increased capillary permeability
3. Increased risk for infection related to loss of skin integrity
4. Acute pain related to burn injury and exposed nerve endings

7. The nurse is preparing the previously burned patient for discharge home. Which of the following statements by the patient would indicate the need for further teaching?

1. "I know I should maintain a progressive exercise program to help increase my strength and endurance."

2. "The hardened areas in my healed scars can be broken down if I massage them daily with lotion or oil."

3. "I can tell that my stretching exercises are being done appropriately when my burn scars start to blanch."

4. "My pressure garments should be removed one to four times a day to allow for adequate circulation."

8. There are many complications associated with burn injuries. Which of the following would be the best indicator of an early complication during the emergency phase of burn care?

1. Blood pressure 118/66
2. Central venous pressure 6
3. Heart rate 114
4. Urine output 30 mL/hr

Answers for review questions appear in Appendix D

KEY TERMS

allograft *p.2260*
autografting *p.2260*
biologic dressing *p.2260*
biosynthetic dressing *p.2260*
chemical burns *p.2236*
donor site *p.2260*
eschar *p.2243*
escharotomies *p.2258*
full-thickness injury *p.2239*

full-thickness skin graft *p.2262*
heterografts *p.2260*
hypertrophic scar *p.2269*
inhalation injury *p.2235*
keloid scar *p.2269*
Lund-Browder formula *p.2245*
meshed skin graft *p.2262*
partial-thickness injury *p.2239*
radiation burns *p.2236*

rule of nines *p.2245*
scald burns *p.2235*
sheet skin grafts *p.2263*
split-thickness skin graft *p.2262*
thermal burns *p.2235*
zone of coagulation *p.2239*
zone of hyperemia *p.2239*
zone of stasis *p.2239*

REFERENCES

Ahrns, K. (2004). Trends in burn resuscitation: Shifting the focus from fluids to adequate end point monitoring, edema control, and adjuvant therapies. *Critical Care Nursing Clinics of North America, 16*(1), 1–25.

American Burn Association. (2002). *Burn care resources: Burn facts.* Retrieved on October 4, 2006, from http://www.ameriburn.org/advocacy/firesafety.html

Andel, H., Kamolz, L., Horauf, K., & Zimpfer, M. (2003). Nutrition and anabolic agents in burned patients. *Burns, 29,* 592–595.

Ballesteros, M. F., Jackson, M. L., & Martin, M. W. (2005). Working towards the elimination of residential fire deaths: The Centers for Disease Control and Prevention Smoke Alarm Installation and Fire Safety Education (SAIFE) program. *Journal of Burn Care & Rehabilitation, 26*(5), 434–439 (11 ref.).

Benson, B. E., Sidor, M. I., Schwartz, R. A., Desposito, F., & Hostetler, M. A. (2006). Burns, electrical. *eMedicine.com.* Retrieved September 9, 2008, from http://www.emedicine.com/ped/topic2734.htm

Borde, V. D., Bernier, J., & Garrel, D. R. (2002). Effects of dietary fatty acids on burn-induced immunosuppression. *Cell Immunology, 220*(2), 116–124.

Burnsurgery.org. (2004). *Burn center transfer criteria.* Retrieved September 18, 2008, from http://www.burnsurgery.org/Modules/initial_mgmt/sec_4.htm

Burn Survivor Resource Center. (2002a). *Chemical burns.* Retrieved October 4, 2006, from http://www.burnsurvivor.com/injury_examples_chemicalburns.html

Burn Survivor Resource Center. (2002b). *Medical care guide: Burn statistics.* Retrieved October 5, 2006, from http://www.burnsurvivor.com/burn_statistics.html

Burn Survivors Throughout the World. (2006). *Rehabilitation of burn scars.* Retrieved October 5, 2006, from http://www.burnsurvivorsttw.org/burns/burnrehab.html

Cancio, L. C., Jimenez-Reyna, J. F., Barbillo, D. J., Walker, S. C., McManus, A. T., & Vaughan, G. M. (2005). One hundred ninety-five cases of high-voltage electrical injury. *Journal of Burn Care & Rehabilitation, 26*(4), 331–340.

Centers for Disease Control and Prevention. (2006). *Skin Cancer: School Health Guidelines.* Retrieved September 18, 2008, from http://www.cdc.gov/healthyyouth/skincancer/guidelines/questions.htm

Chen, G., Xie, W., & Jiang, H. (2001). Clinical observation of the protective effect of oral feeding of glutamine on intestinal mucosal membrane. *Chinese Journal of Burns, 17*(4), 210–211. Retrieved May 1, 2002, from http://firstsearch.oclc.org/WebZ/FSFETCH

Demling, R. H. (2005). The burn edema process: Current concepts. *Journal of Burn Care & Rehabilitation, 26*(3), 200–206.

Demling, R. H., DeSanti, L., Orgill, D. R. (2006a). *Initial management of burn patient.* Retrieved May 11, 2006, from http://www.burnsurgery.org/modules/initial/part_two/sec9.html

Demling, R. H., & DeSanti, L. (2004). Initial management of the burn patient. *Burnsurgery.org.* Retrieved September 18, 2008 from http://www.burnsurgery.org/Modules/initial_mgmt/index_initial.htm

Demling, R. H., & DeSanti, L. (2006b). *Transfer criteria for referral to a burn facility.* Retrieved October 5, 2006, from http://www.burnsurgery.org/modules/initial/part_two/sec9.htm

Demling R. H., DeSanti, L., & Orgill, D. R. (2004). The metabolic response to burn injury and the role of nutritional support. *Burnsurgery.org.* Retrieved October 4, 2005, from http://www.burnsurgery.org/Modules/burnmetabolism/index_metabolism.htm

emedicine Health. (2006). *Chemical burns.* eMedicineHealth.com Retrieved October 5, 2006, from http://www.eMedicineHealth.com/chemical_burns/page6_em.html

Erzurum, V. Z., & Varcellotti, J. (1999). Self-inflicted burn injuries. *Journal of Burn Care & Rehabilitation, 20*(1), 22–24.

Fadaak, H. A. (2000). Gastrointestinal haemorrhage in burn patients: The experience of a burn unit in Saudi Arabia. *Annals of Burns and Fire Disasters, 13*(2).

Fauerbach, J. A., Lawrence, J. W., Munster, A. M., Palombo, D. A., & Richter, D. (1999). Prolonged adjustment difficulties among those with acute post-trauma distress following burn injury. *Journal of Behavioral Medicine, 22*(4), 359–378.

Flynn, M. B. (2002). Burn injuries. In K. McQuillan, K. Von Rueden, R. Hartsock, M. Flynn, & E. Whalen (Eds.), *Trauma nursing: From resuscitation through rehabilitation* (3rd ed., pp. 788–809). Philadelphia: W. B. Saunders.

Gosian, A., & Gamilli, R. L. (2005). A primer in cytokines. *Journal of Burn Care & Rehabilitation, 26*(1), 7–12.

Gottschlich, M., Jenkins, M., Mayes, T., Khoury, R. T., Kagan, R. J., & Warden, G. D. (2002). The 2002 research award. An evaluation of the safety of early vs. delayed enteral support and the effects on clinical, nutrition, and endocrine outcomes after severe burns. *Journal of Burn Care & Rehabilitation, 23*(6), 401–415.

Greenhalgh, D. (2005). Models of wound healing. *Journal of Burn Care & Rehabilitation, 26*(4), 293–305.

Hart, D. W., Wolf, S. E., Zhang, X. J., Chinkes, D. L., Buffalo, M. C., Matin, S. I., et al. (2001). Efficacy of a high-carbohydrate diet in catabolic illness. *Critical Care Medicine, 29*(7), 1321–1324.

Lucile Packard Children's Hospital at Stanford. (2008). *Safety and injury prevention: Fire safety and burns—Injury statistics and incidence rates.* Retrieved September 9, 2008, from http://www.lpch.org/DiseaseHealthInfo/HealthLibrary/safety/firestat.html

Lvsey, S. A., Herndor, D. N., and Hollyoak, M. A. (1995). Transplanted acollular allograft dermal matrix: Potential as a template for the reconstruction of viable dermis. *Transplantation 60*(1), 1–9.

Mabrouk, A. R., Mahmod, O. A., Massoud, K., Magdy, S. M., & Sayed, N. (1999). Suicide by burns: A tragic end. *Burns: Journal of International Society for Burn Injuries, 25*(4), 337–339.

Mandel, J., & Hales, C. A. (2008). *Smoke inhalation.* Retrieved September 9, 2008, from http://www.uptodate.com/patients/content/topic.do?topicKey=~9DITT3s_pPmii9&selectedTitle=1~147&source=search_result

McCall, J. E., & Cahill, T. J. (2005). Respiratory care of the burn patient. *Journal of Burn Care & Rehabilitation, 26*(3), 200–206.

Menchaca-Diaz, J. L., Silva, R. M., Figueiredo, L. F. P., Bugni, G. M., Watanabe, A. Y., Silva, F. J. P., et al. (2003). Bacterial translocation consequential to intestinal bacterial overgrowth provokes aggravation of mortality by sepsis. *Critical Care, 7*(Suppl. 3), P28. Retrieved October 12, 2005, from http://ccforum.com/content/7/S3/P28

Murphy, K. D., Lee, J. O., & Herndon, D. N. (2003). Expert opinion on pharmacotherapy. *Expert Opinion, 4*(3), 369–384.

Murray, C. (2008). Burn wound infections. eMedicine from Web MD. Retrieved on September 18, 2008, from suapple@verizon.net.

National Institutes of General Medical Sciences. (2006). *Fact sheet: Trauma, shock, burn, and injury: Facts and figures. National Institutes of Health.* Retrieved October 5, 2006, from http://www.publications.nigms.nig.gov/factsheets/trauma_burn_facts.html

National Institutes of Health. (2006). *Fact sheet: Burns and traumatic injury.* Retrieved October 5, 2006, from http://www.nih.gov/about/researchresultsforthepublic/BurnsandTraumaticInjury.pdf

Neumeister, M. (2005). Hyperbaric oxygen therapy. *Emedicine.com.* Retrieved October 5, 2006, from http://www.emedicine.com/plastic/topic526.htm

O'Brien, K. A., Weinstock-Zlotnick, G., Sanchez, J., Gorga, D., & Yurt, R. Y. W. (2005). Comparison of positive pressure gloves on hand use in uninjured persons. *Journal of Burn Care & Rehabilitation, 26*(4), 363–370.

Oliver, R. I., Spain, D., & Stadelmann, W. (2005). Burns, resuscitation and early management. *eMedicine.com.* Retrieved August 29, 2005, from http://www.emedicine.com/plastic/topic159.htm

Osborn, K. (2003, May). Nursing burn injuries. *Nursing Management,* 49–56.

Pereira, C. T., Murphy, K. D., & Herndon, D. N. (2005). Altering metabolism. *Journal of Burn Care & Rehabilitation, 26*(3), 197–199.

Porth, C. M. (2007). *Pathophysiology: Concepts of altered health states* (7th ed., pp. 391–397). Philadelphia: Lippincott Williams & Wilkins.

Prensner, J. D., Yowler, C. J., Smith, L. F., Steele, A. L., & Fratianne, R. B. (2001). Music therapy for assistance with pain and anxiety management in burn treatment. *Journal of Burn Care & Rehabilitation, 22*(1), 83–88; discussion 82–83.

Redlick, F., Cooke, A., Gomez, M., Banfield, J., Cartotto, R. C., & Fish, J. S. (2002). A survey of risk factors for burns in the elderly and prevention strategies. *Journal of Burn Care & Rehabilitation, 23*(5), 351–356.

Son, J. T., & Kim, S. H. (2006). The effects of self-selected music on anxiety and pain during burn dressing changes. *Taehan Kanho Hakhoe Chi, 36*(1), 159–168.

Supp, A. P., Neely, A. N., Supp, D. M., Warden, G. D., & Boyce, S. T. (2005). Evaluation of cytotoxicity and antimicrobial activity of Articoat® Burn Dressing for management of microbial contamination of cultured skin substitutes grafted to athymic mice. *Journal of Burn Care & Rehabilitation, 26*(3), 238–246.

Surgical-tutor.org.uk. (2006). *Burns.* Retrieved October 5, 2006, from http://www.surgical-tutor.org.uk/default-home.htm?core/trauma/burns.htm~right

Tadros, T., Traber, D. L., Heggers, J. P., & Herndon, D. N. (2000). Angiotensin II inhibitor DuP753 attenuates burn-and-endotoxin-induced gut ischemia, lipid peroxidation, mucosal permeability, and bacterial translocation. *Annals of Surgery, 231*(4), 566–576.

Tadros, T., Traber, D. L., Heggers, J. P., & Herndon, D. N. (2003). Effects of interleukin-1alpha administration on intestinal permeability and bacterial translocation in burn sepsis. *Annuals of Surgery, 237*(1), 101–109.

Tuan, T., et al. (2003). Increased plasminogen activator inhibitor-1 in keloid fibroblasts may account for their elevated collagen accumulation in fibrin gel cultures. *American Journal of Pathology, 162*(5), 1579–1589.

U.S. Fire Administration. (2006). *Working together for home fire safety.* Retrieved October 5, 2006, from http://www.usfa.fema.gov/downloads/pdf/fswy11.pdf

U.S. Library of Medicine and the National Institutes of Health. (2006). *Dementia.* Retrieved March 9, 2005, from http://www.nlm.nih.gov/medlineplus/ency/article/000739.htm

Van Loey, N., & Van Son, M. (2003). Psychology and psychological problems in patients with burn scars. *American Journal of Clinical Dermatology, 4*(4), 245–272.

Whitehead-Pleaux, A. M., Baryza, M. J., & Sheridan, R. L. (2006). The effects of music therapy on pediatric patients' pain and anxiety during donor site dressing change. *Journal of Music Therapy, 43*(2), 136–153.

Wilkinson, J. M. (2009). *Nursing diagnosis handbook; with interventions and outcomes* (8th ed.). Upper Saddle River, NJ: Prentice Hall Health.

Wischmeyer, P. E., Lynch, J., Liedel, J., Wolfson, R., Riehm, J., Gottlieb, L., et al. (2001). Glutamine administration reduces gram-negative bacteremia in severely burned patients: A prospective, randomized, double-blind trial versus isonitrogenous control. *Critical Care Medicine, 29*(11), 2075–2080.

Wolf, S. E., & Herndon, D. N. (2000). Burns and radiation injuries. In K. L. Mattox, D. V. Feliciano, & E. E. Moore (Eds.), *Trauma* (4th ed., pp. 1137–1151). New York: McGraw-Hill.

Yamamoto, S., Tanabe, M., Wakabayashi, G., Shimazu, M., Matsumoto, K., & Kitajima, M. (2001). The role of tumor necrosis factor-alpha and interleukin-1 beta in ischemia-reperfusion injury of rat small intestine. *Journal of Surgical Residents, 99*(1), 134–141.

Yu, B. H., & Dimsdale, J. E. (1999). Posttraumatic stress disorder in patients with burn injuries. *Journal of Burn Care & Rehabilitation, 20*(5), 426–433; discussion 422–450.

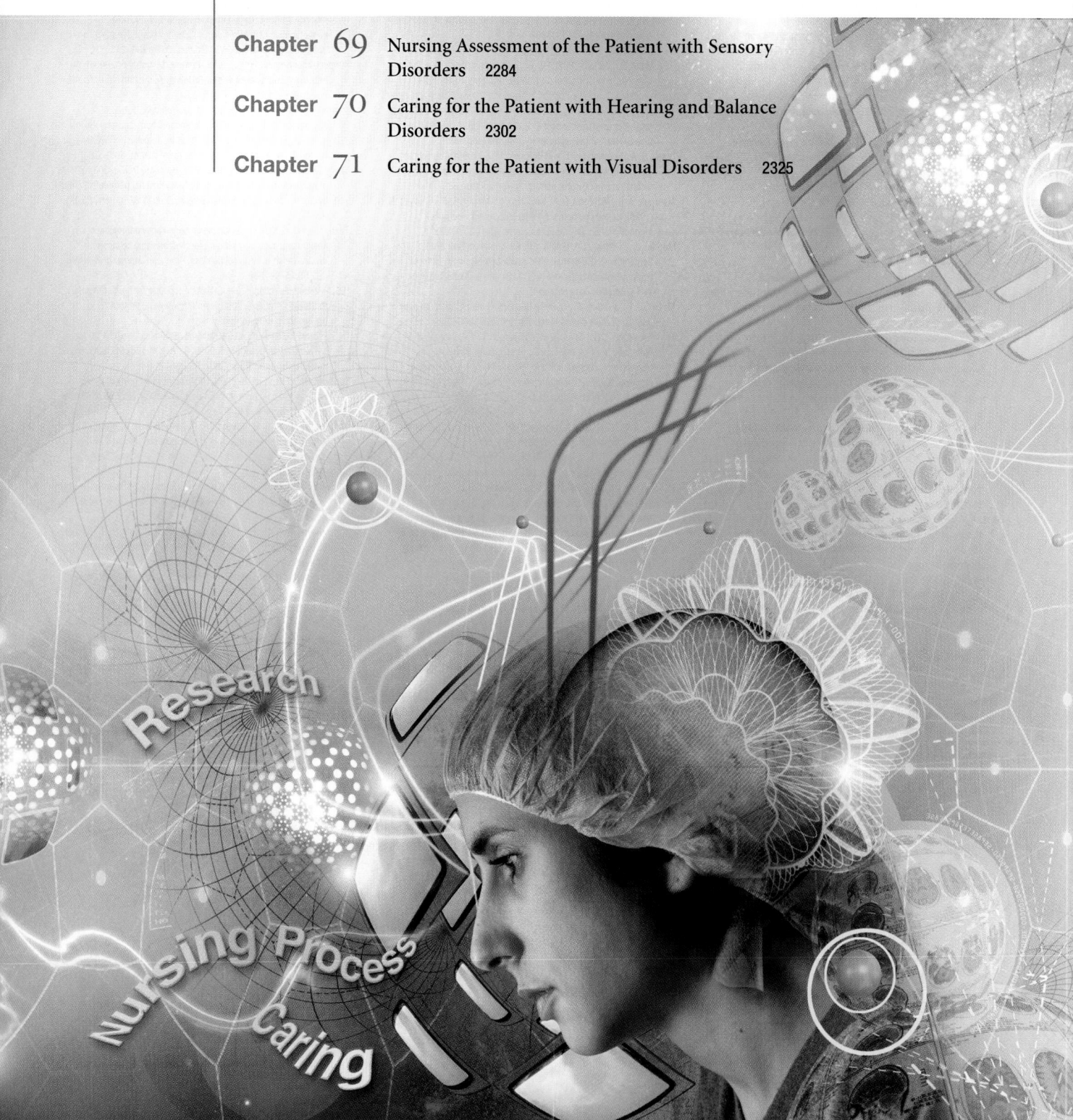

UNIT 15 | Nursing Management of Patients with Sensory Disorders

Research

Nursing Process

Caring

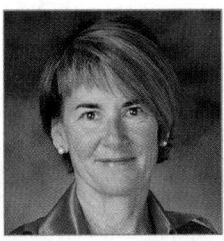

JOYCE My name is Joyce I have been a nurse practitioner specializing in family practice for more than 20 years. After graduating from the University of San Francisco, I worked as a public health nurse for VISTA (Volunteers in Service to America) at a migrant and seasonal farm workers' clinic in Toppenish, Washington. My practice included visiting migrant camps, providing immunizations and antibiotics, checking conditions regarding hygiene, and evaluating the general condition of the camps. During this experience I discovered the existence of nurse practitioners, their role, and their independence—that was what I wanted to become.

As a practicing family nurse practitioner (FNP), I am fortunate to have found a role in the delivery of health care that is completely fulfilling, that allows me to practice independently and utilize the holistic nursing model when providing care. As an FNP I want to know more about patients than just their chief complaints; I want to know about their lives. By delving more deeply into patients lives, I have often found an underlying condition, physical or emotional, that contributes to either the disease state or potential effectiveness of treatment.

In 1992 I received my master's in nursing at Sacramento State University. I received a doctor of education in leadership from St. Mary's College in 2007. While completing my doctorate, I accepted a faculty position at Sacramento Stare University. I am able to continue my practice as an FNP while teaching, pursuing research, and publishing.

It is impossible for me to think of a typical day—they are all so different. As an FNP I care for a wide range of patients, from infants to the elderly, with all systems affected from ENT to GI/GY. I counsel those who have had acute heart attacks and provide reassurance to new mothers that their babies will let them know when they are hungry. Over the years I have seen and cared for hundreds of ENT problems, some very simple, others much more complicated, including multiple sore throats, conjunctivitis, corneal abrasions, tonsillar abscesses, acute otitis media, sinusitis, and the common cold. This can be rather mundane, but then there are conditions that are complicated and frightening due to their potentially troubling lifelong consequences, such as abscessed sinusitis, temporary loss of vision secondary to a corneal burn or significant trauma, and hearing loss due to a medication or trauma. Some ENT complaints are aspects of a larger problem such as a brain mass, an acoustic neuroma, or other neurological condition. Recently, I cared for a deaf couple about to be married, one of whom was receiving a cochlear implant, the other was not. Many implications surrounded this decision—medically, surgically, psychologically, and personally. It was complicated and frightening to them and what this might mean for their marriage.

Navigating through these clinical situations takes **conscientious** patience, **competence, compassion,** and a total **commitment** to the complete health and well-being of each person. One of the most troubling situations I dealt with was the case of JM, a 72-year-old male with a history of upper respiratory complaints and progressively poor generalized health. Over a 2-year period, he was diagnosed with acute and chronic sinusitis, asthma, and GERD (reflux), He was treated with multiple antibiotics, Protein Pump Inhibitors, and nasal and respiratory inhalers. Still the problems persisted. Then his granddaughter noticed his aberrant behavior of swearing and using foul language. Upon reflection, his wife noted other abnormal behavior, such as the inability to remember simple equations or the passwords to his bank accounts. JM was referred to an ENT specialist who found that he had chronic sinusitis that had abscessed into his frontal lobe, causing his confusion and other neurological/cognitive problems. Neurosurgery was performed, but JM experienced a massive cerebral hemorrhage during the procedure and died 4 days later. Recognizing how long the situation was left unaddressed and allowed to progress with a failure of appropriate interventions and referrals that could have possibly changed the clinical outcome or improved the quality of JM's life was frustrating and frightening. It caused me to review my own practice—not just treating symptoms but looking at the person as a whole, the big picture.

Have I listened to the patient? Am I paying attention to what he is worried about? Does she understand the diagnosis and treatment plan? Have I **collaborated** with my patients or have I simply told them what to do? Even after many years of practice, I continue to review my clinical knowledge and my approach to patients and their care. It is my obligation, my **commitment,** to bring to patients the belief that they are in control of their situations. It is not about me—it is about the patient. I must be sure that I am **competent** and **confident** when dealing with health problems, **conscientious** in seeking out consultation if not, and **compassionate** about recognizing the person behind the diagnosis. It is essential that I *always* remember there is a human being at the center and all treatment and care focuses on that center.

> "As a practicing family nurse practitioner (FNP), I am fortunate to have found a role in the delivery of health care that is completely fulfilling, that allows me to practice independently and utilize the holistic nursing model when providing care."

69

Nursing Assessment of the Patient with Sensory Disorders

Arlene McGrory

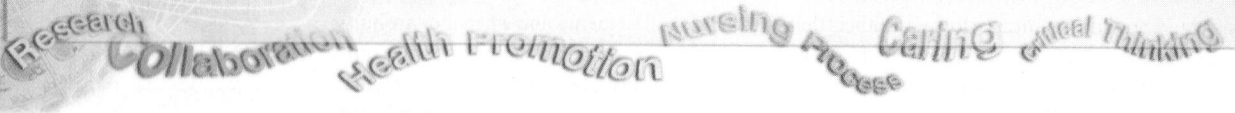

Research   Collaboration   Health Promotion   Nursing Process   Caring   Critical Thinking

THE SPECIALTY of otorhinolaryngology focuses on ear, nose, and throat (ENT) disorders. These disorders are common, may occur at any age, and often require immediate attention. Disorders of the ear, nose, and throat may affect the ability to perceive sound, speak, and breathe. Additionally, some of these disorders can be cosmetically disfiguring and affect body image and ultimately may be socially isolating. Early diagnosis and treatment can help keep people active and get involved in the world normally.

Nurses have numerous opportunities to identify risk factors and encourage healthy behaviors in patients. The modifiable risk factors related to ear, nose, and throat illnesses are primarily environmental, social, and occupational. These risk factors are discussed in the various chapter sections related to ear, nose, and throat conditions. Nurses need to assess patients for these risk factors and educate the patient and family to promote healthy behaviors. Nursing assessment using inspection, palpation, auscultation, and percussion, as well as a review of patients' social and occupational histories and laboratory results, provides information that can help identify conditions.

Anatomy and Physiology of the Ear, Nose, and Throat

The ear, nose, and throat encompass several organs and multiple systems including the integumentary, respiratory, gastroin-

testinal, neurological, endocrine, lymphatic, and circulatory systems. The following sections describe the anatomy and physiology of the ear, nose, and throat.

Ear

The external ear contains the cartilaginous auricle, or pinna. The external ear canal or meatus connects the auricle to the tympanic membrane (Figures 69–1 and 69–2 ■). **Cerumen**, or earwax, lubricates the external ear canal. Fine hair protects the canal from foreign objects. The canal protects the tympanic membrane.

The middle ear includes the tympanic membrane or eardrum, which conducts sound to the ossicles. In the tympanic cavity a small air-filled space in the temporal bone contains the ossicles and oval and round windows. The eustachian tube, the auditory tube from the middle ear to the nasopharynx, maintains equal pressure on both sides of the tympanic membrane.

The malleus, incus, and stapes are the auditory ossicles, which transmit sound waves to the inner ear. The inner ear consists of the bony labyrinth, which includes the vestibule and the utricle and saccule, which are filled with endolymph and are sensory receptors. Semicircular canals contain christa ampullaris receptors. The utricle, saccule, and semicircular canal help equilibrium. The shell-like cochlea is filled with perilymph and endolymph, which transmit sound vibrations. The organ of Corti contains supporting cells and hair cells that transmit

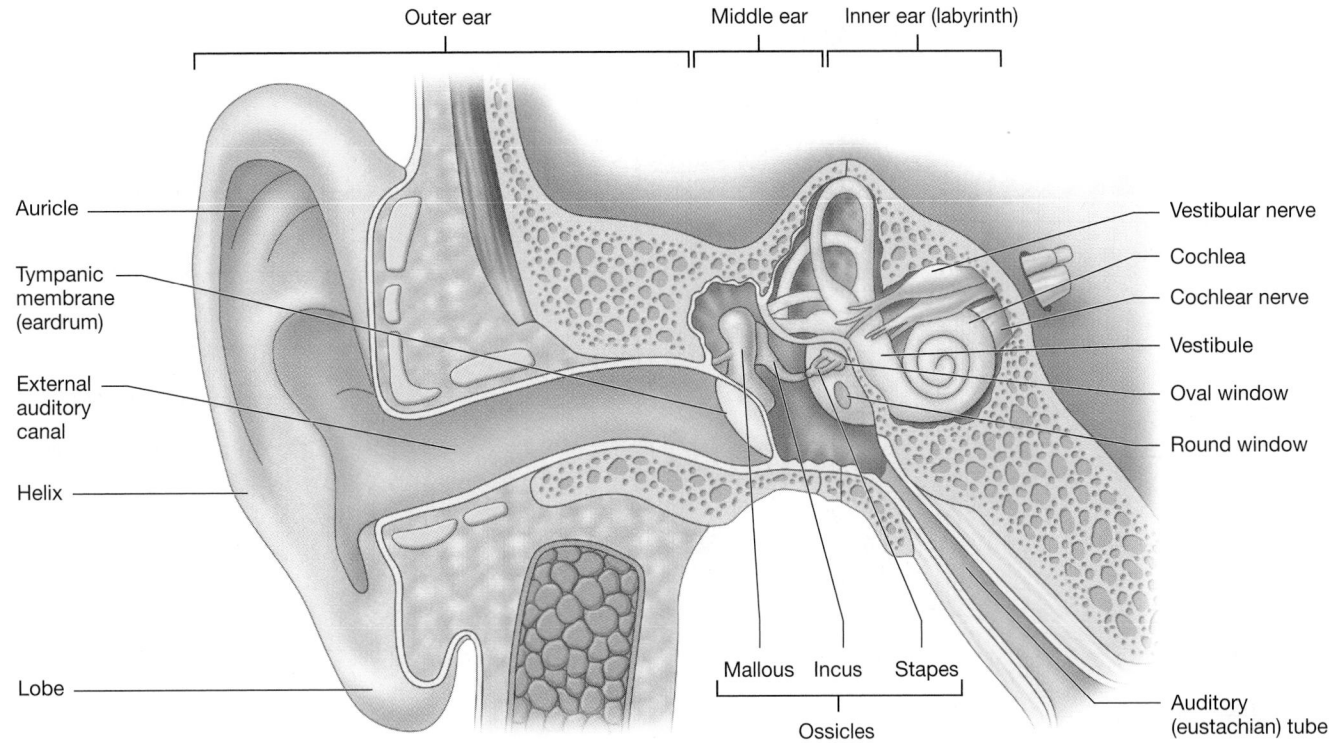

FIGURE 69–1 ■ Outer, middle, and inner ear.
From Lemone, P., and Burke, K. (2003). *Medical–Surgical Nursing: Critical Thinking in Client Care*, 3/e.

Right auricle

FIGURE 69–2 ■ External ear.

sound to the vestibulocochlear nerve (cranial nerve [CN] VIII). Hearing occurs as a result of sound waves vibrating the eardrum, malleus, incus, stapes, and oval window of the inner ear, the perilymph and endolymph of the cochlea, and the hair cells of the organ of Corti. The eighth cranial nerve carries the impulses to the auditory area in the temporal lobes.

Nose

The external nose has a bridge, which includes the nasal septum, tip, and nares or nasal opening (Figure 69–3 ■, p. 2286). Inter-

nally the nose is surrounded superiorly by the olfactory bulb and nerves and frontal sinus, and inferiorly by the hard palate. The interior is open to air and the posterior is surrounded by the sphenoid sinus, pharyngeal tonsil, eustachian tube, nasopharynx, soft palate, oropharynx, and palatine tonsil. The nares are lined with cilia, are highly vascular, and contain mucous membranes with ciliated goblet cells that produce mucus. The olfactory nerve (CN I) in the upper part of the nasal cavities controls the sense of smell. The paranasal sinuses, which include frontal, ethmoid, and sphenoid sinuses, are air cavities that surround the nasal cavity (Figure 69–4 ■, p. 2286). They add resonance to the voice and drain mucus through the nares.

Oral Cavity

The oral cavity includes, from superior to inferior surfaces, the upper lip, gingiva, hard and soft palate, glossopalatine arch, pharyngopalatine arch, palatine tonsil, posterior pharyngeal wall, uvula, and tongue (Figure 69–5 ■, p. 2286). Centermost inside the upper and lower lips, the superior and inferior labial frenulum connects the lips to the gingiva. The gingiva secure the teeth in the mouth. Thirty-two permanent and 20 deciduous teeth, needed for chewing food, are anchored by the gingiva, which is part of the oral mucosa and covers alveolar bone. The tongue is controlled by hypoglossal (CN XII) speech, chewing, and swallowing. The sensory function of the tongue is innervated by the facial nerve (cranial nerve VII) and glossopharyngeal nerve (CN IX). Oral mucosa is pink, moist, and without sores or bleeding.

The pharynx is the tube that extends from the nasopharynx behind the nasal cavity, to the oropharynx part of the oral cavity, to the laryngopharynx. The anterior portion of the laryngopharynx

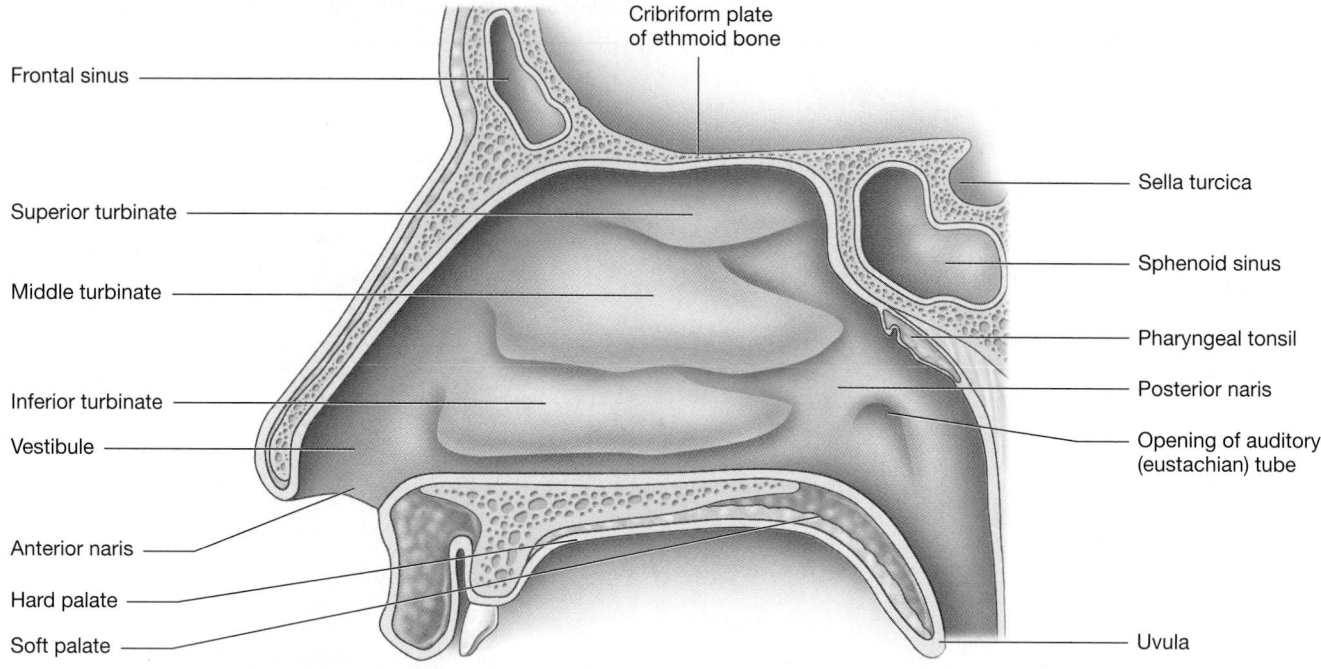

FIGURE 69–3 ■ The nose.

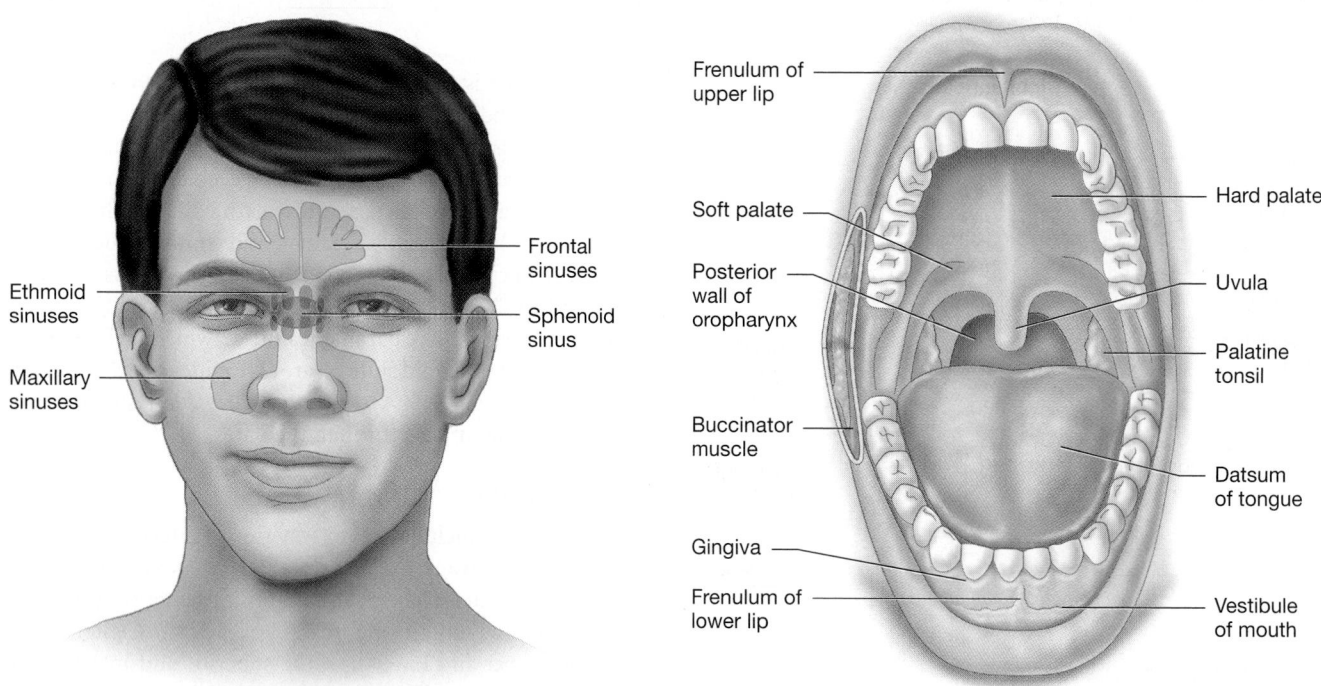

FIGURE 69–4 ■ The sinuses.
From Thompson, J. M. (1993). *Mosby's clinical nursing.* St. Louis: Mosby.

FIGURE 69–5 ■ Structures of the mouth.
From Seidel, H. M., et al. (1991). *Mosby's guide to physical examination,* 2/e, St. Louis: Mosby.

opens onto the larynx, and the posterior portion opens into the esophagus. Both the oropharynx and the laryngopharynx participate in swallowing.

The palatine tonsils are visible on either side of the soft palate. The lingual tonsils are on the base of the tongue. The pharyngeal tonsils or adenoids are behind the nose. The tonsils are lymphatic tissue that helps fight infections. The hard palate is the floor of the nasal cavity. Posterior to the hard palate is the soft palate, which helps prevent aspiration by elevating when swallowing. The uvula is a conelike structure centered on the soft palate that prevents food from entering the nasal passage. Several glands—the salivary, parotid, submandibular, and sublingual glands—and Wharton's duct surround the mouth and drain saliva.

Neck

The neck contains the thyroid gland, which produces thyroid hormone to control metabolism; thyroxine (T_4) and triiodothyronine (T_3); and calcitonin, which decreases calcium and phosphate levels (Figure 69–6 ■). Four parathyroid glands are attached to the thyroid gland posteriorly and serve to increase serum calcium levels. Cervical lymph nodes drain the structures of the head and neck.

The nurse must have a sound working knowledge of the anatomy and physiology of the ear, nose, and throat to be able to understand when the patient has problems with these structures. Along with the nurse's physical assessment skills, diagnostic tests and the patient's current functional abilities will help the interdisciplinary health care team choose interventions.

■ History

In order for the nurse to make an accurate assessment of the patient with an ENT problem, the patient's history needs to be explored. The personal, family, and social aspects of a person's life provide clues to the causes of health problems and the patient's receptivity to the care offered by health care professionals. Chart 69–1 (p. 2288) provides an assessment format that will help keep the nurse focused on the patient's complaint and allow the nurse to systematically assess the patient. Within this framework the patient's functional abilities are also assessed.

Biographic and Demographic History

The biographic information obtained is important in assessing risk for and identifying the presenting problem of patients with ENT problems. Medical, family, and social issues particular to the patient need to be explored. Specific questions are discussed under each organ.

Chief Complaint and Presenting Symptoms

The patient's primary complaint or the reason the person sought health care assistance is the presenting symptom. Examples of primary complaints include pain, breathing difficulties, and pruritus. The nurse's knowledge of the occurrence of diseases and conditions in certain population groups helps to focus the subsequent history.

Common ear problems include conductive deafness, sensorineural hearing loss, and tinnitus. **Conductive hearing loss** results from a lesion between the external auditory canal and the cochlea. **Sensorineural hearing loss** involves defects in the sensory end organ of the cochlea or in nerve transmission to the central nervous system (CNS). Patients can have hearing problems at any age. Knowledge of gender differences also is important. For example, otosclerosis is a familial disorder in which irregular ossification occurs in the stapes of the middle ear causing conductive deafness, sensorineural hearing loss, and tinnitus. It is more common in women than men (Mosby, 2002). Otosclerosis also can be triggered by pregnancy (Sigler, 2002).

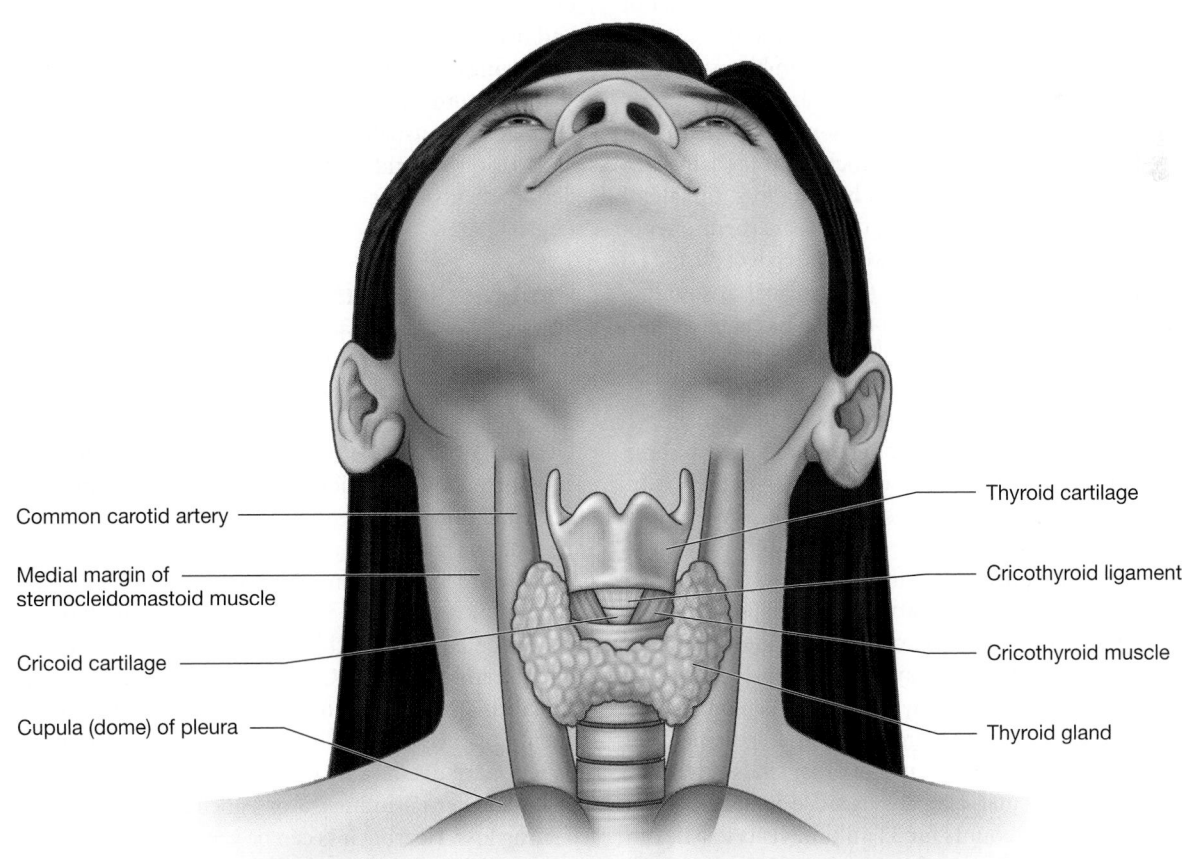

Common carotid artery

Medial margin of sternocleidomastoid muscle

Cricoid cartilage

Cupula (dome) of pleura

Thyroid cartilage

Cricothyroid ligament

Cricothyroid muscle

Thyroid gland

FIGURE 69–6 ■ The neck.

CHART 69–1	Ear, Nose, and Throat Assessment Format			
	Inspection	**Palpation**	**Auscultation**	**Percussion**
Subjective presenting symptom				
History (family, occupational, allergy)				
Current medications				
Ear				
Hearing test results				
Nose and paranasal sinuses				
Mouth				
Lips				
Gingiva and teeth				
Buccal mucosa				
Pharynx and larynx				
Nursing diagnosis				

Age impacts hearing ability. For example, *presbycusis*, hearing loss in the high-frequency range, is the most common sensorineural hearing loss in older people (Heron & Wharrad, 2000; Rabinowitz, 2000). The patient experiencing the gradual hearing loss of aging may limit social interactions as it becomes so difficult to understand the spoken word. During the assessment the nurse should inquire about functional ability and social interactions. Loss of hearing also can be perceived as mental status changes. Nurses need to be more aware of the impact of hearing loss on the elderly (Heron & Wharrad, 2000).

The nurse also should be aware of specific problems with at-risk populations. Acoustic neuromas, which are benign tumors of the Schwann cell sheath, are more common in women ages 40 to 50 years. Ménière's disease is a dysfunction of the labyrinth with symptoms of vertigo (dizziness), hearing loss, unilateral aural fullness, and **tinnitus**, or ringing in the ears (Crummer & Hassan, 2004). It is most common between the ages of 30 and 60 years. Any patient with obstruction of the ear canal, any middle ear disorders, or trauma to the ears or those receiving certain medications can develop tinnitus (Sigler, 2002). Ototoxic drugs are outlined in Chapter 70 ⊘.

Race is also an important consideration when assessing ENT problems, because some ethnic groups are more prone to some medical conditions. Otosclerosis is more common in the southern Indian population and much less common in Asians and blacks (Sigler, 2002).

Epistaxis, nasal bleeding, can occur at any age but is most common in children and in adults over 50 years old. Ten percent of the population experiences epistaxis at least once. It is more prevalent in the winter from inhaling dry air and is of particular concern in patients who have a history of hypertension, hemophilia, or leukemia. In adults nasal fractures are more common in men and are usually from sports injuries, assaults, or other kinds of trauma.

Sinusitis is of particular concern because it occurs at all ages and both sexes. It accounts for 32 million visits to a health care provider each year (National Institutes of Health [NIH], 2006). Smokers have more problems with sinusitis than nonsmokers.

Mouth and pharyngeal and laryngeal conditions occur from infections, tumors, or trauma. These conditions affect a person's ability to breathe and eat. Peritonsillar abscess occurs most often in young adults. Retropharyngeal abscesses are most common in children under 6 years old but are becoming more common in adults (Sigler, 2002). Ludwig's angina, severe cellulitis of the floor of the mouth, occurs as a result of dental disease. Laryngitis can occur from viruses or bacteria, inhaling noxious fumes, excessive use of the voice, or gastric reflux. Patients with head and neck cancer have problems with dysphasia and obstructive sleep apnea (Bailey, 2004; Koliha, 2003).

Vocal cord paralysis occurs more frequently in men than women and is usually the result of thyroid surgery, anterior cervical fusion, carotid endarterectomy, or cancer of the larynx. Elderly patients sometimes have presbylaryngeus, or dysphonia (Sigler, 2002).

Past Medical History

The patient's past medical history provides information about past health-related problems and, in particular, gives clues to the residual problems that may impact current treatment.

Childhood Diseases and Immunizations

The nurse should consider that any adult presenting with an ear, nose, and throat problem may have had a history of problems as a child. The frequency, clinical manifestations, and treatment of ENT disorders are essential information that must be obtained during the assessment. Inquire about any childhood history of ENT problems. Many children are prone to ear infections, sore throats, and tonsillitis. Complications of otitis media, which is either inflammation or infection of the middle ear, include frequent upper respiratory infections and sinus infections. Did the patient have tonsils and adenoids removed? Intrauterine exposure to maternal influenza or rubella can result in congenital hearing loss. Hearing loss can be very isolating and be perceived as mental status change.

Inquire about the presence of genetic diseases, especially those affecting the ear, nose, and throat. Hearing loss in children can occur from infections and genetics. Did the patient have all the childhood illnesses or immunizations? The nurse should inquire about childhood and adult immunizations, including the immunization dates and reactions.

Genetic conditions that affect otolaryngology can be divided into minor and major problems. Major genetic malfunctions include cleft lip and palate, sensorineural hearing impairment, absent or abnormal ears, eye abnormalities, blindness, and microcephaly. Minor genetic problems include high-arched palate, cleft uvula, wide-set eyes, abnormal slant of palpebral fissures, large auricles, and short neck (Jafek & Murrow, 2001).

Previous Illnesses and Hospitalizations

Past illnesses and hospitalizations can give the nurse clues to residual problems and how the patient coped with previous illnesses. In terms of diagnosing problems, the nurse needs to inquire about what has been done thus far. Has the patient had audiologic tests to determine the degree of hearing loss? Has the patient had surgery to correct hearing loss? Sinusitis is a very common condition and many patients have endoscopic sinus surgery for relief of the infection and pain. Has the patient had any cosmetic surgery? The nurse should ask about injuries and accidents, particularly foreign objects lodged in the ear, nose, or throat area. Has the person had any harmful ingestions or falls or been involved in a motor vehicle crash?

Head and neck cancer patients may have had various kinds of surgery, for example, a glossectomy or laryngectomy. Patients with head and neck cancer who have had surgery will need to have a barium swallow to ascertain whether or not the patient can resume normal eating.

Medications

List all current medications including prescribed, over-the-counter (OTC) medications, vitamins, and especially decongestants and sleeping medications. It is important to include systemic medications that may have an effect on the ENT assessment. Many medications are ototoxic and cause permanent bilateral hearing loss with eighth cranial nerve damage and some cause tinnitus (refer to Chapter 70). In particular, patients with compromised renal function are at risk for developing deafness and tinnitus from medications. To minimize this damage, while patients are taking these drugs serum drug levels and serial hearing evaluations should be done. Patients receiving long-term antibiotics can also develop vertigo because of damage to the eighth cranial nerve (Jafek & Murrow, 2001). Medications and chemicals that cause vertigo are outlined in the Risk Factor box in Chapter 70 (p. 2309) . Also ask the patient about the use of herbal and home remedies for ENT problems. Patients who take herbal remedies and OTC products may experience unwanted side effects.

Allergies

All allergies, including medication, food, environmental, chemical sensitivities, and latex allergies should be documented. What are the patient's symptoms when exposed to these allergens? Some common symptoms of allergy experienced by the patient include headache; fatigue; sore mouth or tongue; edema; fluctuating hearing loss; tinnitus; dry, cracking skin; and muscle and joint pain. Conditions that are frequently associated with allergies include chronic sinus disease, recurrent tonsillitis, or ear infections (Jafek & Murrow, 2001).

Cough and Sputum Production

Patients with upper respiratory and sinusitis conditions frequently have copious sputum production and cough from postnasal drip. Any patient with oropharyngeal dysphagia is at risk of aspiration. This kind of patient would cough on attempted swallowing and needs to be referred to a speech therapist (National Guideline Clearinghouse, 2006).

Family Health History

Some ear, nose, and throat conditions are genetically transmitted. Damage to hearing can occur *in utero* from genetic or infectious conditions (influenza or rubella) (Dillon, 2003). Half of the incidence of severe hearing loss occurring in 1 in 1,000 live births comes from genetic causes. It is typically noticed because of impaired speech development. Half the people who have otosclerosis have a family history of the condition (Sigler, 2002). The nurse needs to investigate whether any family members were hard of hearing before 50 years old and, if so, what caused the hearing loss. Have any family members had ear surgery? Do other family members have any type of ear problems?

It may be helpful to draw a genogram of living and dead family members to trace the incidence of any genetically linked conditions. Inquire about illnesses of other family members, including allergies, asthma, diabetes mellitus, and alcohol or other drug abuse.

Social History

Social history and habits include occupational and recreational pursuits, cultural considerations, and environmental exposures. Each of these areas has the potential to impact normal ear, nose, and throat functioning. Each is discussed next.

Occupational and Recreational

Occupational and recreational related ear problems can occur for a variety of reasons. Anyone who experiences high levels of noise occupationally or recreationally without wearing hearing protection risks hearing impairment and potential deafness. The major sources of high levels of noise (90 to 170 dB) include chain saws and other power tools, rock concerts, gunshots, jets, diesel locomotives, motorcycles, and lawn mower engines. One-third of all hearing loss can be attributed to occupational noise exposure (American Academy of Audiology, 2003). Experiencing recreational and occupational noise on an acute or chronic basis can cause bilateral sensorineural hearing loss at higher frequencies (3,000 to 6,000 Hz).

For patients who present with symptoms of sinusitis, the nurse must inquire about occupational exposure and the onset or worsening of symptoms. If the symptoms continue or become intolerable, the patient may need a referral to a career counselor to investigate a job change.

Sinus congestion occurs frequently with airline pilots, flight attendants, swimmers, and divers because the changes in barometric pressure may inhibit the clearance of sinus secretions. Smoking cigars or cigarettes or chewing tobacco increases the chance of precancerous and cancerous lesions on the nose, throat, mouth, pharynx, and larynx. A history of alcohol use is strongly associated with head and neck cancer. Exposure to noxious fumes or chemicals can lead to tumor development. Recreational activities also may increase the risk. For example, swimming can cause bacterial otitis externa, also called swimmer's ear (Smith & Osborne, 2003).

Cultural Considerations

Culture can impact how receptive the patient is to the prescribed medical treatment. Many people in the deaf community refuse genetic services because of a history of stigmatization. For example, at one time in the United States, deaf people were sterilized and prohibited from marrying, and programs were developed to extinguish their language.

Some Native American and Alaskan Indians prefer to use the traditional methods of healing, such as the medicine man, before resorting to Western methods of health care. People of other cultures, such as Asian Americans, Pacific Islanders, and Hispanics, may also prefer to use traditional methods of healing. Chinese patients rarely complain verbally but nonverbal communication, such as leaving uneaten food on a plate, may be used to express their dislike. Chinese people are particularly reluctant to accept surgical procedures (Spector, 2004). This may be seen by practitioners of Western methods of treatment as noncompliance.

In relation to the assessment of the ear, nose, and throat, during history taking the nurse needs to be sensitive to cultural norms. For example, for American Indian and Alaska Native populations note taking during the interview is taboo (Spector, 2004). In this case the nurse needs to directly address the issue with the patient or devise a culturally sensitive method of recording the information.

Environmental Exposures

Patients can be exposed to many allergens such as seasonal pollen in the environment. Environmental chemicals, both those occurring naturally (seasonal pollen) and those produced by industry, can create acute and chronic health hazards. Since the 1970s U.S. industry has produced an excess of 70,000 chemicals that potentially cause ill health (Chalupka, 2001). Nurses need to be more aware of the pervasiveness of these chemicals, their toxic effects, and the symptoms these chemicals produce particularly as they relate to the ear, nose, and throat examination. The *NIOSH Pocket Guide to Chemical Hazards* (U.S. Department of Health and Human Services 1997) can help identify chemical health hazards and symptoms.

In assessing the ear, nose, and throat several chemicals are common irritants. Adult exposure to environmental smoke may cause rhinitis, pharyngitis, and nasal congestion. Volatile organic compounds and formaldehyde can cause tingling in the ears, nose, and throat, rhinitis, epistaxis, and nasal congestion and may exacerbate childhood asthma. Combustion from poorly vented wood stoves and fireplaces, kerosene lamps, and garage exhaust may cause rhinitis, cough, and asthma. Sulfur dioxide gas causes nose and throat irritation (Chalupka, 2001).

Habits

Evaluating the patient's health habits can be an opportunity for health teaching. The nurse should inquire about the use and amount of tobacco products and alcohol ingestion. Does the patient use sunscreen? The nurse should inquire about the use of recreational drugs. A history of recreational drug use, such as cocaine, which is inhaled through the nasal passages, can cause perforation of the septum, bleeding, crusting, and a whistling sound with respiration. The nurse should teach the patient that

using cotton tip applicators, hairpins, paper clips, or other such objects in the ear can damage the tympanic membrane and cause possible acute bacterial otitis externa (Smith & Osborne, 2003).

Travel

Changes in air pressure during airplane travel can cause ear discomfort. Common measures used to prevent this discomfort are to swallow more frequently and/or yawn. Another technique is to pinch the nostrils shut, take a mouthful of air, and force it into the back of your nose and try to blow your thumb and fingers off your nostrils. Subsequently the ears should be cleared and hearing returned. If none of these techniques is successful, the individual may try to use a decongestant or nose spray. Feeding a baby with a bottle or putting a pacifier in the baby's mouth will help the baby's ear pop. Because a cold, sinus infection, or allergy commonly blocks the eustachian tube, postponing the trip until the symptoms are less bothersome may be helpful. Any patient who has undergone ear surgery should consult with their health care provider about a safe time to travel by air (American Academy of Otolaryngology-Head and Neck Surgery, 1993).

Ear

The ears are sensory organs that, in conjunction with the nervous system, provide rich aural stimuli that enhance the quality of our lives. The ability to hear is essential for the normal development and maintenance of speech. The external and middle ear captures, transmits, and amplifies sound. The inner ear's vestibular structures are stimulated by sound waves to assist in balance.

Current Health and Risk Factors

The nurse needs to understand the current health of the patient and any risk factors, that might impact on possible problems of the ear, nose, and throat. Disorders of the external ear occur from obstruction or inflammation. Disorders of the middle ear occur because of abnormal patency, functional or mechanical obstruction, and infection (refer back to Figure 69–1 ■, p. 2285).

Disorders of the middle ear impair hearing, and can cause tinnitus or ringing in the ears. Conductive hearing loss occurs from loss of transmission of sound to the inner ear from diseases such as external ear infections, cerumen impaction, and middle ear effusion or obstruction (Crummer & Hassan, 2004; Marzo, 2003). Sensorineural hearing loss occurs when there is damage to the eighth cranial nerve or the end organ of hearing. This hearing loss can occur in a variety of ways. Presbycusis followed by noise exposure is the primary cause of sensorineural hearing loss followed by noise exposure. Congenital factors such as birth trauma and prenatal infections or exposure to toxic substances also cause sensorineural hearing loss. In addition, neoplastic conditions, acoustic neuromas, Ménière's disease, **ototoxicity** from drugs or other chemicals, infections, and systemic diseases can cause sensorineural hearing loss (Rabinowitz, 2000) (see Chapter 70 ☉).

Disorders of the ear also can be associated with neurological problems. The nurse needs to inquire about a history of meningitis, double vision, numbness in hands or feet, weakness in arms or legs, tingling in the mouth or face, loss of consciousness, fainting, or seizures. When noise-induced hearing loss occurs, the hair cells of the basilar membrane of the cochlea have been damaged.

 **CRITICAL ALERT** *In any patient with sudden hearing loss, the nurse must investigate the possibility of trauma and ask the patient what medications are being taken and for how long.*

Hearing loss can be exacerbated by concurrent exposure to ototoxic solvents or heavy metals (Rabinowitz, 2000). The nurse should be aware of this important modifiable health risk, screen for risk factors, and teach the proper use of hearing protection. Is the patient's workplace very noisy? Does the patient wear any personal protective ear protection? How often does the patient wear earplugs?

Current Issue

What is the patient's current ear problem? The focus of the interview and assessment should be on identifying hearing loss, **otalgia** (ear pain), tinnitus, vertigo, and infection. A risk factor analysis should be done and any acute injury should be assessed.

Hearing Loss

Each year 60,000 people are diagnosed with unilateral hearing loss (Kim & Toriumi, 2003). About 28 million Americans have some hearing loss (Marzo, 2003). The nurse needs to inquire about difficulty hearing high- or low-pitched sounds, or both. Questions included in this assessment include the following:

- Does the patient have difficulty discriminating sounds in a group setting?
- Has the change in hearing been sudden or gradual?
- Do family members complain that the patient cannot hear them?
- What were the events leading to the perception of hearing loss?
- Does the patient perceive distortion in hearing, differences in pitch or sound, fullness or pressure in the ear?
- Has the patient ever had a hearing examination and, if so, why?
- What were the results of the hearing examination?
- Does the patient work in a profession where there is chronic loud noise and, if so, is ear protection worn?

Some occupational pursuits require the use of hearing protection, for example, people working with jet engines. A standard set of hearing tests can be performed depending on the symptoms, as outlined in Chapter 70 ⊕ Diagnostic Tests for Hearing Loss box (p. 2312).

Is the patient wearing a hearing aid and, if so, in one or both ears? Are they turned on? Do the hearing aids help hearing? How old are the batteries? How recently did the patient change batteries? Does the hearing aid cause any irritation of the ear canal? Does the patient have an implantable hearing device? The nurse needs to observe any behavioral cues that may indicate possible hearing loss:

- Irritability
- Difficulty hearing higher frequency consonants (e.g., *sl* or *sh*)
- Complaints about people mumbling or giving inappropriate answers
- Use of a high volume on the television or radio
- Frequently asking for words to be repeated
- Leaning forward or turning head to hear better
- Avoiding group situations or anyplace with increased background noise

- Appearing aloof
- Using a very soft or loud voice.

Otalgia

The nurse needs to inquire about the presence, duration, and intensity of otalgia (ear pain). Is it unilateral or bilateral, constant or intermittent, and where is the location of the pain? Does the patient have a sense of fullness in the ears? Is it worse when moving and relieved by staying still? Does the application of warmth help? Use a pain scale to determine the intensity of pain. Ask about a history of trauma to the ears. What measures have been used to relieve it and have they been successful? Ask if the patient uses a cotton applicator or other implement to clean the ears.

Tinnitus

Tinnitus (ringing in the ears) affects approximately 50 million Americans (Sigler, 2002). It is usually an unwanted, primarily localized, internal auditory perception usually not heard by others. Objective tinnitus can be heard by others and is caused by vascular problems of the carotid arteries or jugular veins. Subjective tinnitus can only be heard by the patient and can be caused by metabolic, pharmacologic, psychogenic, and/or neurological abnormalities (Crummer & Hassan, 2004). The nurse needs to assess when the patient first noticed ringing in the ears and/or any kind of head noise. What is the intensity or frequency? Is the noise high or low pitched, buzzing, humming, or hissing or is it loud and persistent? Is it intermittent or constant, unilateral or bilateral, and what, if anything, relieves the symptoms? Has the patient been taking medications such as aspirin? A thorough history, head and neck exam, and audiometric exams are warranted (Crummer & Hassan, 2004).

Vertigo

Vertigo is the illusion of rotational movement, tilting, or swaying with feelings of imbalance during standing and walking. More than 90 million Americans over the age of 17 years report vertigo to their health care providers (Sandhaus, 2002). It can be a symptom of serious central cerebral dysfunction (acoustic neuroma, brain tumor, or trauma) or a benign peripheral problem (semicircular canals, peripheral nerve). It is a cardinal symptom of vestibular dysfunction.

With objective vertigo the patient perceives moving surroundings and the body stays still. Subjective vertigo is just the reverse, with the perception that the body is moving and the surroundings are still. Nausea and vomiting may persist but loss of consciousness is not usually a problem. Other symptoms that the patient may experience include presyncope, disequilibrium, and light-headedness. Presyncope is a feeling of faintness. Disequilibrium is the feeling of falling. Light-headedness may be psychogenic or idiopathic. Peripheral causes are usually intensely vertiginous, whereas central causes are mildly vertiginous with nystagmus (Sandhaus, 2002). To rule out the possibility of other system involvement, all cranial nerves should be tested. Cardiac rate, rhythm, and orthostatic blood pressure, which can mimic positional vertigo, also should be checked.

The nurse needs to ask the patient to describe the physical sensation of vertigo. Has the patient fallen or been injured because of the vertigo? Does this vertigo happen when changing positions? Is it intermittent or constant? Is there any unsteadiness of gait? It is also important for the nurse to inquire about

MyNursingKit • Video: Eyes, Ears, Nose, Throat

current medications that may cause vertigo (Chapter 70 ☺). The assessment must include an evaluation of both prescription and OTC medications that may cause ototoxicity, which is hearing loss resulting from eighth cranial nerve (vestibulocochlear) damage, and sometimes loss of balance or vertigo. The patient needs to be referred to a health care provider for further testing for causes, such as brain tumors.

Hearing Loss, Tinnitus, Vertigo, and Medications

The combination of vertigo, tinnitus, and hearing loss can be very disabling for a person. Eighty-five percent of patients with tinnitus also have hearing loss. Ototoxic tinnitus can be caused by ACE inhibitors; some anesthetics, such as bupivacaine and lidocaine; and antibiotics, specifically gentamicin, sulfisoxazole, trimethoprim-sulfamethoxazole, and vancomycin (Jafek & Murrow, 2001).

Many patients who take medications, specifically salicylates, erythromycin, and loop diuretics, can develop bilateral and permanent ototoxic hearing loss. Loop diuretics damage stria vascularis in the organ of Corti. Aminoglycosides damage the cochlear hair cells, causing bilateral hearing loss and dizziness. Vancomycin's toxic effect results in high-frequency hearing loss, which may lead to permanent deafness. This occurs due to damage to the auditory receptor cells (Jafek & Murrow, 2001). Note that benign positional vertigo is usually not associated with hearing loss or tinnitus.

Infection or Drainage

The nurse needs to inquire about any spontaneous purulent, clear (cerebrospinal fluid), or bloody drainage. What is the consistency and amount of drainage? Is it unilateral or bilateral, acute or chronic? Does the patient have a fever, recent upper respiratory infection, cough, earache, or other symptoms that would indicate an infection? These questions all help diagnose infection. If present the patient needs referral to a health care provider for further evaluation and treatment.

Barotrauma

Barotrauma, which is physical injury or rupture of the tympanic membrane, results from changing air pressure (Mosby, 2002). The nurse should inquire about any problems with the ears subsequent to diving or an airplane flight. Has the patient had any sports injuries or been involved in a car crash? Air bags deploying in an enclosed space (car windows closed) can cause ear barotrauma.

Physical Examination

Ear conditions do not occur in isolation from the other body systems. For instance, checking the temperature of a patient with complaints of otalgia is important when assessing for infection. Checking the blood pressure and pulse of a patient who has symptoms of possible vestibular dysfunction such as vertigo is important to rule out cardiovascular conditions. All cranial nerves should be checked because their proper functioning or impairment in relation to ear, nose, and throat problems is integral to understanding the other body systems. For example, an abnormality of the facial nerve (CN VII) with asymmetric facial movements can suggest Bell's palsy or a cerebrovascular accident. Chapter 28 ☺ describes the assessment of the cranial nerves.

Inspection and Monitoring

External structures of the ear are inspected visually. The top of the ears should cross a line from the outer canthus of the eye. An auricle below this line or at a posterior angle greater than 10 degrees may indicate chromosomal aberrations. Inspect for size, symmetry, shape, skin color, redness, drainage, scaling or nodules (may be cancer or gout). If drainage is present, is it sanguineous, serous, mixed, purulent, or odiferous? Inspect the mastoid bone for size or color of skin. Note any tenderness.

The inside of the ear is inspected with an otoscope. An otoscopic examination includes inspection of the auditory canal and tympanic membrane. Look for inflammation, exudates, lesions, and foreign bodies. Check for narrowing of the ear canal, nodules, redness, scales, edema, and drainage. Normally the eardrum is slightly conical, shiny, smooth, and pearl gray. Cerumen should be moist and may vary in color from brown to white, but hardened, dry, or foul-smelling cerumen may indicate infection. In a majority of Asians and Native Americans, cerumen is dry, white, and flaky. In African Americans and Caucasians, cerumen is brown, wet, and sticky. Look for the structures of the tympanic membrane, for landmarks indicating the border of the annulus, the light reflex, umbo, the short process, and the long handle of the malleus. Note the color and presence of perforations, bulging, or retraction of the tympanic membrane, dilation of the vessels, bubbles, or fluid. Normal middle ear fluid is thin and amber (Anderson et al., 1998). To test the mobility of the tympanic membrane, a pneumatoscope is used. A **pneumatoscope** is an otoscope with a bulb attachment in which the nurse introduces air in to the ear canal and middle ear. A ruptured tympanic membrane will not move.

Palpation

During the physical assessment gently palpate the auricle (refer back to Figure 69–1 ■, p. 2285), which is the external ear or pinna, with the thumb and forefinger to check for tenderness, pain, or nodules. Palpate the mastoid behind the auricle. It should be smooth, hard, and nontender. Abnormalities of the auricle include Darwin's tubercle (a benign protrusion on the upper part of the helix). Keloid scar formation from ear piercing or trauma is common in African Americans. Sebaceous cysts in the meatus or in back of the auricle can become painful, as well as at nodules along the rim of auricle. Exostoses are benign bony lumps arising from the ear canal near the tympanic membrane. They are more frequent in men than women and originate from irritated periosteum from swimming in cold water (Sigler, 2002). The nurse should palpate the preauricular and postauricular lymph nodes (Jafek & Murrow, 2001).

Hearing Tests

During the nursing assessment the nurse observes for any obvious clues to hearing loss like asking for words to be repeated. If any hearing test abnormalities are found, the patient should be referred to an audiologist for further testing. Hearing acuity is tested to determine the presence of hearing loss and, if present, whether it is conductive or sensorineural. The **Weber test** screens hearing acuity and helps distinguish whether hearing loss is conductive or sensorineural. A tuning fork tapped at the base will emit a vibratory frequency range of 512 to 1,024 Hz, which corresponds to normal speech. When conducting the Weber test, place an activated tuning fork midline on top of the patient's head, bridge of the nose, or the chin. A negative or normal Weber test occurs when the patient perceives sound equally in both ears or "in the middle." Sound that lateralizes to the affected ear is conducted through bone and is a conductive hearing loss from external or middle ear disorders. Sound that lateralizes to the unaffected ear indicates nerve damage or sensorineural hearing loss from inner ear or auditory or brain pathology.

The **Rinne test** is used to measure the conduction of sound by bone. In this text an activated tuning fork is placed on the right and left mastoid bone sequentially. The patient should indicate when the sound is no longer heard. The tuning fork is then placed in front of the auditory canal. Normally air conduction through the external auditory canal is twice as long as with mastoid bone conduction. With a conductive hearing loss, bone conduction is greater than air conduction (Crummer & Hassan, 2004). With the **Schwabach test** the nurse places an activated tuning fork on the mastoid process of the patient and alternately tests for both air and bone conduction. With the **voice whisper test** the examiner stands approximately 1 to 2 feet in back of the patient and whispers several words near each ear. The patient should be able to hear bilaterally and equally.

Vestibular hearing function tests the receptors for the vestibular system, which are located in the semicircular ducts of the inner ear. The vestibular nerve fibers travel in the vestibulocochlear (VIII) cranial nerve to the vestibular nuclei of the oculomotor (III), trochlear (IV), and abducens (VI) cranial nerves. Disorders of the vestibular function can be peripheral, involving the labyrinth, or central, involving the vestibular connections. Abnormal nystagmus, tinnitus, or hearing loss are other common manifestations of vestibular dysfunction. Vestibular function tests are outlined in the Diagnostic Tests for Vestibular Function box in Chapter 70 👁 (p. 2310).

The **caloric test** is used to assess the abnormal nystagmus, tinnitus, or hearing loss that is a result of vestibular dysfunction. This test can differentiate peripheral lesions from eight cranial nerve lesions (Sandhaus, 2002). Warm or cold water is introduced into the ear. The normal response is vertigo and nystagmus within 30 to 60 seconds. When cold water is introduced into the left ear, the normal response is a right beating nystagmus. When warm water is introduced into the left ear, a left beating nystagmus is elicited (Jafek & Murrow, 2001). This test is only done on a person with an intact eardrum and no visible blood or fluid behind the tympanic membrane. A caloric test is done on an unconscious patient to test for severe brainstem injury. A patient with a brain injury does not have nystagmus.

The **Romberg test** assesses the patient's ability to maintain an upright posture when arms are out in front, with eyes open and closed. This is used to test for inner ear balance and the proprioceptive ability of the visual and cerebellar system.

Auscultation

When assessing for objective tinnitus, the nurse can auscultate over the head and neck, periauricular area, orbits, and mastoid and verify for audible sounds (Crummer & Hassan, 2004). If noted this indicates objective tinnitus is present and helps differentiate between subjective and objective tinnitus.

Ear Monitoring Equipment

In addition to the tests and monitoring equipment described earlier, the otoscope also is used to inspect the ear canal and tympanic membrane. Hearing aids remain the most common and effective interventional devices to correct hearing impairments.

Hearing aids should be checked for cleanliness. The audiologist can provide the patient with a small wire brush to remove built-up cerumen. In addition, patients should keep an extra supply of batteries on hand. Indications and types of hearing aids are discussed in detail in Chapter 70 👁 .

Health Promotion

To prevent hearing loss, individuals should avoid exposure to continuous, very loud noises as well as sudden, sharp loud noises. It is important for persons who are exposed to very noisy environments to wear hearing protection to prevent hearing loss. Swimmers may be at risk for frequent ear infections and should be encouraged to wear earplugs when in the water. Patients should be advised not to dry their ears after bathing with an applicator or any other small object. Gently use the end of a towel to remove excess water or use a cotton ball to wick the water out. Some people develop excess cerumen, which can cause temporary hearing loss, and need periodically to have the nurse remove the cerumen by irrigation.

◼ Nose and Paranasal Sinuses

The nose is the external opening of the respiratory system (refer back to Figure 69–3 ◼, p. 2286). It warms, moistens, filters air, and provides a sense of smell. The nasal cavity is surrounded by paranasal sinuses, which lighten the skull, help speaking, and produce mucus (refer back to Figure 69–4 ◼, p. 2286). Obstruction of the nasal passages due to inflammation, infection, or neoplasms can occur.

Current Health and Risk Factors

Proper functioning of the nose and paranasal sinuses is essential for an adequate airway. The nurse assesses these areas both subjectively and objectively, as discussed later. The external disorders of the nose are related to the skin. Chapter 66 👁 discusses skin disorders that occur on the face and nose.

Current Issue

Medical conditions that impair proper nasal airway functioning need immediate attention and include pain, headache, difficulty breathing, bleeding and drainage, trauma, sense of smell, sneezing, and sleep patterns/obstructive sleep apnea. It is important to assess when the symptoms began, what brings them on, whether they are intermittent or constant, and what relieves them.

Pain

The source of pain in the nose or paranasal sinuses may be infection, trauma, or tumor. Poor preventive care of teeth and gums can be a source of infections that can spread to the sinuses and cause pain. Sinusitis or rhinosinusitis is the most common health problem in the United States (Smith & Osborne, 2003). Human immunodeficiency virus (HIV) can cause severe sinusitis from gram-negative and opportunistic infections. Chapter 60 👁 includes a complete description of HIV.

Headache

When the source of the headache is the nose and paranasal sinuses, the nurse should inquire about the frequency, intensity, and duration of the headache that localizes to the sinuses. Inquire if the headache is accompanied by nasal congestion, maxilla or dental pain, fetid breath, fever, or lethargy (Smith & Osborne,

2003). If headaches persist or become worse, the patient needs to be referred for diagnostic testing of the sinus tracks.

Difficulty Breathing

Inquire about the circumstances that occur when the patient has difficulty breathing. In addition to investigating cardiac and respiratory causes, difficulty breathing due to nasal problems can be caused by obstruction, infection, or inflammation. Inquire about a history of allergies, and upper respiratory infections and self or medical treatment. Inflammation and edema from eustachian tubes extending to the nasal mucosa may obstruct airflow between the middle ear and nose. An assessment of the lungs would assist in ruling out pulmonary versus upper airway causes of the shortness of breath.

Bleeding or Drainage

Bleeding or other drainage from the nose needs to be investigated in relation to a primary or secondary cause. Epistaxis, or blood draining from the nose, occurs in approximately 10% of the population at any age (Sigler, 2002). It can be caused by hypertension, malignancy, coagulation defects, or trauma or its causes may be idiopathic. Inquire about clear drainage from the nose, especially if the patient has had recent head trauma, because this might indicate cerebrospinal fluid leak. The nurse needs to evaluate the type, amount, and frequency of nasal drainage as well as any associated symptoms.

Trauma

A history of trauma to the nose such as a fracture may cause a deviated septum, which can obstruct breathing. A deviated septum also may be congenital. The obstruction is typically unilateral, and can be surgically corrected to reopen the nasal passage. Other trauma to the nose includes burns, abrasions, and lacerations. Each of these situations needs to be assessed and appropriate referrals made for treatment.

Sense of Smell

The sense of smell can be partially or completely impaired due to obstruction from trauma, polyps, sinus infections, hormonal disorders, and dental problems. Patients who receive radiation therapy for head and neck cancer also can have diminished sense of smell (National Institute on Deafness and Other Communication Disorders, 2002a). Under normal circumstances, the sense of smell diminishes slightly with age. **Anosmia** is the complete loss of smell. It can be associated with the presence of nasal polyps (Sigler, 2002). To test the sense of smell, use a variety of pungent substances such as cloves and vanilla to assess the olfactory nerve (CN I).

Sneezing

The nurse needs to inquire about a history of upper respiratory infection. Sneezing, particularly at specific times of the year or under specific environmental circumstances, should be investigated for the possibility of allergies or respiratory infection. **Allergic rhinitis** is an inflammation of the nasal mucosa caused by an allergic substance, for example, hay fever or pollen (Tierney, McPhee, & Papadakis, 2001). The nurse needs to inquire if the allergies are related to a specific time of year. Does the patient regularly take medications for allergic rhinitis, sinus infections, stuffy nose, or frequent respiratory infections? Some nasal sprays and decongestants may cause rebound nasal swelling. OTC oral decongestants may have an adverse effect on patients with diabetes, hypertension, hyperthyroidism, and cardiac illnesses.

Sleep Patterns/Obstructive Sleep Apnea

Sleep patterns need to be assessed by the nurse. Disorders of sleep related to the nasal passage range from habitual snoring to **obstructive sleep apnea (OSA)** (Gupta & Reiter, 2004). OSA is defined as brief periods of breathing cessation or a marked reduction in tidal volume with a minimum of five episodes of apnea per hour during sleep accompanied by excessive daytime somnolence (Flemmons, 2002). Patients with severe obesity, cardiac conditions, hypertension, increased neck circumference, craniofacial abnormalities, hypothyroidism, and acromegaly are at increased risk of OSA (Flemmons, 2002; Gupta & Reiter, 2004). The usual treatments include continuous positive airway pressure (CPAP) at night or oral appliances. Additionally, a variety of surgical procedures can be used to relieve OSA, including palatoplasty, septoplasty, tonsillectomy, tracheostomy, and turbinate reduction. Newer innovative technologies include genioglossus or hyoid advancement, tongue-base reduction, and laser palatoplasty (Gupta & Reiter, 2004).

Physical Examination

The nose should be examined for external and internal problems. The sinuses need to be assessed by palpation, inspection with transillumination, and percussion of the frontal and maxillary sinuses. The absence of transillumination reveals mucosal thickening or sinus fullness. Tenderness with gentle percussion reveals fullness in the sinus cavity. These assessments are described later.

Inspection

During the physical exam the nurse inspects the nose for contour, symmetry, and color, and its relationship to other facial structures (Anderson et al., 1998). The face is assessed for the presence of edema around the nose and eyes. The external nose is inspected for deformities, tumors or masses, dryness or ulcerations, and signs of trauma or bleeding. Nostrils should be symmetrical and without nasal flaring, which indicates increased respiratory effort.

To inspect the internal nasal passages, use a penlight, a nasal speculum, or a nasopharyngeal mirror to assess for color abnormalities, lesions, swelling, drainage, and bleeding. The nasal membrane is normally redder than the mouth, but can be pale, edematous, and bluish gray in patients who have allergic rhinitis. Inspect the nasal mucosa for bleeding and the nasal septum for perforation or deviation. To check for patency and airflow, ask the patient to occlude one nare at a time and breathe. Air movement may be impeded if the patient has a deviated septum, polyps, foreign body obstruction, allergies, or an upper respiratory infection. Observe any drainage and note the consistency and any postnasal drip, bleeding, or blood-tinged mucus.

Palpation

The nose and frontal and maxillary paranasal (frontal and maxillary) sinuses are palpated to detect fullness, tenderness, displacement, movement, crepitus, or edema. In a darkened room use a penlight against the patient's cheek to transluminate through the roof of the mouth. Normally a faint glow can be seen through the bones of the sinuses, but with sinusitis there is absent or diminished light transmission. The nurse also needs to palpate the submaxillary and submental lymph nodes for swelling.

Percussion

The nurse percusses the periorbital and nasal sinuses for tenderness. Under normal circumstances these areas should not be painful. Tenderness or pain may indicate an allergic sinusitis, trauma, or an infectious process (Dillon, 2003). Discuss the pain with the patient, identifying specific areas of discomfort, and inquire about any recent injury to the area.

Nose and Paranasal Sinuses Monitoring Equipment

The equipment needed to monitor the nose and paranasal sinuses includes a flashlight to transilluminate the sinuses, an otoscope with a nasal speculum, and an oxygen saturation monitor. The nurse should monitor oxygenation routinely for any patient with a nasal or sinus problem. Oxygen saturation should be maintained between 93% and 100% for individuals with normal lung function. It is important to assess the range within which a particular patient stays. If the oxygen level is not adequate, supplementary oxygen should be provided. In addition, the nose and paranasal sinuses should be monitored for the amount, type, and color of mucous production. Frequently nose and sinus congestion causes pain, and a valid and reliable pain scale should be used on admission and throughout the hospital stay to assess the results of the treatment.

Health Promotion

Sinus pain is a common reason patients self-medicate and visit the doctor. It is important to caution the patient to not self-medicate and to instead consult a health care provider or nurse practitioner regarding appropriate remedies. It may helpful for the patient with chronic sinus congestion to address the possible allergic basis of the sinusitis and try to eliminate or minimize allergen exposure in daily life.

Mouth

The mouth is an integral part of the respiratory and alimentary tract. The mouth is used for eating, speaking, and breathing. The mouth includes the lips, gingiva, buccal mucosa, and tongue.

Current Health and Risk Factors

Good health of the mouth allows people to function at the most basic levels: breathing and eating. A systematic assessment of the mouth can reveal local and systemic problems that need to be addressed. When assessing the mouth the nurse can promote health when observing dental and gingival disease or poorly fitting dentures. In addition, health promotion activities regarding hydration and nutrition can be incorporated into the assessment. The nurse can also assess the patient's self-care abilities. Inquire about how frequently the patient visits the dentist, brushes, and flosses teeth. Refer back to Figure 69–5 ■, p. 2286, which displays the structures of the mouth.

Current Issue

The disorders of the mouth include fetid breath, change in taste, poor dentition, pain, change in voice, infection and inflammation, and trismus. During the assessment the nurse must inquire about the occurrence of any of these problems, how often they occur, and what treatment has been sought.

Fetid Breath

Fetid breath, or halitosis, may be a symptom of tooth decay, poor oral hygiene, gum, and tonsil or sinus disease. Fruity breath commonly occurs with patients who are malnourished or in diabetic ketoacidosis. A musty smell to the breath, or fetor hepaticus, is the result of liver failure and nitrogenous breakdown. The odor of ammonia is caused by end-stage renal disease.

Poor Dentition

The dental assessment includes evaluating the patient for any difficulty with chewing or swallowing. Poorly fitting dentures or orthotic appliances and inadequate dentition can cause difficulty chewing, nutritional problems, and mouth sores. Ask the patient if partial or full dentures are worn. Tooth loss resulting from oral disease may affect normal closure of mouth and jaw alignment. Inquire about dental habits such as flossing of teeth, frequency of brushing, how often the teeth are professionally cleaned, and occurrence of dental caries.

Infection and Inflammation

An infection or inflammation of the pharynx or tonsil can be detected easily by observing the condition of the mucosa, presence of drainage, and pain. A yellow or green streaked posterior pharynx indicates postnasal drainage. A gray membrane is indicative of diphtheria. White exudative patches with a reddened mucosa (exudative pharyngitis) are the result of streptococcal, chlamydial, or gonorrheal bacteria or a virus. Tonsillitis and peritonsillar abscess with erythema and exudates are also visible upon inspection (Dillon, 2003).

Trismus

Trismus is restricted jaw movement from shrinkage of connective tissue in the posterior mandibular or temporomandibular region. It is usually due to radiation treatment for head and neck cancer, trauma, infection, surgery (MedicineNet, 2007) or structural abnormalities, or it may be a symptom of temporomandibular joint syndrome.

Physical Examination

The physical examination of the mouth is essential to understand the systemic problems of the patient as well as local conditions. The mouth reveals much about the overall nutritional state. The National Guidelines box (p. 2296) lists oral assessment guidelines.

Inspection

Inspect the mouth for color, moisture, and lesions and the overall condition of teeth, gingiva, tonsils, uvula, and hard and soft palate. Normally the mouth is pink and moist with intact mucous membranes, no lesions, and no alteration in taste. Inquire whether the patient has experienced a change in taste. Fluid intake and output need to be assessed because signs of dehydration can be observed in the dry mucosa.

 *A healthy oral cavity can reflect general good health. Poor nutrition and hydration are revealed in problems with the gingiva, lips, and tongue.*

Inspect the hard and soft palate for ulcerations or lesions (Chart 69–2, p. 2296). Normally the hard and soft palates are concave and pink. The hard palate has many ridges and the soft

MyNursingKit | Video: Health and Physical Assessment: Mouth/Throat—Oral Examination

NATIONAL GUIDELINES for Oral Assessment

Area to Be Observed	Rating 1 Normal	Rating 2 Mild Abnormality	Rating 3 Severe Abnormality
Voice	Normal	Deep, rasp, hoarse	Difficulty talking, pain
Swallow reflex	Normal	Some pain on swallowing	Unable to swallow
Lips	Smooth, pink, moist	Dry, cracked	Ulcerated or bleeding
Tongue	Pink, moist, papillae present	Coated or loss of papillae with a shiny appearance, with or without redness	Blistered or cracked
Saliva	Watery	Thick	Absent
Mucous membrane	Pink and moist	Reddened or coated, without ulceration	Ulcerated with or without bleeding
Gingiva	Pink, stippled, and firm	Edematous with or without redness	Spontaneous bleeding or bleeding with pressure
Teeth or denture-bearing area	Clean with no debris	Plaque or debris in localized area if teeth are present	Plaque or debris generalized along gum line or denture-bearing area

Source: National Guideline Clearinghouse. (2004). *Nursing management of oral hygiene.* Retrieved February 17, 2007, from http://www.guideline.gov/summary/summary.aspx?doc_id=7153&nbr= 004285&string=ear+AND+nose+AND+throat.

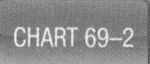

CHART 69–2 Signs and Symptoms of Oral and Pharyngeal Cancer

Sore that bleeds easily and does not heal

Lump or thickening

Red or white patch that persists

Difficulties chewing, swallowing, or moving tongue or jaw—late symptoms

Source: American Cancer Society. (2006). *Cancer facts and figures 2006.* Atlanta, GA: Author.

---

palate is smooth. White patches in the mouth could be *Candida albicans*, streptococcal infection, leukoplakia, or a precancerous condition. Note the color, pigmentation, ulcers, or nodules.

To assess for trismus, ask the patient to open the mouth widely. There should be no restricted jaw movement or pain. Palpate the temporomandibular joint (TMJ) just below the earlobe where the mandible and maxilla join. Assess for sounds or clicks or friction sounds. Assess for pain and restricted jaw movement when opening the mouth. Gently palpate the trachea for deviation, mobility, tenderness, and consistency. Avoid firm palpation, because it will cause gagging. With a folded gauze pad and a tongue blade, inspect the mucosa around the tongue.

Health Promotion

To maintain good oral health, the patient should see the dentist at regular intervals and use good oral hygiene measures. Because the use of tobacco in any form and the excessive use of alcoholic beverages are the primary risk factors in the development of oral cancer, it is important for the nurse to encourage the cessation of tobacco and excessive alcohol use (American Cancer Society, 2006; National Guideline Clearinghouse, 2004).

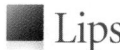 ## Lips

The lips function to keep food and saliva in the mouth during chewing, and they help form words and facial expressions. The proper functioning of the lips reflects the patient's state of health. The lips are a sphincter muscle, the orbicularis oris covered by skin externally and internally by mucous membrane. The sensory receptors in lips help judge the temperature and texture of food.

Current Health and Risk Factors

The lips are an important part of the physical examination of the oral cavity. The lips can develop local problems and can reflect systemic problems. The chief complaint is most frequently related to hydration, ulcerations, lesions, bleeding, and infections.

Hydration

When a person is hydrated their lips are moist and pink to brown in color. Dehydration produces cheilitis or dry and cracked lips. Dehydration can develop from poor intake of fluids, diuretics, sun exposure, or fever.

Color

Lip color may be an indicator of more systemic problems. Cyanosis can indicate hypoxia or vasoconstriction. A cold body temperature also will cause the lips to become cyanotic. Pale lips may be a clinical manifestation of anemia. Reddened lips reveal an infectious or inflammatory disorder.

Ulcerations, Lesions, or Bleeding

Lesions can reveal a generalized inflammatory disorder. Any local lesion on the lip needs to be evaluated for the possibility of basal cell or squamous cell cancer, infections, or nutritional deficiencies. Cheilosis, manifested by increased moisture in the corners of the mouth, reflects a riboflavin deficiency, poorly fitting dentures, or immune deficiencies. Bleeding from the lips can occur as a result of certain drugs that cause a deficiency in clotting mechanisms or from some congenitally acquired conditions that manifest as generalized bleeding disorders.

Infections

Local and systemic infections commonly appear on the lips. A local viral infection called herpes simplex, or a cold sore, can commonly appear on the lips. A chancre on the lips is a painless ulcer of primary syphilis.

Physical Inspection

During the physical exam the color, moisture, swelling, lesions, or other signs of inflammation in and around the lips are assessed. Lips should be moist, pink or darker and have no lesions, bleeding, dryness, or swelling. Local problems that can easily be inspected are asymmetrical lips resulting from a congenital deformity, for example, a cleft lip, or from trauma, paralysis, or surgical intervention. Many systemic problems can be revealed by inspecting the lips. Fissures at the corners of the lips or cheilosis reveals a vitamin B deficiency. Swollen, inflamed lips are a sign of an allergic response called angioedema. Drying and cracking lips or cheilitis (inflammation of the lips) can occur from allergies and lip licking.

Palpation

When palpating the lips for tenderness and consistency, use the gloved thumb and forefinger to gently pull down on the lower lip and pull up on the upper lip. Palpating the lips should reveal soft tissue and the lips should be nontender and have no masses. Abnormal masses or lesions should be noted and followed up.

Health Promotion

Implications for health promotion as it relates to lips should focus on encouraging the patient to use lip gloss with sunscreen protection. Use of any type of tobacco should be avoided because it can cause lip cancer. A patient with cheilosis needs nutritional counseling to improve dietary intake. The use of a daily multivitamin might be helpful. A patient with cyanotic lips may need to be referred to cardiac rehabilitation to maximize cardiac efficiency. A patient with pale lips may need to have a complete physical examination to assess the reason for the anemia.

■ Gingiva and Teeth

Gingiva (gums) is a dense, strong oral mucosa that provides the support for and surrounds the teeth. Adults normally have 28 to 32 teeth if the third and fourth molars have erupted. The teeth function to cut, grind, and chew food. The muscles of mastication are innervated by the trigeminal (CN V) and facial (CN VII) cranial nerves.

Current Health and Risk Factors

The condition of the gingiva and teeth reflects the patient's health habits and nutrition and can reflect the side effects of treatment for some conditions. With the aging process bone resorption and receding and pale gingiva can make the teeth appear larger. The teeth and gingiva can have problems with inflammation and drainage; teeth become loose, broken, or fall out, and gingiva is subject to gingival hypertrophy.

Purulent drainage from the gingiva can occur from an infectious process such as upper respiratory infections or a local abscess. Other inflammations can occur from poorly fitting dentures, leukemia, and HIV. *Candida albicans* can occur with white patches overlying reddened inflamed gingiva (Dillon, 2003). Periodontitis is inflammation of the area around the teeth. Brownish colored gums may reflect Addison's disease. Loose, broken, or missing teeth may result from general poor oral care, poor nutrition, or trauma. Gingival hypertrophy is a painless hyper-

plasia that can occur with pregnancy and some medications including phenytoin and calcium channel blockers (Dillon, 2003).

Physical Examination

The teeth and gingiva are integral to the eating and drinking of fluids. Their poor health can have an impact on overall health. The essential nursing physical assessment of the teeth and gingiva is described next. Referral to dental specialists is appropriate for routine care and treatment.

Inspection

Ask the patient to open his mouth. Does the patient have his own teeth, full dentures, partial dentures, or orthodontic appliances? Count the upper and lower teeth. The 32 teeth (or 28 if the third molars have been extracted) should be white and firmly set in the gingiva, with good occlusion. Are the teeth in good condition or do they have caries? Ask the patient when he last visited the dentist and how often he receives preventive care for his teeth. Observe for exposed root of the tooth from receding gums. If the patient wears dentures, do they fit well? A patient with loose teeth, dental decay, and discolored teeth should be referred to a dentist. The patient's breath should smell fresh.

Observe for redness, tenderness, edema, retraction, discoloration, or easy bleeding of the gingiva. This can represent gingivitis, scurvy, or poorly fitting dentures. Pale mucous membranes can be an indication that the patient is anemic. Oral cancer lesions usually associated with smoking and alcohol use can present on gums. Any lesion should be investigated by the health care provider.

Health Promotion

Dental visits should occur at regular intervals. Patients should be taught to floss their teeth to remove plaque and help with gingival health. A patient with gingival hypertrophy should visit the dentist more frequently and use a soft toothbrush to avoid irritation.

■ Buccal Mucosa

The buccal mucosa consists of the gingiva and the hard and soft palate. The palate forms the roof of the mouth and separates the mouth from the oropharynx. It is divided into the anterior hard palate and the posterior soft palate. The soft palate is flexible with chewing and swallowing and is covered with a thin mucosa membrane that extends to the uvula.

Current Health and Risk Factors

The oral mucosa is easy to assess for local and systemic problems. General nutritional status, infections, tumors, mouth sores, and pain can be easily identified. Normal oral mucosa is pink, moist, and intact and has no lesions. Poor nutritional status is seen in swollen, dry, and red mucosa. Mouth infections can occur especially when there is poor nutrition and inadequate dental care. Patients who use antibiotics or have HIV are susceptible to oral candidiasis, which manifests as white patches on an inflamed mucosa (Dillon, 2003).

Cancer of the mouth can occur on any part of the oral mucosa. The chance of developing oral cancer increases with habitual drinking of alcohol and the use of smoking and chewing tobacco. The symptoms of oral cancer are nonhealing lip or mouth sores, a mass in the mouth or throat, leukoplakia, bleeding, pain or numbness, chronic sore throat, foreign body sensation in the mouth or throat, dysphasia, a voice change, or ear pain (American Cancer Society, 2006).

Leukoplakia is a white adherent mucosal coating, which may lead to cancer. Stomatitis, also called mucositis, can occur as a secondary problem with patients who have decreased immune status, and as a consequence of radiation therapy or chemotherapy from cancer treatment. Canker sores, or herpes simplex, can occur with some frequency in some people.

It is important for the nurse to inquire about the location, duration, and intensity of mouth pain. Does the patient have a sore throat, and dental, jaw, or mouth pain, or any pain opening the jaw? The nurse needs to assess whether or not the patient has trismus which is restricted jaw movement and pain (Dillon, 2003).

Physical Examination

The normal buccal mucosa is moist, color consistent with that of gingiva, intact, and without bleeding or sores. When assessing the mouth the following areas should be evaluated: voice, swallow reflex, lips, tongue, saliva, mucous membrane, gingiva, teeth, or denture-bearing area.

Inspection

Prior to inspecting the mouth the nurse needs to request that the patient remove her dentures or other mouth prosthesis. The palate, dentures, and gingiva were discussed earlier. Inspect the tonsils for the presence or absence of edema, spots, exudates, lesions, or drainage. Tonsils are graded from 1+ (visible), 2+ (between pillars and uvula), 3+ (touching the uvula), to 4+ (one or both tonsils extend to the midline of the oropharynx).

Approximately 1,500 mL of saliva is produced daily by the Wharton's ducts, Stenson's ducts, parotid (beneath each ear), submandibular, sublingual (on the floor of the mouth), and buccal glands (the lips and cheeks). Wharton's ducts contain about 20 papillae and are located at the openings for the submandibular glands at the base of the tongue on either side of the frenulum. They should be patent, be secreting saliva, and be without lesions or inflammation.

Palpation

Palpate the oral mucosa with a gloved hand. Stenson's ducts, the openings for the parotid glands, are found at the second molars. Palpate with a gloved hand the floor of the mouth for swelling or tenderness of the tonsillar and submental lymph nodes. Note any palpable nodules, which may indicate cancer. Palpating the back of the oral cavity with a tongue blade will make the patient gag. This tests the sensory function of the hypoglossal nerve (CN IX) and the motor function of the vagus nerve (CN X).

Health Promotion

The National Guidelines box (p. 2296) recommends best practices for oral health include tooth brushing with fluoridated toothpaste twice a day. Avoid using hydrogen peroxide unless prescribed by a dentist or a health care provider.

■ Tongue

The tongue is a muscular organ essential to speaking and chewing food. The anterior two-thirds of the tongue is covered with papillae, which contain approximately 10,000 taste buds. People identify five different tastes: sweet, bitter, salty, and umami (glutamate found in chicken broth, meat extracts, and some cheeses) (National Institute on Deafness and Other Communication Disorders, 2002b). The intrinsic and extrinsic muscles of the tongue help move food during mastication. The extrinsic muscles are used during swallowing and speech.

Current Health and Risk Factors

The tongue can reflect the general health and local problems. Abnormalities of the tongue include inflammatory or infectious lesions, enlargement, allergic reactions, limited movement, and loss of sense of taste. Glossitis, an inflammation of the tongue, can be caused by chemotherapy or a vitamin B_{12}, iron, or niacin deficiency. *Candida albicans*, or thrush, can cause a thick white coating or redness on the tongue. Thrush can be caused by changes in normal flora from chemotherapy or radiation therapy, AIDS, antibiotic therapy, or alcohol, tobacco, or cocaine use (Dillon, 2003).

An enlarged tongue can occur with myxedema, acromegaly, Down's syndrome, or amyloidosis. Infectious processes such as glossitis can cause enlargement of the tongue. An allergic reaction can cause an enlarged tongue and subsequently compromise the airway.

A tongue that cannot move normally or a tongue paralyzed from trauma to CN XII or syringobulbia will cause difficulty with speaking and eating. A patient who has had a cerebrovascular accident may have limited movements of the tongue.

Sense of Taste

About 200,000 people each year visit health care providers with complaints of problems with their sense of taste. It frequently is associated with problems with their sense of smell. Loss of a sense of taste can be temporary or permanent. A diminished sense of taste is called hypogeusia. A complete loss of a sense of taste is called ageusia. Diminished sense of taste can be congenital, but it usually occurs from a head injury or an illness such as upper respiratory disorder. Exposure to chemicals such as insecticides and some medicines can cause a diminished sense of taste (National Institute on Deafness and Other Communication Disorders, 2002b). Patients who have received radiation therapy for head and neck cancer may have a diminished sense of taste. In addition, taste disorders can occur concurrently with obesity, diabetes, hypertension, malnutrition, Parkinson's disease, Alzheimer's disease, smoking, and Korsakoff's psychosis. The elderly experience changes in taste with less distinct perception of sweetness, reduced saliva, and thinner mucosa (National Institute on Deafness and Other Communication Disorders, 2002b).

Physical Examination

The tongue has multiple functions, each of which needs to be assessed during a physical examination. Changes or abnormalities of the tongue may indicate both a local and systemic disorder. The nurse must document and report changes to the health care provider.

Inspection

The tongue should be midline; the dorsum should be pink, moist, and rough (taste buds) and have no lesions. It should move freely and have symmetrical strength. The ventral surface should have large blood vessels visible, no lesions and no inflammation.

During the assessment the nurse evaluates the patient's ability to speak and swallow. The patient may need referral to a speech therapist who will evaluate and treat the speech deficit. Referral for a swallow study may be necessary if paralysis is present. The risk of aspiration increases with tongue paralysis.

To assess for proper functioning of the hypoglossal nerve (CN XII), ask the patient to stick out her tongue. Observe the dorsal surface for color, hydration, texture, symmetry, fasciculation, atrophy, position in the mouth, and the presence of lesions. There should be no pain, ulcerations, or lesions. The tongue should be pink, moist, symmetrical, and midline. The patient should be able to move the tongue up and down and side to side. Ask the patient to press the tongue against the cheek on each side. Also ask the patient to touch the tip of the tongue to the roof of the mouth. Ask the patient to taste and identify several different kinds of flavors. The ventral surface should be moist, rough from taste buds, have prominent blood vessels, and have no lesions.

Palpation

Palpate the submandibular glands in front of the ear. Use your gloved finger on the outside of the cheek to press against the tongue to assess bilateral tongue strength.

Tongue Monitoring Equipment

The nurse should use a gloved hand and a tongue blade to look carefully at all areas of the tongue. In addition, asking a patient to swallow a small sip of water will help assess swallowing. Listening to the patient speak will help assess speech and tongue movements. Test the patient's taste with sweet, bitter, salty, and many other flavors.

Health Promotion

To prevent allergic reactions to environmental allergens and medications that might cause edema of the tongue, the patient should wear a medic alert bracelet. Patient's who have allergies to bee stings should carry and be given instructions about how to use an EpiPen. A patient who has trouble swallowing because of limited tongue movement needs to be referred to a speech and swallowing therapist to learn techniques to swallow without choking or pocketing food. Any patient with a lesion on the tongue needs to see a health care provider who can diagnose and treat it.

◼ Pharynx and Larynx

The pharynx and larynx integrate components of the respiratory, neurological, lymphatic, endocrine, vascular, and musculoskeletal systems. The larynx includes the supraglottis, glottis, and subglottis, the thyroid cartilage, and vocal cords. The trachea is a flexible cylindrical tube, 2.5 cm by 11 cm, extending in front of the esophagus from the cricoid cartilage to right and left bronchi. The trachea has C-shaped hyaline cartilage rings that protect the airway. The trachea is a passageway for air, and the esophagus is a passageway for food. Thyroid cartilage, cricoid cartilage, and epiglottis surround the larynx.

Current Health and Risk Factors

The patient may present with problems originating in the pharynx or larynx with difficulty speaking, breathing, or having a sense of a lump in his throat. These symptoms can be the result of tumor, infection or inflammation, foreign body, or trauma to the neck and may be very painful. The patient should be encouraged to seek immediate treatment to preserve the airway. The patient's habits are also important to assess, including smoking and/or alcohol intake, because it is frequently associated with cancer of the vocal cord or larynx. A smoking history is expressed as packs per day for a number of years. Alcohol history is expressed as the number of drinks per day, kind of alcohol, and the number of years of drinking. Has the patient had any change in voice recently? Has the patient had any episodes of respiratory distress?

Tumors of the head and neck particularly occur with slow-growing basal cell carcinoma and rapidly invasive squamous cell carcinoma. Inquire about the patient's use of tobacco and ingesting alcohol. Diagnosis and treatment of head and neck cancer are discussed in Chapter 34 🔗. A partial or total laryngectomy is the permanent removal of the voice box. From then on the patient breathes through the neck and will have to learn alternative methods of communication such as esophageal speech.

Neck and throat infections may be life threatening because of the potential to cause airway compromise. Epiglottitis, for example, is an infection of the supraglottic larynx usually caused by *Haemophilus influenzae* type B. Pharyngitis, which may include the tonsils, palate, and uvula, may be caused by bacteria, viruses, and fungi. An infection of the tonsils, tonsillitis, can be caused by bacteria or viruses. Inadequate treatment of tonsillitis may cause a peritonsillar abscess or quinsy sore throat.

A foreign body in the trachea requires emergency treatment. The Heimlich maneuver can be useful in dislodging the foreign body. If unsuccessful, take the patient to the emergency department immediately.

Trauma to the neck can occur from a sports injury or violence or may be work related and it can cause airway compromise and vocal change. Trauma damage requires immobilization, an x-ray, and immediate treatment to preserve the damaged airway.

Change in Voice

Change in the sound of the voice can occur from an infectious process, such as epiglottitis, or from neoplasms and chronic smoking. It also may occur from vocal cord paralysis, which is more common in elderly men than women. Thyroid surgery, anterior cervical fusion or carotid endarterectomy, and cancer of larynx and lung are the most common causes of vocal cord paralysis (Sigler, 2002). Vocal cord paralysis is a particularly important issue because of the potential for dyspnea and stridor to accompany it (Sigler, 2002). Inquire about how long the voice change has been present, whether it is getting worse, and whether there any other associated symptoms. Does the patient have difficulty swallowing food and saliva, which would indicate the presence of a mass? Chart 69–2 (p. 2296) in the chapter outlines the signs and symptoms of oral cancer. The patient's voice should be normal without any hoarseness, be clear and spontaneous, and not have a nasal intonation.

 *The nurse must investigate any changes in voice because they could relate to airway obstruction. The first priority is to assess oxygenation, so begin by checking the oxygen saturation and vital signs. Assess for shortness of breath. Report abnormal assessment findings to the health care provider.*

Physical Examination

The physical examination should address whether the patient has any of the above problems. Knowledge of normal anatomy of the structures of the neck is essential. It takes time and practice to learn how to inspect and palpate the thyroid, carotid artery, and lymph nodes.

Inspection

Observe the trachea for inflammation, pain, excessive salivation or dryness, drainage, masses, and lymphoid tissue in the throat. Inspect the neck in a neutral position and when hyperextended. It should be erect and midline and have no tracheal deviation or visible lumps, bulges, or masses. Involuntary contraction of the neck so that the neck tips to the side is acquired or congenital torticollis. Inspect the lower third of the neck for enlargement of the thyroid. Normally the thyroid is not visible and has no masses, swelling, or hypertrophy. Any enlargements may indicate malignant or benign disorders or infectious processes. Are lymph nodes visible or is the jugular vein distended? Is the patient in any respiratory distress? Does the patient have full range of motion of the neck?

Swallow and gag reflexes are tested with a tongue blade touching the back of the mouth, which causes gagging to occur. To test the glossopharyngeal nerve (CN IX) and vagus nerve (CN X), use a tongue depressor to press down on the tongue when the patient says "aaah." Note the rise and fall of the uvula and check for symmetry, edema, or discharge.

Palpation

Palpate the preauricular, postauricular, tonsillar, submandibular, and submental lymph nodes along the mandible between two fingers to determine the dimension, texture, and consistency. Palpable lymph nodes should be described according to shape, dimension, size, consistency, masses, crepitus, mobility, and tenderness. Palpable lymph nodes should be soft to rubbery, freely mobile, distinct, round, and nontender. Because the thyroid gland moves as a person swallows, ask the patient to swallow while palpating the thyroid gland from the anterior or posterior. An enlarged thyroid gland indicates thyroid disease, and further laboratory tests are warranted. Palpate the trachea for normal midline position and the absence of crepitus. Does the patient complain of any pain during palpation?

Auscultation

If a mass is palpated, auscultate the thyroid gland with the bell of the stethoscope over each lobe to identify a possible bruit. Normally there should be no thyroid sounds. Sounds are sometimes associated with hyperthyroidism (Dillon, 2003). Auscultate the larynx and trachea for breath sounds.

Pharynx and Larynx Monitoring Equipment

Patients who have pharyngeal or laryngeal problems may need to be assessed with a tongue blade and flashlight to inspect for pharyngeal tumors or drainage, and/or to test the gag reflex. Some patients need to have their oxygen saturation monitored. Some patients are dependent on alternative methods of breathing, for example, a patient with a tracheostomy, laryngectomy, or endotracheal or nasopharyngeal tube.

Health Promotion

The most important implication for health promotion measures that patients can take is to avoid the use of any tobacco products and minimize the use of alcohol. Patients who are on antibiotics need to be reminded to complete the cycle of medications. Families need to be taught the Heimlich maneuver.

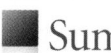 Summary

Diseases of the ear, nose, and throat are some of the most common health problems that bring a patient to seek health care. The nurse has an important role in assessing the potential and actual problems associated with these disorders. Promoting healthy behaviors in relation to the ears, nose, and throat can help reduce the cost of health care. Early treatment can prevent increasing disability.

NCLEX® REVIEW

1. A patient's ear canal is shiny with brown sticky cerumen. The nurse would consider these findings as being:

   1. An infection.
   2. Normal.
   3. Evidence of a foreign body.
   4. Abnormal exudate.

2. A patient begins to sneeze soon after entering an examination room. Which of the following should the nurse ask this patient?

   1. How long have you had a head cold?
   2. How long have you been using nasal sprays?
   3. Has anyone ever told you that you snore when asleep?
   4. Do you think that there is something in the room causing you to sneeze?

3. An elderly patient has several sores on his gums and tells the nurse that he hasn't been to a dentist since he received his dentures. Which of the following should the nurse respond to this patient?

   1. Maybe you should stop wearing the dentures.
   2. Even though you have dentures, seeing a dentist regularly is necessary for good oral health.
   3. I'm sure that you don't miss going to the dentist.
   4. Those sores will heal; just give it some time.

4. An elderly patient sits quietly and does not engage in conversation with those seated nearby. The nurse realizes this patient might be experiencing:

   1. Mental status changes.
   2. Dementia.
   3. Social isolation because of hearing loss.
   4. Antisocial behavior disorder.

5. A patient is unable to hear words that the nurse whispers to the health care provider who is standing about two feet away from the patient. The nurse would interpret this finding as being:

1. Normal.

2. Evidence of hearing loss in the ear closest to the examiner.

3. Evidence of acoustic nerve damage.

4. Evidence of a blocked ear canal.

Answers for review questions appear in Appendix D

KEY TERMS

allergic rhinitis *p.2294*
anosmia *p.2294*
barotrauma *p.2292*
caloric test *p.2293*
cerumen *p.2284*
conductive hearing loss *p.2287*
epistaxis *p.2288*

fetid breath *p.2295*
obstructive sleep apnea (OSA) *p.2294*
otalgia *p.2291*
ototoxicity *p.2290*
pneumatoscope *p.2292*
Rinne test *p.2293*
Romberg test *p.2293*

Schwabach test *p.2293*
sensorineural hearing loss *p.2287*
tinnitus *p.2288*
trismus *p.2295*
vertigo *p.2291*
voice whisper test *p.2293*
Weber test *p.2292*

PEARSON
EXPLORE **mynursingkit**™

MyNursingKit is your one stop for online chapter review materials and resources. Prepare for success with additional NCLEX®-style practice questions, interactive assignments and activities, web links, animations and videos, and more!

Register your access code from the front of your book at
www.mynursingkit.com

REFERENCES

American Academy of Audiology. (2003). *Position statement: Preventing noise-induced occupational hearing loss.* Retrieved February 1, 2004, from http://www.audiology.org/layouts/aaa/login. aspx?ReturnURL=%2fresources% 2fdocumentibray%2fPages%2fHearingConservation.apx

American Academy of Otolaryngology-Head and Neck Surgery. (1993). *Ear, altitude and airplane travel.* Alexandria, VA: Author.

American Cancer Society. (2006). *Cancer facts and figures 2006.* Atlanta, GA: Author.

Anderson, H. G., Cyr, M. M., Guadagnini, J. P., Hickey, M. M., Higgins, T. S., Harris, L. L., et al. (Eds.). (1998). *General history, risk factors, and normal physical assessment.* Huntoon, M. B. (Eds.). (1998) *Core curriculum for otorhinolaryngology and head and neck nursing.*

Bailey, K. (2004). Management of dysphagia in patients with advanced esophageal cancer. *Gastrointestinal Nursing, 2*(2), 18–22.

Chalupka, S. (2001). Essentials of environmental health, enhancing your occupational health nursing practice (part 1), *AAOHN Journal, 49*(3), 137–154.

Crummer, R. W., & Hassan, G. A. (2004). Diagnostic approach to tinnitus. *American Family Physician, 69*(1), 120–127.

Dillon, P. (2003). *Nursing health assessment.* Philadelphia: F. A. Davis.

Flemmons, W. (2002). Obstructive sleep apnea. *New England Journal of Medicine, 347*(7), 498–504.

Gupta, V., & Reiter, E. (2004). Current treatment practices in obstructive sleep apnea and snoring. *American Journal of Otolaryngology, 25*(1), 18–25.

Heron, R., & Wharrad, H. (2000). Prevalence and nursing staff awareness of hearing impairment in older hospital patients. *Journal of Clinical Nursing, 9*(6), 834–841.

Jafek, B. W., & Murrow, B. W. (2001). *ENT secrets* (2nd ed.). Philadelphia: Hanley & Belfus.

Kim, D., & Toriumi, D. (2003) What's new in otolaryngology–head and neck surgery? *Journal of American College of Surgeons, 297*(1), 97–114.

Koliha, C. A. (2003). Obstructive sleep apnea in head and neck cancer patients post treatment . . . something to consider. *ORL-Head and Neck Nursing, 21*(1), 10–14.

Marzo, S. (2003). Implantable hearing devices. *ORL-Head and Neck Nursing, 21*(4), 22–25.

MedicineNet. (2007). *Definition of trismus.* Retrieved on July 22, 2007, from http://www.medterms.com/script/main/art.asp?articlekey= 40739

Mosby *(2002) Mosby's medical, nursing, and allied health dictionary* (5th ed.). (2002). St. Louis: Mosby.

National Guideline Clearinghouse. (2004). *Nursing management of oral hygiene.* Retrieved from http://www.guideline.gov/summary/ summary.aspx?doc_id=7153&nbr=004285&string=ear+AND+ nose+AND+throat

National Guideline Clearinghouse. (2006). *Cough and aspiration of food and liquids due to oral-pharyngeal dysphagia: ACCP evidence-based clinical practice guidelines.* Retrieved February 17, 2007, from http://www.guideline.gov/summary/summary. aspx?ss= 15&doc.id=8664&string=ear+AND+nose+AND+throat

National Institute on Deafness and Other Communication Disorders. (2002a). *Smell and smell disorders fact sheet.* Bethesda, MD: Author.

National Institute on Deafness and Other Communication Disorders. (2002b). *Taste and taste disorders fact sheet.* Bethesda, MD: Author.

National Institutes of Health. (2006). *NIAID fact sheet: Sinusitis.* Retrieved March 24, 2007, from http://www.niaid.nih.gov/factsheets/ sinusitis.htm

Rabinowitz, P. (2000). Noise-induced hearing loss. *American Family Physician, 6*(5), 2749–2756, 2759–2760.

Sandhaus, S. (2002). Stop the spinning: Diagnosing and managing vertigo. *Nurse Practitioner, American Journal of Primary Health Care, 27*(8), 19–25.

Sigler, B. A. (2002). Ear, nose and throat. In J. M. Thompson, G. K. McFarland, J. E. Hirsch, & S. Tucker (Eds.), *Mosby's clinical nursing.* St. Louis: Mosby.

Smith, L., & Osborne, R. (2003). Infections of the head and neck. *Topics in Emergency Medicine, 25*(2), 106–116.

Spector, R. (2004). *Cultural diversity in health and illness* (6th ed.). Upper Saddle River, NJ: Pearson Prentice Hall.

Tierney, L. M., McPhee, S. J., & Papadakis, M. A. (Eds.). (2001). *Current medical diagnosis and treatment.* Stamford, CT: Appleton & Lange.

U.S. Department of Health and Human Services. (1997). *NIOSH pocket guide to chemical hazards.* Washington, DC: Author.

Caring for the Patient with Hearing and Balance Disorders

Barbara Moyer
Kathleen Osborn

With contributions by:
Dawna Martich

Outcome-Based Learning Objectives

After studying this chapter, the learner will be able to:

1. Identify and define the major structures included in the sense of hearing.
2. Compare and contrast the two mechanisms of hearing.
3. Distinguish the three types of hearing loss.
4. Apply health promotion strategies to prevent hearing loss in all age groups.
5. Compare and contrast the three different pathologic causes for a hearing disorder.
6. Discuss discharge priorities for a patient with a hearing disorder.
7. Explain specific aspects of the nursing management for a geriatric patient with a hearing disorder.
8. Apply the nursing process to a patient with a hearing disorder.

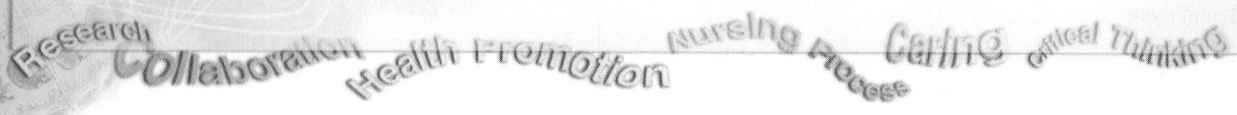

AN INTACT SENSE OF HEARING AND BALANCE is essential to health and daily function. Damage to the ears and accompanying structures will have a negative impact on individuals in all age groups. Identified as being one of the five major senses, hearing is often taken for granted. Many times an alteration in the sense of hearing is not detected until the person is questioned about her voice volume or atypical responses to environmental and verbal stimuli. Loss of hearing may lead to problems in both an individual's professional and personal life, and it also can impact safety. To function in society, one must be able to give and receive information accurately.

Balance also is partially controlled by the ear. A normal functioning inner ear is necessary to maintain body balance. Along with the ear, the joints, the muscles, and the eyes send messages to the cerebellar portion of the brain for coordination and perception. Problems with balance increase the risk for accidental falls, thereby impacting safety.

Anatomy and Physiology of the Ear

The complexities of hearing are best understood when each part of the ear is analyzed (Figure 70–1 ■). The ear is divided into three parts: external/outer, middle, and inner. The external or outer ear

is comprised of some structures visible to the naked eye and others that are not. The pinna, or the most visible portion of the ear, is made up of cartilaginous tissue. The pinna is the portion of the ear that is most easily seen. The pinna collects and directs sound waves into the external auditory ear canal. The ear canal is also made up of cartilaginous material and is relatively short at approximately 1 inch in length. Within this structure sits ceruminous and sebaceous glands that produce cerumen, which is commonly referred to as earwax. The bony portion of the ear canal, which covers the mastoid process, is also considered a structure of the external/outer ear. The tympanic membrane (eardrum), comprised of tissue that makes up the ear canal, is the final structure within this portion of the outer ear anatomy. It is this structure that transmits sounds from the outer to the middle ear.

The middle ear begins from the inner side of the tympanic membrane and extends to the eustachian tube. Within this portion of the ear sit the three auditory bones: the malleus, the incus, and the stapes (Figure 70–1 ■). The malleus is attached to the inner portion of the tympanic membrane. When the tympanic membrane vibrates with sound, so does the malleus. The incus is attached to the malleus and also vibrates in response to sound. The stapes is the structure that separates the middle from the inner ear. The base of the stapes, the footplate, fills the oval

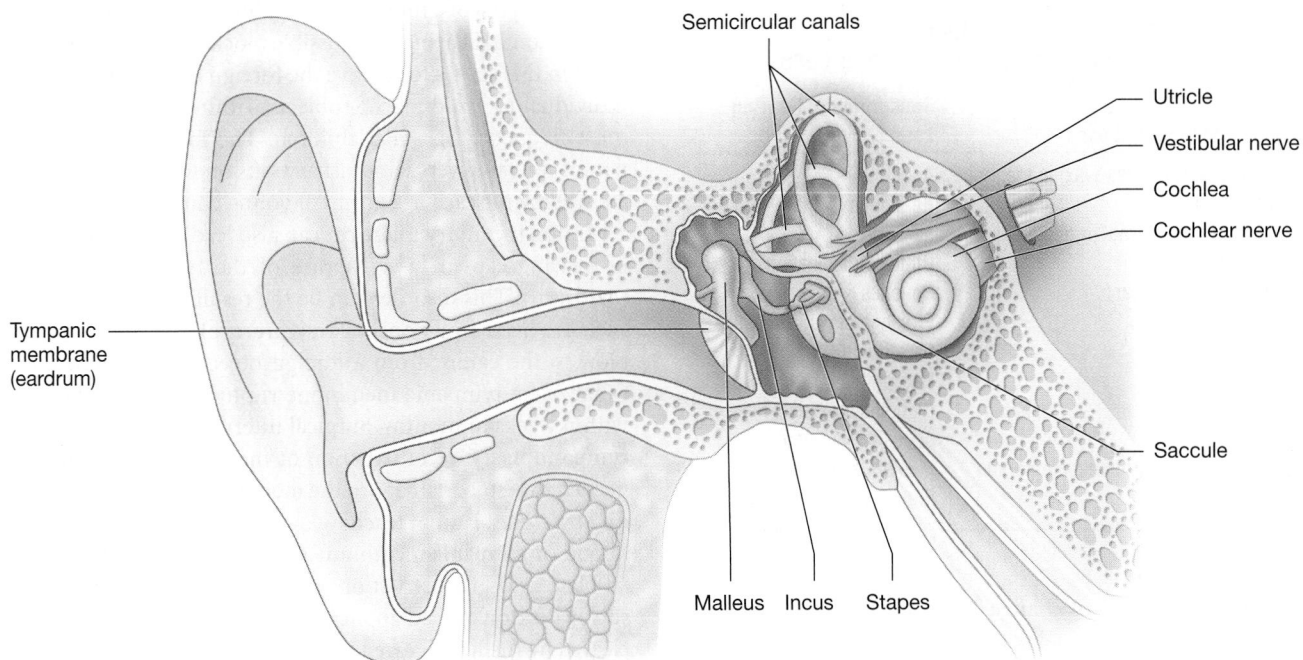

FIGURE 70–1 ■ Anatomical structures of the ear.
Source: AMA's Current Procedural Terminology, Revised 1998 Edition.

window, which leads to the inner ear. The footplate of the stapes fits tightly into a tiny oval window of the bony cochlea that opens into the inner ear. The stapes vibrates and makes the fluid in the inner ear vibrate.

The inner ear includes the cochlea, the vestibular system that contains the bony labyrinth and the semicircular canals, and the acoustic nerve. The cochlea is responsible for hearing, whereas the vestibular system is responsible for balance. The cochlea, shaped like a snail, contains a structure termed the organ of Corti. The small hairs within this organ change sound vibrations into neural signals that are transmitted to the brain via the acoustic nerve. The bony labyrinth consists of the saccule and utricle, organs that provide position sense. Within the inner ear are found the semicircular canals, specifically the horizontal, anterior, and posterior canals, which help with balance and movement. The acoustic nerve consists of two separate parts, the vestibular and cochlear branches. This eighth cranial nerve (CN) controls hearing and equilibrium.

Mechanism of Hearing

There are actually two mechanisms involved with hearing: bone conduction and air conduction. **Bone conduction** is the conduction of sound to the inner ear through the bones of the skull. **Air conduction** begins the process when noise enters the external ear and travels to the middle ear. Once inside the middle ear, the sound is transmitted through the three auditory bones, the malleus, incus, and stapes. Once the sound or noise reaches the stapes, it is then transmitted to the inner ear where it reaches the acoustic nerve and is transmitted to the brain for interpretation. Hearing disorders can be caused by an alteration anywhere within the auditory structures.

■ Etiology and Epidemiology of Hearing Impairment

The most prevalent disorder associated with the structures of the ear is hearing loss. This disorder is estimated to affect approximately 30 million Americans and is considered a chronic health condition seen in all types of people in all age groups, although the percentage of those affected accelerates with age. Also, men are twice as likely as women to have hearing loss (Isaacson, 2005). The degree of hearing loss can range from mild to complete. Causes of this disorder are varied and have distinct types: conductive, sensorineural, or mixed. In **conductive hearing loss**, sound waves cannot reach the inner ear for processing and interpretation. With **sensorineural hearing loss**, the cause is damage to the auditory nerve or possibly damage to the small hair cells within the inner ear. **Mixed hearing loss** refers to both conductive and sensorineural hearing loss caused by a dysfunction of both air and bone conduction processes.

In the case of sensorineural hearing loss caused by noise, the culprit is prolonged exposure to sounds with an elevated decibel level. Typically, exposure to decibel levels of 85 or greater can lead to sensorineural hearing loss (American Academy of Otolaryngology–Head and Neck Surgery [AAO-HNS], 2002). Higher decibel levels cause death of nerve endings in the ear structures. Over time, and if enough of the nerve endings are damaged or destroyed, hearing loss will occur. Nerve endings will not regenerate therefore this type of hearing loss is permanent. Chart 70–1 (p. 2304) describes causes of conductive and sensorineural hearing loss in more detail.

Sounds create vibrations measured in frequencies. A sound with a low frequency vibrates slower than a sound with a high

MyNursingKit | Video: Eyes, Ears, Nose, Throat: Deafness; Deafness Culture

CHART 70–1 Causes of Conductive and Sensorineural Hearing Loss

Conductive Hearing Loss	Sensorineural Hearing Loss
Buildup of cerumen (earwax) in the auditory canal	Aging
Infection of the external or middle ear (otitis media)	Head injury
	Infection
	Ototoxic medications
Fluid in the middle ear	Genetics
A punctured eardrum	Prolonged noise exposure
Edema	Myxedema
Tumors	Labyrinthitis
Foreign body	Diabetes mellitus
Otosclerosis	Acoustic neuroma
Perforation of the tympanic membrane	Ménière's disease
	Presbycusis

frequency. With a loss or change in the nerve endings in the ear structures, the brain is unable to pick up or interpret these frequencies. The first change seen in individuals with sensorineural hearing loss is a loss of high-frequency sounds. This manifests as the inability to interpret or understand the words spoken by females or children in addition to losing the ability to discern the spoken sounds of *s, f, sh, ch, h,* or a soft *c.* The last type of hearing loss, mixed, is caused by both conductive and sensorineural factors.

Pathophysiology and Treatment of Hearing Impairment or Loss

The causes of hearing impairment or loss can be categorized as mechanical, inflammatory, or an obstructive disorder. Causes of mechanical hearing loss include external otitis, exostosis, foreign bodies, trauma, and otosclerosis. **Otitis externa,** or swimmer's ear, is an infection of the skin covering the outer ear canal. External otitis is commonly a bacterial infection caused by *Streptococcus, Staphylococcus,* or pseudomonal types of bacteria. Swimmer's ear is usually caused by excessive water exposure. When water pools in the ear canal (frequently trapped by earwax), the skin becomes soggy, diluting the acidity that normally prevents infection. A cut in the lining of the ear canal also can allow bacteria to penetrate the skin. When this happens bacteria and fungi (from contaminated water or objects placed in the ear) continue to grow and the ear canal gets red and swollen. Diffuse external otitis can lead to irreversible skin conditions, canal stenosis, and deafness.

Exostosis, or surfer's ear, is a condition of the ear canal in which the bony lining under the skin develops a number of lumps that grow into the tube. Exostosis is found among saltwater enthusiasts, usually males 20 to 39 years of age (UCSD Student Health Service, 2007). Possibly due to cold water, the bony portion of the external canal becomes thickened and eventually creates a knoblike projection. Over time, several of these bony growths may close the ear canal causing hearing loss. The condition is painless and may go unnoticed for a number of years until hearing loss becomes obvious. Surgical removal of the outgrowths is necessary to restore hearing.

The lodging of a foreign body within the ear canal also causes a reduction in hearing and possible blockage of cerumen. Treatment in this case is to remove the foreign body and instruct the individual to avoid placing objects within the ear. This occurs most frequently in small children. The nurse should provide parents or caregivers with instructions on what is the appropriate size toy for each age group of young children.

Traumatic injury to the ear can also lead to a mechanical loss of hearing caused by a rupture of the tympanic membrane (eardrum). This disorder can be the result of a sudden trauma such as a head injury or skull fracture, explosive injury, or severe blow to the ear, or from a foreign object pushed into the ear canal. Most tympanic membrane ruptures heal spontaneously within weeks to months. Surgical intervention in the form of a **tympanoplasty,** reconstruction of the tympanic membrane, is needed to restore damage to the membrane and possible middle ear structures. Patient teaching includes ways to reduce the likelihood of tympanic membrane rupture such as protect the ears in blast areas (construction workers), avoid instrumentation such as cotton-tipped applicators, and avoid water sports until cleared by the health care provider.

Another mechanical cause of hearing loss is due to otosclerosis or a primary bone dyscrasia that leads to conductive hearing loss. **Otosclerosis** is a condition in which the structures of the ear begin to harden. Symptoms of this disorder are hearing loss, tinnitus, and dizziness and other sensations of motion. Otosclerosis affects both ears in 80% of patients (Kim, Chang, & Lim, 2000). Also, hearing might appear to be better in noisy environments. Seen as a common cause of conductive hearing loss, treatment options are limited to a **stapedectomy.** A stapedectomy is a surgical procedure in which the innermost bone (stapes) is removed and replaced with a small plastic tube of stainless steel wire (prosthesis) to improve the movement of the sound to the inner ear. Under local or general anesthesia, the surgeon opens the ear canal and uses an operating microscope to separate the stapes from the incus. Next a laser vaporizes the tendon and arch of the stapes bone, which helps remove it from the middle ear. The surgeon opens the window that joins the middle ear to the inner ear and acts as a platform for the stapes bone. Finally, the laser makes a tiny opening and gently clips the prosthesis to the incus bone. This prosthesis bridges the gap between the incus and the inner ear providing sound conduction.

Hearing loss due to an inflammatory process is seen in conditions that cause the accumulation of drainage in the ear canal (otitis external, acute/chronic otitis media), and chronic mastoiditis. When exposed to pathogens, as in otitis externa or media, the individual can usually recall a recent infective process such as the flu or a cold. Possibly the individual might have recently participated in water-related activities. In both diagnoses the patient experiences fullness in the ears with varying degrees of hearing impairment and pain. Depending on the cause, treatment could be with local or systemic antibiotics and instruction to protect the ears. Should the offending organism be isolated to the middle ear area and if the infections reoccur frequently, further treatment may include tube placement or other surgical interventions. The insertion of tubes in the ears, or a **myringotomy,** can be done on an outpatient basis. After creating an incision in the tympanic membrane (eardrum), a small plastic or metal tube is placed through the opening. The purpose of the tube is to ventilate the middle ear and equalize the pressure within the ear and the outside environment. The tubes typically stay in place for 6 to 12 months or until they spontaneously fall out. Anyone with tubes in the ears should avoid getting water inside them. After removal, if the symptoms return, the tubes might need to be reinserted.

An acute or chronic infection of the mastoid process can also lead to changes in hearing and balance referred to as **mastoiditis**. Most often the cause of mastoiditis is a bacterial infection. The individual will experience signs of a systemic infection along with drainage from the ear and subsequent changes in hearing and position sense. Systemic antibiotics are usually the first treatment. However, if chronic mastoiditis occurs, a **mastoidectomy** (removal of the mastoid process) is indicated. This procedure can either be done through the ear or externally through an incision to the occipital bone. Postoperative care depends on the approach used in addition to prevention of infection, maximizing safety, and promoting healing.

An obstruction might be the cause of the change in a person's ability to hear. Examples of such obstructions may include a malignancy within any of the ear structures or a benign acoustic neuroma, described in Chart 70–2 (p. 2306). In the case of a malignancy, surgical intervention and subsequent chemotherapeutic agents may be required. This depends on the type of malignancy following identification of the cause of hearing change. With an acoustic neuroma, treatment begins with surgical removal of the neuroma followed by medications and therapy as prescribed.

Hearing Loss in the Newborn

Hearing loss can have a variety of causes. In the newborn, it can be linked to birth trauma, toxicity, infection, fetal anoxia during delivery, premature or low birth weight, genetics, or an elevated serum bilirubin level. In addition, deafness upon birth has been seen in those women who have been exposed to highly communicable diseases such as rubella and syphilis or who have ingested known **ototoxic** (impairs hearing and balance) medications while pregnant. Ototoxic medications are outlined in Chart 70–3 (p. 2307).

The presence of hearing can be assessed as early as 2 to 3 days of life. Hearing loss is one of the most common developmental abnormalities present at birth. Approximately 1 to 3 infants per 1,000 are born with significant hearing loss. If left undiagnosed, it will impede speech, language, and cognitive developments. Currently 27 states and the District of Columbia have mandatory early hearing screening programs (National Conference of State Legislators, 2007). Individuals with hearing impairment at this early age will face a lifetime of challenges. Learning how to communicate with sign language and lip reading are just two ways to aid the person born without the sense of hearing.

 Sudden hearing loss is considered a medical emergency. Individuals who suddenly lose their hearing should seek immediate medical attention.

Hearing Loss in Children

Otitis media, an inflammation of the middle ear, is the most frequently diagnosed disease in infants and children. The eustachian tube, a passage between the middle ear and the back of the throat, is smaller and more nearly horizontal in children than adults. Thus it is more easily blocked by conditions such as large adenoids and infections. Until this tube changes in size and angle as the child grows, children are more susceptible to otitis media. As mentioned, the three tiny bones in the middle ear carry sound vibrations from the eardrum to the inner ear. When fluid is present, the vibrations are not transmitted. This results in mild or even moderate hearing loss. Generally this type of hearing loss is conductive and temporary. Repeated episodes of otitis media, however, may lead to permanent sensorineural hearing loss. Genetic factors are thought to cause more than 50% of all incidents of congenital hearing loss in children (Smith & Camp, 2007). Some genetic syndromes such as Down syndrome may lead to hearing loss. Finally, there are a variety of conditions that may cause acquired hearing loss (loss after birth). Some examples are ear infections, meningitis, measles, encephalitis, chickenpox, influenza, mumps, head injury, use of ototoxic drugs, and noise exposure.

Hearing Loss in Adults

Hearing loss in adults affects all portions of the ear. Some causes of outer and middle ear sound wave interference are malformation, skull fractures, infections, impacted earwax or foreign objects, a punctured eardrum, or a cyst or tumor. The most common causes of hearing loss in adults are damage to the structures of the inner ear and damage to the auditory nerve that sends those impulses to the brain (University of Iowa Hospital & Clinics, 2006). Other causes are injury, exposure to noise, infection or disease, use of ototoxic drugs (salicylates, aminoglycosides, antibiotics, loop diuretics), tumors, trauma (including acoustic neuroma), and the aging process. Other conditions are otosclerosis and Ménière's disease.

Hearing Loss in Older Adults

Hearing loss is one of the three most common chronic conditions among older adults after high blood pressure and arthritis. Approximately 25% to 40% of adults older than 65 years have some degree of hearing loss, and it is estimated that 40% to 60% of people ages 75 years or older have hearing loss commonly caused by gradual changes in the inner ear (Parmet, Lynm, & Glass, 2003). **Presbycusis** is the loss of hearing that gradually occurs in most individuals as they grow older. Presbycusis is usually a sensorineural hearing disorder. It is most commonly caused by gradual changes in the inner ear as a result of loss of hair cells in the organ of Corti within the ear. The individual might first experience the symptom of **tinnitus**, a constant ringing or roaring within their ears, and then over time the degree of hearing loss will vary. Some individuals might have loss of the middle ranges of hearing. Others might be unable to hear normal conversation in a noisy room. Treatment of this type of loss usually involves a hearing aid.

Hearing loss can also be caused by a virus or bacteria, changes in blood supply to the ear because of heart conditions or stroke, head injuries, tumors, and certain medications previously mentioned. Sometimes presbycusis is a conductive hearing disorder, meaning the loss of sound sensitivity caused by abnormalities of the outer and/or middle ear. Such abnormalities may include reduced function of the tympanic membrane or reduced function of the three tiny bones in the middle ear that carry sound waves from the tympanic membrane to the inner ear.

CHART 70–2 **Common Disorders of the Ear**

Disorder	Cause	Clinical Manifestations	Treatment
External Ear			
Otitis externa (swimmers' ear)	Hot humid environment Water sports Sharp objects that cause open lesions Headphones	Open lesions Itching Pain with movement of tragus Plugged ear Pressure Hearing loss Exudate	Reduce local inflammation and pain Moist heat Topical antibiotics Topical steroids Pain medications Instruct patient not to use cotton-tipped applicators Instruct patient to use earplugs when swimming
Cerumen or foreign body	Cerumen buildup Small objects placed in ear	Pressure Pain Hearing loss	Irrigation Mineral oil
Middle Ear			
Otitis media Acute Chronic Serous	Infectious agent in middle ear causes swelling of mucosa and ossicles If untreated may cause rupture of tympanic membrane	Pressure Pain Hearing is diminished Headache Malaise Fever Nausea Vomiting	Systemic antibiotics Rest Quiet environment Analgesics Antipyretics Antihistamines Myringotomy
Mastoiditis	Complication of otitis media	Swelling behind the ear Pain with movement of tragus, pinna, or head Localized cellulitis	Systemic antibiotics Surgical removal (mastoidectomy) of involved tissue, if no response to antibiotics
Trauma to the tympanic membrane	Complication of infection Rapid changes in middle ear cavity pressure Direct damage with a foreign body (pencil) Slapping of external ear Excessive nose blowing	Hearing loss (transient or permanent) Pain	Avoid inserting objects into the ear Hearing aid Surgical reconstruction of the ossicles and tympanic membrane
Inner Ear			
Tinnitus	Medications Trauma Ménière's disease	Mild ringing to loud roaring that may disturb thought and attention span	Stop medications. No cure if cause cannot be found. Mask sound with noise, music, and background sound during sleep. Ear molds and hearing aids can amplify sounds to drown out tinnitus. Contact American Tinnitus Association for further therapy.
Labyrinthitis	Infection of the labyrinth from a complication of otitis media	Hearing loss on affected side Tinnitus Spontaneous nystagmus to the affected side Vertigo with associated nausea and vomiting	Systemic antibiotics Stay in darkened room Antiemetics Antivertiginous medications
Ménière's disease	Either overproduction or decreased reabsorption of endolymphatic fluid causing a distortion in the inner canal system	Tinnitus Unilateral sensorineural hearing loss Vertigo Clinical manifestations occur in attacks that can last for several days	Instruct to move head slowly to prevent worsening of vertigo Salt and fluid restrictions Stop smoking Antivertiginous medications Antiemetics Mild diuretics Antihistamines Antianxiety medications Labyrinthectomy Endolymphatic decompression
Acoustic neuroma	Benign tumor of CN VIII	Mild vertigo Tinnitus Gradual sensorineural hearing loss	Surgical removal with resultant permanent hearing loss

CHART 70–3	**Ototoxic Medications**

Chemotherapeutic Agents That Can Cause Ototoxicity

Actinomycin	Methchlorethamine
Bleomycin	Methotrexate
Carboplatin	Nitrogen mustard
Cisplatin	Procarbazine
DCM	Vincristine
Fluorouracil	

Antibiotics with a High Potential for Ototoxicity

Amikacin	Lincomycin
Ampicillin	Metronidazole
Capreomycin	Minocycline
Chloramphenicol	Neomycin
Clindamycin	Netilmicin
Colistin	Polymyxin B
Dihydrostreptomycin	Streptomycin
Erythromycin	Tobramycin
Etiomycin	Vancomycin
Gentamicin	Viomycin
Kanamycin	

Antibiotics with a Suspicion for Ototoxicity

Floxins

Diuretics with a High Degree of Ototoxicity

Bumetanide	Furosemide
Diamox	Mannitol
Ethacrynate acid	Torsemide
Ethacrynate sodium	Piretanide

Medications with Quinidine Known to Produce Ototoxicity

Atabrine	Plaquenil
Chloroquine	Quinidex
Lariam (mefloquine)	Quinine sulfate

Ototoxicity Associated with Aspirin and NSAIDs

Advil	Lodine
Aleve	Naprosyn
Anaprox (Naproxen)	Nuprin
Dolobid	Relafen
Feldene	Toradol
Ibuprofen (Motrin)	Voltaren
Indocin	

Ototoxicity Associated with Aspirin

Ascriptin	Empirin
Bufferin	Excedrin
Disalcid	Fiorinal
Ecotrin	Trilisate

Ototoxicity Associated with Analgesics

Hydrocodone with acetaminophen

Exposure to Environmental Chemicals

Butyl nitrite	Mercury
Carbon disulfide	Styrene
Carbon monoxide	Tin
Hexane	Toluene
Lead	Trichloroethylene
Manganese	Xylene

Chemicals

Alcohol	Metals
Aniline dyes	Nicotine
Caffeine	Potassium bromide
Carbon monoxide	Povidone–iodine

Sources: Gale encyclopedia of medicine (3rd ed.). (2006). Farmington Hills, MI: Gale Cengage; http://www.dizziness-and-balance.com; http://www.healthatoz.com; Vestibular Disorders Association (2004, February 16), http://www.vestibular.org.

Noise-Induced Hearing Loss

Noise-induced hearing loss (NIHL) is seen most frequently after an individual has had a prolonged exposure to noise or sound at the level of 85 to 90 dB or a sudden exposure to sound/noise at greater than 90 dB. Often viewed as an occupational hazard, NIHL can occur in anyone who has been exposed to loud noises or sounds. Treatment of NIHL begins with overnight rest. Removing the source of the noise or sound with rest typically restores hearing function. Continuous exposure may cause permanent damage. Individuals who have repeated exposure, such as factory/construction workers, rock musicians, and other individuals exposed to loud sounds on a regular basis, should be counseled to use protective devices. For research about NIHL, see the Evidence-Based Practice box (p. 2308).

Acoustic Neuroma

Acoustic neuroma is a benign tumor of the eighth cranial nerve (Chart 70–2). As the tumor grows it extends from the internal auditory canal to the cerebellopontine angle, the angle between the cerebellum and pons, a common site for the growth of acoustic neuromas, and eventually presses on the brainstem. Clinical manifestations include tinnitus and unilateral sensorineural hearing loss, which may progress to mild vertigo. As the tumor enlarges other cranial nerves are impacted.

After the unilateral hearing loss has been confirmed, definitive diagnosis is made by computed tomography (CT) and magnetic resonance imaging (MRI). Surgical removal via a craniotomy is necessary, with permanent loss of hearing on the affected side.

Balance and Equilibrium

Balance of the body is maintained by the interactions between the eyes, the joints and muscles (proprioceptive system), the brain, and the labyrinth (vestibular apparatus). These structures all function together to maintain position sense and equilibrium.

EVIDENCE-BASED PRACTICE

Noise-Induced Hearing Loss

Clinical Problem

Exposure to excessive loud sounds causes damage to sensitive hair cells in the inner ear and to the nerve of hearing. Every day, people experience sound in the environment such as sounds from television and radio, traffic, and equipment. Normally these sounds are at safe levels that do not affect hearing. When exposed to excessive loud and repetitive loud sounds, the pure force of these vibrations can cause damage to hair cells leading to noise-induced hearing loss (NIHL).

Research Findings

The National Institutes of Health is conducting several research studies on NIHL. One is looking at the effects of noise on hair cells within the ear. Findings thus far support that noise damages these hair cells, leading to a hearing loss. Another study is trying to determine if noise causes a disruption in the blood flow to the cochlea within the ear. Researchers are studying the effects of peripheral vascular disease medication to maintain blood flow to the cochlea while exposed to noise that would otherwise lead to NIHL. Both of these studies are still under investigation.

Implications for Nursing Practice

Nurses should serve as advocates in the prevention, education, identification, and interventions for individuals with NIHL. They also should promote healthy lifestyle practices for all individuals who are at risk for NIHL.

Critical Thinking Questions

1. Identify ways to prevent NIHL.

2. Who is affected by NIHL?

3. What types of activities predispose individuals to the development of NIHL?

Answers to Critical Thinking Questions appear in Appendix D.

Reference

Dangerous decibels. (2007). Retrieved September 26, 2008, from http://www.dangerousdecibels.org.

nystagmus, an oscillation of the eyes that is linked to the body's ability to maintain balance with motion or movement. Treatment includes reducing the motion and possibly using antiemetic (Droperidol) and antivertiginous (Dramamine) medications until the sensation passes.

Labyrinthitis

One of the pathophysiological causes of vertigo is **labyrinthitis** (Chart 70–2, p. 2306). Labyrinthitis, an inflammation of the inner ear, affects both the cochlear and/or vestibular portion of the labyrinth. A recent infection within the sinuses or upper respiratory tract might be the cause. Infection can enter from the meninges, the middle ear, or from the bloodstream. The individual experiences a sudden onset of dizziness and vertigo that might last briefly, such as 3 to 6 days. Seen as self-limiting, the dizziness and vertigo might take up to 6 weeks to resolve. Tinnitus, nausea and vomiting, hearing loss, and spontaneous nystagmus also occur. Meningitis, or infection in the brain, is a complication of labyrinthitis.

If chronic, the individual might need surgical intervention in the form of a labyrinthectomy or **vestibular nerve dissection** to reduce the impulses and remove the subjective sensation of dizziness/vertigo. A **labyrinthectomy** (removal of the labyrinth) will cause total deafness of the affected ear. In the case of a vestibular nerve dissection, the patient will need a craniotomy to access the vestibular nerve. The surgeon will partially sever the nerve. The outcome will be a reduction or removal of the vertigo and hearing loss. Diagnostic tests for vestibular function are outlined in the Diagnostic Tests for Vestibular Function box (p. 2310). Treatments are outlined on Chart 70–2 (p. 2306).

Other infectious causes of balance disorders include the common cold, childhood diseases such as measles and mumps, and more complex diseases such as meningitis, encephalitis, and syphilis. The common cold is discussed in Chapter 34 ☞, and meningitis and encephalitis are discussed in Chapter 29 ☞.

An alternation or change in any one of their functioning will lead to a disorder with balance (Figure 70–2 ■).

Balance Disorders

The primary symptom of a balance disorder is the development of vertigo. Defined as an attack of dizziness, **vertigo** is often described as a "spinning" sensation. This sensation can last from 10 minutes up to several hours or days. Oftentimes, the most comfortable position for a patient experiencing vertigo is lying flat, immobilizing the head. Sudden head movements can precipitate nausea and vomiting. In addition to irritability, the patient might complain of tinnitus and reduced hearing on the involved side. The Risk Factors box outlines the risk factors associated with balance disorders.

The term *motion sickness* is often used to describe the symptoms associated with vertigo. In motion sickness, vertigo is present with nausea and possible vomiting. Motion causes

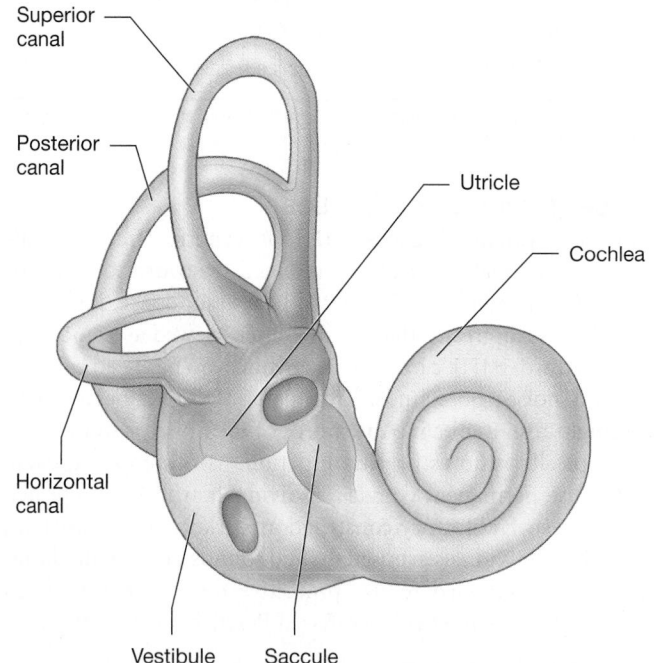

FIGURE 70–2 ■ Anatomical structures of balance.
Source: Balance Disorders (NIH Publication No. 00-4374).

RISK FACTORS Associated with Balance Disorders or Problems

Things to Avoid	Things to Encourage
Driving vehicles if dizzy or unsteady	Change positions slowly
Operating hazardous machinery	Move from lying to upright position in stages
Prolonged periods of standing	Remove throw rugs, litter, and avoid highly polished floors
Exposure to excessive heat or sunlight	Use assistive devices for picking things up from floor
Climbing step ladders	Replace fluids if excess fluid loss
Stooping to pick things up from floor	Take antihypertensive medications after meals
Using over-the-counter medications	Apply nonslip surfaces in bathtub or shower
Using alcohol or drugs that cause vertigo	Provide hand grips in bathroom
Smoking in bed or near oxygen	Provide railings in hallways and stairs
Prolonged bed rest, which causes skeletal muscle weakness and tone	Remove protruding objects (hooks, shelves) from stairway walls
Unsafe conditions while cooking	Wear shoes or slippers with nonskid soles
Increased susceptibility to glare	Install good lighting in hallways or stairs
High heels or unsafe footwear	
Things that cause increased dizziness	
Medications and chemicals that cause vertigo:	Avoid when possible
Alcohol	
Aminoglycosides	
Anticonvulsants	
Antihypertensives	
Cocaine	
Cytotoxic agents	
Furosemide	
Nitroglycerin	
NSAIDs (indomethacin)	
Salicylates	
Tranquilizers	

Ménière's Disease

A second pathologic cause of vertigo, **Ménière's disease**, is defined as a metabolic alteration in the labyrinthine fluid. Individuals with this diagnosis experience a sudden onset of dizziness, nausea, vomiting, giddiness, and hearing loss that can range from several minutes to hours or days in length. Treatment includes medications (Chart 70–3, p. 2307 and in the Pharmacology Summary on p. 2313) and avoidance of tobacco, alcohol, and caffeine. If extremely limiting, surgical intervention includes surgical destruction of the labyrinth with resulting irreversible hearing loss. Another procedure that is done early in the disease is endolymphatic decompression. A small tube is placed in the endolymphatic sac to allow for drainage to reduce vertigo. Treatments are outlined in Chart 70–2 (p. 2306).

Benign Paroxysmal Positional Vertigo

In benign paroxysmal positional vertigo (BPPV) the symptom of dizziness is thought to be due to the formation of otoconia, which are small crystals of calcium carbonate derived from the utricle (Figure 70–1 ■, p. 2303).

Etiology, Epidemiology, and Pathophysiology

The formation occurs due to the utricle being damaged by head injury, infection, or other disorder of the inner ear, or it may have degenerated because of advanced age. Viruses affecting the ear causing vestibular neuritis, minor strokes involving the an-

terior inferior cerebellar artery, and Ménière's disease are significant but unusual causes. BPPV is also common in persons who have been treated with ototoxic medications such as gentamicin (Black, Pesznecker, Homer, & Stallings, 2004). In about 50% of the cases, the cause is idiopathic. BPPV accounts for approximately 20% of all occurrences of dizziness in the general population and about 50% in the older population (Hain, 2007).

Clinical Manifestations

The symptoms of BPPV include dizziness or vertigo, lightheadedness, imbalance, and nausea. Activities that bring on the symptoms of BPPV vary among individuals, although a change in position most commonly precipitates them. It is the change in the position of the head with respect to gravity that causes the vertigo. Getting out of bed and/or rolling over in bed are triggers. As the name implies, BPPV may be present for a few weeks, then stop, then come back again (Hain, 2007).

Diagnostic Procedures

A variety of diagnostic tests are used to help in the diagnosis of hearing and balance disorders. The diagnosis is made based on the patient's medical history, findings on physical examination, and the results of vestibular and auditory tests. The medical history must evaluate the use of ototoxic medications and a review of what triggers the symptoms. It is significant if the dizziness is triggered by lying down or by rolling over in bed.

DIAGNOSTIC TESTS for Vestibular Function

Test	Normal	Expected Abnormality	Hearing Loss
Caloric test (assesses the degree of vestibular and brainstem function, differentiating peripheral lesions from CN VIII lesions) (Sandhaus, 2002) Perform only if tympanic membrane is intact. Irrigate the ear canal with a few drops of cold water.	Nausea, horizontal nystagmus, vertigo toward unirrigated side.	No eye movement (nystagmus) in unconscious patient	Impaired brainstem function
Romberg test (assesses ability to maintain an upright posture when arms are out in front, with eyes open and closed) Stand with feet close together without swaying with eyes open and eyes closed.	Slight swaying is normal. If patient maintains balance, the Romberg test is negative.	Swaying and inability to maintain balance	Impairment in inner ear balance (vestibular nerve [CN VIII] functions), proprioceptive ability, visual, and cerebellar

The Dix-Hallpike test is used to aid the diagnosis. The patient is brought from sitting to a supine position, with the head turned 45 degrees to one side and extended about 20 degrees backward. If the test is positive, the patient will experience a burst of nystagmus (jumping of the eyes). The eyes jump upward as well as twist so that the top part of the eye jumps toward the down side. Electronystagmography (ENG) testing may be needed to look for the characteristic nystagmus (jumping of the eyes) induced by the Dix-Hallpike test and an MRI scan is done if a stroke or brain tumor is suspected (Hain, 2007).

When evaluating a person's ability to hear, three characteristics are assessed: frequency, pitch, and intensity. **Frequency** is the number of sound waves emanating per second and is measured in Hertz (Hz). The ability to hear frequencies from 500 to

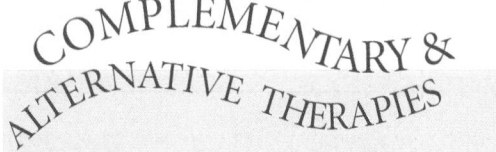

COMPLEMENTARY & ALTERNATIVE THERAPIES T'ai Chi

Description:

T'ai chi chun (TCC), often called just t'ai chi, is an Asian form of exercise that dates back to the 12th century. It is comprised of a series of flowing, graceful movements designed to circulate the body's vital energy, or chi. Those who practice t'ai chi do so to increase their balance, circulation, and overall health. T'ai chi has become a popular method of exercising to maintain good health.

Research Support:

Studies on t'ai chi published from 1996 and 2004 show that it may have the following benefits:

- better balance
- less fear of falling
- greater strength
- greater functional mobility
- increased flexibility
- improved psychological well-being
- better sleep for elderly individuals who are sleep disturbed
- improved cardiovascular functioning

One study examined whether t'ai chi improves balance, muscular strength and endurance, and flexibility in older adults with at least one cardiovascular disease (CVD) risk factor. The study involved 39 older Chinese adults who engaged in a 60-minute t'ai chi class three times per week for 12 weeks. Researchers found that t'ai chi created statistically significant improvements in all balance, muscular strength and endurance, and flexibility measures after 6 weeks. Those improvements also increased further after 12 weeks. Researchers concluded that t'ai chi is a valid intervention for improving balance, upper- and lower-body muscular strength, endurance, and flexibility in older adults (Taylor-Piliae, Haskell, Stotts, & Froelicher, 2006).

The impact of t'ai chi on balance and fear of falling was assessed in another study that used a novel way of involving them in exercise: videoconferencing. A group tele-exercise program was designed so that participants could participate in t'ai chi exercise classes in their own homes through a videoconferencing system. These classes were structured, interactive, and supervised, and were conducted three times per week for 15 weeks. At the completion of the 15-week study, results showed significant improvement in fear of falling and balance (Wu & Keyes, 2006).

References

Kuramoto, A. M. (2006). Therapeutic benefits of t'ai chi exercise: Research review. *Wisconsin Medical Journal, 105*(7), 42–46.

Taylor-Piliae, R. E., Haskell, W. L., Stotts, N. A., & Froelicher, E. S. (2006). Improvement in balance, strength, and flexibility after 12 weeks of t'ai chi exercise in ethnic Chinese adults with cardiovascular disease risk factors. *Alternative Therapies in Health and Medicine, 12*(2), 50–58.

Wu, G., & Keyes, L. M. (2006). Group tele-exercise for improving balance in elders. *Telemedicine Journal and E–Health, 12*(5), 561–570.

Source: Kuramoto, 2006.

2,000 Hz is needed to understand everyday speech. The term **pitch** describes frequency; low pitch is 100 Hz and high pitch is 10,000 Hz.

The **decibel (dB)** is a measurement of loudness or the intensity of sound. Sounds typically range from 0 to 140 dB or greater, with a critical level for hearing being 30 dB. Zero decibel is the sound measurement of slight whispering, whereas the blast of a gun approaches 140 dB.

The various tests used to determine these three components of hearing are outlined in the Diagnostic Tests box (p. 2312). These tests also assist in determining the reason for hearing loss (i.e., conductive versus sensorineural) and the degree of loss.

Medical Management

BPPV is not life threatening and is frequently self-limiting because symptoms often subside or disappear within 2 months of onset (Imai et al., 2005). Therefore, patients can opt to just wait it out. Certain modifications in daily activities may be necessary to cope with the dizziness. For example, instruct the patient to:

- Use two or more pillows at night.
- Avoid sleeping on the "bad" side.
- In the morning get up slowly and sit on the edge of the bed for a minute.
- Avoid bending down to pick up things and extending the head.
- Be careful when lying back such as in the dentist's chair or at a hair salon sink.

Motion sickness medications are sometimes helpful in controlling the nausea associated with BPPV but do not prevent the dizziness.

Some maneuvers will help move the otoconia out of the sensitive part of the ear (posterior canal) to a less sensitive location. The health care provider sequentially moves the head into four positions, staying in each position for roughly 30 seconds. The recurrence rate for BPPV after these maneuvers is about 30% at 1 year; in some instances a second treatment may be necessary. Use of an antiemetic medication prior to the maneuver may be helpful if nausea is anticipated (Hain, 2007). The patient should continue with the daily modifications described above for at least 1 week to avoid provoking head positions that might bring BPPV on again.

If the exercises are ineffective in controlling symptoms, and the symptoms have persisted for a year or longer, a surgical procedure called *posterior canal plugging* may be recommended. This procedure blocks most of the posterior canal's function without affecting the functions of the other canals or parts of the ear. The surgery poses a small risk to hearing—about 3%—but is effective in about 85% to 90% of individuals who have had no response to any other treatment (Shaia et al., 2006). See Complementary & Alternative Therapies box for additional treatment for balance disorders.

Other Causes of Balance Disorders

Other causes for a balance disorder include an intracranial neoplasm (brain tumor) or a cerebrovascular accident (stroke). With a brain tumor, a balance disorder might be one of the first presenting symptoms. The mass will be found while the patient is undergoing a thorough diagnostic evaluation to determine the cause of the balance disorder. In the case of a stroke, a change in balance might also be one of the first presenting symptoms. A

stroke can be caused by either an intracranial hemorrhage or a cerebral embolism. Depending on the location of the bleeding or blood clot, the structure of the cerebrum is affected, tissue displaced, and pressure placed on other brain structures. A change in balance oftentimes will be the first indication of a pending or actual stroke. The causes and treatment of strokes are discussed in detail in Chapter 30 ☍ .

Interventions for Hearing Loss

Treatment of a hearing loss will depend on the underlying cause. This could range from simply removing the cause, as with noise-induced hearing loss or ear canal obstruction, to a surgical procedure. In the case of an infection, antibiotics or a myringotomy might be indicated to treat the infection and drain any fluid and pressure within the middle ear. (The Pharmacology Summary feature, p. 2313 discusses antibiotics and other medications used to treat hearing as well as balance disorders.) Should the cause of hearing loss be due to otosclerosis, a stapedectomy may be the treatment of choice.

Removal of Foreign Body

Foreign bodies of the ear are relatively common in emergency medicine. They are seen most often but not exclusively in children. Various objects may be found, including toys, beads, stones, folded paper, and biologic materials such as insects or seeds. Patients in extreme distress secondary to an insect in the ear require prompt attention. The insect should be killed prior to removal, using mineral oil or 2% lidocaine. Methods of removal consist of irrigation, suction, and instrumentation. Irrigation with water is contraindicated if the tympanic membrane is perforated. Irrigation is also contraindicated for soft objects, organic matter, or seeds, which may swell if exposed to water. Suction is sometimes a useful way to remove foreign bodies. Suction the ear with a small catheter held in contact with the object. Grasp the object with alligator forceps. Place a right-angled hook behind the object and pull it out. Form a hook with a 25-gauge needle to snag and remove a large soft object such as a pencil eraser. It is imperative to avoid any intervention that pushes the object deeper into the ear. After the foreign body is removed, inspect the external ear canal. For most foreign bodies, no medications are needed. However, if infection or abrasion is evident, fill the ear canal several times a day for 5 to 7 days with a combination antibiotic and steroid otic suspension (e.g., Cortisporin).

Removal of Impacted Cerumen

In the event of impacted cerumen, the treatment of choice is removal of the impaction. A health care provider or trained nurse should remove the impaction. Typically this is accomplished by flushing the ear canal with a syringe filled with water that is at or near body temperature. Some health care providers prefer a mixture of hydrogen peroxide and water. The flushing action loosens the impaction from the walls of the canal, and the warm water facilitates drainage from the ear. If the impaction does not clear, the patient is instructed to place mineral oil in the ear three times per day for 2 days. This will soften the dry impacted cerumen, and then the irrigation may be repeated. After removal of the impaction, the patient should be instructed not to insert any objects into the ear canal and to have frequent ear examinations.

DIAGNOSTIC TESTS for Hearing and Balance

Test	Expected Abnormality	Rationale for Abnormality
Voice and watch tick Used to test high-frequency hearing loss The examiner stands 1–2 feet behind and to the side of the patient, while the patient occludes each ear sequentially and the examiner whispers four unrelated words near each ear.	With a hearing abnormality, the patient will not be able to hear words whispered.	If the patient is unable to hear whispering, there is then some degree of hearing loss. The loss of the ability to hear a watch ticking is considered to be a loss of high-frequency sounds.
Weber test (tuning fork test) Used to test sensorineural hearing loss Place an activated tuning fork midline on top of the patient's head, bridge of nose, or chin.	Hear sound in the damaged ear. Hear no sound in the damaged ear.	If the patient has conductive hearing loss, the sound will lateralize to the ear with the loss because the sound is being conducted directly through the bone to the ear. It the patient has sensorineural hearing loss, the sound will lateralize to the hearing ear because nerve damage in the nonhearing ear prevents hearing.
Rinne test (tuning fork test) Used to test conductive hearing loss Place activated tuning fork on the right and left mastoid bone sequentially and in front of each ear.	Hear sound longer through bone. Hear sound longer through air.	This test compares bone conduction with air conduction. If the patient hears sounds longer through bone, then the patient has a conductive hearing loss. If the patient hears sounds longer through the air, then the patient has a sensorineural hearing loss.
Schwabach test (compares the patient's perception of bone conduction to the examiner's) Place an activated tuning fork on the mastoid process of the patient and alternately test for both air and bone conduction.	Diminished—the examiner hears the sound longer than the patient does. Prolonged—the patient hears the sound longer than the examiner does.	Sensorineural loss Conductive loss
ACOUSTIC IMMITTANCE TESTS		
Tympanometry Used to test the flexibility of the tympanic membrane	Tympanic membrane does not move.	Tests for mobility and if there is anything impeding movement of the tympanic membrane and ossicles of the middle ear.
Acoustic reflexes Used to test the flexibility of the stapedius muscle	Stapedius muscle will not contract.	Measures the change in admittance produced by contraction of the stapedius muscle as it responds to an intense sound; stimulation of one ear causes reaction in both ears.
Pure tone audiometry Used to determine type and degree of hearing loss	Unable to hear certain decibel levels.	Provides a record of which decibel levels the patient is unable to hear. This test will not provide the cause of the hearing loss.
Auditory brainstem response Used to test decibel levels of hearing	Cannot hear clicks.	This test measures hearing by measuring the decibel levels the patient hears and if there is anything in the way of nerve pathways.
Electronystagmography Used to test for Ménière's disease	There will be changes in the electrical potentials (waveforms) created by eye movements during spontaneous, positional, or calorically evoked nystagmus.	This test is used to assess the oculomotor and vestibular systems. It is helpful when trying to confirm the diagnosis of Ménière's disease.
Platform posturography Used to test for balance disorders	The patient will not be able to maintain balance or position sense.	Checks for impairments with position sense and balance.
Sinusoidal harmonic acceleration Used to test balance disorders	Eye movements will be uncoordinated.	Another test for balance disorders, this test uses a rotary chair. Through the movements of the chair, the vestibulo-ocular system can be assessed.
Middle ear endoscopy Used to test new-onset hearing loss	Some disorder exists within the middle ear, seen by direct visualization of these structures.	Office procedure to evaluate cause of new-onset hearing loss and to diagnose vertigo.

PHARMACOLOGY Summary of Medications to Treat Select Hearing and Balance Disorders

Medication Category	Action	Application/Indication	Nursing Responsibility
• Isopropyl alcohol drops (dries moisture) • Acetic acid (VoSoL) solution • Antiseptic	Restores acidity and helps keep ear canals dry. Has an antibacterial and antifungal action.	Reduces infection of otitis externa	Dry ears post swimming. Place 1 to 2 drops into each ear after swimming.
• Polymyxin, neomycin, hydrocortisone (Cortisporin, Pediotic) ciprofloxacin (Cipro HC Otic) and ofloxacin (Floxin Otic) • Otic antibiotics	Disrupts cell wall synthesis of susceptible bacteria.	Reduces infection of otitis externa	Note any allergies prior to starting antibiotics. Stop treatment if irritation occurs when using medication. Report any unusual symptoms related to ears or hearing (tinnitus, roaring sounds, loss of hearing acuity, or dizziness).
Amoxicillin (Amoxil) • Cephalosporins, macrolides, trimethoprim-sulfamethoxazole (Bactrim) • Amoxicillin/clavulanic acid (Augmentin) Antibiotic	Disrupts cell wall synthesis of susceptible bacteria.	Acute otitis media	Check for previous allergies to penicillin (amoxicillin) or sulfa (Bactrim). Report any unusual symptoms such as rash, irritation, itching.
Antibiotics • Neomycin, Garamycin, tobramycin, quinolones (Cipro) • IV antibiotics: ampicillin, Unasyn, Ceftin Antibiotic	Disrupts cell wall synthesis of susceptible bacteria.	Chronic otitis media	Note any allergies to specific medications. Report unusual symptoms related to ears or hearing (tinnitus, roaring sounds, loss of hearing acuity, or dizziness).
Steroid eardrops	Has an anti-inflammatory effect on ear canals.	Chronic otitis media	Assess for new onset of ear drainage, earache, erythema, pain, or vertigo. Assess that the ear canal is clear and not impacted with cerumen before medication administration. Consider giving in combination with antibiotics to treat infections. Be aware that steroids may mask infections.
Meclizine (Antivert, Bonine) Antihistamine Antivertigo agent	Long-lasting piperazine antihistamine, structurally and pharmacologically related to cyclizine.	Ménière's disease	Advise caution while driving or engaging in hazardous activities until response to drug is known. Be aware that sedative action may add to that of other central nervous systems (CNS) depressants.
Diphenhydramine (Benadryl) Antihistamine	H_1-receptor antagonist and antihistamine with significant anticholinergic activity.	Ménière's disease	Advise caution while driving or engaging in hazardous activities until response to drug is known. Be aware of additive CNS depressant effects with concurrent use. May cause a drying effect, thus it is important to increase fluid intake if not contraindicated.
Streptomycin IM or gentamicin (transtympanic injection) Aminoglycoside antibiotic Anti-infective	Disrupts cell wall synthesis of susceptible bacteria.	Ménière's disease (selectively destroys vestibular apparatus if vertigo uncontrollable)	Note allergies. Monitor for ototoxicity and hearing problems. Report tinnitus, roaring noises, impaired hearing, sense of fullness in ears. Monitor intake and output to be on alert for nephrotoxicity.

(continued)

PHARMACOLOGY Summary of Medications to Treat Select Hearing and Balance Disorders—*Continued*

Medication Category	Action	Application/Indication	Nursing Responsibility
Diazepam (Valium) Antianxiety CNS agent	Psychotherapeutic agent related to chlordiazepoxide.	Ménière's disease	Monitor for CNS effects such as hypotension, muscular weakness, tachycardia and respiratory depression. Use safety precautions because drowsiness and ataxia may occur. Avoid CNS depressants because of additive effects.
Phenergan (antiemetic)	Long-lasting derivative of phenothiazine with marked antihistamine activity.	Ménière's disease (may be needed to reduce nausea)	Supervise ambulation because sedation and dizziness may occur. Take initial dose 30–60 minutes before anticipated travel. Avoid sunlamps or prolonged exposure to sunlight. Do not take OTC medications without health care provider approval. Avoid CNS depressants because of additive effects. Relieve dry mouth by increasing fluid intake, chewing sugarless gum, or sucking on hard candy.

Assistive Devices

Assistive devices are available for individuals who have partial or total hearing loss. These include phone amplifiers, which allow the caller to speak in a normal tone while amplifying the sound for the person with the hearing impairment. Small portable amplifiers also are available and are carried by those with hearing impairments to assist with communication. Additionally, special apparatus can be connected to doorbells and telephones that cause lights to flash when activated.

The two main types of assistive devices for individuals who have partial or total hearing loss are assistive listening devices (ALDs) and alerting devices (ADs). ALDs help with listening, whereas ADs signal the presence of a sound. Basic ALD systems are devices that amplify the sound, which allow the caller to speak in a normal tone while amplifying the sound for the person with the hearing impairment, or enhancement systems that produce higher frequencies (pitches), which are important for understanding speech through microphones or transmitters. Alerting devices may be modified so that one is alerted when sound devices (telephones, alarm clocks, doorbells) ring. Lamps throughout the house can be made to "flash" when someone rings the doorbell or a small "vibrator" can be placed under a pillow to wake one up in the morning when the alarm goes off.

Hearing Dogs

Hearing guide dogs are specially trained to alert the deaf person or a person with a hearing impairment to ringing doorbells, potential dangers, and other sounds that require a response. The dog alerts the person by physical contact. In public, the dog positions itself between the person with the hearing impairment and possible danger, such as oncoming traffic. Information about qualifying for a dog is obtained through International Hearing Dog Inc., which is a nonprofit organization fully funded by donations. Its mission is to train and place hearing dogs with persons who are deaf or hard of hearing with or without multiple disabilities at no charge to the recipient.

Hearing Aid

A hearing aid is a small electronic sound amplifier that fits either into the external ear canal or just behind the ear. The purpose of the hearing aid is to improve hearing, thereby preventing social isolation and anxiety. The aid can be worn in one or both ears. The patient should be fitted for the hearing aid based on type and degree of hearing loss as determined by a certified licensed audiologist. For sensorineural hearing loss there are aids that will depress the low-frequency sound and enhance the high-frequency sound. The hearing aid will only make sounds louder; it will not help with discriminating words or understanding speech. Hearing aids amplify all sounds including background noise, so the person needs to learn to filter out background noise. Initially, patients are typically encouraged to use the hearing aid for only part of the day and use television/radio to get used to the change in volume. The patient needs to learn to adjust the tone or volume on the aid to achieve the best sound. The newer digital/programmable hearing aids are programmed by the audiologist with a computer, so the sound quality and response time can be adjusted on an individual basis (National Institute on Deafness and Other Communication Disorders [NIDCD], 2002a). These hearing aids are better able to compensate for background noise because they allow amplification at certain programmed frequencies, rather than all of them.

Hearing aids are delicate devices that need careful handling and care in order to work properly. The nurse needs to instruct the patient on care and cleaning requirements for the hearing aid. The following items are typical maintenance tasks for hearing aids:

- Clean the ear mold with mild soap and water.
- Check the battery regularly.

- Clean the hole in the middle of the device.
- Always have an extra battery on hand.
- Avoid spraying hairspray or other beauty products on the hearing aid.
- Turn off the hearing aid when not in use.

The patient also will need instructions about side effects or complications. The patient should contact the health care provider if skin irritation or accelerated cerumen accumulation occurs. If the hearing aid does not improve hearing, the patient may need to try another brand. Chart 70–4 lists the different types of hearing aids.

Cochlear Implants

A cochlear implant is a small, complex electronic device that can help to provide a sense of sound to a person who is profoundly deaf or severely hard of hearing. The intention was for this implant to aid individuals with neurofibromatosis, one of the hereditary forms of deafness, to hear. An implant does not restore or create normal hearing, although it can give a deaf person a useful auditory understanding of the environment and help him or her to understand speech. With a cochlear implant, electrodes are placed in the cochlea and attached to a microphone and signal processor, which are surgically placed under the skin behind the ear. The microphone and signal processor transmit electrical stimuli to the 22 implanted electrodes. The electrical signals stimulate the auditory nerve fibers and then the brain where the sounds are interpreted. Once implanted the patient undergoes extensive cochlear rehabilitation. Several months of training with an audiologist and speech pathologist are needed to learn to interpret the sounds.

Cochlear implants are beginning to be used in children with promising results. A longitudinal study was conducted on 107 children with hearing impairments who received cochlear implants before the age of 7. The findings showed that these children developed communication skills within a few months (NIDCD, 2002b).

Speech Reading and Sign Language

Speech reading, also known as lip reading, uses the eyes to assist with understanding what is being said to the deaf person. There are formal speech reading classes where the deaf person is taught special clues and how to understand body language. The deaf person or someone with a hearing impairment typically understands only a portion of the words, but communication is enhanced.

Sign language is another means of enhancing communication for the deaf person or person with a hearing impairment. American Sign Language is one example of a complex visuospatial language that is used by the deaf community. Sign language is a linguistically complete, natural language that is native to many deaf men and women, as well as some hearing children born into deaf families.

A program designed to test the self-efficacy for health-related behaviors among deaf adults is discussed in the Evidence-Based Practice box.

■ Nursing Management

Preparing to provide care to a patient with a hearing or balance disorder should begin with an assessment of the patient's current status. From this information, the nurse can then determine

---

On Efficacy of Deaf Heart Health Intervention

Clinical Problem
Performing activities of daily living (ADLs) or working in society produces self-perception or task-related problems for culturally deaf individuals.

Research Findings
A quasiexperimental pre/post-test study was performed to test the effectiveness of the Deaf Heart Health Intervention (DHHI) in increasing self-efficacy for health-related behaviors among culturally deaf adults. The DHHI targets modifiable risk factors for cardiovascular disease. A sample of 84 participants completed a time 1 and time 2 data collection process. The sign language version of the Self-Rated Abilities Scale for Health Practice (SRAHP) was used to measure self-efficacy for nutrition, psychological well-being/stress management, physical activity/exercise, and responsible health practices. Total self-efficacy scores were significantly higher in the intervention group than in the comparison group at time 2, controlling for scores at baseline $(F < 1, 81 > = 26.02, p < 0.001)$. Results support the development of interventions specifically tailored for culturally deaf adults to increase their self-efficacy for health behaviors.

Implications for Nursing Practice
Nurses need to be aware of health and mental behaviors that cause problems with self-efficacy among culturally deaf individuals and promote intervention strategies that help improve these individuals.

Critical Thinking Questions

1. What are some health-related behaviors that may increase self-efficacy for culturally deaf adults?

2. Identify ways in which culturally deaf adults can adjust to their environment.

3. What role might school nurses play in helping to identify culturally deaf adolescents?

Answers to Critical Thinking Questions appear in Appendix D.

Reference
Jones, E. G., Renger, R., & Kang, Y. (2007). Research in nursing and health: Self-efficacy for health related behaviors among deaf adults. *Research in Nursing and Health 30*(2), 185–192.

EVIDENCE-BASED PRACTICE

CHART 70–4	Basic Types of Hearing Aids for Sensorineural Hearing Loss
Type	**Description**
In-the-ear	Fit in outer ear; used for mild to severe hearing loss.
Behind-the-ear	Worn behind the ear and connected to a plastic earmold that fits inside the outer ear; used for mild to profound hearing loss.
Canal aids	Fit into the ear canal and used for mild to moderately severe hearing loss.
Body aids	Aid attaches to a belt or pocket and is connected to the ear by a wire; used for profound hearing loss.

Source: Extracted from National Institute on Deafness and Other Communication Disorders at http://www.nidcd.nih.gov/health/hearing/hearingaid.asp.

diagnoses appropriate to address these findings. Examples of nursing diagnoses may include the following:

- *Disturbed Sensory Perception: Auditory*
- *Impaired Social Interaction*
- *Social Isolation*
- *Risk for Loneliness*
- *Ineffective Coping*
- *Impaired Walking*

- *Deficient Knowledge*
- *Anticipatory Grieving*
- *Risk for Situational Low Self-Esteem*
- *Risk for Injury*

From the diagnoses, the nurse can then plan interventions to aid in the care of a patient with special needs. Refer to the Nursing Process: Patient Care Plan for a Hearing or Balance Disorder feature for more information on nursing care for these disorders.

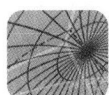

NURSING PROCESS: Patient Care Plan for a Hearing or Balance Disorder

Assessment of Hearing

Subjective Data:
When did you first notice that you had a change in your ability to hear?
Did you have a recent exposure to a loud noise or infection?

Objective Data:
Results of hearing tests.
Test ability to hear at normal voice range.
Test lower and higher pitch.
Speak into both ears to test unilateral verses bilateral hearing loss.

Nursing Assessment and Diagnoses	Outcomes and Evaluation Parameters	Planning and Interventions with *Rationales*
Nursing Diagnoses: *Disturbed Sensory Perception: Auditory* and *Impaired Verbal Communication*	**Outcomes:** Patient/family understand that the disease causes progressive hearing loss. Patient/family understand what treatments will help. **Evaluation Parameters:** Patient can communicate. Assistive devices are helping with hearing and communication.	**Interventions and *Rationales*:** Assess degree of hearing loss. *Helps determine best approach to communicate.* Teach about disease process. *Helps reduce anxiety and stress related to the change or loss in hearing.* Speak clearly and slowly in a normal to deep voice; face the patient when speaking; use touch to gain the patient's attention. *Aids in verbal and nonverbal communication with the patient.* Respond to call light as soon as possible; answer questions; teach about medications/treatments *to decrease fear and anxiety.* Provide emotional support to the member having difficulty coping with the new sensory deficit *to decrease fear and anxiety.* Instruct or reinforce instruction on use of hearing aid. *Aids in retention of training and reinforces the need for using the assistive device for hearing.* Provide sensory stimulation; encourage expressing feelings of concern and loss for hearing deficit; teach to watch for visual cues. *Provides additional support for the patient.*

Assessment of Balance

Subjective Data:
How long have you been experiencing dizziness/vertigo?
Have you fallen?
How long have you been dizzy with walking?
Are you using any hazardous machinery such as a car or equipment at work?
Are you nauseated with the dizziness/vertigo?
Do you drive an automobile?

Objective Data:
Observation of ataxia while ambulating
Observation of bumping into things while ambulating

Nursing Assessment and Diagnoses	Outcome and Evaluation Parameters	Planning and Interventions with *Rationales*
Nursing Diagnoses: *Risk for Falls, Risk for injury,* and *Impaired Walking*	**Outcomes:** Patient will understand that balance disorder is temporary. Patient will participate in rehabilitative activities to maximize position sense. Patient will adhere to medication regime prescribed for balance disorder. **Evaluation Parameters:** Dizziness and vertigo subside. Patient is able to resume normal activities of daily living (ADLs) and lifestyle.	**Interventions and *Rationales*:** Explain the cause for dizziness and vertigo. *Helps the patient understand the reason for the symptoms.* Assist the patient with ambulation and other ADLs *to ensure the patient does not experience any injuries while dizzy.* Utilize safety measures such as keeping bedside rails in elevated position and call light within reach. *Safety precautions.* Teach family how to assist patient with ambulation and ADLs upon discharge *to ensure ongoing safety measures until the dizziness and vertigo subside.*

Discharge Priorities

When planning for discharge from an acute care facility for treatment of a hearing or balance disorder, the nurse is in the best position to help the patient and family with physical, psychological, and future occupational needs. Helping the patient and family deal with the cause of the hearing or balance deficit and identify choices to avoid future problems associated with hearing and balance are the approaches of choice. The Deaf Mental Health Charter (2007) commissioned by the Sign and Mental Health Foundation, London, England, has identified a variety of areas that need implementation to address the types of choices that the deaf community may make. These areas are outlined in the Patient Teaching and Discharge Priorities box.

If discharging a patient from an acute care facility, physical teaching needs might include postoperative wound care, medication therapy, coping, and a return-to-work plan. In the outpatient setting, teaching needs might be focused on adherence to a prescribed medication regime, avoidance of behaviors that caused the hearing/balance disorders, protective devices for the workplace, and other health promotional activities.

Should the hearing or balance disorder lead to a long-term change in the ability to hear, other instructions would include communication instruction such as sign language, use of a hearing aid, suggestions to family for communicating with the family member who has the hearing impairment, and learning to avoid the same exposure that caused the hearing impairment in their loved one.

Health Promotion

The Deaf Community has limited access to health promotion information and care. Health care providers, educators, and policy makers could improve medical care to the Deaf Community by (1) better understanding its culture and language, (2) creating more health education programs specifically for the Deaf Community, (3) developing opportunities for more deaf people and American Sign Language (ASL) users to enter the health professions, and (4) creating incentives for hearing health care professions to become ASL proficient (Sadler, Huang, & Padden et al., 2001).

Neonate/Baby/Childhood

The instructions on how to protect hearing can begin when the mother brings her newborn child to the pediatrician for routine checkups. The infant should be tested for hearing prior to reaching 1 month of age. Children of all ages should be examined immediately if exhibiting symptoms of an ear infection. If left untreated, hearing loss might ensue.

Mothers should be instructed on the risk of using cotton swabs to clean the ears of their children. Alternative methods to clean the ear should be provided such as using a wick to absorb fluid in the

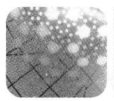

PATIENT TEACHING & DISCHARGE PRIORITIES for the Hearing and Balance Disorders

Need	Teaching
Usable information techniques	Provide access to easily understood information in appropriate formats, such as plain language, visual representation in subtitled DVDs and videos.
	Assist with location of classes for American Sign Language, if applicable.
	Provide for health information or programs (including mental health promotion) that are accessible to the Deaf community. Design these programs in close cooperation with organizations that serve the Deaf community.
Safe environment	The inpatient, outpatient, day services, or work settings need to have services that make the environment safer; for instance, visual fire safety provisions and access to alerting and telephone services, TVs with teletext ability, pagers, and inclusive ways to operate remote door-entry systems.
Communication support	Deaf people who use BSL as their first and preferred form of communication have the right to qualified interpreter support. Deaf people who use English and hearing aids have the right to use lipspeaker-cued speech or speech to text transcription.
Health promotion	Provide access to health information or programs (including mental health promotion) to the deaf community. These programs should be designed in close cooperation with organizations that serve the deaf community. Different means of promotion, such as face-to-face delivery in BSL, may be more effective to reach deaf people.
Assessment, care, and treatment	Deaf people have the right to be assessed by a trained worker who has deaf/deaf blind awareness and skills. Deaf-specific advisory services should be considered. Using these services aims to ensure that deaf persons can fully participate in any assessment and discussion of services.
Placement	Any placement decision should take into account the deaf person's preferred communication method and language.
Advocacy	Deaf people have the right to independent advocacy in health, mental health service, education, employment, and social care. This is to ensure that the deaf person can fully participate in any assessment and discussion of services to make informed choices.
Physical teaching needs	In the outpatient setting, teaching needs might be focused on adherence to prescribed medication regime, avoidance of behaviors that caused the hearing/balance disorders, protective devices for the workplace, and other health promotional activities. If the patient had surgery, include teaching on postoperative wound care, medication therapy, coping, and a return to work plan.

Source: Deaf Mental Health Charter. (2007). *Mental Health Foundation.* Retrieved June 21, 2007, from http://www.mhf.org.uk/our-work/service-development/all-age-groups/deaf-charter. Commissioned by Sign and Mental Health Foundation, London, England.

ear canal. Children should not have small objects as toys for play since these small objects can become lodged within the ear canal. Children also should have their ears protected with earplugs while participating in water activities and with muffs prior to being exposed to loud noises. Even though most, if not all, children experience head colds, if not treated properly, head colds can lead to infections that settle in the ears. Children who experience repeated colds should have an examination of their ears and associated structures to make sure the ears are not becoming affected or damaged from ongoing nasal and sinus inflammation and infection.

Adolescence

Teenagers who frequently listen to loud music can experience a temporary loss of hearing. Over time, this hearing loss can become more permanent. Parents should caution their teenagers to reduce the volume of music to avoid this damaging effect.

Adults

Adults also are at risk for hearing and balance disorders. Causes might include the indiscriminate use of cotton swabs to clean the ear canal and loud noise from factory work, jack hammers, music, explosive devices, automobile engines, and the like. Engaging in water activities or sports also can lead to infections within the ear structures. If not treated, these infections also can lead to hearing loss similar to that which is seen more frequently in children.

Because balance and position sense are intimately related to the structures of the inner ear, changes in balance should not be ignored. Individuals who find they struggle to maintain a sense of balance should seek medical attention. The examination will most likely include a thorough study of the ear structures in efforts to determine the cause of dizziness or vertigo.

Individuals of all ages should learn to protect their ears and hearing by having earplugs for water activities/showers, earmuffs to reduce exposure to loud noises, and common sense to reduce the volume of music or entertainment activities such as television.

Patient, Family, and Community Perspectives

Having a loss of hearing creates unique challenges for the individual. Environmental noise cannot be discerned, leaving the person prone to hazards such as an oncoming automobile or even the warning buzz of a bee. Communities need to provide street warning signs for motorists driving in areas where residents with hearing impairments live. Schools should provide educational programs for students to learn the hazards of hearing impairment and loss. Adults should be encouraged to seek advice for hearing loss and be supported when needing to purchase and care for hearing aids. Those who cannot have their hearing restored through surgery or devices need to be supported with training and education to learn sign language or provided with a telephonic device to aid with communication.

Rehabilitative programs exist for these individuals to help them regain position sense and balance. Individuals with a known balance disorder should be advised to avoid operating motor vehicles or machinery. The Risk Factors box (p. 2309) lists those needs to be included in the rehabilitative programs. The patient's health care provider may need to contact the Department of Motor Vehicles to report the patient's balance disorder. The patient's driver's license could be suspended until the disorder passes and the patient passes a medical clearance prior to resuming the use of a motor vehicle.

■ Collaborative Care

The patient with a hearing or balance disorder may need the aid of additional caregivers. These caregivers include therapists in occupational and physical medicine and speech and hearing. Learning to care for a hearing aid might first be reviewed with an audiologist and then turned over to the nurse for instructional reinforcement. If the patient is experiencing a balance disorder and being treated with rehabilitative services, the nurse's role is to reinforce the instructions provided by the therapist.

■ National Guidelines for Hearing Loss Prevention

A program led by the U.S. Department of Health and Human Services (DHHS), termed *Healthy People 2010,* has identified specific objectives to help with the problem of hearing loss, as outline in the National Guidelines box. The *Healthy People 2010* focus area on vision and hearing stresses the importance of early intervention to protect and conserve the vision and hearing of young children and to mitigate the severity of vision and hearing impairments that can heavily degrade the quality of life of older Americans. The vision and hearing section of the *Healthy People 2010* document (U.S. Department of Health and Human Services, 2000)) stresses the following:

- Increase the proportion of persons who have a hearing examination on schedule.
- Increase the number of persons who are referred by their primary care health care provider for hearing evaluation and treatment.
- Increase the use of appropriate ear protective devices, equipment, and practices.
- Decrease noise-induced hearing loss in children and adolescents ages 17 years and younger.
- Decrease adult hearing loss in the noise-exposed public.

NATIONAL GUIDELINES for *Healthy People 2010*
Objectives for Reducing Hearing Loss

1. Increase the number of newborns having a first hearing examination by 1 month of age. Babies with a hearing loss should have additional testing by 3 months of age. If hearing loss continues, enrollment in a rehabilitative program by 6 months of age.

2. Decrease the number of ear infections in children.

3. Increase the number of Deaf/hard-of-hearing individuals who use adaptive devices such as hearing aids or cochlear implants.

4. Increase the number of individuals who have routine hearing examinations.

5. Increase the number of individuals who are referred by their primary health care provider for a hearing evaluation and treatment.

6. Increase the use of protective devices, such as earplugs or earmuffs, in people of all ages.

7. Reduce the number of individuals of all ages who suffer from noise-induced hearing loss.

Source: U.S. Department of Health and Human Services. (2000). *Healthy people 2010: Understanding and improving health.* Retrieved February 5, 2008, from http://www.healthypeople.gov.

A radiologist-funded group of health care providers has written a set of guidelines to aid in the diagnosis of hearing and balance disorders. These guidelines, entitled the *American College of Radiology Appropriateness Criteria for Vertigo and Hearing Loss* (2008), recommend specific diagnostic tests as a precursor to prescribing treatment for a balance or hearing disorder (see the National Guidelines box). Commonly referred to as national guidelines, this list names specific hearing/balance disorders then states the ideal diagnostic tests that should be used to diagnose the disorder. Tests frequently recommended include an MRI, with and without contrast, a CT scan, with and without contrast, skull films, and tomography. The intention of these diagnostic tests is to first determine or possibly rule out the presence of cerebral pathology as the cause for the change in hearing or balance.

Cultural Considerations

Very few cultural differences are seen in hearing and balance disorders. One interesting difference is with the Vietnamese. These individuals have dry earwax, which is gray in color and brittle to the touch. In a majority of Asians and Native Americans cerumen is dry, white, and flaky. In African Americans and Caucasians cerumen is brown, wet, and sticky (Hunter, 1996; Mitchell, 1997).

Genetic Implications

Congenital hearing loss occurs when a trait found within the chromosomes of both parents passes to the infant. The trait can be dominant, recessive, or sex linked. Congenital conditions that include some degree of hearing impairment are outlined in the Genetic Considerations box.

GENETIC CONSIDERATIONS Related to Hearing and Balance Disorders

Disorder	Results	Ear Structure
Usher syndrome	Balance problems	Inner ear
Treacher Collins syndrome	Bone development	Middle ear
Nonsyndromic deafness	Conductive problems	Inner ear
ESPN	Changes in hairlike projections	Inner ear
Pendred syndrome	Hearing loss and goiter	Inner ear
Neurofibromatosis	Tumor (acoustic neuroma)	Inner ear
Diastrophic dysplasia	Cartilage and bone	External ear
Von Hippel Lindau syndrome	Endolymphatic sac tumors	Inner ear
Jervell and Lange-Nielsen syndrome	Flow of potassium ions	Inner ear
Alport syndrome	Organ of Corti	Inner ear
Crouzon syndrome	Ear canals	Middle and inner
Chromosome 18	Low-set ears	Outer and middle

Source: Genetics Home Reference website: http://ghr.nlm.nih.gov. A Service of U.S. National Library of Medicine.

The risk of giving birth to a child with a hearing deficit depends on the health of the parents and their respective health backgrounds. Histories of known deafness in families should cause those of childbearing years to seek genetic testing and counseling prior to conception. To proceed with the understanding that a child could be born deaf will undoubtedly cause prospective parents much anxiety around the decision to reproduce at all.

Treatment of congenital deafness will vary depending on the underlying congenital cause. As more research is conducted on the different congenital disorders, treatment options will likely expand.

Gerontological Considerations

More often than not, deafness is associated with aging. It is estimated that one-third of adults over the age of 60 have some degree of hearing loss. This percentage increases to approximately 50% of all adults over the age of 85 experiencing an alteration in their ability to hear (NIDCD, 2001).

The causes of hearing loss and balance disorders in the elderly can be from a metabolic disorder, such as type II diabetes mellitus, or from the aging process. In diabetes, the disorder can go undetected for many years. By the time of diagnosis, the patient might already have long-term complications to the nervous system. Included in these complications could be damage to the auditory nerve leading to a change in the ability to hear. The impact of unstable blood glucose levels can also lead to a balance disorder.

Exposure to known ototoxic medications (see Chart 70–3, p. 2307) throughout life could finally manifest in later years. A patient might have ingested a medication that was not known to

NATIONAL GUIDELINES for Vertigo and Hearing Loss

The *American College of Radiology Appropriateness Criteria for Vertigo and Hearing Loss* (2008) provides the radiologic diagnostic tests used to aid in the diagnosis of vertigo and hearing loss. This document addresses the hearing and balance disorders based on presenting symptoms, categorized as variants from normal. With the clinical condition of hearing loss/vertigo the variants are:

1. Sensorineural hearing loss, acute vertigo
2. Sensorineural hearing loss, intermittent vertigo
3. Sensorineural hearing loss, no vertigo
4. Conductive hearing loss, rule out petrous bone abnormality
5. Episodic vertigo, new onset (hours to days)
6. Vertigo, no hearing loss, normal neurological exam
7. Total deafness, cochlear implant candidate, surgical planning
8. Fluctuating hearing loss, history of meningitis or to rule out congenital anomaly.

Based on the patient's presenting hearing or balance disorder, these guidelines are consulted to determine which diagnostic test to perform to aid in the diagnosis of the disorder.

American College of Radiology (2008). Guideline title: Vertigo and hearing loss. Retrieved on September 29, 2008 from http://www.guideline.gov/summary/summary.aspx?ss=15&doc_id=9602&nbr=5123.

be ototoxic until after years of pharmacologic study. Older individuals might be experiencing presbycusis. Because the onset of hearing loss associated with presbycusis is slow and gradual, individuals might not even recognize that their hearing is changing until a significant amount of deterioration has occurred. Oftentimes, the individual finds he can no longer hear high-pitched sounds or voices, particularly with loud or noisy background sounds. The individual might also identify tinnitus, because this symptom is common in those diagnosed with presbycusis as the cause for their hearing deficit/change.

Nursing Assessment of the Elderly

When providing care to an elderly patient with a hearing deficit or balance disorder, the nurse needs to include specific items in the assessment process. First the method of communication must be determined. A loud voice does not ensure successful hearing or comprehension. Depending on the cause and degree of hearing loss, the nurse might simply drop the tone of the voice to be successful with vocal communication with an elderly patient who has a hearing impairment because the loss of high-frequency sounds occurs first.

The review of systems or head-to-toe assessment should include any known cardiac disorders, blood pressure history or known hypertension, and any metabolic disorders such as diabetes. Conditions that involve the arteries and veins such as peripheral vascular disease or atherosclerosis could provide answers for any cause of hearing or balance disorders linked to an alteration in blood flow to the brain.

The reason for the current hospitalization or visit to the health care provider's office should include a reference to any change in hearing or balance. The current blood pressure and pulse should be assessed for possible association with the patient's current cardiovascular status. In addition, assess whether the patient is able to ambulate without assistance or appears wobbly or unbalanced when attempting to walk. This could be linked to a disorder within the ears or balance-related structures.

Questions to the patient about her health should include any history of a cardiovascular accident or transient ischemic attacks. Additionally, ask if the patient has a history of cerebral brain tumors or other diagnosed pathologic conditions that could be linked to the current symptoms of the hearing/balance disorder.

Finally, an assessment of the past medical history of the elderly patient presenting with a hearing or balance disorder should include any and all exposure to communicable diseases that might have been treated with antibiotics that have known ototoxic side effects. An example might be pulmonary tuberculosis that was treated with streptomycin.

Psychosocial and Economic Needs

The elderly patient experiencing a change in hearing or balance might be embarrassed to admit the change. Oftentimes, elderly patients might not have adequate finances to purchase a hearing aid or they might feel that needing such a device is a sign of weakness or aging. Patients who are unstable with ambulation caused by a balance disorder might find they stay close to home to avoid falling. This can lead to social isolation, which in turn can lead to depression. Couple a balance disorder with a hearing loss and an elderly person might become a social recluse, lost in a world of increasing silence. Previous joys found in living might diminish as elderly patients realize that they might be approaching the end of their life.

Medications and Compliance

The medications used to treat hearing and balance disorders can be a hindrance as well as beneficial. Medications to treat other diseases or conditions can have the side effects of hearing disturbance or tinnitus (antibiotics, aspirin) or dizziness (beta blockers, ACE inhibitors). Taking medications to aid with a balance disorder might adversely interact with other prescribed medications (opioids, central nervous system depressants). Depending on the medications and results of combining medications, patients might choose to stop taking some medications in favor of others that have less of an impact on their general sense of well-being.

Laboratory Test Alterations

The elderly patient being evaluated for a hearing or balance disorder will most likely have a complete battery of serum laboratory tests done. The purpose of the findings might be to indicate whether the patient has an electrolyte or blood glucose disorder. An electrolyte disturbance, such as low sodium or low potassium levels, can be associated with light-headedness. A low blood glucose level also can present with light-headedness and lack of coordination. Diagnostic tests to determine the degree of presbycusis (see the Diagnostics Tests box, p. 2312) would undoubtedly reveal the condition and offer the patient treatment choices including a referral for a hearing aid or surgery to replace the stapes.

Prognosis and Complications

Depending on the diagnosis, the prognosis would vary. Should the patient need surgery, such as a stapedectomy, some degree of hearing might be restored. Should the course of treatment include medications and hearing aids, other issues might interfere with the prognosis. If the patient were unable to afford the medications or hearing aid, the situation would continue to exist and possibly worsen in time. Care should be taken to address the needs of the elderly should they hesitate to commit to a referral for a hearing aid.

Caregiver Needs

Needs for those providing care to an elderly individual with a hearing or balance disorder vary. If the elderly person were independent, the caregiver would most likely be able to adjust his own lifestyle and activities to those of the individual to whom he is providing the care. If a balance disorder is added to the mix of other health issues, the caregiver might need additional support. The caregiver might not be able to leave the elderly individual alone due to the risk of falling or injury. Each situation needs to be assessed to determine the best options for both the elderly patient and caregivers alike.

End-of-life Issues

It is often believed that the sense of hearing is the last sense "to go" when an individual is facing an inevitable death. Should this be the case, conversations need to be adjusted accordingly. The nurse's responsibility is to control the environment as much as possible to ensure that no inappropriate conversations occur near the patient.

Research

Research opportunities focus on the causes and treatment of hearing and balance disorders. The Research Opportunities and Clinical Impact box identifies just a few of these opportunities.

Summary

Most nurses will care for an individual with a hearing and balance disorder during the course of their careers. The nurse must be knowledgeable and sensitive to the needs of people with hearing impairments to ensure safety and decrease anxiety. These unique challenges will provide extreme rewards especially when the prescribed therapy restores hearing to someone who might otherwise live the rest of their years in progressive silence.

RESEARCH OPPORTUNITIES AND CLINICAL IMPACT RELATED TO HEARING AND BALANCE DISORDERS

Research Area	Clinical Impact
Hearing aids for sensorineural hearing loss	Improved hearing.
	Three new types of hearing aids designed to help individuals with a sensorineural hearing loss are under investigation: linear peak clipper (PC), compression limiter (CL), and wide dynamic range compressor (WDRC). Researchers have found that all three new hearing aids have increased hearing between 10% and 30% in individuals with sensorineural hearing loss.
Occupational hazard	Research ways to decrease hearing loss due to continuous exposure to loud noise.
Prevent genetic deafness	Normal hearing

Clinical Preparation

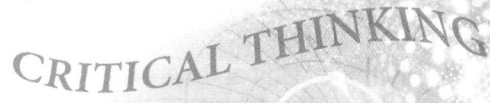

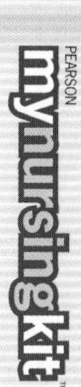

 Read

- History of Current Illness
- Past Medical History
- Physical Exam
- Admitting Medical Orders
- Laboratory Study Results

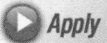 **Document**

- Summary of Hospitalization
- Pathophysiology Form
- Laboratory Values
- Laboratory Results Explanation

Apply

- List of Potential Nursing Diagnoses
- Concept Map
- Critical Thinking Questions

Log on to MyNursingKit.com to download forms you will need and to complete further steps in the Clinical Preparation assignment.

HISTORY OF PRESENT ILLNESS

Mrs. M. is a 78-year-old Caucasian female admitted through the emergency department for substernal chest pain. Even though Mrs. M. was admitted to the hospital with rule-out myocardial infarction, one health issue of concern was her inability to hear or follow simple commands. On closer evaluation it was determined that Mrs. M. had a definite hearing problem, one worthy of more investigation.

Once Mrs. M.'s cardiac status was stabilized, the concern turned to her hearing problem. Mrs. M. stated that she has noticed a progressive decline in her ability to hear, so much so that she has asked her family to provide a telephone with an amplifier so that she can hear conversations better. After an audiology examination conducted several years ago, she was diagnosed with presbycusis in addition to some degree of sensorineural hearing loss, probably due to ototoxic medications.

Medical–Surgical History

Allergies: naproxen sodium, hives

Medications: Lanoxin 0.125 mg po q a.m., aspirin 85 mg po q a.m., Toprox XL 100 mg po daily, Altace 2.5 mg po bid

Previous illnesses: pulmonary tuberculosis, 1944, treated with repeated pneumothorax treatments; history of taking streptomycin in 1955 prophylactically for tuberculosis; diagnosed with type II diabetes mellitus in 1993, diet controlled; progressive alteration in hearing

Surgeries: bilateral knee replacements, 1994

Social History

Family history: parents deceased; husband, two daughters alive/well

Social history: married, lives with husband split-level home

Physical Exam

Elderly white female

Height: 5 ft 3 inches; weight: 154 lbs

Temperature: 98.0°F

Pulse: 64 and regular

Respirations: 18 and regular

Blood pressure: 138/88 right arm

O_2 saturation: 93% on room air

HEENT: uses reading glasses; own teeth/no dentures

Neck: no JVD; carotid pulses present bilaterally

Heart: NSR, rate/rhythm regular

Lungs: present right lobes, reduced left upper lobe

Abdomen: soft, nontender, mildly obese

Extremities: no edema; pedal pulses strong; bilateral scars present over both knees

Neuro: Alert and oriented × 3

CXR: mild cardiomegaly

ECG: changes consistent with mild ischemia

Admitting Medical Orders

Admit to telemetry unit

Cardiology

Condition: stable

Allergies: naproxen sodium, hives

Diagnosis: R/O pending MI; status postcardiac catheterization; 80% blockage of LAD coronary artery; stent placed

Audiology consult

IV: saline lock; flush q8h

Diet: NAS

Oxygen: 2 L NC

Daily weight

I&O

Accu-Chek ac and at bedtime

Sequential compression devices (SCDs) to lower extremities

Bed rest with bathroom privileges

Vital signs and oxygen saturation q4h

Incentive spirometer q2h while awake

Call house officer if: pulse < 60 & > 110/minute; BP < 90 & > 160 systolic; temperature > 38.5; urine output < 30 mL/hr for 2 hours; respiratory rate > 30/minute; oxygen saturation <92%; Accu-Chek < 70 and > 130

Scheduled Medications

Lanoxin 0.125 mg po q a.m.

Aspirin 81 mg po q a.m.

Toprox XL 100 mg po daily

Altace 2.5 mg po bid

Postcatheterization: Plavix 75 mg po q a.m.

Glipizide SR 10 mg po daily

PRN Medications

Nitroglycerin 0.4 mg sublingual prn chest pain q5min × 3

Morphine 0.3–5 mg IV q3–5min; maximum dose 15 mg q3hr prn pain

Phenergan 25 mg IV q6h prn nausea

Mylanta 30 mL q4–6h po prn dyspepsia

Triazolam 0.125–0.25 mg po q noc, prn sleep

Ativan 0.5–2 mg IV q6–8h prn anxiety

Milk of Magnesia 30 mL po daily, prn constipation

Tylenol 650 mg po/PR q4h for pain

Ordered Laboratory Studies

Fasting blood sugar

Hemoglobin A1c

Troponin I q8h × 3

CPK-MB q8h × 3

Basic chemistry panel, CBC, magnesium q a.m.

Lipid panel in a.m.

Ordered Diagnostic Studies

Chest x-ray on admission

12-lead ECG

Echocardiogram

Cardiac catheterization

LABORATORY STUDY RESULTS

Test	Before Heart Catheterization	After Heart Catheterization	Day 2
Sodium	140 mEq/L	138 mEq/L	139 mEq/L
Potassium	4 mEq/L	4.2 mEq/L	4.2 mEq/L
Chloride	101 mEq/L	99 mEq/L	103 mEq/L
Carbon dioxide (CO_2)	22 mEq/L	24 mEq/L	25 mEq/L
Blood urea nitrogen (BUN)	19 mg/dL	18 mg/dL	18 mg/dL
Creatinine	1.2 mg/dL	1.0 mg/dL	1.1 mg/dL
Fasting blood sugar	160 mg/dL		
Hemoglobin A1c	7.0%		
Phosphorus	2.1 mg/dL	3.2 mg/dL	3.7 mg/dL
Calcium	8.1 mg/dL	8.2 mg/dL	8.6 mg/dL
Magnesium	2.0 mEq/L	1.9 mEq/L	2.0 mEq/L
Creatine kinase	4,018 units/L	3,612 units/L	2,000 units/L

Test	Before Heart Catheterization	After Heart Catheterization	Day 2
Relative index	>5.9%	>10.1%	>9.2%
CK–MB	>300.00%	>300.00%	259.7%
Troponin I	>100 ng/mL	80.91 ng/mL	51.00 ng/mL
WBC	11.5/mm³	11.0/mm³	9.3/mm³
RBC	4.21/mm³	4.89/mm³	4.92/mm³
Hemoglobin	12.9 g/dL	11.5 g/dL	12.7 g/dL
Hematocrit	37.5%	36.8%	37.6%
Platelets	262,000/mm³	280,000/mm³	300,000/mm³
Cholesterol	256 mg/dL		
High-density lipoproteins (HDL)	30 mg/dL		
Low-density lipoproteins (LDL)	158 mg/dL		
Very low-density lipoproteins (VLDL)	60%		
Apolipoproteins	152 mg/dL		
Triglycerides	201 mg/dL		

CRITICAL THINKING QUESTIONS

1. Mrs. M. needs to have the television on extremely loud and her roommate is complaining. What can you do to help the situation?

2. Knowing the type of hearing loss Mrs. M. is experiencing, what would be the best treatment for her?

3. Is Mrs. M. a candidate for a hearing aid or cochlear implant? Why?

4. Identify four specific discharge instructions to help the family work with Mrs. M.'s hearing disorder until further treatment is prescribed.

Answers to Critical Thinking Questions appear in Appendix D.

NCLEX® REVIEW

1. A patient tells the nurse that she's had her right eardrum punctured many times when she was a child. The nurse realizes this patient might have difficulty with:
   1. Balance.
   2. Movement.
   3. Sound transmission.
   4. Equilibrium.

2. A patient tells the nurse that she hears better when she isn't wearing a scarf over her head. The nurse realizes this patient is describing which mechanism of hearing?
   1. Bone conduction
   2. Air conduction
   3. Middle ear conduction
   4. Acoustic nerve conduction

3. A young male was brought into the emergency department because he suddenly couldn't hear. Upon examination, it was determined that a small object was lodged deeply into his ear canal. Which type of hearing loss did this patient experience?
   1. Mixed
   2. Acoustic
   3. Conductive
   4. Sensorineural

4. A young mother with a 2-week-old infant tells the nurse that she hopes her baby has good hearing since deafness "runs in her family." Which of the following should the nurse instruct this patient?
   1. The baby can't be tested for hearing until at least the age of 1.
   2. Even if tested, the baby's hearing will change as he grows.
   3. The baby should be tested now.
   4. The baby's sense of hearing hasn't developed yet.

5. A patient is scheduled for a stapedectomy. The nurse realizes this procedure is used to most likely treat which of the following causes of a hearing disorder?
   1. Mechanical
   2. Inflammatory
   3. Obstructive
   4. Mixed

6. The nurse is caring for a patient with a hearing deficit. Which of the following should be included in this patient's discharge planning for environmental safety?
   1. Assist with location for American Sign Language classes
   2. Removal of scatter rugs throughout the home
   3. Mechanism to ensure a visual alert in the event of a home fire
   4. Instruction on electrical cord safety

7. An elderly patient tells the nurse that she has a difficult time hearing. Which of the following should the nurse do to assist this patient's hearing deficit?

1. Shout directly into the patient's ear.

2. Drop the tone of the voice when talking.

3. Clap hands directly into the patient's face to gain the patient's attention.

4. Write everything down for the patient to read.

8. A patient with a new onset of a hearing loss becomes anxious when the nurse begins to leave the room. Which of the following should the nurse do to help this patient?

1. Assure the patient that the call light will be answered as soon as possible.

2. Tell the patient that there are other patients who have more important needs at this time.

3. Suggest that the patient walk in the hall to see other people.

4. Turn on the television for the patient.

Answers for review questions appear in Appendix D

KEY TERMS

acoustic neuroma *p.2307*
air conduction *p.2303*
bone conduction *p.2303*
conductive hearing loss *p.2303*
decibel (dB) *p.2311*
exostosis *p.2304*
frequency *p.2310*
labyrinthectomy *p.2308*
labyrinthitis *p.2308*

mastoidectomy *p.2305*
mastoiditis *p.2305*
Ménière's disease *p.2309*
mixed hearing loss *p.2303*
myringotomy *p.2304*
noise-induced hearing loss (NIHL) *p.2307*
otitis externa *p.2304*
otitis media *p.2305*
otosclerosis *p.2304*

ototoxic *p.2305*
pitch *p.2311*
presbycusis *p.2305*
sensorineural hearing loss *p.2303*
stapedectomy *p.2304*
tinnitus *p.2305*
tympanoplasty *p.2304*
vertigo *p.2308*
vestibular nerve dissection *p.2308*

PEARSON

EXPLORE **mynursingkit**™

MyNursingKit is your one stop for online chapter review materials and resources. Prepare for success with additional NCLEX®-style practice questions, interactive assignments and activities, web links, animations and videos, and more!

Register your access code from the front of your book at
www.mynursingkit.com

REFERENCES

American Academy of Otolaryngology–Head and Neck Surgery. (2002). *Noise and hearing protection.* Retrieved June 25, 2007, from http://www.entnet.org/healthinfo/hearing/noise_hearing.cfm

American College of Radiology. (2008). Guideline title: *Vertigo and hearing loss.* Retrieved on September 29, 2008 from http://www.guideline.gov/summary/summary.aspx?ss=15&doc_id=9602&nbr=5123

Black, F. O., Pesznecker, S. C., Homer, L., & Stallings, V. (2004). Benign paroxysmal positional nystagmus in hospitalized subjects receiving ototoxic medications. *Otol. Neurotol., 25*(3), 353–358.

Deaf Mental Health Charter. (2007). *Mental Health Foundation.* Retrieved June 21, 2007, from http://www.mhf.org.uk/our-work/service-development/all-age-groups/deaf-charter

Hain, T. C. (2007). *Benign paroxysmal positional vertigo.* Retrieved on August 21, 2007, from http://www.dizziness-and-balance.com/disorders/bppv/bppv.html

Holloway, N. M. (2004). *Medical-surgical care planning* (4th ed.). Philadelphia: Lippincott Williams & Wilkins.

Hunter, J. (1996). *Genetics and inheritance.* Retrieved July 2007 from Dartmouth University website: http://www.dartmouth.edu/~cbbc/courses/bio4/bio4-1997/01-Genetics.html

Imai, T., et al. (2005). Natural course of the remission of vertigo in patients with benign paroxysmal positional vertigo. *Neurology, 64,* 920–923.

Isaacson, J. E. (2005). In C. M. Porth (Ed.), *Pathophysiology: Concepts of altered health* (7th ed.). Philadelphia: Lippincott Williams & Wilkins.

Jones, E. G., Renger, R. and Kang, Y. (2007). Self efficacy for health related behaviors among deaf adults. *Research in Nursing and Health. 30*(2), 185–192.

Kim, C. S., Chang, S. O., & Lim, D. (Eds.). (2000). Updates in cochlear implantation. *Advances in Otorhinolaryngology, 57,* 22–27.

Mitchell, R. (1997). *Genetics and inheritance.* Retrieved July 2007 from Dartmouth University website: http://www.dartmouth.edu/~cbbc/courses/bio4/bio4-1997/01-Genetics.html

Kuramoto AM. (2006). Therapeutic benefits of t'ai chi exercise: research review. WMJ. 105(7):42-6.

Murray, R. B. and Zentner, J. P. (2001). *Health promotion strategies through the life span* (7th ed.). New Jersey: Prentice Hall, pages 765–767, 782–783.

National Conference of State Legislators. (2007, May). *50 State summary of newborn hearing screening laws.* Retrieved June 21, 2007, from http://www.ncsl.org/programs/health/hear50.htm

National Institutes on Deafness and Other Communication Disorders. (2001, January). *Hearing loss and older adults* (NIH Publication No. 01-4913). Retrieved June 25, 2007, from http://www.nidcd.nih.gov

National Guidelines Clearinghouse. (1999). ACR Appropriateness Criteria for vertigo and hearing loss. www.guideline.gov

National Health and Nutrition Exam Survey (2004). Retrieved on June 25, 2007 from www.cdc.gov/nchs/nhanes.htm

National Institute of Health. (2000). Clinical advisory: NIDCD/VA clinical trial finding can benefit millions with hearing loss. Retrieved from www.nlm.nih.gov. on June 25, 2007. October 2000.

National Institutes on Deafness and Other Communication Disorders. (2002a, November). *Cochlear implants* (NIH Publication No. 00-4798). Retrieved June 25, 2007, from http://www.nidcd.nih.gov

National Institutes on Deafness and Other Communication Disorders. (2002b, February). *Hearing aids* (NIH Publication No. 99-4340). Retrieved June 25, 2007, from http://www.nidcd.nih.gov

Parmet, S., Lynm, C., & Glass, R. (2003). Adult hearing loss. *Journal of the American Medical Association, 289,* 2020.

Sadler, G. R., Huang, J. T., Padden, C. A., et al. (2001). Accommodating Deaf Patients in Non-Hospital Settings. *Journal of Cancer Education, 16*(2) 105-8.

Sandhaus, S. (2002). Stop the spinning: Diagnosing and managing vertigo. *Nurse Practitioner, American Journal of Primary Health Care, 27*(8), 19–25.

Shaia, W. T., Zappia, J. J., Bojrab, D. I., LaRouere, M. L., Sargent, E. W., & Diaz, R. C. (2006). Success of posterior semicircular canal occlusion and application of the dizziness handicap inventory. *Otolaryngology–Head Neck Surgery, 134*(3), 424–430.

Smith, R. J. H., & Camp, G. V. (2007). *Deafness & hereditary hearing loss: Overview.* Seattle: University of Washington.

UCSD Student Health Service. (2007). Retrieved July 2007 from http://studenthealth.UCSD.edu

University of Iowa Hospital & Clinics. (2006). *Hearing loss in adults.* Retrieved July 2007 from http://www.uihealthcare.com/topics/hearing/hear4685.html

United States Department of Health and Human Services. (2000). *Healthy people 2010: Understanding and improving health.* Retrieved February 5, 2008, from http://www.healthypeople.gov

Caring for the Patient with Visual Disorders

Lucie S. Elfervig

Outcome-Based Learning Objectives

After studying this chapter, the learner will be able to:

1. Identify the normal basic anatomy and physiology of the eye.

2. Perform basic assessment, tests, and examination of the eye in obtaining meaningful data for management and treatment.

3. Describe different types of visual and ocular conditions and problems.

4. Apply nursing diagnoses, nursing process, and patient teaching associated with the visual and ocular problems of adults.

5. Discuss and provide meaningful resources for patients with visual and ocular problems.

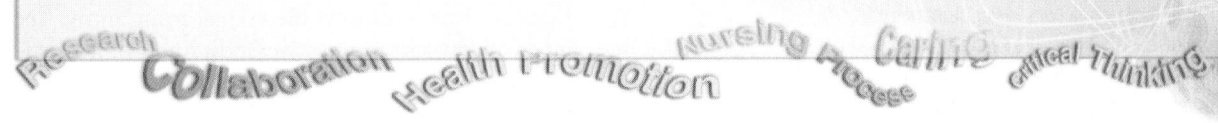

Research · Collaboration · Health Promotion · Nursing Process · Caring · Critical Thinking

THE SENSE of sight is one of the primary means of being active and taking joy in the visual world, being that the other senses seem to direct one toward seeing what is heard, what is touched, what is smelled, and what is tasted. So, truly sight guides most of one's daily activities. The eyes also provide a window or insight into the body's functions. Systemic problems or conditions that have visual or ocular manifestations can be discovered for the first time on an ocular examination. Chart 71–1 (p. 2326) outlines the more common systemic problems that may be manifested through ocular conditions. Often, ocular impairment can be preventable with early recognition and treatment that will save vision and prevent blindness. Visual disorders, depending on the degree of vision loss, can be very disturbing, with a sense of hopelessness, loss, powerlessness, and bereavement for the patient as well as the patient's family. Vision loss may be as minor as a refractive error that can be corrected with glasses, contact lenses, or laser or as severe as ocular trauma with functional vision loss, no light perception, or enucleation. Visual impairment creates both a physical and a psychological adjustment that can limit a patient's activities of daily living (ADL).

Visual assessment is a vital part of the nurse's function in caring for the whole patient and giving reassurance to patients that the nurse is there for their total well-being. Nurses play a key role in assisting, planning, implementing, evaluating, and educating patients and their families in adapting to new cop-

ing skills for everyday changes that can come with visual disorders. This chapter provides an overview of visual disorders for the adult through the aged, clarifying in greater detail the ocular disorders that appear more often today, and how best to evaluate and manage eye and ocular conditions. Many eye professionals perform specific roles in the evaluation, assessment, and treatment of medical and surgical ocular diseases and conditions. Typically health care providers adhere to the vision objectives set forth for the first time in *Healthy People 2010*. These objectives, commonly referred to as *Healthy Vision 2010*, provide a framework to assessment and promotion of ocular health through the chapter. These are detailed in the National Guidelines feature entitled Healthy Vision 2010 for Eye Evaluation (p. 2327).

Anatomy and Physiology Overview

The eyeball and its structures can be examined externally and internally. The orbit and ocular adnexa structures include the orbital contents and walls, eyebrows, eyelashes, eyelids, lacrimal puncta, lacrimal system, and extraocular muscles (Figure 71–1 ■, p. 2326). The eye structures include the canthus, conjunctiva, limbus, sclera, cornea, anterior and posterior chambers, trabecular meshwork, choroid, ciliary body, iris, pupil, lens, vitreous body, and retina.

CHART 71–1 **Ocular Conditions Resulting from Systemic Problems**

Systemic Problem	Ocular Condition
Atopic dermatitis	Keratoconus
	Trichiasis
Cerebrovascular accident (stroke)	Vascular occlusion
	Hemianopia, blindness
Cirrhosis	Xanthelasma
Diabetes mellitus	Rubeosis iridis
	Dot/blot hemorrhages
	Exudates
	Vitreous hemorrhage
Giant cell arteritis	Anterior ischemic optic neuropathy (AION)
	Amaurosis fugax
	Cilioretinal artery occlusion (CAO)
	Cotton-wool spots (CWS)
Gout	Asteroid hyalosis
	Bilateral conjunctival hyperemia
Herpes zoster (shingles)	Disciform keratitis
	Unilateral facial lesions
	Trigeminal dermatomes
Histoplasmosis	Choroiditis
	Peripheral hypopigmented spots
	Choroidal neovascular membrane (CNV)
Hypertension	Hard exudates, edema
	Narrow arterioles
	Cotton-wool spots
Hyperthyroidism (Graves' disease)	Exophthalmos
	Eyelid retraction
	Braley's sign*
Immunosuppressive disease (AIDS)	Cytomegalovirus retinitis
Inflammatory bowel disease	Frequent subconjunctival hemorrhages
	Limbal infiltrates
	Episcleritis
Leukemia	Roth's spots**
	Papilledema
Multiple sclerosis (MS)	Optic nerve edema
	Nystagmus
	Diplopia
Rheumatoid arthritis	Anterior scleritis
	Episcleritis
	Filamentary keratitis
Systemic Lupus Erythematosis (SLE)	Keratoconjunctivitis sicca (KCS)***
	Cotton-wool spots
	Central serous retinopathy (CSR)
Third nerve palsy	Ptosis
	Ophthalmoplegia
Toxoplasmosis	Retinochoroiditis
	Cystoid macular edema (CME)
Usher's syndrome	Posterior subcapsular cataract (PSC)
	Pigmentary retinopathy
	Bull's-eye retinal lesions
	(Other key symptom: deafness)

*Braley's sign: Intraocular pressure increases in an upward gaze, as compared to looking in a normal position.
**Roth's spot: retinal hemorrhage that has a white center.
***Keratoconjunctivitis sicca (KCS): dry eye syndrome.

Sources: Gold, D. H., & Weingeist, T. A. (2001). *Color atlas of the eye in systemic disease.* Philadelphia: Lippincott Williams & Wilkins; Kanski, J. J. (2001). *Systemic diseases and the eye: Signs and differential diagnosis.* London: Mosby International Limited; and Watson, P. G., Hazleman, B. L., Pavesio, C. E., & Green, W. R. (2004). *The sclera & systemic disorders* (2nd ed.). Philadelphia: Butterworth-Heinemann.

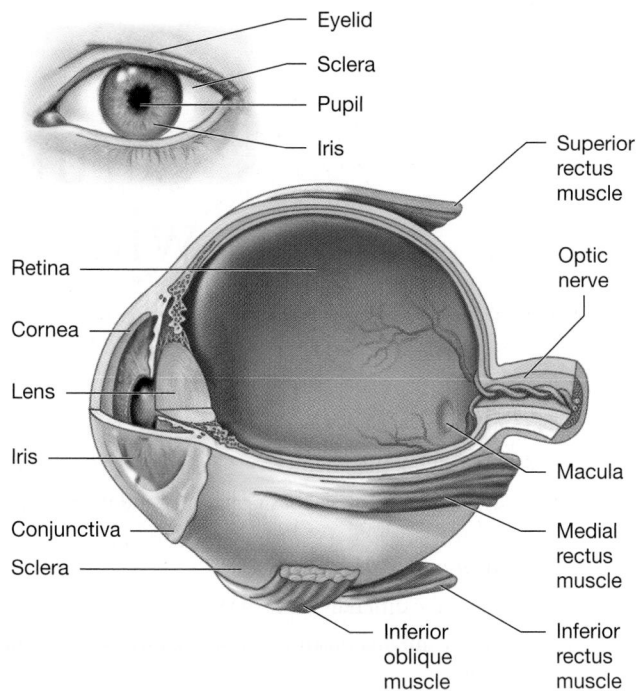

FIGURE 71–1 ■ The human eye.

Orbit and Ocular Adnexa

The eyeball is encased on three sides by the bony cavity called the orbit, which protects the eyeball from injury. The orbit is lined with muscles, connective, and adipose or fat tissue. It is approximately 40 millimeters in all three dimensions (height, width, and depth), like a pear lying on its side. The orbital walls are made up of seven bones that include the frontal, zygomatic, sphenoid, ethmoid, lacrimal, palatine, and maxillary bones. The eyebrow lies over the bony prominence (superior orbital ridge) above the eyelids that acts as a protective ridge from falling debris or foreign objects getting into the eye. The upper and lower eyelashes are the ciliary hairs of the eyelids that help keep debris from falling into the eye. The eyelids contain the ocular glands, which include oil glands (meibomian and glands of Zeis), mucous glands (goblet cells), sweat glands (Moll), and aqueous glands (lacrimal and accessory lacrimal glands of Krause and Wolfring).

The space or exposed area between the upper and lower eyelids is called the interpalpebral fissure. The eyelids have a blink mechanism that operates by the levator palpebrae superioris muscle to protect the anterior portion of the eye and the spreading of tears across the cornea. This blink mechanism is very important to the health of the cornea. Upper and lower lacrimal puncta are the small openings at the nasal end of the upper and lower eyelid margins for the drainage of tears produced by the lacrimal system. The lacrimal gland lies under the upper eyelid skin between the lateral eyebrow edge and outer canthus.

The eyeball is able to move in all cardinal fields of gaze by the six extraocular muscles, which are the four rectus muscles (superior, medial, inferior, and lateral) and two oblique muscles (superior and inferior). The extraocular muscles are innervated by the third, fourth, and sixth cranial nerves, which coordinate the vision of both eyes with the occipital lobe of the brain to view a single image.

MyNursingKit | The American Academy of Opthalmology

HEALTHY VISION NATIONAL GUIDELINES for Eye Evaluation

Healthy Vision 2010 (DHHS, 2000b), objectives provide a way to identify vision and eye problems and an opportunity to improve the vision of all Americans with prevention measures established by the following organizations: the American Academy of Ophthalmology, National Eye Institute, Centers for Disease Control and Prevention's Vision Health Initiative, Glaucoma Foundation, and American Academy of Optometry. The focus of *Healthy Vision 2010* is to make Americans aware of eye diseases that can result in loss of vision and the necessary measures for prevention of eye disease and injury. The promotion of vision health and quality of life for all people, at all stages of life, addresses issues that affect cost, disability, and diseases in vision loss. To achieve its overall prevention goals, *Healthy People 2010* supports comprehensive community-based eye screenings and regular vision checkups—these vary between age and disease entity—with an eye health care provider. Regular eye examinations are a means of prevention, diagnosing eye problems early, as well as treatment for people diagnosed with diabetic retinopathy, cataracts, glaucoma, macular degeneration, and any vision problems that might lead to blindness. *Healthy People 2010* recommends comprehensive programs that must be applied universally to the general population and in a more intensive fashion to selected and indicated persons known to be at high risk for vision impairment; for example, those with diabetes (DHHS, 2000a). *Healthy People 2010* recognizes vision as the primary cue for conducting everyday activities. Vision is instrumental in development, learning, communicating, working, health, and quality of life. Vision loss creates many environmental, social, and psychological challenges for individuals and their families.

Healthy Vision 2010 has 10 main objectives related to vision assessment:

1. *Dilated eye examination.* To detect early diseases and disorders of the eye, because many eye conditions have no signs or symptoms, or warning. This should be done at least every 2 years for adults.

2. *Vision screening for children (under 5 years).* To detect vision problems before beginning school, in an effort to save sight.

3. *Impairment due to refractive errors.* Over 60% of Americans have refractive defects that could benefit from corrective lenses.

4. *Impairment in children and adolescents (under 18 years).* Reduce blindness and visual impairment, especially nearsightedness (myopia), which affects about 25% of schoolchildren.

5. *Diabetic eye disease.* Reduce vision loss and impairment due to diabetic retinopathy. Early diagnosis and treatment can prevent about 90% of vision loss with an annual dilated eye examination. About 50% of patients with diabetes are diagnosed too late for effective treatment.

6. *Reduce visual impairment due to glaucoma.* Optic nerve damage is a major health problem, and left untreated it will lead to blindness. Up to 3 million Americans have glaucoma and as many as 120,000 are blind. Glaucoma is the number-one cause of vision loss in African Americans. Half of the people with glaucoma are not being treated because they are unaware they have this condition; it is known as the silent blinder.

7. *Cataracts.* Reduce vision loss due to cataracts. They can occur in children, but are mostly a problem for adults age 50 and older. Treatment is readily available with surgery and intraocular lens implantation.

8. *Occupational injury.* Reduce vision loss from occupational injury and lost workdays. It is reported that 3 out of every 5 occupational eye injuries are due to not wearing safety goggles or protective eyewear. The Occupational Safety and Health Administration requires that employees be provided with protective eyewear, which can prevent 90% of eye-related accidents.

9. *Protective eyewear.* Increased use of personal protective eyewear for recreation, for hazardous projects at home, and for sports (hockey, racquetball, tennis, baseball, basketball, and paintball), which all bring some risk of eye injury.

10. *Vision rehabilitation.* Increase in the use of services for the visually impaired and the use of adaptive devices in aiding vision.

Nurses need to be knowledgeable of these objectives and guidelines in educating patients and families in the prevention of vision loss, in providing educational materials on eye health, and in promoting early detection and treatment of eye diseases.

Sources: U.S. Department of Health and Human Services (DHHS). (2000a). *Healthy People 2010: Vision and hearing.* Retrieved April 26, 2007, from http://www.healthypeople.gov/document/HTML/Volume2/28Vision.htm; and U.S. Department of Health and Human Services (DHHS). (2000b). *Healthy Vision 2010.* Retrieved April 26, 2007, from http://www.healthyvision.2010.org

Eye Structures

It is necessary to understand the anatomic structure of the eye as a whole in order to identify pathophysiological conditions and their impact on the individual. The basic anatomic structures are explained next.

The temporal and nasal canthi are the outer and inner tissue edges where the upper and lower eyelids meet. The palpebral and bulbar conjunctivas are the mucous membrane lining of the undersurface of the eyelids and eyeball itself, up to the limbal margin, respectively. The fornix or cul-de-sac is the junction where the palpebral and bulbar conjunctivas meet. The limbus or the corneoscleral junction is the margin between the sclera and the cornea. The sclera, which is the white part and the outer protective layer of the eyeball, helps maintain its shape. The cornea, which is the transparent, avascular center at the anterior surface of the eyeball, is the major refractive surface of the eye. The refractive media of the cornea bend light rays to a single focus on the retina. The epithelium is the outermost layer of the cornea that is protected by the tear film layers that also gives the cornea its smooth surface. The tear film is composed of three layers, and if any of the layers is defective, the health of the eye can be compromised. The tears are formed by a natural reflex response or emotional stimulus.

The anterior chamber is the space between the back of the cornea and the front of the iris. The posterior chamber is the space between the back of the iris and the front of the lens. Both these chambers contain aqueous humor, which is a clear fluid that provides nutrients for the eye. The aqueous humor is produced by the ciliary body, which also helps regulate intraocular pressure. The trabecular meshwork is a mesh-like filtering structure located at the iris–scleral junction (limbal region) at the angle in the anterior chamber. The meshwork assists in the regulation of the intraocular pressure of the eye with the filtering and flow of aqueous humor as it drains into the canal of Schlemm at the angle.

Uveal Tract

The uveal tract is composed of the choroid, ciliary body, and iris. The choroid is the middle layer of the eyeball between the retina and the sclera. The choroid contains the major vascular system of the eye that nourishes the outer retina. The ciliary body makes up the ciliary processes and ciliary muscles. The processes produce the aqueous humor that flows through the chambers and can affect the intraocular pressure of the eye. The ciliary muscles control the accommodative ability of the lens by the attachment of the zonular fibers between the lens and ciliary muscles. The ciliary muscle contractions can change the configuration of the trabecular meshwork or canal of Schlemm by increasing aqueous outflow and, in turn, can affect the intraocular pressure of the eye. The iris is a vascular and pigmented fiber that forms the colored portion of the eye that encompasses the pupil. The iris (iris diaphragm) is the division between the anterior and posterior chambers. The pupil is the black middle space of the iris, which constricts and dilates by the sphincter and the dilator muscles, respectively. This allows the refraction of light to enter the eye for vision. The pupils normally react to bright light by constricting, and they are usually equal, round, and accommodative.

Lens

The lens divides the aqueous humor from the vitreous humor or gel. It is the focusing structure of **accommodation** that allows seeing objects at close and at far range. The lens is supported by the zonular fibers that are attached to the ciliary body. It is the one ocular structure that continues to grow with aging.

Vitreous Body

The vitreous body is the largest chamber (roughly two-thirds) of the eye that maintains the shape of the eyeball. The vitreous gel is made up mainly of water with a collagen framework, which includes collagen (structure), hyaluronic acid (which gives the vitreous its viscosity), proteins, and solutes. The collagen network can be aggregated by vitreous collapse due to aging that forms vitreous opacities, which cast shadows on the retina. These shadows are referred to as **floaters**. The posterior and peripheral vitreous interfaces with the retina.

Retina

The retina is composed of 10 thin layers. Two of the major retina layers are the photoreceptor layer and the retinal pigment epithelium. The photoreceptor layer is composed of cones and rods for photopic (day) and scotopic (night) vision. The center of the retina, called the macula, is where the greatest number of cone receptors is located for central and color vision. The rod receptors mainly are in the peripheral retina for side or field vision. The very center of the macula is called the fovea or fovea centralis, where the greatest concentrations of cones are located for the sharpest visual acuity. The two main functions of the retinal pigment epithelium are the metabolism of vitamin A and the absorption of light, which aid in visual acuity by providing nutrients to the photoreceptors.

Other major structures in the retina are the optic disc and vessels. The optic disc is oval or circular, pinkish orange in color, with distinct margins; has a central depression or cup; and is the physiological blind spot on a visual field. The central cup of the disc is where the retinal vessels (arteries and veins)

enter and branch out to form the superior and inferior arcades that are the outer borders of the macula. The optic nerve is an extension of the central nervous system that forms a visual pathway behind the eyes. The pathway crosses at the chiasm where the optic nerve of each eye meets and crosses nasally and uncrosses temporally to form the optic tracts. The optic tracts continue to the lateral geniculate bodies, to the optic radiations, and then to the visual cortex of the occipital lobe of the brain.

Visual Assessment

Visual assessment should follow a thorough health history. Chart 71–2 outlines the categories and assessment of a health and ocular history. The categories include the general medical history, the visual history, and the history of clinical manifestations. It is important to ask the patient specifically about any inherited conditions such as diabetes, hypertension, macular degeneration, glaucoma, or unexplained vision loss. And if an injury has occurred, the nurse needs to make certain to question whether the trauma involved any metal-on-metal contact, as this tends to cause intraocular penetration.

Initial Examination

The initial examination should include the following procedures: visual acuity (VA) at far range (Figure 71–2 ■) and at near range (Figure 71–3 ■), external eye examination, the direct ophthalmoscope examination, and an intraocular pressure reading. For patients that cannot read, use a picture chart to obtain acuity. Chart 71–3 (p. 2330) outlines the steps for visual acuity testing.

The external evaluation can be done with the use of a penlight and visual observation. The components for completing

CHART 71–2	Health and Ocular History Assessment
Category	**Assessment**
General history	Any known allergies (drugs, foods, environment)? Using any prescription or over-the-counter medications? Any recent illnesses or surgeries? Any known medical history (especially diabetes, ulcers, strokes, hypertension, and pulmonary)?
Visual history	Wears glasses, contact lenses, or no correction? Are one or both eyes involved? Using any topical eyedrops or oral eye medications? Vision prior to problem, injury, or trauma (if applicable)? Any vision or eye test already obtained previously? Any prior eye surgery or laser?
History of clinical manifestations	Any signs and symptoms? Duration of signs and symptoms? Time and place of signs and symptoms, problem or injury/what happened? Any penetrating or perforating injury? Any metal?

Eye test chart for 10 feet

Actual size   20 ft. equivalent

$\frac{10}{100}$ K V D $\frac{20}{160}$

$\frac{10}{60}$ Z S H C $\frac{20}{125}$

$\frac{10}{50}$ H S K R N $\frac{20}{100}$

$\frac{10}{40}$ C H K R V D $\frac{20}{80}$

$\frac{10}{30}$ H O N S D C V $\frac{20}{60}$

$\frac{10}{25}$ O K H D N R C S $\frac{20}{50}$

$\frac{10}{20}$ V H D N K U O S R C $\frac{20}{40}$

$\frac{10}{15}$ B D C L K Z V H S R O A $\frac{20}{30}$

$\frac{10}{12}$ H K G B C A N O M P V E S R $\frac{20}{25}$

$\frac{10}{10}$ P K U E O B T V X R M J H C A Z D I $\frac{20}{20}$

$\frac{10}{8}$ D K N T W U L J S P X V M R A H C F O Y Z G $\frac{20}{15}$

FIGURE 71–2 ■ Visual acuity chart for far.

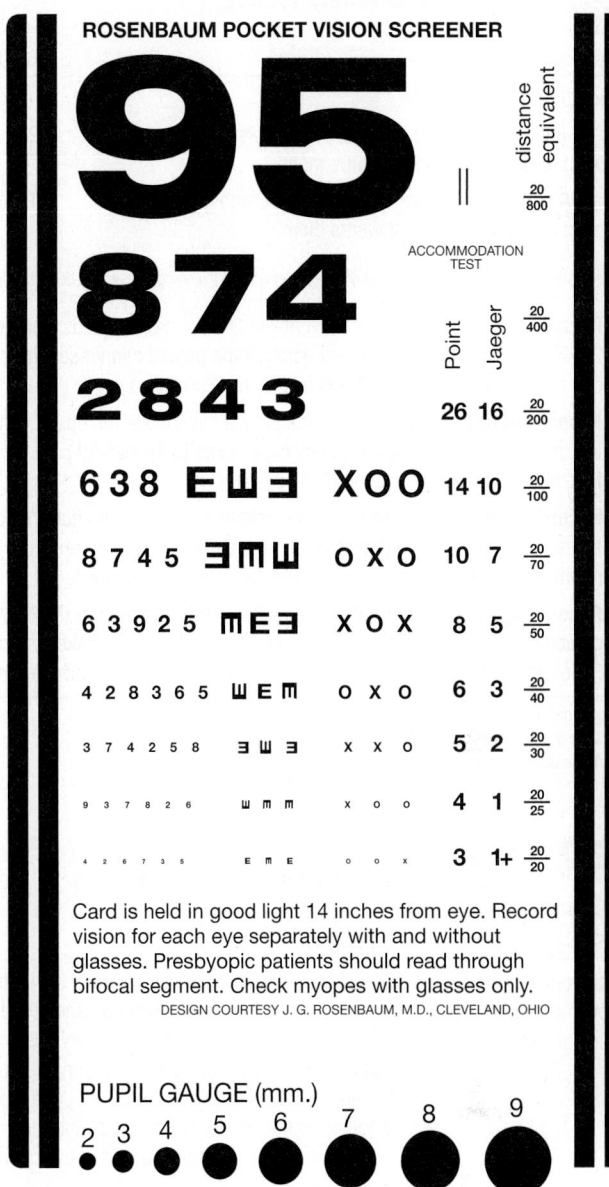

FIGURE 71–3 ■ Visual acuity chart for near.

the external examination and procedures are listed in Chart 71–4 (p. 2330) and Chart 71–5 (p. 2331).

Direct ophthalmoscope examination is used to check the fundus of the eye by viewing through the pupil. During the process, the nurse needs to view the cornea, anterior chamber, lens, and vitreous for clarity; check for any opacity in the visual pathway; and check the optic nerve (disc) for color, shape, and vessels (Figure 71–4 ■, p. 2332). Most medical offices, clinics, ambulatory centers, outpatient facilities, and emergency departments will be equipped with a direct ophthalmoscope.

It also is important to check intraocular pressure (IOP) if one has a tonometer (Figure 71–5 ■, p. 2332), or the nurse may need to gently palpate over the eyelid to indicate whether the eyeball is hard or soft (Figure 71–6 ■, p. 2332).

Diagnostic eye tests are essential for a complete ocular and visual evaluation to decide on the most definitive diagnosis and treatment regimen. Many of the diagnostic tests require anesthetic or dilating eyedrops. These drops are described in the Pharmacology Summary feature (p. 2346). The tests can include preoperative evaluations for cataract surgery for proper lenses implant, assessment of corneal health, visualization for possible retinal opacities and breaks, advancement of glaucoma, and genetic anomalies. Some of these diagnostic tests may include baseline fundus photography, fluorescein angiography, or ultrasonography. Other tests may be necessary to order for a more systemic assessment, such as x-rays, computed tomography (CT) scan, magnetic resonance imaging (MRI), and carotid ultrasound, in addition to specific blood tests and cultural sensitivities. Diagnostic tests that are used to assess ocular and visual health are outlined in the Diagnostic Tests box (p. 2333).

■ Visual Impairment

Visual impairment can be anything from correctable refractive errors, inherited anomalies, acquired visual changes, nutritional deficiencies, to aging changes. Refractive errors are the most

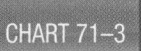

CHART 71–3   Visual Acuity Testing

Types	Distances	Charts
Take Visual Acuity (VA)*		
Far VA (right eye, left eye, and both eyes): with glasses or contact lenses if the patient wears them.	20 feet (6 meters)	Snellen acuity or equivalent distance chart
Near VA (right eye, left eye, and both eyes): with glasses or contact lenses if the patient wears them.	14–16 inches (38–40 centimeters)	Near reading chart

*Test vision with each eye separately: right eye, then left eye (covering the eye not being tested); once vision is obtained with each eye, then test vision with both eyes open.

- **Record VA**—20/20, 20/30, etc. whatever line the patient reads, and document each eye separately and together (e.g., 20/30 right eye, 20/50 left eye, 20/40 both eyes) for far and near acuity. If the patient cannot see the chart at the standard distance, then walk up to the patient with the chart until he can read the largest letter (this is usually the 200 letter).
- **Record Count Fingers (CF)***—If the patient cannot see the nurse's fingers, then the nurse moves her hand and sees whether the patient can detect the motion; the nurse moves increasingly closer to the patient until he sees the nurse's hand moving. For example, the recording might read: CF at 5 feet with right eye, left eye, and both eyes.
- **Record Hand Motion (HM)****—If the patient cannot see the nurse's hand move, then shine a light in the patient's eyes (best to dim the room lights) and see whether he can detect the light; the nurse moves increasingly closer to the patient until the light is perceived. For example the recording might read: HM at 2 feet with right eye, left eye, and both eyes.
- **Record Light Perception (LP) or Record No Light Perception (NLP)*****—If the patient cannot see the nurse's light, then the visual acuity is no light perception (NLP), with right eye or left eye. When doing LPs, make sure the light is bright, room lights are dimmed, and the opposite eye is covered well. For example the recording might read: LP at 3 inches with right eye, left eye, and both eyes.

* At the distance seen (e.g., CF at 5 feet), with right eye, left eye, and both eyes.
** At the distance seen (e.g., HM at 2 feet), with right eye, left eye, and both eyes.
*** At the distance seen (e.g., LP at 3 inches), with right eye, left eye, and both eyes.

CHART 71–4   Ocular and Vision Evaluation Tests

Test	Procedure
Extraocular muscle movement (cardinal fields of gaze)	The patient is seated directly opposite the tester, facing each other about 1 foot apart. The patient is instructed to look at a pen or target that is held in the tester's hand at a distance of 16 inches (40 centimeters). The patient is asked to follow the pen when the tester moves it in the primary position (looking straight ahead) to eight cardinal fields of gaze: from the primary position to look right upward, straight up, left upward, left temporal, left downward, straight down, right downward, and right temporal. The tester is to observe the patient and note whether her eyes move equally together in all fields of gaze, note whether both eyes are symmetrical, and record either as normal or, if any deviation from normal, as minimal (−1), moderate (−2), severe (−3), or total (−4) loss of eye movement.
Cover–uncover test for tropia	The patient is to wear his own corrective lenses, if he has them. Have the patient fixate on a target about 20 feet (6 meters) away for far and 16 inches (40 centimeters) for near; it can be a visual acuity chart, picture chart, E chart, or toy, the smallest line of clear acuity. The tester is to sit in front of the patient, but does not block target view. Note the eye that is fixating, cover that eye with an occluder, and note what the fellow eye does. If the uncovered eye moves to pick up fixation, note the direction it moves—toward the nose, then it was fixated outward, so it is exo; or toward the ear, then it was fixated inward, so it is eso. If the uncovered eye does not move and has steady fixation, no strabismus exists. The eye would move up and down to indicate vertical tropia.
Alternating cover test for phoria	The patient is to wear her own corrective lenses, if she has them. Have the patient fixate on a target about 20 feet (6 meters) away for far and 16 inches (40 centimeters) for near; it can be a visual acuity chart, picture chart, E chart, or toy, the smallest line of clear acuity. The tester is to sit in front of the patient, but does not block target view. Place the occluder in front of the right eye, hold it for about a second or so, and then move it swiftly over the left eye. This alternating cover test is repeated many times. Repeat with the occluder in front of the left eye for a second or so, then move it swiftly over the right eye, and repeat. The tester observes the eye that is just being uncovered to see whether it deviates. If the just uncovered eye moves inward, then it was fixed outward, so it is exo; and if the just uncovered eye moves outward, then it was fixed inward, so it is eso. If the just uncovered eye does not move and has steady fixation, no strabismus exist. The eye would move up and down to indicate vertical phoria.
Confrontation fields (visual field testing)	The tester is comparing the range of the patient's visual field in relation to the tester's visual field, which is assumed normal. The light source should be behind the patient, and the background behind the tester should be dark and uniform. The patient is seated, and the tester sits or stands directly opposite and facing the patient about 2 feet away. The patient's right eye is open and left eye is closed or occluded, while the tester's left eye is open and right eye is closed, and each fixes on the other's open eye. The tester will move her fingers or bright test object from the far periphery and note when it comes into the field of view; the tester and patient should see it at the same time. This is done for the four major quadrants (superior, nasal, inferior, and temporal) and repeated for the patient's left eye. The approximate normal degrees of angle recognition of the test object are 60° superior, 60° nasal, 70° inferior, and 80° temporal. Record results, and if any visual field defects are noted, the patient should be sent in for sophisticated visual field testing.

CHART 71–5	Ocular and Visual Evaluation and Assessment

Examination	Assessment
Initial Examination	
Central visual acuity	Take visual acuity (VA) of each eye separately and together at far and at near, with patient glasses if he wears them: with Snellen acuity chart or reading card; or use a newspaper, read a wall clock, or recognize faces at the bedside or at the doorway. Make some record of visual acuity.
Peripheral visual acuity	Take side vision; see whether the patient can see movement and objects coming in from the periphery. Confrontations can be done here; a visual field (VF) screening test.
Intraocular pressure (IOP)	Check IOP, if one has a tonometer, or may need to gently palpate over the eyelid to indicate whether the eyeball is hard or soft.
External Examination (Observations and Penlight Test)	Observe face and all structure surrounding the eye for any asymmetry or color, size, shape, or expression differences; and overall general appearance.
Eyelids	Does the eyelid close automatically (blink reflex)? Does the eyelid cover the cornea completely when closed? Does the eyelid lag or droop (ptosis)?
Eyelashes	Do the eyelashes curve inward (entropion) or outward (ectropion)? Are there any misaligned or missing lashes (trichiasis)?
Eyeball	Observe for obvious laceration, trauma, bruises, or black eye (ecchymosis). Does the eyeball appear sunken (enophthalmos) or protruding (proptosis)?
Conjunctiva	Observe and check for tearing, itching (pruritus), drainage, injection (hyperemia), swelling (edema), discoloration, lesions, scaling, or irregularities.
Sclera	Observe color (white) and vascular (red).
Cornea	Observe for clarity.
Anterior chamber	Check anterior chamber for whether it is clear and deep, meaning without discharge, deposits, or opaques; pus (hypopyon); or blood (hyphema). Sclera white and conjunctiva clear.
Pupils	Check pupils for size (in millimeters), shape, and whether pupils are equal, round, reactive to light and accommodation (PERRLA).
Iris	Observe color, shape, and size.
Muscles	Check eye mobility by checking the primary and eight cardinal fields of gaze for extraocular muscle function. Check for cross-eyes (exo = out, eso = in) by doing cover eye tests. Draw pictures of what is seen if indicated for documentation.
Direct Ophthalmoscope Examination*	Check for a red reflex, and note whether present or whether a different reflex is noted between the eyes (e.g., leukocoria-white reflex). View for media clarity (cornea, anterior chamber, lens, and vitreous), checking for any opacities or foreign bodies in the visual pathway. Check the optic nerve (disc) for color, shape, vessels, and cup/disc (C/D) ratio. View fovea (central vision area of the macula) for edema, color abnormalities, and foveal reflex (yellowish-orange reflex) to determine whether present or not, and whether there is asymmetry or atrophy.

*See Figures 71–2, 71–3, and 71–4 (pp. 2329 and 2332).

common vision problem in the general population. Four of the leading causes of visual impairment are macular degeneration, diabetic retinopathy, glaucoma, and cataracts. Measuring refractive error is referred to as a manifested refraction (MR) that is performed on a phoropter, a refractive device used to measure the degree of optical correction needed for one's best-corrected visual acuity (BVA) with the use of spherical, cylindrical, and prismatic lenses.

Refraction

Refraction refers to refractive errors or the bending of light rays through different media (cornea, anterior humor, lens, and vitreous humor) as the rays enter the eyes (Miller & Scott, 2004).

Refractive errors now are being referred to as first-order aberrations, with the new wavefront technology able to measure more precisely each layer of the eye and eye structures for more meticulously customized correction (Thall, Thammano, & Miller, 2004). **Aberration** is more ideally defined as any deviation from perfect behavior; in other words, the lower the aberration, the sharper the image (Thall et al., 2004).

Emmetropia

The term for no refractive error or normal vision without any corrective optical devices is **emmetropia**, meaning the eye is able to focus light rays on the retina to form a clear and sharp image on its own. *Surgically induced emmetropia* is a term used to describe

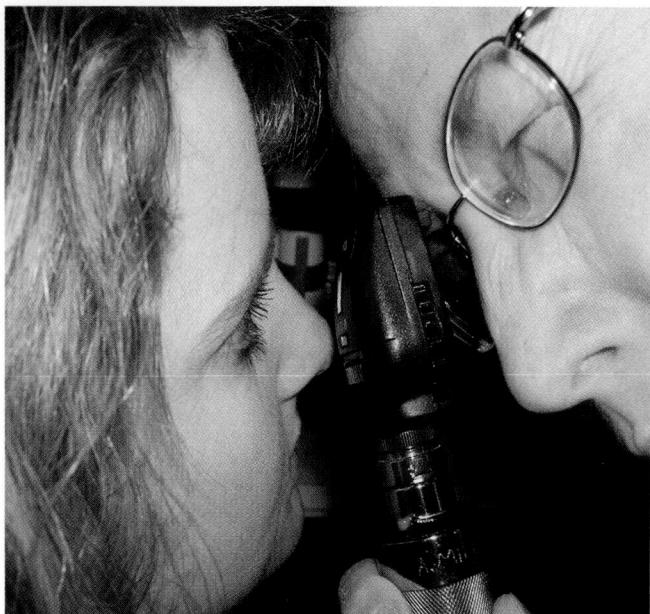

FIGURE 71–4 ■ Direct ophthalmoscope examination.
Source: Kathleen Osborn

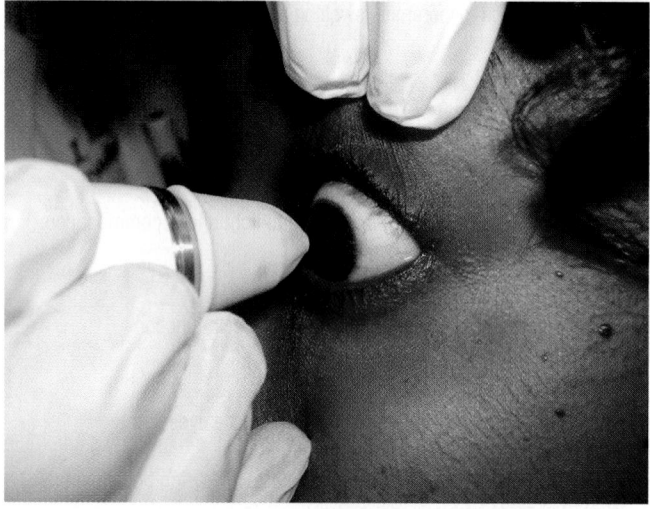

FIGURE 71–5 ■ Application of Tono-Pen for intraocular pressure.
Source: Kathleen Osborn

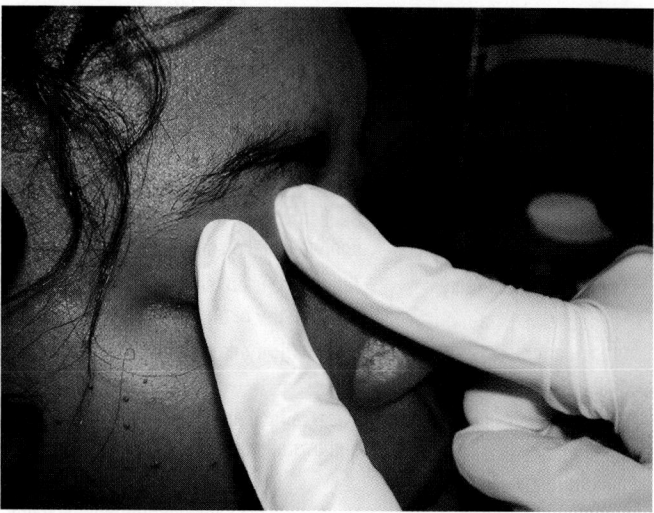

FIGURE 71–6 ■ Palpation of intraocular pressure.
Source: Kathleen Osborn

patients who have had previous refractive surgical correction to create 20/20 visual acuity without any corrective optical devices such as glasses or contact lenses. Refractive surgery is the use of a laser to reshape the corneal curvature to eliminate or to reduce refractive errors. Refractive surgery gradually is becoming the norm, instead of the exception, with the advent of decreased cost, increased advertisement, and social pressure to keep looking youthful. Contact lenses and glasses are becoming less "in vogue," even though they are an alternative to refractive surgery. Potential contraindications that negate refractive surgery may be unrealistic expectations, too high of a refractive or astigmatic error, cornea that is too thin (< 560 micrograms), pupil natural dilation that is too large (> 6.5 to 9 millimeters), severely dry corneas, previous eye surgery, and lack of understanding of the procedure and its risks and benefits (Abad & Azar, 2004). The preoperative refractive laser surgery evaluation may include an extensive interview and

visual/ocular measurements. A number of refractive laser surgical correction procedures are available, depending on the patient and/or surgeon preference and the particular presenting problem.

Ametropia

Ametropia is a general term used to indicate a refractive error that is present, which usually can be corrected with glasses, contact lenses, or possibly refractive surgery. The four most common forms of ametropia are myopia, hyperopia, astigmatism, and presbyopia.

Myopia

Myopia, nearsightedness, is the condition in which distance objects are unclear. The parallel light rays fall in front of the retina, because of a longer axial length of the eyeball, which requires a minus (concave) corrective lens to focus the image on the fovea for sharp vision. Other myopic shifts can be created when a patient with diabetes has elevated blood sugar, which makes the natural crystalline lens swell, or there are nuclear sclerosis cataracts in the elderly. Myopia is the most common ametropia, making up over 80% of the refractive errors in the general population (Abad & Azar, 2004).

Hyperopia

Hyperopia or hypermetropia, farsightedness, is the condition in which near objects are unclear. The parallel light rays fall behind the retina, because of a shorter axial length of the eyeball, which requires a plus (convex) corrective lens to focus the image on the fovea for normal or correct vision.

Astigmatism

Astigmatism, irregular corneal surface or asphericity, means that the refractive power is not homogeneous in all meridians, which prevents light rays from focusing on a single point (AAO-3, 2008–2009). Astigmatism usually can be corrected with the required lens or contact lens correction at a specific optical axis.

Presbyopia

Presbyopia is lack of accommodation, the ability to focus from distance to near images, because of aging. Presbyopia usually requires a plus lens correction, bifocals, or trifocals, depending on

DIAGNOSTIC TESTS for Visual Disorders

Test	Definition
Exophthalmometry	The measuring of the degree the eyeball extends from the edge of the eyelids or protrudes from the orbit (e.g., a sign of hyperthyroidism).
Schirmer's test	The measuring of tear production; to treat variations of dry eye syndrome.
Glare test	The measuring of artificial sunlight's effect at various degrees of bright light intensity (usually three: low, medium, and high); for cataract surgery readiness determination.
Potential acuity meter (PAM)	The measuring of potential visual acuity returns after cataract surgery.
Gonioscopy	Using a microscopic instrument to view and to examine the anterior chamber angle structures for patency or any obstructions.
Visual field (VF) perimetry	The measuring of peripheral or side vision with standard machines or manual screenings for vision loss or blind spots (scotoma).
Glaucoma diagnostic test (GDx)	The measuring of the optic nerve health and glaucomatous changes.
Pachymetry (PACH)	The measuring the thickness of the cornea; used in the treatment of glaucoma and refractive surgery.
Keratometry readings (K-readings)	The measuring of the corneal curvature for detecting astigmatism; used in refractions, refractive surgery, and cataract surgery.
Corneal topography (topo)	The measuring of the corneal layers for use in refractive surgery and treating keratoconus and other corneal anomalies.
Ultrasonography:	The use of high-frequency sound waves to detect and outline intraocular and orbital structures by measuring the distance between them. Changes and opacities can be easily recognized by this method.
• A-scan	Measuring axial length for cataract surgery: distinguish between benign and malignant eye tumors.
• B-scan	Two-dimensional image for viewing intravitreal opacities, detachments, tumors, muscles, and inflammation.
Fundus photography (FP)	The photographs of the posterior pole of the retina.
Fluorescein angiography (FA) or indocyanine green (ICG) angiography	The intravenous injection of a dye into the bloodstream to measure the retinal vascular perfusion, infarcts, stenosis, ischemia, leakages, neovascularizations, avascular obstructions, microaneurysms, and retina defects for the evaluating, diagnosing, monitoring, and treating of ocular diseases.
Optical coherence tomography (OCT)	The viewing and measuring of the retinal layers for edema, holes, degeneration, and other anomalies.
Ophthalmodynamometry (ODN)	The measuring of the blood pressure of the ophthalmic artery by increasing intraocular pressure; and it induces pulsations in the central retinal artery at the optic nerve, to determine carotid artery insufficiency or poor disc perfusion.
Color vision tests	The measuring of color vision for any deficiency, such as the lack of red-green discrimination or blue-yellow discrimination.
Electrophysiology:	The measuring of the visual pathways from the retinal photoreceptors to the visual cortex of the brain.
• Visual evoked potential (VEP)	The measuring of vision potential of seeing (occipital cortex); in diagnosing visual function, unexplained vision loss, retinal vascular diseases, ocular traumatic problems, visual pathway lesions, toxic or nutritional eye diseases, glaucoma, and optic nerve diseases.
• Electro-oculogram (EOG)	The measuring (from cornea to retinal layers) of retinal pigment epithelium functions; in diagnosing ocular melanoma, opacification, retinal toxicities, retinal disorders (especially in macular dystrophies), and inherited retinal diseases (especially Best's disease).
• Electroretinogram (ERG)	The measuring of cone/rod functions (diffuse electrical response generated by the neural to nonneural cells of the retina); in diagnosing intracranial lesions, inherited retinal diseases (e.g., retinitis pigmentosa), retinal vascular diseases, visual opacities/traumatic problems, toxic or nutritional diseases, glaucoma, and unexplained vision loss.
Ophthalmic radiography: • Plain x-ray	Right oblique, left oblique, and lateral views of the affected side for the diagnoses of orbital fractures and tumors are usually sufficient.
• Computed tomography (CT) scan, with and without contrast	For serial section views of the orbit and eye; especially in diagnosing tumors, intraocular masses, orbital disease, intracranial diseases, and bone structure.
• Magnetic resonance imaging (MRI)	For high magnetic field to evaluate the brain, orbit, and eye; giving better definition of tissue and fluid locations, especially edema that involves the orbital area and surrounding tissue.

(continued)

DIAGNOSTIC TESTS for Visual Disorders—*Continued*

Test	Definition
• Carotid ultrasound	Used to determine blockage of the carotid arteries, uses high frequency sound waves to create images of the insides of the carotids to determine whether plaque has formed in the arteries. May also be used with a Doppler to show blood flow through the arteries.
Laboratory tests: • Elevated erythrocyte sedimentation rate (ESR) in temporal arteritis • Normal ESR in anterior ischemic optic neuropathy	Laboratory tests are usually not very significant in the diagnoses of ocular or vision problems. The erythrocyte sedimentation rate (ESR or sed rate) would be one significant blood test used for diagnoses in ophthalmology in relation to temporal arteritis versus anterior ischemic optic neuropathy.

the patient's needs or preferences. As one ages, the nucleus fibers become compressed with additive cortical fibers, resulting in decreasing accommodation (AAO-11, 2008–2009) or a more rigid lens. It generally is during the fourth decade of life that one experiences the loss of elasticity of the natural crystalline lens, which causes the loss of the ability to focus up close, resulting in presbyopia.

Strabismus

Strabismus is a functional misalignment of the extraocular muscles that causes the eyes not to focus together or to a single point. The eye can misdirect in any of the following positions; *eso* meaning toward the nose or medial, *exo* meaning toward the ear or temporal, *hyper* meaning upward or superior, and *hypo* meaning downward or inferior. This is normally a childhood condition, but it can affect one's vision throughout life.

Adult Strabismus

Adult strabismus refers to adults with cross-eyes, those that have lost their ability to fuse. Adult onset of strabismus is usually the result of head trauma and insult to the brain, especially if one is unconscious for a long period of time (AAO-6, 2008–2009). Adults with strabismus will see double (diplopia), because they do not suppress vision. Asthenopia may be another common symptom, which includes eye discomfort on use, such as headache, eyestrain, and brow ache (Pratt-Johnson & Tillson, 2001).

Adult strabismus may be treated with eye muscle exercises, eyeglasses containing prisms, botulinum toxin (Botox) injections, and eye surgery. Eye muscle exercise usually is used when treating a form of adult strabismus, called convergence insufficiency, in which eyes cannot align themselves for close work or reading. These exercises can retrain eyes to focus inward together. Prism eyeglasses can be used to correct mild double vision associated with adult strabismus. Botox injections are an effective treatment when overactive eye muscles are causing strabismus. Eye muscle surgery is the most common treatment; it is used to loosen or tighten the muscles around the eye in order to correct the misalignment.

Diplopia

Diplopia describes double vision, the phenomenon when one object appears as two. Diplopia can be binocular or monocular (AAO-5, 2008–2009). Binocular diplopia can be functional or real. Monocular diplopia usually is an optical or refractive error, and glasses or contact lens correction will solve the problem

(Pratt-Johnson & Tillson, 2001). With functional diplopia, the person is not moving eyes properly for single focus vision (Pratt-Johnson & Tillson, 2001).

Amblyopia

Amblyopia, or more commonly called "lazy eye," is when a person has an eye with decreased or impaired vision with no obvious anatomic explanation. It is usually due to the lack of proper maturation during the growth and development stages, or just to not having the proper refractive correction, meaning no glasses, or the lack of use of correction by patients.

Other possible causes of amblyopia could be toxins, such as poison, alcohol, or tobacco; psychological (hysterical) problems; nutritional (e.g., vitamin B) insufficiency; cataracts (physical occlusion); and strabismic (cross-eyed or wall-eyed) phenomenon (AAO-6, 2008–2009). For all of these reasons and possibly others, the microscopic connections between the brain and visual receptors are not making the necessary links for good visual outcome. Amblyopia usually occurs about age 7 from not using the affected eye, and if not corrected by then, it may become irreversible. One treatment for amblyopia may be occlusion of the normal vision eye, attempting to force the poor vision eye to function properly (Guttman, 2004). Amblyopia does not develop in adulthood from not using an eye for vision.

Phoria

Phoria is a tendency toward a function deviation or defect that results from a break in visual fusion by covering an eye. **Esophoria** is a tendency of the eye to turn inward toward the nose or nasal canthus when that eye is covered or when the eye becomes tired. Exophoria is a tendency of the eye to turn outward toward the ear or temporal canthus when that eye is covered or possibly when the eye becomes tired.

Tropia

Tropia is a definite functional defect that results from a break in visual fusion due to an imbalance or misalignment of the extraocular muscles when both eyes are not covered. Esotropia is misalignment of one eye when it crosses inward toward the nasal canthus and the other eye is in normal alignment whether covered or not (Figure 71–7 ■). Exotropia is misalignment of one eye when it crosses outward toward the temporal canthus and the other eye is in normal alignment whether covered or not. When a tropia is mild, it is difficult at times to distinguish from a phoria; cover tests are very useful in making a distinction.

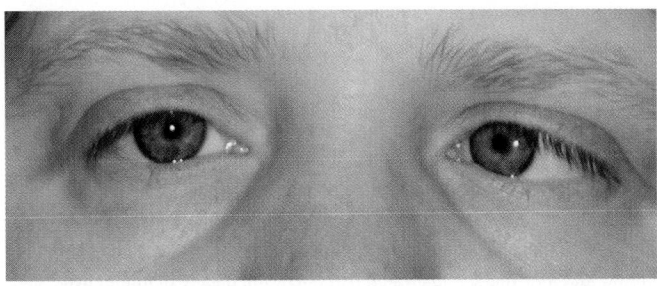

FIGURE 71–7 ■ Esotropia.
Source: Kathleen Osborn

Nystagmus

Nystagmus is an involuntary tremor, oscillation, or jerky movement of the eyeball. Nystagmus usually is divided into two types: sensory and motor. Sensory nystagmus is the result of loss of foveal fixation due to the pathology of the macula, retina, or optic nerve (Pratt-Johnson & Tillson, 2001). This condition or symptom often is seen in albinism due to foveal hypoplasia. Other causes may be congenital cataracts; aniridia (no iris); macular anomalies, optic nerve defect or abnormal rod photoreceptor function; and achromatopsia (color blindness) (Pratt-Johnson & Tillson, 2001). Motor nystagmus is the result of not finding a sensory cause of dysfunction and no obvious foveal organic pathology; it is usually less severe than sensory nystagmus (Pratt-Johnson & Tillson, 2001).

The assessment should include a screening cover eye test to rule out any strabismic tendencies or poor visual acuity. During a cover test, the health care provider directs the patient to focus on a small object both at a distance and close up. Each eye is covered alternately; as the cover paddle is moved from one eye to the other, the health care provider notes how much each eye has to move when uncovered to pick up the fixation target. If the alignment of the eyes is outside normal limits or the patient is experiencing symptoms, the health care provider may recommend treatment.

Easy tests with the use of a direct ophthalmoscope can be performed to gain meaningful information. These include checking the foveal reflexes to see whether they are equally bright in color and checking corneal reflexes to determine whether they are equally aligned. Unequal foveal reflexes may indicate a deviating eyeball, which would be the one with the brighter reflex (Brueckner test). Unequal alignment of corneal reflexes (Hirschberg test) also may indicate a deviation in the visual gaze, meaning the eyes have different fixation points (Pratt-Johnson & Tillson, 2001).

Macular Degeneration

Macular degeneration (MD) is defined as deterioration of the macula, the area of central vision in the posterior pole or retina, causing central acuity loss. Age-related macular degeneration (ARMD or AMD) is the most common cause of vision loss in those over age 60. Vision loss due to aging is a major health problem today, especially with the advent of the baby boomer generation. Vision loss may affect one's cognitive ability with aging; vision and cognition may share a similar nervous system cell loss, as indicated in recent research (Age-Related Eye Disease Study [AREDS] Research Group, 2006; Wong et al., 2002). The Evidence-Based Practice feature (p. 2336) examines the possible link between age-related macular degeneration and cognitive function.

Age-related macular degeneration is progressive, causing atrophic or deteriorating changes of the macula and retinal pigment epithelial (RPE) layer (Elfervig, 1998). The more common risk factors associated with macular degeneration include aging, hypertension, atherosclerosis and cardiovascular disease, smoking, lung conditions, diabetes, hyperlipidemia, hyperopia, light-colored iris, ultraviolet light exposure, and heredity (Rosenfeld & Gorin, 1999). Age-related macular degeneration is classified into two major types, dry and wet, discussed later. The degeneration of the macula occurs with time and can eventually lead to legal blindness. **Legal blindness** is defined as the best-corrected visual acuity of 20/200 of both eyes or worse, or 20 degrees or more of peripheral field loss.

Drusen

Drusen usually is the earliest fundus sign of age-related macular degeneration. **Drusen** (Figure 71–8 ■, p. 2337) is yellowish, round, slightly elevated, different-sized subretinal pigment epithelial deposits in the macula (Maguire, 1999). However, not all drusen are diagnostic of macular degeneration. Over half the population over age 70 has drusen; however, usually only when vision loss is associated with it, is it referred to as a sign of early age-related macular degeneration.

Patients with macular degeneration may notice at first that it is a little more difficult to see with the affected eye while doing close-up work, or that they have trouble seeing at a distance, especially with driving. A frequent symptom is **metamorphopsia**, a condition characterized by vision distortion; that is, when straight lines such as door frames or posts look crooked or irregular. Other symptoms also may include a difference in the sizes and colors of objects between eyes, meaning the loss of **contrast sensitivity (CS)**. The individual may find she is having trouble with daily activities, such as sewing, gardening, reading, watching television, and almost any activity that requires looking directly at some object to accomplish a task or skill. The Amsler grid, as shown in Figure 71–9 ■, (p. 2337) is a self-testing tool for daily use, highly recommended for this population, to notice early macular changes from macular degeneration.

Dry Age-Related Macular Degeneration

Dry age-related macular degeneration (AMD) is referred to as nonexudative, geographic, or atrophic changes in the macula (see Figure 71–8 ■, p. 2337). Dry AMD occurs when the light-sensitive cells in the macula slowly break down, gradually blurring central vision in the affected eye. As it gets worse, an individual may see a blurred spot in the center of vision. Over time, as less of the macula functions, central vision is gradually lost in the affected eye. The most common symptom of dry AMD is slightly blurred vision. One may have difficulty recognizing faces or need more light for reading and other tasks. Dry AMD generally affects both eyes, but vision can be lost in one eye while the other eye seems unaffected. One of the most common early signs of dry AMD is drusen (see Figure 71–8 ■, p. 2337) (National Eye Institute, 2006).

Wet Age-Related Macular Degeneration

Wet age-related macular degeneration is exudative, serous, or neovascular changes in the macula (Figure 71–10 ■, p. 2337). Wet AMD occurs when abnormal blood vessels behind the retina start to grow under the macula. These new blood vessels

Age-Related Macular Degeneration and Cognitive Function

Clinical Problem

Vision loss due to aging is a major health problem today, especially with the aging of those of the baby boomer generation, who are now over 50 years of age. Vision loss may affect one's cognitive ability with aging; vision and cognition may share a similar nervous system cell loss, indicated in other studies (AREDS Research Group, 2006; Wong et al., 2002). Vision loss from age-related macular degeneration (AMD) is the leading cause of visual impairment among people age 60 and older (Singerman et al., 2005). According to the United States Census Bureau (2000), 35 million Americans are age 60 and older; and among these, approximately 14% have some sensory impairment (vision and hearing loss), and about 11% have some mental decline. Evidence has shown that when one cannot visually focus clearly, one cannot think clearly either. Early detection of visual impairment and employing the best current means of prevention, treatment, and stabilization may make the difference between chronicity and quality of life for aging adults both visually and mentally. Nurses must understand how to apply evidence-based findings when managing patients with vision loss, especially older citizens with AMD.

Research Findings

The AREDS Research Group (2006) conducted an investigation into the association between cognitive ability and visual impairment from AMD. These investigators hypothesized that aging of mind and vision are related in functional ability. Participants numbered about 2,900 in taking the AREDS Cognitive Function Battery to identify differences of macular abnormalities from AMD and severity of visual acuity loss. The findings suggested a possible association of advanced AMD with visual acuity loss with decreased cognitive function in older people with vision loss worse than 20/40.

Implications for Nursing Practice

This study clearly indicates a need for nurses to educate patients with AMD to keep regular follow-ups with their vision health care provider in order to maintain good visual acuity and health as long as possible. They should be advised to avoid smoking, to limit exposure to air pollution and ultraviolet rays, and to maintain good general health (stabilize any hypertension and hyperlipidemia) in order to age well. Treatments for AMD may include the use of antioxidants, intravitreal injections, or laser as applicable. Patients that are visually impaired need to be informed about the importance of maintaining cognitive stimulating activity, through regular activity, large print books, and special visual systems. Auto reading books or tapes also may prove to be beneficial in keeping one cognitively active. The relationship between decreased vision and cognitive function may also be based on the fact that visual impairment can affect the quality of interactive experiences of older adults in developing meaningful relationships. The nurse needs to understand the relationship of cognitive functions with decreases in visual function gained from this study (AREDS Research Group, 2006) in order to counsel the patient significantly. Keeping active on a regular basis may enrich mental, physical, and psychosocial well-being.

Critical Thinking Questions

1. In order of priority, what are the most important points to include in an education plan for the patient with visual impairment from AMD?

2. What methods would be effective in increasing compliance with the stabilization of vision loss from AMD?

3. Identify nursing measures that would decrease the risk of vision loss from AMD.

Answers to Critical Thinking Questions appear in Appendix D.

References

Age-Related Eye Disease Study (AREDS) Research Group. (2006). Cognitive impairment in the Age-Related Eye Disease Study. AREDS Report No. 16. *Archives of Ophthalmology, 124*(4), 537–543.

Singerman, L. J., Brucker, A. J., Jampol, L. M., Lim, J. I., Rosenfeld, P., Schachat, A. P., et al. (2005). Neovascular age-related macular degeneration: Roundtable. *Retina, 25*(Suppl. 7), S1–S22.

United States Census Bureau. (2000). Demographic Summary. Retrieved February 2, 2007, from http://www.census.gov/main/www/cen2000.html.

Wong, T., Klein, R., Nieto, F., Moraes, S., Mosley, T., Couper, D., et al. (2002). Is early age-related maculopathy related to cognitive function? The atherosclerosis risk in communities study. *American Journal of Ophthalmology, 134*(12), 828–835.

tend to be very fragile and often leak blood and fluid, which raise the macula from its normal place at the back of the eye. Damage to the macula occurs rapidly, and loss of central vision can develop quickly. An early symptom of wet AMD is that straight lines appear wavy. Wet AMD is also known as advanced AMD (National Eye Institute, 2006).

Disciform Scar

Disciform scar is a chronic sign of age-related macular degeneration formation. Disciform scar is associated with hemorrhage and serous fluid in and beneath the retinal pigment epithelial layer causing retinal pigment epithelium and photoreceptor damage (Martidis & Tennant, 2004). If this goes untreated, the fibrocytes (scar tissue) from the choroid will accumulate between and within the retinal pigment epithelium and photoreceptors. This will develop finally into a disc-shaped scar that results in severe vision loss; it is referred to as the end stage of macular degeneration.

Laboratory and Diagnostic Procedures and Medical Management

Medical management options for dry macular degeneration can include the possibility of doing nothing and letting aging take its course. Management also may include a recommendation of taking antioxidant eye vitamins (Age-Related Eye Disease Study [AREDS] Research Group, 2003) or supplementing one's diet with the consumption of dark-green leafy vegetables, orange/yellow vegetables, and fruits to try to revitalize the aging retina. Of note, antioxidants also are contraindicated for patients on anticoagulants. Chapter 14 🔗 discusses antioxidants.

 CRITICAL ALERT *Patients on blood thinners should not take antioxidant eye vitamins, because antioxidants can improve clotting. Check with the health care provider first before taking.*

Medical management options for wet macular degeneration are nonsteroidal anti-inflammatory medications (D'Amato,

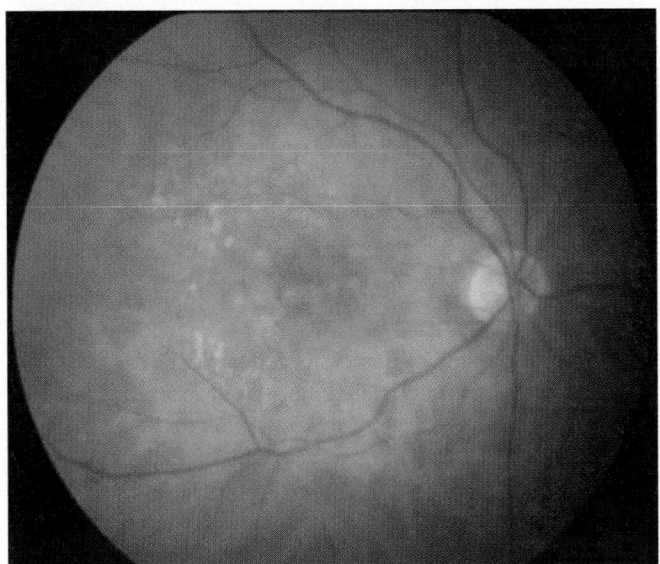

FIGURE 71–8 ■ Dry age-related macular degeneration with drusen.
Source: Kathleen Osborn

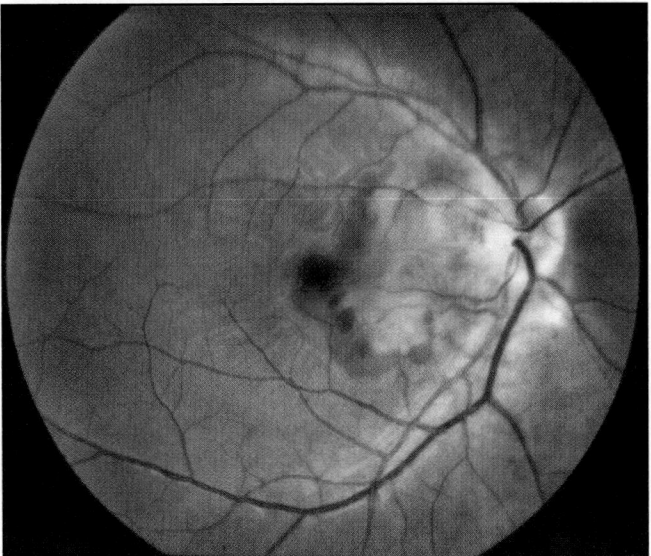

FIGURE 71–10 ■ Wet age-related macular degeneration (choroidal neovascularization).
Source: Kathleen Osborn

Amsler grid testing

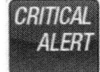

- Hold card about 16 inches away (normal reading distance)
- Use good lighting
- Wearing best corrected glasses for near
- Cover or close left eye
- Look at the center black spot with right eye
- Notice if any irregularities or distortions in the grid lines, such as, missing, crooked or bent, doubled, light gray in color, blotch or gray shaded area
- Cover or close right eye
- Look at the center black spot with left eye
- Repeat: noticing any irregularities or distortions in the grid lines

FIGURE 71–9 ■ Amsler grid.

1999), laser photocoagulation, photodynamic therapy, vitrectomy with choroidal neovascularization removal (Elfervig, 2000b), and intravitreal injection of anti–vascular endothelial growth factor (anti-VEGF) antigen binding drugs (Ferrara,

Damico, Shams, Lowman, & Kim, 2006). The fluorescein angiogram and optical coherence tomography are required diagnostic tests (see the Diagnostic Tests box, p. 2333) to be evaluated for photodynamic therapy and are used to determine who is a good candidate for the procedure.

Photodynamic therapy laser is a clinical procedure that requires an intravenous injection of a special verteporfin dye that is photosensitive, so that the laser beam treats only the leaking blood vessels and not the surrounding retinal tissue. The therapy can be repeated on a 3-month cycle, and it usually takes at least two laser procedures to obtain therapeutic results. After patients have had photodynamic therapy, their eyes and skin are very sensitive to sunlight and they must avoid direct sunlight exposure for 3 to 5 days. Photodynamic therapy (PDT) was once the treatment of choice for wet age-related macular degeneration. Now, it is also being used in combination therapy with anti-VEGF treatments (Dhalla et al., 2006). The day of the laser procedure, patients must wear sunglasses, a long-sleeve shirt, pants, gloves, socks, shoes, and a wide-brimmed hat, so they are protected from direct sunlight. Patients will be monitored by the health care provider every 3 months until the neovascularization is arrested.

CRITICAL ALERT   *Verteporfin dye is a light-activated medication or photosensitive dye used in photodynamic therapy (PDT) with a nonthermal laser. Injection of the dye into the vein makes the eyes and skin photosensitive. On the day of laser surgery, the patient should wear or bring to wear the following after the surgery for the trip home: dark sunglasses, wide-brimmed hat, gloves, long-sleeve shirt, pants, socks, and shoes (no sandals).*

Direct sunlight exposure can result in third-degree burns or severe skin irritation. Avoid sunlight and bright light exposure for 4 to 5 days postsurgery. During daylight, close curtains and window shades; avoid skylights, tanning beds, halogen lights, and dental or surgical appointments or procedures. One can use regular indoor lights, watch television, go to the movies, but must wait until after sundown to go outside to do any chores.

Intravitreal injection of anti-VEGF drugs is becoming the treatment of choice for wet age-related macular degeneration. An injection of the anti-VEGF drug is administered into the vitreous cavity (Eye Tech Study Group [ETSG], 2003; Ferrara et al., 2006). The frequency of the injections is determined by the leakage regression response to the drug found on fluorescein angiography (FA) or optical coherence tomography (OCT). Injections can be as frequent as every 4 to 6 weeks for stabilizing vision and consistent visual acuity improvements (Dhalla et al., 2006; Ruiz-Moreno, Montero, Barile, & Zarbin, 2006).

Nursing Management

The quality of life with central vision loss can significantly affect one's perception with communicating and just getting about on a daily basis. Nursing management of patients with age-related macular degeneration can be complex and multifaceted. Application of the nursing process will facilitate a comprehensive approach to patients' assessment and care. The nursing assessment and management data, which include specific questions to patients that are visually impaired with wet macular degeneration, are found in the Nursing Process: Patient Care Plan for Macular Degeneration feature. This care plan applies the nursing process to the relevant nursing diagnoses and provides a comprehensive care plan for patients that are visually impaired during the early stages of wet macular degeneration.

Collaborative Management

To achieve potential vision restoration and return to society as before, patients with wet macular degeneration need a multidisciplinary team approach, including the ophthalmologist, ophthalmic advance nurse practitioner, nurse, social worker, and optometrist or low vision rehabilitation specialist. To ensure maximum vision potential, vision care is managed by both nurses and the health care provider. As the wet macular degeneration starts to dry and stop leaking, some macular scarring may develop, leaving a degree of visual impairment or possibly legal blindness. The optometrist and low vision rehabilitation specialist will provide the necessary glasses or low vison aids to enhance patients' visual acuity, hopefully to a functional level. Patients will need instructions as well as practice in the best use of vision aids. The social worker is accustomed to helping patients adjust to a new lifestyle with vision deficit.

Health Promotion

Due to the possibility of the loss of independence as a result of legal blindness from age-related macular degeneration (AMD), it is important for the patient to know whether he has a family history of AMD, because this directly affects the patient's quality of life. Regular eye examinations are a means to detect early changes of AMD and to assess the use of eye vitamins and any new investigative findings in the treatment of AMD. Nutritional supplements for age-related macular degeneration are presented in the Complementary & Alternative Therapies box.

Diabetic Retinopathy

Retinopathy generally refers to degenerative changes in the retina. The most common causes of retinopathy result from diabetes mellitus (DM) or diabetes, thus causing weak and leaking blood vessels in the retina. The various stages of diabetic retinopathy include nonproliferative, preproliferative, and proliferative (Bhavsar & Drouilhet, 2006; Elfervig & Elfervig, 2001; Eliott, Lee, & Abrams, 2001; Porth, 2007) (Figure 71–11 ■, p. 2342).

Epidemiology, Etiology, and Risk Factors

Diabetic retinopathy (DR) is the leading cause of legal blindness among young adults and working-age Americans—those

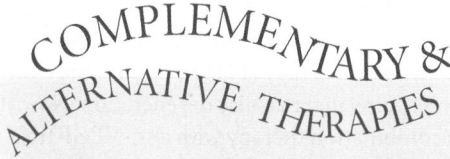

Nutritional Supplements for Age-Related Macular Degeneration

Description:
Age-related macular degeneration (ARMD) is the third most common cause of blindness in the world. ARMD creates partial or complete blindness in thousands of people. Its prevalence is expected to increase as the population ages. A small number of patients experience slowed disease progression from laser therapy and surgery, but these treatments are unlikely to restore lost vision. However, there are many CAM therapies that can improve this condition; the two most common therapies are antioxidants and omega-3 fatty acids ("Nutritional Supplements," 2006).

Research Support:
Studies have shown that dietary intake of omega-3 fatty acids benefits visual development. In addition, several other studies show that omega-3 fatty acids may be useful for conditions of the retina and lens. A Canadian literature review assessed and analyzed the evidence for whether omega-3 fatty acids prevent the development or progression of retinitis pigmentosa. Researchers found six studies published between 1995 and 2004 that met their eligibility criteria. These studies showed that omega-3 fatty acids improved some retinitis pigmentosa outcomes (Hodge et al., 2006).

Another review of published studies examined the role of nutritional and herbal medicines in treating ARMD, cataracts, diabetic retinopathy, and glaucoma. Although the evidence did support the use of certain vitamins and minerals in patients with certain forms of ARMD, it did not support use of these supplements to prevent or treat cataracts, diabetic retinopathy, or glaucoma (West, Oren, & Moroi, 2006).

Another review of literature included eight trials and found one major U. S. trial that showed that antioxidant (beta-carotene, vitamin C, and vitamin E) and zinc supplementation prevented progression to advanced ARMD and loss of visual acuity (Evans, 2006).

References
Evans, J. R. (2006). Antioxidant vitamin and mineral supplements for slowing the progression of age-related macular degeneration. *Cochrane Database of Systematic Reviews, 19*(2), CD000254.

Hodge, W. G., Barnes, D., Schachter, H. M., Pan, Y. I., Lowcock, E. C., Zhang, L., et al. (2006). The evidence for efficacy of omega-3 fatty acids in preventing or slowing the progression of retinitis pigmentosa: A systematic review. *Canadian Journal of Ophthalmology, 41*(4), 481–490.

"Nutritional supplements for macular degeneration." (2006). *Drug Therapy Bulletin, 44*(2), 9–11.

West, A. L., Oren, G. A., & Moroi, S. E. (2006). Evidence for the use of nutritional supplements and herbal medicines in common eye diseases. *American Journal of Ophthalmology, 141*(1), 157–166.

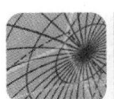

NURSING PROCESS: Patient Care Plan for Macular Degeneration

Assessment of Patient/Family Understanding of Vision Loss

Subjective Data:

Are you taking any eye systemic medications or antioxidant eye vitamins?

Are you on any blood thinners?

Do you smoke?

Do you wear glasses, contact lenses, or use any low vision aids?

Have you had any eye problems or vision problems in the past?

Are you seeing black spots or wavy lines in your vision?

Have you had any eye treatments, surgeries, lasers, or photodynamic therapy?

Do you spend a lot of time outdoors, and do you wear ultraviolet protective glasses or sunglasses?

Does anyone else in the family have macular degeneration?

What is your occupation?

Does it involve one or both eyes?

Have you had any vision or eye tests done?

Has treatment already been started for this problem?

What has your health care provider told you about this disease?

Objective Data:

Distance visual acuity

Near visual acuity

Intraocular pressure

Central blind spot

Eye examination

Vital signs

Interview behavior

Nursing Assessment and Diagnoses	Outcomes and Evaluation Parameters	Planning and Interventions with *Rationales*
Nursing Diagnosis: *Deficient Knowledge* related to macular degeneration	**Outcomes:** Patient/family able to verbalize visual limitations and the necessary lifestyle changes. ***Evaluation Parameters:*** Verbalizes understanding of reason for visual loss. Identifies vision loss. Identifies alternative devices of assistance. Demonstrates ability of skills to use alternative devices.	**Interventions and *Rationales*:** Provide education and resources about vision loss, means of treatment and management, and role in self-care and alternative devices in assisting. *To assess understanding of vision loss by means of care, management, and follow-up.* Encourage self-care in keeping compliant with and proactive in maintaining vision health. *To assess self-care compliance and management.* Educate about and promote normalization with enhancement of skills in self-esteem and socialization, and means to access support systems. *To monitor knowledge of social interaction deficits by assessing means of improvement. To use skills that enhance social interactions.* Provide presence, good listening, and skills in socialization, anxiety reduction, relationship building, and accessing support resources. *To monitor active social encounters.* Provide the necessary means to maintain functional activities as long as possible for a better quality of life. Assess needs in maintaining everyday functional activities. *To mark appliances with Velcro or material that is recognizable to touch for identification.* Assess needs in limiting frustrations. *To provide access to auto reading or large television screens for entertainment enjoyment. To provide magnifier or bright lights for enhancing vision when applicable.* Provide continued independence. *To monitor everyday activities in assessing continued independence.*

Assessment of Patient/Family Coping

Subjective Data:

How are you handling your vision problems?

How long have you had this eye problem?

Do you have any other health or medical problems?

How would you describe your ocular or vision problems, signs, and symptoms?

Who are your support systems?

Objective Data:

Body language

Family support systems

Ability to adjust lifestyle

(continued)

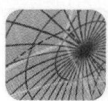

NURSING PROCESS: Patient Care Plan for Macular Degeneration—*Continued*

Nursing Assessment and Diagnoses	Outcomes and Evaluation Parameters	Planning and Interventions with *Rationales*
Nursing Diagnoses: *Anxiety* related to altered self-concept secondary to vision loss, especially centrally, and the fear of becoming legally or totally blind *Ineffective Coping* due to the inability to ask for help related to low self-esteem secondary to vision loss *Interrupted Family Processes* related to the shock of patient's vision loss	**Outcomes:** Experience a reasonable level of anxiety and fear. Evidence of effective family coping. ***Evaluation Parameters:*** Explains levels of anxiety and fear and coping patterns to overcome them. Relates less anxiety and fear after teaching. Expresses an improved level of psychological and physical comfort. Exhibits useful coping mechanisms in managing anxiety and fear. Assertive in asking for assistance when vision is not adequate to perform a given task. Expresses a need for assistance. Obtains the help needed to get the task done. Enjoys family support and meaningful family functions. Identifies altered family processes and reasons why. Exhibits effective family functioning. Comfortable in communicating without the means of observing facial expressions. Expresses self well in communicating with others. Engages sociably. Demonstrates a positive self-image with lifestyle adaptations and the resources of support to assist in keeping a positive attitude. Identifies changes in one's self-esteem. Identifies self in a realistic light with current circumstances. Expresses positive feelings about oneself. Exhibits healthy coping and adaptive skills.	**Interventions and *Rationales:*** Monitor level of anxiety and fear from mild to panic. *To assess for lower levels of anxiety and fear.* Provide reassurance and comfort with presence and active listening. *To observe improved levels of comfort.* Teaching disease process. *To assess less anxiety and fear with understanding.* Educate patient that peripheral vision is not lost with macular degeneration. *To assess improved self-concept with acceptance of vision loss.* Assist and teach patient in using other senses of hearing and touching more effectively to enhance communication skills. *To observe communicating with others well to increase sociability.* Assist patient in not feeling embarrassed or less of a person by teaching effective means of asking for assistance when necessary. *To observe obtaining help when needed with a sense of self-satisfaction of obtained task.* Provide presence, active listening, and emotional support. Teach and provide skills for coping; body image, self-role, self-awareness, and self-concept enhancements; and cognitive rethinking, value clarifications, and support resources. *To monitor positive lifestyle adaptations.*

Assessment of Home Environment

Subjective Data:
What kind of work do you do?
Are you able to perform your activities of daily living (ADL)?

Objective Data:
Home environment
Need for assistance
Financial stability

Nursing Assessment and Diagnoses	Outcomes and Evaluation Parameters	Planning and Interventions with *Rationales*
Nursing Diagnosis: *Impaired Home Maintenance* related to functional ability secondary to vision loss	**Outcomes:** Manage and maintain a clean and safe environment to live. ***Evaluation Parameters:*** Identifies obstacles in home management. Exhibits means to use support system. Exhibits ability to use alternative and adaptive devices that are safe.	**Interventions and *Rationales:*** Assist in family integrity promotion, involvement, mobilization, process, maintenance, and support. *To observe engaging in usual family functions, with acceptance of family support and love.* Assist in providing resources for home cleaning assistance and support system enhancement. *To report factors that are obstacles in home maintenance and management.* *To assess the use of resources for home help by using the necessary devices for a clean and safe home environment.*

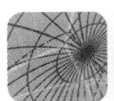

NURSING PROCESS: Patient Care Plan for Macular Degeneration—*Continued*

Assessment of Patient Response to Illness

Subjective Data:
Tell me about your perceptions of your disease.
What impact has this had on your life?
How has it impacted family dynamics and your role in the family?

Objective Data:
Facial expressions
Family relationships
Evidence of making necessary adjustments

Nursing Assessment and Diagnoses	Outcomes and Evaluation Parameters	Planning and Interventions with *Rationales*
Nursing Diagnoses: *Hopelessness* related to vision loss *Powerlessness* related to loss of controls in one's lifestyle secondary to vision loss	**Outcomes:** Express a sense of hope and feelings of hopefulness. Express a sense of power and express control over one's life situations. ***Evaluation Parameters:*** Verbalizes feelings and expresses hope. Identifies the future and sets realistic goals. Exhibits a positive feeling for now and later. Expresses self-confidence and trust of others. Demonstrates self-direction in decision making and problem solving. Identifies factors that can be controlled. Identifies the needs for care, treatment, and future situations in one's life.	**Interventions and *Rationales:*** Instill and provide presence, active listening, emotional and spiritual support, and hope. *To open communications and to facilitate feeling of hopefulness.* Teach and provide skills for behavior modification, coping skills, and crisis intervention. *To assist in setting future realistic goals and the ability to achieve set goals. To observe trust in making informed decisions and using effective problem solving.* Provide presence, and emotional and spiritual support. Teach and provide skills for coping, crisis intervention, decision making, and support system enhancement. *To assess factors of control and power by decision making concerning future care and treatment. To provide the resources of support and assistance, when indicated.*

Assessment of Safety Measures

Subjective Data:
Describe the physical layout of your residence.
How much are you able to get around independently?
What are your support systems?

Objective Data:
Ability to perform ADL
Use of aids such as a cane
Caregiver presence and ability to assist

Nursing Assessment and Diagnoses	Outcomes and Evaluation Parameters	Planning and Interventions with *Rationales*
Nursing Diagnoses: *Risk for Injury* or *Risk for Falls* related to vision loss *Readiness for Enhanced Self-Care* related to vision loss	**Outcomes:** Remain free from injury and falls related to vision loss. Perform self-care adequately in performing all the necessary activities of daily living. ***Evaluation Parameters:*** Identifies potential areas of injury and places of risk. Demonstrates appropriate measures to provide and to maintain safety. Identifies self-care deficits. Exhibits ability to use support systems. Exhibits ability to use necessary adaptive devices. Verbalizes knowledge of the options of antioxidant eye vitamins, when indicated.	**Interventions and *Rationales:*** Educate on visual defects and provide the necessary safety skills and management to prevent injury or falls. *To assess understanding of visual deficits with seeking the means to provide a safe environment to prevent injury or falls.* Provide resources for normal daily activities, self-care needs and tools, and support system information. *To observe self-care using the necessary information for support and resources to perform activities of daily living in maintaining a normal life with known self-care deficits. To provide means to keep an adequate supply of antioxidant eye vitamins, when indicated (contraindicated for smokers and patients on anticoagulants).*

persons under the age of 60—typically affecting individuals in their most productive years (Bhavsar & Drouilhet, 2006). It is the leading cause of blindness for all ages in the United States (Porth, 2007). From the initial diagnosis of diabetes, if occurring during adulthood or at a prepubertal age, patients may have a 5-year so-called "grace period" during which retinopathy usually is not visually detectable. This is referred to as diabetes without ophthalmic complications.

Approximately 16 million Americans have diabetes, with 50% of them not even aware that they have it. Of those that know, only one-half receive appropriate eye care. Thus, it is not surprising that diabetic retinopathy is the leading cause of new blindness in persons aged 25 to 74 in the United States and is responsible for more than 8,000 cases of new blindness each year (Fong et al., 2003). This means that diabetes is responsible for 12% of blindness, and the rate is even higher among certain ethnic groups. An

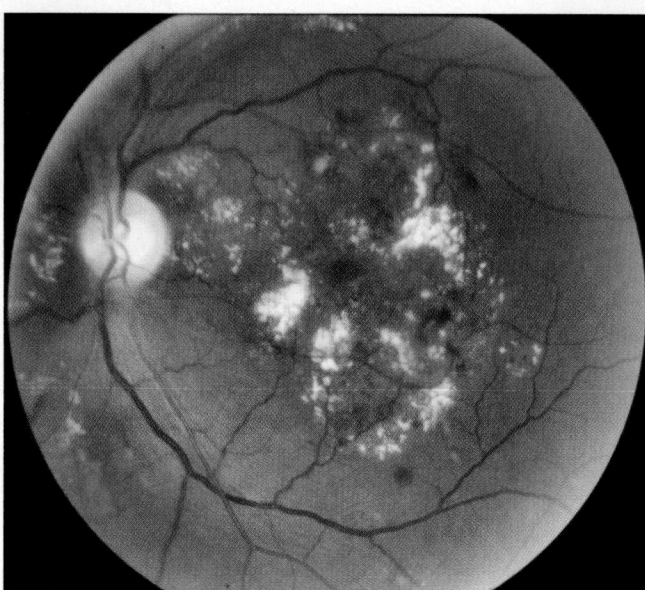

FIGURE 71–11 ■ Diabetic retinopathy.
Source: Kathleen Osborn

increased risk of diabetic retinopathy appears to exist in patients with Native American, Hispanic, and African American heritage (Bhavsar & Drouilhet, 2006). The major risk factors for diabetic retinopathy are years of being diabetic, family history, hyperglycemia, hypertension, hyperlipidemia, smoking, anemia, and renal disease.

Pathophysiology and Clinical Manifestations

Diabetic retinopathy results in edema from leaking capillaries that hemorrhage. Other signs are **cotton-wool spots (CWS)** from ischemic tissue that can advance to neovascularization (Elfervig & Elfervig, 2001). Diabetic retinopathy progresses in stages: from nonproliferative diabetic retinopathy, to preproliferative diabetic retinopathy, proliferative retinopathy, neovascularization of the disc or elsewhere in the retina, vitreous hemorrhage, gliotic (scar) tissue or traction retinal detachment, retinal detachment, or neovascular glaucoma of the iris. Nonproliferative diabetic retinopathy is manifested by cotton-wool spots or soft exudates caused by lack of blood supply to the tissue, **flame-shaped hemorrhages** from the nerve fiber layer of the retina, and dot/blot hemorrhages from the outer plexiform layer of the retina (Rosenblatt & Benson, 2004). Once a person is diagnosed with diabetes mellitus, she should have a baseline dilated eye examination and evaluation. Patients with diabetes usually are followed annually if no signs or symptoms of diabetic retinopathy are present and are seen more often if active diabetic retinopathy is in progress. Sometimes just by getting blood sugar and blood pressure under control, the vessel leakage from diabetes will clear on its own. Thus, it is very important to emphasize good blood sugar and blood pressure controls, and to educate patients about not smoking or giving up smoking. Diabetic retinopathy signs and symptoms can range from none to floating spots, streaks, lines, scattered lights, distortion, hazy and cloudy view, darkness, and poor color vision, depending on the location of the retinopathy in the retina (Elfervig & Elfervig, 2001; Porth, 2007).

Laboratory and Diagnostic Procedures

Fasting glucose and hemoglobin A_{1c} (Hb A_{1c}) are laboratory tests that are performed to help diagnose diabetes. The Hb A_{1c} level also is important in the long-term follow-up care of patients with diabetes and diabetic retinopathy. Controlling diabetes and maintaining the Hb A_{1c} level in the 6% to 7% range are the goals in the optimal management of diabetes and diabetic retinopathy. If these levels are maintained, the progression of diabetic retinopathy is reduced substantially. Fluorescein angiography also is used in the diagnosis and management of diabetic retinopathy (see the Diagnostic Tests box, p. 2333). These scans reveal microaneurysms, blot and dot hemorrhages, areas of nonperfusion, and evidence of collateral vessels that do not leak (Bhavsar & Drouilhet, 2006).

Medical Management

Preventing diabetic retinopathy from developing or progressing is considered the best approach to protecting vision. Therefore, glucose control may retard the progression of retinopathy. Management of hypertension and hyperlipidemia also is important, as these conditions also may contribute to the risk of developing or furthering diabetic retinopathy.

Laser photocoagulation provides the major direct treatment modality for diabetic retinopathy (Bhavsar & Drouilhet, 2006). This laser treatment is applied directly to leaking microaneurysms, and grid photocoagulation with a checkerboard pattern of laser burns is applied to diffuse areas of leakage and thickening. It is not recommended near the disc. Vitrectomy has proved effective in removing vitreous hemorrhage and severing vitroretinal membranes that develop (Porth, 2007).

■ Nursing Management

The nurse has many opportunities for education and intervention with patients and family in preserving vision function and promoting eye health to prevent the advancement of diabetic retinopathy. Nursing management of patients with diabetic retinopathy can be complex and multifaceted. Application of the nursing process facilitates a comprehensive approach to patients' assessment and care.

Assessment and Nursing Diagnoses

Assessment data includes specific questions related to blood sugar and blood pressure controls and vision fluctuation. It also establishes the background of the patient by determining how long the patient has been a diabetic and other contributing factors to the diagnosis of retinopathy. Specific questions might be asked of the patient:

- What type of medication are you on for diabetic control?
- How is your blood glucose and your blood pressure?
- Are you taking any other systemic medications?
- Do you smoke?
- Do you wear glasses, contact lenses, or have you had any eye problems in the past?

From an objective perspective, the nurse should assess the patient for visual acuity, blood sugar, and blood pressure values. An eye examination also is in order as is an assessment of behavioral manifestations.

Nursing diagnoses are developed from the assessment data, and a patient care plan depicts the nursing process used in caring for patients with diabetic retinopathy. In determining diagnoses the nurse must recognize that the patient is undergoing changes in self-perception and in the ability to maintain familiar and constant roles in caring for self and for participating as a member of a social group, e.g., family, friends. Typical diagnoses to be considered are those related to anxiety, ineffective coping, infection potential related to surgery, altered family processes, and impaired home maintenance and self-care deficits along with impaired social interaction.

Outcomes and Evaluation Parameters

Outcomes and evaluation parameters should be focused on the desired response of the patient in adapting to the overall diagnosis of diabetic retinopathy: reduced anxiety and coping patterns. They are demonstrated patient behaviors, both subjective and objective, that indicate the patient is adjusting to the overall diagnosis of diabetic retinopathy.

Planning and Interventions

Planning and nursing interventions focus on communication and education and monitoring the patient's verbal and nonverbal behaviors. For instance, the nurse is responsible for instructing the patient on the relevance of blood sugar to the diagnosis and how to control it. Information on the reduction of risk factors also is shared as is education regarding available resources for maintaining self-care and a safe environment to those with visual defects. Anxiety and comfort levels also are monitored in order to determine on-going patient needs and provide assistance as appropriate.

Collaborative Management

A multidisciplinary team approach consists of the health care provider, internist or endocrinologist, ophthalmologist, ophthalmic advance nurse practitioner, nurses, nutritionist, and optometrist. They all serve to provide comprehensive care to patients with diabetic retinopathy. Management of diabetic retinopathy may include medical controls or surgical intervention, such as laser photocoagulation or surgical vitrectomy (Rosenblatt & Benson, 2004) (Figure 71–12 ▪) by the ophthalmologist. Sometimes just by having the internists adjust patients' medications to stabilize blood sugar and/or blood pressure will negate any need for laser. Severe hypertension or hyperglycemia also can prevent laser treatment, especially if the diastolic blood pressure is above 100 mmHg or the blood sugar is over 300 mg/dL, because the laser is less effective under these conditions. Laser also can be a means to stabilize the fundus for impending vitrectomy, to improve the surgical outcome. It is not uncommon for patients with diabetes who have diabetic retinopathy to have anywhere from three to six laser sessions per eye over their lifetime. The nurse practitioner or nurse can provide the necessary education and follow-up monitoring of patients' progress to assist them in complying with a diabetic regimen. The nutritionist assists with establishing a diet regimen to enhance health and control diabetes. The optometrist provides

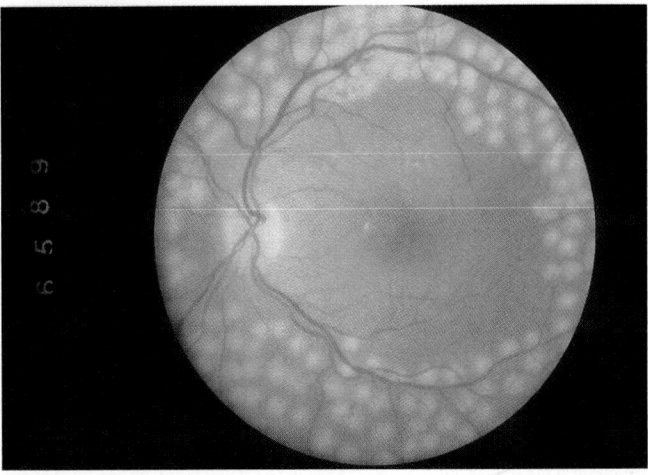

FIGURE 71–12 ▪ Laser photocoagulation.
Source: Kathleen Osborn

visual evaluations between regular health care provider visits and makes the necessary refractive corrections when indicated.

Because blood sugar fluctuation can cause changes in vision, it is recommended that periodic blood sugar checks be established. Hyperglycemia may cause the natural crystalline lens to swell, creating myopic shift and a temporary change in refractive error. Hypoglycemia may cause a cerebral response creating temporary blurred vision, diplopia, drowsiness, faintness, confusion, anxiety, headache, slurred speech, sweating, tremor, seizures, and even coma. It is recommended that the blood sugar be gotten under control and stabilized for at least 6 to 9 weeks before changing glasses or contact lenses. A possible cure for diabetes is islets of Langerhans transplant or pancreatic transplant, which will consequently stop the progression of diabetic retinopathy, but retinopathy damage that is already present, does not reverse. See Chapter 53 ⊕ for more information on diabetes.

Health Promotion

Due to the progressive nature of diabetic retinopathy, especially after the 5-year grace period, health promotion begins as soon as the patient is diagnosed with diabetes. Patient/family education focuses on controlling the blood sugar and risk factors that aggravate the disease progression, such as hypertension, hyperlipidemia, smoking, overeating, and lack of exercise. Education includes all of the latter and possible lifestyle changes and preventive care. It is important for patients to have regular eye examinations annually if no diabetic retinopathy is present and more frequently if diabetic retinopathy is already in progress.

Glaucoma

Glaucoma includes a group of conditions that feature an optic neuropathy accompanied by optic disc cupping and visual field loss. It generally is associated with an increase in intraocular pressure; however, some people with normal intraocular pressure may develop characteristic optic nerve and visual field changes. Glaucoma is a very significant health condition, especially with aging Americans, because its incidence increases with age.

Epidemiology and Etiology

Glaucoma is the second most common form of legal blindness in the United States, and the third most common in the world

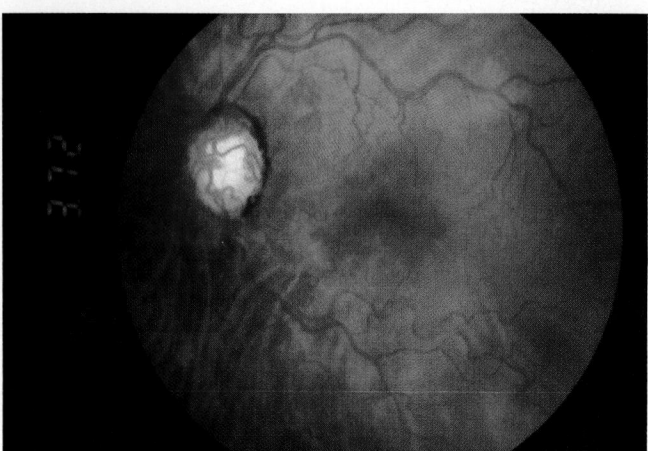

FIGURE 71–13 ■ Glaucoma with collaterals on the disc.
Source: Kathleen Osborn

(Elfervig, 2002a), but with treatment loss of sight can be prevented (Figure 71–13 ■). An estimated 60 million people worldwide have glaucoma. About 6 million people worldwide are blind from glaucoma, including 100,000 Americans, making it the leading cause of blindness in the United States (Porth, 2007). Normal range of intraocular pressure is between 10 and 21 mmHg, but not all persons with elevated intraocular pressure (greater than 22 mmHg) have glaucoma or optic nerve damage (ocular hypertension), and not all persons with normal intraocular pressure are glaucoma free (low- or normal-tension glaucoma) (Elfervig, 2002a).

Pathophysiology

Generally glaucoma is described as open angle or closed angle, depending on its outflow mechanism, and primary or secondary, depending on its etiology. Primary glaucoma infers that it has no relation to other ocular conditions, and secondary glaucoma is the result of another preexisting ocular condition. Aqueous humor, which is produced by the ciliary body and secreted by ciliary processes, flows from the posterior chamber through the pupillary space and is deposited into the anterior chamber. Aqueous humor exits from the anterior chamber in the anterior angle into the trabecular meshwork, Schlemm's canal, intrascleral channels, and through episcleral and conjunctival veins, into venous circulation (AAO-10, 2008–2009). This continuous production and dissemination of aqueous fluid is responsible for maintaining normal intraocular pressure. Glaucoma is the condition that develops when any sequence of the production of aqueous humor or the drainage of aqueous humor does not function properly. This causes aqueous fluid to build up intraocularly, which causes the intraocular pressure to increase in the eye, thus putting pressure on the optic nerve and causing it to atrophy. This can lead to permanent blindness if left untreated (AAO-10, 2008–2009). Ocular changes may include optic nerve neuropathy, retinal ganglion cell dropout, poor optic nerve perfusion, and nerve fiber layer destruction. The retinal ganglion cell layer of the sensory retina is composed of the neurons that project to the vision center of the brain, and the axons converge to form the optic nerve. The ganglion cell normally dies with aging (apoptosis), but glaucoma accelerates this process; and when over half the ganglion cells die, visual acuity loss becomes more apparent (Stewart, 2004).

More recent studies (Walker & Piltz-Seymour, 2004) have illustrated that central corneal thickness, measured with pachometry, can alter intraocular pressure readings. Diurnal intraocular pressure is intraocular pressure that can vary at different times of the day (PDR, 2004a). Intraocular pressure elevation puts pressure on the optic nerve, which can cause destruction of the nerve fiber layer of the retina, possibly causing a permanent vision loss. Hallmark signs of glaucoma are elevated intraocular pressure, visual field defects, optic nerve cupping or notching, and nerve fiber layer hemorrhages.

Open-Angle Glaucoma

Open-angle glaucoma (OAG) is the condition that exists when a patient has an open angle, meaning there is adequate anterior chamber space for proper drainage of aqueous fluid, but elevated intraocular pressure is present. The elevated pressure is due to the increase in aqueous production or the decrease in aqueous drainage due to trabecular meshwork obstruction, canal of Schlemm obstruction, or degenerative changes of the drainage tissue (AAO-10, 2008–2009). Open-angle glaucoma is sometimes referred to as the "silent blinder" or "thief in the night," because patients experience no symptoms in the early stages, and possibly it is first recognized due to noticeable vision loss. Side vision loss usually comes later in the course of the disease. Standard terms for open-angle glaucoma (OAG) are chronic (COAG), primary (POAG), or pigmentary. Pigmentary occurs when pigment pieces of the iris are blocking the drainage canal. Primary open-angle glaucoma, the most common form of glaucoma, occurs when the mechanical blockage may be caused from the iris being too near the Schemm's canal, thus bulging forward and blocking the trabecular meshwork (Zimmerman, Sakiyalak, Krupin, & Rosenberg, 2004). Chronic open-angle glaucoma is long-standing glaucoma.

Ocular Hypertension

Ocular hypertension refers to elevated intraocular pressure with no other signs or symptoms, no damage to the optic nerve, and no visual field loss. Ocular hypertension can be a precursor to impending glaucoma. Treatment includes observation only, unless intraocular pressure becomes unstable, there is a strong family history of glaucoma, or the intraocular pressure starts to elevate. Then medical treatment would indicate the starting of antiglaucoma drops (Walker & Piltz-Seymour, 2004). See the later Pharmacology Summary feature (p. 2346).

Low-Tension Glaucoma

Low-tension glaucoma (LTG), or normal-tension glaucoma (NTG), refers to normal intraocular pressure readings, but even though the pressure is within normal parameters, it is still too high for patients if optic nerve atrophy or visual field loss occurs. This usually results from inadequate blood perfusion to the optic nerve, possibly due to vasospastic etiology, such as in patients that suffer with frequent migraine headaches (Hitchings, 2004).

Secondary Glaucoma

Secondary glaucoma refers to elevated intraocular pressure due to a secondary cause, such as congenital anomalies, hyphema, inflammation (uveitis, iridocyclitis), tumors, drugs (topical steroids), hypermature cataract, or choroidal neovascularization (Choplin & Lundy, 1998). Conditions that interrupt the aqueous fluid drainage system, such as trauma, exophthalmos, or advanced diabetes, can cause structural changes that give rise to elevated intraocular pressure (Choplin & Lundy, 1998).

Acute Angle-Closure Glaucoma

Acute angle-closure glaucoma (AACG) is when the angle in the anterior chamber closes suddenly due to a shallow or narrow anterior angle (which is between the iris and cornea) by iris blockage, thereby preventing aqueous flow through the trabecular meshwork (Elfervig & Elfervig, 2007; Trobe, 2006) and into the canal of Schlemm (Traverso, Bagnis, & Bricola, 2004). This causes the intraocular pressure to rise very high, creating extreme eye pain and pressure with blurry vision, fixed mid-dilated pupil, corneal edema, hyperemia, photophobia, light halos, epiphora, and frontal headaches (Trobe, 2006) that can be accompanied by nausea, vomiting, and abdominal ache (Elfervig & Elfervig, 2007; PDR, 2004a). Typically, the ocular pain alone will motivate patients to seek immediate eye care in the clinic or emergency department.

CRITICAL ALERT

With acute angle-closure glaucoma:
Do not dilate the pupils!
Assess for pupils, hazy cornea, eye pain, and vision loss.
Assess for any systemic symptoms of headache, nausea, or vomiting.
Obtain intraocular pressure frequently, by the nurse, every 20 to 30 minutes until the intraocular pressure is lower, below 30 mmHg, with a health care provider's standing order for proper eye medication and systemic medications for emergency use.

The treatment goal of acute angle-closure glaucoma is to lower intraocular pressure, as quickly as possible, with systemic medications orally or intravenously, as well as topical ophthalmic drops that are ordered by the health care provider. The application of topical ophthalmic antiglaucoma drops, systemic or intravenous carbonic anhydrase inhibitors, or osmotic agents is common treatment, in addition to the administration of topical ophthalmic steroid drops every 10 to 15 minutes for the first hour, then hourly until intraocular pressure is stable (Netland & Allen, 1999). See the later Pharmacology Summary feature (p. 2346). Peripheral iridectomy (PI) or laser iridotomy is the standard immediate surgical procedure to ease high intraocular pressure and relieve blockage (Traverso et al., 2004). Measures are continued and the pressure is checked every 30 to 40 minutes, until it is lowered enough to clear corneal swelling and quiet the anterior chamber. Once the eye is quiet and comfortable, a more extensive ocular examination can be conducted. One means for angle closure to occur is when pupils normally dilate in the dark or at night. This can be intermittent at first, and then suddenly permanent closure may take place (Campbell & Netland, 1998). Other predispositions to angle closure are hyperopia, increased iris thickness with drug dilation, a large natural crystalline lens (cataracts), and a pupillary block that traps aqueous fluid. Sometimes acute angle-closure glaucoma subsides without intervention, but usually medical and surgical intervention is indicated to prevent ocular damage and keep open angle patency.

Clinical Manifestations

The usual onset of glaucoma is asymptomatic, slow, silent, and painless. Some symptoms may be blurred vision or eye ache; but usually by the time these symptoms develop, some permanent optic nerve damage has occurred along with vision loss or insidious visual field defects. The aged, males, and African Americans seem to be at greater risk for open-angle glaucoma (PDR, 2004a). Open-angle glaucoma is one of the major causes of vision loss or legal blindness in the aged, second only to age-related macular degeneration. It usually is bilateral and has a hereditary predisposition, but pressure can vary in each eye. Family history, diabetes, and being very farsighted can put one at greater risk for developing glaucoma.

Laboratory and Diagnostic Procedures

Pachometry is a new device to measure central corneal thickness. It is now used as one of the standard devices in determining accurate intraocular pressure. (See the Diagnostic Tests box, p. 2333.) Average central corneal thickness is about 545 ± 20 micrometers, which has a bearing on the final intraocular pressure recorded for a diagnosis of open-angle glaucoma. If the cornea is too thick, the intraocular pressure reading can be falsely read as too high; or if the cornea is too thin, the intraocular pressure reading can be falsely read as too low (PDR, 2004a; Walker & Piltz-Seymour, 2004). The intraocular pressure is obtained by tonometry reading; that number reading is adjusted according to corneal thickness.

Medical Management

There is no known cure for glaucoma, but it can be well controlled with early diagnosis and treatment. Without treatment glaucoma eventually will cause blindness. Chronic untreated glaucoma can result in a rigid eyeball, sightlessness, and eye pain, and may even require enucleation for a very painful blind eye. The eye health care provider determines the best target pressure as a goal to be reached in conjunction with the extent of optic nerve damage and type of glaucoma. Treatment may include antiglaucoma eyedrops, oral medications, and laser or surgery intervention, depending on the type of glaucoma, the stage of the disease process, and the number of risk factors present. The different types of antiglaucoma eyedrops, categorized in the Pharmacology Summary feature (p. 2346), are usually the first line of therapy. When medical treatment is unsuccessful, intolerable, or patients are noncompliant, surgical options are considered. Surgical and laser options for glaucoma treatment are YAG laser (neodymium: yttrium-aluminum-garnet) for peripheral iridectomy or iridoplasty, laser trabeculoplasty (LTP), laser trabeculectomy, viscocanalostomy, ciliodestructive procedure, or trabeculotomy and trabeculectomy filtering procedure (AAO-10, 2008–2009).

▪ Nursing Management

The nurse plays a major role in educating patients about glaucoma and proper management to prevent the advancement of glaucoma. Nursing management of patients with glaucoma can be complex and multifaceted. Application of the nursing process facilitates a comprehensive approach to patients' assessment and care.

Assessment and Nursing Diagnoses

The assessment data includes specific questions related to intraocular pressure controls and vision fluctuation. Subjective data which the nurse needs to gather include: family history of glaucoma, status of eye exam, any current medications being

PHARMACOLOGY Summary of the Topical Ophthalmic Drops for Diagnostic Procedures and Treatment of Glaucoma

Medication Category	Action	Application/Indication	Nursing Responsibility
Anesthetics			
Proparacaine Tetracaine	Anesthetizes corneal nerves and surrounding tissue (conjunctiva); partial or complete loss of sensation.	*Numbing of the cornea:* Applanation tonometry to check intraocular pressure (IOP) or gonioscopy for glaucoma. Removal of a superficial corneal foreign body or sutures. Perform minor corneal or conjunctival procedures. Schirmer's diagnostic test. Contact lenses fitting. Lacrimal canalicular manipulation. Preop preparation, especially in laser therapy. Trauma evaluation. Dosage: 1 to 2 drops over cornea. Onset: within 12 seconds. Duration: about 10–20 minutes. Reapply as needed.	Assessment of clinical signs of allergic reaction, especially to "caines." Explain that the patient's eye is being numbed. Temporary elimination of blink reflex. May need to patch eye following a procedure for protection. Caution: The patient is not to rub or touch eye for several minutes, until numbing sensation dissipates. Never give a patient numbing drops for self-administration; they can cause serious corneal damage, opacity, and vision loss. Monitor for adverse ocular reactions: corneal edema, redness, burning, stinging, keratitis, and delayed epithelial wound healing.
Fluorescein sodium with topical anesthetic		*Numbing and staining of the cornea:* Applanation tonometry or gonioscopy to check IOP for glaucoma. Access corneal abrasion/injury, herpetic lesions, or foreign body. Access tear flow in lacrimal drainage tests. Assist in contact lenses fitting. Evaluate postop closure of sclerocorneal wound in delayed anterior chamber reformation. Removal of superficial corneal foreign body or sutures. Perform minor corneal or conjunctival procedures.	Explain to patient that her tears and edges of eyelids and lashes will be yellow temporarily; the color washes out with her tears. Make sure the drops are current and have not been contaminated by touching the patient's eyelashes or lids with tip of bottle; fluorescein drops can grow *Pseudomonas* if contaminated. Caution: Topical use only and not to be used for long periods (can delay wound healing if overused). Patients with cardiac disease or hyperthyroidism. Observe for adverse ocular reactions: stinging, burning, redness, keratitis, corneal opacity, decreased vision, and iritis. Observe for adverse systemic reactions: dermatitis and depression (rare).
Mydriatics			
Phenylephrine (Neo-Synephrine)	Contends for binding site on muscarinic receptors with activation of α-adrenoceptors on sympathetically innervated iris dilator muscle, arterioles, and Muller's muscle. Produces pupillary dilation by this stimulation of iris dilator muscle and paralyzes iris sphincter and ciliary muscle.	*Pupillary dilation required:* Diagnostic procedures, fundus examination, uveitis (posterior synechiae), preoperatively for laser therapy, etc. Dosage: 1 to 2 drops 20–30 minutes prior to examination or procedure. Onset: 20–60 minutes. Duration: 3–5 hours.	Assess for clinical signs of allergic reaction. Contraindicated in patients with narrow-angle glaucoma. Caution: topical use only. May cause an exaggerated adrenergic effect if used with monoamine oxidase inhibitor (MAOI) agents (up to 21 days after). Instruct patient to wear sunglasses to block ultraviolet (UV) light exposure. Advise patient that driving with eyes dilated may cause difficulty, especially on a sunny day. Practice good hand hygiene to avoid iatrogenic dilation. Advise of possible additive effect if patient is on tricyclic antidepressants. Observe for adverse ocular reactions: stinging and burning. Observe for adverse systemic reactions: collapse, tremor, palpitation, perspiration, and pallor.

Sources: Elfervig, L. S. (2002b). Pharmacology. In K. Goldblum & P. Lamb (Eds.), *Core curriculum for ophthalmic nursing* (2nd ed.). Dubuque, IA: Kendall/Hunt; PDR. (2004a). *Glaucoma: Disease management guide* (1st ed.). San Francisco: Allergan; and PDR. (2004b). *Physicians' desk reference for ophthalmic medicines* (32nd ed.). Montvale, NJ: Thomson.

Medication Category	Action	Application/Indication	Nursing Responsibility
Cycloplegics Atropine (Atropine Care 1%) Cyclopentolate (Cyclogyl) Homatropine (Equipin) Scopolamine Tropicamide	Blocks postganglionic innervation of ciliary body, longitudinal muscle, and iris sphincter, to produce paralysis of ciliary muscle (blocking accommodation) and iris sphincter (blocking constriction).	*Pupillary dilation required:* Refraction requiring mydriasis and cycloplegia, especially in children, who have a large accommodative ability. Acute inflammation of the anterior uveal tract (relieve iris spasm). Preop or postop mydriasis for iridocyclitis. Optical aid in axial lens opacity. Diagnosis procedures. *Atropine:* Dosage: 1 to 2 drops bid, qid. Onset: 45–120 minutes. Duration: 7–14 days. *Cyclopentolate:* Dosage: 1 to 2 drops. Onset: 30–60 minutes. Duration: 6–24 hours. *Homatropine:* Dosage: 1 to 2 drops. Onset: 30–60 minutes. Duration: 3 days. *Scopolamine:* Dosage: 1 to 2 drops 1 hour before refraction. Onset: 30–60 minutes. Duration: 4–7 days. *Tropicamide:* Dosage: 1 to 2 drops; repeat in 5 minutes as necessary. Onset: 20–40 minutes. Duration: 4–6 hours.	Assess for clinical signs of allergic reaction. Contraindicated in patients with narrow-angle glaucoma. Caution use in Down syndrome patients and the elderly. The darker the iris pigmentation, the greater the dosage for effect. Pressure placed with fingers at the bridge of the nose (lacrimal sac compression) may prevent excess systemic absorption. Instruct patient to wear sunglasses to block UV light exposure. Driving with eyes dilated may cause difficulty, especially on a sunny day. Perform good hand hygiene to avoid iatrogenic dilation. Topical use only. Observe for adverse ocular reactions: redness, conjunctivitis, lid inflammation, dry eyes, edema, and follicles. Observe for adverse systemic reactions: fever, dermatitis, flushing, dry mouth and skin, irritability, tachycardia, urinary retention, loss of coordination, hallucinations, coma, death, progressive respiratory depression, and stroke symptoms (which stop in 7 hours when drop is discontinued).
Miotics Carbachol Pilocarpine	Constricts pupils for ocular hypotension. Cholinergic agonist agents–induce, muscarinic receptor contraction of ciliary muscle in facilitating aqueous outflow, and increases trabecular meshwork outflow to decrease intraocular pressure (IOP).	*Open-angle glaucoma, good second-and third-line therapy.* *Preop and postop IOP controls.* *Acute glaucoma attack prevention in noneffected eye or antidote for mydriasis.* Dosage: 1 to 2 drops tid, qid, or 5–6 times a day, depending on eyedrop selection to the affected eye.	Promote compliance with eyedrops. Assess for relief of elevated intraocular pressure, drug effectiveness. Review patient history, due to contraindications of patients with iritis, conjunctivitis, or keratitis, and post–cataract surgery to prevent posterior synechiae. Inform patient that he may have difficulty with dark adaptation with field of vision reduced. Caution with night driving and working with hazardous equipment in dim light. Instruct to stop use prior to general anesthesia. Assess for clinical manifestation of allergic reaction. Observe for adverse ocular reactions: blurred vision, stinging, red eye, ciliary spasm, and induced myopia. Observe for adverse systemic reactions: sweating, headache, syncope, salivation, arrhythmias, hypotension, asthma, pulmonary distress, cramping, vomiting, diarrhea, and urinary frequency. Observe for systemic toxicity with overdose; antidote atropine.

(continued)

PHARMACOLOGY **Summary of the Topical Ophthalmic Drops for Diagnostic Procedures and Treatment of Glaucoma—*Continued***

Medication Category	Action	Application/Indication	Nursing Responsibility
Beta Blockers			
Nonselective β-adrenergic antagonist: Carteolol (Cartrol) Levobunolol (AKBeta) Metipranolol (Toprol) Timolol (Apo-timol) *Selective β-adrenergic antagonist:* Betaxolol (Betoptic) Levobetaxolol (Betaxon)	Antagonist agents inhibit agonist actions (blockers). β-Adrenergic antagonist affects ocular function by competing with agonist for β-adrenergic receptor binding sites, thereby blocking the effects of sympathetic stimulation. This results in decreased aqueous production and may increase aqueous outflow to decrease IOP.	*Primary open-angle glaucoma (POAG), ocular hypertension, aphakic glaucoma, or secondary glaucoma.* Dosage: 1 drop daily, bid, or tid, depending on eyedrop selection to the affected eye.	Promote compliance with eyedrops. Assess for relief of elevated intraocular pressure, drug effectiveness. Review patient history, due to contraindications of patients with chronic obstructive pulmonary disease (COPD), asthma, sinus bradycardia, overt cardiovascular failure, cardiogenic shock, greater than 1° atrioventricular (AV) block, and patients on catecholamine (reserpine). Selective β-adrenergic antagonist poses less risk of pulmonary adverse effects. May mask hypoglycemia in insulin-dependent diabetes mellitus (IDDM) and clinical signs of hyperthyroidism. Can elevate triglycerides. Protect drops from light. Instruct patient of possible additive effects if on systemic beta-blockers. Assess for clinical manifestation of allergic reaction. Observe for adverse ocular reactions: blurred vision, foreign body sensation, photophobia, ptosis, diplopia, and decreased corneal sensitivity. Observe for adverse systemic reactions: insomnia, arrhythmias, pulmonary distress, and bronchospasm (can cause death).
Alpha₂ Agonists			
Apraclonidine (Iopidine) Brimonidine (Alphagan P)	Mimics endogenous adrenergic compounds. Affects ocular function by select binding to α₂ receptors with sympathetic nervous system influence on aqueous formation, pupil width, and ocular blood flow to decrease IOP from glaucoma by decreasing aqueous production and increasing uveoscleral outflow.	*POAG, ocular hypertension, or preop IOP controls for laser therapy.* Dosage: 1 drop bid, tid, or 1 drop preop and postop laser therapy.	Instruct regarding need for compliance with eyedrops. Assess for relief of elevated intraocular pressure, drug effectiveness. Review patient history, due to contraindications of patients on clonidine and monamine oxidase inhibitors (MAOI) therapy. Can develop a vasovagal response during laser surgery and overreduction in IOP. Caution in patients with cardiovascular disease, renal dysfunctions, hepatic dysfunctions, depression, cerebral insufficiency, or Raynaud's disease. Assess for history of drug allergies prior to administration. Assess for adverse ocular reactions: red eye, mydriasis, upper lid elevation, burning stinging, blurriness, follicles, and itching. Observe for adverse systemic reactions: drowsiness, fatigue, headaches, blood pressure changes, dry mouth, nasal congestion, respiratory, or gastrointestinal (GI) discomforts.

PHARMACOLOGY **Summary of the Topical Ophthalmic Drops for Diagnostic Procedures and Treatment of Glaucoma—*Continued***

Medication Category	Action	Application/Indication	Nursing Responsibility
Prostaglandins Bimatoprost (Lumigan) Latanoprost (Xalatan) Travoprost (Travatan)	Increases uveoscleral outflow, increasing aqueous outflow.	*POAG, ocular hypertension, or elevated IOP lowering.* Dosage: 1 drop daily at bedtime.	Encourage compliance with eyedrops. Assess for relief of elevated intraocular pressure, drug effectiveness. Review patient history, due to contraindications. Inform patient of possible red eye (usually goes away within 8–12 weeks), increased eyelash growth, and discoloration of iris and tissue around the eye. Do not drop over contact lenses. Caution: Patients with pulmonary compromise, renal or liver dysfunctions, uveitis, or iritis; aphakic, pseudophakic, or macular edema; do not use Latanoprost with thimerosal. Assess for clinical manifestation of allergic reaction. Observe for adverse ocular reactions: persistent red eye, hyperpigment of iris and adnexa, increased growth of eyelashes, blurriness, stinging, itching, foreign body sensation, conjunctivitis, and macular edema. Observe for adverse systemic reactions: chest pain, angina, respiratory infection, colds, rash, back pain, and joint pain.
Carbonic Anhydrase Inhibitors (CAIs) Brinzolamide (Azopt) Dorzolamide (Trusopt)	Decreases the pressure in the eyes by reducing how much fluid (aqueous humor) is produced in the eye.	*Glaucoma treatment for IOP lowering.* Dosage: 1 drop bid or tid, depending on eyedrop selection.	Encourage compliance with eyedrops. Assess for relief of elevated intraocular pressure, drug effectiveness. Review patient history, due to contraindications if on sulfa drugs; patients with severe renal failure and hepatic insufficiency may have low levels of electrolytes (sodium [Na] and potassium [K]), hyperchloremic acidosis (especially po CAI medication). Caution: May mask hypoglycemia in IDDM, patients with pulmonary or cardiac disease, and patients on high dose of aspirin. Evaluate for clinical manifestation of allergic reaction. Observe for adverse ocular reactions: blurred vision, foreign body sensation, photophobia, ptosis, diplopia, and decreased corneal sensitivity. Observe for adverse systemic reactions: arrhythmias, pulmonary distress, drowsiness, Na and K imbalance, GI upset, and paresthesia.

taken, and past and present eye problems. The nurse also should assess the patient to determine how one is adapting to the visual problems and what anxieties or fears the patient might be experiencing. Is the patient experiencing feelings of loss of control? From an objective perspective the nurse will assess actual visual acuity, body language for distress, family support systems, and the patient's ability to adjust to lifestyle behaviors.

Nursing diagnoses are developed from the assessment data, and a patient care plan applies the nursing process to the relevant nursing diagnoses and provides a comprehensive approach for caring for patients with glaucoma. Diagnoses may include anxiety and fear based on altered self-concept, potential ineffective coping, pain related to intraocular pressure, and health maintenance issues. The nurse also must consider impaired home maintenance issues, risks for injury or falls, self-care deficits related to vision loss, and feelings of powerlessness related to loss of control.

Outcomes and Evaluation Parameters

Evaluation of the patient's response to treatment and nursing interventions is measured through outcome parameters. The focus of evaluation is the ability of the patient to keep intraocular pressure under control, to maintain a level of anxiety and fear at a reasonable level, and to prevent eye pain. Also noteworthy is the patient's ability to maintain and manage a clean and safe environment in which to live.

Planning and Interventions

Planning and implementation of nursing interventions focus on ways to help the patient achieve desired outcomes. Emphasis should be placed on helping the patient find resources and assistance to manage at home and to resume normal activities. Emotional and spiritual support should be provided as should education and specific instructions on how to care for self. Identification of risk factors and instructions on self-care and community resources also is very important.

■ Collaborative Management

The best results for patients with glaucoma are achieved through a multidisciplinary team approach, including the ophthalmologist, ophthalmic advance nurse practitioner, nurse, and optometrist. Management of glaucoma may include medical controls with the continuous use of eyedrops or surgical intervention by the ophthalmologist. The nurse practitioner or nurse can provide the necessary education and follow-up monitoring of patients' progress to ensure compliance with the glaucoma regimen. Nursing assessment and education include patients' compliance with regular use of eyedrops and follow-up, which is one of the main goals in treating glaucoma. The major reason for the cause of blindness from glaucoma, besides not knowing one has glaucoma, is noncompliance in using eyedrops and not taking glaucoma as a disease seriously. It is imperative that patients understand that the long-term goal of treatment is to lower intraocular pressure to prevent optic nerve damage, and only with continued use of drops can this goal be reached. The new generation of glaucoma eyedrops can lower intraocular pressure with once or twice a day dosage, which eliminates confusion, saves

time, and makes compliance feasible. It is essential to inform patients of potential side effects of the drops and let patients know that some side effects may be only temporary for a couple of months and then dissipate. Patients may need to change eyedrops if side effects are persistent. Eyedrops must be administered properly to gain the full benefit of the medication and prevent waste. Having patients give a return demonstration with artificial tears will allow the nurse to determine patients' ability for self-medication. If multiple drops are prescribed, it is helpful to give patients an index card with the list of drops and when to use them. This will assist patients in preventing drug errors and promoting compliance. The optometrist can provide visual evaluations between regular health care provider visits and make necessary refractive corrections when indicated, thereby, contributing to patients' compliance with eye medications.

Discharge Priorities and Health Promotion

Patient education includes information on risk factors for glaucoma such as family history, myopia, previous eye trauma, low blood pressure, African ancestry, diabetes, longtime exposure to steroids, and aging. On early detection of glaucoma and subsequent treatment to prevent permanent vision loss, health care providers need to focus on patient compliance with glaucoma eyedrops, as outlined in the Pharmacology Summary feature (p. 2346), and regular follow-ups. The patient is taught how to instill eyedrops properly for the full benefit of treatment. Regular eye examination is imperative to know whether treatment prescribed for glaucoma is effective; because no symptoms will occur until vision becomes blurry or lost, and this may not be reversible.

Cataracts

Cataracts are opacity (loss of transparency) of the natural crystalline lens, usually as a result of natural aging, that causes oxidative damage to the lens solubility and increasing cloudiness. The term *phakic* refers to the mature crystalline lens. The crystalline lens is one of the anatomic body structures that continue to grow with the passage of time. Sometimes the lens is compared to an onion with its additive layers; therefore, increased compression and density result in opacity. Cataracts can normally be recognized in adults as early as in the late 20s or early 30s, as the beginning of cataract formation is classified as lenticular changes. Risk factors that may accelerate cataract growth are ultraviolet light, x-ray exposure, smoking, poor diet, diabetes, and corticosteroid therapy. Congenital or traumatic cataracts are the exception to the normal growth phase of cataract formation and may need immediate treatment with surgical removal. Cataracts can be the leading cause of blindness, especially in remote areas of the world, where cataract surgery is not accessible. Cataracts are curable, and if people live long enough, most will experience them at some point in their lifetime.

The onset of the signs and symptoms of cataracts are usually gradual. Patients start to notice that headlights from automobiles look like starbursts. They are bothered with glare, have difficulty reading street signs at night, and experience progressive reading difficulty even with glasses or bifocals. The refractive index changes and the power increases possibly may make patients more nearsighted. This is called a myopic shift and temporarily provides better vision without glasses for the hyperopic or farsighted person.

This is referred to as "second sight" (AAO-11, 2008–2009). Usually cataracts are a painless, progressive loss of vision with aging.

Cataracts are classified according to the opacity formation location in the crystalline lens. The four most basic types of cataract are nuclear, cortical, posterior, and anterior. The other classifications of cataract formations that may be used pertain to specific conditions or inheritance. Chart 71–6 is inclusive of the types of cataract types.

Immature Cataracts

The immature cataract is still in the earlier stages of maturation or ripening, beginning with sectors of opacity and intervening clear areas (AAO-11, 2008–2009) (Figure 71–14 ■). Mature cataracts are easily recognizable with an ophthalmoscope and more definitively with a slit-lamp biomicroscopy. Sometimes the cataract is so dense and noticeable, a penlight will do. *Senile* or *mature cataract* is a term used in describing the later stages of formation and most commonly is reached by the time one reaches 70 to 80 years of age.

Diagnosis is made by a vision test with best-corrected visual acuity of about 20/50 or worse, and a glare test, which mimics sunlight for 20/200 or worse vision, to be considered for cataract surgery. A potential acuity meter (PAM) test also is performed to gauge the approximate visual acuity return after cataract surgery. (See the Diagnostic Tests box, p. 2333.) This may vary depending on whether any other vision problems existed preoperatively; for example, if patients have age-related macular degeneration, diabetic retinopathy, or had previous eye surgery.

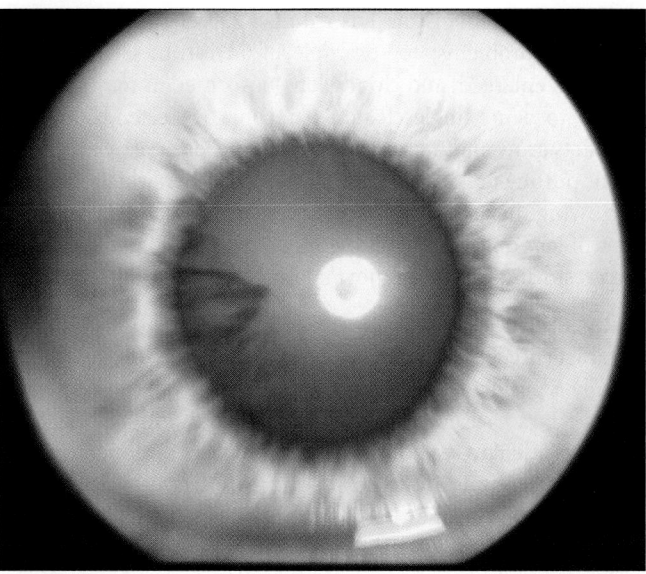

FIGURE 71–14 ■ Nuclear sclerotic with spokes (cortical cataract).
Source: Kathleen Osborn

Cataract Surgical Implications

The decision to operate is ultimately determined by the patient when the individual is no longer able to perform activities of daily living, work, drive a motor vehicle, watch television, read, or use a computer. Cataract removal, with few exceptions, usually is recommended by the time one is past 85 years of age.

CHART 71–6   **Categories of Cataract Types**

Type	Description
Nuclear sclerotic (NS) cataract	The nuclear cataract refers to the thickening or hardening (opacity) of the nucleus or central location of the natural crystalline lens (AAO-11, 2008–2009).
Senile, mature, or brunescent cataract	The advanced stage of cataract formation, when it turns brown in color, is most commonly reached by the time the patient is in his 70s or 80s.
Hypermature or Morgagni's cataract	The nuclear sclerosis has gone past maturity into a liquid state.
Cortical or spokes cataract	The cataract thickening is in the peripheral cortex of the natural lens. The radial opacities look like spokes on a wagon wheel, and visual acuity disturbances come on later, if the nucleus is still clear.
Anterior subcapsular cataract (ASC)	The thickening of the natural lens at the anterior or front capsular surface. This more commonly develops from ocular trauma or uveitis conditions (Streeten, 2000).
Posterior subcapsular (PSC) or cupuliform cataract	The thickening of the crystalline lens at the posterior or back capsular surface. This type of cataract is seen more commonly after long systemic steroid usage or a long period of intraocular inflammation. This can cause more difficulty with reading, and bright lights and glare compound this difficulty (AAO-11, 2008–2009).
Hereditary cataract	The lens opacity that has a genetic precondition that usually develops in the third to fifth decade of life. A precondition may be an autosomal dominant inherited disorder or genetic abnormalities, such as Down syndrome or Marfan's syndrome (AAO-6, 2008–2009).
Traumatic cataract	The opaque lens formation due to trauma to or about the eye. This type of cataract usually develops within a brief period (only months) and affects only the involved eye. Manifested symptoms may be blurry vision, glare, photophobia, pain, and iritis (AAO-11, 2008–2009).
Surgically induced or oil-droplet cataract	The cataract that mimics a tear droplet in the nucleus of the lens, which more commonly develops after a vitrectomy surgery (Eliott, Lee, & Abrams, 2001), especially in younger adults ages 30 to 50. The vision is usually blurry enough to interfere with work performance or activities of daily living. Common complaints are unexplained vision loss, the need for frequent glasses changes, and increasing myopia. Oil droplet describes the appearance of a type of opacity that results.

Sources: American Academy of Ophthalmology (AAO-6). (2008–2009). *Basic and clinical science course: Pediatric ophthalmology and strabismus* (Section 6). San Francisco: Author; American Academy of Ophthalmology (AAO-11). (2008–2009). *Basic and clinical science course: Lens and cataract* (Section 11). San Francisco: Author; Eliott, D., Lee, M. S., & Abrams, G. W. (2001). Proliferative diabetic retinopathy: Principles and techniques of surgical treatment. In S. J. Ryan (Ed.), *Retina* (3rd ed., Vol. 2). St. Louis: Mosby; and Streeten, B. W. (2000). Pathology of the lens. In D. M. Albert & F. A. Jakobiec (Eds.), *Principles & practice of ophthalmology* (2nd ed., Vol. 4). Philadelphia: W. B. Saunders.

Sometimes when one has cataract surgery, it can possibly solve two problems; for example, if an intumescent cataract (swollen, enlarged, and cloudy lens) is formed, it may be a precursor to acute angle-closure glaucoma (Streeten, 2000). As cataracts grow and mature, the crystalline lens enlarges, crowding or putting pressure on the anterior chamber, which results in narrowing the angle. Cataract surgery can solve both the problems of lens opacity and of opening the anterior chamber angle, thus restoring vision and normal intraocular pressure.

Cataract Surgery

Cataract surgery is 98% successful (Streeten, 2000). The surgery usually is performed one eye at a time, and if the fellow eye also needs cataract surgery, it is performed about 6 to 8 weeks later. This is prudent to see how the patient recovers postoperatively. If unforeseen complications do arise from the first cataract surgery, they can be taken into consideration when the fellow eye has cataract surgery. Some conditions that may predispose patients to less than ideal results are age-related macular degeneration, diabetes, Marfan's syndrome, or previous retinal detachment. Before cataract surgery is done, a good dilated eye examination is done, to make sure there are no existing problems. If any problems are present, they will need to be addressed before the surgery is performed; for example, active diabetic retinopathy.

Cataract surgery usually is done in an ambulatory surgery center (ASC) under topical or local anesthesia. The anesthesia may vary depending on the surgeon and patient's preference. Preoperative ophthalmic antibiotic/anti-inflammatory drops for surgical preparation and dilation are administered. Preparation for surgery usually includes lid scrubs, and the facial area around the eyes is cleaned with antiseptic solution and well rinsed prior to surgery. Cataracts usually are removed by phacoemulsification with the use of ultrasonic power to fragment (break up) the lens, and the lens fragments are then aspirated with vacuum and flow irrigation. Extracapsular cataract extraction (ECCE) usually is done with a single small surgical incision near the sclerolimbal margin, called no stitch surgery. Extracapsular cataract extraction is the removal of the entire lens (nucleus and cortex) and the central portion of the anterior capsule, leaving the posterior capsule fully intact. The lens implanted is placed in the lens sulcus. On rare occasions an intracapsular cataract extraction (ICCE) may be the best option. This is when the entire lens with capsule is removed. An artificial lens is surgically implanted, called an intraocular lens (IOL) implant. A posterior chamber intraocular lens (PCIOL) is the most commonly used intraocular lens. An anterior chamber intraocular lens (ACIOL) or sutured intraocular lens is used when a posterior chamber intraocular lens cannot be stabilized due to surgical or ocular complications, such as broken zonules, or other systemic problems, such as Marfan's syndrome. New custom IOL implantations that are now available for patients having cataract removals can correct for accommodation or astigmatism. *Pseudophakic* is the term used after cataract surgery when patients have an intraocular lens implant and no longer have a natural crystalline lens. Aphakic refers to no lens implant or without lens implant after cataract surgery of the natural lens removal. These patients will need to wear thick glasses or contact lenses for best-corrected visual acuity. The goal of the lens implant is to restore best-corrected vision for patients so that pa-

tients do not have to wear glasses or contact lenses. However, unless a multifocal lens implant is used (a combination lens for near and distance vision), patients most often will still need reading glasses for seeing up close.

Secondary intraocular lens implant implies that an intraocular lens is implanted after the primary cataract surgery was performed at an earlier date (AAO-11, 2008–2009). For whatever reason, a primary intraocular lens was never implanted at the time of the original cataract surgery. The secondary intraocular lens implant is placed in the aphakic eye (that without a lens).

On completion of the surgery, eyedrops are put in the surgical eye, followed by the application of an eye patch and shield, and postoperative topical ocular medications are prescribed. See the Pharmacology Summary feature (p. 2346). Patients usually are given a postoperative take-home pack, which may include eye patches, sterile eyewash, sunglasses, topical eye medications or prescriptions, and an analgesic prescription for minor operative discomfort. Patients need to know how to care for the postsurgical eye properly with appropriate cleaning and wearing an eye patch or shield as directed.

Postoperative Cataract Care

Postoperative treatment and follow-up care on postoperative day 1 include removal of the eye patch and shield and assessment of visual acuity and intraocular pressure, followed by slit-lamp biomicroscopy and ophthalmoscopy to check the wound stability and any potential postoperative problems (Oetting, 2001). Depth perception may be temporarily impaired following cataract surgery due to the eye patch, being the first eye done, or being aphakic. Patients that are aphakic will need glasses or contact lenses for corrective vision. It often is recommended to postpone getting new corrective lenses for about 6 to 12 weeks after cataract surgery, thus giving the eyes the needed time to heal completely, and sparing patients the expense of more than one pair of glasses. Patients should be instructed to take it easy for a few days and to use topical ophthalmic antibiotic/anti-inflammatory drops as prescribed, for approximately 4 weeks.

Possible cataract surgery complications may include a dropped natural crystalline lens or intraocular lens implant, surgical astigmatism, and decentered or tilted intraocular lens. These and other complications are outlined in Chart 71–7 (AAO-11, 2008–2009).

◼ Nursing Management

Nursing management for cataract surgery focuses on preparing patients for the procedure by explaining that it is typically an outpatient procedure performed under local or topical anesthesia. Preoperatively, patients are informed by the ophthalmologist and confirmed by the nurse about what a cataract is, the surgical procedure, and the benefits and risks of cataract surgical removal. The nurse should assess understanding, answer misconceptions or questions, and relieve anxieties. Postoperative instructions should be discussed with patients and significant others prior to surgery for understanding. Instruction should include a demonstration of proper eyedrop instillation, with a return demonstration from the person who will be instilling postoperative eyedrops. Assessment of the operative and nonoperative eye prior to surgery should be completed and documented. It is essential to record all current medications, prescription and over

CHART 71–7	Potential Complications Post-Cataract Surgery

Complication	Description
Decentered/tilted intraocular lens	The intraocular lens falls out of central position or tilts in any direction, causing aberrations or less than clear vision. If not a problem, leave well enough alone. If a problem, surgeon may need to go back in to straighten the intraocular lens, suture it in place, or remove it.
Surgical astigmatism	Abnormal curvature of the cornea is induced with sutures; once healed, the sutures can be cut and refractive adjustments made.
Bullous keratopathy	Corneal edema from surgical manipulation and vitreocorneal adherence; complaining of blurry vision, epiphora, and photophobia; treated with topical eye medication (antibiotics).
Hyphema	Blood in the anterior chamber; complaining of blurry vision and pain; treated with topical eye medication and patching, and quiet; check intraocular pressure often.
Glaucoma	Elevated intraocular pressure; complaining of nothing, but noted on intraocular pressure check; may have pain and blurry vision; treated with topical antiglaucoma eye medication, and occasionally oral medication is indicated if intraocular pressure is > 50 mmHg.
Dropped natural lens Dropped intraocular lens	The natural crystalline lens or the intraocular lens implant is dropped in the vitreous; this requires a pars plana vitrectomy with air–fluid–gas exchange to retrieve the lens, usually immediately at the time of surgery or shortly afterward.
Cystoid macular edema	Edema of the choroidal layer in the macula (central vision); treated with topical eye medication and possibly vitrectomy with air–fluid–gas exchange.
Retained crystalline lens material	Lens material in the capsule is an irritant that can become infectious and cause inflammation; complaining of blurred vision and pain. Treat the problem it is causing, or Elschnig's pearls, lens remnants, can be polished.
Vitreous prolapse	If the rupture of the posterior capsule results, this allows vitreous into the anterior chamber, which may cause pupillary block, poor healing, infection, retinal breaks, or retinal detachments; usually this is corrected at the time of surgery with an anterior vitrectomy to remove vitreous from the anterior chamber.
Retinal detachment	Retinal layers detach or separate from their base; complaining of a curtain, a veil, floaters, or light flashes in vision; treated with endolaser or a vitrectomy with air–fluid–gas exchange.
Vitreous hemorrhage	Blood in the vitreous chamber; complaining of blurry vision and floaters; treated with head elevated during rest or sleep, and let the blood settle inferiorly, or may need a vitrectomy with air–fluid–gas exchange.
Uveitis	Inflammation of the uveal tract (iris, ciliary body, and choroid) from surgical trauma or allergy to intraocular lens; complaining of photophobia, epiphora, and pain; treated with topical eye medication (possible mydriatics, antibiotics/anti-inflammatories, or steroids) or intraocular lens removal.
Endophthalmitis	Intraocular infection and inflammation of the eyeball and tissue; complaining of pain, blurred vision, purulent discharge, hypopyon, and corneal edema; treated with intravitreal, fortified topical, topical, and/or oral antibiotics, and may also require a vitrectomy with air–fluid–gas exchange.
Posterior capsular opacity	This is the most common complaint after cataract surgery, because the posterior capsule is left intact. This capsule prevents other potential major complications that could occur if the capsule were opened. Opacity or haziness of the posterior capsule membrane may take place within several weeks to years or may never develop; complaining of hazy or blurry vision and cataract coming back; cannot read or drive; treated with Nd:YAG laser to open the capsule.

Source: Adapted from American Academy of Ophthalmology (AAO-11). (2008–2009). *Basic and clinical science course: Lens and cataract* (Section 11). San Francisco: AAO.

the counter (OTC), with dosage and frequency, especially any anticoagulants, because they may need to be stopped temporarily before and immediately following surgery.

Infections and Inflammation

All structures of the adnexa and eyeball are subject to infection and inflammation. This section covers some of the most common and serious inflammatory conditions. Inflammatory eye conditions usually are very responsive to treatment, and in most cases the eye is restored to normal with little or no treatment. However, some severe eye infections can mean hospitalization and result in the loss of vision and possibly the eye.

Dry Eye Syndrome

Keratoconjunctivitis sicca, or dry eye syndrome (DES), is the result of poor tear production and formation, or excessive evaporation (AAO-8, 2008–2009). With aging, especially with menopausal women, dry eyes can become a chronic problem, with less tear surface tension. This results in tears running down the face instead of adhering to the cornea epithelial surface. Dry eyes also can be a side effect of some systemic medications (e.g., propranolol) or systemic disease (e.g., Sjögren's syndrome) (AAO-8, 2008–2009). Dry eyes give the sensation of a sandpaper or "gritty" feeling in the eye, blurred vision, and difficulty focusing up close. Treatment usually includes frequent use of artificial tear supplements and/or puncta plugs. Patients are instructed on frequent instillation of artificial tears and being consistent with application. If patients find that using the tears once, twice, or a number of times a day provides relief, they are instructed to use the tears the same number of times each day, so as to prevent the eye from drying out completely between applications. Puncta plugs are plastic or collagen devices that are inserted by an eye health care provider into the puncta to obstruct tears from leaving the eye. If dry eyes become so chronic that they result in corneal defects and scarring, surgical intervention may be indicated with various degrees of tarsorrhaphy, which is the suturing of the upper and lower eyelids together, to lessen corneal exposure (AAO-8, 2008–2009). Artificial tears usually are over-the-counter medication, but a new artificial tear by prescription (cyclosporine ophthalmic emulsion) is available that may keep the eye moist for a longer period of time and help increase tear production.

Blepharitis

Blepharitis, or meibomitis, is inflammation of the eyelids, with redness and crustiness (dry flaky dermis). The use of warm compresses and lid scrubs often is adequate treatment. If the condition is more chronic and becomes ulcerative, the addition of antibiotic ointment may be indicated. This is a very common condition in the aged population, in which the meibomian glands build up with a waxy deposit, the tears do not function properly, and dry eyes develop (Lamb, 2002; Rougé, 2004). Patients complain of **foreign body sensation (FBS)**, nasal canthus deposits, itching, tearing, burning, and irritation. This can be difficult to eliminate and usually requires continuous weekly or daily lid scrubs and warm compresses, which are described in Chart 71–8.

Conjunctivitis

Conjunctivitis is inflammation of the conjunctiva, the clear mucous membrane that covers the sclera of the eye (bulbar conjunctiva), the underlining of the eyelids (palpebral conjunctiva), and the space between the lid and globe (forniceal conjunctiva, fornix, or cul-de-sac) (AAO-2, 2008–2009). On an initial evaluation, it is important to try to obtain a culture or cytologic/serologic study on the type of discharge (especially if muco-purulent). The three most common types of conjunctivitis—viral, allergic, and bacterial—are outlined in Chart 71–9.

CHART 71–8	Eyelid Cleaning and Comfort Measure
Warm Compresses	This is the use of a facecloth or washcloth placed in lukewarm water. Fold it in half and place gently over eyelids for 3 to 8 minutes, especially trying to feel the warmth at the margin of the eyelids to dissolve or melt the waxy discharge that collects at the base of the eyelashes.
Eyelid Scrubs	This is the use of baby shampoo or no tears shampoo diluted in warm water (3 drops of shampoo to 125 milliliters of water). Use a Q-tip applicator or the soft edge of a facecloth to scrub eyelid margins gently. Commercial lid scrubs are also available in local pharmacies.

CHART 71–9	Three Most Common Forms of Conjunctivitis			
Form	**Discharge**	**Eyelid Edema**	**Lymph Node**	**Pruritus**
Viral conjunctivitis	Clear, sticky	Minimal	Usually	None
Allergic conjunctivitis	Clear, runny	Moderate to severe	None	Intense
Bacterial conjunctivitis	Purulent	Moderate	None	None

Viral Conjunctivitis

Viral conjunctivitis, commonly referred to as "classic pinkeye," is inflammation caused by an adenovirus. This also is referred to as an epidemic keratoconjunctivitis (EKC) when the inflammation encompasses both the cornea and the conjunctiva (AAO-8, 2008–2009). Initially the inflammation starts unilaterally and quickly spreads bilaterally. After about a week of incubation time, such signs and symptoms as clear mucous sticky discharge, excessive tearing (epiphora), hyperemia, small white conjunctival elevations (follicles), light sensitivity (photophobia), foreign body sensation, conjunctival inflammation and irritation, and tissue edema to the point of a transparent bluish hue (chemosis) develop. Preauricular lymph node enlargement and soreness also can be symptoms of viral conjunctivitis (Elfervig & Elfervig, 2007; Trobe, 2006). Causative agents may include adenovirus, herpes simplex, herpes zoster, or influenza virus (Rubenstein & Jick, 2004). Treatment includes good hand hygiene, which is imperative, plus not sharing washcloths, towels, and pillows due to this condition's extremely contagious nature. Viral conjunctivitis usually will take its course and clear on its own.

Patients can use artificial tears, topical ophthalmic antibiotic/steroid, or decongestant eyedrops for 7 to 10 days. Cold compresses for eye comfort also may help increase the healing time and shorten the disease course. Patients should not return to school or to work if in the active stages for at least 4 days, and possibly a week to 10 days, due to the severity and the epidemic nature of viral conjunctivitis.

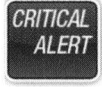 *Viral conjunctivitis is highly contagious. The nurse should use effective hand hygiene frequently, before and after putting in medicated eyedrops. The examination area should be sanitized with antibacterial solutions after examination.*
The patient should be instructed in effective hand hygiene technique and advised not to touch eyes or faces of others, and to keep a distance from others. The patient also should be instructed to use clean sheets and towels and not to share them with others.

Allergic Conjunctivitis

Allergic conjunctivitis, sometimes referred to as hay fever conjunctivitis, is caused by environmental changes and contaminants. This also is referred to as a vernal keratoconjunctivitis when the inflammation involves both the cornea and the conjunctiva during seasonal changes, and appears to be most common in young males (Lamb, 2002; Wu & Ariyasu, 1999). It usually is bilateral, with whitish discharge, hyperemia, swelling, burning, stinging, epiphora, and pruritus (Elfervig & Elfervig, 2007; Trobe,

2006). This commonly is a seasonal occurrence, especially in the spring and fall, and usually reoccurs annually. Symptoms seem to lessen after sleeping and with less environmental exposure by staying indoors. Causative agents may include animal dander, dust, wind, smoke, feathers, ingested foods, makeup, creams, systemic medications, and anything that can cause an allergic response. Medical management includes topical decongestant eyedrops for 7 to 10 days, good hand hygiene, cold compresses, and oral antihistamines. These measures usually will bring the allergies under control. If this is a seasonal episode, using preventive measures such as taking oral antihistamines a couple of weeks prior to the season may abate clinical manifestations. It may be necessary for patients to seek medical evaluation and treatment.

Bacterial Conjunctivitis

Bacterial conjunctivitis usually is unilateral in the early stages, but often becomes bilateral, with mucopurulent discharge, hyperemia, chemosis, eyelid inflammation and irritation (blepharitis), lid crusting, eyelid edema, and eyelids sticking and matting together, especially on awakening in the morning (Elfervig & Elfervig, 2007; Trobe, 2006). The preauricular nodes usually are not enlarged (Trobe, 2006). Causative agents may include *Staphylococcus aureus, Neisseria gonorrhoeae, Streptococcus pneumoniae, Corynebacterium diphtheriae, Haemophilus influenzae, Listeria,* and *Moraxella* (Rubenstein & Jick, 2004). Medical management includes topical ophthalmic antibiotic drops or ointment for 7 to 10 days, warm compresses, and good hand hygiene technique.

Other common infections and inflammations of the eye are outlined in Chart 71–10 (p. 2356) by description, signs, causes, and management. The conditions include subconjunctival hemorrhage, sty, chalazion, pinguecula, pterygium, dendritic keratitis, herpes zoster ophthalmicus, episcleritis, and scleritis.

Uveitis

Uveitis is inflammation of the uvea or uveal tract, which includes inflammation of the iris, the ciliary body, and the choroid. An in-depth medical history is prudent if uveitis is suspected because of endogenous uveitis, meaning the cause originated from systemic conditions, such as arthritis, oncologic causes, infections, or lupus (Nussenblatt & Whitcup, 2004). Other definitive locations are iritis (includes the iris), cyclitis (includes the ciliary body), anterior uveitis or iridocyclitis (includes the iris and ciliary body), or posterior uveitis or choroiditis (includes the choroid) (Elfervig, 2002a). Clinical manifestations may include blurry vision, tearing, floaters, erythema, hyperemia, edema, or photophobia. Eye pain is usually described as dull with an ache inside the eye. Dark glasses do not seem to help the photophobia.

Noticeable ciliary infection signs when observing the eye may include a small, irregular pupil and dilated or engorged episcleral vessels on the sclera (Nussenblatt & Whitcup, 2004). A slit-lamp examination could reveal cells and flare in the anterior chamber. Cells are white blood cells, and flare is protein deposits floating in the aqueous humor (Harper, Chorich, & Foster, 2002). If patients complain of floaters and blurry vision, the adjacent connecting structures may be inflamed: the vitreous (vitritis), the retina (retinitis), or the retina and choroid (retinochoroiditis) (AAO-9, 2008–2009; Elfervig, 2002a).

Medical management usually includes topical antibiotics to treat the infection, topical or periocular injected steroids to treat the inflammation, and topical mydriatic and cycloplegic drops for temporary dilation and paralysis of the ciliary muscle for comfort (Foster & Vitale, 2002). See the Pharmacology Summary feature (p. 2346). The cycloplegic drops will affect accommodation, so if patients do not have reading glasses or bifocals, they may have temporary difficulty reading small print while on these drops (Foster & Vitale, 2002).

Bullous Keratopathy

Bullous keratopathy or Fuchs' dystrophy is edema and degeneration of the corneal epithelium causing scarring and reduced vision that result from membrane endothelial outgrowths into Descemet's corneal layer (Beers & Berkow, 1999). The severity of the condition can result in corneal ulcer from an epithelial infection and may require a corneal graft later. Initially, it may present with guttata, petite whitish hyaline deposits in Descemet's membrane (Wu & Ariyasu, 1999). This also can be a result of surgical trauma. Medical management includes corneal contact lens bandage, hypertonic saline drops, and intraocular pressure–lowering drops, as indicated (Wu & Ariyasu, 1999).

Corneal Ulcer

Cornea ulcers are local necroses of the corneal tissue due to incursion by bacteria, fungi, or viral infections. These invasions can be the result of contact lens overwear, foreign body penetration, wound or trauma, ocular surgical trauma, chronic conjunctivitis or blepharitis, nutritional vitamin A deficiency, entropion, exophthalmos, exposure keratitis, and chronic, severe dry eyes. All of these conditions allow infectious organisms to penetrate the cornea, resulting in degeneration of corneal tissue (Wu & Ariyasu, 1999). The most common invading organisms are *Pseudomonas, Staphylococcus, Streptococcus,* herpesvirus, and *Acanthamoeba* (AAO-8, 2008–2009). Patients may complain of foreign body sensation, epiphora, and blurry vision initially.

On examination with the biomicroscope, a small dull-grayish deposit can be noted in the epithelium, which progresses to a whitish circumscribed opacity in the cornea that necroses into an ulcer. Other ocular signs may be chronic hyperemic eye, **hypopyon** (pus in anterior portion of eye) or corneal neovascularization with later progression (AAO-8, 2008–2009; Elfervig & Elfervig, 2007). A dendritic infiltrate is very diagnostic of a fungal infection (McLeod, 2004). The deeper the ulcer is in the corneal layers, the more severe the disease and complications, and it is considered an urgent condition to be treated aggressively by an ophthalmologist. Medical management options can vary from fortified eyedrops to corneal transplant (penetrating keratoplasty).

Trachoma

Trachoma is chronic inflammation of the conjunctiva that ranges from mild to severe, even scarring. It is caused by repeated invasion of *Chlamydia trachomatis,* which causes chronic infection and inflammation (Rubenstein & Jick, 2004). Ocular manifestations can be follicles, hyperemia, entropion, and trichiasis, and can result in blindness from corneal opacification. This ocular disease is more common in Third World

CHART 71–10 Infections and Inflammations of the Eye

Condition	Description/Sign	Cause/Management
Non-traumatized eye (subconjunctival hemorrhage)	Dilated blood capillaries or small capillary leakage on the sclera or conjunctiva.	Coughing, sneezing, sudden motion, or straining, especially if a patient is on a blood thinner; usually resolves spontaneously.
Hordeolum (sty or stye)	Infection of the eyelid glands. Internal hordeolum is located within the eyelid itself, a pustular infection of the meibomian gland; and external hordeolum is located at the eyelid margin, a pustular infection of the oil glands of Zeis.	Can resolve spontaneously, when warm compresses are applied two to four times a day to the infected area to aid in localization and rupture of the pustule; topical ophthalmic antibiotic ointment and incision and drainage of the pustule also may be indicated if it does not resolve spontaneously.
Chalazion	Inflammation in the meibomian gland of the eyelid; referred to as an internal hordeolum or meibomian cyst. Appears as a raised, round, inflamed (erythematic), and tender area near the lid margin.	Blockage of the sebaceous material in the meibomian gland. Treat with warm compresses and ophthalmic antibiotic ointment. If this becomes a nuisance or interferes with vision, it can be surgically excised.
Pinguecula	Small, yellowish conjunctival elevation at the 3 and 9 o'clock positions on the scleroconjunctival area, which results from prolonged ultraviolet, sunlight, or environmental exposure.	Usually does not cause any symptoms and does not require treatment. If it becomes irritating, use artificial tears.
Pterygium	Yellowish-white triangular growth of conjunctival tissue at the 3 and 9 o'clock positions close to the limbus that results from prolonged ultraviolet exposure and can spread onto the cornea.	If it continues to grow across the cornea, passing the central visual axis causing vision loss, then laser or surgical intervention is indicated. Otherwise, it is just observed, with no treatment, or treated with artificial tears if it becomes irritating.
Herpetic keratitis (dendritic keratitis)	Inflammation of the cornea. Staining of the corneal epithelium reveals a bare branch-like configuration on the cornea (dendrite). Signs and symptoms are photopia, epiphora, foreign body sensation, and hyperemia.	Caused by the herpes simplex virus. Treatment with antiviral drops usually is sufficient, but systemic drugs may be indicated if drops are not effective in clearing the inflammation. Epithelial débridement around the dendrite of loose tissue with a cotton-tip applicator may aid in accelerating the healing process. Atropine Care 1% drops also may help in healing and comfort (AAO-8, 2008–2009).
Herpes zoster ophthalmicus	Varicella-zoster virus (shingles or chickenpox) involves the globe of the eye. Nose lesion (nasociliary nerve affected) can be diagnostic (McLeod, 2004). Signs are eyelid edema, hyperemia, corneal edema, keratitis, and elevated intraocular pressure.	Forehead dermatitis. Infection treated with antiviral oral medications, topical steroid drops, and atropine drops. The intraocular pressure is monitored often until it returns to normal and remains stable. Patients over age 60 may need a short course of oral corticosteroids to prevent acute postherpetic neuralgia or persistent pain (McLeod, 2004).
Episcleritis	Inflammation of the episclera (outermost layer of the sclera); appears with single, large, dilated vessels in the episcleral layer at about the 3 and 9 o'clock positions on the sclera (Goldstein & Tessler, 2004). The patient complains of hyperemia, photophobia, local tenderness, and epiphora.	Treatment may range from nothing and observation; to topical vasoconstrictor, topical steroid drops, or oral nonsteroidal anti-inflammatory drugs to shorten the course of discomfort. It usually is self-limiting and rarely becomes serious (Daly, 2002).
Scleritis	Inflammation of the sclera and deep episclera. This can be serious and vision threatening and is found more commonly in women between 45 and 65 years of age (Daly, 2002). Complaints may be localized eye pain, tenderness, photophobia, epiphora, and hyperemia. The irritated area appears bluish (meaning deep vessel involvement); this can range from being diffuse, nodular, or necrotizing tissue. About 15% of patients develop vision loss within the first year (Beers & Berkow, 1999).	Treatment may include cytotoxic immunosuppression, but usually systemic corticosteroid is the initial treatment of choice. Patients should be closely monitored for hematopoietic, renal, and other organ involvement.

Sources: American Academy of Ophthalmology (AAO-8). (2008–2009). *Basic and clinical science course: External disease and cornea* (Section 8). San Francisco: Author; Beers, M. H., & Berkow, R. (1999). *The Merck manual of diagnosis and therapy* (17th ed.). Whitehouse Station, NJ: Merck Research Laboratories; Daly, S. W. (2002). Scleral disorders. In K. Goldblum & P. Lamb (Eds.), *Core curriculum for ophthalmic nursing* (2nd ed.). Dubuque, IA: Kendall/Hunt; Goldstein, D. A., & Tessler, H. H. (2004). Episcleritis, scleritis, and other scleral disorders. In M. Yanoff & J. S. Duker (Eds.), *Ophthalmology* (2nd ed.). St. Louis: Mosby; and McLeod, S. D. (2004). Infectious keratitis. In M. Yanoff & J. S. Duker (Eds.), *Ophthalmology* (2nd ed.). St. Louis: Mosby.

countries and is the second leading cause of preventable blindness in the world, second only to cataracts (Mayo Clinic, 2006).

Preseptal Cellulitis

Preseptal cellulitis is inflammation of the eyelid tissue in front of the orbital septum and does not involve the eyeball (Elfervig & Elfervig, 2007; Trobe, 2006). It can exhibit the following signs and symptoms of the eyelid: warmth, tenderness, swelling, redness, and chemosis. It usually does not involve problems with eye movement or pain. Patients also may be febrile and irritable from the inflammation and discomfort. Systemic antibiotics and warm compresses for 10 days is the recommended medical treatment.

Orbital Cellulitis

Orbital cellulitis is inflammation of the postseptal orbital tissue from the spread of bacteria from elsewhere (endogenous), usually from the nasal and sinus system, or the traumatic induction of bacteria into the orbit (AAO-7, 2008–2009) (Figure 71–15 ■). The most common causative organisms in adults are staphylococci and streptococci from bacterial sinusitis (Dutton, 2004). Clinical manifestations may include fever, red and edematous eyelids, periocular pain, hypopyon, proptosis, impaired ocular motility, afferent pupillary defect, optic nerve swelling, corneal abscess, decreased vision (can be a rapid onset), hyperemia, and erythema (Elfervig & Elfervig, 2007; Trobe, 2006). Patients should be referred immediately to a health care provider, so that the primary locus of the infection can be identified with thorough examination and history of any trauma, flu or upper respiratory infection, sinusitis, or toothaches. Test requirements may be x-rays, computed tomography (CT) scan, and Gram stain and culture of any discharges from the eye, nose, mouth, or skin. Medical management may involve hospitalization with aggressive intravenous and systemic broad-spectrum antibiotics, topical fortified antibiotic eyedrops and subconjunctival antibiotics, surgical

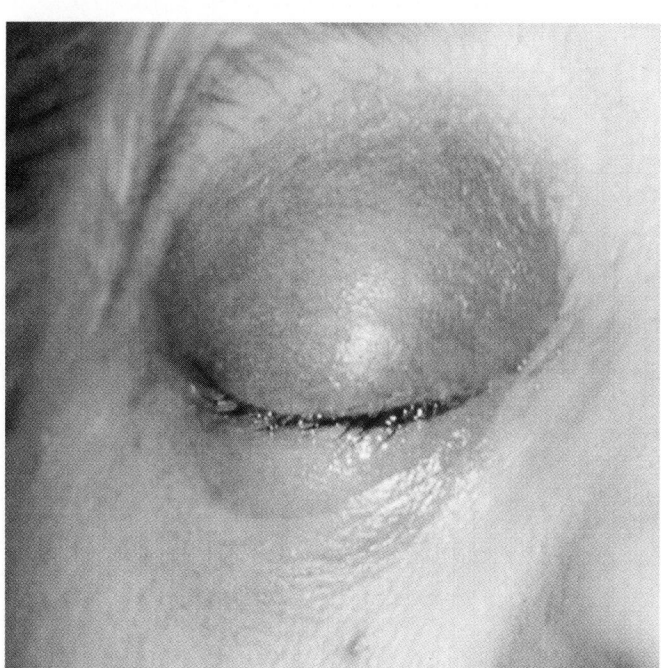

FIGURE 71–15 ■ Orbital cellulitis.
Source: Courtesy of Dr. Elferuiz

débridement/drainage or vitrectomy, whatever is indicated pending culture result. Vision and pupil functions should be checked every 5 to 6 hours. Orbital cellulitis can lead to intracranial abscess and cavernous sinus thrombosis, which when involved has the added symptoms of nausea, vomiting, headache, and possible loss of consciousness, a life-threatening complication. When patients are ready to be discharged, it is very important for them to follow the discharge regimen, or recurrent infection and loss of the eye may develop, which could be life threatening.

Discharge Priorities and Health Promotion

Discharge planning starts with admission to the hospital and is continuous throughout the hospitalization. An organized plan of care with set goals will ensure the highest level of recovery. The ultimate goal is to return patients home with no complications or added problems.

To assist and to augment understanding, an organized and comprehensive instructional plan is necessary with patient brochures and information. The Patient Teaching & Discharge Priorities box (p. 2358) outlines the necessary components of the teaching plan for orbital cellulitis, which includes the healing regimen, risks of recurrent infection and other potential complications, pain management, emotional adjustment, and sensory deprivation or recovery. Discharge instructions include continuous use of systemic antibiotics and topical antibiotic eyedrops or ointment, use of good hygiene technique to prevent reinfection, ways to achieve altered comfort, monitoring the healing process of the eye, health care provider notification of complications, and compliance with follow-up care. Care specialists may include an ophthalmologist, an otolaryngologist, a health care provider, and a nurse consultant.

Endophthalmitis

Endophthalmitis is a mucopurulent intraocular inflammation that occurs most often after intraocular surgery, such as for cataract, glaucoma, strabismus, or penetrating keratoplasty. The incidence of endophthalmitis is approximately 1 in 1,000 population. The exogenous pathogens harbored on the lids and in the conjunctival fornix invade the eye and inflammation results (Elfervig & Elfervig, 1999). Endophthalmitis also can be a consequence following incisive eye trauma, especially by a contaminated foreign body (Elfervig & Elfervig, 1999). It is an infection of the vitreous in combination with the retinal and the uveal layers of the eye. Endophthalmitis is classified as endogenous as the result of hematogenous dissemination of infection from elsewhere in the body, or exogenous as a result of surgery infectivity (more frequent) or acute ocular injury (Campochiaro, 1999). Causes of endophthalmitis can be bacterial (more frequent) or fungal infection (Elfervig & Elfervig, 1999). *Staphylococcus epidermidis* is the most widespread exogenous infecting organism of the eye (Campochiaro, 1999). Fungal endophthalmitis can be the result of *Candida* species and *Aspergillus* species organisms (Seal, Bron, & Hay, 1998). Fungal infections are less common and more endogenous (Hamza, Loewenstein, & Haller, 1999). Endogenous infection is tainted organisms in the blood that settle in the choroid or retina, resulting in retinitis, choroiditis, or chorioretinitis that invades the vitreous chamber, causing an inflammatory reaction and acute endophthalmitis (Hamza et al., 1999).

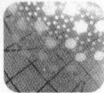

PATIENT TEACHING & DISCHARGE PRIORITIES for Orbital Cellulitis

Need	Teaching

HEALING REGIMEN

Patient/family

Follow antibiotic regimen, as prescribed:
- Daily application of fortified topical antibiotic ointment and drops
- Daily administration of systemic antibiotics
- Daily monitor for signs of improvement.

Perform daily eye patch changes, as indicated by amount of purulent discharge and healing; or the eye may need no patching as healing takes place and there is no discharge or drainage.

Eye shield as a protection and safety measure if eye is not too proptotic.

Monitor visual acuity changes frequently:
- Increased blurriness
- Diplopia
- Any improvements.

Monitor for increase in infection:
- Proptosis (eye bulging out more)
- Corneal dullness and loss of sensitivity
- Increase in swelling
- Appears cross-eyed
- Eye movement impaired
- Pupil size changes
- Increase in erythema or discoloration
- Increase in warmth to touch or pain/soreness.

Observe for any central nerve system involvement:
- Nausea or vomiting
- Febrile
- Level of consciousness decreased
- Headaches.

Maintain quiet and rest at home:
- No going out
- No strenuous activity
- No heavy lifting.

Follow-up appointments:
- Daily to weekly visits to the ophthalmologist
- Follow-up with otolaryngologist if sinus infection involvement.

Family/support system

Assess availability of, knowledge of, and compliance with treatment regimen.

Assess respite needs and resources.

Setting

Assess discharge placement needs.

Assess home environment for need for assistive devices.

Assess for need for professional home health needs.

Assess for a healing environment.

Assess need for follow-up appointments.

RISK OF INFECTION

Patient/family

Assess for clean techniques:
- Use good hand hygiene before changing any dressings or applying topical medications.
- Soiled linens are changed.
- Keep hands clean and fingernails short; do not scratch or rub swollen eyelid, as may introduce germs or break down tender tissue.
- Use protective eye shield or wear gloves when sleeping, if the healing process creates itching and the stimulus to touch eyelid.

Assess for any signs or symptoms of infection increase, and report as needed.

Signs and symptoms include:
- Proptosis (eye bulging out more), increase in swelling of eyelid
- Appears cross-eyed; eye movement impaired; pupil size changes
- Increase in redness or discoloration to eyelid
- Increase in warmth to touch or soreness to eyelid
- Increase in vision blurriness or eye pain
- Nausea or vomiting
- Febrile
- Level of consciousness, if decreased.

Teach clean techniques to minimize the risk of infection.

Describe signs and symptoms that need immediate medical attention.

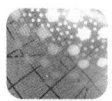

Need	Teaching
Setting	Assess environment for risk factors.
PAIN MANAGEMENT	Assess for altered comfort.
Patient/family	Assess for pain:
	• Increase in redness (hyperemia or injection)
	• Swelling
	• Increase in blurriness of vision
	• Increase in discharge
	• Proptosis does not subside.
	Reduce or relieve discomfort with healing promotion by using warm compresses to eyelid.
	Promote the use of analgesic medication as prescribed for discomfort.
	Encourage the patient that with each day of healing, increased comfort should follow.
Setting	Assess environment for safety and endorsement of therapeutic needs.
EMOTIONAL ADJUSTMENT	Anxiety and fear of going totally blind or of condition being life threatening.
Patient/family	Assist with anxiety coping.
	Answer any questions or concerns truthfully.
	Encourage expression of frustrations and fear of vision loss.
	Encourage frequent family contact and positive support.
	Encourage self-care and individual recovery to normal activity as soon as applicable and safe.
	Express that it is normal to feel some fear and discouragement after discharge.
Setting	Encourage the patient to seek information if there is a lack of understanding.
	Incorporate family and friends for support and interaction.
	Seek spiritual guidance and understanding.
SENSORY DEPRIVATION OR RECOVERY	Monitor whether visual acuity is getting worse or improving.
	Monitor whether mental acuity is declining.
Patient/family	Monitor visual acuity and whether eyelid appears to be healing.
	Monitor mental status:
	• Level of consciousness or awareness.
	Report changes in visual acuity or mental awareness.
	Seek medical attention if visual acuity or mental acuity becomes worse.
	Vision loss may make patient feel isolated and alone.
	Mental awareness or the lack thereof may require further assistance, reevaluation, and immediate follow-up and examination.
	Encourage family interaction frequently.
Setting	Assess environment for injury prevention and needs if vision or mental awareness is impaired.
RISK OF COMPLICATIONS	Potential complications:
	• Blindness, intracranial abscess, cranial nerve palsies, cavernous sinus thrombosis, or meningitis can be fatal.
Patient/family	Should be suspicious of complications if daily improvement is not observed, increased bulging of the eye, or increased globe misalignment.
	Assess for any reinfection of orbit, and report as needed any reoccurring signs and symptoms, or if eye does not appear to be improving.
	Monitor visual acuity changes: increase in blurriness, pain.
	Monitor for increase in infection and clinical deterioration:
	• Progressive proptosis (eye bulging out)
	• Globe displacement
	• Increase in swelling
	• Appears cross-eyed
	• Eye movement impaired
	• Pupil size larger
	• Increase in redness or discoloration
	• Increase in warmth to touch.
	Observe for any central nervous system involvement:
	• Nausea or vomiting
	• Febrile
	• Level of consciousness.
	If unusual signs or symptoms observed, even if not sure what they are, question any problems and notify the health care provider.

(continued)

Need	Teaching
Setting	Hospital.
	Readmission if orbital infection does not start to improve in 24–48 hours.
	Very aggressive treatment with intravenous antibodies.
	Orbital abscess surgical incision and drainage if indicated.
	Culture and sensitivity, Gram stain, computed tomography (CT) scan, x-rays, magnetic resonance imaging (MRI), or lumbar puncture.

Risk factors for the development of endophthalmitis include a possible complication following cataract surgery; which can be related to the patient's history, aseptic technique, or intraocular lens implant (Falk, Beer, & Peters, 2006; Seal et al., 1998). Patients on immunosuppressive therapy also may be at a higher risk for endophthalmitis due to poor wound healing (Seal et al., 1998). Additional risk factors for endophthalmitis include diabetes, torn posterior capsule, iris manipulation, lens fragments in the vitreous, and prolonged surgery time (Montan et al., 1998). The incidence of fungal endophthalmitis increases with immuno-compromised persons and intravenous drug abusers, especially by contaminated needles (Montan et al., 1998).

Clinical Manifestations

Clinical manifestations of endophthalmitis usually are blurred vision (the most general symptom), which can occur rapidly, eye pain, hypopyon (most familiar sign), cells and flare in the anterior chamber, corneal edema, photophobia, conjunctival injection, and chemosis (Elfervig & Elfervig, 2007; Trobe, 2006). Fungal involvement causes a vitreous clouding (poor media clarity) and light perception visual acuity (Hamza et al., 1999).

Diagnostic and Laboratory Procedures and Medical Management

Diagnostic tests may include fluorescein angiography and ultra-sonography (B-scan), which is useful for cloudy media. (See the Diagnostic Tests box, p. 2333.) Anterior chamber and vitreous tap or vitreous biopsy is recommended if a specimen is indicated (Seal et al., 1998). Vitreous and aqueous Gram stain and semiquantitative cultures are essential (Campochiaro, 1999). Certain gram-positive organisms seem to have a better visual prognosis (Campochiaro, 1999).

Aggressive treatment is crucial to avoid a severe and enduring vision loss, thus improving the chances of the visual acuity outcome (Seal et al., 1998). Evisceration often is the treatment of choice for advanced endophthalmitis with severe recurrent mucopurulent infection and no light perception vision. The outcome of surgical management of endophthalmitis has a good prognosis for vision restoration, possibly as high as 20/50 in about half the cases (Falk et al., 2006; Seal et al., 1998). Being aware of early changes in patients' vision or recognizing suspicious complaints, with immediate intervention, especially if endophthalmitis is suspected, can save sight.

Eye Trauma and Injury

Eye injury is a significant and disabling health problem. Injuries to the eye from traumatic events are a common occurrence that should be treated as emergencies requiring immediate attention. In the United States approximately 2.5 million individuals experience an eye injury requiring treatment in an emergency department, inpatient or outpatient facility, or private health care provider's office (Mulrooney, 2006). In persons under 25 years of age, ocular trauma is the number-one cause of vision loss. Fortunately, advances in microsurgical techniques over the past decade have allowed vision to be saved in some of these injured eyes. Common and frequent injuries to the eyes and eyelids are discussed next.

Epidemiology and Etiology

Eye emergencies include cuts, scratches, foreign objects in the eye, burns, chemical exposure, and blunt injuries to the eye or eyelid. Because the eye is easily damaged, any of these conditions can lead to vision loss if left untreated. A recent study estimated that from 2002 to 2003 there were 27,152 injuries in the United States related to the wearing of eyeglasses. The same study concluded that sports-related injuries due to eyeglasses wear were more common in those under the age of 18, and that fall-related injuries due to eyeglasses wear were common in those aged 65 and over (Sinclair, Smith, & Xiang, 2006). On the other hand, eyeglasses have been found to offer protection, resulting in a lower incidence of severe eye injuries to those wearing them (May et al., 2000).

A chemical injury to the eye can be caused by a work-related accident or by common household products, such as cleaning solutions, garden chemicals, solvents, or many other types of chemicals. Fumes and aerosols can also cause chemical burns. With acid burns, the haze on the cornea often clears with a good chance of recovery. However, alkaline substances—such as lime, lye, commercial drain cleaners, and sodium hydroxide found in refrigeration equipment—may cause permanent damage to the cornea. Ongoing damage may occur in spite of prompt treatment. It is important to flush the eye with clean water or saline while seeking urgent medical care. Dust, sand, and other debris can easily enter the eye. Persistent pain and redness indicate that professional treatment is needed. A foreign body may threaten vision if the object enters the eye itself or damages the cornea or lens. Foreign bodies propelled at high speed by machining, grinding, or hammering metal on metal present the highest risk.

Trauma from sports is very common. Some of the more recurrent injuries occur during the following activities: hockey, archery, darts, BB guns, bicycling, sports that involve rackets, baseball, boxing, and basketball. Trauma also may be caused by flying pieces of wood, metal, glass, stone, and other materials. Blunt injury by fist also should be considered, as should road traffic accidents with head and facial trauma. Other causes of intraocular trauma may arise from workplace tools or even common household implements.

A black eye usually is caused by direct trauma to the eye or face. Certain types of skull fractures can result in bruising around the eyes, even without direct trauma to the eye. The bruise is caused by bleeding under the skin. The tissue surrounding the eye turns black and blue, and gradually becomes purple, green, and yellow over several days. The abnormal coloring disappears within 2 weeks. Usually, swelling of the eyelid and tissue around the eye also occurs. Occasionally, serious damage to the eye itself occurs from the pressure of the swollen tissue. Bleeding inside the eye can reduce vision, cause glaucoma, or damage the cornea. Accidents, occupational injuries, sports injuries, and fights are some of the risk factors associated with black eyes.

Pathophysiology with Clinical Manifestations and Medical Management

The actual pathophysiology resulting from an eye injury is dependent on the type of injury. Clinical manifestations, laboratory and diagnostic procedures, and specific medical management also are contingent on the type of injury. The most common types of eye trauma or injury are discussed next.

Chemical Burns

Chemical burns require immediate irrigation by washing the eye continuously for 15 to 25 minutes. If suspicious or aware that the chemical is an *alkali*, the eye should be irrigated for a good 35 plus minutes or more, especially over the cornea. The most common alkaline agents are lye, lime, potash, ammonia, drain cleaners, chemical cleaners and detergents, fertilizers, and industrial solvents (Elfervig & Elfervig, 2007; Trobe, 2006). If litmus paper is available, use it as an indicator, and do not stop irrigating until litmus paper illustrates neutral, pH of 7 to 7.3. It is important to keep in mind that chemical agents can come in many forms: liquid, gas, or solid. Alkali (pH > 7) burns usually are more serious than acid (pH < 7) burns, because an alkali (hydroxyl ions) continues to burn or damage tissue after contact if it is not completely removed or neutralized. The most common offensive acid agents are battery acid and laundry bleach.

In checking for foreign bodies, never remove a penetrating foreign body, and refer the patient immediately to an ophthalmologist. Signs and symptoms might be painful loss of vision with a burning sensation, corneal swelling, excessive tearing, hyperemia, chemosis, photophobia, and blepharospasm. Emergency treatment involves copious irritation that may require flipping the upper lid (Figures 71–16, 71–17, and 71–18 ■) and pulling down the lower lid (fornix), using a lid speculum, or instilling topical ophthalmic anesthetic drops to allow the eye to be open well enough to complete a more effective irrigation. Evaluation of the eye should be done using the format stated in the Visual Assessment section earlier in this chapter. Treatment indications may include topical ophthalmic cycloplegics for comfort, topical ophthalmic antibiotic eyedrops and ointment for infection, topical ophthalmic steroid drops for inflammation, and a sterile eye patch and/or shield, pending the health care provider's orders. Refer back to Charts 71–4 and 71–5 (pp. 2330 and 2331) for ocular and vision evaluation tests and assessment.

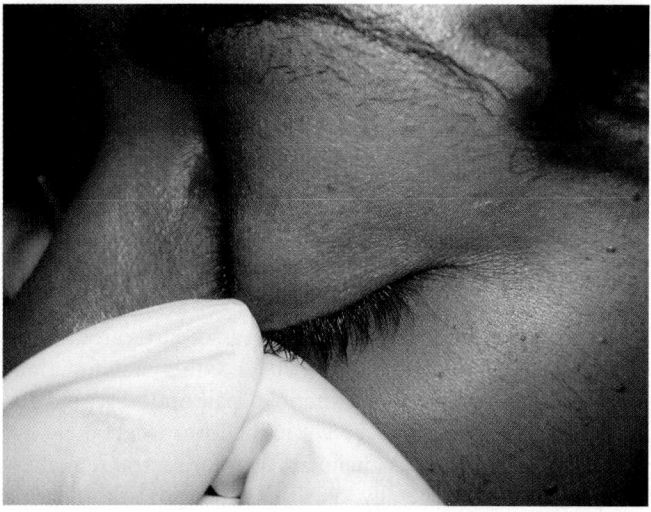

FIGURE 71–16 ■ Demonstration of flipping the upper eyelid. First step, placing finger on eyelid.
Source: Courtesy of Dr. Elferuiz

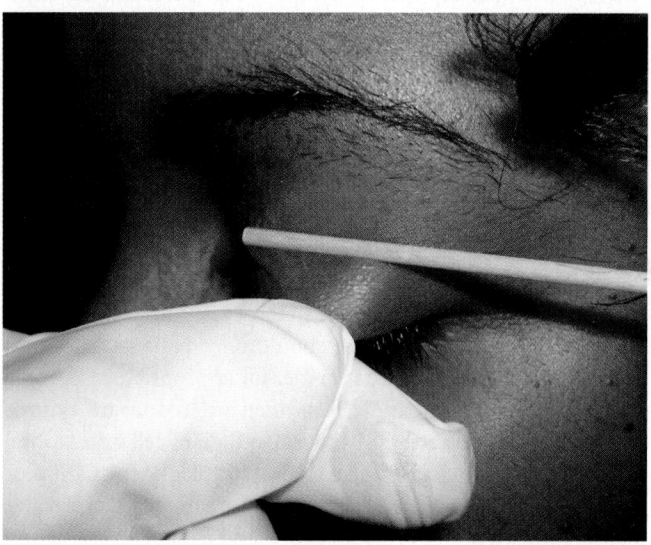

FIGURE 71–17 ■ Demonstration of flipping the upper eyelid. Placing wooden dowel to roll eyelid.
Source: Kathleen Osborn

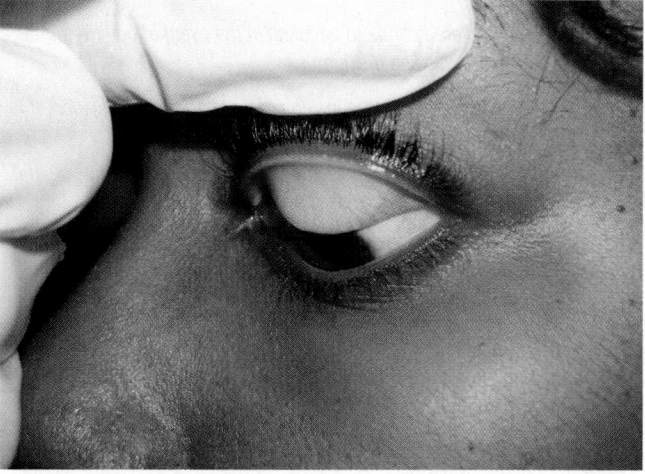

FIGURE 71–18 ■ Demonstration of flipping the upper eyelid. Lid back exposing conjuctivitis.
Source: Kathleen Osborn

 *It is important to keep in mind that chemical agents that may cause burns come in many forms; that is, liquid, gas, or solid. When a chemical burn to an eye occurs, seconds count! The affected eye should be irrigated with copious amounts of water or normal saline for no less than 20 to 35 minutes or until litmus paper pH is neutral. The eyelid may be inverted for better irrigation.*

Central Retinal Artery Occlusion

Central retinal artery occlusion (CRAO) is a vascular infarction to the central retinal artery wherein blockage by an embolus results in acute unilateral vision loss, afferent pupillary defect, and decreased carotid pulse with associated carotid bruit (Elfervig & Elfervig, 2007; Trobe, 2006). Other manifestations may include narrowed retinal arterioles, pale optic disc, and diffused pale posterior retina, except in the fovea where there is a classic "cherry-red spot," a hallmark sign for central retinal artery occlusion that generally vanishes in about 2 weeks (Sharma & Brown, 2001b) with the return of normal color. Emergency measures are taken to decrease intraocular pressure with topical antiglaucoma drops, oral carbonic anhydrase inhibitors, and an anterior chamber tap (paracentesis). Other desperate attempts to restore perfusion to the central retinal artery, but which have not been proven effective, may include trying to restore vasodilation by rebreathing CO_2 (breathing inside a paper bag), using hyperbaric chamber treatment, and performing intermittent digital massage of the globe with the eyelid closed, as soon as possible and best within less than 24 hours (Elfervig & Elfervig, 2007; Trobe, 2006). Once stability is established and the nurse or ophthalmologist is able to take a medical history, it is imperative that the nurse ask about vascular diseases that cause hardening of the arteries and listen with a stethoscope for carotid bruits. The ophthalmologist or nurse should refer patients to the internist or family health care provider for appropriate tests and a complete physical evaluation. Tests often ordered are an erythrocyte sedimentation rate (ESR) to rule out giant cell or temporal arteritis, a carotid ultrasound to check for plaque formation or carotid insufficiency, an echocardiogram for heart and valve malfunctions, a blood pressure check, and a diabetic evaluation (Sharma & Brown, 2001b). Typically, most patients seek medical attention after 24 hours; so for patients with cardiovascular anomalies, instruct them to seek emergency eye care immediately if any of the earlier ocular signs or symptoms occur.

 *Immediate actions to be taken in the event of central retinal artery occlusion include:*

Have patient breathe inside a paper bag for vasodilation, if it is within minutes of the occlusion taking place.

Do an intermittent gentle digital massage of the globe to aid perfusion, if it is within the first 24 hours of occlusion taking place.

Check intraocular pressure, by the nurse.

Assess eye for pain and vision loss.

Access standing orders to obtain an erythrocyte sedimentation rate.

Open Globe

Open globe or ruptured globe refers to an open eyeball with a laceration, penetrating injury, or intraocular foreign body. These ruptures usually are from a blunt trauma, motor vehicle crash, sporting event, fistfight, or high-velocity object creating an open, jagged-edged wound (Elfervig & Elfervig, 2007; Robson, Behrman, & Abbuhl, 2007; Trobe, 2006). Ruptured globe commonly is associated with a dislocated lens, retinal detachment, vitreous hemorrhage, and a wide area of tissue damage. Patients can present with the following ocular signs: **hyphema** (bleeding in the eye), edema, chemosis, acute diffuse subconjunctival hemorrhage, corneal laceration, irregular pupil, and lens cloudiness. Open globes often can have orbital fractures, so it is important to observe for facial hypoesthesia (insensitivity to touch) over the cheek, to palpate gently along the orbital rim for a step-off notch area, and to note whether diplopia is present (Elfervig & Elfervig, 2007; Trobe, 2006). Once the confirmation of ruptured globe is made, immediate surgical priority is instituted. The prognosis is guarded toward expected final visual outcome.

 Immediate actions to be taken in the event of an open globe injury include:

Assess open wounds, intraocular foreign body or protrusion, and support appropriately; and refer immediately to the emergency department.

Obtain visual acuity and assess for other ocular symptoms; if this is not possible, an immediate referral to the emergency department is indicated.

Observe for facial hypoesthesia (loss of sensation).

Obtain a history surrounding the circumstances.

Laboratory and Diagnostic Procedures

Visual acuity is a must and usually is the first test done following an eye injury, using standard visual acuity charts for near and distance acuity, unless other urgent matters preclude doing this test first (see Chart 71–3, p. 2330, for proper testing). It is a good idea to keep a couple of pairs of standard reading glasses (e.g., +2.00 and +3.00) on hand at the clinic or workplace, because often patients forget or lose their glasses. Using a pinhole is one way to take a distance visual acuity without corrective lenses. When standard testing charts are not available, use the best means available to obtain some measure of vision; often a newspaper or book (standard print read at 14 to 16 inches is ~ 20/40 acuity) is used for near vision, and looking out a window at a license plate may work for distance vision. Sometimes one has to be a little inventive when testing for visual acuity. When recording vision results, it is necessary to document devices and materials used for obtaining distance and near vision, especially if one is not using standard equipment (e.g., patient was able to read a license plate appropriately 10 feet away without corrective lenses with each eye separately and together). Any type of acuity should be recorded, whether it is count fingers, hand motion, light perception, or no light perception. Pupil check should be done to see whether pupils are equal, round, and reactive to light and accommodation (PERRLA); and the nurse should be alert to afferent pupillary defect. Normal eyes constrict when light is shined in one of them; if they dilate it may indicate optic nerve injury. If a patient is complaining of minor eye irritation and not a true eye emergency, and if a foreign body is found on evaluation to be an eyelash, dust, or lint that is easily removable with a tissue or irrigation, this can be done by the nurse. It is essential to document the type of foreign body and how it was removed.

◼ Nursing Management

Time is crucial in true eye emergencies, where minutes count. When first assessing eye injuries, it is imperative to provide timely and appropriate triage, treatment, and referral, as this can affect the final visual outcome. When a patient presents with a chemical burn to the eye, copious irrigation of the eyeball, fornix, and facial area with water for the first 15 to 25 minutes is crucial in possibly saving the cornea, and therefore vision, before doing anything else. After the rinsing, an initial evaluation can be made. If the evaluation indicates that it is not a true emergency situation or that an immediate referral is not necessary, and the patient's condition is stable, it is appropriate to take a detailed history to identify the offending chemical and determine whether a neutralizing agent is available. The nurse should record the necessary information, take the visual acuity of both eyes, check pupil responses, and assess how much ocular involvement seems to have taken place. See Charts 71–2, and 71–5 (pp. 2328 and 2331) for assessment protocols. After initial assessment of an eye emergency and initial treatment is instituted, and if no intraocular foreign body is present, the nurse should place a protective shield over the eye, if indicated.

When an intraocular foreign body is present, it is critical to leave the object in place and stabilize it, especially if it is protruding from the eye. The object should not be removed, and the nurse should be very careful not to put pressure on the intraocular foreign body. This provides safety in transportation. It usually is best to keep patients in a sitting position, because lying down or reclining may advance the intraocular foreign body deeper into the eye with the natural force of gravity. The nurse should instruct patients not to eat or drink anything from that time forward, because emergency surgery may be done promptly. Time and contents of the last meal consumed should be documented for the record. Patients' activity should be restricted and patients should be kept comfortable and quiet at all times. The ophthalmologist will perform further evaluation with a complete ocular examination. Be aware that any type of ocular emergency, trauma, injury, intraocular foreign body, or laceration may need tetanus prophylaxis, as indicated. If ordering magnetic resonance imaging (MRI) of patients, there are two things to keep in mind. It should not be done if a metal intraocular foreign body is suspected, because the MRI could move or dislodge the intraocular foreign body, thereby causing more ocular damage. Second, if previous retinal repair surgery was done, it is necessary to check with the patients' ophthalmologist to determine whether an encircling band or scleral buckle was used in the retinal surgical repair; in the past (over 5 years ago), metal clips or staples were used to secure the encircling band or scleral buckle on the retina, and the MRI magnification could remove or dislodge these clips. These metal clips have not been used in retinal repair more recently.

CRITICAL ALERT *Precautions related to magnetic resonance imaging (MRI) of the eye include:*

In the past, an encircling band or scleral buckle in retinal repair surgery was secured with metal clips or clasps.

Patients with a history of retinal repair surgery should check their past medical history or with their surgical ophthalmologist to find out whether they had an encircling band or scleral buckle used in their retinal repair surgery and whether it was secured with metal clips or clasps.

Magnets pull on metal and can pull metal out of position.

MRI magnification can pull out metal intraocular foreign bodies, and surgical metal clips or clasps, thus causing damage to eye tissue.

Eye Urgencies

Some eye injuries are described as urgencies, meaning that treatment is imperative. These conditions include penetrating and perforating trauma, blunt trauma, neovascular glaucoma, **flashes** and floaters, retinal vascular occlusions, and sudden vision loss, when response time could be several minutes, several hours, or even several days. Sudden vision loss can be divided into acute macular hole, retinal occlusions, anterior ischemic optic neuropathy, temporal arteritis, amaurosis fugax, and ocular migraines. A comprehensive discussion of each of these eye urgencies follows.

Penetrating or Perforating Trauma

Penetrating trauma refers to an injury that penetrates or enters the eye, but does not exit the eye. Perforating trauma refers to an injury that goes through the eye completely and exits the eye. Common weapons of injury are knives, scissors, guns, branches/sticks, wood, arrows, darts, and nails. Depending on the seriousness of the trauma, ocular manifestations will vary. Some of the signs and symptoms are epiphora, hyperemia, subconjunctival hemorrhage, hyphema, proptosis, ecchymosis, edema, iris defects, laceration, abnormal intraocular pressure, blurry vision, diplopia, eye pain, and foreign body sensation or actually seeing the intraocular foreign body in the eye. Once the type of wound is confirmed, appropriate management is instituted, and if a penetrating intraocular foreign body is present, surgery probably will be recommended. Treatment also will include topical ophthalmic antibiotics, systemic antibiotics and anti-inflammatory medications, plus a topical ophthalmic mydriatic for comfort (AAO-8, 2008–2009). See the Pharmacology Summary feature (p. 2346).

Blunt Trauma

Blunt trauma refers to an eye injury from a blunt object, such as fists, projectile objects (tennis balls, paintballs), or a motor vehicle crash, which can present with hyphema, chemosis, ecchymosis, edema, subconjunctival hemorrhage, epiphora, decreased vision, photophobia, and any degree of discomfort. Nursing management includes using the same measures as if patients have a ruptured globe. Re-bleeding after an initial hyphema occurs in about 10% of the cases, usually within about 7 to 10 days. Treatment varies with the level of seriousness (AAO-7, 2008–2009). There are many other eye injuries that commonly are seen, such as corneal abrasions, contact lens overwear, and corneal foreign body. These injuries are outlined in Chart 71–11 (p. 2364).

Neovascular Glaucoma

Neovascular glaucoma (NVG) is intraocular pressure elevation due to a new blood vessel growth network within the iris and the trabecular meshwork causing angle closure (Fanous, 2004). Neovascular glaucoma can be an end stage to severe diabetic retinopathy, when blood glucose is uncontrolled, resulting in retinal hypoxia and capillary nonperfusion (AAO-10, 2008–2009). Treatment for neovascular glaucoma has a low success rate, so prevention is the best means of therapy. Laser photocoagulation is one surgical recommendation.

Ocular Flashes and Floaters

Flashes (photopsias) and floaters are symptoms that can occur from many intraocular conditions, but more commonly from posterior vitreous detachment (PVD), vitreous hemorrhage,

CHART 71–11	**Common Ocular Eye Injuries**

Injury	Description	Signs/Symptoms	Assessment
Corneal abrasion	Scratched area of the cornea causing corneal defect.	Foreign body sensation, eye pain, epiphora, photophobia, blurry vision.	Take a good history, evaluate with topical ophthalmic anesthetic drop and fluorescein stains (strips), and examine with a blue (cobalt) light; the abrasion appears yellowish-green in color. Draw a picture of the corneal defect, and invert the upper eyelid to evaluate further for debris or foreign body, if indicated. Seek medical treatment if further evaluation and ophthalmic medications are indicated (Visto, 2000).
Contact lens overwear (superficial punctuate keratitis [SPK] or giant papillary conjunctivitis [GPC])	Result of contact lens abuse, because of sleeping in them too long, poor hygiene of maintaining contact lenses, or wearing damaged or infected lenses.	Above, plus: injection, pruritus, halos, mucous discharge.	Contact lenses need to be removed or—if contaminated with an infection or deposits, or if damaged—thrown away. Stay out of contact lenses for 1 to 2 weeks, or until all eye irritation is cleared. Take a good history; evaluate the eye with topical anesthetic drop and fluorescein stain, and use blue light check for corneal abrasions. Record contact lens type, age, length of time worn, type of cleaning and storage solutions, and last time cleaned. All contact lens wearers should have a pair of backup glasses for such occasions. Depending on the severity and stage of overwear, the patient may need to seek medical treatment (Dabezies et al., 1998).
Corneal foreign body	Small, superficial corneal lesions that give the sensation of having sand or grit in the eye.	Above, plus corneal edema.	Mineral matter can be less irritating, as metal, vegetation, and insects usually cause an inflammatory response, which can result in swelling and infection. Take a good history, and note whether the patient was wearing safety glasses or goggles. Evaluate the eye with topical anesthetic ophthalmic drop and staining; and upper eyelid inverted to check for foreign bodies (if indicated). Management may require irrigation only to remove a minor irritant. If a corneal defect is present, seek medical treatment (Parrish & Chandler, 1998).

Sources: Dabezies, O., Klyce, S., Morgan, J., Hartstein, J., Donshik, P., Boswall, G., et al. (1998). Corneal changes from contact lenses. In H. Kaufman, B. Barron, & M. McDonald (Eds.), *The cornea* (2nd ed.). Boston: Butterworth-Heinemann; Parrish, C. M., & Chandler, J. W. (1998). Corneal trauma. In H. Kaufman, B. Barron, & M. McDonald (Eds.), *The cornea* (2nd ed.). Boston: Butterworth-Heinemann; and Visto, D. A. (2000). Corneal abrasion: To patch or not to patch. *Insight, 25*(1), 4–6.

and retinal breaks or detachments (AAO-12, 2008–2009). (See the Retinal Detachment section later in this chapter.) Photopsias (flashes) are when a person notices a light flashing in the eye, something like a lightbulb when it blows out. Floaters are described as gnats or grayish filament floating in one's line of sight. Photopsias and floaters can be the first warning signs for more serious eye problems and need to be distinguished by a comprehensive dilated eye examination with slit-lamp biomicroscopy and indirect ophthalmoscopy. An ultrasonogram (B-scan) is performed when the fundus cannot be viewed adequately with an indirect ophthalmoscope due to some opacity. Treatment measures are indicated by cause, from observation to surgery.

Retinal Vascular Occlusions

Retinal vascular occlusions include central retinal artery occlusion (CRAO) (see the discussion in the Eye Trauma and Injury section earlier in this chapter). Central retinal vein occlusion (CRVO) is a compression of the central retinal vein that causes a tumultuous blood flow giving rise to thrombosis (AAO-4, 2008–2009). Branch artery occlusion (BAO) refers to an occlusion of the branch artery off the central retinal artery (Sharma & Brown, 2001b). Branch vein occlusion (BVO) is an occlusion of the branch vein off the central retinal vein, commonly the superior temporal vein (Fekrat & Finkelstein, 2001). Occlusion is a stroke to the eye that can cause a sudden loss of vision by ocular vascular infarction to the arterial or venous circulation of the optic nerve, either centrally or peripherally (branch vessels). The blood flow is blocked by an acute vascular plaque or embolus, which creates an ischemic retinal defect. The signs may include a pale or swollen optic disc, nerve fiber layer (NFL) infarctions, retinal apoplexy, cotton-wool spots, or soft exudates, which can cause vision loss and visual field defects (Schachat, 2001). Other signs for a central retinal vein occlusion can be peripapillary flame-shaped hemorrhages or intraretinal hemorrhages; a branch vein occlusion can be flame-shaped or intraretinal hemorrhages and distended vessels off the disc near the superior or inferior arcades. Arterial occlusions will cause white retina, areas of nonperfusion, and arterial attenuation (Schachat, 2001). The longer the occlusion is present, the greater the vision loss. Arteriole occlusions seem to cause more of a permanent or greater vision deficiency. With venous occlusions some vision seems to return with early treatment. One of the most severe complications of central retinal vein occlusion is developing neovascular glaucoma (Clarkson, 2001).

A complete medical evaluation should be done by a health care provider to evaluate for vascular insufficiency, hyperlipidemia, hypertension, or diabetes. It is important to educate known patients with cardiovascular anomalies or arteriosclerosis about seeking eye care immediately if any of the earlier ocular signs or symptoms are manifested. Many patients that have had retinal occlusions state that they experienced a sharp pain or severe headache to the temporal area of the face on the side of the involved eye just minutes to hours before the stroke to the eye and loss of vision occurred. Nursing management includes obtaining a good history and making proper referrals. The oph-

thalmologist or ophthalmic nurse specialist will do an ocular examination and order a fluorescein angiogram and visual field test. (See the Diagnostic Tests box, p. 2333.) The treatment may include systemic anticoagulants, such as an aspirin or pentoxifylline, antiglaucoma ophthalmic drops, laser photocoagulation, or radial optic nerve neurotomy.

Sudden Vision Loss

Sudden loss of visual acuity is a very frightening experience that usually is unexplainable at first to patients. This leaves patients wondering what happened. Some of the ocular problems that can cause a sudden loss of vision are acute macular hole, retinal occlusions, anterior ischemic optic neuropathy, temporal arteritis, amaurosis fugax, and ocular migraines. These ocular conditions are outlined in Chart 71–12 with descriptions and management.

Eyelid Laceration

Eyelid laceration refers to any cut or open wound to the eyelid that has many possible causes such as from an open globe, penetrating trauma, blunt trauma, falls, or motor vehicle crash

---

CHART 71–12 Sudden Vision Loss Eye Problems

Problem	Description/Management
Acute macular hole	A hole in the central area of the retina, where one's 20/20 vision is located, called the fovea. Signs and symptoms include unilateral, painless, and substantial loss in central vision that appears as a round orangish-red spot in the macula. There is a grayish area surrounding the hole, which usually indicates edema and drusen (yellow deposits) may be present. Medical management for a true macular hole probably will mean a vitrectomy with air–fluid–gas exchange and intraocular steroids.
Anterior ischemic optic neuropathy (nonarteritic ischemic optic neuropathy)	An ischemic attack to the optic nerve (ON). Signs and symptoms include unilateral, painless decrease in vision; afferent pupillary defect; disc edema; and normal erythrocyte sedimentation rate (ESR) (which distinguishes this from arteritic ischemic optic neuropathy). No effective management is known at this time. The degree of vision loss depends on the extent of ischemia.
Temporal arteritis (giant cell arteritis or arteritic ischemic optic neuropathy)	A unilateral loss of vision. Signs and symptoms may include altitudinal visual field loss and decreased color vision, afferent pupillary defect, optic nerve swelling, forehead and scalp tenderness, arthritis-type discomfort, painful chewing, loss of weight, and elevated erythrocyte sedimentation rate. This usually occurs in patients around the age of 65. The patient needs a comprehensive medical work-up, a temporal artery biopsy for diagnosis confirmation, erythrocyte sedimentation rate, plus a complete ocular examination with visual field. Medical management with systemic steroid is of an urgent nature to prevent vasculitis and contralateral eye disease, to prevent the possibility of rendering the patient legally blind.
Amaurosis fugax	A transient, sudden, and painless decrease in vision unilaterally is caused by Hollenhorst plaques, which obstruct arterial blood flow to the ophthalmic artery. The temporary or fleeting loss of vision can last from about 30 minutes to hours, and usually gives the patient a panic attack of possibly going blind. On complete ocular examination, the plaques might be visualized in the retinal vasculature coupled with retinal edema, and very rarely for ophthalmic artery stenosis. The eye exam also will include fluorescein angiography and fundus photography. A complete medical and neurological evaluation is indicated to rule out transient ischemic attack (TIA) and carotid stenosis. Medical management may include systemic anticoagulants and hypolipidemic agents, or endarterectomy.
Ocular migraine (occipital lobe ischemia)	A mirage-like image, shimmering edge, heat waves, or smoke-like screen that appears in one's vision, something like an aura. Usually no headache is involved; however, the patient may experience mild discomfort and sudden peripheral vision loss or transient visual obscuration. This visual impairment occurs mainly in the temporal quadrant. The peripheral vision disappears for about 10 to 20 minutes, and vision returns to normal after the episode. No treatment is required if this is a true ocular migraine. Aspirin or acetaminophen may help to prevent the reoccurrence if one is going through a period of ocular migraine episodes and can possibly remove the cause, such as particularly stressful circumstances.

Sources: Arnold, A. C. (2004). Ischemic optic neuropathy, diabetic papillopathy, and papillophlebitis. In M. Yanoff & J. S. Duker (Eds.), *Ophthalmology* (2nd ed.). St. Louis: Mosby; Jabs, D. A. (2001). Rheumatic diseases. In S. J. Ryan (Ed.), *Retina* (3rd ed., Vol. 2). St. Louis: Mosby; Lee, A. G., & Brazis, P. W. (2003). *Clinical pathways in neuro-ophthalmology: An evidence-based approach* (2nd ed.). New York: Thieme; Sharma, S., & Brown, G. C. (2001a). Ocular ischemic syndrome. In S. J. Ryan (Ed.), *Retina* (3rd ed., Vol. 2). St. Louis: Mosby; and Sjaarda, R. N., & Thompson, J. T. (2001). Macular hole. In S. J. Ryan (Ed.), *Retina* (3rd ed., Vol. 3). St. Louis: Mosby.

(AAO-7, 2008–2009). Lid laceration injuries are divided into six levels of severity, which are shown in Chart 71–13 (Elfervig & Elfervig, 2007). Patients should be made aware of the signs and symptoms of a possible infection, such as hyperemia, inflammation, edema, discharge, or pain. The use of ice packs to control hemorrhaging and reduce swelling will offer some comfort. Medical treatment can be as minor as an adhesive butterfly strip, topical antibiotic/anti-inflammatory drops or ointments, and a sterile patch. A patch is contraindicated if an intraocular foreign body is present. Surgical treatment may be the best option when greater tissue is involved with the injury, which may include surgical repair or reconstruction, as indicated according to the level of severity (AAO-7, 2008–2009).

Nurses should educate patients on good hand hygiene before applying eyedrops or ointment to prevent the risk of infection. The nurse should assist in pain management for *Readiness for Enhanced Comfort* and psychological support for *Ineffective Coping* for patients with severe vision losses, those who commonly express *Anxiety* and *Fear*. Patient education is a must to prevent the risk of noncompliance. Education about the prescribed treatment regimen and regular follow-up care should be reinforced by the nurse to promote healing for the best possible visual outcome and patient's hopefulness.

◼ Retinal Detachment

Retinal detachment is the separation of the sensory retinal layers from the retinal pigment epithelium, where subretinal fluid collects in the potential space (AAO-12, 2008–2009). This condition usually requires immediate surgical repair, especially if the macula is still on or intact. If the macula is off or detached and there is choroidal edema, there is time to place patients on steroids for a few of days before surgery. This allows time to decrease the edema and give the retinal tissue time to heal, thus, providing more surgical manipulability and possibly a better surgical outcome.

Clinical manifestations of a retinal detachment vary and are outlined in Chart 71–14. There literally may be no clinical manifestations, or patients may have blurry vision, a shower of floaters, light flashes, and a curtain or veil in the line of vision. It is most likely that patients will not experience pain, but they may experience a panic attack (Steidl & Hartnett, 2003). Primary high-risk factors may include trauma, high myopia, lattice degeneration, retinoschisis, retinopathy, tumors, and post-cataract surgery. Secondary risk factors may include vitreous hemorrhage, diabetic retinopathy, severe uveitis, severe hypertension, Marfan's syndrome, and toxemia from pregnancy. Retinal detachment that involves the macula may be recognizable through a direct ophthalmoscope without dilation and can have a whitish retinal reflex (Figure 71–19 ◼). If the macula is still intact and the retinal detachment is in the periphery, then a dilated eye examination is necessary to view the retinal detachment. An ultrasonogram (B-scan) is indicated for any detachment to view the extent of the detachment, tissue involvement, and location. (See the Diagnostic Tests box, p. 2333.)

CHART 71–13	Lid Laceration Categories
Category	**Involvement**
Superficial	Usually can be treated by a nonophthalmologist with Steri-Strips, butterflies, or Band-Aids.
Full thickness	Lid margin and lid function, and ocular abnormality; be cautious.
Medial one-third of upper and lower lids	May involve the canalicular (tear) system; be cautious.
Deep laceration of upper lid	Ptosis; indicates levator muscle may be involved; be very cautious.
Fat prolapse	Globe penetration, foreign body, and impaired lid function; be cautious.
Loss of tissue	Grafting of the skin or reconstructive surgery may be necessary.

Sources: Elfervig, L. S., & Elfervig J. L. (2007). Recognition and triage of ocular emergencies. *Refinements: Clinical Education Modules for Today's Ophthalmic Team, 2*(1), 1–14. Manuscript updated and submitted for republication; and Green, J. P., Charonis, G. C., & Goldberg, R. A. (2004). Eyelid trauma and reconstruction techniques. In M. Yanoff & J. S. Duker (Eds.), *Ophthalmology* (2nd ed.). St. Louis: Mosby.

CHART 71–14	Clinical Manifestations of a Retinal Detachment
Sign	**Description**
Absence (none)	The patient does not realize anything is wrong when the retinal detachment is so far in the periphery near the ora.
Blurry vision	The patient will notice her central vision is blurry or cloudy; this is because the retinal detachment involves the central macula and edema.
Shower of floaters	The patient will notice black/gray spots or clear ameba-type spots in his vision, which are more noticeable against a light background or blue skies; these are clumps of vitreous proteins or clumps of red blood cells from a hemorrhage.
Flashes of light	The patient will notice flashing lights (like a lightbulb breaking) in her peripheral vision; more common when getting up from a lying position or entering a dark environment. This is usually caused by the vitreous pulling on the retinal sensory layer.
Curtain or veil	The patient will notice a curtain- or a veil-like shape come across his central vision; this is usually the detached retinal flap or retinal layers' separation moving around in the vitreous crossing in the central line of sight. The superior temporal quadrant is the most common location for a retinal detachment, so the patient will notice an inferior nasal flap or vision loss.
No pain	The patient does not experience any pain with a spontaneous retinal detachment, but may panic when noticing vision changes or loss.
Loss of tissue	Grafting of the skin or reconstructive surgery may be necessary.

Source: Adapted from Steidl, S. M., & Hartnett, M. E. (2003). *Clinical pathways in vitreoretinal disease.* New York: Thieme.

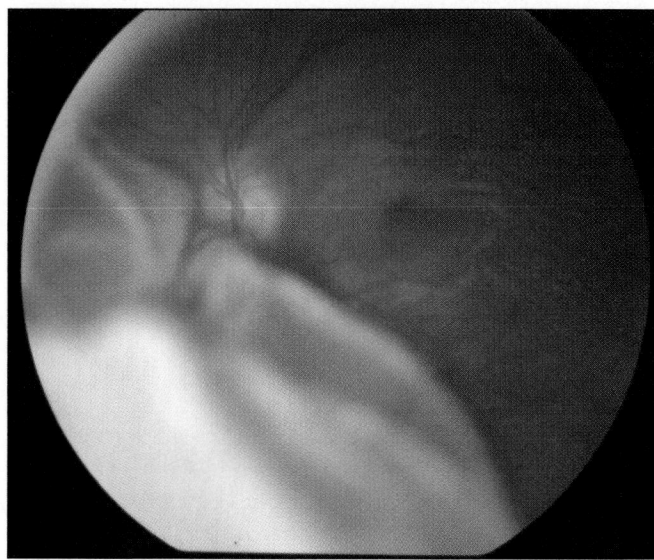

FIGURE 71–19 ■ Retinal detachment with macula off.
Source: Kathleen Osborn

Posterior Vitreous Detachment

Posterior vitreous detachment (PVD) occurs when the vitreous separates from the retinal surface and liquefies (syneresis), usually due to aging and increased axial length of the eye. This occurrence typically starts unilaterally and the fellow eye usually starts later (Hikichi & Yoshida, 2004). Symptoms of only occasional flashes and floaters usually are the most common signs and can be annoying. If the diagnosis proves to be the latter, bilateral PVD, and there are no tears, holes, or detachments located, time would allow the ophthalmologist an opportunity to observe the condition and have patients return to the office in 2 to 3 weeks for a reevaluation. If symptoms increase or become more obvious, patients should be instructed to return to the ophthalmologist's office sooner. Posterior vitreous detachment can also be a procurer of retinal detachments. The vitreous is firmly attached at the vitreous base (near ora serrata), the disc margins, the macula, and large vessel margins; retinal breaks can occur more easily in these areas with a spontaneous or traumatic posterior vitreous detachment (AAO-12, 2008–2009).

Retinal Breaks

Retinal breaks are retinal tears or holes. They can give the same warning signs as a retinal detachment. These patients need to be seen by an ophthalmologist to be evaluated by a dilated fundus examination. If a retinal detachment is highly probable, the patient should be instructed to stay quiet and refrain from straining, lifting heavy objects, or participating in activities. If it is only a small retinal break, it can usually be treated with cryopexy or laser photocoagulation.

Vitreous Hemorrhage

Vitreous hemorrhage is the presence of blood or red blood cells in the vitreous humor or cavity that commonly is caused by diabetic retinopathy, retinal detachment, or trauma. Vision is usually blurry to very poor depending on the degree of blood present, resulting in painless, unilateral vision loss. Vitreous hemorrhages often are observed over time to see whether the blood will reabsorb spontaneously. If it does not reabsorb, surgery may be indicated.

Nonrhegmatogenous and Rhegmatogenous Detachment

The two major types of retinal detachment are nonrhegmatogenous and rhegmatogenous. Nonrhegmatogenous may include serous and traction retinal detachment. Serous detachment occurs from serous leakage (clear fluid) that separates retinal intraocular layers between the retina and retinal pigment epithelium, or separates choroidal intraocular layers between the choroid and sclera, which pulls the retina off as a result of inflammation (Elfervig & Elfervig, 1998). Traction detachment occurs from scar tissue, fibrovascular formation of the vitreous that detaches the retina. This type of detachment is more common in long-standing diabetes with inflammation and with patients that have had previous ocular trauma (Elfervig & Elfervig, 1998). Rhegmatogenous detachment occurs from a break or a tear in the retina. The break or tear can occur when the vitreous degenerates and tugs the retina off by separating its sensory layers (Elfervig & Elfervig, 1998).

Retinal Detachment Surgical Implications

Retinal detachment surgical repairs usually are outpatient procedures that do not require hospitalization. The surgical procedures can be as simple as a cold (cryopexy) or hot laser (photocoagulation), or can be more invasive with pneumatic retinopexy or vitrectomy.

Cryopexy

Cryopexy (cryo) or cryotherapy means basically to fix by freezing, with the use of nitrous oxide (N_2O). Cryopexy is a type of cold laser that seals a retinal hole or retinal tear in the peripheral retina, usually present in an anterior position, meaning between the equator and the ora of the peripheral retina (Williams & Aaberg, 2001). Laser photocoagulation means to seal with light energy that converts to thermal heat. When a retinal hole or retinal tear is too posterior, meaning behind the equator, fundus photocoagulation laser usually is the treatment of choice (Williams & Aaberg, 2001). The photocoagulation laser uses argon or dye to seal the retinal hole or retinal tear. Cryopexy and thermal laser scars are both permanent, leaving a micropigmented or white scarred area in the retina tissue.

Vitrectomy

Vitrectomy is the surgical removal of the vitreous by a pars plana incision and air, gas, or fluid exchange (Charles, 2001). The air, gas, or fluid exchange is to realign and reattach the retina, to keep the retina in its proper anatomic position. A scleral buckle or encircling band sometimes is used during vitrectomy to enforce and stabilize the weak area of the retina, to lessen the chance of a re-detachment (Charles, 2001). A scleral buckle and encircling band are usually permanent and can make the eyeball more myopic, thus changing the refractive error of vision and possibly requiring a change in glasses or the addition of glasses. Once patients have a retinal detachment, they are considered to be at high risk for future retinal detachments, because they are now known to be more prone to them.

■ Eye Tumors or Neoplasms

Tumors of the eye can be life threatening, but many are not and are said to be benign. Medical and surgical treatment should include a good eye examination and observation; and suspicious-looking

CHART 71–15	Signs of Ocular Tumors
Sign	**Ocular Change**
Vision change	The vision becomes less clear or distorted.
Strabismus	An eye being crossed; may complain of diplopia.
Changed moles, freckles, or wart-like lesions	A pigmented area in and around the eye that appears to grow larger and darker.
Periorbital ecchymosis	A dark circle discoloration of the eyelids, around the eyes; the child appears somewhat like a raccoon.
Proptosis	An eye appears to "bug out"; or globe displacement.
Ptosis	An eyelid that droops; look for misalignments.
Subcutaneous mass	A notable growth or elevation noted on the face, adnexa, or eyeball; or palpable nodule.

Sources: American Academy of Ophthalmology (AAO-6). (2008–2009). *Basic and clinical science course: Pediatric ophthalmology and strabismus* (Section 6). San Francisco: Author; Shields, J. A., & Shields, C. L. (1999a). *Atlas of eyelid and conjunctival tumors.* Philadelphia: Lippincott Williams & Wilkins; Shields, J. A., & Shields, C. L. (1999b). *Atlas of intraocular tumors.* Philadelphia: Lippincott Williams & Wilkins; and Shields, J. A., & Shields, C. L. (1999c). *Atlas of orbital tumors.* Philadelphia: Lippincott Williams & Wilkins.

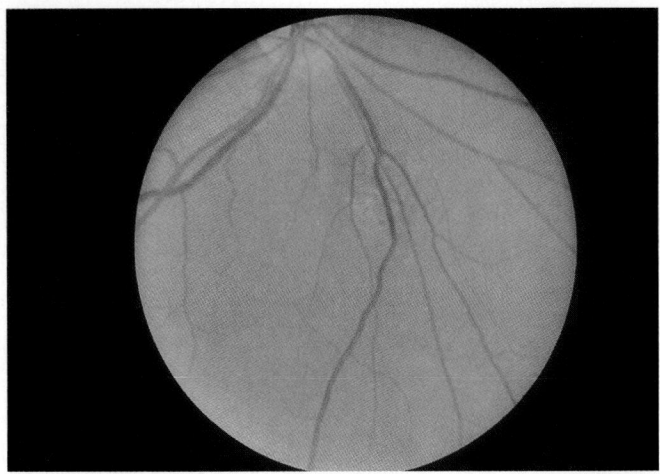

FIGURE 71–20 ■ Choroidal nevus.
Source: Kathleen Osborn

tumors should be biopsied by an ophthalmologist or neuro-ophthalmologist. The eyes and surrounding tissue are subject to both benign and cancerous lesions, but due to the limitations of this chapter they will not be discussed in their entirety. This section covers some of the more common eye neoplasms, which will be divided into benign eye lesions, precancerous eye lesions, and malignant eye lesions. Some signs of an ocular tumor may seem like ordinary ocular changes, but if certain signs are manifested without a reasonable explanation, a neoplasm may be awakening. Chart 71–15 outlines possible signs of ocular tumors.

Benign Eye Tumors

Benign eye lesions are tumors in or around the eyeball that are not cancerous or are nonmalignant and not life threatening. These lesions are sometimes called a nevus, hyperplasia, pigmented hypertrophy, or freckle. Most of the time benign eye tumors just need watching or close observation, but they can be excised if they impair vision or cause significant cosmetic alterations.

Nevus

Nevus, sometimes called a freckle, is a brownish pigmented area of eye tissue that usually is flat or slightly elevated, varies in size and shape, varies in pigment intensity, and can be amelanotic, meaning without pigment or whitish. Nevi often are located near the corneoscleral limbus on the iris, conjunctiva, and eyelid, and on the choroidal retina (Figure 71–20 ■). Nevi rarely have malignant potential (Shields & Shields, 1999a). They usually are just observed unless they change in color or continue to grow, and then further evaluation is warranted with possible treatment.

Hypertrophy of Retinal Pigment Epithelium

Hyperplasia or pigmented hypertrophy of retinal pigment epithelium is a black pigment area or dot in the retina or on the eyelid where pigmented cells have accumulated. This condition

usually is benign and needs only periodic observation, every 1 or 2 years. No treatment is necessary, unless the dot enlarges or changes color, which usually is uncommon.

Lymphoid Hyperplasia

Lymphoid hyperplasia is the proliferation of lymphoid infiltrates with benign lymphocytes and plasma cells that can invade the iris, ciliary body, and choroid, and also can involve conjunctiva and orbit. It is unilateral and occurs largely in adults, and it is manifested in the choroid as circumscribed or diffused yellow thickening, usually accompanied with a secondary retinal detachment (Shields & Shields, 1999a). Treatment is surgical excision, irradiation, and chemotherapy; it is difficult to distinguish benign lymphoid tumors from malignant lymphoid lesions, even on the basis of histological appearance (Green, 2002). Laboratory analysis was done using microscopy, immunophenotyping, and gene rearrangement using the Southern blot technique, necessary for differentiation. DNA-rearrangement analysis allows a very precise determination of the benign and malignant lymphoid infiltrates of the ocular region. These tumors can also generally be distinguished by their signal intensity on T2-weighted images (Abe et. al., 2005).

Papilloma

Papilloma is a frequent benign epithelial growth or lesion (looks like a wart) that usually grows on or near the upper or lower eyelid margins of older adults (Green, 2002). Treatment is observation or cosmetic excision. It generally is the same color as the adjacent skin, and it is formed from small projections of fibrovascular connective tissue lined by hyperkeratotic epidermis (Shields & Shields, 1999a). Papillomatous configurations can be pedunculated (granular and whitish or pigmented), sessile (smooth surface and pinkish), and consist of solitary or multiple benign lesions (Shields & Shields, 1999a).

Seborrheic Keratosis

Seborrheic keratosis is a common benign basal cell papilloma or seborrheic wart cutaneous lesion that is usually a focal, periocular, light-brownish pigmented, discrete, slightly elevated, and placoid lesion (Shields & Shields, 1999a). In African Americans, it is characterized as dermatosis papulosa nigra. Other characteristics are acanthotic (basal cell proliferation) or adenoid (keratin cysts) types (Shields & Shields, 1999a). Treatment is observation or cosmetic excision. Inverted follicular keratosis seen in middle-aged males is a discrete, benign cutaneous nodule that is usually on an eyelid margin as papillomatous (wart like) or pigmented; usually surgical excision is warranted (Shields & Shields, 1999a). *Basosquamous cell acanthoma* may be a more accurate term, because it is not related to hair follicles (Shields & Shields, 1999a).

Xanthelasma

Xanthelasma is a bilateral benign deposit of yellowish-white, slighted elevated lipid plaques in the subcutaneous dermis of the upper and lower eyelids (Green, 2002). Normolipemia or an indication of secondary hyperlipidemia (e.g., such as in patients with diabetes) may be diagnostic of Erdheim-Chester disease (Shields & Shields, 1999a). Xanthelasma is referred to as xanthoma or tuberous xanthoma when the deposits become quite enlarged, which are more indicative of hypercholesterolemia (Shields & Shields, 1999a). These growths are removed only if unattractive and bothersome to patients. Blood cholesterol levels should be checked, because hyperlipidemia may be symptomatic of increasing lipid deposits.

Telangiectasis

Telangiectasis is a small focal red lesion associated with dilated conjunctival capillaries. Small dilated vessels are differentiated from systemic vascular hematoma in Louis-Bar syndrome or Rendu-Osler-Weber syndrome. Parafoveal telangiectasis shows central endothelial degeneration with lipid accumulation within the vessel walls, and advanced degeneration of the pericytes (AAO-4, 2008–2009). Pericytes are the protective basement membrane (mural cells) around ocular and kidney vessels that gives strength and vascular endurance to keep cells from degenerating (AAO-2, 2008–2009). This is why patients with diabetes have increasing vessel leakage (endothelial damage), because the pericyte membrane is absent, which protects the capillary lumen (AAO-12, 2008–2009).

Precancerous Eye Tumors

Precancerous eye lesions are premalignant tumors. The lesions not only can be stable benign tumors but also can continue to grow and develop into cancer or malignant tissue.

Actinic Keratosis

Actinic keratosis (senile or solar keratosis) is a familiar precancerous cutaneous lesion, is caused by repeated exposure to sunlight, and can develop into cutaneous squamous cell carcinoma (Shields & Shields, 1999a). Characteristics may include multiple erythematous, excoriated (scab-like), sessile plaques, or papillary dermis buds (Shields & Shields, 1999a). This commonly is seen in older Caucasians with prolonged sun exposure; for example farmers, fishermen, and carpenters. Treatment is observation, but excision is recommended if it is at all suspicious. Other treatment options are chemotherapy or cryotherapy, especially if keratosis has multiple characteristics.

Melanocytic Nevus

Melanocytic nevus, which can be congenital or acquired, is a benign cutaneous nevus of the eyelid or peripunctal conjunctiva. It can be pigmented or amelanotic, usually does not cause a loss of eyelashes if on the eyelid, and can be a precancerous state to malignant melanoma (Shields & Shields, 1999a). Treatment is

observation, but if it is suspicious, excision is suggested. This can be problematic if much of the eyelid is involved; and a possible radical removal with cosmetic surgery may be indicated, especially if metastasis is suspected (Shields & Shields, 1999a).

Malignant Eye Tumors

Malignant eye lesions are cancerous tumors. They are in or around the eyeball, are local and definite, or can be diffused and life threatening through metastasis.

Basal Cell Carcinoma

Basal cell carcinoma is most commonly eyelid cancer, usually in light-skinned adults in their fifth decade of life or older, most often located in the nasal canthus of the upper cheek (Vaughn, Dortzbach, & Gayre, 2004). Diagnosis is confirmed with a biopsy and surgical excision or radiation. The two most principal types are the noduloulcerative (firm, round nodule with fine dilated capillaries and ulcerated center) and the diffuse morpheaform (hard, pale, flat with undefined margins); but presentations can vary from cystic, pigmented, and other forms (Vaughn et al., 2004). Treatment may include wide excision with frozen section. Surgery may be multiple procedures for a large lesion, which also might include reconstruction and skin grafts. Radiation and cryotherapy may be used if surgical resection is not a good option.

Squamous Cell Carcinoma

Squamous cell carcinoma or Bowen's disease of the eyelid and the conjunctival and lacrimal sacs is clinically presented as an erythematous, crusted, keratotic (horny growth) local lesion (Vaughn et al., 2004). This is common in adults with a history of chronic sun exposure. Treatment of choice is complete surgical excision and eyelid reconstruction, if indicated. Small tissue biopsy may be warranted before extensive surgery for reconfiguration. Management also may include radiotherapy or cryotherapy for nonresectable cases. Metastasis is more common with squamous cell carcinoma compared to basal cell carcinoma.

Intraocular Lymphoid

Intraocular lymphoid is infiltration of malignant lymphocytes of the uveal tract, vitreous, optic nerve, or retina that can be unilateral or bilateral. The most common lymphoid is reticulum cell sarcoma or non-Hodgkin's B-cell lymphoma (Shields & Shields, 1999b). Treatment usually follows along with the systemic course (e.g., leukemia) of management combined with ocular irradiation.

Intraocular Choroidal Metastasis Tumor

Intraocular choroidal metastasis tumor is a secondary cancer arising from another systemic cancer, such as lung or breast carcinoma (Figure 71–21 ■, p. 2370). Typically, it can appear like "leopard skin" over the choroidal retina, which causes changes in the retinal pigment epithelium, secondary retinal detachment, or choroidal detachment (AAO-4, 2008–2009). Treatment of choice usually is chemotherapy or radiation external beam, or plaque. Secondary complications are treated as indicated, such as vitrectomy for a retinal detachment.

Merkel Cell Carcinoma

Merkel cell carcinoma is a primary cutaneous neuroendocrine tumor, which is aggressive and can involve the eyelid and eyebrow as a painless red nodule (Vaughn et al., 2004). Management

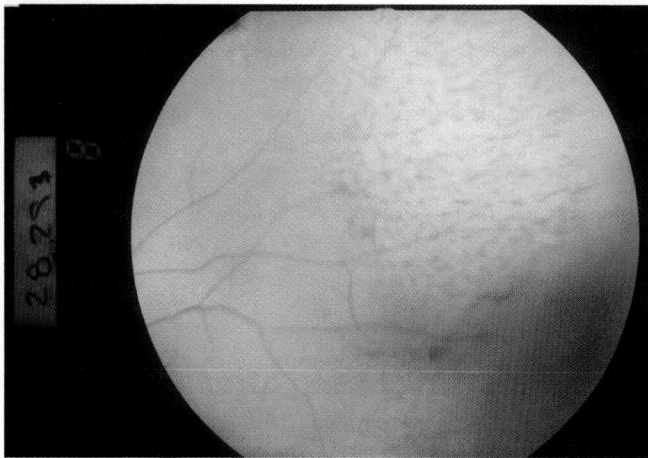

FIGURE 71–21 ■ Metastatic tumor of the choroid.
Source: Kathleen Osborn

requires a wide surgical excision, because this tumor can reoccur and metastasize.

Kaposi's Sarcoma

Kaposi's sarcoma is a malignant vascular tumor seen more commonly in young adults with AIDS (Vaughn et al., 2004). It is a smooth, bluish, subcutaneous eyelid tumor that is commonly associated with immunosuppression and in conjunction with many other cutaneous lesions. Medical management is chemotherapy and radiation.

Orbital Tumors

Orbital tumors are malignant metastatic lesions that have spread to the orbit from the bloodstream. One of the first signs may be proptosis or eye displacement. Other manifestations are pain, diplopia, or edema of the eyelid or conjunctiva. Orbital tumors are diagnostic of carcinomas in adults, in which lesions originate from epithelial structures of the breast, prostate, lung, or other anatomy (Dutton, 2004). Often when an orbital tumor is metastatic in females, they have a history of breast cancer or in males, prostate cancer. Lung cancer also can be the primary site of an orbital metastatic tumor. Findings that will influence treatment options are whether the tumor is benign or malignant, whether it has metastasized, the size and location of the tumor, and whether the tumor is vision threatening or life threatening. Treatment options may include observation, radiation, plaque, or excision, depending on the type of tumor.

■ Nursing Management and Health Promotion

The nurse should instruct patients about risk factors, detection, self-examination, regular follow-up care, and possible treatment options concerning ocular neoplasms. It can be very difficult to distinguish between benign and malignant neoplasms. It always is wise to refer to a health care provider for extensive evaluation if a discoloration, growth, or lesion is noticed on a patient, especially if it is changing in size or color, appears to be growing, has a discharge, or will not heal.

■ Gerontological Considerations

Many ocular and visual changes can occur with aging, and most are normal with passage of time. Descriptions of some of the ocular and visual changes that occur due to aging, and that can affect one's lifestyle significantly, are presented in the Gerontological Considerations box.

■ Cultural Considerations

Culture and geographic locations also can have a significant impact on the types of visual impairment people may manifest or experience. The Cultural Considerations box (p. 2372) outlines some visual disorders that are more common in specific cultures and certain geographic locations due to climate and environmental conditions.

■ Genetic Considerations

Genetics is the study of the gene matrix that makes each person unique and provides the molecules and cellular processes for anatomic description of visual development and outcome. Understanding some of the inherited mutations can assist in the treatment and prognosis of specific visual defects. Descriptions of some of the hereditary conditions that might be factors in visual impairment of adults are presented in the Genetic Considerations box (p. 2372).

■ Ethical Issues

The decision to donate a cornea is a difficult one, fraught with ethical considerations. It is based on the wish to donate an organ in order to benefit another in the restoration of vision. Some are eligible to make this decision; others are not. The ethical issues to be considered are discussed in the Ethical Issues box (p. 2374). The national guidelines that identify donor contraindications for corneal transplants are shown in the National Guidelines box (p. 2374).

■ Research

Research is another mechanism by which to explore and find answers for those that are visually impaired as new devices and clinical outcomes are developed. Vision researchers are striving to meet population needs as well as individual needs. Research topics related to vision research aimed at discovering cures and solutions to visual disorders are outlined in the Research Opportunities and Clinical Impact box (p. 2374).

■ Summary

This chapter has focused on the most common eye disorders, including eye emergencies. The majority of these disorders are treated in an outpatient setting. However, should the need arise or the setting change to inpatient due to geographical circumstances the principles and guidelines set in this chapter are applicable. The clinical preparation vignette is written to assist the learner in caring for a patient with an ocular disorder, but one who also suffers from diabetes, and comprises a very typical situation found by nurses in many settings.

GERONTOLOGICAL CONSIDERATIONS for the Aging Eye

Aging Eye Change	Explanation
Facial Features, Eyebrows, Eyelids, and Eyelashes	
Eyebrow and eyelash pigmentation loss	The eyebrows and eyelashes turn gray to white.
Senile enophthalmos	The recession or sinking of the eyeball into the orbit as a result of the loss of subcutaneous fat, decreased elastic tissue, and decreased muscle tone, but does not affect vision. No intervention necessary.
Ptosis senilis	A pseudoparalytic drooping of the upper eyelid; if it causes a problem by crossing the visual axis, it can be surgically corrected.
Blepharochalasis or dermatochalasis	An atrophy of elastic tissue of the eyelids resulting in the upper eyelid hanging over the eyelid margin or lashes. Redundant eyelid tissue creates wrinkles and folds. If it causes a problem with vision or cosmetically, it can be surgically corrected.
Senile entropion or blepharelosis	The inward turning (inversion) of the eyelid margin; if it causes a problem with irritation or foreign body sensation to the cornea, it can be surgically corrected.
Senile ectropion	The outward turning (eversion) of the eyelid margin; if it causes a problem with dry eye syndrome with the loss of tears and cannot be corrected with artificial tear use, it can be surgically corrected.
Conjunctiva	
Conjunctivochalasis	The loss of transparency and more laxity of the conjunctiva, wherein the bulbar conjunctiva wrinkles into the lower eyelid margin.
Sclera	
Sclera rigidity	The sclera becomes harder or rigid with loss of elasticity. This can also affect accurate intraocular pressure reading with indentation tonometry.
Senile scleral translucency	The sclera thins and becomes more transparent, exhibiting dark-grayish oval areas of the sclera, anterior to muscle insertion.
Scleral lipid deposition	The anterior sclera will appear yellowish due to lipid depositions in the deeper scleral tissue.
Pupil and Iris	
Pupil sclerosis	The pupil size decreases with age (senile miosis) because of pupil sphincter sclerosis, which narrows the visual field and affects peripheral vision to a mild degree. No intervention is usually necessary.
Cornea	
Keratoconjunctivitis sicca or dry eye syndrome	A deficiency of tear production, especially in postmenopausal women, can make the cornea feel gritty or have a foreign body sensation. This is usually relieved with frequent use of artificial tear drops or ointments.
Arcus senilis or gerontoxon	A grayish-white ring that develops at the peripheral edge of the cornea (limbus) from lipoid deposits into the corneal stroma, and does not affect vision; no intervention is required.
Guttata or corneal dystrophy	The thickening of Descemet's membrane (fourth layer of the cornea) with hyaline deposits from the loss of endothelial cells. These cells help maintain the health of the cornea and vision clarity.
Lens	
Cataract	The yellowing or opacity of the natural crystalline lens that is corrected surgically when a cataract is mature. In the meantime, corrective lenses can help; may also notice an alteration in color perception, especially for blues, violets, and greens.
Optic Nerve, Retinal, Vitreous	
Glaucoma	An elevated intraocular pressure due to aging, whereby trabecular meshwork is sluggish due to the loss of elasticity.
Age-related macular degeneration	The degeneration of the macula due to aging; the loss of retinal pigment epithelium and visual function.
Senile circumpapillary choroidal atrophy or peripapillary halo	The degeneration of arterioles in the choriocapillaris causing sclerosis, especially around the optic nerve; usually does not affect vision. No intervention is necessary.
Senile retinoschisis or schisis	A primary, acquired, gradual splitting of the retina into two distinct layers. SR develops from the coalescence of intraretinal microcysts located in an area of peripheral cystoid degeneration near the ora serrata and extends posteriorly and circumferentially. This process leads to the splitting of the retina at the outer plexiform layer or, less commonly, at the inner nuclear layer
Syneresis	Degeneration of the vitreous humor with loss of gel consistency, acts as a precursor to posterior vitreous detachment of gel, which is commonly called floaters. This occurs during the aging process and seldom calls for an intervention unless secondary complications result, such as retinal detachment.

(continued)

GERONTOLOGICAL CONSIDERATIONS for the Aging Eye—*Continued*

Aging Eye Change	Explanation
Vision	
Presbyopia	The loss of accommodation about the fourth decade of life is the loss of the ability to focus up close and necessitates the need for reading glasses or bifocals.
Astigmatism	The cornea can flatten more with age; this changes the corneal curvature and may result in new astigmatism or changes in astigmatism. This can be corrected with lenses.
Stereopsis loss	The loss of depth perception due to light scatter or glare that affects vision performance, causing difficulty with night vision, especially driving and judging heights properly. This can possibly be helped with brighter, nonglare lights and brighter colors, such as reds, oranges, and yellows.

CULTURAL CONSIDERATIONS for Visual Disorders

Culture	Ocular Condition
African Americans	Glaucoma
African Caribbeans	Sickle hemoglobinopathies
Africans, Central Americans, and South Americans	River blindness
Africans, Middle Easterners, Indians, and Southeast Asians	Trachoma
Caucasians	Age-related macular degeneration
Hispanic Americans and African Americans	Diabetic retinopathy
Japanese and Spaniards	Progressive myopia

Source: Yanoff, M., & Duker J. S. (Eds.). (2004). *Ophthalmology* (2nd ed.). St. Louis, MO: Mosby.

GENETIC CONSIDERATIONS in Adults with Visual Impairments

Consideration	Definition
Color blindness:	A hereditary condition that disables vision to distinguish colors.
• Protanomaly	Mild red-green discrimination, deficient red photoreceptors.
• Deuteranomaly	Red-green discrimination; most common form of color blindness (X linked).
• Tritanomaly	Mild blue-green discrimination.
• Protanopia	Severe red discrimination, appearing very dark; no red photoreceptors.
• Deuteranopia	More severe red-green discrimination.
• Tritanopia	Only two cone pigments and no blue photoreceptors.
Refractive errors	The inheritance of hyperopia, myopia, and/or astigmatic refractive errors.
Keratoconus	A hereditary central thinning of the cornea, making it a cone-shaped elevation of the central cornea that is usually progressive and more noticeable in those 20 years or older.
Corneal dystrophy (or Fuchs' dystrophy)	It can be hereditary deterioration of the cornea due to loss of endothelial cells from Descemet's membrane (fourth corneal layer) thickening, and possibly progressing to poor vision and cornea transplant.
Cataracts	A hereditary cataract usually matures faster, and cataract surgery can be necessary as early as in the second to fourth decade of life, instead of the usual sixth to eighth decade of life.
Glaucoma (Mendelian inheritance)	It can be hereditary, causing intraocular pressure elevation, optic nerve atrophy, and poor perfusion of the optic nerve.
Uveitis	It can be hereditary with inflammation of the uveal tract, which includes the iris, ciliary body, and choroid.
Leber's hereditary optic atrophy	A hereditary, rapidly developing bilateral optic nerve degeneration; vision loss usually stabilizes and occurs in males in their 20s and 30s.

GENETIC CONSIDERATIONS in Adults with Visual Impairments—*Continued*

Consideration	Definition
Disorder	
Marfan's syndrome	A hereditary condition whereby the bone structure is very long and thin, especially arms, legs, fingers, and toes. Weak ligaments, bone deformities, and heart disease are prevalent. Those with Marfan's syndrome often are myopic, with large corneas, early cataracts, dislocated lenses, ptosis, strabismus, and choroidal malformations.
Usher's syndrome	A hereditary combination of bilateral deafness and night blindness.
Alport's syndrome	A hereditary combination of kidney disease, deafness, and lens abnormality; such as small and round lenses, early cataracts, and anterior lenticonus (cone-shaped protrusion of the lens).
Joubert syndrome	A hereditary central nerve system defect with severe psychomotor deficiencies, breathing problems, and nystagmus.
Wagner's disease	A hereditary vitreoretinal degeneration syndrome that makes one more prone to retinal tears and detachments. Other ocular signs are myopia, lattice degeneration, strabismus, and cataracts in the teen years.
Stickler syndrome	A hereditary progressive connective tissue disease that causes enlarged and degenerative joints, arthritis, flattened midface, cleft palate, and deafness. Ocular signs are vitreoretinal degeneration, high myopia, and early cataracts.
Grönblad-Strandberg syndrome (pseudoxanthoma elasticum)	A hereditary elastic connective disorder that gives skin a leathery appearance, something like a plucked chicken's skin, with major artery defects. The retinal symptoms are angioid streaks, which are subretinal pigmented lines from cracks in Bruch's membrane that form macular hemorrhages and scars.
Age-related macular degeneration	A deterioration of the macula causing central vision loss and distortion. It is often hereditary, developing as early as in one's 50s.
Kandori's syndrome	A hereditary form of nonprogressive night blindness with numerous irregular and large gray-yellowish flecks in the retina.
Refsum's disease	A hereditary disease that is characterized by footdrop, inability to sleep, increased cerebrospinal fluid, accumulation of fatty acids, and electrocardiogram changes. Ocular signs are poor dark adaptation, constricted visual field, nystagmus, ptosis, and small pupil (miosis).
Retinitis pigmentosa (night blindness)	A hereditary bilateral rod/cone dysfunction with diminished or loss of side vision that can slowly progress to central vision loss and blindness.
Retinoblastoma	A hereditary malignant retinal tumor (most common in childhood); this may be the reason for an adult to have an eye removed or be blind in both eyes. If untreated, it can metastasize to the brain and cause death.
Nursing Assessment	
	Assess family history for glaucoma, cataracts, night blindness, color blindness, or other visual anomalies. Assess family history for other systemic disorders, such as deafness and cutaneous, metabolic, and connective tissue disorders. Assess physically for body asymmetry, deafness, and cutaneous, metabolic, and connective tissue disorders.
Management Issues	
	Question about DNA testing or other genetic testing that has been done in this family. Refer family for genetic counseling and evaluation to discuss inheritance, family risk factors, and gene-based intervention. Provide genetic information, materials, and resources. Provide assessment and understanding of genetic information and inherited conditions. Provide support and coping with new genetic findings. Be a patient advocate in management of care with genetic conditions and others that are predisposed to genetic problems. Being a counselor for the whole family may be indicated, so that the family members understand what genetic traits may be transmitted to the following generations.
Genetic Resources	
	Genetic Alliance[a] Gene Clinic[b] National Organization of Rare Diseases[c] Online Mendelian Inheritance in Man (OMIM)[d] "Genetic Testing for Inherited Eye Disease"[e] *Archives of Ophthalmology:* January and February 2007 issues devoted to ophthalmic genetics for in-depth details on inherited eye diseases and conditions

[a] http://www.geneticalliance.org

[b] http://www.geneclinics.org

[c] http://www.rarediseases.org

[d] http://www.ncbi.nlm.nih.gov/Literature/index.html or http://www.ncbi.nlm.nih.gov/genome/guide/human/

[e] Stone, E. M. (2007). Genetic testing for inherited eye disease. *Archives of Ophthalmology, 125*(2), 205–212.

ETHICAL ISSUES for Corneal Transplants

Approximately 40,000 corneal transplants are done in the United States each year (Rabinowitz, 2005). The decision to donate corneal tissue for transplantation can have ethical considerations. It is important for the family that is being asked to donate a cornea for the benefit of someone else's vision, that the decision be a well-informed one, one that is freely chosen, and one that is compatible with the ethical beliefs of the individuals concerned. It is important for the family members to know that whatever decision they make, to donate or not to donate, they have freedom of choice. Under the circumstances of facing the loss of a loved one, any decision they make is the right decision for them. Usually the decision is one of three choices: Donate all organs, donate only the cornea, or do not donate at all. The two most common reasons not to donate are (1) the fear of something being done before the person is dead, and (2) the fear that the health care provider may hasten the death to benefit another.

Thoughts for Consideration

- Donation is an ethical decision to benefit another person.
- With treatment of the body after death, respect is the greatest issue, especially for psychological, religious, spiritual, moral, and cultural reasons.
- Donation is the last giving act the person donor does to reflect his life.
- The family knows that the loved one still lives on in another person. (NHMRC, 1997)

Sources: American Academy of Ophthalmology (AAO-8). (2008–2009). *Basic and clinical science course: External disease and cornea* (Section 8). San Francisco: Author; National Health and Medical Research Council (NHMRC). (1997). *Donating organs after death: Ethical issues.* Canberra, Australia: Australian Government Publishing Service; and Rabinowitz, Y. (2005, August 29). *Corneal transplants.* Retrieved April 26, 2007, from http://www.laser-prk.com/corneal.htm.

NATIONAL GUIDELINES for Criteria for Donor Contraindications of the Cornea

Acquired or congenital eye disorders that would prevent successful surgical outcome include:

- Active disseminated lymphoma or leukemia
- Active fungal or bacterial endocarditis
- Active intraocular or ocular inflammation
- Active septicemia
- Immunosuppressant diseases (HIV, syphilis, or hepatitis)
- Intrinsic malignancies
- Prior intraocular surgery of donor
- Prior refractive corneal surgery
- Unknown cause of death
- Unknown central nervous system (CNS) disease or CNS infection. (AAO-8, 2008–2009)

Sources: Eye Bank Association of America. (2001). *Frequently asked questions.* Retrieved October 4, 2008, from http://www.rsotresight.org/general/faqs.htm; Main, S. (2005). Regulation of eye banking and uses of ocular tissue for transplantation. *Clinical Laboratory Medicine, 24*(3), 607–624.

RESEARCH OPPORTUNITIES AND CLINICAL IMPACT RELATED TO VISUAL DISORDERS

Research Area	Clinical Impact
Vision Research	
Bradyopsia, light blindness, a new eye disease discovery caused by bright light exposure limiting function visual acuity with 20/20 acuity on Snellen vision chart due to phototransduction failure (Nishiguchi & Dryja, 2004).	Identification of patients that cannot see when moving from the indoors to the outside in bright sunlight or vice versa. They are blind for at least 5–10 seconds and are stopped in their tracks before vision starts to return, but vision is never comfortable. Contrast and swift-moving objects are difficult to track or see.
Diabetic Retinopathy Research	
Anti-VEGF therapy: Lack of oxygen to retinal tissue produces the release of vascular endothelial growth factor (VEGF), which causes blood vessels in the retina to leak, resulting in edema, tissue thickening, and growth of new vessels (Campochiaro, 2004).	Repair the progress of edema and scarring from diabetic retinopathy; to restore and preserve vision.
Oxygen therapy may improve decreased vision from diabetic retinopathy (Nguyen et al., 2004).	Supplement oxygen to prevent the growth of new vessels due to ischemic tissue for long-term vision restoration.
New anti-VEGF therapy: for the treatment of proliferative diabetic retinopathy (PDR) complicated with vitreous hemorrhage (Spaide & Fisher, 2006).	Treat the progress of PDR and vitreous hemorrhage in advanced diabetic retinopathy; to preserve vision.

RESEARCH OPPORTUNITIES AND CLINICAL IMPACT RELATED TO VISUAL DISORDERS—*Continued*

Research Area	Clinical Impact
Cornea Research	
Keratoprostheses, artificial cornea, and polymethymethacrylate (PMMA) device for implantation on the cornea (Alfonso, 2004).	Yield long-term vision restoration and lessen the rejection of donor tissue.
Melanoma Research	
Quality-of-life issues following choroidal melanoma treatment (Collaborative Ocular Melanoma Study—Quality of Life Study Group, 2006; Marr, 2006).	Anxiety of enucleation vs. brachytherapy in the treatment of eye melanoma; enucleation treatment anxiety was less in the long run.
Macular Degeneration Research	
Sunlight exposure and the incidence of macular degeneration that takes away central visual acuity with aging (Tomany, Cruickshanks, Klein, Klein, & Knudtson, 2004).	Prevent damage of the macula by wearing protective eyewear to block ultraviolet light, such as wearing sunglasses and hats to prevent long periods of sunlight exposure to central vision.
Age-related macular degeneration is a potential public health crisis: Antioxidant dietary supplements are a possible means to regress this threat to low vision (AREDS Research Group, 2003).	Supplement of antioxidants or vitamins to diet may slow down or improve macular tissue from breaking down, to restore some degree of healthy tissue function for increased vision.
Macular degeneration being the leading cause of legal blindness in older adults, especially the wet form. Patients may have hope with statin and aspirin therapy to lower the risk of going legally blind (Wilson, Schwartz, Bhatt, McCulloch, & Duncan, 2004).	Taking statin and aspirin could lessen the chances of going legally blind from wet macular degeneration.
Independence and the quality of life with vision loss from age-related macular degeneration and other health morbidity for older adults. The study to address all these areas of impact on one's life (Elfervig, 1997).	With increased vision loss, older adults have more difficulty carrying out activities of daily living, especially shopping, laundry, and handling finances. The more systemic illnesses a person has along with vision loss, the more difficulty with housekeeping, handling finances, and just doing daily chores. Married persons with vision loss and other health problems had greater satisfaction with life than did single persons with the same problems. Patients with macular degeneration can keep active and maintain a good degree of independence, with varying degrees of vision deficiency, if they have proper equipment and home setup, with new learned skills.
Evidence impact of vision-related quality of life (QOL) in patients with age-related macular degeneration (Berdeaux, Nordmann, Colin, & Arnould, 2005; Ferris, 2005).	Preserving minimal visual acuity in the worse eye may contribute to vision-related QOL for the better.

Sources: Age-Related Eye Disease Study (AREDS) Research Group. (2003). Potential public health impact of age-related eye disease study results. *Archives of Ophthalmology, 121*(11), 1621–1624; Alfonso, E. C. (2004). Keratoprostheses: Artificial corneas yield long-term vision. *Ophthalmology Times, 29*(12), 1, 60; Berdeaux, G. H., Nordmann, J. P., Colin, E., & Arnould, B. (2005). Vision-related quality of life in patients suffering from age-related macular degeneration. *American Journal of Ophthalmology, 139*(2), 271–279; Campochiaro, P. A. (2004). Reduction of diabetic macular edema by oral administration of kinase inhibitor. *Investigative Ophthalmology & Visual Science, 45*(3), 922–931; Collaborative Ocular Melanoma Study—Quality of Life Study Group (COMS QOLSG). (2006). Quality of life after iodine 125 brachytherapy vs. enucleation for choroidal melanoma. *Archives of Ophthalmology, 124*(2), 226–238; Elfervig, L. S. (1997). *Functional independence and life satisfaction with vision loss from age-related macular degeneration: A study of older adults.* Doctoral dissertation, Louisiana State University Medical Center, UMI No. 9717113; Ferris, F. L. (2005). Vision-related quality of life in patients suffering from age-related macular degeneration. *Evidence-Based Ophthalmology, 6*(3), 163–164; Marr, B. (2006). Quality of life after iodine 125 brachytherapy versus enucleation for choroidal melanoma five-year results from the collaborative ocular melanoma study: COMS QOLS Reports No. 3. *Evidence-Based Ophthalmology, 7*(3), 154–156; Nguyen, Q., et al. (2004). Supplemental oxygen improves diabetic macular edema: A pilot study. *Investigative Ophthalmology & Visual Science, 45*(2), 617–624; Nishiguchi, K. M., & Dryja, L. (2004, March). New eye disease: Light blindness. *EyeNet,* 13–14; Spaide, R. F., & Fisher, Y. L. (2006). Intravitreal bevacizumab (avastin) treatment of proliferative diabetic retinopathy complicated by vitreous hemorrhage. *Retina, 26*(3), 275–278; Tomany, S. C., Cruickshanks, K. J., Klein, R., Klein, B. E., & Knudtson, M. D. (2004). Sunlight and the 10-year incidence of age-related maculopathy. *Archives of Ophthalmology, 122*(5), 750–757; and Wilson, H. L., Schwartz, D. M., Bhatt, H. R., McCulloch, C. E., & Duncan, J. L. (2004). Statin and aspirin therapy are associated with decreased rates of choroidal neovascularization among patients with age-related macular degeneration. *American Journal of Ophthalmology, 137*(4), 615–624.

Clinical Preparation

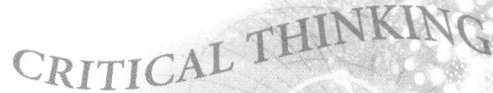

CRITICAL THINKING

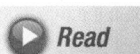 **Read**

- History of Current Illness
- Past Medical History
- Physical Exam
- Admitting Medical Orders
- Laboratory Study Results

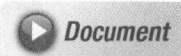 **Document**

- Summary of Hospitalization
- Pathophysiology Form
- Laboratory Values
- Laboratory Results Explanation

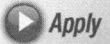 **Apply**

- List of Potential Nursing Diagnoses
- Concept Map
- Critical Thinking Questions

Log on to MyNursingKit.com to download forms you will need and to complete further steps in the Clinical Preparation assignment.

HISTORY OF PRESENT ILLNESS

As the on-coming nurse to a clinic facility, you are presented with the following patient in the examination room as your first patient of the morning. Mrs. M is a 55-year-old executive at a local bank, who presented at the clinic with sudden vision loss in her left eye, seeing darkness with some floaters when she awakened this morning. She arrived at the clinic with her husband, who did the driving, along with her grown daughter.

Medical–Surgical History

Mrs. M's past medical history includes hypertension, hyperlipidemia, and non–insulin-dependent diabetic mellitus for the past 10 years. She is currently taking aspirin, Avapro, Zocor, and Glucotrol; is on a low-salt diabetic diet; and does not smoke. Her only surgery was an appendectomy as a child. She has a family history of diabetes and hypertension, no known vision problems, no known allergies, and she is not on any eyedrops. When asked when she had her last professional eye examination, Mrs. M states she has never had one. Mrs. M states her vision was good until this morning.

Physical Examination

In your findings Mrs. M is 5'2" tall, weighing 175 pounds. She states she did not hit her head or her eye; she just awakened this morning with blurry vision in the left eye. When you shine a penlight in her right eye, you get a bright, clear reflex, and in her left eye you get a dull, flat reflex. Her pupils are equal at 3.5 millimeters, are round, and react to light and accommodation. Her facial features, ocular adnexa, and eyes appear symmetrical: There are no discolorations, no discharges, no pain, no growths, no size difference, and no misalignments; the only asymmetry is that the left eyelid droops slightly. The visual acuity is 20/30 right eye and 20/200 left eye with glasses for both near and far vision. Her blood glucose is checked and found to be 300 mg/dL, and urinalysis showed a trace of protein. Her vital signs are temperature 98°F, pulse 75 beats per minute, respiratory rate 17/minute, and blood pressure 160/100. Mrs. M is referred to a local vitreoretinal ophthalmologist for further evaluation, examination, and treatment.

CRITICAL THINKING QUESTIONS

1. What might be the cause of a sudden vision loss in a patient with diabetes?

2. Besides blood sugar and vital signs checks, what else might you test Mrs. M for; what test might be most diagnostic?

3. What possible treatments may clear Mrs. M's vision?

4. What changes might her health care provider make in Mrs. M's treatment for diabetes?

5. What measures will Mrs. M have to take at home to improve her vision?

Answers to Critical Thinking Questions appear in Appendix D.

NCLEX® REVIEW

1. A patient tells the nurse that she thinks there's something wrong with her vision because she sometimes sees black things "moving" in her vision. The nurse realizes this patient is describing:
   1. Glaucoma.
   2. Cataracts.
   3. Floaters.
   4. Detached retina.

2. While conducting a cover-uncover test for tropia, the nurse notes that a patient's uncovered eye moves toward the nose. This finding would indicate:
   1. The uncovered eye is fixated inward.
   2. The uncovered eye is fixated outward.
   3. The uncovered eye has steady fixation.
   4. Vertical tropia.

3. A patient with a history of head trauma is in need of treatment for adult strabismus. Which of the following would be considered as appropriate for this patient?
   1. Contact lenses
   2. Occlusion of the normal vision eye
   3. Bifocal lenses
   4. Eye muscle surgery

4. The nurse is planning care for a patient with glaucoma. Which of the following should be included in this plan of care?
   1. Diet
   2. The correct use of eyedrops
   3. Control of heart disease
   4. Use of corrective lenses

5. A patient has been diagnosed as being brain dead and the family is not sure if the patient's corneas should be donated. Which of the following can the nurse provide to this patient's family?
   1. Explain that since there is an organ shortage, the family really should donate the patient's corneas.
   2. Explain that whatever decision they make, they have freedom of choice.
   3. Explain to the family that time is of the essence and they need to decide before the patient dies.
   4. They can always visit the person who received the donated corneas.

Answers for review questions appear in Appendix D

KEY TERMS

aberration *p.2331*
accommodation *p.2328*
acute angle-closure glaucoma (AACG) *p.2345*
amblyopia *p.2334*
ametropia *p.2332*
astigmatism *p.2332*
cataracts *p.2350*
central retinal artery occlusion (CRAO) *p.2362*
contrast sensitivity (CS) *p.2335*
cotton-wool spots (CWS) *p.2342*
diabetic retinopathy (DR) *p.2338*

diplopia *p.2334*
drusen *p.2335*
emmetropia *p.2331*
esophoria *p.2334*
flame-shaped hemorrhages *p.2342*
flashes *p.2363*
floaters *p.2328*
foreign body sensation (FBS) *p.2354*
glaucoma *p.2343*
hyperopia *p.2332*
hyphema *p.2362*
hypopyon *p.2355*

legal blindness *p.2335*
macular degeneration (MD) *p.2335*
metamorphopsia *p.2335*
myopia *p.2332*
nystagmus *p.2335*
open globe *p.2362*
phoria *p.2334*
presbyopia *p.2332*
retinal detachment *p.2366*
retinopathy *p.2338*
strabismus *p.2334*
tropia *p.2334*

EXPLORE **PEARSON mynursingkit**™

MyNursingKit is your one stop for online chapter review materials and resources. Prepare for success with additional NCLEX®-style practice questions, interactive assignments and activities, web links, animations and videos, and more!

Register your access code from the front of your book at
www.mynursingkit.com

REFERENCES

Abad, J. C., & Azar, D. T. (2004). Current concepts, classification, and history of refractive surgery. In M. Yanoff & J. S. Duker (Eds.), *Ophthalmology* (2nd ed.). St. Louis: Mosby.

Abe, S., Tamakawa, M., Andoh, M., Kohda, K., Teranishi, C., & Ohta, I. (2005). Lymphoid tumor in the orbit: malignant or benign? MRI, histomorphological and molecular genetic analysis of eight cases. *European Journal of Plastic Surgery, 27*(8), 378–382.

Age-Related Eye Disease Study (AREDS) Research Group. (2003). Potential public health impact of Age-Related Eye Disease Study results. AREDS Report No. 11. *Archives of Ophthalmology, 121*(11), 1621–1624.

Age-Related Eye Disease Study (AREDS) Research Group. (2006). Cognitive impairment in the Age-Related Eye Disease Study. AREDS Report No. 16. *Archives of Ophthalmology, 124*(4), 537–543.

Alfonso, E. C. (2004). Keratoprostheses: Artificial corneas yield long-term vision. *Ophthalmology Times, 29*(12), 1, 60.

American Academy of Ophthalmology (AAO-2). (2008–2009). *Basic and clinical science course: Fundamentals and principles of ophthalmology* (Section 2). San Francisco: Author.

American Academy of Ophthalmology (AAO-3). (2008–2009). *Basic and clinical science course: Optics, refraction, and contact lenses* (Section 3). San Francisco: Author.

American Academy of Ophthalmology (AAO-4). (2008–2009). *Basic and clinical science course: Ophthalmic pathology and intraocular tumors* (Section 4). San Francisco: Author.

American Academy of Ophthalmology (AAO-5). (2008–2009). *Basic and clinical science course: Neuro-ophthalmology* (Section 5). San Francisco: Author.

American Academy of Ophthalmology (AAO-6). (2008–2009). *Basic and clinical science course: Pediatric ophthalmology and strabismus* (Section 6). San Francisco: Author.

American Academy of Ophthalmology (AAO-7). (2008–2009). *Basic and clinical science course: Orbit, eyelids, and lacrimal system* (Section 7). San Francisco: Author.

American Academy of Ophthalmology (AAO-8). (2008–2009). *Basic and clinical science course: External disease and cornea* (Section 8). San Francisco: Author.

American Academy of Ophthalmology (AAO-9). (2008–2009). *Basic and clinical science course: Intraocular inflammation and uveitis* (Section 9). San Francisco: Author.

American Academy of Ophthalmology (AAO-10). (2008–2009). *Basic and clinical science course: Glaucoma* (Section 10). San Francisco: Author.

American Academy of Ophthalmology (AAO-11). (2008–2009). *Basic and clinical science course: Lens and cataract* (Section 11). San Francisco: Author.

American Academy of Ophthalmology (AAO-12). (2008–2009). *Basic and clinical science course: Retina and vitreous* (Section 12). San Francisco: Author.

Arnold, A. C. (2004). Ischemic optic neuropathy, diabetic papillopathy, and papillophlebitis. In M. Yanoff & J. S. Duker (Eds.), *Ophthalmology* (2nd ed.). St. Louis: Mosby.

Beers, M. H., & Berkow, R. (1999). *The Merck manual of diagnosis and therapy* (17th ed.). Whitehouse Station, NJ: Merck Research Laboratories.

Berdeaux, G. H., Nordmann, J. P., Colin, E., & Arnould, B. (2005). Vision-related quality of life in patients suffering from age-related macular degeneration. *American Journal of Ophthalmology, 139*(2), 271–279.

Bhavsar, A. R., & Drouilhet, J. H. (2006). Retinopathy, diabetic, background. *Emedicine.* Retrieved June 16, 2008, from http://www.emedicine.com/oph/topic414.htm

Campbell, D. G., & Netland, P. A. (1998). *Stereo atlas of glaucoma.* St. Louis: Mosby–Year Book.

Campochiaro, P. A. (1999). Acute posterior bacterial endophthalmitis. *Ophthalmology Clinics of North America, 12,* 83–88.

Campochiaro, P. A. (2004). Reduction of diabetic macular edema by oral administration of kinase inhibitor. *Investigative Ophthalmology & Visual Science, 45*(3), 922–931.

Charles, S. (2001). Principles and techniques of vitreous surgery. In S. J. Ryan (Ed.), *Retina* (3rd ed., Vol. 3). St. Louis: Mosby.

Choplin, N. T., & Lundy, D. C. (1998). *Atlas of glaucoma.* London: Martin Dunitz Ltd.

Clarkson, J. G. (2001). Central retinal vein occlusion. In S. J. Ryan (Ed.), *Retina* (3rd ed., Vol. 2). St. Louis: Mosby.

Collaborative Ocular Melanoma Study—Quality of Life Study Group (COMS QOLSG). (2006). Quality of life after iodine 125 brachytherapy vs. enucleation for choroidal melanoma. *Archives of Ophthalmology, 124*(2), 226–238.

Dabezies, O., Klyce, S., Morgan, J., Hartstein, J., Donshik, P., Boswall, G., et al. (1998). Corneal changes from contact lenses. In H. Kaufman, B. Barron, & M. McDonald (Eds.), *The cornea* (2nd ed.). Boston: Butterworth-Heinemann.

Daly, S. W. (2002). Scleral disorders. In K. Goldblum & P. Lamb (Eds.), *Core curriculum for ophthalmic nursing* (2nd ed.). Dubuque, IA: Kendall/Hunt.

D'Amato, R. J. (1999). Pharmacologic therapy: Angiogenesis inhibition. In J. W. Berger, S. L. Fine, & M. G. Maguire (Eds.), *Age-related macular degeneration.* St. Louis: Mosby.

Dhalla, M. S., Shah, G. K., Blinder, K. J., Ryan, E. H., Mittra, R. A., & Tewari, A. (2006). Combined photodynamic therapy with verteporfin and intravitreal bevacizumab for choroidal neovascularization in age-related macular degeneration. *Retina, 26*(9), 988–993.

Dutton, J. J. (2004). Orbital diseases. In M. Yanoff & J. S. Duker (Eds.), *Ophthalmology* (2nd ed.). St. Louis: Mosby.

Elfervig, L. S. (1997). *Functional independence and life satisfaction with vision loss from age-related macular degeneration: A study of older adults.* Doctoral dissertation, Louisiana State University Medical Center, UMI No. 9717113.

Elfervig, L. S. (1998). Age-related macular degeneration. *Nurse Practitioner Forum, 9*(1), 4–6.

Elfervig, L. S. (2000). Photodynamic therapy (PDT). *TNA District 1 Dispatcher, 2*(1), 5.

Elfervig, L. S. (2002a). Uveal disorders (glaucoma). In K. Goldblum & P. Lamb (Eds.), *Core curriculum for ophthalmic nursing* (2nd ed.). Dubuque, IA: Kendall/Hunt.

Elfervig, L. S. (2002b). Pharmacology. In K. Goldblum & P. Lamb (Eds.), *Core curriculum for ophthalmic nursing* (2nd ed.). Dubuque, IA: Kendall/Hunt.

Elfervig, L. S., & Elfervig, J. L. (1998). Retinal detachment. *Insight, 23*(2), 66–70.

Elfervig, L. S., & Elfervig, J. L. (1999). Endophthalmitis. *Insight, 24*(3), 99–103.

Elfervig, L. S., & Elfervig, J. L. (2001). Proliferative diabetic retinopathy. *Insight, 26*(3), 88–93.

Elfervig, L. S., & Elfervig J. L. (2007). Recognition and triage of ocular emergencies. *Refinements: Clinical Education Modules for Today's Ophthalmic Team, 2*(1), 1–14. Manuscript updated and submitted for republication.

Eliott, D., Lee, M. S., & Abrams, G. W. (2001). Proliferative diabetic retinopathy: Principles and techniques of surgical treatment. In S. J. Ryan (Ed.), *Retina* (3rd ed., Vol. 2). St. Louis: Mosby.

Eye Bank Association. (2001). *Frequently asked questions.* Retrieved October 4, 2008, from http://www.restoresight.org/general/faqs.htm

Eye Tech Study Group (ETSG). (2003). Anti-vascular endothelial growth factor therapy for subfoveal choroidal neovascularization secondary to age-related macular degeneration. *American Journal of Ophthalmology, 110*(5), 979–986.

Falk, N. S., Beer, P. M., & Peters, G. B. (2006). Role of intravitreal triamcinolone acetonide in the treatment of postoperative endophthalmitis. *Retina, 26*(5), 545–548.

Fanous, M. M. (2004). Neovascular glaucoma. In M. Yanoff & J. S. Duker (Eds.), *Ophthalmology* (2nd ed.). St. Louis: Mosby.

Fekrat, S., & Finkelstein, D. (2001). Branch retinal vein occlusion. In S. J. Ryan (Ed.), *Retina* (3rd ed., Vol. 2). St. Louis: Mosby.

Ferrara, N., Damico, L., Shams, N., Lowman, H., & Kim, R. (2006). Development of ranibizumab, an anti-vascular endothelial growth factor antigen binding fragment, as therapy for neovascular age-related macular degeneration. *Retina, 26*(8), 859–870.

Ferris, F. L. (2005). Vision-related quality of life in patients suffering from age-related macular degeneration. *Evidence-Based Ophthalmology, 6*(3), 163–164.

Fong, D. S., Aiello, L., Gardner, T. W., et al. (2003). Diabetic retinopathy. *Diabetes Care, 26,* 226–229.

Foster, C. S., & Vitale, A. T. (Eds.). (2002). *Diagnosis and treatment of uveitis.* Philadelphia: W. B. Saunders.

Gold, D. H., & Weingeist, T. A. (2001). *Color atlas of the eye in systemic disease.* Philadelphia: Lippincott Williams & Wilkins.

Goldstein, D. A., & Tessler, H. H. (2004). Episcleritis, scleritis, and other scleral disorders. In M. Yanoff & J. S. Duker (Eds.), *Ophthalmology* (2nd ed.). St. Louis: Mosby.

Green, D. (2002). Neoplastic disorders. In K. Goldblum & P. Lamb (Eds.), *Core curriculum for ophthalmic nursing* (2nd ed.). Dubuque, IA: Kendall/Hunt.

Green, J. P., Charonis, G. C., & Goldberg, R. A. (2004). Eyelid trauma and reconstruction techniques. In M. Yanoff & J. S. Duker (Eds.), *Ophthalmology* (2nd ed.). St. Louis: Mosby.

Guttman, C. (2004). Experience underlines efficacy of full-time occlusion for amblyopia. *Ophthalmology Times, 29*(4), 1, 20.

Hamza, H. S., Loewenstein, A., & Haller, J. A. (1999). Fungal retinitis and endophthalmitis. *Ophthalmology Clinics of North America, 12,* 89–108.

Harper, S. L., Chorich, L. J., & Foster, C. S. (2002). Diagnosis of uveitis. In C. S. Foster & A. T. Vitale (Eds.), *Diagnosis and treatment of uveitis.* Philadelphia: W. B. Saunders.

Hikichi, T., & Yoshida, A. (2004). Time course of development of posterior vitreous detachment in the fellow eye after development in the first eye. *American Journal of Ophthalmology, 111*(9), 1705–1707.

Hitchings, R. (2004). Normal-tension glaucoma. In M. Yanoff & J. S. Duker (Eds.), *Ophthalmology* (2nd ed.). St. Louis: Mosby.

Jabs, D. A. (2001). Rheumatic diseases. In S. J. Ryan (Ed.), *Retina* (3rd ed., Vol. 2). St. Louis: Mosby.

Kanski, J. J. (2001). *Systemic diseases and the eye: Signs and differential diagnosis.* London: Mosby International Limited.

Lamb, P. A. (2002). Conjunctival disorders. In K. Goldblum & P. Lamb (Eds.), *Core curriculum for ophthalmic nursing* (2nd ed.). Dubuque, IA: Kendall/Hunt.

Lee, A. G., & Brazis, P. W. (2003). *Clinical pathways in neuro-ophthalmology: An evidence-based approach* (2nd ed.). New York: Thieme.

Maguire, M. G. (1999). Natural history. In J. W. Berger, S. L. Fine, & M. G. Maguire (Eds.), *Age-related macular degeneration.* St. Louis: Mosby.

Marr, B. (2006). Quality of life after iodine 125 brachytherapy versus enucleation for choroidal melanoma five-year results from the collaborative ocular melanoma study: COMS QOLS Reports No. 3. *Evidence-Based Ophthalmology, 7*(3), 154–156.

Martidis, A., & Tennant, M. T. (2004). Age-related macular degeneration. In M. Yanoff & J. S. Duker (Eds.), *Ophthalmology* (2nd ed.). St. Louis: Mosby.

May, D. R., Kuhn, F. P., Morris, R. E., Witherspoon, C. D., Danis, R. P., Matthews, G. P., et al. (2000). The epidemiology of serious eye injuries from the United States Eye Injury Registry. *Graefe's Archive for Clinical and Experimental Ophthalmology, 238*(2). Retrieved September 24, 2008, from http://www.springerlink.com/content/u0pxmaf7p4hd5vh6/

Mayo Clinic. (2006). Trachoma overview. *Revolution Health.* Retrieved October 5, 2008, from http://www.revolutionhealth.com/condidions/ eye/trachoma/understand-overview?section=s,,,

McLeod, S. D. (2004). Infectious keratitis. In M. Yanoff & J. S. Duker (Eds.), *Ophthalmology* (2nd ed.). St. Louis: Mosby.

Miller, D., & Scott, C. A. (2004). Epidemiology of refractive errors. In M. Yanoff & J. S. Duker (Eds.), *Ophthalmology* (2nd ed.). St. Louis: Mosby.

Montan, P., Koranyi, G., Setterquist, H., Stridh, A., Philipson, B., & Wiklund, K. (1998). Endophthalmitis after cataract surgery: Risk factors relating to technique and events of operation and patient history. *Ophthalmology, 105,* 2171–2175.

Mulrooney, B. C. (2006). Cataract, traumatic. *Emedicine.* Retreived October 2, 2008 from http://www.emedicine.com/oph/TOPIC52.HTM

National Eye Institute. (2006). *Age-related macular degeneration.* Retrieved June 3, 2008, from http://www.nei.nih.gov/health/maculardegen/armd_facts.asp

National Health and Medical Research Council (NHMRC). (1997). *Donating organs after death: Ethical issues.* Canberra, Australia: Australian Government Publishing Service.

Netland, P. A., & Allen, R. C. (Eds.). (1999). *Glaucoma medical therapy: Principles and management.* San Francisco: The Foundation of the American Academy of Ophthalmology.

Nguyen, Q. et al. (2004). Supplemental oxygen improves diabetic macular edema: A pilot study. *Investigative Ophthalmology & Visual Science, 45*(2), 617–624.

Nishiguchi, K. M., & Dryja, L. (2004, March). New eye disease: Light blindness. *EyeNet,* 13–14.

Nussenblatt, R. B., & Whitcup, S. M. (2004). *Uveitis: Fundamentals and clinical practice* (3rd ed.). Philadelphia: Mosby.

Oetting, T. A. (2001). A paradigm shift in cataract surgery: Less for the surgeon to do—More for the nurses and technicians to do. *Insight, 26*(1), 23–30.

Parrish, C. M., & Chandler, J. W. (1998). Corneal trauma. In H. Kaufman, B. Barron, & M. McDonald (Eds.), *The cornea* (2nd ed.). Boston: Butterworth-Heinemann.

PDR. (2004a). *Glaucoma: Disease management guide* (1st ed.). San Francisco: Allergan.

PDR. (2004b). *Physicians' desk reference for ophthalmic medicines* (32nd ed.). Montvale, NJ: Thomson.

Porth, C. M. (2007). *Essentials of pathophysiology: Concepts of altered health states.* Philadelphia: Lippincott Williams & Wilkins.

Pratt-Johnson, J. A., & Tillson, G. (2001). *Management of strabismus and amblyopia: A practice guide* (2nd ed.). New York: Thieme.

Rabinowitz, Y. (2005, August 29). *Corneal transplants.* Retrieved April 26, 2007, from http://www.laser-prk.com/corneal.htm

Robson, J., Behrman, A. J., & Abbuhl, S. (2007). Globe rupture. *Emedicine.* Retrieved June 18, 2008, from http://www.emedicine.com/emerg/TOPIC218.HTM

Rosenblatt, B. J., & Benson, W. E. (2004). Diabetic retinopathy. In M. Yanoff & J. S. Duker (Eds.), *Ophthalmology* (2nd ed.). St. Louis: Mosby.

Rosenfeld, P. J., & Gorin, M. B. (1999). Genetics. In J. W. Berger, S. L. Fine, & M. G. Maguire (Eds.), *Age-related macular degeneration*. St. Louis: Mosby.

Rougé, L. J. (2004, April). Breaking the blepharitis cycle. *EyeNet*, 25–26.

Rubenstein, J. B., & Jick, S. L. (2004). Disorders of the conjunctiva and limbus. In M. Yanoff & J. S. Duker (Eds.), *Ophthalmology* (2nd ed.). St. Louis: Mosby.

Ruiz-Moreno, J. M., Montero, J. A., Barile, S., & Zarbin, M. A. (2006). Photodynamic therapy and high-dose intravitreal triamcinolone to treat exudative age-related macular degeneration: 1-year outcome. *Retina*, 26(6), 602–612.

Schachat, A. P. (2001). Medical retina. In S. J. Ryan (Ed.), *Retina* (3rd ed., Vol. 2). St. Louis: Mosby.

Seal, D. V., Bron, A. J., & Hay, J. (1998). *Ocular infection: Investigation and treatment in practice*. St. Louis: Mosby.

Sharma, S., & Brown, G. C. (2001a). Ocular ischemic syndrome. In S. J. Ryan (Ed.), *Retina* (3rd ed., Vol. 2). St. Louis: Mosby.

Sharma, S., & Brown, G. C. (2001b). Retinal artery obstruction. In S. J. Ryan (Ed.), *Retina* (3rd ed., Vol. 2). St. Louis: Mosby.

Shields, J. A., & Shields, C. L. (1999a). *Atlas of eyelid and conjunctival tumors*. Philadelphia: Lippincott Williams & Wilkins.

Shields, J. A., & Shields, C. L. (1999b). *Atlas of intraocular tumors*. Philadelphia: Lippincott Williams & Wilkins.

Shields, J. A., & Shields, C. L. (1999c). *Atlas of orbital tumors*. Philadelphia: Lippincott Williams & Wilkins.

Sinclair, S. A., Smith, G. A., & Xiang, H. (2006). Eyeglasses-related injuries treated in U.S. emergency departments in 2002–2003. *Ophthalmic Epidemiology*, 13(1), 23–30.

Singerman, L. J., Brucker, A. J., Jampol, L. M., Lim, J. I., Rosenfeld, P., Schachat, A. P., et al. (2005). Neovascular age-related macular degeneration: Roundtable. *Retina*, 25(Suppl. 7), S1–S22.

Sjaarda, R. N., & Thompson, J. T. (2001). Macular hole. In S. J. Ryan (Ed.), *Retina* (3rd ed., Vol. 3). St. Louis: Mosby.

Spaide, R. F., & Fisher, Y. L. (2006). Intravitreal bevacizumab (avastin) treatment of proliferative diabetic retinopathy complicated by vitreous hemorrhage. *Retina*, 26(3), 275–278.

Steidl, S. M., & Hartnett, M. E. (2003). *Clinical pathways in vitreoretinal disease*. New York: Thieme.

Stewart, W. C. (2004). New (pending) glaucoma medical therapy. In M. Yanoff & J. S. Duker (Eds.), *Ophthalmology* (2nd ed.). St. Louis: Mosby.

Stone, E. M. (2007). Genetic testing for inherited eye disease. *Archives of Ophthalmology, 125*(2), 205–212.

Streeten, B. W. (2000). Pathology of the lens. In D. M. Albert & F. A. Jakobiec (Eds.), *Principles & practice of ophthalmology* (2nd ed., Vol. 4). Philadelphia: W. B. Saunders.

Thall, E. H., Thammano, P., & Miller, R. (2004). Perspectives in aberrations of the eye. In M. Yanoff & J. S. Duker (Eds.), *Ophthalmology* (2nd ed.). St. Louis: Mosby.

Tomany, S. C., Cruickshanks, K. J., Klein, R., Klein, B. E., & Knudtson, M. D. (2004). Sunlight and the 10-year incidence of age-related maculopathy. *Archives of Ophthalmology, 122*(5), 750–757.

Traverso, C. E., Bagnis, A., & Bricola, G. (2004). Angle-closure glaucoma. In M. Yanoff & J. S. Duker (Eds.), *Ophthalmology* (2nd ed.). St. Louis: Mosby.

Trobe, J. D. (2006). *The physician's guide to eye care* (3rd ed.). San Francisco: American Academy of Ophthalmology.

U.S. Census Bureau. (2000). Demographic profiles. Retrieved February 2, 2007, from http://www.census.gov/main/www/cen2000.html

U.S. Department of Health and Human Services (DHHS). (2000a). *Healthy People 2010: Vision and hearing*. Retrieved April 26, 2007, from http://www.healthypeople.gov/document/HTML/Volume2/28Vision.htm

U.S. Department of Health and Human Services (DHHS). (2000b). *Healthy Vision 2010*. Retrieved April 26, 2007, from http://www.healthyvision.2010.org

Vaughn, G. J., Dortzbach, R. K., & Gayre, G. S. (2004). Eyelid malignancies. In M. Yanoff & J. S. Duker (Eds.), *Ophthalmology* (2nd ed.). St. Louis: Mosby.

Visto, D. A. (2000). Corneal abrasion: To patch or not to patch. *Insight, 25*(1), 4–6.

Walker, R. S., & Piltz-Seymour, J. R. (2004). When to treat glaucoma. In M. Yanoff & J. S. Duker (Eds.), *Ophthalmology* (2nd ed.). St. Louis: Mosby.

Watson, P. G., Hazleman, B. L., Pavesio, C. E., & Green, W. R. (2004). *The sclera & systemic disorders* (2nd ed.). Philadelphia: Butterworth-Heinemann.

Williams, G. A., & Aaberg, T. (2001). Techniques of scleral buckling. In S. J. Ryan (Ed.), *Retina* (3rd ed., Vol. 3). St. Louis: Mosby.

Wilson, H. L., Schwartz, D. M., Bhatt, H. R., McCulloch, C. E., & Duncan, J. L. (2004). Statin and aspirin therapy are associated with decreased rates of choroidal neovascularization among patients with age-related macular degeneration. *American Journal of Ophthalmology, 137*(4), 615–624.

Wong, T., Klein, R., Nieto, F., Moraes, S., Mosley, T., Couper, D., et al. (2002). Is early age-related maculopathy related to cognitive function? The atherosclerosis risk in communities study. *American Journal of Ophthalmology, 134*(12), 828–835.

Wu, W., & Ariyasu, R. G. (1999). Cornea and external disease. In D. A. Lee & E. J. Higginbotham (Eds.), *Clinical guide to comprehensive ophthalmology*. New York: Thieme.

Yanoff, M., & Duker J. S. (Eds.). (2004). *Ophthalmology* (2nd ed.). St. Louis: Mosby.

Zimmerman, R., Sakiyalak, D., Krupin, T., & Rosenberg, L. F. (2004). Primary open-angle glaucoma. In M. Yanoff & J. S. Duker (Eds.), *Ophthalmology* (2nd ed.). St. Louis: Mosby.

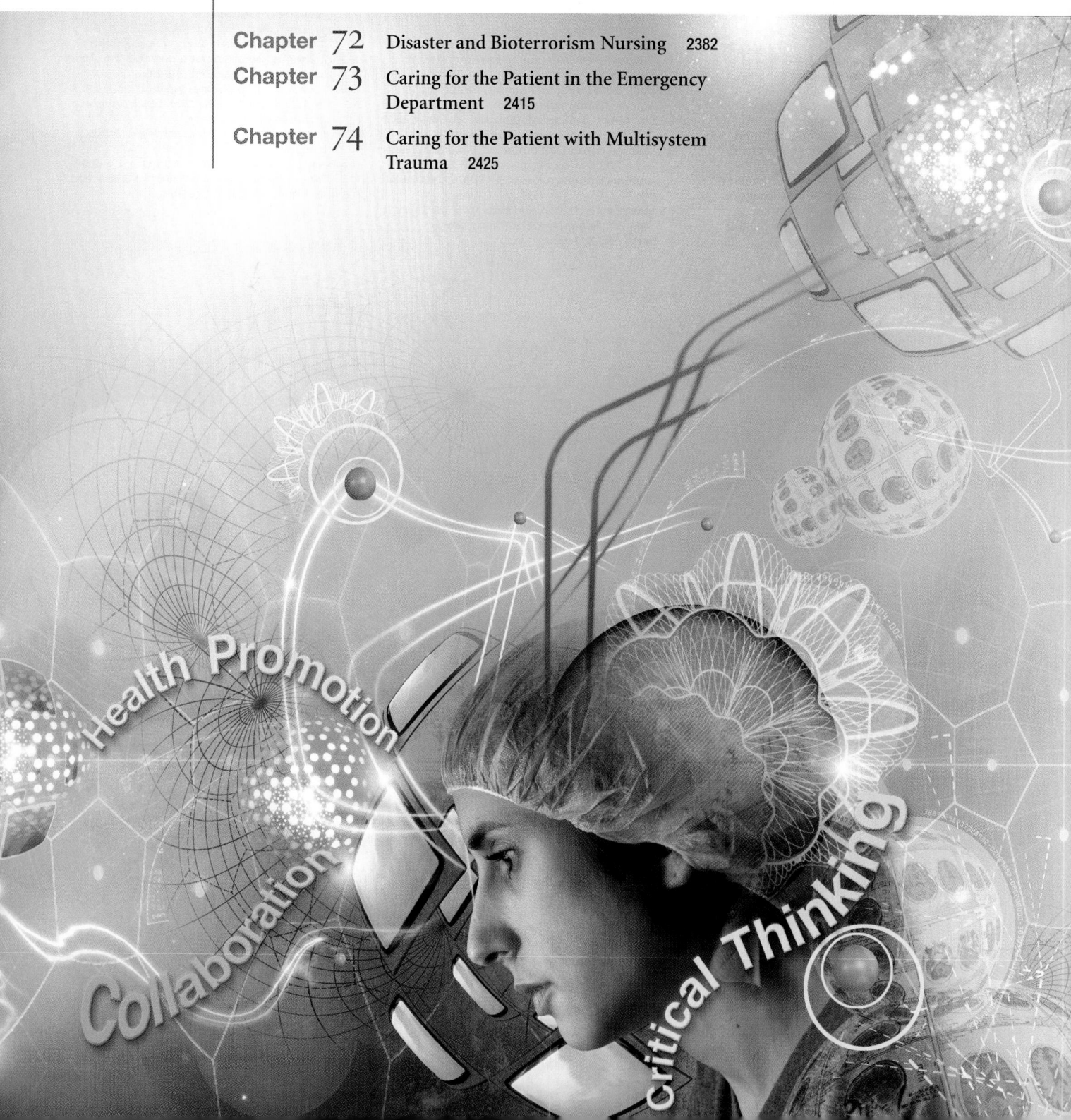

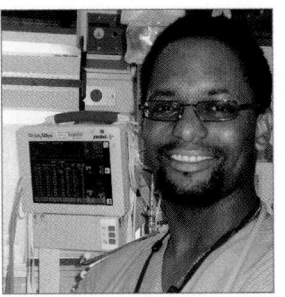

CHRISTOPHER My name is Christopher and I am a registered nurse and part of the specialized and unique staff that make up the Emergency Department (ED) in a large hospital. ED nurses specialize in variety and diversity because our patient population is everybody and everyone. The institution where I work is a Level I trauma teaching hospital in a midsize urban city serving hundreds of patients daily. We never close and offer all specialties of medical care for 24 hours out of every day. We see and do things during our typical workday that cannot be imagined. I function with my peers (physicians, pharmacists, nurses, technicians, respiratory therapists, etc.) in a collaborative effort with the goal of a better outcome for all those we encounter during our day.

Life is unpredictable as is the vast population of patients who visit the ED. With that being said, it is vital as an ED RN that I respond in a predictable, competent, and conscientious way. I have a commitment to those who come to the ED to respond with compassion and competence, doing all that I can to end my patients' "emergencies." As an RN, I am driven by the how and the why: How did this happen? Why did this happen?—two questions that are essentially behind what I and my colleagues do as medical professionals. A patient presents to the department with a chief complaint (CC) and as a collaborative team we attempt to answer the how/why questions. Sometimes the answers are straightforward, sometimes they are incomplete, but we are committed to finding the answer. Regardless of the seriousness of the complaint, the nurses in the ED treat all patients with the same level of comportment and caring.

Consider this example shift report: Today's assignment is the resuscitation room (RR), also known as the Trauma Bay. The RR is usually where patients who are severely ill or injured start for stabilization. It is important for ED nurses to have excellent assessment skills and a strong knowledge base about injury and illness so they can anticipate events that might occur.

The start of the shift is uneventful. One patient is in the RR; a restrained driver of a rollover motor vehicle crash (MVC). The patient is stable: three stable hematocrits, no fractures and some bumps and bruises, soon to be discharged home alive because "seat belts save lives!" I start to check the supplies in the room because it is important to be prepared at all times. The triage nurse tells me that a report has been received from the prehospital providers that they are bringing in a 19-year-old male who was found down at a party and could not be awakened. His level of consciousness is 9 out of 15 on the Glasgow Coma Scale (eyes, 2; verbal, 2; motor, 5) and decreasing. Fundamental to life are the ABCs: A = airway (EMS came in manually ventilating the patient, who is moved from stretcher to bed and the team moves quickly to secure an airway); B = breathing (something the patient is not doing effectively on his own, so he will need to be supported by a ventilator); and C = circulation (the patient's heart rate and blood pressure were within normal limits and not an immediate concern).

Having confidence in your coworkers and your own abilities allows many things to happen at once: The physicians prepare to intubate the patient as intravenous lines are established by the nurses and labs sent. The patient is stabilized with a safe effective airway, and within 25 minutes the patient is back from the CT scanner (no head injury) and moved to another area of the ED to "metabolize to freedom" (the patient's blood alcohol level was over four times the legal limit.)

I work 12-hour shifts. During that time I see and do too many things to begin to list. There are also those days where you feel that despite all of your efforts, something more could have been done. Every day there are emergencies, some are more subjective than others, but it is not my place to judge but to have compassion as I work with the patients. The patient who comes in after an MVC and succumbs to injuries, the patient with an active GI bleed who is stabilized and sent to the ICU, or the patient with just a burning sensation upon urination all receive the same attention and my total commitment.

> "I have a commitment to those who come to the ED to respond with compassion and competence, doing all that I can to end my patients' "emergencies.""

Disaster and Bioterrorism Nursing

Karen Silady

Outcome-Based Learning Objectives

After studying this chapter, the learner will be able to:

1. Define terrorism.
2. Describe the historical use of various agents.
3. Discuss various chemical agents, signs and symptoms, and treatment.
4. Compare and contrast biologic agents, signs and symptoms, and treatment.
5. Delineate the signs and symptoms of radiation illness.
6. Apply the principles of an incident command system in the hospital setting during a WMD event.
7. Describe the role of DMAT, DMORT, and the Strategic National Stockpile.
8. Apply critical incident stress principles to WMD events.

Research Collaboration Health Promotion Nursing Process Caring Critical Thinking

Terrorism is an act, the purpose of which is to disrupt daily life and/or to cause terror and panic. Terrorism is defined by the Federal Bureau of Investigation (FBI) as "the unlawful use of force or violence against persons or property to intimidate or coerce a Government, the civilian population, or any segment thereof, in furtherance of political or social objectives" (FBI, 2006).

The FBI further describes terrorism as "international" when the use of force or violence is committed by a group or individual that is foreign based and/or has some connection to a foreign power, or whose activities cross international boundaries. This can include groups such as al Qaeda in the Middle East, the Irish Republican Army (IRA) in Ireland, the Freedom for the Basque Homeland (Euskadi Ta Askatasuna: ETA) in Spain, and the individual suicide bombers in Israel (FBI, 2006).

Terrorism

Terrorism is defined as "domestic" when the group or individuals operate out of the United States or Puerto Rico without foreign direction and their activities are directed at the U.S. government or the U.S. population This includes such groups as the Ku Klux Klan, Greenpeace, white supremacist groups, the Black Panthers, and lone individuals such as Timothy McVeigh (FBI, 2006).

It is often said that one man's terrorist is another man's freedom fighter. Politics aside, the problem with terrorism for nursing is that it creates large numbers of dead and injured that will require physical as well as psychosocial care. In addition, those who have witnessed the event will also need psychosocial care to deal with what was witnessed.

Targets

Ideal targets for terrorists would be anything and anywhere that large-scale disruption would ensue and are often based on the idealism behind the terrorist group. This includes large gatherings of people; nuclear power plants; chemical plants; federal buildings and other governmental institutions; infrastructure systems such as public utilities; military installations; religious buildings such as churches, synagogues, and mosques; controversial businesses such as abortion clinics; and world headquarters of companies. The point of terrorist events is to attract media attention, increase support for the cause, undermine the government or the agency attacked, influence policy, and create a sense of vulnerability. Occasionally the purpose is solely revenge (Sidell, Patrick, Dashiell, Alibel, & Layne, 2002).

Historical Use of Various Agents

Terrorism is not a new phenomenon, and different agents have been used throughout history.

Chemical Agents

In war and in terrorist events, there are numerous accounts of the use of chemical weapons. The Chinese in 1000 B.C. used arsenic smoke as a weapon (Lee, 2003). During World War I, on April 15, 1915, the Germans released 150 tons of chlorine gas near Ypres, Belgium. Because chlorine is heavier than air, it hugged the ground and settled into the trenches of the allied forces. This characteristic gives chlorine its nickname "the dragon." There were approximately 800 deaths, but psychologically the event was devastating to the 15,000 troops, resulting in a complete retreat. Because the allies had gas masks, chlorine came to be more of a tactical weapon. On June 12, 1917, at a site near Ypres, sulfur mustard was released; sulfur affects the eyes, lungs, and skin. This caused 20,000 casualties and forced the troops to don hot, bulky protective clothing along with the gas masks (Christopher et al., 1997). Mustard was also used by Iraq against Iran from 1980 to 1988 and against Kurdish citizens in Halahja, Iraq, in 1988, resulting in 5,000 deaths (Durham, 2002; U.S. Army Medical Research Institute of Chemical Defense [USAMRICD], 2000).

In 1994 and again in 1995, the Aum Shinrikyo cult released sarin gas into the Tokyo subway system. This was accomplished by carrying dilute sarin in plastic bags and then puncturing the bags with the tip of an umbrella. Sarin is a very potent nerve gas that can cause death in minutes. It was first invented as an insecticide by the Germans in 1937. This incident in Tokyo is the largest disaster caused by a nerve gas during a time of peace (Lee, 2003).

Accidents with respect to chemical agents abound. In Bhopal, India, in 1984 there was the accidental release of 50,000 pounds of methyl isocyanate (composed of phosgene, methylamine, and isocyanate) from a Union Carbide plant, which killed thousands in the initial exposure, with ultimately over 150,000 casualties (Durham, 2002).

Biologic Agents

As long ago as the 6th century B.C., there is documented use of **biologic agents**, bacteria, viruses and toxins, in warfare. The Assyrians poisoned enemy water wells with rye ergot, a fungus that grows on rye. This causes hallucinations and cardiac problems.

During the French and Indian War (1754–1763), Jeffrey Amherst, commander of the British forces in North America, authorized blankets and handkerchiefs used by smallpox victims to be distributed to the Indians who were sympathetic to the French (Christopher, Cieslak, Pavlin, & Eitzen, 1997; Durham, 2002; Kortepeter, 2001). During World War I (1914–1918), there is credible evidence that German agents infected horses and cattle in the United States with glanders (*Burkholderia* [*Pseudomonas*] *mallei*) before the animals were shipped to France. There are multiple allegations of many other biologic agents having been used in a similar fashion during that war (Christopher et al., 1997; Durham, 2002; Kortepeter, 2001).

During World War II (1939–1945), the Japanese had an extensive biologic experimentation program. The program was centered near Pingfang with other sites in Mukden, Changchun, and Nanjing. Agents used included *Yersinia pestis, Vibrio cholerae, Shigella, Neisseria meningitidis,* and *Bacillus anthracis.* It is said that 10,000 prisoners died from infection or execution following infection experimentation. The United States was accused by North Korea, China, and the Soviet Union of using biologic weapons during the Korean War. During the Cold War, there were numerous allegations on all sides regarding the use of and experimentation with biologic agents. Then-President Richard Nixon by executive order terminated the United States offensive biologic weapons program in 1970 (toxins) and 1971 (microorganisms).

During the Vietnam War, pungi sticks were routinely used by the Vietcong. These were sharpened bamboo sticks placed in rice paddies that had been rubbed with human waste to create great infected sores. The famous "yellow rain" from that war caused people and animals to become disoriented and ill, including some fatalities. Although still controversial, it is believed that some of these were clouds of trichothecene toxins (T-2 mycotoxin). Others believe that these were simply large clouds of tropical bee feces (Christopher et al., 1997; Kortepeter, 2001).

In April 1979 in Sverdlovsk (now Yekaterinburg), Russia, there was an accidental release of anthrax from a military microbiology facility secondary to a significant problem with the air filters. At least 77 cases, with 66 deaths, due to inhalation of anthrax were reported in relation to this incident (Christopher et al., 1997; Kortepeter, 2001). In the fall of 1984, there was a large salmonella outbreak in the city of The Dalles, Oregon. It was traced back to a religious commune, the Rajneeshees, who had intentionally contaminated a local salad bar with *Salmonella typhimurium.* This resulted in 751 cases of enteritis and 45 hospitalizations (Christopher et al., 1997; Torok et al., 1997).

The Bulgarian defector Georgi Markov lived in London. He was assassinated in 1978 by Bulgarian agents who had shot him in the leg with a pellet using a spring-loaded weaponized umbrella. The pellet had been hollowed out and filled with ricin, then sealed with wax that melts at body temperature. It is believed that similar weapons have been used in 60 known assassinations (Christopher et al., 1997).

Radiologic Agents

The only known wartime use of nuclear devices was the bombing of Nagasaki and Hiroshima by the United States during World War II (Jacocks, 2003; Udeani & Aguilera, 2002). This is widely accredited with assisting in ending the war.

In 1979 there was a small accidental leak of radiation at the Three Mile Island nuclear power plant in the Unites States from an overheated reactor coil. Over 2,000 lawsuits were filed, although no effects on physical health were ever documented. All the lawsuits were eventually dismissed (Raso, 1999).

On April 26, 1986, the Chernobyl Nuclear Reactor Unit 4 accidentally released a large cloud of radioactivity 80 miles northwest of Kiev in the Ukraine. This cloud was known to have gone over Belorussia, the Baltic republics, and headed toward Scandinavia. Due to many political factors at the time, acknowledgment of the incident by the then–Soviet Union took over 7 days. There are 56 official victims recorded, but virtually no data are available regarding numbers of casualties from this incident (World Nuclear Association, 2008; Jacocks, 2003). Much of what is known regarding radiation injuries comes from the Japanese incidents in World War II, Chernobyl, and Soviet weapons workers who had little to no safety procedures for protection (Jacocks, 2003).

Alexander Litvinenko, a former Russian spy, was poisoned with polonium-210 in the autumn of 2006. It is suspected that he was poisoned while dining in a restaurant in London. He ultimately died of acute radiation sickness (BBC, 2007).

Explosive Agents

The chronicles of war over the centuries are filled with the use of explosive devices since the invention of gunpowder. In the United States, recent incidents include 168 deaths and 759 injured from the bombing of the Alfred P. Murrah Federal Building in Oklahoma City April 19, 1995, by Timothy McVeigh. He made a bomb using items commonly found in home improvement stores (WashingtonPost.com, 1998).

The World Trade Center, which ultimately collapsed when struck by airplanes in the September 11, 2001, terrorist incident, was also bombed in 1993 with 6 deaths and 1,000 injured (Durham, 2002). The September 11, 2001, attack by al Qaeda of flying hijacked planes into the World Trade Center, the Pentagon, and then crashing one plane in Pennsylvania resulted in approximately 3,000 deaths. The 1996 Summer Olympics in Atlanta, Georgia, were rocked by an explosion in Centennial Park killing 1 person and injuring at least 100 (Cable News Network [CNN], 1996).

Worldwide, the recent frequent suicide bombings in Israel have given health care professionals extensive experience in caring for the victims of blast injuries. Frequent worldwide and local threats are defused prior to explosion or injury. A recent event involved police defusing an 8-pound bomb planted at the Pamplona Running of the Bulls festival in Spain in July 2003 by Freedom for the Basque Homeland (Euskadi Ta Askatasuna: ETA) (BBC, 2003).

Planning for Disasters

Dr. Eric Auf der Heide, from the U.S. Department of Health and Human Services, reviewed the literature regarding "lessons learned" from actual disasters and wrote:

> Disaster planning is only as good as the assumptions on which it is based. However, some of these assumptions are derived from a conventional wisdom that is at variance with empirical field disaster research studies. Knowledge of disaster research findings might help planners avoid common disaster management pitfalls, thereby improving disaster response planning. (Auf der Heide, 2006)

He then compared common assumptions about disasters and compared them with research findings, and discussed the implications for planning. Chart 72–1 presents these findings.

National Standards of Nursing Education

There was a time when nursing education regarding terrorism in the United States was considered unnecessary. Because of the events surrounding the September 11, 2001, World Trade Center disaster in New York, this education is now considered core information for all nurses. Since August 29, 2005, the events surrounding Hurricanes Katrina and Rita have forced the nation to focus on disaster response. Although this chapter focuses on terrorism and the issues involved, it is recognized that an all-hazards approach to planning and response is necessary.

In the aftermath of Hurricane Katrina, President George W. Bush, in a speech from Jackson Square in New Orleans in 2005, announced his order to the Department of Homeland Security

to review all emergency plans in every major city in America. The final results of that study were published June 16, 2006, entitled *Nationwide Plan Review Phase 2 Report* (Chertoff, 2006). In this report, 15 major areas of deficiency for state and urban areas were identified, including such things as a clear command structure, care of special needs populations, patient tracking, communication, and the ability to provide care for large numbers of casualties. Regardless of the cause of the catastrophe, whether terrorism or hurricane, the nurse needs to be prepared to work within an alternate structure and care for numerous patients, often with fewer resources.

Gebbie and Qureshi (2002) published a simple set of competencies for working nurses in regard to emergency and disaster preparedness based on previous work done for public health workers in the American Journal of Nursing (Chart 72–2, p. 2386). This has become something of a classic work and is frequently quoted.

The International Nursing Coalition for Mass Casualty Education (**INCMCE**), now called the Nursing Emergency Preparedness Education Coalition (NEPEC), coordinated by Vanderbilt University, consists of representatives from nursing education, nursing organizations, accrediting bodies, and governmental agencies. This coalition has a stated purpose to "assure a competent nurse workforce to respond to mass casualty incidents" (INCMCE, 2003). The INCMCE has published a lengthy document "Educational Competencies for Registered Nurses Responding to Mass Casualty Incidents." This document defines core competencies in the areas of critical thinking, assessment, technical skills, and communication. It describes core knowledge in the areas of health promotion, risk reduction, and disease prevention; health care systems and policies; illness and disease management; information and health care technologies; ethics; and human diversity. It also defines professional role development.

In the post–September 11th environment, multiple agencies and groups have developed educational programs regarding terrorism and health care with varying levels of complexity and varying focus. A recent Google.com search with key words "terrorism education" delivered almost 27 million sites. The vast majority of these programs are still grossly based on a handful of core government/military documents considered by experts to be the most solid sources of information available today about biologic, chemical, and radiologic agents (Chart 72–3, p. 2387).

◼ Types of Events

Because of the massive damage and injury caused, the agents used by many terrorists are termed *weapons of mass destruction* (**WMD**). Although there are numerous acronyms for these agents, the acronym suggested for common use by the Department of Justice is **CBRNE,** which stands for chemical, biologic, radiologic, nuclear, and explosive devices, with incendiary (fire-causing) devices being included under explosive devices. Depending on the agent used and the target, many vectors, or means, of spreading the agent are available. These include spraying devices, letters and packages, contaminated water or food, insects and animals, and the wind. The various agents enter the body in basically one of four ways: ingestion, inhalation, injection, or dermal exposure.

Effective dissemination can be difficult. Many agents must be finely aerosolized and some clump in humid weather. The device

CHART 72–1	**Common Disaster Planning Assumptions versus Research Observations**		
Assumption	**Research Observation**	**Planning Implications**	**Potential Interventions**
Dispatchers will hear of the disaster and send emergency response units to the scene.	Emergency response units, both local and distant, will often self-dispatch.	Effective disaster planning requires planning not only for the jurisdiction but also at the intercommunity level. Plans should anticipate the likelihood that more help than needed will arrive, whether requested or not.	Expect unsolicited responders, and develop a plan for coordinating them. Establish intercommunity or statewide mutual aid plans and training. Use staging or check-in areas outside of rapidly established security perimeters.
Trained emergency personnel will carry out field search and rescue.	Most initial search and rescue is carried out by the survivors themselves.	Planners may incorrectly assume that they will have control over disaster emergency medical service (EMS) responses. Disaster search and rescue is often ad hoc and uncoordinated. Even if they are not part of the planned response, law enforcement officers often become involved in search and rescue. Survivors involved in search and rescue may have the best information on the location of the missing.	Train first responders how to coordinate with survivors carrying out search and rescue. Designate personnel to obtain information from survivors about the location of the missing.
Trained EMS personnel will carry out triage, provide first aid, or stabilize medical care, and if necessary decontaminate casualties before patient transport.	Casualties are likely to bypass on-site triage, first aid, and decontamination stations and go directly to hospitals.	Hospitals should not assume that casualties will be triaged, decontaminated, or given first aid in the field. Patients arriving in private cars may need to be extricated carefully so that injuries are not aggravated.	Develop real-time instructions that can be given to survivors (by commercial radio) on how to protect themselves; give first aid; and deal with contaminated casualties. Provide courses on first aid, search and rescue, and disaster care for the public. Send first responders to hospitals to extricate casualties from private vehicles.
Casualties will be transported to hospitals by ambulance.	Most casualties are not transported by ambulance. Rather, they arrive at hospitals by a variety of nonambulance vehicles (private cars, police vehicles, buses, or on foot).	EMS authorities often have little control over time of transport or hospital destination for disaster casualties. Transport outside of the EMS system also poses challenges for patient tracking.	Educate the public about precautions to take when transporting casualties and about which should not be moved. Establish procedures for collecting information after the fact from hospitals about what casualties they have received.
Casualties will be transported to hospitals appropriate for their needs and in such a manner that no hospital receives a disproportionate number.	Most casualties are transported to the closest or most familiar hospitals.	Although specific hospitals may be designated to receive contaminated casualties, it is the patients who will often choose their destination. Thus, all hospitals must be prepared to do decontamination. Although it may not be possible to prevent inefficient casualty distribution, it may be possible to influence or plan around it.	Consider having ambulances bypass hospitals closest to the disaster. Establish area and intercommunity EMS/hospital mutual aid plans and radio systems so that ambulances can be directed to hospitals best able to treat their patients. Use a "first-wave" protocol to divide initial casualties among area hospitals.

(continued)

CHART 72–1 **Common Disaster Planning Assumptions versus Research Observations—*Continued***

Assumption	Research Observation	Planning Implications	Potential Interventions
Authorities in the field will ensure that area hospitals are promptly notified of the disaster and the numbers, types, and severities of casualties to be transported to them.	Hospital notification of a disaster may be from the first arriving victims or the news media rather than from the authorities in the field. Often, information and updates about incoming casualties are insufficient or lacking.	Initial hospital response may have to depend on the resources in house. Hospital procedures that require time-consuming activities before casualty arrival (donning chemical-resistant suits, etc.) may not be practical.	Base initial hospital response plans on in-house rather than on-call resources. Provide in-house staff with authority to activate and modify the plan. Develop plans for the expedient decontamination of unannounced casualties, which might include the use of fire hoses supplied with warm water, until more sophisticated decontamination equipment can be set up.
The most serious casualties will be the first to be transported to hospitals.	The least serious casualties often arrive first.	Because accurate and timely information from the field is often lacking, emergency departments (EDs) may not know of the more serious patients yet to come. As a result, when these patients arrive, they may find all beds occupied.	Assign field responders to communicate casualty information to hospitals. Hold beds open at hospitals for the possibility of later arriving, more serious casualties.

CHART 72–2 **Emergency and Disaster Preparedness Core Competencies for Nurses**

1. Describe the agency's role in responding to a range of emergencies that might arise.
2. Describe the chain of command in emergency response.
3. Identify and locate the agency's emergency response plan (or the pertinent portion of it).
4. Describe emergency response functions or roles, and demonstrate them in regularly performed drills.
5. Demonstrate the use of equipment (including personal protective equipment) and the skills required in emergency response during regular drills.
6. Demonstrate the correct operation of all equipment used for emergency communication.
7. Describe communication roles in emergency response.
8. Identify the limits of one's own knowledge, skills, and authority, and identify key system resources for referring matters that exceed these limits.
9. Apply creative problem-solving skills and flexible thinking to the situation, within the confines of one's role, and evaluate the effectiveness of all actions taken.
10. Recognize deviations from the norm that might indicate an emergency and describe appropriate action.
11. Participate in continuing education to maintain up-to-date knowledge in relevant areas.
12. Participate in evaluating every drill or response and identify necessary changes to the plan.

ADDITIONAL CORE COMPETENCIES FOR MANAGERS

13. Ensure that there is a written plan for major categories of emergencies.
14. Ensure that all parts of the plan are practiced regularly.
15. Ensure that gaps in knowledge or skills are filled.

Source: Gebbie, K. M., & Qureshi, K. (2002). Emergency and disaster preparedness: Core competencies for nurses. *American Journal of Nursing, 1*(102), 46–51. With permission.

may be technically difficult to use. The so-called "shoe bomber" was caught because he could not get the bomb fuse to light with repeated strikes of his lighter. The agent can potentially be hazardous to the terrorist, requiring extensive protective gear such as with some of the biologic agents.

Identification of an incident can be difficult, especially if the agent is one in which the symptoms have a delayed onset from the time of exposure. Patients will self-present to a variety of health care facilities, so there often is a delay before the event is recognized. It is important to maintain a high index of suspicion.

The key is in recognizing clusters. In chemical events, this would include the symptoms suggestive of the agent (Agency for Toxic Substances and Disease Registry [ATSDR], 2001a, 2001b; Community Research Associates [CRA], 2003: USAMRICD, 2000).

In biologic agents, it is harder to discern initially without a direct clue such as a threatening note or direct identification of munitions or tampering. Biologic clusters are found using usual public health epidemiologic methodology. Clues would include a large epidemic of a particular set of symptoms, more severe symptoms than are usually seen for a particular pathogen, an

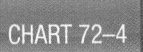

CHART 72–3   Core Sources of Information Regarding Terrorism Response

Agency for Toxic Substances and Disease Registry (ATSDR). (2001). *Managing hazardous materials incidents.* Atlanta, GA: U.S. Department of Health and Human Services.

Three-volume set from the U.S. Public Health Service.

Jacocks, J. (Ed.). (2003). *Medical management of radiological casualties* (2nd ed.). Bethesda, MD: Armed Forces Radiobiology Research Institute.

The armed forces' handbook for nuclear and radiologic agents.

Kortepeter, M. (Ed.). (2001). *USAMRIID's medical management of biological casualties handbook* (4th ed.). Fort Detrick, MD: U.S. Army Medical Research Institute of Infectious Diseases.

The armed forces' handbook for biologic agents.

Sidell, F. R., Patrick, W. C., Dashiell, T. R., Alibek, K., & Layne, S. (Eds.). (2002). *Jane's chem-bio book* (2nd ed.). Alexandria, VA: Jane's Information Group.

A handbook developed by a think tank regarding chemical and biologic agents.

U.S. Army Medical Research Institute of Chemical Defense (USAMRICD). (2000). *Medical management of chemical casualties handbook* (3rd ed.). Aberdeen Proving Ground, MD: Author.

The armed forces' handbook regarding chemical agents.

U.S. Department of Transportation (DOT). (2008). *2008 Emergency response guidebook.** Washington, DC: U.S. Government Printing Office.

The core hazardous materials book used in the United States, Mexico, and Canada.

Websites

http://www.bt.cdc.gov

The Centers for Disease Control and Prevention's website. Is a center of information pertaining to all aspects of terrorism and health care.

http://www.emsa.ca.gov

The California Emergency Medical Services Authority (EMSA) website. Has the entire hospital incident command system (HICS) and training available; free downloading.

*Also available at http://hazmat.dot.gov/pubs/erg/guidebook.htm

CHART 72–4   Personal Protective Equipment Levels

LEVEL A

Highest level of respiratory, skin, and eye

Fully encapsulated chemical-resistant suit

Full face piece and supplied air (self-contained breathing apparatus, or SCBA)

Inner chemical-resistant gloves

Chemical-resistant safety boots

"Moon suit"

LEVEL B

Same respiratory as Level A but less skin

Full face piece and supplied air (SCBA)

Chemical-resistant clothing

Inner and outer chemical-resistant gloves

Chemical-resistant safety boots

Hard hat

LEVEL C

Full face piece with air purifying canister–equipped respirator

Chemical-resistant clothing

Hard hat

LEVEL D

Regular work clothing

Safety shoes

Safety goggles/splash shield

unusual disease or a disease unusual for the region, unusual strains, and a large number of cases of unexplained disease or death. The onset of a biologic agent event would depend on the agent used, especially the incubation period (Kortepeter, 2001). Illness in the animal population often will act as a herald that a significant event is occurring.

Symptoms, clustering, and onset in radiologic incidents depend greatly on the type of radiation involved and the delivery method. A radiological dispersion device (**RDD**), or so-called "dirty bomb," would have a different presentation than a fission device (atomic bomb) (CRA, 2003; Jacocks, 2003). Note that the likelihood of the use of a fission device in a terrorist event is considered very low. Explosions are fairly easy to identify because they create patients with traumatic injuries.

Personal Protective Equipment

Personal protective equipment (**PPE**) is the clothing and equipment that are protective to the person from whatever agent to which one is exposed, be it chemical, biologic, or radiologic. PPE is classified according to the degree of protection it delivers: Level A, Level B, Level C, and Level D (Chart 72–4, and Figures 72–1

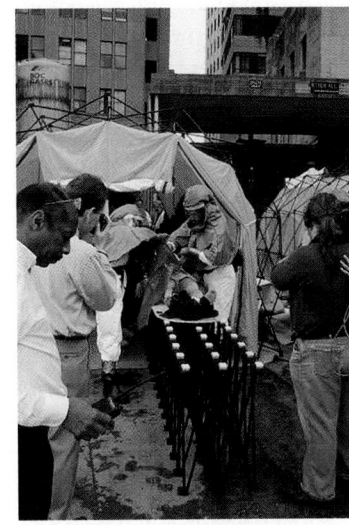

FIGURE 72–1 ■ Decontamination drill in PPE suit.
Source: Photo courtesy of Robert J. McBride RN, New Orleans

and 72–2 ■, p. 2388). Many daily exposures to hazardous materials that are not even related to terrorist events will require personal protection and perhaps even decontamination.

No one suit is protective for all agents. Factors to determine the level of PPE to use include not only the agent but also other practical matters such as the temperature, humidity, body size,

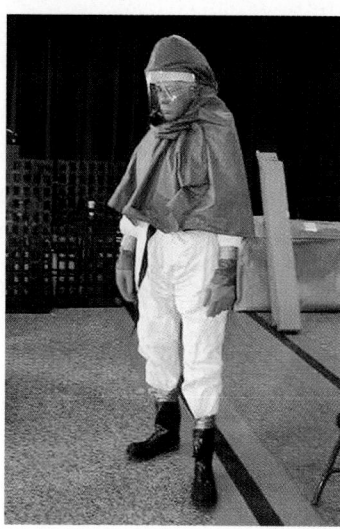

FIGURE 72–2 ■ PPE suit.
Source: Photo courtesy of Robert J. McBride RN, New Orleans

facial hair, and strenuousness of the expected activity. There are many problems with PPE for the user, including hyperthermia, dehydration, and claustrophobia. In addition, there are limited vision, limited dexterity, limited movement, and communication problems. During operations, there need to be preset hand signals indicating distress that can be used by the person in the gear.

Proper donning and doffing of PPE are essential to prevent contamination. Extensive training and practice are required. Proper donning includes such things as correct use of all gear, taping all openings, and checking for breaches in gear before entering contaminated area; there need to be specific checklists for removing protective clothing at the end of an incident or end of a tour of duty. The person in the PPE will require decontamination before being allowed into noncontaminated areas.

While wearing the PPE, there is constant concern about possible breach of protection as well as whether the level of protection is appropriate for the situation. In general, the greater the level of protection, the greater the risk of an adverse effect. There are very specific medical criteria regarding who is allowed to don higher level PPE. Once in the PPE, the safety officer and medical management personnel must monitor the wearer for problems (ATSDR, 2001a, 2001b; Hick et al., 2003; Lehmann, 2002; Sidell et al., 2002; USAMRICD, 2000). The United States Department of Labor, Occupational Safety and Health Administration (OSHA) published the final draft of *OSHA Best Practices for Hospital-Based First Receivers of Victims from Mass Casualty Incidents Involving the Release of Hazardous Substances* in January 2005 (OSHA, 2005). This document contains recommendations for PPE purchasing and training based on a hospital's hazard analysis. Safety concerns for the personnel wearing the PPE are also discussed.

Level A

Level A protection is the highest level of protection for the skin, eyes, mucous membranes, and respiratory system. This is what is commonly referred to as the "moon suit." Level A has a fully encapsulated, vapor-tight, chemical-resistant suit; chemical-resistant boots/shoes with steel toe and shank; chemical-resistant inner

and outer gloves; coveralls; hard hat; two-way communications system; and completely self-contained breathing apparatus (SCBA). There are cooling units available to extend the time a person can tolerate being in these suits as well as lower level suits.

SCBA has a full face piece connected to a compressed air source. Some are closed circuit. This system uses a small tank of supplemental oxygen, and recycled exhaled gases are rebreathed ("rebreather"). The open circuit SCBA has a tank of air, and the exhaled air is released into the atmosphere. SCBAs give the person freedom to travel within the time limit of the air bottle. Supplied air respirators (SARs) have a long hose that attaches the person to a more distant air supply. This system limits the person to an area the length of the air supply hose, but the person has no time limit on air supply. SCBAs and SARs require individual fit testing (ATSDR, 2001a, 2001b; Hick et al., 2003; Sidell et al., 2002; USAMRICD, 2000).

Level B

Level B is similar to Level A except that chemical protective clothing (CPC) is used instead of the fully encapsulating suit. This provides splash protection but is not vapor proof. Chemical protective clothing includes two-piece chemical splash suits, disposable chemical-resistant overalls, and other chemical-resistant clothing. Inner and outer resistant gloves and resistant steel toe and shank boots are used. SCBA is used with a full face shield. Level B is the minimum level recommended for initial entry into sites until the hazard has been identified.

Chemical protective clothing can be affected by chemical degradation of the suit, whereby through aging or contact with a chemical the suit's structural integrity is damaged. Level B does use the self-contained breathing apparatus. Chemicals can eventually permeate protective clothing depending on the exact chemical. Manufacturer's literature will include permeation "breakthrough" times for various chemicals. Penetration of the suit occurs when the integrity is breached; there may be an opening in the suit (such as an untaped zipper), the suit tears, or the suit has a defect (ATSDR, 2001a, 2001b; Hick et al., 2003; Sidell et al., 2002; USAMRICD, 2000).

Level C

By the time patients arrive to a hospital or other health care facility, they will have had a prolonged exposure to the agent and yet are still alive. Many hospitals and health care facilities therefore use a Level B suit with Level C respiratory protection. Level C consists of full face piece with an air purifying canister–equipped respirator and chemical-resistant clothing. This level is used when skin and eye exposures are unlikely, the agent is known, and the criteria for the exact respiratory equipment being used are met.

Air purifying respirators (APRs) and powered air purifying respirators (PAPRs) purify ambient air based on the type of canister and filter connected to the system. PAPRs use a battery-operated blower that delivers essentially decontaminated air at slight positive pressure into a face piece. Both APRs and PAPRs can protect against particulates, some gases, and vapors, depending on the filters, absorbents, and canisters used. When used with high efficiency particulate air filtration (HEPA filters) in combination with organic vapor cartridges, a level of biologic protection can be achieved. Radiologically contaminated particles can also be trapped (ATSDR, 2001a, 2001b; Hick et al., 2003; Sidell et al., 2002; 3M, 2002; USAMRICD, 2000).

Level D

Level D PPE is regular clothing. It affords simple protection, but no respiratory or skin protection. Safety goggles, splash shields, and regular latex-type gloves can be considered part of Level D protection (ATSDR, 2001a, 2001b; Hick et al., 2003; Sidell et al., 2002; USAMRICD, 2000).

Decontamination

Decontamination is the reduction or removal of contaminating agents. In instances of radiologic contamination, the point is to remove the radioactive contaminants. In these cases, the runoff needs to be contained. Decontamination in the hospital or health care setting can involve persons who received "gross" decontamination at the scene prior to arrival and persons who presented to the facility outside of the emergency medical services route without any prior treatment. It is important to recognize that contaminated persons must be fully decontaminated before being admitted to the facility to prevent the facility from being contaminated. The axiom is "there are no patients until they are decontaminated." Victims, first responders from the scene, equipment, and personnel assisting with the process all will undergo decontamination.

Gross decontamination, or field decontamination, is a process whereby the greater part of the agent is removed or washed away. This is usually done by some type of high-volume rinse system such as systems created using fire hoses. It is estimated that 80% of the agent can be removed by simply removing the clothing (ATSDR, 2001a, 2001b; Jacocks, 2003; Medical Center of Louisiana at New Orleans (MCLNO), 2003; Sidell et al., 2002; Texas Engineering Extension Service, National Emergency Response and Rescue Training Center [TEEX], 2003; USAMRICD, 2000).

The area set up for decontamination is outside. In setting up this area, there are three zones: the hot zone, warm zone, and cold zone. It is best if the hospital is upwind of the decontamination area. The **hot zone**, also called the exclusion or red zone, is the area of highest contamination. This is where persons waiting to be decontaminated are staged. There is usually

a triage area set up here to sort those requiring quicker treatment (see the START Triage section later in this chapter), and each person receives a numbered tag. A brief registration is done to collect basic information such as name, date of birth, and social security number. This is logged with the triage number. Many hospitals have prenumbered sets of triage kits with tags, registration sheets, and belongings bags on the disaster cart.

The **warm zone,** or yellow zone, is also referred to as the contamination reduction corridor (Figure 72–3 ■). This is where the actual decontamination process takes place. The **cold zone,** or green zone, is also known as the support zone. The hospital is in the cold zone. No one is allowed into the cold zone without being decontaminated (ATSDR 2001a, 2001b; MCLNO, 2003; Sidell et al., 2002; TEEX, 2003; USAMRICD, 2000). Chart 72–5 outlines the three zones of decontamination.

The decontamination lines are usually divided into male and females, and also into those who are ambulatory and the nonambulatory. The first step is to disrobe completely. Clothing is generally collected in red bags and labeled. Personal belongings, such as watches, wallets, jewelry, and eyeglasses, are usually collected in clear plastic bags and labeled. In the shower area, the person will fully lather up, including in all body creases, the hair, and the genital area. Attention should be directed toward contaminated wounds first, as agents are more rapidly absorbed by broken skin. There has been controversy regarding the best agents for decontamination. Common current consensus is some type of liquid soap or baby shampoo. A 0.5% bleach is still used for some equipment decontamination. For those who are ambulatory, only guidance will be needed in the process of being cleaned. The nonambulatory patients will require physical washing by specially trained personnel in full personal protective gear. Once washing is complete, they will dry off, are given some type of hospital gown or clothing, and are admitted into the cold zone disposition area from where they are sent into the hospital system (ATSDR, 2001a, 2001b; MCLNO, 2003; Sidell et al., 2002; TEEX, 2003; USAMRICD, 2000).

In suspected terrorist events, all of the clothing and personal belongings collected are considered evidence from a crime scene. The Federal Bureau of Investigation (FBI) will confiscate these items as evidence. It is important that these items be handled using usual chain-of-custody procedures. If the personal items can be decontaminated, after the FBI is finished with these items, an effort is made to return them to the correct owner (ATSDR, 2001a, 2001b; MCLNO, 2003; Sidell et al., 2002; TEEX, 2003; USAMRICD, 2000).

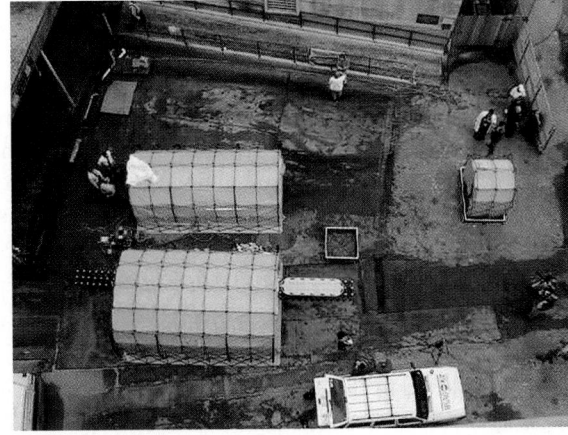

FIGURE 72–3 ■ Decontamination setup.
Source: Photo courtesy of Robert J. McBride RN, New Orleans

CHART 72–5	**Zones of Decontamination**	
Hot Zone	**Warm Zone**	**Cold Zone**
Red	Yellow	Green
Patient entry	Decontamination	Clean treatment area
EMS access	Ambulatory	Clean evacuation
Triage	Nonambulatory	Staging area for personnel
Initial disrobing		
Emergency first aid		

Chemical Agents

Chemical agents are generally considered either industrial or military depending on their use. From here they are further divided based on the military's original view on how these chemicals affect the body. Chemical agents include nerve agents and vesicants, or blistering agents, which are generally considered to be military agents only. Blood agents, choking agents, and irritants are the other categories, and they are mostly toxic industrial chemicals (Chart 72–6).

Spread

Most dissemination of chemical agents is by aerosol. The spread of chemical agents by this method depends on the agent's vapor pressure, how fast it goes from a liquid to a gas at room temperature, and its vapor density, its weight relative to air. High vapor pressure agents evaporate quickly, such as acetone (fingernail polish remover). High vapor density agents, such as chlorine, tend to sink and hug the ground. Low vapor pressure agents and high vapor density agents are said to be **persistent**, that is, they stay around for a long time, creating a hazardous environment for a longer period and thus a longer exposure time. An agent is considered persistent if it lasts longer than 24 hours as a liquid on surfaces. Persistent agents such as mustard and VX become useful in denying access to an area or to materials. Nonpersistent agents, such as sarin (used in the Tokyo attacks) and cyanide, are more useful as tactical agents within a population (ATSDR, 2001a, 2001b; CRA, 2003; Sidell et al., 2002; USAMRICD, 2000).

Nursing Management of the Patient Exposed to Chemical Agents

Nursing management of the patient exposed to chemical agents depends greatly on the agent and the severity of the exposure. Application of the nursing process will facilitate a comprehensive approach to patient assessment and care. Nursing diagnoses depend on the agent and symptoms seen. For all chemical agents, *Risk for Injury* related to gross contamination with chem-

ical will apply. Patient assessment parameters will follow the signs and symptoms expected, based on the class of agent. (A sample Nursing Process: Patient Care Plan for nerve agents is in the Nerve Agents section, p. 2392.)

Collaborative Management

The main categories of nerve agents, vesicants, blood agents, choking agents, and irritants are presented with common signs and symptoms and basic treatment. Much of the care is symptomatic. All patients with chemical exposure require comprehensive care from a health care team including nurses, health care providers, toxicologists, and specialists from all fields, depending on the nature and severity of the injury. Psychological and emotional care of these patients needs to be included while providing physical care.

Routes of Entry

There are several means for chemical agents to be spread. It is important to attempt to identify the route of entry in order to identify other potential patients.

Ingestion

Chemicals can be put in food, medicines, and water or other liquids. Ingestion through the public water supply is a less likely scenario due to dilution and the treatment water receives at the plants. Water wells and individual buildings are considered more likely targets. An example of the oral route was the 1982 episode of product tampering whereby bottles of Tylenol were contaminated with cyanide and seven people died. Although the casualty count was low, it created tremendous terror in the population (ATSDR, 2001a, 2001b; CRA, 2003; USAMRICD, 2000).

Inhalation

Inhalation is considered the most common route for chemicals, as most episodes of chemical agent release will be by aerosol. Many devices can be used for dissemination including mosquito trucks, aerial sprayers such as crop dusters, and various industrial spray equipment pieces including pesticide sprayers, wind dispersion, and using buildings' heating and cooling systems. The new term for this activity is *aerobiology* (ATSDR, 2001a, 2001b; CRA, 2003; USAMRICD, 2000).

Injection

Injection can be by needle or dart or any other sharp object such as broken glass. The number of casualties is low by this method. Other injection methods include the shrapnel from a chemical dispersion devise. The shrapnel containing the chemical in the device would enter the body and be absorbed into the tissue (ATSDR, 2001b; CRA, 2003; USAMRICD, 2000).

Dermal Exposure

Dermal exposure would cause external damage to the skin and eyes. It could then be absorbed through the skin and into the body. This would occur through either an aerosol release or an intention spill. With an aerosol release, the agent would have to have a high vapor density so that it would fall on the intended population. With an intentional spill, the agent would most likely be persistent in nature (ATSDR, 2001b; CRA, 2003; USAMRICD, 2000).

CHART 72–6	**Chemical Agents by Class**
NERVE AGENTS	**CHOKING AGENTS (ASPHYXIATES)**
Sarin (GB)	Ammonia
Soman (GD)	Chlorine
Tabun (GA)	Phosgene
V agent (VX)	
	IRRITANTS
VESICANTS	Mace (CN)
Mustard	Tear gas (CS)
Lewisite	Pepper spray (OC)
Phosgene oxime	
BLOOD AGENTS	
Hydrogen cyanide	
Cyanogen chloride	

Nerve Agents

Nerve agents are the most toxic of the known chemical agents. During World War II, Germany developed many nerve agents but for unknown reasons never used them. The only known use of nerve agents was in the Iran–Iraq War and by terrorists. Nerve agents work in a manner similar to organophosphate insecticides in that they inactivate acetylcholinesterase, thereby increasing the acetylcholine at the receptor site. This process results in an overstimulation at the synapse. The effect on the patient is dose related. The most common routes of exposure are inhaled and topical. The agents are readily absorbed from the skin and eyes.

The signs and symptoms seen, which are the same as with organophosphate poisoning, are remembered by the mnemonic SLUDGEM: salivation, lacrimation, urination, defecation, gastric upset, emesis, and miosis. Often there is a complaint of dim vision. The nerve agents also cause cardiac dysrhythmias, confusion, fasciculations and convulsions, along with unconsciousness. Almost all people affected by a nerve agent will have miosis, and most will have a runny nose and shortness of breath. The combination of pinpoint pupils and muscle fasciculations is the most reliable sign of nerve poisoning (Abramowicz, 2002; Dang, Kare, Schneiderman, & Dang, 2002; McKee et al., 2000; Sidell et al., 2002; USAMRICD, 2000).

The attachment of the nerve agent to the enzyme is permanent unless removed by therapy. Atropine assists with symptomatic relief and is the most common drug used in the treatment of nerve gas exposure. Atropine will help with the muscarinic effects such as rhinorrhea, salivation, sweating, bronchoconstriction, bronchorrhea, nausea, vomiting, and diarrhea. The most common reversal agents are the oximes such as Protopam chloride (2-PAM chloride). Protopam helps with muscle twitching and respirations. Atropine and Protopam are packaged together into what is called a MARK I kit. The MARK I kit is administered intramuscularly via an auto injector. The reversal agents must be used early in the course, because, once aging has occurred, the reversal agent is of no effect. Diazepam can help with the convulsions. With all nerve agents, those who survive need full decontamination. Their clothing must be double sealed in plastic and handled as little as possible to avoid secondary exposure to others (Abramowicz, 2002; ATSDR, 2008; Dang et al., 2002; McKee et al., 2000; Sidell et al., 2002; USAMRICD, 2000).

The remainder of the care is outlined in the Nursing Process: Patient Care Plan for Known Nerve Agent Exposure feature (p. 2392).

Sarin (GB)

Sarin is a clear, colorless, and tasteless liquid that has no odor in its pure form. Sarin easily evaporates into a gas, as occurred in the Tokyo event. Sarin mixes easily with water so it can be used to poison food and water. It is heavier than air, so it tends to sink. Once a person is exposed, sarin will continue to release from a person's clothing for about 30 minutes, causing secondary exposures. Low-dose exposure would produce symptoms within seconds to hours. Even a small drop of sarin can cause sweating and muscle twitching at the site of exposure (Centers for Disease Control and Prevention [CDC], 2006e; Sidell et al., 2002; USAMRICD, 2000).

Soman (GD)

Soman is a clear, colorless, and tasteless liquid. It does have a slightly fruity camphor odor, but this cannot be relied on to provide warning against toxic exposure. It can discolor with aging to a dark brown. Soman is highly volatile and so poses a short-lived threat when released. However, soman is heavier than air and so sinks when released. Soman mixes readily with water, so it also can be used to poison food and water. Soman breaks down slowly in the body; therefore, it has a cumulative effect with repeated exposures (ATSDR, 2001c; CDC, 2006f; Sidell et al., 2002; USAMRICD, 2000).

Tabun (GA)

Tabun is a clear, colorless, and tasteless liquid. It has a slightly fruity odor that cannot be relied on to give warning of exposure. Tabun can become a vapor when heated. It also mixes easily with water and is heavier than air. Compared to sarin, tabun is less volatile and therefore will last longer on surfaces than sarin does (ATSDR, 2001c; CDC, 2006h; Sidell et al., 2002; USAMRICD, 2000).

V Agent (VX)

V agent, more commonly called VX, is the most toxic substance known to man. Less than one drop on the skin can be fatal. It is believed by some that any skin exposure to VX is lethal unless washed off immediately on contamination. VX is an amber-colored, odorless, and tasteless oily liquid and is very persistent. It evaporates at about the same rate as motor oil. VX is primarily a liquid exposure hazard, but when exposed to high heat can become a gas. Although it cannot be mixed as readily into water as the other nerve agents, VX can be used to contaminate water and food sources. VX is heavier than air, so it will sink to low-lying areas. Its persistence and toxicity make it the worst of the nerve agents (ATSDR, 2001c; CDC, 2006i; Sidell et al., 2002; USAMRICD, 2000).

Vesicants

Vesicants are **blister agents** that cause redness and irritation to skin that progresses to partial thickness and often full-thickness blisters. In the eyes, the vesicants can cause irritation and conjunctivitis to corneal burns and blindness. With inhalation, vesicants can cause mucosal sloughing and airway obstruction. In high doses, bone marrow suppression can be seen in 3 to 5 days. Especially after oral ingestion, nausea, vomiting, and diarrhea can occur. Emesis and feces may be blood stained. Systemic absorption from any route can cause symptoms such as headache, nausea and vomiting, leukopenia, and anemia.

With most agents except lewisite, there is an asymptomatic period of hours following exposure. The damage is being done to the tissue; it is the overt signs that are delayed. Complete decontamination is required with clothing being double bagged for protection. If eye exposure is suspected, eye irrigation is recommended. There are numerous reports of apathy, lethargy, and sluggishness in people exposed to mustard after exposure and for a period of time afterward. This phenomenon has not been well studied. There is no specific therapy for vesicant exposure. All treatment is supportive (Abramowicz, 2002; ATSDR, 2001c; CDC, 2006a; McKee et al., 2000; Sidell et al., 2002; USAMRICD, 2000).

Mustard

Mustard has been used as a chemical weapon many times in recent history. Mustard is an oily liquid ranging in color from light yellow to brown. It has an odor like garlic, horseradish, onion, or mustard, from which it derives its name. Odor should not be relied on for detection of exposure. Mustard freezes at 57°F, so it is primarily a liquid hazard, but it is a definite vapor hazard at

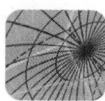

NURSING PROCESS: Patient Care Plan for Known Nerve Agent Exposure

Assessment of Exposure

Subjective Data:

Determine from information sources the agent suspected.

Ask assessment questions of the patient regarding nerve agent symptoms, including dim vision and abdominal discomfort, circumstances of exposure and previous decontamination, and past medical history.

Objective Data:

Assess readiness for decontamination, including equipment and personnel.

Perform pre–personal protective equipment (PPE) assessments of personnel including vital signs and weight.

Perform full patient assessment for nerve agent exposure. (See the Nerve Agents section in this chapter.)

Nursing Assessment and Diagnoses	Outcomes and Evaluation Parameters	Planning and Interventions with *Rationales*
Nursing Diagnosis: *Injury, Risk for* related to gross contamination with chemical	**Outcomes:** The patient is fully decontaminated. No exposures to health care workers or facility. No injury to the health care providers. ***Evaluation Parameters:*** Patient has no chemical left on body as measured with chemical strips or other devices. No increase in symptomatology following decontamination. Health care workers and decontamination workers have no exposure to chemical and no symptoms of chemical exposure or exhaustion. Clean areas maintained. No contamination of the facility.	**Interventions and *Rationales:*** Decontamination area set up into hot, warm, and cold zones, with a triage area in the hot zone as well as re-triage in the cold zone. Areas monitored to maintain zones. Health care workers and other decontamination personnel don full and appropriate PPE prior to contact with contaminated patients. Monitor personnel during decontamination process for signs of agent exposure and heat exhaustion. *To prevent contamination of and injury to personnel.* Fully undress patients and place belongings in clear bags, double bagged, with identification easily seen through bag. *To preserve evidence and prevent secondary exposure.* Fully scrub patients, including creases and hair, using warm soapy water, and rinse. *To remove remaining chemical.* Assess patient prior to decontamination and reassess patient in the cold zone for symptoms of exposure. *To determine severity of symptoms and care needed.*

Assessment of Airway

Subjective Data:

Does the patient complain of shortness of breath (SOB), difficulty breathing, drowning sensation, or weakness?

Objective Data:

Assess for amount of salivation, lacrimation, emesis, rhinorrhea, and bronchorrhea in airways. Assess for fasciculations, level of consciousness and degree of confusion, seizures, respiratory rate, degree of work of breathing, breath sounds, cough effort, vital signs, and skin and nail bed color.

Nursing Assessment and Diagnoses	Outcomes and Evaluation Parameters	Planning and Interventions with *Rationales*
Nursing Diagnosis: *Airway Clearance, Ineffective* related to copious secretions, weakness, depressed level of consciousness, and ineffective cough	**Outcomes:** The patient will maintain a patent airway and adequate gas exchange. ***Evaluation Parameters:*** Clear breath sounds. Clear airways. Pulse oximeter above 95%. Skin warm, dry, and pink with brisk capillary refill.	**Interventions and *Rationales:*** Assess patient for amount and type of secretions. Full respiratory assessment including vital signs, breath sounds, work of breathing, cough effort, skin vital signs, and pulse oximeter. *To determine degree of distress.* Observe for cyanosis, increased confusion, and restlessness. *These are signs of increased hypoxia.* Allow patient to sit in high Fowler's position. *To facilitate respiratory effort and airway clearance.* Suction airways as needed for ineffective/inadequate cough. Endotracheal intubation as indicated. *To maintain clear airway.* Administer oxygen as needed. *To maintain adequate gas exchange.* Administer atropine and Protopam as ordered. *To dry secretions and assist with shortness of breath.* Teach effective coughing techniques such as huff cough. *To improve airway clearance and reduce fatigue from constant coughing.*

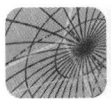

NURSING PROCESS: Patient Care Plan for Known Nerve Agent Exposure—*Continued*

Assessment of Cardiac Status

Subjective Data:
Sensation of palpitations, racing heart, skipping beats.

Objective Data:
Cardiac monitor.
Radial and apical pulse. Blood pressure.
Level of consciousness.

Nursing Assessment and Diagnoses	Outcomes and Evaluation Parameters	Planning and Interventions with *Rationales*
Nursing Diagnosis: *Cardiac Output, Decreased* related to dysrhythmias	**Outcomes:** The patient will have a normal sinus rhythm with adequate cardiac output. *Evaluation Parameters:* Sinus rhythm without ectopy on cardiac monitor. Awake, alert, and oriented level of consciousness.	**Interventions and *Rationales:*** Measure apical and radial pulses and blood pressure, and level of consciousness. *To determine relative perfusion.* Place on cardiac monitor. Monitor with at least 2 leads. *To determine dysrhythmias and need for treatment.* Monitor electrolytes. *Altered electrolytes can affect the cardiac rhythm.*

Assessment of Fluid Status

Subjective Data:
Degree of thirst, headache, amount of cramping, and nausea.
Previous amounts of fluid lost.

Objective Data:
Assess degree of dehydration.
Monitor electrolytes and serum osmolality, physical signs of dehydration, vital signs, and level of consciousness.

Nursing Assessment and Diagnoses	Outcomes and Evaluation Parameters	Planning and Interventions with *Rationales*
Nursing Diagnosis: *Fluid Balance, Readiness for Enhanced* related to copious secretions, high urinary output, vomiting, and diarrhea	**Outcome:** The patient will attain fluid and electrolyte balance. *Evaluation Parameters:* Diarrhea and emesis halted. Intake and output equal. Secretions controlled. Serum osmolality and electrolytes within normal limits. Vital signs within normal limits.	**Interventions and *Rationales:*** Assess hydration status such as oral mucous membrane moisture, intake and output, sunken eyes, skin tenting, thirst, and headache. *To determine degree of dehydration and any improvement in or deterioration of condition.* Strictly monitor intake and output. *To determine fluid balance and any improvement in or deterioration of condition.* Assess vital signs, orthostatic vital signs, cardiac rhythm, and level of consciousness. *To identify signs of hypovolemic shock, perfusion, and electrolyte imbalances.* Monitor serum osmolality and electrolytes when ordered. *To determine replacement needs.* Assess for nausea and administer antiemetics as ordered. *To decrease nausea and vomiting.* Administer atropine and Protopam. *To decrease secretion production and decrease diarrhea and emesis.* Administer normotonic intravenous solutions and oral replacement when tolerating oral fluids. *To replace lost fluids and restore fluid balance.* Administer electrolyte replacement intravenously or orally when tolerated. *To replace lost electrolytes and restore balance.*

Assessment of Coping

Subjective Data:
Assess for feelings of apprehension, fear, uneasiness, palpitations, loss of concentration, degree of sense of threat, feelings of helplessness, powerlessness, increased tension, and worry.

Objective Data:
Assess for decreased concentration, narrow focus.
Signs of tension-reducing behaviors such as biting fingernails, cursing, and rocking.
Altered pitch and tone of voice.
Other typical signs and symptoms—such as increased heart rate, increased respiratory rate, tremor, dry mouth, and increased gastrointestinal symptoms—are not reliable signs due to the nerve agent exposure.

(continued)

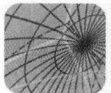

NURSING PROCESS: Patient Care Plan for Known Nerve Agent Exposure—*Continued*

Nursing Assessment and Diagnoses	Outcomes and Evaluation Parameters	Planning and Interventions with *Rationales*
Nursing Diagnosis: *Coping, Ineffective* related to perceived and actual threat from situation, unknown outcome, and possible further danger	**Outcome:** There will be a decrease in the patient's anxiety. *Evaluation Parameters:* The patient will report no sensation of palpitations. Will answer simple questions clearly without lag. Will report a subjective decrease in sensation of anxiety and helplessness and an increased sense of control. Anxiety-reducing behaviors will be greatly decreased or absent, such as no rocking and no nail biting.	**Interventions and *Rationales:*** Use calm, reassuring approach. *To increase confidence in caregiver and reduce anxiety of unknown.* Reassure patient that appropriate medical care is being rendered for condition. Explain procedures and purpose of medications and interventions in simple terms. Explain in simple terms the effects of the nerve agent. *Reduce anxiety by decreasing the fear of the unknown and learning what to expect.* Identify for patient the safety of the facility/situation, if true. *To reassure of current safety.* Stay with patient. If the nurse must leave the patient, the nurse should tell the patient when he will return and do so. *To build a trusting relationship and provide sense of security in care.* Acknowledge patient's fears and anxiety. *To identify feelings as a normal reaction, provide insight into situation, and decrease anxiety.* Teach simple stress reduction exercises such as imagery. *To allow for self-comforting and assist with relaxation.* Administer antianxiety agents if ordered and indicated. *To decrease anxiety and promote rest.*

100°F, which is common in the more arid regions of the world. Because of its chemical properties, mustard is often mixed with other chemicals to keep it liquid at lower temperatures. The effects from mustard are seen anywhere from 2 to 48 hours postexposure. Mustard also has some mild cholinergic properties, which may be responsible for the early gastrointestinal symptoms and the miosis seen (Abramowicz, 2002; ATSDR, 2001c; McKee et al., 2000; CDC, 2006g; Sidell et al., 2002; USAMRICD, 2000).

On the skin, the erythema starts with itching. As the erythema fades, areas of increased pigmentation are left. The erythema usually starts in warm, moist thin-skinned locations such as the axillae, perineum, antecubital fossae, and neck. The blisters usually start 4 to 24 hours postexposure. The vesicles start small and then coalesce to form bullae. These large blisters are usually dome shaped with thin walls, yellowish in color, and surrounded by erythema. The fluid is clear, thin, and straw colored at first. Later, the fluid turns more yellow and tends to coagulate. The fluid does not contain mustard and is not harmful to those exposed. In high-dose exposures, the lesions may develop central necrotic areas, which are extremely slow to heal. These blistered areas are extremely painful, and it takes large doses of narcotics to control the pain. These burns cause less fluid loss than thermal burns, and care must be given to avoid overhydration in fluid resuscitation (ATSDR, 2001c; CDC, 2006g; Sidell et al., 2002; USAMRICD, 2000).

The early respiratory effects are usually irritation or burning of the nares, sinus pain or irritation, nosebleeds, and irritation of the pharynx. Laryngitis with voice changes can occur with a nonproductive cough. Damage to the trachea and upper airways can lead to a productive cough. With the lower airways involved, there is increasing dyspnea and increased sputum production. Signs of a chemical pneumonitis can appear 2 to 3 days postexposure. Pseudomembranes can form from necrosis of the airway mucosa. Death in mustard exposure is usually from respiratory failure (ATSDR, 2001c; CDC, 2006g; Sidell et al., 2002; USAMRICD, 2000).

The eyes are the most sensitive to mustard. Blisters do not form. Usually the symptoms are in a range from conjunctivitis, to photophobia, blepharospasm, pain, and then corneal damage. Severe corneal damage, perforation of the cornea, and scarring can occur, including blindness (ATSDR, 2001c; CDC, 2006g; Sidell et al., 2002; USAMRICD, 2000).

Lewisite

Lewisite is an oily and colorless liquid with the odor of geraniums. It is more volatile than mustard. Lewisite causes stinging and burning on contact in such severity that the person will take immediate steps to remove it. Lewisite also causes more immediate blistering. The blisters tend to be smaller and in clusters, as opposed to large bullae with mustard. There is almost no human data from lewisite; most data are from animal investigations. (ATSDR, 2001c; CDC, 2006b; Sidell et al., 2002; Truab & Hoffman, 2002; USAMRICD, 2000).

Within 5 minutes of exposure, lewisite will cause a grayish area of dead epithelium. Redness and blistering follow rapidly, but do not reach their height for 12 to 18 hours. The lesions have more necrosis and tissue sloughing than those of mustard. With eye exposure, pain and blepharospasm occur on contact. The eyes are often swollen shut within an hour. Because of the extreme irritancy to the respiratory system, the person usually self-limits exposure by masking or exiting the area. There is evidence that third spacing of fluid occurs after a massive exposure causing a hypotensive state called "lewisite shock." British antilewisite agent was created to use topically to limit toxicity of this agent. Although no longer formulated for this use, it is still used in heavy metal poisoning (ATSDR, 2001c; CDC, 2006b; Sidell et al., 2002; USAMRICD, 2000).

Phosgene Oxime

Phosgene oxime is a different chemical from the choking agent phosgene discussed later. Phosgene oxime is solid below 95°F. It is colorless as a solid, but yellow to brown as a liquid, and it can have a peppery or pungent odor. It can be released into food and water. It is not a true vesicant, as it does not cause blisters. Phosgene oxime is known as an urticant or nettle agent, as it causes intense itching and a hive-like rash on contact. There is very little experience with this agent (ATSDR, 2001c; CDC, 2006d; Sidell et al., 2002; Truab & Hoffman, 2002; USAMRICD, 2000).

The liquid or vapor of phosgene oxime causes pain on contact, followed by blanching with an erythematous ring, then wheals within 30 minutes, with later necrosis. The pain can persist for several days. It can cause extreme pain in the eyes. It is very irritating to the airways, causing pulmonary edema after both skin exposure and inhalation (ATSDR, 2001c; CDC, 2006d; Sidell et al., 2002; Truab & Hoffman, 2002; USAMRICD, 2000).

Blood Agents

Blood agents include the gases such as hydrogen cyanide and cyanogen chloride and crystals such as sodium cyanide and potassium cyanide. Although it has a bitter almond odor, only about 50% of the population has the genetic ability to detect it. Cyanide is naturally present in some fruit pits and lima beans. It is used extensively in industry such as in ore extraction and the manufacturing of paper and plastics. It is present when many common household items burn in fires and thus represents a frequent threat to many in the course of daily work, as well as a possible terrorist agent. The primary route of exposure is through inhalation, although liquid is absorbed through the skin, eyes, and oral mucosa. If the exposure was with a liquid, then decontamination is needed. Cyanide acts by blocking the mitochondrial enzyme cytochrome oxidase, which leads to reduced aerobic metabolism. Glucose breakdown continues, resulting in a buildup of pyruvate, which is converted to lactic acid resulting in lactic acidosis and intracellular shortage of adenosine triphosphate (ATP) (ATSDR, 2001c; CDC, 2004; Dang et al., 2002; Martin, 2002; Sidell et al., 2002; USAMRICD, 2000).

In higher concentration exposures to cyanide, death is usually within 3 to 8 minutes. In lower exposures or with ingestion, the onset of symptoms is slower. The initial transient rapid respiratory rate may be followed by apprehension, anxiety, agitation, and vertigo. There can be a feeling of general weakness, nausea with or without vomiting, and muscular trembling. Later respirations slow, with loss of consciousness, convulsions, and apnea with cardiac standstill. Because of the slow onset of symptoms, treatment is possible (ATSDR, 2001c; CDC, 2004; Dang et al., 2002; Sidell et al., 2002; USAMRICD, 2000).

Medical management of cyanide poisoning starts with administration of 100% oxygen. Amyl nitrate by inhalation or sodium nitrate by intravenous injection is used to create methemoglobin,

as cyanide has a higher affinity for methemoglobin. Sodium thiosulfate is administered to convert the cyanide to thiocyanate, which is excreted in the urine. Hyperbaric oxygen treatment has been shown to be efficacious, especially when the patient is cyanotic. Supportive therapy includes intravenous bicarbonate for severe acidosis, vasopressors to support blood pressure, and valium to treat seizures. Long-term disorders of the basal ganglia are often seen after cyanide poisoning (ATSDR, 2001c; CDC, 2004; Dang et al., 2002; Sidell et al., 2002; USAMRICD, 2000).

Choking Agents (Asphyxiates)

Choking agents are also called **asphyxiates** or lung-damaging agents. Inhalation is the usual route of exposure. Initially, irritation of the nasopharynx causes sneezing, pain, and erythema, which are difficult to distinguish from exposure to a riot control agent. Dysphagia, a choking sensation, and a cough often follow. Central airway damage is characterized by signs and symptoms such as hoarseness, stridor, and coarse crackles. Within 2 to 24 hours, signs of pulmonary edema begin, starting with shortness of breath on exertion, wheezes, fine crackles, and large amounts of white to pink frothy sputum. It is important to note that the pulmonary edema is not of cardiac origin, so diuretics are contraindicated. Pulmonary edema within 4 hours of exposure indicates a poor prognosis. Treatment is largely supportive, with oxygen, ventilatory support if indicated, and bronchodilators. Bed rest with absolute minimal activity is a must, as physical activity exacerbates the symptoms. Steroids and ibuprofen have been used for phosgene exposure to decrease inflammation, but their use in other choking agent exposure is unknown. Decontamination is indicated if liquid or solid materials are present (Abramowicz, 2002; Dang et al., 2002; Sidell et al., 2002; USAMRICD, 2000).

Ammonia

At room temperature, anhydrous ammonia is a colorless, highly irritating gas with a strongly pungent odor. It is a common agent in household cleaners and found in fertilizers. In higher concentrations, it is used extensively in industrial settings. It is also a key ingredient in the manufacture of crystal methamphetamine. Anhydrous ammonia is highly irritating to the eyes and respiratory tract, causing lacrimation and rhinorrhea, swelling of the throat and bronchi, coughing, and pulmonary edema. In higher concentrations, it causes chemical pneumonitis and can cause lung hemorrhage. Skin exposure in higher concentrations can cause pain and corrosive injury. For survivors of severe inhalation injuries, residual chronic lung disease is common. Three clinical patterns of presentation are described for phosgene and chlorine depending on the exposure. In the first 3 to 5 days postexposure, there can be a chemical bronchitis and pneumonitis with fever and a high white blood cell count (ATSDR, 2001c, 2004; Sidell et al., 2002; Truab & Hoffman, 2002; USAMRICD, 2000).

Chlorine

Chlorine is a widely recognized odor as it is common in household bleach and swimming pool chemicals. As a gas, it has a yellow-green color and tends to settle on the ground. In mild exposure to chlorine, there is a choking sensation, eye and nose irritation, a cough, and exertional dyspnea. In moderate exposure, there is hoarseness, stridor, and pulmonary edema within 2 to 4 hours. In a severe exposure, respiratory distress at rest and pulmonary edema can occur within 30 to 60 minutes. Copious upper respiratory secretions are present. Sudden death from laryngeal edema, laryngospasm, or bronchospasm can occur. Sodium bicarbonate is sometimes used for the metabolic acidosis seen in massive exposures (ATSDR, 2001c; CDC, 2006a; Sidell et al., 2002; Truab & Hoffman, 2002; USAMRICD, 2000).

Phosgene

Phosgene is a colorless gas that has the odor of newly mown hay, freshly cut grass, or corn but forms a white cloud that hugs the ground. Although highly volatile, phosgene is twice as potent as chlorine. Phosgene is distinguished by its odor and its generalized mucous membrane irritation in high concentrations including causing laryngospasm. With phosgene there is dyspnea, and the onset of pulmonary edema is delayed. In mild exposure, cough, dyspnea, and or chest tightness first occurs. Eye irritation and lacrimation are indicative of moderate phosgene exposure. In severe exposure, the pulmonary edema occurs in about 4 hours with respiratory distress at rest. With phosgene, sudden death may also occur from the laryngeal edema, laryngospasm, or bronchospasm (ATSDR, 2001c; CDC, 2006c; Sidell et al., 2002; Traub & Hoffman, 2002; USAMRICD, 2000).

Irritants

Irritants, commonly known as **riot control agents**, produce transient discomfort and eye closure so that the recipient is temporarily unable to fight or resist. They generally cause pain, burning, lacrimation, or discomfort on exposure to mucous membranes within seconds of exposure, but these effects rarely persist for more than a few minutes. Fresh air is the treatment, but showering will be helpful in alleviating symptoms. Clothing should be double bagged in plastic and handled as little as possible. Large and prolonged doses in contained areas can cause eye injury and respiratory failure (McKee et al., 2000; USAMRICD, 2000).

Tear Gas (CS)

Tear gas is colorless to gray with a sharp, irritating odor some describe as that of hair spray. With exposure to tear gas, there is usually a burning sensation in the nose, rhinorrhea, and sneezing and increased salivation when it contacts the mouth. With inhalation into the airways, there is bronchorrhea, coughing, and a sensation of chest tightness. If there is damaged skin, such as abrasions, there will be a tingling or burning sensation, and sometimes an erythematous reaction. With sustained exposure (hours) in hot and humid conditions, a second-degree–type burn can occur. Nausea and vomiting can also occur (USAMRICD, 2000). Although normally the signs and symptoms are of short duration and severity, there are reports of young, healthy nonsmoking subjects requiring intensive care treatment following exposure for hypoxia, hemoptysis, and pulmonary infiltrates when combined with strenuous exercise (Thomas, 2002).

Mace (CN) is available commercially for self-protection but is otherwise not used. Its effects are similar to those of tear gas (USAMRICD, 2000).

Pepper Spray (OC)

Pepper spray, also known as "oleoresin capsicum," is a suspension of red pepper initially used by the U.S. Postal Service against aggressive dogs. Police use it in riot control situations and to assist in difficult apprehensions. Although there have been many accusations of deaths from pepper spray, the April 2003 report by the Department of Justice, *The Effectiveness and Safety of Pepper Spray*, concluded that no deaths have been caused directly by pepper spray, although there are indications that it has contributed to two deaths (National Institute of Justice, 2003).

Other Agents

It is worth mentioning that the military does have other agents that will most likely never be encountered by the civilian population. Incapacitating agents include BZ from the family benzilates. **Incapacitating agents** cause symptoms that are the opposite of nerve agents, as they decrease the effective acetylcholine at receptor sites. Central nervous system signs and symptoms can include stupor, confusion, and confabulation. Other signs and symptoms include mydriasis, blurred vision, dry mouth, and an initial rapid heart rate followed by a normal or slow heart rate. **Vomiting agents** include diphenylchloroarsine (DA) and diphenylcyanoarsine (DC). They cause a strong pepper-like irritation in the upper respiratory tract, leading to irritation of the eyes, lacrimation, sneezing, cough, nausea, and vomiting. These would most often be used in combination with another agent so as to cause persons to unmask (McKee et al., 2000; Sidell et al., 2002; USAMRICD, 2000).

■ Biologic Agents

Biologic agents include bacteria, viruses, and toxins. Biologic agents are usually in a liquid or dry form. Most agents tend to be off white to amber, brown, or red. This color can easily be changed with the addition of simple food dyes so as to blend these agents into the background of the area of dispersion. Unlike chemical agents, biologic agents are not detectable with the usual five human senses. Because the period of illness is longer than with chemical agents, the impact on health care is much longer and larger than with chemicals. If such an agent were dispersed, there would be waves of patients depending on the incubation and population affected, as opposed to a single influx (Franz et al., 1997; Kortepeter, 2001; Sidell et al., 2002). Chart 72–7 outlines the biologic agents by class: bacteria, viruses, and toxins.

CHART 72–7	**Biologic Agents by Class**
BACTERIA	**VIRUSES**
Anthrax	Dengue fever
Brucellosis	Ebola
Cholera	Rift Valley fever
Glanders	Smallpox
Plague	Venezuelan equine encephalitis (VEE) virus
Q fever	Viral hemorrhagic fever (VHF)
Rickettsia	
Tularemia	**TOXINS**
Typhus	Botulinum
	Ricin
	Saxitoxin
	Staphylococcal enterotoxin B (SEB)
	Trichothecene mycotoxins

Biologic agents are categorized as Category A, B, or C. Category A agents are those that pose the highest risk to national security because they (1) cause high mortality with the potential for major public health effects including special actions for public health preparedness, (2) are easily disseminated or easily spread person to person, and (3) may cause public panic and public disruption. Category A agents include smallpox, anthrax, plague, botulism, tularemia, and viral hemorrhagic fever. Category B agents are moderately easy to disseminate, can cause moderate morbidity and low mortality, and require specific actions and enhancements by the Centers for Disease Control and Prevention (CDC). Category B agents include brucellosis, glanders, ricin, staphylococcal enterotoxin B, and some of the food- and water-borne illnesses such as salmonella, *Shigella*, and *Vibrio*. Category C agents are emerging pathogens that could be engineered in the future because they are readily available, are easily produced and disseminated, and have the potential for high morbidity and mortality. The Category C agents include Hantaviruses, tick-borne encephalitis virus, and yellow fever (CDC, 2006a, 2006j, 2008; House, Graber, & Scheckel, 2003).

Nursing Management of WMD Infection

Nursing management of the patient with an infection from a WMD event is the same as that of any other patient with the same infection. Refer to Chapter 20 ⬤ for the care of the patient with infectious disease. Application of the nursing process will identify an assessment data cluster that will assist in identifying the agent involved.

Collaborative Management

As with other infectious agents, weaponized biologic agents require aggressive infectious disease management. A health care team that includes nurses, health care providers, public health personnel, and infectious disease specialists will be required. When large numbers of patients are involved, public health's role becomes key in managing the spread of the disease. As with chemical agents, psychological and emotional care needs must be included in the comprehensive approach.

Spread

There are multiple routes in which biologic agents can be dispersed.

Aerosol Route

The spread of biologic agents would usually be by an aerosol method. Most biologic agents can be aerosolized to a size of 1 to 10 microns. Particles larger than 15 microns will not stay suspended in the air but will fall out to the ground. Secondary aerosolization occurs when the particles that have fallen to the ground are stirred by currents created by passing people or objects such as cars. Breathing in through the nose filters out only those particles larger than 10 microns (Hagler, 2004). Most aerosolized biologic agents will be taken deeply into the lungs by those exposed (Franz et al., 1997). The aerosols can be created using simple sprayers such as a garden or paint sprayer, crop

duster planes, mosquito trucks, fire extinguishers, all the way to a dispersion bomb, much as with chemical agents. These all take a high level of knowledge and sophistication to create (Franz et al., 1997; Kortepeter, 2001; Sidell et al., 2002).

Oral Route

Foods and fruits can be contaminated either during distribution or in the manufacturing process. Outbreaks of food poisoning at various restaurants or at family picnics are examples of accidental contamination of foods. The oral route was used in the Oregon salad bar incident mentioned earlier (Torok et al., 1997). The accidental contamination of food usually produces few casualties.

Most public-type water supplies are at very low risk for significant contamination due to the chlorination treatment process. Reverse osmosis systems have been shown to be effective against the toxins of ricin, microcystin, T-2 mycotoxin, and saxitoxin. Contamination of a personal water well or single building's water supply at the intake would be a more likely scenario (Sidell et al., 2002).

Injection

The injection route for biologic agents is not a common terrorist method. It is more commonly used in specific assassination attempts, such as that of Georgi Markov (Christopher et al., 1997). It would be possible to contaminate hospital equipment and thus have injection be the vector, but this is unlikely.

Dermal Exposure

Intact skin affords an excellent barrier for most biologic agents, so dermal exposure is not an effective means of transmission for most bacteria and viruses. Open wounds such as paper cuts or other small abrasions will provide a portal of entry. Cutaneous anthrax is commonly acquired this way. Some of the toxins such as T-2 mycotoxin ("yellow rain") are believed to be able to penetrate skin (Sidell et al., 2002).

Vector Transmission

Biologic agents can intentionally be spread with fleas, ticks, and mosquitoes, just as they are in nature. This is a complicated process but is known to have been accomplished. This route is not considered as a likely scenario because other methods are easier and less expensive (Sidell et al., 2002).

Bacteria

Bacteria generally cause disease by invading host organisms and or producing toxins. *Rickettsia* is unique in that these bacteria rarely can grow without a living host cell and yet are most susceptible to antibiotics. Some bacteria form spores that are resistant to heat, cold, drying, chemicals, and radiation and can therefore germinate under favorable conditions (Kortepeter, 2001).

Anthrax

Anthrax, which is spore forming, is caused by *Bacillus anthracis*. The spores are very stable and may remain for years in soil and water. There are three clinical forms of anthrax: cutaneous, inhalation, and gastrointestinal. Anthrax typically has an incubation period of 1 to 5 days. Those with known exposure can receive ciprofloxacin or doxycycline prophylactically. There is a vaccine available used primarily in the active duty military. Treatment is with ciprofloxacin, doxycycline, or penicillin with streptomycin, along with symptomatic treatment (Franz et al., 1997; Hardin, 2002; Inglesby et al., 2002; Kortepeter, 2001; Sidell et al., 2002).

A terrorist attack using anthrax would most likely be with aerosol, resulting in inhalation anthrax, as in the 2001 U.S. Postal Service incidents on the East Coast ("Follow-Up of Deaths," 2003). Following the primary aerosolization, the spores settle onto surfaces and can be resuspended when disturbed. This occurrence is uncertain and depends on many factors. Anthrax is also known as "woolsorter's disease" because it is known to occur in workers handling contaminated wool, hair, and hides. Standard (universal) isolation precautions are adequate for anthrax. There is no indication that health care workers caring for these patients need any type of prophylaxis (Franz et al., 1997; Hardin, 2002; Inglesby et al., 2002; Kortepeter, 2001; Sidell et al., 2002).

Cutaneous Anthrax

Cutaneous anthrax, also known as malignant pustule anthrax, occurs most frequently on the arms and hands of those working with infected livestock. Spores enter through broken skin. The lesions can occur up to 12 days postexposure. The lesion initially appears as a pruritic macule or papule that enlarges to a round ulcer by the second day. Vesicles may appear. The central lesion develops into eschar, which dries and loosens, falling off in 1 to 2 weeks. Painful lymphadenopathy and lymphangitis can occur with some systemic symptoms. Antibiotics do not change the course of the lesion but do help with the systemic symptoms. Especially when treated, death from cutaneous anthrax is rare (Franz et al., 1997; Hardin, 2002; Inglesby et al., 2002; Kortepeter, 2001; Sidell et al., 2002).

Inhalation Anthrax

The initial symptoms of inhalation anthrax are nonspecific and last for a few days or less: cough, dyspnea, fever, headache, chills, diaphoresis, chest pain, weakness, and sometimes abdominal pain. There is usually a short period of improvement followed by the abrupt development of the second phase. The second phase is more severe with fever, more severe dyspnea, shock, and a classic widening mediastinum and pleural effusions. Up to half of the patients develop hemorrhagic meningitis. Inhalational anthrax has a high mortality rate (Franz et al., 1997; Hardin, 2002; Inglesby et al., 2002; Kortepeter, 2001; Sidell et al., 2002).

Gastrointestinal Anthrax

Gastrointestinal anthrax is rare in humans and occurs most frequently by eating the undercooked meat of infected animals. A large amount of anthrax must be ingested to cause the disease. In the oral pharyngeal form, an oral or esophageal ulcer forms along with sepsis, regional lymphadenopathy, and edema. In the lower gastrointestinal tract, the lesions tend to occur in the end of the ileum or in the cecum. It usually presents with nausea and vomiting, and progresses rapidly to bloody diarrhea, acute abdomen, and sepsis. Massive ascites has been known to occur (Franz et al., 1997; Hardin, 2002; Inglesby et al., 2002; Kortepeter, 2001; Sidell et al., 2002).

Brucellosis

Brucellosis, also called "undulant fever," was the first disease weaponized by the United States in 1954. Undulant fever is caused by one of six species of *Brucellae*. Undulant fever has a variable incubation, from 5 to 60 days, but it is believed that the incubation would be shorter if this agent were weaponized for inhalation. Brucellosis typically presents as a nonspecific flu-like illness, with fever, headache, myalgias, arthralgias, back pain, diaphoresis, chills, and general malaise and weakness. Vertebral osteomyelitis, intervertebral disk space infection, paravertebral abscess, and sacroiliac infections are rare but severe complications. Gastrointestinal symptoms occur in 70% of adults. No human vaccine is available. Treatment is with doxycycline plus rifampin or ofloxacin with rifampin. For those with known exposure, prophylaxis is with doxycycline plus rifampin. Trimethoprim-sulfamethoxazole can be substituted for rifampin; however, the relapse rate may reach 30% (Franz et al., 1997; Kortepeter, 2001; Sidell et al., 2002).

Plague

Plague, caused by *Yersinia pestis*, occurs in three forms: bubonic, septicemic, and pneumonic. Plague is spread from rodents to humans by the bite of infected fleas. Incubation is generally 2 to 10 days. As it can be spread person to person, droplet precautions are indicated with pneumonic plague. Bubonic plague requires standard (universal) precautions. Those exposed to plague can receive doxycycline, ciprofloxacin, or tetracycline prophylactically. Plague is usually treated with streptomycin, gentamicin, ciprofloxacin, or doxycycline. Plague meningitis is treated with chloramphenicol. Untreated plague has a high mortality rate (Franz et al., 1997; Inglesby et al., 2000; Kortepeter, 2001; Sidell et al., 2002).

A vaccine did exist at one time. The CDC references a 1982 article from the *Morbidity and Mortality Weekly Report (MMWR)* regarding recommendations for the administration of this vaccine ("Plague Vaccine," 1982). The Computer Sciences Corporation is in clinical trials for a plague vaccine that uses recombinant technology. This vaccine was originally developed by USAMRICD. No results of the clinical trials are yet available (Computer Sciences Corporation, 2008).

Bubonic Plague

The onset of disease is abrupt with fever, chills, weakness, myalgias, headache, and an acutely swollen and painful lymph node near the site of the flea bite. This is called a **bubo** and is normally seen in the lower leg or groin, because the legs are the most common site of flea bites in humans. The bubo is so painful that it usually prevents motion in the affected area. The bubos recede with antibiotic therapy. Incision and drainage of these lesions is contraindicated as that would present an exposure risk to the health care worker. Diagnostic sampling can be done by needle aspiration, which may provide short-term symptomatic relief (Franz et al., 1997; Inglesby et al., 2000; Kortepeter, 2001; Sidell et al., 2002).

Septicemic Plague

Septicemic plague can present primarily or secondary to bubonic plague. Septicemic plague presents similarly to other gram-negative septicemias with high fever, chills, malaise, hypotension, nausea, vomiting, and diarrhea. With plague, purpuric lesions, necrosis of small vessels, gangrene of the nose and fingertips, and disseminated intravascular coagulopathy can occur, from whence it is believed the name the "black death" originated (Franz et al., 1997; Inglesby et al., 2000; Kortepeter, 2001; Sidell et al., 2002).

Pneumonic Plague

Pneumonic plague usually occurs secondary to bubonic or septicemic plague; however, it is expected to be the primary event in a weaponized plague attack that would be in an aerosolized form. The incubation period is usually 1 to 6 days. The onset is acute and fulminant with high fever, chills, headache, malaise, and myalgias followed within 24 hours by a productive cough. Although the sputum is usually bloody, it can be watery or purulent. Abdominal pain, nausea, vomiting, and diarrhea can also be present. The pneumonia progresses rapidly to dyspnea, stridor, and cyanosis with respiratory failure and circulatory collapse (Franz et al., 1997; Inglesby et al., 2000; Kortepeter, 2001; Sidell et al., 2002).

Tularemia

Tularemia is caused by *Francisella tularensis*. It is considered to be one of the more likely biologic choices for weaponization. It is found in a variety of small mammals. Tularemia is known to be spread by ticks, flies, and mosquitoes as well as by contact with or ingestion of infected soil, food, or water. It can be spread in aerosol, as seen in laboratory workers, but no person-to-person spread has been documented. Tularemia has an incubation period of about 3 to 5 days. Prophylaxis for known exposure is with doxycycline, tetracycline, or ciprofloxacin. Treatment of the disease is with streptomycin, gentamicin, or ciprofloxacin. A vaccine has been used in laboratory workers but is not in general release. Standard (universal) isolation precautions are indicated for tularemia (Barrueto & Hoffman, 2002; Dennis et al., 2001; Franz et al., 1997; Kortepeter, 2001; Sidell et al., 2002).

Typhoidal Tularemia

Typhoidal tularemia is seen with inhalation exposure. It has an abrupt onset of fever, body aches (especially the lower back), shaking chills, and sore throat, along with chest pain or tightness and a cough that may or may not be productive. A true and extremely severe pneumonia can develop. Symptoms can be progressive and include nausea, vomiting, diarrhea, and weight loss (Barrueto & Hoffman, 2002; Dennis et al., 2001; Franz et al., 1997; Kortepeter, 2001; Sidell et al., 2002).

Ulceroglandular Tularemia

Ulceroglandular tularemia is characterized by a cutaneous papule, which becomes ulcerative, with regional lymphadenopathy at the inoculation site. The lesion appears at the same time as the general symptoms of fever, chills, headache, and malaise (Barrueto & Hoffman, 2002; Dennis et al., 2001; Franz et al., 1997; Kortepeter, 2001; Sidell et al., 2002).

Oropharyngeal Tularemia

Oropharyngeal tularemia is from drinking contaminated water or eating contaminated food. Occasionally, it can be from inhalation. A stomatitis can develop, but most commonly there is an exudative tonsillitis or pharyngitis, sometimes with ulceration. There is usually pronounced cervical lymphadenopathy (Barrueto & Hoffman, 2002; Dennis et al., 2001; Franz et al., 1997; Kortepeter, 2001; Sidell et al., 2002).

Q Fever

Q fever was first called "query fever" because the cause was unknown. Q fever is caused by the *rickettsia Coxiella burnetii*, which is highly infectious by the aerosol route. The common vectors are cattle, sheep, goats, dogs, cats, and birds. Q fever has an incubation of 2 days to 2 weeks, most commonly 10 to 14 days. Symptoms can be slow or abrupt in onset and usually consist of fever, chills, myalgias, and headache, with fatigue, anorexia, and weight loss less commonly. It can develop into pneumonia. About one-third of the patients with Q fever will develop abnormal liver function tests. Those patients with preexisting valvular heart disease can occasionally develop endocarditis. A vaccine is under development. Q fever is generally treated with tetracycline or doxycycline. For known exposure to Q fever, prophylaxis is tetracycline or doxycycline (Franz et al., 1997; Kortepeter, 2001; Sidell et al., 2002).

Viruses

Viruses have either DNA or RNA as genetic material. Viruses are intracellular parasites and lack a system for their own metabolism. They require a host for replication (Kortepeter, 2001).

Smallpox

Smallpox is caused by the variola virus. There are two forms: variola major: and the less severe variola minor. In 1980 the World Health Organization declared that smallpox had been eradicated. It is estimated that 80% to 90% of adults and 100% of children are highly susceptible to the disease. Monkeypox, cowpox, and vaccinia are of the same genus, but only smallpox is spread person to person, primarily by droplet or aerosol. Smallpox is thought to be the most likely biologic agent to be used in a terrorist attack. Because it is supposed to have been eradicated, a single case of smallpox should be considered suspect and treated as an international emergency, beginning with notification of local health authorities (Franz et al., 1997; Hardin, 2002; Henderson et al., 1999; Kortepeter, 2001; Sidell et al., 2002).

Following exposure, the incubation period varies from 7 to 19 days, with an average of 12 days. Symptoms usually begin abruptly with fever, vomiting, headache, backache, rigors, and malaise. About 15% of patients develop delirium. Two to three days later, oral lesions appear at the same time as a red rash appears on the face, hands, and forearms. It spreads next to the legs and then the trunk. This centrifugal distribution is an important diagnostic feature. The rash begins as macules and progresses quickly to papules and then pustular vesicles. In contrast to varicella (chickenpox), which has multiple crops, smallpox has one crop of lesions. This single crop of lesions remains in roughly the same stage of progression. In the second week after onset, the pustules form scabs that leave depressed, depigmented scars after healing. The virus can be recovered from scabs, so the patient needs to remain isolated and considered infectious until all the scabs separate.

In the event of an outbreak of smallpox, vaccination of all persons is recommended. Even 4 days after true exposure, the vaccine can prevent or decrease the severity of the symptoms. Smallpox vaccine is not without its problems. The smallpox vaccine is actually vaccinia, a related virus. There are side effects including fever and axillary lymphadenopathy all the way to a postvaccine encephalitis. There are 1 to 2 deaths per million vaccinated along with cases of vaccinia and eczema vaccinatum. In the absence of known true exposure, vaccination is contraindicated in the immunosuppressed (including HIV infection), those with a history of or current eczema, or those in current close contact with persons with one of these conditions (Franz et al., 1997; Hardin, 2002; Henderson et al., 1999; Kortepeter, 2001; Neff, Lane, Fulginiti, & Henderson, 2002; Sidell et al., 2002).

As soon as the diagnosis of smallpox is made, droplet isolation of the patient should be instituted (preferably at home), and all household and face-to-face contacts should be vaccinated and placed under surveillance. If there is a large number of cases, cohorting is indicated, including consideration of a cohort health care facility if indicated (Franz et al., 1997; Hardin, 2002; Henderson et al., 1999; Kortepeter, 2001; Sidell et al., 2002).

Venezuelan Equine Encephalitis

Venezuelan equine encephalitis (VEE) virus is a complex group of eight alpha viruses that are mosquito borne. VEE was tested by the United States in the 1950s and 1960s as a biologic weapon. It can be spread in weaponized form as an aerosol or by deliberately infected mosquitoes. It has an incubation of 1 to 6 days followed by sudden onset of symptoms. Symptoms are severe and include spiking high fevers, shaking chills, severe headache, photophobia, and aching in the lumbar region and legs. Nausea, vomiting, diarrhea, cough, and sore throat may follow. The acute phase lasts approximately 24 to 72 hours, with recovery in 1 to 2 weeks. Neurological involvement is rare (0.5% to 4%). There are a variety of investigational vaccines, each specific to one virus but not to all. Treatment for those with uncomplicated VEE includes analgesia for the headache and myalgias. Those with encephalitis may need anticonvulsants and intensive care–level supportive therapy. Universal precautions are used for VEE, except that the patient should be treated in a screened-in area, with residual insecticides, as the patient is an infection reservoir for mosquitoes for at least 5 days after onset of symptoms (Franz et al., 1997; Kortepeter, 2001; Sidell et al., 2002).

Viral Hemorrhagic Fevers

Viral hemorrhagic fevers (VHFs) encompass a large number of RNA viruses. The syndrome is an acute febrile illness characterized by prostration, myalgias, and evidence of vascular involvement such as easy bleeding, petechiae, and postural hypotension. These symptoms can progress to include all organ systems. The mortality rate ranges widely, depending on the disease, with Ebola being approximately 90%, and the rates for yellow fever and Dengue fever being lower. Lassa, Congo-Crimean, Hantaan, Ebola, and Marburg viruses can be spread by aerosol; so full respiratory isolation, including hair, face, eye, and shoe protection, with negative airflow is indicated. Full respiratory protection with high efficiency particulate air (HEPA) filtered respirators, battery-powered air purifying respirators, or a positive pressure–supplied air respirator is indicated when the patient has a prominent cough, vomiting, diarrhea, or hemorrhage. Downstream personnel, such as linen handlers and environmental service workers, must also use full precautions. Prompt burial or cremation with minimal handling of the remains is recommended. Routine (universal) isolation with special attention to proper disposal of sharps is satisfactory for most of the others, as these patients have a large amount of the virus in their blood and secretions. A vaccine is available for yellow fever. There are other vaccines in various stages of testing and development. Ribavirin has been shown to be of some use in Lassa virus, Rift Valley fever, and Congo-Crimean fever (Borio et al., 2002; Franz et al., 1997; Kortepeter, 2001; Sidell et al., 2002).

Toxins

Toxins are produced by living organisms. Except for the mycotoxins, they are generally not active on the skin. Toxins have a variety of chemical properties in that some are easily denatured by heat or light. For some, such as ricin and mycotoxins, very large quantities would be needed for an effective open air attack. The bacterial toxins, such as Botulinum, are the most toxic substances by weight (Kortepeter, 2001).

Botulinum

Botulinum toxin is derived from *Clostridium botulinum* and two other clostridia species. There are seven recognized forms: A, B, C, D, E, F, and G, all of which produce similar symptoms. This is significant in that different antitoxins are available based on species. Botulinum, which causes botulism, is the most potent toxin known to humans, being 15,000 times more toxic than the nerve agent VX. When untreated, there is an approximate 60% mortality rate. Food-borne botulinum is common in improperly prepared canned foods. The mechanism of action is that the botulinum toxin acts to prevent release of acetylcholine presynaptically, thus, interrupting nerve transmission, the opposite of what occurs in chemical nerve agents. Botulinum is best spread through foods, but it can be aerosolized as well. There is no vaccine (Arnon et al., 2001; Franz et al., 1997; Kortepeter, 2001; Sidell et al., 2002).

Botulinum presents 12 to 72 hours postexposure with symptoms of an afebrile, symmetric, and descending paralysis. Ptosis, diplopia, blurred vision, photophobia, and dilated pupils, with trouble talking, swallowing, and an altered voice, are early signs. Mucous membranes are often dry and the patient may complain of a dry mouth and sore throat. The gag reflex may be absent. Paralysis of the respiratory muscles requires intubation and ventilation. There is generalized weakness followed by the descending flaccid paralysis. Sensory symptoms usually do not occur. Intensive nursing care is required for up to 3 months with full recovery taking up to 1 year. The antitoxin must be administered early, as it can neutralize the circulating toxin only in patients with symptoms that are progressing (CDC, 2006k; Franz et al., 1997; Kortepeter, 2001; Sidell et al., 2002).

Staphylococcal Enterotoxin B

Staphylococcal enterotoxin B (SEB) is one of the exotoxins produced by *Staphylococcus aureus*. It is generally spread through food, but it can be weaponized as an aerosol. SEB is one of the most common causes of food poisoning. Exotoxins are actually excreted from the organism. Because SEB's primary site of action is in the intestine, it is called an enterotoxin. Related toxins include toxic shock syndrome toxin-1. When ingested, SEB can cause extremely high fevers, nausea, vomiting, and diarrhea with profound fluid loss. After oral ingestion, onset of symptoms is 1 to 12 hours, usually 3 to 4 hours. With inhalation, onset of symptoms is 3 to 12 hours. When inhaled, SEB causes a sudden onset of high fever, headache, myalgias, chills, a nonproductive cough, dyspnea, and retrosternal chest pain. Severe cases can lead to pulmonary edema, respiratory failure, and death. The fever lasts up to 5 days in the range of 103° to 106° to 108°F. The cough may last 4 weeks. Vaccines are currently under development (Franz et al., 1997; Kortepeter, 2001; Sidell et al., 2002).

Ricin

Ricin is a toxin made from the mash left over when castor beans are processed to make castor oil. It is fairly easy to extract and can be spread in food or aerosolized. It is less potent than many other agents, so it would take large amounts of product to cover a significant area. When injected, as in the Georgi Markov incident in London in 1978 (Christopher et al., 1997), ricin causes severe necrosis of muscles and lymph nodes near the site of injection, with moderate organ failure following. After ingestion of ricin, symptoms would occur in less than 6 hours.

Expected symptoms in ricin poisoning include nausea, vomiting, necrosis of the gastrointestinal epithelium with resultant upper and lower gastrointestinal bleeding, and renal, hepatic, and splenic necrosis and failure. Dehydration, hypotension, hallucinations, and convulsions can occur. Depending on the dose inhaled, symptoms may occur 4 to 8 hours postexposure. With inhalation, the symptoms may include coughing, fever, chest tightness, dyspnea, nausea, and myalgias and arthralgias. The onset of profuse sweating is often the sign of the symptomatology ending. Humans would be expected to develop severe lung inflammation, with progressive respiratory symptoms including cyanosis and pulmonary edema. Management is primarily supportive, although if it is a known ingestion, vigorous gastric lavage and cathartics are recommended. Vaccines are under development (CDC, 2008; Kortepeter, 2001; Sidell et al., 2002).

Trichothecene Mycotoxins

The trichothecene (T-2) mycotoxins are a group of about 40 compounds produced by the mold (fungi) of *Fusarium, Myrothecium, Trichoderma*, and *Stachybotrys* genus and others. They are extremely stable to heat and ultraviolet light, requiring autoclaving at 1500°F for 30 minutes to be inactivated. When one of these molds is baked into bread and ingested, some individuals developed a lethal illness called alimentary toxic aleukia characterized by initial signs of abdominal pain, nausea and vomiting, and diarrhea with prostration. Within days, chills, fever, myalgias, with bone marrow suppression and secondary sepsis occurred. Those that survived to this point then developed painful throat and laryngeal ulcers with petechiae and ecchymosis, bloody diarrhea, hematemesis, hematuria, epistaxis, and vaginal bleeding (Kortepeter, 2001; Sidell et al., 2002).

Mycotoxins can be released by aerosol, commonly called yellow rain. In an air release, the toxins can be inhaled, absorbed through the skin, and ingested. Within minutes of exposure, burning skin, redness, tenderness, and blistering with progression to skin necrosis with leathery blackening and sloughing of large areas of skin occurs. From eye exposure, symptoms of eye pain, redness, lacrimation, blurred vision, and foreign body sensation occur. Nasal contact results in nasal itching and pain, sneezing, epistaxis, and rhinorrhea. Mouth and throat exposure causes pain and blood-tinged saliva and sputum. Tracheobronchial and pulmonary exposure is characterized by dyspnea, wheezing, and coughing. With ingestion, and thus gastrointestinal exposure, nausea, vomiting, and cramping abdominal pain with watery or bloody diarrhea occur. Systemic findings include weakness, prostration, dizziness, ataxia, and loss of coordination. Tachycardia with hypothermia and hypotension follows in fatal

cases. Death may occur in minutes to hours or days. The only treatment is supportive (Kortepeter, 2001; Sidell et al., 2002).

■ Radiologic Agents

The environment holds many sources of radiation. People are exposed to diagnostic x-rays, the sun, luminous paints, ceramics, and cosmetics daily. Radiologic accidents and terrorist incidents are on a much different scale in terms of the amount of radiation received and the type of radiation involved (Jacocks, 2003). **Radiologic agents** include any agent that is a source of alpha, beta, or gamma radiation that can be used as a weapon.

■ Nursing Management of the Patient Exposed to Radiologic Agents

Nursing management of the patient exposed to radiologic agents depends greatly on the dose and severity of the exposure. Application of the nursing process will facilitate a comprehensive approach to patient assessment and care. This again is a situation in which psychological, emotional, and spiritual care are important.

■ Collaborative Management

All patients exposed to radiologic agents require comprehensive care from a health team including nurses, health care providers, various specialists, and radiologists, depending on the systems involved and the severity of the injury.

Devices

Of all the WMD scenarios, according to experts, the least likely is a nuclear blast because of the materials and technology required, as well as the uncontrolled results. This would be an event such as the atomic bombs dropped in Nagasaki and Hiroshima. For radiologic events, a radiological dispersion device (RDD), the so-called dirty bomb, or a simple radiologic device is considered to be more probable. A simple radiologic device is the spread of radioactive material without an explosion. An example is placing a container on a street corner to expose passersby. A radiological dispersion device does not cause a nuclear reaction. It is an explosive device that releases radioactive material into the environment. This type of device mostly creates trauma patients from the explosion, but complicates medical evacuation of the area and care of the victims because of the contamination. The radiologic contamination from an RDD also causes widespread fear, panic, and terror even if it is too low level to cause actual bodily harm (Jacocks, 2003; Udeani & Aguilera, 2002).

In a nuclear explosion there is the blast, an intense shock wave, thermal radiation manifested as heat and light, followed by nuclear radiation. Nuclear blasts create injury just as blasts from conventional weapons do. The heat and light will create thermal burns. The nuclear radiation will cause acute radiation syndrome (Udeani & Aguilera, 2002). The care of these burns and traumatic injuries would be no different than that of those sustained by other means. Burn injuries are covered in Chapter 68 ⊘, and traumatic injuries are covered in Chapter 74 ⊘.

Types of Radiation

Nonionizing radiation is low energy and nonharmful, such as from classroom lights. Ionizing radiation produces charged ions in the material it strikes. The three most common ionizing particles are alpha, beta, and gamma. The radiation absorbed dose (rad) is a measure of energy deposited in matter by the ionizing radiation. This term is being replaced by the international system *gray* (Gy). One gray equals 100 rad. A roentgen-equivalent-man (rem) is a unit that describes the biologic effect of one rad (Jacocks, 2003; Veenema & Karam, 2003).

Exposure

To describe severity of exposure, the measure of a lethal dose is used. An exposure of 350 rad, or 3.5 gray, will cause death in half the people exposed, if no medical care is received, within 60 days. This is referred to as a lethal dose of 50/60 (LD 50/60). With medical treatment the lethal dose can be increased to between 600 and 800 rads. Unlike chemicals, radiation cannot be detected with the five senses. Geiger counters, dosimeters, and various other detection equipment are employed when radiation is suspected (CRA, 2003; Jacocks, 2003; Udeani & Aguilera, 2002).

Ionizing Radiation

Alpha particles are very big and heavy. They penetrate poorly, traveling only 1 to 2 inches. They are easily stopped by a piece of paper or clothing and do not penetrate the dead skin layer. External alpha radiation rarely causes a health risk, although decontamination is necessary. If introduced through broken skin, inhaled, or ingested causing internal contamination, alpha particles can cause extensive damage especially to the kidneys, lungs, liver, and skeletal system (Fell-Carlson, 2003; Jacocks, 2003; Udeani & Aguilera, 2002; Veenema & Karam, 2003). This is the radiation particle in polonium-210, the material found in the former Russian spy Alexander Litvinenko at his death (BBC, 2007).

Beta particles are smaller than alpha particles. Beta particles can travel about 10 feet through the air and can penetrate skin a short distance causing severe burns ("beta burns"). Damage to the eyes can occur from beta particles, and when ingested or inhaled internal injuries can occur. Shielding with heavy clothing, walls, or thin metals is effective protection against penetration of beta particles (Fell-Carlson, 2003; Jacocks, 2003; Udeani & Aguilera, 2002; Veenema & Karam, 2003).

Gamma rays are emitted during nuclear detonation and are present in fallout. Gamma rays can travel several hundred feet in air and travel through tissue to the deep organs. Gamma radiation is also referred to as "penetrating radiation." Because of this penetration, gamma rays are an external and internal hazard. Dense materials such as lead, concrete, and steel can block penetration of gamma rays. Neutrons are also released in nuclear detonations, and they can penetrate thick concrete (CRA, 2003; Fell-Carlson, 2003; Jacocks, 2003; Udeani & Aguilera, 2002; Veenema & Karam, 2003).

Routes of Entry

Gamma radiation can enter the body by penetration, and this is termed irradiation. In this type of exposure, the victim is not radioactive. This is the same process by which diagnostic x-rays are performed.

Radiologic contamination occurs when particulate matter that is radioactive is released. People become contaminated when the material is deposited on the skin, ingested, inhaled, or absorbed in some manner. Internal contamination can lead to incorporation, whereby the radioactive material is assimilated into body tissue. This can cause both immediate and delayed problems.

Alpha and beta particles can be inhaled if they are airborne. Radiation can be injected and ingested. With dermal exposure, radiation can cause an external burn and or be absorbed into the body if the skin is broken.

Radiation exposure depends on the three principles of time, distance, and shielding. The shorter the time of exposure, the less absorption by the tissue. Radiologic exposure follows the inverse square law in relationship to distance, so that if the distance from the source is doubled, the dose rate of exposure is decreased by a factor of 4. If a source has a radiation level of 100 radiation absorbed dose (R/hr) at 1 foot, at 2 feet the radiation would be 25 R/hr, and at 8 feet it would be 1.56 R/hr. Shielding refers to the materials between the person and the source of radiation. The more dense the material, such as lead, the more protection is afforded (CRA, 2003; Jacocks, 2003).

Radiation Exposure

In most hospitals, one of the radiologists is usually the designated radiation safety officer in charge of determining exposure and risk. Most hospitals have Geiger counters readily available to determine the simple presence or absence of a certain level of radiation in the environment. Personnel involved in the care of radiation victims will need dosimeters to determine their exposure. These personnel will more than likely need decontamination. Depending on the severity of the exposure, many different effects can be seen. Those exposed to low-level external contamination may have skin burns that will heal, to no sequelae. These are *not* considered to be at higher risk later for cancer. Many of those with internal contamination will need follow-up monitoring to measure clearance of the radionuclides from the body. These individuals are also not considered to be at higher risk for cancers later in life. Those exposed to higher levels of radiation that have caused symptoms are considered to be at elevated risk for cancer later (Veenema & Karam, 2003).

In lower level radiation exposure, early treatment can be the key to decrease incorporation (the uptake of radiation into the cells of the body) and decrease symptoms and sequelae. Potassium iodide can have a protective effect on the thyroid if taken before, or within 3 to 4 hours after, exposure to a radioactive cloud. It comes in capsules as well as in liquid. It protects the thyroid gland by filling the receptor sites so that radioactive iodines cannot bind (CDC, 2006n).

Prussian blue is a blue dye first produced in 1704 for use in Prussian military uniforms. Prussian blue can be taken to help remove certain ingested radioactive substances. It works by binding to cesium and thallium in the gut, which are then excreted in the stool. Prussian blue reduces cesium's half-life from approximately 110 days to approximately 30 days. It reduces thallium's half-life from approximately 8 days to approximately 3 days. Prussian blue is still commonly available as a dye and as a paint in art stores (CDC, 2006l; Seed, 2002).

Acute Radiation Syndrome

Acute radiation syndrome (ARS) is an acute illness caused by irradiation of the whole body, or at least a significant part of the body. Radiation generates highly reactive free radicals and directly damages proteins, messenger RNA (mRNA), and DNA. In smaller doses, it interferes with cell proliferation whereas in higher doses it causes cell death. Those body tissues with a higher turnover rate are more susceptible to the effects of radiation, such as the bone marrow (Merck Manuals, 2005). Acute radiation syndrome varies in severity based on dose and the age and relative state of wellness of the person exposed. The severity and extent of the symptoms increase and the duration of each phase shortens as the radiation dose goes up. There are four phases to ARS (Jacocks, 2003).

Prodromal Phase

The prodromal phase has an onset of minutes to hours, and lasts from hours to days, depending on the dose of radiation. It is characterized by the relatively rapid onset of nausea, vomiting, and malaise. At higher levels, fever, hypotension, and diarrhea can also be present. Onset of symptoms within 30 minutes of exposure is most likely indicative of a lethal dose. The gastrointestinal symptoms usually resolve within 2 days, but the fatigue and malaise often continue. At higher doses, 200 rads and above, lymphocyte counts will decrease and cognitive impairment can occur (Jacocks, 2003; Udeani & Aguilera, 2002; Veenema & Karam, 2003).

Latent Phase

Following the prodromal phase, there is a transition phase in which the individual will be relatively symptom free. This latent phase varies from no time to 2 weeks, depending on the dose received (Jacocks, 2003).

Illness Phase

In the illness phase, also called the manifest stage, there is overt illness. This phase presents as a hematopoietic (blood-forming) system, gastrointestinal system, central nervous system, or skin syndrome, or a combination of any of these, based on the system injured.

The hematopoietic system shows the earliest indications of the severity of the radiation exposure. There will be a drop in all cell counts due to death of the bone marrow. A depressed immune system, fever, sepsis, and hemorrhage are common. Those with lower level exposure can recover if they receive medical support and their bone marrow regenerates. Medical support includes blood transfusions, protection from infection, and antibiotic therapy. Occasionally, stem cell transplantation is needed (Jacocks, 2003; Udeani & Aguilera, 2002; Veenema & Karam, 2003).

Gastrointestinal symptoms, nausea, vomiting, and diarrhea are usually seen in doses greater than 600 rad and are a result of damage to the epithelial cells lining the small intestine. The symptoms lead to fluid and electrolyte imbalances and opportunistic infections, which can lead to septicemia. Symptomatic care is prescribed including antiemetics, sedatives, fluid replacement, and a bland diet. Persistent high fevers and bloody diarrhea are ominous signs (Jacocks, 2003; Udeani & Aguilera, 2002; Veenema & Karam, 2003).

The central nervous system is one of the most radiation-resistant tissues in the body. Central nervous system symptoms are seen with doses in excess of 1,000 rads. With this level of radiation, there is usually almost immediate nausea, vomiting, disorientation, and seizures from the loss of fluid, electrolytes, edema, and increased intracranial pressure. Death follows within hours to days. Care involves administering sedatives and analgesics to control seizures and anxiety, as this syndrome is fatal (Jacocks, 2003; Udeani & Aguilera, 2002; Veenema & Karam, 2003).

Recovery or Death

Mortality from ARS is directly related to the amount of radiation exposure. Those with a large exposure will usually die within several months of the exposure. The deaths are most commonly related to opportunistic infections as a result of bone marrow destruction. Survivors' recovery phase may last for several months up to two years.

■ Explosions

Injuries from explosions run the gamut of traumatic injuries from extremely minor ones, not needing medical attention, to complete crush and incineration. Blasts cause injuries that are not always described in basic trauma chapters. Although the mechanism of injury for these problems is a blast force, these injuries are treated in the usual manner (CDC, 2006m; Riley, Clark, & Wong, 2002; Udeani & Aguilera, 2002).

Blast Injuries

There are a few injuries specific to blasts. Blasts are divided into high order explosives (HE) and low order explosives (LE), based on the strength of the ordinance (Chart 72–8, p. 2404). The injuries are divided into primary, secondary, and tertiary. Primary blast injuries are usually caused by high order explosives. Primary blast injuries result from the direct effect of increases in atmospheric pressure causing barotrauma. Ruptured eardrums are the most common injury. The most severe injuries are to the lung and include pneumothoraces, contusions, hemorrhage, bronchopleural fistulas, thrombosis, disseminated intravascular coagulation (DIC), and adult respiratory distress syndrome (ARDS). High order explosives can also cause bowel perforation, gastrointestinal bleeding, shearing injuries to the mesentery, rupture of the testicles, and other solid organ damage. Concussion and traumatic brain injury may also result (CDC, 2006m) (Chart 72–9, p. 2404).

Secondary blast injuries are from flying debris. These include minor lacerations, contusions, and abrasions; dust and smoke inhalation; all the way to impaled large foreign objects and being trapped by large pieces of debris. Tertiary blast injuries occur when the person is thrown by the blast through the air and the person strikes another object. Any variety of injuries can be expected (CDC, 2006m; Riley et al., 2002; Udeani & Aguilera, 2002).

■ How These Events Affect the Health Care System

In the after action reports of the Tokyo sarin gas attack, numerous problems with the hospital disaster plan were identified. Although over 4,000 presented for treatment, less than 1,000 were found to have any symptoms. There was no plan for moving casualties, family, and media through the hospital system. People came into the hospital from all three entrances, causing mass chaos. The entire hospital was contaminated, as the agent was not

CHART 72–8	Blast Injury from High Order Explosives

Category	Mechanism	Body Part Affected	Types of Injuries
Primary	Impact of the overpressurization wave with body surfaces	Gas-filled structures the most susceptible: lungs, gastrointestinal (GI) tract, and middle ear	Blast lung Tympanic membrane (TM) rupture and middle ear damage Abdominal hemorrhage and perforation Eye rupture Concussion and traumatic brain injury (TBI)
Secondary	Flying debris and bomb fragments	Any body part	Penetrating ballistic (fragmentation) or blunt injuries Eye penetration (can be occult)
Tertiary	Individual thrown by the blast wind	Any body part	Fracture and traumatic amputation Any blunt traumatic injury Closed and open brain injuries
Quaternary	All explosion-related injuries, illnesses, or diseases not due to primary, secondary, or tertiary mechanisms Includes exacerbation or complications of existing conditions	Any body part	Burns (flash, partial, and full thickness) Crush injuries Closed and open brain injuries Asthma, chronic obstructive pulmonary disease (COPD), or other breathing problems from dust, smoke, or toxic fumes Angina Hyperglycemia, hypertension

Source: Adapted from Centers for Disease Control and Prevention (CDC). (2006, June 14). *Explosions and blast injuries: A primer for clinicians.* Table 1, Mechanisms of blast injury. Retrieved December 12, 2006, from http://www.bt.cdc.gov/masscasualties/explosions.asp.

CHART 72–9	Blast Injuries by System

System	Injury or Condition
Auditory	Tympanic membrane (TM) rupture, ossicular disruption, cochlear damage, foreign body
Eye, orbit, face	Perforated globe, foreign body, air embolism, fractures
Respiratory	Blast lung, hemothorax, pneumothorax, pulmonary contusion and hemorrhage, arteriovenous (AV) fistulas (air embolism), airway epithelial damage, aspiration pneumonitis, sepsis
Digestive	Bowel perforation, hemorrhage, ruptured liver or spleen, sepsis, mesenteric ischemia from air embolism
Circulatory	Cardiac contusion, myocardial infarction from air embolism, shock, vasovagal hypotension, peripheral vascular injury, air embolism–induced injury
Central nervous system (CNS)	Concussion, closed and open brain injury, stroke, spinal cord injury, air embolism–induced injury
Renal	Renal contusion, laceration, acute renal failure due to rhabdomyolysis, hypotension, and hypovolemia
Extremity	Traumatic amputation, fractures, crush injuries, compartment syndrome, burns, cuts, lacerations, acute arterial occlusion, air embolism–induced injury

Source: Adapted from Centers for Disease Control and Prevention (CDC). (2006, June 14). *Explosions and blast injuries: A primer for clinicians.* Table 2, Overview of explosive-related injuries. Retrieved December 12, 2006, from http://www.bt.cdc.gov/masscasualties/explosions.asp.

identified until 3 hours after the event. Although gowns, gloves, and simple masks were available, chemical-resistant personal protective equipment was not accessible. Many hospital workers suffered secondary exposure. The hospital used 700 ampoules of pralidoximine and 2,800 ampoules of atropine. Additional supplies had to be flown in to meet the demand (Lee, 2003).

WMD as Medical Disasters

Routine life in a hospital currently revolves around overcrowding and understaffing with shortages of needed supplies. The addition of a WMD event is expected to break most already overstretched health care systems. WMD events are the ultimate mass casualty incident and are medical disasters. These events overwhelm the hospital's ability to allocate resources because the high number of casualties affects the infrastructure of the health care delivery system. About 80% of victims walk in for health care, and hospitals provide the majority of that care; and yet most disaster plans still rely on field triage to assess and spread out the people needing care. Personal protective equipment (PPE) is a must in all situations. All disaster plans must address mass casualty incidents and WMD, with a structured plan in which there are clear lines of command and communication, and clearly delineated roles; and the media need to be included in the plan. The media can be used to decrease the mass hysteria and get vital information to the public (Compton, Stewart-Craig, & Doak, 1999; Scharoun, Van Caulil, & Liberman, 2002; U.S. General Accounting Office, 2003). President Bush (2002), in the *National Strategy to Combat Weapons of Mass Destruction*, states, ". . . appropriate civilian agencies must possess the full range of operational capabilities to counter the threat and use of WMD by states, and terrorists against the United States, our military forces, and friends and allies." This is a call for action and preparation, including for the health care team.

Specific Problems

According to the August 2003 U.S. General Accounting Office (GAO; in 2004 it became the U.S. Government Accountability Office) report on hospital preparedness, most urban hospitals have plans, or are working on plans, but most do not have the capacity to handle a large increase in patient load. This includes staffing, supplies, equipment, and space. Of particular note were few ventilators, few isolation beds, few PPE suits, and the inability to handle more than 6 patients for decontamination per hour. (The GAO report indicates that 2,700 ventilators are being added to the Strategic National Stockpile.) The tremendous expense for rarely, if ever, used resources was cited as a concern regarding preparation.

In the initial response, quick identification of the agent, isolation, decontamination, and care needed must be identified. The verification and appropriate use of volunteers must be addressed. Health care workers may be reluctant to go to work because of family care issues and fear of exposure to the agent. Identification of the patients present and family and friends searching for loved ones needs an action plan (Compton et al., 1999; Scharoun et al., 2002; U.S. General Accounting Office, 2003). Telephone lines, including cell phones, are usually quickly overwhelmed. Especially because of outside calls, the hospital telephone system is usually unusable. Two-way radios, ham radios, e-mail, and cable television can all be used to facilitate communications (Lenzer, 2003). Initiating the disaster plan, decontamination concerns and protecting personnel, having adequate initial supplies and personnel, and initiating care to the patients, while preserving the crime scene and evidence, presents a daunting task. For adequate preparation, drilling of the disaster plan must be routinely done.

Problems After the Initial Response

Problems after the initial response include continuing with identifying the patients that are present, including full demographic information. Family and friends will be looking for missing loved ones, and there needs to be a communications system for this information. The need for good communication and a functioning communications system cannot be overemphasized. In a WMD event, a large number of patients admitted to the hospital will need ongoing care. Many of the patients will have similar symptoms and require similar care. This will overtax the pharmacy, hospital equipment, and supplies for some time to come. In addition, decontamination of the hospital or parts of the hospital may be necessary (Compton et al., 1999; Scharoun et al., 2002; U.S. General Accounting Office, 2003).

There will be bigger issues of obtaining supplies and adequate staff for the long term. A sample suggestion regarding supplies is that hospitals keep atropine in the dry form, as the usual stock will be almost immediately depleted due to the amounts used. Staff will face long hours, poor work conditions, and tremendous stress and pressure. Along with nurses and health care providers, food service workers, secretaries, maintenance, environmental services, laundry, central supply technicians, and a host of other personnel will be needed. Special attention needs to be paid to the psychological and emotional health of the worker. The stress on the patients, families, and community will all also be factors (Compton et al., 1999; Scharoun et al., 2002; U.S. General Accounting Office, 2003).

■ National Incident Command System

Managing a terrorist event requires the cooperation of multiple agencies working together. To this end, President George W. Bush wrote the February 28, 2003, *Homeland Security Presidential Directive Five (HSPD-5)*, which directs the secretary of the Department of Homeland Security to establish a comprehensive national incident management system (Bush, 2003). Appropriately called the National Incident Management System (NIMS), NIMS provides a framework for all levels of government and local agencies to work together in preparing for, responding to, and recovering from domestic incidents. NIMS is housed in the Federal Emergency Management Agency (FEMA) Emergency Management Institute (EMI). EMI's main goal is emergency management training (Ridge, 2004).

NIMS is based on the **incident command system (ICS)**, initially designed for use at California wildfire sites by its fire departments. NIMS creates a standard but flexible all-hazards organizational structure whereby the various agencies involved can interact and communicate in an organized manner. It is designed to be used in all phases of disaster management: prevention, preparedness, response, recovery, and mitigation (Ridge, 2004). NIMS has an incident commander (IC), one person in charge of the entire operation. The operation itself is broken into four main areas: operations, planning, logistics, and finance, with a "chief" over each division. Those four chiefs report directly to the incident commander. Also reporting directly to the commander are a safety officer, public information officer, and liaison officer. Room is made in the structure for an expert position who would answer directly to the incident commander (Ridge, 2004). Extensive training on the NIMS system is available from FEMA; its website is kept up to date with new training sessions as they are developed.

The incident command system was adapted to the hospital environment initially by the state of California and evolved into what is now called the hospital incident command system (HICS). The new version of HICS was released in October 2006.

Hospital Incident Command System

HICS uses this same structure adapted to a hospital environment. The HICS manual and supporting documents, available free online, contain the structure with all job descriptions, sample policies and procedures, as well as sample documents/tracking sheets, which can be copied and/or adapted for use as needed (CRA, 2003; California Emergency Medical Services Authority [EMSA], 2006). The hospital incident command system naturally fits into the National Incident Command System, which allows the hospital to speak the same language and use the same divisions as all other agencies.

Organization

The hospital incident command system would be used in the hospital any time there is an incident with the potential to overwhelm resources (Figure 72–4 ■, p. 2406). This could include large accidents with multiple victims all the way to massive WMD events. With HICS, the plan is flexible to the situation. Only those positions and functions that are required by the incident need to be

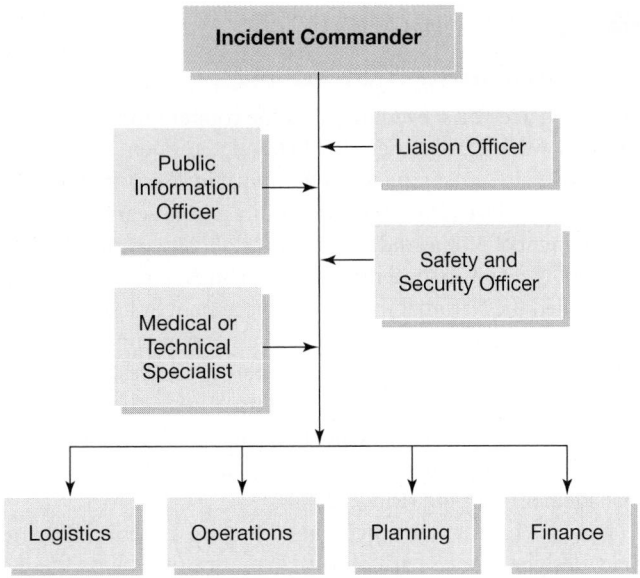

FIGURE 72–4 ■ Hospital incident command system.

activated. Many of the positions can be combined and filled by one person. The plan gives a clear chain of command and clear responsibilities, has a common language and common mission, prioritizes duties, and ensures thorough documentation of actions. The comprehensive documentation allows for a more complete evaluation of the event in the after action sessions. It also improves recovery of expenses while decreasing liability (EMSA, 2006).

HICS uses the same basic structure as NIMS. There is an incident commander (IC) to whom the public information officer, the safety and security officer, the liaison officer, and the section chiefs answer. The incident commander organizes and directs the emergency operations center and gives overall direction for the hospital operations. The public information officer provides information to the media, releases other information as indicated, and assists with communication. The safety and security officer monitors and has authority over the safety of rescue operations and hazardous conditions. This position organizes and enforces scene, facility, and traffic protection and security. The liaison officer functions as the contact person for representatives of other agencies such as the fire department and police departments. As with NIMS, there is room made in the administrative structure for a medical or technical specialist if needed. An example of a needed specialist might be a radiation specialist in the event of a dirty bomb (EMSA, 2006).

Sections

There are four sections: planning, logistics, finance, and operations. The head of each section is a chief. Each section can be further divided if needed. This subdivides the work and allows for a manageable span of management responsibility for each individual (EMSA, 2006).

The planning section ensures the formulation and documentation of an overall response plan and helps to set objectives. It gathers data and status reports from various areas within the hospital to aid in decision making. The planning section is responsible for duties such as providing a situation status report to the hospital and hospital workers every 4 to 6 hours. Planning

also interacts with other sections such as assisting in establishing a plan for medical staff rotation in cooperation with personnel from the operations section.

The logistics section provides the hospital environment and materials to meet all objectives. This includes organizing and directing all operations associated with maintaining the physical environment; adequate food for patients, visitors, and personnel; shelter; and adequate medical and pharmaceutical supplies. This includes such duties as transportation, assessing damaged areas for use or evacuation, communications, and materials supply.

The finance section provides the funding for operations and ensures hospital-wide documentation of activities and expenses to assist with recovery of costs. Large events typically cost millions of dollars in salaries, materials, equipment, and other costs. A single incident can bankrupt a facility without reimbursement. Even federal relief dollars require documentation of expenses for receipt of reimbursement.

The operations section covers much of the day-to-day work of delivering medical care. This includes matching staff to patient needs, organizing inpatient care, and managing the treatment areas such as triage, the emergency department, operating rooms, discharging of patients, and morgue operations (EMSA, 2006).

START Triage

To sort through the massive influx of people during mass casualty incidents, there needs to be a method of identifying those most in need of decontamination and care. The Simple Triage and Rapid Treatment (START) system was designed by Hoag Hospital and the Newport Beach, California, Fire Department for use in multicasualty incidents. It has become the standard method of triage in mass casualty. This method is effective both in the field at the scene of an incident and for sorting at the door of the hospital. START is not designed for use in the pediatric population. A corollary system called "Jump START" has criteria for children based on the same categories (Disaster Management Systems, 2005; Romig, 2008).

The START triage system uses four categories: Red means immediate care needed, with usually two or more systems affected. Yellow means delayed care needed, with usually one system involved. Green means minor care is needed; and black means deceased or that death is expected, with no life-extending care to be delivered (Figure 72–5 ■).

To determine the appropriate category, respirations, perfusion, and neurological status are checked. The first step is to identify the "walking wounded." An announcement is made that all who can walk go to a designated area. These persons are all automatically assigned to the green or minor category. For those left, the airway is opened and respirations are ranked as a red if greater that 30 and the person receives a tag; if respirations are less than 30, no tag is given; and a black tag is given if respirations are zero. Next, major hemorrhage is controlled and perfusion is assessed by checking for a radial pulse, as one must have a blood pressure of at least 80 mmHg to have a radial pulse. If there is no radial pulse, the legs are elevated and a red immediate tag is applied; if there is a pulse, no tag is applied. The last step is to check the neurological status. If the person can answer a simple yes–no question, the tag applied is a yellow delayed tag. If unable to answer, the person receives a red immediate tag.

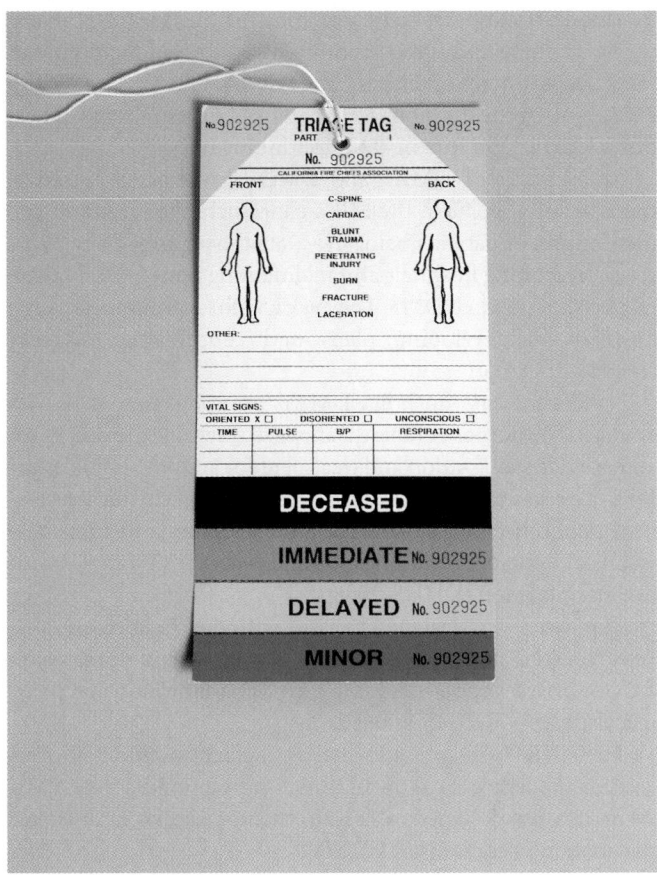

FIGURE 72–5 ■ Triage tag.

For a red tag, the immediate care needed category, classic assessment findings include that respirations are present only after repositioning the airway, respiratory rate is less than 8 or greater than 30, capillary refill is delayed more than 2 seconds, and there may be a significant decrease in level of consciousness. For a yellow tag, the delayed care needed category, the injuries can be controlled or treated for a limited time in the field. Green, the minor care designation, includes those who are ambulatory, with or without minor injuries, that do not require immediate or significant treatment. The black, the deceased or expectant category, is for those with no spontaneous effective respiration after the airway is repositioned (Community Emergency Response Team–Los Angeles [CERT-LA], 2003; Disaster Management Systems, 2005; MCLNO, 2003).

As with any methodology, the START triage system requires practice for proficiency. Some hospitals use START tags on designated days throughout the month during routine operations as a drill for personnel to remain familiar with the tags and system.

■ National Resources

In addition to regional and state supplies, there are national resources available to assist in a disaster situation.

Strategic National Stockpile

The National Pharmaceutical Stockpile program was created in 1999 during the Clinton administration under the auspices of Centers for Disease Control and Prevention (CDC). Its original funding was only $5.2 million per year. The National Pharmaceutical Stockpile program was renamed the **Strategic National Stockpile (SNS)** program and was moved into the new Department of Homeland Security on March 1, 2003. The purpose of the stockpile is to maintain a national repository of pharmaceutical agents, vaccines, medical supplies, and equipment that will be delivered to the site of a large-scale disaster to augment local and state resources in order to decrease morbidity and mortality in the civilian population (Esbitt, 2003; Williams, 2002).

Organization

The Strategic National Stockpile is organized using a five-tiered approach. These are the 12-hour push packs, vendor managed inventory, storage and rapid deployment of vaccines, buying power with surge capacity, and technical assistance. To obtain Strategic National Stockpile assets, the affected state's governor must request the SNS from the CDC. The CDC director will evaluate the request and release the supplies if deemed necessary (CDC, 2005; Esbitt, 2003).

Although the SNS delivers material and technical assistance, the state and local agencies must provide the manpower to use and distribute the materials to the population. There is no charge for the supplies themselves. The state will need nurses, pharmacists, and health care providers for the dispensing sites, but can use nonmedical volunteers to assist with crowd control, move materials, and operate machinery such as forklifts (Esbitt, 2003; Williams, 2002).

Push Packs

Although the 12-hour push pack is less than 4% of the stockpile, it is what is most commonly considered in terms of the SNS. The push packs are so named because they can be shipped within 12 hours of the decision to deploy the assets (Chart 72–10). There are 12 of these located around the United States. Each set consists of 100 containers weighing approximately 50 tons total. Each container is on wheels and is easily moved by one or two people. The containers are designed to fill a 747 cargo jet completely. The receiving site must have about 12,000 square feet of space for storage, repackaging bulk supplies, performing inventory control, and distributing the supplies (Esbitt, 2003; Williams, 2002).

The contents of the push packs are reviewed by content experts frequently and changed based on the current perceived threats. The contents of the push packs include bulk oral antibiotic agents, intravenous and intramuscular medications, analgesics, and other emergency medications. They also include equipment such as pill-counting equipment and an automatic packaging machine. Other supplies include intravenous supplies, airway supplies, and

---

CHART 72–10   **Contents of 12-Hour Push Pack**

Antibiotics and other pharmaceuticals

IV supplies

Airway supplies

Bandage supplies

Pill counting and packaging equipment

Through vendor managed inventory (VMI): vaccines, antivirals/antitoxins

bandaging supplies. It costs about $9 million per month to store and maintain the push packs (Esbitt, 2003; Williams, 2002).

The SNS delivered a team of technical advisers to New York on September 11, 2001, and a 12-hour push pack. The technical advisers arrived 5 hours after deployment and the push pack arrived 7 hours after deployment (Esbitt, 2003). The SNS was most recently deployed to the Gulf Coast region following Hurricanes Katrina and Rita in 2005.

Vendor Managed Inventory

Vendor managed inventory (VMI) is federally owned inventory that is stored by the vendor until needed. Vendor managed inventory is designed to be used to provide specific pharmaceuticals and supplies when the WMD agent is known or for smaller scale events when an entire push pack is not needed. It can also be used to resupply at the scene when a push pack has been deployed. When needed as part of the initial response, the goal is to deliver the VMI within 12 hours. During the anthrax events of 2001, more than 50 requests for antibiotics were filled and shipped to 11 states and the District of Columbia. Each shipment delivery time was less than 5 hours (Esbitt, 2003).

Vaccine and antitoxins are stockpiled using VMI. When shipped, special cooler containers are used to maintain the products at the correct temperature. For smallpox, only the vaccine, diluent, bifurcated needles, and transfer needles are sent. The location must supply items such as gloves, gauze, Band-Aids, sharps containers, and waste bags (Williams, 2002).

The federal government has special prearranged contracts that allow for the purchase of large amounts of supplies and pharmaceuticals should the need arise. In this surge capacity contracting, there are over 97 lines of inventory (Williams, 2002).

Technical Support

A team of advisers, called the Technical Advisory Response Unit (TARU), is 5 to 7 experts in logistics, public health, communications, operations, and emergency response. The TARU can help state and local authorities with receiving, managing, distributing, dispensing, and replenishing the SNS. These units can provide technical assistance with operation of the machinery such as the repackaging unit. They can assist in recovering the support equipment and cargo containers, and in recovering unused SNS assets and materials (Esbitt, 2003).

National Disaster Medical System

Housed in the Department of Health and Human Services, the Office of Preparedness and Response directs and manages the National Disaster Medical System (NDMS), which ensures resources are available after a disaster that overwhelms the local health care resources. Under the National Response Plan, NDMS is responsible for coordinating and managing the federal response to federally declared disasters and major emergencies including natural disasters, technologic disasters, major transportation incidents, and acts of terrorism. Within NDMS are six major divisions: Disaster Medical Assistance Teams (DMATs), Disaster Mortuary Operational Response Teams (DMORTs), National Veterinary Response Teams (NVRTs), National Pharmacy Response Teams (NPRTs), National Nurse Response Teams (NNRTs), and Federal Coordinating Centers (FCCs). All of these teams are made up of volunteers who, when deployed, become federal employees for the duration of their tour. There

is a modest reimbursement. For most of these teams, there is special training and online continuing education requirements (U.S. Department of Health and Human Services [DHHS], 2008a). All of the divisions were deployed in response to Hurricanes Katrina and Rita in 2005 continuing into 2006.

The services of DMAT and DMORT will be discussed in more detail next. First, the FCCs coordinate the reception and distribution of patients being evacuated to an area. They play a role in recruiting hospitals and maintaining non–federal hospital participation in NDMS. They work with local authorities and hospitals in developing plans and coordinating exercises (DHHS, 2008b).

NVRTs are very much like DMAT teams, but they work with animals. The purpose of these teams is to assess the medical needs and provide stabilization and treatment for animals; provide surveillance regarding animal disease, biologic and chemical terrorism, public health assessments, animal decontamination, and technical assistance regarding food and water quality; and provide hazard mitigation (DHHS, 2008b).

The NPRT was designed to assist with the chemical prophylaxis or vaccination if needed for a biologic event. These teams are comprised of pharmacists, pharmacy technicians, and pharmacy students (DHHS, 2008b).

The NNRT will be used when an incident occurs that overwhelms the nation's supply of nurses in responding to a WMD event. It is also designed to assist in chemoprophylaxis or a mass vaccination program (DHHS, 2008b).

Disaster Medical Assistance Teams

The Disaster Medical Assistance Team (DMAT) is part of NDMS (DHHS, 2008b; Dayton DMAT, 2008; Riley, 2003). A **DMAT** is a group of volunteer health care providers, nurses, emergency medical technicians, technical staff, and other health care professionals and support staff designed to provide emergency medical services. They can provide care at a temporary site such as a tent, or at a fixed site such as a hospital. In mass casualty situations, the team can provide triage, medical care, and prepare patients for evacuation. The DMAT may assist overloaded local staff at local health care facilities and/or provide primary health care. When deployed, the team arrives with enough supplies and equipment to sustain itself for 72 hours (Dayton DMAT, 2008; Riley, 2003). Following Hurricanes Katrina and Rita, multiple DMAT teams were deployed to the entire Gulf region. They performed duties ranging from vaccination clinics, to relieving local hospital staff in the hospital, to providing the primary source of medical care in a decimated area.

Types of DMAT Teams

A level 1 DMAT travels with all of its own supplies and equipment, including tents (Figure 72–6 ■). It is fully self-contained for 72 hours. A level 2 DMAT is deployed with another team, or it relieves a level 1 team. It is not considered self-sufficient, as it does not carry its own supplies. A level 3 team has local responsibilities only. There are about 55 DMAT teams. Other specialty teams include burn teams, pediatric teams, veterinary teams, and mortuary teams (Dayton DMAT, 2008; Riley, 2003).

Deployment

DMATs are completely voluntary and used only within the United States. Once activated for deployment, the team member becomes a temporary federal employee. As a federal em-

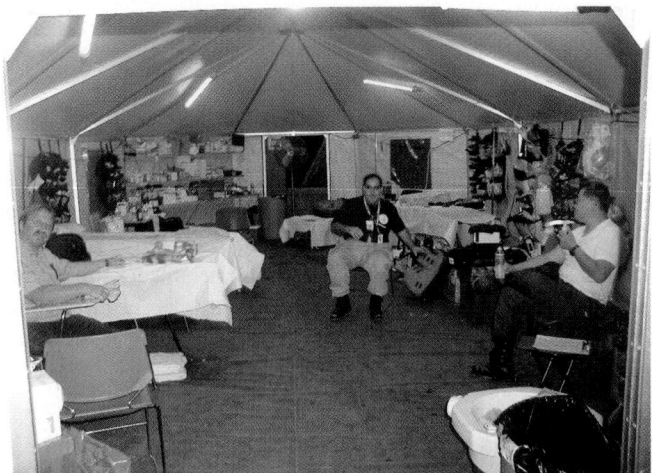

FIGURE 72–6 ■ DMAT tent and team members.
Source: Kathleen Osborn

CHART 72–11	**What Can DMORT Do to Help?**

- Mobile morgue operations
- Forensic examination
- DNA acquisition
- Remains identification
- Search and recovery
- Scene documentation
- Medical/psychological support
- Embalming/casketing
- Family assistance center
- Antemortem data collection
- Postmortem data collection
- Records data entry
- Database administration
- Personal effects processing
- Coordination of release of remains
- Provide a liaison to United States Public Health Service (USPHS)
- Provide communications equipment
- Safety officers and specialists

ployee, any license or certification is automatically recognized in all 50 states. Team members are paid wages, travel is reimbursed, and there is a food stipend. There are meetings and training to attend including such things as setting up the tents, familiarization with the equipment, and learning how to work within the team. Each member is required to provide certain personal gear needed for deployment such as eye and ear protection, leather work gloves, canteen, sleeping bag, camping knife, hand cleanser gel, and toilet paper. Further information on becoming part of a DMAT team is available online (Dayton DMAT, 2008; Riley, 2003).

Disaster Mortuary Operational Response Teams

In large-scale events, along with large numbers of ill or injured people, there will be large numbers of the dead. Management of the dead requires special training and resources. Disaster Mortuary Operational Response Teams (**DMORTs**) are designed to assist with this task. The DMORTs are under the NDMS through OEP in the Department of Health and Human Services in the same manner as the DMAT. DMORTs can provide comprehensive mass fatality management for incidents that overwhelm local resources. As with DMATs, these are volunteers who become temporary federal employees when deployed. As people in the United States expect full identification, federal level assistance is needed in large events due to the tremendous drain on resources and finances (DHHS, 2008b).

Services

DMORT extensive services include mobile morgue operations, forensic exam assistance, DNA acquisition, remains identification, search and recovery, scene documentation, medical and psychological support, embalming and casketing, a family assistance center, antemortem and postmortem data collection, record keeping, processing of personal effects, coordination of release of remains, communication, and safety officers and specialists (Chart 72–11). DMORT teams can identify those requiring decontamination prior to release or autopsy. In identifying remains, they have extensive data gathering, which has helped in identifying even minute remains allowing the family to have closure. Recent missions have included the Space Shuttle *Columbia* disaster and the World Trade Center disaster (DHHS, 2008b; Smith, 2003).

■ Critical Incident Stress Management

The psychological impact of a mass casualty event cannot be overestimated. When the event is deliberate, such as with a terrorist event, the impact is event greater. A common goal of terrorist activity is to threaten the psychological cohesion and well-being of a community. Terrorism is psychological warfare. The psychological casualties of an event will far outweigh the physical casualties by design (Everly, 2003). Persons involved in the incident itself, health care workers, rescuers, as well as the general population will all be affected. Efforts to mitigate the adverse psychological effects of terrorism include providing training and education before incidents occur, providing crisis intervention at the time of the event, and supplying the community with information and assistance following an incident (Everly, 2003).

Stress

Stress is the physical and psychological arousal and response to a perceived or real threat, challenge, or change. When the environment changes, people change (Mitchell & Bray, 1980).

Common Signs of Stress

Common signs of stress are divided into emotional, behavioral, cognitive, and physical indicators. Examples of emotional signs of stress include numbness, anger, grief, depression, feeling overwhelmed, hopelessness, and being overly worried. Behavioral signs include changes in one's ordinary pattern of behavior, changes in eating, decreased personal hygiene, a change in smoking pattern, a change in alcohol use pattern, withdrawal, prolonged silences, and sudden gregariousness not in keeping with one's personality. Cognitive changes include confusion in thinking, difficulty making decisions, disorientation, and memory problems. Physical signs include excessive sweating, dizzy spells, increased heart rate, elevated blood pressure, rapid breathing, tremor, and gastrointestinal disturbances (Everly & Mitchell, 1998a, 1998b; Mitchell & Bray, 1980; Mitchell, Sakraida, & Kameg, 2003). Health care workers must be aware of these signs and look for them in themselves and others. Refer to Chapter 12 🌐 for more about stress and adaptation to it.

Another common reaction to stress is the use of "gallows" or "dark" or "black" humor, especially in the rescuer community. Research has shown that this style is not disrespectful of the injured, the deceased, or their survivors (Maxwell, 2003).

Critical Incident

The stressor, which caused the stress, becomes a **critical incident** when it is an abnormal occurrence that is so markedly distressing and powerful that it overcomes a person's normal feeling of control and coping ability. Critical incident stress is the normal response to an abnormal occurrence. It is the occurrence that is abnormal, not the response (Burns & Rosenberg, 2001; Everly & Mitchell, 1998a, 1998b; Mitchell & Bray, 1980; Mitchell et al., 2003). These incidents disrupt people's lives with strong emotional reactions that have the potential to interfere with their ability to function either at the scene or later. The severity of the reaction is influenced by many things, including any previous exposure to incidents, length of time of exposure, the severity of the exposure (relative horror), perceptions of the events, preexisting coping strategies, other current stressors, well-being at the time of the event, and the available social support (Everly & Mitchell, 1998b; Mitchell et al., 2003).

For health care workers, the critical incident can be further categorized as the incident itself, the professional's performance, and/or the professional's reaction to the event. For health care workers in the aftermath of a WMD incident, the event itself and all the work that follows have the potential to act as a catalyst for a critical incident stress response (Burns & Rosenberg, 2001; Everly & Mitchell, 1998a, 1998b; Mitchell & Bray, 1980; Mitchell et al., 2003).

Crisis Intervention and Critical Incident Stress Management

Crisis intervention is essentially first aid for those in crisis. The goals of crisis intervention are to stabilize and mitigate the signs and symptoms of stress and dysfunction, and to facilitate a return to functioning (Everly, 2000; Everly & Mitchell, 1998a). **Critical incident stress management** is a comprehensive approach to the management of stress and critical incidents. The goal is to reduce and control the harmful effects of stress, maintain health and productivity, and speed recovery from the stressful event. The approach has seven components: preincident preparation, group information briefings (demobilization), defusings, critical incident stress debriefing, individual intervention, family critical incident stress management, and follow-up and referral (Everly & Mitchell, 1998b). The point of all of these interventions is to prevent the development of post-traumatic stress disorder (PTSD), which has been found to be present in roughly 9% of all of those exposed to critical incidents in recent years (Everly & Mitchell, 1998a, 1998b; Mitchell & Bray, 1980; Mitchell et al., 2003).

Health Care Workers

Health care workers usually have a "rescuer" personality. Those who are unable to help with a major effort such as a WMD event,

especially in the early stages, often will feel greater stress. There is a need to do "something," anything (Everly & Mitchell, 1998b; Levenson & Acosta, 2001; Mitchell & Bray, 1980). As time wears on, cumulative stress also becomes a problem for health care workers due to the overwhelming nature of the situation they face each day. For health care workers and other emergency services personnel, there are three common, formalized ways of assisting to increase knowledge and decrease the perceived stress: demobilization, critical incident defusing, and critical incident stress debriefing. It is important to note that these processes are not psychotherapy but rather sessions for information, education, and ventilation (Everly & Mitchell, 1998b; Mitchell et al., 2003).

Demobilization

Demobilization is also called group information briefings and crisis management briefings. These usually occur during rest breaks, at the end of a shift, or in the middle of the event as the event dictates. This provides information and resources to a group that has been affected by an incident. It brings people together, provides rumor control, and addresses possible reactions and self-help guidelines, usually in the form of a little handout. These are typically only a few minutes long (Everly & Mitchell, 1998b).

Critical Incident Defusing

Critical incident defusings are formal sessions that occur within 8 hours of the event. They typically last 20 to 45 minutes. They are done in small groups of 6 to 8 people of similar job descriptions. There is no record made of the proceedings. Often a defusing will negate the need for a formal debriefing. The facilitators introduce themselves and state the ground rules including strict confidentiality. The event, experiences, and reactions are reviewed. Reassurance is given and an assessment is made for the need for more help. The last phase normalizes the experience and teaches some basic stress survival skills (Everly & Mitchell, 1998b).

Critical Incident Stress Debriefing

Critical incident stress debriefing (CISD) is a formal event run by trained counselors. It is held within 72 hours of the event and typically lasts 2 to 3 hours. Again, no record is made of the proceedings and strict confidentiality is enforced. There are seven phases to a CISD.

In the first phase, the interventional team members and facilitators are introduced along with an explanation of the process and expectations. In the fact phase, each participant describes the event from his perspective on a cognitive level. Each describes his role and location during the event. The thought phase allows the participants to describe their cognitive reactions (thoughts) regarding the events and transitions into the emotional reactions. The fourth phase, the reaction phase, tend to be the most powerful and emotional part of the process. Participants describe the most traumatic part for them and their emotional reactions. In the symptom phase, the participants are guided back from a highly charged emotional state to a more cognitive level by being asked to describe some symptoms of stress they have experienced such as insomnia or tremors. The teaching phase is run more by the facilitators, and it serves as a cognitive anchor. Here the facilitators discuss normal stress reactions and provide some stress survival and management tips. This phase continues until the concerns of the group are exhausted. The seventh and last phase is the reentry phase. The session is summarized and any questions are answered. Handouts with stress management information, such as signs of stress and tips for self-care, and community referrals are given to the participants. There is usually a short social time with refreshments, which allows anyone with an individual question for the facilitators to ask the question outside the group. This technique has been employed in hundreds of large and small events worldwide (Chart 72–12) (Everly & Mitchell, 1998b; Mitchell et al., 2003).

Community

Crisis intervention for a community revolves around providing information, education, and direction. After an event, coordination of services for survivors, families, and communities, along with a centralized list of mental health volunteers, is needed. This should be part of the community's disaster plan with advanced coordination as to who responds and when. Within 24 hours, representatives for all the organizations and agencies, such as the state or county department of mental health, critical incident stress management teams, professional organizations, universities, and clergy, need to have a meeting to identify needs, resources, and responsibilities. With its extensive experience in handling disasters, its name recognition, and trust, the American Red Cross makes the ideal organization for handling mental health coordination for the community, as the state and county departments are often overwhelmed with delivery of services (Bowenkamp, 2003).

Considerations in planning and delivering mental health care to the community include assessing school needs, screening of volunteer workers, including any licensure issues, and making assignments based on skills and needs. Clergy may be teamed with mental health professionals and function independently depending on the need. The community may need assistance with day care including pediatric counseling. There needs to be defined support for families when notified of a death. The defusing and debriefing of each of the teams of volunteers and other mental health workers at the end of their shift is a key component of maintaining the workforce. Teams may also be needed to respond to families or persons unable to go to centers for assistance (Bowenkamp, 2003).

Community "town meetings," either in person or through the media, and frequent news bulletins provide relevant operations updates, stress management, and education. These help to provide rumor control and build and aid in community cohesion. These meetings foster personal and community empowerment (Everly, 2003).

Ottenstein (2003) has proposed a protocol for a guided group discussion that could be used in a community group or in a televised group for the community. Participants are encouraged to take notes. The stated goal during the introduction phase is "to help people share each other's fears and coping strategies so that we can learn a new way of coping with those threats and fears." The point is to help the group members understand what they can do to support themselves, their families, and each other.

Discussion topics include how each person attempts to gain control or to eliminate the threat, how people are using coping strategies to deal with the threat, and the use of unhealthy coping strategies such as increased smoking and drinking when under extreme stress. The new safety and security procedures and coping with the frustrations they produce are discussed. Acknowledge that spiritual beliefs can be powerful coping tools for difficult times. The concept of constructive ventilation is explained. Time is then given to allow for the constructive ventilation of feelings and emotions by the participants. Chart 72–13 summarizes self-care tips for stress management. The discussion is then summarized and the leaders teach additional coping strategies based on the ideas and feelings expressed. This protocol was implemented following the September 11, 2001, attacks, the anthrax attacks on the postal system, and the sniper attacks in Maryland and Virginia in 2002.

CHART 72–12 Stages in Critical Incident Stress Debriefing

1. **Introduction.** Introduce intervention team members (facilitators), explain the process, and set expectations. Strict confidentiality is emphasized.

2. **Fact.** Describe on a cognitive level the event from each participant's view.

3. **Thought.** Describe cognitive reactions and transition to emotional reactions.

4. **Reaction.** Identify emotional reactions to the most traumatic aspect.

5. **Symptom.** Identify personal symptoms of distress and transition back to cognitive level.

6. **Teaching.** Provide cognitive anchor. Educate regarding normal reactions and adaptive coping mechanisms.

7. **Reentry.** Clarify and prepare for termination.

CHART 72–13 Self-Care Tips for Stress Management

EXPECT EMOTIONAL REACTIONS

Emotions will vary day to day. They may reemerge weeks to months later.

Do not fight the feelings; they are part of the healing process and will diminish over time.

TAKE CARE OF YOURSELF EMOTIONALLY

Be gentle with yourself and others.

Tell and retell what happened.

Reach out to others for help and support.

Plan extra time to do tasks.

Do not try to make major life decisions at this time.

Try to maintain a normal schedule.

TAKE CARE OF YOURSELF PHYSICALLY

Eat regular meals of nutritious food. Decrease or cut out caffeine, as this will help with decreasing nervousness.

Get regular exercise.

Do activities relaxing for you.

Take rest breaks.

Go to bed for 8 hours each night.

Be wary of alcohol and other drugs, including tobacco. Alcohol is a depressant and interrupts normal sleep cycles.

Give yourself time to heal. If the symptoms do not gradually decrease or they cause you distress, call for assistance.

Source: Adapted from class handouts Critical Incident Stress Management Course # 26128327 May 26 and 27, 2000.

Summary

Regardless whether a disaster is weather related or a terrorist attack, hospitals, cities, counties, states, and the nation must be as prepared as possible. Nurses should know the disaster plan within their facility and where to find information quickly regarding possible substances that the patients may have been exposed to.

NCLEX® REVIEW

1. The student nurse inquires about an example "international" terrorism. The most appropriate response by the nurse would be:
   1. "When an act of terror or violence is generated toward the United States government by a group or an individual from Puerto Rico."
   2. "When a group such as the Ku Klux Klan or the Black Panthers performs terrorist activity against citizens of our own country."
   3. "When the group responsible for committing the violence has connection to a foreign country like al Queda in the Middle East."
   4. "When an individual like Timothy McVeigh uses an unlawful act of violence to destroy or intimidate individuals or the government."

2. The nurse attends a seminar on the use of various biological, chemical, radiological, and explosive agents throughout history. Which of the following statements by the nurse would indicate the need for further instruction?
   1. "The outbreak of an intentionally caused food-borne illness in Oregon during the early 1980s was attributed to *Shigella sonnei*."
   2. "There were never any documented adverse health effects following the Three Mile Island nuclear power leak in the U.S."
   3. "The largest peace-time incident involving a nerve agent occurred when sarin gas was released into the Tokyo subway system."
   4. "One of the earliest documented examples of biologic weapons use occurred in the 6th century B.C. with the Assyrian use of rye ergot."

3. The nurse is caring for the patient with a possible exposure to a biologic agent several days ago. The assessment reveals HR 142, BP 80/53, RR 34 and labored, T 103.2°F with chills, and diaphoresis. The patient complains of headache and chest pain, and chest x-ray reveals a wide mediastinum. Based on these findings, the nurse suspects the patient has contracted:
   1. Septicemic plague.
   2. Undulant fever.
   3. Typhoidal tularemia.
   4. Inhalation anthrax.

4. Which of the following nursing diagnoses would be the priority when caring for the patient with recent known nerve agent exposure?
   1. Ineffective airway clearance related to copious secretions and ineffective cough.
   2. High risk for altered cardiac output related to electrical conduction abnormalities.
   3. Increased risk for fluid and electrolyte imbalance related to vomiting and diarrhea.
   4. Ineffective individual coping related to perceived and actual threat from situation.

5. Approximately 30 minutes after exposure to a radiological leak at an industrial facility, several patients arrive at the emergency department. Upon their arrival at the hospital, the patients are all experiencing nausea, vomiting, diarrhea, fatigue, and hypotension. The nurse understands the patients are in which phase of Acute Radiation Syndrome?
   1. Latent phase
   2. Prodromal phase
   3. Recovery phase
   4. Illness phase

6. Which of the following statements is true regarding the use of the Hospital Incident Command System (HICS)?
   1. The Incident Commander is in charge of all four areas of operations—planning, logistics, safety, and public information.
   2. The plan outlines clearly defined responsibilities and positions that must remain independent of one another and individually run.
   3. This flexible plan allows for only necessary positions and functions to be activated on an as needed basis during the incident.
   4. Media utilization is limited in order to decrease mass hysteria and unwarranted overwhelming of communications.

7. With regard to the Strategic National Stockpile (SNS) the nurse understands that:
   1. It helps augment the local and state resources so as to help decrease the morbidity and mortality in the civilian population following a large-scale disaster.
   2. This program is organized using a four-tiered approach to include medical supplies and equipment, pharmaceutical agents, vaccines, and technical assistance.
   3. The 12-hour push pack is designed to be used to provide pharmaceuticals and medical supplies for treatment of a known agent or for smaller scale events.
   4. A team of logistical and operational experts called the National Disaster Response Unit may be required to assist state and local authorities with supply distribution.

8. Which of the following statements indicates the nurse has a clear understanding of Critical Incident Stress Management as it relates to health care workers?
   1. "Critical Incident Stress Debriefings (CISD) are formal sessions run by trained counselors that are held within 8 hours of a critical event."
   2. "Demobilizations are group briefings that increase knowledge and decrease stress by having each participant describe their cognitive level."
   3. "Group information briefings bring people together in an informal setting to give mutual reassurance and assess the need for more help."
   4. "Critical incident defusings are formal, confidential group sessions where the stressful event and its experiences and reactions are reviewed."

Answers for review questions appear in Appendix D

KEY TERMS

acute radiation syndrome (ARS) *p.2403*
asphyxiates *p.2395*
biologic agent *p.2383*
blister agent *p.2391*
bubo *p.2398*
CBRNE *p.2384*
chemical agent *p.2390*
choking agent *p.2395*
critical incident *p.2410*
critical incident stress debriefing
 (CISD) *p.2410*
critical incident stress management *p.2410*
decontamination *p.2389*
DMAT *p.2408*
DMORT *p.2409*
incapacitating agent *p.2396*
incident command system (ICS) *p.2405*
INCMCE *p.2384*
irritants *p.2396*
nerve agents *p.2391*
persistent *p.2390*
PPE *p.2387*
radiologic agents *p.2401*
RDD *p.2387*
riot control agent *p.2396*
Strategic National Stockpile (SNS) *p.2407*
terrorism *p.2382*
toxin *p.2400*
vesicant *p.2391*
vomiting agent *p.2396*
WMD *p.2384*
zones: cold zone, hot zone, warm
 zone *p.2389*

PEARSON

EXPLORE **mynursingkit™**

MyNursingKit is your one stop for online chapter review materials and resources. Prepare for success with additional NCLEX®-style practice questions, interactive assignments and activities, web links, animations and videos, and more!

Register your access code from the front of your book at
www.mynursingkit.com

REFERENCES

Abramowicz, M. (Ed.). (2002). Prevention and treatment of injury from chemical warfare agents. *The Medical Letter on Drugs and Therapeutics, 44*(1121), 1–4.

Agency for Toxic Substances and Disease Registry (ATSDR). (2001a). *Managing hazardous materials incidents: Vol. I. Emergency medical services: A planning guide for the management of contaminated patients.* Atlanta, GA: U.S. Department of Health and Human Services.

Agency for Toxic Substances and Disease Registry (ATSDR). (2001b). *Managing hazardous materials incidents: Vol. III. Medical management guidelines for acute chemical exposures.* Atlanta, GA: U.S. Department of Health and Human Services.

Agency for Toxic Substances and Disease Registry (ATSDR). (2001c). *Managing hazardous materials incidents: Vol. II. Hospital emergency departments: A planning guide for the management of contaminated patients.* Atlanta, GA: U.S. Department of Health and Human Services.

Agency for Toxic Substances and Disease Registry (ATSDR). (2004, September). *ATSDR Ammonia CAS # 7664-41-7.* Retrieved December 12, 2006, from http://www.atsdr.cdc.gov/tfacts126.pdf

Agency for Toxic Substances and Disease Registry (ATSDR). (2008). *Medical management guidelines for nerve agents: Tabun (GA); sarin (GB); soman (GD); and VX.* Retrieved September 22, 2008, from http://www.atsdr.cdc.gov/MHMI/mmg166.html

Arnon, S. S., Schechter, R., Inglesby, T. V., Henderson, D. A., Bartlett, J. G., Ascher, M. S., et al. (2001). Botulinum toxin as a biological weapon: Medical and public health management. *Journal of the American Medical Association, 285*(8), 1059–1070.

Auf der Heide, E. (2006). The importance of evidence-based disaster planning. *Annals of Emergency Medicine, 47*(1), 34–49.

Barrueto, F., & Hoffman, R. S. (2002). Biological agents: Botulinum, plague, and tularemia. *Resident and Staff Physician, 48*(4), 34–40.

Borio, L., Inglesby, T., Peters, C. J., Schmaljohn, A. L., Hughes, J. M., Jarling, P. B., et al. (2002). Hemorrhagic fever viruses as biological weapons: Medical and public health management. *Journal of the American Medical Association, 287*(18), 2391–2405.

Bowenkamp, C. (2003). Coordination of mental health and community agencies in disaster response. *International Journal of Emergency Mental Health, 2*(3), 159–165.

British Broadcasting Company (BBC). (2003). *ETA suspects held near Pamplona.* Retrieved October 4, 2008, from http://news.bbc.co.uk/2/hi/europe/3068149.stm

British Broadcasting Company (BBC). (2007). *Timeline: Litvinenko death case.* Retrieved October 4, 2008, from http://news.bbc.co.uk/1/hi/uk/6179074.stm

Burns, C., & Rosenberg, L. (2001). Redefining incidents: A preliminary report. *International Journal of Emergency Mental Health, 3*(1), 17–24.

Bush, G. W. (2002, December). *National strategy to combat weapons of mass destruction.* Retrieved October 31, 2003, from http://www.whitehouse.gov/news/releases/2002/12/WMDStrategy.pdf

Bush, G. W. (2003, February 28). *Homeland Security presidential directive/HSPD-5.* Retrieved December 1, 2006, from http://www.whitehouse.gov/news/releases/2003/02/20030228-9.html

Cable News Network (CNN). (1996, July 28). *Games go on after day of shock, grief.* Retrieved December 14, 2006, from http://www.cnn.com/US/9607/27/bomb.probe.pm

California Emergency Medical Services Authority (EMSA). (2006, August). *Hospital incident command system guidebook.* Retrieved December 14, 2006, from http://www.emsa.ca.gov/HICS/files/Guidebook_Glossary.pdf

Centers for Disease Control and Prevention (CDC). (2004, January 27). *Facts about cyanide.* Retrieved December 12, 2006, from http://www.bt.cdc.gov/agent/cyanide/basics/facts.asp

Centers for Disease Control and Prevention (CDC). (2005, April 14). *Strategic national stockpile.* Retrieved December 13, 2006, from http://www.bt.cdc.gov/stockpile/index.asp

Centers for Disease Control and Prevention (CDC). (2006a). *Bioterrorism agents/diseases.* Retrieved December 12, 2006, from http://www.bt.cdc.gov/agent/agentlist-category.asp

Centers for Disease Control and Prevention (CDC). (2006b, February 22). *Facts about lewisite.* Retrieved December 12, 2006, from http://www.bt.cdc.gov/agent/lewisite/basics/facts.asp

Centers for Disease Control and Prevention (CDC). (2006c, February 22). *Facts about phosgene.* Retrieved December 12, 2006, from http://emergency.cdc.gov/agent/phosgene/basics/facts.asp

Centers for Disease Control and Prevention (CDC). (2006d, February 22). *Facts about phosgene oxime.* Retrieved December 12, 2006, from http://www.bt.cdc.gov/agent/phosgene-oxime/basics/facts.asp

Centers for Disease Control and Prevention (CDC). (2006e, February 22). *Facts about sarin.* Retrieved December 12, 2006, from http://www.bt.cdc.gov/agent/sarin/basics/facts.asp

Centers for Disease Control and Prevention (CDC). (2006f, February 22). *Facts about soman.* Retrieved December 12, 2006, from http://www.bt.cdc.gov/agent/soman/basics/facts.asp

Centers for Disease Control and Prevention (CDC). (2006g, February 22). *Facts about sulfur mustard.* Retrieved December 12, 2006, from http://www.bt.cdc.gov/agent/sulfurmustard/basics/facts.asp

Centers for Disease Control and Prevention (CDC). (2006h, February 22). *Facts about tabun.* Retrieved December 12, 2006, from http://www.bt.cdc.gov/agent/tabun/basics/facts.asp

Centers for Disease Control and Prevention (CDC). (2006i, February 22). *Facts about VX.* Retrieved December 12, 2006, from http://www.bt.cdc.gov/agent/vx/basics/facts.asp

Centers for Disease Control and Prevention (CDC). (2006j, February 22). *Fact sheet: Anthrax information for health care providers.* Retrieved December 10, 2006, from http://www.bt.cdc.gov/agent/anthrax/anthrax-hcp-factsheet.asp

Centers for Disease Control and Prevention (CDC). (2006k, April 19). *Botulism facts for health care providers.* Retrieved December 7, 2006, from http://www.bt.cdc.gov/agent/botulism/hcpfacts.asp

Centers for Disease Control and Prevention (CDC). (2006l, May 10). *Prussian blue.* Retrieved December 7, 2006, from http://www.bt.cdc.gov/radiation/prussianblue.asp

Centers for Disease Control and Prevention (CDC). (2006m, June 14). *Explosions and blast injuries: A primer for clinicians.* Retrieved December 12, 2006, from http://www.bt.cdc.gov/masscasualties/explosions.asp

Centers for Disease Control and Prevention (CDC). (2006n, October 11). *Potassium iodide (KI).* Retrieved December 7, 2006, from http://www.bt.cdc.gov/radiation/ki.asp

Centers for Disease Control and Prevention (CDC). (2008, March 5). *Facts about ricin.* Retrieved September 22, 2008, from http://www.bt.cdc.gov/agent/ricin/facts.asp

Chertoff, M. (2006, June 16). *Nationwide plan review phase 2 report.* Retrieved June 20, 2006, from http://www.dhs.gov/xlibrary/assets/Prep_NationwidePlanReview.pdf

Christopher, G. W., Cieslak, J., Pavlin, J. A., & Eitzen, E. M. (1997). Biological warfare: A historical perspective. *Journal of the American Medical Association, 278*(5), 412–417.

Community Emergency Response Team–Los Angeles (CERT-LA). (2003, March 26). *CERT Los Angeles simple triage and rapid treatment.* Retrieved December 1, 2006, from http://www.cert-la.com/triage/start.htm

Community Research Associates (CRA). (2003). *Emergency response to terrorism: Instructor's guide.* Washington, DC: Office for Domestic Preparedness.

Compton, B., Stewart-Craig, E., & Doak, M. (Eds.). (1999). *SBCCOM domestic preparedness training program.* Washington, DC: Science Applications International Corporation.

Computer Sciences Corporation (CSC). (2008). *Department of Defense Joint Vaccine Acquisition Program (U.S.): CSC's DVC edges one step closer to plague vaccine.* Retrieved September 28, 2008, from http://www.csc.com/industries/government/casestudies/1710.shtml

Dang, C., Kare, J., Schneiderman, A., & Dang, A. B. (2002). Chemical warfare agents. *Topics in Emergency Medicine, 24*(2), 25–39.

Dayton Disaster Medical Assistance Team (DMAT). (2008). *Team basics.* Retrieved October 5, 2008, from http://www.daytondmat.com/dmat/dmatinfo.html

Dennis, D. T., Inglesby, T. V., Henderson, D. A., Bartlett, J. G., Ascher, M. S., Eitzen, E., et al. (2001). Tularemia as a biological weapon: Medical and public health management. *Journal of the American Medical Association, 285*(21), 2763–2773.

Disaster Management Systems (DMS). (2005). *All Risk triage tags.* Retrieved December 14, 2006, from http://www.triagetags.com

Durham, B. (2002). The background and history of manmade disasters. *Topics in Emergency Medicine, 24*(2), 1–14.

Esbitt, D. (2003, July–September). The Strategic National Stockpile. *Disaster Management and Response,* 68–70.

Everly, G. S. (2000). The role of pastoral crisis intervention in disasters, terrorism, violence, and other community crises. *International Journal of Emergency Mental Health, 2,* 139–142.

Everly, G. S. (2003). Psychological counterterrorism. *International Journal of Emergency Mental Health, 5*(2), 57–59.

Everly, G. S., & Mitchell, J. T. (1998a). *Assisting individuals in crisis.* Ellicott City, MD: International Critical Incident Stress Foundation.

Everly, G. S., & Mitchell, J. T. (1998b). *Critical incident stress management: The basic course workbook.* Ellicott City, MD: International Critical Incident Stress Foundation.

Federal Bureau of Investigation–Denver (FBI). (2006). *Terrorism.* Retrieved December 12, 2006, from http://denver.fbi.gov/nfip.htm

Fell-Carlson, D. (2003, January 30). Terrorist danger: Nurses must be ready for radiological threat. *Nurseweek,* 22–23.

Follow-up of deaths among U.S. postal service workers potentially exposed to *Bacillus anthracis*—District of Columbia, 2001–2002. (2003). *Morbidity and Mortality Weekly Report, 52*(39), 937–938.

Franz, D. R., Jarling, P. B., Friedlander, A. M., McClain, D. J., Hoover, D. L., Bryne, W. R., et al. (1997). Clinical recognition and management of patients exposed to biological warfare agents. *Journal of the American Medical Association, 278*(5), 399–411.

Gebbie, K. M., & Qureshi, K. (2002). Emergency and disaster preparedness: Core competencies for nurses. *American Journal of Nursing, 1*(102), 46–51.

Hagler, D. A. (2004). Nursing assessment: Respiratory system. In M. K. Lewis, M. M. Heitkemper, & S. R. Dirksen (Eds.), *Medical surgical nursing: Assessment of clinical problems* (pp. 542–565). St. Louis: Mosby.

Hardin, E. (2002). Biologic casualties: Treatment and management. *Topics in Emergency Medicine, 24*(2), 15–24.

Henderson, D. A., Inglesby, T. V., Bartlett, J. G., Ascher, M. S., Eitzen, E., Jarling, P. B., et al. (1999). Smallpox as a biological weapon: Medical and public health management. *Journal of the American Medical Association, 281*(22), 2127–2137.

Hick, J. L., Hanfling, D., Burstein, J. L., Markham, J., Macintyre, A. G., & Barbera, J. A. (2003). Protective equipment for health care facility decontamination personnel: Regulations, risks, and recommendations. *Annals of Emergency Medicine, 42*(3), 370–380.

House, H., Graber, M. A., & Scheckel, S. S. (2003, October). Is your emergency department ready for a terrorist attack? *Emergency Medicine,* 46–51.

Inglesby, T. V., Dennis, D. T., Henderson, D. A., Bartlett, J. G., Ascher, M. S., Eitzen, E., et al. (2000). Plague as a biologic weapon: Medical and public health management. *Journal of the American Medical Association, 283*(17), 2281–2290.

Inglesby, T. V., O'Toole, T., Henderson, D. A., Bartlett, J. G., Ascher, M. S., Eitzen, E., et al. (2002). Anthrax as a biological weapon, 2002: Updated recommendations for management. *Journal of the American Medical Association, 287*(17), 2236–2253.

International Nursing Coalition for Mass Casualty Education (INCMCE). (2003, July). *Educational competencies for registered nurses responding to mass casualty incidents.* Retrieved December 12, 2006, from http://www.incmce.org/competenciespage.html

Jacocks, J. (Ed.). (2003). *Medical management of radiological casualties* (2nd ed.). Bethesda, MD: Armed Forces Radiobiology Research Institute.

Kortepeter, M. (Ed.). (2001). *USAMRIID's medical management of biological casualties handbook* (4th ed.). Fort Detrick, MD: U.S. Army Medical Research Institute of Infectious Diseases.

Lee, E. C. (2003). Clinical manifestations of sarin nerve gas exposure. *Journal of the American Medical Association, 290*(5), 659–662.

Lehmann, J. (2002, September). Considerations for selecting personal protective equipment for hazardous material decontamination. *Disaster Management and Response,* 21–25.

Lenzer, J. (2003). Preparing your emergency department for a disaster: Whether it's bioterrorism or a natural disaster, make sure you're ready. *ACEP 2003 Reference & Resource Guide,* 10–15.

Levenson, R. L., & Acosta, J. K. (2001). Observations from ground zero at the World Trade Center in New York City: Part I. *International Journal of Emergency Mental Health, 3*(4), 241–244.

Martin, C. O. (2002, July). Cyanide toxins. *Emergency Medicine,* 11–13.

Maxwell, W. (2003). The use of gallows humor and dark humor during crisis situations. *International Journal of Emergency Mental Health, 5*(2), 93–98.

McKee, C. B., Collins, L., Keetley, J., Bausum, H., Besch, T., Moss, C., et al. (2000, May). *USACHPPM tech guide 244: The medical NBC battlebook.* Washington, DC: U.S. Army Center for Health Promotion and Preventative Medicine.

Medical Center of Louisiana at New Orleans (MCLNO). (2003, June). *Medical Center of Louisiana, Hazmat decon training: An operations level course. Student handbook.* New Orleans: Author.

Merck Manuals. (2005, November). *Radiation injury.* Retrieved December 7, 2006, from http://www.merck.com/mmpe/print/sec21/ch317/ch317a.html

Mitchell, A. M., Sakraida, T. J., & Kameg, K. (2003). Critical incident stress debriefing: Implications for best practice. *Disaster Management and Response, 1*(2), 46–51.

Mitchell, J. T., & Bray, G. P. (1980). *Emergency services stress.* Upper Saddle River, NJ: Brady/Prentice-Hall.

National Institute of Justice, Office of Justice Programs. (2003, April). *The effectiveness and safety of pepper spray.* Retrieved December 6, 2006, from http://www.ncjrs.org/pdffiles1/nij/195739.pdf

Neff, J. M., Lane, J. M., Fulginiti, V. A., & Henderson, D. A. (2002). Contact vaccinia—Transmission of vaccinia from smallpox vaccination. *Journal of the American Medical Association, 288*(15), 1901–1905.

Occupational Safety and Health Administration. (2005, January). *OSHA best practices for hospital-based first receivers of victims from mass casualty incidents involving the release of hazardous substances.* Retrieved February 1, 2005, from http://www.osha.gov/dts/osta/bestpractices/html/hospital_firstreceivers.html

Ottenstein, R. J. (2003). Coping with threats of terrorism: A protocol for group intervention. *International Journal of Emergency Mental Health, 5*(1), 39–42.

Plague vaccine. (1982, June 11). *Morbidity and Mortality Weekly Report, 31*(22), 301–304. Retrieved December 12, 2006, from http://www.cdc.gov/MMWR/preview/mmwrhtml/00041848.htm (page converted August 5, 1998, last reviewed May 2, 2001)

Raso, J. (1999, March 1). Three Mile Island: A 20th anniversary remembrance. *American Council on Science and Health.* Retrieved December 12, 2006, from http://www.acsh.org/publications/publD.867/pub_detail.asp

Ridge, T. (2004, March 1). *National Incident Management System.* Retrieved December 1, 2004, from http://fema.gov/pdf/emergency/nims/nims_doc_full.pdf

Riley, D., Clark, M., & Wong, T. (2002). World Trade Center terror: Explosion trauma-blast, burns, and crush injury. *Topics in Emergency Medicine, 24*(2), 47–59.

Riley, J. M. (2003, July–September). Providing nursing care with federal disaster relief teams. *Disaster Management and Response,* 76–79.

Romig, L. (2008). *The JumpSTART pediatric MCI triage tool.* Retrieved September 22, 2008, from http://www.jumpstarttriage.com/JumpSTART_and_MCI_Triage.php

Scharoun, K., Van Caulil, K., & Liberman, A. (2002). Bioterrorism vs. health security: Crafting a plan of preparedness. *Health Care Manager, 21*(1), 74–92.

Seed, T. M. (2002). Prevention and treatments: Summary statement. In Proceedings of the International Conference on Low-Level Radiation Injury and Medical Countermeasures. Supplement *to International Journal of AMSUS, 167*(2), 87–93.

Sidell, F. R., Patrick, W. C., Dashiell, T. R., Alibel, K., & Layne, S. (Eds.). (2002). *Jane's chem-bio book* (2nd ed.). Alexandria, VA: Jane's Information Group.

Smith, C. (2003, September 11). *Disaster mortuary operations response team.* Presentation at National Healthcare Profession Preparedness Consortium Health Care Leadership Course, Nobles Training Center, Anniston, AL.

Texas Engineering Extension Service, National Emergency Response and Rescue Training Center (TEEX). (2003). *Emergency medical services (EMS): Operations and planning for WMD incidents. Student manual.* Washington, DC: Office of Preparedness and Emergency Operations.

Thomas, R. J. (2002). Acute pulmonary effects from o-Chlorobenzylidenemalonitrile "tear gas": A unique exposure outcome unmasked by strenuous exercise after a military training event. *Military Medicine, 167*(2), 136–139.

3M. (2002, March). *Technical Data Bulletin #151: PAPR management and planning for first responders.* St. Paul, MN: Author.

Torok, T. J, Tauxe, R. V., Wise, R. P., Livengood, J. R., Sokolow, R., Mauvais, S., et al. (1997). A large community outbreak of salmonellosis caused by intentional contamination of restaurant salad bars. *Journal of the American Medical Association, 278*(5), 389–395.

Truab, S. J., & Hoffman, R. S. (2002). Agents of chemical warfare: I. Vesicant and irritant gases. *Resident and Staff Physician, 48*(6), 22–28.

Udeani, J. C., & Aguilera, P. (2002). Management of nuclear casualties. *Topics in Emergency Medicine, 24*(2), 40–46.

U.S. Army Medical Research Institute of Chemical Defense (USAMRICD). (2000). *Medical management of chemical casualties handbook* (3rd ed.). Aberdeen Proving Ground, MD: Author.

U.S. Department of Health and Human Services (DHHS). (2008a). *National disaster medical systems (NDMS).* Retrieved October 5, 2008, from http://www.hhs.gov/aspr/opeo/ndms/index.html

U.S. Department of Health and Human Services (DHHS). (2008b). *National disaster medical systems (NDMS) response teams.* Retrieved October 5, 2008, from http://www.hhs.gov/aspr/opeo/ndms/teams/index.html

U.S. Department of Transportation (DOT). (2008). *2008 Emergency response guidebook.* Washington, DC: U.S. Government Printing Office. Retrieved September 22, 2008, from http://hazmat.dot.gov/pubs/erg/guidebook.htm

U.S. General Accounting Office (GAO). (2003, August). *Report to congressional committees, hospital preparedness.* Washington, DC: Author.

Veenema, T. G., & Karam, P. A. (2003). Radiation: Clinical responses to radiologic incidents and emergencies. *American Journal of Nursing, 103*(5), 32–40.

WashingtonPost.com. (1998). *Oklahoma bombing chronology.* Retrieved December 12, 2006, from http://www.washingtonpost.com/wp-srv/national/longterm/oklahoma/stories/chron.htm

Williams, W. (2002, November 14). *CDC logistician.* Presentation at National Healthcare Profession Preparedness Consortium Health Care Leadership Course, Nobles Training Center, Anniston, AL.

World Nuclear Association. (2008). *Chernobyl accident.* Retrieved October 4, 2008, from http://www.world-nuclear.org/info/chernobyl/inf07.html

Caring for the Patient in the Emergency Department

Renee Semonin-Holleran

Outcome-Based Learning Objectives

After studying this chapter, the learner will be able to:

1. Explain the practice of emergency nursing.
2. Differentiate among the various components of the triage process and determine each component's relevance.
3. Compare and contrast patient priority categories.
4. Explain the legal issues related to the practice of emergency nursing.
5. Describe preparation for emergency nursing practice.

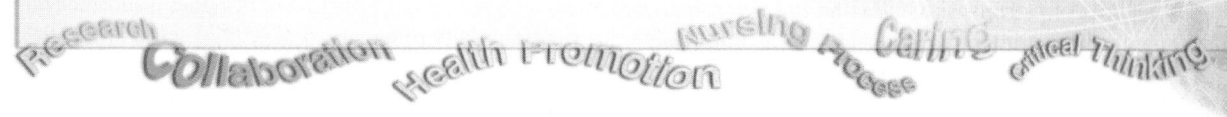

Emergency nursing is described as the care of individuals of all ages who have perceived or actual physical or emotional alterations of health that have not been diagnosed or require further interventions. Emergency nursing care is episodic, may involve primary as well as secondary and tertiary care, and is usually acute or critical in nature (Bonalumi & King, 2007; MacPhail, 2003). Emergency nursing involves care in a variety of areas including the prehospital and hospital environments.

The Emergency Nurses Association (ENA) states that emergency nursing provides care that ranges from birth to death. Emergency nursing also includes injury prevention, women's health, disease management, and providing care aimed at managing life- and limb-threatening emergencies. Unique to emergency nursing practice is the application of the nursing process to patients of all ages who require stabilization and/or resuscitation for a variety of illnesses and injuries (ENA, 1999).

History

Florence Nightingale has long been associated with the origins of emergency nursing when she took nurses out to the field to provide care to wounded soldiers. The care she and her fellow nurses provided on the battlefields demonstrated the value of rapid management of acute patients. As hospitals developed, care that had generally been done by health care providers,

nurses, or even family members in patients' homes was redirected to the hospital.

Emergency nursing and emergency medicine have developed into a specialty during the past 50 years. Care provided to soldiers during the Korean and Vietnam wars demonstrated that rapid and acute care could make a difference in patient outcomes. However, the departments in hospitals that were dedicated to the emergent care of patients were limited. Oftentimes, the emergency department was one room staffed by a nurse who was generally called down from another floor or by the hospital nursing supervisor.

When emergency medicine was recognized as a specialty in the late 1970s, it quickly became one of the fastest growing medical fields. The Emergency Department Nurses Association was established in 1970 by Anita Dorr (Buffalo, New York) and Judith Kelleher (Downey, California). The association's name was later changed to the Emergency Nurses Association. Initially, ENA and the American College of Emergency Physicians shared the same offices. As both associations grew, so did issues between the two groups (Schriver, Talmadge, Chuong, & Hedges, 2003). However, the important issues that face both emergency nurses and health care providers have brought both organizations together. Today emergency medicine and emergency nursing both have specific curricula and clinical requirements. Each also has specialized examinations. For emergency nursing that is the Certified Emergency

Nurse exam or the CEN. For information regarding the exam, go to the Emergency Nurses Association website.

The Role of the Emergency Department

In 2006, more than 119 million visits were made to emergency departments in the United States (National Center for Health Statistics, 2007). Emergency department visits continue to grow, yet emergency departments are closing, initiating ambulance diversions, increasing waiting times, and boarding patients who are critically ill and injured. This overcrowding in emergency departments is occurring because of decreasing numbers of doctors and nurses and limited hospital beds (Institute of Medicine [IOM], 2006; Reeder & Garrison, 2001).

Emergency departments have become the source of care for many types of patients, but particularly for patients who are poor and uninsured. Emergency departments are open 24 hours a day, 7 days a week. Additionally, because of the Emergency Medical Transport and Active Labor Act (discussed later in this chapter), emergency departments cannot refuse to provide a medical screening examination and stabilizing care when patients present for care. The increase in uninsured patients, the open access, and the ability to provide 24-hour-a-day care have stressed the capacity of emergency departments.

Emergency departments must also deal with the challenges of providing care to a more and more diverse patient population. Examples of the types of patients who utilize the emergency department to supply their primary care include illegal immigrants, prisoners, and homeless and underinsured patients. Additionally, the population has become more diverse culturally and care of these patients requires that emergency nurses and health care providers be culturally competent (see the Cultural Considerations box).

In the United States, the emergency department has become the single point of universal access to health care. This will continue to be an important challenge in the practice of emergency nursing, and one for which nursing will need to provide a leadership role in order to solve.

IOM Report and the Future of Emergency Care

In June 2006, the Institute of Medicine released a report on the state of emergency care in the United States. The IOM report recognized many of the challenges that are being faced today by the emergency medical system and its nurses and health care providers. Overcrowding, ambulance diversions, shortage of on-call specialists, lack of emergency preparedness, and deficiencies in pediatric emergency care are some of the issues that were identified. The recommendations summarized in the National Guidelines box have been made to improve emergency care systems in the United States using a multifaceted, multiorganizational approach. The IOM study and these proposals will provide a framework for the delivery of emergency care in the years to come.

Emergency Nursing Roles

The role of the emergency nurse is many and varied. Emergency nursing can be practiced both inside and outside of the hospital. In addition, emergency nurses may be involved in numerous functions within the emergency department including education, prevention, and research. Chart 73–1 summarizes some of the roles of emergency nurses.

Specialty Roles in Emergency Nursing

Emergency care requires a team approach and involves basic and advanced providers. As emergency nursing has evolved, both specialty and advanced practice roles have developed. Many of these roles are governed by specific agencies (e.g., state boards of nursing practice) or national associations (e.g., Sexual Assault Nurse Examiners). Chart 73–2 provides a summary of some of these specialty roles.

Triage

The word *triage* is derived from a French word that means "to sort." In emergency care, **triage** is a process that is used to determine the severity of a patient's illness or injury.

Medical triage evolved during war where battles resulted in lots of casualties and resources were limited. Napoleon's surgeon, Dominique Jean Larrey, has been credited with initiating this concept on the battlefield. Florence Nightingale used the triage concept during the Crimean War. She went out after the daily fighting and sorted out those who might or might not survive and provided much needed care (Thomas, Bernardo, & Herman, 2003).

During the 20th century, battlefield triage consisted of a primary assessment and the performance of critical interventions such as control of bleeding and then rapid transport to MASH units. During the Korean and Vietnam wars, helicopter transport was introduced to enhance the rapidity of patient care (Bracken, 2003).

In the 1960s, as emergency department censuses began to grow, the need for triage was recognized. Initially triage was performed by a physician or nurse physician team. Today, triage is generally performed by experienced emergency department nurses (Gilboy, Travers, & Wuerz, 1999).

Triage is performed in both the prehospital and hospital environments. Triage is a fluid process and is based on the number of patients, the amount of resources available, and the care that is available. Triage is an important component of emergency nursing practice as patient censuses continue to increase and more has to be provided with less.

CULTURAL CONSIDERATIONS for Emergency Care Providers

The cultural competence of emergency care providers should include an awareness of existing racial and ethnic health disparities and recognition of the incidence and prevalence of health problems among diverse populations that may present to the emergency department for care. A culturally competent emergency care provider also possesses the skills to identify and manage racial and ethnic differences in health values, beliefs, and behaviors, incorporating these so that patients receive the best care in the emergency department (Cone, Richardson, Todd, Betancourt, & Lowe, 2003; Lipson & Dibble, 2007).

NATIONAL GUIDELINES Summary of IOM Recommendations for Emergency Care in the United States

Recommendation	Actions
Improve hospital efficiency and patient flow through the emergency department.	Use tools from other disciplines such as engineering and operations research to improve patient flow.
	Establish clinical decision units or 24-hour observation units to hopefully prevent unnecessary admissions.
	Increase use of informational technologies to track and coordinate patient flow.
	Develop standards through accreditation bodies for crowding, boarding, and diversion.
Create a coordinated, regionalized, accountable emergency care system.	Develop regionalized systems that include hospitals, emergency medical services (EMS), and other agencies working together.
	Patients should be taken to the care center that can provide the optimal care, for example, to trauma or stroke centers.
	Develop well-defined standards and performance improvement measures.
Increase funding for emergency care systems.	Fund research to identify best practices.
	Request reimbursement for care of all patients who are treated in the emergency department.
	Acquire funding for disaster preparedness.
Improving pediatric emergency care.	Develop triage and transport protocols designed to provide children with the most appropriate care.
	Educate and train emergency care providers to care for children.
	Include pediatric concerns as part of disaster plans.
	Hire pediatric coordinators in EDs and EMS agencies to ensure that appropriate equipment, training, and services are provided to children.

Source: Institute of Medicine. (2006). *Hospital-based emergency care at the breaking point.* Washington, DC: National Academy of Sciences.

CHART 73–1   Emergency Nursing Roles

Role	Description
Urgent care center nursing	Nurses provide care in free-standing facilities that provide urgent care for minor illnesses and injuries.
Prehospital nursing	Nurses provide care in the prehospital care environment. These nurses are prepared through additional education that is generally regulated by the states in which they practice. For example, some states require nurses to take a prehospital nursing course or become emergency medical technicians (EMTs) or EMT-paramedics.
Transport nursing	Nurses accompany air or ground transport patients. Even though many nurses who perform transport may have emergency nursing experience, transport nurses may also have critical care nursing experience.
Military nurses	Nurses provide care as part of their military service.
Industrial nursing and occupational health nursing	Nurses provide care to specific industries or companies. Basic life support and ACLS are additional responsibilities of many of these nurses.
Correctional nursing	Nurses provide care in prisons and jails.

CHART 73–2   Specialty Roles in Emergency Nursing

Role	Description
Nurse educator	This is a nurse who is responsible for the educational needs of the emergency department. This role may also include patient and community education.
Emergency nurse practitioner (ENP)	ENPs are nurse practitioners who specialize in providing advanced nursing practice. There is no specific certification for emergency nursing, however, many ENPs hold certifications as family nurse practitioners, acute care nurse practitioners, pediatric nurse practitioners, or adult nurse practitioners.
Emergency clinical nurse specialist (ECNS)	A clinical nurse specialist is prepared at either the master's or doctoral level as an expert in emergency nursing. An ECNS may provide direct patient care, provide education, develop and perform research, and serve as a role model and change agent in the emergency department.
Case manager	An emergency case manager can provide care to a single patient or a group of patients. Case managers interact with many departments and outside agencies to assist the patient, families, and emergency department staff with care issues such as home health, drug dependence, and psychiatric problems so that the best and most cost-effective care is given to the patient.

The goals of triage include:

- Early and brief patient assessment
- Determination of the patient's urgency for care
- Documentation of findings
- Control of patient flow through the emergency department
- Assignment of patients to the appropriate care area
- Initiation of diagnostic measures
- Initiation of limited therapeutic interventions
- Infection control
- Promotion of public relations
- Health education for patients and families.

CRITICAL ALERT *An important part of triage is the "intuitiveness" that the emergency nurse may have about the patient. The triage nurse recognizes that there is something wrong. Oftentimes, few data are available to validate these "feelings." However, experienced emergency department nurses are good resources to alert new nurses about how to identify the less obvious indicators that a patient may be in trouble.*

Types of Triage

The type of triage that is used in an emergency department is dependent on several things including patient census, department layout, and number and type of staff. As previously stated, triage is usually performed by an experienced registered nurse. However, other types of triage models are summarized in Chart 73–3.

Components of Triage

Triage begins with an "across the room assessment." This involves what the triage nurse sees, smells, or sometimes even feels when first evaluating the patient. For example:

- Is the patient's airway open or is he drooling?
- Is the patient breathing and, if so, is the breathing effective?
- What is the patient's skin color: normal, pale, flushed?
- Are there any obvious signs of illness or injury?

A minimal amount of information should be gathered about why the patient has presented to the emergency department. Several mnemonics can be used to gather data depending on the patient's chief complaint or reason why she came to the emergency department. Charts 73–4, 73–5, and 73–6 contain mnemonics that can assist with collecting historical data in triage. Even though the CIAMPEDS mnemonic is directed more at collecting data for a pediatric patient, it can easily be adapted for the adult patient as well (ENA, 2004).

A brief, but focused physical assessment should be performed. Objective data can be collected by using a primary assessment that includes airway, breathing, circulation, and disability. The components of the primary assessment are discussed in detail in Chapter 74 🔗.

A secondary assessment may be required in some cases to better differentiate the severity of a patient's condition. The secondary assessment should include exposure with environmental control, a full set of vital signs and family presence, provision of comfort, additional history, and a head-to-toe assessment as needed using inspection, palpation, and auscultation. The components of the secondary survey are discussed in detail in the Chapter 74 🔗.

CHART 73–4	**CIAMPEDS Mnemonic**
C	Chief complaint
I	Immunizations
I	Isolation: exposed to a disease or hazardous material that may put the rest of the department in danger
A	Allergies
M	Medications
P	Parents' or caregivers' impression about the patient
E	Events surrounding the illness or injury
D	Diet
D	Diapers or output
S	Symptoms associated with the chief complaint, for example, fever, nausea, and vomiting

CHART 73–5	**MVIT Mnemonic**
M	Mechanism of injury
V	Vital signs
I	Injury
T	Treatment

CHART 73–6	**AMPLE History Mnemonic**
A	Allergies
M	Medications
P	Past medical history
L	Last meal
E	Everything that is related to the chief complaint

CHART 73–3	**Types of Triage**	
Type of Triage	**Components**	
Traffic director	*Nonprofessional (hospital registrar)* Writes down chief complaint.	
Spot check	*Nurse/health care provider* Evaluates patient. Assigns an urgency category.	
Comprehensive triage	*Registered nurse* Evaluates patient. Assigns an urgency category. Implements interventions (e.g., ordering a radiograph). Administers pain medication.	

Gerontological Considerations

With the aging population, it is important for the emergency department (ED) nurse to be familiar with the unique aspects of elderly assessment and planning of care. At a hospital in Canada that received 51,000 ED visits annually, adults who were 70 years of age or older used approximately 70% of the total bed days, and in 2005, those 75 years of age and older had an ED admit rate of approximately 37%, compared to an average admit rate for all ages of 15% (Sendecki, 2007). For this reason the hospital in Canada developed a course that applied geriatric/geropsychiatric knowledge, skills, and abilities the ED nurse can implement into their daily practice. An example is the need to assess falls as a symptom that requires investigation of root causes, treatment plan follow-up, and risk reduction to prevent another fall. They also assigned a position in the ED for a geriatric emergency nurse (GEN). The focus of the GEN is to identify needs and start a proactive care plan that is used during the patient's admission. The GEN also alerts community care to anticipated needs upon discharge. At the end of a 4-month trial they found that the GEN had seen approximately 25% of all patients who were 75 years of age or older; of those, 50% were admitted to the hospital; and the average length of stay of those who had been assessed by the GEN was 11.5 days, compared with 15.4 for those of the same age group not seen by the GEN (Sendecki, 2007). The ENA has also focused on ED care for elderly patients, as outlined in the Gerontological Considerations box. Chapter 10 provides detailed information regarding the aging patient.

Triage Urgency Categories

Once an initial evaluation has been made related to the patient's physical condition and chief complaint, the triage nurse will assign the patient an urgency category. Urgency categories rate patient acuity and assist in prioritizing care. Generally, an emergent patient is one who has an immediate life-threatening problem, for example, an airway obstruction. An urgent patient can wait a little longer, but would need to be seen as soon as possible. An example is a patient with chest pain, cardiac risk factors, and stable vital signs. Finally, a nonurgent patient can wait for care.

Many emergency departments use a three-level urgency category, but the continued increase in emergency department censuses, the augmented acuity of patients who are being cared for in the emergency department, and the numbers of patients who use the emergency department for primary care have prompted the use of additional levels of urgency. Charts 73–7 and 73–8, respectively, summarize four- and five-level triage urgency scales. There are resources available such as the Emergency Severity Index from the Emergency Nurses Association that describes the use of a five-level triage urgency category.

 Even when patients have been assigned a triage category, their condition may change, so patients who must wait for care must be reassessed at specific intervals. Triage policies and procedures should reflect when this must be done and documented. Unfortunately, patients have suffered significant harm and even death while waiting to be seen!

Disaster Triage

When a disaster occurs (earthquake, tornado, terrorist event), triage is directed at rapidly identifying patient urgency, assigning a category, and rapidly deploying to the most appropriate area for care. However, in a disaster, there may not be enough personnel or resources to care for everyone. In such a case, care may be withheld so that limited resources are used for those who will survive (Delaney & Drummond, 2002).

During a disaster, many emergency departments and community disaster programs use the START (simple triage and rapid treatment) system. This system evaluates respirations, perfusion, and mental status in order to determine who needs immediate transport, who can wait, or who may be unsalvageable. Color codes are used as a method of identification and communication. For example, green may mean that the patient can walk to an area for care (Super, Groth, & Hook, 1994). Refer to Chapter 72 for a detailed description of the START triage system.

Each emergency department and community should have a disaster plan that describes the manner of triage that should be employed during a disaster. The roles of the emergency nurse and other staff members should be practiced on a regularly

GERONTOLOGICAL CONSIDERATIONS in the Emergency Department

The Emergency Nurses Association has developed an online course entitled Geriatric Emergency Nursing Education (GENE). The course covers best practices that can be used to deliver optimal care and respond to the special needs of older adults. The course covers these topics:

- Attitudes and ageism
- Physical and psychological changes
- Atypical presentation of illness
- Triage
- Pain management
- Abuse and neglect
- Palliative care
- Discharge planning.

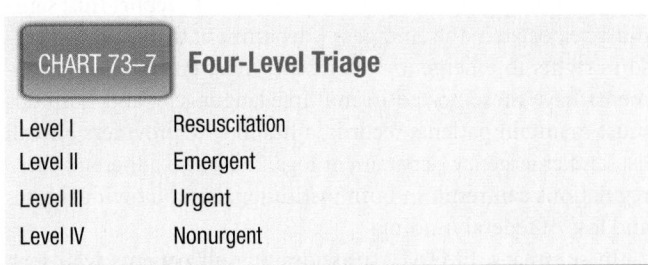

CHART 73–7	**Four-Level Triage**
Level I	Resuscitation
Level II	Emergent
Level III	Urgent
Level IV	Nonurgent

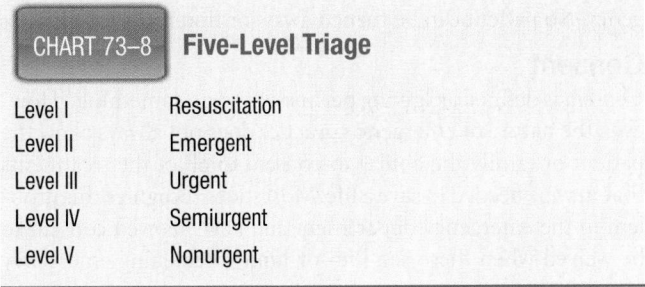

CHART 73–8	**Five-Level Triage**
Level I	Resuscitation
Level II	Emergent
Level III	Urgent
Level IV	Semiurgent
Level V	Nonurgent

scheduled basis. Additional information about disaster management is provided in Chapter 72 🕮 .

Legal Issues

The practice of emergency nursing requires comprehension and understanding of some of the legal issues that impact the emergency department. Three of these issues are discussed here: the Emergency Medical Treatment and Active Labor Act, consent, and evidence collection.

Emergency Medical Treatment and Active Labor Act

The **Emergency Medical Treatment and Active Labor Act (EMTALA)** is a part of the 1986 COBRA laws and the 1990 OBRA amendment that defines the legal responsibilities of Medicare-participating hospitals in treating individuals who present with emergency medical conditions (*Federal Register*, 2003). In summary, EMTALA provides that:

- A hospital is required to perform a medical screening exam to determine if there is an emergency when a patient presents to the emergency department.
- If it is determined that an emergency condition exists, the hospital must provide for further medical examination and treatment as required to stabilize the patient.
- If the hospital does not have the capabilities to provide the care needed, the patient may be transferred.
- An appropriate transfer is one in which the medical benefits outweigh the risk of transport or the patient makes an informed consent for transfer.
- The patient must be transferred with an appropriate level of care provided during the transport process.
- A hospital may never delay an appropriate medical screening examination or further examination or treatment to inquire about the patient's payment method or insurance status.

Also under EMTALA, hospitals that receive patients who may have been inappropriately transferred need to report this; signs must be posted in the emergency department that explain a person's rights to emergency treatment (most emergency departments have these posted in multiple languages); and hospitals must maintain patients records, a health care providers on-call list, and emergency department logs. Failure to adhere to these regulations can result in both institutional and individual fines and loss of federal funding.

In summary, EMTALA provides that all patients who seek treatment in the emergency department have a medical screening and treatment as deemed appropriate based on their emergency. No patient can be turned away for financial reasons.

Consent

Consent is defined as "giving permission to do something." However, the nature of emergency practice does not always allow the patient or family the ability to consent to all of the treatments that may be needed to save a life. Most states recognize this problem in the emergency department and have allowed consent to be waived when there is a life- or limb-threatening emergency (Lee, 2003).

The emergency nurse will generally encounter three types of consent. These include a *general (blanket) consent*, which is usually obtained at registration. This type of consent form will allow for evaluation and treatment, such as radiographs, laboratory tests, and medications. If more invasive tests are needed or the patient must undergo a specific procedure such as a fracture reduction that requires conscious sedation, informed consent should be obtained. *Informed consent* involves the patient stating by signing that he has a full understanding of the procedure, including its risks, and is competent to give consent. Even though the emergency nurse should check to see that a consent form has been signed, it is the health care providers responsibility to obtain informed consent. Finally, *implied consent* allows treatment in an emergency situation based on the presumption that if the patient were able to, she would give permission for treatment (Lee, 2003).

Each state dictates ages of consent, situations that may allow for legal consent despite age (pregnant underaged females), and other interesting nuances related to consent. It is imperative that the emergency nurse be familiar with the applicable state laws and hospital policies related to consent. When in doubt, always safely err on the side of the patient and when possible consult hospital risk management personnel before acting. It is also important to document why decisions were made to prevent any "legal" second-guessing.

Evidence Collection and Preservation

Unfortunately, a major part of emergency nursing practice is caring for the victims of violence. Sexual assault, domestic assault, and motor vehicle crashes are only a few of the examples of the types of patients who may require that the emergency nurse collect and preserve evidence. **Forensic evidence** is something that is legally submitted to a court of law as a means of determining the truth related to an alleged crime (Doyle, 2001). Examples of evidence include clothing, body fluids, bite marks, and photographs of injuries.

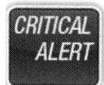 *Every emergency department should have a policy and procedure for the collection and preservation of evidence. Improper collection and preservation could lead to erroneous interpretation of the evidence.*

Evidence must be collected using a specific protocol and procedure that includes how to label the evidence, preserve it, and maintain the chain of custody. Some evidence collection protocols are directed by specific legal agencies or even state agencies. Chart 73–9 contains a summary of procedural steps for evidence collection and preservation in the emergency department (Semonin-Holleran, 2004).

Preparation for Practice

Preparation for practice in the emergency department for new graduates or nurses without emergency experience can be demanding. Nursing care in the emergency department includes learning to manage the care of four or five patients simultaneously; starting all of the patient care, for example, inserting intravenous lines and drawing blood for evaluation; limited and focused patient assessment, oftentimes with little or no patient information; discharge teaching and planning; and care of populations and patient problems not frequently encountered in admitted patients such as acute psychosis, sexual assault, and

CHART 73–9	Collection and Preservation of Evidence and Chain of Custody

1. Identify the indications for evidence collection and consult authorities to ensure that the appropriate evidence is collected and preserved.

2. Obtain and use the appropriate evidence collection kit.

3. Obtain patient consent according to hospital policy and procedure. In some cases consent may not be necessary, for example, in a homicide investigation. Consult appropriate authorities.

4. When collecting evidence, change gloves frequently to prevent cross-contamination.

5. Try not to perform any wound care until photographs have been taken.

6. Place evidence in individual labeled containers.

7. Wet evidence should always be dried before packaging.

8. Always place evidence in a paper bag.

9. Label all evidence with this information:
   a. Patient's name
   b. Source of collection
   c. Date
   d. Time
   e. Person collecting the evidence.

10. Evidence should be sealed with evidence tape. Never lick evidence envelopes.

11. Photographs may be taken by an emergency nurse. They must be labeled and stored in a secured area. Only take photographs if experienced in how to do it properly.

12. Document the evidence collection procedure. Use checklists when available.

13. Place evidence in a secure, locked area until it is released to the appropriate authorities.

14. Maintain the chain of custody, who collected the evidence, anyone who touches or secures it and what is done with the evidence until it is given to law enforcement, for all evidence.

15. Complete the chart and document what was given to authorities and who received the evidence.

---

homelessness. It also requires familiarity with diverse patient populations, varied age groups, and social problems that may never be solved (Proehl, 2002).

Additional education for new orientees to the emergency department should include:

- Advanced Cardiac Life Support (ACLS)
- Trauma Nursing Core Course (TNCC)
- Emergency Nursing Pediatric Course (ENPC).

Nursing care for patients or conditions not frequently encountered by new orientees with their limited experience (e.g., obstetrics and gynecology; eye, ear, nose, and throat; pediatric and psychiatric emergencies) should also be included.

Discharge Priorities

The majority of patients seen in the emergency department are sent home rather than admitted to the hospital. An important part of discharge planning is providing information about how to manage the problem that brought the patient to the emergency department and where the patient should obtain further care.

Discharge instructions should be clear and use terminology that the patient understands. Most educators recommend that discharge instructions be written at a fifth- or sixth-grade level. When possible, they should be translated into a language that the patient or family understands or at a minimum an interpreter should be present when the instructions are given. Illustrations of what is expected (e.g., how to wrap an elastic bandage on an injured extremity) may be of assistance. Instructions must also be age appropriate. This is especially important when medications are being prescribed.

Many commercial programs that provide discharge instructions are available. These instructions can be printed and sent with the patient or, in some cases, they can be accessed online from the patient's home.

Discharge instructions should include information about follow-up care. In some emergency departments, patients may be asked to return; in other EDs, patients may be referred to a health care provider, advanced practitioner, or clinic. It is important to ensure that the patient or family members understand the information that is provided. Asking the patient questions or to do a return demonstration may assist in determining the level of understanding. Some emergency departments have instituted follow-up calls to not only find out about follow-up care, but to check on the patient's status. It is important to allow the patient or family the opportunity to ask questions and feel as comfortable as possible with the prescribed care for their illness or injury.

Health Promotion

Emergency nurses not only play a key role in the management of ill or injured patients, but also in injury and disease prevention. One primary example is through Emergency Nurses CARE (ENCARE). ENCARE was started by two emergency nurses in the 1980s who had become involved in trying to prevent injuries and death from alcohol-related emergencies (ENA Injury Prevention Institute/ENCARE, 2008). Emergency Nurses CARE has now become the Injury Prevention Institute/ENCARE of the Emergency Nurses Association.

ENCARE provides training for volunteer nurses and emergency medical technicians related to specific issues such as injury prevention and public health issues. Currently ENCARE provides five primary education and prevention programs:

- Alcohol Awareness Program
- Bike and Helmet Safety
- Child Passenger Safety
- Gun Safety: It's No Accident
- Healthy Aging: Take Care.

Through the efforts of its many volunteers, ENCARE has reached hundreds of thousands of people throughout the United States.

Much research has been done and is ongoing regarding injury prevention and the best ways to educate communities. Other research opportunities for emergency nursing are included in the Research Opportunities and Clinical Impact feature.

Summary

The practice of emergency nursing involves the care of diverse patient populations in many types of situations. It requires skills that include the ability to identify critically ill and injured patients and start their care from the beginning and patience with difficult societal problems such as caring for the homeless. It also involves ethical challenges as described in the Ethical Issues feature, and the practice of emergency nursing should be evidenced based. The Evidence-Based Practice feature gives an example of evidence-based nursing practice in the emergency department.

Emergency nursing encompasses all aspects of care from pediatric to geriatric, medical to surgical, and to a very diverse population of patients both culturally and economically. It requires excellent assessment and critical thinking skills as well as procedural proficiency. Emergency nursing is a rewarding way to "nurse."

ETHICAL ISSUES Regarding Pain Management in the Emergency Department

Pain is the most common complaint seen in the emergency department. Despite this, only 40% to 60% of the patients are treated for pain. Many patients face **oligoanalgesia**, in which no interventions are provided for pain relief despite patient complaints of pain when they come to the emergency department. Many reasons are cited for this, including fear of "masking" symptoms and concern about the physiological effects of pain medications. Other studies have demonstrated that women and minorities do not receive appropriate pain management. Emergency nurses need to be patient advocates and ensure that a patient's pain is assessed, documented, and managed. Pain management requires a collaborative approach including protocols so that analgesic agents can be administered as soon as possible. All patients should receive pain care (Knox et al., 2007).

EVIDENCE-BASED PRACTICE

Family Presence During Resuscitation in the Emergency Department

Clinical Problem
Should the family be allowed to be present during resuscitation in the emergency department?

Research Findings
In 1982, the Foote Hospital in Michigan surveyed 13 surviving relatives about whether they would have liked to be present during the resuscitation of their family members. Seventy-two percent said that they would have liked to have been present. A program was developed to allow selected "accompanied" family members to be allowed to be present during resuscitation. Seventy family members and 21 physicians, nurses, and others were surveyed after the event. Seventy-six percent of the family members felt that being present assisted them in their grieving process. They also felt that the patient did not die alone and emergency care providers did everything that they could. Staff members, however, felt hampered in their resuscitation efforts and reported increased stress because the patients became more "human" in the presence of family members. No family member interfered with the resuscitation efforts (Doyle et al., 1987).

This landmark study opened the "floodgates" to consider the role of the family in resuscitation. Since 1987, more than 60 papers have been published that address this issue. Families have expressed that they are not concerned about what they may see or hear in the resuscitation area—they just want to be with their family member. More than half of the families felt they had a right to be present and, again, felt that their grieving process was aided. The staff's perspective includes fear of interference from the family and the need to display more professional behaviors during the resuscitation process. Interestingly, physicians are more opposed to family presence than are nurses.

Implications for Nursing Practice
When implementing family presence in the ED during resuscitation, a policy needs to be in place that addresses when it can and cannot be allowed; all staff need to be prepared and trained; well-qualified and trained staff should always accompany the patient; and resources must be available to the staff to help them cope with any issues that may arise (Walker, 2006).

Critical Thinking Questions

1. What should be in place in the emergency department to allow family presence?
   a. A clergy member to provide spiritual care for the patient and family
   b. A policy and procedure that describes how to implement the process
   c. Staff who object to the presence of a family member during resuscitation
   d. Security or police so that the family is kept away during resuscitation

2. Which of the following fears have staff members expressed when allowing a family member to be with a patient during resuscitation?
   a. Fear that the family member may interfere with the resuscitation
   b. Fear that they must see the patient as a human being during the resuscitation
   c. Fear that they must act more professionally during the resuscitation
   d. All of the above

Answers to Critical Thinking Questions appear in Appendix D.

References
Doyle, C., Post, H., Burney, R., Maino, J., Keefe, M., et al. (1987). Family participation during resuscitation: An option. *Annals of Emergency Medicine, 16*, 673–675.

Walker, W. (2006). Witnessed resuscitation: A concept analysis. *International Journal of Nursing Studies, 43*, 377–387.

RESEARCH OPPORTUNITIES AND CLINICAL IMPACT RELATED TO EMERGENCY NURSING

Research Area	Clinical Impact
Physiological Research	
The management of acute and chronic pain in the emergency department	Many patients do not have their pain appropriately managed and frequently present to the emergency department for pain medication.
Use of alternative methods to manage pain in the emergency department	Alternative methods of pain management such as acupuncture, acupressure, and massage could be used by nurses to manage pain in the emergency department.
Development of guidelines to manage shock in the emergency department	Innovative assessment and monitoring methods and treatment therapies would emerge for the management of the patient in shock.
Psychosocial, Ethical, and Legal Research	
Effectiveness of family presence during invasive procedures and resuscitation	Identify how to include the family in the care of their critically ill or injured family member. Assist in end-of-life decision making.
Problem of overcrowding in emergency departments and ambulance diversion by EDs	Learn to manage the limited resources of emergency departments, including nursing staff, in order to meet the needs of all patients, particularly the uninsured and underinsured patients who use the emergency department for their health care.
Effectiveness of follow-up phone calls within 24 hours of a patient visit	Decrease return visits and get patients into the appropriate health care systems, thereby decreasing costs.

NCLEX® REVIEW

1. As it relates to the practice of emergency nursing, the nurse understands that:
   1. It always involves episodic patient care that is usually chronic or critical in nature.
   2. It can describe patient care for perceived, actual, or undiagnosed health problems.
   3. It has long been associated with Judith Kelleher and her care of wounded soldiers.
   4. It is challenged to become culturally competent as the patients become analogous.

2. You are the emergency department nurse responsible for triage. All of the following patients present simultaneously for care. With your triage assessment complete, which patient should be treated first?
   1. A patient complaining of chest pain and shortness of breath with pale, clammy skin, nausea and diaphoresis
   2. A patient with a three centimeter laceration to the right forearm with normal sensation and minimal bleeding
   3. A patient having a possible allergic reaction with facial edema, drooling, stridor, and severe urticaria with pruritis
   4. A patient experiencing increasingly more severe problems urinating and has a large palpable bladder

3. The patient presents to the emergency department with a complaint of nontraumatic back pain for four months that has previously been evaluated by his or her primary care provider. The patient states, "I ran out of my pain medicine last night, and my doctor refuses to call in another prescription." Objective findings are unremarkable. Vital signs are HR 89, BP 130/60, RR 18, T 98.9°F, SpO$_2$ 99%, and pain 5 on a 0–10 scale. Based on the four-level system, how should this patient be categorized at triage?

   1. Level I – Resuscitative
   2. Level II – Emergent
   3. Level III – Urgent
   4. Level IV – Nonurgent

4. The patient presents to the emergency department with a left shoulder dislocation that must be reduced quickly as the radial pulse on the affected side is no longer palpable. The injury occurred 30 minutes prior to arrival, and the patient states he or she is experiencing severe pain. The emergency nurse understands that which of the following consents must be obtained prior to this patient's treatment?
   1. General consent and informed consent
   2. Informed consent and implied consent
   3. Implied consent and blood product consent
   4. Blood product consent and general consent

5. You are orienting a new nurse graduate to the emergency department. Which of the following statements made by the new nurse regarding preparation for emergency nursing would indicate the need for further instruction?
   1. "I am planning on taking additional training to help prepare myself to deal with any potential psychiatric emergencies."
   2. "I am glad that emergency nurses do not have to deal with obstetrical issues because they can call the labor and delivery nurses."
   3. "I will take the Trauma Nursing Core Course soon because I know I need more experience with trauma assessment."
   4. "I now feel more confident in my time management skills when it comes to caring for multiple patients simultaneously."

Answers for review questions appear in Appendix D

KEY TERMS

emergency nursing *p.2415*
Emergency Medical Treatment and Active
   Labor Act (EMTALA) *p.2420*

forensic evidence *p.2420*
oligoanalgesia *p.2422*

triage *p.2416*

PEARSON

EXPLORE mynursingkit™

MyNursingKit is your one stop for online chapter review materials and resources. Prepare for success with additional NCLEX®-style practice questions, interactive assignments and activities, web links, animations and videos, and more!

Register your access code from the front of your book at
www.mynursingkit.com

REFERENCES

Bonalumi, N., & King, D. (2007). Professionalism and leadership. In S. Hoyt and J. Selfridge-Thomas (Eds.), *Emergency nursing core curriculum* (6th ed.). Philadelphia: W. B. Saunders.

Bracken, J. (2003). Triage. In L. Newberry (Ed.), *Sheehy's emergency nursing: Principles and practice* (5th ed.). St. Louis: Mosby.

Cone, D. C., Richardson, L. D., Todd, K., Betancourt, J., & Lowe, R. (2003). Health care disparities in emergency medicine. *Academic Emergency Medicine, 10*(11), 1176–1183.

Delaney, J., & Drummond, R. (2002). Mass casualties and triage at a sporting event. *British Journal of Sports Medicine, 36,* 85–88.

Doyle, C., Post, H., Burney, R., Maino, J., Keefe, M., et al. (1987). Family participation during resuscitation: An option. *Annals of Emergency Medicine, 16,* 673–675.

Doyle, J. S. (2001). *Evidence collection handbook from the Kentucky State Police.* Retrieved October 10, 2008, from http://firearmsid.com/KSP%20Evidence%20Manual/KSP%20Manual%20Main.htm

Emergency Nurses Association. (1999). *Emergency Nurses Association scope of emergency nursing practice.* Des Plaines, IL: Author.

Emergency Nurses Association. (2004). *Emergency nursing pediatric course.* Des Plaines, IL: Author.

ENA Injury Prevention Institute/ENCARE. (2008). *History and background.* Retrieved October 10, 2008, from http://www.ena.org/ipinstitute/history

Federal Register. (2003). Department of Health and Human Services 42 CFR Parts 413,482, and 489 Medicare programs; Clarifying policies related to the responsibilities of Medicare-participating hospitals in treating individuals with emergency medical conditions. Final rule September 9, 2003.

Gilboy, N., Travers, D., & Wuerz, R. (1999). Re-evaluating triage in the new millennium: A comprehensive look at the need for standardization and quality. *Journal of Emergency Nursing, 25*(6), 463–473.

Institute of Medicine. (2006). *Hospital-based emergency care at the breaking point.* Washington, DC: National Academy of Sciences.

Knox, T., Ducharme, J., Choiniere, M., Crandall, C., Fosnocht, D., Homel, P., et al. (2007). Pain in the emergency department: Results of the Pain and Emergency Department Initiative (PEMI) multicenter study. *Journal of Pain, 8*(6), 460–466.

Lee, G. (2003). Legal and regulatory constructs. In L. Newberry (Ed.), *Sheehy's emergency nursing: Principles and practice* (5th ed.). St. Louis: Mosby.

Lipson, J. G., & Dibble, S. L. (Eds.). (2007). *Culture and clinical care.* San Francisco: UCSF Nursing Press.

MacPhail, E. (2003). Overview of emergency nursing. In L. Newberry (Ed.), *Sheehy's emergency nursing: Principles and practice* (5th ed., pp. 1–5). St. Louis: Mosby.

National Center for Health Statistics. (2007). *Emergency department visits.* Retrieved September 10, 2007, from http://www.cdc.gov/nchs/fastats/ervisits.htm

Proehl, J. (2002). Developing emergency nursing competence. *Nursing Clinics of North America, 37*(1), 89–96.

Reeder, T. J., & Garrison, H. G. (2001). When the safety net is unsafe: Real-time assessment of the overcrowded emergency department. *Academic Emergency Medicine, 8*(11), 1070–1073.

Schriver, J., Talmadge, R., Chuong, R., & Hedges, J. (2003). Emergency nursing. *Journal of Emergency Nursing, 29*(5), 431–439.

Semonin-Holleran, R. (2004). Preservation of evidence. In J. Proehl (Ed.), *Emergency nursing procedures.* Philadelphia: W. B. Saunders.

Sendecki, C. (2007). Care of the acutely ill elderly in ER: Growth of the role of geriatric ER nurses. *Outlook* (Fall 2007).

Super, G., Groth, S., & Hook, R. (1994). *START: Simple triage and rapid treatment plan.* Newport Beach, CA: Hoag Memorial Hospital.

Thomas, D. O., Bernardo, L. M., & Herman, B. (2003). *Core curriculum for pediatric emergency nursing.* Boston: Jones and Bartlett Publishers.

Walker, W. (2006). Witnessed resuscitation: A concept analysis. *International Journal of Nursing Studies, 43,* 377–387.

Caring for the Patient with Multisystem Trauma

Cheryl Wraa

Outcome-Based Learning Objectives

After studying this chapter, the learner will be able to:

1. Discuss the correlation between mechanism of injury with patient assessment based on an understanding of the kinematics of trauma.

2. List the priorities of the primary and secondary surveys.

3. Explain the rationale for the tertiary survey.

4. Compare and contrast special considerations experienced during the initial resuscitation.

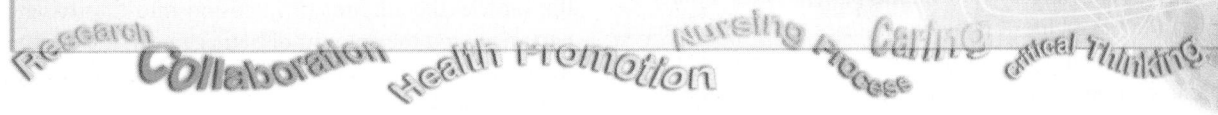

TRAUMATIC INJURY is a major public health problem. It is currently recognized as one of the most important threats to public health and safety in the United States with regard to years of productive life lost, permanent disability, and cost (American College of Surgeons, Committee on Trauma, 2006). In the United States, injury is a leading cause of death regardless of age, race, gender, or economic status (Centers for Disease Control and Prevention [CDC], 2007b). In high-income nations such as the United States, injury is the leading cause of death in the first four decades of life; in low- and middle-income nations it is second only to infectious diseases (Sommers, 2006).

Although traumatic injury is a leading cause of death, many patients survive their injuries but may experience a permanent disability, chronic pain, and a permanent change in their quality of life. The National Trauma Data Bank (NTDB) contains the largest aggregation of data reported from the trauma registries of hospital trauma centers. Their 2006 report reviews combined data from 2001 through 2005. The data show that the majority of injuries are unintentional, with the greatest percentage (41.3%) related to motor vehicle traffic incidents followed by falls (27.2%) (NTDB, 2007). It is important to note that the word *unintentional* is used rather than *accidental*. Throughout the years it has been recognized that the cause of most unintentional injury is the result of poor choices or behaviors, and that these in-

juries may have been preventable. An example of a poor choice is to consume alcohol and then attempt to drive. Alcohol alters a person's judgment and coordination. The following statistics are part of the Emergency Nurses Association (ENA) Injury Prevention Institute/ENCARE *Alcohol Awareness Fact Sheet* (2006a):

- Alcohol-related motor vehicle crashes kill someone every 31 minutes and nonfatally injure someone every 2 minutes.

- Twenty-one-year-olds to 24-year-olds have the highest rate of alcohol impaired driving and the highest percentage of fatal alcohol-related crashes.

- A systematic review of 65 studies on fatal nontraffic injuries, found that intoxication occurred in 31.5% of homicide cases, 31% of unintentional injury deaths, and 22.7% of suicide cases.

Alcohol consumption is also a major factor in family violence, suicides, homicides, and altercations.

Because unintentional injuries are a major source of morbidity and mortality, injury prevention has become a major public health goal. The U.S. Department of Health and Human Services and Public Health Service have developed the *Healthy People 2010: National Health Promotion and Disease Prevention Objectives*. The objectives that pertain to injury and violence prevention are listed in the National Guidelines box (p. 2426).

MyNursingKit | Emergency Nurses Association

NATIONAL GUIDELINES *Healthy People 2010*

Goal: Reduce injuries, disabilities, and deaths due to unintentional injuries and violence.

Objectives:

1. Injury prevention to reduce:
   - Nonfatal head injuries
   - Nonfatal spinal cord injuries
   - Firearm-related deaths
   - Nonfatal firearm-related injuries
   - Child fatality
   - Nonfatal poisonings
   - Deaths from poisoning
   - Deaths from suffocation

2. Unintentional injury prevention to:
   - Reduce deaths from unintentional injuries
   - Reduce nonfatal unintentional injuries
   - Reduce deaths from motor vehicle crashes
   - Reduce pedestrian deaths
   - Reduce nonfatal motor vehicle injuries
   - Reduce nonfatal pedestrian injuries
   - Increase use of safety belts
   - Increase use of child restraints

- Increase motorcycle helmet use
- Establish graduated driver licensing
- Increase bicycle helmet use
- Establish bicycle helmet laws
- Reduce residential fire deaths
- Increase functioning smoke alarms in residences
- Reduce deaths from falls
- Reduce hip fractures
- Reduce drowning
- Reduce dog bite injuries
- Increase injury protection in school sports

3. Violence and abuse prevention to:
   - Reduce homicides
   - Reduce maltreatment and maltreatment fatalities of children
   - Reduce physical assault by intimate partners
   - Reduce rape or attempted rape
   - Reduce sexual assault other than rape
   - Reduce physical assaults
   - Reduce physical fighting among adolescents
   - Reduce weapon carrying by adolescents on school property

---

Kinematics of Injury

Imperative in the care of the trauma patient is the ability to identify and treat all life-threatening injuries quickly. Traumatic injury occurs when a source of energy makes contact with the body and the body cannot tolerate the exposure to that energy. The extent of injury depends on the type and amount of energy force and the tissue response to the force. Newton's first law of motion states that a body at rest remains at rest, and a body in motion remains in motion until acted on by an outside force (Feliciano, Mattox, & Moore, 2008). Force is the result of energy transference. Energy is neither created nor destroyed—it is transferred; and different factors influence the amount of energy the human body absorbs, including:

- The amount of energy absorbed by objects that are struck first (the body of the vehicle for example)
- The amount of energy absorbed by protective devices such as helmets, padded dashboards, and air bags.

The slower the energy force is applied, the less energy transference and degree of destruction.

Injury patterns have been identified through the evaluation of the type of trauma that occurred and the amount of force that was generated. These known patterns assist health care providers to be anticipatory when caring for trauma patients. The predictive patterns of injuries are referred to as **kinematics**.

Motor Vehicle Collisions

As stated, motor vehicle collisions cause some of the most commonly seen injuries. When a patient is admitted due to a motor vehicle crash it is important to try to ascertain the speed the vehicle was traveling and where it impacted an object or was impacted by another vehicle. This will enable the nurse to better understand the amount of energy that was dispersed. Other indicators of the force energy are the amount of damage noted to the vehicle, the amount of intrusion into the passenger compartment, and the amount of damage from the occupant striking parts of the interior such as the steering wheel, dashboard, or windshield.

Frontal Impact

When a vehicle impacts an object or another vehicle head-on, energy is transferred to the vehicle. The front stops and the rear of the automobile continues to move forward until all energy is dispersed. The same principle occurs with the passenger in the vehicle. When the front of the vehicle stops, the body continues to move forward. If the passenger is restrained properly, then the seat belts will absorb most of the energy and prevent the body from colliding with immovable objects such as the windshield. This is also true if the air bag is deployed. A seat belt can impose a load that is 20 to 50 times as great as the weight of the body. The portion of the body that has the ability to receive this load is the pelvis. If the passenger has the belt over the abdomen rather than the pelvis, compression injury may occur to the abdominal organs. Abrasions and/or ecchymosis from the seat belt are important indicators of possible underlying injury (Figure 74–1 ■).

If the passenger is not restrained and the air bag does not deploy, then the body might travel down and under the steering wheel or up and over the steering wheel, incurring injury at the body's point of impact with the vehicle (Figure 74–2 ■). Patterns of injury that are anticipated are:

- Cervical spine fracture
- Traumatic brain injury
- Anterior flail chest
- Myocardial contusion

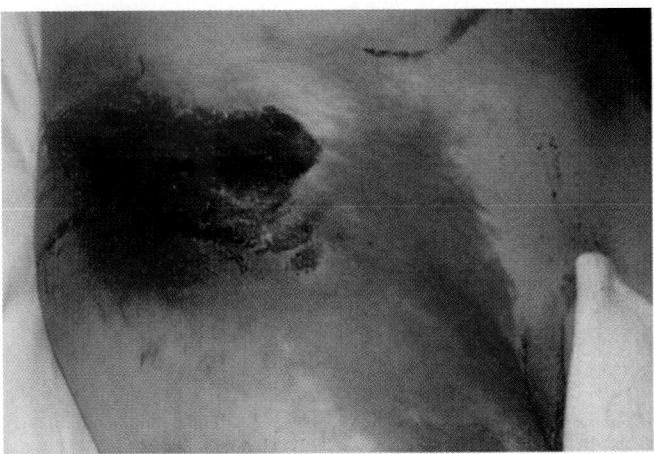
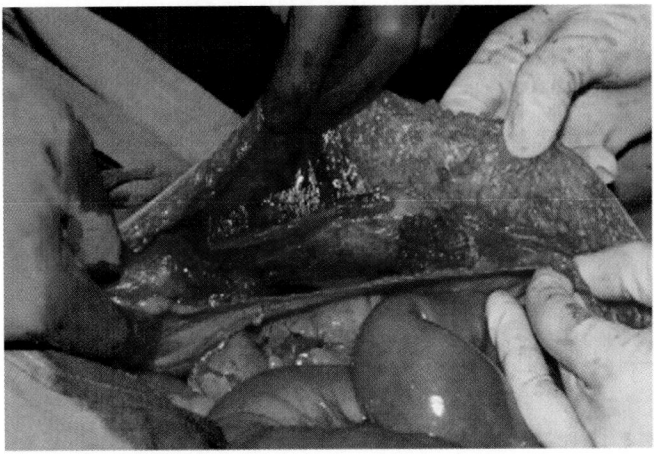

FIGURE 74–1 ■ Sealtbelt injury.
Source: Cheryl Wraa

- Pneumothorax
- Traumatic aortic disruption
- Fractured spleen or liver
- Posterior fracture/dislocation of the hip, knee, and/or ankle (American College of Surgeons [ACS], 2004; Feliciano, Mattox, & Moore, 2008).

Side Impact

As many as 31% of fatalities from motor vehicle crashes are a result of side impact (ACS, 2004). Most injuries from side impact are dependent on whether the vehicle remains in place or moves away from the point of impact. If the vehicle remains in place,

then the amount of damage to the vehicle and intrusion into the passenger compartment signifies the amount of energy that the body may have absorbed. Passengers generally receive most injuries on the same side of the body as the vehicle impact. Patterns of injury that are anticipated are:

- Contralateral neck sprain
- Cervical spine fracture
- Brachial plexus injury
- Lateral flail chest
- Pneumothorax
- Traumatic aortic disruption

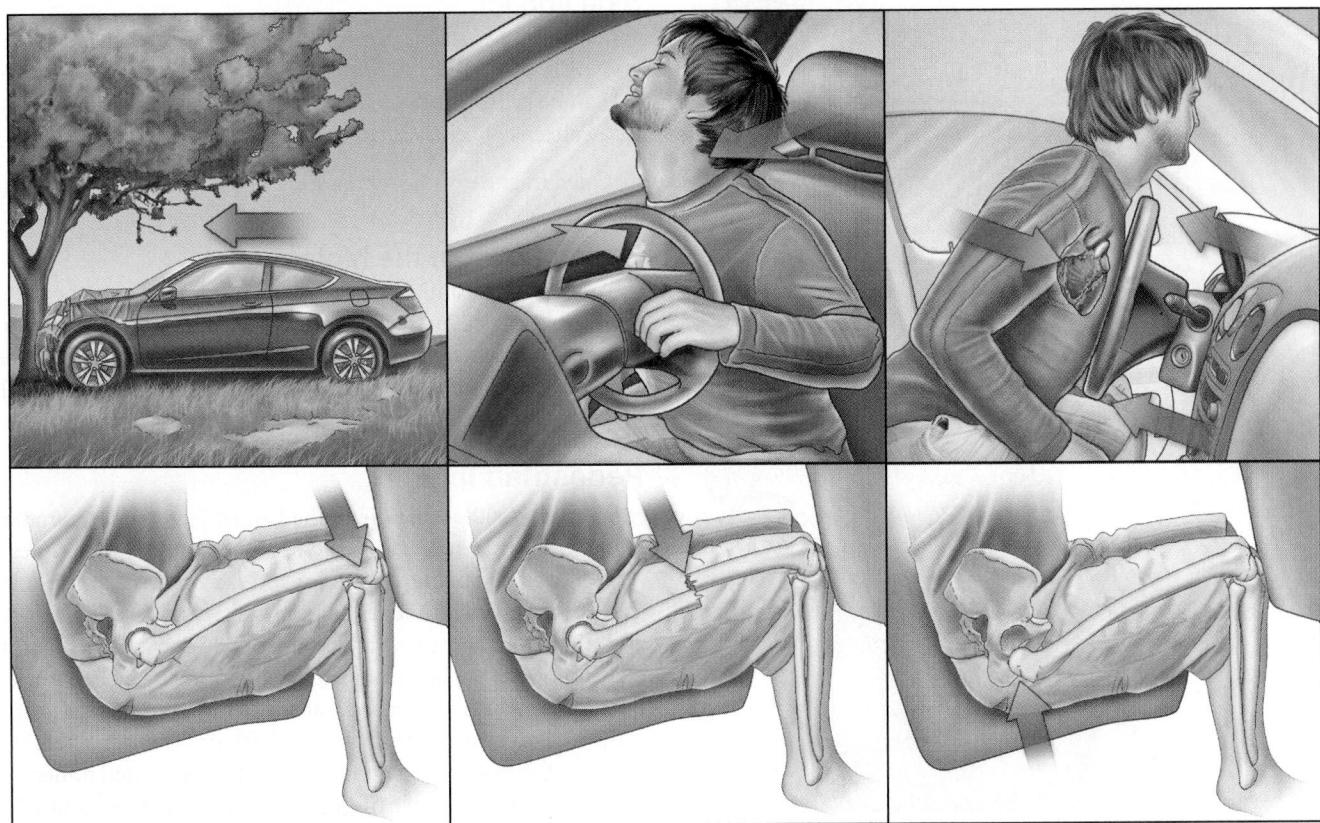

FIGURE 74–2 ■ Unrestrained frontal impact.

- Diaphragmatic rupture
- Fractured spleen/liver and/or kidney depending on the side of impact
- Fractured pelvis or acetabulum (ACS, 2004).

Rear Impact

When a vehicle is struck from behind, the initial impact accelerates the stationary vehicle and may force the vehicle into a frontal collision. If the headrests in the vehicle are not properly positioned, the sudden acceleration may cause hyperextension of the neck. If the vehicle that is hit then stops suddenly from a frontal impact or the driver applying the brakes suddenly, then rapid forward deceleration occurs (Figure 74–3 ■). This increases the chance for passenger injury. Patterns of injury that are anticipated are:

- Cervical spine injury
- Soft tissue injury to the neck (ACS, 2004).

Vehicle Rollover

When a vehicle rolls over it can be difficult to predict the pattern of injury. Injury occurs at the points where the body contacts the vehicle. Generally, this type of mechanism produces more severe injury than other types of crashes because of violent, multiple motions during the rollover. It is important to assess these patients carefully because they have the potential for multiple-system injuries.

Ejection

When a person is ejected from a vehicle, his chance of severe injury increases by more than 300% (ACS, 2004). Ejection occurs when the passenger is thrown from the vehicle, and injury occurs at the body's point of impact. Ejection places the patient at risk for all injury mechanisms and mortality is significantly increased (ACS, 2004).

Motorcycle Crashes

Motorcycle crashes are also common causes of traumatic injuries. Motorcycles do not have the surface area to absorb energy from impacts, therefore, energy is directly absorbed by the rider and injuries are substantially more severe than in vehicle crashes.

Frontal Impact

A motorcycle's center of gravity is located in front of the driver's seat. When a frontal impact occurs, the back of the motorcycle tips upward from the weight under the handlebars. The driver is propelled over the handlebars, but may not be totally ejected due to the back tipping forward. If there is a passenger behind the driver, this person is often catapulted over the driver and fully ejected. Patterns of injury include:

- Fractured femurs, tibias, and fibulas (from the driver's body hitting the handlebars)
- Chest and abdominal injuries (from compression against the handlebars)
- Traumatic brain and cervical spine injury (ACS, 2004).

Side Impact

When a motorcyclist is impacted from the side, that side of the body is unprotected and absorbs all of the energy. The exposed leg can be crushed between the motorcycle and the second object. Patterns of injury include:

- Open fracture of the femur, tibia/fibula, and malleolus (ACS, 2004).

Laying Down of the Motorcycle

If a motorcyclist anticipates a collision, she may use the technique of laying down the bike and sliding off to the side. The energy transference occurs as the body slides away from the bike. Without sufficient protective clothing, abrasions will occur with pieces of asphalt becoming embedded in the abrasions.

Pedestrian Injuries

More than 7,000 people die in the United States each year after being struck by a motor vehicle (ACS, 2004). Injury patterns can be predicted depending on the age and size of the victim and the size of the vehicle. Children tend to freeze and face the vehicle and, therefore, end up with more frontal injuries than adults. Depending on the height of the child and the vehicle bumper, the impact occurs on the chest or the femurs and then the child is thrown backward with the upper back or head impacting the ground. A very small child may be knocked down and under the vehicle due to his center of gravity, size, and weight. Multiple-system trauma should be suspected on any child hit by a vehicle.

Adults usually try to escape being hit and turn away from the vehicle, thus sustaining lateral injuries on the side impacted by

Whiplash

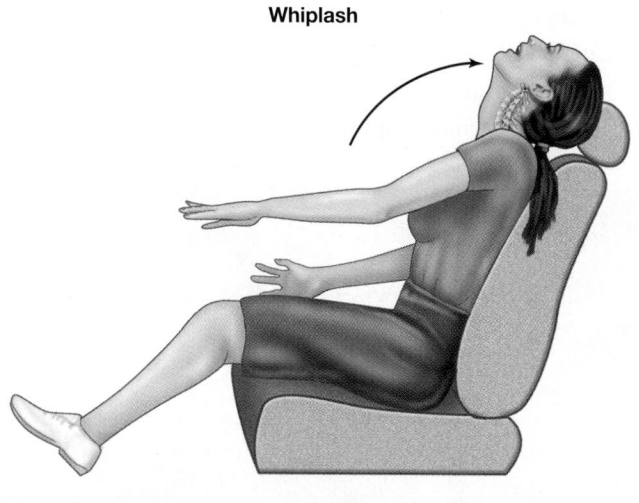

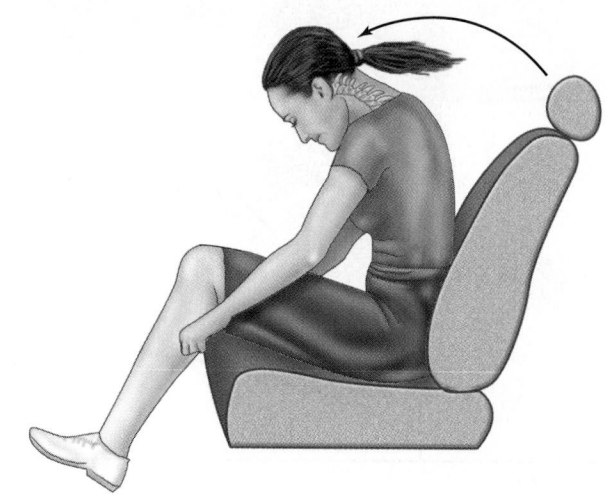

FIGURE 74–3 ■ Rear impact.

RISK FACTORS for Youth Violence

Individual Risk Factors
- History of violent victimization or involvement
- Attention deficits, hyperactivity, or learning disorders
- History of early aggressive behavior
- Involvement with drugs, alcohol, or tobacco
- Low IQ
- Poor behavioral control
- Deficits in social-cognitive or information processing abilities
- High emotional distress
- History of treatment for emotional problems
- Antisocial beliefs and attitudes
- Exposure to violence and conflict in the family

Family Risk Factors
- Authoritarian childrearing attitudes
- Harsh, lax, or inconsistent disciplinary practices
- Low parental involvement
- Low emotional attachment to parents or caregivers
- Low parental education and income

- Parental substance abuse or criminality
- Poor family functioning
- Poor monitoring and supervision of children

Peer/School Risk Factors
- Association with delinquent peers
- Involvement in gangs
- Social rejection by peers
- Lack of involvement in conventional activities
- Poor academic performance
- Low commitment to school and school failure

Community Risk Factors
- Diminished economic opportunities
- High concentrations of poor residents
- High level of transiency
- High level of family disruption
- Low levels of community participation
- Socially disorganized neighborhoods

Source: Centers for Disease Control and Prevention. (2007b). *Injury and violence.* Retrieved April 14, 2007, from http://www.cdc.gov/node.do/id/0900f3ec8000e539.

the vehicle. Approximately 80% of adults hit by a vehicle will have injuries to the lower extremities (Feliciano et al., 2008). Injury patterns include:

- Lower extremity fractures above and below the point of impact
- Fractured pelvis (pedestrian hits the hood of the vehicle or point of impact)
- Head injury (pedestrian falls off hood of vehicle to the ground) (ACS, 2004).

Falls

Falls are the leading cause of death for Americans 65 years of age and older (CDC, 2007a) and will be discussed in detail later in the chapter. The injury from a fall is similar to that of a motor vehicle crash in that it is caused by an abrupt change in velocity. The roof line of a one-story house is usually 15 feet. With falls greater than 15 feet, adults usually land on their feet. If the fall is less than 15 feet, adults will land in the same position at which they fell. Small children have larger heads in proportion to their bodies and therefore, no matter the distance of the fall, they tend to land headfirst.

The severity of the injury also depends on the give of the surface on which the person lands. A soft surface, such as sand, will absorb more energy than cement. Patterns of injury include:

- Calcaneus fractures
- Compression fractures to T_{12}–L_1
- Bilateral wrist fractures (as the body falls forward after the first impact)
- Traumatic brain injury (ACS, 2004).

Penetrating Injuries

Violence is an important public health problem. According to the CDC, in 2004, more than 750,000 persons ages 10 to 24 were

treated in emergency departments for injuries due to violence. During that same year, a nationwide survey of high school students revealed that 33% reported being in a fight one or more times during the preceding year and that 17% of students reported carrying a weapon during the month preceding the survey (CDC, 2007b). The CDC also reported that research on youth violence has shown certain risk factors to be associated with youth violence, as listed in the Risk Factors box.

The severity of injury in penetrating trauma depends on the velocity or speed of the penetrating object. Energy created by the object is dissipated into the surrounding tissues much like a shock wave. Consider the shock wave going through human tissue that is elastic in nature (Figure 74–4 ■). The stress that is imparted to the tissue is dependent on the velocity, or speed, of the object entering the body, the velocity of the waves in the tissue, and the mass or density of the object that entered the body. The larger and faster the article, the more damage to the tissues (ACS, 2004).

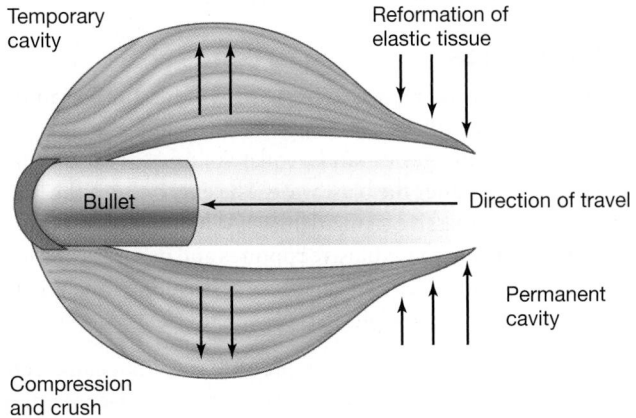

FIGURE 74–4 ■ Cavitation.

Stab Wounds

Stab wounds are low velocity and produce their injury directly as the object penetrates tissue. Knowing the length of the object and how far it entered the body helps the nurse to anticipate what organs might be injured. Also, knowing the position of the attacker and victim can help identify the path of the weapon. Knowing the gender of the attacker may also assist in determining the path of the weapon. Men tend to stab upward and women tend to stab overhand or downward.

Although tissue damage is usually isolated to the area of penetration, a single stab wound may penetrate several body cavities depending on the pathway. During expiration the dome of the diaphragm reaches as high as the fifth rib. Stab wounds to the chest at or below the level of the nipple should be suspect for abdominal injury as well. Also, an attacker may stab the victim only once but move the weapon around causing extensive internal damage to the surrounding structures.

Gunshot Wounds

Every year more than 30,000 Americans are killed with firearms. In the United States, unintentional firearm deaths of children nearly all occur in or around the home. Firearm injuries peak in the 19-year-old age group and then decrease after the age of 22. Serious injuries from a firearm, such as traumatic brain injury, can require a lifetime of care and rehabilitative services that can cost upwards of $1,000,000 over the victim's lifetime (Emergency Nurses Association, Injury Prevention Institute, 2006b; NTDB, 2007).

The severity of the damage caused by a bullet depends on the amount of energy transferred from the bullet to the body. Handguns and some small-caliber rifles are considered medium energy; hunting and assault rifles are considered high energy and, therefore, capable of transferring more energy to the tissue than smaller guns. The degree of deformation of the bullet also influences the degree of tissue damage. Bullets that are constructed of soft lead and flatten on impact, or have a hollow point that "mushrooms" on impact, cause more tissue damage than a full metal jacket bullet due to the increased diameter.

It is important to assess the patient for the number of wounds that are present. It is difficult to determine whether a wound is an entrance or exit wound so the nurse should never assume that the bullet is not still in the body if two wounds are present. Bullets will follow the path of least resistance once they enter the body, so it is almost impossible to truly know the path the bullet has taken from just the external exam.

Blast Injuries

Terrorist activity has increased the chance of blast injury in the United States. In a blast, explosives are detonated and changed to gases. When the gas expands, equal volumes of air are displaced and travel after the blast wave. The energy from the blast wave can cause massive tissue damage. When the blast occurs, the casing that held the explosive ruptures and its pieces become high-velocity projectiles that can cause penetrating injury. Blast injury can occur in three phases:

1. The concussive effects of the pressure wave can cause central nervous system (CNS) injury, rupture of air-containing organs, and tearing of membranes and small vessels.

2. Fragments of glass, rock, and metal debris become high-velocity projectiles that can cause penetrating injury.

3. The victim may be thrown through the air and sustain injury similar to that sustained when ejected from a vehicle or when a person has fallen from a height.

Adequate care of the trauma patient depends on the health care team's ability to quickly identify life-threatening injury and intervene. Understanding kinematics and the subsequent patterns of injury helps the caregivers to be anticipatory and less likely to miss an injury.

■ Initial Assessment of the Trauma Patient

It is important to develop a systematic approach to the trauma patient. Deaths from trauma occur in a trimodal distribution. The first peak of deaths from trauma occurs prior to definitive care at the scene or en route to the medical facility and results from nonsurvivable injuries such as aortic disruption; the second peak occurs within the first few hours after injury and is most commonly due to hemorrhage or severe traumatic brain injury; the third wave occurs days to weeks after the injury and is a result of complications, including infection or multiple organ dysfunction. A systematic, thorough initial assessment and resuscitation will decrease the number of deaths that occur during the second and third peaks by quickly identifying injury and beginning definitive care.

Initial nursing management follows a systematic approach to care and includes a rapid primary survey, resuscitation of vital functions, a detailed secondary survey, and initiation of definitive care. During the initial assessment the health care team must identify injuries, intervene when life-threatening injuries are present, and prioritize care. It is critical for all members of the trauma team to prepare for the arrival of trauma patients and know their role during the initial resuscitation (Figure 74–5 ■). As one member of the team completes the primary and secondary survey, many procedures are done simultaneously such as accessing veins, obtaining blood for tests, and inserting a Foley catheter and gastric tube.

It is important to have one team member who is overseeing the resuscitation and directing the team. This person is usually a trauma surgeon and does not provide direct care unless necessary. Instead, this person observes the resuscitation efforts and correlates all data being obtained to direct the plan of care. The nurse should be familiar with the resuscitation area and the equipment available. We discuss the initial steps of trauma care next.

Primary Survey

The primary survey follows a specific sequence:

A Airway maintenance with cervical spine immobilization

B Breathing and ventilation

C Circulation and hemorrhage control

D Disability (neurological status)

E Exposure/environmental control (e.g., remove all clothing but prevent hypothermia by placing warm blankets on the patient or using ambient warmers).

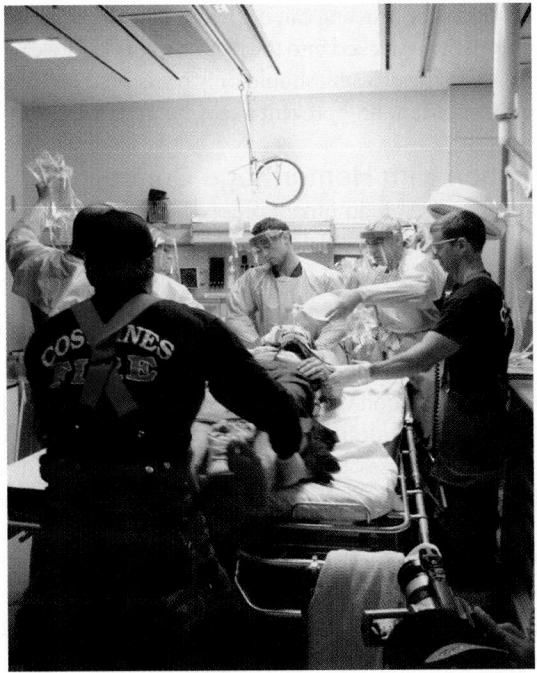

FIGURE 74–5 ■ Trauma team.
Source: Cheryl Wraa

Airway Maintenance

A secure and patent airway is the first priority for the trauma patient. While the airway is assessed, the patient's cervical spine should be maintained in a midline position and not moved (Figure 74–6 ■). The patient's airway should first be assessed for patency. Look for signs of airway obstruction from blood or foreign bodies, facial/mandibular fractures, or tracheal/laryngeal injury that may occlude the airway. If the patient's level of consciousness is such that she would not be able to protect her airway if she began to vomit, then an endotracheal tube should be inserted to protect the airway. Whenever a trauma patient is intubated, it is important to protect the cervical spine by maintaining in-line stabilization during the procedure. All multiple-system trauma patients, particularly with an altered level of consciousness or blunt injury above the clavicle, should be treated as if they have a cervical spine injury until proven otherwise.

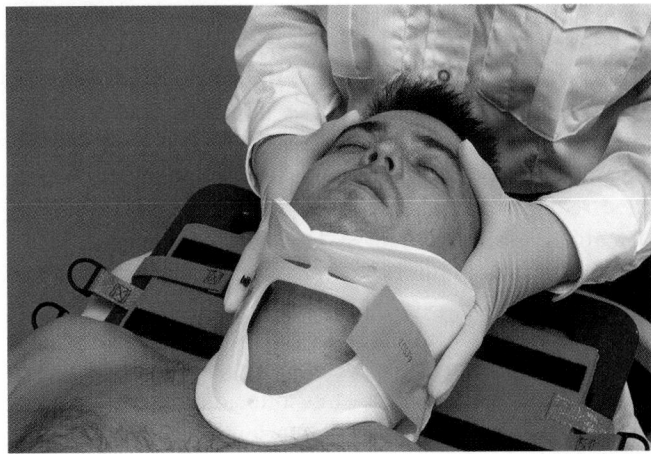

FIGURE 74–6 ■ Cervical stabilization.

 CRITICAL ALERT *Reevaluation of the patient's airway should be done frequently.*

Breathing and Ventilation

Adequate function of the lungs, chest wall, and diaphragm is necessary for adequate ventilation. Expose the chest to visualize and assess chest wall excursion. Listen to breath sounds to identify a pneumothorax or hemothorax. Palpate the chest wall to identify injuries that might compromise ventilation. Injuries that can impair ventilation acutely include **flail chest**, which occurs when two or more ribs are fractured in two or more places and are no longer attached to the thoracic cage, resulting in a free-floating segment. The free-floating segment moves independently from the rest of the chest resulting in paradoxical chest wall movement (Figure 74–7 ■). This can be observed during inspection of the chest. The impaired movement of the chest wall results in decreased tidal volume, vital capacity, and impaired cough leading to hypoventilation and atelectasis.

The amount of energy exerted on the body to cause a flail chest usually will damage the underlying lung tissue, resulting in a **pulmonary contusion**. Pulmonary contusion is initially a hemorrhage followed by alveolar and interstitial edema. The

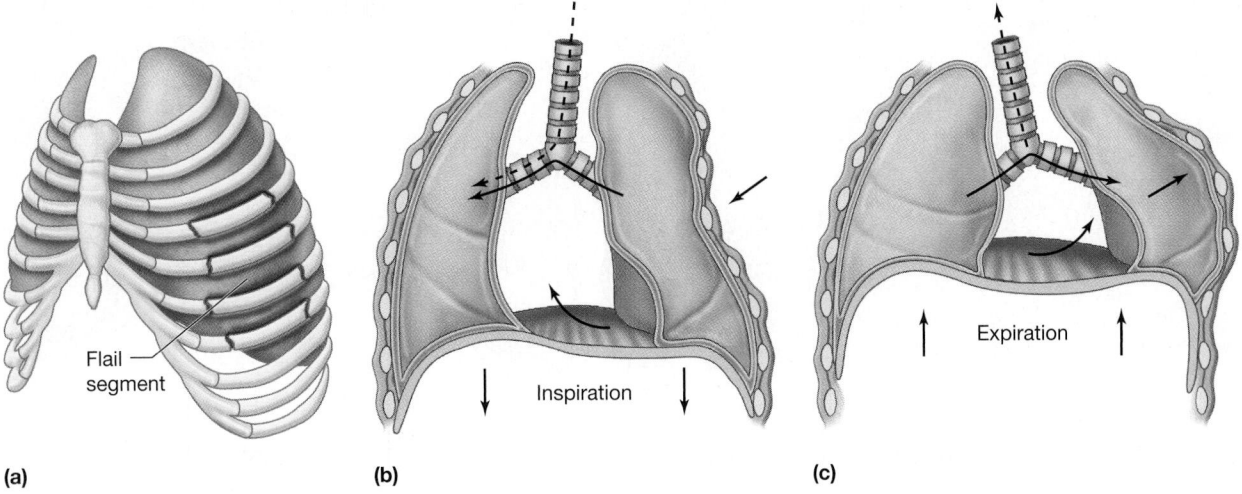

(a)   (b)   (c)

FIGURE 74–7 ■ Flail chest.

edema affects the alveolar-capillary units in the area of the contusion. If the edema increases it can cause decreased compliance and increased pulmonary vascular resistance and can affect pulmonary blood flow. Clinical manifestations may develop over 24 to 48 hours and include moist crackles in the contused lung, cough with blood-tinged sputum, and pulmonary infiltrate on chest radiograph. Pulmonary contusion is the most common, potentially lethal chest injury (Urden, Stacy, & Lough, 2006).

Tension pneumothorax occurs when an injury perforates the chest or pleural space. During inspiration air enters the pleural space and becomes trapped. As more air is trapped, the pressure in the pleural space increases collapsing the lung and causing the mediastinum to shift to the opposite side (Figure 74–8 ). This pressure exerts pressure on the heart and vascular structures in the chest, resulting in decreased cardiac output and venous return. A tension pneumothorax is diagnosed by clinical assessment, and the pressure must be released immediately by venting the chest on the affected side with a large-bore needle or chest tube or the patient will die. Symptoms include severe dyspnea, tachycardia, and hypotension.

A **massive hemothorax** is an accumulation of 1,500 mL or more of blood in the thoracic cavity. This amount of hemorrhage can result from injury to intercostal or internal mammary arteries, lung tissue, the heart, or the great vessels. The patient will present with signs and symptoms of hypovolemic shock with breath sounds diminished or absent over the affected lung. An **open pneumothorax** is an open communication between the atmosphere and intrathoracic pressure and is usually caused by penetrating trauma. This communication with the atmosphere causes an immediate collapse of the lung on the affected side. The patient will present with respiratory distress and as he inspires a sucking sound may be heard as the air moves in and out of the hole in the chest. An occlusive dressing can be placed over the wound to prevent air from being sucked into the pleural cavity until a chest tube can be placed. The dressing should only be secured on three sides to allow air to escape and prevent a tension pneumothorax.

Circulation with Hemorrhage Control

Hemorrhage is the predominant cause of preventable death in the injured patient (ACS, 2004). During the primary survey, hypotension should be considered hypovolemic in origin until proven otherwise. Elements of the primary survey that provide important information to the nurse regarding the patient's circulatory status are level of consciousness, skin color, and pulse. If the patient's circulating blood volume is reduced, the cerebral perfusion may be impaired, resulting in an altered level of consciousness. As blood volume decreases, the body compensates by shunting blood away from the skin to vital organs. This shunting causes the skin to become pale and cool. Pulses should be assessed bilaterally for quality, rate, and regularity. A weak, thready pulse may be a sign of hypovolemia, but may have other causes as well. The absence of central pulses (femoral and carotid pulses) signifies the need for immediate resuscitative measures to restore depleted blood volume and maintain effective cardiac output.

If external hemorrhage is identified, measures to control the bleeding should be taken immediately. The easiest way to do this is to apply direct manual pressure on the wound.

CRITICAL ALERT *Tourniquets should not be used to control bleeding except in unusual circumstances (e.g., traumatic amputation). Tourniquets crush tissues and cause distal ischemia.*

The major sources of occult blood loss are hemorrhage into the chest or abdominal cavities, into the soft tissue surrounding a major long bone fracture, or into the retroperitoneal space

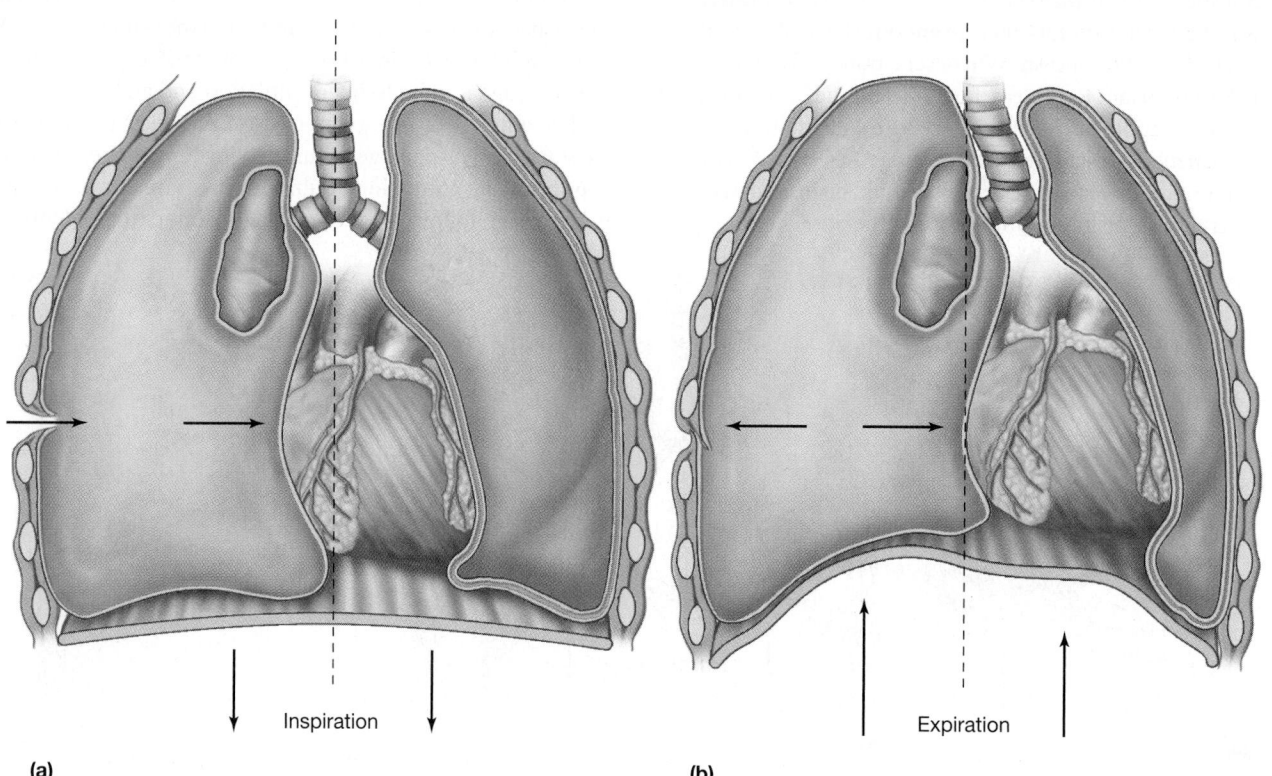

(a)   Inspiration   (b)   Expiration

FIGURE 74–8 ■ Tension pneumothorax.

from a pelvic fracture. Control of bleeding may require immediate operative intervention.

Treatment of hemorrhage consists of administration of fluids, blood, and blood products. Hypovolemic shock is a life-threatening emergency and affects all organ systems of the body by depriving tissue of adequate oxygen and nutrients. For a detailed discussion of shock, refer to Chapter 61 ☞. The initial response of the body to acute blood loss is to decrease circulation to less vital organs such as the kidneys, gastrointestinal tract, and skin in order to preserve circulation to vital organs such as the heart, brain, and lungs. This response is triggered by the decrease in cardiac output and subsequent change in pulse pressure that is sensed by baroreceptors in the aortic arch and atrium of the heart. Neural reflexes then begin a sympathetic outflow to the heart and other organs, which respond by increasing heart rate and initiating vasoconstriction. The activation of the rennin system leads to vasoconstriction and the retention of sodium and water to help replete the vascular volume. The pituitary and the adrenal medulla are stimulated to release adrenocorticotropic hormone, norepinephrine, and epinephrine to enhance the compensatory mechanisms.

The decrease in oxygen and nutrients to the cells causes the body's metabolism to change from aerobic to anaerobic, releasing lactic acid and causing metabolic acidosis. If the blood loss continues, the compensatory mechanisms will fail and damage occurs throughout the body in all systems. Myocardial hypoperfusion and lactic acidosis cause cardiac dysfunction that, in turn, perpetuates the entire process. Hypoperfusion of the brain causes cardiac and respiratory depression and failure of the sympathetic nervous system. As a result of this failure, vasodilation occurs that leads to venous pooling and increased capillary permeability, which causes the leakage of fluid into the interstitial space (third spacing) and the total body edema (anasarca) noted in trauma patients. Irreversible damage at the cellular level occurs because the cell membrane loses integrity. This is primarily due to free radicals, especially reactive oxygen species and reactive nitrogen species. These free radicals lead to oxidation of DNA molecules, fatty acids, and amino acids advancing cell degradation. Because the electrical gradient is lost, the cell swells, the endoplasmic reticulum and mitochondria are damaged, and utilization of oxygen becomes dysfunctional. Ruptured lysosomes release enzymes that digest other cellular structures and cell death occurs, which further enhances the impact of the initial hemorrhage.

Respiratory distress syndrome may result from the increased permeability of the pulmonary capillary membrane, microemboli formation, and pulmonary vasoconstriction. Hypoperfusion and vasoconstriction to the gastrointestinal system cause decreased peristalsis and functioning of the gut. Renal vasoconstriction and hypoperfusion lead to acute tubular necrosis and, if not reversed, to acute renal failure. Disseminated intravascular coagulation (DIC) develops due to hematologic dysfunction, including acidosis, hypoxemia, hypotension, and cessation of capillary blood flow.

The most abundant type of white blood cells are neutrophils. A large amount of the damage from hemorrhagic shock is the result of the formation of reactive oxygen species (ROSs) in neutrophils. Neutrophils fight infection and use ROSs to fight pathogens as they directly break down microbial pathogens. However, ROSs also signal molecules in programmed cell death (apoptotic) pathways. Although ROSs break down pathogens, neutrophils overproduce and accumulate ROSs causing **apoptosis** (programmed cell death in a multicellular organism), which would be expressed in the clinical setting as sepsis.

Recent research into the cellular pathways involved in the inflammatory response to injury and shock is concerned with T-cell proliferation in response to stimulators in the adaptive and innate immune responses. Research has found decreased levels of helper T-cell cytokine production and reduced antibody secretion (Spaniol, Knight, Zebley, Anderson, & Pierce, 2007). The decrease in these specific levels corresponds to the suppressed adaptive immune function that is seen in trauma patients with hemorrhagic shock. Research is focused on which receptors are involved in the reduction of the adaptive immune function and how to activate the receptors to maintain the adaptive immune system function at a level that will prevent infection.

Fluid Resuscitation

Traditionally, the treatment for hemorrhagic shock has been immediate, aggressive infusion of normal saline or Ringer's lactate solution. Current data suggest, however, that although aggressive fluid resuscitation may be useful for patients with isolated extremity, thermal, or head injury, fluid resuscitation should be limited in patients with potentially uncontrollable internal hemorrhage, especially in patients with penetrating truncal injury that will be treated at a trauma center (Pepe, Dutton, & Fowler, 2008). The reason aggressive fluid resuscitation may be harmful is that increasing the mean arterial pressure in a patient who is actively bleeding will lead to increased blood loss. The hemostatic mechanisms of the body are overcome by the artificially elevated blood pressure and formed clots are dislodged. Due to the increased bleeding, more fluids and blood are required and the proinflammatory effects of the products develop. Aggressive infusion of crystalloid in the presence of uncontrolled hemorrhage promotes continued bleeding and increases mortality (Hai, 2004). The amount of initial fluid resuscitation will be determined by the patient's response to fluids. The response should be continually assessed to determine if perfusion is adequate. The nurse must also be aware that many factors including age, comorbidities, and medications can affect a patient's response to fluid resuscitation. The goal is to control the bleeding and promote oxygenation at the cellular level.

There is also an area of concern with the administration of Ringer's lactate solution stimulating apoptosis. A study looking at the initial resuscitation of combat casualties found that the use of Ringer's lactate solution for hemorrhagic shock increased apoptosis in intestinal mucosa, smooth muscle, liver, and lung cells, and caused a severe immunologic response, coagulopathy, and renal failure. This was not observed with the use of plasma, natural colloids, and whole blood during resuscitation (Spaniol et al., 2007).

Blood products are used to restore circulating volume, improve oxygen carrying capacity, and replace coagulation factors. Type-specific blood is preferred, but if needed immediately, type O may be used. Ongoing research indicates that fresh frozen plasma and platelets need to be given early in conjunction with packed red cells to treat coagulopathy (Hess, Holcomb, & Hoyt, 2006; Ketchum, Hess, & Hippala, 2006). Trauma centers are developing guidelines for massive transfusion that reflect this practice. Chart 74–1 (p. 2434) is an example of a guideline for massive transfusion.

CHART 74-1   **Massive Transfusion Guideline**

Purpose: The Massive Transfusion Guideline (MTG) development was a cooperative effort by the Trauma Multidisciplinary Committee at the University of California, Davis Medical Center to provide a standard for efficient and effective procurement and delivery of blood products to patients exhibiting hemorrhagic shock. The term *massive transfusion* is defined as replacement of at least one blood volume (~5 liters in an adult) within the first 12 hours of resuscitation.

MASSIVE TRANSFUSION GUIDELINE PACK

6 units of packed red blood cells (pRBCs)

3 fresh frozen plasma (FFP) Jumbo units (6 units of FFP)

1 plateletpheresis unit (a 6-pack of platelets)

ACTIVATION

The MTGs can be activated in any of the following hospital locations:

Emergency department

Operating room

Critical care unit

Radiology (interventional radiology)

Labor and delivery

- The health care provider caring for the patient (trauma attending or anesthesiologist or direct designee) first determines that massive transfusion is likely to be necessary and notifies the blood bank.
- An order must be placed in the electronic medical record (EMR) for MTGs.

- A properly labeled blood specimen should be sent STAT (ordered in the EMR as "RBC" (red blood cells) if a new patient or "RBC Add-on" if a specimen is 3 days current). A prothrombin time (PT), partial thromboplastin time (PTT), and fibrinogen or thromboelastography (TEG) should also be sent.
- Transfusion of un-crossmatched RBCs should be ongoing until type specific and/or crossmatch compatible RBCs are available.
- FFP should be started as soon as it is determined that more than 3 units of pRBCs are likely to be necessary.
- Upon initiation of MTGs, blood bank personnel will prepare 6 units of pRBCs, and 3 units of FFP Jumbo will be placed into a cooler and delivered to the patient, along with one plateletpheresis not placed in the cooler and instead kept at room temperature. This will be switched out with another cooler prepared in the same manner as above upon return of the first cooler. Subsequent component orders will be repeated until the health care provider caring for the patient determines that the MTG can be discontinued.
- The health care provider initiating the MTGs or a designee must notify the blood bank as soon as possible when the MTGs are no longer needed.
- All blood products should be given via a Level I rapid infuser/fluid warmer or other blood-warming device to prevent hypothermia.
- The patient's medical record number will be held constant throughout the MTGs.

Sources: Hess, J. R., Holcomb, J. B., & Hoyt, D. B. (2006). Damage control resuscitation: The need for specific blood products to treat the coagulopathy of trauma. *Transfusion, 46,* 685–686; Hirshberg, A., Dugas, M., Banez, E. I., Scott, B. G., Wall, M. J. Jr., & Mattox, K. L. (2003). Minimizing dilutional coagulopathy in exsanguinating hemorrhage: A computer simulation. *Journal of Trauma, 54,* 454–463; Ho, A. M., Dion, P. W., Cheng, C. A., et al. (2005). A mathematical model for fresh frozen plasma transfusion strategies during major trauma resuscitation with ongoing hemorrhage. *Canadian Journal of Surgery, 48,* 470–478; Holcomb, J. B., & Hess, J. R. (2006). Early massive trauma transfusion: Current state of the art. *Journal of Trauma, 60*(Suppl), S1–S9; Ketchum, L., Hess, J. R., & Hippala, S. (2006). Indications for early fresh frozen plasma, cryoprecipitate, and platelet transfusion in trauma. *Journal of Trauma, 60*(Suppl.), S51–S58; Malone, D. L., Hess, J. R., & Fingerhut, A. (2006). Massive transfusion practices around the globe and a suggestion for a common massive transfusion protocol. *Journal of Trauma, 60*(Suppl), S91–S96.

Disability

The primary assessment of disability involves a rapid neurological evaluation to establish the patient's level of consciousness. The Glasgow Coma Scale score (see Chart 32–2, p. 841) should be determined at this time. An altered level of consciousness can be indicative of decreased blood volume with poor perfusion, hypoxia, or a traumatic brain injury. Alcohol and mind-altering drugs may alter the level of consciousness, but should never be considered the cause until all other possibilities have been excluded.

Exposure/Environmental Control

The trauma patient should be completely undressed to facilitate a thorough examination. As trauma patients are being examined they should be covered with warm blankets or an external warming device to prevent hypothermia. Intravenous fluids should be warmed prior to infusion to prevent a decrease in a patient's core temperature with the infusion of large amounts of cold solution. Allowing patients to become cold can be very detrimental to their care, as discussed in the Evidence-Based Practice feature.

Adjuncts to the Primary Survey

Monitoring of the patient's physiological parameters is the best way to assess the effectiveness of resuscitation efforts. The patient should be placed on a cardiac monitor. Dysrhythmias may

indicate blunt cardiac injury. Pulseless electrical activity (PEA) may indicate tension pneumothorax, as described earlier in the chapter; profound hypovolemia; and/or **cardiac tamponade**, which is bleeding into the pericardial sac.

As the accumulation of blood increases, it compresses the atria and ventricles decreasing venous return and filling pressure, which leads to decreased cardiac output, myocardial hypoxia, and cardiac failure. The patient with cardiac tamponade presents with findings termed **Beck's triad**. These findings are neck vein distention caused by the elevated central venous pressure, muffled heart sounds, and hypotension. Immediate treatment is required to remove the accumulated blood and relieve the pressure that is being exerted on the heart. This is accomplished either by pericardiocentesis, which involves aspiration via a large-bore needle placed into the pericardial sac, or an emergency surgical thoracotomy to visualize the heart, relieve the accumulated blood, and locate and control the source of bleeding.

Pulse oximetry measures the oxygen saturation of hemoglobin, but does not measure ventilation. Adequacy of ventilation should be monitored by the ventilatory rate and arterial blood gases (ABGs).

Bedside screening radiographs are usually accomplished at this time. As the patient is logrolled off the backboard and

Hypothermia in Trauma Patients

Clinical Problem

Allowing a trauma patient to become cold will contribute to the development of coagulopathy.

Research Findings

Hemorrhage is one of the leading causes of death following trauma. Trauma patients are susceptible to early development of coagulopathy, and patients who are severely injured are coagulopathic on hospital admission. Hypothermia, acidosis, and dilution from standard resuscitation with crystalloid can worsen the presenting coagulopathy and perpetuate bleeding. Rapid diagnosis of coagulopathy, followed by prevention or correction of hypothermia and acidosis should be a priority during the initial assessment and resuscitation (Tieu, Holcomb, & Schreiber, 2007).

Coagulopathy of trauma is a syndrome of bleeding from mucosal lesions, serosal surfaces, and wound and vascular access sites. It is associated with serious injury, hypothermia, acidosis, hemodilution, and occasionally with DIC. The coagulopathy can be largely explained by the effects of cold on platelet function, the effect of pH on coagulation factor activity, and the dilutional effects of resuscitative fluids (Hess & Lawson, 2006).

Hardy, de Moerloose, and Samama (2006) conducted a Medline search for articles on *massive transfusion, transfusion, trauma, surgery, coagulopathy,* and *hemostatic defects.* Experts reviewed the literature. Their principal findings were that coagulopathy results from hemodilution, hypothermia, the use of fractionated blood products, and DIC. In trauma patients, tissue trauma, shock, tissue anoxia, and hypothermia contribute to the development of DIC and microvascular bleeding. Hardy and colleagues compared the clinical significance of the effects of different therapies and stated that maintaining a normal body temperature is a first-line, effective strategy to improve hemostasis during massive transfusion.

The U.S. Army Institute of Surgical Research conducted a study (Martini, Pusateri, Uscilowicz, Delgado, & Holcomb, 2005) to identify the independent contributions of hypothermia and acidosis to coagulopathy in swine. They found that hypothermia caused a delay in the onset of thrombin generation, and acidosis primarily caused a decrease in thrombin generation rates. The results confirmed the need to prevent or correct hypothermia and acidosis.

Implications for Nursing Practice

With the organization of trauma systems, improvements in prehospital care, the development of trauma centers, and the standardization of methods of resuscitation, aggressive resuscitation of patients in extremis has improved over time. Severely traumatized patients may now be in the ICU or operating room before they reach the physiological limit defined as the onset of the triad: hypothermia, acidosis, and coagulopathy. It is important for nurses to understand the triad and the consequences. As stated before, maintaining a normal body temperature is a first-line, effective strategy to improve hemostasis and prevent worsening coagulopathy.

Critical Thinking Questions

1. Which of the following nursing measures would decrease the risk of coagulopathy?
   a. Administering warm intravenous fluids
   b. Covering the patient with a sheet
   c. Administering room temperature intravenous fluids
   d. Covering the patient with warm blankets
   e. a and d
   f. All of the above

2. The nurse understands that prevention of hypothermia is important because:
   a. It increases cardiac output.
   b. It decreases the risk of coagulopathy.
   c. It preserves neurological function.
   d. It increases renal function.

Answers to Critical Thinking Questions appear in Appendix D.

References

Hardy, J. F., de Moerloose, P., & Samama, C. M. (2006). Massive transfusion and coagulopathy: Pathophysiology and implications for clinical management. *Canadian Journal of Anaesthesia, 53*(6 Suppl.), S40–S58.

Hess, J. R., & Lawson, J. H. (2006). The coagulopathy of trauma versus disseminated intravascular coagulation. *Journal of Trauma, 60*(6), S12–S19.

Martini, W. Z., Pusateri, A. E., Uscilowicz, J. M., Delgado, A. V., & Holcomb, J. B. (2005). Independent contributions of hypothermia and acidosis to coagulopathy in swine. *Journal of Trauma, 58*(5), 1002–1009.

Tieu, B. H., Holcomb, J. B., & Schreiber, M. A. (2007). Coagulopathy: Its pathophysiology and treatment in the injured patient. *World Journal of Surgery, 31*(5), 1055–1065.

EVIDENCE-BASED PRACTICE

---

the back is examined, plates may be placed to do chest and abdominal/pelvic radiographs.

Placement of an indwelling urinary catheter and a gastric catheter should be accomplished as part of the resuscitation. Urinary output is an important indicator of the patient's volume status and her response to resuscitation. The placement of an indwelling urinary catheter is contraindicated in patients suspected of having a urethral injury. Signs of possible urethral injury include blood at the urethral meatus, perineal ecchymosis, blood in the scrotum, and a high-riding or nonpalpable prostate, which is identified by manual rectal exam. Placement of a gastric catheter reduces stomach distention and the risk of vomiting and aspiration. If the patient has multiple facial fractures, it may be necessary to place an oral gastric catheter.

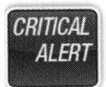 **CRITICAL ALERT** *Never insert a urinary catheter before the genitalia and rectum have been examined.*

The patient's blood pressure should be monitored frequently to observe for changes and/or trends. Remember, blood pressure may be a poor measure of actual tissue perfusion. Return to an adequate hemodynamic state requires more than a normal blood pressure.

If the patient arrived at a nontrauma center, this is the time to consider initiating the transfer process to a designated trauma center for definitive care (ACS, 2004).

Secondary Survey

Following the primary survey and intervention of resuscitative measures with adequate patient response, the secondary survey should be completed. The secondary survey consists of a detailed head-to-toe evaluation of the patient with reassessment of all vital signs and should ideally be performed in 5 to 10 minutes. As with the primary survey, the secondary survey is done in a systematic fashion to reveal all injuries the patient has sustained.

Head and Face

The nurse palpates through the scalp to identify lacerations and possible depressed skull fractures. Observe the face for the development of **Battle's sign**, which is ecchymosis over the mastoid area and is indicative of a basilar skull fracture. Palpate the face for fractures and midface stability. If the midface is unstable, the patient will have difficulty maintaining a patent airway. When the patient lies supine, the midface collapses and occludes the airway.

Eyes

If the patient is responsive, gross visual acuity should be checked along with pupillary size and reactivity to light. Assess for **raccoon eyes**, which are ecchymoses over the orbit of the eyes and are indicative of a basilar skull fracture. Inspect the eye for any foreign bodies, globe injury, or **hyphema**, a collection of blood in the anterior chamber of the eye. The blood is visible and can block vision. If the nurse notes that the patient is wearing contact lenses, these should be removed at this time.

Ears

The ears should be inspected for blood, cerebrospinal fluid (CSF), or brain matter. Remove and save hearing aids.

Nose

Inspect the nose for blood or a CSF leak. An easy way to test for a CSF leak is to use gauze to absorb the bloody fluid. If CSF is mixed with the blood, it will create a gold-colored ring around the blood. This is commonly referred to as the "halo effect." Palpate for crepitus or deformity.

Mouth

Inspect the mouth for loose or broken teeth, tongue lacerations, or expanding intraoral hematomas. Remove dentures at this time.

Neck

While maintaining cervical spine stabilization, the neck should be palpated for spinous process deformity or crepitance. Inspect the anterior neck carefully for expanding hematomas that may compress the trachea. How to evaluate patients with suspected cervical spine trauma is a controversial topic in medicine. The controversy surrounds which patients require radiographs, how much imaging is necessary, and exactly what sort of imaging should be done. The American College of Radiology's (ACR's) expert panel on musculoskeletal imaging has issued recommendations for imaging of patients with suspected cervical spine trauma (ACR, 2007). In summary, the expert panel recommends that patients who are alert, have no loss of consciousness, are not under the influence of drugs or alcohol, have no distracting injuries, have no cervical tenderness, and have no neurological findings do not need imaging. All others should have a computed tomography (CT) scan of the cervical spine that includes sagittal and coronal reconstruction.

The ACR's expert panel also recommend that patients who have symptoms referable to the upper cervical spine and have a negative CT scan, should have a single lateral radiograph to evaluate C_2. This is especially important for patients over the age of 65 because such patients have a higher incidence of C_2 fractures. The guidelines recommend that magnetic resonance imaging (MRI) be reserved for patients who have clinical evidence of spinal cord injury, those suspected of ligamentous instability, and to "clear" patients who remain unconscious after 48 hours.

Chest

Inspect the chest for paradoxical chest movement from a flail segment. Palpate for subcutaneous emphysema and bony tenderness. Auscultate for absent or asymmetric breath sounds.

Abdomen

Inspect the abdomen for ecchymoses and distention. Palpate for tenderness. Many centers now use ultrasound for the **FAST examination**, which refers to *focused assessment with sonography for trauma*. Within minutes the FAST exam can confirm the presence of free fluid within the chest or abdomen, which signifies bleeding and the need for rapid intervention.

Pelvis

The pelvis should be assessed for stability by gently compressing the iliac wings and symphysis pubis. If a caregiver has assessed for stability and states that the pelvis feels unstable, then no one else should compress the pelvis because it may cause more damage to the vessels and tissue. A patient with a major pelvic fracture is at risk for retroperitoneal hemorrhage. A prefabricated pelvic stabilization device or a sheet should be applied to an unstable pelvic fracture that may contribute to hemodynamic instability. This will help to decrease the bleeding and prevent further damage until the pelvic bones can be surgically stabilized (Isenhour & Marx, 2007).

Genitalia

In the male patient, inspect the scrotum for ecchymoses or hematomas and the penile meatus for blood. Assess female patients for vaginal bleeding and obtain a history regarding last menstruation and the chance of pregnancy. A pregnancy test should be performed for any woman of childbearing age.

Extremities

Each extremity should be inspected for deformity and swelling. Palpate for tenderness, crepitus, limited joint movement, and pulses. Whenever an injury is suspected, it is important to assess for circulation, sensation, and motor response distal to the injury. Refer to Chapter 56 for an in-depth review of musculoskeletal trauma.

> **CRITICAL ALERT**　*If an injured extremity is found to be pulseless, notify the trauma team immediately.*

Laboratory and Diagnostic Procedures

Trauma patients are monitored closely during the first 24 hours post injury as not to miss an injury. Diagnostic tests that may be utilized are presented in the Diagnostic Tests feature.

DIAGNOSTIC TESTS for Trauma

Test	Expected Abnormality	Rationale for Abnormality
Hematocrit	Decrease	Initially should obtain a baseline to look for trends downward, signifying ongoing bleeding. Patients requiring crystalloid resuscitation for hemorrhagic shock benefit from serial hematocrit measurement in order to determine the degree of hemodilution and the need for blood transfusion.
White blood cell (WBC) count	Increased	Initially the WBC count will be elevated as part of the body's normal response to trauma. Detection of neutrophilia based on serial evaluations may indicate an inflammatory process in the peritoneal cavity. During the critical care and intermediate phases of care, an elevation in the WBC count can be indicative of a wound infection, pulmonary infection, or sepsis.
Glucose	Decrease or increase	Decrease: used to rule out hypoglycemia in patients with decreased level of consciousness. Increase: stress response from traumatic injury.
Lipase	Increase	Progressive elevation increases suspicion of pancreatic, liver, or bowel injuries.
Arterial blood gases	Metabolic acidosis	Metabolic acidosis is strongly associated with hypoperfusion.
Coagulation studies: International Normalized Ratio (INR) Activated partial thromboplastin time (APT) Partial thromboplastin time (PTT)	Increased	May identify if the patient was on long-term anticoagulation at home. Severe TBI causes the release of tissue thromboplastin, which increases INR. Patients receiving massive blood transfusions require frequent monitoring of clotting factors. Packed RBCs do not contain clotting factors and platelets, so the patient may require FFP to prevent coagulopathy.
Urinalysis	Positive for occult blood Toxicology screening	Signifies injury to urinary tract. A positive toxicology report may help to explain altered mental status. On all female patients of childbearing age, a bedside urine pregnancy test should be performed.
Blood alcohol level and toxicology screening	Elevated blood alcohol and positive toxicology screen	May help to explain altered mental status.
Imaging: Cervical spine Chest Abdomen Pelvis Thoracic spine Lumbosacral spine Injured extremities	Fractures and/or dislocations Pneumothoraxes Hemothoraxes	Helps identify life- or limb-threatening injuries.

■ Nursing Management

During the initial resuscitation, the health care providers present work as a team to evaluate and intervene where necessary. After the initial resuscitation, the nurse has the most consistent contact with the patient and is the team member who will quickly identify trends and changes in the patient condition. The Nursing Process: Patient Care Plan (p. 2438) presents a detailed patient care plan for the trauma patient.

Tertiary Survey

Many trauma patients are unresponsive or confused when they are first evaluated and are unable to furnish valuable medical history data that may affect their care. As thorough as the trauma team may be in evaluating the patient, not all injuries are detected by the primary and secondary survey. For this reason a tertiary trauma survey (TTS) is increasingly being implemented (Petersen, 2004). The TTS is completed within 24 hours of admission as a patient evaluation that identifies and catalogs all injuries after the initial resuscitation and operative intervention. The TTS is repeated when the patient is awake, responsive, and able to communicate and includes a comprehensive review of the medical record, repetition of the primary and secondary surveys, review of all laboratory data, and review of all radiographic studies with an attending radiologist.

Continued reevaluation of the multiple-system trauma patient is key to prevent missed injury and preventable death. A

NURSING PROCESS: Patient Care Plan for Trauma

Assessment of Circulation and Perfusion

Subjective Data:

Where are your injuries?

Do you have any other preexisting health problems?

Do you take any medications that may affect your blood pressure?

Do you take any medications that "thin your blood"?

Objective Data:

Assess:

Level of consciousness

Oxygen saturation

Work of breathing

Peripheral and central pulses: rate and quality

Blood pressure

Respiratory rate

Temperature

Skin color and temperature

Urine output

Nursing Assessment and Diagnoses	Outcomes and Evaluation Parameters	Planning and Interventions with *Rationales*
Nursing Diagnosis: *Tissue Perfusion, Ineffective* related to hypovolemia; interruption of flow: arterial and/or venous	**Outcome:** Patient will maintain adequate tissue perfusion. **Evaluation Parameters:** Vital signs within normal limits. Level of consciousness: awake, alert, and appropriate. Skin: good color, warm and dry. Peripheral pulses strong and equal Urine output of 1 mL kg^{-1} hr^{-1}.	**Interventions and *Rationales:*** Cannulate two veins with large-bore catheters and regulate fluids at appropriate rates. *Adequate fluid and blood administration help maintain perfusion of vital organs.* Apply direct pressure to obvious external bleeding *to slow the loss of blood.* Notify the health care provider immediately of significant drop in blood pressure, urine output, or increased heart rate. *Patient may have a missed injury that requires surgical intervention.*

Assessment of Airway

Subjective Data:

Are you feeling short of breath?

Are you having difficulty breathing?

Is it painful when you take a deep breath or cough?

Objective Data:

Assess breath sounds.

Assess respiratory rate, rhythm, depth, and symmetry.

Monitor oxygen saturation.

Monitor arterial blood gas values.

Nursing Assessment and Diagnoses	Outcomes and Evaluation Parameters	Planning and Interventions with *Rationales*
Nursing Diagnosis: *Airway Clearance, Ineffective* related to edema of the airway, laryngeal spasm, altered level of consciousness, direct trauma, obstruction by secretions, or aspiration of foreign matter	**Outcome:** Patient will maintain a patent airway. **Evaluation Parameters:** Regular rate, depth, and pattern of breathing. Bilateral chest expansion. Effective cough and gag reflex. Absence of stridor or hoarse voice.	**Interventions and *Rationales:*** Open and clear airway. Patient may have debris or blood in mouth from the trauma. Insert oro- or nasopharyngeal airway. Patient may have adequate respiratory drive but needs support to keep airway open. *Prepare to assist with endotracheal intubation. Level of consciousness too low to protect and maintain airway.*

Assessment of Ventilation

Subjective Data:

Are you feeling short of breath?

Are you having difficulty breathing?

Objective Data:

Observe patient for:

Altered chest excursion

Shallow respirations

Nasal flaring

Use of accessory muscles

Increased or decreased respiratory rate

Nursing Assessment and Diagnoses	Outcomes and Evaluation Parameters	Planning and Interventions with *Rationales*
Nursing Diagnosis: *Breathing Pattern, Ineffective* related to chest wall deformity, decreased energy, musculoskeletal impairment, neuromuscular dysfunction, pain	**Outcome:** Patient will demonstrate effective breathing patterns. **Evaluation Parameters:** Uncompromised respiratory status as evidenced by depth of inspiration and ease of breathing; chest expansion symmetric; accessory muscle use not present; adventitious breath sounds not present.	**Interventions and *Rationales:*** Control pain *to allow for optimal chest expansion.* Teach patient how to use the incentive spirometer *to help prevent atelectasis.* Suction as needed *to remove secretions and encourage coughing.* Have patient turn, cough, and deep breathe at least every 2 hours *to mobilize secretions and prevent atelectasis.* Administer oxygen as ordered *to maintain adequate PaO$_2$.*

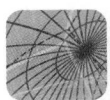

NURSING PROCESS: Patient Care Plan for Trauma—*Continued*

Assessment of Pain

Subjective Data:
On a scale of 1 to 10 with 1 being a little pain and 10 being the worst pain you have ever felt, at what level is your pain?
Do you routinely take pain medication at home? If yes, what is the name of the medication and why do you take it?
Are you allergic to any medications?

Objective Data:
Monitor patient for:
Facial grimacing
Change in breathing pattern
Change in blood pressure and/or pulse rate
Diaphoresis
Agitation

Nursing Assessment and Diagnoses	Outcomes and Evaluation Parameters	Planning and Interventions with *Rationales*
Nursing Diagnosis: *Pain*	**Outcome:** Pain level will be tolerable. **Evaluation Parameters:** Diminished or absent level of pain through patient's self-report. Absence of physiological indicators of pain.	**Interventions and *Rationales*:** **Nonpharmacologic** Reduce lighting and noise. Cultural and spiritual factors such as prayer, ritual, and music can also increase the patient's comfort. *Promotes relaxation and comfort.* **Pharmacologic** Administer intravenous opioid analgesics as prescribed. Assess response. *Intravenous administration is necessary if there is altered tissue perfusion from volume deficit.*

Assessment of Anxiety

Subjective Data:
Ask patient to verbalize thoughts and feelings about the traumatic event.
How do you feel about being in the hospital?

Objective Data:
Observe patient for:
Restlessness
Poor eye contact
Irritability
Hand tremors
Anorexia
Difficulty concentrating

Nursing Assessment and Diagnoses	Outcomes and Evaluation Parameters	Planning and Interventions with *Rationales*
Nursing Diagnoses: *Anxiety and Fear* related to unfamiliar environment, invasive procedures, possible disfigurement, scarring, threat to health status, role functions, or self-concept, loss of control, pain	**Outcome:** Patient will experience decreased anxiety and fear. **Evaluation Parameters:** Ability to verbalize concerns and ask questions. Use of effective coping skills. Decreased fear-related behaviors.	**Interventions and *Rationales*:** Explain all procedures in clear terms. *Increases patient's understanding and alleviates fear of the unknown.* Maintain adequate pain relief. *Pain increases anxiety.* Administer prescribed antianxiety medication *to decrease physiological responses.* Spend therapeutic time with the patient to answer questions. *Anxiety may interfere with understanding of complex explanations.*

Assessment of Nutrition

Subjective Data:
Ask the patient about their appetite and how much of their meal they have eaten.

Objective Data:
24-hour caloric intake
Daily weight
Presence of bowel sounds, nausea and vomiting, or flatus

Nursing Assessment and Diagnoses	Outcomes and Evaluation Parameters	Planning and Interventions with *Rationales*
Nursing Diagnosis: *Nutrition Imbalanced, Risk for Less than Body Requirements* related to decreased appetite secondary to treatments, fatigue, environment, and increased protein and vitamin requirements for healing	**Outcome:** Patient will ingest daily nutritional requirements for activity level and metabolic needs. **Evaluation Parameters:** Maintains adequate weight. Maintains adequate caloric intake.	**Interventions and *Rationales*:** Communicate the need for adequate caloric intake of carbohydrates, fats, protein, vitamins, minerals, and fluids. *Adequate nutrition can reduce the risk of complications and promote healing.* Consult with the nutritionist to establish appropriate daily caloric requirements *to ensure optimal intake.* Offer small frequent meals *to help prevent gastric distention.* Determine the patient's food preferences and arrange to have those foods provided. Encourage family to bring allowed foods from home. Eliminate any offensive odors. Control pain and nausea. Provide a relaxed atmosphere during meals. *Can improve appetite and lead to increased intake.*

study conducted at Harborview Medical Center, University of Washington, Seattle, identified patterns of errors that contributed to inpatient trauma deaths. The study showed important error patterns that included a failure to successfully intubate, secure, or protect the airway; delayed operative or angiographic control of acute abdominal/pelvic hemorrhage; delayed intervention for ongoing intrathoracic hemorrhage; inadequate deep venous thrombosis or gastrointestinal prophylaxis; lengthy initial operative procedures rather than damage control surgery in unstable patients; overresuscitation with fluids; and complications of feeding tubes (Gruen, Jurkovich, McIntyre, Foy, & Maier, 2006). Although preventable deaths will occur, continued reassessment of the multiple-system trauma patient will help to minimize these errors.

Discharge Priorities

Discharge priorities for the trauma patient can be multifactorial depending on the extent of the injuries. When caring for the multiple-system trauma patient, refer to the chapters that concentrate on the specific injury. For example, for multiple extremity fractures refer to the chapter on musculoskeletal injuries (Chapter 55).

Special Considerations

There are clinical situations or conditions that affect the delivery of trauma care. It is important for the nurse to be aware of these special considerations in order to give optimum care to the trauma patient.

End-of-Life Considerations

Trauma care has always focused on curing patients and returning individuals to a quality lifestyle. Unfortunately, trauma patients do die and they and their families may not receive end-of-life care that results in a death that reflects the best interests of the patient and family. One reason this occurs is because the trauma team has been so focused on curative care that it is difficult for them to change to palliative care. It is also a difficult conversation to have with the family because death from injury is usually a sudden event and is emotionally hard to process. According to the American Trauma Society (2003), "Death due to trauma needs to be managed in a manner that is sensitive, caring, and respectful to the patient, the family, and the medical caregivers. For patients with no likelihood of survival, implementation of aggressive resuscitation efforts and transport to a trauma center are empirically and morally questionable. For hospitalized patients, the failure to recognize that curative care is no longer effective and that palliative care needs to be initiated results in less than optimal care for the patient and family and may delay care of other patients who need intensive care to recover" (p. 1).

The need to integrate palliative care into trauma care is an essential part of providing excellent trauma care for all patients and families. To assist nurses caring for trauma patients throughout the continuum of care including end-of-life situations, policies should be in place that assist the trauma team in making the decision to shift from curative to comfort care and that address the changes in the focus of care for dying patients. For an in-depth discussion of end-of-life care, refer to Chapter 17 . The Ethical Issues box further discusses end-of-life care.

> ### ETHICAL ISSUES Related to Trauma Patients and Their Families
>
> One very difficult issue for nurses occurs when a nurse believes that the aggressive curative care being given to a trauma patient is futile or not in the best interest of the patient. The patient may have expressed to his family prior to the trauma that he did not want heroic measures taken if his quality of life would be severely affected. As the nurse it is important to advocate for the patient's wishes. Several steps can be taken by the nurse to clarify the issue. Request a multidisciplinary meeting with the health care team to identify concerns and clarify goals and expected outcomes for the patient. If the team cannot agree on the goals for the patient, an ethics committee consultation can be requested. The nurse can also facilitate a multidisciplinary family conference if there seems to be a conflict between the goals of the team and the expectations of the family. Be respectful of cultural conversational norms, listen to identify concerns, and attempt to match expressed needs with services the nurse can provide or facilitate.

Traumatic Brain Injury

Multiple-system trauma patients who sustain traumatic brain injury (TBI) can be difficult to assess due to their decreased level of consciousness. The patient must be carefully evaluated for injury that may cause hemorrhage because a decrease in the blood pressure is detrimental to cerebral perfusion. Refer to Chapter 29 for an in-depth review of brain injury.

Spinal Cord Injury

Any multiple-system trauma patient must be considered to have a vertebral column injury even if the patient does not have a neurological deficit. If the trauma patient is unconscious, it will be difficult to assess neurological function. For trauma patients, approximately 55% of spinal injuries occur in the cervical region, 15% in the thoracic region, 15% at the thoracolumbar junction, and 15% in the lumbosacral area (ACS, 2004).

It is very important to protect the spine from excessive manipulation. If the patient's spine is protected, a rigid cervical collar is properly placed and manual stabilization is maintained while the patient is logrolled. Then, evaluation of the spine and exclusion of spine injury can be deferred in the presence of systemic instability. If a patient is known to have a neurological deficit and is hypotensive, it should not be assumed that the drop in blood pressure is due to neurogenic shock. All sources of bleeding must be ruled out so as not to miss an injury. Refer to Chapter 32 for an in-depth review of spinal cord injuries.

Trauma in Pregnancy

For any female trauma patient between the ages of 10 and 50, potential for pregnancy should be considered. Because of the significant physiological changes during pregnancy, patterns of injury may be affected. Anatomically, the uterus remains in the pelvis until approximately the 12th week. By 20 weeks gestation, the uterus is at the umbilicus, and it rises to the costal margin at 34 to 36 weeks. As the uterus enlarges the bowel is pushed upward and lies mostly in the upper abdomen. In later pregnancy the bowel is somewhat protected from blunt trauma, but the uterus, placenta, and fetus are at risk. During the third trimester of pregnancy, the uterus is large and thin walled.

In the vertex position the fetal head sits within the pelvis. If the mother sustains a pelvic fracture, the fetus could sustain significant head injury. The placenta has little elasticity, so shearing forces from deceleration (such as a frontal impact crash) could lead to abruption of the placenta from the uteroplacental interface causing bleeding within the uterus. Also, placental vasculature is maximally dilated throughout pregnancy but is very sensitive to catecholamine stimulation. The mother's response to the traumatic injury may cause constriction of the vasculature. Also, an abrupt decrease in the mother's intravascular volume may result in a profound constriction of the uterine vasculature, thus reducing fetal oxygenation even if the mother is exhibiting reasonably normal vital signs.

During pregnancy, plasma volume increases with a smaller increase in red blood cell volume, resulting in a physiological anemia. However, because of the increased plasma volume, a healthy pregnant patient may lose 1,200 to 1,500 mL of blood volume before exhibiting signs of hypovolemia such as tachycardia or hypotension. As stated before, this amount of blood loss can cause fetal distress as evidenced by an abnormal fetal heart rate.

Oxygen consumption is increased during pregnancy. The pregnant trauma patient should always receive supplemental oxygen and be monitored to ensure adequate oxygenation during resuscitation efforts.

Gastric emptying time is prolonged during pregnancy so it should always be assumed that the pregnant woman has a full stomach. To protect the patient from vomiting and possibly aspirating, it is important to place a nasogastric tube early to decompress the stomach.

The pregnant uterus may compress the vena cava and reduce venous return to the heart when the mother is lying supine. Therefore, the mother should be placed on her left side and the uterus displaced manually to the left side to relieve the pressure. If a spinal injury is suspected, the mother can be logrolled 4 to 6 inches to her left and supported with bolstering devices to displace the uterus.

The most important thing to remember when caring for a pregnant trauma patient is that the best treatment for the fetus is the provision of optimum resuscitation of the mother and early assessment and monitoring of the fetus.

Intimate Partner Violence

Statistics regarding intimate partner violence (IPV) are difficult to obtain because the various data sources define IPV differently. Some sources include threats and some only include physical and sexual violence. Also, many incidents are not reported to the police. The CDC (2007c) states that approximately 20% of IPV rapes or sexual assaults, 25% of physical assaults, and 50% of stalkings directed toward women are reported. Even fewer incidents against men are reported. Therefore, available statistics are felt to greatly underestimate the magnitude of the problem. Following are some statistics reported by the CDC (2007c):

- Nearly 5.3 million incidents of IPV occur each year among U.S. women ages 18 and older, and 3.2 million occur among men. Most assaults are relatively minor and consist of pushing, grabbing, shoving, slapping, and hitting.

- In the United States every year, about 1.5 million women and more than 800,000 men are raped or physically assaulted by an intimate partner. This translates into about 47 IPV assaults per 1,000 women and 32 assaults per 1,000 men.

- IPV results in nearly 2 million injuries and 1,300 deaths nationwide every year.

- One study found that 44% of women murdered by an intimate partner had visited an emergency department within 2 years of the homicide. Of these women, 93% had at least one injury visit (Crandall, Nathens, Kernic, Holt, & Rivara, 2004).

- Between 4% and 8% of pregnant women are abused at least once during the pregnancy.

Intimate partner violence can result in death and disability. This type of injury also represents an increasing number of emergency department visits. Aside from sexual violence, physical violence may include the following: scratching, throwing, grabbing, biting, choking, shaking, slapping, punching, burning, use of restraints, and use of a weapon. Indicators that may suggest the presence of domestic violence include:

- Self-blame for injuries
- Injuries inconsistent with stated history
- Frequent emergency department or office visits
- Symptoms suggestive of substance abuse
- Low self-esteem, depression, suicide attempts
- Self-abuse
- Partner insists on being present for interview and examination. May answer questions for patient.

Nutritional Support

The Eastern Association for the Surgery of Trauma (EAST) formed a work group to develop evidence-based guidelines for practice. Understanding the importance of nutrition with regard to healing, the guidelines shown in the National Guidelines for Nutritional Support box (p. 2442) were developed for nutritional support of the trauma patient. The guidelines contain three levels of recommendations:

- **Level I**—The recommendation is convincingly justifiable based on the available scientific information alone.

- **Level II**—The recommendation is reasonably justifiable by available scientific evidence and strongly supported by expert opinion.

- **Level III**—The recommendation is supported by available data but adequate scientific evidence is lacking. The recommendation is useful for educational purposes and in guiding future clinical research.

Gerontological Considerations

Trauma is the seventh leading cause of death in patients 65 years of age or older and accounts for 25% of all injury fatalities (ACS, 2004). Many studies have shown that elderly trauma patients have a higher level of injury-related mortality (Feliciano et al., 2008). This increased risk of death is attributed to preexisting medical conditions that make it difficult for the elderly patient to tolerate changes in their normal physiological parameters during the acute stress of trauma or major surgery. The three leading causes of death in

---

NATIONAL GUIDELINES for Nutritional Support

Route of Nutritional Support

Level I Recommendations:
- Patients with blunt and penetrating abdominal injuries sustain fewer septic complications when fed enterally rather than parenterally.
- Patients with severe head injuries have similar outcomes whether fed enterally or parenterally.

Early versus delayed feedings

Patients with penetrating and blunt injuries to the abdomen who have small bowel access: Enteral feeding can be started in most after resuscitation is complete and hemodynamic stability has been achieved. Gastrointestinal injury below the site of access may slow advancement of tube feedings but is not a contraindication to direct small bowel feedings.

Level I Recommendation:
- Intragastric feedings should be started in burn patients as soon after admission as possible since delayed enteral feeding (>18 hours) results in a high rate of gastroparesis.

Level II Recommendation:
- Patients with severe head injury who do not tolerate gastric feedings within 48 hours of injury should be changed to postpyloric feedings if feasible and safe for the patient.

Level III Recommendations:
- Patients who are incompletely resuscitated should not have direct small bowel feedings instituted due to the risk of gastrointestinal intolerance and possible internal necrosis.
- For patients undergoing laparotomy, direct small bowel access should be obtained and enteral feedings begun, if not contraindicated, within 12 to 24 hours of injury.

Standard versus enhanced nutritional support

Enhanced enteral formulations are defined by the addition of omega 3 fatty acids, nucleotides, arginine, beta carotene, and/or glutamine when adequate calorie/protein requirements are met early in the course of treatment.

Level I Recommendation:
- Use of enhanced enteral nutrition in severely injured patients is beneficial to the trauma patient when given in conjunction with early feeding and adequate protein/calorie support. Level I evidence shows reduced incidence of multisystem organ dysfunction, infectious complications, and overall length of hospital stay.

Source: EAST Practice Management Guidelines Workgroup. (2003). *Practice management guidelines for nutritional support of the trauma patient.* Retrieved October 18, 2008 from http://www.east.org/tpg/nutrition.pdf.

---

the elderly are falls, motor vehicle crashes, and burns (ACS, 2004). Elder abuse also occurs, as discussed in the Gerontological Considerations box.

Key differences between the elderly and younger people include the following:

- Increased incidence of subdural hematoma because of increased dural vein fragility and less elasticity with age. Elderly patients with head injury have a poorer prognosis than younger patients.
- The thorax is less compliant and therefore more susceptible to injury. A simple fall can cause a flail chest.
- Reduced pulmonary reserve occurs with the aging process. Elderly patients will have progressive pulmonary compromise with multiple rib fractures since splinting often leads to ventilatory failure and pneumonia.
- Elderly patients are less able to increase cardiac output on demand due to decreased compliance and a limited degree of compensatory ability. Elderly patients are also more likely to be taking beta-blockers which will blunt the sympathetic nervous system response and not allow the heart rate to increase.
- The aorta of the elder patient is relatively inelastic and more vulnerable to injury.
- Signs of peritoneal irritation are more subtle.
- The elderly are far more susceptible to postoperative complications due to comorbidities.

GERONTOLOGICAL CONSIDERATIONS
Elder Abuse and Neglect

Elder abuse is underreported by patients due to a fear of abandonment and also failure of health care workers to inquire. When screening for suspected abuse, general questions that could be asked are:

- Do you feel safe?
- Are you able to take care of yourself or do you need help?
- Do you live by yourself or with others?
- Who maintains your checkbook?
- Who prepares your meals?

Clinical evidence of abuse/neglect includes:

- Injuries of varying age (as in child abuse)
- Dehydration and malnutrition
- Poor personal hygiene
- Decubitus ulcers
- Unexplained medication overdoses or lack of compliance with medication regimen
- Unexplained venereal disease or genital infection.

Intervention with suspected elder abuse or neglect requires a multidisciplinary team approach. The different disciplines are better able to assess the multifactorial aspects of the situation including physical and mental status, competency, financial status, assistance, and protection with referrals to community agencies for continual monitoring of the situation.

- Osteoporotic bones are more vulnerable to fracture and elderly patients have decreased pain perception, meaning that subtle fractures may be missed.
- Artificial pacemakers and medications such as beta-blockers and calcium channel blockers blunt the usual chronotropic response to hemorrhage.

Falls

According to the CDC (2007a) falls are the leading cause of injuries that result in death among older adults. Falls are also the most common cause of nonfatal injuries. For those that fall, 20% to 30% sustain moderate to severe injuries that decrease their mobility, make it difficult to live alone, and increase the chance of early death. In 2003, approximately 1.8 million people ages 65 and older were treated in emergency departments for nonfatal injuries from falls. For the elderly patient, falls are the most common cause of TBIs (CDC, 2007a).

Prevention efforts are now moving toward fall assessments for elderly patients, which include physical assessment for fall risk and a survey of the patient's home surroundings for hazards. Older patients can take several steps to reduce their risk of falling:

- Exercise regularly to increase strength and improve balance. Research findings have demonstrated the efficacy of t'ai chi exercise to improve balance and decrease falls among older adults (CDC, 2007a).
- Review medications, both prescription and over-the-counter, to reduce side effects and interactions. This should be done by a health care provider.
- Check vision annually.
- Establish adequate lighting throughout the elderly person's residence.
- Reduce hazards in the home that can lead to falls such as throw rugs on which elderly persons could trip.

The National Fire Protection Agency and the CDC have developed a fire and fall prevention program for elders called Remembering When (NFPA, 2003). The program is available in twenty languages and is available on the NFPA website.

Elderly Drivers

Elderly drivers ages 65 and older have a higher crash death rate per mile driven than all others except teen drivers. This age group is the fastest growing segment of the population: By 2020 more than 40 million elderly adults will be licensed to drive (CDC, 2007d). Changes with aging that put the elderly driver at risk are decreases in vision, hearing, cognitive functions, and physical impairments. Research is being conducted to develop risk assessment tools and prevention programs to increase awareness and assist elderly people to be safe drivers.

■ Trauma Rehabilitation

Rehabilitation is the multidisciplinary plan of care that maximizes an impaired individual's function by minimizing the deficits to achieve the highest quality of life possible. Rehabilitation of the trauma patient begins the moment health care services are provided. As the patient stabilizes from the initial resuscitation, the focus changes to recovery and adaptation. Depending on the extent of injury to the patient, the rehabilitation team may consist of many disciplines including health care providers, nurses, social workers, physical therapists, occupational therapists, speech therapists, vocational counselors, and financial counselors, as well as family members. It is important for the patient's goals to be developed by the team because this approach assists with consistency and communication among all team members. The primary nursing objectives during this phase of care are to assist the patient in overcoming or adapting to disabilities. This adaptation involves dealing with psychological as well as physical needs regardless of whether the disability is temporary or permanent.

Health Promotion

One-third to one-half of trauma deaths occur in the prehospital setting before any possibility of treatment (Feliciano et al., 2008). These deaths can only be decreased by prevention efforts. Injury prevention is the key to reducing death caused by trauma and decreasing the severity of injuries and the disability that can arise from a traumatic injury.

Strategies and educational programs to decrease traumatic injury and death include safety-related vehicle design and occupant protection; speed limits; laws and education regarding the use of helmets; laws and education regarding driving under the influence of alcohol or drugs; graduated driver's licensing systems; laws and education regarding smoke detectors; education regarding water temperatures and scald burns; laws regarding the use of flame retardants in children's sleepwear; gun laws; and laws and education regarding domestic violence, child abuse, and elder abuse. Injury prevention programs should be multidisciplinary and reach all members of the community. Many prevention programs are available through national organizations such as the CDC, American Trauma Society, Emergency Nurses Association, and the National Fire Protection Association.

In the United States, one of the most significant improvements in the care of injured patients has been the development of trauma systems (Feliciano et al., 2008). The elements of a trauma system are prehospital care, access to care, hospital care, and rehabilitation, along with prevention, disaster planning, patient education, research, and financial planning. Of great importance for a system's success is having prehospital communications, a transport system, trained personnel, and trained trauma care personnel for all phases of care. It is well known that patients who are severely injured benefit from receiving care at a trauma center due to the rapid response of surgeons and trained health care team members who can evaluate, resuscitate, and operate if necessary.

It has also been shown that patients who have not incurred immediate life-threatening problems also benefit from receiving care at a trauma center. Helling, Nelson, Moore, Kintigh, and Lainhart (2005) completed a retrospective study of 1,592 consecutive trauma patients admitted to the trauma service of an urban trauma center. They found that a large proportion of the patients initially thought to have minor injuries required resources that were available at the trauma center, including specialty care, and intensive care unit, and operating room accessibility. The study revealed that more than one-third of the patients had multiple-system injuries and nearly 20% were considered to have major trauma that required the prioritization of care abilities and expertise ideally found in a trauma center environment.

Statewide trauma system planning can enhance community health through an organized system of injury prevention, acute care, and rehabilitation that is integrated into the public health system throughout a state. The goal of the system is to enhance community health by identifying risk factors in the community and creating solutions to decrease the incidence of injury, to provide access to timely, definitive care for the injured patient, and to decrease overall injury-related morbidity, mortality, and years of life lost through rehabilitation. The U.S. Department of Health and Human Services released the Model Trauma Care System Plan in February 2003 under the Trauma System Agenda for the Future (Cooper, 2008). It was established as a framework for measuring progress in trauma system development and set the standard for systems of trauma care.

Research

Traumatic injury is a major health care and economic issue in the United States. Many trauma patients experience long-term disabilities. Nurses have a responsibility to promote prevention, education, and research that will result in positive patient outcomes. Some examples of needed research are described in the Research Opportunities and Clinical Impact box.

Summary

Improvements in the care of the trauma patient are only a partial solution to this health care issue. Support for aggressive trauma prevention programs is essential to reduce not only the loss of life, but also the economic and emotional effects of traumatic injury. The goal of significantly reducing morbidity and mortality from trauma will be achieved through the influence of prevention campaigns.

RESEARCH OPPORTUNITIES AND CLINICAL IMPACT RELATED TO TRAUMA

Research Opportunities	Clinical Impact
Describe the psychological experiences of trauma patients and families.	Help to define the psychosocial impact of the event and identify the needs.
Many research opportunities involve the nutritional needs of trauma patients:	
Energy prediction equations need to be validated, and standard language and definitions determined.	Nutritional needs could be consistently and accurately defined in multiple settings using objective criteria.
Obese patients have more complications from traumatic injury. Are there specific metabolic or nutritional interventions that might improve prognosis?	Decrease morbidity and mortality in the obese trauma patient population.
Identify physiological parameters to assess pain intensity in comatose patients.	Ensure that adequate pain relief is being accomplished.
Should relatives be present and witness trauma resuscitation?	Allowing relatives to see what is happening, even for a short time, may help to prevent anxiety or terrible imagery.

Clinical Preparation

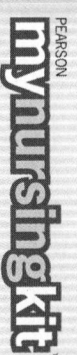

 Read

- History of Current Illness
- Past Medical History
- Physical Exam
- Admitting Medical Orders
- Laboratory Study Results

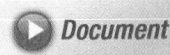 **Document**

- Summary of Hospitalization
- Pathophysiology Form
- Laboratory Values
- Laboratory Results Explanation

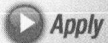 **Apply**

- List of Potential Nursing Diagnoses
- Concept Map
- Critical Thinking Questions

Log on to MyNursingKit.com to download forms you will need and to complete further steps in the Clinical Preparation assignment.

HISTORY OF PRESENT ILLNESS

The patient is an 18-year-old male who was brought into the emergency department by ambulance as a trauma activation. He was in full C-spine precautions including board and collar. The patient was a restrained driver of a vehicle that ran into a tree head-on at approximately 65 miles per hour. There was positive air bag deployment. The patient self-extricated but was unable to ambulate at the scene secondary to left leg pain. A left leg deformity was noted in the field and was splinted. He is amnestic to the event with a Glasgow Coma Scale (GCS) score of 14. He denies abdominal pain, headache, or neck pain. He does complain of severe left leg pain.

Medical–Surgical History

The patient denies any health problems, takes no medications, and states he has no allergies.

Social History

The patient is a freshman at the local college. He does not smoke cigarettes; he drinks beer on the weekends and occasionally smokes marijuana.

Physical Exam

Vital signs on arrival: blood pressure 132/80, heart rate 96, respiratory rate 18, and temperature 36°C. His left thigh, left knee, and left lower leg are tender to palpation with apparent soft tissue swelling. Distal pulses are intact. The left lower extremity is slightly shortened and rotated. Radiographs revealed a left femur and left tibial fracture. A Steinman pin was placed by the orthopedic service for reduction of the femur fracture. C-spine, chest, and pelvic radiographs are normal. CT scan of the abdomen is normal. The patient is admitted to the trauma unit to rule out intra-abdominal injury and will go to the operating room for ORIF of the fractured femur.

Admitting Medical Orders

Service: trauma
Diagnosis: blunt-force trauma, concussion, left femur fracture, left tibial fracture, rule out intra-abdominal injury
Allergies: no known allergies
Vital signs: every 4 hours including oxygen saturation; GCS scale and neurovascular checks to left lower extremity; 20 lb skeletal traction to left lower extremity
Call house officer: temp > 38.5°C, HR > 130 or < 60, RR > 30 or < 12, BP sys > 160 or < 90, O_2 sat < 92%, urine output < 120 mL in 4 hours, change in neurovascular exam to left lower extremity, any Hct result that is 5 less than the baseline ED Hct
Activity: bed rest
Diet: nothing by mouth
IV: D5/0.45NS with 20 mEq KCl at 125 mL/hr
Foley catheter to gravity drainage
I&O: every 4 hours

Respiratory care: use incentive spirometer every hour when awake
DVT prophylaxis: sequential compression device to right lower extremity

Scheduled Medications

Hydromorphine PCA 0.2 mg/mL, incremental dose 0.4 mg, lockout 6 minutes
Docusate 100 mg po twice daily

PRN Medications

Diphenhydramine 25–50 mg IV every 6 hours if needed for itching
Morphine 1–4 mg IV every 3 hours as needed for severe pain
Magnesium hydroxide liquid 30 mL po every 12 hours as needed
Ondansetron 4 mg IV every 12 hours as needed for nausea

Ordered Laboratory Studies

Complete blood count every morning
Hemoglobin and hematocrit every 4 hours
Chemistry panel every other day

LABORATORY STUDY RESULTS

HD1	1030	1245	1510	2200	0400
Hgb	16.4 g/dL	15.4 g/dL	14.7 g/dL	14.4 g/dL	12.6 g/dL
Hct	48.4%	44.9%	43.3%	42.5%	36.8%
WBC	18.1/mm³	21.4/mm³	20.0/mm³	19.2/mm³	13.4/mm³
RBC	5.49/mm³	5.08/mm³	4.93/mm³	4.81/mm³	4.19/mm³
PTT	23.9 seconds				
INR	0.97				
Na	138 mEq/L				
K	3.8 mEq/L				
Cl	102 mEq/L				
CO$_2$	25 mEq/L				
Glucose	145 mg/dL				
CA	8.9 mg/dL				
Lipase	29 U/dL				

CRITICAL THINKING QUESTIONS

1. What is the main purpose of the primary survey?
2. Having heard the history of the incident, what injury patterns would you anticipate?
3. The CT of the abdomen was normal. Does this rule out intra-abdominal injury?
4. What is the importance of warming the patient?

Answers to Critical Thinking Questions appear in Appendix D.

NCLEX® REVIEW

1. A patient comes into the emergency department after sustaining injuries from a rear impact motor vehicle crash. Which of the following injuries is this patient most likely experiencing?
   1. Pelvis
   2. Tibia
   3. Chest
   4. Spinal

2. A patient comes into the emergency department as a victim of an assault. The patient has multiple bleeding head and facial lacerations with draining coming from the right ear. The patient's speech is slurred and he admits to recent alcohol consumption. Which of the following should be the first priority when treating this patient?
   1. Apply direct pressure to the wounds to control the bleeding.
   2. Perform a full neurologic exam and check for "halo effect."
   3. Utilize a rigid cervical collar to stabilize the cervical spine.
   4. Transport the patient to radiology for a CT scan of the head.

3. The nurse is providing care to a trauma patient. When conducting the tertiary trauma survey, the nurse understands that:
   1. It will include a comprehensive medical record review to help ensure all injuries and treatments for the patient with trauma have been properly addressed.
   2. A work group will develop evidence-based guidelines for practice regarding the best and most important nutritional recommendations for the patient with trauma.
   3. This systematic approach to initial trauma assessment helps the health care team identify injuries, provide appropriate interventions, and prioritize patient care.
   4. The multidisciplinary plan of care developed will help increase the patient's quality of life and maximize the impaired patient's function by minimizing any deficits.

4. A patient who has sustained multiple trauma has a low blood pressure with minimal bleeding from skin lacerations. Which of the following should the nurse do?
   1. Insert an indwelling urinary catheter.
   2. Ensure adequate oxygenation.
   3. Assess for bleeding into the chest, abdomen, pelvis, or around long bones.
   4. Ensure adequate cervical spine support precautions.

Answers for review questions appear in Appendix D

KEY TERMS

apoptosis *p.2433*
Battle's sign *p.2436*
Beck's triad *p.2434*
cardiac tamponade *p.2434*
FAST examination *p.2436*

flail chest *p.2431*
hyphema *p.2436*
kinematics *p.2426*
massive hemothorax *p.2432*
open pneumothorax *p.2432*

pulmonary contusion *p.2431*
tension pneumothorax *p.2432*
raccoon eyes *p.2436*
rehabilitation *p.2443*

PEARSON
EXPLORE **mynursingkit**™

MyNursingKit is your one stop for online chapter review materials and resources. Prepare for success with additional NCLEX®-style practice questions, interactive assignments and activities, web links, animations and videos, and more!

Register your access code from the front of your book at
www.mynursingkit.com

REFERENCES

American College of Surgeons. (2004). *Advanced trauma life support for doctors* (7th ed.). Chicago: Author.

American College of Surgeons, Committee on Trauma. (2006). *Resources for optimal care of the injured patient.* Chicago: American College of Surgeons.

American Trauma Society. (2003). *End-of-life issues: Quality, availability, and ethics.* Upper Marlboro, MD: Author.

Centers for Disease Control and Prevention. (2007a). *Falls among older adults.* Retrieved April 14, 2007, from http://www.cdc.gov/ncipc/factsheets/adultfalls.htm

Centers for Disease Control and Prevention. (2007b). *Injury and violence.* Retrieved April 14, 2007, from http://www.cdc.gov/node.do/id/0900f3ec8000e539

Centers for Disease Control and Prevention. (2007c). *Intimate partner violence.* Retrieved April 14, 2007, from http://www.cdc.gov/ncipc/factsheets/older.htm

Centers for Disease Control and Prevention. (2007d). *Older adult drivers.* Retrieved April 14, 2007, from http://www.cdc.gov/ncipc/factsheets/older.htm

Cooper, G. (2008). *HRSA model trauma systems planning and evaluation.* Retrieved on October 17, 2008, from http://www.emsa.ca.gov/systems/files/trauma/ModelTraumaPlan.ppt#256,1,HRSA Model Trauma Systems Planning & Evaluation.

Crandall, M., Nathens, A. B., Kernic, M. A., Holt, V. L., & Rivara, F. P. (2004). Predicting future injury among women in abusive relationships. *Journal of Trauma: Injury, Infection, and Critical Care, 56*(4), 906–912.

Daffner, R. H., Hackno, D. B., Dalinka, M. K., Davis, P. C., Rosnick, C. S., Rubin, D. A., et. al., (2007). Expert panel on musculoskeletal and neurologic imaging. Suspected spine trauma. Renton, VA. American College of Radiology (ACR). Retrieved June 26, 2008, from http://www.guidelines.gov/summary/summary.aspx?doc_id=11597&nbr=006010-strong=recommendations+AND+imaging+AND+patients+AND+s-suspected+AND+cervical+AND+Spine+AND+trauma.

Emergency Nurses Association, Injury Prevention Institute. (2006a). *Alcohol awareness fact sheet.* Retrieved June 26, 2008, from http://www.ena.org/ipinstitute/fact/ENAIPFactSheet-Alcohol.pdf

Emergency Nurses Association, Injury Prevention Institute. (2006b). *Gun safety.* Retrieved June 26, 2008, from http://www.ena.org/ipinstitute/fact/ENAIPFactSheet-GunSafety.pdf

Feliciano, D. V., Mattox, K. L., & Moore, E. E. (2008). *Trauma* (6th ed.). New York: McGraw-Hill Medical.

Gruen, R. L., Jurkovich, G. J., McIntyre, L. K., Foy, H. M., & Maier, R. V. (2006). Patterns of errors contributing to trauma mortality: Lessons learned from 2,594 deaths. *Annals of Surgery, 244*(3), 371–380.

Hai, S. A. (2004). Permissive hypotensive resuscitation: An evolving concept in trauma. *Journal of the Pakistan Medical Association, 54*(8), 434–436.

Hardy, J. F., de Moerloose, P., & Samama, C. M. (2006). Massive transfusion and coagulopathy: Pathophysiology and implications for clinical management. *Canadian Journal of Anaesthesia, 53*(6 Suppl.), S40–S58.

Helling, T. S., Nelson, P. W., Moore, B. T., Kintigh, D., & Lainhart, K. (2005). Is trauma center care helpful for less severely injured patients? *Injury, 36,* 1293–1297.

Hess, J. R., Holcomb, J. B., & Hoyt, D. B. (2006). Damage control resuscitation: The need for specific blood products to treat the coagulopathy of trauma. *Transfusion, 46,* 685–686.

Hess, J. R., & Lawson, J. H. (2006). The coagulopathy of trauma versus disseminated intravascular coagulation. *Journal of Trauma, 60*(6), S12–S19.

Isenhour, J., & Marx, J. (2007). *General approach to blunt abdominal trauma in adults.* Retrieved April 14, 2007, from http://www.UpToDate.com

Ketchum, L., Hess, J. R., & Hippala, S. (2006). Indications for early fresh frozen plasma, cryoprecipitate, and platelet transfusion in trauma. *Journal of Trauma, 60*(Suppl.), S51–S58.

Martini, W. Z., Pusateri, A. E., Uscilowicz, J. M., Delgado, A. V., & Holcomb, J. B. (2005). Independent contributions of hypothermia and acidosis to coagulopathy in swine. *Journal of Trauma, 58*(5), 1002–1009.

National Fire Protection Agency (NFPA). (2003). *Remembering when: a fire and fall prevention program for older adults.* Retrieved October 17, 2008, from http://www.nfpa.org/assets/files/PDF/RememberingWhen.ppt#256

National Trauma Data Bank. (2007). *National Trauma Data Bank report 2006.* Chicago: American College of Surgeons.

Pepe, P. E., Dutton, R. P., & Fowler, R. L. (2008). Preoperative resuscitation of the trauma patient. *Current Opinion in Anaesthesiology, 21*(2), 216–221.

Petersen, V. (2004). *Trauma tertiary surveys what, why, when, how, and who: Detecting missed injuries in the multiply-injured patient.* Retrieved July 22, 2004, from http://www.trauma.org/nurse/tertiarysurvey.html

Sommers, M. S. (2006). Injury is a global phenomenon of concern in nursing science. *Journal of Nursing Scholarship, 38*(4), 314–320.

Spaniol, J. R., Knight, A. R., Zebley, J. L., Anderson, D., & Pierce, J. D. (2007). Fluid resuscitation therapy for hemorrhagic shock. *Journal of Trauma Nursing, 14*(3), 152–160.

Tieu, B. H., Holcomb, J. B., & Schreiber, M. A. (2007). Coagulopathy: Its pathophysiology and treatment in the injured patient. *World Journal of Surgery, 31*(5), 1055–1065.

Urden, L. D., Stacy, K. M., & Lough, M. E. (2006). *Thelan's critical care nursing.* St. Louis: Mosby.

APPENDIX A 2009–2011 NANDA-APPROVED NURSING DIAGNOSES

Activity Intolerance

Activity Intolerance, Risk for

Activity Planning, Ineffective

Airway Clearance, Ineffective

Anxiety

Anxiety, Death

Aspiration, Risk for

Attachment, Parent/Infant/Child, Risk for Impaired

Autonomic Dysreflexia

Autonomic Dysreflexia, Risk for

Bleeding, Risk for

Blood Glucose, Risk for Unstable

Body Image, Disturbed

Body Temperature: Imbalanced, Risk for

Bowel Incontinence

Breastfeeding, Effective

Breastfeeding, Ineffective

Breastfeeding, Interrupted

Breathing Pattern, Ineffective

Cardiac Output, Decreased

Caregiver Role Strain

Caregiver Role Strain, Risk for

Childbearing Process, Readiness for Enhanced

Comfort, Impaired

Comfort, Readiness for Enhanced

Communication: Impaired, Verbal

Communication, Readiness for Enhanced

Confusion, Acute

Confusion, Acute, Risk for

Confusion, Chronic

Constipation

Constipation, Perceived

Constipation, Risk for

Contamination

Contamination, Risk for

Coping: Community, Ineffective

Coping: Community, Readiness for Enhanced

Coping, Defensive

Coping: Family, Compromised

Coping: Family, Disabled

Coping: Family, Readiness for Enhanced

Coping (Individual), Readiness for Enhanced

Coping, Ineffective

Decisional Conflict

Decision Making, Readiness for Enhanced

Denial, Ineffective

Dentition, Impaired

Development: Delayed, Risk for

Diarrhea

Disuse Syndrome, Risk for

Diversional Activity, Deficient

Electrolyte Imbalance, Risk for

Energy Field, Disturbed

Environmental Interpretation Syndrome, Impaired

Failure to Thrive, Adult

Falls, Risk for

Family Processes, Dysfunctional: Alcoholism

Family Processes, Interrupted

Family Processes, Readiness for Enhanced

Fatigue

Fear

Fluid Balance, Readiness for Enhanced

Fluid Volume, Deficient

Fluid Volume, Deficient, Risk for

Fluid Volume, Excess

Fluid Volume, Imbalanced, Risk for

Gas Exchange, Impaired

Grieving

Grieving, Complicated

Grieving, Risk for Complicated

Growth, Disproportionate, Risk for

Growth and Development, Delayed

Health Behavior, Risk-Prone

Health Maintenance, Ineffective

Health Management, Ineffective Self

Health-Seeking Behaviors (Specify)

Home Maintenance, Impaired

Hope, Readiness for Enhanced

Hopelessness

Human Dignity, Risk for Compromised

Hyperthermia

Hypothermia

Identity, Disturbed Personal

Immunization Status, Readiness for Enhanced

Infant Behavior, Disorganized

Infant Behavior: Disorganized, Risk for

Infant Behavior: Organized, Readiness for Enhanced

Infant Feeding Pattern, Ineffective

Infection, Risk for

Injury, Risk for

Insomnia

Intracranial Adaptive Capacity, Decreased

Knowledge, Deficient (Specify)

Knowledge (Specify), Readiness for Enhanced

Latex Allergy Response

Latex Allergy Response, Risk for

Liver Function, Impaired, Risk for

Loneliness, Risk for

Maternal/Fetal Dyad, Risk for Disturbed

Memory, Impaired

Mobility: Bed, Impaired

Mobility: Physical, Impaired

Mobility: Wheelchair, Impaired

Moral Distress

Motility, Dysfunctional Gastrointestinal

Motility, Risk for Dysfunctional Gastrointestinal

Nausea

Neonatal Jaundice

Neurovascular Dysfunction: Peripheral, Risk for

Noncompliance (Specify)

Nutrition, Imbalanced: Less than Body Requirements

Nutrition, Imbalanced: More than Body Requirements

Nutrition, Imbalanced: More than Body Requirements, Risk for

Nutrition, Readiness for Enhanced

Oral Mucous Membrane, Impaired

Pain, Acute

Pain, Chronic

Parenting, Impaired

Parenting, Readiness for Enhanced

Parenting, Risk for Impaired

Perfusion, Ineffective Peripheral Tissue

Perfusion, Risk for Decreased Cardiac

Perfusion, Risk for Impaired Renal

Perfusion, Risk for Ineffective Cerebral Tissue

Perfusion, Risk for Ineffective Gastrointestinal Tissue

Perioperative Positioning Injury, Risk for

Personal Identity, Disturbed

Poisoning, Risk for

Post-Trauma Syndrome

Post-Trauma Syndrome, Risk for

Power, Readiness for Enhanced

Powerlessness

Powerlessness, Risk for

Protection, Ineffective

Rape-Trauma Syndrome

Relationship, Readiness for Enhanced

Religiosity, Impaired

Religiosity, Readiness for Enhanced

Religiosity, Risk for Impaired

Relocation Stress Syndrome

Relocation Stress Syndrome, Risk for

Resilience, Impaired Individual

Resilience, Readiness for Enhanced

Resilience, Risk for Compromised

Role Conflict, Parental

Role Performance, Ineffective

Sedentary Lifestyle

Self-Care, Readiness for Enhanced

Self-Care Deficit: Bathing/Hygiene

Self-Care Deficit: Dressing/Grooming

Self-Care Deficit: Feeding

Self-Care Deficit: Toileting

Self-Concept, Readiness for Enhanced

Self-Esteem, Chronic Low

Self-Esteem, Situational Low

Self-Esteem, Risk for Situational Low

Self-Mutilation

Self-Mutilation, Risk for

Self Neglect

Sensory Perception, Disturbed (Specify: Auditory, Gustatory, Kinesthetic, Olfactory, Tactile, Visual)

Sexual Dysfunction

Sexuality Pattern, Ineffective

Shock, Risk for

Skin Integrity, Impaired

Skin Integrity, Risk for Impaired

Sleep Deprivation

Sleep Pattern, Disturbed
Sleep, Readiness for Enhanced
Social Interaction, Impaired
Social Isolation
Sorrow, Chronic
Spiritual Distress
Spiritual Distress, Risk for
Spiritual Well-Being, Readiness for Enhanced
Spontaneous Ventilation, Impaired
Stress, Overload
Sudden Infant Death Syndrome, Risk for
Suffocation, Risk for
Suicide, Risk for
Surgical Recovery, Delayed
Swallowing, Impaired
Therapeutic Regimen Management: Family, Ineffective

Therapeutic Regimen Management, Ineffective
Therapeutic Regimen Management, Readiness for Enhanced
Thermoregulation, Ineffective
Tissue Integrity, Impaired
Tissue Perfusion, Ineffective (Specify: Cerebral, Cardiopulmonary, Gastrointestinal, Renal)
Tissue Perfusion, Ineffective, Peripheral
Transfer Ability, Impaired
Trauma, Risk for
Trauma, Risk for Vascular
Unilateral Neglect
Urinary Elimination, Impaired
Urinary Elimination, Readiness for Enhanced
Urinary Incontinence, Functional
Urinary Incontinence, Overflow

Urinary Incontinence, Reflex
Urinary Incontinence, Stress
Urinary Incontinence, Urge
Urinary Incontinence, Risk for Urge
Urinary Retention
Ventilatory Weaning Response, Dysfunctional
Violence: Other-Directed, Risk for
Violence: Self-Directed, Risk for
Walking, Impaired
Wandering

Source: NANDA Nursing Diagnoses: Definitions and Classification, 2007–2008. Philadelphia: North American Nursing Diagnosis Association. Used with permission.

APPENDIX B   Standard Precautions

Standard precautions are designed to reduce the risk of transmission of microorganisms from both recognized and unrecognized sources of infection. They are the primary strategies for preventing nosocomial infections within institutions, and are important to protect health care workers as well. Standard precautions apply to (1) blood; (2) all body fluids, secretions, and excretions except sweat, regardless of whether or not they contain visible blood; (3) nonintact skin; and (4) mucous membranes. Standard precautions are applied to all patients receiving care in hospitals, regardless of their diagnosis or presumed infection status. These precautions are specifically designed for hospitals; however, they also may be implemented in extended and long-term care facilities, and to a more limited extent in providing home care or in other community-based care settings.

Hand Washing

- Wash your hands (a) after touching blood, body fluids, secretions, excretions, and contaminated items, whether or not gloves are worn; (b) immediately after removing gloves, even if gloves appear to be intact; (c) between contacts with patients; and (d) when otherwise indicated to prevent transfer of organisms to other patients. You may need to wash your hands between tasks and procedures on the same patient to prevent cross-contaminating different body sites.
- Use soap and warm water for hand washing when hands are visibly dirty or contaminated with blood or other body fluids.
- If hands are not visibly soiled, use an alcohol-based hand rub for routinely decontaminating hands in all other situations.

Gloves

- Wear clean, nonsterile gloves when touching blood, body fluids, secretions, excretions, and contaminated items.
- Put on clean gloves just before touching mucous membranes and nonintact skin.
- Change your gloves between tasks and procedures on the same patient after contacting material that may contain a high concentration of microorganisms.
- Wear gloves for all invasive procedures such as performing venipuncture or other vascular or surgical procedures.
- Wear gloves if you have cuts, scratches, or other breaks in the skin.
- Remove gloves promptly after use, before touching noncontaminated items and surfaces, and before going to another patient; wash hands immediately after removing gloves.

Mask, Eye Protection, Face Shield

Wear a mask and eye protection or a face shield to protect mucous membranes of your eyes, nose, and mouth during procedures and patient care activities that are likely to generate splashes or sprays of blood, body fluids, secretions, or excretions.

Gown

Wear a gown (clean, disposable) to protect your skin and prevent soiling of clothing during procedures and patient care activities that are likely to generate splashes or sprays of blood, body fluids, secretions, or excretions. Remove soiled gowns promptly, washing your hands immediately after gown removal.

Equipment

Handle used patient care equipment that is soiled with blood, body fluids, secretions, and excretions in a way that prevents exposing your skin and mucous membranes, contaminating your clothing, and transferring microorganisms to other patients or environments. Ensure that reusable equipment is cleaned and appropriately reprocessed before using for the care of another patient.

Environmental Control

Follow hospital procedures for routine care, cleaning, and disinfecting environmental surfaces, beds, bed rails, bedside equipment, and other frequently touched surfaces.

Linen

Handle and transport linens soiled with blood, body fluids, secretions, and excretions in a manner that prevents exposing your skin and mucous membranes, contaminating your clothing, and transferring microorganisms to other patients and environments. Place soiled linen in leakage-resistant bags at the location where it is used.

Occupational Health and Bloodborne Pathogens

- Take care to prevent injuries when using needles, scalpels, and other sharps; when handling sharp instruments after procedures; when cleaning used instruments; and when disposing of used needles.
- Never recap used needles, manipulate them using both hands, or handle them in a manner that directs the point of a needle toward any part of your body. If it is necessary to protect the needle prior to disposal, use a one-handed "scoop" technique or mechanical device to hold the needle sheath.
- Do not remove used needles from disposable syringes by hand; do not bend, break, or otherwise manipulate used needles by hand.
- Place used disposable syringes and needles, scalpel blades, and other sharp items in appropriate puncture-resistant containers located as close as practical to the area in which the items were used.
- Place reusable syringes and needles in a puncture-resistant container for transport to the reprocessing area.

- Use mouthpieces, resuscitation bags, or other ventilation devices as an alternative to mouth-to-mouth resuscitation methods whenever possible.

Patient Placement

Place patients who contaminate the environment or who do not (or are not expected to) assist in maintaining appropriate hygiene or environmental control (e.g., an ambulatory, confused patient with fecal incontinence) in a private room.

Sources: Centers for Disease Control and Prevention. (2002). Guidelines for hand hygiene in health-care settings: Recommendations of the Healthcare Infection Control Practices Advisory Committee and the HICPAC/SHEA/APIC/IDSA Hand Hygiene Taskforce. *MMWR, 51*(RR-16), 1–56; Hospital Infection Control Practices Advisory Committee. (1997). Part II. Recommendations for isolation precautions in hospitals. Atlanta: Public Health Service, U.S. Department of Health and Human Services, Centers for Disease Control and Prevention.

APPENDIX C   Units of Measurement in Metric and Household Systems

ABBREVIATIONS

Volume

Metric		Household	
milliliter	mL	microdrop	mcgtt
liter	L	drop	gtt
cubic centimeter	cc	teaspoon	t or tsp
		tablespoon	T or tbs
		fluid ounce	oz
		pint	pt
		quart	qt

Weight

Metric		Household	
microgram	mcg	ounce	oz
milligram	mg	pound	lb
gram	g		
kilogram	kg		

Length

Metric		Household	
centimeter	cm	inch	in
meter	m	foot	ft

Area

Metric	
square meter	m^2

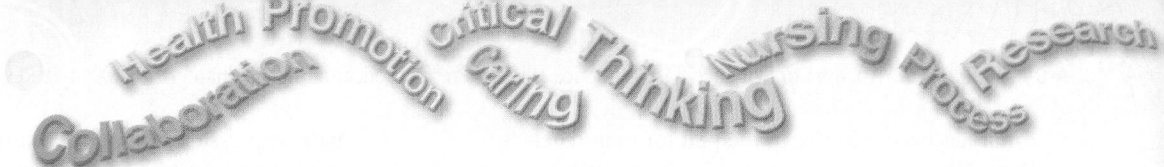

APPENDIX D   Answers to Evidence-Based Practice, Clinical Preparation, and End-of-Chapter NCLEX-Style Review Questions

Evidence-Based Practice Boxes

Chapter 10

Evidence-Based Practice #1 Answers

1. In this scenario, the nurse will need to perform a digital rectal exam to assess for hardened stool in the rectal vault. If the patient is uncooperative, a provider's order for any abdominal x-ray to assess for fecal impaction would be indicated.
2. Because narcotics can cause a slowing of the intestine, with constipation as a result, the nurse will need to consider adding a stool softener or laxative to the patient's medication regimen.
3. Yes, patients often have fecal impaction of stool in the rectum but have small amounts of liquid stool that are expelled around the impaction. The nurse will need to facilitate removal of the hardened stool through the use of either a suppository or an enema or via manual disimpaction, if needed.

Evidence-Based Practice #2 Answers

1. Ask the daughter why she feels her mother should have a mammogram now, when she has refused them in the past. This allows the daughter to verbalize her concerns about her mother, which may reflect the daughter's greater concerns as to her mother's overall medical condition.
2. If the daughter is the patient's appointed spokesperson, share with her your findings. She may already know about the mass and have decided to take no further action, or it may be new information to her. Either way, notify the patient's provider with your findings for further action, if indicated.
3. Call the breast imaging center in advance to determine whether it has the equipment available to accommodate this patient. If the patient is frail, the breast imaging center may want to schedule a longer appointment than usual to give the patient extra time to complete the mammogram.

Evidence-Based Practice #3 Answers

1. The nurse should diplomatically remind the health care provider that Darvocet (propoxyphene) can cause adverse central nervous system effects in the elderly, with little analgesic advantage over acetaminophen. The nurse can suggest a medication more appropriate in this population, such as acetaminophen with a short-acting opiate if necessary for pain control. It is also helpful to know what is available in your facility's emergency medication kit so that you will be able to give a medication without having to order it from the pharmacy and wait for delivery.
2. Diphenhydramine can cause urinary retention, especially in elderly males who may have a baseline prostate hypertrophy. Diphenhydramine should not be used as a sleeping agent; safer alternatives exist. The nurse should notify the health care provider of the patient's symptoms and then discuss a plan of treatment, including addressing the patient's urinary retention as well as insomnia.
3. Her health care provider needs to know about her diazepam use because this medication should be avoided in the elderly due to its extremely long half-life. The nurse needs to discuss with both the patient and the health care provider a plan of care to address the patient's "nerves." Obtaining medications from multiple providers is a dangerous practice, especially for the aging patient.

Chapter 12

1. The perception and chronicity of stress causes a cellular response and an increase in oxidative stress. The cellular response includes a reduction in the number of telomeres and telomerase, a decrease in the ability of the cells to divide, and a decrease in the DNA component, which precipitates genetic damage and eventually cell death. Over time, the tissues comprising the affected cells also die, producing the effects of aging: muscles weaken; skin wrinkles; hair grays; eyesight; hearing; and organs fail; and thinking abilities diminish.
2. Young adults have higher telomerase levels and a greater ability for the enzyme to repair the cell by regenerating telomeres. The telomerase levels decrease with normal aging. This process is accelerated with high levels of chronic psychological stress, thus precipitating premature aging. It is important to know this information to assist in the assessment process. Understanding the age differentiation helps the nurse to know which type of patient is the most vulnerable candidate for cellular response to chronic perceived stress.
3. a. Sleep.
   b. Social connections.
   c. Exercise.
   d. Quiet time alone.
   e. Rest and relaxation.
   f. Meditation/contemplation.
   g. Hobbies.
   h. Nutrition.
   i. Journaling.
   j. Yoga.

Chapter 14

1. Postpyloric placement of a feeding tube into the small bowel can be useful to minimize the risk of high gastric residuals. If it is not contraindicated, elevation of the head of the bed to a 45-degree angle may decrease risk of aspiration.
2. Feedings should not be held until there are two or more consecutive gastric residual volumes greater than 250 mL.

Chapter 15

1. Is this new onset pain?
   What is the patient's perception of discomfort?
   Has this type of pain occurred before?

What has been effective in the past for pain relief?
Drug allergies or unwanted side effects such and nausea and vomiting.
2. Facial grimacing.
Increased movement.
Increased heart rate and blood pressure.
Ask family members and caregivers what the usual response to pain is.

Chapter 17

1. Ask and identify open-ended questions to clarify how they are feeling.
2. Listen carefully to what they are saying. Let them know that you are available to answer questions. Advocate for the patient and family by contacting other members of the health care team as needed.

Chapter 20

1. a. Ensure an adequate diet with vitamins A and C, iron, and zinc.
   b. Avoid exposure to others with infection.
   c. Instruct the patient to wash hands after toileting and before eating.
   d. Report to the surgeon all medications taken.
2. a. Check color; redness may indicate infection.
   b. Check temperature; warmth may indicate infection.
   c. Check for swelling.
   d. Check for drainage from the wound. If present, check the color and amount of drainage.
3. a. Wash hands before and after touching the patient.
   b. Wear gloves when providing wound care.
   c. Keep the patient well hydrated and provide foods that are high in protein.
4. a. Instruct patients to take their prescriptions as directed, including the prescribed frequency and duration.
   b. Educate patients on when antibiotics are appropriate and not appropriate.

Chapter 21

1. Ask the patient an open-ended question to describe what insights have become apparent during the interview.
2. Listen carefully to the story of the patient. Use nonverbal cues to support the patient.

Chapter 23

1. f. b & c
2. a. Slow the transfusion.
   b. Take vital signs and oxygen saturation.
   c. Call the health care provider.

Chapter 25

1. These questions are designed to get one to think about issues that may influence the generalizability of research findings and the need to replicate research studies using subjects of both genders, varying ages, and multiple ethnicities and cultures. In thinking about this study, one might wonder how culture, specifically the Chinese culture, might influence things such as attitudes toward pain and pain expression as well as attitudes toward taking pain medication or using nonpharmacologic therapies for pain control. Culture may also play a role in how the subjects respond to being part of a research study. One needs to know more fully about Chinese culture to theorize about how these research results will generalize to a Western culture. Similarly, it is helpful to know about national health insurance in China. The economics of health care in a country influence aspects of care, such as what kind of preoperative teaching is available, what pain medications are used, how medications are administered, and what nonpharmacologic approaches are covered by the insurance. These may, in turn, influence attitudes.

2. Pain is a subjective experience, and the use of a visual analog scale is a valid and reliable measure of a person's pain experience. The researchers could include objective indices of pain or of physiological stress, with physiological stress serving as a marker for pain. Examples of objective measures might include blood pressure (elevation or changes correlating with pain ratings), heart rate (elevation or correlation with pain rating), respiratory rate (elevation), and plasma cortisol levels (elevation). Objective markers have limitations because they are nonspecific; nevertheless, they could contribute to the discussion of pain reduction. The authors could also use functional performance as indirect markers of pain reduction. Physical performances that often improve with pain relief include ability and distance of ambulation, amount of time spent out of bed, and ability and frequency of deep breathing or ability to perform coughing exercises.

Chapter 26

1. a. Communication with surgical team for timing of antibiotic administration and to maintain surgical asepsis guidelines.
   b. Institute measures to maintain normothermia throughout surgery and postanesthesia care unit.
   c. Develop policies that ensure that standards regarding warning procedures are used by all members of the surgical team.

Chapter 27

1. It is not known which aspects of the protocol accounted for the change in the patient outcomes. One could explain, using Maslow's hierarchy of needs, that the protocol was effective because it helped patients to meet basic needs of comfort: toileting, repositioning, and pain management. These needs were met on a regular basis without the patient having to ask. The protocol also increased patients' sense of personal control over their environment by ensuring that important objects were close by and by giving information about care schedules. Perhaps the consistency of the schedule met higher levels of human need by allowing patients to feel safe and cared for. Several nursing theories can be used to explain the outcomes of this study. Hildegard Peplau's interpersonal relationships theory that puts the nurse–patient relationship at the center of nursing practice or Jean Watson's theory of caring are both appropriate, as are many

nursing theories. Katherine Kolcaba's theory of comfort is particularly relevant to the protocol of nursing rounds. In her theory, enhanced comfort is an immediate and desirable outcome of nursing interventions.

2. It seems as if any number of patient outcomes might be influenced by a nursing round protocol (the protocol used in the study or one that is tailored for specific nursing units). Examples of specific patient outcomes include reduction in urinary or bowel incontinence, reduction in the incidence of decubiti, improved pain management, increased mobility, and increased oral fluid intake.

3. The study could be replicated using a larger number of nursing units and varied types of units (medical, cardiac, oncology, neurology, surgical specialties, etc.). The protocol could be lengthened from the 4 weeks that was used. The nursing rounds protocol could be adapted for specific patient populations (e.g., it could include a reminder to use the incentive spirometry on a surgical unit).

Chapter 29

1. a. Difficulty with concentration.
   b. Family observations of irritability.
   c. Memory impairment.
2. a. A recent motor vehicle accident, with or without loss of consciousness.
   b. Participation in sporting events.
   c. Difficulty in school or work environment.
3. a. Consults for therapies, such as speech and occupational therapies.
   b. Family teaching and support.

Chapter 30

1. The elderly, any patient with uncontrolled hypertension, any patient on Coumadin.
2. Severe headache, difficulty with speech, decreased motor function of either side of the body, sudden loss of consciousness.
3. Close control of blood glucose, careful monitoring of blood pressure, vigilant neurological assessment.

Chapter 31

1. a. Disease process.
   b. Disease and symptom management.
   c. Community resources for assistance at home.
2. a. Verbalize instructions back to the nurse.
   b. Demonstrate the skill back to the nurse.
3. a. Get regular medical checkups.
   b. Get regular physical activity, such as walking.
   c. Use stress management techniques such as pleasurable activities, praying, or meditating.

Chapter 32

1. a. Immobility due to paralysis and spinal precautions.
   b. Ineffective cough.
   c. Use of a cervical orthosis.
   d. Abnormalities in the mechanics of swallowing.
2. a. Frequent coughing with oral intake.
   b. Wet vocal quality.

   c. Difficulty managing oral secretions.
3. a. Sitting patient in an upright position for meals once cleared for activity.
   b. Avoid talking while eating.
   c. Avoidance of large boluses of food at one time.
   d. Monitor patient to ensure that food is cleared from the oropharynx.

Chapter 35

1. a. Most people spend 90% of their time indoors.
2. a. Tobacco smoke must be eliminated from the indoor environment.
3. a. Reducing the exposure to indoor allergens and pollutants will reduce exacerbation of respiratory illness.

Chapter 36

1. c. Confused and not able to cooperate.
2. b. COPD.

Chapter 38

1. a. Has anyone in your family, including parents, grandparents, siblings, aunts, and uncles, ever been diagnosed with AF?
   b. Have you ever been diagnosed with any cardiac disorder, such as heart failure, valve disease, heart attack, or rheumatic fever?
   c. Do you smoke, drink caffeine, or drink alcohol, and if so, in what quantity?
   d. Are you diabetic?
2. a. Report light-headedness, dizziness, shortness of breath, or chest pain to your health care provider as soon as they occur.
   b. Stop smoking and drinking alcohol and caffeine.
   c. Consistently take prescribed medications.
   d. Have family members tested if the AF is genetically induced.

Chapter 40

1. a. Use of interpreters.
   b. Instructions written in native languages.
   c. Use of family or friends who can assist with interpretation.
2. a. Are you noticing any changes in your energy level when performing your daily activities?
   b. Is there a change in the number of hours of sleep needed to feel rested?
   c. Has the need to rest during the day increased recently?
3. a. Statistics about the prevalence of heart disease in women.
   b. The types of clinical symptoms that women experience compared to those experienced by men.
   c. Lifestyle changes that would prevent or slow the progress of heart disease.

Chapter 41

1. a. Understand when it is important to seek medical help for the tachycardia.
   b. How to avoid activities that bring on the tachycardia.

    c. How to slow the heart rate when tachycardia occurs.

    d. List of ideas and activities that would be safe.

2. a. Education about the relationship between tachycardic episodes and the progression of the disease.

    b. Providing alternative activities that interest the young person to decrease the frustration associated with the limitations of the disease.

    c. Evaluate the presence of social support and educate these significant individuals about the need for activity restriction.

3. a. Space activities to allow for periods of rest.

    b. Medicate with antianxiety per orders when necessary.

    c. Control the environment and visitors to diminish stress.

    d. Evaluate current measures and the need for further intervention when necessary.

Chapter 42

1. a. Notify the patient's health care provider.

    b. Ask to talk to another member of the family to see if it is possible to get the patient his medications.

    c. Have the patient explore the possibility of having the medications delivered by the pharmacy.

    d. Ask the patient if he can afford to have a taxi deliver the medications.

2. a. Ask the patient specific questions about her diet, in terms of food types and amounts.

    b. Ask the patient to keep track of the amount of fluids consumed each day.

    c. Discuss with the patient/family the implications associated with failure to comply with therapy.

    d. Ascertain the patient/family understanding of failure to comply with medical management.

    e. Report clinical manifestations to the health care provider.

3. a. Ask the patient about diet, fluid intake, and compliance with medications.

    b. Ask the patient about support system and availability of help with cooking and procurement of medications.

    c. Assess patient motivation with compliance with treatment plan.

    d. Assess patient/family understanding of treatment needs and ability to comply.

Chapter 43

1. Assessment of other risk factors for the development of DVT. Reporting homocysteine and risk factors to the health care provider. Instating health care provider orders to prevent DVT. Assessment for the effectiveness of the interventions.

2. Active and passive range of motion. Foot and ankle exercises. Graduated stocking, pneumatic compression devices.

3. Prevent venous pooling of blood.

Chapter 45

1. A, C, E, F

2. Visual inspection of the oral mucosa.

3. When assessing the oral cavity, the nurse should note any subjective complaints, such as soreness or pain of the lips or gums, reports of increased salivation, toothache, or earache. The objective assessment findings of concern would include indurations or painless ulcer on the lips, ulcerations, areas of thickening, increased salivation, leukoplakia, erythroplakia, rough areas, slurred speech, dysphagia, or difficulty chewing or speaking.

Chapter 46

1. Most medications are metabolized by the liver. Decreased hepatic blood flow and shunting of blood slows the metabolism of medications and creates a higher bioavailability. Also, the shifts in body fluids that occur with decreased serum albumin will change the volume of distribution for the medications.

2. The nurse should check the medication information to see if the pharmacologic half-life is affected by liver failure. Because the metabolism of morphine is greatly affected, the nurse should review the dosage and frequency with the health care team to ensure the safety of the patient.

Chapter 47

1. Nonadherence with fluid restrictions may cause fluid overload with symptoms of shortness of breath, muscle cramping, dizziness, anxiety, panic, pulmonary edema, and hypertension. Nonadherence with dietary restrictions and medication regimens may result in chronically elevated serum levels of phosphate, which contribute to the development of coronary artery disease and the development of secondary hyperparathyroidism.

2. Implement adherence-enhancing interventions with the goal of improving the clinical outcome.

Chapter 49

1. c
2. a
3. a

Chapter 50

1. Meeting the needs of the spouse will improve the quality of life for both the patient and the spouse.

2. d. Involve spouses in medical decision making along with the patient.

Chapter 53

1. The best answer would be "b." This is an adolescent who is not focused so much on the future as on his current lifestyle. It is important to look at what is going on around him to try to find the reason why he is not checking his blood glucose. There may be a variety of reasons as to why he does not test his glucose, including feeling self-conscious about his diabetes. At this point, the nurse can help to explore practical ways to integrate glucose testing into his lifestyle, regardless of whether he really understands the long-term complications or not.

2. The best answer would be "a." The point that you want to emphasize is that regardless of the type of diabetes, the relationship between glucose control and the development of

complications is a primary mediator of complications (chronically elevated blood glucose levels are associated with the development of diabetes-related complications). The nurse may also want to explore whether there are financial or other concerns that are influencing one's ability to check blood glucose levels.

3. Of the two responses, the second is the best. This is because it involves a systematic approach to the problem while recognizing that if the patient and family decide to continue multiple daily injections, the plan will be in place to recognize and prevent hypoglycemia.

Chapter 55

1. Identifying high-risk individuals allows the health care team, patient, and family to develop a plan and implement preventive measures to decrease the chance of a fall and subsequent fracture.

2. Moderate exercise such as walking, swimming, or riding a stationary bike helps to strengthen muscles, slows the loss of calcium from the bone, and helps to maintain balance. Exercise such as yoga helps to strengthen core muscles, which helps with maintenance of balance and flexibility.

Chapter 56

1. The pin site will become infected. Skeletal traction pins are exposed to the environment where they protrude through the skin, and bacteria can travel down to the bone. Moisture creates an area for bacteria, always present at the pin–skin interface, to accumulate and grow.

2. Signs and symptoms of infection include pain, redness, edema, and drainage from the site.

Chapter 57

1. Early control of pain is more effective in controlling pain than is medication administered after pain becomes severe. With amputation, pain normally begins to diminish in intensity 3 or 4 days after surgery.

2. Phantom limb pain is the sensation of pain in the amputated body part. The cause of the phenomenon is unknown, but the perception of pain can interfere with the patient's rehabilitation.

Chapter 58
Critical Thinking Application #1 Answers

1. a. Have the patient take the medication with food.
   b. Encourage small frequent meals.
   c. Drink milk when taking medication.
2. a. Xanthine oxidase inhibitors.
   b. Nonsteroidal anti-inflammatory drugs.
   c. Steroids.
   d. Uricosuric agents.

Critical Thinking Application #2 Answers

1. a. Compliance with multiple treatments, such as medication and lifestyle changes.
   b. What impact can the nursing profession make on improving patient care with gout?
   c. Providing an understanding of the risks and pathophysiology of the disease process.
   d. Teaching the patient ways to improve lifestyle choices and reduce gout attacks.
   e. Educating the patient on medication therapy.

Chapter 60

1. b. Ease of availability and financial resources.
2. a. Diminished or absent diarrhea.
   c. Absence of candidiasis.
   d. No painful swallowing.

Chapter 61

1. a. Hypotension after infusion of 2 liters of isotonic crystalloid infusion.
2. b. Infusing 7 liters of crystalloid solution through a central line.
3. 1. Suctioning blood from the patient's airway.
   2. Initiating a large-caliber IV for fluid resuscitation.
   3. Stabilizing the patient's pelvis with a sheet.
   4. Applying 100% oxygen by mask to the patient.

Chapter 63
Evidence-Based Practice #1 Answers

1. Pain, short duration of inspiration, and frustration.
2. a. Provide patient education regarding the relationship between lung inspiration, oxygenation, and pulmonary complications.
   b. Provide instruction on proper use of IS, including length of inspiration, volume goals, and frequency.
   c. Recruit family to encourage patient.
   d. Provide adequate pain management.
   e. Provide frequent encouragement and progress assessments/reports to patient.
3. a. Lung sounds.
   b. Chest expansion.
   c. Pain level with inspiration.
   d. Oxygenation status.
   e. Incentive spirometry volume and frequency of use.

Evidence-Based Practice #2 Answers

1. a. Assessment.
   b. Regular flushing.
   c. Solution based on clinical assessment.
2. Benefits include prevention of clot formation. However, risks are increased HIT.

Chapter 64

1. a. Understanding at what point during the course of treatment there is a potential to develop fatigue.
   b. Explanation of how the patient may feel as he or she becomes fatigued.
   c. A list of strategies to reduce energy consumption.
   d. Dietary suggestions to optimize nutrition during and after treatment.
2. a. Report presence of fatigue to health care team so that recommendations can be offered.

b. Encourage the patient and family to discuss the impact of fatigue on their daily lives.

c. Referral to social services or psychiatry as needed.

d. Acknowledge the potential for fatigue to alter sexuality.

3. a. Provide information about interventions available to treat fatigue.

b. Accurate assessment and prompt treatment for fatigue.

c. Encourage patients to maintain adequate activity to increase energy stores.

Chapter 67

1. e. All of the above.

2. a. It would combine to form the compound silver chloride and the silver would no longer be bioavailable to perform its function because ionic silver is the element that is effective against bacteria.

3. e. All of the above.

Chapter 68

1. a. Obtain immediate medical care when injuries occur.

b. Understand that there is an increased risk for complications and prolonged hospitalization.

c. Daily foot inspection for breakdown.

d. Avoidance of extreme temperatures when bathing.

e. No exposure to heaters to help keep feet warm.

2. a. Fireplaces.

b. Poorly controlled heaters.

c. Living alone.

d. Confusion and poor memory.

e. Little to no social support.

f. Inadequate nutrition.

g. Inadequate blood sugar control.

3. a. Blood sugar control.

b. Adequate nutritional support.

c. Strict aseptic technique for wound care.

d. Reporting of the first signs of infections.

Chapter 70
Evidence-Based Practice #1 Answers

1. Know which noises can cause damage (those above 85 decibels). Wear earplugs or other hearing protection devices when involved in a loud activity. Be alert to hazardous noise in the environment. Protect children who are too young to protect themselves. Make family, friends, and colleagues aware of the hazards of noise. Have a medical examination by an otolaryngologist, a physician who specializes in diseases of the ears, nose, throat, head, and neck, and a hearing test by an audiologist, a health professional trained to identify and measure hearing loss and to rehabilitate persons with hearing impairments.

2. Everyone is exposed to hazardous sound levels at one time or on a regular basis—individuals of all ages, including children, adolescents, young adults, and older people. Exposure occurs in the workplace, in recreational settings, and at home.

3. A variety of activities can predispose an individual to NIHL. It may occur from only a one-time exposure to loud sound as well as from repeated exposure to sounds at various loudness levels over an extended period of time. Examples of activities are listening to loud iPods, radios, or TV. Examples of workplace noises are jackhammers and explosive sounds. Participation in recreational activities, such as flying loud model airplanes, snowmobiling, go-carting, woodworking, target shooting, and hunting, may even be a factor.

Evidence-Based Practice #2 Answers

1. Culturally deaf adults are at risk for health-related behaviors that address nutrition, psychological well-being, stress management, physical activity and exercise, activities of daily living, and responsible health care practices.

2. Culturally deaf adults may use a variety of interventions to help them adjust to their environments. The following is just a small list of such activities: learning sign language; having communities provide street warning signs for adults with hearing impairments; using devices that help with communication, such as flashing lights for doorbells or visual readings for telephone communication; and participating in educational activities that will inform society of ways to prevent hazards that cause hearing impairment or hearing loss.

3. School nurses not only are helpful in identifying those adolescents with hearing problems through screening programs, but they may act as advocates for educational activities that inform adolescents of hazardous activities that may lead to NIHL.

Chapter 71

1. a. Inform the patient as to what AMD is and how it impacts the vision and general well-being of the patient, with a return demonstration of gained knowledge.

b. Advise patient about possible ways to decrease the advancement of AMD with prevention.

c. Teach the patient about when it is important to seek medical direction for vision changes from AMD, with a return demonstration of information gained.

d. List the problem stages of treatment or management of AMD.

2. a. Educating about the relationship of possible aging, genetics, ultraviolet light, air pollution, smoking, comorbidities, blood thinners, zinc, luteins, antioxidants, and VEGF toward the advancement of AMD.

b. Providing alternative activities that interest older adults to decrease the frustration associated with the limitations of vision with AMD and general well-being.

c. Incorporating a significant other in the relationship and care, depending on the degree of visual impairment, to prevent social isolation.

d. Providing possible activities that would be beneficial and safe in adding to the prevention or stabilization of visual impairment from AMD.

3. a. Educate on maintaining good general health and avoiding comorbidities that may affect or advance a decline in vision health.

b. Educate on self-vision testing, for example, Amsler grid, and coping with vision loss and maintaining quality of life.

c. Control the environment by adding more independence activities with visual impairment.

d. Evaluate current measures and the need for further intervention as needs present.

Chapter 73

1. b. A policy and procedure should be present to assist in the implementation of family presence. Staff members need education and support.

2. d. All of the above.

Chapter 74

1. f. All of the above.
2. b. It decreases the risk of coagulopathy.

Clinical Preparation Boxes

Chapter 14

1. a. Obesity (BMI 33).
   b. Obesity, family history, hypercholesterolemia, hypertension, hyperglycemia, decreased serum HDL cholesterol, sedentary activity level.

2. a. Assess readiness to lose body weight.
   b. Educate on health benefits of losing weight.
   c. Assist in development of short-term goals toward losing 1 to 2 pounds/week:
      • Increase physical activity. Begin with sitting for fewer hours in the day and gradually add activity.
      • Decrease intake by 500 to 100 kcal/day; assist patient with identifying ways to do this, such as decreased intake of alcohol and empty calories (e.g., change cream in coffee to fat-free half and half, snack on fruit instead of chips).
   d. Educate about the DASH diet for hypertension (reduced sodium, saturated fat, and cholesterol; moderate alcohol; adequate dairy; ample fruits, vegetables, and whole grains).
   e. Refer to registered dietitian.

3. a. Fat intake.
   b. Alcohol intake.
   c. Caffeine intake.
   d. Large meals.
   e. Eating large meals late in the evening, close to bedtime (lying flat with increased gastric pressure).
   f. Overweight/obese.

4. Reduced intake of fat, moderating alcohol intake, weight loss.

Chapter 15

1. Sensory, affective, cognitive, and behavioral.
2. Discuss concerns about pain management and discuss reasons for behavior when wife is present.
3. PCA demand doses attempted/given, medication side effects, renal function, patient's current and acceptable level of pain.

Chapter 19

1. This patient has a respiratory acidosis—the $PaCO_2$ is increased and the pH is acid. The HCO_3^- is higher than normal, with a base excess of $+5$.
2. Age, 50 pack/year smoking history, emphysema, history of coronary artery disease.
3. Emphysema and pneumonia.
4. Coughing and deep-breathing exercises. Up in chair and walking at regular intervals.

Chapter 20

1. Room 122—apparent best immune system.
2. Yes—open draining leg wound that is positive for *S. aureus*.
3. Diabetes, living in the woods, age, and smoking.
4. *Body Image, Disturbed.*
   Fatigue.
   Mobility: Physical, Impaired.
   Pain, Acute.
   High Risk for Self-Care Deficit: Toileting.
   Skin Integrity, Impaired.
   Tissue Perfusion, Ineffective, Risk for.

Chapter 21
Part 1

1. *Assessment:* The nurse's initial assessment of Ms. Bell began at the time of her first visit to the health care center. The nurse began to collect the database concerning the characteristics that Ms. Bell was demonstrating. The subjective database suggested depression and distortion of reality concerning her health and work problems. The objective database was anger, agitation, and intolerance for the environment and the reporting of psychosomatic symptoms.
   Related Factors: Ms. Bell has highly ambivalent feelings concerning her family and the loss of employment.
   Nursing Diagnosis: Coping: Family Disabled (Wilkinson, 2005, p. 117).
   Alternative Diagnosis: Management of Therapeutic Regimen: Families/Individual, Ineffective (Wilkinson, 2005, p. 118).
   NOC Outcomes (Wilkinson, 2005):
   • Aggression control.
   • Depression control.
   • Neglect recovery.
   Goals/Evaluation Criteria:
   • Ms. Bell will use *Disabled Family Coping* as demonstrated by satisfactory status in aggression control, depression control, and neglect of recovery.
   • *Family and Individual Coping* with:
     Demonstrates role flexibility.
     Manages problems.
     Receives care and cares for the needs of family members.
     Secures financial stability.
     Asks for assistance when appropriate (Wilkinson, 2005, p. 119).
   NIC Interventions:
   • Coping enhancement: Assist Ms. Bell to adapt to the real and perceived stress and changes that were interfering with her life goals.

- Normalization promotion: Assist Ms. Bell with adaptation to a chronic disease, diabetes mellitus. Encourage her to accept that her life experience is a reality (Wilkinson, 2005).

Nursing Activities:
- Obtain a history of the family's patterns of behavior and changes that have occurred.
- Assess the interaction between Ms. Bell and her family.
- Determine the physical, emotional, educational, and spiritual resources of Ms. Bell.
- Assess Ms. Bell's motivation for resolving the crisis.
- Discuss with Ms. Bell the most effective ways to assist her with becoming familiar with her multiple health needs. Ms. Bell needs referrals to other agencies such as social services, nutrition counseling, support groups, and the Council on Aging.

Part 2

The strategies essential to controlling Ms. Bell's hypertension were an adequate knowledge base of what the disease is, how it may be controlled, the use of lifestyle changes, and weight control. Ms. Bell was encouraged to participate in the plan of care, and her questions can be answered through the use of the office hotline.

Part 3

If Ms. Bell relapses into noncompliance, the nurse will assess the problems interfering with Ms. Bell's following through with her plan of care. With this information, the plan of care can be modified by removing the element that was keeping her from following through. At times, the patient may not understand how and why a particular segment of the plan was important to the management and control of the disease. The use of totally illustrated brochures and conferences within the location may assist in the understanding of hypertension. In addition, the teaching appointments can be recorded on audio tape for the patient's review at home.

2. • Acceptance of the diagnosis of high blood pressure.
   - Enabling Ms. Bell in seeking information about high blood pressure and how the diagnosis is made.
   - Partnership with the nurse as the treatment plan is established, maintained, and revised.
   - Use of the plan and the ability to negotiate changes in the treatment plan as the physiological situation need modification.
   - Understands the reason for keeping appointments with the health care provider. Ms. Bell will report self-screening results at each visit.
   - Ms. Bell monitors herself for the treatment response.
   - Ms. Bell performs self-screening tests such as blood pressure, weight, and glucose monitoring.
   - Ms. Bell seeks to reinforce her lifestyle changes.

3. When the nurse listens to Ms. Bell in a therapeutic manner, the nurse will engage in an assessment of the patterns of communication and as a self-interpreting person. This means listening to the individual for his or her interpretation and the embedded meaning of the situation. This activity, the process of active listening, is "attending to and

attaching significance to a patient's verbal and nonverbal messages" (Wilkinson, 2005, p. 82).

4.

Nursing Assessment of Loss

Nursing Assessment and Diagnoses	Outcomes and Evaluation Parameters	Planning and Interventions with Rationale
Subjective: "I'm standing under a very dark cloud." "How much more can or must I tolerate?"	**Outcome:** Practice effective coping strategies.	**Interventions and Rationales** Discusses importance of participating in the high blood pressure support group in the community.
Objective: Death of husband of 35 years Loss of employment due to downsizing Daughter lives 250 miles away	***Evaluation Parameters:*** Documented improvements in self-reports. States reasons for changes in lifestyle and coping styles.	Discusses changing role in her home, community, and church. Reviews changes in lifestyle.
Nursing Diagnosis: Chronic Losses related to chronic illness and Ineffective Coping with lifestyle related to chronic illness		*Lifestyle changes and modification of role within family, community, and church have positive value in fostering effective coping strategies.*

Chapter 23

1. ASA and Celebrex.
2. Rehydration, undetected bleeding.
3. Transfusion reactions, lung sounds. Identification of patient, vital signs, and signs and symptoms of transfusion reactions.
4. Fluid overload due to his age and cardiac history.
5. History of taking Lopressor, a beta-blocker that decreases heart rate.
6. The Na and Cl levels are elevated (concentrated blood solutes). The BUN is elevated, but the creatinine is normal. Values return to normal after rehydration.
7. To rule out pancreatitis, which can cause GI bleed.
8. Vitamin K absorption by the intestine is decreased in GI bleed, and vitamin K is needed for clotting. Vitamin K affects the part of the clotting cascade that is measured by the PT and INR.

Chapter 27

1. *Pain:* Abdominal incisions are painful, and Mr. Landry's pain ratings show that he is not getting adequate pain relief. Pain is a likely factor in his reluctance to ambulate and to use the incentive spirometer.

   Impaired Gas Exchange: Mr. Landry is on 4 liters of oxygen but has only marginal oxygen saturation. He is not performing deep breathing or coughing as needed to open the airways and alveoli and to clear respiratory secretions.

Fluid Volume, Deficient: Mr. Landry is losing fluid through the NGT and because he has a fever. The low urine output, tachycardia, dry skin, thirst, and vertigo when standing suggest that he is dehydrated.

Anxiety: Mr. Landry demonstrates anxious behaviors and he reports feeling anxious. Anxiety is an uncomfortable state, and it can influence all aspects of his care and recovery.

Activity Intolerance: Mr. Landry has vertigo, tachycardia, and tachypnea with activity.

2. Pain: Evidenced by high pain ratings and reluctance to do IS, cough, and ambulate.

   Atelectasis: Evidenced by fever, crackles, shallow breathing.

   Dehydration: Evidenced by tachycardia, low urine output, warm skin, thirst.

   Orthostatic hypotension: Likely, given his complaints of vertigo on standing.

   Ileus: Evidenced by no passing of flatus (expected finding for the first several days postop following surgery on colon).

   Nausea: Evidenced by complaints of nausea.

   Anemia: Evidenced by a low hematocrit and hemoglobin.

   Vital Signs: Part of routine nursing care. The data are used to monitor for a variety of postoperative complications, including fever, bleeding, dehydration, abnormal cardiac rhythm.

   NPO: To prevent abdominal distention and nausea and vomiting.

   NGT to low continuous suction: Used to decompress the stomach. Prevents abdominal distention until peristalsis returns to the bowel. Abdominal distention would place tension on the sutures.

   IS: A mechanism used to encourage deep breathing. Deep breathing increases lung volumes and stimulates surfactant. This intervention is used to treat hypoxia and to prevent atelectasis and pneumonia.

   Foley: Used to get an accurate, hourly measurement of urine output.

   I&O: Used to estimate fluid balance. Many patients are slightly dehydrated at the end of surgery. In this case, Mr. Landry is continuing to lose fluid as a result of a fever and drainage from the NGT.

   Pneumatic compression boots: Increase venous return from the legs, helping to prevent deep venous thrombus (DVT).

   Ambulate: Ambulation is the single most important intervention to prevent postoperative complications. Ambulation increases respiratory rate, minute ventilation, tidal volume, and inspiratory flow rates, helping to prevent atelectasis and pneumonia. Ambulation increases blood flow to organs and tissues, helping with wound healing, restoring peristalsis, and preventing venous stasis and DVT.

   Cardiac telemetry: Used to monitor for bradycardia and dysrhythmia because Mr. Landry is receiving Metoprolol intravenously.

Dextrose 5% and 0.45 sodium chloride with 20 mEq KCl: This is an isotonic solution used to replace routine fluid loss and to cover fluid loss through the NGT. Mr. Landry requires potassium replacement because he is NPO and unable to replace routine loss of potassium in the urine and additional potassium losses from gastric drainage.

3. The most pressing nursing activities are the treatment of Mr. Landry's pain and nausea. Until pain and nausea are controlled, Mr. Landry will be unable to concentrate on learning to use incentive spirometry or participate in morning care. The nurse should first change the syringe in the PCA pump (this activity is entirely within the nurse's control) to make sure that Mr. Landry has uninterrupted pain medication. Second, the nurse should empty and record urine output and then call the surgeon for the antiemetic. Calling for the antinausea medication is important, but Mr. Landry has been having a low urine output that, if it continues, will require intervention (calling the surgeon and administration of a fluid bolus), and measuring urine output will only take a minute. Third, the nurse calls the surgeon for an antiemetic order (and reports the urine output if low). Once Mr. Landry is comfortable, he should receive teaching on use of the incentive spirometry. A.M. care is important to helping patients feel better, but most patients will decline morning care if they are uncomfortable with either pain or nausea.

4. Treatment for cancer, including colon cancer, depends on the stage of the cancer. Although surgery is a treatment for colon cancer, it is also part of the staging process because the tissue and lymph nodes removed will be examined for evidence of cancer cells. Mr. Landry may need adjunctive treatment (chemotherapy or radiation) once the stage of the cancer is determined. The nurse's best response in this situation is to explore with Mr. Landry his understanding of his disease and the treatment plan. The nurse can help clarify information provided by the surgeon and encourage Mr. Landry to ask the surgeon about questions he has regarding further treatment. The nurse can also help clarify for Mr. Landry the roles of the various people who are or will be involved in his care (e.g., the surgeon, the oncologist, the primary health care provider). The nurse should encourage Mr. Landry to keep the appointment with the oncologist.

Chapter 29

1. An injury to the left temporal area may result in speech difficulties, motor and/or sensory deficits to the right side of the body, and/or confusion.

2. The first sign that Jose's neurological status had changed was when he became restless and agitated and tried to climb over the rails. Though a subtle sign, restlessness and/or agitation may be the first sign that the level of consciousness has deteriorated.

3. The significance of this subtle neurological change is the probability that the size of the subdural hematoma may

be expanding. Subdural hematomas are space-occupying lesions; therefore, an expanding lesion has the potential to increase ICP, with neurological deterioration to follow.

4. With a decrease in the patient's neurological assessment, the nurse might expect the size of the subdural hematoma to have increased, causing more mass effect and increasing ICP.

5. Although the change in the patient's level of consciousness is usually the first sign of neurological deterioration, Jose had other signs to support his decrease in status. His severe headache and projectile vomiting were signs of increasing ICP. He also was more confused than on prior examination. The nurse could expect to see further signs of deterioration if the hematoma is not evacuated. If the hematoma continues to increase in size, without treatment, further deterioration of this patient's neurological condition might occur. An increase in the size of the hematoma would result in increased mass effect and cerebral edema. Clinical manifestations of increasing ICP were discussed earlier in this chapter and include further depression of the level of consciousness, continuing through stupor, lethargy, coma, and possibly death from herniation.

Chapter 30

1. The rupture of an aneurysm with hemorrhage into the subarachnoid space produces severe pain. The complaint of "worst headache of my life" is a hallmark complaint of subarachnoid hemorrhage.

2. Motor and speech deficits in a right-handed person usually indicate a left side lesion; hemiparesis of both upper and lower extremities indicates that the middle cerebral artery probably is affected.

3. The patient showed several signs of decreased neurological function. She was agitated, indicating increased ICP. She also had a decrease in her speech function, indicating decreased blood flow to the left middle cerebral artery territory.

4. Resume triple H therapy: Increase IV fluids; raise blood pressure, including the use of vasopressors, if necessary, for the treatment of vasospasm. Hyponatremia is often seen in the presence of vasospasm and must be corrected. The addition of supplemental salt tablets and hypertonic saline should be administered judiciously to increase serum sodium to a normal level.

Chapter 31

1. Stroke, seizure, CSF leak, infection, and prevention of venous thrombotic events (rate is higher in cases >4 hours).

2. Motor status, for improvement of symptoms—tremor, rigidity, bradykinesia. Also complications from overstimulation of dopaminergic neurons: dyskinesia, dystonia, confusion, hallucination.

3. Depression, anxiety, body image.

4. Orthostatic blood pressures; history of nausea with administration; orders for antiemetic other than prochlorperazine; motor status and mental status.

Chapter 32

1. History of smoking, history of submersion, dyspnea, tachypnea, hypoxia on ABGs. Also, patient has a lower cervical spinal cord injury, which may affect the ability to use respiratory accessory muscles.

2. An order should be obtained for prophylactic anticoagulation therapy such as low-molecular-weight heparin. Antiembolic stockings and pneumatic compression devices should be worn by the patient. Mobilization of the patient should be instituted as soon as the patient is medically stable.

3. Ileus, stress ulcer, constipation, bowel incontinence.

4. Lack of social support, refusal to open eyes, poor interaction with staff, diagnosis of a complete cervical spinal cord injury.

5. Severe hypertension, bradycardia, patient complaint of pounding headache, blurred vision, skin flushing, piloerection, and nasal congestion. Sit the patient upright and place lower extremities in a dependent position. Find and eliminate the cause. Common causes include bladder distention, stool impaction, and pressure ulcer formation. If blood pressure remains elevated, an order for a quick-acting antihypertensive may be needed.

Chapter 34

1. The nurse is responsible for recognizing the frustration and concern that this may cause the patient. The nurse also is responsible for assisting the patient in finding ways to communicate. This may take several forms: having the patient use a chalk board to write on, pantomiming, using signs and symbols that the patient can point to, and assisting the patient in lip reading. If the tracheostomy still is in place, a speaking (flutter) valve may be used to assist the patient in speaking.

2. Maintaining an open airway is the first priority for the nurse and patient. The nurse should instruct the patient on keeping the airway open through suctioning and wound care. It is important to instruct the patient on how to keep the stoma clean and free of crusts. It also is important to reassure the patient that he or she can maintain an open airway and adequate oxygenation by following the instructions for keeping the stoma clean and free of crusts. Normal oxygenation is evidenced by normal oxygen saturation levels, lungs that are clear to auscultation, and unlabored breathing. The patient can be taught to assess these critical elements and take appropriate or emergency action if adequate oxygenation is not present.

It is helpful to remember that the patient has made a difficult decision in opting to have the total larynx removed. The nurse's attitude and approach to helping the patient speak should be one of caring and compassion.

3. The patient is dealing with a major change in self-image and, in all probability, a major change in lifestyle, including recreational activities, at least for the present. The nurse, through his or her attitude and approach to the patient, or demeanor, should convey understanding of the

patient's situation and feelings. For example, if the patient reacts with anger or by withdrawing, the nurse should recognize these symptoms as ones of depression and adjustment to the changes the patient is experiencing; they are not directed at the nurse or other health care providers.

If the patient and/or family members can express their feelings, it is helpful for the nurse to listen, to not pass judgment, and to offer resources that may be available to help the patient adjust. Specifically, relative to comportment, the nurse should assume an interested, unhurried approach to patient care, with the nurse's posture and demeanor communicating interest and concern.

Chapter 35

1. The nurse evaluates the spirometry values when available as a measure of lung function and continues to evaluate all lab values daily. Physical assessments with a focus on respiratory status are done twice a shift. The nurse obtains information related to the home environment, such as the presence of stairs or safety hazards and dust or environmental pollutants, average daily exercise and activities of daily living, support systems, family or significant others, the patient's understanding of the disease and treatments, use of oxygen and use and cleaning of oxygen equipment at home, and financial status and insurance. This information will be needed to individualize the discharge plan and identify teaching needs.

2. A barrel chest is one in which the anterior-posterior (A-P) diameter is twice that of the transverse diameter. The normal chest has an A-P diameter of half of the transverse diameter. This manifestation is caused by inflation of alveoli due to emphysema.

3. Solu-Medrol alleviates symptoms of inflammation and may relieve wheezing and chest tightness. Because it is a glucocorticoid, it raises serum blood sugar. It may also cause retention of sodium, with a lowering of potassium. It causes gastric irritation, so it should be taken with an antacid or food. It also depresses the immune response, so the patient is more prone to infections. In some patients it may cause mood swings.

4. Mr. H and his wife should be given plenty of written material to reinforce teaching content. Blood sugars should be checked at least twice a day with a glucometer. The patient and/or spouse should demonstrate this to the nurse before discharge. Usually, if the glucose reading is consistently above 200 g/dL, the health care provider should be notified. Because prednisone depresses the immune system, the patient should avoid crowds and/or individuals with infections. He should be observed using an inhaler and taught to rinse his mouth after using each medication to prevent thrush. If he experiences side effects such as "feeling hyper," palpitations, or a fast heart rate after using Atovent, he should call his health care provider. He should be taught to take his blood pressure and should be given the acceptable range. This should be 100/70 to 140/80. If he experiences dizziness, weakness, or headache, he should call his provider. In addition, the patient should describe reasons for taking an antibiotic and possible side effects, such as gastrointestinal disorders. A representative from the oxygen company should meet Mr. H in the hospital if possible for an introductory information session on his oxygen prescription and needed equipment and follow-up on teaching at home after discharge.

5. Mr. H should receive a balanced diet and high-protein, high-potassium foods. If he is retaining sodium, this will be restricted in the diet to 1 to 4 grams daily. He must adhere to his diabetic meal plan as well. He should drink 8 to 10 glasses of water daily. Dairy products should be used in moderation because they may interfere with mobilization of secretions. He should use his supplemental oxygen during meals because eating requires energy, and this will support his additional oxygen needs at mealtime. While at home, he should continue this routine. Prednisone and any potential exacerbation of his condition are likely to raise his glucose level, so his general physical condition, diet, exercise, fluid intake, and glucose levels should be continually monitored.

6. Use of continuous therapy can prevent the development of cor pulmonale and pulmonary hypertension. This increases the survival rate and general quality of life because the patient is able to lead a more normal, active life without the onset of these cardiopulmonary complications of COPD.

Chapter 36

1. a. Inability to maintain adequate oxygen levels for normal tissue perfusion.
   b. Increased risk of aspiration.
   c. Two other common complications of NPPV include facial trauma related to the tight-fitting mask and abdominal distention. Chart 36-19 outlines the contraindications for NPPV.

2. a. CPAP mask: Holds airways open in order to increase resistance and increase oxygenation.
   b. BiPAP mask: Has IPAO for inspiratory positive airway pressure and EPAP or expiratory airway pressure. Numerous full masks and nasal masks.
   c. Patients who are on NPPV can communicate and eat and require very little, if any, sedation.
   d. The benefit of NPPV is that Mr. A does not have an endotracheal tube in his throat and the further mortality and morbidity associated with intubation and ventilator-associated pneumonia (VAP) are absent.
   e. Patient comfort and prevention of skin breakdown are the indications for selection.

3. a. The nurse should be aware that the most serious potentially fatal complication of NPPV is aspiration. Therefore, the airway must have frequent assessments.
   b. Continuous heart rate, pulse oximetry (SpO$_2$), and specially trained nurses and respiratory therapists who are experienced with NPPV are essential for these patients.
   c. An NG tube might be considered to empty his stomach and decrease the risk of gastric distention and aspiration of gastric contents.

Chapter 39

1. Hypertension, non–insulin-dependent diabetes, hyperlipidemia, current smoker.
2. Urgent PCI in the setting of AMI is the treatment of choice in eligible patients who can be transported to an appropriate hospital in a timely manner.
3. To inhibit platelet activation resulting from the AMI.
4. Impending cardiogenic shock from the AMI.

Chapter 40

1. Because this patient had a drug-eluting stent placed, it is imperative to have adequate antiplatelet therapy to prevent subacute stent thrombosis, which will then cause a subsequent heart attack, as well as to prevent restenosis.
2. This patient had a STEMI, so it is crucial to follow his cardiac enzymes to know the extent of damage as well as to measure against possible reinfarction.
3. ReoPro will provide maximal protection against platelet activation and aggregation to prevent additional thrombus burden after stent placement. This drug is in the classification of GPIIB/IIIA inhibitors and blocks the final common pathway of the clotting cascade.
4. V_1–V_4.
5. Do a 12-lead ECG, apply oxygen, give nitroglycerin sublingual, and call the doctor. Anticipate changes on the ECG that would be similar to his initial ECG and reflect changes in leads V_1–V_4 representing his left anterior descending artery.

Chapter 41

1. To diagnose problems with heart structure and function in the presence of cardiomegaly in a young person. He has a questionable history of a heart murmur, and he reportedly uses cocaine and drinks alcohol, both of which have an adverse effect on the cardiac structure and function. He will most likely have four-chamber dilation.
2. The patient is complaining of clinical manifestations similar to those of a myocardial infarction; therefore, the enzyme tests are done to rule out a myocardial infarction.
3. To rule out coronary artery disease and any other possible reason for cardiomyopathy.
4. Cardiac dysrhythmias are also frequently associated with cardiomyopathy. Lasix is potassium depleting, thus further increasing the risk of cardiac dysrhythmias.
5. Stop cocaine or alcohol intake due to the increased risk of myocardial ischemia caused by these two substances. Diet and fluid intake changes, medication schedule, and activity restriction. Referral to Alcoholics Anonymous and Narcotics Anonymous; this patient needs to understand that if lifestyle changes do not occur, life expectancy is about 5 years.
6. Forward blood flow and improved pump function as a result of the ACE inhibitors, nitropaste, and Lasix therapy. Decreased preload and afterload will result in decreased cardiac workload and decreased stretch on the myocardial fibers.

Chapter 42

1. • Vital signs every 4 hours, including blood pressure, heart rate, oxygenation saturation, temperature.
   • Medications: simvastatin 20 mg po qhs, levothyroxine 0.125 mg po daily, glipizide 500 mg po bid, furosemide 80 mg po bid, potassium 40 mEq po bid, lisinopril 2.5 mg po daily.
   • Low sodium (<2,000 mg/day), fluid-restricted (<2 liters/day) diet.
   • Intake and output tracking.
   • Blood sugars ac and at bed time.
   • Daily A.M. weights.
2. To assess for an objective measure of fluid volume loss with weight changes in response to diuretic therapy.
3. Day 2 serum potassium.
4. Hypotension, worsened renal function, hyperkalemia.
5. Because the patient is fluid volume overloaded and therefore at risk of further congestion if initiated.

Chapter 43

1. Improved pain management, improved sleep and rest patterns, maintaining skin integrity, preventing injury/infection, improving control of blood sugar, preventing complications of immobility, and emotional and spiritual support.
2. Additional information that would be helpful would include an ankle-brachial index measurement, arterial duplex ultrasonography, and aortic angiogram with run-off.
3. Cigarette smoking is a significant risk factor for developing PAD. Avoiding all nicotine products is essential for the patient with PAD to decrease the risk of complications of vasospasm and poor healing.
4. Angiography of the aorta and lower extremities is performed to visualize anatomy and locate areas of stenosis and/or occlusion. It is an invasive procedure, requiring arterial access and contrast administration.
5. Preventing bleeding from the access site, monitoring for complications, maintaining hydration, providing pain management, accessing neurovascular status of the affected extremity, vital signs, and keeping the affected extremity straight for 4–6 hours.

Chapter 45

1. Aspirin inhibits prostaglandin E_2, which is part of the mucosal barrier that protects the gastric mucosa from the digestive actions of the gastric secretion.
2. Proton pump inhibitors effectively inhibit acid secretion and promote healing of the gastric ulcer.
3. Acute hemorrhage will decrease the hemoglobin, hematocrit, and RBCs and will cause an increase in the release of immature RBCs, as indicated by the increase in the reticulocyte count.

Chapter 46

1. Confusion, irritability, asterixis, and hyperactive reflexes.
2. Continuous damage and regeneration of liver tissue leads to fibrosis and scarring, which can affect liver function and cause structural changes in the liver so that blood and bile

flow is impeded/obstructed, leading to esophageal varices (blood flow) and jaundice (bile). Because the liver function is impaired, the serum albumin may be decreased, contributing to the formation of ascites. The liver converts ammonia to urea and when this function is impaired, ammonia levels increase, leading to neurological symptoms such as irritability, confusion, and asterixis.

3. Ammonia is a by-product of protein metabolism and the liver is unable to convert ammonia to urea, so the diet should provide less protein so that there is less ammonia.

4. Lactulose changes the acidity of the stool, which converts ammonia to ammonium ion, which is not absorbable. It also decreases the number of ammonia-forming bacteria.

Chapter 47

1. The patient was underresuscitated, causing decreased fluid volume. This reduced the perfusion to the kidneys, causing ischemic injury to the tubular epithelium and preventing normal concentration of urine, filtration of waste products, and regulation of acid–base balance, electrolyte hemostasis, and fluid balance.

2. Due to the impaired filtration, the nurse would expect to see elevated serum creatinine, blood urea nitrogen (BUN), potassium, and phosphate.

Chapter 49

1. Donning gloves and assessing the site where the blood is coming from. Observe the site for the amount of drainage, the suture line, and any disrupted sutures or signs of dehiscence. Take a full set of vital signs, including oxygen saturation and temperature, and notify the health care provider if medical intervention is needed. Apply pressure to the oozing incision site with sterile gauze until the oozing has stopped, and then apply a reinforcing dressing to the incision. Maintain very close observation.

   If the nurse chooses to remove the abdominal dressing as top priority, that is an error: The occlusive dressing is adding pressure to the oozing incision and should remain in place.

   If the nurse chooses to leave the patient's bedside, that is an error: Leaving the patient's bedside when vital signs are bordering on shock and she appears very tired, with a bleeding incision, would not be advised.

2. Asking for the health care provider to be notified using the patient call light is a correct action.

   Continue holding pressure on the dressing site.

   Ask another nurse to monitor vital signs and oxygen saturation.

   Apply oxygen to the patient who is hypotensive, tachycardic, or tachypneic.

   Put the head of the bed flat.

   Stay with the patient until the health care provider arrives.

3. **Indicates priorities.

   The incision has just been assessed, so the nurse can wait 30 minutes for the next assessment.

   **The patient has lost a reasonable amount of blood and needs the increased fluids from the IV.

**Oxygen should be applied because the oxygen-carrying capacity has been decreased secondary to drop in hemoglobin and hematocrit.

**The patient is in pain, 7/10, and needs analgesics.

The Unasyn will need to be prepared, so there is leeway before having to give it.

Vital signs are ordered every 4 hours and were done just prior to the retention sutures being inserted.

**CBC is essential due to blood loss.

Calling laboratory results to the health care provider will occur when results received.

**Educating the patient on safety is an important consideration to prevent injury.

**Changing the linens is important because the patient has blood on her sheets, which is unsightly, can increase emotional discomfort, and can cause skin breakdown from the wetness against the patient.

The increased IV rate will take care of fluids temporarily, and the diet change can be implemented at the next meal.

Chapter 50

1. Pain.

2. If the catheter is occluded in any way, the patient will experience increased pain.

3. There is no significance as to the drainage itself because urine often seeps around a suprapubic catheter. There is significance in respect to potential damage to skin tissues from a wet dressing.

4. Low hemoglobin provides decreased oxygen to the patient for healing and it decreases the patient's overall energy level, which can decrease the patient's desire to ambulate and to eat. Oxygen, nutrition, and ambulation contribute to the patient's healing and recovery. The diabetes can alter wound healing, and glucose levels should be kept in good control to increase the ability of the body to heal. Nurses should also track hemoglobin trends to detect internal bleeding. This hemoglobin level is trending downward, and the cause of it needs to be sought.

5. It is not unusual to see a low-grade fever within 24 hours of a significant surgical event. The fever is the body's response to trauma. If the temperature is above 100.4°F or is elevated after 24 hours, it is more indicative of an infection.

Chapter 52

1. Prevailing symptoms include weight gain, constant fatigue, cold intolerance, dry skin, thinning hair, and difficulty concentrating. The patient also expresses that she does not feel as alert as usual and is experiencing a decline in work performance and task completion. These symptoms are indicative of low thyroxine levels and circulating hormone levels and hypothyroidism.

2. A high level of TSH is caused by the pituitary responding to an underproduction of thyroid hormone that, in turn, results in lower thyroxine (T_4). Measurement of the T_4 serum level reflects the amount of unbound thyroxine in the blood and is considered the best clinical measure of thyroxine levels. Low levels of T_4 in the presence of high

levels of TSH indicate that the problem is due to disease of the thyroid gland.

3. The main focus of the plan of care should be symptom management. This includes the following key elements:
   - Instruction in hormone replacement therapy. It is important to understand the prescribed medication and to take it precisely according to directions in order to return the patient to a euthyroid or normal thyroid state.
   - Assessment of fatigue and activity tolerance to determine ability to provide self-care.
   - Assessment of skin, nails, and hair condition because patient is at risk for impaired skin integrity and alopecia.
   - Assessment of bowel function because patient is at risk for constipation and abdominal pain due to the reduced activity (lethargy) and hypometabolic state.
   - Assessment of body temperature and ability to tolerate ambient temperatures. Patient may be prone to hypothermia due to hypometabolic state.
   - Assessment of cognition and thought processes because patient may experience disturbed thought processes due to hypothyroidism. Is patient oriented to time, place, person, and circumstances?

Chapter 53

1. The major biochemical deficits include (1) hyperglycemia, (2) metabolic acidosis, and (3) fluid and (4) electrolyte imbalance.

2. Polyuria, polydipsia, weight loss, and fatigue primarily result from hyperglycemia. The poor skin turgor, dry mucous membranes, and sinus tachycardia primarily result from the fluid imbalance (dehydration). The increasing lethargy, facial flushing, deep rapid breathing, and fruity odor of breath result from the metabolic acidosis (ketosis). The nausea and vomiting are thought to result from the metabolic acidosis (ketosis). The patient's sodium is low and his potassium is high; however, he appears to have no symptoms related to hyponatremia or hyperkalemia.

3. The nursing interventions derived from these treatments include (1) general assessment of patient's response to therapy, (2) evaluation of the patient's response to insulin therapy (e.g., monitoring for changes in blood glucose level; monitoring for signs and symptoms of hypoglycemia; monitoring for correction of metabolic acidosis [ketosis]), (3) evaluating patient's response to fluid replacement, and (4) evaluating the patient's response to electrolyte replacement therapy.

4. Severe DKA is a medical emergency. In terms of clinical signs and symptoms, the most significant difference is that the patient with severe DKA is more likely to present in an obtunded or comatose state. In terms of laboratory values, the most significant differences in the laboratory values between mild and severe DKA are related to the degree of metabolic acidosis: arterial pH < 7.0; serum bicarbonate < 10; anion gap > 12. Although the basic fluid and electrolyte treatments would be the same, the patient may present with more pronounced fluid and electrolyte imbalances (e.g., hyperkalemia, hyperosmolality). The fluid and electrolyte imbalances may reflect renal insufficiency and/or renal failure. As such, the fluid and electrolyte treatment of severe DKA may become highly individualized.

5. The general discharge plan for this patient includes (1) general teaching about the pathophysiology of type 1 diabetes; (2) basic dietary instruction; (3) instruction on insulin injection techniques; (4) instruction on signs and symptoms of hypoglycemia; (5) instruction on blood glucose monitoring—patients should be provided with a meter or provisions should be made to purchase a blood glucose monitor at discharge; and (6) follow-up appointment with health care provider—patient should be given phone number of person to contact for questions prior to appointment.

Chapter 55

1. Other questions may include these: (1) Is there a history of past fractures? (2) How did her accident occur? (3) What type of activities does she participate in at home? (4) Has she had a bone density study? (5) Has she ever taken hormones?

2. This patient is an older adult, which would lead to suspicion of osteoporosis. This patient's risk factors include the following: (1) age, (2) postmenopausal, and (3) family history of fractures. These risk factors would warrant further investigation.

3. Alkaline phosphate is found in the bone, liver, vascular endothelium, lung, kidney, and intestinal mucosa. Increased levels may be a warning sign and indicate the need for further investigation. An elevated alkaline phosphate can be observed when the body attempts to form new bone (i.e., metastatic cancer) (Corbett, 2004).

4. Serum calcium and phosphate.

5. The goal is to restore function and independence. In the acute phase, the goal of medical management would be to align and stabilize the hip fracture. This is achieved through surgical intervention. Older patients are at a greater risk for postop complications (i.e., infection, pulmonary complications, and thrombophlebitis). Following surgery, medical management would direct treatment in the prevention of postop complications and restoring function.

6. Nursing diagnoses:
   a. *Pain* related to edema and inflammatory response.
   b. *Risk for Impaired Skin Integrity* related to immobility.
   c. *Risk for Infection* related to invasive procedure.
   d. *Deficient Knowledge* related to unfamiliarity with surgical procedure.

7. In the postoperative phase it will be important for the nurse to know the patient's past medical–surgical history. It will be important for the patient to understand that her past medical–surgical history may help the team anticipate and prevent problems. Postoperative teaching should focus on reviewing strategies for preventing postop complications. She should be instructed regarding pain medication and the importance of progressively increasing her activity. Physical therapy is critical to her recovery, so reviewing some of the expectations might be helpful. The patient will need to understand that the Foley catheter may remain in her bladder until she is able to ambulate to the bathroom.

Other topics might include the use of TED, sequential decompression devices, incentive spirometry, and an abduction pillow.

Chapter 56

1. Postoperative complications can include hypovolemic shock, compartment syndrome, and rhabdomyolysis. The nurse should complete a neurovascular exam of the injured extremity that consists of assessing the color, temperature, capillary refill, pulses, edema, sensory and motor function, and pain level.

2. The right leg should be elevated and supported in correct anatomic position.

Chapter 57

1. Compartment syndrome pain is not relieved by narcotic pain medication, and the affected part is swollen and tense. Normal postoperative incisional pain is located only in the surgical site and is relieved by administration of pain medication.

2. Immediately upon admission to the nursing unit, the nurse should assess the patient for airway patency, breathing effectiveness, and evidence of bleeding at the surgical site and perform a neurovascular assessment of structures distal to the surgical site.

3. The type of surgical approach impacts the type of precautions necessary after hip replacement surgery. In the posterior approach, body positions that cause backward action or actions that cause the hip joint to swivel inward will stress the prosthesis and increase the potential for dislocation. Posterior hip precautions include not bending forward greater than 90 degrees and not moving the operative leg across the body midline. Anterior hip precautions include not moving the hip backward and not turning the leg and foot outward.

4. Postoperative pulmonary complications are prevented by early ambulation and use of pulmonary exercises such as coughing and deep breathing and use of incentive spirometry every 2 hours while awake.

5. The nurse must determine whether the patient is exhibiting confusion related to hypoxia, pain, infection, or hypotension or as an adverse effect of medications. The nurse should assess the patient's respiratory status, vital signs, and oxygen saturation. If these are within normal parameters, the nurse should determine whether the patient is in pain and medicate the patient if indicated. Medications can contribute to delirium, and the nurse should assess the medications ordered for the postoperative elderly person for their potential to contribute to confusion.

Chapter 58

1. Weight and pain in the toe.
2. Food with increased purines. Foods that should be avoided are organ meats, meat extracts, anchovies, sardines, herring, mackerel, scallops, game meats, and gravy. Patients should consume a moderate amount of protein and limit meat, fish, and poultry to 4 to 6 ounces per day. Diet should include low-fat dairy products, tofu, and eggs. Alcohol consumption should be limited to one drink three times a week, although beer ingestion should be completely discontinued because it has a high purine count and increases gout risks regardless of amount.
3. Excruciating pain in his right great toe. Stress. Weight.
4. With gouty arthritis, there is an imbalance with purine metabolism. Instead of the uric acid crystals being excreted through the kidneys, they accumulate in the joints. These crystals are needle-like, causing excruciating pain, usually in the joints of the elbows, wrists, fingers, knees, ankles, and toes, with 75% of patients affected in the great toe.

Chapter 60

1. Mr. B is relatively young and has symptoms consistent with significant immune insufficiency evidenced by oral and esophageal candidiasis. Mr. B also has HIV risk factors: history of sexually transmitted infection, indicating unprotected sex, multiple partners, and IV drug use. He currently uses alcohol and tobacco, which are gateway drugs for other forms of illegal substance abuse.

2. HIV testing is often very frightening and overwhelming to a patient. Therapeutic communication includes expressing feelings of caring, empathy, and understanding that HIV testing is frightening because the potential diagnosis is very serious. This should be balanced with calm and direct provision of information on the process of testing. Testing information should include information on consent for testing, confidentiality of test results, process of drawing blood and confirming any positive test with a second blood test, importance of testing to enable diagnosis, and appropriate treatment and the availability of antiretroviral medications that can help control the progression of HIV if the test is positive.

3. The CD4 receptor is the small protein found on T-helper cells and other cells that allows the HIV virus into the cell. Because the receptor was first isolated on T-helper cells and is found there in abundance, T-helper cells are also called CD4. HIV infection results in a progressive decline in the number of CD4 T-helper cells. The role of these CD4 cells in the immune response is critical because they initiate and regulate the process of stimulating other cells to initiate the immune response and attack an invading antigen such as virus or bacteria. They also stimulate B cells to make antibodies. Additionally, T-helper 1 cells (CD4) are responsible for the initiation of a response to a tumor or mutant cells. Therefore, when CD4 cells decline with HIV infection, the patient is at great risk of developing opportunistic infections and some cancers, such as lymphoma.

4. Yes, a CD4 count < 200/mL is a category C3 AIDS defining CD4 count according to CDC Guidelines described in Chapter 59, Chart 59–10.

5. Triple antiretroviral therapy, possibly including zidovudine + lamivudine (Combivir) and indinavir (Crixivan). Triple therapy interferes with HIV replication at different points in the replication process, thus more effectively controlling HIV replication and decreasing viral load levels. Additionally, triple therapy has a lower incidence of viral resistance than monotherapy.

Chapter 61

1. David should be assessed for hyperthermia from infection, seizure activity that may result from meningeal irritation, hypotension and hypoxia, and the development of hypotension that will lead to an altered mental status because of altered circulation. This hypotension can result from the sepsis and the body's inflammatory response.
2. Meningitis can be transmitted from droplet contamination from respiratory exposure. Respiratory isolation should be instituted. The nurse and anyone who has contact with David should wash their hands before and after leaving his room. Chemoprophylaxis may be recommended for any close contacts that David may have had. The local health department and college campus should be notified about David's infection in order to ensure that appropriate precautions are taken to prevent further spread of the disease. Some health care providers recommend a prophylactic vaccination of all college students.
3. Toxins from the bacteria causing David's meningitis will cause vasodilation and hypotension. Levophed has been found to be very beneficial in the early management of sepsis to maintain an adequate blood pressure and end-organ perfusion.

Chapter 63

1. Anemia and thrombocytopenia.
2. The low level of reticulocytes shows that erythropoiesis has not accelerated.
3. Petechiae, conjunctival hemorrhage, GI bleeding, positive guaiac.
4. Shortness of breath, pallor, activity intolerance.
5. Bleeding precautions, ambulation with assistance, reinforcement of patient education to prevent additional injury and falls.

Chapter 64

1. Infection, nutritional status, pain, and coping.
2. Calculate the ANC: 1,050.
3. Perform hand hygiene, assess invasive devices for redness and drainage, assess urine for sign of infection, assess for worsening respiratory status, instruct visitors to avoid contact with patient if they are ill, provide private room.
4. Listen attentively, demonstrate compassion and caring, offer resources as needed, collaborate with health care provider to determine further medical interventions.

Chapter 66

1. Hypotension, decreased level of consciousness, increased wound size, fever, renal failure.
2. Spread through breaks in the skin and contaminated hands. Contact isolation, strict aseptic technique.
3. There will be some scarring, but the goal is to return the leg to normal function, and the extent of the injury is still being determined.

Chapter 68

1. Grief, circulation, gas exchange.
2. Increase circulation distal to the burn injury. Loss of circulation and possible loss of limb.

3. Delays wound healing.
4. Fluid resuscitation will decrease these values.

Chapter 70

1. The nurse can contact environmental services/housekeeping to obtain a device that can be attached to the patient's bed to control the volume on the television. The nurse can instruct Mrs. M to place this device close to her best hearing ear so as to hear the television and not disturb the roommate.
2. Mrs. M most likely is experiencing hearing loss from the ototoxic medication streptomycin, which she took in 1955 for tuberculosis treatment. In addition, she was given the diagnosis of presbycusis. The first course of treatment for her hearing disturbance would be a hearing aid.
3. A hearing aid would be the first step to correcting Mrs. M's hearing disturbance. Because she also has some degree of nerve damage, a cochlear implant might be suggested if the hearing aid proves to be nonbeneficial to restoring her hearing.
4. Four specific discharge instructions for the family with regard to Mrs. M's hearing disorder include:
   a. Face Mrs. M when speaking.
   b. Do not shout.
   c. Drop the pitch of the voice.
   d. Speak slowly and enunciate, avoid slurring, avoid speaking rapidly.

Chapter 71

1. Vitreous hemorrhage, proliferative diabetic retinopathy, diabetic retinopathy with macula edema, retinal detachment.
2. Cholesterol, BUN, perfusion time.
3. Blood sugar under control, blood pressure under control, laser photocoagulation, vitrectomy.
4. Insulin dependent, blood sugar control, weight control, blood pressure control, regular eye examination referrals, and regular exercise.
5. Regular dilated eye examinations once a year if there are no vision problems and more often if there are problems, blood sugar and blood pressure controls, diet, exercise, and staying healthy.

Chapter 74

1. To identify and intervene with life-threatening injuries.
2. Patterns of injury that are anticipated are as follows:
   - Cervical spine fracture
   - Traumatic brain injury
   - Anterior flail chest
   - Myocardial contusion
   - Pneumothorax
   - Traumatic aortic disruption
   - Fractured spleen or liver
   - Posterior fracture/dislocation of the hip, knee, and/or ankle.
3. No, the CT will reveal solid organ injury but may not identify bowel injury.
4. Decreased core temperature with an inflammatory response leads to increased coagulopathy.

End-of-Chapter NCLEX-Style Review Questions

Chapter 1

1. Answer: 1. Health promotion and maintenance

   Rationale: Health promotion and maintenance are emphasized in nursing education. Advocacy is a characteristic of the role in which the nurse acts on behalf of patients in order to protect their rights and assist in obtaining information and services. Complementary therapies are strategies used in conjunction with traditional treatment. Physiological adaptation is the management and provision of care to patients with acute, chronic, or life-threatening physical health conditions.

   Congnitive Level: Analysis

   Nursing process: Implementing

   Client needs: Health Promotion and Maintenance

2. Answer: 2. Psychological and spiritual

   Rationale: Adding the aspects of caring enables nursing to meet psychological and spiritual needs. Without caring, nursing is a scientific and technical profession. The physiological needs will be met without the aspects of caring through the utilization of the technical body of knowledge. Ethical and moral needs are personal values.

   Cognitive level: Application

   Nursing process: Assessment

   Client needs: Psychosocial Integrity

3. Answer: 4. Total patient care nursing

   Rationale: Total patient care refers to a delivery model in which the nurse assumes total responsibility for meeting the needs of assigned patients during their time on duty. Functional nursing is an adaptation of the industrial model and is work assignment based on functions and tasks to be completed within a specific time frame. Modular nursing is the utilization of mini teams who stay near the bedside; it involves assigning a wider range of responsibilities. Primary care nursing has a professional nurse assigned to plan and coordinate care from admission to discharge.

   Cognitive level: Application

   Nursing process: Implementation

   Client needs: Safe, Effective Care Environment

4. Answer: 3. Variety of patient diagnoses and complexities of patient care

   Rationale: A variety of patient diagnoses and complexities of patient care require that the staff nurse incorporate organization and coordination into the practice role. The need to support the achievement of practice standards is a nursing administration level responsibility. Patient advocacy would require coordination but not necessarily organization as an inherent role. The nurse manager has 24-hour accountability for the unit.

   Cognitive level: Application

   Nursing process: Implementation

   Client needs: Safe, Effective Care Environment

5. Answer: 1. Cultural encounters

   Rationale: Cultural encounters are the fourth component of Campinha-Bacote's model. Cultural study is a process that would increase cultural knowledge. Cultural diversity refers to the variations among groups of people with respect to habits, values, preferences, beliefs, taboos, behaviors, and social interaction. Culture refers to a complex of learned patterns of behavior, beliefs, and values that can be attributed to a particular group of people.

   Cognitive level: Application

   Nursing process: Evaluation

   Client needs: Psychosocial Integrity

Chapter 2

1. Answer: 2. Advanced beginner

   Rationale: The novice stage begins in the first year of education to become a nurse. The advanced beginner is a new graduate. There is a level of trust in the environment and legitimacy of coworkers' knowledge. There is freedom with learning, mainly because of no responsibility for situations with which they have no experience. Competency is evidenced by exhilaration with good personal performance as opposed to remorse when performance could have been more precise or effective. Proficiency is evidenced by a change in the perspective of a situation or being able to read and respond to a patient's needs. This nurse was functioning at the level of advanced beginner.

   Cognitive level: Analysis

   Nursing process: Evaluation

   Client needs: Physiological Integrity: Physiological Adaptation

2. Answer: 4. The patient's hemoglobin and hematocrit levels are low.

   Rationale: There is a difference between practical knowledge and theoretical knowledge. With practical knowledge, practice is shaped by one's knowledge of the discipline, the science and technology relevant to the situation at hand. Theoretical knowledge is scientific, formal knowledge that is needed prior to the development of practical knowledge. This patient's hemoglobin and hematocrit levels were low, which could mean bleeding. A reduction in hemoglobin means a lesser amount of oxygen will reach the body organs. This patient's condition is changing, even though the vital signs are not yet reflecting the change.

   Cognitive level: Analysis

   Nursing process: Implementation

   Client needs: Physiological Integrity: Physiological Adaptation

3. Answer: 2. Return the patient to the bed.

   Rationale: Clinical knowledge is knowledge necessary to perform proficiently in the clinical setting. Clinical judgment is clinical reasoning, across time, about a particular patient. Techne is something that can be standardized and replicated. Even though the care map states a day 2 total knee replacement patient should be transferred from the bed to a chair with minimal weight bearing, the sudden onset of bright red bleeding would indicate that this patient be immediately returned to bed and be prepared for further intervention. The care map, or standardized care, should not be followed in the best interest of the patient.

Cognitive level: Application

Nursing process: Implementation

Client needs: Physiological Integrity: Physiological Adaptation

4. Answer: 2. Repeat the questions to evaluate the patient's hearing.

Rationale: Phronesis is a form of rationality and skill-based character. It is similar to clinical judgment, which is clinical reasoning across time about a patient. The nurse should determine if the patient understands the health-related questions before assuming the patient is in acute distress or has a worsening condition.

Cognitive level: Analysis

Nursing process: Implementation

Client needs: Physiological Integrity: Reduction of Risk Potential

5. Answer: 3. Further explore the patient's breathlessness.

Rationale: To make good clinical judgments, the nurse must be skillful in moral and clinical perception. Even though conceptual knowledge is needed, it is not sufficient to ensure the nurse will notice and correctly identify a change in a patient's condition even though the nurse may know conceptually what the formal characteristic of the patient condition is in principle. The most important thing for the nurse to do to help this patient is to further explore the patient's breathlessness. Culturing the leg wounds and elevating the legs could theoretically wait until a later time. The patient should not be ambulated to the bathroom but rather should be provided with a bedpan.

Cognitive level: Analysis

Nursing process: Evaluation

Client needs: Physiological Integrity: Physiological Adaptation

Chapter 3

1. Answer: 2. It is a proven process that produces consistent, high-quality results.

Rationale: Best practices are defined as proven processes that produce consistent, high-quality results. Evidence-based practice can be described as an approach that integrates current research evidence with clinical expertise and patient's needs. Benchmarking offers qualitative or quantitative measurement of specific data related to reported outcome information. The Leapfrog Group focuses on collecting data about medical errors and setting standards that will reduce errors.

Cognitive level: Analysis

Nursing process: Planning

Client needs: Safe, Effective Care Environment: Management of Care

2. Answer: 4. Volume

Rationale: Volume for hospitals overall is based on units of services. The overall hospital generally looks at patient days, and departments look at relative statistics for the

type of work they do. Volume is a component of the revenue category. Salaries/wages is a component of controllable operating expenses. Supplies is a component of operating expenses. Overhead is considered an operating expense.

Cognitive level: Application

Nursing process: Planning

Client needs: Safe, Effective Care Environment: Management of Care

3. Answer: 2. Select supplies that can be used over a period of time for less cost.

Rationale: It is important for nurses to take an active role in containing costs through judicial use of supplies. The nurse should select supplies that can be used over a period of time for less cost. Using supplies already charged to another patient is unethical and can lead to contamination issues. Selecting too many supplies or stocking supplies in a patient's room for future use is not a judicial use of supplies.

Cognitive level: Application

Nursing process: Planning

Client needs: Safe, Effective Care Environment: Management of Care

4. Answer: 2. The Joint Commission

Rationale: The Joint Commission conducts accreditation surveys every 3 years. Beginning in 2004 the "tracer" methodology process was implemented that monitors a specific patient through his or her hospitalization and evaluates policies along with the patient's interactions and experience with all services. Effective in 2005, the Commission started making unannounced survey visits. The Occupational Safety and Health Administration (OSHA) is an agency that oversees environmental safety and works through federal and state partnerships to inspect and enforce safety standards in the workplace. The Centers for Disease Control and Prevention (CDC) is an agency that focuses on protecting the health and safety of people within and outside of a health care environment by development and application of disease prevention and control, promotion of environmental health, and education. The state board of nursing is an agency that oversees the practice of professionally licensed care providers by setting specific requirements for initial licensure, ongoing or continuing education hours and courses, the scope of practice for the particular discipline, and the disciplinary action processes.

Cognitive level: Application

Nursing process: Evaluation

Client needs: Safe, Effective Care Environment: Safety and Infection Control

5. Answer: 3. Health care power of attorney

Rationale: A health care power of attorney is a legal document that establishes a surrogate decision maker to make medical treatment decisions for an individual should that individual become incapacitated. A living will is a formal written document that communicates the wishes of the individual about life-sustaining medical treatments should he become terminally ill. An advance directive is instructions about future health care if the patient cannot speak for herself. An oral advance directive includes instructions given to a health care provider during the course of treatment, illness, or stay in the hospital. This directive is documented in the patient's medical record. A written advance directive is a witnessed document, which requires the individual's signature and those of the witnesses.

Cognitive level: Application

Nursing process: Evaluation

Client needs: Safe, Effective Care Environment: Management of Care

Chapter 4

1. Answer: 2. Principlism

   Rationale: Principlism is an emerging theory that incorporates existing ethical principles and attempts to resolve conflicts by applying one or more of the ethical principles. Four principles form the basis for decision making: respect for autonomy, nonmaleficence, beneficence, and justice. In deontology, a sense of duty consists of rational respect for the fulfilling of one's obligations to other human beings, rather than looking at the rewards of one's actions. Rule utilitarianism seeks the greatest happiness for all; it appeals to public agreement as a basis for objective judgment about the nature of happiness. Act utilitarianism tries to determine in a particular situation which course of action will bring about the greatest happiness, or the least harm and suffering, to a single person.

   Cognitive level: Analysis

   Nursing process: Evaluation

   Client needs: Safe, Effective Care Environment: Management of Care

2. Answer: 3. Options

   Rationale: The M stands for massage or identify the issues and all of the people involved. The O stands for examining options. The R stands for resolving the dilemma. The A stands for act by applying the chosen option. And the L stands for look back and evaluate the success of achieving desired outcomes.

   Cognitive level: Application

   Nursing process: Planning

   Client needs: Safe, Effective Care Environment: Management of Care

3. Answer: 2. Social justice model

   Rationale: The social justice model considers broad social issues that may arise within an institution and within this model; many ethics committees hold ethical grand rounds. The autonomy model facilitates decision making for the competent patient. The patient benefit model uses substituted judgment and facilitates decision making for the incompetent patient. Fidelity model does not exist.

   Cognitive level: Application

   Nursing process: Planning

   Client needs: Safe, Effective Care Environment: Management of Care

4. Answer: 1. Read the state nurse practice act.

   Rationale: The state nurse practice act sets educational and examination requirements, provides for licensing by individuals who have met these requirements, defines the functions of each category of nurse, and may include a section on mandatory continuing education hours for renewal of licenses. Reading the organization's standards of patient care and contacting the school in which she earned her nursing education would not be appropriate for the nurse to do. Assuming she can provide all aspects of care is also something this nurse should not do.

   Cognitive level: Analysis

   Nursing process: Assessment

   Client needs: Safe, Effective Care Environment: Management of Care

5. Answer: 4. Tort

   Rationale: Tort law is defined as a wrongful act committed against another person or the person's property. Common law is based on justice, reason, and common sense. It represents law made by judges through decisions in specific cases; these case-by-case decisions are used again and again in similar cases and, thereby, become customary or common to all people living under the authority of the court of law. Civil law starts with abstract rules, which judges must then apply to the various cases before them. Contracts are promises that the law will enforce. Contract law is that which governs the formation of these promises or agreements between two or more parties, in relation to a particular subject.

   Cognitive level: Application

   Nursing process: Planning

   Client needs: Safe, Effective Care Environment: Management of Care

Chapter 5

1. Answer: 1. Case method

   Rationale: The case method of nursing care is one in which the registered nurse is responsible for the patient and has total care responsibility for the patient during the shift worked. Functional nursing is task oriented and nurses perform assigned tasks but are not given a patient assignment. In team nursing, patients are assigned to a team that is led by a registered nurse. In primary nursing, each patient is assigned to a nurse who has 24-hour responsibility for the nursing care provided to a particular patient.

   Cognitive level: Analysis

   Nursing process: Assessment

   Client needs: Safe, Effective Care Environment: Management of Care

2. Answer: 4. Intentional fragmentation of care

   Rationale: The functional nursing model of care is an industrial efficiency model that intentionally fragments care because of the increased number of personnel performing specific tasks for individual patients. Holistic and comprehensive care are characteristics of the case method of care delivery. Maximum use of individual caregivers' strengths for a large number of patients is a characteristic of the team nursing care delivery system. Better care outcomes and greater nurse satisfaction are characteristics of the primary nursing care delivery system.

Cognitive level: Analysis

Nursing process: Assessment

Client needs: Safe, Effective Care Environment: Management of Care

3. Answer: 2. Team

Rationale: Responsibility for the delegation of tasks within team nursing is the same as in the functional nursing care delivery system. In the case method care delivery system, the entire caregiving staff consists of registered nurses. Unlicensed assistive personnel are not used. Within primary nursing, other caregivers are considered associate caregivers and the primary nurse is responsible for delegating responsibilities to these caregivers. Primary care is relationship-based care and is a blend of primary nursing with a professional nursing practice environment.

Cognitive level: Application

Nursing process: Implementation

Client needs: Safe, Effective Care Environment: Management of Care

4. Answer: 1. Highest quality for lowest cost

Rationale: The cost-effective measurement of nursing care delivery systems is difficult to achieve. Identifying the best care for the lowest cost may be deemed a cost-effective choice. The characteristics of job autonomy and nurse accountability are measurements of nurse job satisfaction. Patient acuity is the measurement of patient severity of illness and the amount of nursing care required to care for the patient.

Cognitive level: Analysis

Nursing process: Evaluation

Client needs: Safe, Effective Care Environment: Management of Care

5. Answer: 2. Functional

Rationale: Organizations that follow a functional approach to patient care avoid high labor costs by using lower paid workers and will not change the system to improve coordination and increase costs by adding advanced practice nurses or case managers. In the case method of care delivery, advanced practice nurses and case managers aid in the coordination of care. Advanced practice nurses and case managers are used as consultants within the team nursing care delivery system. Advanced practice nurses are used in the primary nursing care delivery system to add clinical expertise and education; however, the use of case managers is redundant in this model of care delivery.

Cognitive level: Application

Nursing process: Planning

Client needs: Safe, Effective Care Environment: Management of Care

Chapter 6

1. Answer: 3. The Joint Commission

Rationale: Each year the Joint Commission publishes patient safety goals that need to be addressed by health care facilities to improve patient care. They are listed on the Joint Commission website for the current and subsequent years. Medicare and Medicaid do not publish annual patient safety goals but expect organizations to comply with the Joint Commission's goals and standards. State boards of nursing control the practice of nursing by development of state nursing practice acts that establish guidelines to ensure safe practice. The standards set by the practice acts are based on the nursing process, which is a systematic method of planning and providing care to the patient, and requires compliance as evidenced in documentation.

Cognitive level: Analysis

Nursing process: Planning

Client needs: Safe, Effective Care Environment: Management of Care

2. Answer: 2. Draw a single line through the entry, write the word *error,* date, time, and sign the entry.

Rationale: When a documentation error occurs, correct it immediately by drawing a single line through the entry, identify it as an error with the date and time, and sign it. Never try to obliterate the error with ink or correction fluid because this can appear as if the documenter is trying to hide something.

Cognitive level: Application

Nursing process: Implementation

Client needs: Safe, Effective Care Environment: Management of Care

3. Answer: 4. There is a tendency to document everything.

Rationale: A disadvantage to narrative documentation is the tendency to chart everything that happens. The disadvantage of the CBE system is the time it takes to develop the guidelines and standards of care. Listing problems in chronological order is a disadvantage to the problem-oriented system. Having to evaluate each problem once per shift is a disadvantage of the PIE system.

Cognitive level: Application

Nursing process: Implementation

Client needs: Safe, Effective Care Environment: Management of Care

4. Answer: 2. Concept Map

Rationale: The concept map assists the learner in the development of the nursing plan of care using the nursing process. The Kardex contains information regarding the patient's name, age, religion, medical diagnoses, past medical history, surgeries and major procedures since admission, current medications, treatments, diet, intravenous therapy, and diagnostic tests and procedures. The medication administration record includes the usual dose, route, frequency, class, and action of the drug, rationale for administration, side effects with nursing implications, and assessment data that indicate effectiveness. The past medical history is data found within the Kardex.

Cognitive level: Analysis

Nursing process: Planning

Client needs: Safe, Effective Care Environment: Management of Care

Chapter 7

1. Answer: 1. Assessing the wound
   Rationale: Independent activities are those that nurses perform, prescribe, and or delegate based on their education and skills. Examples are assessing, analyzing and diagnosing, planning, implementing, and evaluating. Interdependent activities are those activities that overlap with other health team members, physicians, social workers, pharmacist, nutritionist, and therapists (physical, speech, occupational) and require coordination and planning with these various health team members. Dependent activities are those that are prescribed by the physician and carried out by the nurse. They include implementing the physician's orders to administer medications or treatments.
   Cognitive level: Analysis
   Nursing process: Evaluation
   Client needs: Safe, Effective Care Environment: Management of Care

2. Answer: 1. Assessment
   Rationale: A definition of assessment as it relates to nursing is "the act of reviewing a situation for the purpose of diagnosing the patient's problems." Planning is done after the formulation of nursing diagnoses and is prioritized according to the patient's needs. Implementation is the "doing" or intervening phase of the nursing process. It involves organization and actual delivery of nursing care, which leads to achievement of stated goals and objectives. Evaluation focuses on the patient's behavioral changes and compares them with the criteria stated in the objectives. It consists of both the patient's status and the effectiveness of the nursing care.
   Cognitive level: Application
   Nursing process: Implementation
   Client needs: Health Promotion and Maintenance: Prevention/Early Detection of Health Problems

3. Answer: 3. Psychomotor
   Rationale: To conduct a comprehensive nursing assessment, the nurse must utilize cognitive, affective, and psychomotor skills. Conducting a fingerstick to assess a blood glucose level is utilizing the psychomotor skill. There is no psychosocial skill level utilized to conduct a comprehensive nursing assessment.
   Cognitive level: Analysis
   Nursing process: Implementation
   Client needs: Health Promotion and Maintenance: Prevention/Early Detection of Health Problems

4. Answer: 4. Determining a nursing diagnosis
   Rationale: Goal setting is done during the planning phase of the nursing process. Planning of interventions is done during the planning phase of the nursing process. Nursing diagnoses are clinical judgments about an individual, family, or community response to actual or potential health problems and life processes. Nursing diagnoses are different from collaborative problems such as medical diagnoses because nurses' accountability differs for nursing diagnoses and collaborative problems. Nurses ultimately are accountable for formulating nursing diagnoses and intervening appropriately.
   Cognitive level: Application
   Nursing process: Evaluation
   Client needs: Health Promotion and Maintenance: Prevention/Early Detection of Health Problems

5. Answer: 2. Planning
   Rationale: The use of critical thinking with the nursing process enhances the validity, reliability, and effectiveness of outcomes to patients. It is essential in nursing when the nurse is assessing, diagnosing, implementing, and evaluating the patient and developing the care plan. Getting a better understanding of something or someone else is part of the assessment phase of the nursing process. Reducing the risk of getting undesirable results is part of the implementation phase of the nursing process. Increasing the likelihood of achieving beneficial results is part of the evaluation phase of the nursing process. Making decisions about an action is part of the planning phase of the nursing process.
   Cognitive level: Analysis
   Nursing process: Evaluation
   Client needs: Health Promotion and Maintenance: Prevention/Early Detection of Health Problems

Chapter 8

1. Answer: 3. The effectiveness of a type of wound dressing
   Rationale: Basic research is done to extend the knowledge base in a discipline or to formulate or refine a theory. This would include studying how Orem's theory can be applied to the nursing process. Applied research focuses on finding solutions to existing problems such as wound dressings, side effects of medications, or outcomes of teaching.
   Cognitive level: Analysis
   Nursing process: Planning
   Client needs: Safe, Effective Care Environment: Management of Care

2. Answer: 3. Collect numerical values within a controlled situation.
   Rationale: Quantitative research is characterized by the collection of numerical values, under a controlled situation, that yield data, which can be generalized. Qualitative research describes events as they occur naturally. It is a systematic, subjective approach used to describe life experiences and give them meaning. This type of research uses methods that are more subjective, a smaller sample size, and fewer research controls. The design of the qualitative study tends to evolve over time during the study. Qualitative studies do not follow the same linear progression of quantitative studies; instead, the process tends to resemble a circle more than a line.
   Cognitive level: Analysis
   Nursing process: Implementation
   Client needs: Safe, Effective Care Environment: Management of Care

3. Answer: 4. In a laboratory
   Rationale: Quantitative designs typically are descriptive, correlational, quasi-experimental, and experimental. An

experimental design is used to find the effects of an intervention, is highly controlled, and most often occurs in a laboratory setting.

Cognitive level: Application

Nursing process: Planning

Client needs: Safe, Effective Care Environment: Management of Care

4. Answer: 2. Identify the problem to be studied.

Rationale: The first step in any research process is to identify a researchable problem. A researchable problem is a situation in need of a solution, alteration, or improvement. It is an area of concern for a particular population that requires investigation and that is derived from a topical area. Determining the patients who will participate in the study, assigning data collection roles, and setting the time frame for the study are all steps involved in research but occur later in the process.

Cognitive level: Analysis

Nursing process: Planning

Client needs: Safe, Effective Care Environment: Management of Care

5. Answer: 4. Write out the research problem or question.

Rationale: The research design is the overall plan for the study and should be described in detail. The research design includes data collection methods and methods to analyze the data. It doesn't matter if the research is quantitative or qualitative. The research question or problem statement is the primary guide for the design of the study.

Cognitive level: Application

Nursing process: Planning

Client needs: Safe, Effective Care Environment: Management of Care

Chapter 9

1. Answer: 2. Data about the patient's physical, social, cultural, environmental, and emotional statuses

Rationale: Assessment, the first step of the nursing process, is when the nurse gathers initial data. It is a systematic process that assists the nurse in identifying current health status, actual and potential problems, and areas that need health promotion. It also provides a baseline on which future comparisons can be made. The assessment includes data about the physical, emotional, mental, spiritual, and cultural factors that impact health. It consists of both objective and subjective data.

Cognitive level: Application

Nursing process: Assessment

Client needs: Health Promotion and Maintenance: Prevention/Early Detection of Health Problems

2. Answer: 4. Address the patient including the surname.

Rationale: When beginning the interview, nurses should address patients using their surnames and then introduce themselves and their role in the agency. They should state if they are students. Finally, nurses should tell patients the purpose for the interview.

Cognitive level: Application

Nursing process: Planning

Client needs: Health Promotion and Maintenance: Prevention/Early Detection of Health Problems

3. Answer: 2. What makes you think that you have cancer?

Rationale: The nurse should ask more probing questions in efforts to have the patient explain his or her fears of cancer. Responses that are nonproductive and should be avoided by the nurse include providing false reassurance, using authoritarian language, giving unwanted advice and not allowing patients to make their own decisions, talking too much, using professional jargon that the patient will not understand, and using avoidance language or euphemisms to avoid reality.

Cognitive level: Application

Nursing process: Implementation

Client needs: Health Promotion and Maintenance: Prevention/Early Detection of Health Problems

4. Answer: 3. Inspection

Rationale: Inspection is the deliberate, systematic examination of the patient using both sight and smell. It begins with the first encounter and continues during the entire time the nurse is with the patient. The nurse observes gait, mannerisms, stature, and other physical attributes. The inspection begins by assessing the patient's appearance and comparing the right and left side of the body for symmetry. Palpation uses touch in order to collect data to determine specific characteristics of the body. Such characteristics as temperature, texture, moisture, tenderness, pain, vibrations, and edema are assessed using palpation. Percussion is the creation of sound vibrations by pushing, tapping, or using a device to generate a vibration. The vibrations produced will help in determining position of organ structures. Auscultation is the technique of listening to body sounds. The nurse must use both the unassisted sense of hearing and, where needed, a stethoscope.

Cognitive level: Analysis

Nursing process: Assessment

Client needs: Health Promotion and Maintenance: Prevention/Early Detection of Health Problems

5. Answer: 1. Analysis of the situation

Rationale: The five components of critical thinking related to health assessment include collection of information, analysis of the situation, generation of alternatives, selection of alternatives, and evaluation. Collection of information begins with the interview and continues throughout the entire health assessment. The second skill is analysis of the situation. During this phase the nurse must distinguish normal from abnormal. The patient's age, gender, genetic background, and culture affect the analysis. The nurse must utilize laboratory findings, diagnostic tests, charts, and measures related to development and aging. Generation of alternatives includes identifying options and establishing priorities. It begins with identification of options and then the nurse and patient work together to establish the priorities. The next step is the selection of alternatives. The critical thinking skills needed for this step are the ability to develop outcomes and plans. The outcome is the final result of what the patient will attain, and the plan is the activities that will lead to that outcome. The last step in critical thinking is evaluation. Evaluation requires the nurse to determine if the expected outcomes have been achieved.

Cognitive level: Analysis

Nursing process: Assessment

Client needs: Health Promotion and Maintenance: Prevention/Early Detection of Health Problems

Chapter 10

1. Answer: 3. Point of maximal impulse may be at the sixth left intercostal space, midclavicular line.

    Rationale: Inspiration tends to be shallower in the elderly patient, but accessory muscle use is often noted during expiration. Thus, vital capacity is decreased while residual capacity is increased. The taste sensation is decreased due to the atrophy of papillae on the outer edges of the tongue. Peristalsis decreases in the elderly client, and a decreased thirst sensation may lead to decreased fluid intake. Enlargement or decreased rigidity of the heart muscle may cause displacement of the point of maximal impulse at the fifth or sixth left intercostal space at the midclavicular line.

    Cognitive level: Analysis

    Nursing process: Assessment

    Client needs: Health Promotion and Maintenance; Physiological Integrity

2. Answer: 2. Elderly patients who are hospitalized may be immunized according to the recommendations, as this can decrease both pneumonia and its resultant death rates.

    Rationale: The United States Preventive Services Task Force guidelines do not address the specific needs for the frail patient, those with functional decline, or those with limited life expectancy. The pneumococcal and influenza vaccines may be given at the same time in separate arms because there is no decreased antibody response or increased reaction severity when given together. Doses of the varicella-zoster virus vaccine should be 14 times greater than the vaccine for the varicella virus in order to boost immunity against shingles and its sequelae, such as post-herpetic neuralgia. When elderly patients are already hospitalized, this may provide an opportunity to update them on their immunizations. Studies have shown that vaccinations for older adults are 50% to 60% effective in preventing hospitalizations from pneumonia and 80% effective in preventing death.

    Cognitive level: Analysis

    Nursing process: Assessment

    Client needs: Safe, Effective Care Environment; Health Promotion and Maintenance; Physiological Integrity

3. Answer: 4. As an adjunct for researchers to evaluate the quality of drug prescribing, utilization, and education in the nursing home

    Rationale: The Beers criteria were initially developed to aid researchers in evaluating the quality of prescribing, utilization, and education related to medications in the nursing home setting, but now it includes the identification of medications or medication classes that may be either ineffective or potentially harmful among elderly patients, even in home or community settings. Approximately 5% to 15% of hospital admissions among elderly patients may be linked to adverse drug reactions or toxic drug effects. Polypharmacy includes the administration of excessive amounts of medications or numbers of medications together. Polypharmacy is best prevented by a thorough assessment of medication history. The United States Preventive Services Task Force is a panel of independent preventive and primary care specialists whose purposes include making recommendations about preventive services to be included in routine primary care and documenting evidence for the effectiveness and outcomes of screening, counseling, and preventive medications.

    Cognitive level: Analysis

    Nursing process: Assessment

    Client needs: Safe, Effective Care Environment; Health Promotion and Maintenance; Physiological Integrity

4. Answer: 2. Ensure confidentiality and inquire directly about the contusion.

    Rationale: This scenario suggests possible elder abuse. With any abuse situation, the patient should be ensured confidentiality. It is possible that the incident requires reporting to law enforcement or some other appropriate agency, and nurses should be aware of laws regarding mandatory reporting. The patient is a victim and should not be blamed or accused of causing the event, and a questionable situation of abuse or neglect should never be ignored. It is not the nurse's job to contact the news media or make implications or allegations regarding abuse or neglect cases.

    Cognitive level: Application

    Nursing process: Implementation

    Client needs: Safe, Effective Care Environment; Health Promotion and Maintenance; Physiological Integrity

5. Answer: 3. Residential Care Facility.

    Rationale: Residential care facilities can be covered by some long-term care policies and offer assistance with ADLs and medications. These facilities are not usually medically focused. Skilled nursing care facilities provide long-term intermediate or skilled nursing care and are usually covered by insurance for short periods of time. The types of clients who require 24-hour-a-day supervision, special diets or moderate assistance with ADLs need this type of residence. Adult day care programs may not be covered by insurance and offer few to no health services. Senior supported housing is not covered by insurance and includes low-income housing for seniors that may also include social activities and help with meals and laundry. They offer no health services.

    Nursing process: Analysis

    Category of client need: Safe, effective care environment/ Health promotion and maintenance/Psychosocial integrity

Chapter 11

1. Answer: 4. Patients who know they are heterozygous for coronary artery disease can initiate medications and lifestyle changes to help lower cholesterol.

   Rationale: Although legislation to protect patients with genetic disorders is pending, sometimes insurance and employer discrimination exists. Sometimes patients are afraid that being diagnosed as having or carrying the trait for a disease or disorder will make it more difficult, not easier, to find health coverage or employment. The nurse should be able to counsel the parents who are carriers of phenylketonuria that the disease is autosomal recessive and, thus, the chance of having offspring with the disease is 25%, not 50%. Again, the nurse should be able to counsel the parents of a patient with Turner syndrome, but the nurse should inform them about the monosomy cause. Patients who are heterozygous for coronary artery disease can reduce cholesterol levels by means of appropriate medication and lifestyle regimens.

   Cognitive level: Analysis

   Nursing process: Assessment

   Client needs: Health Promotion and Maintenance; Psychosocial Integrity; Physiological Integrity

2. Answer: 2. "There is always either an abundance or deficiency of genes within the chromosome."

   Rationale: The nurse should always remain professional and never give a nonchalant answer to a patient. It is the nurse's responsibility to appropriately educate the patient. A variation in genes, in combination with environmental factors, causes complex disorders; and gene mutation results from a change in the DNA sequence of an individual gene. Chromosomal disorders are caused by an abundance or deficiency of genes in the chromosome, but there is no abnormality with an individual gene.

   Cognitive level: Analysis

   Nursing process: Implementation

   Client needs: Health Promotion and Maintenance

3. Answer: 1. "The primary function of introns is to code for proteins using transcription and translation."

   Rationale: The upregulation, or increased transcription, of mRNA causes a subsequent increase in activity and production of more proteins. A codon codes for a single amino acid. Through transcription and translation, the amino acid will form a protein. The double-helix shape of DNA is formed by the alignment of purines and pyrimidines that forms two polynucleotide chains. Introns are noncoding regions within the gene. The exons code for proteins using transcription and translation.

   Cognitive level: Analysis

   Nursing process: Implementation

   Client needs: Health Promotion and Maintenance

4. Answer: 2. Cystic fibrosis

   Rationale: A mutant gene located on an autosome instead of the X chromosome is an autosomal disorder. The fact that two copies of the mutation are required for expression instead of one makes the disorder recessive. Marfan syndrome is an autosomal dominant disorder where only one copy of the mutation is required for expression of the disorder or disease. Color blindness is not autosomal at all, but rather it is X-linked. However, the disorder is recessive. Leigh disease follows an atypical pattern of inheritance, in which a defect in mtDNA is inherited maternally. Cystic fibrosis is the only disorder included that is both autosomal and recessive.

   Cognitive level: Analysis

   Nursing process: Assessment

   Client needs: Health Promotion and Maintenance

5. Answer: 3. To assist in identifying disease risk and developing a customized prevention program for some conditions

   Rationale: Carrier genetic tests are done to determine if unaffected or healthy individuals are carriers of disease-causing genes that could be passed to offspring. Genotype is the genetic makeup of the individual and not visible by outward signs. Genomic imprinting is caused by a chromatin alteration that affects gene expression but not DNA sequence. Differences in gene expression between maternal and paternal alleles are often caused by genomic imprinting. Core genetic conditions are screened for in newborns, and prenatal genetic testing is often done when the child is at risk for a genetic disorder. Pedigrees are used by health care professionals such as nurses, physicians, and genetic counselors to help identify disease risk and develop a personalized prevention and treatment program for certain genetic conditions.

   Cognitive level: Application

   Nursing process: Planning

   Client needs: Safe, Effective Care Environment; Health Promotion and Maintenance; Physiological Integrity

Chapter 12

1. Answer: 3. Long commute to work each day

   Rationale: Stress may be caused by internal and external sources. Internal stressors originate within a person. They include lifestyle choices, such as the use of caffeine; an overloaded schedule; negative self-talk, such as self-criticism and overanalyzing; and stressful personality traits, such as being a perfectionist, workaholic, or pleaser. External stressors originate outside the body. They are precipitated by changes in the external environment. They may be triggered by the actual physical environment, the social environment, the organizational environment, major life events, or other catastrophic events such as hurricanes, floods, and fires. Daily hassles, such as commuting long distances, misplacing keys, and experiencing mechanical breakdowns, also act as external stressors.

   Cognitive level: Analysis

   Nursing process: Assessment

   Client needs: Psychosocial Integrity: Coping and Adaptation

2. Answer: 2. Attributed to hardiness

   Rationale: According to the stimulus-based theory of stress, stress is defined as a stimulus, a life event, or a set of circumstances that arouses physiological and/or psychological reactions that result in a disrupted response that may increase the individual's vulnerability to illness. The patient is not demonstrating this response to the stressors. Daily hassles are experiences and conditions of daily living that have been appraised as relevant and harmful or threatening to an individual's well-being. Uplifts, the counterpart to hassles, are defined as positive experiences that are likely to occur in everyday life. This patient is demonstrating hardiness. Some individuals who experience high scores in terms of life-event changes do not experience illness. The hardy person has a clear sense of personal values and goals, a strong tendency toward interaction with the environment, a sense of meaningfulness, and an internal rather than an external locus of control.

Cognitive level: Analysis

Nursing process: Assessment

Client needs: Psychosocial Integrity: Coping and Adaptation

3. Answer: 1. Elevated blood pressure

Rationale: The general adaptation syndrome has three phases: alarm, resistance, and exhaustion. Physical signs and symptoms of the alarm reaction generally are those of the sympathetic nervous system stimulation. They include increased blood pressure, increased heart and respiratory rate, decreased gastrointestinal motility, pupil dilation, and increased perspiration. The patient also may complain of such symptoms as increased anxiety, nausea, fatigue, anorexia, and weight loss. There are fewer signs and symptoms of the resistance stage. The bodily symptoms of the alarm reaction disappear, and resistance rises above normal. Instead of continuing to lose weight, such as occurred in the alarm phase, the person returns to a "normal" weight. In the exhaustion phase, physical symptoms of the alarm reaction may reappear briefly in a final attempt by the body to survive. This is exemplified by a terminally ill person whose vital signs become stronger just before death. The individual in the stage of exhaustion usually becomes ill and may die if assistance from outside sources is not available.

Cognitive level: Analysis

Nursing process: Assessment

Client needs: Psychosocial Integrity: Coping and Adaptation

4. Answer: 3. The additional stresses of daily life add more stress hormones to the body, which can lead to disease.

Rationale: In our modern society with stressful daily events, hassles, and relationships, stress does not always let up. The stress hormones continue to wash through the system at high levels, never leaving the blood and tissues. Long-term activation of the stress system can have hazardous effects on the body, increasing the risk of obesity, heart disease, depression, and a variety of other illnesses. Repressed stressful emotions can predispose to a variety of diseases, from rheumatoid arthritis to cancer.

Cognitive level: Analysis

Nursing process: Evaluation

Client needs: Physiological Integrity: Physiological Adaptation

5. Answer: 4. Improve nutritional intake including foods containing vitamin E

Rationale: Oxidative stress is a physiological response to both internal and external stressors. Although it is not a disease, it is a condition that can lead to or accelerate disease development. Oxidative stress occurs when the available supply of the body's antioxidants is insufficient to handle and neutralize free radicals of different types. Free radicals have useful functions in the body under controlled conditions and it is not wise to strive to remove all free radicals from the body. Water-based foods have not been linked to the formation of free radicals. Ingesting high doses of vitamin C has not proven to effect free-radical production. Oxygen free radicals are neutralized by antioxidants such as vitamin E. Poor nutrition contributes to oxidative stress.

Cognitive level: Application

Nursing process: Planning

Client needs: Physiological Integrity: Physiological Adaptation

6. Answer: 1. Increased heart rate and blood pressure

Rationale: The physiological effects of stressors include increased heart rate, increased blood pressure, loss of appetite, sweating, and dilated pupils. Additional signs are pale skin, increased rate and depth of respirations, decreased urine output, dry mouth, and decreased intestinal peristalsis.

Cognitive level: Analysis

Nursing process: Assessment

Client needs: Physiological Integrity: Physiological Adaptation

Chapter 13

1. Answer: 2. Freud

Rationale: This patient is demonstrating the concept of denial, which is considered an ego defense mechanism within Freud's psychoanalytical theory. Erikson's theory addresses how persons develop across the life span. Maslow's theory focuses on the hierarchy of human needs. Piaget's theory focuses on the cognitive development of children.

Cognitive level: Analysis

Nursing process: Assessment

Client needs: Psychosocial Integrity: Psychosocial Adaptation

2. Answer: 3. Asking the patient if more information is needed to help in the decision-making process

Rationale: Certain actions foster the nurse–patient relationship. Conveying respect for the person's uniqueness, being nonjudgmental, showing attentiveness, and being empathic all create the building blocks of a therapeutic nurse–patient relationship. Patients need to feel safe, secure, and understood. Also pivotal is that the nurse is perceived as knowledgeable, trustworthy, sensitive, and unambiguous. There is also an emphasis on problem solving and a mandatory duty to accountability, responsibility, and confidentiality. Integral to the nurse–patient relationship is the concept of empowerment. When we empower persons, we assist them in developing the resources they need in which to make informed decisions about their health care based on their own priorities. The nurse should ask the patient if more information is needed to help in the decision-making process.

Cognitive level: Analysis

Nursing process: Assessment

Client needs: Psychosocial Integrity: Coping and Adaptation

3. Answer: 2. Sit with the patient and encourage him to explain to the best of his ability.

Rationale: Cultural competence is defined as the nurse continually striving to provide culturally appropriate care to patients and families. Nurses must convey empathy, show respect, build trust, establish rapport, listen actively, provide appropriate feedback, and demonstrate genuine interest. Barriers to effective transcultural communication include nurses' lack of knowledge, bias, ethnocentrism, prejudice, and stereotyping. Language differences, differences in the understanding of terminology, and differences in perceptions and expectations also create barriers.

Cognitive level: Analysis

Nursing process: Implementation

Client needs: Psychosocial Integrity: Coping and Adaptation

4. Answer: 1. I will do my best to learn how to do this. I have to.

Rationale: The nurse must assess the emotional and experiential readiness of the patient or family to learn. The following factors are to be considered when assessing the readiness to learn: level of emotional health, motivation to learn, self-concept and body image, social and economic stability, past experiences with learning, and attitude toward learning. The response that best identifies this patient's readiness to learn is the one that positively shows the patient's willingness to learn the skill.

Cognitive level: Analysis

Nursing process: Assessment

Client needs: Safe, Effective Care Environment: Management of Care

5. Answer: 1. Sit with the patient and be prepared to answer any questions.

Rationale: Nurses are often in contact with individuals and families when they are vulnerable or in crisis and, therefore, nurses become a valuable resource. Early intervention is essential to reduce the effects of the crisis. Providing information and resources sometimes serves to prevent a full-blown crisis from occurring. Rapport needs to be established quickly. It is important to understand the meaning the event has for the patient and, further, to allow for free expression of feelings, which can be cathartic. Once these things are accomplished, the nurse can then help the patient clarify the events of the crisis.

Cognitive level: Application

Nursing process: Implementation

Client needs: Psychosocial Integrity: Coping and Adaptation

Chapter 14

1. Answer: 1. Body mass index (BMI), weight, and waist circumference

Rationale: Anthropometric measurements are physical measurements that include height, weight, BMI, waist circumference, body composition, and measurement of fat and muscle. Food diaries provide valuable information, but are not anthropometric measurements. Blood pressure and pulse are measures of cardiovascular status.

Cognitive level: Application

Nursing process: Implementation

Client needs: Health Promotion and Maintenance

2. Answer: 4. Explain importance of adhering to scheduled mealtimes.

Rationale: The nurse should focus on interventions that will help to interrupt the binge–purge cycle. Regular mealtimes help to establish a pattern and avoid hunger that is brought on by long periods without eating. Finger foods should be avoided because portion control is difficult. Avoiding hunger should be stressed since this can lead to overeating. Regular exercise is encouraged, but excessive exercise may prompt the bulimic patient to view the exercise as a compensation for binging.

Cognitive level: Application

Nursing process: Implementation

Client needs: Physiological Integrity: Reduction of Risk Potential

3. Answer: 3. Maintain your carbohydrate intake by eating noodles, toast, and sports drinks.

Rationale: During periods of illness the need for insulin continues, so the patient should try to maintain a carbohydrate intake of 150 to 200 g/day. Some suggested types of carbohydrates that are easy to digest include ginger ale, cranberry and apple juice, sports drinks, toast, noodles, chicken noodle soup, gelatin, and pudding. Carbohydrates should not be restricted or be sugar free. Insulin is still needed during illness; doses may be adjusted but not stopped.

Cognitive level: Application

Nursing process: Implementation

Client needs: Physiological Integrity: Reduction of Risk Potential

4. Answer: 2. The wound drains large amounts of exudates.

Rationale: A large wound draining large amounts of exudates, which are rich in protein, will contribute to further protein losses. Antibiotic therapy should contribute to protein losses. Dairy products are often high in protein and could help to restore protein levels. A need for surgical debridement indicates there is necrotic tissue in the wound.

Cognitive level: Analysis

Nursing process: Diagnosis

Client needs: Physiological Integrity: Physiological Adaptation

5. Answer: 1. Burn injuries
   Rationale: Patients recovering from burn injuries have a high caloric requirement that often necessitates intermittent enteral feedings, either in addition to oral feedings or as the sole source of nutrition. The other conditions should not require the need for enteral feedings.
   Cognitive level: Application
   Nursing process: Assessment
   Client needs: Physiological Integrity

Chapter 15

1. Answer: 1. Is a common symptom to most illnesses, disease processes, and traumatic injuries
   Rationale: Although pain is recognized by all cultures, the expression and response to that pain can vary greatly among different cultures. Today's health care system can be very unfriendly at times to patients experiencing pain. Many health care providers lack the knowledge to or are unwilling to treat pain. Also, because of the widespread and undertreated nature of pain today, many patients experience significant personal, social, or economic distress. Pain is, however, a common symptom to most illnesses, disease processes, and traumatic injuries.
   Cognitive level: Analysis
   Nursing process: Assessment
   Client needs: Safe, Effective Care Environment

2. Answer: 3. Recognize the fundamental responsibility of all nurses to help alleviate patient suffering and relieve pain.
   Rationale: Chronic nonmalignant pain is not usually proportional to objective disease severity. A ban on opiate use in chronic nonmalignant pain is not ethically acceptable, even when patients are being assessed and treated for concurrent psychiatric disorders. A psychiatric disorder does not mean that these patients are not entitled to pain relief. Patients, their families, and even health care providers may have concerns about dependence or addiction associated with chronic opiate use, and disciplinary actions do exist for some nurses who administer inappropriate amounts of pain-controlling medications. However, being prescribed and receiving opiates for pain control does not subject patients to potential legal sanctions. Nurses do have the legal and ethical responsibility to help alleviate patient pain and suffering.
   Cognitive level: Analysis
   Nursing process: Implementation
   Client needs: Safe, Effective Care Environment

3. Answer: 4. "My pain may last for months, years, or for my whole life."
   Rationale: Pain of short duration with complete resolution is known as transient pain, whereas pain associated with a recent event, such as surgery, illness, or trauma, is acute pain. Recurrent pain is short in duration but recurs after a pain-free period. Chronic pain usually lasts in excess of 3 to 6 months but may last for years or even a lifetime.
   Cognitive level: Analysis
   Nursing process: Evaluation
   Client needs: Health Promotion and Maintenance

4. Answer: 2. The McGill Pain Questionnaire and the patient interview.
   Rationale: The patient's self-report of pain intensity, behavioral assessment, numeric rating system, simple verbal descriptive scale, Critical-Care Pain Observation Tool, and visual analog scale are all examples of unidimensional pain assessment methods. Within the choices given, only the McGill Pain Questionnaire and patient interview are credited with assessing the multidimensional pain experience.
   Cognitive level: Application
   Nursing process: Assessment
   Client needs: Health Promotion and Maintenance

Chapter 16

1. Answer: 2. "There is a potential for the baby to have birth defects."
   Rationale: According to genetic theories, each partner contributes on the genetic level and drug use impacts the sperm and egg health. The husband's cocaine use may impact fetal development; birth defects are more commonly linked to paternal DNA damage than maternal DNA damage. Telling the mother the infant should be fine provides false reassurance. It will not help to use barrier contraception at this point because the fetus has already formed. Sociocultural and environmental factors do have an influence on substance abuse, but the biologic and genetic influence also play a large role and at this point in the pregnancy have the greatest influence.
   Cognitive level: Application
   Nursing process: Implementation
   Client needs: Physiological Integrity

2. Answer: 4. Impulsive and extroverted
   Rationale: A number of personality traits are associated with disruptive substance abuse, including extroversion, impulsivity, social conformism, anxiousness, tenseness, and being less satisfied with present life situation. Being gregarious, quiet, studious, independent, and loyal are not characteristics usually associated with substance abuse.
   Cognitive level: Application
   Nursing process: Assessment
   Client needs: Psychosocial Integrity

3. Answer: 3. Diaphoresis
   Rationale: Symptoms associated with alcohol withdrawal usually develop around 62 hours after the last drink and include elevated temperature, severe diaphoresis, hypertension, and tachycardia. Behavioral symptoms include confusion, agitation and tremors, and altered sensory perception.
   Cognitive level: Analysis
   Nursing process: Assessment
   Client needs: Physiological Integrity

4. Answer: 1. Cardiac arrhythmias
   Rationale: Inhalants and solvents can cause life-threatening arrhythmias, such as ventricular fibrillation. Withdrawal of some amphetamines may cause severe depression and

suicidal tendencies. Methamphetamine withdrawal may produce outbursts of rage. Hallucinations can occur with the use of hallucinogens and alcohol withdrawal.

Cognitive level: Application

Nursing process: Implementation

Client needs: Physiological Integrity

5. Answer: 3. Diazepam, Valium

Rationale: Treatment of PCP intoxication includes the use of diazepam to treat the seizures, muscle spasms, and agitation that occur. Naloxone is the antidote for opiate overdoses. Prochlorperazine is a phenothiazine and would be contraindicated because PCP is an anticholinergic. Amitriptyline, a tricyclic antidepressant, is often used to help a patient withdrawing from cocaine because such patients often experience depression.

Cognitive level: Application

Nursing process: Planning

Client needs: Physiological Integrity

Chapter 17

1. Answer: 1. Integrating the goals and expertise of many different disciplines encourages the development of the most comprehensive plan of care.

Rationale: Patients and their families may receive conflicting information with increasing numbers of medical teams. Advance directives may provide civil and criminal immunity for health care personnel meeting certain conditions, but solely being part of or using an interdisciplinary approach to palliative care does not. Also, the patient's goals of care should guide the utilization of technology in end-of-life care, not vice versa. An interdisciplinary approach does, however, offer the patient the most comprehensive plan of care because of the variety of experience and expertise it brings.

Cognitive level: Application

Nursing process: Implementation

Client needs: Safe, Effective Care Environment; Psychosocial Integrity

2. Answer: 4. "The family usually finds it easier to withdraw life-sustaining treatments than to withhold them."

Rationale: End-of-life, palliative care is always focused on symptomatology rather than cure. All patients have the rights of autonomy, privacy, and decision making regarding their own health care. However, it is often more emotionally difficult for a family to withdraw life-sustaining treatments once they have been initiated than to withhold them.

Cognitive level: Application

Nursing process: Evaluation

Client needs: Safe, Effective Care Environment; Psychosocial Integrity

3. Answer: 2. "By signing the advance directive my appointed family member will have the ability to make health care decisions for me if I become ill."

Rationale: An advance directive directs the health care team in the decision-making process for the incapacitated patient, and the patient's own wishes regarding treatment are followed. The living will, a type of advance directive, also describes the patient's desires for any life-prolonging treatments. Signing the advance directive does not grant proxy for a friend or family member to make health care decisions. Only by signing a medical durable power of attorney may decision-making rights be granted to the person of the patient's choosing.

Cognitive level: Application

Nursing process: Evaluation

Client needs: Safe, Effective Care Environment

4. Answer: 1. "We will continue to increase the pain medication until the symptoms are relieved."

Rationale: Efforts to control pain in the hospice patient are of great importance. Nonpharmacologic methods such as providing room for the patient's family and reducing excess light and noise may help make the patient more comfortable, and concerns surrounding physical or psychological dependencies related to increased opiate or benzodiazepine use are inappropriate. Conversely, when being titrated for pain control in the hospice patient, opiates have no maximum dose. Dosages are continuously titrated to achieve symptom relief.

Cognitive level: Application

Nursing process: Implementation

Client needs: Physiological Integrity

5. Answer: 2. "Some Russians may make their elderly family members a DNR so they will die comfortably and without life-sustaining treatments."

Rationale: Followers of Judaism believe the dying person should not be left alone. Baha'i law forbids the body from being cremated, but in Buddhism organ donation is encouraged and cremation is common. People from South Asia tend to express grief openly, whereas American Indians grieve privately. Russians do tend to encourage DNR orders to promote a comfortable death and prevent artificial life support.

Cognitive level: Analysis

Nursing process: Evaluation

Client needs: Psychosocial Integrity

Chapter 18

1. Answer: 3. Extracellular fluid volume deficit

Rationale: The intracellular fluids (ICFs) are fluids that exist within the cell cytoplasm and nucleus. The extracellular fluids (ECFs) are fluids that exist outside the cell, such as interstitial fluid between cells, fluid in the bloodstream (serum), cerebrospinal fluid (CSF) in the central nervous system, gastrointestinal secretions, sweat, and urine. Two-thirds of the body's water is ICF and one-third is ECF.

Cognitive level: Analysis

Nursing process: Assessment

Client needs: Physiological Adaptation: Physiological Integrity

2. Answer: 2. Prepare to administer a hypotonic intravenous solution.

Rationale: This patient is dehydrated as evidenced by the elevated hemoglobin and serum sodium and potassium levels. A hypertonic solution would exacerbate the dehydration and would not be indicated. The nurse should prepare to administer a hypotonic solution, which has a lower osmolality to hydrate the patient. An isotonic intravenous solution has the osmolality of blood and would most likely not serve to rehydrate the patient very effectively. This patient is dehydrated and a sodium and fluid restriction would be detrimental to this patient's care.

Cognitive level: Analysis

Nursing process: Planning

Client needs: Physiological Integrity: Physiological Adaptation

3. Answer: 1. $Na+$: 115 mEq/L

Rationale: Of the four electrolytes presented, the $Na+$ of 115 is out of range because normal values for sodium are 135 to 145 milliequivalents/liter (mEq/L). Ninety-eight percent of potassium is found within cells. Small amounts are found in blood (3.5 to 5.0 millimoles/liter [mmol/L]) and bone. Ninety-eight percent of calcium in the body is found in the bones and teeth. Two percent is in the blood serum (8.5 to 10.5 mg/dL; 50% ionized and 45% bound to albumin). More than 50% of body magnesium is stored in muscle and bone, and only 1% is in the blood (1.4 to 2.1 mg/dL).

Cognitive level: Analysis

Nursing process: Assessment

Client needs: Physiological Adaptation: Reduction of Risk Potential

4. Answer: 1. Hypokalemia

Rationale: Diarrhea may increase excretion of potassium to 200 mEq/day. Vomiting and/or nasogastric suction can increase loss through GI fluids removed. Typical circumstances leading to hypocalcemia include primary hyperparathyroidism, bone malignancy, and drug toxicity. Hypermagnesemia is often associated with renal failure. Hypophosphatemia causes include vitamin D deficiency, bowel disorders that lead to malabsorption, excessive use of phosphate-binding antacids, alcoholism, or diabetic ketoacidosis.

Cognitive level: Analysis

Nursing process: Assessment

Client needs: Physiological Integrity: Physiological Adaptation

5. Answer: 1. Dependent edema

Rationale: With fluid volume excess, the patient would likely show dependent edema, increased blood pressure, decreased urine output, shortness of breath, and adventitious breath sounds. An example of this condition is a patient with congestive heart failure.

Cognitive level: Analysis

Nursing process: Assessment

Client needs: Physiological Integrity: Physiological Adaptation

6. Answer: 4. Obtain an electrocardiogram

Rationale: Obtaining an ECG is a priority because serum potassium levels greater than 6.0 mEq/L can be life threatening due to the decreased ability of the heart to repolarize as evidenced by the tented T wave, loss of the P wave, and a wide, bizarre QRS with a depressed ST segment. Evaluating the level of consciousness would be associated with hyponatremia; measuring urine output hourly would be fruitless for a patient with renal failure; and the ABGs, although likely abnormal, would not serve as a priority intervention.

Cognitive level: Analysis

Nursing process: Implementation

Client needs: Physiological Integrity: Physiological Adaptation

7. Answer: 3. Eat a balanced diet including tomato juice and potatoes.

Rationale: Discharge teaching of patient/family with regard to hypokalemia includes properly taking potassium supplements such as K-Dur. In addition, increasing potassium-rich foods in the diet and recognizing/reporting increased muscle weakness are critical teaching points. Kayexalate enemas are used for hyperkalemia and, therefore, would not be an appropriate measure.

Cognitive level: Application

Nursing process: Planning

Client needs: Physiological Integrity: Physiological Adaptation

Chapter 19

1. Answer: 1. Increasing

Rationale: Because it is a negative log, as the hydrogen ion concentration increases, the pH decreases. Conversely, as the hydrogen ion concentration goes down, pH goes up. The hydrogen ion is the smallest ionic particle and it is extremely reactive. The hydrogen ion combines with alkali/bases or other negatively charged ions at low concentrations.

Cognitive level: Analysis

Nursing process: Assessment

Client needs: Physiological Integrity: Physiological Adaptation

2. Answer: 3. Increase the secretion of hydrogen ions.

Rationale: The main metabolic acids are lactic acid, pyruvic acid, ketoacids seen in diabetic acidosis, acetoacetic acid, and beta-hydroxybutyric acid. These acids are eliminated by the kidneys or they are metabolized by the liver. The capacity for elimination of these metabolic acids is much less than that of the lungs. In respiratory acidosis and most cases of metabolic acidosis, the kidneys excrete hydrogen ion and conserve bicarbonate to correct the pH.

Cognitive level: Analysis

Nursing process: Assessment

Client needs: Physiological Integrity: Physiological Adaptation

3. Answer: 4. 10 L/min

Rationale: The amount of ventilation is generally quantified by how much air the lungs move in 1 minute, referred to as the minute ventilation. Minute ventilation is the product of respiratory rate and depth, referred to as the tidal volume. Normal resting respiratory rate is about 12 breaths per minute. Normal resting depth tidal volume is about 500 mL. This yields a normal minute ventilation of

6 L/min: 12 breaths/min × 500 mL = 6,000 mL or 6 L. This patient's respiratory rate is 20 breaths per minute. The minute ventilation would be 10 L/min.

Cognitive level: Application

Nursing process: Assessment

Client needs: Physiological Integrity: Physiological Adaptation

4. Answer: 2. Deep rapid respirations

Rationale: In a state of metabolic acidosis, such as that which exists during diabetic ketoacidosis, the medullary centers will stimulate the lungs to increase the minute ventilation to blow off CO_2, even if that level is normal. These rapid, deep respirations, referred to as Kussmaul's respirations, are an attempt to correct the arterial pH by decreasing respiratory acid. This process is referred to as compensation.

Cognitive level: Analysis

Nursing process: Assessment

Client needs: Physiological Integrity: Physiological Adaptation

5. Answer: 1. Ammonia

Rationale: In the face of a high load of metabolic acids, the kidneys also increase their production of the urinary buffer, ammonia. Under normal circumstances, ammonia excretion is about 30 mmol/day, or about 0.5 mmol/kg. This excretion can increase to about 280 mmol/day, but this response takes several days to be completed.

Cognitive level: Analysis

Nursing process: Assessment

Client needs: Physiological Integrity: Physiological Adaptation

6. Answer: 4. pH

Rationale: The steps to analyze an arterial blood gas results are as follows: Step 1: Assess the pH; Step 2: Assess the $PaCO_2$; Step 3: Assess the bicarbonate and the base excess; Step 4: Evaluate compensation.

Cognitive level: Application

Nursing process: Assessment

Client needs: Physiological Integrity: Physiological Adaptation

7. Answer: 3. Place the patient in high Fowler's position.

Rationale: The patient is in respiratory acidosis. The main treatment for respiratory acidosis is correction of the underlying disorder that led to its development. For a patient with pneumonia, this would include antibiotic therapy, improving oxygenation, and management of fever. Placing the patient in high Fowler's position will improve air flow. Breathing into a paper bag and/or giving a sedative are indications of respiratory alkalosis. Sodium bicarbonate administered intravenously is a controversial treatment for metabolic acidosis.

Cognitive level: Analysis

Nursing process: Implementation

Client needs: Physiological Integrity: Physiological Adaptation

8. Answer: 3. Slow, shallow respirations

Rationale: Whenever excretion of CO_2 via the lungs fails to keep up with the body's CO_2 production, respiratory

acidosis will occur such as with a drug overdose. Kussmaul's respirations (rapid, deep breaths) occur with metabolic acidosis, seizures are associated with respiratory alkalosis, and hyperreflexia is a symptom of metabolic alkalosis.

Cognitive level: Analysis

Nursing process: Assessment

Client needs: Physiological Integrity: Physiological Adaptation

9. Answer: 3. "I will take a stress management class or seek counseling."

Rationale: Respiratory alkalosis is characterized by a lower than normal $PaCO_2$ accompanied by an elevated pH. Respiratory rate is a major determinant of the $PaCO_2$ level. Excessively fast or deep ventilation "blows off" the carbon dioxide, decreasing the level and increasing the pH, causing alkalosis. Psychological conditions such as anxiety and panic or severe pain can also cause overventilation. Patients with psychological hyperventilation syndromes should benefit from reassurance and methods to decrease stress.

Cognitive level: Application

Nursing process: Evaluation

Client needs: Physiological Adaptation: Reduction of Risk Potential

Chapter 20

1. Answer: 1. Response of white blood cells to the cellular injury

Rationale: The inflammatory process involves a vascular phase and a cellular phase. The cellular phase includes the responses and actions of the white blood cells. Neutrophils then die, releasing proteolytic enzymes that liquefy the dead cells and bacteria, resulting in the formation of pus. The vascular phase would include such responses as temporary vasoconstriction followed by vasodilation and leakage of fluid into the interstitial space.

Cognitive level: Analysis

Nursing process: Assessment

Client needs: Physiological Integrity: Physiological Adaptation

2. Answer: 1. Inadequate nutrition

Rationale: A balanced diet helps the body maintain an effective immune system by providing the nutrients needed for growth of new, healthy tissue. With age, the immune system weakens as a result of decreasing thymus gland function and some lymphocytes become less responsive in the elderly, while others function normally. A personality disorder or urban living would not necessarily increase risk for infection.

Cognitive level: Application

Nursing process: Assessment

Client needs: Health Promotion and Maintenance: Prevention/Early Detection of Health Problems

3. Answer: 2. Airborne

Rationale: Tuberculosis is spread by airborne transmission, which occurs when the organism is expelled from the infected person and remains suspended in the air in tiny droplets no larger than 5 microns. Contact transmission can occur by direct contact or indirect contact, such as with sneezing or coughing. Vehicle transmission occurs when the organism's life is maintained on something outside the reservoir until it is passed to the susceptible host. Vector-borne transmission occurs when a disease-producing organism is carried by a living intermediate host that transfers the organism to a susceptible host.

Cognitive level: Analysis

Nursing process: Assessment

Client needs: Physiological Integrity: Physiological Adaptation

4. Answer: 4. Wash for at least 15 seconds covering all surfaces.

Rationale: Guidelines for hand washing include the following: Vigorously rub hands together for 15 seconds, generating friction on all surfaces including between the fingers and under fingernails. Wet hands under running water using tepid, not hot, water. Artificial nails are not to be worn due to high risk for microorganism growth. Avoid the use of petroleum-based moisturizers because they can lead to a deterioration of latex gloves.

Cognitive level: Application

Nursing process: Implementation

Client needs: Safe, Effective Care Environment: Safety and Infection Control

5. Answer: 4. *Staphylococcus epidermidis*

Rationale: *Staphylococcus epidermidis* is found commonly on the skin, nasopharynx, and lower GU tract. Infection occurs with indwelling devices that are inserted through the skin, such as catheters. Group A beta-hemolytic streptococci are found in the nose and throat, respiratory secretions, and the hands. This bacteria is the cause of acute pharyngitis, cutaneous impetigo, and systemic infection. *Staphylococcus aureus* is found in the nasopharynx, skin, and clothing. This bacteria can be found in subcutaneous and cutaneous abscesses, and foreign devices such as IVs. *Neisseria meningitidis* is found in the nasopharynx and transported through the respiratory tract; it causes meningitis.

Cognitive level: Analysis

Nursing process: Assessment

Client needs: Physiological Integrity: Physiological Adaptation

6. Answer: 3. Injecting already formed antibodies into the body

Rationale: Active immunization involves the introduction of live, killed, or attenuated toxin of a disease organism into the body. The immune system responds by producing antibodies. Active immunization provides long-term and possibly lifelong immunity. Some vaccines require boosters to maintain the immunity. Examples of active immunizations include measles, mumps, hepatitis B, and hepatitis A. Passive immunity provides immunity for a short period of time, usually around 6 to 12 weeks. This involves already formed antibodies injected into the body. The individual may still have the disease but it will be a less severe case. An example of this type

of immunity is immunoglobulin injections given to people exposed to hepatitis A.

Cognitive level: Analysis

Nursing process: Assessment

Client needs: Health Promotion and Maintenance: Prevention/Early Detection of Health Problems

7. Answer: 2. Increase the proportion of all tuberculosis patients who complete curative therapy within 12 months.

Rationale: Increasing compliance with medication treatment for tuberculosis is an actual *Healthy People 2010* goal. Eradication of the disease is not realistic. No immunization for health care workers is currently available. The rural population is not targeted for focus with avoidance of tuberculosis spread; an overcrowded condition such as that found in urban living is a risk factor however.

Cognitive level: Analysis

Nursing process: Planning

Client needs: Health Promotion and Maintenance: Prevention/Early Detection of Health Problems

8. Answer: 3. Have you received chemotherapy for cancer, psoriasis, or rheumatoid arthritis?

Rationale: The patient should be asked about any preexisting conditions that might affect the immune system such as the use of steroids, chemotherapy, transplants, or other chronic illnesses. Employment history, recreational activities, and exercise routine would not generate information about infectious diseases.

Cognitive level: Analysis

Nursing process: Assessment

Client needs: Health Promotion and Maintenance: Prevention/Early Detection of Health Problems

Chapter 21

1. Answer: 2. Prehypertension

Rationale: The term *prehypertension* describes those individuals with a blood pressure finding on two or more office visits of 130–139/80–89 mmHg as being at twice the risk to develop hypertension as those with lower values. Hypertension stage I is a BP of 140–159 mmHg systolic or 90–99 mmHg diastolic, whereas stage II would be multiple measurements of a systolic pressure greater than 160 mmHg or a diastolic pressure exceeding 100 mmHg.

Cognitive level: Analysis

Nursing process: Diagnosis

Client needs: Physiological Integrity

2. Answers:

1. Cardiac output
2. Peripheral vascular resistance
3. Baroreceptors
4. Chemoreceptors
5. Body fluid volume

Rationale: Cardiac output × peripheral vascular resistance equals blood pressure (CO × PVR = BP). Baroreceptors, located in carotid sinuses and the wall of the left ventricle, monitor arterial BP and counteract rising pressure by vasodilation through stimulation of the vagus nerve. Chemoreceptors regulate ventilation and communicate with the brainstem and cardiovascular centers to cause widespread vasoconstriction. Fluid balance is essential to maintaining normal blood pressure. When hypovolemia and hypervolemia occur, it is reflected in the systemic blood pressure. Adrenocorticotropic hormone (ACTH) functions as an aid to growth and development, not affecting blood pressure.

Cognitive level: Analysis

Nursing process: Evaluation

Client needs: Physiological Integrity

3. Answer: 3. 56-year-old male, African American, insulin-dependent diabetic

Rationale: Age (older than 55 for men and 65 for women) is considered a risk factor for hypertension along with being of male gender. African American individuals have two times greater possibility of developing high blood pressure than Caucasian Americans. Environmental factors such as obesity, cigarette smoking, sedentary lifestyle, use of illegal drugs, and excessive alcohol consumption create risk. Stress such as job stresses, economic position, losses and/or gains of any kind, and many other issues of life are risk factors for hypertension.

Cognitive level: Analysis

Nursing process: Assessment

Client needs: Health Promotion and Maintenance

4. Answer: 3. Not crush, break in half, or chew the extended release form of the drug

Rationale: Instruct the patient taking a sustained-action capsule or tablet, such as nifedipine (Procardia XL), a calcium channel blocker, that it cannot be crushed, broken up, or chewed. Adding potassium would be necessary with a loop diuretic; dry cough is most associated with angiotensin-converting enzyme inhibitors. Beta-adrenergic blocking agents require teaching blood pressure and pulse taking prior to medication. If pulse is below 60, inform the health care provider prior to taking the medication.

Cognitive level: Application

Nursing process: Implementation

Client needs: Safe, Effective Care Environment

5. Answers:
1. Asian populations undergoing Westernization will have significant increases in high blood pressure.
2. Individuals living in the southeastern region of the United States have a higher percentage of high blood pressure.

Rationale: African Americans have a 3 to 4 times higher risk of angioedema and cough attributed to ACE inhibitors than Caucasians. American Indian and Asian populations undergoing Westernization will have significant increases in high blood pressure. Individuals living in the southeastern region (sometimes called the Salt Belt) of the United States have a higher percentage of high blood pressure. Compliance with the DASH diet and exercise to prevent/control hypertension is not culture dependent.

Cognitive level: Application

Nursing process: Evaluation

Client needs: Health Promotion and Maintenance

6. Answers:
1. Developing a diet plan that is low in saturated fats and sodium
2. Eliminating or reducing alcohol consumption to one ounce a day

Rationale: A diet rich in fruits, vegetables, and whole grains and low in sodium and saturated fats is recommended with all stages of hypertension. Alcohol consumption will elevate arterial blood pressure and adds "empty" calories to the patient's diet. A sedentary lifestyle is avoided; aerobic exercise 3 to 5 times per week reduces stress and blood pressure. Smoking cessation is encouraged, not reduction of nicotine. Coping with stress-producing situations is the goal, because total avoidance is not possible. A realistic weight loss goal is 1 to 2 pounds per week.

Cognitive level: Analysis

Nursing process: Planning

Client needs: Health Promotion and Maintenance

7. Answer: 2. Verbalizing the warning signs and symptoms of cerebral vascular accident

Rationale: High blood pressure, referred to as the "silent killer," often goes undetected until signs and symptoms of other organ involvement are present. High blood pressure is the leading contributing cause of cerebral vascular accident; therefore, knowing the warning signs is the priority outcome. Generic brands of antihypertensive drugs are acceptable and a cost-saving method for long-term use. Positive personal relationships help with stress reduction, but are not the priority. Stage II hypertension warrants monitoring of blood pressure more often than once a month.

Cognitive level: Application

Nursing process: Planning

Client needs: Health Promotion and Maintenance

Chapter 22

1. Answer: 3. A midline catheter

Rationale: A midline catheter is the best peripheral vascular access device for parenteral therapy up to 4 weeks. A peripheral short catheter is for infusions that last between 72 and 96 hours. A winged steel infusion set is for infusions of less than 4 hours in duration. A PICC line is a central venous access device and not a peripheral vascular access device.

Cognitive level: Application

Nursing process: Planning

Client needs: Physiological Integrity: Pharmacological and Parenteral Therapies

2. Answer: 4. Secondary administration set

Rationale: A stop cock and extension set are add-on devices that might not be necessary for the infusion of the medication. An elastomeric balloon is a one-time-use device seen most frequently in home care. The secondary administration set is the device used to administer an intravenous medication when the patient is already receiving parenteral therapy. This administration set is piggybacked into the main infusion line.

Cognitive level: Application
Nursing process: Implementation
Client needs: Physiological Integrity: Pharmacologic and Parenteral Therapies

3. Answer: 2. Preserve the patient's right to safe quality care and protect the nurse who administers infusion therapy.

Rationale: The primary goal of the Infusion Nursing Standards of Practice is to preserve the patient's right to safe quality care and protect the nurse who administers infusion therapy. Even though it is important for nurses to follow Standard Precautions, be in compliance with all regulatory agencies, and have adequate skill levels, these are not Standards of Practice of the Infusion Nursing organization.

Cognitive level: Application
Nursing process: Planning
Client needs: Physiological Integrity; Pharmacologic and Parenteral Therapies

4. Answer: 4. Review the procedure with the patient and obtain consent.

Rationale: The first thing the nurse should do is review the procedure with the patient or conduct education. Obtain the patient's consent to have the access device inserted. Once this has been done, the nurse can then gather equipment and prepare flushes all using standard precautions.

Cognitive level: Application
Nursing process: Planning
Client needs: Physiological Integrity: Pharmacologic and Parenteral Therapies

5. Answer: 2. Stop the infusion and remove the catheter.

Rationale: This patient is complaining of an infiltration of the parenteral fluids. The nurse should discontinue the infusion immediately and remove the catheter. The nurse should then elevate the affected extremity to relieve patient discomfort and assist in absorption of excess fluids and improving circulation. The nurse should not take the time to check for a blood return, reposition the catheter, or change the dressing and observe the site.

Cognitive level: Application
Nursing process: Evaluation
Client needs: Physiological Integrity: Pharmacologic and Parenteral Therapies

Chapter 23

1. Answer: 1. Increase plasma colloidal osmotic pressure and plasma volume.

Rationale: Albumin will increase colloidal osmotic pressure and plasma volume. Albumin does not impact platelets or coagulation and does not include red blood cells.

Cognitive level: Analysis
Nursing process: Planning
Client needs: Physiological Integrity: Pharmacologic and Parenteral Therapies

2. Answer: 2. The youngest age for a blood donor is 17.

Rationale: There are specific guidelines for being a blood donor. Vital signs need to be within normal limits. Blood pressure needs to be less than 180/100 mmHg.

Blood count or hemoglobin needs to be greater than 12.4 mg/dL for a female. A blood donor needs to be between the ages of 17 and 65. There are no guidelines or restrictions about family members donating to other family members.

Cognitive level: Application
Nursing process: Implementation
Client needs: Physiological Integrity: Pharmacologic and Parenteral Therapies

3. Answer: 4. Patient provides informed consent for the transfusion.

Rationale: A history of blood transfusion reactions and the patient's circulatory and respiratory status are included in the assessment phase of blood administration. Assembling appropriate equipment is part of the implementation phase of blood administration. The patient providing informed consent for the transfusion is part of the planning phase of blood administration.

Cognitive level: Application
Nursing process: Planning
Client needs: Physiological Integrity: Pharmacologic and Parenteral Therapies

4. Answer: 1. Stop the blood transfusion.

Rationale: Circulatory overload can occur with transfusions when the blood is infused too rapidly or in too large a quantity, causing hypervolemia. High-risk patients include the elderly and those individuals who already have increased circulatory volume or who have a history of heart failure. Clinical manifestations of circulatory overload include dyspnea, tachycardia, distended neck veins, crackles in the lungs, and a rise in blood pressure. If the transfusion is not slowed down or stopped, pulmonary edema will result. Administering an antipyretic or epinephrine and flushing the access device are inappropriate actions.

Cognitive level: Planning
Nursing process: Implementation
Client needs: Physiological Integrity: Pharmacologic and Parenteral Therapies

5. Answer: 2. Stop the transfusion, call for help, and begin life-supporting measures.

Rationale: The sudden onset of chest pain is seen in an acute hemolytic reaction. This is a life-threatening situation. Slowing the transfusion rate and administering epinephrine or antipyretics are not appropriate actions for this level of transfusion reaction.

Cognitive level: Application
Nursing process: Implementation
Client needs: Physiological Integrity: Pharmacologic and Parenteral Therapies

Chapter 24

1. Answer: 2. Help with diagnosis, treatment, and evaluation of care.

Rationale: The three purposes of hemodynamic monitoring are aiding in the diagnosis of various disorders, assisting in guiding therapies to minimize or correct dysfunction, and evaluating the patient's response to therapy. There are noninvasive ways to ensure a correct blood pressure reading. The use of hemodynamic monitoring does not reduce the amount of patient care required. Although hemodynamic monitoring will provide information about the patient's status, it is not used individually to determine if a patient is stable enough for transfer.

Cognitive level: Application

Nursing process: Planning

Client needs: Physiological Integrity: Physiological Adaptation

2. Answer: 3. Find out if the correct type of tubing was used.

Rationale: High-pressure tubing instead of flexible intravenous tubing is necessary to withstand the external pressure exerted by the sleeve and to decrease the distortion of the waveform. The nurse should find out which type of tubing was used.

Cognitive level: Analysis

Nursing process: Assessment

Client needs: Physiological Integrity: Physiological Adaptation

3. Answer: 4. Advance the catheter into the pulmonary artery.

Rationale: This patient is having a pulmonary artery catheter placed. As the pulmonary artery catheter passes through the right ventricle, the tip of the catheter can irritate the ventricle. Patients may exhibit premature ventricular contractions. This rhythm usually ceases when the catheter is advanced into the pulmonary artery or withdrawn from the right ventricle.

Cognitive level: Analysis

Nursing process: Implementation

Client needs: Physiological Integrity: Physiological Adaptation

4. Answer: 4. Compare the result with other measurements.

Rationale: A venous pressure of 2 to 6 mmHg is adequate; however, patients may be hemodynamically stable or unstable with lower or higher pressures. Monitoring the trend in pressure readings, either increasing or decreasing, is of more importance than one observed value. The findings should also be correlated with a patient assessment.

Cognitive level: Application

Nursing process: Assessment

Client needs: Physiological Integrity: Physiological Adaptation

5. Answer: 2. Eliminate any values that differ by 10%.

Rationale: When using the thermodilution method of obtaining a cardiac output, a specified amount of solution, typically 5 to 10 mL, is injected through the proximal injectate port of the PA catheter. This process is commonly referred to as "shooting" a cardiac output. The injectate should be at room temperature when it enters the right atrium and mixes with blood. The cardiac output computer calculates the time required for the solution of a different temperature to reach the thermistor, located at the end of the catheter in the pulmonary artery. The change of temperature occurs over time to produce a cardiac output curve. Hesitation or starting

and stopping during a CO injection would yield an invalid curve. The injectate should be injected smoothly and in less than 4 seconds. Injecting less than or greater than the recommended amount of injectate invalidates the measurement. Any cardiac output value that is questionable based on the curve or two CO measurements that differ by 10% should be discarded.

Cognitive level: Analysis

Nursing process: Evaluation

Client needs: Physiological Integrity: Physiological Adaptation

6. Answer: 1. Fluid volume overload or ventricular failure

Rationale: Excess preload may indicate hypervolemia or ventricular failure. Excessive circulating volume strains the heart and compromises adequate tissue oxygenation. Excess preload increases the workload of the heart and increases myocardial oxygen demands. Diuretics and venodilators are ordered if the cause is hypervolemia. If patients do not respond to diuretic therapy or renal failure is diagnosed, then continuous renal replacement therapy utilizing ultrafiltration or dialysis may be considered. If ventricular failure is determined to be the cause, inotropic medications are prescribed.

Cognitive level: Analysis

Nursing process: Assessment

Client needs: Physiological Integrity: Physiological Adaptation

7. Answer: 4. Closure of the pulmonic valve

Rationale: As the pulmonary artery catheter enters the right atrium, the waveform appears similar to a central venous pressure waveform: the *a* wave correlates with the P wave or atrial contraction (systole); the *c* wave may not be visible on the tracing and reflects retrograde swelling of the tricuspid valve into the right atrium, which occurs during ventricular contraction; and the *v* wave represents atrial diastole and the increased pressure against the closed tricuspid valve in early diastole. As the catheter enters the pulmonary artery, the waveform resembles an arterial pressure waveform with not only systolic and diastolic pressures but also a dicrotic notch. The dicrotic notch represents closure of the pulmonic valve.

Cognitive level: Analysis

Nursing process: Assessment

Client needs: Physiological Integrity: Physiological Adaptation

Chapter 25

1. Answer: 1. Reduce allergic reactions to medications or to latex.

Rationale: Allergies and allergic reactions to medications, chemicals, and foods must always be identified and prominently displayed on the patient's wristband, in the chart, and in the medication record. Patients with histories of allergic reactions have a greater risk of hypersensitivity to anesthesia, so the type of allergic reaction is very important. They also are much more likely to develop latex allergies.

Cognitive level: Application

Nursing process: Planning

Client needs: Physiological Integrity: Reduction of Risk Potential

2. Answer: 3. Antibiotic prophylaxis

Rationale: Patients with valvular disorders may require antibiotic prophylaxis to reduce the risk of bacterial endocarditis. Monitoring fluid and electrolyte status and a BNP level would be indicated for a patient with heart failure.

Cognitive level: Application

Nursing process: Planning

Client needs: Physiological Integrity: Reduction of Risk Potential

3. Answer: 2. Stop all NSAIDs 2 weeks before the scheduled surgery.

Rationale: NSAIDs increase the risk of intraoperative and postoperative bleeding. Aspirin inhibits platelet aggregation and the effect lasts the duration of the thrombocyte life span, 7 to 10 days. Preoperative arterial blood gas and recent hemoglobin A1c level are not indicated for this patient. Routine preoperative electrocardiograms are needed for patients over the age of 55.

Cognitive level: Analysis

Nursing process: Planning

Client needs: Physiological Integrity: Reduction of Risk Potential

4. Answer: 1. Encourage deep breathing and coughing

Rationale: To reduce the risk of pulmonary complications, the patient should be instructed and encouraged to breathe deeply and to cough. Monitoring of oxygen saturation levels would be indicated for a cardiovascular complication. Monitoring intake and output would be indicated for cardiovascular and genitourinary complications. Aspiration precautions would be indicated for a gastrointestinal complication.

Cognitive level: Analysis

Nursing process: Planning

Client needs: Physiological Integrity: Reduction of Risk Potential

5. Answer: 2. Can you explain to me what you mean by cauterized?

Rationale: Preoperative teaching is best accomplished in a calm, quiet, and private environment that facilitates discussion and questions and reduces the patient's anxiety or embarrassment. The nurse needs to be sensitive to the patient's level of anxiety, the patient's ability to understand instructions and express himself, and to cultural issues. Written instructions are important for reinforcing teaching and serving as a reference. When written instructions are given to patients, they should avoid medical jargon, be written at a level that is easy to understand, and be available in various languages. The nurse assesses whether or not a patient is literate in English or in another language before giving written instructions.

Cognitive level: Application

Nursing process: Implementation

Client needs: Physiological Integrity: Basic Care and Comfort

6. Answer: 2. Assess the patient's understanding of the procedure to supplement any areas not reviewed through the Internet.

Rationale: The use of the Internet has altered the amount and focus of preoperative teaching. It may also affect the type and amount of information desired. The best approach for the nurse to take would be to assess the patient's understanding of the procedure and to supplement any areas not reviewed through the Internet. Documenting that the patient had preoperative teaching through the Internet might be appropriate, however the nurse should do more. The nurse should not end the preoperative teaching session or leave the patient with instructions to call the nurse in case of questions.

Cognitive level: Analysis

Nursing process: Implementation

Client needs: Physiological Integrity: Reduction of Risk Potential

Chapter 26

1. Answer: 3. Conduct an interview.

Rationale: Preoperative holding is a semirestricted area usually just inside of the surgical area. This area provides a quiet, calm transition area for the patient to wait immediately before surgery. It provides a shield from the sights and sounds of the busy surgical suite and allows personnel to interview the patient and verify the documentation. Inspecting and ensuring the correct operation of surgical instruments is done in the surgical suite. Inserting an indwelling urinary catheter would be done after anesthesia has been provided to the patient, within the surgical suite.

Cognitive level: Application

Nursing process: Implementation

Client needs: Physiological Integrity: Reduction of Risk Potential

2. Answer: 4. Collaborating with the surgeon and suturing the wound closed

Rationale: The RNFA collaborates with the surgeon and performs the role of first assistant during the operation. This role includes handling tissue, providing exposure, using instruments, suturing the wound closed, and providing hemostasis. The anesthesia care provider administers anesthetic agents. Serving as the patient advocate is the role of the circulating nurse. Providing the surgeon with instruments is a role of the scrub nurse.

Cognitive level: Analysis

Nursing process: Implementation

Client needs: Physiological Integrity: Physiological Adaptation

3. Answer: 2. Anesthesiologist

Rationale: The anesthesiologist is the health care provider who is responsible for maintaining the patient's airway; monitoring and ensuring gas exchanges, respiration, and circulation; estimating and replacing blood and fluid losses; administering medications to maintain hemodynamic stability; managing care in the event of a physiological crisis; and constantly communicating with the surgical and nursing team.

Cognitive level: Application

Nursing process: Implementation

Client needs: Physiological Integrity: Physiological Adaptation

4. Answer: 4. Stop all preparations until it can be verified which knee is the site of surgery.

Rationale: According to the AORN and American College of Surgeons guidelines, if any verification process fails to identify the correct site, all activities should be halted until verification is accurate.

Cognitive level: Application

Nursing process: Planning

Client needs: Physiological Integrity: Reduction of Risk Potential

5. Answer: 2. Examine the leg for possible injury or extent of injury and document the event.

Rationale: The most important role of the perioperative nurse is that of patient advocate. Protecting patients from harm is the essence of the advocacy role of nurses, and it is a critical component for patients whose family members are not readily accessible and whose only possible advocate is the nurse. The essence of the advocacy in the perioperative role is defined as protection, giving a voice, providing comfort, and caring. The nurse should examine the leg for injury and document the event.

Cognitive level: Analysis

Nursing process: Implementation

Client needs: Physiological Integrity: Reduction of Risk Potential

6. Answer: 2. Stop the surgery or deepen the anesthesia.

Rationale: Malignant hyperthermia is an emergency. The surgery should be stopped or the anesthesia deepened. The agent responsible for the hyperthermia should be stopped. Once stabilized, the patient should be transferred to the ICU for postoperative care. Calcium channel blockers should not be administered. One hundred percent oxygen should be delivered to the patient.

Cognitive level: Analysis

Nursing process: Implementation

Client needs: Physiological Integrity: Physiological Adaptation

7. Answer: 4. Respiratory therapist

Rationale: The anesthesiologist heads the anesthesia team and might be assisted by a respiratory therapist, by an anesthesia resident or fellow in a university teaching hospital, or by a certified registered nurse anesthetist (CRNA). The CRNA is an advance practice nurse, educated with a master's degree from an accredited nurse anesthesia educational program. CRNAs administer anesthesia and anesthesia-related care and work under the supervision of the anesthesiologist. The scrub nurse would not be working with the patient's oxygen. The RN first assistant would be assisting the surgeon.

Cognitive level: Analysis

Nursing process: Implementation

Client needs: Physiological Integrity: Reduction of Risk Potential

Chapter 27

1. Answer: 1. Bleeding

Rationale: In the patient who is bleeding postoperatively, initially the heart rate increases in an attempt to maintain a normal cardiac output and blood pressure; thus, it is an early sign of bleeding.

Cognitive level: Analysis

Nursing process: Assessment

Client needs: Physiological Integrity: Physiological Adaptation

2. Answer: 2. Easily arousable and moving all four extremities

Rationale: These activities support the second phase of postanesthesia, which begins when the patient is more alert and functional. The use of an oral airway to maintain an airway would not indicate the patient is ready to be discharged to another inpatient care area. Reduced or lack of motor response of the lower extremities after spinal anesthesia would indicate that the patient has not yet recovered from the anesthesia and should not be transferred to another care area at this time. It would be best to help control the vomiting before transferring the patient to another care area.

Cognitive level: Analysis

Nursing process: Planning

Client needs: Physiological Integrity: Reduction of Risk Potential

3. Answer: 3. Ambulate three times a day.

Rationale: Abdominal distention or a postoperative ileus is common with bowel surgery, anesthesia, narcotics, and decreased mobility. The patient should be kept NPO until flatus returns. If vomiting, the patient should have a nasogastric tube placed and put to suction. The patient should also be ambulated three times a day. The patient should not be given a full diet, should not be placed on a fluid restriction, and should not receive an antiemetic.

Cognitive level: Application

Nursing process: Implementation

Client needs: Physiological Integrity: Physiological Adaptation

4. Answer: 2. Keep the wound open to air and permit the Steri-Strips to fall off on their own.

Rationale: It is theorized that postoperative recovery includes four dimensions: physiological recovery, marked by a return of bodily functions; psychological recovery, a return of well-being; social recovery, a return to social activities and independence; and habitual recovery, a point at which the person returns to a full range of normal activities. Patients need to know that recovery takes time. Staples and sutures are often removed 7 to 10 days after the surgery in a follow-up appointment with the nurse or health care provider. If Steri-Strips cover the wound, they are left in place until they fall off naturally.

Cognitive level: Application

Nursing process: Implementation

Client needs: Physiological Integrity: Reduction of Risk Potential

5. Answer: 3. Nurse's ability to manage postoperative pain

Rationale: A study that looks at nurses' ability to manage postoperative pain would provide a basis for understanding how nurses develop clinical judgment. Factors that influence anxiety levels in the older surgical patient would be a topic of study about the psychological well-being of postoperative patients. Strategies to increase the patient's ability to manage symptoms at home and adjustment of discharge teaching to accommodate cultural differences are both topics of study about how to increase patients' competence in managing their own recovery.

Cognitive level: Analysis

Nursing process: Planning

Client needs: Physiological Integrity: Reduction of Risk Potential

Chapter 28

1. Answer: 1. Central nervous system

Rationale: Neuroglia comprise a major cellular component of the nervous system. Neuroglia do not directly transmit information. There are three main types of neuroglia: oligodendrocytes, astrocytes, and microglia. Oligodendrocytes form the myelin sheath covering many neuronal axons. Multiple sclerosis is a disorder that affects the myelin sheath.

Cognitive level: Analysis

Nursing process: Implementation

Client needs: Physiological Adaptation: Reduction of Risk Potential

2. Answer: 3. Medication history

Rationale: The presenting problem is the reason the individual is seeking care. The presenting problem is followed by the history of the present problem. The nurse should begin with the initial presentation of the symptom and proceed to the present. The medication history should include all medications the patient currently is taking or historically has taken. Herbal, over-the-counter, home remedies, and supplements need to be listed as well as prescribed medications. The past medical history includes major illnesses, including all hospitalizations, surgeries, ambulatory procedures, and both acute and chronic illnesses. In addition, childhood diseases, immunizations, medications, and allergies are explored.

Cognitive level: Application

Nursing process: Assessment

Client needs: Physiological Adaptation: Reduction of Risk Potential

3. Answer: 3. Spinal accessory

Rationale: The spinal accessory nerve has motor function only. This nerve innervates the sternocleidomastoid and trapezius muscles. Damage to this nerve can result in impaired strength in lifting the shoulders, or difficulty in turning the head to either side. The vagus nerve controls swallowing and speaking by innervating the larynx and pharynx. The hypoglossal nerve innervates the tongue. The facial nerve has a sensory and motor function. The facial nerve innervates the sense of taste in the anterior two-thirds of the tongue and the motor functioning of the face.

Cognitive level: Application

Nursing process: Assessment

Client needs: Physiological Adaptation: Reduction of Risk Potential

4. Answer: 1. Level of consciousness

Rationale: The mental status examination assesses the higher cortical functions of thinking and reasoning as well as level of consciousness, orientation, speech and language, memory, attention, fund of knowledge, and abstraction. The Glasgow Coma Scale is the most widely recognized level of consciousness assessment tool and is commonly used in emergency departments, trauma units, and intensive care areas. This tool evaluates three areas: eye opening, verbal response, and best motor response.

Cognitive level: Application

Nursing process: Assessment

Client needs: Physiological Adaptation: Reduction of Risk Potential

5. Answer: 3. Normal

Rationale: Reflexes are graded from 0 to +4. A 0 means there is no muscle reflex response. A +1 indicates a diminished response. A +2 is indicative of a normal reflex response. A +3 is more brisk but can be normal for the patient. A +4 indicates hyperactivity and possibly the presence of disease.

Cognitive level: Analysis

Nursing process: Assessment

Client needs: Physiological Adaptation: Reduction of Risk Potential

6. Answer: 2. Handle of the reflex hammer

Rationale: The Babinski reflex is tested by using a moderately sharp object, such as the handle of a percussion hammer, and stroking the lateral aspect of the sole of the foot from the heel to the ball of the foot, curving medially across the ball. The rubber triangle end of the reflex hammer is used to assess the four major reflex areas. A safety pin is not used to assess reflexes. A cotton swab is used to assess a corneal reflex.

Cognitive level: Application

Nursing process: Planning

Client needs: Physiological Adaptation: Reduction of Risk Potential

7. Answer: 4. Nothing; this can be a normal finding.

Rationale: When assessing cranial nerves III, IV, and VI in an elderly patient, the pupils are generally smaller and reflexes to light and accommodation become slower. This is due to aging changes in the muscles of the pupil sphincter and lens, not neurological changes.

Cognitive level: Analysis

Nursing process: Assessment

Client needs: Physiological Adaptation: Reduction of Risk Potential

Chapter 29

1. Answer: 4. Increasing absorption of CSF

   Rationale: Increased CSF absorption is one mechanism to maintain a constant relationship between the three brain components. Brain tissue does not expand; it is compressed. Autoregulation ensures that the brain receives required sufficient oxygen and glucose to meet metabolic needs; this may be inhibited, but it is not blocked as a normal compensatory mechanism.

   Cognitive level: Application

   Nursing process: Assessment

   Client needs: Physiological Integrity

2. Answer: 3. Complaints of a "different" headache and projectile vomiting

   Rationale: Complaints of a "different" headache and projectile vomiting may be an early indication of increasing ICP. Changes in cranial nerve III, the oculomotor nerve, result in changes in papillary response and are early signs of ICP. Decorticate movements are a late sign. Cushing's triad is a late sign of ICP.

   Cognitive level: Application

   Nursing process: Assessment

   Client needs: Physiological Integrity

3. Answers:
   1. Normocapnia levels ($PaCO_2$ levels of 35–40 mmHg)
   2. Euglycemic levels of 80–120 mg/dL
   3. Normothermia and interventions for body temperatures >99.5°F rectally

   Rationale: Normocapnia levels ($PaCO_2$ levels of 35–40 mmHg) are best for the brain; also good are euglycemic levels of 80–120 mg/dL, because the brain is adversely impacted by both hypoglycemia and hyperglycemia, and normothermia and interventions for body temperatures >99.5°F rectally. Pulse oximetry and supplemental oxygen should be used to maintain saturations of 95% or greater.

   Cognitive level: Analysis

   Nursing process: Assessment

   Client needs: Physiological Integrity

4. Answer: 2. A CAT scan of the head to rule out skull fracture

   Rationale: A CAT scan of the head to rule out skull fracture must be performed before wound closure is undertaken. A complete neurological assessment may indicate symptoms suggestive of a cerebral contusion, but a CAT scan is the diagnostic tool. A cerebral arteriogram is not appropriate in this case because the vessel is outside of the skull. A skull series is used to identify bone placement and continuity and, if a hematoma was suspected, a CAT scan would be the appropriate diagnostic test.

   Cognitive level: Application

   Nursing process: Assessment

   Client needs: Physiological Integrity

5. Answer: 1. In the spinal fluid, protein levels will be high and glucose levels will be low.

   Rationale: With bacterial meningitis, the spinal fluid protein levels will be high and glucose levels will be low. The spinal fluid will be clear in viral meningitis. Option 3 is false. The spinal fluid will be bloody if there has been a bleed within the cranium. If bleeding occurred as a result of the puncture, the fluid would clear.

   Cognitive level: Application

   Nursing process: Application

   Client needs: Physiological Integrity

6. Answer: 3. Benign tumors may be surgically difficult to remove and may compress vital structures.

   Rationale: If the tumor is deep within the brain structure, it may be extremely difficult or impossible to remove surgically. Tumors may not invade surrounding tissue, but their growth will compress them and may interfere with their function. Benign tumors can progress into malignant tumors.

   Cognitive level: Application

   Nursing process: Assessment

   Client needs: Physiological Integrity

7. Answer: 4. A flexible approach due to the changing resistance patterns to specific drugs

   Rationale: Brain tissue has no lymph drainage and this can interfer with clearing drugs and debris. Many chemotherapeutic agents cannot cross the blood–brain barrier. Malignant cells are heterogeneous and their sensitivity to the drugs is variable.

   Cognitive level: Application

   Nursing process: Implementation

   Client needs: Physiological Integrity

8. Answer: 3. Provide answers to questions honestly as they arise, educate them about the treatment plan, and involve them in discussions of the rehabilitation process.

   Rationale: Providing answers to questions honestly as they arise, educating patients and family about the treatment plan, and involving them in discussions of the rehabilitation process is important in keeping families informed and involved and provides as much control as possible and appropriate. The role of the nurse extends beyond teaching about the early detection of cognitive impairment because this would severely limit the family's knowledge and support. The early implementation of rehabilitative therapies does not alter the importance of family teaching. Family teaching should offer encouragement and realistic hope.

   Cognitive level: Application

   Nursing process: Implementation

   Client needs: Physiological Integrity

Chapter 30

1. Answer: 3. The strokes are commonly caused by atherosclerosis.

   Rationale: Eighty percent of all strokes are ischemic in nature and most are caused by atherosclerosis. Hemorrhagic strokes are commonly associated with hypertension. Patients experiencing ischemic strokes are generally older than those experiencing hemorrhagic strokes.

   Cognitive level: Analysis

   Nursing process: Assessment

   Client needs: Physiological Integrity

2. Answers:
   1. Plaque formation that alters the internal diameter of a cerebral artery
   2. Thrombus formation as a result of plaque formation.
   3. Lipohyalinosis, a vascular abnormality, caused by hypertension

   Rationale: Plaque formation that alters the internal diameter in a cerebral artery is a common cause of ischemic stroke. The fragmentation of a clot in the venous system of the leg cannot enter the arterial circulation of the brain unless there is a defect in the heart. The plaque disrupts the integrity of the arterial lining, causing blood to enter the clot and ultimately forming a thrombus. Lipohyalinosis is a process that results in a vascular abnormality in small vessels and is normally associated with hypertension.

   Cognitive level: Application
   Nursing process: Planning
   Client needs: Physiological Integrity

3. Answer: 2. Ischemic cascade further extends the area of infarction.

   Rationale: The ischemic cascade further propagates cerebral edema, cerebral ischemia, cerebral infarction, and cell death. Tissues surrounding the necrotic area have undergone tissue hypoxia and may be viable if perfusion is restored before anoxia occurs. The functional ability of the tissue has not been permanently impaired until cell death occurs. The penumbra is the area surrounding the necrotic core.

   Cognitive level: Application
   Nursing process: Planning
   Client needs: Physiological Integrity

4. Answer: 2. Assessing lung and heart sounds to detect fluid overload

   Rationale: With hypervolemic therapy, plasma expanders may cause pulmonary compromise or congestive heart failure. Cerebral salt wasting is a complication of subarachnoid hemorrhage not associated with vasospasm. The nidus is a concentration of abnormal vessels located at the center of an arteriovenous malformation. Seizures may be generalized or focal depending on the area of the brain involved.

   Cognitive level: Application
   Nursing process: Assessment
   Client needs: Physiological Integrity

5. Answer: 3. Endovascular coiling is associated with the patient being able to return to his activities of normal living and work earlier than patients who had undergone neurosurgical clipping.

   Rationale: Endovascular coiling is associated with a shorter, not longer length of hospital stay. Endovascular coiling, not neurosurgical clipping, is associated with a higher survival and lower morbidity rates 1 year after the procedure. Although the availability of an interventional neuroradiologist is important, if the patient is a candidate for endovascular coiling, this is the option of choice.

Cognitive level: Application
Nursing process: Implementation
Client needs: Physiological Integrity

Chapter 31

1. Answer: 2. Alzheimer's disease

   Rationale: A person with Alzheimer's disease will demonstrate multiple cognitive deficits, including aphasia, apraxia, agnosia, and disturbances with executing functioning. Specific cognitive deficits are not typically seen in multiple sclerosis, Parkinson's disease, or myasthenia gravis.

   Cognitive level: Analysis
   Nursing process: Assessment
   Client needs: Physiological Integrity: Reduction of Risk Potential

2. Answer: 2. Myasthenia gravis

   Rationale: Multiple sclerosis is a neuroimmunologic disease that affects myelin, the protective sheath surrounding nerve fibers. Demyelinating lesions or plaques form along nerve fibers in the brain and spinal cord, producing symptoms related to the location of damage. The brain of a patient with Alzheimer's disease shows a profusion of amyloid plaques and neurofibrillary tangles, which form in the hippocampus and other parts of the brain critical to memory. Myasthenia gravis is a disease of muscle weakness as the result of dysfunction at the neuromuscular junction where the transmission of nerve impulses is blocked. Parkinson's disease is a disease of poor dopamine production, which leads to difficulty with movement, tremor, rigidity, and difficulty maintaining posture.

   Cognitive level: Analysis
   Nursing process: Assessment
   Client needs: Physiological Integrity: Reduction of Risk Potential

3. Answer: 4. Instruct to avoid prolonged exposure to hot temperatures to include showers, baths, and environmental temperatures.

   Rationale: A patient with multiple sclerosis will have episodes of fatigue. Fatigue is exacerbated with exposure to hot temperatures, including showers, baths, and environmental temperatures. The use of assistive devices will decrease fatigue. Voiding patterns will not affect a patient's level of fatigue.

   Cognitive level: Application
   Nursing process: Planning
   Client needs: Physiological Integrity: Reduction of Risk Potential

4. Answer: 2. Increase dietary fiber

   Rationale: Interventions to assist a patient with Parkinson's disease who is experiencing constipation include increasing dietary fluid and fiber and avoiding the use of laxatives. Limiting protein is not recommended to help with constipation. Because protein can interfere with levodopa absorption in a small percentage of patients, patients might be instructed to take levodopa at least 30 minutes before eating or 1 hour after eating.

Cognitive level: Application

Nursing process: Planning

Client needs: Physiological Integrity: Reduction of Risk Potential

5. Answer: 2. Encourage talking about advance directives

Rationale: The physical and mental health of the primary family caregiver is critical to the care of the Alzheimer's patient. One health promotional activity that can optimize both patient and caregiver health is to encourage talking about advance directives for management of advanced stages of AD. Involvement in clinical research studies is often done by patients with Parkinson's disease as a way of advancing science while managing their condition with the latest, most promising treatments. Physical and emotional stress can exacerbate the symptoms of multiple sclerosis, so patients should be instructed to avoid extreme temperatures and exposure to infections. People with ALS do maintain careers and interests; however, referral for psychological and/or spiritual counseling may help the patient and family come to terms with the disease and its prognosis.

Cognitive level: Application

Nursing process: Planning

Client needs: Physiological Integrity: Reduction of Risk Potential

6. Answer: 3. Would you like to talk about things that can help you and your husband?

Rationale: People can live with Parkinson's disease for many years. The chronic and progressive nature of the disease can significantly impact older, spousal caregivers, who may not have the physical strength to handle the weight of a patient with limited mobility. Caregiver stress and burden have been shown to increase as the disease progresses. The nurse should encourage the patient to talk about things that can help both the patient and the husband. Minimizing the patient's concerns would not be an appropriate response. Suggesting the patient discuss the concern with her physician is also not an appropriate response.

Cognitive level: Application

Nursing process: Implementation

Client needs: Physiological Integrity: Reduction of Risk Potential

7. Answer: 4. Impact of meditation and prayer on disease management and experience

Rationale: The impact of meditation and prayer on disease management and experience is a topic that addresses complementary/alternative approaches to neurodegenerative disease processes. Interventions that improve the quality of life focus on quality of life research. Topics about literacy address patient/family education research. Anticipatory grief is a topic within emotional and psychological research.

Cognitive level: Analysis

Nursing process: Planning

Client needs: Physiological Integrity: Basic Care and Comfort

Chapter 32

1. Answer: 4. "A sudden deceleration injury, such as a head-on motor vehicle collision, is frequently the cause of hyperflexion injuries."

Rationale: Hyperextension injuries are caused by a sudden forceful extension of the head and neck, for instance, during a forward fall where the chin or forehead strikes the ground. These injuries can cause spinal ligaments to stretch, can compress the spinal cord, and can fracture the posterior spinous processes, but these injuries usually do not cause dislocations. Axial pressure loaded onto the spine may cause compression injuries, which include vertebral body fractures and spinal cord compression. Rotational injuries are associated with lateral flexion or rotation of the spine, causing posterior ligaments to rupture and facets to dislocate and fracture. Sudden deceleration injury, such as a head-on motor vehicle collision, is often the cause of hyperflexion injuries. These injuries can cause anterior vertebral body fractures and posterior spinal column facet fracture and dislocation.

Cognitive level: Application

Nursing process: Evaluation

Client needs: Safe, Effective Care Environment; Health Promotion and Maintenance; Physiological Integrity

2. Answer: 2. Central cord syndrome

Rationale: Central cord syndrome is often caused by hyperextension injuries, such as a rear-impact motor vehicle collision. This syndrome is caused by central spinal cord damage, which, in turn, causes damage to the more centrally located fibers leading to the upper extremities. The fibers leading to the lower extremities are more laterally located, producing less motor and sensory problems in the lower versus upper extremities. Anterior cord syndrome is caused by direct insult to the anterior portion of the spinal cord. Compression or hyperextension injury may produce this problem, but paralysis and loss of pain and temperature sensations are evident below the level of the injury. Also, light touch, vibration, and proprioception are preserved. Cauda equina syndrome is caused by compression of the lumbar nerve roots below the first lumbar vertebra. The associated signs and symptoms can vary based on the specific nerve root involved, but they often involve motor and sensory loss to the pelvic organs and lower extremities. Brown-Séquard syndrome is usually the result of penetrating trauma that causes hemisection of the spinal cord. The ipsilateral side experiences paralysis and proprioception loss, and the contralateral side experiences pain and temperature sensation loss.

Cognitive level: Analysis

Nursing process: Assessment

Client needs: Physiological Integrity

3. Answer: 3. Use of a reclining wheelchair to gradually progress the patient into an upright position so as not to cause orthostatic hypotension

Rationale: A reclining wheelchair or tilt table gradually places the patient into an upright position, decreasing the development of orthostatic hypotension. The use of an abdominal binder and compression stockings does decrease blood pooling in the peripheral veins, but these interventions are used to help improve venous return to the heart and to prevent orthostatic hypotension as well. A duplex Doppler ultrasound is a highly sensitive screening tool for detecting deep venous thrombosis. It does not dissolve clots. Good nutrition is important is aiding bowel evacuation, but increased caloric, protein, and micronutrient intake is used to aid in wound healing and the promotion of good skin integrity. Increased fiber and fluid intake would help prevent constipation.

Cognitive level: Analysis

Nursing process: Intervention

Client needs: Health Promotion and Maintenance; Physiological Integrity

4. Answer: 1. The patient's family will need ongoing education to help them deal with the stress of any role changes associated with the injury.

Rationale: Role changes within the family are a very real possibility following spinal cord injury, and the family will require ongoing support and education to help deal with this change. Elation and jubilation are not negative emotions; however, patients who experience spinal cord injury often do have negative feelings. They may exhibit denial, anger, grief, hopelessness, and depression. Patients should be encouraged to openly discuss their feelings, but they should also be allowed the opportunity to make their own health care decisions when possible. It is because of the physical challenges caused by the spinal cord injury that the patient usually faces significant psychosocial challenges as well.

Cognitive level: Analysis

Nursing process: Planning

Client needs: Psychosocial integrity

5. Answer: 1. Information regarding support systems that can help the patient and their family adjust to the changes in lifestyle and roles.

Rationale: It is important to put patients and their families in touch with support that can help them cope with the often difficult physical and psychological changes associated with spinal cord injury. Rehabilitative programs that maximize function following spinal cord injury should be multidisciplinary and comprehensive. Infrequent position changes predispose the patient to the development of pressure ulcers, but frequent position changes with good skin care regimens can help with pressure ulcer prevention. Suppository medications, digital bowel stimulation, and disimpaction of stool can aid in the prevention of hyperreflexia.

Cognitive level: Application

Nursing process: Planning

Client needs: Psychosocial Integrity

6. Answer: 4. Ineffective airway clearance related to the loss of spinal innervation of the respiratory and accessory muscles.

Rationale: Airway (with cervical spine immobilization in trauma situations) is always the first priority for any patient. When compared with the other nursing diagnoses listed for this patient, ineffective airway clearance would be the primary diagnosis. *Anxiety* is important and should be attended to, but airway issues should be dealt with first. *Risk for Imbalanced Nutrition* and *Risk for Ineffective Peripheral Tissue Perfusion* are potential problems, and actual problems, such as ineffective airway clearance, should be treated before these other diagnoses are addressed.

Cognitive level: Application

Nursing process: Planning

Client needs: Safe, Effective Care Environment

Chapter 33

1. Answer: 2. Crackles

Rationale: Crackles are sounds caused by fluid in the airways. They are described as intermittent or discontinuous, nonmusical, or popping sounds. They are caused by fluid, inflammation, infection, or secretions. The term *rales* is no longer used to describe fluid effects in the airways. Crackles occur when closed airways snap open during inspiration. Wheezes are high-pitched musical sounds caused by air flowing across strands of mucous, swollen pulmonary tissue that narrows the airway, or from bronchospasm. The term *rhonchi* is no longer used to describe harsh sounds caused by secretions in the airways.

Cognitive level: Application

Nursing process: Assessment

Client needs: Health Promotion and Maintenance: Prevention/Early Detection of Health Problems

2. Answer: 3. It might help to know if there are any recent outbreaks of pulmonary disorders in the area of travel.

Rationale: Area of recent travel may become an important aspect of the history in diagnosing potential respiratory problems. In previous years, the severe acute respiratory syndrome outbreak demonstrated to the world that viral pulmonary disease could be traced to a specific location. Recent travel and area of residence have been demonstrated to be an important factor in the history of respiratory symptoms and should be included in the interview process. The other options would not help in figuring out where the patient might have been exposed to an upper respiratory infection.

Cognitive level: Analysis

Nursing process: Assessment

Client needs: Health Promotion and Maintenance: Prevention/Early Detection of Health Problems

3. Answer: 2. Have you been to any activities or functions around other people with respiratory problems?

Rationale: The social history includes information about the patient's lifestyle and habits that may be relevant to his or her current state of health. Patients who smoke have increased risk for pulmonary disease and patients who have allergies and engage in social activities in the out-of-doors such as golfing may have exacerbations of symptoms after participating in these activities. Also, if patients frequent social events where they may be exposed to people with upper respiratory infections or poor hygienic conditions, they may be predisposed to the development of pulmonary infections. The other choices focus on either the patient's health history, family history, or history of immunizations.

Cognitive level: Application

Nursing process: Assessment

Client needs: Health Promotion and Maintenance: Prevention/Early Detection of Health Problems

4. Answer: 3. Edema indicates heart failure, a common finding in a patient with COPD.

Rationale: Edema of the lower extremities is generally related to right heart or congestive heart failure. Right heart failure and combined left- and right-sided failure are common in patients with COPD. Right-sided failure is caused by pulmonary hypertension. Chronic distention of the lower airways makes forward blood flow more difficult. The right heart hypertrophies in an attempt to increase force of blood through the pulmonary tree. The right heart fails and fluid unable to be accommodated is sequestered in dependent interstitial spaces and causes edema.

Cognitive level: Analysis

Nursing process: Assessment

Client needs: Health Promotion and Maintenance: Prevention/Early Detection of Health Problems

5. Answer: 3. Have an arterial blood gas analysis done to compare the readings.

Rationale: The oxygen saturation measured by infrared technology does not necessarily provide the same values obtained from the calculated oxygen saturation obtained from an ABG. Normal infrared oxygen saturation and ABG saturations range from 95% to 100%. Pulse oximetry probes should not be placed on extremities with automated blood pressure cuffs, hemodialysis fistulas, or arterial lines because these interfere with blood flow. Shock and hypovolemia also cause low-flow states that contribute to inaccurate pulse oximetry readings. Patient movement, ambient light, and venous pulsations may also cause inaccurate readings. If ambient light is interfering with readings (producing results higher than suspected), cover the probe with a towel to see if the result is different. Pulse oximetry does not distinguish methemoglobin or carboxyhemoglobin from oxygen-saturated hemoglobin. Fifty percent carboxyhemoglobin reads as 95%. Patients who have suspected thiocyanate toxicity or inhalation injury should have an ABG analysis to determine respiratory status and oxygen saturation.

Cognitive level: Analysis

Nursing process: Assessment

Client needs: Physiological Integrity: Physiological Adaptation

Chapter 34

1. Answer: 2. Once stable, instruct in the use of a water pik.

Rationale: With mandibular fractures, good oral care is essential for healthy healing and prevention of dental

complications. Patient education should include use of the water pik and dietary requirements. The use of systemic antibiotics to prevent meningitis is indicated in the management of temporal bone fractures. The use of eye protection is indicated in the patient with a temporal bone fracture. Facial nerve injury is seen in temporal bone fractures.

Cognitive level: Application

Nursing process: Planning

Client needs: Physiological Integrity: Reduction of Risk Potential

2. Answer: 2. Administer antibiotics as prescribed.

Rationale: Nursing care of the patient relies heavily on assessment of signs and symptoms, which, in turn, is dependent on obtaining a thorough patient history. The history must include the onset and duration of the symptoms including site of pain or discomfort, redness of eyes, flushing of face across the nose, fever, weakness or fatigue, cough, congestion, sore throat, muscle ache, and sore teeth. It also is important to know if any particular event or incident triggered the patient's symptoms. There is no reason to restrict fluids, maintain on bed rest, or consult with a dentist.

Cognitive level: Application

Nursing process: Planning

Client needs: Physiological Integrity: Reduction of Risk Potential

3. Answer: 4. Avoid exposure to strong perfumes, smoke, and rapid changes in temperature.

Rationale: With allergy injections, the dose is gradually increased to a maintenance concentration, which takes about 5 to 6 months. Patients may receive allergy injections for 3 to 5 years, depending on symptoms. The patient should be instructed to stay away from allergens that create a reaction. This means limiting outdoor exposure. Excessive humidity should be reduced and standing water should be removed. The patient should be instructed to eliminate exposure to smoke, strong perfumes and scents, fumes, rapid changes in temperature, and outdoor pollution for patients with nonspecific triggers.

Cognitive level: Application

Nursing process: Planning

Client needs: Health Promotion and Maintenance: Prevention/Early Detection of Health Problems

4. Answer: 1. Presence of smoke detectors in the home and the type of cooking appliances used

Rationale: Caution should be taken to ensure safety around the home. Smoke detectors and electric appliances rather than gas appliances should be used as should technologies that detect the presence of gas fumes in the home.

Cognitive level: Analysis

Nursing process: Assessment

Client needs: Health Promotion and Maintenance: Prevention/Early Detection of Health Problems

5. Answer: 2. Assess the type of difficulty and provide recommendations accordingly.

Rationale: The nursing process guides the management of patients with sleep apnea. The nurse should first assess the patient's description of "difficulty" and then make suggestions accordingly. The nurse should not alter the patient's prescribed treatment without health care provider involvement and should not recommend changing the use of the CPAP machine or not using the device.

Cognitive level: Application

Nursing process: Implementation

Client needs: Health Promotion and Maintenance: Prevention/Early Detection of Health Problems

6. Answer: 2. Smoking is only one cause for the disease. Others include chronic mouth lesions and poor nutrition.

Rationale: A variety of risk factors are associated with head and neck cancer, although some patients do not have any known risk factors; therefore, it is not possible to know for sure how much they contributed to causing the cancer. Some risk factors include alcohol intake, ultraviolet light exposure, tobacco use, mouth irritation, poor nutrition, HPV infection, immune system suppression, male gender, and exposure to Epstein–Barr virus if a first-generation Asian.

Cognitive level: Application

Nursing process: Implementation

Client needs: Psychosocial Integrity: Coping and Adaptation

7. Answer: 4. Secure the tube ties laterally to the chest with suspended ties.

Rationale: Nursing interventions include securing the airway with the appropriate ties in order to prevent the possibility of the tube being dislodged or accidentally removed. The tracheostomy tube ties should be secured to the chest laterally with suspended ties. Circumferential ties can place pressure on the incision lines or reconstruction flaps or grafts. The ties should be changed every day or when soiled to decrease the possibility of infection. The tracheostomy site should be cleaned on a regular basis such as every 8 hours and more frequently as needed to remove crusts and secretions that could obstruct the airway. If the tracheostomy tube has an inner cannula, it should be changed if disposable or cleaned when every tie tracheostomy care procedure is done.

Cognitive level: Application

Nursing process: Implementation

Client needs: Physiological Integrity: Physiological Adaptation

Chapter 35

1. Answer: 2. An acute asthma attack

Rationale: Asthma is a chronic inflammatory disorder of the airways in which many cells and cellular elements play a role, in particular, mast cells, eosinophils, T lymphocytes, macrophages, neutrophils, and epithelial cells. In susceptible individuals, this inflammation causes recurrent episodes of wheezing, breathlessness, chest tightness, and coughing, particularly at night or in the early morning. These episodes usually are associated with widespread but variable airflow obstruction that is often reversible, either spontaneously or with treatment. The inflammation also causes airway hyperresponsiveness or bronchospasm related to a variety of stimuli.

Cognitive level: Analysis

Nursing process: Assessment

Client needs: Physiological Integrity: Physiological Adaptation

2. Answer: 3. Avoid smoking or environments with smoke.

Rationale: The incidence of community-acquired pneumonia is highest in winter months with smoking being an important risk factor. The nurse should emphasize the importance of rest and a gradual increase in activity to avoid fatigue. Instructions should include ways to maintain resistance to infection with proper nutrition and adequate fluid intake. The patient should also be taught about all medications that will be continued at home.

Cognitive level: Application

Nursing process: Planning

Client needs: Physiological Integrity: Physiological Adaptation

3. Answer: 3. Magnesium sulfate

Rationale: Magnesium sulfate is thought to produce bronchodilation through counteraction of calcium-mediated smooth muscle constriction in the patient with COPD. This is given intravenously. Pancreatic enzymes are provided to the patient with cystic fibrosis because of failure of the pancreas to produce these enzymes. Ibuprofen is often used to reduce inflammation in the patient with cystic fibrosis. Pulmozyme decreases sputum viscosity in cystic fibrosis. Its use also has been shown to improve FEV_1 and decrease incidence of exacerbations.

Cognitive level: Application

Nursing process: Planning

Client needs: Physiological Integrity: Physiological Adaptation

4. Answer: 1. Pain management

Rationale: Rib fractures are treated by controlling the patient's pain. Sedation and pain management allow the patient to begin deep breathing and coughing in order to prevent the development of atelectasis, pneumonitis, and hypoxemia. A chest binder may decrease pain on movement. Usually the pain diminishes by the fifth to the seventh day, and healing occurs in 3 to 6 weeks. The nurse emphasizes pain management and gives specific instructions regarding medications for pain until the pain diminishes.

Cognitive level: Analysis

Nursing process: Planning

Client needs: Physiological Integrity: Physiological Adaptation

5. Answer: 4. Pain associated with the primary diagnosis

Rationale: The patient with lung cancer may complain of hoarseness, dysphagia, or vague complaints that have persisted longer than normally expected. Chest pain, tightness, or an ill-defined sensation of fullness may be experienced. This may be accompanied by pleuritic pain on inspiration or a subscapular pain radiating to the arm.

Cognitive level: Analysis

Nursing process: Assessment

Client needs: Physiological Integrity: Physiological Adaptation

6. Answer: 3. Place of employment 10 to 20 years prior to current admission

Rationale: There is a considerable latency period of about 10 to 20 years for asbestosis between exposure and the development of symptomatology. Those at high risk for this disease are asbestos miners, millers, and those employed in the building trade and shipyards, such as loggers, insulation workers, pipe fitters and steamfitters, sheet metal workers, and welders. Working within the roofing materials industry is linked to silicosis.

Cognitive level: Application

Nursing process: Assessment

Client needs: Physiological Integrity: Reduction of Risk Potential

Chapter 36

1. Answer: 1. Oxygen 2 liters nasal cannula

Rationale: Acute respiratory failure results in a failure of oxygenation or ventilation or both. A failure of oxygenation produces hypoxemia, which is defined as a decreased arterial oxygen tension or pressure in the blood below normal range. The administration of oxygen would be the most effective in treating this type of patient. The patient's arterial saturation of oxygen level of less than 90 while breathing room air is representative of hypoxemic respiratory failure. Correcting and treating hypoxia is always a primary goal. Presenting symptoms in acute respiratory failure are shortness of breath, dyspnea, and increased work of breathing with hypoxemia and should always be addressed initially. Educating the patient and family is always important, but addressing the airway is always a priority.

Cognitive level: Application

Nursing process: Implementation

Client needs: Physiological Integrity: Physiological Adaptation

2. Answer: 3. Pulmonary edema

Rationale: The classic clinical presentation of acute pulmonary edema includes rapidly worsening dyspnea, shortness of breath, tachypnea, agitation, increased crackles, and possibly coarse rhonchi in all lung fields. Pink, frothy sputum may also be present. The other clinical signs are hypertension, tachycardia, and possibly S_3 or S_4 heart sounds. The pathophysiology of acute pulmonary edema and the signs and symptoms of this dysfunction are related to the accumulation of fluid, which prevents adequate gas exchange across the alveolar-capillary membrane. Cardiogenic pulmonary edema is pulmonary edema that results from increased hydrostatic pressures in the pulmonary capillary bed secondary to increased pulmonary venous pressure. Noncardiogenic pulmonary edema is related to injury of the alveolar-capillary membrane from numerous causes. Among the most important causes are sepsis, inflammation, inhaled toxins, and drugs. Usually in noncardiogenic pulmonary edema there is no primary cardiac dysfunction.

Cognitive level: Analysis

Nursing process: Assessment

Client needs: Physiological Integrity: Physiological Adaptation

3. Answer: 4. PCWP > 30 mmHg

Rationale: The patient with noncardiogenic pulmonary edema will develop tachycardia, hypertension, bounding pulses, and a drop in PCWP. If the patient's PCWP increases, the health care provider should be notified because this could indicate the development of cardiogenic pulmonary edema where the PCPW > 18 mmHg.

Cognitive level: Application

Nursing process: Assessment

Client needs: Physiological Integrity: Physiological Adaptation

4. Answer: 3. Arterial blood gases showing respiratory acidosis

Rationale: The hypoxemia of a patient with ARDS quickly becomes refractory to standard oxygen therapies, and the patient will require intubation and mechanical ventilation to maintain oxygenation and ventilation. The arterial blood gases frequently demonstrate respiratory acidosis. The chest x-ray exhibits the bilateral patchy infiltrates that are characteristic of the disease instead of the absence of infiltrates. This "white-out" observed on the chest x-ray can cover the entire lung field as the disease progresses. The vital signs are within normal range and will not usually be noted with a patient who has ARDS.

Cognitive level: Application

Nursing process: Assessment

Client needs: Physiological Integrity: Physiological Adaptation

5. Answer: 2. Remove the patient from the ventilator and use the Ambu bag with 100% oxygen.

Rationale: When the patient is experiencing hypoxia, it is imperative that the nurse remove the patient from the mechanical ventilator and administer 100% oxygen until the problem can be detected. Once the oxygenation returns to an acceptable range, the nurse should continue the assessment process. It is also important for the nurse to listen anteriorly and posteriorly in all lung fields. The importance of this exam cannot be overemphasized. When listening, the nurse should compare the right against the left lung and never listen through clothing or other material. The clinician should listen laterally in order to appreciate certain lung segments that can be heard in this position.

Cognitive level: Application

Nursing process: Implementation

Client needs: Physiological Integrity: Physiological Adaptation

6. Answer: 4. When the patient is removed from the ventilator and the Ambu is used it causes overinflation from the Ambu aggressive rates.

Rationale: Most ventilated patients should have PEEP of at least 5 cm of H_2O to prevent the pressure in the alveoli from dropping to zero at the end of expiration. The nurse can cause auto-PEEP with overaggressive rates with an air-mask-bag unit. The patient is removed from the ventilator for transport or for suctioning. Rapid rates are used to bag the patient instead of the rate that was set on the ventilator. The patient might become hypotensive. Treatment would involve disconnecting the patient from the Ambu or ventilator for a few seconds; this would allow the excess pressure to dissipate. PEEP does not have any correlation with hypovolemia.

Cognitive level: Implementation

Nursing process: Assessment

Client needs: Physiological Integrity: Physiological Adaptation

7. Answer: 1. Auscultate lungs for bilateral breath sounds.

Rationale: The nurse as well as other members of the health care team should verify proper placement of the ET tube. The importance of this exam cannot be overemphasized. When listening, the nurse should compare the right against the left lung and never listen through clothing or other material. The clinician should listen laterally in order to appreciate certain lung segments that can be heard in this position. The endotracheal tube being advanced down the right main stem bronchus preventing air form entering the left lung also could cause the absence of lung sounds on the left, so accurate assessment is very important. Securing the ET tube, assessing oxygen saturation, and obtaining a chest x-ray are all important steps that need to be performed after the initial auscultation of breath sounds.

Cognitive level: Application

Nursing process: Implementation

Client needs: Physiological Integrity: Physiological Adaptation

8. Answer: 4. Applying suction when passing the catheter into the patient's tracheostomy

Rationale: To perform tracheostomy suctioning, the nurse or caregiver should use sterile gloves in order to prevent nosocomial infections. The patient should be oxygenated prior to suctioning and the patient's head should be elevated. The patient should always be preoxygenated to prevent hypoxemia as well. The nurse/caregiver should never suction going into the tracheostomy, only when withdrawing the catheter.

Cognitive level: Application

Nursing process: Evaluation

Client needs: Physiological Integrity: Physiological Adaptation

9. Answer: 2. A patient with a chest tube on the right side with bubbling in the water seal chamber

Rationale: The nurse should initially see the patient with the chest tube. A pleural tube is inserted in the pleural space in order to evacuate the air or blood and allow the lung to reexpand. The pleural tube re-creates the negative pressure in the chest that has been violated by trauma or surgery. A pleural chest tube should not bubble in the water seal chamber.

Cognitive level: Application

Nursing process: Assessment

Client needs: Physiological Integrity

Chapter 37

1. Answer: 2. Waist circumference is 110 cm.

Rationale: The patient already has two of the criteria for the metabolic syndrome: hypertension and hypertriglyceridemia. The third factor is a waist circumference of greater than 102 cm in males and 88 cm in females. The fasting blood sugar would need to be greater than or equal to 110 mg/dL. The HDL would need to be less than 40 mg/dL in males. Random blood sugars are not part of the criteria for metabolic syndrome.

Cognitive level: Application

Nursing process: Assessment

Client needs: Physiological Integrity: Physiological Adaptation

2. Answer: 4. Decongestants

Rationale: Decongestants cause vasoconstriction and can contribute to hypertension and cardiac arrhythmias. The other medications would not present a cardiac risk.

Cognitive level: Application

Nursing process: Assessment

Client needs: Physiological Integrity: Physiological Adaptation

3. Answer: 2. "How many pillows do you sleep on?"

Rationale: The degree of orthopnea is best measured by the number of pillows that are needed to help the patient breathe comfortably. Frequency of waking up could be caused by many factors and is not specific to orthopnea. Palpitations can occur for many reasons or even be normal and do not correlate with orthopnea. Nocturia may indicate congestive heart failure, but does not correlate with a diagnosis of orthopnea.

Cognitive level: Application

Nursing process: Assessment

Client needs: Physiological Integrity: Physiological Adaptation

4. Answer: 2. Systolic dysfunction

Rationale: S_3 sounds are a marker of systolic dysfunction. They are heard early during diastole and are associated with ventricular dysfunction. S_4 sounds are indicative of diastolic dysfunction. Conduction defects are not heard as heart sounds. Alterations in the mitral valve are heard as abnormal S_1 sounds.

Cognitive level: Application

Nursing process: Assessment

Client needs: Physiological Integrity: Physiological Adaptation

Chapter 38

1. Answer: 2. QRS complex 0.10 second

Rationale: The following criteria must be present to be a normal electrocardiogram: P wave has a normal and consistent shape and appears before every QRS complex; there is a 1:1 ratio of P wave to QRS complex; PR interval is between 0.12 and 0.20 second; QRS complex is between 0.06 and 0.12 second; QT interval is between 0.34 and 0.43 second; atrial and ventricular rate is between 60 and 100 beats per minute; and atrial and ventricular rhythm is regular.

Cognitive level: Analysis

Nursing process: Assessment

Client needs: Physiological Integrity: Reduction of Risk Potential

2. Answer: 3. 0.12 second

Rationale: Each "small box" is 0.04 second. This patient's QRS complex should be documented as being 0.12 second.

Cognitive level: Application

Nursing process: Assessment

Client needs: Physiological Integrity: Reduction of Risk Potential

3. Answer: 2. Observe and treat the patient for anxiety.

Rationale: This patient is demonstrating premature atrial contractions (PACs) that started after learning of a stressful and/or anxiety-producing event. This patient should be observed for the frequency of the PACs and the anxiety should be treated. Cardioversion is a treatment for atrial flutter. Calcium channel blockers are used with atrial fibrillation. Carotid artery massage is a treatment used for supraventricular tachycardia.

Cognitive level: Analysis

Nursing process: Planning

Client needs: Physiological Integrity: Physiological Adaptation

4. Answer: 1. Have a serum digoxin level drawn.

Rationale: Because some prescribed medications, such as digoxin, cause significant dysrhythmias, the patient's medical history should be reviewed to determine if the dysrhythmia is medication related. Serum drug levels should be ordered as indicated. ACLS protocols would be indicated in some cases of ventricular dysrhythmias. Magnesium is the treatment of choice for torsade de pointes. Lidocaine is used in the treatment of premature ventricular contractions.

Cognitive level: Analysis

Nursing process: Planning

Client needs: Physiological Integrity: Physiological Adaptation

Chapter 39

1. Answer: 4. False positive

Rationale: Sensitivity describes the ability of a test to identify patients with disease. It may be calculated by dividing the number of true positive tests by the sum of true positives plus false negatives. For example, positive tests in subjects with coronary disease are "true positives," whereas negative tests are "false negatives." Similarly, negative tests in patients who are free of disease are "true negatives," and positive tests in patients without disease are "false positives."

Cognitive level: Application

Nursing process: Implementation

Client needs: Health Promotion and Maintenance: Prevention/Early Detection of Health Problems

2. Answer: 4. Echocardiogram

Rationale: With an echocardiogram, hemodynamic data include the amount and speed of blood flow through the valves, enabling the noninvasive detection and follow-up of stenotic or regurgitant heart valves. TEE is frequently used to detect and assess endocarditis, aortic dissection, intracardiac masses such as thrombi or tumors, valvular pathology, and congenital disorders in both children and adults. MRI can be used to evaluate patients with presumed congenital heart diseases, such as coarctation of the aorta or atrial septal defects. PET scan is the current "gold standard" for assessment of myocardial viability.

Cognitive level: Application

Nursing process: Planning

Client needs: Health Promotion and Maintenance: Prevention/Early Detection of Health Problems

3. Answer: 2. Provide intravenous normal saline prior to the procedure.

Rationale: Patients with preexisting renal failure and a history of anaphylactic reaction to contrast dye must be pretreated before the catheterization. Pretreatment for the patient with a history of anaphylactic reaction to contrast dye includes antihistamines and steroids. In the laboratory the patient will usually be given a mild sedative. Patients with renal failure (serum creatinine ≤1.5 mg/dL) should receive intravenous normal saline for several hours before the procedure.

Cognitive level: Application

Nursing process: Planning

Client needs: Physiological Integrity: Reduction of Risk Potential

4. Answer: 4. Stress test

Rationale: A stress test is contraindicated for myocardial infarction within 2 days, unstable angina, aortic stenosis, uncontrolled dysrhythmias, symptomatic heart failure, active endocarditis, uncontrolled hypertension, any acute disorder that may affect exercise, and the inability to obtain informed consent. The ECG is helpful in determining the overall electrical functioning of the patient's heart. The echocardiogram is useful to determining the patient's ejection fraction in addition to the functioning of other cardiac structures. The PCI can be done to prevent further myocardial damage.

Cognitive level: Analysis

Nursing process: Planning

Client needs: Physiological Integrity: Reduction of Risk Potential

5. Answer: 3. Assess the femoral site.

Rationale: All patients must have a complete nursing assessment, with special emphasis on the cardiovascular system including peripheral pulses and the vascular access site. This assessment includes vital signs, ECG monitoring, and assessment of the vascular access site and pulses distal to the puncture site. Evaluation of the access site includes inspection for any signs of bleeding or swelling and palpation for any tenderness. Diagnosis of suspected arterial injuries is made through a careful physical assessment, and confirmed through noninvasive vascular studies or arteriography. Physical examination of the femoral site is performed assessing for the presence of localized tenderness, bruits, or a pulsatile mass. Hematomas are identified by swelling at the site of the arterial puncture. Large hematomas may need to be assessed by ultrasound to rule out the presence of pseudoaneurysms or arteriovenous fistulas.

Cognitive level: Application

Nursing process: Assessment

Client needs: Physiological Integrity: Reduction of Risk Potential

Chapter 40

1. Answer: 4. "My father died of a heart attack at age 70."

   Rationale: Genetics, sex, and age are nonmodifiable risk factors, or those that cannot be changed. Smoking, hypertension, diabetes, obesity, and a sedentary lifestyle are modifiable risk factors. The patient's smoking and high blood sugars reflect modifiable risk factors. Walking provides exercise to modify the risk factor of a sedentary lifestyle.

   Cognitive level: Application

   Nursing process: Assessment

   Client needs: Physiological Integrity: Reduction of Risk Potential

2. Answer: 3. "Was your pain precipitated by activity?"

   Rationale: Stable angina is frequently precipitated by activity, emotional stress, cold weather, or large meals. Pain lasting 15 minutes would be indicative of a myocardial infarction; angina pain usually lasts 5 to 10 minutes. Anginal pain radiates to the jaw, but not always.

   Cognitive level: Application

   Nursing process: Implementation

   Client needs: Physiological Integrity: Physiological Adaptation

3. Answer: 1. The pain was relieved by taking nitroglycerin.

   Rationale: The three key characteristics of typical angina include pain, pressure, tightness, or heaviness that is substernal, central chest, or in the left arm that is provoked by exertion or emotional stress and that is relieved by nitroglycerin. Angina may be precipitated by eating a large meal, but relief with nitroglycerin provides stronger support for a diagnosis of typical angina. Angina may also cause anxiety and dizziness, but again, these do not provide the best support.

   Cognitive level: Application

   Nursing process: Assessment

   Client needs: Physiological Integrity: Physiological Adaptation

4. Answer: 4. Transmural ischemia

   Rationale: When ischemia traverses the entire width of cardiac muscle, it is called transmural and the ST segment is elevated. The more leads in which the ST segment is elevated indicate greater damage. Mild ischemia of subendocardial injury would be reflected as ST segment depression. Past myocardial infarction damage is diagnosed by the presence of a Q wave.

   Cognitive level: Analysis

   Nursing process: Assessment

   Client needs: Physiological Integrity: Physiological Adaptation

5. Answer: 1. Occurrence of an old myocardial infarction

   Rationale: An old MI is diagnosed when a Q wave is present in the absence of ST elevation, patient symptoms, and blood markers. The Q-wave changes are due to necrosis and are irreversible, so they allow for identification of MIs. They cannot determine how long ago the necrosis occurred, so it would not be safe to conclude the damage was recent. Q waves do not reflect pacemaker function or ventricular hypertrophy.

   Cognitive level: Analysis

   Nursing process: Assessment

   Client needs: Physiological Integrity: Physiological Adaptation

6. Answer: 1. Troponin 1 levels

   Rationale: Troponin 1 levels are specific to cardiac muscle and are released from the myocardial cell within 3 to 12 hours of cellular injury and may stay elevated for 5 to 14 days. Myoglobin levels are not a specific indicator of heart damage and only stay elevated for 24 hours. C-reactive protein is also not specific to cardiac muscle. CK-MB levels are specific to myocardial tissue, but return to normal within 72 hours.

   Cognitive level: Application

   Nursing process: Assessment

   Client needs: Physiological Integrity: Physiological Adaptation

7. Answer: 2. Cardiogenic shock

   Rationale: Cardiogenic shock is an acute condition that must be detected and treated immediately to improve survival. An infarction of greater than 40% of the left ventricle and three-vessel disease place the patient at greater risk to develop cardiogenic shock. Pericarditis is associated with large infarctions and low ejection fractions but is not the highest priority. Dressler's syndrome is indicative of pericarditis that occurs 2 to 12 weeks following an MI. PVCs can occur following any cardiac ischemic event, but are not the highest priority.

   Cognitive level: Analysis

   Nursing process: Planning

   Client needs: Physiological Integrity: Physiological Adaptation

8. Answer: 3. Significant stenosis of the left anterior descending, LAD, and circumflex artery

   Rationale: Class I recommendations indicate a CABG is indicated when the patient has significant stenosis of the proximal LAD and left circumflex artery even though the patient is asymptomatic. A 50% occlusion of the circumflex artery is not part of the criteria. Recent history of angina and heart failure are also not qualifying criteria.

Cognitive level: Application

Nursing process: Assessment

Client needs: Physiological Integrity: Physiological Adaptation

9. Answer: 4. Report the findings to the primary care provider.

Rationale: An output of greater than 100 mL/hr reflects postoperative bleeding and should be reported. Output should continued to be monitored but is not the first priority. Having the patient cough and deep breathe does not address the problem of bleeding. Although the chest tube dressing should be checked, the chest tube output reflects internal bleeding and must be reported immediately.

Cognitive level: Analysis

Nursing process: Implementation

Client needs: Physiological Integrity: Physiological Adaptation

Chapter 41

1. Answer: 3. Mitral stenosis

Rationale: Rheumatic fever produces an inflammatory process that often causes valvular heart damage, leading to stenosis of heart valves. Pericarditis and endocarditis may be experienced during the initial inflammatory process, but should not persist after treatment is done. Pulmonary fibrosis is not caused by rheumatic fever.

Cognitive level: Application

Nursing process: Planning

Client needs: Physiological Integrity: Physiological Adaptation

2. Answer: 2. "I had rheumatic heart disease when I was a child."

Rationale: Aortic stenosis is often caused by rheumatic heart disease, which destroys valve leaflets with calcification and fibrosis, which leads to the stenosis. As the narrowing of the valve increases, clinical manifestations are exhibited; dyspnea is the most frequent complaint and is often accompanied by angina and exertional syncope. Having had a CABG or having a dysrhythmia are not contributing factors for aortic stenosis. Palpitations are associated with mitral valve prolapse and stenosis or aortic regurgitation.

Cognitive level: Application

Nursing process: Assessment

Client needs: Physiological Integrity: Physiological Adaptation

3. Answer: 2. Plan for rest periods throughout the day.

Rationale: Excessive exercise and exertion place demands for increased circulation and oxygen to the heart. Allowing time for rest reduces the workload and therefore oxygen demands on the heart. The valve may not need to be replaced; the patient should be taught to take prophylactic antibiotics before dental work, but not to avoid dental work. An elevated temperature could be a sign of endocarditis, but it is not necessary to take the temperature daily. A diet high in fatty foods should be avoided, but it is not necessary to keep a food diet.

Cognitive level: Application

Nursing process: Implementation

Client needs: Physiological Integrity: Physiological Adaptation

4. Answer: 3. The valve will be repaired, but not replaced.

Rationale: An open procedure involves surgical repair under general anesthesia and cardiopulmonary bypass. Valvuloplasty involves repair of the torn or damaged leaflets, chordae tendineae, or papillary muscle, but the valve is not replaced. Anticoagulation therapy will be needed in the postoperative period to prevent thrombus formation at the surgical site. A valvuloplasty does not guarantee that future repairs or valve replacement will not be necessary.

Cognitive level: Application

Nursing process: Implementation

Client needs: Physiological Integrity: Physiological Adaptation

5. Answer: 4. Supportive therapy with medications

Rationale: Because the prognosis for this type of cardiomyopathy is poor, management is focused at reducing the workload of the heart and diminishing heart failure with use of diuretics, calcium channel blockers, beta-blockers, and antiarrhythmic medications. Alcohol ablation and ICDs are sometimes used in the treatment of hypertrophic cardiomyopathy. Aortic valve repair is not indicated for treatment.

Cognitive level: Application

Nursing process: Planning

Client needs: Physiological Integrity: Physiological Adaptation

6. Answer: 3. "Does the pain become worse if you take a deep breath?"

Rationale: Chest pain associated with pericarditis is often described as sharp and gets worse with deep breathing; it is relieved by sitting up. Anginal pain is not associated with position changes or deep breathing. It is relieved by sitting up, not lying flat. Pericarditis does not occur at any particular time of day and is not associated with palpitations.

Cognitive level: Application

Nursing process: Implementation

Client needs: Physiological Integrity: Physiological Adaptation

Chapter 42

1. Answer: 3. Aortic stenosis

Rationale: Risk factors for heart failure include a history of hypertension, coronary heart disease, obesity, diabetes, and structural and valvular disorders, such as aortic stenosis. Pancreatitis, chronic fatigue syndrome, and pleural effusions are not risk factors for heart failure.

Cognitive level: Application

Nursing process: Assessment

Client needs: Physiological Integrity: Physiological Adaptation

2. Answer: 1. Decreased cardiac output

Rationale: Systolic dysfunction occurs when the ventricle is unable to contract forcefully during systole and often hypertrophies in an effort to compensate. As a result, the percentage of blood ejected from the heart is decreased. Aortic stenosis and mitral regurgitation may contribute to the development of heart failure and may be manifested by the presence of a murmur. Systolic dysfunction primarily affects cardiac output, not heart rate.

Cognitive level: Application

Nursing process: Assessment

Client needs: Physiological Integrity: Physiological Adaptation

3. Answer: 1. Activation of the sympathetic nervous system, SNS

Rationale: Activation of the SNS and RAS systems occurs when cardiac output falls, in an effort to increase blood volume and rate of heart contractility. The parasympathetic system is not activated because this would further decrease the heart rate. Cytokines are also released, not suppressed.

Cognitive level: Application

Nursing process: Assessment

Client needs: Physiological Integrity: Physiological Adaptation

4. Answer: 3. Dyspnea

Rationale: Dyspnea is seen secondary to pulmonary congestion, which occurs most with left-sided heart failure. Fluid accumulates in the pulmonary bed as it backs up from the left ventricle. Right-sided failure causes venous congestion with fluid accumulation in the interstitial spaces, manifested by weight gain, anorexia, nausea, and peripheral edema.

Cognitive level: Application

Nursing process: Assessment

Client needs: Physiological Integrity: Physiological Adaptation

5. Answer: 1. A diagnosis of heart failure can be excluded.

Rationale: The BNP is very useful in ruling out a diagnosis of heart failure if the level is normal. Elevated levels correlate with heart failure, increased risk of mortality, acute MI, PE, and renal failure. Because they are not elevated, the patient does not have long-standing heart failure, cardiac ischemia. Pulmonary tissue damage would not be diagnosed with BNP levels.

Cognitive level: Application

Nursing process: Evaluation

Client needs: Physiological Integrity: Physiological Adaptation

6. Answer: 1. ACE inhibitors and beta-blockers

Rationale: Treatment of stage B heart failure is aimed at reduction afterload with ACE inhibitors and reduction of workload on the heart with beta-blockers, as well as antihypertensives and diuretics. Insertion of a defibrillator may be done for stage C heart failure. A patient with stage D heart failure may need hospice referral.

Cognitive level: Analysis

Nursing process: Application

Client needs: Physiological Integrity: Physiological Adaptation

7. Answer: 2. Medications, activity, weight, diet, and symptoms

Rationale: The most important key concepts that patients with heart failure should learn to incorporate into their daily lives follow the acronym MAWDS: medication, activity, weight, diet, and symptoms. Although finances, psychosocial concerns, social support, and spirituality are also important, they are not the key issues.

Cognitive level: Application

Nursing process: Implementation

Client needs: Physiological Integrity: Physiological Adaptation

8. Answer: 3. Depression and anemia

Rationale: Depression, anemia, renal insufficiency, hypertension, coronary heart disease, and sleep apnea have all been shown to worsen the prognosis of patients with heart failure. Patients with heart failure usually experience hypertension, not hypovolemic shock. Liver failure and DVTs are not identified as factors that will increase mortality of heart failure.

Cognitive level: Application

Nursing process: Assessment

Client needs: Physiological Integrity: Physiological Adaptation

9. Answer: 2. Plans for treatment in the final stages of heart failure

Rationale: Discussion about the level of care should occur ahead of time, not at the time of crisis. The nurse needs to address issues of patient comfort and dignity during the terminal stage of heart failure. In end-stage disease, a heart transplant and surgical interventions are not options. Long-term home care management may not be an option for the family and patient.

Cognitive level: Application

Nursing process: Planning

Client needs: Physiological Integrity: Physiological Adaptation

Chapter 43

1. Answer: 1. Intermittent claudication

Rationale: The risk factors, similar to those of heart disease and stroke, include cigarette smoking, diabetes, hyperlipidemia, hypertension, elevated C-reactive protein, and hyperhomocysteinemia. Intermittent claudication, or exercise-induced leg pain, is the most common symptom of peripheral arterial disease. This pain can occur in the buttocks, hip, thigh, or calf, depending on the portion of the arterial tree affected by atherosclerotic disease. With exercise, such as walking, metabolic demands are increased, and the diseased arteries are unable to deliver the needed oxygen to the muscles or to dispose of the metabolic by-product lactic acid. The buildup of lactic acid causes pain in the affected muscle group of the leg. When the walking ceases, or shortly afterward, the pain resolves and exercise may resume.

Cognitive level: Application

Nursing process: Assessment

Client needs: Physiological Integrity: Physiological Adaptation

2. Answer: 3. Teach importance of regular and structured ambulation.

Rationale: The patient with impaired mobility would benefit from being taught the importance of regular and structured ambulation to enhance circulation and promote collateral development. The use of moist heat would aid in comfort for a venous occlusion. Legs should be kept in the dependent position to enhance arterial perfusion. Cool skin to the touch is one of the six Ps of arterial ischemia and should be reported to a health care professional immediately.

Cognitive level: Application

Nursing process: Planning

Client needs: Physiological Integrity: Physiological Adaptation

3. Answer: 2. Dress warmly in cold weather and limit alcohol intake.

Rationale: Nonpharmacologic management of Raynaud's disease is directed toward avoiding known stressors; controlling exposure to extremes in climate; dressing warmly in cold weather; and limiting tobacco, caffeine, and alcohol intake. Some patients may benefit from learning relaxation techniques. Regular physical exercise is important because it improves circulation and warms the body temperature. Some medications, such as beta-blockers, ergot alkaloids, and hormones, can precipitate episodes of vasospasm. There is no cure for Buerger's disease. The primary treatment is directed toward smoking cessation and avoidance of secondhand smoke.

Cognitive level: Application

Nursing process: Planning

Client needs: Physiological Integrity: Physiological Adaptation

4. Answer: 4. Renal impairment due to alterations in blood flow

Rationale: Interruption in blood flow may occur with the endovascular stent or the open approach and the nurse would monitor urine output and BUN and serum creatinine levels. If an embolus were to follow this procedure, the legs are the most common site for perfusion problems. The insertion site for the stent is through a femoral stick and not through an abdominal incision. The hospital stay for this procedure is shorter than for the traditional surgical approach.

Cognitive level: Application

Nursing process: Assessment

Client needs: Physiological Integrity: Physiological Adaptation

5. Answer: 1. The need for early ambulation, use of compression stockings, and range-of-motion exercises

Rationale: Early ambulation, use of compression stockings, and performance of range-of-motion exercises are important nursing processes for this patient. Patients with a deep venous thrombosis with arterial involvement may still use carefully applied compression stockings. Patients benefit from early ambulation.

Cognitive level: Application

Nursing process: Implementation

Client needs: Physiological Integrity: Physiological Adaptation

6. Answer: 2. The signs and symptoms of bleeding

Rationale: Avoiding foods high in vitamin K is indicated for warfarin sodium therapy. Having an INR drawn is indicated for warfarin sodium therapy. Unfractionated heparin is preferred for patients with kidney failure. When low molecular weight heparin is being administered, the patient should be instructed on signs and symptoms of bleeding.

Cognitive level: Application

Nursing process: Implementation

Client needs: Physiological Integrity: Pharmacologic and Parenteral Therapies

7. Answer: 2. Compression stockings will be worn to decrease venous stasis.

Rationale: Bed rest is recommended for the first 24 hours following surgery. The patient may shower the next day following the procedure. Anticoagulants are not a part of the treatment for varicose veins unless there is a condition that warrants these medications.

Cognitive level: Application

Nursing process: Planning

Client needs: Physiological Integrity; Physiological Adaptation

8. Answer: 1. If an aortic aneurysm is diagnosed that is larger than 6 centimeters, surgery will be performed.

Rationale: The physician will monitor the growth of an AAA and will surgically correct when it has reached 5.5 centimeters. If a patient is on steroids, they are discontinued if possible in the medical management of this patient. The infrarenal area is the most common site for the development of an AAA and is repaired with either the surgical or endovascular option.

Cognitive level: Analysis

Nursing process: Assessment

Client needs: Physiological Integrity: Physiological Adaptation

Chapter 44

1. Answer: 4. Diverticulitis

Rationale: This pain pattern in the adult is suggestive of diverticulitis. The pain of acute appendicitis is predominantly in the right lower quadrant. Intussusception and pyloric stenosis are not seen in the adult.

Cognitive level: Analysis

Nursing process: Assessment

Client needs: Physiological Integrity: Reduction of Risk Potential

2. Answer: 1. Inspection

Rationale: The correct order for examination is inspection, auscultation, percussion, and palpation. Bowel sounds should be auscultated prior to percussion to avoid changing the frequency or rate. Light palpation in all quadrants precedes deep palpation.

Cognitive level: Application

Nursing process: Assessment

Client needs: Health Promotion and Maintenance: Prevention/Early Detection of Health Problems

3. Answer: 4. A full bladder

   Rationale: Percussing the abdomen will elicit different sounds. There should be a hollow sound, similar to that of tapping on a watermelon, over the epigastric area and sometimes over the bowels. If this hollow sound is throughout the entire abdomen, it is called tympany and is indicative of an obstruction or distention of the abdomen. This sound is produced by air in the intestine. The liver and a full bladder give off a dull sound, similar to that when percussing a piece of meat.

   Cognitive level: Application

   Nursing process: Assessment

   Client needs: Health Promotion and Maintenance: Prevention/Early Detection of Health Problems

4. Answer: 3. Inflammatory process in the abdomen

   Rationale: Rebound tenderness describes pain that is more prominent when pressure is released and is indicative of an inflammatory process in the abdomen. A negative obturator's sign is a normal finding and further testing may be warranted depending on the initial complaint. A positive Murphy's sign is seen in inflammation of the gallbladder.

   Cognitive level: Application

   Nursing process: Assessment

   Client needs: Health Promotion and Maintenance: Prevention/Early Detection of Health Problems

5. Answer: 2. Ask the patient what caused the abdominal scar.

   Rationale: When obtaining a medical history from patients with gastrointestinal symptoms, past surgeries play a major role. It is also important to correlate this information with the physical exam. At times, patients will forget a surgery, especially if it was many years ago. Therefore, correlating the history with the scars on the abdomen is a helpful tool. When doing the abdominal examination, confirm which operation relates to which scar. This can also trigger more information from the patient. Pay particular attention to the area around the umbilicus, because laparoscopic scars are small and can be very faint.

   Cognitive level: Application

   Nursing process: Assessment

   Client needs: Physiological Integrity: Reduction of Risk Potential

Chapter 45

1. Answer: 1. Increased salivation and bad breath

   Rationale: Vincent's stomatitis, also known as acute necrotizing stomatitis or trench mouth, is a bacterial infection characterized by erythematous ulceration and necrosis of the gingival margins, red gingival papilla, a purulent gray exudate, increased salivation, bad breath, bleeding gums, and pain. Painful red maculae with erythematous halos are seen in the early stage of contact stomatitis, and ulcers covered with a grayish membrane develop in the ulcerative phase of contact stomatitis. Curd-like patches on the tongue and cheek are characteristic of oral candidiasis.

   Cognitive level: Application

Nursing process: Assessment

Client needs: Physiological Integrity: Physiological Adaptation

2. Answer: 1. Premalignant tissue in the esophagus

   Rationale: With repeated exposure of erosive stomach contents, an inflammatory response is initiated. When the inflammation becomes chronic, normal squamous epithelial cells are replaced with columnar epithelium. This new epithelium is called Barrett's epithelium and is a premalignant tissue that increases the risk of esophageal cancer. Esophageal strictures and fine tears may occur with achalasia. Ulcers and inflamed tissue are associated with exacerbations of GERD.

   Cognitive level: Application

   Nursing process: Assessment

   Client needs: Physiological Integrity: Physiological Adaptation

3. Answer: 4. Biopsy of the small intestine

   Rationale: A biopsy of the small intestine is considered the gold standard and currently the most definitive test to diagnose celiac disease. Stools are not Gram stained. The antigliadin antibody is a new test being used, but still not the most definitive. Gastric pH analysis is done when diagnosing GERD.

   Cognitive level: Analysis

   Nursing process: Implementation

   Client needs: Physiological Integrity: Physiological Adaptation

4. Answer: 3. Malabsorption of nutrients often occurs.

   Rationale: Malabsorption of nutrients is more specific to Crohn's. The inflamed tissue occurs most frequently in the jejunum and ileum, which impairs absorption of nutrients. In ulcerative colitis the inflammation occurs in the rectum and sigmoid colon. The loss of exudates from ulcerated tissues in Crohn's further leads to protein losses. Loose watery stools can occur with both disorders. Abdominal pain is usually present in both conditions. Rectal urgency and incontinence can also occur with both conditions.

   Cognitive level: Application

   Nursing process: Planning

   Client needs: Physiological Integrity: Physiological Adaptation

5. Answer: 3. Drinks citrus juice with meals

   Rationale: Foods with a high acidic content or that are spicy will reduce the lower esophageal sphincter tone, causing reflux of acidic stomach contents into the esophagus. A BMI of 21 is normal; obesity can contribute to reflux. Patients who are lactose intolerant often experience abdominal cramping and bloating after eating, not heartburn. Eating high-fiber foods does not cause GERD.

   Cognitive level: Application

   Nursing process: Assessment

   Client needs: Physiological Integrity: Physiological Adaptation

6. Answers:
   1. Daily alcohol intake
   2. A history of irritable bowel disease (IBD)

Rationale: Recent research indicates that daily alcohol consumption increases the risk for colon cancer. IBD causes a chronic inflammation of the bowel, leading to local tissue injury and cancer. A high-fat diet, not low-fat, causes increased deposition of fatty acids within cell membranes and increases intestinal prostaglandins, which stimulate cell proliferation, contributing to cancer. Intake of folic acid, selenium, vitamin D, and calcium reduce the risk for colon cancer. Daily use of NSAIDs helps to reduce inflammation, which in turn reduces cancer risk.

Cognitive level: Application

Nursing process: Planning

Client needs: Physiological Integrity: Reduction of Risk Potential

7. Answer: 4. Place the tube at the shoulder level of patient.

Rationale: Placing the tube at shoulder level reduces the pull of gravity and fluid into the port. The port should be open and patent to allow for air inflow. The port should never be irrigated or plugged. Placing the patient in a high Fowler's position will not correct the problem if the tube is also not positioned higher.

Cognitive level: Application

Nursing process: Implementation

Client needs: Physiological Integrity: Reduction of Risk Potential

8. Answer: 1. Check for signs of hypoglycemia 2 hours after a meal.

Rationale: When the hyperosmolar load of a meal is dumped into the jejunum, there is a rapid rise in blood sugar followed by a release of excessive amounts of insulin. The insulin then causes a secondary hypoglycemia about 2 to 3 hours after eating. Patients with dumping syndrome should rest or even lie down if tolerated for 30 minutes after a meal; ambulation would not be encouraged. Liquids should be taken between meals to reduce the load entering the jejunum. The diet should be low in simple carbohydrates; protein and fats will help to slow transit time and reduce symptoms.

Cognitive level: Analysis

Nursing process: Implementation

Client needs: Physiological Integrity: Physiological Adaptation

9. Answer: 1. Beefy red and moist

Rationale: A stoma should be pink or beefy red and moist without obvious cyanosis or bleeding. It should extend about 2 to 3 cm from the abdominal wall. A slightly purple or pale pink color could be indicative of impaired circulation to the stoma.

Cognitive level: Application

Nursing process: Planning

Client needs: Physiological Integrity: Physiological Adaptation

Chapter 46

1. Answer: 3. "Have you ever had a tattoo?"

Rationale: Hepatitis C is found predominantly in blood, blood products, and transplanted tissue and it has been transmitted by percutaneous exposures, such as tattooing, body piercing, barbering, and folk medicine practices. Traveling in areas where hepatitis A is endemic and eating uncooked shellfish are risks for exposure to hepatitis A. Sharing utensils with a person infected with hepatitis A put the person at risk for hepatitis A, not hepatitis C.

Cognitive level: Application

Nursing process: Implementation

Client needs: Physiological Integrity: Physiological Adaptation

2. Answer: 4. Constant epigastric pain

Rationale: The prodromal phase of hepatitis occurs between exposure to the virus and appearance of jaundice. Symptoms are often vague and include anorexia, nausea, vomiting, malaise, arthralgias, and mild, but constant abdominal, RUQ or epigastric pain. Hyperthermia, not hypothermia, would occur. Appetite is decreased, not increased. Dark-colored urine would be seen during the icteric phase, as serum bilirubin levels rise.

Cognitive level: Application

Nursing process: Assessment

Client needs: Physiological Integrity: Physiological Adaptation

3. Answer: 1. Peripheral edema

Rationale: An albumin level of 2.5 g/dL reflects hypoalbuminemia, which causes a decrease in colloidal osmotic pressure, leading to leakage of fluid into the tissues and is manifested as ascites or peripheral edema in cirrhosis. Lack of vitamin K and prothrombin production by the liver would cause prolonged blood coagulation. The liver's inability to conjugate bilirubin properly would lead to jaundice. Vitamin A may not be absorbed when bile is not produced or released into the duodenum, which may be seen with gallbladder disease or advanced cirrhosis.

Cognitive level: Application

Nursing process: Assessment

Client needs: Physiological Integrity: Physiological Adaptation

4. Answer: 2. Oxazepam, Serax

Rationale: Serax is a benzodiazepine that is not metabolized by the liver, but is still used cautiously to treat agitation. Lactulose is an osmotic laxative and is given to treat elevated ammonia levels and constipation. Protonix is a proton pump inhibitor given to reduce gastric acidity. Vitamin K is stored in the liver and is given to aid in blood clotting since it may be deficient in the patient with cirrhosis.

Cognitive level: Application

Nursing process: Implementation

Client needs: Physiological Integrity: Physiological Adaptation

5. Answer: 1. Provide supportive and comfort measures to the patient and family.

Rationale: An elevated AFP level is indicative of advanced hepatocellular carcinoma and rapid tumor growth.

Survival rates are short term and so quality of life should be provided with supportive and comfort measures. A TIPS is done to treat portal hypertension and ascites that has been refractory to treatment. Liver transplants are only indicated for small tumors without evidence of spread. Protein restriction is sometimes ordered to treat hepatic encephalopathy associated with cirrhosis, and salt restriction is indicated when ascites is present.

Cognitive level: Application

Nursing process: Implementation

Client needs: Physiological Integrity: Physiological Adaptation

6. Answer: 3. The patient has had rapid weight loss secondary to crash dieting.

Rationale: Risk factors for developing gallstones include obesity, high estrogen states, diabetes, hyperlipidemia, cirrhosis, Crohn's disease, rapid weight loss, and bariatric surgery. A high-fiber diet helps to utilize bile and cholesterol and would not predispose the patient to stones. Some drugs, such as oral contraceptives, clofibrate, and hormone replacement therapy can increase the risk of gallstones, but not aminoglycosides. Native American people have a higher risk; people of northern European descent are at greater risk for osteoporosis.

Cognitive level: Application

Nursing process: Assessment

Client needs: Physiological Integrity: Reduction of Risk Potential

7. Answer: 3. Examine abdomen for rigidity and tenderness.

Rationale: Increasing abdominal pain and tenderness may be a sign of intra-abdominal leak of bile or blood so the patient should first be assessed for abdominal tenderness and rigidity, since the opioid analgesia should have been effective in relieving postoperative pain. Administering a second dose of analgesia without first further assessing the pain could mask the cause of the pain. Ambulating the patient could be done after it has been determined the cause of pain is not peritonitis. A side-lying fetal position is helpful for patients with acute pancreatitis.

Cognitive level: Analysis

Nursing process: Implementation

Client needs: Physiological Integrity: Reduction of Risk Potential

8. Answer: 2. Amylase level is normal.

Rationale: In chronic pancreatitis, amylase levels are not always elevated, whereas amylase is usually always elevated with acute pancreatitis. Stools may be clay colored and the abdomen would be tender in both acute and chronic pancreatitis. The blood sugar would most likely be elevated in chronic pancreatitis due to loss of endocrine function with progressive destruction of the gland.

Cognitive level: Analysis

Nursing process: Assessment

Client needs: Physiological Integrity: Reduction of Risk Potential

9. Answer: 2. Clay-colored stools

Rationale: Jaundice occurs in patients with pancreatic cancer when the bile duct becomes blocked from the tumor.

The bilirubin pigment does not enter the duodenum to be changed and excreted in the stool and so the stools are clay colored. The urine becomes dark, not pale, from the pigment. Patients with pancreatic cancer usually lose, not gain, weight. Easy bruising is seen more with liver cirrhosis and cancer.

Cognitive level: Application

Nursing process: Assessment

Client needs: Physiological Integrity: Physiological Adaptation

10. Answer: 2. Eat a diet low in fat.

Rationale: A low-fat diet is indicated because the pancreas is unable to produce the pancreatic enzyme lipase, which is needed for the breakdown of fats. A replacement enzyme such as Viokase may be prescribed. It is not necessary to avoid all analgesics; acetaminophen may be used, but aspirin is usually contraindicated since it may produce gastric irritation. Abstinence from alcohol is mandatory to prevent future attacks of pancreatitis. Eating utensils can be shared.

Cognitive level: Application

Nursing process: Planning

Client needs: Physiological Integrity: Reduction of Risk Potential

Chapter 47

1. Answer: 3. Sodium level is 152 mg/dL.

Rationale: The elevated sodium level would best substantiate a diagnosis of acute renal failure. In acute renal failure the kidneys are unable to excrete electrolytes properly, resulting in the elevated sodium level. A BUN level of 16 is WNL. A calcium level of 8.7 mg/dL is slightly low. A potassium level of 4.8 is WNL and it would be expected to be elevated in ARF.

Cognitive level: Analysis

Nursing process: Assessment

Client needs: Physiological Integrity: Physiological Adaptation

2. Answer: 3. Casts in the urine

Rationale: Pyelonephritis is a sudden inflammation of the kidney and renal pelvis caused by bacteria. Expected abnormalities in the urine include a low specific gravity, high leukocyte count, and casts in the urine. Counts of 100,000 bacteria or greater are often found. A finding of protein in the urine is associated with hydronephritis and glomerulonephritis.

Cognitive level: Application

Nursing process: Assessment

Client needs: Physiological Integrity: Physiological Adaptation

3. Answer: 3. Congestive heart failure

Rationale: Congestive heart failure causes a decrease in cardiac output, which leads to poor renal perfusion, or blood flow coming into the kidney. Contrast dyes can cause acute tubular necrosis, an intrarenal or intrinsic cause of renal failure. Crushing injuries cause breakdown of muscle cells, which can also cause acute tubular necrosis within the kidney. Urinary calculi are a cause of postrenal failure.

Cognitive level: Application

Nursing process: Assessment

Client needs: Physiological Integrity: Physiological Adaptation

4. Answer: 4. Restrict fluid and salt intake.

Rationale: In chronic renal failure (CRF) the kidneys are unable to excrete sodium and water, leading to fluid retention, which contributes to hypertension and increases the workload of the heart. Applying lotion will help to relieve the dry skin and pruritus associated with CRF, but is not specific to the cardiovascular system. A low-fat, low-sodium diet is indicated. Ankles should be evaluated for edema to identify if fluid is being retained, but this is not the best measure to prevent cardiovascular problems.

Cognitive level: Application

Nursing process: Implementation

Client needs: Physiological Integrity: Physiological Adaptation

5. Answer: 3. Self-catheterization

Rationale: A neobladder is formed by creating an internal urine collection reservoir formed from the small intestine and connected to the urethra. Because the neobladder does not empty fully, self-catheterization should be done twice daily. Kegel exercises are taught as part of bladder training to strengthen the muscles when incontinence is a problem. Crede's method is a done to aid in bladder evacuation by applying manual pressure over the lower abdomen. A stoma wafer change would be necessary if the patient had an ileoconduit done.

Cognitive level: Application

Nursing process: Planning

Client needs: Physiological Integrity: Physiological Adaptation

6. Answer: 3. The leg cramps are because of the extra water and salt that is being removed.

Rationale: One complication of hemodialysis is the onset of muscle cramps, which result from the rapid removal of water and sodium. The muscle cramps are not associated with blood transfusions, infections, or amount of protein ingested.

Cognitive level: Analysis

Nursing process: Implementation

Client needs: Physiological Integrity: Physiological Adaptation

Chapter 48

1. Answer: 2. The uterine lining becomes thicker because of estrogen.

Rationale: The menstrual cycle is a complex physiological process that involves the hypothalamus, pituitary gland, ovaries, and endometrium. The cycle begins with the first day of menses. Menses, or vaginal bleeding, occurs when the thickened endometrial lining that was constructed during the previous cycle is sloughed off or shed. As this occurs, the hypothalamus recognizes a need to secrete gonadotropin-releasing hormone. This hormone stimulates the anterior pituitary to release follicle-stimulating

hormone (FSH), which in turn stimulates a few of the follicles that exist on the ovary. From the follicles that first respond to the FSH, one becomes dominant. This growing follicle produces and secretes estrogen. When estrogen peaks, it signals the anterior pituitary to release luteinizing hormone. When LH peaks, ovulation occurs. The dominant follicle extrudes the ovum. The ovum travels to the fallopian tube and into the uterus. Under the influence of estrogen, the uterine lining has been thickening before ovulation. After ovulation, the lining begins to proliferate, that is, it gets thicker.

Cognitive level: Application

Nursing process: Implementation

Client needs: Health Promotion and Maintenance: Growth and Development Through the Life Span

2. Answer: 1. Any other chronic illnesses such as diabetes

Rationale: Medical comorbidities that may impact the reproductive system would include diabetes, hypertension, hepatitis, and HIV. The male with diabetes or hypertension treated with certain antihypertensive drugs may experience impotence. The childhood disease of concern for men is mumps. This viral illness has the potential to affect the testicles, causing sterility. Sexually transmitted infections do not typically cause impotence. The date of first sexual experience would not contribute to the assessment of the patient's current health concern.

Cognitive level: Application

Nursing process: Assessment

Client needs: Health Promotion and Maintenance: Prevention/Early Detection of Health Problems

3. Answer: 2. Occupations and hobbies

Rationale: There is evidence from cohort and case-control research that cigarette smoking and secondhand smoke increase the risks for cervical cancer. Occupations or hobbies where patients have been exposed to hazardous materials increase the risks of male and female infertility. Ask the patient if she has worked around hazardous materials such as excessive heat, radiation, heavy metals, or organic solvents and how she protects herself. There is no evidence to suggest that the amount of exercise or rest/sleep has an impact on fertility.

Cognitive level: Application

Nursing process: Assessment

Client needs: Health Promotion and Maintenance: Growth and Development Through the Life Span

4. Answer: 1. Smegma, a normal finding

Rationale: The examination of the male external genitalia is completed by inspection followed by palpation. If the male is not circumcised, ask the patient to retract the foreskin so that the glans can be inspected. Lesions that may be seen include chancres or ulcers of syphilis, abnormal contour of the scrotum, cancer, warts, herpetic vesicles, or infestation by lice or other insects in the pubic hair. Smegma or a white, cheesy material is a normal finding under the foreskin. Inflammation of the glans is called balanitis. If the patient has reported discharge, but it is not visible, he should be asked to strip the penis to bring discharge to the meatus for culture.

Cognitive level: Analysis

Nursing process: Assessment

Client needs: Health Promotion and Maintenance: Prevention/Early Detection of Health Problems

5. Answer: 2. Hair loss over the mons and vulva is a normal part of the aging process.

Rationale: Over time, decreased estrogen levels in females will contribute to the loss of muscle mass and bone, and increased fat on the abdomen. The breasts will atrophy as the glandular tissue is replaced by fat. The vulva will lose fat and the mons and vulva will lose hair. There may also be graying of the pubic hair.

Cognitive level: Application

Nursing process: Assessment

Client needs: Health Promotion and Maintenance: Growth and Development Through the Life Span

6. Answer: 2. Routine screening for prostate cancer can lead to unnecessary anxiety.

Rationale: For older men, the United States Preventive Services Task Force has found that there is insufficient evidence to recommend for or against routine screening for prostate cancer with serum levels of prostate specific antigen and digital rectal examination of the prostate. Routine screening has been shown to cause unnecessary anxiety, biopsies, and treatments with severe side effects for a cancer that may never have affected the patient. In addition, there continue to be many false-positive PSAs.

Cognitive level: Analysis

Nursing process: Assessment

Client needs: Psychosocial Integrity; Coping and Adaptation

Chapter 49

1. Answer: 3. Doryx

Rationale: Penicillin G is used to treat syphilis. Flagyl is used to treat trichomoniasis. Cleocin is used to treat bacterial vaginosis. Doryx and Zithromax are both used to treat a chlamydia infection.

Cognitive level: Application

Nursing process: Planning

Client needs: Physiological Integrity: Pharmacologic and Parenteral Therapies

2. Answer: 4. Have children before the age of 30

Rationale: Modifiable risk factors for the development of breast cancer include having no children or having children after the age of 30, both of which will increase the risk. The use of underarm antiperspirants and dietary fat intake are considered uncertain, controversial, or unproven risk factors for the development of the disease.

Cognitive level: Application

Nursing process: Implementation

Client needs: Health Promotion and Maintenance: Prevention/Early Detection of Health Problems

3. Answer: 2. Use a mirror to examine the shape and size of each breast.

Rationale: The nurse should instruct the patient to establish a regular schedule of examining and not just at any time during the month. The patient should use a mirror to examine the shape and size of each breast. The breasts should be examined standing (in front of a mirror and in the shower) and lying down on a flat surface. The nurse should include that many lumps are benign and that early detection increases the survival rate.

Cognitive level: Application

Nursing process: Implementation

Client needs: Health Promotion and Maintenance: Prevention/Early Detection of Health Problems

4. Answer: 2. Decreased estrogen production

Rationale: Fibroid tumors of the uterus, also known as leiomyomas and myomas, occur in more than 30% of women 40 to 60 years of age but are almost always benign. The lesions are growths arising from the tissue of the uterine muscle for unknown reasons. They develop slowly in women ages 25 through 40, and tend to enlarge during pregnancy and after menopause; fibroids often decrease on their own, due to decreased estrogen production. Fibroids often cause no symptoms, so many are undiscovered unless the patient has dysfunctional uterine bleeding, pelvic pain, and infertility or pregnancy loss.

Cognitive level: Analysis

Nursing process: Assessment

Client needs: Physiological Integrity: Reduction of Risk Potential

5. Answer: 2. Methotrexate

Rationale: A pessary is a device that, when inserted into the vagina, will help support the vaginal walls, reducing the bulging into the vagina. It is used for management of pelvic support defects such as cystocele, rectocele, and uterine prolapse. Cystoceles and rectoceles are repaired using a procedure called a colporrhaphy. Medical treatment of ectopic pregnancy is preferred over surgical treatment. Methotrexate, a drug often used in cancer treatment, is the current drug of choice and will act on the ectopic cells as it does in cancer treatment: to destroy the cells. It is given if the ectopic pregnancy is unruptured and the patient is in stable condition. It is given intramuscularly and often as an outpatient procedure. Successful treatment may require more than one dose of methotrexate. If surgery is indicated with a ruptured ectopic pregnancy, it consists of repair of the tube if future pregnancies are desired. Removal of the tube may be necessary if repair is not possible or may be desired if future pregnancies are not planned.

Cognitive level: Analysis

Nursing process: Planning

Client needs: Physiological Integrity: Physiological Adaptation

6. Answer: 1. Type 1 diabetes mellitus

Rationale: Female-related causes of infertility are most commonly related to ovulatory dysfunction. Other causes may include hormone imbalance, ovarian cysts, or pelvic infections. Age has also been associated with fertility difficulties. The woman reaches peak fertility in her early 20s, and the likelihood of conceiving after age 35 or 40 is less than 10% per month. In addition to age-related factors, couples at risk for infertility include those with multiple sexual partners, those with a sexually transmitted infection, endometriosis, men with a history of orchitis or a history of undescended testicles, a past history of diethylstilbestrol exposure for both men and women, and those with chronic diseases such as diabetes or thyroid disorders.

Cognitive level: Analysis

Nursing process: Assessment

Client needs: Health Promotion and Maintenance: Growth and Development Through the Life Span

7. Answer: 2. Ambulate

Rationale: An exploratory laparoscopy is a minimally invasive procedure that involves a small incision through which a laparoscope is inserted that allows visualization of the internal organs and structures to assess for disease processes. Carbon dioxide is instilled into the abdomen to elevate the abdominal wall and create a larger work area. After the procedure, the incision is sutured to secure the edges for healing. The patient may experience shoulder pain as the carbon dioxide dissipates from the abdomen. Instruct the patient to sit up and walk to promote gas diffusion and reduce pain.

Cognitive level: Application

Nursing process: Implementation

Client needs: Physiological Integrity: Physiological Adaptation

8. Answer: 4. Locate a SANE immediately.

Rationale: Readily available rape advocates, specially trained law enforcement personnel, and sexual assault nurse examiners (SANEs) should be involved with the patient from the very beginning of the patient's presentation. The importance of careful and meticulous evidence collection is the second priority after ensuring the patient's safety and treatment of injuries. The victim of a sexual assault must consent to the collection of evidence in total or in part. No unnecessary personnel should be involved in handling evidence.

Cognitive level: Application

Nursing process: Implementation

Client needs: Psychosocial Integrity; Psychosocial Adaptation

Chapter 50

1. Answer: 3. Sexually transmitted infections

Rationale: Infection of the epididymis in men younger than 35 years is more likely to be the result of gonococcal, chlamydial, or ureaplasma organisms. A sports injury does not contribute to this condition, mumps can lead to orchitis, and in older men, infection is more likely to be the result of prostatitis, instrumentation of the urinary system, or a structural lesion such as carcinoma of the testis.

Cognitive level: Application

Nursing process: Assessment

Client needs: Physiologic Integrity: Reduction of Risk Potential

2. Answer: 2. Testicular

Rationale: Cancer that forms in the tissue of the testis usually occurs in men between the ages of 20 and 39. It is the most common form of cancer in white men between the ages of 15 and 34.

Cognitive level: Analysis

Nursing process: Assessment

Client needs: Health Promotion and Maintenance: Prevention/Early Detection of Health Problems

3. Answer: 4. Quantifying the symptoms of benign prostatic hypertrophy

Rationale: The American Urological Association (AUA) has developed a symptom index tool that can be used to quantify the symptoms of benign prostatic hypertrophy (BPH) for each patient. The AUA Symptom Score is used both in diagnosing and monitoring therapeutic response. It is a seven-question exploration of symptoms that the patient can answer while waiting to be seen. The score allows the doctor to match treatment options with the severity of the symptoms for each patient. It would focus on sexual dysfunction, urinary tract malignancy, or incontinence.

Cognitive level: Application

Nursing process: Assessment

Client needs: Physiologic Integrity: Reduction of Risk Potential

4. Answer: 4. Checking the drainage tubing for kinks on a regular basis

Rationale: Postsurgical care following a TURP will include maintenance of continuous bladder irrigation to decrease clot formation and bleeding. A three-way catheter is placed after surgery and a steady flow of saline is used to flush the bladder; the amount is determined by the color of outflow and presence of clots. The nurse should be sure that the catheter is secured to the patient's thigh, rather than the bed rail, with a Velcro strap to prevent injury to the urethra and bladder neck. The irrigation and drainage tubing should be checked often for kinks that would block flow. Clot formation will cause obstruction and fluid retention. If a clot should occlude the catheter, the system can be opened and direct irrigation with saline can be done, but this should be a sterile procedure and avoided unless absolutely necessary.

Cognitive level: Application

Nursing process: Planning

Client needs: Physiological Integrity: Reduction of Risk Potential

5. Answer: 3. *Disturbed Body Image*

Rationale: With orchiectomy, the surgery is quick and recovery usually goes well. The loss of the testicles, however, may have a profound effect on the patient. The loss of masculinity can mean depression due to disturbed body image and function with an empty scrotal sac.

Therefore, risk for infection is minimal, mobility should not be affected, nor would impaired urinary elimination be expected.

Cognitive level: Analysis

Nursing process: Planning

Client needs: Psychosocial Integrity: Coping and Adaptation

6. Answer: 1. Encourage to receive a DRE and PSA test annually.

Rationale: It has been recommended that men older than age 50 receive DRE and PSA tests every year. Testicular self-exam should be primarily focused for males under the age of 40. A man's lifetime risk for prostate cancer is 1 in 6, making this disease the most common cancer in men in the United States and the second leading cause of death.

Cognitive level: Application

Nursing process: Implementation

Client needs: Health Promotion and Maintenance: Prevention/Early Detection of Health Problems

Chapter 51

1. Answer: 4. Insulin is a hormone and works through the bloodstream.

Rationale: Because glands are ductless, hormones are released directly into the circulation. The hormone then travels through the bloodstream where it will exert its action on target cells or receptors. A feedback system is a regulatory system that keeps certain activities of body function within a prescribed range to sustain homeostasis. Feedback systems can be positive or negative. In negative feedback, alterations in hormone levels stimulate a series of changes to return the level to normal.

Cognitive level: Application

Nursing process: Implementation

Client needs: Physiological Integrity: Pharmacologic and Parenteral Therapies

2. Answer: 3. Autocrine functioning

Rationale: The endocrine system's functioning is intimately connected to that of the nervous system. Together, they provide a mechanism for communication between cells and organs. This connection is referred to as neuroendocrine regulation. Hormones also function in other ways. If hormones affect cells within the vicinity of their release, it is known as paracrine functioning. Hormones are said to have autocrine functioning when the hormones produced act on the cells that created them. In basal hormone release, small amounts of hormones are released continuously.

Cognitive level: Application

Nursing process: Implementation

Client needs: Health Promotion and Maintenance: Growth and Development Through the Life Span

3. Answer: 3. Epinephrine

Rationale: The adrenal glands have two distinct layers with specialized functions. The outer layer is known as the adrenal medulla. The adrenal medulla produces the catecholamines epinephrine and norepinephrine, substances that play an important role in the body's physiological response to stress. The adrenal cortex secretes corticosteroids of which there are two types, mineralocorticoids and glucocorticoids.

Cognitive level: Analysis

Nursing process: Assessment

Client needs: Physiological Integrity: Physiological Adaptation

4. Answer: 4. Does anyone in your family have diabetes?

Rationale: Exploration of the patient's history is essential. Questioning should seek to assess the onset, characteristics, and severity of symptoms. Along with a review of the entire medical history, family, occupational, and social histories are evaluated. Disorders of the endocrine system tend to occur in a familial pattern. There is a high correlation of diabetes, thyroid disorders, and obesity among families. Knowing this information should assist the interviewer in targeting a more focused assessment. Dietary patterns and involuntary weight losses and gains should be explored. Exposure to chemicals, use of drugs and alcohol, smoking, coping with stress, and behavioral patterns are all areas to be explored.

Cognitive level: Application

Nursing process: Assessment

Client needs: Physiological Integrity: Physiological Adaptation

5. Answer: 3. It checks for ovarian function and might indicate if you are approaching menopause.

Rationale: FSH controls the growth and maturation of ovarian follicles in women and the production of sperm in men. An increased level is seen in ovarian failure of menopause. Blood tests used for adrenal functioning include ACTH stimulation, serum adrenocorticotropic hormone level, serum cortisol level, and urinary cortisol level. The hormones produced from the thyroid include thyroxine, triiodothyronine, and calcitonin. Growth hormone, from the anterior pituitary gland is responsible for the metabolism of carbohydrates, fats, and protein.

Cognitive level: Application

Nursing process: Implementation

Client needs: Physiological Integrity: Physiological Adaptation

Chapter 52

1. Answer: 2. Enterogastrone

Rationale: Enterogastrone is a hormone produced in the gastrointestinal tract. This hormone inhibits secretion and motility. Progesterone is a hormone produced by the placenta and is responsible for gestational support. Angiotensinogen is a hormone produced by the liver that supports the constriction of blood vessels and raises blood pressure. Calcitriol is a hormone produced by the kidney that stimulates calcium absorption from the gastrointestinal tract.

Cognitive level: Analysis

Nursing process: Assessment

Client needs: Physiological Integrity: Reduction of Risk Potential

2. Answer: 1. Giantism

Rationale: Growth hormone is produced by the anterior pituitary gland. An excessive amount of this hormone can lead to giantism in children and adolescents. Acromegaly is the outcome of an excessive amount of growth hormone in adults. Sheehan's syndrome and infertility are seen when there is an underproduction of growth hormone.

Cognitive level: Analysis

Nursing process: Assessment

Client needs: Physiological Integrity: Physiological Adaptation

3. Answer: 2. Take the medication first thing in the morning on an empty stomach.

Rationale: To ensure maximum absorption of the hormone, it is advised that levothyroxine be taken in the early morning on an empty stomach. Synthetic thyroid hormone can be taken safely concurrently with some medications, but patients taking medications such as anticoagulants, beta-blockers, cholesterol-lowering drugs, or seizure control drugs should check with the pharmacist for potential drug interactions. Although administration of levothyroxine will bring thyroid hormone levels within normal limits, it may suppress TSH, which increases the risk of osteoporosis, a side effect that can be avoided by the ingestion of calcium carbonate. However, if the two preparations are taken together, the calcium can interfere with absorption of thyroid hormone. Patients should be advised to take any over-the-counter vitamins, minerals, and antacids at least 4 hours earlier or later than thyroid hormone. Patients also need to be advised that they will be taking thyroid replacement hormone for life. Symptoms of hypothyroidism gradually fade over a period of 3 to 6 weeks as therapy is initiated.

Cognitive level: Application

Nursing process: Implementation

Client needs: Physiological Integrity: Pharmacologic and Parenteral Therapies

4. Answer: 2. Hyperthyroidism

Rationale: Neurological effects of hyperthyroidism include insomnia, jitteriness, shaking, nervousness, irritability, hand tremors, muscle weakness, myalgia, and muscle cramps. Neurological effects of hypothyroidism include drowsiness, fatigue, mental lethargy, forgetfulness, depression, muscular weakness, emotional lability, and paranoia. Patients with pheochromocytoma may experience hypertension, headache, tachycardia, and palpitations. Diabetes insipidus (DI) is characterized by polyuria and polydipsia. Patients with DI present with dry mucous membranes, poor skin turgor, and other signs of dehydration.

Cognitive level: Analysis

Nursing process: Assessment

Client needs: Physiological Integrity: Physiological Adaptation

5. Answer: 2. Strategies to have access to fluids at all times

Rationale: Discharge priorities focus on patient instruction regarding the nature of the disease and the importance of hydration and strategies to ensure the availability of fluid at all times. Medic alert jewelry and a medical identification card should always be carried by the patient so that the patient's condition is known and in emergency situations the treatment is efficient. Patients should be made aware of community resources, including organizations that promote education and research on diabetes insipidus.

Cognitive level: Application

Nursing process: Planning

Client needs: Physiological Integrity: Physiological Adaptation

6. Answer: 3. Consider the onset of myxedema coma and contact the physician.

Rationale: Hypothyroidism is seen clinically at an increasing rate in women over age 50. Clinical manifestations, unless severe, may be too subtle to easily recognize, thus making diagnosis and intervention more difficult. In rare cases, myxedema coma, a rare life-threatening complication in which there is overwhelming cardiopulmonary failure, may be seen in elderly patients, usually precipitated by some untoward event such as infection, trauma, surgery, or neurological disorder. Patients present with all the usual, but exacerbated and serious symptoms of hypothyroidism, and they typically have body temperatures below normal as well. Hypothermia, with body temperature lower than 35°C (95°F), is a key sign that myxedema coma may be impending.

Cognitive level: Analysis

Nursing process: Implementation

Client needs: Physiological Integrity: Physiological Adaptation

7. Answer: 1. What part of your life is terrible?

Rationale: Improvement in clinical management of endocrine diseases is another important frontier in research. Although medical and surgical interventions, as well as hormone replacement therapy, have reaped big rewards in patient management and outcomes, some patients report decreased quality of life despite treatment. This suggests that although hormone levels may appear to be normal after therapy is initiated in endocrine disease, other complex physiological and psychological factors are at play in restoring patients to optimal health. Nurses in ambulatory clinics could play a role in investigating quality of life issues for patients with endocrine disease.

Cognitive level: Application

Nursing process: Assessment

Client needs: Psychosocial Integrity; Coping and Adaptation

Chapter 53

1. Answer: 2. Approximately 20% of Americans over age 60 have diabetes.

Rationale: Approximately 20.9% of the U.S. population over the age of 60 has diabetes. Type 1 accounts for 5% to 10% of diabetes, with type 2 being the most common form. Native Americans, Mexican Americans, and Native Alaskans have a higher incidence of diabetes than

Caucasians, and the highest incidence worldwide occurs in India and China.

Cognitive level: Analysis

Nursing process: Assessment

Client needs: Health Promotion and Maintenance

2. Answer: 3. Fasting blood sugar (FBS) level is 130 mg/dL.

Rationale: Pre-diabetes is determined in two ways: an FBS above normal (80 to 110 mg/dL) or abnormal results of an oral glucose tolerance test. Diabetes is no longer classified by age or treatment regimens. A patient on an oral hypoglycemic agent is classified as having type 2 diabetes. Gestational diabetes does not ensure the patient has pre-diabetes, but it does place her at an increased risk to develop type 2 diabetes later in life.

Cognitive level: Analysis

Nursing process: Assessment

Client needs: Physiological Integrity: Physiological Adaptation

3. Answer: 3. A toddler with a monozygotic twin who has type 1 diabetes.

Rationale: Type 1 diabetes is frequently diagnosed before the age of 20 and it has many genetic, viral, and autoimmune risk factors. There is a 25% to 50% incidence of type 1 diabetes in monozygotic twins, but only a 6% incidence among dizygotic twins. There is an epidemiologic association between viral infections, such as mumps and rubella, and the development of type 1 diabetes, but not bacterial infections. The offspring of a mother with type 1 diabetes has a 3% risk of developing diabetes.

Cognitive level: Analysis

Nursing process: Assessment

Client needs: Physiological Integrity: Reduction of Risk Potential

4. Answer: 2. Abdominal obesity and decreased HDL level

Rationale: The primary abnormalities associated with metabolic syndrome include central or abdominal obesity, insulin resistance, glucose intolerance (which is often manifested as elevated blood sugar levels), increased triglycerides, decreased HDL cholesterol, and hypertension.

Cognitive level: Application

Nursing process: Evaluation

Client needs: Physiological Integrity: Physiological Adaptation

5. Answer: 2. "Avoid doing any isometric exercises."

Rationale: Isometric exercises can raise intraocular pressure and worsen the proliferative retinopathy, so they should be avoided. A dilated eye exam should be done yearly. Protein does not need to be restricted with retinopathy, but may be restricted if renal impairment is present. An ideal target for blood sugar is 80 to 110 mg/dL.

Cognitive level: Application

Nursing process: Implementation

Client needs: Physiological Integrity: Reduction of Risk Potential

6. Answer: 4. Instruct patient to eat within 20 minutes of taking the medication.

Rationale: Patients should eat within 20 minutes of taking a meglitinide to prevent hypoglycemia. They cause a rapid release of insulin, which can lead to hypoglycemia. They should be given before a meal. It is not necessary to check for sulfa allergies; patients taking sulfonylureas should be checked for sulfa allergies.

Cognitive level: Application

Nursing process: Implementation

Client needs: Physiological Integrity: Pharmacologic and Parenteral Therapies

7. Answer: 3. "Exercise may lower your blood sugar for several hours after completing the activity."

Rationale: During exercise, glucose is transported into the muscle for energy use. Patients taking oral hypoglycemic agents and insulin are at increased risk for hypoglycemia following exercise and this may last for several hours. If the blood sugar is 100 mg/dL or less before starting exercise, the patient should consume carbohydrates. If hypoglycemia occurs, the patient should eat complex carbohydrates that will provide a longer supply of energy.

Cognitive level: Application

Nursing process: Implementation

Client needs: Physiological Integrity: Reduction of Risk Potential

8. Answer: 1. Abdominal bloating and diarrhea

Rationale: Alpha glucosidase inhibitors delay the absorption of carbohydrates in the small intestine, which helps to prevent the normal sharp rise in postprandial blood sugar. They cause a number of gastrointestinal side effects, such as diarrhea, flatulence, bloating, and softer stools. They do not cause an elevated temperature. Tremors, palpitations, and fatigue are associated with hypoglycemia, which is seen more with sulfonylureas and meglitinides.

Cognitive level: Application

Nursing process: Evaluation

Client needs: Physiological Integrity: Pharmacologic and Parenteral Therapies

9. Answer: 1. Face is flushed and red.

Rationale: Patients experiencing DKA often have Kussmaul respirations to help correct the acidotic state; the increased levels of $PaCO_2$ have a vasodilating effect, which causes a red, flushed face. Inelastic skin turgor, lethargy, and hypotension can be seen with both DKA and HHS.

Cognitive level: Analysis

Nursing process: Assessment

Client needs: Physiological Integrity: Physiological Adaptation

10. Answer: 3. A male patient with chronic renal failure (CRF).

Rationale: Factors that have been associated with an increased risk for lower extremity ulcers and amputation include patients who have had diabetes for more than 10 years, male gender, poor glucose control, and the presence of cardiovascular, retinal, or renal complications. According to these risk factors, the male patient with CRF is more at risk than a female with cardiovascular disease. The elderly female has fairly well controlled blood sugar and the patient just diagnosed 2 years ago does not meet these criteria.

Cognitive level: Application

Nursing process: Assessment

Client needs: Physiological Integrity: Reduction of Risk Potential

Chapter 54

1. Answer: 3. Flat

Rationale: The long bones of the body include the femur, tibia, fibula, humerus, radius, ulna, clavicle, metacarpals, metatarsals, and phalanges. The short and irregular bones include those within the vertebral column and the carpal and tarsal bones. The flat bones include the ribs, scapula, sternum, and the ilium.

Cognitive level: Analysis

Nursing process: Assessment

Client needs: Physiological Integrity: Reduction of Risk Potential

2. Answer: 2. Social

Rationale: A social history provides additional information about the patient's lifestyle that may affect his or her potential disorder or complaint. The nurse should consider a variety of questions including "Do you use an assistive device such as a cane, walker, or brace?" Characteristics, lengths, exacerbation or diminishment of symptoms, and what is wrong or feared by the patient define the chief complaint. Demographic data may be helpful in determining causes of injury. Biographical data should include age, gender, culture, and educational background.

Cognitive level: Application

Nursing process: Assessment

Client needs: Physiological Integrity: Reduction of Risk Potential

3. Answer: 3. Inspection

Rationale: When inspecting compare corresponding paired joints for symmetry. The nurse should observe for skin color, scars, shape of the site, deformities, muscle atrophy, masses, or swelling. Palpation is used to determine skin temperature, the presence of any nodules, or muscle or joint tenderness and swelling. The assessment technique of percussion is not used for the musculoskeletal status. Range of motion is used to determine the functionality of joints.

Cognitive level: Application

Nursing process: Assessment

Client needs: Health Promotion and Maintenance: Prevention/Early Detection of Health Problems

4. Answer: 2. Shoulder

Rationale: The nurse should explain that testing the range of motion of the shoulders involves having the patient perform seven movements, one of which is testing for adduction by asking the patient to raise the arms above the head with the palms facing each other. The elbow is not assessed by having the patient raise the arms above the head. The wrist and hands are not assessed by ask-

ing the patient to raise the arms above the head with the palms facing each other.

Cognitive level: Application

Nursing process: Assessment

Client needs: Health Promotion and Maintenance: Prevention/Early Detection of Health Problems

5. Answer: 4. Toes pointing inward

Rationale: A normal finding when assessing the feet would be the toes pointing straight and in alignment with the feet, though some may point slightly inward or slightly outward. Abnormal findings include a great toe that is deviated medially and abducted to the first metatarsal with an inflamed bursa or bunion on the medial side or a hallux valgus; an abnormally high arch or a cavus foot; or a wart located over the thick skin of the sole of the foot or a verruca vulgaris.

Cognitive level: Analysis

Nursing process: Assessment

Client needs: Health Promotion and Maintenance: Prevention/Early Detection of Health Problems

6. Answer: 3. External rotation 45 degrees

Rationale: A normal finding is that the patient is able to externally rotate the hip to 45 degrees. Additional normal findings on assessment of the range of motion of the hip include ability to raise the legs to at least 90 degrees of flexion with the knee straight and 120 degrees of flexion with the knee flexed; adduct leg to 20 to 30 degrees and abduct 45 to 50 degrees; internally rotate to 40 degrees and externally rotate to 45 degrees; hyperextend the leg at least 15 degrees; move the extremities against resistance.

Cognitive level: Analysis

Nursing process: Assessment

Client needs: Health Promotion and Maintenance: Prevention/Early Detection of Health Problems

Chapter 55

1. Answer: 3. Stress and strain

Rationale: Two concepts are important to remember: stress and strain. First, stress results when mechanical force is applied to a stretched or compressed bone. Compressive stressors are those of the body weight pushing the bone down, and tensile stresses are from the muscles pulling the bones away from each other. Strain, the second concept, is expressed in length/original length and results as a force that is applied, causing an amount of deformation in the bone relative to its original length.

Cognitive level: Analysis

Nursing process: Assessment

Client needs: Health Promotion and Maintenance

2. Answer: 2. Diet low in calcium and vitamin D

Rationale: A diet low in calcium and vitamin D is a risk factor for both men and women. Low body weight and low body mass index, along with a history of maternal hip fracture, are risk factors affecting men. Anorexia applies to females only.

Cognitive level: Application

Nursing process: Assessment

Client needs: Health Promotion and Maintenance

3. Answer: 1. "Living at my own home increases my chance of a fracture."

    Rationale: In addition to gender (being a female), another factor that increases the risk of hip fracture is living in institutional care, rather than one's own home. Other factors include significant cognitive impairment, certain medications (e.g., anticonvulsants, corticosteroids), personal history and lifestyle factors, certain medical conditions (e.g., type 2 diabetes in women) and low bone mineral density.

    Cognitive level: Application

    Nursing process: Assessment

    Client needs: Safe, Effective Care Environment

4. Answer: 3. Muscle membranes have a protein deficiency or absence of dystrophin.

    Rationale: Muscular dystrophies are a group of genetic myopathies caused by a protein deficiency in muscle membranes. In other words, a person's DNA is not producing a particular protein named dystrophin that is required by muscles and muscle membranes to function properly. Cardiomyopathy leads to heart failure, which is a major cause of death in patients with muscular dystrophy or respiratory failure. The course of Duchenne muscular dystrophy is progressive and usually fatal in the teens or early 20s. The child/adolescent generally has a normal IQ for age with Becker's dystrophy.

    Cognitive level: Analysis

    Nursing process: Evaluation

    Client needs: Health Promotion and Maintenance

5. Answer: 1. Hypokalemic

    Rationale: Hypokalemic myopathy is common in the elderly and is due to a low serum potassium level caused by long-term diuretic use. Other causes of hypokalemic myopathy include potassium deficiency in the diet, excessive alcohol consumption, aldosteronism, intestinal wasting of potassium (malabsorption), and licorice intoxication.

    Cognitive level: Analysis

    Nursing process: Evaluation

    Client needs: Health Promotion and Maintenance

6. Answer: 4. Subjective symptoms

    Rationale: The diagnosis of fibromyalgia is based on the patient's subjective symptoms, as well as a medical and surgical history. Patients with fibromyalgia do not have any other associated musculoskeletal disorder; therefore, arthritis, inflammations, and bursitis should be ruled out. Depression is not uncommon. Family tendency is not used as a diagnostic tool.

    Cognitive level: Application

    Nursing process: Assessment

    Client needs: Health Promotion and Maintenance

Chapter 56

1. Answer: 2. Prevention of injuries

    Rationale: Prevention is the only method to decrease the effects of injuries to the muscles, tendons, ligaments, and bones. Half of all sports-related injuries are preventable. Education and awareness surrounding protective equipment, safer playing environments, and rules designed to prevent injury are important in reducing the frequency and severity of sports injuries. Stretching, warm-up exercises, and strengthening and balance training regimens are key in preventing sports injuries.

    Cognitive level: Application

    Nursing process: Planning

    Client needs: Health Promotion and Maintenance: Prevention/Early Detection of Health Problems

2. Answer: 4. Ossification

    Rationale: A fracture or break in the bone causes a healing cascade beginning with the blood that leaks out at the fracture site. This hematoma is rich in osteoblasts, which make bone. Clotting factors that remain due to the hematoma initiate the formation of a fibrin meshwork that serves as a framework for the fibroblasts and new capillary buds. During cellular proliferation and callus formation, the osteoblasts, or bone-forming cells, multiply and differentiate into the fibrocartilaginous callus. This process begins distal to the fracture where there is greater blood supply. Within a few days a cartilage "collar" is evident around the fracture site. Initially the callus is soft but within the third to fourth week of fracture healing, the bone calcifies as mineral salts are deposited. Ossification is the final lying down of bone after the fracture has been bridged and the fragments are united. Mature bone replaces the callus, and the fracture site feels firm and appears united on radiograph. It is at this point that a cast may be removed.

    Cognitive level: Analysis

    Nursing process: Assessment

    Client needs: Physiological Integrity: Physiological Adaptation

3. Answer: 3. Decrease the potential for contamination.

    Rationale: The important concept is that all open fractures have the potential to be contaminated and this increases the morbidity and mortality of the injury. The time frames vary by institution but many consider 6 to 8 hours to be the maximum time that a contaminated fracture can wait to be taken to the operating room and be "washed out," often referred to as an I&D (i.e., inspection and debridement). Pain relief, assessing, treating injury to surrounding tissue, and casting of the fracture would follow this goal.

    Cognitive level: Analysis

    Nursing process: Planning

    Client needs: Physiological Integrity: Physiological Adaptation

4. Answer: 1. Monitoring hemodynamic status

    Rationale: The nurse should monitor the patient for signs that would indicate the onset of hypovolemic shock and the need for resuscitative measures. An orthopedic trauma patient who has experienced fractures of the pelvis or long bones is at risk for significant bleeding. The nurse should monitor the patient's hemodynamic status including vital signs and laboratory values. A patient may lose as much as 20% of his or her blood volume before exhibiting signs and symptoms of shock. The nurse should monitor the vital signs for an increase in heart rate, decrease in blood pressure, increase in respiratory rate, and a decrease in urine output. Laboratory results will show a decrease in the hemoglobin and hematocrit. Arranging for traction can be delegated, and explaining care is important, however, this is a psychosocial need that should follow hemodynamic stability. Most patients will require intravenous narcotics, such as a patient-controlled analgesic pump.

Cognitive level: Application

Nursing process: Planning

Client needs: Physiological Integrity: Physiological Adaptation

5. Answer: 2. Dark-colored urine

Rationale: Complications associated with rhabdomyolysis include acute renal failure. This occurs due to renal tubular obstruction from the filtration of the released myoglobin. The patient may also exhibit respiratory distress due to muscle weakness and fluid and electrolyte imbalances. Signs and symptoms of rhabdomyolysis may include pain, tenderness, swelling, bruising, and weakness within the affected muscles. Upon assessment the muscles involved may feel soft and flabby. The patient's urine will also become dark in color, referred to as myoglobinuria, as the renal system attempts to filter the myoglobin. They may also develop systemic symptoms including general malaise, fever, nausea and vomiting, confusion, agitation, and anuria as the acute renal failure progresses.

Cognitive level: Analysis

Nursing process: Assessment

Client needs: Physiological Integrity: Physiological Adaptation

6. Answer: 2. You are experiencing something called phantom sensations.

Rationale: There are as many physical/mobility issues to deal with as there are emotional for the patient with an amputation. The patient may have trouble just looking at it, or may have bizarre sensations such as feeling that the foot is cold or itchy when it is not even there. These are called phantom limb sensations and are not caused by narcotic use. The other responses do not acknowledge the patient's concerns or provide a reason.

Cognitive level: Application

Nursing process: Implementation

Client needs: Psychosocial Integrity; Coping and Adaptation

Chapter 57

1. Answers:
    1. Pain level
    2. Pulse quality
    3. Sensation and movement
    4. Color of extremity
    5. Use of muscles

Rationale: The neurovascular assessment should be performed bilaterally so that the affected extremity can be compared to the unaffected extremity. The neurovascu-

lar assessment includes assessment of the five "Ps": pain, pulse, paresthesia, paralysis, and pallor. A complete assessment of circulation and motor and sensory function must be performed. Neurovascular compromise or deterioration should be reported to the surgeon immediately. The nurse should anticipate performing the neurovascular assessment in conjunction with vital signs. Level of consciousness is part of a neurological assessment.

Cognitive level: Application

Nursing process: Assessment

Client needs: Health Promotion and Maintenance

2. Answer: 4. Use an elevated toilet seat in the main bathroom at home.

Rationale: Discharge teaching should include precautions to avoid adduction, flexion, or any movement that may dislocate the hip prosthesis. Precautions include use of an elevated toilet seat, use of a hip abductor pillow while in bed, not bending the hip greater than 90 degrees, not sitting in low chairs, not twisting or turning the body toward the operative side, not turning the leg or foot inward, and keeping the operative leg straight when getting up using arms to push.

Cognitive level: Application

Nursing process: Planning

Client needs: Physiological Integrity: Reduction of Risk Potential

3. Answer: 1. Ace bandages to wrap around the bivalved cast

Rationale: Treatment of compartment syndrome requires release of the constriction to accommodate swelling. If a cast is causing the restriction, it should be bivalved (cut down both sides) with ace wraps or wide tape placed around it to hold it in place. If the constriction is at the fascia level, the patient will require surgery. If the nurse suspects compartment syndrome is present, the surgeon should be notified immediately to prevent permanent disability or loss of limb. If compartment syndrome in an extremity is suspected, the extremity should not be elevated, but should be maintained at the level of the heart to improve perfusion. As edema and engorgement increase, pain increases and is unrelieved by narcotic pain medication administration.

Cognitive level: Application

Nursing process: Implementation

Client needs: Physiological Integrity: Reduction of Risk Potential

4. Answer: 2. A "reacher" tool

Rationale: It is important for the patient not to bend over or flex the affected extremity. A "reacher" tool can be very helpful for picking up an item off the floor, or overhead to avoid standing on a step stool, which requires flexion. A heel lift boot is used to offset development of pressure ulcers for an immobilized patient and the CPM would be indicated following a total knee replacement. Generally, after hip replacement, the patient would use a walker or cane to assist ambulation and avoid flexion by prolonged sitting rather than a wheelchair.

Cognitive level: Application

Nursing process: Assessment

Client needs: Physiological Integrity: Reduction of Risk Potential

5. Answer: 2. "Every hour 2 mg of morphine is delivered continuously."

Rationale: Patient-controlled analgesia (PCA) or around-the-clock pain medication is often utilized in the early postoperative period. The PCA can be set to deliver a constant or basal rate; in addition, the patient is able to self-administer a preset dose at prescribed intervals to achieve pain control. In this scenario, the patient would receive 2 mg of morphine every hour regardless of intermittent use of the pump.

Cognitive level: Analysis

Nursing process: Evaluation

Client needs: Physiological Integrity: Basic Care and Comfort

Chapter 58

1. Answer: 3. It's a common connective tissue disorder.

Rationale: Common connective tissue disorders include lupus erythematosus, gout, and Lyme disease. A term used to describe rheumatic disease is arthritis. A chronic inflammatory process that affects joints is rheumatoid arthritis. An inflammation associated with psoriasis is psoriatic arthritis.

Cognitive level: Application

Nursing process: Implementation

Client needs: Physiological Integrity: Physiological Adaptation

2. Answer: 4. Prevent deformities

Rationale: During the planning stage, goals for a patient with rheumatoid arthritis include prevention of contractures and deformities and provision of health teaching.

Cognitive level: Application

Nursing process: Planning

Client needs: Physiological Integrity: Physiological Adaptation

3. Answer: 1. Reactive arthritis

Rationale: Reactive arthritis is caused by a reaction to an infection somewhere else in the body. Reactive arthritis most commonly causes secondary conditions such as arthritis, uveitis, and urethritis. Other symptoms that may occur are dactylitis, inflammation of the neck and low back, and painless skin lesions termed circinate balanitis.

Cognitive level: Analysis

Nursing process: Assessment

Client needs: Physiological Integrity: Physiological Adaptation

4. Answer: 3. *Imbalanced Nutrition: More than Body Requirements*

Rationale: For the patient with osteoarthritis, priority nursing diagnoses include *Chronic Pain, Impaired Physical Mobility, Risk for Falls, Disturbed Body Image, Readiness for Enhanced Self-Care, Imbalanced Nutrition: More than Body Requirements,* and *Powerlessness.*

Cognitive level: Application

Nursing process: Planning

Client needs: Physiological Integrity: Physiological Adaptation

5. Answer: 2. Gravies

Rationale: Because gouty arthritis is caused by indulging in foods high in purines, it can be controlled by eating a well-balanced, low-calorie, low-purine diet and by reducing alcohol consumption. Foods to be avoided are alcohol, organ meats, and rich foods such as gravies, dried legumes, and anchovies. These foods will increase uric acid in the blood and can lead to uric acid crystal buildup, most often resulting in uric acid crystals located in the joint of the great toe.

Cognitive level: Application

Nursing process: Implementation

Client needs: Physiological Integrity: Physiological Adaptation

6. Answer: 3. Dermatomyositis

Rationale: Myositis may be triggered by an injury, infection, or an autoimmune disease. Polymyositis consists of muscle weakness. Dermatomyositis has the same symptoms as polymyositis except for a distinctive rash over the face, shoulders, arms, and bony prominences. This purplish blue rash can also appear on the eyelids, bridge of the nose, neck, elbows, knees, knuckles, and upper chest.

Cognitive level: Analysis

Nursing process: Assessment

Client needs: Physiological Integrity: Physiological Adaptation

Chapter 59

1. Answer: 3. Bone marrow

Rationale: Deficiencies in functional bone marrow and stem cells can lead to immune deficiency disorders. Lymph nodes and lymph tissue filter debris from the breakdown of cells, bacteria, virus, and fungal antigens. Adenoids are consolidated lymph tissue located in the throat. They function to remove and filter debris, bacteria, and viruses from the upper airways and mouth. The spleen plays a significant role in immune function as part of the lymphatic system. It is comprised of white and red pulp and is involved in hematologic filtration, sequestering of red and white cells, and immune response.

Cognitive level: Analysis

Nursing process: Assessment

Client needs: Physiological Integrity: Physiological Adaptation

2. Answer: 1. The body reacting to self receptors as an antigen

Rationale: Immune tolerance is defined as the ability of the immune system to tolerate all self antigens while retaining the ability to mount an immune response to non-self antigens. Immune tolerance begins during embryonic development of the immune system. Lymphocytes that react with self antigens are selectively eliminated as the immune system develops. This leaves the newborn with B-cell and T-cell lines that do not attack self antigens. Self antigens include HLAs and MHC, as well as several other antigenic particles that are often cell receptors. When the body reacts to self receptors or other cell parts as an antigen, autoimmune disease may result.

Cognitive level: Analysis

Nursing process: Assessment

Client needs: Physiological Integrity: Physiological Adaptation

3. Answer: 1. Produce antibodies in response to exposure to an antigen

Rationale: Plasma cells are differentiated B cells that are found in the plasma and are responsible for production of specific antibodies. Plasma cells produce the antibodies in response to a primary or initial exposure to an antigen. The most common groups of antibodies, also known as immunoglobulins, include immunoglobulin G (IgG), immunoglobulin A (IgA), immunoglobulin M (IgM), immunoglobulin D (IgD), and immunoglobulin E (IgE). Suppressor T cells, also called CD8 cells, slow or stop the immune response. This downregulation is the primary role of suppressor T cells, and is an important part of regulation of the immune system because the ability to stop the production of antibodies and cell destruction is important once the threat of infection has been overcome. Natural killer cells, also referred to as "null cells," are types of T cells that lack CD4 or CD8 external receptors, but are able to directly kill cells or send cytokine messages to start the process of programmed cell death. T-helper 1 cells help regulate immune activity and produce chemicals called cytokines that stimulate cytotoxic cells to destroy mutant and cancer cells.

Cognitive level: Analysis

Nursing process: Assessment

Client needs: Physiological Integrity: Physiological Adaptation

4. Answer: 3. Complement

Rationale: Complement is a group of small proteins made in the liver and present in blood that can interact with cells and each other for a variety of functions. Complement proteins are important in the inflammatory and immune responses. Tumor necrosis factor is a small peptide that is produced by a variety of cells, including granulocytes and lymphocytes. Interferons are proteins made and released by T cells when the invading organism is a virus. Interleukins are lymphokines, chemical mediators released by lymphocytes, that enable the cells of the immune system to communicate and coordinate the immune response.

Cognitive level: Analysis

Nursing process: Assessment

Client needs: Physiological Integrity: Physiological Adaptation

5. Answer: 2. The vaccine is made from killed flu organisms.

Rationale: Acquired immunity involves lymphocyte cells and chemicals that can confer long-term permanent protection against the disease for which the antibodies have been produced. Immunization is a term often used interchangeably with vaccination or inoculation and involves the process of stimulating the immune system to create active immunity for protection against a disease. A vaccine, a preparation that contains an infectious agent or its components, is administered to stimulate the production of antibodies that can prevent infection or create resistance to infection from that agent. Antigens used in vaccines to stimulate an immune response may be inactivated (whole-killed microorganisms or purified products derived from them), live-attenuated (live virus weakened through chemical or physical processes), or recombinant (artificially manufactured from segments of DNA from different sources). Vaccines against influenza, diphtheria, and tetanus use inactivated antigens. Attenuated vaccines include vaccines for measles, mumps, rubella, polio, yellow fever, and varicella. Vaccines are most commonly administered by needle injections, but also can be given by mouth and by aerosol.

Cognitive level: Application

Nursing process: Implementation

Client needs: Health Promotion and Maintenance: Prevention/Early Detection of Health Problems

6. Answer: 2. Antigen presentation

Rationale: B cells must be activated or told to make specific antibodies; this is accomplished through the mechanism of antigen presentation. When a foreign antigen enters a host, the macrophages found in tissue, or monocytes found in blood, ingest the bacterium or virus and then digest the antigen. The macrophage expresses a portion of the digested antigen on its cell surface in the form of a small protein receptor with a part of the bacterial wall attached. T cells are often found near macrophages and can chemically bind to the receptor and accept the antigen onto their surface. T cells then present the antigen to the B cells that have a receptor to match the shape of the antigen. Linking of the T cell and B cell at the site of the antigen activates the B cell to make the appropriately shaped antibody to attach to the antigens.

Cognitive level: Analysis

Nursing process: Assessment

Client needs: Physiological Integrity: Physiological Adaptation

7. Answer: 2. Decreased primary and secondary production of antibodies

Rationale: The effects of aging on the immune system include decreased percentage of suppressor T cells, which means the body cannot downregulate the immune system as quickly; decreased primary and secondary production of antibodies, which means the body has a reduced response to infectious organisms leading to more severe infection; increased auto-antibody production, which means the body shows evidence of more exacerbations of autoimmune disease; and a delayed hypersensitivity response, which means the body has a decreased allergic response.

Cognitive level: Application

Nursing process: Assessment

Client needs: Physiological Integrity: Physiological Adaptation

8. Answer: 4. The patient is at risk for malnutrition.

Rationale: Fatigue and weight loss may be associated with chronic disease processes. Inadequate nutrition affects the ability of the immune cells to function normally and causes immunosuppression. Rapid and significant weight loss that is unintentional is a serious concern because it is a symptom of malignancy. An unintentional weight loss of 10 pounds or more in a month is also an indicator of a need for a nutritional consult. Lymphedema, or nonpitting edema at the site of lymph nodes, indicates inadequate drainage from lymphatic vessels and excessive accumulation of fluid in the interstitial spaces around the lymph vessels. Percussion is helpful in determining if there is inappropriate fluid or a mass in an organ, indicating disease. Symptoms of infection include redness, inflammation, streaking lines, edema, or drainage. Signs of rash or petechiae indicate an allergic response or infection.

Cognitive level: Analysis

Nursing process: Assessment

Client needs: Physiological Integrity; Basic Care and Comfort

9. Answer: 1. Erythrocyte sedimentation rate

Rationale: The erythrocyte sedimentation rate is a serum test that is used to diagnose acute and chronic inflammation, as well as rheumatoid and autoimmune diseases. In the presence of inflammatory mediators, blood proteins are altered and red blood cells stick together and then fall out of solution when the blood sample is spun. This results in an elevated sedimentation rate. This test is ordered when an autoimmune disease is suspected such as rheumatoid arthritis. A protein called rheumatoid factor is often present in the serum of patient's with rheumatoid disease in greater quantities than individuals without autoimmune diseases. Antinuclear antibodies are immunoglobulins (IgG, IgM, IgA) that react with the nuclear portion of leukocytes, forming auto-antibodies against the host's DNA and ribonucleic acid. The presence of these antibodies is indicative of systemic lupus erythematosus. The enzyme-linked immunosorbent assay and the Western blot tests detect the presence of antibodies created in response to infection with the HIV antigen.

Cognitive level: Analysis

Nursing process: Assessment

Client needs: Physiological Integrity: Reduction of Risk Potential

Chapter 60

1. Answer: 2. Hypersensitive reactions are determined by the type of antigen, the time sequence of the reaction, and the immunological response.

Rationale: When the immune system loses self-tolerance, immune hypersensitivity reactions result. The primary

mechanism of an immune deficiency is a genetic disorder that occurred during the embryonic development of the immune system. Immune deficiency is associated with opportunistic infections.

Cognitive level: Analysis

Nursing process: Assessment

Client needs: Physiological Integrity: Physiological Adaptation

2. Answer: 3. The trigger for an autoimmune response is a self-antigen.

Rationale: The primary trigger for a hypersensitive reaction is an environmental antigen. An alloimmune reaction is triggered by antigens from another individual. The symptoms of different categories of hypersensitive responses vary according to the origin of the antigen.

Cognitive level: Analysis

Nursing process: Assessment

Client needs: Physiological Integrity: Physiological Adaptation

3. Answers:

1. AIDS is a syndrome of opportunistic infections that occurs as a final stage in patients infected with HIV.

2. HIV transmission is limited to contact with infected body fluids that have lymphocytes that can harbor HIV.

Rationale: A syndrome of opportunistic infections, AIDS occurs as a final stage in patients infected with HIV. Transmission of HIV is limited to contact with infected body fluids that have lymphocytes that can harbor HIV. AIDS is the end disease manifestation of HIV. HIV precedes AIDS and is associated with the virus's entry into the host's lymphocytes.

Cognitive level: Analysis

Nursing process: Assessment

Client needs: Physiological Integrity, Physiological Adaptation

4. Answers:

1. Subjective assessment to promote the early detection of infection from any body region.

2. Health care providers and family members wash hands before and after patient contact to reduce the risk of opportunistic infection cross-contamination.

3. Encourage hydration and maintenance of weight to support the immune system.

Rationale: Cultures should be obtained prior to starting antibiotics to ensure the appropriate therapy is initiated in a timely manner.

Cognitive level: Application

Nursing process: Assessment

Client needs: Physiological Integrity: Physiological Adaptation

Chapter 61

1. Answer: 2. Anaphylactic

Rationale: Anaphylactic shock is most likely caused by insect bites, medication allergies, food allergies, latex allergies, and idiopathic reactions. Cardiogenic shock is most often caused by myocardial infarction/contusion, ruptured ventricles or papillary muscles, and cardiomyopathy. Neurogenic shock is most often caused by spinal cord or medulla trauma, anesthetic agents, severe emotional stress, or severe pain. Septic shock is most often caused by bacterial or viral infections, immunosuppression, technological causes, or antibiotic misuse.

Cognitive level: Analysis

Nursing process: Assessment

Client needs: Physiological Integrity: Physiological Adaptation

2. Answer: 1. The stress response

Rationale: Glucose metabolism is impaired in a manner similar to that of oxygen metabolism. The result of this impaired metabolism is insulin resistance. This phenomenon has been observed in patients with sepsis and those who are critically ill or injured. The stress response that is initiated by an illness or injury triggers gluconeogenesis to supply glucose energy to heal. The liver and kidneys produce more glucose in response to epinephrine, norepinephrine, glucagons, and cortisol, which are part of the body's stress response. Insulin resistance is unresponsiveness of anabolic processes to the normal effects of insulin and possibly tissue insensitivity to insulin.

Cognitive level: Analysis

Nursing process: Assessment

Client needs: Physiological Integrity: Physiological Adaptation

3. Answer: 2. Low circulating blood volume or hypoglycemia

Rationale: The brain is dependent on both oxygen and glucose. When either of these is not sufficient, an alteration in cerebral perfusion occurs. The patient will suffer an altered mental status, which will eventually lead to coma and even death.

Cognitive level: Analysis

Nursing process: Assessment

Client needs: Physiological Integrity: Physiological Adaptation

4. Answer: 2. 86-year-old female with abdominal injuries

Rationale: Patient risk factors such as significant injuries, catastrophic illness, age, and allergies must be quickly acknowledged. It is interesting that both the very young and aged share similar risk factors for developing shock including compromised immune systems due to age, fluid shifts, and an integumentary system that may not afford needed protection.

Cognitive level: Analysis

Nursing process: Assessment

Client needs: Physiological Integrity: Physiological Adaptation

5. Answer: 1. Normal saline

Rationale: Fluids that are used for resuscitation include lactated Ringer's solution or normal saline. The type of fluid used will depend on the provider's preference, because at present the research has not clearly defined one more favorably over the other. The initial amount of fluid will range from 2 to 3 liters for an adult if the cause of the shock is unknown. If the patient has sustained blood loss, then administration of blood and blood products will be needed; however, patients who have sustained blood loss greater than 2 liters should not receive excessive fluid resuscitation from either colloids or crystalloids until surgical management of bleeding has been initiated because it dilutes the existing volume and further diminishes oxygen-carrying capacity.

Cognitive level: Application

Nursing process: Implementation

Client needs: Physiological Integrity: Physiological Adaptation

6. Answer: 2. Nitroprusside sodium

Rationale: Dopamine and dobutamine hydrochloride improve cardiac contractility. Nitroprusside sodium and nitrates decrease afterload. Epinephrine and norepinephrine bitartrate increase afterload.

Cognitive level: Application

Nursing process: Planning

Client needs: Physiological Integrity: Physiological Adaptation

7. Answer: 1. Systemic inflammatory response syndrome

Rationale: Systemic inflammatory response syndrome (SIRS) is an organized immune response that can be triggered by infectious or noninfectious clinical insults including burns, pancreatitis, acute respiratory distress syndrome, surgery, and trauma. Sepsis is a clinical syndrome defined as the presence of SIRS associated with a confirmed infectious process. Septic shock is a state of acute circulatory failure characterized by persistent hypotension unexplained by other causes, for example, despite the fact that adequate fluids have been administered. Severe sepsis is defined as sepsis or the presence of a confirmed infection and a systemic inflammatory response, and single or multiple organ failure. The patient is hypotensive, which causes hypoperfusion abnormalities such as arterial hypoxemia, acute oliguria, and coagulation abnormalities.

Cognitive level: Analysis

Nursing process: Assessment

Client needs: Physiological Integrity: Physiological Adaptation

8. Answer: 4. Central venous pressure 10 mmHg

Rationale: Fluid resuscitation should be directed to achieve a central venous pressure reading of 8 to 12 mmHg, a mean arterial pressure of greater than or equal to 65 mmHg, a urine output of greater than or equal to 0.5 mL/kg, and a central venous or mixed venous oxygen saturation of greater than or equal to 70%.

Cognitive level: Analysis

Nursing process: Evaluation

Client needs: Physiological Integrity: Physiological Adaptation

9. Answer: 1. MODS

Rationale: Reperfusion injury, which results from the reestablishment of blood flow after ischemia, causes conversion of the enzyme xanthine dehydrogenase to xanthine oxidase to form oxygen free radicals with oxygen when hypoperfused tissues are reperfused. These oxygen radicals attack already damaged tissues and can lead to MODS.

Cognitive level: Analysis

Nursing process: Assessment

Client needs: Physiological Integrity: Physiological Adaptation

10. Answer: 4. Frequent assessment of vital signs and clinical status

Rationale: Frequent monitoring and assessment to trend changes in vital signs and clinical manifestations will provide the most reliable information about early signs of MODS. Nursing care needs to be focused on decreasing oxygen demand, which includes pain and anxiety management as well as spacing activity to allow for long periods of rest. The nurse should assess for signs of pain and anxiety and medicate as needed. Tachycardia related to pain and anxiety increases oxygen consumption due to the stress imposed on the body by pain. Positioning of the patient is important to prevent the complications that occur with immobility such as skin breakdown, pulmonary congestion, and pooling of blood and secretions. Hypermetabolism causes loss of muscle, so it is important to prevent additional loss of movement. Patients should receive active and passive ROM exercises to retain strength and joint motion.

Cognitive level: Application

Nursing process: Planning

Client needs: Physiological Integrity: Physiological Adaptation

Chapter 62

1. Answer: 1. The stem cell is a primitive cell located in the bone marrow that is the precursor of red blood cells, white blood cells, and platelets.

Rationale: Stem cells are primitive cells located in the bone marrow that are the precursor to all blood lines. When stimulated these cells undergo a series of cell divisions and differentiations to become the appropriate respective cell in a process known as hematopoiesis. However, when the bone marrow has been destroyed, as with certain diseases or medications, the liver and spleen can produce blood cells in a process known as extramedullary hematopoiesis. Although the blood is considered to be a type of connective tissue, it has two important functions. The first is to transport oxygen, nutrition, secretory products, and waste products, but the second is to house and transport the immunologic products that are critical to the body's defense against infections. The proportion of red bone marrow diminishes and is replaced by yellow bone marrow as the patient ages. However, in the healthy individual the active red bone marrow can replace the fatty yellow bone marrow if an increase in blood cell production is required.

Cognitive level: Analysis

Nursing process: Assessment

Client needs: Health Promotion and Maintenance; Physiological Integrity

2. Answer: 3. "The cells of the reticuloendothelial system facilitate blood clotting and initiate the inflammatory and immune responses."

Rationale: White blood cells are only found in small amounts in the blood unless they are needed. Instead, they can be found in the bone marrow, lungs, liver, spleen, and lymph nodes as developing and mature cells. Reticulocytes are small, immature red blood cells that are released whenever there is an increased demand for red cells. The red blood cells, or erythrocytes, are responsible for transporting, maintaining the chemical integrity of, and distributing oxygen-carrying hemoglobin to the body's tissues. One function of the reticuloendothelial system is to provide phagocytic cells for the inflammatory and immune responses, but these cells do not facilitate blood clotting.

Cognitive level: Application

Nursing process: Evaluation

Client needs: Physiological Integrity; Physiological Adaptation

3. Answer: 4. MCH, MCV, MCHC

Rationale: The PT (prothrombin time) and aPTT (activated partial thromboplastin time) are useful coagulation studies, and the PLT determines the numbers of platelets. The HGB (hemoglobin) and HCT (hematocrit) can be reduced with anemia, but this does not help classify the type of anemia. The ANC (absolute neutrophil count) is helpful when measuring the proportion of white blood cells that are available for an initial immune response. Red blood cell (RBC) count alone is not a reliable indicator of RBC function or adequacy. The RDW (red blood cell distribution width) measures the consistency of RBC size, and the white blood cell (WBC) count determines the number of leukocytes. The MCH (mean corpuscular hemoglobin), MCV (mean corpuscular volume), and MCHC (mean corpuscular hemoglobin concentration) are used primarily for the classification of anemia and delineating the likely cause.

Cognitive level: Application

Nursing process: Planning

Client needs: Physiological Integrity

4. Answer: 1. HCT 28%

Rationale: A HCT level of 28% is dangerously low for any patient and should immediately be reported to the health care provider. The other values, PLT 400,000/μL, WBC 10,000/μL, and MCH 30 pg/dL, are all within normal limits for either a male or female patient.

Cognitive level: Application

Nursing process: Analysis

Client needs: Health Promotion and Maintenance; Physiological Integrity

5. Answer: 2. An increase in the total white blood cell count because of the proliferation of juvenile band and immature blast cells

Rationale: A shift to the left indicates that the total white blood cell count has increased because of the proliferation of juvenile band and immature blast cells. This phenomenon is the result of bone marrow stimulation to release large amounts of leukocytes, usually in response to severe infection. The absolute neutrophil count (ANC) measures the proportion of white blood cells that are available for use in a first response immune reaction. The mean corpuscular hemoglobin (MCH) and mean corpuscular hemoglobin concentration (MCHC) measure the hemoglobin proportion in an erythrocyte, indicating the efficacy of interaction between the hemoglobin molecule and the red cell. Numerous clotting studies are used to indicate problems within the clotting cascade, and these are not related to a shift to the left.

Cognitive level: Analysis

Nursing process: Assessment

Client needs: Physiological Integrity

6. Answer: 2. Vascular contraction, intrinsic adenosine diphosphate release, prothrombin conversion into thrombin, fibrinogen conversion into fibrin

Rationale: The first step in primary hemostasis is vascular contraction, followed by platelet adhesion and formation of a soft aggregate plug, respectively. The initial platelets that respond to the site of insult release intrinsic adenosine diphosphate, which causes more platelets to aggregate together. Once the short-lived primary hemostasis has occurred, secondary hemostasis begins through either the intrinsic or extrinsic pathway. During these mechanisms Factor XII activates Factor XI; active Factor VII and active Factor XI start a cascade of events that eventually activate Factor X; and active Factor X, along with Factor III, Factor V, Ca^{2+}, and platelet thromboplastic factor, activates prothrombin activator. Also, prothrombin activator converts prothrombin into thrombin, and thrombin converts fibrinogen into fibrin.

Cognitive level: Analysis

Nursing process: Assessment

Client needs: Physiological Integrity

7. Answer: 3. "What medications are you currently taking?"

Rationale: Medications that are myelosuppressive in nature or those that affect bleeding times, such as aspirin, can suppress or alter blood cell production or function, respectively. The patient's allergies to shellfish or IV contrast material are irrelevant to hematologic function. Cholecystectomy, assuming minimal blood loss or complications, is also unrelated to hematologic function. A widened pulse pressure or tachycardia may indicate compensatory mechanisms during states of hypoxia, such as with anemia, but heart disease is not known to cause or be caused by a primary hematologic issue.

Cognitive level: Application

Nursing process: Assessment

Client needs: Health Promotion and Maintenance

Chapter 63

1. Answer: 3. Reduction in hematopoietic stem cells

Rationale: Hematopoietic stem cells (HSCs) reside largely in the spongy bone marrow of the femurs, hips, ribs, sternum, and other long bones, while a small volume of HSCs circulates in the peripheral blood. HSCs may be thought of as the common ancestor cell of all of the blood cell lines. Although HSCs eventually give rise to mature red blood cells, platelets, and white cells, they themselves do not possess the full capabilities of oxygen transportation, clotting, or immune response associated with their more mature progeny, the erythrocytes, platelets, and leukocytes.

Cognitive level: Analysis

Nursing process: Assessment

Client needs: Physiological Integrity: Reduction of Risk Potential

2. Answer: 1. Reduced red blood cell production

Rationale: Dietary elements play a key role in red blood cell production. Deficiencies in any of these elements can negatively affect erythropoiesis. This blood cell development is highly dependent on sufficient quantities of metals such as iron, cobalt, and manganese, vitamins B_{12}, B_6, C, E, folate, riboflavin, pantothenic acid, and thiamin, amino acids, and carbohydrates. Although cellular growth requires all of these elements, vitamin B_{12}, folate, and iron play particularly pivotal roles in erythropoiesis. Folate and vitamin B_{12} are required for the extensive DNA synthesis that occurs with erythropoiesis. All proliferating cells require iron, but the iron requirements of erythroid cells in the late basophilic erythroblast through reticulocyte stages, when hemoglobin is synthesized and accumulates, are much greater than for all other cell types. Disease such as megaloblastic anemia and iron deficiency anemia result when sufficient supplies do not exist to support erythropoiesis.

Cognitive level: Analysis

Nursing process: Assessment

Client needs: Physiological Integrity: Reduction of Risk Potential

3. Answer: 4. Glossitis

Rationale: Because the highly efficient iron storage system provides a rich reservoir for active metabolic needs, early iron deficiency anemia often does not produce bothersome symptoms. As with all anemia, the severity of the symptoms correlates with the degree of hemoglobin deficiency, which in turn correlates with the volume of total iron body stores. As erythropoiesis becomes increasingly hampered, the patient may present with the general manifestations of anemia such as fatigue, pallor, shortness of breath, cold intolerance, headache, and activity intolerance. When iron stores fall critically low as to impact epithelial cell production, the patient may present with symptoms uniquely indicative of iron deficiency anemia including pica or clay eating, glossitis or tongue inflammation, gastric atrophy, stomatitis, ice eating or pagophagia, and leg cramping.

Cognitive level: Application

Nursing process: Assessment

Client needs: Physiological Integrity: Physiological Adaptation

4. Answer: 2. RBC mass being lost at the same rate as total blood volume

Rationale: For sudden blood loss, hematocrit values may not accurately indicate the severity of the problem because RBC mass is lost at the same rate as total blood volume, thus the percentage of RBCs in the blood is unaffected. After 2 to 3 days when then body is able to initiate the compensatory mechanism of increasing plasma volume, RBCs become diluted as reflected by decreasing erythrocyte, hemoglobin, and hematocrit values.

Cognitive level: Analysis

Nursing process: Assessment

Client needs: Physiological Integrity: Physiological Adaptation

5. Answer: 4. Frequent skin and oral mucosa assessment

Rationale: Nursing interventions for a patient with thrombocytopenia should focus on reducing the risk for bleeding. This would include assessing the color and presence of blood in the urine and stool. Additional interventions would include frequent vital signs, breath sounds, and abdominal and neurological assessments.

Cognitive level: Application

Nursing process: Planning

Client needs: Physiological Integrity: Physiological Adaptation

6. Answer: 3. Persistent and last for days or weeks

Rationale: The hallmark clinical presentation of hemophilia is prolonged bleeding and inability to form clots in response to injury, both of which can appear and persist for days to weeks. For patients with severe disease completely lacking any Factor VIII or Factor IX, such bleeding can have serious life-threatening consequences. Distinguished from the disease of primary hemostasis, which causes increased bruising and superficial hemorrhages in the integumentary, people with hemophilia typically suffer from bleeding deep in the tissues. Typically, bleeding sites include joints and organs. If left uncontrolled the internal bleeding can cause severe pressure on closed compartments. Serious consequences of internal bleeding into closed spaces include increased intracranial pressure, hemiarthrosis leading to compartment syndrome, and oropharyngeal bleeding. The eventual sequelae following each of these situations can cause lifetime disability. Increased intracranial pressure can cause ischemia and brain tissue damage. Bleeding into the joints predisposes the patient to arthritis, synovial tissue damage, and joint malformation. Oropharyngeal bleeding may occlude the airway so severely as to require intubation.

Cognitive level: Analysis

Nursing process: Planning

Client needs: Physiological Integrity: Physiological Adaptation

Chapter 64

1. Answer: 2. Instruct in the avoidance of tobacco, excessive alcohol, and a high-fat diet.

Rationale: The risk factors for the development of cancer can be divided into endogenous and exogenous causes. Endogenous causes include increasing incidence with age, an occasional genetic link, and the need for immunocompetence to identify antigens. Exogenous causes include exposure to drugs, chemicals, and tobacco smoke; a diet high in fat and low in fiber; multiple sex partners; large consumption of ethyl alcohol; exposure to ultraviolet and ionizing radiation; and exposure to viruses that have been linked to cancer. The effects of psychosocial stress have yet to be linked specifically to the development of cancer.

Cognitive level: Application

Nursing process: Implementation

Client needs: Health Promotion and Maintenance: Reduction of Risk Potential

2. Answer: 3. Angiogenesis

Rationale: Mechanisms of metastasis include angiogenesis, migration, cell attachment, cell invasion, and growth factors. Angiogenesis is the creation of new blood vessels due to migration and proliferation of endothelial cells from existing blood vessels. New blood vessels provide nutrients, protein growth factors, and oxygen to the tumor mass.

Cognitive level: Application

Nursing process: Implementation

Client needs: Physiological Integrity: Physiological Adaptation

3. Answer: 2. Prostate

Rationale: The treatment for prostate cancer includes surgery or a radical prostatectomy, radiotherapy to include external beam or brachytherapy, cryotherapy, chemotherapy, and expectant management or "watchful waiting."

Cognitive level: Analysis

Nursing process: Assessment

Client needs: Physiological Integrity: Physiological Adaptation

4. Answer: 3. Use strict aseptic technique when caring for venous access devices.

Rationale: The patient with cancer is at risk for the development of an infection. Care for this patient should include the avoidance of rectal procedures, including taking rectal temperatures. Foods that could harbor bacteria should be avoided such as raw meat and fresh fruits and vegetables. Intramuscular injections should be avoided. Strict aseptic technique should be used at all times when caring for venous access devices, urinary catheters, and other monitoring devices.

Cognitive level: Application

Nursing process: Planning

Client needs: Physiological Integrity: Reduction of Risk Potential

5. Answer: 1. Cluster care activities to increase rest periods.

Rationale: Many patients who receive radiotherapy experience fatigue. The exact causative mechanism is unknown, although it is thought to be due to the result of tumor breakdown, which releases by-products into the bloodstream. Another explanation for the development of fatigue is the increase in basal metabolic rate consuming the body's energy stores. Fatigue typically begins during the third or fourth week of treatment and will gradually wane once the treatment is over. The loss of energy and feeling of tiredness tend to be cumulative and have a significant impact on patients' quality of life. Patient education regarding the side effects of radiation begins before treatment and needs to continue once it is over. Teaching patients that side effects should be expected may decrease their fear that treatment is ineffective. Nursing care needs to be designed with energy conservation in mind. Clustering patient care activities together will allow for prolonged periods of rest for patients who are experiencing fatigue. Teaching patients and their caregivers these principles will assist the patient in coping with the tiredness experienced with fatigue while at home.

Cognitive level: Application

Nursing process: Implementation

Client needs: Physiological Integrity: Physiological Adaptation

6. Answer: 3. Alter the immunologic relationship between the tumor and the patient.

Rationale: Biotherapy is known as treatment with agents whose origin, mostly mammal, is from biologic sources and/or affecting biologic responses. Biotherapy has emerged since the 1980s as another treatment option for patients with cancer who are receiving high-dose chemotherapy and transplantation. Nurses caring for patients receiving biotherapy need to possess an understanding of the immune system before they can begin to comprehend the rationale behind this unique treatment modality and the primary agents currently used. Although the mechanism of action varies with each type of biologic response modifier, the goal is the same: to destroy or halt the malignant growth of a tumor. A therapeutic effect is accomplished by altering the immunologic relationship between the tumor and the patient.

Cognitive level: Analysis

Nursing process: Planning

Client needs: Physiological Integrity: Physiological Adaptation

Chapter 65

1. Answer: 4. Vitamin D deficiency

Rationale: Functions of the skin include retarding the loss of body heat and fluids, assisting in the control of body temperature, functioning as an excretory organ, and functioning as a synthesizer of vitamin D when sunlight reacts with cholesterol.

Cognitive level: Analysis

Nursing process: Assessment

Client needs: Health Promotion and Maintenance: Prevention/Early Detection of Health Problems

2. Answer: 3. Biographic and demographic data

Rationale: Biographic and demographic data include data such as the patient's name, address, telephone number, Social Security number, contact person, age, gender, race or ethnic origin, marital status, birthplace, occupation, level of education, and religious affiliation. Examples of biographic and demographic data that may be significant to assessment of the skin include travel to different environments such as when camping or travel to rural areas of the world. The patient's current issue or the reason for seeking health care is referred to as the chief complaint. The reason for obtaining information about the past medical history is to identify the patient's entire past relevant health problems. Past illnesses could possibly have some effect on the patient's current health. The nursing assessment includes questions about major illnesses such as diabetes, cardiovascular disease, and infectious diseases. Patients with diabetes are prone to skin breakdown and delayed wound healing. Patients with cardiovascular disease may have clubbed nail beds. Infectious diseases such as cellulitis have skin manifestations, which assist with the diagnosis.

Cognitive level: Application

Nursing process: Assessment

Client needs: Health Promotion and Maintenance: Prevention/Early Detection of Health Problems

3. Answer: 4. Social history

Rationale: Social history includes use of alcohol or street drugs that can have adverse effects on the condition of the patient's skin. The presence of certain cutaneous lesions in a patient should prompt an investigation into the patient's drinking and drug habits. If drug use is suspected due to the presence of a cutaneous lesion, the nurse needs to inquire about skin popping. Skin popping is a technique used by individuals to administer illicit drugs. Skin popping is a significant risk factor in skin and soft tissue infections, which are common among injection drug users.

Cognitive level: Application

Nursing process: Assessment

Client needs: Physiological Integrity: Physiological Adaptation

4. Answer: 3. Inspect and palpate the skin at the same time.

Rationale: The assessment should proceed in an orderly fashion, beginning with an examination of the most frequently exposed areas such as the face, hands, arms, legs, and feet. The nurse inspects the skin while the patient is in a sitting or lying position with all clothes removed except an examination or hospital gown. The nurse will inspect and palpate simultaneously.

Cognitive level: Application

Nursing process: Assessment

Client needs: Health Promotion and Maintenance: Prevention/Early Detection of Health Problems

5. Answer: 4. Normal findings

Rationale: The nail surface is normally slightly curved with the posterior and lateral folds smooth and rounded. The nail edges should be smooth, rounded, and clean. The normal nail bed angle is 160 degrees. The nail base is firm to palpation. A nail bed with greater than a 160-degree angle suggests a clubbed nail. Clubbing of nails indicates a state of chronic hypoxia and is often seen with congenital and adult heart disease and chronic obstructive pulmonary disease. The surface of the nail should be smooth and nonbrittle, with no splitting. Pits, transverse grooves, or lines may indicate a nutritional deficiency. Patients with arterial insufficiency may have thickened, ridged nails.

Cognitive level: Application

Nursing process: Assessment

Client needs: Health Promotion and Maintenance: Prevention/Early Detection of Health Problems

6. Answer: 3. Keloid

Rationale: A fissure is a linear crack or break from the epidermis to the dermis. A scale is an abundance of dry or oily keratinized cells. A keloid results from the overproduction of scar tissue that extends laterally beyond the initial wound; it is usually raised and smooth in appearance. A cherry angioma is a distinct benign vascular lesion.

Cognitive level: Analysis

Nursing process: Assessment

Client needs: Physiological Integrity: Reduction of Risk Potential

7. Answer: 4. Vitiligo

Rationale: Jaundice is a yellowish discoloration of the skin, sclera, and mucous membranes that is often associated with increased amounts of bilirubin in the blood. Pallor is paleness of the skin that occurs when the red-pink tones from the oxygenated hemoglobin in the blood are lost. Petechiae are pinpoint purpuric lesions of the skin. Vitiligo is the absence of pigmentation in a circumscribed area.

Cognitive level: Analysis

Nursing process: Assessment

Client needs: Physiological Integrity: Reduction of Risk Potential

Chapter 66

1. Answer: 1. Atopic dermatitis

Rationale: Atopic dermatitis is characterized by severe itching. Treatment involves controlling the aggravating factors and treating the rash. It is important to moisturize the skin to maintain the skin barrier. Bathing should be held to a minimum; however, when bathing, the patient should use tepid water and mild, unscented soap such as Cetaphil or Dove.

Cognitive level: Analysis

Nursing process: Implementation

Client needs: Physiological Integrity: Basic Care and Comfort

2. Answer: 2. Eat foods high in vitamin C, iron, and zinc.

Rationale: The nurse should instruct the patient to maintain a high-calorie, high-protein, well-balanced diet. Include vitamin C, iron, and zinc in the diet. Avoid foods that cause hypersensitivity reactions.

Cognitive level: Application

Nursing process: Implementation

Client needs: Physiological Integrity: Physiological Adaptation

3. Answer: 4. Instruct in the use of sunscreen.

Rationale: The sun, along with other pollutants in the air, can irritate and damage the skin, with most of the damage occurring before the age of 18. Nearly 80% of this

damage can be prevented if sunscreen is applied properly in those first 18 years of life.

Cognitive level: Application

Nursing process: Implementation

Client needs: Health Promotion and Maintenance: Prevention/Early Detection of Health Problems

4. Answer: 1. Rub the medication into wet skin thoroughly.

Rationale: Topical corticosteroids should be applied in a thin layer and rubbed in thoroughly on wet skin. Retinoic acid can be irritating to the skin and produce phototoxicity. Systemic antihistamines can cause drowsiness.

Cognitive level: Application

Nursing process: Implementation

Client needs: Physiological Integrity: Pharmacologic and Parenteral Therapies

5. Answer: 1. Signs of infection

Rationale: The focus of nursing care is to prevent problems or recognize complications early so they can be successfully treated. The nurse must assess the patient frequently, noting changes in skin color, texture, wound size, drainage, and temperature. Analysis of the data collected during assessment will provide a basis for determining a treatment plan and assessing response to treatment. Patients with skin disorders may develop problems with hydration, fluid balance, or nutrition. Fluid loss through wounds leads to dehydration and electrolyte imbalances. The skin also provides protection against infection, so when its barrier is broken, infection becomes more likely. It is very important to assess for signs of infection both in the wound and systemically. Clinical manifestations of infection include fever, increased redness or drainage, increased pain, changes in odor or color of drainage, increased white blood cell count, and increased tissue erosion. If the infecting organism is contagious, such as occurs with staphylococcus, isolation procedures may be needed.

Cognitive level: Application

Nursing process: Assessment

Client needs: Physiological Integrity: Reduction of Risk Potential

6. Answer: 3. There are light materials that you could wear to protect your arms while still enjoying the summer activities.

Rationale: Psychological assessment needs to be uppermost in the mind of the nurse as care is given to patients with skin disorders. The appearance of the skin affects self-esteem and body image. Skin disorders can cause the patient to withdraw from social situations. Society can be unkind to people who have scars or rashes with an unpleasant appearance. Some individuals may withdraw from the patient, fearing the disorder is contagious. Patients should be provided with an open, supportive environment in which they are comfortable voicing their concerns.

Cognitive level: Application

Nursing process: Implementation

Client needs: Psychosocial Integrity: Coping and Adaptation

7. Answer: 2. This is a normal part of aging.

   Rationale: Many anatomic changes occur during the aging process: Skin loses elasticity and water content; the texture and turgor of the skin change; the retaining ligaments of the soft tissue of the face weaken; the face loses volume as a result of decreased subcutaneous adipose stores and muscle mass; facial bones undergo resorption; the eye orbit changes shape, allowing for positional changes of the eye globe; the face becomes elongated and flattened; and smoking, genetics, and sun exposure contribute to the loss of skin elasticity and wrinkle formation.

   Cognitive level: Application

   Nursing process: Implementation

   Client needs: Health Promotion and Maintenance: Growth and Development Through the Life Span

Chapter 67

1. Answer: 3. Proliferation

   Rationale: Homeostasis is the tendency of the human body to maintain stability, and maintaining stability is the first reaction when a wound occurs. The inflammatory phase of wound healing begins at the time of the injury or surgery. The purpose of this critical phase is to prepare the site for growth of new tissue. The proliferative phase is the next phase in the healing process. Reconstruction occurs at this phase. It can last up to 3 weeks after the inflammatory phase in a normal, healthy person. Growth factors originating from injured vessels stimulate the formation of vascular buds and regrowth of vascular loops. Stimulated endothelial cells multiply and form tubular structures, differentiating into arterioles or venules, a process referred to as angiogenesis. These new blood vessels can begin to form in a wound within 3 days of injury, provided there is sufficient blood circulation to the wound bed. Remodeling, the third and final phase of wound healing, occurs after the wound is closed. It begins about 3 weeks after the injury and can still be in progress from 6 months to 2 years later.

   Cognitive level: Analysis

   Nursing process: Assessment

   Client needs: Health Promotion and Maintenance: Prevention/Early Detection of Health Problems

2. Answer: 3. Using the clock face method

   Rationale: A sinus tract is an area, sometimes referred to as a tunnel, where there is nonhealed detached tissue under intact skin. Sinus tracts are measured in centimeters. Referring to location, the area of tunneling is defined on a clock face with 12 o'clock being the head of the body. For example, if a wound located on the anterior aspect of the leg has tunneling on the medial side of the left leg, the measurement would be x amount of centimeters at the 9 o'clock position. There is also a measurement for undermining. Undermining is like a cliff without tissue below and more broad than a sinus tract. It is measured from each point or side using the clock face method. The surface area of the wound is the length multiplied by the width in centimeters squared (cm^2). The volume is the length multiplied by the width and the depth in centimeters cubed (cm^3).

   Cognitive level: Application

   Nursing process: Assessment

   Client needs: Physiological Integrity: Physiological Adaptation

3. Answer: 2. Use the rule of 30 to reposition the patient every two hours.

   Rationale: Positioning is important in the prevention of pressure ulcers. The goal is to get the patient mobile and active as soon as possible; however, when mobility is physically impossible, the patient's position should be changed a minimum of every 2 hours. A sufficient number of people should be available to move the patient so that shearing and friction during movement can be avoided. Assistive devices such as transfer boards or mechanical lifts may be helpful to minimize tissue injury during movement. The "rule of 30" is used for positioning. This rule states that the head of the bed should be elevated 30 degrees or less and the body placed in a 30-degree laterally inclined position when placed on either side. These positions avoid pressure directly over the trochanter and promote improved circulation to the skin over the sacrum and ischial tuberosities. Pillows or foam wedges may be used to keep the patient properly positioned. The prone position may also be used if the patient is able to tolerate it. Attention should be focused on maintaining proper alignment so that functional ability can be maintained.

   Cognitive level: Application

   Nursing process: Planning

   Client needs: Physiological Integrity: Reduction of Risk Potential

4. Answer: 3. Apply a moisture barrier and secure with gauze.

   Rationale: Compression is used for venous wounds. Surgery is indicated for arterial wounds. Debridement is appropriate for wounds with eschar. Appropriate care for a skin tear wound includes avoiding the use of adhesive dressings or tapes, applying a moisture barrier, wrapping a gauze bandage around the extremity, using hydrogel sheet dressings or foam, and/or using zinc-impregnated gauze and cotton.

   Cognitive level: Application

   Nursing process: Implementation

   Client needs: Physiological Integrity: Physiological Adaptation

5. Answer: 1. Autolytic debridement

   Rationale: Autolytic debridement allows the body to utilize its phagocytes to destroy the necrotic tissue. This is often a preferred method of debridement for those persons for whom daily or more frequent dressing changes would be a hardship; that is, patients who are critically ill and cannot be turned. Autolytic debridement is a slow and nonaggressive treatment. Sharp debridement is done with a scalpel, scissors, or nippers. Anesthetics or the operating room may be required depending on wound size and depth. Mechanical debridement is the dislodging of necrotic tissue, which is accomplished by wet-to-dry dressings, the whirlpool, or pulse lavage. Enzymatic debridement is chemically induced by prescriptive ointments that contain papain-urea or collagenase, which penetrates the slough and eschar causing them to soften and "melt down." Once softened, the slough and eschar are mechanically debrided.

Cognitive level: Analysis

Nursing process: Planning

Client needs: Physiological Integrity: Physiological Adaptation

6. Answer: 2. Tell me why you think the wound is ugly.

Rationale: Depression can occur when a patient has a wound. It may affect the way she sees herself or the way she perceives that others see her, especially if the wound is easily visible. Not only does the patient have an emotional response to her wound, but almost everyone the patient encounters has an emotional response to her wound. Wounds are perceived as unpleasant, disgusting, scary, and a nuisance. Depression may affect the patient's ability to perform the daily activities she desires to do, and it may limit patient independence. It can be very costly for the treatments and medications. The patient may have to wear some special type of shoe or device that makes her self-conscious. The nurse needs to assess the patient for her feelings about her wound and associated treatment. Empathize with the patient, and try to devise a plan that is least intrusive and yet realistic.

Cognitive level: Application

Nursing process: Assessment

Client needs: Psychosocial Integrity: Coping and Adaptation

7. Answer: 2. Healing rate

Rationale: Poor nutrition will negatively impact the healing rate of a wound. Wound dressings impact the risk of infection. Mechanisms to preventing scar formation impact wound appearance. Appropriate pain management impacts the patient's comfort level.

Cognitive level: Analysis

Nursing process: Evaluation

Client needs: Physiological Integrity: Physiological Adaptation

Chapter 68

1. Answer: 3. Major burn injury

Rationale: This patient has experienced a major burn injury. The classifications are minor, moderate, and major, not medium. Electrical burns and burns involving the feet are always considered major injuries, even though the dermal injuries only appeared as 2% or less.

Cognitive level: Application

Nursing process: Assessment

Client needs: Physiological Integrity

2. Answer: 4. "Liquid at 140°F requires five minutes to cause a full-thickness burn."

Rationale: Liquids at 120°F require 5 minutes to cause a full-thickness burn. At 140°F liquids can cause a burn injury in 5 seconds or less. Sunscreens help prevent radiation burns from the sun and help decrease the risk of skin cancers. Children's sleepwear should be made from fire retardant materials, and every home should have smoke alarms that are clean and in working order.

Cognitive level: Application

Nursing process: Evaluation

Client needs: Safe and Effective Care Environment

3. Answer: 1. "With bacterial translocation the gastrointestinal mucosal atrophy that occurs causes intraluminal bacteria to migrate to extraluminal sites."

Rationale: Paralytic ileus and gastrointestinal mucosal atrophy are not uncommon with severe burn injuries. This allows opportunity for the intraluminal bacteria to migrate to extraluminal sources in a process called bacterial translocation. Decreased cardiac output can occur early after a burn injury because of the vasoconstriction caused by the sympathetic nervous system. When damaged erythrocytes and muscle tissue cause the release of excess hemoglobin and myoglobin, respectively, the liver is unable to handle this increased load. Therefore, these substances must be excreted through the urine and can clog the renal tubules, causing renal failure. Leukocytes are not transfused, although their stores may be depleted within 48 hours following a burn. Decreased circulating iron causes a resultant low red blood cell count, and it is not uncommon to replace red blood cells or platelets in patients with major burns.

Cognitive level: Application

Nursing process: Assessment

Client needs: Physiological Integrity

4. Answer: 2. The acute care period

Rationale: The emergency and resuscitative periods are the same and include the initial treatment with airway and hemodynamic stabilization with fluid resuscitation. The rehabilitative period begins when the open burn wound size is less than 20% and the patient is at his or her highest level of functioning since admission. This phase focuses on physical and psychological restoration, including increased strength, function, flexibility, and cosmetic restoration. The acute care period begins once the patient is hemodynamically stable. The focus is on wound care, prevention of infection and other complications, and pain control.

Cognitive level: Analysis

Nursing process: Implementation

Client needs: Physiological Integrity

5. Answer: 1. A 35-year-old with a history of migraines and 40% TBSA full-thickness thermal burns to the neck, left upper extremity, and circumferentially around the chest. Vital signs are HR 116, BP 90/68, RR 26 and shallow, SpO$_2$ 90%.

Rationale: The 35-year-old patient has a major burn injury. The size and location of the burn, as well as the circumferential nature of the wound, have the potential to cause increased morbidity and mortality in this patient. The vital signs reflect possible cardiopulmonary

compromise. The 70-year-old patient is older and has a chronic medical condition, but partial-thickness wounds of less than 15% and full-thickness wounds of less than 1% are considered minor. Also, the burns do not involve the head, neck, chest, hands, feet, or perineum nor are the vital signs abnormal. The 12-year-old patient is younger, but not an infant or young child. A partial-thickness burn of 20% is moderate, and it is important to note that while the injury to the foot is significant, it is not full thickness nor would it take precedence over an injury that could compromise airway, breathing, or circulation. The history of astigmatism is unremarkable to the emergent burn treatment, and the vital signs are normal. The 44-year-old patient does have a significant chronic medical condition, as exemplified by the blood pressure reading. However, an 8% full-thickness injury and 15% partial-thickness injury are moderate injuries. It is also important to note that none of the burns are classified as circumferential.
Cognitive level: Analysis
Nursing process: Planning
Client needs: Physiological Integrity

6. Answer: 2. Fluid volume deficit related to increased capillary permeability
Rationale: After airway and breathing, the priority during emergency care is cardiovascular assessment with fluid resuscitation. Therefore, of the choices given, fluid volume deficit would be the priority nursing diagnosis during the emergency phase. Altered skin integrity is addressed during the emergency phase, but it is the basis for care during the acute care phase. Acute pain should certainly be addressed, but it will not take precedence over fluid volume deficit. A potential problem, such as high risk for infection, will also be attended to after actual problems.
Cognitive level: Application
Nursing process: Planning
Client needs: Physiological Integrity

7. Answer: 4. "My pressure garments should be removed one to four times a day to allow for adequate circulation."
Rationale: Exercise programs for burned patients should be progressive in nature so as to improve strength and endurance. These programs may also include stretching exercises to elongate shortened tissues. These exercises are providing adequate stretch when the burn scar blanches. Also beneficial to helping healed burn wounds is scar massage. The massage should be performed daily, from one to four times a day. The massage helps improve the cosmetic appearance and hypertrophy of the scar, as well as increase circulation and possibly range of motion. Pressure garments should be worn continuously for 23 hours a day, not removed several times to promote circulation.
Cognitive level: Analysis
Nursing process: Evaluation
Client needs: Physiological Integrity

8. Answer: 3. Heart rate 114
Rationale: The heart rate is tachycardic, indicating possible hypovolemia. The blood pressure appears normal, but this is a poor early indicator because the increased systemic vascular resistance that occurs causes the blood pressure to be maintained regardless of volume status. A central venous pressure of 6 indicates adequate fluid volume, as does a urine output of 30 mL/hr.
Cognitive level: Analysis
Nursing process: Assessment
Client needs: Physiological Integrity

Chapter 69

1. Answer: 2. Normal
Rationale: The inside of the ear is inspected with an otoscope. An otoscopic examination includes inspection of the auditory canal and tympanic membrane. Look for inflammation, exudates, lesions, and foreign bodies. Check for narrowing of the ear canal, nodules, redness, scales, edema, drainage, and foreign objects. Normally the eardrum is slightly conical, shiny, smooth, and pearl gray. Cerumen should be moist and may vary in color from brown to white, but hardened, dry, or foul-smelling cerumen may indicate infection. In a majority of Asians and Native Americans, cerumen is dry, white, and flaky. In African Americans and Caucasians, cerumen is brown, wet, and sticky.
Cognitive level: Analysis
Nursing process: Assessment
Client needs: Health Promotion and Maintenance: Prevention/Early Detection of Health Problems

2. Answer: 4. Do you think that there is something in the room causing you to sneeze?
Rationale: The nurse needs to inquire about a history of upper respiratory infection. Sneezing, particularly at specific times of the year or under specific environmental circumstances, should be investigated for the possibility of allergies or respiratory infection. Allergic rhinitis is an inflammation of the nasal mucosa caused by an allergic substance, for example, hay fever or pollen. The nurse needs to inquire if the allergies are related to a specific time of year. Does the patient regularly take medications for allergic rhinitis, sinus infections, stuffy nose, or frequent respiratory infections? Some nasal sprays and decongestants may cause rebound nasal swelling. Over-the-counter oral decongestants may have an adverse effect on patients with diabetes, hypertension, hyperthyroidism, and cardiac illnesses.
Cognitive level: Analysis
Nursing process: Assessment
Client needs: Health Promotion and Maintenance: Prevention/Early Detection of Health Problems

3. Answer: 2. Even though you have dentures, seeing a dentist regularly is necessary for good oral health.
Rationale: Poorly fitting dentures or orthotic appliances and inadequate dentition can cause difficulty chewing,

nutritional problems, and mouth sores. To maintain good oral health, the patient should see the dentist at regular intervals and use good oral hygiene measures.

Cognitive level: Analysis

Nursing process: Assessment

Client needs: Health Promotion and Maintenance: Prevention/Early Detection of Health Problems

4. Answer: 3. Social isolation because of hearing loss

Rationale: Age impacts hearing ability. For example, presbycusis, hearing loss in the high-frequency range, is the most common sensorineural hearing loss in older people. The patient experiencing the gradual hearing loss of aging may limit social interactions as it becomes so difficult to understand the spoken word. During the assessment the nurse should inquire about functional ability and social interactions. Loss of hearing also can be perceived as mental status changes. Nurses need to be more aware of the impact of hearing loss on the elderly.

Cognitive level: Analysis

Nursing process: Assessment

Client needs: Psychosocial Integrity: Coping and Adaptation

5. Answer: 1. Normal

Rationale: With the voice whisper test the examiner stands approximately 1 to 2 feet in back of the patient and whispers several words near each ear. The patient should be able to hear bilaterally and equally.

Cognitive level: Analysis

Nursing process: Assessment

Client needs: Health Promotion and Maintenance: Prevention/Early Detection of Health Problems

Chapter 70

1. Answer: 3. Sound transmission

Rationale: The tympanic membrane or eardrum, comprised of tissue that makes up the ear canal, is the final structure within this portion of the outer ear anatomy. It is this structure that transmits sounds from the outer to the middle ear. The cochlea is responsible for hearing, whereas the vestibular system is responsible for balance. Within the inner ear are found the semicircular canals, specifically the horizontal, anterior, and posterior canals, which help with balance and movement. The acoustic nerve consists of two separate parts, the vestibular and cochlear branches. This eighth cranial nerve controls hearing and equilibrium.

Cognitive level: Analysis

Nursing process: Assessment

Client needs: Health Promotion and Maintenance: Prevention/Early Detection of Health Problems

2. Answer: 2. Air conduction

Rationale: There are actually two mechanisms involved with hearing: bone conduction and air conduction. Bone conduction is the conduction of sound to the inner ear through the bones of the skull. Air conduction begins the process when noise enters the external ear and travels to the middle ear. Once inside the middle ear, the sound is transmitted through the three auditory bones, the malleus, incus, and stapes. Once the sound or noise reaches the stapes, it is then transmitted to the inner ear where it reaches the acoustic nerve and is transmitted to the brain for interpretation. Hearing disorders can be caused by an alteration anywhere within the auditory structures.

Cognitive level: Analysis

Nursing process: Assessment

Client needs: Health Promotion and Maintenance: Prevention/Early Detection of Health Problems

3. Answer: 3. Conductive

Rationale: In conductive hearing loss, sound waves cannot reach the inner ear for processing and interpretation. With sensorineural hearing loss, the cause is damage to the auditory nerve or possibly damage to the small hair cells within the inner ear. Mixed hearing loss refers to both conductive and sensorineural hearing loss caused by a dysfunction of both air and bone conduction processes. Acoustic hearing loss would refer to a damaged acoustic nerve.

Cognitive level: Analysis

Nursing process: Assessment

Client needs: Health Promotion and Maintenance: Prevention/Early Detection of Health Problems

4. Answer: 3. The baby should be tested now.

Rationale: Within the *Healthy People 2010* "Objectives for Reducing Hearing Loss," it is recommended that newborns should have a first hearing examination by 1 month of age. Babies with a hearing loss should have additional testing by 3 months of age. And if hearing loss continues, the baby should be enrolled in a rehabilitative program by 6 months of age. Hearing loss in the newborn can be linked to birth trauma, toxicity, infection, fetal anoxia during delivery, premature or low birth weight, genetics, or an elevated serum bilirubin level. In addition, deafness upon birth has been seen in those women who have been exposed to highly communicable diseases such as rubella and syphilis or who have ingested known ototoxic medications while pregnant. The presence of hearing can be assessed as early as 2 to 3 days of life. Hearing loss is one of the most common developmental abnormalities present at birth. If left undiagnosed, it will impede speech, language, and cognitive developments. Individuals with hearing impairment at this early age will face a lifetime of challenges. Learning how to communicate with sign language and lip reading are just two ways to aid the person born without the sense of hearing.

Cognitive level: Analysis

Nursing process: Assessment

Client needs: Health Promotion and Maintenance: Prevention/Early Detection of Health Problems

5. Answer: 1. Mechanical

Rationale: The causes of hearing impairment or loss can be categorized as mechanical, inflammatory, or an obstructive disorder. One mechanical cause of hearing loss is due to otosclerosis or a primary bone dyscrasia that leads to conductive hearing loss. Otosclerosis is a condition in which the structures of the ear begin to harden. Seen as a common cause of conductive hearing loss, treatment options are limited to a stapedectomy.

Cognitive level: Analysis

Nursing process: Assessment

Client needs: Physiological Integrity: Physiological Adaptation

6. Answer: 3. Mechanism to ensure a visual alert in the event of a home fire

Rationale: The home needs to have services or mechanisms that make the environment safer; for instance, visual fire safety provisions and access to alerting and telephone services, and TVs with teletext ability.

Cognitive level: Application

Nursing process: Planning

Client needs: Health Promotion and Maintenance: Prevention/Early Detection of Health Problems

7. Answer: 2. Drop the tone of the voice when talking.

Rationale: When providing care to an elderly patient with a hearing deficit or balance disorder, the nurse needs to include specific items in the assessment process. First the method of communication must be determined. A loud voice does not ensure successful hearing or comprehension. Depending on the cause and degree of hearing loss, the nurse might simply drop the tone of the voice to be successful with vocal communication with an elderly patient who has a hearing impairment because the loss of high-frequency sounds occurs first.

Cognitive level: Application

Nursing process: Implementation

Client needs: Physiological Integrity: Reduction of Risk Potential

8. Answer: 1. Assure the patient that the call light will be answered as soon as possible.

Rationale: The nurse should implement strategies to reduce the patient's anxiety such as responding to the call light as soon as possible, answering questions, teaching about medications/treatments, and providing emotional support to the patient having difficulty coping with the new sensory deficit.

Cognitive level: Application

Nursing process: Implementation

Client needs: Psychosocial Integrity: Coping and Adaptation

Chapter 71

1. Answer: 3. Floaters

Rationale: The vitreous body is the largest chamber of the eye that maintains the shape of the eyeball. The vitreous gel is made up mainly of water with a collagen framework, which includes collagen, hyaluronic acid, proteins, and solutes. Due to aging, the collagen network can be aggregated by vitreous collapse that forms vitreous opacities, which cast shadows on the retina. These shadows are referred to as floaters.

Cognitive level: Analysis

Nursing process: Assessment

Client needs: Health Promotion and Maintenance: Prevention/Early Detection of Health Problems

2. Answer: 2. The uncovered eye is fixated outward.

Rationale: When conducting the cover–uncover test for tropia, the patient is to wear his own corrective lenses, if he has them. Have the patient fixate on a target about 20 feet away for far and 16 inches for near; it can be a visual acuity chart, picture chart, E chart, or toy. The tester is to sit in front of the patient, but does not block target view. Note the eye that is fixating cover that eye with an occluder, and note what the fellow eye does. If the uncovered eye moves to pick up fixation, note the direction it moves: If toward the nose, then it was fixated outward, so it is exo; if toward the ear, then it was fixated inward, so it is eso. If the uncovered eye does not move and has steady fixation, no strabismus exists. The eye would move up and down to indicate vertical tropia.

Cognitive level: Analysis

Nursing process: Assessment

Client needs: Health Promotion and Maintenance: Prevention/Early Detection of Health Problems

3. Answer: 4. Eye muscle surgery

Rationale: Adult strabismus may be treated with eye muscle exercises, eyeglasses containing prisms, botulinum toxin (Botox) injections, and eye surgery. Eye muscle exercise usually is used when treating a form of adult strabismus, called convergence insufficiency, in which eyes cannot align themselves for close work or reading. These exercises can retrain eyes to focus inward together. Prism eyeglasses can be used to correct the mild double vision associated with adult strabismus. Botox injections are an effective treatment when overactive eye muscles are causing strabismus. Eye muscle surgery is the most common treatment; it is used to loosen or tighten the muscles around the eye in order to correct the misalignment.

Cognitive level: Analysis

Nursing process: Planning

Client needs: Psychosocial Integrity: Coping and Adaptation

4. Answer: 2. The correct use of eyedrops

Rationale: Nursing assessment and education include patient compliance with regular use of eyedrops and follow-up, which is one of the main goals in treating glaucoma. The major reason for the cause of blindness from glaucoma, besides not knowing one has glaucoma, is noncompliance in using eyedrops and not considering glaucoma to be a serious disease. It is imperative that patients understand that the long-term goal of treatment is to lower intraocular pressure to prevent optic nerve damage, and only with continued use of drops can this goal be reached. Patient education includes information on risk factors for glaucoma such as family history, myopia, previous eye trauma, low blood pressure, African ancestry, diabetes, longtime exposure to steroids, and aging. The patient is taught how to instill eyedrops properly for the full benefit of treatment.

Cognitive level: Application

Nursing process: Planning

Client needs: Physiological Integrity: Physiological Adaptation

5. Answer: 2. Explain that whatever decision they make, they have freedom of choice.

Rationale: The decision to donate corneal tissue for transplantation can have ethical considerations. It is important for the family that is being asked to donate a cornea for the benefit of someone else's vision that the decision be a well-informed one, one that is freely chosen, and one that is compatible with the ethical beliefs of the individuals concerned. It is important for the family members to know that whatever decision they make, to donate or not to donate, they have freedom of choice. Under the circumstances of facing the loss of a loved one, any decision they make is the right decision for them. Usually the decision is one of three choices: Donate all organs, donate only the cornea, or do not donate at all. The two most common reasons not to donate are (1) the fear of something being done before the person is dead, and (2) the fear that the health care provider may hasten the death to benefit another. Thoughts that the family should consider include these: Donation is an ethical decision to benefit another person; with treatment of the body after death, respect is the greatest issue, especially for psychological, religious, spiritual, moral, and cultural reasons; donation is the last giving act the person donor does to reflect his life; and the family knows that the loved one still lives on in another person.

Cognitive level: Application

Nursing process: Implementation

Client needs: Psychosocial Integrity: Coping and Adaptation

Chapter 72

1. Answer: 3. "When the group responsible for committing the violence has connection to a foreign country like al Queda in the Middle East."

Rationale: Terrorist acts use force, destruction, and violence to coerce and intimidate and cause disruption, terror, and panic. When the group or individual is operating independently from within the United States or Puerto Rico with acts of terrorism that are directed at the U.S. government or its population, then it is said to be an act of "domestic" terrorism. Terrorist acts committed across international boundaries or by groups with foreign ties are said to be acts of "international" terrorism.

Cognitive level: Analysis

Nursing process: Assessment

Client needs: Safe and Effective Care Environment

2. Answer: 1. "The outbreak of an intentionally caused foodborne illness in Oregon during the early 1980s was attributed to *Shigella sonnei*."

Rationale: In 1979 the nuclear power plant at Three Mile Island in the United States did experience an accidental radiation leak. However, there were never any effects on physical health reported. In both 1994 and 1995, sarin gas was released into the Tokyo subway system by the Aum Shinrikyo cult, making the resultant disaster the largest peace-time event involving nerve gas. Rye ergot was used in the 6th century B.C. by the Assyrians who would use it to poison the water wells of their enemies. In 1984, in The Dalles, Oregon, a religious group known as the Rajneeshees intentionally contaminated a salad bar at a local restaurant with *Salmonella typhimurium*.

Cognitive level: Analysis

Nursing process: Evaluation

Client needs: Safe and Effective Care Environment

3. Answer: 4. Inhalation anthrax

Rationale: Although the patient clearly has an infectious process manifesting with signs of shock, tachypnea, dyspnea, and fever with chills, the complaint of chest pain with radiologic confirmation of a widened mediastinum several days following possible biologic agent exposure are classic for inhalation anthrax. Septicemic plague may also present with signs of sepsis or septic shock, but it also usually includes gastrointestinal symptoms such as vomiting and diarrhea. Also known as the "Black Death," septicemic plague causes purpuric lesions, distal gangrene, and disseminated intravascular coagulopathy. Undulant fever is also called brucellosis. It presents much like the flu, with generalized body aches, fever, headache, and malaise. Patients may also have gastrointestinal symptoms. The onset of typhoidal tularemia is abrupt and progressive. Patients may experience fever, chills, and chest pain, but they usually also have severe body aches, low back pain, sore throat, and pneumonia. They may also have nausea, vomiting, diarrhea, and weight loss.

Cognitive level: Analysis

Nursing process: Assessment

Client needs: Physiological Integrity

4. Answer: 1. Ineffective airway clearance related to copious secretions and ineffective cough

Rationale: Although all of the nursing diagnoses are appropriate for the patient with known nerve agent exposure, the priority for any patient is airway. Nursing diagnoses that relate to actual problems would always take precedence over potential problems, such as increased risk for altered cardiac output or for fluid and electrolyte imbalance. Also, physiological issues should be addressed prior to any psychosocial problems this patient may be experiencing.

Cognitive level: Application

Nursing process: Planning

Client needs: Physiological Integrity

5. Answer: 2. Prodromal phase

Rationale: The prodromal phase is the initial phase after exposure and has an onset of minutes to hours and lasts from hours to days. In this phase the onset of symptoms is rapid and may include nausea, vomiting, and fatigue. Fever, hypotension, and diarrhea may occur with high-level exposure. The rapid onset in this case, within half an hour, is bleak. The latent phase follows the prodromal phase, and during this time, the patient is relatively symptom free. Once the patient has recovered from an exposure, the acute symptoms should not occur. The illness phase is marked by overt illness. Signs and symptoms may be more systemic, involving the hematopoietic, gastrointestinal, central nervous, and dermatologic systems in any combination.

Cognitive level: Analysis

Nursing process: Assessment

Client needs: Safe, Effective Care Environment/ Physiological Integrity

6. Answer: 3. This flexible plan allows for only necessary positions and functions to be activated on an as-needed basis during the incident.

Rationale: The Incident Commander is in charge of four areas: operations, planning, logistics, and finance. Although the HICS plan does outline a clear chain of command and responsibilities for each position involved, the positions do not have to have a sole commander nor must they remain independent of other positions. If needed, the positions may be combined under the leadership of one individual. Media use is very helpful if the HICS is activated. Its utilization can decrease mass hysteria by increasing public awareness of the situation. The plan is flexible, allowing for only necessary positions and functions to be activated on an as-needed basis during the incident.

Cognitive level: Analysis

Nursing process: Planning

Client needs: Safe and Effective Care Environment

7. Answer: 1. It helps augment the local and state resources so as to help decrease the morbidity and mortality in the civilian population following a large-scale disaster.

Rationale: The SNS maintains a national repository of pharmaceutical agents, vaccines, and medical supplies and equipment to be delivered to an area after a large-scale disaster. It helps augment the local and state resources so as to help decrease morbidity and mortality in the civilian population. This program is organized with a five-tiered approach that includes 12-hour Push Packs, vendor-managed inventory (VMI), storage of and rapid vaccine deployment, buying power with surge capacity, and technical assistance. The 12-hour Push Packs can be shipped within 12 hours of the decision to do so. They contain critical supplies and pharmaceuticals that might be needed in the event of a large-scale disaster. The VMI is designed to be used to provide pharmaceuticals and medical supplies for treatment of a known agent or for smaller scale events. The Technical Advisory Response Unit is a group of logistical, public health, communications, operations, and emergency preparedness experts who assist state and local authorities with supply receiving, distribution, dispensing, and replenishing.

Cognitive level: Analysis

Nursing process: Planning

Client needs: Physiological Integrity

8. Answer: 4. "Critical incident defusings are formal, confidential group sessions where the stressful event and its experiences and reactions are reviewed."

Rationale: Critical incident stress debriefings are formal sessions run by trained counselors that are held within 72 hours of a critical event. Group information briefings are also called demobilizations. This is a short informal meeting that helps with rumor control, possible reactions, and self-help guidelines. The fact phase of CISD allows for each participant to describe the stressful event from his or her own perspective on a cognitive level. Critical incident defusings give mutual reassurance and assess the need for more help. Critical incident defusings are formal, confidential group sessions where the event and its experiences and reactions are reviewed. Each session consists of six to eight people with similar job descriptions, and each session lasts 20 to 45 minutes.

Cognitive level: Analysis

Nursing process: Evaluation

Client needs: Safe and Effective Care Environment

Chapter 73

1. Answer: 2. It can describe patient care for perceived, actual, or undiagnosed health problems.

Rationale: Emergency nursing does involve episodic patient care, but the care is usually acute or critical in nature. Florence Nightingale has long been associated with the origins of emergency nursing because of her care of wounded soldiers out in the field. Judith Kelleher and Anita Dorr are credited with establishing the Emergency Department Nurses Association in 1970. The patients seeking emergency care are becoming increasingly diverse in culture and ethnicity. Thus, it is important for emergency nurses to also become more educated about, sensitive to, and competent in these diversities and how they affect patient care. Emergency nursing is patient care for perceived, actual, or undiagnosed physical and mental health conditions.

Cognitive level: Analysis

Nursing process: Assessment

Client needs: Safe and Effective Care Environment

2. Answer: 3. A patient having a possible allergic reaction with facial edema, drooling, stridor, and severe urticaria with pruritus

Rationale: Patients requiring immediate airway or cervical spine intervention are always identified and treated first in the emergency department. The patient having an allergic reaction is demonstrating signs of possible airway obstruction (i.e., facial edema, drooling, and stridor). This patient should be treated first among the other patients listed. The patient with chest pain and shortness of breath has signs of a possible cardiac or respiratory event that would require urgent intervention without delay in care, but issues pertaining to airway or cervical spine would be treated emergently. The patients with the urinary condition and the laceration also need intervention, but they are not experiencing life-threatening issues at this time and would be treated after the patients with the airway problem and the cardiopulmonary event, respectively.

Cognitive level: Application
Nursing process: Planning
Client needs: Physiological Integrity

3. Answer: 4. Level IV – Nonurgent

Rationale: The patient's complaint is nontraumatic and chronic, having been an issue for 4 months. Also, the patient has sought previous medical treatment from his or her primary care provider, who now refuses to give the patient access to more prescription analgesics, and the triage assessment is benign. Because the patient's condition does not require immediate resuscitative efforts nor is the patient unstable, categorizing him or her as a Level I or Level II, respectively, would be inappropriate. The Level III category would also be incorrect in this case, because the patient does not have an urgent problem that requires timely intervention. Level IV, nonurgent, is the best choice for this patient in the four-level triage system.

Cognitive level: Application
Nursing process: Evaluation
Client needs: Physiological Integrity

4. Answer: 1. General consent and informed consent.

Rationale: Both general and informed consents should be obtained prior to this patient's treatment. The general consent would be for any treatment, such as evaluation by the staff, and noninvasive procedures, such as radiographs. The informed consent would be for the procedures of conscious sedation and reduction of the dislocation. This consent states that the patient has been fully informed about these procedures and their risks. Implied consent is used only in emergency situations when it is presumed that the patient would give permission for treatment if she or he were able. Blood product consent would be used prior to administration of any blood or blood products.

Cognitive level: Application
Nursing process: Implementation
Client needs: Physiological Integrity

5. Answer: 2. "I am glad that emergency nurses do not have to deal with obstetrical issues because they can call the labor and delivery nurses."

Rationale: Emergency nurses must be prepared for all types of emergencies, including obstetrical issues. Additional preparation for new graduates or nurses who are new to the field of emergency nursing should include instruction in psychiatric emergencies and trauma assessment. The Trauma Nursing Core Course is just one course that is recommended for these nurses. Time management and the ability to care for multiple patients simultaneously are also learned skills that are imperative to emergency nursing.

Cognitive level: Analysis
Nursing process: Evaluation
Client needs: Safe and Effective Care Environment

Chapter 74

1. Answer: 4. Spinal

Rationale: Spinal cord injury is commonly noted in patients following rear-impact motor vehicle crashes.

Cognitive level: Analysis
Nursing process: Assessment
Client needs: Physiological Integrity: Physiological Adaptation

2. Answer: 3. Utilize a rigid cervical collar to stabilize the cervical spine.

Rationale: When assessing and treating patients with trauma, the priorities of the primary survey must be recognized. The first priority is airway with simultaneous cervical spine immobilization. A rigid cervical collar is one way to stabilize the cervical spine in an emergent situation. Controlling bleeding should be performed during the circulation portion of the primary survey. This falls after the priority of airway and cervical spine treatment. A neurological exam would come after dealing with airway, cervical spine, and circulation. Although the patient may need a CT scan to determine if there is a head injury, this is not a priority initially. This intervention would be a portion of the secondary survey that is performed after the primary survey is complete.

Cognitive level: Application
Nursing process: Assessment
Client needs: Health Promotion and Maintenance: Prevention/Early Detection of Health Problems

3. Answer: 1. It will include a comprehensive medical record review to help ensure all injuries and treatments for the patient with trauma have been properly addressed.

Rationale: The tertiary trauma survey includes a comprehensive medical record review, repetition of the primary and secondary surveys, and reviews of all lab and radiologic results to help ensure that all injuries and treatments for the patient with trauma have been properly addressed. It is done within 24 hours of admission and repeated once the patient is awake, responsive, and able to communicate and helps to make certain that all injuries have been properly identified, catalogued, and treated. The Eastern Association for the Surgery of Trauma formed a work group to develop evidence-based guidelines for practice regarding the best and most important nutritional recommendations for the patient with trauma. The primary and secondary surveys provide a systematic approach to initial trauma assessment, helping the health care team identify injuries, provide appropriate interventions, and prioritize patient care. Trauma rehabilitation is a multidisciplinary plan of care developed to help increase the patient's quality of life and maximize the impaired patient's function by minimizing any deficits.

Cognitive level: Analysis
Nursing process: Planning
Client needs: Health Promotion and Maintenance: Prevention/Early Detection of Health Problems

4. Answer: 3. Assess for bleeding into the chest, abdomen, pelvis, or around long bones.

Rationale: Hemorrhage is the predominant cause of preventable death in the injured patient. During the primary survey, hypotension should be considered hypovolemic in origin until proven otherwise. If external hemorrhage is identified, measures to control the bleeding should be taken immediately. The easiest way to do this is to apply direct manual pressure on the wound. The major sources of occult blood loss are hemorrhage into the chest or abdominal cavities, into the soft tissue surrounding a major long bone fracture, or into the retroperitoneal space from a pelvic fracture. Control of bleeding may require immediate operative intervention.

Cognitive level: Application

Nursing process: Assessment

Client needs: Physiological Integrity: Physiological Adaptation

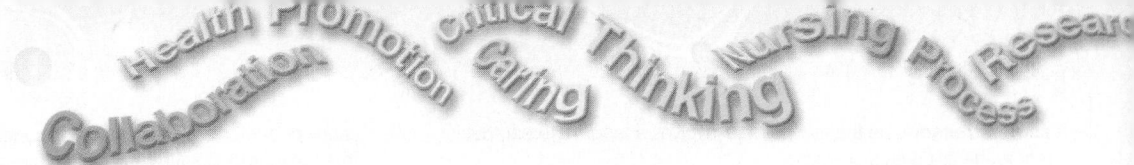

GLOSSARY

12-lead ECG Standard surface ECG with 12 leads, 3 bipolar and 9 unipolar.

2,3-diphosphoglycerate (2,3-DPG) Substance produced by red blood cells during hypoxic states that sustains the deoxyhemoglobin configuration.

abdominojugular reflux An indicator of jugular venous distention that becomes visible as a result of the displacement of excess blood volume when the upper abdominal region is compressed.

abduction Movement of a body part away from the midline (center) of the body.

aberration Deviation from the normal.

ablation Destruction of a specific area of the myocardium through localized delivery of chemicals or electrical energy.

abortion The ending of a pregnancy before the age of fetal viability.

absolute iron deficiency Physiological state indicating insufficient amounts of total body iron.

absolute neutrophil count (ANC) A useful measurement that reveals that proportion of the white blood cells that can be utilized in first-response immune interactions; the most accurate measurement of circulating neutrophils within white blood cells.

absolute refractory period Period of time during which a cardiac cell is unable to respond to any stimulus and cannot spontaneously depolarize. Corresponds with the beginning of the QRS complex and ends at the peak of the T wave on an ECG tracing.

absorption The process by which a medication leaves the site of administration to cross membranes as it journeys to the site of action.

academic nurse educator A nurse who is responsible for designing, implementing, evaluating, and revising academic and continuing education programs for nurses.

accessory muscles The sternocleidomastoid, scalene, and trapezius muscles, which are normally not necessary to respiration, but are utilized by patients who require extra effort to move air in and out of the lungs.

accommodation (1) Process a child goes through to modify existing schema because the incorporation of new knowledge does not fit into existing schema. (2) The ability of the lens to focus up-close or near; to focus a clear image on the retina.

accreditation Process of evaluating an organization against performance standards.

acculturative stress Job-related stress that is exacerbated by cultural differences such as diverse assumptions, values, and beliefs among the participants.

acetylcholine A neurotransmitter critical to the process of memory formation.

achalasia A motor disorder of the esophagus that is characterized by failure of the lower esophageal sphincter to relax properly and by impaired peristalsis.

achlorhydria Lack of hydrochloric acid in the stomach.

acids Compounds in solution that have a pH of less than 7.40. They form hydrogen ion in solution and are proton donors.

acne vulgaris A chronic skin disorder with an increased production of sebum from the sebaceous glands and the formation of comedones that plug the pores.

acoustic neuroma A benign tumor of the eighth cranial (acoustic) nerve.

acquired immunity Type of immunity that occurs after birth and includes antibodies, immune-competent T cells and B cells, and cytokines that act to remove antigens that are considered non-self.

acquired immunodeficiency syndrome (AIDS) The disease resulting from infection by the human immunodeficiency virus; manifested by loss of T cells and opportunistic infections.

acromegaly A hypermetabolic condition of the pituitary gland, characterized by enlargement of the extremities, particularly the hands, feet, and other body parts such as the face, in which excess pituitary hormones (somatotropin and growth hormone) are secreted.

actinic keratosis A skin disorder caused by the sun that leads to proliferation of abnormal, dystrophic cells.

action potential Response of the resting membrane potential to a stimulus that exceeds the membrane threshold value. Carries signals along the muscle cell and conveys information from one cell to another, resulting in cardiac muscle depolarization.

active acquired immunity Type of immunity that involves the production of antibodies by the immune system in response to specific foreign antigens, such as bacteria. This immunity is considered acquired because the body develops the ability to regulate the immune system and produce antibodies after birth and after exposure to antigens in the environment, such as bacteria or viruses.

active immunization Immunization that involves the introduction of a live, killed, or attenuated toxin of a disease organism into the body. The immune system responds by producing antibodies.

activity theory of aging Theory of aging based on the premise that decreased activity later in life leads to meaninglessness and life dissatisfaction, and maintaining activity tends to increase life satisfaction.

acuity The measurement of severity of illness in a patient and the amount of nursing care required to care for the patient.

acute angle-closure glaucoma (AACG) Disorder characterized by the angle in the anterior chamber closing suddenly as a result of iris blockage; prevents aqueous flow through the trabecular meshwork, causing the intraocular pressure to rise suddenly, usually to greater than 40 mmHg.

acute bronchitis Inflammation of the tracheobronchial tree, usually in association with a respiratory infection.

acute care nurse A nurse who works with patients experiencing sudden illness or trauma, usually in the prehospital, hospital, or emergency department.

acute coronary syndrome (ACS) Syndrome collectively described by unstable angina, non–ST segment elevation myocardial infarction (MI), and ST segment elevation MI.

acute graft rejection A type IV cell-mediated immune response that occurs between 2 weeks and 1 month after transplant. This occurs when a recipient's T cells are activated against unmatched HLA antigens in the transplanted tissue.

acute lung injury (ALI) Sometimes used when referring to acute respiratory distress syndrome, but is less severe.

acute pain Pain of relatively short duration that coincides with injury, surgery, or illness.

acute pulmonary edema An abnormal accumulation of fluid in the lungs.

acute radiation syndrome An acute illness caused by irradiation of the whole body. The phases of the illness are prodromal, latent, illness, and recovery or death.

acute respiratory distress syndrome (ARDS) A progressive form of respiratory failure that leads to alveolar capillary inflammation and damage.

acute respiratory failure (ARF) A condition defined as a failure of gas exchange.

acute retroviral syndrome A group of generalized symptoms seen in some individuals during the period of primary infection with the human immunodeficiency virus (1 to 3 months). Symptoms include fever, malaise, lymphadenopathy, and skin rash.

acute stress A reaction to an immediate threat; commonly triggers the fight-or-flight response.

acute stressor One that is brief and involves a tangible threat that is readily identified as a stress.

acute wounds Recent wounds that are either traumatic or iatrogenic in etiology that progress through the stages of wound healing normally.

adaptation A reaction to stress that signifies that the person is able to cope with the stressor or change.

adapter Portion of a catheter that is used to affix infusion equipment to a vascular access device. Also known as the *hub*.

Addisonian crisis (adrenal crisis) A rare, life-threatening disease in which a deficiency of adrenal hormones is exacerbated by stress or trauma.

Addison's disease A rare condition caused by severe or total deficiency of hormones produced by the adrenal cortex.

add-on devices Any extra equipment such as filters, stopcocks, extensions, connectors, and injection ports or caps added to the primary intervenous set.

adduction Movement of a body part toward the midline (center) of the body.

adenomatous polyps Polyps that result from a mutation on chromosome 5. They are long thin projections of tissue arising from the mucosal epithelium and are considered premalignant tissue. Most colorectal cancers develop from this type of polyp.

adjuvant medications Medications that are not primarily indicated for treatment of pain, but are used to augment pain relief medications.

administration set Infusion-specific tubing that delivers parenteral fluid via a sterile pathway from its container to the patient via a vascular access device.

adrenal insufficiency Condition in which the body fails to produce an adequate amount of adrenal hormones.

advanced practice nurse (APRN) A nurse who has been trained to practice beyond the scope defined for a registered nurse by the state nurse practice act. Advanced practice nurses are qualified through postgraduate education and practice through the use of standardized procedures or by indirect supervision of a physician.

advanced practice nursing Specialized type of nursing practice in which nurses diagnose and treat illnesses and provide health care. Most advanced practice nurses are also certified to prescribe medication.

adventitious breath sounds Abnormal lung sound indicating a pathologic process.

adverse drug event (ADE) Noxious and unintended patient event caused by a drug accompanied by various symptoms, signs, and laboratory abnormalities.

adverse drug reaction (ADR) *See* adverse drug event (ADE).

aerophagia The swallowing of air; may lead to intestinal bloating.

affective dimension of pain Describes the emotions patients assign to their pain.

affective learning Involves changes in attitudes, values, and feelings.

afferent Ability to transport toward a center; for example, a sensory nerve that carries impulses from the peripheral nervous system to the central nervous system.

afterload The amount of pressure or resistance the ventricles must overcome to eject blood during systole.

agglutination The surrounding and attaching of antibodies to an antigen, causing the antigens to clump together and stimulate the immune cells to locate the complex and consume it or destroy it.

aging The process of growing old and maturing.

agonist Opioid that is often referred to as morphine-like, or as a mu agonist, because it binds to the mu, kappa, and delta receptors of cells located in the central nervous system, peripheral nervous system, and the gastrointestinal tract.

agonist-antagonist Opioid that is a kappa- or mu-receptor partial agonist; generally considered to be less efficacious than a pure mu agonist.

AIDS indicator conditions Indicates an HIV-infected individual has been diagnosed with opportunistic infections such as *Pneumocystis carinii* pneumonia or AIDS-defining cancer, such as Kaposi's sarcoma, or that the individual's CD4 count has fallen below 200 mL/µL.

air conduction Process of sound waves reaching the inner ear for interpretation.

air embolism Obstruction of a blood vessel by an air bubble.

air-mask-bag unit (AMBU) A device used to deliver oxygen via a mask when a patient is not adequately ventilating or oxygenating.

airway obstruction Obstruction that occurs most often because medications used in anesthesia cause the muscles to relax.

akinesia Condition characterized by areas of abnormal heart contractility where there is loss of or no muscle movement.

alanine aminotransferase (ALT) An enzyme released from hepatocytes when liver injury occurs.

albumin A commercially prepared product that is derived from the plasma portion of blood.

aldosterone A hormone secreted by the adrenal cortex in response to the conversion of angiotensinogen to angiotensin II. Aldosterone causes sodium reabsorption from the renal tubules and thus causes the body to retain water.

alkaline phosphatase (ALP) An enzyme found mostly in the liver and bone. It is released when liver injury or inflammation occurs and when abnormal osteoblastic activity is present in the bone.

alkalis Compounds in solution that have a pH of greater than 7.40, which is caused by either an increase of base/alkali or a loss of acid. There is more base and less acid, thus raising the 20:1 ratio of bicarbonate to carbonic acid.

allele An alternate or variant form of a gene. On a gene pair, one allele is inherited from the father and the other allele from the mother. The maternal and paternal alleles may be identical or homozygous or they may be different forms of the same gene (heterozygous).

Allen's test Test performed prior to arterial line insertion to test the patency of the palmar arch.

allergen An antigen, or protein, from the external environment. Common allergens include dust, food, pollen, and pet dander.

allergic rhinitis Inflammation of the nasal mucosa caused by an allergic substance such as pollen.

allergy A form of type I hypersensitivity reaction that occurs when an external antigen, or allergen, attaches to IgE antibodies. IgE antibodies attach to mast cells and result in degranulation and release of histamine. Symptoms are the result of the activity of histamine.

allogeneic bone marrow Bone marrow from a histocompatible donor.

allograft Grafting of skin to a wound that was harvested from human cadavers.

allograft valve A valve obtained from human cadaver donations; used primarily to replace the aortic and pulmonic valves. Also called a *homograft valve*.

alloimmune response A hypersensitivity response of the immune system to antigens from another human; usually occurs when tissue is transplanted or grafted.

allopathic medicine Method of treating disease with remedies that produce effects different from those caused by the disease itself.

alopecia Loss of hair, which can be a result of familial patterns of baldness, disease, medications, or a pathologic condition.

alpha-amylase An enzyme mainly in the pancreas; aids in the digestion of carbohydrates.

alternative therapy A therapy used instead of conventional or mainstream therapy. Also called *unconventional therapy*.

alveolar ventilation (V_A) The cumulative gas exchange that takes place within each alveolus.

Alzheimer's disease (AD) A chronic, progressive, irreversible brain disorder found most frequently in adults age 65 and older.

amblyopia Disorder in which a person has an eye with decreased or impaired vision with no obvious anatomic explanation, usually from childhood. Also known by the lay term *lazy eye*.

ametropia A general term used to indicate a refractive error that can usually be corrected with glasses, contact lenses, or possibly refractive surgery.

amputation Surgical removal of an anatomic part.

amyotrophic lateral sclerosis (ALS) A rare, progressive neurological disease characterized by loss of motor neurons.

anal canal The last part of the large intestine situated between the rectum and the anus. It is about 2.5 to 4 cm long.

analog A compound that is structurally similar to another with some slight differences in composition.

analytical preciseness Measure of how findings emerge from the data, how the data collection process is made flexible, and how themes emerge from the data.

anaphylaxis A severe form of type I hypersensitivity response that is systemic. Symptoms can include hives, severe bronchoconstriction, and loss of airway.

anasarca Total body edema.

anatomic dead space Area in the transporting airways or upper airways and bronchi that results when no gas exchange occurs. The amount of the tidal volume taken in that remains in the trachea and bronchi. The amount of anatomic dead space can be estimated as 1 mL per pound of ideal body weight. A person with an ideal body weight of 150 pounds has an anatomic dead space of about 150 mL.

androgenetic alopecia Physiological baldness in which androgen levels are normal; however, there is a genetic predisposition to balding.

androgenic alopecia Loss of hair related to excessive androgen production that causes a decrease in size of the hair follicles, leading to hair loss in central and frontal areas.

andropause A decrease in testosterone associated with aging.

anemia Disorder that results when the total body red blood cell volume is decreased; usually measured by hemoglobin, hematocrit, and red blood cell count.

anemic hypoxia Physiological state of decreased oxygen availability due to decreased concentration of hemoglobin or red blood cells.

anergy Impaired or absent ability to react to common antigens.

aneuploidy Having too many or too few chromosomes in a cell or any number other than 46 chromosomes in somatic or body cells or other than 23 chromosomes in germ cells or the eggs and sperm.

aneurysm Localized diseased segment of an artery that becomes thin and dilated because of degenerative changes in the tunica media layer.

angina pectoris Transient chest pain due to myocardial ischemia.

angiogenesis Process in which stimulated endothelial cells multiply and form tubular structures differentiating into arterioles or venules.

anion A negatively charged ion.

anion gap Represents the concentration of all unmeasured anions in plasma. It is comprised of negatively charged proteins as well as the acid anions produced during metabolism such as lactate. It is calculated by subtracting the sum of the chloride and bicarbonate levels from the sodium level, and its reference range is 8 to 16 mEq.

anisocoria Inequality of the size of the pupils; may be congenital or associated with aneurysms, head trauma, diseases of the nervous system, brain lesion, paresis, or locomotor ataxia.

ankle-brachial index (ABI) Ratio of arterial pressure at the ankle to the pressure at the brachial artery; used to predict the severity of peripheral arterial disease that may be present. A decrease in the ABI result with exercise is a sensitive indicator that significant pulmonary arterial disease is probably present.

ankylosing spondylitis A type of arthritis that affects the spine and the sacroiliac joint.

annuloplasty A surgery done to correct valve regurgitation by repairing the enlarged annulus.

annulus The fibrous ring at the junction of the cardiac valve leaflets and the muscular wall.

anorexia Loss of appetite.

anorgasmia Difficulty reaching orgasm.

anosmia The loss or impairment of the sense of smell.

antagonist Substance that displaces and replaces an opioid at the receptor, reversing the opioid's pharmacologic effect and side effects such as respiratory depression.

anterior circulation Describes the areas of the brain supplied by the right and left carotid arteries and their branches, including circulation in the arteries in the anterior portion of the circle of Willis.

anteriorly Front plane of the body.

anthropometric measurements Any physical measurement of the body.

antibody Proteins made by B cells and found in the plasma that are capable of attaching to antigens and stimulating immune responses.

antidiuretic hormone (ADH) A small peptide molecule released by the pituitary gland at the base of the brain. It has an antidiuretic action that prevents the production of dilute urine.

antigen Any foreign substance (bacterium, virus, protein) that elicits an immune response.

antigen–antibody complex The attachment of the FAB portion of an antibody to an antigen, resulting in the stimulation of a strong immune response; each FAB portion of the antibody is specifically shaped for only one type of antigen. Attracts other phagocytic cells such as neutrophils and macrophages to help eliminate the antigen; stimulates creation of B memory cells for long-term protection.

antigenicity The ability of a pathogen to elicit an immune defense in its host. It affects the ability of the host to develop a long-term immunity.

anti-infectives Drugs that are used to treat infections and include antibiotics, antivirals, and antifungals.

antiplatelet therapy Therapy that inhibits platelet adhesion and aggregation.

antrum Any nearly closed cavity or chamber.

anuria Total loss of urine production.

aortic coarctation Narrowing of the lumen of the aorta.

aortic dissection (AD) Weakening of the layers inside the aorta, which can result in tears in the aortic wall and leakage of blood into the chest or abdomen.

aortic valve regurgitation Incomplete closure of the aortic valve, which causes blood to regurgitate back into the left ventricle through a valve; results from abnormal valve cusps or aortic root.

aortic valve stenosis A narrowing of the aortic valve orifice, which results in an obstruction to blood flow from the left ventricle to the aorta during systole.

apathetic Indifferent; showing a lack of emotion.

aphasia The disorder of speech and language due to cerebral dysfunction. The three primary aphasic deficits are in comprehension of spoken language, expressive language, and naming.

apheresis A technology in which the blood of a donor or patient is passed through a machine that separates out one specific particle and returns the remainder of the blood to circulation.

aphonic Without a voice.

aphthous stomatitis (contact stomatitis) A common ulcerative condition limited to the oral cavity. Also known as *canker sores*.

apnea Cessation of airflow for more than 10 seconds.

apoptosis Programmed cell death in a multicellular organism; process by which cells can self-destruct when infected or mutated.

applied research Research that focuses on finding solutions to existing problems.

apudomas A rare tumor of the islets of Langerhans in the pancreas.

areflexia Loss of reflexive activity.

arrhythmogenic right ventricular cardiomyopathy (ARVC) An electrical disturbance that develops when the muscle tissue in the right ventricle is replaced with fibrous scar and fatty tissues.

arterial line An indwelling catheter inserted into an artery in order to monitor blood pressure.

arterial-venous shunts Shunts placed using surgical anastomosis of venous and arterial structures to facilitate dialysis procedures.

arteriosclerosis Thickening, reduced elasticity, and calcification of arterial walls.

arteriovenous malformation (AVM) A mass of abnormal blood vessels in which arterial blood flows directly into the venous system.

arthrodesis Surgical fusion of bone.

arthroplasty Restoration of a joint either by total joint replacement surgery or by resurfacing bone and removing damaged bone and cartilage.

artifact An ECG pattern from sources outside the heart; creates an abnormal pattern on ECG graph paper. This interference causes the baseline or isoelectric line to become fuzzy; this fuzzy baseline is referred to as 60 cycle.

asbestosis Diffuse lung fibrosis caused by exposure to asbestos.

ascites An abnormal intraperitoneal accumulation of fluid containing large amounts of protein and electrolytes.

aspartate aminotransferase (AST) An enzyme found in the liver, heart, skeletal muscle, and kidneys that is released when cellular injury occurs.

asphyxiates Chemical agents that cause injury, illness, and death by damaging the lungs. Also called *choking agents*.

assault Any action that places another person in apprehension of being touched in a manner that is offensive, insulting, or physically injurious without consent or authority.

assessment The act of evaluating or appraising.

assignment The transfer of a task and the accountability for the outcome.

assimilation Incorporation of new concepts into existing schemas.

assisted living A residential setting in which patients are provided long-term assisted care.

assistive device Device required by a patient to assist with ambulation (e.g., cane, crutches, walker).

associate caregiver An LVN/LPN or unlicensed assistive personnel assigned to provide care to patients according to the plan established by the primary nurse.

associate nurse A registered nurse who assists the primary nurse during off-duty hours and provides care consistent with the plan developed by the primary nurse.

asterixis A flapping tremor of the hands when the arms are outstretched; believed to be caused by the accumulation of substances normally detoxified by the liver.

asthma A disease with multiple precipitating factors resulting in reversible airflow obstruction.

astigmatism An optical defect.

asymmetry Unequal.

asystole Complete termination of ventricular activity with no measurable cardiac electrical activity. Represents cardiac standstill from massive cardiac muscle damage.

ataxia A failure of muscle coordination, resulting in loss of balance and coordination, as well as speech difficulties including dysarthria or slurred and scanning speech.

atelectasis Collapse or airless condition of the alveoli caused by hypoventilation and obstruction of airways by secretions.

atherogenesis The development of atherosclerosis.

atheroma Condition characterized by an accumulation in the inner lining of an artery of a plaque of cholesterol and other constituents.

atherosclerosis A type of arteriosclerosis; the most common etiologic process that causes reduced myocardial blood flow.

atopic dermatitis A chronic inflammatory skin disorder characterized by dry skin related to water loss in the epidermis and decreased skin lipid levels.

atrial dysrhythmia Dysrhythmia that generally results from an irritable focus in the atria that fires off an electrical impulse before the SA node has had a chance to fire in a normal fashion. Results in a P-wave configuration on the ECG that is different from that of a normal P wave; however, the QRS complex is normal.

atrial fibrillation A disorganized, very rapid, and irregular atrial rhythm resulting in an irregular ventricular rhythm. The rhythm is usually described as either course or fine fibrillation.

atrial flutter A rapid, regular atrial rhythm with a rate of about 300 beats per minute. Only a fraction of the impulses are transmitted through the AV node as a protective mechanism. Most of the atrial beats fall during the refractory period of the AV node so they are not conducted.

atrial kick Atrial contraction, which augments the blood supply going to the ventricles and ultimately cardiac output.

atrial natriuretic peptide (ANP) A hormone secreted by the right atrium in response to fluid overload that causes the excretion of sodium, which results in loss of the excess fluid; however, most regulation of excess volume is through decreased aldosterone secretion.

atrioventricular (AV) node Node located on the floor of the right atrium just above the tricuspid valve. The AV node has three regions: the AV junctional tissue between the atria and the node; the nodal area between the junctional tissue and the bundle of His; and the AV junction, the region where the AV node joins the bundle of His.

atrophy A reduction in the size of a cell and tissues or in muscle size.

auscultation Technique of listening to the sounds produced by different body areas.

autoantibodies An antibody produced in response to a self protein. Antinuclear antibodies, antibodies that bind to the nucleus of cells and result in cell destruction, are one example of autoantibodies.

autoantibody tests Tests that measure the amount or presence of antibodies to self proteins. Examples include the antinuclear antibody test and anti-IgG serum test.

autocrine functioning Secretion of cells that act to influence only their own growth.

autograft valve Valve obtained from the patient's own pulmonic valve and pulmonary artery. Also called *autologous valve*.

autografting Grafting of the patient's own skin to somewhere else on the patient's body.

autoimmune diseases Diseases that result from hypersensitivity responses and produce tissue damage and destruction. Examples include Goodpasture's syndrome and systemic lupus erythematosus; in both of these diseases, tissue is damaged by the production of antibodies to self-antigens.

autoimmune hemolytic anemia Red blood cell disorder characterized by destruction of cells by antibodies of the host.

autoimmune response Occurs when the body fails to recognize self cells or proteins and mounts an immune response against the self. Autoantibodies result in immune complexes that stimulate phagocytosis and destruction of cells and tissue.

autologous BMT Procedure in which bone marrow is collected from the patient and frozen. It is then reinfused into the patient following high-dose chemotherapy, with or without radiation.

autologous transfusion The process of collecting and reinfusing a patient's own blood.

automated external defibrillator (AED) A small, lightweight device that can recognize and treat ventricular fibrillation.

automaticity Ability of pacemaker cells to generate their own electrical impulses without depending on nervous system stimulation external to the heart.

autonomic hyperreflexia A syndrome characterized by severe hypertension, bradycardia, vasoconstriction below the level of injury, and vasodilation above the level of injury resulting from unchecked stimulation of the sympathetic nervous system triggered by a noxious stimulus.

autonomy Personal freedom to make choices or decisions.

autoregulation The ability of the brain to change its vessel size to accommodate changes in intracranial pressure.

autosomal dominant inheritance A Mendelian pattern of inheritance in which an affected individual has one copy of a mutant allele and one normal allele. Individuals who have autosomal dominant disorders have a 50–50 chance of passing the mutant allele and disorder to their children. This is in contrast to autosomal recessive disorders in which the individual must have two copies of the mutant allele.

autosomal recessive inheritance A Mendelian pattern of inheritance in which an affected individual receives two copies of a mutant allele, one from each parent, or the phenotype is expressed only when two copies of the mutant allele are present.

autosome A single chromosome from any 1 of 22 pairs of the chromosomes that is not a sex chromosome (XX or XY). Disorders caused by mutation in an autosomal gene or gene pair shows autosomal inheritance.

AV dissociation Independent function of the atria and the ventricles.

avascular necrosis (AVN) Condition in which bone tissue dies due to a temporary or permanent loss of blood supply to the bone.

avulsion fracture Fracture that occurs when a ligament is pulled away from its attachment point at the bone and takes a small piece of the bone with it.

azotemia An increase in blood urea nitrogen (BUN) caused when the kidneys are unable to excrete normally.

B cells White blood cells that are produced in the bone marrow and develop into plasma cells that are responsible for the creation and release of antibodies and development of long-term immune protection.

B lymphocytes Type of white blood cell that make antibodies against antigens, perform the role of antigen in presenting cells, and eventually develop into memory cells after activation by antigen interaction.

Bachmann bundle Part of the electrical conduction system of the heart composed of a group of interatrial fibers contained in the left atrium that conduct electrical impulses from the SA node to the left atrium.

bacterial meningitis Inflammation of the meninges caused by a bacterial pathogen.

bacterial phlebitis Inflammation of a vein associated with an infectious process.

bacterial vaginosis (BV) The most common bacterial infection in women of childbearing age. The cause is not clearly understood.

barium enema Type of enema used to obtain an x-ray of the large intestines. Radiographs are taken after the patient receives barium sulphate through an enema tube.

barotrauma Alveoli damage caused by the increased pressure resulting from use of a ventilator. Physical injury or rupture of tympanic membrane, resulting from changing air pressure.

Barrett's epithelium Columnar epithelial tissue that replaces the normal squamous epithelium in the esophagus after prolonged exposure to gastric juice. It is resistant to gastric acid, supports the healing of the esophagus, and is premalignant.

basal skull fracture A fracture of the skull that extends into the base of the skull.

base excess Part of the blood gas report, this is a calculated value that is based on the bicarbonate and carbon dioxide levels and the hematocrit. It expresses the number of milliequivalents of bicarbonate per liter of extracellular fluid that one has too much of (a base excess) or too little of (a base deficit). It is used as a guide by clinicians as they consider how much bicarbonate to administer to a patient with a severe metabolic acidosis.

basement membrane A thin, acellular layer between the dermis and epidermis that acts as scaffolding for the epidermis. Blood supply and nutrients reach the epidermis by passing through the basement membrane.

bases Compounds that combine with hydrogen ion in solution. A proton acceptor.

basic human needs As defined by Abraham Maslow, needs on the first four rungs of Maslow's hierarchy.

basic research Research undertaken to extend the knowledge base in a discipline or to formulate or refine a theory.

basophil A component of the white blood cell differential; actual function is not well known.

battery Contact with another or with another's immediate "personage" (clothes, car keys, cane, purse, etc.) without consent or authority; the touching of another without permission.

Battle's sign Bogginess of the temporal or postauricular region of the head, which indicates fracture of the basilar area of the skull.

Beck's triad Classic assessment findings for the patient with cardiac tamponade, consisting of decreased blood pressure, muffled heart sounds, and jugular venous distention.

behavioral dimension of pain Includes responses to pain that may be situational, developmental, or learned.

beneficence The ethical duty to do good.

benign Lacking malignant cells.

benign prostatic hyperplasia (BPH) Term applied to age-related benign enlargement of the prostate gland where there is no cancerous growth involved.

berry aneurysm Saccular-shaped aneurysm.

bevel The slanted or angled part of a needle or stylet.

Bier block Process in which an IV catheter is inserted in the extremity at the most distal site possible. A pneumatic tourniquet is applied proximal to the surgical site and inflated higher than the patient's systolic blood pressure. When a local anesthetic (lidocaine) is injected intravenously, the obstruction of blood by the tourniquet prevents it from leaving the surgical area.

bigeminy Premature ventricular contraction that occurs every other beat.

bile A substance produced in the liver containing bile salts, cholesterol, bilirubin, electrolytes, and water. It is concentrated and stored in the gallbladder, where it is released in response to a meal to aid in the emulsification and absorption of dietary fat.

bile canaliculi Small channels adjacent to the hepatocytes that move bile toward the common bile duct.

biliary dyskinesia Motility disorders of the gallbladder.

bilirubin A product in the breakdown of hemoglobin. It is conjugated by the hepatocytes and is excreted in bile.

binge-eating disorder (BED) Disorder characterized by the same type of binge eating as bulimia nervosa, but without the compensatory purging.

bioavailable Pertaining to a molecular form that can be readily used by the body.

bioavailable testosterone Free testosterone and testosterone that is loosely bound to albumin.

biologic agent Viruses, bacteria, and toxins that can be weaponized to cause disease, illness, and/or death.

biologic aging theory General theory of aging comprised of programmed theories and error theories. *See* error theories of aging *and* programmed theory of aging.

biologic dressing Heterografts such as pigskin or allografts obtained from living or deceased humans.

biologic valve Valve obtained from other species, most commonly from pigs (porcine valves), although cow valves (bovine) also are used. Also referred to as *xenografts*.

biopsy A portion of tissue examined for the presence of abnormal cells.

biosynthetic dressing A combination of biologic and synthetic materials that are effective as temporary covering for a variety of wounds.

biotherapy Treatment with agents whose origin, mostly mammal, is from biologic sources and/or affecting biologic responses.

biotransformation The process of changing a medication's structure in preparation for elimination. Metabolism occurs primarily in the liver, but also in the kidneys and, to a very small degree, other organ systems. Once a medication is metabolized, it is no longer the same and effectively discontinues its pharmacologic activity.

BiPAP Stands for *bi-level positive airway pressure*, which is a breathing apparatus that helps people get more air into their lungs. The air is delivered through a mask that can be set at two different pressures, one for inhaling (IPAP or inspiratory positive airway pressure) and another for exhaling (EPAP or expiratory airway pressure).

biphasic defibrillation Defibrillation procedure that delivers a charge in one direction for half of the shock and in the opposite direction for the second half.

bipolar lead ECG leads that have electrodes with opposite polarity, one positive and one negative.

biventricular heart failure A global inability of the heart muscle to pump blood effectively from both ventricles, compromising forward flow leading to right and left heart failure symptoms.

blackouts Amnesia for short-term events; can occur in patients with alcohol abuse problems.

bladder suspension A procedure designed to correct urinary incontinence. It is done to suspend the bladder and correct urinary incontinence that is often caused by weakened ligaments due to childbirth. Also called a *Burch procedure*.

blepharoplasty Surgical procedure to fix ptosis or drooping of the eyelid.

blister agent Chemical agent that can cause redness and irritation of the skin and blistering. Also called a *vesicant*.

blood pressure The pressure created by blood circulating through the arteries and veins and the chambers of the heart.

blood transfusion The process of infusing blood products in order to restore circulating volume and therefore increase oxygen carrying capacity.

blunt percussion Technique of placing the palm of the nondominant hand over a body area (such as the kidney) and striking the palm with the closed fist of the dominant hand.

bone conduction Process of sound vibrations reaching the inner ear for interpretation.

bone marrow transplantation Procedure in which hematopoietic cells from the bone marrow of one person are transferred into another person; used to treat a variety of diseases.

Botox Botulism toxin that has been purified and is injected into the lower esophageal sphincter to relax the muscle.

Bouchard's nodes Hard, painless nodules at the joints of the fingers; may indicate osteoarthritis (progressive loss of cartilage at a joint). Bouchard's nodes are found over the proximal interphalangeal joints.

boutonnière deformity Flexion of the proximal interphalangeal joint.

Bowman's capsule A thin, double-walled capsule encasing the glomerulus.

brachytherapy The use of localized radiation within the coronary artery to increase the size of the lumen of the artery.

bradykinesia Slowed movement; primary symptom of Parkinson's disease.

bradypnea A respiratory rate of less than 12 breaths per minute.

brain abscess A localized infection carried from other sites of the body and extending into the cerebral tissue.

breach of confidentiality Failure to prevent the disclosure of all or parts of a patient's medical record without the proper authority to do so.

breakthrough pain A transitory exacerbation of pain that occurs on a background of otherwise stable pain in a patient receiving chronic opioid therapy.

breast cancer The formation of a malignant glandular tumor, which over time destroys normal breast tissue and can spread to other parts of the body.

Brief Pain Inventory (BPI) Questionnaire that asks multiple questions regarding pain and its impact on patient function and addresses the multidimensionality of the pain experience.

bronchial breath sounds Breath sounds normally heard over the right or left bronchus of the lung.

bronchovesicular breath sounds Breath sounds normally heard between the bronchus and the smaller airways.

bruits The sound heard with a stethoscope of blood flowing through a narrowed blood vessel that is outside of the heart.

bubo Acutely swollen and usually painful lymph node seen in plague near the site of the flea bite.

Buck's boots traction A foam boot used for traction.

buffer A compound that minimizes the change in hydrogen ion concentration (and also the pH) when ions are added to or removed from solution. Think of a buffer as a sponge. When there is too much hydrogen ion, the sponge soaks up the extra. When the level of hydrogen ion is decreased, the sponge can be squeezed out to return hydrogen ions to the blood.

bundle branch block Discontinuity of conduction (complete or incomplete) in one branch of the bundle of His that affects normal transmission of the impulse through the ventricles. When one bundle is blocked, the ventricles depolarize asynchronously. Characterized by a delay of excitation to one ventricle; therefore, an abnormal spread of electrical activity through the ventricles occurs.

bundle of His Part of the conduction system that lies on top of the interventricular septum, between the right and left ventricles; it contains pacemaker cells. Also referred to as the *common bundle*.

bursae Sac containing synovial fluid that cushions joints during movement.

burst fracture Fracture that occurs when an axial load is placed on the spine and vertebrae.

cachexia Wasting of skeletal muscle and adipose.

café-au-lait spot Pigmented macules that are light brown in color.

calciphylaxis A condition during severe serum calcium excess, as in renal failure, in which calcium is deposited into the soft tissues of the body. This can be reflected in irregular purple lesions on the lower extremities that may lead to necrosis and gangrene.

calcium The most abundant cation in the body, primarily found in bones and teeth. Serum calcium plays a role in neuromuscular transmission (including cardiac) and cell membrane permeability. Normal serum levels are 8.5 to 10.5 mg/dL, 50% ionized and 40% bound to albumin.

caloric test Assesses abnormal nystagmus, tinnitus, or hearing loss as a result of vestibular dysfunction from eighth cranial nerve lesions by inserting water into the ear.

cancellous (trabecular) bone Bone with a hard outer casing and an interior that is porous, spongy, and meshwork-like in structure.

cancer Common term for all malignant neoplasms.

cancer pain Pain associated with malignancy; can be acute and chronic in nature.

candidiasis A common fungal infection caused by the *Candida* species of fungus; more commonly known as a yeast infection.

capnography Use of a device to measure exhaled or end-tidal carbon dioxide.

capture Term used to indicate that sufficient voltage has been put out by a pacemaker to make a myocardial contraction occur.

caput medusae A term used to describe the engorged, tortuous, and visible blood vessels radiating from the umbilicus in patients with severe liver disorders. In mythology, Medusa's hair was a tangle of snakes.

carbon dioxide An atmospheric gas composed of one carbon atom and two oxygen atoms. Produced as a by-product of metabolism, carbon dioxide can be thought of as a potential acid because, when it is dissolved in water, it forms carbonic acid.

carbon monoxide poisoning Occurs when an individual breathes carbon monoxide fumes that have built up in an enclosed space.

carbonic acid A weak acid formed by water reacting with carbon dioxide. If carbonic acid loses one proton, it becomes the bicarbonate ion.

carboxypeptidase An enzyme that breaks away the end amino acids on protein molecules.

carbuncle An infection of the skin composed of a cluster of boils caused by *Staphylococcus aureus*.

carcinoembryonic antigen (CEA) A glycoprotein found in embryonic gastrointestinal epithelium, but also found in tumors of the adult gastrointestinal tract. It is used to detect colon cancer, most specifically adenocarcinoma.

carcinogenesis Pertaining to the production of cancer.

carcinoma *in situ* Disorder in which neoplasms have not invaded the basement membrane of the epithelial site, thus the surrounding tissues are left untouched by malignant cells.

cardia The upper orifice of the stomach connecting with the esophagus.

cardiac catheterization A term used to describe a variety of invasive procedures used to identify atherosclerotic disease as well as provide anatomic and hemodynamic information about the heart and great vessels using radiopaque catheters.

cardiac conduction system Conduction system unique to the myocardium that is composed of specialized cells that enable it to generate and transmit action potentials without stimulation from the nervous system. The specialized cells are concentrated in the sinoatrial and atrioventricular nodes, and the Purkinje network.

cardiac depolarization Muscle contraction of the heart resulting from electrolyte exchange in the cardiac cells.

cardiac index (CI) Individualized measurement of cardiac output by taking into account the body surface area.

cardiac output (CO) The amount of blood leaving the left ventricle per minute.

cardiac pacemaker An electronic device that is capable of delivering an electrical stimulus to the heart.

cardiac repolarization Process whereby a depolarized cell is polarized, causing a return to the resting membrane potential. Also referred to as the recovery phase that every cardiac cell must go through in order to be ready to accept another stimulus.

cardiac resynchronization therapy (CRT) Therapy that uses atrial-synchronized biventricular pacemakers.

cardiac risk factors Habits, lifestyles, and/or genetic factors that predispose an individual to the development of coronary artery disease.

cardiac tamponade Bleeding into the pericardial sac. As the accumulation of blood increases, it compresses the atria and ventricles decreasing venous return and filling pressure, which leads to decreased cardiac output, myocardial hypoxia, and cardiac failure.

cardioesophageal Pertaining to the junction of the esophagus and the stomach.

cardiogenic embolism Blood clots from cardiac sources.

cardiogenic pulmonary edema (CPE) An abnormal accumulation of fluid in the lungs caused by cardiac failure; results from increased hydrostatic pressures in the pulmonary capillary bed secondary to increased pulmonary venous pressure.

cardiomegaly Enlargement of the heart.

cardiomyopathies (CMPs) Diseases of the myocardial muscle fibers that result in progressive structural and functional abnormalities of the myocardium.

cardioversion The timed delivery of an electrical current to depolarize cardiac muscle in order to terminate tachyarrhythmias, atrial tachycardia, rapid atrial fibrillation, atrial flutter, and junctional tachycardia.

caring The core of nursing; constitutes the essence of nursing regardless of the level at which nursing is practiced.

carotid endarterectomy (CEA) Surgical procedure to correct carotid stenosis by opening the carotid artery, removing plaque, and restoring blood flow in the lumen.

carpal tunnel syndrome Compression of the median nerve in the carpal tunnel, just below the palm dorsally.

carrier People or animals that do not have symptoms of infection but carry an active pathogenic microorganism.

case management An approach to coordinating care for patients in the hospital or in an outpatient setting.

case manager A person who collaboratively plans, coordinates, and evaluates services for cost effectiveness, but does not provide direct patient care.

case method A nursing care delivery system in which total patient care is delivered by a registered nurse who has shift responsibility for the patient.

cast A rigid circumferential encasement device made of plaster or fiberglass.

cataracts The opacity of the natural crystalline lens.

catheter A device that is introduced through the skin, into the vascular network, for the purpose of infusing parenteral solutions and medications.

catheter embolism Occurs when a piece of catheter is fractured and enters the circulatory system. The catheter may block a major vein, causing loss of circulation, or may travel to the heart, causing cardiac irritability and cardiac arrest.

cation A positively charged ion. Major cations affecting cardiac function are potassium (K), sodium (Na), and calcium (Ca).

cauda equina syndrome The bundle of nerve roots in the lower portion of the spinal canal, below the conus medullaris, which when compressed or inflamed causes symptoms of pain, altered reflexes, decreased strength, and decreased sensation. When extreme, can cause paralysis of the lower extremities, bowel and bladder dysfunction, and loss of the Achilles reflex; most commonly seen with large disk herniations at L_4/L_5, causing mass effect on the nerve roots as they descend through the spinal canal.

cavernous malformation Low-flow, cluster-type nodular lesion, not separated by brain tissue.

CBRNE Acronym suggested for common use by the Department of Justice to describe weapons of mass destruction. The acronym stands for chemical, biologic, radiologic, nuclear, and explosive devices.

CD4+ T cells T lymphocytes with cluster of differentiation 4 (CD4) receptors. The HIV particle can attach and enter T-helper (CD4) cells via the CD4 receptor.

celiac disease An autoimmune disorder involving a sensitivity to gluten, a protein found in wheat, that results in an immune-mediated response that causes a histologic change in the villi of the small intestine, resulting in malabsorption.

celiac sprue A lifelong condition affecting the small intestine in which the villi morphology is damaged because of the presence of gluten in the diet.

cell-mediated immune response Immune responses that are initiated through specific antigen recognition by the T cells; important in identifying and destroying cells that are already infected and providing protection against fungi, and has major involvement in rejection of transplant tissues, tumor immunity, and hypersensitivity reactions.

cellulitis A diffuse inflammatory process of the dermis and subcutaneous tissue layers characterized by erythema, edema, and pain; usually caused by staphylococcus or streptococcus infections.

Centers for Disease Control and Prevention (CDC) Agency under the U.S. Department of Health and Human Services whose function is to protect the health and safety of the public with regard to disease prevention and control.

central retinal artery occlusion (CRAO) Blockage of the central retinal artery, usually by an embolism. Its symptom is sudden, painless, unilateral blindness.

central vascular access device (CVAD) A vascular access device that is inserted into a centrally located vein with the tip residing in the vena cava.

central venous pressure (CVP) Measurement of venous return to the right atrium after insertion of a central venous catheter.

centromere The narrowed portion near the center of a human chromosome where the two sister chromatids or spindle traction fibers attach during mitosis or meiosis.

cerebral aneurysm A balloon-like outpouching, or widening, of an artery.

cerebral blood flow (CBF) The measurement of blood flow in the brain.

cerebral edema An increase in water content of the brain; swelling.

cerebral infarction A condition in which brain tissue dies due to lack of oxygen.

cerebral ischemia A condition in which brain tissue is oxygen deprived.

cerebral perfusion pressure (CPP) The pressure gradient that drives cerebral blood flow.

cerebral salt wasting Electrolyte abnormality characterized by loss of sodium and loss of extracellular fluid volume.

certified nurse midwife (CNM) An advanced practice nurse with postgraduate training and state certification to deliver healthy babies without direct supervision by a physician.

certified registered nurse anesthetist (CRNA) An advanced practice nurse with postgraduate training and state certification to administer anesthesia without direct supervision by a physician.

cerumen Earwax.

chain of infection Consists of a causative agent, reservoir, portal of exit, mode of transmission, portal of entry, and susceptible host.

Chance fracture A fracture through the body and posterior elements of the vertebrae of the spine; caused by forward flexion, causing a distraction injury.

chancres Ulcers of syphilis.

chancroid A bacterial, sexually transmitted infection that is rare outside of the tropics.

chemical agent Chemicals that can be used as weapons to cause injury, illness, and death. They are roughly divided by their mechanism of action into blood agents, blister agents, choking agents, irritants, and nerve agents.

chemical burns Burns that occur when the skin is in contact with caustic chemical compounds such as strong acids, alkalis, or organic compounds.

chemical phlebitis Inflammation of a vein associated with infusates of varying ranges of pH or osmolarities.

chemotaxis The movement of white blood cells to an area of inflammation or infection in response to the release of chemical mediators from neutrophils, macrophages, T cells, and injured tissue.

chief complaint Information about what brought the patient to the health care provider in the patient's own words.

chlamydia Most frequently reported sexually transmitted infection in the United States. It is caused by *Chlamydia trachomatis* and is treatable with antibiotics.

chloride A primary anion in extracellular fluid; its normal serum level is 95 to 108 mEq/L. Chloride is usually found in combination with sodium to create electrical neutrality in the body; it assists in the reabsorption of sodium in the kidneys and combines with hydrogen ion to form hydrochloric acid for digestion.

choking agent Chemicals that cause injury, illness, and death by damaging the lungs. Also called an *asphyxiate*.

cholangiocarcinoma Cancer of the gallbladder.

cholecystectomy Surgical removal of the gallbladder either through an open incision or with a laparoscope.

cholecystitis Inflammation of the gallbladder; most commonly caused by gallstones.

cholecystokinin A hormone secreted by the gastrointestinal mucosa that stimulates the gallbladder to eject bile and the pancreas to secrete alkaline fluid.

choledocholithiasis A gallstone in the common bile duct.

cholelithiasis Disorder in which stones form in the gallbladder that may be composed of cholesterol or calcium.

cholesterol A steroid molecule produced primarily by the liver that is essential for the formation and maintenance of cell membranes.

cholinergic crisis A life-threatening condition associated with myasthenia gravis; results from excess acetylcholine.

chromosomal disorder Condition caused by an abnormal chromosome makeup in which there is duplication, loss, or rearrangement of chromosomal material.

chromosome Threadlike structures in the nucleus of a cell that contain the genes. Chromosomes occur in pairs, with a typical human cell containing 46 chromosomes: 22 pairs of autosomes, and 2 sex chromosomes.

chronic bronchitis Hypersecretion of mucus and chronic productive cough that continues at least 3 months of the year for at least 2 consecutive years.

chronic graft rejection Occurs months to years after graft transplant and involves the slow, progressive failure of a transplanted organ.

chronic lymphocytic thyroiditis An autoimmune condition characterized by high titers of the circulating antibodies thyroid peroxidase and thyroglobulin that destroy thyroid cells and may lead to hypothyroidism. It is the most common thyroid disease in the United States. Also known as *Hashimoto's thyroiditis*.

chronic obstructive pulmonary disease (COPD) A disease state characterized by airflow limitation that is not fully reversible.

chronic pain Pain that does not resolve within the expected time frame, and is persistent beyond 3 to 6 months.

chronic stress Stress that occurs on a daily basis and is the result of an ongoing situation.

chronic wounds Wounds that do not follow the expected sequence of repair in a timely and uncomplicated manner.

Chvostek's sign Spasm of facial muscles; latent tetany, which can be demonstrated by tapping the inferior portion of the zygoma resulting in facial spasms.

chyle Lymphatic system drainage; a milky fluid comprised of serous fluid, white cells, and fatty acids, arising from the interstitial fluid of the gastrointestinal tract. It contains a high proportion of fat and proteins.

chyle leak A disruption in the lymph system into the tissues of the neck and chest.

chymotrypsin An enzyme that aids in the breakdown of large protein molecules by breaking the interior bonds of the amino acids.

circadian rhythm Pertinent to events that occur at approximately 24-hour intervals.

circinate balanitis Inflammation surrounding the circular muscle around the penis.

circulating nurse Nurse in the operating room whose duties are performed outside the sterile field. They encompass responsibilities of nursing care management within the operating room to create and maintain a safe, comfortable environment for surgery.

cirrhosis An inflammatory disease of the liver in which normal structure and function are disrupted.

civil law Rules and regulations that form the bases of legal actions; branch of law that pertains to contracts, torts, patents, and the like.

clinical judgment A complex skill involving several cognitive phases and integrative processes; clinical reasoning across time about a particular patient.

clinical knowledge Knowledge necessary to perform proficiently in the clinical setting, including recognizing signs and symptoms, applying skilled know-how in titrating an intravenous rate, recognizing signs of physiological distress and changes in patient's vital signs, and using clinical judgment.

clinical nurse leader (CNL) An advanced practice nurse with postgraduate training with the responsibility to integrate care among other disciplines and manage care at the bedside.

clinical nurse specialist (CNS) An advanced practice nurse with postgraduate training in a clinical disease specialty. The CNS may schedule clinic visits with patients, provide specialized inpatient or nurse education, or case manage a group of patients.

coal miner pneumoconiosis A chronic lung disease leading to pulmonary fibrosis. It is caused by inhalation of coal dust.

code of ethics A formal statement by a group that expresses the group's ideals, values, and ethical principles, which have been agreed on by the group's members to reflect their moral judgments and serve as a standard for their professional actions.

codon The sequence of three nucleotides in mRNA that specifies a single amino acid.

cognitive dimension of pain Includes the impact of personal beliefs, attitudes, and meanings attached to pain.

cognitive reappraisal The process of allowing for changes in the person's evaluation of an event or a relabeling of the cognitive appraisal.

coiling An endovascular procedure in which an aneurysm is filled with a soft coil. Also referred to as a *GDC (Guglielmi detachable coil)*.

collaborative problems Problems that are identified by other health care workers, such as physicians, in contrast to nursing problems, which are identified by nurses. The nurse is accountable for monitoring for changes in the status of the problem and initiating the appropriate interventions.

collagen synthesis Multistep process in which fibrin proteins form a matrix to support the newly forming tissue.

colon The large intestine from the end of the ileum to the anal canal that surrounds the anus.

colon cancer Disease in which malignant tissue arises from the cells in the colon; it is frequently associated with adenomatous polyps. When there is an allelic deletion on chromosomes 5, 17, or 18, the transformation from normal to malignant colon tissue is promoted.

colonoscopy Visualization of the lower gastrointestinal tract, usually through the insertion of an endoscope through the anus.

colposcopy A test in which the health care provider looks at the cells of the cervix through a special magnifying scope that is placed near the opening of the speculum that is inserted into the vagina.

comminuted skull fracture The fragmented interruption of the skull resulting from multiple linear fractures.

commissure The site where cardiac valve leaflets meet each other.

commissurotomy Surgical procedure used to separate fused heart valve leaflets.

common law System of law derived from principles rather than rules and regulations; consists of principles based on justice, reason, and common sense.

community-acquired infection An infection acquired outside a health care facility.

community-based care A setting for practice outside of acute care institutional walls. Care is directed toward individuals and families within any community setting and is designed to assist patients as they move among health care settings. Also describes a philosophy of care in settings that reflect *how* nursing care is provided, not *where*.

community health nursing Type of nursing practice for registered nurses who work in various health district programs. RNs provide follow-up care, immunizations, health education, and referrals of clients to appropriate agencies for assistance.

compact (cortical) bone Bone that is resistant to compression, is dense, and is laid down in concentric layers.

compartment syndrome An acute problem following injury or surgery caused when pressure within the muscles builds to dangerous levels. The resulting increased pressure within the fascial compartment impairs blood supply.

compensation Correction of the blood pH by the system that is *not* the cause of abnormal levels of carbon dioxide or bicarbonate. For example, when an excess of metabolic acid leads to metabolic acidosis, the lungs increase their ventilation to "blow off" carbon dioxide and reduce its level below normal, thus helping bring the pH back toward normal. Metabolic compensation for a respiratory problem is slower; it takes days to weeks to retain the bicarbonate.

complement A group of proteins in the blood that stimulates the inflammatory response and serves as a primary chemical mediator of the antigen–antibody reactions of the B-cell immune response.

complementary therapy A therapy used in addition to a conventional therapy.

complete spinal cord injury Permanent loss of all neurological function below the level of injury.

comprehensive exam A head-to-toe assessment usually performed on new patients who will be seen on a routine basis by various clinicians.

compression injuries Injuries that occur when pressure is applied to the spinal cord as a result of mass effect from bone fragments, disk herniation, tumor, abscess, or blood clot.

Compromised Family Coping Nursing diagnosis that refers to the inability of a family to function optimally.

concentric When referring to coronary artery stenosis, the term used to describe a lesion that occupies the whole circumference.

concussion A recognized collection of symptoms that result from a mild head injury.

conductive hearing loss Type of hearing loss in which sound waves cannot reach the inner ear for processing and interpretation; caused by diseases such as external ear infections.

conductivity Ability of the cardiac cell to accept and then transmit a stimulus to other cardiac cells.

configuration Refers to the pattern of arrangement or position of lesions.

congenital Present at birth or prenatally.

conjugate gaze Paired or joined eyes moving in tandem in the cardinal fields of gaze.

conscious A mental state that encompasses all things that are easily remembered.

conscious sedation A minimally depressed level of consciousness and satisfactory analgesia that allows the patient to retain the ability to maintain an airway independently and to respond to physical stimulation and verbal commands, obtained through the administration of a combination of pharmacologic agents.

constrictive pericarditis Occurs when the pericardial layers adhere to each other as a result of fibrosis of the pericardial sac.

contact dermatitis An inflammation of the skin related to exposure to an irritant or allergen in the environment.

continent ileostomy (Kock ileostomy or Kock pouch) During ileostomy surgery, the procedure in which the terminal ileum is folded back on itself and the inner wall removed, thereby forming a reservoir and a nipple valve that prevents leakage of fecal contents through the stoma.

continuity theory of aging Theory of aging based on the premise that successful aging is obtained by maintaining values, habits, and behaviors from adult life.

continuous passive motion device Machine into which an extremity is placed to perform continuous passive range of motion.

continuous positive airway pressure (CPAP) Procedure that delivers air into a patient's airway through a specially designed nasal mask or pillows.

continuous subcutaneous infusion (CSI) The uninterrupted infusion of small-volume parenteral medication via the subcutaneous route.

continuous subcutaneous insulin infusion (CSII) A method of exogenous insulin delivery that uses an external "insulin pump," which allows for programmed delivery of insulin into subcutaneous tissue.

contractility A mechanical function that enables the cardiac cells to shorten and cause the muscle to contract in response to an electrical stimulus. Also referred to as *rhythmicity*.

contrast sensitivity (CS) The function of being able to distinguish subtle gradations of grayish patterns between targets and background.

contusion An injury to soft tissue caused by trauma; a bruise.

convalescent phase In viral hepatitis, the phase that occurs approximately 6 to 8 weeks after exposure to the virus and lasts up to 10 weeks when liver function returns to normal. Also called the *recovery phase*.

convenience sampling Type of statistical sampling in which the most available persons or units are selected for inclusion in the study; the researcher has no control over the characteristics of the sample. Also referred to as *accidental sampling*.

coping A compensatory process with physiological and psychological components that allows the individual to adapt to a stressor.

cor pulmonale Enlargement of the right ventricle in response to pulmonary hypoxia; literally means "heart of the lungs."

coronary artery disease (CAD) A progressive atherosclerotic disorder of the coronary arteries that results in narrowing or complete occlusion of the vessel lumen.

correlational research design Research conducted to examine linear relationships between two or more variables.

corticosteroids A class of synthetic steroid hormones that decreases the inflammatory response and suppresses immune activity; used to prevent graft rejection. Examples include Solu-Medrol, Solu-Cortef, hydrocortisone, dexamethasone, and prednisone.

cosmetic surgery Surgery performed for the primary purpose of improving physical appearance.

cotton-wool spots (CWS) Soft exudates that appear as white cotton spots in the nerve fiber layer of the retina; caused by lack of blood supply to the tissue.

counterregulatory hormones Hormones that antagonize the actions of insulin. Examples include glucagon, cortisol, growth hormone, and catecholamines.

crackles When auscultating the lungs, common abnormal, short popping sounds heard on inspiration; caused by the movement of fluid or exudates.

C-reactive protein (CRP) A protein released from the liver in response to local inflammation or tissue injury; useful as a marker for inflammation and colon cancer.

creatinine kinase (CK) An enzyme found in high concentrations in the heart and skeletal muscle and in smaller concentrations in the brain.

cremasteric reflex Condition in which testicles rise in the scrotum to the abdominal cavity when the thigh is stroked or the room is cold.

crepitus Abnormal sounds (grating, snapping, crackling, rattling) emanating from a joint while in movement.

cretinism Condition caused by the congenital absence or atrophy of the thyroid gland, resulting in hypothyroidism and characterized by mental deficiency, large tongue, puffy facial features, and dwarfism.

criminal law Law pertaining to conduct that is offensive or contrary to the public good, such as murder, theft, and rape.

crisis The occurrence of an event or series of events that creates a situation that is perceived as threatening.

critical incident A stressful incident that is so markedly distressing and powerful as to overcome a person's normal feelings of control and coping.

critical incident stress debriefing (CISD) Formal event run by trained counselors to assist those involved in a critical incident to better cope with the incident.

critical incident stress management A comprehensive approach to the management of stress and critical incidents.

critical pathways Comprehensive plans of care for specific patient situations or disease processes. Critical pathways include nursing interventions, medical interventions, and expected timelines for patient outcomes.

critical thinking A purposeful, two-dimensional, goal-directed process that is context bound. Two dimensions are necessary for the development of critical thinking: the cognitive, which is reflective, reasoned thinking, and the affective, which is open-mindedness to divergent perspectives and an inquisitive spirit.

Crohn's disease An inflammatory bowel disease that involves all layers (transmural) of the intestinal wall and can occur anywhere from the mouth to the anus, but commonly affects the ileum.

cross-linking theory of aging Theory of aging based on the premise that the binding of glucose to protein causes various problems. Also referred to as the *glycosylation theory of aging*.

cryoprecipitates Clotting factors used to treat bleeding associated with hemophilia and disorders that cause a depletion of the clotting factors.

cryptorchidism Undescended testicle(s).

cultural competence The ongoing practice of knowing, respecting, and incorporating the values of others; being open to the cultural beliefs and behaviors of others.

cultural diversity Variety and differences in the customs and practices of defined social groups; refers to the variation among groups of people with respect to the habits, values, preferences, beliefs, taboos, and rules determined to be appropriative for individual and social interaction.

culture Learned patterns of behavior, beliefs, and values that can be attributed to a particular group of people.

curative procedures Surgeries performed for the primary purpose of curing a condition.

Cushing's syndrome A hypermetabolic state in which there is a chronic excess of corticosteroid hormones for a variety of reasons.

Cushing's triad Combination of widening pulse pressure, bradycardia, and irregular respiratory patterns; may indicate increasing intracranial pressure.

cyanosis Bluish-tinged skin or mucous membranes due to deoxygenated hemoglobin in blood vessels close to the skin.

cystic fibrosis (CF) A chronic disease in which the process of transportation of salt and water across cell membranes is disturbed, leading to production of unusually thick mucus that blocks bodily passages, particularly in the digestive and respiratory systems. This disorder affects all exocrine glands.

cystocele Occurs when the wall between the bladder and the anterior vagina weakens, often as a result of childbirth, and the bladder protrudes into the vaginal vault.

cytogenetics A specialization of genetics that involves the study of chromosomes.

cytokines Chemical signals released by white blood cells (predominately T cells) that act as messages between cells and instruct immune cells to proliferate, differentiate, or alter activities; more than 100 different cytokines have been identified.

cytotoxic edema The accumulation of intracellular water, causing brain swelling.

dactylitis A uniform swelling of the soft tissues between the metacarpophalangeal and interphalangeal joints.

DASH diet A diet low in saturated fat, cholesterol, and total fat. There are two versions of the DASH plan: Plan 1 limits the patient to 2,000 mg of sodium per day; plan 2 limits the patient to 1,500 mg of sodium per day.

data saturation Sampling to the point at which no new information is obtained and redundancy is achieved.

dawn phenomenon Situation in which a patient has fasting hyperglycemia that is not related to nocturnal hypoglycemia and rebound hyperglycemia.

dead space The portion of the tidal volume that does not reach the alveoli of the lungs or take part in the exchange of oxygen and carbon dioxide.

dead space ventilation (V_D) The portion of the tidal volume that is not participating in gas exchange.

decannulation Term used to refer to the process of weaning a patient toward the goal of removing a tracheotomy tube.

decerebrate posturing The characteristic posture of an individual with decerebrate rigidity. The extremities are stiff and extended, and the head is retracted.

decibel (dB) A measurement of sound. Sounds typically range from 0 to 140 dB or greater.

decontamination The reduction or removal of contaminating agents.

decorticate posturing The characteristic posture of a person with a lesion at or above the upper brainstem. The person is rigidly still with arms flexed, fists clenched, and legs extended.

deep venous thrombosis (DVT) The formation of a blood clot within a deep vein, commonly in the thigh or calf.

defamation of character Publication of anything that is injurious to the good name or reputation of another or that tends to bring another's reputation into question.

defibrillation Basically the same as cardioversion in that electrical voltage is delivered to cause depolarization of the myocardium to terminate unwanted rhythms, except it is done in an emergency situation when sudden cardiac arrest has occurred.

degenerative joint disease Progressive loss of cartilage at a joint.

delayed hypersensitivity reaction Occurs when the immune system responds to an antigen over several hours to days. An example is contact dermatitis.

delegation The assignment of work to others while maintaining accountability for the outcome of the work.

deletion The loss of a chromosome or DNA segment of any length.

delirium A disturbance in consciousness resulting in decreased attention and a change in cognition, or development of a perceptual disturbance that develops over a short period of time and tends to fluctuate throughout the day.

delirium tremens (DTs) Tremor and clouding of consciousness that can accompany physiological withdrawal from alcohol.

dementia A general term for brain dysfunction characterized by a decline in cognition and memory that causes loss of ability to carry out activities of daily living and communicate with others, ultimately resulting in death.

deontological theories In ethics, theories that derive norms and rules from the duties human beings owe one another by virtue of commitments that are made and roles that are assumed.

deoxyhemoglobin Configuration of hemoglobin stimulated by hypoxic states and characterized by rapid release of oxygen to peripheral tissues.

deoxyribonucleic acid (DNA) A complex protein present in the chromosomes of the nuclei of cells that is the basis of heredity and the carrier of genetic information for all organisms except RNA viruses.

dependent activities Activities prescribed by the physician and carried out by the nurse; includes implementing the physician's orders to administer medications or treatments.

depressed skull fracture Displacement of a comminuted skull fracture.

dermabrasion Process of removing the epidermis and upper dermis of the skin so that the skin can regenerate into a smooth surface.

dermatofibromas Common, fibrous, tumor-like nodules of the skin.

dermatomyositis Progressive inflammatory muscle condition that occurs with inflammatory skin changes.

dermatophyte A fungus parasite on the skin.

descriptive research design Type of research question, design, and data analysis that will be applied to a given topic.

descriptive vividness In qualitative research, the practice of describing the site, participants, experience of collecting data, and the thinking of the research so clearly that the reader has a sense of personally experiencing the event.

desensitization The process of introducing small amounts of a triggering allergen to an allergic individual in increasing amounts over time. The goal is to reduce the severity of the allergic response.

desquamation Shedding of the outer layer of epidermis (skin or mucosa).

developmental stressor Stressor that occurs during specific periods of the life span, for examples, as a child, adolescent, young adult, middle adult, or older adult.

Diabetes Control and Complications Trial (DCCT) A landmark research study in the United States and Canada which demonstrated that intensive management of type 1 diabetes (aimed at normal blood glucose levels) resulted in decreased occurrence and progression of development of microvascular complications (i.e., retinopathy, neuropathy, nephropathy).

diabetes insipidus (DI) A hypometabolic disorder of the adrenal gland in which there is excretion of a large volume of dilute urine due to deficiency of antidiuretic hormone (ADH) or an inability of the kidneys to respond to ADH.

Diabetes Prevention Program (DPP) A major clinical research trial of patients with pre-diabetes that clearly demonstrated that lifestyle modification was superior to pharmacologic therapy with metformin (an oral diabetes medication) in preventing diabetes.

diabetic ketoacidosis (DKA) An acute emergent complication of diabetes (usually type 1 diabetes) primarily characterized by hyperglycemia, dehydration, and metabolic acidosis.

diabetic peripheral neuropathy (DPN) A chronic complication of diabetes in which the nerves outside of the spinal cord are damaged. Diabetic peripheral neuropathy is associated with numbness, weakness, burning pain (which often worsens at night), and loss of reflexes in the extremities.

diabetic retinopathy (DR) Disorder characterized by weakened and damaged blood vessels (capillaries) that result in edema from leaking capillaries that hemorrhage.

diagnostic procedures Surgeries performed for the purpose of diagnosing a condition.

dialysis catheter A large-bore vascular access device used as a temporary means to facilitate dialysis procedures; its configuration is similar to that of a pheresis catheter.

diaphysis Shaft of a long bone, between both metaphysis.

diascopy Examination of superficial skin lesions with a diascope.

diastolic A blood pressure reading of the minimum pressure in the arteries, which occurs just prior to the next cycle of ventricular ejection of blood; reflects cardiac relaxation.

diastolic dysfunction Impaired relaxation, preventing the heart from filling appropriately at normal preload pressures.

differentiation Maturation process of blood cells during which cell generations gain increasing specialization; begins with the hematopoietic stem cell and goes to the fully mature peripheral cell.

diffuse axonal injury (DAI) A primary injury of diffuse white matter that results in tearing or shearing of axons and small blood vessels.

diffusion The movement of molecules from an area of high concentration to an area of low concentration in liquids, gases, and solids.

dilated cardiomyopathy A disorder of the myocardium characterized by dilation and impaired contraction of one or more ventricles; the most common form of cardiomyopathy.

diploid The number of chromosomes in most cells except the gametes. The diploid number in humans is 46.

diplopia Seeing double vision, when one object appears as two.

direct inguinal hernia Occurs when abdominal contents herniate through a weak point in the fascia of the abdominal wall and into the inguinal canal.

direct percussion Technique of using gentle tapping to illicit the presence or absence of fluid, which results in a dull sound; used to examine such areas as the sinuses.

direct question Question used to elicit specific information and to clarify specific details; for example, "Is the pain sharp or dull?"

discrete lesion An individual or separate lesion.

disengagement theory of aging Theory of aging based on the premise that age-related changes bring about a mutual and reciprocal withdrawal of the individual from society.

diskectomy Surgery to remove a diseased disk.

dislocation Displacement of a bone from its normal position in a joint.

dissecting aortic aneurysm A localized dilation of the aorta that has a longitudinal dissection between the outer and middle layers of the vascular wall.

distribution (1) A description of the lesions on the skin according to location or body region affected. (2) The process of moving a medication into the bloodstream and the extracellular and intracellular compartments, as well as in the compartment that is the site of absorption.

diverticular disease Disease in which abnormal saclike outpouchings (diverticula) of the intestinal wall occur anywhere in the gastrointestinal tract except the rectum, but usually occurring in the distal large intestine.

diverticulitis Inflammation of a diverticulum.

diverticulosis The presence of one or more diverticula.

DMAT Acronym for disaster medical assistance team. A group of volunteer health care professionals and ancillary staff that can provide emergency medical services and relief in times of disaster.

DMORT Acronym for disaster mortuary operations response team. A team of volunteers that can assist with handling mass casualties in time of disaster.

doll's eye reflex *See* oculocephalic reflex.

donor site An area on the body where skin is surgically harvested to use for covering burn wounds.

dopamine A neurotransmitter necessary for ease of movement; loss of dopamine is a key factor in Parkinson's disease.

Dressler's syndrome Condition characterized by fever, pericarditis, chest pain, and pericardial and pleural effusions. Believed to be an autoimmune response, it occurs in 5% to 15% of patients 1 to 4 weeks after a myocardial infarction.

Dreyfus model of skill acquisition A learning model based on determining the level of practice evident in particular situations. It elucidates strengths as well as problems. In this model, situated practice capacities are described rather than traits or talents of the practitioners.

drip factor The number of drops equal to 1 mL of fluid.

drusen Yellowish, round, slightly elevated, different-sized subretinal pigment epithelial deposits in the macula.

dual-channel pump Pole-mounted electronic infusion devices that have multiple channels for infusion within a single device.

dullness A high-pitched tone of short duration that is soft in quality. It is heard over the large organs such as the liver and kidney.

duodenal ulcer An erosion of the duodenal lining resulting from *Helicobacter pylori* infection and hypersecretion of acid and pepsin.

Dupuytren's contracture Difficulty or an inability to extend the ring or fifth finger.

durable power of attorney for health care (DPAHC) A document that allows a patient to appoint a decision maker in the case of future incapacity. The DPAHC specifically states which powers the patient gives to the surrogate. The appointed person responsible for making medical decisions does not need consent from other family members or friends.

dwell The time period during which an infusion catheter remains in place.

dynamic response test A test to assess whether a transducer system is accurately transmitting pressures.

dysconjugate gaze Eyes moving separately from each other in the cardinal fields of gaze.

dyskinesia Involuntary, writhing movements that may involve limbs, trunk, face, and neck; results from overstimulation of dopamine receptors. Condition characterized by areas of abnormal heart contractility where muscle movement is impaired.

dysmenorrhea Painful menstruation.

dyspareunia Painful intercourse; can be a result of several factors such as endometriosis or menopause.

dysphagia Difficulty swallowing.

dysphoria An exaggerated feeling of depression and unrest without apparent cause; a mood of general dissatisfaction, restlessness, anxiety, discomfort, and unhappiness.

dysplasia Change in the appearance of cells after they have been subjected to chronic irritation.

dyspnea Subjective feeling of shortness of breath or difficulty breathing.

dysrhythmia A heartbeat originating from a site other than the primary cardiac pacemaker tissue. The terms *dysrhythmia*, *arrhythmia*, and *ectopic focus* all mean the same thing and are used interchangeably.

eccentric When discussing plaque buildup in a coronary artery, the term used to describe a lesion that occupies part of a vessel wall.

ecchymosis A lesion that is initially dark red or purple, but gradually fades to yellowish green before it disappears.

ECG single photon emission computed tomography (SPECT) A nuclear medicine technique that uses radiopharmaceuticals, a rotating camera, and a computer to produce images representing slices through the body in different planes.

ECG waveform Movement away from the baseline, or the isoelectric line, on an ECG tracing on graph paper.

echocardiography The noninvasive assessment of the structures and function of the heart and great vessels utilizing high-frequency (ultrasound) sound waves.

ectopic Implantation of the products of conception outside the uterine endometrium.

ectopic focus A heartbeat originating from a site other than the primary cardiac pacemaker tissue. Also called *dysrhythmia*.

edema Accumulation of fluid in the intercellular spaces that causes swelling of tissue.

efferent Ability to transport away from a central organ or section; conducts impulses from the brain or spinal cord to the periphery. In the nervous system, efferent nerves are known as motor or effector neurons that carry nerve impulses *away* from the central nervous system to effectors such as muscles or glands.

ego Mediates the drives of the id with a dose of reality.

ego defense mechanisms Utilized to alleviate anxiety by denying, distorting, and misinterpreting reality.

ejection fraction (EF) The amount of blood ejected from the left or right ventricle; calculated by comparing end-diastolic volume to stroke volume.

elastomeric balloon A portable, disposable mechanical infusion device that requires no power source to function.

elective procedures Procedure for which the timing is determined by the patient and the surgeon. A total knee replacement scheduled in advance is an example of an elective surgery.

electrocardiogram Surface recording of the electrical activity of the heart.

electrode An adhesive pad that contains conducting gel and is connected to a cardiac monitor by lead wires. Electrodes serve as sensing devices to detect changes in electrical activity of the heart. Electrodes must be placed in certain positions in order for the ECG machine to have a clear picture of the electrical impulse, and they must have a positive, a negative, and a ground lead.

electrolytes Ionized minerals (calcium, chloride, magnesium, phosphorus, potassium, and sodium) serving as energy transfer mechanisms in combinations of positive charges (cations) or negative charges (anions).

electromyelogram (EMG) A graphic recording that tests the contraction of muscles that have been electrically stimulated.

electron beam computed tomography (EBCT) Procedure that uses an electron gun and a stationary tungsten target to rapidly (about 90 seconds) acquire multiple images of the heart during a single breath hold.

electroneutrality The principle that asserts that the sum of all positive or cationic charges in plasma must equal the sum of all negative or anionic charges. The primary cations measured in venous plasma are sodium and potassium. The main anions are chloride and bicarbonate or serum carbon dioxide.

electronic infusion device (EID) An infusion device that can be portable, or pole mounted; requires a power supply (i.e., batteries or electric current) to function; used to control delivery of parenteral solutions or medications.

electrophysiology study (EPS) An invasive procedure that involves placing multiple multipolar catheter electrodes into the venous and sometimes the arterial side of the heart in order to evaluate the electrical activity of the heart and to identify areas of initiation and propagation of dysrhythmias.

elemental iron Amount of iron in a food substance that is available for absorption from the digestive tract.

elimination The process of excretion from the body that is generally accomplished in the renal system. Elimination can occur after medications are metabolized or medications may be eliminated in their primary form.

emancipated minors Persons under the legal age of adulthood who are no longer under the control and regulation of their parents and who may give valid consent for medical procedures.

embolectomy Mechanical removal of a clot in a blood vessel.

embolization Endovascular procedure in which an aneurysm is obliterated by filling it with a glue-type substance.

emergency doctrine Allows implied consent for treatment to exist in true emergency situations in which an individual is in danger of loss of life or limb.

Emergency Medical Treatment and Active Labor Act (EMTALA) A part of the 1986 COBRA laws and the 1990 OBRA amendment that defines the legal responsibilities of Medicare-participating hospitals in treating individuals who present with emergency medical conditions; ensures that patients have access to emergency services regardless of their ability to pay.

emergency nursing The care of individuals of all ages with perceived or actual physical or emotional alterations of health that are undiagnosed or require further interventions.

emergent (emergency) surgery Surgery that must be performed suddenly without advanced planning.

emmetropia The condition of the normal eye when parallel rays are focused exactly on the retina and vision is perfect. Normal refractive error or vision without any corrective optical devices.

emphysema A disease of the airways that involves destruction of the alveolar walls.

empiric therapy Therapy that is begun before culture results are available; physicians determine if empiric therapy is necessary based on the severity of the infection.

encephalitis Inflammation of brain tissue.

endocrine Glands that secrete directly into the bloodstream.

endoleaks Continued leakage of blood into the aneurysmal sac.

endometriosis Condition in which endometrial-like cells are found outside of the uterus. During the menstrual cycle, these cells respond to hormone production and may swell and bleed. In response, the body will surround these lesions with scar tissue, which can form adhesions on the area of attachment.

end-organ perfusion The blood perfusion of the end organs such as the integumentary system.

endorphins Endogenous, morphine-like substances that reduce or inhibit pain perception in the descending pathways.

endoscopic retrograde cholangiopancreatography (ERCP) Radiograph following injection of a radiopaque material into the papilla of Vater.

endoskeletal Pertaining to the cartilaginous and bony skeleton of the body.

endotoxins Produced by live bacteria and released when the bacteria are killed.

endotracheal tube Tube used to deliver oxygen that is placed in the trachea.

end-stage renal disease (ESRD) A patient is considered to have end-stage renal disease when the loss of filtration ability reaches approximately seven-eighths, at which point the survival of the patient depends on dialysis or, if an acceptable candidate, a kidney transplant.

engraftment Establishment of new bone marrow.

enkephalins Pentapeptides produced in the brain that act as an opiate.

enteral nutrition Use of the gastrointestinal tract for feeding.

enthesitis Upon palpitation, discomfort at the site of the attachment of bone to the tendon.

enzyme immunoassays (EIAs) Laboratory tests of blood to determine whether or not antibodies are present. A specific enzyme is used to link to antibodies, in this case, HIV antibodies. A positive test indicates antibodies are present.

eosinophil Acts as a phagocyte in inflammatory conditions, particularly allergic reactions.

ependymomas Tumors originating from the ependymal cells of the cerebral ventricles.

epididymitis Inflammation of the long, tubular structure that connects and carries sperm from the testicle to the vas deferens.

epidural anesthesia A type of regional anesthesia in which an anesthetic agent is injected in the epidural space.

epidural hematoma (EDH) Bleeding into the space between the skull and the dura.

epiglottitis Infection and inflammation of the epiglottis and surrounding supraglottic structures often resulting in airway obstruction. Usually caused by *Haemophilus influenzae* type B.

epiphysis The end of the bone beyond the physis.

epistaxis Bleeding from the nose.

epithelialization Process by which a wound closes from its margins, covering the defect with a layer of new skin.

erectile dysfunction (ED) The inability to achieve or maintain an erection sufficient to allow intercourse.

error theories of aging Theory of aging based on the premise that environmental factors negatively impact the human body, causing destruction and damage.

erysipelas A form of cellulitis characterized by inflammation and redness of the skin due to group A hemolytic streptococci.

erythrocyte Red blood cell.

erythropoiesis Process of red blood cell development.

erythropoietic stem cell (proerythroblast) The earliest of four stages in development of the normoblast. Ancestor cell giving rise to red blood cells.

erythropoietin Hormone that stimulates the production of red blood cells.

escape Term that applies to the emergence of a pacemaker that is lower in the heart and sustains a heart rate when the SA node fails.

eschar Nonviable burned tissue.

escharotomies Incisions made through burn tissue to relieve the constricting effects of the edema that accompanies circumferential injuries.

esophageal cancer Cancer that occurs anywhere in the esophagus, but more often occurs in the middle and distal portions; is usually squamous cell carcinoma.

esophageal varices Varicose veins in the distal esophagus that result most often from portal hypertension, a complication of cirrhosis of the liver.

esophagus The muscular tube that carries swallowed foods and liquids from the pharynx to the stomach.

esophoria Inward deviation of the eye.

ethical decision making Evaluating the principles and values of all persons involved in a decision before coming to a conclusion.

ethical dilemma A situation that involves two or more unfavorable alternatives to a given situation.

ethics Discipline relating to moral actions and moral values.

ethnography A form of research that focuses on the sociology of meaning through field observation and description of a sociocultural phenomenon.

ethos Notions of what counts as good nursing or good scientific practice.

euphoria An exaggerated feeling of well-being.

eustress Stress associated with positive events.

euthymia Normal, nondepressed, reasonably positive mood.

euthyroid Appearing to function as a normal thyroid gland.

euvolemia Term used when the body is in a state of equal fluid balance, without fluid retention.

evaluation Focuses on a patient's behavioral changes and compares them with criteria stated in predetermined patient outcomes. Evaluation is ongoing through all phases of the nursing process.

evidence-based practice (EBP) A problem-solving approach to clinical decision making that incorporates a search for the best and latest evidence, clinical expertise, and assessment, and a patient's preferences and values within a context of caring. This decision-making approach integrates clinical expertise with the best available evidence from systematic research in contrast to opinion-based health care decision making that is based primarily on values and resources.

excitability Ability of an electrical cell to respond to a stimulus. All cardiac cells possess this property. Also referred to as *irritability*.

exercise testing A cardiovascular stress test combining exercise (either physical or pharmacologic) and electrocardiographic and blood pressure monitoring, typically to evaluate patients with suspected coronary artery disease.

exocrine pancreas The portion of the pancreas that secretes enzymes for digestion into the duodenum.

exon The portion of a gene that contains the code for producing the gene's protein.

exophthalmos Abnormal protrusion of the eyeball; may be due to thyrotoxicosis, tumor of the orbit, orbital cellulitis, leukemia, or aneurysm.

exostosis A condition of the ear canal in which the bony lining under the skin develops a number of lumps that grow into the tube. Also called *surfer's ear*.

exotoxins Proteins released by bacterial cells during growth; they have very specific actions. Exotoxins modify cell enzymes and functions, leading to cell death or dysfunction. They are usually named for the site they affect.

experience An active process of gaining knowledge and skill, not just a passage of time.

experiential learning Requires a turning around of preconceptions, or an adding of nuances to one's understanding. Experiential learning requires openness and responsiveness by the learner to improve practice over time.

experimental research design Type of research in which the researcher attempts to maintain control over all factors that may affect the results of an experiment. In so doing, the researcher attempts to determine or predict what may occur when a hypothesis is tested and conclusions are drawn between independent and dependent variables.

exploratory surgery Surgery performed for the purpose of identifying abnormalities when the diagnosis of a condition is not established beforehand.

expressivity The degree or amount of symptomology to which an individual with a genotype is affected. For example, two individuals may have the same genotype, but one may have all of the symptoms of the disorder, while the second one has relatively few symptoms.

extension set Tubing that adds length and/or access ports to an administration set.

external fixation A treatment in which the bones or bone ends of a fracture are held in place by skeletal pins. The pins are screwed into the bone and attached to a frame worn on the outside of the body.

external locus of control An orientation in which a person believes that events in his or her life are controlled more by fate, luck, and external circumstances.

external stressor Stressor that originates outside the body.

extra-axial tumors Tumors originating from the supporting structures of the brain.

extracellular fluid (ECF) Fluid between the cells (interstitial fluids) and in plasma (serum).

extravasation Inadvertent administration of a vesicant solution or medication into surrounding tissues.

Factor VIII A clotting factor that may be administered intravenously for the treatment of hemophilia A.

false imprisonment The unjustified detention or confinement of a person without legal warrant.

familial intracranial aneurysms The presence of proven aneurysms in two or more family members among first- and second-degree relatives.

fascicles Anterior and posterior pathways that branch off the heart's left bundle branch. The anterior fascicle carries electrical impulses to the anterior wall of the left ventricle. The posterior fascicle spreads electrical impulses to the posterior ventricular wall.

fasciculation Involuntary contraction or twitching of a group of muscles or muscle fibers, visible under the skin.

fasciotomy Incisions made to release skin and muscle coverings.

FAST examination Focused assessment with sonography for trauma.

fast-tracking Term used to describe a situation in which a patient is transferred from the operating room to the postanesthesia care unit (PACU) phase II, bypassing PACU phase I. Fast-tracking is possible when surgical techniques are minimally invasive and anesthesia is of a short duration.

fat embolus Fat that enters the circulatory system after the fracture of a long bone.

ferritin A form of iron in the body acting as a supply reservoir.

fetal alcohol syndrome (FAS) Physical and mental defects found in babies of women who consumed alcohol during pregnancy.

fetid breath Halitosis or foul or putrid breath.

fever of unknown origin (FUO) A fever that lasts 2 weeks or more without identification of the cause.

fibroblasts Small cells that migrate along the fibrin network to produce the connective tissue and collagen fibers.

fibrocystic breast An increase in glandular and fibrous tissues in the breast; characterized by small, nodular cysts that are palpable in the breast.

fibroid tumor Growths arising from the tissue of the uterine muscle; they develop slowly in women ages 25 through 40 years of age.

fibrous cap A dense connective tissue matrix in the inner lining of an artery that is formed when smooth muscle cells secrete collagen, elastin, and glycosaminoglycans.

fidelity In ethics, keeping one's promises or commitments.

fill time Period of time needed for blood to enter the heart between contractions.

filter Add-on device used to screen particulate matter, bacteria, and toxins from the infusion system.

filtration The movement of molecules from an area of higher concentration through permeable membranes to an area of lower concentration as a result of hydrostatic pressure.

first-degree AV block Conduction disturbance in which electrical impulses flow normally from the SA node through the atria, but are delayed at the AV node. This results in a prolongation of conduction rather than an actual block. Due to this delay, the PR interval is greater than 0.20 second, making it abnormal.

Fisher grading scale Grading scale for subarachnoid hemorrhage referring to the amount of blood on a CT scan.

fissure Deep linear crack or furrow in the continuity of the epidermis.

fistula Dehiscent wound that traverses between two different tissue planes; a communication between two areas such as the oral cavity and the skin.

flail chest Occurs when a person sustains two or more rib fractures in two or more places such that the ribs are no longer attached to the thoracic cage, resulting in a free or floating segment of chest wall. As a result, during spontaneous ventilation the floating segment moves in the opposite direction or paradoxically to the chest wall. This condition is almost always associated with pulmonary contusion.

flame-shaped hemorrhages Retinal hemorrhages that occur in the nerve fiber layer.

flare A round area of redness surrounding the wheal of an allergic reaction on the skin.

flashback chamber Small space located after the hub of the catheter and attached to the stylet; used to collect blood.

flashes Sudden bright light noticed by a person; flashes appear as sparks or minuscule strands of light, almost like streaks of lightning across the sky that occur when the vitreous gel bumps, rubs, or tugs against the retina.

flatness A soft, high-pitched tone of short duration. It is heard over muscle and bone.

flexible sigmoidoscopy A sigmoidoscope that uses fiber optics to inspect the sigmoid colon.

floaters Deposits of various size, shape, consistency, refractive index, and motility within the eye's vitreous humor, which is normally transparent.

flow control device Device used to regulate fluid administration.

flushing Procedure performed to maintain device patency and prevent mixing of incompatible solutions or medications.

focused exam An exam performed in emergent or urgent situations that focuses on a specific problem.

folate Naturally occurring, water-soluble form of vitamin B critical for red blood cell formation.

folliculitis Inflammation of the hair follicles.

Folstein Mini-Mental State Exam A common screening tool used by clinicians to evaluate dementia.

foreign body sensation (FBS) A feeling in the eye of a "gritty" feeling, as if something is in the eye.

forensic evidence Something that is legally submitted to a court of law as a means of determining the truth related to an alleged crime.

foreseeability of harm Concept that certain actions are known to cause or create specific outcomes.

for-profit (proprietary) organization Organization that focuses on making a profit from operations and distributing those profits to the owners or investors in the organization.

fraction of inspired oxygen (FiO₂) The amount expressed as a number of oxygen in a gas mixture, 0 (0%) to 1 (100%). For example the FiO_2 of normal room air is 0.21 (21%).

fractures Discontinuities in bone that may be complete or incomplete.

fragment antigen binding (FAB) portion The section of an antibody that is capable of being shaped to receive a specific antigen. DNA within B cells is capable of creating many millions of combinations of FAB portions of antibodies to match an antigen and help protect the body against an invasion by pathogens.

fragment crystalline (FC) portion The section of an antibody that is capable of attaching to the cell membrane of infected or mutant cells or of foreign pathogens (bacteria, viruses) and assisting macrophages to eliminate them.

Frank-Starling law The ability of muscle fibers to stretch to accommodate filling during diastole.

free radical theory of aging Theory of aging that postulates that aging changes are caused by free radical reactions that cause cells and organs to lose function and reserve energy.

fremitus Tactile vibration felt over airways.

frequency The number of sound waves emanating per second; measured in hertz (Hz). Hearing frequencies from 500 to 2,000 Hz are needed to understand everyday speech.

fresh frozen plasma A process in which the plasma portion of blood is separated from the cells and frozen until needed. Units of fresh frozen plasma are used to increase the level of clotting factors in patients with demonstrated deficiency.

friable Easily damaged.

frozen RBCs Red blood cells coated in glycerol prior to freezing and then washed after thawing to remove the glycerol prior to administration. This is a method of storage.

full-thickness injury An injury that extends into the underlying structures and organs.

full-thickness skin graft Grafting of skin that is surgically removed by excising the entire thickness of the donor skin to the level of the subcutaneous tissue, typically 0.025 to 0.30 inch thick.

functional iron deficiency Physiological state characterized by failure to supply enough iron for erythropoiesis despite sufficient quantities.

functional nursing A task-oriented nursing care delivery system in which individual caregivers are not given patient assignments but are expected to perform specific assigned tasks within their capability for all patients in a given area.

furuncle A boil or a walled-off, deep, painful, firm inflammation of the skin that contains pus.

fusiform aneurysms Elliptically shaped aneurysm.

gait Walking.

galactogenesis Formation of breast milk from nutrients available from the bloodstream.

galactorrhea The spontaneous flow of milk in a breast unassociated with childbirth or nursing.

gamete Reproductive cell, ovum or sperm, with the haploid chromosome number.

gamma-glutamyltransferase (GGT) An enzyme found mostly in the liver that is released when cellular damage occurs.

gastric carcinoma Cancer in the stomach, most commonly in the antrum and distal portions; is usually an adenocarcinoma.

gastric outlet obstruction Results from edema, inflammation, or scarring and obstructs the flow of gastric contents from the stomach to the duodenum. Also called *pyloric obstruction*.

gastric ulcer An erosion of the stomach lining that develops most often in the antrum, which is adjacent to the body of the stomach. It is not associated with increased acid secretion, but rather, with a defect in the mucosal barrier to hydrogen ions, allowing the ions to permeate the mucosa.

gastroduodenostomy (Billroth I) A partial gastrectomy in which the lower portion of the stomach is removed and the remainder is anastomosed with the duodenum.

gastroesophageal reflux The backflow of gastric contents into the lower end of the esophagus.

gastroesophageal reflux disease (GERD) A common condition in which acid from the stomach flows back into the esophagus, causing discomfort and, in some cases, damage to the esophageal lining.

gastrojejunostomy (Billroth II) Procedure in which a larger distal portion of the stomach is removed than with the gastroduodenostomy (Billroth I) procedure, and the remainder is anastomosed to the jejunum.

gastroparesis Delayed emptying of food from the stomach into the small bowel.

gate control theory Proposes that the spinal cord has a gating mechanism that either permits or inhibits the transmission of pain information to the brain.

gating Dividing the cardiac cycle into segments so that images viewed in cine mode allow the clinician to evaluate wall motion and systolic thickening in all areas of the left ventricle.

gauge Needle or catheter size.

gene The functional unit of heredity that occupies a certain position on a chromosome and is passed from parent to offspring. Genes consist of DNA and most contain information for making a specific protein.

gene mutations Abnormal genes inherited from parents.

gene therapy Therapy that involves adding a functional gene or group of genes to a cell by gene insertion to correct a hereditary disorder.

general adaptation syndrome (GAS) Physical response to stress as defined by Selye. GAS is composed of three stages: alarm reaction, stage of resistance, and stage of exhaustion.

general anesthesia The production of complete unconsciousness, muscular relaxation, and absence of pain sensation.

genetic variance Variation in genotype that is associated with phenotype.

genital herpes An incurable condition caused primarily by the herpes simplex virus; it can be treated with antiviral drugs.

genital warts Sexually transmitted, cauliflower-like growths in the genital, anal, and vaginal areas. Also called *human papillomavirus*.

genome All of the DNA in an organism or cell to include the 44 autosomes, 2 sex chromosomes, and the mitochondrial DNA.

genomic imprinting Genetic inheritance process in which both maternal and paternal alleles are present, but one allele is expressed and the other remains silent.

genomics The field of genetics concerned with structural and functional studies of the genome.

genotype The genetic makeup of an individual that is not evident as outward or visible characteristics.

germ line cells The sex cell or gamete (egg or spermatozoan).

gerontological nurse practitioner (GNP) A registered nurse with a master's degree from a nurse practitioner program specializing in the care of older adults.

gestational diabetes mellitus (GDM) A specific type of diabetes that occurs during pregnancy in women who had no history of diabetes prior to the pregnancy.

gigantism Condition brought on by overproduction of pituitary growth hormone in youth before the long bones have closed. Characterized by abnormal height.

gingival hyperplasia Excessive proliferation of normal cells of the gingiva.

glaucoma A group of diseases of the optic nerve involving loss of retinal ganglion cells in a characteristic pattern of optic neuropathy. Raised intraocular pressure is a significant risk factor for developing glaucoma (above 22 mmHg).

glomerulus A compact tuft of capillaries in which blood is filtered.

glucagon A hormone produced by the alpha cells of the pancreas. Glucagon has several actions, the most important of which is (along with insulin) maintaining blood glucose levels within a normal range. In diabetes, elevated levels of glucagon contribute to hyperglycemia and ketosis.

gluconeogenesis The formation of glucose from noncarbohydrate organic molecules (i.e., lactate, glycerol, and amino acids); is a function of the liver.

glucose-6-phosphate dehydrogenase (G6PD) deficiency The most common enzyme deficiency contributing to hemolytic anemia. Enzymatic deficiencies in erythrocytes increase the red blood cell's sensitivity and susceptibility to oxidative stress. Deficiencies in the enzyme are genetically encoded and relatively common especially in persons of African American and Mediterranean descent.

glutamate An excitatory neurotransmitter implicated in cell death.

glycated serum proteins (GSPs) A test of short-term blood glucose control (14 to 20 days) obtained by measuring the glycosylation of total serum proteins or glycosylation of albumin. The most widely used method to measure GSPs is the hemoglobin A_{1c} (HbA_{1c}) test. A normal HbA_{1c} is less than 6%. This test is also known as glycated hemoglobin or glycosylated hemoglobin, and is frequently is referred to as "A1C."

glycogen A starch polysaccharide that is stored in the liver and muscles of humans and can be hydrolyzed to glucose.

glycogenolysis The conversion of glycogen to glucose.

glycolysis A biochemical pathway that results in the generation of high-energy compounds (e.g., ATP and NADH).

goal A broad statement of purpose that describes the aim of nursing care.

goiter Abnormal enlargement of the thyroid gland.

goitrogen A substance in a food or a drug that inhibits the production of thyroid hormone.

goniometer Used for measuring a patient's range of motion.

gonorrhea A sexually transmitted infection that is caused by the bacterium *Neisseria gonorrhoeae*, which infects the warm moist environment of the reproductive tract, along with any other mucous membranes in the body.

Gottron's sign Reddish raised rash or papules over the knuckles.

gouty arthritis Condition in which there is an imbalance in purine metabolism, which increases uric acid in the joints by the formation of uric acid crystals.

gouty joint Inflammation of the big toe, dorsum, ankles, heels, or elbows.

graduated compression stockings Elastic stockings that apply varying degrees of pressure on the lower leg with the greatest exertion of pressure at the ankle and the lowest pressure at the thigh (or knee in shorter stockings).

graft versus host disease (GVHD) An alloimmune response in which the grafted tissue initiates an immune response against tissue of the host or recipient of the grafted tissue. An example of graft versus host disease is seen in transplanted bone marrow.

granulation tissue Tiny, round granule-like nodules that become beefy, red, and moist because of the dense revascularization process.

granulocyte White blood cell with numerous granules in the cytoplasm; granulocytes are divided into neutrophils, eosinophils, and basophils.

graph paper Paper specifically designed and used to measure various calculations related to the electrical activity of the heart; it is arranged as a series of horizontal and vertical lines and is standardized to allow for consistency in ECG tracing analysis.

Graves' disease A hypermetabolic condition caused by an autoimmune disease in which the thyroid gland produces too much thyroid hormone.

grounded theory The idea that conclusion of a qualitative study should be grounded in the data, that is, based on direct and careful observations of everyday life within the group.

growth factors A group of extracellular polypeptides (secreted by platelets and macrophages) that affect cell growth, reproduction, movement, or function.

growth needs The top levels of Maslow's hierarchy associated with psychological needs.

gynecomastia Male breast enlargement due to a hormonal imbalance.

hairy tongue A condition in which the tongue is covered with hairlike papilla due to the overgrowth of the fungus *Candida albicans* or *Aspergillus niger*.

haploid The number of chromosomes in an egg or sperm cell; it is half the diploid number.

hardiness Condition in which a person has a clear sense of personal values and goals, a strong tendency toward interaction with the environment, a sense of meaningfulness, and an internal rather than an external locus of control. It is a mediating factor in how people respond to stress.

Hashimoto's thyroiditis An autoimmune condition characterized by high titers of the circulating antibodies thyroid peroxidase and thyroglobulin that destroy thyroid cells and may lead to hypothyroidism. It is the most common thyroid disease in the United States. Also known as *chronic lymphocytic hypothyroidism*.

hassles Experiences and conditions of daily living that have been appraised as relevant and harmful or threatening to an individual's well-being.

Haversian canals Canals located in cortical bone; they contain one or two capillaries and nerve fibers that serve as the transport system for nutrients.

health care delivery system System that provides client-centered, comprehensive, interdisciplinary, integrated, and accessible health care that meets the needs of the clients.

Health Insurance Portability and Accountability Act (HIPAA) A federal law designed to improve the portability of health care coverage for people who lose or change employment, to simplify the administrative process through the use of electronic transactions, and to ensure the privacy of membership information.

health maintenance organization (HMO) Organization that provides coverage for medical care and controls costs through utilization review and management and by restricting access to a specific network of providers.

heart failure A complex and debilitating clinical syndrome in which there is loss or dysfunction of the cardiac muscle or an inability of the ventricle to fill or eject blood.

heaves Palpable sustained lifts of the chest wall due to forceful cardiac contractions.

Heberden's nodes Hard, painless nodules at the joints of the fingers; may indicate osteoarthritis. Heberden's nodes are found over the distal interphalangeal joints.

Helicobacter pylori (H. pylori) A bacterium that infects the stomach and duodenum and is associated with peptic ulcers.

hematocrit The ratio of the volume of erythrocytes (red blood cells) to that of the whole blood.

hematology The branch of biology (physiology), pathology, clinical laboratory, internal medicine, and pediatrics that is concerned with the study of blood, the blood-forming organs, and blood diseases.

hematoma An area of swelling or mass of blood confined to an organ, tissue, or space, due to a broken blood vessel.

hematopoiesis The formation and development of blood cells.

hematopoietic stem cell (HSC) Bone marrow cell that is the precursor to all hematologic cell types.

hematuria The presence of blood in the urine.

heme iron Form of dietary iron that is common in red meats and fish.

hemodynamic monitoring The monitoring of pressures and blood flow within the cardiovascular system.

hemoglobin The oxygen carrying pigment of the erythrocytes, formed by the developing erythrocyte in bone marrow.

hemoglobin A$_{1c}$ (HbA$_{1c}$) test Refers to a series of stable minor hemoglobin components formed nonenzymatically from the glycosylation of the hemoglobin molecule. The amount of HbA$_{1c}$ is directly proportional to the ambient glucose concentration, providing an estimation of blood glucose control during the previous 2 to 3 months. Sometimes also referred to as *glycohemoglobin, glycosylated hemoglobin,* or *A1C.*

hemoglobinopathies Red blood disorders characterized by abnormal hemoglobin.

hemolytic anemia Group of diseases characterized by increased red blood cell destruction.

hemophilia Genetic disorder resulting from mutated genes controlling Factors VIII or Factor IX; characterized by uncontrolled bleeding.

hemoptysis Coughing up of blood from the lower respiratory tract.

hemosiderin A form of iron in the body acting as a supply reservoir.

hemosiderin staining Occurs when the heme part of the red blood cell is deposited in the tissues as red blood cells get trapped and accumulate due to venous congestion. As the red blood cell dies, the heme is deposited and a brownish hue staining color results.

hemostasis Cessation of bleeding; a complex process that changes blood from a fluid to a solid state. Hemostasis occurs in two phases: primary and secondary. Primary hemostasis is characterized by vascular contraction, platelet adhesion, and formation of a soft aggregate plug. Secondary hemostasis is responsible for stabilizing the soft clot and maintaining vasoconstriction.

hemothorax Partial or complete collapse of the lung due to blood in the pleural space.

heparin-induced thrombocytopenia (HIT) Drug-induced, immune-mediated thrombocytopenia; caused by exposure to heparin therapy.

hepatic artery catheter A catheter inserted into the hepatic artery for targeted antineoplastic therapies.

hepatic encephalopathy A result of an increased level of circulating neurotoxins. The most abundant neurotoxin is ammonia and is the end product of protein digestion.

hepatic first pass Refers to the reduction of a medication's effect due to partial metabolism in the liver prior to distribution to the ultimate site of action.

hepatitis A virus (HAV) An RNA virus that causes hepatitis and is transmitted mainly through contaminated food and water.

hepatitis B virus (HBV) A DNA virus that causes hepatitis and is transmitted sexually and parenterally.

hepatitis C virus (HCV) An RNA virus that causes hepatitis and is transmitted mainly parenterally. The majority of the cases develop chronic hepatitis.

hepatitis D virus (HDV) An RNA virus that occurs only in the presence of HBV.

hepatitis E virus (HEV) An RNA virus that is transmitted mostly through the fecal–oral route and is endemic in Southeast Asia and parts of Africa.

hepatocellular Pertaining to the cells of the liver.

hepatojugular reflux An increase in jugular venous pressure when pressure is applied over the abdomen; is suggestive of right-sided heart failure.

hepatorenal syndrome Syndrome characterized by azotemia occurring in a patient with liver failure.

hepcidin Hormone produced in the liver that is responsible for iron supply regulation.

hereditary spherocytosis (HS) Hemolytic anemia disorder characterized by insufficient red blood cell membrane proteins.

hernia Protrusion of an anatomic structure through the wall that normally contains it.

herniation The displacement of brain structures under pressure, causing compression and damage of brain tissue.

herpetic stomatitis Inflammation of the oral cavity caused by the herpes simplex virus.

heterografts Biologic dressing made from animals such as pigs.

heterotropic ossification (OS) The development of bone tissue in areas where bone tissue is not normally present.

heterozygous Having two different alleles for a given gene, one inherited from each parent.

heuristic relevance Discovering or revealing a relationship that may lead to additional development along a particular line of research.

hiatal hernia Protrusion of the upper portion of the stomach into the thorax through the esophageal hiatus.

high-altitude pulmonary edema (HAPE) Type of pulmonary edema that develops in persons who rapidly ascend to heights greater than 2,500 to 3,000 meters (8,202 to 9,842 feet).

high density lipoprotein A type of lipoprotein that binds to cholesterol to transport it back to the liver; lipoproteins may actually remove excess cholesterol from plaque in the arteries.

highly active antiretroviral drug therapy (HAART) Combination therapy has the greatest effect in controlling HIV proliferation and minimizing the development of drug resistance. Antiretroviral drugs are grouped according to the mechanism of action against HIV.

hirsutism Abnormal growth of hair, especially in women.

histamine A protein produced by mast and other cells. Release of histamine results in vasodilation and bronchoconstriction. Symptoms associated with histamine release include shortness of breath, wheezing, itching, and hives.

histamine$_2$ (H$_2$)-receptor blockers Drugs that block the H$_2$-receptors located in the gastrointestinal tract and reduce acid secretion.

HIV antibody positive status An individual's status when enough HIV antibodies have been produced in response to infection by the HIV virus to be measured by antibody serology, usually after 3 weeks to 3 months. Symptoms may or may not be present.

hoarseness Condition that occurs when the normal vibration of the vocal cords is disrupted.

holding area A physical space located adjacent to the operating room where patients wait prior to an operation.

holism An idea based on the premise that the whole is more than the sum of its parts.

Holter monitoring Ambulatory electrocardiogram monitoring for an extended period of time.

homeostasis The tendency toward stability within an organism; it is the first reaction toward that stability when a wound occurs.

homograft valve *See* allograft valve.

homologous transfusion The process of collecting blood from a donor for transfusion into other individuals who are in need of blood.

homozygous Having identical alleles at a given location.

honeymoon period A transient period of time when newly diagnosed patients with type 1 diabetes have restoration of insulin production and thus a reduced requirement for exogenous insulin.

horizontal organization model Service structure of hospitals aligned to form a multihospital system; focuses on traditional acute care services.

hospice Palliative care and support services for patients with terminal illnesses and their families.

hospitalist Physician who concentrates her or his practice in the acute care environment.

host versus graft disease (HVGD) A type of alloimmune hypersensitivity response that involves transplanted organs or tissues; occurs when a recipient's immune system reacts against the foreign antigens on the cells of the graft.

human genome The complete DNA sequence that contains the entire genetic information for a human.

Human Genome Project (HGP) An international research project to map each human gene and completely sequence human DNA.

human immunodeficiency virus (HIV) The infective agent responsible for causing AIDS; HIV is a retrovirus that infects CD4 T cells and fatally impairs immune function. Two specific strains of HIV have been identified: HIV type 1 and HIV type 2.

human leukocyte antigens (HLAs) Genetic protein markers on the cell wall of white blood cells that alert the immune system to the appropriateness of a cell belonging to the system. HLAs can differentiate self from non-self. There are six different HLA markers: HLA-A, HLA-B, HLA-C, HLA-D, HLA-DR, and HLA-DQ. Each of these markers is capable of creating multiple different antigen subtype combinations. HLA matching between donor and recipient is key to preventing transplant graft rejection.

human papillomavirus (HPV) *See* genital warts.

humoral immune response Mechanism by which organisms gain immunity to previously encountered substances; involves B lymphocytes and antibody-mediated immunity. The term *humoral* comes from the Greek word "humor," which means body fluids; B cells are in the plasma.

Hunt-Hess classification Grading scale for subarachnoid hemorrhage.

hydrocele Swelling of the scrotum caused by fluid collection.

hydrogen ion A single, charged atomic proton that is not orbited by any electrons. It is the smallest ionic particle and is extremely reactive.

hydronephrosis Collection of urine in the pelvis of the kidney from obstructed outflow.

hydroxyapatite Inorganic hexagonal matrix of bone composed of calcium and phosphorus.

hyperacute rejection Occurs within the first hours after transplant when the recipient has a preexisting antibody to the antigen in the graft tissue. Blanching of the graft is one of the earliest signs of rejection.

hyperbaric oxygen therapy (HBOT) Refers to intermittent treatment of the entire body with 100% oxygen at greater than normal atmospheric pressures.

hypercarbic drive The stimulus for ventilation that occurs when elevated levels of carbon dioxide alter the pH of the blood and cerebrospinal fluid, making them more acid. Central chemoreceptors located in the brainstem react to this change in the pH and stimulate the body to breathe more deeply and more rapidly. It is the strongest stimulus of ventilation.

hypercatabolism Metabolic state in which degradation of protein stores is elevated.

hypercholesterolemia An increased cholesterol level in the blood.

hyperflexion injuries Increased flexion of a joint from trauma.

hyperglycemia Elevated blood glucose levels.

hypergranulation The formation of soft, pink fleshy projections as the body attempts to heal an enlarged wound track.

hyperkalemia An excess of potassium in the blood.

hyperlipidemia An elevated cholesterol and/or triglyceride level in the blood that is a modifiable risk factor for the development of coronary artery disease.

hypermetabolism Metabolic state in which resting energy expenditure is elevated.

hyperopia A defect in vision caused by an imperfection in the eye (often the eyeball is too short).

hyperosmolar hyperglycemic nonketotic syndrome (HHS) An emergent complication of diabetes characterized by serum hyperosmolarity, hyperglycemia, and dehydration.

hyperparathyroidism A hypermetabolic condition in which the parathyroid gland produces an excess of parathyroid hormone.

hyperplasia An increase in the number of new cells in an organ or tissue.

hyperpnea Refers to both the increased rate and depth of respiration associated with metabolic acidosis. It is sometimes referred to as *Kussmaul's breathing*.

hyperreflexia Exaggeration of the deep tendon reflexes.

hyperresonance A loud, low tone of longer duration than resonance. It is heard when air is trapped in a space such as the lungs.

hypertensive crisis A rare, sometimes fatal, occurrence that is characterized by the sudden onset of a diastolic blood pressure reading of 120 to 130; the clinical manifestation indicates target organ vascular damage and the presence of retinal exudates and hemorrhages.

hypertensive encephalopathy A very dangerous state of multifocal cerebral ischemia due to a severe acutely or subacutely elevated blood pressure.

hyperthyroidism A hypermetabolic condition in which the thyroid gland produces and the body responds to an excess production of thyroid hormones.

hypertonic Term used to identify a solution that contains a higher concentration of electrolytes than that found in body cells. If such a solution is allowed to enter the bloodstream, the osmotic pressure difference between the blood and the cells will cause water to flow out of the cells, which will then shrink.

hypertonic formula An enteral or parenteral nutrition formula with an osmolality, or concentration, that is greater than that of the body's plasma.

hypertrophic cardiomyopathy A disorder of the sarcomere, the contractile element of the cardiac muscle; characterized by left ventricular and occasionally right ventricular hypertrophy, with greater hypertrophy occurring in the septum. Also referred to as *idiopathic hypertrophic subaortic stenosis (IHSS)*.

hypertrophic scar Scar tissue that is an overgrowth of dermal tissue that remains within the boundaries of the wound.

hypertrophy An increase in the size of an organ caused by an increase in the size of the cells and tissues rather than the number of cells.

hyperventilation A state that exists when there is a lower than normal level of carbon dioxide in the blood. Also referred to as *hypocapnia*.

hyphema A collection of blood cells in the anterior chamber of the eye.

hypoalbuminemia Refers to low serum albumin, which most often results from liver damage.

hypochromic Term describing red blood cells that are paler in color than normal, suggesting iron deficiencies.

hypodermoclysis Continuous subcutaneous infusion of a large volume of isotonic parenteral fluids for purposes of rehydration.

hypoglycemia Decreased blood glucose levels.

hypoglycemic unawareness Condition that results from altered counterregulation, particularly deficient glucagon and epinephrine responses to hypoglycemia. This results in a loss of autonomic nervous system symptoms; for instance, tachycardia, palpitations, and tremors are absent. Patients are unaware that they are hypoglycemic and, without treatment, can progress rapidly into severe hypoglycemia.

hypokinesia Condition characterized by areas of abnormal heart contractility where muscle movement is hypoactive.

hypokinetic dysarthria Speech difficulty as a result of slowed, rigid muscles of tongue, mouth, and throat; associated with Parkinson's disease.

hypomimia Decreased facial expression due to rigid facial muscles.

hypoparathyroidism A hypometabolic condition in which the parathyroid gland fails to produce adequate parathyroid hormone.

hypophonia Soft, muffled voice.

hypopituitarism A hypometabolic condition in which the secretion of pituitary hormones is inadequate.

hypopnea A reduction but not complete cessation of airflow to less than 50% of normal.

hypopyon White layer of inflammatory cells in the anterior chamber.

hypospadias Opening of the urinary meatus on the ventral or bottom of the penis, between the penis and scrotum.

hypothalamic–pituitary–adrenal (HPA) axis A feedback loop by which signals from the brain trigger the release of hormones needed to respond to stress. Because of its function, the HPA axis also is referred to as the *stress circuit*.

hypothermia A core body temperature of less than 96.8°F (36°C) or a condition, regardless of body temperature, in which a person experiences shivering, peripheral vasoconstriction, piloerection, and feelings of cold.

hypothesis A statement that predicts a certain relationship between two or more variables.

hypothyroidism A metabolic condition in which the thyroid gland fails to produce adequate thyroid hormones.

hypotonia The absence of muscle tone, resulting in flaccidity of the muscles.

hypotonic Term used to identify a solution in which the concentration of electrolyte is below that found in body cells. In this situation osmotic pressure leads to the migration of water into the cells in an attempt to equalize the electrolyte concentration inside and outside the cell walls.

hypoventilation Decreased ventilation, which causes an increased $PaCO_2$; exists when there is a higher than normal level of carbon dioxide in the blood. Also referred to as *hypercapnia*.

hypoxemia Insufficient oxygen content in the blood.

hypoxia Physiological state of decreased blood oxygen levels.

hypoxic drive The stimulus to ventilation that occurs when peripheral chemoreceptors located in the carotid arteries and the aorta sense a decrease in the oxygen concentration in the blood.

hypoxic hypoxia Physiological state of decreased oxygen availability due to cardiac or pulmonary causes.

hysterectomy A surgical procedure to remove the uterus.

iatrogenic wounds Include intravenous puncture sites, incisions, radiation-induced skin damage, and grafts that occurred while a patient was in the hospital.

icteric phase The phase of acute hepatitis in which jaundice occurs, usually 1 to 2 weeks after the prodromal phase.

id Represents all of a person's biological and psychological drives.

IgE antibodies A class of antibodies produced by the B-lymphocyte plasma cells in response to exposure to a foreign antigen or allergen. They create an antibody–antigen complex that connects to receptors on mast cells and causes degranulation of mast cells and release of histamine; they are the major factor in type I hypersensitivity reactions.

ileal pouch anal anastomosis (IPAA) Procedure in which the entire colon, including the rectum, is removed and a pouch formed from the terminal ileum, which is then attached to the anus.

ileostomy Procedure in which a stoma is formed from the ileum. In a permanent ileostomy, the entire colon is removed and fecal material is collected in an external collection bag.

ileus A condition in which peristalsis does not return as expected postoperatively and the bowel remains hypoactive.

iliopsoas Refers to three muscles of the abdomen—psoas major, psoas minor, and iliacus—that pass from the abdomen through the pelvis and are partially responsible for hip flexion.

immediate hypersensitivity reaction An excessive response of the immune system that occurs in seconds to hours after exposure to an antigen. A systemic anaphylaxis is one example of an immediate hypersensitivity reaction response.

immune complex A substance formed when antibodies attach to antigens to destroy them.

immune deficiencies Deficiencies that occur when all or some part of the immune system fails to develop or is damaged through disease processes and, thus, cannot mount an appropriate immune response. There are two types, primary and secondary.

immune hypersensitivity response Occurs when the immune system overresponds to an antigen, either from the environment, from the individual himself, or from another individual. Disorders fall into three broad categories based on the type of triggering antigen, and include allergy, autoimmune, and alloimmune reactions.

immune tolerance The ability of the immune system to differentiate self from non-self and tolerate all self-antigens while retaining the ability to mount an immune response to non-self-antigens.

immunity The protective process of response to a foreign substance.

immunization The process of stimulating the immune system to create active immunity for protection against a disease by injection with a live or killed vaccine. Often used interchangeably with *vaccination* or *inoculation*.

immunoglobulin A diverse group of plasma proteins, made of polypeptide chains; one of the primary mechanisms for protection against diseases.

immunologic theory of aging Theory of aging based on the premise that the aging body is less able to distinguish its own cells from foreign cells.

impaired fasting glucose (IFG) A category of pre-diabetes in which the fasting glucose level is >100 mg/dL but <126 mg/dL.

impaired glucose tolerance (IGT) A category of pre-diabetes in which the blood glucose level following an oral glucose load of 75 grams is >140 mg/dL but <200 mg/dL.

impaired wound healing The disruption of the normal biochemical repair or regeneration process.

impetigo A common, contagious skin infection caused by *Staphylococcus aureus* and/or group A beta-hemolytic streptococcus that is characterized by vesicles that rupture and form yellow crusts.

implantable cardioverter defibrillator (ICD) Device that can automatically terminate the potentially lethal dysrhythmias of ventricular tachycardia and ventricular fibrillation. Currently these devices are incorporated into cardiac pacemakers.

implanted port A surgically placed central vascular access device; a chambered device comprised of a reservoir and an attached catheter; used for long-term or chronic infusion therapies.

implementation The "doing" or intervening phase of the nursing process.

implied consent Permission that is inferred by a person's conduct or by law.

impotence Refers to problems associated with ejaculation or orgasm, in addition to erectile dysfunction.

incapacitating agent Chemical agents that decrease acetylcholine at nerve synapses. They work in the opposite manner of nerve agents.

incidence The number of newly diagnosed cases of cancer in a specific time period in a defined population.

incident command system (ICS) A system of policies and procedures within a framework that allows for safe and effective management during a disaster.

INCMCE Acronym for International Nursing Coalition for Mass Casualty Education.

incomplete spinal cord injury Preservation of some degree of motor and/or sensory function below the level of a spinal injury.

incretin mimetics A class of medications that enhances glucose-dependent insulin secretion from the pancreatic β-cell resulting in a reduction in postprandial glucose levels. The incretins suppress elevated glucagon levels, promoting satiety, decreasing food intake, and slowing gastric emptying.

independent activities Activities that nurses perform, prescribe, and or delegate based on their education and skills. Assessing, analyzing, diagnosing, planning, implementing, and evaluating are independent activities.

independent practice association (IPA) Organization that contracts on the behalf of individuals or groups of physicians to provide health care to members of a health maintenance organization.

indirect calorimetry The measurement of energy expenditure by measuring oxygen intake and carbon dioxide output.

indirect inguinal hernia Occurs when abdominal contents protrude through the deep inguinal ring.

indirect percussion Technique that involves using the hyperextended middle finger of the nondominant hand (pleximeter) and then the finger tip of the middle finger of the dominant hand (plexor) to strike the pleximeter by using a wrist action that will elicit a sound.

Ineffective Coping Nursing diagnosis that refers to an inability to manage internal or environmental stressors appropriately as a result of inadequate physical, psychological, behavioral, or cognitive resources.

infarction An area of dead tissue.

infective endocarditis An infection of the cardiac endocardial layer of the heart, which may include one or more heart valves, the mural endocardium, and/or a septal defect; previously known as bacterial endocarditis.

infectivity The ability of a pathogen to enter a host and then live and grow within that host.

infiltration Inadvertent administration of a nonvesicant solution or medication into surrounding tissues.

inflammation A defensive mechanism of the body that is intended to neutralize, control, or eliminate an offending agent to prepare a site for repair. It is a nonspecific response that is meant to serve a protective function.

inflammatory bowel disease (IBD) An immunologic disease that results in idiopathic intestinal inflammation; includes Crohn's disease and ulcerative colitis.

inflammatory phase A phase of wound healing that begins at the time of the injury or surgery. The purpose of this phase is to prepare the site for growth of new tissue.

influenza A contagious disease that is caused by the influenza virus. Also known as the *flu*.

informatics The theory, science, and practice of the use of computer and informational technologies to store, retrieve, transmit, and manipulate data.

information technology Refers to those systems, including software programs and computer hardware, used to manage and process information.

informed consent Doctrine that mandates that individuals must be fully appraised of the nature, risks, benefits, alternative therapies, and potential consequences of procedures and therapies in health care settings.

infradian rhythm Rhythmic repetition of cycles lasting for more than a 24-hour period; an example is the female menstrual cycle.

infusate Parenteral fluid or medication.

inhalation injury Inhalation of smoke, causing injury to the lungs.

injection port or cap Device that allows entrance to a catheter's fluid pathway.

insensible fluid loss Water lost from the body carried as vapor in exhaled gases and evaporated from the body as sweat.

insomnia Difficulty falling or remaining asleep.

inspection The deliberate, systematic examination of a patient using both sight and smell.

Institute of Medicine (IOM) Organization that provides unbiased, evidence-based, authoritative information on medicine and health to policy makers, professionals, and the public at large in an effort to improve health.

insulin A hormone produced by the beta cells of the pancreas that has multiple effects. Insulin is necessary for glucose transport into insulin-sensitive tissues and storage of carbohydrates, fats, and proteins.

insulin resistance Unresponsiveness of anabolic processes to the normal effects of insulin and possibly tissue insensitivity to insulin.

intentional torts Wrongful conduct that is intentional in nature and designed to cause harm or damage to another.

interdependent activities Activities that overlap with other health care team members, physicians, social workers, pharmacists, nutritionists, and therapists, and require coordination and planning with those various team members.

interface pressure The pressure between a bony prominence and a surface such as a hospital bed or seating surface.

interferon (IFN) Protein made and released by T cells when the invading organism is a virus; functions to protect other cells from viral attack and stimulates the immune response; also inhibits the growth of certain tumor cells.

interleukin (IL) Chemical message produced by lymphocytes that enables the cells of the immune system to communicate and stimulate or slow an immune response. The various types of IL include IL-1 and IL-6, which are pro-inflammatory and stimulate B-cell production, whereas others, such as IL-12 and IL-13, help slow and inhibit the immune and inflammatory responses.

intermittent claudication (IC) Exercise-induced leg pain.

intermittent pneumatic compression devices Devices used to apply intermittent compression of the calf muscle, thereby increasing venous return.

internal locus of control An orientation in which a person believes that events in his or her life are controlled by his or her own actions and decisions.

internal stressor Stressor that originates within a person.

interphalangeal joint Joints between the fingers.

interstitial fluid Fluid between cells, but not in serum.

intervention An action designed to facilitate achievement of desired patient outcomes. It must be purposeful, must be supported by a rationale, and involve organization and actual delivery of nursing care, which ideally leads to achievement of stated patient goals and objectives.

intestinal obstruction The impairment of the forward movement of intestinal contents by mechanical causes (tumors), adhesions, or functional causes (surgery, anesthesia, medications); can occur anywhere from the pylorus to the rectum.

intra-atrial pathways Part of the electrical conduction system of the heart that consists of the internodal pathways and the Bachmann bundle.

intra-axial tumors Tumors originating from glial cells; found mostly in white matter.

intracellular fluid (ICF) Fluid contained within the cells.

intracranial pressure (ICP) The pressure exerted by cerebrospinal fluid within the ventricles.

intramedullary (I-M) rodding A method of fracture fixation that entails sliding a metal rod down the medullary canal of a long bone.

intraoperative During surgery.

intraosseous therapy Administration of parenteral fluids via the bone marrow; used in emergent situations when vascular access is not available.

intraspinal catheter A catheter used to access the intraspinal route.

intrathecal anesthesia A type of anesthesia in which a local anesthetic agent is inserted into the spinal fluid by penetrating the spinal dura.

intrathecal therapy Delivery of parenteral medications into the cerebrospinal fluid.

intrinsic factor (IF) Chemical secreted by the gastric mucosa required for vitamin B_{12} absorption.

intrinsic pathway Also known as the contact activation pathway, describes the clotting cascade branch initiated by the contact between circulating plasma proteins and the negatively charged surface of the injured subendothelial layer.

intron A noncoding segment of DNA that is transcribed into nuclear RNA, but removed in the subsequent processing into mRNA.

intussusception The slipping of one part of an intestine into another part just below it.

invasion of privacy Violation of the right to protection against unreasonable and unwarranted interference with one's solitude.

invasiveness Degree to which an organism can spread through the body.

ion Electrically charged components derived from the molecules of electrolytes. When placed in water the molecules dissociate into charged components or ions, producing positively and negatively charged ions.

iron deficiency anemia (IDA) Most common cause of anemia resulting from insufficient iron in the diet.

irregularly-irregular rhythm Heartbeats that occur when the R-to-R intervals exhibit no regularity in their distance from each other.

irritants Agents that generally cause pain, burning, lacrimation, or discomfort upon exposure to mucous membranes. Also called *riot control agents*.

ischemia Tissue hypoxia resulting from reduced blood flow to the tissues.

ischemia cascade A series of events that occurs as a compensatory mechanism in response to cerebral hypoxia. Also called *ischemic cascade*.

ischemia reperfusion injury A multifactorial process that occurs when anaerobic metabolism is initiated by hypoperfusion and hypoxia that leads to an oxygen deficit in endothelial, parenchymal, or immune competent cells.

ischemic cascade *See* ischemia cascade.

isoelectric line Straight line on the ECG graph paper that marks the beginning and ending point of all waves. Also referred to as the *baseline*.

isotonic Having the same osmolality as blood (275 to 295 mOsm/kg of body weight).

isotonic formula An enteral or parenteral nutrition formula with an osmolality, or concentration, that is approximately equal that of the body's plasma.

J point On an ECG tracing, the point at which the QRS meets the ST segment.

Joint Commission The accrediting body for hospitals and health care organizations; it is an independent, private, not-for-profit organization.

jugular venous distention (JVD) Increased blood pressure in the jugular vein that reflects the volume and pressure of venous blood, when volume overload is present.

jugular venous pressure (JVP) An indication of the hemodynamic events of the right atrium; derived from measurement of the pulsations of the right internal jugular vein.

junctional dysrhythmia Dysrhythmia resulting from an irritable focus in the junctional tissue that fires off before the SA node has had a chance to, or because the SA node has failed to fire. Three typical junctional dysrhythmias are junctional escape rhythm, premature junctional contraction, and junctional tachycardia.

junctional escape rhythm Dysrhythmia that occurs when the SA node fails to produce an impulse, or when the SA node's rate of firing falls below the intrinsic rate of the AV node. When this occurs, the AV node assumes the role of pacemaker.

justice In ethics, states that people should be treated fairly and equally.

Kaposi's sarcoma A malignancy involving the endothelial layer of blood and lymphatic vessels. Kaposi's is the most common cancer associated with AIDS.

karyotype A set of photographed, banded chromosomes of an individual, arranged from largest to smallest.

keloid scar Hypertrophic scar tissue that extends beyond the wound edges.

ketogenesis Condition in which an excessive amount of ketones are produced during diabetic ketoacidosis (DKA); is the cause of metabolic acidosis during DKA.

kinematics The predictive patterns of injuries.

KUB Abbreviation for kidney-ureter-bladder radiograph, and is also known as a "plain film of the abdomen." The radiograph helps to determine position, size, and structure of the kidneys and urinary tract. It is useful in evaluating for the presence of calculi and masses. This is also an excellent test for intestinal obstruction because it shows the air in the colon nicely.

Kupffer cells Cells that line the liver sinusoids and are phagocytic.

Kussmaul's respirations Deep, sighing respirations. Also called *hyperpnea*.

kyphosis Curvature of the spine that creates a stooped-over "humpback" appearance.

L'Hermite's sign Electric shock-like sensation throughout the body, elicited by flexing the neck.

labyrinthectomy Surgical procedure in which the labyrinth is excised to eradicate vertigo; results in complete hearing loss to the ear.

labyrinthitis Organ of balance within the middle ear.

lactase An enzyme that breaks down lactose, a sugar found in milk.

lactation Breast-feeding.

lactic dehydrogenase (LDH) An intracellular enzyme present in many cells, but high concentrations are found in the liver. The enzyme is released in response to liver injury.

lactose intolerance Results from a deficiency of lactase, the enzyme responsible for the breakdown of lactose, at the brush border of the small intestine, resulting in malabsorption.

lacunar stroke Thrombosis of a small penetrating artery, resulting in ischemia and infarction of deep white matter of the brain.

lamellar bone Mature bone.

laminectomy The removal of a vertebral posterior arch intended to remove a lesion or herniated disk.

laryngeal spasm An abnormal reflexive response to a laryngeal insult.

laryngectomy A permanent surgical airway with removal of the larynx, usually for cancer.

laryngitis Inflammation of the larynx and/or vocal cords.

laryngopharyngeal reflux disease (LPRD) Inflammation of the laryngopharynx as a result of gastric reflux into the pharynx and larynx.

laryngospasm Occurs when the muscles of the larynx contract forcefully, causing a closure or partial closure of the airway.

latent autoimmune diabetes in adults (LADA) An autoimmune form of diabetes that affects adults.

law Rules and regulation by which a society is governed.

lead axis Refers to the imaginary line drawn between the positive and negative electrodes.

leading health indicators Ten indicators from *Healthy People 2010* that reflect major public health concerns: (1) physical activity, (2) overweight and obesity, (3) tobacco use, (4) substance abuse, (5) responsible sexual behavior, (6) mental health, (7) injury and violence, (8) environmental quality, (9) immunization, and (10) access to health care.

Leapfrog Group A coalition of public and private organizations that provides health care benefits. The coalition provides public information on medical errors, health care standards, and health care provider quality performance measures.

left-sided heart failure An abnormal cardiac condition characterized by the impairment of the left side of the heart and elevated pressure and congestion in the pulmonary veins and capillaries.

left ventricular ejection fraction (LVEF) The proportion of blood ejected during each ventricular contraction compared with the total ventricular filling volume.

legal blindness The best-corrected visual acuity of 20/200 or a visual field of 20 degrees or less in both eyes.

leukemia Malignancy of the hematopoietic system.

leukocyte White blood cell.

leukocyte-poor RBCs A unit of packed red blood cells that had most of the white blood cells removed as soon as the blood was taken from the donor (i.e., prior to storage).

leveling Positioning of a transducer system in line with the chamber being monitored.

levodopa Precursor to dopamine; key drug used to treat Parkinson's disease.

licensed vocational/practical nurse (LVN/LPN) A nurse with 1 to 2 years of technical training to provide basic care.

licensure Process for approving a health care organization to provide medical care or services. Also refers to the certification process for professionals.

ligament A strong fibrous band of connective tissue.

limits of formalization In philosophy, the inability to make explicit or formal all elements of a social practice.

linear lesion Lesion that forms a line.

linear skull fracture A simple break in the continuity of the skull with no displacement of bone.

lipase An enzyme secreted by the pancreas that hydrolyzes triglycerides, cholesterol, and phospholipids.

lipodystrophy Abnormal deposition of adipose in the body.

lipohyalinosis Coating of the walls of small arteries with a lipid substance, causing narrowing of the arterial lumen.

lipolysis Breakdown of triglycerides to free fatty acids and glycerol.

lipoma Benign tumor consisting of fat cells.

liposuction Common type of cosmetic surgery, the purpose of which is to remove subcutaneous fat.

literature review A search of the latest research articles and scholarly studies.

lithotomy Position in which the patient lies on the back with the legs flexed at the hips and knees and the legs spread widely at the hip.

living wills A form of an advanced directive that describes a patient's preferences in case he or she becomes incapacitated. They usually describe what level of life-prolonging interventions the patient would or would not want and under what circumstances they should be completed, withheld, or withdrawn.

local adaptation syndrome (LAS) A local response to a stressor that proceeds through the same three stages as the general adaptation syndrome: alarm, resistance, and exhaustion.

locus of control The perception a person has about how much control he or she exerts over the events that happen in his or her life.

long-term care insurance Private insurance that covers the expenses of nursing care in a variety of settings, depending on the policy.

lordosis Excessive inward curvature of the spine.

low density lipoproteins A type of lipoprotein that transports cholesterol and triglycerides from the liver to peripheral tissues.

lower esophageal sphincter (LES) An area at the distal end of the esophagus that prevents the movement of gastric juice into the esophagus.

Ludwig's angina A deep neck infection involving the sublingual, submandibular, and submental spaces; usually the result of a dental abscess.

Luer-Lok™ Screw-type locking mechanism used to prevent accidental separation of infusion equipment.

lumen The bore or internal opening of a catheter.

lumpectomy Removal of a cancerous growth and a small amount of surrounding normal tissue.

Lund-Browder formula Formula for determining burn size that divides the body into percentage areas.

lung abscess An area of pulmonary infection with parenchymal necrosis.

Lyme disease A bacterial infection that affects the organs and joints; transmitted by black-legged ticks.

lymph nodes Lymph tissue that filters debris from the breakdown of cells, bacteria, viruses, and fungal antigens located throughout the body.

lymphangitis An acute inflammation of the lymphatic channels.

lymphatic system The circulatory system of the immune system that is comprised of the lymph vessels, lymph nodes, and lymph tissue and functions to drain lymph fluid (chyle) from throughout the body and return it to venous circulation in the chest.

lymphedema Edema due to the obstruction of the lymphatics.

lymphocyte Mature white cell; the two types of lymphocytes are T lymphocytes (T cells) and B lymphocytes (B cells).

lymphogranuloma venereum (LGV) A sexually transmitted infection caused by *Chlamydia trachomatis*. It is a rare condition, with only 200 cases reported each year.

lymphokines Cytokines that are made by lymphocytes; act as chemical messengers between cells and instruct immune cells to proliferate, differentiate, or alter activities. The major lymphokines are interleukins and interferons.

lymphoma Malignancy of the lymphatic system.

macrocephalic Abnormally large head size; found in acromegaly, hydrocephalus, rickets, osteitis deformans, leontiasis ossea, myxedema, leprosy, and pituitary disturbances.

macronutrients Nutritional components such as protein, carbohydrates, and fat that are needed in large quantities by living organisms.

macrovascular Pertaining to the large blood vessels of the arterial and venous system (e.g., coronary arteries).

macular degeneration (MD) The deterioration and mottling of the macula through the course of time.

magnesium An intracellular cation primarily in muscle and bone (only 1% is in the blood; 1.8 to 2.4 mg/dL).

magnet hospital A hospital designated by the American Nurses Credentialing Center as meeting the standards that result in excellence in delivery of nursing services and promoting a professional practice environment.

magnetic resonance cholangiopancreatography (MRCP) A noninvasive imaging test used to detect bile duct stones and pancreatic duct obstruction.

magnetic resonance imaging (MRI) Technique that uses radiofrequency pulses from a large, powerful magnet to temporarily disrupt the normal spin of certain atoms within the body. When the pulses are stopped, the atoms emit small amounts of energy while returning to their original spin; this energy can be imaged and recorded as high-resolution images that allow detailed noninvasive assessment of the both cardiac anatomy and physiology.

malabsorption The failure of the small intestine to absorb nutrients from digested food.

maladaptive coping mechanisms Those responses to stress that are not effective.

maldigestion The failure of chemical processes such as inadequate pancreatic enzymes or bile salts.

malignant Containing cancerous cells.

malignant hyperthermia (MH) A rare but life-threatening metabolic complication of anesthesia that usually occurs during the induction phase but could occur anytime during surgery. Certain people have a genetic predisposition to this illness. Immediate attention is vital to the recovery of the patient, and intensive care monitoring is mandatory following its occurrence.

malnutrition The physical consequences resulting from underconsumption of energy or nutrients compared to recommended amounts.

malpractice Professional misconduct; failure to meet the standards of care that a reasonably prudent member of the profession would employ.

mammography A low-dose x-ray procedure that allows visualization of the internal structure of the breast.

mandatory reporter A person required by law to report allegations and/or suspicions of abuse.

masked facies Immobile, expressionless facial appearance commonly seen in Parkinson's disease.

massive hemothorax An accumulation of 1,500 mL or more of blood in the thoracic cavity.

mastalgia Breast pain.

mastectomy Removal of the entire breast (total) or a modified radical mastectomy, which is removal of the entire breast along with the surrounding lymph nodes.

mastitis Inflammation of the breast tissue; occurs most frequently in breast-feeding women. Microorganisms invade the tissue through some portal of entry, such as a crack, fissure, or duct.

mastoidectomy Surgical procedure in which the mastoid process is excised in the event of infection.

mastoiditis Infection of the mastoid bone.

mature minors Persons under the legal age of adulthood who are legally able to give valid informed consent.

maturity onset diabetes of the young (MODY) Diabetes that has early onset (usually before the age of 25); it is inherited in an autosomal dominant manner and more closely resembles type 2 diabetes rather than type 1.

McGill Pain Questionnaire (MPQ) Assesses pain intensity, character, and location of pain using a body diagram, and also the duration of the pain experience.

mean arterial pressure (MAP) The average pressure in the arteries during one cardiac cycle.

mean corpuscular hemoglobin (MCH) Amount of hemoglobin per red blood cell.

mean corpuscular hemoglobin concentration (MCHC) Concentration of hemoglobin in each red blood cell.

mean corpuscular volume (MCV) Measure of the size of a red blood cell.

mechanical infusion device (MID) Infusion system that does not rely on an external power source.

mechanical phlebitis Inflammation of a vein associated with a catheter, its insertion, and the selected insertion site.

mechanical valves Commercially manufactured heart valves.

Medicaid Federally aided, but state-operated and -administered, program for providing medical care to qualifying low-income individuals.

medical durable power of attorney (MDPA) A document that sets out wishes for health care if an individual becomes too ill to make those decisions; a trusted person is designated to make health care decisions.

medical nutrition therapy (MNT) Meal planning approaches for patients with diabetes that combine clinical evidence, cultural, social, and ethnic approaches, and patient motivation.

medical record The legal document for all information regarding a patient's hospital course and evidence for the extent of care provided and the outcome of that care.

Medicare Federally sponsored health insurance program for people over age 65, some individuals with disabilities who are younger than age 65, and patients with end-stage renal disease. Medicare consists of Part A, hospital insurance, and Part B, general medical insurance and other options. Medicare also administers its own managed care plan.

medication nurse A registered nurse assigned the specific task of giving all patient medications under a functional nursing care delivery system.

medication reconciliation Process of identifying an accurate list of all medications the patient is taking, and using this list to provide correct medications for the patient anywhere in the health care system.

megakaryocytic stem cells Ancestor cells form giving rise to platelets.

megaloblast Large, immature red blood cells.

megaloblastic anemia Anemia resulting from impaired DNA synthesis of the red blood cells' ancestor cells.

melena Black or maroon, sticky, foul-smelling feces resulting from the digestion of blood.

menarche Beginning of menstruation or first menses.

Ménière's disease Inner ear disorder that affects hearing and balance.

meningiomas Tumors originating from the meninges.

meningismus Meningeal irritation.

menorrhagia Heavy bleeding during a menstrual period.

meshed skin graft Procedure of cutting holes in harvested skin, which allows it to be stretched over a greater surface area.

messenger ribonucleic acid (mRNA) RNA containing genetic information that is transcribed from DNA and translated to produce polypeptides.

metabolic equivalent (MET) A measure of oxygen consumption. One MET is the energy requirement for a person at rest while sitting: around 3.5 mL of oxygen per kilogram of body weight per minute.

metabolic syndrome The diagnosis given when a patient has a cluster of cardiac risk factors, including having three out of the five following conditions: abdominal obesity, high triglycerides, low HDL-C, high blood pressure, and high fasting glucose (≥100 mg/dL).

metabolism All energy and material transformations that occur within a living cell.

metacarpophalangeal joints Joints at the knuckles.

metamorphopsia Condition characterized by vision distortion, that is, when straight lines, such as door frames or posts, look crooked or irregular.

metaphysis An area of widening between the diaphysis and physis.

metaplasia Cell transformation in which a highly specialized cell changes into a less specialized cell.

metastasis The spread of cancerous cells beyond the tumor to distant sites.

metastatic tumors Tumors that originate somewhere else in the body and migrate to another organ.

metered-dose inhaler (MDI) A device that helps deliver a specific amount of medication to the lungs, usually by supplying a short burst of aerosolized medicine that is inhaled by the patient. It is commonly used to treat asthma, chronic obstructive pulmonary disease, and other respiratory disorders.

metered-volume chamber set An administration set comprised of tubing, a semirigid metered chamber, and an access spike to be inserted in the fluid container.

methodological congruence Congruence among four dimensions of a research study: documentation rigor, procedural rigor, ethical rigor, and auditability.

metrorrhagia Bleeding between menstrual periods.

microalbuminuria Small amounts of protein (30 to 299 mg/24 hours) in the urine.

microcephalic Abnormal smallness of the head, often seen in mental retardation.

microcytic Term describing red blood cells that are smaller in size than normal.

micrographia Small, cramped handwriting.

micronutrients Nutritional components such as vitamins or minerals that are needed in small quantities by living organisms.

microvascular Pertaining to the small blood vessels of the arterial and venous system.

midline (ML) catheter A flexible catheter measuring not more than 8 inches with the distal tip dwelling in the basilica, cephalic, or brachial veins, level with the axilla and distal to the shoulder.

mild cognitive impairment (MCI) A term used to describe memory loss that appears greater than what is expected for a patient's age.

millivolts A unit of electrical voltage or potential difference equal to one-thousandth of a volt.

minute ventilation (V_E) A measurement of how much air the lungs move in 1 minute; it is equal to respiratory rate times tidal volume. A normal resting respiratory rate and a normal resting tidal volume of about 500 mL yield a normal minute ventilation of 6 L/min.

missense mutation A mutation that changes a codon specific for one amino acid to specify a different amino acid.

mitral valve prolapse Occurs when one or more of the valve leaflets bulge or prolapse into the left atrium during systole. This prolapse of the valve results in valve regurgitation.

mitral valve regurgitation An inability of the mitral valve to close due to an abnormality in the structure and function of the valve.

mitral valve stenosis Occurs when the mitral valve assumes an abnormal funnel shape due to thickening and shortening of the valve structures as a result of calcification. Contractures develop between the junctions or commissures (leaflets) of the valve. The stenosis narrows the opening of the valve, which obstructs blood flow from the left atrium to the left ventricle.

mixed hearing loss Type of hearing loss that is both conductive and sensorineural in cause.

mixed venous oxygen saturation Measurement of venous oxygen content in the pulmonary artery; used to assess oxygen consumption and metabolic needs of the tissues.

Mobitz I/Wenckebach One of the two types of second-degree block that occurs in the AV node, a progressive prolongation of the electrical impulse delay in the AV node until there is a complete loss of the QRS complex and, thus, no ventricular contraction. Depicted on an ECG tracing as a progressive lengthening of the PR interval until the P wave does not progress through the conduction system, resulting in a dropped QRS complex.

Mobitz II/second-degree block Periodic blocking of sinus impulses at the AV node, the bundle of His, or bundle branches. Occurs when there is an intermittent interruption in the electrical conduction system near or below the AV node and is a more serious dysrhythmia than either first-degree AV block or Mobitz I/ Wenckebach. This dysrhythmia indicates an increased risk of progression to third-degree, or complete, heart block.

mode of transmission Means by which an organism travels from a reservoir to a susceptible host.

modeling The process by which bone growth occurs and where there is a higher rate of bone formation relative to bone loss.

molecular mimicry A process in which peptides from proteins, such as viruses, become structurally similar to self-peptides and activate T-cell autoimmunity.

molimenal Symptoms of menstruation.

MONA A protocol for empirical treatment of patients with suspected myocardial infarction. Cited in the Advanced Cardiac Life Support guidelines, the mnemonic stands for *m*orphine, *o*xygen, *n*itroglycerin, and *a*spirin.

monocyte The largest of the white blood cells and makes up about 3% to 8% of the total leukocyte count. Monocytes are a part of the reticuloendothelial (or mononuclear phagocytic) system, whose function is to engulf and digest microbes and other foreign substances. Monocytes migrate from the blood to various tissues where they mature into macrophages, working to kill invading antigens.

monophasic defibrillation Traditional means by which electrical voltage is delivered to patients in ventricular tachycardia and fibrillation.

monosomy A chromosomal constitution in which one member of the chromosome pair is missing.

Monro-Kellie doctrine Doctrine that provides the foundation for understanding the implications of increased intracranial pressure. Incompressible structures within the cranial vault are in a state of volume equilibrium, such that any increase of the volumes of one component (i.e., blood, CSF, or brain tissue) must be compensated by a decrease in the volume of another. If this cannot be achieved then pressure will rise and once the expandable reserve of the intracranial space is exhausted then small changes in volume can lead to precipitous increases in pressure.

moral agency The ability to affect and influence situations.

MORAL model An ethical decision-making model based on a series of five steps that represent the acronym MORAL: *m*assage the dilemma; *o*utline the options; *r*esolve the dilemma; *a*ct by applying the chosen option; and *l*ook back and evaluate.

morality A code of conduct held to be authoritative in matters of right and wrong.

morphologic classification Classification of skin lesions in terms of type of lesion (primary, secondary, or vascular), size, shape or configuration, color, texture, elevation or depression, and pedunculation.

mortality The number of deaths from cancer in a specific period of time and within an identified population.

mosaicism Nondisjunction of a pair of chromosomes that occurs in a mitotic division after formation of the zygote, and leads to an individual with at least two cell lines differing in genotype or karyotype, derived from a single zygote.

mucormycosis A fungal infection often seen in the sinuses of patients with diabetes who do not have good glycemic control.

multichannel pump Electronic infusion device often used in critical care areas; used to administer multiple parenteral therapies simultaneously.

multiflow adapter Add-on device used to facilitate multiple administrations of fluids and medications via a single vascular access device.

multiple organ dysfunction syndrome (MODS) Diagnosed when two or more organ systems fail.

multiple sclerosis (MS) Disease in which the immune system attacks the nerve tissues in the central nervous system, causing damage to the neurons, which disrupts the body's ability to send signals and causes symptoms. Believed to be an autoimmune disease.

multislice helical CT Detailed, noninvasive imaging of the heart using 16-slice helical scanners, accompanied by ECG gating and iodinated contrast. This device can scan the entire volume of the heart, proximal great vessels, and the coronary arteries with a single 25-second breath hold.

murmurs Abnormal heart sounds produced by turbulent blood flow.

muscle atrophy Shortening of a muscle attached to a joint.

mutation A permanent structural change in DNA.

myasthenia gravis A chronic autoimmune neuromuscular disorder in which acetylcholine receptors at the neuromuscular junction are destroyed.

myasthenic crisis A life-threatening exacerbation of myasthenia gravis that requires mechanical ventilation.

myelin A soft, white coating that surrounds and protects nerve fibers. Myelin also helps nerve fibers conduct electrical impulses.

myeloid progenitor cell Ancestor cell that gives rise to granulocytes and monocytes.

myelopathy Motor, sensory, and reflex abnormalities due to an abnormality of the spinal cord.

myocardial hibernation Condition in which myocardial tissue undergoes cellular structural changes and progressive apoptosis (cell death) in response to prolonged cardiac ischemia.

myocardial infarction (MI) The loss of myocytes or myocardial cell death as a result of prolonged ischemia.

myocardial perfusion Blood flow to the heart muscle.

myocardial perfusion imaging (MPI) Use of a radioactive tracer and a gamma camera to detect blood flow to the myocardium.

myocardial stunning A temporary dysfunction that occurs in response to artery occlusion of short duration (artery spasm) or transient global hypoperfusion during a limited low-flow state such as shock.

myocardial viability Term applied to areas of the myocardium that appear to have normal functioning as well as areas that appear dysfunctional (hibernating or stunned) that might improve with revascularization.

myocarditis A focal or diffuse inflammation of the myocardium or heart muscle; an uncommon disorder that is frequently associated with pericarditis.

myocutaneous flap A piece of tissue, muscle or skin, used in reconstructive surgery; may be used for reconstructing breasts, large lateral temporal, scalp, or intraoral defects, and defects involving the trunk and chest wall.

myoglobin A heme-containing, oxygen-binding protein that is exclusive to striated and nonstriated muscle. Because of its very small molecular weight, it is released into interstitial fluid as early as 2 hours following damage to muscle tissue.

myopia Individuals see nearby objects clearly, but distant objects appear blurred.

myositis An uncommon disease in which the immune system inflames the body's own healthy muscle tissue.

myringotomy Surgical procedure in which tubes are placed in the ears to facilitate drainage and prevent the buildup of pressure within the inner ear and prevent ear infections.

myxedema A long-term consequence of hypothyroidism in which the facial features are coarsened and changed by puffiness, periorbital edema, and a mask-like appearance.

myxedema coma A rare, life-threatening complication of hypothyroidism.

nadir The point at which the lowest blood count is reached.

nasal polyps Small saclike growths inside the nasal cavity and sinuses.

national standards of care Statements of actions consistent with minimum safe professional conduct under specific medical conditions as determined by professional medical organizations.

natural immunity Type of immunity that is the responsibility of a group of body organs, cells, and chemicals that are present at birth or shortly after.

near drowning Condition that connotes survival for at least 24 hours after submersion.

neck dissection Surgical procedure to remove nodal disease in conjunction with the central part of the cancer surgery.

necrotizing fasciitis (NF) An infection of the superficial fascia or the connective tissue surrounding muscle and subcutaneous tissue leading to necrosis.

needleless system Components of infusion equipment that do not use needles.

negative deflection Any waveform that goes below the isoelectric line on ECG graph paper.

negative feedback A compensatory mechanism by which homeostasis is achieved in which the endocrine glands respond to a decrease in hormone levels, leading to gland stimulation and increased hormone production. When a normal level of hormone is reached, it feeds back to suppress the stimulating hormone and a normal state occurs.

negative pressure pulmonary edema (NPPE) A disorder caused by attempts to ventilate a person with an apparent airway obstruction. Also called *postobstruction pulmonary edema* and *airway obstruction pulmonary edema*.

negligence Failure to exercise the degree of care that a person of ordinary prudence would exercise under the same or similar conditions.

neoantigens Antigens created by the developing fetal immune system while it is in the process of eliminating autoreactive lymphocytes.

neoplasm New growth.

nephron The functional unit of the kidney.

nerve agents Chemicals that inactivate acetylcholinesterase at the receptor site. They cause symptoms of SLUDGE'M (*s*alivation, *l*acrimation, *u*rination, *d*efecation, *g*astric upset, *e*mesis, and *m*iosis).

network sampling Type of sampling in which participants refer other participants to the study. Also referred to as *snowball sampling*.

neurofibromatosis An autosomal dominant inherited disorder characterized by the formation of tumors of the peripheral nerves over the entire body.

neurogenic pulmonary edema (NPE) A rare type of pulmonary edema that develops after a neurological insult to the central nervous system.

neurogenic shock Occurs in spinal cord injuries above T_6 thoracic spine and results in interruption of the sympathetic change, causing bradycardia, hypotension, and vasodilation of the peripheral vascular system.

neuromatrix theory Addresses the brain's role in pain perception as well as other multiple determinants.

neuron A nerve cell; the structural and functional unit of the nervous system.

neuropathic pain Pain resulting from injury or dysfunction in one or more nerves.

neuroprotection Therapies used to arrest the sequence of events that occur during the ischemic cascade.

neutralization Action of antibodies that involves the process of changing the charge or shape of the antigen and blocking its ability to attach to another cell.

neutrophil Primary phagocytic defense; responds to bacteria, inflammation, injury, infection, and foreign objects.

nevi Well-circumscribed malformations of the skin. Also known as *moles*.

New York Heart Association (NYHA) classification system A functional classification system that categorizes cardiac patients' subjective degree of symptoms into NYHA classes I through IV.

nidus Refers to the focus of an arteriovenous malformation.

nits The eggs of a louse.

nociception The process by which tissue damage (noxious stimuli) activates sensory neurons to send a pain message to the central nervous system, resulting in a nociceptive pain response; literally means "pain sense."

nociceptive pain Pain resulting from the process of nociception.

nocturia The need to get up at night to urinate.

nodes (bundles) Special cells and fibers that make up the electrical conduction system of the heart.

nodules Small aggregation of cells formed in response to injury or inflammation.

noise-induced hearing loss (NIHL) Hearing loss caused by noises or sounds at a high decibel level for long periods of time.

noncardiogenic pulmonary edema (NCPE) An abnormal accumulation of fluid in the lungs caused by a noncardiac etiology.

noncoring needle Type of access needle required to access an implanted port or reservoir; used to prevent accidental coring of the port's septum.

nondisjunction The failure of two members of a chromosome pair to separate during meiosis or mitosis, resulting in daughter cells with either a missing or extra chromosome.

nonexperimental research design Research design in which the researcher collects data without introducing an intervention.

nongranulocyte White blood cell that is produced in the bone marrow and develops into a lymphocyte or monocyte; does not contain granules in its cytoplasm.

nonheme iron Form of dietary iron available in vegetables, cereals, and fortified food.

nonintentional torts Actions that result in harm to another, but intent is lacking; often synonymous with carelessness.

noninvasive positive pressure ventilation (NPPV) Procedure for delivering breaths to a patient without placement of an artificial airway, such as an endotracheal or tracheostomy tube.

nonmaleficence The duty to do no harm.

nonprobability sampling Type of sampling in which elements and participants are selected by nonrandom methods.

nonsense mutation A single base substitution in DNA that results in a chain-termination codon.

nontunneled and noncuffed device Type of central vascular access device; inserted by a puncture directly through the skin and to the intended location without passing through subcutaneous tissue.

normal sinus rhythm (NSR) A regular heart rate between 60 and 100 beats per minute that has all of the normal components of one cardiac cycle (PQRST) and normal time intervals between the waveforms.

normoglycemia Normal blood glucose levels.

normothermia A normal body temperature.

nosocomial infection An infection that occurs in a hospitalized patient.

not-for-profit organization Organization that reinvests profits from operations back into the organization.

notifiable disease Any of certain diseases or conditions that must be reported to local, county, or state public health departments.

noxious stimuli Tissue damage that activates sensory neurons to send a pain message to the central nervous system, resulting in a nociceptive pain response.

NSTEMI Non–ST segment elevation myocardial infarction is the result of transient subtotal occlusion of a coronary artery with reduced coronary blood flow resulting from plaque disruption and ensuing pathophysiological processes. Serum blood markers and persistent ECG changes are present with NSTEMI.

numeric rating scale (NRS) A horizontal line marked with the numbers 0 to 10 from left to right with three interval descriptors of pain located along the scale: "no pain," "moderate pain," and "worst pain."

nurse–patient relationship The means for applying the nursing process. It is the mechanism by which the nurse works with the patient.

nurse practice acts State guidelines that define the practice of nursing and give guidance in terms of scope of practice issues; they are designed to ensure safe practice.

nurse practitioner (NP) An advanced practice nurse with postgraduate training who is licensed by the state to provide basic medical care under standardized procedures.

nursing care delivery systems A set of concepts based on principles that involve clinical decision making, work allocation, communication, and management.

nursing diagnosis The end product of the nursing assessment. Describes an actual or potential health problem, based on gathered data, that a nurse can legally manage.

nursing process A thinking/doing approach to patient care that provides the nurse with a systematic means of identifying, preventing, and treating actual and potential health problems.

Nursing's Agenda for the Future The American Nurses Association statement outlining issues related to nursing practice. Issues include an expanded role for registered nurses and advanced practice nurses in the delivery of basic and primary health care, obtaining federal funding for nurse education and training, and helping to change and improve the health care workplace.

nutritional imbalance A deficiency or excess of one or more essential nutrients, resulting from inadequate nutrition or too much nutrition.

nystagmus A constant, involuntary tremor, oscillation, or jerky movement of the eyeball; the movement may be in any direction.

objective data Behaviors, activities, and events that can be observed or measured by another person using the senses of observation, palpation, auscultation, percussion, and smell. Objective data are factual: They can be seen, heard, touched, smelled, or tasted.

obstructive sleep apnea (OSA) Disorder of sleep with habitual snoring characterized by brief periods of breathing cessation or a marked reduction in tidal volume with a minimum of five episodes per hour during sleep with excessive daytime somnolence.

occupational asthma Occurs when a worker experiences asthmatic symptoms upon exposure to substances that trigger an asthma attack.

Occupational Safety and Health Administration (OSHA) Agency under the U.S. Department of Labor whose function is to inspect and enforce safety standards in the workplace.

oculocephalic reflex Reflex eye movement that stabilizes images on the retina during head movement by producing an eye movement in the direction opposite to the head movement that maintains the visual field or a more-or-less steady gaze. Also called *doll's eye reflex.*

oculovestibular reflex Reflex that stabilizes images on the retina during head movement by producing an eye movement in the direction opposite that of the head movement.

odontoid process The toothlike projection of C_2 (cervical spine), which sits behind the anterior portion of the ring of C_1.

oligoanalgesia Results when a patient complains of pain, but no interventions are provided for pain relief.

oliguria Decreased urine output of less than 400 mL in a 24-hour period.

Ommaya reservoir Nonvascular infusion device inserted with the catheter tip residing in the ventricles of the brain; used to deliver targeted therapies (i.e., pain and antineoplastic therapies) or to obtain cerebrospinal fluid.

oncosis Cell swelling as a result of changes in membrane permeability.

oncotic pressure In the circulatory system, the term refers to a form of osmotic pressure exerted by proteins in blood plasma that normally tends to pull water into the circulatory system. Also referred to as *colloid osmotic pressure.*

on–off phenomena Abrupt fluctuations in movement ability associated with Parkinson's disease.

open-ended questions Questions that ask for narrative information by stating a topic in general terms; for example, "What brought you to the hospital?"

open globe An open eyeball with a laceration, penetrating injury, or intraocular foreign body; usually results from blunt trauma or projectile injury.

open pneumothorax An open communication between the atmosphere and intrathoracic pressure; usually caused by penetrating trauma.

open reduction internal fixation (ORIF) A treatment in which a fracture is exposed by an incision in the skin directly over the fracture. Implants such as plates (strips of metal), screws, and wires are placed directly on or in the bone to anatomically stabilize a fracture.

opportunistic infections (OIs) Infections from microorganisms that are not usually considered pathogens, but cause disease if the immune system is impaired.

opsonization A chemical coating of an antigen by cytokines or antibodies that makes that cell more attractive to phagocytes.

oral cancer Cancer that arises from the flat cells that line the oral cavity and is slow growing; most often squamous cell carcinoma.

oral candidiasis An overgrowth of the yeast-like fungus *Candida albicans.*

oral glucose tolerance test (OGTT) A test in which the glycemic response to a prescribed dose of oral glucose is used to determine glucose tolerance status (i.e., normal glucose tolerance, impaired glucose tolerance, or diabetes).

orchiectomy Surgical removal of the testes.

orchiopexy Surgical fixation of a testis.

orchitis Inflammation of one or both testes.

orthopnea Shortness of breath relieved by sitting or standing erect.

osmolality Number of molecules of solute per kilogram of water.

osmosis The movement of water from one compartment of low solute concentration through a semipermeable membrane into a second compartment with high solute concentration.

osmotic diuresis Excessive urination caused by the presence of certain substances (such as glucose) in the renal tubules.

osteitis fibrosa cystica A complication of hypoparathyroidism in which the bone softens and becomes deformed or forms cysts.

osteoarthritis (OA) Chronic condition that accompanies aging, affecting the weight-bearing joints most commonly; is the most common form of arthritis.

osteoblasts Any cells that form bone within the body.

osteoclasts Large cells formed in bone marrow and originating from macrophage-like cells; designed to absorb and remove unwanted bone tissue, causing the bone to be "remodeled" or "destroyed."

osteocytes Mature osteoblasts that maintain the bony matrix and participate in the dynamic task of releasing calcium into the bloodstream.

osteoid Type I collagen and noncollagenous protein osteocalcin.

osteology The study of bones and the bone structure of the human body.

osteolysis Destruction of implanted synthetic or cement components of repaired bone segments.

osteonecrosis The death of bone tissue.

osteoporosis A skeletal disease that is characterized by low bone mass and deterioration of the bone tissue. This continued deterioration results in bone fragility and susceptibility to fractures.

otalgia Ear pain.

otitis externa Inflammation/infection of the external ear canal.

otitis media Inflammation/infection of the middle ear.

otolaryngology (otorhinolaryngology) The study of ear, nose, and throat disorders.

otosclerosis Abnormal bone growth within the middle ear that causes hearing loss.

ototoxic Something that, if ingested, causes damage to the auditory nerve, affecting hearing.

ototoxicity Harmful effect on the eighth cranial nerve or organs of hearing and balance.

outcome Individual, measurable patient objective; measurable criterion that indicates the patient's care objectives have been met; a change in patient behavior that results from nursing interventions.

outcome standards Quality standards that focus on whether the services provided by an organization make any difference to patients or to the health status of the patient population.

overnutrition The physical consequences resulting from overconsumption of energy or nutrients compared to recommended amounts.

over-the-needle peripheral-short catheter A catheter with a stylet needle housed in the catheter lumen.

oxidative stress Stress to the cells caused by a decrease in the removal of or an overproduction of oxygen free radicals, common in physiological disorders of the critically ill; the imbalance between reactive oxygen species and the body's defense system.

oxytocin Peptide hormone produced in the hypothalamus but secreted by the posterior pituitary gland. It causes uterine contraction and stimulates breast milk production.

P wave Part of the cardiac cycle; represents atrial contraction or depolarization on an ECG tracing.

pacemaker cell Cardiac cell found in the electrical conduction system, which lies in the heart wall and septum. It generates and conducts impulses.

pacemaker sensitivity Amount of electrical activity the pacemaker will sense or "hear"; measured in millivolts (mV).

packed RBCs Red blood cells that have had the plasma portion of the blood removed by a centrifuge process.

pain An unpleasant sensory and emotional experience associated with actual or potential tissue damage, or described in terms of such damage.

palliative The alleviation (not curative) of suffering from symptoms.

palliative care Comprehensive care focused on alleviating suffering and promoting the quality of remaining life of patients living with a chronic life-threatening or terminal illness; allows patients and families to guide treatment and set goals for care.

palliative procedures Surgeries performed for the primary purpose of alleviating symptoms rather than affecting a cure.

palpation Technique of using touch to collect data to determine specific characteristics of the body.

palpitations An awareness of the beating of the heart.

pancarditis Inflammation of all three layers of the heart: the endocardium, myocardium, and pericardium.

pancreatic beta cells Cells in the pancreatic islets of Langerhans that produce insulin.

pancreatic insufficiency A deficiency of pancreatic enzymes resulting in malabsorption of nutrients.

pancreatic polypeptide A complex peptide hormone secreted by the pancreatic islet cells whose role is not completely understood.

pancreaticoduodenal (Whipple) resection A radical surgical procedure to treat pancreatic cancer that involves removal of the head of the pancreas, the duodenum, the distal portion of the stomach, part of the jejunum, and the lower half of the common bile duct.

pancreatitis Inflammation of the pancreas.

panendoscopy Surgical procedure to evaluate the upper aerodigestive tract, locate the organ of origin, and obtain a cellular diagnosis.

panhypopituitarism Condition in which there is inadequate secretion of all of the hormones of the anterior pituitary.

paracentesis Removal of ascites fluid from the abdomen.

paracrine functioning Bioregulation of one cell type that influences the activity of an adjacent cell type by secreting chemicals that diffuse into the tissue and act specifically on cells in that area.

paraphimosis Condition in which the foreskin is retracted, but cannot be returned to its normal position covering the glans.

paraplegia Paralysis of the lower half of the body including both lower extremities and loss of bowel and bladder function.

parenteral Term used to describe fluids and medications that are administered via routes other than the alimentary canal.

parenteral nutrition Provision of nutrients and energy by means of intravenous access, without use of the gastrointestinal tract.

paresthesia An abnormal physical sensation such as prickling, tingling, or numbness.

Parkinson's disease (PD) A disease of the basal ganglia characterized by a slowing down in the innervation and executive of movement, increased muscle tone rigidity, tremors at rest, and impaired postural reflexes.

paronychia Inflammation of the folds of tissue surrounding the fingernail.

paroxysmal junctional tachycardia (PJT) An irritable focus in the AV junction that assumes the pacemaker role by discharging impulses more rapidly than the SA node. Begins and ends abruptly.

partial-thickness injury Injury in which the epidermis and part of the dermis are destroyed.

passive immunization Immunization that provides immunity for a short period of time, usually around 6 to 12 weeks; involves the injection of already formed antibodies into the body.

paternalism In ethics, policy that allows one to make decisions for another.

pathogenicity Disease-causing potential of a microorganism, the number of invading microorganisms, and the host defenses.

pathologic dead space A portion of the tidal volume that does reach the alveoli, but does not take place in gas exchange. Various lung pathologies and disease conditions can increase this dead space amount and affect the lungs' ability to oxygenate and ventilate.

pathologic fractures Fractures that occur without trauma due to bone thinning.

patient care plan A documented record of the nursing process, a plan designed to incorporate the patient's identified problems, outcomes, and actions to be implemented by the nurse.

patient-centered care An innovative approach to the planning, delivery, and evaluation of health care that is based on mutually beneficial partnerships among health care patients, families, and providers.

patient-controlled analgesia (PCA) pump A computerized machine that is attached to a patient's intravenous line and allows the patient to control the amount of medication that is administered based on his or her pain level.

pattern theory a group of theories that asserts that pain receptors share nerve pathways with other sensory pathways and that the intensity of the stimulus determines the frequency of firing of the receptor.

pediculosis Infestation with lice.

pedigree A diagram that shows the heredity of a particular trait or genetic disorder through many generations of a family.

pelvic inflammatory disease (PID) An infection of the internal reproductive organs, including the fallopian tubes. It is a very common and a very serious complication of many sexually transmitted infections.

The highest risk for the development of PID is seen in women of childbearing age who are sexually active.

penectomy Removal of part of or the entire penis.

penetrance The proportion of individuals with a genotype known to cause a genetic disorder who have signs and symptoms of the disorder.

peptic ulcer A generic term used for any ulceration in the digestive surfaces of the upper GI tract.

percussion Technique of either pushing, tapping, or using a device to generate a sound vibration. The vibrations produced will help in determining position of organ structures.

percutaneous angioplasty The use of mechanical widening when opening blood vessels other than coronary arteries.

percutaneous coronary intervention (PCI) The use of devices to either remove plaque or alter its morphology in the catheterization laboratory, including atherectomy devices, lasers, and intracoronary stents.

percutaneous transluminal coronary angioplasty (PTCA) Treatment of coronary artery disease (CAD) using expandable balloons to crack (tear or rupture) atherosclerotic plaque, thereby enlarging the lumen of the coronary artery.

percutaneously Passing through the skin.

perfusion The movement of blood carrying oxygen.

pericardial effusion An excess buildup of pericardial fluid that is a threat to normal cardiac function. The fluid buildup is the result of an accumulation of infectious exudates or toxins and/or blood.

pericardial friction rub A grating, scraping, squeaking, or a crunching sound that is the result of friction between the roughened, inflamed layers of the pericardium.

pericardial window An opening in the pericardial sac that allows fluid from effusion and tamponade to drain.

pericardiectomy Removal of the pericardial sac to allow fluid to drain from around the heart.

pericarditis Inflammation of the pericardial sac due to an inflammatory process in which the two layers of the pericardium become inflamed and roughened, causing fluid to build up.

perimenopause The time during which periods may increase, decrease, and become irregular as the function of the ovaries waxes and wanes.

perioperative A broad term that refers to the time period surrounding a surgical procedure. It includes the preoperative, intraoperative, and postoperative time periods.

perioperative blood salvage The process of collecting and reinfusing blood lost during both the intraoperative and early postoperative periods.

periosteum Fibrous membrane that covers bone.

peripheral arterial disease (PAD) Disease that affects the arteries of the extremities.

peripheral blood stem cell (PBSC) transplantation Transplantation of stem cells located in peripherally circulating blood.

peripheral nerve block An anesthesia technique in which a local anesthetic is injected into or around a nerve plexus to produce anesthesia of a selected area without inducing a systemic effect.

peripheral parenteral nutrition (PPN) Provision of nutrition intravenously through a peripheral vein.

peripheral-short catheter Type of vascular access device used for short-term infusion therapies.

peripheral vascular resistance The resistance in the pulmonary vasculature.

peripherally inserted central catheter (PICC) Central vascular access device that is inserted into an extremity, typically in the antecubital fossa, and advanced until the tip is positioned in the vena cava.

peristalsis A progressive wavelike movement that occurs involuntarily in hollow tubes of the body.

peritonsillar abscess A rare complication of tonsillitis in which the infection spreads to the tissue around the tonsillar capsule.

perivascular Situated around a blood vessel.

pernicious anemia Anemia caused by insufficiencies in intrinsic factor.

persistent The ability of a chemical agent to remain in an area. In general, the agent would have a low vapor pressure and a high vapor density.

pessary A device that, when inserted into the vagina, will help support the vaginal walls, reducing the bulging of those walls into the vagina.

Peyronie's disease Condition in which plaque forms on the erectile tissue of the penis, primarily in middle-aged or older men.

pH An indicator of hydrogen ion concentration; the negative logarithm of the hydrogen ion concentration expressed in nanomoles per liter. A normal pH of 7.4 is equivalent to 40 nmol/L of hydrogen ion (or 0.0004 mEq/L).

phagocytes Granulocytes, macrophages, and lymphocytes, which are attracted to an injured site by the complement factors and antigens.

phagocytosis The process by which phagocytes absorb and enzymatically degrade foreign matter and devitalized tissue.

phantom limb pain Pain appearing to come from an amputated limb.

pharmacogenetics Area of biochemical genetics concerned with drug responses and their genetically controlled variations.

pharmacogenomics The application of genomic information or methods to pharmacogenetics problems.

pharyngitis Inflammation of the pharynx caused by upper respiratory infection, which causes a sore throat.

pharyngoesophageal Pertaining to the pharynx and the esophagus.

phenomenology A qualitative research method that describes the meaning of a lived experience through the perspective of the participant.

phenotype Observable characteristics of an organism produced by the organism's genotype interacting with the environment.

pheochromocytoma A tumor (usually benign) that originates from the adrenal medulla.

pheresis catheter Central vascular access device used for plasma exchange therapies.

phimosis The inability to retract the foreskin over the penile glans.

phlebostatic axis Reference point used to level transducers.

phoria A tendency toward a functional deviation or defect that results from a break in visual fusion by covering an eye. Latent deviation meaning that the deviation is not apparent unless fusion of the eyes is broken.

phosphorus An abundant mineral used in all sources of energy (ATP, ADP, and AMP). Eighty percent is found bound to calcium in the bone as calcium phosphate. Normal serum levels are 2.5 to 4.5 mg/dL.

photodermatitis A common, inflammatory adverse reaction to sunlight in which the individual sunburns more easily than usual or develops papular or vesicular lesions with exposure to the sun.

phronesis A form of rationality and skill-based character that is similar to clinical judgment.

physes Growth plates.

physiological stress Metabolic conditions characterized by hypermetabolism and hypercatabolism.

pilosebaceous follicles A sebaceous cyst containing hair follicles.

pilot study A small preliminary study prior to conducting a larger study.

pitch Describes frequency; low pitch is 100 Hz and high pitch is 10,000 Hz.

pitting An indention that remains for a short time after pressing edematous skin with the finger.

planning Determining how expected patient outcomes can be achieved through nursing interventions by establishing priorities of care.

plasma The protein portion of blood that remains when cells have been removed.

plasma cells Differentiated B cells that are found in the plasma and are responsible for production of specific antibodies or immunoglobulins.

plasmapheresis A treatment used in some autoimmune diseases that involves removing blood from the body and filtering antibodies out of the plasma. The red blood cells and fluids are returned to the body. The removal of antibodies decreases immune stimulation and helps control clinical symptoms of some autoimmune diseases.

platelet Thrombocyte of blood that is small and colorless with no nucleus, which assists in blood clotting by adhering to other platelets and to damaged epethelium. Also called *blood platelet, thrombocyte.*

pleasure principle The principle of tension reduction.

pleural effusion Abnormal accumulation of fluid in the pleural space.

pleural friction rubs Harsh leathery sound created from inflamed pleural surfaces rubbing against each other.

pneumatoscope An otoscope with a bulb attachment that can be used to introduce air into the ear canal and middle ear to test for ruptured tympanic membrane.

***Pneumocystis carinii* pneumonia (PCP)** An opportunistic fungal respiratory infection that can be seen in severely immune-compromised hosts.

pneumonia An inflammatory process that results in edema of interstitial lung tissue and extravasation of fluid into the alveoli, thus causing hypoxemia.

pneumothorax Partial or complete collapse of the lung.

point mutation A single nucleotide base-pair change in DNA.

polycythemia vera A hematocrit value that is elevated beyond normal values; frequent occurrence in chronic hypoxemia.

polymorphism A common variation in the sequence of DNA among individuals seen in more than 1% of the population.

polypharmacy The administration of many drugs together; also, the administration of excessive medications.

polysomnography Multichannel electrophysiological recording used to detect disturbances of breathing during sleep.

population Entire aggregation of cases in which a researcher is interested.

population-based care Care focused on aggregates and communities. A population is a collection of individuals who have in common one or more personal or environmental characteristics. As an aggregate, the members are defined in terms of geography, special interest, disease state, or other common characteristics.

portal hypertension Increased pressure in the hepatic circulation that is a complication of cirrhosis.

portal of entry The path by which an infective organism enters a susceptible host.

portal of exit Path in the chain of infection that allows a causative agent to escape from a reservoir.

positive deflection Any waveform that goes above the isoelectric line on ECG graph paper.

positive feedback Process by which a deviation from normal is reinforced or accelerated, producing an increased stimulus. For example, uterine contraction stimulates oxytocin secretion, which brings about increased contractions and increased oxytocin.

positive pressure infusion pump Electronic infusion device used to administer parenteral fluids and medications under preset pressures.

postacute withdrawal syndrome (PAWS) An enduring physical remnant of neurotransmitter production and/or receptor site damage. The mood is affected, as are interpersonal interactions and cognitive skills.

postanesthesia care unit (PACU) A physical space located adjacent to the operating room where patients are monitored closely as they recover from anesthesia.

postconcussion syndrome A condition that may follow mild head injury.

posterior circulation Refers to circulation in the arteries in the posterior portion of the circle of Willis.

posteriorly Back plane of the body.

postoperative blood salvage The process of salvaging blood in which blood is obtained from mediastinal and chest tubes, and then reinfused.

It is used following major surgeries, typically cardiovascular, thoracic, and some orthopedic procedures.

post-test probability The likelihood that a disease is actually present in a patient after testing (a positive test indicates disease).

postural instability Diminished postural reflexes, which contribute to difficulty maintaining balance.

potassium An intracellular cation with 98% found within cells. Small amounts are in blood (3.5 to 5.0 mEq/L) and bone. Its function is to maintain intracellular osmolality and participate in cellular depolarization and repolarization.

power analysis A research design's ability to detect relationships that exist among variables.

PPE Acronym for personal protective equipment, which is designed to protect the wearer from various hazards.

PR interval Part of the cardiac cycle; represents time from atrial depolarization to ventricular depolarization on an ECG tracing. Sometimes referred to as the *PRI* or *PR segment*.

practical knowledge Knowledge shaped by one's familiarity with the discipline and practice of the science and technology relevant to the situation at hand.

precipitation One of the actions of antibodies; occurs when an immune complex falls or precipitates out of circulation and is more easily located by neutrophils and monocytes for phagocytosis.

pre-diabetes A condition of glucose intolerance ranging between normal glucose tolerance and overt diabetes.

predictive accuracy Ability of a diagnostic test to predict the presence or absence of disease.

preferred provider organization (PPO) Organization that provides health care coverage through a coordinated plan for medical care that includes a network of contracted providers.

prehypertension A term used to describe those individuals who have a blood pressure finding on two or more office visits of 130 to 139/80 to 89 mmHg. These individuals are at twice the risk of developing hypertension as those with lower values.

preload The volume of blood in the ventricle at the end of diastole.

premature atrial contraction (PAC) An ectopic focus in the atria that occurs early, before the next expected SA impulse, causing depolarization and contraction of the atrial muscle.

premature junctional contraction (PJC) Dysrhythmia that originates in the AV junction. It discharges before the next expected sinus impulse and activates the ventricles in a normal manner. Due to retrograde conduction, the P wave is inverted and may appear before, buried, or after the QRS complex on an ECG tracing.

premature ventricular contraction (PVC) An irritable focus within the ventricle that discharges before the next sinus impulse; thereby, stimulating the ventricle directly and causing a contraction, which is followed by a full compensatory pause. Each contraction is an individual beat, not a rhythm.

premenstrual dysphoric disorder (PMDD) A severe form of premenstrual syndrome that includes five or more symptoms of depression for most of the time during the last week of the luteal phase and begins to remit within a few days after onset of the follicular phase of the menstrual cycle.

premenstrual syndrome (PMS) A complex, often misunderstood condition, involving physical, psychological, and behavioral symptoms associated with the menstrual cycle.

preoperative health evaluation An evaluation done within 30 days of a planned operation and must be documented in the patient's chart per the Joint Commission requirements.

presbycusis Hearing loss caused by changes in the middle and inner ear due to the aging process.

presbyopia Condition where the eye exhibits a progressively diminished ability to focus on near objects with age; also recognized as a symptom of aging.

pressure ulcer A localized injury to the skin and/or underlying tissue usually over a bony prominence, as a result of pressure or pressure in combination with shear and/or friction.

pretest probability The likelihood that a disease is actually present in a patient before testing.

prevalence The measurement of all cancer cases at a designated point in time.

priapism A persistent erection.

PRICE Acronym for *protection* (immobilize and prevent weight bearing), *rest*, *ice*, *compression*, and *elevation*.

primary adrenal insufficiency Condition in which 90% of the adrenal gland has been destroyed, resulting in an absence of adrenal hormones.

primary appraisal The process of evaluating the significance of a transaction as it relates to a person's well-being, based on Lazarus's theory of stress.

primary biliary cirrhosis An autoimmune disease in which there is inflammation and destruction of the intrahepatic biliary system, resulting in fibrosis.

primary immune deficiency Results from genetic abnormalities in immune system development and causes partial or total immune system dysfunction.

primary immune response The first exposure to a specific antigen; results in creation of B memory cells, which provide lifelong protection against the specific antigen.

primary injury Refers to mechanical injury to the brain.

primary intention A wound that is surgically closed or one with smooth, closely aligned margins.

primary lesion Lesion that results from the initial reaction to a pathologic condition.

primary nursing A primary nursing care delivery system is a system in which a registered nurse providing direct care to the patient has 24-hour responsibility for the planning, implementation, and outcomes of patient care.

primary set Infusion set with a single fluid pathway from the fluid container to a vascular access device.

primary tumors Tumors that are at the original site where it first arose. For example, a primary brain tumor is one that arose in the brain as opposed to one that arose elsewhere and metastasized to the brain.

principlism An emerging theory in ethics that incorporates the various ethical principles in attempting to resolve conflicts in clinical settings.

probability sampling Type of sampling that involves random selection when choosing the elements and participants.

process standards Quality standards that focus on whether the activities within an organization are being conducted appropriately.

prodromal phase The phase of acute hepatitis that occurs between exposure to the virus and the appearance of jaundice. It is characterized by fatigue, anorexia, malaise, nausea, vomiting, and a headache; often mistaken for the flu.

progenitor cells In development, a parent cell that gives rise to a distinct cell lineage by a series of cell divisions. Like stem cells, progenitor cells have a capacity to differentiate into a specific type of cell. In contrast to stem cells, however, they are already far more specific: They are pushed to differentiate into their "target" cell.

progesterone Steroid hormone produced by the ovaries and the placenta. It is responsible for uterine changes in the second half of the menstrual cycle.

programmed theory of aging Theory of aging based on the premise that aging follows a biological timetable.

prolactin Peptide hormone produced by the anterior pituitary gland. Stimulates breast development and breast milk during and after pregnancy.

prolapse Condition in which the uterus is unable to remain high in the vaginal canal and begins to protrude into the vagina; can occur if the structures supporting the uterus are weakened during childbirth.

proprioception The awareness of posture, movement, and changes in equilibrium and the knowledge of position, weight, and resistance of objects in relation to the body.

proptosis A downward displacement of the eyeball in exophthalmic goiter or in inflammatory conditions of the orbit.

prostaglandin A long-chain fatty acid that regulates platelet aggregation and controls inflammation.

prostatectomy Removal of the prostate and seminal vesicles.

prostatitis Inflammation of the prostate gland.

protein C A normal component of the coagulation system.

protein-calorie malnutrition Physical state resulting from the underconsumption of energy and protein specifically.

proteinuria The presence of protein in the urine.

proton pump inhibitor (PPI) Drug that blocks the proton pump in the stomach, thus reducing gastric acid secretion.

psoriasis A chronic, noncontagious inflammatory skin disorder; characterized by erythematous papules and plaques with silver-white scales that are sharply demarcated and the result of hyperproliferation of keratinocytes.

psoriatic arthritis An inflammatory process associated with psoriasis.

psychogenic polydipsia Condition in which excessive thirst occurs for psychogenic, rather than organic, reasons.

psychomotor learning Learning that occurs when a physical skill has been acquired.

psychosocial theories of aging Theories of aging that describe the changes that take place emotionally and socially as one enters the later years of life.

ptosis Drooping of the upper eyelid, generally due to paralysis.

pulmonary artery catheter (PAC) A flow-directed, balloon-tipped catheter used to measure intracardiac pressures.

pulmonary artery occlusion pressure (PAOP) Pressure obtained by inflating the balloon on a pulmonary artery catheter at the end of expiration to reflect left ventricular end-diastolic pressure.

pulmonary contusion Occurs when blunt thoracic trauma is applied through the chest wall to the parenchyma, causing disruption of alveolar capillary networks and usually resulting in hypoxemia; initially a hemorrhage into the lung tissue followed by alveolar and interstitial edema.

pulmonary embolism (PE) The presence of a thrombus or blood clot in the pulmonary vessels, which obstructs blood flow and impedes gas exchange.

pulmonic valve regurgitation The inability of the pulmonic valve to completely close, causing blood to regurgitate back into the right ventricle.

pulmonic valve stenosis A narrowing of the cardiac valve orifice that restricts blood flow due to an inability of the valve to completely open, thus, obstructing blood from the right ventricle from flowing into the pulmonary vasculature during systole.

pulse pressure The difference between the systolic and diastolic pressure, which is about 40 mmHg.

pulseless electrical activity (PEA) Absence of a detectable pulse and blood pressure in the presence of electrical activity in the heart as evidenced by some type of ECG rhythm other than ventricular fibrillation or ventricular tachycardia. It is not an actual rhythm, but represents a clinical condition wherein the patient is clinically dead, despite the fact that some type of organized rhythm appears on the ECG monitor.

pulsus paradoxus A greater than 10 mmHg drop in systolic blood pressure during inspiration.

Purkinje network fibers Part of the cardiac conduction system; a network of fibers that carries impulses directly to the ventricular muscle cells. Ventricular contraction is facilitated by the rapid spread of the electrical impulse through the left and right bundle branches, the Purkinje network fibers, and the ventricular muscle.

purposive sampling Type of sampling that implies that certain people or elements are deliberately selected for the study.

pyloric stenosis Narrowing of the pyloric orifice. In adults, frequently results from peptic ulcer disease, malignant compression of the gastric outlet, or pneumatosis intestinalis.

QRS complex Part of the cardiac cycle; represents ventricular contraction or depolarization on an ECG tracing.

QT interval Part of the cardiac cycle; is measured from the Q wave to the end of the T wave. The normal QT interval is 0.34 to 0.43 second.

quadrigeminy Premature ventricular contraction that occurs every fourth beat.

quadriplegia (*Latin*) Paralysis of all four extremities.

qualitative research A systematic, subjective approach used to describe life experiences and give them meaning.

quality Refers to characteristics of and the pursuit of excellence.

quality in fact Conforming to standards and meeting one's own expectations.

quality in perception Meeting the customer's expectations.

quality of care The degree to which health services for individuals and populations increase the likelihood of desired health outcomes and are consistent with current professional knowledge.

quantitative research Research characterized by the collection of numerical values, under a controlled situation, that yield data, which can be generalized.

quasi-experimental research design A study with an intervention, but one in which it is difficult to manipulate or control the setting, subjects, or variables, as is needed for a true experimental study.

quasi-intentional torts Volitional actions that result in harm to another, but intent is lacking.

quota sampling Type of sampling in which participants are selected by a researcher in a nonrandom manner using prespecified characteristics of the sample to increase their representation.

raccoon eyes Ecchymosis over the orbit of the eyes that is indicative of a basilar skull fracture. Also called *raccoon sign*.

radiation Waves and particles of energy. Radiation causes mutation of cells' DNA, which can weaken the cells' defense against a carcinogen or cause cell death.

radiation burns Burns that usually result from overexposure to the sun or are associated with radiation treatment for cancer.

radiologic agents Agents that are a source of alpha, beta, or gamma radiation that can be used as a weapon.

random assignment Subjects are randomly assigned to treatment versus control groups.

range of motion (ROM) Movement of a joint within its normal range.

rate of living theory of aging Considered one of the oldest theories on aging, it is based on the belief that individuals possess a finite amount of some "vital substance." When that substance is consumed, the individual dies.

rationality The ability to reason across time when changes in the patient's condition occurs. It includes noticing subtle changes, not limited to explicit vital signs and may not show up immediately in the vital sign trends.

RDD Acronym for radiation dispersal device, a device that can release radiation into the environment.

reactive arthritis A type of arthritis caused by a reaction to an infection somewhere else in the body. Also called *Reiter's syndrome* or *undifferentiated spondyloarthropathy*.

reactive oxygen species (ROS) Intermediary products, or species, that are produced in the metabolic production of energy; occur when oxygen is used to oxidize molecules and generate energy. A phenomenon that occurs during oxidative stress development and a major contributing factor in diseases in patients who are critically ill.

receptors Structure in a cell membrane or within a cell that combines with a hormone to alter an aspect of the functioning of the cell.

reconstructive surgery Surgery performed for the purpose of rebuilding tissues or body structures to achieve a more normal function and appearance.

rectocele Occurs when the posterior vaginal wall is weakened and the rectum bulges into the vagina.

rectum The lower part of the large intestine between the sigmoid colon and the anal canal.

recurrent pain Acute pain that completely resolves, leaving the patient free from pain for a period of time before the pain reoccurs.

red blood cell (RBC) A type of blood cell that transports oxygen and carbon dioxide. Also called an *erythrocyte*.

red blood cell distribution width (RDW) A direct measurement of the homogeneity (consistency) of red blood cell size.

refeeding syndrome Syndrome consisting of metabolic disturbances that arise from reinstitution of nutrition to patients who are severely malnourished.

refractory period Period of time that ensures the cardiac muscle is totally relaxed before another action potential or depolarization can be initiated.

regional anesthesia The production of insensibility of a part by interrupting the sensory nerve conductivity of any region of the body by local injection of a medication.

regional (locality) rule Existence of a prevailing community standard.

registered nurse (RN) An individual licensed by the state to practice nursing in accordance with the nurse practice act.

rehabilitation The multidisciplinary plan of care that maximizes an impaired individual's function by minimizing the deficits to achieve the highest quality of life possible.

relative refractory period Period when depolarization is almost complete, and corresponds with the top and the downslope of the T wave on an ECG tracing.

remodeling The fourth and final phase of wound healing that begins about 3 weeks after the injury and can still be in progress 6 months to 2 years later.

renal calculi Kidney stones.

renin An enzyme produced in the kidneys that converts angiotensinogen to angiotensin, which is an enzyme that helps elevate blood pressure.

repatriation Return of patients from one health care setting to another appropriate level of care or to a contracted institution.

reperfusion injury Injury to the cells after blood supply to an ischemic area is restored.

research A formal, systematic, and organized method of answering a question, solving a problem, validating and redefining existing knowledge, and developing new knowledge.

research critique A critical appraisal of a piece of completed research.

research design Overall plan or blueprint for a study; guides an investigator in planning and implementing a study.

research problem A situation or circumstance that requires a solution to be described, explained, or predicted.

research process Process of undertaking discrete steps to conduct a research study. Includes identifying a researchable problem, completing a literature review, creating the theoretical/conceptual framework, selecting an appropriate design, and collecting, analyzing, and distributing data/findings.

research purpose A concise, clear statement of the specific goal or aim of the study that is generated from the problem.

research question A research problem stated in an interrogative form.

research utilization (RU) The purposeful application of research findings to the clinical setting to improve patient care.

reservoir A place where an organism can survive and may or may not multiply.

resonance A low-pitched, clear, hollow tone of long duration. It is commonly heard over the lungs.

respect for others In ethics, the highest principle because it incorporates all other principles.

respiratory quotient (RQ) Ratio between carbon dioxide produced and oxygen consumed per molecule of fat, carbohydrate, and protein. Fat has an RQ of 0.7, protein 0.8, and carbohydrate 1.0.

restenosis Accumulation of smooth muscle cells at the site of the original percutaneous coronary intervention that occurs because of an artery's response to injury.

resting membrane potential The difference in electrical charge, or voltage, between the inside and outside of a cardiac cell.

restrictive cardiomyopathy A disorder characterized by endometrial scarring that usually affects one or both ventricles and restricts filling of blood, resulting in systolic dysfunction. The ventricle has normal wall thickness, but the walls are rigid, producing elevated filling pressures and dilated atria.

rete pegs Protrusions in the fifth layer of the epidermis that extend down into the dermis and help anchor the epidermis to the dermis. Also called *epidermal ridges*.

reticular activating system (RAS) Network of neurons that is involved with arousal and consciousness.

reticulocyte A biconcave, immature red blood cell disk without a nucleus.

reticuloendothelial system (RES) Part of the immune system; consists of the phagocytic cells located in reticular connective tissue, primarily monocytes and macrophages.

retinal detachment The separation of the sensory retinal layers from the retinal pigment epithelium, where subretinal fluid collects in the potential space.

retinopathy Degenerative changes in the retina.

retrograde ejaculation Backward ejaculation of semen into the bladder.

retroperitoneal space Area behind the peritoneum and outside the kidney.

reverse transcriptase An enzyme present is some classes of virus, including HIV, that is capable of replicating DNA from RNA, the reverse of normal replication of DNA.

Rh factor A protein substance made up of numerous complex antigens. When it is present on the surface of red blood cells, the person is Rh positive (Rh+); if not present, the person is Rh negative (Rh-). Also called *factor D*.

rheumatic fever A pharyngeal infection caused by Lancefield group A beta-hemolytic streptococci. In 3% of the cases it leads to rheumatic heart disease.

rheumatic heart disease An inflammatory disease of the heart that causes long-term damage, scarring, and malfunction of the heart valves.

rheumatoid arthritis (RA) Chronic inflammatory process that affects the peripheral joints and surrounding muscles, ligaments, tendons, and blood vessels.

rhinitis A collection of symptoms predominantly in the nose and eyes that occur after exposure to airborne particles of dust, dander, or the pollens of certain seasonal plants in people who are allergic to these substances.

rhinoplasty Plastic surgery of the nose.

rhytidectomy Surgical excision of skin to eliminate wrinkles of the face.

right-sided heart failure An abnormal cardiac condition characterized by impairment of the right side of the heart and congestion and elevated pressure in the systemic veins and capillaries.

rigidity Abnormal stiffness or inflexibility associated with Parkinson's disease.

Rinne test A hearing test that measures conduction of sound by bone when placing an activated tuning fork on the right and left mastoid sequentially.

riot control agent Agents that generally cause pain, burning, lacrimation, or discomfort upon exposure to mucous membranes. Also called an *irritant*.

risk management A comprehensive program for identifying and evaluating potential risks to the health care organization. Risks can be illness or injury related as well as financial.

robotics Electromechanical devices that are computer controlled and used to perform surgical tasks.

rolling (paraesophageal) hernia A protrusion of the greater curvature of the stomach through the esophageal hiatus.

Romberg test Assesses inner ear balance, proprioceptive ability, and visual and cerebellar system function by asking the patient to maintain an upright posture when arms are held out in front, with eyes open and eyes closed.

rotational injuries Injuries resulting from extreme lateral flexion or flexion-rotation of the spine, causing disruption of the posterior spinal ligaments and spinal instability.

rule of nines Divides the body into seven areas, which represent 9% or multiples of 9% of the body surface area; used to determine burn size.

S_3 (third heart sound) Abnormal third heart sound in the cardiac cycle; often heard when the ventricles are volume overloaded.

S_4 (fourth heart sound) Abnormal fourth heart sound heard in the cardiac cycle; often heard with heart failure and hypertension.

salience Having some things stand out as more or less important in a practical situation, it is a form of practical knowledge that is learned from many concrete clinical experiences in which a range of relevant clinical issues stand out as high priority.

same-day admission A hospital process in which the patient is not hospitalized prior to a surgical procedure but instead reports directly to the reception area of the operating room from home.

sample A portion selected from a population and interpreted to represent that population; a subset of the population.

sampling Process of selecting a portion of the population to represent the entire population.

scabies Contagious skin disease caused by a mite; commonly found in underdeveloped countries and places where there is overcrowding and poor hygiene.

scald burns Type of thermal injury that occurs from contact with hot foods or liquids, including steam.

schema Coordinated patterns of recurring actions that are created for the purpose of organizing and interpreting information.

Schilling test Procedure to identify anemia due to malabsorption.

Schwabach test Tests hearing for air and bone conduction by using an activated tuning fork on the mastoid process.

schwannomas Tumors of the Schwann cells (nerve sheath tumor).

sclerosing cholangitis An inflammatory disorder of the biliary tract that leads to fibrosis and strictures in the biliary system.

sclerotherapy A treatment for esophageal varices in which a bleeding vessel is sclerosed with a chemical agent.

scoliosis Lateral curvature of the spine.

scope of practice Refers to legally permissible boundaries of practice for a given health care profession.

scrub nurse Nurse in the operating room who works directly with the surgeon within the sterile field, passing instruments, sponges, and other items needed during the surgical procedure.

seborrheic keratosis A benign epidermal lesion seen predominantly in the middle-aged and elderly populations.

secondary adrenal insufficiency Condition in which the pituitary gland has insufficient secretion of ACTH, resulting in insufficient cortisol production by the adrenal glands.

secondary appraisal The process of evaluating the significance of a transaction between the person and his or her environment as it relates to available coping resources and options.

secondary immune deficiencies Impaired immune responses that result from a nongenetic cause such as aging, malnutrition, malignancies, immunosuppressive drug therapy, and infections such as the human immunodeficiency virus.

secondary immune response Second exposure to a specific antigen that triggers a stronger and quicker immune response than the first exposure, with production of greater amounts of antibodies due to the presence of memory B cells; results in a milder set of clinical symptoms or no observable response to the pathogen because the immune system quickly eliminates the pathogen.

secondary injury The body's response that can result from a primary injury.

secondary intention In the granulation process, healing that occurs when major tissue defects gradually close by epithelialization and contracture formation, and then form scar tissue.

secondary lesion Lesion that results from a change in the primary lesion or external trauma to the primary lesion.

secondary set Infusion set used to administer supplemental infusion therapies via the primary infusion system.

second-impact syndrome A condition characterized by a second concussion that occurs before the brain completely recovers from the first concussion.

secretion The active process of moving substances, such as H+ ion, from the blood into the tubular fluid against the concentration gradient.

self-antigen Receptors on cells that are recognized as unique to that individual.

self-sheathing Engineered safety mechanism in which a needle is encased in a protective chamber.

senile purpura A type of hemorrhaging under the skin that occurs most frequently in the elderly because their blood vessels are thinner and more fragile than those of younger people.

sense of coherence (SOC) Refers to how an individual sees the world and one's life in it.

sensitivity Describes the ability of a test to identify patients with disease; calculated by dividing the number of true positive tests by the sum of true positives plus false negatives.

sensitization The process of producing antibodies to an antigen present in the body.

sensorineural hearing loss Type of hearing loss attributed to damage to the eighth cranial nerve.

sensory dimension of pain Includes consideration of the location, intensity, quality, and temporal patterns of pain.

sentinel event Unexpected occurrence that has the potential to, or actually does, result in death or serious physical or psychological injury. Serious injury specifically includes loss of limb or function.

sepsis Clinical syndrome that is defined by the presence of infection and a systemic inflammatory response.

septic arthritis The most destructive form of acute arthritis; can result from trauma, direct inoculation of bacteria during joint surgery, spread of infection from another part of the body (hematogenous), or when an infection from an adjacent bone extends through the cortex into the joint space. Also called *nongonococcal bacterial arthritis*.

septic shock In adults, septic shock refers to a state of acute circulatory failure characterized by persistent hypotension unexplained by other causes. In pediatric patients, septic shock is defined as a tachycardia with signs of decreased perfusion. Hypotension is a late sign in children.

septum Material covering a portal; access point of an implanted port or reservoir, usually made of compressed silicon.

sequelae Residual problems that result from an illness.

seroma A mass caused by the accumulation of serum within a tissue or organ. It is similar to a hematoma except that instead of a collection of blood it is a collection of serous fluid.

serum immunoglobulin G (IgG) An antibody produced by the body that is an indicator of long-term immunity or resolving infection.

serum immunoglobulin M (IgM) An antibody produced by the body in response to an antigen; usually present during the acute phase of an infection.

setting The environment or place (locale) in which research is conducted; may be classified as natural, partially controlled, or highly controlled.

severe sepsis Sepsis with one or more organ system dysfunction.

sex chromosome One of the two chromosomes that determine an individual's genetic sex. The two kinds of sex chromosomes are X and Y. Normal females possess two X chromosomes and normal males one X and one Y.

sheet skin grafts Split-thickness grafts that have not been meshed.

shingles A viral infection that occurs because of the reactivation of latent varicella zoster virus or the virus that causes chickenpox. Also known as *herpes zoster*.

short bowel syndrome Syndrome in which the surface of the small intestine is reduced as a result of surgical resection of the small bowel, typically because of tumors, Crohn's disease, infarction, trauma, or radiation.

shunt A hole or passage that allows movement of fluid from one part of the body to another. Pulmonary shunts exist when there is normal perfusion to an alveolus, but ventilation fails to supply the perfused region.

sick role A set of expectations that people who are ill must meet and which society, including caregivers, expects of them.

sick sinus syndrome (SSS) Term that encompasses a broad range of abnormalities, including disorders of impulse generation and conduction, failure of pacemakers, and a susceptibility to paroxysmal or chronic atrial tachycardia. Also referred to as *sinoatrial disease* and *sinoatrial dysfunction*, a disorder in which the SA node is severely depressed due to heart disease or drugs.

sickle cell anemia Chronic erythrocyte disorder characterized by misshapen "sickle-shaped" red blood cells resulting from malfunctioning hemoglobin molecules.

silicosis Disease that results from exposure to free crystalline silica in mines, foundries, blasting operations, stone, clay, and glass manufacturing.

simple random sampling Type of sampling strategy in which each person in a population has an equal chance of being selected for a study.

simple verbal descriptive scale (SVDS) Scale that uses a horizontal line marked with the numbers 0 to 10 from left to right, but also includes interval descriptors of "no pain," "mild," "discomforting," "distressing," "horrible," or "excruciating pain."

single-gene disorder A disorder due to one or a pair of mutant alleles at a single locus.

sinoatrial (SA) node Part of the electrical conduction of the myocardium; located in the upper posterior portion of the right atrial wall near the opening of the vena cava. The SA node is commonly referred to as the primary pacemaker of the heart.

sinus arrest Momentary cessation of sinus impulse formation, causing a pause in the cardiac rhythm followed by spontaneous resumption of electrical activity. This dysrhythmia may be referred to as sinus pause, and is reflected as an absence of the PQRST complex on an ECG tracing and an absence of cardiac output.

sinus arrhythmia/dysrhythmia Dysrhythmia resembling normal sinus rhythm except for a slight irregularity in the heart rhythm.

sinus bradycardia Situation in which the SA node is firing at a heart rate of less that 60 beats per minute. Often called *sinus brady*.

sinus tachycardia Rapid firing of the sinus node at rates of more than100 beats per minute at rest. There may be a compensatory response to a decreased cardiac output state.

sinusitis Infection or inflammation of the sinuses.

situational stressor Stressor that is unpredictable and may occur at any time during life; such stressors can be positive or negative. The effect of the situational stressor may vary depending on the developmental stage of the individual experiencing the stress.

Sjögren's syndrome An autoimmune disease in which the immune system attacks and destroys the glands that produce tears and saliva.

skeletal traction Treatment that entails placement of a skeletal pin through the bone which is then attached to a weighted cord to maintain proper alignment of the fractured bone.

skills of involvement The skills of perceiving relevant changes or nuances in clinical situations; these skills are experientially learned and form part of a nurse's practical clinical knowledge.

skin testing Introduction of small amounts of various allergens into the skin of an allergic individual through either intradermal injection or a scratch or "prick test" technique to evaluate for a triggering allergen. Individuals sensitive or capable of producing immediate IgE response to allergens will show a wheal and flare when the allergen is introduced in a skin test.

skin traction Treatment that uses straps or foam boots secured to the lower extremity attached to a weighted cord that is pulling no more than 6 pounds to maintain proper alignment of the fractured bone.

sleep apnea A disorder in which a person stops breathing for more than 10 seconds, typically more than 20 to 30 times in an hour. The three main types of sleep apnea are central, obstructive, and a combination of central and obstructive.

sliding (direct) hiatal hernia Occurs when a portion of the fundus of the stomach moves upward through the esophageal hiatus into the thoracic cavity.

sodium Most numerous cation in extracellular fluid (ECF); maintains ECF volume through osmotic pressure, assists acid–base balance, and conducts nerve impulses via sodium channels. Normal blood values are 135 to 145 mEq/L.

sodium bicarbonate A base or alkali that removes hydrogen ion when added to the blood.

solar lentigo Lesions that develop due to a familial tendency and chronic sun exposure in Caucasians older than 60 years of age. They are macules that are darker and larger than freckles and do not fade during winter. Commonly referred to as *age spots* or *liver spots*.

Somogyi effect A response to the use of exogenous insulin, which results in nocturnal hypoglycemia. The hypoglycemia is accompanied by release of counterregulatory hormones; as a result patients awake in the morning with elevated blood glucose levels. This is often referred to as *rebound hyperglycemia*.

specific gravity (SG) An estimate of the solute concentration in a volume of liquid measured with a hydrometer which compares the liquid to an equal amount of distilled water. Normal urine values are 1.016 to 1.022.

specificity Describes the frequency with which a test is normal in subjects who are free of disease; calculated by dividing the number of true negatives in the population by the sum of true negatives plus false positives.

specificity theory Theory asserting that pain is directly related to the degree of injury. Once a noxious stimulus has occurred, the message is carried directly to the pain centers in the brain.

spermatocele Painless, sperm-containing cysts found on the testicle.

spermatogenesis Production of mature male germ cells.

Spetzler-Martin AVM grading scale A scale to grade arteriovenous malformations (AVMs) based on the degree of surgical difficulty in removing them.

spinal anesthesia An anesthesia technique in which a local anesthetic is injected into the subarachnoid space and directly into the cerebrospinal fluid. Also called *intrathecal anesthesia*.

spinal cord injury (SCI) Injury to the spinal cord that results in impairment or loss of motor, sensory, and autonomic functions.

spinal precautions Methods of immobilizing the spine and moving patients to prevent or avoid additional spinal injury. Spinal precautions are initiated at the trauma scene and maintained until spinal injury has been ruled out or appropriate treatment strategies have been implemented.

spinal shock A period of flaccid paralysis and absent reflexes lasting up to 6 weeks after spinal cord injury.

split-thickness skin graft Grafting of a partial layer of skin, including the epidermis and part of the dermis.

spondylitic disease A condition consisting of inflammation and degenerative changes of the spine including formation of osteophytes, calcification and hypertrophy of the ligaments, and degeneration of the intervertebral disks.

sprain An injury to a ligament.

spring-coil container Mechanical infusion device with a combination of a spring coil and collapsible disk; used to deliver small-volume parenteral solutions or medications.

spring-coil syringe Mechanical infusion device that uses a syringe to deliver parenteral solutions or medications.

ST segment Interval between the end of the QRS complex and the beginning of the T wave on an ECG tracing. Represents the time during which the ventricles have been completely depolarized and are beginning ventricular repolarization. Normally is isoelectric on ECG graph paper.

stage 1 hypertension A blood pressure of 140 to 159 mmHg systolic or 90 to 99 mmHg diastolic measured during multiple office visits following the guidelines for obtaining accurate blood pressure measurements.

stage 2 hypertension A blood pressure of greater than 160 mmHg systolic or greater than 100 mmHg diastolic measured during multiple office visits following the guidelines for obtaining accurate blood pressure measurements.

staghorn calculus A calculus or stone that remains in the renal pelvis and becomes so large that it fills the pelvis completely, blocking the flow of urine.

staging The portion of the tumor classification system that describes the extent of the tumor and evidence of metastasis throughout the body.

standards of care General standards of care and guidelines for nursing practice formulated in 1991 by the American Nurses Association.

standards of nursing practice Authoritative statements by which the nursing profession describes the common level of performance or care by which the quality of practice can be determined and responsibilities for which its practitioners are accountable.

standards of professional performance Standards that address the professional nursing role with regard to education, ethics, research, collegiality, and resource utilization.

stapedectomy Removal of the stapes bone and its replacement to restore hearing.

statistical significance A term indicating that the results from an analysis of sample data are unlikely to have been caused by chance, at some specified level of probability.

steady state Dynamic balance of the body's internal environment, even in the presence of change.

steatorrhea Feces that have a high fat content. The stool is typically foul-smelling, greasy, and floats.

stem cell Primitive cell in the bone marrow from which mature blood cells derive.

STEMI Acronym for ST segment elevation myocardial infarction; refers to myocardial injury associated with ST segment elevation on the ECG. ST segment elevation means that myocardial tissue is undergoing severe anoxia and cellular damage, in most cases resulting from complete coronary artery blockage from thrombotic occlusion over an underlying plaque lesion.

stenosis Narrowing of the lumen of a blood vessel.

stent A device used to secure a widened arterial lumen; it is inserted permanently inside the coronary artery, compressing plaque and providing structural support of the vessel. The two general type of stents are bare-metal stents, which do not have a coating, and drug-eluting stents, which are "coated" with medications, including heparin and various immunosuppressant agents, in such a manner that the medications diffuse (elute) into the vessel wall over a period of weeks to months.

Stevens-Johnson syndrome (SJS) A severe, acute, self-limiting skin reaction to infection or to certain medications; affects the epidermal layer of the skin and mucous membranes.

stomatitis Generalized inflammation of the oral mucosa; it is classified according to the etiology.

stopcock Manually operated add-on device used to direct the flow of an infusate.

strabismus A condition in which an individual's eyes do not look at the same object together. Also referred to as *cross-eyed*.

strain An injury to the muscle belly or its tendon attachment to bone.

strategic national stockpile (SNS) A national repository of pharmaceutical agents, vaccines, medical supplies, and equipment that can be delivered to the site of a large-scale disaster to augment local and state resources in order to reduce the morbidity and mortality in the civilian population.

stratified random sampling Type of sampling that gives individuals within designated categories an equal chance of selection. The population is first divided into two or more strata or subpopulations. The goal is to enhance representation.

stress An organism's response to stimulation or change; a state produced by a change in the environment that may be perceived as challenging, threatening, or damaging to the person's dynamic balance or equilibrium. These changes may be real or perceived, and they activate an organism's attempts to cope by means of neural and endocrine mechanisms.

stress perception Recognition of a stressor by the brain.

stress response Activation of physiological fight-or-flight-or-fright systems within the body.

stressor A stimulus that activates a stress response.

stridor A raspy noise heard in the upper airway as a result of air attempting to move through a narrowed opening.

stroke Syndrome characterized by a set of neurological deficits that fit a known vascular region.

stroke volume (SV) The amount of blood leaving a ventricle with each contraction.

structure standards Quality standards that focus on the internal characteristics of an organization and its personnel.

subarachnoid hemorrhage (SAH) A condition characterized by bleeding into the space below the arachnoid space.

subchondral bone The smooth tissue at the ends of bones that is covered with cartilage.

subconscious A mental state that encompasses things that have been forgotten but can easily be brought to consciousness.

subcutaneous emphysema Air that escapes into the subcutaneous tissue.

subcutaneous nodules Small, nontender swellings found over bony prominences on the hands and feet.

subdural hematoma (SDH) Bleeding between the dura and the arachnoid layers of the meninges.

subjective data Data that consists of information the patient or caretaker tells the nurse; information that can be perceived only by the patient and not by the observer.

substance abuse Repeated use of a substance despite significant and repeated negative substance-related consequences.

substance dependence A pattern of substance use that is continued despite significant consequences, usually with physiological tolerance effects and a withdrawal syndrome if the substance is withdrawn.

substance intoxication Reversible substance-specific changes in thinking, emotions, behavior, and/or physiological functions caused by recent substance ingestion.

substance withdrawal A substance-specific mental disorder that follows the cessation or reduced intake of a substance that has regularly been used to induce a state of intoxication.

substance withdrawal syndrome The symptoms that occur when drug use is reduced or discontinued.

substantia nigra Structure located in the midbrain beneath the basal ganglia.

substituted judgment A subjective determination of what a person would have chosen to do had that person been capable of making his or her opinion known.

sudden cardiac death (SCD) Type of cardiac arrest most often associated with abrupt coronary artery occlusion from plaque disruption over severely stenotic lesions in the setting of poorly developed collateral circulation.

superego An extension of the ego that represents an individual's early moral training and ideal values imparted by societal norms.

suppurative Pertaining to the formation of pus.

supraventricular tachycardia (SVT) Tachycardia that is generated somewhere above the ventricles. The term encompasses all fast rhythms with normal QRS complexes and heart rates greater than 100 beats per minute. Rhythms included in this category include sinus tachycardia, premature atrial tachycardia, and paroxysmal junctional tachycardia. This term may be used when it is impossible to identify the source of the tachycardia.

surfactant Surface-active agent that promotes alveolar stability.

surveillance The systematic and continuous assessment of patients for the recognition and management of potentially catastrophic events.

survival Observation of persons with cancer over time and the likelihood of their dying over several time periods; a link between incidence and mortality data.

Swan-Ganz catheter A pulmonary artery catheter that is inserted into the pulmonary artery via the right atrium and ventricle; used to measure cardiac output and pulmonary artery pressure and to infuse fluids.

sympathectomy Excision of a portion of the sympathetic division of the autonomic division of the autonomic nervous system.

synapse The space between the junction of two neurons in a neural pathway where the termination of the axon of one neuron comes into proximity with the cell body or dendrites of another.

syncope Temporary dizziness or loss of consciousness caused by low blood pressure and insufficient blood flow.

syndrome of inappropriate antidiuretic hormone (SIADH) A hypermetabolic state of the adrenal glands in which antidiuretic hormone is produced in excess, leading to the retention of fluid and hyponatremia.

syphilis A sexually transmitted infection (STI) that is caused by the *Treponema pallidum* bacterium; has been called the "great imitator" because its symptoms often mimic those of other STIs.

systemic inflammatory response (SIRS) A systemic response of the immune system that can be triggered by both infectious and noninfectious causes.

systemic lupus erythematosus (SLE) An example of a systemic type III hypersensitivity autoimmune disease characterized by damage to joints and soft organs as a result of the effects of autoantibodies and antibody–antigen activity (immune complex responses).

systemic vascular resistance The arterial systolic pressure; normal SVR is 900 to 1,400 · dyn s/cm⁵.

systolic A blood pressure reading of the maximum pressure in the aorta and major arteries, which occurs when the left ventricle contracts and ejects blood onto the central vascular system.

systolic dysfunction Impaired ventricular function with volume overload and decreased contractility.

T cells White blood cells that are vital to initiating and regulating an immune response; produced in the bone marrow and mature and differentiate into various types of T cells in the thymus and other lymphatic tissue such as CD4 (cluster of differentiation, a type of receptor), CD8, T-memory, and T-suppressor cells. They are a crucial part of the immune response because they function as the regulatory cells of the immune system and are responsible for initiating and controlling immune processes such as phagocytosis, cytokine/lymphokine secretion, and activation of B cells.

T lymphocyte Lymphocytes that, when active, divide rapidly and secrete small proteins called cytokines that regulate or assist in the immune response.

T wave Represents ventricular recovery or repolarization in the cardiac cycle; often referred to as the resting phase of the cycle.

tachypnea Rapid respiratory rate.

tau A specialized protein that is a key component of the neurofibrillary tangles associated with Alzheimer's disease.

teaching Any deliberate act that involves the planning, implementation, and evaluation of instructional strategies that meet expected learner outcomes.

team nursing A nursing care delivery system in which a group of RNs, LVNs/LPNs, and unlicensed assistive personnel are assigned shift responsibility for a group of patients, with the RN assuming a leadership role in accordance with the nurse practice act.

techne Something that can be standardized and replicated.

telemedicine Systems or programs that use video or computer-based equipment to link providers or monitor patients electronically.

teleological theories Theories that derive norms or rules for conduct from the consequences of actions; looks merely at consequences to determine the rightness or wrongness of an action.

telomere The tip or end of each chromosome arm.

temporary transvenous pacing Procedure that involves insertion of a pacemaker wire through a major vein, such as the internal jugular, subclavian, or femoral. The pacemaker wire is then advanced into the heart for pacing.

tenosynovitis An infection of the flexor tendon sheaths.

tension pneumothorax Occurs when an injury perforates the chest or pleural space. During inspiration air enters the pleural space and becomes trapped. As more air is trapped, the pressure in the pleural space increases, collapsing the lung and causing the mediastinum to shift to the opposite side.

terrorism An act designed to disrupt daily life and cause terror and panic. The definition according to the FBI is "The unlawful use of force or violence against persons or property to intimidate or coerce a government, the civilian population, or any segment thereof, in furtherance of political or social objectives."

tertiary or third intention Healing that occurs in wounds that have not been sutured in a timely manner or have broken down and been sutured later.

testicular torsion Twisting of the spermatic cord.

tetraplegia (_Greek_) Paralysis of both upper and lower extremities.

thalassemia Class of hematologic disorders characterized by genetic inheritance of a mutated hemoglobin-coding gene; characterized by increased hemolysis.

T-helper cells A type of T cell that is identified and named by the kind of receptor that is on its surface, a CD4 receptor (cluster of differentiation receptor 4). T-helper cells regulate immune function by stimulating B lymphocytes to produce antibodies and chemically stimulate the cell-mediated response to viral and mutant cells.

theoretical connectedness Requires that the theoretical schema developed for the study be clearly expressed, logically consistent, reflective of the data, and compatible with the practice of nursing.

therapeutic alliance An alliance that involves the nurse and the patient consciously working together to reach mutually agreed-on goals.

therapeutic communication Purposeful communication that is designed to convey openness and caring.

therapeutic lifestyle changes (TLC) Dietary modifications recommended for treatment and prevention of disease.

thermal burns Injury from flames; the most common type of burn injury.

thermistor Thermometer imbedded in a pulmonary artery catheter that is used to detect core temperatures.

third-degree AV block (complete block) Independent excitation and contraction of the atria and ventricles due to the inability of any atrial impulses to reach the ventricles. The top and the bottom of the heart are not communicating; they are each beating independently. This dysrhythmia is referred to as AV dissociation because of the independent function of the atria and the ventricles.

threshold Point at which a stimulus will produce a cell response or depolarization.

thrills Palpable vibratory sensations from turbulent blood flow across cardiac valves due to cardiac murmurs.

thromboangiitis obliterans (TAO) A chronic inflammatory vascular occlusive disease most common in men who smoke. Also known as _Buerger's disease_.

thrombocyte Platelet.

thrombopoietin Hormone produced by the liver and kidneys; responsible for stimulating thrombopoiesis.

thrombus Blood clot that forms in a blood vessel and remains at the site of formation.

through-the-needle peripheral-short catheter Vascular access device in which the catheter is inserted into the vein by threading it through the lumen of an introducer.

thyroid storm A life-threatening, hypermetabolic condition in which excess production of thyroid hormones causes serious cardiac disorders.

thyroidectomy Full or partial surgical removal of the thyroid gland.

thyroiditis Inflammation of the thyroid gland.

thyromegaly Abnormal growth of thyroid tissue.

thyrotoxicosis A critical, hypermetabolic condition in which excess production of thyroid hormones threatens physiological stability and well-being.

tinnitus A buzzing, roaring, or ringing in the ears.

tissue factor (TF) Cytokine that is important in immune function and inflammation; released by a variety of injured tissue cells, macrophages, and platelets; stimulates platelets to stick together and form the beginning of a clot to stop bleeding when injury occurs.

tissue-specific antigens Proteins located in the cell membrane of some tissues such as blood, nerves, lungs, and kidneys that are involved in type II tissue-specific–mediated hypersensitivity reactions.

tolerance Physiological habituation to a substance, resulting in the need for progressively greater amounts to achieve intoxication and/or a diminished effect from continued use of the same amount of the substance.

toll receptors Part of the natural immune response; microcellular receptors on the surface of many types of immune and tissue cells that are able to initiate immune responses when pieces of bacterial cell walls attach to them. Functions include stimulation of a cell to release tumor necrosis factor or start the process of programmed cell death (apoptosis).

tomography Imaging technology that displays images of a single plane (slice) of the heart.

tonsillitis An acute or recurrent infection of the tonsils.

tophi Accumulation of uric acid crystals in the cartilage of the earlobe.

torsade de pointes Form of ventricular tachycardia in which the QRS complexes have varying morphology or shape and width. This dysrhythmia resembles a turning about or twisting motion along the baseline or isoelectric line and tends to recur repeatedly.

tort law A brand of civil law concerning legal wrongs committed by one person against another or against another's property.

total joint replacement A diseased or injured joint that is surgically removed, and replaced with an orthosis.

total parenteral nutrition (TPN) Provision of nutrition intravenously via a central vein.

total patient care Another name for the case method of nursing care delivery.

toxic epidermal necrolysis (TEN) Part of the same syndrome of diseases as Stevens-Johnson syndrome, but it is a more severe form of the disorder and is life threatening with more extensive skin detachment.

toxin Material produced by living organisms that has chemical properties that can cause injury, illness, and death.

tracheal breath sounds Breath sounds auscultated over the trachea; they are normally loud and high pitched.

tracheal deviation Shifting of the tracheal position to the right or left of midline due to the push or pull of thoracic structures.

tracheostomy Refers to the making of a semipermanent or permanent opening into the trachea, and to the opening itself.

tracheotomy A temporary surgical airway into the trachea.

transcription Formation of an RNA molecule on a DNA template in the cell nucleus.

transcutaneous electrical nerve stimulation (TENS) Low-voltage electrical stimulation through the skin; used to relieve pain.

transcutaneous pacing (TCP) Procedure that delivers an electrical stimulus directly through the chest wall.

transduction The transmission of pain from the periphery to the central nervous system.

transection Cutting across.

transesophageal echocardiography (TEE) Echocardiogram performed using a miniaturized transducer advanced down the esophagus. Because the esophagus passes directly behind the posterior surface of the heart, TEE affords excellent views of the posterior structures of the heart and great vessels.

transesophageal ultrasound A diagnostic test that uses an ultrasound device that is passed into the esophagus of a patient to create a clear image of the heart muscle and other parts of the heart.

transferrin Protein concentrated in the small intestine; responsible for transportation of iron from the gut to target cells.

transfusion-related acute lung injury (TRALI) A serious, life-threatening clinical syndrome that is a complication of blood transfusions. It is thought to be caused by the presence of granulocyte antibodies and biologically active lipids in the donor plasma to which the recipient reacts.

transient ischemia attack (TIA) An episode of neurological deficits resulting from temporary ischemia that produces strokelike symptoms but no lasting damage. It occurs when the blood supply to part of the brain is briefly interrupted. Also referred to as a *warning stroke* or *mini-stroke*.

transient pain Acute pain that is brief and then resolves completely such as is the case in a needlestick for phlebotomy or an intramuscular injection.

translation Formation of a polypeptide chain from its mRNA template.

translocation A chromosome aberration that results from a transfer of a segment of one chromosome to another chromosome.

traumatic brain injury (TBI) An acute brain disorder characterized by an injury to the brain secondary to trauma.

traumatic wounds Abrasions, blisters, cuts, bites, stab wounds, gunshot wounds, and first- and second-degree burns.

tremors Involuntary muscle movements of a body part or limb.

triage A process that is used to determine the severity of a patient's illness or injury.

trichomoniasis A sexually transmitted protozoan infection caused by *Trichomonas vaginalis*.

tricuspid valve regurgitation Inability of a heart valve to completely close, resulting in a backflow of blood from the right ventricle to the right atrium.

tricuspid valve stenosis Obstruction of blood flow between the right atrium and the right ventricle due to a narrowed valve orifice.

trigeminy Premature ventricular contraction that is evidenced every third beat.

triglycerides A form of fat derived from fats in food and produced by the body from other sources such as carbohydrates.

triple-H therapy A triad of medical treatments for vasospasm (hemodilution, hypervolemia, and hypertension).

trismus Restricted movement of the jaw.

trisomy The state of having three representatives of a given chromosome instead of the usual pair.

tropia Deviation of an eye from the normal position with respect to the line of vision when the eyes are open.

Trousseau's sign Contraction of the muscles when the nerves are mildly compressed; for example, inflating a blood pressure cuff and keeping it above systolic will induce carpal spasms.

trypsin A pancreatic enzyme that hydrolyzes the interior bonds of large protein molecules.

tumor necrosis factor (TNF) A small peptide produced by a variety of cells, including granulocytes and lymphocytes; critical in the stimulation of the initial inflammatory response, specifically the activity of macrophages and granulocytes; also stimulates cells to initiate programmed apoptosis when mutations occur, which is important in inhibiting tumor development and growth.

tunica adventitia The outer layer of an artery; flexible stratum that consists of fibrous tissue made of collagen and elastic fibers surrounded by collagen bundles.

tunica intima Layer of an artery that consists of a monolayer of connecting endothelial cells and a lamina of connective tissue and smooth muscle cells.

tunica media The middle layer of an artery that consists of multiple layers of smooth muscle cells and connective tissue made up of elastic fibers, collagen, and proteoglycans.

tunneled and cuffed device Long-term central vascular access device whose proximal end is tunneled subcutaneously from the insertion site and the remaining length is brought out through the skin at an exit site.

turgor The elasticity and mobility of the skin; reflects the skin's hydration status.

tympanic membrane Eardrum.

tympanoplasty Surgical repair of the eardrum or bones of the middle ear in an effort to restore hearing.

tympany (1) A high-pitched, drum-like tone of medium duration. It is commonly heard over the air-filled intestines. (2) Abdominal distention with gas.

type 1 diabetes mellitus Type of diabetes characterized by the destruction of pancreatic beta cells.

type 2 diabetes mellitus Type of diabetes characterized by insulin resistance and decreased insulin secretion.

type A blood Blood type for an individual with A antigen.

type AB blood Blood type for an individual with both A and B antigens.

type B blood Blood type for an individual with B antigen.

type I (IgE-mediated) allergic reactions Involve the production of antigen-specific IgE antibodies after exposure to a foreign antigen or allergen; most common of the immune hypersensitivity disorders.

type II (tissue-specific–mediated) hypersensitivity reactions Involve IgG and IgM antibody–antigen immune complexes; tissue-specific antigens on the surface of cells are not recognized as self by the immune system and are attacked and damaged or destroyed. Only tissues with the specific antigens are involved.

type III (immune complex–mediated) hypersensitivity reactions Involve IgG and IgM antibody–antigen immune complexes; differentiated from type II reactions in that such reactions are soluble in plasma and circulate in the blood and are not localized at a tissue-specific surface. The traveling antibody–antigen complexes can deposit in tissue or joints and precipitate phagocytosis and inflammation. Multiple body systems/locations can be involved and a variety of clinical symptoms may be observed.

type IV (cell-mediated) hypersensitivity reactions T-cell–mediated immune response, instead of an antibody response as is the case with type I, II, and III hypersensitivity reactions. Additionally, the response is delayed, with the onset of symptoms 24 to 48 hours after antigen exposure. One example of a type IV hypersensitivity response is poison ivy reaction.

type O blood Blood type for an individual with neither A or B antigens.

type-specific hypersensitivity reactions Four specific mechanisms of overreactive immunologic response (types I, II, III, and IV) to environmental allergens, self-antigens, or antigens from another human.

U wave Follows the T wave in the cardiac cycle and is present only in some people on an ECG tracing.

ulcerative colitis (UC) Disorder that involves chronic inflammation of the mucosal and submucosal layers of the colon and rectum.

unconscious A mental state that encompasses all of those things that cannot be remembered or brought to conscious thought.

undernutrition Synonym for *malnutrition*.

unipolar lead Lead with one positive electrode and one indifferent zero reference point; consists of standard leads and augmented limb leads. The leads provide the five frontal plane leads of a 12-lead ECG.

United Kingdom Prospective Diabetes Study (UKPDS) A large clinical research study in Great Britain of patients with type 2 diabetes which concluded that tight glucose control (i.e., maintaining blood glucose levels close to normal ranges) results in decreased microvascular complications.

unlicensed assistive personnel Health care personnel who are not licensed; they may be technicians or certified nurses' aides or nursing assistants.

Unna's boot A rigid bandage that prevents edema while promoting healing; it is worn for several days at a time. Commonly used to treat venous ulcers.

unstable angina A transitory syndrome falling between stable angina and myocardial infarction wherein thrombus forms in an area of arterial stenosis, but is subsequently fully or partially lysed by endogenous antithrombotic mechanisms.

uplifts Positive experiences that are likely to occur in everyday life.

urgent procedures Surgeries that must be performed sooner rather than later.

urticaria Raised, erythematous, intensely pruritic plaques or wheals that are surrounded by a white halo. Also known as *hives*.

U.S. Preventive Services Task Force (USPSTF) A group of health care experts that makes recommendations for appropriate preventive services and screening exams in adults ages 65 and over.

vaccine A preparation that contains an infectious agent (live or killed) or its components; administered to stimulate the production of antibodies that can prevent infection or create resistance to infection from that agent; a type of acquired artificial immunity.

vaginismus Condition in which the vaginal muscles at the introitus contract very tightly, making vaginal penetration painful.

values Freely chosen beliefs or attitudes about the worth of an individual or object.

valvular regurgitation Inability of a heart valve to completely close, resulting in a backflow of blood through the incompetent valve orifice into the previous chamber.

valvuloplasty A surgical procedure to repair torn or damaged leaflets, chordae tendineae, or papillary muscle.

variables Attributes of a person or object that vary, that is, take on different values. Examples include body temperature, age, and blood pressure.

variant, Prinzmetal, or vasospastic angina Condition characterized by a vasospasm occurring at a single or multiple sites in major coronary arteries and their large branches.

varicocele Varicosities of the veins of the scrotum.

varicose veins Dilated, tortuous, superficial veins most commonly seen in the lower extremities.

vascular access device (VAD) A catheter, tube, or device inserted into the vascular system.

vascular lesion Lesions that appear as red or purple pigmented.

vasectomy Male sterilization surgery.

vasodilator A substance that causes the dilation of blood vessels.

vasodilatory cascade A series of events triggered by hypoxia, resulting in increased intracranial pressure.

vasogenic edema A condition characterized by an alteration in vascular permeability with disruption of the blood–brain barrier.

vasospasm Refers to the transient narrowing of an artery, causing decreased blood flow.

venous thromboembolism (VTE) Includes the disorders of deep venous thrombosis and pulmonary embolism.

ventilated-associated pneumonia (VAP) Pneumonia that develops in mechanically ventilated patients after more than 48 hours of intubation, with no clinical evidence of pneumonia at the time of intubation.

ventilation The movement of air between the atmosphere and the alveoli accomplished by respirations or the ability of the lungs to remove carbon dioxide.

ventilation/perfusion mismatching (V/Q) Usually there is a near equal relationship of ventilation ($\dot{V}$) to perfusion ($\dot{Q}$) in the lungs. The formula $\dot{V}/\dot{Q}$, where ventilation is 4 L/min and perfusion is 5 L/min, explains this relationship. Normal ventilation to perfusion equals 4/5 or 0.8.

ventral hernia A hernia through the abdominal wall.

ventricular dysrhythmia Dysrhythmia that originates in the ventricle and is caused by ectopic or irritable foci in the wall of the ventricle. These are the most serious types of dysrhythmias.

ventricular fibrillation (VF) Dysrhythmia marked by rapid, disorganized depolarization of the ventricles. There are no organized electrical impulses or coordinated atrial or ventricular contractions or palpable pulse.

ventricular tachycardia (VT) Life-threatening excitable ventricular focus arising from the tissue distal to the bifurcation of the bundle of His. It discharges repetitively, acting as the dominant pacemaker. When present, three or more premature ventricular contractions occur in a row at a rate of 130 to 250 beats per minute.

veracity In ethics, truth-telling.

verrucae Viral epidermal eruptions caused by human papilloma virus. Also known as *warts*.

vertically integrated models Organizational service structure of hospitals and related health care services aligned along a continuum of care. This model includes the integration of physician, hospital, and ancillary services. Integrated systems can offer a broad range of services pre- and post-hospitalization from primary care to long-term care.

vertigo Subjective sensation of spinning; dizziness; the illusion of rotational movement, tilting, and swaying with feelings of imbalance during standing or walking; symptom of a balance disorder.

vesicant (1) Chemical agent that can cause redness and irritation of the skin and blistering. Also called a *blistering agent*. (2) Parenteral solution or medication known to cause tissue damage and possible necrosis if infiltrated.

vesicular breath sounds Breath sounds normally heard over most of the chest wall from the movement of air in small airways distal to the bronchioles.

vestibular nerve dissection Surgical procedure to cut the vestibular nerve in the event of constant vertigo or dizziness.

viability The ability of a pathogen to survive outside of its host.

Vincent's stomatitis An acute bacterial infection of the gingiva oral mucous membranes caused most often by the bacteria *Borrelia vincentii*. Also known as *acute necrotizing stomatitis* or *trench mouth*.

viral hepatitis Inflammation of the liver caused by several viruses: HAV, HBV, HCV, HDV, and HEV.

viral load The number of HIV viral particles in a sample of blood, expressed as *copies*. Used to monitor the virulence of HIV infection. Levels of >100,000 copies indicate increased risk of AIDS-related illness.

viral meningitis Inflammation of the meninges due to a viral pathogen.

Virchow's triad The three factors that contribute to thrombosis: damage to the venous wall, a change in flow, and blood hypercoagulability.

virulence Related to the severity of disease a pathogen is capable of causing; virulence can vary depending on the ability of the host to mount an immune response. It is expressed as the number of cases of infection that are serious or produce a disability in all those infected.

visual analog scale (VAS) Does not have numeric intervals; rather it uses "no pain" and "pain as bad as it can possibly be" as descriptors at either end of a horizontal line measuring 10 cm in length.

vital signs Temperature, pulse, respirations, blood pressure, and pain level. Used to monitor patients for infection and hemodynamic changes.

vitamin B$_{12}$ (cobalamin) Essential nutrient found in animal proteins; responsible for the activation of folate iron.

vitiligo Condition leading to a localized loss of melanocytes and, thus, patches of depigmentation.

voice whisper test A hearing test in which the examiner stands 1 to 2 feet in back of the patient and whispers.

volumetric pump Electronic infusion device that calculates the volume of solution delivered based on the amount displaced in the set's reservoir.

volutrauma Similar to barotrauma, but the lung damage is caused by increased volume that causes overdistention of alveoli.

vomiting agent Chemical agents that cause vomiting.

von Willebrand's disease Most common inherited bleeding disorder; characterized by deficiencies in von Willebrand factor.

wandering atrial pacemaker A pacemaker from at least three different sites above the bundle of His. Pacemaker sites may include the SA node, the AV junction, an atrial ectopic site, or any combination of these areas.

washed RBCs Red blood cells that have undergone a washing process that increases the removal of immunoglobulins and proteins that cause reactions. The use of washed RBCs is indicated when previous transfusion reactions have occurred.

wasting syndrome Involves the loss of lean tissue from increased protein metabolism, changes in metabolic rate, and anorexia and diarrhea. It is a hallmark of AIDS-related disease.

wear-and-tear theory of aging Theory of aging based on the premise that exposure to internal and external stressors results in the death of cells.

Weber test A hearing screening test that distinguishes whether hearing loss in an ear is conductive or sensorineural.

Western blot (WB) A specific and sensitive serum test that measures the presence of antibodies to HIV; generally done as a confirmation test when enzyme immunoassay tests for HIV are positive.

wheal A small, round, serous-filled raised blister on the skin that is the result of exposure to an allergen.

wheezes High-pitched musical sounds created by air moving over mucous strands.

white blood cell (WBC) A type of blood cell involved in protecting the body against foreign matter.

white coat phenomenon Phenomenon that occurs when a patient's blood pressure is susceptible to elevation as a result of apprehension and anxiety in a health care provider's office or during any other stressful situation.

whole blood Blood that is obtained from a donor, processed, and infused into a recipient.

wild type A normal allele of a gene or its normal phenotype.

window period The time between actual HIV infection and when HIV tests can detect the presence of the virus or antibodies to the virus in blood; usually 1 to 6 months.

winged steel infusion set A metal needle manufactured with flexible plastic attachments to facilitate insertion technique; used for phlebotomy procedures or for single-dose parenteral administrations and infusions of less than 4 hours duration.

withdrawal Uncomfortable and maladaptive physiological, cognitive, emotional, and behavioral changes associated with lowered blood or tissue concentrations of a substance after an individual has established some tolerance toward it, usually through heavy recent use.

WMD Acronym for weapons of mass destruction, which are agents that can cause massive damage and injury.

Wolff-Parkinson-White (WPW) syndrome AV conduction disorder characterized by two AV conduction pathways. This disorder generates an accessory conduction pathway.

wound dehiscence The separation of sutures or staples along the incision in a previously closed wound.

wound evisceration The protrusion of organs from a wound site.

xerosis A skin condition characterized by dry, pruritic, cracked, or fissured skin with scaling and flaking.

X-linked dominant Disorder in which a trait is dominant if it is phenotypically expressed in heterozygotes due to one or more genes located on the X chromosome.

X-linked recessive Disorder in which a trait is recessive if the trait is expressive only in homozygotes due to one or more genes located on the X chromosome.

Y set Devices used for administration of two or more infusates simultaneously. Access to the multiflow adapter is usually via a cap that maintains sterility of the fluid pathway.

zone of coagulation Area where the amount of injury to the tissue is the greatest.

zone of hyperthermia The outermost portion of an injured area where cell damage is minor.

zone of stasis Area surrounding the zone of coagulation that has potentially viable but injured cells.

zones; hot zone, warm zone, cold zone The hot zone, also called the exclusion or the red zone, is the area of highest contamination in a decontamination area. The warm zone, or yellow zone, is also called the contamination reduction corridor, and this is where actual decontamination takes place. The cold zone, or green zone, is also known as the support zone. No one is allowed in the cold zone without first being decontaminated. Those waiting to be decontaminated would be in the hot zone as well as the triage area.

zygote Fertilized egg.

INDEX

M

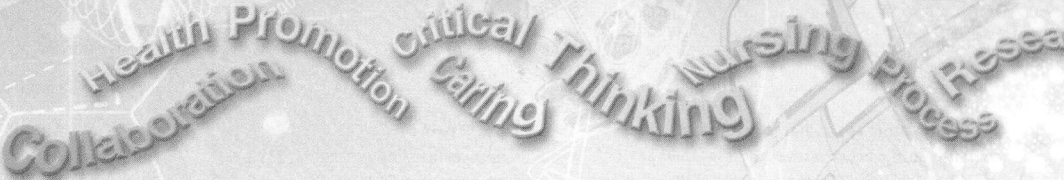

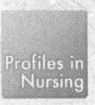

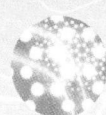

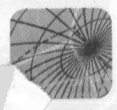

NURSING PROCESS: PATIENT CARE PLAN

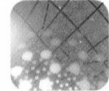

PATIENT TEACHING & DISCHARGE PRIORITIES

RISK FACTORS